Textbook of Pediatric Infectious Diseases

Textbook of Pediatric Infectious Diseases

Edition

4

Volume 1

Ralph D. Feigin, M.D.
President and Chief Executive Officer, Baylor College of Medicine
J. S. Abercrombie Professor and Chairman
Department of Pediatrics, and
Distinguished Service Professor
Baylor College of Medicine
Physician-in-Chief
Texas Children's Hospital
Pediatrician-in-Chief
Ben Taub General Hospital
Chief, Pediatric Service
The Methodist Hospital
Houston, Texas

James D. Cherry, M.D., M.S.C.
Professor of Pediatrics
University of California at Los Angeles
School of Medicine
Chief, Division of Infectious Diseases
UCLA Children's Hospital
Los Angeles, California

W.B. SAUNDERS COMPANY
A Division of Harcourt Brace & Company
Philadelphia London Toronto Montreal Sydney Tokyo

W.B. SAUNDERS COMPANY
A Division of Harcourt Brace & Company

The Curtis Center
Independence Square West
Philadelphia, Pennsylvania 19106

Library of Congress Cataloging-in-Publication Data

Textbook of pediatric infectious diseases / [edited by] Ralph D. Feigin, James D. Cherry.—4th ed.

p. cm.

Includes bibliographical references and indexes.

ISBN 0–7216–6448–2

1. Communicable diseases in children. I. Feigin, Ralph D. II. Cherry, James D. (James Donald). [DNLM: 1. Communicable Diseases—in infancy & childhood. WC 100 T355 1998]

RJ401.T49 1998

618.92′9—dc20

DNLM/DLC 96–26904

TEXTBOOK OF PEDIATRIC INFECTIOUS DISEASES

ISBN 0–7216–7162–4 Volume 1
0–7216–7163–2 Volume 2
0–7216–6448–2 Set

Printed in the United States of America.

Last digit is the print number: 9 8 7 6 5 4 3 2 1

To our wives—Judith *and* Jeanne
our children—Susan, Michael, and Debra, *and*
James, Jeffrey, Susan, and Kenneth
and our grandchildren—Rebecca, Matthew, and Sarah, *and* Ferguson

CONTRIBUTORS

❑ ❑ ❑

Richard D. Aach, B.A., M.D.
Professor, Vice Chairman, and Associate Dean, Case Western Reserve University School of Medicine; Director, Department of Medicine, Mt. Sinai Medical Center, Cleveland, Ohio
Viral Hepatitis Due to Hepatitis Viruses A–E and GB Virus; Cholangitis and Cholecystitis

John G. Aaskov, B.Sc., Ph.D., FRCPath
Senior Lecturer—Immunology, School of Life Science, and Director, WHO Collaborating Centre for Arbovirus Reference and Research, Queensland University of Technology, Brisbane, Queensland, Australia
Alphaviruses; Flaviviruses

Walid Abuhammour, M.D.
Assistant Professor of Pediatrics, Wayne State University School of Medicine; Infectious Diseases Physician, Children's Hospital of Michigan, Detroit, Michigan
Antimicrobial Prophylaxis

David W. K. Acheson, M.D.
Assistant Professor of Medicine, Tufts University School of Medicine; Member, Division of Geographic Medicine and Infectious Diseases, Department of Medicine, New England Medical Center, Boston, Massachusetts
Diarrhea- and Dysentery-Causing Escherichia coli

Christoph Aebi, M.D.
Infectious Disease Fellow, Department of Pediatrics, University of Texas Southwestern Medical Center, Dallas, Texas
Flaviviruses

Laura K. Aguilar, M.D., Ph.D.
Pediatric Resident, Baylor College of Medicine, Texas Children's Hospital, Houston, Texas
Diphtheria

Joshua J. Alexander, M.D., FAAP, FAAPMR
Assistant Professor, Department of Physical Medicine and Rehabilitation and Department of Pediatrics, University of North Carolina School of Medicine, Chapel Hill, North Carolina
Otitis Externa

Miriam J. Alter, Ph.D.
Chief, Epidemiology Section, Hepatitis Branch, Centers for Disease Control and Prevention, Atlanta, Georgia
Hepatitis C Virus

Marvin E. Ament, M.D.
Professor of Pediatrics, University of California, Los Angeles, School of Medicine; Chief, Division of Pediatric Gastroenterology and Nutrition, UCLA Medical Center, Los Angeles, California
Esophagitis

Donald C. Anderson, M.D.
Professor of Pediatrics, Baylor College of Medicine, Houston, Texas; Vice President, Discovery Research Council, Pharmacia & Upjohn Inc., Kalamazoo, Michigan
Leptospirosis; Pneumocystis carinii *Pneumonia*

Marsha S. Anderson, M.D.
Fellow, Pediatric Infectious Disease, University of Colorado, The Children's Hospital, Denver, Colorado
Meningococcal Disease

Stephen S. Arnon, M.D.
Senior Investigator and Chief, Infant Botulism Prevention Program, California Department of Health Services, Berkeley, California
Infant Botulism

Antonio C. Arrieta, M.D.
Associate Director, Pediatric Infectious Diseases, Children's Hospital of Orange County, Orange, California
Urinary Tract Infections

Jane T. Atkins, M.D.
Assistant Professor, Pediatrics, University of Texas–Houston Health Science Center, Houston, Texas
Cryptosporidiosis, Cyclospora *Infection, Isosporiasis, and Microsporidiosis*

Robert L. Atmar, M.D.
Assistant Professor, Departments of Medicine and Microbiology & Immunology, Division of Molecular Virology, Baylor College of Medicine; Assistant Attending, Section of Infectious Diseases, Department of Medicine, Ben Taub General Hospital, Houston, Texas
Coronaviruses

Carol J. Baker, M.D.
Professor of Pediatrics and Microbiology & Immunology and Head, Section of Infectious Diseases, Department of Pediatrics, Baylor College of Medicine; Attending Physician, Infectious Diseases Service, Texas Children's Hospital, Houston, Texas
Cervical Lymphadenitis; Group B Streptococcal Infections

Stephen J. Barenkamp, M.D.
Associate Professor of Pediatrics, St. Louis University School of Medicine; Director, Division of Pediatric Infectious Diseases, Cardinal Glennon Children's Hospital, St. Louis, Missouri
Other Haemophilus *Species*

John G. Bartlett, M.D.
Professor of Medicine, Johns Hopkins University School of Medicine; Chief, Division of Infectious Diseases, Johns Hopkins Hospital, Baltimore, Maryland
Mediastinitis

Robert D. Basow, M.D.
General Pediatrics, Southboro, Massachusetts
Streptobacillus moniliformis *(Rat-Bite Fever);* Spirillum minus *(Rat-Bite Fever)*

Craig W. Beachler, M.D.
Retired; former Active Staff, Washington Hospital, Fremont, California
Nonvenereal Treponematoses

William R. Beisel, M.D., F.A.C.P.
Adjunct Professor, Department of Molecular Microbiology and Immunology, The Johns Hopkins School of Hygiene and Public Health, Baltimore, Maryland
Metabolic Response of the Host to Infections

Beth P. Bell, M.D., M.P.H.
Medical Epidemiologist, Hepatitis Branch, National Center for Infectious Diseases, Centers for Disease Control and Prevention, Atlanta, Georgia
Hepatitis A Virus

Michael L. Bennish, M.D.
Associate Professor of Pediatrics, Medicine, and Community Health, Tufts University School of Medicine; Member, Division of Geographic Medicine and Infectious Diseases, Department of Medicine, New England Medical Center, Boston, Massachusetts
Cholera

David I. Bernstein, M.D.
Professor of Pediatrics, University of Cincinnati; Associate Director, Division of Infectious Diseases, Children's Hospital Medical Center, Cincinnati, Ohio
Rotaviruses

Alison A. Bertuch, M.D., Ph.D.
Postdoctoral Fellow, Hematology-Oncology Section, Department of Pediatrics, Baylor College of Medicine; Postdoctoral Fellow, Texas Children's Cancer Center; Texas Children's Hospital, Houston, Texas
Bacterial Skin Infections

Charles D. Bluestone, M.D.
Eberly Professor of Pediatric Otolaryngology, University of Pittsburgh School of Medicine; Director, Department of Pediatric Otolaryngology, Children's Hospital of Pittsburgh, Pittsburgh, Pennsylvania
Otitis Media

Michael D. Blum, M.D.
Director, Vaccine Infectious Diseases Clinical Research, Merck & Company, Inc., West Point, Pennsylvania
Aspergillus *Infections*

Robert Bortolussi, M.D.
Professor of Pediatrics and Associate Professor of Microbiology, Dalhousie University; Chief of Research and Pediatric Infectious Disease Specialist, IWK–Grace Health Centre, Halifax, Nova Scotia, Canada
Listeriosis

John A. Bosso, Pharm.D.
Professor of Pharmacy and Pediatrics, Colleges of Pharmacy and Medicine, Medical University of South Carolina; Clinical Specialist in Pediatrics, Children's Hospital, Charleston, South Carolina
Fundamentals of Pharmacokinetics, Anti-infective Pharmacodynamics, and Therapeutic Drug Monitoring

Kenneth M. Boyer, M.D.
Professor and Associate Chairman, Department of Pediatrics, Rush Medical College; Director, Section of Pediatric Infectious Diseases, Rush-Presbyterian-St. Luke's Medical Center; Director, Pediatric HIV Programs, Cook County Hospital, Chicago, Illinois
Nonbacterial Pneumonia; Bartonella *(Cat-Scratch Disease);* Borrelia *(Relapsing Fever); Toxoplasmosis*

Michael T. Brady, M.D.
Professor of Pediatrics and Preventive Medicine, College of Medicine, The Ohio State University; Physician Director of HIV Program and Physician Director of Department of Epidemiology, Children's Hospital, Columbus, Ohio
Pseudomonas *and Related Species*

William J. Britt, M.D.
Professor of Pediatrics and Microbiology, University of Alabama School of Medicine; Staff Physician, Children's Hospital, Birmingham, Alabama
Slow Viruses

David A. Bruckner, Sc.D.
Professor, Department of Pathology and Laboratory Medicine, University of California, Los Angeles, School of Medicine; Chief, Clinical Microbiology, UCLA Medical Center, Los Angeles, California
Nomenclature of Aerobic and Anaerobic Bacteria

Yvonne J. Bryson, M.D.
Professor of Pediatrics, University of California, Los Angeles, School of Medicine, and Member, Division of Infectious Diseases, UCLA Children's Hospital, Los Angeles, California
Antiviral Agents

Karina M. Butler, M.B., B.Ch., D.C.H.
Consultant in Pediatric Infectious Diseases, Our Lady's Hospital for Sick Children, The Children's Hospital and the Eastern Health Board, Dublin, Ireland
Cervical Lymphadenitis

Carrie L. Byington, M.D.
Assistant Professor, Departments of Pediatrics and Infectious Diseases, University of Utah School of Medicine and Health Sciences Center, Salt Lake City, Utah
Streptobacillus moniliformis *(Rat-Bite Fever);* Spirillum minus *(Rat-Bite Fever)*

Enrique Caceres, M.D.
Fellow, Pediatric Infectious Diseases, University of Texas–Houston Health Science Center, Houston, Texas
Bacillus cereus; Vibrio parahaemolyticus; *Cryptosporidiosis,* Cyclospora *Infection, Isosporiasis, and Microsporidiosis*

Judith R. Campbell, M.D.
Assistant Professor of Pediatrics, Baylor College of Medicine; Attending Physician, Texas Children's Hospital and Ben Taub Hospital, Houston, Texas
Parotitis

Kathleen A. Campbell, M.D.
Houston Pediatric Associates, Houston, Texas
Coagulase-Positive Staphylococcal Infections

K. Lynn Cates, M.D.
Associate Professor of Pediatrics, Division of Infectious Diseases, Case Western Reserve University, Rainbow Babies and Children's Hospital, Cleveland, Ohio
Immunologic and Phagocytic Responses to Infection; Immunomodulating Agents

Mariam R. Chacko, M.D., M.B., B.S.
Associate Professor, Department of Pediatrics, Baylor College of Medicine; Staff, Texas Children's Hospital, Houston, Texas
Gynecologic Infections in Childhood and Adolescence; Calymmatobacterium granulomatis; Trichomonas *Infections*

Louisa E. Chapman, M.D., M.S.P.H.
Clinical Assistant Professor, Emory University School of Medicine; Medical Epidemiologist, Retrovirus Diseases Branch, Division of AIDS, STD, and TB Laboratory Research, National Center for Infectious Diseases, Centers for Disease Control and Prevention, Atlanta, Georgia
Hantaviruses

Ronni M. Chen, M.D.
Pediatric Ophthalmologist, Kantor Eye Institute, Sarasota; Brandon Eye Clinic, Brandon; and Eye Institute of West Florida, Largo, Florida
Ocular Infections

P. Joan Chesney, M.D.
Professor of Pediatrics, University of Tennessee, Memphis; Active Member, Le Bonheur Children's Medical Center, Memphis, Tennessee
Toxic Shock Syndrome

H. Fred Clark, D.V.M., Ph.D.
Research Professor of Pediatrics, Department of Pediatrics, University of Pennsylvania School of Medicine, Philadelphia, Pennsylvania
Rabies Virus

Thomas G. Cleary, M.D.
Professor of Pediatrics and Director, Pediatric Infectious Diseases, University of Texas–Houston Health Science Center, Houston, Texas
Approach to Patients with Gastrointestinal Tract Infections and Food Poisoning; Bacillus cereus; Shigella; Salmonella; Vibrio parahaemolyticus; Campylobacter jejuni; *Cryptosporidiosis,* Cyclospora *Infection, Isosporiasis, and Microsporidiosis*

Armando G. Correa, M.D.
Assistant Professor of Pediatrics, Baylor College of Medicine; Attending Physician, Texas Children's Hospital and Ben Taub General Hospital, Houston, Texas
Acinetobacter

J. Thomas Cross, Jr., M.D., M.P.H.
Assistant Professor, Division of Infectious Diseases, Department of Internal Medicine and Pediatrics, Louisiana State University School of Medicine and Medical Center—Shreveport, Shreveport, Louisiana
Fungal Meningitis; Other Mycobacteria

Adnan S. Dajani, M.D.
Professor of Pediatrics, Wayne State University School of Medicine; Director, Division of Infectious Diseases, Children's Hospital of Michigan, Detroit, Michigan
Antimicrobial Prophylaxis

Toni Darville, M.D.
Assistant Professor of Pediatrics, University of Arkansas for Medical Sciences; Assistant Professor of Pediatrics, Department of Pediatric Infectious Diseases, Arkansas Children's Hospital, Little Rock, Arkansas
Nocardia

Jeffrey P. Davis, M.D.
Chief Medical Officer and State Epidemiologist for Communicable Diseases, Bureau of Public Health, Wisconsin Division of Health; Adjunct Professor, Departments of Pediatrics and Preventive Medicine, University of Wisconsin Medical School, Madison, Wisconsin
Toxic Shock Syndrome

Gail J. Demmler, M.D.
Associate Professor, Departments of Pediatrics and Pathology, Baylor College of Medicine; Director, Diagnostic Virology Laboratory, Texas Children's Hospital; Attending Physician, Texas Children's Hospital and Ben Taub General Hospital, Houston, Texas
Human Papillomaviruses; Cytomegaloviruses

Penelope H. Dennehy, M.D.
Associate Professor of Pediatrics, Brown University School of Medicine; Associate Director, Division of Pediatric Infectious Diseases, Rhode Island Hospital, Providence, Rhode Island
Active Immunizing Agents

Rosamond Dewart, B.A.
Chief, Travelers' Health Section, Program Operations Branch, Division of Quarantine, National Center for Infectious Diseases, Centers for Disease Control and Prevention, Atlanta, Georgia
Health Information for International Travel

Elliot C. Dick, Ph.D.
Professor of Preventive Medicine (Retired), University of Wisconsin Medical School, Madison, Wisconsin
Rhinoviruses; Coronaviruses

Philip R. Dodge, M.D.
Emeritus Professor of Pediatrics and of Neurology, Washington University School of Medicine; Lecturer in Pediatrics, St. Louis Children's Hospital, St. Louis, Missouri
Parameningeal Infections; Transverse Myelitis or Myelopathy

Desmond F. Duff, M.B., FRCPI, FAAP
Consultant Paediatric Cardiologist, Our Lady's Hospital for Sick Children, Dublin, Ireland
Myocarditis

Lisa M. Dunkle, M.D.
Executive Director, HIV Clinical Research, Bristol-Myers Squibb Pharmaceutical Research Institute, Wallingford, Connecticut
Anaerobic Infections

Paul H. Edelstein, M.D.
Professor of Pathology and Laboratory Medicine, University of Pennsylvania School of

Medicine; Director of Clinical Microbiology, University of Pennsylvania Medical Center, Philadelphia, Pennsylvania
Legionnaires' Disease, Pontiac Fever, and Related Illnesses

Jane C. Edmond, M.D.
Assistant Professor, Department of Ophthalmology, Baylor College of Medicine and Texas Children's Hospital, Houston, Texas
Ocular Infections

Morven S. Edwards, M.D.
Professor of Pediatrics, Baylor College of Medicine; Attending Physician, Texas Children's Hospital and Ben Taub General Hospital, Houston, Texas
Anthrax; Rickettsial Diseases; Animal Bites

B. Keith English, M.D.
Associate Professor, Department of Pediatrics, University of Tennessee College of Medicine; Chief, Division of Infectious Diseases, Le Bonheur Children's Medical Center, Memphis, Tennessee
Enterococcal and Viridans Streptococcal Infections

George D. Ferry, M.D.
Professor of Pediatrics, Baylor College of Medicine; Chief, Gastroenterology and Nutrition Clinic, Texas Children's Hospital, Houston, Texas
Antibiotic-Associated Colitis; Viral Hepatitis Due to Viruses Other than Hepatitis Viruses A–E; Cholangitis and Cholecystitis

Randall G. Fisher, M.D.
Fellow, Pediatric Infectious Diseases, Vanderbilt University Medical Center and Pediatric Infectious Disease Clinic, Vanderbilt University Hospital, Nashville, Tennessee
Miscellaneous Gram-Positive Cocci; Citrobacter; Enterobacter; Klebsiella; Morganella morganii; Proteus; Providencia; Serratia; *Miscellaneous Enterobacteria;* Vibrio vulnificus; *Miscellaneous Non-Enterobacteriaceae Fermentative Bacilli;* Alcaligenes; Eikenella corrodens; Flavobacterium; Stenotrophomonas (Xanthomonas) maltophilia; Erysipelothrix rhusiopathiae

Coy D. Fitch, M.D.
Drefs Professor and Chairman, Department of Internal Medicine, St. Louis University School of Medicine, St. Louis, Missouri
Malaria

Patricia M. Flynn, M.D.
Associate Professor, Department of Pediatrics, University of Tennessee—Memphis; Associate Member, Department of Infectious Diseases, St. Jude Children's Research Hospital, Memphis, Tennessee
Candidiasis

Thomas R. Flynn, D.M.D.
Assistant Professor, Department of Dentistry, Albert Einstein College of Medicine, Yeshiva University; Associate Attending Physician, Montefiore Medical Center, New York, New York
Infections of the Oral Cavity

John P. Fox, M.D., Ph.D. (Deceased)
Formerly Professor Emeritus of Epidemiology, School of Public Health and Community Medicine, University of Washington, Seattle, Washington
Epidemiology of Infectious Diseases

David W. Fraser, M.D.
Adjunct Professor of Medicine, University of Pennsylvania School of Medicine, Philadelphia, Pennsylvania
Public Health Considerations

Lisa M. Frenkel, M.D.
Associate Professor, Department of Pediatrics, Division of Infectious Diseases, University of Washington School of Medicine

and Children's Hospital and Medical Center, Seattle, Washington
Dientamoeba fragilis *Infection*

Richard A. Friedman, M.D.
Associate Professor of Pediatrics, Baylor College of Medicine; Chief, Arrhythmia and Pacing Services, and Chief, Pediatric Cardiology Outpatient Clinic, Texas Children's Hospital, Houston, Texas
Infectious Pericarditis; Myocarditis

David R. Fulton, M.D.
Professor of Pediatrics, Tufts University School of Medicine; Chief, Pediatric Cardiology, Floating Hospital for Children, Boston, Massachusetts
Noninfectious Carditis

Stacey E. Gallas, M.D.
Private Practice, Houston, Texas
Viral and Fungal Skin Infections

Lynne S. Garcia, M.S., M.T., F(AAM)
Manager, Brentwood Facility, UCLA Clinical Laboratories, Department of Pathology and Laboratory Medicine, UCLA Medical Center, Los Angeles, California
Classification/Nomenclature of Human Parasites

W. Lance George, M.D.
University of California, Los Angeles, School of Medicine; Director, Ambulatory Services, West Los Angeles VA Medical Center, Los Angeles, California
Peritonitis and Intra-abdominal Abscess; Retroperitoneal Infection; Clostridial Intoxication and Infection

Michael A. Gerber, M.D.
University of Connecticut School of Medicine, Farmington; Director, Division of Pediatric Infectious Diseases, Connecticut Children's Medical Center, Hartford, Connecticut
Group A, Group C, and Group G Beta-Hemolytic Streptococcal Infections

Anne A. Gershon, M.D.
Professor of Pediatrics, Columbia University College of Physicians and Surgeons; Attending Physician, Babies' and Children's Hospital, New York, New York
Varicella-Zoster Virus

Mark A. Gilger, M.D.
Assistant Professor of Pediatrics, Baylor College of Medicine; Attending Physician in Gastroenterology and Nutrition, Texas Children's Hospital, Houston, Texas
Whipple Disease; Helicobacter pylori

Daniel G. Glaze, M.D.
Associate Professor, Department of Pediatrics, Section of Neurology; Department of Neurology, Section of Neurophysiology, Baylor College of Medicine, Houston, Texas
Guillain-Barré Syndrome

W. Paul Glezen, M.D.
Professor and Head, Preventive Medicine Section, Departments of Microbiology and Immunology and Pediatrics, Baylor College of Medicine; Adjunct Professor of Epidemiology, School of Public Health, University of Texas Health Science Center; Attending Pediatrician, Harris County Hospital District and Ben Taub General Hospital; Courtesy Staff in Infectious Diseases, Texas Children's Hospital, Houston, Texas
Rhinoviruses; Influenza Viruses

Mary P. Glodé, M.D.
Professor of Pediatrics, University of Colorado Health Sciences Center and the Children's Hospital, Denver, Colorado
Meningococcal Disease

Donald A. Goldmann, M.D.
Professor of Pediatrics, Harvard Medical School; Associate in

Infectious Diseases; Hospital Epidemiologist; Chief, Charles Janeway Medical Service; Director, Bacteriology Laboratory, Children's Hospital, Boston, Massachusetts
Nosocomial Infections; Prevention and Control of Nosocomial Infections in Hospitalized Children

Ellie J. C. Goldstein, M.D.
Clinical Professor of Medicine, University of California, Los Angeles, School of Medicine, Los Angeles; Director, R. M. Alden Research Laboratory, Santa Monica–UCLA Medical Center, Santa Monica, California
Human Bites

Maria D. Goldstein, M.D.
Clinical Associate Professor of Pediatrics, University of New Mexico Health Science Center; District Health Officer, New Mexico Department of Health, Public Health Division, Albuquerque, New Mexico
Plague (Yersinia pestis)

Henry F. Gomez, M.D.
Assistant Professor, Pediatrics, University of Texas–Houston Health Science Center, Houston, Texas
Shigella; Salmonella

Edmond T. Gonzales, Jr., M.D.
Professor of Urology, Scott Department of Urology, Baylor College of Medicine; Head, Department of Surgery, and Chief, Urology Service, Texas Children's Hospital, Houston, Texas
Renal Abscess; Prostatitis

Charles Grose, M.D.
Professor of Pediatrics and Professor of Microbiology, University of Iowa College of Medicine; Director of Infectious Diseases, Department of Pediatrics, University of Iowa Hospital, Iowa City, Iowa
Bacterial Myositis and Pyomyositis; Human Herpesviruses 6, 7, and 8

William C. Gruber, M.D.
Associate Professor, Vanderbilt University School of Medicine; Attending Physician, Vanderbilt University Medical Center, Nashville, Tennessee
Miscellaneous Gram-Positive Cocci; Erysipelothrix rhusiopathiae; *Miscellaneous Gram-Positive Bacilli;* Citrobacter; Enterobacter; Klebsiella; Morganella morganii; Proteus; Providencia; Serratia; *Miscellaneous Enterobacteria;* Vibrio vulnificus; *Miscellaneous Non-Enterobacteriaceae Fermentative Bacilli;* Alcaligenes; Eikenella corrodens; Flavobacterium; Stenotrophomonas (Xanthomonas) maltophilia

Duane J. Gubler, Sc.D.
Adjunct Professor, Department of International Health, Johns Hopkins University School of Hygiene and Public Health, Baltimore, Maryland; Department of Microbiology, Colorado State University, Fort Collins, Colorado; Director, Division of Vector-Borne Infectious Diseases, National Center for Infectious Diseases, Centers for Disease Control and Prevention, Fort Collins, Colorado
Flaviviruses

Roberto A. Guerrero, M.D.
Fellow, Pediatric Gastroenterology and Nutrition, Baylor College of Medicine, Houston, Texas
Whipple Disease

Laura T. Gutman, M.D.
Associate Professor of Pediatrics and Director, Duke STD Program, Duke University Medical Center, Durham, North Carolina
Sexually Transmitted Diseases; Gonorrhea; Syphilis

Caroline Breese Hall, M.D.
Professor of Pediatrics and Medicine in Infectious Diseases, University of Rochester Medical School and Strong Memorial Hospital, Rochester, New York
Parainfluenza Viruses; Respiratory Syncytial Virus

Scott B. Halstead, B.A., M.D.
Senior Scientist, Department of Molecular Microbiology and Immunology, School of Hygiene and Public Health, Baltimore; Scientific Director, Infectious Diseases, Naval Medical Research and Development Command, Bethesda, Maryland
Alphaviruses; Flaviviruses

Margaret R. Hammerschlag, M.D.
Professor of Pediatrics and Medicine, State University of New York Health Science Center at Brooklyn; Co-Director, Pediatric Infectious Diseases, University Hospital of Brooklyn and Kings County Hospital Center, Brooklyn, New York
Peritonsillar, Retropharyngeal, and Parapharyngeal Abscesses; Chlamydia *Pneumonia*

Paul E. Hammerschlag, M.D., F.A.C.S.
Clinical Associate Professor of Otolaryngology, Department of Otolaryngology, New York University School of Medicine; Associate Attending, Tisch Hospital, New York University Medical Center, and Bellevue Hospital, New York, New York
Peritonsillar, Retropharyngeal, and Parapharyngeal Abscesses

I. Celine Hanson, M.D.
Associate Professor of Pediatrics, Baylor College of Medicine and Texas Children's Hospital, Allergy/Immunology Section, Houston, Texas
Chronic Bronchitis; AIDS and Other Acquired Immunodeficiency Diseases

Rick E. Harrison, M.D.
Associate Clinical Professor of Pediatrics, University of California at Los Angeles School of Medicine; Co-Director, Pediatric Intensive Care Unit, and Medical Director, Pediatric Transplant Services, UCLA Medical Center, Los Angeles, California
Tetanus

Ulrich Heininger, M.D.
Assistant Professor of Pediatrics, School of Medicine, Friedrich-Alexander University Nürnberg-Erlangen; Attending Physician, Division of Pediatric Infectious Diseases, Universitätsklinik für Kinder und Jugendliche, Erlangen, Germany
Pertussis and Other Bordetella *Infections*

Gloria P. Heresi, M.D.
Assistant Professor, University of Texas–Houston Health Science Center, Houston, Texas
Campylobacter jejuni

Peter W. Hiatt, M.D.
Assistant Professor of Pediatrics and Director, Cystic Fibrosis Center, Baylor College of Medicine; Director, Infant Pulmonary Function Laboratory, Texas Children's Hospital, Houston, Texas
Cystic Fibrosis; Adult Respiratory Distress Syndrome in Children

Sheila M. Hickey, M.D.
Assistant Professor of Pediatrics, Division of Infectious Diseases, University of New Mexico Health Sciences Center; Attending Physician, Children's Hospital of New Mexico, Albuquerque, New Mexico
Antibacterial Therapeutic Agents

Harry R. Hill, M.D.
Professor of Pediatrics and Pathology, Head, Division of Clinical Immunology and Allergy, University of Utah School of Medicine, Salt Lake City, Utah
Immunomodulating Agents

Peter J. Hotez, M.D., Ph.D.
Associate Professor of Pediatrics, Yale University School of Medicine, New Haven, Connecticut
Amebiasis; Blastocystis hominis *Infection;* Entamoeba coli *Infection;* Balantidium coli; *Parasitic Nematode Infections*

Dexter H. Howard, Ph.D.
Professor Emeritus, Microbiology and Immunology, University of California, Los Angeles, School of Medicine, Los Angeles, California
Classification of Fungi

Walter T. Hughes, M.D.
Professor of Pediatrics, University of Tennessee College of Medicine; Arthur Ashe Chair for Pediatric AIDS Research, St. Jude Children's Research Hospital, Memphis, Tennessee
Candidiasis; Cryptococcosis; Pneumocystis carinii *Pneumonia*

W. Charles Huskins, M.D.
Instructor in Pediatrics, Harvard Medical School; Assistant in Infectious Diseases, Children's Hospital, Boston, Massachusetts
Nosocomial Infections; Prevention and Control of Nosocomial Infections in Hospitalized Children

Sandy T. Hwang, M.D.
Fellow, Division of Pediatric Gastroenterology and Nutrition, Baylor College of Medicine, Houston, Texas
Viral Hepatitis Due to Viruses Other than Hepatitis Viruses A–E

Stanley L. Inhorn, M.D.
Professor of Pathology and Laboratory Medicine and Preventive Medicine, University of Wisconsin Medical School; Pathology Staff, University Hospital, and Clinics Medical Director, Wisconsin State Laboratory of Hygiene, Madison, Wisconsin
Rhinoviruses; Coronaviruses

Richard F. Jacobs, M.D.
Professor of Pediatrics, University of Arkansas for Medical Sciences; Chief, Division of Pediatric Infectious Disease, Arkansas Children's Hospital, Little Rock, Arkansas
Lung Abscess; Other Mycobacteria; Nocardia; Actinobacillus actinomycetemcomitans; *Actinomycosis; Fungal Meningitis; Pleural Effusions and Empyema*

Karl M. Johnson, M.D.
Adjunct Professor, Microbiology, Montana State University, Bozeman, Montana
Arenaviral and Filoviral Hemorrhagic Fevers

Erica E. Jost, M.D., M.P.H.
Clinical Assistant Professor of Pediatrics, Brown University School of Medicine; Assistant Physician, Division of Pediatric Infectious Diseases, Rhode Island Hospital, Providence, Rhode Island
Active Immunizing Agents

David P. Jubelirer, M.D.
Associate Clinical Professor of Pediatrics, University of Oklahoma–Tulsa Medical School, Tulsa, Oklahoma
Infectious Pericarditis

Edward L. Kaplan, M.D.
Professor of Pediatrics, University of Minnesota Medical School; Professor, Division of Epidemiology, School of Public Health, University of Minnesota, Minneapolis, Minnesota
Group A, Group C, and Group G Beta-Hemolytic Streptococcal Infections

Sheldon L. Kaplan, M.D.
Professor and Vice-Chairman for Clinical Affairs, Department of Pediatrics, Baylor College of Medicine; Chief, Infectious Diseases Service, Texas Children's Hospital, Houston, Texas
Microbial Virulence Factors; Pyogenic Liver Abscess; Bacteremia and Septic Shock; Arthropods; Use of the Bacteriology, Mycology, and Parasitology Laboratories

Michael Katz, M.D.
Reuben S. Carpentier Professor, Emeritus, of Pediatrics;

Professor, Emeritus, of Public Health, College of Physicians and Surgeons, Columbia University, New York; Vice President for Research, March of Dimes Birth Defects Foundation, White Plains, New York
Parasitic Nematode Infections

James P. Keating, M.D.
Professor of Pediatrics, Washington University School of Medicine, St. Louis, Missouri
Reye Syndrome; Giardiasis

William A. Kennedy, M.D.
Assistant Professor of Pediatrics and Assistant Professor of Microbiology and Immunology, Dalhousie University, Halifax, Nova Scotia, Canada
Listeriosis

Gerald T. Keusch, M.D.
Professor of Medicine, Tufts University School of Medicine; Chief, Division of Geographic Medicine and Infectious Diseases, Department of Medicine, New England Medical Center, Boston, Massachusetts
Diarrhea- and Dysentery-Causing Escherichia coli; *Cholera*

Jerome O. Klein, M.D.
Professor of Pediatrics, Boston University School of Medicine; Director, Division of Pediatric Infectious Diseases, Boston Medical Center, Boston, Massachusetts
Otitis Media; Bacterial Pneumonias

Mark W. Kline, M.D.
Associate Professor of Pediatrics, Baylor College of Medicine; Attending Physician, Texas Children's Hospital, Houston, Texas
Cystic Fibrosis; Congenital Immune Deficiency

Steve Kohl, M.D.
Professor of Pediatrics, University of California, San Francisco; Chief of Pediatric Infectious Diseases, Attending Pediatrician, Moffitt Long Memorial Hospital and San Francisco General Hospital, San Francisco, California
Herpes Simplex Virus

Heidi M. Kokkinos, B.S., M.T.(ASCP)
Clinical Laboratory Scientist, University of California, Los Angeles, Medical Center, Clinical Microbiology, Los Angeles, California
Classification of Fungi

Peter J. Krause, M.D.
Professor of Pediatrics, University of Connecticut School of Medicine, Farmington; Attending Physician, Division of Pediatric Infectious Diseases, Connecticut Children's Medical Center, Hartford, Connecticut
Babesiosis

Paul Krogstad, B.S., M.S., M.D.
Assistant Professor of Pediatrics, University of California, Los Angeles, School of Medicine, and Member, Division of Infectious Diseases, UCLA Children's Hospital, Los Angeles, California
Osteomyelitis and Septic Arthritis

Thomas L. Kuhls, M.D.
Associate Professor, University of Oklahoma College of Medicine; Attending Physician, Children's Hospital of Oklahoma, Oklahoma City, Oklahoma
Appendicitis and Pelvic Abscess; Pancreatitis; Kingella

Timothy R. La Pine, M.D.
Fellow, Division of Neonatology, Department of Pediatrics, University of Utah School of Medicine, Salt Lake City, Utah
Immunomodulating Agents

Ching C. Lau, M.D., Ph.D.
Assistant Professor, Department of Pediatrics, Baylor College of Medicine, Houston, Texas
Tularemia

Robert J. Leggiadro, M.D.
Clinical Professor of Pediatrics, New York University School of Medicine, New York; Chairman, Department of Pediatrics, St. Vincent's Medical Center of Richmond, Staten Island, New York
Other Campylobacter *Species*

Diana Lennon, M.B.Ch.B, FRACP
Professor of Community Paediatrics, University of Auckland School of Medicine, South Auckland Division; Paediatrician in Infectious Diseases, Starship Children's Hospital, Auckland, New Zealand
Acute Rheumatic Fever

Moise L. Levy, M.D.
Associate Professor of Dermatology/Pediatrics, Baylor College of Medicine; Chief, Dermatology Service, Texas Children's Hospital, Houston, Texas
Viral and Fungal Skin Infections

Karen Lewis, M.D.
Pediatric Infectious Disease Consultant, Phoenix Children's Hospital, Phoenix, Arizona
Mastoiditis

Christine A. Lindsay, Pharm.D.
Clinical Assistant Professor, University of Texas School of Pharmacy, Austin; Clinical Coordinator, Children's Medical Center of Dallas, Dallas, Texas
Fundamentals of Pharmacokinetics, Anti-infective Pharmacodynamics, and Therapeutic Drug Monitoring

Martin I. Lorin, M.D.
Professor of Pediatrics, Baylor College of Medicine; Attending Physician, Texas Children's Hospital, Houston, Texas
Fever: Pathogenesis and Treatment; Fever Without Localizing Signs and Fever of Unknown Origin

Harold S. Margolis, M.D.
Chief, Hepatitis Branch, National Center for Infectious Diseases, Centers for Disease Control and Prevention, Atlanta, Georgia
Hepatitis A Virus; Hepatitis C Virus

Melvin I. Marks, M.D.
Professor and Vice Chair, Department of Pediatrics, University of California, Irvine; Executive Director, Memorial Miller Children's Hospital, Long Beach, California
Urinary Tract Infections

Edward O. Mason, Jr., Ph.D.
Professor of Pediatrics, Microbiology, and Immunology, Baylor College of Medicine; Director, Infectious Disease Laboratory, Texas Children's Hospital, Houston, Texas
Use of the Bacteriology, Mycology, and Parasitology Laboratories; Use of the Serology Laboratory

Eric E. Mast, M.D., M.P.H.
Chief, Surveillance Unit, Epidemiology Section, Hepatitis Branch, Centers for Disease Control and Prevention, Atlanta, Georgia
Hepatitis C Virus

David O. Matson, M.D., Ph.D.
Associate Professor of Pediatrics, Eastern Virginia Medical School; Attending Physician, Children's Hospital of The King's Daughters and Sentara Norfolk General Hospital, Norfolk, Virginia
Caliciviruses, Including Hepatitis E Virus

Suzanne Maxson, M.D.
Pediatric Infectious Diseases, Cook Children's Medical Center, Fort Worth, Texas
Actinobacillus actinomycetemcomitans; *Actinomycosis*

George H. McCracken, Jr., M.D.
Professor of Pediatrics, The Sarah M. and Charles E. Seay Chair in Pediatric Infectious Diseases, University of Texas Southwestern Medical Center; Attending Physician, Children's Medical Center, Dallas, Texas
Perinatal Bacterial Diseases; Antibacterial Therapeutic Agents

James E. McJunkin, M.D.
Professor of Pediatrics, Robert C. Byrd Health Sciences Center of West Virginia, Charleston Division; Medical Staff, Pediatrics, Charleston Area Medical Center, Women and Children's Division, Charleston, West Virginia
California/La Crosse Encephalitis

Kelly T. McKee, Jr., M.D., M.P.H.
Chief, Preventive Medicine Service, Womack Army Medical Center, Ft. Bragg, North Carolina
Hantaviruses

Rima L. McLeod, M.D.
Jules and Doris Stein Research to Prevent Blindness Professor, Departments of Visual Sciences, Medicine, and Pathology, University of Chicago Pritzker School of Medicine; Attending Physician, University of Chicago Hospitals and Michael Reese Hospital and Medical Center, Chicago, Illinois
Toxoplasmosis

Marian E. Melish, M.D.
Professor of Pediatrics, Tropical Medicine, and Medical Microbiology, John A. Burns School of Medicine, University of Hawaii; Infectious Diseases Consultant and Attending Pediatrician, Kapiolani Medical Center for Women and Children, Honolulu, Hawaii
Bacterial Skin Infections; Kawasaki Disease; Coagulase-Positive Staphylococcal Infections

Joseph L. Melnick, Ph.D., M.D.(Hon.), D.Sc.
Distinguished Service Professor, Division of Molecular Virology, Baylor College of Medicine, Houston, Texas
Nomenclature and Classification of Viruses

Wayne M. Meyers, M.D., Ph.D., D.Sc.(Hon.)
Research Affiliate, Tulane Regional Primate Research Center, Tulane University, Covington, Louisiana; Chief, Mycobacteriology Branch, and Registrar, Leprosy Registry, American Registry of Pathology, Armed Forces Institute of Pathology, Washington, D.C.
Leprosy

James N. Miller, Ph.D.
Professor of Microbiology and Immunology, University of California, Los Angeles, School of Medicine, Los Angeles, California
Nonveneral Treponematoses

Marjorie J. Miller, Dr.P.H.
Senior Specialist, Clinical Virology, Clinical Laboratories–Microbiology, UCLA Medical Center, Los Angeles, California
Use of the Diagnostic Virology Laboratory

Linda L. Minnich, M.S., S.M.(HAM)
Clinical Virologist, Charleston Area Medical Center, Charleston, West Virginia
California/La Crosse Encephalitis

Sudipta L. Misra, M.B., B.S., M.D., D.M.
Resident, Department of Pediatrics, Maimonides Medical Center, Brooklyn, New York
Esophagitis

Lynne M. Mofenson, M.D.
Associate Branch Chief for Clinical Research, Pediatric, Adolescent, and Maternal AIDS Branch, Center for Research for Mothers and Children, National Institute of Child Health and Human

Development, National Institutes of Health, Rockville, Maryland
Human Retroviruses

David M. Morens, A.B., M.D.
Professor and Head, Epidemiology Program, School of Public Health, University of Hawaii; Professor of Tropical Medicine, School of Medicine, University of Hawaii; Director of Laboratories, Diamond Head Health Center; Staff Physician, Tripler Army Medical Center, Honolulu, Hawaii
Kawasaki Disease

Edward A. Mortimer, Jr., M.D.
Elisabeth Geverance Prentiss Professor Emeritus, Department of Epidemiology and Biostatistics, School of Medicine, Case Western Reserve University; Associate Pediatrician, University Hospitals of Cleveland, Cleveland, Ohio
Epidemiology of Infectious Diseases

Mark S. Munsey, M.S.
Manager, Clinical Operations, Sepracor Pharmaceuticals, Inc., Marlborough, Massachusetts
Other Anaerobic Infections

Anita Newman, M.D., FACS
Attending Staff Surgeon, Children's Hospital of Los Angeles, Los Angeles, California
Sinusitis; Mastoiditis

Karin Nielsen, M.D., M.P.H.
Clinical Instructor, University of California at Los Angeles School of Medicine; Member, Division of Infectious Diseases, UCLA Children's Hospital, Los Angeles, California
Hepatitis B and D Viruses

Michael R. Nihill, M.D., M.B., B.S., M.S., MRCP
Professor, Department of Pediatrics, Baylor College of Medicine; Consultant, Pediatric Cardiology, Texas Children's Hospital, Methodist Hospital, and Harris County Hospital District, Houston, Texas
Infectious Pericarditis

James C. Overall, Jr., M.D.
Professor of Pediatrics and Pathology, University of Utah School of Medicine; Medical Director, Diagnostic Virology Laboratory, Associated Regional and University Pathologists; Consultant in Pediatric Infectious Diseases, Primary Children's and University of Utah Medical Centers, Salt Lake City, Utah
Viral Infections of the Fetus and Neonate

Kelvin S. Panesar, M.D.
Pediatric Pulmonology Fellow, Baylor College of Medicine, Houston, Texas
Interaction of Infection and Nutrition

Christian C. Patrick, M.D., Ph.D.
Associate Professor, Department of Pediatrics, The University of Tennessee, Memphis, College of Medicine; Director of Academic Programs, Director of Clinical Microbiology and Molecular Microbiology, and Associate Member, St. Jude Children's Research Hospital, Memphis, Tennessee
Opportunistic Infections in the Compromised Host; Coagulase-Negative Staphylococcal Infections

Eric M. Pearlman, M.D., Ph.D.
Resident in Pediatric Neurology, Johns Hopkins University School of Medicine, Baltimore, Maryland
Bacterial Meningitis Beyond the Neonatal Period

Georges Peter, M.D.
Professor of Pediatrics, Brown University School of Medicine; Director, Division of Pediatric Infectious Diseases, Rhode

Island Hospital, Providence, Rhode Island
Active Immunizing Agents

C. J. Peters, M.D.
Chief, Special Pathogens Branch, Centers for Disease Control and Prevention, Atlanta, Georgia
Hantaviruses

Larry K. Pickering, M.D.
Professor of Pediatrics, Eastern Virginia Medical School; Director, Center for Pediatric Research, Children's Hospital of The King's Daughters, Norfolk, Virginia
Approach to Patients with Gastrointestinal Tract Infections and Food Poisoning

Joseph F. Piecuch, D.M.D., M.D.
Clinical Professor, Department of Oral and Maxillofacial Surgery, University of Connecticut School of Dental Medicine, Farmington, Connecticut
Infections of the Oral Cavity

Francisco P. Pinheiro, M.D., Ph.D.
Advisor on Viral Diseases, Pan American Health Organization, World Health Organization, Communicable Diseases Program, Division of Disease Prevention and Control, Washington, D.C.
Other Bunyaviruses

William W. Pinsky, M.D.
Associate Dean for Clinical Affairs, Wayne State University School of Medicine; Senior Vice President for Clinical Affairs and Managed Care, Detroit Medical Center, Detroit, Michigan
Infectious Pericarditis

Stanley A. Plotkin, M.D.
Professor Emeritus of Pediatrics, University of Pennsylvania School of Medicine; Professor Emeritus, Wistar Institute, Philadelphia, Pennsylvania; Medical and Scientific Director, Pasteur Mérieux Connaught, Marnes-La-Coquette, France
Rabies Virus

Scott L. Pomeroy, M.D., Ph.D.
Assistant Professor of Neurology, Harvard Medical School; Assistant in Neurology, Boston Children's Hospital, Boston, Massachusetts
Parameningeal Infections; Transverse Myelitis or Myelopathy

Joan S. Purcell, M.D.
Assistant Professor, Department of Obstetrics and Gynecology/ Pediatrics, University of Texas Medical Branch, Galveston, Texas
Trichomonas *Infections*

Jack S. Remington, M.D.
Professor of Medicine, Division of Infectious Diseases, Stanford University School of Medicine; Chairman, Department of Immunology and Infectious Diseases, Marcus A. Krupp Research Chair, Research Institute, Palo Alto Medical Foundation, Palo Alto, California
Toxoplasmosis

Angela Restrepo-Moreno, Ph.D.
Head of the Mycology Laboratory, Corporación para Investigaciones Biológica, Medellin, Colombia
Paracoccidioidomycosis

Michael G. Rinaldi, Ph.D.
Professor of Pathology, Medicine, Microbiology, and Clinical Laboratory Sciences, Director, Fungus Testing Laboratory, University of Texas Health Science Center at San Antonio; Chief, Clinical Microbiology Laboratories, Director, Department of Veterans Affairs, Mycology Reference Laboratory, Audie L. Murphy Division,

South Texas Veterans Health Care System, San Antonio, Texas
Antifungal Agents

John W. Rippon, Ph.D.
Retired; formerly Associate Professor Emeritus of Medicine/Dermatology, University of Chicago Pritzker School of Medicine, Chicago, Illinois
Miscellaneous Mycoses

Judith L. Rowen, M.D.
Assistant Professor, Department of Pediatrics, Infectious Diseases Division, University of Texas Medical Branch, Galveston, Texas
Group B Streptococcal Infections

Xavier Sáez-Llorens, M.D.
Professor of Pediatrics and Infectious Diseases, University of Panama School of Medicine, Panama City; Chief, Pediatric Infectious Disease Division, Hospital del Niño, Panama City, Panama
Perinatal Bacterial Diseases

Pablo J. Sánchez, M.D.
Associate Professor of Pediatrics, Divisions of Neonatal-Perinatal Medicine and Pediatric Infectious Diseases, The University of Texas Southwestern Medical Center at Dallas; Attending Physician, Parkland Memorial Hospital, Children's Medical Center, and St. Paul's Medical Center, Dallas, Texas
Miscellaneous Infections of the Newborn

Jane G. Schaller, M.D.
Professor of Pediatrics, Tufts University School of Medicine; Pediatrician-in-Chief, The Floating Hospital, New England Medical Center, Boston, Massachusetts
Noninfectious Carditis

Ann O. Scheimann, B.S., M.D.
Assistant Professor, Pediatric Gastroenterology and Nutrition, Baylor College of Medicine, Houston, Texas
Cholangitis and Cholecystitis

Kenneth O. Schowengerdt, M.D.
Assistant Professor of Pediatrics (Cardiology), Baylor College of Medicine; Associate in Pediatric Cardiology, Texas Children's Hospital, Houston, Texas
Myocarditis

Gordon E. Schutze, M.D.
Associate Professor of Pediatrics and Pathology, University of Arkansas for Medical Sciences and Arkansas Children's Hospital, Little Rock, Arkansas
Blastomycosis

James S. Seidel, M.D., Ph.D.
Professor of Pediatrics, University of California, Los Angeles, School of Medicine, Los Angeles; Chief, Division of General and Emergency Pediatrics, Harbor-UCLA Medical Center, Torrance, California
Naegleria, Acanthamoeba *and Leptomyxid Ameba*

Craig N. Shapiro, M.D.
Deputy Chief, Epidemiology Section, Hepatitis Branch, National Center for Infectious Diseases, Centers for Disease Control and Prevention, Atlanta, Georgia
Hepatitis A Virus

Eugene D. Shapiro, M.D.
Professor of Pediatrics and of Epidemiology, Yale University School of Medicine and Children's Clinical Research Center; Attending Pediatrician, Children's Hospital at Yale–New Haven, New Haven, Connecticut
Epidemiology and Biostatistics

William T. Shearer, M.D., Ph.D.
Professor of Pediatrics and of Microbiology and Immunology,

Baylor College of Medicine; Chief, Allergy and Immunology Service, Texas Children's Hospital, Houston, Texas
Chronic Bronchitis; Congenital Immune Deficiency; AIDS and Other Acquired Immunodeficiency Diseases

Ziad M. Shehab, M.D.
Professor of Clinical Pediatrics and Pathology, The University of Arizona, Tucson, Arizona
Coccidioidomycosis

Jerry L. Shenep, M.D.
Professor, Department of Pediatrics, University of Tennessee, Memphis, College of Medicine; Associate Member, Department of Infectious Diseases, St. Jude Children's Research Hospital, Memphis, Tennessee
Enterococcal and Viridans Streptococcal Infections

W. Donald Shields, M.D.
Professor of Neurology and Pediatrics, University of California, Los Angeles, School of Medicine; Chief, Division of Pediatric Neurology, UCLA Children's Hospital, Los Angeles, California
Encephalitis and Meningoencephalitis

Robert E. Shope, M.D.
Professor of Pathology, Center for Tropical Diseases, University of Texas Medical Branch, Galveston, Texas
Other Bunyaviruses

Raymond G. Slavin, M.D.
Professor of Internal Medicine and Microbiology, St. Louis University School of Medicine; Director, Division of Allergy and Immunology, St. Louis University Health Sciences Center, St. Louis, Missouri
Hypersensitivity Pneumonitis and Chronic Interstitial Pneumonitis

Karen S. Slobod, M.D., C.M.
Assistant Professor, University of Tennessee, Memphis, College of Medicine; Assistant Member, St. Jude Children's Research Hospital, Memphis, Tennessee
Opportunistic Infections in the Compromised Host

Arnold L. Smith, B.S., M.S., M.D.
Professor and Chairman, Department of Molecular Microbiology, University of Missouri School of Medicine, Columbia, Missouri
Indigenous Flora; Osteomyelitis and Septic Arthritis; Meningococcal Disease

Margaret H. D. Smith, M.D.
Faculty, Tulane University Medical School, New Orleans, Louisiana
Tuberculosis

Steven L. Solomon, M.D.
Assistant Clinical Professor, Division of Infectious Disease, Emory University School of Medicine; Chief, Special Studies Activity, Hospital Infections Program, National Center for Infectious Diseases, Centers for Disease Control and Prevention, Atlanta, Georgia
Public Health Considerations

Jeffrey R. Starke, M.D.
Associate Professor of Pediatrics, Baylor College of Medicine; Director, Infection Control, Texas Children's Hospital, Houston, Texas
Infective Endocarditis; Tuberculosis

Barbara W. Stechenberg, M.D.
Associate Professor of Pediatrics, Tufts University School of Medicine, Boston; Vice Chairman and Director of Pediatric Infectious Diseases, Department of Pediatrics, Baystate Medical Center Children's Hospital, Springfield, Massachusetts
Eosinophilic Meningitis; Moraxella catarrhalis; *Diphtheria;* Pasteurella multocida; *Bartonellosis;* Borrelia *(Lyme Disease)*

Paul G. Steinkuller, M.D.
Assistant Professor, Department of Ophthalmology, Baylor College of Medicine; Chief of Ophthalmology, Texas Children's Hospital, Houston, Texas
Ocular Infections

E. Richard Stiehm, M.D.
Professor of Pediatrics and Chief, Division of Immunology, Department of Pediatrics, University of California, Los Angeles, School of Medicine; Attending Pediatrician, UCLA Children's Hospital, UCLA Medical Center, Los Angeles, California
Passive Immunization

Alan D. Strickland, B.S., M.S., M.D., D.Chem.
Staff Researcher, Discovery Group, Freeport, Texas
Amebiasis

Ciro V. Sumaya, M.D., M.P.H.T.M.
Professor of Pediatrics and Pathology, Division of Infectious Diseases, and Associate Medical Dean, University of Texas Health Science Center; Attending Physician, Medical Center Hospital and Santa Rosa Children's Hospital, San Antonio, Texas
Chronic Fatigue Syndrome; Epstein-Barr Virus

Mary E. Sutton, M.D.
Instructor in Neurology, Harvard Medical School and Boston Children's Hospital, Boston, Massachusetts
Parameningeal Infections; Transverse Myelitis or Myelopathy

David W. Teele, B.A., M.D.
Professor of Paediatrics, Christchurch School of Medicine, University of Otago; Clinical Director, Department of Paediatrics, Christchurch Hospital, Christchurch, New Zealand
Pneumococcal Infections

Robert B. Tesh, B.S., M.S., M.D.
Professor of Pathology and Professor of Microbiology and Immunology, Center for Tropical Diseases, University of Texas Medical Branch, Galveston, Texas
Other Bunyaviruses

Margaret A. Tipple, M.D.
Medical Officer, Office of Health and Safety, Centers for Disease Control and Prevention, Atlanta, Georgia
Health Information for International Travel

Richard G. Topazian, D.D.S.
Professor, Department of Oral and Maxillofacial Surgery, University of Connecticut School of Dental Medicine, Farmington, Connecticut
Infections of the Oral Cavity

Michael F. Tosi, M.D.
Associate Professor of Pediatrics, Case Western Reserve University; Rainbow Babies and Childrens Hospital, Cleveland, Ohio
Immunologic and Phagocytic Responses to Infection

Jeffrey A. Towbin, M.D.
Associate Professor of Pediatrics (Cardiology), Molecular and Human Genetics, Baylor College of Medicine; Pediatric Cardiologist and Director, Heart Failure Clinic, Texas Children's Hospital, Houston, Texas
Myocarditis

Amelia P. A. Travassos da Rosa, Pharmacist
Chief, Arbovirus Service, Instituto Evandro Chagas, Fundação Nacional de Saude, Ministry of Health, Belem, Para, Brazil
Other Bunyaviruses

Theodore F. Tsai, M.D., M.P.H.
Medical Officer, Centers for Disease Control and Prevention, Ft. Collins, Colorado
Orbiviruses and Coltiviruses; Alphaviruses; Flaviviruses; California/La Crosse Encephalitis

Jerrold A. Turner, M.D.
Professor of Medicine and Microbiology and Immunology, University of California, Los Angeles, School of Medicine, Los Angeles; Chief, Section of Parasitic Diseases; Associate Medical Director; and Director of Medical Education, Harbor–UCLA Medical Center, Torrance, California
Cestodes; Trematodes

Jesus G. Vallejo, M.D.
Assistant Professor of Pediatrics, Section of Infectious Disease, Baylor College of Medicine, Houston, Texas
Myocarditis

Jorge Vargas, M.D.
Associate Professor of Pediatrics, University of California at Los Angeles School of Medicine and Division of Pediatric Gastroenterology and Nutrition, UCLA Children's Hospital, Los Angeles, California
Hepatitis B and D Viruses

Pedro F. C. Vasconcelos, M.D.
Infectologist, Arbovirus Service, Instituto Evandro Chagas, Fundação Nacional de Saude, Ministry of Health, Belem, Para, Brazil
Other Bunyaviruses

Ellen R. Wald, M.D.
Professor of Pediatrics and Otolaryngology, University of Pittsburgh School of Medicine; Division Chief, Allergy, Immunology, and Infectious Diseases, Children's Hospital of Pittsburgh, Pittsburgh, Pennsylvania
Uvulitis; Infections in Day Care Environments

Joel I. Ward, M.D.
Professor of Pediatrics, University of California at Los Angeles School of Medicine; Chief, Pediatric Infectious Disease; Director, UCLA Center for Vaccine Research; Harbor–UCLA Medical Center, Torrance, California
Haemophilus influenzae

Richard L. Ward, Ph.D.
Professor of Pediatrics, University of Cincinnati School of Medicine and Children's Hospital Medical Center, Cincinnati, Ohio
Rotaviruses

Louis Weinstein, M.D., Ph.D.
Retired; former lecturer in Medicine, Harvard Medical School, Cambridge; Senior Consultant in Medicine, Brigham and Women's Hospital, Boston, Massachusetts
Tetanus

Robert C. Welliver, M.D.
Professor of Pediatrics, Division of Infectious Diseases, and Co-Director, Division of Infectious Diseases, State University of New York and Children's Hospital, Buffalo, New York
Bronchiolitis and Infectious Asthma

J. Gary Wheeler, M.D.
Associate Professor, Department of Pediatrics, Divisions of Allergy, Clinical Immunology, and Infectious Diseases, University of Arkansas for Medical Sciences; Attending Staff, Arkansas Children's Hospital, Little Rock, Arkansas
Pleural Effusions and Empyema; Lung Abscess

Bernhard L. Wiedermann, M.D.
Associate Professor of Pediatrics, The George Washington University School of Medicine and Health Sciences; Attending in Infectious Diseases and Director, Pediatric Residency Training Program, Children's National Medical Center, Washington, DC
Microbial Virulence Factors; Miscellaneous Causes of Myositis; Aspergillus *Infections; Histoplasmosis; Sporotrichosis; Zygomycosis*

Murray Wittner, M.D., Ph.D.
Professor of Pathology and Parasitology, Albert Einstein College of Medicine; Director, Parasitology and Tropical Diseases Clinic and Laboratory, Jacobi Medical Center, Bronx, New York
Leishmaniasis; Trypanosomiasis

Charles R. Woods, Jr., M.D.
Assistant Professor of Pediatrics, Bowman Gray School of Medicine, Wake Forest University, and Brenner Children's Hospital, Winston-Salem, North Carolina
Gynecologic Infections in Childhood and Adolescence; Other Yersinia *Species*

Edward J. Young, M.D.
Professor of Medicine and Professor of Microbiology and Immunology, Baylor College of Medicine; Chief of Staff, Veterans Affairs Medical Center, Houston, Texas
Brucellosis

Kenneth M. Zangwill, M.D.
Assistant Professor of Pediatrics, Harbor–UCLA Medical Center, University of California at Los Angeles School of Medicine; Member, Division of Infectious Diseases and UCLA Center for Vaccine Research, Harbor–UCLA Medical Center, Los Angeles, California
Haemophilus influenzae

PREFACE

❑ ❑ ❑

Despite the dramatic reduction in morbidity and mortality rates related to infectious diseases that followed the introduction of antimicrobial therapy, as well as active and passive immunization efforts, infectious diseases remain the leading cause of morbidity in infants and children. Children experience an average of six respiratory infections per year, requiring visits to a physician that outnumber the visits made for the purpose of well-child care. Infectious diseases also are the most common cause of school absenteeism.

The first edition of our text was written because we and many of our colleagues were concerned that no single reference existed that comprehensively covered infectious diseases in children. With each subsequent edition, including this one, our goal has been to provide comprehensive coverage of all subjects pertinent to the study of infectious diseases in children. Any attempt to summarize our present understanding of infectious diseases for serious students of the subject is a formidable task. In many areas, new information is accruing so rapidly that material becomes dated before it can appear in a text of this magnitude. Nevertheless, we have endeavored with the help of our many colleagues to provide the most comprehensive and up-to-date discussion of this field.

To provide a text as comprehensive and authoritative as possible, we have enlisted contributions from a large number of individuals, whose collective expertise is responsible for whatever success we may have had in meeting our objective. We offer our deepest appreciation to the 224 fellow contributors from universities or institutions in 10 countries for their professional expertise and devoted scholarship. Their cooperation and willingness to work with us leave us deeply in their debt.

Once again, infectious diseases are discussed according to organ systems that may be affected as well as individually by microorganisms. In all sections in which diseases related to specific agents are discussed, emphasis has been placed to the greatest extent possible on the specificity of clinical manifestations that may be related to the organism causing disease. Detailed information regarding the best means to establish a diagnosis and explicit recommendations for therapy are provided.

The entire text has been revised extensively. This edition also presents a new format for the discussion of infections caused by specific microorganisms. In the past, the various organisms causing disease were alphabetized within each section, offering the reader no particular advantage, as reference to the index still was required to locate a subject by specific page number.

In this edition, the infections with specific microorganisms have been reorganized to more appropriately emphasize the common features that may relate specific microorganisms to each other. Thus, all gram-positive coccal organisms are presented sequentially, followed by gram-negative cocci, gram-positive bacilli, enterobacteria, gram-negative coccobacilli, Treponemataceae, anaerobic bacteria, etc.

In addition, special sections of the text have been devoted to discussions of each of the following: microbial virulence factors; immunologic and phagocytic responses to infection; metabolic response of the host to infections; interaction of infection and nutrition; pathogenesis and treatment of fever; indigenous flora in host economy and pathogenesis; epidemiology of infectious diseases; congenital immune deficiency; AIDS and other acquired immunodeficiency diseases; opportunistic infections in the compromised host; Kawasaki disease; chronic fatigue syndrome; health information for the international traveler; nosocomial infections; prevention and control of infections in hospitalized children; pharmacology and pharmacokinetics of infectious agents; antibacterial, antiviral, antifungal, and antiparasitic agents; public health considerations; infections in day care environments; and use of the bacteriology, mycology, parasitology, virology, and serology laboratories.

A new section on immunomodulating agents and their potential use in the treatment of infectious diseases has been included because information on this subject has become most extensive since the publication of the last edition. Specific sections also are devoted to human bites and animal bites. In addition, the subject of biostatistics as applicable to the subspecialty of infectious diseases has been included for the first time. Other sections that make their first appearance as complete chapters include esophagitis; Whipple disease; infectious hepatitis due to viruses other than hepatitis viruses A through E; *Arcanobacterium haemolyticum; Erysipelothrix rhusiopathiae; Vibrio parahaemolyticus; Acinetobacter; Alcaligenes; Eikenella corrodens; Flavobacterium; Stenotrophomonas (Xanthomonas) maltophilia; Calymmatobacterium granulomatis; Kingella;* caliciviruses, including hepatitis E virus; and orbiviruses and coltiviruses. A chapter also has been devoted to the appropriate and inappropriate uses of prophylactic antimicrobial agents.

This book could not have been brought to fruition without the help and assistance of many individuals whose names do not appear in the text. Words are inadequate to convey our gratitude appropriately; we hope that they know they have our heartfelt thanks.

We would like to single out certain individuals for specific mention. We cannot adequately convey our appreciation for the thousands of hours devoted by Pamela Berea, who edited and also proofread every word of the text that was submitted, either in typed format or on computer disk, as well as the galley and page proofs of this manuscript. We are equally indebted to Mary Campbell, who spent an equivalent amount of time and who was specifically responsible for the coordination of the editorial effort, correspondence with our contributors and with the publisher, and coordination of the manuscript preparation process. We also appreciate the assistance provided to Mary Campbell and to the Editors by Carol Collins, Leslie Spring, Ruthi Stevens, and Sue Yancey, as well as the help provided by Carrel Briley and Sheila Walton.

We also appreciate the help and support of Judith Fletcher, Melissa Messersmith, Sandra Won and Michael Carcel (both formerly of W.B. Saunders), and Tom Stringer at W.B. Saunders, as well as the advice and editorial guidance of Lisette Bralow, who has helped us with every edition of this book.

Finally, we would like to thank the Baylor College of Medicine and Texas Children's Hospital in Houston, Texas, and the University of California School of Medicine at Los Angeles and the UCLA Children's Hospital for providing an environment that is supportive of intellectual pursuits.

RALPH D. FEIGIN, M.D.
JAMES D. CHERRY, M.D.

CONTENTS

❑ ❑ ❑

Color plates appear on pp. 724–729 and 2443–2446.

Volume 1

Part

1

HOST-PARASITE RELATIONSHIPS AND THE PATHOGENESIS OF INFECTIOUS DISEASES

Part

2

INFECTIONS OF SPECIFIC ORGAN SYSTEMS

SECTION ONE

UPPER RESPIRATORY TRACT INFECTIONS

SECTION TWO
LOWER RESPIRATORY TRACT INFECTIONS

SECTION THREE
INFECTIONS OF THE HEART

SECTION TWELVE
SYSTEMIC INFECTIOUS DISEASES

SECTION THIRTEEN
INFECTIONS OF THE FETUS AND NEWBORN

SECTION FOURTEEN
INFECTIONS OF THE COMPROMISED HOST

SECTION FIFTEEN
UNCLASSIFIED INFECTIOUS DISEASES

Part 3
INFECTIONS WITH SPECIFIC MICROORGANISMS

SECTION SIXTEEN
BACTERIAL INFECTIONS

❑ ❑ ❑

SUBSECTION ONE
GRAM-POSITIVE COCCI

Volume 2

❑ ❑ ❑

SUBSECTION FIVE
GRAM-NEGATIVE COCCOBACILLI

Part
5
THERAPEUTICS

Part
6
PREVENTION OF INFECTIOUS DISEASES

SECTION TWENTY-FIVE
OTHER PREVENTIVE CONSIDERATIONS

Part 7

GUIDES TO THE DIAGNOSIS OF INFECTION

Part 8

BIOSTATISTICS APPLICABLE TO THE SUBSPECIALITY OF INFECTIOUS DISEASES

DRUG NOTICE

Pediatric infectious diseases is an ever-changing field. Standard safety precautions must be followed, but as new research and clinical experience broaden our knowledge, changes in treatment and drug therapy become necessary or appropriate. Readers are advised to check the product information currently provided by the manufacturer of each drug to be administered to verify the recommended dose, the method and duration of administration, and contraindications. It is the responsibility of the treating physician relying on experience and knowledge of the patient to determine dosages and the best treatment for the patient. Neither the Publisher nor the editor assumes any responsibility for any injury and/or damage to persons or property.

THE PUBLISHER

PART 1

HOST-PARASITE RELATIONSHIPS AND THE PATHOGENESIS OF INFECTIOUS DISEASES

1

MICROBIAL VIRULENCE FACTORS

Bernhard L. Wiedermann and Sheldon L. Kaplan

Virulence refers to the ability of a microorganism to overcome defense capabilities of the host and cause clinical disease. Many different factors, both microbial and host related, ultimately are responsible for the frequency and severity of disease production; a number of excellent review articles have discussed these topics.[12, 21, 25, 80, 92, 96, 97, 124, 157] This chapter serves as an introduction to some of the common pathogens in pediatric infections for which specific microbial features are thought to confer significant pathogenicity.

In most of the examples discussed here, there is no clear "proof" that these specific properties indeed are necessary and/or sufficient for the production of disease. Most of the evidence supporting a role for these factors in clinical illness is "circumstantial," that is, it is more difficult to prove that a specific microbial trait causes disease than to prove that a given organism is responsible for a disease process. Most of the data concerning microbial virulence factors center around three main types of information: (1) the presence of a particular factor in organisms commonly producing disease and its absence in normally nonpathogenic agents; (2) attenuation of virulence of mutants lacking these features compared with the parent organism; and (3) in some cases, the ability of specific therapy aimed at the virulence factor to prevent or minimize disease in infection produced experimentally. Further elucidation of virulence mechanisms in infectious diseases holds great promise for the development of novel therapeutic interventions.

Some pathogenic microorganisms possess several different factors that seem to confer increased virulence; a cluster of these factors occurring in the same organism has been termed a virulence clone. For example, Scandinavian studies have shown that uropathogenic strains of *Escherichia coli* tend to belong to a limited number of serogroups and have the ability to produce similar fimbriae, hemolysins, and colicins.[109, 210] They also tend to display similar numbers of plasmids and similar outer-membrane protein electrophoretic patterns, suggesting a common evolutionary origin. The O1:K1:H7 clone may have particular significance for uropathogenicity, although it is not known whether this clone is pervasive outside of Scandinavian pyelonephritic strains.[72, 109]

One of the difficulties in studying microbial virulence factors is the ability of individual strains to vary in their ability to express the putative factors; study of the mechanisms governing expression of virulence factors may provide greater insight into developing treatment or prevention strategies. Many organisms appear to control expression of virulence factors in response to environmental signals. For example, *Bordetella pertussis* has a portion of its genome, the *bvg* locus (also called the *vir* locus), that appears to control expression of several virulence determinants.[124] In response to low temperature, the presence of magnesium sulfate, or the presence of nicotinic acid in the environment, *B. pertussis* fails to produce adenylate cyclase, dermonecrotic and pertussis toxins, and hemolysin, and an avirulent phenotype is produced. This phase variation can be caused by a frame shift mutation in an open-reading frame of *bvg*.[194] The protein products of the *bvg* locus have similarities to other signal transduction proteins in other prokaryotic systems and thus may have far-reaching applications for clinical medicine.[9, 21]

For the purpose of this discussion, infection can be considered to occur in five major stages[183]: (1) An organism must come into contact with the host, usually at a mucosal surface, and adhere at this site. (2) Subsequently, proliferation of the organism occurs at this local site, allowing the numbers of organisms to increase in order to cause disease. (3) There may appear then a stage of local tissue damage. (4) Toxins may be produced, which can act locally or systemically. (5) This is followed by tissue invasion and dissemination of the organism to other parts of the body. It should be noted that not all stages of infection are necessary for disease production by some pathogens. The remainder of this discussion consists of selected examples of these processes that appear to be significant factors in the production of infectious diseases in children.

ADHERENCE

Many pathogenic microorganisms are thought to be aided in their ability to produce disease by the presence of certain adhesive or adherence properties that allow a pathogen to gain a "foothold" on the mucosal surfaces of the host. In many instances, these adhesive organelles are host-cell–specific, that is, they may allow attachment only to certain types of cells within the body and thus may help dictate the type of illness produced. Antimicrobial therapy is known to exert profound effects on the adherence of microorganisms in certain situations.[8, 94, 161, 176, 189, 196, 208] In particular, antibiotic concentrations below that necessary to inhibit bacterial growth still may prevent adhesion to mucosal surfaces and thus may become an important treatment strategy.

Fimbriae are filamentous organelles present on the surface of many bacterial cells that most often function as adhesive structures (Fig. 1–1). Pili are defined most appropriately as a subtype of fimbriae involved in genetic conjugation between bacteria. However, the term "pili" often has been used interchangeably with "fimbriae," a convention that will be continued in this discussion.

Escherichia coli

Microbial adherence properties are believed to be quite important in the pathogenesis of urinary tract infection caused by certain strains of *E. coli*. Svanborg-Eden and colleagues[199] provided evidence that *E. coli* strains that cause pyelonephritis tend to adhere to human uroepithelial cells in greater numbers than do strains isolated from the urine of asymptomatic patients. This observation was extended to comparison of isolates from patients with different clinical forms of urinary tract infections.[198] Thus, *E. coli* isolates from the urine of children with pyelonephritis showed a mean adherence of 31 bacteria per cell in an in vitro assay, compared with 19 bacteria per cell in isolates from patients with acute cystitis, 8 bacteria per cell in isolates from individuals with asymptomatic bacteriuria, and about 5 bacteria per cell when fecal *E. coli* isolates from normal children were tested. It was shown later that this uropathogenic adhesive property

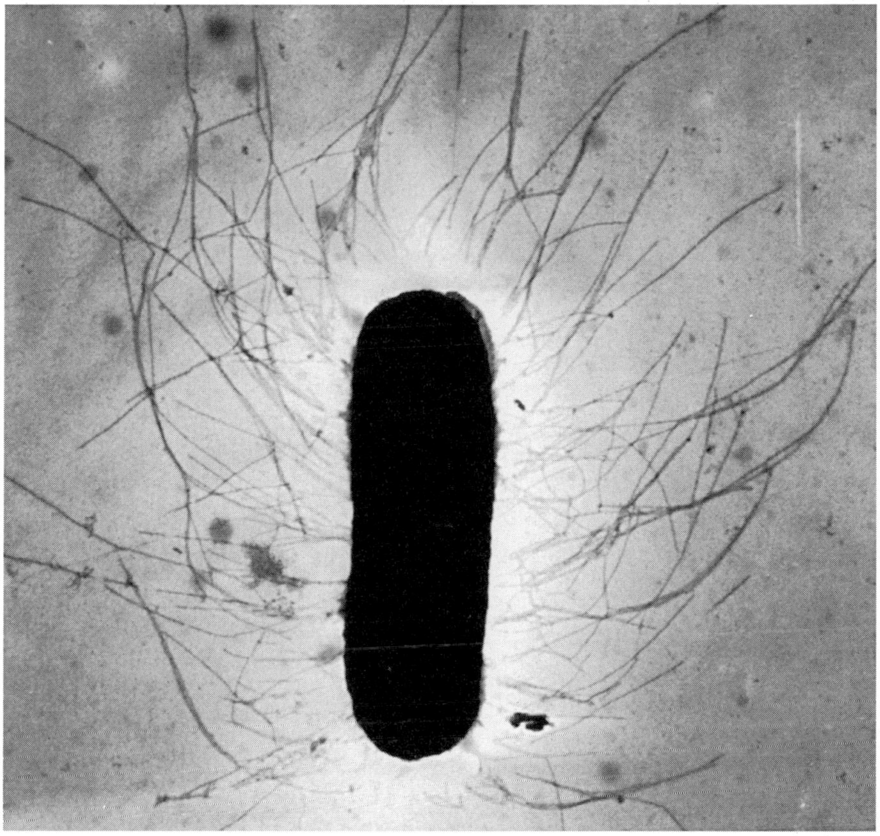

FIGURE 1–1. *Transmission electron micrograph of piliated* Escherichia coli. *(×36,800.) (Courtesy of James Barrish, Department of Pathology, Texas Children's Hospital, Houston, TX.)*

in *E. coli* is determined by the presence of P pili on the cell's surface.

E. coli may express several different types of pili.[90, 129] P pili constitute a class of surface structures responsible for adhesion in uropathogenic strains. In addition to binding to uroepithelial cells, these organelles also mediate adherence to human red blood cells carrying the P blood group antigen.[81] Binding is not inhibited by D-mannose; thus, these organelles are termed mannose-resistant (or nonmannose-sensitive) pili.[209] The receptors on the host cell that mediate this binding belong to the globoseries family of glycolipids.[102, 200, 201] Evidence for this phenomenon stems from the following facts: (1) binding of P-piliated *E. coli* to target cells occurs only when those cells possess a globoseries glycolipid; (2) adhesion can be inhibited by preincubation of target cells with the glycolipid; and (3) host cells that normally would not bind to P-piliated *E. coli* can be made to do so by coating the cells with glycolipid prior to incubation with bacteria.[201] Also, pyelonephritogenic strains tend to have multiple copies of the *pap* operon, encoding for P pili, compared with asymptomatic bacteriuria isolates.[144] In contrast to P pili, binding of type 1, or mannose-sensitive, pili is inhibited by D-mannose. These pili have a less certain role in virulence than do mannose-resistant pili.[90]

S pili in *E. coli* bind to sialic acid–containing glycoconjugates and may enhance virulence for production of meningitis, as shown in an infant rat model.[165] Neonatal rat brain has been shown to have a high density of receptors for this adhesin.[105] Pili (or possibly nonpilus adhesins) with binding specificity for the Dr blood group antigen, termed X adhesins in earlier literature, are thought to be prevalent among strains causing cystitis.[131]

Further studies also have demonstrated that there may be variability in *E. coli* adhesion to epithelial cells from different individuals. Schaeffer and colleagues[166] have shown that adherence of a standard *E. coli* strain to vaginal epithelial cells is greater in a population of women with recurrent urinary tract infection than in healthy controls and that the avidity of adherence can vary significantly from day to day in some women. The authors suggested that these were important host factors in determining the incidence of urinary tract infection in their patients.

Further evidence for the importance of P pili in the pathogenesis of urinary tract infection was demonstrated in a study utilizing transformed fecal *E. coli* isolates that contained recombinant plasmids encoding different adhesins. In one study utilizing recombinant DNA technology, a nonpiliated, nonpathogenic *E. coli* strain was made to express P pili by means of recombination with a plasmid carrying genetic information that encoded P-pilus production from a uropathogenic strain. The expression of P fimbriae seemed to be associated with an increased ability of the *E. coli* isolate to multiply and persist within renal tissue of mice after transurethral inoculation with organisms.[60] However, the uropathogenicity of this recombinant strain did not appear to be as great as that seen with the parent P-piliated strain isolated from a patient with pyelonephritis, suggesting that pili are not the only determinants of pathogenicity. Furthermore, Andersson and colleagues[7] have suggested that P pili are not in themselves sufficient for establishing persistent infections in human volunteers.

One other study from Sweden serves to place the importance of P pili in clinical perspective. In this survey of 174 girls with 606 episodes of urinary tract infection (pyelonephritis, cystitis, or asymptomatic bacteriuria), globoseries glycolipid-specific adhesive properties were more common in *E. coli* isolates from girls with pyelonephritis and no vesicoureteral reflux than in pyelonephritis patients with reflux.[107]

Overall, a lower frequency of virulence-associated properties (O antigen type, hemolysin production, serum resistance, and mannose-resistant globoside-specific adhesins) was noted in *E. coli* isolates from girls with pyelonephritis and reflux, with cystitis, or with asymptomatic bacteriuria than in girls with nonreflux pyelonephritis. Thus, certain host factors, particularly the presence of reflux shown in this study, may be more important than bacterial virulence properties in disease production. Preventive therapy for urinary tract infection by means of interference with the attachment of uropathogenic *E. coli* to uroepithelial cells has been suggested as one strategy for management of patients with recurrent infections. Although in vitro results with some agents are encouraging,[26, 222] further understanding of the importance of host factors is needed before the clinical relevance of this approach can be appreciated.

Adherence mechanisms also seem to be an important factor in diarrheal disease caused by *E. coli*. In humans, two plasmid-mediated colonization factor antigens (CFA-1 and CFA-2) are mannose-resistant pili, which are distinct antigenically from P pili and permit adhesion to enterocytes.[90] An enterotoxigenic *E. coli* isolate possessing CFA-1 was shown in an infant rabbit model to exhibit a greater ability to proliferate within the gastrointestinal tract and to produce a higher rate of diarrheal disease than was a toxin-producing CFA-1–deficient mutant of the same strain.[45] Studies with the same organisms in human volunteers produced similar results.[164] Thus, in this instance, adherence factors appear to be necessary for a toxin-producing organism to cause disease. Enteropathogenic *E. coli* produce bundle-forming pili, which appear to help aggregate enteropathogenic *E. coli* into infectious bundles that adhere to the intestinal surface.[55] Additionally, *E. coli* possessing nonpilus-mediated enterocyte adhesion, the so-called enteroadherent *E. coli*, may be important causes of acute and chronic diarrhea in humans.[28, 99, 114, 158]

Neisseria gonorrhoeae

One of the most striking associations of adherence capabilities with virulence occurs in *Neisseria gonorrhoeae*. Pili of *N. gonorrhoeae* appear to adhere preferentially to human buccal and genital tract epithelial cells, as well as to spermatocytes, compared with red or white blood cells or other tissues.[139, 202] Loss of pili is accompanied by decreased virulence in experimental animals. Virulent *N. gonorrhoeae* also may possess one of a family of outer-membrane proteins, termed type II, which mediate adhesion.[202] Infection can be produced in human volunteers given *N. gonorrhoeae* possessing pili, but it cannot be accomplished with transformants that lack this property.[89] Antibodies found in genital secretions of patients with gonorrhea interfere with these adhesive properties and appear to be directed against pilus antigens.[207] The adhesion factor known as outer-membrane protein II or opacity factor is produced by gonococcal isolates isolated from human volunteers after experimental inoculation with protein II–negative strains, suggesting that a shift to protein II production aids in establishment of infection.[172, 203]

Meningeal Pathogens

Adherence mechanisms also may be important for the determination of virulence in meningeal pathogens. *Neisseria meningitidis* isolates obtained from the nasopharynx of carriers or from the blood or cerebrospinal fluid of patients with meningococcal disease tend to be piliated when grown under appropriate conditions, and the presence of pili correlates with the in vitro adherence to human buccal epithelial cells.[190] In an adenoid organ culture system without immersion in media (thus allowing for an air–mucosal surface interface), piliated strains of *N. meningitidis* were associated with more adherence to mucosa and tissue tropism for nonciliated cells containing microvilli than was a nonpiliated variant.[151] Also, ciliated cells showed more damage when infected by piliated strains.

Approximately 15 per cent of nasopharyngeal *Haemophilus influenzae* type b isolates from patients with systemic *H. influenzae* diseases are highly piliated (>95 per cent of organisms with pili) and adhere to human buccal epithelial cells, but systemic isolates generally do not possess pili or adherence properties.[113] These pili recognize the Anton blood group antigen on red blood cells; the receptor on epithelial cells for α-fimbriae contains a sialyl-lactosyl-ceramide structure.[211, 212] Pili may play a role in mediating attachment of *H. influenzae* to the nasopharynx in the early stages of disease.[4, 83]

The role of *Streptococcus pneumoniae* adherence to respiratory epithelial cells in the pathogenesis of systemic infection is unclear. Most studies have examined bacterial strains or respiratory cells in relation to otitis media.[6, 187] In some studies, strains recovered from blood or cerebrospinal fluid cultures adhered less well in vitro to human pharyngeal cells than did those recovered from cultures of the nasopharynx.[5] It has been proposed that pneumococcal adhesins may link the organism to GlcNAc β 1-3 Gal or GalNAc β 1-4 Gal sequences of glycolipids found in the respiratory tract.[137]

Streptococci

Gram-positive bacteria possess adherence properties not mediated by pili. In a series of elegant experiments, Ofek, Simpson, Beachey, and others have determined that the lipoteichoic acid (LTA) component of the group A streptococcal cell wall mediates adherence of these organisms to human epithelial cells.[3, 13, 14, 125, 181] Fibronectin, a glycoprotein found on cell surfaces and many other areas of the body, appears to function as the receptor for LTA adhesion. Fibronectin treatment of group A streptococci blocks adherence to epithelial cells, and the binding of fibronectin to streptococci is inhibited by LTA.[2, 14, 180] Other adhesins of *Streptococcus pyogenes* may include M protein, a fibronectin-binding protein. Hasty and associates[62] have proposed that a two-step model of adhesion of streptococci to substrata first involves a relatively weak and reversible link (LTA) that facilitated a more specific adherence process that essentially is irreversible. The hyaluronic acid capsule of *S. pyogenes* also appears to play an important role in colonization and infection of the pharynx, perhaps by protecting the organism from phagocytosis.[218]

There also appears to be significant host variation in the avidity of binding of streptococci to epithelial cells. For example, pharyngeal epithelial cells obtained from infants bind only about 50 per cent as do cells from adult donors, and studies suggest that this is because of a lower number or an unfavorable arrangement of LTA-binding sites on infant epithelial cells.[132] Furthermore, rheumatic fever–associated strains of group A streptococci adhere better to pharyngeal cells of rheumatic fever patients than to cells from normal individuals, suggesting a role for adherence in the pathogenesis of rheumatic fever.[173] Further understanding of these host-pathogen relationships may reveal new avenues for therapy or for identification of persons at risk for the development of rheumatic fever.

Other streptococci also possess adhesive properties. Extracellular dextran production appears to be an important virulence factor for the production of dental caries by mediating adhesion to dental surfaces.[213] Dextran production also allows for adherence of alpha-streptococci to cardiac valves.[150, 167] In an animal model of bacterial endocarditis, dextran-positive alpha-streptococci produced higher rates of disease than did the identical organisms after removal of dextran by treatment with dextranase. Similarly, transformants of these strains, which have lost the ability to produce dextran, have attenuated virulence in experimental endocarditis,[167] and strains producing larger amounts of dextran are more virulent than those producing lesser amounts.[36] The ability to aggregate platelets also may contribute to the virulence of *Streptococcus sanguis* to cause endocarditis.[108]

In newborns, adherence also may play a role in the pathogenesis of group B streptococcal infection. In one study, type III group B streptococcal isolates were found to adhere in greater numbers to the buccal epithelial cells of infants being treated for invasive group B streptococcal disease than to cells from age-matched controls.[20] Both groups demonstrated higher adherence rates than did cells from healthy adults. These findings suggested that at least for type III group B streptococci, adherence mechanisms may be important virulence determinants.

Respiratory Pathogens

Bacterial adherence may be an important factor in the colonization of the respiratory tract that precedes the development of clinical pneumonia. Human buccal epithelial cells appear to contain binding sites for some gram-negative bacilli, and the introduction of other factors, such as smoking or significant underlying disease, may cause more of these sites to be available for binding to bacteria.[46, 65, 75, 76] Although the precise mechanisms responsible for these observations are unknown, it appears to involve a loss of cell surface fibronectin with a concomitant increase in salivary protease activity.[74, 221] More recent attention has been turned to developing a better understanding of the epithelial cell receptors for adhesion of respiratory pathogens. A variety of glycosphingolipids have been identified as receptors for different pathogens, with the carbohydrate sequence GalNAc β 1-4 Gal being identified as highly important in some studies but not in others.[11, 73, 95] Type 3 fimbriae, demonstrating mannose-resistant hemagglutination of tannic acid–treated erythrocytes, may be important virulence factors in nosocomial pneumonia caused by *Klebsiella* or *Enterobacter* species.[67]

Respiratory disease caused by *Mycoplasma pneumoniae* also may involve adherence mechanisms in the pathogenesis of infection.[29] Attachment of *M. pneumoniae* to erythrocytes and to lung fibroblasts in tissue cultures appears to be accomplished by means of an organized terminal, or tip, structure.[52, 106, 153] However, loss of virulence of an *M. pneumoniae* isolate has been associated with loss of adhesive capacity but retention of the tip structure, indicating that this structure by itself does not confer adherence or virulence properties.[106]

Fungi

Adherence to epithelial and endothelial surfaces also plays an important role for colonization and ultimately infection by certain yeasts.[214] The mechanism of adhesion by *Candida* species has been elucidated especially well by Hostetter and associates,[70] who have demonstrated that *Candida* species contain a transmembrane protein integrin analogue that recognizes the C3 ligand iC3b and is related closely to mammalian integrins (Mac-1, CD11b, or CR3). The expression of this integrin analogue is increased in vitro by high concentrations of glucose or hydrocortisone, conditions associated with clinical infections caused by *Candida* species. Furthermore, the frequency by which the integrin analogue is expressed by various species of *Candida* mirrors the order of isolation of these species causing human infection (e.g., *Candida albicans* → *Candida tropicalis* → *Torulopsis glabrata).*[71] Because iC3b is secreted by epithelial cells and can block adhesion of *Candida* species to epithelial and endothelial cells, one key step in adherence of these organisms to epithelial and endothelial cells is the interaction of the *Candida* integrin analogue and the iC3b ligand on the cell surfaces. Other adherence mechanisms proposed for *Candida* species involve fibronectin and lectin-like proteins.

Organisms Causing Foreign Body Infections

The pathogenesis of infections associated with foreign bodies appears to depend, in part, on adherence properties of certain bacteria. The lipoteichoic acid component of *Staphylococcus aureus* mediates binding of bacteria to fibronectin-containing receptors on epithelial cells in a manner similar to that of group A streptococci.[24, 149] Although the clinical significance of this fact is not appreciated fully, there may be a role for this relationship in the pathogenesis of foreign body infection. One study of this phenomenon utilized a protein A–deficient strain of *S. aureus*, which did not exhibit protein A–mediated binding to immunoglobulins, in an animal model of foreign body infection.[215] Subcutaneous implantation of polymethyl-methacrylate coverslips into guinea pigs was found to be associated with increased *S. aureus* adherence when compared with unimplanted coverslips. This adherence could be blocked by pretreating the coverslips with fibronectin antibodies. Also, unimplanted coverslips demonstrated increased adherence with *S. aureus* when coated with purified fibronectin prior to exposure to bacteria.

Some strains of *Staphylococcus epidermidis* adhere to foreign bodies by production of an exopolysaccharide matrix, or slime factor, which may be important in infections involving intravascular or peritoneal dialysis catheters.[27, 90, 111, 138, 140] *Pseudomonas aeruginosa*[148] and *C. albicans*[159] also possess similar adherence mechanisms, which may be important factors in catheter-related infections due to these agents. Certain Enterobacteriaceae adhere easily to Dacron materials and may be important in the pathogenesis of vascular graft infections[195]; one group has postulated a role for bacterial adherence in the pathogenesis of middle ear infections in the presence of myringotomy tubes.[86]

LOCAL PROLIFERATION

In most instances, it is not sufficient for an organism merely to attach to mucosal or other surfaces in order to cause disease. Usually, other virulence factors must be expressed so that the microbial agent can persist, and in some cases proliferate, before producing clinical illness. This particularly is important in mucosal sites subjected to "cleansing" processes, such as coughing, sneezing, ciliary motile forces, and peristalsis. Colonization can be said to occur when these normal processes are overcome to the extent that a microorganism is able to persist in the environment indefinitely.

Bacteriocins

Most microorganisms colonizing mucosal surfaces are considered nonpathogenic bacteria, or normal flora. Pathogenic organisms often must compete with these bacteria for essential nutrients in order to survive in the environment. One way in which this is thought to occur is by the production of bacteriocins, which are antibiotic-like toxins synthesized by some bacteria. These protein or protein complex compounds exert toxic effects on bacteria in a variety of ways. Some, such as colicins E2 and E3 and cloacin DF 13, enzymatically disrupt nucleic acids of some bacteria, causing breakdown of ribosomal function and protein synthesis. Others, such as colicins A, E1, Ia, Ib, and K, appear to disrupt transmembrane electrical potential by interfering with a variety of cellular functions.[91] All bacteriocins seem to have in common a protective mechanism that confers immunity on the bacterium producing the toxin, possibly by concomitant production of an "immunity protein."[91] Although no proof exists of the role of bacteriocins in the production of clinical disease, these compounds may become important as therapeutic tools in infectious diseases requiring heavy mucosal colonization for pathogenicity, such as for dental caries.[66, 205]

Siderophores

Ferric iron is required for the growth of most aerobic bacteria and is in short supply in the host. Pathogenic microorganisms must compete with other organisms for the available iron present at mucosal sites (and elsewhere in the body). The supply is limited at mucosal surfaces by the presence of iron-binding proteins, such as lactoferrin, which can inhibit the growth of some bacteria both by direct bactericidal activity and by their iron-sequestering properties.[10, 217] Most bacteria requiring iron for growth have developed mechanisms for extracting iron from the environment, principally by producing their own iron-chelating proteins, called siderophores.[48] Siderophores may be important virulence factors for some organisms.

Although no definite proof exists that these iron-sequestering mechanisms are required virulence factors for any human or animal infection, circumstantial evidence suggests that this is true. For example, most pathogenic *Neisseria* are able to utilize lactoferrin as a sole source of iron, whereas nonpathogenic species generally cannot.[122] Also, siderophore production appears to correlate with pathogenicity in experimental gonococcal infections.[49] Aerobactin, an *E. coli* siderophore, appears to confer virulence for both urinary and blood stream infections.[79, 134] The virulence-associated plasmids Col V in *E. coli*[219] and JM1 in the fish pathogen *Vibrio anguillarum*[32] appear to confer significant iron-sequestering properties on these bacteria. *P. aeruginosa* produces a siderophore, pyoverdine, in the iron-deprived environment of the lung in cystic fibrosis patients,[59] and yersiniabactin, a siderophore isolated from *Yersinia enterocolitica*, may confer increased lethality in a mouse model.[64] Further examination of plasmid-mediated iron-binding systems in other organisms may provide more definitive conclusions concerning the role of siderophore production in microbial virulence.

Immunoglobulin A Proteases

The discovery in 1973 of microbial human IgA protease activity in fecal samples from patients with hepatic cirrhosis[119] has led to extensive investigations of the ability of various microorganisms to produce IgA proteases. The finding that *N. meningitidis* and *N. gonorrhoeae* are able to produce this enzyme, whereas nonpathogenic *Neisseria* lack this property, has led to speculation that IgA protease activity may act as a virulence factor. *Haemophilus aegyptius, H. influenzae, S. pneumoniae*, and several *Bacteroides, Capnocytophaga*, and *Streptococcus* species thought to be important in the production of periodontal disease are the only other bacteria that have been shown to have the ability to produce IgA proteases.[93, 128, 143] For *H. influenzae*, protease production appears to aid in colonization and entry into mucosal cells.[186]

It has been postulated that IgA proteases might be able to enhance microbial virulence by inhibiting the antiadhesive activity of secretory IgA against certain bacteria at the mucosal surface. However, it has been shown subsequently that bacterial IgA proteases are active in cleaving only the IgA1 isotype and are inactive against IgA2. Because both isotypes are present in human secretions, it is unclear whether cleavage of only the IgA1 isotype could interfere significantly with local immune mechanisms. Further examination of the possible role of bacterial IgA proteases in infection has been hindered by the fact that these enzymes are active only against human, gorilla, and chimpanzee IgA, and thus no easily studied animal model has been developed.[93]

LOCAL TISSUE DAMAGE

Cutaneous Infections

Cellulitis caused by *S. pyogenes* or *S. aureus* is one of the most common infections in children. When the skin is altered by abrasion, laceration, or sutures or other foreign material, the barriers to infection are reduced. Enzymes such as hyaluronidase, produced by both *S. aureus* and *S. pyogenes*, are thought to aid the spread of infection locally across tissue planes. Hyaluronic acid, a mucopolysaccharide component of the extracellular ground substance of connective tissue, is hydrolyzed by hyaluronidase.[82] Antibody to hyaluronidase develops after infection due to either of these organisms but is not protective. Other extracellular enzymes such as deoxyribonuclease also may contribute to the ability of these organisms to cause local infections. Although these two microorganisms produce a number of extracellular toxins, how these products contribute to virulence is not understood. For example, the α-toxin of *S. aureus* is a protein of 26,000 to 39,000 molecular weight that interacts with cell membranes to generate aqueous transmembrane pores that disrupt normal calcium ion influx into cells.[17] *S. aureus* α-toxin also induces prostacyclin and platelet-activating factor generation by an enhanced permeability of endothelial cells, interleukin-1β (IL-1β) released from human monocytes, and leukotriene formation in polymorphonuclear leukocytes.[197] It can lyse red blood cells (more so in rabbits than in humans), is associated with destruction of corneal tissues in the rabbit, and also has some neurotoxic activity.[22] In addition, *S. aureus* β-toxin is damaging to cell membranes, is cytotoxic to a wide variety of cell types, and has been shown to be a sphingomyelinase.[155]

S. aureus isolates recovered from patients with septic arthritis or osteomyelitis often have a collagen-binding protein called "collagen adhesin" on their surface. Collagen adhesin mediates attachment of *S. aureus* to cartilage.[204] In a murine model of septic arthritis, *S. aureus* isolates with the collagen adhesin are more likely to cause septic arthritis than are strains lacking this factor.[136a]

Pseudomonas aeruginosa and Related Organisms

P. aeruginosa produces several proteases that may be important in the pathogenesis of local disease caused by this organism.[147, 220] Elastase is a protease produced by *P. aeruginosa* that causes hemorrhagic lesions in pulmonary parenchyma after direct instillation of the organism into the trachea of rabbits.[57] In a guinea pig model of pneumonia, Blackwood and associates[18] showed that strains of *P. aeruginosa* deficient in elastase were less virulent and more easily cleared than were strains producing this enzyme adequately. Elastase is not required for *P. aeruginosa* infection of the cornea in mice.[133]

The presence of *Burkholderia cepacia* in sputum has been associated with clinical deterioration in patients with cystic fibrosis, but there is debate as to its causal role in this process.[54] Under selected growth conditions in vitro, some strains of *B. cepacia* produce proteases and lipases that could accelerate lung destruction.[118]

Clostridium perfringens

Clostridium perfringens produces a number of toxins, some of which may be important in the pathogenesis of local infection.[63, 156, 182] *C. perfringens* α-toxin is a phospholipase C that hydrolyzes sphingomyelin and lecithins and thus is active against membranes from a wide variety of cell types. It is thought to be a virulence factor for infections of muscle, such as gas gangrene associated with *C. perfringens*. β-toxin causes the necrotic enteritis known as darmbrand or pigbel. ϵ- and ι-toxins also have biologic activity but are of unclear clinical significance.

Enterotoxins

Enterotoxins are examples of toxins that act locally to cause disease and are well-characterized virulence factors. The *Vibrio cholerae* toxin is one of the most intensively studied and best understood toxins produced by a microorganism. As is true for many bacterial toxins, the cholera toxin is composed of subunits.[123, 188] Subunit B binds to a specific cholera toxin receptor on intestinal epithelium. GM_1 ganglioside is the major cell membrane–binding site for cholera toxin.[43] Subunit A of the cholera toxin is responsible for the adenosine diphosphate ribosylation of a component of the adenyl cyclase system, an activity that increases intracellular cyclic adenosine monophosphate concentrations and results in efflux of sodium, chloride, and water. The heat-labile enterotoxin produced by enterotoxigenic *E. coli* is similar in structure and mechanism of action to cholera toxin and has GM_1 cell membrane receptors as well. The heat-stable enterotoxin of *E. coli* activates guanylate cyclase activity with a resultant increase in intracellular levels of cyclic guanosine monophosphate.

Systemic Bacterial Toxins

Diphtheria, botulinum, tetanus, and cholera toxins and the enterotoxins of *E. coli* are intracellular-acting toxins composed of subunits.[43, 123] One protein moiety (fragment B) subunit is responsible for binding to specific receptors of cell membranes. The membrane receptors for these and other toxins have been described in detail by Eidels and colleagues.[43] The second protein moiety (fragment A) interacts with an intracellular target to exert its activity. Diphtheria toxin inhibits protein synthesis within the cell by inactivating a protein called elongation factor 2 (EF2), which is essential for protein synthesis. In vitro, the inhibition of EF2 by diphtheria toxin will destroy a susceptible cell within 24 hours. Diphtheria and other toxins can inhibit or inactivate EF2 by catalyzing the transfer of the adenosine diphosphoribose moiety of NAD to a single amino acid residue of EF2, an adenosine diphosphate ribosylation process similar to the mechanism by which many bacterial toxins exert their intracellular actions.[97] The myocarditis and neuritis associated with *Corynebacterium diphtheriae* are caused by diphtheria toxin.

Tetanus toxin or tetanospasmin is elaborated within a wound by the *Clostridium tetani* organism. Tetanus toxin also is a subunit toxin that by mechanisms still unclear blocks the release of the inhibitory neurotransmitter glycine into the synaptic cleft within the central nervous system.[123] By blocking the release of inhibitory neurotransmitters, there is continual stimulation of the motor neurons, which results in tetany.

Clostridium botulinum can produce several immunologically distinct toxins, of which serotypes A, B, and E most commonly produce disease in humans.[43, 123] This subunit toxin is absorbed from the gastrointestinal tract into the systemic circulation, through which it reaches and binds to susceptible cells. The toxin somehow inhibits release of acetylcholine at neuromuscular junctions, resulting in a flaccid paralysis.

Group II strains of *S. aureus* can produce a toxin, exfoliatin, that is responsible for the staphylococcal scalded skin syndrome. This toxin causes a cleavage of the epidermis within the stratum granulosum layer, a process leading to bullous formation.[120] Exfoliatin is a protein of 25,000 to 30,000 daltons, but its mechanism of action is unknown.

A toxin produced by some *S. aureus* strains, designated toxic shock syndrome toxin–1 (TSST-1), is responsible for the clinical manifestations associated with toxic shock syndrome (TSS), although not exclusively.[16, 136] *S. aureus* isolates recovered from patients with TSS are significantly ($p < .001$) more likely to produce TSST-1 than are the control *S. aureus* strains.[171] In nonmenstrual TSS, TSST-1 is less prevalent among *S. aureus* isolates, but other staphylococcal enterotoxins, particularly enterotoxin B, may be of pathogenetic significance in strains lacking TSST-1.[31, 169] TSST-1 production appears to depend on low levels of magnesium in the environment, which is of interest because some high-absorbancy tampons bind magnesium ions.[88] Although the mechanism by which TSST-1 exerts its action to cause TSS is unknown, TSST-1 also is a microbial superantigen that can stimulate large numbers of T cells bearing the Vβ2 chain, leading to massive cytokine release associated with TSS.[170] TSST-1 also contributes to the ability of *S. aureus* to cause arthritis in a murine model that is related to the increased IL-2 receptor expression within arthritic joints.[1]

The streptococcal TSS is similar clinically to TSS but occurs with infection by toxin-producing strains of group A *Streptococcus*.[192] Pyrogenic exotoxin A has been associated highly with group A streptococcal strains causing this syndrome in the United States; this toxin produces a similar illness in experimental animals.[101] Streptococcal pyrogenic exotoxins B and C also have been implicated in some cases of streptococcal TSS.[191] Streptococcal pyrogenic exotoxin B is an extracellular cysteine protease that can cleave inactive human IL-1β precursor to produce biologically active IL-1β, which might contribute to the pathogenesis of streptococcal TSS.[85] Streptococcal pyrogenic exotoxins and other extracellular products may act as superantigens that lead to a strong proliferation of T lymphocytes and excessive production of inflammatory cytokines, similar to TSST-1.[126] However, in patients with streptococcal TSS, there is a depletion of specific Vβ-bearing T cells (a finding supporting the superantigen theory of pathogenesis) that is not correlated with any streptococcal M or T serotype or with known streptococcal pyrogenic exotoxin genes.[216]

Bacterial Toxins of Unclear Significance

Many microorganisms produce toxins whose role in the pathogenesis of disease has not been defined precisely. For example, *P. aeruginosa* produces toxin A, which also inhibits the protein synthesis of cells by inactivating EF2 by adenosine diphosphate ribosylation. This toxin is elaborated by the majority of clinical isolates in vitro and in some animal studies has been correlated with virulence.[98] Cross and colleagues[34] have presented evidence to support the role of toxin A in the pathogenesis of *P. aeruginosa* infections in humans. The production of toxin A was associated significantly ($p < .05$) with mortality in a group of patients with *P. aeruginosa* bacteremia. Patients infected with toxin A–producing *P. aeruginosa* also develop antibodies to toxin A, which may be protective.[147, 148]

Certain pneumococcal proteins may contribute to the pathogenesis of systemic disease due to *S. pneumoniae*. Pneumolysin, a 53-kDa polypeptide hemolysin, is produced by almost all clinical isolates of *S. pneumoniae* and is a member of the family of thiol-activated cytolysins but is not secreted outside the cytoplasm. Pneumolysin can interfere with phagocytosis, activate complement, and disrupt human respiratory epithelium, as well as lower ciliary beat frequency.[137, 152, 211] Isogenic pneumolysin-negative mutants are associated with slower growth in tissues and blood, less acute sepsis, and less severe pulmonary inflammation than is the parent wild-type serotype 2 pneumococcus in a mouse model.[15, 23] Recombinant pneumolysin results in a brisk inflammatory response when injected intracisternally into rabbits. However, parameters of meningeal inflammation are the same in rabbits after intracisternal inoculation with the parent or isogenic pneumolysin-deficient pneumococcal strain.[51] Loss of pneumolysin production is associated with a reduction in virulence of *S. pneumoniae* in a rabbit model of intracorneal infection.[78] Other proteins considered potentially important are autolysin, neuraminidase, and hyaluronidase.

The role of endotoxin in the pathogenesis of septic shock is discussed in Chapter 72.

INVASION OF HOST TISSUES

Bacterial Meningitis

Highly encapsulated organisms, such as *N. meningitidis, S. pneumoniae,* and *H. influenzae* type b, common inhabitants of the nasopharynx, are among the most common organisms causing bacteremic illnesses in children. The manner in which these and other microorganisms invade the epithelial or mucosal barriers of the host is poorly understood, and only recently has some progress been made regarding this matter. McGee and colleagues[117] have described mechanisms by which *N. gonorrhoeae* and *N. meningitidis* invade mucosal cells in tissue culture. After attachment to nonciliated cells of the mucosa of the human fallopian tube, *N. gonorrhoeae* organisms were observed to be entrapped by microvilli, pulled into a membrane-bound vesicle within the cytoplasm, and transported to the base of the cell. Gonococci then were noted in subepithelial tissues, probably after exocytosis. Similarly, *N. meningitidis* attaches to nonciliated mucosal cells of human nasopharyngeal origin. Meningococci entered the cells after entrapment by microvilli and subsequently could be found in the subepithelial tissue. Shaw and Falkow[175] have shown that gonococcal entry into tissue culture cells is inhibited by cytochalasin D, suggesting that this is a microfilament-dependent process. Whether this series of events occurs in the human host is speculative, and the microbial factors associated with this mechanism of tissue invasion remain to be identified.

How *H. influenzae* type b invades the nasopharyngeal mucosa is unknown. In the infant rat model of *H. influenzae* type b bacteremia and meningitis, a prior insult to the nasal epithelium, be it mechanical, chemical, or viral, results in a reduction in the intranasal dose of organisms required to develop bacteremia.[121, 130] Both *H. influenzae* type b itself and its lipopolysaccharide have been associated with various effects on tracheal mucosa in vitro (ciliostasis, loss of cilia, and damage to and sloughing of epithelial cells).[38, 77] Whether these different insults simply mechanically disrupt epithelial barriers or potentiate the ability of microorganisms to invade is not understood. It is of interest that children frequently have signs and symptoms suggestive of a viral upper respiratory infection prior to the diagnosis of bacterial meningitis and may have a virus isolated from their nasopharynx at admission.[84] In a human nasopharyngeal organ culture system, *H. influenzae* type b that are added can be seen invading the mucosal surface at sites of epithelial cell separation.[47] Once past the mucosal barriers, it appears *H. influenzae* type b may penetrate mucosal or submucosal blood vessels directly in order to enter the blood stream.[160]

The ability to shift from a piliated to a nonpiliated phase may be an important virulence factor for some bacteria. Guerina and associates[58] fed *E. coli* in a piliated state (more than 90 per cent of the organisms had nonmannose-sensitive pili) to neonatal rats. Although the oral cavity became colonized with piliated *E. coli*, only nonpiliated strains of *E. coli* were isolated from the blood cultures of bacteremic animals. Thus, these *E. coli* were able to undergo a phase shift in vivo from a piliated to a nonpiliated state, which may be advantageous to the survival of the organism once it has invaded beyond mucosal barriers. For example, heavily piliated *E. coli* were more susceptible to phagocytosis than were less piliated isolates in one study.[179] In addition, piliated *Salmonella typhimurium* isolates are cleared more readily than are nonpiliated variants after perfusion of the murine liver in vitro.[103] The authors postulated that mannose-sensitive pili may mediate trapping of the organisms within the liver.

H. influenzae type b isolated from blood, cerebrospinal fluid, or other sterile body fluids generally are not piliated or only demonstrate very few pili on their surface by electron microscopy and adhere poorly to human buccal epithelial cells.[100] Nasopharyngeal strains of *H. influenzae* type b from some patients have been shown to be highly piliated and to adhere readily to buccal epithelial cells.[113] However, blood and cerebrospinal fluid isolates from these same patients are not adherent to buccal epithelial cells and rarely are piliated.[100, 141] In an animal model of *H. influenzae* type b meningitis, infant rats were inoculated intranasally with piliated strains of *H. influenzae* type b meningitis.[83] As seen with the *E. coli* studies mentioned earlier, nonpiliated *H. influenzae* type b strains were recovered from blood or cerebrospinal fluid cultures. Virtually nothing is known about the mechanisms by which *S. pneumoniae* can invade host tissues.

Shigellosis

A necessary factor for the pathogenesis of *Shigella* gastroenteritis is the ability of the organism to penetrate the intestinal mucosa. Noninvasive strains of *Shigella dysenteriae* type I cannot penetrate guinea pig eye conjunctivae (Sereny test) or rabbit ileal loops and have an opaque colonial morphology compared with invasive strains, which are translucent.[53, 104] Furthermore, virulent *Shigella sonnei* strains are characterized by the production of smooth colonies having the somatic antigen form I, which corresponds to the O side chains of its lipopolysaccharide. Avirulent *S. sonnei* strains lack this form I antigen and have a rough colonial morphology. A 120-megadalton plasmid is necessary for the expression of the form I antigen by *S. sonnei* and thus is considered to be a virulence factor.[163] Additional studies have demonstrated the requirement for a high-molecular-weight plasmid for invasiveness (as assessed by the Sereny test) in all *Shigella* strains (*S. sonnei, S. flexneri, S. dysenteriae,* and *S. boydii*), as well as for enteroinvasive strains of *E. coli*.[61, 177, 178]

DISSEMINATION

Once an organism invades past mucosal or epithelial barriers, factors that promote the microorganism's ability to disseminate within the host are considered determinants of virulence. Many of these factors are associated with the capability of the organism to resist the defenses of the host.

Encapsulation

One major factor that clearly is associated with the development of bacteremia and dissemination is encapsulation with a polysaccharide. The three major microorganisms causing bacterial meningitis in children are *H. influenzae* type b, *N. meningitidis,* and *S. pneumoniae,* all highly encapsulated organisms. Numerous studies have confirmed the importance of polysaccharide capsules in the pathogenesis of systemic infections due to these pathogens.

Although *H. influenzae* either may be unencapsulated (nontypable) or may have a capsule composed of one of six distinct polysaccharides (a, b, c, d, e, and f), strains possessing the type b capsule account for approximately 95 per cent of isolates associated with systemic disease in children.[112] In contrast, nontypable (unencapsulated) strains of *H. influenzae* frequently are associated with localized infections such as otitis media or sinusitis. Thus, the capsular polysaccharide of *H. influenzae* type b, polyribose-ribitol-phosphate, is considered a major virulence factor, and antibody to polyribose-ribitol-phosphate is protective against this organism.

Strains of *N. meningitidis* isolated from blood or cerebrospinal fluid usually possess a polysaccharide capsule that allows the organism to be serogrouped (A, B, C, D, X, Y, Z, W135, and 29E). These polysaccharide capsules also are distinct chemically and immunologically. Serogroup B is responsible for the majority of endemic meningococcal infections. *N. meningitidis* strains isolated from the nasopharynx of individuals without systemic infection are likely to be unencapsulated and thus cannot be grouped.

In addition to the polysaccharide capsule, meningococci can be subdivided further into serotypes based on outer-membrane protein and lipopolysaccharide patterns.[40] Salit and Tomalty[162] compared the relative virulence among seven isolates of *N. meningitidis* recovered from the nasopharynx of carriers and eight isolates from the blood or cerebrospinal fluid of patients with meningococcal infections in a neonatal mouse model. Seven of the cerebrospinal fluid or blood isolates and none of the carrier isolates were serotype 2. Four isolates in both groups were serogroup B, and all but one of the disease-associated isolates were encapsulated. All disease-associated isolates consistently resulted in bacteremia, with the percentage of bacteremic animals ranging from 31 to 64 per cent (mean, 39 per cent). Carrier strains were associated with bacteremia in only 0 to 15 per cent (mean, 3 per cent) of instances ($p < .001$). The authors did not speculate on the reasons for these differences.

Group B *Streptococcus* is another encapsulated microorganism that is an especially important pathogen in the neonate. The organisms can be classified into seven capsular polysaccharide groups: Ia, Ib/c, Ia/c, II, III, IV, and V. As with the other encapsulated bacteria previously discussed, the capsule of group B *Streptococcus* appears to be related closely to the invasive potential of this organism.[42, 46, 105] Type III group B *Streptococcus* organisms fail to activate the alternate complement pathway that is related to the presence of terminal sialic acid residues that appear more readily when the organism is grown in human serum compared with broth media.[110, 142]

E. coli organisms possess capsular polysaccharides that are termed K antigens, of which more than 100 different types have been identified. However, approximately 80 per cent of the *E. coli* strains isolated from the cerebrospinal fluid of neonates with meningitis are of the K1 type.[33, 154, 168] In newborn rats, K1 strains of *E. coli* are more virulent than non-K1 strains after intraperitoneal injection.[19] In addition, *E. coli* K1 strains producing greater amounts of polysaccharide caused greater mortality than did low-polysaccharide-producing strains; the high-producing strains also required the classic complement pathway for opsonization compared with low-polysaccharide producers, which could be opsonized efficiently by the alternative complement pathway. Stevens and colleagues[193] demonstrated that the degree of in vitro opsonophagocytosis of *E. coli* K1 was related inversely to the K1 polysaccharide content. Other studies have shown that K1 *E. coli* are resistant to the killing of normal human serum and polymorphonuclear leukocytes, whereas most non-K1 *E. coli* are not. Thus, there is sufficient evidence to suggest that the K1 capsular polysaccharide is important in the pathogenesis of infection due to *E. coli*. Similarly, virulent *Salmonella typhi* strains possess a polysaccharide antigen designated the Vi antigen. The Vi antigen is a polymer of *N*-acetyl galactosaminuronic acid and appears to block antibody directed against lipopolysaccharide. In animal models, *S. typhi* strains lacking the Vi antigen are less virulent than Vi-positive strains.[68]

The capsular polysaccharide of the anaerobic microorganism *Bacteroides fragilis* is an important virulence factor for this organism.[87] In animal models of intra-abdominal abscesses, gelatin capsules are implanted into the peritoneal cavity of rats. The rats develop acute peritonitis and subsequently intra-abdominal abscesses. Rats implanted with an unencapsulated strain of *B. fragilis* require an accompanying aerobic microorganism, such as *E. coli*, before abscesses develop. However, for encapsulated *B. fragilis*, an additional aerobic organism is not necessary for the development of intra-abdominal abscesses.

Other organisms possessing capsules that are antiphagocytic include *Klebsiella pneumoniae, S. aureus*, group A streptococci, *Pasteurella multocida*, and *Cryptococcus neoformans*. Presumably, these capsules interfere with either recognition of or binding to critical surface antigens by opsonins, and this prevents attachment by the membrane of the polymorphonuclear leukocyte.[185] The capsule also seems to inhibit activation of the alternate complement pathway by underlying surface structures, a process that could lead to complement deposition on the surface membrane of the microorganism.

Other Cell Surface Structures

Other noncapsular components of the bacterial surface appear to convey resistance to host defenses. The M proteins of group A streptococci are cell surface antigens that appear to have antiphagocytic properties. Group A streptococci possessing M protein are phagocytized less easily than M protein–negative strains, and enzymatic removal of the M protein allows phagocytosis to proceed more readily.[69] Many *S. aureus* strains have protein A as a part of the cell wall. The Fc portion of IgG binds specifically to protein A; therefore, IgG molecules attached by their Fc portion to protein A would not be available for binding to specific Fc receptors on the surface of the phagocyte, and antibody-dependent phagocytosis would be inhibited. In vitro studies demonstrate that protein A–poor strains of *S. aureus* are phagocytized more readily by polymorphonuclear leukocytes after opsonization by the alternative complement pathway than are protein A–rich strains.[184] Strains of *S. aureus* deficient in protein A also more efficiently activate the alternative complement pathway than do protein A–rich strains. What actual role protein A has in promoting *S. aureus* infections is unknown. The glycocalyx of *Proteus mirabilis* may aid in formation of struvite urinary calculi in urinary tract infections, further impairing host defense capabilities.[41]

Alginate production by *P. aeruginosa* is responsible for the mucoid appearance of colonies of this organism isolated from the sputum of cystic fibrosis patients. A large body of evidence suggests that alginate is an important virulence factor in this clinical setting, allowing the organism to evade host defenses.[54, 115] Alginate, when combined with the highly sulfonated mucin in the cystic fibrotic airway, aids in the formation of microcolonies that resist mucociliary clearance, and alginate impairs phagocytosis in vitro. Control of alginate production occurs through a variety of genetic loci and appears to respond to environmental stimuli, particularly when nutrients are limited.[39]

Lipopolysaccharide

Another important virulence factor that has been correlated with the capacity of a gram-negative organism to cause systemic disease is the composition of the lipopolysaccharide. *E. coli* can be classified into numerous O antigen types that are based on lipopolysaccharide antigens. Among 119 *E. coli* isolates from adults with bacteremia, approximately 50 per cent were found in 1 of only 7 of the 71 O antigen types tested.[116] *E. coli* serotypes O2, O4, and O6 are encountered most frequently in adult bacteremias. Not only are certain *E. coli* O serotypes more commonly encountered in bacteremic adults, but also O-typable strains in general are more resistant to serum bactericidal effects than are non–O-typable or autoagglutinable strains. It is of interest that different *E. coli* O serotypes (O4, O7, O8, and O16) predominate among *E. coli* associated with neonatal bacteremia or meningitis.[145]

Pluschke and associates[146] employed the infant rat model to investigate the relative virulence of *E. coli* K1 isolates on the basis of O antigen types. After atraumatic oral feeding, all three O serotypes (O1:K1, O7:K1, and O18:K1) successfully colonized the intestinal tract of the infant rats. Although 10 per cent of the animals fed O7:K1 and O18:K1 serotypes developed bacteremia, only 1.1 per cent of the rats fed the O1:K1 serotype became bacteremic. The *E. coli* O7:K1 and O18:K1 strains were found to be serum-resistant, whereas the O1:K1 strains were noted to be killed by serum. The authors were able to explain these differences by demonstrating that although all three *E. coli* K1 serotypes were resistant to alternate complement pathway activity, *E. coli* O1:K1 could be killed efficiently by the classic complement pathway in the absence of specific antibody. In contrast, *E. coli* O7:K1 and O18:K1 serotypes were killed effectively by the classic complement pathway only in the presence of specific antilipopolysaccharide antibody. The chemical composition rather than the chain length of the lipopolysaccharides seemed to mediate these differences.

The role of lipopolysaccharide in the pathogenesis of infections due to *P. aeruginosa* has been examined by comparing the relative virulence of lipopolysaccharide mutants with strains possessing complete lipopolysaccharide structures. Cryz and colleagues[35] determined that mutant *P. aeruginosa* strains lacking complete lipopolysaccharide structures did not differ from strains with complete lipopolysaccharide in regard to serum resistance or the production of toxin A, alkaline protease, and elastase. However, in the murine burn wound model, *P. aeruginosa* mutants with short or no O side chains were 1000-fold less virulent than strains possessing a complete core and O side chains. The mechanism of the enhanced virulence of the complete lipopolysaccharide was not readily explicable.

Other studies have shown that a change or reduction in the O side chains of lipopolysaccharide is accompanied by an increased susceptibility to serum for gram-negative enterics, such as *Salmonella* species.[206] Similar increases in serum sensitivity have been noted for changes in lipopolysaccharide mutants of *N. gonorrhoeae*.[127] The explanation for this increased susceptibility to serum killing appears to be that the mutant lipopolysaccharide strains activate the classic complement pathway in the absence of antibody.[174] Alteration in the lipopolysaccharide of *H. influenzae* type b also appears to affect virulence.

OTHER VIRULENCE FACTORS ASSOCIATED WITH DISSEMINATION

E. coli organisms possessing the Col V plasmid particularly are virulent for experimental animals, and loss of the Col V plasmid results in diminished virulence. There is a relationship between the presence of the Col V plasmid and increased resistance to serum killing and to a more efficient mechanism of iron sequestration that also enhances virulence.[44] Davies and colleagues[37] reported that a significantly greater ($p < .01$) percentage of *E. coli* strains isolated from the blood (31.6 per cent) or urine (26.2 per cent) of hospitalized patients with urinary tract infections produced colicin V, a bacteriocin encoded by Col V, than did fecal *E. coli* strains (13.6 per cent). Therefore, Col V–associated determinants also appear to be virulence factors in human infections.

Microorganisms have developed many other mechanisms for evading phagocytes, and these probably are important virulence factors. Chemotaxis of polymorphonuclear leukocytes is inhibited by a variety of substances associated with organisms such as *Capnocytophaga*, *S. aureus*, and enterotoxigenic *E. coli*. Other organisms may alter polymorphonuclear leukocyte membrane fluidity or metabolism, which inhibits the ability of the polymorphonuclear leukocytes to ingest and kill. *S. pneumoniae, S. pyogenes, S. aureus*, and other pathogens have toxins (i.e., leukocidins) that can destroy polymorphonuclear leukocytes. *Listeria monocytogenes* secretes a hemolysin, listeriolysin, which is correlated with the ability of this organism to escape phagocytic vacuoles and allow intracytoplasmic growth.[30] The interested reader can refer to several comprehensive reviews on the subject of microbial evasion of host defenses.[56, 89, 185]

References

1. Abdelnour, A., Bremell, T., and Tarkowski, A.: Toxic shock syndrome toxin 1 contributes to the arthritogenicity of *Staphylococcus aureus*. J. Infect. Dis. *170*:94, 1994.
2. Abraham, S. N., Beachey, E. H., and Simpson, W. A.: Adherence of *Streptococcus pyogenes, Escherichia coli,* and *Pseudomonas aeruginosa* to fibronectin-coated and uncoated epithelial cells. Infect. Immun. *41*:1261–1268, 1983.
3. Allan, M. L., and Beachey, E. H.: Excretion of lipoteichoic acid by group A streptococci: Influence of penicillin on excretion and loss of ability to adhere to human oral mucosal cells. J. Clin. Invest. *61*:671–677, 1978.
4. Anderson, P. W., Pichichero, M. E., and Connor, E. M.: Enhanced nasopharyngeal colonization of rats by piliated *Haemophilus influenzae* type b. Infect. Immun. *48*:565–568, 1985.

5. Andersson, B., Eriksson, B., Falsen, E., et al.: Adhesion of *Streptococcus pneumoniae* to human pharyngeal epithelial cells in vitro: Differences in adhesive capacity among strains isolated from subjects with otitis media, septicemia, or meningitis or from healthy carriers. Infect. Immun. *32*:311–317, 1981.
6. Andersson, B., Gray, B. M., Dillon, H. C., et al.: Role of adherence of *Streptococcus pneumoniae* in acute otitis media. Pediatr. Infect. Dis. J. *7*:476, 1988.
7. Andersson, P., Engberg, I., Lidin-Janson, G., et al.: Persistence of *Escherichia coli* bacteriuria is not determined by bacterial adherence. Infect. Immun. *59*:2915, 1991.
8. Andreana, A., Perna, P., Utili, R., et al.: Increased phagocytosis and killing of *Escherichia coli* treated with subinhibitory concentrations of cefamandole and gentamicin in isolated rat livers. Antimicrob. Agents Chemother. *25*:182–186, 1984.
9. Arico, B., Miller, J. F., Roy, C., et al.: Sequences required for expression of *Bordetella pertussis* virulence factors share homology with prokaryotic signal transduction proteins. Proc. Natl. Acad. Sci. U. S. A. *86*:6671, 1989.
10. Arnold, R. R., Cole, M. F., and McGhee, J. R.: A bactericidal effect for human lactoferrin. Science *197*:263–265, 1977.
11. Baker, N., Hansson, G. C., Leffler, H., et al.: Glycosphingolipid receptors for *Pseudomonas aeruginosa*. Infect. Immun. *58*:2361, 1990.
12. Beachey, E. H.: Bacterial adherence: Adhesin-receptor interactions mediating the attachment of bacteria to mucosal surfaces. J. Infect. Dis. *143*:325–345, 1981.
13. Beachey, E. H., and Ofek, I.: Epithelial cell binding of group A streptococci by lipoteichoic acid or fimbriae denuded of M protein. J. Exp. Med. *143*:759–771, 1976.
14. Beachey, E. H., and Simpson, W. A.: The adherence of group A streptococci to oropharyngeal cells: The lipoteichoic acid adhesin and fibronectin receptor. Infection *10*:107–111, 1982.
15. Benton, D. A., Everson, M. P., and Briles, D. E.: A pneumolysin-negative mutant of *Streptococcus pneumoniae* causes chronic bacteremia rather than acute sepsis in mice. Infect. Immun. *63*:448, 1995.
16. Bergdoll, M. S., and Schlievert, P. M.: Toxic shock syndrome toxin. Lancet *2*:691, 1984.
17. Bhakdi, S., and Tranum-Jensen, J.: Alpha-toxin of *Staphylococcus aureus*. Microbiol. Rev. *55*:733, 1991.
18. Blackwood, L. L., Stone, R. M., Iglewski, B. H., et al.: Evaluation of *Pseudomonas aeruginosa* exotoxin A and elastase as virulence factors in acute lung infection. Infect. Immun. *39*:198–201, 1983.
19. Bortolussi, R., Ferrieri, P., Bjorksten, B., et al.: Capsular K1 polysaccharide of *Escherichia coli*: Relationship to virulence in newborn rats and resistance to phagocytosis. Infect. Immun. *25*:293–298, 1979.
20. Broughton, R. A., and Baker, C. J.: Role of adherence in the pathogenesis of neonatal group B streptococcal infection. Infect. Immun. *39*:837–843, 1983.
21. Brunham, R. C., Plummer, F. A., and Stephens, R. S.: Bacterial antigenic variation, host immune response, and pathogen-host coevolution. Infect. Immun. *61*:2273, 1993.
22. Callegan, M. C., Engel, L. S., Hill, J. M., et al.: Corneal virulence of *Staphylococcus aureus*: Roles of alpha toxin and protein A in pathogenesis. Infect. Immun. *62*:2478, 1994.
23. Canvin, J. R., Marvin, A. P., Sivakumaran, M., et al.: The role of pneumolysin and autolysin in the pathology of pneumonia and septicemia in mice infected with a type 2 pneumococcus. J. Infect. Dis. *172*:119, 1995.
24. Carruther, M. M., and Kabat, W. J.: Mediation of staphylococcal adherence to mucosal cells by lipoteichoic acid. Infect. Immun. *40*:444–446, 1983.
25. Cassell, G. H.: Microbial surfaces: Determinants of virulence and host responsiveness. Rev. Infect. Dis. *10*(Suppl. 2):S273, 1988.
26. Chan, R. C. Y., Reid, G., Irvin, R. T., et al.: Competitive exclusion of uropathogens from human uroepithelial cells by *Lactobacillus* whole cells and cell wall fragments. Infect. Immun. *47*:84–89, 1985.
27. Christensen, G. D., Simpson, W. A., Bisno, A. L., et al.: Adherence of slime-producing strains of *Staphylococcus epidermidis* to smooth surfaces. Infect. Immun. *37*:318–326, 1982.
28. Clausen, C. R., and Christie, D. L.: Chronic diarrhea in infants caused by adherent enteropathogenic *Escherichia coli*. J. Pediatr. *100*:358–361, 1982.
29. Collier, A. M.: Attachment by mycoplasmas and its role in disease. Rev. Infect. Dis. *5*(Suppl. 4):S685–S691, 1983.
30. Conlan, J. W., and North, R. J.: Roles of *Listeria monocytogenes* virulence factors in survival: Virulence factors distinct from listeriolysin are needed for the organism to survive an early neutrophil-mediated host defense mechanism. Infect. Immun. *60*:951, 1992.
31. Crass, B. A., and Bergdoll, M. S.: Toxin involvement in toxic shock syndrome. J. Infect. Dis. *153*:918, 1986.
32. Crosa, J. H., and Hodges, L. L.: Outer membrane proteins induced under conditions of iron limitation in the marine fish pathogen *Vibrio anguillarum* #775. Infect. Immun. *31*:223–227, 1981.
33. Cross, A. S., Gemski, P., Sadoff, J. C., et al.: The importance of the K1 capsule in invasive infections caused by *Escherichia coli*. J. Infect. Dis. *149*:184–193, 1984.
34. Cross, A. S., Sadoff, J. C., Iglewski, B. H., et al.: Evidence for the role of toxin A in the pathogenesis of infection with *Pseudomonas aeruginosa* in humans. J. Infect. Dis. *142*:538–546, 1980.
35. Cryz, S. J., Pitt, T. L., Furer, E., et al.: Role of lipopolysaccharide in virulence of *Pseudomonas aeruginosa*. Infect. Immun. *44*:508–513, 1984.
36. Dall, L. H., and Herndon, B. L.: Association of cell-adherent glycocalyx and endocarditis production by viridans group streptococci. J. Clin. Microbiol. *28*:1698, 1990.
37. Davies, D. L., Falkiner, F. R., and Hardy, K. G.: Colicin V production by clinical isolates of *Escherichia coli*. Infect. Immun. *31*:574–579, 1981.
38. Denny, F. W.: Effect of a toxin produced by *Haemophilus influenzae* on ciliated respiratory epithelium. J. Infect. Dis. *129*:93–100, 1974.
39. Deretic, V., Schurr, M. J., Boucher, J. C., et al.: Conversion of *Pseudomonas aeruginosa* to mucoidy in cystic fibrosis: Environmental stress and regulation of bacterial virulence by alternative sigma factors. J. Bacteriol. *176*:2773, 1994.
40. DeVoe, I. W.: The meningococcus and mechanisms of pathogenicity. Microbiol. Rev. *46*:162–190, 1982.
41. Dumanski, A. J., Hedelin, H., Edin-Liljegren, A., et al.: Unique ability of the *Proteus mirabilis* capsule to enhance mineral growth in infectious urinary calculi. Infect. Immun. *62*:2998, 1994.
42. Durham, D. L., Mattingly, S. J., Doran, T. I., et al.: Correlation between the production of extracellular substances by type III group B streptococcal strains and virulence in a mouse model. Infect. Immun. *34*:448–454, 1981.
43. Eidels, L., Proia, R. L., and Hart, D. A.: Membrane receptors for bacterial toxins. Microbiol. Rev. *47*:596–620, 1983.
44. Elwell, L. P., and Shipley, P. L.: Plasmid-mediated factors associated with virulence of bacteria to animals. Annu. Rev. Microbiol. *34*:465–496, 1980.
45. Evans, D. G., Silver, R. P., Evans, D. J., et al.: Plasmid-controlled colonization factor associated with virulence in *Escherichia coli* enterotoxigenic for humans. Infect. Immun. *12*:656–667, 1975.
46. Fainstein, V., and Musher, D. M.: Bacterial adherence to pharyngeal cells in smokers, nonsmokers, and chronic bronchitis. Infect. Immun. *26*:178–182, 1979.
47. Farley, M. M., Stephens, D. S., Kaplan, S. L., et al.: Pilus- and non-pilus mediated interactions of *Haemophilus influenzae* type b with human erythrocytes and human nasopharyngeal mucosa. J. Infect. Dis. *161*:274, 1990.
48. Finkelstein, R. A., Sciortino, C. V., and McIntosh, M. A.: Role of iron in microbe-host interactions. Rev. Infect. Dis. *5*(Suppl. 4):S759–S777, 1983.
49. Finkelstein, R. A., and Yancey, R. J.: Effect of siderophores on virulence of *Neisseria gonorrhoeae*. Infect. Immun. *32*:609–613, 1981.
50. Franson, T. R., Sheth, W. K., Rose, H. D., et al.: Scanning electron microscopy of bacteria adherent to intravascular catheters. J. Clin. Microbiol. *20*:500–505, 1984.
51. Friedland, I. R., Paris, M. M., Hickey, S., et al.: The limited role of pneumolysin in the pathogenesis of pneumococcal meningitis. J. Infect. Dis. *172*:805, 1995.
52. Gabridge, M. G., Taylor-Robinson, D., Davies, H. A., et al.: Interaction of *Mycoplasma pneumoniae* with human lung fibroblasts: Characterization of the in vitro model. Infect. Immun. *25*:446–451, 1979.
53. Gemski, P., Takeuchi, A., Washington, O., et al.: Shigellosis due to *Shigella dysenteriae*. 1. Relative importance of mucosal invasion versus toxin production in pathogenesis. J. Infect. Dis. *126*:520–530, 1972.
54. Gilligan, P. H.: Microbiology of airway disease in patients with cystic fibrosis. Clin. Microbiol. Rev. *4*:35, 1991.
55. Girón, J. A., Ho, A. S. Y., and Schoolnik, G. K.: An inducible bundle-forming pilus of enteropathogenic *Escherichia coli*. Science *254*:710, 1991.
56. Gotschlich, E. C.: Thoughts on the evolution of strategies used by bacteria for evasion of host defenses. Rev. Infect. Dis. *5*(Suppl. 4):S778–783, 1983.
57. Gray, L., and Kreger, A.: Microscopic characterization of rabbit lung damage produced by *Pseudomonas aeruginosa* proteases. Infect. Immun. *23*:150–159, 1979.
58. Guerina, N. G., Kessler, T. W., Guerina, V. J., et al.: The role of pili and capsule in the pathogenesis of neonatal infection with *Escherichia coli* K1. J. Infect. Dis. *148*:395–405, 1983.
59. Haas, B., Kraut, J., Marks, J., et al.: Siderophore presence in sputa of cystic fibrosis patients. Infect. Immun. *59*:3997, 1991.
60. Hagberg, L., Hull, R., Hull, S., et al.: Contribution of adhesion to bacterial persistence in the mouse urinary tract. Infect. Immun. *40*:265–272, 1983.
61. Hale, T. L., Sansonetti, P. J., Schad, P. A., et al.: Characterization of virulence plasmids and plasmid-associated outer membrane proteins in *Shigella flexneri, Shigella sonnei,* and *Escherichia coli*. Infect. Immun. *40*:340–350, 1983.
62. Hasty, L. D., Ofek, I., Courtney, H. S., et al.: Multiple adhesins of streptococci. Infect. Immun. *60*:2147, 1992.
63. Hatheway, C. L.: Toxigenic clostridia. Clin. Microbiol. Rev. *3*:66, 1990.
64. Heesemann, J., Hantke, K., Vocke, T., et al.: Virulence of *Yersinia enterocolitica* is closely associated with siderophore production, expression of an iron-repressible outer membrane polypeptide of 65000 Da and pesticin sensitivity. Mol. Microbiol. *8*:397, 1993.
65. Higuchi, J. H., and Johanson, W. G.: The relationship between adherence of *Pseudomonas aeruginosa* to upper respiratory cells in vitro and susceptibility to colonization in vivo. J. Lab. Clin. Med. *95*:698, 1980.
66. Hillman, J. D., Johnson, K. P., and Yaphe, B. I.: Isolation of a *Streptococcus mutans* strain producing a novel bacteriocin. Infect. Immun. *44*:141–144, 1984.

67. Hornick, D. B., Allen, B. L., Horn, M. A., et al.: Fimbrial types among respiratory isolates belonging to the family Enterobacteriaceae. J. Clin. Microbiol. *29*:1795, 1991.
68. Hornick, R. B., Greisman, S. E., Woodward, T. E., et al.: Typhoid fever: Pathogenesis and immunologic control, Part I. N. Engl. J. Med. *283*:686–691, 1970.
69. Horwitz, M. A.: Phagocytosis of microorganisms. Rev. Infect. Dis. *4*:104–123, 1982.
70. Hostetter, M. K.: Adhesins and ligands involved in the interaction of *Candida* spp. with epithelial and endothelial surfaces. Clin. Microbiol. Rev. *7*:29, 1994.
71. Hostetter, M. K.: Yeast as metaphor. Pediatr. Res. *36*:692, 1994.
72. Jantausch, B. A., Wiedermann, B. L., Hull, S. I., et al.: *Escherichia coli* virulence factors and 99mTc-dimercaptosuccinic acid renal scan in children with febrile urinary tract infection. Pediatr. Infect. Dis. J. *11*:343, 1992.
73. Jimenez-Lucho, V., Ginsburg, V., and Krivan, H. C.: *Cryptococcus neoformans, Candida albicans,* and other fungi bind specifically to the glycosphingolipid lactosylceramide (GalB1-4GlcB1-1Cer), a possible adhesion receptor for yeasts. Infect. Immun. *58*:2085, 1990.
74. Johanson, W. G.: Prevention of respiratory tract infection. Am. J. Med. *76*(5A):69–77, 1984.
75. Johanson, W. G., Higuchi, J. H., Chaudhuri, T. R., et al.: Bacterial adherence to epithelial cells in bacillary colonization of the respiratory tract. Am. Rev. Resp. Dis. *121*:55–63, 1980.
76. Johanson, W. G., Woods, D. E., and Chaudhuri, T: Association of respiratory tract colonization with adherence of gram-negative bacilli to epithelial cells. J. Infect. Dis. *139*:667–673, 1979.
77. Johnson, A. P., Clark, J. B., and Osborn, M. F.: Scanning electron microscopy of the interaction between *Haemophilus influenzae* and organ cultures of rat trachea. J. Med. Microbiol. *16*:477–482, 1983.
78. Johnson, J. K., Hobden, J. A., O'Callaghan, R. J., et al.: Confirmation of the role of pneumolysin in ocular infections with *Streptococcus pneumoniae*. Curr. Eye Res. *11*:1221, 1992.
79. Johnson, J. R., Moseley, S. L., Roberts, P. L., et al.: Aerobactin and other virulence factor genes among strains of *Escherichia coli* causing urosepsis: Association with patient characteristics. Infect. Immun. *56*:405, 1988.
80. Jones, C. H., Jacob-Dubuisson, F., Dodson, K., et al.: Adhesin presentation in bacteria requires molecular chaperones and ushers. Infect. Immun. *60*:4445, 1992.
81. Kallenius, G., Mollby, R., Svenson, S. B., et al.: The P antigen as receptor for the hemagglutination of pyelonephritic *Escherichia coli*. FEMS Microbiol. Lett. *4*:297–302, 1980.
82. Kaplan, M. H., and Tennenbaum, M. J.: *Staphylococcus aureus*: Cellular biology and clinical application. Am. J. Med. *72*:248–258, 1982.
83. Kaplan, S. L., Mason, E. O., and Wiedermann, B. L.: Role of adherence in the pathogenesis of *Haemophilus influenzae* type b infection in infant rats. Infect. Immun. *42*:612–617, 1983.
84. Kaplan, S. L., Taber, L. H., Frank, A. L., et al.: Nasopharyngeal viral isolates in children with *Haemophilus influenzae* type b meningitis. J. Pediatr. *99*:591–593, 1981.
85. Kapur, V., Majesky, M. W., Li, L.-L., et al.: Cleavage of interleukin 1β (IL-1β) precursor to produce active IL-1β by a conserved extracellular cysteine protease from *Streptococcus pyogenes*. Proc. Natl. Acad. Sci. U. S. A. *90*:7676, 1993.
86. Karlan, M. S., Skobel, B., Grizzard, M., et al.: Myringotomy tube materials: Bacterial adhesion and infection. Otolaryngol. Head Neck Surg. *88*:783–795, 1980.
87. Kasper, D. L., Onderdonk, A. B., Polk, B. F., et al.: Surface antigens as virulence factors in infections with *Bacteroides fragilis*. Rev. Infect. Dis. *1*:278–288, 1979.
88. Kass, E. H., Schlievert, P. M., Parsonnet, J., et al.: Effect of magnesium on production of toxic-shock-syndrome toxin-1: A collaborative study. J. Infect. Dis. *158*:44, 1988.
89. Kellogg, D. S., Peacock, W. L., Deacon, W. E., et al.: *Neisseria gonorrhoeae*. I. Virulence genetically linked to colonial variation. J. Bacteriol. *85*:1274, 1963.
90. Klemm, P.: Fimbrial adhesins of *Escherichia coli*. Rev. Infect. Dis. *7*:321–340, 1985.
91. Koninsky, J.: Colicins and other bacteriocins with established modes of action. Annu. Rev. Microbiol. *36*:125–144, 1982.
92. Kopecko, D. J., and Formal, S. B.: Plasmids and the virulence of enteric and other bacterial pathogens. Ann. Intern. Med. *101*:260–262, 1984.
93. Kornfeld, S. J., and Plaut, A. G.: Secretory immunity and the bacterial IgA proteases. Rev. Infect. Dis. *3*:521–534, 1981.
94. Kristiansen, B.-E., Rustad, L., Spaune, O., et al.: Effect of subminimal inhibitory concentrations of antimicrobial agents on the piliation and adherence of *Neisseria meningitidis*. Antimicrob. Agents Chemother. *24*:731–734, 1983.
95. Krivan, H. C., Roberts, D. D., and Ginsburg, V.: Many pulmonary pathogenic bacteria bind specifically to the carbohydrate sequence Ga1NAcB1–4Gal found in some glycolipids. Proc. Natl. Acad. Sci. U. S. A. *85*:6157, 1988.
96. Kroll, J. S.: Bacterial virulence: An environmental response. Arch. Dis. Child. *66*:361, 1991.
97. Krueger, K. M., and Barbieri, J. T.: The family of bacterial ADP-ribosylating exotoxins. Clin. Microbiol. Rev. *8*:34, 1995.
98. Kwiatkowska-Patzer, B., Patzer, J. A., and Heller, L. J.: *Pseudomonas aeruginosa* exotoxin A enhances automaticity and potentiates hypoxic depression of isolated rat hearts. Proc. Soc. Exp. Biol. Med. *202*:377, 1993.
99. La Croix, J., Delaze, G., Gosselin, F., et al.: Severe protracted diarrhea due to multi-resistant adherent *Escherichia coli*. Am. J. Dis. Child. *138*:693–696, 1984.
100. Lampe, R. M., Mason, E. O., Kaplan, S. L., et al.: Adherence of *Haemophilus influenzae* to buccal epithelial cells. Infect. Immun. *35*:166–172, 1982.
101. Lee, P. K., and Schlievert, P. M.: Quantification and toxicity of group A streptococcal pyrogenic exotoxins in an animal model of toxic shock syndrome–like illness. J. Clin. Microbiol. *27*:1890, 1989.
102. Leffler, H., and Svanborg-Eden, C.: Chemical identification of a glycosphingolipid receptor for *Escherichia coli* attaching to human urinary tract epithelial cells and agglutinating human erythrocytes. FEMS Microbiol. Lett. *8*:127–134, 1980.
103. Leunk, R. D., and Moon, R. J.: Association of type 1 pili with the ability of livers to clear *Salmonella typhimurium*. Infect. Immun. *36*:1168–1174, 1982.
104. Levine, M. M., DuPont, H. L., Formal, S. B., et al.: Pathogenesis of *Shigella dysenteriae* 1 (Shiga) dysentery. J. Infect. Dis. *127*:261–270, 1973.
105. Levy, N. J., Nicholson-Weller, A., Baker, C. J., et al.: Potentiation of virulence of group B streptococcal polysaccharides. J. Infect. Dis. *149*:851–860, 1984.
106. Lipman, R. P., and Clyde, W. A.: The interrelationship of virulence, cytoadsorption and peroxide formation in *Mycoplasma pneumoniae*. Proc. Soc. Exp. Biol. Med. *131*:1163–1167, 1969.
107. Lomberg, H., Hellstrom, M., Jodal, U., et al.: Virulence-associated traits in *Escherichia coli* causing first and recurrent episodes of urinary tract infection in children with or without vesicoureteral reflux. J. Infect. Dis. *150*:561–569, 1984.
108. Manning, J. E., Hume, E. B. H., Hunter, N., et al.: An appraisal of the virulence factors associated with streptococcal endocarditis. J. Med. Microbiol. *40*:110, 1994.
109. Marild, S., Jodal, U., Orskov, I., et al.: Special virulence of the *Escherichia coli* 01:K1:H7 clone in acute pyelonephritis. J. Pediatr. *115*:40, 1989.
110. Marques, M. B., Kasper, D. L., Pangburn, M. K., et al.: Prevention of C3 deposition by capsular polysaccharides is a virulence mechanism of type III group B streptococci. Infect. Immun. *60*:3986, 1992.
111. Marrie, T. J., Noble, M. A., and Costerton, J. W.: Examination of the morphology of bacteria adhering to peritoneal dialysis catheters by scanning and transmission electron microscopy. J. Clin. Microbiol. *18*:1388–1398, 1983.
112. Mason, E. O., Kaplan, S. L., Lamberth, L. B., et al.: Serotype and ampicillin susceptibility of *Haemophilus influenzae* causing systemic infections in children: 3 years of experience. J. Clin. Microbiol. *15*:543–546, 1982.
113. Mason, E. O., Kaplan, S. L., Wiedermann, B. L., et al.: Frequency and properties of naturally occurring adherent piliated strains of *Haemophilus influenzae* type b. Infect. Immun. *49*:98–103, 1985.
114. Mathewson, J. J., Johnson, P. C., DuPont, H. L., et al.: A newly recognized cause of traveler's diarrhea: Enteroadherent *Escherichia coli*. J. Infect. Dis. *151*:471–475, 1985.
115. May, T. B., Shinabarger, D., Maharaj, R., et al.: Alginate synthesis by *Pseudomonas aeruginosa*: A key pathogenic factor in chronic pulmonary infections of cystic fibrosis patients. Clin. Microbiol. Rev. *4*:191, 1991.
116. McCabe, W. R., Kaijser, B., Olling, S., et al.: *Escherichia coli* in bacteremia: K and O antigens and serum sensitivity of strains from adults and neonates. J. Infect. Dis. *138*:33–41, 1978.
117. McGee, Z. A., Stephens, D. S., Hoffman, L. H., et al.: Mechanisms of mucosal invasion by pathogenic *Neisseria*. Rev. Infect. Dis. *5*(Suppl. 4):S708–S714, 1983.
118. McKenney, D., and Allison, D. G.: Effects of growth rate and nutrient limitation on virulence factor production in *Burkholderia cepacia*. J. Bacteriol. *177*:4140, 1995.
119. Mehta, S. K., Plaut, A. G., Calvanico, N. J., et al.: Human immunoglobulin A: Production of an Fc fragment by an enteric microbial proteolytic enzyme. J. Immunol. *114*:1274–1276, 1973.
120. Melish, M. E., and Glasgow, L. A.: The staphylococcal scalded-skin syndrome: Development of an experimental model. N. Engl. J. Med. *282*:1114–1119, 1970.
121. Michaels, R. H., Myerowitz, R. L., and Klaw, R.: Potentiation of experimental meningitis due to *Haemophilus influenzae* by influenza A virus. J. Infect. Dis. *135*:641–645, 1977.
122. Mickelsen, P. A., Blackman, E., and Sparling, P. F.: Ability of *Neisseria gonorrhoeae, Neisseria meningitidis,* and commensal *Neisseria* species to obtain iron from lactoferrin. Infect. Immun. *35*:915–920, 1982.
123. Middlebrook, M. L., and Dorland, R. B.: Bacterial toxins: Cellular mechanisms of action. Microbiol. Rev. *48*:199–221, 1984.
124. Miller, J. F., Mekalanos, J. J., and Falkow, S.: Coordinate regulation and sensory transduction in the control of bacterial virulence. Science *243*:916, 1989.
125. Miorner, H., Johansson, G., and Kronvall, G.: Lipoteichoic acid is the major cell wall component responsible for surface hydrophobicity of group A streptococci. Infect. Immun. *39*:336–343, 1983.
126. Mollick, J. A., Miller, G. G., Musser, J. M., et al.: A novel superantigen

isolated from pathogenic strains of *Streptococcus pyogenes* with aminoterminal homology to staphylococcal enterotoxins B and C. J. Clin. Invest. *92*:710, 1993.

127. Morse, S. A., and Apicella, M. A.: Isolation of lipopolysaccharide mutant of *Neisseria gonorrhoeae*: An analysis of the antigenic and biologic differences. J. Infect. Dis. *145*:206–216, 1982.
128. Mortensen, S. B., and Kilian, M.: Purification and characterization of an immunoglobulin A1 protease from *Bacteroides melaninogenicus*. Infect. Immun. *45*:550–557, 1984.
129. Mühldorfer, I., and Hacker, J.: Genetic aspects of *Escherichia coli* virulence. Microb. Pathogen. *16*:171, 1994.
130. Myerowitz, R. L., and Michaels, R. H.: Mechanism of potentiation of experimental *Haemophilus influenzae* type b disease in infant rats by influenza A virus. Lab. Invest. *44*:434–441, 1981.
131. Nowicki, B., Svanborg-Eden, C., Hull, R., et al.: Molecular analysis and epidemiology of the Dr hemagglutinin of uropathogenic *Escherichia coli*. Infect. Immun. *57*:446–451, 1989.
132. Ofek, I., Beachey, E. H., Eyal, F., et al.: Postnatal development of binding of streptococci and lipoteichoic acid by oral mucosal cells of humans. J. Infect. Dis. *135*:267–274, 1977.
133. Ohman, D. E., Burn, R. P., and Iglewski, B. H.: Corneal infections in mice with toxin A and elastase mutants of *Pseudomonas aeruginosa*. J. Infect. Dis. *142*:547–555, 1980.
134. Opal, S. M., Cross, A. S., Gemski, P., et al.: Aerobactin and α-hemolysin as virulence determinants in *Escherichia coli* isolated from human blood, urine, and stool. J. Infect. Dis. *161*:794, 1990.
135. Parkkinen, J., Korhonen, T. K., Pere, A., et al.: Binding sites in the rat brain for *Escherichia coli* S fimbriae associated with neonatal meningitis. J. Clin. Invest. *81*:860, 1988.
136. Parsonnet, J.: Mediators in the pathogenesis of toxic shock syndrome: Overview. Rev. Infect. Dis. *11*(Suppl. 1):S263, 1989.
136a. Patti, J. M., Bremell, T., Krajewska-Pietrasik, D., et al.: The *Staphylococcus aureus* collagen adhesin is a virulence determinant in experimental septic arthritis. Infect. Immun. *62*:152, 1994.
137. Paton, J. C., Andrew, P. W., Boulnois, G. J., et al.: Molecular analysis of the pathogenicity of *Streptococcus pneumoniae*: The role of pneumococcal proteins. Annu. Rev. Microbiol. *47*:89, 1993.
138. Patrick, C. C., Hetherington, S. V., Roberson, P. K., et al.: Comparative virulence of *Staphylococcus epidermidis* isolates in a murine catheter model. Pediatr. Res. *37*:70, 1994.
139. Pearce, W. A., and Buchanan, T. M.: Attachment role of gonococcal pili: Optimum conditions and quantitation of adherence of isolated pili to human cells in vitro. J. Clin. Invest. *61*:931–943, 1978.
140. Peters, G., Locci, R., and Pulverer, G.: Adherence and growth of coagulase-negative staphylococci on surfaces of intravenous catheters. J. Infect. Dis. *146*:479–482, 1982.
141. Pichichero, M. E., Anderson, P., Loeb, M., et al.: Do pili play a role in pathogenicity of *Haemophilus influenzae* type b? Lancet 2:960–962, 1982.
142. Platt, M. W., Correa, N., Jr., and Mold, C.: Growth of group B streptococci in human serum leads to increased cell surface sialic acid and decreased activation of the alternative complement pathway. Can. J. Microbiol. *40*:99, 1994.
143. Plaut, A. G.: The IgA1 proteases of pathogenic bacteria. Annu. Rev. Microbiol. *37*:603–622, 1983.
144. Plos, K., Carter, T., Hull, S., et al.: Frequency and organization of pap homologous DNA in relation to clinical origin of uropathogenic *Escherichia coli*. J. Infect. Dis. *161*:518, 1990.
145. Pluschke, G., and Achtman, M.: Degree of antibody independent activation of the classical complement pathway by K-1 *Escherichia coli* differs with O antigen type and correlates with virulence of meningitis in newborns. Infect. Immun. *43*:684–692, 1984.
146. Pluschke, G., Mercer, A., Kusecek, B., et al.: Induction of bacteremia in newborn rats by *Escherichia coli* K1 is correlated with only certain O (lipopolysaccharide) antigen types. Infect. Immun. *39*:599–608, 1983.
147. Pollack, M., and Young, L. S.: Protective activity of antibodies to exotoxin A lipopolysaccharide at the onset of *Pseudomonas aeruginosa* septicemia in man. J. Clin. Invest. *63*:276–286, 1979.
148. Pollack, M.: The virulence of *Pseudomonas aeruginosa*. Rev. Infect. Dis. *6*(Suppl. 3):S617–S626, 1984.
149. Proctor, R. A., Mosher, D. F., and Olbrantz, P. J.: Fibronectin binding to *Staphylococcus aureus*. J. Biol. Chem. *257*:14788–14794, 1982.
150. Ramirez-Ronda, C. H.: Adherence of glucan-positive and glucan-negative streptococcal strains to normal and damaged heart valves. J. Clin. Invest. *62*:805–814, 1978.
151. Rayner, C. F. J., Dewar, A., Moxon, E. R., et al.: The effect of variations in the expression of pili on the interaction of *Neisseria meningitidis* with human nasopharyngeal epithelium. J. Infect. Dis. *171*:113, 1995.
152. Rayner, C. F. J., Jackson, A. D., Rutman, A., et al.: Interaction of pneumolysin-sufficient and -deficient isogenic variants of *Streptococcus pneumoniae* with human respiratory mucosa. Infect. Immun. *63*:442, 1995.
153. Razin, S., Bonai, M., Gamliel, H., et al.: Scanning electron microscopy of mycoplasmas adhering to erythrocytes. Infect. Immun. *30*:538–546, 1980.
154. Robbins, J. B., McCracken, G. H., Gotschlich, E. C., et al.: *Escherichia coli* K1 capsular polysaccharide associated with neonatal meningitis. N. Engl. J. Med. *290*:1216–1220, 1974.
155. Rogolsky, M.: Nonenteric toxins of *Staphylococcus aureus*. Microbiol. Rev. *43*:320–360, 1979.
156. Rood, J. I., and Cole, S. T.: Molecular genetics and pathogenesis of *Clostridium perfringens*. Microbiol. Rev. *55*:621, 1991.
157. Roth, J. A.: Virulence Mechanisms of Bacterial Pathogens. Washington, DC, American Society for Microbiology, 1988.
158. Rothbaum, R. J., Giannella, R. A., and Partin, J. C.: Diarrhea caused by adherent enteropathogenic *E. coli*. J. Pediatr. *101*:486, 1982.
159. Rotrosen, D., Gibson, T. R., and Edwards, J. E.: Adherence of *Candida* species to intravenous catheters. J. Infect. Dis. *147*:594, 1983.
160. Rubin, L. G., and Moxon, E. R.: Pathogenesis of bloodstream invasion with *Haemophilus influenzae* type b. Infect. Immun. *41*:280–284, 1983.
161. Salit, I. E.: Effect of subinhibitory concentrations of antimicrobials on meningococcal adherence. Can. J. Microbiol. *29*:369–376, 1983.
162. Salit, I. E., and Tomalty, L.: Experimental meningococcal infection in neonatal mice: Differences in virulence between strains isolated from human cases and carriers. Can. J. Microbiol. *30*:1042–1045, 1984.
163. Sansonetti, P. J., Kopecko, D. J., and Formal, S. B.: *Shigella sonnei* plasmids: Evidence that a large plasmid is necessary for virulence. Infect. Immun. *34*:75–83, 1981.
164. Satterwhite, T. K., DuPont, H. L., Evans, D. G., et al.: Role of *Escherichia coli* colonisation factor antigen in acute diarrhoea. Lancet 2:181–184, 1978.
165. Saukkonen, K. M. J., Nowicki, B., and Leinonen, M.: Role of type 1 and S fimbriae in the pathogenesis of *Escherichia coli* 018:K1 bacteremia and meningitis in the infant rat. Infect. Immun. *56*:892, 1988.
166. Schaeffer, A. J., Amundsen, S. K., and Jones, J. M.: Effect of carbohydrates on adherence of *Escherichia coli* to human urinary tract epithelial cells. Infect. Immun. *30*:531–537, 1980.
167. Scheld, W. M., Valone, J. A., and Sande, M. A.: Bacterial adherence in the pathogenesis of endocarditis: Interaction of bacterial dextran, platelets, and fibrin. J. Clin. Invest. *61*:1394–1404, 1978.
168. Schiffer, M. S., Oliveira, E., Glode, M. P., et al.: A review: Relation between invasiveness and the K1 capsular polysaccharide of *Escherichia coli*. Pediatr. Res. *10*:82–87, 1976.
169. Schlievert, P. M.: Staphylococcal enterotoxin B and toxic-shock syndrome toxin–1 are significantly associated with nonmenstrual TSS. Lancet *1*:1149, 1986.
170. Schlievert, P. M.: Role of superantigens in human disease. J. Infect. Dis. *167*:997, 1993.
171. Schlievert, P. M., and Kelly, J. A.: Staphylococcal pyrogenic exotoxin type C: Further characterization. Ann. Intern. Med. *96*:982–986, 1982.
172. Schneider, H., Cross, A. S., Kuschner, R. A., et al.: Experimental human gonococcal urethritis: 250 *Neisseria gonorrhoeae* MS11mkC are infective. J. Infect. Dis. *172*:180, 1995.
173. Selinger, D. S., Julie, N., Reed, W. P., et al.: Adherence of group A streptococci to pharyngeal cells: A role in the pathogenesis of rheumatic fever. Science *201*:455–457, 1978.
174. Shafer, W. M., Joiner, K., Guymon, L. F., et al.: Serum sensitivity of *Neisseria gonorrhoeae*: The role of lipopolysaccharide. J. Infect. Dis. *149*:175–183, 1984.
175. Shaw, J. H., and Falkow, S.: Model for invasion of human tissue culture cells by *Neisseria gonorrhoeae*. Infect. Immun. *56*:1625, 1988.
176. Shibl, A. M.: Effect of antibiotics on adherence of microorganisms to epithelial cell surfaces. Rev. Infect. Dis. *7*:51–65, 1985.
177. Silva, R. M., Toledo, M. R. F., and Trabulsi, L. R.: Plasmid-mediated virulence in *Shigella* species. J. Infect. Dis. *146*:99, 1982.
178. Silva, R. M., Toledo, M. R. F., and Trabulsi, L. R.: Correlation of invasiveness with plasmid in enteroinvasive strains of *Escherichia coli*. J. Infect. Dis. *146*:706, 1982.
179. Silverblatt, F. J., Dreyer, J. S., and Schauer, S.: Effect of pili on susceptibility of *Escherichia coli* to phagocytosis. Infect. Immun. *24*:218–223, 1979.
180. Simpson, W. A., and Beachey, E. H.: Adherence of group A streptococci to fibronectin on oral epithelial cells. Infect. Immun. *39*:275–279, 1983.
181. Simpson, W. A., Ofek, I., Sarasohn, C., et al.: Characteristics of the binding of streptococcal lipoteichoic acid to human oral epithelial cells. J. Infect. Dis. *141*:457–462, 1980.
182. Smith, L. D. S.: Virulence factors of *Clostridium perfringens*. Rev. Infect. Dis. *1*:254–260, 1979.
183. Sparling, P. F.: Bacterial virulence and pathogenesis: An overview. Rev. Infect. Dis. *5*(Suppl. 4):S637–S646, 1983.
184. Spika, J. S., Verbrugh, H. A., and Verhoeft, J.: Protein A effect on alternative complement activation and opsonization of *Staphylococcus aureus*. Infect. Immun. *34*:455–460, 1981.
185. Spitznagel, J. K.: Microbial interactions with neutrophils. Rev. Infect. Dis. *5*(Suppl. 4):S806–S822, 1983.
186. St. Geme, J. W., III, de la Morena, M. L., and Falkow, S.: A *Haemophilus influenzae* IgA protease-like protein promotes intimate interaction with human epithelial cells. Mol. Microbiol. *14*:217, 1994.
187. Stenofors, L.-E., and Räisänen, S.: Abundant attachment of bacteria to nasopharyngeal epithelium in otitis-prone children. J. Infect. Dis. *165*:1148, 1992.
188. Stephen, J., and Pietrowski, R. A.: Bacterial Toxins. Washington, DC, American Society for Microbiology, 1983.
189. Stephens, D. S., Krebs, J. W., and McGee, Z. A.: Loss of pili and decreased attachment to human cells by *Neisseria meningitidis* and *Neisseria gonor-*

rhoeae exposed to subinhibitory concentrations of antibiotics. Infect. Immun. *46*:507–513, 1984.

190. Stephens, D. S., and McGee, Z. A.: Attachment of *Neisseria meningitidis* to human mucosal surfaces: Influences of pili and type of receptor cell. J. Infect. Dis. *143*:525–532, 1981.
191. Stevens, D. L.: Streptococcal toxic-shock syndrome: Spectrum of disease, pathogenesis, and new concepts in treatment. Emerg. Infect. Dis. *1*:69, 1995.
192. Stevens, D. L., Tanner, M. H., Winship, J., et al.: Severe group A streptococcal infections associated with a toxic shock–like syndrome and scarlet fever toxin A. N. Engl. J. Med. *321*:1, 1989.
193. Stevens, P., Chu, C. L., and Young, L. S.: K-1 antigen content and the presence of an additional sialic acid–containing antigen among bacteremic K-1 *Escherichia coli*: Correlation with susceptibility to opsonophagocytosis. Infect. Immun. *29*:1055–1061, 1980.
194. Stibitz, S., Aaronson, W., Monack, D., et al.: Phase variation in *Bordetella pertussis* by frameshift mutation in a gene for a novel two-component system. Nature *338*:266, 1989.
195. Sugarman, B.: In vitro adherence of bacteria to prosthetic vascular grafts. Infection *10*:13–16, 1982.
196. Sugarman, B., and Donta, S. T.: Effect of antibiotics on the adherence of Enterobacteriaceae to human buccal cells. J. Infect. Dis. *140*:622–625, 1979.
197. Suttorp, N., Buerke, M., and Tannert-Otto, S.: Stimulation of PAF-synthesis in pulmonary artery endothelial cells by *Staphylococcus aureus* alpha-toxin. Thromb. Res. *67*:243, 1992.
198. Svanborg-Eden, C., Eriksson, B., Hanson, L. A., et al.: Adhesion to normal human epithelial cells of *Escherichia coli* from children with various forms of urinary tract infection. J. Pediatr. *93*:398–403, 1978.
199. Svanborg-Eden, C., Hanson, L. A., Jodal, U., et al.: Variable adherence to normal human urinary tract epithelial cells of *Escherichia coli* strains associated with various forms of urinary tract infection. Lancet 2:490–492, 1976.
200. Svanborg-Eden, C., Hull, R., Falkow, S., et al.: Target cell specificity of wild-type *E. coli* and mutants and clones with genetically defined adhesins. Prog. Food Nutr. Sci. *7*:75–89, 1983.
201. Svenson, S. B., Hulterg, H., Kallenius, G., et al.: P-fimbriae of pyelonephritogenic *Escherichia coli*: Identification and chemical characterization of receptors. Infection *11*:73–79, 1983.
202. Swanson, J.: Gonococcal adherence: Selected types. Rev. Infect. Dis. 5(Suppl. 4):S678–S684, 1983.
203. Swanson, J., Barrera, O., Sola, J., et al.: Expression of outer membrane protein II by gonococci in experimental gonorrhea. J. Exp. Med. *168*:2121, 1988.
204. Switalski, L. M., Patti, J. M., Butcher, W. G., et al.: A collagen receptor on *Staphylococcus aureus* collagen adhesin is a virulence determinant in experimental septic arthritis. Infect. Immun. *62*:152, 1994.
205. Takoda, K., Ikeda, T., Mitsui, I., et al.: Mode of inhibitory action of a bacteriocin produced by *Streptococcus mutans* C3603. Infect. Immun. *44*:370–378, 1984.
206. Taylor, P. W.: Bactericidal and bacteriolytic activity of serum against gram-negative bacteria. Microbiol. Rev. *47*:46–83, 1983.
207. Tramont, E. C., Ciak, J., Boslego, J., et al.: Antigenic specificity of antibodies in vaginal secretions during infection with *Neisseria gonorrhoeae*. J. Infect. Dis. *142*:23–31, 1980.
208. Vaisanen, V., Lounatmaa, K., and Korhonen, T. K.: Effects of sublethal concentrations of antimicrobial agents on the hemagglutination, adhesion, and ultrastructure of pyelonephritogenic *Escherichia coli* strains. Antimicrob. Agents Chemother. *22*:120–127, 1982.
209. Vaisanen, V., Tallgren, L. G., Makela, P. H., et al.: Mannose-resistant hemagglutination and P antigen recognition are characteristic of *Escherichia coli* causing primary pyelonephritis. Lancet 2:1366–1369, 1981.
210. Vaisanen-Rhen, V., Elo, J., Vaisanen, E., et al.: P-fimbriated clones among uropathogenic *Escherichia coli* strains. Infect. Immun. *43*:149, 1984.
211. van Alphen, L., Levene, C., den Broek, L. G., et al.: Combined inheritance of the epithelial cell and erythrocyte receptors for *Haemophilus influenzae*. Infect. Immun. *58*:3807, 1990.
212. van Alphen, L., Poole, J., Geelen, L., et al.: Three erythrocyte and epithelial cell receptors for *Haemophilus influenzae* are expressed independently. Infect. Immun. *55*:2355, 1987.
213. Van Houte, J.: Bacterial adherence in the mouth. Rev. Infect. Dis. 5(Suppl. 4):S659–S669, 1983.
214. Vartivarian, S. E.: Virulence properties and nonimmune pathogenetic mechanisms of fungi. Clin. Infect. Dis. *14*(Suppl 1):S30, 1992.
215. Vaudaux, P., Suzuki, R., Waldvogel, F. A., et al.: Foreign body infection: Role of fibronectin as a ligand for the adherence of *Staphylococcus aureus*. J. Infect. Dis. *150*:546–533, 1984.
216. Watanabe-Ohnishi, R., Low, D. E., McGeer, A., et al.: Selective depletion of Vβ-bearing T cells in patients with severe invasive group A streptococcal infections and streptococcal toxic shock syndrome. J. Infect. Dis. *171*:74, 1995.
217. Weinberg, E. D.: Iron and infection. Microbiol. Rev. *42*:45–66, 1978.
218. Wessels, M. R., and Bronze, M. S.: Critical role of the group A streptococcal capsule in pharyngeal colonization and infection in mice. Proc. Natl. Acad. Sci. U. S. A. *91*:12238, 1994.
219. Williams, P. H.: Novel iron uptake system specified by Col V plasmids: An important component in the virulence of invasive strains of *Escherichia coli*. Infect. Immun. *26*:925–932, 1979.
220. Woods, D. E., and Sokol, P. A.: Role of *Pseudomonas aeruginosa* extracellular enzymes in lung disease. Clin. Invest. Med. *9*:108, 1986.
221. Woods, D. E., Straus, D. C., Johanson, W. G., et al.: Role of salivary protease activity in adherence of gram-negative bacilli to mammalian buccal epithelial cells in vivo. J. Clin. Invest. *68*:1435–1440, 1981.
222. Zafriri, D., Ofek, I., Adar, R., et al.: Inhibitory activity of cranberry juice on adherence of type 1 and type P fimbriated *Escherichia coli* to eucaryotic cells. Antimicrob. Agents Chemother. *33*:92, 1989.

2

IMMUNOLOGIC AND PHAGOCYTIC RESPONSES TO INFECTION

Michael F. Tosi and K. Lynn Cates

This chapter provides an overview of immunologic and phagocytic responses to infection by examining host interactions with pathogens, normal host defense mechanisms, immature host responses of neonates, specific immunodeficiency states, and components of the immunologic evaluation relevant to the practice of pediatric infectious diseases. It is intended to supply sufficient information to permit recognition of the usual clinical presentations of common immunodeficiency disorders and to familiarize the reader with general principles of immunologic evaluations and management of patients with immune disorders. For greater depth and detail, readers are encouraged to refer to the excellent reviews cited.

Host-Parasite Interactions

GENERAL ASPECTS OF THE IMMUNE SYSTEM AND HOST-PARASITE INTERACTIONS

Humans constantly are exposed to a daunting number and diversity of microorganisms that can cause infection. Many organisms that usually coexist harmoniously with the human host on the skin or on mucous membranes of the oral cavity, upper airways, or lower gastrointestinal tract may invade and become pathogens if the delicate balance of the commensal relationship is disrupted. Other organisms are more invasive, and they overtly attack the host's normal surface barriers and internal defense mechanisms. The human host has evolved a complex array of protective mechanisms designed to defend itself against these continuous microbial challenges.[463] In order to understand the pathogenesis, pathology, and natural history of infectious diseases, one must be familiar with the features of infectious agents that confer virulence, which are addressed in other parts of this book. However, it is equally important to understand the elements of the host's response that contribute to containment, elimination, and protection against subsequent infection with these agents. Furthermore, it is important to recognize that host responses not only may contribute to the pathophysiology of disease but also may injure the host in other ways.

It is traditional to view the organization of the immune system in separate arms or compartments, such as complement, phagocytes, cell-mediated immunity, and humoral immunity.[117, 275] An alternative approach is to divide host responses into two larger categories: the earlier and more phylogenetically primitive, nonspecific mechanisms of response to infection, such as complement activation and phagocytic response, and the later, more deliberate, persistent, and highly evolved responses, such as antibody production and cell-mediated immunity, that exhibit an extraordinarily diverse range of specificities. An advantage of viewing the immune system in a compartmentalized fashion is the ability to dissect and consider separate cellular and biochemical mechanisms in the host response to infection. However, one must not neglect the vital concept that the different arms of the immune system engage in numerous and complex interactions that are critical to the optimal function of each individual compartment of the system and to the diversity of the immune response. For example, opsonization of encapsulated bacteria by complement proceeds most efficiently in the presence of specific anticapsular antibodies that can activate the classic pathway of complement.[55, 82, 249] Opsonization itself is a prelude to the efficient attachment and engulfment of microorganisms by phagocytes, which express receptors for antibodies and opsonic complement fragments.[2, 55, 435] Mononuclear phagocytes present processed peptide antigens to T cells.[285] T-cell help is essential for effective stimulation of production of antibodies against protein antigens, and they secrete cytokines that profoundly may influence responses of B cells, phagocytes, and other cells.[285]

The characteristic features of different kinds of infections are determined by specific interactions of microbial virulence mechanisms with host cells and proteins. Virulence tactics commonly employed by organisms include adherence to host cell surfaces, internalization within or invasion of host cells, production of toxins, elaboration of surface barriers such as bacterial polysaccharide capsules, usurpation of host synthetic mechanisms, and direct inhibition of specific host defense mechanisms.[223] The successful evolution of host strategies to protect against microbial attack has resulted in defenses designed to interfere with or to counteract many of these modes of microbial virulence. In recent years, some of humanity's oldest microbial enemies (e.g., smallpox, poliomyelitis, measles) systematically have been, or are being, eradicated. In the meantime, previously unrecognized pathogens such as HIV-1 and Ebola virus have emerged, some of which are being perceived as new plagues on humankind. Unfortunately, many of our oldest nemeses (e.g., tuberculosis, malaria) have not been brought under control, and some remain serious problems throughout the world. Continued study of microbial pathogenesis and immunologic mechanisms is needed to provide the foundation for developing innovative approaches to support and augment human evolutionary adaptations to microbial challenges.

MAIN FEATURES OF HOST RESPONSES TO SPECIFIC CLASSES OF INFECTIOUS AGENTS

Viruses

Viruses are obligate intracellular parasites that consist of genetic material in the form of either DNA or RNA that usually is surrounded by a protein coat and may or may not be bound by a lipid envelope.[303] Diseases caused by viruses are remarkably diverse, ranging from mild and merely inconvenient to rapidly fatal and from acute or brief to chronic or lifelong. However, certain features are common to the pathogenesis of most viral infections. First, viruses must enter host cells in order to replicate. It is presumed that entry is initiated by attachment of a virus surface protein to a specific receptor molecule on the host cell. The exact viral ligand or host cell receptor has been identified in only a few viruses. For example, rhinovirus has evolved a protein that binds to human intercellular adhesion molecule-1 (ICAM-1),[207] which is expressed on both respiratory epithelium and vascular endothelium (see later), and HIV-1 can bind to CD4 on T lymphocytes.[131, 255] After the virus has entered the host cell, the cellular synthetic machinery is redirected to the synthesis of viral components. As with other proteins made by the host cell, a portion of viral protein is processed into peptides and presented on the infected cell surface by major histocompatibility complex (MHC) class I molecules (see later). The host mechanisms most important in defense against the majority of viral pathogens include the production of specific neutralizing antibodies against viral surface proteins, the development of specific CD8+ cytotoxic T-cell responses that eliminate infected cells, and the production of interferons (IFNs) that disrupt viral replication.[285] Other host defenses also may exhibit antiviral activity, although the importance of some of these mechanisms in protection against viral infection in humans has not been established as firmly. For example, it is possible that natural killer (NK) cells mediate the destruction of infected host cells[285] and that antibody-dependent cellular cytotoxicity (ADCC) may ensue after IgG antibodies bind to viral antigens on the infected cell, permitting subsequent attachment of NK cells or cytotoxic T cells via IgG Fc receptors.[169] IFNs and other cytokines may enhance NK and ADCC activity, and cytokines such as tumor necrosis factor–alpha (TNF-α) may exert cytotoxic actions on cells infected with certain viruses.[285] Furthermore, it has been demonstrated that opsonic complement components bound to viral surfaces can interfere with cell attachment and that the late complement components of the membrane attack complex (MAC) can lyse enveloped viruses.[55]

Bacteria

The human host is colonized with a large variety of bacteria at skin and mucous membrane surfaces.[325] The integrity of these mechanical barriers ordinarily prevents systemic invasion of local commensal bacteria.[93] In addition, in healthy hosts, circulating polymorphonuclear leukocytes (PMNs) help keep the resident flora in check by leaving the blood stream at the mucosal sites containing the highest bacterial burdens, such as the oral cavity and the lower intestine.[27] This phenomenon helps account for the increased risk of local and systemic infection due to oral and intestinal organisms in patients with severe neutropenia, including those who receive prolonged chemotherapy for malignancies, and in patients with phagocytic migratory function disorders, such as leukocyte adhesion deficiency syndromes.[27] Important host defenses against most bacteria that invade the human host from without include the complement system, specific antibodies that promote both the opsonic and the bacteriolytic functions of complement, and phagocytes.[2, 27, 55, 249, 435]

Fungi

Host defense mechanisms against fungi are less well understood than those directed at bacteria and viruses. However, phagocytic and cell-mediated immunity appear to be most important.[159, 181] The relative value of these factors appears to depend on the specific organisms involved, as is demonstrated by clinical observations in patients with isolated defects of one or the other. Severe mucosal infections caused by *Candida* species are common in patients with cell-mediated immune deficits, such as HIV infection, the DiGeorge anomaly (see later), chronic mucocutaneous candidiasis, and some forms of severe combined immune deficiency, as well as in patients with disorders of leukocyte migration.[27, 159] Disseminated candidiasis more often is attributed to iatrogenic factors, such as prolonged antimicrobial therapy and indwelling vascular catheters, and patients with malignancies, complicated postsurgical courses, and burns appear to be at increased risk. Although neutrophils from patients with myeloperoxidase deficiency kill *Candida* organisms more slowly than do those from normal persons, these patients usually do not develop *Candida* infections, suggesting that this aspect of neutrophil function is not critical.[27, 159, 280] In contrast with *Candida, Aspergillus* infections are not as great a problem for patients with cell-mediated immune defects as they are for patients with defects in phagocytic host defenses, such as chemotherapy-induced neutropenia, or genetic defects in phagocyte killing such as chronic granulomatous disease (CGD).[53, 189] Fungi such as *Histoplasma* and *Cryptococcus,* like *Candida,* tend to cause severe infections in patients with defects in cell-mediated immunity, although phagocytes clearly are required for most effective clearance of these organisms.[144, 456] The role of antibodies and complement in protection from fungi probably is to provide opsonic activity to enhance phagocyte function.[146]

Features of Normal Immune Function

The ability of the immune system to respond effectively to a remarkably broad range of microbial pathogens and their antigens depends on aggressive, early responses that may be nonspecific and relatively short-lived or more deliberate, long-lasting, and specific and designed to confer protection against subsequent exposure. Although the arms of the immune system will be discussed separately, some of the intricate interactions among the different facets of the immune system previously noted will be addressed. It will be apparent that a degree of redundancy is inherent to the system, so that if one host mechanism fails or is inefficient in protecting against a particular pathogen, another may be able to help contain the microbe initially, provide long-term immunity, or do both.

CELL-MEDIATED IMMUNITY

Cell-mediated immunity provides several important functions in defense of the host against pathogenic microorganisms, including T-cell help for antibody production, cytokine production for the stimulation and regulation of immune responses, and cytotoxic T-cell activity against cells infected with viruses.[31, 149, 285, 344] The development of cell-mediated immunity requires complex interactions between T cells and antigen-presenting cells (APCs) via several types of surface molecules on the respective cell surfaces. These include the interaction between an antigen-specific T-cell receptor (TCR) on the lymphocyte and a peptide antigen presented by the APC; they are represented schematically in Figure 2–1. Other pairs of accessory cell-surface molecules (not depicted) that enhance interactions between T cells and APCs include CD40 ligand/CD40, lymphocyte function to associated antigen 1 (LFA-1)/ICAM-1, and CD28/B7. These are addressed in detail elsewhere.[285]

Antigen Presentation

For the immune system to respond specifically to microbial protein antigens, the antigens must be digested into smaller peptides within an APC.[285] These peptides are presented at

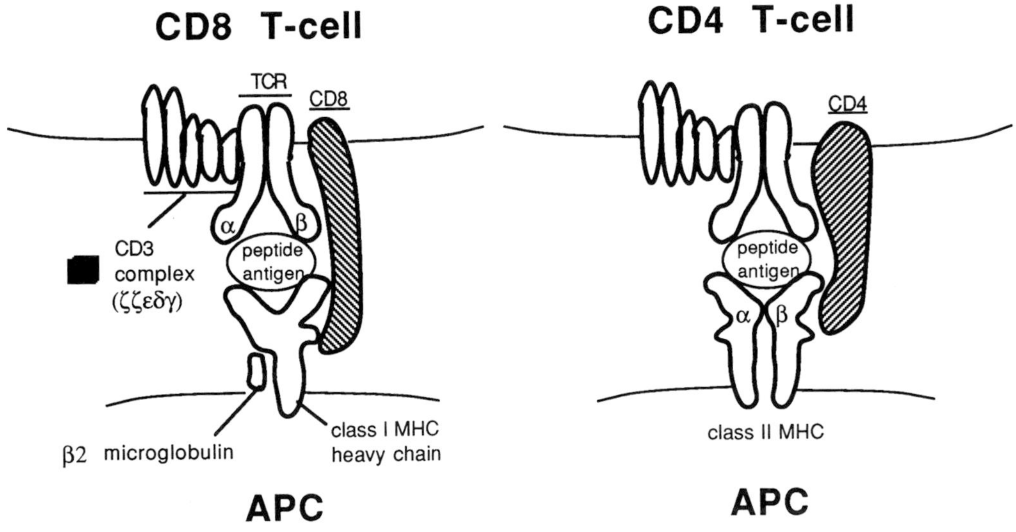

FIGURE 2–1. *Principal cell surface interactions between CD8 and CD4 T lymphocytes and peptide antigens complexed with major histocompatibility complex (MHC) class I and class II molecules, respectively. CD3 (composed of five subunits) is associated closely with the T-cell receptor (TCR), which recognizes a specific peptide presented on MHC molecules. Class I and class II MHC determinants are recognized by CD8 and CD4, respectively. Additional or accessory interactions are discussed in the text. (From Lewis, D. B., and Wilson, C. B.: Developmental immunology and role of host defenses in neonatal susceptibility to infection.* In *Remington, J. S., Klein, J. O. [eds.]: Infectious Diseases of the Fetus and Newborn Infant. 4th ed. Philadelphia, W. B. Saunders, 1995, p. 22.)*

the surface of the APC by MHC molecules. There they can be recognized and bound by T cells bearing receptors with the appropriate antigen specificity. Different mechanisms of foreign peptide antigen presentation are involved, depending on the type of APC and the type of infecting agent. The corresponding processes in development of immune responses to polysaccharide antigens are poorly understood.

Class I Major Histocompatibility Complex

The class I MHC molecule presents antigenic peptides to CD8+ T lymphocytes.[327, 421] It consists of a heavy chain that contains the peptide-binding domain, or cleft, and a transmembrane domain, and it exhibits genetic polymorphism. The class I MHC molecule also has a small extracellular subunit, β_2-microglobulin, whose association with the heavy chain is essential for effective antigen presentation.[66, 285, 362] The three major types of class I MHC heavy chains in humans, HLA-A, -B, and -C, are encoded on chromosome 6 and have at least 22, 31, and 12 different alleles, respectively.[466] This polymorphism permits a great diversity in the peptide-binding repertoire in individuals and within populations. A restricted degree of polymorphism would result in limitations in the ability to present a broad range of antigenic peptides and has been invoked as a possible explanation for the predisposition of certain populations with restricted MHC polymorphism, such as Native Americans, to develop severe infections.[67]

Because class I MHC molecules ordinarily bind peptides derived from proteins recently synthesized de novo within the cell, under normal circumstances they provide an opportunity for cells to express their antigenic identity as "self."[168, 432] However, because viral pathogens use host cell synthetic mechanisms, peptide antigens processed from newly synthesized viral proteins in infected cells also are presented by class I MHC.[167] With few exceptions, such as neurons, virtually all cells in the human host express class I MHC molecules, which they use to present peptide antigens at their surfaces.[130] A portion of newly synthesized cellular proteins is processed into peptides by enzymes at an incompletely defined cytoplasmic site in the cell called the proteasome.[198] These peptides actively are transported into the endoplasmic reticulum, where they are bound in the peptide-binding cleft of MHC class I.[285] The characteristics of peptides that bind class I MHC are relatively restricted. Thus, not all peptide sequences exhibit antigenic potential. Suitable peptides usually are 8 to 10 amino acids in length, and they must contain certain amino acids at specific positions on the peptide in order to be able to bind within the peptide-binding groove or cleft of the MHC class I molecule.[239, 285] Allelic variants of MHC class I require different amino acids at these "anchor" positions for binding to occur.[184] The other amino acids of the peptide may be more variable and probably constitute the antigenic determinants that interact with specific TCRs.[65, 184, 285]

Class II Major Histocompatibility Complex

The immune system includes several cell types that often are called professional APCs. These are bone marrow–derived cells, such as mononuclear phagocytes, B lymphocytes, and dendritic cells, including specialized tissue-specific dendritic cells such as the Langerhans cells of the skin.[122] Dendritic cells, the most efficient APCs for primary activation of naive T cells, are macrophage-like cells that take up and process antigens in tissues and then migrate to local lymph nodes or to the spleen, where they are likely to come in contact with T cells specific for the presented antigens.[155, 293, 363, 421] One important feature of these professional APCs is their expression of class II MHC molecules in addition to class I MHC.[129] Class II MHC molecules are composed of an alpha and a beta chain, which together form the peptide-binding cleft.[83, 374] Class II MHC molecules present peptides derived from proteins that are internalized during phagocytosis of microorganisms or endocytosis.[211, 240, 285] The peptide-binding cleft is configured to accommodate peptides from 13 to 17 amino acids in length, somewhat longer than those bound by class I MHC.[240, 374] There are three major types of class II MHC alpha and beta chains, HLA-DR, -DP, and -DQ, each exhibiting a high degree of polymorphism.[295] In uninflamed tissue, expression of class II MHC is relatively restricted to professional APCs. However, cytokines such as IFN-γ and TNF-α that may be present in an inflammatory milieu can induce MHC class II expression in a much broader distribution of cell types, including endothelial cells, epithelial cells of various organs, and eosinophils.[285] The peptide-binding function of MHC class II highly depends on its dissociation from a separate smaller molecule known as the invariant chain.[361, 425] Because the peptide-binding cleft of MHC class II in the endoplasmic reticulum is bound by the invariant chain, it cannot bind antigenic peptides.[361, 425] In contrast, the endoplasmic reticulum appears to be a major site of peptide binding for MHC class I.[285, 361, 425] Available evidence suggests that after being processed through the Golgi, MHC class II enters an endosomal/lysosomal compartment where dissociation of the invariant chain occurs, permitting binding of antigenic peptides derived from internalized proteins.[361, 425] The class II MHC/peptide complex then moves to the cell surface, where it interacts principally with CD4+ T cells.[156, 291]

Figure 2–2 depicts the essential features of the conventional peptide antigen presentation pathways that involve class I and class II MHC described earlier. Alternative mechanisms have been documented by which class I MHC may present peptides derived from exogenous proteins and class II MHC may present peptides from newly synthesized proteins.[285] The importance of these unconventional pathways of antigen presentation in the immune response is not fully understood.

T Lymphocytes

All lymphocytes have their origins in the pluripotent stem cells of the bone marrow. The development of T lymphocytes, or T cells, begins when the most immature cell committed to the T-cell lineage, the prothymocyte, leaves the marrow and enters the subcapsular region of the thymus.[154, 458] This initiates three stages of thymocyte development.[285] In stage I thymocytes, by mechanisms that are poorly understood, the thymic environment induces the rearrangement of TCR V (variable), D (diversity), and J (joining) gene segments (see later) with the eventual expression of mature alpha-beta TCRs complexed with CD3. This transition, along with the co-expression of both CD4 and CD8 and migration to the thymic cortex, marks the cell as a stage II thymocyte. Stage II thymocytes undergo processes of both positive and negative selection in which their TCR specificity is screened. The mechanism by which this screening takes place is the subject of intense investigation and theoretical controversy, and there are a number of excellent treatises and reviews on the subject.[112, 253, 298, 359] Thymocytes that do not pass this dual screening procedure receive signals that induce programmed cell death (apoptosis).[318] Thymocytes that do pass this screening process probably are those whose TCR specificities and affinities are perceived as optimizing the repertoire for distinguishing self from nonself and eliminating TCR rearrangements that result in undesirably high self-reactivity.

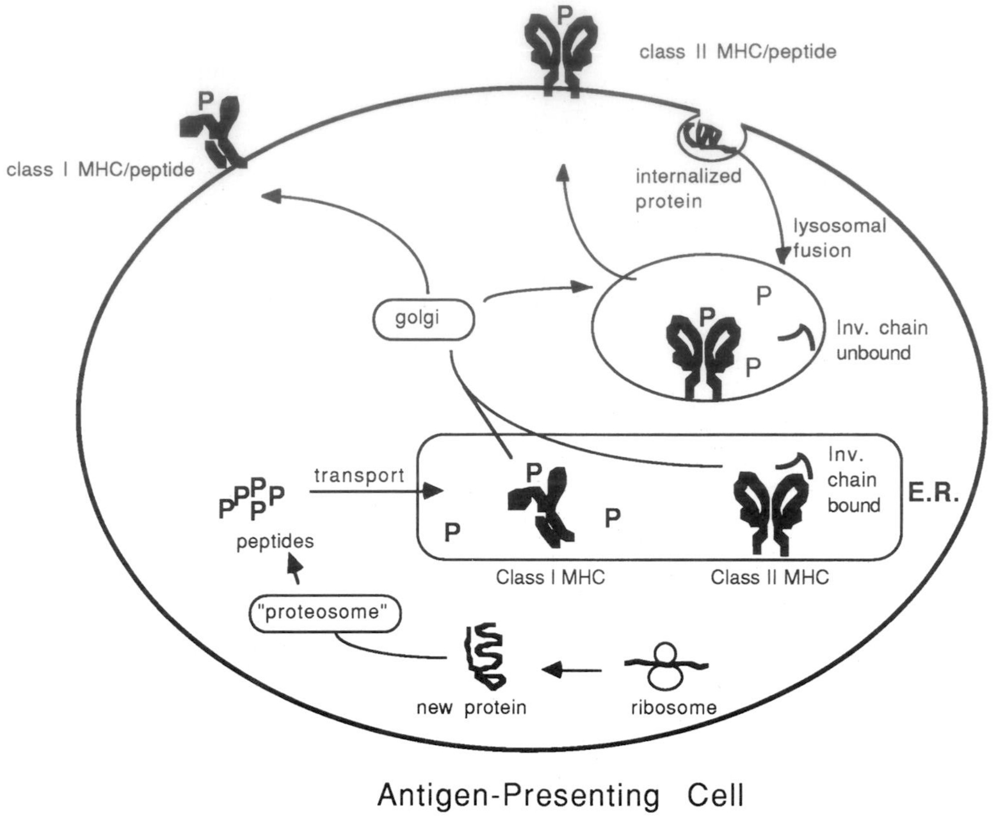

FIGURE 2–2. *Conventional pathways for peptide antigen presentation by class I and class II MHC molecules. In the antigen-presenting cell, a proportion of newly synthesized proteins undergoes proteolysis into peptides by enzymes that constitute the "proteasome." The peptides actively are transported into the endoplasmic reticulum (E.R.), where those with the appropriate length and sequence bind to MHC class I molecules. MHC class II cannot bind peptides in the E.R. because of interference by the associated "invariant chain." The class I MHC/peptide complex is transported via the Golgi to the cell surface, where it may be recognized by CD8+ lymphocytes. Class II MHC molecules pass via the Golgi to a lysosomal compartment, where conditions favor the release of the invariant chain. This permits class II MHC to bind peptides derived from internalized proteins that have entered the lysosomal compartment via fusion of endosomes or phagosomes with the lysosome. The lysosome translocates to the cell surface, where the class II MHC/peptide complex may be recognized by CD4+ lymphocytes.*

These cells, now stage III or medullary thymocytes, account for only about 5 per cent of the original stage II thymocytes, and they express either CD4 or CD8, not both.[445] The next step in T-cell maturation is the release of these mature thymocytes into the periphery, where the CD4+ cells serve as the main source of interleukin-2 (IL-2) and provide help for B-cell antibody production and CD8+ cells engage in cytotoxic activity.[285] The present and subsequent discussion of T cells and TCRs specifically relates to T cells that express TCRs composed of alpha and beta chains, or alpha-beta T cells. T cells of a distinct type, gamma-delta T cells, are far less numerous in most tissues (intestinal epithelium is a notable exception), exhibit much less TCR diversity than do alpha-beta T cells, may not require an intact thymus for development, and have been implicated in host responses to some intracellular bacterial pathogens, including *Listeria* and mycobacteria.[90, 251, 285]

Antigen specificity of alpha-beta T cells resides in their TCRs, which are integral membrane proteins with structural homology with immunoglobulins. TCR diversity results from a rearrangement of V, D, and J segments. These gene segments are dispersed widely on chromosome 7, and there are up to 100 different V segments, one D segment, and as many as 100 different J segments in the complete germ line configuration of the TCR genes.[460] Rearrangement of these gene segments into a mature VDJ sequence requires the action of a recombinase enzyme complex formed by two proteins, RAG-1 and RAG-2. This enzyme effects the deletion of intervening DNA so that a single VDJ sequence (or VJ in the case of the alpha chain) is formed.[336, 383] Thus, part of TCR diversity is the result of all of the possible combinations of V, D, and J segments. However, because of the imprecise action of the recombinase enzyme complex, the degree of diversity is much greater. The variability in the number of nucleotides deleted during rearrangement results in a tremendous increase in diversity of the possible sequences of TCR antigen-binding domains.[174] Additionally, thymocytes undergoing TCR gene rearrangement express the enzyme "terminal deoxytransferase," which appears to add nucleotides at random to extend segments during rearrangement.[174, 395] It has been estimated that as many as 10^{15} different TCR specificities theoretically could result from the various mechanisms that influence TCR segment rearrangement.[133] The basic structure of TCR is similar to that of antibody molecules, and the generation of diversity within the antigen-binding regions of antibodies is similar to that of TCR.

B LYMPHOCYTES AND IMMUNOGLOBULIN

B Lymphocytes

B lymphocytes (B cells) are effectors of humoral immunity in that they are responsible for the production of immunoglobulin.[81, 285, 334] Like T cells, they are derived from pluripotent stem cells. The earliest recognizable precursors of B cells are pro-B cells, whose surfaces bear the pan-B marker CD19. The next precursors are pre-B cells, which differ from pro-B cells in that they can produce mu heavy chain and are more numerous. Pre-B cells make up approximately 5 per cent of bone marrow cells. Pre-B proliferation is stimulated by IL-7 made by bone marrow stromal cells, and pre-B maturation into B cells capable of producing immunoglobulin depends on pre-B expression of a tyrosine kinase, *atk* or *btk*.[214, 433, 434, 443]

The transition from pre-B to mature B cells is marked by the expression of cell-surface immunoglobulin and the resulting ability to recognize and bind antigen. B lymphocytes constitute approximately 20 per cent of circulating lymphocytes and lymphocytes in peripheral lymphoid tissues, such as the lymph nodes, spleen, bone marrow, tonsils, and intestines.[81]

B cells can be identified by the presence of surface immunoglobulin and the pan-B differentiation markers CD19 and CD20 using flow cytometry. Other surface markers vary among individual B cells but may include Fc receptors and the complement receptors CR1, CR2, and CR3.[81, 285]

B-cell activation is induced by recognition and binding of specific antigens to B-cell surface immunoglobulins. Activation leads to increased expression of receptors that bind cytokines (e.g., IL-2, IL-4, IL-6) or T cells and to B-cell clonal proliferation and differentiation into memory B cells and plasma cells. Some data suggest that B-cell differentiation into memory B cells is favored by exposure to the CD40 ligand on dendritic cells in lymphoid organs. In contrast, differentiation into plasma cells is favored by exposure to CD23, IL-1α, IL-6, and IL-10.[285, 288] Plasma cells differ from B cells in that they no longer have surface immunoglobulin expression and they are capable of secreting large amounts of antibody. In fact, they are responsible for most immunoglobulin production. Plasma cells are found in bone marrow, liver, peripheral lymph nodes, and lymphatic tissue in the respiratory and gastrointestinal tracts.

The B-lymphocyte response to some antigens, particularly polysaccharide antigens, proceeds largely without T-lymphocyte involvement and is called T-independent. There are two types of T-independent antibody responses, thymus-independent type 1 (TI-1) and thymus-independent type 2 (TI-2). TI-1 antigens can bind to B cells and activate them directly without the help of T cells (e.g., fixed *Brucella abortus*). TI-2 antigens also can activate B cells directly, but antibody response to TI-2 antigens may be enhanced by the presence of T-cell help, and the isotype produced in response to TI-2 antigens depends on T-cell help. TI-2 antigens consist of repeating identical subunits, such as large polysaccharides (e.g., *Haemophilus influenzae* type b capsular polysaccharide).[218, 285]

The B-cell response to other kinds of antigens, particularly protein antigens such as tetanus and diphtheria toxoids, depends on T-cell help and, therefore, is called T-dependent. B cells efficiently can process and present antigen to CD4+ T cells they encounter in the lymph nodes and spleen. B-cell surface immunoglobulin binds to the T-dependent antigen, the immunoglobulin-protein complex is internalized and processed, and then it is presented to the T cell bound to B-cell surface class II MHC molecules. It is felt that because antigen binding to B-cell surface immunoglobulin is of relatively high affinity, B cells may permit T-cell activation by relatively small amounts of antigen. T cells appear to be stimulated more vigorously by B cells when the B cells present familiar, rather than new, antigens.[166, 186]

T-cell help is provided by both cell surface–associated signals and the release of soluble cytokines. T-cell surface CD40-ligand, which is expressed transiently on activated T cells, binds CD40 on B cells and is important in the T-dependent B-cell response to protein antigens and isotype switching.[35, 326] The cytokine IL-4 stimulates switching to IgG1 and IgE, and IL-10 promotes switching to IgA.[138, 275, 353]

Immunoglobulin

Immunoglobulin molecules may be bound to the surface of B cells, as has been discussed, or free in the circulation, mucosal secretions, or tissues. Free immunoglobulin binds to specific antigens and functions in host defense against infection by opsonizing pathogens for ingestion and killing by phagocytes, fixing complement, neutralizing viruses and toxins, and participating in the formation of immune complexes.

Immunoglobulin molecules are composed of two identical heavy and two identical light chains as illustrated in Figure 2–3.[218, 285] The two heavy chains and the heavy and light chain pairs are bridged by disulfide bonds and noncovalent forces. The carboxyl terminus of the immunoglobulin molecule is the heavy chain constant, or Fc, region. The amino acid sequence of this region determines the nine immunoglobulin isotypes: IgM, IgG1, IgG2, IgG3, IgG4, IgA1, IgA2, IgD, and IgE. The constant region is encoded by V, D, J, and constant (C) regions on chromosome 14.[59, 218, 285, 449] The Fc region is important in phagocytosis of opsonized organisms because it can bind to leukocyte Fc receptors itself or it can participate in complement activation and help direct the deposition of complement on the organism's surface.

The two kinds of light chains, kappa and lambda, are determined by different constant regions. They are encoded by V, J, and C genes on chromosomes 2 and 22, respectively. Each immunoglobulin molecule has a pair of either kappa or lambda light chains.

The amino terminus is the variable, or Fab, region of the immunoglobulin molecule. It serves as the antigen recognition and binding site. Like the TCR, the Fab region consists of two identical heavy and light chain pairs. Diverse antigen specificity results from the variable nature of recombinase-mediated DNA rearrangements of the three hypervariable complementarity-determining regions (CDR1, CDR2, and CDR3) and the four framework regions.[283] The imprecision of the joining process leads to the generation of more than 10^{12} antigenic specificities, many of which are nonfunctional. Further differences in specificity result from differences in approximation of the three CDRs with relationship to each other in the three-dimensional structure of the antigen recognition site, or binding cleft.[312] Somatic mutation, particularly

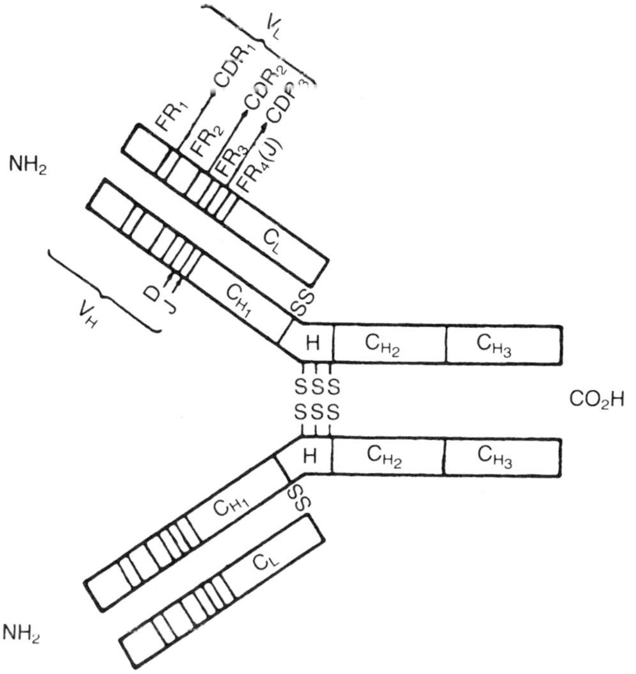

FIGURE 2–3. *Structure of an immunoglobulin molecule. That of IgG is shown. (From Lewis, D. B., and Wilson, C. B.: Developmental immunology and role of host defenses in neonatal susceptibility to infection.* In *Remington, J. S., Klein, J. O. [eds.]: Infectious Diseases of the Fetus and Newborn Infant. 4th ed. Philadelphia, W. B. Saunders, 1995, p. 37.)*

of the three hypervariable regions of the heavy and light chains, generates immunoglobulin with higher-affinity antigen-combining regions.[277, 328]

The ability of immunoglobulin molecules to recognize the three-dimensional structure of intact antigens such as microbial surface capsular polysaccharides or proteins differentiates them from TCRs, which usually only recognize processed peptide antigens.[302]

All immunoglobulin is derived from B cells expressing surface IgM. B cells change immunoglobulin isotype when they differentiate into plasma cells, which produce only one class or subclass of immunoglobulin each. Isotypes other than IgM are the result of isotype switching (e.g., from IgM to IgG) by replacing a part of the constant region of the immunoglobulin heavy chain with another isotype-specific segment. The Fab, or variable antigen-recognizing, region remains unchanged, and, thus, there is no change in antigen specificity. As already noted, isotype switching primarily depends on cytokines and T cells. Specific cytokines have roles ranging from permitting (e.g., IL-4) or augmenting to preventing (e.g., IFN-γ) isotype switching.

IgG and IgG Subclasses

IgG is a monomeric molecule with a molecular weight of approximately 150,000.[218, 285] IgG accounts for about 80 per cent of circulating immunoglobulin. It also is the predominant isotype in the tissues because its monomeric structure permits it to penetrate much more readily than polymeric immunoglobulins such as IgM and IgA. For the same reason, IgG is the only immunoglobulin type that crosses the placenta to the fetus (see later). IgG is composed of the subclasses IgG1, IgG2, IgG3, and IgG4. The half-life of IgG1, IgG2, and IgG4 ordinarily is 23 days, and that of IgG3 is 9 days. In circumstances of hypoimmunoglobulinemia or hyperimmunoglobulinemia, the half-life of IgG often increases or decreases, respectively.

Initial exposure to most antigens induces an IgM and then an IgG response consisting of IgG1 and IgG3. IgG2 and IgG4 usually are produced during the secondary immune response. Formation of specific IgG can signal the formation of memory B cells and, thus, may reflect long-term, potentially lifelong immunity.

The functions of IgG in host defense against infection include opsonization, complement fixation, toxin and viral neutralization, and antibody-dependent cytolysis. IgG binds antigen via its Fab region and to phagocytes and some other cells via its Fc region. IgG1, IgG2, and IgG3, but not IgG4, can trigger complement activation by the classic pathway by binding to C1q. They also help localize complement deposition on the surface of organisms by directing it to specific antigens (e.g., capsules versus outer-membrane proteins or lipopolysaccharides).

Different subclasses of antibody are associated with defense against different kinds of organisms. For example, IgG1 is formed in response to protein antigens such as tetanus toxoid.[415] In adults, the main antibody response to polysaccharides is IgG2, whereas in infants and IgG2-deficient persons, it is IgG1 predominantly.[17] IgG3 appears to be the most important subclass for viral neutralization.

IgM

Free IgM usually exists as a pentamer consisting of five monomeric paired heavy and light chains stabilized by a single J chain.[218, 285] Its half-life is approximately 7 days, and its molecular weight is 900,000. A hexameric IgM consisting of six monomeric heavy and light chains, but no J chain, is less prevalent but fixes complement more efficiently than does the pentameric form.[355] Most IgM is found in the circulation.

The IgM response is the earliest of the isotype responses, appearing within the first few days of infection, but it is transient. The formation of an IgM response in the absence of an IgG response to infection is not associated with the formation of memory B cells. Therefore, an isolated IgM response suggests transient immunity.

The main functions of IgM in host defense include fixing complement, opsonizing organisms for ingestion by phagocytes, and agglutinating them for clearance by the reticuloendothelial system. Each of these activities is enhanced by the polymeric structure of the IgM molecule, which gives it more binding sites and permits more avid binding.

IgA

IgA exists in monomeric circulating and polymeric secretory forms and has a half-life of about 7 days.[125, 218, 285] Its molecular weight ranges from 160,000 for the serum form to 500,000 for secretory IgA. Both forms are produced mainly by plasma cells that have migrated to mucosal sites. The two subclasses of IgA, IgA1 and IgA2, differ in the composition of their heavy chains. Approximately 90 per cent of IgA in the circulation is IgA1, whereas about 60 per cent of IgA in secretions is IgA2. IgA1, but not IgA2, is cleaved by bacterial proteases.

Secretory IgA is made up of two to three IgA molecules joined by a stabilizing J segment that is secreted by plasma cells and a secretory component produced by mucosal epithelial cells. The secretory component permits delivery of IgA to mucosal surfaces. Secretory IgA is found in all mucosal secretions, and it provides host defense at mucosal surfaces by preventing adherence of bacteria and neutralizing viruses.

IgA can activate the alternative pathway of complement, but, because it does not bind C1q, it cannot activate the classic pathway. It also can act as an opsonin or stimulate phagocyte superoxide production and, in the presence of lysozyme and complement, may have some bactericidal activity.

IgE

The IgE molecule has a molecular weight of 200,000 and a half-life of only 2.3 days.[218, 285] Most IgE is produced by plasma cells in lymphoid tissue near gastrointestinal and respiratory mucosal surfaces and released into the circulation. IgE also is found on mast cells and basophils. Serum IgE levels normally are low but tend to be higher in persons with a history of allergies.

The main function of IgE is to trigger immediate hypersensitivity reactions. Mast cells are activated when IgE bound to them by specific receptors is cross-linked by specific antigens. IgE-stimulated release of inflammatory mediators may permit increased influx of other immune factors such as IgG, complement, and cells including phagocytes, lymphocytes, and other eosinophils. IgE may aid toxin neutralization by enhancing the penetration of IgG antibody into the region. Persons with intestinal parasites have elevated serum levels of IgE, suggesting that it may play a role in protecting against parasitic disease. Potential functions of IgE could include directly damaging the parasites, preventing them from attaching and invading, or opsonizing them for phagocytosis and killing by macrophages whose surfaces contain Fc receptors specific for IgE. The IgE response to intestinal parasites also may protect by triggering release of mast cell contents to stimulate a local inflammatory response that results in expulsion of the parasite from the gastrointestinal tract.

IgD

IgD has a molecular weight of approximately 180,000 and a half-life of 2.8 days.[218, 285] It is present in most normal adult serum and secretions in low concentrations. Although some antigenic specificity for IgD has been demonstrated, its function in host defense is unclear. It cannot bind to phagocytes or fix complement. The most important function of IgD appears to be as an antigen receptor on the membrane of B lymphocytes, where it appears to be involved in regulating the development of normal B-cell antibody response.

COMPLEMENT

The complement system consists of more than 30 different free and membrane-bound activation and regulatory proteins. It has multiple key roles in the clearance of invading microbes, including opsonization, killing, and modulating the inflammatory and immune responses.[54, 143, 158, 160, 176, 244, 247, 248, 317] Complement and antibody often act in synergy in host defense against infection. Traditionally, they have been known as the heat-labile and heat-stable factors, respectively, which contribute to serum opsonic and bactericidal activity. The complement response to the initial encounter with an organism usually occurs earlier than that of antibody because it is nonspecific and can be initiated before specific antibody can be produced. Once specific antibody is available, it serves to activate complement more efficiently and to direct complement binding to locations on the microbial surface that support the most proficient execution of its effector functions, such as opsonization and killing.

Approximately 90 per cent of complement proteins are synthesized in the liver, but some components can be produced locally by tissue mononuclear phagocytes and fibroblasts.[113, 345] In healthy persons, the majority of complement is found in the circulation; less than 10 per cent is in mucosal secretions, and little is detectable in cerebrospinal fluid. Circulating complement levels vary over time, particularly in the presence of inflammation. The inflammatory response may lead to increases in levels of those complement components such as C3 that are acute-phase reactants or to decreases in individual components and total complement activity as a result of consumption.

The importance of normal complement component levels and activity in host defense has been well established and is based primarily on the increased susceptibility of patients with complement disorders to recurrent and severe infections.[141–143, 158, 244, 247] Although the complement response to infection usually is beneficial to the host, it also may be associated with adverse clinical manifestations, such as septic shock and acute respiratory distress syndrome.[171, 451]

Complement Activation

Complement proteins are activated in a cascade fashion by either the classic or the alternative pathway as shown in Figure 2–4. The complement cascade beyond C3 proceeds identically whether C3 is activated initially by the classic or the alternative pathway because their C3 convertases, C4b2a and C3bBb, respectively, cleave the C3 molecule at exactly the same location, producing C3a, which is released into the environment, and C3b. Cleavage and activation of C3 lead to a conformational change in C3b that transiently renders its reactive thioester group capable of forming covalent ester or amide bonds with acceptor molecules.[235, 274] If the acceptor molecules are situated on the surface of a microorganism, C3b (or its cleavage product iC3b) can act as an opsonin to promote phagocytosis, or it can initiate activation of the terminal complement proteins C5 through C9 by complexing with the classic and alternative pathway C3 convertases to form the C5 convertases, C4b2a3b and C3bBb3b, respectively. C5 convertases cleave C5 and begin the formation of the MAC. The MAC consists of one molecule each of C5b, C6,

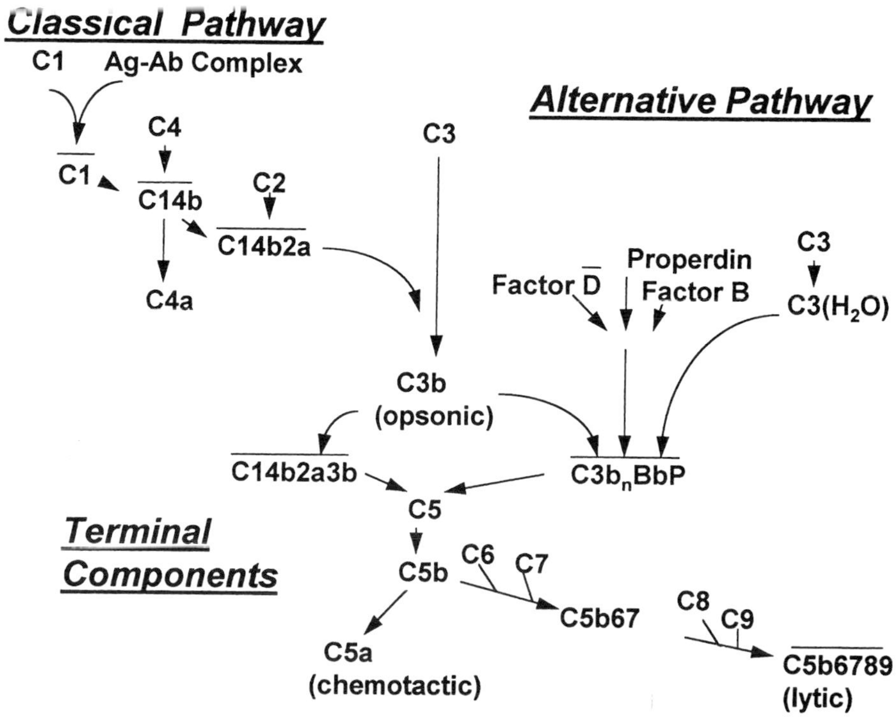

FIGURE 2–4. *Complement activation. The classic and alternative pathways intersect at C3. This is followed by activation of the terminal components, which generate the membrane attack complex (C5b6789). Enzymatically active proteases, which serve to cleave and activate subsequent components, are shown with an overbar. (From Lewis, D. B., and Wilson, C. B.: Developmental immunology and role of host defenses in neonatal susceptibility to infection. In Remington, J. S., Klein, J. O. [eds.]: Infectious Diseases of the Fetus and Newborn Infant. 4th ed. Philadelphia, W. B. Saunders, 1995, p. 64.)*

C7, and C8 and several molecules of C9. It can insert into the outer membrane of target cells, such as erythrocytes and gram-negative bacteria, and cause cell death and lysis.[248]

Ordinarily, the classic pathway is activated by IgM or IgG (IgG1>IgG3>IgG2) antibody-coated targets, such as microorganisms or antigen-antibody complexes.[143] IgM activates complement more efficiently than IgG because only one molecule of polymeric IgM is required, compared with at least two molecules of IgG.[120] IgG4, IgA, IgD, and IgE do not activate complement.

Classic pathway activation is initiated when C1q binds directly to an immunoglobulin molecule on the surface of an organism or, less often, to a surface molecule of the organism itself. C1r and C1s are activated and bound to C1q sequentially, forming C1qrs. This enzyme complex can cleave multiple molecules of C4 and C2 into two fragments each. The C4a and C2b fragments are released into the environment, whereas C4b and C2a remain bound to each other on the surface of the organism to form the classic pathway C3 convertase, C4b2a. C4bC2a can cleave and activate C3 and localize C3b binding to specific sites on the target surface.

In contrast with classic pathway activation, alternative pathway activation usually does not depend on the presence of specific antibody. It can be initiated by microbial surface macromolecules (e.g., polysaccharide, lipopolysaccharide, teichoic acid), although, as noted earlier, specific antibody increases alternative pathway efficiency and directs the location of C3b binding.[248]

Because the classic and alternative pathways differ in their requirements for antibody, the classic pathway usually contributes substantially more to host defense in immune individuals, whereas the alternative pathway is more important in protection of nonimmune persons, such as premature infants who have low levels of transplacentally acquired antibody and older infants and young children whose maternal antibody has waned but who have not produced their own specific antibodies yet.

C3 is activated continuously by C3 convertases and a low-level process called C3 tick-over, and, thus, C3b always is available to bind to microbial surfaces and initiate the alternative pathway.[342] The alternative pathway protein, factor B, has structural and functional similarities to C2, including the ability to bind to surface-bound C3b. Once bound to C3b, factor B undergoes proteolytic cleavage by factor D to release a small soluble fragment, Ba, leaving the larger fragment, Bb, associated with C3b. C3bBb, the alternative pathway C3 convertase, is analogous to the classic pathway C3 convertase, C4b2a. Properdin stabilizes the C3bBb complex, and C3bBb cleaves and activates more C3 molecules, creating the C3 amplification loop (see Fig. 2–4).[170, 173] Alternative pathway activation of C3 by this mechanism is several times less efficient than that of the classic pathway, but it is vital to host defense because it virtually is the only way a nonimmune person can activate C3 until a specific antibody response can be mounted.[140, 173]

The overwhelming majority of microorganisms in nature are not pathogenic, at least in part because their surfaces can activate the alternative pathway in the absence of antibody. Nonpathogenic organisms have surfaces that are classified as activator (protective, receptive, permissive) surfaces because they can bind C3b and protect it from inactivation by regulatory factors. Organisms with activator surfaces support deposition of multiple molecules of C3b by the alternative pathway amplification loop and, thus, are susceptible to complement-mediated opsonization and killing even in the absence of specific antibody.

Organisms whose surfaces do not support activation of the alternative pathway unless specific antibody is available, such as those with surface sialic acid, are some of the most successful pathogens in infants and young children. They include K1 *Escherichia coli*, groups A and B streptococci, *Streptococcus pneumoniae, Neisseria meningitidis, H. influenzae* type b, and some salmonellae.[97, 248] Their surfaces facilitate degradation of C3b to iC3b and thus fail to establish the amplification loop.

Several factors help distinguish activator from nonactivator surfaces. These include their chemical nature and the presence or absence of complement regulatory proteins.[173, 342] For example, most human cells are nonactivators by virtue of their surface sialic acid, which promotes preferential C3b binding to factor H over factor B, rendering C3b susceptible to cleavage into iC3b by factor I, the C3b inactivator. iC3b has opsonic activity but does not support continued activation of the alternative pathway amplification loop; therefore, fewer molecules of C3b are deposited on the cell surface. Organisms with surface sialic acid mimic nonactivator host cells. They include K1 *E. coli*, types Ia and III group B streptococci, and groups B and C *N. meningitidis*. It should be noted that specific antibody against these organisms permits activation of the alternative as well as the classic pathways of complement on their surfaces and correlates with protection.

Other mechanisms that prevent uncontrolled complement activation on cell surfaces include inhibition of alternative pathway C3 convertase, C3bBb, formation by cell-membrane complement receptor 1 (CR1) and decay-accelerating factor, and prevention of the formation of the membrane attack complex by cell-membrane CD59 and C8 binding protein (C8bp).[269]

Complement may be activated and bound to cell surfaces but not be able to carry out its effector functions if it is bound in the wrong location.[82, 202, 234] For example, C3b bound to pneumococcal cell wall underneath a thick polysaccharide capsule is not accessible to CRs on phagocytes and, therefore, does not promote effective opsonophagocytosis. Similarly, complement-mediated killing of some strains of *Salmonella* is prevented when the MAC is bound to long lipopolysaccharide molecules distant from the organism's cell membrane.[248, 249]

Effector Functions of Complement in Host Defense

All complement effector functions in host defense against infection require activation of the complement cascade through at least C3. The cascade needs to be activated only through C3 for effective opsonization, stimulation of leukocytosis, and immune regulation. Activation through C5 is required to produce a normal inflammatory response, including recruitment of phagocytes to sites of inflammation, and activation through C8 is needed for formation of the MAC.

Opsonic Activity

Complement opsonic activity is essential for effective removal of organisms from the circulation by macrophages in the liver and spleen and from other sites by neutrophils and tissue macrophages.[70] Opsonins facilitate recognition, binding, ingestion, and killing of microorganisms by phagocytes. Opsonization particularly is important for protection against gram-positive bacteria and fungi because their thick cell walls prevent them from being killed by the MAC.

As noted earlier, activation of C3 leads to a conformational change in C3b that permits its reactive thioester to bind covalently with acceptor molecules on microbial surfaces, where it can serve as an opsonin. C3b also can be cleaved by inactivators such as factor I and CR1 to form iC3b, which appears to be a more efficient opsonin than C3b.[202, 235] Some organisms, including certain serotypes of pneumococci, have surfaces that support degradation of differing amounts of surface-bound C3b to iC3b.[234] Surface-bound C3b and iC3b permit microbes to be recognized by circulating and tissue phagocytes by interacting with the phagocyte surface complement receptors, CR1 (CD35) and CR3 (CD11b/CD18), respectively. These interactions lead to binding, ingestion, and intracellular killing of the organisms.[202, 235, 274]

Antibodies also are important opsonins in that they facilitate more rapid complement activation and more effective localization of C3b binding to the surface of the organism. In the absence of specific antibody, complement deposition on the surface of the target is random and effector functions such as opsonization are not carried out as successfully.

Inflammation

The cleavage products of several complement proteins contribute to the development of an inflammatory response. C3e stimulates an increase in the number of circulating granulocytes, and C5a serves as a potent stimulus for monocyte, neutrophil, and eosinophil adherence to endothelial cells and migration toward sources of C5a gradients. C5a also upregulates phagocytes' expression of CR1 and CR3 and stimulates them to release stored enzymes and other granular contents that also are important mediators of inflammation, aggregation, and production of microbicidal oxidants. C5a-induced neutrophil aggregation and stasis in the pulmonary circulation are the basis of the respiratory distress syndrome associated with sepsis.[451]

The anaphylotoxins, C4a, C3a, and C5a, induce release of histamine from mast cells and basophils, causing increased vascular dilatation and permeability, which, in turn, permit local influx of other inflammatory mediators.[238] In this way, they help produce the hallmark clinical manifestations of inflammation, swelling, and erythema. When large quantities of anaphylotoxins are released rapidly, they can contribute to septic shock.[171] Carboxypeptidase treatment of C4a, C3a, and C5a destroys their anaphylatoxin activity, but the C5a cleavage product $C5a_{des\ arg}$ maintains some chemoattractant and phagocyte activating activity.[234]

Cidal Activity

Complement can act directly on certain bacteria to kill them. As noted earlier, C5b and the terminal complement proteins C6, C7, C8, and C9 form the MAC, which can kill and lyse target cells such as gram-negative bacteria by penetrating their outer membranes.[248] The C5b-C8 complex serves as a polymerization site for several molecules of C9. Although C9 is not essential to membrane penetration, its presence as poly-C9 allows it to proceed more efficiently.[424] Electron microscopy of the MAC demonstrates that it is composed of a ring-like structure at the outer surface of the target cell membrane and a perpendicular cylindrical component that penetrates the cell membrane. As has been noted, the MAC cannot penetrate the thick cell walls of gram-positive bacteria and fungi and, therefore, cannot kill these organisms directly.

The MAC can lyse some virus-containing host cells and some viruses themselves.[121] In addition, C1 and C4 can enhance virus neutralization by antibody.

Immune Regulation

Complement is involved in the regulation of several facets of the immune response, both directly by binding to CR1, CR2, and CR3 on the surfaces of T cells, B cells, and other cells involved in antigen recognition and indirectly by stimulating the synthesis and release of cytokines.[165] For example, the C3b cleavage product, C3dg, when covalently bound to antigen, brings the antigen close to B cells by binding to B-cell CR2 (CD21).[63, 75, 143, 335] Complement decreases the amount of antigen required to induce an immune response and increases the efficiency of the process by facilitating antigen presentation and localization. C3 also appears to be required for antigenic localization within germinal centers, and it is involved in anamnestic responses and isotype switching. The importance of complement in the immune response has been demonstrated by the finding that C1-, C2-, C4-, and C3-deficient animals have decreased antibody responses that can be restored by providing the missing protein. In addition, patients have been described who have complement deficiencies and low levels of IgG4 and IgG2.[63, 75, 143, 335]

PHAGOCYTES

Since Metchnikoff's earliest observations of host cells attacking foreign bodies in starfish,[304] phagocytes have been recognized as an important component in defense of the host. The most abundant phagocyte in the human host is the neutrophil, or PMN. Although there are some important differences between PMN and other phagocytes, including monocytes, eosinophils, and tissue macrophages, the PMN is an excellent prototype for the discussion of phagocyte function in general.

All phagocytes, including PMN, have their origins in myeloid stem cells of the bone marrow. Differentiation into the various end-stage cells is regulated by specific growth factors and cytokines.[42, 286] The determinants of release of mature PMN from the bone marrow into the systemic circulation are poorly understood. It has been suggested that as granulocytes mature in the marrow they gradually reduce the number of their surface receptors that bind bone marrow stromal components, such as haemonectin.[96] After a critical point during differentiation, stromal binding is reduced enough to permit release of the cells into the circulation.

Once in the circulation, the normal half-life of PMNs is approximately 8 to 12 hours.[448] In the absence of active infection, most PMNs leave the circulation via the gingival crevices and the lower gastrointestinal tract, sites at which the large populations of resident flora produce a continuous stimulation for recruitment of PMNs.[299] That patients with neutropenia, such as that due to chemotherapy for malignancies, develop necrotic gingivitis and ileocolitis is evidence for the importance of the continuous vascular egress of PMNs at these mucosal sites for maintenance of the integrity of these tissues.

The professional circulating phagocyte has three main functions in defense of the human host: (1) migration to the site of infection, (2) recognition and ingestion of invading microorganisms, and (3) killing and digestion of these organisms. When the normal barriers of the skin and mucous membranes are breached by microorganisms, interactions between microbial components and cellular and humoral constituents of the tissues result in production of mediators that initiate the recruitment of PMNs into these tissues.

Phagocyte Recruitment

The first stage in the recruitment of phagocytes from the circulation into infected tissue is the activation of endothelial cells that line nearby capillaries and postcapillary venules.[94, 399] Various mediators, including cytokines, fragments of complement components, eicosanoid compounds, and microbial products, are elaborated as a result of interactions between the invading microbe and tissue proteins and resident cells. These mediators, including IL-1 and TNF-α, diffuse from the site of production and act on the nearby endothelial cells to up-regulate their expression of adhesion molecules that will interact with circulating phagocytes.[398] The first adhesion molecules to be up-regulated are members of the selectin family, P-selectin and E-selectin, which engage in carbohydrate-mediated interactions with their corresponding ligands on circulating PMNs.[62, 271] Expression of P-selectin is up-regulated in a matter of minutes because it resides presynthesized within the cell in rapidly translocatable membrane compartments, or Weibel-Palade bodies.[62] Within 3 to 6 hours of stimulation of the endothelial cells, they begin to up-regulate expression of E-selectin because of new synthesis.[62] The principal carbohydrate moiety responsible for binding to P-selectin and E-selectin is sialyl Lewis X, an oligosaccharide that is presented on several glycoproteins on PMNs, including L-selectin.[62, 271] The circulating PMNs constitutively express L-selectin, and early selectin-mediated interactions result in a progressively slower "rolling-like" behavior of leukocytes along the endothelial luminal surface, the first adhesive phase of leukocyte recruitment.[62, 94, 399] Within 6 to 12 hours of endothelial stimulation, expression of adhesion molecules of the immunoglobulin supergene family becomes up-regulated. The most important of these is ICAM-1.[194, 396, 399] As the movement of PMNs along the endothelial surface becomes progressively slower, there is time for the PMNs themselves to become activated by locally produced mediators and chemoattractants, and they increase the expression and/or binding activity of the β_2 integrins LFA-1 and macrophage antigen 1 (Mac-1) that interact with ICAM-1 and related molecules on the endothelial cells.[30, 396, 398, 399, 413] Both LFA-1 and Mac-1 at the surface of the PMN undergo a conformational activation that increases their binding avidity.[145, 442] Additionally, there is a large storage pool of Mac-1 inside the cell in at least two separate membrane compartments. It is translocated to the cell surface, rapidly increasing the Mac-1 surface expression approximately 10-fold over baseline levels.[30, 34, 57, 72, 73] This second phase of adhesion mediated by integrin-ICAM interactions results in firm PMN adhesion to the endothelium and is required for transendothelial migration, or extravasation, of the PMNs.[30, 94, 396, 398] Platelet–endothelial cell adhesion molecule 1 (PECAM-1) on PMNs interacts with PECAM-1 on endothelial cells, further promoting transendothelial migration.[12] Cytokines such as TNF-α play some role in the activation of PMNs, but activation of PMNs for this second phase of recruitment occurs principally via chemoattractant agents (e.g., C5a), N-formyl bacterial oligopeptides, leukotrienes (e.g., LTB_4), and chemokines (e.g., IL-8) that diffuse from the site of infection and bind to specific PMN receptors.[152, 319] The receptors for these chemoattractants share a seven-transmembrane domain structure and similar intracellular G protein–dependent signaling mechanisms.[195, 319] They constitute the main sensory mechanisms of the PMNs responsible for inducing increased adhesion and permitting spatial orientation and migration toward the source of a chemoattractant gradient. This migration of PMNs depends on the adhesive interactions described earlier, the ability of the cell to deform to permit passage between endothelial cells, the ability of the PMN to sense and orient within a chemoattractant gradient, and the active movement of adhesion sites in the plane of the membrane by the cytoskeletal contractile elements of the cell.[29, 30, 416, 467] A scheme for PMN recruitment to infected tissue is presented in Figure 2–5. The molecular interactions that mediate PMN-

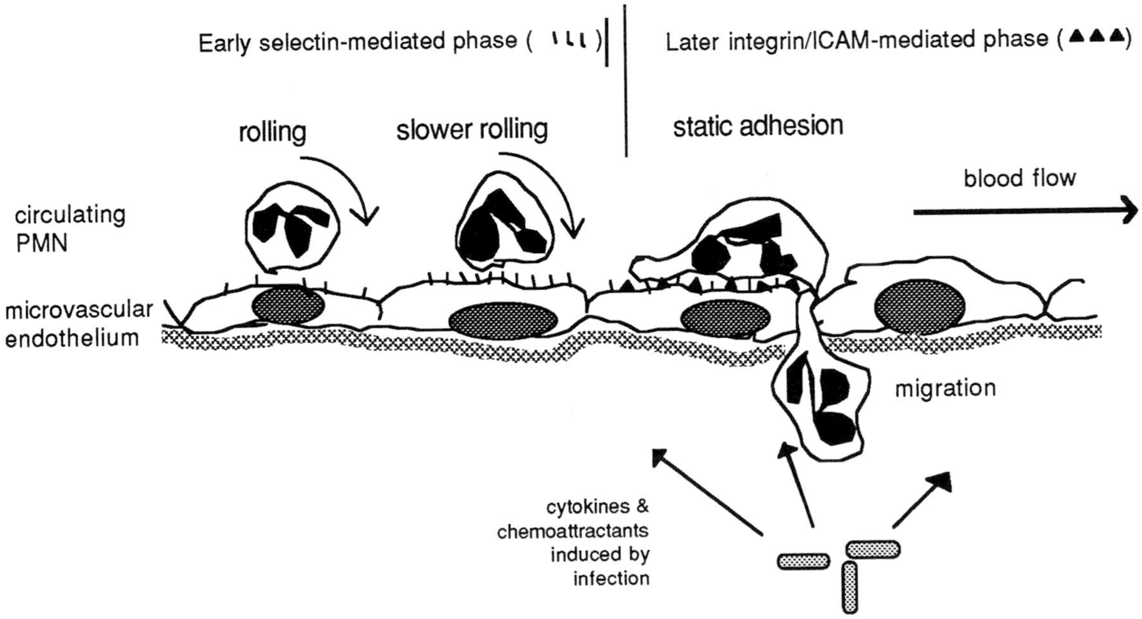

FIGURE 2–5. *Events during polymorphonuclear leukocyte (PMN) recruitment to infected sites. Interactions between microorganisms at the infected site and host cells and proteins result in elaboration of mediators that diffuse to local microcirculation and stimulate the endothelial cells. This induces new surface expression of P-selectin and E-selectin, as well as intercellular adhesion molecule 1 (ICAM-1). The endothelial selectins bind with constituitively expressed carbohydrate ligands of L-selectin on circulating PMNs and slow the passage of the PMNs through the microvessels. As the PMNs take longer to pass through the vessel, they become activated by other mediators diffusing from the infected site and increase their expression and binding activity of the β_2 (CD11/CD18) integrins, macrophage antigen 1 and lymphocyte function–associated antigen 1 (LFA-1). Interactions between these integrins and ICAM-1 (and ICAM-2 in the case of LFA-1) lead to tight adhesion and spreading on the endothelial surface and migration between endothelial cells in response to the gradient of chemoattractants produced at the infected site. Interactions between platelet–endothelial cell adhesion molecule 1 on the PMNs and endothelial cells also contribute to transendothelial migration.*

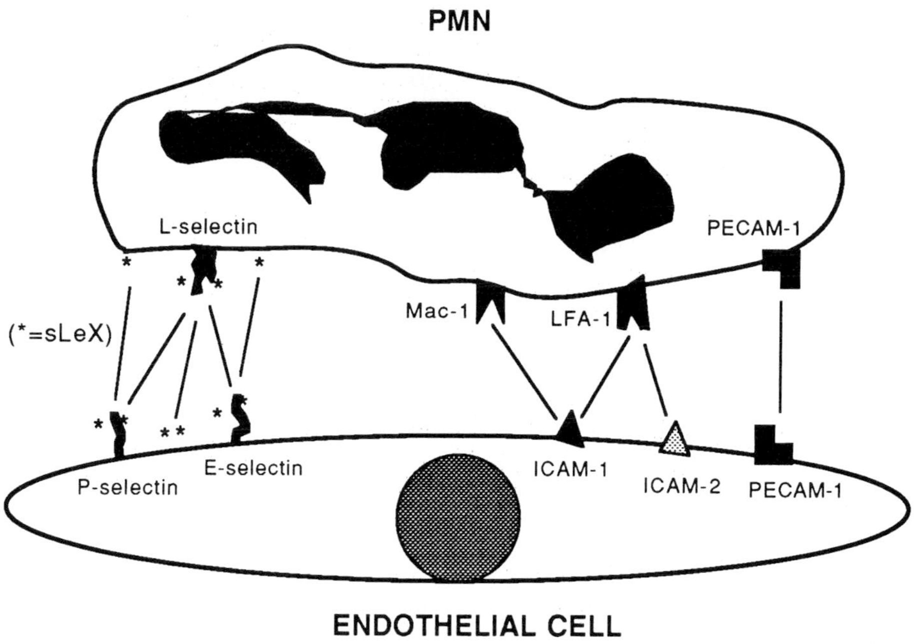

FIGURE 2–6. *Molecular interactions that mediate polymorphonuclear leukocyte (PMN)-endothelial adhesion. The selectins, P-selectin and E-selectin on endothelium and L-selectin on leukocytes, bind to oligosaccharide moieties, including sialyl Lewis X (sLeX), that decorate the corresponding selectins, as well as other molecules on the opposite cell. These interactions mediate the early phase of adhesion in leukocyte recruitment. The* β_2 *integrins macrophage antigen 1 (Mac-1) (CD11b/CD18) and lymphocyte function–associated antigen 1 (LFA-1) (CD11a/CD18) on PMNs both bind intercellular adhesion molecule 1 (ICAM-1) on endothelial cells. LFA-1 also binds ICAM-2, which is expressed constitutively on endothelium. Platelet–endothelial cell adhesion molecule 1 (PECAM-1) molecules interact with each other and are expressed on both PMNs and endothelial cells.*

endothelial adhesion during the recruitment process are depicted in Figure 2–6.

Phagocytosis

After the migrating phagocyte reaches an infected site, its next task is to recognize and ingest, or phagocytose, the invading microbes. A process that greatly facilitates recognition and phagocytosis is opsonization, or coating of the microorganism with serum proteins, especially IgG antibodies and fragments of the third component of complement.[249, 427] PMNs and other phagocytes express specific receptors for the Fc portions of IgG and IgA and the two major opsonic fragments of C3, C3b, and iC3b.[55, 418, 435] It is possible for phagocytosis to occur in the absence of opsonization, and some PMN surface molecules have been implicated in this process.[379] However, nonopsonic phagocytosis generally is inefficient compared with opsonin-dependent phagocytosis, and only the latter is addressed here.

Opsonin Receptors

CR1 is the main phagocyte receptor for C3b.[55, 172] It is expressed on most phagocytic cells, including PMNs. For circulating PMNs, only about 10 per cent or less of the cells' CR1 is expressed on the cell surface. Most of the CR1 resides within the cells, stored in the membrane of small, irregular, low-density secretory vesicles.[54] When PMNs are activated by chemoattractants or other stimuli, these intracellular stores of CR1 rapidly are translocated to the cell surface.[54, 55, 57, 172] Internalization of the receptor also occurs,[54, 56] but the net effect of stimulation in the short term is to increase greatly the amount of CR1 available on the PMN surface for interaction with bound C3b on microorganisms.[54, 55] CR3 is the main PMN receptor for iC3b.[55] Like CR1, 90 per cent or more of the cell content of CR3 is contained in intracellular membrane storage compartments that are translocated rapidly to the cell surface upon cell activation.[27, 55, 57, 331] It is useful and interesting to recall that CR3 is identical to the adhesion-mediating integrin Mac-1 (CD11b/CD18).[27, 55] This integrin contains distinct extracellular binding domains for iC3b and its counter-receptor, ICAM-1.[27, 33] Thus, CR3 serves important functions relevant to both cell recruitment and phagocytosis. Although CR1 and CR3 clearly play important roles in phagocytosis, engagement of complement receptors alone results in relatively inefficient phagocytosis compared with the combined effects of ligation of receptors for both complement fragments and opsonizing antibodies, especially IgG.[55, 249, 435]

Phagocytic cells may express up to three different types of IgG Fc receptors, or FcγRs.[169, 435] FcγRI (CD64) is a high-affinity receptor that is expressed mainly on mononuclear phagocytes, but PMNs exposed to IFN-γ may be induced to synthesize and express this receptor.[435] The two FcγRs ordinarily expressed on PMN are FcγRII (CD32) and FcγRIII (CD16).[428, 435] FcγRII is a 40-kDa molecule conventionally anchored in the cell membrane. It exhibits polymorphisms that determine preferences for binding of certain IgG subclasses.[435] FcγRII appears to be important in direct activation of PMN oxidative burst activity.[428, 435] Its expression on PMNs is constitutive and relatively stable to proteolysis and most cell perturbations.[428, 429] FcγRIII is expressed on PMNs as a 50- to 70-kDa glycolipid-anchored molecule, although it is anchored conventionally on NK cells and macrophages.[435] On the surface of circulating PMNs, it is about seven times more abundant than FcγRII.[428] Additionally, there is an intracellular translocatable storage pool that contains about twice the amount of FcγRIII expressed on the surface of circulating PMNs.[429] When PMNs are activated, there is both shedding of this receptor from the cell surface and translocation of stored receptors from intracellular pools to the cell-surface membrane.[429] FcγRIII appears to be more involved in binding of multivalent IgG than in direct generation of intracellular signals. However, binding of multivalent IgG ligand via FcγRIII appears to facilitate binding of ligand to FcγRII, suggesting a cooperative role for the former in producing cell activation by the latter.[379, 380, 428] FcγRIII also may play a more direct role in mediating IgG-dependent degranulation and phagocytosis.[380, 435]

Additional Fc receptors are expressed on phagocytes for IgA. Such receptors might be expected to play an important role at the mucosal surface, where IgA is prominent in secretions, although they also may play a role at other tissue sites. The best-characterized phagocyte IgA receptor, FcαR, is the receptor for monomeric IgA, CD89.[313] This receptor is expressed on most classes of phagocytes and has been shown to promote phagocytosis and killing of IgA-opsonized bacteria.[236, 237]

Ingestion

The engagement of phagocyte receptors with opsonins on microbes results in the local activation of cytoskeletal contractile elements with the simultaneous extension of pseudopods around the microbe and invagination of the membrane at the site of initial receptor engagement. This in turn permits the ligation of additional opsonin-receptor pairs with further activation and eventual engulfment of the microbe. This engulfment is complete when the membrane compartment surrounding the organism is sealed to form a phagosome. This progressive engagement of opsonin-receptor pairs with eventual engulfment has been called the zipper hypothesis of phagocytosis[417] and is depicted schematically in Figure 2–7. One interesting exception to this conventional mode of ingestion of microorganisms is the progressive spiraling engulfment of *Legionella pneumophila* by mononuclear phagocytes, first described by Horwitz.[233]

Phagocyte Microbicidal Mechanisms

The PMN has a varied arsenal it can use to kill microorganisms after they have been ingested. This intracellular killing usually occurs after the phagosome containing the organism fuses with one or more types of lysosomal granules that carry these microbicidal weapons. The contents of the different types of PMN granules, which contain many of the PMN's microbicidal molecules either free within granules or anchored in the granular membrane, are listed in Table 2–1. Killing mechanisms of PMNs usually are categorized as either oxygen-dependent or oxygen-independent.[366] The oxygen-dependent microbicidal mechanisms of PMNs and other phagocytes depend fundamentally on the activity of a complex enzyme known as NADPH oxidase, whose function is to convert molecular oxygen (O_2) into superoxide anion (O_2^-).[38, 109] This enzyme, in its active state, is assembled from

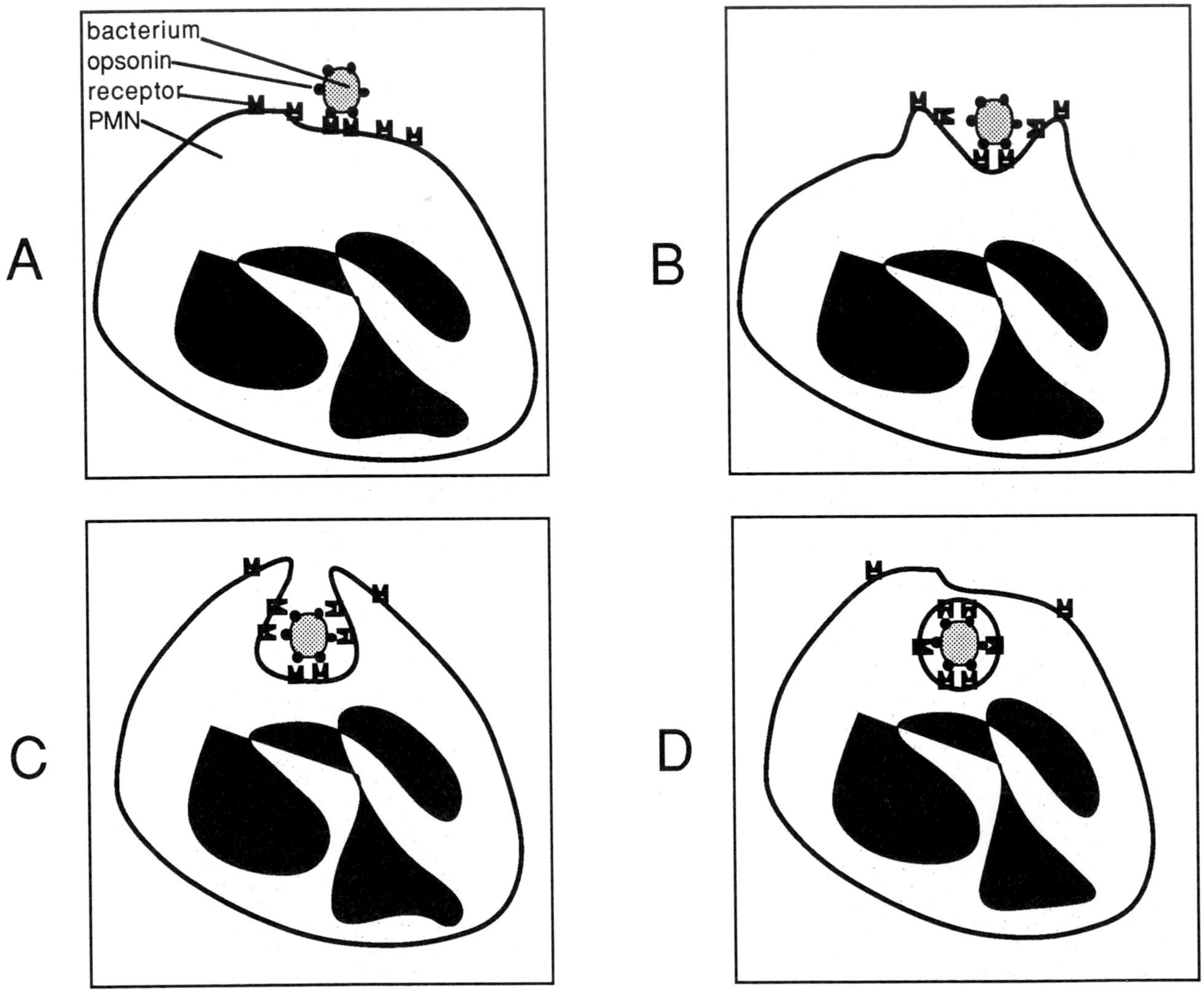

FIGURE 2–7. *Opsonin/receptor-mediated phagocytosis. Phagocytes such as PMNs that reach the site of bacterial infection exhibit enhanced recognition, attachment, and ingestion of bacteria that have been coated with opsonic C3 fragment, IgG, or both via specific receptors on the PMN surface. Binding of the opsonized bacteria to opsonin receptors (A) activates contractile elements of the cytoskeleton to produce an invagination at the initial site of attachment and to extend membrane pseudopods around the organism (B). This, in turn, allows engagement of additional opsonin-receptor pairs, as the organism becomes engulfed (C). Finally, the plasma membrane fuses to create the phagosome (D), which soon will fuse with lysosomal granules, exposing the bacterium to the microbicidal components of the phagocyte.*

TABLE 2–1. Stored Contents of Neutrophil Granules and Vesicles

Primary (Azurophilic) Granules	Secondary (Specific) Granules[a]	Tertiary Granules[b]	Secretory Vesicles[c]
Elastase Cathepsin G Myeloperoxidase Defensins Bactericidal/permeability-increasing protein "p15s" Other cationic proteins Lysozyme	Lactoferrin Vitamin B_{12}–binding protein Lysozyme Gelatinase	Gelatinase	Alkaline phosphatase

Selected membrane-bound proteins in intracellular granules and vesicles: f-met-leu-phe receptor[a, b, c]
type 1 complement receptor (CR1)[c]
CD11b/CD18 (CR3, Mac-1)[a, b, c]
cytochrome b_{558}[a, b, c]
type III Fcγ receptor (CD16)[?, c]

six or more components that include a cytochrome (α and β subunits), a flavoprotein, and a quinone that all are associated with the cell membrane and at least two cytoplasmic proteins, 47_{phox} and 67_{phox} ("phox" for phagocyte oxidase), that assemble with the membrane components to form the active enzyme complex.[37, 71, 109] It is the genetic absence or dysfunction of one or another of these oxidase subunits that results in CGD of childhood (see later). The oxidative reactions downstream from the formation of superoxide anion are summarized in Figure 2–8. Each of the oxidant products derived from these reactions exhibits some degree of microbicidal activity.[366] The spontaneous or catalyzed dismutation of superoxide anion results in the formation of hydrogen peroxide (H_2O_2), a compound commonly used in weak solutions to disinfect wounds. The subsequent interaction between hydrogen peroxide and a halide anion (usually Cl^-) in the presence of myeloperoxidase results in the formation of hypochlorite (OCl^-), the basis of common household bleach, another compound with well-recognized microbicidal activity. These oxidants are relatively short-lived and, except for hypochlorite, have relatively weak microbicidal activity. However, hypochlorite interacts with ammonium (NH_4^+) and amino groups on peptides and proteins to form various chloramines (NH_3Cl, RNH_2Cl), which are much more stable compounds with potent microbicidal activity.[209] Additional reactions include the direct interaction between superoxide

1. $2O_2 + NADPH \xrightarrow{\text{NADPH oxidase}} 2O_2^- + NADP^+ + H^+$

2. $2O_2^- + 2H^+ \xrightarrow[\text{catalyzed by dismutase}]{\text{spontaneous or}} H_2O_2 + O_2$

3. $H_2O_2 + H^+ + Cl^- \xrightarrow{\text{myeloperoxidase}} H^+ + OCl^- + H_2O$

4. $H^+ + OCl^- + RNH_2 \longrightarrow RNHCl + H_2O$

FIGURE 2–8. *Major reactions in the evolution of oxygen-dependent polymorphonuclear leukocyte microbicidal activity. The conversion of molecular oxygen to superoxide anion (O_2^-) by NADPH oxidase is the initial event in the sequence of production of antimicrobial oxidants. Shown in order are the subsequent reactions for production of hydrogen peroxide (H_2O_2), hypochlorite (OCl^-), and chloramines (RNH_2Cl).*

anion and hydrogen peroxide in the presence of catalytic iron to form hydroxyl radical (•OH) in the Haber-Weiss reaction.[366] Thus, PMNs can generate a diverse array of oxidant-free radicals, a number of which have potent antimicrobial activity.

The major sources of oxygen-independent microbicidal activity in PMNs reside with a group of proteins and peptides stored within the primary (azurophilic) granules. Lysozyme is contained in both the primary and the secondary (specific) granules of PMN.[411] It cleaves important carbohydrate linkages in the peptidoglycan structures of bacterial cell walls. Its microbicidal activity is greatest when it acts in concert with the complement MAC.[249] The primary granules contain several cationic proteins that exhibit well-documented microbicidal activity. A 59-kDa protein, bactericidal/permeability-increasing protein, is active against only gram-negative bacteria.[453] Its action appears to require hydrophobic insertion of one segment of the protein into the bacterial outer membrane, resulting in increased permeability and death of the organism. A group of arginine- and cysteine-rich 3- to 4-kDa peptides known as defensins display microbicidal action against a wide range of pathogenic organisms, including both gram-negative and gram-positive bacteria, fungi, chlamydiae, and enveloped viruses.[190, 282] At least two other groups of related microbicidal peptides or proteins have been identified in PMNs and include a group called p15s and a 37-kDa cationic protein.[187, 281, 284] Although not all of the mechanisms of these proteins and peptides have been elucidated fully, there is evidence that some of them may interact with each other synergistically, markedly increasing overall microbicidal activity.[283]

CYTOKINES AND RELATED MEDIATORS THAT REGULATE HOST RESPONSES

A heterogeneous group of soluble small polypeptide or glycoprotein mediators, often collectively called cytokines, form part of a complex network that helps regulate the immune and inflammatory responses. Included in this group of mediators, whose molecular weight ranges from about 8 to about 45 kDa, are the ILs, INFs, growth factors, and chemokines. Cells of the immune system as well as many other cell types in the host may release cytokines, respond to cytokines via specific cytokine receptors, or both, depending on the specific molecule in question. A list of cytokines and related molecules that play a role in immune function, with selected characteristics, is provided in Table 2–2.[267, 285, 349] New cytokines are being discovered and characterized regularly, and the range of sources and effects of cytokines and their inter-relationships are of such complexity that they cannot be addressed here in great detail. Several excellent reviews are available,[131, 287, 367] and the use of cytokines as immunomodulating agents is discussed in Chapter 236. Two specific cytokines, IL-1 and TNF-α, are of such broad and fundamental importance in acute host responses to infection that they warrant specific discussion here.

IL-1 and TNF-α are small polypeptides that exhibit a broad range of effects on immunologic responses, inflammation, metabolism, and hematopoiesis.[61, 148] Many of the well-characterized inflammatory and systemic responses of mammalian hosts to bacterial endotoxin or lipopolysaccharide are mediated by IL-1 and TNF-α.[61, 148] IL-1 has been known by various names in the past but originally was described as endogenous pyrogen, referring to its ability to produce fever in experimental animals.[148] TNF-α, originally named cachectin after the wasting syndrome it produced when injected chronically in mice, produces some of the same effects produced by IL-1.[61, 148] Many of the physiologic changes associated with gram-negative sepsis can be reproduced by injecting experimental animals with these cytokines in the absence of microorganisms. Depending on the doses injected, these effects may include fever, hypotension, and either neutrophilia or leukopenia.[61, 148] Both IL-1 and TNF-α, as well as lipopolysaccharide itself, stimulate inflammatory responses in infected tissue by inducing expression of adhesion molecules of both endothelial cells and leukocytes, stimulating recruitment of leukocytes by inducing release of the chemokine IL-8 and, in the case of TNF-α, activating granulocytes for phagocytosis, degranulation, and oxidative burst activity.[61, 148] For some systemic actions, notably the production of hemodynamic shock, IL-1 and TNF-α are synergistic. Both IL-1 and TNF-α induce production of IL-6, a somewhat less potent cytokine that exhibits some of the same activities as IL-1 and TNF-α.[148]

TABLE 2–2. Important Features of Human Cytokines and Growth Factors

	Molecular Weight (kDa)	Main Cellular Source(s)	Main Biologic Effects
IL-1	17	Mo, TL, BL, NK, PMN, other cell types	Broad range of cellular activation in inflammatory and immune responses
IL-2	15	TL, BL, NK	TL, BL proliferation and activation; enhances TL and NK cytotoxicity
IL-3	14–28	TL	General stimulation of hematopoiesis
IL-4	20	TL, BL, Mast, Mo	TL, BL proliferation; BL isotype switching; stimulates IgE synthesis; enhances MHC class II expression
IL-5	18/18 homodimer	TL	Stimulation of Eo production
IL-6	21	TL, BL, Mo	Broad inflammatory activity; stimulates BL differentiation and megakaryocyte production
IL-7	25	Stromal cells of marrow and thymus	TL, BL growth and differentiation
IL-8	8	Mac, Mo, Endo, Epi, PMN, Eo	Activation and chemotaxis of PMN, Eo
IL-9	39	TL	Mast cell growth and differentiation; growth of activated TL
IL-10	19	TL, BL, Mast, Mac, (Epi)	Broad anti-inflammatory actions; inhibits synthesis of several other cytokines (TNF, IL-2, IL-3, IFN-γ)
IL-11	20	Stromal cells of marrow	General stimulation of hematopoiesis; BL growth and differentiation
IL-12	35/40 heterodimer	BL, Mo	Stimulation of TL growth; induction of IFN-γ production; enhancement of TL and NK cytotoxicity
IL-13	10–17	TL	BL proliferation and isotype switching; enhances MHC class II expression; inhibits production of cytokines by Mac
IFN-α	18–20	Mo, TL	Interference with viral replication; increases MHC class I expression
IFN-β	23	Epi, Fibro	Similar to IFN-α
IFN-γ	20	TL, NK	Similar to IFN-α, IFN-β; stimulates Mac inflammatory functions
TNF-α	17	Mo, Mac, TL, NK	Broad inflammatory effects; fever; cachexia; stimulates catabolism; activation of leukocytes and Endo
GM-CSF	14–35	TL, BL, Mo, PMN, Eo, Fibro, Mast, Endo	Growth of PMN, Eo, Mo, and Mac precursors; enhances leukocyte function
G-CSF	19	Mo, Epi, Fibro	Enhances production and function of granulocytes
M-CSF	20–25 and 35–40 (distinct homodimers)	Mo, TL, BL, Endo, Fibro	Promotes Mo production; stimulates Mo and Mac functions

TL, T lymphocyte; BL, B lymphocyte; Mo, monocyte; Mac, macrophage; PMN, polymorphonuclear leukocyte; Eo, eosinophil; NK, natural killer cell; Mast, mast cell; Epi, epithelial cell; Endo, endothelial cell; Fibro, fibroblast; IL, interleukin; IFN, interferon; GM-CSF, granulocyte macrophage colony-stimulating factor; TNF, tumor necrosis factor; MHC, major histocompatibility complex.

IL-1 and TNF-α act on a wide range of cell types via specific receptors.[148] The importance of effects mediated by IL-1 and TNF-α in the pathophysiology of septic shock has prompted much active research aimed at blocking their effects in order to reduce morbidity and mortality. Naturally occurring soluble antagonists of IL-1 and TNF-α include IL-1 receptor antagonist (IL-1ra) and soluble TNF-α receptor (sTNF-λR). Monoclonal antibodies against TNF-α have shown promise in vitro and in animal models of septic shock.[1, 41, 148, 180] However, one of the main impediments to the clinical success of such agents to date is that the processes they inhibit often are well under way by the time treatment can be initiated, and they are far more effective at preventing the effects of cytokines than reversing them. Additionally, because cytokines have beneficial effects in the host response as well as pathologic effects, it may be difficult to discern clearly the overall effects of inhibiting their actions.[148] More recent attempts to address the issue of the timing of intervention have been directed at the intracellular signaling mechanisms activated through the TNF-α receptor. One example is the administration of lipophilic inhibitors of protein tyrosine kinases, enzymes that propagate the cellular signals via TNF-α receptors.[441] In experimental animals, one of these agents was found to enhance survival, even when the agent was administered 2 hours after systemic injection with endotoxin, whereas other strategies only showed benefit if used prior to, or simultaneous with, endotoxin administration.[441] The role of TNF-α and IL-1 in the inflammatory response in bacterial meningitis has prompted investigations aimed at better understanding and modifying this response, which appears to be responsible for some of the important sequelae of this disease.[447]

Clinical Conditions Associated with Deficient Host Responses to Infection

IMMATURE HOST RESPONSES OF THE NEWBORN INFANT

A mild febrile respiratory illness in a 10-month-old infant might prompt little more than gentle reassurance over the telephone from the child's pediatrician. However, if the patient is an infant in the first few weeks of life, the physician's response is likely to include an evaluation for systemic bacterial infection and administration of parenteral antibiotics in the hospital until a serious infection can be ruled out.[257] Similarly, the appearance of a few cutaneous perioral vesicles characteristic of herpes simplex virus in an older infant usually evokes little concern and no specific treatment. In contrast, the same condition in the first 3 weeks of life is likely to lead to a prolonged hospitalization for antiviral therapy because of the risk of developing serious central nervous system or disseminated infection.[457] It is well recognized that newborn infants are much more susceptible to serious disease from many types of organisms than are older children and adults. This predisposition to infection is even more profound in infants born prematurely.[100, 285] The basis for this special vulnerability of the neonate is complex and encompasses all arms of the immune system. It is of such importance that the clinical approach to infections in infants during the first month of life usually is far more aggressive than that in older children.

Cell-Mediated Immunity

Antigen presentation per se, via the mechanisms discussed earlier, appears to be relatively intact in the newborn infant. Expression of class I and class II MHC molecules has been documented in a broad range of fetal tissues by 12 weeks' gestation,[230, 337] and levels of expression are sufficient to mediate normal MHC class II–restricted antigen presentation by neonatal monocytes to maternal or paternal CD4+ T cells, as well as to induce vigorous rejection of allogeneic fetal tissue by CD8+ cytotoxic T cells.[217, 229]

By about 20 weeks' gestation, the fetal repertoire of diversity of TCRs has developed fully.[440] At the time of birth, although most basic functions of cell-mediated immunity are present, there is a high proportion of immature T cells in the peripheral circulation, which can be identified by their co-expression of CD4 and CD8.[285] This phenotype typifies type II thymocytes, which usually are not found in the periphery in older persons.

Neonatal T cells appear to be relatively deficient in most of their major functions, including CD8+ T-cell–mediated cytotoxicity, delayed hypersensitivity, and T-cell help for B-cell differentiation.[285] Diminished cytokine production by neonatal T cells likely accounts for much of this deficiency.[285] In turn, the relatively naive status of most neonatal T cells may account for reduced cytokine production because memory T cells are much more efficient in all of these functions.[285]

B Cells and Antibody

B Cells

Pre-B cells are found in the fetal liver and omentum by 8 weeks' and in the fetal bone marrow by 13 weeks' gestation.[191, 285, 405] Pre-B cells with surface IgM have been detected as early as 10 weeks' gestation. After 30 weeks' gestation and delivery, pre-B cells are seen only in the bone marrow. Mature B cells are present in the circulation by the eleventh week and have reached adult levels in the bone marrow, blood, and spleen by the twenty-second week of gestation.[136, 191, 405]

Fetal B cells express only IgM, whereas most adult B cells express both IgM and IgD. Neonatal B cells may express three immunoglobulin isotypes (e.g., different combinations of IgG, IgA, IgM, and IgD) on their surfaces.[191, 210] Data from experiments in mice suggest that exposing B cells with surface IgM, but not IgD, to antigens leads to anergy, or B-cell inactivation. It has been speculated that the absence of surface IgD on fetal B cells contributes to the induction of tolerance to self and, possibly, maternal antigens in utero. In addition, the fetus has a higher proportion of the functionally immature CD5+, or B1, cells than adults. These cells produce autoantibodies and, thus, may play a role in the development of tolerance to self antigens, maternal antigens, or both.[47]

Although germinal centers are not present in lymphoid tissue at birth, they begin to develop in the first few months of life concomitant with the infant's exposure to antigens.[426] Despite conflicting in vitro data, neonatal T-cell help for B cells probably is comparable with that of adult T cells, as is reflected by the excellent T-dependent antibody response of the newborn to immunization with protein antigens such as tetanus toxoid.[216] However, neonatal T-cell help is associated with secretion of IgM alone, not other isotypes, possibly because neonatal T cells have diminished production of cytokines critical for promoting isotype switching. Indeed, addition of cytokines such as IL-2, IL-4, and IL-6 helps overcome neonatal B-cell dysfunction in vitro.[285]

In contrast with adult B cells, neonatal B cells cannot respond to polysaccharides without T-cell help.[302] It is of

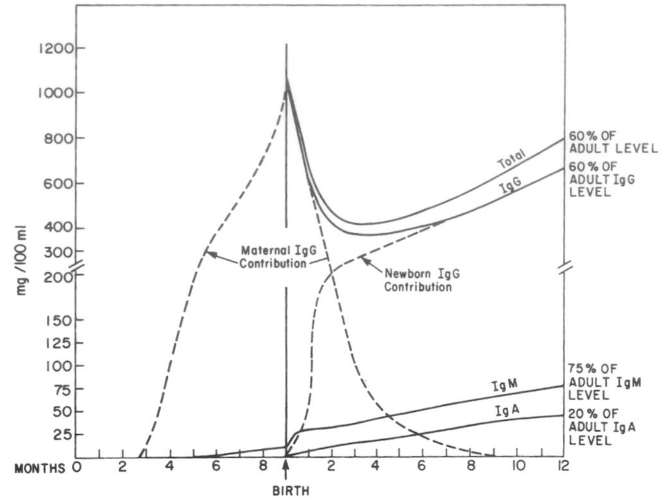

FIGURE 2–9. *Immunoglobulin (IgG, IgM, and IgA) levels in the fetus and infant in the first year of life. The IgG of the fetus and newborn infant solely is of maternal origin. The maternal IgG disappears by 9 months of age, by which time endogenous synthesis of IgG by the infant is well established. The IgM and IgA of the neonate are synthesized entirely endogenously, for maternal IgM and IgA do not cross the placenta. (After Braun, J., and Stiehm, E. R.: The B-lymphocyte system. In Stiehm, E. R. [ed.]: Immunologic Disorders in Infants and Children. 4th ed. Philadelphia, W. B. Saunders, 1996, p. 67.)*

interest, however, that neonatal T cells can produce soluble factors that help adult, but not neonatal, B cells respond to pneumococcal polysaccharide.[358]

Antibody

Maternal IgG accounts for the vast majority of the newborn's immunoglobulin because almost none is made by the healthy fetus, and IgG is the only isotype of maternal immunoglobulin that crosses the placenta.[260, 296] Maternal transport of IgG can be detected as early as 8 weeks' gestation, and the newborn's IgG level is directly proportional to gestational age, reaching 100 mg/dL by 17 to 20 weeks' gestation and 50 per cent of the maternal level by 30 weeks' gestation (Fig. 2–9).[44, 100, 285] By term, the infant has 5 to 10 per cent more IgG than the mother because maternal antibody is transported not only passively but also actively via trophoblast Fc receptors.[436] Trophoblast Fc receptors have higher affinity for IgG1 and IgG3 than for IgG2 and IgG4, and so more of those subclasses are transported from the mother.[161, 279] Thus, newborns may have relatively higher levels of IgG1 and IgG3 than IgG2 and IgG4 compared with adults, and term newborns' IgG1 levels may be higher than their mothers'.

By approximately 2 months of chronologic age, approximately half of the term infant's quantitative IgG is of maternal and half is of infant origin. The physiologic nadir of IgG in all infants is about 3 to 4 months of age and ranges from less than 100 mg/dL in very low-birth-weight preterm infants to about 400 mg/dL in term infants (see Fig. 2–9, Table 2–3).[44, 100] Maternal IgG essentially is gone by about 12 months of age, at which time infant levels are approximately 60 per cent of adult levels. Production of IgG1 and IgG3 matures more rapidly than that of IgG2 and IgG4, reaching adult levels by approximately 8 years of age, versus 10 and 12 years of age, respectively.[333]

Little IgM, IgA, IgE, or IgD is produced by the fetus, and none is transported from the mother.[285] The presence of IgM levels greater than 20 mg/dL at birth suggests an intrauterine infection. Serum IgA levels at birth in both preterm and term infants usually are less than 5 mg/dL and consist of both IgA1 and IgA2. Secretory IgA is not detectable until after birth but usually is present within the first few weeks of life. IgM and IgA reach approximately 60 and 20 per cent of adult levels by 1 year of age, respectively (see Fig. 2–9). Secretory IgA reaches adult levels by 6 to 8 years of age.[213, 285]

The IgG transferred from the mother to the fetus has been demonstrated to protect the newborn from many infectious agents, including viruses such as varicella, polio, measles, mumps, and rubella and bacteria such as tetanus, diphtheria, *H. influenzae* type b, and group B *Streptococcus.*[115] However, the infant is not protected by the mother if she does not have specific IgG antibody, even if she is immune to a given organism. For example, the mother may have low or absent levels of circulating IgG antibody but good memory B cells capable of mounting a booster response. In this case, the mother is protected, but she cannot transfer protection to her infant. Similarly, because no IgM is transferred to the fetus, the mother cannot defend her newborn effectively against many gram-negative enteric organisms, even if she is immune.[117, 402]

The concept of passive transfer of protective IgG is being used to develop vaccines for maternal immunization before or during pregnancy so that passive transfer of vaccine-induced antibody will result in protection during the neonatal period. Examples of organisms for which such strategies

TABLE 2–3. Levels of Immunoglobulins in Sera of Normal Subjects, by Age

Age (Months)	IgG (mg/dL)	IgM (mg/dL)	IgA (mg/dL)	Total Immunoglobulin (mg/dL)
Newborn	1031 ± 200*	11 ± 5	2 ± 3	1044 ± 201
1–3	430 ± 119	30 ± 11	21 ± 13	481 ± 127
4–6	427 ± 186	43 ± 17	28 ± 18	498 ± 204
7–12	661 ± 219	54 ± 23	37 ± 18	752 ± 242
13–14	762 ± 209	58 ± 23	50 ± 24	870 ± 258
25–36	892 ± 183	61 ± 19	71 ± 37	1024 ± 205

*Values were derived from measurements made in 296 children and 30 adults. Levels were determined by the radial diffusion plate method using specific rabbit antisera to human immunoglobulins.

Values are ± 1 SD.

Modified from Stiehm, E. R., and Fudenberg, H. H.: Serum levels of immune globulins in health and disease: A survey. Pediatrics *37*:715–727, 1966. Reproduced with permission of Pediatrics.

are being investigated include group B *Streptococcus, H. influenzae* type b, meningococcus, pneumococcus, rotavirus, and respiratory syncytial virus.[43, 164, 241]

It has been documented that the fetus can respond to antigenic stimulation in the form of maternal immunization with tetanus toxoid vaccine and be primed for a secondary antibody response to repeat immunization after birth.[196, 197] Some, but not all, fetuses near term also can make IgM and IgA antibody to organisms such as the TORCH (toxoplasmosis, rubella, cytomegalovirus, herpes) agents.[162, 208, 321] The amount of fetal antibody produced in response to intrauterine antigenic stimulation is proportional to gestational age.[137, 414]

The most hypervariable region of the immunoglobulin molecule, CDR3 ($>10^{14}$ peptides in adults), is shorter in the fetus than in the adult. The result is that the diversity of the repertoire of fetal B-cell clones with different antigenic specificity is decreased markedly.[285] In the neonatal period, the repertoire for IgM and IgA, but not IgG, is more diverse because of more V, D, and J genes and longer CDR3 regions.[315]

Maternal antibody inhibits the infants' ability to respond to vaccines against certain organisms such as measles, but it does not prevent them from mounting protective immune responses to most normal childhood vaccine antigens, such as tetanus, diphtheria, polio, hepatitis B, and *H. influenzae* type b.[115] In general, neonates have protective responses to T-dependent antigens, even though they may produce less antibody to some antigens than do older infants and adults.[13, 132, 139, 177, 402, 403]

The newborn infant's response to TI-1 antigens is slightly decreased and to TI-2 antigens is poor.[199] The antibody response to most TI-2 antigens, including the polysaccharide capsules of group B streptococci, pneumococci, and *H. influenzae* type b, is not mature until 18 to 24 months of age, although infants as young as 3 months of age can respond to group A meningococcal polysaccharide.[400] In contrast, in the first few weeks of life, infants mount excellent antibody responses to T-independent polysaccharide antigens that have been rendered T-dependent by covalent conjugation of the polysaccharide to a protein carrier (e.g., *H. influenzae* type b).[7]

It has been proposed that immunologic tolerance may be induced in infants by early exposure to some antigens. The subject remains controversial, but some data suggest that immunization to pertussis in the newborn period results in lower levels of antibody to subsequent doses of vaccine than does initially immunizing at 1 month of age.[46, 346, 352] There is no evidence, however, that tolerance is induced by administration of tetanus, diphtheria, or oral polio vaccines in the newborn period.[139, 385]

The response of premature infants to most routine childhood vaccines, including diphtheria, tetanus, pertussis, and oral and inactivated polio, is comparable with that of 2-month-old term infants.[8, 60, 98, 285, 403] It has been well documented, however, that premature infants do not respond well to hepatitis B vaccine for reasons that are unclear.[116, 273]

The data are conflicting, but small-for-gestational-age infants may have somewhat lower total levels of IgG at birth than do normally grown newborns,[161, 393, 464] possibly because of placental insufficiency. Their response to most routine vaccines is good, but it may be slightly decreased to inactivated polio vaccine.[101]

Complement

Complement proteins do not cross the placenta, but studies of mothers with congenital complement component deficiencies and mother-infant pairs discordant for variants of individual components, as well as studies of fetal tissues, have provided evidence for fetal synthesis of complement beginning as early as 5½ weeks' gestation. Most complement proteins are present by 10 weeks' gestation.[9, 114, 261] Levels of complement activity and of individual complement components vary significantly among infants, but, in general, classic pathway hemolytic activity of term neonates ranges from 50 to 80 per cent of maternal values (Table 2–4). Because serum complement levels are elevated during pregnancy, term neonates' levels are about 60 to 90 per cent of normal adult values.[158, 175, 178, 244, 465] Alternative pathway hemolytic activity is decreased more consistently than is classic pathway activity and ranges from about 50 to 70 per cent of normal adult values at term (see Table 2–4).[6, 157, 329, 393, 420] Complement activity usually is lower in premature than in term infants, with hemolytic activity of both pathways, as well as serum levels of most complement proteins, usually corresponding directly with gestational age.[157] However, complement levels are not proportional to weight in term infants. Small-for-gestational-age infants have complement levels comparable with those of babies of the same gestational age who appropriately have grown.[329, 393]

Some studies have found a correlation between infection and complement levels in the newborn period. One study from Japan demonstrated higher CH_{50} and Clq (C4 and C3 levels) in infants of less than 34 weeks' gestation with amnionitis than in those without.[95] Other studies have revealed lower complement levels in infected newborns due to increased complement activation.[157, 158, 420]

Hemolytic activity of both the classic and the alternative pathway rises rapidly and reaches adult levels by 3 to 6 months of age and by approximately 6 to 18 months of age, respectively.[175, 178]

In addition to hemolytic activity, complement-mediated opsonic and bactericidal activity is decreased in newborn sera and generally correlates with C3 and factor B levels.[158] Studies of opsonic and bactericidal activity of newborn sera

TABLE 2–4. Summary of Published Complement Levels in Neonates

Complement Component	Mean Percentage of Adult Levels	
	Term Neonate	*Preterm Neonate*
CH_{50}	56–90 (4)*	45–71 (3)
AP_{50}	49–65 (3)	40–51 (2)
C1q	65–90 (3)	27–58 (2)
C4	60–100 (4)	42–91 (3)
C2	76–100 (2)	96 (1)
C3	60–100 (5)	39–78 (4)
C5	75 (1)	—
C6	47 (1)	—
C7	67 (1)	—
C8	20 (1)	—
C9	<20 (2)	—
B	35–59 (8)	36–50 (3)
P	33–71 (5)	13–65 (2)
H	61 (1)	—
C3bi	55 (1)	—

*Number of studies.

Data reproduced from Lewis, D. B., and Wilson, C. B.: Developmental immunology and role of host defenses in neonatal susceptibility to infection. *In* Remington, J. S., and Klein, J. O. (eds.): Infectious Diseases of the Fetus and Newborn Infant. 4th ed. Philadelphia, W. B. Saunders, 1995, p. 65.

have been reviewed in detail elsewhere.[158, 244, 247, 285] Levels of individual complement proteins do not correlate always with their functional activity.[192, 235, 461] Zach and Hostetter[465] reported not only that total C3 levels were decreased as measured by enzyme-linked immunosorbent assay but also that C3 thioester reactivity was decreased and that it correlated with gestational age. Because the opsonic function of C3 is mediated by its thioester, such a defect may contribute to the newborn's deficiency in functional complement activity.

Although complement levels and activity are decreased substantially in most newborn infants, these abnormalities are relatively mild compared with those seen in hereditary complement deficiencies, and they do not predispose to infection necessarily. For example, several studies have demonstrated that maternally derived type-specific antibodies are sufficient to overcome relative deficiencies in complement and other host defenses in the newborn. This phenomenon underscores the need to verify the information derived from in vitro studies with clinical observations before drawing firm conclusions about the importance of individual host defense mechanisms in protection against specific pathogens.

Phagocytes

The newborn infant exhibits both quantitative and qualitative deficits in phagocytic defenses. Although the number of circulating PMNs usually does not differ greatly from that in older children and adults, under conditions of stress, including systemic infection, the release of marrow reserves of PMNs is impaired markedly.[104] In fact, whereas the ratio of marrow neutrophil reserves to circulating cells in older persons is nearly 15:1, in the newborn infant this ratio is between 2:1 and 3:1.[104, 294] Thus, neutropenia is more likely during severe systemic infections in the newborn than in older children and adults.[103] The resulting deficiency in PMNs available for delivery to infected sites under conditions of stress is a stark disadvantage for the neonate in containing bacterial and fungal infections. Distinct from this quantitative deficiency in marrow reserves of PMNs, there are important functional impairments that also are important in understanding neonatal phagocytic defenses.

The most important and best-documented functional impairments of neonatal PMNs are related to defective adherence and chemotaxis.[24, 26, 27, 265, 309] A number of specific structural, functional, and biochemical abnormalities have been documented, any or all of which may contribute to the overall impairment in adhesion and migration of these cells.[227] Impaired adhesion of neonatal PMNs to endothelial cells and other biologic substrates has been linked with deficiencies in the expression or function of the β_2 integrins Mac-1 (CD11b/CD18) and LFA-1 (CD11a/CD18).[4, 27, 30, 84, 250, 300] The most evident deficiency in this regard is the diminished level of surface expression of Mac-1 on stimulated neonatal PMNs, although expression on resting PMNs is similar to that of adults.[84, 250] The deficiency in stimulated Mac-1 surface expression can be explained principally by the observation that the total cell content of Mac-1 in PMNs from term neonates is only about 60 per cent of that in adult PMNs.[4] The total PMN content of Mac-1 at the time of birth is related directly to gestational age, and PMNs from very early premature infants (less than 30 weeks' gestation) may contain less than 20 per cent of the Mac-1 content of adult PMNs.[300] The PMN content of LFA-1, which is normal at term, appears to be reduced in infants born prior to 35 weeks' gestation.[300] Thus, the neonatal defect in PMN adherence and migration appears to be even more profound in very premature neonates. Several other defects of neonatal PMNs that are likely to influence chemotaxis have been documented. These include defective redistribution of surface adhesion sites,[24] impaired uropod formation during stimulated shape change,[26] reduced cell deformability,[310] impaired microtubule assembly,[26] deficient F-actin polymerization,[212, 228, 377] reduced lactoferrin content and release,[26] reduced ability to effect membrane depolarization and intracellular calcium ion transients,[376] and impaired uptake of glucose during stimulation by chemoattractants.[5] The relative importance of each of these individual impairments to the overall deficiency in chemotaxis by neonatal PMNs remains to be determined.

Evidence suggests that the number and binding efficiencies of receptors for chemoattractants, including C5a and synthetic bacterial peptides such as the formyl peptide N-f-met-leu-phe, are normal.[24, 376, 419] Phagocytosis and microbicidal activity of neonatal PMNs has been found in several studies to be similar to that of adult PMNs.[305, 306] However, in some studies in which the assay conditions are designed to expose a potential defect in these functions (e.g., limiting concentrations of opsonins and high bacterial inocula), defects in phagocytosis and killing have been documented.[305, 306] It is not clear whether these potential deficiencies play a role in impaired neonatal phagocyte defenses in vivo.

PRIMARY/HERITABLE IMMUNOLOGIC DEFICIENCIES

Physicians who care for children often are faced with the problem of a child who has a predilection for recurrent infections. Most of these children are normal infants or toddlers who have been exposed to a succession of common respiratory infections when they entered day care or a similar setting for the first time.[117] Fortunately for most of these children, repeated exposure elicits relative immunity to many or most of the infectious agents. It is an important challenge for the physician to identify those infants and children who do not fit into the normal pattern but who are unusually susceptible to infection with respect to frequency, severity, type of causative agent, and response to appropriate treatment. This challenge usually falls to the pediatrician or family physician because, with few exceptions, the primary immune deficiencies present during infancy and early childhood.[117]

As suggested earlier, the infant or toddler who experiences even six to eight presumed viral upper respiratory infections during the course of a winter season, without other complications, ordinarily would not be considered at high risk for an immunodeficiency. In contrast, a child who had experienced five episodes of acute otitis media in the last 4 months, several episodes accompanied by sinusitis or pneumonia, has displayed reasonable cause for suspicion of a humoral immunodeficiency.[117] For certain organisms, infection in the healthy host is so decidedly uncommon that even a single episode should prompt a high suspicion of impaired host defenses. *Pneumocystis carinii* pneumonia strongly suggests a severe defect of T-cell number or function.[117] Similarly, lymphadenitis or osteomyelitis caused by gram-negative enteric bacilli points to a defect of phagocytic killing, such as CGD.[245] The discussion of specific immunologic defects and their infectious consequences will focus on well-characterized prototypic disorders within each class of primary defects but includes comments on other related disorders.

Antibody Deficiencies

Humoral immunity is provided by antibody and plays an important role in host defense against most pathogens, as is illustrated by the finding that patients with significant antibody deficiencies develop recurrent and sometimes life-threatening infections.[117, 125, 334] They particularly are prone to otitis media, sinusitis, bronchitis, pneumonia, sepsis, and meningitis. Antibodies participate in complement-dependent and complement-independent opsonization, bactericidal activity, virus and toxin neutralization, and the formation of immune complexes that can be cleared by the reticuloendothelial system.[218, 285] The role of different immunoglobulin isotypes and subclasses has been elucidated by the nature of infections found in patients with selective deficiencies and is outlined later.

X-Linked Agammaglobulinemia

X-linked agammaglobulinemia (XLA), first described by Bruton, is a primary immunodeficiency disorder of the B-cell lineage and is the most serious disorder of humoral immunity.[85, 278, 334, 367] It is characterized by absent or severely decreased numbers of circulating B lymphocytes and absent or extremely low levels of all classes of circulating immunoglobulins. It is caused by several different mutations in the gene encoding for a B-cell specific tyrosine kinase, *Btk*, which maps to the long arm of the X chromosome at Xq22.[433, 443] This abnormality in kinase activity results in an arrest in the development of B cells, usually at the pre-B stage, and, thus, there are few B cells or their progeny (e.g., plasma cells) in the circulation or lymphoid tissues.[201]

Most persons with XLA develop chronic or recurrent pyogenic bacterial sinopulmonary or gastrointestinal infections, and they may have recurrent skin infections.[85, 278, 334, 367] Systemic disease, such as sepsis, and serious focal infections resulting from bacteremia, such as meningitis, osteomyelitis, and septic arthritis, do not occur as frequently as respiratory and gastrointestinal infections but are more common and more severe than in normal hosts. The causative agents of most of these infections are *S. pneumoniae* and both type b and nontypable *H. influenzae*, but *Staphylococcus aureus* and *Pseudomonas aeruginosa*, as well as other gram-negative organisms, may be implicated. The most troublesome gastrointestinal infections in XLA are caused by *Salmonella, Campylobacter,* and chronic infestation with *Giardia lamblia.* Although there is no increased susceptibility to most viruses, these patients have been found to have unusually severe or chronic enterovirus infections that can be manifested by chronic meningoencephalitis, dermatomyositis, hepatitis, or a combination thereof, and several patients with XLA have developed vaccine-related paralytic poliomyelitis after receiving the live oral polio vaccine.[278]

The only abnormality on physical examination that is not related directly to infections is a paucity of normal B-cell–containing lymphoid tissues, such as tonsils, adenoids, and peripheral lymph nodes.[334] Patients who are diagnosed and treated early in life have normal physical examination, growth, and development.

Infants with XLA have normal levels of serum IgG at birth, and they are protected from infections during the first few weeks of life by passively transferred maternal antibodies. Most patients present at about 4 to 12 months of age when maternal antibody levels have declined, but, occasionally, the diagnosis is not established until 5 years of age.

Older persons with XLA have low serum levels of IgG, IgM, IgA, and IgE. The diagnosis can be confirmed by studying lymphocyte markers.[334] There is a lack of circulating cells that stain for surface immunoglobulin or with B-cell specific monoclonal antibodies against CD19, CD20, or both. The number and function of T lymphocytes are normal in XLA. It may be difficult to establish the diagnosis in the newborn period because maternally derived immunoglobulin bestows normal IgG levels. However, if there are other reasons to suspect this diagnosis, such as a newborn male with a documented family history, the diagnosis can be made by the striking decrease in circulating B cells.

Advances in genetic techniques have enabled maternal carrier detection.[118] In contrast with carriers of some other X-linked genetic diseases, X chromosome inactivation is not random in carriers of this disorder. Instead of the two populations of B cells in normal persons, B lymphocytes of XLA carriers express only one population of B cells, those with the normal allele on the X chromosome, suggesting that B cells with the mutant allele are at a selective disadvantage and do not develop. Prenatal diagnosis is made by linkage analysis of amniotic fluid cells or quantitation of fetal circulating B cells.

The prognosis for patients with XLA has improved markedly with earlier diagnosis, high-dose intravenous immunoglobulin (IVIG) therapy, and aggressive use of antibiotics.[334] Before the availability of IVIG, most patients who survived to the third decade of life had chronic lung disease from pulmonary infections and hearing loss from recurrent otitis media.[278]

IgG Subclass Deficiency

Persons with IgG subclass deficiencies have levels of one or more IgG subclass that are more than two standard deviations below normal for age, normal to slightly decreased total IgG, normal levels of other immunoglobulin isotypes, and, often, a poor antibody response to certain antigens.[58, 218, 220–222, 314, 334, 339, 340, 386–392] Patients with IgG subclass deficiency who also have IgM and IgA deficiency may have another immunodeficiency disorder such as common variable immunodeficiency (CVI).

Patients with individual or combined deficiencies of IgG1, IgG2, and IgG3 may be at increased risk for infection, particularly if the deficiency is associated with an abnormal antibody response to antigenic stimulation.[58, 218, 220–222, 314, 334, 339, 340, 386–392] The most common kinds of infections in patients with IgG subclass deficiency are upper respiratory. Ordinarily, these patients do not have life-threatening systemic infections.

Deficiency of IgG1, because it accounts for about 60 per cent of total IgG, is most likely to be associated with hypogammaglobulinemia G, and it usually is associated with other subclass deficiencies.[17, 339, 389–391] IgG1-deficient persons may have recurrent pulmonary infections that can lead to chronic lung disease.

IgG2 deficiency is associated with normal total serum IgG levels and is more likely to be symptomatic if it is accompanied by IgG4 or IgA deficiency. As would be expected, patients with IgG2 deficiency have poor antibody responses to polysaccharide, but not protein, antigens. Their infections primarily are localized to the respiratory tract, but some patients have been reported to have recurrent meningococcal meningitis or disseminated pneumococcal disease.

IgG3 deficiency has been associated with low total levels of serum IgG and recurrent respiratory infections, which also may lead to chronic pulmonary disease.[334]

IgG4 deficiency is difficult to diagnose because many normal persons have low serum levels of IgG4 and most normal infants have no detectable IgG4.[334] IgG4 deficiency appears to be of clinical significance, however, if it is associated with IgG2 and IgA deficiency.

The treatment for children with IgG subclass deficiency usually is individualized according to the frequency and severity of symptoms. Noninvasive infections usually can be treated successfully with appropriate antibiotics. Patients with more severe presentations may benefit from IVIG therapy, but those who also are IgA-deficient should be followed closely for the formation of anti-IgA antibodies and treated only with IgA-depleted IVIG preparations. Individuals with IgG2 deficiency should be immunized with vaccines consisting of polysaccharides conjugated to protein carriers, such as *H. influenzae* type b conjugates, and, when they become available, pneumococcal and meningococcal conjugates.

Hyper-IgM Syndrome

Immunoglobulin deficiency with increased IgM is characterized by low levels of IgG, IgA, and IgE but normal to increased levels of IgM in the circulation and normal numbers of circulating B cells.[330, 334] Their IgM is polyclonal and consists of both kappa and lambda light chains. The disorder is caused by an intrinsic T-cell abnormality that alters switching from IgM to other isotypes. The defect has been localized to the X chromosome on the gene encoding the CD40 ligand CD40L (gp39), a protein expressed transiently on activated T cells.[14, 35] In normal persons, CD40 on the surface of B cells interacts with CD40 ligand on activated T cells to cause B-cell differentiation into memory B cells and switching from IgM to other isotypes. B cells from patients with the hyper-IgM syndrome only make IgM antibody, and their B cells only express surface IgM and IgD. Other cells have surface CD40, and, therefore, immunologic abnormalities such as the neutropenia and the increased incidence of infections caused by *P. carinii* and of malignancies in patients with the hyper-IgM syndrome may be the result of impaired cell interactions via CD40.

Clinically, the hyper-IgM syndrome is manifested by recurrent bacterial infections, particularly respiratory, beginning after maternal immunoglobulin levels fall off over the first few months of life.[329, 334] Such persons are susceptible to the same kinds of recurrent pyogenic infections that are associated with other immunoglobulin deficiencies, as well as to infections with organisms more commonly encountered in patients with T-cell defects (e.g., *P. carinii*).[45] Some patients with this syndrome have recurrent diarrhea due to *G. lamblia* and *Cryptosporidium* that is severe enough to require parenteral nutrition. Life-threatening peritonsillar and peritracheal soft tissue infections also have been observed.

Physical examination is normal except for the sequelae of infections and lymphoid hyperplasia, which probably is caused by constant antigenic stimulation. Arthritis and arthralgia may be the result of chronic infection or the production of autoantibodies. Some patients have large verruca vulgaris lesions.

The diagnosis of X-linked hyper-IgM syndrome is established by demonstrating the inability of activated CD4+ T cells to express CD40 ligand (gp39), using either a soluble form of the physiologic receptor for the CD40 ligand (a recombinant of CD40, CD40-Ig) or a monoclonal antibody that recognizes the extracellular domain of CD40 ligand and flow cytometry. The diagnosis is confirmed by demonstration of a mutation within the CD40 ligand gene. About half of patients also have persistent or cyclic neutropenia. Those with autoantibodies may have thrombocytopenia, hemolytic anemia, nephritis, hypothyroidism, or arthritis, as noted earlier.

Inheritance of the hyper-IgM syndrome usually is X-linked, although its occurrence in females suggests the possibility of autosomal recessive or autosomal dominant inheritance.

Treatment of patients with the hyper-IgM syndrome with IVIG usually results in marked clinical improvement.[45] It also may be necessary to treat those who have neutropenia with granulocyte colony-stimulating factor and those with arthritis or other autoimmune symptoms with steroids. Hyper-IgM patients usually do not do as well as those with XLA because, in addition to their immunoglobulin deficiency, they have an increased incidence of neutropenia, autoimmune disease, and malignancy. Gene therapy may prove to be useful in the future.

IgA Deficiency

IgA deficiency is the most common immunodeficiency, occurring in about 1 in 400 to 1 in 800 people. All of the functions of serum IgA can be performed by IgG and IgM.[125, 334] Thus, although deficiencies of secretory IgA may lead to recurrent respiratory or gastrointestinal tract infections, deficiency of serum IgA usually is not associated with increased susceptibility to systemic infections.[22] IgA deficiency has been associated with many other conditions, including recurrent infections, IgG2 deficiency, a family history of immunodeficiency (e.g., relatives with CVI), autoimmune disorders, and malignancy.[21] Recurrent infections are most likely to occur in the subset of IgA-deficient patients who also have IgG2 deficiency.[125, 339] The infections usually are relatively mild and involve the upper respiratory and gastrointestinal tracts. Chronic gastrointestinal disease can be caused by *G. lamblia* infections, nodular lymphoid hyperplasia, lactose intolerance, malabsorption, ulcerative colitis, regional enteritis, or autoimmune disorders (e.g., chronic hepatitis, cirrhosis, pernicious anemia). About 20 per cent of IgA-deficient patients have allergy, and many have elevated levels of IgE.[125] Food allergy is common and may be the result of abnormal processing of antigen at the mucosal surface. Other autoimmune diseases that are associated with IgA deficiency include rheumatoid arthritis, systemic lupus erythematosus, thyroiditis, Still disease transfusion reactions, pulmonary hemosiderosis, myasthenia gravis, and vitiligo.[125]

IgA deficiency appears to be inherited sporadically, but familial cases have been described.[22, 125]

Serum IgA levels less than 5 mg/dL can be clinically significant because patients with levels this low who receive transfusions may make antibody against donor IgA and have severe reactions when transfused again.[384] IVIG reactions also may occur because IVIG preparations contain varying amounts of IgA. IgA-depleted preparations are available and usually are well tolerated, even in patients with high titers of anti-IgA antibodies.[126]

IgE Deficiency

The clinical significance of selective IgE deficiency is unclear because it has been described in healthy persons. Some patients with profound antibody and cellular immunodeficiencies lack serum IgE, but several partial cellular immunodeficiency syndromes are characterized by elevated levels of IgE (e.g., DiGeorge anomaly, Wiskott-Aldrich syndrome, Hodgkin disease).[218, 334] The absence of IgE does not correlate with an enhanced susceptibility to infection in developed countries but has not been investigated in the developing world.

Transient Hypogammaglobulinemia of Infancy

Hypogammaglobulinemia is a normal physiologic phenomenon occurring in all infants beginning about 3 to 4 months of age when maternal antibody wanes and infant synthesis of immunoglobulin has not compensated yet.[218, 285, 334] The syndrome of transient hypogammaglobulinemia of infancy can be differentiated from physiologic hypogammaglobulinemia by the fact that immunoglobulin levels of normal infants begin to rise by about 6 months of age, whereas those of infants with transient hypogammaglobulinemia of infancy do not begin to increase until between 18 and 36 months of age.[218, 285, 334] Infants suspected of having this syndrome should be evaluated for XLA and CVI (see later) and followed closely until their immunoglobulin levels rise to the normal range.

Antibody Deficiency with Normal or Elevated Levels of Immunoglobulins

Some persons with normal levels of all circulating immunoglobulin isotypes are at increased risk of infection.[16, 18, 334] The cause of this disorder remains poorly defined but may be related to an inability to respond to specific antigens or the induction of tolerance by exposure to certain antigens too early in development, or it merely may reflect a delay in the development of the immune system in some persons. The most common infections in these patients are recurrent sinopulmonary infections and, occasionally, recurrent pneumococcal sepsis.[18] Such persons can be identified by their inability to make antibody in response to stimulation with specific antigens. They do not have abnormal total serum immunoglobulin classes or subclasses or B- or T-cell quantity or function. They can respond to some, but not all, antigenic stimulation. Therefore, it is important to test them with a variety of stimuli. A good way to test for this syndrome is to immunize with protein antigens, such as tetanus and diphtheria toxoids, and with polysaccharide antigens, such as pneumococcal and *H. influenzae* type b capsular polysaccharide vaccines. Patients who can respond to protein, but not polysaccharide, antigens also respond to polysaccharide antigens that have been conjugated, or covalently coupled, to proteins.

Treatment with IVIG may help prevent recurrent infections in these patients, although the dose of IVIG is unclear because they have normal levels of immunoglobulin.

Defects of Cell-Mediated Immunity: DiGeorge Anomaly

The prototype of a pure T-cell defect, DiGeorge anomaly, is characterized clinically by congenital heart disease (usually involving the aortic arch), hypocalcemic tetany, unusual facial features, and recurrent infections.[147] In the classic or complete form of this disorder, there is absence or hypoplasia of the thymus and parathyroid glands, cardiac or aortic arch deformities, and a stereotypical constellation of abnormal facial features.[147, 266, 423] Although the condition usually is considered to be associated with immune deficiency because of the thymic hypoplasia, only about 25 per cent of patients actually exhibit an immunologic defect.[51] The term partial DiGeorge syndrome sometimes has been used to describe patients with the typical constellation of anatomic findings but without immune deficiency or similar patients with mild immunologic impairment.[232] The current designation of this disorder as an anomaly rather than a syndrome stems from the observation that although the characteristic features of this disorder stem from abnormal development of the same embryonic tissue (the branchial arches with contributions from cephalic neural crest tissue), the causes of this abnormal development are diverse, including disorders exhibiting classic Mendelian inheritance patterns, teratogenic influences, and chromosomal abnormalities, especially specific deletions of chromosome 22.[205, 206, 232, 270]

DiGeorge anomaly usually first is recognized by the presence of unusual but characteristic facial features, hypocalcemic tetany in the first 2 days of life, or the presence of serious cardiovascular manifestations, most commonly associated with an interrupted aortic arch or truncus arteriosus.[232, 289] Because of the serious nature of the cardiovascular defect, many patients with DiGeorge anomaly do not survive long enough for the immune defect to become a clinical problem.[232] However, with improvements in aggressive surgical approaches to the heart defects, more of these infants are surviving long enough to display manifestations of the immune deficiency that results in an increased frequency and severity of viral and fungal infections, as well as *P. carinii* pneumonia. In such patients, management often includes prophylaxis against the pneumonia, periodic immunoglobulin infusions, and avoidance of live virus vaccines.[232] Transplantation of fetal or postnatal thymic tissue has corrected the immunologic problem for the long term in about one-third of such attempts.[200, 232] More recently, HLA-matched bone marrow transplantation has been successful in a few cases.[71, 200, 232]

Combined Defects of Cellular and Humoral Immunity

Severe Combined Immunodeficiency Disease

Severe combined immunodeficiency (SCID) describes a heterogeneous group of heritable immune deficiencies that involve serious impairments of both cellular and humoral immunity. SCID has a number of different forms, which have been reviewed in detail elsewhere.[232] Although the mode of inheritance has been determined in several of these, the specific nature of the defect has been defined in only a few. All forms of SCID are characterized by severe deficiencies in both humoral and cell mediated immunity, with recurrent severe infections by a wide range of viral, bacterial, and fungal organisms. Long-term management of patients with SCID involves modalities employed in both T- and B-cell disorders, including prophylaxis against PCP, avoidance of live viral vaccines, and immunoglobulin replacement therapy.[232] Bone marrow transplantation successfully has corrected the defect in a number of cases. Adenosine deaminase deficiency is a form of SCID that is of particular interest in that it is the first heritable disorder for which gene therapy has shown clear promise of correcting the disease.[68]

Common Variable Immunodeficiency

CVI is described as a poorly defined group of combined immunodeficiencies that differ from most other primary immunodeficiencies in that they most often present in the second or third decade of life, although they may present at any age.[124, 219, 368] These patients have normal or only somewhat decreased numbers of circulating B cells; low, but not absent, levels of IgG, IgM, and IgA; poor responsiveness to antigens; and abnormal T-lymphocyte function.[177]

Although both T- and B-cell abnormalities often can be demonstrated, the clinical presentation usually is comparable with that in patients with humoral or B-cell defects (i.e., recurrent bacterial sinopulmonary infections).[124, 219, 368] Occasionally, however, in addition to the organisms causing infections in patients with XLA, these patients also have infections with organisms more common in persons with T-lymphocyte abnormalities, such as *P. carinii, Mycoplasma pneumoniae*, recurrent herpes simplex virus, and herpes zoster virus infections. Chronic gastrointestinal problems may be due to *G. lamblia* or other intestinal pathogens. CVI patients are prone to nodular lymphoid hyperplasia, autoimmune diseases, and malignancies. CVI occasionally has been reported to be familial, and it has been described in families with IgA deficiency.

Patients with CVI usually can benefit from therapy with IVIG. Patients who go untreated often develop chronic lung disease.

Complement Deficiencies

Excellent reviews of complement deficiencies are available elsewhere.[141–143, 158, 244, 247, 371] Approximately 0.03 per cent of the general population have complement deficiencies resulting from acquired or congenital abnormalities of single or multiple complement components or regulatory proteins.

The most common complement deficiencies are acquired and are transient. These include the relative complement deficiencies in infants (see earlier) and that result from complement consumption in various inflammatory states, such as connective tissue disorders and acute or chronic infections.[141–143, 158, 244, 247] Acquired complement deficiencies usually are associated with low levels of more than one complement component.[143] These deficiencies generally are not absolute and are of questionable clinical significance in host defense against infection.

In contrast, congenital or hereditary deficiencies more often are manifested by abnormality of a single complement protein. Deficiencies of individual components may have profound clinical implications, however, because they have been well documented to predispose to life-threatening infections. Most primary complement abnormalities (C1q dysfunction and C1rs, C4, C2, C3, C5, C6, C7, C8, and C9 deficiencies) are inherited as autosomal codominant traits.[143] Most secondary complement deficiencies are caused by complement consumption, decreased synthesis, or increased catabolism.

Activation and binding of C3 is an absolute requirement for complement participation in host defense and immunoregulation by either the classic or the alternative pathway. Therefore, it is not surprising that the most serious complement deficiency state is the total absence of C3.[143] Patients with C3 deficiency have abnormal opsonization (including immune complex processing), inflammatory responses, leukocytosis, phagocyte recruitment to sites of microbial invasion, bactericidal activity, and immune regulation.

Congenital C3 deficiency is rare and results from decreased production of C3.[176, 371] Patients with deficiencies of factors H and I have low, but detectable, levels of C3. Absence of either of these regulatory factors allows continuous activation of the alternative pathway and uncontrolled C3 consumption. Similarly, complement nephritic factors permit continued C3 consumption by stabilizing the C3 convertases.

Patients with C3 deficiency caused by any of these mechanisms have increased susceptibility to infections, particularly those caused by encapsulated bacteria, such as pneumococci, meningococci, and *H. influenzae* type b. The infections usually are localized to the respiratory tract (otitis, sinusitis, bronchitis, and pneumonia), but C3-deficient patients also are predisposed to sepsis and meningitis.[143, 176, 371] The clinical presentation of their infections is similar to that of patients with agammaglobulinemia.[143] In addition, most C3-deficient persons develop collagen vascular disease.[143, 176, 371]

Patients with homozygous or heterozygous deficiency of the early classic pathway proteins, C1, C2, and C4, are more prone to develop collagen vascular disease than infections. However, approximately 20 per cent of patients with homozygous deficiency of early components have problems with recurrent or severe infections that are similar to those seen in C3 deficiency.[143, 176, 371] As could be anticipated, these patients do not have as serious or as frequent problems with infections as do patients with alternative pathway deficiencies because they always can protect themselves via the alternative pathway whether or not they have specific antibody to the infecting organism. Their predilection to collagen vascular disease probably is caused, at least in part, by abnormal solubilization and removal of immune complexes. Although there have been reports that deficiency of one of the isotypes of C4 (C4B) is associated with increased susceptibility to infection caused by encapsulated organisms, subsequent studies have not confirmed this finding.[64, 99, 372]

Patients with C3, C4, C2, or CR3 deficiency have decreased antibody response and incomplete switching from IgM to IgG, whereas patients with deficiency of the terminal components have normal antibody responses.[332, 335]

Deficiencies of alternative pathway proteins predispose to serious, often fatal, infections because of the lack of ability to respond promptly to organisms not previously encountered.[143] Although the classic pathway is intact, patients with alternative pathway deficiencies often succumb before they have the opportunity to make the specific antibody required for its activation.

No homozygous factor B–deficient patients have been reported. Most cases of properdin deficiency are X-linked and have been associated with fulminant, usually fatal, meningococcal infection.[142] Factor D deficiency is rare but appears to predispose to recurrent neisserial infection.[258]

There also is an increased risk of systemic neisserial disease, both meningococcal and gonococcal (but particularly meningococcal), in patients with deficiency of the terminal complement proteins C5, C6, C7, and C8.[141] Because C9 is not absolutely required for bacteriolysis (it just makes it occur faster), C9 deficiency is associated with a relatively smaller increased risk of infection than is deficiency of other terminal components. C9 deficiency is present in approximately 0.1 per cent of the population in Japan. In a study performed there, the risk of meningococcal diseases was increased 5000-fold in C7-deficient and 700-fold in C9-deficient persons.[320]

The rate of infection is higher in patients with C5 deficiency than in those with deficiencies of other terminal proteins because C5 is an important chemoattractant and thus is critical for leukocyte recruitment to sites of microbial invasion as well as for bactericidal activity.[141]

The incidence of collagen vascular disease also appears to be increased in patients with terminal component deficiencies, although it should be noted that many patients have undergone complement testing because of collagen vascular disease, and so the denominator is not available.[143]

At least one episode of meningococcal disease occurs in approximately 60 per cent of persons who have been identified as having C5, C6, C7, C8, or properdin deficiency, and 75 to 85 per cent of documented bacterial infections in complement-deficient persons are meningococcal.[143, 176, 371] It is of interest that there are differences in the patterns of meningococcal disease between persons with complement component deficiencies and normal hosts. First, meningococcal disease occurs in individuals who are older (mean, 17 vs. 3 years), and a higher proportion of disease is caused by groups Y, W135, and X in complement-deficient than in normal persons.[143] Furthermore, the mortality rate is much lower than in normal persons.

The presence of severe meningococcal infections in males,

particularly in skipped generations, suggests X-linked properdin deficiency, whereas meningococcal disease in persons older than 10 years of age and caused by unusual serogroups (Y, W135, and X) suggests terminal component deficiency (deficiency is detected in 5 to 10 per cent and 31 per cent with first or sporadic and recurrent episodes of disease, respectively).[141, 143]

Complement abnormalities may be quantitative or qualitative. Thus, it is important to determine both the total amount of individual complement proteins and their functional activity.[143] The most commonly employed test of complement function measures total hemolytic complement (CH_{50}). This assay quantitates activation of complement by the classical pathway using antibody-coated sheep erythrocytes as the target cells for MAC cytolysis. A normal CH_{50} reflects a normal quantity and function of classic pathway proteins (C1, C4, C2), C3, and terminal components through C8. A normal CH_{50} is possible in the absence of C9. The alternative pathway proteins can be measured in a similar assay employing rabbit erythrocytes instead of antibody-coated sheep cells because the surface of rabbit erythrocytes, unlike sheep cells, does not contain sialic acid and, therefore, permits continuous activation of C3 by the alternative pathway amplification loop.

Indications for performing complement evaluations include recurrent serious bacterial infections, one episode of meningococcal disease, or recurrent systemic gonococcal infections.[143] Deficiencies of classical pathway components, C3, and terminal components can be detected by a CH_{50} that is a functional assay. Alternative pathway testing is not performed routinely and always should be sent to reference laboratories. It is important to note that quantitative C3 and C4 assays, which are widely available in routine laboratories, do not detect functional abnormalities or deficiencies of other complement proteins. In general, quantitation of individual proteins other than C3 or C4 should be performed in reference laboratories in consultation with an immunologist or expert on complement.

Replacement of missing complement proteins has been attempted with fresh frozen plasma but usually has not been successful. It generally is not practical because of the short half-life of most of the components,[48, 135, 183, 272, 373] and if the patient is completely lacking a given protein, there is a risk of developing antibodies to it and thus causing reactions to later therapy or transfusions.

Disorders of Phagocyte Function

General Features of Phagocyte Disorders

Our most frequent reminder of the importance of an adequate supply of well-functioning phagocytes comes from patients who develop neutropenia after chemotherapy for malignancies. The high risk of bacterial and fungal infections in these patients mainly is the result of a lack of circulating neutrophils available for delivery to infected tissue.[348] Qualitative disorders of phagocyte function discussed in this section result in similar susceptibilities to these infections, either because the circulating cells are unable to migrate to an infected site or because, even having migrated to the infected tissue, they are unable to engage in normal microbicidal function. There is some overlap among the types of infectious complications associated with disorders of migration versus killing. However, as a rule, defects of neutrophil migration tend to be associated with infections at skin and mucous membrane sites. In contrast, killing defects are more likely to result in infections of soft tissues and internal organs, although skin infections are not uncommon.

Intrinsic Disorders of Cell Migration

Type 1 Leukocyte Adhesion Deficiency

In the late 1970s and the first half of the ensuing decade, several reports described patients with recurrent bacterial infections, diminished neutrophil motility, and delayed separation of the umbilical cord.[3, 28, 29, 32, 76, 123, 179, 215] The neutrophils of these patients were discovered to be markedly deficient in adherence to both natural and artificial surfaces, response to complement-opsonized particles, and expression of surface glycoproteins in the molecular weight range of 150 to 180 kDa. The deficient glycoproteins were found to be members of a family of heterodimeric glycoproteins, LFA-1, Mac-1, and pl50,95, each defined by its own unique alpha subunit, CD11a, CD11b, and CD11c, respectively, but sharing a common 95-kDa beta subunit designated CD18.[28, 29, 33, 412] These proteins, also called the β_2 leukocyte integrins, were identified as critical determinants of adhesion-dependent functions on neutrophils and other phagocytic cells, and their absence appeared to be directly responsible for the striking adherence-dependent defects that characterized the function of leukocytes from patients with this disorder.[28, 29, 33, 412] Variously called Mac-1 deficiency, MO1 deficiency, LFA-1 deficiency, CD11/CD18 deficiency, or CR3 deficiency, this disorder, now usually called type 1 leukocyte adhesion deficiency (LAD-1), is an autosomal recessive disorder with a defect in the β_2 integrin subunit, CD18, localized to chromosome 21.[30, 33, 412] It has been identified in approximately 100 persons worldwide and encompasses a broad ethnic diversity.[30, 33] Patients may exhibit a moderate or severe phenotype, depending on the extent of the defect in protein expression.[29, 30] The documented mutations of the β_2 subunit (CD18) that result in LAD-1 have been diverse, ranging from complete absence to truncations or extensions of the molecule, small deletions, and point mutations.[30, 33]

Patients with LAD-1 develop recurrent necrotic skin and soft tissue infections without pus formation, and they exhibit poor wound healing.[29, 30] They develop a severe generalized form of gingivitis/periodontitis, often losing most or all of their primary and secondary dentition along with some of their alveolar bone.[29, 30] They also may develop enterocolitis much like that of neutropenic patients.[29, 30] Delayed separation of the umbilical cord, presumably due to an impaired inflammatory response, is a common feature of the more severe phenotype of this disorder,[29, 30] but this finding alone in infants without infectious complications or other characteristic features is of doubtful significance.[459] Pronounced leukocytosis is a common feature of LAD-1, even in the absence of active infection.[29, 30] The reason for this is not clearly understood, but the fact that LAD-1 neutrophils are incapable of normal egress from the circulation via the oral cavity or lower intestinal tract may provide an important part of the explanation for the high circulating neutrophil counts.

Functional studies of neutrophils from patients with LAD-1 reveal a marked impairment of adherence-dependent functions that require the β_2 integrins, including attachment to various surfaces, orientation in a chemotactic gradient, chemotaxis through nitrocellulose filters or under agarose gels, aggregation, phagocytosis of iC3b-opsonized particles, degranulation or activation of the oxidative metabolic burst in response to such particles, and recruitment of PMNs in vivo to Rebuck skin windows or dermal suction blisters.[28–30, 91] In contrast, neutrophil functions that are independent of CD11/CD18-mediated interactions, including degranulation or oxidative burst activation in response to soluble stimuli or polarized shape change in suspension in response to chemoattractants, are normal.[28–30] PMNs and NK cells from patients with LAD-1 exhibit impaired ADCC for virus-infected target cells, suggesting that CD11/CD18-mediated cell-cell adhesion is essential for normal killing of virus-infected cells by this mechanism[259] and that the increased severity of viral infections in a few of the most severely affected patients could be related to defective ADCC. The specific diagnosis of LAD usually is made by demonstrating absent or markedly deficient expression of the CD11/CD18 family of glycoproteins on circulating leukocytes by immunofluorescence, gel electrophoresis, or other techniques.[28–30, 33]

Careful attention to skin and oral hygiene, aggressive management of infections, and meticulous local care of wound sites are important in the care of patients with LAD-1 or any serious disorder of neutrophil migration. Prophylactic antibiotics, usually trimethoprim-sulfamethoxazole, have been used in many of these patients, but their efficacy has not been well established. Granulocyte transfusions have been employed with some success to treat severe infections in a few patients with LAD-1.[30, 76] Bone marrow transplantation with HLA-matched allogeneic marrow has led to mixed results, from complete correction of the phagocytic defect to death 9 months after transplantation from graft-versus-host disease.[30, 179] The human CD18 gene has been cloned and sequenced, and human LAD-1 cells have been corrected successfully in vitro with the normal CD18 complementary DNA carried by retrovirus vectors, hinting at the future promise of gene therapy for patients with LAD-1.[224] The development of genetic knockout mice deficient in CD18 may provide a useful model for studying gene therapy in vivo, as well as for helping to elucidate features of the underlying deficiency itself.[264]

Type 2 Leukocyte Adhesion Deficiency

In 1992, a pair of unrelated patients were reported, both products of consanguineous matings, who exhibited clinical characteristics virtually identical to those described for LAD-1.[185] However, expression of the β_2 (CD18) integrins on leukocytes was normal. In addition to defects in neutrophil motility, these children exhibited short stature, psychomotor retardation, and the Bombay (hh) erythrocyte phenotype (homozygous for absence of the H antigen). Phagocytosis by PMNs was normal. These two patients are not sufficient to permit a firm conclusion regarding the underlying nature of this defect. However, current evidence suggests that the most likely explanation is a defect in an enzymatic fucosylation system resulting in the absence of fucosyl residues on sialyl Lewis X, the tetrasaccharide moiety that serves as an important ligand for members of the selectin family of adhesion molecules.[185, 271, 446] In vivo and in vitro studies comparing the adhesive functions of PMNs from LAD-1 and this new disorder, now called LAD-2, have provided elegant validation of the two-stage model of adherence for recruitment of leukocytes in vivo, with the initial selectin-mediated "rolling" stage (deficient in LAD-2) required first in order for the second integrin-mediated "firm adhesion and extravasation" stage (deficient in LAD-1) to occur.[446] A deficiency in either mechanism results in defective delivery of PMNs to infected sites and is manifested clinically as a form of LAD. The other somatic and neurologic features of LAD-2 may be related to more widespread consequences of a generalized defect in fucosylation of glycoproteins.[271]

Specific Granule Deficiency

Several patients with hereditary specific granule deficiency have been reported, beginning with Spitznagel's original description in 1972.[78, 188, 410] These persons exhibited recurrent and severe infections, primarily of the skin and mucous membranes, sometimes involving the lung and, in one patient, the mastoid. Normal human neutrophils contain both azurophilic (primary) granules and specific (secondary) granules whose contents have been summarized previously. Lactoferrin released from specific granules reduces the negative surface charge of the plasma membrane, contributing to nonspecific adhesiveness of the cell.[188] The specific granule membrane also contains some of the intracellular store of preformed Mac-1 (CD11b/CD18) that is mobilized to the plasma membrane upon stimulation by chemoattractants or other stimuli that induce granule secretion.[55, 73] Thus, specific granule deficiency results in marked impairment of adhesion and migration of neutrophils, probably on the basis of both diminished intracellular pools of adhesive proteins and the inability to effect the change in surface charge caused by lactoferrin. This, in turn, leads to the recurrent skin and mucous membrane infections due to *S. aureus*, gram-negative bacilli, and *Candida* that characterize the natural history of patients with this disorder.[78, 188, 410] Specific granule deficiency is presumed to be of genetic origin and probably is autosomal recessive in its mode of inheritance because both males and females are represented equally. The small number of reported cases has made this difficult to confirm. Specific granule deficiency may be diagnosed in a person with recurrent skin and mucous membrane infections whose neutrophils exhibit the characteristic absence of specific granules on Wright stain, as well as a marked impairment of chemotaxis in vivo and in vitro.

Chédiak-Higashi Syndrome

Chédiak-Higashi syndrome is a complex, rare autosomal recessive disorder characterized by partial oculocutaneous albinism, recurrent pyogenic infections, peripheral neuropathy, and neutropenia.[69] The illness also may involve an accelerated lymphoproliferative phase.[69] Granular cells, including neutrophils, contain giant lysosomal granules that are the apparent result of spontaneous intracellular fusion of azurophilic granules and, to a lesser extent, specific granules.[69] Corresponding disorders of intracellular pigment granules and vesicle trafficking in axons account for the albinism and other manifestations of this disease.[69] Similar disorders have been described in Aleutian mink, beige mice, albino Hereford cattle, and albino whales.[69] Patients with Chédiak-Higashi syndrome develop recurrent skin and mucosal infections, most often due to *S. aureus,* that are characteristic of those observed in defects of phagocyte migration.[27, 69, 110] There is a consistent defect in cell migration that appears to be related to abnormal regulation of microtubule polymerization upon stimulation by chemoattractant agents.[69, 110] The possible role of intracellular levels of cyclic adenosine monophosphate and guanylic acid in this microtubule abnormality has been suggested,[80] but the relationship between cyclic nucleotides and the microtubule dysfunction in Chédiak-Higashi syndrome has not been established. Ascorbic acid has been shown in at least one study to normalize both the elevated levels of cyclic adenosine monophosphate and the number of microtubules present within the cell.[80] Studies of two brothers with Chédiak-Higashi syndrome demonstrated abnormally increased tyrosinylation of the alpha subunit of tubulin.[69, 322] Phagocytosis is normal, but killing of ingested bacteria is defective or delayed. The reason for this deficient or delayed killing is uncertain but may involve defective phagolysosomal fusion or abnormalities in levels of microbicidal defensins, which also are stored in primary granules.[190] The diagnosis of Chédiak-Higashi syndrome usually is established clinically on the basis of partial oculocutaneous albinism and recurrent pyogenic infections. A Wright stain demonstrating giant lysosomal granules and laboratory studies showing defective cell migration are confirmatory.

Actin Dysfunction

Filamentous actin constitutes the main contractile mechanism of neutrophils for migration and phagocytosis.[416] Described in a single patient,[79] neutrophil actin dysfunction has been characterized by recurrent skin infections caused by *S. aureus* and *Candida albicans*. Biopsies of infected skin lesions in this young child demonstrated necrotic tissue with a notable absence of neutrophils. In vivo and in vitro studies revealed severely impaired neutrophil chemotaxis and phagocytosis. The capacity for polymerization of actin from cell extracts also was diminished markedly. It is of interest that PMNs from family members of this patient also were found to be deficient in the CD11/CD18 family of glycoproteins that are the basis of LAD-1.[407, 408] The nature of this association is uncertain.

Glycogen Storage Disease Type 1B

Beaudet and colleagues[52] first reported the association of recurrent infection, neutropenia, and impaired neutrophil migration with glycogen storage disease (GSD) type 1B, a metabolic disorder characterized by defective microsomal transport of glucose-6-phosphate. In 1985, Ambruso and coworkers[19] reviewed the features of 21 patients with GSD type 1B, 15 of whom suffered from frequent infections, especially of the skin and subcutaneous tissues. Osteomyelitis, pneumonitis, sinusitis, and septicemia also were reported. Seventeen of these 21 patients were found to have serum inhibitors of myeloid stem-cell proliferation, which were presumed to account for their chronic neutropenia. Impaired neutrophil motility was found in 8 of 11 patients in whom this was evaluated. Assays of neutrophil microbicidal capacity generally were normal. A specific relationship between the underlying metabolic defect in GSD type 1B and the mechanism of impaired cell motility has not been established. However, glucose has been found to be an important energy source for chemotaxis,[452] and it is interesting to note that the uptake of glucose by PMNs in response to chemoattractant stimulation is impaired in GSD type 1B as well as in neonates, both examples of patients with impaired PMN migration.[4, 49]

Extrinsic or Secondary Defects of Polymorphonuclear Leukocyte Migration

Defective Neutrophil Chemotaxis Associated with Serum Inhibitors of Cell Function

A number of investigators have reported the presence of inhibitors of PMN chemotaxis in the serum of patients with recurrent infection.[263, 316, 397, 406, 438, 450] In most cases, the pathophysiologic mechanisms of these inhibitors are unknown. In many of the patients described, other associated immunologic disorders could account for at least part of the increased susceptibility to infection. However, in each case, the patient's neutrophils exhibited diminished chemotaxis in the presence of autologous serum or plasma, whereas identical assays in the presence of control serum or plasma resulted in a normal chemotactic response. Most such inhibitors appear to be immunoglobulins or immunoglobulin-like molecules.

Hyper-IgE Syndrome

In 1966, Davis and colleagues[134] described two young girls with coarse facial features, reddish hair, fair skin, severe eczema, dystrophic nails, staphylococcal skin abscesses, and recurrent sinopulmonary infections. The absence of classic signs of inflammation accompanying the staphylococcal abscesses led to their being characterized as cold abscesses. The term Job syndrome was suggested, referring to the similar biblical affliction. Additional patients were described with a similar disorder, first associated by Buckley[86] with very high serum IgE levels, including a patient who exhibited a defect in neutrophil chemotaxis reported in 1973 by Clark and associates.[108] Subsequent reports of similar patients have demonstrated that there are certain features common to all of the patients with the disease now called hyper-IgE syndrome. These consistent features include a history of staphylococcal infections of the skin and sinopulmonary tract beginning in infancy or early childhood and serum levels of IgE that are greater that 2000 IU/mL.[89, 151, 226] Other characteristic, but variable, features of this disorder include coarse facies, cold abscesses of the skin and subcutaneous tissues, a chronic eczematoid rash, eosinophilia, and mucocutaneous candidiasis.[151] Comprehensive reviews have provided detailed characterizations of the abnormalities of patients with this disorder,[87, 151] the underlying basis of which remains undefined.[88, 193] Consistent abnormalities of cell-mediated immune functions in patients with hyper-IgE syndrome suggest that the pathogenic basis involves a defect of T-cell regulation. Documented abnormalities include diminished reactivity to *Candida* and tetanus toxoid in delayed hypersensitivity skin testing, decreased in vitro lymphocyte proliferative responses to these antigens, and reduced numbers of T cells with the CD45RO memory T-cell phenotype.[88, 105, 151]

Some patients with hyper-IgE syndrome may have a defect in neutrophil chemotaxis.[151] The defect, if observed, usually is intermittent. In several cases, the presence of a serum inhibitor of chemotaxis has been recognized.[151] Donabedian and Gallin[150] demonstrated an inhibitor of granulocyte chemotaxis in supernatants from cultured peripheral blood monocytes from patients with hyper-IgE syndrome. The persistence of infectious complications in this disorder at times when chemotaxis has been found to be normal, as well as the presence of large purulent collections within cold abscesses, raises doubt about the significance of a chemotactic disorder in explaining the markedly increased susceptibility of these patients to recurrent infections.

Impaired Generation of Serum-Derived Chemotaxins

A deficiency in the host's ability to produce chemotaxins derived from serum components may have profound consequences for the recruitment of PMNs to an infected site. The most important serum-derived chemotaxin is the fragment of the fifth component of complement, C5a, and its des-arg form. Several kindreds have been described with either absent or defective C5.[369] The chemoattractant activity measured in activated normal serum virtually is absent in C5-deficient serum.[370] The risk of developing systemic *Neisseria* infections due to deficient activation of the lytic terminal complement sequence appears far more significant than any phagocytic recruitment defect caused by impaired production of chemotaxins.[55, 176] Patients with C3 deficiency also have impaired chemotaxigenesis because C5 cannot be activated. Host impairment usually is more severe because of the importance of C3 in opsonization, as well as its role in the activation of the remainder of the complement cascade.[371] As noted earlier, newborn infants also are relatively deficient in chemotaxigenesis because of immature levels of many of the complement components.[261]

Other Secondary or Poorly Defined Disorders of Polymorphonuclear Leukocyte Migration

Patients with protein-calorie malnutrition have defective PMN chemotaxis that appears to be based on systemic preactivation of circulating cells due to chronic low-level endotoxemia that results from impaired intestinal mucosal integrity.[256] Shwachman-Diamond syndrome, in addition to pancreatic insufficiency, neutropenia, and growth retardation, also is associated with defective PMN migration.[11] Two kindreds with congenital ichthyosis and an associated defect of PMN migration have been described.[308] Patients with severe thermal injuries develop an acquired form of specific granule deficiency with impaired PMN migration beginning about 14 days after injury.[188] Children with juvenile periodontitis of various types may exhibit reduced PMN chemotaxis.[437] In some of these patients, this has been associated with gingival infections due to *Capnocytophaga,* an anaerobic gram-negative organism that can elaborate factors that markedly impair PMN migration.[394] However, in one such patient the diagnosis was LAD-1, a finding that raises some uncertainty about the role of *Capnocytophaga* in such disorders (Tosi, M. F., Shurin, S. B., and Smith, C. W., unpublished data). Several reports have been published of a poorly defined disorder of neutrophil migration called lazy leukocyte syndrome,[10, 307] which is characterized by recurrent staphylococcal skin infections, rhinitis, gingivitis, stomatitis, neutropenia despite adequate marrow precursors, and diminished in vivo and in vitro migration of neutrophils.

Defects in Phagocyte Microbicidal Activity

As described earlier, the broad array of available phagocyte microbicidal mechanisms may be divided into oxygen-dependent and oxygen-independent mechanisms. To date, no isolated deficiency of a specific oxygen-independent microbicidal mechanism has been described. Thus, this section is concerned mainly with the known deficiencies of oxygen-dependent microbicidal mechanisms of phagocytes, especially CGD, the prototypical defect in this group. PMN migration usually is normal in these intracellular killing defects. Monocytes and the fixed phagocytes of the reticuloendothelial system generally share in the deficient microbicidal activity.

Chronic Granulomatous Disease

CGD was one of the earliest syndromes of phagocyte dysfunction to be characterized[354] and probably is the most extensively studied among individual phagocyte defects. It is recognized now to be a family of biochemically and genetically heterogeneous disorders of distinct components of the phagocyte NADPH oxidase complex.[107, 128, 189] Thus, CGD results in the inability of phagocytes to generate superoxide anion and other reactive oxygen species.[189] Organisms that produce catalase pose a special problem for patients with CGD.[153, 189, 245, 276] This encompasses a broad range of pathogens that includes staphylococci, gram-negative enteric bacteria, *Pseudomonas* species, yeast, fungi, *Nocardia,* and numerous other pathogenic species.[153, 189, 245, 276] Most microorganisms produce H_2O_2, which can be used by the CGD phagocyte as an effective microbicidal weapon because it feeds into the sequence of oxidant reactions downstream from the defective oxidase enzyme (see Fig. 2–8).[366] Because catalase is an enzyme that degrades H_2O_2 to oxygen and water, organisms that produce catalase are able to survive within these deficient cells.[189, 245, 366] Infections with catalase-negative bacteria, such as *S. pneumoniae, H. influenzae,* and *N. meningitidis,* do not occur with increased frequency in CGD patients,[189] and these organisms are killed normally in vitro by CGD phagocytes. Phagocyte functions not directly related to oxidative mechanisms of intracellular killing, including adherence, chemotaxis, phagocytosis, and degranulation, usually are normal in CGD patients.[40, 311, 354, 404]

The genetic defect in CGD may be inherited by either X-linked recessive or autosomal recessive mechanisms.[107, 128] In the female obligate carriers of X-linked CGD, the proportion of cells that express the defect usually is about 50 per cent, depending on the proportion of cells in which random inactivation of the normal versus the affected X chromosome occurs.[292] In most of the autosomal recessive forms of CGD, the quantity of the cytochrome in cells is normal, but there is a deficiency in one of two cytosolic proteins of 47 kDa and 67 kDa, each of which is a critical component of the fully assembled NADPH oxidase complex.[37, 107, 109] In a study of 94 patients with CGD from several centers,[107] 51 per cent had the X-linked form with absent cytochrome b, 33 per cent had an autosomal recessive form with absence of the 47-kDa protein, 5 per cent had autosomal recessive disease with absence of the 67-kDa protein, 5 per cent had X-linked recessive cytochrome-positive disease with present but functionally defective cytochrome b, and 5 per cent had autosomal recessive cytochrome-negative CGD, probably due to a defect in synthesis of the cytochrome b alpha chain. Each of these genetically distinct defects results in defective function of the oxidase and the characteristic CGD phenotype.

Patients with CGD experience recurrent serious bacterial and fungal infections, usually beginning in the first few months of life. *S. aureus* and gram-negative bacilli are the most common causes of infection in CGD patients, but fungi, especially *Aspergillus* species, also are prominent etiologic agents.[189, 276, 357] Lymphadenopathy associated with lymphadenitis and chronic suppuration with poor healing is a common presenting feature of CGD. Granuloma formation at infected sites is one of the histologic hallmarks of this disorder.[189, 245, 357] Pulmonary infections and their complications have been the reported cause of death in up to 50 per cent of CGD patients in some series. These infections often are protracted and respond slowly to appropriate antibiotic therapy.[246, 357] Progression to lung abscess, empyema, or both occurs in about 20 per cent of CGD patients with pneumonia.[246] Liver abscesses occur in about half of patients with CGD and may be recurrent.[106, 351] The hepatosplenomegaly common in CGD patients may result from these infections but probably is more likely to result from chronic infections at various sites with systemic lymphoid hyperplasia.[189, 245, 357] Osteomyelitis occurs in about one-third of CGD patients.[189, 245, 357] In contrast with normal children, in whom this infection usually involves the metaphyseal area of long bones, CGD patients more often develop infections of the small bones of the hands and feet. As with normal children, *S. aureus* is the most common etiologic agent, but gram-negative bacilli, *Nocardia,* and *Aspergillus* are among other important etiologic agents in CGD.[189, 422] Skin infections in CGD may include pyoderma, purulent dermatitis, and cutaneous or subcutaneous abscesses and often are preceded by a chronic eczematoid skin rash.[189, 357] However, skin infections are somewhat less of a problem in CGD patients than in patients with leukocyte migration defects.

Although localized infections are the rule in CGD patients, these patients also may develop septicemia.[189, 245, 357] The most common cause of septicemia in most series has been *Salmonella,* but other gram-negative enteric bacilli also have been prominent.[245, 276] Of note, *S. aureus,* the single most common etiologic agent of localized infections in CGD, is a relatively uncommon cause of septicemia in these patients.[357] Infections sometimes seen in CGD patients include recurrent urinary tract infections in about 6 to 8 per cent of patients; ocular infections with conjunctivitis, blepharitis, or both in about 20 per cent of patients; and, rarely, chorioretinitis.[189, 297, 357] Acute pericarditis with or without myocardial abscess also has been reported.[189, 268]

Granuloma formation adjacent to hollow viscera in CGD patients has been found to produce clinically significant obstruction. Reported examples of this problem include obstruction of the gastric outlet, esophagus, small intestine, and ureters.[20, 102, 153] This complication usually responds to treatment with corticosteroids.[102]

CGD should be suspected in patients with a history of recurrent indolent infections caused by catalase-positive organisms such as those described earlier, especially if granulomas are found in biopsy specimens of lymph nodes or other tissues. Confirmation of the diagnosis usually rests on the demonstration of an absent oxidative metabolic burst in the patient's phagocytes. This can be detected by the slide nitroblue tetrazolium test (Fig. 2–10) or by other measurements of oxidative burst activity, such as cytochrome reduction, lucigenin- or luminol-enhanced chemiluminescence, oxygen consumption, hydrogen peroxide production, and flow cytometry of cells loaded with oxidant-sensitive fluorescent dyes.[15, 38, 50, 301, 365, 431] Prenatal diagnosis has been achieved by the use of the slide nitroblue tetrazolium test with blood from placental vessels obtained at fetoscopy.[324]

The management of patients with CGD traditionally has relied on antibiotic prophylaxis, usually with trimethoprim-sulfamethoxazole or an oral antistaphylococcal agent, and an aggressive approach to the specific diagnosis and treatment of acute infections.[357] Granulocyte transfusions have been reported to be at least partially beneficial in a few cases.[92, 111] Bone marrow transplantation has met with limited success, with only one successful long-term engraftment among four separate attempts in different patients.[203, 252, 356, 455] The definition of the molecular basis for CGD and the cloning of the genes responsible for the various forms of this defect have led to correction of some forms of the defect in cultured cells and the development of animal models of CGD in mice,[243, 290, 338, 350, 444] both of which are crucial steps in developing gene therapy for patients with this disorder in the future. The most important recent development in the treatment of patients with CGD is the use of IFN-γ. A multicenter study demonstrated that daily subcutaneous injections of this agent reduced the requirement for hospitalization of CGD patients for serious infections by about two-thirds.[242] The mechanism by which IFN-γ exerts this beneficial effect has not been determined. This treatment carries some mild systemic side effects,[242] but it has become part of the standard regimen for managing most patients with CGD.

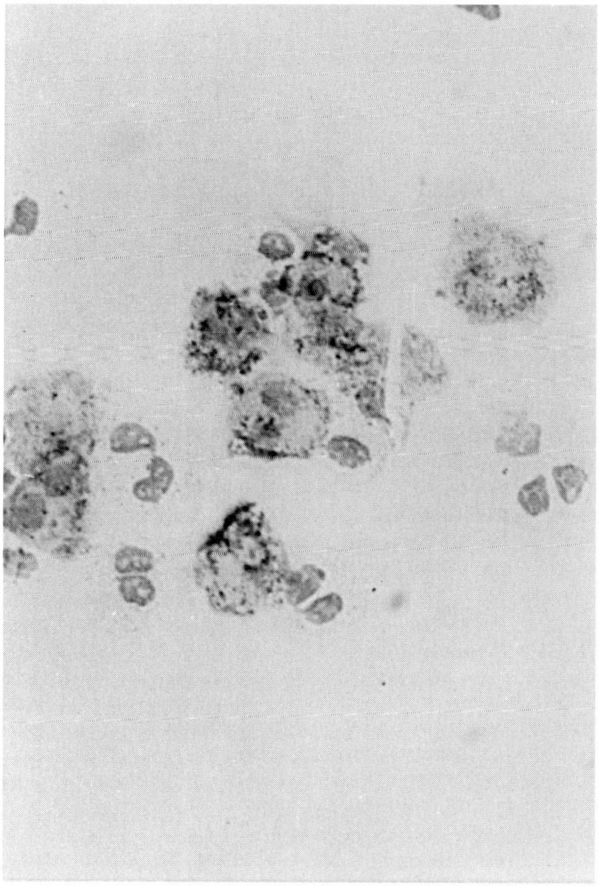

FIGURE 2–10. *Photomicrograph of a slide nitroblue tetrazolium (NBT) test of polymorphonuclear leukocytes (PMNs) isolated from the blood of a maternal carrier of X-linked recessive chronic granulomatous disease (CGD). Because of random inactivation of either the normal or the affected X chromosome in maternal carriers of this disorder, approximately one-half of the PMNs exhibit the granular blue-black staining characteristic of the oxidative reduction of NBT by normal PMNs. In contrast, the remaining PMNs, which express the NADPH oxidase defect of CGD, are visible principally by their nuclear counterstain.*

Deficiencies of Glucose-6-Phosphate Dehydrogenase and Glutathione Peroxidase

The normal activity of the NADPH oxidase enzyme complex depends on the continued availability of NADPH to reduce molecular oxygen to form superoxide anion.[36, 109, 366] The primary source of NADPH for this enzyme is the hexose monophosphate shunt. It is provided with the hexose substrate, 6-phosphoglucose, by the enzyme glucose-6-phosphate dehydrogenase, which also generates NADPH in a coupled reaction.[366] The reactions of the hexose monophosphate shunt itself are coupled to two other enzymes, glutathione reductase and glutathione peroxidase, which recycle oxidized and reduced glutathione.[366] The absence of any of these three enzymes results in a lack of available NADPH to drive the NADPH oxidase. Thus, deficiencies in any of these other three enzymes should result in a phagocyte killing defect similar to CGD. Patients with deficiencies of glucose-6-phosphate dehydrogenase or glutathione peroxidase have been described with functional oxidative metabolic defects and presentations that are clinically indistinguishable from CGD, caused by defects in the NADPH oxidase itself.[39, 375] Glucose-6-phosphate dehydrogenase deficiency usually involves erythrocytes and is associated with hemolytic anemia, especially in conjunction with the administration of sulfonamides.[119, 204] Only when the defect also involves myeloid cells and is severe or complete (<5 per cent of normal enzyme levels) is the CGD-like disorder manifested.[39, 375] A partial deficiency of glutathione reductase has been reported, with hemolytic anemia and early cataracts, but no increased incidence of infection was noted.[364]

Glutathione Synthetase Deficiency

Glutathione, along with glutathione peroxidase and glutathione reductase, the two enzymes involved in its recycling between oxidized and reduced forms, constitutes a protective mechanism in PMNs against membrane damage mediated by reactive oxygen intermediates formed during PMN activation.[364] Thus, the synthesis of an adequate supply of glutathione is critical to these cells. Two brothers with glutathione synthetase deficiency who presented with neutropenia, hemolytic anemia, acidosis, 5-oxyprolinuria, and recurrent infection were reported by Spielberg and colleagues.[77, 409] The

PMNs from these patients exhibited elevated cytosolic hydrogen peroxide levels, diminished oxidative microbicidal activity, and impaired microtubule assembly. Antioxidant therapy with vitamin E normalized the in vitro abnormalities of the patients' PMNs, and there was no further difficulty with recurrent infections.[77] This suggested that vitamin E protected the cell membranes by scavenging excess hydrogen peroxide produced during PMN activation and thus prevented or minimized oxidant-induced membrane damage.

Myeloperoxidase Deficiency

Congenital deficiency of neutrophil myeloperoxidase (MPO), once thought to be a relatively rare disorder, has come to be recognized as the single most common heritable disorder of neutrophil function. However, its clinical significance remains in doubt. Population surveys made possible with the advent of automated flow cytochemical techniques have indicated an incidence of MPO deficiency of about 1 in 2000 persons.[323, 343] Approximately one-half of these patients have complete absence of this neutrophil enzyme, and the remainder have a partial deficiency. The precise mode of inheritance of this defect has not been established, but MPO is known to be a product of a single gene on chromosome 17.[439] The reaction of MPO with hydrogen peroxide and chloride, causing the formation of hypochlorite, is one of the most effective microbicidal mechanisms of neutrophils, and cells from some patients with MPO deficiency have been found to exhibit delayed killing of *C. albicans* and *S. aureus*.[280] MPO deficiency rarely has been associated with unusual infectious complications, except in patients with diabetes mellitus.

IMPORTANT EXAMPLES OF SECONDARY IMMUNODEFICIENCY (NOT INCLUDING HIV INFECTION)

Asplenia

Fulminant infections can occur in patients who have anatomic or functional asplenia.[381] The mortality rate from these infections in asplenic persons ranges from 40 to 80 per cent.[462] The most common pathogens are encapsulated bacteria, including *S. pneumoniae* (50 to 70 per cent), *H. influenzae,* and *N. meningitidis*.[462] They can cause fulminant, often fatal, disease characterized by rapid onset of shock. Malaria, babesiosis, and viral infections also are more severe in asplenic persons. Infections can occur at any time but are most common within the first 2 years after splenectomy.

Both the liver and the spleen are important in phagocytic clearance of bacteria from the circulation, and the spleen is an important site for antibody production. The spleen is relatively more important than the liver in processing antigen in the naive host. The younger the person is when splenic function is lost, the higher the risk for serious infection. Thus, young children who become asplenic are much more susceptible to fulminant infection than are adults, because adults are more likely to have encountered antigens before splenectomy than are children. Persons whose indication for splenectomy is thalassemia or Hodgkin disease are at higher risk of dying of overwhelming infection than are those who have functional asplenia from sickle-cell disease. Patients who undergo spleen removal for spherocytosis or idiopathic thrombocytopenia have a lower risk of infection. The lowest-risk group consists of adults whose spleens are removed surgically after trauma, who are at little or no increased risk of infection.

Congenital asplenia usually is associated with complex congenital cardiac disease and occasionally with structural abnormalities of the gastrointestinal or genitourinary tracts. Thus, asplenia should be suspected in any patient with congenital heart disease and sepsis. Asplenia also should be suspected in patients with increased numbers of circulating pitted erythrocytes that contain Howell-Jolly bodies.

Elective splenectomy for conditions such as hereditary spherocytosis should be delayed as long as possible, and splenic repair or subtotal splenectomy should be performed whenever possible after trauma. Asplenic persons are managed using prophylactic antibiotics until at least 5 years of age.[115] They also should be immunized against encapsulated organisms at the appropriate ages (e.g., *H. influenzae* type b conjugate vaccine beginning at 2 months and pneumococcal and meningococcal polysaccharide vaccines at 2 years).[115] Patients should be warned about their increased risk of serious infections due to malaria and babesiosis.

Sickle-Cell Disease

Immunodeficiency in sickle-cell disease patients is due, in large part, to their functional asplenia.[381] Part of the risk of infection stems from local infarction and tissue necrosis due to sickling, which causes sludging and resultant tissue hypoxia. The reticuloendothelial system also may be obstructed by having to deal with chronic hemolysis. Patients with sickle-cell disease are protected partially from *Plasmodium falciparum* malaria but have a high incidence of fulminant sepsis and meningitis caused by encapsulated organisms (e.g., *S. pneumoniae, H. influenzae* type b, *N. meningitidis*) and *Salmonella*.[182] The relative risk of pneumococcal meningitis in children with sickle-cell disease is approximately 500 times that of normal children. *Salmonella* infections often are associated with osteomyelitis or meningitis.[163]

Patients with sickle-cell disease seem to have normal antibody response to most antigens, including age-appropriate responses to vaccines. A deficiency in heat-labile opsonic activity has been reported and may be due to a defect in the alternative pathway of complement. Indeed, there have been reports of patients with sickle-cell disease who have deficiencies of factor B, but sickle-cell disease patients have normal CH_{50} and normal levels of properdin, C3, and factor I.

Patients with sickle-cell disease should be managed with prophylactic antibiotics until at least 5 years of age and should be immunized against *H. influenzae* type b, pneumococci, and meningococci at the appropriate ages.[115]

Cystic Fibrosis

Cystic fibrosis is an autosomal recessive disorder caused by mutations in both alleles of the gene encoding the protein called cystic fibrosis transmembrane conductance regulator.[454] Most patients with cystic fibrosis develop chronic endobronchial infection with *P. aeruginosa* of the mucoid phenotype. This infection is accompanied by an intense chronic airway inflammation with an exuberant influx of neutrophils that leads to destruction and fibrosis of lung and airway tissue.[262] No systemic disorder of immunity has been documented in cystic fibrosis, but local factors in the airway inflammatory milieu, especially neutrophil-derived proteases such as elastase, contribute to secondary impairments in opsonic and phagocytic host defenses by cleaving opsonic antibody and complement fragments, as well as important phagocytic receptors for these opsonins.[430]

Both the early pathogenesis of the unique chronic endobronchial infection in cystic fibrosis and its relationship to the underlying genetic defect have remained obscure. However, several possible explanations have been offered. A reduction in cell surface sialic acid on cystic fibrosis epithelial cells unmasks the glycoprotein asialo-GM-1, which appears to function as an epithelial receptor for adhesion by *P. aeruginosa* and may promote airway colonization.[378] Additionally, it has been suggested that airway epithelial cells normally internalize *P. aeruginosa* before being sloughed and cleared by mucociliary action and that this internalization may be deficient in cystic fibrosis epithelial cells.[347] Finally, there is evidence that microbicidal peptides of or related to the defensin family, released from airway epithelial cells as a local defense mechanism, may be inactivated by abnormal salt concentrations at the airway epithelial surface, thereby thwarting an important first line of local antibacterial defense.[401] These proposed mechanisms are not mutually exclusive, and none has been proved conclusively to explain the pathogenesis of infection in the airways of cystic fibrosis patients. Currently, they are the subject of intensive investigation.

Evaluation for Immunodeficiency in the Child with Recurrent or Severe Infections

Most immunodeficiency disorders can be diagnosed readily by employing a methodical process that begins with careful analysis of the child's presenting history and physical examination.[117, 125, 143, 231, 334, 381, 382, 463] This information serves as the foundation for a rational laboratory evaluation. It is important to bear in mind that it is normal for children to have several infections every year. Normal children who are exposed to other children, particularly older school age siblings or classmates, develop approximately one infection per month. The overwhelming majority of infections in immunocompetent children are characterized by being mild and localized to the gastrointestinal or upper respiratory tracts, and they either are self-limited or respond rapidly to conventional therapy. Immunocompromised hosts tend to have more frequent, severe, and unusual infections that may not respond readily to appropriate therapy.

HISTORY

A detailed history alone is sufficient to determine whether or not an immunologic evaluation should be pursued in many children who have recurrent or severe infections. If tests for immunity are indicated, the history also serves as a guide to the types of studies that should be performed initially. Table 2–5 provides a list of historical information that is valuable in assessing the likelihood of immunodeficiency. Whenever possible, the child's complete medical records (including growth charts) should be obtained, particularly if several physicians have provided care, because the history often is complicated, and incomplete or inaccurate information may be misleading.

The age of onset of suspicious infections usually helps in defining the underlying problem. For example, children with isolated immunoglobulin deficiencies tend to do well during the first few months of life because they are protected by maternal antibody.[285] They usually start developing serious infections later in the first year of life. Those with cell-mediated or phagocytic disorders may begin developing infections in the newborn period (see earlier). In contrast, healthy children who have been cared for at home by their mothers and who have no siblings often have relatively few infections in the first few years of life but may present for immunologic evaluation when they develop recurrent infections beginning the first few weeks after entering day care, nursery school, or kindergarten.

TABLE 2–5. History in the Evaluation of the Child with Recurrent or Severe Infections

Age at onset of infections
Number, frequency, and periodicity of infections
Nature of infections
Location on body
Organism(s)
Severity
Duration
Nature and duration of therapy
Response to therapy
Hospitalizations
Surgery
Growth pattern
Separation of umbilical stump
Periodontal disease
Allergies
Immunizations
Exposures
Contagious diseases in family, school, or community
Number and ages of siblings
Parents' occupations
Babysitting or day care arrangements
Foreign travel
Parental smoking
Wood furnaces
Family history (especially in males)
Immunodeficiency
Recurrent, severe, or unusual infections
Cause of early deaths
Autoimmune disease
Allergy
Consanguinity
Days of school missed (and why)

The number, nature, and severity of infections help in determining how aggressively to pursue an immunologic evaluation. Certain clinical presentations of disease and causative organisms are associated with a high likelihood of an immunodeficiency. Antibody or complement deficiencies, or functional asplenia, should be suspected in children with recurrent or life-threatening infections such as sepsis and meningitis caused by encapsulated organisms (e.g., *S. pneumoniae, H. influenzae* type b).[85, 143, 247, 278, 334, 367] Complement deficiencies should be considered in persons with recurrent or severe neisserial disease.[143] CGD should be suspected in the presence of tissue infections such as liver abscess, lymphadenopathy, pneumonia, or osteomyelitis caused by *S. aureus*, unusual gram-negative bacteria such as *Serratia marcescens*, or *Aspergillus* species.[189] *P. carinii* infection suggests a T-cell deficiency, either hereditary or due to HIV infection. In contrast, recurrent or even severe infections with group A *Streptococcus* have not been associated with immunodeficiency. Also, recurrent urinary tract infections usually are associated with anatomic abnormalities of the urinary tract and not immunodeficiency.

An essential part of the history is documentation of the child's growth pattern. Children who are thriving, particularly those older than 2 years of age, are much less likely to have serious immune disorders than are those with failure to thrive.

The immunization history should be documented carefully because it may prove to be useful in evaluating the child's ability to mount an antibody response to specific vaccine antigens. The history of recent live viral immunization should be obtained in children who have clinical presentations compatible with polio or measles because infection caused by vaccine strains of these viruses is the first indication of immunodeficiency in some children.

Exposures to contagious diseases may lead to recurrent and, occasionally, even severe infections in persons with normal host defenses. Children who never leave the house may have recurrent infections from organisms brought home by older siblings, other relatives, or neighbors. Certainly it must be assumed that children who attend day care facilities or schools constantly are being exposed to common infections. Familiarity with community patterns of disease such as prevalent clinical manifestations of enterovirus infection or the beginning of croup, respiratory syncytial virus, influenza, or rotavirus seasons can be used to reassure families of normal children with frequent mild infections. It also should be borne in mind that environmental pollutants, such as cigarette smoke and wood-burning stoves, also have been associated with an increased risk of acute lower respiratory illnesses in children.[360]

Because many immunodeficiencies are hereditary, a detailed family history should be obtained that includes questions about the presence of immunodeficiency, recurrent or severe infections, contributing factors to any early deaths, the gender of affected persons, and consanguinity. A history of recurrent or severe infections in more than one male relative is highly suspicious of a familial immunodeficiency disorder. Autoimmune diseases may suggest a familial disorder of complement or cell-mediated immunity.[143]

A thorough history of school absenteeism and the reasons the child stays home may be helpful in differentiating medical from psychosocial problems in older children who present for evaluation for recurrent infections, particularly when symptoms are unusual or inconsistent with physical findings. Prolonged absences for vague problems with no physical findings, particularly in the presence of normal growth, are less likely to be caused by infections than are those characterized by well-defined physical or laboratory findings and poor growth.

In general, recurrent severe infections beginning before the age of 1 year, failure to thrive, invasive disease caused by encapsulated or unusual organisms, or family histories of such infections should prompt an immunologic evaluation.

PHYSICAL EXAMINATION

Physical examination may provide valuable clues as to the nature of the immune disorder. In certain cases, such as some patients with the hyper-IgE syndrome[89, 226] and the DiGeorge anomaly[147] who exhibit the characteristic facies, it may be diagnostic.[89, 226]

As noted earlier, one of the most obvious signs that a child may have a serious underlying medical problem is failure to thrive. Every immunologic evaluation *must* include documentation of current growth parameters and a comparison with past growth.

Many immunodeficiency disorders have dermatologic manifestations. Eczematoid rashes are seen in patients with the hyper-IgE syndrome and CGD.[89, 189, 226] CGD also is characterized by slow wound healing and the development of hypertrophic scars.[189] Patients with Chédiak-Higashi syndrome have partial albinism.[69] Severe gingival disease and early loss of teeth are prominent clinical features in disorders of neutrophil migration, such as LAD.[27]

The chest should be evaluated for physical signs of active disease, such as rales and rhonchi, as well as evidence of chronic infection, such as an increased anterior-posterior diameter. Pneumonia, bronchitis, bronchiectasis, and scarring can occur with most immunodeficiencies but are associated most frequently with immunoglobulin deficiencies.[85, 218, 334]

Cardiac abnormalities may suggest immunodeficiency disorders such as the DiGeorge anomaly,[147] and situs inversus should alert the clinician to the possibility of Kartagener syndrome.[117]

Although hepatosplenomegaly may be found in many types of immunodeficiency disease, it is more common in patients with disorders of phagocyte function.

LABORATORY STUDIES

The laboratory evaluation should be guided by the history and physical findings. Relatively simple and inexpensive screening tests often can help narrow the differential diagnosis and streamline the evaluation. One of the first tests that should be performed is a complete blood count with differential and evaluation of the blood smear. This simple test can detect several immunologic abnormalities, including neutropenia, lymphopenia associated with HIV-1 or forms of SCID, the abnormal neutrophil granules associated with the Chédiak-Higashi syndrome, Howell-Jolly bodies found with asplenia, and some malignancies. Chest radiographs should be examined for thymic tissue, mediastinal lymphadenopathy, pneumonia, bronchiectasis, and other evidence of pulmonary infections. Consideration also should be given to evaluating patients with chronic pulmonary disease for cystic fibrosis with a sweat chloride test.

Quantitative immunoglobulin levels provide a useful screening test for evaluating patients with suspected humoral immune deficiency. It should be remembered, however, that IgG2 deficiency often is not reflected in the IgG level because it makes up such a relatively small proportion of total IgG. Thus, patients with suspected humoral immune deficiency usually should be tested for IgG subclass, as well as quantitative IgG, IgA, and IgM deficiency. IgE levels may be helpful in establishing the diagnosis of the hyper-IgE syndrome, although an elevated IgE level is much more common in patients with allergies than immunologic abnormalities. Immunoglobulin levels may be extremely elevated in children with HIV-1 infection.

Humoral immunity in children who have normal quantitative immunoglobulin and IgG subclass levels but who continue to have frequent sinopulmonary infections that do not respond well to appropriate medical and surgical management (e.g., ventilation tubes) also can be evaluated by measuring antibody responses to specific antigens such as tetanus and diphtheria toxoids and *H. influenzae* type b and meningococcal and pneumococcal capsular polysaccharides. Antibody levels can be measured before immunization and approximately 1 to 2 months after immunization to evaluate the child's ability to respond to different kinds of antigens (i.e., T-cell–dependent antigens such as diphtheria and tetanus toxoid or T-cell–independent antigens such as plain pneumococcal capsular polysaccharide vaccine).

The complement system should be evaluated in persons with recurrent or life-threatening neisserial disease, including recurrent systemic gonorrhea infections and sporadic meningococcal disease. The best screening test is the CH_{50}. A normal CH_{50} reflects a normal quantity and function of classic pathway proteins (C1, C4, C2), C3, and terminal components through C8, as noted earlier.[143] The alternative pathway proteins can be measured in a similar assay employing rabbit erythrocytes instead of antibody-coated sheep cells. Alternative pathway deficiencies are extremely rare; therefore, demonstration of a normal CH_{50} generally is a sufficient indicator of normal complement activity. An abnormal CH_{50} should be repeated immediately, being careful that the specimen is handled correctly. Complement abnormalities may be quantitative or qualitative. Thus, if the repeat CH_{50} remains low, it is important to determine both the serum levels of individual complement proteins and their functional activity, as has been discussed.

Delayed hypersensitivity skin testing with antigens such as *Candida* is useful to assess cell-mediated immunity. T-lymphocyte subset quantitation may be helpful in diagnosing such conditions as SCID and HIV, but more sophisticated testing of lymphocyte function such as mitogen and antigen stimulation should be performed in patients with recurrent or severe fungal infection. These studies should be directed by an immunologist.

Similarly, suspected phagocyte function disorders should be evaluated in consultation with experts in phagocyte function because lack of proper standardization and expertise often leads to misleading results from commercial laboratories. Phagocyte function studies should be directed toward adherence and migration in patients with recurrent skin and mucosal infections and persistent leukocytosis suggestive of a leukocyte adhesion defect. Tests of oxidative metabolic activity and killing should be performed in patients with unusual gram-negative or *Aspergillus* tissue infections suggestive of CGD.

Management of Immunodeficiency Disorders

Proper management of immunodeficiency disorders (as described earlier) can enhance markedly both the quality of life and life expectancy. Although some children with immunodeficiency disorders have serious problems with autoimmune disease, malignancy, or both, the vast majority of morbidity and mortality results from infections. Therefore, this discussion is limited to the general principles of managing infectious complications of immunodeficiency.

EDUCATION

After thorough characterization of the immunologic abnormality, the first step in management is to educate the family and, when he or she is old enough, the patient as to environmental risks, how to take medications, and precisely when and where to seek medical care. Families of patients with inherited disorders (e.g., CGD) should receive genetic counseling and be offered the option of prenatal screening if it is available for the disease in question.

EVALUATION FOR INFECTION

Patients with known immunodeficiency disorders should be evaluated promptly and thoroughly for unexplained fevers or any other indication of infection. Immunodeficient persons are susceptible to a wide variety of pathogens, their responses to appropriate therapy may be slow, and they often require prolonged treatment. Thus, every effort should be made to identify the infecting organism so that treatment can be specific. Unless the pathogen is known, extended courses of empiric broad-spectrum coverage may be required, and this can lead to superinfection due to multiply resistant pathogens.

TREATMENT

Disease-specific therapy already has been discussed. In general, patients with immunodeficiency who are susceptible to bacterial infections should be treated empirically and aggressively with antibiotics at the first indication of infection. Antifungal therapy should be added empirically in patients with increased risk of fungal infection (e.g., patients with cell-mediated immune and neutrophil disorders) if there is not a prompt response to antibacterial therapy. Once a definitive diagnosis has been made, treatment should be tailored to the pathogen. The duration of therapy must be individualized, but, in general, patients with abnormal immune systems should be treated longer than normal hosts who have comparable infections.

Bone marrow transplants have been successful in a few patients with specific immunologic disorders, including SCID, Wiskott-Aldrich syndrome,[341] and CGD.[232, 455] Gene therapy suggests new possibilities for correcting certain immunologic defects. It already has demonstrated substantial promise in adenosine deaminase deficiency,[68] and it is under active investigation for the correction of the phagocyte defect in CGD.[290, 388]

PREVENTION

Patients and household members should be immunized with appropriate vaccines as soon as possible after diagnosis of immunodeficiency.[115] It should be borne in mind that although many immunodeficient patients, such as those with XLA, cannot respond to immunizations, immunization of household members and other close contacts with vaccines may reduce the patients' likelihood of infection. Patients with complement deficiencies, asplenia, and sickle cell disease should be immunized with vaccines directed against encapsulated organisms, such as meningococci, pneumococci, and *H. influenzae.* However, it should be remembered that these persons may not have normal responses to immunization, and, therefore, if it is possible, their antibody responses to these vaccines should be measured; if they are low, these persons should receive extra doses of the vaccines.

Selected patients with recurrent or particularly severe bacterial or fungal infections may require prophylactic antibacterial or antifungal therapy. The benefits of long-term antimicrobial therapy must be weighed carefully, however, against the risks of rapid emergence of multiply resistant organisms.

As has been discussed, IFN-γ reduces the incidence and severity of infections in patients with CGD.[242] Further understanding of the role of cytokines in host defense may permit them to be used more widely for modulating abnormal responses to infection (see Chapter 236, Immunomodulating Agents).

References

1. Abraham, E., Wunderink, R., Silverman, H., et al.: Efficacy and safety of monoclonal antibody to human tumor necrosis factor-α in patients with sepsis syndrome. J. A. M. A. *273*:934–941, 1995.
2. Abramson, J. S., Wheeler, J. G., and Quie, P. G.: The polymorphonuclear leukocyte system. *In* Stiehm, E. R. (ed.): Immunologic Disorders in Infants and Children. 4th ed. Philadelphia, W. B. Saunders, 1996, pp. 94–112.

3. Abramson, J. S., Mills, E. L., Sayer, M. K., et al.: Recurrent infections and delayed separation of the umbilical cord in an infant with abnormal phagocytic cell locomotion and oxidative response during opsonized particle phagocytosis. J. Pediatr. *99*:887–894, 1981.
4. Abughali, N., Berger, M., and Tosi, M. F.: Deficient total cell content of CR3 (CD11b) in neonatal neutrophils. Blood *83*:1086–1092, 1994.
5. Abughali, N., Dubyak, G., and Tosi, M. F.: Impairment of chemoattractant-stimulated hexose uptake in neonatal neutrophils. Blood *82*:2182–2187, 1993.
6. Adamkin, D., Stitzel, A., Urmson, J., et al.: Activity of the alternative pathway of complement in the newborn infant. J. Pediatr. *93*:604–608, 1978.
7. Adderson, E. E., Schackelford, P. G., Quinn, A., et al.: Restricted Ig H chain V gene usage in the human antibody response to *Haemophilus influenzae* type b capsular polysaccharide. J. Immunol. *147*:1667–1674, 1991.
8. Adenyi-Jones, S. C. A., Faden, H., Ferdon, M. B., et al.: Systemic and local immune responses to enhanced-potency inactivated poliovirus vaccine in premature and term infants. J. Pediatr. *120*:686–689, 1992.
9. Adinolfi, M.: Human complement. Onset and site of synthesis during fetal life. Am. J. Dis. Child. *131*:1015–1023, 1977.
10. Aggarwal, J., Khan, A. J., Diamond, S., et al.: Lazy leukocyte syndrome in a black infant. J. Natl. Med. Assoc. *77*:928–931, 1985.
11. Aggett, P. J., Harries, J. T., Harvey, B. A. M., et al.: An inherited defect of neutrophil mobility in Shwachman syndrome. J. Pediatr. *94*:391–394, 1979.
12. Albelda, S. M., Muller, W. A., Buck, C. A., et al.: Molecular and cellular properties of PECAM-1 (endoCAM/CD31): A novel vascular cell-cell adhesion molecule. J. Cell Biol. *114*:1059–1068, 1991.
13. Alford, C. A., Stagno, S., and Reynolds, D. W.: Diagnosis of chronic perinatal infections. Am. J. Dis. Child. *129*:455–463, 1975.
14. Allen, R. C., Armitage, R. J., Conley, M. E., et al.: CD40 ligand gene defects responsible for X-linked hyper-IgM syndrome. Science *259*:990–993, 1993.
15. Allen, R. C., and Loose, L. D.: Phagocytic activation of a luminol-dependent chemiluminescence in rabbit alveolar and peritoneal macrophages. Biochem. Biophys. Res. *69*:245–252, 1976.
16. Ambrosino, D. M., Siber, G. R., Chilmonczyk, B. A., et al.: An immunodeficiency characterized by impaired antibody responses to polysaccharides. N. Engl. J. Med. *316*:790–793, 1987.
17. Ambrosino, D. M., Sood, S. K., Lee, M. C., et al.: IgG1, IgG2, and IgM responses to two *Haemophilus influenzae* type b conjugate vaccines in young infants. Pediatr. Infect. Dis. J. *11*:855–859, 1992.
18. Ambrosino, D. M., Umetsu, D. T., Siber, G. R., et al.: Selective defect in the antibody response to *Haemophilus influenzae* type b in children with recurrent infections and normal serum IgG subclass levels. J. Allergy Clin. Immunol. *81*:1175–1179, 1988.
19. Ambruso, D. R., Edward, R. B., McCabe, M. D., et al.: Infectious and bleeding complications in patients with glycogenosis 1b: Relationship to neutrophil and platelet function. Am. J. Dis. Child. *139*:691–697, 1985.
20. Ament, M. E., Ochs, H. D., and Davis, S. D.: Structure and function of the gastrointestinal tract in primary immunodeficiency syndromes: A study of 39 patients. Medicine *52*:227–248, 1973.
21. Ammann, A. J., and Hong, R.: Selective IgA deficiency and autoimmunity. Clin. Exp. Immunol. *7*:833–838, 1970.
22. Ammann, A. J., and Hong, R.: Selective IgA deficiency: Presentation of 30 cases and a review of the literature. Medicine *60*:223–236, 1971.
23. Anderson, D. C., Freeman, K. B., Hughes, B. J., et al.: Secretory determinants of impaired adherence and mobility of neonatal PMNs. Pediatr. Res. 19:257A, 1985.
24. Anderson, D. C., Hughes, B. J., and Smith, C. W.: Abnormal mobility of neonatal polymorphonuclear leukocytes. Relationship to impaired redistribution of surface adhesion sites by chemotactic factor or colchicine. J. Clin. Invest. *68*:863–874, 1981.
25. Anderson, D. C., Wibble, L. J., Hughes, B. J., et al.: Cytoplasmic microtubules in polymorphonuclear leukocytes: Effects of chemotactic stimulation and colchicine. Cell *31*:719–729, 1982.
26. Anderson, D. C., Hughes, B. J., Wible, L. J., et al.: Impaired motility of neonatal PMN leukocytes: Relationship to abnormalities of cell orientation and assembly of microtubules in chemotactic gradients. J. Leukocyte Biol. *36*:1–15, 1984.
27. Anderson, D. C., Rothlein, R., Martin, S. D., et al.: Impaired transendothelial migration of neonatal neutrophils: Abnormalities of MAC-I (CD11/CD18) dependent adherence reactions. Blood *76*:2613–2621, 1990.
28. Anderson, D. C., Schmalstieg, F. C., Arnaout, M. A., et al.: Abnormalities of polymorphonuclear leukocyte function associated with a heritable deficiency of high molecular weight surface glycoproteins (gp 138): Common relationship to diminished cell adherence. J. Clin. Invest. *74*:546–557, 1984.
29. Anderson, D. C., Schmalsteig, F., Finegold, M. J., et al.: The severe and moderate phenotypes of heritable MAC-1, LFA-1, P150,95 deficiency: Their quantitative definition and relation to leukocyte dysfunction and clinical features. J. Infect. Dis. *152*:668–689, 1985.
30. Anderson, D. C., Smith, C. W., and Springer, T. A.: Leukocyte adhesion deficiency and other disorders of leukocyte motility. *In* Scriver, C. R., Beaudet, A. L., Sly, W. S., et al. (eds.): The Metabolic Basis of Inherited Disease. New York, McGraw-Hill, 1989, pp. 2751–2777.
31. Arai, K.-I., Lee, F., Miyajima, A., et al.: Cytokines: Coordinators of immune and inflammatory responses. Annu. Rev. Biochem. *59*:783–836, 1990.
32. Arnaout, M. A., Pitt, J., Cohen, H. J., et al.: Deficiency of a granulocyte membrane glycoprotein (gp 150) in a boy with recurrent bacterial infections. N. Engl. J. Med. *306*:693–699, 1982.
33. Arnaout, M. A.: Structure and function of the leukocyte adhesion molecules CD11/CD18. Blood *75*:1037–1050, 1990.
34. Arnaout, M. A., Wang, E. A., Clark, S. C., et al.: Human recombinant GM-CSF increases cell to cell adhesion and surface expression of adhesion-promoting surface glycoproteins on mature granulocytes. J. Clin. Invest. *78*:597–601, 1986.
35. Aruffo, A., Farrington, M., Hollenbaugh, D., et al.: The CD40 ligand, gp39, is defective in activated T cells from patients with X-linked hyper-IgM syndrome. Cell *72*:291–300, 1993.
36. Babior, B. M.: The nature of the NADPH oxidase. *In* Gallin, J. I., and Fauci, A. S. (eds.): Advances in Host Defense Mechanisms. New York, Raven Press, 1983, pp. 91–119.
37. Babior, B. M., Kipnes, R. S., and Curnutte, J. T.: Biological defense mechanisms: The production by leukocytes of superoxide, a potential bactericidal agent. J. Clin. Invest. *52*:741–744, 1973.
38. Babior, B. M., Rosin, R. E., McMurrich, B. J., et al.: Arrangement of the respiratory burst oxidase in the plasma membrane of the neutrophil. J. Clin. Invest. *67*:1724–1730, 1981.
39. Baehner, R. L., Johnston, R. B., and Nathan, D. G.: Comparative study of the metabolic and bactericidal characteristics of severely glucose-6-phosphate dehydrogenase-deficient polymorphonuclear leukocytes and leukocytes from children with chronic granulomatous disease. J. Reticul. Soc. *12*:150–160, 1972.
40. Baehner, R. L., Karnovsky, M. J., and Karnovsky, M. L.: Degranulation of leukocytes in chronic granulomatous disease. J. Clin. Invest. *48*:187–192, 1969.
41. Bagby, G. J., Plessala, K. J., Wilson, L. A., et al.: Divergent efficacy of antibody to tumor necrosis factor-α in intravascular and peritonitis models of sepsis. J. Infect. Dis. *163*:83–88, 1991.
42. Bainton, D. F.: Developmental biology of neutrophils and eosinophils. *In* Gallin, J. I., Goldstein, I. M., Snyderman, R. (eds.): Inflammation: Basic Principles and Clinical Correlates. 2nd ed. New York, Raven Press, 1992, pp.303–324.
43. Baker, C. J., and Edwards, M. S.: Group B streptococcal infections. *In* Remington, J. S., Klein, J. O. (eds.): Infectious Diseases of the Fetus and Newborn Infant. 4th ed. Philadelphia, W. B. Saunders, 1995, pp. 980–1054.
44. Ballow, M., Cates, K. L., Rowe, J. C., et al.: Development of the immune system in very low birth weight (less than 1500 g) premature infants: Concentrations of plasma immunoglobulins and patterns of infections. Pediatr. Res. *20*:899–904, 1986.
45. Banatvala, N., Davies, J., Kanariou, M., et al.: Hypogammaglobulinaemia associated with normal or increased IgM (the hyper IgM syndrome): A case series review. Arch. Dis. Child. *71*:150–152, 1994.
46. Baraff, L. J., Leake, R. D., Burstyn, D. G., et al.: Immunologic response to early and routine DTP immunization in infants. Pediatrics *73*:37–42, 1984.
47. Barbouche, R., Forveille, M., Fischer, A., et al.: Spontaneous IgM autoantibody production *in vitro* by B lymphocytes of normal human neonates. Scand. J. Immunol. *35*:659–667, 1992.
48. Barrett, D. J., and Boyle, M. D. P.: Restoration of complement function in vivo by plasma infusion in factor I (C3b inactivator) deficiency. J. Pediatr. *104*:76–81, 1984.
49. Bashan, N., Potashnik, R., Hagay, Y., et al.: Impaired glucose transport in polymorphonuclear leukocytes in glycogen storage disease 1b. Inherit. Metab. Dis. *10*:234–239, 1987.
50. Bass, D. A., Parce, J. W., Dechatelet, L. R., et al.: Flow cytometric studies of oxidative product formation by neutrophils: A graded response to membrane stimulation. J. Immunol. *130*:1910–1917, 1983.
51. Bastian, J., Law, S., Vogler, L., et al.: Prediction of persistent immunodeficiency in the DiGeorge anomaly. J. Pediatr. *115*:391–396, 1989.
52. Beaudet, A. L., Anderson, D. C., Michels, V. V., et al.: Neutropenia and impaired neutrophil migration in type 1B glycogen storage disease. J. Pediatr. *97*:906–910, 1980.
53. Bennett, J. E.: *Aspergillus* species. *In* Mandell, G. L., Bennett, J. E., and Dolin, R. (eds.): Principles and Practice of Infectious Diseases. 4th ed. New York, Churchill Livingstone, 1995, pp. 2306–2311.
54. Berger, M., and Frank, M. M.: The serum complement system. *In* Stiehm, E. R. (ed.): Immunologic Disorders in Infants and Children. 4th ed. Philadelphia, W. B. Saunders, 1996, pp. 133–158.
55. Berger, M., O'Shea, J., Cross, A. S., et al.: Human neutrophils increase expression of C3bi as well as C3b receptors upon activation. J. Clin. Invest. *74*:1566–1571, 1984.
56. Berger, M., Wetzler, E., August, J. T., et al.: Internalization of Type 1 complement receptors and de novo multivesicular body formation during chemoattractant-induced endocytosis in human neutrophils. J. Clin. Invest. *94*:1113–1125, 1994.
57. Berger, M., Wetzler, E. M., Wallis, R. S.: Tumor necrosis factor is the major monocyte product that increases complement receptor expression on mature human neutrophils. Blood *71*:151–158, 1988.
58. Berman, S., Lee, B., Nuss, R., et al.: Immunoglobulin G, total and subclass,

in children with or without recurrent otitis media. J. Pediatr. *121*:249–251, 1992.
59. Berman, J. E., Mellis, S. J., Pollock, R., et al.: Content and organization of the human Ig V_H locus: definition of three new V_H families and linkage to the Ig C_H locus. EMBO J. *7*:727–738, 1988.
60. Bernbaum, J. C., Daft, A., Anolik, R., et al.: Response of preterm infants to diphtheria-tetanus-pertussis immunizations. J. Pediatr. *107*:184–188, 1985.
61. Beutler, B., and Cerami, A.: The biology of cachectin/TNF-α primary mediator of the host response. Annu. Rev. Immunol. *7*:625–655, 1989.
62. Bevilacqua, M. P., and Nelson, R. M.: Selectins. J. Clin. Invest. *91*:379–387, 1993.
63. Bird, P., and Lachmann, P. J.: The regulation of IgG subclass production in man: Low serum IgG4 in inherited deficiencies of the classical pathway of C3 activation. J. Immunol. *18*:1217–1222, 1988.
64. Bishof, N. A., Welch, T. R., and Beischel, L. S.: C4B deficiency: A risk factor for bacteremia with encapsulated organisms. J. Infect. Dis. *162*:248–250, 1990.
65. Bjorkman, P. J., Saper, M. A., Samraoui, B., et al.: The foreign antigen binding site and T cell recognition regions of class I histocompatibility antigens. Nature *329*:512–518, 1987.
66. Bjorkman, P. J., Saper, M. A., Samraoui, B., et al.: Structure of the human class I histocompatibility antigen, HLA-A2. Nature *329*:506–512, 1987.
67. Black, F. L.: Why did they die? Science *258*:1739–1740, 1992.
68. Blaese, R. M.: Development of gene therapy for immunodeficiency: adenosine deaminase deficiency. Pediatr. Res. *33*:S49–S55, 1993.
69. Blume, R. S., and Wolff, S. M.: The Chediak-Higashi syndrome: Studies in four patients and a review of the literature. Medicine *51*:247–280, 1972.
70. Bohnsack, J. F., and Brown, E. J.: The role of the spleen in resistance to infection. Annu. Rev. Med. *37*:49–59, 1986.
71. Borregaard, N., Heiple, J. M., Simons, E. R., et al.: Subcellular localization of the b-cytochrome component of the human neutrophil microbicidal oxidase: Translocation during activation. J. Cell Biol. *97*:52–61, 1983.
72. Borregaard, N., Kjeldsen, L., Lollike, K., et al.: Granules and vesicles of human neutrophils. The role of endomembranes as source of plasma membrane proteins. Eur. J. Haematol. *51*:318–322, 1993.
73. Borregaard, N., Kjeldsen, L., Sengelov, H., et al.: Changes in subcellular localization and surface expression of L-selectin, alkaline phosphatase, and Mac-1 in human neutrophils during stimulation with inflammatory mediators. J. Leukoc. Biol. *56*:80–87, 1994.
74. Borzy, M. S., Ridgway, D., Noya, F. J., et al.: Successful bone marrow transplantation with split lymphoid chimerism in DiGeorge syndrome. J. Clin. Immunol. *9*:386–392, 1989.
75. Bottger, E. C., and Bitter-Suermann, D.: Complement and the regulation of humoral immune responses. Immunol. Today *8*:261–264, 1987.
76. Bowens, T. S., Ochs, H. D., Altman, L. C., et al.: Severe recurrent bacterial infections associated with defective adherence and chemotaxis in two patients with neutrophils deficient in cell-associated glycoproteins. J. Pediatr. *101*:932–940, 1982.
77. Boxer, L. A., Coates, T. D., Haak, R. A., et al.: Lactoferrin deficiency associated with altered granulocyte function. N. Engl. J. Med. *307*:404–410, 1982.
78. Boxer, L. A., Hedley-Whyte, E. T., and Stossel, T. P.: Neutrophil actin dysfunction and abnormal neutrophil behavior. N. Engl. J. Med. *29*:1093–1099, 1974.
79. Boxer, L. A., Oliver, J. M., Spielberg, S. P., et al.: Protection of granulocytes by vitamin E in glutathione synthetase deficiency. N. Engl. J. Med. *301*:901–905, 1979.
80. Boxer, L. A., Wantanbe, A. M., Rister, M., et al.: Correction of leukocyte function in Chediak-Higashi syndrome by ascorbate. N. Engl. J. Med. *295*:1041–1045, 1976.
81. Braun, J., and Stiehm, E. R.: The B-lymphocyte system. *In* Stiehm, E. R. (ed.): Immunologic Disorders in Infants and Children. 4th ed. Philadelphia, W. B. Saunders, 1996, pp. 35–74.
82. Brown, E. J.: Interaction of gram-positive microorganisms with complement. Curr. Top. Microbiol. Immunol. *121*:159–197, 1985.
83. Brown, J. H., Jardetzky, T., Saper, M. A., et al.: A hypothetical model of the foreign antigen binding site of class II histocompatibility molecules. Nature *353*:845–850, 1988.
84. Bruce, M. C., Baley, J. E., Medvik, K. A., et al.: Impaired surface membrane expression of C3bi but not C3b receptors on neonatal neutrophils. Pediatr. Res. *21*:306–311, 1987.
85. Bruton, O. C.: Agammaglobulinemia. Pediatrics *9*:722–728, 1952.
86. Buckley, R. H.: Disorders of the IgE system. *In* Stiehm, E. R. (ed.): Immunologic Disorders in Infants and Children. 4th ed. Philadelphia, W. B. Saunders, 1996, pp. 409–422.
87. Buckley, R. H., and Becker, W. G.: Abnormalities in the regulation of human IgE synthesis. Immunol. Rev. *41*:288–314, 1978.
88. Buckley, R. H., Schiff, S. E., and Hayward, A. R.: Reduced frequency of CD45RO$^+$ T lymphocytes in blood of hyper IgE syndrome patients. J. Allergy Clin. Immunol. *87*:313–321, 1991.
89. Buckley, R. H., Wray, B. B., and Belmaker, E. Z.: Extreme hyperimmunoglobulinemia E and undue susceptibility to infection. Pediatr. *49*:59–70, 1972.
90. Bucy, R. P., Chan, C.-L., and Cooper, M. D.: Tissue localization and CD8 accessory molecule expression of Tγδ cells in humans. J. Immunol. *142*:3045–3049, 1989.
91. Buescher, E. S., Gaither, T., Nath, J., et al.: Abnormal adherence-related function of neutrophils, monocytes, and EB virus-transformed B cells in a patient with C3bi receptor deficiency. Blood *65*:1382–1390, 1985.
92. Buescher, E. S., and Gallin, J. I.: Leukocyte transfusions in chronic granulomatous disease. N. Engl. J. Med. *307*:800–803, 1982.
93. Burnett, G. W., and Scherp, H. W.: Oral Microbiology and Infectious Disease. Baltimore, Williams & Wilkins, 1968.
94. Butcher, E. C.: Leukocyte-endothelial cell recognition: Three (or more) steps to specificity and diversity. Cell *67*:1033–1036, 1991.
95. Cabau, N., Levy, F. M., Zivy, D., et al.: Evolution of titre of serum IgG in newborn. Med. Microbiol. Immunol. *162*:251–258, 1974.
96. Campbell, A. D., Long, M. W., and Wicha, M. S.: Haemonectin, a bone marrow adhesion protein specific for cells of granulocyte lineage. Nature *329*:744, 1987.
97. Cates, K. L., and Levine, R. P.: C3 binding to bacterial surfaces. *In* Cabello, F., and Pruzzo, C. (eds.): Bacteria, Complement, and the Phagocytic Cell. NATO ASI SERIES. New York, Springer-Verlag, 1988, pp. 109–128.
98. Cates, K. L., Goetz, C., Rosenberg, N., et al.: Longitudinal development of specific and functional antibody in very low birth weight premature infants. Pediatr. Res. *23*:14–22, 1988.
99. Cates, K. L., Densen, P., Lockman, J. D., et al.: C4B deficiency is not associated with meningitis or bacteremia with encapsulated bacteria. J. Infect. Dis. *165*:942–944, 1992.
100. Cates, K. L., Rowe, J. C., and Ballow, M.: The premature infant as a compromised host. Curr. Prob. Pediatr. *13*:1–63, 1983.
101. Chandra, R. K.: Fetal malnutrition and postnatal immunocompetence. Am. J. Dis. Child. *29*:450–454, 1975.
102. Chin, T. W., Stiehm, E. R., Faloon, J., and Gallin, J. I.: Corticosteroids in treatment of obstructive lesions of chronic granulomatous disease. J. Pediatr. *111*:349–352, 1987.
103. Christensen, R. D., Shigeoka, A. O., Hill, H. R., et al.: Neutrophil and bone marrow exhaustion in human and experimental neonatal sepsis. Pediatr. Res. *14*:806–808, 1980.
104. Christensen, R. D.: Hematopoiesis in the fetus and neonate. Pediatr. Res. *26*:531–535, 1989.
105. Church, J. A., Frenkel, L. D., and Wright, D. C.: T lymphocyte dysfunction, hyperimmunoglobulinemia E, recurrent bacterial infections, and defective neutrophil chemotaxis in a negro child. J. Pediatr. *88*:982–984, 1976.
106. Chusid, M. J.: Pyogenic hepatic abscess in infancy and childhood. Pediatrics *62*:554–559, 1978.
107. Clark, R. A., Malech, H. L., Gallin, J. I., et al.: Genetic variants of chronic granulomatous disease: Prevalence of deficiencies of two cytosolic components of the NADPH oxidase system. N. Engl. J. Med. *321*:647–652, 1989.
108. Clark, R. A., Root, R. K., Kimball, H. R., et al.: Defective neutrophil chemotaxis and cellular immunity in a child with recurrent infection. Ann. Intern. Med. *78*:515–519, 1973.
109. Clark, R. A., Leidal, K. G., Pearson, D. W., et al.: NADPH oxidase of human neutrophils. J. Biol. Chem. *262*:4065–4074, 1987.
110. Clark, R. A., and Kimball, H. R.: Defective granulocyte chemotaxis in the Chédiak-Higashi syndrome. J. Clin. Invest. *50*:2645–2652, 1971.
111. Cohen, M. S., Isturiz, R. E., and Malech, H. L.: Fungal infection in chronic granulomatous disease: The importance of the phagocyte in defense against fungi. Am. J. Med. *71*:59–66, 1981.
112. Cohn, M.: The a priori principles which govern immune responsiveness. *In* Cellular Basis of Immune Modulation. New York, Liss, 1989, pp. 11–44.
113. Colten, H. R.: Complement biogynthesis. Clin. Immunol. Allergy *5*:287–300, 1985.
114. Colten, H. R., and Goldberger, G.: Ontogeny of serum complement proteins. Pediatrics *64*(Suppl.):775–780, 1979.
115. Committee on Infectious Diseases: 1994 Red Book: Report of the Committee on Infectious Diseases. 23rd ed. Elk Grove Village, IL, American Academy of Pediatrics, 1994.
116. Committee on Infectious Diseases: Update on timing of hepatitis B vaccination for premature infants and for children with lapsed immunization. Pediatrics *94*:403–404, 1994.
117. Conley, M. E., and Stiehm, E. R.: Immunodeficiency disorders: General considerations. *In* Stiehm, E. R. (ed.): Immunologic Disorders in Infants and Children. 4th ed. Philadelphia, W. B. Saunders, 1996, pp. 201–252.
118. Conley, M. E., and Puck, J. M.: Carrier detection in typical and atypical X-linked agammaglobulinemia. J. Pediatr. *112*:688–694, 1988.
119. Cooper, M. R., DeChatelet, L. R., and McCall, C. E.: Complete deficiency of leukocyte glucose-6-phosphate dehydrogenase with defective bactericidal activity. J. Clin. Invest. *51*:769–778, 1972.
120. Cooper, N. R.: The classical complement pathway: Activation and regulation of the first complement component. Adv. Immunol. *37*:151–216, 1985.
121. Cooper, N. R., and Nemerow, G. R.: Complement-dependent mechanisms of virus neutralization. *In* Ross, G. D. (ed.): Immunobiology of the Complement System. Orlando, Academic Press, 1986, pp. 139–162.
122. Croft, M., Duncan, D. D., and Swain, S. L.: Response of naive antigen-specific CD4$^+$ T cells *in vitro*: Characteristics and antigen-presenting cell requirements. J. Exp. Med. *176*:1431–1437, 1992.
123. Crowley, C. A., Curnutte, J. T., Roskin, R. E., et al.: An inherited abnormal-

ity of neutrophil adhesion. Its genetic transmission and its association with a missing protein. N. Engl. J. Med. *302*:1163–1168, 1980.

124. Cunningham-Rundles, C.: Clinical and immunologic analyses of 103 patients with common variable immunodeficiency. J. Clin. Immunol. *9*:22–33, 1989.
125. Cunningham-Rundles, C.: Disorders of the IgA system. *In* Stiehm, E. R. (ed.): Immunologic Disorders in Infants and Children. 4th ed. Philadelphia, W. B. Saunders, 1996, pp. 423–442.
126. Cunningham-Rundles, C., Zhou, Z., Mankarious, S., et al.: Long-term use of IgA depleted intravenous immunoglobulin in immunodeficient subjects with anti-IgA antibodies. J. Clin. Immunol. *13*:272–278, 1993.
127. Cunningham-Rundles, S., Cunningham-Rundles, C., Ma, D. I., et al.: Impaired proliferative response to B lymphocyte activators in common variable immunodeficiency. J. Clin. Immunol. *1*:65–72, 1981.
128. Curnutte, J. T.: Classification of chronic granulomatous disease. Hematol. Oncol. Clin. North Am. *2*:241–252, 1988.
129. Daar, A. S., Fuggle, S. V., Fabre, J. W., et al.: The detailed distribution of MHC class II antigens in normal human organs. Transplantation *38*:293–298, 1984.
130. Daar, A. S., Fuggle, S. V., Fabre, J. W., et al.: The detailed distribution of HLA-A, B, C antigens in normal human organs. Transplantation *38*:287–292, 1984.
131. Dalgleish, A., Beverly, P., Clapham, P., et al.: The CD4 (T4) antigen is an essential component of the receptor for the AIDS retrovirus. Nature *312*:763–767, 1984.
132. Dancis, J., Osburn, J. J., and Kunz, H. W.: Studies of immunology of the newborn infant. IV. Antibody formation in the premature infant. Pediatrics *12*:151–156, 1953.
133. Davis, M. D., and Bjorkman, P. J.: T-cell antigen receptor genes and T-cell recognition. Nature *334*:395–402, 1988.
134. Davis, S. D., Schaller, J., and Wedgewood, R. J.: Job's syndrome: Recurrent "cold" staphylococcal abscesses. Lancet *1*:1013–1015, 1966.
135. Davis, A. E., III: C1 inhibitor and hereditary angioneurotic edema. Annu. Rev. Immunol. *6*:595–628, 1988.
136. DeBiagi, M., Andreani, M., and Centis, F.: Immune characterization of human fetal tissues with monoclonal antibodies. Prog. Clin. Biol. Res. *193*:89–94, 1985.
137. Decoster, A., Darcy, F., Caron, A., et al.: Anti-P30 IgA antibodies as prenatal markers of congenital toxoplasma infection. Clin. Exp. Immunol. *87*:310–315, 1992.
138. Defrance, T., Vanbervliet, F., Briere, F., et al.: Interleukin 10 and transforming growth factor β cooperate to induce anti-CD40-activated naive human B cells to secrete immunoglobulin A. J. Exp. Med. *175*:671–682, 1992.
139. Dengrove, J., Lee, E. J., Heiner, D. C., et al.: IgG and IgG subclass specific antibody responses to diphtheria and tetanus toxoids in newborns and infants given DTP immunization. Pediatr. Res. *20*:735–739, 1986.
140. Densen, P., McRill, C., and Ross, S. C.: The contribution of the alternative and classical complement pathways to gonococcal killing and C3 fixation. *In* Poolman, J. T., Zanen, H. C., Meyer, T. F., et al. (eds.): Gonococci and Meningococci. Dordrecht, The Netherlands, Kluwer Academic Publishers, 1988, pp. 693–697.
141. Densen, P.: Human complement deficiency states and infection. *In* Whaley, K., Loos, M., and Weiler, J. M. (eds.): Complement in Health and Disease. Dordrecht, The Netherlands, Kluwer Academic Publishers, 1993, pp. 173–197.
142. Densen, P., Weiler, J. M., Griffiss, J. M., et al.: Familial properdin deficiency and fatal meningococcemia. Correction of the bactericidal defect by vaccination. N. Engl. J. Med. *316*:922–926, 1987.
143. Densen, P.: Complement. *In* Mandell, G. L., Bennett, J. E., Dolin, R. (eds.): Principles and Practice of Infectious Diseases. 4th ed. New York, Churchill Livingstone, 1995, pp. 58–78.
144. Diamond, R. D.: *Cryptococcus neoformans*. *In* Mandell, G. L., Bennett, J. E., Dolin, R. (eds.): Principles and Practice of Infectious Diseases. 4th ed. New York, Churchill Livingstone, 1995, pp. 2331–2340.
145. Diamond, M. S., and Springer, T. A.: A subpopulation of Mac-1 (CD11b/CD18) molecules mediates neutrophil adhesion to ICAM-1 and fibrinogen. J. Cell. Biol. *120*:545–556, 1993.
146. Diamond, R. D., Root, R. K., and Bennett, J. E.: Factors influencing killing of *Cryptococcus neoformans* by human leukocytes in vitro. J. Infect. Dis. *163*:1108–1113, 1972.
147. DiGeorge, A. M.: A new concept of the cellular basis of immunity (discussion). J. Pediatr. *67*:907–908, 1965.
148. Dinarello, C. A.: Role of interleukin-1 and tumor necrosis factor in systemic responses to infection and inflammation. *In* Gallin, J. I., Goldstein, I. M., Snyderman, R. (eds.): Inflammation: Basic Principles and Clinical Correlates. 2nd ed. New York, Raven Press, 1992, pp. 211–232.
149. Doherty, P. C., Allan, W., and Eichelberger, M.: Roles of αβ-γδ T cell subsets in viral immunity. Annu. Rev. Immunol. *10*:123–151, 1992.
150. Donabedian, H., and Gallin, J. I.: Mononuclear cells from patients with the hyperimmunoglobulin E-recurrent infection syndrome produce and inhibitor of leukocyte chemotaxis. J. Clin. Invest. *69*:115–124, 1982.
151. Donabedian, H., and Gallin, J. I.: The hyperimmunoglobulin E recurrent infection (Job's) syndrome: A review of the NIH experience and the literature. Medicine *62*:195–207, 1983.
152. Donabedian, H., and Gallin, J. I.: Deactivation of human neutrophil chemotaxis by chemoattractants: Effect on receptors for the chemotactic factor f-met-leu-phe. J. Immunol. *127*:839–844, 1981.
153. Donowitz, G. R., and Mandell, G. L.: Clinical presentation and unusual infections in chronic granulomatous disease. *In* Gallin, J. I., and Fauci, A. S. (eds.): Advances in Host Defense Mechanisms. New York, Raven Press, 1983, pp. 55–75.
154. Donskoy, E., and Goldschneider, I.: Thymocytopoiesis is maintained by blood-borne precursors throughout postnatal life. A study of parabiotic mice. J. Immunol. *148*:1604–1612, 1992.
155. Douglas, S. D., and Yoder, M. C.: The mononuclear phagocyte and dendritic cell systems. *In* Stiehm, E. R. (ed.): Immunologic Disorders in Infants and Children. 4th ed. Philadelphia, W. B. Saunders, 1996, pp. 113–132.
156. Doyle, C., and Stominger, J. L.: Interaction between CD4 and class II MHC molecules mediates cell adhesion. Nature *330*:256–259, 1987.
157. Drew, J. H., and Arroyave, C. M.: The complement system of the newborn infant. Biol. Neonate *37*:209–217, 1980.
158. Edwards, M. S.: Complement in neonatal infections: An overview. Pediatr. Infect. Dis. *5*:S168–S170, 1986.
159. Edwards, J. E.: *Candida* species. *In* Mandell, G. L., Bennett, J. E., Dolin, R. (eds.): Principles and Practice of Infectious Diseases. 4th ed. New York, Churchill Livingstone, 1995, pp. 2289–2306.
160. Eichenfield, L. F., and Johnston, R. B., Jr.: Secondary disorders of the complement system. Am. J. Dis. Child. *143*:595–602, 1989.
161. Einhorn, M. S., Granoff, D. M., Nahm, M. H., et al.: Concentrations of antibodies in paired maternal and infant sera: Relationship to IgG subclass. J. Pediatr. *111*:783–788, 1987.
162. Enders, G.: Serologic test combinations for safe detection of rubella infections. Rev. Infect. Dis. *7*:S113–S122, 1985.
163. Engh, C. A., Hughes, J. L., Abrams, R. C., et al.: Osteomyelitis in the patient with sickle-cell disease. J. Bone Joint Surg. *53*:1–15, 1971.
164. Englund, J. A., Glezen, W. P., Turner C., et al.: Transplacental antibody transfer following maternal immunization with polysaccharide and conjugate *Haemophilus influenzae* type b vaccines. J. Infect. Dis. *171*:99–105, 1995.
165. Erdei, A., Fust, G., and Gergely, J.: The role of C3 in the immune response. Immunol. Today *12*:332–337, 1991.
166. Eynon, E. E., and Parker, D. C.: Small B cells as antigen-presenting cells in the induction of tolerance to soluble protein antigens. J. Exp. Med. *175*:131–138, 1992.
167. Falk, K., Rotzschke, O., Deres, K., et al.: Identification of naturally processed viral nonapeptides allows their quantification in infected cells and suggests an allele-specific T cell epitope forecast. J. Exp. Med. *174*:425–434, 1991.
168. Falk, K., Rotzschke, O., Stevanovic, S., et al.: Allele-specific motifs revealed by sequencing of self-peptides eluted from MHC molecules. Nature *351*:290–296, 1991.
169. Fanger, M., Shen, L., Graziano, R., Guyre, P.: Cytotoxicity mediated by human Fc receptors for IgG. Immunol. Today *10*:92–99, 1989.
170. Fearon, D. T., and Austen, K. F.: Properdin: Binding to C3b and stabilization of the C3b-dependent C3 convertase. J. Exp. Med. *142*:856–863, 1975.
171. Fearon, D. T., Ruddy, S., Schur, P. H., et al.: Activation of the properdin pathway of complement in patients with gram-negative bacteremia. N. Engl. J. Med. *292*:937–940, 1975.
172. Fearon, D. T., and Collins, L. A.: Increased expression of C3b receptors on polymorphonuclear leukocytes induced by chemotactic factors and by purification procedures. J. Immunol. *130*:370–375, 1983.
173. Fearon, D. T., and Austen, K. F.: The alternative pathway of complement—A system for host resistance to microbial infection. N. Engl. J. Med. *303*:259–263, 1980.
174. Ferguson, S. E., and Thompson, C. B. A.: A new break in V(D)J recombination. Curr. Biol. *3*:51–53, 1993.
175. Ferriani, V. P. L., Barbosa, J. E., and de Carvelho, I. F.: Serum haemolytic classical and alternative pathways of complement in infancy: Age-related changes. Acta Paediatr. Scand. *79*:322–327, 1990.
176. Figueroa, J. E., and Densen, P.: Infectious diseases associated with complement deficiencies. Clin. Microbiol. Rev. *4*:359–395, 1991.
177. Fink, C. W., Miller, W. E., Dorward, B., et al.: The formation of macroglobulin antibodies. II. Studies on neonatal infants and older children. J. Clin. Invest. *41*:1422–1428, 1962.
178. Fireman, P., Zuchowski, D. A., and Taylor, P. M.: Development of the human complement system. J. Immunol. *103*:25–31, 1969.
179. Fisher, A., Trung, P. H., Descamps-Latsdra, B., et al.: Bone marrow-transplantation for inborn error of phagocytic cells associated with defective adherence, chemotaxis, and oxidative response during opsonized particle phagocytosis. Lancet *2*:473–475, 1983.
180. Fisher, C. L., Dhainaut, J. F., Opal, S. M., et al.: Recombinant human interleukin-1 receptor antagonist in the treatment of patients with severe sepsis. J. A. M. A. *271*:1836–1843, 1994.
181. Fleishmann, J., and Lehrer, R. I.: Phagocytic mechanism in host response. *In* Howard, D. H. (ed.): Fungi Pathogenic for Humans and Animals, Part B2. New York, Marcel Dekker, 1985, pp. 123–149.
182. Fleming, A. F., Storey, J., Molineaux, L., et al.: Abnormal haemoglobins in the Sudan savanna of Nigeria: I. Prevalence of haemoglobins and

relationships between sickle cell trait, malaria, and survival. Ann. Trop. Med. Parasitol. *73*:161–172, 1979.

183. Frank, M. M., Gelfand, J. A., and Atkinson, J. P.: Hereditary angioedema: The clinical syndrome and its management. Ann. Intern. Med. *84*:580–593, 1976.
184. Fremont, D. H., Matsumura, M., Stura, E. A., et al.: Crystal structures of two viral peptides in complex with murine MHC class I H-2K^b. Science *257*:919–934, 1992.
185. Frydman, M., Etzioni, A., Eidlitz-Markus, T., et al.: Rambam-Hasharon syndrome of psychomotor retardation, short stature, defective neutrophil motility, and Bombay phenotype. Am. J. Med. Genet. *44*:297–302, 1992.
186. Fuchs, E. J., and Matzinger, P. B.: Cells turn off virgin but not memory T cells. Science *258*:1156–1159, 1992.
187. Gabbay, J. E., and Almeida, R. P.: Antibiotic peptides and serine protease homologs in human polymorphonuclear leukocytes: Defensins and azurocidin. Curr. Opin. Immunol. *5*:97–102, 1993.
188. Gallin, J. I., Fletcher, M. P., Seligmann, B. E., et al.: Human neutrophil-specific granule deficiency: A model to assess the role of neutrophil-specific granules in the evolution of the inflammatory response. Blood *59*:1317–1329, 1982.
189. Gallin, J. I., Buescher, E. S., and Seligmann, B. E.: Recent advances in chronic granulomatous disease. Ann. Intern. Med. *99*:657–674, 1983.
190. Ganz, T., Selsted, M. E., Szklarek, D., et al.: Defensins: Natural peptide antibiotics of human neutrophils. J. Clin. Invest. *76*:1427–1435, 1985.
191. Gathings, W. E., Lawton, A. R., and Cooper, M. D.: Immunofluorescent studies of the development of pre-B cells, B lymphocytes and immunoglobulin isotype diversity in humans. Eur. J. Immunol. *7*:804–810, 1977.
192. Geelan, S. P. M., Bazemer, A. C., Gerards, L. J., et al.: Deficiencies in opsonic defense to pneumococci in the human newborn despite adequate levels of complement and specific IgG antibodies. Pediatr. Res. *27*:514–518, 1990.
193. Geha, R. S., Reinherz, E., Leung, D., et al.: Deficiency of suppressor T cells in the hyperimmunoglobulin E syndrome. J. Clin. Invest. *68*:783–791, 1981.
194. Gelfand, E. W., and Finkel, T. H.: The T-lymphocyte system. *In* Stiehm, E. R. (ed.): Immunologic Disorders in Infants and Children. 4th ed. Philadelphia, W. B. Saunders, 1996, pp. 14–34.
195. Gerard, C., and Gerard, N.: C5a anaphylatoxin and its seven transmembrane-segment receptor. Annu. Rev. Immunol. *12*:775–808, 1994.
196. Gill, T. J., III, Karasic, R. B., Antoncic, J., and Rabbin, B. S.: Long-term follow-up of children born to women immunized with tetanus toxoid during pregnancy. Am. J. Reprod. Immunol. *25*:69–71, 1991.
197. Gill, T. J., Repetti, C. F., Metlay, L. A., et al.: Transplacental immunization of the human fetus to tetanus by immunization of the mother. J. Clin Invest. *72*:987–996, 1983.
198. Goldberg, A. L., and Rock, K. L.: Proteolysis, proteasomes and antigen presentation. Nature *357*:375–379, 1992.
199. Golding, B., Muchmore, A. V., and Blaese, R. M.: Newborn and Wiskott-Aldrich patient B cells can be activated by TNP-*Brucella abortus*: Evidence that TNP-*Brucella abortus* behaves as a T-independent type 1 antigen in humans. J. Immunol. *133*:2966–2971, 1984.
200. Goldsobel, A. B., Haas, A., and Stiehm, E. R.: Bone marrow transplantation in DiGeorge syndrome. J. Pediatr. *111*:40–44, 1987.
201. Good, R. A.: Studies on agammaglobulinemia: II. Failure of plasma cell formation in the bone marrow and lymph nodes of patients with agammaglobulinemia. J. Lab. Clin. Med. *46*:167–181, 1955.
202. Gordon, D. L., and Hostetter, M. K.: Complement and host defense against microorganisms. Pathology *18*:365–375, 1986.
203. Goudemand, J., Anssens, R., Delmas-Marsalet, Y., et al.: Essai de traitement d'un cas de granulomatose familiale chronique par greffe de moelle osseuse allogenique. Arch. Fr. Pediatr. *33*:121–129, 1976.
204. Gray, G. R., Klebanoff, S. J., Stamatoyannopoulos, G., et al.: Neutrophil dysfunction, chronic granulomatous disease, and nonspherocytic haemolytic anemia caused by complete deficiency of glucose-6-phosphate dehydrogenase. Lancet 2:530–534, 1973.
205. Greenberg, F., Elder, F. F. B., Haffner, P., et al.: Cytogenic findings in a prospective series of patients with DiGeorge anomaly. Am. J. Hum. Genet. *43*:605–611, 1988.
206. Greenberg, F., Crowder, W. E., Paschall, V., et al.: Familial DiGeorge syndrome and associated partial monosomy of chromosome 22. Hum. Genet. *65*:317–319, 1984.
207. Greve, J. M., Davis, G., Meyer, A. M., et al.: The major human rhinovirus receptor is ICAM-1. Cell *56*:839–847, 1989.
208. Griffiths, P. D., Stagno, S., Pass, R. F., et al. Congenital cytomegalovirus infection: Diagnostic and prognostic significance of the detection of specific immunoglobulin M antibodies in cord serum. Pediatrics *69*:544–550, 1982.
209. Grisham, M. B., Jefferson, M. M., Melton, D. F., and Thomas, E. L.: Chlorination of endogenous amines by isolated neutrophils. Ammonia-dependent bactericidal, cytotoxic, and cytolytic activities of the chloramines. J. Biol. Chem. *259*:10404–10413, 1984.
210. Gupta, S., Rahwa, R., O'Reilly, R., et al.: Ontogeny of lymphocyte subpopulations in human fetal liver. Proc. Natl. Acad. Sci. U. S. A. *73*:919–922, 1976.
211. Harding, C. V., Collins, D. S., Slot, J. W., et al.: Liposome-encapsulated antigens are processed in lysosomes, recycled, and presented to T cells. Cell *64*:393–401, 1991.
212. Harris, B. H., Shalit, M., and Southwick, F. S.: Diminished actin polymerization by neutrophils from newborn infants. Pediatr. Res. *33*:27–31, 1992.
213. Haworth, J. C., and Dilling, L.: Concentration of gamma A-globulin in serum, saliva, and nasopharyngeal secretions of infants and children. J. Lab. Clin. Med. *67*:922–933, 1966.
214. Hayashi, S.-I., Kundisada, T., Ogawa, M., et al.: Stepwise progress of B lineage differentiation supported by interleukin 7 and other stromal cell molecules. J. Exp. Med. *171*:1683–1695, 1990.
215. Hayward, A. R., Leonard, J., Wood, C. B. S., et al.: Delayed separation of the umbilical cord, widespread infections and defective neutrophil mobility. Lancet *1*:1099–1101, 1979.
216. Hayward, A. R.: Development of lymphocyte responses and interactions in the human fetus and newborn. Immunol. Rev. *57*:39–60, 1981.
217. Heath, W. R., Kane, K. P., Mescher, M. F., et al.: Alloreactive T cells discriminate among a diverse set of endogenous peptides. Proc. Natl. Acad. Sci. U. S. A. *88*:5101–5105, 1991.
218. Heinzel, F.: Antibodies. *In* Mandell, G. L., Bennett, J. E., Dolin, R. (eds.): Principles and Practice of Infectious Diseases. 4th ed. New York, Churchill Livingstone, 1995, pp. 36–57.
219. Hermaszewski, R. A., and Webster, A. D. B.: Primary hypogammaglobulinaemia: A survey of clinical manifestations and complications. Q. J. Med. *86*:31–42, 1993.
220. Herrod, H. G.: Management of the patient with IgG subclass deficiency and/or selective antibody deficiency. Ann. Allergy *70*:3–11, 1993.
221. Herrod, H. G., Gross, S., and Insel, R.: Selective antibody deficiency to *Haemophilus influenzae* type b capsular polysaccharide vaccination in children with recurrent respiratory tract infection. J. Clin. Immunol. *9*:429–434, 1989.
222. Herrod, H. G.: Clinical significance of IgG subclasses. Curr. Opin. Pediatr. *5*:696–699, 1993.
223. Hewlett, E. L.: Toxins and other virulence factors. *In* Mandell, G. L., Bennett, J. E., Dolin, R. (eds.): Principles and Practice of Infectious Diseases. 4th ed. New York, Churchill Livingstone, 1995, pp. 2–10.
224. Hibbs, M. L., Wardlaw, A. J., Stacker, S. A., et al.: Transfection of cells from patients with leukocyte adhesion deficiency with an intergrin B subunit (CD18) restores lymphocyte function-associated antigen-1 expression and function. J. Clin. Invest. *85*:674–681, 1990.
225. Hill, H. R.: Clinical disorders of leukocyte functions. *In* Snyderman, R. (ed.): Current Topics in Immunology. New York, Plenum Press, 1984, pp. 345–393.
226. Hill, H. R., and Quie, P. G.: Raised serum IgE levels and defective neutrophil chemotaxis in three children with eczema and recurrent bacterial infections. Lancet *1*:183–187, 1974.
227. Hill, H. R.: Biochemical, structural, and functional abnormalities of polymorphonuclear leukocytes in the neonate. Pediatr. Res. 22:375–382, 1987.
228. Hilmo, A., and Howard, T. H.: F-Actin content of neonate and adult neutrophils. Blood *69*:945–951, 1987.
229. Hoffman, A. A., Hayward, A. R., Kurnick, J. T., et al.: Presentation of antigen by human newborn monocytes to maternal tetanus toxoid specific T-cell blasts. J. Clin. Immunol. *1*:217–221, 1981.
230. Hofman, F. M., Danilovs, J. A., and Taylor, C. R.: HLA-DR (Ia)-positive dendritic-like cells in human fetal nonlymphoid tissues. Transplantation *27*:590–594, 1984.
231. Holland, S. M., and Gallin, J. I.: Evaluation of the patient with suspected immunodeficiency. *In* Mandell, G. L., Bennett, J. E., Dolin, R. (eds.): Principles and Practice of Infectious Diseases. 4th. ed. New York, Churchill Livingstone, 1995, pp. 149–158.
232. Hong, R.: Disorders of the T-cell system. *In* Stiehm, E. R. (ed.): Immunologic Disorders in Infants and Children. 4th ed. Philadelphia, W. B. Saunders, 1996, pp. 339–408.
233. Horwitz, M. A.: Interactions between *Legionella pneumophilia* and human mononuclear phagocytes. *In* Thornsberry, C., Balows, A., Feeley, J. C., et al. (eds.): Legionella. Proceeding of the 2nd International Symposium. Washington, D. C., American Society for Microbiology, 1984, pp. 159–166.
234. Hostetter, M. K.: Serotypic variations among virulent pneumococci in deposition and degradation of covalently bound C3b: Implications for phagocytosis and antibody production. J. Infect. Dis. *153*:682–693, 1986.
235. Hostetter, M. K., Kreuger, R. A., and Schmeling, D. J.: The biochemistry of opsonization: Central role of the reactive thiolester of the third component of complement. J. Infect. Dis. *150*:653–661, 1984.
236. Hostoffer, R. W., Krukovets, I., and Berger, M.: Enhancement by tumor necrosis factor-a of Fca receptor expression and IgA-mediated superoxide generation and killing of *Pseudomonas aeruginosa* by polymorphonuclear leukocytes. J. Infect. Dis. *170*:82–87, 1994.
237. Hostoffer, R. W., Krukovets, I., and Berger, M.: Increased FcαR expression and IgA-mediated function on neutrophils induced by chemoattractants. J. Immunol. *150*:4532–4540, 1993.
238. Hugli, T. E.: Structure and function of the anaphylatoxins. Springer Semin. Immunopathol. *7*:193–220, 1984.
239. Hunt, D. F., Henderson, R. A., Shababowitz, J., et al.: Characterization of peptides bound to the class I MHC molecule HLA-A2.1 by mass spectrometry. Science *255*:1261–1263, 1992.
240. Hunt, D. F., Michel, H., Dickinson, T. A., et al.: Peptides presented to the

immune system by the murine class II major histocompatibility complex molecule I-A[d]. Science *256*:1817–1820, 1992.
241. Insel, R. A., Amstey, M., Woodin, K., et al.: Maternal immunization to prevent infectious diseases in the neonate or infant. Int. J. Technol. Assess. Health Care *10*:143–153, 1994.
242. International Chronic Granulomatous Disease Cooperative Study Group: A controlled trial of interferon gamma to prevent infection in chronic granulomatous diseases. N. Engl. J. Med. *324*:509–516, 1991.
243. Jackson, S. H., Gallin, J. I., and Holland, S. M.: The $p47_{phox}$ mouse knockout model of chronic granulomatous disease. J. Exp. Med. *182*:751–758, 1995.
244. Johnston, R. B., Jr.: The complement system in host defense and inflammation: The cutting edges of a double edged sword. Pediatr. Infect. Dis. J. *12*:933–941, 1993.
245. Johnston, R. B., and Baehner, R. L.: Chronic granulomatous disease: Correlation between pathogenesis and clinical findings. Pediatrics *48*:730–737, 1971.
246. Johnston, R. B., and Newman, S. L.: Chronic granulomatous disease. Pediatr. Clin. North Am. *24*:365–376, 1977.
247. Johnston, R. B., Jr.: Disorders of the Complement System. *In* Stiehm, E. R. (ed.): Immunologic Disorders in Infants and Children. 4th ed. Philadelphia, W. B. Saunders, 1996, pp. 133–158.
248. Joiner, K. A.: Complement evasion by bacteria and parasites. Ann. Rev. Microbiol. *42*:201–230, 1988.
249. Joiner, K. A., Brown, E. J., and Frank, M. M.: Complement and bacteria: Chemistry and biology in host defense. Ann. Rev. Immunol. *2*:461–491, 1984.
250. Jones, D. H., Schmalsteig, F. C., Dempsey, K., et al.: Subcellular distribution and mobilization of Mac-1 (CD11b/CD18) in neonatal neutrophils. Blood *75*:488–498, 1990.
251. Kabelitz, D.: Function and specificity of human γδ-positive T cells. Crit. Rev. Immunol. *11*:281–303, 1992.
252. Kamani, N., August, C. S., Douglas, S. D., et al.: Transplantation in chronic granulomatous disease. J. Pediatr. *105*:42–46, 1984.
253. Kappler, J. W., Roehm, N., and Marrack, P.: T cell tolerance by clonal elimination in the thymus. Cell *49*:273–280, 1987.
254. Kew, R. R., and Wester, R. O.: Ge-globulin (vitamin D-binding protein) enhances the neutrophil chemotactic activity of C5a and C5a des arg. J. Clin. Invest. *82*:364–369, 1988.
255. Klatzman, D., Champagne, E., Chamaret, S., et al.: T-lymphocyte T4 molecule behaves as a receptor for human retrovius LAV. Nature *312*:767–770, 1984.
256. Klein, R. B., Fisher, T. J., Gard, S. E., et al.: Decreased mononuclear and polymorphonuclear chemotaxis in human newborn infants and young children. Pediatrics *60*:467–472, 1977.
257. Klein, J. O., and Marcy, S. M.: Bacterial sepsis and meningitis. *In* Remington, J. S., and Klein, J. O. (eds.): Infectious Diseases of the Fetus and Newborn Infant. 4th ed. Philadelphia, W. B. Saunders, 1995, pp. 835–890.
258. Kluin-Nelemans, H. C., van Velzen-Blad, H., van Helden, H. P. T., et al.: Functional deficiency of complement factor D in a monozygous twin. Clin. Exp. Immunol. *58*:724–730, 1984.
259. Kohl, S., Springer, T. A., Shmalsteig, F. C., et al.: Defective natural killer cytotoxicity and polymorphonuclear leukocyte antibody-dependent cellular cytotoxicity in patients with LFA-1/OKM-1 deficiency. J. Immunol. *133*:2972–2981, 1984.
260. Kohler, P. F., and Farr, R. S.: Elevation of cord over maternal IgG immunoglobulin—Evidence for an active placental IgG transport. Nature *210*:1070–1071, 1966.
261. Kohler, P. F.: Maturation of the human complement system. I. Onset of the time and site of fetal C1q, C4, C3 and C5 synthesis. J. Clin. Invest. *52*:671–677, 1973.
262. Konstan, M., and Berger, M.: Infection and inflammation in the lung in cystic fibrosis. *In* Davis, P. (ed.): Cystic Fibrosis. New York, Marcel Dekker, 1993, pp. 221–276.
263. Kramer, N., Perez, H. D., and Goldstein, I. M.: An immunoglobulin (IgG) inhibitor of polymorphonuclear leukocyte motility in a patient with recurrent infection. N. Engl. J. Med. *303*:1253–1258, 1980.
264. Kraus, J. C., Mayo-Bond, L., Rogers, C. E., et al.: An in vivo animal model of gene therapy for leukocyte adhesion deficiency. J. Clin. Invest. *88*:1412–1417, 1991.
265. Krause, P. J., Maderazo, E. G., and Scroggs, M.: Abnormalities of neutrophil adherence in newborns. Pediatrics *69*:184–187, 1982.
266. Kretschmer, R., Say, B., Brown, D., et al.: Congenital aplasia of the thymus gland (DiGeorge's syndrome). N. Engl. J. Med. *279*:1295–1301, 1968.
267. Kunkel, S. L., and Strieter, R. M.: Cytokine networking in lung inflammation. Hosp. Pract. *25*:63–76, 1990.
268. Lababidi, Z., Hakami, N., and Almond, C.: Chronic granulomatous disease associated with acute pericarditis with tamponade. Missouri Med. *74*:170–171, 1970.
269. Lachmann, P. J.: The control of homologous lysis. Immunol. Today *12*:312–315, 1991.
270. Lammer, E. J., and Opitz, J. M.: The DiGeorge anomaly as a developmental field defect. Am. J. Med. Genet. 2(Suppl.):113–127, 1986.
271. Lasky, L. A.: Selectins: Interpreters of cell-specific carbohydrate information during inflammation. Science *258*:964–969, 1992.
272. Lassiter, H. A., Wilson, J. L., Feldhoff, R. C., et al.: Supplemental complement component C9 enhances the capacity of neonatal serum to kill multiple isolates of pathogenic *Escherichia coli*. Pediatr. Res. *35*:389–396, 1994.
273. Lau, Y.-L., Tam, A. Y. C., and Ng, K. W.: Clinical laboratory observations. Response of preterm infants to hepatitis B vaccine. J. Pediatr. *121*:962–965, 1992.
274. Law, S. K., Lichtenberg, N. A., and Levine, R. P.: Covalent binding and hemolytic activity of complement proteins. Proc. Natl. Acad. Sci. U. S. A. *77*:7194–7198, 1980.
275. Lawton, A. R., Cooper, M. D.: Development and function of the immune system. *In* Stiehm, E. R. (ed.): Immunologic Disorders in Infants and Children. 4th ed. Philadelphia, W. B. Saunders, 1996, pp. 1–13.
276. Lazarus, G. M., and Neu, H. C.: Agents responsible for infection in chronic granulomatous disease of childhood. J. Pediatr. *86*:415–417, 1975.
277. Lebecque, S. G., and Gearhart, P. J.: Boundaries of somatic mutation in rearranged immunoglobulin genes: 5′ boundary is near the promoter, and 3′ boundary is > 1 kb from V(D)J gene. J. Exp. Med. *172*:1717–1727, 1990.
278. Lederman, H. M., and Winkelstein, J. A.: X-linked agammaglobulinemia: An analysis of 96 patients. Medicine *64*:145–156, 1985.
279. Lee, S. I., Heiner, D. C., and Wara, D.: Development of serum IgG subclass levels in children. Monogr. Allergy *19*:108–121, 1986.
280. Lehrer, R. I., and Cline, M. J.: Leukocyte myeloperoxidase deficiency and disseminated candidiasis: The role of myeloperoxidase in resistance to candida infection. J. Clin. Invest. *48*:1478–1488, 1969.
281. Lehrer, R. I., and Ganz, T.: Antimicrobial polypeptides of human neutrophils. Blood *76*:2169–2181, 1990.
282. Lehrer, R. I., Lichtenstein, A. K., and Ganz, T.: Defensins: Antimicrobial and cytotoxic peptides of mammalian cells. Annu. Rev. Immunol. *11*:105–128, 1993.
283. Levy, O., Ooi, C. E., Weiss, J., et al.: Individual and synergistic effects of rabbit granulocyte proteins on *Escherichia coli*. J. Clin. Invest. *94*:672–682, 1994.
284. Levy, O., Weiss, J., Zarember, K., et al.: Antibacterial 15-kDa protein isoforms (p15s) are members of a novel family of leukocyte proteins. J. Biol. Chem. *268*:6058–6063, 1993.
285. Lewis, D. B., and Wilson, C. B.: Developmental immunology and role of host defenses in neonatal susceptibility to infection. *In* Remington, J. S., and Klein, J. O. (eds.): Infectious Diseases of the Fetus and Newborn Infant. 4th ed. Philadelphia, W. B. Saunders, 1995, pp. 20–98.
286. Lieschke, G. J., and Burgess, A. W.: Granulocyte colony-stimulating factor and granulocyte-macrophage colony-stimulating factor, parts I and II. N. Engl. J. Med. *327*:28–35, 99–106, 1992.
287. Liles, W. C., and Van Voorhis, W. C.: Review: Nomenclature and biologic significance of cytokines involved in inflammation and the host immune response. J. Infect. Dis. *172*:1573–1580, 1995.
288. Liu, Y.-J., Cairns, J. A., Holder, M. J., et al.: Recombinant 25-kDa CD23 and interleukin 1α promote the survival of terminal center B cells: Evidence for bifurcation in the development of centrocytes rescued from apoptosis. Eur. J. Immunol. *21*:1107–1114, 1991.
289. Lodewyk, H. S., Van Mierop, M. D., and Kutsche, L. M.: Cardiovascular anomalies in DiGeorge syndrome and importance of neural crest as a possible pathogenic factor. Am. J. Cardiol. *58*:133–137, 1986.
290. Lomax, K. J., Leto, T. L., Nunoi, H., et al.: Recombinant 47-kilodaltor cytosol factor restores NADPH oxidase in chronic granulomatous disease. Science *245*:809, 1989.
291. Long, E. O.: Antigen processing for presentation to $CD4^+$ T cells. New Biol. *4*:274–282, 1992.
292. Lyon, M. F.: Some milestones in the history of X-chromosome inactivation. Annu. Rev. Genet. *26*:17–28, 1992.
293. Macatonia, S. E., Knight, S. C., Edwards, A. J., et al.: Localization of antigen on lymph node dendritic cells after exposure to the contact sensitizer fluorescein isothinocyanate. J. Exp. Med. *166*:1654–1667, 1987.
294. Manroe, B., Weinberg, A. G., Rosenfeld, C. R., et al.: The neonatal blood count in health and disease. I. Reference values for neutrophilic cells. J. Pediatr. *64*:60–64, 1979.
295. Marsh, S. G. E., and Bodmer, J. G.: HLA class II nucleotide sequences. Hum. Immunol. *31*:207–227, 1991.
296. Martensson, L., and Fudenberg, H. H.: Gm genes and gamma G-globulin synthesis in the human fetus. J. Immunol. *94*:514–520, 1965.
297. Martyn, L. J., Lischner, H. W., and Pileggi, A. J.: Chorioretinal lesions in familial chronic granulomatous disease of childhood. Trans. Am. Ophthalmol. Soc. *69*:84–112, 1971.
298. Matzinger, P.: Tolerance, danger and the extended family. Annu. Rev. Immunol. *12*:991–1045, 1994.
299. Mauer, A. M., Athens, J. W., Ashenbrucker, H., et al.: Leukokinetic studies. II. A method for labeling granulocytes in vitro with radioactive di-isopropylfluorophosphate (DFP32). J. Clin. Invest. *39*:1482–1489, 1960.
300. McEvoy, L. T., Zakem-Cloud, H., and Tosi, M. F.: Total cell content of CR3 (CD11b/CD18) and LFA-1 (CD11a/CD18) in neonatal neutrophils: Relationship to gestational age. Blood *87*:3929–3933, 1996.
301. McPhail, L. C., DeChatelet, L. R., and Shirley, P. S.: Deficiency of NADPH oxidase activity in chronic granulomatous disease. J. Pediatr. *90*:213–217, 1977.

302. Melchers, F., and Anderson, J. B.: Cell activation: Three steps and their variations. Cell *37*:715–720, 1984.
303. Melnick, J. L.: Nomenclature and classification of viruses. *In* Feigin, R. D., and Cherry, J. D. (eds.): Textbook of Pediatric Infectious Diseases. 3rd ed. Philadelphia, W. B. Saunders, 1992, pp. 1374–1389.
304. Metchnikoff, E.: Immunity in Infectious Diseases. (F. G. Binnie.) London, Cambridge University Press, 1905.
305. Miller, M. E.: Phagocytosis in the newborn infant: Humoral and cellular factors. J. Pediatr. *74*:255–259, 1969.
306. Miller, M. E.: Phagocytic function in the neonate: Selected aspects. Pediatrics *64*:S709–S712, 1979.
307. Miller, M. E., Oski, F. A., and Harris, M. B.: Lazy leukocyte syndrome: A new disorder of neutrophil function. Lancet *1*:665–669, 1971.
308. Miller, M. E., Norman, M. E., Koblenzer, P. J., et al.: A new familial defect of neutrophil movement. J. Lab. Clin. Med. *82*:1–8, 1973.
309. Miller, M. E.: Chemotactic function in the human neonate: Humoral and cellular aspects. Pediatr. Res. *5*:487–492, 1971.
310. Miller, M. E.: Developmental maturation of human neutrophil motility and its relationship to membrane deformity. *In* Bellanti, J. A., Dayton, D. H. (eds.): Phagocytic Cell in Host Resistance. New York, Raven Press, 1975, pp. 295–314.
311. Mills, E. L., and Quie, P. G.: Congenital disorders of the functions of polymorphonuclear neutrophils. Rev. Infect. Dis. *2*:505–517, 1980.
312. Milstein, C.: From antibody structure to immunological diversification of immune response. Science *231*:1261–1268, 1986.
313. Monteiro, R. C., Cooper, M. D., Kubagawa, H.: Molecular heterogeneity of Fcα receptors detected by receptor-specific monoclonal antibodies. J. Immunol. *148*:1764–1771, 1992.
314. Morell, A., Skvaril, F., and Hitzig, W. H.: IgG subclass: Development of the serum concentrations in "normal" infants and children. J. Pediatr. *80*:960–964, 1972.
315. Mortari, F., Wang, J.-Y., and Schroeder, H. W., Jr.: Human cord blood antibody repertoire. Mixed population of V_H gene segments and CDR3 distribution in the expressed Cαγ repertoires. J. Immunol. *150*:1348–1357, 1993.
316. Moy, J. N., Nelson, R. D., Richards, K. L., and Hostetter, M. K.: Identification of an IgA inhibitor of neutrophil chemotaxis and its membrane target for the metabolic burst. Immunology *69*:257–262, 1990.
317. Muller-Eberhard, H. J.: Complement: Chemistry and pathways. *In* Gallin, J. I., and Snyderman., R. (eds.): Inflammation: Basic Principles and Clinical Correlates. 2nd ed. New York, Raven Press, 1992, pp. 33–61.
318. Murphy, K. M., Heimberger, A. B., and Loh, D. Y.: Induction by antigen of intrathymic apoptosis of $CD4^+$ $CD8^+$ TCR^{lo} thymocytes *in vivo*. Science *250*:1720–1723, 1990.
319. Murphy, P. M.: The molecular biology of leukocyte chemoattractant receptors. Annu. Rev. Immunol. *12*:593–633, 1994.
320. Nagata, M., Hara, T., Aoki, T., et al. Inherited deficiency of ninth component of complement: An increased risk of meningococcal meningitis. J. Pediatr. *114*:260–264, 1989.
321. Naot, Y. D., Desmonts, G., and Remington, J. S.: IgM enzyme-linked immunosorbent assay test for the diagnosis of congenital *Toxoplasma* infection. J. Pediatr. *98*:32–36, 1981.
322. Nath, J., Flavin, M., and Gallin, J. I.: Tubulin tyrosinolation in human polymorphonuclear leukocytes: Studies in normal subjects and in patients with Chédiak-Higashi syndrome. J. Cell Biol. *95*:519–526, 1982.
323. Nauseef, W. M., Root, R. K., and Malech, H. L.: Biochemical and immunologic analysis of hereditary myeloperoxidase deficiency. J. Clin. Invest. *71*:1297–1307, 1983.
324. Newburger, P. E., Cohen, H. J., Rothchild, S. B., et al.: Prenatal diagnosis of chronic granulomatous disease. N. Engl. J. Med. *300*:178–181, 1979.
325. Noble, W. C.: Skin microbiology: Coming of age. J. Med. Microbiol. *17*:1–12, 1984.
326. Noelle, R. J., Ledbetter, J. A., and Aruffo, A.: CD40 and its ligand, an essential ligand-receptor pair for thymus-dependent B-cell activation. Immunol. Today *13*:431–433, 1992.
327. Norment, A. M., Salter, R. D., Parham, P., et al.: Cell-cell adhesion mediated by CD8 and MHC class I molecules. Nature *336*:79–81, 1988.
328. Nossal, G. J. V.: The molecular and cellular basis of affinity maturation in the antibody response. Cell *68*:1–2, 1992.
329. Notarangelo, L. D., Chirico, G., Chiara, A., et al.: Activity of classical and alternative pathways of complement in preterm and small for gestational age infants. Pediatr. Res. *18*:281–285, 1984.
330. Notarangelo, L. D., Duse, M., and Ugazio, A. G.: Immunodeficiency with hyper-IgM (HIM). Immunodefic. Rev. *3*:101–122, 1992.
331. O'Shea, J. J., Brown, E. J., Seligmann, B. E., et al.: Evidence for distinct intracellular pools of receptors for C3b and C3bi in human neutrophils. J. Immunol. *134*:2580–2587, 1985.
332. Ochs, H. D., Wedgwood, R. J., Heller, S. R., et al.: Complement, membrane glycoproteins and complement receptors: Their role in regulation of the immune response. Clin. Immunol. Immunopathol. *40*:94–104, 1986.
333. Ochs, H. D., and Wedgwood, R. J.: IgG subclass deficiencies. Annu. Rev. Med. *38*:325–340, 1987.
334. Ochs, H. D., and Winkelstein, J.: Disorders of the B-cell system. *In* Stiehm, E. R. (ed.): Immunologic Disorders in Infants and Children. 4th ed. Philadelphia, W. B. Saunders, 1996, pp. 296–338.
335. Ochs, H. D., Nonoyama, S., Zhu, Q., et al.: Regulation of antibody responses: The role of complement and adhesion molecules. Clin. Immunol. Immunopathol. *67*:S33–S40, 1993.
336. Oettinger, M. A., Schatz, D. G., Gorka, C., et al.: RAG-1 and RAG-2, adjacent genes that synergistically activate V(D)J recombination. Science *248*:1517–1523, 1990.
337. Oliver, A. M., Sewell, H. F., Abramovich, D. R., et al.: The distribution and differential expression of MHC class II antigens (HLA-DR, DP, and DQ) in human fetal adrenal, pancreas, thyroid and gut. Transplant Proc. *21*:651–652, 1989.
338. Orkin, S. H.: Molecular genetics of chronic granulomatous disease. Annu. Rev. Immunol. *7*:277–307, 1989.
339. Oxelius, V.-A., Laurell, A. B., Linquist, B., et al.: IgG subclasses in selective IgA deficiency. N. Engl. J. Med. *304*:1476–1477, 1981.
340. Oxelius, V.-A.: IgG subclass levels in infancy and childhood. Acta Paediatr. Scand. *68*:23–27, 1979.
341. Ozsahin, H., Le Deist, F., Benkerrou, M., et al.: Bone marrow transplantation in 26 patients with Wiskott-Aldrich syndrome from a single center. J. Pediatr. *129*:238–244, 1996.
342. Pangburn, M. K.: The alternative pathway. *In* Ross, G. D. (ed.): Immunobiology of the Complement System. Orlando, Academic Press, 1986, pp. 45–62.
343. Parry, M. F., Root, R. K., Metcalf, J. A., et al.: Myeloperoxidase deficiency: Prevalence and clinical significance. Ann. Intern. Med. *95*:293–301, 1981.
344. Paul, W. E.: Pleiotropy and redundancy: T cell-derived lymphokines in the immune response. Cell *57*:521–524, 1989.
345. Perlmuter, D. H., and Colten, H. R.: Molecular immunobiology of complement biosynthesis: A model of single-cell control of effector-inhibitor balance. Annu. Rev. Immunol. *4*:231–251, 1986.
346. Peterson, J. C., and Peterson, J. C.: Immunization in the young infant. Response to combined vaccines: I-IV. Am. J. Dis. Child. *81*:484–491, 1951.
347. Pier, G. B., Grout, M., Zaidi, T. S., et al.: Role of mutant CFTR in hypersusceptibility of cystic fibrosis patients to lung infections. Science *271*:64–67, 1996.
348. Pizzo, P. A., Robechaud, K. J., Gill, F. A., et al.: Empiric antibiotic and antifungal therapy for cancer patients with prolonged fever and granulocytopenia. Am. J. Med. *72*:101–111, 1982.
349. Plaeger, S. F.: Principal human cytokines. *In* Stiehm, E. R. (ed.): Immunologic Disorders in Infants and Children. 4th ed. Philadelphia, W. B. Saunders, 1996, pp. 1063–1065.
350. Pollack, J. D., Williams D. A., Gifford, M. A., et al.: Mouse model of X-linked chronic granulomatous disease, an inherited defect in phagocyte superoxide production. Nat. Genet. *9*:202–209, 1995.
351. Preimesberger, K. F., and Goldberg, M. E.: Acute liver abscess in chronic granulomatous disease of childhood. Radiology *110*:147–150, 1974.
352. Provenzano, R. W., Wetterlow, L. H., and Sullivan, C. L.: Immunization and antibody response in the newborn infant. N. Engl. J. Med. *273*:959–965, 1965.
353. Purkerson, J., and Isakson, P.: A two-signal model for regulation of immunoglobulin isotype switching. FASEB J. *6*:3245–3252, 1992.
354. Quie, P. G., White, J. G., Holmes, B., et al.: In vitro bactericidal capacity of human polymorphonuclear leukocytes: Diminished activity in chronic granulomatous disease of childhood. J. Clin. Invest. *46*:668–679, 1967.
355. Randall, T. D., Kings, L. B., and Corley, R. B.: The biological effects of IgM hemamer formation. Eur. J. Immunol. *20*:1971–1979, 1990.
356. Rappeport, J. M., Newburger, P. E., Goldblum, R. M., et al.: Allogeneic bone marrow transplantation for chronic granulomatous disease. J. Pediatr. *101*:952–955, 1982.
357. Regelmann, W., Hays, N., and Quie, P. G.: Chronic granulomatous disease: Historical perspective and clinical experience at the University of Minnesota Hospitals. *In* Gallin, J. I., Fauci, A. S. (eds.): Advances in Host Defense Mechanisms. Vol. 3. New York, Raven Press, 1983, pp. 3–23.
358. Rijkers, G. T., Dollekamp, E. G., and Zegers, B. J. M.: The *in vitro* B-cell response to pneumococcal polysaccharides in adults and neonates. Scand. J. Immunol. *25*:447–452, 1987.
359. Robey, E. A., Fowlkes, B. J., Gordon, J. W., et al.: Thymic selection in CD8 transgenic mice supports an instructive model for commitment to a CD4 or CD8 lineage. Cell *64*:99–107, 1991.
360. Robin, L. F., Lees, P. S. J., Winget, M., et al.: Wood-burning stoves and lower respiratory illnesses in Navajo children. Pediatr. Infect. Dis. J. *15*:859–865, 1996.
361. Roche, P. A., and Cresswell, P.: Invariant chain association with HLA-DR molecules inhibits immunogenic peptide binding. Nature *345*:615–618, 1990.
362. Rock, K. L., Gamble, S., Rothstein, L., et al.: Dissociation of β_2-microglobulin leads to the accumulation of a substantial pool of inactive class I MHC heavy chains on the cell surface. Cell *85*:611–620, 1991.
363. Romani, N., Koide, S., Crowley, M., et al.: Presentation of exogenous protein antigens by dendritic cells to T cell clones: Intact protein is presented best by immature, epidermal Langerhans cells. J. Exp. Med. *169*:1169–1178, 1989.
364. Roos, D., Weening, R. S., Voteman, A. A., et al.: Protection of phagocytic leukocytes by endogenous glutathione: Studies in a family with glutathione reductase deficiency. Blood *53*:851–857, 1979.
365. Root, R. K., Metcalf, J., Oshino, N., et al.: H_2O_2 release from human

granulocytes during phagocytosis. I. Documentation, quantitation, and some regulating factors. J. Clin. Invest. *55*:945–955, 1975.
366. Root, R. K., and Cohen, M. S.: The microbicidal mechanisms of human neutrophils and eosinophils. Rev. Infect. Dis. *3*:565–598, 1981.
367. Rosen, F. S., Cooper, M. D., and Wedgwood, R. J.: The primary immunodeficiencies. N. Engl. J. Med. *311*:235–242, 1984.
368. Rosen, F. S., and Janeway, C. A.: The gamma globulins: III. The antibody deficiency syndromes. N. Engl. J. Med. *275*:769–775, 1966.
369. Rosenfield, S. I., Kelly, M. E., and Leddy, J. P.: Hereditary deficiency of the fifth component of complement in man. I. Clinical, immunochemical, and family studies. J. Clin. Invest. *57*:1626–1634, 1976.
370. Rosenfield, S. I., Baum, J., Steigbigel, R. T., et al.: Hereditary deficiency of the fifth component of complement in man. II. Biological properties of C5-deficient human serum. J. Clin. Invest. *57*:1635–1643, 1976.
371. Ross, S. C., and Densen, P.: Complement deficiency states and infection: Epidemiology, pathogenesis, and consequences of neisserial and other infections in an immune deficiency. Medicine *63*:243–273, 1984.
372. Rowe, P. C., McLean, R. H., and Wood, R. A.: Association of homozygous C4B deficiency with bacterial meningitis. J. Infect. Dis. *160*:448–451, 1989.
373. Ruddy, S., Carpenter, C. B., Chin, K. W., et al.: Human complement metabolism: An analysis of 144 studies. Medicine *54*:165–178, 1975.
374. Rudensky, A. Y., Preston-Hurlburt, P., et al.: Sequence analysis of peptides bound to MHC class II molecules. Nature *353*:622–627, 1991.
375. Rutenberg, W. D., Yang, M. C., Doberstyn, B., et al.: Multiple leukocyte abnormalities in chronic granulomatous disease: A familial study. Pediatr. Res. *11*:158–163, 1977.
376. Sacchi, F., and Hill, H. R.: Defective membrane potential changes in neutrophils from human neonates. J. Exp. Med. *160*:1247–1252, 1984.
377. Sacchi, F., Augustine, N. H., and Hill, H. R.: Abnormality in actin polymerization associated with defective chemotaxis in neutrophils from neonates. Int. Arch. Allergy Appl. Immunol. *84*:32–39, 1987.
378. Saiman, L., and Prince, A.: *Pseudomonas aeruginosa* pili bind to asialoGM1 which is increased on the surface of cystic fibrosis epithelial cells. J. Clin. Invest. *92*:1875–1880, 1993.
379. Salmon, J. E., Kapur, S., and Kimberly, R. P.: Opsonin-independent ligation of Fcγ receptors; the 3G8-bearing receptors on neutrophils mediate the phagocytosis of concanavalin A-treated erythrocytes and non-opsonized *E. coli*. J. Exp. Med. *166*:1798–1813, 1987.
380. Salmon, J. E., Edberg, J. C., and Kimberly, R. P.: Fcγ receptor III on human neutrophils: Allelic variants have functionally distinct capacities. J. Clin. Invest. *85*:1287–1295, 1990.
381. Sandberg, E. T., Kline, M. W., and Shearer, W. T.: The secondary immunodeficiencies. *In* Stiehm, E. R. (ed.): Immunologic Disorders in Infants and Children. 4th ed. Philadelphia, W. B. Saunders, 1996, pp. 553–601.
382. Schaffer, F. M., and Ballow, M.: Immunodeficiency: The office work-up. J. Respir. Dis. *16*:523–546, 1995.
383. Schatz, D. G., Oettinger, M. A., and Schlissel, M. S.: V (D) J recombination: Molecular biology and regulation. Annu. Rev. Immunol. *10*:359–384, 1992.
384. Schmidt, A. P., Taswell, H. F., and Gleich, G. J.: Anaphylactic transfusion reaction associated with anti-IgA antibody. N. Engl. J. Med. *280*:188–193, 1969.
385. Schoub, B. D., Johnson, S., McAnerney, J., et al.: Monovalent neonatal polio immunization—A strategy for the developing world. J. Infect. Dis. *147*:836–839, 1988.
386. Schur, P. H., Rosen, F., and Norman, M. E.: Immunoglobulin subclasses in normal children. Pediatr. Res. *13*:181–183, 1979.
387. Schur, P. H.: IgG subclasses. A historical perspective. Monogr. Allergy *23*:1–11, 1988.
388. Shackelford, P. G., Polmar, S. H., Mayus, J. L., et al.: Spectrum of IgG2 subclass deficiency in children with recurrent infections: Prospective study. J. Pediatr. *108*:647–653, 1986.
389. Shackelford, P. G., Granoff, D. M., Polmar, S. H., et al.: Subnormal serum concentrations of IgG2 in children with frequent infections associated with varied patterns of immunologic dysfunction. J. Pediatr. *116*:529–538, 1990.
390. Shackelford, P. G., Granoff, D. M., Madassery, J. V., et al: Clinical and immunologic characteristics of healthy children with subnormal serum concentrations of IgG2. Pediatr. Res. *27*:16–21, 1990.
391. Shackelford, P. G., and Granoff, D. M.: IgG subclass composition of the antibody response of healthy adults, and normal or IgG2-deficient children and to immunization with *H. influenzae* type b polysaccharide vaccine or Hib PS-protein conjugate vaccines. Monogr. Allergy *23*:269–281, 1988.
392. Shackelford, P. G.: IgG subclasses: Importance in pediatric practice. Pediatr. Rev. *14*:291–296, 1993.
393. Shapiro, R., Beatty, D. W., Woods, L. I., et al.: Serum complement and immunoglobulin values in small-for-gestational-age infants. J. Pediatr. *99*:139–141, 1981.
394. Shurin, S. B., Socransky, S. S., Sweeney, E., and Stossel, T. P.: A neutrophil disorder induced by *Capnocytophaga*, a dental micro-organism. N. Engl. J. Med. *301*:849–854, 1979.
395. Siu, G., Kronenberg, M., Strauss, E., et al.: The structure, rearrangement and expression of D_β gene segments of the murine T-cell antigen receptor. Nature *311*:344–350, 1984.
396. Smith, C. W., Marlin, S. D., Rothlein, R., et al.: Cooperative interaction of LFA-1 and Mac-1 with intercellular adhesion molecule-1 in facilitating adherence and transendothelial migration of human neutrophils *in vitro*. J. Clin. Invest. *83*:2008–2017, 1989.
397. Smith, C. W., Hollers, J. C., Dupree, E., et al.: A serum inhibitor of leukotaxis in a child with recurrent infections. J. Lab. Clin. Med. *79*:878–883, 1972.
398. Smith, C. W., Rothlein, R., Hughes, B. J., et al.: Recognition of an endothelial determinant for CD18-dependent human neutrophil adherence and transendothelial migration. J. Clin. Invest. *82*:1746–1756, 1988.
399. Smith, C. W.: Molecular determinants of neutrophil adhesion. Am. J. Respir. Cell. Mol. Biol. *2*:487–489, 1990.
400. Smith, D. H., Peter, G., Ingram, D. L., et al.: Responses of children immunized with the capsular polysaccharide of *Haemophilus influenzae*. Pediatrics *52*:637–644, 1973.
401. Smith, J. J., Travis, S. M., Greenberg, E. P., et al.: Cystic fibrosis airway epithelia fail to kill bacteria because of abnormal airway surface fluid. Cell *86*:1–20, 1996.
402. Smith, R. T., Eitzman, D. V., Catlin, M. E., et al.: The development of the immune response. Pediatrics *33*:163–183, 1964.
403. Smolen, P., Bland, R., Heiligenstein, E., et al.: Antibody response to oral polio vaccine in premature infants. J. Pediatr. *103*:917–920, 1983.
404. Snyderman, R., Pike, M. C., and Altman, L. C.: Abnormalities of leukocyte chemotaxis in human disease. Ann. N. Y. Acad. Sci. *256*:386–388, 1975.
405. Solvason, N., and Kearney, J. F.: The human fetal omentum: A site of B cell generation. J. Exp. Med. *175*:397–404, 1992.
406. Soriano, R. B., South, M. A., Goldman, A. S., and Smith, C. W.: Defect of neutrophil motility in a child with recurrent bacterial infections and disseminated cytomegalovirus infection. J. Pediatr. *83*:951–955, 1973.
407. Southwick, F. S., Howard, T. H., Holbrook, T., et al.: The relationship between CR3 deficiency and neutrophil actin assembly. Blood *73*:1973–1979, 1989.
408. Southwick, F. S., Holbrook, T., Howard, T., et al.: Neutrophil actin dysfunction is associated with a deficiency of Mol. Clin. Res. *34*:533A, 1986.
409. Spielberg, S. P., Boxer, L. A., Oliver, J. M., et al.: Oxidative damage to neutrophils in glutathione synthetase deficiency. Br. J. Haematol. *42*:215–223, 1979.
410. Spitznagel, J. K., Cooper, M. R., McCall, A. E., et al.: Selective deficiency of granules associated with lysozyme and lactoferrin in human polymorphs with reduced microbicidal capacity. J. Clin. Invest. *51*:93A, 1972.
411. Spitznagel, J. K., Dalldorf, F. G., Leffell, M. S., et al.: Character of azurophil and specific granules purified from human polymorphonuclear leukocytes. Lab. Invest. *30*:774–785, 1974.
412. Springer, T. A., Thompson, W. S., Miller, J., et al.: Inherited deficiency of the Mac-1, LFA-1, P150,95 glycoprotein family and its molecular basis. J. Exp. Med. *160*:1901–1918, 1984.
413. Springer, T. A., and Anderson, D. C.: The importance of adherence, chemotaxis, and migration into inflammatory sites: Insights from an experiment of nature. *In* Evered, D., Nugent, J., and O'Connor, M. (eds.): Biochemistry of Macrophages. Ciba Foundation Symposium. London, 118 Pittman, 1986, pp. 102–126.
414. Stepick-Biek, P., Thulliez, P., Araujo, F. G., et al.: IgA antibodies for diagnosis of acute congenital and acquired toxoplasmosis. J. Infect. Dis. *162*:270–273, 1990.
415. Stevens, R., Dichek, D., Keld, B., et al.: IgG_1 is the predominant subclass of *in Vivo*- and *in Vitro*-produced anti-tetanus toxoid antibodies and also serves as the membrane IgG molecule for delivering inhibitory signals to anti-tetanus toxoid antibody-producing B cells. J. Clin. Immunol. *3*:65–69, 1983.
415a. Stiehm, E. R., and Fudenberg, H. H.: Serum levels of immune globulins in health and disease: A survey. Pediatrics *37*:715–727, 1966.
416. Stossel, T. P.: The mechanical responses of white blood cells. *In* Gallin, J. I., Goldstein, I. M., and Snyderman, R. (eds.): Basic Principles and Clinical Correlates. New York, Raven Press, 1992, pp. 459–475.
417. Stossel, T. P.: Phagocytosis: Recognition and ingestion. Semin. Hematol. *12*:83, 1975.
418. Stossel, T. P.: Evaluation of opsonic and leukocyte function with a spectrophotometric test in patients with infection and with phagocytic disorders. Blood *42*:121–130, 1973.
419. Strauss, R. G., and Snyder, E. L.: Chemotactic peptide binding by intact neutrophils from human neonates. Pediatr. Res. *18*:63–66, 1984.
420. Strunk, R. C., Fenton, L. J., and Gaines, J. A.: Alternative pathway of complement activation in full term and premature infants. Pediatr. Res. *13*:641–643, 1979.
421. Swain, S.: T cell subsets and the recognition of MHC class. Immunol. Rev. *74*:129–142, 1983.
422. Tack, K. J., Rham, F. S., Brown, B., et al.: Aspergillus osteomyelitis: Report of four cases and review of the literature. Am. J. Med. *73*:295, 1982.
423. Taitz, L. S., Zarate-Salvador, C., and Schwartz, E.: Congenital absence of the parathyroid and thymus glands in an infant (III and IV pharyngeal pouch syndrome). Pediatrics *38*:412–418, 1966.
424. Taylor, P. W.: Bactericidal and bacteriolytic activity of serum against gram-negative bacteria. Microbiol. Rev. *47*:46–83, 1983.
425. Teyton, L., O'Sullivan, D., Dickson, P. W., et al.: Invariant chain distinguishes between the exogenous and endogenous antigen presentation pathways. Nature *348*:39–44, 1990.

426. Timens, W., Boes, A., Rozeboom-Uiterwijk, T., and Poppema, S.: Immaturity of the human splenic marginal zone in infancy. Possible contribution to the deficiency infant immune response. J. Immunol. *143*:3200–3206, 1989.
427. Tosi, M. F., Anderson, D. C., Barrish, J., et al.: Effect of piliation on interactions of *Haemophilus influenzae* type b with human polymorphonuclear leukocytes. Infect. Immun. *47*:780–785, 1985.
428. Tosi, M., and Berger, M.: Functional differences between the 40 kDa and 50 to 70 IgG Fc receptors on human neutrophils revealed by elastase treatment and antireceptor antibodies. J. Immunol. *141*:2097–2103, 1988.
429. Tosi, M. F., and Zakem, H.: Surface expression of Fcγ receptor III (CD16) on chemoattractant-stimulated neutrophils is determined by both surface shedding and translocation from intracellular storage compartments. J. Clin. Invest. *90*:462–470, 1990.
430. Tosi, M. F., Zakem, H., and Berger, M.: Neutrophil elastase cleaves C3bi on opsonized *Pseudomonas* as well as CR1 on neutrophils to create a functionally important opsonin-receptor mismatch. J. Clin. Invest. *86*:300–308, 1990.
431. Tosi, M. F., and Hamedani, A.: A rapid, specific assay for superoxide release from phagocytes in small volumes of whole blood. Am. J. Clin. Pathol. *97*:566–573, 1992.
432. Townsend, A., and Bodmer, H.: Antigen recognition by class I-restricted T lymphocytes. Annu. Rev. Immunol. *7*:601–624, 1989.
433. Tsukada, S., Saffran, D. C., Rawlings, D. J., et al.: Deficient expression of a B cell cytoplasmic tyrosine kinase in human X-linked agammaglobulinemia. Cell *72*:279–290, 1993.
434. Uckun, F. M., Dibirdik, I., Smith R., et al.: Interleukin 7 receptor ligation stimulates tyrosine phosphorylation, inositol phospholipid turnover, and clonal proliferation of human B-cell precursors. Proc. Natl. Acad. Sci. U. S. A. *88*:3589–3593, 1991.
435. Unkeless, J. C.: Function and heterogeneity of human Fc receptors for immunoglobulin G. J. Clin. Invest. *83*:355–361, 1989.
436. van de Winkel, J. G. J., and Anderson, C. L.: Biology of human immunoglobulin G Fc receptors. J. Leuk. Biol. *49*:511–524, 1991.
437. Van Dyke, T. E., Horoszewicz, H. U., and Genco, R. J.: The polymorphonuclear leukocyte (PMNL) locomotor defect in juvenile periodontitis: Study of random migration, chemokinesis and chemotaxis. J. Peridontol. 53:682, 1982.
438. Van Epps, D., Palmer, D. L., and Williams, R. C.: Characterization of serum inhibitors of neutrophil chemotaxis is associated with anergy. J. Immunol. *113*:189–200, 1974.
439. van Tuinen, P., Johnson, K. R., Ledbetter, S., et al.: Localization of myeloperoxidase to the long arm of human chromosome 17: Relationship to the 15:17 translocation of acute promyelocytic leukemia. Oncogene *1*:319–326, 1987.
440. Vanderkerckhove, B. A. E., Baccala, R., Jones, D., et al.: Thymic selection of the human T-cell receptor Vβ repertoire in SCID-hu mice. J. Exp. Med. *176*:1619–1624, 1992.
441. Vanichkin A., Patya, M., Gazit, A., et al.: Late administration of lipophilic tyrosine kinase inhibitor prevents lipopolysaccharide and *Escherichia coli*–induced lethal toxicity. J. Infect. Dis. *173*:927–933, 1996.
442. Vedder, N. B., and Harlan, J. M.: Increased surface expression of CD11b/CD18 (Mac 1) is not required for stimulated neutrophil adherence to cultured endothelium. J. Clin. Invest. *81*:676–682, 1988.
443. Vetrie, D., Vorechovsky, I., Sideras, F., et al.: The gene involved in X-linked agammaglobulinemia is a member of the *src* family of protein-tyrosine kinases. Nature *361*:226–233, 1993.
444. Volpp, B. D., Nauseef, W. M., Donelson, J. E., et al.: Cloning of the cDNA and functional expression of the 47 kilodalton cytosolic component of the human neutrophil respiratory burst oxidase. Proc. Natl. Acad. Sci. *86*:7195–7199, 1989.
445. von Boehmer, H., Teh, H. S., and Kisielow, P.: The thymus selects the useful, neglects the useless and destroys the harmful. Immunol. Today *10*:57–61, 1989.
446. von Andrian, U. H., Berger, E. M., Ramezani, L., et al: In vivo behavior of neutrophils from two patients with distinct inherited leukocyte adhesion deficiency syndromes. J. Clin. Invest. *91*:2893–2897, 1993.
447. Waage, A., Halstensen, A., and Espevik, T.: Association between tumor necrosis factor in serum and fatal outcome in patients with meningococcal disease. Lancet *1*:355–357, 1987.
448. Walker, R. I., and Willemze, R.: Neutrophil kinetics and the regulation of granulopoiesis. Rev. Infect. Dis. *2*:282–292, 1980.
449. Walter, M. A., Surti, U., Hofker, M. H., et al.: The physical organization of the human immunoglobulin heavy chain gene complex. EMBO J. *9*:3303–3313, 1990.
450. Ward, P. A., and Schlegel, R. J.: Impaired leukotactic responsiveness in a child with recurrent infection. Lancet *2*:344–347, 1969.
451. Weaver, L. J., Craddock, P. R., and Jacob, H. S.: Association of complement activation and elevated plasma-C5a with adult respiratory distress syndrome. Pathophysiological relevance and possible prognostic value. Lancet *1*:947–949, 1980.
452. Weisdorf, D. J., Craddock, P. R., and Jacob, H. S.: Granulocytes utilize different energy sources for movement and phagocytosis. Inflammation *6*:245–251, 1982.
453. Weiss, J., Victor, M., and Elsbach, P.: Role of charge and hydrophobic interactions in the action of the bactericidal/permeability-increasing protein of neutrophils on gram-negative bacteria. J. Clin. Invest. *71*:540–549, 1983.
454. Welsh, M. J., and Smith, A. E.: Molecular mechanisms of CFTR chloride channel dysfunction in cystic fibrosis. Cell *73*:1251–1254, 1993.
455. Westminster Hospitals Bone-Marrow Transplant Team. Bone marrow transplant from an unrelated donor for chronic granulomatous disease. Lancet *1*:210–213, 1977.
456. Wheat, L. J., Connolly-Stringfield, P. A., and Baker, R. L.: Disseminated histoplasmosis in the acquired immune deficiency syndrome: Clinical findings, diagnosis and treatment, and review of the literature. Medicine *69*:361–374, 1990.
457. Whitley, R. J., and Arvin, A. M.: Herpes simplex virus infections. *In* Remington, J. S., Klein, J.O. (eds.): Infectious Diseases of the Fetus and Newborn Infant. 4th ed. Philadelphia, W. B. Saunders, 1995, pp. 354–376.
458. Williams, G. T., Kingston, R., Owen, M. J., et al.: A single micromanipulated stem cell gives rise to multiple T-cell receptor gene rearrangements in the thymus *in vitro*. Nature *324*:63–64, 1986.
459. Wilson, C. B., Ochs, H. D., Almquiest, J., et al.: When is umbilical cord separation delayed? J. Pediatr. *107*:292–293, 1985.
460. Wilson, R. K., Lai, E., Concannon, P., et al.: Structure, organization and polymorphism of murine and human T-cell receptors αβ chain gene families. Immunol. Rev. *101*:149–172, 1988.
461. Winkelstein, J. A., Kurlandsky, L. E., and Swift, A. J.: Defective activation of the third component of complement in the sera of newborn infants. Pediatr. Res. *13*:1093–1096, 1979.
462. Winkelstein, J. A., Lambert, G. H., and Swift, A.: Pneumococcal serum opsonizing activity in splenectomized children. J. Pediatr. *87*:430–433, 1975.
463. Yang, K. D., and Hill, H. R.: Immune responses to infectious diseases: An evolutionary perspective. Pediatr. Infect. Dis. J. *15*:355–364, 1996.
464. Yeung, C. Y., and Hobbs, J. R.: Serum-gamma G-globulin levels in normal, premature, post-mature and "small-for-dates" newborn babies. Lancet *1*:1167–1170, 1968.
465. Zach, T. L., and Hostetter, M. K.: Biochemical abnormalities of the third component of complement in neonates. Pediatr. Res. *26*:116–120, 1989.
466. Zemmour, J., and Parham, P.: HLA class I nucleotide sequences. Hum. Immunol. *31*:195–206, 1991.
467. Zigmond, S. H.: Ability of polymorphonuclear leukocytes to orient in gradients of chemotactic factors. J. Cell Biol. *75*:606–616, 1977.

3

METABOLIC RESPONSE OF THE HOST TO INFECTIONS

William R. Beisel

Although infectious microorganisms constitute a continuing threat at all ages of life, they are particularly dangerous in neonatal infants and young children. Despite the availability of modern sanitation, public health measures, vaccines, and antibiotics, it is characteristic for most children to suffer a sizable number of discrete episodes of acute infection before reaching adulthood. Depending upon their severity and duration, infectious illnesses can interrupt normal growth patterns. More importantly, if closely spaced in time, a series of infections can initiate a downhill health spiral, leading to malnutrition, chronic debilitation, immune system dysfunction, and death.[9, 10, 69, 70, 109] This possibility is of greatest concern in newborn infants and weanling children, especially those in Third World areas.

The human host normally protects itself against invading microorganisms by maintaining a broad array of general defensive mechanisms and immunologic responses. This array includes the initiation of acute-phase reactions triggered by the release of proinflammatory cytokines from macrophages, monocytes, and other cells.[8–10, 32] The resulting nonspecific defensive measures typically include fever and anorexia, slow-wave sleep, accelerated production of phagocytic cells, hormonal responses, and the participation of many biochemical pathways and molecular mechanisms within body cells.[5–10, 141] The acute-phase reaction produces relatively stereotyped patterns of transient metabolic sequelae (diagrammed in Fig. 3–1), which accompany and follow most acute, generalized infectious illnesses and some localized ones.[60] It is important for a pediatrician to anticipate these metabolic changes in order to recognize dangerous complications, such as hypoglycemia and electrolyte imbalance, that may occur during an acute infection.

The array of metabolic changes depicted in Figure 3–1 typically is shared as a group of common responses during all generalized acute infectious diseases.[5–10, 141] Similar changes are seen during other types of disease or trauma, whenever they are accompanied by fever or inflammatory reactions.[60] These common acute-phase responses are composed of a hypermetabolic admixture of anabolic and catabolic components. Each centigrade degree of fever causes basal cellular oxygen consumption to increase about 13 per cent.[8] The resultant increase in cellular energy expenditure comes at a time when food intake and intestinal absorption are diminished by anorexia and, at times, by vomiting and diarrhea. In the absence of an adequate intake of nutrients, body energy needs are met, for the most part, by the oxidation of metabolic substrates that are derived from nutrient stores already contained within body tissues. The hypermetabolic effects of acute fever are fueled primarily by carbohydrate (some of it derived from the metabolism of amino acids),[8] but if infectious illnesses become subacute or chronic, body fats then become the important, sustaining fuel.

Generalized acute-phase metabolic responses may be modified by a number of factors, such as the severity of an infectious process, its duration, and its possible progression to a subacute or chronic disease.[5–10, 15] The age and sex of the patient, the presence of genetic resistance (or susceptibility) factors or partial immunity, the adequacy of nonspecific defensive mechanisms and de novo immune responsiveness, the preexisting nutritional status of the child, and the presence or absence of other diseases all combine to modify host metabolic responses through their diverse influence on the infectious process per se.

Superimposed upon this general array of common host metabolic responses are additional metabolic changes that occur when an infectious process becomes localized within certain anatomic sites or organ systems. As examples, diarrhea during gastrointestinal infections can lead to fluid and electrolyte depletion; hepatic infections can lead to derangements of carbohydrate and amino acid metabolism; and central nervous system infections that cause neuronal destruction are accompanied by muscle paralysis and atrophy. Other infections localized within the cranial vault often produce an inappropriate secretion of antidiuretic hormone and problems of dangerous overhydration in children.[10] The development of shock syndromes during infectious diseases imposes additional metabolic derangements because of progressive stagnant hypoxia.[5, 115]

The total number of discrete metabolic responses known to occur during acute and chronic infectious illnesses continues to expand.[5] Accordingly, the most widely recognized of these multiple responses will be grouped for discussion into major categories, which include changes in nitrogen, amino acid, carbohydrate, lipid, electrolyte, vitamin, and trace element metabolism. The important initiating and control mechanisms provided by cytokines and the endocrine system also will be discussed.

Importantly, each of the many individual metabolic changes during infection must be interpreted in a manner that reflects its longitudinal development and progression over a period of time and its relationship to the evolving phases of the infectious process.[6] Thus, some metabolic changes may be detected during the incubation period; many other responses occur at the onset of fever; and still other phenomena develop during the recovery phase of illness or later during convalescence.

NITROGEN METABOLISM

Fever and its accompanying hypermetabolic state, as induced by acute-phase responses during infectious illnesses, trigger a complex assortment of changes in protein, amino acid, and nitrogen metabolism.[15] Although the catabolic destruction of skeletal muscle protein is most obvious clinically, important anabolic events occur simultaneously. These involve the synthesis of new proteins and cells that are of special importance in host defense mechanisms. Increases in whole-body protein turnover involve both catabolic and anabolic events in chronic infections also, as demonstrated by recent leucine kinetic studies in patients with human immunodeficiency virus infections.[67]

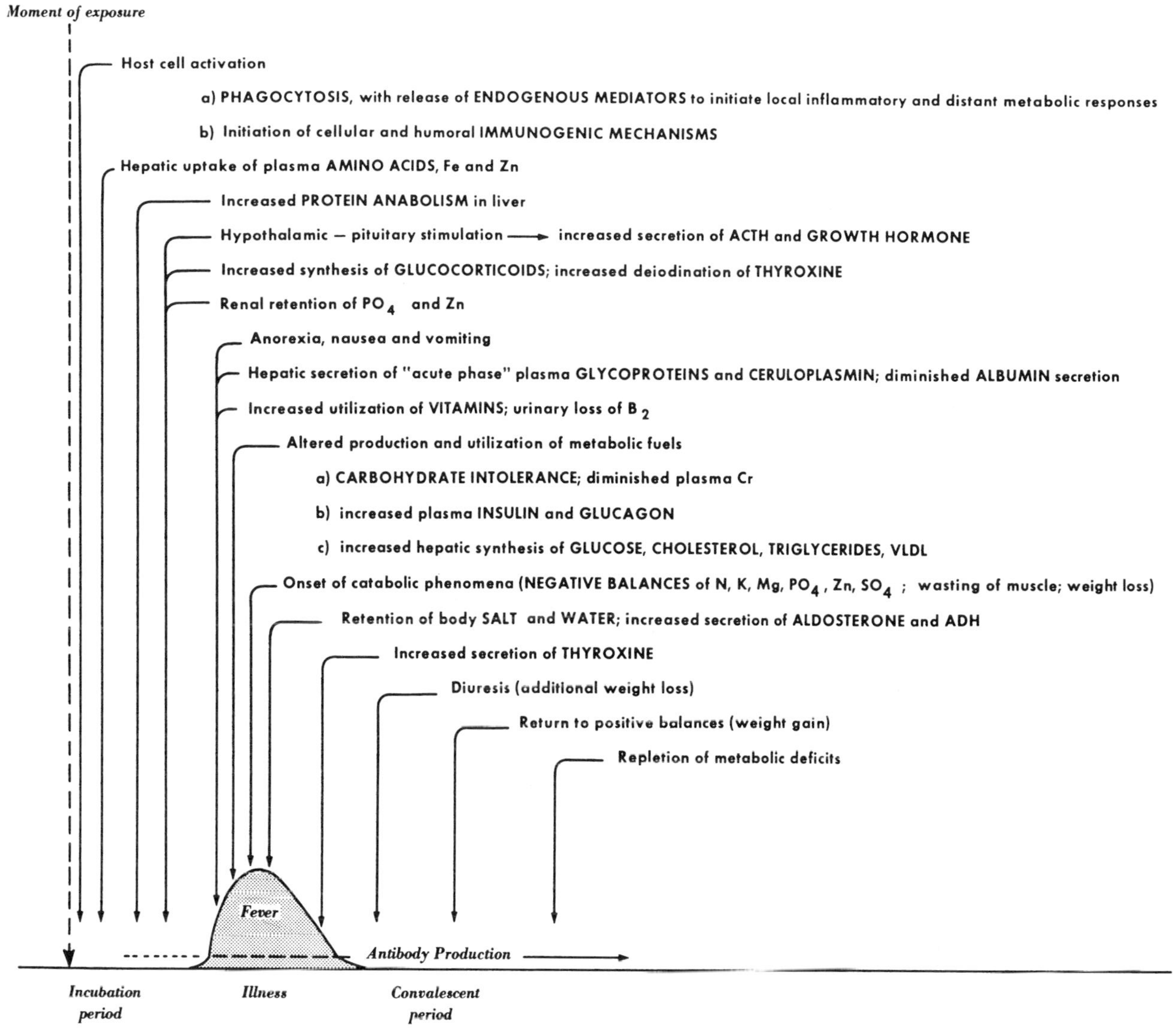

FIGURE 3–1. *Onset time of various host metabolic responses in relation to the sequential phases of a "model" acute, self-limited, generalized infectious illness. (From McKigney, J. I., and Munro, H. N. (eds.): Nutrient Requirements in Adolescence. Cambridge, MA, MIT Press, 1976, p. 250.)*

Nitrogen Balance Studies

Because the ability of body cells to synthesize new proteins is a fundamental necessity for maintaining all known host defensive mechanisms, including the immunologic ones, it is important to understand the changes that take place in the nitrogen metabolism of an infected person.[92] When the availability of free amino acids within body pools is restricted by diet or disease, the catabolism of certain existing body proteins (chiefly the contractile proteins of skeletal muscle) generates the free amino acids required to synthesize new body proteins with higher priorities, in terms of the many new proteins needed for defensive purposes. Information about these metabolic responses has been gained through the quantitative analysis of proteins and other nitrogen-containing compounds in tissues, body fluids, and excretions and through kinetic studies with tagged molecules.[67, 81, 88, 103, 129]

One useful approach has been the measurement of nitrogen balance throughout the sequential course of an infectious process.[5, 15, 92] Daily measurements of nitrogen intake and all nitrogen losses via different routes are obtained to determine whether the body is losing or retaining nitrogen. Other investigative techniques then are needed to provide specific information about the molecular mechanisms involved in producing any observed changes in nitrogen balance. Nevertheless, the use of balance techniques has provided information concerning the typical losses of body nitrogen and muscle mass during acute generalized infections (Fig. 3–2). Quantitation of these catabolic losses provides an important framework of reference for more detailed studies of changes in nitrogen metabolism.

A comprehensive series of nitrogen balance studies was obtained in young adult male volunteers subjected to different kinds of experimentally induced infections during the course of studies to test vaccine efficacy.[15] Extensive normal baseline data were obtained on each volunteer prior to the time of his or her inoculation with or exposure to infectious bacteria, viruses, or rickettsia. By making longitudinal serial measurements throughout the course of the infectious process, it was possible to obtain a comprehensive, prospective evaluation of metabolic balance changes in nitrogen and other elements.[15]

Nitrogen balances did not change from baseline values during the incubation periods of the infectious diseases stud-

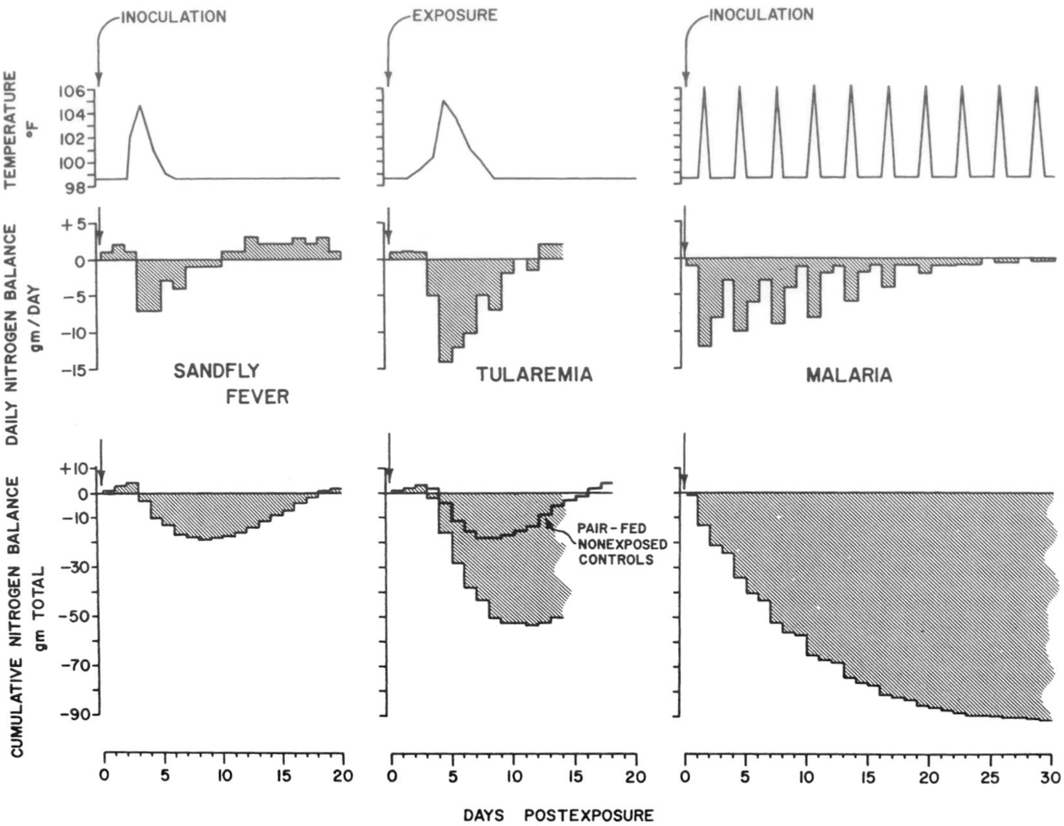

FIGURE 3–2. *Comparisons between the occurrence of fever (top) and changes in daily nitrogen balance (middle) and cumulative nitrogen (bottom) in patients with viral, bacterial, and generalized parasitic infections. Cumulative balance values for pair-fed healthy control subjects show the amounts of body nitrogen loss that can be ascribed to diminished food intake during infection. (From McKigney, J. I., and Munro, H. N. (eds.): Nutrient Requirements in Adolescence. Cambridge, MA, MIT Press, 1976, p. 261.)*

ied (see Fig. 3–2). Only after symptoms and fever had begun did the body begin to lose nitrogen. These losses persisted for a period encompassing the acute illness. Then, in convalescence, the subjects began to retain nitrogen so that gradually, over a period of several weeks, body nitrogen losses were regained. Similar nitrogen balance studies were conducted in healthy control volunteers who were not infected.[11, 12, 15] Instead, these controls were subjected to (1) partial food deprivation to mimic the anorexia-induced reduction in dietary intake measured in the patients with infection; (2) a 24-hour exposure to artificially induced high environmental temperatures to produce an increase in body temperature comparable to that seen in patients with infection; (3) treatment with antibiotic therapy in courses identical to those given to patients with infections; or (4) treatment with oral hydrocortisone using sequentially changing daily doses to mimic the measured adrenal responses of infected subjects.

These balance studies showed that the major losses in body nitrogen resulted from the combined effects of a reduced intake of food plus a continued (or even increased) loss of nitrogen via the urine.[15] In contrast, simple starvation produced a prompt decrease in the daily losses of nitrogen via the urine. Thus, a patient with an acute infectious illness differed markedly from someone subjected only to simple dietary deprivation. Urinary nitrogen losses did not decline appreciably, or they increased in the presence of fever, whether the fever was due to an active infection or to an artificial increase in environmental temperatures.[12] The control studies also showed that the negative nitrogen balances during infection were not caused by adrenal glucocorticoid hormones or the antibiotics used in therapy.[11, 15] Rather, by terminating infection quickly, antibiotics helped to reverse the loss of body nitrogen, thereby allowing a more rapid restoration of nitrogen stores.

Because the loss of sizable quantities of nitrogen has important nutritional consequences, the same balance data were used to determine patterns of cumulative loss of body nitrogen.[5, 6, 15] As shown in Figure 3–2, total losses of body nitrogen grew progressively larger as the acute febrile phase of illness continued; the cumulative total loss of body nitrogen then persisted throughout early convalescence. When nitrogen balances finally became positive, nitrogen was recovered over a period of weeks as body stores were accumulated slowly.

Studies performed in adult patients suffering from infections such as tuberculosis and malaria suggested that the depletion of body stores of protein nitrogen did not continue unabated during subacute or chronic infections.[54] Rather, a new state of relative nitrogen equilibrium became established as chronically ill patients lapsed into a cachectic state. Total body nitrogen in such chronically ill patients was neither gained nor lost. Vital body processes continued to function for extended periods, despite the presence of cachexia and markedly depleted body nitrogen stores.[8] This was a hazardous state at best, comparable with the threat faced by infants and children with severe protein-energy malnutrition, children who constantly faced the additional threat of developing dangerous new or superimposed infectious diseases.[69, 70, 86, 109]

Only a limited amount of nitrogen balance data have been collected in children suffering from acute febrile infections. These data tend to reflect closely the patterns of change described in adults, with one major exception. Adults normally are in a state of nitrogen equilibrium, with neither a net gain nor a net loss over time, whereas healthy infants and children are consistently in positive balance because they must retain nitrogen to meet their needs for normal growth.

Few prospective measurements are available to document the changes in nitrogen balance throughout an entire infectious process in children. However, in 1926, Beck[4] in Germany reported a series of metabolic balance studies conducted in healthy infants inoculated with vaccinia virus. One study was begun in a child exposed to varicella 15 days before the onset of pustules; another study was begun in an infant exposed to measles virus 14 days prior to the onset of clinical illness. The grouped nitrogen balance data from the vaccinated infants are shown in Figure 3–3. Despite the development of a short-lived fever in this relatively mild infection, the infants maintained their usual food intake. Thus, the vaccinated infants did not go into negative nitrogen balance, and their rate of growth barely was slowed.[4] In measles or varicella, illness was of greater severity, and a transient period of negative nitrogen balance was recorded. Similarly, Viteri and Béhar[127] measured nitrogen balance during childhood infections or after administration of live vaccines. Nitrogen loss varied with the severity of the illness. Wilson and colleagues[143] reported nitrogen balance changes in hospitalized children who were convalescing from kwashiorkor when they developed varicella. There was a reduction in nitrogen retention, and some children developed negative balances. Despite efforts to maintain a constant dietary intake, the children consumed less food during the infection.

Acute nondiarrheal infections typically do not cause an increased loss of fecal nitrogen; however, if diarrhea is present during an illness, fecal losses of nitrogen and other nutrients can occur.[86, 107] Nitrogen losses also can occur through

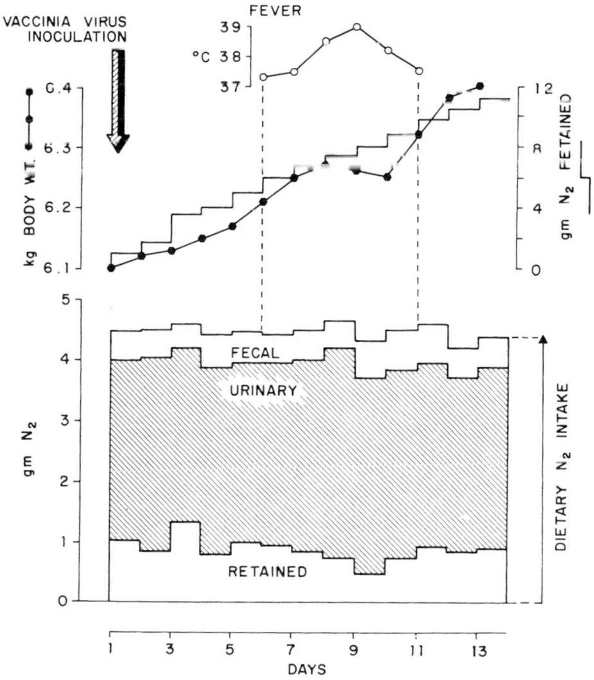

FIGURE 3–3. *Sequential measurements of body weight and cumulative nitrogen balance (top) and daily nitrogen balance (bottom) in a group of five healthy infants inoculated with vaccinia virus. Nitrogen intake values (plotted upward from baseline) and fecal and urinary losses (plotted downward from intake) reveal that the growing infants continued to retain nitrogen despite brief periods of fever. (Drawn from numerical data published by Beck.[4])*

sweat, exudates, blood loss (from illness or from laboratory tests), sputum, gaseous exchanges, or sites of surgical drainage.[12, 15]

The absolute loss of body nitrogen, as measured by metabolic balance techniques during infection, also can be used as a guide for estimating the absolute losses from the body of other intracellular elements, such as potassium, magnesium, phosphate, and, to a lesser degree, sulfur and zinc.[5, 15] By using the ratios present in normal skeletal muscle of nitrogen to potassium and of nitrogen to magnesium, measured losses of body nitrogen during infection can be used to estimate concomitant losses of potassium and magnesium from the body. Similarly, a ratio of nitrogen to phosphorus in skeletal muscle can be used to estimate inorganic phosphate losses during infection, provided that corrections first are made to account for any phosphate losses originating from demineralized bone. Calculations such as these suggest that the absolute losses of body nitrogen during infection are derived primarily from intracellular sources because they correlate in both timing and magnitude with losses of the other principal intracellular elements.[15]

In contrast to infection-induced losses of intracellular elements, the losses of extracellular ions, sodium and chloride, follow an independent course during infection, and calcium losses are minimal in acute infection in the absence of long-term bed rest or paralysis with body immobilization.[15, 139]

Urinary Excretion of Nitrogen-Containing Compounds

The onset of fever typically is accompanied by an increased urinary loss of creatinine. This usually is followed within a day by increased losses of urea and ammonia.[15] Although alpha-amino nitrogen losses may increase transiently at the onset of fever in some infections, this excretion tends to be lower than baseline measurements during the remainder of illness and throughout convalescence. When measured prospectively, excretion of urinary alpha-amino nitrogen or most individual free amino acids did not change appreciably during sandfly fever, a mild virus infection.[130] In contrast, there were increased urinary losses of 3-methylhistidine and phenylalanine. The increased loss of phenylalanine appeared to reflect its increased concentrations in plasma.[131] Studies using radioactive compounds in rats suggested that most of the excess urea excreted during an acute infection was generated by the deamination of endogenous amino acids derived principally from skeletal muscle.[5]

Increased excretion of one of the amino acids, 3-methylhistidine, serves to indicate the extent of skeletal muscle catabolism. This amino acid cannot be reutilized after its release from contractile proteins.[65, 147]

Uric acid excretion may increase during febrile periods, but the greatest changes have been reported during infectious mononucleosis.[84] Uric acid losses are ascribed to an accelerated turnover of nucleic acids and enhanced purine degradation.

An increased excretion of urinary diazo reactants is common during most acute infectious illnesses, especially typhoid fever. These reactants include metabolites, such as kynurenine, 3-hydroxy-kynurenine, *o*-amino-hippuric acid, xanthurenic acid, and anthranilic acid, which are created during the accelerated hepatic metabolism of tryptophan via the kynurenine pathway.[99]

A sudden, dramatic increase in urinary nitrate excretion occurs during acute infections. This increase is a reflection of the cytokine-stimulated production of nitric oxide as a host defensive measure.[33, 119, 122, 128]

METABOLISM OF FREE AMINO ACIDS

The distribution, utilization, and metabolism of free amino acids undergo profound alterations during the course of acute infectious illness. Measurements in patients show patterns of change that can be explained by studies performed in experimental laboratory animals.[35, 94, 95, 132] As some proteins are produced, others are degraded, and many of the released amino acids are redistributed throughout the body before they are reutilized.

A diminution in the concentration of most free individual amino acids in plasma may begin even before the onset of symptoms. Hypoaminoacidemia generally persists throughout the febrile period of illness, the largest decreases occurring in the branched-chain amino acids, leucine, isoleucine, and valine.[81] The decline primarily is due to an accelerated uptake of free amino acids by the liver. This increased flux from plasma to liver has been shown to occur in several species of animals during a variety of infections.[81] The amino acids that enter the liver are used for a variety of purposes. Amino acids may be metabolized to other compounds, oxidized, or reutilized for the synthesis of new proteins. Interleukin-6 appears to trigger many of the alterations in hepatic protein and amino acid metabolism during acute infection.[8, 113]

Amino acids become important sources of energy during the hypermetabolic phase of acute infections. Some amino acids are oxidized directly in muscle, while others are transformed progressively into glucose and glucagon. Gluconeogenic amino acids, such as alanine, are deaminated, and their carbon skeletons are used as the principal substrate for producing glucose, while their nitrogen is used to create urea for excretion.

A complete spectrum of amino acids is required for the synthesis of new body proteins generated during infection, including hepatic enzymes,[100] such as tryptophan oxygenase and tyrosine transaminase, and the lipoproteins and glycoproteins released into the plasma.[5, 92, 93] This group of glycoproteins constitutes the "acute-phase reactants," which include alpha$_1$-antitrypsin, amyloid, alpha$_1$-acid glycoprotein, haptoglobin, C-reactive protein, fibrinogen, the third component of complement, and ceruloplasmin.

These acute-phase reactant proteins are produced in excess during infections, even in protein-deficient children who exhibit acute kwashiorkor.[90] Some of the potentially beneficial functions attributed to acute-phase reactants include an amplification of both humoral and cell-mediated immunity, antiproteinase effects that could limit or contain harmful enzymes liberated during inflammatory reactions, oxidase activities, and the detoxification of free hemoglobin.[92]

In addition to the accelerated synthesis of proteins within the liver, infection increases the production of phagocytic and lymphoid cells. There also is a need for producing increased quantities of such diverse proteins as the cytokines, complement and kinin components, fibronectin, and the several classes of immunoglobulins. All of these requirements involve the need for free amino acids.

Proinflammatory cytokines and interferon-γ stimulate the production of nitric oxide from arginine, its sole precursor.[33, 128] Among its many important biologic effects, nitric oxide is a highly potent microbicidal, parasiticidal, and tumoricidal agent.[119] The importance of nitric oxide in these roles may rival that of free oxygen radicals in potency and effectiveness.[122] This newly recognized host defense agent is generated when cytokine-induced nitric oxide synthase initiates the oxygenation of one of arginine's guanido nitrogen groups to produce citrulline and nitric oxide.[119]

Amino Acid Availability

In the presence of anorexia and a diminished intake of food nutrients, the body is faced in large measure with the task of supplying its increased amino acid needs from endogenous sources. The principal sources of potentially available endogenous amino acids are the proteins of somatic tissues, including skeletal muscle and skin. The free amino acid pool contains the equivalent of about 12.5 g of protein in a normal adult man, an amount that represents only 0.1 per cent of total body protein.[129] Because the normal turnover of protein in a healthy adult is about 200 to 250 g each day, the free amino acid pool must be resupplied continually from endogenous as well as exogenous sources. During infections, the absorption of individual amino acids from the intestine may be depressed and delayed[75] or increased,[28] depending on the infection studied. Protein synthesis is not stopped entirely within body somatic tissues during an infection but is slowed markedly. At the same time, the rates of degradation of somatic proteins are accelerated, so that there is a net loss of muscle, skin, and other somatic proteins through catabolic wasting. Catabolic degradation of skeletal muscle protein can be initiated by interleukin-1,[3, 8, 25, 32] which triggers muscular proteases via the intracellular production of prostaglandin E_2. The body appears to sacrifice contractile proteins of skeletal muscle to obtain the free amino acids needed for higher priority requirements.

Some of the amino acids liberated during muscle protein catabolism are lost directly to the plasma. Others, such as the branched-chain group, are utilized in situ as sources of energy for muscle fibers; after oxidation, their amino groups are used to manufacture new glutamine and alanine, which can be used elsewhere for gluconeogenesis.[65] Because they can be oxidized within skeletal muscle, the rate of release of the branched-chain amino acids from muscle is decreased; this exaggerates the decline in their concentrations in plasma.[5, 81, 129] Some of the free amino acids liberated within muscle are retained within contractile cells and reutilized for the slowed but continuing process of muscle protein anabolism.

This catabolic breakdown of somatic protein to supply amino acids for use in other parts of the body is a highly visible clinical phenomenon. In this regard, the proteins of skin, skeletal muscle, and other somatic structures appear to constitute the principal body pool of "labile" nitrogen, which is called upon to maintain protein homeostasis and the physiologic functions of visceral tissues during periods of infectious illness or other stresses. Because infants and small children have very little muscle protein (and thus, a very small "bank" of readily available amino acids), the infection-induced need for free amino acids puts these youngsters at a special disadvantage.

To study the complex interrelationships in amino acid metabolism, workers have used isotopes to measure the simultaneous rates of anabolism and catabolism in the protein of skeletal muscle and other tissues of experimental animals during infection.[103] In addition, clinically useful estimates of skeletal muscle degradation can be obtained in patients through the quantitative daily measurement of 3-methylhistidine excretion into urine. More than 90 per cent of the total body content of 3-methylhistidine is associated with the peptide chains of actin in all muscle and of myosin in white muscle fibers.[147] This unique amino acid is formed in situ through the transmethylation of histidine, but only after the histidine first has been incorporated into the amino acid structure of myofibrillar proteins. When released, 3-methylhistidine cannot be reutilized by the body and instead is lost via the urine. The increase in excretion of 3-methylhistidine during acute infections is in keeping with other estimates of skeletal muscle wasting. The degree of proteolysis during severe surgical sepsis also has been quantified by measuring the differences between concentrations of glucose, lactate, free fatty acids, ketones, and alanine in femoral arterial and venous blood.[88] Neither free fatty acid nor ketone utilization was increased during acute fevers, but an increased oxidation of glucose and of amino acids derived from protein was used to fuel cellular hypermetabolism. Although infection stimulates a sizable increase in the rates of body protein synthesis, the acceleration of protein catabolism is increased even further, and the body suffers a net loss of somatic proteins and even some visceral ones.[129]

Phenylalanine is one of the amino acids released by the accelerated catabolism of somatic proteins. However, only relatively limited amounts of phenylalanine can be utilized for the synthesis of new proteins or for its conversion into tyrosine.[129, 131] Accordingly, phenylalanine concentrations in the circulating free amino acid pool tend to rise rather than fall during periods of fever. These increases occur coincidentally with the typical declines in plasma values for tyrosine and most other free amino acids. The exaggerated phenylalanine-to-tyrosine ratio can be useful for evaluating these opposing changes during febrile illnesses. An increase in this ratio thus serves as a useful clinical index of the severity of infection-induced alterations in amino acid metabolism.[129] During infections of great severity and those with hepatocellular dysfunction, hypoaminoacidemia may be replaced by an excessive accumulation of many other free amino acids in plasma.[5, 115, 141]

Free tryptophan, also liberated from degrading protein, undergoes an accelerated metabolism via several different metabolic pathways in the liver.[5, 78, 79, 94] In response to the increased hepatic availability of tryptophan or the increased synthesis of tryptophan oxygenase, or both, excess tryptophan enters the kynurenine pathways, where it is converted into different diazo-reactant compounds and pyrimidine nucleotides.[94] At the same time, tryptophan enters other pathways, leading possibly to increased synthesis of serotonin or indoleacetic acid.[99]

CARBOHYDRATE METABOLISM

During the febrile phase of infectious illnesses, carbohydrate metabolism provides much of the additional energy needed by body cells. An increased demand for metabolizable energy is met by a resetting of the endocrine control mechanisms to permit a marked acceleration of the synthesis and release of glucose from the liver.[29, 41, 142] Although some glucose is derived from hepatocellular glycogen, the majority of the additional requirements for glucose during acute infections are met through an acceleration of the hepatic gluconeogenic mechanisms. Recycled lactate and amino acids, especially those with gluconeogenic potential, such as alanine, are the principal substrates used by the liver for increasing its output of newly synthesized glucose; glycerol (derived from the metabolism of triglyceride lipids) and pyruvate also are used.[65]

Early in acute infectious illnesses, basal blood glucose concentrations tend to become somewhat elevated. Insulin-requiring diabetic patients often develop glycosuria at the onset of febrile infections, and more insulin must be given to maintain their control. The tendency for acute infections to be accompanied by an early modest hyperglycemia also is seen in laboratory animals. Modest hyperglycemia often is noted in animals after an injection of bacterial endotoxin.[19, 72]

Although an early hyperglycemic response appears to be the initial change in carbohydrate metabolism, the ability of the body to sustain an accelerated production of glucose may be lost. Hypoglycemia then may emerge as an important clinical problem. Hypoglycemia generally results from one of two major pathogenic mechanisms: a diminished availability of substrate molecules required for gluconeogenesis or a failure of the metabolic mechanisms needed to produce hepatic glucose. Carbohydrate pathway defects at the molecular level have not been found in overwhelming bacterial infections in laboratory animals.[48, 85] Therefore, carbohydrate depletion during overwhelming or terminal infections can be ascribed to substrate nonavailability. However, if hepatic cells are injured during an infectious disease, such as viral hepatitis, hypoglycemia can result from a failure of gluconeogenic processes.[5, 36, 107]

The depletion of substrate for adequate gluconeogenesis occurs primarily as a dangerous clinical complication of neonatal sepsis. Infants are born with only minimal amounts of skeletal muscle protein. Because muscle contains the principal "labile nitrogen" pool for supplying amino acids that can be converted into glucose, neonatal infants lack a sufficient quantity of potential substrate molecules for sustaining long-term gluconeogenesis. Newborn infants especially are prone to develop severe hypoglycemia whenever a septic process becomes established.[146] On the other hand, hypoglycemia that results from a breakdown of hepatic gluconeogenic mechanisms occurs primarily when liver cells are damaged by an infectious or toxemic process. Thus, hypoglycemia can become an important complicating factor in severe viral hepatitis, yellow fever, or endotoxemia during gram-negative sepsis.[36, 72] These conditions can cause hepatocellular damage and a breakdown of enzyme-synthesizing mechanisms within the liver.[72]

A change in glucose tolerance can be detected within hours after the onset of a febrile infection.[102, 111] Baseline blood glucose values may be elevated somewhat, and glucose disappearance is slowed moderately as a component aspect of a febrile illness. Under these circumstances, the pancreatic islets produce insulin in excess quantities. Despite an increase in plasma insulin concentrations, glucose disappearance rates are slowed; these combined metabolic changes resemble those caused by mild insulin resistance.

Bacterial and viral infections also cause an increased secretion of pancreatic glucagon,[102, 105] which, together with catecholamine release during infection,[45, 47, 142] provides hormonal stimuli for accelerating gluconeogenesis within the liver. These hormonal stimuli initiate their hepatic effects during infection by activating adenylate cyclase.[29] The unusual simultaneous increase in basal concentrations of both insulin and glucagon in plasma results from direct cytokine stimulation of pancreatic islet cells.[8, 40, 145] Because of these hormonal changes and high plasma glucocorticoid values in severe bacterial sepsis, infusions of glucose may fail to suppress hepatic gluconeogenesis.[65, 66] The resultant increase in glucose pool size helps to explain the apparent slowing of glucose disappearance and the occurrence of hyperinsulinemia during infections.

Certain viral infections in children seem prone to initiate acute juvenile-type, insulin-requiring diabetes mellitus. Although the evidence for a viral etiology of diabetes has not been established fully in humans, there are epidemiologic suggestions that juvenile diabetes may develop several months after certain viral illnesses, especially mumps, coxsackievirus B (type 4) infection, rubella, or cytomegalovirus infection.[83] Additional epidemiologic evidence is based on a tendency for new cases of juvenile-type diabetes to appear in clusters.

Susceptibility to juvenile diabetes also may be influenced

by genetic make-up. A high incidence of human leukocyte antigen types B8 and Bw15 has been detected in juvenile diabetics.[108] Studies in laboratory animals suggest that genetically susceptible species may have virus receptor sites on their insulin-producing beta cells. These receptors in species with high-risk haplotypes allow viruses to be adsorbed by the pancreatic beta cells, with subsequent destruction of insulin-producing cells.

The cytokine granulocyte colony-stimulating factor influences the uptake of glucose by phagocytic cells, as well as their mobilization during inflammatory reactions.[62] Glucose availability contributes directly to the respiratory burst that accompanies phagocytosis, as well as to the production of the myeloperoxidase enzymes needed to kill engulfed organisms.

LIPID METABOLISM

As shown in Table 3–1, numerous changes in lipid metabolism have been documented during infection. In contrast to the relatively stereotyped patterns of change in nitrogen and amino acid metabolism and in the accelerated production of glucose, responses involving body lipids are more variable from infection to infection. Plasma lipid changes also may be biphasic during the course of a single infection.

This complexity results in part from the multiple factors that control the metabolism of lipids during infectious illnesses,[5, 115] including the need for hepatic synthesis of serum lipoproteins, variations in the production and utilization of free fatty acids and ketones as sources of cellular energy, and variable changes in rates of uptake or release of lipids from body fat depots.[5, 115]

Lipids have another function that is of major importance during acute-phase reactions. This function involves the cytokine-stimulated use of polyunsaturated fatty acids localized within cell walls to serve as precursor molecules for various families of eicosanoids (prostaglandins, prostacyclines, thromboxanes, and lipoxines). These eicosanoid lipids, in turn, trigger many of the diverse cellular responses seen during infection, inflammation, and immune responses.[58, 104]

TABLE 3–1. Basic Mechanisms Leading to Observed Effects of Infection on Lipid Metabolism of the Host

Effects Associated with the Presence of Invading Microorganisms

1. Direct effects
   a. Microorganism use of host lipids for replication
   b. Disruption of host cell metabolism by intracellular microorganisms
   c. Localized destruction of fat cells by the infectious process
2. Indirect effects
   a. Alterations in host metabolism caused by bacterial exotoxins, endotoxins, or bacterial enzymes
   b. Activation of lipases and other lipid-affecting enzymes within host phagocytes

Effects Secondary to Development of Generalized Illness Due to Infection

1. Decreased dietary fat intake
2. Interference with intestinal digestion and absorption of lipids
3. Alterations in lipid transport
   a. Changing concentrations of lipid transport proteins
   b. Decreased lipoprotein lipase activity (caused by tumor necrosis factor), which allows triglycerides to accumulate in plasma
4. Altered lipid metabolism within host cells caused by proinflammatory cytokines
   a. Activation of cell wall phospholipases by proinflammatory cytokines
   b. Creation, from cell wall polyunsaturated fatty acids, of intracellular arachidonic and/or eicosapentanoic acids
   c. Transformation of arachidonic and eicosapentanoic acids into various eicosanoids (prostaglandins, prostacyclines, thromboxanes, and lipoxanes)
5. Other alterations of lipid metabolism within host cells
   a. Altered rates of hormone-mediated lipolysis within fat depots
   b. Accelerated fatty acid synthesis within the liver
   c. Depressed hepatic ketogenesis
   d. Altered rates of lipid uptake and use by peripheral tissues
6. Participation of newly formed eicosanoids in inflammatory and immunologic responses, as well as in the coagulation mechanisms
7. Effects related to the prior nutritional status of the patient
8. Terminal pathologic hyperlipidemic effects associated with gram-negative sepsis and hypotensive shock

Plasma Lipids and Lipoproteins

Because the concentrations of individual lipid moieties in plasma depend on the algebraic summation of both input and removal rates, the mechanisms that control the release or uptake of individual lipids must be studied throughout the course of various kinds of infectious illnesses.

Cholesterol concentrations have been reported to increase, to decrease, or to remain unchanged.[5] Mild virus infections often are associated with a transient decline in serum cholesterol values. When longitudinal studies were conducted during the course of experimentally induced sandfly fever in young adult male volunteers, plasma values for total and esterified cholesterol, phospholipids, and free fatty acids all declined in conjunction with, or immediately prior to, the onset of fever.[63] This decline in concentration included both the cholesterol and protein components of the low-density beta-lipoproteins. In contrast, the plasma triglyceride values showed a biphasic pattern of change: an initial decline was followed by an early convalescent-period rise above baseline control concentrations. A depression of total serum cholesterol values also has been reported during pneumococcal pneumonia, cholera, tuberculosis, and malaria. However, when studied in rhesus monkeys experimentally infected with *Streptococcus pneumoniae* or *Salmonella typhimurium*, rates of [^{3}H] mevalonic acid incorporation into free cholesterol were accelerated,[37] and there was no evidence for an inhibition of squalene synthesis or its conversion to cholesterol. In contrast, the synthesis of cholesterol was blocked partially when monkeys with diet-induced hypercholesterolemia were subjected to a pneumococcal infection.[37]

Marked increases in the concentrations of total serum lipids and triglycerides are found consistently in patients with infections caused by gram-negative bacilli,[5, 55, 115] but this response is minimized or fails to occur in patients with viral or gram-positive coccal infections. A similar difference has been noted in monkeys studied during either *S. pneumoniae* or *S. typhimurium* infection.[56] Tumor necrosis factor, a proinflammatory cytokine with a unique additional function that inhibits the enzyme lipoprotein lipase, appears to be of central importance in accounting for these differences.[55]

Although a release of tumor necrosis factor from activated macrophages may occur in many infections, its release is stimulated markedly by bacterial endotoxins released during gram-negative infections.[8, 74] Hypertriglyceridemia during

S. typhimurium infection in monkeys was generated by tumor necrosis factor–induced mechanisms that reduced both the clearance of lipids from plasma and the activity of heparin-sensitive plasma lipoprotein lipase. Hypertriglyceridemia during pneumococcal infections was far less severe than that observed during gram-negative infections. After endotoxin administration,[55] hypertriglyceridemia developed chiefly as the result of an impaired lipid disposal mechanism, again, secondary to tumor necrosis factor release from macrophages.[8] There also was an acceleration in the rate of hepatic production of triglycerides from free fatty acid precursors.

Lipids and Energy Metabolism During Infection

Cellular energy requirements during chronic infections in laboratory animals appear to be met largely through the catabolism of body fat stores.[67] In contrast, fat wasting does not seem to be as prominent during rapidly lethal bacterial infections. Ketogenesis also seems to be blunted during acute infections.[85] Free fatty acid concentrations in plasma normally are increased by the actions of catecholamines, growth hormone, and glucagon, which are increased during infection.[5] On the other hand, concomitantly high concentrations of plasma insulin apparently serve to inhibit both lipolysis and ketogenesis.[5, 85] The contribution of free fatty acids to energy production during infection thus is influenced by the interplay of these hormones, the availability of glucose, and the functional capacity of the liver to take up fatty acids and convert them to triglycerides.[37, 38, 40, 41]

Finally, brown fat is believed to contribute importantly to heat production in newborn infants via sympathetic nerve activation of this tissue. Because a number of viruses are known to proliferate in brown fat,[116] fever during neonatal viral infections may involve brown fat thermogenesis.

Acute infectious illnesses produce surprisingly few effects upon the intestinal absorption of fat, although this may be reduced somewhat during intestinal infections and parasitemic or enterotoxemic illnesses.[91, 107] Lipid precursors needed for the replication of microorganisms within host tissues must be supplied from metabolic pools within the host. For example, malarial parasites obtain their structural lipids from red blood cell precursors; lipid-containing viruses appear to obtain the lipid components needed for their assembly from lipid-rich membranes already present within host cells.

Lipid Metabolism and Host Defensive Measures

Rapid metabolic responses by cell wall lipids play a major role in initiating a panoply of intracellular events during acute-phase reactions. The attachment of proinflammatory cytokines to cell wall receptors triggers the conversion of polyunsaturated fatty acid in cell wall membranes to a variety of biologically active eicosanoids. Lipids of various eicosanoid families then become the messenger molecules that are responsible for many of the acute-phase metabolic and cellular responses[8, 32] that occur during infection. These short-lived eicosanoids are biopotent at nanomolar to picomolar concentrations. In addition to their importance within lymphocytes of the immune system, eicosanoid lipids transmit stimulatory or inhibitory signals between other cells and tissues in both health and disease.[58, 104] Although they do not initiate disease processes, various eicosanoid lipids, i.e., prostaglandins, leukotrienes, prostacycline, lipoxines, and thromboxanes, are important components of the pathogenic progression of infectious diseases.[58, 104]

Eicosanoids also have important effects on other white blood cells and platelets, as well as on such diverse organs as the brain, lungs, stomach, and kidneys. These eicosanoids appear to be components of complex, often overlapping, regulatory mechanisms that interconnect the immune system, the central nervous system, the endocrine glands, and the functions of many other organs and tissues. These homeostatic (and at times pathogenic) mechanisms are characterized by numerous duplications, amplifications, checks and balances, and feedback control loops.

Biochemical details now are well established concerning the intracellular synthesis of individual eicosanoids from both *n*-3 and *n*-6 polyunsaturated fatty acid precursors.[58, 104] After cytokines interact with cell wall receptors, they activate cell membrane phospholipase enzymes. These enzymes initiate the release (into the cell interior) of arachidonic acid from cell wall (*n*-6) polyunsaturated fatty acid or eicosapentanoic acid from (*n*-3) polyunsaturated fatty acid. These first steps of eicosanoid synthesis can be blocked by adrenocorticoid hormones. In target cells having cyclooxygenase enzymes, arachidonic acid is oxygenated into 4-series leukotrienes, 2-series prostaglandins, or thromboxanes and prostacyclin. On the other hand, if a cell possesses lipooxygenase enzymes, arachidonic acid is oxygenated into the sometimes less potent 5-series leukotrienes, 3-series prostaglandins, or lipoxins.[104] The highly active eicosanoid molecules are degraded rapidly. Importantly, synthesis of prostaglandins of both the 2- and 4-series can be blocked by certain nonsteroidal anti-inflammatory drugs, e.g., aspirin, indomethacin, and ibuprofen.[58, 104]

Other fatty acids may participate in defense mechanisms of the host and, on occasion, even may be involved in pathogenic events of a harmful nature. An increase in the fat content of vital organs is common in patients dying of severe bacterial infections; fatty metamorphosis especially is prominent in the liver, kidney, and heart.[53] Hyperlipemia in gram-negative septicemia may be accompanied by fat embolization to the lungs. Other deleterious actions of body lipids involve the liberation of phospholipids from platelets and their subsequent participation in the activation of the blood-clotting cascade leading to disseminated intravascular coagulation.

ELECTROLYTE AND ACID-BASE METABOLISM

Many of the life-threatening medical emergencies faced by infants and children with acute infectious diseases involve problems in the areas of salt and water or acid-base balance. Some infections cause severe overhydration, and others produce dehydration with hypovolemic shock. Pathogenic mechanisms that come into play during various infections can lead to metabolic alkalosis or acidosis, to respiratory alkalosis or acidosis, or to complex admixtures of these pathophysiologic perturbations.[8, 16]

The onset of fever typically is accompanied by tachypnea and accelerated respiratory gas exchange, which leads in turn to an exaggerated loss of dissolved carbon dioxide from blood and a state of uncompensated respiratory alkalosis.[5] Alkalosis may persist as long as febrile tachypnea lasts and gas exchange within the alveoli remains unimpeded.

Conversely, infections that produce extensive pulmonary consolidation can impair carbon dioxide exchange and cause respiratory acidosis. Respiratory acidosis also is a complication in patients whose pulmonary musculature no longer can function effectively, as in those with poliomyelitis, tetanus, botulism, or respiratory distress syndrome.

Metabolic acidosis generally develops whenever an infectious disease process becomes severe. With the hypotension, vascular stasis, and cellular anoxia seen during gram-negative sepsis, the generation of excessive lactic acid and other acidic metabolic products exceeds the capacity of the body's buffering systems.[5, 115]

Diarrheal diseases can be accompanied by two other forms of metabolic acid-base derangement.[16, 107, 134] Toxigenic diarrhea characterized by high-volume stool loss, such as seen in Asiatic cholera or *Escherichia coli* enterotoxemia, causes an excessive loss of fecal bicarbonate and an alkaline stool, with a resultant decline in blood pH. Bicarbonate is secreted actively in the lower ileum and cannot be reabsorbed completely by the colonic mucosa if there are high-volume losses of watery stool.[16] In contrast, diarrhea accompanied by only low-volume stool losses, as in rotavirus infections,[107] tends to be associated with an acid stool associated with an exaggerated loss of fecal potassium rather than bicarbonate. If fecal potassium losses persist chronically over a long period or occur rapidly as part of the massive fluid loss of acute secretory diarrheas, such as in pediatric cholera, body potassium can be depleted severely. The loss of cellular potassium then can produce metabolic alkalosis, cardiac arrhythmia, paralytic ileus, and weakness in children and the occurrence of hypokalemic vacuolization in cells of the myocardium and renal tubular epithelium. Even if fluid balance is restored promptly in these patients, a prolonged state of metabolic alkalosis can persist until body potassium stores are replenished.

The importance of diarrheal diseases in infants and small children is great, with an estimated 2 to 3 million deaths worldwide each year.[86] Life-threatening dehydration can result from the loss of body water and electrolytes during high-volume diarrhea. Because massive diarrhea produces an isoosmotic loss of body water and electrolytes, the fluid losses come from the extracellular rather than the intracellular space.[134] The circulating blood becomes thick and viscous because of a relative increase in hematocrit values and a progressive concentration of serum proteins, which can increase to more than twice their normal values. Despite serious dehydration, concentrations of plasma sodium remain relatively normal, when expressed in terms of plasma water.[134] This type of acute, massive diarrhea can lead to the rapid onset of hypovolemic shock, renal failure, and death.

Dehydration usually does not become a problem in infectious diseases that lack protracted vomiting, diarrhea, or prominent sweat loss. Instead, severe generalized infections in children may be accompanied by some retention of body water and salt. Soon after the onset of a febrile illness, the adrenal secretion of aldosterone increases,[11, 14] and this mineralocorticoid stimulates the renal retention of sodium and chloride. These electrolytes virtually may disappear from the urine during a severe febrile illness. Retention of salt tends to be accompanied by a retention of body water throughout the period of illness.[5] Generalized edema is an infection-induced manifestation of kwashiorkor and also can be seen during severe infections in well-nourished children. Accumulations of excess water and salt typically are excreted after the acute phase of illness by a transient period of diuresis during the early convalescent period.

Some infections, particularly those that become localized within the central nervous system, also are complicated by an inappropriate secretion of antidiuretic hormone from the posterior pituitary.[34, 140] The ensuing retention of body water may dilute the sodium and chloride in plasma. Sodium redistribution also may contribute to the development of hyponatremia during infections. Sodium may begin to accumulate within body cells, apparently because the sodium pumping mechanisms in extracellular membranes may fail to maintain internal electrolyte homeostasis.[5] This form of sodium sequestration is evidence of severe illness. It is not reversed easily and may be a major complication in patients with severe infections, such as meningococcemia or Rocky Mountain spotted fever.

VITAMIN METABOLISM

Although few measurement data are available concerning infection-induced changes in vitamin metabolism, it generally is believed that the utilization or metabolism of most vitamins is accelerated.[13, 126] Scattered reports suggest that infectious diseases in humans may be followed by classic scurvy, beriberi, pellagra, or xerophthalmia.[109]

Recent attention has focused on vitamin A, which once was termed the anti-infection vitamin. Declining plasma concentrations of vitamin A during childhood infections are accompanied or perhaps caused by a marked urinary loss of this vitamin.[1, 121] Not only does the heightened vitamin A deficiency induced by infection contribute to the subsequent development of ocular and conjunctival pathologies, but also subclinical deficiencies of vitamin A and their associated immunologic dysfunctions can heighten the mortality associated with childhood infections,[110] as shown most dramatically in measles.[118]

Depressed plasma concentrations of several other vitamins also have been reported.[5] In addition to the urinary losses of vitamin A,[1, 121] increased excretion of urinary riboflavin and vitamin C may occur in conjunction with negative nitrogen balance.[13]

Vitamins are known to participate in metabolic processes activated during host defensive mechanisms.[8] The rapid synthesis of steroid hormones by the adrenal cortex is accompanied by a decline in the adrenal content of vitamin C. The B-group vitamins, vitamin C, and folate all participate in the metabolism of activated phagocytic cells.

Controversy continues to exist over whether massive daily doses of vitamin C can suppress or prevent the common cold and other viral respiratory infections. More that two decades ago, the American Academy of Pediatrics Committee on Drugs failed to find sufficient scientific evidence to support Pauling's claim,[26] but new data subsequently were introduced.[50] Concentrations of vitamin C in neutrophils decline during infectious diseases. Vitamin C is recognized for its importance in the locomotive activity of phagocytic cells, as well as its contributions to the immune system.[2]

Intestinal parasites, such as tapeworms, may take up sufficient vitamin B_{12} from the succus entericus to diminish B_{12} absorption and lead to the development of megaloblastic anemia. The intestinal absorption of fat-soluble vitamins and folate also may be impaired for a time in children with enteric infections or parasitic diseases.[68]

TRACE ELEMENT METABOLISM

As outlined in Table 3–2, infectious illnesses often are accompanied by changes in the plasma concentration of several of the trace elements. The most consistent responses include a decrease in the plasma concentrations of iron and zinc and an increase in plasma copper.[5] This triad of trace element changes has been reported in bacterial, viral, rickettsial, and parasitic infections. In acute viral hepatitis, however, serum iron values tend to increase in the second and third weeks of illness. Hepatitis also is associated with an unusual change in the binding of zinc to various ligands.[52] Early after the

TABLE 3–2. Infection-Related Changes in Trace Elements

Trace Element	Observed Change During Infection	Suggested Pathophysiologic Mechanisms
Iron	Hyposideremia (common)	Flux of iron into liver and reticuloendothelial system cells
		Increased synthesis of ferritin
		Sequestration of iron in tissue stores
		Diminished iron absorption
	Anemia	Accelerated red blood cell destruction
		Direct blood loss
		Inhibition erythropoiesis
	Reduced serum iron-binding capacity	Reduced synthesis of transferrin
	Hypersideremia (selective)	Hepatocyte damage during hepatitis
Zinc	Hypozincemia	Accelerated flux of zinc into liver
		Hepatic synthesis of additional metallothioneins
		Negative body balance of zinc
	Hyperzincuria	Hepatitis-induced inhibition of zinc binding to plasma proteins
Copper	Hypercupremia	Accelerated hepatic synthesis and release of ceruloplasmin
Chromium	Hypochromia	Unknown
Manganese	Hypermanganemia	Hepatocyte damage during hepatitis
Cobalt	Hypercobaltemia	Hepatocyte damage during hepatitis
	Macrocytic anemia	Intestinal parasitic competition for available vitamin B_{12}
Gallium	Hypergallemia	Hepatocyte damage during hepatitis
	Accumulation in sites of localized infection	Unknown
Iodine	Accelerated deiodination of thyroid hormones	Increased cellular metabolic rates
		Increased iodine availability for cellular bactericidal functions

acute onset of jaundice, plasma zinc is found to be bound almost entirely as microligands to small molecules, such as the amino acids. This phenomenon contrasts with the normal propensity for about 95 per cent of plasma zinc to bind predominantly as a macroligand with either albumin or alpha$_2$-macroglobulin. In any event, plasma zinc is sequestered rapidly in the liver, where it becomes tightly bound during acute infections to newly synthesized metallothioneins.[117]

Changes in Iron Metabolism

With the exception of acute viral hepatitis, an abrupt depression in serum iron concentrations has been observed in virtually all infections in which iron values have been measured, with pyogenic infections causing the greatest effects. This hypoferremia has been ascribed primarily to an accelerated flux of iron from plasma into the liver, where it becomes localized in reticuloendothelial cells and hepatocytes. There the iron becomes sequestered as intracellular hemosiderin molecules or as a complex with ferritin.[8] Tumor necrosis factor and interleukin-1 appear to trigger this sequestration of iron by inducing the formation of ferritin,[21] some of which may be found in plasma. Plasma ferritin values provide a valuable clue concerning the quantities of body iron available in storage depots. Once iron has become sequestered, it is not released readily until the infection is terminated.

During both acute and chronic infections, there appears to be an inhibition of the normal mechanisms that allows for the continuing release from tissue stores of the iron needed for use in erythropoiesis. Thus, if an infection persists for a prolonged period, anemia may develop. Although the "anemia of infection" resembles iron deficiency anemia in its peripheral manifestations, it develops in the presence of adequate quantities of iron in storage sites and cannot be reversed by the therapeutic administration of iron.[8]

Other factors that influence iron metabolism during infection include an accelerated destruction of red blood cells and their direct loss in diseases in which hemolysis or bleeding is a factor. Excessive laboratory testing of blood samples can occur. In malaria, for example, serum iron values tend to decline, despite the unusually large amounts of hemoglobin released from parasitized red blood cells. The released hemoglobin rapidly complexes with haptoglobin and is taken up by reticuloendothelial cells.[82] As in other forms of hemolytic anemia, a depression of serum haptoglobin values in malaria can serve as an index of the severity of red blood cell destruction.

An inhibition of iron absorption in the intestinal tract also can contribute to an infection-induced depression of serum iron values.[137] Studies using radioactive iron showed that a febrile illness or the febrile response of infants or young children to immunization could depress intestinal iron absorption for several days.[18]

The abrupt fall in serum iron concentration, which can reach virtually undetectable values, takes place without any appreciable change in total serum iron-binding capacity. Although serum transferrin concentrations decline along with those of albumin during severe protein deficiency states, they decline only slowly, if at all, during acute infections. The combination of a normal iron-binding capacity and a markedly depressed serum iron concentration in previously well-nourished children results in an increase in the serum concentration of unsaturated transferrin.[8] Unsaturated transferrin may serve an important host defensive role by competing with siderophores of bacteria, which need to acquire iron for their growth and replication.[136] Because of its high affinity constant for iron, unsaturated transferrin serves as an important potential mechanism for inhibiting bacterial replication.

Increased concentrations of serum iron have been reported during bacillary dysentery, typhoidal infections, and, most commonly, acute viral hepatitis. The increase in serum iron concentrations is delayed in hepatitis until several weeks after the initial appearance of jaundice; this increase may be large enough virtually to saturate the iron-binding capacity of serum. An impairment of mechanisms accounting for the normal daily hepatic removal of iron from serum has been thought to explain the hyperferremia noted during infections associated with liver cell dysfunction. An alternative hypothesis suggests that hepatitis-induced hyperferremia is caused by an escape of iron from the damaged hepatocytes. The latter explanation also is used to explain the reported increase in concentrations of serum manganese, gallium, and cobalt during acute hepatitis.[5]

Changes in Zinc Metabolism

Zinc concentrations decline during various infectious diseases, as they do during a large variety of other diseases characterized by the presence of an inflammatory process.[5, 93] Zinc values, however, rarely fall as low as iron values. This difference apparently is due to the large amount of plasma zinc that is bound tightly to alpha$_2$-macroglobulin. This plasma protein remains relatively constant during periods of infection.[5]

Like iron, zinc appears to move into the liver at an accelerated rate during acute infections. This increased flux of zinc from serum to liver appears to be triggered by the action of proinflammatory cytokines released from activated monocytes and macrophages.[5, 8] The hepatic uptake and sequestration of zinc are associated with an increased synthesis of zinc-binding metallothioneins within the hepatic cells.[117] The reason for this flux of zinc from serum to liver has not been explained in terms of host defense.

Body balances of zinc are believed to become negative during infectious diseases because of a combination of factors, including a reduction in dietary zinc intake, a diminished absorption from the intestinal tract, and a concomitant continuation (or increase) of zinc losses via the urine and possibly via the feces and sweat. During acute infectious hepatitis, there is a marked increase in the urinary loss of zinc. This loss is due to enhanced glomerular filtration and excretion of zinc microligands.[52] The increased formation of zinc microligands with amino acids, such as histidine and cysteine, permits plasma zinc to be excreted from the body via the urine. It is not known whether an increased binding of zinc to amino acid microligands occurs during infections other than acute hepatitis; this phenomenon was not detected during sandfly fever.

Changes in Copper Metabolism

Plasma copper concentrations increase in virtually all infections. This increase appears to accompany the accelerated synthesis and release from the liver of ceruloplasmin, the copper-binding protein of plasma. The increase in plasma ceruloplasmin resembles that of other acute-phase reactant proteins produced by the liver during inflammatory states when triggered by interleukin-6 and other proinflammatory cytokines.[8] Increases in ceruloplasmin and copper occur somewhat later than the abrupt depressions in serum iron and zinc. The increase in copper values tends to persist somewhat longer than the changes in zinc and iron, apparently as a result of the relatively long in vivo half-disappearance time of ceruloplasmin from plasma. Body balances of copper have not been studied during an infectious illness.

PROINFLAMMATORY CYTOKINES

The generalized metabolic and physiologic responses to febrile infections are initiated and sustained by a unique control mechanism. This mechanism involves the secretion by various body cells of hormone-like cytokines (mainly monokines and lymphokines).[32] The cytokines include interleukins, interferons, colony-stimulating factors, and tumor necrosis factor. Cytokines also function during localized infections.[98]

Complex cytokine interactions during illness only now are being unraveled.[8, 32] Cytokines are not classified as hormones because they are produced by a variety of different cells located throughout the body, rather than by anatomically distinct glands, because cytokines are effective at far lower concentrations than hormones, and because their interacting array of checks and balances is far more complex than that of hormones. Although cytokines are not components of either the central nervous or endocrine systems, they interact with and trigger responses by both of these major regulatory control systems.[8, 93]

Proinflammatory cytokines (which include interleukins-1, -6, and -8 and tumor necrosis factor) initiate and orchestrate the highly complex but relatively stereotyped admixture of concomitant anabolic and catabolic events that make up the generalized host response to febrile infections. Individual components of this generalized response form distinct patterns. Some metabolic responses begin during the incubation period, some at the onset of fever, some late in fever, and some during convalescence.[5–10] No matter which type of microorganism causes an acute, generalized, febrile infection, the onset of most metabolic, biochemical, or physiologic responses seems to occur at relatively consistent, predictable times. These many responses can be categorized temporally by their relationships to the time of onset of clinical symptoms and fever.[8] In fact, virtually every metabolic or biochemical process is influenced in some manner by the body's response to an acute infection. The duration and magnitude of individual components of the generalized response show some variability from infection to infection. More must be learned about how the cytokines influence this variability in host metabolic responses.

In today's terminology, this overall response is termed an acute-phase response, an acute-phase reaction, or the systemic inflammatory response syndrome. This acute-phase response may accompany other severe medical and surgical problems, in addition to infection.[60]

This complex response, which also activates complement and stimulates the immune system, appears to help defend the body.[8, 60] But on the darker side, acute-phase responses generate important nutritional costs,[5, 8, 106] costs that can produce severe, life-threatening malnutrition. In addition, acute-phase responses that become excessive or overly prolonged can lead to hypotensive shock, multiple organ dysfunction, and death.[32, 64, 88, 106]

Acute-phase responses are initiated and controlled by the proinflammatory cytokines.[32, 49, 51, 57, 64, 114, 120, 138] The cytokine interferon-α also can contribute to the wasting syndrome of acute infections.[27] The acute-phase reaction may be modified somewhat by bacterial endotoxins, which uniquely stimulate an exaggerated release of tumor necrosis factor, a cytokine that inhibits lipoprotein lipase enzymes, to account for the high plasma concentrations of triglycerides that develop during gram-negative sepsis.[8, 55]

The primary control mechanisms that initiate acute-phase responses normally exist in a standby mode but can be turned on whenever necessary. This is accomplished by the activation of macrophages, blood monocytes, or other body cells and by the subsequent rapid release of proinflammatory cytokines.[8, 32, 74] Many diverse types of stimuli can activate these cells, including the phagocytosis of microorganisms, tissue debris, or other particulate matter; the effects of polynucleotides, certain drugs and chemicals, antigen-antibody complexes, and bacterial toxins; and the actions of other cytokines. During infectious illnesses, proinflammatory cytokines can be detected in body fluids, body secretions, urine, and stools.[42, 71, 98, 101]

After their release from producing cells, proinflammatory cytokines circulate via the plasma or diffuse through tissue fluids to stimulate cell populations in many locations throughout the body. These cytokines have multiple, often overlapping actions, and they stimulate the release of companion cytokines. Interleukin-1 previously was termed endogenous pyrogen, leukocytic endogenous mediator, and lymphocyte-activating factor,[32] and tumor necrosis factor once was called cachectin. Proinflammatory cytokines stimulate the hypothalamic temperature-regulating center to initiate fever,[8, 32] endocrine glands to secrete hormones, the liver to take up amino acids and trace elements and to synthesize many different proteins,[8, 93, 114] the pancreatic islets to release both insulin and glucagon,[40, 145] and the muscle cells to catabolize contractile proteins.[3, 25] These cytokines also stimulate the bone marrow to produce and release neutrophils[93] and synovial cells and fibroblasts to activate collagenase.[32] Marrow stimulation involves the effect of interleukin-1 on progenitor cells[80] as well as its ability to trigger the release of various colony-stimulating cytokines.[8, 46, 80] In this regard, interleukin-1 has been found to be identical with hematopoietin.[80] Importantly, the proinflammatory cytokines also activate the immune system and cause certain subsets of T lymphocytes to secrete interleukins-2, -3, -4, and -5.[8, 32]

Proinflammatory cytokines are thought to function, after attachment to their specific cell wall receptors, by activating phospholipase A_2 within the cell walls, thus leading to the intracellular release of arachidonic and/or eicosapentanoic acids from cell wall polyunsaturated fatty acid phospholipids.[32] Subsequent responses by the cytokine-stimulated cell then are determined by the intracellular enzymes that can metabolize these acids to one of many possible eicosanoids.

Control Mechanisms for Proinflammatory Cytokine Actions

Like those of hormones, proinflammatory cytokine actions are regulated by a number of checks and balances. To act on a cell, a cytokine first must attach itself to a protein receptor on an exterior cell wall. However, cells produce other similar receptor proteins that then are released to float free in plasma.[61, 89] Freely circulating receptors can intercept and inactivate their matching cytokine.[39, 43] Other unique plasma protein molecules, receptor antagonists, also are produced.[124] These can attach to and block the cellular receptors for specific cytokines.[61, 89] Cytokine inhibitor proteins have been identified.[23, 125] Other cytokines, such as interleukins-4 and -10, can suppress the cellular production of proinflammatory cytokines.[30, 44, 61, 97, 123] Cytokine stimulation of cortisol release has complex feedback effects, for cortisol can block the intracellular formation of eicosanoids stimulated by the cytokines. On the other hand, cortisol and epinephrine also can stimulate the production of cytokines.[64]

Cytokine Detection in Biologic Fluids

Individual components of this complex cytokine system of checks and balances now can be measured in body fluids, and their relationships can be studied throughout the course of an acute-phase reaction.[20, 22, 32, 57, 61, 120, 125] These cytokines and their free receptors can be found in mucosal fluids as well as in plasma.[87, 96, 101] Cytokine measurements may have diagnostic and prognostic value.[22, 114] As an example, identification of interleukin-8 in amniotic cord sera was reported to be a specific marker for preterm chorioamnionitis.[114]

Raqib and colleagues[101] described longitudinal measurements of cytokines and receptor antagonists in the plasma and stools of patients with acute shigellosis. Concentrations of tumor necrosis factor–α; interleukins-1β, -6, and -8; and interleukin-1 receptor antagonist in stools were quite high when shigellosis patients first were seen and gradually returned to normal values during the next 2 weeks.[101] We still do not understand fully the pathogenic or physiologic effects of these interacting molecules in either systemic or localized diseases.

HORMONAL RESPONSES

Infectious illnesses are accompanied by a variety of endocrine responses, which especially include increased secretion of the hormones that regulate carbohydrate and energy metabolism and those that influence salt and water retention. These hormonal responses are secondary to and often are initiated by the primary release of proinflammatory cytokines from activated cells.

In addition to their participation in physiologic responses, endocrine functions also may be affected by pathologic complications of an infectious process that results in the direct destruction or dysfunction of hormone-producing cells. The adrenal glands may be destroyed if tubercle bacilli localize in these glands or if hemorrhagic necrosis becomes a complication of such infections as acute meningococcemia. Pancreatic islet cells may be destroyed during viral infections of experimental animals, and the same pathogenic possibility may initiate insulin-requiring diabetes in children. Thyroid function may be impaired after viral infections that trigger an autoimmune thyroiditis, and gonadal tissues may be the site of localization and destruction by the mumps virus.

Pituitary Gland Functions

Secretion of certain of the trophic hormones produced by the anterior pituitary is increased during periods of infection. An increase in adrenocorticotropic hormone production (stimulated by proinflammatory cytokines) triggers an increased secretion of several adrenocorticoids. Plasma concentrations of growth hormone generally are increased in acute infections in which this hormone has been measured,[17, 102] but the increases do not seem to correlate directly in timing or magnitude with the presence or severity of fever.[5, 6] This increase in plasma growth hormone may be due, in part, to its production by mononuclear leukocytes.[135] Plasma concentrations of growth hormone rise rapidly in a somewhat paradoxical manner if an intravenous infusion of glucose is given to patients or laboratory animals with an acute infection.[102] Thyroid-stimulating hormone, on the other hand, does not respond during the early phases of an acute febrile illness but may increase during the convalescent period. No increases in the gonadotropic hormones have been documented during infection. A release of several anterior pituitary hormones can be stimulated by fever-producing doses of bacterial endotoxin. Such responses have been used in the clinical testing of anterior pituitary function.[59, 77]

As described in the earlier discussion of salt and water imbalances, inappropriate secretion of antidiuretic hormone may occur in patients with severe infectious diseases.[34] Such a phenomenon also seems to be a characteristic response in patients whose infectious process becomes localized within the cranial vault.

Adrenal Functions

Although the adrenocortical hormones are known to influence the ability of a patient to respond to stressful situations, relatively few data define the duration and magnitude of the adrenal response or characterize the spectrum of specific steroid hormones produced in excess.[14, 76] Available data suggest that acute generalized infections typically are accompanied by a transient increase in the adrenal output of glucocorticoid hormones that is of short duration. Although these responses generally are limited in magnitude, they serve to maintain a relatively constant concentration of cortisol in plasma throughout the early periods of fever.[14] The usual diurnal decline in plasma 17-OH corticosteroid values fails to occur during the afternoon and evening hours if fever is present. Cortisol-binding proteins have not been observed to change in plasma during periods of acute infection.[11] Thus, the plasma concentrations of unbound, physiologically active cortisol are maintained at or somewhat higher than the normal peak early morning values throughout the initial period of a febrile illness.[11, 14] The total increase in glucocorticoid secretion rates during early illness ranges from two to five times normal values in infections that have been studied. Lesser degrees of increase have been noted in the adrenocortical output of pregnanetriol and the weak ketosteroid androgens.[14] If an infectious illness becomes chronic, adrenal output generally returns to or even below baseline values, and diminished adrenal responsiveness to adrenocorticotropic hormone may develop.

Extremely high concentrations of plasma 17-OH corticosteroids may develop during gram-negative septicemia or prior to death in patients with other severe acute infections.[73, 76] These high terminal values may be ascribed to failures in the hepatic clearance of cortisol from plasma and the metabolic pathways for converting cortisol to water-soluble metabolites; high plasma values are not the result of an extraordinary increase in adrenal secretion rates.[73] In a detailed study of adrenal function in children with meningitis, Migeon and coworkers[76] reported a maximum average increase in cortisol secretion rate of approximately threefold during uncomplicated aseptic or bacterial meningitis. This was accompanied by a threefold increase in the excretion of urinary 17-OH corticosteroids during the first few days of illness. On admission to the hospital, the plasma cortisol concentrations of these children ranged from high normal to twice normal values. On the other hand, severely ill patients who were dying of adrenal hemorrhage generally had values that were depressed or absent.

Mechanisms by which relatively small increases in adrenal glucocorticoid secretion might serve to protect the host have not been defined as yet. However, the ability of the liver to produce some of its proteins during infection is known to be dependent on the permissive presence of glucocorticoid hormones.[14]

The increase in aldosterone production appears to lag somewhat behind the increase in cortisol production during acute infections and then persists longer. Aldosterone increases stimulate the intense retention of sodium and chloride by the kidney during acute infections.[11]

The adrenomedullary secretion of catecholamines may increase in severe infectious diseases.[47, 142] High plasma epinephrine and norepinephrine values develop in gram-negative sepsis and bacterial meningitis. The catecholamine response contributes importantly to the acceleration of gluconeogenesis during infection.

Carbohydrate-Regulating Hormones

Hormones that serve in the normal regulation of carbohydrate metabolism also participate in the host response to infection. In addition to the heightened secretion of the glucocorticoids, catecholamines, and growth hormone, the major pancreatic hormones insulin and glucagon both circulate in increased concentrations in the plasma of patients with acute infectious diseases.[142] The combined effect of these hormonal actions is to accelerate the production of glucose within the liver and to stimulate the release of glucose from stored glycogen. These actions cause the glucose pool size to increase two- or threefold to provide an important source of metabolizable energy during the early febrile periods of acute infections.

Intravenous glucose tolerance tests performed early in the course of febrile infections in young adult subjects[102, 111] led to an exaggerated increase of plasma insulin concentrations in both magnitude and duration, to an appropriate decline in elevated fasting concentrations of plasma glucagon, and to a paradoxical stimulation of growth hormone release. Extreme hyperinsulinism also was observed after glucose infusions given to dogs with endotoxic shock.[19]

The modest increase in fasting plasma insulin concentrations during infections appears to account for an inhibition of both ketogenesis and fat depot lipolysis, two responses that would be expected to occur because of concomitant starvation or semistarvation. The simultaneous combination of high fasting plasma glucagon and insulin values and their effects on both the liver and peripheral fat depots and somatic tissues thus help to explain the observed differences between the anorexia-induced semistarvation of infectious illnesses and the starvation due simply to food deprivation.

Thyroid Hormones

Thyroid hormones do not seem to initiate or sustain the hypermetabolic response to fever. Nevertheless, both thyroxine (T_4) and triiodothyronine (T_3) are deiodinated at accelerated rates within the body tissues, especially the liver, during the early phases of infections studied in humans and experimental animals.[31, 133, 144] This acceleration in the metabolism of peripheral thyroid hormones accounts for an early decline in serum protein-bound iodine values.[112] Only after an infectious illness has progressed for several days does the thyroid gland hormone output appear to increase. This increase in thyroid secretion then persists into early convalescence, so that for a time the production of thyroid hormones exceeds apparent body requirements. As a result, protein-bound iodine values in serum are increased in the convalescent period. This sequence of events produces a biphasic response pattern with an initial decrease and a late increase in concentrations of thyroid hormones. Serum concentrations of "reverse T_3" (Rt_3) increase during febrile illnesses.[24] Because Rt_3 has an apparent role in regulating the peripheral cellular actions of T_4 and T_3, its function during acute infectious illness remains to be elucidated.

In patients studied during falciparum malaria infection, serum T_3 values declined abruptly, whereas serum T_4 values were stable or increased slightly.[133] The decline in serum T_3 concentrations was accompanied by reciprocal increases in Rt_3. The slowing of T_4 turnover during malaria may be due to an impaired ability of hepatocytes to metabolize or deiodinate T_4. Hypothalamic suppression early in malaria appears to result in a decreased release of thyroid-stimulating hormone from the anterior pituitary and a secondary decrease in T_4 and T_3 secretion from the thyroid gland.

References

1. Alvarez, J. O., Salazar-Lindo, E., Kohatsu, J., et al.: Urinary excretion of retinol in children with acute diarrhea. Am. J. Clin. Nutr. *61*:1273–1276, 1995.
2. Anderson, R., Smit, M. J., Joone, G. K., et al.: Vitamin C and cellular immune functions. Ann. N.Y. Acad. Sci. *587*:34–48, 1990.
3. Baracos, V., Rodeman, H. P., Dinarello, C. A., et al.: Stimulation of muscle protein degradation and prostaglandin E_2 release by a leukocytic pyrogen: A mechanism for increased degradation of muscle protein during fever. N. Engl. J. Med. *308*:553–558, 1983.
4. Beck, O.: Weitere untersuchungen zum fieberstoffwechsel des säuglings: Die qualitätiven veranderungen des stickstoffwechsels im fieber. Jahrb. Kinderh. *112*:184–216, 1926.
5. Beisel, W. R.: Metabolic effects of infection. Prog. Food Nutr. Sci. *8*:43–75, 1984.
6. Beisel, W. R.: The influence of infection or injury on nutritional requirements during adolescence. *In* McKigney, J. I., and Munro, H. N. (eds.): Nutrient Requirements in Adolescence. Cambridge, MA, MIT Press, 1976.
7. Beisel, W. R.: Nutrition, infection, specific immune responses, and nonspecific host defenses: A complex interaction. *In* Watson, R. R. (ed.): Nutrition, Disease Resistance and Immune Function. New York, Marcel Dekker, 1984, pp. 3–34.
8. Beisel, W. R.: Nutrition and infection. *In* Linder, M. C. (ed.): Nutritional Biochemistry and Metabolism. 2nd ed. New York, Elsevier Science Publishing Co., 1991, pp. 508–542.
9. Beisel, W. R.: Infection-induced malnutrition: From cholera to cytokines. Am. J. Clin. Nutr. *62*:813–819, 1995.
10. Beisel, W. R., Blackburn, G. L., Feigin, R. D., et al.: Proceedings of a workshop: Impact of infection on nutritional status of the host. Am. J. Clin. Nutr. *30*:1203–1371, 1439–1566, 1977.
11. Beisel, W. R., Bruton, J., Anderson, K. D., et al.: Adrenocortical responses during tularemia in human subjects. J. Clin. Endocrinol. Metab. *27*:61–69, 1967.
12. Beisel, W. R., Goldman, R. F., and Joy, R. J. T.: Metabolic balance studies during induced hyperthermia in man. J. Appl. Physiol. *24*:1–10, 1968.
13. Beisel, W. R., Herman, Y. F., Sauberlich, H. E., et al.: Experimentally induced sandfly fever and vitamin metabolism in man. Am. J. Clin. Nutr. *25*:1165–1173, 1972.
14. Beisel, W. R., and Rapoport, M. I.: Inter-relations between adrenocortical functions and infectious illness. N. Engl. J. Med. *280*:541–546, 569–604, 1969.
15. Beisel, W. R., Sawyer, W. D., Ryll, E. D., et al.: Metabolic effects of intracellular infections in man. Ann. Intern. Med. *67*:744–779, 1967.
16. Beisel, W. R., Watten, R. H., Blackwell, Q., et al.: The role of bicarbonate pathophysiology and therapy in Asiatic cholera. Am. J. Med. *35*:58–66, 1963.
17. Beisel, W. R., Woeber, K. A., Bartelloni, P. J., et al.: Growth hormone response during sandfly fever. J. Clin. Endocrinol. Metab. *28*:1220–1223, 1968.
18. Beresford, C. H., Neale, R. J., and Brooks, O. G.: Iron absorption and pyrexia. Lancet *1*:568–575, 1971.
19. Blackard, W. G., Anderson, Jr., J. H., and Spitzer, J. J.: Hyperinsulinism in endotoxin shock dogs. Metabolism *25*:675–684, 1976.
20. Brown, C. C., Poli, G., Lubaki, N., et al.: Elevated levels of tumor necrosis factor-α in Zairian neonate plasmas: Implications for perinatal infection with the human immunodeficiency virus. J. Infect. Dis. *169*:975–980, 1994.
21. Campbell, C. H., Solgonick, R. M., and Linder, M. C.: Translational regulation of ferritin synthesis in rat spleen: Effects of iron and inflammation. Biochem. Biophys. Res. Commun. *160*:453–549, 1989.
22. Casey, L. C., Balk, R. A., and Bone, R. C.: Plasma cytokine and endotoxin levels correlate with survival in patients with sepsis syndrome. Ann. Intern. Med. *119*:771–778, 1993.
23. Chang, D.-M., and Shaio, M.-F.: Production of interleukin-1 (IL-1) and IL-1 inhibitor by human monocytes exposed to dengue virus. J. Infect. Dis. *170*:811–817, 1994.
24. Chopra, I. J., Chopra, U., Smith, S. R., et al.: Reciprocal changes in serum concentrations of 3,3′5′-triiodothyronine (reverse T_3) and 3,3′5-triiodothyronine (T_3) in systemic illnesses. J. Clin. Endocrinol. Metab. *11*:1043–1049, 1975.
25. Clowes, G. H. A., Jr., George, B. C., Villee, C. A., Jr., et al.: Muscle proteolysis induced by a circulating peptide in patients with sepsis or trauma. N. Engl. J. Med. *308*:545–552, 1983.
26. Committee on Drugs, American Academy of Pediatrics: Vitamin C and the common cold. Nutr. Rev. *32*(Suppl.):39–40, 1974.
27. Constans, J., Pellegrin, I., Pellegrin, J. L., et al.: Plasma interferon-α and the wasting syndrome in patients with the human immunodeficiency virus. Clin. Infect. Dis. *20*:1069–1070, 1995.
28. Cook, G. C.: Increased glycine absorption rate associated with acute bacterial infections in man. Br. J. Nutr. *29*:377–386, 1973.
29. Curnow, R. T., Rayfield, E. J., George, D. T., et al.: Altered hepatic glycogen metabolism and glucoregulatory hormones during sepsis. Am. J. Physiol. *230*:1296–1301, 1976.
30. Derkx, B., Marchant, A., Goldman, M., et al.: High levels of interleukin-10 during the initial phase of fulminant meningococcal septic shock. J. Infect. Dis. *171*:229–232, 1995.
31. DeRubertis, F. R., and Woeber, K. A.: Accelerated cellular uptake and metabolism of L-thyroxine during acute *Salmonella typhimurium* sepsis. J. Clin. Invest. *52*:78–87, 1973.
32. Dinarello, C. A.: The proinflammatory cytokines interleukin-1 and tumor necrosis factor and treatment of the septic shock syndrome. J. Infect. Dis. *163*:1177–1184, 1991.
33. Drapier, J.-C., Wietzerbin, J., and Hibbs, J. B., Jr.: Interferon-gamma and tumor necrosis factor induct the L-arginine–dependent cytotoxic effector mechanism in murine macrophages. J. Immunol. *18*:1587–1592, 1988.
34. Feigin, R. D., and Kaplan, S.: Inappropriate secretion of antidiuretic hormone (ADH) in children with bacterial meningitis. Am. J. Clin. Nutr. *30*:1482–1484, 1977.
35. Feigin, R. D., Middelkamp, J. N., and Reed, C. A.: Murine myocarditis due to coxsackie B_3 virus: Blood amino acid, virologic, and histopathologic correlates. J. Infect. Dis. *126*:574–584, 1972.
36. Felig, P., Brown, W. V., Levine, R. A., et al.: Glucose homeostasis in viral hepatitis. N. Engl. J. Med. *283*:1436–1440, 1970.
37. Fiser, R. H., Denniston, J. C., and Beisel, W. R.: Infection with *Diplococcus pneumoniae* and *Salmonella typhimurium* in monkeys: Changes in plasma lipids and lipoproteins. J. Infect. Dis. *125*:54–60, 1972.
38. Fiser, R. H., Denniston, J. C., Kastello, M. D., et al.: Cholesterogenesis during acute infection in chronically hypercholesterolemic rhesus monkeys. Proc. Soc. Exp. Biol. Med. *140*:314–318, 1972.
39. Frieling, J. T. M., van Deuren, M., Wijdenes, J., et al.: Circulating interleukin-6 receptor in patients with sepsis syndrome. J. Infect. Dis. *171*:469–472, 1995.
40. George, D. T., Abeles, F. B., Mapes, C. A., et al.: Effect of leukocytic endogenous mediators on endocrine pancreas secretory responses. Am. J. Physiol. *233*:E240–E245, 1977.
41. George, D. T., Rayfield, E. J., and Wannemacher, R. W., Jr.: Altered glucoregulatory hormones during acute pneumococcal sepsis in the rhesus monkey. Diabetes *23*:544–549, 1974.
42. Girardin, E., Grau, G. E., Dayer, J.-M., et al.: Tumor necrosis factor and interleukin-1 in the serum of children with severe infectious purpura. N. Engl. J. Med. *319*:397–400, 1988.
43. Godfried, M. H., vad der Poll, T., Weverling, G. J., et al.: Soluble receptors for tumor necrosis factor as predictors of progression to AIDS in asymptomatic human immunodeficiency virus type 1 infection. J. Infect. Dis. *169*:739–745, 1994.
44. Gómez-Jimenez, J., Martin, M. C., Sauri, R., et al.: Interleukin-10 and the monocyte/macrophage induced inflammatory response in septic shock. J. Infect. Dis. *171*:172–475, 1995.
45. Griffiths, J., Groves, A. C., and Leung, F. Y.: Hypertriglyceridemia and hypoglycemia in gram-negative sepsis in the dog. Surg. Gynecol. Obstet. *136*:897–903, 1973.
46. Groofman, J. E., Molina, J.-M., and Scadden, D. T.: Hematopoietic growth factors. N. Engl. J. Med. *321*:1449–1459, 1989.
47. Groves, A. C., Griffiths, J., Leung, F., et al.: Plasma catecholamines in patients with serious postoperative infection. Ann. Surg. *178*:102–107, 1973.
48. Guckian, J. C.: Role of metabolism in pathogenesis of bacteremia due to *Diplococcus pneumoniae* in rabbits. J. Infect. Dis. *127*:1–8, 1973.
49. Halstensen, A., Ceska, M., Brandtzaeg, P., et al.: Interleukin-8 in serum and cerebrospinal fluid from patients with meningococcal disease. J. Infect. Dis. *167*:471–475, 1993.
50. Hemiliä, H., and Herman, Z. S.: Vitamin C and the common cold: A retrospective analysis of Chalmer's review. J. Am. College Nutr. *14*:116–123, 1995.
51. Heney, D., Lewis, I. J., Evans, S. W., et al.: Interleukin-6 and its relationship to C-reactive protein and fever in children with febrile neutropenia. J. Infect. Dis. *165*:886–890, 1992.
52. Henkin, R. I., and Smith, F. R.: Zinc and copper metabolism in acute viral hepatitis. Am. J. Med. Sci. *264*:401–409, 1972.
53. Hirsch, R. L., MacKay, D. G., Travers, R. I., et al.: Hyperlipidemia, fatty liver, and bromsulfophthalein retention in rabbits injected intravenously with bacterial endotoxins. J. Lipid Res. *5*:563–568, 1964.
54. Howard, J. E., Bigham, Jr., R. S., and Mason, R. E.: Studies on convalescence. V. Observations on the altered protein metabolism during induced malarial infections. Trans. Assoc. Am. Physicians *59*:242–247, 1946.
55. Kaufmann, R. L., Matson, C. F., and Beisel, W. R.: Hypertriglyceridemia produced by endotoxin: Role of impaired triglyceride disposal mechanisms. J. Infect. Dis. *133*:548–555, 1976.
56. Kaufmann, R. L., Matson, C. F., Rowberg, A. H., et al.: Defective lipid disposal mechanisms during bacterial infection in rhesus monkeys. Metabolism *25*:615–624, 1976.

57. Keuter, M., Dharmana, E., Gasem, M. H., et al.: Patterns of proinflammatory cytokines and inhibitors during typhoid fever. J. Infect. Dis. *169*:1306–1311, 1994.
58. Kinsella, J. E., Lokesh, B., Broughton, S, et al.: Dietary polyunsaturated fatty acids and eicosanoids: Potential effects on the modulation of inflammatory and immune cells: an overview. Nutrition *6*:22–44, 1990.
59. Kohler, P. O., O'Malley, B. W., Rayford, P. L., et al.: Effect of pyrogen on blood levels of pituitary trophic hormones: Observations of the usefulness of the growth hormone response in the detection of pituitary disease. J. Clin. Endocrinol. Metab. *27*:219–226, 1967.
60. Koj, A.: The role of interleukin-6 as the hepatocyte stimulating factor in the network of inflammatory cytokines. Ann. N.Y. Acad. Sci. *557*:1–8, 1989.
61. Kuhns, D. B., Alvord, W. G., and Gallin, J. I.: Increased circulating cytokines, cytokine antagonists, and E-selectin after intravenous administration of endotoxin in humans. J. Infect. Dis. *171*:145–152, 1995.
62. Lang, C. H., Bagby, G. J., and Dobrescu, C.: Effect of granulocyte colony-stimulating factor on sepsis-induced changes in neutrophil accumulation and organ glucose uptake. J. Infect. Dis. *166*:336–342, 1992.
63. Lees, R. S., Fiser, R. H., Beisel, W. R., Jr., et al.: Effects of an experimental viral infection on plasma lipid and lipoprotein metabolism. Metabolism *21*:825–833, 1972.
64. Liao, J., Keiser, J. A., Scales, W. E., et al.: Role of epinephrine in TNF and IL-6 production from isolated rat liver. Am. J. Physiol. *268*:R896–R9901, 1995.
65. Long, C. L., Haverberg, L. N., Young, V. R., et al.: Metabolism of 3-methylhistidine in man. Metabolism *24*:929–935, 1974.
66. Long, C. L., Kinney, J. M., and Geiger, J. W.: Nonsuppressibility of gluconeogenesis by glucose in septic patients. Metabolism *25*:193–201, 1976.
67. Macallan, D. C., McNurlan, M. A., Milne, E., et al.: Whole-body protein turnover from leucine kinetics and the response to nutrition in human immunodeficiency virus infection. Am. J. Clin. Nutr. *61*:818–826.
68. Mahalanabis, D., Jalan, K. N., Maitra, T. K., et al.: Vitamin A absorption in ascariasis. Am. J. Clin. Nutr. *29*:1372–1375, 1976.
69. Mata, L. J.: Malnutrition-infection interactions in the tropics. Am. J. Trop. Med. Hyg. *24*:564–574, 1975.
70. Mata, L. J., Kronmal, R. A., Urrutia, J. J., et al.: Antenatal events and postnatal growth and survival of children: Prospective observation in a rural Guatemalan village. *In* White, P. L., and Selvey, N. (eds.): Proc. Western Hemisphere Nutrition Congress IV. Acton, MA, Publishing Sciences Group, 1975.
71. Maury, C. P. J., Salo, E., and Pelekonen, P.: Circulating interleukin-1β in patients with Kawasaki disease. N. Engl. J. Med. *319*:1670–1671, 1988.
72. McCallum, R. E., Seale, T. W., and Stith, R. D.: Influence of endotoxin treatment on dexamethasone induction of hepatic phosphoenolpyruvate carboxykinase. Infect. Immun. *39*:213–219, 1983.
73. Melby, J. C., and Spink, W. W.: Comparative studies on adrenal cortical function and cortisol metabolism in healthy adults and in patients with shock due to infection. J. Clin. Invest. *37*:1791–1798, 1958.
74. Michie, H. R., Manogue, K. R., Spriggs, D. R., et al.: Detection of circulating tumor necrosis factor after endotoxin administration. N. Engl. J. Med. *318*:1481–1486, 1988.
75. Migasena, P., and Maegraith, B. G.: Intestinal absorption in malaria. I. The absorption of an amino acid (AIB-I ^{14}C) across the gut membrane in normal and in *Plasmodium knowlesi*–infected monkeys. Ann. Trop. Med. Parasitol. *63*:439–448, 1969.
76. Migeon, C. J., Kenny, F. M., Hung, W., et al.: Study of adrenal function in children with meningitis. Pediatrics *40*:163–183, 1967.
77. Moberg, G. P.: Site of action of endotoxins on hypothalamic-pituitary-adrenal axis. Am. J. Physiol. *220*:397–400, 1971.
78. Moon, R. J., Tremblay, E. S., and Morris, K. M.: Distribution and metabolism of ^{14}C-tryptophan in normal and endotoxic-poisoned mice. Infect. Immun. *8*:604–611, 1973.
79. Morris, K. M., and Moon, R. J.: Quantitative analysis of serotonin biosynthesis in endotoxemia. Infect. Immun. *10*:340–346, 1974.
80. Morrissey, P. J., and Mochizuki, D. Y.: Interleukin is identical to hematopoietin 1: Studies on its therapeutic effects of myelopoiesis and lymphopoiesis. Biotherapy *1*:263–271, 1989.
81. Moyer, E. D., and Powanda, M. C.: Amino acid metabolism during infectious illness. *In* Powanda, M. C., and Canonico, P. G. (eds.): Infection: The Physiologic and Metabolic Responses of the Host. Amsterdam, Elsevier/North Holland, 1981.
82. Murphy, S. G., Klainer, A. S., and Clyde, D. F.: Characterization and pathophysiology of serum glycoprotein alterations in malaria. J. Lab. Clin. Med. *79*:55–61, 1972.
83. Nelson, P. G., Pyke, D. A., and Gamble, D. R.: Viruses and the aetiology of diabetes: A study in identical twins. Br. Med. J. *4*:249–251, 1975.
84. Nessan, V. J., Geerken, R. C., and Ulvilla, J.: Uric acid excretion in infectious mononucleosis: A function of increased purine turnover. J. Clin. Endocrinol. Metab. *38*:652–654, 1974.
85. Neufeld, H. A., Pace, J. A., Kaminski, M. Y., et al.: A probable endocrine basis for the depression of ketone bodies during infections or inflammatory state in rats. Endocrinology *107*:596–601, 1980.
86. Nichols, B. L., and Soriano, H. A.: A critique of oral therapy of dehydration due to diarrheal syndromes. Am. J. Clin. Nutr. *30*:1457, 1977.
87. Noah, T. L., Henderson, F. W., Wortman, I. A., et al.: Nasal cytokine production in viral acute upper respiratory infection of childhood. J. Infect. Dis. *171*:584–592, 1995.
88. O'Donnell, T. F., Jr., Clowes, G. H. A., Jr., Blackburn, G. L., et al.: Proteolysis associated with a deficit of peripheral energy fuel substrates in septic man. Surgery *80*:192–200, 1976.
89. París, M. M., Friedland, I, R., Ehertt, S., et al.: Effect of interleukin-1 receptor antagonist and soluble tumor necrosis factor receptor in animal models of infection. J. Infect. Dis. *171*:161–169, 1995.
90. Patwardhan, V. N., Maghrabi, R. H., Mousa, W., et al.: Serum glycoproteins in protein-calorie deficiency disease. Am. J. Clin. Nutr. *24*:906–912, 1971.
91. Pawlowski, Z. S.: Implications of parasite-nutrition interactions from a world perspective. Fed. Proc. *43*:256–260, 1984.
92. Powanda, M. C.: Change in body balance of nitrogen and other key nutrients: Description and underlying mechanism. Am. J. Clin. Nutr. *30*:1254–1268, 1977.
93. Powanda, M. C., and Beisel, W. R.: Hypothesis: Leukocyte endogenous mediator/endogenous pyrogen/lymphocyte-activating factor modulates the development of nonspecific and specific immunity and affects nutritional status. Am. J. Clin. Nutr. *35*:762–768, 1982.
94. Powanda, M. C., Dinterman, R., Wannemacher, R. W., Jr., et al.: Tryptophan metabolism in relation to amino acid alterations during typhoid fever. Acta Vitaminol. Enzymol. *29*:164–168, 1975.
95. Powanda, M. C., Wannemacher, R. W., Jr., and Cockerell, G. L.: Nitrogen metabolism and protein synthesis during pneumococcal sepsis in rats. Infect. Immun. *6*:266–271, 1972.
96. Proud, D., Gwaltney, J. M., Jr., Hendley, J. O., et al.: Increased levels of interleukin-1 are detected in nasal secretions of volunteers during experimental rhinovirus colds. J. Infect. Dis. *169*:1007–1013, 1994.
97. Puccetti, P., Mencacci, A., Cenci, E., et al.: Cure of murine candidiasis by recombinant soluble interleukin-4 receptor. J. Infect. Dis. *169*:1325–1331, 1994.
98. Ramsey, K. H., Schneider, H., Cross, A. S., et al.: Inflammatory cytokines produced in response to experimental human gonorrhea. J. Infect. Dis. *172*:186–191, 1995.
99. Rapoport, M. I., and Beisel, W. R.: Studies of tryptophan metabolism in experimental animals and man during infectious illness. Am. J. Clin. Nutr. *24*:807–814, 1971.
100. Rapoport, M. I., Lust, G., and Beisel, W. R.: Host enzyme induction of bacterial infection. Arch. Intern. Med. *121*:11–16, 1968.
101. Raqib, R., Wretlind, B., Anderson, J., et al.: Cytokine secretion in acute shigellosis is correlated to disease activity and directed more to stool than to plasma. J. Infect. Dis. *171*:376–384, 1995.
102. Rayfield, E. J., Curnow, R. T., George, D. T., et al.: Impaired carbohydrate metabolism during a mild viral illness. N. Engl. J. Med. *289*:618–621, 1973.
103. Reiss, E.: Protein metabolism in infection. I. Change in certain visceral proteins studies with glycin-N^{15}. Metabolism *8*:151–159, 1959.
104. Robinson D. R.: Lipid mediators of inflammation. Rheum. Dis. Clin. North Am. *13*:385–405, 1987.
105. Rocha, D. M., Santeusanio, F., Faloona, G. R., et al.: Abnormal pancreatic alpha-cell function in bacterial infections. N. Engl. J. Med. *288*:700–703, 1973.
106. Roubenoff, R., Roubenoff, R. A., Cannon, J. C., et al.: Rheumatoid cachexia: Cytokine-driven hypermetabolism accompanying reduced body cell mass in chronic inflammation. J. Clin. Invest. *93*:2379–2386, 1994.
107. Sack, D. A., Rhoads, M., Molla, A., et al.: Carbohydrate malabsorption in infants with rotavirus diarrhea. Am. J. Clin. Nutr. *36*:1112–1118, 1982.
108. Sasazuki, T., McDevitt, H. O., and Grumet, F. C.: The association between genes in the major histocompatibility complex and disease susceptibility. Ann. Rev. Med. *28*:425–452, 1977.
109. Scrimshaw, N. S., Taylor, C. E., and Gordon, J. E.: Interactions of Nutrition and Infection. Geneva, World Health Organization, 1968.
110. Semba, R. D.: Vitamin A, immunity, and infection. Clin. Infect. Dis. *19*:489–499, 1994.
111. Shambaugh, G. E., III, and Beisel, W. R.: Insulin response during tularemia in man. Diabetes *16*:369–376, 1967.
112. Shambaugh, G. E., III, and Beisel, W. R.: Early alterations in thyroid hormone physiology during acute infection in man. J. Clin. Endocrinol. Metab. *27*:1667–1673, 1967.
113. Shaw, A. R.: Molecular biology of cytokines: An introduction. *In* Thompson, A. W. (ed.): The Cytokine Handbook. New York, Academic Press, 1991, pp. 19–42.
114. Shimoya, K., Matsuzaki, N., Taniguchi, T., et al.: Interleukin-8 in cord sera: A sensitive and specific marker for the detection of preterm chorioamnionitis. J. Infec. Dis. *165*:957–969, 1992.
115. Siegel, J. H., Cerra, F. B., Coleman, B., et al.: Physiological and metabolic correlations in human sepsis. Surgery *86*:163–193, 1979.
116. Smith, R. E., and Horwitz, B. A.: Brown fat and thermogenesis. Physiol. Rev. *49*:330–425, 1969.
117. Sobocinski, P. Z., Canterbury, W. J., Mapes, C. A., et al.: Involvement of hepatic metallothioneins in hypozincemia associated with bacterial infection. Am. J. Physiol. *234*:E399–E406, 1978.
118. Sommer, A.: Vitamin A, infectious disease, and childhood mortality: A 2c solution? J. Infect. Dis. *167*:1003–1007, 1993.

119. Stamler, J. S., Singel, D. J., and Loscaizo, J.: Biochemistry of nitric oxide and its redox-activated forms. Science *258*:1891–1902, 1992.
120. Steinmetz, H. T., Herbertz, A., Bertram, M., et al.: Increase in interleukin-6 serum level preceding fever in granulocytopenia and correlation with death from sepsis. J. Infect. Dis. *171*:225–228, 1994.
121. Stephensen, C. B., Alvarez, J. O., Kohatsu, J., et al.: Vitamin A is excreted in the urine during acute infection. Am. J. Clin. Nutr. *60*:388–392, 1994.
122. Stuehr, D. J., and Nathan, C. F.: Nitric oxide: A macrophage product responsible for cytostasis and respiratory inhibition of tumor target cells. J. Exp. Med. *169*:1543–1555, 1989.
123. te Vede, M., Huijbens, R. J. F., Heije, K., et al.: Interleukin-4 (IL-4) inhibits secretion of IL-1 beta, tumor necrosis factor alpha, and IL-6 by human monocytes. Blood *76*:1392–1397, 1990.
124. van der Poll, T., van Deventer, S. J. H., ten Cate, H., et al.: Tumor necrosis factor is involved in the appearance of interleukin-1 receptor antagonist in endotoxemia. J. Infect. Dis. *169*:665–667, 1994.
125. van Deuren, M., van der Ven-Jongekrijg, J., and Demacker, P. M. N.: Differential expression of proinflammatory cytokines and their inhibitors during the course of meningococcal infections. J. Infect. Dis. *169*:157–161, 1993.
126. Vitale, J. J.: The impact of infection on vitamin metabolism: An unexplored area. Am. J. Clin. Nutr. *30*:1473–1477, 1977.
127. Viteri, F. E., and Béhar, M.: Efectos de diversas infecciones sobre la nutricion del prescolar especialmente el saramp ión. Bole. Ofic. Sanit. Panam. *78*:226–240, 1975.
128. Wagner, D. A., and Tannenbaum, S. R.: Enhancement of nitrate biosysthesis by *Escherichia coli* lipopolysaccharide. *In* McGee, P. N. (ed.): Nitrosamines and Human Cancer. Cold Springs, Cold Springs Harbor Laboratories, 1982, pp. 437–441.
129. Wannemacher, R. W., Jr.: Key role of various individual amino acids in host response to infection. Am. J. Clin. Nutr. *30*:1269–1280, 1977.
130. Wannemacher, R. W., Jr., Dinterman, R. E., Pekarek, R. S., et al.: Urinary amino acid excretion during experimentally induced sandfly fever in man. Am. J. Clin. Nutr. *28*:110–118, 1975.
131. Wannemacher, R. W., Jr., Klainer, A. S., Dinterman, R. E., et al.: The significance and mechanism of an increased serum phenylalanine-tyrosine ratio during infection. Am. J. Clin. Nutr. *29*:997–1006, 1976.
132. Wannemacher, R. W., Jr., Powanda, M. C., and Dinterman, R. E.: Amino acid flux and protein synthesis after exposure of rats to either *Diplococcus pneumoniae* or *Salmonella typhimurium*. Infect. Immun. *10*:60–65, 1974.
133. Wartofsky, L., Burman, K. D., Dimond, R. C., et al.: Studies on the nature of thyroidal suppression during acute falciparum malaria: Integrity of pituitary response to TRH and alterations in serum T_3 and reverse T_3. J. Clin. Endocrinol. Metab. *44*:85–90, 1977.
134. Watten, R. H., Morgan, F. M., Songkhla, Y. N., et al.: Water and electrolyte studies in cholera. J. Clin. Invest. *38*:1879–1889, 1959.
135. Weigent, D. A., Baxter, J. B., Wear, W. E., et al.: Production of immunoreactive growth hormone by mononuclear leukocytes. FASEB J. *2*:2812–2818, 1988.
136. Weinberg, E. D.: Iron and susceptibility to infectious disease. Science *184*:952–956, 1974.
137. West, H. D., Jackson, A. H., Elliott, R. R., et al.: The utilization of ingested iron in disease. South. Med. J. *45*:629–633, 1952.
138. Westendorp, R. G. J., Langermans, J. A. M., de Bel, C. E., et al.: Release of tumor necrosis factor: An innate host characteristic that may contribute to the outcome of meningococcal disease. J. Infect. Dis. *171*:1057–1060, 1995.
139. Whedon, G. D., and Shorr, E.: Metabolic studies in paralytic acute anterior poliomyelitis. II. Alterations in calcium and phosphorus metabolism. J. Clin. Invest. *36*:966–981, 1957.
140. White, M. G., Carter, N. W., Rector, F. C., et al.: Pathophysiology of epidemic St. Louis encephalitis. Ann. Intern. Med. *71*:691–702, 1969.
141. Wiles, J. B., Cerra, F. B., Siegel, J. H., et al.: The systemic septic response: Does the organism matter? Crit. Care Med. *8*:55–60, 1980.
142. Wilmore, D. W., Long, J. M., Mason, A. D., Jr., et al.: Catecholamines: Mediator of the hypermetabolic response to thermal injury. Ann. Surg. *180*:653–669, 1974.
143. Wilson, D., Bressani, R., and Scrimshaw, N. S.: Infection and nutritional status. I. The effect of chicken pox on nitrogen metabolism in children. Am. J. Clin. Nutr. *9*:154–158, 1961.
144. Woeber, K. A.: Alterations in thyroid hormone economy during acute infection with *Diplococcus pneumoniae* in the rhesus monkey. J. Clin. Invest. *50*:378–387, 1971.
145. Yelish, M. R., and Filkins, J. P.: Mechanism of hyperinsulinemia in endotoxicosis. Am. J. Physiol. *239*.E156–E161, 1980.
146. Yeung, C. Y.: Hypoglycemia in neonatal sepsis. J. Pediatr. *77*:812–817, 1970.
147. Young, V. R., Alexis, S. D., Maliga, B. S., et al.: Metabolism of administered 3-methylhistidine: Lack of muscle transfer ribonucleic acid charging and quantitative excretion as 3-methylhistidine and its *N*-acetyl derivative. J. Biol. Chem. *247*:3592–3600, 1972.

4

INTERACTION OF INFECTION AND NUTRITION

Ralph D. Feigin and Kelvin S. Panesar

The introduction to the World Health Organization (WHO) report on nutrition and infection, published in 1965, stated:

> The concept that malnutrition could make man more susceptible to infectious disease and also alter the course and outcome of the resulting illness has long been current in the history of medicine and public health. Circumstantial evidence is plentiful, principally based on clinical experience. Well controlled observations have been few, and hence clear proof in support of the concept has been slow to accumulate. It has been much easier to demonstrate that infection is often directly responsible for lowering the state of nutrition.[222]

Nevertheless, the combination of malnutrition and infection is responsible for 40,000 deaths per day in children of the Third World. This problem has been termed "silent genocide" by WHO officials and is the most underreported health problem facing humans. An acute infection has been incriminated frequently as the event precipitating kwashiorkor.[8, 9, 74, 91, 133, 157, 196] Generally, viral diseases such as measles, varicella, hepatitis, and herpes simplex are prevalent in patients with protein-calorie malnutrition.[8, 9, 74, 133, 196] Infection with *Mycobacterium*, *Salmonella*, and other bacteria that reside intracellularly also occurs frequently in the malnourished individual.[157] *Pneumocystis carinii* infection occurs commonly in children compromised by malignancy or by inherited or acquired immunodeficiency disorders; the occurrence of the infection in malnourished individuals has been highlighted.[91] In the village setting of the studies, the severity of these infections has been influenced strongly by the nutritional status of the host.

The association of malnutrition with infection has been documented repeatedly. The devastating effects of long-term semistarvation in infants and small children were described with deep emotion by physicians trapped in the Jewish ghetto of Warsaw by the prolonged Nazi siege.[24, 219] They wrote, "By the time the older children became sick, the younger ones were already dead. After two years, most of the children we saw were over five years old; later we seldom saw children under eight." These physicians described gross and microscopic evidence of lymphoid tissue atrophy and the disappearance of delayed hypersensitivity reactions and acute inflammation, as well as the disappearance of clinical allergies, blood eosinophils, and gastric acid in the severely malnourished. More recent data also support the concept that malnutrition makes people more susceptible to infection. Metabolic, biochemical, and clinical evidence has accumulated that strongly supports the concept that nutrition affects profoundly the progress of infection within the host. The normal host response to infection is detailed in Chapter 3. It is clear that virtually every normal metabolic or endocrine function is altered in some manner by the presence of an infectious illness.

Traditionally, clinical inquiries into the interaction of nutrition and infection have focused on the patient with protein-calorie malnutrition. Nutrition is a critical determinant of immunocompetence and risk of illness. Young children with protein-calorie malnutrition exhibit increased morbidity and mortality due largely to infectious diseases.[41] Undernourished individuals have impaired immune responses. In addition, there is a clear overlap between protein-calorie malnutrition and isolated deficiencies of single nutrients.

In light of the well-recognized biologic synergism between malnutrition and infection, it is notable that malnutrition has not received comparable attention in child health and survival strategies. This may be due in part to the fact that mortality statistics gathered from health facilities in developing countries report only the proximate cause of death (usually infectious diseases), such that only the severe cases of nutritional deficiency are recorded as nutritional causes of death.[150]

PROTEIN-CALORIE MALNUTRITION

Protein-calorie malnutrition is a term used to describe a wide range of clinical conditions resulting from mild to severe undernutrition. The conditions of kwashiorkor and marasmus represent manifestations of protein-calorie malnutrition, while mild forms may be detected primarily by poor growth. Marasmus is characterized by severe wasting, whereas kwashiorkor is manifested by the presence of edema. Both cases appear to be related to consumption of a diet deficient in both protein and calories, but infections also play an important role. In marasmus, the prognosis on refeeding is relatively good, whereas treatment of kwashiorkor is more difficult and the prognosis often is poor.[79] The United Nations has estimated that nearly 184 million children in the world suffer from varying degrees of growth retardation due to undernutrition. When total energy consumption is low, amino acids from dietary protein are used for energy rather than for protein synthesis and growth. Tomkins and Watson[201] described the malnutrition-infection complex as the most prevalent public health problem in the world today. Inadequate diet, including insufficient intake of energy stores, protein, and micronutrients (such as iron, vitamins, and minerals), leads to weight loss, retarded growth rate, diminished immunity, and mucosal damage. These factors exacerbate the incidence, severity, and duration of infectious diseases. This, in turn, leads to the loss of nutrients, malabsorption, altered metabolism, and loss of appetite that leads to further inadequate dietary intake.[19, 142]

In 1992, the extent of malnutrition in developing countries was estimated in the United Nations Second Report on the World Nutrition Situation.[1] This report shows the extent of undernutrition in the 1988–1990 period. The report estimates that 786 million people (approximately 20 per cent of the world's population) suffer from malnutrition. Nearly 184 million (approximately 34 per cent) of the world's children younger than 5 years of age had a weight of 2 standard deviations below the reference standard. Four hundred million (approximately 45 per cent) of the world's women between 15 and 49 years of age were below 45 kg. The data for underweight women are important: there is a relationship between malnutrition in mothers and the birth weight of the child, and low birth weight is related to increased risk of infant mortality. Although the data show that hundreds of millions of people suffer from varying degrees of undernutrition, the United Nations data indicate that fewer adults and children were malnourished in the 1988–1990 period than in the 1974–1976 period.[142]

It is well known that various infectious diseases interfere with or influence the responses of host defense. Metabolic responses of the host to infection include increased utilization of proteins, carbohydrates, lipids, minerals, electrolytes, trace elements, vitamins, and hormones. The normal host response to infection, however, is one in which an immediate and marked stimulus for protein anabolism is initiated. The chemical changes in protein-calorie malnutrition include low serum albumin, low concentrations of essential amino acids in serum, generalized amino aciduria, lower glycosylated hemoglobin levels, and decreased activity of many enzymes. Reduction in the activity of diphosphopyridine nucleotide, cytochrome *c* reductase, plasma esterase, and leukocyte pyruvic kinase has been documented. Thus, the patient with kwashiorkor, depleted of amino acids and protein, is unable to initiate the necessary anabolic response when challenged by infection. This appears to alter the capacity to resist the debilitating effects of infection. Decreased activity of the various enzymes that help to resist infection and the inability to synthesize new enzymes necessary for energy-producing reactions in the body impose an additional burden on the individual with protein-calorie malnutrition. If the diet is insufficient to permit replacement of calories and protein, the individual becomes progressively depleted with each episode of infection. Repeated episodes of infection may be a major factor in precipitating frank kwashiorkor in children on a borderline diet with regard to protein and calories. In addition to these nonspecific responses, specific types of immunity as well as different organ systems are affected by protein-calorie malnutrition.

Postmortem studies have confirmed that acute bacterial infections are the major cause of death in severe protein-calorie malnutrition. Septicemia is the most dreaded infectious complication of protein-calorie malnutrition and has been reported in up to 31 per cent of hospitalized patients. Gram-negative enteric bacilli are the organisms encountered most frequently; less frequent agents include *Haemophilus influenzae, Shigella flexneri, Pseudomonas aeruginosa, Corynebacterium diphtheriae, Streptococcus, Staphylococcus aureus,* and *Neisseria* species. Tuberculosis is more frequent, is more virulent, spreads faster, and reinfects more readily in people with protein-calorie malnutrition. The rate of urinary tract infections in malnourished children is increased significantly; gram-negative enteric bacilli are the organisms encountered most frequently. Diarrhea is common in malnourished children, with the most common cause being enteric pathogens such as *Salmonella enteritidis*, enteropathogenic *Escherichia coli*, and nontyphi *Salmonella*.[177]

In almost all cases of severe protein-calorie malnutrition, there often is biochemical and/or clinical evidence of micronutrient deficiencies, for example, vitamin A deficiency or iron deficiency anemia. There is little evidence that any one micronutrient deficiency is the main cause of protein-calorie malnutrition or by itself is responsible for the edema of kwashiorkor.

Although protein is an essential and important nutrient, protein-calorie malnutrition is associated more often with deficient food intake than with protein intake. When commonly consumed cereal-based diets meet caloric needs, they *usually* will meet protein needs, especially if the diet also provides modest amounts of legumes and vegetables. In terms of control and prevention of protein-calorie malnutrition, improving the quantity and quality of food consumed, immunization, providing oral rehydration therapy for diarrhea, early treatment of common diseases, regular deworming, and attention to the underlying causes of protein-calorie malnutrition, such as poverty and inequity, will help to prevent this highly prevalent condition.[119]

In Utero

The medical literature reports widespread occurrence of infant low birth weight throughout the nations of the world in which malnutrition is prevalent. Hytten,[94] discussing the relationship of maternal diet to the size of the infant body, called attention to the fact that dietary status in pregnancy is only part of the broad environmental picture. He emphasized that the mother's nutrition throughout life may be as important as nutrition during pregnancy in ensuring the birth of an infant of normal size. The well-fed mother deprived of food during pregnancy may have been able to lay down a sufficient energy reserve to protect the fetus during intrauterine life despite deficiencies in day-to-day intake. Clearly, however, severe nutritional deprivation during pregnancy may affect the size and vitality of the fetus.

Smith[180] described conditions in Rotterdam and The Hague from September 1944 to May 1945, during which time the average adult food intake fell to 730 cal/day. This period of deprivation lasted at least 5 but not more than 8 months. Pregnancies that ended just prior to the relief of the famine had begun under good nutritional circumstances. Pregnancies beginning during the famine terminated after relief had been provided. No significant increase in prematurity was noted. In Rotterdam, infants who were conceived before the hunger period but born during the famine were shorter, and their weight was, on the average, 240 g less than expected. The effects of underfeeding occurred primarily during the late stages of pregnancy.

Effects much more severe were reported by Antonov[6] during the siege of Leningrad, where hardships of all types may have been greater and of longer duration. This situation may be closer to conditions in many parts of the world where nutrition prior to conception and perhaps throughout life may be suboptimal. During the most severe period of hunger in Leningrad, the stillbirth rate rose significantly and the prematurity rate was greater than 40 per cent. Birth weights were less than normal, physiologic weight loss in the first few days of postnatal life was greater and of longer duration, and infant morbidity and mortality were high. Severe malnutrition in the mother decidedly affected the development of the fetus and the vitality of the newborn child. Short maternal stature, which is influenced by biosocial factors, large family size, malnutrition, and chronic disease, frequently becomes intergenerational. For example, women who were growth retarded as newborns tend to give birth to infants who are also growth retarded, which may be a reflection of poor maternal nutritional status during childhood and adolescence.[124]

There also is evidence that infection during pregnancy is common in the areas of the world where malnutrition is prevalent. In a prospective study in four Guatemalan villages, venous blood was obtained from infants within 3 days of birth for measurement of serum immunoglobulin concentration. Fifteen per cent of the samples had concentrations of IgM in excess of 19 mg/dL.[132] Twelve per cent of village women who were tested serologically throughout pregnancy for cytomegalovirus, herpes simplex, rubella, syphilis, and *Toxoplasma* showed seroconversion during pregnancy to one of these agents.

Infant size at birth correlates with neonatal survival to a greater extent than does the quality of extrauterine life. Village infants who were small for gestational age at birth had a greater risk of subsequent malnutrition and infection than did term infants with an adequate birth weight. Infants with low birth weight (predominantly small for gestational age) had higher rates of infection with *Shigella*, *Entamoeba histolytica*, and *Giardia* in the first month of life and also exhibited higher occurrences of diarrhea and oral candidiasis in the first 6 months of life than did term infants.

It is apparent that maternal malnutrition prior to or during pregnancy and maternal infection during pregnancy may act alone or in concert to influence the size, gestational age at birth, and vitality of the fetus. To the extent that the fetus is affected, it can be concluded that the interaction of nutrition and infection begins in utero. Brabin[23] has suggested that folacin deficiency in pregnant women enhances maternal immunosuppression, which predisposes to prolonged parasitemia and heavier placental parasitization. If the folacin requirements of the growing fetus are not satisfied, the ontogenetic development of the fetal immune system will be deranged and consequently the child will be more susceptible to malaria as well as other infections. Prenatal nutritional deprivation in animal models impairs T-cell–dependent immune responses of the first- and second-generation offspring.[30] Maternal malnutrition results in impaired placental function and chronic vascular insufficiency, which in turn leads to symmetric growth retardation. As nutritional deprivation becomes more severe, first weight, then length, and finally brain mass is affected. Acute placental insufficiency results in asymmetric growth retardation. When the nutritional insult occurs late in pregnancy, when length velocity is declining and weight velocity is increasing, the amount of muscle, fat, and hepatic glycogen is affected adversely. This type of growth retardation is seen in postmature infants, and in these infants, placental function no longer is adequate to meet fetal needs and the fetus must mobilize its own fat and carbohydrate stores.[124]

Even in the industrialized countries, it often is very difficult to provide enteral nourishment to very low birth weight infants because of systemic illnesses, such as respiratory distress syndrome and gastrointestinal tract immaturity. Many of these infants ultimately will develop clinical and biochemical signs of malnutrition during the early postnatal period that may compromise an already inadequate immune system and alter host susceptibility to infection. Animals malnourished in utero demonstrate retarded growth and functional development in rapidly growing tissues, such as the central nervous system. Reduction in spleen, thymus, and body weights has been noted in rats after intrauterine protein-calorie deprivation. After nutritional restoration in these animals, thymic tissue remained depleted of lymphocytes and significantly reduced in weight. Newborn infants may develop similar long-term immunologic defects after in utero or early postnatal malnutrition. Low birth weight infants born to malnourished mothers demonstrate decreased thymus and spleen size as well as diminished cell-mediated immune responses, reduced transfer of maternal-fetal IgG, and decreased number of T lymphocytes. Infants with fetal growth retardation have demonstrated diminished neutrophil chemotaxis, abnormal nitroblue tetrazolium oxidative reduction, and deficient microbicidal activity.[31, 70]

After birth, nutritional deprivation may create the environment for frequent episodes of infection. Mechanisms responsible for the increased number and severity of infections in the malnourished host will be detailed below. Infections commonly are accompanied by anorexia, vomiting, marked reduction in food intake, impaired digestion, and malabsorption.[122] The increased loss of nitrogen, amino acids, electrolytes, vitamins, and so on, and the increased energy expenditure required during an infection are detailed in Chapter 1. The repetitive infections experienced by children in parts of the world where malnutrition also is prevalent may predispose to protein-calorie malnutrition, even in individuals whose birth weight and baseline nutritional status were adequate. In many instances, it is impossible to determine whether the malnutrition or the infection was the event that initiated the ultimate deterioration of the patient.

THE IMMUNE SYSTEM AND THE MALNOURISHED HOST

Mucosal Immunity

The first barrier to potential pathogens is the physical integrity of the skin and mucous membranes. The interstitial space in the submucosa of the respiratory and gastrointestinal tracts contains IgA-secreting plasma cells. Secretory IgA, a dimeric form, appears to be produced locally and not derived from intravascular sources. This IgA may bind to the mucosa and serve as a proteolytic resistant "antiseptic paint." Diminished secretory IgA may be noted in malnutrition.[179, 192] This, in turn, may increase host susceptibility to infection by permitting increased penetration of infectious agents into the circulation. Interferon-γ is a major cytokine produced by mucosal T lymphocytes that, in addition to its immunoregulatory properties, has been shown in vitro to decrease the expression of secretory components by mucosal epithelial cells and may modulate permeability and barrier functions of mucosal epithelium.[127, 183]

Furthermore, deficiencies in protein, vitamin A, B complex, ascorbic acid, and zinc are associated frequently with tissue changes that contribute to diminution in host resistance to infection. Severe protein malnutrition and xerophthalmia have been shown to suppress significantly the secretion of lysozyme into the tears of children.[213] This impairs host defense against the bacteria that are destroyed by lysozyme. Large visible epithelial lesions may be caused by dietary deficiencies. Examples include the metaplastic hyperkeratosis due to avitaminosis A; the dermatitis, cheilitis, and angular stomatitis from riboflavin and pyridoxine deficiency; the mucosal atrophy and dermatosis of pellagra; the spongy gums and subcutaneous hemorrhages of scurvy; and the atrophy of skin and gastrointestinal mucosa of severe protein deficiency. As adjuncts to structural integrity and secretory IgA, mononuclear cells have an important role in mucosal immunity. Malnourished children have a reduced number of lymphocytes and plasma cells in the interstitial space. Migration of lymphoblasts from the mesentery also is decreased.[39] In the gut, for example, Peyer patches contain antigen-primed lymphocytes that start to differentiate and proliferate after activation. These activated lymphocytes interact with T cells of perifollicular zones and subsequently enter the circulation to reach the central immune organs, such as the spleen, bone marrow, and possibly thymus, where they experience further clonal expansion. Eventually, these become IgA-producing cells that re-enter the circulation and by a selective homing process deliver specific immunity to the mucosa of the gut, as well as to salivary, lacrimal, bronchial, and lactating mammary glands. Homing of these IgA-producing cells is a selective process that involves special corresponding binding sites on lymphocytes and endothelial venule cell membranes of lymph nodes and lymphoid mucosal tissue. This is known as the common mucosal immune system, which provides a reservoir of antigen-committed lymphocytes.[155] This system provides effective protection for both the nursing mother and her infant, since the microbial environment is similar for both.

Humoral Immunity

A number of studies of B-cell function have been performed in patients with protein-calorie malnutrition. Serum immunoglobulins may be normal or elevated.[182] Cohen and Hansen[45] showed that children with protein-calorie malnutrition who were infected synthesized gamma-globulin at three times the rate of uninfected malnourished individuals, thus documenting the fact that synthesis of gamma-globulin was not rate limited in malnutrition at the expense of other protein synthesis, such as that of albumin. In protein-calorie malnutrition, antibody affinity is decreased, which may explain the higher frequency of antigen-antibody complexes found in malnourished patients. As opposed to serum antibody responses, secretory IgA antibody levels are minimal after parenteral immunization with viral vaccines, which may have important implications, such as increased risk for septicemia.[44]

In protein-calorie malnutrition, the most dramatic change in humoral immunity concerns IgE. Serum IgE concentrations in healthy, well-nourished children are extremely low. Significant elevations of serum IgE in malnourished children have been reported in the absence of allergy or parasitic infections, possibly due to imbalance in T-lymphocyte regulation of IgE-producing B-cell function. It is, therefore, possible that the defect in cell-mediated immunity in patients with protein-calorie malnutrition could initiate an exaggerated IgE response during infections with respiratory pathogens, such as respiratory syncytial virus or parainfluenza virus, and also increase the risk for severe bronchiolitis.[111]

Antibody production after immunization with antigen remains the best functional measure of humoral immunity. Much of the data on specific serum antibody responses in human malnutrition are conflicting. Antibody response to tetanus and diphtheria toxoids is normal; however, the responses to immunization with viral antigens are variable. Responses to yellow fever vaccine, hepatitis, and killed influenza A have been reported to be impaired in protein-calorie malnutrition. There is a diminished antibody response to such polysaccharide antigens as killed typhoid vaccine (polysaccharide typhoid O antigen) in protein-calorie malnutrition. The degree of malnutrition may be a critical host determinant; for example, mild protein-calorie malnutrition had no impact on the response to a meningococcal group C polysaccharide vaccine.[76] However, the serum antibody response is relatively well preserved to many protein antigens. Tetanus toxoid, for example, induces protective levels of antibody even in children with severe protein-calorie malnutrition. This diminished antibody response to polysaccharide antigens may be due to a selective impact of protein-calorie malnutrition on the IgG subclasses that contain antibody to polysaccharide antigens, IgG2, and IgG4.[111] It is possible that impairment of IgG subclasses in protein-calorie malnutrition would affect the patient's ability to resist encapsulated organisms negatively. However, further studies investigating the relationship between IgG subclasses and protein-calorie malnutrition are needed.

The balance between T and B cells in the peripheral blood appears to be disturbed in malnutrition.[95] Several investigations have reported decreased numbers of spontaneous sheep erythrocyte rosette-forming cells (generally considered to be T lymphocytes) and normal to increased numbers of Fc and C3 rosette-forming cells (B lymphocytes). Because similar observations have been made in patients with chronic infections, it is impossible to determine at present whether these findings are manifestations of malnutrition per se or whether they can be explained by chronic infection in the malnourished individual.

The role of nucleotides has been studied for their effects on the humoral system. In vitro studies have shown that the immunomodulating actions of polynucleotides on the humoral immune response may depend on the nature of the antigen (T-cell–dependent versus T-cell–independent) and on the presence or absence of antigen stimulus. In vitro studies using murine spleen cells, primed with T-cell–dependent antigens, showed an increase in numbers of antibody-producing cells when functional nucleotides in the form of RNA were introduced to a nucleotide-free culture. However, this result was not seen when T-cell–independent antigens were used to prime the murine spleen cells. It is, therefore, speculated that polynucleotides modulate humoral immune responses to T-cell–dependent, but not T-cell–independent, antigens. Using in vivo studies, activated helper T cells do not appear to increase specific antibody responses further in the presence of polynucleotides. In addition, the presence of polynucleotides also has been shown to suppress *moderately* the proliferation of helper T cells, as well as nonspecific IgM and IgG production. However, when murine spleen cells were stimulated with these antigens, the number of antigen-specific immunoglobulin-secreting cells increased significantly in the presence of polynucleotides. In this way, polynucleotides suppress nonspecific activation of T cells in the presence of antigen stimulus, and they may increase specific antibody responses mainly through affecting resting T cells.[103] These findings suggest an important role for dietary nucleotides in maintaining optimal humoral immune response.

Complement System

The proteins of the complement system appear to be quite sensitive to nutritional stress. Seth and Chandra[172] noted increased opsonic activity in patients with protein-calorie malnutrition. Serum complement, however, as required for chemotaxis and opsonization, was low. Sirisinha and associates[178] reported low serum concentrations of all complement components (as best documented in reductions of C3, factor B, and total hemolytic activity)[43] except C4 in malnourished children. Patients with kwashiorkor had lower levels than did children with marasmus. The genesis of hypocomplementemia is unclear. Electrophoretically distinct C3 breakdown products have been detected in one study as well as increased titers of immunocoagglutinin, an antibody directed to the C423b complex of activated complement. Activation of the complement pathway may be a consequence of infection, however. Complement serum concentrations drop in the malnourished individual, in part as a result of a consumption complementopathy. Restoration of the components occurs only after several weeks of optimal nutrition. Complement-derived chemotactic factors as well as opsonic factors also are depressed. These functional deficits may contribute to an enhanced susceptibility to infection.

Complement, specifically C3, plays an important role in linking humoral immunity and cellular immunity. In a study of malnourished patients hospitalized in San Juan de Dios General Hospital of Guatemala City, Sakamoto and colleagues[165] found that during nutritional rehabilitation the complement system (CH_{50} and C3 levels) recovered more rapidly than after delayed-type hypersensitivity skin testing. This suggests that the complement system is more effective in host defense during the early stage of nutritional recovery than is cellular immunity. Complement activity appears to be preserved better in severe protein-calorie malnutrition than is cell-mediated immunity, even though complement serum concentrations are maintained at lower levels than in well-nourished controls. In animal studies, both well-nourished and malnourished rats respond to injections with *Staphylococcus aureus* with elevated serum complement concentrations (peak concentrations of complement were seen at 2 days after inoculation). Restoration of complement levels were observed in the well-nourished and nutritionally rehabilitated rats after 7 to 14 days; however, malnourished rats were unable to mount a second response during the later stages of *S. aureus* infection. This second complement response appeared as early as 1 week after initiation of nutritional rehabilitation in malnourished rats.[166] This may suggest a decreased ability to synthesize complement de novo in malnutrition; additional studies are needed to ascertain whether or not a similar response is noted in human malnutrition.

Cellular Immunity

The cellular immune system (T-cell system) appears to be the component of the immune system that is affected most significantly in patients with malnutrition. These children are much more susceptible to tuberculosis, measles, disseminated herpes simplex, hepatitis, and *Pneumocystis carinii*; prevention of disease due to these organisms requires optimal function of the cellular immune system. Histologic studies of lymphoid tissues show severe depletion of T-cell areas in malnourished hosts.[136] Some studies suggest that the defect involves a failure of maturation of T cells. In malnutrition, there are a decrease in circulating lymphocytes bearing mature T-cell markers, normal numbers of B cells, and an increase in null cells. These null cells, if incubated with thymic factors, further differentiate into T cells. Subsequent studies have shown decreased thymic factor activity in protein-calorie malnutrition as an important cause for this delayed T-cell differentiation. There also is a decrease in the deoxynucleotidyl transferase activity that is a feature of lymphocyte immaturity. Cell sorting by use of fluorescein-labeled monoclonal antibodies shows that the number of helper CD4+ cells is decreased markedly, often to less than 40 per cent of controls. There is little change in the number of suppressor T cells; thus, the helper/suppressor ratio is decreased significantly. Lymphocyte proliferation and synthesis of DNA also are reduced, especially in the presence of autologous plasma cell cultures, which may be related to inhibitory factors as well as to lack of essential nutrients in the plasma of malnourished patients.[43, 44] McFarlane[135] reported that skin transplants in malnourished rats were rejected; thus, all aspects of cell-mediated immunity may not be impaired simultaneously or to the same extent. Kelly and associates[108] showed that temporary energy restriction in overweight women caused a significant decrease in the number of circulating natural killer cells, as well as a reduction of serum levels of IgG, IgA, and C3, which also is seen in protein-calorie malnutrition.

Chandra[35] also observed that malnourished children had a decreased ability to respond to tuberculin antigen (purified protein derivative) after bacille Calmette-Guérin (BCG) immunization, and, in most cases, they could not be sensitized to dinitrochlorobenzene. Smythe and associates[182] reported similar findings in malnourished children and also noted that there was lymphocyte depletion in the thymus gland of 118 children, 14 to 47 months of age, at necropsy. At the time of death, 47 of these children had kwashiorkor and 23 were marasmic. Seth and colleagues[174] studied 172 preschool children with varying nutritional status and evaluated cell-mediated immune response after BCG immunization. They found that even severely malnourished children were able to evoke a response 8 weeks after BCG immunization. Bhaskaram and coworkers[18] showed that malnutrition did not influence the ability of BCG-vaccinated children to localize tuberculosis infection; however, malnourished children who did not receive the vaccine had a significantly greater incidence of systemic tuberculosis infection than did BCG-vaccinated malnourished children.

Production of mediators (migration inhibition factor, lymphotoxin, interferon, etc.) by the lymphocytes of malnourished subjects has not been studied extensively. Schlesinger and associates[168] measured interferon production by lymphocytes from nine marasmic infants and from three healthy control children. Interferon production was induced in leukocyte cultures by stimulation with Newcastle disease virus. Interferon production was decreased significantly in marasmic infants. Kramer and Good[115] reported that protein-deficient guinea pigs immunized with BCG vaccine produced equivalent amounts of migration inhibition factor, compared with controls, even when dietary protein was reduced to a level of 3 per cent.

Good and colleagues[72] have evaluated many aspects of the effect of nutritional status (including chronic protein deficiency) on cellular immune functions, including tumor immunity in animal models. In the absence of infection, their results document an enhancement of cell-mediated immunity in chronic protein deficiency. The mechanism for this is unclear. It is possible that the stress of chronic protein deficiency may produce an adaptive response that includes increased thymic hormone output. This may enhance differentiation of precursor cells into mature immunocompetent cells, or it may select populations of T cells that are more immunocompetent. The significance of these findings in humans is unclear.

The role of dietary nucleotides in immune function also has been reviewed. In vitro assays show a down-regulation of T-cell– but not B-cell–mediated responses during nucleotide restriction. In vivo, splenic lymphocytes from nucleotide-free hosts display decreased interleukin-2 (IL-2) production and a decreased number of helper-inducer T cells. Nucleotide supplementation resulted in recovery of proliferative response to mitogens, increased numbers of helper-inducer T cells, and increased IL-2 production. Kulkarni and associates[116] showed significant suppression of delayed-type cutaneous hypersensitivity response (used as a function to estimate cellular immunity) to purified protein derivative, sheep red blood cells, and dinitrofluorobenzene in mice that were fed a nucleotide-free diet. This suppressed delayed-type cutaneous hypersensitivity response was reversed by RNA or uracil supplementation to the nucleotide-free diet. In a study by Rudolph and coworkers,[171] lymphocytes from the spleen, thymus, and bone marrow of nucleotide-free mice showed significantly increased deoxynucleotidyl transferase activity, indicating immature T lymphocytes. During dietary nucleotide restrictions, T-cell deficiency may be secondary to deficiencies of IL-2 and IL-3 activity in animal models.[117] These studies suggest that dietary nucleotides may be a major contributor to the changes in cellular immunity seen in protein-calorie malnutrition.

Thymus

The morphologic response of the thymus in malnutrition has been reviewed by Dourov.[56] As early as 1845, Simon recognized that the thymus was an "early critical barometer of nutrition." In protein-calorie malnutrition, the severe nutritional defect leads to thymic atrophy and fibrotic changes. The thymic cortex is affected sooner than is the medulla in malnutrition. In contrast to the atrophy of liver, kidney, or cardiac muscle, thymic atrophy is characterized more by a loss of cells rather than a decrease in cell size. Histologically, there is a loss of corticomedullary differentiation and fewer lymphoid cells, and Hassall bodies are enlarged, degenerated, and occasionally calcified. These histologic changes are noted after 5 days of starvation and can be reversed after 6 days of refeeding. However, in contrast to other organs, thymic tissue does not regain normal size after refeeding. Histopathologic studies show an increase in the extracellular matrix–containing network in thymuses of 19 malnourished children at necropsy. The enhancement of thymic extracellular matrix in malnourished people corresponds positively with the degree of thymocyte depletion.[128]

The biochemical cause of thymic atrophy has yet to be elucidated fully. In general, stress-induced immunodepression appears to be adrenal mediated. It has been hypothesized that some of the thymic atrophy can be attributed to the action of glucocorticoids. The stress of malnutrition has been associated with an increase of serum glucocorticoids. In addition, the reduced serum protein in malnutrition leads to a lowered binding capacity for steroids and an increase in the metabolically active form. Schlesinger and associates[169] found elevated levels of norepinephrine in the thymuses of rats with protein-calorie malnutrition. This may have important functional implications in early regulation of development of the cellular immune response because T-cell response takes place in the thymus.

Functional changes resulting from thymic atrophy also are under investigation. Thymic factors, such as thymosin and thymopoietin, have been incubated with isolated T cells from malnourished children, resulting in a normalization of the maturational characteristics of the lymphocytes.[96, 145] These observations were confirmed when the results were controlled for infection and zinc content.[97] A study in Bolivian children hospitalized for severe protein-calorie malnutrition showed a high degree of T-lymphocyte immaturity that correlated with severe involution of the thymus, regardless of the clinical form of protein-calorie malnutrition. This high percentage of circulating immature T lymphocytes was concomitant with a decrease in mature T lymphocytes and a slight increase in cytotoxic T-cell subpopulations. After in vitro incubation with thymulin, mature T lymphocytes increased, with a concomitant decrease in immature T lymphocytes.[148]

Phagocytosis

Phagocyte function can be divided into three main phases: (1) adherence and chemotaxis; (2) recognition, opsonization, and engulfment; and (3) postphagocytic events, which include (a) formation of phagocytic vacuoles or phagosomes, followed by fusion of lysosomes with phagosomes and degranulation of lysosomal enzymes; (b) microbicidal activity; and (c) associated metabolic changes.[79] Phagocytosis and intracellular microbicidal activity of polymorphonuclear leukocytes and macrophages are critical host functions in the defense against pathogens. These functions depend upon various components of the complement system, antibodies against surface microbial antigens, and possibly acute-phase reactions, such as that of C-reactive protein. The initiators of the acute inflammatory response are humoral factors that have chemotactic and vasoactive properties. The surface constituents of some microorganisms resist phagocytosis; for this reason, humoral factors are required for opsonization.

For appropriate phagocytic function, adequate pool sizes of neutrophils and mononuclear phagocytes are required at inflammatory sites. The bone marrow also needs to have an adequate capacity to mobilize these cells. There is a significant reduction in neutrophil pool sizes in healthy newborn infants. Protein deprivation in mice results in a marked decrease in colony-forming units in the spleen, causing alterations in precursor cell pool sizes. The numbers of circulating phagocytes are normal or increased in protein-calorie malnutrition; however, lymphocyte pool sizes in humans have not been studied thoroughly.[79]

In malnourished individuals, defects in phagocytosis and killing have been identified, but these deficits are subtle rather than gross. Schopfer and Douglas[170] investigated the polymorphonuclear leukocyte function of 46 children with kwashiorkor. Chemotactic response was reduced at early intervals (30, 60, and 120 minutes) and reached values achieved by controls only after 180 minutes, which suggests an early migration defect. It should be emphasized that the intensity of the early cellular response may be of greater importance to the host than may the later response, which may approach that seen in normal individuals. In the presence of normal serum, the internalization of particles or organisms is normal. Serum from malnourished patients is deficient in opsonic activity; therefore, the kinetics of microbial ingestion may be affected adversely. Decreased ingestion, however, actually might improve intracellular killing of those organisms taken into phagolysosomes. Studies of opsonization and phagocytosis of cells in malnourished animals and humans indicate that neutrophil membrane receptors for Fc-IgG and complement (C3b) are intact; however, kinetic studies show a defect in opsonization that likely is related to complement deficiencies in malnourished children.[78] There is no evidence for any abnormalities in lysosomal fusion or degranulation in leukocytes of malnourished hosts.

Schopfer and Douglas[170] also noted that polymorphonuclear leukocytes from children with kwashiorkor did not kill *Candida albicans* intracellularly as well as did control cells. Enzymatic studies of resting cells and lactate production, hexose monophosphate shunt activity during phagocytosis, and morphologic events were not impaired. However, de la Fuente and Munoz[54] showed a decrease in nitroblue tetrazolium reduction in stimulated (latex beads present) and nonstimulated (latex beads absent) macrophages from both young and old mice with protein-calorie malnutrition. Because the nitroblue tetrazolium dye reduction test in nonstimulated phagocytes is an indirect measure of intracellular hexose monophosphate shunt activity, protein-calorie malnutrition may interfere with this metabolic pathway. Studies from children with kwashiorkor show diminished neutrophil iodination during phagocytosis.[78] This suggests an abnormality in the myeloperoxidase-halide–mediated system in malnutrition. Seth and Chandra[173] previously had noted that intracellular bactericidal killing was impaired in patients with kwashiorkor. Fibronectin is a glycoprotein secreted by hepatocytes and macrophages; the levels of immunoreactive fibronectin are an indirect measure of opsonic activity. Starvation in rats as well as protein-calorie malnutrition in infants is associated with reduced levels of fibronectin. These levels of fibronectin increase to greater than normal values after nutritional rehabilitation.[78]

Another example of the detrimental synergistic effects of humoral and cellular immunity in the undernourished host is the delayed development of a granuloma in response to pathogens such as *Mycobacterium tuberculosis*, for which the granuloma is a critical host-defense response.

Neutrophil adhesion is a prerequisite for cell migration and locomotion. Research has shown that neutrophils from malnourished children have enhanced baseline adhesion; however, after stimulation with chemotactic factors, the adherence response is decreased and neutrophil chemotaxis is diminished. After nutritional recovery, the abnormal adherence is reversed and chemotactic activity improves.[5, 79]

Experimental Viral Infection

The effect of malnutrition on experimental viral infection has been studied, but results have not been uniform. Many investigators have concluded that starved, fasted, or underfed animals are more resistant to viral infections than are normal animals and that the severity of viral infection is decreased.[14, 51, 159, 188, 190, 214, 215] Most of these studies were published before 1950, and clinical criteria were utilized in evaluating the severity of viral infection. Despite reports by some investigators that the severity of viral infection is enhanced in protein-deficient animals, the concept that healthy animals are more susceptible than are their malnourished counterparts to experimental viral infection has gained broad acceptance.[106, 171] This antagonistic effect of malnutrition on viral infection was attributed by some investigators to starvation of the virus at the cellular level, with restriction of viral replication.[15, 68] The studies of Woodruff and Kilbourne[221] cast doubt on this prevailing concept and support the theory that protein-calorie malnutrition is as detrimental to the response of the host to viral infection as it is to bacterial infection. Their studies demonstrate convincingly an increased severity of infection with coxsackievirus B3 in male albino mice that were subjected to sustained postweaning undernutrition. Severity of infection was proportional to the magnitude of malnutrition. Virus persisted in the heart, spleen, pancreas, and liver of severely malnourished animals, and mortality was highest in these groups. If a quantitatively optimal diet was fed to previously malnourished mice at the time of infection, they were protected from further viremia and death. Mice maintained on a severely restricted diet up to and after viral challenge developed no detectable serum neutralizing antibodies, whereas those fed an optimal diet did. Normal serum antibodies were found, however, even in moderately[220] malnourished animals, even when their susceptibility to viral infection was increased. Furthermore, if severely malnourished mice were returned to a normal diet at the time of viral inoculation, they were protected to a significant extent from the development of serious visceral lesions. This protection occurred before serum neutralizing antibody titer reached control levels. Thus, serum neutralizing antibody may not correlate necessarily with recovery from the viral infection.

These findings are in agreement with those of Keet and Thom[107] and may explain the particular susceptibility of the malnourished host to infection with viruses, *Mycobacterium*, and other organisms for which protection heavily is dependent upon competent T-cell function.

Measles

Measles probably is the most extreme example of a childhood disease that is relatively benign in urban Western populations but associated with high mortality rates in developing nations. This difference can be attributed to many factors, including vaccination patterns, concurrent disease, and available medical care. However, one of the most important causes of this differential mortality is varying nutritional status. There are several mechanisms by which measles influences the nutritional and immune status. Like any other febrile illness, measles contributes to severe reduction in food intake, vomiting, and increased metabolic losses. Measles also can produce a viral enteritis that results in excessive nitrogen loss due to a protein-losing enteropathy. Measles induces prolonged immunosuppression characterized by a decrease in the number of circulating T cells and impaired proliferation of T lymphocytes that has been shown to last for nearly 6 months after measles infection.

A study in India revealed a close association between protein-calorie malnutrition and measles. It was observed that nearly 25 per cent of children hospitalized for severe protein-calorie malnutrition had an episode of measles in the preceding 3 to 6 months.[19] In a prospective study carried out in the urban slums of Hyderabad, measles was associated with a significant weight loss of 2 to 12 per cent of the initial body weight in children younger than 5 years of age. These children also were shown to have retarded growth up to 6 months after the initial infection. Nearly 4 per cent of children who had measles developed clinical signs of kwashiorkor or marasmus within 3 to 6 months after measles. All children manifesting clinical signs of severe protein-calorie malnutrition in the postmeasles period were undernourished before contracting the infection, which points to the importance of the nutritional status as a major determinant of the severity of nutritional deficiencies and growth failure that occurs in the postmeasles period.[19]

In the malnourished host, the epithelial surfaces are affected severely, with eye and mouth involvement, laryngitis, bronchopneumonia, and gastroenteritis. These children carry and transmit the virus three times longer than does a child with normal nutritional status. They are more susceptible to viral and bacterial superinfection. A study in Nigeria found a mortality rate of 26 per cent.[61]

Respiratory complications accounted for more than 90 per cent of deaths. Some of the severe manifestations of measles are explained by a deficit of vitamin A. As mentioned previously, vitamin A contributes to mucosal immunity through maintenance of epithelial surfaces. It is responsible also for the synthesis of the ground substance of the corneal stroma. The striking occurrence of postmeasles blindness in approximately 1 per cent of all children with measles in developing countries also supports the critical role of vitamin A metabolism in the malnourished host. It is well documented that hyporetinemia is extremely common in children with severe measles.[160] The relationship between cause and effect is unclear. In the case of malnutrition, exhaustion of hepatic stores accounts for decreased retinol and may predispose to severe measles. Alternatively, hepatic stores of retinol may be mobilized inadequately during severe measles. Prophylactic treatment with vitamin A in children with severe measles has been shown to reduce respiratory and gastrointestinal symptoms as well as death, especially in children younger than 2 years of age.[46, 93]

Vaccination is an extremely important tool in preventing measles and its associated infections. Often, tuberculosis and malnutrition are considered as contraindications for measles vaccination. Unlike the natural measles infection, the attenuated virus has no immunosuppressive effect and is thus unlikely to activate latent tuberculosis.[19] Several studies in undernourished children have shown high rates of seroconversion to the measles vaccine, except in cases of severe protein-calorie malnutrition, thus indicating the efficacy of immunization against measles in undernourished children.[16, 50]

HIV and Malnutrition

During the past decade, AIDS has become one of the most pressing public health problems in the world. More than 1 million Americans are infected with HIV. Infection with HIV has a devastating effect on nutritional status. Weight loss is an almost universal feature of this infection, and patients may lose 30 to 50 per cent of their body mass before succumbing to their disease. Weight loss contributes to an accelerated deterioration and also may be used to predict the time of death in patients with HIV infection. Weight loss in AIDS patients is not constant but appears to be episodic and related to intercurrent opportunistic infections. In the absence of such infections, AIDS patients can maintain body weight for indefinite periods.[73] Clinically, malnutrition appears as the last stage in pediatric AIDS and is associated with a very poor prognosis, with a case-fatality rate higher than 90 per cent.[153]

Protein-calorie malnutrition is a common occurrence in AIDS patients and is considered a predominant cause of morbidity in AIDS. In HIV-positive patients with advanced disease, the total body potassium (an index of body cell mass) is reduced when compared with that of controls. AIDS patients have been shown to have total body nitrogen depletion, which could be correlated to total body potassium depletion.

The development of protein-calorie malnutrition in AIDS patients is multifactorial. Alterations in food intake may occur as a result of pathologic lesions in the upper gastrointestinal tract or central nervous system. Food intake can be inhibited indirectly by malabsorption or systemic infections that release factors that inhibit appetite. Nutrient malabsorption is common in AIDS patients and may be occult or clinically severe. Protozoal infections can disrupt mucosal architecture in the small intestine, resulting in severe malnutrition. Systemic infection or other severe inflammatory disorders lead to derangements of intermediary metabolism and protein wasting, even in the presence of adequate nutrients. Investigators of energy metabolism in HIV-infected people have produced conflicting results. In some studies, the resting energy expenditure was increased, and in others it was decreased. Nevertheless, the role of resting energy expenditure is critical to understanding weight loss in HIV infection. The hypermetabolism noted with cachexia is associated with a disproportionate loss of lean body mass compared with extracellular water and body fat. Hypometabolism is an appropriate compensatory response to malnutrition, which is characterized by increased losses of body fat and extracellular water, with relative sparing of lean body mass.[73, 112]

Several cytokines such as interferon-α, IL-6, and tumor necrosis factor (TNF) are involved in nutrition and intermediary metabolism. Both animal and human studies have correlated cytokine levels with anorexia, cachexia, and altered lipid metabolism. Serum levels of interferon-α are increased in some AIDS patients and are correlated significantly with elevated serum triglyceride levels. Other studies of HIV-positive people have noted increased levels of IL-1, TNF, and IL-6, which are involved in the acute-phase response to stress.

Gastrointestinal dysfunction, especially malabsorption, is prevalent in patients with advanced HIV infection. Often, there are no identifiable pathogens. In these patients, villous abnormalities are frequent and small intestine dysfunction can be demonstrated by abnormal D-xylose absorption tests, Schilling tests, ^{14}C-glycocholate absorption, and the presence of steatorrhea.[73, 140] Small intestine pathology or pancreatic insufficiency may lead to fat malabsorption, weight loss, and depletion of fat-soluble vitamins.[118] Hypochlorhydria has been found in almost 75 per cent of AIDS patients and can allow for enteric infections as well as reduced absorption of micronutrients, such as folate and iron. Lactose malabsorption is a common finding and is more severe in symptomatic than asymptomatic HIV-infected children.[223] Subclinical malabsorption may play a role in early HIV disease, whereas overt malabsorption is more frequent in advanced HIV infection.

The Task Force on Nutrition Support in AIDS (1989) recommended that AIDS patients consult a registered dietician for nutritional assessment, which would include diet history, calculation of nutrient intake, and assessment of the degree of malnutrition. Nutrition intervention should begin early in the course of HIV infection in the hopes of stabilizing weight loss, which may improve the survival of AIDS patients. Patients who are unable to consume at least two-thirds of their nutrient needs orally (food and oral supplements) may need more aggressive specialized nutritional support. Specific dietary interventions include maximizing intake of high-calorie, nutrient-dense foods as well as vitamin and mineral supplements, especially vitamins A, E, and C, riboflavin, vitamins B_6 and B_{12}, zinc, and selenium. In addition, dietary counseling should emphasize the importance of daily ingestion of a full complement of amino acids. When a patient cannot consume enough energy from food alone, high-calorie liquid supplements (1.0 to 2.0 kcal/mL) and snacks can be incorporated into the diet. If adequate nutritional status cannot be maintained orally, enteral supplementation, such as nasogastric or nasoenteric tube feedings, should be used for short-term diets. If tube feeding regimens are required for longer than 1 month, a percutaneous endoscopic gastrostomy, surgical gastrostomy, or jejunostomy tube should be placed. In order to maximize absorption and minimize diarrhea, formulas that have low residue or low lactose and that contain peptides and medium-chain triglycerides should be used. If the patient has intractable diarrhea or impaired function of the gastrointestinal tract or if nutrient needs are not met via enteral nutrition, home total parenteral nutrition can be used long term if the patient has a reasonable prognosis. Parenteral nutrition therapy may be complicated by metabolic abnormalities (hypertriglyceridemia, hyperglycemia, fluid and electrolyte imbalance) and problems related to catheters, such as infection, hemorrhage, and pneumothorax. AIDS is an ultimately fatal disease and should be regarded as a chronic process. There are no standard nutritional recommendations for AIDS patients because of the heterogeneous nature of the complications of this disease. The ultimate benefits of nutritional supplementation are still being evaluated in order to improve nutritional status and immune function in AIDS patients.[13, 73]

Bacterial Infection

Bacteremia, the most dreaded infective complication of severe malnutrition, varies in incidence between different studies from 2 to 31 per cent. Most commonly, bacteremia is caused by gram-negative enteric bacilli, especially *Salmonella* and *Escherichia coli,* as well as the common organisms that infect normal hosts. The case fatality rate for severely malnourished children is significantly higher than for other children. A number of reports have been published indicating a high incidence of urinary tract infections in malnourished children. Freyre and associates[69] studied 200 malnourished children with 118 well nourished controls. The incidence of bacteriuria and pyuria was found to be equally common in both groups, and the authors felt that the incidence of other infections in severely malnourished children appeared to be due largely to the same microorganisms that cause infections in well-nourished children.

Parasitic Infection

Parasitic disease in humans has been estimated to affect more than 1 billion people, particularly children who are living in developing countries in Africa, Asia, and Latin America. It also is in these areas where protein-calorie malnutrition from its mildest to the most severe forms (kwashiorkor and marasmus) is endemic. Unfortunately, the same conditions of poverty, overcrowding, poor environment, and inadequate sanitation that are associated with parasitic infections also are associated with people who are at the highest risk for malnutrition. There are periods during human development, such as infancy, childhood, pregnancy, and lactation, when nutrient needs are increased and the consequences of inadequate nutrient intake more readily are definable. A particularly vulnerable time for children appears to be after 4 to 6 months of age up until about 5 years. This is the period when the transition from breast feeding to a home diet occurs and the exposure to disease in the environment increases. Parasitic diseases may reduce intake, interfere with absorption from the intestine, or cause increased losses of nutrients from the body. In addition, women who are nourished poorly may produce more low birth weight babies (less than 2500 g at birth) who are less likely to survive compared with larger neonates. There is evidence to suggest that parasitic infections in humans may reduce voluntary food intake compared with those who are uninfected. The mechanism whereby food intake is reduced in parasitic infections is related to significant immunologic responses in the host, an important outcome of which is anorexia. Injections of IL-1 are accompanied by reduced food intake in chicks.[193] Zwingenberger and associates[224] found elevated levels of tumor necrosis factor and cachectin in humans infected with *Schistosoma mansoni,* which normalized after treatment.

Some parasitic infections cause diarrhea, such as *Giardia intestinalis,* which may reduce fat absorption. *Ascaris lumbricoides* infection has been shown to reduce the absorption of fat in experimental animals and children and is associated with diminished vitamin A and carotenoid levels in children. Parasitic infection also can increase body nitrogen losses through increased intestinal losses of mucus or albumin, through blood loss, or by interfering with protein absorption.

Schistosoma hematobium causes urinary schistosomiasis and is endemic in 52 African and eastern Mediterranean countries. *S. mansoni* and *S. japonicum* cause intestinal schistosomiasis.

S. mansoni is endemic in Africa, the Middle East, and a few countries in South America and the Caribbean. Schistosomiasis is of major importance in tropical areas because it causes granuloma formation and both reversible and irreversible damage to the urinary and intestinal tracts. Schistosomiasis has been implicated as a major contributor to the two most important forms of malnutrition in the Third World: protein-calorie malnutrition and iron-deficiency anemia. Both the larval and adult stages of the infection can alter nutritional status, either by reducing food and nutrient intake or by increasing nutrient excretion (mainly via blood loss, vomiting, diarrhea) or by altering nutrient metabolism within the body. Two major features of *S. hematobium* infection are hematuria and proteinuria. Hematuria and dysuria, the two most common symptoms, are detectable in 70 per cent of infected persons. In Zambian children as well as Gambian children and adults, infected subjects had mean hemoglobin levels 0.9 g/dL lower than those of uninfected subjects, whereas heavily infected Egyptian children had mean hemoglobin levels 1.3 g/dL lower than those of uninfected children. *S. hematobium* infection may cause splenomegaly and hepatomegaly. The nutritional significance of these is unknown. Splenomegaly may be related to increased destruction of erythrocytes and can predispose to anemia, whereas hepatomegaly may alter nutrient metabolism.

Also found in a small number of cases is a mild degree of periportal fibrosis due to schistosomal hepatic fibrosis. Both hepatomegaly and splenomegaly are reversible with adequate treatment.[194]

The daily urinary protein losses in urinary schistosomiasis are on the average of 1 g per day when compared in multicultural studies. *S. mansoni* infection is associated with blood loss in the stool. Farid and associates[62] estimated the daily fecal blood loss in seven chronically infected Egyptian patients to be equivalent to 3.3 mg of iron per day (range, 0.6 to 6.7 mg per day). The iron losses are sufficient to produce anemia if persistent, and the daily intake of iron is not adequate. Cross-cultural studies involving children with *S. mansoni* infection revealed no difference in anthropomorphic measurements between infected and uninfected children; however, severe infection resulted in significantly lower height for age and skin fold thickness than did lighter or no infection. *S. japonicum* effects are similar to those of *S. mansoni*; however, they tend to be more severe because *S. japonicum* produces 10 times as many eggs per worm pair as does *S. mansoni*. Multiple cross-cultural studies in the Philippines and China report that the presence and intensity of *S. japonicum* infection are related directly to reduced arm circumference, skin fold thickness, height, weight, and weight-for-height ratios.[194]

Hookworms and *Trichuris* species are associated with significant intestinal blood losses. Foo[67] showed that children with hookworm infection were on average 1 kg lighter and 2.4 cm shorter than were their uninfected counterparts. These children also had hemoglobin levels 1.1 g/dL lower than those of hookworm-free children. *Ascaris lumbricoides* infection has been shown to interfere with the absorption of fat and is associated with reduced weight and height, decreased vitamin A and carotenoid concentrations, and reduced serum concentrations of albumin and vitamin C.[87] *Giardia intestinalis* is known to cause significant diarrhea, which may reduce fat absorption. Both *G. intestinalis* and *A. lumbricoides* reduce intestinal lactose activity, resulting in lactose intolerance. *Strongyloides stercoralis* infection is associated with a protein-losing enteropathy resulting in significant hypoalbuminemia. To a lesser degree, *G. lamblia* has been associated with a protein-losing enteropathy without hypoalbuminemia.[194]

Obesity

In industrialized countries, the burden of morbidity and mortality continues to shift toward chronic diseases. Research has focused on the effects of surfeit nutrition, especially obesity.

In 1971, Tracey and associates[202] studied two matched groups of children aged 3 months to 2 years. One group contained children whose weight was above the 90th percentile. Children whose weight was between the 25th and 75th percentiles constituted the second group. Data from 120 children of the overweight group were analyzed. Forty-seven of these children experienced at least one respiratory infection during the trial period. One baby in the overweight group died after an acute episode of bronchiolitis. Twenty-three of 103 children in the control group had a respiratory infection during the trial period, and no deaths were noted. A significantly ($p < .01$) greater number of children who were obese experienced respiratory disease than did control children, suggesting that obesity in infants and children may be a factor that predisposes to acute respiratory disease. In 1981, Chandra[35] examined the immunocompetence of obese children, adolescents, and adults. Approximately one-third of the obese group showed a variable impairment of cell-mediated immune responses as well as a reduction of intracellular bacterial killing by polymorphonuclear leukocytes. The obese group had moderately low concentrations of serum zinc and iron, and therapy with these micronutrients for 4 weeks resulted in improvement in immunologic responses.

A variety of cell-mediated immune responses have been evaluated in genetically obese mice. There is a decrease in the number of mononuclear cells and T lymphocytes in the thymus and spleen, with a corresponding decrease in the size of these organs. There is a significantly lower response of lymphocytes to T-cell mitogens, which is shown to increase by about 190 per cent of baseline levels after weight reduction with a very low-calorie diet.[297] There also is a significant decrease in natural killer cell activity. When obese mice were immunized with lymphoma cells, the cytotoxic response of spleen cells was markedly lower than that of lean controls.[42] However, the generation of cytotoxic T lymphocytes after stimulation is normal if sensitization is carried out in vitro. This suggests that the microenvironment of obese animals, which includes hyperlipidemia, hyperglycemia and altered levels of insulin, glucagon, cortisol, and adrenocorticotropic hormone, may be responsible for impaired cellular responses. When lymphocytes from obese and lean mice are sensitized in vitro rather than in vivo, they perform similarly. Furthermore, spleen cells from obese mice are similar in their ability to those of lean mice to produce a graft-versus-host reaction in F1 hybrid mice.[191]

Obese adolescents and adults show a greater risk of sepsis and wound infections after surgery than do lean control subjects.[63, 191, 210] Obese people show a slight impairment of delayed cutaneous hypersensitivity responses, decreased lymphocyte response to mitogens, reduced bactericidal capacity of neutrophils, and reduced helper T-cell populations. Boeck and associates[21] reported that obese patients had little or no detectable plasma TNF compared with control subjects. Animal studies have shown that elevated levels of TNF are associated with insulin resistance; however, most of the obese patients in the study had significant insulin resistance. These findings may reflect a refractive state in obesity where TNF production is down-regulated. Kolterman and colleagues[112] reported reduced release of migration inhibition factor by stimulated lymphocytes from moderately obese nonhyperglycemic subjects to 36 per cent of the level of normal weight controls. Migration inhibition factor is a cytokine that acts to concentrate macrophages in an area of infection.

When dogs were fed a high-calorie diet by Newberne,[143] a greater susceptibility to distemper virus and a shorter survival time were noted than in control animals fed a normal diet. Swiss mice made obese by high-fat diets are less resistant to infection by *Salmonella typhimurium* (which provokes both cellular and humoral responses) and *Klebsiella pneumoniae* (which provokes primarily a humoral response) when compared with Swiss mice fed a standard laboratory diet.[191]

The effect of excess protein in the human diet is unknown. An increased susceptibility to infection and increased mortality rates have been reported in animals. Several investigators have observed an increased susceptibility to *Salmonella gallinarum* infection in chickens.[22, 86, 181] When chickens on a high-protein diet were infected with Newcastle disease agent, mortality and morbidity were greater than those noted in control groups.[22, 189]

High-fat diets show consistently depressed host resistance to tuberculosis and malaria in rats and to pneumococcal infections in chickens.[129] Erickson and associates[59, 60] discovered that high levels of dietary fat, particularly polyunsaturated fat, suppressed the response of lymphocytes to T-cell mitogens. Lymphocytes from animals that were maintained on diets devoid of essential fatty acids showed significant depression of activity in response to supplemental essential fatty acids. Animal models also have demonstrated the adverse effects of excess cholesterol. Fiser and coworkers[65] found that monkeys that were rendered hypercholesterolemic developed altered humoral and cellular immune function. Hypercholesterolemia alters murine host defenses against group B coxsackieviruses.[123] Mice rendered hypercholesterolemic died, whereas uninfected hypercholesterolemic animals and infected animals with normal nutrition all survived. These lines of evidence suggest that any deviation from normal nutritional status may enhance the susceptibility of the host to infection.

Breast Feeding

The nutritional, immunologic, psychosocial, and child-spacing benefits of breast feeding are recognized universally. According to numerous reports, breast-fed infants appear to be less susceptible than do bottle-fed infants to certain infections. The protective effect is most evident for upper respiratory infections, otitis media, and gastroenteritis. In underdeveloped countries, breast milk clearly offers a protective effect against infection. In highly developed countries, the anti-infective properties of breast milk have been subject to great debate. There are many agents present in human milk that could be important in imparting protection to the infant. These include lysozyme, lactoperoxidase, lactoferrin, interferon, complement components, immunoglobulins, leukocytes, lipids, and retinol. These anti-infective factors transmitted by breast milk protect primarily by noninflammatory mechanisms. These anti-infective proteins act to reduce the risk of mucosal infection in the gut. These proteins are thought to escape digestion in young infants as a result of low acid, reduced protease activity in gastric and pancreatic secretions, and the presence of protease inhibitors in breast milk. It has not been established fully whether anti-infective proteins can resist endogenous digestive mechanisms in older children. Studies in Gambia have suggested that at least 30 per cent of ingested secretory IgA escapes digestion in children who are old enough to have developed considerable digestive capacity, whereas more than 98 per cent of lactoferrin appears to be degraded.[154] Cruz and colleagues[47] have suggested that neither nutritional status nor ethnicity affects levels of immunologic components in human milk. The most important to the newborn infants may be secretory IgA, which is found in high concentration in colostrum and early milk. IgA possesses virus-neutralizing and antibacterial properties and is capable of activating the alternate complement pathway, thus providing local protection in the gastrointestinal tract. The effect against otitis media may be the result of transmission of humoral or cellular immune components to the infant or the result of position during bottle feeding. Bottle-fed infants may have a predisposition to otitis media due to the position in which they are fed. The benefits of breast feeding may reduce illness severity and resulting hospitalization. Specifically, morbidity from certain infections, such as bronchiolitis, pneumonia, roseola infantum, and septicemia, may be reduced.

Breast milk contains amylase, bile salt–stimulated lipase, and bile salt–stimulated esterase. These digestive enzymes are present in measurable quantities after 6 months of lactation. Children whose digestive functions are compromised by malnutrition, small bowel overgrowth, and disease may benefit from the addition of breast milk enzymes. For example, bile-stimulated lipase, unlike pancreatic lipase, requires only low concentrations of bile salts for activation and completely digests triglycerides to glycerol and free fatty acids. Colostrum and early milk contain hormones and growth factors such as epidermal growth factor, prostaglandins, insulin, and thyroid hormones thay may benefit children whose gut integrity has been compromised by malnutrition and gastrointestinal disease.[154] However, it is not clear whether these components are present in significant amounts to have any physiologic effect after the first few months of lactation.

The antimicrobial system in human milk constitutes a complex group of biochemical agents that differ widely in structure but have a common effect at the site of mucosa. Lactoferrin is an iron-binding glycoprotein that competes with siderophilic bacteria for ferric iron and thus interferes with the multiplication of organisms. In addition to its antimicrobial effects, lactoferrin may have a positive influence on cell growth and a negative effect on inflammation. Lysozyme is found in relatively high concentrations in external secretions, including human milk, and lyses susceptible bacteria by hydrolyzing beta-1,4 linkages between *N*-acetylmuramic acid and 2-acetylamino-2-deoxy-D-glucose residues in cell walls. Lysozyme is relatively resistant to digestion by trypsin and denaturation due to acid. Secretory IgA comprises more than 90 per cent of the immunoglobulins in human milk and is formed by two intricate processes. The first process is the entero-broncho-mammary pathway, during which mature IgA-producing plasma cells populate the subepithelial zones via migration of B lymphocytes. The second process involves the binding of IgA to polymeric immunoglobulin receptors (membrane-bound secretory component) located on the basolateral plasma membranes of epithelial cells of the mammary gland. The polymeric IgA is complexed with the major fragment of the receptor and is transported through the epithelial cell subsequently secreted into the milk. These processes may be regulated by cytokines and hormones produced late in pregnancy or during lactation. Fibronectin is a high-molecular-weight protein that facilitates the uptake of particulates by phagocytic cells. Human milk also is rich in carbohydrate moieties that interfere with the binding of pathogenic bacteria onto epithelial cells. Human milk provides certain oligosaccharides that promote the growth of *Bifidobacterium* and lactobacilli in the lower intestinal tract, which in turn produce acetic acid, which inhibits the multiplication of bacterial pathogens such as *E. coli*, *Salmonella*, and *Shigella*. Also, some antimicrobial agents, such as lactoferrin and lysozyme, double as anti-inflammatory agents.[71]

Epidemiologic studies of the association between infections and breast feeding have come under great scrutiny. Strong evidence has shown that in developing countries infant morbidity is reduced by breast feeding.[114] The consequences of breast feeding on mortality have been documented in Brazil, where a population-based case-control study found that human milk without supplements reduced the risk of death from diarrhea and respiratory infections.[209] The effect was most pronounced in the first 2 months of life.

Less agreement exists on the evidence for a similar effect in highly developed countries. Bauchner and associates[11] presented a meta-analysis of the association between breast feeding and infections in industrialized countries. Examination of 20 studies found only 6 that met strict methodologic standards. These investigators concluded that the evidence supports only a minimally protective effect of breast feeding.

In 1990, a group from Denmark reported their results after following 500 infants prospectively for the first year of life.[163] They were unable to document a protective effect of breast feeding against infectious illness. These results conflict with earlier studies with larger sample sizes that supported an association between breast feeding and fewer infectious episodes.[33, 36, 48, 64, 147, 212] These differences highlight the importance of environmental factors, such as socioeconomic status, parental education, exposure in day care centers, and parental smoking, on the incidence of infectious disease in infants.

Breast feeding also has distinct advantages over bottle feeding, even in situations in which infection is not an important factor. In a study of 101 children with atopic asthma, only one breast-fed infant displayed clinical manifestations, compared with 11 children when human milk was substituted with cow's milk or soy protein. Although evidence is inconclusive, breast feeding is believed to provide protection against obesity, arteriosclerosis, celiac disease, and other metabolic disorders.[104]

There are circumstances, however, in which breast feeding is contraindicated (e.g., mothers who are sputum-positive for *M. tuberculosis* or who are carriers of hepatitis B virus). Breast milk also has been implicated in the transmission of rubella, cholera, Q fever, HIV, human T-cell lymphotropic virus 1, and cytomegalovirus in selected individuals. Human milk also can transmit environmental toxins, such as polychlorinated biphenyl compounds and DDT. Toxic side effects can occur in nursing infants secondary to passive excretion of medicines taken by the mother.[57] On balance, breast milk clearly is preferable except in unusual circumstances and serves to help diminish the role of infection during infancy.

SINGLE NUTRIENTS

There are many barriers to analyzing the clinical significance of single nutrients in maintaining normal immune function. First, nourishment is a combination event, and nutrient-nutrient interaction can be of major consequence. Competition for transport may affect absorption or excretion in both intracellular and extracellular environments. Second, a hierarchy exists for some nutrient requirements. If an element subserves several functions, as does iron, the prerequisite amount may vary with the function. Third, experimental animal models do not allow always for extrapolation to human medicine. Most species, with the notable exception of the guinea pig, make indigenous vitamin C, and no animal model exists for studying cobalamin deficiency. Finally, infection can affect body stores of essential nutrients. Transient malabsorption of folic acid and vitamin B_{12} has been noted during and after recovery from acute intestinal infections.[137] The urinary excretion of the group B vitamins and vitamin C also has been observed to change during hepatitis and tuberculosis.

Chandra[38] has suggested a framework for micronutrient evaluation. Alterations in immune responses occur early in the course of reduced intake. These alterations predict the risk of infection and mortality. In the case of many nutrients, excessive intake also is associated with immune abnormalities.

Iron deficiency probably is the most prevalent nutritional deficiency recognized in the United States today and results in systemic disease involving all cell systems. There is no reason to believe that the function of iron is any less critical when the host is infected. On the other hand, iron may stimulate the growth of the pathogen with which the host is infected, may inhibit bactericidal proteins, and may enhance bacterial metabolism.[216] Iron in fluids such as plasma, milk, nasal secretions, and saliva is to a greater or lesser extent unavailable to many bacteria and fungi because of the presence of the iron-binding proteins transferrin and lactoferrin.[120, 123, 131, 202] These proteins combine with two atoms of iron per molecule. The percentage of saturation of transferrin with iron in plasma correlates directly with the ability of the sera to support the growth of various microorganisms. When levels of saturation increase, sera can support additional bacterial growth. Microorganisms produce iron chelators known as *siderophores.* If the supply of iron in the host is so high that the physiologic processes to withhold it are exceeded, the invading microbes can obtain iron for growth.[175] Bactericidal capacity of leukocytes in iron deficiency is reduced, which may be due to deficient function of iron-dependent myeloperoxidase and cytochrome enzymes.[42] The administration of iron to animals by the intravenous, intramuscular, or intraperitoneal route reduces the LD_{50} for *Pseudomonas aeruginosa, Salmonella typhosa*, streptococci, *Klebsiella pneumoniae, S. typhimurium*, and *Listeria monocytogenes*.[216]

Secondary bacterial infection occurs commonly in patients with bartonellosis and malaria,[121] and bacterial infection, particularly due to the *S. pneumoniae* and *Salmonella,* is more frequent in individuals with sickle cell anemia.[10, 98, 121] This evidence has been cited by some investigators to support the concept that iron during infection is detrimental to the host. Clearly, this is not justified, for patients with these diseases are known to have other deficits that intrinsically contribute to an increased propensity for infection. Thus, it is impossible specifically to attribute an increased incidence of bacterial infection in these individuals to an increase in free iron.

The administration of iron intramuscularly to children with kwashiorkor has resulted in overwhelming infection and death. Clinicians in these cases concluded that iron therapy should be deferred until transferrin synthesis was restored by protein nutrition. Similarly, the bacteriostatic action of human milk upon coliform bacteria has been neutralized by iron supplementation. However, no evidence exists that gradual oral replenishment of iron predisposes children to infection.

Excess iron in specific tissues may benefit the host by preventing the pathogen from producing factors of virulence. Retention of iron in the reticuloendothelial system may enable macrophages to detoxify bacterial toxins. Iron in monocytes may enhance antibacterial activity of these cells.[132] Iron also may activate lysosomal hydrolases.[98] Thus, free iron may be detrimental to the host during bacterial infection, but iron within cells, particularly in selected tissue, appears to be beneficial to the host.

One situation frequently cited to demonstrate that iron deficiency states are protective of the host is that of malaria. It was noted initially by field researchers in malaria-endemic countries that treatment of iron deficiency, especially with parenteral iron, often was associated with an increase in the incidence of smear-positive malaria. Other studies have manipulated iron availability by using desferrioxamine, which is an iron chelator. Both in vitro and in vivo, desferrioxamine inhibits the growth of malaria parasites. The effect of desferrioxamine appears to be directly on parasitized erythrocytes, which behave as if they contain a chelation-labile iron pool.[110]

MacKay[126] reported that iron-supplemented infants in the 1920s had fewer episodes of bronchitis and gastroenteritis than did control groups; it was her impression that the rate of recovery was better in the iron-fortified children than in the control group. In these studies, however, retrospective control data were utilized, thereby introducing the variable of annual differences in the prevalence of infectious disease. Differences in infection rates were modest and not subjected to statistical evaluation. In another study, the frequency of respiratory infection was significantly less in infants in Chicago's inner city who were given an iron-fortified formula than in those who were not.[4] Criteria for the diagnosis of respiratory infection were not defined in this study, and precautions to minimize bias on the part of observers were not taken. In addition, intervals between patient examinations exceeded those that are optimal for reliable recall of illness.

In a study in Colombia in which iron deficiency was severe, medical care alone had no impact on the morbidity and mortality caused by infectious disease.[7] Mortality was unchanged in groups given nutritional supplements and medical care. Supplemented groups experienced an impressive reduction in enteric infections. The relative contributions of iron and other supplements in decreasing morbidity could not be ascertained.

Cellular development of lymphoid tissues has been shown to be diminished in iron deficiency. Splenic and thymic tissue from iron-deficient rat pups showed histologic evidence of decreased lymphopoiesis. Lymphoid tissue from iron-deficient rats shows reduced cellularity and deranged histology, which suggests a reduced capacity for immunocompetence.[175]

It is known that lymphocyte transformation is decreased in iron-deficient patients.[152] The production of migration inhibitory factor also is diminished in individuals with iron deficiency when contrasted with the host whose serum iron concentration is normal.[102] Impaired delayed cutaneous hypersensitivity responses, decreased in vitro lymphocyte response to mitogens, and reduced number of circulating T cells are seen in humans suffering from iron deficiency.[53] The rate at which granulocytes killed staphylococci also was decreased in 819 iron-deficient patients studied by Joynson and coworkers.[102] In severely iron-deficient rats, there is an increased number of phagocytes in whole blood, but granulocytic activity as measured by nitroblue tetrazolium dye reduction is decreased significantly.[175] In iron-deficient patients studied by Macdougall and associates,[125] impaired leukocyte responsiveness, decreased bactericidal capacity, increased IgA, and increased C3 concentrations were observed. Restoration of normal bactericidal function 4 to 7 days after the initiation of iron therapy and prior to any increase in hemoglobin concentrations was noted, suggesting that tissue iron depletion rather than anemia was an etiologic factor in depressing bactericidal function.

Studies have shown that humoral immunity also is affected by iron deficiency. Five days after injection with sheep red blood cells, the production of IgM and IgG by splenocytes from experimental rats was significantly lower in severe and moderate iron deficiency. It also was shown that plasma IgG was not affected by either severe or moderate iron deficiency, while plasma IgM was lower in severe but not moderate iron deficiency. Although circulating plasma immunoglobulin may be normal in iron deficiency anemia, iron deficiency may result in diminished antibody production. Natural killer cell activity is impaired significantly in both moderate and severe iron deficiency when compared with controls. IL-1 production is impaired in moderate and severe iron deficiency. This can affect cell-mediated immunity adversely and alter humoral immunity and bacterial killing by neutrophils, which is under partial control by IL-1.[170]

It is clear that the interactions of iron, the host, and the microorganism are important. Low levels of iron-binding protein as noted during malnutrition appear to be detrimental to the survival of the host during infection. Similarly, depletion of tissue levels of iron as noted in iron deficiency may be detrimental to optimal performance of the inflammatory and immune systems. To date, there have been no serial studies in which alterations in immune response have been measured during transition from a state of good nutrition to one of poor nutrition, for assessment of the point at which iron deprivation interferes with immunologic states.

The suggestion that iron deficiency protects humans against infection cannot be supported. The diverse role of iron in multiple enzyme systems, both mammalian and bacterial, is understood best in a hierarchy of function in which optimal activity of the different systems may be at different elemental concentrations.

The role of selenium in the prevention of infections in humans still is controversial. Deficiency has been associated with generalized immunosuppression. Neutrophil function, antibody production, and lymphocyte proliferation all are affected. In Keshan, China, selenium deficiency has been implicated in the pathogenesis of a dilated cardiomyopathy. A similar cardiomyopathy has been noted in AIDS.

In the tissues and cells of the immune system, selenium has three major functions: reduction of organic and inorganic peroxides, metabolism of hydroperoxides, and modulation of the respiratory burst. People with symptomatic HIV infection possess less plasma and erythrocyte selenium in addition to decreased glutathione peroxidase activity. Although decreased glutathione peroxidase activity may be due to protein-calorie malnutrition or reduced selenium intake, supplemental nutrition may assist the impaired immune system in AIDS patients. Glutathione peroxidase and phospholipid hydroperoxide glutathione peroxidase are selenium-containing enzymes that catalyze the reduction of peroxides formed from general metabolism, drugs, and other initiators of free radical chain reactions. Both glutathione peroxidase and phospholipid hydroperoxide glutathione peroxidase have been implicated as being responsible for the reduction of prostaglandin G_2 in the arachidonic acid cascade, leading to the synthesis of thromboxane A_2, prostacyclin, and prostaglandins. One or both of the selenium enzymes are involved in the reduction of 5-HPETE, 12-HPETE, and 15-HPETE in the synthesis of leukotrienes and lipoxins. Research also has demonstrated reduction of eicosanoid biosynthesis in the absence of selenium and glutathione peroxidase. The third major role of selenium and the glutathione peroxidases is to modulate the production of the oxidizing products of the respiratory burst: O_2^-, H_2O_2, CLO^-, and chloramines, which are used in the phagolysosome to lyse and destroy phagocytized cells. Selenium deficiency in experimental animals is associated with decreased glutathione peroxidase activity in phagocytic cells, release of increased amounts of H_2O_2 by macrophages and peritoneal granulocytes, and increased superoxide formation in macrophages.[10, 187]

Zinc participates in wound healing and is a cofactor for DNA and RNA synthesis and for some aspects of amino acid and protein metabolism.[152] Zinc deficiency in humans has been associated with poor growth and development, impaired wound healing, and impaired sensory perception. The low levels of zinc in acrodermatitis enteropathica may be related to the serious infections that are noted frequently.[34] Zinc deficiency in mothers may be associated with an increased risk of congenital anomalies in the fetus.

Zinc deficiency is associated with altered humoral responses, such as distorted serum immunoglobulin profiles, as well as impaired antibody production to sheep red blood cells in neonatal mice. Repletion with zinc results in normalization of IgM and elevated IgG responses. Cell-mediated immunity also is altered by zinc deficiency. Delayed hypersensitivity to skin test antigen often is compromised in zinc-deficient states. Patients maintained on parenteral hyperalimentation lacking in zinc showed reduced T-lymphocyte proliferation in response to mitogen phytohemagglutinin, which markedly increased after zinc repletion.[176] Deficiencies in zinc also are associated with reduction in thymulin activity, decreased proliferation of lymphocytes exposed to mitogens, and slower neutrophil chemotaxis. These changes are reversed with the zinc supplementation.[40] Zinc also activates

B cells to secrete immunoglobulin. Oversupplementation of zinc has been shown to cause a suppressive effect on lymphocyte proliferation, as well as reduced chemotactic and phagocytic activities.[49]

Copper is essential for the production of red blood cells and also facilitates absorption of iron from the gastrointestinal tract. It also is critical for several oxidative enzyme systems. Copper deficiency has been shown to cause anemia of varying degrees, incoordination of movement, and gross ataxia in neonates of many species, as well as defects in connective tissue formation. In animal models, the reduced microbicidal activity of granulocytes is attributed to the role of copper in superoxide dismutase and cytochrome *c* oxidase enzyme systems. Copper deficiency is associated with the depressed function of the reticuloendothelial system, reduced microbicidal activity of granulocytes, decreased response of splenic lymphocytes to T- and B-cell mitogens, and impaired natural killer cell cytotoxicity in animal models.[176] Neutropenia has been documented in children with a copper-deficient diet. Patients with Menkes kinky hair syndrome, a progressive brain disease in infants in which copper transport is impaired, are characterized by many of the abnormalities described in various animals who have experimental copper deficiency. These children commonly succumb to pneumonia and other infections.

The role of chromium in disease control remains undefined. Excess amounts adversely affect macrophage and lymphocyte cultures.[70, 211] Deficiency is characterized by impaired glucose utilization.[149] Chromium acts as a cofactor for the potentiation of insulin at the cellular level.[137] The role of chromium in impaired glucose homeostasis in kwashiorkor has been documented.[28]

Manganese is another essential trace element necessary for optimal growth. It affects the primary sites of chondroitin sulfate synthesis. In humans, a manganese deficiency state is characterized by weight loss, transient dermatitis, occasional nausea and vomiting, changes in hair color, hypocholesterolemia, and teratogenicity.

Lymphocyte and neutrophil functions in iodine deficiency are diminished. Iodide interacts with neutrophil peroxidases to form the halide-superoxide system, which is modulated by the amount of thyroid hormone, which supplies the iodide molecule. In hypothyroid patients, the bactericidal activity is decreased and restored after treatment with thyroid hormone.[40]

Two of the fat-soluble vitamins, A and E, have recognized effects on immune system function. Before the discovery of antibiotics, it was noted that urinary tract infections in children responded to vitamin A therapy. In the modern era, vitamin A deficiency is well documented to be a major determinant of respiratory and diarrheal disease in the Third World. Vitamin A levels in the serum have been used as markers of malnutrition; however, the independent effects of its deficiency are significant. The worldwide ramifications have been reviewed.[218] It is estimated that improving the vitamin A status of all children who are deficient will prevent approximately 1 to 3 million deaths each year, curtailing the incidence and/or severity of infectious episodes, especially respiratory and diarrheal infections.[92]

An important role of vitamin A is for cellular differentiation of epithelial surfaces. In both animals and humans, vitamin A deficiency is associated with keratinizing metaplasia of mucus-secreting epithelial surfaces, particularly of the respiratory, gastrointestinal, and genitourinary tracts, as well as corneal tissues. This histopathologic alteration is conducive to an overgrowth of bacteria and secondary infections of loculated areas obstructed by keratinized debris.

A Bitot spot is a triangular patch of xerotic conjunctiva characteristic of xerophthalmia and is composed largely of keratin debris and a heavy growth of *Xerosis bacillus*, a saprophytic diphtheroid. In a malnutrition ward in Bangladesh, 78 per cent of xerophthalmic children had bacteriuria determined by urine culture obtained via bladder tap, compared with 17 per cent of nonxerophthalmic malnourished peers.[25] It also has been demonstrated that there is an inverse relationship between the level of retinol in the serum of study children and the proportion of bacteria that adheres to cells obtained by nasopharyngeal lavage.[37, 186]

Immune changes in patients with vitamin A deficiency are characterized by reduced thymic weight, reduced immunoglobulin production, decreased T-helper cell activity, decreased lymphocyte proliferation, and increased bacterial binding to epithelial cells.[44] Vitamin A deficiency also is characterized by reduced phagocytosis and diminished nitroblue tetrazolium dye reduction. Lysozyme is a vitamin A–dependent glycoprotein; the activity of this protein is decreased markedly in vitamin A deficiency.[217] It is clear, however, that children in the Third World frequently are caught in a vicious cycle in which infection leads to vitamin A deficiency, which in turn increases the risk of subsequent infection. The impact that vitamin A supplementation will have on childhood morbidity and mortality depends on several factors, including the prevalence and severity of deficiency, aggravating conditions (e.g., protein-calorie malnutrition), associated nutrient defects, virulence of the infectious agents to which they are exposed, and adequacy of supplementation.[185] Carotenoids also have important immunoregulatory functions involving T and B lymphocytes, natural killer cells, and macrophages.[42]

Several studies have shown that vitamin E deficiency impairs both cellular and humoral immunity in different animal models. In humans, vitamin E deficiency impairs T-cell–mediated function, which is reversible by vitamin E supplementation. Supplementation in an amount 2 to 10 times greater than at present recommended significantly increased humoral and cell-mediated immune responses and phagocytic functions in laboratory animals and humans.[199] Vitamin E enhances immune responses and phagocytosis by acting as an antioxidant to prevent lipid peroxidation of cell membranes. Rapidly proliferating cells of the stimulated immune and phagocytic systems particularly are prone to peroxidative damage by free radicals, peroxides, and superoxides. The antioxidant effect also modulates the biosynthesis and activity of prostaglandins, thromboxane, and leukotrienes.[199]

Nockels showed that vitamin E–supplemented chickens and turkeys had a decreased incidence of *E. coli* infections.[144] Moderate amounts of vitamin E also have been shown to heighten humoral responses. This immunomodulation is synergistic with selenium[81] and copper.[199] Zinc deficiency, even when marginal, can decrease markedly vitamin E serum concentrations.[161]

Concentrations of vitamins A, B_6, and C have been reported to be lower than normal during acute bacterial and viral infections, and reduced concentrations of folic acid in blood and serum have been found in infants with diarrhea or acute bacterial infection,[134] as well as in adults with tuberculosis or malaria.[162, 202] Severe xerophthalmia has been noted in vitamin A–deficient Indian children. Often, this was preceded by diarrhea, measles, or a respiratory infection. Xerophthalmia may be precipitated by a fall in serum vitamin A and retinal-binding protein concentrations during the course of the infection. Altered concentrations of circulating vitamins during infection have been attributed to several mechanisms, including impaired absorption from the gastrointestinal tract, liver cell damage, and altered rates of vitamin excretion. Transient malabsorption of folic acid and vitamin

B_{12} has been noted during and after recovery from acute intestinal infections, including cholera and salmonellosis.[122] The urinary excretion of the group B vitamins and vitamin C also has been observed to change during hepatitis and tuberculosis.[82, 100]

Vitamin B_6 deficiency has been shown to impair both humoral and cell-mediated immunity in rodents. In humans consuming a low vitamin B_6 diet or treatment with deoxypyridoxine (vitamin B_6 antagonist), there is a decreased number of circulating lymphocytes as well as reduced antibody production and a mild decrease in the percentage of helper T cells.[138] Lymphocyte differentiation and maturation are altered, and delayed-type hypersensitivity responses are reduced.[158] The thymus is smaller and thymic hormone activity is decreased in vitamin B_6 deficiency. In addition, vitamin B_6 deficiency is associated with delayed rejection of allografts and diminished T-lymphocyte cytotoxicity.[42] Vitamin D serves both as an immunoregulatory hormone and as a lymphocyte-differentiating hormone in addition to its classic role of mineral homeostasis. 1,25-Dihydroxyvitamin D_3 functions in the manner of a steroid hormone in many different cell types. Lymphocytes possess receptors for 1,25-$(OH)_2$-vitamin D_3, and an extensive number of RNA polymerase II–transcribed genes that govern oncogene and lymphokine expression are regulated by this vitamin/hormone.[12]

The possibility that vitamin C may be important in preventing upper respiratory infections has received widespread publicity in both the medical and lay press. Host susceptibility to infection clearly is increased in scurvy. Chalmers[29] reported, however, after a review of 14 clinical trials of ascorbic acid in the prevention and treatment of the common cold, that differences between supplemented and nonsupplemented subjects were minor and insignificant. Nevertheless, in most studies, the severity of symptoms was worse in patients who received placebo. Miller and colleagues[139] performed a double-blind co-twin controlled study on 44 monozygotic twins of school age. During the 5-month study period, no statistically significant difference in the number or severity of illness episodes was noted between the recipients of vitamin C and a placebo control group. Several studies have shown a consistent decrease in the duration of the common cold episodes; although most of the results are not statistically significant, all of them point consistently in the same direction.[97]

A study involving 674 Marine recruits reported that the administration of vitamin C had no effect on the frequency of the common cold.[151] It is clear that administration of ascorbic acid is not a panacea for upper respiratory infections. Physiologic quantities of ascorbic acid are necessary for normal metabolism of lipids and iron, and the side effects are few unless pharmacologic doses are ingested. Lack of vitamin C clearly is detrimental; excess intake is of no proven value. One of the major functions of vitamin C is as an antioxidant that protects the $alpha_1$ proteinase inhibitor from inactivation by free radical products of the respiratory burst. $Alpha_1$ proteinase inhibitor is present in plasma, where it reacts with elastase, thus protecting the extracellular space from escaped proteases from damaged cells. The concentration of intracellular vitamin C is approximately 50 times that found in plasma, which suggests that vitamin C may protect intracellular regions from oxidants that leak into the cytoplasm. Leukocytes from vitamin C–deficient guinea pigs show significantly diminished chemotaxis; in vitro, neutrophil chemotaxis is stimulated significantly by 2 to 5 mM of vitamin C (concentration of vitamin C in human plasma is 0.01 to 0.15 mM). Vitamin C deficiency also is associated with impaired phagocytic activity. Vitamin C may be important to the phagocytic and chemotactic response due to modulation of tubulin tyrosinolation by an antioxidant effect. Microtubule organization depends on the redox state of the cell and is responsible for phagocytosis and locomotion.[83]

Tropical pyomyositis is a hematogenous pyogenic infection characterized by abscess formation in various muscle tissues. Osawa[146] first suggested that thiamine deficiency may predispose to the occurrence of tropical pyomyositis. Muscle tissue generally is quite resistant to infection. Lack of thiamine may change the biochemical milieu of the muscle, rendering it more susceptible to infection.

Recent developments in the field of malnutrition and infection support the concept that malnutrition impairs the response of the host to infection; some of the mechanisms have been suggested. Experimental animal studies demonstrate an enhanced susceptibility to infection with any deviation from optimal nutrition. The critical studies not available are those that might inform us about the import of specific deficiencies of elements, vitamins, lipids, proteins, and so on, upon host resistance. Do selected deficiencies have an adverse impact upon one or two areas of host resistance, or do they have broad effects? Combinations of less severe nutrient deficiencies must be studied for us to ascertain whether the effects are synergistic.

EFFECT OF MALNUTRITION ON RESISTANCE TO INFECTION

When malnutrition diminishes resistance to infection or when infection aggravates malnutrition, the relationship between the two can be described as synergistic. In other situations, malnutrition impedes the multiplication of the agent more than it diminishes resistance of the host. In this case, the interaction between infection and malnutrition can be considered somewhat antagonistic. Vitamin A deficient patients have been reported to have a higher incidence of tuberculosis, bronchitis, otitis media, urinary tract infections, and bronchopneumonia. Protein deficiency leaves patients more susceptible to typhus, hepatitis, amebic dysentery, diarrheal disease, and tuberculosis. An increased frequency of pharyngitis and upper respiratory infections has been observed in subjects on a pantothenic acid–deficient diet for 35 days. It seems reasonable to assume that most deficiency states decrease host resistance to infection.

Copper-deficient patients are more susceptible to bronchopneumonia and bacterial sepsis, especially with *E. coli*. Copper-deficient animals show increased mortality when exposed to *Salmonella typhimurium, Listeria monocytogenes*, and coxsackievirus B. The biochemical lesion underlying impaired immunocompetence in copper deficiency has not been defined.

DIARRHEAL AND RESPIRATORY DISEASE

Disease of the intestinal tract is the most obvious link between the mutually aggravating conditions of infection and malnutrition. Historically, diarrhea has been a primary cause of childhood morbidity and mortality in developing countries. Poor nutrition increases susceptibility to diarrhea, and, in turn, diarrhea contributes to deteriorating nutrition.[88] Steps to improve overall general nutrition and to provide oral rehydration therapy in acute situations can contribute to decreasing diarrheal disease and its effects. Overcrowding and poor sanitation, conditions that coexist with poverty, also act synergistically with malnutrition to enhance the risk and morbidity of diarrhea.[167]

Nonenteral infections such as pneumonia, septicemia, and meningitis, as well as severe dehydration, measles infection, and severe protein-calorie malnutrition, are major risk factors for mortality in diarrheal diseases. Measures such as correction of fluid and electrolyte imbalance, treatment of associated infections, and nutritional restitution have been shown to reduce the risk of mortality of diarrhea.[163, 200] Several studies have suggested that breast feeding and immunization against major pathogens (measles, rotavirus, cholera) serve a protective role in reducing the incidence of morbidity and mortality from diarrhea.[26, 90, 209] Important steps such as improving water quality and availability, ensuring proper food and personal hygiene, control of zoonotic reservoirs, and improving waste disposal and sanitation will minimize transmission of pathogens to those individuals at risk.[89, 184]

Gracey[75] has suggested that protein-calorie malnutrition predisposes to chronic diarrhea in malnourished children by causing changes in the intestinal mucosa. The changes include thinning of the gut wall, flattening of the intestinal villi, inflammatory infiltration of the lamina propria, and alteration of the enterocytes from columnar to cuboidal or squamous. The gastric mucosa also is abnormal in malnourished states. Chronic gastritis has been noted in Indonesian children in association with a reduction of secretion of gastric acid. This, in turn, may lead to heavy bacterial infestation of the upper gut. Steatorrhea in malnutrition results from bile salt pool depletion and impaired micelle formation. Carbohydrate intolerance and malabsorption occur partly due to bacterial overgrowth. In a study done by Black and coworkers[20] in Bangladesh, malnutrition was a determining factor in the duration of diarrhea but not in the incidence of diarrhea caused by *E. coli* and *Shigella*.

The mechanisms of nutrient loss in diarrhea that lead to malnutrition include maldigestion resulting in insufficient breakdown of substrates, malabsorption characterized by inefficient uptake, and excessive wastage of nutrients from the body. All three of these mechanisms act synergistically with viral, bacterial, and parasitic agents to exacerbate the ill effects of malnutrition on the individual.[89, 184] Nutritional restitution is of vital importance and a key factor in survival. This may be initiated via oral feedings or by a modified parenteral route in those children who are unable to tolerate oral feedings.[200]

In the underdeveloped world, acute respiratory infections rank with diarrheal disease as the leading causes of morbidity and mortality. In developing countries, acute respiratory infections account for about 28 per cent of childhood deaths and are even more frequent than are diarrheal episodes. Acute lower respiratory infections, such as pneumonia and bronchiolitis, are more prevalent in developing countries; the annual incidence of pneumonia for children younger than 5 years of age in industrialized countries is 3 to 4 per cent, compared with 10 to 20 per cent in most developing countries. The link between malnutrition and pneumonia has been recognized for years.[204] Malnourished infants are 10 to 20 times as likely to contract pneumonia as children with normal weight for age.[90] Severe complications, such as empyema and bronchiectasis, also are more likely in the face of nutritional deficiencies. A community-based study in the Philippines clearly demonstrated that malnutrition was the most important determinant of mortality associated with respiratory disease.[205] Such evidence supports WHO recommendations that in areas of prevalent malnutrition the use of antibiotic therapy be determined on the basis of clinical signs that can be recognized by minimally trained health care workers.[198] The presentation of a child with cough, chest indrawing, inability to drink, or a respiratory rate of more than 50 breaths per minute meets the requirement for antimicrobial therapy.

The World Bank Health Sector Review on Acute Respiratory Infections suggested that the five most cost-effective interventions to reduce mortality from respiratory infections are case management, breast feeding promotion, vaccination against childhood communicable diseases, reduction of malnutrition, and pneumococcal vaccination. Reduction in malnutrition probably is the most important preventive intervention because mortality is correlated directly to nutritional status. Other studies also have stressed the importance of vitamin A supplementation in malnourished children, improving access to health care services, adequate housing, and proper waste management in reducing the transmission and development of acute respiratory diseases in children.[90, 206, 207, 208]

BURNS, INFECTION, AND NUTRITION

In the United States, it is estimated that each year about 2.5 million people seek medical care for burns. More than 100,000 people are hospitalized with burns each year, and 12,000 burn victims die of their injuries.[60] Over the past 50 years, great strides have been made in the treatment and management of patients who have suffered thermal injuries. There has been a marked decrease in burn mortality, particularly in patients younger than the age of 35 years. From 1942 to 1952, a 50 per cent total body surface burn killed nearly half of the people younger than 35 years of age, whereas now a 98 per cent body surface area burn kills only half the young people who receive it.[84]

Infection always has been the predominant determinant of wound healing, incidence of complications, and outcome of burn patients. The incidence of infectious complications in burn patients is increased in proportion to the fraction of the body surface injured. The direct effects of heat on skin and underlying tissue make the burn wound particularly susceptible to infection. The denatured protein in burn-injured tissue serves as a rich medium for microbial growth and proliferation. The thermal thrombosis that renders the eschar avascular further promotes infection by precluding delivery of the cellular components of the host defense system and limiting delivery of blood-borne antibiotics to the infected wound site. Further microbial proliferation occurs at the interface between viable tissue and the eschar; this is known as the *subeschar space*. If host defenses are adequate, the eschar is sloughed; however, microbial invasion of the viable tissue occurs if host defenses are deficient.

Infection remains the most common cause of morbidity and mortality in burn patients, even though the incidence of the burn wound infection has been reduced significantly since the introduction of topical antibiotics. Pneumonia is the most frequent infection occurring in burn patients, with bronchopneumonia being the most common form of this infection. Other infectious complications, such as suppurative thrombophlebitis and septicemia, have been decreasing in incidence due to improvements in patient management, wound care, and infection control.[156]

Recently, a larger role to the development of sepsis has been attributed to the gastrointestinal tract. The gastrointestinal barrier is normally highly effective in containing its flora. However, the stress of thermal injury as well as other stresses that can occur in burn patients, such as major trauma, surgery, malnutrition, or immunosuppression, can result in breakdown of the barrier followed by translocation. Translocation is the passage of inert particles and microorganisms across the intestinal wall. It is well known that burn wounds are colonized by gram-negative organisms, which are more likely to originate from the gastrointestinal tract hematogenously than from the skin. Alteration of the indigenous microbial flora has been shown to increase translocation markedly. The flora of gastrointestinal tract can be altered by stress of injury, antibiotics, and composition of enteral feedings. Healthy rats fed a normal enteral diet showed no translocation, while rats given parenteral nutrition displayed bacterial overgrowth and increased incidence of translocation. In addition, dietary fiber preserves mucosal architecture and is associated with a decrease in bacterial translocation. Bacterial translocation can be prevented by supplementing total parenteral nutrition solution with glutamine.[27, 58]

Major thermal injury is associated with extreme hypermetabolism and catabolism. These conditions occur shortly after successful resuscitation from the shock phase of the burn injury.[203] It has been shown that translocation of bacteria and their toxins from ischemic bowel in burn injury causes a massive release of cytokines and inflammatory mediators from macrophages in the splanchnic area. These factors include IL-1, IL-6, TNF, prostanoids, free radicals, endotoxins, catecholamines, cortisol, and glucagon.[52] This hypermetabolic state is characterized by elevated cardiac output, increased energy expenditure, erosion of lean body mass, negative nitrogen balance, and abnormal substrate production. In addition, gluconeogenesis, glucose oxidation, and plasma clearance of glucose are accelerated.[203]

The release of cytokines and inflammatory mediators after thermal injury also results in the alteration of the immune system. Depressed cytotoxic activity of T cells, decreased ratio of helper to suppressor T lymphocytes, suppressed stimulation of lymphocyte proliferation by hemagglutinin, and suppressed mixed lymphocyte responses have been present after thermal injury. Phagocytes show depressed phagocytic activity, reduced intracellular killing, and increased superoxide formation. Decreased serum concentrations of immunoglobulins, activation of complement with release of anaphylatoxins, and formation of membrane attack complexes leading to inflammation and cytolysis are the sequelae of altered humoral immunity after burn injuries in children and adults.[80]

Over the past 15 years, the role of nutrition in maintaining immunocompetence and modulating hypermetabolism in burned patients has become increasingly important. The use of early enteral nutrition when combined with early excision of nonviable tissue has resulted in reduced energy requirements in burned children.[85] Providing proper nutrition by the enteral route when possible may satisfy caloric needs, regulate microflora, and maintain the integrity of the mucosa of the gut, but it also may blunt the hypermetabolic response following thermal injury.[58, 99] New therapeutic modalities, such as glutamine and xanthine oxidase inhibitors, soon may become available to protect and treat the compromised gastrointestinal barrier. Routine antimicrobial prophylaxis is not recommended, but short-term perioperative prophylaxis is used in many centers. Selective bowel decontamination with aztreonam has been shown to decrease burn wound colonization with gram-negative bacteria.[130] Several studies have suggested that growth hormone treatment accelerates donor site wound healing and promotes protein anabolism in severely burned children.[141] Many immunoprotective measures, such as intravenous immunoglobulins, specific tetravalent *Pseudomonas* immunoglobulins, recombinant granulocyte colony-stimulating factor, neutrophil transfusions, plasmapheresis, and opsonin replacement using fresh-frozen plasma, have been described anecdotally; however, their efficacy has not been proved in larger clinical trials.[55, 80] The patient who is inflicted by thermal injury faces impaired metabolism, nutrition, and immunocompetence. Critical factors focusing on maintaining adequate nutrition, modulating hypermetabolism, restoring proper immune function, wound coverage, and controlling infection will need to be assessed continually in order to lessen the morbidity and mortality in these patients.

PROPHYLAXIS AND IMMUNIZATION

With the exception of severe protein-calorie malnutrition, it appears that nutritional deprivation has but a minor suppressive effect upon humoral immunity.

The link between malnutrition and infection must be seen from both biologic and social viewpoints. Strategies for improving the control of disease in the developing world have been reviewed by Keusch and Scrimshaw.[109] Immediate interventions include immunizations, oral rehydration programs, promotion of breast feeding, adequate weaning foods with increased protein, continued feeding during infection, nutrient fortification, and growth monitoring. Complex measures such as improved sanitation and general education are important long-term goals. Although data are far from complete, it appears from general information that virtually every immunization program among populations with malnourished children has been successful.[95] Unfortunately, adequate studies to define the extent of immunization failure in malnourished populations have not been performed. Studies in Haiti have suggested that immunization schedules can be adjusted in less developed countries to maximize the beneficial effect.[89] Their observations confirmed that immunologic response is independent of nutritional status. The most important factor for seroconversion is the absence of passively acquired maternal antibodies. Tuberculosis is associated with a high mortality rate in developing countries. BCG vaccination does not offer absolute protection against this disease. Seth and associates[174] evaluated cell-mediated immune responses after BCG immunization in Indian school children with varying nutritional status. Demonstration of normal cell-mediated immune responses correlated positively with adequate nutrition. Cell-mediated immune responses to purified protein derivative waned more rapidly in malnourished than in normal individuals. These studies suggest that the timing of reimmunization with BCG must be planned on an individual basis in relation to the nutritional status of the child. Of even greater import, no data are available to answer important questions: (1) What are possible harmful effects of live viral vaccines in the malnourished child? (2) Does administration of live attenuated viruses in the malnourished child lead to the development of slow, persistent infection?

Several studies were undertaken to find the effect of protein-calorie malnutrition on the immune response to immunization. Several investigators have concluded that the immune response to immunization remains unimpaired in balanced mild to moderate malnutrition; however, severe forms of protein-calorie malnutrition may affect negatively the ability to seroconvert after immunization, especially when maintained for long periods.[2, 3, 50, 172] These results suggest that immunization of the mild to moderately malnourished child may afford him or her comparable degrees of protection as the well-nourished child. The severely malnourished child, however, may have minimal, if any, response to immunization. Further research is needed to improve the immune response after vaccinations in children with severe protein-calorie malnutrition.

One form of immunologic reconstitution has been attempted in malnourished children to determine whether the frequency and severity of infectious episodes could be affected. Jose and associates[101] gave transfer factor to 40 Australian aboriginal children, 2 to 46 months of age, who were hospitalized with acute infection. Many also suffered from protein-calorie malnutrition. These and a control group of 35 children were followed for at least 12 months. Children treated with transfer factor experienced significantly fewer episodes of diarrheal disease, but no protection against chest, middle ear, or skin infection could be demonstrated. Flo and associates[66] showed that malnourished rats, after oral immunization with cholera toxin, had diminished levels of total IgA in intestinal fluid as well as an impaired ability to neutralize cholera toxin in vitro when compared with well-nourished controls. In this study, there were no observed differences in serum levels of total IgA between well-nourished and malnourished rats. This suggests that oral immunizations have a diminished capacity to evoke an immune response when compared with systemic immunizations, which may reflect impaired mucosal immunity in severe malnutrition.

CONCLUSION

Attempts to reduce the mortality and morbidity referable to infection in the malnourished individual must be predicated upon a more comprehensive understanding of this process than that which is at present available; the need for further research is clear. In the interim, every effort must be expended to control infection and improve nutrition throughout the world. This requires education, abolition of poverty, improvement in sanitation, improved prenatal care to reduce the incidence of prematurity, and either greater access to appropriate food supplies or education directed toward improving the utilization of food of appropriate nutritional quality when it already is available.

References

1. ASCC/SCN: Second Report on the World Nutrition Situation. Vol. 1. Global and Regional Results. Geneva, ACC/SCN Secretariat, W.H.O., 1992.
2. Adeiga, A., et al.: Evaluation of immune response in infants with different nutritional status: Vaccinated against tuberculosis, measles, and poliomyelitis. J. Trop. Pediatr. *40*:345–350, 1994.
3. Ahmed, F., Jones, D. B., and Jackson, A.: Effect of under-nutrition on the immune response to rotavirus infection in mice. Ann. Nutr. Metab. *34*:21–31, 1990.
4. Andelman, M. B., and Sered, B. R.: Utilization of dietary iron by term infants: A study of 1048 infants from a low socioeconomic population. Am. J. Dis. Child. *111*:45–55, 1966.
5. Anderson, D. C., Krishna, G. S., Hughes, J. B., et al.: Impaired polymorphonuclear leukocyte motility in malnourished infants: Relationship to functional abnormalities of cell adherence. J. Lab. Clin. Med. *101*:881–895, 1983.
6. Antonov, A. N.: Children born during the siege of Leningrad in 1942. J. Pediatr. *30*:250–259, 1947.
7. Arbeter, A., Echeverri, L., Franco, D., et al.: Nutrition and infection. Fed. Proc. *30*:1421–1428, 1971.
8. Ascoli, W., Guzman, M. A., Scrimshaw, N. S., et al.: Nutrition and infection: Field study in Guatemalan villages, 1959–1964. IV. Death of infants and preschool children. Arch. Environ. Health *15*:439–449, 1967.
9. Ascoli, W., and Mata, L. J.: Studies of diarrheal disease in Central America. VII. Treatment of preschool children with paramycin and sulfamethoxypyridazine under field conditions in a Guatemalan highland village. Am. J. Trop. Hyg. *14*:1057–1061, 1965.
10. Barrett-Connor, E.: Bacterial infection and sickle cell anemia: An analysis of 250 infections in 166 patients and a review of the literature. Medicine (Baltimore) *50*:97–112, 1971.
11. Bauchner, H., Leventhal, J. M., and Shapiro, E. D.: Studies of breast-feeding and infections. J.A.M.A. *256*:887–892, 1986.
12. Beisel, W. R.: Vitamins and the immune system. Ann. N. Y. Acad. Sci. *585*:5–8, 1990.
13. Bell, S. J., Mascioli, E. A., Forse, R. A., et al.: Nutrition support and the human immunodeficiency virus (HIV). Parasitology *107*:S53–S67, 1993.
14. Bendinelli, M., Ruschi, A., and Santopadre, G.: Replicazione virale e produzione di interferone intopi a dieta carente infettai con virus mengo. Riv. Ital. Ig. *25*:191–204, 1965.
15. Beveridge, W. I. B.: Immunity to viruses. *In* Betts, A. O., and York, C. J. (eds.): Viral and Rickettsial Infections of Animals. Vol. 1. New York, Academic Press, 1967.
16. Bhaskaram, P., Madhusudan, J., Radhakrishna, K. V., et al.: Immunological response to measles vaccination in poor communities. Hum. Nutr. Clin. Nutr. *40C*:295–300, 1986.
17. Bhaskaram, P.: Infections and malnutritions among poor children. Indian J. Pediatr. *54*:535–545, 1987.
18. Bhaskaram, P., Hemalatha, P., and Rao, K. V.: BCG vaccination in malnourished child population. Indian Pediatr. *29*:39–44, 1992.
19. Bhaskaram, P.: The vicious cycle of malnutrition-infection with special reference to diarrhea, measles, and tuberculosis. Natl. Inst. Nutr. Indian Council Med. Res. *29*:805–813, 1992.
20. Black, R. E., Brown, K. H., and Becker, S. B.: Malnutrition is a determining factor in diarrheal duration, but not incidence, among young children in a longitudinal study in rural Bangladesh. Am. J. Clin. Nutr. *37*:87–94, 1984.
21. Boeck, M.A., Chin, C., and Cunningham-Rundles, S.: Altered immune function in a morbidly obese pediatric population. Ann. N. Y. Acad. Sci. *587*:253–256, 1990.
22. Boyd, F. M., and Edwards, H. M., Jr.: The effect of dietary protein on the course of various infections in the chick. J. Infect. Dis. *112*:53–56, 1963.
23. Brabin, B. J.: Hypothesis: The importance of folacin in influencing susceptibility to malarial infection in infants. Am. J. Clin. Nutr. *35*:146–151, 1982.
24. Braude-Heller, A., Ratbalsam, I., and Elbinger, R.: Clinical aspects of hunger disease in children. *In* Winick, M. (ed.): Hunger Disease. New York, John Wiley & Sons, 1959, pp. 45–68.
25. Brown, K. H., Gaffar, A., and Alamgir, S. M.: Xerophthalmia, protein-calorie malnutrition, and infections in children. J. Pediatr. *95*:651–656, 1979.
26. Brown, K. R., Black, G., Lopez, R., et al.: Infant feeding practices and their relationship with diarrheal and other diseases in Huascar (Lima), Peru. Pediatrics *83*:31–40, 1989.
27. Burke, D. J., Alverdy, J. C., Aoys, E., et al.: Glutamine supplemented total parenteral nutrition improves gut immune function. Arch. Surg. *124*:1396, 1989.
28. Carter, J. P., Kattab, A., Abd-el-hadi, K., et al.: Chromium (3) in hypoglycemia and in impaired glucose utilization in kwashiorkor. Am. J. Clin. Nutr. *21*:195–202, 1968.
29. Chalmers, T. C.: Effects of ascorbic acid on the common cold. Am. J. Med. *58*:532–536, 1975.
30. Chandra, R. K.: Antibody formation in first and second generation offspring of nutritionally deprived rats. Science *190*:289–290, 1975.
31. Chandra, R. K.: Fetal malnutrition and postnatal immunocompetence. Am. J. Dis. Child. *129*:450–454, 1975.
32. Chandra, R. K.: Serum thymic hormone activity in protein-energy malnutrition. Clin. Exp. Immunol. *38*:228–230, 1979.
33. Chandra, R. K.: Prospective studies of the effect of breastfeeding on incidence of infection and allergy. Acta Paediatr. Scand. *68*:691–694, 1979.
34. Chandra, R. K.: Acrodermatitis enteropathica: Zinc levels and cell-mediated immunity. Pediatrics *66*:789–791, 1980.
35. Chandra, R. K.: Immune response in overnutrition. Cancer Res. *41*:3795–3796, 1981.
36. Chandra, R. K.: Breast feeding, growth and morbidity. Nutr. Res. *1*:25–31, 1981.
37. Chandra, R. K.: Increased bacterial binding to respiratory epithelial cells in vitamin A deficiency. Br. Med. J. *297*:834–835, 1988.
38. Chandra, R. K.: Micronutrients and immune functions. Ann. N. Y. Acad. Sci. *585*:9–16, 1990.
39. Chandra, R. K., and Wadhwa, M.: Nutritional modulation of intestinal mucosal immunity. Immun. Invest. *18*:119–126, 1989.
40. Chandra, R. K.: Micronutrients and immune functions. Ann. N. Y. Acad. Sci. *587*:9–16, 1990.
41. Chandra, R. K.: Immunocompetence is a sensitive and functional barometer of nutritional status. Acta Paediatr. Scand. *374*(Suppl.):S129–S132, 1991.
42. Chandra, R. K.: Nutrition and immunity: Lessons from the past and new insights into the future. Am. J. Clin. Nutr. *53*:1087–1101, 1991.
43. Chandra, R. K.: Nutrition and immunoregulation: Significance for host resistance to tumors and infectious diseases in humans and rodents. J. Nutr. *122*(Suppl. 3):754–757, 1992.
44. Chandra, R. K.: Nutition and immunity: Part I: Effects of nutrition on the immune system. Nutrition *10*:207–210, 1994.
45. Cohen, S., and Hansen, J. D. L.: Metabolism of albumin and γ-globulin in kwashiorkor. Clin. Sci. *23*:351–359, 1962.
46. Coutsoudis, A., Broughton, M., and Coovadia, H. M.: Vitamin A supplementation reduces measles morbidity in young African children: A randomized, placebo-controlled, double-blind trial. Am. J. Clin. Nutr. *54*:890–895, 1991.
47. Cruz, J. R., Arevalo, C., and Hanson, L. A.: Effects of ethnicity on immunologic components in human milk. *In* Hamosh, M., and Goldman, A. S. (eds.): Human Lactation. 2. Maternal and Environmental Factors. New York, Plenum Press, 1986, pp. 569–579.

48. Cunningham, A. S.: Morbidity in breast fed and artificially fed infants. J. Pediatr. *95*:685–689, 1979.
49. Cunningham-Rundels, S., et al.: Physiological and pharmacological effects of zinc on immune response. Ann. N. Y. Acad. Sci. *587*:113–122, 1990.
50. Dao, H., Delisle, H., and Fournier, P.: Anthropometric status, serum prealbumin level, and immune response to measles vaccination in Mali children. J. Trop. Pediatr. *38*:179–184, 1992.
51. Davies, W. L., Smith, S. C., Pond, W. L., et al.: Effect of dietary restriction on susceptibility of mice to infection with Theiler's GDVII virus. Proc. Soc. Exp. Med. *72*:528–531, 1949.
52. Deitch, E. A.: The management of burns. N. Engl. J. Med. *323*:1249–1243, 1990.
53. Delafuente, J. C.: Nutrients and immune response. Rheum. Dis. Clin. North Am. *17*:203–211, 1991.
54. de la Fuente, M., and Munoz, M. L.: Impairment of phagocytic process in macrophages from young and old mice by protein malnutrition. Ann. Nutr. Metab. *36*:41–47, 1992.
55. Derganc, M.: Present trends in fluid therapy, metabolic care, and prevention of infection in burned children. Crit. Care Med. *21*:S395–S399, 1993.
56. Dourov, N.: Thymic atrophy and immune deficiency in malnutrition. Curr. Top. Pathol. *75*:127–150, 1986.
57. Edelman, R.: Infant nutrition and immunity. Ann. N. Y. Acad. Sci. *587*:232–235, 1990.
58. Epstein, M. D., Banducci, D. R., and Manders, E. K.: The role of the gastrointestinal tract in the development of burn sepsis. Plast. Reconstr. Surg. *90*:524–530, 1992.
59. Erickson, K. L.: Dietary fat modulation of immune response. Int. J. Immunopharmacol. *8*:529–543, 1986.
60. Erickson, K. L., Adams, D. A., and Scibienski, R. J.: Dietary fatty acid modulation of murine B-cell responsiveness. J. Nutr. *116*:830–1840, 1986.
61. Fagbule, D., and Orifunmishe, F.: Measles and childhood mortality in semi-urban Nigeria. Afr. J. Med. Sci. *17*:181–185, 1988.
62. Farid, Z., Bassily, S., Schulert, A. R., et al.: Blood loss in chronic *S. mansoni* infection in Egyptian farmers. Trans. R. Soc. Trop. Med. Hyg. *61*:289–314, 1967.
63. Fasol, R., Schindler, M., Schumacher, B., et al.: The influence of obesity on perioperative morbidity: Retrospective study of 502 aortocoronary bypass operations. Thorac. Cardiovasc. Surg. *40*:126–129, 1992.
64. Fergusson, D. M., Horwood, L. J., Shannon, F. T., et al.: Infant health and breast feeding during the first 16 weeks of life. Aust. Pediatr. J. *14*:254–258, 1978.
65. Fiser, R. H., Jr., Denniston, J. C., McGann, V. G., et al.: Altered immune functions in hypercholesterolemic monkeys. Infect. Immun. *8*:105–109, 1973.
66. Flo, J., Roux, M., and Massouh, E.: Deficient induction of the immune response to oral immunization with cholera toxin in malnourished rats during suckling. Infect. Immun. *62*:4948–4954, 1994.
67. Foo, L.: Hookworm infection and protein-energy malnutrition: Transverse evidence from two Malaysian ecological groups. Trop. Geogr. Med. *42*:8–12, 1990.
68. Foster, C., Jones, J. H., Henle, W., et al.: Comparative effects of vitamin B_1 deficiency and restriction of food intake on the response of mice to the Lansing strain of poliomyelitis virus, as determined by the paired feeding technique. J. Exp. Med. *80*:257–264, 1944.
69. Freyre, E. A., Rondon, O., Bedoya, J., et al.: The incidence of bacteriuria and pyuria in Peruvian children with malnutrition. J. Pediatr. *83*:57–61, 1973.
70. Gallagher, K., Matarazzo, W., and Gray, I.: Trace metal modification of lymphocyte transformation in vitro. Fed. Proc. *37*:377, 1978.
71. Goldman, A. S., and Goldblum, R. M.: Human milk: Immunologic-nutritional relationships. Ann. N. Y. Acad. Sci. *587*:236–245, 1990.
72. Good, R. A., Fernandes, E. J., Yunis, W. C., et al.: Nutritional deficiency, immunologic function and disease. Am. J. Pathol. *84*:599–614, 1976.
73. Gorbach, S. L., Knox, T. A., and Roubenoff, R.: Interactions between nutrition and infection with human immunodeficiency virus. Nutr. Rev. *51*:226–234, 1993.
74. Gordon, J. E., Ascoli, W., Mata, L. J., et al.: Nutrition and infection: Field study in Guatemalan villages, 1959–1964. Arch. Environ. Health *16*:424–437, 1968.
75. Gracey, M.: Chronic diarrhoea in protein-energy malnutrition. Paediatr. Indones. *21*:235–239, 1981.
76. Greenwood, B. M., Bradley, A. K., Blakebrough, I. S., et al.: The immune response to a meningococcal polysacchride vaccine in an African village. Trans. R. Soc. Trop. Med Hyg. *74*:340–346, 1980.
77. Halsey, N. A., Boulos, R., Mode, F., et al.: Response to measles vaccine in Haitian infants 6 to 12 months old: Influence of maternal antibodies, malnutrition, and concurrent illnesses. N. Engl. J. Med. *313*:544–549, 1985.
78. Harris, M. C., and Douglas, S. D.: Nutritional influence on neonatal infections in animal models and man. Ann. N. Y. Acad. Sci.. *587*:246–255, 1990.
79. Harris, M. C., and Douglas, S. D.: Nutritional modulation of phagocyte function with special emphasis on the newborn. Indian J. Pediatr. *57*:147–158, 1990.
80. Heideman, M., and Bengtsson, A.: The immunologic response to thermal injury. World J. Surg. *16*:53–56, 1992.
81. Heinzerling, R. H., Nockels, C. F., Quarles, C. L., et al.: Protection of chicks against *E. coli* infections by dietary supplementation with vitamin E. Proc. Soc. Exp. Biol. Med. *146*:279–283, 1974.
82. Heise, F. H., and Martin, G. J.: Ascorbic acid metabolism in tuberculosis. Proc. Soc. Exp. Biol. Med. *34*:642–644, 1936.
83. Hemila, H.: Vitamin C and the common cold. Br. J. Nutr. *67*:3–16, 1992.
84. Herndon, D. N.: The 1994 Presidential address: Accepting the challenge. J. Burn Care Rehabil. *15*:463–469, 1994.
85. Hildreth, M. A., Herndon, D. N., Desai, M. H., et al.: Current treatment reduces calories required to maintain weight in pediatric patients with burns. J. Burn Care Rehabil. *11*:405–409, 1990.
86. Hill, C. H., and Garren, H. W.: Protein levels and survival time of chicks infected with *Salmonella gallinarum*. J. Nutr. *43*:28–32, 1961.
87. Hlaing, T.: Ascariasis and childhood malnutrition. Parasitology *107*:S125–S136, 1993.
88. Ho, M. S., Glass, R. I., Pinsky, P. F., et al.: Diarrheal deaths in American children: Are they preventable? J. A. M. A. *260*:3281–3285, 1988.
89. Hodges, M.: Diarrhoeal disease in early childhood: Experiences from Sierra Leone. Parasitology *107*:S37–S51, 1993.
90. Huffman, S. L., and Martin, L.: Child nutrition, birth spacing, and child mortality. Ann. N. Y. Acad. Sci. *585*:236–247, 1990.
91. Hughes, W. T., Price, R. A., Sisko, F., et al.: Protein-calorie malnutrition. Am. J. Dis. Child. *128*:44–52, 1974.
92. Humphrey, J. H., West, K. P., Jr., and Sommer, A.: Vitamin A deficiency and attributable mortality among under-5-year-olds. Bull. W. H. O. *70*:225–232, 1992.
93. Hussey, G. D., and Klein, M.: A randomized, controlled trial of vitamin A in children with severe measles. N. Engl. J. Med. *323*:160–164, 1990.
94. Hytten, S. E.: Nutritional aspects of foetal growth. *In* Nutrition and Early Growth, Sixth International Congress of Nutrition. Edinburgh, Churchill Livingstone, 1964.
95. Immune response in the malnourished child. Subcommittee on Interactions of Nutrition and Infection. Committee on International Nutrition Programs. The National Health Research Council, National Academy of Science, May 1976.
96. Jackson, T. M., and Zaman, S. N.: The in vitro effect of the thymic thymopoietin on a subpopulation of lymphocytes from severely malnourished children. Clin. Exp. Immunol. *39*:717–721, 1980.
97. Jambon, B., Ziegler, O., Maire, B., et al.: Thymulin (facteur thymique serique) and zinc contents of the thymus glands of malnourished children. Am. J. Clin. Nutr. *48*:335–342, 1988.
98. Janoff, A.: The role of iron in macrophages. J. Theoret. Biol. *7*:168–170, 1964.
99. Jenkins, M. E., Gottschlich, M. M., and Warden, G. D.: Enteral feeding during operative procedures in thermal injuries. J. Burn Care Rehab. *15*:199–205, 1994.
100. Jones, P. N., Mills, E. H., and Capps, R. B.: The effect of liver disease on serum vitamin B_{12} concentrations. J. Lab. Clin. Med. *49*:910–922, 1957.
101. Jose, D. G., Ford, G., Ford, W., et al.: Therapy with parent's lymphocyte transfer factor in children with infection and malnutrition. Lancet *1*:263–265, 1976.
102. Joynson, D. H., Walker, D. M., Jacobs, A., et al.: Defect of cell-mediated immunity in patients with iron-deficiency anaemia. Lancet *2*:1058–1059, 1972.
103. Jyonouchi, H.: Nucleotide actions on humoral immune responses. J. Nutr. *124*(Suppl. 1):138S–143S, 1994.
104. Kacew, S.: Adverse effects of drugs and chemicals in breast milk on the nursing infant. J. Clin. Pharmacol. *33*:213–221, 1993.
105. Kasa, R. M.: Vitamin C: From scurvy to common cold. Am. J. Med. Tech. *49*:23–26, 1983.
106. Katz, M., and Plotkin, S. A.: Enhanced severity of experimental herpes simplex infection in mice fed a protein-free diet. J. Nutr. *93*:555–560, 1967.
107. Keet, M. P., and Thom, H.: Serum immunoglobulins in kwashiorkor. Arch. Dis. Child. *44*:600–603, 1969.
108. Kelly, D. S., Daudu, P. A., Branch, L. B., et al.: Energy restriction decreases number of circulating natural killer cells and serum levels of immunoglobulins in overweight women. Eur. J. Clin. Nutr. *48*:9–18, 1994.
109. Keusch, G. T., and Scrimshaw, N. S.: Selective primary health care: Strategies for control of disease in the developing world. XXIII. Control of infection to reduce the prevalence of infantile and childhood malnutrition. Rev. Infect. Dis. *8*:273–287, 1986.
110. Keusch, G. T.: Micronutrients and susceptibility to infection. Ann. N. Y. Acad. Sci. *587*:181–187, 1990.
111. Keusch, G. T.: Nutritional effects of response of children in developing countries to respiratory tract pathogens: Implications for vaccine development. Rev. Infect. Dis. *13*(Suppl. 6):S486–S491, 1991.
112. Kolterman, O. G., Olefsky, J. M., Kurahara, C., et al.: A defect in cell-mediated immune function in insulin-resistant diabetic and obese subjects. J. Lab. Clin. Med. *96*:535–543, 1980.
113. Kotler, D. P.: Nutritional effects and support in the patient with acquired immunodeficiency syndrome. J. Nutr. *122*(Suppl. 3):723–727, 1992.
114. Kovar, M. G., Serdula, M. K., Marks, J. S., et al.: Review of the epidemiologic evidence for an association between infant feeding and infant health. Pediatrics *74*:615–638, 1984.

115. Kramer, T. R., and Good, R. A.: Effects of protein insufficient diets on the ability of guinea pigs to produce antigen specific MIF. Fed. Proc. *34*:829, 1975.
116. Kulkarni, A. D., Fanslow, W. C., Rudolph, F. B., et al.: Immunohemopoietic effects of dietary nucleotide restriction in mice. Transplantation *53*:467–472, 1992.
117. Kulkarni, A. D., Rudolph, F. B., and Van Buren, C. T.: The role of dietary sources of nucleotides in immune function: A review. J. Nutr. *124*(Suppl. 8):1442S–1446S, 1994.
118. Lake-Bakaar, G., Quadros, E., Beidas, S., et al.: Gastric secretory failure in patients with acquired immunodeficiency syndrome (AIDS). Ann. Intern. Med. *109*:502–504, 1988.
119. Latham, M. C.: Protein-energy malnutrition: Its epidemiology and control. J. Environ. Pathol. Toxicol. Oncol. *10*:168–169, 1990.
120. Laurell, C. B.: Metal-binding plasma proteins and cation transport. *In* Putnam, F. W. (ed.): The Plasma Proteins, I. New York, Academic Press, 1960, pp. 229–264.
121. Lehmann, H., Huntsman, R. G., and Ager, J. A. M.: The hemoglobinopathies and thalassemia. *In* Stanbury, J. B., Wyngaarden, J. B., and Fredrickson, D. S. (eds.): The Metabolic Basis of Inherited Disease. 2nd ed. New York, McGraw-Hill, 1966, pp. 1100–1136.
122. Lindenbaum, J.: Malabsorption during and after recovery from acute intestinal infection. Br. Med. J. *2*:326–329, 1965.
123. Loria, R. M., Kibrick, S., and Madge, G. E.: Infection of hypercholesterolemic mice with Coxsackievirus B. J. Infect. Dis. *133*:655–662, 1976.
124. Luke, B.: Nutritional influences on fetal growth. Clin. Obstet. Gynecol. *37*:538–549, 1994.
125. Macdougall, L. G., Anderson, R., McNab, G. M., et al.: The immune response in iron-deficient children: Impaired cellular defense mechanisms with altered humoral components. J. Pediatr. *86*:833–843, 1975.
126. MacKay, H. M.: Anaemia in infancy: Its prevalence and prevention. Arch. Dis. Child. *3*:117–144, 1928.
127. Madara, J. L., and Stafford, J.: Interferon-gamma directly affects barrier function of cultured intestinal epithelial monolayers. J. Clin. Invest. *83*:724–727, 1989.
128. Madi, K., Maeda, C. T., and Savino, W.: Thymic extracellular matrix in human malnutrition. J. Pathol. *171*:231–236, 1993.
129. Maki, P. A., and Newberne, P. M.: Dietary lipids and immune function. J. Nutr. *122*(Suppl. 3):610–614, 1992.
130. Manson, W. L., Dijkema, H., and Klasen, J.: Alteration of wound colonization by selective intestinal decontamination in thermally injured mice. Burns *16*:166–168, 1990.
131. Masson, P. L., and Heremans, J. F.: Studies on lactoferrin, the iron-binding protein of secretions. *In* Peeters, H. (ed.): Protides of the Biological Fluids. Vol. 14. Amsterdam, Elsevier, 1967, pp. 115–124.
132. Mata, L. J.: Malnutrition-infection interactions in the tropics. Am. J. Trop. Med. Hyg. *24*:564–574, 1975.
133. Mata, L. J., Urrutia, J. J., and Gordon, J. E.: Diarrhoeal disease in a cohort of Guatemalan village children observed from birth to age two years. Trop. Geogr. Med. *19*:247–257, 1967.
134. Matoth, Y., Zamir, R., and Bar-shani, S.: Studies on folic acid in infancy. II. Folic and folinic acid blood levels in infants with diarrhea, malnutrition and infection. Pediatrics *33*:694–699, 1964.
135. McFarlane, H.: Cell-mediated immunity in protein-calorie malnutrition. Lancet 2:1146–1147, 1971.
136. McMurray, D. N.: Cell-mediated immunity in nutritional deficiency. Prog. Food Nutr. Sci. *8*:193–228, 1984.
137. Mertz, W.: Chromium occurrence and function in biological systems. Physiol. Rev. *49*:163–239, 1969.
138. Meydani, S. N., Hayek, M., and Coleman, L.: Influence of vitamins E and B_6 on immune response. Ann. N. Y. Acad. Sci. *585*:125–137, 1990.
139. Miller, J. Z., Nance, W. E., Norton, J. A., et al.: Therapeutic effect of vitamin C: A co-twin control study. J.A.M.A. *237*:248s–251s, 1977.
140. Miller, T. L., Orav, E. J., Martin, S. R., et al.: Malnutrition and carbohydrate malabsorption in children with vertically transmitted human immunodeficiency virus 1 infection. Gastroenterology *100*:1296–1302, 1991.
141. Muller, M. J., and Herndon, D. N.: The challenge of burns. Lancet *343*:216–220, 1994.
142. Nesheim, M. C.: Human nutrition needs and parasitic infections. Parasitology 107:S7–S18, 1993.
143. Newberne, P. M.: Overnutrition on resistance of dogs to distemper virus. Fed. Proc. *25*:1701–1710, 1966.
144. Nockels, C. F.: Protective effects of supplemental vitamin E against infection. Fed. Proc. *38*:2134–2138, 1979.
145. Olusi, S. O., Thurman, G. B., Goldstein, A. L.: Effect of thymosin on T-lymphocyte rosette formation in children with kwashiorkor. Clin. Exp. Immunopathol. *15*:687–691, 1980.
146. Osawa, Y.: Ueber die Entstenung der Polymositis acuta purulenta in Japan. Beitr. Klin. Chirg. *146*:621–653, 1929.
147. Paine, R., and Coble, R. J.: Breast-feeding and infant health in a rural US community. Am. J. Dis. Child. *136*:36–38, 1980.
148. Parent, G., Chevalier, P., Zalles, L., et al.: In vitro lymphocyte-differentiating effects of thymulin (Zn-FTS) on lymphocyte subpopulations of severely malnourished children. Am. J. Clin. Nutr. *60*:274–278, 1994.
149. Pekarek, R. S., Hauer, E. C., Rayfield, E. J., et al.: Relationship between serum chromium concentrations and glucose utilization in normal and infected subjects. Diabetes *24*:350–353, 1975.
150. Pelletier, D. L., Frongillo, E. A., Jr., Schroeder, D. G., et al.: A methodology for estimating the contribution of malnutrition to child mortality in developing countries. J. Nutr. *124*(Suppl. 10):2106S–2122S, 1994.
151. Pitt, M. A., and Costrini, A. M.: Vitamin C prophylaxis in Marine recruits. J.A.M.A. *241*:908–911, 1979.
152. Powanda, M. C., Cockerell, G. L., Moc, J. B., et al.: Induced metabolic sequelae of tularemia in the rat: Correlation with tissue damage. Am. J. Physiol. *229*:479–483, 1975.
153. Prazuck, T., Tall, F., Nacro, B., et al.: HIV infection and severe malnutrition: A clinical and epidemiological study in Burkina Faso. AIDS *7*:103–108, 1993.
154. Prentice, A.: Breast feeding and the older infant. Acta Paediatr. Scand. Suppl. *374*:78–88, 1991.
155. Prindull, G., and Ahmad, M.: The ontogeny of the gut mucosal immune system and the susceptibility to infections in infants of developing countries. Eur. J. Pediatr. *152*:786–792, 1993.
156. Pruit, B. A., and MacManus, A. T.: The changing of epidemiology of infection in burn patients. World J. Surg. *16*:57–66, 1992.
157. Purtilo, D. T., and Connor, D. H.: Fetal infections in protein-calorie malnourished children with thymolymphatic atrophy. Arch. Dis. Child. *50*:149–152, 1975.
158. Rall, L. C., and Meydani, S. N.: Vitamin B_6 and immune competence. Nutr. Rev. *51*:217–225, 1993.
159. Rasmussen, A. F., Jr., Waisman, H. A., Elvehjem, C. A., et al.: Influence of the level of thiamine intake on the susceptibility of mice to poliomyelitis virus. J. Infect. Dis. *74*:41–47, 1944.
160. Reddy, V., Bhaskaram, P., Raghuramulu, N., et al.: Relationship between measles, malnutrition, and blindness: A prospective study in Indian children. Am. J. Clin. Nutr. *44*:924–930, 1986.
161. Rivlin., R. S.: The clinical significance of micro-nutrients in relation to immune functions. Ann. N. Y. Acad. Sci. *585*:55–57, 1990.
162. Roberts, P. D., Hoffbrand, A. V., and Mullin, D. L.: Iron and folate metabolism in tuberculosis. Br. Med. J. 2:198–202, 1966.
163. Rubin, D. H., Leventhal, J. M., Krasilnikoff, P. A., et al.: Relationship between infant feeding and infectious illness: A prospective study of infants during the first year of life. Pediatrics *85*:464–471, 1990.
164. Sachdev, H. P. S., Kumar, S., Singh, K. K., et al.: Risk factors for fatal diarrhea in hospitalized children in India. J. Pediatr. Gastroenterol. Nutr. *12*:76–81, 1991.
165. Sakamoto, M.: The sequence of recovery of the complement systems and phytohemagglutinin skin reactivity in malnutrition. Nutr. Res. *2*:137–145, 1982.
166. Sakamoto, M., and Nishioka, K.: Complement system in nutritional deficiency. World Rev. Nutr. Diet *67*:114–139, 1992.
167. Sallon, S., El-Shawwa, R., Khalil, M., et al.: Diarrhoeal disease in children in Gaza. Ann. Trop. Med. Parasitol. *88*:175–182, 1994.
168. Schlesinger, L. A., Olbaum, L., Grez, L., et al.: Cell mediated immune studies in marasmic children from Chile: Delayed hypersensitivity, lymphocyte transformation and interferon production. *In* Suskind, R. M. (ed.): Malnutrition and the Immune Response. New York, Raven Press, 1977, pp. 91–98.
169. Schlesinger, L., Munoz, C., Arevalo, M., et al.: Depressed immune response in malnourished rats correlates with increased thymic noradrenaline level. Int. J. Neurosci. *77*:229–236, 1994.
170. Schopfer, K., and Douglas, S. D.: Neutrophil function in children with kwashiorkor. J. Lab. Clin. Med. *88*:450–461, 1976.
171. Scrimshaw, N. S.: Nutrition and infection. Prog. Food Nutr. Sci. *1*:393–420, 1975.
172. Semba, R., Muhilal, Scott, A., et al.: Depressed immune response to tetanus in children with vitamin A deficiency. J. Nutr. *121*:101–107, 1992.
173. Seth, V., and Chandra, R. K.: Opsonic activity, phagocytosis, and bactericidal capacity of polymorphs in undernutrition. Arch. Dis. Child. *47*:282–284, 1972.
174. Seth, V., Kukreja, R. K., Saundaram, K. R., et al.: Waning of cell mediated immune response in preschool children given BCG at birth. Indian J. Med. Res. *76*:710–715, 1982.
175. Sherman, A. R.: Influence of iron on immunity and disease resistance. Ann. N. Y. Acad. Sci. *587*:140–146, 1990.
176. Sherman, A. R.: Zinc, copper, and iron nutriture and immunity. J. Nutr. *122*(Suppl. 3):604–609, 1992.
177. Shimeles, D., and Lulseged, S.: Clinical profile and pattern of infection in Ethiopian children with severe protein-energy malnutrition. East Afr. Med. J. *71*:264–267, 1994.
178. Sirisinha, S., Edelman, R., Suskind, R., et al.: Complement and C3-proactivator levels in children with protein-calorie malnutrition and effect of dietary treatment. Lancet *1*:1016–1020, 1973.
179. Sirisinha, S., Suskind, R., Edelman, R., et al.: Secretory and serum IgA in children with protein calorie malnutrition. Pediatrics *55*:166–170, 1975.
180. Smith, C. A.: The effect of wartime starvation in Holland upon pregnancy and its product. Am. J. Obstet. Gynecol. *53*:599–608, 1947.
181. Smith, H. W., and Chubb, L. G.: The effect of feeding different levels of protein concentrates on the susceptibility of chickens to *Salmonella gallinarum*. J. Comp. Pathol. *67*:10–20, 1957.
182. Smythe, P. M., Brereton-Stiles, G. G., Crace, H. J., et al.: Thymolymphatic

deficiency and depression of cell-mediated immunity in protein-calorie malnutrition. Lancet *2*:939–943, 1971.
183. Sollid, L. M., Kvale, D., Brandtzaeg, P., et al.: Interferon-gamma enhances expression of secretory component, the epithelial receptor for polymeric immunoglobulins. J. Immunol. *138*:4303–4306, 1987.
184. Solomons, N. W.: Pathways to the impairment of human nutritional status by gastrointestinal pathogens. Parasitology *107*:S19–S35, 1993.
185. Sommer, A: Vitamin A status, resistance to infection and childhood mortality. Ann. N. Y. Acad. Sci. *585*:17–23, 1990.
186. Sommer, A: Vitamin A: Its effect on childhood sight and life. Nutr. Rev. *52*:S60–S66, 1994.
187. Spallholz, J. E., et al.: Advances in understanding selenium's role in the immune system. Ann. N. Y. Acad. Sci. *587*:123–139, 1990.
188. Sprunt, D. H.: Effect of undernourishment on the susceptibility of rabbit to infection with vaccinia. J. Exp. Med. *75*:297–304, 1942.
189. Squibb, R. L.: Nutrition and biochemistry of survival during Newcastle disease virus infection. III. Relation of dietary protein to nucleic and free amino acids of avian liver. J. Nutr. *82*:427–431, 1964.
190. Squibb, R. L., and Grun, J.: Effect of nutritional status on resistance to infection in the avian species. Fed. Proc. *25*:1695–1700, 1966.
191. Stallone, D. D.: The influence of obesity and its treatment on the immune system. Nutr. Rev. *52*:37–50, 1994.
192. Steihm, E. D.: Humoral immunity in malnutrition. Fed. Proc. *39*:3093–3097, 1980.
193. Stephenson, L.: The impact of schistosomiasis on human nutrition. Parasitology *107*:S107–S123, 1993.
194. Sullivan, P. B., Marsh, M. N., Phillips, M. B., et al.: Prevalence and treatment of giardiasis in chronic diarrhoea and malnutrition. Arch. Dis. Child. *65*:304–306, 1990.
195. Sullivan, P. B., Lunn, P. G., Northrop-Clewes, C. A., et al.: Parasitic infection of the gut and protein-losing enteropathy. J. Pediatr. Gastroenterol. Nutr. *15*:404–407, 1992.
196. Suskind, R. M., Olson, L. C., and Olson, R. E.: Protein calorie malnutrition and infection with hepatitis-associated antigen. Pediatrics *51*:525–530, 1973.
197. Tanaka, S., Inoue, S., Isoda, F., et al.: Impaired immunity in obesity: Suppressed but reversible lymphocyte responsiveness. Int. J. Obes. Relat. Metab. Dis. *17*:631–636, 1993.
198. Technical Advisory Group on Acute Respiratory Infections: A programme for controlling acute respiratory infections in children: A memorandum from a WHO meeting. Bull. W. H. O. *62*:47–58, 1984.
199. Tengerdy, R. P.: The role of vitamin E in immune response and disease resistance. Ann. N. Y. Acad. Sci. *585*:24–33, 1990.
200. Thapa, B. R: Intractable diarrhoea of infancy and its management: Modified cost effective treatment. J. Trop. Pediatr. *40*:157–161, 1994.
201. Tomkins, A., and Watson, F.: Malnutrition and infection, a review. United Nations Administrative Commitee on Coordination, Subcommittee on Nutrition. Geneva, ACC/SCN, W. H. O., 1989.
202. Tracey, V. V., De, N. C., and Harper, J. R.: Obesity and respiratory infection in infants and young children. Br. Med. J. *1*:16–18, 1971.
203. Tredget, E. E., and Yu, Y. M.: The metabolic effects of thermal injury. *16*:68–79, 1992.
204. Tunbridge, W. M., and Wicks, A. C.: A review of bronchopneumonia in African children. Cent. Afr. J. Med. *13*:229–234, 1967.
205. Tupasi, T. E., Velmonte, M. E., Sanvictores, M. E., et al.: Determinants of morbidity and mortality due to acute respiratory infections: Implications for intervention. J. Infect. Dis. *157*:615–623, 1988.
206. Tupasi, T. E., deLeon, L. E., Lupsia, S., et al.: Community based studies of acute respiratory tract infections in young children. Rev. Infect. Dis. *12*:S940–S949, 1990.
207. Tupasi, T. E., Lucerno, M. G., Magdangal, D. M., et al.: Etiology of acute lower respiratory tract infection in children from Alabang. Metro Manila *12*:S929–S939, 1990.
208. Vathanophas, K., Sangchai, R., Raktham, S., et al.: A community-based study of acute respiratory tract infection in Thai children. Rev. Infect. Dis. *12*:S957–S965, 1990.
209. Victora, C. G., Vaughan, J. P., Lombardi, C., et al.: Evidence for protection by breast-feeding against infant deaths from infectious diseases in Brazil. Lancet *2*:319–322, 1987.
210. Vinton, A. L., Traverso, L. W., and Jolly, P. C.: Wound complications after modified radical mastectomy compared with tylectomy with axillary lymph node dissection. Am. J. Surg. *161*:584–588, 1991.
211. Waters, M. D., Gardner, D. E., Arany, C., et al.: Metal toxicity for rabbit alveolar macrophages in vitro. Environ. Res. *9*:32–47, 1975.
212. Watkins-Leeder, S. R., and Corkhill, R. T.: The relationship between breast and bottle-feeding and respiratory illness in the first year of life. J. Epidem. Comm. Health. *33*:180–182, 1979.
213. Watson, R. R.: Nutrition, disease resistance and age. Food Nutr. News *51*:1–6, 1979.
214. Weaver, H. M.: Resistance of cotton rats to the virus of poliomyelitis as affected by intake of vitamin B complex, partial inanition and sex. Am. J. Dis. Child. *69*:26–32, 1945.
215. Weaver, H. M.: Resistance of cotton rats to virus of poliomyelitis as affected by intake of vitamin A, partial inanition and sex. J. Pediatr. *28*:14–23, 1946.
216. Weinberg, E. D.: Roles of iron in host-parasite infections. J. Infect. Dis. *124*:401–410, 1971.
217. West, C. E., Rombout, J. H. W. M., Zijpp, A. J. V. D., et al.: Vitamin A and immune function. Proc. Nutr. Soc. *50*:251–262, 1991.
218. West, K. P., Howard, G. R., and Sommer, A.: Vitamin A and infection: Public health implications. Ann. Rev. Nutr. *9*:63–86, 1989.
219. Winick, M. (ed.): Hunger Disease: Studies by the Jewish Physicians in the Warsaw Ghetto. New York, John Wiley and Sons, 1959.
220. Woodruff, J. F.: The influence of quantitated post-weaning undernutrition on coxsackievirus B3 infection of adult mice. II. Alteration of host defense mechanisms. J. Infect. Dis. *121*:164–181, 1970.
221. Woodruff, J. F., and Kilbourne, E. D.: The influence of quantitated post-weaning undernutrition on coxsackievirus B3 infection of adult mice. I. Viral persistence and increased severity of lesions. J. Infect. Dis. *121*:137–163, 1970.
222. World Health Organization: Nutrition and infection: Report of a WHO Expert Committee. W. H. O. Tech. Rep. Ser. *314*:5–30, 1965.
223. Zuin, G., Fontana, M., Monti, S., et al.: Malabsorption of different lactose loads in children with human immuno-deficiency virus infection. J. Pediatr. Gastroenterol. Nutr. *15*:408–412, 1992.
224. Zwingenberger, K., Irschick, E., Vergetti, G., et al.: Tumor necrosis factor in hepatosplenic schistosomiasis. Scand. J. Immunol. *31*:205–211, 1990.

5

FEVER: PATHOGENESIS AND TREATMENT

Martin I. Lorin

Fever is defined as a centrally mediated elevation of body temperature in response to a stress or insult. Defining the limits of "normal" body temperature, however, is more difficult. Generally, the accepted range of rectal temperature is from 36.1 to 37.8° C (97° to 100° F).[32, 45] Children tend to have higher body temperatures than adults. It is well recognized that young children can have rectal temperatures as high as 38.5° C (101° F) late in the afternoon (at the zenith of the circadian rhythm) or after physical activity.[50] Clearly, a body temperature slightly above an arbitrary upper limit of 37.8° C (100° F) does not always imply a pathologic process. The important distinction between fever and heat illness is described below.

TEMPERATURE REGULATION

Humans, like other mammals, are homeothermic, which means that body temperature normally is maintained within a relatively narrow range, despite significant fluctuations in energy intake and expenditure and despite widely varying environmental temperatures. Body temperature is controlled by an elaborate thermoregulatory system that modulates heat production and heat loss so that core temperature is maintained within normal limits. Numerous studies have confirmed that the thermoregulatory center is located in the preoptic region of the anterior hypothalamus (PAOH).[12, 25, 65] In the laboratory animal, destruction of this region of the brain renders the animal incapable of properly controlling body temperature.[65] Profound changes in body temperature have been induced by injecting epinephrine, norepinephrine, and serotonin into the hypothalamus or lateral ventricles of the cat.[85] It is believed that there are separate, discrete anatomic regions within the PAOH that sense and compute core temperature (the *thermostat*), provide a reference point for normal temperature (the *set-point*), control heat production (the *heat gain center*), and dissipate heat (the *heat loss center*).[12]

Heat production is dependent on both metabolic and physical activity. Basal metabolic rates vary, with the highest rates occurring in the smallest individuals, whose surface area is great compared with body mass. A variety of factors, such as age, thyroid status, environmental temperature, and ingestion of food, influence basal metabolic rate. Physical activity and exercise markedly increase heat production by muscles. The release of catecholamines during exposure to cold increases oxygen consumption and heat production by 20 to 40 per cent.[68] Shivering further increases heat production by muscles.

The newborn infant has a special heat-producing mechanism in the form of brown fat, which possesses a dense population of mitochondria and lipid vacuoles; the metabolic rate of this unique tissue exceeds that of the heart or liver,[26] and doubling of basal metabolic rate is possible without shivering (nonshivering thermogenesis).[76] The skin overlying brown fat frequently has a higher temperature than the rectum.[34]

Heat is lost through radiation, evaporation, convection, and conduction. Generally, 60 per cent of total body heat loss occurs by radiation. Loss by radiation depends on differences in the temperature of the surfaces radiating toward each other and on the size of the surfaces involved.[68] The ratio of surface area to body mass is greatest during the neonatal period, resulting in relative temperature instability during this period of life. Skin temperature is affected by the rate of blood flow, and changes in perfusion of the skin represent the principal mechanism by which heat loss by radiation can be increased or decreased.

One of the most labile methods of heat loss is evaporation. Insensible water loss equals 750 to 800 mL/m^2/24 hr,[85] and considerable energy is lost during the process of evaporation. Evaporation of 1 mL of water requires 0.58 kcal of heat.[68] One-quarter of all heat loss occurs by evaporation.[31, 68] Increased heat loss during exercise is accomplished primarily by radiation (cutaneous vasodilation) and by evaporation (sweating), which can dissipate as much as 1700 kcal/hr.[68] Evaporation is aided by convection, for sweat must evaporate rather than fall from the skin to dissipate heat. Heat lost by convection depends on the movement of air across the body surface; the rate of heat loss is directly proportional to the velocity of air current and the amount of surface area exposed.

In the case of an individual who is standing, little heat is lost by conduction because only the feet are in contact with external objects. In contrast, for a child lying in contact with cold objects, conduction loss is much greater. When a child is being bathed or sponged, conduction becomes the major mechanism of heat loss. Conduction also is a critical process by which heat within the body moves to the surface.[34]

Body temperatures tend to be higher in children than in adults. The decrease to adult levels begins at about 1 year of age and continues through puberty, stabilizing at 13 to 14 years of age in girls and at 17 to 18 years of age in boys.[4, 14] Maximum daily body temperature for most children occurs between 1700 and 1900 hours, whereas minimum temperature is noted in most individuals between 0 and 0600 hours. This circadian rhythm is not very evident in the first few months of life, but it is well established by the second birthday and tends to be more pronounced during childhood than during adulthood.

PATHOGENESIS OF FEVER

Fever, in contradistinction to heat illness, is a centrally regulated rise of body temperature in response to some pathologic stimulus. Considerable evidence suggests that the PAOH acts as if the set-point had been raised, modulating the heat gain center upward and the heat loss center downward until heat gain and heat loss again are in balance, but at a higher temperature.[22, 56, 60, 62]

The febrile response is mediated by a group of low-molecular-weight proteins (originally called "endogenous pyrogens"), which are produced by polymorphonuclear leukocytes and most other phagocytic cells derived from bone marrow precursors.[2, 13, 37, 40] It now is believed that a number of cytokines, especially interleukin-1, interleukin-6, and tumor necrosis factor, all act as endogenous pyrogens directly in the PAOH to elevate the set-point.[52, 72] In contrast, exogenous pyrogens, such as endotoxin, have no effect when injected directly into the PAOH of animals. They are believed to produce fever by acting on circulating leukocytes, which, in turn, produce cytokines. The almost immediate febrile response to intravenously injected interleukin-1 and the delay in response of several hours to similar injections of endotoxins are compatible with this hypothesis.

The mechanisms of pyrogen production and release have been elucidated partially.[2, 93] Pyrogen-producing cells contain a nonpyrogenic precursor molecule that must be converted to a pyrogenically active form. Data indicate that mediators released by activated blood and tissue macrophages have a variety of diverse metabolic and physiologic actions that prepare the individual to handle stress or to combat infection.[6, 20, 27] In addition to fever, these responses include the production and release from bone marrow of neutrophils, the hepatic synthesis of metal-binding proteins and the subsequent sequestration of iron and zinc, the production of acute-phase proteins, and the acceleration of skeletal muscle proteolysis, which generates free amino acids needed for host defenses. The fact that some of these mediator-induced changes can be demonstrated in cultured cells or tissue preparations indicates that these effects are independent of the fever itself.

The mechanism of fever has been studied in few human diseases. Persistent fever in patients with typhoid fever has been attributed to endogenous pyrogen mobilized from various sites of inflammation.[43] The cause of fever in noninfectious diseases, such as sickle cell crises and inflammatory bowel disease, remains unclear. Because these disorders are associated with inflammation, it is probable that fever in these patients also reflects a response to the release of cytokines from inflammatory cells.

A variety of disorders associated with antigen-antibody reactions can induce fever in humans. Antibodies to Rh-positive cells, for example, have been implicated as the cause of fever after transfusion of blood that is not compatible with that of the recipient. These reactions produce immune lysis of erythrocytes and may liberate antigen-antibody complexes, which, in turn, activate the production of endogenous pyrogens by host leukocytes.[78] It also has been shown that fever associated with hypersensitivity to penicillin is the result of the interaction of antigen-antibody complexes with leukocytes, which then release endogenous pyrogen.[18] Autoimmune destruction of host tissue has been suggested as the cause of fever in individuals afflicted with collagen vascular diseases.[69] It is believed that the common denominator in all these conditions is the release of cytokines from activated macrophages in the blood or the reticuloendothelial system. Both cellular and humoral immune reactions appear capable of inducing the release of pyrogenic cytokines.[2]

Fever is a common finding in children with cancer. It has been suggested that pyrogenic substances may be released from sites of tissue destruction or inflammation or from cells that have been stimulated by autoimmune factors induced by malignant cells.[2] Pyrogenic material may be secreted by the tumor itself, for substances similar to the originally described endogenous pyrogen have been recovered from the urine of febrile patients with Hodgkin disease and from tissue extracts obtained from a human hypernephroma.[18]

There are a few childhood disorders in which cytokines appear to play no role in the production of fever. In children with familial dysautonomia (Riley-Day syndrome), fever primarily reflects an abnormality of the hypothalamic receptors or of the peripheral cutaneous nervous system as it modulates blood flow. In the child with thyroid storm or the rare youngster with a pheochromocytoma, fever is a direct result of peripheral activation of the thermoregulatory mechanisms that increase body temperature or reduce heat loss rather than an effect on the thermoregulatory center itself.

It is unclear if these conditions should be classified as fever or as heat illness.

DISTINCTION BETWEEN FEVER AND HEAT ILLNESS

The distinction between fever and heat illness is important, not only in regard to understanding the pathophysiology of elevated body temperature but also because treatment of the two conditions is very different (Table 5–1). Although the term *fever* often is applied loosely to all types of elevated body temperature, its use is limited more precisely to those conditions in which the elevated temperature results from a thermoregulated response controlled by the PAOH. That this response is controlled centrally has been documented amply.[23, 28, 83] The apparent upper limit of the febrile response is further evidence of its thermoregulated nature. Core temperatures above 41.1° C (106° F), even in severe, untreated infections, are seen only rarely,[33] and temperatures above this level generally reflect involvement of the central nervous system or a component of heat illness.

The term *heat illness,* in contrast to *fever,* refers to situations in which either environmental stresses exceed the ability of the central thermoregulatory mechanism to maintain normal body temperature or internal factors impair the body's ability to dissipate metabolic heat. The salient feature in heat illness is that the body temperature is elevated, despite the fact that the set-point in the PAOH is normal.[83] In victims of heat illness, core temperatures higher than 43.4° C (110° F) have been recorded.

Examples of heat illness include hyperthyroidism (increased heat production) and anhidrotic ectodermal dysplasia (impairment of sweating and evaporative heat loss). A variety of pharmacologic agents, both medical drugs (anticholinergics and phenothiazines) and street drugs (LSD and PCP), can cause heat illness by impairing the central or peripheral regulation of heat dissipation. Heat stroke and malignant hyperthermia are two especially dangerous forms of heat illness that carry a high mortality.

Although there are no data to indicate that elevated body temperatures in the range seen with fever cause any permanent tissue damage, it is clear that the marked elevation of temperature accompanying heat illness can have devastating effects on various tissues and organs.[82] Whereas the need to treat fever symptomatically can be debated, restoration of normal body temperature in heat illness is mandatory. Because the basic derangement in fever is an elevation of the set-point in the PAOH, drugs such as acetaminophen and ibuprofen, which restore the set-point to normal, are rational and effective modes of therapy. In heat illness, in contrast, the set-point is normal and administration of these agents is useless. The most effective therapy for heat illness is the prompt reduction of body temperature by external cooling. At the same time, all possible measures should be taken to correct the basic derangement itself. Time is of the essence in treating heat stroke and malignant hyperthermia. External cooling must be accomplished by such heroic measures as immersion in ice water or ice water sponging; cooling blankets and tepid sponges are inadequate.

MEASUREMENT OF BODY TEMPERATURE

In ordinary clinical practice, core temperature is measured best by use of a rectal thermometer. Generally, rectal temperature is about 1° F higher than oral temperature and 2 to 2½° F higher than axillary temperature. Oral temperature can be influenced by the immediately prior ingestion of hot or cold liquids or solids and by tachypnea.[86] In the newborn infant, axillary temperature may be less reliable as a means of detecting fever than was thought previously.[57]

Electronic thermometers achieve a steady-state reading in less than 30 seconds, compared with 2 to 4 minutes for the mercury rectal thermometer. The electronic thermometer appears to be sufficiently accurate for routine clinical use, although the lack of calibration facilities on most models is worrisome. These instruments are practical for hospital, clinic, and office use; their role in the home remains to be

TABLE 5–1. Characteristics of Fever Compared with Heat Illness

	Examples	Mechanism of Temperature Elevation	Need to Reduce Body Temperature to Normal	Treatment
Fever	Infection, malignancy, trauma	Centrally thermoregulated in response to elevation of set-point in PAOH*	Optional	Acetaminophen or ibuprofen
Heat illness	Hyperthyroidism, atropine poisoning, heat stroke, malignant hyperthermia	Increased heat production or decreased heat loss	Mandatory	External cooling

*PAOH, preoptic region of the anterior hypothalamus.

defined. Devices that measure skin temperature by the use of temperature-sensitive liquid crystals are appealing but inaccurate. Studies have shown that these devices frequently underestimate core temperature,[66, 74] which is not surprising because skin temperature may be normal or even low in the early stages of fever, when perfusion of the skin is decreased.

The infrared ear thermometer (IET) has been gaining popularity for hospital, office, and home use, despite considerable concern over the level of accuracy of these devices. These instruments *estimate* the temperature of the tympanic membrane, which is assumed to be in closer equilibrium with core temperature than is either oral or rectal temperature. Although some studies have shown sufficient correlation with rectal temperature to justify clinical use,[48] other studies have found the correlation to be inadequate.[36] Hooker[42] reported that the IET failed to identify 5 of 15 febrile patients, and Freed and Fraley[36] found poor correlation with rectal temperatures. It appears that not all IETs are equally accurate; the very low priced models especially are suspect. However, one major problem that remains unresolved in the clinical evaluation of IETs is the arbitrary use of rectal temperature as the gold standard. It is clear that at times of rapid change in body temperature, rectal temperature can lag behind core temperature. In these situations, tympanic membrane temperature may be a more accurate reflection of core temperature than is rectal measurement. When tympanic membrane temperature and rectal temperature disagree, one cannot always assume that the tympanic temperature is in error.

At this time, it would seem that the IET is ideal for situations in which measurement of rectal temperatures is inconvenient or contraindicated (e.g., major trauma, neutropenia, rectal inflammation) and the use of the oral thermometer is impractical. Use of the IET in other situations is a matter of personal preference. It would be wise not to rely on the IET in neonates, very young infants, or other patients in whom small differences from rectal temperature would be important. It is important that personnel using IETs be familiar with the proper use of the instrument, especially in regard to any "offset" switches that allegedly convert the actual reading to a figure "equal" to oral or rectal temperature.

SYMPTOMATIC THERAPY OF FEVER

If and when fever should be treated symptomatically are important but still incompletely answered questions. It is disappointing that despite the clinical frequency of fever and the ubiquity of fever in the laboratory animal and despite data indicating that fever is part of an integrated defense mechanism rather than an incidental biologic response, for the majority of clinical situations we still do not know whether fever is beneficial, harmful, or neutral.[1, 2, 6, 27, 28, 32, 50] Clearly, there are conditions in which fever has a beneficial role and others in which it is detrimental. In most cases of acute, self-limited febrile illness in the otherwise well child, the most compelling reasons for treatment are relief of discomfort and alleviation of parental anxiety. Schmitt[73] aptly has dubbed this parental attitude *fever phobia*.

Possible Beneficial Effects of Fever

In a few specific situations, the high temperature of fever directly may impair the reproduction or even the survival of an invading microorganism. Some species of gonococci and some treponema are killed by temperatures of 40° C (104° F) or higher.[7, 47] Prior to the antibiotic era, favorable effects of fever therapy were noted in cases of neurosyphilis and gonococcal urethritis, and there are data to suggest that fever may impair the growth of some types of pneumococci and some viruses.[16, 41, 77, 90] Kluger and associates[39, 51] have provided evidence that many pathogenic bacteria require more iron at higher temperatures and that, in association with fever, there is both a decrease in serum iron and an increase in serum ferritin, diminishing the amount of free iron available to bacteria at the very time when they need it most. These investigators have proposed that the simultaneous rise in body temperature and decrease in free serum iron represent a coordinated host defense.

Modest elevation of body temperature has been associated with acceleration of a variety of immunologic responses, including phagocytosis, leukocyte migration, lymphocyte transformation, and increased interferon production.[3, 10, 67, 71] Whether these quantitatively small changes clinically are significant remains unclear. Several laboratory studies of bacterial infections in cold-blooded animals (goldfish and lizards) have shown improved survival with moderate elevation of body temperature.[11, 24] In a study of rabbits infected with *Pasteurella multocida*, Vaughn and Kluger[88] found that the best survival rates were associated with moderate elevations of body temperature in the range of about 4.5° F above baseline.

Possible Adverse Effects of Fever

Although the above data indicate that fever, especially moderate fever, may enhance the immunologic response, there also are data suggesting that fever, especially high fever, can impair the immunologic response. Ellingson and Clark[35] and Austin and Truant[3] reported that the in vitro phagocytosis of staphylococci by polymorphonuclear leukocytes decreased at temperatures of 40° C (104° F) or higher. Although Roberts and Steigbigel[67] found enhancement of lymphocyte transformation to mitogen at 38.5° C (101.3° F), they noted decreased cell viability and decreased function at 40° C (104° F). Several studies have found an increased mortality associated with fever in infected animals, especially those with endotoxin shock. In 1909, Ruata[70] reported that guinea pigs with gram-negative sepsis kept at an increased ambient temperature had a higher mortality than did similarly infected animals maintained at ordinary ambient temperatures. In a study of pneumococcal peritonitis in rabbits receiving suboptimal doses of penicillin, prevention of fever by shearing the animals' fur decreased the mortality rate.[49] In the Vaughn and Kluger[88] study with rabbits infected with *P. multocida* cited above, body temperatures above 38.9° C (102° F) were associated with increased mortality.

Systematic studies of the effect of controlled euthermia during clinical infection in patients have not been carried out. Metabolic studies during experimental human infection suggest that maintenance of euthermia rather than hyper- or hypothermia may be most beneficial.[5]

Although the metabolic effects of fever are well tolerated by the normal child, there are clinical conditions in which these metabolic changes may be deleterious. Fever increases the basal metabolic rate by 10 to 12 per cent for each degree of centigrade temperature elevation and is accompanied by proportionate increases in oxygen consumption, carbon dioxide production, and requirements for fluid and calories. The need for free water is increased significantly because of increased insensible water loss from the skin and respiratory tract. Fever and the associated metabolic changes stress the cardiopulmonary system. Although fever appears to have little or no effect on normal pulmonary vasculature, in dogs it has been found to enhance hypoxia-induced pulmonary vasoconstriction.[8]

Fever can precipitate febrile seizures in the susceptible child between the ages of 6 months and 5 years. It has been estimated that as many as 2 to 4 per cent of all children in this age group will experience at least one seizure in association with fever.[56] In addition, fever is associated with other neurologic manifestations—irritability, delirium, disorientation, and hallucinations. Finally, it should be noted that although there are no data to suggest that the temperature elevations usually associated with fever cause damage to the brain, there are experimental animal data indicating that fever can enhance the effects of injury on the brain. Clasen and associates[19] induced a standardized insult to the brains of monkeys in the laboratory. Half of the animals were kept at normal body temperature, the other half at a core temperature of 40° C (104° F) for 2 hours. The investigators found that the hyperthermic animals had increased edema and hemorrhage in the injured hemisphere.

Finally, it should be noted that in certain situations reduction of fever can make it easier to evaluate the patient. Disorientation, tachypnea, and tachycardia all may disappear with restoration of normal body temperature, alleviating concern about meningitis, pneumonia, and heart disease, respectively.

THE TREATMENT OF FEVER

The decision to treat fever symptomatically should be individualized for each patient. In general, there appears to be no compelling reason to treat all fevers or always to reduce body temperature completely to normal. It seems reasonable to treat fever when it is making the patient uncomfortable and to treat fever in children who are susceptible to febrile seizures either because of their age or because of a history of prior convulsions. Patients who are critically ill, as well as patients with presumed sepsis or septic shock, should be maintained in a euthermic state. Patients at risk of cardiac or respiratory failure; patients with neurologic disease or injury; and patients with disturbed or precarious fluid, electrolyte, or metabolic status also probably will benefit from reduction of fever. Finally, it appears advisable to treat children with high fever—40° C (104° F) or higher.

Once the decision has been made to treat fever symptomatically, there are several options that need to be considered in regard to the mode of treatment. Because fever is the result of an elevation of the set-point in the PAOH, the most rational method of treating fever is to restore this set-point to normal, and, fortunately, there are drugs such as aspirin, acetaminophen, and ibuprofen that accomplish exactly that. These agents lower the set-point to normal by interfering with the synthesis of prostaglandins in the PAOH.

Aspirin and ibuprofen inhibit prostaglandin synthetase in a wide variety of tissues in addition to the central nervous system, and for this reason these agents have a long list of side effects, even in therapeutic dosage. Gastritis and gastrointestinal upset,[59] gastrointestinal bleeding,[9] and impaired platelet aggregation[63, 87] have been well documented with ordinary, short-term therapeutic administration of these medications. Bronchospasm occurs in almost a third of children with asthma after a single dose of aspirin[64] and has been shown to be a direct pharmacologic effect rather than an allergic phenomenon.[91] Additionally, therapeutic doses of aspirin have been shown—both in laboratory animals[15] and in patients[84]—to increase the leakage of pulmonary capillaries and to favor the formation of pulmonary edema. In vitro suppression of immunologic responses has been reported,[61] and ordinary doses of aspirin were shown to prolong the nasal shedding of rhinovirus in human subjects.[79] Because of the apparent relationship between aspirin and Reye syndrome,[38, 55, 80] aspirin no longer is recommended for simple antipyresis in children.

Acetaminophen, in contrast to aspirin and ibuprofen, is almost totally free of side effects when used in ordinary therapeutic doses.[21, 53] In addition, the excretion of acetaminophen is less rate limited than that of aspirin, and therefore there is less tendency for acetaminophen to accumulate with moderate overdose.

Ibuprofen appears to decrease fever at about the same rate as acetaminophen. Although the nadir of temperature after ibuprofen administration is statistically significantly lower than after acetaminophen administration, the absolute difference is small and of no clinical significance.[46, 75, 89, 92] Currently, there are no published studies with a rescue strategy and therefore no proof that ibuprofen is effective in patients whose fever fails to respond to acetaminophen. The antipyretic effect of ibuprofen is about 2 hours longer than that of acetaminophen, i.e., 6 versus 4 hours.

Theoretically, ibuprofen shares most of the side effects of aspirin, other than an association with Reye syndrome. A large, multicenter study of ibuprofen versus acetaminophen in more than 700 pediatric and family medicine practices found no cases of Reye syndrome or acute renal failure and a negligible incidence (7.2/100,000) of gastrointestinal hemorrhage in the ibuprofen group.[54] None of the cases of gastrointestinal hemorrhage required transfusion.

In view of the increased cost and potential toxicity of ibuprofen compared with acetaminophen and the questionable need to reduce fever maximally in most cases, acetaminophen remains the drug of choice for the routine treatment of fever. One potential advantage of ibuprofen is that in overdose it has less severe toxic effects than does acetaminophen. The major causes of morbidity and mortality in ibuprofen poisoning are acute renal failure and central nervous system changes, including apnea. All of these are managed more easily than acute hepatic failure, which can occur with severe acetaminophen poisoning. However, current packaging has made serious acetaminophen poisoning infrequent with the pediatric preparations of this drug.

Although antipyretic agents frequently are prescribed on the basis of age, the physician should be aware of the correct dosage based on weight.[17, 29, 30]

In the well-hydrated child with normal liver and renal function, acetaminophen appears safe in doses up to 15 mg/kg every 4 hours, although the package insert recommends a maximum of five doses per 24 hours. Because acetaminophen has a prolonged half-life in the newborn period and because there are few data regarding the kinetics of acetaminophen in the first few months of life, it is advisable that it be used with caution in this age group, and then only in either reduced dosage or decreased frequency. The maximum dose for older children generally is presumed to be 600 mg every 4 hours.

The recommended dosage of ibuprofen is 5 mg/kg every 6 hours for temperatures of 38.9° C (102° F) or lower and 10 mg/kg every 6 hours for temperatures higher than 38.9° C. However, because there is no reason to use ibuprofen for temperatures of 38.9° C or lower, there really is little rational for the lower dose. There are no published data regarding either combined or alternating use of ibuprofen and acetaminophen, and therefore such practice cannot be recommended. It is reasonable to switch to ibuprofen for those patients whose response to acetaminophen is judged to be inadequate.

Although restoration of the hypothalamic set-point by pharmacotherapy is the most rational way to treat fever, external cooling (as by sponging with cold, cool, or tepid water) can be effective in reducing fever and restoring body temperature to normal.[44, 81] Ice water sponging has a more rapid cooling effect than does tepid water sponging, but the associated discomfort makes it undesirable.[81] Water in the range of 29.4 to 32° C (85 to 90° F) generally is preferable. The addition of alcohol to the sponge water is contraindicated because absorption of alcohol through the skin and by inhalation of fumes can result in central nervous system depression.[58] In the hospitalized patient, a cooling blanket may be more convenient. External cooling especially is effective in infants and young children because of their relatively large surface areas.

Because external cooling alone does not restore the PAOH set-point to normal, it is best combined with the use of acetaminophen. This may be the optimal approach in children with very high fevers or in cases in which it is desirable to reduce fever quickly. In a few situations, sponging alone may be indicated, for example, for very young infants, children with hepatic failure, and children with allergy to both acetaminophen and ibuprofen.

References

1. Atkins, E.: Fever: New perspectives on an old phenomenon. N. Engl. J. Med. *308*:958–960, 1983.
2. Atkins, E., and Bodel, P.: Fever. N. Engl. J. Med. *286*:27–34, 1972.
3. Austin, T. W., and Truant, G.: Hyperthermia, antipyretics and function of polymorphonuclear leukocytes. Can. Med. Assoc. J. *118*:493–495, 1978.
4. Bayley, N., and Stolz, H. R.: Maturational changes in rectal temperatures of 61 infants from 1 to 36 months. Child Dev. *8*:195–206, 1937.
5. Beisel, W. R., Sawyer, W. D., Ryll, E. D., et al.: Metabolic effects of intracellular infections in man. Ann. Intern. Med. *67*:744–779, 1967.
6. Beisel, W. R.: Mediators of fever and muscle proteolysis. N. Engl. J. Med. *308*:586–588, 1983.
7. Bennett, I. L., Jr., and Nicastri, A.: Fever as a mechanism of resistance. Bacterial. Rev. *24*:16–34, 1960.
8. Benumof, J. L., and Wahrenbock, E. A.: Dependency of hypoxic pulmonary vasoconstriction on temperature. J. Appl. Physiol. *42*:56–58, 1977.
9. Bergman, G. E., Philippidis, P., and Naiman, J. L.: Severe gastrointestinal hemorrhage and anemia after therapeutic doses of aspirin in normal children. J. Pediatr. *88*:501–503, 1976.
10. Bernheim, H. A., Bodel, P. T., Askenase, P. W., et al.: Effects of fever on host defense mechanisms after infection in the lizard, *Dipsosaurus dorsalis*. Br. J. Exp. Pathol. *59*:76–84, 1978.
11. Bernheim, H. A., and Kluger, M. J.: Fever: Effect of drug-induced antipyresis on survival. Science *193*:237–239, 1976.
12. Bligh, J.: Temperature Regulation in Mammals and Other Vertebrates. New York, American Elsevier Publishers, 1973, pp. 38–39.
13. Bodel, P., and Atkins, E.: Release of endogenous pyrogen by human monocytes. N. Engl. J. Med. *276*:1002–1008, 1967.
14. Bosma, J. F., and Kelley, V. C.: Body temperature regulation in health and diseases. *In* Kelley, V. C. (ed.): Practice of Pediatrics. Vol. 1. Hagerstown, MD, Hoeber Medical, 1967, pp. 7–8.
15. Bowers, R. E., Brigham, K. L., and Owen, P. J.: Salicylate pulmonary edema: The mechanism in sheep and review of the clinical literature. Am. Rev. Respir. Dis. *115*:261–268, 1977.
16. Carmichael, L. E., Barnes, F. D., and Percy, D. H.: Temperature as a factor in resistance of young puppies to canine herpesvirus. J. Infect. Dis. *120*:669–678, 1969.
17. Cashman, T. M., Starns, R. J., Johnson, J., et al.: Comparative effects of naproxen and aspirin on fever in children. J. Pediatr. *95*:626–629, 1979.
18. Ciba Foundation Symposium: Pyrogens and Fever. *In* Wolstenholme, G. E. W., and Birch, J. (eds.): London, Churchill Livingstone, 1971.
19. Clasen, R. A., Pandolfi, S., Laing, I., et al.: Experimental study of relation of fever to cerebral edema. J. Neurosurg. *41*:576–581, 1974.
20. Clowes, G. H. A., Jr., George, B. C., Villee, C. A., Jr., et al.: Muscle proteolysis induced by a circulating peptide in patients with sepsis or trauma. N. Engl. J. Med. *308*:545–552, 1983.
21. Committee on Drugs, American Academy of Pediatrics: Commentary on acetaminophen. Pediatrics *61*:108–112, 1978.
22. Cooper, K. E., Cranston, W. I., and Snell, E. S.: Temperature regulation during fever in man. Clin. Sci. *27*:345–356, 1964.
23. Cooper, K. E.: The body temperature "set-point" in fever. *In* Bligh, J., and Moore, R. E. (eds.): Essays on Temperature Regulation. New York, American Elsevier Publishers, 1972, p. 150.
24. Covert, J. B., and Reynolds, W. W.: Survival value of fever in fish. Nature *267*:43–45, 1977.
25. Cranston, W. I.: Central mechanisms of fever. Fed. Proc. *38*:49–51, 1979.
26. Dawkins, M. J. R., and Hull, D.: Brown adipose tissue and the response of newborn rabbits to cold. J. Physiol. *172*:216–238, 1964.
27. Dinarello, C. A.: Interleukin-1 and the pathogenesis of the acute-phase response. N. Engl. J. Med. *311*:1413–1418, 1984.
28. Dinarello, C. A., Cannon, J. G., and Wolff, S. M.: New concepts on the pathogenesis of fever. Rev. Infect. Dis. *10*:168–189, 1988.
29. Done, A. K.: Treatment of fever in 1982: A review. Am. J. Med. *14A*:27–35, 1983.
30. Done, A. K., Yaffe, S. J., and Clayton, J. M.: Aspirin dosage for infants and children. J. Pediatr. *95*:617–625, 1979.
31. DuBois, E. F.: Basal Metabolism in Health and Disease. 3rd ed. Philadelphia, Lea & Febiger, 1936.
32. DuBois, E. F.: Fever and the Regulation of Body Temperature. Springfield, IL, Charles C Thomas, 1948.
33. DuBois, E. F.: Why are fever temperatures over 106° F rare? Am. J. Med. Sci. *217*:361–368, 1949.
34. Eiler, D. M., and Stetson, J. B.: Fever: A physiological view. Int. Anesthesiol. Clin. *5*:359–379, 1967.
35. Ellingson, H. V., and Clark, P. F.: The influence of artificial fever on mechanisms of resistance. J. Immunol. *43*:65–83, 1942.
36. Freed, G. L., and Fraley, J. K.: Lack of agreements of tympanic membrane temperature assessments with conventional methods in a private practice setting. Pediatrics *89*: 384–386, 1992.
37. Gander, G. W., and Goodale, F.: The role of granulocytes and mononuclear leucocytes in fever. *In* Lomax, P., Schonbaum, E., and Jacob, J. (eds.): Temperature Regulation and Drug Action. Basel, S. Karger, 1975, pp. 51–58.
38. Glick, T. H., Likosky, W. H., Levitt, L. P., et al.: Reye's syndrome: An epidemiologic approach. Pediatrics *46*:371–377, 1970.
39. Grieger, T. A., and Kluger, M. J.: Fever and survival: The role of serum iron. J. Physiol. (Lond.) *279*:187–196, 1978.
40. Hahn, H. H., Char, D. C., Postel, W. B., et al.: Studies on the pathogenesis of fever. XV. The production of endogenous pyrogen by peritoneal macrophages. J. Exp. Med. *126*:385–394, 1967.
41. Hoekelman, R. A.: Take two aspirin and call me in the morning: Salicylate use and Reye's syndrome. Am. J. Dis. Child *136*:973–974, 1982.
42. Hooker, E. A.: Use of tympanic thermometers to screen for fever in patients in a pediatric emergency department. South. Med. J. *86*:856-858, 1993.
43. Hornick, R. B., Greisman, S. E., Woodward, T. E., et al.: Typhoid fever: Pathogenesis and immunologic control (first of two parts). N. Engl. J. Med. *283*:686–691, 1970.
44. Hunter, J.: Study of antipyretic therapy in current use. Arch. Dis. Child. *48*:313–315, 1973.
45. Ivy, A. C.: What is normal or normality? Q. Bull. Northwestern Univ. Med. Sch. *18*:22–32, 1944.
46. Kauffman, R. E., Sawyer, L. A., Scheinbaum, M. L.: Antipyretic efficacy of ibuprofen vs acetaminophen. Am. J. Dis. Child. *146*:622–625, 1992.
47. Kendell, H. W.: Fever Therapy. Springfield, IL, Charles C Thomas, 1935, pp. 67–83.
48. Kennedy, R. D., Fortenberry, J. D., Surratt, S. S., et al.: Evaluation of an infrared tympanic membrane thermometer in pediatric patients. Pediatrics *85*:854–858, 1990.
49. Klastersky, J., and Kass, E. H.: Effect of suppression of fever on mortality rate in experimental pneumococcal sepsis. Clin. Res. *17*:370, 1969.
50. Kluger, M. J.: Fever, Its Biology, Evolution and Function. Princeton, Princeton University Press, 1979, p. 31.
51. Kluger, M. J., and Rothenberg, B. A.: Fever and reduced iron: Their interaction as a host defense response to bacterial infection. Science *203*:374–376, 1979.
52. Kluger, M. J.: Fever revisited. Pediatrics *90*:846–850, 1992.
53. Koch-Weser, J.: Acetaminophen. N. Engl. J. Med. *295*:1297–1300, 1976.
54. Lesko, S. M., and Mitchell, A. A.: An assessment of the safety of pediatric ibuprofen: A practitioner-based randomized clinical trial. J. A. M. A. *273*:929–933, 1995.
55. Linneman, C. C., Jr., Shea, L., Kauffman, C. A., et al.: Association of Reye's syndrome with viral infection. Lancet *2*:179–182, 1974.
56. Lorin, M. I.: The Febrile Child: Clinical Management of Fever and Other Types of Pyrexia. New York, John Wiley & Sons, 1982, pp. 153, 226–227.
57. Mayfield, S. R., Bhatia, J., Nakamara, K. T., et al.: Temperature measurement in term and preterm neonates. J. Pediatr, *104*:271–275, 1984.
58. McFadden, S. W., and Haddow, J. E.: Coma produced by topical application of isopropanol. Pediatrics *43*:622–623, 1969.
59. Miller, R. R., and Jack, H.: Acute toxicity of aspirin in hospitalized medical patients. Am. J. Med. Sci. *274*:271–279, 1977.
60. Nakayama, T., et al.: Thermal stimulation of electrical activity of single units of the preoptic region. Am. J. Physiol. *204*:1122–1126, 1963.
61. Opelz, G., and Terasaki, P. I.: Suppression of lymphocyte transformation by aspirin. Lancet *2*:478–480, 1973.
62. Palmes, E. D., and Park, C. R.: The regulation of body temperature during fever. Arch. Environ. Health. *11*:749–759, 1965.
63. Pearson, H.: Comparative effects of aspirin and acetaminophen on hemostasis. Pediatrics *62*(Suppl.):926–929, 1978.
64. Rachelefsky, G. S., Coulson, A., Siegel, S. C., et al.: Aspirin intolerance in chronic childhood asthma: Detected by oral challenge. Pediatrics *56*:443–448, 1975.
65. Reaves, T. A., and Hayward, J. N.: Hypothalamic and extrahypothalamic

thermoregulatory centers. *In* Lomax, P., and Schonbaum, E. (eds.): Body Temperature. New York, Marcel Dekker, 1979, p. 58.
66. Reisinger, K. S., Kao, J., and Grant, D. M.: Inaccuracy of the Clinitemp skin thermometer. Pediatrics *64*:4–6, 1979.
67. Roberts, N. J., and Steigbigel, R. T.: Hyperthermia and human leukocyte function: Effects on response of lymphocytes to mitogen and antigen and bactericidal capacity of monocytes and neutrophils. Infect. Immun. *18*:673–679, 1977.
68. Roe, C. F.: Fever and energy metabolism in surgical disease. Monogr. Surg. Sci. *3*:85–132, 1966.
69. Root, R. K., and Wolff, S. M.: Pathogenetic mechanisms in experimental immune fever. J. Exp. Med. *128*:309–323, 1968.
70. Ruata, G. Q.: L'influenza del caldo umido sulle infezioni. Bull. Sci. Med. Bologna *9*:59–110, 1909.
71. Ruiz-Gomez, J., and Isaacs, A.: Interferon production by different viruses. Virology *19*:8–12, 1963.
72. Saper, C. B., and Breder, C. D.: The neurologic basis of fever. N. Engl. J. Med. *330*:1880–1886, 1994.
73. Schmitt, B. D.: Fever phobia: Misconception of parents about fever. Am. J. Dis. Child. *134*:176-181, 1980.
74. Scholenfield, J. H., Gerber, M. A., and Dwyer, P.: Liquid crystal forehead temperature strips: A clinical appraisal. Am. J. Dis. Child. *136*:198–201, 1982.
75. Sidler, J., Frey, B., and Baerlocher, K: A double-blind comparison of ibuprofen and paracetamol in juvenile pyrexia. Br. J. Clinic. Pract. *70*(Suppl):22–25, 1990.
76. Silverman, W. A., and Sinclair, J. C.: Temperature regulation in the newborn infant. N. Engl. J. Med. *274*:92–94, 1966.
77. Small, P. M., Tauber, M. G., Hackbarth, C. J., et al.: Influence of body temperature on bacterial growth rates in experimental pneumococcal meningitis in rabbits. Infect. Immun. *52*:484–487, 1986.
78. Snell, E. S., and Atkins, E.: The mechanism of fever. *In* Bittar, E. E. (ed.): The Biological Basis of Medicine. Vol. 2. London, Academic Press, pp. 397–419, 1968.
79. Stanley, E. D., Jackson, G. G., Panusarn, C., et al.: Increased viral shedding with aspirin treatment of rhinovirus infection. J. A. M. A. *231*:1248–1251, 1975.
80. Starko, K. M., Ray, C. G., Dominguea, L. B., et al.: Reye's syndrome and salicylate use. Pediatrics *66*:859–864, 1980.
81. Steele, R. W., Tanaka, P. T., Lara, R. P., et al.: Evaluation of sponging and of oral antipyretic therapy to reduce fever. J. Pediatr. *77*:824–829, 1970.
82. Stine, R. J.: Heat illness. J. A. C. E. P. *8*:154–160, 1979.
83. Stitt, J. T.: Fever versus hyperthermia. Fed. Proc. *38*:39–43, 1979.
84. Sutcliffe, J.: Pulmonary oedema due to salicylates. Br. J. Radiol. *28*:314–316, 1955.
85. Talbot, N. B., Richie, R. H., and Crawford, J. D.: Metabolic Homeostasis: A Syllabus for Those Concerned with the Care of Patients. Cambridge, Harvard University Press, 1959.
86. Tandberg, D., and Sklar, D.: Effect of tachypnea on the estimation of body temperature by an oral thermometer. N. Engl. J. Med. *308*:945–946, 1983.
87. Van Daele, M. C., and De Gaetano, G.: Purpura and acetylsalicylic acid therapy. Acta Paediatr. Scand. *60*:203–208, 1971.
88. Vaughn, L. K., and Kluger, M. J.: Fever and survival in rabbits infected with *Pasteurella multocida*. J. Physiol. (Lond.) *282*:243–251, 1978.
89. Walson, P. D., Galletia, G., Chomile, F., et al.: Comparison of multidose ibuprofen and acetaminophen therapy in febrile children. Am. J. Dis. Child. *146*:626-632, 1992.
90. Walter, D. L., and Boring, W. D.: Factors influencing host-virus interactions. III. Further studies on the alteration of Coxsackie virus infection in adult mice by environmental temperature. J. Immunol. *80*:39–44, 1958.
91. Weinberger, M.: Analgesic sensitivity in children with asthma. Pediatrics *62*(Suppl.):910–915, 1978.
92. Wilson J. T., Brown, R. D., Kearns, G. L., et al.: Single dose, placebo-controlled comparative study of ibuprofen and acetaminophen antipyresis in children. Pediatrics *119*: 803–811, 1991.
93. Wood, W. B., Jr.: The pathogenesis of fever. *In* Mudd, S. (ed.): Infectious Agents and Host Reactions. Philadelphia, W. B. Saunders, 1970, pp. 146–162.

6

INDIGENOUS FLORA

Arnold L. Smith

Indigenous flora and *normal flora* are the terms used to describe the microorganisms (bacteria, yeast) that are found in various locations on individuals who are "normal" and "healthy." Humans have evolved with this flora, the overwhelming majority of which does not have an immediately apparent classic symbiotic relationship. There are, however, benefits to the individual's having an indigenous flora. This most obviously is seen in experiments with germ-free animals. Animals delivered and reared in a germ-free environment are agammaglobulinemic, they have a very thin lamina propria, and their intestinal epithelial cell renewal rate is 50 per cent that of conventionally reared animals.[6] Their mucosa almost totally is devoid of lymphocytes, and surprisingly the germ-free animals live almost twice as long as conventionally reared animals. However, death, when it occurred in germ-free animals, frequently was due to intestinal obstruction secondary to gastrointestinal atonia.

In spite of the longer natural life of germ-free animals, they are exquisitely susceptible to infections: most experiments have used enteric pathogens. For example, the LD_{50} for *Salmonella typhimurium* in mice usually is about 10^6 colony-forming units. However, in experimental animals whose normal flora is ablated (by germ-free approach or treatment with an antibiotic), the LD_{50} is approximately 10 organisms.[3]

The normal flora appears to prime the host immune system with the M cells in Peyer patches processing antigens derived from normal flora to which then humoral and secretory antibodies are made. For example, blood group antibodies arise because of the immune response to antigenically cross-reacting normal flora.[7]

GENERAL COMPOSITION

The exact bacterial genera and even species vary throughout the body (Table 6–1). It has been estimated that there are approximately 10^{14} bacterial cells on and in the average adult body: this exceeds the total number of human cells 100-fold. The indigenous flora differs markedly between the various anatomic sites. For example, the skin and the gastrointestinal tract commensals differ, and there are differences between early infancy and adulthood. The variation in the specific species of bacteria colonizing various sites is due to differences in pH and temperature, the existence of an oxidative or reductive environment, the amount of water present, the nutrient level, and the organism's resistance to locally produced nonspecific antibacterial compounds. In addition, the presence or absence of age-specific eukaryotic cell-surface ligands also determines whether or not a specific bacterial species can adhere to and colonize that epithelium. These eukaryotic ligands are important in that virtually all of the epithelia colonized with indigenous flora (except skin and

TABLE 6–1. Indigenous Flora

Site	Infant	(Density)*	Adult	(Density)*
Skin	*Staphylococcus epidermidis*	(10^5)	*S. epidermidis*	(10^5)
			Propionibacterium acnes	
Mouth/oropharynx	*Streptococcus salivarius*	(10^5)	*S. salivarius*	(10^6)
	Haemophilus influenzae		*Streptococcus mutans*	(10^7)
			Streptococcus mitis	
			Anaerobes	
Small intestine	Jejunum	($<10^3$)	*Lactobacillus*	
	Ileum	(10^7)	*Streptococcus*	
			Actinomyces	
Colon	*Bifidobacterium*	(10^{10})	*Bacteroides*	(10^{10})
	(Lactobacillus bifidus)		*Bifidobacterium*	
			Peptostreptococcus	
			Clostridium	
			Enterococcus	
			Enterobacteriaceae	
Vagina	Diphtheroids		*Lactobacillus acidophilus*	(10^8)
	S. epidermidis		*S. epidermidis*	
			Candida	
Urethra	*S. epidermidis*	(10^4)	Enterobacteriaceae	(10^4)

*Per gram or milliliter.

vagina) have a continued flow of secretions that mechanically can wash away the colonizing bacteria.[1] In addition, in certain anatomic locales, the normal low-level secretion of mucin also entraps surface bacteria, permitting them to be expelled from that locale. Mucin binding appears to be primarily a protective effect because infection (high bacterial density accompanied by inflammation) of a mucosal surface invariably is accompanied by increased mucin secretion.

SITES OF INDIGENOUS FLORA

The "normal" flora is present on the skin, in the mouth, and in the upper respiratory tract; is most numerous in the gastrointestinal tract; and also is present in the genital urinary tract and in some individuals in the eye. Normal flora is not present in blood or body fluids (cerebrospinal fluid, urine, bile, or synovia).

Tears contain several antibacterial substances that, in addition to instigating the flushing action of the flowing system, all decrease the number of bacteria. About one-third of conjunctival cultures are sterile. *Staphylococcus epidermidis* is recovered frequently enough to merit its designation as a commensal of conjunctiva, but it is not clear whether it is present transiently from adjacent skin. Other genera that probably are true commensals are *Neisseria*, *Moraxella*, and *Haemophilus*.[17]

BACTERIAL COMPOSITION AT SPECIFIC LOCATIONS

Skin

The skin is a reservoir for a diverse microbial flora whose composition depends on the degree of moisture and the relative amount of sebum present. In the newborn infant, the bacteria rarely are detected on skin except around the anus and around the anterior nares. In these locations, the nares often yield *Staphylococcus aureus*, and the perianal skin reflects the fecal flora. At the onset of puberty, *Propionibacterium acnes* is detected on the skin with increasing frequency. Adult frequencies of isolation of *P. acnes* are obtained at about 16 years of age. *P. acnes* is a microaerophilic gram-positive rod that grows in the sebum and breaks down skin lipids to fatty acids. Thus, it is most numerous in the parts of the body where there are hair follicles, to which sebaceous glands commonly drain. *P. acnes* is resistant to the bactericidal effects of skin lipids and their acidic breakdown products, whereas other organisms that land on the skin may be susceptible. It is very difficult to decontaminate the skin of an adult because of the subsurface (sebaceous gland) reservoir of *P. acnes*.[15]

Gram-negative bacteria are an extraordinarily rare skin commensal. When they are detected, they most commonly are found in the moist intertriginous areas. They are killed readily by drying. *Enterobacter*, *Klebsiella*, and *Escherichia coli* are gram-negative bacteria that can be found on the skin.[15]

Respiratory Tract

The respiratory tract is covered by a variety of epithelium consisting of stratified squamae in the most anterior part of the nasopharynx (within the nasal cavity). Pseudostratified ciliated columnar epithelium lines the respiratory portion of the nasopharynx, but then a predominant lymphoepithelial tissue is found in the posterior oropharynx. The lower respiratory tract (below the larynx) is assumed to be free of commensal flora. In reality, commensal oral pharyngeal bacteria are aspirated into the lower respiratory tract in low numbers, probably daily. However, they do not colonize that anatomic locale but are cleared by host defense mechanisms.

The oropharynx of the normal adult has large concentrations of fibronectin on and between the epithelial cells. Fibronectin, in addition to being an intracellular cement, also is a ligand for gram-positive bacteria. Streptococcal species are the most prevalent commensal adhering to fibronectin. Approximately 25 to 30 per cent of normal individuals carry *S. aureus* in the anterior part of the nasopharynx. This organism colonizes the sebaceous glands around hair follicles in the anterior nares. In the oral pharynx are numerous bacterial genera, primarily *Streptococcus*, nonpathogenic *Neisseria*, and *Branhamella*, as well as potentially pathogenic organisms, such as *Haemophilus influenzae, Neisseria meningitidis,* and *Streptococcus pneumoniae*.[12]

There also is a specific microflora associated with teeth. *Streptococcus* species (*S. sanguinis, S. oralis, S. gordonae,* and *S. mitis*) are some of the first colonizers of the tooth surface that adhere to the glycoprotein pellicle from saliva. These bacteria have the ability to coaggregate, i.e., adhere to each other and to other bacterial genera. This is the phenomenon in which bacterial interactions form microcolonies on the surface of the tooth. For example, *Actinomyces naeslundii* has adhesins for *S. sanguinis* and *S. gordonae*. All of these species reach high concentrations in expectorated saliva, which usually contains a mixed flora with 10^8 organisms/mL. Most of these salivary bacteria are derived from the various epithelial surfaces. The bacterial plaque developing on teeth may contain as many as 10^{11} streptococci/g in addition to the coaggregating bacteria: *Veillonella, Bacteroides, Treponema, Fusobacterium, Clostridium,* and *Peptostreptococcus*. The anaerobes are more prevalent in the gingival creases because of oxygen sensitivity.

Gastrointestinal Tract

The gastrointestinal tract consists of the esophagus, stomach, small intestine, and colon. The esophagus normally has minimal resident flora, as does the stomach: less than 1000 bacteria/mL of luminal fluid.[16] Organisms swallowed from the mouth are killed quickly by the digestive enzymes and acid in the stomach. Immediately after a meal, gastric contents can contain up to 10^6 bacteria/g, but then after digestion, the density (in the ingested food) again decreases to a level of less than 1000/mL.[8] An exception to this general rule is the potential for *Helicobacter pylori* to infect the stomach and upper duodenum and produce ulcers.[11] This bacterium manages to survive in this hostile environment by producing a cloud of ammonia that neutralizes the gastric acid.[5]

Aspirates of duodenal or jejunal fluid in most individuals contain some streptococci, lactobacilli, and a rare *Bacteroides*. These are present in densities of 1000 organisms/mL or less. Bacterial densities exceeding 10^5/mL in small bowel fluid usually indicate some intrinsic abnormality of the gastrointestinal tract: a blind loop, achlorhydria, or some malabsorption syndrome. In these latter instances, the "indigenous flora" that grows to the increased density is thought to be pathogenic, compromising the absorption of vitamin B_{12}. Further along the jejunum and ileum, bacterial density progressively increases, so that at the ileocecal junction, bacterial density is approximately 10^7 organisms/mL. The same organisms predominate (i.e., streptococci, *Bacteroides*, and lactobacilli).[8]

The colon carries the most prolific flora in the body: 25 to 30 per cent of the weight of feces is bacteria, and more than 90 per cent of these bacteria are anaerobes. If one assumes that the average bacterial volume is 1 μm^3, the absolute packing density of bacteria is approximately 10^{12} organisms/mL. The bacterial density in the colon approaches this, with values routinely measured at 10^{11} organisms/g of feces. The ratio of anaerobes to aerobes is thought to be 1000:1, with approximately 300 different anaerobic species being present in fecal contents.[8, 9]

Genitourinary Tract

The distal portion of both the male and female urethra has colonizing bacteria, as does the vaginal mucosa. The bladder, ureters, and kidneys and their contained fluid normally are sterile. The indigenous flora on the most distal portion of the urethra consists of skin bacteria (*S. epidermidis* and streptococci), *Mycobacterium smegmatis,* and *Bacteroides* and *Fusobacterium* in the anaerobic crevices.

The vaginal flora usually consists of diphtheroids, lactobacilli, *S. epidermidis, Enterococcus faecalis,* micrococci, and various anaerobic streptococci.[5] In sexually active individuals, *Ureaplasma, Chlamydia,* and occasionally *Gardnerella vaginalis* are found.[19]

ACQUISITION OF INDIGENOUS FLORA BY THE NEWBORN

Skin

The normal term fetus does not have indigenous flora. At the time of birth, the infant acquires (most often in the oropharynx and external auditory canal) those organisms present in the mother's vagina. Infants delivered by cesarean section acquire bacteria from fomites and from the hands of hospital personnel. One of the many reasons that infants born by cesarean section have a higher incidence of neonatal infection is that they first encounter and acquire nosocomial organisms, rather than the "protective" lactobacilli and streptococci. In rare instances, these organisms (*Neisseria gonorrhoeae, Streptococcus agalactiae, H. influenzae*) potentially are pathogenic to the infant. The child's skin is unremarkable until the he or she reaches puberty. At that time, *P. acnes* first is isolated.[13] These are anaerobic gram-positive rods that grow in subsurface sebum and have the ability to metabolize skin lipids to fatty acids. The latter products (fatty acids) can elicit inflammation, leading to the association of *P. acnes* and clinical syndrome of acne.

Oropharynx

Because the neonate's oral cavity lacks teeth, the organisms with ligands for the tooth pellicle are absent. Thus, *Streptococcus salivarius,* which has tropism for the tongue, is the most prevalent oral organism. Shortly after birth, the infant's oropharynx contains the same organisms found in the mother's vagina: lactobacilli, micrococci, streptococci, staphylococci, and rare corynebacteria, as well as some yeast. Among the streptococci are microaerophilic and aerobic species. These bacteria decrease in density during the first 5 days after birth but subsequently are replaced by the bacteria present in the mouth of the mother, transmitted by kissing or hand-to-mouth contact. Occasionally present at lower frequency are *Actinomyces,* lactobacilli, corynebacteria, and *Fusobacterium*. Both *Prevotella* and *Treponema* increase in frequency during adolescence.[18]

Gastrointestinal Tract

There is considerable controversy regarding the indigenous bacterial flora in the feces of infants in the first several months of life. The initial observations made some years ago indicated that the breast-fed baby had a bacterial population distinct from the bottle-fed infant.[21] The statement commonly was made that in the breast-fed infant, 99 per cent of the organisms present in feces are of the genus *Bifidobacterium,* an anaerobic gram-positive rod. Human milk, which is high in lactose and low in buffering capacity in comparison with cow's milk, was responsible for this condition because *Bifidobacterium* ferments lactose to yield acetic acid. *Bifidobacterium* grows optimally at an acid pH (5.0 to 5.5). In contrast, infants fed cow's milk, which has a greater buffering capacity, tend to have less acidic stools and were said to have a flora similar to that found in the colon of the adult. However, in more recent years, the lactose concentration of commercially available formula has increased and the protein and phosphate concentration has decreased in order to mimic the composition of human milk. Thus, in several studies, there was no difference in the populations of bacteria in the feces of formula- or breast-fed infants.[2, 20] The only consistent distinction found in contemporary studies by Stark and Lee[20] was that *Clostridium* always was more infrequent and present in lower density in breast-fed infants.[20] Infants who are hospitalized are inoculated with a variety of potentially pathogenic organisms (e.g., *Candida albicans*, *S. epidermidis*, various Enterobacteriaceae). Most often these potential pathogens are introduced by the hands of the hospital personnel.[10, 14] Fomites, intravascular cannulae, endotracheal tubes, and suction catheters occasionally can inoculate hospitalized infants.[4]

SUMMARY

Indigenous flora is acquired by the infant primarily from the mother. The composition of the flora is dependent upon the local physical-chemical environment, intrinsic properties of the microbe, and the host physiology. Indigenous flora is of benefit to the infant through augmentation of nonspecific host defenses and stimulation of the immune system. Its presence is "protective" to the infant.[9] Ablation of the normal flora in general has an adverse effect on the child.

References

1. Beachey, E. H.: Bacterial adherence: Adhesion-receptor interactions mediating the attachment of bacteria to mucosal surfaces. J. Infect. Dis. *143*:325–345, 1981.
2. Benno, Y., Sawada, K., and Mitsuoka, T.: The intestinal microflora of infants: Composition of fecal flora in breast-fed and bottle-fed infants. Microbiol. Immunol. *28*:975–986, 1984.
3. Bohnhoff, M., Miller, C. P., and Martin, J. R.: Resistance of the mouse's intestinal tract to experimental *Salmonella* infection. J. Exp. Med. *120*:805–816, 1964.
4. Fierer, J., Taylor, P. M., and Gezon, H. M.: *P. aeruginosa* epidemic traced by delivery room resuscitation. N. Engl J. Med *176*:991–996, 1967.
5. Goldacre, M., Watt, B., and Loudon, N.: Vaginal microbial flora in young women. Br. Med. J. *1*:1450–1462, 1979.
6. Gordon, H. A., and Pesti, L.: The quotobiotic animal as a tool in the study of host-microbial relationships. Bacteriol. Rev. *35*:390–429, 1971.
7. Hanson, L. A., Ashrof, R., Cruz, J. R., et al.: Immunity related to exposition and bacterial colonization of the infant. Acta Paediatr. Scand. *365*:38–45, 1990.
8. Hentges, D. J. (ed.): Human Intestinal Microflora in Health and Disease. New York, Academic Press, 1983.
9. Hentges, D. J.: The protective function of the indigenous intestinal flora. Pediatr. Infect. Dis. *45*:217–220, 1986.
10. Knittle, M. A., Eitzman, D. V., and Baer, H.: Role of hand contamination of personnel in the epidemiology of gram-negative nosocomial infections. J. Pediatr. *86*:433–439, 1975.
11. Lee, A., Fox, J., and Hazell, S.: Pathogenicity of *Helicobacter pylori*. Infect. Immun. *B1*:1601–1610, 1993.
12. Marsh, P., and Martin, M.: Oral Microbiology. 2nd ed. Washington, D.C., ASM Press, 1984.
13. Matts, M.: Carriage of *Corynebacterium acnes* in school children in relation to age and race. Br. J. Dermatol. *91*:557–561, 1974.
14. Mayhall, C. G., Lamb, A., Bitar, C. M., et al.: Nosocomial infection in a neonatal unit: Identification of risk factors. Infect. Control *1*:239–246, 1980.
15. Noble, W. C.: Microbiology of Human Skin. London, Lloyd-Luke, 1981.
16. Savage, D. C.: Microbial ecology of the gastrointestinal tract. Ann. Rev. Microbiol. *31*:1077–1033, 1977.
17. Smith, A. L.: Acute bacterial conjunctivitis. *In* Year Book of Pediatrics. Chicago, Year Book Medical Publishers, 1988, pp. 389–392.
18. Socransky, S. S., and Mangoniello, S. D.: The oral microbiota of man from birth to senility. J. Periodontol. *42*:485–496, 1971.
19. Spiegel, C. A.: Bacterial vaginosis. Clin. Microbiol. Rev. *4*:485–502, 1991.
20. Stark, P. L., and Lee, A.: The microbial ecology of the large bowel of breast-fed and formula-fed infants during the first year of life. J. Med. Microbiol. *15*:189–203, 1982.
21. Tissier, H.: Reparation des microbes dans l'imtistin du nourrisson. Annal Institut Pasteur *19*:109–123, 1905.

7

EPIDEMIOLOGY OF INFECTIOUS DISEASES

Edward A. Mortimer, Jr., and John P. Fox

Epidemiology is concerned primarily with describing and explaining the occurrence of disease in populations. This chapter is a general review of epidemiology as it relates to infectious diseases of pediatric importance. Readers concerned with the epidemiology of a particular disease should consult the appropriate chapter for the available relevant information. This chapter will help readers to recognize that nearly all the information presented is epidemiologically relevant and to understand why.

Physicians who engage in pediatric practice, teaching, or research in the area of pediatric infectious disease or in public health require competence in epidemiology in order to understand the mechanisms of infection, modes of transmission, and approaches to control. Epidemiology, which comprises principles and methods, must be meshed with biostatistics and with more content-oriented sciences, including but not limited to clinical medicine, microbiology, pathophysiology, immunology, demography, and sociology.

Epidemiology may be considered in a general sense to be of three types: descriptive, analytic or causative, and experimental. All three are of importance in infectious disease.

Descriptive epidemiology provides accounts of the health experiences of populations, including morbidity and mortality. The data are of two types: incidence and prevalence. *Incidence* data consist of the numbers of new cases of, or deaths from, a given disorder that occurs in a defined population for a period that may be measured from days to years. Sequential temporal comparisons often are included for assessing trends. Incidence data, as measures of the impact of a disorder, frequently are useful for setting public health priorities.

Prevalence data describe the existing number of cases of a disorder at a single moment in time. Prevalence data are largely applicable to chronic disorders such as diabetes mellitus, tuberculosis, or HIV infection and have no utility when applied to acute disorders, such as measles, or murder. Additionally, in studies of infectious disease, the prevalence of serologic markers may be used to estimate the immune status of a population or the proportion of a group that has had prior experience with an infection. For certain infections such as tuberculosis and diphtheria, skin testing may serve as a substitute for serologic testing.

Analytic, or *causative*, epidemiology searches for clues to the cause of disease. It is based on the simple principle that disease does not occur at random in the population and classically considers time, person, and place. In other words, there are differences between those who acquire a given disorder and those who do not. Identification of those differences may lead to ascertaining causation and to means of control. These differences may be inherent in the individuals themselves and include biologic characteristics (e.g., hereditary, such as race; acquired, such as immunity) and lifestyle. They may be external, largely comprising environmental risk factors for disease, including in the instance of infectious disease various factors that influence the likelihood of exposure to the agent, such as geography, weather, contact with vectors (including other humans), and social and economic conditions. In studies of infectious disease, there is considerable overlap between descriptive and analytic epidemiology for the simple reason that differences in disease distribution by person, place, and time often are obvious in descriptive data and provide clues for further pursuit.

Analytic epidemiologic studies of infectious disease, as well as those related to other types of conditions, generally fall into three categories. The least frequently employed but nonetheless useful category is the cross-sectional study. Such studies can be conducted in either of two ways. First, one might examine apparently comparable populations with differing prevalence rates of a given infection for characteristics that might explain these different rates. Alternatively, if this disorder sufficiently is prevalent, one can determine rates of disease in those with and those without the suspected risk factor. A classic example is the relationship of sickle-cell trait to resistance to *Plasmodium falciparum* malaria, which was looked at both ways.[1] In studies of variations in the prevalence of the sickle-cell gene in Africa, it was noted that the trait appeared to be more prevalent in areas with a high incidence of malaria. Based on this observation, other studies were conducted that showed that in hyperendemic areas, individuals with the sickle-cell trait might have some resistance to malarial infection, thus permitting selective survival in malarial areas. This observation led to studies of the mechanism of this phenomenon and of certain other erythrocyte characteristics, including blood subgroups, that influenced malarial infection.

The second type of causative or analytic epidemiologic study employed in infectious diseases is the prospective study, sometimes called the cohort study. In this type of study, rates of infection and routes of transmission may be determined by examining subsequent rates of infection in groups of individuals with differences in exposure, which may be measured by timing, duration, intimacy of contact, or disparate sources or avenues of potential transmission. The classic studies of the transmission of group A streptococcal infections in military recruits constitute an excellent example. One particular finding was that transmission of infection from individuals with streptococcal pharyngitis to others in military barracks occurred at rates inversely related to distances between bunks, which established that transmission largely was by intimate respiratory contact with droplets containing hundreds or thousands of organisms, rather than by airborne droplet nuclei.[71] In other studies, the same group showed that fomites, naturally contaminated with streptococci, did not participate in transmission of infection.[60]

Studies of the transmission of staphylococci to newborn infants are another example of prospective epidemiologic studies in infectious disease. In the 1950s, outbreaks of staphylococcal disease, sometimes severe, occurred in newborn nurseries. In an effort to determine how these organisms were transmitted to babies by personnel or other infants, advantage was taken of nurseries with persistently high rates of colonization of infants.[54] Two types of prospective studies were conducted. One consisted of instituting measures that prevented transmission by all but one or two routes, thus permitting assessment of the importance of the unblocked routes in transmission. The other method was the reverse; one or another suspected route of transmission was blocked, and subsequent colonization of infants was monitored. These studies showed that transmission of organisms from personnel who were carriers or from previously colonized infants primarily occurred by the hands of personnel.

Another type of analytic epidemiologic study useful in infectious disease is the retrospective or case-control study. In the aforementioned prospective type of study, the investigator starts with individuals who are exposed to a given agent and, for comparison purposes, a similar group of unexposed individuals. The outcome measure of the study is infection or no infection. In contrast, in a retrospective study, the populations under study are made up of groups who already have the disorder in question. For comparison, similar control subjects who do not have the disease are recruited. From all individuals in both groups, historical data about prior exposure, experience, and characteristics are obtained, usually by interview but sometimes by laboratory methods such as serology. Thus, in a retrospective study, the investigator starts with diseased individuals and searches for exposures; in a prospective study, the investigator starts with exposures and monitors for infection.

Retrospective studies are of particular utility when the disease is relatively uncommon because a prospective study might require an unwieldy number of subjects. A retrospective study obviously is preferable when there is no prior information about the probable cause or source of the disease. For this reason, retrospective studies sometimes are designated as "fishing expeditions." A disadvantage of retrospective studies is that they do not provide an estimate of the true risk or rate of disease occurring after exposure, i.e., the proportion of exposed individuals who actually develop the disorder in question. The reason for this is that the study addresses subjects who already have the disease, and rarely, if ever, is it possible to estimate the size of the exposed population from which those subjects were drawn. Instead, a retrospective study provides only an odds ratio, which is the relative probability of exposed individuals acquiring the disease, compared with that of those who have not been exposed. The odds ratio is, however, a reasonable approximation of the relative risk as determined by prospective studies.

The third type of epidemiologic study useful in infectious disease is *experimental epidemiology* (the clinical trial). Clinical trials generally are employed to determine the efficacy of preventive or therapeutic measures. As such, they often require prior information derived from analytic epidemiologic studies as well as from other basic and clinical sciences. Sometimes studies that are, in effect, clinical trials may provide useful information regarding the cause or routes of transmission of infection, as with studies of staphylococcal transmission in nurseries.

To assess the efficacy of therapeutic or preventive measures, experimental epidemiologic studies require comparison groups of individuals who do not receive the measure in question or, sometimes, are given an older or alternative modality. There are rare exceptions; no one would have advocated a randomized, controlled trial of streptomycin in tuberculous meningitis when the first anecdotal reports of cures appeared for the simple reason that without treatment the disease universally was fatal.

However, most clinical trials are not undertaken in situations in which the untreated group uniformly experiences an unambiguous outcome. Moreover, even when the outcome measure is a condition that reasonably is clear-cut, such as varicella, a trial of a preventive vaccine usually requires unimmunized controls because attack rates may vary from place to place and year to year, intensities of exposure may be different, and some subjects already may be immune.[73]

In a controlled clinical trial, it is important that the treatment and control groups be as nearly similar as possible in terms of characteristics that may affect the outcome. Clinical trials designed to assess the efficacy of therapeutic or preventive measures must take into consideration many such factors. These usually include age, sex, socioeconomic status, general health, and likelihood of exposure. Therefore, in any trial, efforts should be made to balance treated and untreated subjects in terms of recognized factors. However, not all variables that may inject bias into the results of a clinical trial necessarily are known or recognized in advance. Accordingly, to ensure insofar as possible that these characteristics are distributed approximately equally between the two groups, the process of randomization almost always is necessary. Additionally, true randomization must occur; methods employing odd versus even record numbers or birth dates, alternate days of the week, and the like are inappropriate. The optimum method is a system of random numbers, as published in most textbooks of biostatistics.

Randomization avoids selection bias, best defined as underlying differences between the treatment and control groups, whether internal (inherent) or external, such as likelihood of exposure. Avoidance of selection bias is of paramount importance for any type of comparative study, in analytic epidemiologic studies as well as in experimental epidemiologic studies.

Two other types of bias must be avoided: confounding bias and ascertainment bias. Confounding bias best is defined as a factor that appears more often in either the treated or control group and is likely to influence the outcome. Obviously, confounding bias in some instances is a form of selection bias. Nonetheless, specific forms of confounding bias may be found in clinical trials. If a study attempted to assess the value of steroids in the treatment of certain severe infections, the study might be confounded if the two groups received different antibiotics.

Very important is the potential for ascertainment bias. Put rather simply, ascertainment bias occurs in analytic epidemiologic studies and in experimental epidemiology. When ascertainment bias derives from recounting of events by the study subjects, it usually is referred to as reporting or recall bias. Many examples exist. In a retrospective (case-control) epidemiologic study, the affected individuals for obvious reasons may exert more diligence than may healthy controls in pursuing factors that they feel, or are led to believe, might have an effect on the development of their disorders or on the outcome. The potential for this type of recall bias was of particular concern in the studies that eventually pointed to salicylates as risk factors for Reye syndrome. Reporting bias also is a potential problem in experimental epidemiology, particularly when the outcome of the therapeutic or preventive measure under assessment depends on reporting of symptoms by subjects. If, for example, the study subjects anticipate a beneficial effect from a vaccine against the common cold, recipients may tend to ignore or fail to report minor symptoms after immunization (the placebo effect).

The other form of potential ascertainment bias has to do with observations by investigators. Those who pursue the assessment of the efficacy of a new preventive or therapeutic measure in infectious disease as a rule would not do so unless they subscribe to the belief that the measure in question might offer more benefit than might other approaches. Therefore, it is important to ensure that the subtle but nonetheless human characteristic of anticipating the hoped-for outcome does not influence observation of outcomes in analytic or experimental epidemiologic studies. In analytic studies that look for clues to causation, particularly retrospective studies, it is of paramount importance that prior exposures of cases and controls be pursued with equal vigor.

For these reasons, comparative epidemiologic studies, whether analytic or experimental, usually require "blinding" of the investigators and of the subjects. Depending on the nature of the investigation, studies may be single-, double-, or triple-blind. In single-blind studies, the study subjects are unaware of their status as members of the treated or control groups. In double-blind studies, not only the subjects but also the investigators lack such knowledge. In triple-blind studies, those responsible for the analyses are blinded, as are the subjects and the researchers. Blinding of those who conduct the analyses, whether they are examining clinical or laboratory data, may have consequences when the data are subject to some interpretation.

These principles apply to all epidemiologic studies, not just to studies of infectious disease. They are applicable to the study of cardiovascular disease, cancer, and all of the other ills that affect humans. However, in infectious disease, there are three additional factors that contribute uniquely to who is and who is not affected: (1) the cause is a specific external agent (the infecting organism); (2) transmission of the organism to the host is required; and (3) there are certain host factors, such as immunity to infection or disease caused by many of these agents. Recognition of these factors (the infecting agent, transmission, and immunity) evolved gradually over many years. Before considering variations in person, place, and time, it is useful to consider these special features of infectious disease causation.

HISTORICAL PERSPECTIVES

Epidemiology evolved from the study of the great epidemic diseases, such as plague, cholera, and smallpox. The periodic waves of these diseases, associated with high mortality, stimulated the first serious efforts to explain disease occurrence on the basis of other than supernatural or divine forces.

Fundamental to such explanations was the concept of contagion. This long had been implicit in attitudes toward victims of leprosy, exemplified by such early Christian practices as conducting antemortem funerals for lepers, who then were given a bell and cup and forbidden further human contact or, more drastically, were buried alive or burned at the stake.[64] However, an Italian physician-poet, Girolamo Fracastoro (1478–1553), was the first to voice this concept formally, first in a poem *(Syphilides, sine Morbi Gallici, libre tres)* in which he dubbed syphilis the "French disease" and later in the book *De Res Contagiosa* (published in 1546), in which he expressed the complete idea of infection transferred by minute, invisible particles.[66]

During the next two centuries, Fracastoro was forgotten, and views like those of Thomas Sydenham (1624–1689) prevailed.[20] This notable English physician, who introduced laudanum (derived from opium) as a pain killer and recognized the efficacy of Peruvian bark (quinine) in malaria, revived the hippocratic idea of "epidemic constitutions" (of atmospheric nature), which, by grafting onto existing illness, gave all concurrent illnesses the character reflecting the then prevailing "constitution." These views persisted in colonial America, where they were expounded by such eminent persons as Noah Webster (of dictionary fame) and Dr. Benjamin Rush of Philadelphia.

Nonetheless, by the mid-eighteenth century, the theory of contagion had gained acceptance for particular diseases, including measles, syphilis, and smallpox. Indeed, it is alleged to have been exploited in an early act of biologic warfare; Massachusetts colonists reportedly presented the blankets of smallpox victims as gifts to the Indians, who then suffered a decimating epidemic.[23]

The true origin of the concept of immunity is uncertain, but it was applied first in relation to smallpox. Variolation (inoculation of young people with lesion material expected to induce modified but immunizing disease) was practiced in China as early as the eleventh or twelfth century and in England and the American colonies in the early eighteenth century. Also popular in rural England at this time was the belief that cowpox, the minor disease acquired from afflicted cattle, induced immunity to smallpox. This was verified by Jenner (reported in 1798) and resulted in general acceptance of cowpox vaccine (vaccinia) to protect against smallpox.

Implicit in the concept of contagion as formulated by Fracastoro in 1546 was the germ theory of disease. This was stated explicitly in 1855 by John Snow, an English anesthesiologist who took up cholera epidemiology as an avocation. Snow argued that the causative agent of cholera was a living cell that multiplied with great rapidity but was too small to be seen under the microscopes then in use.[68] It remained for Louis Pasteur (1822–1895) to validate the germ theory formally by showing that the microorganisms responsible for fermentation were not generated spontaneously but came from the air.[58] On this basis, Lord Lister revolutionized surgery by using carbolic acid to combat atmospheric germs and to minimize "putrefication" in surgical procedures.[66]

In Pasteur's wake, bacteria were cultured with great frequency from ill persons and, all too often, erroneously identified as causal agents. Robert Koch (1843–1910), who first isolated the bacterial causes of tuberculosis and cholera, also was the first to introduce scientific rigor to the proof of primary causation. His famed "postulates," to be satisfied before a causal relation between a bacterium and a disease could be accepted, required that (1) the presence of the agent be demonstrated in every case by its recovery in pure culture; (2) the agent not be found in cases of other disease; (3) once isolated, the agent be capable of reproducing the disease in experimental animals; and (4) the agent be recovered in pure culture from such experimental disease.[31] Koch's postulates since have been modified, in large part to meet problems posed by viruses. As obligate intracellular parasites, viruses cannot be "cultivated in pure culture." Also, they often are host-specific and will not produce disease in an animal model. Thus, other considerations have been invoked as elements of proof. These include the significance of recovery of the agent from the diseased tissues, the demonstration of a rise in titer of specific antibody in temporal relation to the disease, and, most conclusive, the specific preventive effect of vaccines containing the viral antigen.[37] One further situation, not recognized by Koch, is that infections with true pathogens do not always cause disease. Indeed, we now recognize pathogenicity (defined as the proportion of infections that result in disease) as an important characteristic of infectious disease agents.

DISEASE CAUSATION

General Concepts

Causation of infectious diseases is simple conceptually and relatively well understood. It is defined in terms of the primary cause and the contributing factors (or secondary causes). The former is the specific microorganism (disease agent) without which the particular disease cannot occur. The contributing factors affect the likelihood that infection will occur and help determine that disease will result, given infection. Because identification of the causative agent in a comparatively few instances has led to the development of effective means for specific protective immunization (diphtheria and tetanus toxoids, vaccines against polio and measles), it is common to overemphasize the importance of the primary cause. Here it is important to note that infection and disease are not synonymous, although infection obviously is necessary for disease to occur. *Infection* denotes colonization, multiplication, and, indeed, completion of the entire pathogenetic process of the organism in the host, usually including induction of an immune response, but without producing recognizable pathologic and clinical manifestations. *Disease* is present when pathologic and clinical changes occur with infection. Many examples exist of infections that may or may not produce disease in the host, such as poliomyelitis, mumps, and influenza; moreover, disease, when it occurs, varies in severity among infected people. Some infections, of course, produce full-blown disease in all infected susceptibles; measles is an example. Simple *colonization*, in contrast to infection and disease, is a state in which the organism parasitizes the host at an appropriate site, replicates, and often persists but fails to proceed further with the processes of infection and disease, including the induction of immunity. The *carrier state*, in which the organism persists over time and can be infective for others, may occur after colonization, infection, or disease.

Many contributing factors, largely related to the host and to the conditions of exposure, determine whether colonization takes place and whether the subsequent processes of infection and disease occur. These contributing or risk factors are many and various and from the standpoint of the host may include, but are not limited to, age; sex; race; immune status; the general state of health, including underlying diseases; and genetic constitution. Similarly, non-host contributing factors may be many, including climate, the presence of vectors, sanitation, intimacy of exposure, and socioeconomic conditions. These contributing factors vary among infectious diseases and are discussed with the specific diseases.

Agent Factors

Disease agents can be described collectively as invading, living parasites. They belong to one of four classes of organisms: (1) higher parasites (parasites, for short), which are multicellular animals (metazoa) including mites and helminths (worms) or single-celled animals (protozoa) such as amebae and the malarial parasites; (2) fungi; (3) bacteria, including two groups of obligate intracellular parasites—rickettsiae and chlamydiae; and (4) viruses. In other chapters, specific pathogens belonging to these groups are described with respect to their distinguishing characteristics and the diseases they cause. Our interest here is in indicating what attributes of living parasites are significant epidemiologically. Properties directly important to disease occurrence are those that relate to the perpetuation of the agent as a species, that govern the type of contact required to infect humans, and that determine the production of disease. Also important are characteristics useful in classification and specific identification of agents. Some of the important attributes are "intrinsic," in that they can be described after appropriate direct examination of the agent. Others can be described only on the basis of the behavior of the agents in the host; hence, they are "host-related."

Intrinsic Properties

Classification of agents is important because knowledge of well-known agents, such as polioviruses, may help predict critical properties of similarly classified but less well-studied agents, such as the numerous other enteroviruses. Precise identification of agents is basic to the specific recognition of infections and related disease. Both are dependent on intrinsic properties, including morphology (which alone provides the basis for identifying most higher parasites), chemical composition (the type of nucleic acid is important to viral classification), and antigenic character. The last is central to specific identification of agent isolates and of antibodies induced by infection. Requirements for growth or replication provide keys to the identification of some bacteria (e.g., sugar fermentation) and of many viruses that replicate optimally or only in cultures of certain types of cells incubated at specified temperatures. For example, rhinoviruses replicate best in human diploid cells incubated at 33° C.

Many infectious agents possess intrinsic markers that can distinguish strains within species. They also may assist in tracking down the source of infection. Thus, within poliovirus serotypes, strains from a common source can be identified by their distinctive antigenic character, for example, vaccine-like strains recovered from family contacts of vaccinated infants. More sophisticated techniques, such as nucleotide sequencing of wild polioviruses or outer-membrane serotyping of meningococci of the same group, permit epidemiologic tracing of various strains of the same organism worldwide. Similarly, sporadic cases of typhoid fever may be traced to a common carrier by the vulnerability of the isolated bacteria to lysis with a particular type of bacteriophage. Such markers also may be related to the pathogenicity of strains. Thus, infection with a temperate bacteriophage renders *Corynebacterium diphtheriae* toxigenic and so identifies pathogenic strains.

Several intrinsic properties relate to transmission and long-term survival of infectious agents. Persistence in the free state outside of the host depends on requirements for replication (viruses replicate only within the cells of their hosts, whereas the nutrient requirements of bacteria often exist in food or milk) and on viability under natural conditions of temperature, moisture, and radiation. The ability of agents to persist determines whether transmission requires direct contact, as with influenza viruses, or can involve indirect mechanisms operating over longer periods. Examples include polioviruses, typhoid bacilli, and the bacterial cause of legionellosis.

The spectrum of animals and arthropods that an agent can parasitize (the host range) helps determine the possibilities for successful links in the transmission and reservoir mechanisms. The broader the range, the greater the possibilities. Agents utilizing arthropod vectors include St. Louis encephalitis virus and *Rickettsia prowazekii* (the cause of epidemic typhus). The former can infect many avian and mammalian species, as well as a wide range of mosquitoes, whereas the latter is restricted largely to the louse vector and the human host. Among agents requiring no vector, many infect only humans (diphtheria bacillus, measles virus), whereas others have multiple natural hosts (rabies virus, most of the *Salmonella* group of bacteria).

Elaboration of exotoxins is an intrinsic attribute of many bacteria and contributes in varying degrees to disease pathogenesis and, indirectly, to immunity in many infections. Another attribute, which can operate in two opposing ways, is susceptibility to chemotherapeutic agents or antibiotics. Successful treatment may shorten the period of communicability, as in streptococcal infections, but may lead to relaxed precautions against infection; syphilis and gonorrhea are notable examples.

Instability of some intrinsic attributes, reflecting emergence of genetically different populations because of mutations, selective pressures, gene or plasmid transfer between bacteria, or genetic recombination, can be of great importance. One example is resistance to chemotherapeutic or antibiotic agents that may result from selective pressure (the probable explanation for the rapid acquisition by gonococci of sulfanilamide resistance) or plasmid transfer between enteric bacteria of resistance to antibiotics. Such resistance currently is of increasing importance, as exemplified by the appearance of multidrug-resistant *Mycobacterium tuberculosis* and penicillin-resistant pneumococci. Change in antigenic character can diminish the effectiveness of immunity and complicate specific recognition of infection. Influenza A virus is the classic example of this, with periodic major changes in either or both critical surface antigens—hemagglutinin and neuraminidase—associated with pandemic disease and progressive minor change in the hemagglutinin in the interpandemic period. The major changes are thought to result from genetic recombination occurring when a human strain and an animal strain concurrently infect a single human or animal host. The resulting recombinant strain presumably possesses the infectivity for humans of the human strain and one or both surface antigens of the animal strain. The lesser interpandemic antigenic drift probably results from selective pressure as the virus replicates in partially immune human hosts. Finally, the emergence of new diseases, such as St. Louis encephalitis, which first affected humans in Paris, Illinois, in 1932, or of a known disease in a new reservoir, possibly exemplified by sylvatic plague in the United States, can be the result of adaptation of the agent to a new host.

Host-Related Properties

As already noted, some epidemiologically important properties of infectious agents can be defined only with reference to specific hosts. These include infectivity, pathogenicity, virulence, and immunogenicity.

Infectivity (ability to invade and multiply in a host) is measured conceptually in terms of the minimum number of infective particles required to establish an infection. This number, which can vary from one host to another and within the same host with portal of entry and host age, can be determined only experimentally. Hence, except for relatively benign agents such as rhinoviruses or vaccine strains of polioviruses with which challenge of human volunteers is permissible, infectivity of agents for humans must be inferred from the facility with which they spread in populations or, more directly, from the frequency with which infection develops in exposed susceptible individuals within a reasonable incubation period (the *secondary attack rate*). By this latter measure, measles, varicella, and polioviruses are highly infective; rubella, mumps, and rhinoviruses are of intermediate infectivity; and typhoid and tubercle bacilli are of relatively low infectivity. However, it is important to recognize that infectivity and, indeed, pathogenicity may vary among strains of the same organism. As examples, the infectivity of group A streptococci is related directly to the amount of M protein in the cell wall, and strains of *Staphylococcus aureus* that appear identical in the laboratory may differ strikingly in both infectivity and virulence. Additionally, there is some evidence that strains of influenza A may vary in infectivity and virulence independent of preexisting immunity in the host.

Pathogenicity (ability to induce disease) is measured in

terms of the proportion of infections that result in disease. This ordinarily can be determined readily by studies of the occurrence and outcome of naturally occurring infections in humans. Although this proportion may be affected by the size of the infecting dose and by a number of host factors, including age, commonly prevalent agents can be ordered in a gradient of pathogenicity on the basis of the usual outcome of infection. Highly pathogenic agents include typhoid bacilli, rabies, measles, varicella, and rhinoviruses. Those of intermediate pathogenicity include rubella, mumps, and adenoviruses; polioviruses and the tubercle bacillus are of low pathogenicity.

Virulence, offered as a synonym for pathogenicity in medical dictionaries, is defined more usefully as a measure of the severity of the disease that does occur. Various criteria may be employed: days confined to bed, serious sequelae such as persisting paralysis, and death. The measure of virulence is the number of severe cases over the total number of cases, which, when death is the criterion, becomes the familiar *case-fatality rate*. With this as our measure, the viral agents previously mentioned fall into a very different gradient from that based on pathogenicity. Rabies virus (with a case-fatality rate of 100 per cent) and AIDS (with a case-fatality rate of 80 per cent) qualify as highly virulent, and only poliovirus (with a case-fatality rate of 7 to 10 per cent for paralytic disease) can be classed as moderately virulent. Measles, with an occasional death from encephalitis or other complication, is far down the scale but still ahead of mumps, varicella, nonfetal rubella, and rhinoviruses, for which case-fatality is near zero.

Immunogenicity (ability to induce specific immunity) is measured best in terms of the degree and duration of resistance conferred by infection. Although agents may differ in respect to the immunogenicity of their intrinsic protective antigens, more important factors are the sites of primary infection and disease and the amount of antigen formed during infection to stimulate host response. Superficial sites, such as the respiratory mucosa, are guarded chiefly by secretory antibody, which is poorly persistent; agents such as rhinoviruses, which replicate only at such sites, are relatively ineffective stimulants of systemic immune response. The amounts of the respective toxins released during clinical tetanus and diphtheria usually do not induce satisfactory immunity. In contrast, systemic viral infections, as with measles and yellow fever viruses, induce solid and long-lasting immunity.

The Agent-Host Relation

How the host contributes to the survival of the agent as a species is of interest here. At the minimum, the infected host provides a shelter in which the agent can multiply and from which it may spread. Key questions are how long the agent can persist in the host and over what period and by what avenues it can escape. We shall consider escape in relation to modes of transmission in a later section. Discussed here are the time relations and descriptive terms of different phases of infection. These are suggested schematically in Figure 7–1.

When the agent is not recoverable readily but perhaps is hidden within host cells or at some other site, infection is termed *latent*. Conversely, when the agent is being shed, as in feces or respiratory secretions, or can be recovered from blood or tissues, infection is said to be *patent*. Infections necessarily are latent at first (the *latent period*) and become patent when the agent has multiplied sufficiently for shedding to begin. The *period of communicability* commonly begins soon after initial shedding and continues as long as the level of shedding is sufficient for transmission. Rapidity of disease spread thus is related to the length of the latent period, which almost always is shorter (sometimes much shorter) than the better known *incubation period* (time until disease develops). Indeed, the period of communicability has no consistent relation to either the occurrence or duration of disease.

Persistence in the host is important to the agent for as long as escape remains possible. The period of persistence (Fig. 7–1) varies widely among agents. Infection terminates completely within 2 to 3 weeks with many, such as most respiratory viruses, and after a few months with some, such as polio- or adenoviruses. Truly persistent lifelong infections may become permanently latent (associated with lifelong immunity, as with measles); may remain permanently patent (about 3 per cent of typhoid cases, numerous hepatitis B virus infections); may be intermittently patent (herpesvirus infections); or, after years of latency, may recrudesce with both patency and associated disease (tuberculosis, Brill disease due to *R. prowazekii*, herpes zoster due to varicella-zoster virus).

Reservoirs of Infectious Agents

Reservoir is defined here as the total mechanism responsible for perpetuation of an agent species. With the possible exception of agents such as tetanus spores that virtually have indefinite potential for survival in the environment, the reservoir is a continuing chain of transmission from one host to another (host now including both vertebrate and invertebrate species). Chains with long links, requiring infrequent transmissions, especially are favorable to agent species survival.

Among agents for which man is the only natural vertebrate host, a number of contrasting patterns exist. By far the most common is exemplified by infections with most respiratory viruses, characterized by short latent periods (1 to several

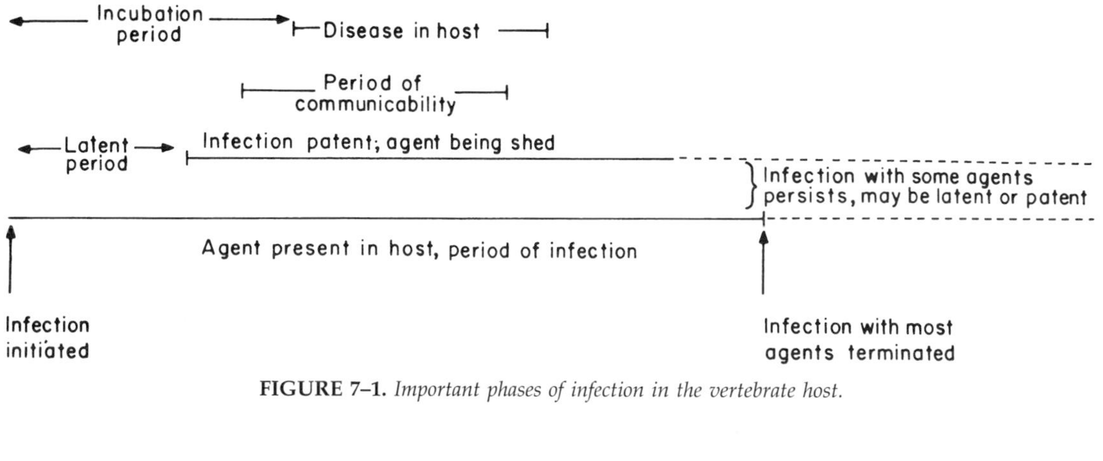

FIGURE 7–1. *Important phases of infection in the vertebrate host.*

days) and relatively short periods of communicability (rarely longer than 1 week). Thus, the links are short, and frequent transmissions are necessary. At the other extreme are long-persisting infections associated with continuous (typhoid carriers, hepatitis B virus, HIV) or intermittent (herpes simplex virus) patency or shedding. The links in this case may be as long as the postinfection life of the host and make possible generation-to-generation transmission. This also may occur via congenital infection, as in mice infected with lymphocytic choriomeningitis virus. Possible or probable examples of this in humans include cytomegalovirus and hepatitis B virus infections. Long links also occur in persistent infections that, after many years of latency, recrudesce to cause disease and renewed shedding (varicella-zoster virus and *R. prowazekii*). Basically similar patterns are known or presumed to exist in the case of zoonotic agents pathogenic for humans and their natural lower vertebrate hosts. Examples include *Brucella* and such arenaviruses as lymphocytic choriomeningitis virus and Machupo virus of Bolivian hemorrhagic fever.

When infection of invertebrate (vector) hosts constitutes a link in the chain of transmission, a wide range of reservoir patterns is possible. The simplest involves those agents for which humans are the only natural vertebrate hosts (malarial parasites, *R. prowazekii*, the several dengue viruses), with the chain formed of alternating links of human and vector infection. More commonly, the basic reservoir is a similar alternating chain primarily involving lower vertebrate hosts, with humans an opportunistic and usually blind-end host. Examples include murine typhus rickettsiae and plague bacillus (both cycling primarily in rats and rat fleas), Lyme disease, and various arboviruses (yellow fever, St. Louis encephalitis). In the case of the latter, the relatively broad vertebrate (numerous avian and mammalian species) and invertebrate (various mosquito species) host range results in very complex patterns that, in a given area, are defined by the prevalent susceptible host species. With some interesting exceptions to be mentioned shortly, the links in these chains are defined temporally by the persistence of patent infection in the vertebrate host and the relatively short life span of the invertebrate host. In temperate regions, where vector abundance is highly seasonal, how many agents survive over winter is a still unanswered question.

Several aspects of infection of the invertebrate (vector) host are important. Typically, infection is acquired in a blood meal and endures for (and does not influence) the life span of the arthropod. Thus, hibernating arthropods may constitute the long link in the chain by which the agent survives the winter. In at least two cases, infection kills the vector: *R. prowazekii* in the body louse and plague bacilli in the rat flea. As with malaria, infection of the arthropod also may permit completion of an essential stage in the developmental cycle of the agent. Finally, transmission of infection from arthropod to arthropod may constitute alternate or necessary links in the chain. Transovarial transmission of *Rickettsia tsutsugamushi* (scrub typhus) in mites is essential because the individual mite feeds only once, during the larval stage, on vertebrate hosts. Transovarial transmission also occurs in ticks infected with *Rickettsia rickettsii* (Rocky Mountain spotted fever) and in *Aedes triseriatus* mosquitoes infected with La Crosse virus (California encephalitis), in both cases affording an overwintering mechanism. Venereal transmission of La Crosse virus between mosquitoes also has been demonstrated.[70]

Finally, the inanimate environment can play a role in the reservoir mechanism. This occurs with bacteria that can multiply in the free state (salmonellae and staphylococci in food) and with agents endowed with unusual survival capacity (tetanus bacillus and *Histoplasma capsulatum*, both of which form highly resistant spores). It also occurs when a brief sojourn under proper environmental conditions is required for a necessary stage in the life cycle, e.g., hookworm eggs from human feces must hatch into larvae to become infectious.

Transmission Mechanisms

Transmission, in this context, is defined as the transport of an agent from one vertebrate host to another. It involves escape from the source host and conveyance to and entry into the recipient host. The basic interdependence of these sequential steps results in their usual correspondence, as illustrated in Table 7–1, together with specific disease examples. Although humans are the usual or only source for most agents of human disease, lower vertebrates serve as the major or only (rabies virus) source for some pathogens.

The basic concepts presented in Table 7–1 are fairly self-evident, but some definitions and special comments may be helpful. *Fomites* are intimate personal articles, such as handkerchiefs, playthings, and eating utensils. *Direct contact* includes not only physical contact (shaking hands, kissing, sexual intercourse) but also, in practice, short-range (within 10 feet) airborne transmission by heavy droplets that contain hundreds or thousands of organisms and descend rapidly to the ground or floor. As an example, these heavy droplets are the primary route of transmission of group A streptococcal pharyngitis.[71]

Indirect transmission for respiratory and some other infections includes acquisition of organisms from dust (such as tubercle bacilli), from fomites (inanimate objects in the environment such as bedding), and from airborne droplet nuclei (small droplets containing only one or a few organisms that promptly dry, float in the air for long periods, and may be wafted for moderately long distances, such as between rooms or floors in a hospital). Transmission by airborne droplet nuclei is limited to highly infectious agents, such as varicella; because respiratory colonization with group A streptococci requires a large inoculum, airborne droplet nuclei play no role in their transmission. Other forms of indirect transmission include inanimate vectors, such as food, milk, and water, which are frequent vehicles for spread, particularly of intesti-

TABLE 7–1. Typical Correspondence Between Escape from Host, Conveyance, and Portal of Entry

Agent Shed Via	How Conveyed	Portal of Entry	Disease Example
Respiratory secretions	Airborne droplets, fomites, direct contact	Respiratory	Common cold, influenza
Feces	Food, fomites, water, flies	Oral	Poliomyelitis, typhoid
Blood	Arthropod vector	Skin, via insect bite	Typhus, dengue, malaria
Lesion exudate	Direct contact, sexual intercourse, fomites, flies	Skin, genital or ocular mucous membrane	Carbuncles, syphilis, trachoma, inclusion conjunctivitis

nal infections. Another source of indirect transmission is the animate vector, which either may function as a vehicle for transport (as with flies that carry organisms from feces to food) or actually may be infected. In the latter case, multiplication and transformation in the vector are required for transmission, as with African trypanosomiasis and the tsetse fly.

Conveyance ends when the agent reaches a portal of entry, which, to be effective, must provide ready access to a tissue in which the pathogen can lodge and multiply. For a given agent, a particular portal (nasal or genital mucosa, oral) often is obligatory or usual, but alternate portals may be possible. For instance, rhinoviruses replicate only in the nasal mucosa, whereas typhus rickettsiae typically enter through skin broken by a louse bite but also can infect via ocular or respiratory mucous membranes.

Host Factors

As suggested in considering why paralytic poliomyelitis occurs, a number of biologic and behavioral characteristics of the human host influence the occurrence of infection and of resulting disease. In this section, we shall consider biologic and behavioral factors separately and systematically. Although the host characteristics to be considered are of widely differing natures, they operate by influencing one or more of the following: degree of exposure, innate susceptibility to infection, and the likelihood of specific immunity. Although much of the discussion will focus on the individual human host, it should be remembered that factors that influence individuals also affect whole human populations.

Infection of the Host

Before considering specific factors, it is helpful to review the initiation, course, and possible consequences to the host of infection. A key principle to be emphasized is the usual existence of a gradient of response to exposure and infection. Because of this, the occurrence of characteristic overt disease is a notably unreliable measure of the extent of activity of a disease agent. Thus, given exposure, infection may not occur; given infection, disease may not result, and given disease, it may range from trivial to the fully developed syndrome "characteristic" of the agent.

An inadequate challenge dose, an unsuitable portal of entry, or specific host immunity may explain failure of infection to occur. Whether infection causes disease and the extent, nature, and outcome of resulting disease are determined partly by host-related properties of the agent (pathogenicity and virulence) and partly by host defense mechanisms, a variety of which confront the infectious agent that has reached a site of primary infection. Bacteria and other extracellular parasites stimulate an inflammatory response at the site in an effort to localize the invaders by a retaining fibrin network, and the invaders are destroyed by congregating numerous phagocytic cells. Organisms that escape are confronted with gauntlets of sinusoidal passages lined by phagocytic cells in regional (lymph nodes) and blood stream (bone marrow, spleen, and liver) filters.

A further line of defense develops with the immune response to infection. Developing antibody combines with perninting extracellular organisms to render them more vulnerable to phagocytosis and digestion. The initial presence of specific antibody would, of course, have prevented or greatly limited invasion of the host. Viruses and other intracellular parasites are vulnerable to antibody while extracellular, as during invasion, but are unaffected once they have gained entrance into cells. Indeed, in the case of some viruses (lymphocytic choriomeningitis virus in the mouse is a model), the cell-mediated component of immune response may play a role in the pathogenesis of disease rather than as an aid in defense. Fortunately, viruses do remain vulnerable to the inhibitory action of interferon, a low-molecular-weight protein elaborated by virus-infected cells.

Several aspects of the outcome of infection are important. The first is survival of the host. Death is an obviously unsatisfactory outcome not only for the host but also for the many agents whose survival as a species depends on the host. The remaining aspects relate to the surviving host. Was recovery from disease complete, or were there permanent sequelae? If the latter, were they stationary (as paralysis due to polioviruses) or potentially progressive (rheumatic heart disease due to streptococcal infection, pulmonary tuberculosis)? Another aspect, persistence of the agent, was discussed previously under agent-host relations. The final aspect is the state of postinfection resistance. If this is incomplete, the recovered host may experience reinfection, with or without disease, and again become a source of infection for others.

Biologic Factors

Biologic factors include characteristics such as age, sex, and race (ethnic group), which are so important and easily ascertained that determining their relation to disease occurrence is a usual first step in an epidemiologic description. They also include other factors such as genetic make-up, general health status, and specific immunity.

The influence of *age* is illustrated best by means of common diseases such as varicella, measles, and mumps (before the advent of vaccines). All three occur predominantly in young children, who are affected because of their usual lack of immunity and their high risk of exposure to their age peers, among whom most infections occur. Older people are very likely to be immune and, unless they are parents of young children, are unlikely to be exposed to infected individuals. Age also is related often to the outcome of infections in nonimmune individuals. Demonstration of this requires that all infections be recognized and classified according to the occurrence and severity of resulting disease. When many or most infections are subclinical (as with polioviruses), the increase in case fatality with age is apparent immediately, but special studies are required to show that the proportion of infections that resulted in disease also increased with age. In contrast, the case-fatality rate for pertussis is highest in young infants. With measles and varicella viruses, infections at any age usually result in characteristic disease, but, as exemplified by measles encephalitis, the frequency of serious disease rises with age.

That *sex* is a factor is indicated by the fact that with a few notable exceptions, such as acute respiratory disease in women, diseases typically are somewhat more frequent in males than in females. The question, with respect to any particular disease, is whether these differences between sexes reflect innate differences in susceptibility to disease or are due to sex-associated differences in play habits and occupation that affect the degree of exposure or host stress. Typical, for example, is the increased intrahousehold exposure of mothers and older girls who nurse ill family members. Antibody prevalence studies in the prevaccine era indicate that boys and girls had the same risk of infection with polioviruses, but the sex ratio for paralytic polio was 1.3:1.0 (male versus female). In those older than 20 years of age, this was reversed. Possible explanations are the greater stress among boys (due to more strenuous play) and women (associated with child-bearing and rearing of children).

The incidence of many diseases varies greatly between

groups defined by *race* or *ethnic group*. These are explained most often by socioeconomically determined differences in environmental factors related to degree of exposure and resulting prevalence of immunity or, in more recent times, similarly determined differences in health awareness affecting acceptance of vaccines. However, ethnic groups share many genetically determined traits that may include heightened susceptibility or resistance to specific disease agents. Thus, selective pressures may be invoked to explain the greater resistance of whites (exposed for countless centuries) to tuberculosis and the heightened resistance of blacks to malaria.

Genetically determined susceptibility or resistance also may be manifested by differences in disease occurrence between families or kinships of the same ethnicity. However, before such differences can be attributed to genetic factors, adequate account must be taken of the many environmental influences that affect families as groups, including common exposures, diet, education, and economic status. The classic twin studies of Kallman and Reisner[41] clearly demonstrated a genetic contribution to the occurrence of tuberculosis. Similarly conclusive data for other infectious diseases are almost nonexistent, although the operation of genetic factors in humans must be presumed from observations in animal models, such as the classic work of Webster, who, by selective inbreeding, developed strains of mice susceptible or resistant to specific neurotropic viruses.[72] The genetic control of immune response, also demonstrated in the mouse model, provides a probable explanation, the operation of which in humans is suggested strongly by studies showing a relation of human leukocyte antigen specificities to chronic hepatitis B antigenemia.[35]

General health status includes physiologic state, nutritional status, presence of intercurrent disease, and stress. The importance of such factors is, in many cases, commonly accepted, although rarely documented by well-controlled studies. Infancy, during which immune mechanisms are immature, is a period of special vulnerability to many infectious diseases. Puberty, associated with rapid growth and change in endocrine balance, is a period of vulnerability to acne and tuberculosis. Pregnancy predisposes to both tuberculosis and paralytic poliomyelitis.

Gross protein malnutrition causes definite impairment of cell-mediated immune response[42] and correspondingly increased susceptibility to bacterial and parasitic infection. Viral infections are less influenced by immune response but may depress response (and so further increase susceptibility) to concurrent other infections, thus perhaps explaining the high mortality associated with measles in malnourished infants. Whereas a current viral infection, by an interfering effect, may induce temporary resistance to a second virus, preexisting or intercurrent disease more commonly decreases host resistance to infection. Thus, diabetics especially are vulnerable to bacterial infections; measles and pertussis may reactivate quiescent tuberculosis; and, perhaps of greatest importance, otherwise benign respiratory viral infections, notably influenza, may pave the way for serious bacterial pneumonia. Furthermore, AIDS enhances the susceptibility to and severity of tuberculosis, toxoplasmosis, and other infections.

Finally, stress induced by widely divergent stimuli (including strong emotions, physical exertion, trauma, or excessive heat or cold), according to Selye,[65] may operate through a pituitary-adrenocortical hormonal path to decrease resistance to infections. Widely accepted examples include physical exertion, child-bearing, and rearing of children as factors predisposing to paralytic poliomyelitis and both pregnancy and rapid growth during puberty as causes of reactivation of quiescent tuberculosis.

Immunity and *immune response* are discussed elsewhere, but some general comments are appropriate here. In discussing infection in the host, immune response was considered as a potential mechanism of defense and, thus, significant in relation to the course and outcome of infections. Although clearly important in recovery from bacterial infection, antibody response is of questionable significance in viral infections because viruses within cells are inaccessible to antibody, and, by the time antibody appears, many or most susceptible cells have been infected already. Nonetheless, the importance of antibody in viral infections is suggested by the great vulnerability of immunodeficient children to vaccine strains of poliovirus and by the sometimes beneficial effect of passive immunotherapy in progressive vaccinia and herpes zoster. Cell-induced immune response may play a greater role in pathogenesis of disease (tuberculosis, lymphocytic choriomeningitis virus infection in mice) than in recovery from infection.

Immunity to a specific agent usually develops after natural infection, may be induced by vaccine, or may be acquired passively, as from mothers by infants or via injected gammaglobulin, in which case it is of relatively short duration. A key point is that *immunity* is a relative term. At its maximum (exemplified by postinfection immunity to measles), protection against infection virtually is absolute. At the other extreme (exemplified by many respiratory viral infections), susceptibility to infection persists or wanes as with pertussis, although severity of related disease may be reduced. In most instances, protection appears to be mediated by antibody, although the possible contribution of cell-mediated immunity has not been well evaluated.

To the extent that immunity protects the individual against infection or acts to minimize shedding of the agent when infection occurs, the immune host can play no part in the spread of an infectious agent in the population. This suggests that if a sufficient proportion of a population were immune, a contact-transmitted agent could not spread and any nonimmune members would be spared exposure. The obvious question, then, is: What proportion must be immune to achieve effective *herd immunity*? Unfortunately, as explained in a review of this problem,[25] there is no practical answer to the question. The underlying concept is valid only in homogeneous, randomly mixing populations in which all possible pairs of individuals have the same probability of making effective contact. In real life, this situation does not exist and is approximated only in small, closed groups. Whether an agent can spread is not determined by the proportion of immune individuals but by the number (not the proportion) of susceptible individuals and the opportunity for contact between them. Thus, even though measles vaccine has been used extensively in the United States, outbreaks of measles continue to occur in segments of the population, often defined by race and low economic status, that failed to accept vaccine. Indeed, a major outbreak of measles with approximately 30,000 cases occurred in 1989 and 1990 in the United States.[3]

Human Behavior

Governed largely by habits of the individual and the customs and culture of groups, human behavior greatly influences exposure to and modes of transmission of disease agents. Cultural factors also underlie attitudes toward preventive and curative practices. These relations are so self-evident for the most part that no detailed discussion is needed.

Water is a potential vehicle for many agents. When commonly imbibed without boiling, as in the United States, community water systems constitute potential channels for transmission that, fortunately, usually are guarded well. Unfortunately, occasional operational failures occur, as exemplified by a failure of a water quality monitoring device in a filtration plant that resulted in an outbreak of *Cryptosporidium* diarrhea affecting an estimated 403,000 persons in Milwaukee in 1993.[49] Foods and milk likewise are excellent vehicles for disease transmission, especially those items that are consumed raw or after minimal cooking. Well-known examples include trichinosis from undercooked pork, fish tapeworm from raw fish (a delicacy in Scandinavia and parts of the Orient), and various forms of food poisoning due to bacterial contamination during handling, poor refrigeration, and inadequate cooking. In recent years, outbreaks of bloody diarrhea, often associated with the hemolytic-uremic syndrome, due to *Escherichia coli* O157:H7 have occurred as a result of improperly prepared products of bovine orgin, particularly ground beef.[33] Of special interest to pediatricians is the fallacious belief that raw milk possesses nutritive values (and flavor) that are lost in pasteurization. The result is "certified" milk that, although produced under carefully controlled conditions, has been a frequent vehicle of streptococci, salmonellae, and other agents of serious disease, including *E. coli* O157:H7.

Closely related to water and foods is the disposal of human excreta. Casual defecation near habitations (as by young children) or in or near running water (a cultural compulsion in India) leads to dissemination of enteric pathogens by filth flies and by water. Use of human feces (night soil) in the Orient and elsewhere to fertilize crops commonly eaten raw, such as strawberries and lettuce, has an obvious similar potential.

Many more individual types of behavior also are important. Infrequent bathing and laundering of clothes favor infestation with body lice. Inadequate clothing increases exposure to arthropod vectors and, as in young children lightly clad for summer weather, facilitates their exchange of feces. Going barefoot provides exposure to hookworm larvae. Hand washing minimizes the role of hands in indirect transmission of both enteric (fecal) and respiratory (nasal secretion) pathogens. Rhinovirus infections result from inserting contaminated fingers into the nose and eyes.[34] Intimate personal contact (hand shaking, kissing, sexual intercourse, and play between young children) fosters the spread of a wide variety of agents. Even recreation, such as travel, picnics, and camping, may lead to unusual exposures to disease agents. Sexual behavior is associated with the transmission of a number of infections, including HIV, syphilis, gonorrhea, group B streptococci, and hepatitis B. Finally, education and individual temperament influence utilization of health services and conscious avoidance of obvious health hazards.

Environmental Factors

The environment in concept embraces all that is external to the individual human host. It is convenient to recognize three broad environmental areas: *physical*, which includes geologic and climatologic or meteorologic features; *biologic*, comprising all flora and fauna, which additionally include all living microbial pathogens; and *socioeconomic*, which extends to encompass the interrelations of humans. Identification and evaluation of the contribution of environmental factors often are difficult. Their multiplicity and the fact that they typically operate in an interrelated manner complicate the appraisal of their individual contributions. Also, environmental factors often act through very indirect paths, and some have the potential to affect the agent, the host, and the agent-host relationship. Thus, solar radiation is lethal for many pathogens in the free state, helps humans to synthesize vitamin D, and can provoke recrudescence of a latent herpes simplex virus infection to cause recurrent fever blisters. Finally, the capacity of people to modify adverse environmental conditions beneficially is another important factor.

The contribution of environmental factors to disease occurrence is complex. Here only a few selected examples will be used to illustrate how environmental factors influence the occurrence of infectious diseases.

Geographic and Geologic Factors

Dr. Jacques May was a pioneer in the field of geographic epidemiology, or medical geography.[51] Although many pathogens, dependent on humans for their survival, are active wherever people congregate in sufficient numbers, many others occur only in certain geographic areas. From a practical standpoint, knowledge of the geographic distribution of such diseases is important in preparing travelers to minimize exposure to agents prevalent at their destinations. However, Dr. May's (and our) greater interest is in the factors that influence disease distribution and how they act.

Spread of disease agents on a global scale requires their transport. This obviously is influenced by distance alone and by geographic features—mountain ranges, oceans, rivers—that assist or impede travel. The importance of these factors declines as the extent and speed of travel increase but remains substantial, especially in developing countries. The minimal effect of geographic barriers in containing highly infective agents is exemplified by pandemic influenza, which in 1957 and again in 1968 emerged in the Orient and rapidly spread throughout the world.

More importantly, geography acts indirectly by determining other aspects of the environment. Climate is determined largely by latitude, longitude, altitude, and relation to bodies of water and mountain ranges and, in turn, greatly influences the biologic environment and human activity. Geography, together with geologic factors, also influences the socioeconomic environment. The natural paths of travel (including waterways), natural harbors, and the location of mineral deposits help determine where populations will concentrate. Water supply, dependent in part on geologic formations, is a factor limiting population size and, together with fossil fuels and mineral deposits, influences the type, extent, and location of industrial development. Soil types vary greatly in their ability to hold and purify water and in their capacity to support vegetation, which, in turn, influences the type and abundance of animal life. Thus, soil is a determinant of the type and importance of agriculture and a major factor influencing the biologic environment.

Climate

The term *climate* describes the typical annual pattern, with its seasonal variation, of climatologic conditions in a specified region. These conditions (climatologic factors) include solar radiation, temperature, humidity, barometric pressure, winds, precipitation (and drought), and lightning. These factors can affect infectious disease agents directly. Many microbial agents in the free state are vulnerable to excessive heat and radiation and uncontrolled drying. The life cycles and reservoir mechanisms of many pathogens, including higher parasites, are dependent on appropriate temperature and humidity. Maturation and hatching of hookworm larvae from ova deposited in the soil require both warmth and reasonable humidity, and the multiplication of malarial parasites and arboviruses in their mosquito vectors and the very abundance of the vectors are favored by warm temperatures.

The usual seasonal variation in incidence of specific infectious diseases suggests important influences of climatologic factors, but how they operate may be hard to determine. Overall, respiratory infections are more frequent in the colder months, but within this period (roughly October through mid-May), there are great variations in the relative prevalences of the many respiratory pathogens. Rhinoviruses, for example, peak in the early fall and spring, and influenza viruses are most active in midwinter. Parainfluenza virus infections usually peak in the fall. Increased congregation of people indoors clearly facilitates transmission, and fluctuations in temperature and humidity not only affect the viability of agents in airborne droplet nuclei or on fingers or fomites but also may affect host susceptibility to infection. Enterically transmitted infections are most frequent in the warmer months, presumably largely because of season-related changes in host behavior. Thus, the outdoor play of scantily clad children facilitates the spread of skin infection and fecally shed agents, such as enteroviruses. Rotavirus infections are an exception, being most frequent in colder months. More completely understood are the seasonal patterns of infections spread by arthropod vectors, reflecting seasonal variations in the abundance and activity of both the vectors and the various lower vertebrate host species, which together constitute the reservoir mechanisms of the specific disease agents. Indeed, climate overall, as a major determinant of the biologic environment, helps determine both the abundance and particular species of flora and fauna in a given area.

Longer-term changes in climate have been associated with changes in patterns of infection. As an example, the hantavirus outbreak in the southwestern United States in 1993 has been attributed to unusually heavy precipitation in the spring of 1993 after 6 years of drought, resulting in marked proliferation of the deer mouse population, the reservoir of the virus.[74]

Of current concern is the gradual increase in global temperatures.[59] The geographic distribution of malaria is dependent on environmental temperature, and year-to-year variations associated with climatic changes in affected areas in Africa have been observed. In the Western Hemisphere, dengue and arboviral encephalitides, among other mosquito-born disorders, have shown year-to-year variations in incidence dependent on temperature growth and humidity. In another vein, the reproduction of toxin-producing marine algae and *Vibrio cholerae* is enhanced by warmer sea water, and this may have been responsible for recent outbreaks of disorders attributable to these organisms. These short-term, climate-related variations in the distribution of infections may presage longer-term shifts in affected geographic areas as the atmosphere warms, as a result of which, for example, temperate areas may experience infections ordinarily associated with tropical or subtropical regions.

Biologic Environment

As living entities, microbial pathogens and higher parasites by definition are included in the biologic environment, as are the vertebrate and invertebrate species involved in the transmission and reservoir mechanisms of numerous agents. For some, including malarial parasites, dengue viruses, and epidemic typhus rickettsiae, humans are the only important vertebrate host, but transmission is by arthropod vectors. For others, referred to as zoonoses, the vertebrate reservoir hosts are subhuman. Some of these, including the rickettsiae of Rocky Mountain spotted fever and murine typhus, the plague bacillus, and the many arboviruses, require arthropod vectors for transmission, whereas others are spread directly from their natural vertebrate hosts (various salmonellae, rabies virus, and the agents of psittacosis and trichinosis).

Although bacterial and fungal pathogens are classified as plants (viruses are unassigned), the direct contribution of the biologic environment to disease occurrence chiefly involves fauna. Plant and animal life also act in less direct and often interrelated ways. Human susceptibility to infection is affected by nutritional states to which both flora and fauna contribute. The nature and abundance of plant life and its seasonal stage of development determine the number and species of wildlife present. Thus, grassy plains favor herbivores, and fruits and berries attract many birds. Arthropod vectors often depend on plants for breeding sites (tree holes, plant axils) and utilize foliage for shelter from predators and for resting in a suitable microclimate. The steel-belted radial automobile tire has changed the geographic distribution of at least one type of arthropod-borne viral disease: La Crosse encephalitis.[18] Used casings are difficult to recycle because of the steel belting and are discarded in waste dumps, often in large piles. Rain water accumulates in the casings, forming a favorable environment for breeding mosquitoes, which also serve as vehicles for transportation of infected larvae from one area to another. Animals provide them with blood meals that often contain infectious agents. The biologic environment also influences people's recreational activities (hunting, bird watching) and, by determining the type and importance of agriculture, their occupation and economy.

Socioeconomic Environment

This difficult-to-define sector depends on the density and distribution of populations; the available natural resources; the level of social, political, cultural, and scientific development; and, most importantly, the interrelations of people. Socioeconomic factors typically affect health by indirect means, and because they often closely are interrelated, evaluation of the impact of individual factors is very difficult.

The relation of population distribution and density to the occurrence of infectious diseases is substantial. Increasing density favors the spread of infectious agents to humans from both human and nonhuman sources; hence, the occurrence of related disease and development of immunity. In large and dense populations, agents such as measles virus typically infect in early childhood and persist because a sufficient number of new susceptible individuals are added continuously by birth. In smaller populations, the agents are unable to persist and are reintroduced at unpredictable intervals, so that "childhood" diseases long may be delayed. Populations of urban and rural areas differ not only in relative density but also in other important ways. Exposure to zoonotic agents, especially those prevalent in wildlife and livestock, is greater in rural areas, although rats and stray dogs may abound in city slums. Environmental sanitation (protection of water and milk supplies, safe disposal of sewage) often is a personal problem for rural residents but is handled by cooperative efforts in urban populations. Also, the relative importance of schools and school buses in facilitating exchange of infectious agents is greater in rural areas, where isolation of farm residents otherwise restricts contacts between young children.

The basic population unit is the household, membership in which has similar implications for health in both rural and urban areas. Family members are similar genetically; share a common diet and economic status; are subject to the same cultural, religious, and educational influences; and are exposed to a common local physical and biologic environment. Most important for contact-transmitted diseases, intrafamilial contacts are prolonged and increase in intimacy with household crowding. Prolonged contact especially is important for persisting infections, such as herpes simplex and tuberculosis. Family size, regardless of the degree of crowding, particularly is important for acute infections because it determines the number of potential introducers who bring home infections acquired elsewhere. The likelihood of exposure in early childhood thus increases with family size. Except for early infancy, a period of special vulnerability to some agents (respiratory syncytial virus, pertussis), early exposure is beneficial because most resulting infections are less apt to have serious consequences.

A population with a highly developed *social and political structure*, through its capacity for cooperative action, enjoys many advantages that directly or indirectly benefit health. These include provision of both preventive and curative health services, effective environmental sanitation, and well-developed educational facilities. Education, of course, closely relates to personal health practices that are based on understanding what individuals should do to minimize disease hazards. Schools, where the educational process begins, have been identified already as important in the exchange of disease agents between children, especially those spread by contact and airborne droplet nuclei. This is offset in part by the benefits derived from school-based immunization programs.

Economic status affects the occurrence of diseases indirectly through its relation to adequacy of housing, nutrition, level of education, and availability and use of health services. It also is related closely to occupation, which may be associated with exposure to specific infections, such as Rocky Mountain spotted fever (cattle and sheep herders in the West) and ornithosis (workers in poultry-processing plants).

DISEASE OCCURRENCE IN POPULATIONS

Patterns of disease occurrence that are not random but instead reflect the influences of underlying causes (risk factors) not only help predict future disease occurrence but also provide important clues to understanding causation.

Describing the pattern of disease occurrence begins with definition and classification of disease in the individual so that cases can be identified and counted reliably. Next, we must develop ways to express the occurrence of disease in defined populations quantitatively. The full description results from the composite answers to three questions: Who is attacked? Where does disease occur? When does it occur?

Infection and Disease in the Individual

Epidemiologic interest focuses on the specific etiologic identification of infection and disease, terms that, it must be stressed, are not synonyms. Technically, any deviation from normal function or state constitutes disease. Because virtually all infections cause at least some deviation from the normal state (such as change in white cell pattern in the blood and mobilization of such cells at the site of infection), they do in fact cause disease. Practically, however, many infections result in no clinical evidence of disease and are important to the individual only because they induce immunity. Because subclinical infections help define the overall pattern of occurrence of infection and often play a significant role in its spread, their recognition is important epidemiologically. Unfortunately, subclinical infections go unrecognized except when healthy persons are observed for infection in longitudinal or case-control studies.

Thus, only infections resulting in disease usually come to our attention. To the extent that they are recognized etiologically, they provide the earliest and most available indicator of the pattern of infection in the population.

With a few exceptions, such as measles and chickenpox, the resulting clinical syndromes are not pathognomonic and confront the clinician with the familiar problem of differential diagnosis. Basically, clinical manifestations depend more on the site(s) of disease than on the infecting agent. Because the number of possible disease targets in the body is small and the number of potential agents is large, reasonably distinct clinical entities may be caused by any of several agents. Notable examples include "common colds," some 40 per cent of which are caused by rhinoviruses and 60 per cent by any of many other viruses, and aseptic meningitis, which may be due to mumps virus or to any of some 70 enteroviruses. Also, infection with a specific agent may have several possible clinical outcomes. Infections with polioviruses usually (perhaps 80 per cent) are subclinical but can result in brief febrile illness (about 15 per cent), in aseptic meningitis (4 to 5 per cent), or in classic paralytic disease (<1 per cent). Response to agents with multiple potential targets varies even more widely. Group B coxsackieviruses, for example, can cause such disparate entities as acute upper respiratory disease, aseptic meningitis, polio-like paralytic disease, myocarditis (often fatal in infants), and epidemic pleurodynia (Bornholm disease).

Knowledge of the agents active in the community when a given illness occurs helps narrow the differential diagnosis, but confirmed etiologic diagnosis requires laboratory assistance. This usually takes the form of identifying the agent by culture, by direct visualization in specimens related to the disease site, by antigen detection by probes or other techniques, or by demonstration of specific antibody response in tests of "acute" and "convalescent" serum pairs. Diagnosis is most secure when both approaches suggest infection with the same agent. Although demonstration of the agent in relation to the disease site carries special weight (for example, in a pharyngeal swab specimen from a respiratory illness), its presence could be the result of preexisting persisting infection unrelated to the current illness. Antibody response, indicative of newly acquired infection, excludes the latter possibility.

Describing Infection and Disease in Populations

At this point, it is necessary to introduce and define terms and quantitative expressions commonly employed in describing the occurrence of infection and disease in populations. First, however, we must consider briefly the availability and reliability of the relevant information.

Sources of Information

There are many sources of data regarding the incidence of infectious diseases. These include United States Vital Statistics, which tabulates only fatal cases; the Centers for Disease Control and Prevention, which receives reports of specific notifiable diseases from state health departments and summarizes them in the *Morbidity and Mortality Weekly Report;* and state and local health departments. Unfortunately, these vary in their completeness by source and by disease because of underreporting, subjects who are not seen, and errors in diagnosis. Among the different states, there are some variations in reporting requirements and, indeed, adherence to these requirements by providers. Reporting is most complete for uncommon but characteristic disorders of unusual interest, particularly if they are severe or fatal and require hospitalization, such as rabies, anthrax, trichinosis, plague, and diphtheria. Reporting is enhanced by outbreaks, as with measles and classic pertussis in recent years. Some notifiable infections, such as leptospirosis and atypical pertussis in partially immune persons, often are unrecognized and therefore not reported. Even after the advent of penicillin until about 25 years ago, scarlet fever was a reportable disease in many areas. Because some health departments continued to subject affected households to useless or outmoded stringent control measures, such as quarantine or cremating the child's doll in the furnace, some physicians simply treated the patient with antibiotics and ignored reporting requirements. Today physicians occasionally fail to report venereal diseases to avoid embarrassment to patients. Another source of data, often useful in certain areas, are state health department laboratories, which perform specific microbiologic or serologic tests for providers.

Infectious diseases that are not notifiable by law pose a difficult problem. Although necessarily limited in scale, longitudinal studies of defined populations of families have yielded valuable information. Examples include the Cleveland Family Study conducted by Dingle and colleagues[21]; the Tecumseh, Michigan, study of respiratory illnesses directed by Monto and associates[52, 53]; and the New York and Seattle Virus Watch studies.[17, 22, 26–30, 69] Finally, well-designed serosurveys make possible reliable estimates of rates of prior infection with agents that induce long-persisting antibody.

International data on the incidence of infectious diseases are less precise except in well-developed countries, such as the United Kingdom and Canada. For the developing world, the World Health Organization and the United Nations International Children's Emergency Fund provide estimates of the incidences of morbidity and mortality from various infectious diseases in different nations based on local reports, which are not collected systematically necessarily. Continuing collection of such data is important for monitoring the effects of the Expanded Program on Immunization, which is directed at controlling the major vaccine-preventable diseases of childhood. More difficult to develop are definitive data about the incidence and causation of the respiratory and diarrheal diseases that are estimated to kill up to 6 million children annually in the developing world (about 5 per cent of the yearly birth cohort).

Of maximum importance is a disease definition that is as useful as possible, which means that the sensitivity and specificity of the definition should be so balanced that as many cases of the disease as possible are identified, while confusion that occurs when other disorders with overlapping manifestations meet criteria that are too nonspecific is avoided. An optimum disease definition particularly is important in developing approaches to preventive measures, in searching for clues to causation of a new disease, in enabling comparisons among different studies, and in clinical trials of prophylactic or therapeutic measures. A well-known example of a useful disease definition is the Jones criteria for the diagnosis of rheumatic fever, established in 1944 at the request of the National Research Council in an effort to bring order out of chaos at a time when the disease was a major problem in both the civilian and military populations.[40] These criteria were modified in 1955 to enhance their specificity by making evidence of a prior group A streptococcal infection a sine qua non for the reason that too many cases of polyarthritis of other causes met the original criteria.[2]

Recognizing the importance of standardized diagnostic criteria for surveillance of infectious diseases of public health importance, in 1990 the Centers for Disease Control and Prevention published case definitions for reportable infections.[9] Optimum utilization of these criteria and reporting of confirmed and probable cases to proper authorities are of particular importance currently when, for a variety of reasons, some formerly well-controlled contagious diseases are recrudescent. All states mandate reporting of contagious diseases of major public health importance, particularly those of childhood such as measles and poliomyelitis; for uncommon disorders, such as listeriosis, and for some common disorders that are differentiated less readily etiologically, such as influenza, requirements for reporting vary.[16]

Definitions of Terms and Rates

Two commonly employed (and often misused) terms—*incidence* and *prevalence*—have significantly distinct meanings. *Incidence* refers to new occurrences of infection or disease in a population during a specified period, commonly a year, whereas *prevalence* refers to the state (infected, ill, immune) of individuals in a population at a specified point in time (point prevalence).

To describe variations in occurrence over limited periods within a single population such as a city or a state, simple *numerical incidence* (number of cases or infections) often is employed, for example, daily or weekly (during an epidemic), monthly (to reflect seasonal patterns), or annually (to compare successive years). However, comparisons between different populations or subgroups within a population or at widely separated times in the same population require use of the *incidence rate,* or *attack rate.* This is defined as follows:

Number of new occurrences (cases, infections) within a specified period/population at midperiod × 100; 1000; 10,000; etc.

Thus, if 10,000 cases of influenza occurred in a city of 200,000 people in a year, the incidence (or attack) rate would be expressed as 5 per 100 per year.

Unlike *incidence,* which is useful for both acute and persistent conditions, *prevalence* is employed usefully only in describing states of relatively long duration (months or years), such as immunity, persisting infection, and chronic disease. Thus, in relation to an acute disease such as influenza, we speak of the incidence of disease and the prevalence of immunity (reflected by antibody). Because most interest is in comparisons of different populations or population subgroups, prevalence is expressed customarily as the *prevalence rate.* This is defined as follows:

Number of persons (infected, ill, or immune) at a given point in time/population at that time × 100; 1000; 10,000; etc.

For infections transmitted by contact, the frequency with which infection or disease occurs among exposed susceptible persons provides a measure of the infectivity of the agent. This frequency, called the *secondary attack rate,* is defined as follows:

Number of contacts becoming infected or ill within the maximum incubation period/total number of "susceptibles" exposed × 100

The secondary attack rate is applied usefully only to relatively closed groups, households, or classrooms, where exposure safely can be presumed for all members. The first, or primary, case is the presumed source of exposure; other cases occurring within less than the minimum incubation period are called *coprimary cases.* In calculating the secondary attack rate, primary and coprimary cases are excluded from both numerator and denominator. Subsequent cases occurring within the maximum incubation period constitute the secondary cases. Those developing later are excluded as derived from outside sources or from tertiary spread. The exclusion of immune individuals from the denominator is feasible only for diseases (measles, chickenpox) sufficiently characteristic clinically that the history serves to identify them. Although immune individuals are not identifiable readily in the case of common respiratory diseases, the secondary attack rate based on all exposed members of the group still remains a useful tool. Its usefulness decreases, however, when the period of communicability of the primary case (as with *Mycoplasma pneumoniae*) is longer than the incubation period because distinction between secondary and tertiary cases becomes difficult.

Finally, the occurrence of death due to a specific disease is expressed in two different ways. One, the *cause-specific mortality rate*, is defined as follows:

Number of deaths from the disease in a given year in a population/total population at midyear × 100,000

This is a measure of the effect of the disease on the population. The potential significance of the disease to the affected individual is suggested by the *case-fatality rate* (or *ratio*), which is defined as follows:

Number of deaths from the disease within a specified period/number of cases in the same period × 100

Relating Infection and Disease to Personal Characteristics

A multiplicity of attributes may serve to distinguish one person from another. Some are determined at conception: age, sex, ethnicity, genetic make-up, and birth order. Others, far more numerous, are acquired subsequently. These may be biologic (specific immunity, nutritional state), behavioral (smoking, dietary, recreational habits), or socioeconomic (occupation, educational level, marital status). As indicated in discussing host factors in disease causation, many of these attributes relate to exposure to disease agents or to susceptibility or resistance to the effects of such agents and hence to the occurrence and severity of disease.

Relative Usefulness and Importance of Attributes

Personal attributes vary in both usefulness and importance in describing the occurrence of infection and disease. Usefulness depends chiefly on the ease and reliability with which the prevalence of an attribute in the population can be determined. Although almost any potentially relevant attribute of an individual patient can be identified, it is not very useful for purposes of description unless we can estimate how many people in the population also possess the attribute. From census data or other accessible records, numbers of people in groups defined by age, sex, race, occupation, or marital status can be estimated easily. However, special surveys would be necessary to estimate the prevalence of specific immunities or of possibly significant exposures, such as to household pets.

The importance of personal characteristics to disease description varies in two ways. One is in the degree of association that exists between an attribute and a specific disease. For example, age is associated strongly with disease due to prevalent contagious agents, whereas sex usually is not. The second way is in the independence or relative interdependence of attributes as variables. Inherent characteristics, such as age, sex, and ethnic origin, are independent of one another, whereas acquired attributes rarely are. As examples, the nature of interpersonal contacts, degree of personal hygiene, and usual forms of recreation are associated closely with age or sex, or both. The common interdependence of attributes means that before making inference from a particular association, one should explore association with other, possibly correlated attributes. Some examples will emerge in the following discussion of a few of the most commonly used characteristics.

Age Patterns

Occurrence of infection and disease in general is so strongly related to age that, until possible differences in age distribution are taken into account, differences in occurrence between population subgroups defined by other attributes cannot be interpreted meaningfully. Fortunately, age as an attribute is ascertained easily and reliably for both affected individuals and the total membership of the relevant population. Description of the age pattern involves only computing a series of *age-specific rates* for sequential age groups, usually defined in intervals of 5 years or multiples thereof (0 to 4, 5 to 9, 10 to 19, etc.). For conditions of pediatric concern, the use of single-year intervals (<1, 1, 2, 3, and 4 years) to cover early childhood may be more informative. Affected persons in an age group form the numerator, and all persons in the population in that age group serve as the denominator. Rates so computed describe the age profile of immunity at a specified point in time (age-specific antibody prevalence rates), of new infections or disease (age-specific incidence rates), or of deaths due to a disease (disease- and age-specific mortality rates).

Age-specific incidence rates for acute infectious diseases indicate the risk of disease in each age group and, depending on the disease agent, reflect more or less accurately the underlying age-specific infection rates. Reasons that disease and infection rates may differ can be illustrated by comparing measles and polioviruses. Measles infection usually results in typical disease, and the concordance between the two rates is very close. In the case of polioviruses (in the period before vaccines were available), not only was the proportion of subclinical infections high overall, but also it varied inversely with age.

Age-Adjustment of Rates

The need to take age distribution into account when comparing disease in different populations is indicated when (1) the rates vary with age and (2) the distributions of the populations by age differ substantially. For example, from published United States mortality data for 1983 and 1984, one can compare pneumonia and influenza mortality rates for Alaska and Florida. During those years, there were 89 deaths so recorded in 986,000 Alaskans at risk for an annual mortality rate of 9.0 per 100,000. In contrast, in sunny Florida, there were 4703 deaths from pneumonia and influenza among the 21,792,000 residents at risk for those 2 years, for a rate of 21.6 per 100,000, nearly two and one half times that of Alaska. These are what are called *crude mortality rates*. However, in this instance, these rates are misleading for the reasons that the likelihood of death from pneumonia and influenza increases with age, and the age distributions of the populations of these two states differ strikingly. Indeed, national death rates from these infections are nearly 10-fold greater in people 65 to 74 years of age, compared with those 55 to 64 years of age. For those years, 17.5 per cent and 3.0 per cent of the Florida and Alaska populations, respectively, were 65 years or older. In order to make a valid comparison of the pneumonia and influenza mortality rates for these two states, it is necessary to perform age adjustment, a relatively simple process that will not be detailed here because the method can be found in available texts of biostatistics and epidemiology. Rather simply, what is done is to determine mortality rates for specific age groups (usually 5 or 10 years) for the two populations and calculate the deaths that would be expected in a common (or standard) population for the same age groupings, using the age-specific rates of the populations being compared, in this instance those of Alaska and Florida. Summation of these expected deaths permits calculation of the rates that would have occurred in the standard population if the age-specific rates of Alaska applied and if those of Florida applied. In this example, the age-adjusted mortality rate for pneumonia and influenza for Alaska is 35.2 per 100,000 and that for Florida 21.8, nearly the reverse of the crude rates. (The combined population of the two states was used as the standard.) It should be noted that these age-adjusted rates are not true rates; they are used for comparison. Although often applicable to infectious disease, age-adjusted rates are required almost always for comparisons of morbidity and mortality from chronic diseases.

Sex Patterns

Because sex is a readily ascertained characteristic of the membership of populations, the occurrence of infections and disease in relation to sex is described easily. Its simplest form is the *sex ratio*, the ratio of cases in males to cases in females. This is meaningful only when, as in childhood, the population is about equally divided by sex. Although males exceed females at birth (106:100), the death rates for males exceed those for females at all ages (average, 1.5:1). From about 20 years of age on, females outnumber males, the difference increasing with age. This means that, in comparing sex-specific rates, age adjustment is necessary or, better yet, the age profiles for the sexes should be compared directly so that important differences in the contour can be seen. This is illustrated in Table 7–2, which records the age- and sex-specific occurrence of a polio-like disease of still unknown etiology in Iceland in 1948 and 1949.[67] In this case, the male and female age distributions sufficiently are similar that the unadjusted sex-specific rates can be compared, suggesting that the risk for females was about 1.6 times that for males. However, direct comparison of the corresponding age-specific rates reveals the additional, possibly important fact that the female-male risk ratio for 20 years of age or older (2.05:1) was appreciably greater than that for the younger population (1.2:1).

Ethnic or Racial Patterns

A third attribute by which members of the population can be grouped in describing disease occurrence is race or ethnic origin, the usefulness of which has decreased with the increasing frequency of mixed marriages. The United States census classification is based on information collected as to race and native origin. People of mixed racial parentage are classified by the race of the nonwhite parent or, if both are nonwhite, by that of the father. People of foreign birth are classified by country. Native-born children of foreign-born parents are identified as "foreign stock" and grouped according to parental origin. Thus, census data provide estimates of population subgroups belonging to several "races" (white, black, Native American, Chinese, Japanese) or "foreign stocks" (including both foreign-born and first-generation).

Among such population subgroups, differences in the occurrence of many infections and other diseases have been noted. Knowledge of such differences is useful in case-finding and organizing the application of specific preventive measures. Explanation of the differences is essential to understanding disease causation but often leads to controversy. Subgroups defined by ethnicity possess some similarity in genetic constitution that may determine susceptibility or resistance to specific agents. They also may be affected distinctively by environmental factors because of voluntary or involuntary differences in behavior and pattern of living. The excess occurrence of tuberculosis in black Americans, potentially explainable on the basis of genetic or environmental factors, is a typically controversial phenomenon.

TABLE 7–2. Epidemic Neuromyasthenia in Akureyri, Iceland, 1948 to 1949, by Age and Sex

Age Group (years)	Population		Rate per 100	
	Male	*Female*	*Male*	*Female*
0–4	425	395	0.24	1.26
5–9	313	310	2.88	2.90
10–19	673	687	11.74	13.25
20–29	534	559	5.06	11.99
30–39	455	499	5.49	10.82
40+	939	1098	2.88	5.37
Total	3339	3548	5.12	8.29

Adapted from Sigurdsson, B., Sigurjonsson, J., Sigurdsson, J. H., et al.: A disease epidemic in Iceland simulating poliomyelitis. Am. J. Hyg. *52*:222–238, 1950. © 1950, The Johns Hopkins University Press.

Disease Patterns in Kinships

Genetically determined susceptibility and resistance to specific infectious agents have not yet been associated clearly with recognized genetic markers, such as human leukocyte antigen type, which could serve as a basis for defining population subgroups. Hence, most efforts to look for genetic influences have been studies of disease occurrence in people of differing degrees of relationship within kinships or in the total memberships of different kinships. An example of the former is the classic study of Kallman and Reisner,[41] who found that, within the immediate families of tuberculosis patients who were one of a pair of twins, disease prevalence was related directly to degree of genetic similarity, highest in monozygotic co-twins, next in siblings (including dizygotic co-twins), and least in spouses. The latter approach is illustrated incompletely by a study in South Bend, Indiana, in which it was found that the frequency of paralytic poliomyelitis in the preceding 5 years was significantly greater in the close kinships of current-year polio patients than in the community at large.[62] Unfortunately, the investigator ignored the probability that the close relatives were subject to the same influences related to socioeconomic status and standards of hygiene that helped select the propositi patients from the community population in the first place.[32] To complete the study, the close kinships of healthy control propositi (matched with the patients for age, sex, and socioeconomic status) should have been observed similarly.

Family Episodes of Infection and Disease

With respect to contact-transmitted infectious diseases, the family is more important as the basic epidemiologic subgroup of a population than for its shared genes. Indeed, as described elsewhere in some detail,[24] the continuing observation of family units for episodes of infection and related illness has contributed significantly to knowledge of the epidemiology of widely prevalent disease agents. In the earliest family studies, illness (typically acute upper respiratory) provided the only indication of infection, and all illnesses constituting an apparent family episode were assumed to be caused by the same, albeit unknown, agent. In more recent studies, such as the Virus Watch programs in New York and Seattle,[17, 22, 26–30, 69] the available methodology made it possible to monitor family members for specific infections revealed by virus isolation and/or antibody response, whether related to illness or not.

The situation in all family studies begins with one member's infection, acquired from outside the house. That member then exposes his or her fellow family members. The introductory infection and any infections in those exposed constitute a family episode that is described basically in terms of the times of onset of the related infections and the identities (age, sex, position in the family) of the introducer and both the infected and uninfected contacts. Analysis of cumulated episodes of common respiratory illness, observed in the early studies, identified children as the most frequent introducers (hence important in community spread). The age of the introducers varied with the setting: school age in rural England,[46] 6 years of age or younger in Cleveland,[21] and preschool age in London.[6] Analysis also yielded estimates of cross-infection risks within the family, expressed in terms of secondary attack rates among specified members (for example, younger children) exposed to specified introducers (for example, a school child or a parent). In general, risk of contacts was related inversely by age overall, reflecting the influence of immunity, and to intimacy of within-family contact (ready exchange between spouses and between children nearest in age). Finally, the time relation between onset of illness in the introducer and onset in those exposed serves to define the range of incubation periods.

Studies of the Virus Watch type make it possible to identify and analyze family episodes caused by specific viruses (influenza A) or groups of viruses (adeno- or rhinoviruses), including both subclinical and overt infections. Analysis of the episodes can yield additional information concerning such critical aspects as mode and duration of agent shedding; the spectrum of clinical response to infection, including the proportion that is subclinical; and the significance of prior immunity in the face of close exposure, as measured by the frequency and clinical consequences of reinfections that result. Results of the analysis of adenovirus episodes are illustrative.[27] Virus appears regularly in the feces and less often (about 50 per cent) in the pharynx, and shedding may be abortive (a few days only) or continue intermittently for many months. Overall, half of infections are subclinical, and illness, typically febrile and respiratory, is more common with pharyngeal excretion (65 per cent) than with only fecal shedding (31 per cent). Immunity is 85 per cent protective against infection; reinfections that do occur usually are subclinical. Young children and especially infants younger than 2 years of age are the usual introducers, and within-family spread depends more on duration than on mode of virus excretion by the introducer.

Socioeconomic Patterns

The foregoing illustrates the use and usefulness of several family-related attributes and of immunity. The use of other acquired attributes in describing disease occurrence is either quite limited or self-evident. A partial exception is *socioeconomic status*, which covers a complex of attributes, including levels of education and income and, less tangibly, "social standing." The problem is to discover a useful single indicator. One possibility is area of residence as classified by median income or measures that reflect housing standards, such as type of plumbing and average number of persons per room. Relevant data are available for census tracts, which have proved useful when tracts are reasonably homogeneous.

However, occupation of the head of a household appears to be the one attribute most closely reflecting socioeconomic status. On this basis, the British have defined five broad social classes that directly apply to employed adults and can be extended to cover their dependents. These, in descending order, are professional, intermediate, skilled, partly skilled, and unskilled occupations. For use in the United States, based on census-recorded occupations, these have been translated as follows:

I. Professional workers
II. Nonfarm technical, administrative, and managerial workers
III. Clerical, sales, and skilled workers
IV. Semiskilled workers
V. Nonfarm laborers

Farm workers of whatever level are included in a sixth group as agricultural workers.

Relating Infection and Disease to Place

Place is of interest, epidemiologically, when occupied by humans and, unless indicated as relating to work, recreation, or travel, refers here to residence. Place usually is classified geographically (hemisphere, continent, nation) but also can be classified usefully by environmental characteristics, such as climate, altitude, stage of economic development, population density, and urban or rural nature. Variations in disease occurrence with place reflect parallel variations in the operation of causative factors and raise an important general question. Are these factors to be found in the characteristics of the physical and biologic environment inherent to place or in the characteristics of the inhabitants? The former is suggested when age-adjusted risk of disease increases for immigrants and decreases for emigrants, when risk does not vary among ethnic groups present, and when similar ethnic groups in other places enjoy a lower risk. As a cautionary note, in seeking to explain disease variation with place, one must consider possible differences in reliability and completeness of recognition and reporting of disease.

Global Variation

On the global scale, the World Health Organization collects and publishes information concerning disease occurrence derived from statistics compiled routinely within nations for morbidity from notifiable infectious diseases and for causes of death. Unfortunately, great variations between nations in the quality and availability of medical care and other health services result in corresponding variations in the reliability and completeness of the data collected by the World Health Organization. Generally speaking, basic demographic data and the quality and availability of health services are equally good in well-developed countries, so that specific disease rates can be compared. In less-developed countries, demographic data often are inaccurate and medical services are inconstant in quality and concentrated in urban populations within which their availability varies with economic status. Thus, many illnesses and deaths are unattended medically, especially in rural areas, and births commonly are attended by midwives. Because infant deaths are reported more completely than are births, infant mortality rates notably are unreliable.

Fortunately, with respect to infectious and parasitic diseases, knowledge of disease frequency is less important than is qualitative knowledge of disease distribution and spread. Such knowledge guides the application and enforcement of international control measures and is the basis for advice by physicians to prospective foreign travelers. Important diseases such as yellow fever, plague, and cholera, because of their case-fatality rate and characteristic clinical picture, almost certainly will come to attention when substantial numbers of cases occur. However, knowledge of such occurrence may not be made generally or promptly available. For example, some countries, hopeful that a new outbreak (perhaps of cholera) will be controlled soon, may withhold information to avoid discouraging economically important tourists.

Two additional considerations are relevant to evaluating the disease hazards of foreign travel. One is the fact that recognized disease occurrence in the indigenous population may be an inaccurate index of risk to a newcomer. Particular agents, such as polioviruses and hepatitis A virus, may be so prevalent that infections in natives occur so early in life that they usually are subclinical. The second consideration is the nature of the proposed travel. The usual tourist or business traveler chiefly visits larger population centers and popular tourist attractions where the most important hazards are pathogens transmitted by food or water. Those whose activities will bring them into more intimate contact with the people and the biologic environment (Peace Corps workers, military personnel) may encounter additional hazards, such as rabies and the locally prevalent arthropod-transmitted pathogens.

As suggested in considering geographic influences on disease occurrence, the distribution of many diseases is influenced by relevant environmental factors rather than political boundaries. Hence, in depicting (or predicting) the global distribution of a particular disease, it is useful to identify regions defined by the presence of factors believed to be important to disease occurrence. This particularly is relevant for underdeveloped regions where recognition (and reporting) of disease is unreliable. Thus, the presence of *R. prowazekii* (epidemic typhus) can be predicted safely where heavy clothing is worn but laundered infrequently because of a cool climate and poverty, a combination engendering heavy infestation with the louse vector. Such conditions prevail in underdeveloped areas in the temperate zone and at higher altitudes in the tropics and subtropics. Other examples include murine typhus, to be expected in poorly developed tropical and subtropical areas where warm temperatures ensure that domestic rats harbor an abundance of fleas, and rabies, inevitably present where stray dogs are abundant because of lack of controls and cultural attitudes.

There are important exceptions to the foregoing rule, represented by regions possessing the requisite environmental setting but, fortunately, not yet invaded by the expected disease agent. Recognition of the vulnerability of such regions motivates rigorous efforts to keep the specific agents from entering. A notable example is the Indian subcontinent, which remains free of yellow fever virus despite an overabundance of susceptible humans and monkeys and of an efficient vector, the *Stegomyia* mosquito. Less widely recognized, the Pacific coastal region of the United States possesses the requisite setting (potentially effective mosquito vectors and susceptible lower vertebrate hosts) to maintain the virus of Japanese B encephalitis, which is widely prevalent along the Asian rim of the Pacific Ocean.

For the great majority of agents pathogenic for humans, the chief environmental requisite is a susceptible human population, and most such agents already exist wherever population size and density are sufficient for them to persist. Thus, concern about global spread is limited to a few important pathogens such as the cholera vibrio and influenza virus.

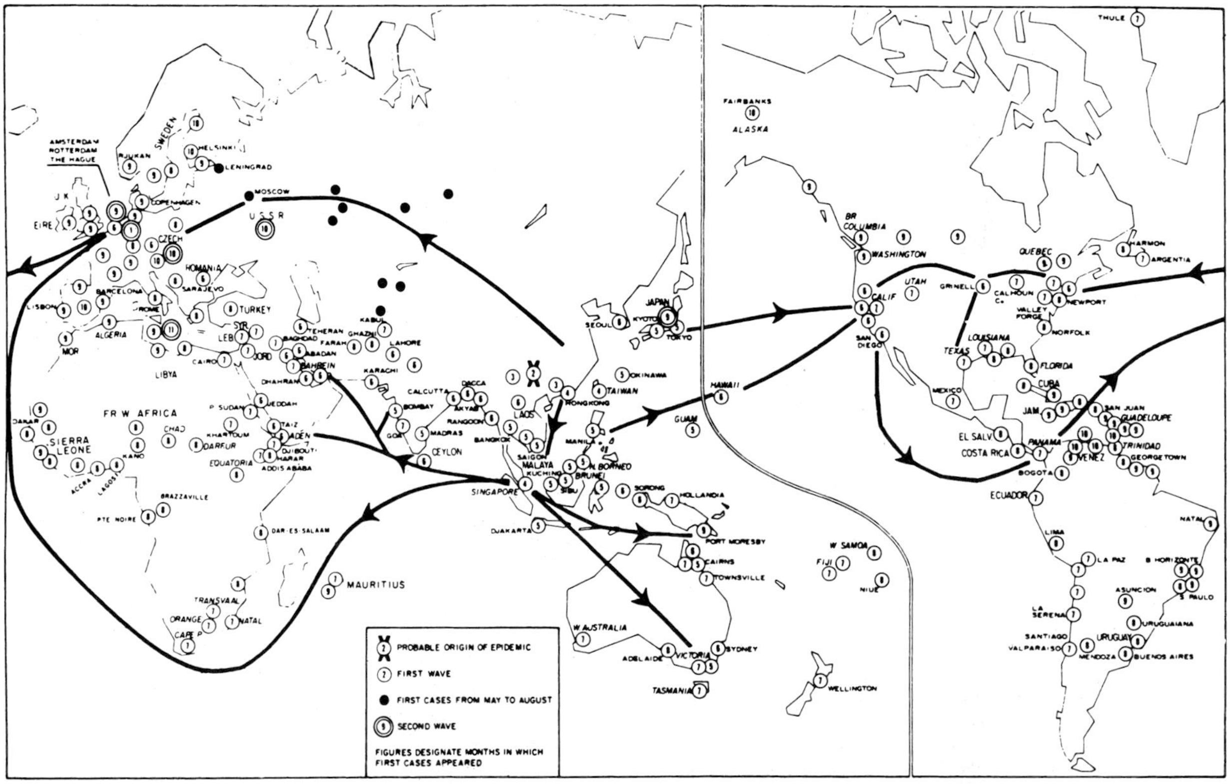

FIGURE 7–2. *Progress of Asian influenza pandemic, February 1957 to January 1958. (Influenza Surveillance Unit: The epidemiology of Asian influenza, 1957–1960. National Communicable Disease Center. From the Centers for Disease Control and Prevention.)*

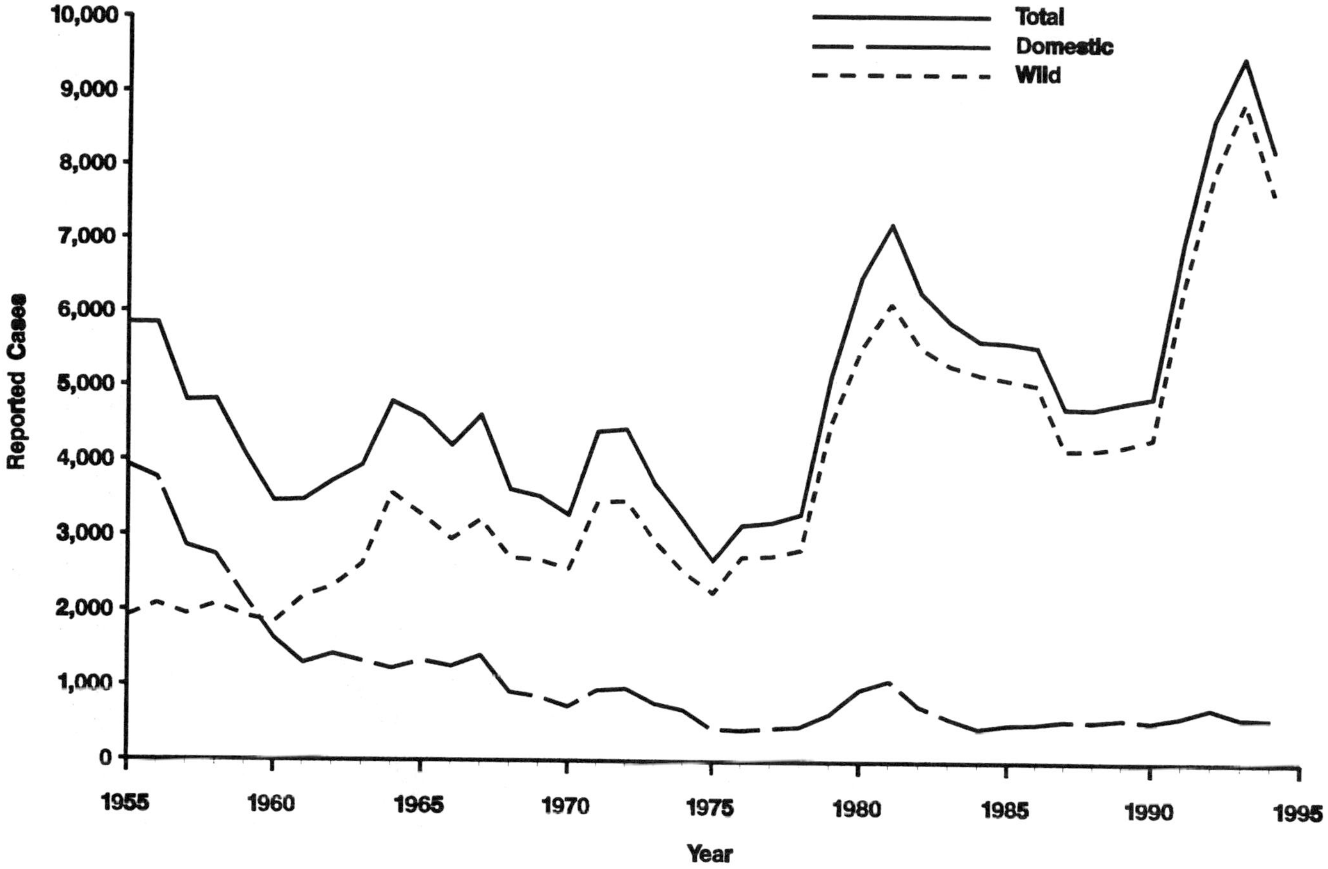

FIGURE 7–3. *Cases of rabies in wild and domestic animals by year, United States and Puerto Rico, 1955 to 1994. (From Centers for Disease Control and Prevention: Summary of notifiable diseases, United States. M. M. W. R. 43:3–80, 1994.)*

(Smallpox now is of no concern because its eradication has been achieved.) Cholera is a special case in that its spread also depends on poor sanitation. Thus, neither persistence nor even limited spread should follow its introduction into highly developed areas. However, although no recognized persistence has followed recent invasions of southern Europe, endemic cholera has existed since at least 1973 in the Louisiana and Texas bayou regions, with inadequately cooked shellfish the source of reported cases.[4] Influenza A virus continues as a major, and so far unstoppable, threat by virtue of its ability to emerge at 10- to 12-year intervals in a new antigenic coat, which largely negates the preexisting widespread immunity. Pandemics emerged in 1957, 1968, and 1977 in the Far East and rapidly spread in both directions around the world. The progress of the 1957 Asian strain is charted in Figure 7–2.

Variations Within Nations

Our concern here is with nations large enough to have substantial variation in environmental factors inherent in place. We will assume (as may be done safely in the case of developed nations such as the United States) that data for different parts of the country can be compared. Because they pose somewhat different problems, we will consider separately what might be called "diseases in nature" communicable to humans and those diseases and disease agents that persist in humans alone.

Among the more important diseases in nature encountered in the United States are rabies, Rocky Mountain spotted fever, and encephalitis caused by one of four arboviruses. On the national level, of most interest are variations in the relative, rather than absolute, risk of infection; simple numerical incidence, rather than rates, often is used to depict disease distribution. This particularly is well illustrated for rabies, which is more important in the United States for the threat it poses (and the drastic treatment required when exposure is suspected) than for the very few human cases that occur.

Data on rabies in animals and humans in the United States are collected by the Centers for Disease Control and Prevention. During the 20 years from 1975 to 1994, there was more than a threefold increase in animal rabies, from 2627 to 8147 cases annually (Fig. 7–3).[11] As indicated in the figure, this increase is limited to wild animals, which account for nearly 95 per cent of animal rabies. The small number of cases in domestic animals, which usually results from wild animals, constitutes a hazard to humans because of close contact. At present in the United States, most human cases result from either bats or domestic animals.

In recent years, an increase in raccoon rabies has occurred, accounting for more than half of all animal rabies in 1993.[44] An epizootic of raccoon rabies that began in the Southeast has spread to northeastern states in the past 15 years and threatens to spread westward into Ohio and other midwestern states. Figure 7–4 shows the geographic distribution of animal rabies in the United States in 1988, and Figure 7–5 shows the shifts that occurred during the ensuing 5 years. Molecular typing techniques, as shown in Figure 7–5, have enabled tracing of animal-specific variants of rabies virus, thus facilitating the orgin and spread of outbreaks in animals. Except for bat rabies, which is distributed widely nationwide, there is very little geographic overlap among other animals

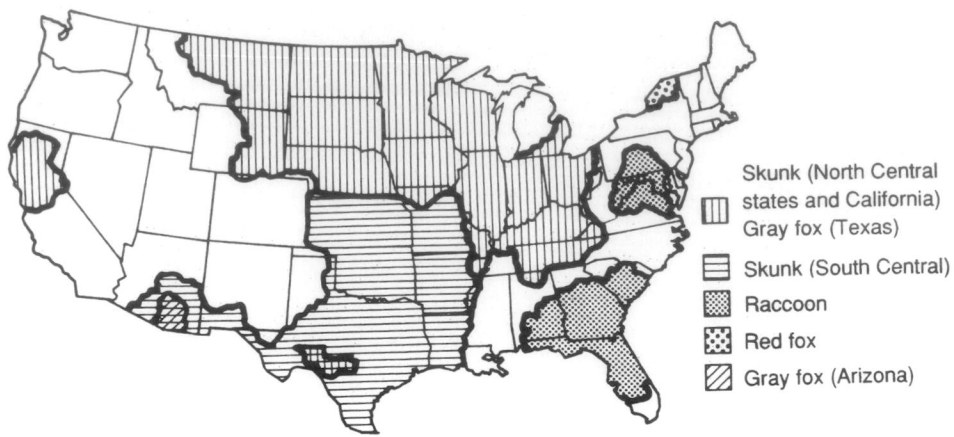

FIGURE 7–4. *Distribution of rabies cases in animals, by geographic divisions, in the United States and United States Territories in 1988. (From Centers for Disease Control: Rabies surveillance, United States, 1988. M. M. W. R. 38:1–21, 1988.)*

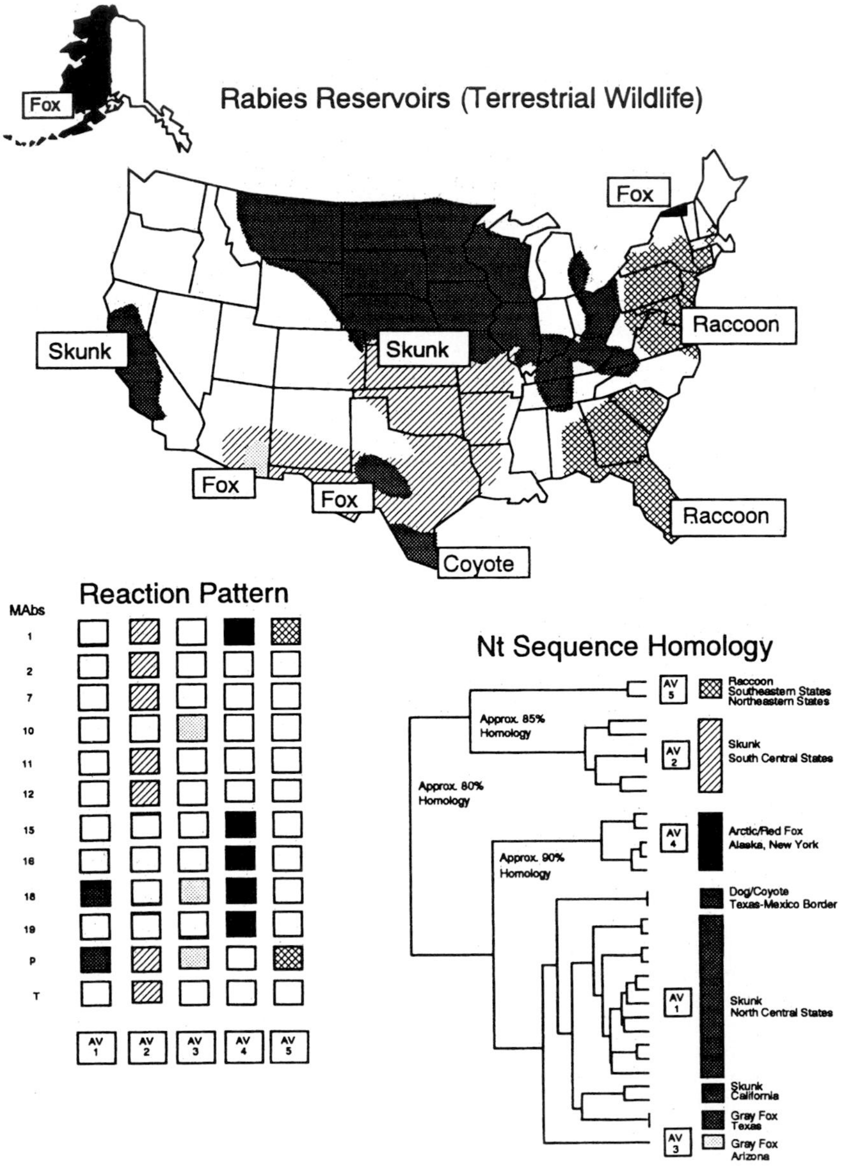

FIGURE 7–5. *Distribution of five distinct rabies variants and their antigenic and genetic patterns and the wild animals primarily affected in the United States, 1988. The filled boxes represent negative reactions by direct immunofluorescence of infected brain material. (From Krebs, J. W., Strine, T. W., Smith, J. S., et al.: Rabies surveillance in the United States during 1993. J. Am. Vet. Med. Assoc. 205:1695–1709.)*

and their specific strains. In addition, this technique has been used to identify the source of strains affecting humans when there is no history of animal bite or other contacts.

The increase in animal rabies is of some concern. Control is difficult if not impossible, and the cost of rabies control in humans and domestic animals is high. During the 10 years from 1986 to 1995, there were 21 cases of human rabies in the United States, but 14 of these were in 1993 to 1995.[11] It is too early to say whether this small increase is of consequence.

The rickettsiae causing Rocky Mountain spotted fever exist in nearly every state, but the frequency of disease is dictated more by the numbers and density of humans living in suburban and rural areas, where the agent persists in a tick–lower vertebrate reservoir, than by the level of infection among the tick vectors. Of the 465 cases reported in 1994, 48 per cent occurred in the South Atlantic coastal states (Maryland through Florida) and 14 per cent in the West South Central area (Arkansas, Louisiana, Oklahoma, and Texas).[11] Only 13 cases were reported from the Mountain region for which the disease was named, in spite of the prevalence of infected ticks.

Four viruses—St. Louis encephalitis, California encephalitis, and western and eastern equine encephalitis—account for more than 99 per cent of all arbovirus encephalitis in the United States. The yearly number of cases between 1964 and 1983 varied widely, from 70 in 1972 and 1979 to 2113 in 1975 (mean, 285), and similar variation occurred in cases of St. Louis encephalitis (range, 5 in 1973 to 1815 in 1975; mean, 181) and western equine encephalitis (range, 0 in 1980 to 172 in 1965; mean, 28). Eastern equine encephalitis was less variable (range, 0 to 14; mean, 5), and California encephalitis was least so (range, 30 to 160; mean, 69). Geographic patterns also exhibit some yearly variation, but St. Louis encephalitis is distributed most widely, overlapping significantly with western equine encephalitis in the West and with eastern equine encephalitis in the Southeast. California encephalitis is concentrated in the upper Midwest.

Infections entirely dependent on humans also do not occur uniformly throughout the United States. The differences largely are temporal. For example, the periodic waves of influenza often are evident first along the East Coast, whereas the 2- to 3-year cycling of measles in metropolitan areas is not synchronized nationally but determined in each area by the local build-up of susceptible individuals. However, there are significant regional differences in the long-term frequency of diseases such as poliomyelitis in the prevaccination era (higher in the North than in the South) and viral hepatitis.

Figure 7–6 shows the incidence rates for hepatitis A and B by states and territories for 1994.[11] For hepatitis A, there are striking geographic differences that are not explained entirely. Different geographic rates for hepatitis B are explained largely by intravenous drug use and male homosexual activity.

Local Patterns of Infection and Disease

"Local" units of population for which demographic data readily are available in the United States include "large" units, such as counties, metropolitan areas, and large cities, which contain smaller units (smaller cities and towns [within counties] and census tracts [within metropolitan areas and large cities]). The smaller units, including unincorporated areas within counties, often can be characterized by variables (urban or rural nature, population density, socioeconomic status, racial or ethnic group) that may help explain observed differences in the occurrence of specific infections and related diseases.

Particularly in relation to outbreaks of acute infectious diseases, spot maps commonly are used to show the local distribution of individual cases. Placing of new pins (a different color each week) to mark the residences of newly reported cases serves to visualize the outbreak's geographic progression. The final distribution of the pins may help to identify a major source of infection. A classic example is the 1854 outbreak of cholera in the Golden Square district of London in which the clustering of residences of fatal cases helped Snow incriminate the Broad Street pump as the source.[68] Sometimes, place of work is a better guide to source of infection than is place of residence. In another classic study, of murine typhus in Montgomery, Alabama, in the early 1920s, the residences of cases (Fig. 7–7) were scattered widely, whereas the work places (Fig. 7–8) were concentrated in relation to feed stores and food-handling businesses, all heavily rat-infested. This led Maxcy to studies demonstrating the basic role of rats and rat fleas in this disease.[50]

Figure 7–9 shows the spot map technique in conjunction with census tract information to illustrate and interpret the change in pattern of poliomyelitis in Kansas City, Missouri, related to the introduction of Salk vaccine in 1955. Cases in the 1946 and 1952 epidemics were scattered widely and, especially in 1952, involved many in the higher-income population in the southwestern part of the city. Vaccine acceptance by the white population was much greater than by the black population, among whom cases in the 1959 epidemic were concentrated sharply. Census tract information also was used in explaining the occurrence of cases of St. Louis encephalitis in the 1964 epidemic in Houston, Texas.[48] Cases tended to cluster in the central area, and the incidence per 100,000 was highest (36.0) in the nonwhite areas; elsewhere, it varied inversely with the socioeconomic level of areas: upper, 11.3; middle, 21.0; and lower, 30.1. However, when census tracts were divided into a central zone and four concentric surrounding zones, incidence rates by zone dropped sharply with increasing distance from the center (from 78.7 in the central zone to 5.4 in the most peripheral) while within each zone rates did not vary appreciably between tracts grouped by socioeconomic level. Thus, distance of residence from the city center (where environmental conditions favored an abundance of vector mosquitoes), rather than race or social class, proved to be the critical determinant.

Temporal Patterns of Infection and Disease

In discussing variations in occurrence of infection and disease with person and place, time was specified or implied. Similarly, in considering variations with time, the populations involved must be defined by place, at least. Because temporal variations in observed effect must reflect parallel variations in the activity of causes, time is another important variable in seeking to identify causative factors.

Definitions

The unit of time employed can vary from hours to decades to centuries. In describing acute outbreaks, the units are short—hours for food poisoning, days or weeks for most infectious diseases—whereas long-term time trends are described in longer units of years or decades. Comparisons extending over one or more decades may be complicated by changes in diagnostic standards and reporting, as occurred with reporting poliomyelitis in the United States, which was extended in the 1940s to include both minor paralysis and nonparalytic disease.

Finally, the meanings of two words commonly employed

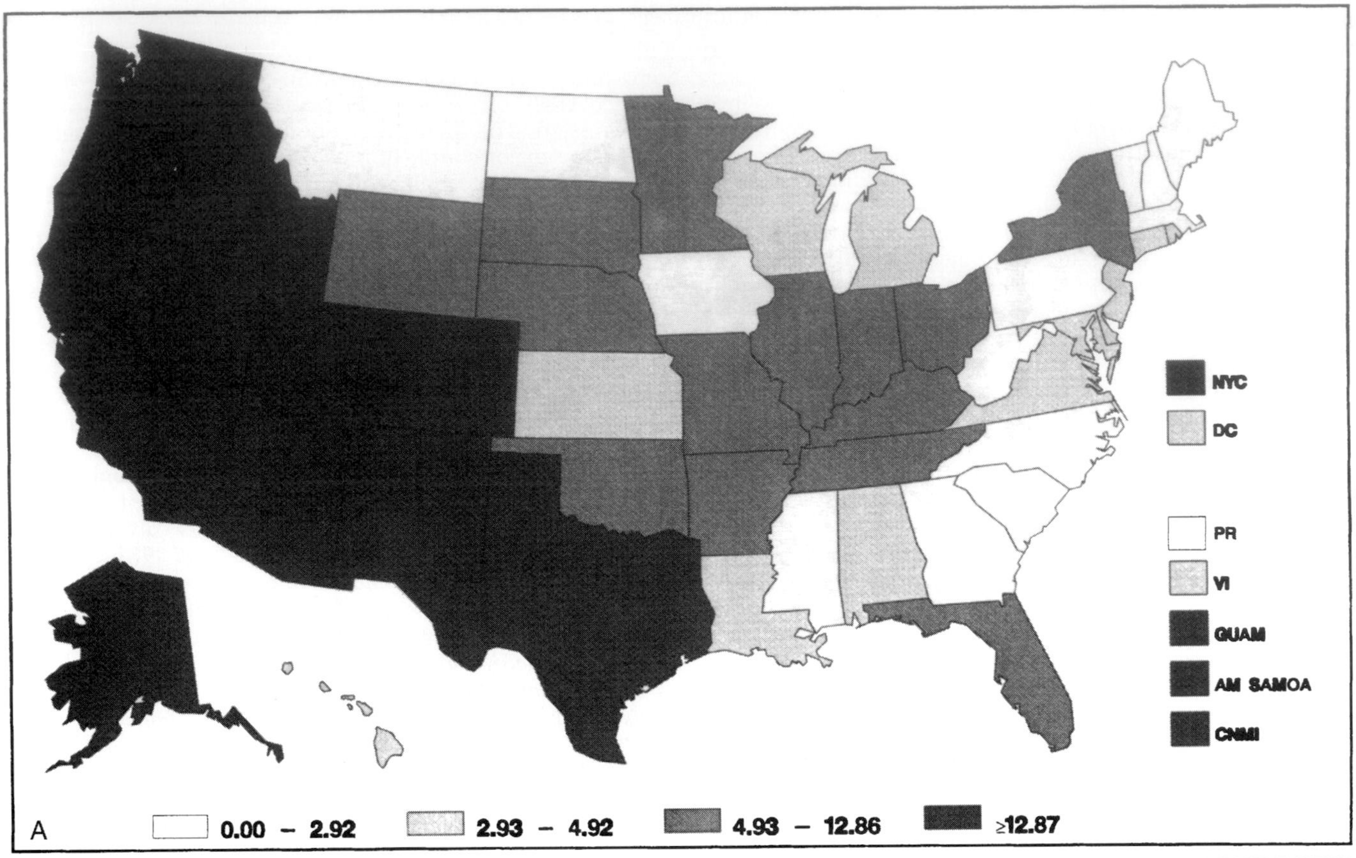

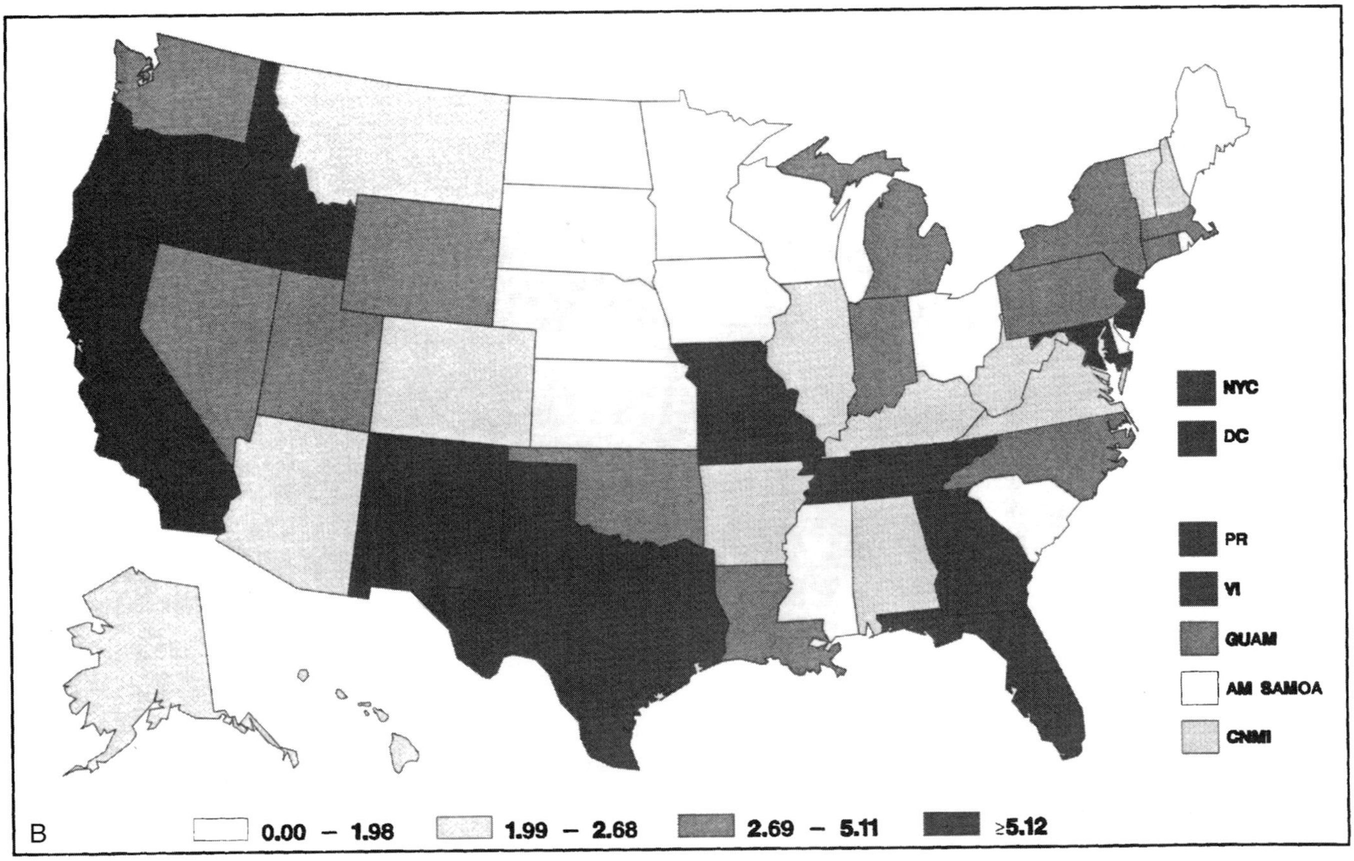

FIGURE 7–6. *Cases of hepatitis A and B per 100,000 population for each state and territory, United States, 1994. (From Centers for Disease Control and Prevention: Summary of notifiable diseases, United States, M. M. W. R. 43:3–80, 1994.)*

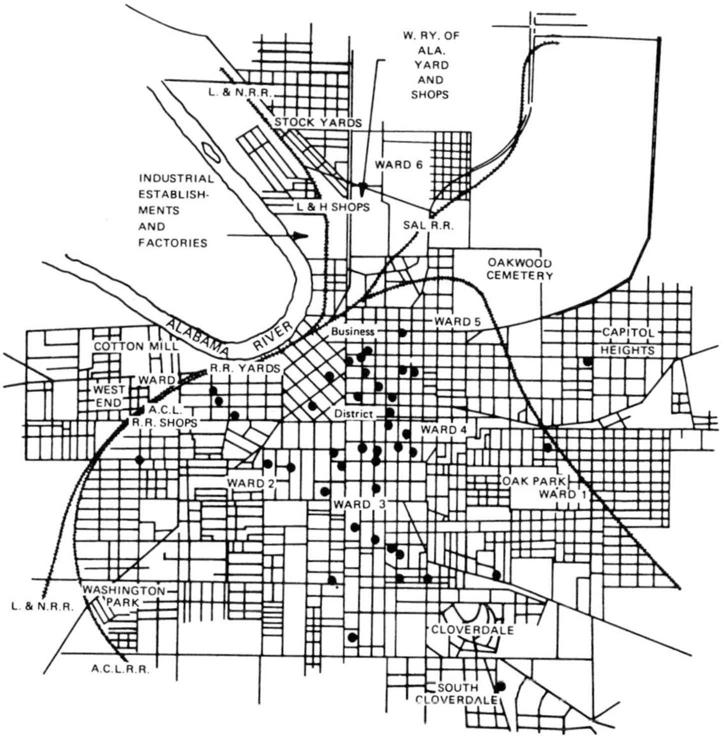

FIGURE 7–7. *Cases of mild typhus (Brill disease) in Montgomery, Alabama, 1922 to 1925, spotted according to residence. (From Maxcy, K. F.: An epidemiological study of endemic typhus [Brill disease] in the southeastern United States. Public Health Rep. 41:2967–2995, 1926.)*

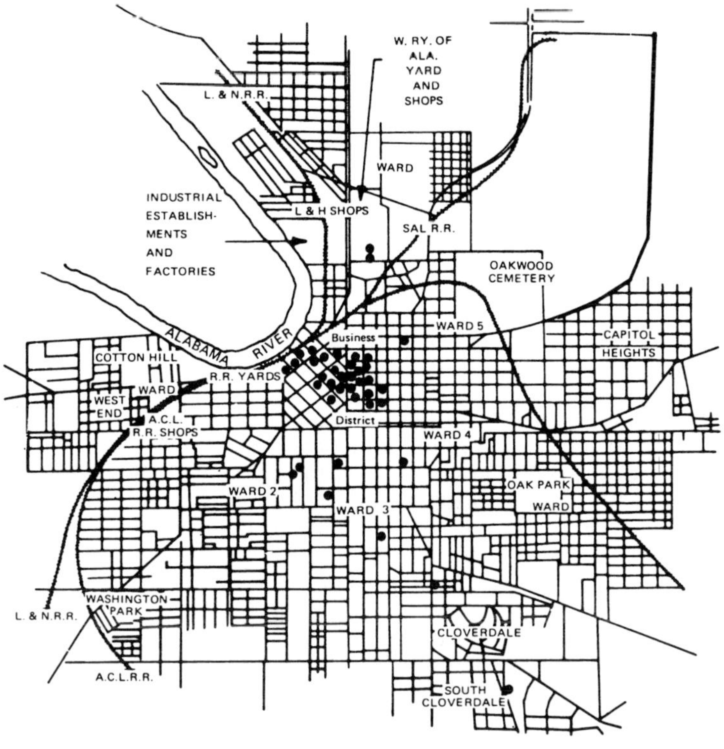

FIGURE 7–8. *Cases of mild typhus (Brill disease) in Montgomery, Alabama, 1922 to 1925, spotted according to place of employment or, if unemployed, according to place of residence. (From Maxcy, K. F.: An epidemiological study of endemic typhus [Brill disease] in the southeastern United States. Public Health Rep. 41:2967–2995, 1926.)*

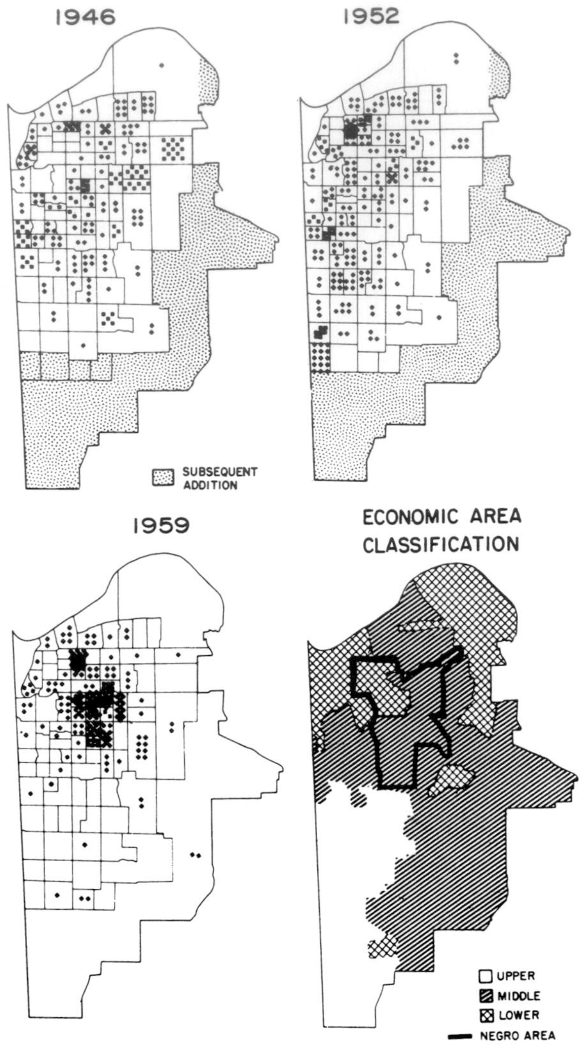

FIGURE 7–9. *Distribution of reported poliomyelitis cases, by census tract, Kansas City, Missouri, epidemic years 1946, 1952, and 1959. (From Chin, T. D. Y., and Marine, W. W.: The changing patterns of poliomyelitis observed in two urban epidemics, Kansas City and Des Moines, 1959. Public Health Rep. 76:553–563, 1961.)*

to describe the occurrence of disease over time in a given area should be stated clearly. *Endemic* refers to diseases regularly present. The usual frequency, including expected seasonal variations, is called the *endemic level*. The term *epidemic* often is applied indiscriminately (and sometimes incorrectly) to any large clustering of cases in time and place. More precisely, it applies to any number of cases, small or large, representing a significant excess over the usual or endemic level.

This principle underlies the familiar monitoring of influenza in the United States by the Centers for Disease Control and Prevention, based on deaths due to influenza and pneumonia. This is illustrated in Figure 7–10, in which the weekly ratios of pneumonia and influenza deaths to total deaths observed from September 1980 to August 1983 are compared with the ratios expected on the basis of the time series method* and "epidemic threshold," which depicts the upper 95 per cent confidence limit. When the observed value exceeds the expected for 2 successive weeks, an influenza epidemic is indicated. On this basis, epidemics began in week 50 of 1980 and week 3 of 1983.

In practice, especially at the local level, health authorities use the term *outbreak* rather than *epidemic* (unless the number of cases is very large) to minimize public alarm. The term *pandemic* is used to describe excess disease occurring in many countries, as did influenza in 1957 and 1968.

*This method, which replaced the regression method of Serfling in 1980, is described in some detail by Choi and Thacker.[14, 15]

Time Clusters

Concern here is with the recognition and interpretation of events (infections and disease) occurring with some frequency within a limited period, i.e., clustering in time. A selected series of examples will serve to illustrate the more important possibilities.

An important determinant of clustering of infections is the incubation (or latent) period. Infection resulting from a known exposure is manifested within a predictable range of time by initiation of shedding of the agent and onset of disease (if it occurs). For simplicity, we will speak only of disease hereafter because it provides the only readily recognizable indication of infection. Although the average incubation period of a given disease is remarkably constant, the usual range broadens as the incubation period increases. This range can be estimated by cumulating cases of which the time of exposure is known precisely or approximately and, taking this as day 0 on the time axis, plotting the day of onset of each case. The width of the resulting cluster provides an estimate of the range of incubation periods. The best estimate is obtained by using only cases with single, clearly timed exposures, such as when contact with the source case occurred only once, as during a playmate's birthday party.

A more readily obtained but less precise estimate is that derived from the cumulative analysis of family episodes of a disease, based on the assumption that the initial or primary case is the source of subsequent disease in family contacts. Because the primary case is infectious for several days, on any of which effective exposure may occur, the onsets of secondary cases will cluster over a range that, in theory, may reflect the true range plus the period of infectivity of the primary case.

Knowledge of the range of incubation periods has several practical implications. For contagious diseases, it can be used to distinguish true secondary cases that occur in families from others arising from extrafamilial sources (those with onsets too soon after that of the primary are called *coprimary cases*) or representing a second generation of spread within the family (*tertiary cases*). It also determines for how long after known exposure contacts should be observed or possibly held in quarantine for development of resulting disease. For poorly contagious diseases, such as typhoid fever, or for noncontagious diseases, such as food poisoning, the distribution of onsets in an outbreak can be used to distinguish between "point" epidemics (common time and place of exposure) and outbreaks reflecting exposure to a possibly continuing source. In the former case, the onsets will fall within the usual range of incubation periods. Furthermore, when the point source is not obvious, investigation can be focused on the interval defined by subtracting the shortest incubation period from the date of onset of the first case and the longest period from the date of onset of the last case.

An example is the occurrence in 1939 of 13 cases of typhoid fever in Schenectady, New York. The onsets of the first and last cases were June 5 and June 29, respectively. Assuming the usual range of incubation periods to be 5 to 30 days, the critical period was calculated to be May 29 to May 31, within which occurred a church-sponsored Memorial Day picnic at

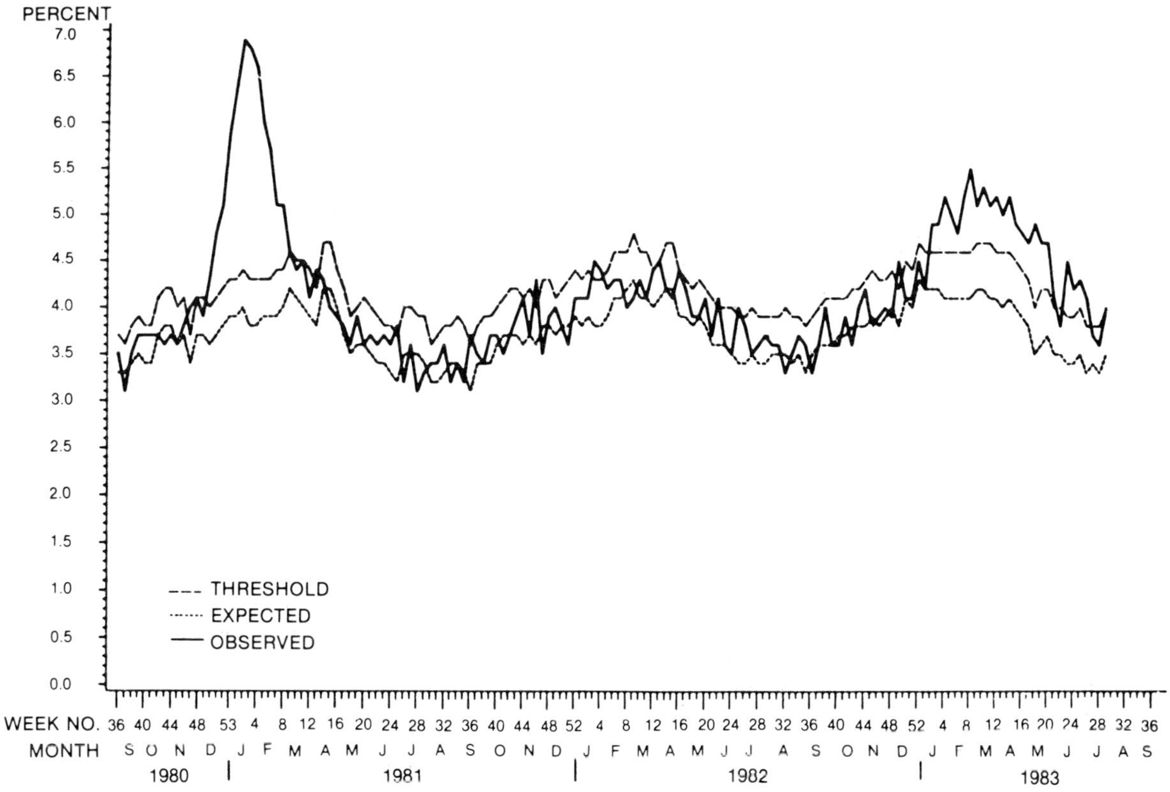

FIGURE 7–10. *Percentage of deaths attributable to pneumonia and influenza in 121 United States cities, 1980 to 1983. (From Centers for Disease Control: Annual Summary, 1982. M. M. W. R. 31[No. 54], December 1983.)*

which, it was discovered, salad prepared by an unrecognized typhoid carrier was served.

The concept of an incubation period has additional useful applications. By taking the onsets of paralytic poliomyelitis as day 0 and looking backward on the time axis, "provoking" factors, such as irritant inoculations, were identified by the clustering of their times of occurrence. Similarly, by setting time of vaccination at day 0, the cumulated experience of those vaccinated can be (and has been) analyzed for identification of adverse effects of specific vaccines, recognized as such because they cluster in time. Such evidence, for example, led to the recognition of poliomyelitis disease caused by both inactivated (Salk) and live virus (Sabin) polio vaccine and, in 1976, was an important point in linking swine influenza vaccine to the Guillain-Barré syndrome.[45]

Short-Term Patterns

EPIDEMICS. "Point" epidemics, as noted, have a duration limited by the range of the period of incubation of the particular disease because no secondary spread of the agents occurs. Concern here is with the much more common outbreaks or epidemics that extend over longer periods. On the basis of the agents and the mechanisms of transmission, three distinct types can be recognized.

The first consists typically of outbreaks of poorly contagious or noncontagious disease, reflecting the new but persisting activity of a source that must be identified and terminated quickly. One example of such a "continuing source" type of outbreak was a community-wide outbreak of salmonellosis in Madeira, California, in 1965, which was traced quickly to the water supply.[63] Unrecognized typhoid carriers working as food handlers and shellfish harvested from sewage-polluted waters and contaminated with hepatitis A virus have provided many other examples of outbreaks requiring prompt and careful epidemiologic investigation to identify the sources.

The element of contagion distinguishes the second type of epidemic, in which disease spreads from person to person. Such epidemics generally are self-limited, and the curve describing them often resembles the bell-shaped curve of a normal distribution. Modification of this curve as in abrupt decline from the peak is the expected result of successful control efforts, evaluation of which often is controversial. As discussed in more detail elsewhere,[25] epidemics of contagious disease arise where the persisting or newly introduced agent exists in a population containing sufficient susceptible individuals who make contact with one another adequate to permit transfer of infection from each new case to, on the average, more than one susceptible individual. When this average falls below 1, the curve declines, and when the probability of successful transfer of infection approaches 0, the epidemic terminates (typically, well before the supply of susceptible individuals has been exhausted).

Many reasons underlie this decline and termination of transmission. They include seasonal changes in environmental factors affecting agent viability, such as temperature and humidity, and in host behavior, affecting intimacy of contact, such as indoor school versus outdoor play, as well as the progressive conversion of susceptible individuals to immune individuals. If one assumes constant units on the time axis, the slope of the ascending limb of the epidemic curve is determined by the incubation period (interval between successive cases) and factors influencing transmission (infectivity of the agent, frequency of adequate contact between susceptibles). In the absence of effective control measures, the duration of epidemics of a particular disease depends on the size of the susceptible population and the persistence of favorable environmental factors.

Epidemics of "diseases in nature" constitute the third type. Because susceptible individuals usually are abundant in the exposed human population, these epidemics typically reflect increases in the number of sources of infection in nature. With zoonoses such as arbovirus encephalitis, the initiation, slope of the curve, and duration of the epidemic are determined by the number of susceptible lower vertebrate hosts, the seasonally determined abundance of the vector mosquitoes, and the length of the extrinsic incubation period in the vector. Thus, epidemics due to western equine encephalitis virus tend to begin earlier and progress more rapidly than do those due to St. Louis encephalitis virus, even when both agents utilize the same host and vector species, as in California. This is at least in part because the extrinsic incubation period is much shorter for western equine encephalitis than for St. Louis encephalitis.

SEASONAL AND CYCLIC VARIATIONS. Predictable periodic variations in disease take two forms—seasonal and cyclic—neither of which is understood completely in the case of agents infecting only humans.

Seasonal variation presumably reflects the influence on the activity of the agent of changes in temperature, precipitation, and length of days. It is understood readily with respect to diseases in nature that depend on lower vertebrate hosts and arthropod vectors, the abundance and activity of which are determined seasonally. Similarly, the increased occurrence in the warmer months of bacterial enteric infections (spread by indirect means) is explainable largely by more rapid bacterial growth in unrefrigerated milk and food, the increase in abundance of filth flies, and lowered sanitary precautions associated with summer recreational activities.

However, mode of transmission is only a partial determinant of seasonal pattern. Thus, although the enteroviruses (including polio), the rotaviruses causing acute gastroenteritis, and hepatitis A virus all spread chiefly by fecal-oral mechanisms (both direct and indirect), the seasonal patterns are distinctly different (late summer and fall for the enteroviruses and late winter for the rotaviruses and hepatitis A virus). Similarly, although infections with agents present in respiratory secretions and spread by airborne mechanisms or contaminated fomites are infrequent in the summer when contacts among susceptible children often are out of doors, their seasonal peaks occur at significantly different times. The respiratory disease season coincides roughly with the school year. Rhinoviruses are most active in the early fall and late spring. Parainfluenza virus types 1 and 2 peak in the fall. The annual peaks of respiratory syncytial virus vary among fall, winter, and spring. Mumps peaks in late fall, influenza in late winter or early spring, and measles typically in the spring. As suggested by London and Yorke,[47, 77] differences in incubation period and infectivity at least partly are responsible for these differences in pattern.

Plotting variation over a series of years will reveal for some diseases a roughly regular cyclic variation. In larger metropolitan areas, the usual biennial measles epidemic shows as an enlarged annual wave. Before 1950, deaths due to meningococcal meningitis occurred on a nationwide basis in cycles of 7 to 9 years, a phenomenon presumably terminated by the advent of sulfonamides and antibiotics. Figure 7–6 depicts the similar cyclic occurrence of viral hepatitis (all forms but type A probably predominating) in 1952 to 1968, with peaks in 1954 and 1961 representing the crest of waves preceded by progressive build-ups and followed by progressive declines in the yearly seasonal highs and lows. From 1968 on, types B and non-A, non-B hepatitis contributed increasingly to total viral hepatitis, the curve for which was influenced little by one additional cycle of type A hepatitis, which peaked in 1970. Such cyclic patterns are believed to result in part from the fact that the degree of depletion of susceptible individuals during annual waves is inconstant, for reasons that, with respect to measles, are discussed in considerable detail by London and Yorke.[47, 77] Pandemic influenza A, which provides the most dramatic example of cycling (10- to 12-year intervals), is explainable on a very different basis, namely, a major change in the antigenic character of the agent, the probable mechanism for which was discussed previously.

Long-Term Trends

Except for poliomyelitis during the first half of the twentieth century, clearly defined long-term trends in the occurrence of infectious diseases in the United States usually have been downward, and in no case has the description or understanding of the mechanisms posed a major difficulty. In the case of poliomyelitis, the increase in the rate of paralytic disease beginning about 1880 is attributable to a number of factors, including improved sanitation, which resulted in an expanding proportion of older children and young adults without previous exposure to the causative viruses. In young infants, the vast majority of poliovirus infections are benign but produce long-lasting immunity; the older an individual who becomes infected, the more likely is paralysis. Thus, the incidence of paralytic disease is related inversely to the level of sanitation as long as there is an opportunity for introduction of the virus into an area. In the United States, the increase in paralytic disease with epidemics continued unabated (with an apparent sharp increase around 1940 due to changes in reporting criteria) until the widespread use of poliovirus vaccines. The post-1955 decline in poliomyelitis, the much earlier decline in pertussis and diphtheria, the disappearance of smallpox, and the more recent marked declines in measles and rubella all are attributable chiefly to widespread use of effective specific vaccines. Similarly, the disappearance of indigenous malaria and the decline to a negligible level of rabies in humans reflect the application of a variety of effective control measures.

Since 1900, infectious disease mortality has decreased markedly in the United States.[55] For example, mortality due to infection in infants decreased about 95 per cent between 1900 and 1973 and that in chidren 1 to 14 years of age, 99 percent.[55] In adults, infectious disease mortality rates declined markedly as well. Much of this decline can be attributable to nonmedical measures (socioeconomic changes, improved sanitation, smaller famiies, and the like). With some exceptions, such as bacterial meningitis, smallpox, and poliomyelitis, newer measures, such as antibiotics and vaccines, played a lesser role in reducing mortality (although not morbidity; measles and pertussis mortality, for example, declined strikingly before the advent of the vaccines, but their incidence rates did not).

However, for reasons that are not entirely clear, there is strong evidence of a recent increase in mortality from infectious diseases in the United States.[61] Data were obtained from the National Center for Health Statistics for the years 1980 to 1992 and showed a 39 per cent increase in age-adjusted infectious disease mortality during that period. The increase in crude mortality rates, which reflects better the burden on the health care system, was 58 per cent. The most important contributors to this increase were respiratory infections, AIDS, and sepsis. There was a decrease in mortality in children younger than 5 years of age. There was a more than sixfold increase in the 25- to 44-year-old population (presumably attributable in large part to AIDS), and a 25 per cent increase in those 65 years of age or older. Although these data are subject to the well-known physician-related inaccuracies of death certificates, there is no doubt that there has been a considerable increase in mortality from infectious diseases. Infectious diseases are not disappearing despite earlier trends, and these data reinforce the need for surveillance.

These phenomena warrant three unrelated final comments. First, as successful vaccines become available and are used widely, the disease under attack is reported far more completely. In the case of measles, it was estimated that before vaccine was available, only about 10 per cent of cases were reported. No recent national estimates are available, but as of 1984 it was probable that less than 5 per cent were reported. In New York City, 56 per cent of about 1000 patients seen at or admitted to 12 hospitals were reported during a widely publicized 1991 epidemic.[19] Second, the widespread use of effective vaccines may alter the epidemiology of their target infections in ways that may not be anticipated if, in contrast to smallpox, the disease is not eradicated. Note, for example, the shift in the age incidence of pertussis in recent years with peaks in infants and young adults. This shift is unlikely to be an artifact of enhanced reporting; instead, it probably represents waning immunity in persons vaccinated in childhood as a consequence of diminished disease frequency and lack of exposure and transmission to infants. Whether a similar phenomenon contributes to the recent recrudescence of measles and a shift in its age distribution, along with other factors, is unknown. Third, although age-adjusted incidence rates typically (and necessarily) are used in describing changes in disease occurrence over long periods, they have little meaning as disease becomes very infrequent, possibly verging on disappearance. At this point, interest focuses on the actual number and distribution of cases, each of which requires explanation (as with paralytic poliomyelitis) or institution of rigorous, localized control measures (as would result with malaria, yellow fever, or smallpox).

Emerging Infections

Although two decades ago it might have been said that most infectious disorders had been explored thoroughly epidemiologically and that little was left to do, this is no longer the case. Indeed, infectious disease epidemiology has become increasingly challenging, and in many ways the problems are more complex and necessitate greater cooperation with additional disciplines, such as microbiology and molecular biology. In part, this is because of the so-called *emerging infections,* a term that has come into vogue in recent years and refers to two different groups of disorders. The first is associated with the appearance of previously unrecognized or possibily heretofore nonexistent infections in humans. Well-known examples are legionellosis, AIDS, Lyme disease, hemorrhagic colitis due to *E. coli* O157:H7, Ebola virus infection, and hantavirus infection. The other group includes previously recognized human infections that exhibit changes in epidemiologic behavior or biologic characteristics that enhance their transmission or virulence. These changes usually can be attributed to external influences, such as altered demographics, including increasing population and rural-urban migration, international travel, new technology or technologic failure, changes in land use, adaptation of infecting organisms to various influences, and inadequate or underused public health measures.[38] To this list should be added changes in host factors, such as immune defenses. Obviously, there is not a clear dividing line between new infections and old ones with new behavior. However, examples of those with new behavior include multidrug-resistant tuberculosis, penicillin-resistant pneumococcal infections, invasive group A streptococcal (popularly known as flesh-eating bacteria) infections, the staphylococcal toxic shock syndrome, cryptosporidiosis, LaCrosse encephalitis, and a number of infections that are fostered by immunosuppression or various therapeutic measures, such as antibiotics and catheters.

These emerging infections are not minor threats. Although in some instances, relatively small populations have been affected to date, the potential for widespread disease of epidemic or even pandemic proportions exists. This potential can be expected to increase because the demographic and other conditions that have predisposed to the emergence of these infections continue to grow and intensify. Accordingly, it is imperative that maximum efforts be made to reverse this process. To achieve this goal requires worldwide collaborative efforts among various disciplines, including epidemiology, microbiology, entomology, immunology, clinical medicine, demography, nutrition, sanitation, and even political science, to list only a few.

In recent years, infectious disease epidemiologic surveillance has been enhanced by the development of sophisticated techniques for so-called *molecular epidemiology.* These techniques enable the identification of subtypes of specific organisms. Each of the three well-known strains of poliovirus can be subtyped on the basis of genetic variations, providing a means of tracing the spread of infection with remarkable precision.[43] For example, a 1992 outbreak of type 3 poliovirus infection in a religious group opposed to vaccination in the Netherlands was shown to be most likely due to a strain of virus from the Indian subcontinent.[57] In addition, the identical strain produced illness in the religious groups of the same denomination in Alberta, Canada, undoubtedly because of travel-related contact. These techniques also are used to distinguish wild poliovirus strains from those of vaccine origin.[76] Parenthetically, it should be noted that immune responses to poliovirus vaccine are not affected by these molecular variations. Other well-known recent applications of molecular epidemiology include characterization of the hantavirus that produced illness in the southwestern United States,[56] the worldwide epidemiology of variants of HIV,[36] and the spread of animal species–specific strains of rabies virus in the United States.[44]

The responsibilities of epidemiologists regarding emerging infections may be described in three categories. The first is that of surveillance, including the recognition of the appearance of a previously unrecognized infection or a new variant of an existing disease. Optimum surveillance requires systematic observations and specific diagnostic criteria to ensure precision. Recent examples of such criteria include those for AIDS,[10] the streptococcal toxic shock syndrome,[5] and the recognition of drug-resistant pneumococci.[39] An important part of surveillance is to determine who, when, and where: who is affected (age and other personal characteristics, contact with others who are ill, etc.); when the disorder occurs (year-to-year variations, season, temporal course of the outbreak, etc.); and where (geographic locations, urban or rural, local ecology, etc.). Second, an important task is to use surveillance and other data to develop understanding of the epidemiology of the infection, which often provides leads to the etiology, pathogenesis, and approaches to control. The third role of epidemiology is that of monitoring the effects of various control measures, including, for example, assessment of the safety and efficacy of anticipated new vaccines such as those for rotavirus enteritis, malaria, and AIDS.

The increasing magnitude and speed of international travel enhance the likelihood of global spread of disease and complicate approaches to prevention or containment of epidemic infections. Moreover, many of the emerging infections are not limited geographically by their ecologic requirements, as largely is the case with schistosomiasis. Thus, the nations of the world increasingly are dependent on each other for surveillance, a task that is not accomplished easily given the logistics; costs (in the face of other needs and priorities, particularly of many developing countries); and the required standardization, collaboration, communication, coordination, and centralized resource for assembly and analysis of surveillance. Although the World Health Organization, the Pan American Health Organization, the United States military and the Public Health Service, and various other organizations do maintain surveillance systems and laboratories in various parts of the world, these efforts at present are considered to be inadequate except for some infections and in some areas. Accordingly, the development of comprehensive national and worldwide surveillance systems has been urged strongly.[12, 38]

References

1. Allison, A. C.: Protection afforded by sickle-cell trait against subtertian malarial infection. Br. Med. J. *1*:290–294, 1953.
2. American Heart Association: Committee Report: Jones criteria (revised) for guidance in the diagnosis of rheumatic fever. Circulation *32*:664–668, 1965.
3. Atkinson, W. L., Orenstein, W. A., and Knugman, S.: The resurgence of measles in the United States, 1989–1990. Ann. Rev. Med. *43*:451–163, 1992.
4. Blake, P. A., Allegra, D. T., Snyder, J. D., et al.: Cholera: A possible endemic focus in the United States. N. Engl. J. Med. *302*:305–309, 1980.
5. Breiman, R. F., Davis, J. P., Facklam, R. R., et al.: The Working Group on Severe Streptococcal Infections: Defining the group A streptococcal toxic shock syndrome. J. A. M. A. *269*:390–391, 1993.
6. Brimblecombe, F. S. W., Cruickshank, R., Masters, P. L., et al.: Family studies of respiratory infections. Br. Med. J., *1*:119–128, 1958.
7. Centers for Disease Control: Annual summary 1982. M. M. W. R. *31*:1–149, 1983.
8. Centers for Disease Control: Rabies surveillance, United States, 1988. M. M. W. R. *38*(55-1):1–21, 1988.
9. Centers for Disease Control: Case definitions for public health surveillance. M. M. W. R. *39*(RR-13):1–43, 1990.
10. Centers for Disease Control and Prevention: 1993 revised classification system for HIV infection and expanded case definition for AIDS among adolescents and adults. M. M. W. R. *41*:1–19, 1992.
11. Centers for Disease Control and Prevention: Summary of notifiable diseases, United States. M. M. W. R. *43*:3–80, 1995, and *44*:3–87, 1996.
12. Centers for Disease Control and Prevention: Addressing emerging infectious disease threats: A prevention strategy for the United States. Atlanta, U.S. Department of Health and Human Services, Public Health Service, 1994.
13. Chin, T. D. Y., and Marine, W. W.: The changing patterns of poliomyelitis observed in two urban epidemics, Kansas City and Des Moines, 1959. Public Health Rep. *76*:553–563, 1961.
14. Choi, K., and Thacker, S. B.: An evaluation of influenza mortality surveillance, 1962–1979. I. Time series forecasts of expected pneumonia and influenza deaths. Am. J. Epidemiol. *113*:216–226, 1981.
15. Choi, K., and Thacker, S. B.: An evaluation of influenza mortality surveillance, 1962–1979. II. Percentage of pneumonia and influenza deaths as an indicator of influenza activity. Am. J. Epidemiol. *113*:227–235, 1981.
16. Chorba, T. L., Berkelman, R. L., Safford, S. K., et al.: Mandatory reporting of infectious diseases by clinicians. J. A. M. A. *262*:3018–3026, 1989.
17. Cooney, M. K., Hall, C. E., and Fox, J. P.: The Seattle Virus Watch. III. Evaluation of isolation methods and summary of infections, detected by virus isolations. Am. J. Epidemiol. *96*:286–305, 1972.
18. Craig, G. B., Jr.: Biology of *Aedes triseriatus*: Some factors affecting control. *In* Calisher, C. H., and Thompson, W. H. (eds.): California Serogroup Viruses. Proceedings of an International Symposium. New York, Alan R. Liss, 1983, pp. 329–341.
19. Davis, S.: Unpublished data presented to Advisory Committee on Immunization Practices. Centers for Disease Control, June 3, 1991.
20. Dewhurst, K.: Dr. Thomas Sydenham (1624–1689). Berkeley and Los Angeles, University of California Press, 1966.
21. Dingle, J. H., Badger, G. R., and Jordan, W. S., Jr.: Illness in the Home. Cleveland, The Press of Western Reserve University, 1964.
22. Elveback, L. R., Fox, J. P., Ketler, A., et al.: The Virus Watch Program: A continuing surveillance of viral infections in metropolitan New York families. III. Preliminary report on association of infections with disease. Am. J. Epidemiol. *83*:436–454, 1966.
23. Fothergill, L. C.: Biological warfare and its defense. Public Health Rep. *72*:865–871, 1957.
24. Fox, J. P.: Family-based epidemiology studies. The Second Wade Hampton Frost Lecture. Am. J. Epidemiol. *99*:165–179, 1974.
25. Fox, J. P., and Elveback, L. R.: Herd immunity: Changing concepts. *In* Notkins, A. L. (ed.): Viral Immunology and Immunopathology. New York, Academic Press, 1975, pp. 273–290.
26. Fox, J. P., Elveback, L. R., Spigland, I., et al.: The Virus Watch Program: A continuing surveillance of viral infections in metropolitan New York families. I. Overall plan, methods of collecting and handling information, and a summary report of specimens collected and illnesses observed. Am. J. Epidemiol. *83*:289–412, 1966.
27. Fox, J. P., Hall, C. E., and Cooney, M. K.: The Seattle Virus Watch. VII. Observations of adenovirus infections. Am. J. Epidemiol. *105*:362–386, 1977.
28. Fox, J. P., Hall, C. E., Cooney, M. K., et al.: The Seattle Virus Watch. II. Objectives, study population and its observation, data processing and summary of illnesses. Am. J. Epidemiol. *96*:270–285, 1972.
29. Fox, J. P., Hall, C. E., Cooney, M. K., et al.: Influenza virus infections in Seattle families, 1975–1979. I. Study design, methods and the occurrence of infections by time and age. Am. J. Epidemiol. *116*:212–227, 1982.
30. Fox, J. P., Hall, C. E., Cooney, M. K., et al.: Influenza virus infections in Seattle families, 1975–1979. II. Pattern of infection in invaded households and relation of age and prior antibody to occurrence of infection and related illness. Am. J. Epidemiol. *116*:228–242, 1982.
31. Frobisher, M.: Fundamentals of Microbiology. 7th ed. Philadelphia, W. B. Saunders, 1962, p. 354.
32. Gelfand, H. M.: Inheritance of susceptibility to poliomyelitis. N. Engl. J. Med. *258*:964–965, 1958.
33. Griffin, P. M., and Tauxe, R. V.: The epidemiology of infections caused by *Escherichia coli* 0157:H7, other enterohemorrhagic *E. coli* and the associated hemolytic-uremic syndrome. Epidemiol. Rev. *13*:60–98, 1991.
34. Gwaltney, J. M., Jr., and Hendley, J. O.: Rhinovirus transmission: One if by air, two if by hand. Am. J. Epidemiol. *107*:357–361, 1978.
35. Hillis, W. D., Hillis, A., Bias, W. B., et al.: Association of hepatitis B surface antigenemia with HLA locus B specificities. N. Engl. J. Med. *296*:1310–1314, 1977.
36. Hu, D. J., Dondero, T. J., Rayfield, M. A., et al.: The emerging genetic diversity of HIV: The importance of global surveillance for diagnostics, research, and prevention. J. A. M. A. *275*:210–215, 1996.
37. Huebner, R. J.: The virologist's dilemma. Ann. N. Y. Acad. Sci. *67*:430–438, 1957.
38. Lederberg, J., Shope, R. E., and Oaks, S. C., Jr., (eds.): Emerging Infections: Microbial Threats to Health in the United States. Washington, D. C., National Academy Press, 1992.
39. Jernigan, D. B., Cetron, M. S., and Breiman, R. F.: Minimizing the impact of drug-resistant *Streptococcus pneumoniae* (DRSP). J. A. M. A. *275*:206–209, 1996.
40. Jones, T. D.: Diagnosis of rheumatic fever. J. A. M. A. *126*:481–484, 1944.
41. Kallman, F. J., and Reisner, D.: Twin studies on the significance of genetic factors in tuberculosis. Am. Rev. Tuberculosis *47*:549–574, 1943.
42. Katz, M., and Stiehm, E. R.: Host defense in malnutrition. Pediatrics *59*:490–495, 1977.
43. Kew, O. M., Mulders, M. N., Lipskaya, G. Y., et al.: Molecular epidemiology of polioviruses. Semin. Virol. *6*:401–414, 1995.
44. Krebs, J. W., Strine, T. W., Smith, J. S., et al.: Rabies surveillance in the United States during 1993. J. Am. Vet. Med. Assoc. *205*:1695–1709, 1994.
45. Langmuir, A. D., Bregman, D. J., Kurland, L. T., et al.: An epidemiologic and clinical evaluation of Guillain-Barré syndrome reported in association with the administration of swine influenza vaccines. Am. J. Epidemiol. *119*:841–879, 1984.
46. Lidwell, O. M., and Sommerville, T.: Observations on the incidence and distribution of the common cold in a rural community during 1948 and 1949. J. Hyg. Camb. *59*:365–381, 1961.
47. London, W. P., and Yorke, J. A.: Recurrent outbreaks of measles, chickenpox and mumps. I. Seasonal variation in contact rates. Am. J. Epidemiol. *98*:453–468, 1973.
48. Luby, J. P., Miller, G., Gardner, P., et al.: The epidemiology of St. Louis encephalitis in Houston, Texas, 1964. Am. J. Epidemiol. *86*:584–597, 1967.
49. MacKenzie, W. R., Hoxie, N. J., Proctor, M. E., et al.: A massive outbreak in Milwaukee of *Crytosporidum* infection transmitted through the public water supply. N. Engl. J. Med. *331*:161–167, 1994.
50. Maxcy, K. F.: An epidemiological study of endemic typhus (Brill's disease) in the southeastern United States. Public Health Rep. *41*:2967–2995, 1926.
51. May, J. M.: The ecology of human disease. *In* Studies in Medical Geography, No. 1. New York, MD Publications, 1958.
52. Monto, A. S., and Cavallaro, J. J.: The Tecumseh study of respiratory illness. II. Patterns of occurrence of infection with respiratory pathogens, 1965–1969. Am. J. Epidemiol. *94*:280–289, 1971.
53. Monto, A. S., Napier, J. A., and Metzner, H. L.: The Tecumseh study of respiratory illness. I. Plan of study and observations on syndromes of acute respiratory disease. Am. J. Epidemiol. *94*:269–279, 1971.
54. Mortimer, Jr., E. A.: Hospital staphylococcal infections: Interruption of transmission as a means of control. Med. Clin. North Am. *47*:1247–1256,1963.
55. Mortimer, Jr., E. A.: Immunization against infectious disease. Science *200*:902–907, 1978.
56. Nichol, S. T., Spiropoulou, C. F., Morzunov, S., et al.: Genetic identification

of a hantavirus associated with an outbreak of acute respiratory illness. Science *262*:914–917, 1993.
57. Oostvogel, P. M., van Wijngaarden, J. K., van der Avoort, H. G. A. M., et al.: Poliomyelitis outbreak in an unvaccinated community in the Netherlands, 1992–1993. Lancet *344*:665–670, 1994.
58. Pasteur, L.: The physiological theory of fermentation. *In* Eliot, C. (ed.): Scientific Papers. New York, P. F. Collier and Sons, 1910, pp. 289–381.
59. Patz, J. A., Epstein, P. R., Burke, T. A., et al.: Global climate change and emerging infectious diseases. J. A. M. A. *275*:217–223, 1996.
60. Perry, W. D., Siegel, A. C., Rammelkamp, C. H., Jr., et al.: Transmission of group A streptococci. I. The role of contaminated bedding. Am. J. Hyg. *66*:85–101, 1957.
61. Pinner, R. W., Teutsch, S. M., Simonsen, L., et al.: Trends in infectious disease mortality in the United States. J. A. M. A. *275*:189–193, 1996.
62. Reedy, J. J.: Recessive inheritance of susceptibility to poliomyelitis in fifty pedigrees. J. Hered. *48*:37–44, 1957.
63. Renteln, H. A., and Hinman, A. R.: A waterborne epidemic of gastroenteritis in Madeira, California. Am. J. Epidemiol. *86*:1–10, 1967.
64. Rosen, G.: A History of Public Health. New York, MD Publications, 1958, pp. 62–64.
65. Selye, H.: The Physiology and Pathology of Exposure to Stress. Montreal, Acta Inc., 1950.
66. Sigerist, H. E.: The Great Doctors. New York, W. W. Norton, 1933, pp. 100–108 and 375–379.
67. Sigurdsson, B., Sigurjonsson, J., Sigurdsson, J. H., et al.: A disease epidemic in Iceland simulating poliomyelitis. Am. J. Hyg. *52*:222–238, 1950.
68. Snow on Cholera, being a reprint of two papers by John Snow, M. D., together with a biographical memoir by B. W. Richardson and an introduction by Wade Hampton Frost. New York, Commonwealth Fund, 1936.
69. Spigland, I., Fox, J. P., Elveback, L. R., et al.: The Virus Watch Program: A continuing surveillance of viral infections in metropolitan New York families. II. Laboratory methods and a preliminary report on infections revealed by virus isolation. Am. J. Epidemiol. *83*:413–435, 1966.
70. Thompson, W. H., and Beaty, B. J.: Venereal transmission of La Crosse (California encephalitis) arbovirus in *Aedes triseriatus* mosquitoes. Science *196*:530–531, 1977.
71. Wannamaker, L. W.: The epidemiology of streptococcal infections. *In* McCarty, M. (ed.): Streptococcal Infections. New York, Columbia University Press, 1954, p. 157.
72. Webster, L. T.: Experimental epidemiology. Medicine *25*:77–109, 1946.
73. Weibel, R. E., Neff, B. J., Kuter, B. J., et al.: Live attenuated varicella virus vaccine: Efficacy trial in healthy children. N. Engl. J. Med. *310*:1409–1415, 1984.
74. Wenzel, R. P.: A new hantavirus infection in North America. N. Engl. J. Med. *330*:1004–1005, 1994.
75. Winslow, C. E. A.: The Colonial era and the first years of the Republic (1606–1799): The pestilence that walketh in darkness, No. 1. *In* Top, F. H. (ed.): The History of American Epidemiology. St. Louis, C. V. Mosby, 1954, pp. 31–44.
76. Yang, D.-F., De, L., Holloway, B. P., et al.: Detection and identification of vaccine-related polioviruses by the polymerase chain reaction. Virus Res. *20*:159–179, 1991.
77. Yorke, J. A., and London, W. P.: Recurrent outbreaks of measles, chickenpox and mumps. II. Systematic differences in contact rates and stochastic effects. Am. J. Epidemiol. *98*:469–482, 1973.

PART 2

INFECTIONS OF SPECIFIC ORGAN SYSTEMS

SECTION ONE

UPPER RESPIRATORY TRACT INFECTIONS

8

THE COMMON COLD

James D. Cherry

The common cold is an acute, communicable, viral disease characterized by nasal stuffiness, sneezing, coryza, throat irritation, and no or minimal fever. Although "URI" (upper respiratory infection) and "nasopharyngitis" are used frequently as synonyms for "the common cold" by physicians and other health workers, the practice should be discouraged; URI is much too broad a term, and pharyngitis is not present in the majority of colds. To add to the confusion regarding terminology, "a cold" frequently has an even more inclusive connotation to the lay person.

HISTORY

Although the common cold undoubtedly has had an impact on the events of history, the specific symptom complex in ancient times was overshadowed by more severe contagious problems (influenza, plague, smallpox), as well as by septic diseases (otitis, mastoiditis, pneumonia) that were complications of upper respiratory viral infections. The name "common cold" most certainly arose from the fact that the onset of symptoms included the feeling of chilliness on exposure to cold. This association was perceived as a cause-and-effect relationship. It is of interest that more than 200 years ago Benjamin Franklin pointed out that colds were caught from other people rather than by exposure to cold.[78]

In 1914, Kruse[67] demonstrated that colds could be transmitted by the nasal instillation in healthy adults of Berkefeld-filtered nasal washings from ill persons and that the causative agent was smaller than common bacteria. These findings were confirmed clearly in 1930 by Dochez and associates.[31] The way was paved for more extensive study of respiratory viral infections when in 1933 Smith and colleagues[89] reported the isolation and cultivation of an influenza A virus from a human.

The greatest contribution to our present understanding of the common cold has been the use of human volunteers under carefully controlled conditions. The Common Cold Research Unit at Salisbury, England, was established in 1946,[2, 96] and volunteer studies at this institution as well as those performed in the United States[13, 23, 27, 47–49, 52–54, 64, 72] during the last 50 years are responsible for our present understanding of colds in adults.

Although studies of respiratory illness in children also have been extensive, controlled volunteer trials have not been performed. Pediatric studies have been most useful in delineating the spectrum of clinical manifestations by age group and seasonal prevalence rates of the different respiratory viruses.

ETIOLOGIC AGENTS

Initial investigations into the etiology of the common cold were based on the theme that there was one etiologic agent to be discovered. Subsequent studies revealed that many different groups of viruses were involved etiologically and that within each group there frequently were many types. The agents associated with colds are presented in Table 8–1. Each of these agents is covered more fully in other chapters; in this chapter, only an overview will be presented. As a group, rhinoviruses are the most common cause of colds in children as well as adults. Also of major importance in the etiology of colds are reinfections with parainfluenza viruses and respiratory syncytial virus. Although the quantitative contribution of coronaviruses to colds in children is not known as yet, it is probable that they are significant contributors.

Enteroviruses and adenoviruses have been implicated frequently in upper respiratory illnesses, but in most instances the illnesses do not conform to those of strictly defined colds. Reoviruses cause colds, but their contribution to the overall incidence is unknown. Other agents, such as *Mycoplasma pneumoniae, Coccidioides immitis, Histoplasma capsulatum, Bordetella pertussis, Chlamydia psittaci,* and *Coxiella burnetii,* also have been associated with illnesses with initial cold-like symptoms.

TABLE 8–1. Infectious Agents Associated with the Common Cold

Category	Agents
Common viruses that usually cause the common cold	Rhinoviruses Parainfluenza viruses Respiratory syncytial virus Coronaviruses
Common infectious agents that occasionally cause illness with common cold symptoms	Adenoviruses Enteroviruses Influenza viruses Reoviruses *Mycoplasma pneumoniae*
Illnesses with initial symptoms suggestive of the common cold	*Coccidioides immitis* *Histoplasma capsulatum* *Bordetella pertussis* *Chlamydia psittaci* *Coxiella burnetii*

TABLE 8–2. Comparative Incidence of Upper Respiratory Infection by Age: London, 1952–1953, Seattle, 1965–1969, and Cleveland, 1948–1950

London		Seattle		Cleveland	
Age (Years)	*Illnesses/Person/ Year*	*Age (Years)*	*Illnesses/Person/ Year*	*Age (Years)*	*Illnesses/Person/ Year*
		<1	3.5	<1	6.9
0–4	5.0	1	3.8	1	8.3
		2–5	3.7	2–5	8.3
5–9	3.6	6–9	2.7	6–9	6.1
10–16	4.1	10–19	1.6	10–11+	5.5
Adult	2.9	Adult	2.9	Adult	4.8

Data modified from Brimblecombe et al.,[11] Fox et al.,[40] and Badger et al.[5]

EPIDEMIOLOGY

The common cold is an exceedingly frequent illness of childhood. In spite of the fact that more than 100 serologically different viral types cause this illness, there is a general predictability of incidence and seasonal occurrence. Although numerous epidemiologic studies have been conducted on the occurrence of respiratory illnesses, it is difficult to calculate a precise incidence of the common cold because criteria of disease classification have been different. The findings in three carefully done studies are presented in Table 8–2. In a wide range of family life settings, the average number of colds per year in children is three to eight.[5–11, 40] In the family setting, adults have on the average about one half the number of colds as do their children. The conventional spread of colds has its initial focus in the school.[5, 8, 11] School age children become infected and introduce secondary infections in the home. Under these conditions, the secondary attack rate is highest in other school age children and preschool age children. Generally, the secondary attack rate in adult family members is about one half that of the children. The introduction of infection into the family by adults is unusual. The present trend toward day care centers and preschool programs has increased primary infections in these younger children and has made them the source from which secondary family infections frequently occur. Close personal contact between children is necessary for the transmission of viruses that cause colds. In the typical pediatric practice office setting, no increased risk of the acquisition of respiratory illnesses by well babies has been demonstrated.[71]

Among children, boys tend to have more colds than girls.[5, 11] On the other hand, in the conventional family setting, mothers tend to have at least one more cold a year than their spouses.[5, 11, 40, 41] The usual incubation period of colds is 1 to 5 days.

In all nonisolated populations, colds are more frequent during the winter months than during the summer time.[30, 42, 73, 96] This seasonal discrepancy in incidence is as apparent in areas of relatively high wintertime mean temperatures as it is in locations with extremely low temperatures. In the tropics, colds are more prevalent during the rainy season.

Colds occur throughout the world. However, in isolated populations in which the number of people is few (such as members of antarctic exploration teams and isolated island communities), colds do not occur unless introduced by a visiting person.[58]

Although colds can be produced regularly in volunteers, the method of transmission of viruses, which results in colds under natural circumstances, is far from clear.[12, 14, 23, 26, 27, 29, 47, 49, 52, 56, 64, 65, 72, 83, 96] In people infected with respiratory viruses that cause colds, the greatest concentration of virus is in the nasal secretions. Children tend to have greater concentrations of virus than do adults, and they tend to shed virus for longer periods. Neither secretions related to coughing nor saliva contains appreciable amounts of virus and therefore is an unlikely source of contagion. During the process of talking, little virus is disseminated into the air. The greatest amount of virus from an infected individual is contributed to the surrounding environment by sneezing, nose blowing, and the general contamination of external surfaces (including the sufferer's hands) with nasal secretions. The route of acquisition of virus is by the nose and possibly the conjunctiva. With these facts in mind, it is easy to see that a susceptible individual can become infected by the inhalation of virus in droplet nuclei (small particles) resulting from a sneeze, by the direct nasal hit of virus containing large droplets from a sneeze, by nose blowing, or by the inoculation of virus (usually by the fingers of the recipient) from nasal secretions from disseminators that have been transmitted directly or indirectly. In children, it is most likely that spread either involves close contact with large droplets of nasal secretions containing virus that are applied to the nose from the hands of the future host or occurs by close-range airborne acquisition.

As all readers of this chapter are aware, there is considerable folklore related to the catching of a cold. However, all available evidence to date indicates that cold weather per se, chilling, wet feet, and drafts neither cause nor increase the susceptibility of persons to colds.[32, 64]

PATHOPHYSIOLOGY

The pathophysiology of human infections with viruses that cause colds is presented in the sections of this book covering the individual infectious agents. Here, a general overview is presented.

Few studies on the pathophysiology of respiratory infections have been done in children; therefore, the material presented in this section has been derived mainly from studies in adults.[4, 21, 33, 76, 82, 86, 96, 102]

The clinical syndrome of the common cold can occur in association with more than 100 different viral types and in many instances can occur with either a primary infection or a reinfection with a particular viral type.

Although it is possible that the primary site of virus inoculation in some colds is on the conjunctival surface, the vast majority result from inhalation or self-inoculation of virus onto the nasal mucosa. After virus acquisition, infection of the cells of the local respiratory epithelium occurs. This infection varies in the degree of cytopathology on the basis of the viral agent. The infection spreads locally, resulting in an increase in nasal secretions with an increased protein content. Symptoms (nasal stuffiness and throat irritation followed by sneezing) begin on the second or third day and are caused by both cellular damage and irritation. Virus shedding is at its maximum in 2 to 7 days, although some shedding may continue for another 2 weeks. Hilding[57] examined biopsy specimens, scrapings, and smears of nasal secretions and noted that initially there was submucosal edema followed by shedding of the ciliated epithelial cells. By the fifth day, the epithelial damage had reached its maximum, with regeneration over the next 10 days. Winther and associates[100] performed similar studies and noted the sloughing of epithelial cells, but they found that the epithelial lining remained continuous with normal cell borders. On the second day of disease, there was an increase in the number of neutrophils in the epithelium and in the lamina propria. Epithelial mast cells were not involved in the inflammation. The nasal discharge during the second to the seventh day is mucopurulent, owing to its content of desquamated epithelial cells and also polymorphonuclear leukocytes.

In experimental rhinovirus colds in adults, little or no discernible damage to the nasal epithelium has been demonstrated.[50, 101, 102] Recently, Arruda and associates[4] noted in adults infected with rhinovirus types 14 and 39 that virus replicates in both ciliated and nonciliated cells in the nasopharynx and that only a very small proportion of the cells were infected.

Because damage to the nasal epithelium is not noted in rhinovirus colds, it appears that cell death is not the cause of symptomatology. Naclerio and colleagues[74] and Proud and associates[81] have found that kinins are generated locally and their concentrations correlate with the severity of symptoms. More recently, it has been noted that interleukin-1 (IL-1) may contribute to the pathogenesis of rhinovirus infections.[82]

In studies in children with acute URIs, it was found that IL-1B, IL-8, IL-6, and tumor necrosis factor–α were elevated markedly in nasal lavage fluid.[76]

Pedersen and colleagues[77] studied nasal mucociliary transport in naturally acquired colds and noted that transport was reduced markedly during the acute illness and that slight impairment remained for about 1 month. They point out that because some children have four to six colds during a winter season, these children may have constantly impaired mucociliary transport.

Although viremia has been noted during infections with some of the viruses that cause colds, viremia is not a known occurrence during the typical common cold. The infection is restricted to the epithelial surfaces of the upper respiratory air passages, including the sinuses and the eustachian tubes. With infection, local interferon is produced and presumably has a major role in controlling the infection.[19] Serum antibody and secretory antibody regularly result from infection. The role of cell-mediated factors in both immunity and disease pathogenesis of colds is unknown. Levandowski and associates[69] noted in rhinovirus-challenged volunteers that total T cells and particularly T-helper cells were depressed. The magnitude of this finding correlated with progression of infection and symptoms. In a more recent study in which volunteers received rhinovirus type 39, Skoner and associates[86] found a slight increase in both T-helper (CD4+) and T-suppressor (CD8+) cells during illness.

The role of antibody (both serum and secretory) in the protection against reinfection and clinical colds is complicated. High levels of both secretory and serum antibodies appear to be protective against reinfections.[17, 18, 38, 60–63, 68, 87, 94] Clinically abortive colds probably are reinfection colds with early antibody recall. Fleet and colleagues[38] have demonstrated a short-lived heterologous resistance to rhinovirus colds, which probably is not due to interferon or antibody.

Unexplained constitutional factors also appear to control the clinical manifestations of colds.[84] Although studies have demonstrated genetic disease susceptibility patterns related to tissue types, no studies relating to common respiratory infections have been done.[22] In experimental coronavirus infections in adults, clinical severity correlated with detectable IgE in nasal secretions.[15] This finding suggests that atopy may be related to symptomatology in colds caused by coronaviruses.

Although clinical symptomatology and virologic data suggest that colds are upper respiratory diseases, studies of pulmonary function have indicated occult lower respiratory tract involvement.[3, 20, 79]

CLINICAL PRESENTATION

Because the common cold is caused by more than 100 different viral types, there could be considerable variation in the clinical manifestations. As indicated in the beginning of this chapter, the limits of illness to be considered under the diagnosis of the common cold arbitrarily but rigidly have been set. It is disappointing to note that although many comprehensive studies of respiratory viral illnesses of children have been done, little attention has been given to the details of URI.

Illness in children must be considered under two categories: that of infants and that of older children. The latter is similar to illness in adults. In studies involving 100 young adults, Jackson and colleagues[63] noted that virtually all complained of nasal discharge, nasal obstruction, and sore throat; about 80 per cent had malaise, postnasal discharge, headache, and cough; slightly less than 50 per cent reported a feverish feeling and chilliness; and about 25 per cent noted burning eyes and nasal membranes and muscle aching. In older children, the onset of illness is heralded by dryness and irritation in the nose and a scratchy feeling in the throat.[75] The initial symptoms are followed within a few hours by sneezing and watery nasal discharge; chilly feelings and occasionally muscular aches also are noted. Other complaints include headache, general malaise, anorexia, and low-grade fever.

After a variable period of from 1 to 3 days, the illness changes; the nasal secretions become thicker and frequently develop a purulent appearance. Persistent nasal discharge, associated with the trauma of repeated blowing of the nose, leads to excoriation around the nose. Nasal obstruction leads to mouth breathing, which causes drying of the throat, increasing the discomfort in the throat. The usual duration of illness is about 7 days, but lingering cough and nasal discharge may persist for 2 weeks or more.

In infants, the manifestations of illness may be more varied. The onset of illness is more likely to be associated with fever than in the older child, and this can be in the 38° to 39° C (100.4° to 102.2° F) range. Nasal manifestations in infants are similar to those in older children, but the only other manifestations are irritability and restlessness. Occasionally, coryza is the only symptom. Nasal obstruction may interfere significantly with both feeding and sleeping. Vomiting and diarrhea also may occur.

DIFFERENTIAL DIAGNOSIS

Because the clinical entity "the common cold" is a somewhat arbitrary grouping of signs and symptoms limited to anatomic boundaries and is caused by many different viral types, the approach to the differential diagnosis must consider both clinical and etiologic criteria. There are many upper respiratory illnesses caused by a large number of infectious agents that should not be confused with colds. For example, a common cold diagnosis should not be considered if there is objective pharyngitis, other enanthema, or evidence of obstructive airway disease.

The common cold is an acute, self-limited disease, and therefore the diagnosis should not be considered in a child who has persistent nasal signs or symptoms. Subacute or chronic illness should suggest the possibility of adenoiditis or sinusitis.

The most important differential diagnostic considerations are those clinical entities of noninfectious etiology. Allergic rhinitis is a particularly important prospect in the child with "recurrent colds." Careful attention to family history, a search for allergies, the presence or absence of nasal eosinophilia, and the serum IgE value will help confirm or exclude this consideration.

Although not reported particularly in pediatric patients, mental stress can lead to vasomotor responses and rhinitis in some susceptible persons. Chemical irritants can cause cold-like symptoms, and the clinical response varies greatly among different individuals. Early symptoms of many illnesses, such as pertussis, epiglottitis, measles, and diphtheria, are those of a cold, but in a short period, the more serious nature of the actual illness will be apparent.

SPECIFIC DIAGNOSIS

The epidemiologic history is the single, most important aspect of specific diagnosis. In children, if exposure history is requested, a contact usually is uncovered. If strict attention to clinical criteria of the common cold has been adopted, routine laboratory study is unnecessary. There frequently is the urge to take a throat culture to rule out the possibility of group A streptococcal infection. Usually, this is unnecessary because nasal symptomatology is not a characteristic of acute streptococcal illness except in infancy and pharyngitis is not within the limits of the diagnosis of the common cold. The white blood cell count also is of little use.

Specific diagnosis can be made by the isolation of virus from the nasal secretions. This is done best by either a nasal wash technique[51] or a nasopharyngeal swab. With laboratory techniques of diagnostic virologic facilities such as those in many university hospitals, parainfluenza viruses, respiratory syncytial virus, and most rhinoviruses and influenza viruses will be recovered. Direct antigen detection techniques can be used to identify infections due to respiratory syncytial virus, parainfluenza viruses, adenoviruses, and influenza viruses. Coronaviruses and some rhinoviruses and influenza strains can be recovered only by special laboratory techniques.

TREATMENT

Although literally hundreds of cold remedies are available, few offer any benefit to the pediatric patient, and many may be harmful.[43, 44, 59, 88] No clinically available antiviral agents are active against the viruses that cause colds.

In the approach to the child with a cold, it is best to assume that no therapy whatsoever is indicated in the majority of cases. Then, specific symptomatic care can be added in the individual case when it is needed. Many children as well as adults feel miserable when they have a cold, and therefore therapy with an analgesic often is useful. Although aspirin has been the recommended analgesic in the past, more recent studies have implicated it as an etiologic factor in influenza-associated Reye syndrome. Because it is difficult clinically to differentiate influenza viral infections from other respiratory viral infections, it is prudent to use acetaminophen rather than aspirin. The dose per single administration of acetaminophen by year of age is the following: younger than 1 year, 60 mg; 1 to 3 years, 60 to 120 mg; 3 to 6 years, 120 mg; 6 to 12 years, 150 to 300 mg; older than 12 years, 325 to 650 mg. Administration may be repeated three to four times daily in young children and every 4 hours in older children. Acetaminophen rarely should be given to infants younger than 6 months of age.

In adult volunteers with rhinovirus infections, it was found that acetaminophen was associated with suppression of the serum neutralizing antibody response, and there was an increase in nasal symptoms when compared with subjects who received a placebo.[46] In another adult volunteer study, naproxen administration resulted in a reduction in headache, malaise, myalgia, and cough when compared with placebo.[92]

Relief of nasal obstruction is the most important therapeutic consideration in young children. Locally applied or orally administered, systemically active decongestants are used frequently, but neither their true efficacy nor their adverse effects have been evaluated carefully. It is clear that excessive use of sprays and drops with vasoconstrictive drugs can lead to rebound obstruction, which actually prolongs the illness. The associated drying effect of the orally administered vasoconstrictive drugs can be expected to be deleterious to normal clearance mechanisms. In young infants, sympathomimetic-antihistamine mixtures in oral drop dosage form particularly are dangerous because respiratory depression may occur.[44] If vasoactive drugs are used, their use should be restricted to times when maximum benefit will occur (i.e., bedtime) and they should be discontinued within 3 days.

The use of isotonic saline drops and gentle aspiration can be very effective in the temporary relief of nasal obstruction in the infant. Also useful is the general humidification of room air, as this moisture tends to dilute tenacious nasal mucus so that its elimination is facilitated.

Antibiotics have no place in the routine therapy of common colds,[45, 70, 90] nor do antihistamines.[99] Occasionally in children, persistent cough during convalescence is a problem of such magnitude that it disturbs sleep. In such cases, the judicious use of codeine or other remedies at bedtime is indicated.

In more recent years, the greatest controversy related to the common cold has been over the efficacy of vitamin C, both prophylactically and therapeutically. In two carefully controlled volunteer studies, the administration of 3 g of ascorbic acid per day did not prevent or alter the symptomatology of experimental colds.[85, 98] In addition, during the last 15 years, there have been several large controlled trials in which vitamin C and placebo preparations have been used to prevent and to treat colds.[1, 16, 24, 25, 34, 66, 80] In some of these studies a degree of benefit was reported, whereas in others no efficacy was noted. It is most probable that the reported benefits are a result of statistical artifacts and placebo effect due to poor study design rather than specific pharmacologic drug effects. However, it is probable that the antihistaminic action of vitamin C[97, 103] afforded relief to some persons with allergic rhinitis who thought that their illnesses were colds. Because there are many toxic effects of ascorbic acid[9] and its use in respiratory illnesses at best is questionable, it would seem unwarranted to give children vitamin C in excess of normal daily requirements.

Intranasally administered alpha-2 interferon has been shown to be effective in the prevention of rhinovirus colds in controlled clinical trials.[91] However, the effect is variable, and adverse effects of the medication are common.[93] Intranasal alpha-2 interferon was not effective in the treatment of naturally occurring colds but demonstrated some benefit in experimental coronavirus colds.[55, 95]

Zinc lozenges have been used to treat the common cold, but in two controlled studies no benefit was found.[36] It also has been observed that the intranasal administration of nedocromil sodium had a beneficial effect in rhinoviral infections in adult volunteers.[10]

In one study, it was found that adults who took sauna baths once or twice a week had fewer colds than had a nonsauna bathing control group.[35] In another study, volunteers with colds did not benefit from inhaling heated vapor.[39]

PROGNOSIS

The prognosis of common colds in children is excellent. However, secondary complications do occur, and frequently these need careful and prolonged therapy. The most common complications are otitis media, sinusitis, bacterial adenoiditis, bacterial pharyngitis, and lower respiratory bacterial infections.

PREVENTION

It is clear from studies in isolated populations that once a particular respiratory viral infection has run through the entire group, no further respiratory viral illnesses can occur until a new infected person enters the population. From this type of evidence it would seem that quarantine or isolation-type practices could prevent colds. However, the average urban society of today is so complex that prevention through isolation procedures is impractical. Therefore, efforts to control the spread of respiratory virus should be minimal and practical. However, for children with undue susceptibility to complications, contact with crowds or with infected children and adults should be avoided.

The use of virucidal nasal tissues has been shown to reduce the spread of rhinovirus colds in human volunteers markedly and also to reduce modestly colds in the family setting.[28, 37]

References

1. Anderson, T. W., Beaton, G. H., Corey, P. N., et al.: Winter illness and vitamin C: The effect of relatively low doses. Can. Med. Assoc. J. *112*:823–826, 1975.
2. Andrewes, C. H.: The natural history of the common cold. Lancet *1*:71–75, 1949.
3. Aquilina, A. T., Hall, W. J., Douglas, R. G., Jr., et al.: Airway reactivity in subjects with viral upper respiratory tract infections: The effects of exercise and cold air. Am. Rev. Resp. Dis. *122*:3–10, 1980.
4. Arruda, E., Boyle T. R., Winther, B., et al: Localization of human rhinovirus replication in the upper respiratory tract by in situ hybridization. J. Infect. Dis. *171*:1329–1333, 1995.
5. Badger, G. F., Dingle, J. H., Feller, A. E., et al.: A study of illness in a group of Cleveland families. II. Incidence of the common respiratory diseases. Am. J. Hyg. *58*:31–40, 1953.
6. Badger, G. F., Dingle, J. H., Feller, A. E., et al.: A study of illness in a group of Cleveland families. III. Introduction of respiratory infections into families. Am. J. Hyg. *58*:41–46, 1953.
7. Badger, G. F., Dingle, J. H., Feller, A. E., et al.: A study of illness in a group of Cleveland families. IV. The spread of respiratory infections within the home. Am. J. Hyg. *58*:174–178, 1953.
8. Badger, G. F., Dingle, J. H., Feller, A. E., et al.: A study of illness in a group of Cleveland families. V. Introductions and secondary attack rates as indices of exposure to common respiratory diseases in the community. Am. J. Hyg. *58*:179–182, 1953.
9. Barness, L. A.: Safety considerations with high ascorbic acid dosage. Ann. N.Y. Acad. Sci. *258*:523–528, 1975.
10. Barrow, G. I., Higgins, P. G., Al-Nakib, W., et al.: The effect of intranasal nedocromil sodium on viral upper respiratory tract infections in human volunteers. Clin. Exper. Allergy *20*:45–51, 1989.
11. Brimblecombe, F. S. W., Cruickshank, R., Masters, P. L., et al.: Family studies of respiratory infections. Br. Med. J. *1*:119–128, 1958.
12. Buckland, F. E., and Tyrrell, D. A. J.: Experiments on the spread of colds. I. Laboratory studies on the dispersal of nasal secretion. J. Hyg. Camb. *62*:365–377, 1964.
13. Bush, R. K., Busse, W., Flaherty, D., et al.: Effects of experimental rhinovirus 16 infection on airways and leukocyte function in normal subjects. J. Allergy Clin. Immunol. *61*:80–87, 1978.
14. Bynoe, M. L.: The common cold. Practitioner *197*:739–746, 1966.
15. Callow, K. A., Tyrrell, D. A. J., Shaw, R. J., et al.: Influence of atopy on the clinical manifestations of coronavirus infection in adult volunteers. Clin. Allergy *18*:119–129, 1988.
16. Carr, A. B., Einstein, R., Lai, L. Y. C., et al.: Vitamin C and the common cold: Using identical twins as controls. Med. J. Aust. *2*:411–412, 1981.
17. Cate, T. R., Couch, R. B., and Johnson, K. M.: Studies with rhinoviruses in volunteers: Production of illness, effect of naturally acquired antibody, and demonstration of a protective effect not associated with serum antibody. J. Clin. Invest. *43*:56–67, 1964.
18. Cate, T. R., Rossen, R. D., Douglas, R. G., Jr., et al.: The role of nasal secretion and serum antibody in the rhinovirus common cold. Am. J. Epidemiol. *84*:352–363, 1966.
19. Cate, T. R., Douglas, R. G., Jr., and Couch, R. B.: Interferon and resistance to upper respiratory virus illness. Proc. Soc. Exp. Biol. Med. *131*:631–636, 1969.
20. Cate, T. R., Roberts, J. S., Russ, M. A., et al.: Effects of common colds on pulmonary function. Am. Rev. Resp. Dis. *108*:858–865, 1973.
21. Cherry, J. D.: Newer respiratory viruses: Their role in respiratory illnesses of children. Adv. Pediatr. *20*:225–289, 1973.
22. Cherry, J. D.: Comments. Pediatr. Res. *11*:250–251, 1977.
23. Couch, R. B., Cate, T. R., Douglas, R. G., Jr., et al.: Effect of route of inoculation on experimental respiratory viral disease in volunteers and evidence for airborne transmission. Bacteriol. Rev. *30*:517–529, 1966.
24. Coulehan, J. L., Eberhard, S., Kapner, L., et al.: Vitamin C and acute illness in Navajo schoolchildren. N. Engl. J. Med. *18*:973–977, 1976.
25. Coulehan, J. L.: Ascorbic acid and the common cold: Reviewing the evidence. Postgrad. Med. *66*:153–160, 1979.
26. D'Alessio, D. J., Peterson, J. A., Dick, C. R., et al.: Transmission of experimental rhinovirus colds in volunteer married couples. J. Infect. Dis. *133*:28–36, 1976.
27. D'Allessio, D. J., Meschievitz, C. K., Peterson, J. A., et al.: Short-duration exposure and the transmission of rhinoviral colds. J. Infect. Dis. *150*:189–194, 1984.
28. Dick, E. C., Hossain, S. U., Mink, K. A., et al.: Interruption of transmission of rhinovirus colds among human volunteers using virucidal paper handkerchiefs. J. Infect. Dis. *153*:352–356, 1986.
29. Dick, E. C., Jennings, L. C., Mink, K. A., et al.: Aerosol transmission of rhinovirus colds. J. Infect. Dis. *156*:442–448, 1987.
30. Dingle, J. H., Badger, G. F., Feller, A. E., et al.: A study of illness in a group of Cleveland families. I. Plan of study and certain general observations. Am. J. Hyg. *58*:16–30, 1953.
31. Dochez, A. R., Shibley, G. S., and Mills, K. C.: Studies in the common cold. IV. Experimental transmission of the common cold to anthropoid apes and human beings by means of a filtrable agent. J. Exp. Med. *52*:701–716, 1930.
32. Douglas, R. G., Jr., Lindgren, K. M., and Couch, R. B.: Exposure to cold environment and rhinovirus common cold: Failure to demonstrate effect. N. Engl. J. Med. *279*:742–747, 1968.
33. Douglas, R. G., Jr.: Pathogenesis of rhinovirus common colds in human volunteers. Ann. Otol. Rhinol. Laryngol. *79*:563–571, 1970.
34. Elwood, P. C., Hughes, S. J., and St. Leger, A. S.: A randomized controlled trial of the therapeutic effect of vitamin C in the common cold. Practitioner *218*:133–137, 1977.
35. Ernst, E., Pecho, E., Wirz, P., Saradeth, T.: Regular sauna bathing and the incidence of common colds. Ann. Med. *22*:225–227, 1990.
36. Farr, B. M., Conner, E. M., Betts, R. F., et al.: Two randomized controlled trials of zinc gluconate lozenge therapy of experimentally induced rhinovirus colds. Antimicrob. Agents Chemother. *31*:1183–1187, 1987.
37. Farr, B. M., Hendley, J. O., Kaiser, D. L., et al.: Two randomized controlled trials of virucidal nasal tissues in the prevention of natural upper respiratory infections. Am. J. Epidemiol. *128*:1162–1172, 1988.
38. Fleet, W. F., Couch, R. B., Cate, T. R., et al.: Homologous and heterologous resistance to rhinovirus common cold. Am. J. Epidemiol. *82*:185–196, 1965.
39. Forstall, G.J., Macknin, M.L., Yen-Lieberman, B.R., Medendorp, S.V.: Effect of inhaling heated vapor on symptoms of the common cold. J. A. M. A. *271*:1109–1111, 1994.
40. Fox, J. P., Hall, C. E., Cooney, M. K., et al.: The Seattle virus watch. II. Objectives, study population and its observation, data processing and summary of illnesses. Am. J. Epidemiol. *96*:270–285, 1972.
41. Foy, H. M., Cooney, M. K., Hall, C., et al.: Case-to-case intervals of rhinovirus and influenza virus infections in households. J. Infect. Dis. *157*:180–182, 1988.
42. Frost, W. H., and Gover, M.: The incidence and time distribution of common colds in several groups kept under continuous observation. *In*

Maxcy, K. F. (ed.): Papers of Wade Hampton Frost. New York, Commonwealth Fund, 1941, pp. 359–392.

43. Gadomski, A., Horton, L.: The need for rational therapeutics in the use of cough and cold medicine in infants. Pediatrics *89*:774–776, 1992.
44. Goldbloom, R. B.: Nasopharyngitis (the common cold). *In* Gellis, S. S., and Kagan, B. M. (eds.): Current Pediatric Therapy. 11th ed. Philadelphia, W. B. Saunders Co., 1984, p. 93.
45. Gordon, M., Lovell, S., and Dugdale, A. E.: The value of antibiotics in minor respiratory illness in children: A controlled trial. Med. J. Aust. *1*:304–306, 1974.
46. Graham, N. M. H., Burrell, C. J., Douglas, R. M., et al.: Adverse effects of aspirin, acetaminophen, and ibuprofen on immune function, viral shedding, and clinical status in rhinovirus-infected volunteers. J. Infect. Dis. *162*:1277–1282, 1990.
47. Gwaltney, J. M., Jr., Moskalski, P. B., and Hendley, J. O.: Hand-to-hand transmission of rhinovirus colds. Ann. Intern. Med. *88*:463–467, 1978.
48. Gwaltney, J. M., Jr., Moskalski, P. B., and Hendley, J. O.: Interruption of experimental rhinovirus transmission. J. Infect. Dis. *142*:811–815, 1980.
49. Gwaltney, J. M., Jr., and Hendley, J. O.: Transmission of experimental rhinovirus infection by contaminated surfaces. Am. J. Epidemiol. *116*:828–833, 1982.
50. Gwaltney, J. M., Jr., Hendley, J. O., Simon, G., et al.: Rhinovirus infections in an industrial population. I. The occurrence of illness. N. Engl. J. Med. *275*:1261–1268, 1966.
51. Hall, C. B., and Douglas, R. G., Jr.: Clinically useful method for the isolation of respiratory syncytial virus. J. Infect. Dis. *131*:1–5, 1975.
52. Hall, C. B., Douglas, R. G., Jr., Schnabel, K. C., et al.: Infectivity of respiratory syncytial virus by various routes of inoculation. Infect. Immun. *33*:779–783, 1981.
53. Hayden, F. G., and Gwaltney, J. M., Jr.: Intranasal interferon $\gamma 2$ for prevention of rhinovirus infection and illness. J. Infect. Dis. *148*:543–550, 1983.
54. Hayden, F. G., and Gwaltney, J. M., Jr.: Intranasal interferon $\alpha 2$ treatment of experimental rhinoviral colds. J. Infect. Dis. *150*:174–180, 1984.
55. Hayden, F. G., Kaiser, D. L., and Albrecht, J. K.: Intranasal recombinant alfa-2b interferon treatment of naturally occurring common colds. Antimicrob. Agents Chemother. *32*:224–230, 1988.
56. Hendley, J. O., Wenzel, R. P., and Gwaltney, J. M., Jr.: Transmission of rhinovirus colds by self-inoculation. N. Engl. J. Med. *288*:1361–1364, 1973.
57. Hilding, A.: The common cold. Arch. Otolaryngol. *12*:133–150, 1930.
58. Holmes, M. J., and Allen, T. R.: Viral respiratory diseases in isolated communities: A review. Br. Antarct. Surv. Bull. *35*:23–31, 1973.
59. Hutton, N., Wilson, M. H., Mellits, E. D., et al.: Effectiveness of an antihistamine-decongestant combination for young children with the common cold: A randomized, controlled clinical trial. J. Pediatr. *118*:125–130, 1991.
60. Jackson, G. G., Dowling, H. F., and Anderson, T. O.: Neutralization of common cold agents in volunteers by pooled human globulin. Science *128*:27–28, 1958.
61. Jackson, G. G., Dowling, H. F., Anderson, T. O., et al.: Susceptibility and immunity to common upper respiratory viral infections: The common cold. Ann. Intern. Med. *53*:719–730, 1960.
62. Jackson, G. G., Dowling, H. F., Akers, L. W., et al.: Immunity to the common cold from protective serum antibody: Time of appearance, persistence and relation to reinfection. N. Engl. J. Med. *266*:791–796, 1962.
63. Jackson, G. G., Dowling, H. F., and Muldoon, R. L.: Present concepts of the common cold. Am. J. Public Health *52*:940–945, 1962.
64. Jackson, G. G.: Understanding of viral respiratory illnesses provided by experiments in volunteers. Bacteriol. Rev. *28*:423–430, 1964.
65. Jennings, L. C., Dick, E. C., Mink, K. A., et al.: Near disappearance of rhinovirus along a fomite transmission chain. J. Infect. Dis. *158*:888–892, 1988.
66. Karlowski, T. R., Chalmers, T. C., Frenkel, L. D., et al.: Ascorbic acid for the common cold: A prophylactic and therapeutic trial. J. A. M. A. *231*:1038–1042, 1975.
67. Kruse, W.: Die erreger von husten und schnupfen. München Med. Wochenschr. *61*:1547, 1914.
68. Lefkowitz, L. B., Jr., Jackson, G. G., and Dowling, H. F.: The role of immunity in the common cold and related viral respiratory infections. Med. Clin. North Am. *47*:1171–1184, 1963.
69. Levandowski, R. A., Ou, D. W., and Jackson, G. G.: Acute-phase decrease of T lymphocyte subsets in rhinovirus infection. J. Infect. Dis. *153*:743–748, 1986.
70. Lexomboon, U., Duangmani, C., Kusalasai, V., et al.: Evaluation of orally administered antibiotics for treatment of upper respiratory infections in Thai children. J. Pediatr. *78*:771–778, 1971.
71. Lobovitz, A. M., Freeman, J., Goldmann, D. A., et al.: Risk of illness after exposure to a pediatric office. N. Engl. J. Med. *313*:425–428, 1985.
72. Meschievitz, C. K., Schultz, S. B., and Dick, E. C.: A model for obtaining predictable natural transmission of rhinoviruses in human volunteers. J. Infect. Dis. *150*:195–201, 1984.
73. Monto, A. S., Cavallaro, J. J., and Keller, J. B.: Seasonal patterns of acute infection in Tecumseh, Mich. Arch. Environ. Health *21*:408–417, 1970.
74. Naclerio, R. M., Proud, D., Lichtenstein, L. M., et al.: Kinins are generated during experimental rhinovirus colds. J. Infect. Dis. *157*:133–142, 1988.
75. Nelson, W. E.: Infections of the upper respiratory tract. *In* Nelson, W. E. (ed.): Textbook of Pediatrics. 6th ed. Philadelphia, W. B. Saunders, 1954, pp. 770–786.
76. Noah, T. L., Henderson, F. W., Wortman, I. A., et al.: Nasal cytokine production in viral acute upper respiratory infection of childhood. J. Infect. Dis. *171*:584–592, 1995.
77. Pedersen, M., Sakakura, Y., Winther, B., et al.: Nasal mucociliary transport, number of ciliated cells, and beating pattern in naturally acquired common colds. Eur. J. Resp. Dis. *64*(Suppl. 128):355–364, 1983.
78. Pepper, W.: The Medical Side of Benjamin Franklin. Philadelphia, W. J. Campbell, 1911, pp. 50–51, 60–65, 72–73.
79. Picken, J. J., Niewoehner, D. E., and Chester, E. H.: Prolonged effects of viral infections of the upper respiratory tract upon small airways. Am. J. Med. *52*:738–746, 1972.
80. Pitt, H. A., and Costrini, A. M.: Vitamin C prophylaxis in marine recruits. J. A. M. A. *241*:908–911, 1979.
81. Proud, D., Naclerio, R. M., Gwaltney, J. M., et al.: Kinins are generated in nasal secretions during natural rhinovirus colds. J. Infect. Dis. *161*:120–123, 1990.
82. Proud, D., Gwaltney, J. M., Hendley, J. O., et al.: Increased levels of interleukin-1 are detected in nasal secretions of volunteers during experimental rhinovirus colds. J. Infect. Dis. *169*:1007–1013, 1994.
83. Reed, S. E.: An investigation of the possible transmission of rhinovirus colds through indirect contact. J. Hyg. Camb. *75*:249–258, 1975.
84. Sargent, F., Lombard, O. M., and Sargent, V. W.: Further studies on stability of resistance to the common cold: The importance of constitution. Am. J. Hyg. *45*:29–32, 1947.
85. Schwartz, A. R., Togo, Y., Hornick, R. B., et al.: Evaluation of the efficacy of ascorbic acid in prophylaxis of induced rhinovirus 44 infection in man. J. Infect. Dis. *128*:500–505, 1973.
86. Skoner, D. P., Whiteside, T. L., Wilson, J. W., et al.: Effect of rhinovirus 39 infection on cellular immune parameters in allergic and nonallergic subjects. J. Allergy Clin. Immunol. *92*:732–743, 1993.
87. Smith, C. B., Purcell, R. H., Bellanti, J. A., et al.: Protective effect of antibody to parainfluenza type I virus. N. Engl. J. Med. *275*:1145–1152, 1966.
88. Smith, M. B. H., and Feldman, W.: Over-the-counter cold medications: A critical review of clinical trials between 1950 and 1991. J. A. M. A. *269*:2258–2263, 1993.
89. Smith, W., Andrewes, C. H. and Laidlaw, P. P.: A virus obtained from influenza patients. Lancet *2*:66–68, 1933.
90. Soyka, L. F., Robinson, D. S., Lachant, N., et al.: The misuse of antibiotics for treatment of upper respiratory tract infections in children. Pediatrics *55*:552–556, 1975.
91. Sperber, S. J., and Hayden, F. G.: Chemotherapy of rhinovirus colds. Antimicrob. Agents Chemother. *32*:409–419, 1988.
92. Sperber, S. J., Hendley, J. O., Hayden, F. G., et al.: Effects of naproxen on experimental rhinovirus colds: A randomized, double-blind, controlled trial. Ann. Intern. Med. *117*:37–41, 1992.
93. Tannock, G. A., Gillett, S. M., Gillett, R. S., et al.: A study of intranasally administered interferon A (rIFN-alpha 2A) for the seasonal prophylaxis of natural viral infections of the upper respiratory tract in healthy volunteers. Epidemiol. Infect. *101*:611–621, 1988.
94. Tremonti, L. P., Lin, J. S. L., and Jackson, G. G.: Neutralizing activity in nasal secretions and serum in resistance of volunteers to parainfluenza virus type 2. J. Immunol. *101*:572–577, 1968.
95. Turner, R. B., Felton, A., Kosak, K., et al.: Prevention of experimental coronavirus colds with intranasal alpha-2b interferon. J. Infect. Dis. *154*:443–447, 1986.
96. Tyrrell, D. A. J.: Common Colds and Related Diseases. Baltimore, Williams & Wilkins, 1965.
97. Valic, F., and Zuskin, E.: Pharmacological prevention of acute ventilatory capacity reduction in flax dust exposure. Br. J. Ind. Med. *30*:381–384, 1973.
98. Walker, G. H., Bynoe, M. L., and Tyrrell, D. A. J.: Trial of ascorbic acid in prevention of colds. Br. Med. J. *1*:603–606, 1967.
99. West, S., Brandon, B., Stolley, P., et al.: A review of antihistamines and the common cold. Pediatrics *56*:100–107, 1975.
100. Winther, B., Brofeldt, S., Christensen, B., et al.: Light and scanning electron microscopy of nasal biopsy material from patients with naturally acquired common colds. Acta Otolaryngol. (Stockh.) *97*:309–318, 1984.
101. Winther, B., Farr, B., Turner, R. B., et al.: Histopathologic examination and enumeration of polymorphonuclear leukocytes in the nasal mucosa during experimental rhinovirus colds. Acta Otolaryngol. (Suppl.) (Stockh.) *413*:19–24, 1984.
102. Winther, B.: Effects on the nasal mucosa of upper respiratory viruses (common cold). Danish Med. *41*:193–204, 1994.
103. Zuskin, E., Lewis, A. J., and Bouhuys, A.: Inhibition of histamine-induced airway constriction by ascorbic acid. J. Allergy Clin. Immunol. *51*:218–226, 1973.

9

INFECTIONS OF THE ORAL CAVITY

Thomas R. Flynn, Joseph F. Piecuch,
and Richard G. Topazian

Although most infections of the oral cavity in children are odontogenic and may be treated simply with local measures, their occasional spread to adjacent or distant fascial spaces or to the maxilla and mandible may result in life-threatening complications. Consequently, careful attention should be given to such infections, including liberal use of the dental consultation.[13, 45]

MICROBIOLOGIC CONSIDERATIONS IN DENTAL INFECTIONS

Normal Flora

That the oral cavity provides an environment favorable to the growth of microorganisms is substantiated by reports of bacterial counts in the range of 10^8 to 10^{11} organisms/mL of saliva.[3, 6] More than 30 species of bacteria normally can be identified in saliva in varying proportions, depending on a dynamic interaction of different microbial ecosystems, including the tongue, the gingival crevice, and the presence of plaque.[42, 48] Age, anatomic relationships, eruption of teeth, presence of decayed teeth, diet, oral hygiene, antibiotic therapy, systemic disease, cancer chemotherapy,[43] and hospitalization all can modify the microbial population. In the older literature, emphasis was placed on the role of *Streptococcus* and *Staphylococcus* species in producing odontogenic infections, to the exclusion of most anaerobic bacteria. This emphasis probably was the result of failure to culture satisfactorily for anaerobic organisms, and it now is well known that the ratio of anaerobic to aerobic organisms ranges from 3:1 to 10:1.[3, 7]

The nomenclature of the oral flora is changing rapidly, owing to the improved understanding of the genetic makeup of these bacteria provided by molecular biology techniques. Table 9–1 summarizes nomenclatural changes among selected members of the oral flora.[8, 51, 52]

The flora of children is quite similar to that of adults, with several exceptions. At birth, the oral cavity is sterile, but colonization with *Streptococcus salivarius* is rapid. This organism has been found in 80 per cent of cultures taken from 1-day-old infants.[53] The percentage of *Streptococcus* species decreases from 98 per cent at day 1 to 70 per cent at 4 months[40] as other organisms become established. *Staphylococcus* species, *Neisseria, Veillonella, Actinomyces, Nocardia, Fusobacterium, Bacteroides, Corynebacterium, Candida,* and a variety of coliforms gradually become established by 1 year. As eruption of the deciduous dentition occurs, anaerobic organisms become well established in the gingival crevice, yet the spirochetes, *Bacteroides melaninogenicus,* and related oral anaerobes, which commonly are associated with the gingival crevice in adults, appear to be present in fewer numbers prior to age 13 to 16 years.[6, 53] Eruption of deciduous teeth also is associated with the establishment of *Streptococcus mutans* and *Streptococcus sanguis,* which adhere to the enamel surface.

Pathogenic Organisms

Not all residents of the oral flora are pathogens. In the odontogenic infections caries and periodontal disease, there appears to be a progression from initiating infections caused by oral streptococci toward a predominance of oral anaerobes in the more severe and long-standing infections. For example, caries is initiated primarily by *S. mutans,* a member of the alpha-hemolytic *Streptococcus* viridans group. As tooth decay progresses toward the dental pulp, *Lactobacillus* and *Actinomyces* species join the carious milieu. Severe pulpal infections are caused generally by a combination of these same oral facultative streptococci plus obligate anaerobes, such as *Porphyromonas endodontalis,* formerly classified as *B. melaninogenicus.*[56]

Periodontal infections also are polymicrobial, with gram-positive aerobes, primarily streptococci, predominating in gingivitis and with the gram-negative anaerobic rods predominating in bone-destroying periodontitis. Juvenile periodontitis (formerly called periodontosis), a particularly aggressive periodontal infection in children and adolescents, shows a predominance of *Actinobacillus actinomycetemcomitans* in its cultivable flora.

Orofacial odontogenic infections that spread beyond the teeth and alveolar processes are polymicrobial, yielding on average four to six isolates per case.[5, 29, 41] Severe orofacial infections have been associated statistically with *Fusobacterium nucleatum.*[20] The concept of the progression from aerobic streptococci to anaerobic gram-negative rods in orofacial infections is supported further by studies that have found a predominance of streptococci in early infections (in the first

TABLE 9–1. Terminology Changes for Selected Oral Pathogens

Older Terminology	Current Terminology
Streptococcus viridans	*Streptococcus anginosus* *Streptococcus intermedius* *Streptococcus constellatus* *Streptococcus mutans* *Streptococcus sanguis* *Streptococcus mitis* *Streptococcus salivarius* *Streptococcus vestibularis*
Streptococcus milleri	*Streptococcus anginosus* *Streptococcus intermedius* *Streptococcus constellatus*
Bacteroides melaninogenicus	*Prevotella melaninogenica* *Prevotella intermedia* *Porphyromonas asaccarolyticus* *Porphyromonas gingivalis* *Porphyromonas endodontalis* *Capnocytophaga* species
Streptococcus faecalis	*Enterococcus faecalis*
Streptococcus faecium	*Enterococcus faecium*
Peptococcus species	*Peptostreptococcus* species

TABLE 9–2. Most Frequent Pathogens Isolated from Orofacial Infections in Two Studies

	Per Cent of Cases	
Microorganism	***Lewis et al.****	***Heimdahl et al.*†**
Streptococcus milleri	50	31
Peptostreptococcus species	64	31
Other anaerobic streptococci	8	38
Bacteroides (Prevotella) oralis	40	9
Bacteroides (Prevotella) gingivalis	28	‡
Bacteroides (Porphyromonas) melaninogenicus	24	26
Fusobacterium species	14	45

*Data from Lewis, M. A. O., MacFarlane, T. W., and McGowan, D. A.: Quantitative bacteriology of acute dento-alveolar abscesses. J. Med. Microbiol. *21*:101–104, 1986.

†Data from Heimdahl, A., Von Konow, L., Satoh, T., et al.: Clinical appearance of orofacial infections of odontogenic origin in relation to microbiological findings. J. Clin. Microbiol. *22*:299–302, 1985.

‡This organism was not reported in this study.

3 days of symptoms) and a predominance of anaerobes in late infections.[29] Table 9–2 lists the frequency with which the major pathogens in orofacial infections were isolated in two studies.[20, 29]

Infections originating from nonodontogenic causes (facial trauma, surgical manipulation, tonsillitis) are included in most studies of soft tissue and fascial space infections, and contamination from the skin or oropharynx might allow for aerobic organisms, such as *Staphylococcus aureus* and aerobic *Streptococcus* species, to become established.[6] In contradistinction, infections originating solely from the dental periapical tissues are much more likely to be predominantly anaerobic.

A pitfall in the identification of organisms as described in the older literature was the failure to culture satisfactorily for anaerobic organisms. The more current literature recognizes this fact.[30, 41] The preponderance of anaerobic organisms in odontogenic infections mandates the use of both anaerobic and aerobic culturing techniques in those situations in which cultures are indicated.

ANATOMIC CONSIDERATIONS

Most severe orofacial infections develop consequent to dental infection, periapical, periodontal, or pericoronal. Spread occurs along anatomic pathways of least resistance.[3, 7, 21, 28, 55] Periodontal and pericoronal infections rarely have major sequelae because they generally drain from the gingival sulcus along the surface of the tooth into the oral cavity. On the other hand, infections associated with the root apices generally are confined within the bony alveolar process (Fig. 9–1). Should spontaneous intraoral drainage occur through either the periodontium or the pulp chamber, further spread through the marrow spaces is unlikely. If such drainage does not occur, spread through bone (osteomyelitis) or perforation of the cortical plate of the affected jaw may take place. Infections associated with root apices in close proximity to the buccal cortical plate generally spread buccally, whereas those close to the lingual or palatal cortical plate or to the maxillary sinus will spread in those directions (Fig. 9–2).

Once penetration of the cortical plate occurs, infection will involve the adjacent soft tissues and may manifest either as cellulitis or as a soft tissue abscess, which eventually may perforate mucous membrane or skin as a sinus tract (Fig. 9–3).

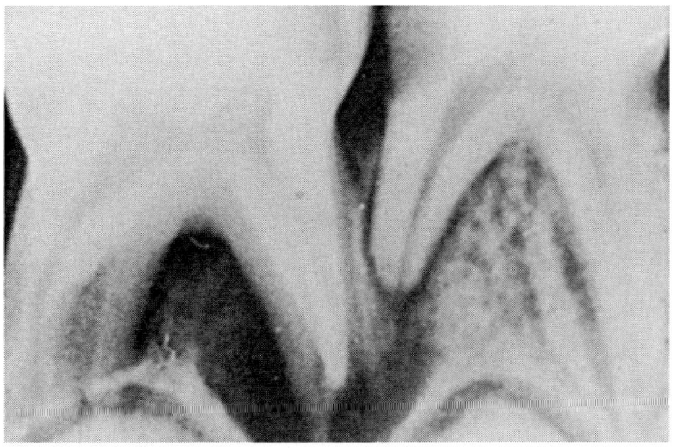

FIGURE 9–1. *Radiolucency representing a chronic periapical abscess involving the mesial root of the deciduous second molar and the distal root of the deciduous first molar. The developing mandibular bicuspids are seen inferior to the deciduous roots. The cause of the abscess is the deep carious lesions in both teeth, which appear to have penetrated the pulp chambers.*

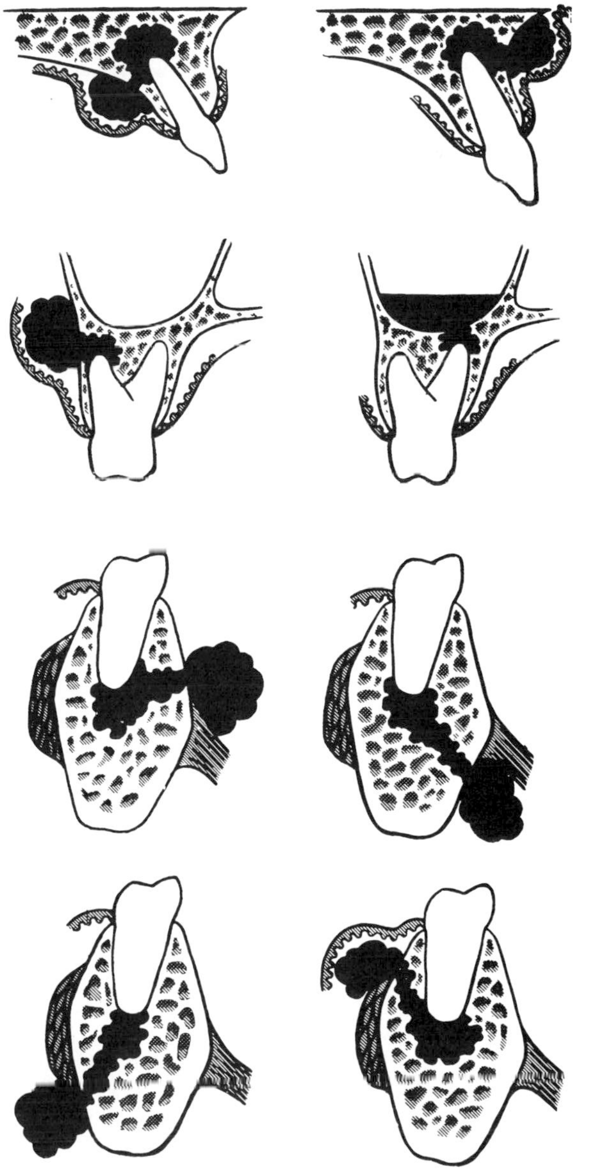

FIGURE 9–2. *Possible pathways of spread of periapical infection. (From Shafer, W. G., Hine, M. K., and Levy, B. M.: Textbook of Oral Pathology. 2nd ed. Philadelphia, W. B. Saunders, 1963.)*

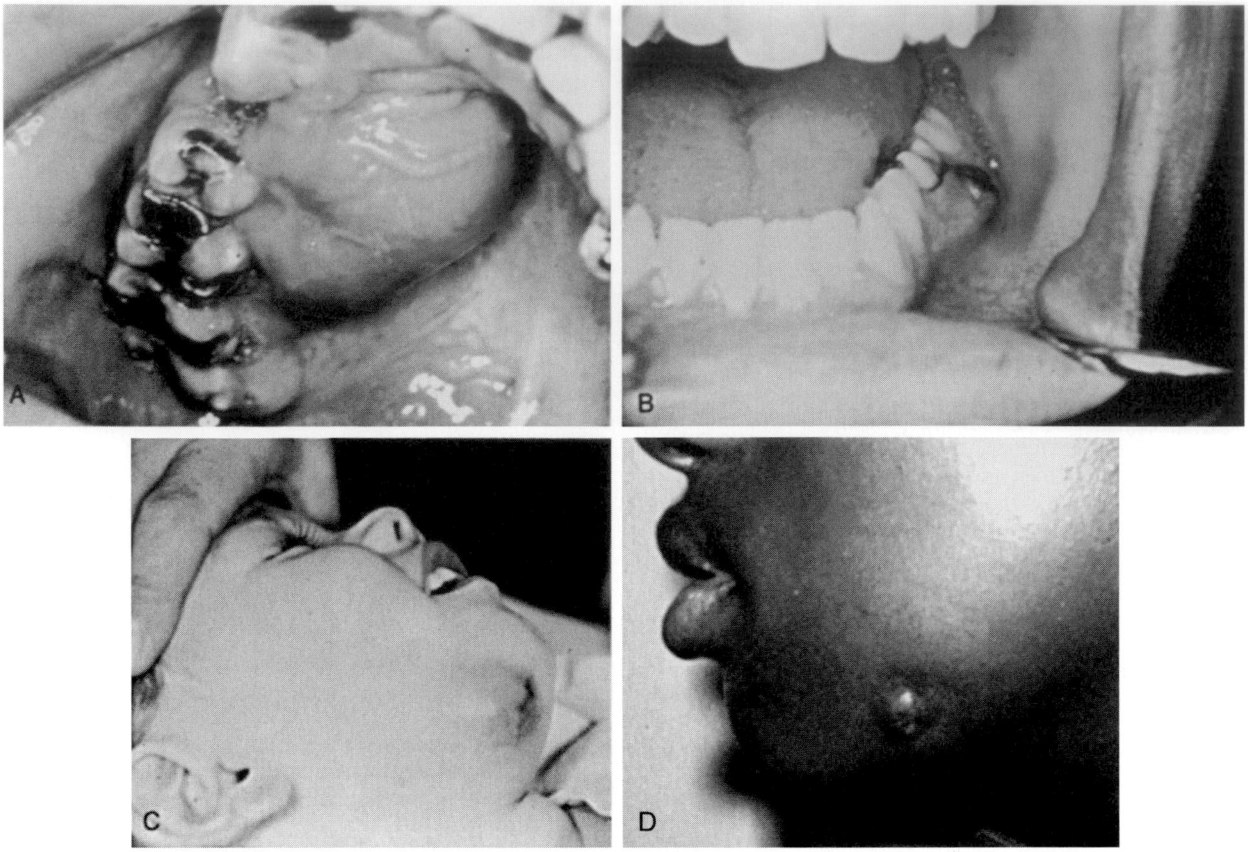

FIGURE 9–3. *Spread of odontogenic infection.* A, *Palatal abscess resulting from infected first premolar.* B, *Intraoral mucosal fistula from periapical abscess of mandibular left first molar.* C, *Soft tissue infection secondary to periapical abscess.* D, *Draining cutaneous sinus tract from a chronically infected lower molar in an adolescent female. (*A *from Piecuch, J.: Odontogenic infections. Dent. Clin. North Am. 26:129–145, 1982;* D *from Flynn T. R., and Topazian, R. G.: Infections of the oral cavity.* In *Waite, D. E. (ed.): Textbook of Practical Oral and Maxillofacial Surgery. Philadelphia, Lea & Febiger, 1987.)*

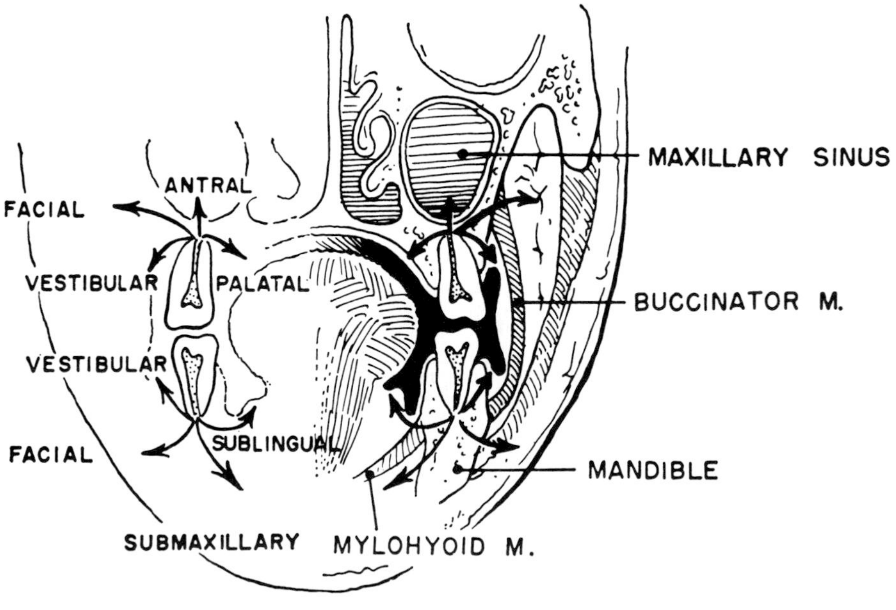

FIGURE 9–4. *Common pathways of spread of periapical infection. (From Kruger, G.: Textbook of Oral Surgery. 4th ed. St. Louis, C. V. Mosby, 1980.)*

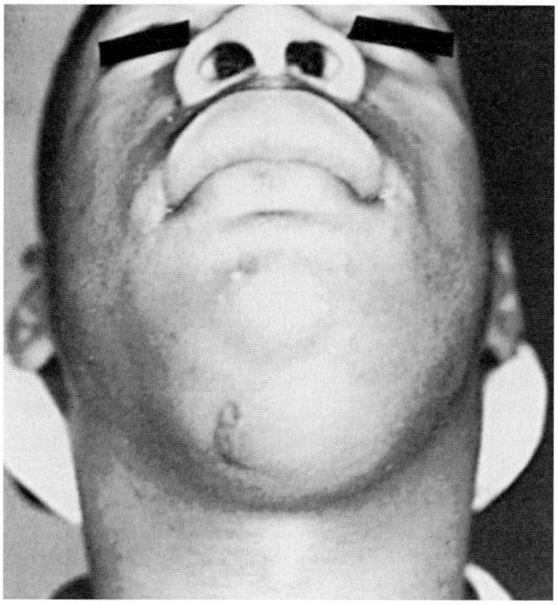

FIGURE 9–5. *Submental space abscess.*

Perforation of periapical infections through bone follows a typical pattern that results from the position of the root apices in relation to the bony cortex and to muscle attachments (Fig. 9–4). Infections involving maxillary anterior teeth and buccal roots of maxillary posterior teeth generally perforate labially or buccally, whereas those involving palatal roots of posterior teeth perforate palatally or, rarely, into the maxillary sinus. The presence of the buccinator muscle attachment superior to the root apices usually confines these infections and fistulas to the oral cavity. In children, however, maxillary root apices often are superior to the buccinator, and infections may spread to the buccal or infraorbital space or to the periorbital tissues. They eventually may drain through the skin.

Mandibular incisor or canine tooth infections may spread either labially or lingually because the alveolar process is thin in this area. Labial perforation, which is more common, may be confined intraorally if the root apices are superior to the origin of the mentalis muscle but may spread extraorally if the apices are inferior to the mentalis attachment (Fig. 9–5). Mandibular premolar and first molar infections often perforate buccally, whereas the second and third molars perforate lingually.

When spread of mandibular infections occurs lingually, the relationship of the tooth apices to the mylohyoid muscle origin is significant (Fig. 9–6). From the first molar forward, the dental root apices are superior to the mylohyoid, and these infections will localize intraorally in the floor of the mouth (sublingual space). The apices of the second and third molars generally are inferior to the mylohyoid, and so the submandibular space will be involved, with an extraoral presentation. As in maxillary infections, the relationship of the buccinator muscle to the root apices will determine whether the infection spreads intraorally or extraorally.

Two fascial spaces commonly associated with odontogenic infections are the submandibular and masticator spaces.[15, 16, 28] The submandibular space is formed within the superficial layer of deep cervical fascia inferior to the mylohyoid muscle and inferomedial to the mandible. Anteriorly and posteriorly, it is limited by the bellies of the digastric muscle. Within this space lies the submandibular gland and portions of the facial artery and anterior facial vein. This space is closely approximated to the sublingual and masticator spaces. Infections of the submandibular space may originate in these adjacent spaces as well as from mandibular posterior teeth.

The masticator space also is formed within the superficial

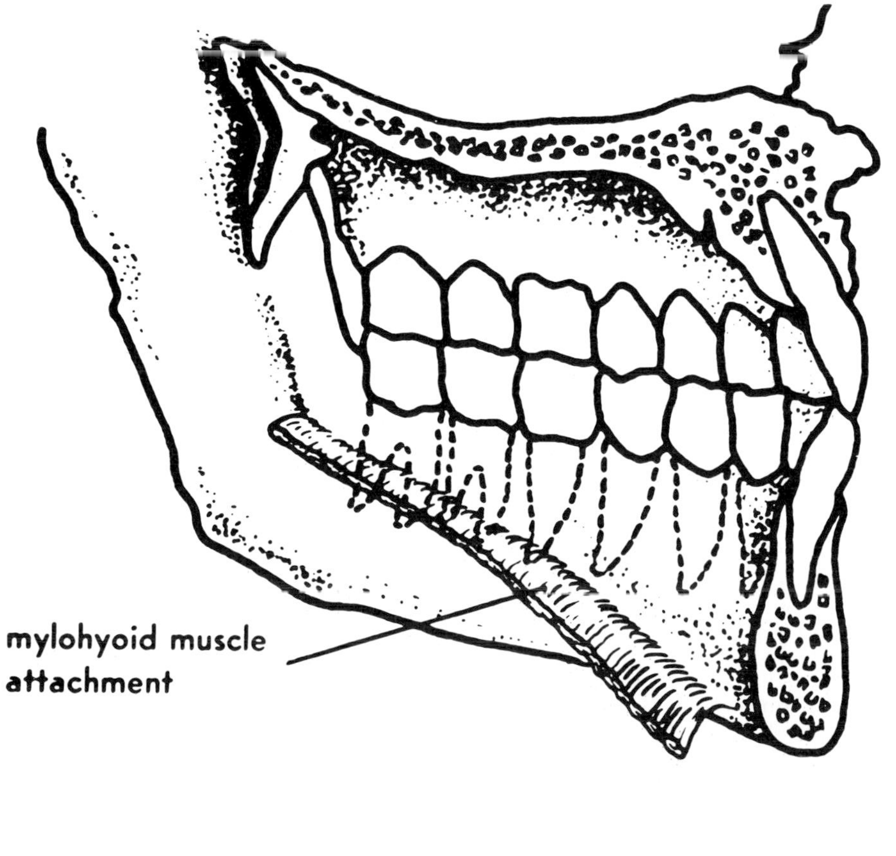

FIGURE 9–6. *Relation of tooth apices to the origin of mylohyoid muscle. (From Waite, D.: Textbook of Practical Oral Surgery. Philadelphia, Lea & Febiger, 1978.)*

layer of deep cervical fascia. Its name is appropriate, as its contents include the masseter, internal and external pterygoid, and temporalis muscles, as well as the mandibular ramus and the inferior alveolar neurovascular bundle. Adjacent are the submandibular, lateral pharyngeal, and retropharyngeal spaces. Infections of the masticator space may originate in adjacent spaces or spread to it from periapical or pericoronal infections of the mandibular second and third molars and maxillary third molar.

TREATMENT OF ODONTOGENIC INFECTIONS

Patients with odontogenic infections may present with symptoms ranging from minor to life-threatening. Too often a patient may be given a thorough systemic and extraoral head and neck evaluation while the intraoral search for the etiologic agent is overlooked.

Thorough oral examination begins with an evaluation of the degree of mandibular opening. Interincisal distance on wide opening extends up to 40 mm or more, even in young children. Painful limitation of oral opening, or trismus, is associated with inflammation of the muscles of mastication and indicates spread of the infection to the masticator space. If associated with a high fever, this can represent a serious turn of events. Teeth are inspected visually for caries by percussion for tenderness and by electrical sensitivity or hot and cold stimulation for the pulpal pain response. Gingival tissues are probed for periodontal defects, and salivary glands are palpated for tenderness and milked to observe for purulent discharge from the duct orifices.

General Therapeutic Principles

As with infections elsewhere in the body, the principles of treatment of oral infections involve surgical drainage and antibiotics. Surgical drainage may comprise standard incision and drainage of an orofacial swelling or, in the case of localized periapical infection, may involve endodontic drainage through the pulp or extraction of the offending tooth.

Surgical treatment of odontogenic infections is primary. Dodson and colleagues,[10] in a review of head and neck infections requiring hospitalization of children, found that facial infections of the regions at or above the level of the upper lip and teeth most frequently were upper respiratory or sinus related, and lower face infections primarily were odontogenic. Upper face infections resolved without surgery in 65 per cent of cases, and lower face infections resolved without surgery in only 25 per cent of cases. Odontogenic infections almost always required some sort of surgical intervention. This finding may be due to the fact that the portal of entry in respiratory infections is through the surface mucosa, whereas the tooth roots carry the invading bacterial pathogens deep into the bone of the jaw, through which the surrounding deep fascial spaces become infected. Respiratory pathogens frequently are viral, and odontogenic infections almost uniformly are bacterial, which may explain the propensity of odontogenic infections to form abscesses that need to be drained. Odontogenic infections treated only with antibiotics almost always recur in worse form than their previous manifestation. On the other hand, the indications for antibiotics in addition to appropriate dental surgical therapy are fever, trismus, lymphadenopathy, osteomyelitis, and immune system compromise. Minor infections localized to the alveolar processes can be treated by tooth extraction, gingival curettage, or root canal therapy, with or without intraoral incision and drainage, without the use of antibiotics in the nonimmunocompromised individual.

Antibiotic selection for odontogenic infections, although ultimately based on Gram stain and aerobic and anaerobic cultures, generally is begun empirically prior to availability of culture results. Penicillin G or V is the logical first choice, based on its lack of toxicity, bactericidal nature, and the sensitivity of most streptococci and oral anaerobes to this drug. Antibiotic sensitivity studies, however, indicate that the oral anaerobes now are largely resistant to erythromycin.[44] Other studies suggest that orofacial infections in hospitalized patients harbor penicillinase-producing organisms in 33 per cent of cases,[5] whereas those infections not requiring hospitalization yield penicillin-resistant organisms in only 9 per cent of cases.[13] Clindamycin remains highly effective against the likely oral pathogens, including streptococci and the oral anaerobes; its association with *Clostridium difficile* colitis and its effectiveness in severe orofacial infections indicate that it should be reserved, in this era of increasing microbial resistance to antibiotics, for the most severe cases.

The aforementioned considerations suggest that the empiric antibiotic of choice in early and mild odontogenic infections should be penicillin or erythromycin in penicillin allergy and penicillin or clindamycin in severe or chronic cases. Table 9–3 lists the authors' recommendations for empiric antibiotic therapy in odontogenic infections.

Second-line antibiotics in odontogenic infections are the cephalosporins, whose effectiveness against the oral anaerobes has been waning, and metronidazole, which is effective against obligate anaerobes only. The safety and effectiveness of metronidazole in children, however, have not been established.

Other considerations that may be of importance in antibiotic selection for individual cases are as follows: (1) *Eikenella corrodens*, an occasional pathogen in odontogenic infections, is uniformly resistant to clindamycin, which may explain the lack of effectiveness of clindamycin in some cases. (2) Some cephalosporins do not cross the blood-brain barrier in high concentrations, which may be a factor in antibiotic selection for odontogenic infections that are approaching the cranial cavity. Penicillin is able to cross the blood-brain barrier when the meninges are inflamed. Metronidazole crosses the blood-brain barrier, and therefore its use may be justified in severe odontogenic infections approaching the brain in children. Ceftazidime is one cephalosporin that crosses the blood-brain barrier well. (3) Tetracycline is incorporated permanently into newly formed dentin, thereby causing permanent disfiguring discoloration of the dentition. Therefore, it should not be

TABLE 9–3. Empiric Antibiotics of Choice for Odontogenic Infections

Type of Infection	Antibiotic of Choice
Mild or early infections	Penicillin
	Cephalexin (or other first-generation cephalosporin)
	Erythromycin
Penicillin allergy	Erythromycin
	Cephalexin (if the penicillin allergy was not the anaphylactoid type)
	Clindamycin
Severe or chronic infections	Penicillin
	Clindamycin
	Penicillin + metronidazole
Penicillin allergy	Clindamycin
	Ceftazidime (if penicillin allergy was not the anaphylactoid type)

used in children until at least 9 years of age, when all but the third molar teeth will have full crown formation. (4) β-Lactamase inhibitors used in combination with β-lactam antibiotics may improve their effectiveness against resistant anaerobes, although the effectiveness of these drugs in odontogenic infections has not been studied. (5) Staphylococci are uncommon pathogens in odontogenic infections, and coverage for staphylococci is not indicated in empiric therapy for these infections, although their role in upper respiratory and sinus infections is well known.

If clinical signs or Gram stain suggests the presence of *S. aureus*, a penicillinase-resistant antimicrobial, such as oxacillin or dicloxacillin, may be added to the penicillin, pending the results of the culture. Alternatively, a first-generation cephalosporin, such as cephalexin, cephalothin, or cefazolin, may be used.

Nursing Bottle Caries

Nursing bottle caries is a pattern of tooth decay affecting mainly the primary upper incisors and frequently the upper and lower primary molars in children of bottle feeding age. It is caused by a practice of putting the child to bed with a nursing bottle filled with a sugar-containing drink, such as milk, fruit juice, or a soft drink. The child sucks on the bottle intermittently during sleep, when salivary secretion is low, and the sugar-containing liquid stays in the mouth for extended periods. This provides an excellent environment for the growth of caries-producing organisms, such as *S. mutans*. Nursing bottle caries can destroy virtually the entire primary dentition of a child as it erupts. Pediatric physicians and dentists therefore should instruct parents to avoid putting their child to bed with a nursing bottle or, if they must do so, to use only water in the bedtime drink.

Periapical Abscess

Extension of microorganisms through the root apex will lead to the formation of an abscess. Early in this process, the acute abscess is indistinguishable clinically and radiographically from an acute pulpitis, particularly because radiographic evidence of bone destruction may take from 7 to 14 days or more to develop. Sensitivity to heat stimulus (relieved by cold), exquisite sensitivity to percussion, and tenderness to finger pressure on the alveolar process are indications that the tooth has become abscessed. Electric pulp testing may be diagnostic if the tooth shows no response to the electrical stimulus, but a positive pain response may be equivocal in multirooted teeth. Chronic abscesses are diagnosed more easily by looseness of the tooth, the presence of suppuration from draining sinus tracts or from the gingival crevice (see Fig. 9–3), and the presence of a radiolucency on the radiographs (see Fig. 9–1). Depending on the path of least resistance, fluctuant areas may be noted in the buccal or lingual mucosa. Spread through the tissues, or cellulitis, may lead to the classic presentation of swollen face, pain, elevated temperature, and malaise.

In 1951, Krogh[25] demonstrated a 3 per cent complication rate when 2626 infected teeth were removed at the time of initial presentation. In 1975, Martis and Karakasis[36] published a similar study in which they treated 1376 acute dentoalveolar abscesses by immediate extraction. A 3 per cent complication rate was found in this study as well. A complication was defined as further extension of the infection, requiring additional treatment. Hall and associates[18] published a report in 1968 in which 350 patients with odontogenic cellulitis were divided randomly into two groups. The first group had extractions carried out on the day of initial presentation, whereas the second group waited (with antibiotics) until the fourth day for surgical treatment to be performed after "localization" had occurred. The investigators' observations showed that in neither group did extraction spread the cellulitis. In addition, those with earlier extractions recovered more rapidly, whereas those with delayed treatment had a greater need for incision and drainage, which was twice as likely to be extraoral than intraoral. In 1978, Martis and colleagues[37] showed in a series of more than 2000 patients that extraction without antibiotics in the presence of periapical infection led to the same complication rate as extraction of noninfected teeth.

When faced with the prospect of early relief of symptoms as well as a 97 per cent chance that extraction (or occasionally root canal treatment) will cure the infection, it is clear that early surgical intervention is mandatory. The use of antibiotics must be determined on an individual basis according to principles outlined previously.

Periodontal Infections

Surrounding the teeth is a distinctive, pink-colored keratinized mucosa, the gingiva (Fig. 9–7*A*). Normal gingiva is attached firmly to the alveolar bone and extends between the teeth as the interdental papilla. A thin cuff of free (nonattached) gingiva surrounds each tooth, and the resulting crevice between the free gingiva and the tooth normally is 1 to 3 mm in depth. It is represented by a thin roll of tissue along each tooth in the illustration.

Accumulation of food deposits and bacteria in the gingival crevice may result in gingivitis, a localized inflammation of the free gingiva that presents as an erythematous, nonpainful swelling of the interdental papillae. In severe cases (Fig. 9–7*B*), the gingival architecture may become distorted, and accumulations of plaque are evident. Although gingivitis is prevalent at all ages, affecting more than 50 per cent of children[39] and almost all adults to some degree, it often is most severe in compromised hosts, including diabetics and immunosuppressed patients. Poor oral hygiene is the usual etiology of gingivitis, and this condition generally responds to dental scaling and improved oral hygiene.

In adolescents as well as in adults, gingivitis may progress to periodontitis, a progressively severe infection that is characterized by hypertrophied gingivae, tooth mobility due to irreversible resorption of alveolar bone, and a purulent exudate. Unfortunately, this insidious condition usually is painless and may progress for years before being recognized. Localized periodontal treatment and meticulous oral hygiene may arrest the condition.

A rare variant, juvenile periodontitis,[27] usually is localized to the molar and incisor regions of younger, otherwise healthy children. Deep gingival pocketing and severe bone resorption are characteristic of this process and may result in loss of the dentition in these areas. The etiology is thought to involve the presence of a gram-negative anaerobe, *A. actinomycetemcomitans*, and localized bacterial inhibition of leukocyte function. Tetracycline in older patients has been useful in combination with periodontal surgery and meticulous home care.

Acute necrotizing ulcerative gingivitis (Fig. 9–7C) is a specific infection caused by fusiform bacilli and spirochetes. Synonyms include trench mouth and Vincent infection. Erythema at the tips of the interdental papillae soon is supplanted by frank ulceration and foci of spontaneous bleeding. A pseudomembranous necrotic exudate forms along the mar-

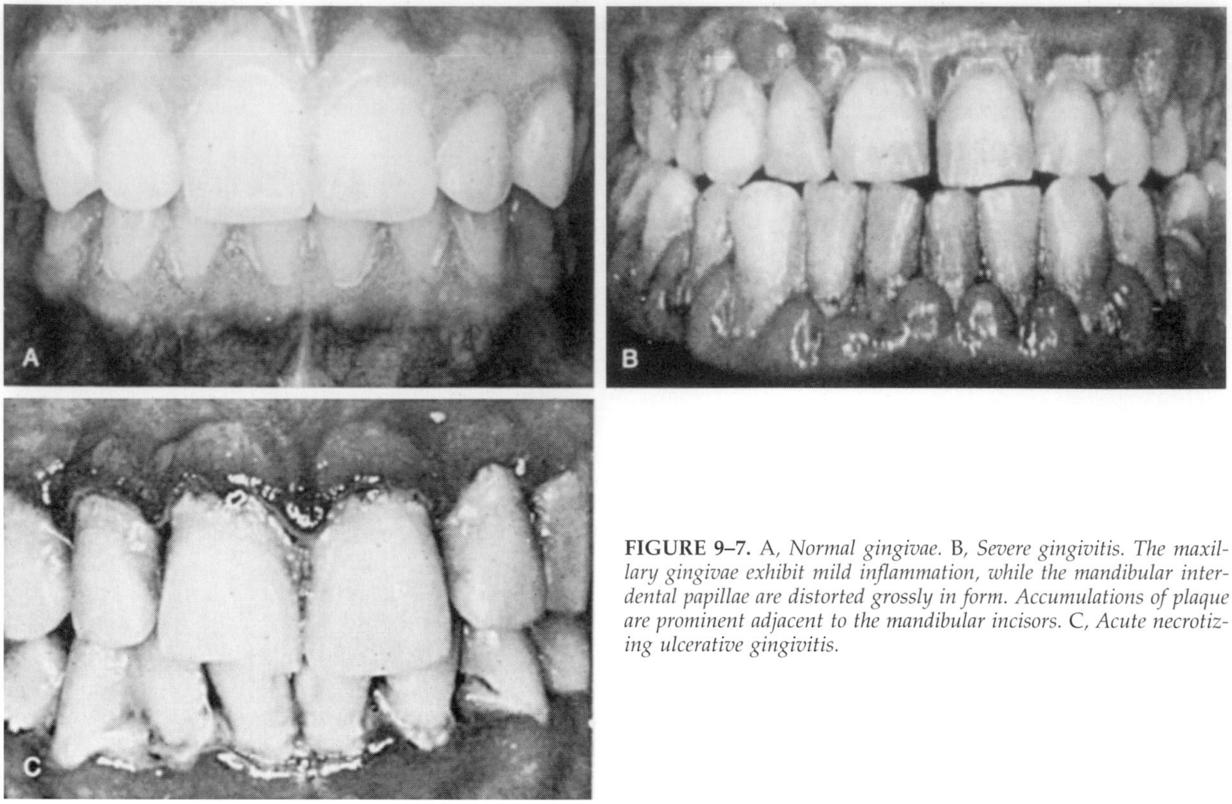

FIGURE 9–7. A, *Normal gingivae.* B, *Severe gingivitis. The maxillary gingivae exhibit mild inflammation, while the mandibular interdental papillae are distorted grossly in form. Accumulations of plaque are prominent adjacent to the mandibular incisors.* C, *Acute necrotizing ulcerative gingivitis.*

ginal gingivae and the interdental papillae. The papillae later become blunted. Acute necrotizing ulcerative gingivitis is characterized by pain, foul breath and taste, thick ropy saliva, malaise, and occasionally fever. Theories suggest a concomitant viral etiology. Treatment consists initially of penicillin therapy followed within a few days by localized gingival curettage and oral rinses with 0.5 per cent hydrogen peroxide or 0.12 per cent chlorhexidine.[32] It should be noted, however, that the safety and effectiveness of chlorhexidene in children have not been established yet.

Pericoronitis

Impaction of microorganisms and debris under the soft tissue overlying the crown of a tooth, often a mandibular third molar, or any erupting permanent tooth leads to the development of inflammation. Drainage usually occurs spontaneously from under the flap, thus localizing the problem. Blockage of natural drainage may lead to spread of infection to adjacent soft tissues and fascial spaces (Fig. 9–8).

The periodontal pathogens usually are the causative organisms in pericoronitis and include the *Prevotella* and *Porphyromonas* species and oral spirochetes, such as *Treponema denticola*. These usually are sensitive to penicillin. Pericoronitis most frequently occurs about the posterior portion of the crown of the lower third molar because it erupts during adolescence. In most cases, partial eruption of the third molar is caused by insufficient length of the horizontal ramus of the mandible to house all of the teeth. Therefore, part of the third molar is trapped under the oral mucosa covering the buccinator muscle and the superior pharyngeal constrictor because they form the most anterior portion of the oropharynx. In cases in which there is insufficient room for the eruption of the third molar, the pericoronitis will become recurrent or chronic, and the impacted third molar should be removed.

Lower third molars lie in proximity to the pterygomandibular space, a portion of the masticator space. When these infections spread to involve this space, trismus results, which obscures the infection to clinical examination. Therefore, the presence of trismus with a history of pain in the third molar region is an ominous sign of infection involving the masticator space, which, although not manifested by external facial swelling, may begin to involve the deeper parapharyngeal spaces. These infections may become life-threatening. The lower third molar is the most frequent offending tooth in severe odontogenic infections requiring hospitalization, and these infections occur most frequently in adolescence and young adulthood.[19]

A variety of treatment modalities are applicable to pericoronitis, including local incision and drainage as well as extraction of the tooth.[37, 49] Penicillin is used if fever or trismus is present. Resolution of symptoms should occur in less than 1 week.

Oral Manifestations of HIV Infection in Children

The most common oral lesions associated with perinatally acquired HIV infection in children are oral candidiasis, parotid salivary gland enlargement, herpes simplex virus gingivostomatitis, and caries.[24] In contradistinction to adult HIV infection, HIV-associated periodontitis and gingivitis are much less common. Neoplastic oral manifestations of HIV infection, such as Kaposi sarcoma, and non-Hodgkin lymphoma have not been reported, and hairy leukoplakia is quite rare.[26] In contrast to adults, children infected with HIV have a greater susceptibility to bacterial infections, especially

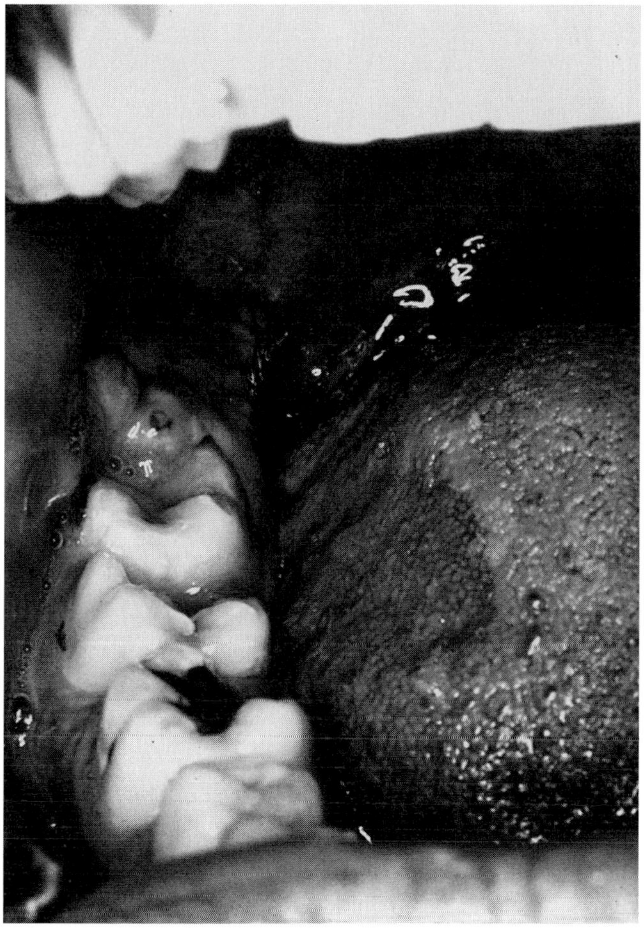

FIGURE 9–8. *Pericoronitis.*

with encapsulated organisms, such as *Streptococcus pneumoniae* and *Haemophilus influenzae*. Septicemia from an oral focus of infection can become a life-threatening problem in the HIV-infected child, and therefore optimum oral health must be established and vigorously maintained in these children.[26] Routine use of chlorhexidene gluconate 0.12 per cent mouthrinse may be helpful in minimizing gingivitis, candidiasis, and bacterial superinfections of the oral cavity, although its safety and effectiveness have not been demonstrated in children yet.

Oral candidiasis most frequently is of the pseudomembranous type, which is seen in the oral cavity as a creamy white plaque that is rubbed off easily, leaving exposed a reddened surface mucosa. Because oral candidiasis is rare in normal children after 6 months of age, persistence of oral candidiasis for 2 months or more in a child older than 6 months of age who has not received antibiotic therapy in the past 2 weeks is suggestive of HIV infection. Persistent oral candidiasis indicates acquired immunodeficiency category P-2D3 (symptomatic infection with secondary infectious diseases) in the Centers for Disease Control and Prevention classification of HIV infection in children younger than 12 years of age.[24]

Oral candidiasis was associated with a decreased survival time in a study of 99 children with perinatally acquired HIV infection. The median time from birth to the first lesion of oral candidiasis was 2.4 years, and median time from lesion to death was 3.4 years, with a relative hazard rate of 14.2.[23]

Treatment of oral candidiasis lesions is difficult due to frequent recurrence of oral fungal infection with resistant biotypes of *Candida albicans* or colonization by related but more resistant species, such as *Candida krusei*, *Candida parapsilosis*, and *Candida guilliermondi*. Treatment regimens may progress from nystatin to clotrimazole, fluconazole, and amphotericin B, depending on the extent of disease, clinical response, and culture and sensitivity results.[35] It should be noted that sudden onset of rampant dental caries has been associated with prolonged oral use of sucrose-containing antifungal antibiotic preparations.[60]

Parotid salivary gland enlargement, which may be painful and become secondarily infected, has been reported in 14 to 30 per cent of HIV-infected children. The enlargement appears to be due to infiltration of the glands by T8 lymphocytes and has been associated with increased survival time. The median time from birth to development of parotid enlargement was 4.6 years and from lesion to death was 5.4 years, with a relative hazard rate of 0.38.[23]

Herpes simplex virus infections, although common in normal children, appear to be particularly severe and recur more often in HIV-infected children. The lesions appear first as multiple clustered vesicles on the lips or keratinized oral mucosa, which soon rupture to leave painful irregular oral ulcers or crusted labial ulcers. Fever and dysphagia may warrant hospital admission for hydration, nutrition, and therapy with parenteral acyclovir. Less severe cases may be treated with oral acyclovir.

Dental caries is increased in pediatric HIV cohorts. The cause of this finding is not clear. It may be due to xerostomia secondary to parotid enlargement in some cases, prolonged use of sucrose-containing antifungal agents in others, and nursing bottle caries in still others. The association of nursing bottle caries with pediatric HIV infection may be due to their common increased prevalence in urban dwellers with limited economic resources, although nursing bottle caries also is found frequently in children with other chronic diseases.[60]

COMPLICATIONS OF ODONTOGENIC INFECTIONS

Fascial Space Infections

Spread of infection to the fascial spaces may result in dramatic facial swelling and high fever and, if untreated, may result in respiratory embarrassment. The characteristics of the more common fascial space infections related to odontogenic infection are described here.

Infraorbital space infections generally are related to maxillary anterior teeth and are well localized to the infraorbital fossa by the levator labii superioris and levator anguli oris muscles. Facial swelling lateral to the nose is prominent as decreased mobility of the upper lip due to inflammation of these muscles. If fluctuant, intraoral incision and drainage with placement of a small Penrose drain for 1 to 2 days generally are sufficient treatment. Antibiotics are indicated for all fascial space infections.

Trismus is the hallmark of masticator space infection. It is caused by spasm in the muscles of mastication, which define this large potential space. The resulting inability to open the mouth hinders access to the airway for endotracheal intubation. In addition, abscesses of the masticator space may rupture into the oropharynx, causing aspiration of pus, or they may pass easily around the medial pterygoid muscle to involve the lateral pharyngeal and retropharyngeal spaces. Figure 9–9 shows a 6-year-old boy whose lower primary molar abscesses spread to involve the buccal, pterygomandibular, and lateral pharyngeal spaces. Extraoral and intraoral drainage, prolonged intubation, and extraction of the offending teeth were required.

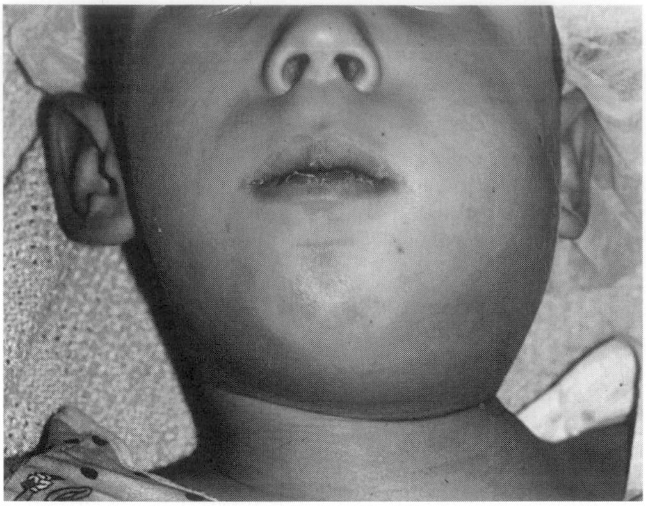

FIGURE 9–9. *Lateral pharyngeal space abscess in a 6-year-old boy. Note the swelling above the hyoid bone and anterior to the sternocleidomastoid muscle. There also is swelling in the buccal and submandibular spaces.*

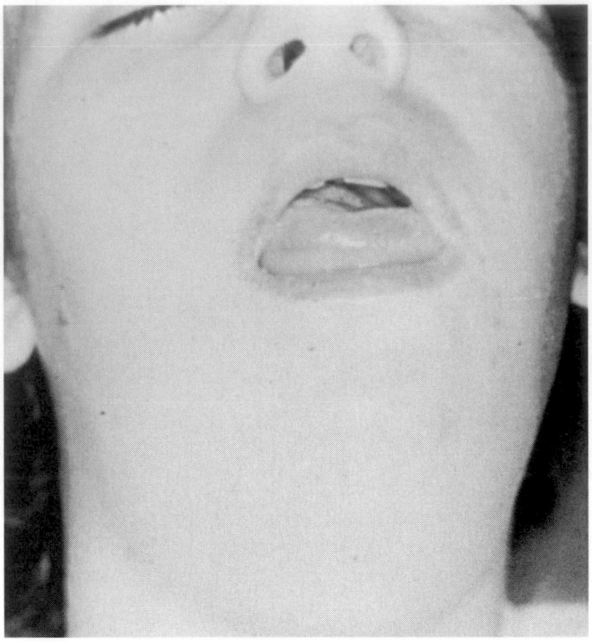

FIGURE 9–11. *Ludwig angina.*

Infections of the submandibular space (Fig. 9–10) may be localized unilaterally or may involve bilateral structures. Treatment of submandibular space infection is by means of extraoral incision and drainage.

First described in 1836, Ludwig angina consists of infection of the sublingual and submandibular spaces bilaterally and is characterized by hard, brawny swelling and a minimum of suppuration. The tongue often is edematous and raised to the roof of the mouth, with little mobility (Fig. 9–11). Airway obstruction should be considered imminent, and indeed, the greatest cause of death in Ludwig angina is blockage of the airway by soft tissue swelling, pus, or blood, which occurred in more than 50 per cent of its victims in the pre-antibiotic era.[17] Today, death is rare, although the need for tracheostomy or prolonged endotracheal intubation is common. The cause of this infection often is odontogenic infection but also may include laceration of the floor of the mouth and mandibular fracture. Usually a disease of middle-aged people, it is rare in children but may occur in greater frequency in the immunologically compromised.[14] Surgical drainage of all four spaces is indicated, accompanied by vigorous antibiotic therapy.

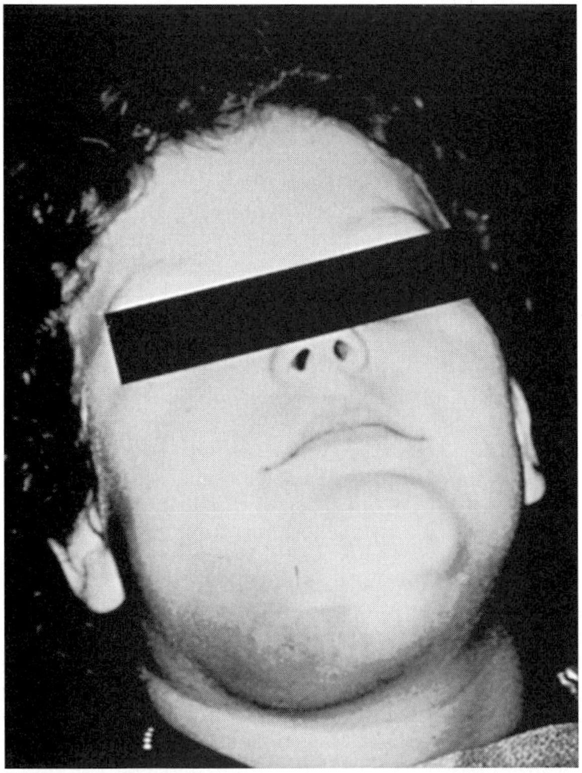

FIGURE 9–10. *Submandibular space abscess.*

Necrotizing Fasciitis

Necrotizing fasciitis causes a frightening loss of skin and underlying tissues that has received considerable notoriety in the press. Cervicofacial necrotizing fasciitis often is odontogenic and typically causes a superficially spreading cellulitis that follows the platysma muscle from the cheek down the entire neck to the anterior chest wall (Fig. 9–12*A*). Figure 9–12*B* illustrates such a swelling in an 8-year-old boy. The presumptive cause was odontogenic infection of the primary molars, which caused a high fever and a rapidly progressive cellulitis extending from the cheek to the chest. The cause of these infections often is group A streptococci, but a wide variety of microorganisms may be involved. Therefore, wide-spectrum antibiotic therapy is indicated empirically, along with hydration, transfusions if necessary, and support of electrolyte balance, especially with calcium, which may be sequestered by necrotic fat molecules.[1]

Odontogenic Sinusitis

A significant percentage of cases of sinusitis are odontogenic, especially in adults, because the maxillary sinus follows the erupting permanent tooth roots into the alveolar process. This pneumatization of the alveolar process progresses throughout life and is accelerated by loss of the upper posterior teeth. Periapical upper posterior dental infections

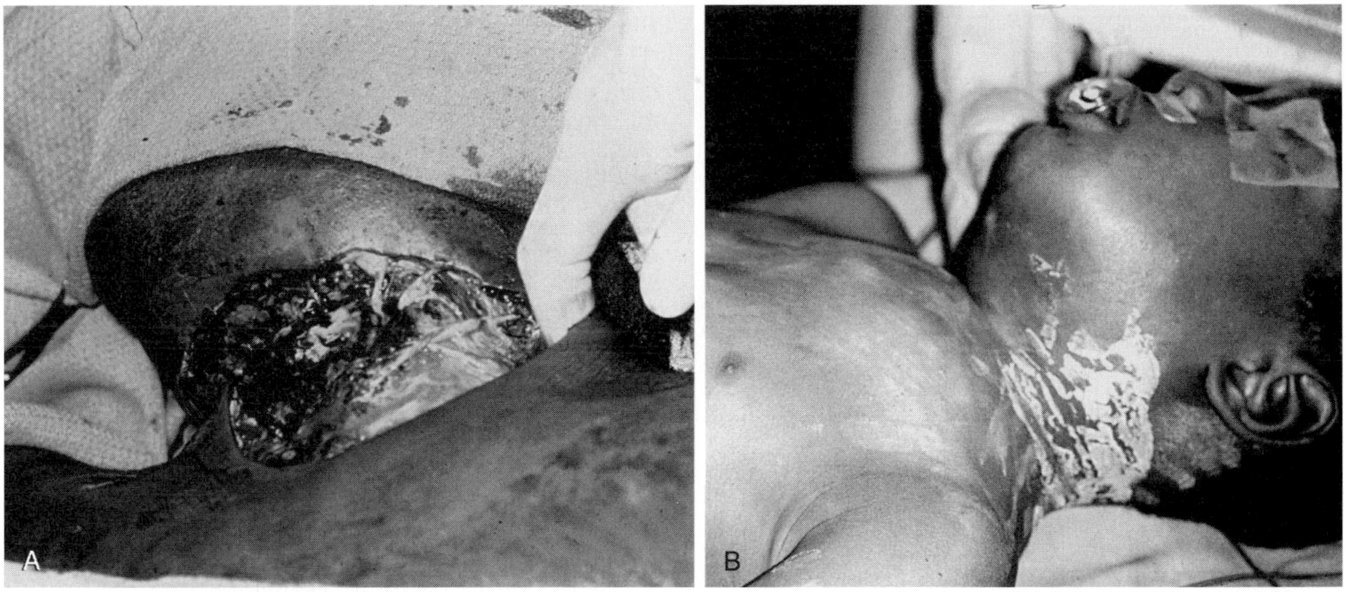

FIGURE 9–12. A, *Surgical débridement of necrotic skin and platysma muscle of the left neck of a diabetic female with necrotizing fasciitis. Note how easily blunt finger dissection can undermine the skin in the plane of the necrotic platysma muscle.* B, *Necrotizing fasciitis in an 8-year-old boy. Note the swelling extending from the buccal space down the neck and onto the anterior chest wall, following the extent of the platysma muscle. The chalky material on the posterior neck is calamine lotion placed by the patient's mother for vesicles that resembled poison ivy.*

occasionally will rupture through the maxillary sinus floor to involve the paranasal sinuses. Therefore, dental infection should be eliminated in the complete treatment of severe recurrent sinusitis in children.

Figure 9–13 illustrates a case of left pansinusitis, including ethmoiditis and a subperiosteal orbital abscess in a 9-year-old boy associated with infected upper primary molars. His treatment involved a team approach of the dental and otolaryngology services for tooth extraction, incision and drainage of the buccal and infraorbital spaces, endoscopic sinus surgery, and external drainage of the orbital abscess.

Haemophilus influenzae Buccal Cellulitis

Occasionally, a child will present with an acute buccal space swelling and cellulitis with no clinically apparent odontogenic cause. There usually is a history of recent upper respiratory infection or sinusitis. The pathogenic sinus flora, especially *H. influenzae*, sometimes has been cultured from these infections, which may have started by migration of these organisms through emissary veins piercing the thin cortical bone overlying the lateral surface of the maxillary sinus. Unless the infection is severe, incision and drainage usually are not necessary, and treatment with antibiotics directed to the flora of sinusitis is successful.[58]

Orbital and Intracranial Complications

Odontogenic infections that spread to involve the orbit and the brain are rare. Orbital and intracranial abscesses may, however, have an odontogenic origin, and therefore the dental condition of patients with these conditions should be evaluated by a dentist. Probably no more than 5 to 10 per cent of orbital cellulitis is odontogenic in origin.[22, 61] This infection generally is unilateral and is characterized by proptosis, chemosis, lid edema, and restriction of extraocular motion secondary to edema.[46] No nerve palsies or visual changes are present. Treatment includes surgical drainage, antibiotics, and elimination of the dental infection.

Cavernous sinus thrombosis, which may be difficult to differentiate clinically from orbital cellulitis, is considerably more serious because microorganisms proliferate intracranially. The risk of death is high. Characteristics include bilateral involvement, with rapid progression from one eye to the other, proptosis, chemosis, and lid edema. Extraocular movements are limited because of inflammation of the third, fourth, and sixth cranial nerves. Systemic signs of meningeal irritation and funduscopic evidence of obstruction of the retinal veins also are present.[7, 46, 55] Treatment includes high doses of parenteral antibiotics, elimination of the causative dental pathosis, and incision and drainage of infected fascial spaces.

Brain abscess and subdural empyema are rare today, compared with several decades ago. Of the large series of brain abscess cases reported, 0 to 4 per cent of cases have been attributed to dental etiologies.[33, 59] However, all of the studies in which the individual case histories are described disclose a pansinusitis intervening between the dental infection and the brain.[34, 50] Therefore, odontogenic brain abscesses appear to occur by direct extension through the paranasal sinuses, usually to the frontal lobe via the frontal sinuses. On the other hand, odontogenic cavernous sinus thrombosis appears to be propagated by an ascending thrombophlebitis.

OSTEOMYELITIS OF THE JAWS IN CHILDREN

Osteomyelitis of the jaws in children usually results from periodontal or, more commonly, periapical infection. Open fracture of the jaws with delayed treatment also is a significant cause of osteomyelitis. Extension from contiguous infections, such as otitis, parotitis, and mastoiditis, occurs much less often.

Osteomyelitis of the jaws occurring in children must be viewed with great concern because it may result in the following problems: (1) the loss of primary and permanent

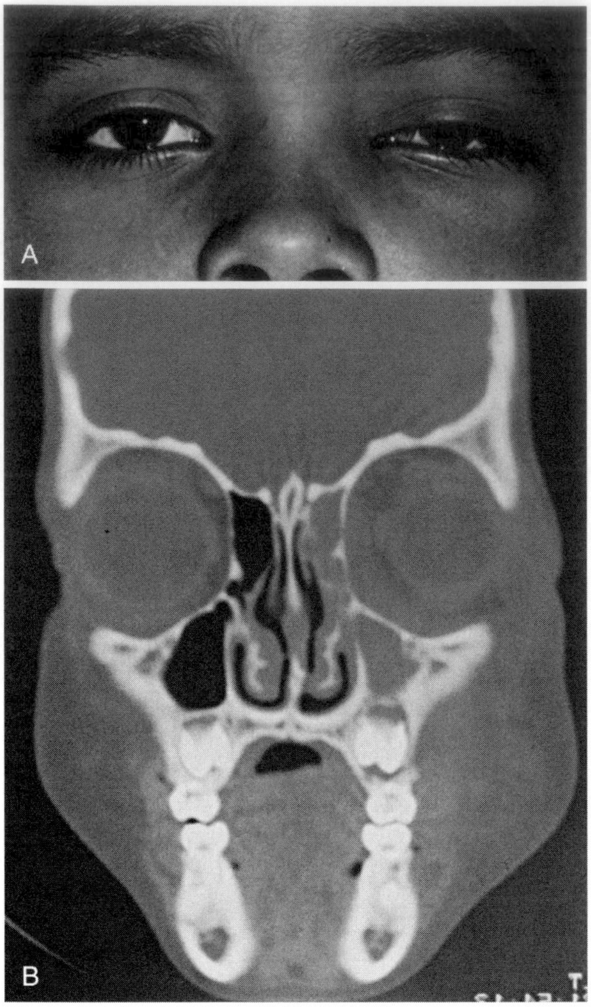

FIGURE 9–13. A, *A 9-year-old boy with a left pansinusitis and an abscess of the upper left first primary molar. Note the left periorbital discoloration and swelling, with partial ptosis and displacement of the globe laterally.* B, *Computed tomographic scan of the same patient. Note the left maxillary sinus opacification in close proximity to the infected tooth, the opacification of the ethmoid sinuses, elevation of the periosteum away from the medial orbital wall, and displacement of the globe laterally within the orbit.*

teeth; (2) sequestration of segments of the jaws; (3) growth defects, such as mandibular hypoplasia, asymmetry, and ankylosis[12]; (4) disfiguring facial scars and cutaneous fistulas; and (5) lesions suggestive of malignancy, which require open biopsy. For these reasons, osteomyelitis of the jaws in children should be diagnosed rapidly and treated aggressively. A useful classification of this disease is shown in Table 9–4.[57]

TABLE 9–4. Osteomyelitis of the Jaws

Suppurative	Nonsuppurative
Acute suppurative	Chronic sclerosing
Chronic suppurative	Facial sclerosing
Primary	Diffuse sclerosing
Secondary	Garré sclerosing
Infantile	Actinomycotic
	Radiation osteomyelitis and necrosis

Predisposing Factors

Preexisting systemic disease with accompanying alteration of host resistance plays a major role in the initiation of osteomyelitis of the jaws. This includes such conditions as uncontrolled diabetes, agranulocytosis, leukemia, sickle-cell disease, and febrile illnesses. Conditions that alter the vascularity of bone and thus the ability to combat infections, including bone tumors, fibrous dysplasia, Paget disease, and radiation to the jaws, also are important predisposing conditions. Major maxillofacial injuries resulting in open fractures of the jaws, especially those that are not treated immediately, are an important cause of osteomyelitis.

Microbiology

Because the etiology of osteomyelitis of the jaws includes causes other than purely odontogenic infections, the bacterial spectrum is broad.

Most instances of osteomyelitis of the jaws are caused by aerobic streptococci (alpha-hemolytic streptococci, *Streptococcus* viridans group), anaerobic streptococci, and other anaerobes, particularly peptostreptococci, fusobacteria, and *Bacteroides* and related genera.[44] Only occasional cases are caused by *S. aureus*, with entry through the skin as the probable route. Other bacteria involved include oral anaerobes, aerobic and microaerophilic cocci, and gram-negative organisms. Specific forms of osteomyelitis are caused by *Actinomyces israelii*, *Treponema pallidum*, and *Mycobacterium tuberculosis*. *Salmonella* organisms have been associated with osteomyelitis of the jaws in sickle-cell anemia.[9]

Clinical Findings

Osteomyelitis involves the mandible far more frequently than the maxilla because the relatively poor blood supply to the mandible comes primarily from one major vessel and the periosteal blood supply. There are four major forms of the disease that may be distinguished clinically: (1) acute suppurative; (2) secondary chronic, the form that begins as an acute osteomyelitis and becomes chronic; (3) primary chronic, the form that has no acute phase and always has appeared to be a low-grade infection; and (4) nonsuppurative osteomyelitis. Those most often seen in children are the acute suppurative, the secondary chronic, and one nonsuppurative form, Garré sclerosing osteomyelitis. These conditions are described in some detail.

Suppurative Osteomyelitis

Suppurative osteomyelitis usually begins with deep, intense pain in the jaws, high intermittent fever, and an obvious etiology—most often a deeply carious or discolored tooth. Occasionally in the early stages, mental nerve paresthesia is present. Over the course of several days, facial swelling develops, and in 10 to 14 days, teeth begin to loosen, pus exudes around the gingival sulcus, and multiple mucosal or cutaneous sinus tracts form. In addition to the draining sinuses, a firm cellulitis is present in the soft tissues accompanied by trismus and cervical lymphadenopathy. There is a leukocytosis, ranging typically from 8000 to 15,000 cells/mm^3, although it ordinarily does not reach the levels that are seen in acute osteomyelitis of the long bones. After 10 days to 2 weeks, radiographs may show scattered areas of bone destruction suggestive of a moth-eaten appearance (Fig. 9–14), and periosteal reaction characterized by the laying down

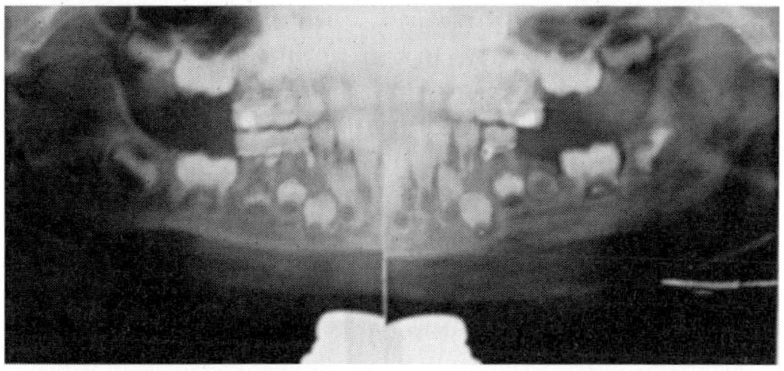

FIGURE 9–14. *Radiograph of the jaws of a 4-year-old girl with suppurative osteomyelitis of the left mandible. The film shows marked destruction of the body and ramus of the mandible.*

of new bone commonly is seen. Smears of specimens and cultures should be taken whenever possible, including cultures of bone sequestra. Interpretation of cultures must be made with caution because of the possibility of skin and oral contaminants in the specimen.

Initially, antibiotics dose-adjusted for age should be given empirically using a regimen described in Table 9–5. As results from smears and culture are obtained, antibiotics may be changed, unless the infection is responding favorably, in which case no change should be made. The involved tooth should be removed as early as possible to allow for drainage and to provide material for culture.

Antibiotic therapy should be continued for at least 2 to 4 weeks after all symptoms subside. If the infection persists, repeated cultures should be obtained and the antibiotic changed if necessary. The greater vascularity of the jaws may explain their more rapid response to antibiotic therapy and surgery, compared with long bones. Therefore, the duration of intravenous antibiotic therapy in osteomyelitis of the jaws may not need to be as prolonged as in that of the long bones. Consideration should be given to sequestrectomy, saucerization, and/or the placement of closed wound irrigation and suction. Saucerization involves the removal of teeth in the immediate area and removing the overlying buccal plate of bone, allowing access to the medullary portion and sequestra that may be present. Occasionally, it is necessary to place catheters via an extraoral approach for closed irrigation and suction. This permits instillation of antibiotics, allowing direct contact with the bone. Hyperbaric oxygen treatment may be considered in chronic cases refractory to antibiotic treatment.[38]

Infantile Osteomyelitis

Osteomyelitis of the jaws in the newborn is uncommon but worthy of special mention because of its serious sequelae. It occurs most often a few weeks after birth and usually involves the maxilla. It is not odontogenic in origin but is thought to arise from neonatal trauma to oral tissues; hematogenous spread from skin, middle ear, mastoid, or tonsils; or from an infected nipple.[47] Clinically, the patient presents with a facial cellulitis centered about the orbit (Fig. 9–15). Irritability and malaise precede cellulitis and are followed by marked elevation in temperature, anorexia, and dehydration. Extraorally, inner canthal swelling, palpebral edema with closure of the eye, conjunctivitis, and proptosis may be seen together with a purulent discharge from the nose or from the inner canthus. Oral examination shows swelling of the maxilla on the affected side extending to both the buccal and the palatal regions, with fluctuance often present with multiple sinus tracts. *S. aureus* is the organism usually found. Aggressive, prompt treatment must be undertaken to prevent permanent optic damage, neurologic complications, loss of tooth buds and bone, and extension to the dural sinuses. Intravenous penicillin and a penicillinase-resistant penicillin should be given simultaneously with surgical drainage of all fluctuant areas, repeated Gram smears, and culture and sensitivity testing. Antibiotics should be continued orally for 2 to 4 weeks after all signs of the infection have disappeared. If sequestra form, these should be removed conservatively. It should be noted that tooth buds may be lost, and surviving teeth may be deformed or discolored after eruption.

Garré Sclerosing Osteomyelitis

This condition, also known as chronic nonsuppurative sclerosing osteomyelitis and proliferative osteomyelitis of Garré,[4] is notable because of the similarity of some of its characteristics to those of other neoperiostoses. It is characterized by a localized, hard, nontender swelling of the mandible (Fig.

TABLE 9–5. Recommended Antibiotic Regimen for Osteomyelitis of the Jaws

Empiric Therapy	
Regimen I	1. Aqueous penicillin, 250,000 units/kg/24 hr in 6 divided doses IV with: 2. Oxacillin, 200 mg/kg/24 hr in 4 divided doses IV. When patient has been asymptomatic for 48 to 72 hours, switch to regimen II.
Regimen II	1. Penicillin V, 50 mg/kg/24 hr in 6 divided doses p.o. with: 2. Dicloxacillin, 75 mg/kg/24 hr in 4 divided doses p.o. for an additional 2 to 4 weeks
Initial Therapy with Gram Stain Results	
Smear Suggestive of Staphylococcal Infection	
Regimen III	Oxacillin, 200 mg/kg/24 hr in 4 divided doses IV. When patient has been asymptomatic for 48 to 72 hours, switch to regimen IV.
Regimen IV	Dicloxacillin, 75 mg/kg/24 hr in 4 divided doses p.o. for an additional 2 to 4 weeks
Smear Suggestive of Anaerobic Infection	
Regimen V	Aqueous penicillin, 250,000 units/kg/24 hr in 6 divided doses IV. When patient has been asymptomatic for 48 to 72 hours, change to penicillin V, 50 mg/kg/24 hr in 6 divided doses p.o. for 2 to 4 weeks
Smear Suggestive of Both Staphylococcal and Anaerobic Organisms	
Regimen I Initially	
Therapy in Cases of Allergy to Penicillin (in Order of Preference)	
	1. Clindamycin, 30 mg/kg/24 hr in 3 divided doses IV, then: Clindamycin, 30 mg/kg/24 hr in 3 divided doses p.o. 2. Cephalosporin: Cefazolin, 80 mg/kg/24 hr in 4 divided doses IV Cephalexin, 50 mg/kg/24 hr in 4 divided doses p.o.

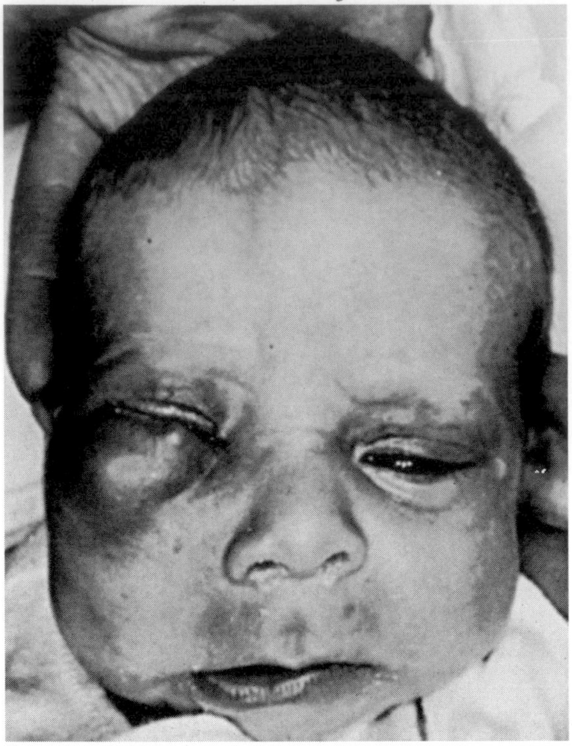

FIGURE 9–15. *Characteristic clinical picture of a 3-week-old child with infantile osteomyelitis. (Courtesy of Dr. M. Michael Cohen, Sr.)*

9–16). Lymphadenopathy, hyperpyrexia, and leukocytosis are not present. It is associated commonly with a carious tooth, usually the lower first molar (Fig. 9–17), and a history of a past toothache. It also may be associated with a recent dental extraction or an infected flap of tissue over an erupting tooth.[31] Radiographs are quite impressive, showing a focal area of well-calcified bone proliferation that is smooth and that often has a laminated or onion-peel appearance (Fig. 9–18). Garré osteomyelitis is thought to be a response to a low-grade stimulus, such as a dental infection, that influences

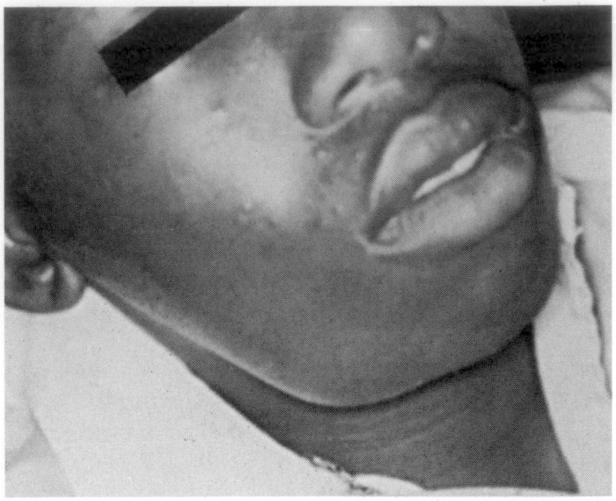

FIGURE 9–16. *Enlargement of the right side of the mandible in a 12-year-old patient with Garré sclerosing osteomyelitis. The swelling is hard and nontender.*

the potentially active periosteum of young individuals. Its appearance resembles that of infantile cortical hyperostosis (Caffey disease), osteosarcoma, and Ewing sarcoma and must be distinguished from these.[11] Treatment consists of extraction or endodontic therapy of the involved tooth, with continued clinical and radiographic follow-up of the patient to ensure that the new bone formation does not progress. Ordinarily, remodeling occurs over time, but biopsy should be performed to rule out neoplasm if the lesion does not regress. No antibiotic therapy is necessary.

HERPES SIMPLEX VIRUS INFECTIONS

Herpes simplex virus type 1 infections[54] are manifested commonly as herpetic gingivostomatitis. Five stages of infection have been identified: (1) primary mucocutaneous infection, (2) acute infection of ganglia, (3) establishment of latency, (4) reactivation, and (5) recurrent infection.

Primary infection is established by direct contact either with people who have draining lesions or with an asymp-

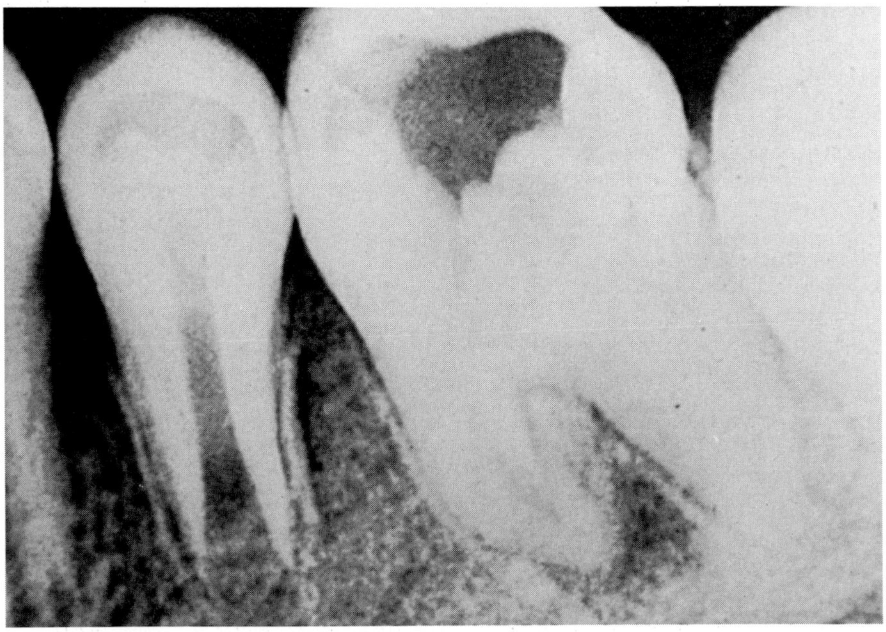

FIGURE 9–17. *Radiograph of a deeply carious lower first molar tooth with periapical spread of infection. This is the usual cause of Garré osteomyelitis.*

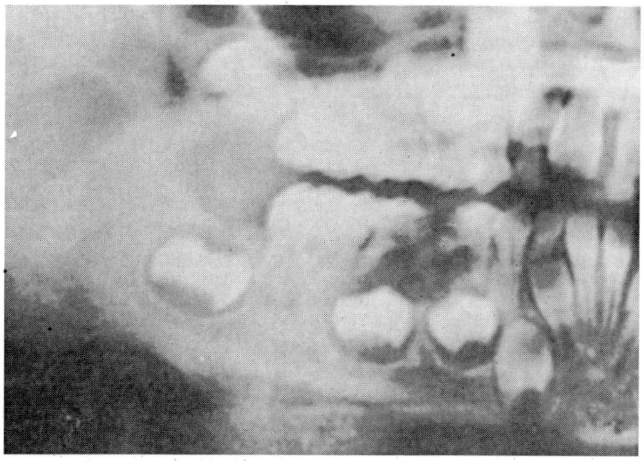

FIGURE 9–18. *Characteristic radiograph of Garré osteomyelitis showing the laminated or onion-peel appearance of the mass. (Courtesy of Dr. Larry J. Peterson.)*

tomatic carrier who may continue to shed the virus, despite the lack of symptoms. The highest incidence of primary infection appears to be between the ages of 2 and 4 years. Infants are protected by maternal antibodies. A series of 19,000 children with gingivostomatitis recorded by Jauretic in 1966 contained no cases in infants younger than 6 months of age. There appears to be no seasonal variation or male/female difference in incidence.

The incubation period is thought to be approximately 6 days, followed by the development of small vesicles that may coalesce to form larger lesions or ulcers. In severe cases, the lips, gingivae, oral mucosa, and pharynx all may be involved. Many patients with primary herpes labialis may be asymptomatic, however, and may not develop symptoms. Healing occurs in 1 to 2 weeks, with gradual crusting of the lesions followed by re-epithelialization.

Latency is thought to continue throughout life, with reactivation occurring at various times, possibly triggered by actinic radiation and emotional or physical stress. Recurrent disease is manifested by vesicles at the mucocutaneous border, which are painful for about 2 days, followed by crusting and complete healing in 7 to 8 days.

See Chapter 163 (Postnatal Herpes Simplex Virus Infection) for methods of diagnosis and treatment.

Up to 50 per cent of the adult population in industrialized countries and a higher percentage in less developed nations may suffer from recurrent herpes labialis. Surprisingly, many, if not most, adults who suffer from recurrent "cold sores" are not aware that they can transmit the disease and should be counseled in this regard. Likewise, medical, dental, and nursing personnel also should be advised that occurrence of cutaneous lesions (the "herpetic whitlow") is not unknown after direct contact of the practitioners' fingers with lesions during the physical examination.

References

1. Balcerak, R. J., Sisto, J. M., and Bosack, R. C.: Cervicofacial necrotizing fasciitis: Report of three cases and literature review. J. Oral Maxillofac. Surg. *46*:450–459, 1988.
2. Barkin, R., Bonis, S., Elzhammer, R., et al.: Ludwig's angina in children. J. Pediatr. *87*:563–565, 1975.
3. Bartlett, J. G., and Gorbach, S. L.: Anaerobic infections of the head and neck. Otolaryngol. Clin. North Am. *9*:655–678, 1976.
4. Benca, P. G., Mostofi, R., and Kuo P.: Proliferative periostitis (Garré's osteomyelitis). Oral Surg. *63*:258–260, 1987.
5. Brook, I., Frazier, E. H., and Gher, M. E.: Aerobic and anaerobic microbiology of periapical abscess. Oral Microbiol. Immunol. *6*:123–125, 1991.
6. Busch, D. E.: Anaerobes in infections of the head and neck and ear, nose, and throat. Rev. Infect. Dis. *6*:S115–S122, 1984.
7. Chow, A. W., Roser, S. M., and Brady, F. A.: Orofacial odontogenic infections. Ann. Intern. Med. *88*:392–402, 1978.
8. Coykendall, A. L.: Classification and identification of the viridans streptococci. Clin. Microbiol. Rev. *2*:315–328, 1989.
9. Daramola, J. O.: Massive osteomyelitis of the mandible complicating sickle cell disease: Report of case. J. Oral Surg. *39*:144–146, 1981.
10. Dodson, T. B., Perrott, D. H., and Kaban, L. B.: Pediatric maxillofacial infections: A retrospective study of 113 patients. J. Oral Maxillofac. Surg. *47*:327–330, 1989.
11. Eversole, L. R., Lieder, A. S., Gorwin, J. O., et al.: Proliferative periostitis of Garré: Its differentiation from other neoperiostoses. J. Oral Surg. *37*:725–731, 1979.
12. Fisher, A. D.: Osteomyelitis of the mandible in a child. J. Oral Surg. *353*:60–63, 1977.
13. Gilmore, W. C., Jacobus, N. V., Gorbach, S. L., et al.: A prospective double-blind evaluation of penicillin versus clindamycin in the treatment of odontogenic infections. J. Oral Maxillofac. Surg. *46*:1065–1070, 1988.
14. Goldberg, M. H., and Topazian, R. G.: Odontogenic infection and deep fascial space infection of dental origin. *In* Topazian, R. G., and Goldberg, M. H. (eds.): Oral and Maxillofacial Infections. 3rd ed. Philadelphia, W. B. Saunders, 1994, pp. 198–250.
15. Granite, E. L.: Anatomic considerations in infections of the face and neck. J. Oral Surg. 34:34–44, 1976.
16. Grodinsky, M., and Holyoke, E.: The fascia and fascial spaces of the head and neck and adjacent regions. Am. J. Anat. *63*:367–407, 1938.
17. Gross, S., and Nieburg, P.: Ludwig's angina in childhood. Am. J. Dis. Child. *131*:291–292, 1977.
18. Hall, H. D., Gunter, Jr., J. W., Jamison, H. C., et al.: Effect of time of extraction on resolution of odontogenic cellulitis. J. Am. Dent. Assoc. *77*:626–631, 1968.
19. Haug, R. H., Hoffman, M. J., and Indresano, A. T.: An epidemiologic and anatomic survey of odontogenic infections. J. Oral Maxillofac. Surg. *49*:976–980, 1991.
20. Heimdahl, A., Von Konow, L., Satoh, T., et al.: Clinical appearance of orofacial infections of odontogenic origin in relation to microbiological findings. J. Clin. Microbiol. *22*:299–302, 1985.
21. Howe G: Orofacial infections and their management. *In* Howe, G. (ed.): Minor Oral Surgery. Bristol, John Wright & Sons, 1966.
22. Kaban, L., and McGill, T.: Orbital cellulitis of dental origin: Differential diagnosis and the use of computed tomography as a diagnostic aid. J. Oral Surg. *38*:682–685, 1980.
23. Katz, M. H., Mastrucci, M. T., Leggott, P. J., et al.: Prognostic significance of oral lesions in children with perinatally acquired human immunodeficiency virus infection. Am. J. Dis. Child. *147*:45–48, 1993.
24. Ketchem, L., Berkowitz, R. J., McIlveen, L., et al.: Oral findings in HIV-seropositive children. Pediatr. Dent. *12*:143–146, 1990.
25. Krogh, H. W.: Extraction of teeth in the presence of acute infections. J. Oral Surg. *9*:136–151, 1951.
26. Leggott, P. J.: Oral manifestations of HIV infection in children. Oral Surg. *73*:187–192, 1992.
27. Lesco, B., and Brownstein, M. P.: Recognition of periodontal disease in children. Pediatr. Clin. North Am. *29*:457–474, 1982.
28. Levitt, G. W.: Cervical fascia and deep neck infections. Otolaryngol. Clin. North Am. *9*:703-716, 1976.
29. Lewis, M. A. O., MacFarlane, T. W., and McGowan, D. A.: Quantitative bacteriology of acute dento-alveolar abscesses. J. Med. Microbiol. *21*:101–104, 1986.
30. Lewis, M. A. O., MacFarlane, T. W., McGowan, D. A., et al.: Assessment of the pathogenicity of bacterial species plated from acute dentoalveolar abscesses. J. Med. Microbiol. *27*:109–116, 1988.
31. Lichty, G., Langlais, R. P., and Aufdemorte, T.: Garré's osteomyelitis: Literature review and case report. Oral Surg. *50*: 309–313, 1980.
32. Magnusson, B. O., Matsson, L., and Modeen, T.: Gingivitis and periodontal disease in children. *In* Magnusson, B. O., Koch, B., and Poulsen, S. (eds.): Pedodontics: A Systematic Approach. Copenhagen, Munksgaard, 1981.
33. Mampalam, T. J., and Rosenblum, M. L.: Trends in the management of bacterial brain abscesses: A review of 102 cases over 17 years. Neurosurgery *23*:451–458, 1988.
34. Maniglia, A. J., Goodwin, W. J., Arnold, J. E., et al.: Intracranial abscesses secondary to nasal, sinus, and orbital infections in adults and children. Arch. Otolaryngol. Head Neck Surg. *115*:1424–1429, 1989.
35. Marchisio, P., and Principi, N.: Treatment of oropharyngeal candidiasis in HIV-infected children with oral fluconazole. Eur. J. Clin. Microbiol. Infect. Dis. *13*:338, 1994.
36. Martis, C. S., and Karakasis, D. T.: Extractions in the presence of acute infections. J. Dent. Res. *54*:59–61, 1975.
37. Martis, C. S., Karabouta, I., and Lazaridis, N.: Extraction of impacted mandibular wisdom teeth in the presence of acute infection. Int. J. Oral Surg. *7*:541–548, 1978.
38. Marx, R., Johnson, R., and Kline, S.: Prevention of osteoradionecrosis: A randomized prospective clinical trial of hyperbaric oxygen vs. penicillin. J. Am. Dent. Assoc. *111*:49–54, 1985.

39. Massler, M.: Epidemiology of gingivitis in children. J. Am. Dent. Assoc. *45*:319, 1952.
40. McCarthy, C., Snyder, M. G., and Parker, R. B.: The indigenous oral flora of man. I. The newborn to one-year-old infant. Arch. Oral Biol. *10*:61–70, 1975.
41. Moenning, J., Nelson, C., and Kohler, R.: The microbiology and chemotherapy of odontogenic infections. J. Oral Maxillofac. Surg. *43*:976–985, 1989.
42. Morhert, R. E., and Fitzgerald, R. J.: Nutritional determinants of the ecology of the oral flora. Dent. Clin. North Am. *42*:473–489, 1976.
43. O'Sullivan, E. A., Duggal, M. S., Bailey, C. C., et al.: Changes in the oral microflora during cytotoxic chemotherapy in children being treated for acute leukemia. Oral Surg. *76*:161–168, 1993.
44. Peterson, L. J.: Microbiology of head and neck infections. Oral Maxillofac. Clin. North Am. 3:247, 1991.
45. Piecuch, J. F.: Odontogenic infections. Dent. Clin. North Am. *26*:129–145, 1982.
46. Price, C. D., Hameroff, S. B., and Richards, R. D.: Cavernous sinus thrombosis and orbital cellulitis. South. Med. J. *64*:1243–1247, 1971.
47. Raymon, Y., Oberman, M., Horowitz, I., et al.: Osteomyelitis of the maxilla in the newborn. Int. J. Oral Surg. 6:90–94, 1977.
48. Rogers, A. H.: The oral cavity as a source of potential pathogens in focal infection. Dent. Clin. North Am. *42*:245–248, 1976.
49. Rud, J.: Removal of impacted lower third molars with acute pericoronitis and necrotizing gingivitis. Br. J. Oral Surg. *7*:153–160, 1970.
50. Schwaber, M. K., Pensak, M. L., and Bartels, L. J.: The early signs and symptoms of neurotologic complications of chronic suppurative otitis media. Laryngoscope *99*:373–375, 1989.
51. Shah, H. N., and Collins, D. M.: *Prevotella*, a new genus to include *Bacteroides melaninogenicus* and related species formerly classified in the genus *Bacteroides*. Int. J. Systemat. Bacteriol. *40*:205–208, 1990.
52. Shah, H. N., and Collins, D. M.: Proposal for reclassification of *Bacteroides asaccharolyticus, Bacteroides gingivalis, and Bacteroides endodontalis* in a new genus, *Porphyromonas*. Int. J. Systemat. Bacteriol. *38*:128, 1988.
53. Socransky, S., and Manganiello, S.: The oral microbiota of man from birth to senility. J. Periodontol. *42*:485–496, 1971.
54. Straus, S. E. (moderator): Herpes simplex virus infection: Biology, treatment, prevention. NIH Conference. Ann. Intern. Med. *103*:404, 1985.
55. Summers, G. W.: The diagnosis and management of dental infections. Otolaryngol. Clin. North Am. 9:717–728, 1976.
56. Sundqvist, G.: Taxonomy, ecology, and pathogenicity of the root canal flora. Oral Surg. *78*:522–530, 1994.
57. Topazian, R. G.: Osteomyelitis of the jaws. *In* Topazian, R. G. and Goldberg, M. H. (eds.): Oral and Maxillofacial Infections. 3rd ed. Philadelphia, W. B. Saunders, 1994, pp. 251–288.
58. Topazian, R. G.: Uncommon infections of the oral and maxillofacial regions. *In* Topazian, R. G., and Goldberg, M. H. (eds.): Oral and Maxillofacial Infections. 3rd ed. Philadelphia, W. B. Saunders, 1994, pp. 407–429.
59. Traub, W. H.: Brain abscess and acute purulent meningitis: Recent developments in clinical microbiology. *In* Schiefer, W., Klinger, M., and Brock, M. (eds.): Brain Abscess and Meningitis: Subarachnoid Hemorrhage: Timing Problems. New York, Springer-Verlag, 1981.
60. Valdez, I. H., Pizzo, P. A., and Atkinson, J. C.: Oral health of pediatric AIDS patients: A hospital-based study. J. Dent. Child. *61*:114–148, 1994.
61. Woods, R.: Pyogenic dental infections: A ten-year review. Aust. Dent. J. *23*:107–111, 1978.

10

Pharyngitis (Pharyngitis, Tonsillitis, Tonsillopharyngitis, and Nasopharyngitis)

James D. Cherry

Pharyngitis is an inflammatory illness of the mucous membranes and underlying structures of the throat. The clinical diagnostic category includes tonsillitis, tonsillopharyngitis, and nasopharyngitis; inflammation frequently also involves the nasopharynx, uvula, and soft palate. Illness usually is acute but also may be subacute or chronic. To diagnose pharyngitis requires objective evidence of inflammation (erythema, exudate, or ulceration). The symptom of sore throat invariably accompanies pharyngitis, but it should not be used as the sole criterion; sore throat is a common complaint of children with colds in whom no objective evidence of pharyngeal inflammation is present.

Although the clinical finding of pharyngitis suggests an almost exclusive group A streptococcal etiology to many physicians, etiologic considerations should include a multitude of viruses, bacteria, and other infectious and noninfectious agents.

Etiologically, pharyngitis is subdivided conveniently into two categories: illness with nasal symptomatology (nasopharyngitis) and illness without nasal involvement (pharyngitis or tonsillopharyngitis). In acute illness, nasopharyngitis nearly always is of viral etiology, whereas pharyngitis without nasal signs has diverse etiologic possibilities, including bacteria, viruses, fungi, and other infectious agents. Here, nasopharyngitis and pharyngitis without nasal involvement are considered separately.

HISTORY

Although throat inflammation undoubtedly has been a physical finding of disease throughout human existence, only in relatively recent years has attention been given to pharyngitis as a primary complaint. The throat findings of diphtheria were mentioned in the third century A.D.,[133] and Vincent angina was noted in the military before the Christian era,[36] but group A streptococcal infection and pharyngitis were not clearly associated until World War II.[24, 112] Although Glover and Griffith[48] in 1931 mentioned streptococcal tonsillitis, the major reference to streptococci in the preantibiotic era was in association with scarlet fever, erysipelas, and suppurative processes.[18]

NASOPHARYNGITIS

Etiologic Agents

Etiologic agents of nasopharyngitis, categorized by type of lesion, frequency and season of occurrence, and duration of illness, are listed in Table 10–1. The relative importance of nasal and pharyngeal manifestations also is presented.

Although Table 10–1 shows three bacterial agents and one rickettsia, the overwhelming majority of nasopharyngitis occurrence is because of viral infections. The specific infectious agents are discussed fully in their respective sections of this book; therefore, only an overview is presented here.

Adenoviruses are the most common cause of nasopharyngitis, with types 1, 2, 3, 4, 5, 6, 7, 7a, 9, 14, and 15 accounting for the majority of illnesses.[8, 27, 68, 92, 104, 123, 127, 138] Nasopharyngitis also is common with influenza and parainfluenza viral infections.[6, 56, 62, 63, 68, 69, 98, 101–103, 110, 111, 118, 130] Although rhinoviral

TABLE 10–1. Etiologic Agents of Nasopharyngitis

Etiologic Agent and Reference	Type of Pharyngeal Lesion*			Relative Importance of Nasal and Pharyngeal Symptoms†		Frequency of Pharyngitis‡	Main Season	Duration of Pharyngitis
	Erythematous	*Follicular*	*Exudative*	*Nasal*	*Pharyngeal*			
Bacteria								
Corynebacterium diphtheriae[149]	+++		++++	+	+++	+	Fall, winter, spring	Acute, subacute
Haemophilus influenzae[142]	++			++	++	+	Fall, winter, spring	Acute, subacute
Neisseria meningitidis[124]	++			+	+++	+	Fall, winter, spring	Acute, subacute
Viruses								
Adenoviruses[8, 27, 71, 92, 104, 123, 127, 138]	++++	++++	++	+	+++	++++	All seasons	Acute
Enteroviruses (polio, coxsackieviruses A and B, echovirus)[17, 26, 71, 72, 92, 120, 121, 143]	+++		+	+	+++	+++	Summer, fall	Acute
Influenza A and B[71, 102, 110, 118, 130]	+++			+	+++	++	Fall, winter	Acute
Parainfluenza 1–4[6, 56, 62, 63, 69, 98, 101, 103, 111, 117, 130]	++		+	+++	+	++	Fall, winter, spring	Acute
Respiratory syncytial[16, 61, 63, 87, 103]	++			+++	+	+	Fall, winter, spring	Acute
Rhinoviruses[58, 71]	+			+++	+	+	Fall, winter, spring	Acute
Rotaviruses[55, 80, 87, 113]	++			++	++	++	Fall, winter, spring	Acute
Rickettsia								
Coxiella burnetii[67]	++			++	++	+	All seasons	Acute

*Pluses indicate the relative degree and severity of the lesion (++++, most marked; +, minimal).
†Each +, 25%.
‡++++, 76–100%; +++, 51–75%; ++, 26–50%; +, 1–25%.

and respiratory syncytial viral infections are common in children and both always have nasal manifestations (coryza), the occurrence of objective pharyngeal manifestations is uncommon.[16, 58, 61–63, 68, 87, 103] Respiratory symptoms with cough, nasal discharge, and pharyngitis frequently occur in children with rotaviral gastroenteritis.[55, 80, 113]

Epidemiology

Nasopharyngitis is a common illness of childhood. It tends to be most prevalent in young children, in association with primary infections with respiratory viruses. Nasal symptoms with enteroviruses are less common in school age children than in preschool age children. In contrast, older children rarely have pharyngitis with respiratory syncytial, parainfluenza, and rhinoviral infections. Nasopharyngitis due to adenoviral infection particularly is frequent in the adolescent and young adult in military training.[27, 123, 138]

Nasopharyngitis is more common during the cold weather months (see Table 10–1). There is no apparent sex predilection. The method of transmission is similar to that of other respiratory viral infections (see Chapter 8).

Pathophysiology

The pathophysiology of nasopharyngitis is presented in the common cold chapter (Chapter 8) and in the pharyngitis section of this chapter, as well as in the chapters discussing the individual viral agents. In nasopharyngitis associated with *Haemophilus influenzae* and *Neisseria meningitidis*, it is quite probable that the nasal symptomatology results from a concomitant respiratory viral infection.[18]

Clinical Presentation

Because nasopharyngitis is caused by many different etiologic agents, it is reasonable to expect varied clinical manifestations. These differences are highlighted in Table 10–1. Fever occurs in nearly all cases of nasopharyngitis. With adenoviral and influenza viral disease, the pharyngeal findings are most prominent, whereas with the other respiratory viruses, coryza is more notable than pharyngeal complaints. In adenoviral infections, follicular pharyngitis is the rule, and exudate is common. In contrast, the other respiratory viruses usually present with only pharyngeal erythema. Nasopharyngitis of a viral etiology most often is an acute, self-limited disease lasting from 4 to 10 days. In general, adenoviral illnesses tend to be more prolonged than those resulting from the other respiratory viruses. Other symptomatology in nasopharyngitis is related to the causative virus. For example, parainfluenza and respiratory syncytial viral infections also might have lower respiratory tract findings (laryngotracheitis, pneumonia, or bronchiolitis), and influenza might be associated with more severe, generalized complaints.

Although respiratory symptoms in association with rotavirus gastroenteritis have been noted frequently, there has been little careful clinical study of the respiratory manifestations. Lewis and associates,[80] in a careful study, observed a statistically significant occurrence of nasal discharge, cough, and red throat in children with rotavirus diarrhea when compared with children with diarrhea due to other causes.

Nasopharyngitis with *H. influenzae* and *N. meningitidis* infections has been noted mainly in people with septicemia and meningitis. Usually, the nasal symptomatology (coryza) preceded the pharyngitis and the severe systemic disease by a few to several days. In Q fever, the predominant finding is pneumonia. With diphtheria, the exudative pharyngitis and constitutional symptoms are most prominent.

Differential Diagnosis and Treatment

See the following section.

PHARYNGITIS, TONSILLITIS, AND TONSILLOPHARYNGITIS

Etiologic Agents

Etiologic agents of pharyngitis categorized by type of lesion, frequency of occurrence, and duration of illness are presented in Table 10–2. A great number of diverse possibilities exist for the differential diagnosis of pharyngitis. The specific agents or factors are presented in their respective sections of this book, and therefore only an overview is given here.

As with all infectious diseases, etiologic prevalence depends upon multiple factors (status of the host, age, season, environment, exposure, and type of lesion), and these must be considered in each individual case. In otherwise healthy children, the following infectious agents account for more than 90 per cent of acute infections with pharyngeal involvement: *Streptococcus pyogenes*; adenoviruses; influenza viruses A and B; parainfluenza viruses 1, 2, and 3; Epstein-Barr virus; enteroviruses; and *Mycoplasma pneumoniae*.[1, 6, 8, 9, 17, 20, 26, 27, 30, 33, 47, 51, 56, 60, 62, 63, 69, 71, 72, 91–93, 98, 101–104, 110, 111, 117–121, 123, 125, 127, 128, 138, 139, 143]

Although it is suggested frequently[18] that the group A streptococcus is the only worthy bacterial consideration in the etiology of pharyngitis, the data in Table 10–2 indicate broader possibilities. For example, when streptococci with β-hemolysis recovered from children and adolescents with pharyngitis are typed, group B, C, and G strains occasionally are found.[5, 21, 23, 44, 59, 134, 135] Turner and associates[135] found that of the group C streptococci, only *Streptococcus equisimilis* caused pharyngitis; *Streptococcus anginosus* (*Streptococcus milleri*) was part of the normal oropharyngeal flora.

Laboratory accidents have provided evidence that *H. influenzae* can cause pharyngitis,[100, 141] and children with systemic illnesses due to *H. influenzae* and *N. meningitidis* frequently have an associated marked pharyngitis.[122, 142, 146] *Arcanobacterium haemolyticum* and *Corynebacterium ulcerans* occasionally cause an illness mimicking diphtheria.[11, 54, 70, 74, 84, 105] *A. haemolyticum* also causes an illness that has been confused with streptococcal scarlet fever.[35, 70, 82, 84]

Because anaerobic microorganisms are universal constituents of the normal throat flora, it frequently is difficult to assign etiologic significance to these agents in throat infections. However, at present it seems clear that Vincent stomatitis and angina are the results of mixed infections with anaerobes.[37, 49, 83, 137] More recently, Brook and Gober[10] noted a significant association between encapsulated organisms of the *Bacteroides melaninogenicus* group and acute tonsillitis in children. It is my impression that acute and subacute infections with anaerobes account for a number of pharyngeal infections in adolescents in which cultures do not reveal group A streptococci and infectious mononucleosis tests are negative. Gonococcal and treponemal infections should be considered in sexually active or known exposed teenagers and other children.[13, 25, 38, 66, 145]

Adenoviral types 1, 2, 3, 4, 5, 6, 7, 7a, 9, 11, 14, 15, and 16 are the most common causes of pharyngitis in young children, and they also are prominent etiologic agents in older children and adolescents.[8, 14, 27, 29, 92, 95, 104, 123, 127, 138] Pharyngeal involvement in parainfluenza viral infections frequently is overshadowed by other respiratory symptomatology (e.g., cough, coryza) and in enteroviral infections by systemic complaints (e.g., fever, exanthem, meningitis).[1, 6, 17, 26, 56, 62, 63, 69, 72, 92, 98, 101, 103, 111, 117, 120, 121, 125, 130, 143] An enteroviral etiology should be suspected when small ulcerative lesions are noted that involve the soft palate and uvula, as well as the posterior pharyngeal wall (see Chapter 12). Infection with Epstein-Barr virus causes infectious mononucleosis with pharyngeal involvement similar to that resulting from group A streptococcal infection.[60, 139] The clinical manifestations of Epstein-Barr virus are age related: young children rarely have marked pharyngeal involvement.

Acquired cytomegalovirus infection causes an infectious mononucleosis–like syndrome, but pharyngitis is less common than it is in Epstein-Barr virus mononucleosis.[75] Primary as well as recurrent herpes simplex virus infections occasionally have pharyngeal manifestations.[15, 18, 33, 92] However, many illnesses that are ascribed clinically to herpes simplex virus actually are misidentified instances of aphthous stomatitis. Virtually all instances of herpes simplex virus infections with pharyngitis also will reveal lesions in the anterior mouth and externally around the mouth. Although Koplik spots are known universally as the enanthem of measles, many physicians are unaware of the diffuse nature of the associated measles pharyngitis.[19]

The role of *Chlamydia* species in the cause of pharyngitis is not clear. Grayston and associates[52, 53] noted the occurrence of pharyngitis in adolescents and young adults infected with *Chlamydia pneumoniae*.[52, 53] In a study in children, IgM antibody to *Chlamydia trachomatis* was found in children with pharyngitis.[57] Because there is cross-reactivity between *C. trachomatis* and *C. pneumoniae*, it is likely that the illnesses studied were caused by the latter agent rather than *C. trachomatis*. Ogawa and colleagues[99] noted prolonged and recurrent tonsillitis associated with sexually transmitted *C. trachomatis*.

Relatively mild pharyngitis occurs in young children with *M. pneumoniae* infections, and in older children, pharyngeal involvement is more pronounced.[20, 47, 51, 63] In young adult volunteers, *Mycoplasma hominis* was noted to cause pharyngitis.[94] Although lower respiratory tract findings and systemic complaints are most marked in Q fever, moderate subjective and mild objective evidence of pharyngitis also is noted.[32, 67] Exudative pharyngeal involvement with *Candida* species is common.[78, 124] *Candida* infection is most common in children whose normal throat flora has been disrupted and in children who have a compromised immunologic response.

Recurrent aphthous stomatitis usually involves the anterior oral cavity but is noted occasionally with extensive pharyngeal and soft palate lesions.[50, 115] Although L-forms of *Streptococcus sanguis* can be recovered consistently from the lesions of this disease,[50] their role in the etiology is unclear. In Behçet syndrome, the ulcerative lesions are subacute or chronic and usually not associated with surrounding pharyngeal inflammation.[85] In Kawasaki disease (mucocutaneous lymph node syndrome), the pharyngeal mucosa is deeply erythematous.[90]

Pharyngeal involvement is common in noninfectious illnesses in which host resistance has been altered. The lesions usually are ulcerative, but secondary bacterial or fungal overgrowth can lead to marked erythematous and exudative findings.

Epidemiology

Pharyngitis is common in children and, as noted in Table 10–2, is the result of many different infectious agents. In general, bacterial pharyngitis is more common in the cold weather seasons; an enteroviral etiology is most common in the summer and fall. Viral pharyngitis tends to occur relatively more frequently in younger children than does bacterial disease.[29] There is no apparent sex predilection.

TABLE 10–2. Etiologic Agents of Pharyngitis

Etiologic Agent or Factor	Type of Lesion*					Frequency of Occurrence†	Duration of Pharyngitis
	Erythematous	Follicular	Exudative	Ulcerative	Petechial		
Bacteria							
Streptococcus pyogenes[9, 30, 33, 47, 91, 93, 119, 128]	+ + + +	+ +	+ + +		+ + +	+ + + +	Acute
Other streptococci (groups B, C, and G)[2, 21–23, 44, 59, 134, 135]	+ + +	+	+ +			+ +	Acute
Corynebacterium diphtheriae[88, 119, 149]	+ + +		+ + + +			+	Acute
Corynebacterium pyogenes[140]	+ + + +		+ + + +			+	Acute
Corynebacterium ulcerans[82, 105, 132]	+ + + +		+ + +			+	Acute
Arcanobacterium haemolyticum[4, 11, 35, 54, 70, 74, 84]	+ + + +	+ +	+ + +			+	Acute
Mixed anaerobes (*Bacteroides* species, *Peptostreptococcus, Fusobacterium* species)[10, 12, 37, 49, 83, 137]	+ + +		+	+ + + +		+ +	Subacute
Actinomyces species[37]	+			+		+	Chronic
Francisella tularensis[65, 136, 147]	+ + + +		+ + +			+	Acute
Haemophilus influenzae[100, 129, 141, 142, 146]	+ +					+ +	Acute, subacute
Legionella pneumophila[96]	+ + + +					+	Acute
Neisseria meningitidis[122]	+ +		+			+ +	Acute
Neisseria gonorrhoeae[66, 145]	+ +		+			+	Acute, subacute, chronic
Leptospira spp.[64, 106]	+ + + +					+	Acute
Treponema pallidum[13, 25, 38]	+	+		+		+	Subacute
Borrelia species[77]	+ + + +					+	Acute
Streptobacillus moniliformis[109]	+					+	Acute
Yersinia enterocolitica[114, 131]	+ + + +		+ +			+	Acute
Yersinia pseudotuberculosis[116]							
Streptococcus pneumoniae[86]	+			+		+	Acute
Salmonella typhi[3, 97]	+					+	Acute
Chlamydia							
Chlamydia pneumoniae[52]	+ + + +					+ +	Acute
Chlamydia trachomatis[99]	+ +	+	+			+	Acute recurrent
Viruses							
Adenoviruses[8, 27, 92, 95, 104, 123, 138]	+ + + +	+ + + +	+ +			+ + + +	Acute
Influenza A and B[102, 110, 118, 130]	+ + +					+ + +	Acute
Parainfluenza 1–4[6, 56, 62, 63, 69, 98, 101, 103, 111, 117, 130]	+ +					+ + +	Acute
Respiratory syncytial[16, 61–63, 87, 103]	+ +					+	Acute
Enteroviruses (polio, coxsackieviruses A and B, echovirus)[1, 17, 26, 72, 92, 120, 121, 125, 143]	+ + +		+	+ +		+ + +	Acute
Epstein-Barr[60, 139]	+ + +	+	+ + + +		+ +	+ + +	Acute, subacute
Reoviruses[79, 148]	+ +					+	Acute
Cytomegalovirus[7, 75]	+					+	Acute
Herpes simplex[15, 18, 33, 92, 144]	+ +		+ +	+ + + +		+ +	Acute
Measles[19]	+ + +				+	+ +	Acute
Rubella[19, 39]					+ +	+	Acute
Rhinoviruses[58]	+					+	Acute
Mycoplasma							
Mycoplasma pneumoniae[20, 47, 51, 63]	+ +	+	+			+ +	Acute
Mycoplasma hominis[94]	+		+			+	Acute
Rickettsia							
Coxiella burnetii[32, 67]	+ +					+	Acute
Fungi							
Candida species[78, 124]	+		+ + + +			+ + +	Acute, subacute, chronic
Parasites							
Toxoplasma gondii[76]	+					+	Acute
Recognized illnesses of uncertain etiology							
Aphthous stomatitis[50, 115]	+			+ + + +		+ +	Acute recurrent
Behçet syndrome[85]	+			+ + + +		+	Chronic recurrent
Kawasaki disease[90]	+ +					+	Acute
Stevens-Johnson syndrome[19]	+		+	+ + + +		+	Acute
Illness in which host factors or therapeutic agents are primary causes (neutropenia, other immunodeficiencies, cancer, chemotherapeutic agents, generalized neoplastic disease)[19]	+			+ + + +		+ +	Chronic

*Pulses indicate the relative degree and severity of the lesion (+ + + +, most marked; +, minimal).
†+ + + +, 76–100%; + + +, 51–75%; + +, 26–50%; +, 1–25%.

The majority of diseases associated with pharyngitis require close person-to-person contact for spread. Pathogens are transmitted directly by close-range airborne dissemination or indirectly by the hands of the future host. Several food-borne outbreaks of streptococcal pharyngitis have been reported.[34, 40] Prechewing of food by adults also may be a cause of streptococcal pharyngitis in infants.[126]

Pathophysiology

The pathology and pathophysiology of diseases in which pharyngitis is prominent are presented in the chapters of this book on specific infectious agents (in particular, Chapters 86, 160, and 170).

Clinical Presentation

The clinical findings in pharyngitis are highlighted in Table 10–2. Manifestations related to individual pathogens are detailed in the chapters of this book dealing with the specific agents. The onset of pharyngitis usually is sudden and accompanied by fever and the complaint of sore throat. Frequently, parents will observe that the child's breath is not normal and that the throat and particularly the tonsils are red. Other initial complaints include headache, nausea, vomiting, and, sometimes, abdominal pain. Anorexia is the rule, as is some degree of lessened activity. Parents also report frequently that the child's cervical lymph nodes are enlarged and tender.

Physical examination usually substantiates the parents' observations—the child is febrile with moderate to severe pharyngeal erythema and some degree of cervical adenitis. As noted in Table 10–2, the pharyngeal response is varied. With acute common infections, the basic lesion is erythema. Associated with erythema can be follicular, ulcerative, and petechial lesions and/or generalized or circumscribed exudative areas. Follicular lesions are most characteristic of adenoviral infections, whereas exudative lesions are most common in group A streptococcal infections and in infectious mononucleosis. Meland and associates[89] noted that the absence of cough and the presence of swollen lymph nodes had the highest specificity in predicting a streptococcal cause of pharyngitis. Ulcerative lesions are observed most frequently in enteroviral infections (see Chapter 170). Petechiae on the soft palate frequently are seen in group A streptococcal infections but also are common in infectious mononucleosis, measles, and rubella.

Occurrences of pharyngitis in children almost entirely are acute, self-limited diseases; those of viral etiology last 4 to 10 days, and those caused by group A streptococci, if untreated, last slightly longer. Subacute and chronic pharyngeal disease is not common in children, but the etiologic possibilities are numerous (see Table 10–2).

DIFFERENTIAL DIAGNOSIS

As noted in Table 10–2, the differential considerations in pharyngitis are numerous, as in nasopharyngitis (see Table 10–1). Although there is considerable overlap in the spectrum of illness in pharyngeal infections, many clues help in ruling in or out certain diagnostic possibilities. The diagnosis of pharyngitis requires carefully eliciting epidemiologic and other historical data (i.e., exposure, season, incubation period, age of patient, associated clinical findings), in addition to the observation of pharyngeal physical findings.

The overwhelming majority of acute instances of nasopharyngitis are of viral etiology (see Table 10–1), with adenoviruses accounting for the greatest number of cases. Nasopharyngitis also occurs during epidemic influenza A and B and parainfluenza 1 and 2 and with sporadic parainfluenza 3 infections. In all cases, proper epidemiologic and historical data should be elicited so that early diphtheria and other unusual but treatable illnesses are not diagnosed incorrectly. Retrospective study has indicated that nasopharyngitis occasionally occurs in severe infections from *H. influenzae* and meningococci, so the possibility of these infections should be considered when the epidemiology suggests it.

Although the majority of cases of pharyngitis without nasal symptomatology are caused by viral infections, the number of other etiologic possibilities is great. Unfortunately, the all-too-frequent approach by many physicians is to consider all pharyngitis as being of bacterial origin and to treat it with antibiotics. Initial consideration in the child with pharyngitis should be the duration of illness. Subacute, chronic, and recurrent problems (see Table 10–2) generally suggest more unusual problems and require a more deliberate approach.

In all instances of acute pharyngitis, streptococcal disease must be ruled out.

SPECIFIC DIAGNOSIS

The epidemiologic history and careful clinical categorization are the most important aspects of specific diagnosis. The most pressing diagnostic need in upper respiratory infections in everyday pediatric practice is the distinction of bacterial from viral disease—who and who not to treat with antibiotics. An approach to the problem is presented in Table 10–3.

The child with the common cold, herpangina, or pharyngoconjunctival fever has a viral disease and does not need therapy with antibiotics. In most instances, when these clinical diagnoses are apparent, throat cultures for bacterial pathogens are not necessary. The child with severe acute pharyngitis with exudate and fever and cervical lymphadenitis also is treated easily because the majority of these children have disease resulting from group A streptococci.

Only a relatively small number of children have illnesses at the extremes of those in Table 10–3. Indeed, most of the illnesses seen routinely by the physician dealing with children fall into the large middle area, "Never-Never Land." On clinical grounds, there is no certain way to make an etiologic diagnosis and specifically to rule out infection due to *S. pyogenes*. Therefore, until recently, the usually recommended approach to management of pharyngitis and nasopharyngitis was to obtain a throat culture to determine whether group A streptococci were present. Several rapid tests for the detection of group A streptococci have become available that make the immediate diagnosis and treatment of streptococcal pharyngitis possible in the practice setting.[28, 41–43, 81, 107] In general, these rapid tests have high specificity, but sensitivity is less than optimal. Therefore, if early treatment is desirable today, a reasonable approach to the diagnosis of streptococcal pharyngitis is to carry out a rapid test. If the test is positive, specific therapy is instituted. In the case of a negative rapid test, a routine throat culture is performed, and therapy is withheld pending the culture results.[108]

There is a question regarding whether early treatment of streptococcal pharyngitis is desirable.[31, 45, 46, 107, 108] Certainly in the public clinic, where follow-up of children with positive throat cultures often is difficult, immediate diagnosis and treatment are important. However, as Pichichero and associates[107] and El-Daher and colleagues[31] have shown, early treatment may result in a decreased desirable antibody response,

TABLE 10–3. Treatment Considerations in Upper Respiratory Tract Infections

Clinical Entity	Etiology
Common cold, herpangina, pharyngoconjunctival fever	Viral, 100%
Never-Never Land	
↓	↓
Marked pharyngitis with exudate and fever and cervical lymphadenitis	Bacterial, 70%

Modified from Cherry, J. D.: Newer respiratory viruses: Their role in respiratory illness of children. *In* Schulman, I., et al. (eds.): Advances in Pediatrics, Vol. 20. © 1973, Year Book Medical Publishers, Inc., Chicago. Used by permission.

thus allowing reinfection with type-specific organisms. Therefore, in settings in which the communication between physicians and parents is satisfactory, it seems advisable in many instances to withhold the institution of treatment for a day or two. Gerber and associates[45, 46] argue against this approach because immediate therapy can reduce the risk of transmission of infection, and they challenge the interpretation of the findings of Pichichero and colleagues and El-Daher and coworkers.[31, 45, 46]

Cultures for other pathogens should be reserved for unusual situations, such as persistent symptomatology, indicative epidemiology, or other pertinent historical data. Because *H. influenzae* and *Streptococcus pneumoniae* frequently are part of the normal flora, their isolation is not always etiologically significant. However, if cultures reveal predominant growths of either, it is quite likely that they are contributing to the disease process, and antibiotic therapy directed at them will benefit the patient.[18, 86, 146] When the possibility of disease because of anaerobic agents exists, a Gram-stained smear from an exudative area may be rewarding. When the pharyngeal findings are unique or when many cases of a similar illness are observed, a viral culture from the throat is indicated.

TREATMENT

The specific treatment of diseases with nasopharyngitis and pharyngitis is presented in chapters of this book that deal with the individual pathogens. Although there are a multitude of proprietary remedies available for respiratory infections, and sore throat specifically, none have a place in the care of the pediatric patient. Particularly to be condemned are throat lozenges that contain a large number of useless ingredients, many potentially harmful. Antibiotic-containing lozenges particularly are to be condemned because they may allow streptococcal disease to go unrecognized. Antiseptic mouthwashes have no value, and decongestants and antihistamines have no proven efficacy and frequently lead to troublesome side effects.

Because children with pharyngitis frequently feel bad, therapy with an analgesic is reasonable. Formerly, aspirin was the analgesic usually recommended. However, because aspirin is an etiologic factor in influenza-associated Reye syndrome and because it is difficult clinically to differentiate influenza viral infections from other respiratory viral infections, it is prudent to use acetaminophen rather than aspirin. The dose per single administration of acetaminophen by year of age is as follows: younger than 1 year, 60 mg; 1 to 3 years, 60 to 120 mg; 3 to 6 years, 120 mg; 6 to 12 years, 150 to 300 mg; older than 12 years, 325 to 650 mg. Administration may be repeated three or four times daily in young children and every 4 hours in older children. Acetaminophen rarely should be given to infants younger than 6 months of age. In young children, careful attention to adequate hydration particularly is necessary.

PROGNOSIS

Almost all occurrences of nasopharyngitis and pharyngitis are self-limited, and the overall prognosis is excellent. However, a constant vigil for streptococcal and other more serious diseases is necessary. Failure to diagnose and treat group A streptococcal infections, syphilis, and other more unusual infections can lead to serious short- and long-term difficulties.

PREVENTION

Because pharyngitis and nasopharyngitis are caused by infections with a large number of different respiratory pathogens, there is no practical specific approach to prevention. On occasion, streptococcal disease can be prevented by the judicious use of prophylactic penicillin. For young children or others with undue susceptibility to serious disease with common respiratory pathogens, reduction in contact situations (e.g., day care centers) is prudent.

References

1. Ager, E. A., Felsenstein, W. C., Alexander, E. R., et al.: An epidemic of illness due to Coxsackievirus group B, type 2. J. A. M. A. *187*:251–256, 1964.
2. Arditi, M., Shulman, S. T., Davis, A. T., et al.: Group C β-hemolytic streptococcal infections in children: Nine pediatric cases and review. Rev. Infect. Dis. 2:34–45, 1989.
3. Ash, I., McKendrick, G. D. W., Robertson, M. H., et al.: Outbreak of typhoid fever connected with corned beef. Br. Med. J. 1:1474–1478, 1964.
4. Banck, G., and Nyman, M.: Tonsillitis and rash associated with *Corynebacterium haemolyticum*. J. Infect. Dis. *154*:1037–1039, 1986.
5. Benjamin, J. T., and Perriello, V. A., Jr.: Pharyngitis due to group C hemolytic streptococci in children. J. Pediatr. *89*:254–256, 1976.
6. Bisno, A. L., Barratt, N. P., Swanston, W. H., et al.: An outbreak of acute respiratory disease in Trinidad associated with para-influenza viruses. Am. J. Epidemiol. *91*:68–77, 1970.
7. Bonkowsky, H. L., Lee, R. V., and Klatskin, G.: Acute granulomatous

hepatitis: Occurrence in cytomegalovirus mononucleosis. J. A. M. A. *233*:1284–1288, 1975.
8. Brandt, C. D., Kim, H. W., Vargosko, A. J., et al.: Infections in 18,000 infants and children in a controlled study of respiratory tract disease: I. Adenovirus pathogenicity in relation to serologic type and illness syndrome. Am. J. Epidemiol. *90*:484–500, 1969.
9. Breese, B. B.: Streptococcal pharyngitis and scarlet fever. Am. J. Dis. Child. *132*:612–616, 1978.
10. Brook, I., and Gober, A. E.: *Bacteroides melaninogenicus*: Its recovery from tonsils of children with acute tonsillitis. Arch. Otolaryngol. *109*:818–819, 1983.
11. Carlson, P., Kontianinen, S., Renkonen, O. V., et al.: *Arcanobacterium haemolyticum* and streptococcal pharyngitis in Army conscripts. Scand. J. Infect. Dis. *27*:17–18, 1995.
12. Carrie, S., Fenton, P. A.: Necrobacillosis: An unusual case of pharyngotonsillitis. J. Laryngol. Otol. *108*:1097–1098, 1994.
13. Catalano, P. M., and Schragger, A. H.: Early and latent syphilis. Arch. Dermatol. *92*:433–435, 1965.
14. Centers for Disease Control: Adenovirus type 16—Long Island, New York. M. M. W. R. *28*:530–532, 1979.
15. Cesario, T. C., Poland, J. D., Wulff, H., et al.: Six years' experience with herpes simplex virus in a children's home. Am. J. Epidemiol. *90*:416–422, 1969.
16. Chanock, R. M., Parrott, R. H., Vargosko, A. J., et al.: Respiratory syncytial virus. Am. J. Public Health *52*:918–925, 1962.
17. Cherry, J. D., and Jahn, C. L.: Herpangina: The etiologic spectrum. Pediatrics *36*:632–634, 1965.
18. Cherry, J. D.: Newer respiratory viruses: Their role in respiratory illness of children. Adv. Pediatr. *20*:225–290, 1973.
19. Cherry, J. D.: Personal observations.
20. Cherry, J. D., and Welliver, R. C.: *Mycoplasma pneumoniae* infections of adults and children. West. J. Med. *125*:47–55, 1976.
21. Chretien, J. H., McGinniss, C. G., Thompson, J., et al.: Group B beta-hemolytic streptococci causing pharyngitis. J. Clin. Microbiol. *10*:263–266, 1979.
22. Cimolai, N., Elford, R. W., Bryan, L., et al.: Do the β-hemolytic non-group A streptococci cause pharyngitis? Rev. Infect. Dis. *10*:587–601, 1988.
23. Cimolai, N., Morrison, B. J., MacCulloch, L., et al.: Beta-haemolytic non-group A streptococci and pharyngitis: A case-control study. Eur. J. Paediatr. *150*:776–779, 1991.
24. Commission on Acute Respiratory Diseases: Endemic exudative pharyngitis and tonsillitis: Etiology and clinical characteristics. J. A. M. A. *125*:1163–1169, 1944.
25. Conant, M. A., and Lane, B.: Secondary syphilis misdiagnosed as infectious mononucleosis. Calif. Med. *109*:462–464, 1968.
26. Cramblett, H. G., Moffet, H. L., Black, J. P., et al.: Coxsackievirus infections: Clinical and laboratory studies. J. Pediatr. *64*:406–414, 1964.
27. Dascomb, H. E., and Hilleman, M. R.: Clinical and laboratory studies in patients with respiratory disease caused by adenoviruses (RI-APC-ARD agents). Am. J. Med. *Aug.*:161–174, 1956.
28. Denny, F. W.: Current problems in managing streptococcal pharyngitis. J. Pediatr. *111*:797–806, 1987.
29. Douglas, R. M., Miles, H., Hansman, D., et al.: Acute tonsillitis in children: Microbial pathogens in relation to age. Pathology *16*:79–82, 1984.
30. Dyment, P. G., Klink, L. B., and Jackson, D. W.: Hoarseness and palatal petechiae as clues in identifying streptococcal throat infections. Pediatrics *41*:822–823, 1968.
31. El-Daher, N. T., Hijazi, S. S., Rawashedeh, N. M., et al.: Immediate vs. delayed treatment of group A beta-hemolytic streptococcal pharyngitis with penicillin V. Pediatr. Infect. Dis. J. *10*:126–130, 1991.
32. Eshchar, J., Waron, M., and Alkan, W. J.: Syndromes of Q fever. J. A. M. A. *195*:146–149, 1966.
33. Evans, A. S., and Dick, E. C.: Acute pharyngitis and tonsillitis in University of Wisconsin students. J. A. M. A. *190*:699–708, 1964.
34. Farley, T. A., Wilson, S. A., Mahoney, F., et al.: Direct inoculation of food as the cause of an outbreak of group A streptococcal pharyngitis. J. Infect. Dis. *167*:1232–1235, 1993.
35. Fell, H. W. K., Nagington, J., Naylor, G. R. E., et al.: *Corynebacterium haemolyticum* infections in Cambridgeshire. J. Hyg. Camb. *79*:269–275, 1977.
36. Finegold, S. M., Bartlett, J. G., Chow, A. W., et al.: Management of anaerobic infections. Ann. Intern. Med. *83*:375–389, 1975.
37. Finegold, S. M., and Rosenblatt, J. E.: Practical aspects of anaerobic sepsis. Medicine *52*:311–322, 1973.
38. Fiumara, N. J., and Berg, M.: Primary syphilis in the oral cavity. Br. J. Vener. Dis. *50*:463–464, 1974.
39. Forchheimer, F.: The enanthem of German measles. Phila. Med. J. *II*:15–17, 1898.
40. Fries, S. M.: Diagnosis of group A streptococcal pharyngitis in a private clinic: Comparative evaluation of an optical immunoassay method and culture. J. Pediatr. *126*:933–936, 1995.
41. Gallo, G., Berzero, R., Cattai, N., et al.: An outbreak of group A food-borne streptococcal pharyngitis. Eur. J. Epidemiol. *8*:292–297, 1992.
42. Gerber, M. A.: Comparison of throat cultures and rapid strep tests for diagnosis of streptococcal pharyngitis. Pediatr. Infect. Dis. *8*:820–824, 1989.
43. Gerber, M. A., Spadaccini, L. J., Wright, L. L., et al.: Latex agglutination tests for rapid identification of group A streptococci directly from throat swabs. J. Pediatr. *105*:702–705, 1984.
44. Gerber, M. A., Randolph, M. F., Martin, N. J., et al.: Community-wide outbreak of group G streptococcal pharyngitis. Pediatr. *87*:598–603, 1991.
45. Gerber, M. A.: Effect of early antibiotic therapy on recurrence rates of streptococcal pharyngitis. Pediatr. Infect. Dis. J. *10*:S56–S60, 1991.
46. Gerber, M. A., Randolph, M. F., DeMeo, K. K., et al: Lack of impact of early antibiotic therapy for streptococcal pharyngitis on recurrence rates. J. Pediatr. *117*:853–858, 1990.
47. Glezen, W. P., Clyde, W. A., Jr., Senior, R. J., et al.: Group A streptococci, mycoplasmas, and viruses associated with acute pharyngitis. J. A. M. A. *202*:455–460, 1967.
48. Glover, J. A., and Griffith, F.: Acute tonsillitis and some of its sequels: Epidemiological and bacteriological observations. Br. Med. J. *Sept. 19*:521–527, 1931.
49. Gorbach, S. L., and Bartlett, J. G.: Anaerobic infections (three parts). N. Engl. J. Med. *290*:1177–1184, 1237–1245, 1289–1294, 1974.
50. Graykowski, E. A., Barile, M. F., Lee, W. B., et al.: Recurrent aphthous stomatitis: Clinical, therapeutic, histopathologic, and hypersensitivity aspects. J. A. M. A. *196*:637–644, 1966.
51. Grayston, J. T., Alexander, E. R., Kenny, G. E., et al.: *Mycoplasma pneumoniae* infections: Clinical and epidemiologic studies. J. A. M. A. *191*:369–374, 1965.
52. Grayston, J. T., Campbell, L. A., Kuo, C. C., et al.: A new respiratory tract pathogen: *Chlamydia pneumoniae* strain TWAR. J. Infect. Dis. *161*:618–625, 1990.
53. Grayston, J. T.: *Chlamydia pneumoniae* (TWAR) infections in children. Pediatr. Infect. Dis. J. *13*:675–685, 1994.
54. Green, S. L., and LaPeter, K. S.: Pseudodiphtheritic membranous pharyngitis caused by *Corynebacterium hemolyticum*. J. A. M. A. *245*:2330–2331, 1981.
55. Gurwith, M., Wenman, W., Hinde, D., et al.: A prospective study of rotavirus infection in infants and young children. J. Infect. Dis. *144*:218–224, 1981.
56. Harris, D. J., Wulff, H., Ray, C. G., et al.: Viruses and disease: II. An outbreak of parainfluenza type 2 in a children's home. Am. J. Epidemiol. *87*:419–425, 1968.
57. Harrison, H. R., Magder, L. S., Boyce, W. T., et al.: Acute *Chlamydia trachomatis* respiratory infection in childhood: Serologic evidence. Am. J. Dis. Child. *140*:1068–1071, 1986.
58. Higgins, P. G., Ellis, E. M., Woolley, D. A., et al.: Viruses associated with acute respiratory infections in Royal Air Force personnel. J. Hyg. Camb. *68*:647–654, 1970.
59. Hill, H. R., Caldwell, G. G., Wilson, E., et al.: Epidemic of pharyngitis due to streptococci of Lancefield group G. Lancet *16*:371–374, 1969.
60. Hoagland, R. J.: Clinical manifestations of infectious mononucleosis: A report of two hundred cases. Am. J. Med. Sci. *240*:21–28, 1960.
61. Hoekstra, R. E., Herrmann, E. C., Jr., and O'Connell, E. J.: Virus infections in children: Clinical comparison of overlapping outbreaks of influenza A2/Hong Kong/68 and respiratory syncytial virus infections. Am. J. Dis. Child. *120*:14–16, 1970.
62. Holzel, A., Parker, L., Patterson, W. H., et al.: Virus isolations from throats of children admitted to hospital with respiratory and other diseases, Manchester 1962–4. Br. Med. J. *1*:614–619, 1965.
63. Horn, M. E. C., Brain, E., Gregg, I., et al.: Respiratory viral infection in childhood: A survey in general practice, Roehampton 1967–1972. J. Hyg. Camb. *74*:157–168, 1975.
64. Humphrey, T., Sanders, S., and Stadius, M.: Leptospirosis mimicking MLNS. J. Pediatr. *91*:853–854, 1977.
65. Jacobs, R. F., Condrey, Y. M., and Yamauchi, T.: Tularemia in adults and children: A changing presentation. Pediatrics *76*:818–822, 1985.
66. Jamsky, R. J.: Gonococcal tonsillitis: Report of a case. Oral Surg. *44*:197–200, 1977.
67. Johnson, J. E., III, and Kadull, P. J.: Laboratory-acquired Q fever: A report of fifty cases. Am. J. Med. *41*:391–403, 1966.
68. Jordan, W. S., Jr.: Acute respiratory diseases of viral etiology: I. Ecology of respiratory viruses—1961. Am. J. Pub. Health *52*:897–945, 1962.
69. Kapikian, A. Z., Chanock, R. M., Reichelderfer, T. E., et al.: Inoculation of human volunteers with parainfluenza virus type 3. J. A. M. A. *178*:537–546, 1961.
70. Karpathios, T., Drakonaki, S., Zervoudaki, A., et al.: *Arcanobacterium haemolyticum* in children with presumed streptococcal pharyngotonsillitis or scarlet fever. J. Pediatr. *121*:735–737, 1992.
71. Kellner, G., Popow-Kraupp, T., Kundi, M., et al.: Contribution of rhinoviruses to respiratory viral infections in childhood: A prospective study in a mainly hospitalized infant population. J. Med. Virol. *25*:455–469, 1988.
72. Kibrick, S.: Current status of Coxsackie and ECHO viruses in human disease. Prog. Med. Virol. *6*:27–70, 1964.
73. Komaroff, A. L., Aronson, M. D., Pass, T. M., et al.: Serologic evidence of chlamydial and mycoplasmal pharyngitis in adults. Science *222*:927–928, 1983.
74. Kovatch, A. L., Schuit, K. E., and Michaels, R. H.: *Corynebacterium hemolyt-*

icum peritonsillar abscess mimicking diphtheria. J. A. M. A. *249*:1757–1758, 1983.

75. Lajo, A., Borque, C., Del Castillo, F., et al.: Mononucleosis caused by Epstein-Barr virus and cytomegalovirus in children: A comparative study of 124 cases. Pediatr. Infect. Dis. J. *13*:56–60, 1994.
76. Lascari, A. D., and Bapat, V. R.: Syndromes of infectious mononucleosis. Clin. Pediatr. *9*:300–305, 1970.
77. Le, C. T.: Tick-borne relapsing fever in children. Pediatrics *66*:963–966, 1980.
78. Lehner, T.: Oral thrush, or acute pseudomembranous candidiasis: A clinicopathologic study of forty-four cases. Oral Surg. *18*:27–37, 1964.
79. Lerner, A. M., Cherry, J. D., Klein, J. O., et al.: Infections with reoviruses. N. Engl. J. Med. *267*:947–952, 1962.
80. Lewis, H. M., Parry, J. V., Davies, H. A., et al.: A year's experience of the rotavirus syndrome and its association with respiratory illness. Arch. Dis. Child. *54*:339–346, 1979.
81. Lieu, T. A., Fleisher, G. R., and Schwartz, J. S.: Cost-effectiveness of rapid latex agglutination testing and throat culture for streptococcal pharyngitis. Pediatrics *85*:246–256, 1990.
82. Lipsky, B. A., Goldberger, A. C., Tompkins, L. S., et al.: Infections caused by nondiphtheria corynebacteria. Rev. Infect. Dis. *4*:1220–1235, 1982.
83. Macdonald, J. B., Socransky, S. S., and Gibbons, R. J.: Aspects of the pathogenesis of mixed anaerobic infections of mucous membranes. J. Dent. Res. *42* (Suppl. 1):529–544, 1963.
84. Mackenzie, A., Fuite, L. A., Chan, F. T. H., et al.: Incidence and pathogenicity of *Arcanobacterium haemolyticum* during a 2-year study in Ottawa. Clin. Infect. Dis. *21*:177–181, 1995.
85. Mamo, J. G., and Baghdassarian, A.: Behcet's disease: A report of 28 cases. Arch. Ophthalmol. *71*:4–14, 1964.
86. Markowitz, M.: Cultures of the respiratory tract in pediatric practice. Am. J. Dis. Child. *105*:12–18, 1963.
87. Maynard, J. E., Fletz, E. T., Wulff, H., et al.: Surveillance of respiratory virus infections among Alaskan Eskimo children. J. A. M. A. *200*:927–931, 1967.
88. McCloskey, R. V., Eller, J. J., Green, M., et al.: The 1970 epidemic of diphtheria in San Antonio. Ann. Intern. Med. *75*:495–503, 1971.
89. Meland, E., Digranes, A., and Skjaerven, R.: Assessment of clinical features predicting streptococcal pharyngitis. Scand. J. Infect. Dis. *25*:177–183, 1993.
90. Melish, M. E., Hicks, R. M., and Larson, E. J.: Mucocutaneous lymph node syndrome in the United States. Am. J. Dis. Child. *130*:599–607, 1976.
91. Moffet, H. L., Cramblett, H. G., and Smith, A.: Group A streptococcal infections in a children's home: II. Clinical and epidemiologic patterns of illness. Pediatrics *33*:11–17, 1964.
92. Moffet, H. L., Siegel, A. C., and Doyle, H. K.: Nonstreptococcal pharyngitis. J. Pediatr. *73*:51–60, 1968.
93. Mortimer, E. A., Jr., and Boxerbaum, B.: Diagnosis and treatment: Group A streptococcal infections. Pediatrics *36*:930–932, 1965.
94. Mufson, M. A.: *Mycoplasma hominis 1* in respiratory tract infections. Ann. N. Y. Acad. Sci. *174*:798–808, 1970.
95. Nakayama, M., Miyazaki, C., Ueda, K., et al.: Pharyngoconjunctival fever caused by adenovirus type 11. Pediatr. Infect. Dis. J. *11*:6–9, 1992.
96. Nigro, G., Pastoris, M. D., Fantasia, M. M., et al.: Acute cerebellar ataxia in pediatric legionellosis. Pediatrics *72*:847–849, 1983.
97. Nourmand, A., and Ziai, M.: Typhoid and paratyphoid fever in children. Review of symptoms and therapy in 165 cases. Clin. Pediatr. *8*:235–238, 1969.
98. Numazaki, Y., Yano, N., Shigeta, S., et al.: Studies on parainfluenza virus infections among infants and children in Sendai: II. Serologic and epidemiologic investigation. Japan J. Microbiol. *12*:343–351, 1968.
99. Ogawa, H., Hashiguchi, K., and Kazuyama, Y.: Prolonged and recurrent tonsillitis associated with sexually transmitted Chlamydia trachomatis. J. Laryngol. Otol. *107*: 27–29, 1993.
100. Park, W. H., and Cooper, G. V.: Accidental inoculation of influenza bacilli on, the mucous membranes of healthy persons with development of infection in at least one: Persistence of type characteristics of the bacilli. J. Immunol. *6*:81–85, 1921.
101. Parrott, R. H., Vargosko, A., Luckey, A., et al.: Clinical features of infection with hemadsorption viruses. N. Engl. J. Med. *260*:731–738, 1959.
102. Parrott, R. H., Kim, H. W., Vargosko, A. J., et al.: Serious respiratory tract illness as a result of Asian influenza and influenza B infections in children. J. Pediatr. *61*:205–213, 1962.
103. Parrott, R. H.: Viral respiratory tract illnesses in children. Bull. N. Y. Acad. Med. *39*:629–648, 1963.
104. Pereira, M. S.: Adenovirus infections. Postgrad. Med. J. *49*:798–801, 1973.
105. Pers, C.: Infection due to *Corynebacterium ulcerans* producing diphtheria toxin: A case report from Denmark. Acta Pathol. Microbiol. Immunol. Scand. *95*:361–362, 1987.
106. Peter, G.: Leptospirosis: A zoonosis of protean manifestations. Pediatr. Infect. Dis. *1*:282–288, 1982.
107. Pichichero, M. E., Disney, F. A., Talpey, W. B., et al.: Adverse and beneficial effects of immediate treatment of group A beta-hemolytic streptococcal pharyngitis with penicillin. Pediatr. Infect. Dis. *6*:635–643, 1987.
108. Pichichero, M. E., Disney, F. A., Green, J. L., et al.: Comparative reliability of clinical, culture, and antigen detection methods for the diagnosis of group A beta-hemolytic streptococcal tonsillopharyngitis. Pediatr. Annals *21*: 798–805, 1992.
109. Place, E. H., and Sutton, L. E.: Erythema arthriticum epidemicum (Haverhill fever). Arch. Intern. Med. *54*:659–684, 1934.
110. Podosin, R. L., and Felton, W. L., II: The clinical picture of Far East influenza occurring at the Fourth National Boy Scout Jamboree: Report of 616 cases. N. Engl. J. Med. *258*:778–782, 1958.
111. Poland, J. D., Wulff, H., Welton, E. R., et al.: Viruses and disease: Studies in a children's home. Am. J. Epidemiol. *84*:92–102, 1966.
112. Rantz, L. A., Boisvert, P. J., and Spink, W. W.: Hemolytic streptococcic and nonstreptococcic diseases of the respiratory tract: A comparative clinical study. Arch. Intern. Med. *78*:369–386, 1946.
113. Rodriguez, W. J., Kim, H. W., Arrobio, J. O., et al.: Clinical features of acute gastroenteritis associated with human reovirus-like agent in infants and young children. J. Pediatr. *91*:188–193, 1977.
114. Rodriguez, W. J., Controni, G., Cohen, G. J., et al.: *Yersinia enterocolitica* enteritis in children. J. A. M. A. *242*:1978–1980, 1979.
115. Rogers, R. S., III: Recurrent aphthous stomatitis: Clinical characteristics and evidence for an immunopathogenesis. J. Invest. Dermatol. *69*:499–509, 1977.
116. Saari, T. N., and Triplett, D. A.: *Yersinia pseudotuberculosis* mesenteric adenitis. J. Pediatr. *85*:656–659, 1974.
117. Saliba, G. S., Glezen, W. P., and Chin, T. D. Y.: Etiologic studies of acute respiratory illness among children attending public schools. Am. Rev. Respir. Dis. *95*:592–602, 1967.
118. Schmidt, J. P., Metcalf, T. G., and Miltenberger, F. W.: An epidemic of Asian influenza in children at Ladd Air Force Base, Alaska, 1960. J. Pediatr. *61*:214–220, 1962.
119. Schmidt, W. C., and Rammelkamp, C. H., Jr.: Bacterial infections of the nasopharynx, with particular reference to the prevention of rheumatic fever and glomerulonephritis. Pediatr. Clin. *Feb.*:139–154, 1957.
120. Scott, T. F. McNair: Clinical syndromes associated with entero virus and reo virus infections. Adv. Virus Res. *8*:165–197, 1962.
121. Siegel, W., Spencer, F. J., Smith, D. J., et al.: Two new variants of infection with Coxsackievirus group B, type 5, in young children: A syndrome of lymphadenopathy, pharyngitis and hepatomegaly or splenomegaly, or both, and one of pneumonia. N. Engl. J. Med. *268*:1210–1216, 1963.
122. Smith, H. W., Thomas, L., Dingle, J. H., et al.: Meningococcic infections: Report of 43 cases of meningococcic meningitis and 8 cases of meningococcemia. Ann. Intern. Med. *20*:12–32, 1944.
123. Sohier, R., Chardonnet, Y., and Prunieras, M.: Adenoviruses: Status of current knowledge. Prog. Med. Virol. *7*:253–325, 1965.
124. Solomon, P.: Oral moniliasis complicating combined broad spectrum-antibiotic and antifungal therapy. N. Engl. J. Med. *265*:847–848, 1961.
125. Steigman, A. J., Lipton, M. M., and Braspennickx, H.: Acute lymphonodular pharyngitis: A newly described condition due to Coxsackie A virus. J. Pediatr. *61*:331–336, 1962.
126. Steinkuller, J. S., Chan, K., and Rinehouse, S. E.: Prechewing of food by adults and streptococcal pharyngitis in infants. J. Pediatr. *120*:563–564, 1992.
127. Sterner, G.: Adenovirus infection in childhood: An epidemiological and clinical survey among Swedish children. Acta Paediatr. *142*:5–30, 1962.
128. Stillerman, M., and Bernstein, S. H.: Streptococcal pharyngitis: Evaluation of clinical syndromes in diagnosis. Am. J. Dis. Child. *101*:476–489, 1961.
129. Stollerman, G. H.: Sore throat: A diagnostic and therapeutic dilemma. J. A. M. A. *189*:145–146, 1964.
130. Sutton, R. N. P.: Respiratory viruses in a residential nursery. J. Hyg. Camb. *60*:51–67, 1962.
131. Tacket, C. O., Davis, B. R., Carter, G. P., et al.: *Yersinia enterocolitica* pharyngitis. Ann. Intern. Med. *99*:40–42, 1983.
132. Tomlinson, A. J. H.: Human pathogenic coryneform bacteria: Their differentiation and significance in public health today. J. Appl. Bacteriol. *29*:131–137, 1966.
133. Top, F. H., Sr.: Diphtheria. *In* Top, F. H., Sr., and Wehrle, P. F. (eds.): Communicable and Infectious Diseases. St. Louis, C. V. Mosby, 1972, pp. 190–207.
134. Turner, J. C., Hayden, G. F., Kiselica, D., et al.: Association of group C beta-hemolytic streptococci with endemic pharyngitis among college students. J. A. M. A. *264*: 2644–2647, 1990.
135. Turner, J. C., Fox, A., Fox, K., et al.: Role of group C beta-hemolytic streptococci in pharyngitis: Epidemiologic study of clinical features associated with isolation of group C streptococci. J. Clin. Microbiol. *31*: 808–811, 1993.
136. Tyson, H. K.: Tularemia: An unappreciated cause of exudative pharyngitis. Pediatrics *58*:864–866, 1976.
137. Uohara, G. I., and Knapp, M. J.: Oral fusospirochetosis and associated lesions. Oral Surg. *24*:113–123, 1967.
138. Van Der Veen, J.: The role of adenoviruses in respiratory disease. Am. Rev. Resp. Dis. *88*:167–180, 1963.
139. Veltri, R. W., Sprinkle, P. M., and McClung, J. E.: Epstein-Barr virus associated with episodes of recurrent tonsillitis. Arch. Otolaryngol. *101*:552–556, 1975.
140. Von Graevenitz, A.: Which bacterial species should be isolated from throat cultures? Eur. J. Clin. Microbiol. 2:1–3, 1983.

141. Walker, J. E.: Infection of laboratory worker with bacillus influenzae. J. Infect. Dis. 43:300–305, 1928.
142. Walker, S. H.: The respiratory manifestations of systemic *Hemophilus influenzae* infection. J. Pediatr. 62:386–392, 1963.
143. Ward, R.: Poliomyelitis. Pediatr. Clin. North Am. 7:947–963, 1960.
144. Wat, P. J., Strickler, J. G., Myers, J. L., et al.: Herpes simplex infection causing acute necrotizing tonsillitis. Mayo Clin. Proc. 69:269–271, 1994.
145. Wiesner, P. J., Tronca, E., Bonin, P., et al.: Clinical spectrum of pharyngeal gonococcal infection. N. Engl. J. Med. 288:181–185, 1973.
146. Willard, C. Y., and Hansen, A. E.: Bacterial flora of the nasopharynx in children: Influence of respiratory infections and previous antimicrobial therapy. Am. J. Dis. Child. 97:318–325, 1959.
147. Wills, P. I., Gedosh, E. A., and Nichols, D. R.: Head and neck manifestations of tularemia. Laryngoscope 92:770–773, 1982.
148. Zalan, E., Leers, W. D., and Labzoffsky, N. A.: Occurrence of reovirus infection in Ontario. Can. Med. Assoc. J. 87:714–715, 1962.
149. Zalma, V. M., Older, J. J., and Brooks, G. F.: The Austin, Texas, diphtheria outbreak: Clinical and epidemiological aspects. J. A. M. A. 211:2125–2129, 1970.

11

HERPANGINA

James D. Cherry

Herpangina is a fairly frequent, acute febrile illness that occurs in the summer and fall in temperate climates and is characterized by papular, vesicular, and ulcerative lesions on the anterior tonsillar pillars, soft palate, tonsils, pharynx, and posterior buccal mucosa. It is caused by many different enteroviruses.

HISTORY

Zahorsky[38, 39] generally is credited with the identification and characterization of the disease spectrum of herpangina. In his first paper in 1920 entitled "Herpetic Sore Throat," he presented the findings in 82 cases. In 1924, he introduced the name "herpangina" so that the clinical entity would not be confused with other diseases of the mouth and throat. In both papers, Zahorsky notes that Moro in 1906 previously had referred to a similar illness. Johnsson and Lindahl[13] also reported that similar syndromes had been observed by Trousseau in 1906 and Marfan in 1924, as well as by Moro in 1906. In 1939, Levine and associates[19] described epidemic herpangina in three summer camps, and in 1940, Breese[4] reported 28 cases that he observed during the summers of 1938 and 1940. In 1951, Huebner and associates[12] and Parrott and colleagues[27] clearly established the etiologic relationship of coxsackieviruses A to herpangina. In 1965, Cherry and Jahn[6] noted from the literature as well as from their own observations that herpangina resulted from infection with many echoviruses and coxsackieviruses B, as well as coxsackieviruses A.

ETIOLOGIC AGENTS

Virologic studies in the early 1950s that utilized suckling mice inoculation clearly indicated that several coxsackieviruses A were the cause of epidemic herpangina.[12, 14, 15, 27, 32, 36] In subsequent years, tissue culture techniques became widely used in diagnostic virology, and many studies revealed additional enteroviral types in association with herpangina.[6] It is of interest that, except for the initial interest in herpangina in 1950, careful study of the etiology of epidemic disease has not been carried out. Most herpangina virus/illness associations that have been made over the last 35 years have resulted from secondary findings in other investigations.[1–3, 7–11, 16–18, 20–24, 26, 28–31] A listing of viral agents associated with herpangina is presented in Table 11–1. It is obvious that in recent years coxsackieviruses B have been implicated most frequently. It must be pointed out, however, that diagnostic studies utilizing suckling mice inoculation only rarely have been performed during the last 25 years. As noted in Table 11–1, herpes simplex virus also can cause a clinical picture suggestive of herpangina.[8, 22] Indeed, Zahorsky[38] suggested that the cause of poliomyelitis also could be etiologic in herpangina because a similar enanthem had been observed in both sporadic and epidemic poliomyelitis.

EPIDEMIOLOGY

See sections on coxsackieviruses and echoviruses in Chapter 169.

PATHOPHYSIOLOGY

The pathophysiology of coxsackievirus and echovirus infections is presented in their respective sections in Chapter 169. However, specific experimental data related to herpangina are presented by Simkova and Petrovicova.[33] In rhesus monkeys, they found that oropharyngeal lesions typical of herpangina developed in 2 to 7 days after oral, intravenous, or subcutaneous administration of coxsackievirus A4. These studies indicate that the oropharyngeal lesions are the result of multiplication of virus at the secondary infection site after viremia rather than a primary manifestation of initial cellular involvement.

CLINICAL MANIFESTATIONS

Although Zahorsky[38, 39] and others[12, 27] have considered herpangina as a specific febrile disease, it would seem more appropriate to restrict the term "herpangina" to the characteristic oropharyngeal lesions. Herpangina is one of the protean manifestations of enteroviral infections, and it can occur in association with exanthem, meningitis, and other clinical constellations.

The onset of herpangina is typical of the majority of enteroviral infections and is characterized by the sudden awareness of fever.[4, 27, 38, 39] There usually is no characteristic prodrome, but young children may be irritable and occasionally listless and anorexic for a few hours before the febrile state is recognized. The initial temperature can be quite variable, with a

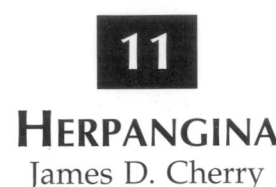

TABLE 11–1. Etiologic Agents Found in Association with Sporadic or Epidemic Herpangina

Virus	Occurrence		Reference
	Epidemic	Sporadic	
Coxsackievirus A			
1	+		14, 35, 36
2	+		14, 32, 35, 36
3	+		14, 32, 35, 36
4	+		14, 32, 35, 36
5	+		5, 14, 35, 36
6	+		14, 32, 35, 36
7		+	14, 29
8	+		14, 32, 35, 36
9		+	6, 14, 17, 29
10	+		14, 32, 35, 36
16		+	6, 14
22	+		14, 35, 36
Coxsackievirus B			
1	+	+	6, 10, 20, 29, 35, 36
2		+	1, 10, 14, 21, 29, 35, 36
3		+	9–11, 14, 18, 25, 29, 35–37
4		+	2, 3, 6, 7, 10, 14, 28, 29, 35, 36
5		+	2, 10, 14, 29, 31, 35, 36
Echovirus			
6		+	14
9		+	6, 14, 16, 29, 31
11		+	23, 34
16	+	+	14, 26
17		+	6
22		+	23
25	+		24
Herpes simplex		+	8, 22

range from normal to 41° C (106° F). In general, the temperature tends to be higher in younger patients. Breese[4] noted that the most common temperature in young children was between 39.5° and 40° C (103° and 104° F). Older children frequently complain of headache and backache. Vomiting occurs in about 25 per cent of children younger than 5 years of age. In one outbreak of illness due to coxsackievirus A4,[8] initial symptoms were anorexia and drooling (100 per cent); sore throat (50 per cent); coryza (45 per cent); headache (18 per cent); and vomiting, diarrhea, or both (36 per cent).

In the majority of instances of herpangina, the oropharyngeal lesions are present on the first examination at the time of or shortly after fever is noted. In the coxsackievirus A4 outbreak described by Forman and Cherry,[8] the enanthem was not observed until 24 to 48 hours after the initial nonspecific symptoms. The characteristic lesions in herpangina are small (1 to 2 mm) vesicles and ulcers. These lesions apparently start as papules, become vesicular, and then ulcerate in a short, but variable, period. In my experience, the most commonly observed lesions are ulcers. Breese[4] noted in a number of children seen early in the illness that a petechial appearance preceded the typical vesicular ulcerative enanthem.

The lesions usually are discrete, with an average of 5 per patient; some patients will have only 1 or 2 lesions, whereas others may have 14 or more. When seen early, the vesicular lesions are observed to enlarge from 1 to 2 mm to 3 to 4 mm over a 2- to 3-day period.[27] Each vesicular and ulcerative lesion is surrounded by an erythematous ring that varies in size up to 10 mm in diameter. The most common site of the lesions is the anterior tonsillar pillars. Lesions also occur on the soft palate, uvula, tonsils, pharyngeal wall, and, occasionally, the posterior buccal surfaces. In some cases, additional lesions have been noted on the dorsum or tip of the tongue. However, by definition, cases in which the primary involvement is on the tongue or anterior mouth and in which the lesions are of a general size greater than 5 mm are not considered to be herpangina.

Aside from the specific lesions, the remainder of the throat appears normal, minimally injected, or erythematous. Although occasionally noted in association with aseptic meningitis or other more severe enteroviral illness, most cases of herpangina are mild and without complication. The usual duration of signs and symptoms is 3 to 6 days.

Routine laboratory study is of little value in herpangina. The total white blood cell count may be normal or slightly elevated; the differential count most often is normal.

DIFFERENTIAL DIAGNOSIS

The classic appearance of the oropharynx in herpangina makes diagnosis easy. It can be differentiated clearly from bacterial pharyngitis on clinical grounds, so bacterial cultures seldom are necessary. The follicular lesions of adenoviral infections can be confused with it, but these frequently are exudative, not ulcerative, and associated with a more marked, generalized, erythematous pharyngitis than is herpangina. Additional differential considerations are presented elsewhere (see Chapters 10 and 169).

SPECIFIC DIAGNOSIS

In most instances, a clinical diagnosis is all that is necessary. However, because herpangina is a good indicator of enteroviral disease in a community, submission of throat or rectal specimens to a viral diagnostic center can be rewarding.

TREATMENT, PROGNOSIS, AND PREVENTION

No treatment is necessary other than attention to hydration and observation for signs of more severe enteroviral illness. Except in rare instances (associated myocarditis, encephalitis), the prognosis is excellent. No general preventive measures are necessary, but it would seem wise not to expose young children unnecessarily to persons known to be afflicted.

References

1. Ager, E. A., Felsenstein, W. C., Alexander, E. R., et al.: An epidemic of illness due to Coxsackie virus group B, type 2. J. A. M. A. *187*:251–256, 1964.
2. Artenstein, M. S., Cadigan, F. C., Jr., and Buescher, E. L.: Epidemic Coxsackie virus infection with mixed clinical manifestations. Ann. Intern. Med. *60*:196–203, 1964.
3. Artenstein, M. S., Cadigan, F. C., Jr., and Buescher, E. L.: Clinical and epidemiological features of Coxsackie group B virus infections. Ann. Intern. Med. *63*:597–603, 1965.
4. Breese, B. B., Jr.: Apthous pharyngitis. Am. J. Dis. Child. *61*:669–674, 1941.
5. Chawareewong, S., Kiangsiri, S., Lokaphadhana, K., et al.: Neonatal herpangina caused by Coxsackie A-5 virus. J. Pediatr. *93*:492–494, 1978.
6. Cherry, J. D., and Jahn, C. L.: Herpangina: The etiologic spectrum. Pediatrics *36*:632–634, 1965.

7. Felici, A., and Gregorig, B.: Contribution to the study of diseases in Italy caused by the Coxsackie B group of viruses. II. Epidemiological, clinical and virological data obtained in the course of a summer outbreak caused by Coxsackie B4 virus. Arch. Ges. Virusforsch. *9:*317–328, 1959.
8. Forman, M. L., and Cherry, J. D.: Enanthems associated with uncommon viral syndromes. Pediatrics *41:*873–882, 1968.
9. Glick, S. M., and Stroud, R.: An unusual case of Coxsackie B infection. Arch. Intern Med. *109:*97–101, 1962.
10. Hable, K. A., O'Connell, E. J., and Herrmann, E. C., Jr.: Group B coxsackieviruses as respiratory viruses. Mayo Clin. Proc. *45:*170–176, 1970.
11. Hierholzer, J. C., Mostow, S. R., and Dowdle, W. R.: Prospective study of a mixed coxsackie virus B3 and B4 outbreak of upper respiratory illness in a children's home. Pediatrics *49:*744–752, 1972.
12. Huebner, R. J., Cole, R. M., Beeman, E. A., et al.: Herpangina: Etiological studies of a specific infectious disease. J. A. M. A. *145:*628–633, 1951.
13. Johnsson, T., and Lindahl, J.: Herpangina: A clinical and virological study. Arch. Ges. Virusforsch. *2:*96–109, 1953.
14. Kibrick, S.: Current status of Coxsackie and ECHO viruses in human disease. Prog. Med. Virol. *6:*27–70, 1964.
15. Kravis, L. P., Hummeler, K., Sigel, M. M., et al.: Herpangina: Clinical and laboratory aspects of an outbreak caused by Group A Coxsackie viruses. Pediatrics *11:*113–119, 1953.
16. Lepow, M. L., Carver, D. H., and Robbins, F. C.: Clinical and epidemiologic observations on enterovirus infection in a circumscribed community during an epidemic of ECHO 9 infection. Pediatrics *26:*12–26, 1960.
17. Lerner, A. M., Klein, J. O., Levin, H. S., et al.: Infections due to Coxsackie virus group A, type 9, in Boston, 1959, with special reference to exanthems and pneumonia. N. Engl. J. Med. *263:*1265–1272, 1960.
18. Lerner, A. M., Klein, J. O., and Finland, M.: Infection with Coxsackie virus group B, type 3, with vesicular eruption: Report of two cases. N. Engl. J. Med. *263:*1305, 1960.
19. Levine, H. B., Hoerr, S. O., and Allanson, J. C.: Vesicular pharyngitis and stomatitis: An unusual epidemic of possible herpetic origin. J. A. M. A. *112:*2020–2022, 1939.
20. McLean, D. M., Coleman, M. A., Larke, R. P. B., et al.: Viral infections of Toronto children during 1965. I. Enteroviral disease. Can. Med. Assoc. J. *94:*839–843, 1966.
21. Marchessault, V., Pavilanis, V., Podoski, M. O., et al.: An epidemic of aseptic meningitis caused by Coxsackie B type 2 virus. Can. Med. Assoc. J. *85:*123–126, 1961.
22. Marks, M. I.: Herpangina and pleurodynia associated with herpes simplex virus. Pediatrics *48:*305–307, 1971.
23. Moore, M.: Enteroviral disease in the United States, 1970–1979. J. Infect. Dis. *146:*103–108, 1982.
24. Moritsugu, Y., Sawada, K., Hinohara, M., et al.: An outbreak of type 25 Echovirus infections with exanthem in an infant home near Tokyo. Am. J. Epidemiol. *87:*599–608, 1968.
25. Nakayama, T., Urano, T., Osano, M., et al.: Outbreak of herpangina associated with Coxsackievirus B3 infection. Pediatr. Infect. Dis. *8:*495–498, 1989.
26. Neva, F. A., Feemster, R. F., and Gorbach, I. J.: Clinical and epidemiological features of an unusual epidemic exanthem. J. A. M. A. *155:*544–548, 1954.
27. Parrott, R. H., Ross, S., Burke, F. G., et al.: Herpangina: Clinical studies of a specific infectious disease. N. Engl. J. Med. *245:*275–280, 1951.
28. Ray, C. G., Plexico, K. L., Wenner, H. A., et al.: Acute respiratory illness associated with Coxsackie B4 virus in children. Pediatrics *39:*220–226, 1967.
29. Reinhard, K. R.: Ecology of enteroviruses in the western Arctic. J. A. M. A. *183:*410–418, 1963.
30. Sabin, A. B.: Role of ECHO viruses in human disease. *In* Rose, H. M. (ed.): Viral Infections of Infancy and Childhood. Symposium No. 19, Section on Microbiology, New York Academy of Medicine. New York, Hoeber–Harper, 1960, pp. 78–100.
31. St. Geme, J. W., Jr., and Prince, J. T.: Vesicular pharyngitis associated with Coxsackie virus group B, type 5. N. Engl. J. Med. *265:*1255–1256, 1961.
32. Scott, T. F. M.: Clinical syndromes associated with entero virus and reo virus infection. Adv. Virus Res. *8:*165–197, 1962.
33. Simkova, A., and Petrovicova, A.: Experimental infection of rhesus monkeys with Coxsackie A 4 virus. Acta Virol. *16:*250–257, 1972.
34. Suzuki, N., Ishikawa, K., Horiuchi, T., et al.: Age-related symptomatology of ECHO 11 virus infection in children. Pediatrics *65:*284–286, 1980.
35. Wenner, H. A.: The enteroviruses. Am. J. Clin. Pathol. *57:*751–761, 1972.
36. Wenner, H. A.: Virus diseases associated with cutaneous eruptions. Prog. Med. Virol. *16:*269–336, 1973.
37. Winsser, J., and Altieri, R. H.: A three-year study of Coxsackie virus, group B, infection in Nassau County. Part I. Fecal studies of patients. Am. J. Med. Sci. *247:*269–273, 1964.
38. Zahorsky, J.: Herpangina: A specific infectious disease. Arch. Pediatr. *41:*181–184, 1924.
39. Zahorsky, J.: Herpetic sore throat. South. Med. J. *13:*871–872, 1920.

12

PHARYNGOCONJUNCTIVAL FEVER

James D. Cherry

Pharyngoconjunctival fever is an acute, communicable disease syndrome characterized by fever, pharyngitis, and conjunctivitis. It is caused by several serologic types of adenovirus; illness is both epidemic and sporadic.

HISTORY

Shortly after the first isolation of adenoviruses in tissue culture by Rowe and associates[50] in 1953, the clear association of infection with certain adenoviral types and the syndrome of fever, pharyngitis, and conjunctivitis was established.[48] For an approximate 5-year period after the discovery of the adenoviral etiology of pharyngoconjunctival fever, the literature contained numerous confirmatory reports from throughout the world.[1, 3, 6–8, 11, 14, 16, 18, 19, 22–25, 28–33, 35–38, 43–46, 53, 55–57, 59, 61–63, 65, 66] In almost all reports, the association of swimming and the contraction of the syndrome was noted. It would appear from a quick perusal of the reports that both the syndrome and the etiologic agents were new discoveries. However, epidemics of pharyngoconjunctival fever–like illness have been noted throughout this century. Béal[4] in 1907 in France perhaps was the first to note the syndrome. In the 1920s, epidemics of febrile disease with conjunctivitis associated with swimming in public pools and lakes were noted in Germany[47] and the United States.[2] It is quite probable that "swimming bath conjunctivitis," as described by Derrick[13] in 1943, was due to adenoviral infection; an epidemic of conjunctivitis studied by Cockburn and associates[11] in Greeley, Colorado, in 1951 was proved later to have been due to adenovirus type 3.

During the last 28 years, there have been relatively few reports of pharyngoconjunctival fever.[9, 12, 15, 20, 21, 26, 27, 41, 42, 44, 49, 51, 52, 58, 60, 64, 67, 70] My experience suggests that this is not because of a decrease in prevalence of the syndrome but to a general disinterest in the differential diagnosis of viral respiratory disease.

ETIOLOGIC AGENTS

In epidemic pharyngoconjunctival fever, the most likely etiologic agent is adenovirus 3.[3, 5, 6, 8, 11, 20, 22, 24, 29, 32–34, 38, 41, 42, 45, 48, 55, 61, 70] The next most prevalent adenoviruses association with epidemic disease is type 7.[9, 14, 18] One or more epidemics also have been noted with adenoviruses 2, 4, 7a, 11, and 14.[1, 6, 12, 15, 16, 44 61, 63, 70] Sporadic occurrences of pharyngoconjunctival fever have been observed in association with infections with adenoviruses 1, 2, 3, 4, 5, 6, 7, 7a, 8, 14, 19, and 13/30 (an intermediate type).[6, 7, 21, 22, 26–28, 31, 35–37, 43, 51, 52, 56–60, 62, 64, 67]

EPIDEMIOLOGY

Pharyngoconjunctival fever occurs in large community-wide epidemics, in focal outbreaks, and as sporadic cases. Most major community epidemics have occurred in the summertime and have been centered around public swimming facilities. Two community outbreaks involving primarily swimmers have occurred in the wintertime.[9, 20] In swimming-associated outbreaks, it is probable that infection occurs by conjunctival inoculation of adenoviruses from contaminated water. To date, however, the virus has been recovered from the incriminated water in only two outbreaks.[12, 42] In one outbreak, adenovirus type 4 was recovered from water samples on two occasions 14 days apart.[12] More recently, an adenovirus type 3 was recovered from a pool in which 681 campers had symptoms.[42] In this outbreak, both the frequency of swimming and the history of towel sharing increased the risk of illness. An adenovirus type 3 also was recovered from a sewage outlet area in a lake that was close to a swimming beach.[38]

The incubation period of swimming-associated infections is about 5 to 7 days.[5, 20, 33, 63] Secondary cases regularly occur in contacts (most often family members) of swimming-acquired cases. In these instances, the incubation period frequently is slightly longer (9 days).[3, 20] However, this may be due to a delay in the time of spread of the virus to the contact rather than an actual prolongation of incubation. Secondary cases probably result from large-droplet respiratory spread to the conjunctiva or the upper respiratory tract, or both. An alternative method would be the contamination of the recipient's hands with eye discharge and then autoinoculation of the conjunctiva.

In nonswimming-associated outbreaks of adenoviral respiratory illness with appropriate serotypes, conjunctivitis only rarely occurs.[8, 19, 26, 31, 37, 59] This fact, in conjunction with the finding that in volunteers[6, 54, 66] pharyngoconjunctival fever occurred after conjunctival administration of virus but not after nasopharyngeal application, would suggest that for the syndrome to occur the conjunctiva must be inoculated directly. After conjunctival inoculation, pharyngeal spread and systemic illness occur. However, after direct respiratory inoculation, the conjunctiva does not become involved unless respiratory secretions containing virus are applied to the conjunctiva, presumably by autoinoculation. Hospital outbreaks of pharyngoconjunctival fever–like illnesses have been reported.[17, 39] Most instances have occurred in intensive care units. An outbreak of pharyngoconjunctival fever also has been noted in a day care center.[10]

Although some early epidemic investigations suggested that boys were more susceptible to disease than were girls,[18, 61] the incidence of pharyngoconjunctival fever in children in fact does not differ by sex.[5, 57] In some cultures, boys had more exposure to swimming and therefore had more illness. In an outbreak that occurred in children hospitalized in Japan for long-term treatment of bronchial asthma, the attack rate was 68.2 per cent in boys and only 6.3 per cent in girls. This sex difference was attributed to the fact that the boys and girls took separate daily communal baths. Secondary cases in adult family members are more common in mothers than in fathers, presumably because of greater contact with the children.[5, 20]

PATHOPHYSIOLOGY

The route of infection with adenoviruses that are capable of causing pharyngoconjunctival fever determines the pathologic manifestations.

Conjunctival biopsy specimens in volunteer studies revealed an inflammatory response with lymphocytic infiltration of the submucosal layer.[6, 7] Biopsy material from palatine tonsils of infected volunteers revealed both hypertrophy and hyperplasia of the lymphoid tissue with congestion and edema of the surrounding connective tissue.

CLINICAL PRESENTATION

By definition, pharyngoconjunctival fever is a syndrome characterized by fever, pharyngitis, and conjunctivitis. During epidemics, all children and adults who have the same infection do not have the complete syndrome triad. Some patients have only pharyngitis, and some have only conjunctivitis. For purposes of this discussion, all descriptions of frequency of signs and symptoms are calculated from the starting point of 100 per cent fever, pharyngitis, and conjunctivitis.

The frequencies of specific signs and symptoms are presented in Tables 12–1 and 12–2.[7, 9, 18, 24, 33, 35, 36, 41, 48, 53, 54, 61] Although some patients have noted mild prodromal symptoms of headache and malaise, the usual onset of illness is abrupt, with sore throat, generalized aches and pains, eye irritation, or pain and fever. Throat complaints vary from mild to severe sore throat. In some patients, only a dry, scratchy feeling is reported; others have noted the feeling of a foreign body. On examination, the tonsils and pharyngeal lymphoid tissue are hypertrophied. The degree of pharyngeal redness and infection varies considerably from patient to

TABLE 12–1. Relative Frequency of Symptoms in Epidemic Pharyngoconjunctival Fever

Symptoms	Frequency*
Throat complaints	+ + + +
Soreness	+ + + +
Cough	+ +
Foreign body sensation	+ +
Dry feeling	+
Eye complaints	+ + +
Aching or soreness	+ + +
Burning sensation	+ +
Lacrimation	+
Photophobia	+
Nasal complaints	+ + +
Coryza	+ +
Stuffiness and/or blockage	+ +
Sneezing	+
Epistaxis	+
Other complaints	+ + + +
Headache	+ + + +
Anorexia	+ + +
Malaise	+ +
Generalized aches and pains	+ +
Nausea	+ +
Vomiting	+
Diarrhea	+
Abdominal pain	+

Data from references 7, 9, 18, 24, 33, 35, 36, 41, 48, 53, 54, 61.
*+ + + +, 76 to 100 per cent; + + +, 51 to 75 per cent; + +, 26 to 50 per cent; +, 1 to 25 per cent.

TABLE 12–2. Relative Frequency of Signs in Epidemic Pharyngoconjunctival Fever

Signs	Frequency*
Throat findings	+ + + +
Erythema and injection	+ + + +
Hypertrophied lymphatic tissue	+ + + +
Follicular exudate	+ +
Eye findings	+ + + +
Erythema and injection of palpebral and bulbar conjunctiva	+ + + +
Edema	+ + +
Granular and follicular involvement	+ +
Eyes unequally affected	+ +
Superficial punctate keratitis	+
Lymph node enlargement	+ + + +
Cervical	+ + + +
Preauricular	+
Generalized	+
Fever	+ + + +
≥39° C (≥102.2° F)	+ + +
Other	
Flushed face	+ + +
Enlarged liver and/or spleen	+

Data from references 7, 9, 18, 24, 33, 35, 36, 48, 53, 54, 61.
*+ + + +, 76 to 100 per cent; + + +, 51 to 75 per cent; + +, 26 to 50 per cent; +, 1 to 25 per cent.

patient. About one-third of those affected will have follicular exudative lesions that cannot be differentiated from streptococcal disease on clinical grounds. Follicular lesions also have been noted on the soft palate, and the papillae of the tongue may be hypertrophied.

Hypertrophy of the adenoids occurs, which results in nasal blockage. Coryza is common. Posterior nasal discharge is common and leads to cough in many instances. In some investigations, epistaxis has occurred in as many as 20 per cent of the cases.[53, 61]

In general, complaints related to the conjunctivitis are fewer than might be suggested by the usual physical appearance. Most patients note some aching or soreness; photophobia and lacrimation are unusual. The appearance of the palpebral conjunctiva usually is granular. The lesions may be almost microscopic or as large as 2 to 3 mm in diameter. Hemorrhages occasionally are noted on the bulbar surface. Frequently, involvement starts in one eye and does not involve the other eye until 2 or 3 days later. Occasionally, the involvement is restricted to one eye.

Some degree of anterior and posterior cervical lymphadenopathy occurs in most patients. Preauricular involvement is surprisingly infrequent when the degree of eye involvement is taken into consideration. Generalized lymphadenopathy is observed in 10 to 20 per cent of affected patients, and liver and spleen enlargement is frequent.

The majority of patients complain of generalized symptoms, but the degree varies considerably among those affected. Temperature higher than 39° C (102.2° F) occurs in more than 50 per cent of the patients, and headache is the rule. General malaise and anorexia are common; gastrointestinal symptoms occur in about 25 per cent of cases. Vomiting and diarrhea are most common in the younger age groups.

Compared with other respiratory viral infections, the duration of illness with pharyngoconjunctival fever is relatively long. In the majority of patients, the fever is sustained or remittent for 3 to 4 days and then gradually returns to normal over 24 to 48 hours. About 10 per cent of patients will have fever that lasts longer than 7 days. Throat and eye findings usually are improved considerably by the seventh day of illness, but these findings, as well as nasal complaints, fatigue, and headache, may persist for 14 days.

Early in the illness, the total white blood count is within normal limits or slightly elevated, with a normal differential count or one with a slight increase in polymorphonuclear leukocytes. During convalescence, many patients have a moderate leukopenia with an equal number of lymphocytes and polymorphonuclear cells. Smears from affected conjunctivae usually do not reveal abnormal cytology.

DIFFERENTIAL DIAGNOSIS

Because the symptom triad of fever, pharyngitis, and conjunctivitis virtually is unique to pharyngoconjunctival fever, the differential diagnosis should be easy. The only difficulty on clinical grounds is in trying to assign a specific type of adenovirus. In general, major epidemic disease is most likely to be due to type 3 or 7; sporadic cases can occur with types 1 to 8, 14, 19, and 13/30. There are no known differences in manifestations by different adenoviral types.

Of some concern in the differential diagnosis is picornavirus epidemic conjunctivitis (acute hemorrhagic conjunctivitis).[40, 68, 69] Two enteroviruses (coxsackievirus A24 and enterovirus 70) have been implicated etiologically in several extensive disease outbreaks. Affected patients have had severe conjunctivitis with preauricular lymphadenitis, but fever and pharyngitis have not been prominent, associated signs. However, in one outbreak, 23 per cent of those studied had upper respiratory tract symptoms.[40]

Generalized diseases that on occasion might be confused with pharyngoconjunctival fever include leptospirosis, psittacosis, *Mycoplasma pneumoniae* infection, Q fever, Newcastle disease virus infection, and prodromal measles. Of these illnesses, all but Newcastle disease virus infection have generalized symptomatology that is disproportionately more important than either conjunctivitis or pharyngitis. Human infection with Newcastle disease virus easily could be confused on clinical grounds with pharyngoconjunctival fever. However, a history of exposure to chickens or other fowl should aid in diagnosis.

Of more difficulty in differential diagnosis are illnesses usually characterized by either pharyngitis or conjunctivitis. On occasion, infections with influenza viruses, parainfluenza viruses, enteroviruses (other than coxsackievirus A24 and enterovirus 70), and Epstein-Barr virus are confusing. Although eye complaints do occur in these illnesses, severe conjunctivitis usually does not occur.

The differential diagnosis of conjunctivitis includes bacterial infections caused by *Haemophilus influenzae, Streptococcus pneumoniae, Streptococcus pyogenes,* and *Neisseria gonorrhoeae.* In all of these infections, purulent discharge is greater than that usually observed in pharyngoconjunctival fever. *Chlamydia trachomatis* infections perhaps are the most troublesome in the differential diagnosis. In the past, many cases of swimming pool conjunctivitis were attributed to chlamydial infections. It is probable that many of such reported cases in reality were adenoviral infections. *C. trachomatis* infections can be diagnosed by the demonstration of characteristic inclusions in Giemsa-stained scrapings from the palpebral conjunctivae, by direct immunofluorescence, by enzyme immunoassay, or by culture. Epidemic adenoviral keratoconjunctivitis is another differential diagnostic consideration. Other differential diagnostic possibilities that should cause no difficulty include cat-scratch fever, tularemia, and allergic conjunctivitis.

SPECIFIC DIAGNOSIS

In most instances, a clinical diagnosis is all that is necessary. Specific viral diagnosis can be accomplished with ease in any routinely equipped diagnostic virology laboratory. Diagnosis can be made by virus isolation in tissue culture or by direct antigen detection by indirect immunofluorescence or enzyme-linked immunosorbent assay.[10, 47] Cultures from the conjunctivae generally are more diagnostically specific than are those from the throat. The recovery of an adenovirus (particularly type 2) from the throat in an isolated case does not indicate necessarily an etiologic role for the recovered virus. An adenoviral etiology also can be verified by studying paired serum samples for a titer rise to the adenoviral group antigen.

TREATMENT

Generally, no treatment is necessary or effective in pharyngoconjunctival fever. If conjunctivitis persists and becomes purulent, an investigation for bacterial pathogens and appropriate topical antimicrobial therapy are indicated. Steroid-containing ophthalmic ointments should be avoided.

PROGNOSIS

The prognosis generally is excellent. Although superficial keratitis occasionally occurs, permanent scarring is not a problem. Sinusitis, otitis media, and bacterial conjunctivitis are rare secondary complications that, if untreated, can result in long-term difficulties.

PREVENTION

Volunteer studies clearly have indicated that infection and presumable resultant antibody are protective against future disease. Therefore, protection theoretically could be achieved through immunization, but priority to study and implement an immunization program is low. Because the major cause of pharyngoconjunctival fever due to adenoviruses is swimming in contaminated water, discretion in bathing locations is advised. Swimming pool water should be chlorinated adequately, and pool filtration systems should be inspected daily. Ill persons should be excluded from swimming pools during their illness and for a period of up to at least 2 weeks after recovery.

References

1. Albano, A., Salvaggio, L., and Morrone, G.: Episodio epidemico de febbre faringocongiuntivale da adenovirus di tipo 2. Boll. Ist Sieroterap. Milan. *40*:580–584, 1961.
2. Bahn, C. A.: Swimming bath conjunctivitis. New Orleans Med. Surg. J. *79*:586–590, 1927.
3. Barr, J., Kjellén L., and Svedmyr, A.: Hospital outbreak of adenovirus type 3 infections: A clinical and virologic study on 38 patients partly involved in a nosocomial outbreak. Acta Pediatr. *47*:365–382, 1958.
4. Béal, R.: Sur une forme particul ière de conjonctivité aigue avec follicules. Annales D'oculistique January, 1–33, 1907.
5. Bell, J. A., Rowe, W. P., Engler, J. I., et al.: Pharyngoconjunctival fever: Epidemiological studies of a recently recognized disease entity. J. A. M. A. *157*:1083–1092, 1955.
6. Bell, J. A., Ward, T. G., Huebner, R. J., et al.: Studies of adenoviruses (APC) in volunteers. Am. J. Public Health *46*:1130–1146, 1956.
7. Bell, J. A.: Clinical manifestations of pharyngoconjunctival fever. Am. J. Ophthalmol. *43*:11–14, 1957.
8. Bell, T. M., Turner, G., MacDonald, A., et al.: Type-3 adenovirus infection. Lancet *2*:1327–1329, 1960.
9. Caldwell, G. G., Lindsey, N. J., Wulff, H., et al.: Epidemic of adenovirus type 7 acute conjunctivitis in swimmers. Am. J. Epidemiol. *99*:230–234, 1974.
10. Chomel, J. J., Szymczyszyn, P., Honneger, D., et al.: An epidemic of adenovirus type 1 conjunctivitis. Pediatr. Infect. Dis. J. *8*:885–886, 1989.
11. Cockburn, T. A., Rowe, W. P., and Huebner, R. J.: Relationship of the 1951 Greeley, Colorado, outbreak of conjunctivitis and pharyngitis to type 3 APC virus infection. Am. J. Hyg. *63*:250–253, 1956.
12. D'Angelo, L. J., Hierholzer, J. C., Keenlyside, R. A., et al.: Pharyngoconjunctival fever caused by adenovirus type 4: Report of a swimming pool–related outbreak with recovery of virus from pool water. J. Infect. Dis. *140*:42–47, 1979.
13. Derrick, E. H.: Swimming-bath conjunctivitis, with a report of 3 probable cases and a note on its epidemiology. Med. J. Aust. *2*:334–336, 1943.
14. Duxbury, A. E., McCutchan, R., White, J., et al.: Epidemic adenovirus infection in a Victorian migrant centre presenting as pharyngoconjunctival fever. Med. J. Aust. *2*:413–417, 1960.
15. Ellis, A. W., McKinnon, G. T., Lewis, F. A., et al.: Adenovirus type 4 in Melbourne, 1969–1971. Med. J. Aust. *1*:209–211, 1974.
16. Epshtein, F. G., Agarkova, L. G., Dreizin, E. Y., et al.: Acute respiratory diseases in children caused by adenovirus of 7a type. Sov. Med. *2*:81–85, 1962.
17. Faden, H., Gallagher, M., Ogra, P., et al.: Nosocomial outbreak of pharyngoconjunctival fever due to adenovirus type 4: New York. M. M. W. R. *27*:49, 1978.
18. Forssell, P., Lapinleimu, K., Strandstrom, H., et al.: Febrile pharyngitis and conjunctivitis: An epidemic associated with APC virus infection. Ann. Med. Exp. Biol. Fenn. *34*:287–292, 1956.
19. Forssell, P., Halonen, H., Stenstrom, R., et al.: An adenovirus epidemic due to types 1 and 2. Ann. Pediatr. Fenn. *8*:35–44, 1962.
20. Foy, H. M., Cooney, M. K., and Hatlen, J. B.: Adenovirus type 3 epidemic associated with intermittent chlorination of a swimming pool. Arch. Environ. Health *17*:795–802, 1968.
21. Foy, H. M., and Grayston, J. T.: Adenoviruses. *In* Evans, A. S. (ed.): Viral Infections of Humans: Epidemiology and Control. New York, Plenum Medical Book Company, 1976.
22. Fukumi, H., Nishikawa, F., Nakamura, K., et al.: Studies on the adenovirus as an etiological agent of pharyngoconjunctival fever. Jpn. J. Med. Sci. Biol. *10*:79–85, 1957.
23. Fukumi, H., Nishikawa, F., Nakamura, K., et al.: Further studies of the cases associated with adenoviruses. Jpn. J. Med. Sci. Biol. *10*:407–418, 1957.
24. Fukumi, H., Nishikawa, F., Mizutani, H., et al.: An epidemic of adenovirus type 3 infections among school children in an elementary school in Tokyo. Jpn. J. Med. Sci. Biol. *11*:129–140, 1958.
25. Fukumi, H., Nishikawa, F., Takemura, M., et al.: Isolation of adenovirus possessing both the antigens of types 3 and 7. Jpn. J. Med. Sci. Biol. *14*:173–181, 1961.
26. Harris, D. J., Wulff, H., Ray, C. G., et al.: Viruses and disease. III. An outbreak of adenovirus type 7a in a children's home. Am. J. Epidemiol. *93*:399–402, 1971.
27. Herrmann, E. C., Jr.: Experiences in laboratory diagnosis of adenovirus infections in routine medical practice. Mayo Clin. Proc. *43*:635–644, 1968.
28. Huebner, R. J., Rowe, W. P., and Chanock, R. M.: Newly recognized respiratory tract viruses. Ann. Rev. Microbiol. *12*:49–76, 1958.
29. Jansson, E., Wager, O., Forssel, P., et al.: Epidemic occurrence of adenovirus type 7 infection in Helsinki. Ann. Paediatr. Fenn. *8*:24–34, 1962.
30. Jones, B. R.: Sporadic ocular disease associated with adenovirus infection in London. Proc. R. Soc. Med. *50*:758–760, 1957.
31. Jordan, W. S., Jr., Badger, G. F., Curtiss, C., et al.: A study of illness in a group of Cleveland families. X. The occurrence of adenovirus infections. Am. J. Hyg. *64*:336–348, 1956.
32. Kaji, M., Kimura, M., Kamiya, S., et al.: An epidemic of pharyngoconjunctival fever among school children in an elementary school in Fukuoka prefecture. Kyushu J. Med. Sci. *12*:1–8, 1960.
33. Kaji, M., Kamiya, S., Tatewaki, E., et al.: An epidemic of pharyngoconjunctival fever in Moji, Kyushu. Kyushu J. Med. Sci. *12*:241–249, 1961.
34. Kawana, R., Kaneko, M., Matsumoto, I., et al.: An outbreak of pharyngoconjunctival fever due to adenovirus type 3. Jpn. J. Microbiol. *10*:149–157, 1966.
35. Kendall, E. J. C., Riddle, R. W., Tuck, H. A., et al.: Pharyngoconjunctival fever: School outbreaks in England during the summer of 1955 associated with adenovirus types 3, 7, and 14. Br. Med. J. *2*:131–136, 1957.
36. Kimura, S. J., Hanna, L., Nicholas, A., et al.: Sporadic cases of pharyngoconjunctival fever in Northern California, 1955–1956. Am. J. Ophthalmol. *43*:14–16, 1957.
37. Kjellén, L., Sterner, G., and Svedmyr, A.: On the occurrence of adenoviruses in Sweden. Acta Paediatr. *46*:164–176, 1957.
38. Kjellén, L., Zetterberg, B., and Svedmyr, A.: An epidemic among Swedish children caused by adenovirus type 3. Acta Paediatr. *46*:561–568, 1957.
39. Larsen, R. A., Jacobson, J. T., Jacobson, J. A., et al.: Hospital-associated epidemic of pharyngitis and conjunctivitis caused by adenovirus (21/H21 + 35). J. Infect. Dis. *154*:706–709, 1986.
40. Lim, K. H., and Yin-Murphy, M.: An epidemic of conjunctivitis in Singapore in 1970. Singapore Med. J. *12*:247–249, 1971.
41. Martone, W. J., Hierholzer, J. C., Keenlyside, R. A., et al.: An outbreak of

adenovirus type 3 disease at a private recreation center swimming pool. Am. J. Epidemiol. *111*:229–237, 1980.
42. McMillan, N. S., Martin, S. A., Sobsey, M. D., et al.: Outbreak of pharyngoconjunctival fever at a summer camp: North Carolina, 1991. M. M. W. R. *41*:342–343, 1992.
43. Merchant, R. K., Rowe, W. P., Kasel, J. A., et al.: Pharyngoconjunctival fever due to type 1 adenovirus: Report of three cases. N. Engl. J. Med. *258*:131–133, 1958.
44. Nakayama, M., Miyazaki, C., Ueda, K., et al.: Pharyngoconjunctival fever caused by adenovirus type 11. Pediatr. Infect. Dis. J. *11*:6–9, 1992.
45. Oker-Blom, N., Wager, W., Strandström, H., et al.: Adenoviruses associated with pharyngoconjunctival fever: Isolation of adenovirus type 7 and serological studies suggesting its etiological role in an epidemic in Helsinki. Ann. Med. Exp. Biol. Fenn. *35*:342–351, 1957.
46. Ormsby, H. L., and Aitchison, W. S.: The role of the swimming pool in the transmission of pharyngeal-conjunctival fever. Can. Med. Assoc. J. *73*:864–866, 1975.
47. Paderstein, R.: Was ist schwimmbad-konjunktivitis? Klin. Monat. Augenh. *74*:634–642, 1925.
48. Parrott, T. H., Rowe, W. P., Huebner, R. J., et al.: Outbreak of febrile pharyngitis and conjunctivitis associated with type 3 adenoidal-pharyngeal-conjunctival virus infections. N. Engl. J. Med. *251*:1087–1090, 1954.
49. Player, V., and Westmoreland, D.: Rapid diagnosis of adenovirus pharyngoconjunctival fever: Use of a monoclonal antibody-based ELISA test during an outbreak. J. Virol. Methods *24*:307–312, 1989.
50. Rowe, W. P., Huebner, R. J., Gilmore, L. K., et al.: Isolation of a cytopathogenic agent from human adenoids undergoing spontaneous degeneration in tissue culture. Proc. Soc. Exp. Biol. Med. *84*:570–573, 1953.
51. Schaap, G. J. P., DeJong, J. C., Van Bijsterveld, O. P., et al.: A new intermediate adenovirus type causing conjunctivitis. Arch. Ophthalmol. *97*:2336–2338, 1979.
52. Schwartz, H. S., Vastine, D. W., Yamashiroya, H., et al.: Immunofluorescent detection of adenovirus antigen in epidemic keratoconjunctivitis. Invest. Ophthalmol. *15*:199–207, 1976.
53. Sobel, G., Aronson, B., Aronson, S., et al.: Pharyngoconjunctival fever. Am. J. Dis. Child. *92*:596–612, 1956.
54. Sohier, R., Chardonnet, Y., and Prunieras, M.: Adenoviruses: Status of current knowledge. Progr. Med. Virol. *7*:253–325, 1965.
55. Sterner, G.: Infections with adenovirus type 7 in children and their relationship to acute respiratory disease. Acta Paediatr. *48*:287–298, 1959.
56. Sterner, G., Gerzen, P., Ohlson, M., et al.: Acute respiratory illness and gastroenteritis in association with adenovirus type 7 infections. Acta Paediatr. *50*:457–468, 1961.
57. Sterner, G.: Adenovirus infection in childhood: An epidemiological and clinical survey among Swedish children. Acta Paediatr. *51*:1–30, 1962.
58. Sutton, R. N. P., Pullen, H. J. M., Blackledge, P., et al.: Adenovirus type 7; 1971–74. Lancet *2*:987–991, 1976.
59. Tyrrell, D. A. J., Balducci, D., and Zaiman, T. E.: Acute infections of the respiratory tract and the adenoviruses. Lancet *2*:1326–1330, 1956.
60. Van Bijsterveld, O. P., DeJong, J. C., Muzerie, C. J., et al.: Pharyngoconjunctival fever caused by adenovirus type 19. Ophthalmologica *177*:134–139, 1978.
61. Van Der Veen, J., and Van Der Ploeg, G.: An outbreak of pharyngoconjunctival fever caused by types 3 and 4 adenovirus at Waalwijk, the Netherlands. Am. J. Hyg. *68*:95–105, 1958.
62. Van Der Veen, J.: The role of adenoviruses in respiratory disease. Am. Rev. Resp. Dis. *88*:167–180, 1963.
63. Van Horne, R. G., Saslaw, S., Anderson, G. R., et al.: An intrafamilial epidemic of pharyngoconjunctival fever. Arch. Intern. Med. *99*:70–73, 1957.
64. Vastine, D. W., Schwartz, H. S., Yamashiroya, H. M., et al.: Cytologic diagnosis of adenoviral epidemic keratoconjunctivitis by direct immunofluorescence. Invest. Ophthalmol. *16*:195–200, 1977.
65. Wallis, A. L.: An unusual epidemic. Lancet *2*:290–291, 1955.
66. Ward, T. G., Huebner, R. J., Rowe, W. P., et al.: Production of pharyngoconjunctival fever in human volunteers inoculated with APC viruses. Science *122*:1086–1087, 1955.
67. Ward, T. G.: Viruses of the respiratory tract. Progr. Med. Virol. *15*:126–158, 1973.
68. Yin-Murphy, M., and Lim, K. H.: Picornavirus epidemic conjunctivitis in Singapore. Lancet *1*:857–858, 1972.
69. Yin-Murphy, M.: Simple tests for the diagnosis of picornavirus epidemic conjunctivitis (acute haemorrhagic conjunctivitis). Bull. W. H. O. *54*:675–679, 1976.
70. Yodfat, Y., and Nishmi, M.: Successive overlapping outbreaks of febrile pharyngitis and pharyngoconjunctival fever associated with adenovirus types 2 and 7, in a kibbutz. Israel J. Med. Sci. *10*:1505–1509, 1974.

13

UVULITIS

Ellen R. Wald

Infections of the uvula have been reported infrequently in the medical literature. When the uvula is the most inflamed structure in the posterior pharynx of a febrile child, acute infection should be suspected. Other causes of uvulitis include trauma (from instrumentation), inhalant irritation (from cannabis use), vasculitis, and allergy.[1, 4, 5]

ETIOLOGY

The bacterial agents that cause uvulitis in children include *Haemophilus influenzae* type b and *Streptococcus pyogenes*.[6] Uvulitis caused by *H. influenzae* may occur concurrently with epiglottitis or as an isolated infection.[8, 11] Uvulitis caused by *S. pyogenes* appears always to occur in concert with pharyngitis. Other bacterial causes have not been reported; no search for viral agents has been conducted. Several cases of uvulitis caused by *Candida albicans* have been described in immunocompetent toddlers.[7]

In adults, two cases of uvulitis caused by *Streptococcus pneumoniae* have been reported. In each patient, there was an associated epiglottitis.[3, 10]

EPIDEMIOLOGY

The epidemiology of uvulitis is the epidemiology of its two etiologic agents: *S. pyogenes* and *H. influenzae* type b. As such, it occurs in the school age child between 5 and 15 years of age (the so-called streptococcal age group) in association with pharyngitis. Similarly, it can be seen in the *H. influenzae* age group (3 months to 5 years) if a child has not received the now routine and universally recommended conjugate vaccine to prevent infections caused by *H. influenzae* type b. Cases of uvulitis in association with epiglottitis have been reported from the United States (New Jersey, Pennsylvania, Illinois),[3, 6, 9] as well as from England.[2] Infections caused by *S. pyogenes* and *H. influenzae* primarily occur in the winter and spring, but both types can occur throughout the year.

PATHOGENESIS

Uvulitis is an acute cellulitis characterized by dramatic swelling and erythema. Infection of the uvula probably arises from direct invasion by *S. pyogenes* or *H. influenzae* type b, both being recognized as normal nasopharyngeal flora. In the latter case, epiglottitis also may arise by direct extension,

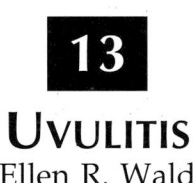

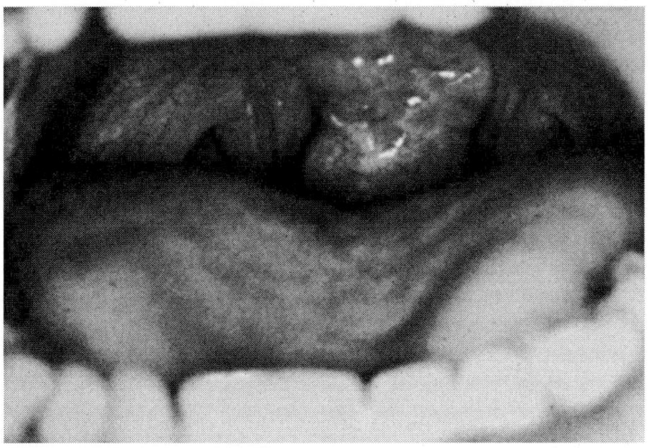

FIGURE 13–1. *Swollen (two to three times normal size) and erythematous uvula in patient without epiglottitis or pharyngitis.*

and the bacteremia may result secondarily from either the uvula or the epiglottis as a primary site of infection.

Uvulitis that is noninfectious may result from injury, chemical irritation, or allergic inflammation. A child ultimately diagnosed to have Kawasaki disease presented with uvulitis.[5]

CLINICAL MANIFESTATIONS

In a review of five patients with streptococcal uvulitis, there was an associated pharyngitis in all.[6] The patients presented with low-grade fever and sore throat. Three of the five patients experienced a choking or gagging sensation in the pharynx that induced coughing and spitting; one of these patients also presented with drooling. Although pharyngitis was noted on physical examination, the swelling and erythema of the uvula were most dramatic (Fig. 13–1). None of the patients had evidence of respiratory distress.

In patients with uvulitis and epiglottitis,[3, 6] the presentation usually is typical for epiglottitis, with sudden onset of high fever, dysphagia, and increasing respiratory distress. However, Rapkin[9] reported a case of uvulitis/epiglottitis in which the epiglottitis initially was unsuspected. Lateral neck radiography (performed to evaluate the possibility of a retropharyngeal abscess) belatedly alerted the clinicians to the correct diagnosis.

In patients with uvulitis and no epiglottitis, the presentation may be similar to that of epiglottitis (acute onset of fever, odynophagia, and drooling) or less specific, with fever and irritability or decreased appetite.[8, 11] The diagnosis in the latter cases is provided by physical examination of the oropharynx, which shows a swollen and erythematous uvula (see Fig. 13–1).

DIAGNOSIS

The diagnosis of streptococcal uvulitis is suspected when a school age child presents with low-grade fever, pharyngitis, and uvulitis. The diagnosis is confirmed by the recovery of *S. pyogenes* from a surface culture of the throat or uvula or both.

The diagnosis of uvulitis caused by *H. influenzae* is suspected in a highly febrile infant or preschool age child who has uvular inflammation on physical examination. Lateral neck radiography must be performed to evaluate the possibility of epiglottitis, unless there are obvious signs of upper respiratory obstruction, in which case immediate endoscopy is warranted. If epiglottitis is discovered, the airway must be secured and appropriate parenteral antimicrobials initiated after blood and surface cultures are obtained. Any surface culture obtained to search for *H. influenzae* must be plated onto chocolate agar. After appropriate cultures are obtained, parenteral antimicrobials should be initiated, as in other bacteremic *H. influenzae* infections.

DIFFERENTIAL DIAGNOSIS

The differential diagnosis of the patient with acute onset of fever, dysphagia, and drooling includes herpes simplex gingivostomatitis, uvulitis, epiglottitis, severe pharyngitis, and peritonsillar or retropharyngeal abscess. Although it is appropriate to be extremely cautious in examining the pharynx of any patient with suspected epiglottitis, some children will tolerate attempted visualization of the oral cavity without undue upset. Instrumentation with a tongue blade should be avoided. If the examination does not show gingivostomatitis or peritonsillar abscess, lateral neck radiography should be performed. If epiglottitis or retropharyngeal abscess is confirmed, airway management and antimicrobials are indicated for the former, incision and drainage and antimicrobials for the latter. If the lateral neck is normal and the uvula is inflamed, uvulitis with or without pharyngitis is confirmed.

TREATMENT

Management of uvulitis is guided primarily by the associated pharyngitis or epiglottitis, if either is present. In the case of streptococcal pharyngitis, penicillin therapy for 10 days is most appropriate. These patients usually can be treated orally with penicillin V, 25 to 50 mg/kg/day, administered three times daily.

In the case of uvulitis/epiglottitis, management of the airway is most important. This can be accomplished by nasotracheal intubation or tracheotomy. Appropriate parenteral antibiotic therapy usually is initiated.

In the case of uvulitis without epiglottitis, antimicrobial therapy appropriate for bacteremic *H. influenzae* type b is necessary. In geographic areas where β-lactamase–producing *H. influenzae* is rare, ampicillin at 200 mg/kg/day in four divided doses is satisfactory. In geographic areas where β-lactamase–producing *H. influenzae* organisms are prevalent, an advanced-generation cephalosporin, such as cefotaxime at 200 mg/kg/day in four divided doses or ceftriaxone at 100 mg/kg/day in one dose or two divided doses, is appropriate. In a patient with serious penicillin hypersensitivity, chloramphenicol at 75 mg/kg/day in four divided doses also is a satisfactory regimen. After the patient has defervesced and has improved clinically, an oral antimicrobial agent can be substituted. The results of blood and surface cultures now can guide therapy. For an ampicillin-sensitive *H. influenzae* infection, amoxicillin at 40 mg/kg/day in three divided doses should be prescribed to complete a 7- to 10-day course of treatment. For β-lactamase–producing *H. influenzae,* a variety of oral agents can be prescribed, including cefixime at 10 mg/kg in a single daily dose, cefuroxime at 30 mg/kg/day in two divided doses, sulfamethoxazole-trimethoprim at 40/8 mg/kg/day in two divided doses, erythromycin-sulfisoxazole at 50/150 mg/kg/day in four divided doses, or amoxicillin–potassium clavulanate at 40 mg/kg/day of amoxicillin in three divided doses.

Resolution was prompt in the two cases of uvulitis allegedly due to *C. albicans;* one child was treated with topical nystatin, and the other improved spontaneously.[7]

References

1. Butterton, J. R., and Clawson-Simons, J.: Hymenoptera uvulitis. N. Engl. J. Med. *317*:1291, 1987.
2. DeNavasquez, S.: Acute laryngitis and septicemia due to *H. influenzae* type b. Br. Med. J. 2:187–188, 1942.
3. Gorfinkel, H. J., Brown, R., and Kabins, S. A.: Acute infectious epiglottitis in adults. Ann. Intern. Med. *70*:289–294, 1969.
4. Guarisco, J. L., Cheney, M. L., LeJeune, F. E., Jr., et al.: Isolated uvulitis secondary to marijuana use. Laryngoscope *98*:1309–1312, 1988.
5. Kazi, A., Gauthier, M., Lebel, M. H., et al.: Uvulitis and supraglottitis: Early manifestations of Kawasaki disease. J. Pediatr. *120*:564–567, 1992.
6. Kotloff, K. L., and Wald, E. R.: Uvulitis in children. Pediatr. Infect. Dis. 2:392–393, 1983.
7. Krober, M. S., and Weir, M. R.: Acute uvulitis apparently caused by *Candida albicans*. Pediatr. Infect. Dis. J. *10*:73, 1991.
8. Li, K. I., Kiernan, S., and Wald, E. R.: Isolated uvulitis due to *Hemophilus influenzae* type b. Pediatrics *74*:1054–1057, 1984.
9. Rapkin, R. H.: Simultaneous uvulitis and epiglottitis. J. A. M. A. *43*:1843, 1980.
10. Westerman, E. L., and Hutton, J. P.: Acute uvulitis associated with epiglottitis. Arch. Otolaryngol. Head Neck Surg. *112*:448–449, 1986.
11. Wynder, S. G., Lampe, R. M., and Shoemaker, M. E.: Uvulitis and *Hemophilus influenzae* bacteremia. Pediatr. Emerg. Care 2:23–25, 1986.

14

PERITONSILLAR, RETROPHARYNGEAL, AND PARAPHARYNGEAL ABSCESSES

Paul E. Hammerschlag and Margaret R. Hammerschlag

A deep neck abscess is a collection of pus in a potential space bounded by fascia.[6] These potential spaces are areas of least resistance to the spread of infection. An infection may begin with a minimal area of cellulitis and progress to a deep neck abscess, which then may extend to invade adjacent potential spaces; these frequently encompass vital structures in the neck. Destruction or dysfunction of these structures represents the major complications of deep neck infections.[28]

EPIDEMIOLOGY OF HEAD AND NECK SPACE INFECTIONS IN CHILDREN

Data concerning the frequency of head and neck space infections in children are limited. A survey conducted by the American Academy of Otolaryngology found the incidence of peritonsillar abscesses to be approximately 30 per 100,000 person years, or about 45,000 cases annually in the United States and Puerto Rico.[13] A retrospective study from the Children's Hospital of Pittsburgh identified 117 children with head and neck space infections seen between 1986 and 1992.[45] Peritonsillar space infections (cellulitis and abscesses) were the most frequent, accounting for 61 (49 per cent) of the cases, followed by retropharyngeal space infections with 27 (22 per cent) of the cases. There were only three (2 per cent) parapharyngeal space infections seen during the period of the study. Broughton[13] reported seeing 14 pediatric patients, 15 months to 17 years of age, with retropharyngeal and parapharyngeal space infections over a 9-year period at the University of Kentucky Medical Center. The patients seen at Pittsburgh ranged from 1 month to 18 years of age, with a mean age of 7.8 years.[5]

Peritonsillar abscesses are rare in young children. They are most common in late adolescence and the early part of the second decade. The mean age of the children with peritonsillar infection in Pittsburgh was 11 years, whereas the mean age of the patients with retropharyngeal space infections was 4 years. This is similar to a mean age of 4.5 years reported by Thompson and associates[44] in 1988. Retropharyngeal abscesses have been reported to occur more frequently in young children.

All of the peritonsilllar infections were associated with tonsillitis, and 15 per cent had antecedent infectious mononucleosis shown by positive monospot tests. Results of a meta-analysis of 15 previously reported series of patients with peritonsillar abscess reported by Herzon[22] found prior tonsillar infection rates ranging from 11 to 56 per cent, with an overall rate of 36 per cent. The relatively high incidence of peritonsillar abscess reported in the Academy of Otolaryngology study raised the possiblity that the decreasing rate of tonsillectomy might increase the risk of developing peritonsillar abscess.[22]

PERITONSILLAR ABSCESS (QUINSY)

A peritonsillar abscess (quinsy) is circumscribed medially by the fibrous wall of the tonsil capsule and laterally by the superior constrictor muscle. Pus may be localized in the superior pole, midpoint, or inferior pole or, rarely, dispersed, with multiple loculations in the peritonsillar space. The superior pole is the most common location; the frequency ranges from 41.2 to 70 per cent, with the remaining inferior locations accounting for the balance.[7, 9]

The etiology of peritonsillar abscesses is not constant; they may follow any "virulent" tonsillitis, with extension through the fibrous tonsil capsule.

Clinical Manifestations

The recent history may include a sore throat with occasional unilateral pain, malaise, low-grade pyrexia, chills, diaphoresis, dysphagia, reduced oral intake, trismus, and a muffled "hot potato voice." Trismus results from irritation and reflex spasm of the internal pterygoid muscle. Sixty-three per cent of the children with peritonsillar infection from the Pittsburgh series had trismus.[45] Impaired palatal motion from edema contributes to the muffled voice.

On physical examination, there is minimal to moderate toxicity, dehydration, and drooling. Inspection of the oropharynx may be compromised by trismus. The soft palate is displaced toward the unaffected side, is swollen and red, and frequently contains a palpable fluctuance. The edematous uvula is pushed across the midline. The displaced tonsil and its crypts rarely are coated with exudate. The breath is fetid, and there is ipsilateral, tender, cervical adenopathy. Indirect laryngoscopy reveals supraglottic and lateral pharyngeal edema.

The white blood cell count is elevated, with a predominance of polymorphonuclear leukocytes.

Studies have suggested that intraoral sonography can differentiate peritonsillar abscess fron peritonsillar cellulitis, eliminating the need for blind aspiration of the tonsillar fossa in cases that are clinically equivocal.[14]

Treatment

Aspiration of the fluctuant mass with an 18-gauge needle commonly confirms the diagnosis of peritonsillar abscess, especially if the pus is located in the superior pole. Pus in locations other than the superior pole may be neither accessible to aspiration intraorally nor drained by this route. An "acute quinsy tonsillectomy" with the medial wall of the abscess removed is the ideal procedure to provide adequate drainage at that site.[15] Peritonsillar abscess is an accepted indication for a tonsillectomy to prevent its recurrence; acute tonsillectomy also saves the patient the burden of repeat hospitalization. Patients treated with immediate tonsillectomy were hospitalized approximately half as long as those treated with incision and drainage.[29, 33] The patients also reported more rapid relief of pain with the acute tonsillectomy. The risk of this procedure was not greater than that associated with delayed tonsillectomy. In addition, the patient morbidity caused by two hospitalizations involving two surgical procedures is reduced by a "quinsy tonsillectomy."[4, 8, 9]

Studies have suggested that many peritonsillar abscesses can be managed by simple needle aspiration combined with antibiotic therapy on an outpatient basis.[10, 22, 38, 40, 42, 45, 46] An extensive meta-analysis of 10 previous studies conducted from 1961 through 1994 involving 496 patients with peritonsillar abscess found an overall success rate of needle aspiration of 94 per cent (range, 85 to 100 per cent).[22] This compares favorably with the success rate reported for incision and drainage. Intraoral sonography also can be used to monitor patients' responses after treatment.[1, 13]

A high recurrence rate of peritonsillar abscesses has not been documented well, although it is a commonly accepted clinical observation. The meta-analysis reported by Herzon[22] of 19 studies from the United States, Europe, and Israel involving 1399 patients found recurrence rates of peritonsillar abscess of 10 to 15 per cent. The rates of recurrence appear to be lower in the United States (0 to 17 per cent) than in the series reported from Europe and Israel (3 to 22 per cent). A retrospective analysis of 290 patients treated for peritonsillar abscess found that patients who had a history of recurrent tonsillitis prior to developing the abscess had a fourfold greater rate of recurrences than those with no history (40 versus 9.6 per cent).[25] It was recommended that patients with a history of recurrent tonsillitis prior to admission be treated with tonsillectomy.[25]

The incidence of abscess within the contralateral peritonsillar capsule is variable, with a range of 2 to 24 per cent.[25] Thus, bilateral tonsillectomies often are advocated.

Pre- and postoperatively (tonsillectomy or incision and drainage), the patient should be treated with appropriate antibiotics until asymptomatic. Irrigation with warm saline every 2 hours aids in débriding the area, may reduce the peritonsillar edema, and provides some symptomatic relief.

Untreated peritonsillar abscess may point, with spontaneous rupture, or extend to the pterygomaxillary space with potentially fatal complications.

PTERYGOMAXILLARY ABSCESS (PHARYNGOMAXILLARY, LATERAL, AND PHARYNGEAL SPACE ABSCESSES)

The potential pterygomaxillary space is an inverted conical cavity (Fig. 14–1*B*) lying along an oblique axis roughly parallel to the ramus of the mandible (Fig. 14–1*C*). The base of the skull at the jugular foramen forms the base of the "cone," and its apex is at the bone (Fig. 14–1*B*). The buccopharyngeal fascia, lateral to the superior pharyngeal constrictor, delineates the medial boundary, and the parotid gland and its partially dehiscent deep layer of the superficial cervical fascia form the lateral wall of this cone. The internal pterygoid muscle and mandible demarcate the cone on its anterolateral aspect. The pterygomaxillary space is contiguous with the peritonsillar, submandibular, and retropharyngeal spaces—all potential avenues of egress for an extending pterygomaxillary space abscess (Fig. 14–1*A*).

The posterior portion of the cone contains the contents of the carotid sheath (carotid artery and internal jugular vein), the cranial nerves IX through XII, and the cervical sympathetic chain. Anterior are the internal pterygoid muscle and fatty connective tissue.

Involvement of these structures determines the clinical manifestations and complications of the pterygomaxillary space abscess. An abscess in the posterior compartment may show medial displacement of the lateral pharyngeal wall and parotid space induration and swelling, with variable overlying facial nerve weakness, carotid artery erosion and hemorrhage,[26] internal jugular vein thrombosis, decreased gag reflex and dysphagia, ipsilateral vocal cord paralysis, weakness of the ipsilateral trapezius muscle, ipsilateral lingual deviation, and Horner syndrome from cervical sympathetic chain involvement.[15]

Extension of the abscess into the anterior compartment causes trismus from irritation of the internal pterygoid muscle. Induration at the angle of the jaw and medial displacement of the tonsil and pharyngeal wall also occur with an anterior compartment abscess.

By the time a patient with an abscess seeks medical attention, the source of the pterygomaxillary space infection may be unclear. Reports indicate variable etiologies: incompletely or inadequately treated bacterial pharyngitis, tonsillitis,[3] peritonsillar abscess, dental infections, bacterial parotitis, mastoiditis (Bezold abscess from a mastoid tip infection traveling along the digastric muscles), petrositis, cervical adenitis with suppuration, cervical vertebral tubercular adenitis in the adult,[5, 35] and a foreign body.[15, 16] Local anesthetic infiltration for dental procedures and for management of posttonsillectomy bleeding has been implicated in case reports. There are a few reported cases of pterygomaxillary abscesses in children, and these tend to occur in later childhood and adolescence. Only three cases of parapharyngeal abscess and cellulitis were reported in the Pittsburgh series.[45]

Clinical Manifestations

In addition to the preceding description, there may be complaints of tender cervical swelling, induration and erythema of the side of the neck, sore throat, dysphagia, trismus, hoarseness, malaise, chills, and diaphoresis.

There is a variable low-grade pyrexia with occasional temperature spikes. Examination discloses variable toxicity, respiratory tract distress, laryngeal edema, medial displacement of the lateral pharyngeal wall and inferior tonsil pole, trismus, and, infrequently, drooling. Indirect laryngoscopy may

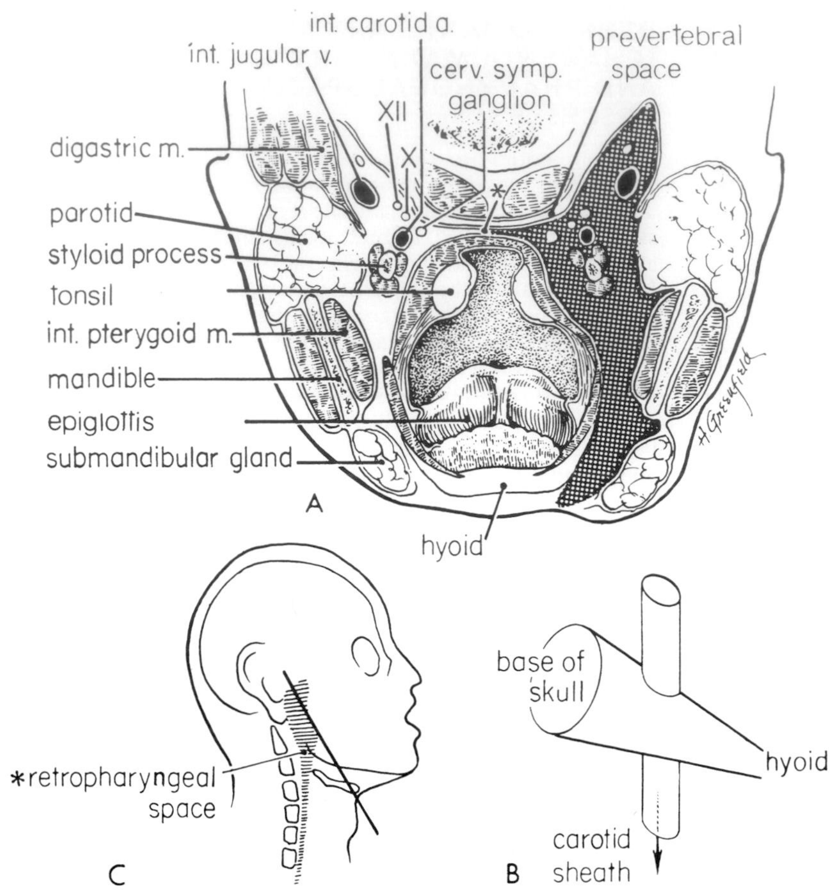

FIGURE 14–1. A, *Oblique transverse section of the oropharynx posterosuperiorly and the hypopharynx anteroinferiorly. Depicted are a peritonsillar abscess on the right and a pterygomaxillary space abscess on the left. The asterisk indicates the retropharyngeal space.* B, *The "cone" of the potential pterygomaxillary space with its carotid sheath.* C, *The vertical dimensions of the retropharyngeal space. The black oblique line represents the level of the drawing in* A.

document ipsilateral vocal cord paralysis and obliteration of the pyriform sinus. On palpation of the neck, there is a tender, high cervical mass, initially diffuse and later fluctuant. Pharyngeal blood clots may presage carotid artery erosion. Bleeding from or blood clots in the external auditory canal have been noted in patients with carotid artery erosion and dissection of the abscess through the junction of the bony and cartilaginous external auditory canal.

A submental vertex skull radiograph shows ipsilateral pharyngeal fullness (Fig. 14–2). An anteroposterior view (preferably with a copper grid) of the upper airway demonstrates ipsilateral edema and obliteration of the pyriform sinus (Fig. 14–3).

The complications of pterygomaxillary abscesses are related to the structures involved: involvement of the carotid artery can produce hemiplegia from emboli; internal jugular vein thrombosis with cephalad extension may lead to a cavernous sinus thrombosis, whereas inferior extension leads to internal jugular vein thrombosis. Internal jugular vein thrombosis is characterized by spiking temperature, toxicity with intense diaphoresis, headaches, and increased intracranial pressure. Occasionally, there are septic pulmonary emboli. A Queckenstedt maneuver during a lumbar puncture may verify an internal jugular vein thrombosis.

Extension into the retropharyngeal region by a pterygomaxillary abscess may lead to a posterior mediastinitis. Airway obstruction secondary to laryngeal edema and aspiration pneumonia from suppuration of the abscess into the pharynx have been reported.

Initially, the pterygomaxillary abscess may be difficult to differentiate from a peritonsillar abscess, but the latter usually is less toxic and has a distinct, soft, palatal fluctuance.

Treatment

Intravenous antibiotic therapy with incision and drainage is the primary treatment. An otolaryngologic consultation

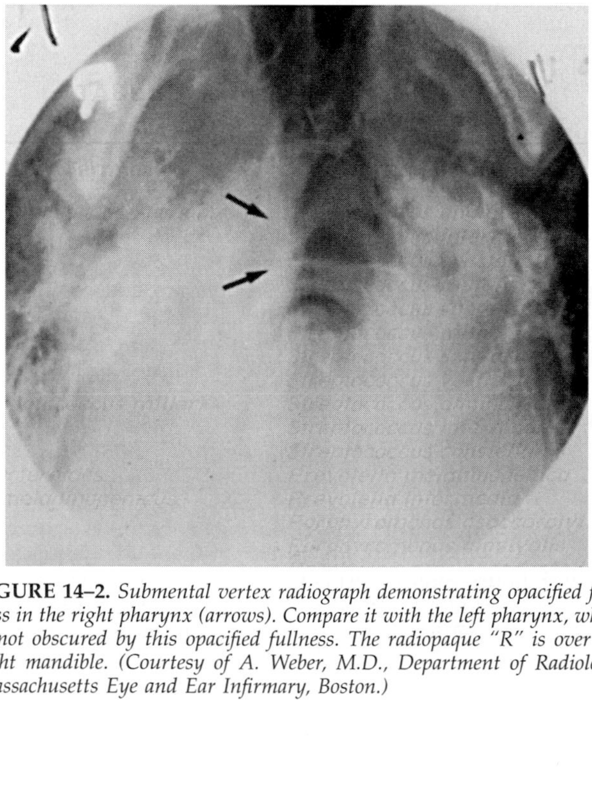

FIGURE 14–2. *Submental vertex radiograph demonstrating opacified fullness in the right pharynx (arrows). Compare it with the left pharynx, which is not obscured by this opacified fullness. The radiopaque "R" is over the right mandible. (Courtesy of A. Weber, M.D., Department of Radiology, Massachusetts Eye and Ear Infirmary, Boston.)*

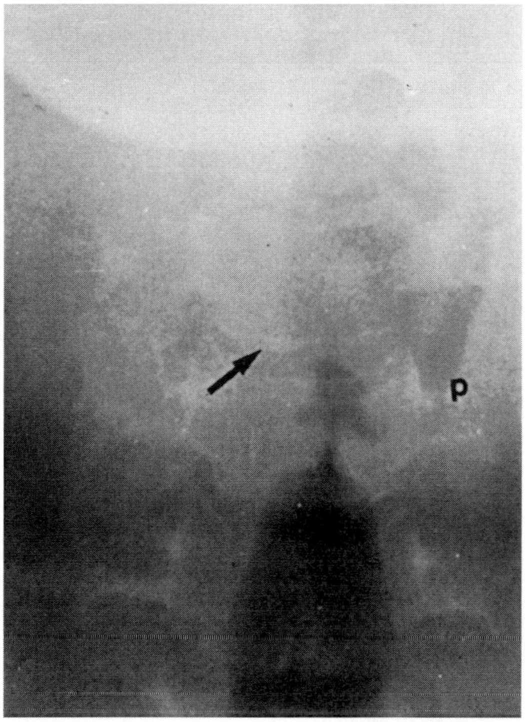

FIGURE 14–3. *Anteroposterior view of the upper airway. Note the obliteration of the right pyriform sinus by an opacity (arrow); left pyriform sinus is designated by "p." The vocal cords and the ventricles are well visualized here.*

should be obtained for this potentially complex surgery of the neck. The incision should be external, with sufficient exposure to provide immediate access to the common carotid artery for ligation, should there be carotid artery erosion.[30] An intraoral drainage and incision procedure is to be condemned because rapid access to the vital structures of the neck is not possible with this approach. Use of computed tomography has made it possible for some patients with parapharyngeal abscesses to be managed with needle aspiration and antibiotics. However, the number of reported cases is small and usually analyzed with cases of retropharyngeal abscess.[13, 18, 27] De Marie and colleagues[31] reported eight patients with parapharyngeal abscesses who were managed with computed tomography–guided selective needle aspirations; two of the patients were 10 and 17 years of age, respectively. Two patients developed complications of mediastinitis, pleuritis, and pericarditis, requiring more extensive drainage procedures.

RETROPHARYNGEAL ABSCESS (POSTERIOR VISCERAL SPACE, RETROVISCERAL SPACE, AND RETROESOPHAGEAL SPACE ABSCESSES)

The anterior wall of the retropharyngeal space is the middle layer of the deep cervical fascia, which abuts the posterior esophageal wall (the superior pharyngeal constrictor muscle). The deep layer of the deep cervical fascia circumscribes the posterior wall of this potential space. Inferiorly, these two fasciae fuse to limit the depth of this pocket at a level between the first and second thoracic vertebrae. A retropharyngeal abscess can erode inferiorly through the junction of these fasciae to extend posteriorly into the prevertebral space (see Fig. 14–1*A*). Subsequently, pus in the prevertebral space can descend inferiorly below the diaphragm to the psoas muscles.

The retropharyngeal space contains two paramedial chains of lymph nodes that receive drainage from the nasopharynx, adenoids, and posterior paranasal sinuses. These structures are prominent in early childhood and atrophy at puberty.[21] Retropharyngeal abscesses are most common in young children and are thought to be secondary to suppurative adenitis of these retropharyngeal nodes.[3] Other sources of infection are penetrating foreign bodies, endoscopy, trauma, pharyngitis, vertebral body osteomyelitis, petrositis, and dental procedures.[45] In one series of 17 cases of retropharyngeal abscesses presenting to the Children's Hospital, Denver, 7 children (41 per cent) had perforations of their hypopharynx or esophagus, including 2 neonates (most likely associated with attemps at intubation).[34] In the Pittsburgh series, 63 per cent of the children with retropharyngeal abscess had antecedent tonsillitis, pharyngitis, or viral upper respiratory tract infection.[45] Two children had previous trauma. However, no details on the type of trauma were given. In adults, tuberculosis and syphilis were common causes of retropharyngeal abscesses in the preantibiotic era.[36]

Clinical Manifestations

The symptoms of retropharyngeal abscess frequently begin insidiously after mild antecedent infection. Airway stridor from edema, cellulitis, or an obstructing mass is common. Laryngeal edema may cause dyspnea and tachypnea. Dysphagia, drooling, and odynophagia may occur. There is no trismus, but a stiff neck secondary to muscle tenderness may be present along with an ipsilateral tender cervical adenopathy. Thirty-three per cent of the 27 children with retropharyngeal abscess in the Pittsburgh series had torticollis or limitation of neck motion.[45] In the adult, the symptoms may be milder. Complaints of chest pain, by an adult, may reflect mediastinal extension.

Early in the course, there is midline or unilateral swelling of the posterior pharynx. Later, gentle palpation may demonstrate a large fluctuant mass in the posterior pharynx. Vigorous palpation is to be avoided because the abscess may rupture into the upper airway.

Posterior pharyngeal edema and a convex mass containing air may be demonstrated by a lateral neck radiograph. Cervical vertebrae frequently are retroflexed secondary to distentions by the abscess (Figs. 14–4 and 14–5). As with other abscesses, the white blood count is increased, with a predominance of granulocytes.

Treatment

Administration of intravenous antibiotics and incision and drainage are the treatment of choice. If the mass is small, a peroral incision with the patient in the Rose position (supine with the neck hyperextended) may provide some drainage, but there is a slight risk of aspiration. If the mass is large or if there is persistent fever after peroral drainage, an external incision is preferred. A tracheotomy may be required if there is risk of compromising the airway.

Posterior mediastinitis can result from the spread of infection from the retropharyngeal area into the prevertebral space. Other complications may be seen when the abscess extends to the parapharyngeal space and involves the great vessels and cranial nerves.

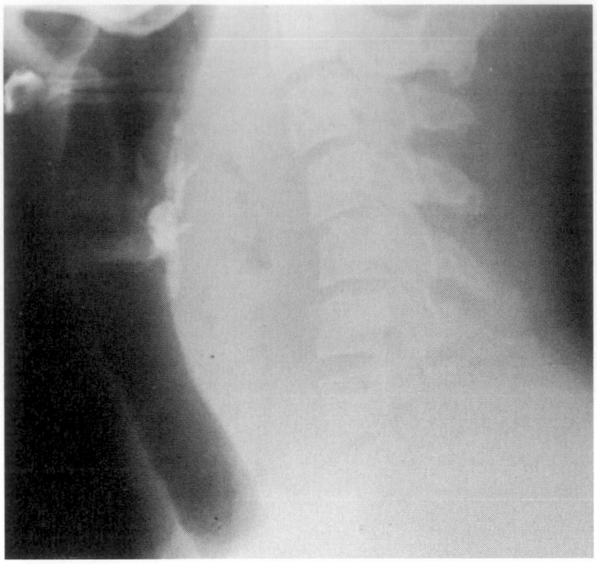

FIGURE 14–4. *Lateral neck radiograph demonstrating a retropharyngeal abscess containing gas and causing convexity of the cervical vertebrae.*

The computed tomographic scan has made the diagnosis and management of deep neck space infections more precise.[18, 27, 43] In contrast to conventional radiologic studies, the computed tomographic scan distinguishes cellulitis of the neck, which usually does not require surgical treatment, from a deep neck abscess, which requires surgical drainage. With its ability to define differences in tissue density, computed tomographic scanning permits accurate determination of the extent of the abscess and its extension and involvement of adjacent spaces.[18, 27, 43] When there is more than one space involved, accurate assessment of these spaces may ensure sufficient surgical drainage. Vascular structures can be identified as well as potential complications, such as venous thrombosis. Gas also may be detected by computed tomography (Fig. 14–6).

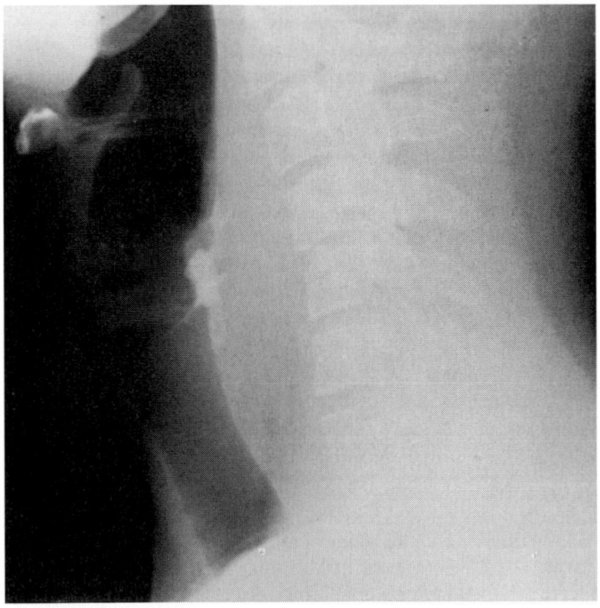

FIGURE 14–5. *The patient shown in Figure 14–4, 48 hours after incision and drainage. Note the reduced size in the retropharyngeal area and the lack of gas.*

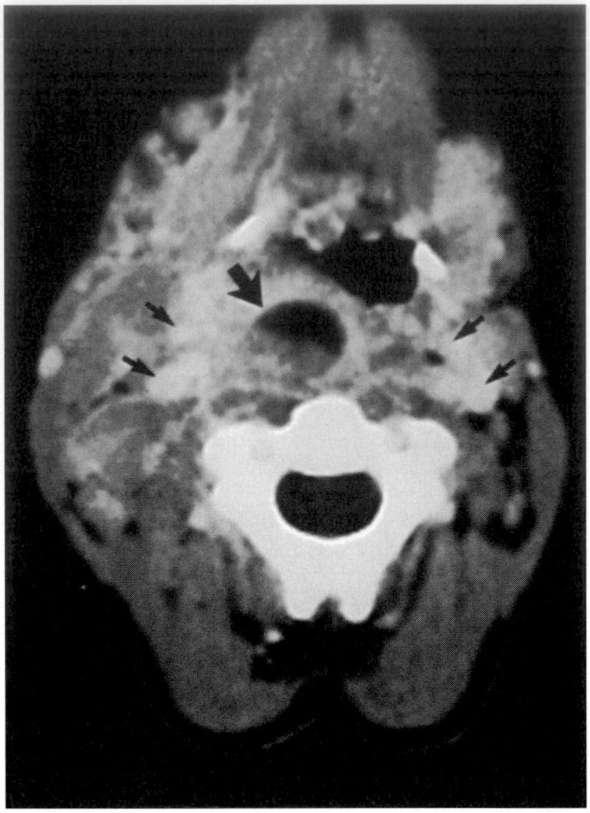

FIGURE 14–6. *Axial computed tomographic scan from a patient with a retropharyngeal abscess at the level of the base of the tongue demonstrating the abscess with its rim containing gas (large arrow). The patient is supine, with the gas displaced superiorly. The great vessels are lateral to the abscess (small arrows).*

There now are more extensive data on the use of computed tomographic scanning in the diagnosis of deep neck infections. A 10-year retrospective study from the Massachusetts Eye and Ear Infirmary compared preoperative computed tomographic scans with intraoperative findings in 38 patients who underwent surgical exploration of the parapharyngeal or retropharyngeal space within 48 hours of the scans. Overall, the intraoperative findings confirmed the computed tomographic scan interpetation in 76.3 per cent of the patients.[27] Five of the 38 (13.2 per cent) patients had computed tomographic scans indicative of abscesses that were not confirmed at surgery. Exploration of the parapharyngeal or retropharyngeal space revealed cellulitis. The false-negative rate was 10.5 per cent. The sensitivity of computed tomographic scanning for detection of parapharyngeal or retropharyngeal space abscess was 87.9 per cent. Similar findings were reported in the Pittsburgh series; the sensitivity of computed tomographic scanning for differentiating an abscess from cellulitis was 91 per cent.[45] There were three cases in which the radiologist's blinded computed tomographic scan interpetation did not correlate with the operative findings. Two patients with false-positive interpretations had retropharyngeal infections and underwent needle aspiration. The positive predictive value of computed tomographic scans in detection of abscess versus cellulitis was 83 per cent. These findings have important implications when considering whether patients should be managed by needle aspiration or by incision and drainage. Broughton[13] described the experience at the University of Kentucky Medical Center, where 8 of 14 patients with deep neck infections seen over a 9-year period were treated successfully by antibiotics alone. All were reported to have small abscesses on computed tomographic scan. However, it is possible that some only had cellulitis. Fifteen of the children in the Pittsburgh study with parapharyngeal and/or retropharyngeal space infections underwent surgical intervention: 11 (73 per cent) underwent incision and drainage, and 4 (27 per cent) underwent needle aspiration.[45] All had a sucessful outcome. Twelve (44 per cent) of the children with retropharyngeal infections were treated with intravenous antibiotics alone, and all did well.

MICROBIOLOGY OF DEEP NECK ABSCESSES

Group A streptococci *(Streptococcus pyogenes)* and *Staphylococcus aureus* have been considered to be the organisms most frequently associated with pharyngeal space infections. However, studies have demonstrated the presence of oral anaerobes in these infections; these organisms may be responsible for the gas seen on lateral neck radiographs (see Fig. 14–4). This is not surprising because the main portals of entry for pharyngeal space infections are the nasopharynx, oropharynx, paranasal sinuses, mastoid, and lower molars, all areas that are colonized with anaerobes.

The most complete microbiologic data available are from studies of peritonsillar abscesses. Flödstrom and Hallander[20] in 1976 reported the results of bacterial cultures on aspirates of pus from 37 patients with peritonsillar abscesses. The ages of the patients were not given. Group A streptococci were isolated from 17 of these patients, whereas 15 had an increase in their antistreptolysin O or anti-DNAase titers. Anaerobes were found in 28 of the cultures, including those of eight patients, that also disclosed the presence of streptococci. The most common anaerobic species isolated were fusobacteria (13), peptostreptococci (16), and *Bacteroides* species (18). Among the aerobic organisms, *S. aureus* was isolated four times and *Haemophilus influenzae* twice. There were no isolates of aerobic gram-negative enteric organisms. Sprinkle and associates[41] reported similar data in six patients 18 months to 21 years of age. Group A streptococci were isolated from two of the six patients. Four of the patients grew anaerobes, including *Bacteroides fragilis, Bacteroides melaninogenicus,* and *Fusobacterium necrophorus.*

Jokipii and colleagues[23] performed semiquantitative cultures of aspirated pus from 42 peritonsillar abscesses and found similar results. Group A streptococci were the most frequently isolated aerobic bacteria and were isolated in pure culture 4 of 10 times. Anaerobes were more abundant than aerobes; the most important species were *Bacteroides, Peptostreptococcus,* and *Fusobacterium,* both in frequency and quantitatively. Most of the infections were polymicrobial, with two to seven bacteria in 83 per cent of the specimens. Three studies from the United States and Finland have reported similar findings.[12, 24, 40] The pathogenic role of anaerobic bacteria in peritonsillar abscesses has been reinforced by reports of complications due to fusobacterial infection in children.[37, 39] *Fusobacterium* and *Bacteroides* species have been associated with septic thrombophlebitis and pulmonary emboli from the jugular veins.

Several studies of the microbiology of retropharyngeal and parapharyngeal abscesses in children have been reported. Not surpisingly, the organisms isolated are similar to those found in peritonsillar abscesses, but with a higher number of anaerobic species. Brook[11] examined aspirated pus from 14 children 1 to 6 years of age (median age, 3 years, 2 months) with retropharyngeal abscesses. Anaerobes were isolated from all patients, and they were the only organisms isolated in two patients (14 per cent) and were mixed with aerobes in the remainder (86 per cent). The predominant anaerobic species were *Bacteroides, Peptostreptococcus,* and *Fusobacterium.* The predominant aerobic species were alpha- and gamma-hemolytic streptococci, *S. aureus, Haemophilus* species, and group A beta-hemolytic streptococci. Seventy-one per cent of the isolates were beta-lactamase–positive, including all isolates of the *S. aureus* group, 6 of 18 of the *B. melaninogenicus* group (33 per cent), and 2 of 3 of the *Bacteroides oralis* group. Dodds and Maniglia[17] reported the results of cultures from nine retropharyngeal and three parapharyngeal abscesses from children and adolescents. The organisms isolated were similar to those reported by Brook,[11] but the microbiology was not as complete because this was a retrospective study and all specimens may not have been processed for anaerobic culture. Streptococcal species were the most frequent isolates, followed by *S. aureus* and *H. influenzae.* There was one isolate each of *F. necrophorum, Escherichia coli,* and *Klebsiella pneumoniae.*

Asmar performed cultures on material from 17 children with retropharyngeal abscesses; viridans streptococci were isolated from 11 of the abscesses, followed by *S. aureus* (8) and group A streptococci (6).[2] The most frequently identified anaerobes were *Peptostreptococcus* species. Overall, there were 45 aerobic and 18 anaerobic species identified.

Tuberculosis of the cervical spine eroding through the cervical vertebrae is a rare cause of retropharyngeal abscess.[36] There also is one report of atypical mycobacteria causing a retropharyngeal abscess in a similar clinical setting.

Barratt and colleagues[3] reported one case of retropharyngeal abscess caused by *Coccidioides immitis* in a 24-year-old woman with Hodgkin disease. The infection also was secondary to cervical vertebral osteomyelitis.

Because a large variety of organisms can be found in pharyngeal space infections, obtaining adequate cultures is of the greatest importance. The optimal material for culture is an aspirate of the pus obtained at operation. Throat swabs or swabs of the abscess obtained after drainage usually are inadequate because of contamination with normal oropharyngeal flora. The pus, when obtained, can be transported in a capped syringe if anaerobic transport media are not available. Most pathogenic obligate anaerobes can survive in a purulent exudate, despite extended periods of air exposure.[19] A Gram stain of the exudate will provide important clues to the bacterial etiology. A Gram stain showing a mixture of organisms suggests a mixed aerobic-anaerobic infection.

Use of a beta-lactamase–resistant antibiotic may be necessary in the treatment of deep neck abscesses because of the presence of beta-lactamase–producing bacteria, including *S. aureus* and *Bacteroides* species.[11, 12, 45] Drugs that may be effective include ampicillin-sulbactam, expanded-spectrum cephalosporins (may not cover *S. aureus*), oxacillin or nafcillin, and ticarcillin–clavulanic acid. These may need to be used in combination with clindamycin or metronidazole, which may be particularly useful for *B. fragilis.* Erythromycin is less satisfactory because it has less activity against *B. fragilis* and *Fusobacterium.* The routine use of aminoglycoside antibiotics is not indicated because aerobic gram-negative enteric rods rarely are found in these infections. Antibiotic therapy, however, is effective only in conjunction with adequate surgical drainage.

References

1. Ahmed, K., Jones, A. S., and Shah, K.: The role of ultrasound in the management of peritonsillar abscess. J. Laryngol. Otol. *108*:610–612, 1994.
2. Asmar, B. I.: Bacteriology of retropharyngeal abscess in children. Pediatr. Infect. Dis. J. *9*:595–596, 1990.

3. Barratt, G. E., Koopmann, C. F., and Coulthard, S. W.: Retropharyngeal abscess: A ten year experience. Laryngoscope *94*:455–463, 1984.
4. Bateman, G. H., and Kodicek, J.: Primary quinsy tonsillectomy. Ann. Otol. Rhinol. Laryngol. *68*:315–321, 1959.
5. Beck, A. L.: Deep neck infection. Ann. Otol. Rhinol. Laryngol. *56*:722–765, 1947.
6. Beck, A. L.: Deep neck infection. Ann. Otol. Rhinol. Laryngol. *56*:439–481, 1947.
7. Beeden, A. G., and Evans, J. N. G.: Quinsy tonsillectomy: A further report. J. Laryngol. Otol. *84*:443–448, 1970.
8. Bonding, P.: Tonsillectomy à chaud. J. Laryngol. Otol. *81*:1171–1182, 1973.
9. Brandon, Jr., E. C.: Immediate tonsillectomy for peritonsillar abscess. Trans. Am. Acad. Ophthalmol. Otolaryngol. *77*:412–416, 1973.
10. Brodsky, L., Sobie, S. R., Korwin, D., et al.: A clinical prospective study of peritonsillar abscess in children. Laryngology *98*:780–783, 1988.
11. Brook, I.: Microbiology of retropharyngeal abscesses in children. Am. J. Dis. Child. *141*:202–204, 1987.
12. Brook, I., Frazier, E. H., and Thompson, D. H.: Aerobic and anaerobic microbiology of peritonsillar abscess. Laryngoscope *101*: 289–292, 1991.
13. Broughton, R. A.: Nonsurgical management of deep neck infections in children. Pediatr. Infect. Dis. J. *11*:14–18, 1992.
14. Buckley, A. R., Moss, E. H., and Blokmanis, A.: Diagnosis of peritonsillar abscess: Value of intraoral sonography. Am. J. Roentgenol. *162*:961–964, 1994.
15. Chassaignae, E.: Traite Pratique de la Suppuration et du Drainage Chirurgal. Vol. II. Paris, Masson, 1859.
16. Danforth, H. B., and Brown, A. K., Jr.: A foreign body etiology of pterygomaxillary space abscess. Laryngoscope *73*:1485, 1963.
17. Dodds, B., and Maniglia, A. J.: Peritonsillar and neck abscesses in the pediatric age group. Laryngoscope *98*:956–959, 1988.
18. Endicott, J. N., Nelson, R. J., and Saraceno, C. A.: Diagnosis and management decisions in infections of the deep fascial spaces of the head and neck utilizing computerized tomography. Laryngoscope *92*:630–633, 1982.
19. Finegold, S. M.: Anaerobic Bacteria in Human Disease. New York, Academic Press, 1977, pp. 129–141.
20. Flödstrom, A., and Hallander, H. O.: Microbiological aspects of peritonsillar abscesses. Scand. J. Infect. Dis. *8*:157–160, 1976.
21. Grodinsky, M.: Retropharyngeal and lateral pharyngeal abscesses: An anatomic and clinical study. Ann. Surg. *110*:177–199, 1939.
22. Herzon, F. S.: Peritonsillar abscess: Incidence, current management practices, and a proposal for treatment guidelines. Laryngoscope *105*:1–17, 1995.
23. Jokipii, A. M. M., Jokipii, L., Sipila, P., et al.: Semiquantitative culture results and pathogenic significance of obligate anaerobes in peritonsillar abscesses. J. Clin. Microbiol. *26*:957–961, 1988.
24. Jousimies-Somer, H., Savolainen, S., Makitie, A., et al.: Bacteriologic findings in peritonsillar abscesses in young adults. Clin. Infect. Dis. *16*:S292–298, 1993.
25. Kronenberg, J., Wolf, M., and Leventon, G.: Peritonsillar abscess: Recurrence rate and the indication for tonsillectomy. Am. J. Otolaryngol. *8*:82–84, 1987.
26. Langenbrunner, D. J., and Dajani, S.: Pharyngomaxillary space abscess with carotid artery erosion. Arch. Otolaryngol. *94*:447–457, 1971.
27. Lazor, J. B., Cunningham, J., Eavey, R. D., et al.: Comparison of computed tomography and surgical findings in deep neck infections. Otolaryngol. Head Neck Surg. *111*:746–750, 1994.
28. Leavitt, G. W.: Cervical fascia and deep neck infections. Otolaryngol. Clin. North Am. *9*:703–716, 1976.
29. Lee, K. J., Traxler, J. H., Smith, A. W., et al.: Tonsillectomy: Treatment of peritonsillar abscess. Trans. Am. Acad. Ophthalmol. Otolaryngol. *77*:417–421, 1973.
30. Liston, R. L.: On a variety of false aneurysm. Br. Foreign Med. Rev. *15*:155–161, 1843.
31. de Marie, S., Tham, R., van der Mey, A. G. L., et al.: Clinical infections and nonsurgical treatment of parapharyngeal space infections complicating throat infection. Rev. Infect. Dis. *11*:975–982, 1989.
32. Mattucci, K., and Samet, C.: Pterygomaxillary space abscess. N.Y. State J. Med. *74*:1409–1412, 1974.
33. McCurdy, J. A., Jr.: Peritonsillar abscess. Arch. Otol. *103*:414–415, 1977.
34. Morrison, J. E., Jr., and Pashley, N. R.: Retropharyngeal abscess in children: A 10-year review. Pediatr. Emerg. Care *4*:9–11, 1988.
35. Mosher, H. P.: The submaxillary fossa approach to deep pus in the neck. Trans. Am. Acad. Ophthalmol. Otolaryngol. *34*:19–36, 1926.
36. Neumann, J. L., and Schlueter, D. P.: Retropharyngeal abscess as the presenting feature of tuberculosis of the cervical spine. Am. Rev. Resp. Dis. *110*:508–511, 1974.
37. Oleske, J. M., Starr, S. E., and Nahmias, A. J.: Complications of peritonsillar abscess due to *Fusobacterium necrophorum*. Pediatrics *57*:570–571, 1976.
38. Ophir, D., Bawnik, J., Porat, M., et al.: Peritonsillar abscess: A prospective evaluation of outpatient management by needle aspiration. Arch. Otolaryngol. *114*:661–663, 1988.
39. Rubinstein, E., Onderdonk, A. B., and Rahal, J. J.: Peritonsillar infection and bacteremia caused by *Fusobacterium gonidiaformans*. J. Pediatr. *85*:673, 1974.
40. Savolainen, S., Jousimies-Somer, H. R., Makitie, A. A., et al.: Peritonsillar abscess. Arch. Otolaryngol. Head Neck Surg. *119*:521–524, 1993.
41. Sprinkle, P. M., Veltri, R. W., and Kantor, C. M.: Abscesses of the head and neck. Laryngoscope *84*:1142–1148, 1974.
42. Stringer, S. P., Schaefer, S. D., and Close, L. G.: A randomized trial for outpatient management of peritonsillar abscess. Arch. Otolaryngol. *114*:278–298, 1988.
43. Thawley, S. E., Godo, M., and Fuller, T. R.: Computerized tomography in the evaluation of head and neck lesions. Laryngoscope *88*:451–459, 1978.
44. Thompson, J. W., Cohen, S., R., and Reddix, P.: Retropharyngeal abscess in children: A retrospective and historical analysis. Laryngoscope *98*:589–592, 1988.
45. Ungkanont, K., Yellon, R. F., Weissman, J. L., et al.: Head and neck space infections in infants and children. Otolaryngol. Head Neck Surg. *112*:375–382, 1995.
46. Weinberg, E., Brodsky, L., Stanievich, J., et al.: Needle aspiration of peritonsillar abscess in children. Arch. Otolaryngol. Head Neck Surg. *119*:169–172, 1993.

15

CERVICAL LYMPHADENITIS

Karina M. Butler and Carol J. Baker

Cervical lymphadenopathy is enlargement of the lymph nodes in the neck. Cervical lymphadenitis implies that there is inflammation of a node or nodes. The inflammatory response by the host is triggered by some form of injury or invasion proximal to the involved lymph node or nodes. The nodes become affected secondarily by drainage through connecting afferent lymphatic channels. The injury may be acute or chronic, infectious or noninfectious. Proper anatomic definition of the inflamed node or nodes,[47] combined with a knowledge of the structures of the head and neck drained by them, may allow identification of a portal of entry for infectious agents, the most common cause of cervical lymphadenitis in infants and children.

Figure 15–1 illustrates those regional lymph nodes commonly affected in infants and children with cervical adenitis. The *superficial cervical* lymph nodes lie on top of the sternocleidomastoid muscle along the course of the external jugular vein. They receive afferents from the superficial tissues of the neck, mastoid, superficial parotid (preauricular) nodes, and submaxillary glands. Their efferents terminate in the upper deep cervical lymph nodes. The *mastoid* lymph nodes overlie the mastoid process of the temporal bone and receive drainage from the parietal scalp and inner surface of the pinna. The *occipital* lymph nodes lie on the upper part of the trapezius and receive afferents from the occipital scalp and superficial portions of the upper posterior neck. Their efferents terminate in the deep cervical glands, as do those from the mastoid nodes. The *deep cervical* lymph nodes lie deep to the

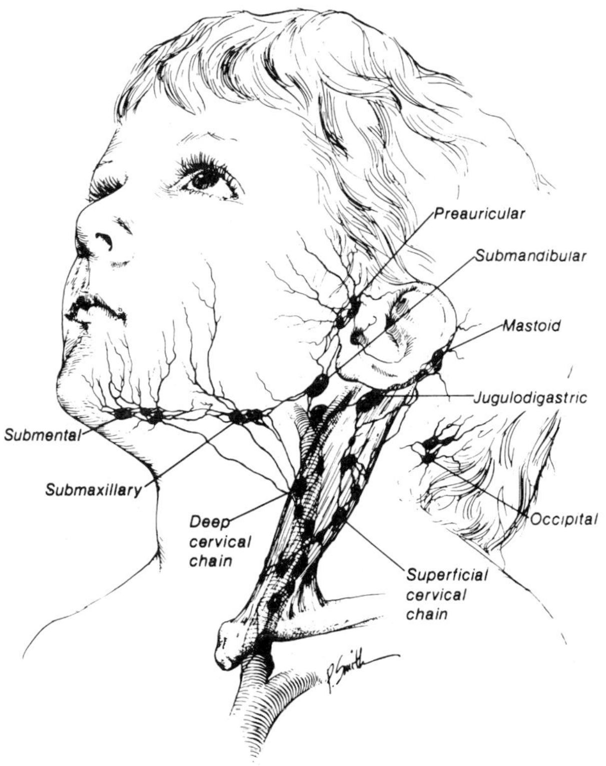

FIGURE 15–1. *The lymphatic drainage and lymph nodes involved in infants and children with cervical lymphadenitis.*

sternomastoid muscle along the whole length of the internal jugular vein and are divided into upper and lower groups. The *jugulodigastric* gland, a member of the upper group, lies at the angle of the jaw below the posterior belly of the digastric muscle. The lymphoid tissue of the palatine tonsil is drained into this gland; thus, it frequently becomes enlarged in patients with "tonsillitis" or with tuberculous infection originating from the tonsils. The larynx, trachea, thyroid gland, and esophagus drain into the lower deep cervical glands. The *submental* lymph nodes, which lie between the digastric muscles below the myohyoid, receive superficial and deep drainage from the anterior tongue, lower lip, and chin, from both sides of the midline. They send efferents to the submandibular and upper deep cervical glands. The *submandibular* lymph nodes lie adjacent to the submandibular salivary gland and receive rather wide, superficial drainage from the lateral aspect of the lower lip, the vestibule of the nose, the cheeks, the medial parts of the eyelids, and the forehead. Deep drainage to these nodes arises from the posterior part of the mouth, gums, teeth, and tongue as well as from superficial and submental lymph nodes.

Because the majority of the lymphatic drainage of the head and neck goes to the submaxillary and deep cervical nodes, these glands are involved in more than 80 per cent of cases of cervical adenitis in young children. Submental and superficial cervical lymphadenitis is observed less frequently.

EPIDEMIOLOGY

The epidemiology of infectious cervical adenitis is that of its infectious agents. Although cervical lymphadenitis can be a manifestation of focal viral infections of the oropharynx or respiratory tract, often it is part of a more generalized reticuloendothelial response to systemic infection. Viruses commonly associated with prominent cervical adenitis include Epstein-Barr virus (EBV), cytomegalovirus (CMV), and HIV. In HIV-infected children, cervical adenitis either may herald or may be a part of the more generalized lymphadenopathy associated with this infection. Although human herpesvirus 6 (HHV-6), the cause of roseola in infants (exanthem subitum), is associated with the development of a mononucleosis syndrome and cervical adenopathy in adults,[2] lymphadenitis is not a prominent feature in children with primary infection.[34] The epidemiology of cervical adenitis varies with age, geographic location, and socioeconomic status. In general, lower socioeconomic status is associated with a higher incidence of infection in younger children.

When bacterial in origin, with the exception of group A streptococci and *Mycobacterium tuberculosis*, the agents isolated from these glands are those normal inhabitants of the nose, mouth, pharynx, and skin—*Staphylococcus aureus*, anaerobes, atypical mycobacteria, *Actinomyces israelii*—and person-to-person transmission does not occur. In contrast, both group A streptococci and *M. tuberculosis* infection of cervical lymph nodes results from contact with human infection by way of airborne droplets. Except in neonates, where male dominance has been reported in cases due to group B streptococci,[7] infectious lymphadenitis has no sexual or seasonal predilection.[9, 27] Any age group may be affected. In neonates, *S. aureus* and group B streptococci are the most common pathogens. Suppurative cervical lymphadenitis due to *Staphylococcus epidermidis* in an otherwise healthy infant has been reported.[68] Nonetheless, despite the high frequency of nasal colonization by this organism, it remains a rare etiologic agent. Some studies[27, 81, 90] indicate that *S. aureus* has the leading role in infancy, whereas in childhood either group A streptococci or *S. aureus* is equally likely to be pathogenic. Other reports have varied regarding the relationship between age and probable etiologic agent.[9, 17] Together, *S. aureus* and *S. pyogenes* accounted for 65 to 89 per cent of consecutive cases in prospectively evaluated series.[9, 27, 90]

The epidemiology of bacterial lymphadenitis varies by geographic location. Resurgence of infection with *Yersinia pestis* in the southwestern United States means that, in areas where it is endemic, it also must be considered in the differential diagnosis. Furthermore, epidemic diphtheria, reported in the Russian Federation in 1990, has spread to several countries of the former Soviet Union and must be added to the list of possible causes of cervical lymphadenitis in that area.[25]

The distinctive epidemiologic features of mycobacterial infection are summarized in Table 15–1. Scrofula caused by *M. tuberculosis* is a relatively rare disease. When it does occur, it usually affects adults and older children. In contrast, children

TABLE 15–1. Differentiation of *Mycobacterium tuberculosis* and Atypical Mycobacterial Cervical Adenitis

	Atypical MCA	*M. tuberculosis*
Age	1–6 years	All ages
Race	White	Black, Asian
Exposure to tuberculosis	Absent	Present
Abnormal chest radiographs	Never	Often
Residence	Suburban	Urban
PPD-S > 15 mm	Uncommon	Often
Bilateral involvement	Rare	Not uncommon

PPD-S, purified protein derivative–S.

with atypical mycobacterial infection almost always are 1 to 6 years of age, live in suburban or rural communities, and have no history of contact with *M. tuberculosis*.[13, 26, 28, 31, 44, 77, 84, 88] Whereas *M. tuberculosis* is an infection acquired primarily by inhalation, both the gastrointestinal tract and the respiratory tract may serve as the primary portal of entry for atypical mycobacteria.[31, 59, 65] There appears to be an ethnic predilection for atypical infection to occur in whites and for tuberculous infections to occur in blacks and Asians.

The advent of the HIV pandemic has had a major impact on the nature and frequency of mycobacterial infections. There has been a marked increase in the incidence of tuberculous infection in HIV-infected adults and a similar trend in HIV-infected children. Annualized case rates for tuberculosis in HIV-infected children have increased from 58 per 100,000 during the years 1981 to 1985 to 478 per 100,000 during the years 1990 to 1992.[33] The increase in cases is not confined just to HIV-infected children. The increased prevalence of tuberculous infection in the community means that all children are at increased risk of exposure to an infectious adult.[14] Of additional concern is the frequency with which drug-resistant tuberculosis is being detected in children, with up to 15 per cent of isolates resistant to isoniazid and rifampin.[33] *Mycobacterium avium-intracellulare* and *Mycobacterium scrofulaceum* are the usual causes of atypical mycobacterial lymphadenitis in children.[88] However, a report from Australia advises that *Mycobacterium haemophilum* now must be added to the list of responsible agents.[6] Furthermore, because of its fastidious growth requirements, it may be responsible for many of the cases of culture-negative tuberculous lymphadenitis. Cervical lymphadenitis due to *Mycobacterium chelonae* is rare, usually involves the submandibular glands, and typically occurs where there is an antecedent history of dental pathology.[4]

Cervical lymphadenopathy often is the direct result of infection with HIV per se. However, the development of acute tender adenitis in an HIV-infected child should provoke a search for another etiology. Although the typical childhood pathogens remain the most common invaders in this setting, as in other immunocompromised children, more unusual opportunists also should be sought.

Cat-scratch disease is a common cause of lymphadenitis in children and young adults.[15] In 1988, English and associates[29] first isolated a pleomorphic gram-negative bacillus, later identified as *Afipia felis*, from lymph nodes of patients with cat-scratch disease. It now is recognized that *Bartonella henselae* (formerly called *Rochalimaea henselae*), a morphologically similar but genetically distinct pleomorphic gram-negative bacillus, causes most cat-scratch disease.[1]

The cervical nodes are the second most common site of cat-scratch disease involvement. Although unusual and severe manifestations of this infection have been described in adult patients with AIDS,[40, 49, 70] for the most part it remains a mild, self-limited infection in children and adolescents, showing no ethnic group predilection. Seasonal variation with an increased incidence in fall, winter, and early spring does occur in temperate zones. A history of animal contact with cats usually can be elicited.[20] The importance of bites and scratches by kittens in transmitting this disease has been well defined.[55] However, the absence of a history of traumatic contact with cats in a substantial number of cases has raised the possibility that other modes of transmission exist. Zangwill and associates[91] have suggested that fleas might serve as vectors of transmission. Their hypothesis is strengthened by the detection of *Bartonella* DNA by polymerase chain reaction in collections of fleas from cats owned by two infected patients.[91]

PATHOPHYSIOLOGY

Although cervical lymphadenitis is a common entity in pediatric clinical practice, little information exists regarding its pathogenesis. Viral cervical adenitis either may be part of a local response to viruses invading the oropharynx or respiratory tract (e.g., adenoviruses, coxsackieviruses) or may be part of a more generalized reticuloendothelial response to systemic viral infection (e.g., EBV, CMV, HHV-6, HIV). Infection attributed to group A streptococci and *S. aureus* is presumed to enter the cervical lymphatics from the oropharynx and anterior nares, respectively. In the patient with group A streptococcal pharyngitis or tonsillitis, whether infection remains localized at the pharyngotonsillar tissues or spreads to cervical lymph nodes and results in suppuration primarily is a function of host defense. For example, although peak attack rates for group A streptococcal pharyngitis are observed among school age children, suppurative cervical adenitis rarely occurs. In contrast, infants and children younger than 3 years of age rarely have group A streptococci isolated from throat cultures, but this is the age group more commonly afflicted with suppurative cervical lymphadenitis.[64]

In infections attributed to *S. aureus*, colonization of the anterior nares is believed to be a prerequisite for cervical lymphadenitis. Reports by Brook and Winter[15, 16] concluded this because organisms of identical phage types were isolated from the anterior nares and the cervical abscesses of their patients. An investigation of children in St. Louis found no such correlation between isolates from nasal and cervical node cultures.[9] The role of *S. aureus* as a primary pathogen has been the subject of some debate. Thirty per cent of aspirates in most series yield mixed cultures of *S. aureus* and group A streptococci, and there frequently are significant elevations of antistreptolysin O titer in the sera of patients whose lymph nodes yielded a pure culture of *S. aureus*. In a California study, 65 per cent of patients had node aspirates yielding a pure culture of *S. aureus* and 41 per cent of these exhibited an immune response to one or more of the extracellular antigens of group A streptococci.[90] Similarly, the finding that despite the high prevalence of penicillin resistance among *S. aureus* many children improve with penicillin or ampicillin treatment suggests that, although streptococci and staphylococci may coexist in these nodes, staphylococci may play a subsidiary role as secondary invaders. Most children with isolates of *S. aureus* from suppurative lymph nodes show no evidence of coexistent streptococcal infection or viral upper respiratory infection. In this more common circumstance, it is apparent that *S. aureus* has the capacity to be a primary invader.

Recovery of anaerobic bacteria from cervical nodes suggests invasion of the lymphatics by normal mouth flora, often as a result of local tissue destruction by periodontal disease.[17] The delineation of the pathophysiology of cervical lymphadenitis of diverse bacterial etiology will require an understanding of the interaction between a given microorganism (inoculum size, elaboration of extracellular enzymes, ability to adhere to epithelium) and the host (humoral and surface immune capacity, degree of trauma, and so on).

CLINICAL PRESENTATION

The clinical manifestations of cervical lymphadenitis vary considerably but are consistent with the diverse etiologies associated with cervical node enlargement in infants and children. It is useful to categorize the mode of presentation as either acute or subacute and chronic, for, although the boundaries are ill defined and there is much overlap, common etiologies tend to fall fairly consistently within one or another category. Cervical lymphadenitis of acute onset may be categorized further as either bilateral or unilateral. In most situations, acute, bilateral cervical adenitis is either part of a generalized reticuloendothelial response to a systemic infection or a localized reaction to acute pharyngitis. Presence or absence of associated features (i.e., pharyngitis, enanthems or exanthems, generalized adenopathy, hepatosplenomegaly, and so on) aids in the differentiation.

Acute unilateral cervical lymphadenitis is caused by streptococcal or staphylococcal infection in 53 to 89 per cent of cases.[9, 27, 37, 90] In newborns, *S. aureus* is the most common cause and clinical features are similar to those seen in older children. Group B streptococci has been described as causative in a "cellulitis-adenitis" syndrome in infancy.[7] These infants differ from those with staphylococcal adenitis in that they are younger, more often are male, and have a greater incidence of systemic symptoms, irritability, and anorexia, and 94 per cent have associated bacteremia. The typical patient presents with fever, facial or submandibular cellulitis, and ipsilateral otitis media.[7]

The patient with disease attributed to *S. aureus* or group A streptococci typically is 1 to 4 years of age (70 to 80 per cent of cases), and the male:female ratio is equal. Clinically, there is little that helps to differentiate streptococcal from staphylococcal infections. Cervical adenitis can occur as part of the "streptococcosis" syndrome of infancy, with an onset heralded by coryza, an irregular low-grade fever, nasal discharge with excoriation and crusting around the nares, vomiting, and loss of appetite. Lymph node enlargement occurs within a few days of onset and resolves, as do other symptoms, without treatment within 6 to 8 weeks.[64] Suppuration of cervical glands may occur at any time during this interval, but this is uncommon if antimicrobial therapy is given early in the illness. Group A streptococci also should be suspected as a cause of cervical adenitis in the patient with typical vesiculopustular or crusted lesions of impetigo involving the face or scalp.

Systemic symptoms in children with staphylococcal or streptococcal cervical adenitis usually are minimal or absent unless associated with cellulitis, metastatic foci of infection, or bacteremia. The primary site of lymph node involvement by frequency is submandibular (50 to 60 per cent), upper cervical (25 to 30 per cent), submental (5 to 8 per cent), occipital (3 to 5 per cent), and lower cervical (2 to 5 per cent).[9, 27, 89] Involved nodes generally vary in size from 2.0 to 6.0 cm in diameter, and one-fourth to one-third become fluctuant. Patients with lymphadenitis due to *S. aureus* are more likely to have suppuration and a longer duration of symptoms prior to diagnosis than those with disease caused by other bacterial agents.[9, 81] Among patients who develop suppurative adenitis, 86 per cent do so within 2 weeks of onset[89] (Fig. 15–2). Approximately one-third of patients in one study had concomitant lymphadenopathy at other anatomic sites.[9] A history of recent upper respiratory tract symptoms, including sore throat (40 per cent), earache or coryza (16 per cent), and impetigo (32 per cent), is frequent, as are signs of pharyngitis, tonsillitis, and/or otitis media.[9, 27] However, these do not help to delineate etiology. Hepatomegaly or splenomegaly is rare and, if present, should suggest bacteremia or generalized disease processes (infectious mononucleosis, reticuloendotheliosis, tuberculosis, HIV infection, and so on).

Kawasaki disease may present as a febrile illness associated with bilateral or unilateral cervical lymphadenopathy and often is confused with the more common acute pyogenic infections.[86] Other features (conjunctivitis, oral manifestations, changes in the peripheral extremities, polymorphic erythematous rash) are required criteria for the diagnosis.[57] Although originally called *mucocutaneous lymph node syndrome*, unilateral lymph node enlargement of at least 1.5 cm is an inconsistent feature.[10, 57] Lymphadenopathy usually subsides when the fever subsides, although in some cases it may follow a more chronic course.

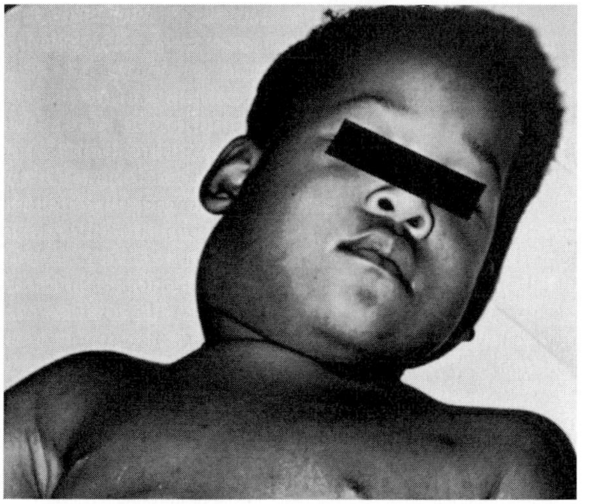

FIGURE 15–2. *A 2-year-old boy with fever and unilateral inflammation of the cervical lymph nodes of 2 days' duration. Needle aspirate culture of this nonfluctuant node grew* Staphylococcus aureus. *Antistaphylococcal therapy resulted in complete resolution of adenitis without surgical drainage.*

The rapid development of painful lymphadenitis, quickly succeeding the sudden onset of fever, chills, weakness, and headache, is one of the classic presentations of infection caused by *Yersinia pestis* (bubonic plague). The groin is the site most often involved. However, other locations, including the cervical area, may be affected. Rapid diagnosis and treatment are critical because infection can be fulminant.

In cases of diphtheria, cervical adenopathy develops secondary to infection of the posterior structures of the mouth and proximal pharynx. A whitish-gray membrane covers the mucosal surfaces. In severe cases, the cervical adenopathy, which typically is bilateral, can result in a "bull neck" appearance.

Careful physical examination of the head and neck, particularly areas drained by affected lymph nodes, may yield important clues about etiology. The presence of periodontal disease is associated with a higher incidence of anaerobic organisms causing adenitis[16]; the history or presence of tick bites suggests the possibility of tularemia[78]; and the presence of papular or pustular lesions, suggesting an inoculation site, raises the possibility of rarer causes of infection, including *Nocardia*, actinomycosis, sporotrichosis, plague, and cutaneous diphtheria, as well as cat-scratch disease.

Mycobacterial infections, cat-scratch disease, and toxoplasmosis are among the more common entities presenting as subacute or chronic lymphadenitis. The epidemiologic and clinical features that aid in the differentiation of typical and atypical mycobacterial infections are summarized in Table 15–1. The clinical manifestations virtually are identical[13, 24, 58] (Fig. 15–3). Typically, the child presents with a history of painful cervical node swelling. The submandibular cervical nodes usually are involved in atypical mycobacterial infection,[3, 13, 54, 69, 71, 83, 88] whereas other cervical nodes are involved more frequently with *M. tuberculosis*.[3, 13, 39, 54, 71] As the infection progresses, the skin overlying the node may develop a

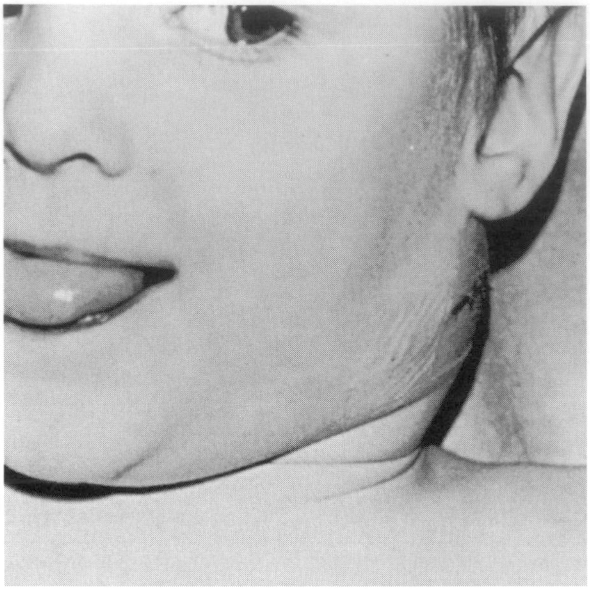

FIGURE 15–3. *A 4-year-old boy who had bilateral nontender enlargement of lymph nodes of 6 weeks' duration without other symptoms. Purified protein derivative–S resulted in 18-mm induration, excisional biopsy acid-fast stain was positive, and cultures grew* Mycobacterium tuberculosis.

pinkish discoloration caused by increased vascularity, although there is no increase in skin temperature. This finding may be followed by adherence of the skin to the underlying mass. If left untreated, fluctuance and spontaneously draining sinus tracts may develop.

The patient with *M. tuberculosis* is more likely than one with atypical mycobacterial disease to be older than 4 years of age and to have generalized lymphadenopathy (10 to 20 per cent of cases), bilateral node enlargement (10 per cent of cases), a history of exposure to tuberculosis (93 per cent of cases), and an urban residence.[13, 54, 62] However, there are no differences as they relate to duration of adenopathy, fever, and presence or absence of constitutional symptoms. An abnormal chest roentgenogram has been noted in 28 to 71 per cent of cases due to *M. tuberculosis*,[22, 71, 72, 79, 84] in contrast to the 98 to 100 per cent of normal chest roentgenograms found in patients with atypical mycobacterial disease.[31, 69, 71, 83] In a summary of 447 reported childhood cases of atypical mycobacterial infections from 15 countries, Lincoln and Gilbert[46] detected only six cases of bilateral cervical node involvement, four with abnormal chest roentgenograms and none with nodal enlargement other than cervical. Similar findings have been reported by others.[69, 83] Intradermal testing with purified protein derivative–S uncommonly produces more than 15 mm of induration at 48 hours in the child with atypical mycobacterial infection, but reactions between 5 and 15 mm are relatively common.[51]

Cat-scratch disease may present days to weeks after the initial inoculation. Characteristically, a history of contact with a cat or kitten or a scratch will be present. Later, when the primary lesion may have healed, tender regional adenopathy appears. Although axillary nodes most frequently are affected, 25 per cent of children have isolated cervical node involvement. Constitutional symptoms, present early in the course of the illness, usually are mild and may have resolved by the time the adenitis appears. Fever is observed in one-fourth of patients and, if present, has a mean duration of 5 to 7 days.[50] Nodes suppurate in one-tenth to one-third of patients.[20, 23] Rare manifestations include Parinaud syndrome,[21] encephalopathy,[48] exanthems[20] (usually of the erythema nodosum type), and osteolytic lesions.[22]

Acquired toxoplasmosis may present as regional lymphadenopathy, frequently with posterior cervical node involvement.[56, 66, 82] Most children exhibit few if any constitutional symptoms. The characteristic location combined with a history of exposure to cats or of eating undercooked meats should raise this diagnostic possibility, and the diagnosis then may be confirmed by appropriate serologic testing. This is an uncommon etiology for cervical adenopathy in children living in the United States.

A rare disorder of unknown etiology that also may present as painless cervical adenopathy, with or without fever, is subacute necrotizing lymphadenitis (Kikuchi lymphadenitis). A disorder recognized most frequently in young women, it invariably runs a benign course with spontaneous resolution over 3 to 4 months.[18, 30, 74, 85] It remains to be determined if it is infectious in nature, perhaps the result of infection with a single novel agent or a nonspecific host response to any of a variety of agents. Finally, when presented with a history of subacute or chronic lymphadenitis, careful physical examination should be undertaken to exclude obvious local causes (i.e., seborrhea, head lice, *Tinea capitis*, and chronic otitis media) before an extensive diagnostic work-up is initiated.

DIFFERENTIAL DIAGNOSIS

Cervical swellings are encountered frequently in pediatric practice, and most of these represent lymph nodes. When considering the diagnostic possibilities in patients with cervical lymphadenitis, one first must ascertain whether or not the pathologic process actually involves a lymph node, then whether or not its cause is infectious, and, if infectious, the likely etiologic agent. The duration of the cervical swelling aids in the differential diagnosis because most tumors or developmental anomalies have been noted for weeks. Rapid enlargement may occur in the latter, but usually this occurs as the result of secondary infection. Location is a most helpful clue because midline masses rarely represent lymph nodes and the most common neck masses of congenital origin (thyroglossal duct cyst, branchial cleft cyst, and cystic hygromas) all have characteristic anatomic locations.

Of the midline masses, thyroglossal duct cysts by far are the most common.[41, 63] These may occur anywhere from the foramen caecum to the thyroid, are midline, and move on tongue protrusion. They may have an associated sinus tract, midline or just lateral to it, from which cloudy mucus sometimes can be expressed. They may become infected secondarily, but, in the noninfected state, they are nontender, smooth, and round with well-defined margins. Thyroglossal duct cysts must be differentiated from other midline masses, including epidermoid cysts, lipomas, thyroid tumors, and the rare midline lymph node.

The second most common benign congenital neck mass is the branchial cleft cyst. This usually arises from the second branchial cleft and lies at the anterior border of the sternocleidomastoid muscle. Although such cysts usually manifest themselves as skin dimples, they may become infected secondarily and present as inflammatory swellings or draining sinus tracts. A careful examination should detect a sinus tract. Branchial cleft cysts can present at any age but usually do so during early school age.

Cystic hygromas, considerably less common than thyroglossal duct or branchial cleft cysts, are the third most frequent cause of congenital neck masses. These arise from lymphatics derived from either the jugular vein or mesenchymal tissue. They may occur elsewhere but most commonly are found posterior to the sternocleidomastoid muscle in the supraclavicular fossa. Most present in the first 2 years of life, many being noted at birth or soon thereafter. They are soft, compressible tumors that transilluminate well, and, although benign in themselves, they may cause symptoms through pressure exerted on surrounding structures. Confusion may arise when cystic hygromas increase in size in association with an upper respiratory tract infection. The latter causes increased lymph flow, so that the hygroma persists while other lymph nodes decrease in size after resolution of the infection. In most circumstances, palpation and transillumination readily distinguish these congenital malformations.

These four cervical masses—thyroglossal duct cysts, thyroid tumors, branchial cleft cysts, and cystic hygromas—accounted for 63.7 per cent of lesions in children with persistent cervical masses reported by Moussatos and Baffes.[58] Other lesions included neurogenic tumors, parotid tumors, and miscellaneous benign tumors (12.3 per cent). The remainder of masses represented lymph nodes. As a rule, masses located completely anterior to the sternocleidomastoid muscle are benign. The exception to this is the thyroid tumor.[58] Malignancies that mimic cervical lymph nodes usually are located in the posterior triangle or are multiple masses extending across both the anterior and posterior triangles. In contrast, about 50 per cent of masses in the posterior triangle represent malignancies, and most of these are of lymphoid origin. Whereas most cysts and tumors present as solitary, unilateral, nontender masses, lymph nodes of noninfectious etiology frequently are multiple and bilateral, although they may be mildly tender.

Noninfectious chronic inflammatory involvement of cervical lymph nodes may represent a variety of uncommon, usually benign, but sometimes malignant entities (Table 15–2). Fifty per cent of malignant neck masses in children are caused by lymphomas, Hodgkin and non-Hodgkin. Neuroblastoma is the second most common malignancy, accounting for 15 per cent. The likelihood of a given diagnosis is age-dependent, with neuroblastoma being more common than Hodgkin disease in the younger age groups.[37] Thyroid tumors are the third most frequent neck malignancies. Other entities to be included in the differential diagnosis include leukemia,[19] metastatic carcinoma,[58] phenytoin (Dilantin)–induced pseudolymphoma,[19] serum sickness,[19] storage disorders (Gaucher disease, Niemann-Pick disease), collagen vascular disease,[19] sarcoidosis,[38] sinus histiocytosis with massive lymphadenopathy,[8, 67] reticuloendotheliosis or histiocytosis X,[19] and postvaccinal lymphadenitis.[61] Except for malignancies, these disease entities almost always are associated with lymphadenopathy that is not limited to the cervical region and have a variety of clinical and laboratory findings that allow the correct diagnosis to be made.

A large number of infectious agents have been reported in association with cervical adenitis in infants and children (Table 15–3). Among patients evaluated prospectively with needle aspirate cultures of affected lymph nodes, *S. aureus* or group A streptococci are the organisms isolated most commonly.[9, 17, 27, 81, 90] No significant difference has been reported that will distinguish between patients with adenitis attributed to streptococci or staphylococci with respect to sex, ethnicity, dental problems, symptoms, presence of fever, or site or size of lymph nodes. However, in those patients from whom *S. aureus* is isolated, a longer duration of disease prior to diagnosis, a larger percentage of fluctuant lymph nodes,[9, 81] and a tendency toward slower resolution are found.[27] Most patients with bacterial cervical lymphadenitis, including those with mycobacterial infection, are from 1 to 6 years of age. Older children are more likely to have negative lymph node aspirate cultures.[9, 77, 81]

TABLE 15–2. Etiology of Cervical Adenitis: Noninfectious

	Isolated Cervical	Cervical Associated with Generalized Adenopathy
Malignancy		
Hodgkin disease	+	+
Non-Hodgkin lymphomas	+	+
Rhabdomyosarcoma	+	−
Neuroblastoma	+	+
Leukemia	+	+
Metastatic carcinoma	+	−
Thyroid tumors	+	−
Drugs		
Isoniazid	−	+
Phenytoin (Dilantin)	−	+
Serum sickness	−	+
Collagen Vascular Disease		
Juvenile rheumatoid arthritis	−	+
Systemic lupus erythematosus	−	+
Miscellaneous		
Sarcoidosis	−	+
Reticuloendotheliosis	−	+
Sinus histiocytosis with massive lymphadenopathy	+	+
Histiocytosis X	−	+
Postvaccinial	+	−
Storage disorders	−	+
Kawasaki disease	+	+
Masses Simulating Adenopathy		
Cystic hygroma	+	−
Branchial cleft cyst	+	−
Thyroglossal duct cyst	+	−
Epidermoid cyst	+	−
Sternocleidomastoid tumor	+	−

Anaerobes rarely were associated with cervical adenitis in early studies.[9, 27] Proper bacteriologic techniques for the isolation of these fastidious organisms allowed Brook[17] to report anaerobes alone in 18 per cent and mixed anaerobic and aerobic bacteria in 20 per cent of patients, suggesting that anaerobic organisms may play a more significant role in the etiology of cervical lymphadenitis than recognized previously. Therefore, the older child with "negative" cultures, especially the one with poor dental hygiene or periodontal disease, may have anaerobic infection, as did the 9-year-old boy in Figure 15–4. Needle aspiration of this cervical mass yielded *Peptococcus, Peptostreptococcus, Bacteroides fragilis,* and viridans streptococci. Resolution of the lymphadenitis was prompt after incision and drainage and penicillin therapy. Dental disease or manipulation also should suggest the possibility of cervicofacial actinomycosis (lumpy jaw). These patients have a submandibular mass and frequently a fistula from the skin to the oral cavity.[11]

Less commonly occurring bacteria,[45] as well as viruses, fungi, and parasites, can cause cervical lymphadenitis in children, but in these patients there usually is less evidence of acute inflammation, with or without adenopathy at additional sites, as well as historical and physical findings that suggest unusual causes of cervical lymph gland enlargement.

SPECIFIC DIAGNOSIS

A detailed history to ascertain preceding dental problems, presence of skin lesions, animal exposure (including expo-

TABLE 15–3. Etiology of Cervical Adenitis: Infectious

	Isolated Cervical	Cervical Associated with Generalized Adenopathy
Bacterial		
Staphylococcus aureus	+	−
Group A streptococci	+	+
Mycobacterium tuberculosis	+	+
Atypical mycobacteria	+	−
Bartonella henselae	+	−
Gram-negative enterics	+	−
Anaerobes	+	−
Haemophilus influenzae	+	−
Yersinia pestis	−	+
Actinomyces israelii	+	−
Diphtheria	+	−
Tularemia	+	−
Brucellosis	−	+
Syphilis	+	+
Viral		
Measles	+	+
Rubella	+	+
Epstein-Barr virus	+	+
Herpes simplex	+	−
Human herpesvirus 6	+	+
Cytomegalovirus	+	+
Mumps	+	−
Varicella	+	+
HIV	+	+
Fungal		
Histoplasmosis	+	+
Cryptococcus	+	−
Aspergillosis	+	−
Candida	+	−
Sporotrichosis	+	−
Parasitic		
Toxoplasma gondii	+	+

sure to fleas and ticks), duration of illness, presence of associated symptoms, contact with tuberculosis, presence of risk factors for HIV infection, drug usage (especially Dilantin) or other unusual ingestions (undercooked meat, unpasteurized dairy products), recent travel outside the geographic region of residence, and sites of occult infection drained by the affected node may yield important diagnostic clues in the patient with cervical lymphadenitis. Physical examination should include careful inspection for the presence of dental disease, noncervical lymphadenopathy, hepatosplenomegaly, and oropharyngeal or skin lesions.

In the acute stage of cervical lymphadenitis, needle aspiration of the affected node is a valuable diagnostic tool. Sixty to eighty-eight per cent of patients with acute cervical lymphadenitis subjected to needle aspiration of the affected node for bacterial and mycobacterial culture have an etiologic agent recovered.[9, 17, 39, 90] Only inflamed nodes should be aspirated, but these need not be fluctuant. No serious complications of this procedure have been recorded. The largest or most fluctuant node should be selected and the skin cleansed and anesthetized. Skin anesthesia can be induced effectively using a topical anesthetic cream, e.g., lidocaine-prilocaine (EMLA), placed on the selected aspiration site under an occlusive dressing 30 to 45 minutes prior to the procedure. An 18- or 20-gauge needle attached to a 20-mL syringe is used. If no material is aspirated, 1 to 2 mL of sterile *nonbacteriostatic* saline is injected into the node and it is reaspirated. The aspirate should be inoculated directly from the syringe onto aerobic (including chocolate agar) and anaerobic media, as well as onto Sabouraud agar (fungi) and into a broth media suitable for the early detection of mycobacteria, such as the Bactec radiometric assay. In this latter system, the release of labeled carbon dioxide in an automated ion chamber system can detect mycobacteria as early as 12 to 17 days after inoculation of the broth.[76] Gram and acid-fast stains are mandatory, and their reading will serve as a guide to initial antimicrobial therapy. Thioglycolate broth and anaerobically incubated blood agar plates are incapable of providing optimal conditions for the isolation of many anaerobic bacteria.[9] Therefore, optimal methods for cultivation of fastidious anaerobes should be employed because anaerobic organisms may be recovered in up to 20 per cent of cases.[17] Cultures of infected skin lesions and exudates on tonsils also should be performed but not to the exclusion of needle aspiration.

Isolation of group A streptococci from the throat or skin cultures of a patient with lymphadenitis does *not* confirm the etiology of the lymph node inflammation. Patients have been noted to have isolation of group A streptococci from throat and of *S. aureus* from lymph node aspirate cultures.[9, 64] Intradermal skin testing for tuberculosis with purified protein derivative (5 TU) tuberculin should be carried out. Induration of 15 mm or greater is suggestive of infection with *M. tuberculosis,* whereas reactions of 5 to 14 mm may be caused by either a tuberculous or nontuberculous mycobacterial infection.[51] In an attempt to develop a rational approach to the use and interpretation of differential skin testing, Huebner and associates,[36] using standardized tuberculous (purified protein derivative–T) and nontuberculous mycobacterial antigens, studied 144 children with chronic cervical adenopathy, of whom 123 had mycobacterial culture results available. The low incidence of tuberculosis within the study population (four cases) prevented an interpretation regarding the utility of these antigens in distinguishing disease caused by *M. tuberculosis* from that caused by other mycobacteria. Children with culture-confirmed mycobacterial lymphadenopathy had significantly larger reactions to nontuberculous mycobacterial antigens than did those with microscopy-negative and culture-negative results. The study was terminated prematurely

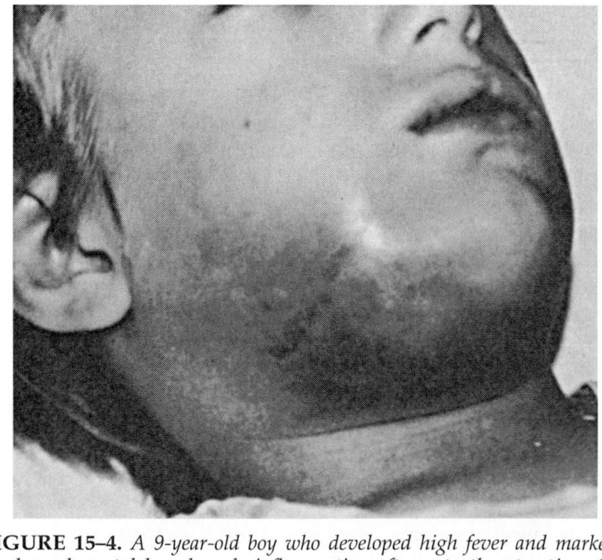

FIGURE 15–4. *A 9-year-old boy who developed high fever and markedly tender submental lymph node inflammation after a tooth extraction. Cultures from this fluctuant mass grew three anaerobes and viridans streptococci.*

because of an unacceptably high incidence of a blistering skin reaction to nontuberculous mycobacterial antigens.

Intradermal skin testing, using a crude extract from affected nodes, historically has been used to establish the diagnosis of cat-scratch disease.[20] However, a diagnosis usually is reached based on the presence of regional adenopathy, a history of cat exposure (particularly if there is a history of a scratch or a primary skin lesion), and negative laboratory studies for other causes of lymphadenopathy. *B. henselae*, the more common etiologic agent of this disease, can be isolated from blood if lysis-centrifugation blood cultures or the Bactec blood culture system is used. Isolates then may be identified using a commercially available system (Microscan Rapid Anaerobe Panel, Baxter, Sacramento, CA).[1] Serologic methods for the detection of IgG antibodies to *B. henselae* are available.[1, 91] In a minority of cases, lymph node biopsy is undertaken to exclude other, more serious, pathologies; the characteristic histopathologic features confirm the diagnosis. Even so, skin or lymph node biopsy is not advocated in the patient with typical cat-scratch disease.

If after the aforementioned evaluation the etiology of the adenitis remains uncertain or the lymphadenopathy has persisted with no detectable response to antimicrobial therapy, a more intense diagnostic evaluation is indicated. Studies may include a complete blood count; a venereal disease research laboratory test; serology for EBV, CMV, HHV-6, HIV, histoplasmosis, coccidioidomycosis, toxoplasmosis, tularemia, *B. henselae,* and *Brucella;* and a roentgenogram of the chest. If the diagnosis remains in doubt and the node persists, enlarges, is hard, or is fixed to the adjacent structures, biopsy *should* be performed. Biopsy material should be submitted for the studies outlined earlier for lymph node aspirate cultures as well as for routine histology; Giemsa, periodic acid–Schiff, and methenamine silver stains; and, in select cases only, viral cultures. If the histology reveals noncaseating granulomas and the child has a history of cat exposure, the most likely diagnosis is cat-scratch disease[50, 53] and serologic testing is indicated. Sarcoidosis involving lymph nodes would have a similar histology but is rare in children and a condition in which isolated cervical node involvement has not been observed.[38, 75]

Older children are more likely to have negative cultures of lymph node aspirates[9, 81] and to be more frequent candidates for excisional lymph node biopsy. They also are more likely to have lymphomas. Thus, it is important that appropriate tissue be excised, especially from adolescents, so that precise diagnostic interpretation can be made. This can be facilitated by the proper selection of a lymph node to be biopsied; intact removal of the node chosen; and proper fixation, cutting, and staining of the specimen.[18] If only one node or one anatomic group of nodes is enlarged, the largest node should be excised. If several groups of lymph nodes are involved, the site for biopsy should be selected according to the likelihood of diagnostic yield. Biopsies from the lower neck and supraclavicular area have the highest yield.[42] Other areas, including the upper cervical, submandibular, axillary, and parotid lymph nodes, are much more likely to be affected by reactive hyperplasia, which may or may not be related to the underlying disease process. If lymphoma is suspected, needle biopsies or frozen sections are contraindicated.[12, 19]

Even under optimal conditions, many reactive processes have been noted to simulate lymphoma, including rheumatoid arthritis, toxoplasmosis, Dilantin-induced adenopathy, dermatopathic adenitis, and infectious mononucleosis.[19] A thorough history and appropriate serologic studies should be able to exclude reactive processes known to simulate lymphoma.

TREATMENT

Optimal management of the child with cervical lymphadenitis depends on an accurate assessment of the underlying etiology. Because almost all cases are associated with infectious agents, every effort should be made to ascertain the etiologic agent so that specific therapy can be initiated. Aspiration of the affected lymph node for Gram and acid-fast stains will serve as a guide for initial therapy, and culture and antimicrobial susceptibility will form the basis for prescribing specific treatment in patients with bacterial lymphadenitis.[9, 27] However, when the patient presents with typical findings of acute bacterial lymphadenitis, empiric therapy may be undertaken without prior needle aspiration. In this situation, close follow-up is essential because failure to show some clinical response after 48 hours of therapy is an indication for this diagnostic procedure to be performed.

Acute suppurative cervical lymphadenitis most frequently is caused by infection with *S. aureus* or group A streptococci.[9, 16, 27, 73, 81, 90] In nodes that progress to abscess formation, *S. aureus* is the single most frequent agent isolated[9, 27, 73] and drainage is mandatory. Ultrasound evaluation of the involved nodes is useful to detect suppuration within the gland and, thus, the need for drainage. Because of the frequency of infection caused by *S. aureus* or group A *Streptococcus*, empiric antimicrobial therapy should be directed against these two agents. Penicillinase-resistant penicillins should be used. If the patient requires parenteral therapy, oxacillin or nafcillin (150 mg/kg/day) may be used, or, when oral therapy is deemed to be adequate, cloxacillin (50 mg/kg/day) or dicloxacillin (25 mg/kg/day) is recommended. Augmentin, the fixed combination of amoxicillin and clavulanic acid, provides good activity against methicillin-susceptible staphylococci and streptococci and has an expanded spectrum of activity against the oral anaerobic organisms. These features, combined with its palatability, make it an attractive alternative to the traditional penicillinase-resistant penicillins. However, clavulanate-associated diarrhea can be problematic in some children. In penicillin-allergic patients, cephalosporins may be used: cefazolin (100 mg/kg/day) for parenteral use and cephalexin (25 to 50 mg/kg/day) for oral use. Once-daily ceftriaxone (50 to 100 mg/kg/day) is an attractive and effective alternative to the parenteral antibiotics that require more frequent administration. Cefixime is *not* active against *S. aureus* and is not a suitable agent for the empiric treatment of bacterial adenitis. Clindamycin (30 mg/kg/day) for parenteral or oral use also has good antistaphylococcal and anaerobic activity. Antibiotic therapy may need to be modified if there is an obvious primary focus of infection suggesting a different etiologic agent. For example, in the patient with periodontal or dental disease, adequate anaerobic activity is mandatory and therapy with penicillin V (50 mg/kg/day), augmentin (40 mg/kg/day), or clindamycin (30 mg/kg/day) should be initiated, pending results of cultures.

Patients with marked lymph node enlargement, moderate-to-severe systemic symptoms, or concomitant cellulitis frequently require parenteral therapy for the first few days. This allows for a high concentration of the drug within the inflamed tissue and may promote more rapid localization, especially in patients with staphylococcal adenitis. Although the use of parenteral drugs has to be individualized, most infants and children with staphylococcal or streptococcal lymphadenitis respond to orally administered antimicrobials.

Adenitis caused by group A streptococci should be treated with penicillin G (100,000 IU/kg/day) or penicillin V (50 mg/kg/day) for a total of 10 days. In the child with penicillin allergy, erythromycin ethyl succinate (40 mg/kg/day) or cephalexin (25 to 50 mg/kg/day) may be used. Both drugs have been demonstrated to be effective in the treatment of cervical lymphadenitis.[9, 15] Treatment should be continued for at least 10 days or approximately 5 days after signs of local inflammation and systemic toxicity have disappeared, whichever is the longer. If required, analgesics should be given and not overlooked in infants and children too young to verbalize their discomfort. The average duration of antibiotic therapy is 10 days, unless abscess formation occurs late in the first or early in the second week of treatment.[15] In this situation, incision and drainage are indicated,[9, 16, 27] and therapy should be continued until resolution of the acute process occurs, usually within another 5 to 7 days.

Some clinical improvement is to be expected within 48 hours after initiation of therapy, and this will be manifested by a decrease in inflammation and tenderness of the lymph node as well as a fall in the maximum daily temperature. The size of the lymph node may not show evidence of regression at this stage, and total resolution of fever should not be expected. It is important to record accurate measurements of the node at the time of presentation because a subjective evaluation is an unreliable indicator of lymph node evolution during therapy. If no clinical improvement is noted by 48 hours, needle aspiration is recommended. Furthermore, the history and physical examination should be reassessed and a more detailed laboratory evaluation initiated. Regression of lymph node size is slow, usually requiring 4 to 6 weeks or more. Persistence of significant enlargement beyond 6 to 8 weeks, even in the face of good initial response to antimicrobial therapy, demands that an underlying disorder be excluded. Once signs of acute inflammation have resolved, prolonged antimicrobial therapy is of little value because penetration of antimicrobials through the fibrous capsule of the node is poor.[15] Spontaneous regression occurs in most patients, although this may require several weeks. Uncommonly, reactivation of inflammation may occur and a meticulous search for an untreated primary source of bacterial infection, such as a secondarily infected dermatitis, infestation, a foreign body, or dental abscess, should be undertaken. Re-treatment should include specific measures to eliminate the predisposing condition.

If Gram stain of the lymph node aspirate suggests a microorganism other than *S. aureus* or group A streptococci, initial antimicrobial therapy should be directed at the most likely agent until culture results are known. Because attempts to perform careful Gram stains and careful anaerobic cultures of lymph node aspirates in most reported series have been limited, the large number of infants and children with sterile aspirates may be attributed, in part, to a failure to isolate fastidious anaerobes indigenous to the mouth. These microorganisms should respond to penicillin G therapy. For penicillin-resistant organisms, clindamycin is a useful alternative drug. In the first 2 months of life, group B streptococci as well as *S. aureus* are important pathogens to consider in selecting initial therapy. Penicillinase-resistant penicillins are active against both agents. If group B streptococci are isolated, penicillin G can be substituted. Final bacteriologic identification and antimicrobial susceptibility tests should be the ultimate guide to specific antimicrobial therapy in all patients. Treatment of cervical lymph node infections associated with rarely encountered bactéria, fungi, and parasites listed in Table 15–3 is discussed under those specific disease entities.

Although controversy exists as to whether cervical adenitis associated with *M. tuberculosis* in a child is truly a localized process, only rarely do patients have disseminated infection.[28, 33, 60] When infection is not localized, pulmonary or hilar lymph node involvement is common.[28, 39, 62, 90] A 6-month regimen of isoniazid (10 mg/kg/day), rifampin (15 to 20 mg/kg/day), and pyrazinamide (30 mg/kg/day) or, in the child older than 10 years of age, ethambutol (15 to 25 mg/kg/day to a maximum of 1500 mg) currently is recommended for the treatment of uncomplicated intrathoracic pulmonary tuberculosis or isolated cervical lymphadenitis in children.[5] Triple therapy is given daily for the first 2 months of therapy, after which isoniazid and rifampin are administered, either daily or on a twice-weekly basis, for the following 4 months. In areas where multiple drug resistance in *M. tuberculosis* is prevalent, an additional agent is added for initial treatment. Detailed discussion of the treatment of tuberculosis in children is provided in Chapter 101. Response to antituberculous therapy is usual, with rapid resolution of symptoms and marked regression of lymph nodes within 3 months. However, nodes remain palpable for months because scarring and fibrosis are regular accompaniments to resolution of disease. Draining sinuses, a common complication of lymph node aspiration or incision and drainage prior to the advent of effective antituberculous chemotherapy, no longer develop.[62]

Cervical lymphadenitis attributed to atypical mycobacteria is much more common in the young child than that caused by *M. tuberculosis.* These microorganisms demonstrate in vitro resistance to commonly employed antituberculous drugs. Resistance particularly is common among Runyon groups II and III mycobacteria (*M. scrofulaceum* and *M. intracellulare,* respectively). Surgical excision is the treatment of choice for nontuberculous mycobacterial lymphadenitis,[52] and total removal of all the visibly affected nodes is recommended.[3, 24, 35, 69, 88] When this is impossible or when it would result in considerable cosmetic problems, thorough curettage has been found to be effective.[60] Antituberculous therapy generally has been ineffective.[54] Rifabutin, an analogue of rifampin, and the new macrolides clarithromycin and azithromycin each exhibit activity against *M. avium-intracellulare* and offer renewed optimism for the medical treatment of lymphadenitis caused by this agent. The successful treatment of a child with *M. avium* complex parotid lymphadenitis using a combination of clarithromycin and ethambutol has been reported.[32]

Cat-scratch disease usually is a benign, self-limited disorder requiring no specific therapy. Antimicrobials have no proven efficacy, but agents such as trimethoprim-sulfamethoxazole or rifampin for young children and ciprofloxacin for adolescents are recommended by some experts. If the lymph node progresses to fluctuance, needle aspiration may hasten resolution and also relieve discomfort. Surgical excision may be required in a minority of patients who have persistence despite needle aspiration or who develop draining sinuses.

PROGNOSIS

With effective antimicrobial therapy, complete resolution of cervical lymphadenitis due to *S. aureus*, group A streptococci, and *M. tuberculosis* is the rule. Delay in diagnosis or initiation of therapy may prolong the clinical course and even may result in complications or sequelae, such as sinus tracts (mycobacteria),[13, 62] abscess formation,[15, 26] cellulitis or bacteremia *(S. aureus* and *S. pyogenes),*[9] acute glomerulonephritis (group A streptococci),[27] disseminated disease *(M. tuberculosis),*[39] or even mycotic carotid artery aneurysm.[87] Except for abscess formation, these complications are rare. Although lymph node infection caused by *S. aureus* is more likely to result in abscess formation, at least one study has noted a significantly greater duration of infection prior to treatment in patients in whom *S. aureus* was isolated from the abscess cavity cultures.[9] The extracellular products of this organism (coagulase, fibrinolysin, hyaluronidase, and so on) in part explain its propensity for abscess formation, which may occur in 50 to 70 per cent of patients.[16, 27, 89] Even in patients whose course is complicated by suppuration, appropriate drainage in conjunction with specific antimicrobial therapy results in prompt resolution of signs and symptoms, and only rarely will relapse occur. Today, it is uncommon to recommend surgical excision of affected nodes, with the exception of disease due to atypical mycobacteria, for which surgical excision remains the treatment of choice. Antimicrobial therapy has been responsible for the disappearance of those events commonly associated with cervical adenitis historically: thrombosis of the internal jugular vein, rupture of the carotid artery, generalized septic embolic phenomena, mediastinal abscess, purulent pericarditis, and even death.[43, 80, 89]

With the advent of effective antituberculous agents, the prognosis for tuberculous cervical adenitis also is excellent. With surgical excision early in the course of lymphadenitis caused by atypical mycobacterial infection, resolution can be anticipated.[69] Persistent and recurrent disease is the most frequent complication encountered.[88] Cat-scratch disease usually is a benign, self-limited disorder only rarely requiring therapeutic intervention, such as needle aspiration, to relieve pain.

PREVENTION

Appropriate medical and, occasionally, surgical therapy of predisposing conditions (e.g., dental caries, abscess, and/or group A streptococcal pharyngitis or nasopharyngitis, purulent otitis media, impetigo, other infections involving the face and scalp) and minimizing the exposure of infants and children to adults with active tuberculosis should reduce the incidence of cervical lymphadenitis. Some authors suggest that decreased exposure to animals may result in fewer infections,[9] especially for adenitis attributed to toxoplasmosis or cat scratches.[23, 66]

References

1. Adal, K. A., Cockerell, C. J., and Petri, W. A., Jr.: Cat scratch disease, bacillary angiomatosis, and other infections due to *Rochalimaea*. N. Engl. J. Med. *330*:1509–1515, 1994.
2. Akashi, K., Eizuru, Y., Sumiyoshi, Y., et al.: Brief report: Severe infectious mononucleosis–like syndrome and primary human herpes 6 infection in an adult. N. Engl. J. Med. *329*:168–171, 1993.
3. Altman, R. P., and Margileth, A. M.: Cervical lymphadenopathy from atypical mycobacteria: Diagnosis and surgical treatment. J. Pediatr. Surg. *10*:419–422, 1975.
4. Alvi, A., and Myssiorek, D.: *Mycobacterium chelonae* causing recurrent neck abscess. Pediatr. Infect. Dis. J. *12*:617–618, 1993.
5. American Academy of Pediatrics: Tuberculosis. *In* Peter, G. (ed.): 1994 Red Book: Report of the Committee on Infectious Diseases. 23rd. ed. Elk Grove Village, IL, American Academy of Pediatrics, 1994, p. 489.
6. Armstrong, K. L., James, R. W., Dawson, D. J., et al.: *Mycobacterium haemophilum* causing perihilar or cervical lymphadenitis in healthy children. J. Pediatr. *121*:202–205, 1992.
7. Baker, C. J.: Group B streptococcal cellulitis-adenitis in infants. Am. J. Dis. Child. *136*:631–633, 1982.
8. Bankaci, M., Morris, R. F., Stool, S. E., et al.: Sinus histiocytosis with massive lymphadenopathy: Report of its occurrence in two siblings with retropharyngeal involvement in both. Ann. Otol. Rhinol. Laryngol. *87*:327–331, 1978.
9. Barton, L. L., and Feigin, R. D.: Childhood cervical lymphadenitis: A reappraisal. J. Pediatr. *84*:846–852, 1974.
10. Bell, D. M., Morens, D. M., Holman, R. C., et al.: Kawasaki syndrome in the United States. Am. J. Dis. Child. *137*:211–214, 1983.
11. Bennhoff, D. F.: Actinomycosis: Diagnostic and therapeutic considerations and a review of 32 cases. Laryngoscope *94*:1198–1217, 1984.
12. Betsill, W. L., Jr., and Hajdu, S. I.: Percutaneous aspiration biopsy of lymph nodes. Am. J. Clin. Pathol. *73*:471–479, 1980.
13. Black, B. G., and Chapman, J. S.: Cervical adenitis in children due to human and unclassified mycobacteria. Pediatrics *33*:887–893, 1984.
14. Braun, M. M., and Cauthen, G.: Relationship of the human immunodeficiency virus epidemic to pediatric tuberculosis and bacillus Calmette-Guérin immunization. Pediatr. Infect. Dis. J. *11*:220–220, 1992.
15. Brook, A. H., and Winter, G. B.: Cervico-facial suppurative lymphadenitis due to staphylococcal infection in childhood. Br. J. Oral Surg. *8*:257–263, 1971.
16. Brook, A. H., and Winter, G. B.: Staphylococcal cervico-facial lymphadenitis in children. Lancet *2*:660–661, 1972.
17. Brook, I.: Aerobic and anaerobic bacteriology of cervical adenitis in children. Clin. Pediatr. *19*:693–696, 1980.
18. Buckley, J. G., Hinton, A., and Allen, C.: Kikuchi's disease: Apparent malignancy of a neck mass. J. Laryngol. Otol. *102*:941–944, 1988.
19. Butler, J. J.: Non-neoplastic lesions of lymph nodes of man to be differentiated from lymphomas. Natl. Cancer Inst. Monogr. *32*:233–249, 1969.
20. Carithers, H. A.: Cat-scratch disease: An overview based on a study of 1200 patients. Am. J. Dis. Child. *139*:1124–1133, 1985.
21. Carithers, H. A.: Oculoglandular disease of Parinaud: A manifestation of cat-scratch disease. Am. J. Dis. Child. *132*:1195–1200, 1978.
22. Carithers, H. A.: Cat-scratch disease associated with an osteolytic lesion. Am. J. Dis. Child. *137*:968–970, 1983.
23. Carithers, H. A., Carithers, C. M., and Edwards, R. O., Jr.: Cat-scratch disease: Its natural history. J. A. M. A. *207*:312–316, 1969.
24. Castro, D. J., Hoover, L., Castro, D. J., et al.: Cervical mycobacterial lymphadenitis. Arch. Otolaryngol. *111*:816–819, 1985.
25. Centers for Disease Control and Prevention: Diphtheria epidemic: New independent states of the former Soviet Union. M. M. W. R. *44*:177–181, 1995.
26. Chapman, J. S., and Guy, L. R.: Scrofula caused by atypical mycobacteria. Pediatrics *23*:323–331, 1959.
27. Dajani, A. S., Garcia, R. E., and Wolinsky, E.: Etiology of cervical lymphadenitis in children. N. Engl. J. Med *268*:1329–1333, 1963.
28. Davis, S. D., and Comstock, G. W.: Mycobacterial cervical adenitis in children. J. Pediatr. *58*:771–778, 1961.
29. English, C. K., Wear, D. J., Margileth, A. M., et al.: Cat-scratch disease: Isolation and culture of the bacterial agent. J. A. M. A. *259*:1347–1352, 1988.
30. Fujimori, T., Shioda, K., and Sussman, E. B.: Subacute necrotising lymphadenitis: A clinicopathologic study. Acta Pathol. Jpn. *31*:791–797, 1981.
31. Gill, M. J., Fanning, E. A., and Chomyc, S.: Childhood lymphadenitis in a harsh northern climate due to atypical mycobacteria. Scand. J. Infect. Dis. *19*:77–83, 1987.
32. Green, P. A., von Reyn, C. F., and Smith, R. P., Jr.: *Mycobacterium avium* complex parotid lymphadenitis: Successful therapy with clarithromycin and ethambutol. Pediatr. Infect. Dis. J. *12*:615–617, 1993.
33. Gutman, L. T., Moye, J., Zimmer, B., et al.: Tuberculosis in human immunodeficiency virus–exposed or –infected United States children. Pediatr. Infect. Dis. J. *13*:963–968, 1994.
34. Hall, C. B., Long, C. E., Schnabel, K. C., et al.: Human herpesvirus-6 infection in children. N. Engl. J. Med. *331*:432–438, 1994
35. Harris, B. H., Webb, W., Wilkinson, A. H., et al.: Mycobacterial lymphadenitis. J. Pediatr. Surg. *17*:589–590, 1982.
36. Huebner, R. E., Schein, M. F., Cauthen, G. M., et al.: Usefulness of skin testing with mycobacterial antigens in children with cervical lymphadenopathy. Pediatr. Infect. Dis. J. *11*:450–456, 1992.
37. Jaffe, B. F.: Pediatric head and neck tumors: A study of 178 cases. Laryngoscope *83*:1644–1651, 1973.
38. Kendig, E. L., Jr.: The clinical picture of sarcoidosis in children. Pediatrics *54*:289–292, 1974.
39. Kent, D. C.: Tuberculous lymphadenitis: Not a localized disease process. Am. J. Med. Sci. *254*:866–873, 1967.
40. Koehler, J. E., LeBoit, P. E., Egbert, B. M., et al.: Cutaneous vascular lesions and disseminated cat-scratch disease in patients with the acquired immunodeficiency syndrome (AIDS) and AIDS-related complex. Ann. Intern. Med. *109*:449–455, 1988.
41. Knight, P. J., Hamoudi, A. B., and Vassy, L. E.: The diagnosis and treatment of midline neck masses in children. Surgery *93*:603–611, 1983.
42. Knight, P. J., Mulne, A. F., and Vassy, L. E.: When is lymph node biopsy indicated in children with enlarged peripheral nodes? Pediatrics *69*:391–396, 1982.
43. Kratz, R. C., Stine, F. A., Grover, J. W., et al.: Suppurations of the neck. Arch. Otolaryngol. *70*:692–695, 1959.
44. Lai, K. K., Stottmeier, K. D., Sherman, I. H., et al.: Mycobacterial cervical lymphadenopathy: Relation of etiologic agents to age. J. A. M. A. *251*:1286–1288, 1984.
45. Lampe, R. M., Baker, C. J., Septimus, E. J., et al.: Cervicofacial nocardiosis in children. J. Pediatr. *99*:593–595, 1981.
46. Lincoln, E. M., and Gilbert, L. A.: Disease in children due to mycobacteria other than *Mycobacterium tuberculosis*. Am. Rev. Resp. Dis. *105*:683–714, 1972.
47. Lockhart, R. D., Hamilton, G. F., and Fyfe, F. W.: Anatomy of the Human Body. Philadelphia, J. B. Lippincott, 1959, pp. 662–664.
48. Lyon, L. W.: Neurologic manifestations of cat-scratch disease: Report of a case and review of the literature. Arch. Neurol. *25*:23–27, 1971.
49. Marasco, W. A., Lester, S., and Parsonnet, J.: Unusual presentation of cat

scratch disease in a patient positive for antibody to the human immunodeficiency virus. Rev. Infect. Dis. *11*:793–803, 1989.
50. Margileth, A. M.: Cat scratch disease: Nonbacterial regional lymphadenitis: The study of 145 patients and a review of the literature. Pediatrics *42*:803–818, 1968.
51. Margileth, A. M.: The use of purified protein derivative mycobacterial skin test antigens in children and adolescents: Purified protein derivative skin test results correlated with mycobacterial isolates. Pediatr. Infect. Dis. *2*:225–231, 1983.
52. Margileth, A. M.: Management of nontuberculous (atypical) mycobacterial infections in children and adolescents. Pediatr. Infect. Dis. *4*:119–121, 1985.
53. Margileth, A. M.: Cat-scratch disease update. Am. J. Dis. Child. *138*:711–713, 1984.
54. Margileth, A. M., Chandra, R., and Altman, R. P.: Chronic lymphadenopathy due to mycobacterial infection: Clinical features, diagnosis, histopathology, and management. Am. J. Dis. Child. *138*:917–921, 1984.
55. Margileth, A. M., Wear, D. J., Hadfield, T. L., et al.: Cat-scratch disease: Bacteria in skin at the primary inoculation site. J. A. M. A. *252*:928–931, 1984.
56. McCabe, R. E., Brooks, R. G., Dorfman, R. F., et al.: Clinical spectrum in 107 cases of toxoplasmic lymphadenopathy. Rev. Infect. Dis. *9*:754–774, 1987.
57. Melish, M. E., Hicks, R. V., and Reddy, R.: Kawasaki syndrome: An update. Hosp. Pract. *17*:99–105, 1982.
58. Moussatos, G. H., and Baffes, T. G.: Cervical masses in infants and children. Pediatrics *32*:251–256, 1963.
59. O'Brien, R. J., Geiter, L. J., and Snider, D. E., Jr.: The epidemiology of nontuberculous mycobacterial diseases in the United States. Am. Rev. Resp. Dis. *135*:1007–1014, 1987.
60. Olson, N. R.: Nontuberculous mycobacterial infections of the face and neck: Practical considerations. Laryngoscope *91*:1714–1726, 1981.
61. Omokoku, R., and Castells, S.: Post-DPT inoculation cervical lymphadenitis in children. N. Y. State J. Med. *81*:1667–1668, 1981.
62. Ord, R. J., and Matz, G. J.: Tuberculous cervical lymphadenitis. Arch. Otolaryngol. *99*:327–329, 1974.
63. Pounds, L. A.: Neck masses of congenital origin. Pediatr. Clin. North Am. *28*:841–844, 1981.
64. Powers, G. F., and Boisvert, P. L.: Age as a factor in streptococcosis. J. Pediatr. *25*:481–504, 1944.
65. Prince, D. S., Peterson, D. D., Steiner, R. M., et al.: Infection with *Mycobacterium avium* complex in patients without predisposing conditions. N. Engl. J. Med. *321*:863–868, 1989.
66. Rafaty, F. M.: Cervical adenopathy secondary to toxoplasmosis. Arch. Otolaryngol. *103*:547–549, 1977.
67. Rosai, J., and Dorfman, R. F.: Sinus histiocytosis with massive lymphadenopathy: A newly recognized benign clinicopathological entity. Arch. Pathol. *87*:63–70, 1969.
68. Ryan-Poirier, K., and Patrick, C. C.: Cervical adenitis caused by *Staphylococcus epidermidis*. J. Clin. Microbiol. *31*:426–427, 1993.
69. Schaad, U. B., Votteler, T. P., McCracken, G. H., et al.: Management of atypical mycobacterial lymphadenitis in childhood: A review based on 380 cases. J. Pediatr. *95*:356–360, 1979.
70. Schlossberg, D., Morad, Y., Krouse, T. B., et al.: Culture-proved disseminated cat-scratch disease in acquired immunodeficiency syndrome. Arch. Intern. Med. *149*:1437–1439, 1989.
71. Schroder, K. E., Elverland, H. H., Mair, I. W. S., et al.: Granulomatous cervical lymphadenitis. J. Otolaryngol. *8*:127–131, 1979.
72. Schuit, K. E., and Powell, D. A.: Mycobacterial lymphadenitis in childhood. Am. J. Dis. Child. *132*:675–677, 1978.
73. Scobie, W. G.: Acute suppurative adenitis in children: Review of 964 cases. Scott. Med. J. *14*:352–354, 1969.
74. Shirakusa, T., Eimoto, T., Kikuchi, M., et al.: Histiocytic necrotizing lymphadenitis. Postgrad. Med. J. *64*:107–109, 1988.
75. Siltzbach, L. E., and Greenberg, G. M.: Childhood sarcoidosis: A study of 18 patients. N. Engl. J. Med. *279*:1239–1244, 1968.
76. Sommers, H. M., and Good, R. C.: Mycobacterium. *In* Lennette, E. H., Balows, A., Hausler, W. J., Jr., et al. (eds.): Manual of Clinical Microbiology. 4th ed. American Society for Microbiology, 1985, pp. 216–240.
77. Spark, R. P., Fried, M. L., Bean, C. K., et al.: Nontuberculous mycobacterial adenitis of childhood. Am. J. Dis. Child. *142*:106–108, 1988.
78. Speert, D. P., Britt, W. J., and Kaplan, E. L.: Tick-borne tularemia presenting as ulcerative lymphadenitis. Clin. Pediatr. *18*:239–241, 1979.
79. Starke, J. R., and Taylor-Watts, K. T.: Tuberculosis in the pediatric population of Houston, Texas. Pediatrics *84*:28–35, 1989.
80. Stuteville, O. H.: Otorhinolaryngologic surgery: The spread of infections in the head and neck. J. Int. Coll. Surg. *29*:750–754, 1958.
81. Sundaresh, H. P., Kumar, A., Hokanson, J. T., et al.: Etiology of cervical lymphadenitis in children. Am. Fam. Physician *24*:147–151, 1981.
82. Thomaidis, T., Anastassea-Vlachou, K., Mandalenaki-Lambrou, C., et al.: Chronic lymphoglandular enlargement and toxoplasmosis in children. Arch. Dis. Child. *52*:403–407, 1977.
83. Thompson, J. N., Watanabe, M. J., Greene, G. R., et al.: Atypical mycobacterial cervical adenitis: Clinical presentation. Laryngoscope *90*:287–294, 1980.
84. Tomblin, J. L., and Roberts, F. J.: Tuberculous cervical lymphadenitis. Can. Med. Assoc. J. *121*:324–330, 1979.
85. Turner, R. R., Martin, J., and Dorfman, R. F.: Necrotizing lymphadenitis: A study of 30 cases. Am. J. Surg. Pathol. *7*:115–123, 1983.
86. Waggoner-Fountain, L. A., Hayden, G. F., and Hendley, J. O.: Kawasaki syndrome masquerading as bacterial lymphadenitis. Clin. Pediatr. *34*:185–189, 1995.
87. Wells, R. G., and Sty, J. R.: Cervical lymphadenitis complicated by mycotic carotid artery aneurysm. Pediatr. Radiol. *21*:402–403, 1991.
88. Wolinsky, E.: Mycobacterial lymphadenitis in children: A prospective study of 105 nontuberculous cases with long-term follow-up. Clin. Infect. Dis. *20*:954–963, 1995.
89. Wright, N. L.: Cervical infections. Am. J. Surg. *113*:379–386, 1967.
90. Yamauchi, T., Ferrieri, P., and Anthony, B. F.: The aetiology of acute cervical adenitis in children: Serological and bacteriological studies. J. Med. Microbiol. *13*:37–43, 1980.
91. Zangwill, K. M., Hamilton, D. H., Perkins, B. A., et al.: Cat scratch disease in Connecticut: Epidemiology, risk factors, and evaluation of a new diagnostic test. N. Engl. J. Med. *329*:8–13, 1993.

16

PAROTITIS

Judith R. Campbell

Parotitis, inflammation of the parotid gland, is caused by a variety of infectious agents and noninfectious systemic illnesses. Several definitions are used to describe the clinical presentations and etiologic processes that lead to parotid gland swelling and inflammation. *Suppurative parotitis*, first described in the 1800s, is a serious bacterial infection in neonates and postsurgical patients.[25] *Epidemic parotitis*, particularly prevalent in the prevaccine era, primarily was due to mumps virus infection.[29] In the postvaccine era, this form of parotitis also is due to other viral pathogens and therefore is referred to as *viral parotitis*. Rarely, a more indolent, slowly progressive, granulomatous infection may occur that is referred to as *granulomatous parotitis*. *Recurrent parotitis of childhood* is a unique illness that is characterized by multiple episodes of acute and subacute parotid gland swelling. The histologic findings in this disease include architectural changes in the ducts and chronic inflammation. Many noninfectious systemic illnesses cause persistent or recurrent parotid gland swelling and inflammation; this is referred to as *chronic parotitis*.

PATHOPHYSIOLOGY

Despite the various agents that cause parotitis, involvement of the gland mainly occurs by three mechanisms. The most common is a localized infection limited to the gland and surrounding structures. Parotitis may be a manifestation of a systemic infection, as in mumps, or rarely may develop secondary to hematogenous seeding during transient bacteremia. There are several common contributing factors and pathophysiologic mechanisms that lead to swelling of the gland. The parotid is well encapsulated and consists of a superficial and a deep lobe that are separated by the facial nerve. The parotid duct (Stensen duct) traverses the buccal soft tissue anteriorly and exits opposite the second upper molar. Thin, watery secretions from the parotid gland cleanse the ductal system and have some bacteriostatic properties, thereby preventing accumulation of bacteria and debris.[19] Factors that predispose individuals to the development of parotitis include side effects of certain drugs and diseases that lead to dehydration, xerostomia, or ductal obstruction (Table 16–1).[19, 25] Decreased salivary flow allows retrograde migration of bacteria. Stasis in the ductal system, due to ductal ectasia, inflammation, calculi, or strictures, allows proliferation of bacteria and inflammation within the gland.

ETIOLOGY

Infectious parotitis may be caused by aerobes, anaerobes, mycobacteria, and viruses (Table 16–2). In all age groups, *Staphylococcus aureus* is the most common organism associated with suppurative parotitis.[23, 25] Gram-negative pathogens (*Escherichia coli* and *Pseudomonas* species) also may cause suppurative parotitis, particularly in neonates and debilitated or hospitalized patients.[16, 24, 25] The role of anaerobic organisms in this infection has become apparent, especially when poor oral hygiene and oral pathology are associated features.[4, 5, 20] In cases of recurrent parotitis of childhood, *Streptococcus* species are the most commonly isolated bacteria.[21, 23] Granulomatous parotitis most often is due to *Mycobacterium tuberculosis* and may occur in the absence of systemic or disseminated tuberculous disease.[19, 22, 27] Other causes of granulomatous parotitis include *Mycobacterium avium-intracellulare, Actinomyces* species, and gram-negative intracellular organisms (*Francisella tularensis* and *Brucella* species).[12, 19] In the postvaccine era, the most common viral cause of parotitis still is the paramyxovirus mumps virus. However, coxsackieviruses, Epstein-Barr virus, influenza A virus, parainfluenza viruses, herpes simplex virus, cytomegalovirus, and lymphocytic-choriomeningitis virus all have been implicated in cases of parotitis.[1, 2, 14, 15, 18, 19]

CLINICAL PRESENTATION AND DIAGNOSIS

A detailed history and physical examination are critical in assisting the clinician in determining the most likely etiology of parotid gland swelling. One should determine the onset and duration of symptoms, their periodicity, and the character of salivary secretions. In addition, the presence of a systemic disease must be excluded. Examination of the parotid gland is achieved best by simultaneous palpation of the intraoral and extraoral salivary structures. Gentle external pressure should be applied to the gland and the parotid duct examined for evidence of purulent secretions or surrounding erythema.

Suppurative parotitis occurs most commonly in neonates or patients with dehydration, poor oral hygiene, malnutrition, or any medication or disease that decreases salivary secretions. Most often the disease is unilateral; however, bilateral suppurative parotitis may occur in as many as 17 per cent of cases.[25] The disease is characterized by acute onset of pain, swelling, warmth, and induration of the involved gland. Associated physical findings may include fever, trismus, malaise, and cervical adenitis. In suppurative parotitis, the Gram stain and culture (aerobic and anaerobic) of purulent material from the duct can provide a specific microbiologic diagnosis. In addition, elevation of the white blood cell count with a neutrophil predominance may help differentiate this form of parotitis from viral parotitis and parotid disease of a noninfectious etiology.

Mumps is the most common form of viral parotitis and is characterized by a prodrome of fever, malaise, anorexia, and headache. Usually, the following day, unilateral or bilateral earache and parotid tenderness develop. The gland or glands enlarge over the subsequent 2 to 3 days, and the orifice of the Stensen duct is erythematous and swollen, yet secretions from the duct are clear. At the point of maximal swelling, the angle of the jaw is obliterated and the earlobe lifted upward and out. The other salivary glands are involved in up to 10 per cent of cases.[21] Rare systemic manifestations of mumps infection include epididymo-orchitis, meningitis, meningoencephalitis, and oophoritis. Other viral agents may produce similar clinical manifestations and can be differentiated from mumps only by culture and hemagglutination-inhibition, complement-fixation, or enzyme-linked immunosorbent assay serology. In viral parotitis, the white blood cell count may be normal, slightly elevated, or depressed, with a lymphocytic predominance.

Granulomatous parotitis typically presents as a painless, slowly enlarging mass without surrounding inflammation. It may be misdiagnosed as a slow-growing tumor until the correct diagnosis often is made by biopsy and culture. Both *M. tuberculosis* and *M. avium-intracellulare* may cause infection in the parenchyma of the gland or in intraglandular or peri-

TABLE 16–1. Predisposing Factors for Parotitis

Drug-Induced Xerostomia	Disease-Related Xerostomia	Obstruction
Anticholinergics	Sjögren syndrome	Dental appliances
Antihistamines	Diabetes mellitus	Oral tumors
Antidepressants	Chronic liver disease	Radiation therapy
Phenothiazines	Cystic fibrosis	Trauma
Beta blockers		
Diuretics		
General anesthesia		

TABLE 16–2. Parotitis: Infectious Etiologies

Aerobic Bacteria	**Mycobacteria**
Staphylococcus aureus	*Mycobacterium tuberculosis*
Alpha-hemolytic streptococci	*Mycobacterium avium-intracellulare*
Streptococcus pneumoniae	Other mycobacteria
Streptococcus pyogenes	**Viruses**
Haemophilus species	Mumps
Pseudomonas aeruginosa	Coxsackie A and B
Escherichia coli	Echoviruses
Proteus species	Epstein-Barr
Salmonella species	Influenza A
Anaerobic Bacteria	Parainfluenza 1 and 3
Peptostreptococcus species	Cytomegalovirus
Prevotella species	Herpes simplex type 1
Fusobacterium species	Lymphocytic-choriomeningitis
Actinomyces species	HIV

glandular lymph nodes.[22] Clinical evidence of systemic tuberculous disease usually is absent. Actinomycosis of the parotid gland causes a slowly enlarging, nodular, nontender gland; however, associated oral or cervicofacial infection usually is present. Fistulas draining yellow or white material with sulfur granules are common.[12]

Recurrent parotitis of childhood is a rare disease, with onset typically before 10 years of age and a peak incidence around 6 years of age.[9, 21] Some authors hypothesize that an underlying congenital abnormality, such as sialectasia, is a common predisposing feature. Clinically, these children experience repeated episodes of fever, pain, and unilateral swelling of the parotid gland. Purulent material often can be expressed from the Stensen duct and, when cultured, often yields streptococcal organisms. Several authors have noted that recurrences become less frequent with increasing age and that the disease tends to cease at the onset of puberty or early adulthood.[9, 21]

HIV has been identified as a cause of chronic parotid enlargement and inflammation. Parotid enlargement may be present in as many as 20 to 50 per cent of children with HIV infection and AIDS.[17, 28, 30] The parotid gland is the only salivary gland that contains lymphoid tissue within the capsule; therefore, enlargement of these lymph nodes may result in parotid enlargement. Intraparotid and periparotid lymph nodes usually have the follicular hyperplasia that has been observed histologically in cervical and other nodes from patients infected with HIV. In addition, the immunocompromised state of patients with AIDS may predispose them to infection of the parotid gland with other agents, such as cytomegalovirus, Epstein-Barr virus, and bacterial agents.[26, 31]

DIFFERENTIAL DIAGNOSIS

Parotitis most often is diagnosed based on clinical presentation, microbiology, serology, and response to empiric therapy. Currently, sialography and computed tomography of the gland are useful in evaluating for anatomic defects, calculi, or abscess formation; however, sialograms are contraindicated in the setting of acute infection.

Noninfectious causes of parotid swelling and inflammation include collagen vascular diseases (Sjögren syndrome and systemic lupus erythematosus), metabolic disorders (hepatic disease, hyperlipoproteinemia, hyperuricemia), endocrine disorders (diabetes mellitus, hypothyroidism), tumors, leukemic infiltration, drugs (antineoplastic chemotherapy), and poisons (iodine).[19, 21, 23] Sjögren syndrome, the most common cause of noninfectious parotitis, is due to lymphocyte-mediated destruction of the exocrine glands.[11, 23] Patients with this disease have diminished or absent glandular secretions and mucosal dryness; therefore, xerostomia and keratoconjunctivitis sicca are prominent clinical features. In addition, the parotid glands are enlarged bilaterally, are firm, and have an irregular contour. Sialography reveals sialectasia, and saliva from these patients has unique biochemical characteristics. Antibodies to nuclear antigens SS-A and SS-B can be detected in the sera of patients with Sjögren syndrome.[23] It is important to remember that patients with chronic noninfectious parotitis have changes in the ductular architecture or strictures that can predispose them to episodes of infectious parotitis.

TREATMENT

Treatment of parotitis includes rehydration, parotid massage, discontinuation of any medications that diminish salivary flow, and sialalogues (e.g., lemon drops, hard candy, chewing gum), which increase salivary flow.[3, 19, 23, 25] In cases of suspected suppurative parotitis, a broad-spectrum antibiotic regimen that is effective against *S. aureus*, *Streptococcus* species, gram-negative organisms, and anaerobes should be administered empiricially, pending specific culture results. Antibiotic regimens frequently employed include penicillinase-resistant penicillins, first-generation cephalosporins, and clindamycin in combination with an aminoglycoside.[3] If the patient has been hospitalized for a prolonged period or if the predominant organisms on Gram stain of the purulent discharge are gram-negative, ceftazidime should be considered as initial empiric therapy.[23, 25] The treatment of viral parotitis consists of antipyretics, analgesia, and hydration. In cases of mycobacterial infection, excision of the gland may be required, in addition to specific antimycobacterial therapy.[22, 27] Reports have described successful treatment of parotitis due to atypical mycobacteria with clarithromycin and azithromycin.[10] In contrast, actinomycosis of the parotid gland is managed medically with penicillin G.[12] Children with recurrent parotitis should be treated with antibiotics during acute episodes, but chronic suppressive antimicrobial therapy is not recommended. Only 10 to 20 per cent of these patients will require surgical excision of the gland for persistence of symptoms beyond puberty.[7]

COMPLICATIONS

With improved fluid management of postsurgical patients and the use of broad-spectrum antimicrobial agents, complications secondary to infectious parotitis now are rare. In neonates or immunocompromised patients, sepsis may be a severe complication of this infection. Abscess formation may result from delayed or ineffective therapy. The most serious and rare complication is extension to other structures of the head and neck and along fascial planes to the face, external auditory canal, jugular vein, mandible, and even the mediastinum.

PREVENTION

Suppurative parotitis can be prevented in postsurgical patients by maintaining adequate hydration and good oral hygiene. The most common form of viral parotitis, mumps, can be prevented by appropriate vaccination. However, in the mid-1980s, a relative resurgence of mumps in previously vaccinated populations was noted.[6, 13] It is expected that the current recommendation to revaccinate children with measles-mumps-rubella vaccine at 11 or 12 years of age will reduce the occurrence of mumps in previously vaccinated children.[8]

References

1. Arditi, M., Langman, C. B., Christensen, M., et al.: Probable herpes simplex virus type 1–related acute parotitis, nephritis and erythema multiforme. Pediatr. Infect. Dis. J. *7*:427–429, 1988.
2. Brill, S. J., and Gilfillan, R. F.: Acute parotitis associated with influenza type A: A report of twelve cases. N. Engl. J. Med. *296*:1391–1392, 1977.
3. Brook, I.: Diagnosis and management of parotitis. Arch. Otolaryngol. Head Neck Surg. *118*:469–471, 1992.
4. Brook, I., and Finegold, S. M.: Acute suppurative parotitis caused by anaerobic bacteria: Report of two cases. Pediatrics *62*:1019–1020, 1978.
5. Brook, I., Frazier, E. H., and Thompson, D. H.: Aerobic and anaerobic microbiology of acute suppurative parotitis. Laryngoscope *101*:170–172, 1991.
6. Cochi, S. L., Preblud, S. R., and Orenstein, W. A.: Perspectives on the

relative resurgence of mumps in the United States. Am. J. Dis. Child. *142*:499–507, 1988.
7. Cohen H.A., Gross S., Nussinovitch M., et al.: Recurrent parotitis. Arch. Dis. Child. *67*:1036–1037, 1992.
8. Committee on the Control of Infectious Diseases, American Academy of Pediatrics 1994 Red Book: Report of the Committee on the Control of Infectious Diseases. 23rd ed. Evanston, IL, American Academy of Pediatrics, 1994.
9. Ericson, S., Zetterlund, B., and Öhman, J.: Recurrent parotitis and sialectasis in childhood: Clinical, radiologic, immunologic, bactetriologic, and histologic study. Ann. Otol. Rhinol. Laryngol. *100*:527–535, 1991.
10. Green, P. A., Fordham von Reyn, C., and Smith, Jr., R. P.: *Mycobacterium avium* complex parotid lymphadenitis: Successful therapy with clarithromycin and ethambutol. Pediatr. Infect. Dis. J. *12*:615–617, 1993.
11. Hearth-Holmes, M., Baethge, B. A., Abreo, F., et al.: Autoimmune exocrinopathy presenting as recurrent parotitis of childhood. Arch. Otolaryngol. Head Neck Surg. *119*:347–349, 1993.
12. Hensher, R., and Bowerman, J.: Actinomycosis of the parotid gland. Br. J. Oral Maxillofac. Surg. *23*:128–134, 1985.
13. Hersh, B. S., Fine, P. E. M., Kent, W. K., et al.: Mumps outbreak in a highly vaccinated population. J. Pediatr. *119*:187–193, 1991.
14. Jantausch, B. A., Wiedermann, B. L., and Jeffries, B.: Parainfluenza virus type 2 meningitis and parotitis in an 11-year-old child. South. Med. J. *88*:230–231, 1995.
15. Krilov, L. R., and Swenson, P.: Acute parotitis associated with influenza A infection. J. Infect. Dis. *152*:853, 1985.
16. Leake, D., and Leake, R: Neonatal suppurative parotitis. Pediatrics *46*:203–207, 1970.
17. Lepage, P., Van de Perre, P., and Van Vliet, G., et al.: Clinical and endocrinologic manifestations in perinatally human immunodeficiency virus type 1–infected children aged 5 years or older. Am. J. Dis. Child *145*:1248–1251, 1991.
18. Lewis, J. M., and Utz, J. P.: Orchitis, parotitis and meningoencephalitis due to lymphocytic-choriomeningitis virus. N. Engl. J. Med. *265*:776–780, 1961.
19. Loughran, D. H., and Smith L. G.: Review: Infectious disorders of the parotid gland. N. J. Med. *85*:311–314, 1988.
20. Matlow, A., Korentager, R., Keystone, E., et al.: Parotitis due to anaerobic bacteria. Rev. Infect. Dis. *10*:420–423, 1988.
21. Myer, C., and Cotton, R. T.: Salivary gland disease in children: A review. Part 1: Acquired non-neoplastic disease. Clin. Pediatr. *25*:314–322, 1986.
22. O'Connell, J. E., George, M. K., Speculand, B., et al.: Mycobacterial infection of the parotid gland: An unusual cause of parotid swelling. J. Laryngol. Otol. *107*:561–564, 1993.
23. Pou, A. M., Johnson, J. T., and Weissman, J.: Management decisions in parotitis. Compr. Ther. 21:85–92, 1995.
24. Pruett, T. L., and Simmons, R. L.: Nosocomial gram-negative bacillary parotitis. J. A. M. A. *251*:252–253, 1984.
25. Raad, I. I., Sabbagh, M. F., and Caranasos, G. J.: Acute bacterial sialadenitis: A study of 29 cases and review. Rev. Infect. Dis. *12*:591–601, 1990.
26. Redleaf, M. I., Bauer, C. A., and Robinson, R. A.: Fine-needle detection of cytomegalovirus parotitis in a patient with acquired immunodeficiency sydrome. Arch. Otolaryngol. Head Neck Surg. *120*:414–416, 1994.
27. Rowe-Jones, J. M., Vowles, R., Leighton, S. E. J., et al.: Diffuse tuberculous parotitis. J. Laryngol. Otol. *106*:1094–1095, 1992.
28. Schuval, S. J., Bonagura, V. R., and Ilowite, N. T.: Rheumatologic manifestations of pediatric human immunodeficiency virus infection. J. Rheumatol. *20*:1578–1582, 1993.
29. Simpson, R. E. H.: Infectiousness of communicable diseases in the household (measles, chickenpox, and mumps). Lancet 2:549–554, 1952.
30. Sperling, N. M., and Lin, P.-T.: Parotid disease associated with human immunodeficiency virus infection. Ear Nose Throat J. *69*:475–477, 1990.
31. Stellbrink, H.-J., Albrecht, H., and Greten, H.: Pneumococcal parotitis and cervical lymph node abscesses in an HIV-infected patient. Clin. Invest. *72*:1037–1040, 1994.

17

SINUSITIS

James D. Cherry and Anita Newman

Sinusitis is an inflammation of the mucosal lining of one or more of the paranasal sinuses. Although this inflammation of sinus mucosa most probably occurs to some degree with every upper respiratory tract infection that produces rhinitis, there apparently is a spontaneous resolution of the vast majority of these episodes. It has been estimated that 0.5 to 10 per cent of upper respiratory infections are complicated by acute sinusitis.[23, 117] The higher incidence noted in the more recent report may be due to a heightened awareness of the illness and improved sinus imaging. However, the growing number of children in day care has led to a real increase in the incidence of upper respiratory tract infections.[117, 121] In addition, recognition that sinus infection negatively can affect the health of the growing numbers of children with chronic pulmonary disease has increased the interest in this disease.[70]

When considering a diagnosis of sinusitis in a child, the major problem is to distinguish simple upper respiratory tract infection or allergic inflammation from secondary bacterial infection of the sinuses. Sometimes symptoms and signs of sinusitis occur simultaneously with rhinitis, but most often they occur after rhinitis. Infection in the sinuses usually persists after the preceding rhinitis has resolved. Sinusitis is classified by the duration of clinical symptoms: acute (up to 3 weeks), subacute (3–10 weeks), and chronic (>10 weeks).

HISTORY

Purulent sinusitis and its relationship to orbital inflammation have been known for more than 2000 years.[49] Nathaniel Highmore, a seventeenth century English physician and anatomist, is given credit for the separation of dental and antral disease.[85] John Hunter indicated the importance of surgical drainage in purulent sinusitis and suggested perforating the partition between the maxillary antrum and the nose.[85] During the first half of the twentieth century, sinusitis was responsible for considerable morbidity and mortality, and surgical care of sinusitis frequently was lifesaving. Since the advent of antibiotics, sinusitis has had a lower medical profile. However, interest in this topic has increased. The advent of the newer surgical techniques of functional endoscopic sinus surgery that now have been applied to children, improved diagnostic imaging studies, and the greater social importance of upper respiratory tract infections through missed work time for parents when they must seek treatment[70] are just some of the factors involved.

ANATOMY

All the paranasal sinuses develop as outpouchings of the nasal cavity. Three shelf-like structures, the inferior, middle, and superior turbinates, are on the lateral nasal wall. The superior turbinate is not well developed in the first year of life.[131] Beneath each turbinate is the corresponding meatus into which the sinuses open; that is, the frontal, maxillary, and anterior ethmoid sinuses open into the middle meatus. The sphenoid and posterior ethmoid cells open high in the nasal vault into the superior meatus.[118]

The maxillary sinuses develop early in the second trimester of fetal life as lateral outpouchings in the posterior aspect of the middle meatuses. They are present at birth,[3, 73, 97, 131] with floors barely below the attachment of the inferior turbinates.[118] They expand rapidly by 4 years of age.[131] Ultimately, at full size, the lateral borders of the maxillary sinuses reach the lateral orbital rims. The position of the floors of the sinuses is determined by the eruption of the dentition.[118] The ostia of the maxillary sinuses are located high on the medial walls of the sinuses. This impedes gravitational drainage of secretions; ciliary activity is required to move secretions from the body of the maxillary sinuses through the ostia into the nose.[118]

The ethmoid sinuses develop in the fourth month of gestation[118] and are present at birth.[73, 97, 131] They are not a single large cavity but a grouping of cells, 3 to 15 in number, each with its own opening or ostium. They have a honeycombed radiographic appearance and are small anteriorly and large posteriorly. The walls of the ethmoid labyrinth are thin, especially the lateral walls bordering on the orbits; they are referred to as the *lamina papyracea*.[118]

Development of the frontal sinuses is variable. In adults, 80 per cent have bilateral frontal sinuses, 1 to 4 per cent have agenesis of the frontal sinuses, and the remainder have unilateral hypoplasia. The position of the frontal sinuses is supraorbital after 4 years of age, but they are not distinguished radiographically from the ethmoid sinuses until 6 to 8 years of age. The frontal sinuses do not reach adult size for another 8 to 10 years.[118]

The onset of development of the sphenoid sinuses occurs within the first 2 years of life, but they remain rudimentary until about 6 years of age. They have reached their permanent size, although not their permanent shape, by 12 years of age.[131]

Although the full development of the sinuses may take 20 years, by 12 years of age the nasal cavity and the paranasal sinuses nearly have completed their development and have reached adult proportions.[131] Sinus disease in postpubertal adolescents is similar to that in adults.

The mucosal lining of all the paranasal sinuses is composed of ciliated columnar epithelium and goblet cells.[100] It is continuous and similar to that lining the nasal cavity, except that the mucosa in the nose is thicker and contains more glands. The epithelium of all the paranasal sinuses and nasal cavity is covered in part by a mucus blanket.

PATHOPHYSIOLOGY

The pathogenesis of sinus infection undoubtedly is similar to that of otitis media. The middle ear, with its extension, the eustachian tube, and the paranasal sinuses normally are sterile, but their contiguous areas (nasopharynx and nose) have a dynamic microbial flora. Under normal conditions, ciliary function with mucus flow can be expected to keep the sinuses clear of pathogens. The cilia within the sinuses propel the mucus toward their respective ostia, and from there nasal ciliary action moves the mucus blanket posteriorly toward the pharynx. However, insults that damage the ciliary epithelium and affect the morphology, number, and function of cilia or those that alter the production or viscosity of the mucus blanket lead to obstruction of the flow of mucus. This allows the inoculation of large numbers of pathogens into the sinuses, which can lead to infection. Once instituted, sinus infection is complicated further by inflammatory obstruction of the ostium leading to the nose.

Recurrent chronic sinusitis implies a problem with local mucociliary defense, a defect in systemic immunity, or a fixed anatomic sinus obstruction. Often, the predisposing factors work in tandem, as in a child with a septal deformity and a viral illness.[70] In chronic sinusitis, the mucosa is thickened, and there is marked edema, vessel dilatation, and infiltration of inflammatory cells.[112] Goblet cells are decreased in density, and seromucous glands are increased in density compared with their presence in normal sinuses. The single most important factor leading to purulent sinus infection in children as well as in adults is upper respiratory viral infection.[19, 26, 70, 117]

Wald and colleagues[117] in a prospective study involving a large number of children younger than 3 years of age demonstrated a doubling of the rate of sinusitis (defined as upper respiratory symptoms persisting longer than 15 days) among children in a day care setting compared with children not in day care. The differences presumably were due to increased exposure to viral respiratory illnesses. Radiographic studies in children with acute colds regularly indicate abnormalities of the maxillary sinuses, suggesting that the infection involves these areas.[72] These asymptomatic sinus opacifications may persist for 2 weeks after the symptoms of the upper respiratory illness have resolved.[22, 63, 118] Viral infection that involves the sinuses rarely is differentiated from its primary manifestation, such as the common cold, nasopharyngitis, and influenza, and recovery is the rule. However, if the effect of the viral infection on the mucosal surface is severe and is associated with the inoculation of one or more pathogenic bacterial agents and obstruction of an ostium, then disease will occur.

The mechanisms by which upper respiratory viral infections set the stage for secondary bacterial infection in the sinuses are complex. Recent data indicate that the symptoms in upper respiratory viral infections are due not to extensive damage to ciliated nasal epithelium but to aspects of the host response[4, 45, 77, 79, 82, 86, 87, 130] (see Chapter 8).

Other irritants can set the stage for sinus infection. For example, swimming in ocean, lake, or chlorinated pool water can lead to sinus involvement. Drying of the nasal mucosa, which is common during the winter in cold climates, may be a precipitating factor. Children with respiratory allergies are prone to sinusitis,[34, 88–90] and allergy probably is the second most prevalent predisposing factor in childhood sinusitis, acting via mucosa congestion and perhaps depressing local and systemic immune responses.[70, 101] Richards and colleagues[93] reported a diagnosis of atopy in 62 per cent of a selected cohort of pediatric patients who had documented recurrent sinusitis and were referred to allergy clinics in Los Angeles, California. Dental infections or extractions also can lead to maxillary sinusitis if the tooth root is adjacent to the maxillary sinus floor.[20]

Sudden change in pressure, as with diving or during descent in an airplane, physically can overcome local mucociliary defense mechanisms and lead to the sudden onset of acute sinusitis.[70] Defects of ciliary function, such as those occurring in the immotile cilia syndrome and Kartagener syndrome, predispose the child to chronic sinusitis.[27, 54, 61, 90, 97, 105] Refractory sinusitis also is common in children with primary and acquired immunodeficiency diseases.[18, 70, 74, 98, 102, 113] A growing population of immunocompromised children undergoing treatment for malignancies and organ transplants as well as young patients with maternally transmitted and blood-transmitted acquired immunodeficiency syndrome constitute another growing population with a potential for difficult-to-manage sinusitis. Finally, anatomic obstruction due to septal deformities, craniofacial anomalies, foreign bodies, adenoidal hypertrophy, or nasal masses/polyps predisposes children to sinusitis. Nasal polyps in young children usually are not due to allergies and therefore should constitute an indication for a cystic fibrosis evaluation.[70]

Immunologic mechanisms clearly are important in the pathogenesis of sinus infections, as indicated by the high prevalence of chronic sinus infections in children with immunodeficiencies.[18, 70, 74, 98, 102, 113] Sinus and nasal mucus contains immunoglobulins (IgA, IgG, and IgM) and lysozymes.[16, 96] Secretory IgA, which is produced locally, is the predominant immunoglobulin in nasal mucus.[47] IgG antibodies in nasal mucus result from passive leakage from plasma cells in the epithelium and submucosa and from the serum.[12] In general, with increasing age and resulting from previous exposures, these immunoglobulins develop species- and type-specific antibodies that block epithelial colonization by specific microorganisms.

Shapiro and associates[102] studied 61 children with refractory sinusitis and found that 34 had abnormal immunologic studies. Abnormal findings included poor response to pneumococcal type 7 antigen after immunization, IgG 3 subclass deficiency, low serum IgA or IgG values, and elevated serum IgE values.

ETIOLOGY

Although the majority of studies on the etiology of sinusitis have involved adults, adequate pediatric data are available. The findings in studies of adults appropriately can be applied to adolescents as well. Despite the relatively large number of etiologic studies, many workers persist in their opinion that the cause of sinusitis is obscure.[29] This is fostered by the fact that in many studies culture techniques did not allow for exclusion of the nasal flora.

It is important here to examine the results of anterior nasal cultures from normal persons and from those with respiratory illnesses to clear up confusion regarding the make-up of normal flora. During early investigations of the common cold, Shibley and associates[103] noted that in a group of 13 people followed for 4 to 9 months, neither *Haemophilus influenzae* nor hemolytic streptococci were obtained from nasal culture when the subjects were well. However, when their study subjects were ill with colds, *H. influenzae* was recovered from 9 per cent of the cultures and hemolytic streptococci from 6 per cent. In a study of 500 consecutive medical patients, Jacobson and Dick[55] noted in all but two instances that the recovery of pneumococci and hemolytic streptococci from the nose correlated with nasal or sinus disease. Studies in children have disclosed more varied results. Dunlap and Harvey[26] and Harvey and Dunlap[48] were able to recover *H. influenzae*, pneumococci, and hemolytic streptococci from the noses of normal children with some consistency. However, they were interested in carriage and spread of organisms, and therefore the state of well-being of their subjects was not delineated clearly.

Orobello and colleagues[80] found that cultures of ipsilateral middle meatus correlated well with maxillary (83 per cent) and ethmoid (80 per cent) sinus cultures. However, nasopharyngeal cultures correlated less well, with only 45 and 40 per cent of maxillary and ethmoid sinus cultures, respectively, being similar.

Yang[132] studied children in a day nursery and noted that neither pneumococci nor *H. influenzae* could be recovered from the noses of well children. Hays and Mullard[51] only rarely could find *Streptococcus pneumoniae*, beta-hemolytic streptococci, or *H. Influenzae* in nose cultures from normal children. In an extensive study, Box and associates[11] noted pneumococci in nasal specimens of 38 per cent of children without respiratory illness, but in only 3 per cent was the growth of great magnitude (>100 colonies per plate). In the same study, *Haemophilus* species and beta-hemolytic streptococci were recovered from 14 per cent and 1 per cent, respectively, of the cultured specimens from noses. In comparison, in the same study, pneumococci and *Haemophilus* species were recovered from 57 and 25 per cent, respectively, of the cultures of patients with respiratory illness.

In a study carried out in the Finnish military, nasal cultures from 183 healthy recruits revealed the following frequencies of specific organisms: *H. influenzae,* 4 per cent; *S. pneumoniae,* 1 per cent; *Moraxella catarrhalis,* 3 per cent; and *Streptococcus pyogenes,* 0 per cent.[59] In contrast, in 185 recruits with acute maxillary sinusitis, the percentages of nasal isolates for the same organisms were 61, 25, 7, and 6 per cent, respectively. In 91 per cent of cases in which a sinus aspirate culture yielded an isolate, the same organism was found in a nasal sample. Similar results have been obtained in other studies performed in adults with acute sinusitis, in which nontypable *H. influenzae* and *S. pneumoniae* account for approximately 74 per cent of all bacterial strains recovered in sinus aspirates.[29, 46] In all studies, *Staphylococcus aureus* clearly is part of the normal nasal flora. It is present in well or sick children about 50 per cent of the time.

To summarize, it can be stated that finding pneumococci, *H. influenzae, M. catarrhalis,* or *S. pyogenes* in the nose of a normal child is unusual and should suggest a nasal or paranasal infectious illness. However, the recovery of *S. aureus* cannot be correlated with disease.

A review of many reports of children indicates that *S. pneumoniae, H. influenzae,* and *M. catarrhalis* are the most common etiologic agents in acute and subacute ethmoid and maxillary sinusitis.[36, 49, 51, 53, 54, 69, 73, 115, 119, 120, 123, 124, 128] In one of the studies[124] of sinus aspirates from 50 children, *S. aureus* was not isolated from the maxillary sinus. One study of pediatric patients with chronic sinusitis suggested an increased importance of anaerobes and staphylococcal species.[15] In other studies in children with chronic sinusitis who have undergone surgery, a predominance of coagulase-negative staphylococci, viridans streptococci, and *S. aureus* was noted.[75, 80] Several studies[36, 49, 128] documenting that *S. pneumoniae, H. influenzae,* and *M. catarrhalis* were the most common etiologic agents were concerned primarily with orbital involvement; between 50 and 85 per cent of cases of orbital cellulitis had radiographic evidence of sinusitis. Orbital complications of ethmoiditis primarily affect children. *Staphylococcus* species, *S. pneumoniae,* and other streptococci have been found in children with orbital involvement from ethmoiditis[3] or frontal sinusitis.[35]

In Table 17–1, etiologic agents of sinusitis are listed by age of patient and type of illness. It is clear that in all age groups and in acute, subacute, and chronic disease, *H. influenzae* and *S. pneumoniae* are the principal pathogens in the vast majority of cases. It also is clear that a large number of different bacterial species have been recovered from the sinuses of affected patients. In young children, more than 90 per cent of all cases of sinusitis are caused by five organisms: *H. influenzae, S. pneumoniae, M. catarrhalis, S. aureus,* and *S. pyogenes.* In the adolescent, the same organisms, plus largely penicillin-sensitive anaerobes, account for most cases. As noted in Table 17–1, a vast array of gram-negative enteric and other bacilli has been recovered from patients with sinusitis, in most instances from those who have had various forms of antibiotic therapy prior to culture. It also is important to note that organisms previously considered to be nonpathogens, such as *Staphylococcus epidermidis,* have been implicated etiologically.

Although clinically recognized sinusitis has been rare in patients with *Mycoplasma pneumoniae* infection, Griffin and

TABLE 17–1. Etiologic Agents in Sinusitis Analyzed by Patient Age and Type of Illness

	Frequency				Age Group (years)		
	Overall	*Acute*	*Subacute*	*Chronic*	*≤5*	*6–12*	*>12*
Aerobic bacteria							
Haemophilus influenzae	++++	++++	++++	++++	++++	++++	++++
Streptococcus pneumoniae	++++	++++	++++	++++	++++	++++	++++
Moraxella catarrhalis	+++	+++	++	+	+++	+	+
Staphylococcus aureus	++	+	+	++	++	++	++
Streptococcus pyogenes	++	++	++	++	+	++	+
Alpha- and nonhemolytic streptococci	+		+	+			+
Staphylococcus epidermidis	+		+	+		+	+
Alcaligenes species	+			+			+
Escherichia coli	+			+			+
Klebsiella pneumoniae	+			+			+
Pseudomonas aeruginosa	+			+			+
Other*	+			+			+
Anaerobic bacteria							
Peptococcus species	++	+	+	++		+	++
Peptostreptococcus species	++	+	+	++			++
Bacteroides species	++	+	+	++			++
Veillonella	++	+	+	++			++
Other†	+		+	+			+
Mycoplasma							
Mycoplasma pneumoniae	+	+					+
Other							
L-forms	+			+			+
Mixed: aerobes and anaerobes	++	+	+	++			++
Mixed: *Haemophilus influenzae* with other organisms	++	+	+	++		+	++
Other‡	+	+		+		+	+

**Serratia*, diphtheroids, *Enterococcus* species, *Neisseria* species, *Haemophilus* species, *Proteus* species, *Acinetobacter, Citrobacter* species, *Eikenella corrodens*.
†*Fusobacterium* species, *Bifidobacterium, Propionibacterium*.
‡Rhinovirus, adenovirus, *Aspergillus* species, other fungi.
Data from references 5, 10, 14, 15, 17, 25, 29, 31, 32, 39, 58, 59, 64, 69, 81, 90, 91, 107, 108, 111, 114, 115, 119, 120, 123–125.

Klein[40] noted radiographic evidence of sinusitis in about two thirds of a group of Navy recruits with *M. pneumoniae* pneumonia. In adults with chronic suppurative maxillary sinusitis, mycoplasmas have been sought but not recovered.[10, 39, 109] Bhattacharyya and colleagues[10] noted L-forms in 21 per cent of all sinuses in patients with chronic disease.

Fungal diseases of the sinuses have been well described in adults.[126] *Aspergillus* species are the most common fungal causes of sinusitis. It has been suggested that many cases of chronic sinusitis from which a microorganism is not recovered may be due to *Aspergillus* species infections.[60] The presence of eosinophils, Charcot-Leyden crystals, and hyphae found retrospectively, and not noted on the original examination, in mucus recovered from sinuses suggests that some cases of chronic sinusitis may represent *Aspergillus* hypersensitivity. This allergic aspergillosis in the sinuses is similar to allergic bronchopulmonary aspergillosis. In a series of six patients who were 8 to 16 years of age and had allergic aspergillosis sinusitis, all presented with nasal polyposis and facial deformity, indicating advanced disease.[71] Mucormycosis, an infection caused by *Zygomycetes* (formerly *Phycomycetes*) is an infection seen in immunocompromised children and adults.[66] *Drechslera, Bipolaris*, and *Curvalaria lunata* have been added to the list of fungi that can cause sinusitis in children.[9, 32, 106]

Although sinusitis has been reported as a complication of Epstein-Barr virus infection, the sinus infections appear to be a complication of steroid treatment and not specifically the viral infection.[37]

EPIDEMIOLOGY

Although sinus involvement is common with respiratory viral infection, the identification of sinusitis as a specific illness in previously healthy children is uncommon. In a survey of all office visits, totaling 2613, Breese and colleagues[13] noted only six children (0.23 per cent) in whom the initial diagnosis was sinusitis. The true incidence of sinusitis in childhood is unknown. In 1989, Wald and colleagues[119] estimated that between 0.5 and 5 per cent of upper respiratory tract infections are complicated by acute sinusitis. More recent estimates by the same authors have been as high as 10 per cent.[117] The most recent estimates of greater incidence could be related to a heightened awareness and concern for lost work days by working parents, a possible correlation between pulmonary problems in an increasing number of children with chronic lung disease, better imaging techniques, increased interest in endoscopic sinus surgery, more disease because of more exposure due to more children in day care,[70] and an increased recognition or perhaps incidence of allergy-related illness.[92, 93] Seasonal prevalence has not been studied, but it is reasonable to assume that disease would increase during the cold-weather months because this is the time of greatest respiratory viral activity. Cases in older children also can be expected to occur more frequently in association with swimming.

Although it is not well documented, sinusitis appears to be more of a problem in geographic areas where marked temperature changes occur. In children, sinusitis appears to be more common in boys than in girls.[50, 73] Host factors are important in sinusitis because the illness is more common in allergic children, in children with chronic ear infections, and in patients with cystic fibrosis and Kartagener syndrome.[54, 78, 97] Although there appears to be an association between sinus disease and asthma, there still is controversy regarding whether or not sinusitis and other upper airway stimuli can induce asthma.[33, 93, 133] However, a review of hospital admissions of patients with status asthmaticus at the Childrens Hospital of Los Angeles showed a marked increase in admissions in recent years, and sinusitis was diagnosed in 23 per cent.[92] Children with various immunologic defects frequently have sinusitis.

Sinusitis is noncontagious person-to-person, but point-source outbreaks are possible from swimming in heavily contaminated water.

CLINICAL PRESENTATION

The clinical symptomatology of sinusitis varies by age. Older children and adolescents have localized complaints similar to those of adults, whereas in young children, the findings are related less clearly to the sinuses. Table 17–2 presents the overall frequencies of symptoms, signs, and laboratory findings for acute, subacute, and chronic disease.

TABLE 17–2. Clinical Findings in Acute, Subacute, and Chronic Sinusitis of Children

	Per Cent Occurrence	
	Acute and Subacute Sinusitis	*Chronic Sinusitis*
Symptoms		
Fever	50	20
Rhinorrhea	80	80
Cough (persistent and evening)	50	90
Pain/headache	30	30
Sore throat	20	20
Periorbital swelling	30	0
Vomiting	20	10
Allergic history	20	40
Malodorous breath	20	20
Signs		
Rhinorrhea	80	80
Temperature ≥38.3° C (≥101° F)	20	0
Sinus tenderness	20	10
Otitis media	40	60
Posterior pharyngeal pus	0	10
Transillumination positive	30	10
Periorbital swelling	30	0
Malodorous breath	20	20
Laboratory		
Abnormal radiographs	100	100
Maxillary	90	90
Ethmoid	40	40
Frontal and sphenoid	10	10
Unilateral	70	10
Bilateral	30	90
Erythrocyte sedimentation rate elevation	50	10
White blood cell count elevation with an increased percentage of band form neutrophils	40	10

Data from references 1, 7, 50, 52, 56, 61, 62, 73, 78, 90, 93, 97, 107, 120.

In young children, disease involves only the ethmoid and maxillary sinuses. In these children, illness frequently has its onset after an upper respiratory viral infection. However, there may be a period of general improvement between the acute respiratory illness and the symptoms related to sinus infection. The most prominent symptom in all children, and particularly in those younger than 10 years of age, is persistent rhinorrhea. The discharge frequently is purulent, but it can be serous or even watery on occasion. Associated with rhinorrhea is cough, which becomes more prominent with increasing duration of disease. The cough particularly is troublesome at night because it is due to the stimulation by the sinus drainage as it traverses the pharyngeal wall. The posterior drainage also occasionally causes vomiting. Fever is of variable occurrence in sinusitis and, in a general way, is related inversely to both age and duration of illness. Malodorous breath often is reported by parents. The first evidence of illness in some children is fever and periorbital swelling. In most instances, periorbital cellulitis is a manifestation of ethmoid sinusitis.

Although facial pain and headache are frequent complaints of sinus disease in adults, these complaints have been noted only in about one third of the cases in children and are unusual in the young child. The main symptom in the older child and adolescent is rhinorrhea. However, in the older patient with more chronic disease, the nasal symptomatology may be minimal or absent. The complaint of troublesome postnasal drip is frequent.

Physical signs in sinusitis also differ by age. Nasal discharge is the most frequent finding in all age groups. However, young children are more likely to have a serous or watery discharge than are adolescents. Temperature elevation is more common in acute disease and in association with orbital cellulitis. Sinus tenderness, common in older patients, is noted only rarely in children. Particularly significant is tenderness with percussion of the upper molars. Examination of the throat frequently will reveal free exudate. Occasionally, the breath is malodorous.

The ears are abnormal in almost half of all patients with sinusitis. In acute disease in young children, this can be acute otitis media, but usually the findings are more suggestive of serous disease. Acute sinusitis frequently is unilateral, whereas chronic disease more often is bilateral.

Children with chronic sinusitis frequently will have only minimal complaints. The parent will note that the child does not feel well and frequently will report that the child has had a persistent respiratory infection for months. In a series of children with chronic (>3 months) upper respiratory complaints who were referred to allergy clinics, 60 per cent had sinusitis.[78] In this study, the combination of moderate to severe rhinorrhea and cough with minimum sneezing was reported to have a specificity of 95 per cent and a sensitivity of 38 per cent in predicting the presence of chronic sinusitis. In the referred children in this study, sinusitis was found in 63 per cent of atopic children and in 75 per cent of nonatopic children.

Laboratory studies other than cultures and radiography are not very useful in the evaluation of the child with sinusitis. Herz and Gfeller[52] noted that in their study erythrocyte sedimentation rates were elevated in only about one half of the patients, and leukocytosis occurred in only one third. In general, younger children with orbital cellulitis and ethmoid sinusitis are more likely to have both elevated sedimentation rates and white blood cell counts.

DIFFERENTIAL DIAGNOSIS

Differential considerations in sinusitis are not many and are more concerned with whether sinus involvement in a particular child is the primary event or a secondary problem related to a more general host defect. Children with recurrent and chronic sinusitis should be evaluated for respiratory allergy, cystic fibrosis, immunologic deficiency, and Kartagener and other immotile-cilia syndromes.

Foreign bodies in the nose can be mistaken for sinusitis, as can cysts in the maxillary antra. Nasal structural defects (congenital and acquired), such as palatal clefts, unilateral choanal atresia, nasal polyps, and septal deviation, can be confused with sinusitis, but more commonly these problems are predisposing factors in sinus infections.

Dental infections frequently are mistaken for maxillary sinus disease. However, dental infections can lead by direct extension to sinus involvement. Primary infections in the region of the eye also occur without sinus disease. In young children, a chronic infection of the adenoids can be confused clinically with sinusitis. Infections with *Bordetella pertussis* can be confused with subacute sinusitis.

SPECIFIC DIAGNOSIS

Although persistent nasal symptomatology and the presence of other clinical findings as listed in Table 17–2 indicate a diagnosis of sinusitis, the only certain way to make the diagnosis is by obtaining roentgenograms and cultures reflecting sinus flora. Although it has been suggested by some that maxillary sinus roentgenograms frequently are abnormal in normal children,[72, 104] other data indicate that abnormal roentgenograms are infrequent in normal children older than 1 year of age.[63] During infancy, the maxillary sinuses are so small that minimal mucosal edema may "opacify" a sinus on a radiograph. In young children, roentgenographic examination should consist of two views: lateral and Waters. In older children, Caldwell and basal projections also should be performed. It should be pointed out that roentgenograms in acute upper respiratory viral infections as a rule will be abnormal; these are not false-positive roentgenograms but are the result of viral infections. However, from a therapeutic point of view, sinus roentgenograms usually should not be obtained unless nasal symptomatology in an upper respiratory illness has not shown signs of improvement after 5 to 7 days.

Plain film radiographic examination rapidly is being supplanted by computed tomography (CT) and magnetic resonance imaging (MRI) for the diagnosis of sinusitis. Many endoscopic sinus surgeons consider CT to be a mandatory part of the preoperative evaluation. MRI is useful in cases that may be complicated by orbital or intracranial extension. The high prevalence of incidental sinus opacification in asymptomatic infants and children noted radiographically has been confirmed by CT studies.[22, 38] Since the advent of MRI, it has become evident that a significant number of incidental sinus abnormalities also occur in adults. These findings in both children and adults may be from subclinical or resolving respiratory infections or due to unrecognized allergies.[21]

CT has been recognized widely as the standard for the diagnosis of paranasal sinus disease. In particular, coronal thin-section images offer excellent delineation of lesions in the osteomeatal complex.[134] Axial images are useful for the evaluation of periorbital and intraorbital complications.[30] In some institutions, a so-called "screening CT" of the sinuses is performed with a limited number of slices.[43] It can be offered at a cost and radiation exposure that are similar to those associated with plain film studies but with much greater accuracy. Unfortunately, all young children and infants require sedation for CT, which limits its suitability.

Which radiographic technique (plain radiography, CT, or MRI) is selected for evaluation of the child with presumed sinusitis should be determined by availability of techniques and the expertise of the radiologist, as well as clinical symptoms. Roentgenograms, in most instances, should not be obtained early in the illness of children with uncomplicated upper respiratory complaints because of the high incidence of transient abnormalities.[2] Radiography is indicated in children with continuing symptoms of sinusitis after extensive medical therapy or in children with possible complications of sinusitis. If available, CT is optimal.[2] In the absence of low-cost screening CT, plain radiography should be the initial imaging study in most children who have symptoms of sinus disease.[21] Children who have periorbital swelling or proptoses should undergo immediate contrast-enhanced CT studies in both axial and coronal planes. If symptoms or CT findings suggest intracranial extension, MRI should be performed.[2, 21]

Although ultrasonography would appear to offer an alternative to sinus roentgenography, there is some question about its dependability unless there is one normal air-filled maxillary sinus or one opacified maxillary sinus for comparison.[120, 125] The hallmark of specific diagnosis in sinusitis is similar to that of other infectious diseases: the culture of infected material. This erroneously is considered by many physicians as an impossible task because of the inability to obtain material directly from the sinuses of children. However, as discussed in the section on etiology, properly performed nasal culture will reveal the causative organism in the majority of instances. Nasal culture should be taken from the region of the maxillary ostium in the middle meatus. It is important to point out that cultures should be obtained from this area and not from the nasopharynx. Wald and associates[125] found no correlation between bacteria isolated directly from the maxillary sinuses and nasopharyngeal and throat culture isolates. Best results are obtained when a vasoconstrictor, such as 0.25 per cent phenylephrine hydrochloride, is administered first and the culture is obtained with a wire-cotton swab under direct vision. With this technique, material frequently can be obtained as it comes from the sinus ostium. Bilateral cultures always should be obtained. In serious cases, such as children with neurologic complications, or in treatment failures, antral puncture for culture can be lifesaving. Anaerobic as well as aerobic culture should be performed on any material recovered by antral puncture.

TREATMENT

Acute and Subacute Sinusitis

The successful treatment of acute and subacute sinusitis in children primarily depends upon the administration of an appropriate antibiotic, in adequate dosage, for a sufficient period. In most instances, therapy should be instituted prior to obtaining the results of cultures. Antibiotic selection in this situation is not a great problem in children because the etiologic agent is *H. influenzae*, *S. pneumoniae*, *M. catarrhalis*, *S. aureus*, or *S. pyogenes* in more than 90 per cent of acute cases.

Initial antibiotic selection should be based upon the severity of the clinical illness, and it must take into consideration the antibiotic resistance patterns of the common causative organisms, as well as the cost and ease of administration of the treatment regimen. Today, about 35 per cent of nontypable *H. influenzae* and 85 per cent of *M. catarrhalis* strains produce β-lactamases and are resistant to amoxicillin.[24] In addition, between 15 and 25 per cent of *S. pneumoniae* strains have either intermediate (10 to 20 per cent) or complete (3 to 5 per cent) penicillin resistance.[8]

In the mildly ill child, the use of amoxicillin (50 mg/kg/24 hours every 6 hours) is a reasonable initial choice; this will be adequate for most *Streptococcus* species infections and the majority of *H. influenzae* infections.[24, 120, 122] Only *S. aureus* and *M. catarrhalis* will be treated inadequately by this regimen, and culture results and therapeutic response quickly will indicate a need for a change. Because of the high incidence of β-lactamase–producing *H. influenzae* and *B. catarrhalis* in some communities, consideration may be given to the use of amoxicillin–clavulanate potassium (amoxicillin 50 mg/kg/24 hours every 6 hours), trimethoprim-sulfamethoxazole (trimethoprim 10 to 20 mg/kg/24 hours, every 8 to 12 hours), or an oral cephalosporin (e.g., cefaclor, cefuroxime, cefixime, cefpodoxime proxetil, loracarbef) in the mild or moderately ill child.

The seriously ill child should be hospitalized, and therapy for β-lactamase–producing staphylococci and highly resistant pneumococci should be implemented, in addition to coverage for amoxicillin-resistant *H. influenzae* and *M. catarrhalis.* This coverage is achieved best with vancomycin (40 mg/kg/24 hours every 6 hours) and cefotaxime (100 to 200 mg/kg/24 hours every 6 hours) or ceftriaxone (100 mg/kg/24 hours every 12 hours). Therapy should be adjusted on the basis of clinical response and culture results. The dosage and duration of antimicrobial therapy in sinusitis are critical. Penicillins penetrate the sinuses relatively poorly.[6, 28, 44, 57, 67] The duration of therapy should be a minimum of 10 days.

The relief of obstruction at the sinus ostia and the establishment of drainage are time-honored principles of therapy. To achieve these goals, locally applied and systemically active vasoconstrictive drugs are used. However, there is no evidence of their therapeutic effectiveness to date. The beneficial effects of oral, systemically active, vasoconstrictive drugs are hampered by the fact that their drying effect may be deleterious to the mucus blanket. Topical vasoconstrictor drugs (e.g., phenylephrine hydrochloride) are plagued by rebound vasodilation. We believe these drugs should be used rarely in acute disease; their main use is to relieve pain due to obstruction, and they should be used only for 2 to 3 days.

Chronic and Recurrent Sinusitis

Allergic disorders are common in chronic and recurrent sinusitis.[70, 116] Children should be evaluated for allergy, and when identified, specific treatment should be employed. Specific allergens and irritants should be avoided (via air filtering, removal of pets, avoidance of tobacco smoke, etc.), and pharmacologic management should be implemented.

Nasal saline washes (twice daily in each nostril) are useful because they liquefy secretions and enhance mucociliary transport, which improves sinus drainage and ventilation. Antihistamines may be useful if allergic rhinitis is a contributing factor to the chronic sinus infection. Anti-inflammatory agents also may be useful. In selected cases, either topically applied corticosteroids or cromolyn sodium may be beneficial. Corticosteroids should be used carefully because their use on occasion can lead to superinfection in the sinuses with *Pseudomonas* species, other highly resistant gram-negative bacilli, or fungi. For effective corticosteroid use, Wald[116] suggests using a topical decongestant first so that the steroid preparation can reach the affected areas better.

In chronic or recurrent disease, antimicrobial treatment should be based upon culture and sensitivity data. Specific antimicrobial agents are the same as those employed in acute and subacute disease, but treatment should be prolonged for 3 weeks or more and for 7 days after the resolution of symptoms. *Aspergillus* species, *Bipolaris,* and other fungal infections require prolonged therapy with an antifungal agent to which the specific agent is susceptible. Itraconazole, ketoconazole, and fluconazole all have been effective in selected cases. Allergic aspergillosis of the sinuses can be managed with topical steroids without specific antifungal therapy (see Chapter 28).

In the past, surgical therapy for sinusitis in children was of questionable benefit. Surgical therapy included diagnostic and therapeutic irrigation; permanent drainage procedures in children with complications of sinusitis and in those who had immune defects; and such procedures as adenoidectomy, septoplasty, and turbinectomy to relieve anatomic obstructions in order to improve nasal/sinus ventilation. In one uncontrolled study of children with otitis media with effusion and sinusitis, the sinusitis was improved 6 months after adenoidectomy in 56 per cent of children, whereas only 24 per cent of similar children who were not operated on had similar improvement.[110]

Until recently, creating nasoantral windows was the most common major surgical procedure for chronic sinusitis in children.[41, 76] However, long-term success with this procedure was poor because of the high rate of closure of the windows. A new interest in sinus surgery has resulted from the introduction of endoscopic techniques. Although there is considerable controversy regarding the use of these techniques in children, several studies have found endoscopic surgery to be safe and effective.[42, 65, 68, 84, 94]

The goal of functional endoscopic sinus surgery is to remove obstruction at the ostiomeatal complex where the mucociliary flow from the frontal, maxillary, and ethmoid sinuses converges.[65, 94] This results in improved drainage and a restoration of normal physiologic function of the frontal, maxillary, and ethmoid sinuses. Surgery involves an anterior ethmoidectomy and enlargement of the natural ostium of the maxillary sinus. Follow-up surgery 2 to 3 weeks after the initial surgery is necessary to remove crusts, blood clots, granulative tissue, and adhesions.

In a study of 210 children with a history of chronic sinusitis for 3 months or longer, functional endoscopic sinus surgery resulted in successful outcomes in 165 (79 per cent).[65] The follow-up period was from 3 to 36 months (mean, 18 months), and all of the infections in these children had failed to respond to prior extensive medical management. In this series, no major complications occurred.

Functional endoscopic sinus surgery should be considered for children with chronic or recurrent sinusitis that has failed extensive, prolonged, and adequate medical management. This management includes specific antimicrobial therapy for specific organisms identified by culture, the diagnosis and treatment of allergic and other contributing conditions, and a trial of prophylactic antimicrobial agents.

Orbital and intracranial abscesses and cavernous sinus thrombosis secondary to sinus infection require emergency surgery, which often is lifesaving.[95, 99, 127, 129] Cellulitis, osteomyelitis, and meningitis also frequently require surgery if they do not respond to antimicrobial therapy.[95] Surgery in these cases involves drainage of the sinuses/abscesses. This can be accomplished by an external surgical incision. Newer endoscopic techniques may allow for intranasal drainage and avoidance of facial scars.[3] Surgical procedures also may be indicated in the child with acute or chronic disease resulting from an identified underlying problem, such as an immunologic deficiency.

PROGNOSIS

The prognosis of identified and adequately treated sinusitis in otherwise normal children is excellent. However, all too frequently, children suffer with subnormal health because sinusitis goes unrecognized; it partially may be treated because of other clinical impressions, and this contributes to the chronicity of the problem. Sinusitis is likely to be recurrent in children with a history of previous chronic disease and in children with repeated adverse exposure, such as swimming in contaminated or irritating water. Children with allergic respiratory disease also are likely to have frequent recurrences. Sinusitis in the immunocompromised child frequently is resistant to cure; long-term continuous therapy can be of benefit in such patients, however.

Serious complications occur in untreated sinusitis. These include meningitis; osteomyelitis; cavernous sinus thrombosis; and epidural, subdural, brain, and orbital abscesses.[99, 127, 129] Signs and symptoms of neurologic involvement in sinusitis frequently call for aggressive surgical management of the sinusitis as well as the intra- and paracranial lesions.

Paranasal sinusitis also has been noted on occasion to cause bronchial asthma.[83, 89] Its successful treatment has resulted in clearing of the asthma.

PREVENTION

Sinusitis, as such, is not preventable in the majority of instances. However, in some individuals, change of lifestyle can do much to improve the situation. For example, sinusitis in some children clearly is related to their swimming habits and therefore can be controlled by elimination of swimming or perhaps by the use of nose plugs. Good allergic management including intranasal corticosteroid or cromolyn therapy will prevent sinus disease in certain atopic children. Relief of nasal airway obstruction due to allergic rhinitis, enlarged adenoids, or other anatomic problems also should help to prevent sinusitis. Early attention to persistent nasal discharge also can be expected to lessen the damage associated with sinus infection.

References

1. Alfaro, V. R.: Nasal sinus disease in children. Pediatr. Clin. North Am. *9*:1061–1072, 1962.
2. April, M. M., Zinreich, J., Baroody, F. M., et al.: Coronal CT scan abnormalities in children with chronic sinusitis. Laryngoscope *103*:985–990, 1993.
3. Arjmand, E. M., Lusk, R. P., and Muntz, H. R.: Pediatric sinusitis and subperiosteal orbital abscess formation: Diagnosis and treatment. Otolaryng. Head Neck Surg. *109*:886–894, 1993.
4. Arruda, E., Boyle, T. R., Winther, B., et al.: Localization of human rhinovirus replication in the upper respiratory tract by in situ hybridization. J. Infect. Dis. *171*:1329–1333, 1995.
5. Axelsson, A., and Brorson, J. E.: The correlation between bacteriological findings in the nose and maxillary sinus in acute maxillary sinusitis. Laryngoscope *88*:2003–2011, 1973.
6. Axelsson, A., Grebelius, N., Jensen, C., et al.: Treatment of acute maxillary sinusitis. IV. Ampicillin, cephradine and erythromycin estolate with and without irrigation. Acta Otol. *79*:466–472, 1975.
7. Axelsson, A., and Runze, U.: Symptoms and signs of acute maxillary sinusitis. Otol. Rhinol. Laryngol. *38*:298–308, 1976.
8. Baquero, F., and Loza, E.: Antibiotic resistance of microorganisms involved in ear, nose and throat infections. Pediatr. Infect. Dis. J. *13*:S9–S14, 1994.
9. Berry, A. J., Kerkering, T. M., Giordano, A. M., et al.: Phaeohyphomycotic sinusitis. Pediatr. Infect. Dis. *3*:150–152, 1984.
10. Bhattacharyya, T. K., Mehra, Y. N., and Agarwal, S. C.: Incidence of bacterial, L-form and mycoplasma in chronic sinusitis. Acta Otol. *74*:293–296, 1972.
11. Box, Q. T., Cleveland, R. T., and Willard, C. Y.: Bacterial flora of the upper respiratory tract. I. Comparative evaluation by anterior nasal, oropharyngeal, and nasopharyngeal swabs. Am. J. Dis. Child. *102*:293–301, 1961.
12. Brandtzaeg, P.: Mucosal immunology: With special reference to specific immune defence of the upper respiratory tract. Otorhinolaryngology *50*:225–235, 1988.
13. Breese, B. B., Disney, F. A., and Talpey, W.: The nature of a small pediatric group practice: Part I. Pediatrics *38*:264–277, 1966.
14. Brook, I.: Beta-lactamase–producing bacteria in head and neck infection. Laryngoscope *98*:428–431, 1988.
15. Brook, I.: Bacteriologic features of chronic sinusitis in children. J. A. M. A. *246*:967–969, 1981.
16. Carenfelt, C., Lundberg, C., and Karlen, K.: Immunoglobulins in maxillary sinus secretion. Acta Otol. *82*:123–130, 1976.
17. Carenfelt, C., and Lundberg, C.: Purulent and nonpurulent maxillary sinus secretions with respect to pO2, pCO2, and pH. Acta Otol. *84*:138–144, 1977.
18. Cherry, J. D.: Infection in the compromised host. *In* Stiehm, E. R. (ed.): Immunologic Disorders in Infants and Children. 4th ed. Philadelphia, W. B. Saunders, 1996, pp. 975–1013.
19. Colman, B. H.: Sinusitis. Practitioner *215*:725–731,1975.
20. Dawes, J. D. K.: Diagnosis and treatment of sinusitis. Br. Med. J. *1*:843–845, 1966.
21. Diament, M. J.: The diagnosis of sinusitis in infants and children: X-ray, computed tomography, and magnetic resonance imaging: Diagnostic imaging of pediatric sinusitis. J. Allergy Clin. Immunol. *90*:442–444, 1990.
22. Diament, M. J., Senac, M. O., Jr., Gilsanz, V., et al.: Prevalence of incidental paranasal sinuses opacification in pediatric patients: A CT study. J. Comput. Assisted Tomogr. *11*:426–431, 1987.
23. Dingle, J. H., Badjer, D. F., and Jordan, W. S., Jr.: Patterns of Illness: Illness in the Home. Cleveland, Western Reserve University, 1964, p. 347.
24. Doern, G. V.: Resistance among problem respiratory pathogens in pediatrics. Pediatr. Infect. Dis. J. *14*:420–423, 1995.
25. Dudley, J. P., Goldstein, E. J. C., George, W. L., et al.: Sinus infection due to *Eikenella corrodens*. Arch. Otol. *104*:462–463, 1978.
26. Dunlap, M. B., and Harvey, H. S.: Host influence on upper respiratory flora. N. Engl. J. Med. *255*:640–646, 1956.
27. Eliasson, R., Mossberg, B., Camner, P., et al.: The immotile cilia syndrome: A congenital ciliary abnormality as an etiologic factor in chronic airway infections and male sterility. N. Engl. J. Med. *297*:1–6, 1977.
28. Eneroth, C. M., Lundberg, C., and Wretlind, B.: Antibiotic concentrations in maxillary sinus secretions and in the sinus mucosa. Chemotherapy *21*(Suppl. 1):1–7, 1975.
29. Evans, F. O., Jr., Sydnor, J. B., Moore, W. E. C., et al.: Sinusitis of the maxillary antrum. N. Engl. J. Med. *293*:736–739, 1975.
30. Fernbach, S. K., and Naidich, T. P.: CT diagnosis of orbital inflammation in children. Neuroradiology *22*:7–13, 1981.
31. Frederick, J., and Braude, A. I.: Anaerobic infection of the paranasal sinuses. N. Engl. J. Med. *290*:135–137, 1974.
32. Frenkel, L. M., Kuhls, T. L., Nitta, K., et al.: Recurrent bipolaris sinusitis following surgical and antifungal therapy. Pediatr. Infect. Dis. *6*:1130–1132, 1987.
33. Friday, G. A., and Fireman, P.: Sinusitis and asthma: Clinical pathogenic relationships. Clin. Chest Med. *9*:557–565, 1988.
34. Friedman, R., Ackerman, M., Wald, E., et al.: Asthma and bacterial sinusitis in children. J. Allergy Clin. Immunol. *74*:185–189, 1984.
35. Garcia, C. E., Cunningham, M. J., Randall, A. C., et al.: The etiologic role of frontal sinusitis in pediatric orbital abscesses. Am. J. Otolaryngol. *14*:449–452, 1993.
36. Gellady, A. M., Shulman, S. T., and Ayoub, E. M.: Periorbital and orbital cellulitis in children. Pediatrics *61*:272–277, 1978.
37. Givner, L. B., McGehee, D., Taber, L. H., et al.: Sinusitis, orbital cellulitis and polymicrobial bacteremia in a patient with primary Epstein-Barr virus infection. Pediatr. Infect. Dis. *3*:254–156, 1984.
38. Glasier, C. M., Archer, D. P., and Williams, K. D.: Incidental paranasal sinus abnormalities on CT of children: Clinical correlation. Am. J. Neuroradiol. *7*:861–864, 1986.
39. Gnarpe, H., and Lundberg, C.: L-phase organisms in maxillary sinus secretions. Scand. J. Infect. Dis. *3*:257–259, 1971.
40. Griffin, J. P., and Klein, E. W.: Role of sinusitis in primary atypical pneumonia. Clin. Med. *78*:23–27, 1971.
41. Gross, C. W.: Surgical management: An otolaryngologist's perspective. Pediatr. Infect. Dis. *4*:567, 1985.
42. Gross, C. W., Gurucharri, M. J., Lazar, R. H., et al.: Functional endonasal sinus surgery (FESS) in the pediatric age group. Laryngoscope *99*:272–275, 1989.
43. Gross, C. W., McGeady, S. J., Kerut, T., et al.: Limited-slide CT in the evaluation of paranasal sinus disease in children. Am. J. Roentgenol. *156*:367–369, 1991.
44. Gullers, K., Lundberg, C., and Malmborg, A. S.: Penicillin in paranasal sinus secretions. Chemotherapy *14*:303–307, 1969.
45. Gwaltney, M. J., Jr., Hendley, J. O., Simon, G., et al.: Rhinovirus infections in an industrial population. I. The occurrence of illness. N. Engl. J. Med. *275*:1261–1268, 1966.
46. Hamory, B. H., Sande, M. A., Sydnor, A., Jr., et al.: Etiology and antimicrobial therapy of acute maxillary sinusitis. J. Infect. Dis. *139*:197–202, 1979.
47. Hansson, L. A., Ahlstedt, S., Andersson, B., et al.: Mucosal immunity. Ann. N. Y. Acad. Sci. *409*:1–21, 1983.
48. Harvey, H. S., and Dunlap, M. B.: Seasonal prevalence of upper respiratory pathogens. N. Engl. J. Med. *264*:684–686, 1961.

49. Hawkins, D. B., and Clark, R. W.: Orbital involvement in acute sinusitis: Lessons from 24 childhood patients. Clin. Pediatr. *16*:464–471, 1977.
50. Haynes, R. E., and Cramblett, H. G.: Acute ethmoiditis: Its relationship to orbital cellulitis. Am. J. Dis. Child. *114*:261–267, 1967.
51. Hays, G. C., and Mullard, J. E.: Can nasal bacterial flora be predicted from clinical findings? Pediatrics *49*:596–599, 1972.
52. Herz, G., and Gfeller, J.: Sinusitis in paediatrics. Chemotherapy *23*:50–57, 1977.
53. Holdaway, M. D., and Turk, D. C.: Capsulated *Haemophilus influenzae* and respiratory tract disease. Lancet *1*:358–360, 1967.
54. Hoshaw, T. C., and Nickman, N. J.: Sinusitis and otitis in children. Arch. Otol. *100*:194–195, 1974.
55. Jacobson, L. O., and Dick, G. F.: Normal and abnormal bacterial flora of the nose. J. A. M. A. *117*:2222–2225, 1941.
56. Jaffe, B. F.: Chronic sinusitis in children: Comments on pathogenesis and management. Clin. Pediatr. *13*:944–948, 1974.
57. Jeppesen, F., and Illum, P.: Concentration of ampicillin in antral mucosa following administration of ampicillin sodium and privampicillin. Acta. Otol. *73*:428–432, 1972.
58. Jousimies-Somer, H. R., Savolainen, S., and Ylikoski, J. S.: Bacteriological findings of acute maxillary sinusitis in young adults. J. Clin. Microbiol. *26*:1919–1925, 1988.
59. Jousimies-Somer, H. R., Savolainen, S., and Ylikoski, J. S.: Comparison of the nasal bacterial floras in two groups of healthy subjects and in patients with acute maxillary sinusitis. J. Clin. Microbiol. *27*:2736–2743, 1989.
60. Katzenstein, A. L., Sale, S. R., and Greenberger, P. A.: Pathologic findings in allergic aspergillus sinusitis. Am. J. Surg. Pathol. *7*:439–443, 1983.
61. Kern, E. B.: Sinusitis. J. Allergy Clin. Immunol. *73*:25–31, 1984.
62. Kogutt, M. S., and Swischuk, L. E.: Diagnosis of sinusitis in infants and children. Pediatrics *52*:152–156, 1973.
63. Kovatch, A. L., Wald, E. R., Ledesma Medina, J., et al.: Maxillary sinus radiographs in children with nonrespiratory complaints. Pediatrics *73*:306–308, 1984.
64. Krajina, Z., Koskovic, F., and Babic, I.: The bacteriology of the respiratory tract in various pathological conditions. Acta Otol. *67*:453–459, 1969.
65. Lazar, R. H., Ramzi, R. Y., and Gross, C. W.: Pediatric functional endonasal sinus surgery: A review of 210 cases. Head and Neck *14*:92–98, 1992.
66. Lehrer, R. I., Howard, D. H., Sypherd, P. S., et al.: Mucormycosis. Ann. Intern. Med. *93*:93–108, 1980.
67. Lundberg, C., and Malmburg, A. S.: Studies of antibiotics in sinus secretions. Rhinology *9*:166–168, 1971.
68. Lusk, R. P., and Muntz, H. R.: Endoscopic sinus surgery in children with chronic sinusitis: A pilot study. Laryngoscope *100*:654–658, 1990.
69. Lystad, A., Berdal, P., and Lund-Iversen, L.: The bacterial flora of sinusitis with an in vitro study of the bacterial resistance to antibiotics. Acta Otol. *188*(Suppl.):390–399, 1963.
70. Manning, S. C.: Pediatric sinusitis. Otolaryngol. Clin. North Am. *26*:623–638, 1993.
71. Manning, S. C., Vuitch, F., Weinberg, A. G., et al.: Allergic aspergillosis: A newly recognized form of sinusitis in the pediatric population. Laryngoscope *99*:681–685, 1989.
72. Maresh, M. M., and Washburn, A. H.: Paranasal sinuses from birth to late adolescence. II. Clinical and roentgenographic evidence of infection. Am. J. Dis. Child. *60*:841–861, 1940.
73. McLean, D. C.: Sinusitis in children: Lessons from 25 patients. Clin. Pediatr. *9*:342–345, 1970.
74. Mofenson, L. M., Korelitz, J., Pelton, S., et al.: Sinusitis in children infected with human immunodeficiency virus: Clinical characteristics, risk factors, and prophylaxis. Clin. Infect. Dis. *21*:1175–1181, 1995.
75. Muntz, H. R., and Lusk, R. P.: Bacteriology of the ethmoid bullae in children with chronic sinusitis. Arch. Otolaryngol. Head Neck Surg. *117*:179–181, 1991.
76. Muntz, H. R., and Lusk, R. P.: Nasal antral windows in children: A retrospective study. Laryngoscope *100*:643–646, 1990.
77. Naclerio, R. M., Proud, D., Lichtenstein, L. M., et al.: Kinins are generated during experimental rhinovirus colds. J. Infect. Dis. *157*:133–142, 1988.
78. Nguyen, K. L., Corbett, M. L., Garcia, D. P., et al.: Chronic sinusitis among pediatric patients with chronic respiratory complaints. J. Allergy Clin. Immunol. *92*:824–830, 1993.
79. Noah, T. L., Henderson, F. W., Wortman, I. A., et al.: Nasal cytokine production in viral acute upper respiratory infection of childhood. J. Infect. Dis. *171*:584–592, 1995.
80. Orobello, P. W., Park, R. I., Belcher, L. J., et al.: Microbiology of chronic sinusitis in children. Arch. Otolaryngol. Head Neck Surg. *117*:980–983, 1991.
81. Palva, T., Grumlaut-Onroos, J. A., and Palva, A.: Bacteriology and pathology of chronic maxillary sinusitis. Acta Orol. *54*:159–175, 1962.
82. Pedersen, M., Sakakura, Y., Winther, B., et al.: Nasal mucociliary transport, number of ciliated cells, and beating pattern in naturally acquired common colds. Eur. J. Resp. Dis. *128*(Suppl.):355–364, 1983.
83. Phipatanakul, C. S., and Slavin, R. G.: Bronchial asthma produced by paranasal sinusitis. Arch. Otol. *100*:109–112, 1974.
84. Poole, M. D.: Pediatric sinusitis is not a surgical disease. Ear Nose Throat J. *71*:622–623, 1992.
85. Proctor, D. F.: The historical background of modern otolaryngology. *In* Ravitch, M. M. (ed.): The Nose, Paranasal Sinuses and Ears in Childhood. Springfield, Charles C. Thomas, 1963, pp. 3–19.
86. Proud, D., Naclerio, R. M., Gwaltney, J. M., et al.: Kinins are generated in nasal secretions during natural rhinovirus colds. J. Infect. Dis. *161*:120–123, 1990.
87. Proud, D., Gwaltney, J. M., Hendley, J. O., et al.: Increased levels of interleukin-1 are detected in nasal secretions of volunteers during experimental rhinovirus colds. J. Infect. Dis. *169*:1007–1013, 1994.
88. Rachelefsky, G. S., Katz, R. M., and Siegel, S. C.: Chronic sinusitis in children with respiratory allergy: The role of antimicrobials. J. Allergy Clin. Immunol. *69*:382–387, 1982.
89. Rachelefsky, G. S., Katz, R. M., and Siegel, S. C.: Chronic sinus disease with associated reactive airway disease in children. Pediatrics *73*:526–529, 1984.
90. Rachelefsky, G. S., Katz, R. M., and Siegel, S. C.: Chronic sinusitis in the allergic child. Pediatr. Clin. North Am. *35*:1091–1101, 1988.
91. Rantanen, T., and Arvilommi, H.: Double-blind trial of doxycycline in acute maxillary sinusitis: A clinical and bacteriological study. Acta Otol. *76*:58–62, 1973.
92. Richards, W.: Hospitalization of children with status asthmaticus: A review. Pediatrics *84*:111–118, 1989.
93. Richards, W., Roth, R., and Church, F.: Underdiagnosis and undertreatment of chronic sinusitis in children. Clin. Pediatr. *30*:88–92, 1991.
94. Rosenfeld, R. M.: Pilot study of outcomes in pediatric rhinosinusitis. Arch. Otol. Head Neck Surg. *121*:729–736, 1995.
95. Rosenfeld, R. A., and Rowley, A. H.: Infectious intracranial complications of sinusitis, other than meningitis, in children: 12-year review. Clin. Infect. Dis. *18*:750–754, 1994.
96. Rossen, R. D., Butler, W. T., Cate, T. R., et al.: Protein composition of nasal secretion during respiratory virus infection. Proc. Soc. Exp. Biol. Med. *119*:1169–1176, 1965.
97. Rulon, J. T.: Sinusitis in children. Postgrad. Med. *48*:107–112, 1970.
98. Rynnel-Dagoo, B., Forsgren, J., Freijd, A., et al.: Rationale for antibiotic therapy in pediatric ear, nose and throat infections: Immunologic issues. Pediatr. Infect. Dis. J. *13*:15–20, 1994.
99. Sable, N. S., Hengerer, A., and Powell, K. R.: Acute frontal sinusitis with intracranial complications. Pediatr. Infect. Dis. *3*:58–61, 1984.
100. Schenck, N. L., and Rauchbach, E.: Frontal sinus disease. IV. Cellular response to experimentally induced infection. Laryngoscope *86*:1726–1733, 1976.
101. Shapiro, G. G.: The role of nasal airway obstruction in sinus disease and facial development. J. Allergy Clin. Immunol. *82*:935–940, 1988.
102. Shapiro, G. G., Virant, F. S., Furukawa, C. T., et al.: Immunologic defects in patients with refractory sinusitis. Pediatrics *87*:311–316, 1991.
103. Shibley, G. S., Hanger, F. M., and Dochez, A. R.: Studies in the common cold. I. Observations of the normal bacterial flora of nose and throat with variations occurring during colds. J. Exp. Med. *43*:415–431, 1926.
104. Shopfner, C. E., and Rossi, J. O.: Roentgenogram evaluation of the paranasal sinuses in children. Am. J. Roentgenol. *118*:176–186, 1973.
105. Shurin, P. A.: Etiology and antimicrobial therapy of paranasal sinusitis in children. Ann. Otol. Rhinol. Laryngol. *90*(Suppl.):72–74, 1981.
106. Sobol, S. M., Love, R. G., Stutman, H. R., et al.: Phaeohyphomycosis of the maxilloethmoid sinus caused by *Drechslera spicifera*: A new fungal pathogen. Laryngoscope *94*:620–627, 1984.
107. Sparrevohn, U. R., and Buch, A.: The bacteriology of maxillary sinusitis. I. Technique. Acta. Otol. *34*:425–436, 1946.
108. Spector, S. L., English, G. M., McIntosh, K., et al.: Adenovirus in the sinuses of an asthmatic patient with apparent selective antibody deficiencies. Am. J. Med. *55*:227–231, 1973.
109. Sprinkle, P.: Current status of mycoplasmatales and bacterial variants in chronic otolaryngic disease. Laryngoscope *82*:737–747, 1972.
110. Takahashi, H., Fujita, A., and Hanjo, I.: Effect of adenoidectomy on otitis media with effusion, tubal function, and sinusitis. Am. J. Otol. *10*:208–213, 1989.
111. Tinkelman, D. G., and Silk, H. J.: Clinical and bacteriologic features of chronic sinusitis in children. Am. J. Dis. Child. *143*:938–941, 1989.
112. Tos, M., and Mogensen, C.: Mucus production in chronic maxillary sinusitis. Acta Otol. *97*:151–159, 1984.
113. Umetsu, D. J., Ambrosino, D. M., Quinti, I., et al.: Recurrent sinopulmonary infection and impaired antibody response to bacterial capsular polysaccharide antigen in children with selective IgG subclass deficiency. N. Engl. J. Med. *313*:1247–1251, 1985.
114. Urdal, K., and Berdal, P.: The microbial flora in 81 cases of maxillary sinusitis. Acta Otol. *37*:20–25, 1949.
115. Van Cauwenberge, P., Verschraegen, G., and Van Renterghem, L.: Bacteriological findings in sinusitis (1963–1975). Scand. J. Infect. Dis. *9*:72–77, 1976.
116. Wald, E. R.: Chronic sinusitis in children. J. Pediatr. *127*:339–347, 1995.
117. Wald, E. R., Guerra, N., and Byers, C.: Upper respiratory tract infection in young children: Duration of and frequency of complications. Pediatrics *87*:129–133, 1991.
118. Wald, E. R.: Rhinitis and acute and chronic sinusitis. *In* Bluestone, C. D., Stool, S. E., and Scheetz, M. D. (eds.): Pediatric Otorhinolaryngology. 2nd ed. Philadelphia, W. B. Saunders, 1990, pp. 729–944.

119. Wald, E. R., Byers, C., Guerra, N., et al.: Subacute sinusitis in children. J. Pediatr. 115:28–32, 1989.
120. Wald, E. R.: Sinusitis in children. Pediatr. Infect. Dis. 7:S150–S153, 1988.
121. Wald, E. R., Dashefky, B., Byers, C., et al.: Frequency and severity of infections in day care. J. Pediatr. 112:540–546, 1988.
122. Wald, E. R., Chiponis, D., and Ledesma-Medina, J.: Comparative effectiveness of amoxicillin and amoxicillin-clavulanate potassium in acute paranasal sinus infections in children: A double-blind, placebo-controlled trial. Pediatrics 77:795–800, 1986.
123. Wald, E. R.: Epidemiology, pathophysiology and etiology of sinusitis. Pediatr. Infect. Dis. 4:S51–S81, 1985.
124. Wald, E. R., Reilly, J. S., Casselbrant, M., et al.: Treatment of acute maxillary sinusitis in childhood: A comparative study of amoxicillin and cefaclor. J. Pediatr. 104:297–302, 1984.
125. Wald, E. R., Milmoe, G. J., Bowen, A. D., et al.: Acute maxillary sinusitis in children. N. Engl. J. Med. 304:749–754, 1981.
126. Washburn, R. G., Kennedy, D. W., Begley, M. G., et al.: Chronic fungal sinusitis in apparently normal hosts. Medicine 67:231–247, 1988.
127. Wassermann, D.: Acute paranasal sinusitis and cavernous sinus thrombosis. Arch. Otol. 86:99–103, 1967.
128. Watters, E. C., Wallar, P. H., Hiles, D. A., et al.: Acute orbital cellulitis. Arch. Ophthalmol. 94:785–788, 1976.
129. Whitaker, C. W.: Intracranial complications of ear, nose, and throat infections. Laryngoscope 81:1375–1380, 1971.
130. Winther, B.: Effects on the nasal mucosa of upper respiratory viruses (common cold). Danish Med. Bull. 41:193–204, 1994.
131. Wold, G., Anderhuber, W., and Kuhn, F.: Development of the paranasal sinuses in children: Implications for paranasal sinus surgery. Ann. Otol. Rhinol. Laryngol. 102:705–711, 1993.
132. Yang, H.S.: Nasal flora of the children in a day nursery. Am. J. Dis. Child. 61:262–272, 1941.
133. Zimmerman, B., Stringer, D., Feanning, S., et al.: Prevalence of abnormalities found by sinus x-ray in childhood asthma: Lack of relation to severity of asthma. J. Allergy Clin. Immunol. 80:268–273, 1987.
134. Zinreich, S. J., Kennedy, D. W., Rosenbaum, A. E., et al.: Paranasal sinuses: CT imaging requirements for endoscopic surgery. Radiology 163:769–775, 1987.

18

OTITIS EXTERNA

Ralph D. Feigin and Joshua J. Alexander

Otitis externa is a common finding in children, especially during the summer. Approximately 5 to 20 per cent of patients visiting their physician during the summer months in tropical and subtropical areas have infection of the external ear.[31] The precise cause of otitis externa is unknown. The disease seems to be multifactorial in etiology and involves an interaction of host and environmental factors.

ETIOLOGY

The external auditory canal has many features designed to protect the surface epithelium from invading pathogens. Hairs located on the outer one-third of the canal actively push debris toward the opening of the external auditory meatus. The continuous flow of epithelium from the tympanic membrane to the external meatus, coupled with the rolling motion of the lateral external auditory canal, also serves to facilitate the movement of debris toward the external auditory meatus. Apocrine and sebaceous glands produce cerumen, which provides an acid pH medium that acts as a chemical barrier against infection. Factors that disrupt these natural protective mechanisms produce conditions that are favorable for the development of otitis externa. These include high temperature and humidity, increased sweating,[15] allergy, stress, trauma, removal of cerumen, alkaline pH, environmental bacterial contamination, and maceration.[31]

Swimming has been associated with the development of otitis externa. Prolonged immersion, frequent showering and hair washing,[28] repeated ear cleansing, and use of cotton swabs and cerumen scoops can lead to the complete removal of the acid medium required to protect the epithelium. Maceration of the skin follows, permitting bacteria to enter. Divers have a higher degree of skin trauma and maceration and also have a higher rate of otitis externa than do other individuals.[30, 34, 39] The use of occlusive head gear, such as diver's hoods and ear plugs, is associated with increased bacterial colonization of the external ear.[5] At this time, no direct relationship exists between bacterial colonization of the external auditory canal and otitis externa. However, the combination of prolonged immersion and occlusion may predispose the diver to an increased risk of otitis externa.

Several studies have shown that the incidence of otitis externa increases as the bacterial counts in the water increase. Among nondiving children on an Israeli kibbutz using a highly contaminated swimming pool (>3000 bacteria/100 mL water), the rate of otitis externa was as high as 36 per cent.[34] Investigators found an association between the degree of *Pseudomonas* colonization in five Ontario lakes and the incidence of otitis externa.[32] Other investigators, however, have reported no correlation between bacterial counts of the water in which an individual is immersed and extent of infection.[7] Many believe that the hot, humid summer weather is the cause of "swimmer's ear."

Children with chronic serous otitis media may have an increased incidence of otitis externa. Continuous negative pressure causes abnormal desquamation of epithelium and accumulation of wax in the canal, often leading to maceration of the skin as a result of water trapped in the debris. Restoration of normal ear pressure in 15 patients who suffered from chronic otitis externa resulted in marked improvement of the symptoms and clinical findings.[17]

Several additional factors may predispose children to otitis externa. Impacted cerumen can trap water in the proximal part of the canal, leading to maceration of the underlying skin. Cleansing the ear with soapy water often replaces the acid medium with an alkaline film. Contact dermatitis related to hairsprays, shampoo, hearing aids, or earrings; antibiotics prescribed for the treatment of otitis externa; and bacteria present in the canal secondary to chronic draining otitis media may cause otitis externa. Otitis externa in an infant has been associated with a bath sponge contaminated by *Pseudomonas aeruginosa*.[33] Other factors that predispose children to otitis externa include (1) a congenitally narrow external auditory meatus, (2) acquired narrowing of the external auditory canal or meatus secondary to inflammation, (3) small external auditory canals in certain disorders due to chromosomal defects (e.g., Down syndrome), (4) bathing with immersion of the ears in bath water, and (5) infection transmitted by or from the hands to the ears. Many systemic illnesses also have been associated with infection. These include anemia, vitamin deficiencies, seborrhea, psoriasis, Langerhans' cell histiocytosis, and anxiety (neurodermatitis). Even relapsing acute myelogenous leukemia may present as otitis externa.[25]

BACTERIOLOGY

In approximately 30 per cent of normal individuals, the external canal is sterile. *Staphylococcus epidermidis* can be recovered from the external auditory canal in 50 per cent of individuals; in 3 per cent, *Staphylococcus aureus* may be recovered.[37] As many as 31 per cent of normal patients have fungi, *Aspergillus niger* or *Candida albicans* as part of the normal flora of the external ear.[35]

The pathogens cultured most frequently from patients with otitis externa are *S. aureus* and *P. aeruginosa*, the latter being more prominent in tropical climates. *Proteus vulgaris*, diphtheroids, *Escherichia coli*, *Klebsiella* species, *Peptostreptococcus* species, and *Bacteroides* species are other agents that have been implicated in the etiology of this disease process.[6, 10, 15, 24, 31, 40]

CLINICAL MANIFESTATIONS

According to Senturia and colleagues,[31] otitis externa may be divided into three stages: preinflammatory, acute, and chronic. During the preinflammatory stage, the lipid cover is removed, leading to maceration and pruritus. As the patient scratches in an attempt to relieve the discomfort, he or she often traumatizes the skin, predisposing it to bacterial invasion. On examination, the canal may appear to be normal.

The acute stage also may be divided into three stages. In mild disease, the canal is erythematous and edematous. There often is a clear, odorless discharge and exfoliative debris in the canal. In moderate otitis externa, itching and pain are prominent. The lumen is occluded partially with seropurulent debris. There also may be mild periauricular edema. Severe disease with marked periauricular edema and complete obliteration of the canal causes intense pain upon chewing and movement of the tragus. Examination of the external auditory canal of patients with chronic otitis reveals thickened edematous skin with eczematous gray, brown, or greenish secretion.

DIAGNOSIS AND DIFFERENTIAL DIAGNOSIS

Most patients present for evaluation of ear pain, which may vary in intensity from mild to severe. Often there is marked tenderness with movement of the tragus. The skin of the ear canal is attached directly to the periosteum and perichondrium. Edema in the canal compresses the nerves directly against bone. Because the skin of the auricle is connected directly to the canal epithelium, any movement of the auricle is transmitted to the canal, causing pain secondary to nerve compression. In chronic cases, itching, tinnitus,[1] hearing loss (conductive), and/or a feeling of fullness may bring the patient to the physician. A caseous discharge may or may not be present. Hearing usually is normal if the canal is clear and can be evaluated by tuning fork, tympanography, or audiography.

The differential diagnosis of otitis externa includes both benign and malignant conditions. The list includes furunculosis, foreign bodies, suppurative and nonsuppurative otitis media, bullous myringitis, herpes zoster oticus,[15] mastoiditis, benign necrotizing otitis externa,[38] malignant otitis externa, and various malignancies.[20]

Furunculosis usually is found in the outer one-half of the canal, where sebaceous glands and/or hair follicles become obstructed and infected, most commonly by *S. aureus*.[15] Physical examination reveals a "localized" area of infection. Pain usually is relieved after incision and drainage of the abscess with a No. 11 blade and/or 18-gauge needle.[26]

Children commonly place small objects in the external canal. Foreign bodies may incite a localized inflammatory reaction secondary to trauma. These objects usually can be removed with careful use of a cerumen scoop under otoscopic or microscopic guidance or by saline lavage. Local or general anesthesia may be required to remove an object trapped at the isthmus.

Acute otitis media generally causes ear pain that is not exacerbated by movement of the tragus. Discharge is not present unless the tympanic membrane has erupted. When the tympanic membrane perforates, bloody discharge often is present, and the intensity of the pain diminishes substantially. Once the discharge is removed from the canal, the tympanic membrane can be examined. It often is erythematous and inflamed. These patients generally are febrile to 40° to 40.5° C (104° to 105° F) and have an elevated white blood cell count. Commonly, tympanometry will demonstrate a type B tracing.[40] Appropriate oral antibiotic therapy is indicated.

Bullous myringitis may involve both the tympanic membrane and the external canal. Serous or hemorrhagic blebs cause severe pain. Fever generally is absent, and hearing is not affected unless the child also has otitis media. The blebs may need to be incised if pain is severe.

Herpes zoster oticus (Ramsey Hunt syndrome) is a cranial neuritis caused by varicella-zoster virus. It is manifested by a vesicular eruption on the pinna and external auditory meatus, severe otalgia, and ipsilateral facial paralysis. Diagnosis is made by viral culture of an open vesicle, and treatment consists of topical and intravenous acyclovir.[15]

Acute mastoiditis causes sagging of the posterior canal wall that may look like simple edema. These patients have extreme tenderness over the mastoid process and usually have minimal tragal and auricular tenderness. Swelling may blunt the postauricular crease and cause anterior deviation of the auricle. Mastoid radiography should distinguish a case of severe otitis externa from mastoiditis, whereas computed tomography and magnetic resonance imaging help define deep tissue inflammation or abscess.[16]

Benign necrotizing otitis externa is a relatively rare condition that can present with otorrhea, pruritus of the ear, and mild otalgia. It is characterized by the development of an avascular bony sequestration in the tympanic plate and can be treated by long-term conservative management or surgery.[38]

Malignant external otitis is not seen commonly in the pediatric age group, except in children with chronic illness or malnourishment[11] or those who are immunosuppressed.[27] It occurs most frequently in the elderly diabetic population and is caused most commonly[15] by *P. aeruginosa*. The infection begins in the canal, often after minor trauma, and spreads rapidly to involve the soft tissue, cartilage, bone, nerves, and parotid gland. Pain is severe, and discharge is copious. In contrast to simple otitis externa, edema and active granulation tissue are found in the canal. Movement of the temporomandibular joint and palpation below the external canal cause extreme pain. Patients who develop facial paralysis, which is more common in children than in adults with this condition, have an ominous prognosis. An erythrocyte sedimentation rate appears to be a sensitive index for malignant otitis externa,[15] and a ^{99}Tc bone scan may be helpful in early[15] detection of the osteomyelitis that is associated with this condition.[9] Complications of malignant external otitis noted in children are stenosis of the external auditory canal, auricular cartilage deformity, tympanic membrane necrosis,[11] and sensorineural hearing loss.[36] A positive bone scan itself, however, should not be considered to be diagnostic of malignant external otitis, because positive scans have been noted in children with severe otitis externa.[21] A biopsy specimen also should be sent for histopathology to rule out a primary or metastatic malignancy.[15] Malignancy also may masquerade as otitis externa. Squamous cell carcinoma is the most common presentation; however, basal cell carcinoma and adenocarcinoma as well as metastatic lymphoma can be found in the external canal. Ear canal malignancy may present with a bloody discharge, deafness, and/or a nonhealing ulcer or otalgia. Malignancy should be considered if the pain is out of proportion to the degree of skin involvement.

TREATMENT

The goal of treatment is to relieve pain, cleanse the canal, restore the protective epithelial barrier, and prevent reinfection. In the preinflammatory stage, the canal can be flushed with 3 per cent hypertonic saline or Burow solution (two tablets in 1 pint of water) three times daily. The canal should be dried with a cotton swab after each irrigation. If no infection is present, topical corticosteroid creams, such as Benisone, Kenalog, or Tridesilon, may be used three times each day. If the canal is infected, Neosporin-G Cream, three times per day, may be provided. Acetic acid (VōSol) should be used to restore the acid pH 1 or 2 weeks after this treatment.

In contrast to the preinfected stage, irrigation should be avoided when the canal is infected mildly. Cortisporin solution or suspension (a mixture of polymyxin, neomycin, and hydrocortisone in an acid pH medium that is active against both staphylococci and gram-negative rods) should be used four times daily. It is important to remember that hypersensitivity to neomycin may occur, complicating the existing otitis externa. This hypersensitivity may be masked by the steroid application when moderate or severe infection is found.

If the external ear canal is very swollen and painful, Burow solution, acetic acid, or Cortisporin may be placed in the canal on a cotton wick in an attempt to reduce swelling. Anodynes also may be used as needed. It is important to take a culture of the canal prior to the initiation of therapy. After the swelling has decreased, colistin sulfate or clindamycin drops should be used until the patient has been symptom-free for 1 to 2 weeks. In children who have indwelling tympanostomy tubes, local therapy should be used with care because direct contact with the otic nerves could cause permanent damage.

Analgesics as well as antibiotic coverage with tetracycline (in children older than 8 years of age), ampicillin, or cephalosporins may be indicated, especially if the child is febrile. Cellulitis that accompanies otitis externa is secondary to gram-positive organisms that usually respond to these antibiotics. Systemic therapy with oxacillin or nafcillin may be required in patients with severe chondritis associated with otitis media when chondritis is caused by *S. aureus*. Therapy with an appropriate aminoglycoside or ciprofloxacin if the patient is 18 years or older[12] should be considered when otitis is caused by *P. aeruginosa*. For the duration of therapy, the patient should be advised to avoid showers and excessive exercise. Severely infected external auditory canals may require drainage of abscesses that may be present. This should be done only after 24 hours of antibiotic coverage. In cases in which anaerobic bacteria are isolated or their presence is suspected, the use of imipenem, cefoxitin, or the combination of amoxicillin or ticarcillin and clavulanic acid may be warranted.[6]

Fungal disease is managed best by careful cleansing with hydrogen peroxide[2] and thorough drying followed by[23] treatment of the canal by the physician once a day for 3 days with *m*-cresyl acetate.[31] Other treatment regimens include sulfanilamide powder insufflated into the canal to form a thin layer. Usually, one treatment is sufficient.[19] Gentian violet, Burow solution, 5-fluorocytosine,[18] 3 per cent iodochlorhydroxyquin (Vioform), 2 per cent ketoconazole cream,[13] nystatin-triamcinolone (Mycolog-II) ointment,[23] clotrimazole (Lotrimin) drops, thimerosal (Merthiolate),[29] and tolnaftate also may be effective.[8, 22]

Finally, the rare case of otitis externa caused by Langerhans' cell histiocytosis may be treated successfully with topical 20 per cent nitrogen mustard otic drops.[14]

PREVENTION

Patients with a history of otitis externa related to water activities should minimize exposure to water by using earplugs when bathing or swimming. After prolonged swimming, acetic acid (2 per cent) drops may decrease recurrence of otitis externa by neutralizing the alkaline effects of pool water.[2, 15]

References

1. Agius, A. M., Pickles, J. M., and Burch, K. L.: A prospective study of otitis externa. Clin. Otol. *17*:150–154, 1992.
2. Biedlingmaier, J. F.: Two ear problems you may not need to refer. Postgrad. Med. *96*:141–148, 1994.
3. Bierel, J. F. (ed.): Logan Turner's Disease of Nose and Throat. Boston, Wright, 1982, pp. 338–344.
4. Bressler, K.: Ear foreign-body removal: A review of 98 consecutive cases. Laryngoscope *103*:367–370, 1993.
5. Brook, I., and Coolbaugh, J. C.: Changes in the bacterial flora of the external ear canal from the wearing of occlusive equipment. Laryngoscope *94*:963–964, 1984.
6. Brook, I., Frazier, E. H., and Thompson, D. H.: Aerobic and anaerobic microbiology of external otitis. Clin. Infect. Dis. *15*:955–958, 1992.
7. Calderon, R. L., and Ad Mood, E. W.: Epidemiological assessment of water quality and "swimmer's ear." Arch. Environ. Health *37*:300–305, 1982.
8. Caruso, V. G., and Meyerhopt, W. L.: Trauma and infection of the external ear. *In* Paparella, M. M., and Shumrick, D. A. (eds.): Otolaryngology II. Philadelphia, W. B. Saunders, 1980, pp. 1345–1349.
9. Cohen, D., Friedman, P., and Eilon, A.: Malignant external otitis versus acute external otitis. J. Laryngol. Otol. *101*:211–215, 1987.
10. Dibb, W. L.: Microbial aetiology of otitis externa. J. Infect. *22*:233–239, 1991.
11. Evans, P., and Hofmann, L.: Malignant external otitis: A case report and review. Am. Fam. Physician *49*:427–431.
12. Gehanno, P.: Ciprofloxacin in the treatment of malignant external otitis. Chemotherapy *40*(Suppl. 1):35–40, 1994.
13. Gintautiene, K., Lamarca, C., Duvalsaint, F., et al.: Effect of ketoconazole on external otitis. Proc. West. Pharmacol. Soc. *34*:351–352, 1991.
14. Hadfield, P. J., Birchall, M. A., and Albert, D. M.: Otitis externa in Langerhans' cell histiocytosis: The successful use of topical nitrogen mustard. Int. J. Pediatr. Otorhinolaryngol. *30*:143–149, 1994.
15. Hirsch, B.: Infections of the external ear. Am. J. Otolaryngol. *13*:145–155, 1992.
16. Hopkin, R. J., Bergeson, P. S., Pinckard, R. C., et al.: Otitis externa posing as mastoiditis. Arch. Pediatr. Adolesc. Med. *148*:1346–1349, 1994.
17. Khalifa, M. S., Abdel Nabi, E. A., and Labib, K. L.: Middle ear pressure changes in relation to recurrent otitis externa. J. Laryngol. Otol. *98*:241–242, 1984.
18. Kintzel, P., Trausch, D. E., and Copfer, A. L.: Otic administration of amphotericin B 0.25% in sterile water. Ann. Pharmacother. *28*:333–335, 1994.
19. Kopstein, E.: Otitis externa: Unorthodox but effective treatments. Laryngoscope *94*:1248, 1984.
20. Lee, K. J.: Differential Diagnosis Otolaryngology. New York, Arco, 1978, pp. 110–114.
21. Levin, W. J., Shary, J. H., III, Nichols, L. T., et al.: Bone scanning in severe external otitis. Laryngoscope *96*:1193–1195, 1986.

22. Liston, S. L., and Siegel, L. G.: Tinactin in the treatment of fungal otitis externa. Laryngoscope *96*:699, 1986.
23. Lucente, F. E.: Fungal infections of the external ear. Otolaryngol. Clin. North Am. *26*:995–1006, 1993.
24. Mugliston, T., and O'Donoghue, G.: Otomycosis: A continuing problem. J. Laryngol. Otol. *99*:327–333, 1985.
25. Padmore, R. F., Bedard, Y., and Chapnick, J.: Relapse of acute myelogenous leukemia presenting as acute otitis externa. Cancer *53*:569–572, 1984.
26. Potsic, W. P.: Office pediatric otology. Otolaryngol. Clin. North Am. *25*:781–789, 1992.
27. Rubin, J., Yu, V. L., and Stool, S. E.: Malignant external otitis in children. J. Pediatr. *113*:965–970, 1988.
28. Russell, J. D., Donnelly, M., McShane, D. P., et al.: What causes acute otitis externa? J. Laryngol. Otol. *107*:898–901, 1993.
29. Schneider, M. L.: Merthiolate in treatment of otomycosis. Laryngoscope *91*:1194–1195, 1981.
30. Senturia, B. H., and Carr, C. D.: Studies of the factors considered responsible for diseases of the external ear. Laryngoscope *68*:2052–2077, 1958.
31. Senturia, B. H., Morris, D. M., and Lucente, F.: Disease of the External Ear: An Otologic-Dermatologic Manual. New York, Grune & Stratton, 1980, pp. 31–59.
32. Seyfried, P., and Cook, R. J.: Otitis externa infections related to *Pseudomonas aeruginosa* levels in 5 Ontario lakes. Can. J. Public Health *75*:83–91, 1984.
33. Sheth, K. J., Miller, R. J., Sheth, N. K., et al.: *Pseudomonas aeruginosa* otitis externa in an infant associated with a contaminated infant bath sponge. Pediatrics *77*:920–921, 1986.
34. Simchen, E., Franklin, D. D., and Hillel, S.: "Swimmer's ear" among children of kindergarten age and water quality of swimming pools in 11 kibbutzim. Israel J. Med. Sci. *20*:584–588, 1984.
35. Singer, D. E., Freenan, E., Hoffert, W. R., et al.: Otitis externa: Bacteriological and mycological studies. Ann. Otol. Rhinol. Laryngol. *24*:317–330, 1952.
36. Sobie, S., Brodsky, L., and Stanievich, J. F.: Necrotizing external otitis in children: Report of two cases and review of the literature. Laryngoscope *97*:598–601, 1987.
37. Stewart, J. D.: Chronic exudative otitis. J. Laryngol. Otol. *65*:24–32, 1951.
38. Wormold, P. J.: Surgical management of benign necrotizing otitis externa. J. Laryngol. Otol. *108*:101–105, 1994.
39. Wright, D. N., and Alexander, J. M.: Effect of water on the bacterial flora of swimmer's ears. Arch. Otolaryngol. *99*:15–18, 1974.
40. Yelland, M.: Otitis externa in general practice. Med. J. Aust. *156*:325–330, 1992.

19

Otitis Media

Jerome O. Klein and Charles D. Bluestone

The term *otitis media* denotes inflammation of the mucoperiosteal lining of the middle ear. *Acute otitis media* is the rapid onset of signs and symptoms of acute infection within the middle ear. *Otitis media with effusion* is an inflammation of the middle ear in which a collection of liquid is present in the middle ear space and there are no signs or symptoms of acute infection. *Middle ear effusion* is liquid in the middle ear. The effusion may be serous, a thin, watery liquid; mucoid, a thick, viscid, mucus-like liquid; purulent; or a combination of these. Fluctuating or persisting loss of hearing is present in most patients who have middle ear effusion; hearing impairment is the most frequent complication of acute otitis media or otitis media with effusion. Suppurative complications of otitis media occur when there is extension of inflammation and infection beyond the mucoperiosteal lining of the middle ear (e.g., mastoiditis, epidural abscess).

INCIDENCE AND EPIDEMIOLOGY OF ACUTE OTITIS MEDIA

Acute otitis media is one of the most common infectious diseases of childhood. A survey of diagnoses made in office practices in the United States in 1990 identified 24.5 million visits at which the principal diagnosis was otitis media; diagnoses of otitis media had increased from 9.91 million visits recorded in 1975.[123] In Boston, Teele and associates[140] found that approximately 33 per cent of pediatric office visits for illness of any kind were attributable to acute otitis media or otitis media with effusion. The same group of investigators reported that, by 1 year of age, 62 per cent of children had at least one episode of acute otitis media, and 17 per cent had three or more episodes.[141] By 3 years of age, greater than 80 per cent of children had at least one episode of acute otitis media, and 46 per cent had three or more episodes. A similar preponderance of cases of acute otitis media during the first or second year of life with a decline in incidence rate thereafter has been reported by investigators from locations as diverse geographically as Finland,[107, 127] Sweden,[64] Cleveland, Ohio,[85] Huntsville, Alabama,[62] and Galveston, Texas.[12] The results of these studies suggest that by 3 years of age, children may be categorized into three groups of approximately equal size relative to acute infections of the middle ear: one group is free of ear infections; a second group may have occasional episodes of otitis media usually associated with infections of the respiratory tract; and a third group is otitis-prone, subject to repeated (three or more) episodes of acute infection.

Host Risk Features (Table 19–1)

The peak age-specific attack rate occurs between 6 and 18 months of age. The frequent occurrence of otitis media in otherwise healthy infants is in part a reflection of the fact that the eustachian tube of the young child is shorter, wider, straighter, and more horizontal than that of the older child. Thus, organisms from the nasopharynx reach the middle ear more readily than they do in older individuals. By 3 years of age, the incidence of acute otitis media decreases because of changes in the anatomy and physiology and maturing immune mechanisms. Children who have had little or no experience with otitis media by age 3 years are unlikely to develop problems with middle ear infections unless some predisposing factor occurs, such as tumor or fracture of a facial bone or acquired immune deficiency.

Acute otitis media, like most bacterial infections in children, appears to occur more commonly in boys than in girls.[141] A genetic predisposition to acute otitis media is suggested by data indicating that there is familial aggregation; histories of severe and recurrent ear infections in siblings and parents are frequent in families with an otitis-prone child.[41, 141] Although prematurity has not been associated previously with predisposition to middle ear infection, a study from the Netherlands suggests that a gestational age of younger than 33 weeks and very low birth weight (<1500 g) are risk factors

TABLE 19–1. Risk Features for Severe and Recurrent Acute Otitis Media

Male gender
Familial aggregation: disease in siblings and parents
Very low birth weight (<1500 g) and gestational age younger than 33 weeks
Early onset of disease
Race: Native American, Alaskan Eskimo, Australian Aborigine
Poverty: crowded living conditions, poor sanitation, lack of access to medical care
Prone sleeping position
Use of pacifier
Not breast-fed
Group day care
Exposure to smoke and environmental antigens
Congenital or acquired immunodeficiency

for recurrent otitis media.[33] Age at first episode of acute otitis media is associated significantly with recurrent episodes.[141]

Predisposing factors for race and ethnicity may be difficult to separate from poor social and economic conditions. Particularly high rates of the disease have been observed among Eskimos,[68, 108, 116] Native Americans,[132] and Australian aboriginal children.[94] Factors of poverty predisposing to respiratory infections and otitis media include crowded living conditions, poor sanitation, and limited access to medical care.[88]

Although most children with recurrent and severe otitis media have no obvious predisposing factor, a small number have altered host defenses, including anatomic changes (e.g., cleft palate or uvula, submucous cleft), alterations of normal physiologic defenses (e.g., patulous eustachian tube, barotrauma), and congenital or acquired immunologic deficiencies (e.g., immunoglobulin deficiency, chronic granulomatous disease, malignancy). Active middle ear disease is a constant event in children with cleft palate.[100, 101] Children with acquired immunodeficiency syndrome have a higher age-specific incidence of otitis media beginning at 6 months of age, compared with uninfected children.[6] Nasotracheal intubation has been identified as a factor in the development of acute otitis media and otitis media with effusion in neonates and older children.[10, 32, 105]

Environmental Risk Factors (see Table 19–1)

An increased incidence of respiratory infections including otitis media in group day care compared with home care has been documented in the United States,[54, 96, 118] Sweden,[56] and Finland.[3, 126] A survey of children in Memphis, Tennessee, found that those in day care experienced more episodes of otitis media and were also more likely to have placement of ventilation tubes.[7] By the second year of life, 21 per cent of Pittsburgh, Pennsylvania, children observed from birth who were in group day care (seven children or more) had surgical procedures for middle ear disease (almost all were myringotomy and placement of tubes), compared with only 3 per cent of children in home care.[149] The increase in incidence of otitis media from 9.91 million office visits in 1975 to 24.5 million office visits in 1990 is associated with increased usage of group day care for young infants.[123]

Children who are breast-fed have fewer incidents of ear disease than do infants who are bottle-fed. In a Boston, Massachusetts, study,[141] breast feeding for 3 months or more was associated with decreased risk of acute otitis media in the first year of life. Although bottle-fed infants are placed in a reclining or horizontal position and the breast-fed infant is held in a vertical position, the data suggest that a constituent of breast milk is the important factor and not position during feeding. Of children with cleft palate who were provided breast milk or formula in a similar container, those who received breast milk had fewer cases of middle ear effusion.[102]

Sleep position and use of a pacifier have been identified as risk features in two recent studies. More episodes of acute otitis media were identified in children who slept prone (compared with those who slept supine) in an investigation of 14,000 infants in Bristol, England.[42] Use of a pacifier increased the risk of recurrent acute otitis media in Finnish children attending day care centers.[96a] More than three episodes of acute otitis media occurred in 29.5 per cent of children younger than 2 years of age using pacifiers and in 20.6 per cent of those not doing so; in children 2 to 3 years of age, the incidence of recurrent acute otitis media was 30.6 per cent and 13.2 per cent, respectively. Although data from these studies need to be corroborated, suggesting to parents that infants sleep in the supine position and limiting use of a pacifier may be opportunities to decrease the incidence of acute otitis media.

Allergy to environmental antigens plays a role in congestion of the mucosa of the eustachian tube. Smoke exposure can result in goblet cell hyperplasia, mucus hypersecretion, ciliostasis, and decreased mucociliary transport.[145] The availability of a biochemical marker, cotinine, in saliva, serum, or urine has made documentation of passive exposure to tobacco smoke more reliable than that provided by history alone. High concentrations of serum cotinine were associated by Etzel and colleagues[34] with increased incidence of acute otitis media and increased duration of middle ear effusion.

Studies in both the United Kingdom and the United States demonstrate seasonal variation in the occurrence of acute otitis media. The pattern within a period of a year is sinusoidal, with the peak incidence in December through March and lowest incidence in July through September.[63, 91] These findings do not correlate with general climatic conditions because the United States studies were performed in Texas and Washington, D. C., and the United Kingdom study in northern England. The incidence, however, coincides with the peak incidence of respiratory infections in both countries.

ETIOLOGIC AGENTS

The microbiologic causes of otitis media have been documented by appropriate cultures of middle ear effusions obtained by needle aspiration. Many bacteriologic studies of acute otitis media have been performed, and the results are consistent in demonstrating the importance of *Streptococcus pneumoniae* and *Haemophilus influenzae* and a minor role for *Moraxella catarrhalis* and group A streptococci. These bacterial pathogens also may be present in fluids obtained from children with otitis media with effusion. Respiratory viruses alone or in combination with bacteria have been identified in 17 per cent of middle ear fluids of children with acute otitis media.[112] *Chlamydia trachomatis* is responsible for some episodes of otitis media in infants 6 months of age or younger.

Bacteria may be isolated from middle ear fluid in about two-thirds of patients with acute otitis media (Table 19–2). The isolates obtained by needle tympanocentesis in studies of acute otitis media in children during the period 1985 to 1992 are shown in Table 19–2. The most common bacterial pathogen recovered from the middle ear of patients in each study was *S. pneumoniae*, which was found in 27 to 52 per cent of cases. Nontypable strains of *H. influenzae* were iso-

TABLE 19–2. Bacterial Pathogens Isolated from Middle Ear Aspirates in Infants and Children with Acute Otitis Media (Percentage of Children with Pathogen 1985–1992*)

	Mean	Range
Streptococcus pneumoniae	38	27–52
Haemophilus influenzae	27	16–52
Moraxella catarrhalis	10	2–15
Group A *Streptococcus*	3	0–11
Staphylococcus aureus	2	0–16
Miscellaneous bacteria	8	0–24
None or nonpathogens	28	12–35

*Percentage greater than 100 because of nontypable pathogens per middle ear effusion.

From Bluestone, C. D., and Klein, J. O.: Otitis Media in Infants and Children. 2nd ed. Philadelphia, W. B. Saunders, 1995.

lated in 16 to 52 per cent of cases. *M. catarrhalis* (previously *Branhamella catarrhalis*) accounted for 2 to 15 per cent of cases of acute otitis media.[146] Concomitant isolation of two or more organisms in the same effusion occurs in up to 7 per cent of cases. Disparate results of cultures in children with bilateral acute otitis media occur in about 20 per cent of cases.[104]

Relatively few pneumococcal serotypes are responsible for most otitis media caused by *S. pneumoniae*. The most common types, in order of decreasing frequency, are 19, 23, 6, 14, 3, and 18.[49, 67] All of these serotypes are included in the currently available polysaccharide pneumococcal vaccines.

Most *H. influenzae* isolated from middle ear fluid are nontypable.[59, 60, 130] In unimmunized children, type b strains may be responsible for about 10 per cent of children with *Haemophilus* otitis, and about one-quarter of these children have or develop bacteremia or meningitis.[51] Previously thought to be limited to preschool children, *H. influenzae* now is known to cause otitis media in older children and adolescents.[119, 121] Thirty per cent or more of *H. influenzae*[15] and at least 75 per cent of *M. catarrhalis*[74, 125, 146] isolated from middle ear fluids produce beta-lactamase.

Several clinical situations warrant special consideration: (1) the occurrence of purulent conjunctivitis in association with acute otitis media (conjunctivitis-otitis syndrome) usually is attributable to nontypable *H. influenzae*[19, 20]; (2) acute otitis media is common among children hospitalized in intensive care units, and the bacteriology may be reflective of the hospital environment[32]; (3) early recurrences of acute otitis media (within 1 month) represent reinfection more often than relapse[24]; and (4) children with tympanostomy tubes may develop acute otitis media caused by organisms associated with otitis externa (e.g., *Staphylococcus aureus, Pseudomonas aeruginosa, Staphylococcus epidermidis*).[117]

The bacteriology of otitis media with effusion mimics that of acute otitis media.[44, 45, 92, 110, 122, 133] In contrast, the etiologic agents of chronic suppurative otitis media with persistent perforation include *P. aeruginosa, S. aureus*, anaerobic bacteria, and enteric gram-negative bacilli.[21, 69, 99] *Mycobacterium tuberculosis* is a rare, but important cause of chronic suppurative otitis media with persistent perforation.[151]

Bacteria found in middle ear aspirates usually are present in the nasopharynx of children with acute otitis media, but multiple pathogens may be present in the nasopharynx that are not present in the middle ear.[35] Although not useful for specific microbiologic diagnosis of acute otitis media, nasopharyngeal cultures are of value for monitoring antibiotic susceptibility patterns of bacterial pathogens associated with acute otitis media. Several investigators have noted quantitative differences in the nasopharyngeal flora of patients with and without otitis media, and these differences may play a role in the pathogenesis of middle ear disease. Long and colleagues[79] described a significant association between the recovery of abundant *H. influenzae* ($\geq$50 per cent total colony count) from the nasopharynx and bacteriologically confirmed otitis media. An additional finding was that a semiquantitative nasopharyngeal culture was sensitive and specific in predicting the middle ear pathogen. Similar nasopharyngeal colonization rates for *S. pneumoniae* occur in ill and healthy children.[55, 78, 79] Gray and coworkers[49] have correlated the occurrence of acute otitis media with nasopharyngeal acquisition of new serotypes of *S. pneumoniae*.

Sterile cultures are noted after needle tympanocentesis in about one-third of patients with acute otitis media. This in part may reflect limitations of bacterial culture methods because antigen detection tests often indicate the presence of pneumococcal capsular polysaccharide in sterile middle ear fluid.[75, 81]

The clinical history suggests that viral infection is an initiating event of acute otitis media by producing congestion of the mucosa of the upper respiratory tract. In addition, epidemiologic data support an association between viral respiratory infection and the occurrence of acute otitis media.[53] Infection with respiratory syncytial virus, influenza viruses, and adenoviruses was associated with a greater risk of otitis media than was infection with other viruses. In contrast to this epidemiologic association is the low viral isolation rate from middle ear fluid in patients with otitis media. A virus was isolated from only 29 of 663 (4.4 per cent) specimens obtained by tympanocentesis and reviewed by Klein and Teele in 1976.[73] A higher virus identification rate in middle ear fluid has been reported using culture and antigen detection.[27, 70, 115] Ruuskanen and colleagues[112] summarized eight studies published between 1982 and 1990 using immunoassay or isolation; virus was identified in middle ear fluids in 17 per cent of the samples: as a single agent in 6 per cent and in combination with a bacterial pathogen in 11 per cent. Viruses identified in middle ear fluids have included respiratory syncytial virus, influenza viruses, adenoviruses, parainfluenza viruses, enteroviruses, and rhinoviruses. Concomitant isolation of viral and bacterial pathogens from middle ear fluid appears to be common.[27, 115]

A role for *Mycoplasma pneumoniae* in the etiology of otitis media was suggested by the observation of myringitis in nonimmune adults inoculated with the organism.[111] A subsequent study attempted to isolate the organism from middle ear fluid in patients with otitis media but was successful in only 1 of 771 patients.[73] This study suggests that mycoplasmas are an infrequent cause of acute otitis media.

C. trachomatis has been implicated as a cause of acute otitis media. Tipple and colleagues[143] recovered *C. trachomatis* from 3 of 11 middle ear specimens in infants with chlamydial pneumonia. Each of the patients had clinical findings consistent with acute otitis media. Chang and associates[26] isolated *C. trachomatis* from 3 of 26 unselected patients with otitis media. In contrast, Hammerschlag and coworkers[50] failed to recover the organism from any of 68 patients with otitis media. Thus, *C. trachomatis* may play a limited role in acute otitis media during the first months of life. In contrast, *Chlamydia pneumoniae* is rare as a cause of respiratory disease in children younger than 5 years of age.[98] The organism was isolated from the middle ear fluid of a patient with otitis media with effusion, but a prospective study of 75 children 6 months to 12 years of age referred for myringotomy or placement of tympanostomy tubes failed to identify *C. pneumoniae* in the middle ear fluids.[47]

Although *S. pneumoniae* and *H. influenzae* are responsible for most cases of bacterial otitis media, *M. catarrhalis* and group A streptococci are responsible for some cases and should be considered in choosing appropriate antimicrobial agents. The incidence of acute otitis media due to *M. catarrhalis* was noted to be as high as 22 and 27 per cent in 1983 reports from Pittsburgh[74] and Cleveland,[125] respectively, but in most studies is less than 10 per cent. A majority of strains of *M. catarrhalis* isolated from middle ear fluids produce beta-lactamase, and some patients fail to improve if they are treated with a beta-lactamase–susceptible drug.

During the preantibiotic era, otitis due to group A streptococci frequently was associated with scarlet fever and often was of a severe and destructive form. In recent years, group A streptococci have been isolated frequently in some studies from Scandinavia but have been infrequent in most studies from the United States.

Tuberculous otitis was an occasional cause of severe middle ear disease at the turn of the century in the United States and Western Europe and still occurs in developing countries. Otitis due to *M. tuberculosis* is characterized by a painless, watery otorrhea through single or multiple perforations of the tympanic membrane.[128]

Other bacteria are responsible for occasional cases of acute otitis media, including *S. aureus* (which is infrequent in the United States but appears to be the etiologic agent in up to 10 per cent of cases in Japan[4]), gram-negative enteric bacilli (responsible for about 20 per cent of otitis media in neonates but rare in older infants), anaerobic bacteria, *Clostridium tetani*, and *Corynebacterium diphtheriae*.

Etiology in the Neonate

Clinical investigators have performed needle tympanocentesis to isolate bacterial pathogens causing otitis media in the first 6 weeks of life. A total of 169 infants were included in four of these studies.[9, 14, 124, 142] Bacteria were isolated from middle ear fluid in 68 per cent of cases. As in older children, *S. pneumoniae* and *H. influenzae* were the most frequently isolated organisms. Other than the more frequent occurrence of disease caused by gram-negative enteric organisms (about 20 per cent of cases) and the occasional isolation of other neonatal pathogens (e.g., group B streptococci), the bacteriology of otitis media in this age group was similar to that in older children.

PATHOGENESIS

The pathogenesis of otitis media is likely to follow the following sequence of events in most children. The patient has an antecedent event (usually caused by an upper respiratory viral infection) that results in congestion of the respiratory mucosa throughout the respiratory tract, including the nose, nasopharynx, eustachian tube, and middle ear; congestion of the mucosa in the eustachian tube results in obstruction of the narrowest portion of the tube, the isthmus. The obstruction results in negative pressure in the middle ear and then development of middle ear effusion. The secretions of the mucosa of the middle ear, which usually drain through the eustachian tube, now have no egress and accumulate in the middle ear. The effusion may be asymptomatic, i.e., lacking the signs and symptoms of acute infection, which is termed *otitis media with effusion*. If pathogenic bacteria that colonize the nasopharynx are present in the middle ear after obstruction of the eustachian tube has taken place, the organisms multiply, resulting in an acute suppurative infection, an abscess, characterized by signs and symptoms of acute infection, such as fever and otalgia.[16, 17, 46, 114] For children with recurrent episodes of acute otitis media or otitis media with effusion, anatomic or physiologic abnormalities of the eustachian tube appear to be predisposing factors. It also is possible that there are subtle changes in immune response that predispose to frequent episodes of otitis media. There is experimental evidence that virus-induced impairments in neutrophil migration and bacterial killing also may be important in the pathogenesis of acute otitis media.[2]

With growth of the skull and change in the position, length, and width of the eustachian tube over time, the predilection to otitis media in accompanying acute infections of the upper respiratory tract in the first 3 years of life diminishes and the patient has fewer episodes of acute otitis media. Children younger than 3 years of age with similar respiratory infections are predisposed to have the complication of acute infection of the middle ear, whereas the older children challenged by the same microorganism have the signs of the upper respiratory infection but need not have the complicating ear infection.

The pathogenesis of persistent middle ear effusion or otitis media with effusion remains uncertain. An effective antimicrobial agent sterilizes the acute bacterial infection of acute otitis media. The middle ear effusion, now sterile, may persist for weeks to months. The median duration of middle ear effusion after acute otitis media is approximately 23 days (Fig. 19–1). The type of antibacterial drug used does not appear to alter the duration of fluid in the middle ear after acute infection.

PATHOPHYSIOLOGY

Tympanic Membrane

In the presence of otitis media, changes in the tympanic membrane occur rapidly. The presence of congested blood vessels, edema (which obscures normal landmarks), and bulging or sagging of Shrapnell membrane indicate not only a myringitis (inflammation of the tympanic membrane) but also the presence of fluid in the middle ear space. Blebs that appear on the surface epithelium are a consequence of acute otitis media or edema or hydropic degeneration of the membrane.

Inflammation may occur on outer epithelial or inner mucosal sides of the fibrous layer (middle layer) of the drum. In

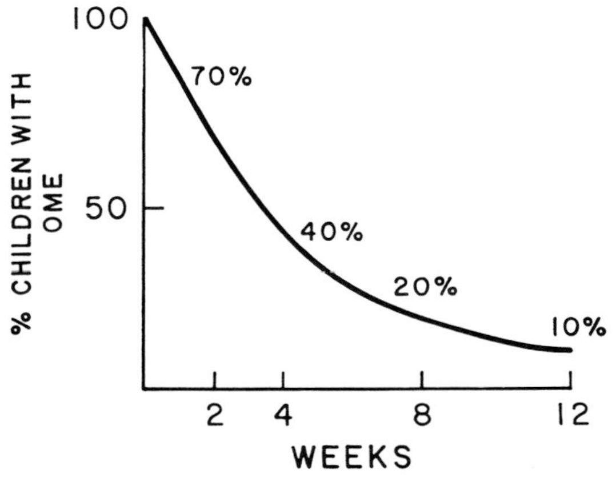

FIGURE 19–1. *Persistence of middle ear effusion after onset of acute otitis media. (Modified from Teele, D. W., Klein, J. O., and Rosner, B. A.: Epidemiology of otitis media in children. Ann. Otol. Rhinol. Laryngol. 89:5–6, 1980; in Bluestone, C. D., and Klein, J. O.: Otitis Media in Infants and Children. 2nd ed. Philadelphia, W. B. Saunders, 1995.)*

severe cases, infection may involve the fibrous layer itself. The membrane thickens as a result of edema and infiltration of polymorphonuclear leukocytes. All three layers of the drum may undergo dissolution, due to pressure necrosis resulting from the expanding middle ear abscess or thrombophlebitis of tympanic veins, with resulting perforation. With evacuation of the contents of the middle ear abscess, healing may be rapid, and the perforation usually heals within a few days. In the process of healing, metaplasia of the epithelium, hyaline degeneration, calcium deposition, and scar formation may occur. Occasionally, when a perforation is close to the margin of the annulus or occurs in Shrapnell membrane, the skin of the external auditory canal and the surface squamous epithelium of the tympanic membrane may grow through the aperture and invade the middle ear. This may lead to formation of a cholesteatoma (epidermal inclusion cyst). Even if the perforation heals, a differential in air pressure across the tympanic membrane caused by malfunction of the eustachian tube may result in resorption of air in the middle ear cavity and negative pressure in the middle ear. This causes retraction of Shrapnell membrane or the atrophic scar into the middle ear or mastoid attic.

Eustachian Tube

The eustachian tube is about 3.8 cm long in the adult. It opens in the fossa of Rosenmüller and then extends upward, backward, and laterally to open in the upper anterior wall of the tympanic cavity (protympanum). In the child, the tube is shorter, straighter, and more patulous. The eustachian tube is composed of two portions: the cartilaginous portion extending into the nasopharynx and the bony portion originating in the middle ear. The upper third of the tube is bony; the middle ear opening is the widest; and the medial end (the part joining the cartilaginous eustachian tube), or isthmus, is the narrowest (2.4 mm and 0.3 mm). Pneumatic peritubal air cells arising from the middle ear cavity surround it and can extend to the petrous apex. The internal carotid artery lies anteromedial to this region (Fig. 19–2).

The lower two-thirds of the eustachian tube is a narrow, slit-like, fibrocartilaginous passage. It makes a 160-degree angle with the bony portion at its junction. The cross-section of the tube looks like a shepherd's crook, with a cartilaginous superior and medial surface and a fibrous lateral surface.

Three muscles are associated with the eustachian tube. The tensor tympani muscle lies on top of it; the levator palatini muscle lies under it; and the tensor palatini muscle arises on the tube, scaphoid fossa, and spine of sphenoid and then courses around the hook of the hamulus and forms an aponeurosis with its mate (from the opposite side) in the soft palate. This is the only muscle that acts directly on the eustachian tube.

The eustachian tube area, protympanum, and hypotympanum are lined by ciliated columnar epithelium with goblet cells or secretory cells (respiratory epithelium, schneiderian epithelium). The epithelium is continuous with the upper airway system and paranasal sinuses. This area also contains a well-defined subepithelial connective tissue layer, which thins out and may be absent nearing the antrum and mastoid air cell system. The movement of the cilia and "mucous blanket" always is toward the eustachian tube and nasopharynx. The tube is surrounded by a plexus of lymphoid channels. It has an arterial supply from a branch of the middle meningeal or accessory meningeal artery and from branches of the artery of the pterygoid canal. The nerve supply is from the tympanic plexus (IX) (sensory) and sphenopalatine ganglion (sympathetics and parasympathetic palatine fiber).

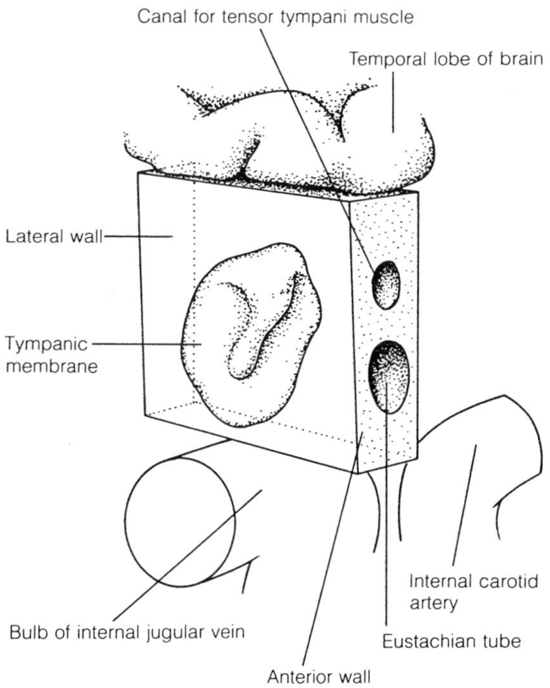

FIGURE 19–2. *The middle ear. (From Klein, J. O., and Daum, R. S.: The Diagnosis and Management of the Patient with Otitis Media. Copyright Biomedical Information Corporation, New York, 1985.)*

Whereas the bony portion is rigid and patulous, the medial two-thirds normally is held closed by elastic recoil of the fibrocartilaginous tissue. Thus, contraction of the tensor palatini muscle that inserts in the anterolateral wall opens the tube on swallowing. On the average, the adult swallows once per minute awake and once every 5 minutes asleep. Suckling children usually swallow five times per minute.

Mucus and ciliary action flow from the middle ear to the eustachian tube. The eustachian tube acts as a unidirectional valve that favors outflow from the middle ear to the pharynx. Reverse flow can be induced by an increase in pressure in the nasopharynx (Valsalva, barotrauma). Thus, during occlusion of the eustachian tube, the oxygen and carbon dioxide (and other gases) are absorbed from the middle ear by diffusion into the rich vasculature, and a negative pressure is created. A patent eustachian tube is a critical prerequisite for subsidence of middle ear disease.

CLINICAL PRESENTATION

Children with acute otitis media may have nonspecific signs and symptoms, including fever, irritability, headache, apathy, anorexia, vomiting, and diarrhea. Signs of respiratory viral infection, including cough and coryza, usually are present before the specific signs of ear infection occur. Fever occurs in about one-third[120] to two-thirds[95] of children with otitis media.

Specific signs and symptoms associated with otitis media and its complications and sequelae include the following.

Otalgia, or ear pain, is the most common complaint of infants and children with acute otitis media. The symptom is suggested in young infants who are pulling at the ear or excessively irritable. Some infants will not have earache; Hayden and Schwartz[53] identified absence of ear pain in approximately one-fifth of 335 consecutively diagnosed episodes of otitis media, usually among children older than 2 years of age.

Otorrhea is discharge from the middle ear through a perforation in the tympanic membrane or from the external auditory canal when inflamed. The acute perforation usually is central in the membrane. Relief of the pressure on the tympanic membrane results in immediate relief of pain and usually a decrease in temperature. Because the tympanic membrane has a dense network of blood vessels, rapid repair of the membrane occurs, and the perforation usually is inapparent within 24 to 72 hours. If the tympanic membrane seals and mucous membrane infection still is present, fluid may reaccumulate with renewed acute signs of otitis media.

Hearing loss occurs whenever fluid fills the middle ear space, whether the fluid is associated with acute infection or with otitis media with effusion. When fluid fills the middle ear space, the median hearing loss is 25 dB (the equivalent of having plugs in the ear canals).[39]

Vertigo occurs but is not a common complaint of children with otitis media. Vertigo is more common in unilateral than bilateral disease and also may be due to labyrinthitis. Older children describe a feeling of spinning, whereas younger children may not be able to verbalize these symptoms but manifest disequilibrium by falling or stumbling.

Tinnitus is an uncommon complaint in children, but when it does occur, the symptom often is due to otitis media and eustachian tube dysfunction.

Swelling about the ear, especially in the postauricular area, may be a sign of mastoiditis.

Facial paralysis in children occurs as a complication of acute otitis media or chronic otitis media with perforation of the tympanic membrane or as a result of an enlarging cholesteatoma.

Conjunctivitis has been associated with acute otitis media due to nontypable strains of *H. influenzae*. The conjunctivae are injected with tearing or purulent discharge.[20]

Craniofacial anomalies, such as cleft palate, mandibulofacial dysostosis, and Down syndrome, may predispose to frequent ear disease. Hypernasal speech suggests velopharyngeal insufficiency.

OTOSCOPY

Examination of the ear should begin with observation of the auricle and the external auditory meatus. Palpation of the periauricular areas should be performed to indicate presence of periostitis or diffuse external otitis. The ear canal should be examined for inflammation or cerumen that obstructs vision of the tympanic membrane.

For proper assessment of the tympanic membrane and its mobility, a pneumatic otoscope in which the diagnostic head has a secure seal should be used. The speculum should have the largest lumen that comfortably can fit in the child's cartilaginous external auditory meatus. The important landmarks of the tympanic membrane that can be visualized with the otoscope are indicated in Figure 19–3. The otoscopic examination should include observation of these conditions of the tympanic membrane:

1. *Position:* normal is slightly convex; bulging indicates increased pressure from positive air pressure or fluid; a retracted drum indicates negative pressure with or without effusion; fullness of the tympanic membrane is apparent initially in the posterosuperior portion of the pars tensa and the pars flaccida because these two areas are the most highly compliant parts of the membrane.

2. *Appearance and color:* the normal color is pearly gray and translucent; any congestion of the mucous membrane of the middle ear will be reflected in congestion of the vessels of the tympanic membrane and appear pink or with congested vessels; a blue discoloration suggests blood in the middle ear associated sometimes with basal skull fracture; the inflamed middle ear mucosa usually is reflected in a bright red tympanic membrane.

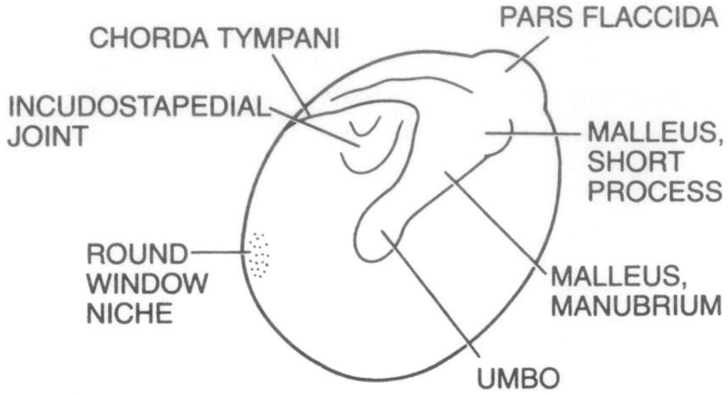

FIGURE 19–3. *Important landmarks of the tympanic membrane that usually can be visualized with the otoscope. (From Bluestone, C. D., and Klein, J. O.: Otitis Media in Infants and Children. 2nd ed. Philadelphia, W. B. Saunders, 1995.)*

3. *Integrity of the membrane:* all four quadrants of the tympanic membrane should be inspected for presence or absence of perforation, retraction pockets, or cholesteatoma.

4. *Mobility:* application of positive and negative pressures by the pneumatic otoscope enables the viewer to determine the presence of an air- (rapid excursion of the membrane on positive and negative pressures) or fluid-filled space (limited or no excursion of the membrane); a middle ear with negative pressure will not respond to otoscopic negative pressure, and a middle ear with high positive pressure will not respond to otoscopic positive pressure (Fig. 19–4).

Tympanometry

Tympanometry measures the compliance of the tympanic membrane (Fig. 19–5).[22, 30, 36, 87, 109] Under normal circumstances, the pressure in the middle ear virtually is the same as the external ambient pressure; the eustachian tube functions to equate middle ear pressure to atmospheric pressure. If for any reason there is a pressure differential across the tympanic membrane, stress will be applied to the drum. Middle ear compliance therefore varies as a function of the pressure differential across the tympanic membrane. Where there is blockage of the eustachian tube with no fluid in the middle ear, the tympanometry curve will have a shape similar to that observed on a normal tympanogram, but the point of maximal compliance will be shifted to the negative pressure side. This is because maximal compliance is reached when the tympanic membrane reaches a peak of compliance, i.e., when external canal pressure is reduced to the same level as in the middle ear.

If there is ossicular discontinuity or a flaccid or atrophic tympanic membrane, the drum is highly compliant, and a highly peaked tympanogram is obtained. Abnormal tympanograms obtained in the presence of fluid in the middle ear are characterized by:

1. Reduced height of the curve, i.e., the middle ear has reduced compliance.

2. Shift to negative pressure sides of the curve and point of maximal compliance, i.e., eustachian tube blockage.

3. A flat curve without definite peak, the most characteristic feature.

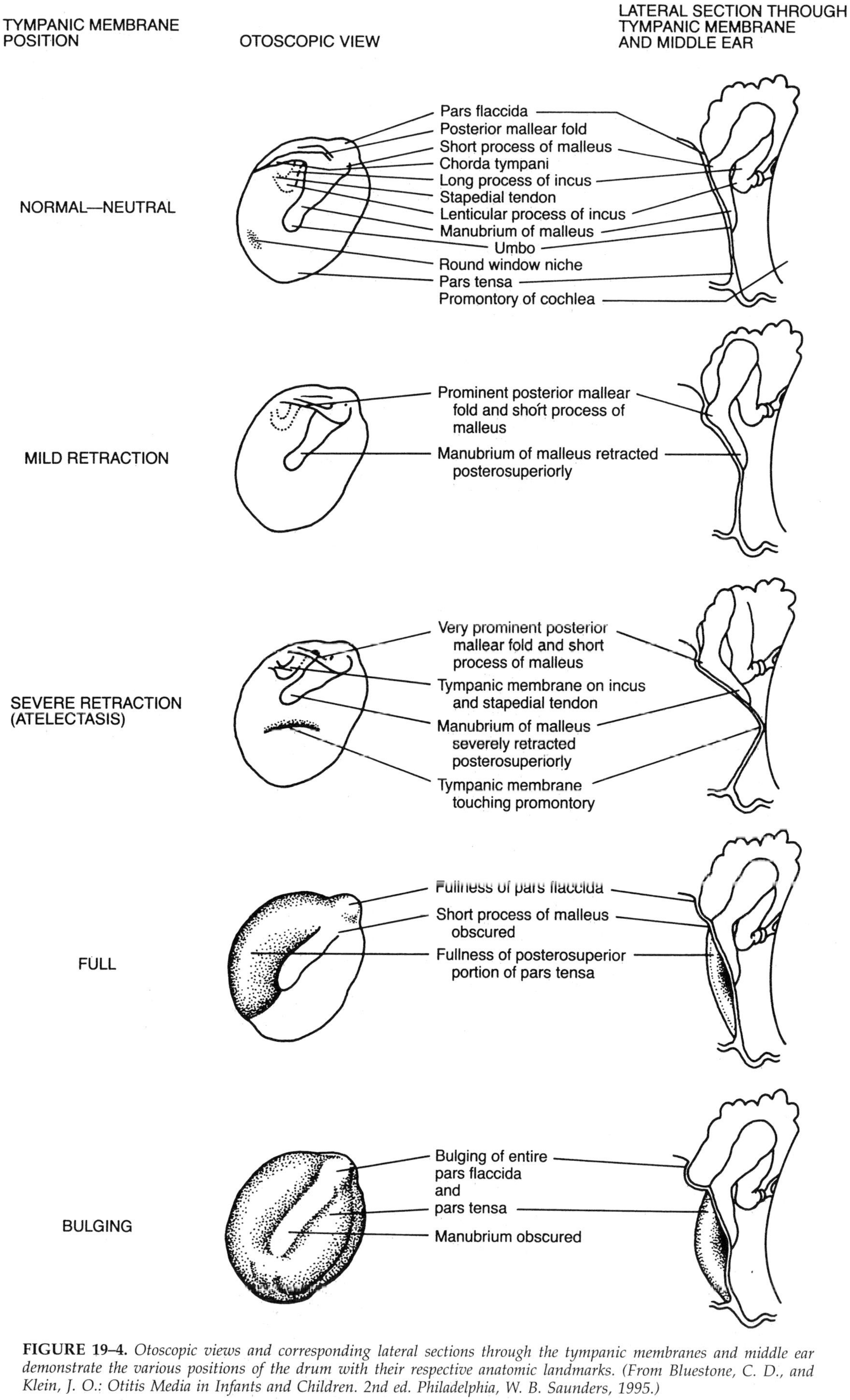

FIGURE 19–4. *Otoscopic views and corresponding lateral sections through the tympanic membranes and middle ear demonstrate the various positions of the drum with their respective anatomic landmarks. (From Bluestone, C. D., and Klein, J. O.: Otitis Media in Infants and Children. 2nd ed. Philadelphia, W. B. Saunders, 1995.)*

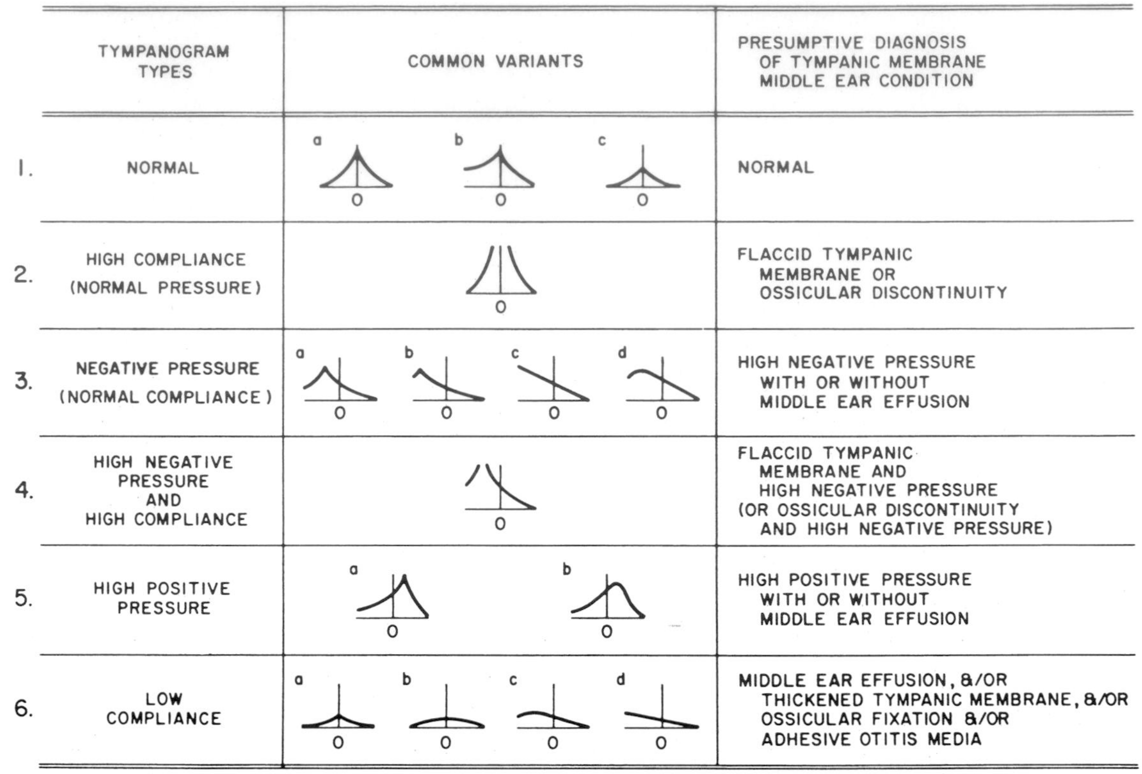
TYMPANOGRAM TYPES
COMMON VARIANTS
PRESUMPTIVE DIAGNOSIS OF TYMPANIC MEMBRANE MIDDLE EAR CONDITION
1.
NORMAL
a
b
c
0
NORMAL
2.
HIGH COMPLIANCE (NORMAL PRESSURE)
0
FLACCID TYMPANIC MEMBRANE OR OSSICULAR DISCONTINUITY
3.
NEGATIVE PRESSURE (NORMAL COMPLIANCE)
a
b
c
d
0
HIGH NEGATIVE PRESSURE WITH OR WITHOUT MIDDLE EAR EFFUSION
4.
HIGH NEGATIVE PRESSURE AND HIGH COMPLIANCE
0
FLACCID TYMPANIC MEMBRANE AND HIGH NEGATIVE PRESSURE (OR OSSICULAR DISCONTINUITY AND HIGH NEGATIVE PRESSURE)
5.
HIGH POSITIVE PRESSURE
a
b
0
HIGH POSITIVE PRESSURE WITH OR WITHOUT MIDDLE EAR EFFUSION
6.
LOW COMPLIANCE
a
b
c
d
0
MIDDLE EAR EFFUSION, &/OR THICKENED TYMPANIC MEMBRANE, &/OR OSSICULAR FIXATION &/OR ADHESIVE OTITIS MEDIA

FIGURE 19–5. *Tympanogram types related to presumptive conditions of the middle ear. (From Bluestone, C. D., and Klein, J. O.: Otitis Media in Infants and Children. 2nd ed. Philadelphia, W. B. Saunders, 1995.)*

Although tympanometry with the electroacoustic impedance bridge has proved to be a satisfactory method for detecting the presence of fluid in the middle ear cavity, there are technical difficulties in obtaining accurate readings in infants and children, including requirement for a secure seal of the probe in the ear canal, the need for a period of quiet to obtain an accurate reading, and decreased accuracy in infants younger than 7 months of age (because of the highly compliant external auditory canals).[103] In addition, only a few of many instruments currently on the market in the United States have data about sensitivity and specificity based on tympanometric patterns of otoscopic results prior to myringotomy.[38, 97] Less persuasive data are available from studies correlating tympanometry and otoscopy findings.[22, 28, 36, 87, 109]

Acoustic Reflectometry

The acoustic otoscope, or reflectometer (MDI Instruments, Woburn, MA), is a hand-held instrument that utilizes a microphone in the probe tip placed in the opening of the child's external ear canal. The tip measures the level of transmitted and reflected sound from an 80-dB sound source that varies from 2000 to 4500 Hz in a 100-msec period. Acoustic energy is reflected back toward the probe tip from the ear canal and eardrum. The operating principle is based on the fact that a sound wave in a closed tube will be reflected when it strikes the end of the tube. Sound reflectivity is measured in units that indicate the status of a fluid- or air-filled middle ear.[29] Babonis and associates[5] found that tympanometry and reflectometry had comparable accuracy in predicting middle ear effusion documented by myringotomy. Acoustic reflectometry has some technical advantages when compared with tympanometry; accurate readings can be obtained in crying children, and a secure seal of the probe tip in the ear canal is not required. More data are required comparing results of otoscopy, tympanometry, and acoustic reflectometry validated by aspirating the middle ear contents to determine presence of an air- or fluid-filled space.

Audiometric Tests

Audiometric testing may be employed to measure auditory acuity and evaluate conductive hearing losses, but assessment of hearing is not an accurate method for identifying middle ear effusion. Hearing loss is the most prevalent complication of otitis media and is present uniformly whenever fluid fills the middle ear. The audiogram usually reveals a mild to moderate conductive hearing loss (median is 27 dB).[39] Eustachian tube obstruction early in the clinical course of otitis media results in absorption of gases from the middle ear and drum retraction. The reduced compliance of the drum results in increased stiffness in the ossicular chain system. The audiogram reveals a low-frequency conductive hearing loss. As serous effusion appears and the middle ear fills with serum and pus, the ossicular system has an increased mass applied to it and the audiogram flattens out, giving a high-frequency conductive hearing loss.

Tympanocentesis and Myringotomy

Tympanocentesis, a needle aspiration of the middle ear effusion, is used primarily for diagnosis of presence or absence of an effusion and for microbiologic study. Because cultures of the upper respiratory tract are of limited value in providing specific microbiologic diagnosis of otitis media, only materials obtained by aspiration of the middle ear abscess can be considered a true reflection of the etiology of acute otitis media. Myringotomy is an incision in the anterior lower quadrant of the tympanic membrane for therapeutic drainage.

Tympanocentesis or myringotomy should be considered in patients who at onset appear toxic or are seriously ill, in patients who are toxic after initiation of antimicrobial therapy, in the presence of suppurative complications (including mastoiditis and meningitis), and in the immunologically deficient patient in whom an unusual organism may be present.

Radiography

Roentgenographic evaluation of the temporal bone is indicated when complications or sequelae of otitis media are suspect or present. Plain radiographs are of limited value in the diagnosis of osteitis of the mastoid or cholesteatoma; computed tomography and magnetic resonance imaging are more precise and should be obtained if a suppurative intratemporal or intracranial complication is suspected.

DIFFERENTIAL DIAGNOSIS

Inflammation or foreign body in the external ear canal may produce ear pain simulating that of acute otitis media. When external otitis or furunculosis of the external canal is present, there often is severe itching in the ear canal and pain elicited by manipulation of the pinna. The canal may be narrowed and so tender that otoscopic examination is not possible.

An erythematous tympanic membrane may be due to an upper respiratory tract infection with congestion of the mucosa lining the entire respiratory tract, including the middle ear. A "red drum" also may be produced by trauma or aggressive examination of the external canal and may appear suddenly in the crying child.

Otalgia may be associated with infections of the tonsils, adenoids, teeth, nasopharynx, hypopharynx, or larynx. Tumors in those regions can refer pain to the ipsilateral ear along the tenth cranial nerve. Lymphomas, leukemias, and rhabdomyosarcomas involving the palate, nasopharynx, or base of the skull eventually will occlude one or both eustachian tubes, producing serous effusions and otalgia.

Acute otitis media must be differentiated from an acute exacerbation of an unrelated disease in a patient with persistent middle ear effusion. Because fluid persists for weeks to months after each episode of acute otitis media, an intercurrent infection, not associated with middle ear disease, may be misdiagnosed as acute otitis media because of the presence of acute systemic signs of an infectious illness plus a middle ear effusion. This event may be one of the frequent reasons for overdiagnosis of acute otitis media. At present, there is no readily available technique, other than tympanocentesis, to distinguish a relapse of acute otitis media, from a new and recurrent episode of acute otitis media, from an intercurrent and unrelated infection associated with persistent middle ear effusion.

OTITIS MEDIA WITH EFFUSION

The presence of a relatively asymptomatic middle ear effusion has many synonyms, such as secretory, nonsuppurative, and serous otitis media, but the most acceptable term is *otitis media with effusion*. After every episode of acute otitis media, fluid persists in the middle ear for weeks to months[139] (see Fig. 19–1); in a study of Boston children, 70 per cent of the patients still had effusion at 2 weeks; 40 per cent had it at 1 month; 20 per cent at 2 months, and 10 per cent at 3 months. Similar results of persistent middle ear effusion after an episode of acute otitis media have been noted in all other clinical studies of acute otitis media. The incidence or prevalence of otitis media with effusion that is unrecognized by parents and therefore not brought to medical attention has been studied extensively.[25, 37, 106] The prevalence of effusion varied with age and the time of year. Incidence of otitis media with effusion peaked during the second year of life and was more prevalent in winter than in summer months.[37, 106, 136] In some children, the duration of otitis media with effusion may be as short as 1 or several days.[13] Because hearing loss is present whenever fluid fills the middle ear space, physicians are concerned about the many children with prolonged time spent with effusion, the accompanying hearing loss, and possible adverse effects on speech, language, and cognitive development.

The pathogenesis of otitis media with effusion remains uncertain. Although appropriate antibacterial agents are effective in sterilizing the middle ear effusion in acute otitis media, the drugs do not rid the ear of the fluid. At some later point, bacteria may re-enter the fluid-filled middle ear space. Bacteria can be recovered from one-third to one-half of specimens obtained at the time of myringotomy or tympanostomy tube insertion.[44, 45, 92, 110, 122] The bacteriology in such cases has mimicked closely the bacteriology of acute otitis media, with *S. pneumoniae* and *H. influenzae* being the predominant organisms isolated. The significance of this finding at present is unknown. The bacteria merely may colonize middle ear fluid without producing inflammation, or they may play a role in the production or persistence of middle ear fluid. In addition to live bacteria, nonviable bacteria, pneumococcal capsular polysaccharide, and endotoxin have been found in chronic middle ear effusions.[31, 44, 75]

Much attention has been given to the nature and composition of the middle ear effusion. The presence of biologic mediators of inflammation in the middle ear fluid has been demonstrated[11, 76, 120]; these include chemotactic factors, macrophage-inhibiting factors, activated complement, histamine, prostaglandins, leukotrienes,[65, 66, 93] and immune complexes.[148] Elevated levels of IgA, IgE, IgM, and IgG also have been noted in serous effusions.

Clinical evaluation depends on otologic examination and audiologic and tympanometric testing. Symptoms of this disease include conductive deafness that usually is fluctuant and may be position-dependent. The patient may have a dull earache or a sensation of fullness in the ear. The eardrum usually is dull with a poor light reflex and may be retracted. Color may be pale pink or ground glass in appearance.

COMPLICATIONS AND SEQUELAE: INTRATEMPORAL (Fig. 19–6)

Intracranial suppurative complications of otitis media, including meningitis, brain abscess, and lateral sinus thrombosis, are relatively uncommon today in developed countries. Intratemporal complications that occur within the aural cavity and adjacent structures of the temporal bone are more common. These include acute and chronic perforation of the tympanic membrane, chronic suppurative otitis media, mastoiditis, cholesteatoma and retraction pocket, adhesive otitis media, tympanosclerosis, and ossicular discontinuity and fixation. The most frequent complication is hearing loss

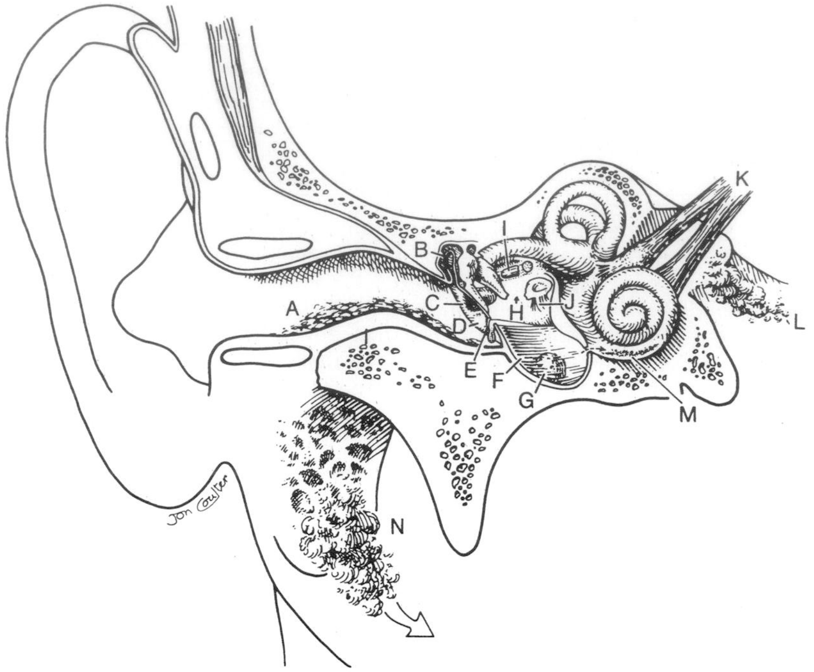

FIGURE 19–6. *Intratemporal complications and sequelae of otitis media include the following:* A, *Infectious eczematoid dermatitis.* B, *Cholesteatoma.* C, *Retraction pocket of tympanic membrane.* D, *Tympanosclerosis.* E, *Perforation of tympanic membrane.* F, *Chronic suppurative otitis media.* G, *Cholesterol granuloma.* H, *Ossicular discontinuity.* I, *Facial paralysis.* J, *Adhesive otitis media with fixation of the ossicles.* K, *Hearing loss.* L, *Petrositis.* M, *Labyrinthitis.* N, *Mastoiditis with extension into the neck (Bezold abscess). (From Teele, D. W., Klein, J. O., Rosner, B. A., et al.: Otitis media with effusion during the first three years of life and development of speech and language. Pediatrics 74:282–287, 1984. Reproduced with permission of Pediatrics.)*

that occurs whenever the middle ear cavity is filled with fluid.

Hearing Loss

Fluctuating or persisting loss of hearing is present in most children who have middle ear effusion; impairment of hearing is the most prevalent complication of otitis media with effusion. Audiograms of children with middle ear effusion usually reveal a mild to moderate conductive loss in the range of 15 to 40 dB.[39] With such deficits, the softer speech sounds and voiceless consonants may be missed. The hearing loss is not influenced by the quality of fluid in the middle ear; ears with thin fluids are impaired to the same degree as those with fluids of glue-like consistency.[23, 150] The hearing impairment usually is reversed with resolution of the effusion. Uncommonly, permanent conductive hearing loss occurs due to irreversible changes from the inflammatory reaction, resulting in adhesive otitis media or ossicular discontinuity. High negative pressure in the middle ear or atelectasis in the absence of effusion also may cause conductive loss.

Sensorineural hearing loss after acute otitis media may occur due to the effect of increased tension and stiffness of the round-window membrane and is reversible. A permanent sensorineural loss may occur as a result of spread of infection or products of inflammation through the round-window membrane.[80]

Effects of Otitis Media on Development of the Child

Children with severe or recurrent otitis media have prolonged time spent with middle ear effusion. Hearing impairment accompanies the effusion in most children. If the hearing impairment occurs at a time of rapid intellectual growth, the result may be impaired development of speech, language, and cognitive abilities (Fig. 19–7). Because language acquisition is dynamic during infancy, any problems in receiving or interpreting sound signals might have a significant effect on development of speech and language. Softer speech sounds and voiceless consonants, in particular, may be missed or confused when effusion is present in the middle ear. Although many studies have been performed and are reviewed in a recent clinical practice guideline (*Otitis Media with Effusion in Young Children*) published by the Agency for Health Care Policy and Research of the U. S. Department of Health and Human Services,[134] the limitations of design of many of the studies and inconsistencies of the results limit conclusions about the effect of otitis media on development. The interested reader should consult the guideline for a valuable review and extensive bibliography. Nevertheless, it is possible that many infants and young children with recurrent otitis media and prolonged time spent with middle ear effusion have substantive loss in potential for development of speech, language, and cognitive abilities. Selected references about long-term outcomes of otitis media include studies by Gravel and Wallace,[48] Teele and colleagues,[138] and Friel-Patti and associates.[40]

Perforation of the Tympanic Membrane

Acute perforation (not due to trauma) usually is secondary to acute otitis media but also may occur during the course

MIDDLE EAR EFFUSION

↓

CONDUCTIVE HEARING LOSS

↓

DECREASED PERCEPTION OF LANGUAGE

↓

IMPAIRED DEVELOPMENT OF SPEECH AND LANGUAGE

LOWER SCORES ON TESTS OF COGNITIVE ABILITIES

POOR PERFORMANCE IN SCHOOL

FIGURE 19–7. *Long-term sequelae of middle ear effusion. (From Bluestone, C. D., and Klein, J. O.: Otitis Media in Infants and Children. 2nd ed. Philadelphia, W. B. Saunders, 1995.)*

of otitis media with effusion. The perforation occurs because of pressure of the expanding middle ear contents on the membrane resulting in local ischemia and tissue damage, usually in the central portion of the membrane. With rupture, the middle ear contents are discharged into the external ear canal with instant relief of pain and defervescence in acute infection. Because the membrane is highly vascular, the perforation may seal quickly and not be evident within hours to days. If the mucous membrane of the middle ear remains inflamed, fluid may reaccumulate behind the resealed tympanic membrane.

Chronic perforation may occur after an acute episode, spontaneous extrusion, or removal of a tympanostomy tube. If squamous epithelium grows at the edges of the perforation, healing may be prevented and the perforation will persist. The term *chronic suppurative otitis media* is limited to a stage of ear disease in which there is chronic inflammation of the middle ear and mastoid and in which a nonintact tympanic membrane (due to perforation or tympanostomy tube) and otorrhea are present. Mastoiditis usually is present, and a cholesteatoma may have formed.

Cholesteatoma

The cholesteatoma usually is a cystic structure lined by squamous epithelium resting on a fibrous strand. The contents of the cyst are the products of desquamation, keratinization, and pus formulation. Cholesteatoma may invade, causing local bone erosion and destruction of the ossicular chain. Aural cholesteatomas can be classified as congenital or acquired.

A congenital cholesteatoma is a congenital rest of epithelial tissue and appears as a white cyst-like structure within the middle ear or temporal bone.

Acquired cholesteatoma may be secondary to implantation of epithelial tissue or may be a sequela of otitis media or a retraction pocket, or both. Implantation cholesteatoma may develop either from epithelium that has migrated through a perforation of the tympanic membrane or from intra-aural epithelium remaining after middle ear or mastoid surgery. Infection caused by such organisms as *S. aureus, P. aeruginosa, Proteus* species, nonhemolytic streptococci, and *Aspergillus* may be present. The process of alternating infection and healing will cause the advancement of squamous epithelium into the middle ear and antrum.[36, 77, 113] The persistent infection also stimulates proliferation of the mucoperiosteum of the attic region, thus creating an accelerated tissue growth (increased production of collagenase) and a destructive and expansive process. It is characterized by a foul smell, pus, squames, and bone destruction.

Management of cholesteatoma is surgical removal of the entire cyst. Antimicrobial therapy may be necessary if secondary infection is present.

Adhesive Otitis Media

Adhesive otitis media is a result of healing after chronic inflammation of the middle ear and mastoid. Fibrous tissue proliferates in the muscosal lining and may impair movement of the ossicles and result in conductive hearing loss. Adhesive changes may bind the eardrum to the ossicles and surrounding middle ear structures and cause resorption of the ossicles.

Tympanosclerosis

Tympanosclerosis, or scarring of the tympanic membrane, may be a sequela of chronic middle ear inflammation or trauma. White plaques are present in the tympanic membrane, with nodular deposits in the submucosal layers. The histopathology is marked by hyaline degeneration resulting from a healing reaction characterized by fibroblastic invasion of the submucosa followed by thickening and fusion of the fibers.

Ossicular Discontinuity and Fixation

Ossicular chain abnormalities, including osteitis, may be secondary to chronic inflammation in the middle ear or the presence of a retraction pocket or cholesteatoma. The long process of the incus most commonly is involved. Erosion of the blood supply, cholesteatoma, or adhesive otitis media may be the cause of the bone erosion and disarticulation. Conductive hearing loss is present to a varying degree. Diagnosis may be assisted by computed tomography or magnetic resonance imaging.

Mastoiditis

At birth, the mastoid consists of a single cell, the antrum, connected to the middle ear by a small channel, the aditus ad antrum. Pneumatization of the mastoid bone takes place soon after birth and usually is extensive by 2 years of age. It is likely that whenever there is acute otitis media, there is some degree of mastoiditis. With healing of the middle ear infection, healing of the mastoid also takes place. In a small number of cases, mastoid disease progresses with hyperemia and edema of the mucosal lining of the pneumatized cells; accumulation of serous and then purulent exudates in the cells; demineralization of the cellular walls and necrosis of bone; and, finally, formation of abscess cavities due to coalescence of adjacent cells after destruction of the cell walls. Pus may escape into contiguous areas, including the posterior cranial fossa, the middle cranial fossa, the sigmoid and lateral sinuses, the canal of the facial nerve, the semicircular canals, and the petrous tip of the temporal bone.

Signs of acute mastoiditis with periostitis include fever, otalgia, postauricular erythema, tenderness, and slight swelling. The pinna may be displaced inferiorly and anteriorly.

Initial management of acute mastoiditis includes parenteral antibiotics and myringotomy to provide drainage of the middle ear and mastoid contents. Surgical drainage of the mastoid should be performed if the symptoms of the acute infection, including fever and otalgia, persist. If the infection progresses, causing destruction of the bony trabeculae, a mastoid empyema, mastoidectomy should be performed to prevent spread of the infection to adjacent structures.

Petrositis

Petrositis occurs when there is extension of suppurative infection from the middle ear and mastoid into the petrous portion of the temporal bone. Signs of petrositis include pain behind the eye, deep ear pain, persistent ear discharge, and sixth nerve palsy. The triad of pain behind the eye, aural discharge, and sixth nerve palsy is known as Gradenigo syndrome. Management is similar to that described above for mastoiditis.

Labyrinthitis

Spread of acute otitis media into the cochlear and vestibular apparatus through the round (less commonly, the oval) window results in inflammation of the labyrinth. The signs of labyrinthitis include sudden, progressive, or fluctuating sensorineural hearing loss or vertigo in association with otitis media or mastoiditis. Signs of suppurative labyrinthitis (in the absence of meningitis) warrant aggressive otologic surgery and parenteral antimicrobial therapy.

Facial Paralysis

Facial paralysis may occur as a sequela of acute otitis media because of exposure of the facial nerve in the middle ear cleft due to a bony dehiscence. The palsy usually is unilateral. The paralysis usually resolves with medical therapy for acute otitis media, but if there is persistent paralysis of the facial nerve, decompression may be necessary.

COMPLICATIONS AND SEQUELAE: INTRACRANIAL (Fig. 19–8)

The middle ear and mastoid air cells are adjacent to the dura of the posterior and middle cranial fossa, the sigmoid venous sinus of the brain, and the inner ear. Suppuration in the middle ear or mastoid may spread to these structures, producing suppurative complications, such as meningitis, extradural abscess, subdural empyema, focal encephalitis, brain abscess, and lateral sinus thrombosis. Intracranial complications should be suspected when the child with acute or chronic otitis media develops persistent and severe headache, severe otalgia, and change in affect or level of responsiveness. Conversely, children with diagnosed intracranial infection, such as meningitis, should have middle ear or mastoid disease assessed as the origin of the central nervous system disease.

Intracranial extension of infection from the middle ear into the intracranial area may occur because of any of the following:

1. Progressive thrombophlebitis, permitting infection to spread through the intact bone.
2. Erosion of the bony walls of the middle ear or mastoid.
3. Extension along preformed pathways, such as the round window, deshiscent sutures, skull fractures, and congenital or surgically acquired bony dehiscences.

The microbiology, pathogenesis, diagnosis, and management of intracranial complications of otitis media and mastoiditis are discussed extensively elsewhere (see Chapters 20, 38, 39, and 43).

MANAGEMENT OF ACUTE OTITIS MEDIA

Management of acute otitis media focuses on the choice of an appropriate antimicrobial agent. Decongestants and antihistamines may provide some comfort for the patient who has congestion of the upper respiratory tract but provide no benefit in terms of earlier resolution of the middle ear infection. The antimicrobial agent should have a spectrum of activity that includes *S. pneumoniae* and *H. influenzae* and has documented clinical and microbiologic efficacy, limited side effects, availability in a convenient dosage schedule, palatability when provided in suspension, and reasonable cost.

The patient treated with appropriate antimicrobial therapy should have substantial resolution of signs and symptoms within 72 hours and absence of signs of relapse, recurrence, or suppurative sequelae.

The United States Food and Drug Administration has approved 13 products for treatment of acute otitis media (Table 19–3). The manufacturers have provided data indicating clinical efficacy for otitis media, but many of the published studies included sample sizes that were too small to show differences between the new and the standard agent adequately. The data available show no major clinical advantage for any one drug. Amoxicillin remains the current drug of choice because it continues to be effective, safe, and relatively inexpensive. The current incidence of amoxicillin-resistant *H. influenzae* and *M. catarrhalis* due to production of beta-lactamase or penicillin-resistant *S. pneumoniae* does not require a change in recommendations for otitis media in most communities.

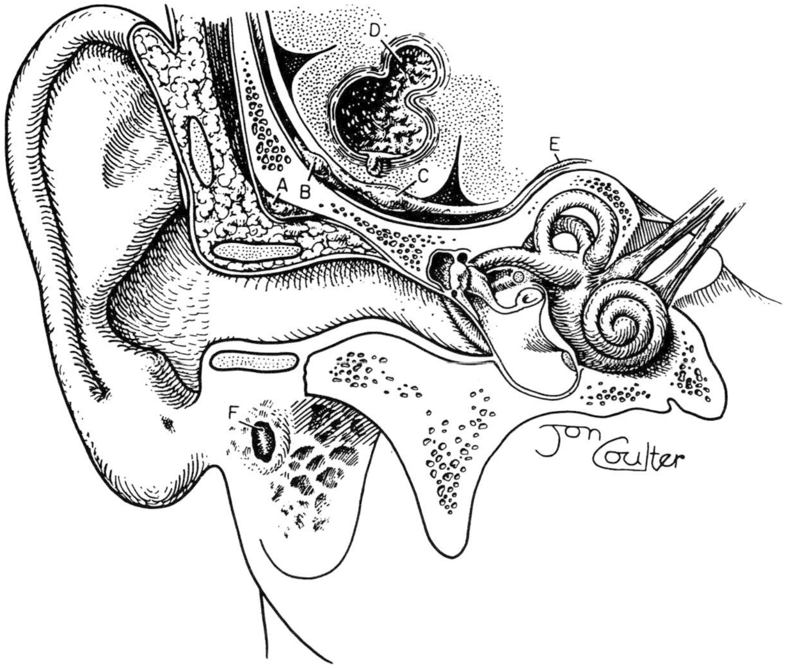

FIGURE 19–8. *Suppurative complications of otitis media and mastoiditis.* A, *Subperiosteal abscess.* B, *Extradural abscess.* C, *Subdural empyema.* D, *Brain abscess.* E, *Meningitis.* F, *Lateral sinus thrombosis. (From Bluestone, C. D., and Klein, J. O.: Otitis Media in Infants and Children. 2nd ed. Philadelphia, W. B. Saunders, 1995.)*

TABLE 19–3. Daily Dosage Schedule for Antimicrobial Agents Useful in Otitis Media*

Agent	Dosage/24 Hours
Penicillin G (benzathine salt)†	600,000 units in 1 dose for 30-kg child 1,200,000 units in 1 dose for >30-kg child
Amoxicillin	40 mg/kg in 3 doses
Amoxicillin-clavulanate	40 mg/kg in 3 doses
Cefprozil	30 mg/kg in 2 doses*
Cefpodoxime	10 mg/kg in 2 doses
Cefaclor	40 mg/kg in 2–3 doses
Cefixime	8 mg/kg in 1–2 doses
Cefuroxime axetil	30 mg/kg in 2 doses
Loracarbef	30 mg/kg in 2 doses
Erythromycin-sulfisoxazole	50 mg/kg erythromycin 150 mg/kg sulfisoxazole in 4 doses
Clarithromycin	In 2 doses
Azithromycin	10 mg/kg in 1 dose
Trimethoprim-sulfamethoxazole (TMP-SMZ)	8 mg TMP, 40 mg SMZ in 2 doses

*Approved for use in the United States for treatment of acute otitis media (January 1996).

†Intramuscular route; all others are oral.

From Bluestone, C. D., and Klein, J. O.: Otitis media, atelectasis, and eustachian tube dysfunction. *In* Bluestone, C. D., Stool, S. E., and Kenna, M. A. (eds.): Pediatric Otolaryngology, 3rd ed. Philadelphia, W. B. Saunders, 1996, p. 512.

If the physician has experienced an increased number of failures with amoxicillin or laboratory tests indicate a large proportion of beta-lactamase–producing strains, other regimens that are beta-lactamase stable, such as amoxicillin-clavulanate, a cephalosporin, or a sulfonamide, would be appropriate. If highly resistant *S. pneumoniae* becomes prevalent, beta-lactam drugs may not be effective and physicians will be dependent on results of contemporary antibiotic susceptibility patterns to indicate optimal therapy.

Diffusion of Antimicrobial Agents into Middle Ear Fluids

Most antimicrobial agents of value for treatment of acute otitis media achieve significant concentrations in middle ear fluid. The concentrations are, in general, parallel to, although lower than, concentrations of drug in serum. Purulent fluids have higher concentrations of drug than do mucoid or serous fluids. Penicillins and cephalosporins achieve concentrations in middle ear fluids that are approximately one-fifth to one-third of the levels present in serum. Sulfonamides and erythromycin achieved middle ear concentrations that were approximately 50 per cent of serum concentrations. An extensive review of concentrations achieved in middle ear fluids is provided in the textbook *Pediatric Otolaryngology,* edited by Bluestone, Stool, and Kenna.[18]

Sterilization of Middle Ear Fluids by Antimicrobial Agents

To define the ability of antimicrobial agents to eradicate bacterial pathogens from middle ear fluids of children with acute otitis media, investigators have used serial aspirates of the infected fluids.[58, 61, 86, 90] The initial aspirate identifies the bacterial pathogen of the acute middle ear infection; the second aspirate, days after initiation of therapy, defines the ability of the drug to eradicate the infection. The results of these tests generally are consistent with data available from in vitro assays of the drugs against the major bacterial pathogens and the concentrations of drug achieved in the middle ear fluids.[71] Pneumococcal infections were sterilized by most penicillins, cephalosporins, and macrolides; failure rates of 10 per cent or more were identified only in infections treated with cefaclor, cefixime, and cefpodoxime; sulfonamides alone were ineffective, but trimethoprim-sulfamethoxazole was effective. When infection due to *H. influenzae* was present, amoxicillin was effective if the organism did not produce beta-lactamase but failed when a beta-lactamase organism was the pathogen. Failure rates in excess of 20 per cent were evident for the cephalosporins, cefaclor, and cefprozil and for the macrolides erythromycin and clarithromycin.

Sterilization of Middle Ear Fluids Without Antibacterial Agents

Using the same technique of dual aspirates to identify the microbiologic efficacy of antibacterial drugs, Howie[57] identified sterilization of infected middle ear fluids without drugs. A placebo replaced active therapy in the dual aspirate study: 2 to 7 days after the initial aspirate identified the presence of pneumococci or *H. influenzae,* 19 per cent of the pneumococci and 48 per cent of the *Haemophilus* strains no longer were present. The differential clearing of the bacteria with persistence of most pneumococci but resolution of half of the infections due to nontypable *H. influenzae* is likely to be associated with some immune or bacteriostatic factor in the middle ear inflammatory exudate that acts to inhibit growth of these organisms. These data of spontaneous resolution need to be considered in evaluating the efficacy of new and old antibacterial drugs.

Dosage Schedules

Dosage schedules of the antimicrobial agents of value for therapy of acute otitis media have been determined on the basis of studies of the pharmacokinetics and results of clinical trials (Table 19–3).

Duration of Therapy

Duration of therapy is based on clinical trials and tradition. Most clinical trials and standard pediatric practice include a 10-day course of an antimicrobial agent. The United States Food and Drug Administration recently approved a 5-day schedule of once-a-day azithromycin administered orally based on studies comparing the clinical efficacy of 5-day azithromycin with 10-day amoxicillin-clavulanate courses.[89] These data suggest that short courses of therapy may be appropriate for many children with acute otitis media, although some children (likely those with severe and recurrent disease) will require more prolonged schedules.

Clinical Course After Initiation of Therapy

The clinical course of a child who receives appropriate antimicrobial therapy includes significant resolution of acute signs within 48 to 72 hours. Instructions to the parent should indicate the need to contact the physician if the signs or symptoms worsen at any time or are unimproved at 72 hours. Persistent ear pain or systemic signs, such as fever, signal the need for re-evaluation to examine for other foci of infections, to determine the need for another antimicrobial agent, or to perform tympanocentesis or myringotomy to incise and drain the middle ear abscess and culture the fluid to identify the pathogen. If a new antibiotic is needed, one with beta-lactamase stability and activity against penicillin-resistant pneumococci (if such information is available from local surveillance studies) should be chosen.

Follow-up visits should be made to determine that the child has recovered from the acute infection and to diagnose persistent middle ear effusion if it is present. The utility of the traditional 10- to 14-day visit was reassessed by Hathaway and coworkers[52] and Mandel and colleagues[83]; the investigators concluded that the follow-up visit can be extended to 4 to 6 weeks after onset of treatment in those children whose parents believed the disease had resolved at 10 to 14 days. For those who still had signs or symptoms of disease (other than persistent middle ear effusion), the 10- to 14-day visit was recommended.

Visits at 4 to 6 weeks and repeated at 1-month intervals if effusion is present are of value in determining the duration of middle ear effusion after the acute episode and identifying children who may be candidates for placement of tympanostomy tubes.

Symptomatic Therapy

Antipyretics, analgesics, and local heat usually are helpful in the child with an acute painful and febrile episode. An oral decongestant, such as pseudoephedrine hydrochloride, may relieve nasal congestion, and antihistamines may help patients with known or suspected nasal allergy. The efficacy of antihistamines and decongestants for resolution of middle ear effusion is unproven.

MANAGEMENT OF OTITIS MEDIA WITH EFFUSION

The following options have been investigated for management of the child with prolonged middle ear fluid or with otitis media with effusion:

1. Another 10-day course of a broad-spectrum antimicrobial agent that has activity against beta-lactamase–producing organisms because bacterial pathogens are found in approximately one-quarter of patients with otitis media with effusion; a meta-analysis of blinded studies identified resolution of effusion in 14 per cent of cases.[135]
2. Myringotomy or myingotomy and tympanostomy tubes to drain the middle ear fluid, aerate the middle ear space, and permit the middle ear mucosa to return to normal.[84]
3. Adenoidectomy with or without tonsillectomy for children who have recurrences after an initial placement of tympanostomy tubes.[43]
4. Steroid therapy alone or with an antibiotic has been demonstrated to be effective in some children with otitis media with effusion. Berman[8] recommended a regimen of prednisone, 1 mg/kg/day (given orally in two doses), for 7 days with an antibiotic for 14 to 21 days. Children without a history of varicella infection who have been exposed to the virus in the month before treatment should not receive prednisone because of the risk of disseminated disease. The guidelines published by the Agency for Health Care Policy and Research concluded that the data were insufficient in sample size or duration of observation to recommend use of steroids for otitis media with effusion.[136]

Topical or systemic nasal decongestants, antihistamines, and anti-inflammatory agents,[1, 147] alone or in combination, have been found to be of limited or no value in the management of otitis media with effusion.

We favor an initial course of a broad-spectrum antibiotic for children with 3 or more months of otitis media with effusion. If the effusion does not resolve, use of tympanostomy tubes is the most efficient method for management of prolonged middle ear effusion. The use of tympanostomy tubes first was suggested more than 100 years ago by Politzer, but the procedure did not become readily available until it was reintroduced by Armstrong in 1954. Myringotomy and placement of ventilating tubes result in the following immediate benefits to the patient with otitis media with effusion: the effusion is drained, and the fluid-filled space is aerated; the middle ear secretions, which constantly are being formed by the secretory cells of the mucosa, are drained; the chronically diseased mucosa (characterized by hypertrophic secretory cells) returns to normal; the hearing impairment due to the middle ear fluid disappears; concern for effects of hearing loss on development of speech and cognitive abilities is diminished; and the child who was not responsive or attentive (a condition often unrecognized as hearing impairment by the parent) now is more social and more involved with siblings, parents, and playmates. The procedure may be disadvantageous for the following reasons: general anesthesia is required; the cost is significant; and, although uncommon, there may be sequelae, such as persistent otorrhea, permanent perforation, scarring of the membrane, and cholesteatoma.

Current recommendations for pediatric otitis media with effusion include follow-up visits for 1 to 2 months after the acute episode. When the effusion persists for 3 or more months, the child should receive medical treatment with a course of antibiotics (2 to 3 weeks) or in conjunction with a 7-day regimen of prednisone. If the effusion fails to resolve with medical management, the child should be referred to an otolaryngologist for consideration of placement of tympanostomy tubes.

PREVENTION

Advising Parents

Parents of children who have severe and recurrent otitis media or risk factors for middle ear infections should be advised of measures that may reduce the incidence of infection, such as breast feeding; enrolling children in small, rather than large, group day care centers; and reducing exposure to tobacco smoke. In addition, data about the risks for recurrent otitis media of the prone sleeping position and use of a pacifier, although requiring corroboration, may be added to the parent discussion. Physicians also may advise parents that the seasonal incidence of otitis media suggests that their child's condition is expected to improve in late spring and summer and that aggressive measures of management, including chemoprophylaxis and surgery, may be postponed until the course of disease has been determined in the next respiratory season.

Pneumococcal Vaccine

Each pneumococcal antigen in the currently available 23-type polysaccharide vaccine produces an independent antibody response. In children 2 years of age or older and adults, antibody develops in about 2 weeks. Studies of polysaccharide vaccines in Finland and the United States have indicated that the vaccines are effective in prevention of type-specific pneumococcal otitis media if an adequate immune response occurs, but the number of types producing an adequate response in children younger than 2 years of age is limited.[82, 131, 137] Administration of vaccine in older children may provide protection against some types (more with each year the child is older) and be of value for the child who continues to have severe and recurrent otitis media after 2 years of age. Conjugate pneumococcal vaccines containing capsular polysaccharide conjugated to a protein carrier produce a significant immune response in infants as young as 2 months of age and now are in clinical trials.

Chemoprophylaxis

Chemoprophylaxis has been successful in reducing the number of new symptomatic episodes of acute otitis media in children who have a history of recurrent infections. The results of 15 reports of controlled clinical trials of modified courses of antimicrobial agents compared with those in which placebo or historical controls were used have been reviewed.[72] The majority of studies used a sulfonamide or a broad-spectrum penicillin. All of the reports indicated benefit to the enrollees in reduction of new episodes when they were compared with controls: amoxicillin efficacy varied from 44 to 67 per cent, and sulfonamide efficacy ranged from 40 to 88 per cent (although the efficacy of sulfonamides was reported as only 8 per cent in one study).

We recommend the following protocol based on the results of these studies. Criteria for enrollment include three documented episodes of acute otitis media in 6 months or four episodes in 12 months. Because children who have episodes of acute infection early in life or have siblings with severe and recurrent ear infections are prone to otitis, prophylaxis also should be considered for children who have one episode in the first 6 months of life plus a family history of ear infections or who have two episodes in the first year of life.

A sulfonamide or amoxicillin is the agent used most often and provides the advantages of demonstrated efficacy, safety, and low cost. The drug is administered at one-half the therapeutic dose (administered once a day); amoxicillin is given at a dose of 20 mg/kg, and sulfisoxazole is given at a dose of 50 mg/kg.

Chemoprophylaxis should be provided during the fall, winter, and early spring months (when respiratory tract infections are most frequent) for a period of up to 6 months.

Children, when free of signs of acute infection, should be examined at approximately 2-month intervals to determine if middle ear effusion is present. Management of prolonged middle ear effusion should be considered separately from prevention of recurrences of acute infection.

Acute infections are expected to occur, although at a lower rate, during the course of prophylaxis. The infection should be treated with the alternative regimen; a cephalosporin or amoxicillin/clavulanate would be suitable alternatives, irrespective of the prophylactic agent used.

References

1. Abramovich, S., O'Grady, J., Fuller, A., et al.: Naproxen in otitis media with effusion. J. Laryngol. Otol. *100*:263–266, 1986.
2. Abramson, J. S., Giebink, G. S., Mills, E. L., et al.: Polymorphonuclear leukocyte dysfunction during influenza virus infection in chinchillas. J. Infect. Dis. *143*:836–845, 1981.
3. Alho, O. P., Koivu, M., Sorri, M., et al.: Risk factors for recurrent acute otitis media and respiratory infection in infancy. Int. J. Pediatr. Otorhinolaryngol. *19*:151–161, 1990.
4. Baba, S.: Recent aspects of clinical bacteriology in otitis media. Presented at Presymposium on Management of Otitis Media, Kyoto, January 12, 1985.
5. Babonis, T. R., Weir, M. R., and Kelly, P. C.: Impedance tympanometry and acoustic reflectometry at myringotomy. Pediatrics *87*:475–480, 1991.
6. Barnett, E. D., Klein, J. O., Pelton, S. I., et al.: Otitis media in children born to human immunodeficiency virus–infected mothers. Pediatr. Infect. Dis. J. *11*:360–364, 1992.
7. Bell, D. W., Gleiber, D. W., Mercer, A. A., et al.: Illness associated with child day care: A study of incidence and cost. Am. J. Public Health *79*:479–484, 1989.
8. Berman, S.: Otitis media in children. N. Engl. J. Med. *332*:1560–1565, 1995.
9. Berman, S. A., Balkany, T. J., and Simmons, M. A.: Otitis media in infants less than 12 weeks of age: Differing bacteriology among in-patients and out-patients. J. Pediatr. *93*:453–454, 1978.
10. Berman, S. A., Balkany, T. J., and Simmons, M. A.: Otitis media in the neonatal intensive care unit. Pediatrics *62*:168, 1978.
11. Bernstein, J. M.: Biologic mediators of inflammation in middle ear effusion. Ann. Otol. Rhinol. Laryngol. *85*(Suppl. 25):90–96, 1976.
12. Biles, R. E., Bufler, P. A., and O'Donnell, A. A.: Epidemiology of otitis media: A community study. Am. J. Public Health *70*:593–598, 1980.
13. Birch, L., and Elbrond, O.: Daily impedance audiometric screening of children in a day-care institution: Changes through one month. Scand. Audiol. *14*:5–8, 1985.
14. Bland, R. D.: Otitis media in the first six weeks of life: Diagnosis, bacteriology and management. Pediatrics *49*:187–197, 1972.
15. Bluestone, C. D.: Management of otitis media in infants and children: Current role of old and new antimicrobial agents. Pediatr. Infect. Dis. *7*:S129–S136, 1988.
16. Bluestone, C. D., and Beery, Q. C.: Concepts on the pathogenesis of middle-ear effusions. Ann. Otol. Rhinol. Laryngol. *85*:182–186, 1976.
17. Bluestone, C. D., Cantekin, E. I., and Beery, Q. C.: Effect of inflammation on the ventilatory function of the eustachian tube. Laryngoscope *87*:493–507, 1977.
18. Bluestone, C. D., Stool, S. E., and Kenna, M. A. (eds.): Pediatric Otolaryngology. Vol. 1, 3rd ed. Philadelphia, W. B. Saunders, 1996, pp. 515–517.
19. Bodor, F. F.: Systemic antibiotics for treatment of the conjunctivitis–otitis media syndrome. Pediatr. Infect. Dis. *8*:287–290, 1989.
20. Bodor, F. F., Marchant, C. D., Shurin, P. A., et al.: Bacterial etiology of conjunctivitis–otitis media syndrome. Pediatrics *76*:26–28, 1985.
21. Brook, I.: Prevalence of beta-lactamase–producing bacteria in chronic suppurative otitis media. Am. J. Dis. Child. *139*:280–283, 1985.
22. Brooks, D. N.: Hearing screening: A comparative study of an impedance method and pure tone testing. Scand. Audiol. *2*:67–72, 1973.
23. Brown, D. T., Marsh, R. R., and Potsic, W. P.: Hearing loss induced by viscous fluids in the middle ear. Int. J. Pediatr. Otorhinolaryngol. *5*:39–46, 1983.
24. Carlin, S. A., Marchant, C. D., Shurin, P. A., et al.: Early recurrences of otitis media: Reinfection or relapse? J. Pediatr. *110*:20–25, 1987.
25. Casselbrant, M. D., Brostoff, L. M., Cantekin, E. I., et al.: Otitis media with effusion in preschool children. Laryngoscope *95*:428–436, 1985.
26. Chang, M. J., Rodriguez, W. J., and Mohla, C.: *Chlamydia trachomatis* in otitis media in children. Pediatr. Infect. Dis. *1*:95–97, 1982.
27. Chonmaitree, T., Howie, V. M., and Truant, A. L.: Presence of respiratory viruses in middle ear fluids and nasal wash specimens from children with acute otitis media. Pediatrics *77*:698–702, 1986.
28. Coffey, Jr., J. D., Martin, A. D., and Booth, H. N.: *Neisseria catarrhalis* in exudative otitis media. Arch. Otolaryngol. *86*:403–406, 1967.
29. Combs, J. T.: Two useful tools for exploring the middle ear. Contemp. Pediatr. *10*:60–75, 1993.
30. Cooper, Jr., J. E., Gates, G. A., Owen, J. H., et al.: An abbreviated impedance bridge technique for school screening. J. Speech Hear. Disord. *40*:260–269, 1975.
31. DeMaria, T. F., Prior, R. B., Briggs, B. R., et al.: Endotoxin in middle ear effusions from patients with chronic otitis media with effusion. *In* Lim, D. J., Bluestone, C. D., Klein, J. O., et al. (eds.): Recent Advances in Otitis Media with Effusion. Philadelphia, Decker, 1984, pp. 123–125.
32. Derkay, C. S., Bluestone, C. D., Thompson, A. E., et al.: Otitis media in the pediatric intensive care unit: A prospective study. Otolaryngol. Head Neck Surg. *100*:292–299, 1989.
33. Engel, J. A. M., Anteunis, L. J. C., Hendriks, J. J. T., et al.: Epidemiological aspects of otitis media with effusion in infancy. *In* Abstracts of the Sixth International Symposium on Recent Advances in Otitis Media, Fort Lauderdale, June 4–8, 1995, p. 15.
34. Etzel, R. A., Pattishall, E. N., Haley, N. J., et al.: Passive smoking and middle ear effusion among children in day care. Pediatrics *90*:228–232, 1992.
35. Faden, H., Stanievich, J., Brodsky, L., et al.: Changes in nasopharyngeal flora during otitis media of childhood. Pediatr. Infect. Dis. J. *9*:623, 1990.
36. Fernandez, C., Lindsay, J. R., and Moskowitz, M.: Some observations on the pathogenesis of middle ear cholesteatoma. Arch. Otolaryngol. *69*:537–546, 1959.
37. Fiellau-Nikolajsen, M.: Tympanometry in three-year-old children. II. Seasonal influence on tympanometric results in nonselected groups of three-year-old children. Scand. Audiol. *8*:181–185, 1979.
38. Finitzo, T., Friel-Patti, S., Chinn, K., et al.: Tympanometry and otoscopy

prior to myringotomy: Issues in diagnosis of otitis media. Int. J. Pediatr. Otorhinolaryngol. *24*:101–110, 1992.

39. Fria, T. J., Cantekin, E. I., and Eichler, J. A.: Hearing acuity of children with otitis media with effusion. Arch. Otolaryngol. Head. Neck Surg. *111*:10–16, 1985.
40. Friel-Patti, S., Finitzo-Hieber, T., Conti, G., et al.: Language delay in infants associated with middle ear disease and mild fluctuating hearing impairment. Pediatr. Infect. Dis. *1*:104–109, 1982.
41. Fry, J., Dillane, J. B., Jones, R. F. M., et al.: The outcome of acute otitis media. Br. J. Prev. Soc. Med. *23*:205–209, 1969.
42. Gannon, M. M., Haggard, M. P., Golding, J., et al.: Sleeping position: A new environmental risk factor for otitis media? *In* Abstracts of the Sixth International Symposium on Recent Advances in Otitis Media. Fort Lauderdale, June 4–8, 1995, p. 24.
43. Gates, G. A., Avery, C. A., Prihoda, T. A., et al.: Effectiveness of adenoidectomy and tympanostomy tubes in the treatment of chronic otitis media with effusion. N. Engl. J. Med. *317*:1444–1451, 1987.
44. Giebink, G. S., Juhn, S. K., Weber, M. L., et al.: The bacteriology and cytology of chronic otitis media with effusion. Pediatr. Infect. Dis. *1*:98–103, 1982.
45. Giebink, G. S., Mills, E. L., Huff, J. S., et al.: The microbiology of serous and mucoid otitis media. Pediatrics *63*:915–919, 1979.
46. Giebink, G. S., and Quie, P. G.: Otitis media: The spectrum of middle ear inflammation. Annu. Rev. Med. *29*:285–306, 1978.
47. Goo, Y. A., Hori, M. K., Voorhres, J. H., Jr., et al.: Failure to detect *Chlamydia pneumoniae* in ear fluids from children with otitis media. Pediatr. Infect. Dis. J. *14*:1000–1001, 1995.
48. Gravel, J. S., and Wallace, I. F.: Listening and language at 4 years of age: Effects of early otitis media. J. Speech Hear. Res. *35*:588–595, 1992.
49. Gray, B. M., Converse, G. M., III, and Dillon, H. C., Jr.: Serotypes of *Streptococcus pneumoniae* causing disease. J. Infect. Dis. *140*:979–983, 1979.
50. Hammerschlag, M. R., Hammerschlag, P. E., and Alexander, E. R.: The role of *Chlamydia trachomatis* in middle ear effusions in children. Pediatrics *66*:615–617, 1980.
51. Harding, A. L., Anderson, P., Howie, V. M., et al.: *Hemophilus influenzae* isolated from children with otitis media. *In* Sell, S. H., and Karzon, D. T. (eds.): *Hemophilus influenzae*. Nashville, Vanderbilt University Press, 1973.
52. Hathaway, T. J., Katz, H. P., Dershewitz, R. A., et al.: Acute otitis media: Who needs post-treatment follow-up? Pediatrics *94*:143, 1994.
53. Hayden, G. F., and Schwartz, R. H.: Characteristics of earache among children with acute otitis media. Am. J. Dis. Child. *139*:721–723, 1985.
54. Henderson, F. W., Collier, A. M., Sanyal, M. A., et al.: A longitudinal study of respiratory viruses and bacteria in the etiology of acute otitis media with effusion. N. Engl. J. Med. *306*:1377–1383, 1982.
55. Hendley, J. O., Sande, M. A., Stewart, P. M., et al.: Spread of *Streptococcus pneumoniae* in families: Carriage rates and distribution of types. J. Infect. Dis. *132*:55–68, 1975.
56. Hesselvik, L.: Respiratory infections among children in day nurseries. Acta Paediatr. Scand. *74*(Suppl.):33–103, 1949.
57. Howie, V. M.: Eradication of bacterial pathogens from middle ear infections. Clin. Infect. Dis. *14*(Suppl. 2):209–210, 1992.
58. Howie, V. M.: Otitis media. Pediatr. Rev. *18*:320–323, 1993.
59. Howie, V. M., and Ploussard, J. H.: Bacterial etiology and antimicrobial treatment of exudative otitis media: Relation of antibiotic therapy to relapses. South. Med. J. *64*:233–239, 1971.
60. Howie, V. M., Ploussard, J. H., and Lester, Jr., R. L.: Otitis media: A clinical and bacteriological correlation. Pediatrics *45*:29–35, 1970.
61. Howie, V. M., and Ploussard, J. H.: The "in vivo sensitivity test:" Bacteriology of middle ear exudate during antimicrobial therapy in otitis media. Pediatrics *44*:940–944, 1969.
62. Howie, V. M., Ploussard, J. H., and Sloyer, J.: The "otitis-prone" condition. Am. J. Dis. Child. *129*:676–678, 1975.
63. Howie, V. M., and Schwartz, R. H.: Acute otitis media: One year in general pediatric practice. Am. J. Dis. Child. *137*:155–158, 1983.
64. Ingvarsson, L., Lundgren, A., and Oloffson, B.: Epidemiology of acute otitis media in children: A cohort study in an urban population. *In* Lim, D. J., Bluestone, C. D., Klein, J. O., et al. (eds.): Recent Advances in Otitis Media with Effusion. Philadelphia, Decker, 1984, pp. 19–22.
65. Jung, T. T. K., Smith, D. M., Juhn, S. K., et al.: Prostaglandins and otitis media: Studies in the chinchilla. Otolaryngol. Head Neck Surg. *88*:316–323, 1980.
66. Jung, T. T. K., Juhn, S. K., and Michael, A. F.: Localization of prostaglandin-forming cyclooxygenase in middle ear and external canal tissue. Otolaryngol. Head Neck Surg. *91*:187–192, 1983.
67. Kamme, C., Ageberg, M., and Lundgren, K.: Distribution of *Diplococcus pneumoniae* types in acute otitis media in children and influence of the types on the clinical course in penicillin V therapy. Scand. J. Infect. Dis. *2*:183–190, 1970.
68. Kaplan, G. J., Fleshman, J. K., Bender, T. R., et al.: Long-term effects of otitis media: A 10-year cohort study of Alaskan Eskimo children. Pediatrics *52*:577–585, 1973.
69. Kenna, M. A., and Bluestone, C. D.: Microbiology of chronic suppurative otitis media in children. Pediatr. Infect. Dis. *5*:223–225, 1986.
70. Klein, B. S., Dollete, F. R., and Yolken, R. H.: The role of respiratory syncytial virus and other viral pathogens in acute otitis media. J. Pediatr. *101*:16–20, 1982.
71. Klein, J. O.: Microbiologic efficacy of antibacterial drugs for acute otitis media. Pediatr. Infect. Dis. *12*:973–975, 1993.
72. Klein, J. O.: Preventing recurrent otitis: What role for antibiotics? Contemp. Pediatr. *11*:44–60, 1994.
73. Klein, J. O., and Teele, D. W.: Isolation of viruses and mycoplasmas from middle ear effusions: A review. Ann. Otol. Rhinol. Laryngol. *85*(Suppl. 25):140–144, 1976.
74. Kovatch, A. L., Wald, E. R., and Michaels, R. H.: β-lactamase–producing *Branhamella catarrhalis* causing otitis media in children. J. Pediatr. *102*:261–263, 1983.
75. Leinonen, M. K.: Detection of pneumococcal capsular polysaccharide antigens by latex agglutination, counterimmunoelectrophoresis, and radioimmunoassay in middle ear exudates in acute otitis media. J. Clin. Microbiol. *11*:135–140, 1980.
76. Lim, D. J., Bluestone, C. D., Saunders, W. H., et al.: Report of research committee on middle ear effusions. Ann. Otol. Rhinol. Laryngol. *85*(Suppl. 25):1–295, 1976.
77. Lim, D. J., and Saunders, W. H.: Acquired cholesteatoma: Light and electron microscopic observations. Ann. Otol. Rhinol. Laryngol. *81*:1–11, 1972.
78. Loda, F. A., Collier, A. M., Glezen, W. P., et al.: Occurrence of *Diplococcus pneumoniae* in the upper respiratory tract of children. J. Pediatr. *87*:1087–1093, 1975.
79. Long, S. S., Heuretig, F. M., Teter, M. J., et al.: Nasopharyngeal flora and acute otitis media. Infect. Immun. *41*:987–991, 1983.
80. Lundman, L., Juhn, S. K., Bagger-Sjoback, D., et al.: Permeability of the normal round window membrane to *Haemophilus influenzae* type b endotoxin. Acta Otolaryngol. *112*:524–529, 1992.
81. Luotonen, J., Herva, E., Karma, P., et al.: The bacteriology of acute otitis media in children with special reference to *Streptococcus pneumoniae* as studied by bacteriological and antigen detection methods. Scand. J. Infect. Dis. *113*:177–183, 1981.
82. Makela, P. H., Leinonen, M., Pukander, J., et al.: A study of the pneumococcal vaccine in prevention of clinically acute attacks of recurrent otitis media. Rev. Infect. Dis. *3*(Suppl.):124–133, 1981.
83. Mandel, E. M., Casselbrant, M. L., Rockette, H. E., et al.: Efficacy of 20- vs. 10-day antimicrobial treatment for acute otitis media. Pediatrics *96*:5–13, 1995.
84. Mandel, E. M., Rockette, H. E., Bluestone, C. D., et al.: Myringotomy with and without tympanostomy tubes for chronic otitis media with effusion. Arch. Otolaryngol. Head Neck Surg. *115*:1217–1224, 1989.
85. Marchant, C. D., Shurin, P. A., Turczyk, V. A., et al.: Course and outcome of otitis media in early infancy: A prospective study. J. Pediatr. *104*:826–831, 1984.
86. Marchant, C. D., Shurin, P. A., Turcyzk, V. A., et al.: A randomized controlled trial of cefaclor compared with trimethoprim-sulfamethoxazole for treatment of acute otitis media. J. Pediatr. *105*:633–638, 1984.
87. McCandless, G. A., and Thomas, G. K.: Impedance audiometry as a screening procedure for middle ear disease. Trans. Am. Acad. Ophthalmol. Otolaryngol. *78*:98–102, 1974.
88. McEldowney, D., and Kessner, D. M.: Review of the literature: Epidemiology of otitis media. *In* Gloric, A., and Gerwin, K. S. (eds.): Otitis Media. Springfield, IL, Charles C Thomas, 1972.
89. McLinn, S.: Double blind and open label studies of azithromycin in the management of acute otitis media in children: A review. Pediatr. Infect. Dis. J. *14*:S62–S66, 1995.
90. McLinn, S. E.: Cefaclor in treatment of otitis media and pharyngitis in children. Am. J. Dis. Child. *134*:560–563, 1980.
91. Medical Research Council Working Party Report: Acute otitis media in general practice. Lancet 2:510–514, 1957.
92. Meyerhoff, W. L., and Giebink, G. S.: Pathology and microbiology of otitis media. Laryngoscope *92*:273–277, 1982.
93. Mogi, G.: Secretory IgA and antibody activities in middle ear effusions. Ann. Otol. Rhinol. Laryngol. *85*(Suppl. 25):97–102, 1976.
94. Morris, P. S.: A systematic review of otitis media in Australian Aboriginal children. *In* Abstracts of the Sixth International Symposium on Recent Advances in Otitis Media, Fort Lauderdale, June 4–8, 1995, p. 11.
95. Mortimer, E. A., Jr., and Watterson, R. L., Jr.: A bacteriologic investigation of otitis media in infancy. Pediatrics *17*:359–366, 1956.
96. Murwitz, E. S., Gunn, W. J., Pinsky, P. F., et al.: Risk of respiratory illnes associated with day-care attendance: A nationwide study. Pediatrics *87*:62–69, 1991.

96a. Niemela, M., Uhari, M., and Mottonen, M: A pacifier increases the risk of recurrent acute otitis media in children in day care centers. Pediatrics *96*:884–888, 1995.

97. Nozza, R. J., Bluestone, C. D., Kardatzke, D., et al.: Towards the validation of aural acoustic immittance measures for the diagnosis of middle ear effusion in children. Ear Hearing *13*:442–453, 1992.
98. Ogawa, H., Fujisawa, T., and Kazuyama, Y.: Isolation of *Chlamydia pneumoniae* from middle ear aspirates of otitis media with effusion: A case report. J. Infect. Dis. *162*:1000–1001, 1990.
99. Papastavros, T., Giamarellou, H., and Varlejides, S.: Role of aerobic and

anaerobic microorganisms in chronic suppurative otitis media. Laryngoscope *96*:438–442, 1986.

100. Paradise, J. L., and Bluestone, C. D.: Early treatment of the universal otitis media of infants with cleft palate. Pediatrics *53*:48–54, 1974.
101. Paradise, J. L., Bluestone, C. D., and Felder, H.: The universality of otitis media in 50 infants with cleft palate. Pediatrics *44*:35–42, 1969.
102. Paradise, J. L., Elster, B. A., and Tan, L.: Evidence in infants with cleft palate that breast milk protects against otitis media. Pediatrics *94*:853, 1994.
103. Paradise, J. L., Smith, C. G., and Bluestone, C. D.: Tympanometric detection of middle ear effusion in infants and young children. Pediatrics *56*:198–210, 1976.
104. Pelton, S. I., Teele, D. W., Shurin, P. A., et al.: Disparate cultures of middle ear fluids in bacterial otitis media. Am. J. Dis. Child. *134*:951–953, 1980.
105. Persico, M., Barker, G. A., and Mitchell, D. P.: Purulent otitis media: A "silent" source of sepsis in the pediatric intensive care unit. Otolaryngol. Head Neck Surg. *93*:330, 1985.
106. Poulsen, G., and Tos, M.: Screening tympanometry in newborn infants and during the first six months of life. Scand. Audiol. *7*:159–166, 1978.
107. Pukander, J., Luotonen, J., Sipila, M., et al.: Incidence of acute otitis media. Acta Otolaryngol. *93*:447–453, 1982.
108. Reed, D., and Brody, J.: Otitis media in urban Alaska. Alaska Med. *8*:64–67, 1966.
109. Renvall, U., and Holmquist, J.: Tympanometry revealing middle ear pathology. Ann. Otol. Rhinol. Laryngol. *85*(Suppl. 25):209–215, 1976.
110. Riding, K. H., Bluestone, C. D., Michaels, R. H., et al.: Microbiology of recurrent and chronic otitis media with effusion. J. Pediatr. *93*:739–743, 1978.
111. Rifkind, D. R., Chanock, R., Kranetz, H., et al.: Ear involvement (myringitis) and primary atypical pneumonia following inoculation of volunteers with Eaton agent. Am. Rev. Respir. Dis. *85*:479–489, 1962.
112. Ruuskanen O., Arola, M., Heikkinen, T., et al.: Viruses in acute otitis media: Increasing evidence for clinical significance. Pediatr. Infect. Dis. J. *10*:425, 1991.
113. Ruedi, L.: Cholesteatoma formation in the middle ear in animal experiments. Acta Otolaryngol. *50*:233–242, 1959.
114. Sanyal, M. A., Henderson, F. W., Stempel, E. C., et al.: Effect of upper respiratory tract infection on eustachian tube ventilatory function in the preschool child. J. Pediatr. *97*:11–15, 1980.
115. Sarkkinen, H., Ruuskanen, I., Meurman, O., et al.: Identification of respiratory virus antigens in middle ear fluids of children with acute otitis media. J. Infect. Dis. *151*:444–448, 1985.
116. Schaefer, O.: Otitis media and bottle feeding. An epidemiological study of infant feeding habits and incidence of recurrent and chronic middle ear disease in Canadian Eskimos. Can. J. Public Health *62*:478–489, 1971.
117. Schneider, M. L.: Bacteriology of otorrhea from tympanostomy tubes. Arch. Otolaryngol. Head Neck Surg. *115*:1225–1226, 1989.
118. Schwartz, B., Giebink, G. S., Henderosn, F. W., et al.: Respiratory infections in day care. Pediatrics *84*:1018–1020, 1994.
119. Schwartz, R. H., and Rodriguez, W. J.: Acute otitis media in children eight years old and older: A reappraisal of the role of *Hemophilus influenzae*. Am. J. Otolaryngol. 2:19–21, 1981.
120. Schwartz, R. H., Rodriguez, W. J., Brook, I., et al.: The febrile response in acute otitis media. J. A. M. A. *245*:2057–2058, 1981.
121. Schwartz, R. H., Rodriguez, W. J., Khan, W. N., et al.: Acute purulent otitis media in children older than 5 years: Incidence of *Hemophilus* as a causative organism. J. A. M. A. *238*:1032–1033, 1977.
122. Senturia, B. H.: Classification of middle ear effusion. Ann. Otol. Rhinol. Laryngol. *79*:358–370, 1970.
123. Schappert, S. M.: Office visits for otitis media: United States, 1975–90. From Vital and Health Statistics of the Centers for Disease Control/ National Center for Health Statistics *214*:1–18, 1992.
124. Shurin, P. A., Howie, V. M., Pelton, S. I., et al.: Bacterial etiology of otitis media during the first 6 weeks of life. J. Pediatr. *92*:893–896, 1978.
125. Shurin, P. A., Marchant, C. D., Kim, C. H., et al.: Emergence of beta-lactamase–producing strains of *Branhamella catarrhalis* as important agents of acute otitis media. Pediatr. Infect. Dis. *2*:34–38, 1983.
126. Sipila, M., Karma, P., Pukander, J., et al.: The Bayesian approach to the evaluation of risk factors in acute and recurrent acute otitis media. Acta Otolaryngol. *106*:94–101, 1988.
127. Sipila, M., Pukander, J., and Karma, P.: Incidence of acute otitis media up to the age of 1½ years in urban infants. Acta Otolaryngol. *104*:138–145, 1987.
128. Skolnik, P. R., Nadol, J. B., Jr., and Baker, A. S.: Tuberculosis of the middle ear: Review of the literature with an instructive case report. Rev. Infect. Dis. *8*:403, 1986.
129. Skoner, D. P., Stillwagon, P. K., Casselbrandt, M. L., et al.: Inflammatory mediators in chronic otitis media with effusion. Arch. Otolaryngol. Head Neck Surg. *114*:1131–1133, 1988.
130. Sloyer, J. L., Jr., Cate, C. C., Howie, V. M., et al.: Immune response to acute otitis media in children. II. Serum and middle ear fluid antibody in otitis media due to *H. influenzae* J. Infect. Dis. *132*:685–688, 1975.
131. Sloyer, J. L., Jr., Ploussard, J. H., and Howie, V. M.: Efficacy of pneumococcal polysaccharide vaccine in preventing acute otitis media in infants in Huntsville, Alabama. Rev. Infect. Dis. *3*(Suppl.):119–123, 1981.
132. Spivey, G. H., and Hirschhorn, N.: A migrant study of adopted Apache children. Johns Hopkins Med. J. *140*:43–46, 1977.
133. Sriwardhana, K. B., Howard, A. J., and Dunkin, K. T.: Bacteriology of otitis media with effusion. J. Laryngol. Otol. *103*:253–256, 1989.
134. Stool, S. E., Berg, A. O., Berman, S., et al.: Otitis Media with Effusion in Young Children: Clinical Practice Guideline. Number 12. AHCPR Publication No. 94-0622. Rockville, MD, Agency for Health Care Policy and Research, Public Health Service, U.S. Department of Health and Human Services, July 1994.
135. Stool, S. E., Berg, A. O., Berman, S., et al.: Otitis Media with Effusion in Young Children: Clinical Practice Guideline. Number 12. AHCPR Publication No. 94-0622. Rockville, MD, Agency for Health Care Policy and Research, Public Health Service, U.S. Department of Health and Human Services, July 1994, p. 48.
136. Stool, S. E., Berg, A. O., Berman, S., et al.: Otitis Media with Effusion in Young Children: Clinical Practice Guideline Number 12. AHCPR Publication No. 94-0622. Rockville, MD, Agency for Health Care Policy and Research, Public Health Service, U.S. Department of Health and Human Services, July 1994, p. 52.
137. Teele, D. W., Klein, J. O., the Greater Boston Collaborative Otitis Media Study Group, et al.: Use of pneumococcal vaccine for prevention of recurrent acute otitis media in infants in Boston. Rev. Infect. Dis. *3*(Suppl.):113–118, 1981.
138. Teele, D. W., Klein, J. O., Chase, C., et al.: Otitis media in infancy and intellectual ability, school achievement, speech, and language at age 7 years. J. Infect. Dis. *162*:685–694, 1990.
139. Teele, D. W., Klein, J. O., and Rosner, B. A.: Epidemiology of otitis media in children. Ann. Otol. Rhinol. Laryngol. *89*(Suppl. 68):5–6, 1980.
140. Teele, D. W., Klein, J. O., Rosner, B., et al.: Middle ear disease and the practice of pediatrics. J. A. M. A. *249*:1026–1029, 1983.
141. Teele, D. W., Klein, J. O., Rosner, B., et al.: Epidemiology of otitis media during the first seven years of life in children in greater Boston: A prospective cohort study. J. Infect. Dis. *160*:83–94, 1989.
142. Tetzlaff, T. R., Ashworth, C., and Nelson, J. D.: Otitis media in children less than 12 weeks of age. Pediatrics *59*:827–832, 1977.
143. Tipple, M. A., Beem, M. O., and Saxon, E. M.: Clinical characteristics of the afebrile pneumonia associated with *Chlamydia trachomatis* infection in infants less than 6 months of age. Pediatrics *63*:192–197, 1979.
144. Tos, M., Poulson, G., and Hancke, A. B.: Screening tympanometry during the first year of life. Acta Otolaryngol. *88*:388–394, 1979.
145. U.S. Department of Health and Human Services: The health consequences of smoking: A report from the Surgeon General. Department of Health. Human Services Publication (DHS)84-50205. Rockville, MD, Office on Smoking and Health, 1984, p. 292.
146. Van Hare, G. F., Shurin, P. A., Marchant, C. D., et al.: Acute otitis media caused by *Branhamella catarrhalis*: Biology and therapy. Rev. Infect. Dis. *9*:16–27, 1987.
147. Varsano, I. B., Volovitz, B. M., and Grossman, J. E.: Effect of naproxen, a prostaglandin inhibitor, on acute otitis media and persistence of middle ear effusion in children. Ann. Otol. Rhinol. Laryngol. *98*:389–392, 1989.
148. Veltri, R. W., and Sprinkle, P. M.: Secretory otitis media: An immune complex disease. Ann. Otol. Rhinol. Laryngol. *85*(Suppl. 25):135–319, 1976.
149. Wald, E. R., Dashefsky, B., Byers, C., et al.: Frequency and severity of infections in day care. J. Pediatr. *112*:540–564, 1988.
150. Weiderhold, M. L., Zajtchuk, J. T., Vap, J. G., et al.: Hearing loss in relation to physical properties of middle ear effusions. Ann. Otol. Rhinol. Laryngol. *85*:185–189, 1980.
151. Yaniv, E.: Tuberculous otitis: An underdiagnosed disease. Am. J. Otolaryngol. *8*:356–360, 1987.

20

MASTOIDITIS

Karen Lewis, Anita Newman, and James D. Cherry

Mastoiditis, a suppurative infection of the mastoid air cells, is a potential complication of all cases of otitis media due to the continuity of the mucoperiosteal lining of the mastoid with that of the middle ear.[21] The spectrum of disease in mastoiditis ranges from asymptomatic cases with apparent spontaneous resolution to progressive disease with life-threatening complications.[10] Since the advent of antibiotic therapy, mastoiditis is seen much less frequently, but the frequency of complications remains the same.[20, 64] With mastoiditis occurring less commonly, physicians are less apt to consider the diagnosis, especially when the clinical picture has been masked by antibiotic therapy or when the process is chronic and of low grade. Proper antibiotic therapy, often accompanied by surgical drainage, can halt and prevent serious complications if mastoiditis is diagnosed early enough.

HISTORY

Prior to the advent of antibiotics, mastoiditis was a frequent complication of otitis media that could be treated only by expectant waiting or surgery.[30, 32] When surgery was used, many patients with mastoiditis were able to be cured by simple mastoid drainage alone, with a mortality rate quoted at 2 per cent.[32] However, intracranial complications of mastoiditis carried a very grave prognosis. In the preantibiotic era, between 1928 and 1933, 25 of every 1000 deaths at Los Angeles County Hospital in California were caused by intracranial complications of otitis media, such as meningitis, venous sinus thrombosis, and brain abscess. In contrast, between 1949 and 1954, only 2.5 per 1000 deaths at the same hospital were caused by complications of otitis or mastoiditis. The use of antibiotics in treating mastoiditis at first led to a marked decrease in the surgical approach to treatment of this illness.[10, 64] However, the realization that infection can persist and complications of mastoiditis can occur even while the patient is receiving antibiotic therapy has resulted in the present-day combined approach of antibiotics and surgery.[24, 40, 43]

BACTERIOLOGY

The bacteriology of acute mastoiditis differs somewhat from that of acute otitis media (Table 20–1). In acute otitis media, *Streptococcus pneumoniae* is the most frequent pathogen isolated (30 per cent), with *Haemophilus influenzae* being the second most common (22 per cent), *Moraxella catarrhalis* being the third most common (7 per cent), and group A beta-hemolytic streptococci being a distant fourth (2 per cent) (see Chapter 19). However, studies on acute mastoiditis (defined as symptoms of less than 1 month's duration) show that whereas *S. pneumoniae* still is the first most common isolate, *Streptococcus pyogenes* and *Staphylococcus aureus* are the second and third most common isolates, respectively.[20, 24, 26, 40, 43] *H. influenzae* has been isolated from the middle ear of patients with mastoiditis but less often than one would expect, given its frequent recovery in acute otitis media without mastoiditis. Gram-negative bacteria, enterococci, anaerobes, and *Mycobacterium tuberculosis* also have been isolated occasionally in patients with acute mastoiditis.

Chronic mastoiditis has a different bacteriologic spectrum than acute mastoiditis. Aerobic cultures of chronic mastoiditis and chronic otitis media both show predominantly *S. aureus* and gram-negative bacilli, especially *Pseudomonas aeruginosa*.[7, 15, 48] In addition, a wide variety of anaerobic organisms can be isolated from an infected mastoid and middle ear.[7, 15] Brook[7] studied the aerobic and anaerobic bacteriology of chronic otitis media (of at least 3 months' duration) in 24 children. Anaerobic isolates alone were found in 17 per cent, aerobic organisms alone in 4 per cent, and mixed aerobic and anaerobic infections in 79 per cent. All cases had from two to seven different bacterial isolates. *Peptococcus* species, *Actinomyces* species, and *Bacteroides melaninogenicus* were the anaerobic organisms isolated most commonly. Of note is that 17 patients were infected with β-lactamase–producing organisms (i.e., *S. aureus* or *B. melaninogenicus, Bacteroides fragilis*, or other *Bacteroides* species that were resistant to ampicillin).

M. tuberculosis currently is an uncommon cause of mastoiditis in the United States but still is a cause of chronically draining ears in lower socioeconomic groups or immigrants from endemic areas.[38] Case reports of mastoiditis implicate such organisms as nontuberculous mycobacteria,[42] *Aspergillus fumigatus*,[22] *Paragonimus*-like trematodes,[44] *Nocardia asteroides*,[36] *Actinomyces* species,[54] *Blastomyces dermatitidis*,[28] and *Histoplasma capsulatum*.[36] *Pneumocystis carinii* otitis media and mastoditis have occurred as the first manifestation of AIDS.[19]

ANATOMY AND PATHOPHYSIOLOGY

The mastoid process comprises the posterior part of the temporal bone and, as such, is adjacent to many important structures. Within the mastoid is an interconnecting system of air cells divided by bony septa that drain superiorly into the middle ear by way of a narrow aditus.[6, 21] Only the superior portion of the mastoid air space, the antrum, is present at birth; pneumatization of the mastoid starts soon after birth and usually is pneumatized well by 2 years of age.[6, 32] Structures lying anteromedially to the mastoid process include the middle ear and ossicles, the facial nerve, the posterior bony wall of the external auditory canal, the jugular vein, and the internal carotid artery. Posteromedially, the mastoid borders the posterior cranial fossa and the sigmoid sinus. Superiorly, the mastoid borders the middle cranial fossa. Medially, the mastoid cortex encases the cochlea and semicircular canals. The soft tissues and muscles of the lateral neck are located inferiorly. Any or all of these adjacent structures can be affected by extension of a suppurative process in the mastoid.

A certain amount of mastoid inflammation accompanies all cases of otitis media because the mastoid air spaces are continuous with the middle ear cavity and both are lined by a continuous mucoperiosteum.[6, 21] The first stage of an ear and mastoid infection is associated with hyperemia of the middle ear and the mastoid air cell mucosa. If the infection persists, an exudative stage develops, with serum, fibrin,

TABLE 20–1. Summary of Bacterial Isolates from the Middle Ear, Subperiosteal Abscess, or Mastoid of Children with Mastoiditis in Five Studies

	Acute Mastoiditis				Chronic Mastoiditis
Isolates	***Ginsburg et al.***[20]	***Hoppe et al.***[26]	***Ogle and Lauer***[43]	***Nadal et al.***[40]	***Brook***[7]
Streptococcus pneumoniae	14	13	7	9	1
Streptococcus pyogenes	8	4	3	4	2
Staphylococcus aureus	8	2	2	4	8
Haemophilus influenzae	1		3	1	—
Pseudomonas species	2		1	3	7
Other gram-negative bacilli	1	1	—	1	7
Anaerobes	2		3	2	61
Mycobacterium tuberculosis	1		—		—
Staphylococcus epidermidis	1	2	5		—
Streptococcus viridans	1		1		—
Candida albicans	—		1		—
Other	4*		2†		4‡
Total no. of patients	57	28	30	54	24

**Eikenella corrodens*, microaerophilic streptococci, nonenterococcal group D streptococci, group D streptococci.
†*Morganella morganii*, nonhemolytic streptococci.
‡Alpha-hemolytic streptococci.

polymorphonuclear cells, and red blood cells accumulating in the middle ear and mastoid. The accumulation of purulent exudate increases the middle ear pressure, eventually resulting in perforation of the tympanic membrane, followed by mucopurulent drainage from the middle ear and mastoid air cells. Some children also will have such marked mucoperiosteal swelling that the drainage of pus from the mastoid is blocked. The pus under pressure creates an environment of local acidosis, hypoxia, and ischemia, causing decalcification and resorption of the bony septa. The term *coalescent mastoiditis* is applied to this process because with the destruction of the bony septa, the mastoid air cells coalesce into large cavities. Osteomyelitis of the adjacent bone may develop, with subsequent bony erosion and eventual extension of the infection into surrounding structures.[6, 21]

Congenital and acquired cholesteatomas often are associated with chronic ear infections.[47, 48, 51, 61] Acquired cholesteatomas are the product of keratinizing squamous epithelium that has invaded the middle ear cavity. The accumulation of exfoliated keratin from the cholesteatoma may block the drainage of pus from the mastoid air cells, thus contributing to the development of mastoiditis.[51] Cholesteatomas also may cause slow, insidious erosion of underlying bone, predisposing to extramastoid spread of infection months or years later.[21, 48]

CLINICAL PRESENTATION

The classic presentation of acute mastoiditis is a febrile child with ear pain, postauricular swelling, and postauricular tenderness developing days to weeks after the beginning of acute otitis media.[20, 40, 43] If antibiotics were used to treat the otitis media, the child may have appeared to improve, only to become ill again while still receiving therapy or once the antibiotics were stopped; conversely, the child may not have responded to the antibiotics at all. Examination of the tympanic membrane in acute mastoiditis usually will be abnormal.[20, 24, 40] Early in the course of illness, periosteal inflammation will produce swelling and tenderness and sometimes redness over the mastoid process.[6, 20] Palpable postauricular fluctuance occurs later when pus from the mastoid air cells breaks through the underlying bony cortex and forms a subperiosteal abscess.[23] In children older than 1 year of age, the most common area where fluctuance is felt lies behind the ear, where it pushes the earlobe up and out; however, in children younger than 1 year of age, the fluctuance often may present above the ear, pushing the pinna down and out.[20]

Chronic mastoiditis is a much more indolent disease process than acute mastoiditis. It develops when there has been long-standing middle ear disease, usually over months to years.[48] Fever and postauricular swelling may or may not be present. Persistent or intermittent mucopurulent drainage from a previously perforated eardrum is very suggestive of chronic mastoiditis. Hearing loss and ear pain also may accompany chronic mastoiditis.[48] All of these symptoms can be mild enough to be ignored until serious intracranial suppuration occurs. Persistent ear drainage, persistent ear pain, or an otitis media nonresponsive to antibiotics should prompt a search for mastoiditis.

COMPLICATIONS

Complications of mastoiditis include subperiosteal abscess,[23] Bezold abscess,[17] facial nerve paralysis,[57] meningitis,[10, 20] brain abscess,[10, 20] cerebellar abscess,[6] epidural abscess,[6] subdural empyema, labyrinthitis,[21] venous sinus thrombophlebitis,[13] bacteremia,[10, 37] benign intracranial hypertension, osteomyelitis of the temporal bone with occasional extension to adjacent bones,[6, 21] hearing loss,[45] septic pulmonary emboli,[27] and cerebrospinal fluid otorrhea.[21]

Subperiosteal abscesses appear as a behind-the-ear fluctuant mass that obscures the postauricular sulcus. They occur when pus in the mastoid breaks through the bony cortex or extends along vascular channels and dissects under the overlying periosteum.[23]

A Bezold abscess develops when a mastoid infection erodes through the bony cortex on the inner surface of the mastoid process and dissects down the tissue planes to form a deep neck abscess. Fluctuance over the mastoid is not felt. Rather, there are swelling and tenderness below the mastoid process and under the sternocleidomastoid muscle.[17]

The facial nerve runs close to the mastoid and the middle

ear, making it vulnerable to injury when there is extension of mastoid or middle ear infections.[21] Pressure and inflammation on the facial nerve from symptomatic or asymptomatic mastoiditis can lead to transient or permanent facial nerve paralysis that usually is unilateral, although bilateral facial palsy from mastoiditis can occur.[6, 57]

Because the temporal bone that houses the mastoid air cells comprises the floor of the middle and posterior cranial fossa, bony erosion from osteomyelitis, preexisting bony defects, or spread of infection along vascular channels can allow for intracranial spread of mastoid infections into the middle and posterior cranial fossae. The infection may remain confined to the extradural space as an extradural abscess or may penetrate the dura and produce a subdural empyema, a brain abscess, a cerebellar abscess, or meningitis.[6, 21]

Invasion of infection into the bony labyrinth through the oval or round window will trigger a labyrinthitis, with initial tinnitus, hearing loss, nausea, and dizziness progressing to severe vertigo, ear pain, vomiting, nystagmus, and balance difficulties.[21]

Intracranial venous sinus thrombophlebitis is a rare but potentially fatal complication of mastoiditis.[6, 21, 55] The lateral aspect of the sigmoid sinus is formed by the temporal bone. Therefore, venous sinus thrombophlebitis results when an underlying mastoiditis extends through the temporal bone in close proximity to the lateral or sigmoid venous sinus. A perisinus abscess initially is formed, followed by a mural thrombus in the sinus wall. The thrombus eventually may occlude the entire sinus, or it may suppurate and spread along the sinus, resulting in septicemia, increased intracranial pressure, septic emboli, and extension of infection to other intracranial structures.[13, 18] The classic findings of a septic thrombosis of the lateral sinus are spiking fevers, shaking chills, and tenderness along the jugular vein associated with acute or chronic otitis. However, when only a perisinus abscess is present or if the patient partially is being treated with antibiotics, the only symptoms may be a low-grade fever and headache.[1, 55]

Benign intracranial hypertension can be seen in association with lateral sinus obstruction secondary to mastoiditis and is termed *otitic hydrocephalus.* On rare occasions, otitic hydrocephalus can be seen with mastoiditis in the absence of lateral sinus thrombosis. The decreased venous drainage caused by the venous sinus obstruction results in increased intracranial pressure, headache, papilledema, and sixth nerve palsy without enlarged ventricles or a space-occupying lesion.[1, 21]

Conductive hearing loss occurs when the middle ear mastoid infection is severe enough to damage or destroy the ossicles. Tuberculous mastoiditis classically presents with marked conductive hearing loss that often is not reversible.

Osteomyelitis secondary to mastoiditis can spread to adjacent bones. Involvement of the petrous portion of the temporal bone produces a syndrome that was described by Gradenigo in 1907 with a triad of abducens paralysis or paresis, severe pain in the distribution of the trigeminal nerve, and suppurative otitis media; additional cranial nerve deficits also may occur. Antibiotics may mask the classic signs of petrositis and allow progression to severe intracranial complications such as meningitis and epidural abscess. Petrositis only may be suspected when antibiotic and surgical management for mastoiditis fails to control chronic ear drainage.[21]

M. tuberculosis mastoiditis is uncommon but should be considered in children who have chronic ear discharge in spite of antibiotic therapy. Children can go for months or years with chronic draining ears before the diagnosis of tuberculous mastoiditis is considered.[8, 38] Children from lower socioeconomic homes, immigrants from endemic areas, or children with tuberculosis contacts in the family are at risk. The classic presentation in the preantibiotic era was an afebrile young child with painless persistent watery ear drainage, an enlarged preauricular lymph node, a history of tuberculosis contact, and often facial nerve paralysis.[52, 60]

However, tuberculous mastoiditis not always is painless.[63] Sometimes the diagnosis first is suspected only when a mastoidectomy wound does not heal.[34, 48] Early in the disease, physical examination may reveal small yellow spots (caseating granulomas) on a thickened and hyperemic tympanic membrane. These coalesce early and produce tympanic membrane perforations.[34] The discharge through these perforations initially is watery, but later it becomes purulent.[33] Pale, avascular granulation tissue is abundant throughout the middle ear and mastoid and often is seen in the external auditory canal and around the tympanic membrane perforation.[52, 63] Both pre- and postauricular, nontender, enlarged lymph nodes may be present,[33, 36] and early and severe hearing loss is a characteristic problem.[63] Often, there will be evidence of tuberculosis elsewhere in the body.[63] A 5–tuberculin unit purified protein derivative skin test usually, but not always, is positive.[38]

DIFFERENTIAL DIAGNOSIS

Postauricular swelling, a chronically draining ear, or radiographic evidence of mastoid abnormalities also can appear in other disease entities. Postauricular lymphadenopathy can occur secondary to a scalp infection, causing postauricular swelling. However, the swelling would be discrete, would not displace the pinna, and would not obliterate the postauricular sulcus.[20] Mumps can cause parotid swelling, pushing the earlobe up and out, but the swelling is over the parotid gland rather than located postauricularly. Histiocytosis,[35] acute lymphocytic leukemia,[39] acute myelogenous leukemia,[56] Burkitt lymphoma,[62] aneurysmal bone cysts,[12] and other benign and malignant tumors of the mastoid bone[11] also can present with symptoms clinically suggestive of mastoiditis. An underaerated and sclerotic mastoid seen by radiography can result from repeated but resolved middle ear infections.[9] Serous otitis media may cause clouding of the involved mastoid on radiographs without a concomitant mastoid infection.[4] Kawasaki disease may mimic acute mastoiditis with postauricular lymph node swelling and ear pain.[49] Children with severe and recurrent ear infections may have an underlying congenital or acquired immunodeficiency.

SPECIFIC DIAGNOSIS

The diagnosis of mastoiditis can be made on clinical grounds alone when a child has an acute episode of fever, otitis media, and posterior auricular tenderness and fluctuance. It is much more difficult to suspect mastoiditis when there is no swelling and tenderness over the mastoid process, such as when an infection has been masked by antibiotic treatment or when it has extended to an area other than over the mastoid process. Mastoiditis needs to be considered in all cases of otitis media not responding to antibiotics and in all intracranial suppurative diseases that do not have an apparent focus.

Obtaining an aspirate from the middle ear is an important part of properly diagnosing and managing mastoiditis. Gram stains of aspirates from the middle ear are quite accurate and, as such, can help in the initial selection of antibiotic therapy in chronic mastoiditis. Brook[7] found that in 24 children with tympanocentesis, half of the Gram stains showed a complete correlation with subsequent culture results and a partial correlation in the other half (one bacterial species was not seen). Leukocytes were seen on all the Gram stains. In addition, cultures from the middle ear accurately reflect mastoid disease.[20, 37]

Ginsburg and associates[20] compared the results of cultures of middle ear aspirates and mastoid cultures in 16 of their patients with acute mastoiditis and found that the same bacterial species was isolated from both sites. A sterile aspiration through an intact tympanic membrane gives the most accurate culture information. If the tympanic membrane is perforated, the purulent drainage may be contaminated by colonizing ear canal flora. However, an aspirate for culture generally should be obtained from the ear drainage, preferably from as close to the perforation as possible. Aspiration of postauricular fluctuance also is useful in identifying the responsible organism(s).[23, 43] In addition, specimens should be obtained directly from the mastoid at surgery. All of these should be sent for both aerobic and anaerobic cultures with proper anaerobic transport technique. If the child has had a chronic ear infection or if the child is in a high-risk population for acquiring tuberculosis, mycobacterial stains and cultures also should be obtained, and a purified protein derivative should be placed.

A lumbar puncture should be performed if the clinical presentation is suggestive of meningeal irritation; a computed tomographic (CT) scan should precede the lumbar puncture if there is papilledema or a suggestion of focal intracranial extension. Lymphocytosis of the cerebrospinal fluid suggests a parameningeal focus of infection. An immunologic evaluation should be considered if a child has had recurrent episodes of otitis media leading to mastoiditis.

Peripheral white blood cell counts in mastoiditis may be normal or elevated, often with an increase in band-form neutrophils.[24, 40] The erythrocyte sedimentation rate often is elevated in acute mastoiditis, but in chronic mastoiditis, it usually is within normal limits.[45]

The radiographic changes seen in mastoiditis begin with clouding or haziness of the mastoid air cells on the radiograph.[20, 21] Persistent infection causes resorption of the thin bony septa dividing the air cells; consequently, there is loss of the normal trabeculations seen in the mastoid, because the air cells coalesce.[4] Further infection produces bony destruction or local sclerosis. The radiograph in Figure 20–1 shows opacification of the right mastoid and loss of the fine bony septa of the mastoid air cells secondary to mastoiditis. However, mastoiditis can be present without any evidence by standard radiographs.[37, 43, 61]

Clouding of the mastoid air cells can occur in serous otitis media as well as in mastoiditis.[4]

Mastoiditis often can be diagnosed on clinical findings alone. However, when radiologic confirmation is needed, a CT scan of the temporal bone often will show mastoid abnormalities that are not seen by standard radiographs. The CT scan is the radiographic modality of choice to assess temporal bone pathology.[31] Early in the course of mastoiditis, nonspecific clouding of the middle ear and mastoid is seen. With time, there are necrosis and coalescence of the bony septa. Other CT findings in mastoiditis include hypoaeration of the mastoid and adjacent bony destruction.

CT scans with contrast also are useful in the search for intracranial complications of mastoiditis, such as venous sinus thrombosis and brain abscess.[16, 21, 31] Figure 20–2 shows a CT scan of a child with unilateral mastoiditis complicated by lateral sinus thrombosis and elevated intracranial pressure. At times, magnetic resonance imaging can be better at assessing the spread of infection outside of the temporal bone.[21, 31, 58]

Technetium bone scanning is not useful routinely for diagnosing mastoiditis, but it may be helpful in identifying mastoid inflammation that is not identifiable by CT scan or regular radiographs.[31, 37, 59]

TREATMENT

The pediatrician and the otolaryngologist should work together on the management of a child with suspected or proven mastoiditis, because all children with mastoid infections are potential surgical candidates. Some kind of drainage for the middle ear should be provided early in the course of therapy, for both therapeutic and diagnostic purposes. This could consist of tympanocentesis with subsequent tympanostomy tubes[20, 40, 43] or a myringotomy.[24] A specific etiologic diagnosis is more important today than in the past because of the increasing incidence of infections due to penicillin-resistant pneumococci and methicillin-resistant, coagulase-negative and coagulase-positive staphylococci.[3, 25, 41, 46]

If the patient has an acute onset of posterior auricular swelling and tenderness with minimal or no posterior auricular fluctuance and no signs of intracranial complications, he

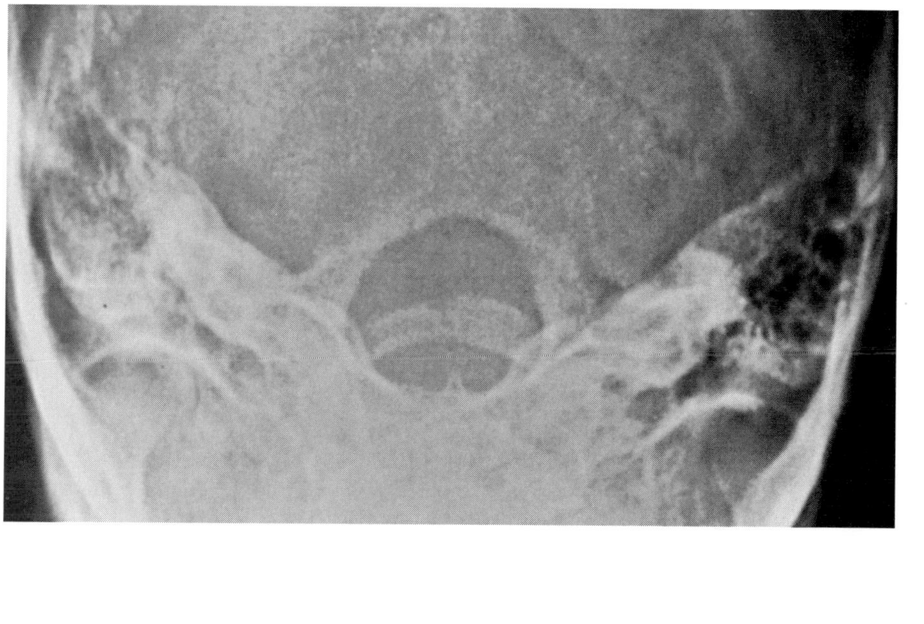

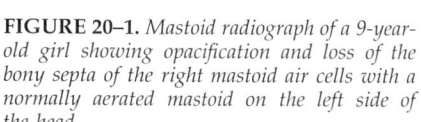

FIGURE 20–1. *Mastoid radiograph of a 9-year-old girl showing opacification and loss of the bony septa of the right mastoid air cells with a normally aerated mastoid on the left side of the head.*

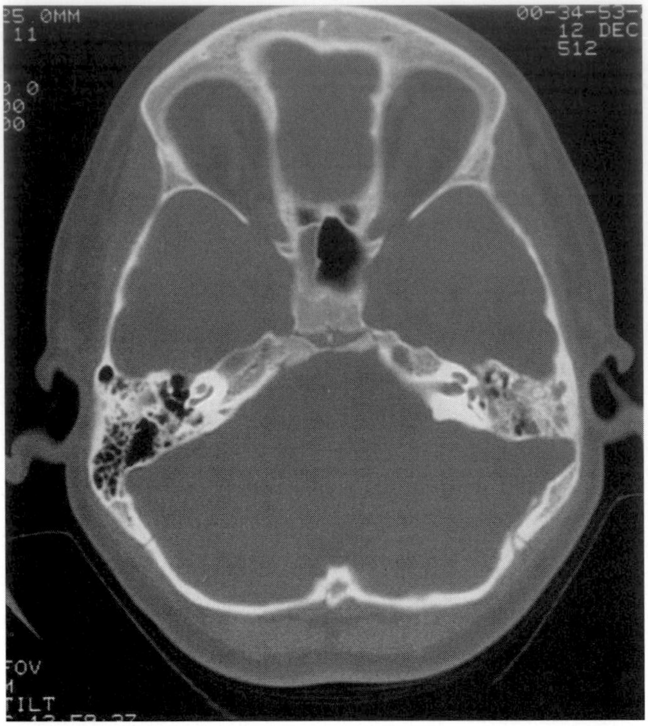

FIGURE 20–2. *Computed tomographic scan of the head of a 12-year-old boy with left lateral sinus thrombosis and increased intracranial pressure complicating left mastoiditis. The left mastoid air cells are opacified with marked loss of the fine bony septa, in contrast to the right mastoid air cells.*

or she is likely to respond to antibiotic therapy alone.[24, 40, 43] Indications for surgical intervention include postauricular fluctuance; a history of chronic ear drainage with postauricular swelling or bony changes on radiographs; facial nerve palsy; nausea, vomiting, and vertigo suggestive of labyrinthitis; meningitis; brain abscess; venous sinus thrombosis with or without intracranial hypertension; epidural or subdural empyema; and petrositis. In addition, if the patient initially is treated medically, a mastoidectomy is indicated if there is progression of postauricular swelling or fluctuance or persistence of fever, ear pain, or purulent ear drainage while the child is receiving parenteral antibiotics.[21, 24, 40, 43]

The initial choice of antibiotics for mastoiditis must be made empirically, based on the knowledge of the most likely organisms. Because acute mastoiditis most often is caused by *S. pneumoniae* or *S. pyogenes* and less often by *S. aureus* and *H. influenzae,* oxacillin (150 mg/kg/day divided every 6 hours) and cefotaxime (150 to 200 mg/kg/day divided every 6 hours) can be recommended. However, in severe infections with possible central nervous system involvement, it often is desirable initially to administer vancomycin (40 mg/kg/day intravenously every 6 hours) instead of oxacillin because of the possibility of resistant pneumococci or staphylococci. In cases of chronic mastoiditis in which symptoms have been present for more than 1 month, *S. aureus,* gram-negative bacilli (especially *P. aeruginosa),* and anaerobes occur more frequently. Therefore, a broad-spectrum combination of intravenous antibiotics is recommended: a penicillinase-resistant penicillin, such as oxacillin (150 mg/kg/day divided every 6 hours), for staphylococcal coverage; an aminoglycoside, such as gentamicin (7.5 mg/kg/day divided every 8 hours), for gram-negative bacillary coverage; and a semisynthetic penicillin, such as mezlocillin (200 to 300 mg/kg/day divided every 6 hours), which is synergistic with gentamicin against *P. aeruginosa* and which is effective against many but not all anaerobes. The antibiotics then can be adjusted based on the identification and sensitivities of the organisms isolated from the pretherapy cultures.

The approach to antibiotic therapy of both acute and chronic bacterial mastoiditis should conform to the principles of therapy for osteomyelitis. Treatment is begun initially with intravenous antibiotics. Intracranial extension of infection or mastoiditis with an organism for which there is no effective oral antibiotic (such as *P. aeruginosa*) requires long-term intravenous antibiotic therapy. Otherwise, once the patient has responded well clinically, oral antibiotic therapy can be considered. Total length of therapy should be for a minimum of 3 weeks and possibly longer, depending on the severity of illness, the causative organism, and the clinical response. Optimally, the causative organisms and their sensitivities should be known, and there needs to be an oral agent to which the organisms are sensitive. An oral regimen should not be attempted if vomiting or diarrhea is present, because this would prevent adequate oral absorption. When the causative organism is known, documentation of adequate antibiotic serum levels is done by substituting the oral antibiotic for the scheduled intravenous antibiotic dose. After the child has received at least three oral doses, a peak serum level should be drawn. If adequate blood levels (10 times the MIC of the organism) are obtained and there is reasonable assurance that the child will be given the antibiotic, the child may be treated as an outpatient for a minimum of 3 weeks of total therapy, with weekly follow-up visits to assess continued clinical response and compliance with the oral antibiotic regimen. Following the sedimentation rate may be helpful in monitoring the treatment. The oral antibiotic should be given strictly every 6 hours rather than four times a day in order to ensure round-the-clock therapeutic drug levels.

No study has examined the optimal antituberculous chemotherapy for mastoiditis. If *M. tuberculosis* mastoiditis is probable or diagnosed, antituberculous chemotherapy should be started as recommended for tuberculosis of the bone[2] (see Chapter 101).

If fever, purulent ear drainage, or ear pain persist in spite of antibiotic therapy and surgery, further evaluation is needed to search for either resistant organisms or a persistent site of infection that requires additional surgical drainage.

PROGNOSIS

The prognosis of mastoiditis depends on the extent of the infection and the causative organism. Mastoiditis that is treated adequately early in the course of the illness before the onset of intracranial extension has a very good prognosis. Facial nerve paralysis is reversible early on,[52, 57] and benign intracranial hypertension resolves with treatment of the mastoiditis.[21] Permanent neurologic deficits and death are possible if the mastoiditis extends to cause meningitis, brain abscesses, epidural abscess, subdural empyema, or venous sinus thrombophlebitis. Symptoms of mastoiditis may recur if antibiotic therapy is not of sufficient duration or if surgical débridement of an infected bone or of an infected cholesteatoma is not adequate.

Sensorineural and conductive hearing deficits are reversible early on in mastoiditis; however, chronic infection may produce irreversible hearing loss.

PREVENTION

Early adequate antibiotic treatment of otitis media will reduce a child's risk of developing mastoiditis significantly.

In addition, rapid treatment of known mastoiditis along with early investigation of persistent ear drainage, persistent ear pain, or an otitis media that is not responding to antibiotic management will decrease the risk of suppurative complications associated with mastoiditis.

References

1. Alford, B. R., and Cohn, A. M.: Complications of suppurative otitis media and mastoiditis. *In* Paparella, M. M., and Shumrick, D. A. (eds.): Otolaryngology. 2nd ed. Philadelphia, W. B. Saunders, 1980, pp. 1490–1509.
2. American Academy of Pediatrics: Tuberculosis. *In* Peter G. (ed.): 1994 Red Book: Report of the Committee on Infectious Diseases. 23rd ed. Elk Grove Village, IL, American Academy of Pediatrics, 1994, pp. 480–500.
3. Archer, G. L., and Climo, M. W.: Antimicrobial susceptibility of coagulase-negative staphylococci. Antimicrob. Agents Chemother. *38*:2231–2237, 1994.
4. Bloch, C., and Feuerstein, S. S.: Serous otitis media and mastoiditis: Their radiologic and clinical manifestations. Mt. Sinai J. Med. *43*:27–42, 1976.
5. Bluestone, C. D., and Klein, J. O.: Intracranial suppurative complications of otitis media and mastoiditis. *In* Bluestone, C. D., and Stool, S. E. (eds.): Pediatric Otolaryngology. Philadelphia, W. B. Saunders, 1983, pp. 565–576.
6. Bluestone, C. D., and Klein, J. O.: Otitis Media in Infants and Children. Philadelphia, W. B. Saunders Co., 1988, pp. 233–244.
7. Brook, I.: Aerobic and anaerobic bacteriology of chronic mastoiditis in children. Am. J. Dis. Child. *135*:478–479, 1981.
8. Buchanan, G., and Rainer, E. H.: Tuberculous mastoiditis. J. Laryngol. Otol. *102*:440–446, 1988.
9. Caffey, J., and Silverman, F. N. (eds.): Pediatric X-ray Diagnosis. 5th ed. Chicago, Year Book Medical Publishers, 1967, pp. 107–113.
10. Davison, F. W.: Otitis media: Then and now. Laryngoscope *65*.142–151, 1955.
11. De, S. K., and Dey, D. D.: Tumours of the mastoid temporal bone. J. Laryngol. Otol. *102*:582–587, 1988.
12. deVries, E. J., Kamerer, D. B., and Rafalko, D.: Aneurysmal bone cyst masquerading as acute mastoiditis. Otolaryngol. Head Neck Surg. *100*:613–616, 1989.
13. Doyle, K. J., and Jackler, R. K.: Otogenic cavernous sinus thrombosis. Otolaryngol. Head Neck Surg. *104*:873–877, 1991.
14. Feigin, R. D., Kline, M. W., Hyatt, S. R., et al.: Otitis media. *In* Feigin, R. D., and Cherry, J. D. (eds.): Textbook of Pediatric Infectious Diseases. 3rd. ed. Philadelphia, W. B. Saunders, 1992, pp. 175–189.
15. Finegold, S. M.: Anaerobic infections in otolaryngology. Ann. Otol. Rhinol. Laryngol. *90*(Suppl. 84):13–16, 1981.
16. Fritsch, M. H., Miyamoto, R. T., and Wood, T. L.: Sigmoid sinus thrombosis diagnosis by contrasted MRI scanning. Otolaryngol. Head Neck Surg. *103*:451–456, 1990.
17. Gaffney, R. J., O'Dwyer, T. P., and Maguire, A. J.: Bezold's abscess. J. Laryngol. Otol. *105*:765–766, 1991.
18. Garcia, R. D. J., Baker, A. S., Cunningham, M. J., et al.: Lateral sinus thrombosis associated with otitis media and mastoiditis in children. Pediatr. Infect. Dis. J. *14*:617–623, 1995.
19. Gherman, C. R., Ward, R. R., and Bassis, M. L.: *Pneumocystis carinii* otitis media and mastoiditis as the initial manifestation of the acquired immunodeficiency syndrome. Am. J. Med. *85*:250–252, 1988.
20. Ginsburg, C. M., Rudoy, R., and Nelson, J. D.: Acute mastoiditis in infants and children. Clin. Pediatr. *19*:549–553, 1980.
21. Glasscock, M. E., and Shambaugh, Jr., G. E. (eds.): Surgery of the Ear. Philadelphia, W. B. Saunders, 1990, pp. 85–103, 110–121, 170–178, 217–222, 249–275.
22. Hall, P. J.: *Aspergillus* mastoiditis. Otolaryngol. Head Neck Surg. *108*:167–170, 1993.
23. Hawkins, D. B., and Dru, D.: Mastoid subperiosteal abscess. Arch. Otolaryngol. *109*:369–371, 1983.
24. Hawkins, D. B., Dru, D., House, J. W., et al.: Acute mastoiditis in children: A review of 54 cases. Laryngoscope *93*:568–572, 1983.
25. Hofmann, J., Cetron, M. S., Farley, M. M., et al.: The prevalence of drug-resistant *Streptococcus pneumoniae* in Atlanta. N. Engl. J. Med. *333*:481–486, 1995.
26. Hoppe, J. E., Koster, S., Bootz, F., et al.: Acute mastoiditis: Relevant once again. Infection 22:178–182, 1994.
27. Hughes, C. E., Spear, R. K., Shinabarger, C. E., et al.: Septic pulmonary emboli complicating mastoiditis: Lemierre's syndrome revisited. Clin. Infect. Dis. [illegible], 1994.
28. Istorico, L. J., Sanders, M., Jacobs, R. F., et al.: Otitis media due to blastomycosis: Report of two cases. Clin. Infect. Dis. *14*:355–358, 1992.
29. Jazrawy, H., Wortzman, G., Kassel, E. E., et al.: Computed tomography of the temporal bone. J. Otolaryngol. *12*:37–44, 1983.
30. Keeler, J. C.: Modern Otology. Philadelphia, F. A. Davis, 1930, pp. 417–481.
31. Kenna, M. A.: Treatment of chronic suppurative otitis media. Otolaryngol. Clin. North Am. *27*:457–471, 1994.
32. Levine, M.: Practical Otology. Philadelphia, Lea & Febiger, 1938, pp. 216–238, 267–284.
33. Lincoln, E. M., and Sewell, E. M.: Tuberculosis in children. New York, McGraw-Hill, 1963, pp. 216–223.
34. Lucente, F. E., Tobias, G. W., Parisier, S. C., et al.: Tuberculous otitis media. Laryngoscope *88*:1107–1116, 1978.
35. McCaffrey, T. V., and McDonald, T. J.: Histiocytosis X of the ear and temporal bone: Review of 22 cases. Laryngoscope *89*:1735–1742, 1979.
36. Meyerhoff, W. L.: Granulomas and other specific diseases of the ear and temporal bone. *In* Paparella, M. M., and Shumrick, D. A. (eds.): Otolaryngology. 2nd ed. Philadelphia, W. B. Saunders, 1980, pp. 1548–1575.
37. Moloy, P. J.: Anaerobic mastoiditis: A report of two cases with complications. Laryngoscope *92*:1311–1315, 1982.
38. Mumtaz, M. A., Schwartz, R. H., Grundfast, K. M., et al.: Tuberculosis of the middle ear and mastoid. Pediatr. Infect. Dis. *2*:234–236, 1983.
39. Nabors, M. W., Narayan, R. K., and Poplack, D. G.: Intracranial and otological presentation of acute lymphocytic leukemia. Neurosurgery *17*:309–312, 1985.
40. Nadal, D., Herrmann, P., Baumann, A., et al.: Acute mastoiditis: Clinical, microbiological, and therapeutic aspects. Eur. J. Pediatr. *149*:560–564, 1990.
41. Nelson, C. T., Mason, Jr., E. O., and Kaplan, S. L.: Activity of oral antibiotics in middle ear and sinus infections caused by penicillin-resistant *Streptococcus pneumoniae*: Implications for treatment. Pediatr. Infect. Dis. J. *13*:585–589, 1994.
42. Nylen, O., Alestig, K., Fasth, A., et al.: Infections of the ear with nontuberculous mycobacteria in three children. Pediatr. Infect. Dis. J. *13*:653–656, 1994.
43. Ogle, J. W., and Lauer, B. A.: Acute mastoiditis. Am. J. Dis. Child. *140*:1178–1182, 1986.
44. Oyediran, A. B. O. O., Fajemisin, A. A., Abioye, A. A., et al.: Infection of the mastoid bone with a *Paragonimus*-like trematode. Am. J. Trop. Med. Hyg. *24*:268–273, 1975.
45. Palva, T., and Pulkkinen, K.: Mastoiditis. J. Laryngol. Otol. *72*:573–588, 1959.
46. Pikis, A., Akram, S., Donkersloot, J. A., et al.: Penicillin-resistant pneumococci from pediatric patients in the Washington, D. C., area. Arch. Pediatr. Adolesc. Med. *149*:30–35, 1995.
47. Primrose, W. J., and Cinnamond, M. J.: Acute mastoid abscess and cholesteatoma. Int. J. Pediatr. Otorhinolaryngol. *12*:229–235, 1987.
48. Procter, B.: Chronic otitis media and mastoiditis. *In* Paparella, M. M., and Shumrick, D. A. (eds.): Otolaryngology. 2nd ed. Philadelphia, W. B. Saunders, 1980, pp. 1455–1489.
49. Puczynski, M. S., Stankiewicz, J. A., and Ow, P. E.: Mucocutaneous lymph node syndrome mimicking acute coalescent mastoiditis. Am. J. Otol. *7*:71–73, 1986.
50. Rathore, M. H., and Kline, M. W.: Community-acquired methicillin-resistant *Staphylococcus aureus* infections in children. Pediatr. Infect. Dis. J. *8*:645–647, 1989.
51. Shaffer, H. L., Gates, G. A., and Meyerhoff, W. L.: Acute mastoiditis and cholesteatoma. Otolaryngology *86*:394–399, 1978.
52. Singh, B.: Role of surgery in tuberculous mastoiditis. J. Laryngol. Otol. *105*:907–915, 1991.
53. Stanley, R. J., McCaffrey, T. V., and Weiland, L. H.: Fungal mastoiditis in the immunocompromised host. Arch. Otolaryngol. Head Neck Surg. *114*:198–199, 1988.
54. Tarabichi, M., and Schloss, M.: Actinomycosis otomastoiditis. Arch. Otolaryngol. Head Neck Surg. *119*:561–562, 1993.
55. Teichgraeber, J. F., Per-Lee, J. H., and Turner, J. S.: Lateral sinus thrombosis: A modern perspective. Laryngoscope *92*:744–751, 1982.
56. Todd, N. W., and Bowman, C. A.: Acute myelogenous leukemia presenting as atypical mastoiditis with facial paralysis. Int. J. Pediatr. Otorhinolaryngol. *7*:173–177, 1984.
57. Tovi, F., and Leiberman, A.: Silent mastoiditis and bilateral simultaneous facial palsy. Int. J. Pediatr. Otorhinolaryngol. *5*:303–307, 1983.
58. Tovi, F., and Hirsch, M.: Computed tomographic diagnosis of septic lateral sinus thrombosis. Ann. Otol. Rhinol. Laryngol. *101*:79–81, 1991.
59. Tovi, F., and Gatot, A.: Bone scan diagnosis of masked mastoiditis. Ann. Otol. Rhinol. Laryngol. *101*:707–709, 1992.
60. Turner, A. L.: Tuberculosis of the middle ear cleft in children. J. Laryngol. Rhinol. Otol. *30*:209–247, 1915.
61. Venezio, F. R., Naidich, T. P., and Shulman, S. T.: Complications of mastoiditis with special emphasis on venous sinus thrombosis. J. Pediatr. *101*:509–513, 1982.
62. Welling, D. B., and McCabe, B. F.: American Burkitt's lymphoma of the mastoid. Laryngoscope *97*:1038–1042, 1987.
63. Windle-Taylor, P. C., and Bailey, C. M.: Tuberculous otitis media: A series of 22 patients. Laryngoscope *90*:1039–1044, 1980.
64. Zoller, H.: Acute mastoiditis and its complications: A changing trend. South. Med. J. *65*:477–480, 1972.

21

EPIGLOTTITIS (SUPRAGLOTTITIS)

James D. Cherry

Epiglottitis (supraglottitis) is an illness characterized by inflammation and edema of the epiglottis and frequently also the eryepiglottic folds and ventricular bands at the base of the epiglottis.[36] It usually is caused by *Haemophilus influenzae* type b, and it mainly is a disease of children. The illness is characterized by rapid onset and progression, and without treatment, death occurs due to obstruction of the airway. Epiglottitis in children is a pediatric otolaryngologic emergency.

HISTORY

The early history of epiglottitis is obscure, probably because of the importance of diphtheritic croup.[37] In 1887, Baron[8] described in detail a 30-year-old woman with epiglottitis who recovered after treatment with hot poultices and steam with tincture of benzoin. In 1900, Theisen[165] described three cases in the United States. It was not until the early 1940s that acute epiglottitis became recognized as a definite clinical entity caused by *H. influenzae* type b.[2, 16, 151] In 1948, Rabe,[125] in a study of 347 children with "infectious croup," presented evidence for the division of the clinical illness into three etiologic categories: diphtheritic croup, viral croup, and *H. influenzae* type b croup (acute epiglottitis).

The 1990s represent a new era in epiglottitis due to the dramatic decrease in incidence because of the widespread use of *H. influenzae* type b conjugate vaccines.[3, 30, 62, 68, 173, 181]

EPIDEMIOLOGY

In the prevaccine era, the epidemiology of invasive *H. influenzae* type b disease varied markedly among different population groups.[180, 181] Epiglottitis also varied by population group, but this variation was not related necessarily to the rate of overall *H. influenzae* type b invasive disease in the population. For example, among Alaskan Eskimos and Navajo Native Americans, whose risk for invasive *H. influenzae* type b disease is 4 to 10 times that of most other American populations, epiglottitis was not recognized among 295 patients with invasive *H. influenzae* type b illness.[43, 180]

Of *H. influenzae* type b invasive disease, the percentage of cases of epiglottitis varies markedly among different localities. For example, in Israel, only 0.3 per cent of invasive *H. influenzae* type b infections were epiglottitis, whereas in Ireland; Wales; northeast England; Sydney, Australia; and Denmark, the percentage of epiglottitis cases varied between 16 and 32 per cent.[44, 60, 77, 90, 114, 124] In Minnesota and Dallas County, Texas, only 6 per cent and 3 per cent, respectively, of invasive *H. influenzae* type b infections were epiglottitis.[120] In contrast with these findings in the United States, Europe, and Australia, the most common manifestation of invasive *H. influenzae* type b infection in Sweden is epiglottitis.[40, 169] In Sweden, the incidence of epiglottitis in children 14 years of age or younger in 1981 to 1983 was 10 per 100,000 per year. The incidence in Minnesota and Dallas County, respectively, in children 5 years of age or younger was 5.4 and 4.4 cases per 100,000 per year.[119] In St. Louis, Missouri, the yearly rate in children 16 years of age or younger was calculated to be 6 per 100,000.[38]

In children in the United States, the peak occurrence of epiglottitis occurred during the third year of life, and 72 per cent of all cases occurred in children from 1 to 5 years of age.[12, 15, 17, 41, 57, 79] The disease is more common in boys than in girls; in eight studies with 611 cases, 58 per cent were boys.[12, 15–17, 41, 57, 79, 118]

In specific geographic areas, there have been marked differences in the yearly percentage of cases of epiglottitis, but no intercity, national, or international cycles of illness have been demonstrated.[12, 15, 41, 57, 79, 118] Seasonal prevalence varies by locality but is not marked. The greatest number of cases in three studies occurred in the winter and spring,[17, 79, 118] whereas Baxter[15] observed more cases during the summer and in November and Cohen and Chai[41] found no seasonal pattern.

Epiglottitis is a disease that most commonly occurs in temperate climates.[59, 82] In several U.S. military hospitals, there was a wide geographic variation in incidence; no cases were found among 4625 admissions at Gorgas Hospital in Panama, whereas 1 of 600 admissions to Elmendorf Hospital in Alaska was for epiglottitis.[12]

Epiglottitis also occurs in adults, but it is less common than in children.[63, 112, 161, 171] Rates in Rhode Island, Denmark, Finland, and northern California were 1.0, 0.9, 0.2, and 1.8 per 100,000 per year, respectively.

In the present *H. influenzae* type b conjugate vaccine era, the incidence of epiglottitis is dropping, as it is for all invasive disease due to *H. influenzae*.[3, 30, 68, 173, 181] In northern Finland, the incidence in children 4 years of age or younger fell from 7.6 per 100,000 prior to 1988 to 0 per 100,000 after 1988.[3] At the Children's Hospital of Philadelphia, Pennsylvania, the average annual incidence of epiglottitis declined from 10.9 per 10,000 admissions before 1990 to 1.8 per 10,000 admissions from 1990 through 1992.[68] In this study, it was noted also that the median age of patients increased from 35.5 months before 1990 to 80.5 months in the post-1989 period.

ETIOLOGY

Acute supraglottitis almost always is caused by *H. influenzae* type b in children. Lemierre and colleagues[101] and Sinclair[151] first called attention to "*H. influenzae* type b laryngitis." This variant of laryngitis was characterized by marked swelling of the epiglottis and arytenoid regions, high fever, and shock. All 10 children described by Sinclair[151] had *H. influenzae* type b bacteremia. Rabe[125] recognized a form of "croup" associated with epiglottitis and *H. influenzae* type b bacteremia; 25 of 28 blood cultures (89 per cent) yielded this organism. Table 21–1 summarizes 34 pediatric series with reported blood culture data. In children, 1570 of 2279 (69 per cent) had blood cultures performed; *H. influenzae* type b was isolated from 1191 of 1570 (76 per cent).

As the clinical entity gained recognition, the frequency with which blood cultures were obtained and the yield of *H. influenzae* type b increased. During 17 years of experience with epiglottitis in Denver, Colorado,[118] 40 per cent of all

TABLE 21–1. Etiology of Epiglottitis in Children

Author and Year of Study		Number of Patients	Number of Patients Having Blood Cultures (%)	Patients with Blood Cultures Yielding *H. influenzae* Type b (%)	Other Bacteria Isolated from Blood (%)*
Sinclair[151]	1941	10	10 (100)	10 (100)	None
Rabe[125]	1948	28	28 (100)	25 (89)	None
Berenberg and Kevy[17]	1958	42	16 (38)	11 (69)	*S. pneumoniae*
Vetto[177]	1960	37	2 (5)	2 (100)	None
Margolis et al.[111]	1972	15	15 (100)	13 (87)	None
Johnson et al.[79]	1974	55	33 (60)	20 (61)	None
Bass et al.[12]	1974	97	6 (6)	1 (17)	*S. aureus*
Milko et al.[116]	1974	41	33 (80)	33 (100)	None
Branefors-Helander and Jeppsson[26]	1975	15	14 (93)	13 (93)	None
Margolis et al.[110]	1975	32	32 (100)	30 (94)	None
Battaglia and Lockhart[13]	1975	40	40 (100)	13 (33)	None
Rapkin[126]	1975	4	4 (100)	4 (100)	None
Smith and Ingram[155]	1975	8	8 (100)	8 (100)	None
Benjamin and O'Reilly[16]	1976	61	51 (84)	36 (71)	None
Molteni[118]	1976	72	29 (40)	10 (34)	None
Breivik and Klaastad[27]	1978	27	9 (33)	5 (56)	*S. aureus*
Cohen and Chai[41]	1978	147	49 (33)	28 (57)	*H. influenzae*, not type b
Faden[57]	1979	48	56 (98)	48 (86)	*S. pneumoniae*†
Bottenfield et al.[25]	1980	24	22 (92)	18 (82)	None
Briggs and Altenau[28]	1980	53	44 (83)	30 (68)	*H. influenzae* type a *H. influenzae*, nontypable *H. parainfluenzae*
Baugh and Baker[14]	1982	24	22 (92)	18 (82)	None
Broughton and Warren[31]	1984	24	19 (80)	19 (100)	None
Drake-Lee et al.[54]	1984	25	19 (76)	19 (100)	None
Sly et al.[154]	1984	171	89 (52)	71 (80)	None
Claesson et al.[40]	1984	211	85 (40)	74 (81)	*H. parainfluenzae*
McGregor et al.[113]	1985	31	31 (100)	19 (61)	None
Vernon and Sarnaik[176]	1986	60	56 (93)	54 (96)	None
Gerber and Pfenninger[65]	1986	137	126 (92)	83 (66)	None
Hodge and Ganzel[76]	1987	25	24 (96)	14 (58)	None
Blackstock et al.[21]	1987	14	12 (86)	10 (83)	None
Bull et al.[33]	1988	349	234 (67)	187 (80)	None
Brilli et al.[29]	1989	41	41 (100)	39 (95)	None
Losek et al.[107]	1990	169	169 (100)§	131 (78)	*Bacillus* species *S. pneumoniae* *S. aureus*‡
Gorelick and Baker[68]	1994	142	142 (100)	95 (67)	None
		2279	1570 (69)	1191 (76)	12 (1)

*Each organism represents one patient.
†One patient had *S. pneumoniae* and *H. influenzae* type b bacteremia.
‡One patient had *S. aureus* and *H. influenzae* type b bacteremia.
§Only patients with blood cultured and no prior antibiotic treatment reported.

blood cultures yielded *H. influenzae* type b; however, 70 per cent yielded this organism during the last 5 years of the study.

Supraglottitis with bacteremia due to other organisms in children is rare. In this regard, *Streptococcus pneumoniae*[17, 57, 107]; *Staphylococcus aureus* (including one case in a 5-day-old baby)[10, 27, 55, 107]; *Haemophilus parainfluenzae*[28, 168]; group A,[94, 103] group B,[106] and group C[7, 145] streptococci; *Pseudomonas aeruginosa*[95] (in a patient with severe combined immunodeficiency syndrome); untypable and type a *H. influenzae*[28]; and *Bacillus* species[107] have been implicated. *Candida tropicalis* was isolated from the blood of a 3½-year-old girl with supraglottitis who had been the recent recipient of an autologous bone marrow transplant.[178]

In adults, *H. influenzae* type b also is the major cause of epiglottitis, but other organisms are more common in adults than in children.[8, 26, 36, 39, 45, 58, 63, 73, 81, 88, 91, 112, 132, 150, 158, 161, 169] Daum and Smith[48] reviewed 474 published cases of epiglottitis in adults in which 293 had blood cultures performed and 79 of those cultures (27 per cent) yielded *H. influenzae*. Forty-three of these positive cultures were type b, thirty-five isolates were not typed, and one isolate was not type b. Trollfors and associates[169] in Sweden found that blood cultures were obtained from 185 of 356 (52 per cent) adult patients, and *H. influenzae* was isolated from 53 per cent of them. Of these, 53 were type b, and the type of the remaining 45 was not known.

S. pneumoniae was reported to be isolated from the blood

of 18 adults with supraglottitis, 10 of whom were receiving immunosuppressive therapy or were infected with HIV 1,[20, 26, 78, 86, 88, 99, 125, 133, 134, 148] and *H. parainfluenzae* was isolated from the blood of 5 patients.[39, 61, 108, 142, 182] Case reports have attested that other pathogens occasionally are implicated. *Pasteurella multocida* was isolated from the blood of one patient who received dialysis at home.[80] *Kingella kingae* was isolated from the blood of one adult with embryonal cell carcinoma, granulocytopenia, and supraglottitis.[85] *Klebsiella pneumoniae* was isolated from the blood of one adult with supraglottitis and acute lymphocytic leukemia and from an epiglottic abscess of another,[157] and *Aspergillus flavus* was isolated from tissue obtained from an epiglottic biopsy.[24] One adult with diabetes had an epiglottic abscess from which group B *Streptococcus* was isolated.[130] Group A streptococci were isolated from the blood of a 30-year-old postpartum female[129] and from epiglottic tissue post mortem in a 50-year-old man.[135] Fatal epiglottitis with contiguous abscess formation in the soft tissues of the neck was associated with group F streptococcal bacteremia in a 58-year-old woman.[135] In another adult, swelling of one side of the epiglottis and an aryepiglottic fold was associated with a parapharyngeal abscess; *Fusobacterium necrophorum* was isolated from the blood and abscess of this patient.[105] A homosexual man, HIV status unknown, had *Bacteroides melaninogenicus* recovered from an epiglottic abscess at a time when *Bacteroides urolyticus* was recovered from his blood.[50] *Vibrio vulnificus* was isolated from the blood of a man with β-thalassemia and supraglottitis after contact with a pet fish.[115] Macneil and colleagues[109] described an adult known to have an epiglottic cyst who subsequently developed supraglottitis. After initiation of ampicillin and cefotaxime, aspiration of the cyst yielded purulent material containing gram-negative rods; *Bacteroides fragilis* was isolated on culture.

The presence of any pathogen in the upper airway cannot be distinguished from asymptomatic colonization. However, direct culture of the epiglottis, trachea, or nasopharynx may yield a preponderance of *H. influenzae* type b. Berenberg and Kevy[17] isolated *H. influenzae* type b from 11 of 12 epiglottic swabs. Branefors-Helander and Jeppsson[26] isolated *H. influenzae* type b from 10 of 11 epiglottic swabs from children and from 6 of 10 adults. Other investigators found *H. influenzae* type b in tracheal, pharyngeal, or epiglottic cultures with varying frequency, ranging from 0 per cent in 17 adults[73] to 94 per cent in 32 children.[110] *S. aureus, S. pneumoniae,* group A streptococci, and *Candida albicans* all have been isolated from the airways of patients with epiglottitis, but their etiologic role was not established. *Haemophilus paraphrophilus*[83] was recovered from the epiglottic surface of a single patient, as was *Moraxella catarrhalis* in another patient.[175]

The possibility that supraglottitis could be caused by a virus has been noted: a 16-month-old child with type 1 herpes simplex virus stomatitis complicated by stridor and respiratory distress had an epiglottis and aryepiglottic folds that were edematous and covered with vesicular lesions resembling those in the oral mucosa.[23] Additionally, parainfluenza type 3 and influenza type B viruses were isolated from the nasopharynx of two children with supraglottic inflammation.[71]

Epiglottitis also can result from noninfectious causes. Hot foods can cause thermal epiglottitis, as can poisoning with cocaine alkaloid.[15, 88, 92]

ANATOMY (Fig. 21–1)

The thin, elastic, leaf-like epiglottic cartilage is attached to the anterior surface of the thyroid cartilage via the thyroepiglottic ligament. The hypoepiglottic ligament also provides

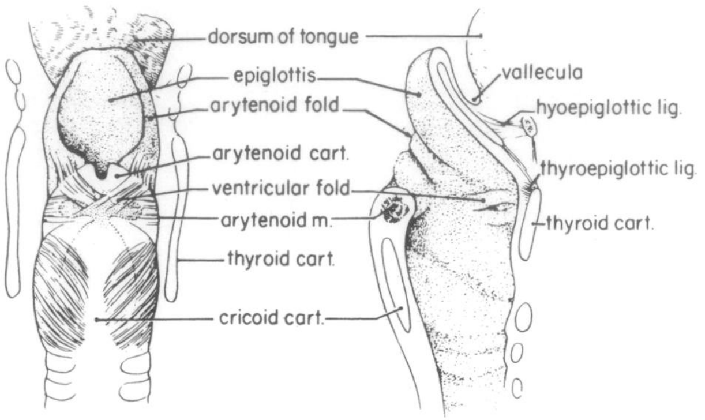

FIGURE 21–1. *Anatomic relationships of the supraglottic larynx. Left, posterior view; right, sagittal view.*

support, anchoring the epiglottis to the hyoid bone. The superior aspect of the epiglottis arches slightly posteriorly. Stratified squamous epithelium covers the anterior surface of the epiglottis and the superior third of the posterior portion; respiratory epithelium covers the remaining posterior surface. The stratified squamous epithelium is loosely adherent, creating a large potential space for the accumulation of inflammatory cells and edema fluid.

The aryepiglottic folds arise from the epiglottis and terminate posteriorly near the paired arytenoid cartilages. These structures commonly are involved in the supraglottic infection and occasionally are the site of serious disease without epiglottitis per se.[15] Immediately anterior to the epiglottis are the valleculae epiglotticae, where saliva pools before deglutition.

PATHOPHYSIOLOGY

Supraglottic cellulitis with marked edema involving the epiglottis, the aryepiglottic folds, ventricular bands, and arytenoids is the hallmark of this illness. As the edema increases, the epiglottis curls posteriorly and inferiorly. Inspiration tends to draw the inflamed supraglottic ring into the laryngeal inlet, while expiration is unopposed.[146] This "ball-valve" mechanism is thought to produce slight hypoxia without hypercapnia.[137] Microscopically, there is diffuse infiltration with polymorphonuclear leukocytes, hemorrhage, edema, and fibrin deposition; this can progress to microabscesses with *H. influenzae* type b occasionally seen in the tissue.[82, 132] Frank abscess formation has been documented in adults.[105, 109, 130, 135, 157, 183, 188] Infection of the supraglottic larynx may spread inferiorly to involve the paraglottic space,[74] but as a rule, there is neither upward extension into the laryngeal lymphatics nor downward extension into the subglottic region.[16, 82]

Infection of the supraglottic structures probably arises from direct invasion by *H. influenzae* type b with subsequent bacteremia. The bacteremia appears to be relatively short in duration and of low concentration. This is suggested by several observations: (1) the serum concentration of the capsular polysaccharide is directly proportional to the concentration and duration of bacteremia,[138] (2) children with epiglottitis have less *H. influenzae* type b capsular polysaccharide in their sera than patients with meningitis,[179] and (3) the density of *H. influenzae* type b in blood is significantly lower in patients with epiglottitis than in patients with meningitis.[98, 136, 159] In 23 patients with epiglottitis, the geometric mean number of organisms was 123 cfu/mL, whereas the geometric mean number in 43 patients with meningitis was 2203 cfu/mL ($p < .001$).[98]

What predisposes the epiglottitis to infection is unknown. It is possible that mild trauma to the epiglottis during food intake occurs. This could result in damage to the mucosal surface, which in turn could allow the invasion of organisms that already were present in the upper respiratory tract. It also seems possible that a viral infection could damage the mucosal surface so that secondary bacterial infection could occur.

Acute-phase sera in most children with epiglottitis lack specific bactericidal and hemagglutinating antibody; seroconversion regularly occurs after infection.[26, 110]

Conflicting evidence exists relating to a possible genetic difference between patients with *H. influenzae* type b epiglottitis and other individuals.[4, 70, 163, 188] Whisnant and associates[188] surveyed human leukocyte antigens (HLA) and erythrocytic antigens among 30 children with epiglottitis and 20 patients with meningitis. HLA-A11 was found in 17 and 3 per cent of the patients with meningitis and epiglottitis, respectively ($p < .01$). HLA-B5 occurred in 13 and 3 per cent of patients with epiglottitis and meningitis, respectively ($p < .05$), while B40 occurred more often (23 versus 10 per cent) in patients with meningitis than in those with epiglottitis ($p < .05$). Moreover, the frequency of A28 and B17 antigens was higher among the patients with epiglottitis than in uninfected controls.[188] However, the results of another study did not confirm these observations.[70]

The distribution and frequency of MNS erythrocyte antigens in patients with epiglottitis may differ from those observed in others. For example, the NNSS genotype occurred in 6.4 per cent of patients with epiglottitis and 0.5 per cent of healthy controls ($p < .0002$),[188] but this difference was not confirmed.[70] However, the results of two studies suggest that the MNS's genotype occurs less often in patients with *H. influenzae* type b meningitis than in patients with epiglottitis.[70, 188] In one study, white children with *H. influenzae* type b meningitis lacked G2m(n), an allotype antigen of IgG2 subclass heavy chains, more frequently than controls.[4] But in another study in a white population in Finland, this was not noted.[162] The frequency of the Km(1) immunoglobulin allotype in children with epiglottitis did not differ significantly from the prevalence of that marker in blacks or whites. However, in blacks with *H. influenzae* type b meningitis, the Km(1) marker occurred less frequently in patients than in controls.[70]

The identification of one outer-membrane protein subtype of *H. influenzae* type b that was associated relatively infrequently with epiglottitis suggests that there may be isolate-specific differences in the propensity of *H. influenzae* type b to cause epiglottitis.[160]

CLINICAL MANIFESTATIONS

The classic onset of epiglottitis in children is abrupt, and disease progression is rapid; careful history on occasion will reveal the occurrence of a trivial antecedent upper respiratory tract infection.[12, 13, 16, 17, 26, 29, 41, 57, 73, 79, 81, 103, 107, 110, 111, 118, 122, 125, 152, 177, 187] The total duration of illness before hospitalization usually is less than 24 hours and occasionally as short as 2 hours. In one study in which 142 medical records of children with epiglottitis were reviewed, it was found that the duration of illness before tracheotomy was 12 hours or less in 73 per cent and more than 24 hours in only four patients.[41]

The most common presentation of acute epiglottitis in children includes the sudden onset of fever, severe sore throat, dysphagia, and drooling. Airway obstruction always occurs and is rapidly progressive. It is manifested by distress on inspiration, a choking sensation, irritability, restlessness, and anxiety. The speech is muffled or thick sounding, but hoarseness usually does not occur. The child usually insists on sitting up with a characteristic posture with the arms back, the trunk leaning forward, the neck hyperextended, and the chin pushed forward. This posture increases the diameter of the obstructed airway.

In contrast with that in acute laryngotracheitis, in which marked inspiratory stridor occurs, the degree of observed stridor in epiglottitis often is not severe. This apparent lack of respiratory distress often leads the unwary physician to underestimate the severity of the child's illness. With progression, the air exchange becomes progressively worse, and hypoxia, hypercapnia, and acidosis develop. These findings cause increased irritability, restlessness, and disorientation, and if an artificial airway is not established, the child will experience a sudden cardiorespiratory arrest.

Fever occurs in virtually all children, with most temperatures between 38.8° and 40.0° C (101.8° and 104° F). Blood leukocyte counts almost always are elevated; the mean total count in five studies was about 20,000 cells/mm^3.[17, 41, 79, 185] The differential cell count reveals an increased percentage of neutrophils and band forms; most patients will have absolute band counts that are more than 500 cells/mm^3.

The clinical picture of epiglottitis in adults is more indolent than it is in children.[73, 191] In two studies, an average of 1 to 3 days elapsed before medical aid was sought. The mean temperature was 38.2° C (100.7° F), and some patients were afebrile; the temperature range was 36.6° to 40.0° C (97.8° to 104° F). Blood leukocyte counts averaged 17,000/mm^3 (range, 8000 to 32,000/mm^3). Sore throat and dysphagia were universal. Zwahlen and Regamy[191] reviewed the clinical features of 100 reported adult cases of epiglottitis. Of these, 78 per cent had dyspnea; 49 per cent, dysphonia; 41 per cent, cyanosis; and 38 per cent, stridor. Forty-six per cent had edema of the neck. A precordial purring or fluttering sensation was described by one adult patient.[139]

DIFFERENTIAL DIAGNOSIS

The hallmark of the successful management of acute epiglottitis is an awareness of the condition and an understanding of the rapidity of its progression. A correct early diagnosis frequently is lifesaving. Acute epiglottitis must be differentiated from seven other conditions with symptoms of acute upper airway obstruction. Aspects of the differential diagnosis are presented in the text in Chapter 22 and in Table 22–5.

In epiglottitis, the important differential points are a lack of a croupy cough; the presence of a swollen, cherry-red epiglottis; the sitting posture of the child with the chin pushed forward and, also, a reluctance or refusal to lie down; and the relatively greater apprehension and anxiety of the child than the degree of chest retraction suggests. In contrast, the child with acute laryngotracheitis will have a normal epiglottis on examination; will always have a typical barking cough; will be comfortable in a supine position; and frequently will appear to have only minimal apprehension, in spite of retractions in which the sternum appears to be indenting 2 inches or more.

Acute angioneurotic edema that involves the epiglottis can mimic acute epiglottitis. However, in this condition, the temperature usually is normal and the patient will be less toxic appearing. This condition usually is brought on by a specific allergic reaction after the ingestion of a food or medicine.

Supraglottitis should be considered in children with uvulitis because their clinical features may overlap and both infections may be present. Concomitant uvulitis and epiglottitis were described with *H. influenzae* type b bacteremia in children[89, 128] and *S. pneumoniae* bacteremia in an adult.[186] Isolated uvulitis has been associated with *H. influenzae* type b bacteremia and group A beta-hemolytic streptococcal pharyngitis.[89, 104] Uvulitis in the absence of epiglottitis was described in a child with odynophagia, drooling, and *H. influenzae* type b bacteremia.[104]

A foreign body lodged in a vallecula, the larynx, or penetrating posterior pharyngeal tissues may mimic the signs and symptoms of acute supraglottitis.[184] Very rarely, a paravertebral collection of pus, from cervical osteomyelitis or parapharyngeal abscess, can spread anteriorly and produce acute "croup." Congenital anomalies and laryngeal papillomas can be excluded by their chronic course. *Candida albicans* has caused neonatal laryngeal obstruction without radiologic epiglottitis.[123]

Infection of supraglottic structures by *Mycobacterium tuberculosis* is less common than glottic involvement; tuberculous laryngitis is exceedingly rare in children and always is associated with pulmonary lesions.[56] The onset is considerably more insidious than *H. influenzae* type b supraglottitis. Nasopharyngeal diphtheria may mimic acute epiglottitis and may be associated with a serosanguineous nasal discharge.

Chronic epiglottic enlargement with edema was observed in two children with cancer who had received radiotherapy to the neck. Their clinical features were not confused with those of acute supraglottitis, although one patient had dysphagia and snored.[190] Severe, chronic inflammatory epiglottitis with associated granulomatous lymphangitis was found on histologic examination of tissue obtained from a 19-month-old black child who had epiglottic enlargement without erythema for 3 months.[184] "Tuberculoid" granulomatous lesions were seen at histologic examination of an epiglottic biopsy obtained from a 22-year-old man, HIV status unknown, who presented with weight loss, sore throat, and dysphonia of 1 month's duration.[117] The epiglottitis and aryepiglottic folds of this patient were erythematous and edematous.

Lymphangiectasis of the epiglottis produced airway obstruction with stridor and intermittent cyanosis in a 4-month-old white boy. Histologically, the epiglottis consisted of multiple, dilated lymphatic vessels lined by a single layer of epithelial cells with no discernible wall. The stroma contained scattered lymphocytes and a few neutrophils. This lesion spontaneously regressed, and the child was normal at 1 year of age.[172]

SPECIFIC DIAGNOSIS

The clinical picture of sore throat, dysphagia, drooling, anxiety, and inspiratory distress without significant stridor and the characteristic sitting position should suggest the presumptive diagnosis in most cases. The definitive anatomic diagnosis is made by the visualization of the epiglottis and the etiologic diagnosis by culture of an organism from the blood or the surface of the epiglottitis. An *H. influenzae* type b etiology also can be established by the demonstration of antigenemia or antigenuria.[155, 179]

In the typical case, the epiglottis is fiery-red and greatly swollen. In children, the epiglottis can be seen by simple depression of the tongue with a tongue blade. In older children and adults, indirect or direct laryngoscopy usually is necessary to confirm the diagnosis. On occasion, the obstruction is due to swelling of the ventricular bands and the aryepiglottic folds, so that the epiglottis may appear relatively normal.

There is major controversy relating to the safety of using a tongue depressor in examining a child with suspected epiglottitis because sudden cardiorespiratory arrest has been noted to occur. However, most instances of cardiorespiratory arrest that I am aware of occurred after the child was forced into a supine position rather than because of the examination itself. In many instances, patients with presumptive epiglottitis can be examined in an upright position with a tongue blade or by the use of indirect laryngoscopy.

Case management should be individualized. In the child with moderate or advanced disease, the clinical diagnosis should be apparent without an intraoral examination. In this situation, intraoral examination should not be done, but the child should be prepared for the establishment of an airway. This preparation should be rapid but controlled so that intubation can be performed in an operating room.

The diagnosis of epiglottitis can be established by the classic appearance on a lateral neck radiograph (Fig. 21–2).[126, 185] However, it is my opinion that this radiographic procedure rarely is necessary; all too often it leads to a delay in the necessary definitive therapy.[41, 82, 116] The use of the lateral neck radiograph should be reserved for subacute cases in which the specific diagnosis after clinical examination is not clear.

The lateral film of the neck, delineating the soft tissues, taken with the patient upright, gives the best view of the upper airway anatomy (see Fig. 21–2). The hypopharynx is dilated; normal cervical lordosis may be replaced by a straight or kyphotic contour. The valleculae are narrowed

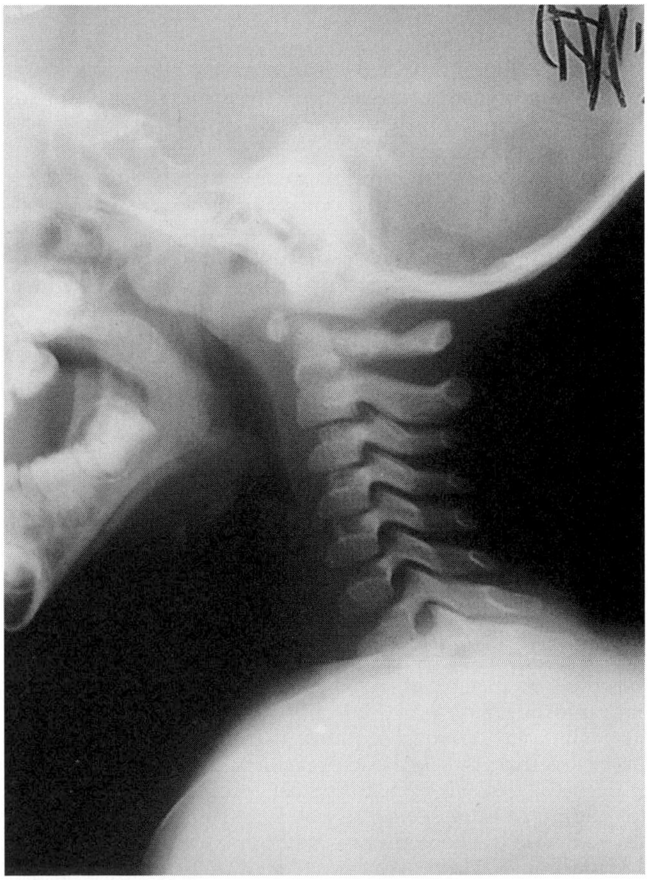

FIGURE 21–2. *A lateral neck radiograph from a child with acute epiglottitis showing the swollen epiglottis (thumb sign) encroaching upon the airway. (Courtesy of Dr. Ines Bouchat.)*

and may be obliterated. A thickened mass of tissue stretching from the valleculae to the arytenoids emphasizes the appropriateness of the term "supraglottitis." In adults with epiglottitis, the width of the epiglottis and aryepiglottic folds uniformly exceeds 8 and 7 mm, respectively.[144]

When performed, radiography of the neck in the anteroposterior projection usually reveals that tracheal narrowing is absent. However, some children with acute supraglottitis have localized subglottic narrowing indistinguishable from that found in acute laryngotracheitis.[147, 153]

All patients with suspected epiglottitis should have a blood culture, and a culture should be obtained from the surface of the epiglottis when an artificial airway is established. Today, cultures are of increasing importance due to the changing epidemiology of *H. influenzae* type b infection and the resulting increased likelihood of the illness being due to an organism other than *H. influenzae* type b. A white blood cell count with a differential also may provide useful information. In children who have received antimicrobial treatment prior to cultures, it is worthwhile to perform a direct antigen test for *H. influenzae* type b on the blood and urine.

TREATMENT

The treatment of acute epiglottitis should be relatively simple in that there are only two main aspects of therapy: an airway must be established, and an appropriate antimicrobial agent needs to be administered. However, in the past, the mortality rate due to epiglottitis has varied from 0 to 32 per cent.[41, 73] This suggests major differences in the implementation of treatment.

Most deaths occur in transit to the hospital or within the first few hours after arrival. Once the diagnosis is suspected, the patient should be attended constantly by individuals skilled in resuscitation with appropriate equipment for airway stabilization and ventilatory support. Delays of 2 or 3 hours have proved fatal; every effort should be made to reduce the time needed to secure a patient's airway and initiate antibiotic therapy. Prior to this, unnecessary stress should be avoided. In most cases, radiographic confirmation should be omitted. Blood tests, extensive history taking, and transport delay should be eliminated.

Medical centers and pediatric services that have planned protocols for the diagnostic investigation and treatment of patients with suspected acute epiglottitis generally have better morbidity and mortality statistics than services that do not. Pediatricians, radiologists, otolaryngologists, and anesthetists all may contribute to the assessment and management of a case; roles and responsibilities of each service that have been defined in advance minimize confusion and make the institution of care easier.

Securing the Airway

In general, the cornerstone of all management plans is the establishment of an airway in all children in whom the diagnosis of epiglottitis is made.[36]

In 1938, Sinclair[151] recognized that tracheostomy was lifesaving. Berenberg and Kevy[17] advocated hospitalization for all patients with epiglottitis but tracheostomy only "if necessary." However, Bass and associates[12] have a compelling argument for routine tracheostomy. Among 83 patients with documented epiglottitis, 11 of whom were adults, these authors noted that 16 of 83 (19 per cent) had life-threatening obstruction when first seen. An additional 14 (17 per cent) progressed to this point within 6 hours of admission; 9 of 83 (11 per cent) required emergency tracheostomy while hospitalized. Of these nine, two died and one suffered anoxic brain damage. All nine were being monitored carefully, with bedside tracheostomy equipment available and trained personnel nearby. Six of the adults required tracheostomy for survival.[12] Margolis and colleagues[111] noted that elective tracheostomy, performed at the time of diagnosis, eliminated fatalities in 15 consecutive patients. This observation was in contrast to four deaths in 20 patients observed until tracheostomy "was required."

A large body of literature attests to the safety and efficacy of nasotracheal intubation as a replacement for tracheostomy,[13, 42, 75, 96, 111, 122, 127, 141, 149, 164, 166] which has a complication rate of 50 per cent.[164, 187] Biologically inert tubes, with their decreased risk of complicating subglottic stenosis,[149] and the recollection that endotracheal tube insertion was universal before tracheostomy[116] was an accepted procedure led to the routine use of nasotracheal intubation in this disease. Nasotracheal intubation requires a shorter duration of airway maintenance: 32 patients with epiglottitis managed with tracheostomy had a mean duration of intubation of 7.5 days and a mean hospitalization of 8.8 days. In contrast, a nasotracheal tube was used for a mean of 38 hours with a 6.5-day hospitalization in five patients.[116] Diaz and Lockhart[51] managed 104 patients with nasotracheal intubation. The mean intubation time was 53 ± 14.9 hours; seven patients (6.8 per cent) extubated themselves, and two required reintubation. Laryngeal edema occurred in three patients (2.9 per cent) who had been intubated. In two, subglottic granulations required excision.

It is my belief, as well as that of Daum and Smith,[48] that the argument for performing elective tracheostomy or, preferably, intubation in all children with supraglottitis is compelling, and the procedure should be performed immediately after diagnosis. Whether this "stimulus-response" approach is necessary for adults with epiglottitis is controversial.[11, 62, 73, 146, 150] Mayo Smith and associates[112] compared selected clinical features in adults with epiglottitis at the time of diagnosis who died or received an artificial airway with those of adults who recovered without airway intervention. Few differences emerged. Patients who died or who were managed with airway intervention had respiratory distress and bacteremia more often than those who recovered without airway intervention. Obviously, the presence of bacteremia was not known upon presentation. Moreover, the mortality among all adults managed expectantly was 4.6 per cent, a figure comparable with the mortality (6.1 per cent) in children in a series reported prior to recommendations for routine securing of the airway at diagnosis.[34, 112] The preponderance of evidence until very recently has been that securing the airway in all adults with supraglottitis via nasotracheal intubation should reduce mortality.[6, 9, 11, 12, 18, 19, 45, 88, 112] However, Frantz and associates[63] reported an analysis of 129 cases of acute epiglottitis in adults in which no deaths occurred in the cohort and 85 per cent were managed without airway intervention.

To aid in intubation and reduce long-term sequelae, most investigators have advocated using a nasotracheal tube that is 0.5 to 1.0 mm smaller than that predicted by the patient's age.[75, 116, 141] Recommendations for tube size are shown in Table 21–2.[102, 149]

Published criteria for extubation (summarized in reference 13) include those based on duration of therapy and those based on daily examination of the epiglottis and supraglottic structures by direct laryngoscopy[49] or fiberoptic bronchoscopy.[121, 174]

Long-term complications appear rarely with nasotracheal intubation. Thirty-three children with epiglottitis managed

TABLE 21–2. Size of Nasotracheal Tubes Recommended for Children with Acute Supraglottitis[103, 150]

Age	Size (mm)
Birth–6 mo	3.0
6 mo–3 yr	3.5
3 yr–5 yr	4.0
Older than 5 yr	4.5

with nasotracheal intubation (mean duration of intubation, 55 hours) were evaluated 1 to 8 years later. By history and measurement of peak expiratory flow rates, no complications were found.[141] Although additional long-term data are necessary to ensure absence of residua, elective nasotracheal intubation appears to be the procedure of choice.

Several reports documented the recognition of idiopathic pulmonary edema *prior* to[100] or, more commonly, after[22, 49, 53, 64, 84, 156, 167] insertion of an endotracheal tube to relieve laryngeal obstruction due to epiglottitis. One hypothesis to explain this phenomenon is that airway obstruction produces markedly negative intrapleural pressure with increased venous return to the right side of the heart with decreased left ventricular output and increased pulmonary blood volume.[97] These changes increase the pulmonary microvascular pressure and produce pulmonary hyperemia and edema. Endotoxemia may play a role in altering vascular permeability but is not necessary for recognition of this complication of airway obstruction because abrupt onset of pulmonary edema was described when airway obstruction caused by croup, foreign body, and malignant neoplasm was relieved acutely.[32] The frequency of pulmonary edema complicating intubation in supraglottitis was about 9 per cent,[153] and it has occurred in an adult.[131] Continuous positive airway pressure in all intubated patients with epiglottitis probably will provide prophylaxis against this complication,[51, 64] but controlled data are lacking.

Antibiotics

The mainstay of antibiotic therapy for acute epiglottitis in recent years has been ceftriaxone (50 to 100 mg/kg/day given every 12 hours intravenously) or cefotaxime (100 to 200 mg/kg/day given every 6 hours intravenously) because virtually all cases in both children and adults have been due to *H. influenzae* type b. However, in the present conjugate vaccine era, the incidence of all invasive *H. influenzae* type b disease has decreased dramatically. Therefore, in previously vaccinated children, the etiology may be due to another organism. Culture results today have added significance because one possible etiology that would require a change in therapy would be *S. aureus*.

No controlled data exist regarding the duration of antimicrobial administration, but a course of 7 days seems appropriate. In the event that group A streptococci are isolated from the airway, penicillin is the drug of choice. A semisynthetic penicillinase-resistant penicillin or vancomycin should be used for *S. aureus*, whereas erythromycin is indicated for *Corynebacterium diphtheriae*.

Other Supportive Measures

Some authors have advocated steroid therapy on the basis of anecdotal experience in patients with epiglottitis, but no controlled data exist to support its use and such therapy may be hazardous: among 91 patients with epiglottitis who received steroid therapy, 4 patients (4 per cent) had evidence of bleeding from the gastrointestinal tract sufficient in 2 to require transfusion,[52] a phenomenon observed by others.[93] Therapy with racemic epinephrine is without benefit.

Expert respiratory nursing care is essential. Inadvertent extubation must be avoided, particularly in the first 24 hours. Judicious use of sedatives that do not depress respiration appreciably (e.g., chloral hydrate) may be appropriate.

COMPLICATIONS

Extraepiglottic complications are not very common in children with acute epiglottitis. In one study involving 72 children with epiglottitis, it was noted that 25 per cent had pneumonia, 25 per cent had cervical adenitis, 8 per cent had tonsillitis, and 5 per cent had otitis media.[118] The other common invasive manifestations of *H. influenzae* type b infections (meningitis, arthritis, and cellulitis) rarely are found in conjunction with epiglottitis.[118, 140]

PREVENTION

Prophylaxis of Household Contacts

Household contacts of patients with *H. influenzae* type b infection are at increased risk for *H. influenzae* type b infection.[69] Whether an increased risk occurs in day care contacts is unresolved.[47] Although contacts of patients with *H. influenzae* type b epiglottitis younger than 5 years of age are colonized less frequently than contacts of patients with other *H. influenzae* type b invasive infections,[46] secondary disease was described in household contacts when an index patient had epiglottitis.[1, 66, 67, 170] Secondary *H. influenzae* type b epiglottitis was described in a child[1] and two adults who were household contacts of a patient with *H. influenzae* type b meningitis.[66, 67] *H. influenzae* type b epiglottitis occurred in two siblings[72] who presented within 1 day. Thus, it has been assumed that household contacts exposed to individuals with invasive *H. influenzae* type b infections are at a risk for secondary disease similar to that of those contacts exposed to patients with other invasive infections.

Rifampin prophylaxis, 20 mg/kg/day (600 mg/dose maximum) for 4 days, is recommended for all members of a patient contact group when the index patient has *H. influenzae* type b epiglottitis and there is at least one contact 4 years of age or younger in the contact group.[5]

The recognition that adults occasionally may acquire secondary infection, particularly epiglottitis, when exposed to children with invasive *H. influenzae* type b infection has prompted some experts to extend prophylaxis to all patient contact groups, regardless of the presence of one or more contacts 4 years of age or younger. All experts, however, recommended that adults and older children be made aware of the signs and symptoms of *H. influenzae* type b disease, particularly when their patient contact group would not receive prophylaxis under current guidelines.

Haemophilus influenzae Type b Vaccines

All children younger than 5 years of age should be immunized with a conjugate *H. influenzae* type b vaccine according to the recommendations of the Committee on Infectious Diseases of the American Academy of Pediatrics and the Advisory Committee on Immunization Practices of the Centers for Disease Control and Prevention using a vaccine-specific appropriate vaccination schedule.[5, 35]

References

1. Addy, M. G., Ellis, P. D. M., and Turk, D. C.: Haemophilus epiglottitis: Nine recent cases in Oxford. Br. Med. J. *1*:40–41, 1972.
2. Alexander, H. E., Ellis, C., and Leidy, C.: Treatment of type-specific *H. influenzae* infections in infancy and childhood. J. Pediatr. *20*:673–698, 1942.
3. Alho, O.-P., Jokinen, K., Pirila, T., et al.: Acute epiglottitis and infant conjugate *Haemophilus influenzae* type b vaccination in northern Finland. Arch. Otolaryngol. Head Neck Surg. *121*:898–902, 1995.
4. Ambrosino, D. M., Schiffman, G., Gottschlich, E. C., et al.: Correlation between G2m(n) immunoglobulin allotype and human antibody response and susceptibility to polysaccharide encapsulated bacteria. J. Clin. Invest. *75*:1953–1942, 1985.
5. American Academy of Pediatrics: *Haemophilus influenzae* infections. *In* Peter, G. (ed.): 1994 Red Book: Report of the Committee on Infectious Diseases. 23rd ed. Elk Grove Village, IL, American Academy of Pediatrics, 1994, pp. 203–217.
6. Andreassen, U. K., Husum, B., Tos, M., et al.: Acute epiglottitis in adults: A management based on a 17-year material. Acta Anaesthesiol. Scand. *28*:155–157, 1984.
7. Barnham, M., Kerby, J., Chandler, R. S., et al.: Group C streptococci in human infection: A study of 308 isolates with clinical correlations. Epidemiol. Infect. *102*:379–390, 1989.
8. Baron, B. J.: Comments on a case of extremely acute edematous laryngitis. Br. Med. J. *2*:1328, 1887.
9. Bass, J. W.: Routine tracheotomy for epiglottitis: What are the odds? J. Pediatr. *83*:510–511, 1973.
10. Bass, J. W.: Personal communication, 1977.
11. Bass, J. W.: Response to CPC. N. Engl. J. Med. *298*:342–343, 1978.
12. Bass, J. W., Steele, R. W., and Wiebe, R. A.: Acute epiglottitis: A surgical emergency. J. A. M. A. *229*:671–675, 1974.
13. Battaglia, J. D., and Lockhart, C. H.: Management of acute epiglottitis by nasotracheal intubation. Am. J. Dis. Child. *129*:334–336, 1975.
14. Baugh, R., and Baker, S. R.: Epiglottitis in children: Review of 24 cases. Otolaryngol. Head Neck Surg. *90*:157–162, 1982.
15. Baxter, J. D.: Acute epiglottitis in children. Laryngoscope *77*:1358–1367, 1967.
16. Benjamin, B., and O'Reilly, B.: Acute epiglottitis in infants and children. Ann. Otol. *85*:565–572, 1976.
17. Berenberg, W., and Kevy, S.: Acute epiglottitis in childhood: A serious emergency, readily recognized at the bedside. N. Engl. J. Med. *258*:870–874, 1958.
18. Bishop, M. L.: Epiglottitis in the adult. Anesthesiology *55*:701–702, 1981.
19. Bishop, M. J., and Weymuller, E. A.: Adult epiglottitis revisited. Anesthesiology *57*:545–546, 1982.
20. Black, M. J., Harbour, J., Remsen, K. A., et al.: Acute epiglottitis in adults. J. Otolaryngol. *10*:23–27, 1981.
21. Blackstock, D., Adderley, R. J., and Steward, D. J.: Epiglottitis in young infants. Anesthesiology *69*:97–100, 1987.
22. Blankson, V. N.: Pulmonary edema complicating epiglottitis. J. Med. Soc. N. J. *80*:939–941, 1983.
23. Bogger-Goren, S.: Acute epiglottitis caused by herpes simplex virus. Pediatr. Infect. Dis. *6*:1133, 1987.
24. Bolivar, R., Gomez, L. G., Luna, M., et al.: Aspergillus epiglottitis. Cancer *51*:367–370, 1983.
25. Bottenfield, G. W., Arcinue, E. L., Sarnaik, A., et al.: Diagnosis and management of acute epiglottitis: Report of 90 consecutive cases. Laryngoscope *90*:822–825, 1980.
26. Branefors-Helander, P., and Jeppsson, P. H.: Acute epiglottitis: A clinical, bacteriological and serological study. Scand. J. Infect. Dis. *7*:103–111, 1975.
27. Breivik, H., and Klaastad, O.: Acute epiglottitis in children. Br. J. Anaesth. *50*:505–509, 1978.
28. Briggs, W. H., and Altenau, M. M.: Acute epiglottitis in children. Otolaryngol. Head Neck Surg. *88*:665–669, 1980.
29. Brilli, R. J., Benzing, G., and Cotcamp, D. H.: Epiglottitis in infants less than two years of age. Pediatr. Emerg. Care *5*:16–21, 1989.
30. Broadhurst, L. E., Erickson, R. L., and Kelley, P. W.: Decreases in invasive *Haemophilus influenzae* diseases in US Army children, 1984 through 1991. J. A. M. A. *269*:227–231, 1993.
31. Broughton, S. J., and Warren, R. E.: A review of *Haemophilus influenzae* infections in Cambridge 1975–1981. J. Infect. *9*:30–42, 1984.
32. Burtner, D. D., and Goodman, M.: Anesthetic and operative management of potential upper airway obstruction. Arch. Otolaryngol. *104*:657–661, 1978.
33. Butt, W., Shann, F., Walker, C., et al.: Acute epiglottitis: A different approach to management. Crit. Care Med. *16*:43–47, 1988.
34. Cantrell, R. W., Bell, R. A., and Morioka, W. T.: Acute epiglottitis: Intubation versus tracheostomy. Laryngoscope *88*:994–1005, 1978.
35. Centers for Disease Control: Immunization Practices Advisory Committee: *Haemophilus* b conjugate vaccine for prevention of *Haemophilus influenzae* type b disease among infants and children 2 months of age and older. M. M. W. R. *40*(RR-1):1–7, 1991.
36. Cherry, J. D.: Acute epiglottitis, laryngitis, and croup. *In* Remington, J. S., and Swartz, M. N. (eds.): Current Clinical Topics in Infectious Diseases. New York, McGraw-Hill, 1981, pp. 1–30.
37. Cherry, J. D.: Croup. *In* Kiple, K. F. (ed.): The Cambridge World History of Human Disease. Cambridge, Cambridge University Press, 1993, pp. 654–657.
38. Cherry, J. D.: Unpublished data, 1973.
39. Chow, A. W., Bushkell, L. L., Yoshikawa, T. T., et al.: *Haemophilus parainfluenzae* epiglottitis with meningitis and bacteremia in an adult. Am. J. Med. Sci. *267*:365–368, 1974.
40. Claesson, B., Trollfors, B., Ekström-Jodal, B., et al.: Incidence and prognosis of acute epiglottitis in children in a Swedish region. Pediatr. Infect. Dis. *3*:534–538, 1984.
41. Cohen, S. R., and Chai, J.: Epiglottitis: Twenty-year study with tracheotomy. Ann. Otol. *87*:461–467, 1978.
42. Coker, S. B., and Scherz, R. G.: Safe alternative to tracheostomy in acute epiglottitis. Am. J. Dis. Child. *129*:136, 1975.
43. Coulehan, J. L., Michaels, R. H., Hallowell C., et al.: Epidemiology of *Haemophilus influenzae* type b disease among Navajo Indians. Public Health Rep. *99*:404–409, 1984.
44. Dagan, R., and the Israeli Pediatric Bacteremia and Meningitis Group: A two-year prospective, nationwide study to determine the epidemiology and impact of invasive childhood *Haemophilus influenzae* type b infection in Israel. Clin. Infect. Dis. *15*:720–725, 1992.
45. Darnell, J. C.: Acute epiglottitis in adults: Report of a case and review of the literature. J. Indiana State Med. Assoc. *69*:21–23, 1976.
46. Daum, R. S., Glode, M. P., Goldmann, D. A., et al.: Rifampin chemoprophylaxis for household contacts of patients with invasive infections due to *Haemophilus influenzae* type b. J. Pediatr. *98*:485–491, 1981.
47. Daum, R. S., Granoff, D. M., Gilsdorf, J., et al.: *H. influenzae* type b infections in day care attendees: Implications for management. Rev. Infect. Dis. *8*:46–55, 1986.
48. Daum, R. S., and Smith, A. L.: Epiglottitis (Supraglottitis). *In* Feigin, R. D., and Cherry, J. D. (eds.): Textbook of Pediatric Infectious Diseases. 3rd ed. Philadelphia, W. B. Saunders, 1992, pp. 197–209.
49. Davis, H. W., Gartner, J. C., Galvis, A. G., et al.: Acute upper airway obstruction: Croup and epiglottitis. Pediatr. Clin. North Am. *28*:859–880, 1981.
50. Devita, M. A., and Wagner, I. J.: Acute epiglottitis in the adult. Crit. Care Med. *14*:1082–1083, 1986.
51. Diaz, J. H., and Lockhart, C. H.: Early diagnosis and airway management of acute epiglottitis in children. South. Med. J. *75*:399–403, 1982.
52. DiTirro, F. R., Silver, M. H., and Hengerer, A. S.: Acute epiglottitis: Evolution of management in the community hospital. Int. J. Pediatr. Otorhinolaryngol. *7*:145–152, 1984.
53. Donnelly, J., Overtun, J. H., and Mellis, C. M.: Pulmonary oedema following relief of epiglottitis. Anaesth. Intensive Care *9*:290–291, 1981.
54. Drake Lee, A. B., Broughton, S. J., and Grace, A.: Children with epiglottitis. Br. J. Clin. Prac. *38*:218–220, 1984.
55. Dudley, J. P.: Supraglottitis and *Hemophilus parainfluenzae*: Pathogenic potential of the organism. Ann. Otol. Rhinol. Laryngol. *96*:400–402, 1987.
56. Dworetzky, J. P., and Risch, O. C.: Laryngeal tuberculosis: A study of 500 cases of pulmonary tuberculosis with a resume based on twenty-eight years of experience. Ann. Otol. Rhinol. Laryngol. *50*:745–761, 1941.
57. Faden, H. S.: Treatment of *Haemophilus influenzae* type b epiglottitis. Pediatrics *63*:402–407, 1979.
58. Farley, M. M., Stephens, D. S., Brachman, P. S., Jr., et al.: Invasive *Haemophilus influenzae* disease in adults: A prospective, population-based surveillance. Ann. Intern. Med. *116*:806–812, 1992.
59. Fearon, B. W., and Bell, R. D.: Acute epiglottitis: A potential killer. Can. Med. Assoc. J. *112*:760–766, 1975.
60. Fogarty, J., Moloney, A. C., and Newell, J. B.: The epidemiology of *Haemophilus influenzae* type b disease in the Republic of Ireland. Epidemiol. Infect. *114*:451–463, 1995.
61. Fontanarosa, P. B., Polsky, S. S., and Goldman, G. E.: Adult epiglottitis. J. Emerg. Med. *7*:223–231, 1989.
62. Frantz, T. D., and Rasgon, B. M.: Acute epiglottitis: Changing epidemiologic patterns. Otolaryngol. Head Neck Surg. *109*:457–460, 1993.
63. Frantz, T. D., Rasgon, B. M., and Quesenberry, C. P., Jr.: Acute epiglottitis in adults: Analysis of 129 cases. J. A. M. A. *272*:1358–1360, 1994.
64. Galvis, A. G., Stool, S. E., and Bluestone, C. D.: Pulmonary edema following relief of acute upper airway obstruction. Ann. Otol. *89*:124–128, 1980.
65. Gerber, A. C., and Pfenniger, J.: Acute epiglottitis: Management by short duration of intubation and hospitalisation. Intensive Care Med. *12*:407–411, 1986.
66. Glode, M. P., Halsey, N. A., Murray, M., et al.: Epiglottitis in adults: Association with *Haemophilus influenzae* type b colonization and disease in children. Pediatr. Infect. Dis. *3*:548–551, 1984.
67. Glode, M. P.: Post exposure prophylaxis for bacterial meningitis. *In* Sande, M. A., Smith, A. L., and Root, R. K. (eds.): Bacterial Meningitis. New York, Churchill Livingstone, 1985.
68. Gorelick, M. H., and Baker, M. D.: Epiglottitis in children, 1979 through

1992: Effects of *Haemophilus influenzae* type b immunization. Arch. Pediatr. Adolesc. Med. *148*:47–50, 1994.
69. Granoff, D. M., and Daum, R. S.: Spread of *Haemophilus influenzae* type b: Recent epidemiologic and therapeutic considerations. J. Pediatr. *97*:854–860, 1980.
70. Granoff, D. M., Pandey, J. P., Boies, E., et al.: Response to immunization with *Haemophilus influenzae* type b polysaccharide-pertussis vaccine and risk of *Haemophilus* meningitis in children with the Km(1) immunoglobulin allotype. J. Clin. Invest. *74*:1708–1714, 1984.
71. Grattan-Smith, T., Forer, M., Kilham, H., et al.: Viral supraglottitis. J. Pediatr. *110*:434–435, 1987.
72. Handler, S. D., Plotkin, S. A., Potsic, W. P., et al.: *Haemophilus influenzae* epiglottitis occurring concurrently in two siblings. Clin. Pediatr. *21*:634–635, 1982.
73. Hawkins, D. B., Miller, A. H., Sachs, G. B., et al.: Acute epiglottitis in adults. Laryngoscope *83*:1211–1220, 1973.
74. Healy, G. B., Hyams, V. J., and Tucker, G. F.: Paraglottic laryngitis in association with epiglottitis. Ann. Otol. Rhinol. Laryngol. *94*:618–621, 1985.
75. Heldtander, P., and Lee, P.: Treatment of acute epiglottitis in children by long-term intubation. Acta Otolaryngol. *75*:379–381, 1973.
76. Hodge, K. M., and Ganzel, T. M.: Diagnostic and therapeutic efficiency in croup and epiglottitis. Laryngoscope *97*:621–625, 1987.
77. Howard, A. J., Dunkin, K. T., Musser, J. M., et al.: Epidemiology of *Haemophilus influenzae* type b invasive disease in Wales. Br. Med. J. *303*:441–445, 1991.
78. Isenberg, D. A., Lipkin, D. P., Mowbray, J. F., et al.: Fatal pneumococcal epiglottitis in lupus overlap syndrome. Clin. Rheum. *3*:529–532, 1984.
79. Johnson, G. K., Sullivan, J. L., and Bishop, L. A.: Acute epiglottitis: Review of 55 cases and suggested protocol. Arch. Otolaryngol. *100*:333–337, 1974.
80. Johnson, R. H., and Rumans, L. W.: Unusual infections caused by *Pasteurella multocida*. J. A. M. A. *237*:146–147, 1977.
81. Johnstone, J. M., and Lawy, H. S.: Acute epiglottitis in adults due to infection with *Haemophilus influenzae* type b. Lancet *2*:134–136, 1967.
82. Jones, H. M.: Acute epiglottitis: A personal study over twenty years. Proc. R. Soc. Med. *63*:706–712, 1970.
83. Jones, R. N., Slepack, J., and Bigelow, J.: Ampicillin-resistant *Haemophilus paraphrophilus* laryngoepiglottitis. J. Clin. Microbiol. *4*:405–407, 1976.
84. Kanter, R. K., and Watchko, J. F.: Pulmonary edema associated with upper airway obstruction. Am. J. Dis. Child. *138*:356–358, 1984.
85. Kennedy, C. A., and Rosen, H.: *Kingella kingae* bacteremia and adult epiglottitis in a granulocytopenic host. Am. J. Med. *85*:701–702, 1988.
86. Kessler, H. A., Schade, R., and Trenhome, G. M.: Acute pneumococcal epiglottitis in immunocompromised adults. Scand. J. Infect. Dis. *12*:207–210, 1980.
87. Kharasch, S., Vinci, R., and Reece, R.: Esophagitis, epiglottitis, and cocaine alkaloid ("crack"): "Accidental" poisoning or child abuse? Pediatrics *86*:117–119, 1990.
88. Khilanani, U., and Khatib, R.: Acute epiglottitis in adults. Am. J. Med. Sci. *287*:65–70, 1984.
89. Kotloff, K. L., and Wald, E. R.: Uvulitis in children. Pediatr. Infect. Dis. *2*:392–393, 1983.
90. Kristensen, K., Kaaber, K., Ronne, T., et al.: Epidemiology of *Haemophilus influenzae* type b infections among children in Denmark in 1985 and 1986. Acta Paediatr. Scand. *79*:587–592, 1990.
91. Kristensen, K.: *Haemophilus influenzae* type b infections in adults. Scand. J. Infect. Dis. *21*:651–653, 1989.
92. Kulick, R. M., Selbst, S. M., Baker, M.D., et al.: Thermal epiglottitis after swallowing hot beverages. Pediatrics *81*:441–444, 1988.
93. Kyrcz, R. W., and Indyk, D.: Atypical acute epiglottitis with gastrointestinal bleeding. J. Fam. Pract. *27*:102–103, 1988.
94. Lacroix, J., Ahronheim, G., Arcand, P., et al.: Group A streptococcal supraglottitis. J. Pediatr. *109*:20–24, 1986.
95. Lacroix, J., Ahronheim, G., and Girouard, G.: *Pseudomonas aeruginosa* supraglottitis in a six-month-old child with severe combined immunodeficiency syndrome. Pediatr. Infect. Dis. *7*:739–741, 1988.
96. Lacroix, J., Blanc, V. F., Weber, M., et al.: Étude de 100 cas consécutifs d'epiglottite aiguë. L'Union Médicale du Canada *111*:774–779, 1982.
97. Lang, S. A., Duncan, P. G., Shephard, D. A. E., et al.: Pulmonary edema associated with airway obstruction. Can. J. Anaesth. *37*:210–218, 1990.
98. La Scolea, L. J., Rosales, S. V., Welliver, R. C., et al.: Mechanisms underlying the development of meningitis or epiglottitis in children after *Haemophilus influenzae* type b bacteremia. J. Infect. Dis. *151*:1162–1165, 1985.
99. Lederman, M. M., Lowder, J., and Lerner, P. I.: Bacteremic pneumococcal epiglottitis in adults with malignancy. Am. Rev. Respir. Dis. *125*:117–118, 1982.
100. Lee, S. C., Meislin, H., and Iserson, K. V.: Epiglottitis presenting as acute pulmonary edema. Ann. Emerg. Med. *14*:60–63, 1985.
101. Lemierre, A., Meyer, A., and Laplane, R.: Maladies infectieuses: Les septicemies à bacille de Pfeiffer. Ann. Méd. *39*:97–119, 1936.
102. Levison, H., Tabachnik, E., and Newth, C. J. L.: Wheezing in infancy, croup and epiglottitis. Curr. Probl. Pediatr. *12*:1–65, 1982.
103. Lewis, J. K., Gartner, J. C., and Galvis, A. G.: A protocol for management of acute epiglottitis. Clin. Pediatr. *17*:494–496, 1978.
104. Li, K. I., Kiernan, S., Wald, E. R., et al.: Isolated uvulitis due to *Haemophilus influenzae* type b. Pediatrics *74*:1054–1057, 1984.
105. Lindquist, J. R., Franzen, R. E., and Ossoff, R. H.: Acute infectious supraglottitis in adults. Ann. Emerg. Med. *9*:256–259, 1980.
106. Lipson, A., Kronick, J. B., Tewfik, L., et al.: Group B streptococcal supraglottitis in a 3-month-old infant. Am. J. Dis. Child. *140*:411–412, 1986.
107. Losek, J. D., Dewitz-Zink, B. A., Melzer-Lange, M., et al.: Epiglottitis: Comparison of signs and symptoms in children less than 2 years old and older. Ann. Emerg. Med. *19*:55–58, 1990.
108. Mace, S. E.: Acute epiglottitis in adults. Am. J. Emerg. Med. *3*:543–550, 1985.
109. Macneil, A., Campbell, A. M., and Clark, L. J.: Adult acute epiglottitis in association with infection of an epiglottic cyst. Anaesth. Intensive Care *17*:211–212, 1989.
110. Margolis, C. Z., Colletti, R. B., and Grundy, G.: *Haemophilus influenzae* type b: The etiologic agent in epiglottitis. J. Pediatr. *87*:322–323, 1975.
111. Margolis, C. Z., Ingram, D. L., and Meyer, J. H.: Routine tracheotomy in *Hemophilus influenzae* type b epiglottitis. J. Pediatr. *81*:1150–1153, 1972.
112. Mayo Smith, M. F., Hirsch, P. J., Wodzinski, S. F., et al.: Acute epiglottitis in adults. N. Engl. J. Med. *314*:1133–1139, 1986.
113. McGregor, A. R., Dawson, K. P., and Abbott, G. D.: Acute epiglottitis in childhood, Christchurch 1970–84. N. Z. Med. J. *98*:1011–1013, 1985.
114. McIntyre, P. B., Leeder, S. R., and Irwig, L. M.: Invasive *Haemophilus influenzae* type b disease in Sydney children 1985–1987: A population-based study. Med. J. Aust. *154*:832–837, 1991.
115. Mehtar, S., Bangham, L., Kalmanovitch, D., et al.: Adult epiglottitis due to *Vibrio vulnificus*. Br. Med. J. *296*:827–828, 1988.
116. Milko, D. A., Marshak, G., and Striker, T. W.: Nasotracheal intubation in the treatment of acute epiglottitis. Pediatrics *53*:674–677, 1974.
117. Mitchell, D. B., and Drake-Lee, A. B.: Chronic non-specific granulomatous epiglottitis. J. Laryngol. Otolaryngol. *99*:1305–1308, 1985.
118. Molteni, R. A.: Epiglottitis: Incidence of extraepiglottis infection: Report of 72 cases and review of the literature. Pediatrics *58*:526–531, 1976.
119. Murphy, T. V., Osterholm, M. T., Pierson, L. M., et al.: Prospective surveillance of *Haemophilus influenzae* disease in Dallas County, Texas, and in Minnesota. Pediatrics *79*:173–180, 1987.
120. Murphy, T. V., Granoff, D. M., Pierson, L. M., et al.: Invasive *Haemophilus influenzae* type b disease in children $<$5 years of age in Minnesota and in Dallas County, Texas, 1983–1984. J. Infect. Dis. 165(Suppl. 1):S7–S10, 1992.
121. Nussbaum, E.: Fiberoptic laryngoscopy as a guide to tracheal extubation in acute epiglottitis. J. Pediatr. *102*:269–270, 1983.
122. Oh, T. H., and Motoyama, E. K.: Comparison of nasotracheal intubation and tracheostomy in management of acute epiglottitis. Anaesthesiology *46*:214–216, 1977.
123. Perrone, J. A.: Laryngeal obstruction due to *Monilia albicans* in a newborn. Laryngoscope *80*:288–291, 1970.
124. Quigley, C., Kaczmarski, E. B., Jones, D. M., et al.: *Haemophilus influenzae* type b disease in north-west England. J. Infect. *26*:215–220, 1993.
125. Rabe, E. F.: Infectious croup: III. *Hemophilus influenzae* type b croup. Pediatrics *2*:559–566, 1948.
126. Rapkin, R. H.: The diagnosis of epiglottitis: Simplicity and reliability of radiographs of the neck in the differential diagnosis of the croup syndrome. J. Pediatr. *80*:96–98, 1972.
127. Rapkin, R. H.: Nasotracheal intubation in epiglottitis. Pediatrics *56*:110–112, 1975.
128. Rapkin, R. H.: Simultaneous uvulitis and epiglottitis. J. A. M. A. *243*:1843, 1980.
129. Richens, J., and Montgomery, J.: Acute epiglottitis (supraglottitis) in the puerperium caused by infection with group A *Streptococcus*. Papua New Guinea Med. J. *31*:293–294, 1988.
130. Ridgeway, N. A., Verghese, A., Perlman, P. E., et al.: Epiglottic abscess due to group B *Streptococcus* communication. Ann. Otol. Rhinol. Laryngol. *93*:277–278, 1984.
131. Rivera, M., Hadlock, F. P., and O'Meara, M. I.: Pulmonary edema secondary to acute epiglottitis. A. J. R. Am. J. Roentgenol. *132*:991–992, 1979.
132. Robbins, J. P., and Fitz-Hugh, G. S.: Epiglottitis in the adult. Laryngoscope *81*:700–706, 1971.
133. Rose, F. B., Garman, R. F., Falkenberg, K. J., et al.: Adult epiglottitis, cellulitis and *Streptococcus pneumoniae* bacteremia. Scand. J. Infect. Dis. *14*:301–302, 1982.
134. Rothstein, S. G., Persky, M. S., Edelman, B. A., et al.: Epiglottitis in AIDS patients. Laryngoscope *99*:389–392, 1989.
135. Russell, G. A., Gresham, G. A., and Wight, D. G. D.: Acute epiglottitis in adults not due to *Haemophilus*. J. Laryngol. Otol. *99*:1035–1038, 1985.
136. Santosham, M., and Moxon, E. R.: Detection and quantitation of bacteremia in childhood. J. Pediatr. *91*:719–721, 1977.
137. Scheidemandel, H. H. E., and Page, R. S.: Special considerations in epiglottitis in children. Laryngoscope *85*:1738–1745, 1975.
138. Scheifele, D. W., Daum, R. S., Syriopoulou, V., et al.: Comparison of two antigen detection techniques in a primate model of *H. influenzae* type b infection. Infect. Immun. *26*:827–831, 1979.
139. Schiffman, F. J., and Lichtman, H. C.: Paroxysmal precordial purring sign in epiglottitis. Lancet *335*:609, 1990.
140. Schuh, S., Huang, A., and Fallis, J. C.: Atypical epiglottitis. Ann. Emerg. Med. *17*:168–170, 1988.

141. Schuller, D. E., and Birch, H. G.: The safety of intubation in croup and epiglottitis: An eight-year follow-up. Laryngoscope *85:*33–46, 1975.
142. Schultes, A., and Agia, G. A.: Acute *Hemophilus parainfluenzae* epiglottitis in an adult. Postgrad. Med. *75:*207–211, 1984.
143. Schultz, R. L., and Morrison, W. V.: Short term intubation in children with acute epiglottitis. South. Med. J. *75:*158–160, 1982.
144. Schumaker, H. M., Doris, P. E., and Birnbaum, G.: Radiographic parameters in adult epiglottitis. Ann. Emerg. Med. *13:*588–590, 1984.
145. Schwartz, R. H., Knerr, R. J., Hermansen, K., et al.: Acute epiglottitis caused by β-hemolytic group C streptococci. Am. J. Dis. Child. *136:*558–559, 1982.
146. Scully, R. E., Galdabini, J. J., and McNeely, B. U.: Presentation of case. N. Engl. J. Med. *297:*878–883, 1977.
147. Shackelford, G. D., Siegel, M. J., and McAlister, W. H.: Subglottic edema in acute epiglottitis in children. Am. J. Roentgenol. *131:*603–605, 1978.
148. Shalit, M., Gross, D. J., and Levo, Y.: Pneumococcal epiglottitis in systemic lupus erythematosus on high-dosage corticosteroids. Ann. Rhem. Dis. *41:*615–616, 1982.
149. Shann, F. A., Phelan, P. D., Stocks, J. G., et al.: Prolonged nasotracheal intubation of tracheostomy in acute laryngotracheobronchitis and epiglottis? Aust. Paediatr. J. *11:*212–217, 1975.
150. Shih, L., Hawkins, D. B., and Stanley, Jr., R. B.: Acute epiglottis in adults: A review of 48 cases. Ann. Otol. Rhinol. Laryngol. *97:*527–529, 1988.
151. Sinclair, S. E.: *Haemophilus influenzae* type b in acute laryngitis with bacteremia. J. A. M. A. *117:*170–173, 1941.
152. Singer, J. I., and McCabe, J. B.: Epiglottitis at the extremes of age. Am. J. Emerg. Med. *6:*228–231, 1988.
153. Slovis, T. L., and Arcinue, E.: Subglottic edema in acute epiglottitis in children. Letter. Am. J. Roentgenol. *132:*500, 1979.
154. Sly, P. D., Landau, L. I., and Wagener, J. S.: Acute epiglottitis in childhood: Report of an increased incidence in Victoria. Aust. N. Z. J. Med. *14:*131–134, 1984.
155. Smith, E. W. P., and Ingram, D. L.: Counterimmunoelectrophoresis in *Haemophilus influenzae* type b epiglottitis and pericarditis. J. Pediatr. *85:*571–573, 1975.
156. Soliman, M. G., and Richer, P.: Epiglottitis and pulmonary edema in children. Can. Anaesth. Soc. J. *25:*270–276, 1978.
157. Stanley, R. E., and Liange, T. S.: Acute epiglottitis in adults (the Singapore experience). J. Otolaryngol. *102:*1017–1021, 1988.
158. Stuart, M. J., and Hodgetts, T. J.: Adult epiglottitis: Prompt diagnosis saves lives. Br. Med. J. *308:*329–330, 1994.
159. Sullivan, T. D., La Scotea, L. J., and Neter, E.: Relationship between the magnitude of bacteremia and the clinical disease. Pediatrics *69:*669–702, 1982.
160. Takala, A., Eskola, J., Bol, P., et al.: *Haemophilus influenzae* type b strains of outer membrane subtypes 1 and 1c cause different types of invasive disease. Lancet *2:*647–649, 1987.
161. Takala, A., Eskola, J., and Alphen, L.: Spectrum of invasive *Haemophilus influenzae* type b disease in adults. Arch. Intern. Med. *150:*2573–2576, 1990.
162. Takala, A. K., Sarvas, H., Kela, E., et al.: Susceptibility to invasive *Haemophilus influenzae* type b disease and the immunoglobulin G2m(n) allotype. J. Infect. Dis. *163:*637–639, 1991.
163. Tejani, A., Mahadevan, R., Dobias, B., et al.: Occurrence of HLA types in *H. influenzae* type b disease. Tissue Antigens *17:*205–211, 1981.
164. Templer, J. W.: Trauma to the larynx and cervical trachea. *In* English, G. M. (ed.): Otolaryngology. Hagerstown, MD, Harper & Row, 1976.
165. Theisen, D. F.: Angina epiglottidea anterior: Report of three cases. Albany Med. Ann. *21:*395–405, 1900.
166. Tos, M.: Nasotracheal intubation instead of tracheotomy in acute epiglottitis in children. Acta Otolaryngol. *75:*382–383, 1973.
167. Travis, K. W., Todres, I. D., and Shannon, D. C.: Pulmonary edema associated with croup and epiglottitis. Pediatrics *59:*695–698, 1977.
168. Trollfors, B., Brorson, J. E., Clarsson, B., et al.: Invasive infections caused by *Haemophilus* species other than *Haemophilus influenzae* infection. Infection *13:*12–14, 1985.
169. Trollfors, B., Nylen, O., and Strangert, K.: Acute epiglottitis in children and adults in Sweden 1981–1983. Arch. Dis. Child. *65:*491–494, 1990.
170. Trollfors, B.: Invasive *Haemophilus influenzae* infections in household contacts of patients with *Haemophilus influenzae* meningitis and epiglottitis. Acta Paediatr. Scand. *80:*795–797, 1991.
171. Tveteras, K., and Kristensen, S.: Acute epiglottitis in adults: Bacteriology and therapeutic principles. Clin. Otolaryngol. *12:*337–343, 1987.
172. Tyler, D. C., and Haas, J. E.: Airway obstruction due to epiglottic lymphangiectasis: A case report. Int. J. Pediatr. Otorhinol. *6:*285–289, 1983.
173. Valdepena, H. G., Wald, E. R., Rose, E., et al.: Epiglottitis and *Haemophilus influenzae* immunization: The Pittsburgh experience: A five-year review. Pediatrics *96:*424–427, 1995.
174. Vauthy, P. A., and Reddy, R.: Acute upper airway obstruction in infants and children: Evaluation by the fiberoptic bronchoscope. Ann. Otol. Rhinol. Laryngol. *89:*417–418, 1980.
175. Vernham, G. A., and Crowther, J. A.: Acute myeloid leukaemia presenting with acute *Branhamella catarrhalis* epiglottitis. J. Infect. *26:*93–95, 1993.
176. Vernon, D. D., and Sarnaik, A. P.: Acute epiglottitis in children: A conservative approach to diagnosis and management. Crit. Care Med. *14:*23–25, 1986.
177. Vetto, R. R.: Epiglottitis: A report of thirty-seven cases. J. A. M. A. *173:*990–994, 1960.
178. Walsh, T. J., and Gray, W. C.: *Candida epiglottitis* in immunocompromised patients. Chest *91:*482–485, 1987.
179. Ward, J. I., Siber, G. R., Scheifele, D. W., et al.: Rapid diagnosis of *Haemophilus influenzae* type b infections by latex particle agglutination and counterimmunoelectrophoresis. J. Pediatr. *93:*37–42, 1978.
180. Ward, J. I., Lum, M. K. W., Margolis, H. S., et al.: *Haemophilus influenzae* disease in Alaskan Eskimos: Characteristics of a population with an unusual incidence of invasive disease. Lancet *1:*1281–1285, 1981.
181. Ward, J.: *Haemophilus influenzae. In* Feigin, R. D., and Cherry, J. D. (eds.): Textbook of Pediatric Infectious Diseases. 4th ed. Philadelphia, W. B. Saunders, 1998.
182. Warner, J. A., and Finlay, W. E. I.: Fulminating epiglottitis in adults: Report of three cases and review of the literature. Anaesthesia *40:*348–352, 1985.
183. Warshawski, J., Havas, T. E., McShane, D. P., et al.: Adult epiglottitis. J. Otolaryngol. *15:*362–364, 1986.
184. Watts, Jr., F. B., and Slovis, T. L.: The enlarged epiglottis. Pediatr. Radiol. *5:*133–136, 1977.
185. Weber, M. L., Desjardins, R., Perreault, G. et al: Acute epiglottitis in children: Treatment with nasotracheal intubation: Report of 14 consecutive cases. Pediatrics *57:*152–155, 1976.
186. Westerman, E. L., and Hutton, J. P.: Acute uvulitis associated with epiglottitis. Arch. Otolaryngol. Head Neck Surg. *112:*448–449, 1986.
187. Wetmore, R. F., and Handler, S. D.: Epiglottitis: Evolution in management during the last decade. Ann. Otol. *88:*822–826, 1979.
188. Whisnant, J. K., Regentine, G. N., Gralnick, M. A., et al.: Host factors and antibody response in *Haemophilus influenzae* type b meningitis and epiglottitis. J. Infect. Dis. *133:*448–455, 1976.
189. Wolf, M., Strauss, B., Kronenberg, J., et al.: Conservative management of adult epiglottitis. Laryngoscope *100:*183–185, 1990.
190. Yousefzadeh, D. K., Tewfik, H. H., and Franken, E. A.: Epiglottic enlargement following radiation treatment and head and neck tumors. Pediatr. Radiol. *10:*165–168, 1981.
191. Zwahlen, A., and Regamy, C.: Les épiglottites aiguës de l'adulte. Schweiz. Med. Wochenschr. *108:*447–482, 1978.

22

CROUP (LARYNGITIS, LARYNGOTRACHEITIS, SPASMODIC CROUP, LARYNGOTRACHEOBRONCHITIS, BACTERIAL TRACHEITIS, AND LARYNGOTRACHEOBRONCHOPNEUMONITIS)

James D. Cherry

Croup is a term used to identify several different respiratory illnesses characterized by varying degrees of inspiratory stridor, cough, and hoarseness resulting from obstruction in the region of the larynx. The etiology of croup syndromes is diverse, and the consideration of noninfectious possibilities in the differential diagnosis is of major importance. A classification of etiologic considerations in supraglottic, laryngeal, and infraglottic acute obstructions is presented in Table 22–1.

Epiglottitis (discussed in Chapter 21) and diphtheria (presented in Chapter 95) are mentioned here only for historical perspective and as a consideration in differential diagnosis. Croup is presented under the subheadings of laryngitis, laryngotracheitis, spasmodic croup, laryngotracheobronchitis, bacterial tracheitis, and laryngotracheobronchopneumonitis.

HISTORICAL ASPECTS

The word *croup* is derived from the Anglo-Saxon word *Kropan,* to cry aloud.[22] Until the twentieth century, most croup-like illnesses were thought to be diphtheria. Diphtheritic croup is an ancient disease that has been traced to the time of Homer. The historical trail of diphtheria disappeared in the fifth century and did not reappear until 1100 years later. In the sixteenth century, epidemics were noted in Europe. Top[174] credits Bretonneau for differentiating diphtheritic croup from spasmodic croup in 1826. In the twentieth century, the history of croup is marked by three important events: (1) the rapid decline in incidence of diphtheria associated with the use of toxoid, (2) the introduction and widespread use of antibiotics, and (3) the advent of tissue culture techniques, resulting in the establishment of viruses as etiologic agents. After these three events, there was a prevalent academic view that all croup was of viral etiology, and bacteria generally were dismissed as causative agents.[29, 50, 144] However, a careful review of many publications from the first half of the twentieth century clearly indicates a causative role for several bacteria in addition to *Corynebacterium diphtheriae* in croup.[7, 13, 14, 35, 36, 54, 63, 81, 86, 115, 126, 131, 147, 148] During the last two decades, bacterial croup (bacterial tracheitis) was rediscovered.[23, 24, 27, 40, 44, 45, 49, 51, 53, 66, 69, 71, 87, 91, 105, 106, 116, 120, 125, 127, 159, 166, 167, 171, 182, 188]

In the 1940s, Davison separated spasmodic croup from other, more severe forms of croup.[36] The clinical and pathologic aspects of this entity were poorly defined, and today it often is not separated clinically from more severe forms of croup.

TERMINOLOGY

The terminology and classification of infectious illnesses involving the larynx and infraglottic region have evolved over time. Unfortunately, classifications often have mixed etiologic systems with anatomic systems and therefore have led to confusion. For example, croup often has been presented in articles under the heading of laryngotracheobronchitis when the authors really were discussing laryngotracheitis.[88, 107, 117, 139, 149, 154, 172] The term *membranous croup* has been used as the title for papers dealing with bacterial croup.[40, 69] This is confusing because historically membranous croup was diphtheria. Also, many papers dealing with bacterial croup have been titled bacterial tracheitis.[27, 44, 45, 49, 51, 53, 87, 91, 105, 106, 125, 159, 182, 188] This seems inappropriate because the majority of cases of bacterial croup seen today have lower respiratory tract involvement as well as tracheal findings. Table 22–2 lists the classifications and definitions used in this chapter.

In the present era, there has been a general decline in the physician's knowledge of the clinical symptomatology of croup and the relationship of history and physical findings to the needs of therapy and general prognosis.

ETIOLOGY

The etiologic agents in laryngitis, spasmodic croup, laryngotracheitis, laryngotracheobronchitis, and laryngotracheo-

TABLE 22–1. Clinical Considerations in Acute Supraglottic, Laryngeal, and Infraglottic Obstructions

Infectious
Acute epiglottitis
Laryngitis
Laryngeal diphtheria
Laryngotracheitis
Laryngotracheobronchitis
Laryngotracheobronchopneumonitis
Bacterial tracheitis
Spasmodic croup
Mechanical
Foreign body
Secondary to trauma resulting from intubation
Allergic
Acute angioneurotic edema

Data from references 23, 24, 29, 55, 57, 127, 142.

TABLE 22–2. Classification and Definition of Infectious Illnesses Involving the Larynx and Infraglottic Region[24, 34, 55, 126]

Category	Other Terms	Definitions
Laryngitis		Inflammation of the larynx resulting in hoarseness; usually occurs in older children and adults in association with common upper respiratory viral infection
Laryngeal diphtheria	Membranous croup, true croup, diphtheritic croup	Infection involving the larynx and other areas of the upper and lower airway due to *Corynebacterium diphtheriae,* resulting in a gradually progressive obstruction of the airway and associated inspiratory stridor
Laryngotracheitis	False croup, virus croup, acute obstructive subglottic laryngitis	Inflammation of the larynx and trachea usually caused by infection with parainfluenza and influenza viruses; occasionally secondary bacterial infection
Laryngotracheobronchitis and laryngotracheobronchopneumonitis	Membranous laryngotracheobronchitis, pseudomembranous croup	Inflammation of the larynx, trachea, and bronchi, and/or lung; usually similar in onset to laryngotracheitis but more severe illness; bacterial infection frequently has causative role
Bacterial croup	Bacterial tracheitis, membranous croup, membranous tracheitis, membranous laryngotracheo-bronchitis, pseudomembranous croup	A severe form of laryngotracheitis, laryngotracheobronchitis, or laryngotracheobronchopneumonitis due to bacterial infection
Spasmodic croup	Spasmodic laryngitis, catarrhal spasm of the larynx, subglottic allergic edema	An illness characterized by the sudden onset at night of inspiratory stridor; associated with mild upper respiratory infection without inflammation or fever but with edema in the subglottic region

Modified from Cherry, J. D.: Acute epiglottitis, laryngitis, and croup. *In* Remington, J. S., and Swartz, M. N. (eds.): Current Clinical Topics in Infectious Diseases. Vol. 2. New York, McGraw-Hill, 1981. Reproduced with permission of The McGraw-Hill Companies.

bronchopneumonitis are presented by frequency and severity of illness in Table 22–3. Laryngitis is a common manifestation of infection with many respiratory viruses in older children, adolescents, and adults. Outbreaks of laryngitis in closed population groups (such as boarding schools and military training camps) most frequently are caused by adenovirus types 4 and 7, and community outbreaks most often are noted in association with epidemic influenza. Sporadic instances of laryngitis most often are due to adenoviral infections. Laryngitis also has been reported in association with group A streptococcal infections; interestingly, the incidence of this association has varied from 2 to 40 per cent.[11, 122, 179]

It generally is accepted today that both acute laryngotracheitis and spasmodic croup, which rarely are differentiated clinically, are caused by infection with many different viruses. Although there have been a large number of studies of respiratory viral infections, there has been almost no attempt to delineate the differences in etiologic spectrum by severity of illness.

Parainfluenza virus type 1 is the most common cause of acute laryngotracheitis and is responsible for frequent and clearly delineated winter epidemics. Croup with parainfluenza type 2 virus seldom is severe but on occasion is related to small outbreaks. Parainfluenza virus type 3 is a frequent cause of sporadic but severe illness.

The most severe laryngotracheitis has been noted in association with influenza A viral infections (both H2N2 and H3N2 subtypes). Both respiratory syncytial virus and several different adenoviruses frequently are isolated in croup. Generally, these illnesses are not severe, but occasionally lower respiratory involvement is a problem. Laryngeal, tracheal, and bronchial involvement is common in measles.[26] Although rhinoviruses, *Mycoplasma pneumoniae*, enteroviruses, herpes simplex virus, and reoviruses have been associated with croup, they generally cause only minimal distress.

Bacteria, other than *Haemophilus influenzae* in epiglottitis and *C. diphtheriae* in membranous croup, until relatively recently generally were dismissed as causative agents in croup.[29, 50, 144] However, a careful review of many publications on laryngotracheobronchitis from the first half of the twentieth century indicates a role for several common bacterial pathogens.[7, 13, 14, 27, 36, 37, 44, 51, 54, 63, 66, 81, 86, 115, 126, 131, 147, 148, 166, 171, 182] Almost two decades ago, bacterial croup was rediscovered,[87] and since then there have been several reports of this illness.[40, 45, 49, 53, 69, 71, 91, 105, 106, 116, 120, 125, 127, 159, 167, 188] In the reports from the preantibiotic era, *Streptococcus pyogenes* was the pathogen implicated most commonly. In more recent reports, *Staphylococcus aureus* has been the most common agent. Other important bacteria are *Streptococcus pneumoniae* and *H. influenzae*. More recently, *Moraxella catarrhalis* has been found to be the causative agent in several cases.[53, 91, 188] *Cryptosporidium* also has been recovered from the trachea of an infant with a subacute illness.[70] It seems likely in most instances that bacterial croup is the result of bacterial superinfection in viral disease.[16, 27, 49, 69, 83, 106, 116, 125, 127, 130]

EPIDEMIOLOGY

Croup accounts for about 15 per cent of lower respiratory tract disease seen in pediatric practice. In a large 11-year study in a pediatric practice in Chapel Hill, North Carolina, Denny and associates[43] noted the incidence of croup by age and sex. Their data are presented in Table 22–4. The highest attack rate occurred in children 7 to 36 months of age. Few cases occurred after the sixth birthday. Hoekelman[74] studied

TABLE 22–3. Etiologic Agents in Laryngitis, Spasmodic Croup, Laryngotracheitis, Laryngotracheobronchitis, and Laryngotracheobronchopneumonitis Presented by Frequency and Severity of Illness

Category	Etiologic Agents	Frequency*	Associated with Outbreaks	Severity†	References
Laryngitis	Adenoviruses				
	Types 4 and 7	+ + + +	Yes	+ to + + +	33, 77, 164, 179
	Types 2, 3, 5, 8, 11, 14, and 21	+ + +	No	+ to + + +	
	Influenza viruses types A and B	+ + + +	Yes	+ to + + + +	5, 77, 132, 179
	Parainfluenza viruses				
	Type I	+ +	Yes	+ to + + +	
	Types 2 and 3	+	Yes	+ to + +	
	Rhinoviruses and respiratory syncytial virus	+ +	No	+ to + +	77, 138, 146, 179
	Enteroviruses	+	No	+	77, 179
	Staphylococcus pyogenes	+ to + + +	Yes	+ to + +	11, 122
Laryngotracheitis and spasmodic croup	Parainfluenza viruses	+ + + +		+ to + + +	9, 18–20, 25, 41, 43, 60, 61, 64, 72, 76, 78, 99, 103, 108, 109, 111, 124, 132, 136, 137, 140, 180
	Type 1	+ + + +	Yes		
	Type 2	+ +	Yes		
	Type 3	+ +	No		
	Influenza viruses	+ +			15, 18, 19, 25, 41, 43, 52, 56, 60, 64, 78, 79, 108, 111, 124, 132, 136, 137, 140, 180
	Type A	+ + +	Yes	+ to + + + +	
	Type B	+	Yes	+ to + +	
	Respiratory syncytial virus	+ +	No	+ to + +	17–20, 25, 41, 43, 60, 61, 64, 78, 99, 109, 121, 136, 137, 139, 175, 181, 185, 189
	Measles virus	+ +	Yes	+ to + + +	26
	Adenoviruses	+ +	No	+ to + +	10, 18–20, 25, 41, 64, 76, 78, 99, 103, 108, 109, 124, 136, 137, 139, 162, 175 180, 181
	Unspecified types and types 1, 2, 3, 5, 6, and 7				
	Rhinoviruses	+	No	+	25, 60, 64, 108, 124
	Mycobacterium pneumoniae	+	No	+ +	18, 20, 25, 41–43, 64, 78, 109
	Enteroviruses	+	No		19, 25, 30, 60, 61, 64, 78, 85, 108, 121, 163, 175, 185
	Coxsackievirus type A9	+	No	+	
	Coxsackievirus types B4 and B5	+	No	+	
	Echoviruses types 4, 11, and 21	+	No	+	
	Herpes simplex viruses	+	No	+	78, 83, 124, 163
	Reoviruses	+	No	+	189
Laryngotracheobronchitis and laryngotracheobronchopneumonitis	Parainfluenza viruses types 1, 2, and 3	+	No	+ + +	13, 61, 65, 76, 109, 117, 134, 136
	Influenza types A and B				
	Staphylococcus aureus,	+	No	+ + +	52, 56, 79, 137
	S. pyogenes, Streptococcus pneumoniae, and *Haemophilus influenzae*	+ +	No	+ + + +	7, 13, 14, 36, 37, 40, 45, 49, 54, 63, 69, 71, 81, 86, 87, 91, 105, 106, 115, 116, 126, 127, 131, 147, 148, 159
	Other bacteria	±	No	+ + + +	53, 69, 71, 91, 105, 120, 188
	Cryptosporidium	±	No	+ +	70

*+ + + +, most frequent; + + +, frequent; + +, occasional; +, rare; ±, questionable.
†+ + + +, most severe; + + +, severe; + +, not severe; +, minimal distress.

TABLE 22–4. Incidence of Croup by Patient Age and Sex, Chapel Hill, NC, 1964 to 1975

Age (Years)	Incidence/100 Children/Year (M/F)	Incidence by Sex (M/F)
0–½	2.76/2.01	1.37
½–1	4.95/2.86	1.73
1–2	5.60/3.66	1.53
2–3	3.55/2.63	1.35
3–4	2.55/1.60	1.59
4–5	1.69/1.16	1.46
5–6	1.15/0.92	1.25
6	0.47/0.44	1.07
All ages	1.82/1.27	1.43

From Denny, F. W., Murphy, T. F., Clyde, W. A., Jr., et al.: Croup: An 11-year study in a pediatric practice. Pediatrics *71*:871–876, 1983. Used by permission.

the occurrence of illness prospectively in 246 full-term, first-born, well babies during their first year of life. Three infants (1.2 per cent) had croup during the study year. The analysis of a pediatric practice in which there were about 3000 active records and about 10,000 yearly visits of children younger than 5 years of age disclosed five cases of croup in a group of 50 consecutive hospitalized patients.[12]

Although croup occurs occasionally in older children, the majority of cases occur within the first 3 years of life. A review of 211 children hospitalized for croup over a 2-year period at Cardinal Glennon Memorial Hospital for Children in St. Louis showed 26 per cent of those cases in children younger than 1 year of age and 73 per cent in those younger than 3 years of age.[59] Similar age data have been observed by others.[43, 50, 55, 149, 153]

Croup is decidedly more common in boys than in girls (see Table 22–4). In our studies, two of every three hospitalized children were boys.[59] Berg,[8] Kravitz,[100] and Rosales and Davenport[149] noted similar sex-related illness ratios. The 3-year seasonal pattern of croup as manifested by emergency room visits at Cardinal Glennon Memorial Hospital for Children is presented in Figure 22–1. In each of the years, late fall–early winter peaks occurred. In the Chapel Hill studies, it was noted that there was an increase in the number of croup cases beginning in September, with a peak in October and November, and then a decrease over the next 7-month period.[43] In a 2-year emergency room study in Toronto involving 1700 cases, it was found that the peak month of visits and hospital admissions was October.[153] Epidemic peaks of acute laryngotracheitis reflect community-wide activity with parainfluenza 1 and 2 viruses or influenza A or B outbreaks.[43, 65]

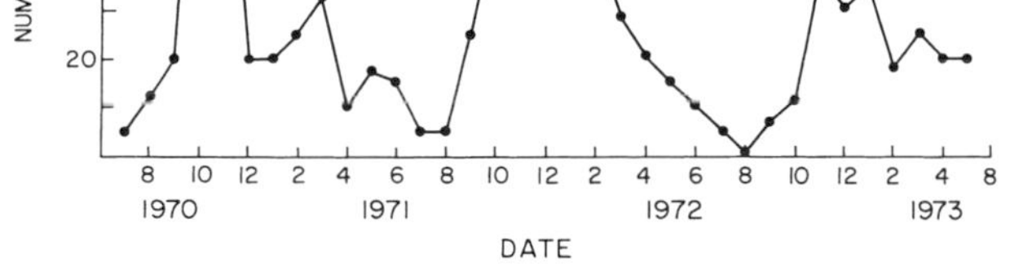

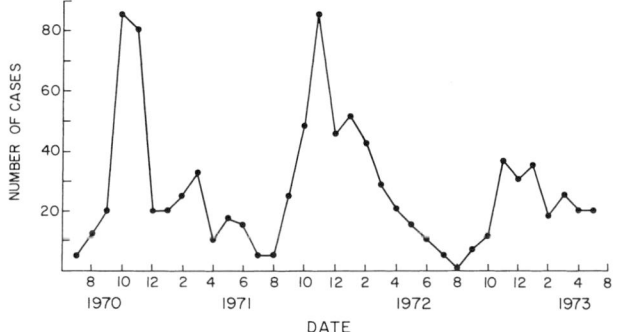

FIGURE 22–1. *Seasonal occurrence of croup, Cardinal Glennon Memorial Hospital for Children Emergency Room, July 1970 to June 1973.*

In the Toronto study, the time of the visit to the emergency room was analyzed.[153] The peak number of visits occurred between 10:00 P.M. and 4:00 A.M. During this period, about 17 per cent of those children seen were admitted to the hospital. In contrast, of children seen between 12:00 P.M. and 6:00 P.M., about 50 per cent were admitted to the hospital.

Because croup is caused by the same viruses that cause other respiratory illnesses, it is probable that the method of spread is similar for all (see discussion of the common cold in Chapter 8). In children, most spread involves close person-to-person contact, with large droplets of virus-containing nasal secretions being applied to the nose from the hands of the future host or by close-range airborne acquisition. Parainfluenza viruses are common causes of colds in adults, so older persons with relatively trivial illnesses may be the source of the more severe childhood croup.

PATHOPHYSIOLOGY

Acute Laryngitis, Laryngotracheitis, Laryngotracheobronchitis, and Laryngotracheobronchopneumonitis

Although the eventual site of clinically important pathology in laryngotracheitis is within the larynx and trachea, the initial acquisition of infection is similar to that of other respiratory viral infections and occurs within the upper air passages, including the nasal and pharyngeal epithelial surfaces. After virus acquisition, infection of the cells of the local respiratory epithelium occurs, spreading locally to involve the larynx and trachea. The initial symptomatology of nasal stuffiness and throat irritation reflects the primary sites of involvement.

Studies in organ culture systems have shown that several respiratory viruses inhibit tracheal ciliary function and eventually lead to marked destruction of the epithelium as well as evidence of viral infection in the lamina propria.[97, 145]

Laryngoscopic studies in acute laryngotracheitis reveal redness and swelling of the lateral walls of the trachea, just below the vocal cords.[35, 36, 169] Because the subglottic trachea is surrounded by a firm cartilaginous ring, the inflammatory swelling can occur only by encroaching on the patency of the airway; the subglottic space often is reduced to a slit 1 to 2 mm wide.

As the disease progresses, the tracheal lumen becomes further obstructed by a fibrinous exudate, and its surface is covered by pseudomembranes made up of the exudative material. The vocal cords frequently are swollen, and their mobility is impaired.

Histologic study of postmortem material from the larynx and trachea reveals marked edema and cellular infiltration in the lamina propria, submucosa, and adventitia. The cellular infiltrate includes histiocytes, lymphocytes, plasma cells, and polymorphonuclear leukocytes.[13, 14, 123, 131, 148]

From the older literature, it seems apparent that the classic laryngotracheobronchitis and the same disease with pneumonia represent the extension of disease from the trachea to the bronchi and alveoli. The progressive obstructive disease with exudate and pseudomembrane obstruction at the bronchial and bronchiolar levels usually is the result of secondary bacterial involvement. In bacterial croup, the tracheal wall is infiltrated with inflammatory cells, and there are ulceration and microabscess formation.[106]

More recent studies have suggested that in uncomplicated croup there may be failure of gas exchange within the lung in addition to hypoxia resulting from subglottic tracheal obstruction.[128, 172]

Because parainfluenza viral infections are common in young children and because only a small number get croup, it is probable that host factors are important in the pathogenesis. Welliver and associates[184] found that children with croup caused by parainfluenza viruses were much more likely to have virus-specific IgE antibody in their secretions than children with parainfluenza infections who did not have croup. In the same study, it was found that illness severity correlated directly with the specific IgE antibody titer. In another study, Welliver and colleagues[183] found that lymphocytes from children with croup showed greater stimulation on exposure to parainfluenza virus antigen than those from children with noncroup upper respiratory parainfluenza viral infections. In the same croup patients, the investigators also found a diminished histamine-induced suppression of lymphocyte reactivity to parainfluenza viral antigens. These findings suggest a defect in suppressor function in patients with croup.

Bacterial Tracheitis

As pointed out earlier, the bronchi and lungs also usually are involved in bacterial tracheitis, and this illness is due to secondary bacterial infection in viral laryngotracheitis, laryngotracheobronchitis, or laryngotracheobronchopneumonitis.[2, 21–24, 27, 40, 44, 45, 49, 53, 66, 71, 87, 91, 105, 106, 127, 130, 159, 167] In addition to the findings in laryngotracheitis of viral origin, there is thick pus within the lumen of the trachea and lower air passages as well.[71, 91, 105, 116] Also, there are ulcerations, pseudomembranes, and microabscesses.

Spasmodic Croup

Spasmodic croup is somewhat of an enigma because it occurs in association with respiratory viral infections similar to those that cause more severe laryngotracheitis. Using direct laryngoscopy, Davison[35] noted that the subglottic tissues in spasmodic croup showed noninflammatory edema. Although definitive proof is lacking, it is reasonable to assume that in spasmodic croup there is no direct viral involvement of the tracheal epithelium and that the obstruction is the result of the relatively sudden occurrence of a noninflammatory edema within the submucosa of the subglottic trachea. The reason for this sudden edematous swelling is unknown, but it is readily reversible; the tendency for its occurrence appears to run in families. Hide and Guyer[73] noted that children who had recurrent croup were more likely to have a family history of allergy compared with children who did not have recurrent croup.

Studies by Zach[190] suggest that children with recurrent croup have a hyperreactivity airway disorder and a tendency toward low serum IgA levels.

CLINICAL PRESENTATION

Acute Laryngitis

Clinical characteristics of laryngitis are presented in Table 22–5. Laryngitis mainly is a disease of older children, adolescents, and adults that is disturbing but self-limited. The specific clinical manifestation is hoarseness. Other symptoms depend on the causative infectious agent. Adenoviruses and influenza viruses cause the most severe instances of laryngitis. With these viruses, fever is usual, and sore throat, headache, muscle aches and pains, and prostration are common. In contrast, patients with laryngitis resulting from rhinoviral, parainfluenza viral, or respiratory syncytial viral infections have minimal or no fever and few systemic complaints. They usually have pronounced nasal symptomatology (coryza and stuffiness), however.

Occasionally, hoarseness may persist, which may be a result of secondary bacterial infection of the upper respiratory tract.

Acute Laryngotracheitis

Although the clinical spectrum of acute laryngotracheitis varies considerably, its manifestations usually are significantly different from those of the other acute diseases, with obstruction in the region of the larynx (see Table 22–5). Onset of illness usually is not alarming and suggests the onset of a cold. Initial symptoms are nasal complaints and include dryness, irritation, and coryza. Ordinary cough and the complaint of sore throat are frequent. Fever is a usual occurrence within the first 24 hours, which is not true of the common cold. After a period as short as a few hours but usually after 12 to 48 hours, upper airway obstructive signs and symptoms are seen. The cough first becomes "croupy" (sounding like a barking seal), then gradually there is increasing evidence of respiratory stridor (difficulty associated with inspiration). Examination at this time reveals a child with a hoarse voice, coryza, a normal or minimally inflamed pharynx, and a slightly increased respiratory rate with a prolonged inspiratory phase. Fever ranging between 37.8° and 40.5° C (100° and 105° F) nearly always is observed.

The speed of progression and final degree of upper airway obstruction are quite variable. Some children will have hoarseness and barking cough but no other evidence of obstruction; in these cases, the symptoms last for about 3 to 7 days, with a gradual return to normal. In other cases, the obstruction is progressive and leads to severe respiratory distress with supra- and infraclavicular and sternal retractions, cyanosis of varying degrees, and apprehension. With hypoxia, the cardiac rate increases and the child becomes restless. Without intervention, asphyxial death will occur rapidly in some children. In others, the problem of hypoxia is more prolonged, and respiratory fatigue may lead to the patient's demise. The duration of illness in the severely affected child, regardless of therapy, rarely is less than 7 days and frequently is as long as 14 days.

Laboratory study in acute laryngotracheitis is of only minimal value. The white blood cell count frequently is elevated above 10,000 cells/mm^3, and the number of polymorphonuclear cells predominates.[25, 129] Very high white blood cell counts (>20,000) with a large number of band-form neutrophils should suggest bacterial superinfection or the possibility of acute epiglottitis. The posteroanterior chest radiograph reveals the subglottic narrowing, and a lateral neck roentgenogram indicates the size of the epiglottitis.

Acute Laryngotracheobronchitis and Laryngotracheobronchopneumonitis (Bacterial Tracheitis) (see Table 22–5)

Laryngotracheobronchitis and laryngotracheobronchopneumonitis are far less common than laryngotracheitis and spasmodic croup; however, these illnesses are more common than generally realized.[23, 27, 40, 44, 45, 49, 53, 66, 69, 71, 87, 91, 105, 106, 116, 120, 125, 167, 188] These entities may be looked upon as an extension of acute laryngotracheitis, as numerous descriptions in the literature suggest.[7, 13, 14, 36, 37, 54, 63, 81, 91, 115, 131, 143, 144, 147, 148] The severity of the illness is due to secondary bacterial infection. Initial symptoms and signs are similar to those of laryngotracheitis. Usually, the afflicted child will have mild to moderately severe illness for 2 to 7 days and then suddenly become markedly worse. Occasionally, both upper and lower airway obstructions appear to occur simultaneously. In many children, the distress from tracheal obstruction is of such magnitude that the symptoms and signs of lower respiratory involvement go unnoticed. Symptoms and signs associated with extension of disease to the bronchi, bronchioles, and lung substance include rales, air trapping, wheezing, and a further increase in the respiratory rate. Obstruction in these illnesses usually is of such a degree that either intubation or tracheostomy is necessary.

Several instances of laryngotracheobronchopneumonitis with toxic shock syndrome have been observed.[21, 130, 160, 167] In general, the children with these staphylococcal infections initially have the onset of croup, then develop the more severe manifestations of bacterial tracheitis, and finally develop the exanthem and other manifestations of toxic shock syndrome. An infant with both tracheitis and supraglottitis due to *M. catarrhalis* has been reported.[2] Other findings in laryngotracheobronchitis and laryngotracheobronchopneumonitis are presented in Table 22–5.

Spasmodic Croup (see Table 22–5)

In recent years, the clinical entity of spasmodic croup has been incorporated by many in the overall diagnosis of croup. Although in some instances it is difficult at the onset to distinguish mild cases of laryngotracheitis from spasmodic croup, it clearly is important from the prognostic and therapeutic perspectives to delineate the two entities.

Spasmodic croup occurs in children 3 months to 3 years of age. The onset always is at night, and the characteristic presentation occurs in a child who previously was thought to be well or to have had a very mild cold with coryza as the only symptom. The child awakens at night with sudden dyspnea, croupy cough, and inspiratory stridor. There is no fever. The symptoms apparently are the result of sudden subglottic edema; relief is brought about easily by general reassurance and moist air administration. The occurrence of spasmodic croup tends to run in families, with repeated attacks occurring in some children. After one attack, the child is quite likely to have another attack the same evening as well as on three or four successive evenings. These can be prevented by employing mild sedation at bedtime and ensuring adequate humidification of the bedroom air.

DIFFERENTIAL DIAGNOSIS

The therapeutic approaches to the various acute obstructions in the region of the larynx vary markedly. Therefore, correct diagnosis is essential and frequently lifesaving. Table 22–5 lists the differential points of eight conditions with symptoms and signs of acute upper airway obstruction.

The most frequent serious differential diagnostic problem is the recognition of acute epiglottitis and its separation from the less fulminant laryngotracheitis. In epiglottitis, the important differential points are lack of a croupy cough; the presence of a swollen, cherry-red epiglottis; the sitting posture of the child with the chin pushed forward and, also, a reluctance or refusal to lie down; and the relatively greater apprehension and anxiety of the patient than the degree of chest retraction suggests. In contrast, the child with acute laryngotracheitis will have a normal epiglottis on examination, will always have a typical barking cough, will be comfortable in a supine position, and frequently will appear to have only minimal apprehension, in spite of retractions in which the sternum appears to be indenting 2 inches or more.

Early in the course of epiglottitis, the diagnosis can be confirmed only by the observation of the epiglottis, and this can be performed without difficulty.[112] Later in the disease, the posture of the child and the history of rapidly progressing disease make the differential from laryngotracheitis readily apparent, so that examination of the epiglottis directly (a dangerous procedure if the child is forced to lie down) or indirectly by a lateral neck radiograph rarely is indicated and usually is contraindicated.

Laryngotracheobronchitis and laryngotracheobronchopneumonitis can be recognized by signs of lower respiratory involvement (rales, air trapping, wheezing, and pulmonary infiltrates on the radiograph). Bacterial disease should be suspected in laryngotracheobronchitis and laryngotracheobronchopneumonitis and when symptoms and signs worsen in laryngotracheitis. A lateral radiograph can be useful in the evaluation because it may reveal soft tissue densities within the trachea.

Lateral neck and chest radiographs are regarded by many physicians as definitive tests to rule in or out epiglottitis and laryngotracheitis. However, in a careful study by Stankiewicz and Bowes,[161] the sensitivity and specificity of both radiographs were low.

Although a rarity today, laryngeal diphtheria always should be considered and ruled out in croup. Important in this regard are the immunization history, pharyngeal evidence of diphtheria, the relative slowness of disease progression, and a greater degree of hoarseness due to direct laryngeal membrane formation.

Spasmodic croup rarely should be confused with acute laryngotracheitis, but a perusal of the literature indicates that the two entities both are considered most commonly as laryngotracheitis. This is unfortunate because prognostic and therapeutic considerations for the two entities are different. Spasmodic croup always is of sudden onset at night, occurs without fever, and is relieved by simple therapeutic modalities.

The possibility of foreign body and angioneurotic edema always must be considered in upper airway obstructive disease. Differential points are presented in Table 22–5. Rarely, acute upper airway obstruction occurs in adolescents as a result of psychogenic and emotional factors.[62, 95, 152]

SPECIFIC DIAGNOSIS

The epidemiologic history frequently is important in specific diagnosis. Bacterial cultures from the throat, laryngeal region, and blood are helpful in diagnosing epiglottitis and also important in laryngotracheitis, laryngotracheobronchitis, and laryngotracheobronchopneumonitis when secondary infection is suspected. The white blood cell count should be obtained because it can be helpful when secondary bacterial infection is considered.

A specific etiologic diagnosis can be made by the isolation of virus or its identification by a direct antigen test from a nasopharyngeal specimen. The diagnostic virologic facilities of many medical centers enable the identification of parainfluenza viruses, respiratory syncytial viruses, adenoviruses, most rhinoviruses, and influenza viruses.

TREATMENT

The treatment of croup has created considerable controversy over the last 55 years: tracheostomy versus no tracheos-

TABLE 22–5. Differential Diagnosis of Acute Obstruction in the Region of the Larynx

Category	Acute Epiglottitis	Laryngeal Diphtheria	Laryngitis	Acute Laryngotracheitis	Laryngotracheo-bronchitis and Laryngotracheo-bronchopneumonitis (Including Bacterial Tracheitis)	Spasmodic Croup	Foreign Body	Acute Angioneurotic Edema
Common age of occurrence	1 to 8 years	All ages	Older children and adults	3 months to 3 years	3 months to 3 years	3 months to 3 years	All ages	All ages
Past and family history	Not contributory	No or inadequate immunization	Not contributory	Family history of croup	May be family history of croup	Family history of croup; perhaps previous attack	Occasional history of ingestion	Allergic history; perhaps previous attack
Prodrome	Occasioncl coryza	Usually pharyngitis	Usually stuffy nose or coryza	Usually coryza	Usually coryza	Minimal coryza	None	Occasionally cutaneous allergic manifestations
Onset (time to full-blown disease)	Rapid; 4 to 12 hours	Slowly for 2- to 3-day period	Variable; 12 hours to 4 days	Moderate but variable; 12 to 48 hours	Usually gradually progressive; 12 hours to 7 days	Sudden; always at night	Usually sudden	Rapid
Symptoms on presentation								
Fever	Yes; usually 39.5° C (103° F)	Yes; usually 37.8° to 38.5° C (100° to 101° F)	Yes; 37.8° to 39.4° C (100° to 103° F) with adenoviral and influenza viral infections; usually minimal with other viruses	Yes; quite variable, 37.8° to 40.5° C (100 to 105° F)	Yes; quite variable, 37.8° to 40.5° C (100 to 105° F)	No	No, unless secondary infection	No
Hoarseness and barking cough	No	Yes	Yes	Yes	Yes	Yes	Usually no	No
Dysphagia	Yes; usually severe	Usually yes	No	No	No	No	Frequently yes	Yes
Inspiratory stridor	Yes; moderate to severe	Yes; minimal to severe	No	Yes; minimal to severe	Yes; usually severe	Yes; moderate	Variable	Yes
Toxic appearance	Severe	Usually no	No	Usually minimal	Usually moderate; may be severe	No	No	No

Signs on presentation								
Oral cavity	Pharyngitis and excessive salivation	Membranous pharyngitis	Normal or mild to moderate pharyngitis	Usually minimal pharyngitis	Usually minimal pharyngitis	Normal	Normal	Pale appearance
Epiglottis	Cherry-red and swollen	Usually normal; may contain membrane	Normal	Normal	Normal	Normal	Normal	Swollen and pale
Roentgenogram	Swollen epiglottis on lateral film	Not useful	Not useful	Subglottic narrowing on P-A film	Subglottic narrowing on P-A film; irregular soft-tissue densities within trachea on lateral film	Not useful	May reveal foreign body	Swollen epiglottis on lateral film
Laboratory								
Leukocyte count	Usually markedly elevated with increased percentage of band forms	Usually elevated with increased percentage of band forms	Usually normal	Mildly elevated with >70% polymorphonuclear cells	Variable; usually mildly elevated with 70% polymorphonuclear cells; may be increased band count	Normal	Normal, unless secondary infection	Normal; sometimes eosinophilia
Bacteriology	Throat and blood cultures yield *Haemophilus influenzae* type b	Smear and culture from membrane reveal organism	Usually normal flora in throat; occasionally *Staphylococcus pyogenes* in throat	Only important if secondary infection suspected	Normal throat flora; tracheal culture often yields *S. pyogenes, Staphylococcus aureus, Streptococcus pneumoniae,* or *H. influenzae*	Normal flora	Only important if secondary infection suspected	Normal flora
Clinical course	Rapidly progressive; cardiorespiratory arrest will occur within hours if not treated	Slowly progressive obstruction of the airway	Hoarseness persists at a constant degree about 4 to 7 days; occasionally persists 2 to 3 weeks	Variable speed of progression of obstruction; usually does not require surgical intervention	Degree of obstruction usually severe; persists 7 to 14 days; frequently requires surgical intervention	Symptoms of short duration with treatment; repeat attacks common	Variable depending upon size and substance of foreign body	Variable; sometimes leads to rapid asphyxia without therapy

Data from references 35, 36, 40, 49, 58, 69, 71, 87, 105, 106, 119, 173.

tomy, intubation versus tracheostomy, warm versus cold humidification, antibiotics versus no antibiotics, steroids versus no steroids, sedation versus no sedation, and racemic epinephrine therapy versus mist therapy alone. Few of these controversies have been resolved scientifically, but the passage of time has lessened the importance of some of the discrepant opinions.

Of most importance in the evaluation of therapeutic modalities and the specific approach to therapy in croup is accurate differential diagnosis. Unfortunately, a look at the most important controversy (the use of steroids) would indicate that in most instances cases of spasmodic croup, in which a favorable outcome invariably can be expected, were not separated clinically from cases of laryngotracheitis, in which the outcome is less predictable.

Acute Laryngotracheitis

In managing acute laryngotracheitis, each case must be treated individually: one child will need minimal simple therapy (i.e., mist therapy), whereas another will require consideration of all modalities. In all children with acute laryngotracheitis, attention should be given to the anxiety and apprehension of the patient and parents and to the immediate institution of mist therapy. The parents should be reassured immediately, and it is important not to separate the child from them. Physical examination should be performed rapidly by one physician and all but absolutely necessary procedures deferred. The early institution of mist therapy will do much to relieve anxiety, but a parent should be at the bedside because mist tents can be frightening to a child.

The judicious use of sedatives also is useful in relieving apprehension and anxiety. Sedatives should not be used continuously or in dosages that will suppress respirations, however.

Mist therapy is the cornerstone of croup management. Nebulization in laryngotracheitis will prevent desiccation of the inflamed epithelial surfaces and help prevent inspissation of secretions and exudate.[133] The viscosity of the exudate will be reduced, thus allowing its easier removal by coughing.[46] Mist therapy also may stimulate nasal and laryngeal receptors that cause slowing of the respiratory rate, which will benefit the child with croup.[151]

Contrary to popular belief, the temperature of the nebulized air need not be cold but should be comfortable to the child. Prior to the availability of the current generation of humidification devices, steam was the usual method of supplying moisture. In the enclosed environment, this often led to excessive temperatures, which caused distress to the child. Excessively cold moist air is equally distressing.

Oxygen should be administered to the child who is hypoxemic from respiratory distress. The studies of Newth and associates[128] and Taussig and colleagues[172] indicate that mild hypoxemia is more common than clinically realized. The drying effect of oxygen is counterproductive to the removal of tracheal exudate, so its use should not be routine.

Since 1952, there have been numerous communications in the English medical literature on the use of corticosteroids in croup. The majority of these reports contain testimonial information reporting the efficacy of one steroid preparation or another. There also have been nine double-blind, controlled studies.[47, 48, 85, 98, 102, 104, 157, 165, 168] Eden and Larkin[48] noted in 1964 no difference between control and methylprednisolone therapy in a study of 50 children with acute croup. In 1967, Eden and colleagues[47] studied another 50 patients and could find no benefit from dexamethasone when compared with a control preparation. Sussman and colleagues[168] also could not demonstrate any benefit from dexamethasone therapy. In contrast to these three studies, Skowron and others[157] noted a slight benefit regarding duration of stridor, retractions, fever, and hospital days in a group receiving dexamethasone. However, they suggested that steroids should not be used routinely in laryngotracheitis because the overall benefits were minimal and there is a potential risk in steroid administration. In 1969, James[85] noted that dexamethasone-treated patients recovered from their obstructive symptoms more quickly than the control group. In another study involving 30 children, Leipzig and associates[104] concluded that dexamethasone in an adequate dose (0.3 mg/kg initially and repeated in 2 hours) given intramuscularly hastens the recovery from uncomplicated croup. Unfortunately, this study and its predecessors have major inadequacies in design.[24, 177] In a study with 72 children, Koren and colleagues[98] noted that dexamethasone did not offer any benefit to patients with laryngotracheitis but did decrease significantly the respiratory rate in children with spasmodic croup compared with placebo-treated controls. Although these latter findings were statistically significant, the benefits were not clinically significant.

Two additional modest studies of the use of dexamethasone in croup were published as well as a meta-analysis of the evidence from the various randomized trials and a set of related editorials and a review.[4, 90, 102, 155, 158, 165] Kuusela and Vesikari[102] concluded that dexamethasone was beneficial in acute spasmodic croup, and Super and associates[165] concluded that dexamethasone is beneficial in reducing the overall severity of moderate to severe acute laryngotracheitis during the first day of treatment.

The meta-analysis suggested that the use of steroids in children hospitalized with croup resulted in a significantly increased number with clinical improvement 12 hours and 24 hours after treatment and a reduced incidence of endotracheal intubation than occurred in the controls.[90] In this analysis, it also was noted that improvement at 12 hours was greater in those children who received higher initial doses of steroid (≥125 mg of cortisone) than those who received lower doses. Two additional studies suggesting a beneficial effect of the use of systemic steroids in croup were published as well as two studies indicating benefit from the use of nebulized budesonide.[32, 80, 96, 114] Based on the meta-analysis cited earlier and other studies, reviews on the management of croup recommend the use of systemic steroids in the treatment of croup.[3, 31, 38, 39, 82, 156]

In the past when I reviewed the data on the use of steroids in croup, it concerned me that the specific clinical entity that was being treated was poorly defined and that there was no evidence that steroids worked in any illness other than spasmodic croup.[24] Today, my analysis of the available data results in the same conclusion: there is no evidence of benefit from the use of steroids except in spasmodic croup, which readily responds to treatment with moist air. Of most concern to me today is the fact that risks of steroid use have not been evaluated and because sample sizes in available studies cannot be studied by meta-analysis.

I have seen two children develop lower respiratory tract complications during steroid treatment for croup. In one case, an adenoviral pneumonia worsened, and in the second case, bacterial tracheitis with pneumonia occurred. Interestingly, in the study of Super and colleagues,[165] there were two steroid-treated patients who developed pneumonia during therapy; none of the controls developed pneumonia.

Burton and associates[16] reported the occurrence of *Candida* laryngotracheitis as a complication of steroid and antibiotic treatment in a child with croup.[16]

In summary, the use of a single dose of a systemic steroid,

such as intramuscular dexamethasone (0.6 mg/kg), or the limited use of nebulized budesonide probably is quite safe and may be useful in the child with more severe spasmodic croup. Steroids should not be used in laryngotracheobronchitis, laryngotracheobronchopneumonitis, or epiglottitis.

Because laryngotracheitis is a disease of viral etiology, it seems apparent that antibiotic therapy would not be indicated and consequently not employed. However, in our analysis of more than 200 hospitalized children with laryngotracheitis, we noted that antibiotics had been administered to 85 per cent.[59] A review of the records in many instances revealed that the physician had given antibiotic therapy because the possibility of epiglottitis had not been ruled out adequately. In several instances, the epiglottis had been observed and thought to be somewhat reddened and/or questionably enlarged.

A second consideration in regard to antibiotic therapy in croup is the fact that the most dramatic reduction in mortality coincides with the introduction and widespread use of antibiotics. In my opinion, many of the croup deaths in the preantibiotic era were caused by secondary bacterial infections. Although antibiotic usage contributed to the reduction in croup deaths, other factors may be important. At about the same time that antibiotics were introduced, disease caused by *S. pyogenes* decreased in incidence and severity. Reasons for the decreased frequency of streptococcal disease were not clear.

The majority of patients with laryngotracheitis today do not need antibiotic therapy. However, in severe cases in which the consideration of bacterial sepsis cannot be ruled out, antibiotic therapy should be employed. The pathogens to consider include pneumococci, group A streptococci, *S. aureus*, and *H. influenzae*. In patients with laryngotracheitis in whom persistent fever or changing signs occur, secondary infection should be considered. In these instances, appropriate cultures should be obtained prior to therapy (see the section on laryngotracheobronchitis for specific antibiotic therapy).

The use of nebulized racemic epinephrine, which was introduced by Jordan[88] in 1966 and popularized by Jordan and other members of the Utah group,[1, 89] has been adopted widely throughout the United States and elsewhere.[93, 101, 107, 119, 150, 154] The usual method of nebulization of racemic epinephrine is by intermittent positive-pressure breathing (IPPB), and in several series, the use of this form of therapy was associated with a marked reduction in tracheostomies.

In 1973, Gardner and associates[58] performed the first double-blind, controlled study in which racemic epinephrine was nebulized by a compressor without IPPB. They found that saline-treated patients responded as well to therapy as did the racemic epinephrine recipients. In retrospect, this study can be criticized because the investigators failed to differentiate spasmodic croup from laryngotracheitis. In 1975, Taussig and associates[172] reported a small but carefully conducted study with IPPB and racemic epinephrine, in which they noted acute improvement in all cases, recurrence of symptoms in 2 hours, and no change in partial pressure of oxygen with clinical improvement; 24 to 36 hours after therapy, treated and untreated children were clinically similar. In another significant study that involved children hospitalized with severe croup without improvement after admission to a high-humidity mist room, Westley and colleagues[186] showed that racemic epinephrine therapy caused definite short-term improvement in children when compared with saline treatment. This study particularly is important because a parainfluenza viral etiology was documented in more than 65 per cent of the study's subjects, and all cases clearly were laryngotracheitis and not spasmodic croup.

In summary, the following points can be made about the use of racemic epinephrine in the treatment of croup: (1) the majority of children with croup will respond to moist air alone; (2) the general improvement in outcome in croup (decreased numbers of tracheostomies) is for the most part the result of the greater attention to therapy rather than the result of racemic epinephrine treatment; (3) significant rebound follows racemic epinephrine therapy, so that it frequently needs to be repeated many times; (4) in the hospitalized child with severe acute laryngotracheitis, it should be used when tracheotomy is possibly necessary. Tracheotomy can be prevented in some cases. The most important issue today regarding the use of racemic epinephrine is whether it can be used safely for outpatient therapy.[28, 92, 141] In the past, most experts advised against the use of racemic epinephrine in the outpatient setting because of the known rebound that occurs. Some data suggest that with careful observation for a sufficient period (at least 2 hours) after administration, patients can be managed safely and hospitalizations decreased.[28, 92, 141]

The establishment of a mechanical airway seldom is necessary in laryngotracheitis today. The planned procedure has a better outcome than the procedure performed under emergency conditions. Traditionally, tracheostomy was the preferred method when a mechanical airway was needed.[6, 57, 191] However, it has been demonstrated that when careful attention to tube size and other aspects of placement and maintenance is given, nasotracheal intubation compares favorably with tracheostomy.[6, 191] The management of the child with a mechanical airway requires trained pediatric intensive care physicians and the facilities of an adequately staffed intensive care unit.

Two antiviral drugs have activity against viruses that cause laryngotracheitis.[68, 84, 113, 170, 187] Amantadine is approved for use in treating influenza A viral infections, and ribavirin is active against parainfluenza viruses, influenza A and B viruses, and respiratory syncytial virus (see Chapter 233, Antiviral Agents; Chapter 181, Influenza Viruses). At present, it would seem reasonable to consider amantadine in the therapy of severe croup that occurs during documented epidemics caused by influenza A virus. However, few trials of this mode of therapy have been conducted in children, and it has not been demonstrated to be beneficial to adults with pulmonary complications of influenza. Ribavirin is approved for use in the United States for patients with respiratory syncytial viral infection. It has been shown to be modestly effective in influenza and respiratory syncytial viral infections when administered by special small-particle aerosol generators.

Laryngotracheobronchitis and Laryngotracheobronchopneumonitis (Bacterial Tracheitis)

In general, all the treatment considerations discussed for laryngotracheitis, except steroids and racemic epinephrine by aerosol, apply to laryngotracheobronchitis and laryngotracheobronchopneumonitis. Most importantly, however, because most patients have bacterial disease, antibiotics should be administered to all patients after appropriate cultures. Empiric therapy should be directed against *S. aureus*, *S. pyogenes*, *S. pneumoniae*, and *H. influenzae*. At present, initial treatment with oxacillin (150 mg/kg/day every 6 hours intravenously) and a third-generation cephalosporin, such as cefotaxime (150 mg/kg/day every 6 hours intravenously), is reasonable. The physician should be aware of the possibility of a methacillin-resistant staphylococcus. In severe cases, vancomycin (40 mg/kg/day intravenously every 6 hours) may be used instead of oxacillin.

Most children with advanced laryngotracheobronchitis or laryngotracheobronchopneumonitis will need the placement of a mechanical airway. Whenever possible, this should be done electively rather than as an emergency procedure.

Spasmodic Croup

The major problem in the therapy of spasmodic croup is overtreatment. Many physicians are unfamiliar with the benign nature of this disease and will institute IPPB, steroids, and other unnecessary therapies. Spasmodic croup will respond to the administration of moist air in all instances. Another mode of therapy is the administration of syrup of ipecac in a subemetic dose. My experience with this latter therapy has been favorable, but most children have vomited in spite of low dosage.

Further attacks of spasmodic croup the same evening or during the next few nights can be prevented by the use of mild sedation at bedtime.

Laryngitis

Patients with laryngitis should rest their voices as much as possible. Increased fluid intake and the use of a vaporizer will help liquefy secretions and should provide symptomatic relief. Because group A streptococcal infection is a cause of laryngitis, culture should be carried out. If positive, penicillin or a suitable alternative antimicrobial agent should be administered. In children and adolescents with prolonged hoarseness, sinusitis should be considered. Radiographs of the sinuses and a quantitative culture from the nose should be obtained in search of a predominant abnormal bacterial flora. If either is positive, therapy with appropriate antibiotics is indicated. If laryngeal symptoms are persistent, the child should undergo laryngoscopic examination and other appropriate studies to exclude tumor, foreign body, and other chronic diseases.

PROGNOSIS

The prognosis of acute laryngotracheitis has improved markedly over the last 50 years. Today, a child with croup only rarely requires a mechanical airway, and virtually all deaths should be preventable. The child should be observed for the following complications: hypoxemia and cardiorespiratory failure, pulmonary edema,[176] pneumothorax and pneumomediastinum, mechanical problems due to tracheotomies and nasotracheal tubes, and secondary bacterial infections.

Two studies have noted that children with a history of croup have a higher prevalence of increased bronchial reactivity than children without a history of croup.[67, 110]

PREVENTION

At present, acute laryngotracheitis is not preventable. Trials with attenuated parainfluenza viral vaccines were not effective.[178] The widespread use of influenza vaccines could reduce the incidence of croup due to influenza A and B viruses.

References

1. Adair, J. C., Ring, W. H., Jordan, W. S., et al.: Ten-year experience with IPPB in the treatment of acute laryngotracheobronchitis. Anesth. Analg. *50*:649–655, 1971.
2. Alligood, G. A., and Kenny, J. F.: Tracheitis and supraglottis associated with *Branhamella catarrhalis* and respiratory syncytial virus. Pediatr. Infect. Dis. *8*:190, 1989.
3. American Academy of Pediatrics: Parainfluenza. *In* Peter, G. (ed.): 1994 Red Book: Report of the Committee on Infectious Diseases. 23rd ed. Elk Grove Village, IL, American Academy of Pediatrics, 1994, pp. 341–342.
4. Anonymous: Steroids and croup. Lancet 2:1134–1136, 1989.
5. Banatvala, J. E., Reiss, B. B., Anderson, T. B., et al.: Asian influenza in 1963 in two general practices in Cambridge, England. Can. Med. Assoc. J. *93*:593–597, 1965.
6. Barker, G. A.: Current management of croup and epiglottitis. Pediatr. Clin. North Am. *26*:565–579, 1979.
7. Baum, H. L.: Acute laryngotracheobronchitis. J. A. M. A. *91*:1097–1102, 1928.
8. Berg, R. B.: Weight and sex of children hospitalized with infectious croup: An analysis of 850 cases. Pediatrics *31*:18–21, 1963.
9. Bisno, A. L., Barratt, N. P., Swanston, W. H., et al.: An outbreak of acute respiratory disease in Trinidad associated with para-influenza viruses. Am. J. Epidemiol. *91*:68–77, 1970.
10. Brandt, C. D., Kim, H. W., Vargosko, A. J., et al.: Infections in 18,000 infants and children in a controlled study of respiratory tract disease. I. Adenovirus pathogenicity in relation to serologic type and illness syndrome. Am. J. Epidemiol. *90*:484–500, 1969.
11. Breese, B. B.: Diagnosis of streptococcal pharyngitis. *In* Breese, B. B., and Hall, C. B. (eds.): Beta Hemolytic Streptococcal Diseases. Boston, Houghton Mifflin, 1978, pp. 79–96.
12. Breese, B. B., Disney, F. A., and Talpey, W.: The nature of a small pediatric group practice. Part I. Pediatrics *38*:264–277, 1966.
13. Brennemann, J., Clifton, W. M., Frank, A., et al.: Acute laryngotracheobronchitis. Am. J. Dis. Child. *55*:667–695, 1938.
14. Brighton, G. R.: Laryngotracheobronchitis. Ann. Otol. Rhinol. Laryngol. *49*:1070–1082, 1940.
15. Brocklebank, J. T., Court, S. D. M., McQuillin, J., et al.: Influenza-A infection in children. Lancet *2*:497–500, 1972.
16. Burton, D. M., Seid, A. B., Kearns, D. B., et al.: *Candida laryngotracheitis*: A complication of combined steroid and antibiotic usage in croup. Int. J. Pediatr. Otorhinol. *23*:171–175, 1992.
17. Chanock, R. M., Parrott, R. H., Johnson, K. M., et al.: Myxoviruses: Parainfluenza. Am. Rev. Respir. Dis. *88*(Part 2):152–166, 1962.
18. Chanock, R., Chambon, L., Chang, W., et al.: WHO respiratory disease survey in children: A serological study. Bull. W. H. O. *37*:363–369, 1967.
19. Chanock, R. M., and Parrott, R. H.: Acute respiratory disease in infancy and childhood: Present understanding and prospects for prevention: E. Mead Johnson Address, October 1964. Pediatrics *36*:21–39, 1965.
20. Chapman, R. S., Henderson, F. W., Clyde, W. A., Jr., et al.: The epidemiology of tracheobronchitis in pediatric practice. Am. J. Epidemiol. *114*:786–797, 1981.
21. Chenaud, M., Leclerc, F., and Martinot, A.: Bacterial croup and toxic shock syndrome. Eur. J. Pediatr. *145*:306–307, 1986.
22. Cherry, J. D.: Croup. *In* Kiple, K. F. (ed.): The Cambridge World History of Human Disease. Cambridge, Cambridge University Press, 1993, pp. 654–657.
23. Cherry, J. D.: Acute epiglottitis, laryngitis and croup. *In* Remington, J. S., and Swartz, M. N. (eds.): Current Clinical Topics in Infectious Diseases. New York, McGraw-Hill, 1981, pp. 1–30.
24. Cherry, J. D.: The treatment of croup: Continued controversy due to failure of recognition of historic, ecologic, etiologic and clinical perspectives. J. Pediatr. *94*:352–354, 1979.
25. Cherry, J. D.: Newer respiratory viruses: Their role in respiratory illnesses of children. *In* Schulman, I. (ed.): Advances in Pediatrics. Vol. 20. Chicago, Year Book Medical Publishers, 1973, pp. 225–289.
26. Cherry, J. D.: Measles. *In* Feigin, R. D. and Cherry, J. D. (eds.): Textbook of Pediatric Infectious Diseases. 4th ed. Philadelphia, W. B. Saunders, 1998.
27. Conley, S. F., Beste, D. J., and Hoffmann, R. G.: Measles-associated bacterial tracheitis. Pediatr. Infect. Dis. J. *12*:414–415, 1993.
28. Cornell, H. M., and Bolte, R. G.: Outpatient use of racemic epinephrine in croup. Am. Fam. Phys. *46*:683–684, 1992.
29. Cramblett, H. G.: Croup: Present day concept. Pediatrics *25*:1071–1076, 1960.
30. Cramblett, H. G., Moffett, H. L., Black, J. P., et al.: Coxsackie virus infections: Clinical and laboratory studies. J. Pediatr. *64*:406–414, 1964.
31. Cressman, W. R., and Myer, C. M., III: Diagnosis and management of croup and epiglottitis. Pediatr. Clin. North Am. *41*:265–276, 1994.
32. Cruz, M. N., Stewart, G., and Rosenberg, N.: Use of dexamethasone in the outpatient management of acute laryngotracheitis. Pediatrics *96*:220–223, 1995.
33. Dascomb, H. E., and Hilleman, M. R.: Clinical and laboratory studies in patients with respiratory disease caused by adenoviruses (R1-APC-ARD agents). Am. J. Med. *21*:161, 1956.
34. Davison, F. W.: Inflammatory diseases of the larynx of infants and small children. Ann. Otol. Rhinol. Laryngol. *76*:753, 1967.
35. Davison, F. W.: Acute laryngeal obstruction in children. J. A. M. A. *171*:1301–1305, 1959.
36. Davison, F. W.: Acute obstructive laryngitis in children. Penn. Med. J. *53*:250–254, 1950.

37. Davison, F. W.: Acute laryngotracheobronchitis: Further studies on treatment. Arch. Otolaryngol. *47*:455–464, 1948.
38. Dawson, K., Cooper, D., Cooper, P., et al.: The management of acute laryngo-tracheo-bronchitis (croup): A consensus view. J. Pediatr. Child Health *28*:223–224, 1992.
39. DeBoeck, K.: Croup: A review. Eur. J. Pediatr. *154*:432–436, 1995.
40. Denneny, J. C., and Handler, S. D.: Membranous laryngotracheobronchitis. Pediatrics *70*:705–707, 1982.
41. Denny, F. W., and Clyde, W. A., Jr.: Acute lower respiratory tract infections in nonhospitalized children. J. Pediatr. *108*:635–646, 1986.
42. Denny, F. W., Clyde, W. A., Jr., and Glezen, W. P.: *Mycoplasma pneumoniae* disease: Clinical spectrum, pathophysiology, epidemiology, and control. J. Infect. Dis. *123*:74–92, 1971.
43. Denny, F. W., Murphy, T. F., Clyde, W. A., Jr., et al.: Croup: An 11-year study in a pediatric practice. Pediatrics *71*:871–876, 1983.
44. Donnelly, B. W., McMillan, J. A., and Weiner, L. B.: Bacterial tracheitis: Report of eight new cases and review. Rev. Infect. Dis. *12*:729–735, 1990.
45. Dudin, A. A., Thalji, A., and Rambaud-Cousson, A.: Bacterial tracheitis among children hospitalized for severe obstructive dyspnea. Pediatr. Infect. Dis. *9*:293–295, 1990.
46. Dulfano, M. J., Adler, K., and Wooten, O.: Physical properties of sputum. IV. Effects of 100 per cent humidity and water mist. Am. Rev. Respir. Dis. *107*:130–132, 1972.
47. Eden, A. N., Kaufman, A., and Yu, R.: Corticosteroids and croup: Controlled double-blind study. J. A. M. A. *200*:403–404, 1967.
48. Eden, A. N., and Larkin, V. D. P.: Corticosteroid treatment of croup. Pediatrics *33*:768–769, 1964.
49. Edwards, K. M., Dundon, M. C., and Altemeier, W. A.: Bacterial tracheitis as a complication of viral croup. Pediatr. Infect. Dis. *2*:390–391, 1983.
50. Eichenwald, H. F.: Respiratory infections in children. Hosp. Pract. *11*:81–90, 1976.
51. Eid, N. S., and Jones, V. F.: Bacterial tracheitis as a complication of tonsillectomy and adenoidectomy. J. Pediatr. *125*:401–402, 1994.
52. Eller, J. J., Fulginiti, V. A., Plunket, D. C., et al.: Attack rates for hospitalized croup in children in a military population: Importance of A2 influenza infection. Pediatr. Res. *6*:386, 1972.
53. Ernst, T. N., and Philp, M.: Bacterial tracheitis caused by *Branhamella catarrhalis*. Pediatr. Infect. Dis. *6*:574, 1987.
54. Everett, A. R.: Acute laryngotracheobronchitis: An analysis of 1,175 cases with 98 tracheotomies. Laryngoscope *61*:113–123, 1951.
55. Fearon, B.: Acute obstructive laryngitis in infants and children. Hosp. Med. *4*:51–67, 1968.
56. Forbes, J. A.: Severe effects of influenza viral infection. Med. J. Aust. *44*:75–79, 1958.
57. Fried, M. P.: Controversies in the management of supraglottitis and croup. Pediatr. Clin. North Am. *26*:931–942, 1979.
58. Gardner, H. G., Powell, K. R., Roden, V. J., et al.: The evaluation of racemic epinephrine in the treatment of infectious croup. Pediatrics *52*:68–71, 1973.
59. Gardner, H. G., Powell, K. R., and Cherry, J. D.: Unpublished data, 1973.
60. Gardner, P. S., McQuillin, J., McGuckin, R., et al.: Observations on clinical and immunofluorescent diagnosis of parainfluenza virus infections. Br. Med. J. *2*:7–12, 1971.
61. Gardner, P. S.: Virus infections and respiratory disease of childhood. Arch. Dis. Child. *43*:629–645, 1968.
62. Geist, R., and Tallett, S. E.: Diagnosis and management of psychogenic stridor caused by a conversion disorder. Pediatrics *86*:315–317, 1990.
63. Gittens, T. R.: XXXIII. Laryngitis and tracheobronchitis in children: Special reference to nondiphtheritic infections. Ann. Otol. Rhinol. Laryngol. *41*:422–438, 1932.
64. Glezen, W. P., Loda, F. A., Clyde, W. A., Jr., et al.: Epidemiologic patterns of acute lower respiratory disease of children in a pediatric group practice. J. Pediatr. *78*:397–406, 1971.
65. Glezen, W. P., Loda, F. A., and Denny, F. W.: The parainfluenza viruses. *In* Evans, A. S. (ed.): Viral Infections of Humans: Epidemiology and Control. New York, Plenum Publishing, 1976, pp. 337–349.
66. Gold, S. M., Shott, S. R., and Myer, C. M., III: Radiological case of the month. Arch. Pediatr. Adolesc. Med. *150*:97–98, 1996.
67. Gurwitz, D., Corey, M., and Levison, H.: Pulmonary function and bronchial reactivity in children after croup. Am. Rev. Respir. Dis. *122*:95–99, 1980.
68. Hall, C. B., McBride, J. T., Walsh, E. E., et al.: Aerosolized ribavirin treatment of infants with respiratory syncytial viral infection: A randomized double-blind study. N. Engl. J. Med. *308*:1443–1447, 1983.
69. Han, B. K., Dunbar, J. S., and Striker, T. W.: Membranous laryngotracheobronchitis (membranous croup). A. J. R. Am. J. Roentgenol. *133*:53–58, 1979.
70. Harari, M. D., West, B., and Dwyer, B.: *Cryptosporidium* as cause of laryngotracheitis in an infant. Lancet *1*:1207, 1986.
71. Henry, R. L., Mellis, C. M., and Benjamin, B.: Pseudomembranous croup. Arch. Dis. Child. *58*:180–183, 1983.
72. Herrmann, E. C., Jr., and Hable, K. A.: Experiences in laboratory diagnosis of parainfluenza viruses in routine medical practice. Mayo Clin. Proc. *45*:177–188, 1970.
73. Hide, D. W., and Guyer, B. M.: Recurrent croup. Arch. Dis. Child. *60*:585–586, 1985.
74. Hoekelman, R. A.: Infectious illness during the first year of life. Pediatrics *59*:119–121, 1977.
75. Holdaway, M. D.: Croup and epiglottitis: Diagnosis and action. Drugs *13*:452–457, 1977.
76. Holzel, A., Parker, L., Patterson, W. H., et al.: Virus isolations from throats of children admitted to hospital with respiratory and other diseases, Manchester 1962–4. Br. Med. J. *1*:614–619, 1965.
77. Hope-Simpson, R. E., and Higgins, P. G.: A respiratory virus study in Great Britain: Review and evaluation. Prog. Med. Virol. *11*:354–407, 1969.
78. Horn, M. E. C., Brain, E., Gregg, I., et al.: Respiratory viral infection in childhood: A survey in general practice, Roehampton 1967–1972. J. Hyg. Camb. *74*:157–168, 1975.
79. Howard, J. B., McCracken, G. H., Jr., and Luby, J. P.: Influenza A_2 virus as a cause of croup requiring tracheotomy. J. Pediatr. *81*:1148–1150, 1972.
80. Husby, S., Agertoft, L., Mortensen, S., et al.: Treatment of croup with nebulised steroid (budesonide): A double-blind, placebo-controlled study. Arch. Dis. Child. *68*:352–355, 1993.
81. Hyde, C. I., and Ruchman, J.: Acute infectious edematous laryngitis in which recovery followed tracheotomy. Arch. Pediatr. *48*:124–129, 1931.
82. Infectious Diseases and Immunization Committee, Canadian Paediatric Society: Steroid therapy for croup in children admitted to hospital. Can. Med. Assoc. J. *147*:429–430, 1992.
83. Inglis, A. F., Jr.: Herpes simplex virus infection: A rare cause of prolonged croup. Arch. Otolaryngol. Head Neck Surg. *119*:551–552, 1993.
84. Jackson, G. G., and Stanley, E. D.: Prevention and control of influenza by chemoprophylaxis and chemotherapy: Prospects from examination of recent experience. J. A. M. A. *235*:2739–2742, 1976.
85. James, J. A.: Dexamethasone in croup: A controlled study. Am. J. Dis. Child. *117*:511–516, 1969.
86. Johnson, M. C.: Acute laryngotracheobronchitis in infants: Report of three cases. Arch. Otolaryngol. *17*:230–234, 1933.
87. Jones, R., Santos, J. I., and Overall, J. C., Jr.: Bacterial tracheitis. J. A. M. A. *242*:721–726, 1979.
88. Jordan, W. S.: Laryngotracheobronchitis: Evaluation of new therapeutic approaches. Rocky Mt. Med. J. *63*:69, 1966.
89. Jordan, W. S., Graves, C. L., and Elwyn, R. A.: New therapy for postintubation laryngeal edema and tracheitis in children. J. A. M. A. *212*:585–588, 1970.
90. Kairys, S. W., Olmstead, E. N., and O'Connor, G. T.: Steroid treatment of laryngotracheitis: A meta-analysis of the evidence from randomized trials. Pediatrics *83*:683–693, 1989.
91. Kasian, G. F., Bingham, W. T., Steinberg, J., et al.: Bacterial tracheitis in children. Can. Med. Assoc. J. *140*:46–50, 1989.
92. Kelley, P. B., and Simon, J. E.: Racemic epinephrine use in croup and disposition. Am. J. Emerg. Med. *10*:181–183, 1992.
93. Kepes, E. R., Martinez, L. R., Andrews, I. C., et al.: Racemic epinephrine in postintubation laryngeal edema. N. Y. State J. Med. *72*:583–584, 1972.
94. Kibrick, S.: Current status of coxsackie and ECHO viruses in human disease. Prog. Med. Virol. *6*:27–70, 1964.
95. Kissoon, N., Kronick, J. B., and Frewen, T. C.: Psychogenic upper airway obstruction. Pediatrics *81*:714–717, 1988.
96. Klassen, T. P., Feldman, M. E., Watters, L. K., et al.: Nebulized budesonide for children with mild to moderate croup. N. Engl. J. Med. *331*:285–289, 1994.
97. Klein, J. D., and Collier, A. M.: Pathogenesis of human parainfluenza type 3 virus infection in hamster tracheal organ culture. Infect. Immunol. *10*:883–888, 1974.
98. Koren, G., Frand, M., Barzilay, Z., et al.: Corticosteroid treatment of laryngotracheitis vs spasmodic croup in children. Am. J. Dis. Child. *137*:941–944, 1983.
99. Korppi, M., Halonen, P., Kleemola, M., et al.: The role of parainfluenza viruses in inspiratory difficulties in children. Acta Paediatr. Scand. *77*:105–111, 1988.
100. Kravitz, H.: Sex distribution of hospitalized children with acute respiratory diseases, gastroenteritis and meningitis. Clin. Pediatr. *4*:484–491, 1965.
101. Kristjansson, S., Berg-Kelly, K., and Winso, E.: Inhalation of racemic adrenaline in the treatment of mild and moderately severe croup: Clinical symptom score and oxygen saturation measurements for evaluation of treatment effects. Acta Paediatr. *83*:1156–1160, 1994.
102. Kuusela, A. L., and Vesikari, T.: A randomized double-blind, placebo-controlled trial of dexamethasone and racemia epinephrine in the treatment of croup. Acta Paediatr. Scand. *77*:99–104, 1988.
103. Laxdal, O. E., Robertson, H. E., Braaten, V., et al.: Acute respiratory infections in children. I. An intensive study of etiology in an open community. Can. Med. Assoc. J. *88*:1049–1054, 1963.
104. Leipzig, B., Oski, F. A., Cummings, C. W., et al.: A prospective randomized study to determine the efficacy of steroids in treatment of croup. J. Pediatr. *94*:194–196, 1979.
105. Liston, S. L., Gehrz, R. C., and Jarvis, C. W.: Bacterial tracheitis. Arch. Otolaryngol. *107*:561–564, 1981.
106. Liston, S. L., Gehrz, R. C., Siegel, L. G., et al.: Bacterial tracheitis. Am. J. Dis. Child. *137*:764–767, 1983.

107. Lockhart, C. H., and Battaglia, J. D.: Croup (laryngotracheal bronchitis) and epiglottitis. Pediatr. Ann. *6*:262–269, 1977.
108. Loda, F. A., Clyde, W. A., Jr., Glezen, W. P., et al.: Studies on the role of viruses, bacteria, and *M. pneumoniae* as causes of lower respiratory tract infections in children. J. Pediatr. *72*:161–176, 1968.
109. Loda, F. A., Glezen, W. P., and Clyde, W. A., Jr.: Respiratory disease in group day care. Pediatrics *49*:428–437, 1972.
110. Loughlin, G. M., and Taussig, L. M.: Pulmonary function in children with a history of laryngotracheobronchitis. J. Pediatr. *94*:365–369, 1979.
111. Macasaet, F. F., Kidd, P. A., Bolano, C. R., et al.: The etiology of acute respiratory infections. III. The role of viruses and bacteria. J. Pediatr. *72*:829–839, 1968.
112. Mauro, R. D., Poole, S. R., and Lockhart, C. H.: Differentiation of epiglottitis from laryngotracheitis in the child with stridor. Am. J. Dis. Child. *142*:679–682, 1988.
113. McClung, H. W., Knight, V., Gilbert, B. E., et al.: Ribavirin aerosol treatment of influenza B virus infection. J. A. M. A. *249*:2671–2674, 1983.
114. McDonogh, A. J.: The use of steroids and nebulised adrenaline in the treatment of viral croup over a seven-year period at a district hospital. Anaesth. Intensive Care *22*:175–178, 1994.
115. McNab, J. C. G.: Acute streptococcal infection of the trachea in an infant, aged fifteen months. J. Laryngol. *30*:337–338, 1915.
116. McKenzie, M., Norman, M. G., Anderson, J. D., et al.: Upper respiratory tract infection in a 3-year-old girl. J. Pediatr. *105*:129–133, 1984.
117. McLean, D. M., Roy, T. E., O'Brien, M. J., et al.: Parainfluenza viruses in association with acute laryngotracheobronchitis, Toronto, 1960–61. Can. Med. Assoc. J. *85*:290–294, 1961.
118. Meade, R. H., III: Laryngeal obstruction in children. Pediatr. Clin. North Am. *9*:233–262, 1962.
119. Melnick, A., Berger, R., and Green, G.: Spasmodic croup in children: Personal experiences with intermittent positive pressure breathing in therapy. Clin. Pediatr. *11*:615–617, 1972.
120. Miller, B. R., Arthur, J. D., Parry, W. H., et al.: Atypical croup and *Chlamydia trachomatis*. Lancet *1*:1022, 1982.
121. Miller, D. G., Gabrielson, M. O., and Horstmann, D. M.: Clinical virology and viral surveillance in a pediatric group practice: The use of double-seeded tissue culture tubes for primary virus isolation. Am. J. Epidemiol. *88*:245–256, 1968.
122. Mogabgab, W. J.: Beta-hemolytic streptococcal and concurrent infections in adults and children with respiratory disease, 1958 to 1969. Am. Rev. Resp. Dis. *102*:23–34, 1970.
123. Morgan, E. A., and Wishart, D. E. S.: Laryngo-tracheobronchitis: A statistical review of 549 cases. Can. Med. Assoc. J. *56*:8–15, 1947.
124. Mufson, M. A., Krause, H. E., Mocega, H. E., et al.: Viruses, *Mycoplasma pneumoniae* and bacteria associated with lower respiratory tract disease among infants. Am. J. Epidemiol. *91*:192–202, 1970.
125. Naqvi, S. H., and Dunkle, L. M.: Bacterial tracheitis and viral croup. Pediatr. Infect. Dis. *3*:282–283, 1984.
126. Neffson, A. H.: Acute laryngotracheobronchitis: A 25-year review. Am. J. Med. Sci. *208*:524–547, 1944.
127. Nelson, W. E.: Bacterial croup: A historical perspective. J. Pediatr. *105*:52–55, 1984.
128. Newth, C. J. L., Levison, H., and Bryan, A. C.: The respiratory status of children with croup. J. Pediatr. *81*:1068–1073, 1972.
129. Nichol, K. P., and Cherry, J. D.: Bacterial-viral interrelations in respiratory infections of children. N. Engl. J. Med. *277*:667–672, 1967.
130. Nijssen-Jordan, C., Donaldson, J. D., and Halperin, S. A.: Bacterial tracheitis associated with respiratory syncytial virus infection and toxic shock syndrome. Can. Med. Assoc. J. *142*:233–234, 1990.
131. Orton, H. B., Smith, E. L., Bell, H. O., et al.: Acute laryngotracheobronchitis: Analysis of sixty-two cases with report of autopsies in eight cases. Arch. Otolaryngol. *33*:926–960, 1941.
132. Paisley, J. W., Bruhn, F. W., Lauer, B. A., et al.: Type A2 influenza viral infections in children. Am. J. Dis. Child. *132*:34–36, 1978.
133. Parks, C. R.: Mist therapy: Rationale and practice. J. Pediatr. *76*:305–313, 1970.
134. Parrott, R. H.: Viral respiratory tract illnesses in children. Bull. N. Y. Acad. Med. *39*:629–648, 1963.
135. Parrott, R. H., Kim, H. W., Vargosko, A. J., et al.: Serious respiratory tract illness as a result of Asian influenza and influenza B infections in children. J. Pediatr. *61*:205–213, 1962.
136. Parrott, R. H., Vargosko, A. J., Kim, H. W., et al.: Acute respiratory diseases of viral etiology. III. Myxoviruses: Para influenza. Am. J. Public Health *52*:907–917, 1962.
137. Parrott, R. H., Vargosko, A. J., Kim, H. W., et al.: Clinical syndromes among children. Am. Rev. Respir. Dis. *88*:73–76, 1962.
138. Person, D. A., and Herrmann, E. C., Jr.: Experiences in laboratory diagnosis of rhinovirus infections in routine medical practice. Mayo Clin. Proc. *45*:517, 1970.
139. Plachtova-Pecenkova, I., Brockova, M., Fecova, D., et al.: Note on the aetiology of acute laryngotracheobronchitis in children: Findings in the autumn of 1965 and the spring of 1966. J. Hyg. Epidemiol. Microbiol. Immunol. *12*:227–237, 1968.
140. Poland, J. D., Welton, E. R., and Chin, T. D. Y.: Influenza virus B as a cause of acute croup syndrome. Am. J. Dis. Child. *107*:54, 1964.
141. Prendergast, M., Jones, J. S., and Hartman, D.: Racemic epinephrine in the treatment of laryngotracheitis: Can we identify children for outpatient therapy? Am. J. Emerg. Med. *12*:613–616, 1994.
142. Rabe, E. F.: Infectious croup. I. Etiology. Pediatrics *2*:255–265, 1948.
143. Rabe, E. F.: Acute inflammatory disorders of the larynx and laryngotracheal area. Pediatr. Clin. North Am. *4*:169–182, 1957.
144. Rabe, E. F.: Infectious croup. II. "Virus" croup. Pediatrics *2*:415–427, 1948.
145. Reed, S. E., and Boyde, A.: Organ cultures of respiratory epithelium infected with rhinovirus or parainfluenza virus studied in a scanning electron microscope. Infect. Immunol. *6*:68–76, 1972.
146. Reilly, C. M., Hoch, S. M., Stokes, J., Jr., et al.: Clinical and laboratory findings in cases of respiratory illness caused by coryzaviruses. Ann. Intern. Med. *57*:515–525, 1962.
147. Richards, L.: Fulminating laryngo-tracheo-bronchitis. Ann. Otol. Rhinol. Laryngol. *42*:1014–1040, 1933.
148. Richards, L.: A further study of the pathology of acute laryngo-tracheobronchitis in children. Ann. Otol. Rhinol. Laryngol. *47*:326–341, 1938.
149. Rosales, J. K., and Davenport, H. T.: Acute laryngotracheobronchitis and epiglottitis. Can. Anaesth. Soc. J. *9*:467–478, 1962.
150. Rull, J., and Hargitai, R.: Laryngitis subglottica kezelese mikronephrin tulnyomasos belelegeztetesevel. Orvosi Hetilap *115*:2727–2731, 1974.
151. Sasaki, C. T., and Suzuki, M.: The respiratory mechanism of aerosol inhalation in the treatment of partial airway obstruction. Pediatrics *59*:689–694, 1977.
152. Schalen, L., and Andersson, K.: Differential diagnosis and treatment of psychogenic voice disorder. Clin. Otolaryngol. *17*:225–230, 1992.
153. Sendi, K., Crysdale, S., and Yoo, J.: Tracheitis: Outcome of 1,700 cases presenting to the emergency department during two years. J. Otolaryngol. *21*:20–24, 1992.
154. Singer, O. P., and Wilson, W. J.: Laryngotracheobronchitis: 2 years' experience with racemic epinephrine. CMA J. *115*:132–134, 1976.
155. Skolnik, N. S.: Treatment of croup: A critical review. Am. J. Dis. Child. *143*:1045–1049, 1989.
156. Skolnik, N.: Croup. J. Fam. Pract. *37*:165–170, 1993.
157. Skowron, P. N., Turner, J. A. P., and McNaughton, G. A.: The use of corticosteroid (dexamethasone) in the treatment of acute laryngotracheitis. Can. Med. Assoc. J. *94*:528–531, 1966.
158. Smith, D. S.: Corticosteroids in croup: A chink in the ivory tower? J. Pediatr. *115*:256–257, 1989.
159. Sofer, S., and Chernick, V.: Increased need for tracheal intubation for croup in relation to bacterial tracheitis. Can. Med. Assoc. J. *128*:160–161, 1983.
160. Solomon, R., Truman, T., and Murray, D. L.: Toxic shock syndrome as a complication of bacterial tracheitis. Pediatrics *4*:298–299, 1985.
161. Stankiewicz, J. A., and Bowes, A. K.: Croup and epiglottitis: A radiologic study. Laryngoscope *95*:1159–1160, 1985.
162. Sterner, G., Gerzen, P., Ohlson, M., et al.: Acute respiratory illness and gastroenteritis in association with adenovirus type 7 infections. Acta Paediatr. *50*:457–468, 1961.
163. Stott, E. J., Bell, E. J., Eadie, M. B., et al.: A comparative virological study of children in hospital with respiratory and diarrhoeal illnesses. J. Hyg. Camb. *65*:9–23, 1967.
164. Stuart-Harris, C. H.: The adenoviruses and respiratory disease in man. Lectures on the Scientific Basis of Medicine *8*:148–164, 1958–59.
165. Super, D. M., Cartelli, N. A., Brooks, L. J., et al.: A prospective randomized double-blind study to evaluate the effect of dexamethasone in acute laryngotracheitis. J. Pediatr. *115*:323–329, 1989.
166. Suresh, G. K., Dhawan, A., and Kohli, V.: Tracheal diphtheria mimicking bacterial tracheitis. Pediatr. Infect. Dis. J. *11*:502, 1992.
167. Surh, L., and Read, S. E.: Staphylococcal tracheitis and toxic shock syndrome in a young child. J. Pediatr. *105*:585–587, 1984.
168. Sussman, S., Grossman, M., Magoffin, R., et al.: Dexamethasone (16, alpha-methyl, 9, alphafluoroprednisolone) in obstructive respiratory tract infections in children: A controlled study. Pediatrics *34*:851–855, 1964.
169. Szpunar, J., Glowacki, J., Laskowski, A., et al.: Fibrinous laryngotracheobronchitis in children. Arch. Otolaryngol. *93*:173–178, 1971.
170. Taber, L. H., Knight, V., Gilbert, B. E., et al.: Ribavirin aerosol treatment of bronchiolitis associated with respiratory syncytial virus infection in infants. Pediatrics *72*:613–618, 1983.
171. Tan, A. K. W., and Manoukian, J. J.: Hospitalized croup (bacterial and viral): The role of rigid endoscopy. J. Otolaryngol. *21*:48–53, 1992.
172. Taussig, L. M., Castro, O., Beaudry, P. H., et al.: Treatment of laryngotracheobronchitis (croup): Use of intermittent positive-pressure breathing and racemic epinephrine. Am. J. Dis. Child. *129*:790–793, 1975.
173. Temple, A. R.: Recent advances in diagnosis and management of croup. J. Fam. Pract. *2*:85–89, 1975.
174. Top, F. H., Sr.: Diphtheria. *In* Top, F. H., Sr., and Wehrle, P. F. (eds.): Communicable and Infectious Diseases. St. Louis, C. V. Mosby, 1972, pp. 190–207.
175. Toth, M., and Major, V.: Virological investigation of hospitalized cases of pseudocroup and acute laryngotracheobronchitis. Acta Microbiol. *12*:189–200, 1965.
176. Travis, K. W., Todres, I. D., and Shannon, D. C.: Pulmonary edema associated with croup and epiglottitis. Pediatrics *59*:695–698, 1977.

177. Tunnessen, W. W., Jr., and Feinstein, A. R.: The steroid-croup controversy: An analytic review of methodologic problems. J. Pediatr. *96*:751–756, 1980.
178. Tyeryar, F. J., Jr., Richardson, L. S., and Belshe, R. B.: Report of a workshop on respiratory syncytial virus and parainfluenza viruses. J. Infect. Dis. *137*:835–846, 1978.
179. Tyrrell, D. A. J.: Common Colds and Related Diseases. Baltimore, Williams & Wilkins, 1965, pp. 1–197.
180. Vargosko, A. J., Chanock, R. M., Huebner, R. J., et al.: Association of type 2 hemadsorption (parainfluenza 1) virus and Asian influenza A virus with infectious croup. N. Engl. J. Med. *261*:1–9, 1959.
181. Vihma, L.: Surveillance of acute viral respiratory diseases in children. Acta Paediatr. Scand. *192*(Suppl.):8–53, 1969.
182. Walker, P., and Crysdale, W. S.: Croup, epiglottitis, retropharyngeal abscess, and bacterial tracheitis: Evolving patterns of occurrence and care. Int. Anesth. Clin. *30*:57–70, 1992.
183. Welliver, R. C., Sun, M., and Rinaldo, D.: Defective regulation of immune response in croup due to parainfluenza virus. Pediatr. Res. *19*:716–720, 1985.
184. Welliver, R. C., Wong, D. T., Middleton, E., Jr., et al.: Role of parainfluenza virus–specific IgE in pathogenesis of croup and wheezing subsequent to infection. J. Pediatr. *101*:889–896, 1982.
185. Wenner, H. A., Christodoulopoulou, G., Weston, J., et al.: The etiology of respiratory illnesses occurring in infancy and childhood. Pediatrics *31*:4–17, 1963.
186. Westley, C. R., Cotton, E. K., and Brooks, J. G.: Nebulized racemic epinephrine by IPPB for the treatment of croup: A double-blind study. Am. J. Dis. Child. *132*:484–487, 1978.
187. Wilson, S. Z., Gilbert, B. E., Quarles, J. M., et al.: Treatment of influenza A (H1N1) virus infection with ribavirin aerosol. Antimicrob. Agents Chemother. *26*:200–203, 1984.
188. Wong, V. K., and Mason, W. H.: *Branhamella catarrhalis* as a cause of bacterial tracheitis. Pediatr. Infect. Dis. *6*:945–946, 1987.
189. Wulff, H., Kidd, P., and Wenner, H. A.: Etiology of respiratory infections: Further studies during infancy and childhood. Pediatrics *33*:30–44, 1964.
190. Zach, M. S.: Airway reactivity in recurrent croup. Eur. J. Respir. Dis. *128*(Suppl.):81–88, 1983.
191. Zulliger, J. J., Schuller, D. W., Beach, T. P., et al.: Assessment of intubation in croup and epiglottitis. Ann. Otol. Rhinol. Laryngol. *91*:403–406, 1982.

SECTION TWO

LOWER RESPIRATORY TRACT INFECTIONS

❑ ❑ ❑

23

ACUTE BRONCHITIS

James D. Cherry

Bronchitis is a common diagnosis in pediatric practice, although little unanimity exists among physicians regarding its exact clinical constellation, and in the true pathologic sense, it probably never occurs as an isolated entity. Acute bronchitis is a febrile illness with cough, rhonchi, and referred breath sounds.[13] Asthmatic bronchitis (infectious asthma), similar to acute bronchitis but with associated wheezing and expiratory distress, is discussed in Chapter 25. Pathologically, the clinical illness of acute bronchitis reflects acute inflammatory disease of the larger air passages, including the trachea and the large and medium-sized bronchi.[21]

ETIOLOGY

The various infectious agents incriminated in acute bronchitis are presented in Table 23–1. Infections with adenoviruses, influenza viruses, parainfluenza viruses, respiratory syncytial virus, and *Mycoplasma pneumoniae* account for the overwhelming majority of cases of acute bronchitis in children. These viruses, plus many rhinoviruses and a few enteroviruses, account for virtually all cases in the United States today.

Of the adenoviruses, type 7 has been associated most commonly with acute bronchitis in children. However, in military recruits, including adolescents, adenovirus types 4 and 7 cause epidemic acute respiratory disease, in which bronchitis is a usual occurrence.[18, 55]

Influenza A virus infection is a common cause of severe acute bronchitis. This is most apparent at the time of antigenic shift of influenza A virus subtype and pandemic disease. Acute bronchitis due to influenza A virus also is a regular occurrence between pandemics in new susceptibles (young children) in the population. Influenza B virus also is an important cause of bronchitis, and in one large longitudinal study, it was a more common causative agent than influenza A virus.[11]

All cases of measles involve the bronchi; but fortunately, measles has been an uncommon disease since the widespread use of vaccines. Of the parainfluenza viruses, type 3 most commonly is associated with acute bronchitis. Respiratory syncytial virus is a common cause of acute bronchitis, particularly in the very young child.

Of the bacterial agents listed in Table 23–1, only *Bordetella pertussis* and *Haemophilus influenzae* clearly can be incriminated. When sought, *M. pneumoniae* is a surprisingly common cause of bronchitis. *Chlamydia pneumoniae* has been found to be the cause of bronchitis in adolescents and young adults.[27]

EPIDEMIOLOGY

The epidemiology of the common viruses that are associated with bronchitis is presented in Section 17. Chapman and associates[11] published the results of a study of acute bronchitis in a single private group pediatric practice in Chapel Hill, North Carolina. The study occurred over a 104-month period, during which there were 5489 episodes of lower respiratory illness. Of these illnesses, 40.1 per cent were acute bronchitis. The bronchitis attack rate was highest during the second year of life (6.71 per cent), and then it decreased gradually to about 2.0 per cent in teenagers. In contrast with the age-specific attack rates, the ratio of bronchitis cases to all lower respiratory illness cases increased with age. In the first year of life, the ratio was 0.29, and in children 12 years of age or older, it was 0.69.

During the first 6 years of life, respiratory syncytial virus and parainfluenza virus type 3 were the most common etiologic agents noted in the Chapel Hill study. During the first 2 years of life, adenoviruses also were associated commonly with bronchitis. After age 6, *M. pneumoniae* and influenza A and B viruses were the most common etiologic agents. In a study of cough illnesses of 6 days' duration or longer in university students, it was found that 15 of 31 students with laboratory evidence of *B. pertussis* infection were considered by their primary care providers to have bronchitis.[39]

The incidence of acute bronchitis peaks in the winter months, declines to midsummer, and rises again through the fall. Attack rates generally are higher in boys than in girls.[11, 33, 56] A sex difference is most pronounced during the first 6 years of life.

PATHOPHYSIOLOGY AND PATHOLOGY

Because acute bronchitis is an illness characterized by clinical features and one not usually associated with death, knowledge of its pathophysiology and pathology is meager. The general pathophysiology of human infections with viruses and *M. pneumoniae* that cause acute bronchitis is presented more completely in the sections of this book related to the individual infectious agents.

In virtually all cases of acute bronchitis, there is in addition evidence of upper respiratory viral infection (pharyngitis and/or rhinitis). Tracheal and bronchial infection apparently is the result of distal spread. In bronchitis, the clinical features result from damage to the ciliated epithelium of the lower trachea and the large and medium-sized bronchi.[21] Although the cytopathology of the different infectious agents is different,[60] the resulting obstruction of the air passages leads to

TABLE 23–1. Infectious Agents Associated with Acute Bronchitis

Agent	Importance in Causation*	References
Viruses		
Adenovirus types 1–7, 12	+++	1, 2, 4, 8–10, 14, 19, 22, 23, 30, 31, 35, 46, 50, 53, 56, 57, 59
Enterovirus	+	25, 30, 31, 50
Coxsackieviruses B	+	8
Echoviruses 8, 12, 14	+	54
Polioviruses	+	22, 54
Herpes simplex	+	22, 50, 54
Influenza	+++	1, 5, 7–11, 14, 19, 23, 25, 52, 54
A	++	5, 8, 10, 11, 25, 30, 31, 52, 54
B	++	8, 10, 11, 25, 30
C	+	1
Measles	+	14, 21, 44
Mumps	+	54
Parainfluenza	+++	1, 5, 8–11, 14, 22–25, 28, 30, 35, 50, 52, 54, 57
1	++	8–11, 19, 25, 28
2	++	5, 8–10, 25, 28
3	+++	1, 2, 5, 8–11, 19, 25, 28, 31, 52
4	+	24
Respiratory syncytial	+++	1–3, 7–11, 14, 19, 22, 23, 25, 29–32, 38, 47, 50, 51, 53, 54, 57
Rhinoviruses	++	8, 14, 22, 23, 25, 30, 31, 43, 49, 50
Bacteria		
Bordetella pertussis	+	21
Bordetella parapertussis	±	
Haemophilus influenzae	+	35, 58
Moraxella catarrhalis	+	17, 26
Streptococcus pneumoniae	±	35
Streptococcus pyogenes	±	35, 42, 50
Other		
Chlamydia psittaci	+	10
Chlamydia pneumoniae	+	27
Mycoplasma pneumoniae	+++	8–11, 14, 19, 25, 30, 45

*+++, very common; ++, common; +, rare; ±, of questionable etiologic significance.

similar symptomatology. The duration of symptoms depends to some extent on the specific initial infectious agent and, in cases of prolonged illness, on secondary bacterial infection.

It is intriguing to note that in acute bronchitis the larynx and subglottic trachea are not involved prominently; conversely, today bronchial involvement is seen only occasionally in croup.

CLINICAL PRESENTATION

Initial manifestations of acute bronchitis are upper respiratory in nature and, depending on the etiologic agent, either predominantly are nasal, as in the common cold, or show additional objective evidence of pharyngitis, as in nasopharyngitis. Fever usually is present, varying from 37.8° to 39° C (100° to 103° F) on most occasions. Cough always is present, and its onset can be insidious or abrupt. Initially, the cough is dry and harsh and often brassy in younger children. As the illness progresses, the cough becomes looser. In older children, purulent sputum is raised and expectorated. In younger children, the swallowing of often tenacious sputum frequently leads to gagging and vomiting. Older children may complain of chest pain resulting from coughing.

On initial physical examination, a variable degree of rhinitis usually is present; many patients will have diffuse pharyngeal erythema. As the disease progresses, these upper respiratory signs generally decrease. Examination of the chest reveals rhonchi and referred breath sounds. Coarse, changing rales are noted frequently.

In the usual case of acute bronchitis, the illness can be separated into three phases: a 1- to 2-day prodromal period when fever and upper respiratory symptoms predominate, a 4- to 6-day period of marked tracheobronchial symptomatology with some fever and general discomfort, and a recovery period that may last 1 or 2 weeks and is characterized by cough and expectoration.

Occasionally, the recovery period particularly is distressing and is associated with a low-grade fever, suggesting secondary bacterial infection. Bronchitis caused by *C. pneumoniae* often is insidious in onset and frequently is associated with or preceded by pharyngitis.[27, 34] Illness persists for several weeks but responds to appropriate antibiotic therapy.

Laboratory study in acute bronchitis is of limited use. Children in whom throat cultures reveal pathogenic bacteria in predominant growth tend to have more severe illness than children with only viral infections.[12, 40] The white blood cell count usually is greater than 10,000 cells/mm^3, and about a third of the cases have a predominance of neutrophils.[40] The chest radiograph is normal unless there is associated pulmonary involvement.

DIFFERENTIAL DIAGNOSIS AND SPECIFIC DIAGNOSIS

Because acute bronchitis is a clinical entity caused by multiple etiologic agents, the differential aspect of diagnosis of most difficulty is the selection of the specific infectious cause. Also of importance is the separation of acute, self-limited bronchitis from chronic, more serious problems such as cystic fibrosis, allergic respiratory disease, and sinusitis.

An epidemiologic history frequently can help in assigning a particular virus, *M. pneumoniae, C. pneumoniae,* or *B. pertussis* as the presumptive etiologic agent. For example, if epidemic bronchiolitis is occurring in the community, respiratory syncytial virus would be a likely cause. Similarly, predictions of causation by influenza virus, parainfluenza virus, adenoviruses, *M. pneumoniae, C. pneumoniae,* or *B. pertussis* can be made through clinical epidemiologic observations. Specific etiologic diagnosis can be made through the isolation of an organism or its identification by a direct antigen test from the nasopharyngeal secretions. Serologic study on paired sera may be useful for the diagnosis of *M. pneumoniae, C. pneumoniae,* and *B. pertussis.*

Children with protracted illnesses or febrile exacerbations should be examined by culture and radiograph for secondary bacterial infection of the tracheobronchial tree or the lungs, or both. Children with chronic recurrent illnesses should be tested for cystic fibrosis, allergic conditions, and anatomic problems, such as gastroesophageal reflux and tracheoesophageal fistula.

TREATMENT

Treatment of acute bronchitis is distinguished more by what *not* to do than by specific modalities. In the majority of mild cases, no specific therapy is indicated.

For the many children who feel miserable during the initial phases of acute bronchitis, analgesic therapy may be useful.

Formerly, aspirin was the recommended analgesic. However, because studies have implicated aspirin as an etiologic factor in influenza-associated Reye syndrome and because it is difficult clinically to differentiate influenza viral infections from other respiratory viral infections, it is prudent to use acetaminophen rather than aspirin. The dose per single administration of acetaminophen by year of age is the following: younger than 1 year, 60 mg; 1 to 3 years, 60 to 120 mg; 3 to 6 years, 120 mg; 6 to 12 years, 150 to 300 mg; older than 12 years, 325 to 650 mg. Administration may be repeated three or four times daily in young children and every 4 hours in older children. Acetaminophen rarely should be given to infants younger than 6 months of age.

As a result of widespread advertising, it is common in acute bronchitis to use an array of cold remedies, which contain various combinations or antihistamines, decongestants, and antitussives. None have been demonstrated useful in acute bronchitis, and in certain stages of illness, they may aggravate the recovery process. Repeated bouts of coughing occasionally result in emesis, exhaustion, or insomnia, and the careful use of antitussive agents (codeine or dextromethorphan) can be useful.[16] Cough suppressants should be used with caution when a cough is productive, however.

Fluids should be encouraged to prevent overall dehydration and to decrease the viscosity of new secretions. Mist therapy also will help in thinning the exudate-containing respiratory secretions.[20, 41]

In severe cases of acute bronchitis, treatment with specific antiviral agents should be considered. When influenza A virus is the likely etiologic agent, amantadine therapy may be of benefit. In situations involving hospitalized children with illness due to respiratory syncytial virus, parainfluenza viruses, or influenza viruses, treatment with ribavirin by small-particle aerosol should be considered (see Section 17, Viral Infections [Chapter 181, Influenza Viruses; Chapter 182, Parainfluenza Viruses; Chapter 185, Respiratory Syncytial Virus]; Chapter 233, Antiviral Agents).

As noted in Table 23–1, most cases of acute bronchitis are caused by viruses, so antibiotic therapy would appear not to be indicated. However, in cases in which fever returns or no trend toward recovery is seen by the sixth or seventh day of illness, the possibility of secondary bacterial infection should be considered. The association of sinusitis or a throat culture with a predominant growth of a respiratory pathogen (*Streptococcus pneumoniae, Streptococcus pyogenes, Moraxella catarrhalis, H. influenzae*) is an indication for therapy. Infection with *M. pneumoniae* also should be treated, but unlike treatment of pneumonia, the therapy usually will not show an impressive response. Bronchitis due to *C. pneumoniae* should be treated with erythromycin (50 mg/kg/day divided every 6 hours) for 10 to 14 days.[27]

PROGNOSIS

The prognosis in acute bronchitis usually is excellent. Although the duration of cough can be disturbing to both parent and child, full recovery is the rule. Several studies suggest that lower respiratory illness in the first few years of life may be associated with persistent respiratory symptoms and with abnormalities in lung function in later life.[6, 15, 36, 37] Although none of these studies specifically has followed children with acute bronchitis, the findings in other illnesses (bronchiolitis and croup) indicate a need to follow children with episodes of acute bronchitis carefully as well.

PREVENTION

At present, there is no practical method of prevention of acute bronchitis in children. However, because the majority of cases result from infections with common respiratory viruses, the development of vaccines could be expected to be helpful.

References

1. Aitken, C. J. D., Moffat, M. A. J., and Sutherland, J. A. W.: Respiratory illness and viral infection in an Edinburgh nursery. J. Hyg. (Camb.) *65*:25–36, 1967.
2. Avila, M. M., Carballal, G., Rovaletti, H., et al.: Viral etiology in acute lower respiratory infections in children from a closed community. Am. Rev. Respir. Dis. *140*:634–637, 1989.
3. Berglund, B., and Strahlmann, C. H.: Respiratory syncytial virus infections in hospitalized children: Evaluation of the virus isolation and complement-fixation techniques in the virological diagnosis: Clinical and epidemiological characteristics. Acta Paediatr. Scand. *56*:1–10, 1967.
4. Brandt, C. D., Kim, H. W., Vargosko, A. J., et al.: Infections in 18,000 infants and children in a controlled study of respiratory tract disease. I. Adenovirus pathogenicity in relation to serologic type and illness syndrome. Am. J. Epidemiol. *90*:484–500, 1969.
5. Brocklebank, J. T., Court, S. D. M., McQuillin, J., et al.: Influenza A infection in children. Lancet *1*:497–500, 1972.
6. Burrows, B., Knudson, R. J., and Lebowitz, M. D.: The relationship of childhood respiratory illness to adult obstructive airway disease. Am. Rev. Respir. Dis. *115*:751–760, 1977.
7. Caul, E. O., Waller, D. K., Clarke, S. K. R., et al.: A comparison of influenza and respiratory syncytial virus infections among infants admitted to hospital with acute respiratory infections. J. Hyg. (Camb.) *77*:383–392, 1976.
8. Chanock, R. M., and Parrott, R. H.: Acute respiratory disease in infancy and childhood: Present understanding and prospects for prevention: E. Mead Johnson Address, October 1964. Pediatrics *36*:21–39, 1965.
9. Chanock, R. M., Mufson, M. A., and Johnson, K. M.: Comparative biology and ecology of human virus and mycoplasma respiratory pathogens. Prog. Med. Virol. *7*:208–252, 1965.
10. Chanock, R., Chambon, L., Chang, W., et al.: WHO respiratory disease survey in children: A serological study. Bull. W. H. O. *37*:363–369, 1967.
11. Chapman, R. S., Henderson, F. W., Clyde, W. A., Jr., et al.: The epidemiology of tracheobronchitis in pediatric practice. Am. J. Epidemiol. *114*:786–797, 1981.
12. Cherry, J. D., Diddams, J. A., and Dick, E. C.: Rhinovirus infections in hospitalized children: Provocative bacterial interrelationships. Arch. Environ. Health *14*:390–396, 1967.

13. Cherry, J. D.: Newer respiratory viruses: Their role in respiratory illnesses of children. *In* Schulman, I. (ed.): Advances in Pediatrics. Vol. 20. Chicago, Year Book Medical Publishers, 1973, pp. 225–290.
14. Cherry, J. D.: Personal observations.
15. Colley, J. R. T., Douglas, J. W. B., and Reid, D. D.: Respiratory disease in young adults: Influence of early childhood lower respiratory tract illness, social class, air pollution, and smoking. Br. Med. J. *8*:195–198, 1973.
16. Committee on Drugs: Use of codeine- and dextromethorphan-containing cough syrups in pediatrics. Pediatrics *62*:118–122, 1978.
17. Darelid, J., Lofgren S., and Malmvall BE: Erythromycin treatment is beneficial for longstanding *Moraxella catarrhalis* associated cough in children. Scand. J. Infect. Dis. *25*:323–329, 1993.
18. Dascomb, H. E., and Hilleman, M. R.: Clinical and laboratory studies in patients with respiratory disease caused by adenoviruses (RI-APC-ARD agents). Am. J. Med. *21*:161–174, 1956.
19. Denny, F. W., and Clyde, W. A., Jr.: Acute lower respiratory tract infections in nonhospitalized children. J. Pediatr. *108*:635–646, 1986.
20. Dulfano, M. J., Adler, K., and Wooten, O.: Physical properties of sputum. IV. Effects of 100 per cent humidity and water mist. Am. Rev. Respir. Dis. *107*:130–132, 1973.
21. Edwards, G.: Acute bronchitis: Aetiology, diagnosis, and management. Br. Med. J. *1*:963–966, 1966.
22. Gardner, P. S.: Virus infections and respiratory disease of childhood. Arch. Dis. Child. *43*:629–645, 1968.
23. Gardner, P. S.: How etiologic, pathologic, and clinical diagnoses can be made in a correlated fashion. Pediatr. Res. *11*:254–261, 1977.
24. Gardner, S. D.: The isolation of parainfluenza 4 subtypes A and B in England and serological studies of their prevalence. J. Hyg. (Camb.) *67*:545–550, 1969.
25. Glezen, W. P., Loda, F. A., Clyde, W. A., Jr., et al.: Epidemiologic patterns of acute lower respiratory disease of children in a pediatric group practice. J. Pediatr. *78*:397–406, 1971.
26. Gottfard, P., and Brauner, A.: Children with persistent cough: Outcome with treatment and role of *Moraxella catarrhalis*? Scand. J. Infect. Dis. *26*:545–551, 1994.
27. Grayston, J. T., Campbell, L. A., Kuo, C. C., et al.: A new respiratory tract pathogen: *Chlamydia pneumoniae* strain TWAR. J. Infect. Dis. *161*:618–625, 1990.
28. Herrmann, E. C., Jr., and Hable, K. A.: Experiences in laboratory diagnosis of parainfluenza viruses in routine medical practice. Mayo Clin. Proc. *45*:177–188, 1970.
29. Hilleman, M. R.: Respiratory syncytial virus. Am. Rev. Respir. Dis. *88*(Suppl.):181–189, 1963.
30. Horn, M. E. C., Brain, E., Gregg, I., et al.: Respiratory viral infection in childhood: A survey in general practice, Roehampton 1967–1972. J. Hyg. (Camb.) *74*:157–168, 1975.
31. Kellner, G., Popow-Kraupp, T., Kundi, M., et al.: Contribution of rhinoviruses to respiratory viral infections in childhood: A prospective study in a mainly hospitalized infant population. J. Med. Virol. *25*:455–469, 1988.
32. Kim, H. W., Arrobio, J. O., Brandt, C. D., et al.: Epidemiology of respiratory syncytial virus infection in Washington, D.C. I. Importance of the virus in different respiratory tract disease syndromes and temporal distribution of infection. Am. J. Epidemiol. *98*:216–225, 1973.
33. Kravitz, H.: Sex distribution of hospitalized children with acute respiratory diseases, gastroenteritis and meningitis. Clin. Pediatr. *4*:484–491, 1965.
34. Kuo, C. C., Jackson L. A., Campbell, L. A., et al.: *Chlamydia pneumoniae* (TWAR). Clin. Microbiol. Rev. *8*:451–461, 1995.
35. Laxdal, O. E., Robertson, H. E., Braaten, V., et al.: Acute respiratory infections in children. I. An intensive study of etiology in an open community. Can. Med. Assoc. J. *88*:1049–1054, 1963.
36. Lebowitz, M. D., and Burrows, B.: The relationship of acute respiratory illness history to the prevalence and incidence of obstructive lung disorders. Am. J. Epidemiol. *105*:544–554, 1977.
37. Leeder, S. R., Woolcock, A. J., and Blackburn, C. R. B.: Prevalence and natural history of lung disease in New South Wales schoolchildren. Int. J. Epidemiol. *3*:15–23, 1974.
38. McClelland, L., Hilleman, M. R., Hamparian, V. V., et al.: Studies of acute respiratory illnesses caused by respiratory syncytial virus. 2. Epidemiology and assessment of importance. N. Engl. J. Med. *264*:1169–1175, 1961.
39. Mink, C. A. M., Cherry, J. D., Christenson, P., et al.: A search for *Bordetella pertussis* infection in university students. Clin. Infect. Dis. *14*:464–471, 1992.
40. Nichol, K. P., and Cherry, J. D.: Bacterial-viral interrelations in respiratory infections of children. N. Engl. J. Med. *277*:667–672, 1967.
41. Parks, C. R.: Mist therapy: Rationale and practice. J. Pediatr. *76*:305–313, 1970.
42. Pereira, M. S.: Adenovirus infections. Postgrad. Med. J. *49*:798–801, 1973.
43. Person, D. A., and Herrmann, E. C., Jr.: Experiences in laboratory diagnosis of rhinovirus infections in routine medical practice. Mayo Clin. Proc. *45*:517–526, 1970.
44. Robbins, F. C.: Measles: Clinical features. Am. J. Dis. Child. *103*:266–273, 1962.
45. Saliba, G. S., Glezen, W. P., and Chin, T. D. Y.: *Mycoplasma pneumoniae* infection in a resident boys' home. Am. J. Epidemiol. *86*:408–418, 1967.
46. Similä, S., Jouppila, R., Salmi, A., et al.: Encephalomeningitis in children associated with an adenovirus type 7 epidemic. Acta Paediatr. Scand. *59*:310–316, 1970.
47. Spence, L., and Barratt, N.: Respiratory syncytial virus associated with acute respiratory infections in Trinidadian patients. Am. J. Epidemiol. *88*:257–266, 1968.
48. Sterner, G., Gerzen, P., Ohlson, M., et al.: Acute respiratory illness and gastroenteritis in association with adenovirus type 7 infections. Acta Paediatr. *50*:457–468, 1961.
49. Stott, E. J., Eadie, M. B., and Grist, N. R.: Rhinovirus infections of children in hospital: Isolation of three possibly new rhinovirus serotypes. Am. J. Epidemiol. *90*:45–52, 1969.
50. Stuart-Harris, C. H.: The present status of the respiratory viruses and acute respiratory disease in man. Israel J. Med. Sci. *2*:255–268, 1966.
51. Suto, T., Yano, N., Ikeda, M., et al.: Respiratory syncytial virus infection and its serologic epidemiology. Am. J. Epidemiol. *82*:211–224, 1965.
52. Sutton, R. N. P.: Respiratory viruses in a residential nursery. J. Hyg. Camb. *60*:51–67, 1962.
53. Toth, M., Barna, M., and Voltay, B.: Aetiology of acute respiratory diseases in infants and children. Acta Paediatr. Hung. *6*:367–374, 1965.
54. Urquhart, G. E. D., Moffat, M. A. J., Calder, M. A., et al.: An aetiological study of respiratory infection in children, Edinburgh City Hospital, 1961–1963. J. Hyg. (Camb.) *63*:187–199, 1965.
55. Van der Veen, J.: The role of adenoviruses in respiratory disease. Am. Rev. Respir. Dis. *88*:167–180, 1963.
56. Van Lierde, S., Corbeel, L., and Eggermont, E.: Clinical and laboratory findings in children with adenovirus infections. Eur. J. Pediatr. *148*:423–525, 1989.
57. Vihma, L.: Surveillance of acute viral respiratory diseases in children. Acta Paediatr. Scand. *192*(Suppl.):7–53, 1969.
58. Walker, S. H.: The respiratory manifestations of systemic *Hemophilus influenzae* infection. J. Pediatr. *62*:386–392, 1963.
59. Yodfat, Y., and Nishmi, M.: Successive overlapping outbreaks of febrile pharyngitis and pharyngoconjunctival fever associated with adenovirus types 2 and 7, in a Kibbutz. Israel J. Med. Sci. *10*:1505–1509, 1974.
60. Zinserling, A.: Peculiarities of lesions in viral and mycoplasmal infections of the respiratory tract. Virchows Arch. [A] *356*:259–273, 1972.

24

CHRONIC BRONCHITIS

I. Celine Hanson and William T. Shearer

Chronic bronchitis is reported widely in the adult literature and classically described as "a clinical disorder characterized by excessive mucus production in the bronchial tree with manifestation, i.e., cough, present on most days for a maximum of 3 months in the year and not less than 2 successive years."[1] For most pediatricians and in the pediatric literature, the clinical entity of chronic bronchitis is ill defined and most commonly synonymous with asthmatic bronchitis.[32] Lack of uniform or standardized definitions of chronic bronchitis leads to wide discrepancies in reported prevalences (Table 24–1), and the listed etiologic agents often overlap with those agents presumed to be responsible for acute or asthmatic

TABLE 24–1. Prevalence of Childhood Bronchitis

Reference	Study	Prevalence of Bronchitis
Bland et al.[3]	1974—Kent schoolchildren (acute and chronic)	5.5%
Burrows and Lebowitz[6]	1975—Arizona children (chronic)	7.1%
Burrows et al.[5]	1977—Arizona retrospective questionnaire (chronic)	46.4%
Kubo et al.[18]	1978—Japanese children (chronic and recurrent)	1.4%
Peat et al.[25]	1980—Sydney schoolchildren (acute and chronic)	20.0%

Modified from Morgan, W. T., and Taussig, L. M.: The chronic bronchitis complex in childhood. Pediatr. Clin. North Am. *37*:851–864, 1984.

bronchitis. The pathology of the disease entity also is unclear. Bronchoscopy of pediatric patients with chronic bronchitis has revealed findings not dissimilar to those noted in children with asthma, which reflects the inclusion of asthma in the spectrum of the chronic bronchitis complex.[22] Pediatric bronchoscopic evaluation yields heterogeneous histomorphic findings (granulocyte and mononuclear cell predominance at lavage and biopsy) that are distinct from findings in adults with chronic bronchitis.[30]

DIFFERENTIAL DIAGNOSIS

Because chronic bronchitis is accepted by most as a complex of symptoms characterized by persistent cough with or without wheezing,[6, 18, 22] it is imperative that the physician address those diseases that include chronic bronchitis with consideration of the spectrum of signs and symptoms with which they may present. Table 24–2 includes a list of illnesses that are associated with recurrent lower respiratory tract illnesses or chronic cough for more than 3 months. Heading the list is asthma,[10, 34] defined as reversible obstructive airways disease with a significant inflammatory component leading to increased edema and mucus production, as discussed in Chapter 25. Recurrent episodes of acute bronchitis often are interpreted as chronic bronchitis, although the intermittent nature of these episodes and absence of a persistent cough usually distinguish this group of patients clinically.[4, 13] Specific viral infections (rhinovirus, parainfluenza virus) in children with or without allergic rhinitis may provoke airway hyperreactivity and late asthmatic reactions, which may be confused symptomatically with chronic bronchitis.[7, 19] Persistent lower tract infections (i.e., *Chlamydia*, pertussis, and *Mycobacterium*) frequently present with the complex of symptoms described and are evaluated best with chest roentgenographs in a search for enlarged hilar nodes or interstitial lung infiltrates. Respiratory tract secretions for appropriate bacterial and viral culture and serum for determinations of antibacterial antibodies should be obtained. In the case of tuberculosis, a delayed hypersensitivity skin test for *Mycobacterium tuberculosis* antigen should be applied.

Cystic fibrosis, the most common inherited lethal condition in Caucasians, with an incidence of approximately 1/2000 births, is manifested by failure to thrive, steatorrhea, nasal polyps, and recurrent lower respiratory tract symptoms and identified easily by abnormally elevated chloride levels (>60 mEq/L) as measured by the sweat iontophoresis test.[16]

Primary ciliary dyskinesia encompasses the immotile cilia disorders and Kartagener syndrome (rhinosinusitis, bronchitis and/or bronchiectasis, and situs inversus). Patients with these illnesses suffer from defects in mucociliary transport, as evidenced by a decrease in ciliary beat frequency. Electron microscopy of bronchial cilia shows structural defects classically with absent dynein arms.[27] The diagnosis is made by bronchial or in some cases nasal turbinate biopsy.

The primary immune disorders most frequently associated with recurrent sinopulmonary infections include selective IgA deficiency,[9] hypogammaglobulinemia (both primary and secondary), IgG subclass deficiencies, and ataxia telangiectasia. Selective IgA deficiency, the most commonly encountered form of the immunodeficiency, with an incidence of 1:500, is accompanied by a propensity for atopy and an increase in associated autoimmune disease (most often rheumatoid arthritis and systemic lupus erythematosus). The diagnosis is made readily by evaluation of quantitative serum immunoglobulins defining IgA levels of less than 10 mg/dL. IgG subclass deficiencies have been detected most recently in patients with depressed IgA levels (i.e., <60 mg/dL)[24] and, in addition, are linked to recurrent infections, particularly otitis, sinusitis, and recurrent lower respiratory tract infections.[29] The patient with ataxia telangiectasia has both depressed serum IgA concentrations and marked dysfunction of the swallowing mechanism, leading to recurrent lower respiratory tract infections probably secondary to recurrent aspiration. These patients are identified by the classic telangiectases of the skin and conjunctiva in association with aberrant and progressively deteriorating neurologic symptoms and immunodeficiency (depressed IgA and IgE and aberrant T-cell–mediated immunity). Some of these patients have depressed IgG subclasses (IgG2, IgG4) as well.[24] Graft-versus-host disease affecting the lungs has been described in immunocompromised patients after bone marrow transplantation.[2] The lesion is caused by chronic pulmonary lymphocytic infiltrates and pulmonary fibrosis mimicking the symptom

TABLE 24–2. Conditions Associated with Chronic Cough (3 Months or Longer) or Lower Respiratory Tract Illness

I. Asthma
II. Recurrent episodes of bronchitis (*Chlamydia*, pertussis, mycobacteria)
III. Cystic fibrosis
IV. Primary ciliary dyskinesia
  A. Kartagener syndrome
  B. Immotile cilia syndrome
V. Immunodeficiency
  A. Selective IgA deficiency
  B. Subclass of IgG deficiency
  C. Hypogammaglobulinemia (primary and secondary)
  D. Ataxia telangiectasia
  E. Graft-versus-host disease status after bone marrow transplant
  F. Prematurity
  G. HIV infection
VI. Anatomic lesions
  A. Foreign body
  B. Status after esophageal atresia repair
  C. Mediastinal tumors
  D. Congenital heart disease
VII. Irritants
  A. Milk aspiration (gastroesophageal reflux, tracheoesophageal fistula)
  B. Tobacco smoke
  C. Pollution
  D. Occupational exposure

Modified from Morgan, W. T., and Taussig, L. M.: The chronic bronchitis complex in childhood. Pediatr. Clin. North Am. *37*:851–864, 1984.

complex of chronic bronchitis and often is indistinguishable radiographically or clinically from those infections that characteristically are pathogenic (i.e., *Pneumocystis carinii, Candida albicans, Aspergillus*).

Secondary immune disorders (prematurity and pediatric HIV infection) also may be associated with significant sinopulmonary infections. Premature infants with attendant severe respiratory distress syndrome requiring positive-pressure ventilation may develop bronchopulmonary dysplasia (BPD). Diagnostic criteria include (1) hypoxia requiring oxygen supplementation, (2) characteristic diffuse interstitial markings on chest roentgenograph, and (3) clinical signs of pulmonary disease (tachypnea, intercostal retractions).[26] In one series, more than 60 per cent of surviving BPD children were documented to have significant pulmonary disease and associated morbidity, i.e., increased hospitalizations.[28] Continued improved care for premature infants and resultant decreased mortality may increase the population of infants afflicted with BPD. Pediatric HIV infection is estimated to affect 1200 to 1800 U.S. infants annually and is associated with serious lower respiratory tract illness.[12] In particular, lymphoid interstitial pneumonitis and/or pulmonary lymphoid hyperplasia reported in 25 per cent of all children with AIDS may produce chronic cough, sputum production, and hypoxia. Definitive diagnosis is by biopsy. Characteristic roentgenographic findings of diffuse bilateral interstitial or nodular infiltrates in an HIV-infected infant without known infectious etiologies may lead to a presumptive diagnosis. Lower respiratory tract infections (viral, bacterial, fungal) are common in children with AIDS: *P. carinii* pneumonia was reported in 38 per cent of cases, pulmonary candidiasis was noted in 4 per cent of cases, and recurrent bacterial infections were reported in 21 per cent of cases.[12] The diagnosis of HIV infection is by viral diagnostic assays (HIV culture, polymerase chain reaction, p24 antigen, immune complex–dissociated p24 antigen) for perinatally exposed infants younger than 18 months of age and by serology (enzyme-linked immunosorbent assay and confirmational assays [Western blot analysis, indirect fluorescent antibody assay]) for perinatally exposed infants 18 months of age or older.[8]

Anatomic lesions that lead to pulmonary obstructive airway disease can simulate the complex of chronic bronchitis. The infant with chronic cough, poor feeding habits, and failure to thrive should undergo evaluation for gastroesophageal reflux or a tracheoesophageal fistula, which most easily are identified by barium swallow or pH probe monitoring. Mediastinal tumors can produce extrinsic obstruction, leading to recurrent cough and wheezing. Congenital heart disease should be considered in this patient group and can be evaluated with chest roentgenography, electrocardiography, and echocardiography.

Respiratory tract irritants have been implicated as a cause of chronic cough, as documented in adult populations of industrial European nations.[15, 21, 33] It is of note that nonindustrial, rural communities, such as the forest zone of Nigeria, report virtually no chronic bronchitis, whereas metropolitan New York reports an increased risk for both upper and lower respiratory tract infections in both adults and children who reside in those parts of the city with the highest ambient air levels of sulfur dioxide and particulate air pollution.[20] A correlation between tobacco smoking and reduced ventilatory capacity in adults has been reported by many investigators. Peat and associates[25] described teenagers in Sydney, Australia, with recurrent episodes of bronchitis with worsened lung function when coupled with tobacco smoking. There has been some evidence that children who acquire an upper respiratory tract infection and are exposed chronically to parental smoking, especially maternal smoking, are at greater risk for development of lower respiratory tract disease and wheezy bronchitis than are children whose parents do not smoke.[3, 14, 23] These data should prompt the physician to obtain a smoking history not only for the patient but also for other household members. Occupational exposures long have been cited for exacerbating pulmonary diseases and possibly causing persistent lower respiratory tract irritation presenting as chronic cough. Classic examples of dust exposure leading to increased risk are described in coal miners in Great Britain, foundry workers in the Rhine-Ruhr area of Germany, and potters in West Virginia; it also is well known that tobacco smoking accentuates the irritant effect of occupational exposure for these adult patients.

EPIDEMIOLOGY AND ETIOLOGY

Differentiating the impact of clinical, social, and environmental factors on lower respiratory tract disease, including chronic bronchitis, has been problematic and led to conflicting outcomes in epidemiologic assessments.[5, 11, 17, 31] In addition, the lack of a standardized definition of chronic bronchitis in the pediatric literature leads to confusing data when attempting to appreciate the prevalence or etiology of the disease complex.[22, 32] In Table 24–1, the information from Kubo and associates[18] separates acute recurrent bronchitis, asthmatic bronchitis, and chronic bronchitis, leading to a drop in the prevalence from a proposed 46.4 per cent (in the Arizona questionnaire) to 1.4 per cent.[22] There also is considerable overlap in evaluating etiologic agents for chronic bronchitis. The same viral agents proposed as the exacerbating factors of asthmatic bronchitis (see Chapter 25) are implicated in exacerbations of chronic bronchitis.[13, 18] They include rhinoviruses, parainfluenza viruses, respiratory syncytial virus, influenza A and B viruses, adenoviruses, and enteroviruses. For a group of 40 pediatric patients with chronic bronchitis and exacerbations of cough and fever, predominant bacterial pathogens isolated from washed sputum are listed in Table 24–3 and include *Haemophilus influenzae, Streptococcus pneumoniae,* and *Staphylococcus aureus*.[18] These bacteria also are implicated as etiologic agents in the triggering of asthmatic bronchitis. Treatment of exacerbations of chronic bronchitis with antibiotic therapy usually is effective in reducing sputum volume and purulence but shows no parallel elimination of the cultured microorganisms.

TREATMENT

When a specific diagnosis is found in association with chronic cough or wheezing, therapy is directed toward the

TABLE 24–3. Dominant Pathogens in Washed Sputum of Chronic Bronchitis (40 Cases)

	No. of Cases
Haemophilus influenzae and *Streptococcus pneumoniae*	21 (52.5%)
Haemophilus influenzae	17 (42.5%)
Staphylococcus aureus	2 (5.0%)
Superinfection with gram-negative rods	
Pseudomonas aeruginosa	4
Klebsiella pneumoniae	2
Escherichia coli	1
Enterobacter cloacae	1

From Kubo, S., Funabashi, S., Uehara, S., et al.: Clinical aspects of "asthmatic bronchitis" and chronic bronchitis in infants and children. J. Asthma Res. *15*:99–132, 1978.

primary disease entity as well as the clinical presentation of cough. Hence, bronchodilators (theophylline preparations, beta-adrenergic agents, cromolyn sodium, corticosteroids) are used, when appropriate, for the treatment of chronic cough associated with asthma. Appropriate positioning techniques (prone 30 degrees), feeding schedules, and medications (bethanecol, etc.) are indicated in the approach to infants with gastroesophageal reflux. The patient with hypogammaglobulinemia or an IgG subclass deficiency can be aided with supplemental intravenous immunoglobulin preparations currently commercially available (100 to 400 mg/kg/dose every 2 to 4 weeks) in an attempt to decrease incidence of infections.

It is imperative that those patients with such chronic pulmonary diseases as cystic fibrosis, asthma, or ciliary dyskinesias understand the pulmonary irritant effect of tobacco smoking, dust exposure, and air pollution. A change of occupation may be essential for their well-being. It also is imperative to stress the irritant effect of parental smoking on the already compromised pulmonary function of the child. Antibiotic therapy for chronic bronchitis usually is reserved only for those patients with severe illness in whom the likelihood of secondary bacterial infection is great. In these instances, therapy usually consists of ampicillin (75 mg/kg/24 hours), erythromycin (40 mg/kg/24 hours), or, in adolescents, tetracycline (25 to 50 mg/kg/24 hours). For the patient receiving methylxanthine therapy, it is important to remember that certain antibiotics, e.g., erythromycin, lead to elevated serum concentrations of theophylline, which makes toxicity more likely. As with patients who have obstructive lung disease, attention must be aimed at careful and sequential monitoring of pulmonary function. The prognosis for chronic bronchitis is varied and is dependent on the specific etiology of this syndrome.

References

1. American Thoracic Society: Chronic bronchitis, asthma, and pulmonary emphysema. Thorax *15*:762–768, 1980.
2. Beschorner, W. E., Saral, R., Hutchins, G. M., et al.: Lymphocytic bronchitis associated with graft-versus-host disease in recipients of bone marrow transplants. N. Engl. J. Med. *299*:1030–1036, 1978.
3. Bland, M., Bewley, B. R., and Rollard, V.: Effects of children's and parents' smoking on respiratory symptoms. Arch. Dis. Child. *53*:100–105, 1974.
4. Boule, M., Gaultier, C., Tournier, G., et al.: Lung function in children with recurrent bronchitis. Respiration *38*:127–134, 1979.
5. Burrows, B., Knudsen, R. J., and Lebowitz, M. D.: The relationship of childhood respiratory illness to adult obstructive airway disease. Am. Rev. Respir. Dis. *115*:751–759, 1977.
6. Burrows, B., and Lebowitz, M. D.: Characteristics of chronic bronchitis in a warm dry region. Am. Rev. Respir. Dis. *112*:365–370, 1975.
7. Busse, W. W.: Respiratory infections: Their role in airway responsiveness and the pathogenesis of asthma. J. Allerg. Clin. Immun. *85*:671–684, 1990.
8. Centers for Disease Control and Prevention: 1994 revised classification system for human immunodeficiency virus infection in children less than 13 years of age. M. M. W. R. *43*:1–17, 1994.
9. Chipps, B. E., Talama, R. C., and Winklestein, J. A.: IgA deficiency, recurrent pneumonia, and bronchiectasis. Chest *73*:519–526, 1978.
10. Cloutier, M. M., and Laughlin, G. M.: Chronic cough in children: A manifestation of airway hyperreactivity. Pediatrics *67*:6–12, 1981.
11. Dodge, R., Burrows, B., Lebowitz, M. D., et al.: Antecedent features of children in whom asthma develops during the second decade of life. J. Allerg. Clin. Immun. *92*:744–749, 1993.
12. Hanson, I. C.: Respiratory infections in HIV-infected children. Immun. Allerg. Clin. North Am. *13*:205–217, 1993.
13. Horn, M. E. C., and Gregg, I.: Role of viral infection and host factors in acute episodes of asthma and chronic bronchitis. Chest *63*:44–85, 1973.
14. Irvine, D., Brooks, A., and Walker, R.: The role of air pollution, smoking, and respiratory illnesses in childhood in the development of chronic bronchitis. Chest *77*:251–253, 1980.
15. Irwin, R. S., Corrao, W. M., and Pratter, M. R.: Chronic persistent cough in the adult. Am. Rev. Respir. Dis. *123*:413–417, 1981.
16. Klein, R. B., and Huggins, B. W.: Chronic bronchitis in children. Semin. Respir. Med. *9*:13–22, 1994.
17. Kolnaar, B. G. M., Van den Bosch, W. J. H. M., Van den Hoogen, H. J. M., et al.: The clustering of respiratory diseases in early childhood. Fam. Med. *26*:106–110, 1994.
18. Kubo, S., Funabashi, S., Uehara, S., et al.: Clinical aspects of "asthmatic bronchitis" and chronic bronchitis in infants and children. J. Asthma Res. *15*:99–132, 1978.
19. Lemanske, R. F., Dick, E. C., Swenson, C. A., et al.: Rhinovirus upper respiratory tract infection increases airway hyperreactivity and late asthmatic reactions. J. Clin. Invest. *83*:1–10, 1989.
20. Love, G. T., Lan, S. P., Shy, C. M., et al.: The incidence and severity of acute respiratory illness in families exposed to different levels of air pollution, New York metropolitan area 1971–1972. Arch. Environ. Health *36*:66–74, 1981.
21. Monto, A. S., and Ross, H.: Acute respiratory illness in the community: Effect of family composition, smoking, and chronic symptoms. Br. J. Prev. Soc. Med. *31*:101–108, 1977.
22. Morgan, W. T., and Taussig, L. M.: The chronic bronchitis complex in childhood. Pediatr. Clin. North Am. *31*:851–864, 1984.
23. Neuspiel, D. R., Rush, D., Butler, N. R., et al.: Parental smoking and postinfancy wheezing in children: A prospective cohort study. Am. J. Public Health *79*:168–171, 1989.
24. Oxelius, V. A.: Quantitative and qualitative investigations of serum IgG subclasses in immunodeficiency diseases. Clin. Exp. Immunol. *36*:112–116, 1979.
25. Peat, J. K., Woolcock, A. J., Leider, S. R., et al.: Asthma and bronchitis in Sydney school children. I. Prevalence during a six-year study. Am. J. Epidemiol. *111*:721–727, 1980.
26. Redding, G. J., Brown, G. F., Jacobs, M., et al.: Bronchopulmonary dysplasia (BPD). Pediatr. Pulmonol. *3*(Suppl.):3–13, 1989.
27. Rossman, C. M., Forrest, J. B., Ruffin, R. E., et al.: Immotile cilia syndrome in persons with and without Kartagener's syndrome. Am. Rev. Respir. Dis. *121*:1011–1016, 1980.
28. Rozycki, H. J., and Kirkpatrick, B. V.: New developments in bronchopulmonary dysplasia. Pediatr. Ann. *22*:532–538, 1993.
29. Schur, P. H., Borel, H., Gelfand, E. W., et al.: Selective gamma-G globulin deficiencies in patients with recurrent pyogenic infections. N. Engl. J. Med. *283*:631–634, 1970.
30. Smith, T. F., Ireland, T. A., Zaatari, G. S., et al.: Characteristics of children with endoscopically proved "chronic bronchitis." Am. J. Dis. Child. *139*:1039–1044, 1985.
31. Strachan, D. P., Seagrott, V., and Cook, D. G.: Chest illness in infancy and chronic respiratory disease in later life: An analysis by month of birth. Intern. J. Epidemiol. *23*:1060–1068, 1994.
32. Taussig, L. M., Smith, S. M., and Blumenfeld, R.: Chronic bronchitis in childhood: What is it? Pediatrics *67*:1–5, 1981.
33. Wanner, H. U.: Effects of atmospheric pollution on human health. Experientia *49*:754-758, 1993.
34. Williams, H., and McNicol, K.: Prevalence and natural history of wheezing bronchitis and asthma in children: An epidemiological study. Br. Med. J. *4*:321–325, 1969.

25

BRONCHIOLITIS AND INFECTIOUS ASTHMA

Robert C. Welliver

Both bronchiolitis and infectious asthma (the latter condition also being referred to as *asthmatic bronchitis* or *wheezy bronchitis,* among other terms) are common illnesses of children, characterized by symptoms of upper respiratory tract infection and signs of obstructive airway disease. Bronchiolitis and infectious asthma often are considered distinct entities, and it certainly is true that not all infants who develop bronchiolitis will have infectious asthma in later life. Nevertheless, further study seems to indicate that the two are quite similar in terms of clinical presentation, pathologic findings, and mechanisms of pathogenesis. Differences between the two, in terms of etiologic agents that precipitate illness episodes or in terms of response to therapy, are more a function of patient age (i.e., older or younger than 3 years of age in particular) than of any underlying disease process. *Infectious asthma* therefore will be considered as a term defining the occurrence of repeated episodes of bronchiolitis, and the two conditions will be discussed together.

DEFINITION

Bronchiolitis is an acute communicable disease predominantly presenting in infancy and characterized by cough, coryza, fever, expiratory wheezing, grunting, tachypnea, retractions, and air trapping. The age at which the first (and the most severe) episodes most commonly occur is 2 to 6 months. *Infectious asthma* is a term generally used to refer to infection-induced wheezing occurring beyond infancy. Nevertheless, a given patient may experience bronchiolitis during the first months of life and a recurrent episode caused by the same virus in the second year, suggesting an identical underlying nature of the two illnesses.

HISTORY

Although all practicing pediatricians today are familiar with the term *bronchiolitis* and associate it with an acute clinical illness with the signs and symptoms of obstructive emphysema, it is surprising to note that it has been recognized in the medical literature for only a relatively brief period.

In the early years of the twentieth century, the term *capillary bronchitis* was used to describe an inflammatory illness of the smallest alveoli.[59] However, it was pointed out that the condition could not be distinguished clinically from pneumonia, and there was doubt whether the pathologic entity (bronchiolitis) ever occurred separately from pneumonia. In the eleventh edition of *Holt's Diseases of Infancy and Childhood*[76] in 1940, capillary bronchitis is discussed only briefly and is considered under pneumococcal pneumonia. Not until the sixth edition of the *Textbook of Pediatrics*[174] in 1954 was acute bronchiolitis listed as a heading; even at this time it was associated with interstitial pneumonitis.

In contrast to the delayed textbook recognition of bronchiolitis, good clinical descriptions were presented in journals. In 1941, Hubble and Osborn[80] published "Acute Bronchiolitis in Children," in which an epidemic of bronchiolitis involving 50 hospitalized children was described. Pratt[138] in 1944 and Nelson and Smith[125] in 1945 presented excellent clinical papers. Studies in the late 1950s and early 1960s established the etiologic association of respiratory syncytial virus and other viruses with acute bronchiolitis.[7, 24–27, 142, 149]

ETIOLOGIC AGENTS

It clearly has been established that respiratory syncytial virus is the major cause of bronchiolitis in infancy and virtually the only etiologic consideration when the disease is epidemic.[7, 8, 11, 21, 23–28, 46, 54, 88, 100, 101, 107, 120, 132, 133, 141, 149, 167] In sporadic instances of bronchiolitis, other infectious agents have been found in etiologic association. The relative frequency of infectious agents in the overall etiology of bronchiolitis is presented in Table 25–1. These data were compiled from 12 reports in which respiratory illness in children was observed over an extended period and, in most instances, a large number of clinical illness categories were being studied. In the nonepidemic situation, more than 50 per cent of the isolates or instances of serologic evidence of infection are infectious agents other than respiratory syncytial virus. During epidemics in the colder months, virologic and serologic study indicates a respiratory syncytial viral etiology in 80 per cent or more of the cases and especially in severe cases. In contrast, sporadic disease rarely is associated with a better than 50 per cent association of infectious agent and illness, despite the fact that infections undoubtedly are the cause of sporadic, as well as epidemic, bronchiolitis.[117]

Children surviving infantile bronchiolitis often have recurrent episodes of wheezing that, on clinical grounds, also seem to be precipitated by upper respiratory infections. Studies designed to determine the infectious agents responsible for these repeated wheezing episodes have yielded variable results, presumably because they involve patients of different ages followed during different seasons of the year.[9, 106, 113–116]

TABLE 25–1. Infectious Agents Associated with Acute Bronchiolitis

Infectious Agent	Relative Frequency (%)	
Respiratory syncytial virus		50
Parainfluenza viruses		25
Type 1	(8)	
Type 2	(2)	
Type 3	(15)	
Adenoviruses		5
Mycoplasma pneumoniae		5
Rhinoviruses		5
Influenza viruses		5
Type A	(3)	
Type B	(2)	
Enteroviruses		2
Herpes simplex virus		2
Mumps virus		<1

From references 21, 23, 25, 46, 54, 88, 100, 107, 120, 132, and 167.

TABLE 25–2. Principal Agents Recovered from Children of Different Ages with Wheezing Precipitated by Infection

Agent*	Frequency of Isolation of Each Age Group†			
	0–2 years	*2–5 years*	*5–9 years*	*9–15 years*
Respiratory syncytial virus	+ + + +	+ + +	+ +	+ +
Adenoviruses	+ +	+ +	+	0
Parainfluenza viruses	+ +	+ +	+ +	+ +
Rhinoviruses	+	+ to + +	+ + to + + +	+ + to + + +
Mycoplasma pneumoniae	+	+ +	+ + +	+ + + +

*Other agents that more rarely precipitate wheezing include enteroviruses, herpes simplex virus, cytomegalovirus, coronaviruses, influenza viruses, mumps virus, varicella-zoster virus, *Bordetella pertussis,* and *Coxiella burnetii.*

†+ + + +, very common; + + +, common; + +, occasional; +, uncommon.

See references 9, 47, 48, 58, 71, 77, 106, 113, 114, 116, and 154.

A comprehensive study based on more than a decade of observation of children from birth through 15 years of age[71] has revealed that viruses and *Mycoplasma pneumoniae* are the most common etiologic agents (Table 25–2). Respiratory syncytial virus is the most common cause of recurrent, wheezing-associated respiratory illness occurring in young children, including those who previously experienced bronchiolitis, which strongly suggests the identical nature of infection-related wheezing episodes occurring in children of different ages. With increasing patient age, rhinoviruses and *M. pneumoniae* account for the majority of infection-induced wheezing episodes. The parainfluenza viruses are important causes of such wheezing episodes throughout childhood, and adenoviruses are common causes in infancy. Respiratory syncytial virus remains an important cause of wheezing in adolescents[71] and can cause airway obstruction in very elderly individuals.[176]

The role of bacterial agents as primary agents, synergistically active participants, or secondary invaders in bronchiolitis has interested investigators for many years. It can be stated definitively that currently there is no evidence of a primary role for bacteria in bronchiolitis of infants.[7, 100] The data on synergistic viral-bacterial infections are equivocal. Wood and colleagues[190] in 1954 and Sell[154] in 1960 reported studies in which bacteriologic and serologic evidence tended to associate *Haemophilus influenzae* infections with bronchiolitis. Some of the children from these studies later were shown serologically to have had respiratory syncytial virus infection.[29] Later studies showed evidence of mixed viral-bacterial infections in bronchiolitis[107, 127] and other lower respiratory illnesses.[127] It should be noted, however, that these mixed infections were found no more commonly among bronchiolitis patients than among patients with mild upper respiratory tract disease, whereas respiratory syncytial virus was recovered 10 times as often from patients with lower respiratory tract disease than from patients with upper respiratory tract disease alone.[107] Therefore, a role of any significance for mixed viral-bacterial infection in bronchiolitis of infancy is unlikely. Bacterial superinfection is uncommon in bronchiolitis, as is discussed later in this chapter (see Complications and Prognosis).

The association of asthma and infectious illnesses has been appreciated throughout the twentieth century. Initial reports tended to relate bacterial agents to wheezing; as early as 1909, Carmalt-Jones[20] reported improvement of patients with asthma in association with injections of a bacterial vaccine. Throughout the first half of the twentieth century, "bacterial allergy" was the main consideration in infection-related wheezing, and controversy raged about the therapeutic merits of bacterial vaccines.[5, 45] In spite of the widespread use of bacterial vaccines in the treatment of infectious asthma, there is no evidence that bacterial organisms of the normal flora precipitate asthmatic attacks.[5, 39, 45, 67, 105, 118, 119, 175] However, in children with sinus infections with *Streptococcus pneumoniae* and/or *H. influenzae,* eradication of the infection may result in marked improvement of the asthma. Antibiotic therapy of bacterial sinusitis itself certainly is justified. Nevertheless, therapeutic trials of antibiotics for either infantile bronchiolitis[44] or recurrent episodes of wheezing[79] have not yielded beneficial results. The routine use of antibiotics either prophylactically or therapeutically in acute wheezing episodes in children cannot be defended.

EPIDEMIOLOGY

Bronchiolitis predominantly is a disease of infancy (although similar disease occurring in older children arbitrarily may be referred to as another diagnostic entity). In a study involving 1148 children, the peak age of incidence was between 2 and 6 months, with more than 80 per cent of the cases occurring during the first year of life.[133] In pediatric practice, Breese and associates[12] noted in a review of their practice that of 50 children hospitalized with medical illnesses, 2 had bronchiolitis. In a much larger study of families in the Houston area, rates of respiratory syncytial virus infection were 68.8 per 100 children in the first year of life and 82.6 per 100 children in the second year, including many reinfections. Lower respiratory illness due to respiratory syncytial virus was noted in 22.4 of 100 children in the first year of life. Of all respiratory syncytial virus infections occurring before 12 months of age, one-third were accompanied by lower respiratory illness. Although the attack rate of respiratory syncytial virus decreases with age, the frequency with which lower respiratory disease occurs among those infected remains relatively constant (Table 25–3), at least for the first 4 years of life.[56] In the Tucson area, a study of 1179 children enrolled in a health maintenance organization found that the rate of lower respiratory illness in the first year of life was 32.9 episodes per 100 children; 60 per cent of these episodes were diagnosed as bronchiolitis.[192]

Studies in the Washington, D.C., area[88] estimated the risk of hospitalization for bronchiolitis among infants aged 0 to 12 months to be 10 per 1000. A combined study involving 10 centers in Great Britain[31] concluded that the frequency of hospitalization for lower respiratory tract disease (predominantly wheezing) due to respiratory syncytial virus was 1 per 114 infants younger than 1 year of age and 1 per 476 children younger than 5 years of age. Peak rates of hospitalization were observed for children from 1 to 3 months of age

TABLE 25–3. Attack Rates of Respiratory Syncytial Virus

Age (mo.)	Child Years	Infections per 100 Child Years	LRI per 100 Child Years	LRI per 100 Infections
0–12	125	68.8	22.4	32.6
13–24	92	82.6	13.0	15.8
25–36	65	46.2	10.8	23.3
37–48	39	33.3	7.7	23.1

LRI, lower respiratory tract infections.
From Glezen, W. P., Taber, L.H., Frank, A. L., et al.: Risk of primary infection and reinfection with respiratory syncytial virus. Am. J. Dis. Child. *140*:543–546, 1986.

(1 in 56). Environmental factors are a major determinant of the risk of hospitalization for lower respiratory illness due to respiratory syncytial virus, with the incidence of hospitalization for infants 1 to 3 months of age residing in rural, urban, or heavily industrialized areas of Great Britain being 1 in 80, 1 in 60, and 1 in 40, respectively. The same figures for all children younger than 5 years of age were 1 in 714, 1 in 588, and 1 in 227.[31] Studies completed in North Carolina[71] in which the incidence of all respiratory infection–associated wheezing (both requiring hospitalization or mild enough to permit outpatient management) was determined in a group practice showed that the incidence of such illness was 11.4 cases per 100 children in the first year of life, 6.0 per 100 children in the second year, and 1.3 per 100 children in elementary school.

Epidemic bronchiolitis due to respiratory syncytial virus is markedly seasonal, with peak activity in the period from January to May and virtually no activity from August to October.[88] In contrast to the number of bronchiolitis cases due to respiratory syncytial virus, a small number of sporadic cases due to other agents are seen throughout the whole year. In their study of 1179 cases, Kim and associates[88] noted that 77 per cent of the cases of respiratory syncytial virus infection occurred between December and June. The lowest incidence occurred in August (2 per cent).

Bronchiolitis is more common in boys: the male to female ratio is about 1.5:1.[93] In older children, wheezing due to viral and mycoplasma infections remains more common in males (male to female ratio, 1.35:1) until 9 years of age, when the incidence becomes equal for the sexes.[71]

CLINICAL PRESENTATION

Acute bronchiolitis is most common in infants 2 to 12 months of age. In most instances, the patient's history reveals exposure to an adult or older child with a common cold or other relatively trivial respiratory infection. Occasionally, as in the day care setting, the child will have been exposed to other children with more marked respiratory illness. After exposure, the incubation period is about 4 to 6 days. The initial signs include copious nasal discharge (often serous in the early stage), cough, irritability, poor feeding, and vomiting in some cases. Fever usually is present, with rectal temperatures ranging from normal to 40.6° C (105.4° F) (mean, 39° C [102° F]).[141] Nasal congestion with tenacious secretions and progressive cough and dyspnea dominate the clinical picture. Symptoms usually progress in severity over a 3- to 7-day period, with the time of the onset of wheezing often recognizable from the caretaker's description of the illness. A few cases progress either more insidiously or, less commonly, more rapidly. At the time of hospital admission, all patients have cough and evidence of respiratory distress. Examination reveals fever in 50 to 80 per cent of cases. The pulse is rapid, and the respiratory rate usually is between 40 and 80 breaths per minute. The breathing is labored, with flaring of the alae nasae; grunting; and supraclavicular, subcostal, and intercostal retractions. The degreee of retraction of the lower chest wall may be a particularly accurate indicator of severity of illness. Wheezing often is audible without a stethoscope, and the chest is full. Hyperresonance may be noted on percussion, and auscultation generally reveals harsh rhonchi, high-pitched expiratory wheezes, or fine inspiratory rales. Occasionally, wheezing is not audible, despite other evidence of airway obstruction. A prolonged expiratory phase of breathing is noted. Cyanosis occurs in about one-fourth of the cases.

Other findings include a mild conjunctivitis in one-third of the cases, pharyngitis of varied severity in about one-half of the affected infants, and otitis media in 5 to 15 per cent of the cases. The abdomen frequently appears distended, and the liver and spleen usually are palpable. The latter organs are not enlarged but are pushed down because of emphysema and the flattened diaphragm.

The hospital course of bronchiolitis is variable and somewhat affected by the therapy employed. Significant improvement was noted in one-half of the cases within 2 days in one large study.[1] In the same study, about one-third of the cases had a gradual course without evidence of clear-cut improvement at any one time; 71 per cent of the patients were afebrile by the third hospital day. In another study performed more than 25 years later,[57] the average duration of symptoms was 3.4 days. Longer stays were required for infants with initial oxygen saturations of less than 90 per cent and those younger than 6 weeks of age at the onset of illness. Reasonable criteria for admission in otherwise healthy infants therefore would seem to include hypoxia (oxygen saturation of less than 90 to 92 per cent), age younger than 6 weeks, and a degree of respiratory distress sufficient to reduce fluid intake to inadequate levels. Other criteria include apnea, immunodeficiency, and the presence of significant underlying heart or lung disease. Most patients can be discharged from the hospital within 2 to 3 days after admission, although mild wheezing still may be present.

In 121 hospitalized patients, the total white blood cell count was less than 12,500/mm^3 in 74 per cent, and in only 15 determinations were there more than 60 per cent neutrophils.[1] In another study, Portnoy and colleagues[137] noted a mean leukocyte count of 16,000/mm^3 in children with lower respiratory tract disease, including bronchiolitis, as well as an increased percentage of band form neutrophils when compared with that of a control group. As in most infections, eosinophil counts in peripheral blood are reduced at the time of acute respiratory syncytial virus infection. Nevertheless, eosinophil counts still are greater in infants with respiratory syncytial virus bronchiolitis (particlarly in males) than in infants with upper respiratory illness alone due to respiratory syncytial virus.[52]

Abnormalities of blood gas tensions and pH occur and relate to the severity of disease. Hypoxemia is common; clinical cyanosis is not a reliable index of arterial oxygen tension (PaO_2).[34, 142, 161] The respiratory rate is related inversely to the PaO_2 except when respiratory failure is imminent. In mild to moderate cases, carbon dioxide retention does not occur because the alveoli that are functioning can compensate for alveoli that are not ventilated. In severe disease, the blood pH is low and the $PaCO_2$ is elevated.[37, 157] The technique of pulse oximetry has obviated the need for arterial blood gas sampling, except in severe cases where hypercarbia is a concern.

In certain patients, clinical findings (such as the degree of chest wall retractions and wheezing) often are out of proportion to the degree of hypoxia as measured by pulse oximetry.[121, 179] These infants with marked dyspnea must be evaluated carefully because respiratory failure may occur precipitously despite their relatively reassuring oximetry readings. A more meaningful scoring system to assess severity of illness has been developed.[60]

The roentgenographic appearance of the chest in bronchiolitis varies considerably.[92] Anteroposterior films may be normal in mild cases. In moderate to severe illness, radiographs often appear exceptionally clear because of hyperinflation. The diaphragms often are flattened or depressed. The costophrenic angle is less acute, and the hilar vascular shadows are stretched out. Frequently, areas of atelectasis give the appearance of pneumonitis, although true consolidation (as suggested by this appearance) is uncommon. The heart usually appears small, and the liver and spleen are pushed down by the depressed diaphragms.

On the lateral roentgenogram, the diaphragm is depressed markedly, and frequently there is reversal of the normal convexity. The anteroposterior diameter of the chest is increased.

With recurrent wheezing episodes, the prodrome may be considerably shorter in duration with little or no fever. Coryza may become progressively less noticeable or may even be absent in older children. In these afebrile children with brief prodromes, differentiation of infection-induced wheezing from more conventional asthma becomes essentially impossible clinically.[184]

TABLE 25–4. Factors Associated with an Increased Risk and Severity of Bronchiolitis and of Postbronchiolitic Morbidity

Factor	Increase in Frequency	Increase in Severity	Increase in Later Morbidity
Crowding	+ + +	+ + +	?
Passive smoking	+ + +	+ + +	+ +
Male gender	+	+ +	+ +
Absence of breast feeding	+	+	?
Family history of asthma	+/−	+/−	+/−
Personal atopy	−	−	+ + +
Congenitally small airways	+ +	?	−
Airway reactivity	−	+	+ +
RSV-specific IgE response	+ +	+ +	+ +

+ + +, implies strong relationship; + +, implies moderate relationship; +, implies weak relationship; +/−, implies controversial relationship; −, implies no relationship; ?, implies unknown relationship; RSV, respiratory syncytial virus.

From references 15, 31, 55, 62, 71, 94, 103, 109, 110, 159, 173, 181, 183, 185, 186, 192, 193, 196, and 197.

PATHOPHYSIOLOGY

The pathophysiology of bronchiolitis deservedly has been the focus of numerous investigations. Several original theories now can be discounted reliably, whereas others deserve further study. Pathologic examinations of the lung in bronchiolitis reveal necrosis of the respiratory epithelium with destruction of the ciliated layer; mononuclear cell invasion of the peribronchial tissues; edema of the submucosa and adventitia; and obstruction of small airways with dense plugs of mucus, fibrin, and alveolar debris. An associated interstitial pneumonitis may occur, and patchy areas of atelectasis are common.[2, 188] Recovery apparently is complete histologically,[188] although mucus plugging of the airway still was prominent in the airway of an infant 5 weeks after an acute episode of bronchiolitis. This infant had experienced a full clinical recovery (despite the persistent mucus plugging in some areas of the lung) before eventually dying of acute pneumococcal pneumonia.[123]

Infants particularly are prone to the development of severe illness as a result of infection of the small airways for many reasons, including the obviously small airway diameters. The infant lung is deficient in collateral alveolar ventilation through the pores of Kohn, which develop only in later life.[108] Therefore, atelectatic areas cannot be re-expanded readily. Other studies have demonstrated that the small airways in children younger than the age of 5 years contribute five- to sevenfold more to total airway resistance than do small airways of adults.[75] Therefore, viral infections involving small airways in young children would be much more likely to present as a serious clinical illness than would similar infections in adults. Nevertheless, most infants infected with respiratory syncytial virus do not develop lower respiratory illness, which suggests that host or environmental factors may be involved in determining the pathogenesis of respiratory syncytial virus infection. A list of environmental factors is presented in Table 25–4, and potentially important host factors are described later.

It has been demonstrated that certain infants, who apparently are in normal health, have relatively smaller airways than other infants on pulmonary function testing. When followed prospectively, these infants are somewhat more likely to develop wheezing early in life than are infants with larger airways.[109] Therefore, the presence of congenitally smaller airways may place infants at greater risk for bronchiolitis. These abnormalities of lung function no longer are associated with an increased risk of wheezing after 3 years of age. Instead, evidence of atopy then becomes the principal risk factor for recurrent wheezing.[110]

Several studies have demonstrated that the airways of infants are intrinsically more reactive to bronchospastic stimuli than airways of older children,[97, 173] particularly children from families with asthma.[196] How long this increased reactivity persists is unknown, but infants infected while airways are overly reactive to irritative stimuli presumably would be more likely to develop obstructive airway disease. In later childhood, repeated viral infections are necessary to sustain this increased reactivity.[178] Viral infections that clinically appear to be restricted to the upper respiratory tract in adults and children nevertheless result in transient, increased constrictive responses of the airway to a variety of stimuli, including histamine, irritants, and other agents (airway hyperreactivity), as well as small airway dysfunction.[3, 33, 41, 99] It has been postulated that these constrictive responses after infection occur as a result of denudation of airway epithelium with exposure and subsequent activation of airway irritant receptors, thereby effecting bronchoconstriction through stimulation of the parasympathetic nervous system.[41] Whether these changes could account for the severe degree of airway obstruction observed in bronchiolitis is in doubt, in that the abnormalities are relatively mild in comparison with the markedly increased reactivity that is observed in asthmatic individuals after exposure to allergens. Also, these virus-induced changes were observed in all infected individuals, including those who did not experience wheezing at the time of the virus infection. However, if airways already are hyperreactive in infants, either on a hereditary basis or as a result of a preceding viral infection, then the subsequent stimulus of respiratory syncytial virus infection may be sufficient to cause airway obstruction.

Immunologic deficits might be expected to lead to more severe forms of virus-induced respiratory illness. However, studies of the antibody response to respiratory syncytial virus infection both in serum and in respiratory secretions show that the response is similar among patients with bronchiolitis or simple upper respiratory illness alone due to this agent.[86, 182] Antibody-directed cellular cytotoxicity expressed against tissue culture cells infected with respiratory syncytial virus also is similar in patients with all forms of illness due to this agent.[84, 151] Also, although it has been shown that cells infected with respiratory syncytial virus can activate complement via both classical and alternate pathways,[163] currently available studies suggest that in vivo activation of the complement cascade occurs with equal frequency among patients with all forms of illness due to the virus.[85] Finally, when studied during the acute illness, cell-mediated immune responses (measured by lymphoproliferation) to respiratory syncytial virus and parainfluenza virus[152, 180] are greater among patients with bronchiolitis than among those with upper respiratory illness alone due to these agents. Cytotoxic T-lymphocyte activity is not detected easily in infants with bronchiolitis,[4] but there is no evidence for a deficiency of cytotoxic activity among these patients. In infants with the acquired immunodeficiency syndrome, respiratory syncytial virus infection may be unusually persistent, but bronchiolitis apparently is no more severe than in immunologically normal infants.[22, 90] Therefore, immunologic deficiency apparently can be excluded as a potential contributing factor in bronchiolitis.

Immunologic hypersensitivity, on the other hand, often has been suggested as playing a role in the development of severe bronchiolitis. Original field trials demonstrated that a formalin-inactivated respiratory syncytial virus vaccine induced humoral and cell-mediated immune responses to the virus. Nevertheless, vaccinated subjects manifested more severe forms of illness than unvaccinated controls when subjects in each group subsequently were infected naturally.[87] The resulting disease in vaccine recipients was quite similar in form to bronchiolitis occurring after natural respiratory syncytial virus infection, but there was an increased rate of hospitalization and two deaths in vaccinated individuals. Therefore, some form of hypersensitivity apparently was induced by vaccination.

Other studies of unvaccinated, naturally infected infants also suggest that immunologic sensitization to respiratory syncytial virus plays a role in disease pathogenesis. In one study, infants with fatal respiratory syncytial virus pneumonia had abundant virus but little immunoglobulin present in lung tissues, whereas infants with bronchiolitis had demonstrable immunoglobulin but no detectable virus.[50] It should be noted that this study included an extremely small number of patients. The concept that serum IgG antibody to respiratory syncytial virus, acquired either by vaccination or transplacentally, might sensitize the host has been dispelled by results of studies demonstrating that severe bronchiolitis may occur in the absence of circulating antibody[133] and that titers of maternal antibody actually correlate with protection against infection due to the virus.[55, 129]

Support for the concept that cell-mediated immune sensitization to respiratory syncytial virus may play a role in the pathogenesis of bronchiolitis comes from the results of several studies. Cell-mediated immune responses to viral antigen were greater among recipients of an inactivated respiratory syncytial virus vaccine than among control subjects who previously had experienced natural infection.[89] Exaggerated cell-mediated immune responses also were observed among infants younger than 6 months of age at the time of infection with respiratory syncytial virus (the group at the highest risk for bronchiolitis), in comparison with infants infected at a later age.[152] Finally, studies of infants acutely infected with respiratory syncytial virus[180] and parainfluenza virus have demonstrated enhanced cell-mediated immune responses among patients with bronchiolitis in comparison with upper respiratory illness alone due to either agent. The exact mechanism by which cell-mediated hypersensitivity might contribute to bronchiolitis requires further investigation. Mice infused with cytotoxic T lymphocytes previously sensitized to respiratory syncytial virus (by restimulation of cells with respiratory syncytial virus in vitro) develop much more severe lung pathology and exhibit higher death rates after respiratory syncytial virus infection than do mice infected without previous infusion of sensitized cells.[98] These results have not been confirmed in humans, partly because of the difficulty in demonstrating cytotoxic T lymphocytes in the peripheral blood of acutely infected subjects. An effect related to an exaggerated release of lymphokines also is possible. Lymphokines released by activated T lymphocytes (interleukins-3 and -5, among others) are capable of activating eosinophils and mast cells to release inflammatory factors.[42]

Immediate hypersensitivity to viral antigens has received much consideration as a potential contributing factor in bronchiolitis. The relationship of a family history of asthma to the development of bronchiolitis in infancy remains controversial.[94, 159, 164, 197] However, production of virus-specific IgE and subsequent release of mediators of bronchoconstriction have been documented in infants hospitalized with bronchiolitis due to respiratory syncytial virus and the parainfluenza viruses.[15, 181, 183, 184] In bronchiolitis caused by respiratory syncytial virus, the quantities of virus-specific IgE produced and histamine present in respiratory secretions correlate with the severity of illness, as measured by degree of arterial oxygen tension.[183] Leukotriene C_4 is a product of mast cells and eosinophils and is a potent stimulant of airway smooth muscle constriction and mucus secretion. This mediator is released into the airway in acute bronchiolitis,[177] as is histamine,[183] and both histamine and prostaglandins are found in increased concentrations in serum.[160] A possible role for eosinophils in the pathogenesis of bronchiolitis is supported by the finding of increased concentrations of eosinophil cationic protein in secretions of infants with bronchiolitis and an overall correlation of concentrations of this protein with the degree of hypoxia.[51, 52] Peripheral blood eosinophil counts are depressed during the acute phase of most infectious diseases, including respiratory syncytial virus infection. Nevertheless, eosinophil counts in peripheral blood are higher in infants with bronchiolitis than in those with upper respiratory illness only, particularly in males.[52] This is of interest because males generally have more severe forms of bronchiolitis. Therefore, there is reasonable evidence that the development of more severe forms of respiratory syncytial virus bronchiolitis may be a result of immunologic hypersensitivity responses occurring in the lung, particularly IgE-mediated hypersensitivity. Interestingly, eosinophils were observed in the lung tissues at autopsy in the two infants who developed fatal respiratory syncytial virus bronchiolitis after receiving the formalin-inactivated vaccine mentioned earlier.[87] This suggests that IgE-mediated hypersensitivity may have played a role in the adverse responses to that vaccine, as well as in the pathogenesis of bronchiolitis itself.

Other studies have identified potential mechanisms by which viral infections may precipitate airway obstruction in subjects with airways prone to constriction, although their actual role in expression of clinical illness remains to be defined. Immune complexes of respiratory syncytial virus and its antibody stimulate metabolism of granulocyte arachidonic acid to bronchoactive metabolites such as thromboxanes.[43] Viral infections induce beta-adrenergic blockade in granulocytes of asthmatic individuals,[17] although it is not known whether such changes also occur in cells in the respiratory tract that regulate airway diameter. Exposure of leukocytes to viral antigens in vitro enhances basophil histamine release upon appropriate stimulation.[18, 82] Finally, damage to the respiratory epithelium may have an enhancing effect on the magnitude of the IgE response to inhaled antigens[53]; thus, viral infections could contribute in this way to the development of wheezing.

It now is well known that children with histories of bronchiolitis manifest an increased frequency of airway hyperreactivity when tested many years after even a single episode of bronchiolitis. In some studies, these lung findings appear to be independent of a familial predisposition to asthma or to personal evidence of atopy.[61, 62, 83, 138, 158] In contrast, other studies suggest that recurrent wheezing after bronchiolitis and abnormalities of lung function are correlated with family histories of asthma (although not necessarily atopic disease in general) and personal evidence of atopy, such as the presence of cutaneous hypersensitivity to multiple allergens.[102, 103, 185, 197] Passive exposure to cigarette smoke also may contribute to long-term morbidity.[102, 103, 185, 193] Although it cannot be excluded that damage from the original viral infection leads to this observed increase in airway reactivity, results of in vitro tracheal organ cultures[72] and histopathologic studies in infants recovering from bronchiolitis[188] demonstrate that respiratory syncytial virus infection is confined to the superficial epithelium, and complete healing without residua is the rule. Therefore, it may seem more reasonable to conclude that airway hyperreactivity already was present at the time of the bronchiolitis episode, rather than being a result of infection. The demonstration of hyperreactive airways in the majority of normal infants strengthens this hypothesis.[97]

A unifying concept of the pathogenesis of bronchiolitis can be formulated incorporating the aforementioned findings. Bronchiolitis may occur as a result of infection in early life of individuals whose airways are hyperreactive and in those with congenitally smaller airways. Mild forms of illness occur in those individuals who are not additionally immunologically hypersensitive to viral antigen. In contrast, both severe forms of bronchiolitis and recurrent episodes of wheezing occur, according to currently available data, in those individuals who manifest IgE-mediated hypersensitivity to one or more viral antigens, possibly in addition to having increased airway reactivity. Increased airway reactivity is an inheritable trait, frequently acquired in association with a tendency to atopy,[10] and associated with abnormalities of lung function in asthmatics. Passive smoking and exposure to allergens may sustain increased airway reactivity in later childhood. The concept of increased airway reactivity as a fundamental defect in bronchiolitis therefore may explain the frequency of repeated wheezing episodes, the long-term abnormalities of pulmonary function, and the possible association of bronchiolitis with atopy.

DIFFERENTIAL DIAGNOSIS

All too frequently all infantile respiratory distress occurring after the immediate newborn period is considered to be bronchiolitis.[194] However, the list of causes of infantile dyspnea confused with bronchiolitis can be shortened considerably if the cardinal characteristic of bronchiolitis (lower airway obstruction) versus upper airway obstruction is considered—expiratory distress versus inspiratory distress. Recognition of upper airway obstructive disease should cause little difficulty, because the problem is one of distress with inspiration rather than air trapping. Illnesses that cause lower airway obstructive disease and diseases that suggest this problem are listed in Table 25–5.

TABLE 25–5. Differential Diagnostic Considerations in Acute Bronchiolitis and Infectious Asthma

Allergic
Asthma
Allergic pneumonias (allergic aspergillosis, etc.)
Anatomic
Vascular ring, lung cysts, lobar emphysema
Pneumothorax, hydrothorax, chylothorax
Foreign body
Circulatory Failure
Congenital and acquired heart disease
Anemia
Nephritis
Infections
Viral, chlamydial, rickettsial, mycoplasmal, bacterial, and fungal pneumonias
Migrating parasites
Irritants
Inhalation of toxic substance (chlorine gas, etc.)
Aspiration pneumonia
Gastroesophageal reflux
Metabolic
Poisons (salicylate, etc.)
Acidosis

The differential diagnosis of allergic disease causes the most difficulty. Generally, the first episode of allergic respiratory disease, when it occurs in association with infection, cannot be separated from bronchiolitis by any objective measures. Anatomic defects such as vascular rings can cause obstruction of the airway at many locations; thus, inspiratory, expiratory, or combination distress can occur. Frequently, a child with a defect will not have any difficulty until the occurrence of a trivial respiratory infection, which complicates the diagnostic picture.

Foreign bodies should be considered even in very young infants. Gastroesophageal reflux has become recognized as a frequent cause of wheezing in young infants. Because of its obvious therapeutic implications, bacterial pneumonia is the most important differential consideration, although wheezing occurs very infrequently in association with bacterial pneumonia.[106, 107]

SPECIFIC DIAGNOSIS

Because bronchiolitis and infectious asthma are clinical diseases with arbitrary boundaries and multiple etiologic agents, it is difficult to outline a method for specific diagnosis. When illness is epidemic, it virtually is assured that respiratory syncytial virus is the cause. History and appropriate laboratory studies and radiographs should be used to rule out the other differential possibilities that are listed in Table 25–5.

A specific etiologic diagnosis can be made by the isolation of virus from the nasopharynx. The diagnostic virologic facilities of many medical centers enable the isolation in tissue culture of respiratory syncytial virus, parainfluenza and influenza viruses, adenoviruses, rhinoviruses, enteroviruses, and herpesviruses. The use of the shell vial technique has been applied to respiratory syncytial virus infection with success.[162] The polymerase chain reaction technique also shows promise in amplification of small quantities of respiratory syncytial virus RNA from clinical specimens.[134] However, rapid detection of viral antigen of respiratory syncytial virus directly in nasopharyngeal secretions by commercially available (e.g., enzyme-linked immunosorbent assay) or fluorescent antibody techniques currently is the method of choice in most laboratories, for several reasons. The accuracy of these techniques probably is superior to that of standard cell culture, antigens remain stable under transport conditions that inactivate live virus, and results are available several days earlier than by cell culture. Infections with influenza and parainfluenza viruses and adenoviruses also can be identified by rapid detection techniques, and reliable commercial kits permitting simultaneous testing for each of these agents are available.

TREATMENT

The cornerstone of therapy for bronchiolitis is the administration of oxygen, because sicker patients usually are hypoxemic.[40, 157] Oxygen saturation should be maintained at 92 per cent or higher. Usually an oxygen concentration of 40 per cent will achieve this goal, and the patient's respiratory status can be monitored by pulse oximetry; however, blood gas determinations should be obtained when indicated by clinical findings (i.e., increasing respiratory rate, cyanosis, agitation). It is common practice to place children with bronchiolitis in tents and administer mist vigorously. Although oxygen should be humidified, the use of mists and aerosols except to deliver specific antiviral therapy is discouraged; mist can act as an irritant, causing reflex bronchoconstriction,[172] and the water usually does not reach the lower airways.[6]

Although dehydration is a potential problem in children with bronchiolitis because of vomiting and lack of intake, care must be taken not to overhydrate such patients. Because edema is an important part of the pathology of bronchiolitis, excess water can contribute to airway obstruction.

Beta-adrenergic bronchodilators have been employed frequently in bronchiolitis. Slight improvements in air flow, in oxygenation, and in clinical illness scores have been reported,[66, 91, 96, 147] but these effects are not likely to be meaningful clinically; hospitalization is not prevented, and hospital stays are not shortened. In one study, oral and aerosolized beta-adrenergic agents were compared with inactive substances given by the corresponding route. The degree of improvement was the same in all four groups.[49] Combinations of salbutamol and dexamethasone also have no objective effect.[170]

In the past, epinephrine often was administered subcutaneously to older infants in an attempt to differentiate allergic disease from true bronchiolitis. This approach rarely was successful either in differentiating one illness from the other or in improving the condition of the patient. However, one study suggested that aerosolized racemic epinephrine produced greater improvement than the use of beta-adrenergic aerosols alone.[148] Aerosolized sympathomimetic drugs are used frequently in older children with wheezing presumed to be caused by viral infections, with somewhat better results than in infants.[78, 96, 135, 147] Nevertheless, there is no evidence that this form of therapy reduces the need for hospitalization of these patients. In summary, trials of beta-adrenergic aerosols (and perhaps intravenous aminophylline) should be attempted in all seriously ill patients,[13, 40] although persistence with either of these approaches in the absence of an initial response may prove harmful.[81, 128] Aerosols of ipratropium also have been administered in bronchiolitis, without observable benefit.[153]

Possible explanations for poor responses to bronchodilators include a paucity of beta-adrenergic receptors in infancy[143]; decreased amounts of smooth muscle capable of responding to bronchodilators surrounding the terminal airways[140]; the nature of the airway obstruction itself (intense mucus plugging)[188]; and, presumably, persistence of virus in the airway, stimulating continued inflammation and/or release of bronchoconstrictive mediators.

Corticosteroids have been employed repeatedly in bronchiolitis. Controlled studies have failed to reveal any therapeutic advantage or harmful effects.[34, 35, 95, 104, 195] Corticosteroids seemingly have no place in the management of the moderately ill child with bronchiolitis, although it has never been determined if intervention with corticosteroids early in the course of bronchiolitis could prevent eventual hospitalization. In the child with life-threatening disease, corticosteroids need not be withheld because of fear of complications. There is evidence that administration of corticosteroids may be useful in prevention of recurrent attacks of bronchiolitis.[14, 19]

Early experience with the antiviral substance ribavirin in bronchiolitis suggested that mild subjective benefits as well as improvement in oxygenation occurred after near-continuous aerosol administration of this compound.[63, 64, 84, 145, 168] The degree of improvement in those treated with ribavirin was not marked. Furthermore, no study demonstrated whether the administration of ribavirin could prevent deaths, avoid the need for mechanical ventilation, or shorten hospital stays. Perhaps the most convincing study suggesting a beneficial effect of ribavirin involved the use of the drug in patients already receiving mechanically assisted ventilation. In this study, ribavirin recipients had a shorter duration of assisted ventilation, oxygen therapy, and hospitalization.[161] Controls in this study received water by aerosol, although inhalation of hypotonic solutions can provoke bronchospasm in certain individuals.[117] A subsequent study in a similar patient population, but using saline as a control substance, found only trends in favor of ribavirin that were not statistically significant.[111]

Ribavirin is quite expensive and is difficult to use because of the need for prolonged aerosol administration. Although the drug is hygroscopic and may precipitate in ventilatory circuits of mechanical ventilators, it can be administered safely to infants on mechanically assisted ventilation if plugging of the circuits is prevented by the use of filters.[131] Because ribavirin is teratogenic in rodents, concern has arisen regarding the safety of health care workers exposed to aerosols of the drug.[68, 144] Ribavirin has not been detected in plasma or urine samples of health care providers caring for patients receiving ribavirin by aerosol. Although absorption probably occurs in these workers, the amount absorbed is negligible. Women who already are pregnant may be excused from caring for patients receiving ribavirin, but further measures do not seem justifiable at this time. In summary, it is not possible to exclude completely a beneficial effect of ribavirin in patients with severe bronchiolitis, but the drug does not appear to be of benefit from a cost-effectiveness standpoint in those with any less severe degree of illness.

Other approaches to therapy of respiratory syncytial virus infection include the use of interferon-α[30] or vitamin A.[170] Data obtained to this point are inconclusive. A hyperimmune human immunoglobulin preparation containing a very high titer of neutralizing antibody against respiratory syncytial virus has been tested both in the prevention and treatment of respiratory syncytial virus infection in high-risk populations.[60, 69] The results of the prophylaxis study were positive, as discussed later. However, initial analysis of the data did not reveal a significant therapeutic effect of this compound once respiratory syncytial infection was established.

Because bronchiolitis is a viral disease, antibiotics are not useful or necessary. Unfortunately, in many instances, the radiographic picture is suggestive of pneumonia and the blood leukocyte count is elevated; the physician therefore feels compelled to administer antibiotics. There is no evidence of harm from this course of action, although overuse of potentially toxic antibiotics such as chloramphenicol should be resisted because bacterial infection of the lung is quite rare in bronchiolitis, even when infiltrates are present on chest radiographs. Institution of antibiotics should be considered during the course of therapy when a change in illness suggests the possibility of secondary bacterial infection. Cultures should be obtained (blood, tracheal aspirate) prior to therapy. When therapy is to be administered at the time of admission because of the possibility of pneumonia, the usual etiologic agents should be considered *(S. pneumoniae* and *H. influenzae)* and ampicillin or amoxicillin employed. When secondary infection is a possibility, *Staphylococcus aureus* and other hospital-associated organisms must be considered. Secondary bacterial infection occurred in no more than 7 of 565 (1.2 per cent) children with respiratory syncytial virus infection.[65]

The child with bronchiolitis generally will be more comfortable in the supine position with the head end of the crib slightly elevated. Infant seats are used frequently but are not optimal because the child's head tends to fall to the side or forward, which constricts the upper airway. The sitting position also causes a possibly deleterious upward pressure on the diaphragm.

If respiratory failure occurs (virtually absent inspiratory breath sounds, severe inspiratory retractions, cyanosis in 40 per cent oxygen, decreased or absent response to painful stimuli, and a $PaCO_2$ of ≥65 torr), ventilatory assistance, such as nasotracheal intubation, neuromuscular blockade, and positive pressure ventilation,[37, 130, 156] is indicated.

PREVENTION

The development of a method to prevent respiratory syncytial virus infection remains a high priority. Initially, a formalin-inactivated respiratory syncytial virus vaccine was prepared in a similar fashion to the early poliovirus vaccine. This vaccine was ineffective and in fact enhanced the severity of subsequent respiratory syncytial virus–related illness in vaccinees.[87] Later, a live, temperature-sensitive vaccine was developed by adapting respiratory syncytial virus to grow at low temperatures in cell culture. This attenuated vaccine was designed to grow at the lower temperatures of the upper respiratory tract but would be inactived at the higher temperatures in the lung. In initial field trials, the vaccine strain caused febrile respiratory illnesses in seronegative vaccinees but did not replicate adequately in seropositive subjects.[28] Further trials of temperature-sensitive mutant respiratory syncytial virus strains as vaccines currently are in progress. Another vaccine candidate consists of a purified preparation of the respiratory syncytial virus fusion protein, the protein responsible for fusion of the viral and host epithelial cell lipid membranes. This vaccine apparently is effective in previously infected children older than 18 months of age[174] but is ineffective in its current formulation in younger children.

In contrast to the largely negative experience with vaccine development, protection against serious illness due to respiratory syncytial virus infection has been achieved using a pooled preparation of human serum obtained from donors with very high titers of neutralizing antibody against respiratory syncytial virus.[60] This compound, when administered during the respiratory syncytial virus season on a monthly basis to infants and young children with a history of birth at less than 32 weeks' gestation or to those with bronchopulmonary dysplasia, caused a marked reduction in the severity of illness, rates of hospitalization, and duration of stays in the intensive care unit. A similar benefit could not be demonstrated in patients with underlying congenital heart disease. These trials presently are being repeated using a monoclonal antibody against the respiratory syncytial virus fusion protein.

COMPLICATIONS AND PROGNOSIS

Virtually all cases of bronchiolitis in healthy children resolve without acute complications. In the experience of the author, secondary bacterial infection in bronchiolitis now is extremely rare, although during the 1950s and early 1960s, when epidemic staphylococcal disease was prevalent, severe staphylococcal pneumonia sometimes occurred in patients originally presenting with bronchiolitis. Certainly, the appearance of a pleural effusion in bronchiolitis is an indication for prompt thoracentesis for exclusion of bacterial superinfection.

Scott and colleagues[150] noted minor electrocardiographic abnormalities in 2 per cent of 188 children with bronchiolitis.

The overall mortality in bronchiolitis is determined largely by the presence of underlying illness. Henderson and Rosenzweig[70] in 1951 and Dennis and associates[36] in 1960 noted a 2 per cent mortality during extensive studies of hospitalized cases in Detroit and Oakland. Heycock and Noble[74] noted a 5.5 per cent death rate during an 8-year period in which 1230 cases were reviewed. During a 5-year study period, Ackerman[1] observed no deaths in 207 cases, but two deaths occurred after the study. More recently, a multicenter study in Great Britain[31] estimated the minimum mortality due to respiratory syncytial virus infection in infancy at 0.5 per cent. Deaths should occur rarely, except in infants with severe underlying cardiac or pulmonary disease and in the absence of mechanisms for providing assisted ventilation. Mortality rates in infants with underlying cardiac or pulmonary disease are in the range of 3 to 5 per cent, even with modern methods of supportive care.[122]

The relationship of bronchiolitis to the subsequent development of asthma long has been controversial. As many as 50 per cent of patients with bronchiolitis have recurrent episodes of wheezing. Results of early studies revealed that evidence of an atopic disposition in bronchiolitis patients or in their families was correlated highly with the occurrence of wheezing in later childhood,[38, 44, 47, 146, 187, 197] but subsequent studies, particularly from Great Britain,[139, 158, 159] have found no such correlation. Titers of total serum IgE[136] and peripheral blood eosinophil counts[155] have some predictive value for recurrent wheezing after bronchiolitis. Also, pulmonary function tests performed in former bronchiolitis patients up to 12 years after an episode of bronchiolitis reveal an increased frequency of airway hyperreactivity in response to challenge with exercise or chemical agents, increased residual volume–to–total lung capacity ratios, reduced expiratory air flow at low lung volumes, and even abnormally low arterial oxygen tensions.[61, 83, 139, 158, 165, 171, 189] Although these abnormalities are observed commonly in individuals with asthma, they could not be explained in several of the above studies simply by the presence of a personal or family history of atopy.[62, 139, 158] Some factor other than atopy partially must determine the apparent sequelae of bronchiolitis.

Damage to the airway from the initial respiratory syncytial virus infection is one possible contributing factor. McConnochie and Roghmann[102] evaluated several epidemiologic factors and found that although exposure to cigarette smoke in the home in childhood and personal evidence of allergy were factors strongly predictive of recurrent wheezing, these factors did not account for all the recurrent episodes (airway reactivity was not assessed). These authors postulated that some long-term effect of bronchiolitis itself partially determined the risk of recurrent wheezing. However, when studied directly, long-term morbidity after bronchiolitis does not appear to be related to the severity of the initial episode of bronchiolitis or to the age of the infant at the time of the original infection,[61, 62, 139, 158] making it unlikely that the nature of the initial illness contributes substantially. Passive exposure to cigarette smoke, both during pregnancy and throughout childhood, also is a recognized risk factor for the development of bronchiolitis and recurrent wheezing after bronchiolitis.[102, 110, 185, 193]

Both the long-term pulmonary function abnormalities and the propensity for recurrent wheezing after bronchiolitis can be explained by the theory that bronchiolitis patients are born with hyperreactive airways that are prone to episodic obstruction. In follow-up studies performed at the author's institution,[185] recurrent wheezing at age 8 years was associated with comparatively greater reactivity of airways to provocholine challenge, and virtually all airway dysfunction measured was at least partially reversible with bronchodilators. These results suggest that increased airway reactivity contributes substantially to long-term abnormalities seen after bronchiolitis. Increased airway reactivity on a congenital basis cannot be the sole explanation. Factors such as exposure to cigarette smoke in infancy and childhood,[169, 193] atopic predisposition,[103, 185] and other considerations also play a role in the development of recurrent wheezing after bronchiolitis, but their effects may be mediated by sustaining hyperreactivity of the airway.

The overall outlook for infantile bronchiolitis generally is excellent. In a follow-up study conducted at the author's institution,[185] severe lung disease was not observed in former bronchiolitis patients. Oxygen saturations all were greater than 95 per cent, and at least some of the air flow obstruction present at age 7 to 9 years was reversible with a single bronchodilator treatment. It should be noted that single episodes of infantile bronchiolitis (in the absence of passive smoke exposure and without recurrent wheezing episodes) have not been associated with abnormalities of lung function or airway hyperreactivity in later childhood.[83, 166, 178] The natural history of postbronchiolitic wheezing in childhood is for episodes of wheezing to become progressively milder,[61, 102, 139, 158] and the frequency of postbronchiolitic wheezing eventually falls to essentially the same rate as that of children who did not experience bronchiolitis in infancy.[73, 102] Nevertheless, the overall prognosis is not entirely benign, and exposure to noxious environmental elements may result in an accelerated deterioration of lung function in later life.[32, 187, 191] The combination of respiratory tract illness in early life and subsequent cigarette smoking especially may be harmful.[16] It seems important that individuals who develop bronchiolitis in infancy should avoid smoking in later life, as well as occupations that are associated with exposure to irritants in the air.

References

1. Ackerman, B. D.: Acute bronchiolitis: A study of 207 cases. Clin. Pediatr. *1*:75–81, 1962.
2. Adams, J. M., Imagawa, D. T., and Zike, K.: Epidemic bronchiolitis and pneumonitis related to respiratory syncytial virus. J. A. M. A. *176*:1037–1039, 1961.
3. Aquilina, A. T., Hall, W. J., Douglas, G., et al.: Airway reactivity in subjects with viral upper respiratory tract infections: The effects of exercise and cold air. Am. Rev. Respir. Dis. *122*:3–10, 1980.
4. Bangham, R. M., Cannon, M. J., Karzon, D. T., et al.: Cytotoxic T-cell response to respiratory syncytial virus in mice. J. Virol. *56*:55–59, 1985.
5. Barr, S. E., Brown, H., Fuchs, M., et al.: A double-blind study of the effects of bacterial vaccine on infective asthma. J. Allergy *36*:47–61, 1965.
6. Bau, S. K., Aspin, N., Wood, D. E., et al.: The measurement of fluid deposition in humans following mist tent therapy. Pediatrics *48*:605–612, 1971.
7. Beem, M., Wright, F. H., Fasan, D. M., et al.: Observations on the etiology of acute bronchiolitis in infants. J. Pediatr. *61*:864–869, 1962.
8. Beem, M., Wright, F. H., Hamre, D., et al.: Association of the chimpanzee coryza agent with acute respiratory disease in children. N. Engl. J. Med. *263*:523–530, 1960.
9. Berkovich, S., Millian, S. J., and Snyder, R. D.: The association of viral and mycoplasma infections with recurrence of wheezing in the asthmatic child. Ann. Allergy *28*:43–49, 1970.
10. Boushey, H. A., Holtzman, M. J., Sheller, J. R., et al.: Bronchial hyperreactivity. Am. Rev. Respir. Dis. *121*:389–413, 1980.
11. Brandt, C. D., Kim, H. W., Arrobio, J. O., et al.: Epidemiology of respiratory syncytial virus infection in Washington, D.C. III. Composite analysis of eleven consecutive yearly epidemics. Am. J. Epidemiol. *98*:355–364, 1973.
12. Breese, B. B., Disney, F. A., and Talpey, W.: The nature of a small pediatric group practice: Part 1. Pediatrics *38*:264–277, 1966.
13. Brooks, L. J., and Cropp, G. J. A.: Theophylline therapy in bronchiolitis: A retrospective study. Am. J. Dis. Child. *135*:934–936, 1981.
14. Brunette, M. G., Lands, L., and Thibodeau, L. P.: Childhood asthma: Prevention of attacks with short-term corticosteroid treatment of upper respiratory tract infection. Pediatrics *81*:624–629, 1988.
15. Bui, R. H. D., Molinaro, G. A., Kettering, J. D., et al.: Virus-specific IgE and IgG_4 antibodies in serum of children infected with respiratory syncytial virus. J. Pediatr. *110*:87–90, 1987.
16. Burrows, B., Knudson, R. J., and Lebowitz, M. D.: The relationship of childhood respiratory illness to adult obstructive airway disease. Am. Rev. Respir. Dis. *115*:751–760, 1977.
17. Busse, W. W.: Decreased granulocyte response to isoproterenol in asthma during upper respiratory infections. Am. Rev. Respir. Dis. *115*:783–791, 1977.
18. Busse, W. W., Swenson, C. A., Borden, E. C., et al.: Effect of influenza A virus on leukocyte histamine release. J. Allergy Clin. Immunol. *71*:382–388, 1983.
19. Carlsen, K. H., Leegaard, J., Larsen, S., et al.: Nebulised beclomethasone dipropionate in recurrent obstructive episodes after acute bronchiolitis. Arch. Dis. Child. *63*:1428–1433, 1988.
20. Carmalt-Jones, D. W.: The treatment of bronchial asthma by a vaccine. Br. Med. J. 2:1049–1050, 1909.
21. Caul, E. O., Waller, D. K., Clarke, S. K. R., et al.: A comparison of influenza and respiratory syncytial virus infections among infants admitted to hospital with acute respiratory infections. J. Hyg. (Camb.) *77*:383–392, 1976.
22. Chandwani, S., Borkowsky, W., Krasinski, K., et al.: Respiratory syncytial virus infection in human immunodeficiency virus-infected children. J. Pediatr. *117*:251–254, 1990.
23. Chanock, R., Chambon, L., Chang, W., et al.: WHO Respiratory Disease Survey in Children: A serologic study. Bull. W. H. O. *37*:363–369, 1967.
24. Chanock, R. M., Parrott, R. H., Vargosko, A. J., et al.: IV. Respiratory syncytial virus. Am. J. Public Health *52*:918–925, 1962.
25. Chanock, R. M., Mufson, M. A., and Johnson, K. M.: Comparative biology and ecology of human virus and mycoplasma respiratory pathogens. Prog. Med. Virol. *7*:208–252, 1965.
26. Chanock, R. M., and Parrott, R. H.: Acute respiratory disease in infancy and childhood: Present understanding and prospects for prevention. Pediatrics *36*:21–39, 1965.
27. Chanock, R. M., Kim, H. W., Vargosko, A. J., et al.: Respiratory syncytial virus. I. Virus recovery and other observations during a 1960 outbreak of bronchiolitis, pneumonia, and minor respiratory diseases in children. J. A. M. A. *176*:647–653, 1961.
28. Chanock, R. M. and Murphy, B. R.: Use of temperature-sensitive and cold-adapted mutant viruses in immunoprophylaxis of acute respiratory tract disease. Rev. Infect. Dis. *2*:421–431, 1980.
29. Cherry, J. D.: Newer respiratory viruses: Their role in respiratory illness of children. Adv. Pediatr. *20*:225–290, 1973.
30. Chipps, B. E., Sullivan, W. F., and Portnoy, J. M.: Alpha-2a-interferon for treatment of bronchiolitis caused by respiratory syncytial virus. Pediatr. Infect. Dis. J. *12*:653–658, 1993.
31. Clarke, S. K. R., Gardner, P. S., Poole, P. M., et al.: Respiratory syncytial virus infection: Admissions to hospital in industrial, urban, and rural areas. Br. Med. J. *2*:796–798, 1978.
32. Colley, J. R. T., Douglas, J. W. B., and Reid, D. D.: Respiratory disease in

young adults: Influence of early childhood lower respiratory tract illness, social class, air pollution, and smoking. Br. Med. J. *3*:195–198, 1973.
33. Collier, A. M., Pimmel, R. L., Hasselblad, V., et al.: Spirometric changes in normal children with upper respiratory infections. Am. Rev. Respir. Dis. *117*:47–53, 1978.
34. Connolly, J. H., Field, C. M. B., Glasgow, J. F. T., et al.: A double blind trial of prednisolone in epidemic bronchiolitis due to respiratory syncytial virus. Acta Paediatr. Scand. *58*:116–120, 1969.
35. Dabbous, I. A., Tkachyk, J. S., and Stamm, S. J.: A double blind study on the effects of corticosteroids in the treatment of bronchiolitis. Pediatrics *37*:477–484, 1966.
36. Dennis, J. L., Palmer, W. M., and Cleveland, R. W.: Bronchiolitis in infants: Problem in practice. J. A. M. A. *172*:688–691, 1960.
37. Downes, J. J., Wood, D. W., Striker, T. W., et al.: Acute respiratory failure in infants with bronchiolitis. Anesthesiology *29*:426–434, 1968.
38. Eisen, A. H., and Bacal, H. L.: The relationship of acute bronchiolitis to bronchial asthma: A 4 to 14 year followup. Pediatrics *31*:859–861, 1963.
39. Eisen, A. H.: The role of infection in allergic disease. Pediatr. Clin. North Am. *16*:67–83, 1969.
40. Ellis, E. F.: Therapy of acute bronchiolitis. Pediatr. Res. *11*:263–264, 1977.
41. Empey, D. W., Laitinen, L. A., Jacobs, L., et al.: Mechanisms of bronchial hyperreactivity in normal subjects after upper respiratory tract infection. Am. Rev. Respir. Dis. *113*:131–139, 1976.
42. Fabian, I., Kletter, Y., Mor, S., et al.: Activation of human eosinophil and neutrophil functions by haematopoietic growth factors: Comparisons of IL-1, IL-3, IL-5 and GM-CSF. Br. J. Haematol. *80*:137–143, 1992.
43. Faden, H., Kaul, T. N., and Ogra, P. L.: Activation of oxidative and arachidonic acid metabolism in neutrophils by respiratory syncytial virus antibody complexes: Possible role in disease. J. Infect. Dis. *148*:110–116, 1983.
44. Field, C. M. B., Connolly, J. H., Murtagh, G., et al.: Antibiotic treatment of epidemic bronchiolitis: A double-blind trial. Br. Med. J. *1*:83–85, 1966.
45. Fontana, V. J., Salanitro, A. S., Wolfe, H. I., et al.: Bacterial vaccine and infectious asthma. J. A. M. A. *193*:895–900, 1965.
46. Foy, H. M., Cooney, M. K., Maletzky, A. J., et al.: Incidence and etiology of pneumonia, croup and bronchiolitis in preschool children belonging to a prepaid medical care group over a four-year period. Am. J. Epidemiol. *97*:80–92, 1973.
47. Freeman, G. L., and Todd, R. H.: The role of allergy in viral respiratory tract infections. Am. J. Dis. Child. *104*:330–334, 1962.
48. Freeman, G. L.: Wheezing associated with respiratory tract infections in children. Clin. Pediatr. *5*:586–592, 1966.
49. Gadomski, A. M., Aref, G. H., Badr El Din, O., et al.: Oral versus nebulized albuterol in the management of bronchiolitis in Egypt. J. Pediatr. *124*:131–138, 1994.
50. Gardner, P. S., McQuillin, J., and Court, S. D. M.: Speculation on pathogenesis in death from respiratory syncytial virus infection. Br. Med. J. *1*:327–332, 1970.
51. Garofalo, R., Kimpen, J. L. L., Welliver, R. C., et al.: Eosinophil degranulation in naturally acquired respiratory syncytial virus infection. J. Pediatr. *120*:28–32, 1992.
52. Garofalo, R., Dorris, A., Ahlstedt, S., et al.: Peripheral blood eosinophil counts and eosinophil cationic protein content of respiratory secretions in bronchiolitis: Relationship to severity of disease. Pediatr. Allergy Immunol. *5*:111–117, 1994.
53. Gershwin, L. J., Osebold, J. W., and Zee, Y. C.: Immunoglobulin E-containing cells in mouse lung following allergen inhalation and ozone exposure. Int. Arch. Allergy Appl. Immunol. *65*:266–277, 1981.
54. Glezen, W. P., Loda, F. A., Clyde, W. A., Jr., et al.: Epidemiologic patterns of acute lower respiratory disease of children in a pediatric group practice. J. Pediatr. *78*:397–406, 1971.
55. Glezen, W. P., Paredes, A., Allison, J. E., et al.: Risk of respiratory syncytial virus infection for infants from low-income families in relationship to age, sex, ethnic group, and maternal antibody level. J. Pediatr. *98*:708–715, 1981.
56. Glezen, W. P., Taber, L. H., Frank, A. L., et al.: Risk of primary infection and reinfection with respiratory syncytial virus. Am. J. Dis. Child. *140*:543–546, 1986.
57. Green, M., Brayer, A. F., Schenkman, K. A., et al.: Duration of hospitalization in previously well infants with respiratory syncytial virus infection. Pediatr. Inf. Dis. J. *8*:601 605, 1989.
58. Gregg, I.: The role of viral infection in asthma and bronchitis. *In* Proudfoot, A. T. (ed.): Symposium on Viral Diseases. Edinburgh, T. A. Constable Ltd., 1975, pp. 82–98.
59. Griffith, J. P. C., and Mitchell, A. G.: The Diseases of Infants and Children. Vol. II. Philadelphia, W. B. Saunders, 1927, pp. 274–355.
60. Groothuis, J. R., Simoes, E. A. F., Levin, M. J., et al.: Prophylactic administration of a respiratory syncytial virus immune globulin to high-risk infants and young children. N. Engl. J. Med. *329*:1524–1530, 1993.
61. Gurwitz, D., Mindorff, C., and Levison, H.: Increased incidence of bronchial reactivity in children with a history of bronchiolitis. J. Pediatr. *98*:551–555, 1981.
62. Hall, C. B., Hall, W. J., Gala, C. L., et al.: Long-term prospective study in children after respiratory syncytial virus infection. J. Pediatr. *105*:358–364, 1984.
63. Hall, C. B., McBride, J. T., Walsh, E. E., et al.: Aerosolized ribavirin treatment of infants with respiratory syncytial viral infection. N. Engl. J. Med. *308*:1443–1447, 1983.
64. Hall, C. B., McBride, J. T., Gala, C. L., et al.: Ribavirin treatment of respiratory syncytial virus infection in infants with underlying cardiopulmonary disease. J. A. M. A. *254*:3047–3051, 1985.
65. Hall, C. B., Powell, K. R., Schnabel, K. C., et al.: Risk of secondary bacterial infection in infants hospitalized with respiratory syncytial viral infection. J. Pediatr. *113*:266–271, 1988.
66. Hammer, J., Numa, A., and Newth, C. J. L.: Albuterol responsiveness in infants with respiratory failure caused by respiratory syncytial virus infection. J. Pediatr. *127*:485–490, 1995.
67. Hampton, S. F., Johnson, M. C., and Galakatos, E.: Studies of bacterial hypersensitivity in asthma. I. The preparation of antigen of *Neisseria catarrhalis*, the induction of asthma by aerosols, the performance of skin and passive transfer tests. J. Allergy *34*:63–95, 1963.
68. Harrison, R., Bellows, J., Rempel, D., et al.: Assessing exposures of health-care personnel to aerosols of ribavirin: California. M. M. W. R. *37*:560–563, 1988.
69. Hemming, V. G., and Prince, G. A.: Immunoprophylaxis of infections with respiratory syncytial virus: Observations and hypothesis. Rev. Infect. Dis. *12*:S470–S475, 1990.
70. Henderson, A. T., and Rosenzweig, S.: Bronchiolitis in infancy: Clinical study with special emphasis on the cardiac complications. U. S. Armed Forces Med. J. 2:943–952, 1951.
71. Henderson, F. W., Clyde, W. A., Jr., Collier, A. M., et al.: The etiologic and epidemiologic spectrum of bronchiolitis in pediatric practice. J. Pediatr. *95*:183–190, 1979.
72. Henderson, F. W., Hu, S. C., and Collier, A. M.: Pathogenesis of respiratory syncytial virus infection in ferret and fetal human tracheas in organ culture. Am. Rev. Respir. Dis. *118*:29–37, 1978.
73. Henderson, F. W., Stewart, P. W., Burchinal, M. R., et al.: Respiratory allergy and the relationship between early childhood lower respiratory illness and subsequent lung function. Am. Rev. Respir. Dis. *145*:283–290, 1992.
74. Heycock, J. B., and Noble, T. C.: 1,230 cases of acute bronchiolitis in infancy. Br. Med. J. *5309*:879–881, 1962.
75. Hogg, J. C., Williams, J., Richardson, J. B., et al.: Age as a factor in the distribution of lower-airway conductance and in the pathologic anatomy of obstructive lung disease. N. Engl. J. Med. *282*:1283–1287, 1970.
76. Holt, L. E., and Howland, J.: Diseases of the lungs: Peculiarities of the thorax in children. *In* Holt, L. E., and McIntosh, R. (eds.): Holt's Diseases of Infancy and Childhood. 11th ed. New York, D. Appleton-Century Co., 1940, pp. 498, 513.
77. Horn, M. E. C., Brain, E., Gregg, I., et al.: Respiratory viral infection in childhood: A survey in general practice, Roehampton 1967–1972. J. Hyg. (Camb.) *74*:157–168, 1975.
78. Horn, M. E. C., Brain, E. A., Gregg, I., et al.: Respiratory viral infection and wheezy bronchitis in childhood. Thorax *34*:23–28, 1979.
79. Horn, M. E. C., Reed, S. E., and Taylor, P.: Role of viruses and bacteria in acute wheezy bronchitis in childhood: A study of sputum. Arch. Dis. Child. *54*:587–592, 1979.
80. Hubble, D., and Osborn, G. R.: Acute bronchiolitis in children. Br. Med. J. *1*:107–110, 1941.
81. Hughes, D. M., Lesouef, P. N., and Landau, L. I.: Effect of salbutamol on respiratory mechanics in bronchiolitis. Pediatr. Res. *22*:83–86, 1987.
82. Ida, S., Hooks, J. J., Siraganian, R. P., et al.: Enhancement of IgE-mediated histamine release from human basophils by viruses: Role of interferon. J. Exp. Med. *145*:892–906, 1977.
83. Kattan, M., Keens, T. G., Lapierre, J. G., et al.: Pulmonary function abnormalities in symptom-free children after bronchiolitis. Pediatrics *59*:683–688, 1977.
84. Kaul, T. N., Welliver, R. C., and Ogra, P. L.: Development of antibody dependent cell-mediated cytotoxicity in the respiratory tract after natural infection with respiratory syncytial virus. Infect. Immun. *37*:492–498, 1982.
85. Kaul, T. N., Welliver, R. C., and Ogra, P. L.: Appearance of complement components and immunoglobulins on nasopharyngeal epithelial cells following naturally acquired infection with respiratory syncytial virus. J. Med. Virol. *9*:149–158, 1982.
86. Kaul, T. N., Welliver, R. C., Wong, D. T., et al.: Secretory antibody response to respiratory syncytial virus infection. Am. J. Dis. Child. *135*:1013–1016, 1981
87. Kim, H. W., Canchola, J. G., Brandt, C. D., et al.: Respiratory syncytial virus disease in infants despite prior administration of antigenic inactivated vaccine. Am. J. Epidemiol. *89*:422–434, 1969.
88. Kim, H. W., Arrobio, J. O., Brandt, C. D., et al.: Epidemiology of respiratory syncytial virus infection in Washington, D.C. I. Importance of the virus in different respiratory tract disease syndromes and temporal distribution of infection. Am. J. Epidemiol. *98*:216–225, 1973.
89. Kim, H. W., Leikin, S. L., Arrobio, J., et al.: Cell-mediated immunity to respiratory syncytial virus induced by inactivated vaccine or by infection. Pediatr. Res. *10*:75–78, 1976.
90. King, J. C., Jr., Burke, A. R., Clemens, J. D., et al.: Respiratory syncytial virus illnesses in human immunodeficiency virus– and noninfected children. Pediatr. Infect. Dis. J. *12*:733–739, 1993.

91. Klassen, T. P., Rowe, P. C., Sutcliffe, T., et al.: Randomized trial of salbutamol in acute bronchiolitis. J. Pediatr. *118*:807–811, 1991.
92. Koch, D. A.: Roentgenologic considerations of capillary bronchiolitis. Am. J. Roentgenol. Rad. Ther. Nucl. Med. *82*:433–436, 1959.
93. Kravitz, H.: Sex distribution of hospitalized children with acute respiratory diseases, gastroenteritis and meningitis. Clin. Pediatr. *4*:484–491, 1965.
94. Laing, I., Riedel, F., Yap, P. L., et al.: Atopy predisposing to acute bronchiolitis during an epidemic of respiratory syncytial virus. Br. Med. J. *284*:1070–1072.
95. Leer, J. A., Jr., Green, J. L., Heimlich, E. M., et al.: Corticosteroid treatment in bronchiolitis: A controlled, collaborative study in 297 infants and children. Am. J. Dis. Child. *117*:495–502, 1969.
96. Lenney, W., and Milner, A. D.: Alpha and beta adrenergic stimulants in bronchiolitis and wheezy bronchitis in children under 18 months of age. Arch. Dis. Child. *53*:707–709, 1978.
97. Lesouef, P. N., Geelhoed, G. C., Turner, D. J., et al.: Response of normal infants to inhaled histamine. Am. Rev. Respir. Dis. *139*:62–66, 1989.
98. Liew, F. Y., and Russell, S. M.: Inhibition of pathogenic effect of effector T cells by specific suppressor T cells during influenza virus infection in mice. Nature *304*:541–543, 1983.
99. Little, J. W., Hall, W. J., Douglas, R. G., et al.: Airway hyperreactivity and peripheral airway dysfunction in influenza A infection. Am. Rev. Respir. Dis. *118*:295–303, 1978.
100. Loda, F. A., Clyde, W. A., Jr., Glezen, W. P., et al.: Studies on the role of viruses, bacteria, and *M. pneumoniae* as causes of lower respiratory tract infections in children. J. Pediatr. *72*:161–176, 1968.
101. Loda, F. A., Glezen, W. P., and Clyde, W. A., Jr.: Respiratory disease in group day care. Pediatrics *49*:428–437, 1972.
102. McConnochie, K. M., and Roghmann, K. J.: Bronchiolitis as a possible cause of wheezing in childhood: New evidence. Pediatrics *74*:1–10, 1984.
103. McConnochie, K. M., and Roghmann, K. J.: Wheezing at age 8 and 13 years: Changing importance of bronchiolitis and passive smoking. Pediatr. Pulmonol. 6:138–146, 1989.
104. McGeorge, M.: Severe obstructive bronchiolitis in infancy: Treatment with hydrocortisone. Clin. Pediatr. *3*:11–18, 1964.
105. McIntosh, K.: Bronchiolitis and asthma: Possible common pathogenic pathways. J. Allergy Clin. Immunol. *57*:595–604, 1976.
106. McIntosh, K., Ellis, E. F., Hoffman, L. S., et al.: The association of viral and bacterial respiratory infections with exacerbations of wheezing in young asthmatic children. J. Pediatr. *82*:578–590, 1973.
107. Macasaet, F. F., Kidd, P. A., Bolano, C. R., et al.: The etiology of acute respiratory infections. III. The role of viruses and bacteria. J. Pediatr. *72*:829–839, 1968.
108. Macklin, C. C.: Alveolar pores and their significance in the human lung. Arch. Pathol. *21*:202, 1936.
109. Martinez, F. D., Morgan, W. J., Wright, A. L., et al.: Diminished lung function as a predisposing factor for wheezing respiratory illness in infants. N. Engl. J. Med. *319*:1112–1117, 1988.
110. Martinez, F. D., Wright, A. L., Taussig, L. M., et al.: Asthma and wheezing in the first six years of life. N. Engl. J. Med. *332*:133–138, 1995.
111. Meert, K. L., Sarnaik, A. P., Gelmini, M. J., et al.: Aerosolized ribavirin in mechanically ventilated children with respiratory syncytial virus lower respiratory tract disease: A prospective, double-blind, randomized trial. Crit. Care Med. *22*:566–572, 1994.
112. Miller, D. G., Gabrielson, M. O., and Horstmann, D. M.: Clinical virology and viral surveillance in a pediatric group practice: The use of double-seeded tissue culture tubes for primary virus isolation. Am. J. Epidemiol. *88*:245–256, 1968.
113. Minor, T. E., Baker, J. W., Dick, E. C., et al.: Greater frequency of viral respiratory infections in asthmatic children as compared with their non-asthmatic siblings. J. Pediatr. *85*:472–477, 1974.
114. Minor, T. E., Dick, E. C., De Meo, A. N., et al.: Viruses as precipitants of asthmatic attacks in children. J. A. M. A. *227*:292–298, 1974.
115. Minor, T. E., Dick, E. C., Baker, J. W., et al.: Rhinovirus and influenza type A infections as precipitants of asthma. Am. Rev. Respir. Dis. *113*:149–153, 1976.
116. Mitchell, I., Inglis, J. M., and Simpson, H.: Viral infection as a precipitant of wheeze in children: Combined home and hospital study. Arch. Dis. Child. *53*:106–111, 1978.
117. Moler, F. W., Bandy, K. P., and Custer, J. R.: Ribavirin therapy for acute bronchiolitis: Need for appropriate controls. J. Pediatr. *119*:509, 1991.
118. Mueller, H. L.: The dual role of infection in asthma of childhood. Postgrad. Med. *50*:225–229, 1971.
119. Mueller, H. L., and Lanz, M.: Hyposensitization with bacterial vaccine in infectious asthma: A double-blind study and a longitudinal study. J. A. M. A. *208*:1379–1383, 1969.
120. Mufson, M. A., Krause, H. E., Mocega, H. E., et al.: Viruses, *Mycoplasma pneumoniae* and bacteria associated with lower respiratory tract disease among infants. J. Epidemiol. *91*:192–202, 1970.
121. Mulholland, E. K., Olinsky, A., and Shann, F.: Clinical findings and severity of acute bronchiolitis. Lancet *335*:1259–1261, 1990.
122. Navas, L., Wang, E., de Carvalho, V., et al.: Improved outcome of respiratory syncytial virus infection in a high-risk hospitalized population of Canadian children. J. Pediatr. *121*:348–354, 1992.
123. Neilson, K. A., and Yunis, E. J.: Demonstration of respiratory syncytial virus in an autopsy series. Pediatr. Pathol. *10*:491–502, 1990.
124. Nelson, W. E.: Viral or probable viral infections. *In* Nelson, W. E. (ed.): Pediatrics. 6th ed. Philadelphia, W. B. Saunders, 1954, pp. 823–828, 1438–1446.
125. Nelson, W. E., and Smith, L. W.: Generalized obstructive emphysema in infants. J. Pediatr. *26*:36–55, 1945.
126. Neuzil, K. M., Gruber, W. C., Chytil, F., et al.: Safety and pharmacokinetics of vitamin A therapy for infants with respiratory sncytial virus infections. Antimicrob. Agents Chemother. *39*:1191–1193, 1995.
127. Nichol, K. P., and Cherry, J. D.: Bacterial-viral interrelations in respiratory infections of children. N. Engl. J. Med. *277*:667–672, 1967.
128. O'Callaghan, C., Milner, A. D., and Swarbrick, A.: Paradoxical deterioration in lung function after nebulised salbutamol in wheezy infants. Lancet *2*:1424–1425, 1986.
129. Ogilvie, M. M., Vathenen, S., Radford, M., et al.: Maternal antibody and respiratory syncytial virus infection in infancy. J. Med. Virol. *7*:263–271, 1981.
130. Outwater, K. M., and Crone, R. K.: Management of respiratory failure in infants with acute viral bronchiolitis. Am. J. Dis. Child. *138*:1071–1075, 1984.
131. Outwater, K. M., Meissner, C., and Peterson, M. B.: Ribavirin administration to infants receiving mechanical ventilation. Am. J. Dis. Child. *142*:512–515, 1988.
132. Parrott, R. H.: Viral respiratory tract illnesses in children. Bull. N.Y. Acad. Med. *39*:629–648, 1963.
133. Parrott, R. H., Kim, H. W., Arrobio, J. O., et al.: Epidemiology of respiratory syncytial virus infection in Washington, D.C. II. Infection and disease with respect to age, immunologic status, race and sex. Am. J. Epidemiol. *98*:289–300, 1973.
134. Paton, A. W., Paton, J. C., Lawrence, A. J., et al.: Rapid detection of respiratory syncytial virus in nasopharyngeal aspirates by reverse transcription and polymerase chain reaction amplification. J. Clin. Microbiol. *30*:901–904, 1992.
135. Phelan, P. D., and Williams, H. E.: Sympathomimetic drugs in acute viral bronchiolitis: Their effect on pulmonary resistance. Pediatrics *44*:493–497, 1969.
136. Polmar, S. H., Robinson, L. D., Jr., and Minnefor, A. B.: Immunoglobulin E in bronchiolitis. Pediatrics *50*:279–284, 1972.
137. Portnoy, B., Hanes, B., Salvatore, M. A., et al.: The peripheral white blood count in respirovirus infection. J. Pediatr. *68*:181–188, 1966.
138. Pratt, E. L.: Acute bronchiolitis in infants. Med. Clin. North Am. *28*:1098–1107, 1944.
139. Pullan, C. R., and Hey, E. N.: Wheezing, asthma, and pulmonary dysfunction 10 years after infection with respiratory syncytial virus in infancy. Br. Med. J. *284*:1665–1669, 1982.
140. Reid, L.: Influence of the pattern of structural growth of lung on susceptibility to specific infectious diseases in infants and children. Pediatr. Res. *11*:210–215, 1977.
141. Reilly, C. M., Stokes, J., Jr., McClelland, L., et al.: Studies of acute respiratory illnesses caused by respiratory syncytial virus. 3. Clinical and laboratory findings. N. Engl. J. Med. *264*:1176–1182, 1961.
142. Reynolds, E. O. R.: Bronchiolitis. *In* Kendig, E. L., Jr. (ed.): Disorders of the Respiratory Tract in Children. Philadelphia, W. B. Saunders, 1967, pp. 272–282.
143. Roan, Y., and Galant, S. P.: Decreased neutrophil beta adrenergic receptors in the neonate. Pediatr. Res. *16*:591–593, 1982.
144. Rodriguez, W. J., Bui, R. H. D., Connor, J. D., et al.: Environmental exposure of primary care personnel to ribavirin aerosol when supervising treatment of infants with respiratory syncytial virus infections. Antimicrob. Agents Chemother. *31*:1143–1146, 1987.
145. Rodriguez, W. J., Kim, H. W., Brandt, C. D., et al.: Aerosolized ribavirin in the treatment of patients with respiratory syncytial virus disease. Pediatr. Infect. Dis. J. *6*:159–163, 1987.
146. Rooney, J. C., and Williams, H. E.: The relationship between proved viral bronchiolitis and subsequent wheezing. J. Pediatr. *79*:744–747, 1971.
147. Rutter, N., Milner, A. D., and Hiller, E. J.: Effect of bronchodilators on respiratory resistance in infants and young children with bronchiolitis and wheezy bronchitis. Arch. Dis. Child. *50*:719–722, 1975.
148. Sanchez, I., De Koster, J., Powell, R., et al.: Effect of racemic epinephrine and salbutamol on clinical score and pulmonary mechanics in infants with bronchiolitis. J. Pediatr. *122*:145–151, 1993.
149. Sandiford, B. R., and Spencer, B.: Respiratory syncytial virus in epidemic bronchiolitis of infants. Br. Med. J. *5309*:881–882, 1962.
150. Scott, L. P., III, Gutelius, M. F., and Parrott, R. H.: Children with acute respiratory tract infections: An electrocardiographic survey. Am. J. Dis. Child. *119*:111–113, 1970.
151. Scott, R., DeLandazuri, M. O., Gardner, P. S., et al.: Human antibody-dependent cell-mediated cytotoxicity against target cells infected with respiratory syncytial virus. Clin. Exp. Immunol. *28*:19–26, 1977.
152. Scott, R., Kaul, A., Scott, M., Chiba, Y., et al.: Development of in vitro correlates of cell-mediated immunity to respiratory syncytial virus infection in humans. J. Infect. Dis. *137*:810–817, 1978.
153. Seidenberg, J., Masters, I. B., Hudson, I., et al.: Effect of ipratropium

bromide on respiratory mechanics in infants with acute bronchiolitis. Aust. Paediatr. J. *23*:169–172, 1987.
154. Sell, S. H. W.: Some observations on acute bronchiolitis in infants. Am. J. Dis. Child. *100*:31–39, 1960.
155. Simon, G., and Jordan, W. S., Jr.: Infectious and allergic aspects of bronchiolitis. J. Pediatr. *70*:533–538, 1967.
156. Simpson, H., Matthew, D. J., Habel, A. H., et al.: Acute respiratory failure in bronchiolitis and pneumonia in infancy: Modes of presentation and treatment. Br. Med. J. 2:632–636, 1974.
157. Simpson, H., Matthew, D. J., Inglis, J. M., et al.: Virological findings and blood gas tensions in acute lower respiratory tract infections in children. Br. Med. J. *2*:629–632, 1974.
158. Sims, D. G., Downham, M. A. P. S., Gardner, P. S., et al.: Study of 8-year-old children with a history of respiratory syncytial virus bronchiolitis in infancy. Br. Med. J. *1*:11–14, 1978.
159. Sims, D. G., Gardner, P. S., Weightman, D., et al.: Atopy does not predispose to RSV bronchiolitis or postbronchiolitic wheezing. Br. Med. J. *282*:2086–2088, 1981.
160. Skoner, D. P., Fireman, P., Caliguiri, L., et al.: Plasma elevations of histamine and a prostaglandin metabolite in acute bronchiolitis. Am. Rev. Respir. Dis. *142*:359–364, 1990.
161. Smith, D. W., Frankel, L. R., Mathers, L. H., et al.: A controlled trial of aerosolized ribavirin in infants receiving mechanical ventilation for severe respiratory syncytial virus infection. N. Engl. J. Med. *325*:24–29, 1991.
162. Smith, M. C., Creutz, C., and Huang, Y. T.: Detection of respiratory syncytial virus in nasopharyngeal secretions by shell vial technique. J. Clin. Microbiol. *29*:463–465, 1991.
163. Smith, T. F., McIntosh, K., Fishaut, M., et al.: Activation of complement by cells infected with respiratory syncytial virus. Infect. Immun. *33*:43–48, 1981.
164. Stempel, D. A., Clyde, W. A., Jr., Henderson, F. W., et al.: Serum IgE levels and the clinical expression of respiratory illnesses. J. Pediatr. *97*:185–190, 1980.
165. Stokes, G. M., Milner, A. D., Hodges, I. G. C., et al.: Lung function abnormalities after acute bronchiolitis. J. Pediatr. *98*:871–874, 1981.
166. Strope, G. L., Stewart, P. W., Henderson, F. W., et al.: Lung function in school-age children who had mild lower respiratory illnesses in early childhod. Am. Rev. Respir. Dis. *144*:655–662, 1991.
167. Sturdy, P. M., McQuillin, J., and Gardner, P. S.: A comparative study of methods for the diagnosis of respiratory virus infections in childhood. J. Hyg. (Camb.) *67*:659–670, 1969.
168. Taber, L. H., Knight, V., Gilbert, B. E., et al.: Ribavirin aerosol treatment of bronchiolitis associated with respiratory syncytial virus infection in infants. Pediatrics *72*:613–618, 1983.
169. Tager, I. B., Weiss, S. T., Munoz, A., et al.: Longitudinal study of the effects of maternal smoking on pulmonary function in children. N. Engl. J. Med. *309*:699–703, 1983.
170. Tal, A., Bavilski, C., Yohai, D., et al.: Dexamethasone and salbutamol in the treatment of acute wheezing in infants. Pediatrics *71*:13–18, 1983.
171. Taussig, L. M.: Clinical and physiologic evidence of the persistence of pulmonary abnormalities after respiratory illnesses in infancy and childhood. Pediatr. Res. *11*:216–218, 1977.
172. Taussig, L. M.: Mists and aerosols: New studies, new thoughts. J. Pediatr. *84*:619–622, 1974.
173. Tepper, R. S., Rosenberg, D., and Eigen, H.: Airway responsiveness in infants following bronchiolitis. Pediatr. Pulmonol. *13*:6–10, 1992.
174. Tristram, D. A., Welliver, R. C., Mohar, C. K., et al.: Immunogenicity and safety of respiratory syncytial virus subunit vaccine in seropositive children 18–36 months old. J. Infect. Dis. *167*:191–195, 1993.
175. Twarog, F. J., and Colten, H. R.: Rational management of allergic disease: The role of immunotherapy. Pediatrics *60*:320–323, 1977.
176. Vikerfors, T., Grandien, M., and Olcen, P.: Respiratory syncytial virus infections in adults. Am. Rev. Respir. Dis. *136*:561–564, 1987.
177. Volovitz, B., Welliver, R. C., DeCastro, G., et al.: The release of leukotrienes in the respiratory tract during infection with respiratory syncytial virus: Role in obstructive airway disease. Pediatr. Res. *24*:504–507, 1988.
178. Voter, K. Z., Henry, M. M., Stewart, P. W., et al.: Lower respiratory illness in early childhood and lung function and bronchial reactivity in adolescent males. Am. Rev. Respir. Dis. *137*:302–307, 1988.
179. Wang, E. E. L., Milner, R. A., Navas, L. et al.: Observer agreement for respiratory signs and oximetry in infants hospitalized with lower respiratory infections. Am. Rev. Respir. Dis. *145*:106–109, 1992.
180. Welliver, R. C., Kaul, A., and Ogra, P. L.: Cell-mediated immune response to respiratory syncytial virus infection: Relationship to the development of reactive airway disease. J. Pediatr. *94*:370–375, 1979.
181. Welliver, R. C., Kaul, T. N., and Ogra, P. L.: The appearance of cell-bound IgE in respiratory-tract epithelium after respiratory-syncytial-virus infection. N. Engl. J. Med. *303*:1198–1202, 1980.
182. Welliver, R. C., Kaul, T. N., Putnam, T. I., et al.: The antibody response to primary and secondary infection with respiratory syncytial virus: Kinetics of class-specific responses. J. Pediatr. *96*:808–813, 1980.
183. Welliver, R. C., Wong, D. T., Sun, M., et al.: The development of respiratory syncytial virus-specific IgE and the release of histamine in nasopharyngeal secretions after infection. N. Engl. J. Med. *305*:841–846, 1981.
184. Welliver, R. C., Wong, D. T., Middleton, E., Jr., et al.: Role of parainfluenza virus-specific IgE in pathogenesis of croup and wheezing subsequent to infection. J. Pediatr. *101*:889–896, 1982.
185. Welliver, R. C., and Duffy, L.: The relationship of RSV-specific immunoglobulin E antibody responses in infancy, recurrent wheezing, and pulmonary function at age 7–8 years. Pediatr. Pulmonol. *15*:19–27, 1993.
186. Williams, H., and McNicol, K. N.: Prevalence, natural history, and relationship of wheezy bronchitis and asthma in children: An epidemiological study. Br. Med. J. *4*:321–325, 1969.
187. Wittig, H. J., Cranford, N. J., and Glasner, J.: The relationship between bronchiolitis and childhood asthma: A follow-up study of 100 cases of bronchiolitis in infancy. J. Allergy *30*:19–23, 1959.
188. Wohl, M. E. B., and Chernick, V.: Bronchiolitis. Am. Rev. Respir. Dis. *118*:759–781, 1978.
189. Wohl, M. E. B., Stigol, L. C., and Mead, J.: Resistance of the total respiratory system in healthy infants and infants with bronchiolitis. Pediatrics *43*:495–509, 1969.
190. Wood, S. H., Buddingh, G. J., and Abberger, B. F., Jr.: An inquiry into the etiology of acute bronchiolitis of infants. Pediatrics *13*:363–372, 1954.
191. Woolcock, A. J., Leeder, S. R., Peat, J. K., et al.: The influence of lower respiratory illness in infancy and childhood and subsequent cigarette smoking on lung function in Sydney schoolchildren. Am. Rev. Respir. Dis. *120*:5–14, 1979.
192. Wright, A. L., Taussig, L. M., Ray, C. G., et al.: The Tucson children's respiratory study. II. Lower respiratory illness in the first year of life. Am. J. Epidemiol. *129*:1232–1246, 1989.
193. Wright, A. L., Holberg, C., Martinez, F. D., et al.: Relationship of parental smoking to wheezing and nonwheezing lower respiratory tract illnesses in infancy. J. Pediatr. *118*:207–214, 1991.
194. Wright, F. H., and Beem, M. O.: Diagnosis and treatment: Management of acute viral bronchiolitis in infancy. Pediatrics *35*:334–337, 1965.
195. Yaffe, S. J., Weiss, C. F., Cann, H. M., et al.: Should steroids be used in treating bronchiolitis? Pediatrics *46*:640–642, 1970.
196. Young, S., Le Souf, P., Geelhoed, G. et al.: The influence of a family history of asthma and parental smoking on airway responsiveness in early infancy. N. Engl. J. Med. *324*:1168–1174, 1991.
197. Zweiman, B., Schoenwetter, W. F., Pappano, J. E., Jr., et al.: Patterns of allergic respiratory disease in children with a past history of bronchiolitis. J. Allergy Clin. Immunol. *48*:283–289, 1971.

26

NONBACTERIAL PNEUMONIA

Kenneth M. Boyer

Nonbacterial pneumonias are the most frequent pulmonary infections encountered in pediatrics.[35, 36, 41, 47, 53, 70, 71, 82, 83, 86, 113, 117, 134, 137, 140, 143, 166, 169, 172, 177, 181, 218] A number of terms are used for these conditions, based on their causes, clinical presentations, or histologic features. Although their connotations differ, viral pneumonia, atypical pneumonia, infant pneumonitis, and interstitial pneumonia frequently are encountered. The varied causes, excluding bacteria and fungi, cover a broad taxonomic spectrum. With improvement in microbiologic techniques, the number of known causative agents continues to increase. Defining etiology once was in the province of the epidemiologist and virologist, but a sufficient body of knowledge has accumulated to permit informed diagnostic judgment by the practicing physician and rapid specific diagnosis by the clinical microbiology laboratory. Although most nonbacterial pneumonias have a good prognosis, they occasionally are life-threatening. Therapy directed against the causative agent may shorten the course or avert serious complications. Occasionally, it is lifesaving.

The features of infection by the more common nonbacterial causes of pneumonias are covered in greater detail in other chapters of this book (see Sections 13, 14, 17, 18, 19, 20, 22). This chapter provides an overview of pneumonia syndromes caused by viruses, mycoplasmas, and chlamydiae, as well as by *Coxiella burnetti* and *Pneumocystis carinii.*

HISTORICAL ASPECTS

The development of systematic bacteriology in the late nineteenth century led to the widespread belief that pneumonias were bacterial infections with differences in presentation (broncho, lobular, lobar) that primarily were the result of differences in anatomic localization. During the 1918 influenza pandemic, most postmortem examinations of pneumonia patients revealed numerous bacteria in the lungs. A variety of different species were identified, not exclusively *Haemophilus influenzae*, the organism at that time regarded as the cause of influenza. In a few cases in which no bacteria were found, Goodpasture[87] and Winternitz and colleagues[224] found distinctive histopathologic lesions in the lung that prompted the conclusion that they were induced by a nonbacterial agent. The isolation of influenza A virus by Smith and associates[209] in 1933, therefore, altered the prevailing bacteriologic and anatomic concepts of pneumonia and ushered in a new era of etiologic diagnosis of respiratory syndromes.

The first isolation of influenza virus, and the subsequent isolation of *Chlamydia psittaci* (psittacosis) and *C. burnetii* (Q fever), involved transmission of infection to experimental animals such as ferrets and chick embryos. The development of tissue culture techniques in the 1950s enabled a number of other common respiratory viruses to be identified—adenoviruses, parainfluenza viruses, respiratory syncytial virus (RSV), enteroviruses, and rhinoviruses. The major etiologic agent of primary atypical pneumonia had been passed to experimental animals in the 1940s but was not identified definitely as a mycoplasma until 1962.[41]

In the 1960s and 1970s, the most valuable studies of nonbacterial respiratory infections in pediatrics were comprehensive longitudinal investigations in which epidemiologic and clinical patterns of illness were defined. These studies established that the majority of lower respiratory tract infections in infants and young children are caused by nonbacterial agents, principally respiratory viruses and *Mycoplasma pneumoniae.* The attention of current investigators increasingly is directed at developing methods for rapid diagnosis, chemotherapy, and prevention, although new agents—for example, *Chlamydia trachomatis* and *Chlamydia pneumoniae*—continue to be associated with distinctive pediatric pneumonia syndromes.

ETIOLOGY

Three *Mycoplasma* species, one *Rickettsia* species, three *Chlamydia* species, one protozoan parasite, and at least 14 different virus groups have been associated with pneumonia syndromes in children. The overall importance of these agents is not measured simply by their incidence. Some agents, although quite common, generally give rise to relatively mild illness; others, less frequently encountered, characteristically may cause serious disease. In Table 26–1, the major agents in various age groups are presented by their overall frequency, their typical degree of severity, and their mode of access to the lung. Although the incidence data are representative of a number of major epidemiologic studies,[35, 36, 41, 47, 54, 62, 69–71, 82, 83, 86, 113, 134, 137, 143, 146, 166, 169, 172, 177, 181, 218] it should be recalled that the maximum proportion of pneumonias of proven cause in such studies has been about 50 per cent. Possible explanations for the high proportion of cases of unknown cause include bacterial etiology[161]; late collection of viral cultures and sera[70]; suboptimal storage, transport, or cultivation of specimens[83, 193]; and as yet unidentified agents.

RSV generally is accepted as the most frequent agent in pediatric pneumonias, particularly those associated with bronchiolitis.[15, 18, 23, 25, 107, 118, 124, 152, 165, 210, 217] Although infection with this virus is quite common in all age groups, lower respiratory tract involvement especially is prominent in infancy.

The three parainfluenza viruses (para 1, para 2, and para 3) are second only to RSV as causes of lower respiratory tract disease in infants and younger children. Para 3 is the most frequent of these agents in pneumonia[81, 85, 112, 179]; infection by para 1 and para 2 generally produces laryngotracheitis.

Influenza A and B viruses are not as prevalent overall as RSV and parainfluenza viruses, but during periods of epidemic spread they may become predominant isolates in hospitalized children with lower respiratory tract diseases.[13, 24, 86, 125, 176, 180, 201]

Adenoviruses are common isolates in children with pneumonia[4, 7, 17, 22, 26, 38, 82, 108, 110, 111, 119, 170, 185, 214, 227] and pertussis syndrome.[22, 49, 171, 173] Their overall impact in causation of nonbacterial pneumonia in children probably is somewhat less than that of the aforementioned agents; however, a number of fatal illnesses have been reported. Their common asymptomatic carriage and potential for endogenous activation by unrelated illnesses can make proof of causation difficult.[68, 171] Of the 49 known adenoviruses, types 1, 2, 3, 4, 5, 7, 14, 21, and 35 clearly have been associated with pneumonia.[22, 126] In certain aboriginal populations, such as the Maori, Native American, and Inuit, adenoviruses commonly produce severe infection.[109, 130] In military recruits, adenoviruses are second to *M. pneumoniae* as a cause of atypical pneumonia.[55]

Rhinoviruses[13, 78, 182, 191, 215] have been associated less frequently with pneumonia, although upper respiratory infection with the multiple serotypes of these organisms is frequent. Some degree of lower respiratory involvement by rhinoviruses also is indicated by their documented role in exacerbations of asthma[162] and bronchitis.[157] Among the enteroviruses, primary virus pneumonia has been documented best with coxsackieviruses A9[135] and B1,[58] although coxsackieviruses A16, B4, and B5 and echoviruses 9, 11, 19, 20, and 22 also have been reported.[41, 95, 205] Coronaviruses have been implicated as causes of pneumonia in a few seroepidemiologic studies, but tissue culture recovery of these agents has been rare.[123, 154]

Pneumonia is the most frequent serious complication of measles. Kohn and Koiransky[128] demonstrated by careful radiographic study that 55 per cent of routine measles cases had pulmonary infiltrates early in the illness, suggesting viral, rather than bacterial, causation. Secondary bacterial pneumonia in measles is due to the common respiratory pathogens: *Streptococcus pneumoniae, H. influenzae, Streptococcus pyogenes,* and *Staphylococcus aureus.* Progressive, fatal, primary measles pneumonia (Hecht giant-cell pneumonia) occurs in immunocompromised patients, particularly those

TABLE 26–1. Etiologic Agents in Nonbacterial Pneumonia

Etiologic Agents	Frequency*			Usual Degree of Severity†			Mode of Access to Lung
	0–3 mo	*4 mo–5 yr*	*6–16 yr*	*0–3 mo*	*4 mo–5 yr*	*6–16 yr*	
Virus							
Respiratory syncytial virus	+ + +	+ + + +	+	+ +	+ +	−	Respiratory
Parainfluenza viruses							
Type 1	+	+ +	+	+ +	+ +	+	Respiratory
Type 2	+	+	+	+ +	+ +	+	Respiratory
Type 3	+ +	+ + +	+ +	+ +	+ +	+	Respiratory
Influenza viruses							
Type A	+ +	+ + +	+ + +	+ +	+ +	+	Respiratory
Type B	+ +	+ +	+	+ +	+ +	+	Respiratory
Adenoviruses‡	+	+ +	+ +	+ + +	+ +	+	Respiratory
Rhinoviruses§	+	+	+	−	+ +	+	Respiratory
Enteroviruses¶	+	+	+	+ +	+ +	+	Respiratory (hematogenous)
Coronaviruses	−	+	+	−	+ +	+	Respiratory
Measles virus	+	+ +	+ +	+ + +	+ +	+ +	Respiratory (hematogenous)
Rubella virus	+	−	−	+ +	−	−	Hematogenous
HIV	+	+ +	+	+ +	+ +	+ +	Hematogenous
Varicella-zoster virus	+	+	+	+ + +	+ + +	+ + +	Hematogenous (respiratory)
Cytomegalovirus	+ + +	+	+	+ +	+ + +	+ + +	Hematogenous (respiratory)
Epstein-Barr virus	−	+	+ +	−	+ +	+	Hematogenous (respiratory)
Herpes simplex virus	+ +	+	+	+ + + +	+ + +	+ + +	Hematogenous (respiratory)
Mycoplasmas							
Mycoplasma pneumoniae	−	+	+ + + +	−	+ +	+	Respiratory
Mycoplasma hominis	?	−	−	?	−	−	Respiratory
Ureaplasma urealyticum	?	−	−	?	−	−	Respiratory
Chlamydiae							
Chlamydia pneumoniae	?	?	+ + +	?	?	+	Respiratory
Chlamydia psittaci	+	+	+	−	+ +	+ +	Respiratory
Chlamydia trachomatis	+ + + +	−	−	+ +	−	−	Respiratory
Rickettsiae							
Coxiella burnetii	−	+	+	−	+ +	+ +	Respiratory (hematogenous)
Protozoa							
Pneumocystis carinii	+	+ +	+	+ + +	+ + +	+ + +	Respiratory

*+ + + +, most frequent; + + +, frequent; + +, infrequent; +, rare; −, no reported cases; ?, uncertain.
†+ + + +, often fatal; + + +, severe; + +, usually hospitalized; +, home management; −, no reported cases; ?, uncertain.
‡Types 1, 2, 3, 4, 5, 7, 14, and 21.
§90 or more types known.
¶Coxsackieviruses A9, A16, B1, B4, and B5; echoviruses 9, 11, 19, 20, and 22.

with hematologic malignancy and AIDS.[129, 147, 203, 204] The typical measles rash often is absent. Persons immunized with killed measles virus vaccine during the 1960s can experience an unusual nodular pneumonia, along with vasculitis of the distal extremities, when infected with wild measles virus. Although rare, atypical measles remains important because its pathogenetic mechanism has implications for development of new vaccines.[73]

Viruses that may attack the lungs by hematogenous spread include varicella-zoster virus (VZV), Epstein-Barr virus (EBV), rubella virus, cytomegalovirus (CMV), herpes simplex virus (HSV), and HIV. Rubella virus, CMV, and HSV may cause interstitial pneumonia in the congenitally or perinatally infected infant.[8, 104, 229, 230] CMV and VZV are causes of life-threatening pneumonia in the immunocompromised host.[114, 186, 223] Pneumonia has been noted in association with primary EBV infections.[5, 61] Pulmonary infiltration also is a component of the fatal X-linked lymphoproliferative syndrome caused by EBV.[189] One of the characteristic features of HIV infection in children is lymphocytic interstitial pneumonitis, an indolent but progressive process that occurs in about a quarter of children who develop AIDS.[196] Both HIV RNA and EBV DNA have been demonstrated in the lung tissue of affected children.[6] The relative contributions of the two agents to the pathogenesis of lymphocytic interstitial pneumonitis are not understood clearly, although EBV is suspected to be the trigger.[122]

Of the 15 known *Mycoplasma* species that infect humans, only *M. pneumoniae* is a well-established cause of pneumonia. In children younger than 2 years of age, infection is common but pneumonia is unusual. In children older than 5 years of age, *M. pneumoniae* is the most common etiology of nonbacterial pneumonia.[43, 70] Studies have associated genital mycoplasmas, in particular *Ureaplasma urealyticum* and *Mycoplasma hominis,* with congenital and perinatally acquired pneumonia. However, proof of causation is not secure.[30, 31]

Three *Chlamydia* species have been associated with pneumonia. *Chlamydia psittaci* is the well-recognized cause of psittacosis (ornithosis). *C. trachomatis,* the established agent of inclusion blenorrhea in the neonate, causes a characteristic afebrile pneumonitis syndrome in infants 4 to 14 weeks of age.[16] In urban areas in the United States where the condition has been studied carefully—Chicago, Seattle, San Francisco, and Birmingham—it is the most frequent cause of pneumonia in that age group.[57, 106] *C. pneumoniae* was isolated first in 1965 and recognized as a cause of pneumonia in 1986.[89] It now is emerging as one of the more frequent causes of pneumonia in older children and young adults.[90, 198]

Of the rickettsiae, only *C. burnetii* is associated with pneumonia, in the form of Q fever. This infection may be severe but, owing to its restricted ecologic niche, is rare in children.

P. carinii, a protozoan parasite, is an important cause of pneumonia in the compromised host,[114, 186, 223] although its incidence in children receiving chemotherapeutic regimens for malignancy has been reduced dramatically by the use of trimethoprim-sulfamethoxazole (TMP-SMX) prophylaxis.[115] *P. carinii* is an established cause of pneumonia in premature and debilitated infants[76] and, with *C. trachomatis,* CMV, and genital mycoplasmas, has been associated with the afebrile pneumonitis syndrome of infancy.[57, 184, 212, 213] It is the most frequent cause of death in infants with HIV infection, although the incidence in this population will be affected by earlier diagnosis and more aggressive chemoprophylactic use of TMP-SMX.[34, 206]

EPIDEMIOLOGY

The major contributors to the overall epidemiology of nonbacterial pneumonias in children are RSV, parainfluenza viruses, *M. pneumoniae,* and, to a lesser extent, influenza viruses A and B.[54] Because of their brief incubation periods and high degree of communicability, these agents often spread through communities in well-defined waves (Fig. 26–1).[81, 83] During intervals between epidemics, RSV, para 1 and 2, and influenza viruses A and B rarely are isolated. Between peaks, *M. pneumoniae* and para 3 tend to persist endemically. During respiratory disease seasons in the colder months, an interference phenomenon has been noted whereby peaks of infection by particular agents seldom occur simultaneously (Fig. 26–2).[83]

Annual incidence rates of childhood pneumonia show a rough inverse correlation with age, ranging from 40 per 1000 in children younger than 5 years of age to 7 per 1000 in adolescents 12 to 15 years of age.[70, 169] RSV is the most common etiologic agent in children younger than 5 years of age; *M. pneumoniae* is most common in those who are older than that age.[70] Most studies have shown a male predominance in pediatric lower respiratory infections on the order of 1.25 to 1. Increased rates of lower respiratory infections in lower socioeconomic groups correlate best with family size, a reflection of environmental crowding.[83]

Pregnancy, chronic lung disease, valvular heart disease, and neuromuscular conditions in adults predispose to greater severity of viral, particularly influenzal, pneumonia.[142] In children, congenital heart disease and bronchopulmonary dysplasia are associated with greater severity of viral pneumonia, particularly with RSV.[144] Pulmonary deterioration in patients with cystic fibrosis has been shown to be accelerated by respiratory viral infection.[220] In treated hematologic malignancy, marrow transplantation, and immunosuppressed states, common respiratory viruses have been recognized increasingly as causes of severe pneumonia and respiratory failure.[102, 105] Children with these underlying conditions also are prone to serious pulmonary infection with such agents as measles virus, VZV, and CMV, which have the capacity for hematogenous dissemination and viral latency. Pediatric HIV infection has added a new category of immunocompromised children susceptible to these pathogens as well as the common bacterial agents of pneumonia. Profoundly immunocompromised patients, as in severe combined immunodeficiency disease, are prone to progressive as well as prolonged pulmonary disease caused by common respiratory viruses.[120]

Transmission of the more common agents of lower respiratory tract disease most often is by means of droplet spread resulting from relatively close contact with a source case. Direct inoculation at the alveolar level probably does not occur in most cases because of the extremely small size of aerosolized particles necessary to accomplish this. Studies of nosocomially transmitted RSV infections have shown the importance of adults with relatively trivial upper respiratory infection as intermediates in transmission to susceptible young infants.[98] School age children often introduce respiratory viral agents into households, resulting in secondary infections in parents and younger siblings.[83] The increasing

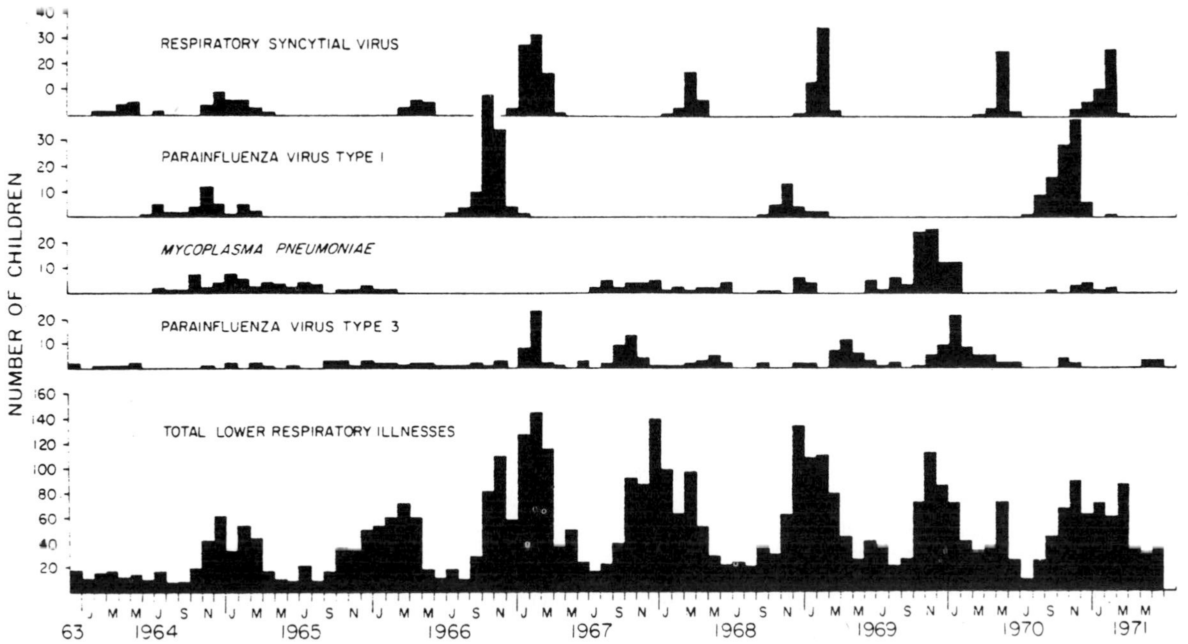

FIGURE 26–1. *Number of isolations, according to month, of four major respiratory pathogens from children with lower respiratory illnesses in Chapel Hill, North Carolina. (From Glezen, W. P., and Denny, F. W.: Epidemiology of acute lower respiratory disease in children. N. Engl. J. Med. 288:500, 1973. Reprinted with permission from the New England Journal of Medicine.)*

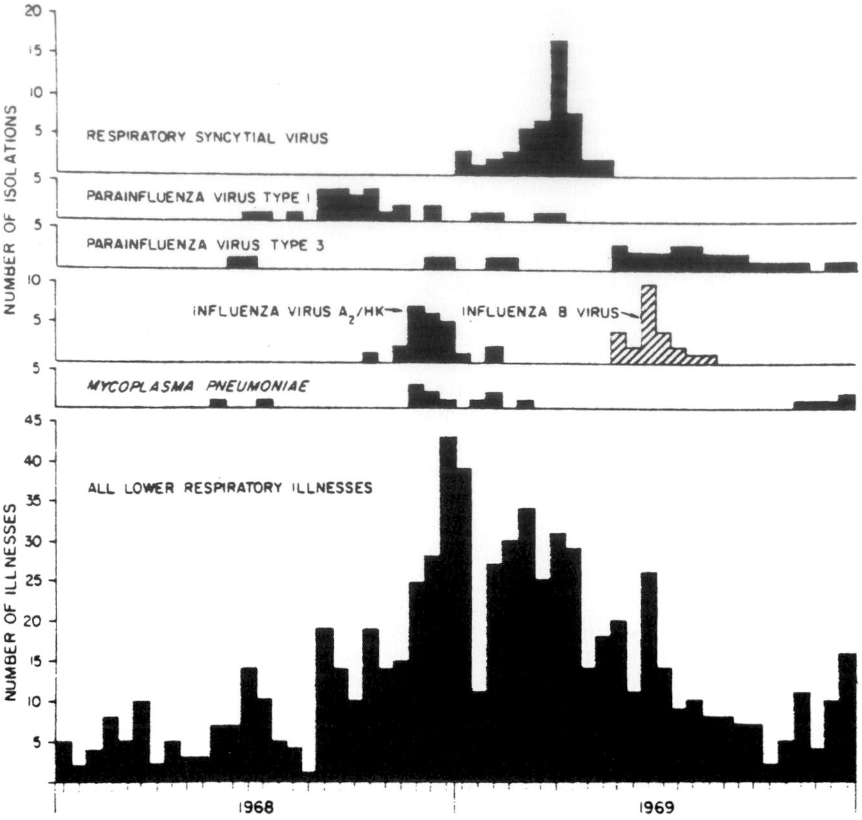

FIGURE 26–2. *Weekly isolations, in 1968 and 1969, of respiratory pathogens from children with lower respiratory illnesses in Chapel Hill, North Carolina. (From Glezen, W. P., and Denny, F. W.: Epidemiology of acute lower respiratory disease in children. N. Engl. J. Med. 288:500, 1973. Reprinted with permission from the New England Journal of Medicine.)*

use of group day care by working parents has been associated with enhanced transmission of a number of respiratory pathogens[44, 139] and certainly has extended "school age" to a younger group of children.

PATHOGENESIS AND PATHOLOGY

After inoculation of the upper respiratory tract, viral agents that cause pneumonia proliferate and spread by contiguity to involve lower and more distal portions of the respiratory tract. Infected epithelium loses its ciliary appendages, rounds up, and sloughs into the air passages, resulting in stasis of mucus and accumulation of cellular debris.[1, 29, 231] When infection extends to the terminal airways, alveolar lining cells lose their structural integrity, resulting in loss of surfactant production, hyaline membrane formation, and pulmonary edema. Inflammatory response at the site of tissue damage results in mononuclear infiltration of submucosal and interstitial structures, which further contributes to narrowing of air passages and alveolocapillary block of gas exchange. Relative expiratory obstruction results in hyperinflation and "air trapping." Complete obstruction or stop-valve mechanisms result in atelectasis. Ventilation-perfusion mismatch further exacerbates hypoxia.

The relative rarity of fatal outcome in common nonbacterial pneumonias has resulted in a relatively narrow view of their characteristic pathology, limited largely to autopsy studies of overwhelming illnesses in infants and military recruits. The pathology associated with infection by RSV, adenoviruses, and influenza virus A has been studied most extensively in humans. Studies of the pathology of RSV, parainfluenza virus, and *Mycoplasma* infections have been aided by animal model systems such as mice,[88] the Syrian hamster,[84] and the cotton rat.[93]

Five major pathologic expressions have been described in fatal human infections, any or all of which may be present in a given case: acute bronchiolitis, necrotizing bronchiolitis, interstitial pneumonia, alveolar pneumonia, and diffuse alveolar damage. Acute bronchiolitis is characterized by relatively superficial and reversible destruction of ciliated respiratory epithelium, with accompanying mononuclear infiltration. Necrotizing bronchiolitis extends to the deeper submucosal layers lining the respiratory tract and may not be as readily reversible. It is associated particularly with adenovirus pneumonia.[14] Interstitial pneumonia is a diffuse process in which the inflammatory mononuclear response predominantly involves the peribronchial alveolar septa. In alveolar pneumonia, the alveoli are filled with degenerating lining cells and mononuclear or polymorphonuclear inflammatory cells with or without hyaline membranes. Hyaline membranes consist of fibrin deposits triggered by local release of tissue factor–factor VII complex as well as inhibitors of fibrinolysis.[19] When hyaline membranes are present, the process is described as diffuse alveolar damage. It is the histopathologic hallmark of the acute phase of the adult respiratory distress syndrome.[194, 195] Acute bronchiolitis and interstitial pneumonia are observed in most cases of fatal nonbacterial pneumonia, regardless of cause.[1] Alveolar pneumonia may reflect bacterial superinfection, adult respiratory distress syndrome, or agonal changes associated with intensive ventilator support and oxygen toxicity.

Three important factors that influence the pathologic expression of nonbacterial pneumonias in children are anatomy, preexisting pulmonary disease, and immunity. In the young infant, the small caliber of the terminal airways and the absence of interconnections between alveolar spaces (pores of Kohn) contribute to wheezing and lobular atelectasis.[168, 225] Preexisting pulmonary disease—for example, bronchopulmonary dysplasia—is characterized by emphysema, squamous metaplasia of the tracheobronchial tree, hypertrophied goblet cells, and enhanced airway smooth muscle reactivity. Inability to clear the excessive secretions triggered by infection in patients with bronchopulmonary dysplasia often leads to bronchospasm, atelectasis, and respiratory failure.

Immunopathologic mechanisms have been invoked to explain the disparities in clinical expression of infection by RSV and *M. pneumoniae* between infants and older children.[37, 155] Interaction between RSV-infected epithelial cells and specific IgE, leading to histamine release, has been postulated as an immune mechanism for bronchospasm in RSV disease.[221] Cumulative immunity after repeated natural infections by *M. pneumoniae* may account for the more impressive clinical expression of illness in older children and adults.[66] Specific cell-mediated immunity, detectable at low levels in young children but increased in adults, probably contributes to pathogenesis.

Opportunistic nonbacterial pathogens generally take advantage of the defects in cell-mediated immunity induced by immunosuppressive therapy or HIV infection. A variety of unique pathologic expressions of viral pneumonia may ensue in these circumstances, including giant-cell pneumonia (leukemia or HIV infection with superimposed measles),[147, 203, 204] lymphoid interstitial pneumonitis or pulmonary lymphoid hyperplasia (HIV with associated EBV infection),[6, 196] and graft-versus-host disease (bone marrow allograft with associated CMV infection).[60, 216, 223]

CLINICAL PRESENTATION

Acute nonbacterial pneumonia in the infant or young child generally follows 1 or 2 days of coryza, decreased appetite, and low-grade fever. Onset generally is gradual, with increasing fretfulness, respiratory congestion, vomiting, cough, and fever. In the very young infant, fever may be minimal and apneic spells the most prominent (and frightening) presenting complaint.[27] The most reliable physical findings are those of respiratory distress: tachypnea (respiratory rate ≥ 50/minute[40]), tachycardia, nasal flaring, and retractions, but without the stridor characteristic of upper airway obstruction. In the patient with atelectasis or air trapping, grunting may be present. Cyanosis generally accompanies apneic spells or coughing attacks but may be present at rest in advanced disease or when underlying chronic cardiopulmonary conditions are present.

Other physical findings are quite variable and in fact may be normal. Wheezing is present in infants with associated bronchiolitis or bronchospasm. Hyperresonance may be noted if air trapping is present. Diminished local percussion or breath sounds may indicate lobar consolidation or atelectasis. In interstitial pneumonia, fine crackling rales may be present diffusely or locally. Also important in initial assessment is an evaluation of the young child's state of hydration because increased insensible losses from fever and hyperventilation, coupled with anorexia, can result in significant fluid deficits.

The afebrile pneumonitis syndrome of young infants, in contrast to the usual acute viral pneumonias affecting this age group, is subacute to chronic in its development and is nonseasonal. Characteristic features include the absence of fever, a "staccato" cough pattern (individual coughs separated by inspirations), and diffuse rales on auscultation.[16] Radiographic findings usually consist of interstitial infiltrates with subsegmental atelectasis. Hypergammaglobulinemia and mild eosinophilia are frequent laboratory abnormalities.

Most infants with HIV/AIDS who develop *P. carinii* pneumonia have a progressive febrile course leading to respiratory failure over 1 to 3 weeks. Typical upper respiratory symptoms may be absent, and there may be failure to respond to conventional antibiotic therapy. When pneumonia actually is detected by chest radiograph, the severity of involvement may not be appreciated because abnormalities often are subtle early in the course. However, even with mild radiographic abnormalities, hypoxia may be obvious and severe. Often, it is the discovery of HIV seropositivity that first raises this diagnostic possibility. An important observation is the fact that *P. carinii* pneumonia may develop in infants with HIV/AIDS whose CD4 lymphocyte counts are in the "normal" range.[206]

Nonbacterial pneumonia in the older child and adolescent occurs clinically more nearly like that in an adult. Premonitory complaints generally include such systemic symptoms as malaise, myalgia, and anorexia in addition to upper respiratory symptoms. "Chilliness" may occur, but rigors generally are absent. Cough generally is irritative and nonproductive. Temperature higher than 39° C (102.2° F) is unusual. Although tachypnea, flaring, and retractions generally are present, they may be less apparent than in the infant or young child. Findings on examination of the chest are more reliable than in infancy and may include local percussion dullness or diminished breath sounds and local or diffuse fine rales. Because apnea is rare in older patients, cyanosis is an ominous sign of advanced disease and respiratory failure. Although mild dehydration often is present, it generally is not evident on examination. Nonspecific rash suggests a viral or mycoplasmal cause.[12]

Radiologic findings in nonbacterial pneumonias are variable according to age and infecting agents.[50, 51, 150, 175, 192, 207] In the infant and young child, bilateral air trapping and perihilar infiltrates are the most frequent findings. Patchy areas of consolidation may represent lobular atelectasis or alveolar pneumonia. In the older child and adolescent, lobar involvement more frequently is definable, but typically the affected areas are not consolidated completely. Although lobar consolidation may occur in nonbacterial pneumonias, this finding should be distinguished from atelectasis and is more consistent with a bacterial etiology. Similarly, although small pleural effusions may be detected in decubitus films in nonbacterial pneumonias,[87] effusions are much more suggestive of bacterial etiology.

Peripheral leukocyte counts are quite variable in nonbacterial pneumonia.[70, 172, 188] Portnoy and associates[188] noted that the median leukocyte count in a group of patients with lower respiratory disase was 14,465/mm^3, and Nichol and Cherry[172] observed that counts 10,000/mm^3 or higher with 70 per cent or more neutrophils were common in children hospitalized for viral respiratory illness. Leukocytosis is most frequent in children with influenza and parainfluenza pneumonias.[70] Gram stains of sputum or tracheal secretions in nonbacterial pneumonias tend to show epithelial cells as the predominant cell type, with a mixed bacterial population representing the patient's pharyngeal flora. A predominance of neutrophils may be seen, but this generally reflects bacterial superinfection or preexisting chronic pulmonary disease.

DIFFERENTIAL DIAGNOSIS

In the differential diagnosis of nonbacterial pneumonias, the following factors need to be considered: status of the host—normal or compromised; the environment—animate (human and other animal exposure) or inanimate; the age of the patient; and, finally, the season. In certain epidemiologic settings, the diagnosis of a nonbacterial pneumonia may be made with relative certainty. Often, however, this category of pulmonary infection is a diagnosis of exclusion. The major conditions to be differentiated include noninfectious pulmonary diseases; bacterial pneumonias amenable to conventional antibiotics; and the more unusual bacterial, fungal, or parasitic infections that may require specialized forms of therapy.

Noninfectious conditions that may simulate nonbacterial pneumonia are summarized in Table 26–2. These conditions particularly are relevant to consider in the child with persistent or recurrent pulmonary disease. The line of demarcation between infectious and noninfectious conditions is not always sharp. In the child with sickle-cell anemia, for example, pulmonary vascular occlusive crisis presents with fever, leukocytosis, and patchy pulmonary infiltrates (the acute chest syndrome).[11, 187] Differentiation from pneumococcal, *Haemophilus,* or mycoplasal pneumonia, to which the child with sickle-cell anemia has increased susceptibility, may be difficult or impossible. Early recognition of noninfectious conditions either mimicking or underlying pneumonia may prevent recurrence or improve prognosis. Aspiration resulting from gastroesophageal reflux, for example, is a relatively common correctable cause of recurrent diffuse pneumonia.[45] Early recognition and treatment of cystic fibrosis as an underlying condition have clear beneficial effects in reducing irreversible pulmonary damage.[174]

Pneumonias caused by pyogenic bacteria classically are lobar in distribution and exhibit consolidation on roentgenogram. Atelectasis, on the other hand, is common in viral pneumonia and must be distinguished from true consolidation. Pleural effusions, circular infiltrates, consolidations with convex margins, and pneumatoceles all favor bacterial etiology. In the young child, high fever associated with significant leukocytosis also favors a bacterial etiology.[153] A number of other laboratory investigations, such as erythrocyte sedimentation rate, C-reactive protein, and reduction of nitroblue tetrazolium by leukocytes, frequently are positive in bacterial respiratory infection.[63, 149] In our opinion, however, these tests add little to a careful initial clinical examination, roentgenographic findings, a differential white count, and, if accessible, a Gram stain of tracheal secretions in excluding a bacterial cause.[151] Specific detection techniques for bacterial antigens, used with urine or respiratory secretions, occasionally are helpful. However, false-negative results occur frequently. Thus, bacterial etiology cannot be excluded with certainty.[117, 197]

Positive cultures of blood, pleural fluid, or lung aspirates provide definite evidence of the etiology of bacterial pneumonia. Because of the common asymptomatic carriage of potential pulmonary pathogens in children, however, the diagnostic value of upper respiratory bacterial cultures is debated.[12, 82, 138] In the child with a suspected nonbacterial pneumonia, the finding of "normal flora" in nasopharyngeal or endotracheal secretions is reassuring. In the child who is not doing well, a predominant pathogen in such cultures can be helpful in selecting or altering antimicrobial therapy.[20, 41]

Among the less common causes of pneumonia, tuberculosis should never be forgotten. Tuberculin testing should be included in the initial evaluation and especially is important in children residing in urban areas, recent immigrants, and Native Americans. Fungal pneumonia, particularly coccidioidomycosis, histoplasmosis, and blastomycosis, should be considered in children residing in or visiting endemic areas. Often, a suggestive history may be elicited, such as exposure to excavations (back-yard swimming pools, geologic or archeologic "digs"), clean-up chores in old sheds and barns, and exposure to dust storms. Erythema nodosum and eosinophilia are common clinical clues to these entities. Immunodiffusion serologic testing often yields the diagnosis. Other fungal pneumonias, such as aspergillosis and cryptococcosis, occur in the setting of immunosuppression. These conditions, coupled with the possibilities of *Pneumocystis,* fungal, resistant bacterial, and CMV pneumonia, warrant the use of bronchoalveolar lavage or open lung biopsy as a definitive approach to diagnosis in the compromised host.[72, 226] In an appropriate epidemiologic setting, progressive pneumonia should prompt serologic testing for HIV. Pulmonary disease at present is the most common defining condition in pediatric AIDS.[196] Pulmonary paragonimiasis, due to the lung fluke *Paragonimus westermani,* has been recognized as a cause of chronic pneumonia in Indochinese refugees in the United States.[28]

SPECIFIC DIAGNOSIS

The means for virologic isolation are available in most major medical centers and public health laboratories. With the possible exceptions of HSV and adenoviruses, respiratory viruses rarely are carried asymptomatically. Thus, identification of an agent in upper respiratory secretions is strong evidence for its causative role in pneumonia. Conventional

TABLE 26–2. Noninfectious Conditions that May Simulate Nonbacterial Pneumonia in Children

Technical	Damage by physical agents	Collagen disease (SLE, JRA)
Poor inspiratory film	Lipoid pneumonia	Sarcoidosis
Underpenetrated film	Kerosene pneumonia	Neoplasm
Physiologic	Near-drowning	Histiocytosis X
Prominent thymus	Smoke inhalation	Bronchogenic cyst
Breast shadows	Iatrogenic pulmonary damage	Vascular ring
Chronic pulmonary disease	Drugs (bleomycin, nitrofurantoin)	Pulmonary sequestration
Asthma	Radiation pneumonitis	Congenital lobar emphysema
Bronchiectasis	Graft-versus-host disease	Alpha$_1$-antitrypsin deficiency
Bronchopulmonary dysplasia	Atelectasis	Allergic alveolitis
Pulmonary fibrosis	Mucus plug	Dusts (farmer's lung)
Cystic fibrosis	Foreign body	Molds (allergic aspergillosis)
Recurrent aspiration	Congestive heart failure	Excreta (pigeon-breeder's lung)
Gastroesophageal reflux	Pulmonary infarction	Pulmonary hemosiderosis
Tracheoesophageal fistula	Sickle vaso-occlusive crisis	Desquamative interstitial pneumonitis
Cleft palate	Fat embolism	Adult respiratory distress syndrome
Neuromuscular disorders	Pleural effusion	
Familial dysautonomia	Pleural reaction	

SLE, systemic lupus erythematosus; JRA, juvenile rheumatoid arthritis.

virologic techniques provide the most sensitive and specific means of identification (see Chapter 244). However, most of the common respiratory viral pathogens, as well as chlamydiae and mycoplasmas, now are identified readily using "rapid" techniques. The available methods and reagents are expanding rapidly; they include fluorescent antibody techniques, enzyme-linked immunosorbent assay, direct DNA probes, and the polymerase chain reaction.[39, 59, 77, 136, 163] Clinical specimens may be tested directly or after preincubation in tissue culture systems. In the individual case, serologic diagnosis of acute respiratory viral infection is, in general, less satisfactory than is virologic diagnosis. The difficulties with serology relate to timing of specimens, choice of antigens to test, and variation in quality and specificity of available reagents.

On the other hand, laboratory facilities for the actual isolation of chlamydiae, mycoplasmas, and rickettsiae are available less readily to the clinician. Thus, serologic techniques are important means of specific diagnosis. Acute-phase reactants (e.g., cold agglutinins in *M. pneumoniae* infection) are of greatest diagnostic help during acute illness but are not present invariably. Serologic tests also can be helpful in diagnosis of chlamydial infant pneumonitis—high levels of IgG-specific antibodies uniformly are found at presentation.[16] *Pneumocystis* infection usually is diagnosed by visualizing organisms in silver-stained specimens obtained by bronchoscopy with bronchoalveolar lavage or by open lung biopsy, although noninvasive diagnosis by serologic and molecular biologic techniques currently is under investigation.[135a, 183, 213]

Because of the epidemiologic behavior of nonbacterial respiratory infections, a reasonable guess as to the specific cause often can be made, based on such factors as age, season, and associated clinical features. If the presence of a particular nonbacterial agent in a community can be established by isolation or serologic means, however, the probability of other patients with similar manifestations having illness caused by that agent is increased greatly. Regional viral surveillance programs, such as those carried on in Rochester[97] and Houston,[80] can be particularly helpful to the practicing pediatrician in this regard.

TREATMENT

Therapy for nonbacterial pneumonia primarily is expectant and supportive. However, the list of specific therapies available for these conditions continues to increase (see Sections 13, 14, 17, 18, 19, 20, 22; Chapter 233). Rapid etiologic diagnosis permits appropriate use of these therapies, particularly for hospitalized patients and compromised hosts. Although they shorten the course of illness, they frequently have less dramatic therapeutic effect than specific antibiotic therapy of bacterial infections.

The course of uncomplicated viral pneumonia is not influenced by the administration of antibiotics. However, in the vast majority of cases in which pulmonary involvement is uncovered, antibiotic therapy is employed because bacterial disease cannot be ruled out with certainty. In all but the most mild cases, this approach is both reasonable and practical. It is important, however, that antibiotic therapy in routine cases be appropriate for the most common bacterial pathogens (*S. pneumoniae* and *H. influenzae*). In the immunocompromised host or when secondary infection is a possibility, *S. aureus* (including methicillin-resistant strains) and other hospital-associated and opportunistic pathogens must be considered.[142]

In fulminant viral pneumonia due to varicella in the compromised host, specific antiviral chemotherapy with acyclovir may be lifesaving, but it should be recalled that as many as half of the patients with this condition have complicating bacterial sepsis that requires antibiotic therapy as well.[64] Treatment with amantadine and rimantadine should be considered for children with viral pneumonia in the context of a community epidemic of influenza A. Treatment for lymphocytic interstitial pneumonia in pediatric AIDS includes antiretroviral therapy, with prednisone pulses used for increasing hypoxia.[156] Progressive CMV interstitial pneumonia in bone marrow or solid organ transplant recipients is treated best with ganciclovir and intravenous immunoglobulin, ideally with high-titer antibody activity.[60]

TMP-SMX and pentamidine are equally effective for treatment of *P. carinii* pneumonitis, but the former is the drug of choice because of its lower toxicity. TMP-SMX may be given orally (20 mg/kg/day of the TMP component divided every 6 hours) or intravenously (15 mg/kg/day divided every 8 hours). Pentamidine should be reserved for patients who are intolerant of TMP-SMX. Atovaquone is a future therapeutic option, pending more complete information on its pharmacokinetic profile in pediatrics. Completion of a course of therapy with any agent should transition directly to long-term chemoprophylaxis.

Inhalational administration of the antiviral compound ribavirin has been used successfully to treat viral pneumonias caused by RSV and influenza.[79, 100, 127] Anecdotal experience and in vitro activity suggest that it also may be beneficial in parainfluenza and measles virus infection.[9] Early studies indicated that ribavirin was of particular value in the treatment of RSV infection in nonventilated infants with underlying cardiopulmonary disease[101] and in previously normal infants with RSV pneumonia and respiratory failure.[208] However, several multicenter re-evaluations of ribavirin therapy in RSV-infected infants with and without respiratory failure have yielded equivocal results.[132, 158, 164, 222] These observations, coupled with the high cost of the drug,[65] concerns about its possible teratogenicity in medical personnel,[2] and the complexity of its administration during mechanical ventilation,[52] have led to reassessments of its use and a change in American Academy of Pediatrics recommendations from "should be used"[2] to "may be considered."[3]

Bronchospasm is present in a substantial proportion of nonbacterial pneumonias. Airway reactivity may be preexisting or arise as part of the pathogenesis of the pneumonia itself. Intervention, particularly with inhaled bronchodilators, has become a part of routine management of any patient with wheezing, regardless of age or mechanism, in most hospitals. Rigorous pulmonary function studies have shown that only about half of previously normal infants with RSV-associated respiratory failure respond to inhaled albuterol.[103] However, in several double-blind controlled trials, inhaled albuterol and racemic epinephrine both have shown statistically significant overall benefits.[159, 190, 199, 202] Other studies in mildly ill infants using albuterol and ipratropium have been less convincing.[74, 219] Interestingly, none of the available studies of ribavirin therapy for RSV bronchiolitis and pneumonia have controlled for the effects of concomitant inhaled bronchodilator therapy.

The use of systemic corticosteroids in nonbacterial pneumonia should be approached with great caution. In patients with preexisting asthma or bronchopulmonary dysplasia and acute deterioration triggered by pneumonia, steroids are a noncontroversial element of treatment. In adult AIDS patients with rapidly progressive *P. carinii* pneumonia, short-course steroid therapy clearly is beneficial.[21, 75] Comparable data do not exist for pediatric HIV/AIDS patients. In infants and children without preexisting lung disease, steroid therapy of viral bronchiolitis with or without concomitant pneumonia has shown neither consistent benefit nor harm.[133, 211] The value of steroids probably strikes a balance between their anti-inflammatory effects in short-term use and their immunosuppressive effects with more prolonged administration.

Other key elements of supportive therapy include maintaining adequate hydration, providing high humidity, maintaining oxygenation and ventilation, mobilizing lower respiratory secretions, and, particularly in young infants, continuous monitoring of respiration. Because of increased insensible losses due to fever, hyperventilation, and anorexia, mild dehydration frequently is observed initially, and continuing losses are to be expected during the acute phase of illness. Thus, restoration of deficits and adequate maintenance of fluid intake are desirable. Maintenance of nutrition often is difficult when respiratory distress is present—oral feeding is limited or contraindicated. Parenteral nutrition through peripheral veins is adequate during acute self-limited pneumonias. Situations involving more prolonged hospitalization or mechanical ventilation should lead to early consideration of central alimentation.

The therapeutic benefits of mist tents are debated because negligible amounts of nebulized water actually reach the bronchiolar level.[178] However, high humidity is required to prevent the drying effects of supplemental oxygen therapy; by slowing evaporation, it probably also serves to reduce the viscosity of mucus secretions and the magnitude of insensible fluid losses. Mobilization of respiratory secretions by means of vibration and postural drainage is indicated in nonbacterial pneumonias complicated by atelectasis[141] but is not helpful in the absence of excessive secretions or mucus plugging.[167] Progression of infiltrates and hypoxia occasionally are secondary to pulmonary edema and may necessitate diuretic therapy.

Because of ventilation-perfusion abnormalities and alveolocapillary block, most children with nonbacterial pneumonia have some degree of hypoxemia. In the child with respiratory distress, provision of supplemental oxygen reduces anxiety and ventilation rates. Increases in inspired oxygen to approximately 30 per cent are provided easily by nasal cannulae, which are the most convenient means of administration. More severe respiratory distress or cyanosis requires documentation of respiratory status by means of arterial blood gas determination and more exact regulation of inspired oxygen administered by mask or hood. Noninvasive monitoring by means of oximetry can reduce the need for frequent blood gas sampling and arterial lines.[99] Consistent oxygen saturations of 95 per cent or more should be the target. In respiratory failure, mechanical ventilation may be required to maintain oxygenation and prevent carbon dioxide retention.[56, 94, 148] In this instance, management in an intensive care unit setting is mandated, with invasive monitoring of gas exchange.

Apnea and bradycardia occur commonly in young infants with respiratory syncytial, parainfluenza, and influenza viral pneumonia.[27, 46] This complication particularly is frequent in infants with a history of premature birth. Although the mechanism for these episodes is uncertain, continuous cardiorespiratory monitoring of any young infant with viral pneumonia is prudent.

Acetaminophen should be used to control high fever and will benefit the patient in terms of comfort as well as reducing oxygen and nutritional requirements. Expectorants, antihistamines, and cough suppressants, although widely prescribed for upper respiratory infections of children and adults, probably have no place in the acute management of nonbacterial pneumonias. In convalescence, persistent irritative cough that interferes with sleep may be alleviated by judicious use of codeine or dextromethorphan.[48]

PROGNOSIS

In the preantibiotic era, pneumonia (of which the majority of cases were "bronchopneumonia") was the most frequent cause of death in children. At present, a fatal outcome is rare but always a possibility. It is most likely to occur in young infants or compromised hosts.

The incidence of long-term complications of nonbacterial pneumonias is unknown. It is likely, however, that these conditions play a role in development of some cases of bronchiectasis, chronic pulmonary fibrosis, desquamative interstitial pneumonitis, bronchiolitis obliterans, and unilateral hyperlucent lung (Swyer-James syndrome). These complications are well-documented sequelae of measles and adenoviral and influenza viral pneumonia.[121, 130, 131, 145] They are most frequent today in children who have survived complex and prolonged hospitalization involving aggressive ventilator management of respiratory failure.[194, 195]

At a minimum, children with pneumonia should be reevaluated clinically 2 to 3 weeks after diagnosis. Provided the child is asymptomatic, has returned to normal activities, and has a benign physical examination, a follow-up x-ray is not required.[92] Repeated chest radiographs are necessary for children with complicated clinical courses, underlying pulmonary disease, or prior episodes of pneumonia or if signs or symptoms of respiratory difficulty persist at the time of follow-up. It should be recognized that about 20 per cent of even uncomplicated pneumonias will show persistent x-ray abnormalities at 3 to 4 weeks after diagnosis, but a selective approach to follow-up films permits early recognition of atelectasis, unresolved infiltrates, or progressive disease.

PREVENTION

Nosocomial spread of respiratory viruses occurs readily in pediatric wards and involves intermediate carriage by medical personnel who have acquired mild upper respiratory infections.[96] A reasonable approach to interdicting nosocomial transmission is to group patients with pneumonia and exclude personnel with symptomatic respiratory illness from ward duties.

For the common viral causes of pneumonia, vaccines at present are available only for influenza and adenoviruses. Annual influenza vaccination using "split-product" vaccines is recommended for children with chronic respiratory disease, HIV/AIDS, and other conditions predisposing to pneumonia.[33] Adenoviral vaccines have been used widely in the military but are not recommended for use in pediatrics. Attenuated, inactivated, and subunit vaccines against RSV, para 3, and *M. pneumoniae* have received considerable investigative effort but have not yet proved to be effective.[116, 167a]

Intramuscular passive immunizations with pooled immunoglobulin and varicella-zoster immunoglobulin are established postexposure measures to prevent measles and varicella pneumonia, respectively, in compromised hosts. RSV-specific intravenous immunoglobulin has been shown to be of value in preventing RSV lower respiratory tract morbidity in infants with prematurity or cardiac disease.[91] Despite the complexity of its administration, this product now is entering clinical use. Others, such as "humanized" monoclonal antibodies and specific Fab immunoglobulin fragments produced by recombinant DNA technology, currently are under study.[10, 228]

P. carinii pneumonia can be prevented in pediatric patients with hematologic malignancy or HIV/AIDS by prophylactic administration of TMP-SMX. This medication has become a part of routine management of these conditions and has reduced dramatically the incidence of *P. carinii* infection.[32, 34, 115] Unless HIV infection reasonably can be excluded using multiple HIV cultures or polymerase chain reaction, seropositive HIV-exposed infants should receive chemoprophylaxis from 4 to 6 weeks of age up to 12 months of age, regardless of immune status. Seropositive children 1 to 5 years of age should receive prophylaxis if their CD4 count is less than 500 cells/μL or their CD4 percentage is less than 15. The criterion for prophylaxis in older children and adults is a CD4 count of less than 200 cells/μL or a percentage less than 15. The recommended dosage of TMP-SMX is 150 mg/M^2/day of TMP divided in two doses on 3 successive days each week.[34]

Opportunistic CMV pneumonia, a major hazard in seronegative high-risk premature infants and recipients of allogeneic bone marrow transplants, can be prevented effectively by the exclusive use of CMV-seronegative blood products.[230] In marrow transplant recipients who are seropositive and thus at risk for reactivation disease, prophylactic acyclovir, ganciclovir, and intravenous immunoglobulin have been shown to reduce rates of infection and interstitial pneumonia.[160, 200, 216]

References

1. Aherne, W., Bird, T., Court, S. D. M., et al.: Pathological changes in virus infection of the lower respiratory tract in children. J. Clin. Pathol. *23*:7–18, 1970.
2. American Academy of Pediatrics, Committee on Infectious Diseases: Use of ribavirin in the treatment of respiratory syncytial virus infection. Pediatrics *92*:501–504, 1993.
3. American Academy of Pediatrics, Committee on Infectious Diseases: Reassessment of the indications for ribavirin therapy in respiratory syncytial virus infection. Pediatrics *97*:137–140, 1996.
4. Andiman, W. A., Jacobson, R. I., and Tucker, G.: Leukocyte-associated viremia with adenovirus type 2 in an infant with lower-respiratory-tract disease. N. Engl. J. Med. *297*:100–101, 1977.
5. Andiman, W. A., McCarthy, P., Markowitz, R. I., et al.: Clinical, virologic, and serologic evidence of Epstein-Barr virus infection in association with childhood pneumonia. J. Pediatr. [illegible], 1981.
6. Andiman, W. A., Eastman, R., Martin, K., et al.: Opportunistic lymphoproliferations associated with Epstein-Barr viral DNA in infants and children with AIDS. Lancet 2:1390–1393, 1985.
7. Angella, J. J., and Connor, J. D.: Neonatal infection caused by adenovirus type 7. J. Pediatr. *72*:474–478, 1968.
8. Ballard, R. A., Drew, W. L., Hufnagle, K. G., et al.: Acquired cytomegalovirus infection in preterm infants. Am. J. Dis. Child. *133*:482–485, 1979.
9. Banks, G., and Fernandez, H.: Clinical use of ribavirin in measles: A summarized review. *In* Smith, R. A., Knight, V., and Smith, J. A. D. (eds.): Clinical Applications of Ribavirin. New York, Academic Press, 1984, pp. 203–209.
10. Barbas, C. F., Crowe, J. E., Cababa, D., et al.: Human monoclonal Fab fragments derived from a combinatorial library bind to respiratory syncytial virus F glycoprotein and neutralize infectivity. Proc. Natl. Acad. Sci. U. S. A. *89*:10164–10168, 1992.
11. Barrett-Connor, E.: Acute pulmonary disease and sickle cell anemia. Am. Rev. Resp. Dis. *104*:159, 1971.
12. Barrett-Connor, E.: The nonvalue of sputum culture in the diagnosis of pneumococcal pneumonia. Am. Rev. Respir. Dis. *103*:845–848, 1971.
13. Bauer, C. R., Elie, K., Spene, L., et al.: Hong Kong influenza in a neonatal unit. J. A. M. A. *223*:1233–1235, 1973.
14. Becroft, D. M. O.: Histopathology of fatal adenovirus infection of the respiratory tract in young children. J. Clin. Pathol. *20*:561–569, 1967.
15. Beem, M., Wright, F. H., Hamre, D., et al.: Association of the chimpanzee coryza agent with acute respiratory disease in children. N. Engl. J. Med. *263*:523–530, 1960.
16. Beem, M., and Saxon, E.: Respiratory-tract colonization and a distinctive pneumonia syndrome in infants infected with *Chlamydia trachomatis*. N. Engl. J. Med. *296*:306–310, 1977.
17. Benyesh-Melnick, M., and Rosenberg, H. S.: The isolation of adenovirus type 7 from a fetal case of pneumonia and disseminated disease. J. Pediatr. *64*:83–87, 1964.
18. Berkovich, S., and Taranko, L.: Acute respiratory illness in the premature nursery associated with respiratory syncytial virus infections. Pediatrics *34*:735–760, 1964.
19. Bertozzi, P., Astedt, B., Zenzius, L., et al.: Depressed bronchoalveolar urokinase activity in patients with adult respiratory distress syndrome. N. Engl. J. Med. *322*:890–897, 1990.
20. Boyer, K. M., and Cherry, J. D.: Pneumonias in children. Curr. Top. Pediatr. *1*:169–182, 1979.
21. Bozzette, S. A., Sattler, F. R., Chin, J. et al.: A controlled trial of early adjunctive treatment with corticosteroids for *Pneumocystis carinii* pneumonia in the acquired immunodeficiency syndrome. N. Engl. J. Med. 323:1451–1457, 1990.
22. Brandt, C. D., Kim, H. W., Vargosko, A. J., et al.: Infections in 18,000 infants and children in a controlled study of respiratory tract disease. I. Adenovirus pathogenicity in relation to serologic type and illness syndrome. Am. J. Epidemiol. *90*:484–500, 1969.
23. Brandt, C. D., Kim, H. W., Arrobio, J. O., et al.: Epidemiology of respiratory syncytial virus infection in Washington, DC. III. Composite analysis of eleven consecutive yearly epidemics. Am. J. Epidemiol. *98*:355–364, 1973.
24. Brocklebank, J. T., Court, S. D. M., McQuillin, J., et al.: Influenza-A infection in children. Lancet 2:497–500, 1972.
25. Brodie, H. R., and Spencer, L. P.: Respiratory syncytial virus infections in children in Montreal: A retrospective study. Can. Med. Assoc. J. *109*:1199–1201, 1973.
26. Brown, R. S., Nogrady, M. B., Spence, L., et al.: An outbreak of adenovirus type 7 infection in children in Montreal. Can. Med. Assoc. J. *108*:434–439, 1973.
27. Bruhn, F. W., Mokrohisky, S. T., and McIntosh, K.: Apnea associated with respiratory syncytial virus infection in young infants. J. Pediatr. *40*:382–386, 1977.
28. Burton, K., Yogev, R., London, N., et al.: Pulmonary paragonimiasis in Laotian refugee children. Pediatrics *70*:246–248, 1982.
29. Carson, J. L., Collier, A. M., and Hu, S. S.: Acquired ciliary defects in nasal epithelium of children with acute viral upper respiratory infections. N. Engl. J. Med. *312*:463–468, 1985.
30. Cassell, G. H., Waites, K. B., Crouse, D. T., et al.: Association of *Ureaplasma urealyticum* infection of the lower respiratory tract with chronic lung disease and death in very-low-birthweight infants. Lancet 2:240–245, 1988.
31. Cassell, G. H., Waites, K. B., and Crouse, D. T.: Mycoplasmal infections. *In* Remington, J. S., and Klein, J. O. (eds.): Infectious Diseases of the Fetus and Newborn Infant. 4th ed. Philadelphia, W. B. Saunders, 1995, pp. 619–655.
32. Centers for Disease Control: Guidelines for prophylaxis against *Pneumocystis carinii* pneumonia for children infected with human immunodeficiency virus. M. M. W. R. *40*(RR-2):1–13, 1991.
33. Centers for Disease Control: Prevention and control of influenza: Recommendations of the Immunization Practices Advisory Committee. M. M. W. R. *39*(RR-7):1–15, 1990.
34. Centers for Disease Control and Prevention: 1995 revised guidelines for prophylaxis against *Pneumocystis carinii* pneumonia for children infected with or perinatally exposed to human immunodeficiency virus. M. M. W. R. *44*(RR-4):1–11, 1995.
35. Chanock, R. M., and Parrott, R. H.: Acute respiratory disease in infancy and childhood: Present understanding and prospects for prevention. Pediatrics *36*:21–39, 1965.
36. Chanock, R. M., Mufson, M. A., and Johnson, K. M.: Comparative biology and ecology of human virus and mycoplasma respiratory pathogens. Progr. Med. Virol. *7*:208–252, 1965.
37. Chanock, R. M., Kapikian, A. Z., Mills, J., et al.: Influence of immunological factors in respiratory syncytial virus disease. Arch. Environ. Health *21*:347–356, 1970.
38. Chany, C., Lepine, P., Lelong, M., et al.: Severe and fatal pneumonia in infants and young children associated with adenovirus infections. Am. J. Hyg. *67*:367–378, 1958.
39. Chao, R. K., Fishaut, M., Schwartzman, J. D., et al.: Detection of respiratory syncytial virus in nasal secretions from infants by enzyme-linked immunosorbent assay. J. Infect. Dis. *139*:483–486, 1979.
40. Cherian, T., John, T. J., Simoes, E., et al.: Evaluation of simple clinical signs for the diagnosis of acute lower respiratory tract infection. Lancet 2:125–128, 1988.
41. Cherry, J. D.: Newer respiratory viruses: Their role in respiratory illnesses of children. Adv. Pediatr. *20*:225–290, 1973.
42. Cherry, J. D., Hurwitz, E. S., and Welliver, R. C.: *Mycoplasma pneumoniae* infections and exanthems. J. Pediatr. *87*:369–373, 1975.
43. Cherry, J. D., and Welliver, R. C.: *Mycoplasma pneumoniae* infections of adults and children. West. J. Med. *125*:47–55, 1976.
44. Child Day Care Infectious Disease Study Group: Public health considerations of infectious diseases in child day care centers. J. Pediatr. *105*:683–701, 1984.
45. Christie, D. L., O'Grady, L. R., and Mack, D. V.: Incompetent lower esophageal sphincter and gastroesophageal reflux in recurrent acute pulmonary disease of infancy and childhood. J. Pediatr. *93*:23–27, 1978.
46. Church, N. R., Anas, N. G., Hall, C. B., et al.: Respiratory syncytial

virus–related apnea in infants: Demographics and outcome. Am. J. Dis. Child. *138*:247–250, 1984.
47. Claesson, B. A., Trollfors, B., Brolin, I., et al.: Etiology of community-acquired pneumonia in children based on antibody responses to bacterial and viral antigens. Pediatr. Infect. Dis. J. *8*:856–862, 1989.
48. Committee on Drugs: Use of codeine and dextromethorphan-containing cough syrups in pediatrics. Pediatrics *62*:118–122, 1978.
49. Connor, J. D.: Evidence for an etiologic role of adenoviral infection in pertussis syndrome. N. Engl. J. Med. *283*:390–394, 1970.
50. Conte, P., Heitzman, E. R., and Marakarian, B.: Viral pneumonia: Roentgen pathological correlations. Radiology *95*:267–272, 1970.
51. Courtnoy, I., Lande, A. E., and Turner, R. B.: Accuracy of radiographic differentiation of bacterial from nonbacterial pneumonia. Clin. Pediatr. *28*:261–264, 1989.
52. Demers, R. R., Parker, J., Frankel, L. R., et al.: Administration of ribavirin to neonatal and pediatric patients during mechanical ventilation. Respir. Care *31*:1188–1196, 1986.
53. Dennehy, P. H., and McIntosh, K.: Viral pneumonia in childhood. *In* Weinstein, L., and Fields, B. N. (eds.): Seminars in Infectious Disease. V. Pneumonias. New York, Thieme-Stratton, 1983, pp.
54. Denny, F. W.: The replete pediatrician and the etiology of lower respiratory tract infections. Pediatr. Res. *3*:463–470, 1969.
55. Dingle, J., and Langmuir, A. D.: Epidemiology of acute respiratory disease in military recruits. Am. Rev. Respir. Dis. *97*:1–65, 1968.
56. Downes, J. J., Wood, D. W., Striker, T. W., et al.: Acute respiratory failure in infants with bronchiolitis. Anesthesiology *29*:426–434, 1968.
57. Dworsky, M., and Stagno, S.: Newer agents causing pneumonitis in early infancy. Pediatr. Infect. Dis. *1*:188–195, 1982.
58. Eckert, H. L., Portnoy, B., Salvatore, M. A., et al.: Group B coxsackie virus infection in infants with acute lower respiratory disease. Pediatrics *39*:526–531, 1967.
59. Eisenstein, B. J.: The polymerase chain reaction: A new method of using molecular genetics for medical diagnosis. N. Engl. J. Med. *322*:178–183, 1990.
60. Emanuel, D., Cunningham, I., Jules-Elysee, K., et al.: Cytomegalovirus pneumonia after bone marrow transplantation sucessfully treated with the combination of ganciclovir and high-dose intravenous immune globulin. Ann. Intern. Med. *109*:777–782, 1988.
61. Evans, A. S.: Infectious mononucleosis in University of Wisconsin students: Report of a five-year investigation. Am. J. Hyg. *71*:342–362, 1960.
62. Evans, A. S.: Epidemiological concepts and methods. *In* Evans, A. S. (ed.): Viral Infections of Humans: Epidemiology and Control. New York, Plenum Publishing, 1976, pp. 1–32.
63. Feigin, R. D., Shackelford, P. G., Choi, S. C., et al.: Nitroblue tetrazolium dye test as an aid in the differential diagnosis of febrile disorders. J. Pediatr. *78*:230–237, 1971.
64. Feldman, S., Hughes, W. T., and Daniel, C. B.: Varicella in children with cancer: Seventy-seven cases. Pediatrics *56*:388–397, 1975.
65. Feldstein, T. J., Swegarden, J. L., Atwood, G. F., et al.: Ribavirin therapy: Implementation of hospital guidelines and effect on usage and cost of therapy. Pediatrics *46*:14–17, 1995.
66. Fernald, G. W., and Clyde, W. A.: Pulmonary immune mechanisms in *Mycoplasma pneumoniae* disease. *In* Kirkpatrick, C. H., and Reynolds, H. Y. (eds.): Immunologic and Infectious Reactions in the Lung. New York, Marcel Dekker, 1976, pp. 101–130.
67. Fine, N. L., Smith, L. R., and Sheedy, P. F.: Frequency of pleural effusions in mycoplasmal and viral pneumonias. N. Engl. J. Med. *283*:790–793, 1970.
68. Fox, J. P., Brandt, C. D., Wasserman, F. E., et al.: The Virus Watch Program: A continuing surveillance of viral infections in metropolitan New York families. VI. Observations of adenovirus infections, virus excretion patterns, antibody response, efficiency of surveillance, patterns of infection, and relation to illness. Am. J. Epidemiol. *89*:25–50, 1969.
69. Fox, J. P., and Hall, C. E.: Viruses in Families. Surveillance of Families as a Key to Epidemiology of Virus Infections. Littleton, MA, PSG Publishing, 1980.
70. Foy, H. M., Cooney, M. K., McMahon, R., et al.: Viral and mycoplasmal pneumonia in a prepaid medical care group during an eight-year period. Am. J. Epidemiol. *97*:93–102, 1973
71. Foy, H. M., Cooney, M. K., Maletzky, A. J., et al.: Incidence and etiology of pneumonia, croup and bronchiolitis in preschool children belonging to a prepaid medical care group over a four-year period. Am. J. Epidemiol. *97*:80–92, 1973.
72. Frankel, L. R., Smith, D. W., and Lewiston, N. J.: Bronchoalveolar lavage for diagnosis of pneumonia in the immunocompromised child. Pediatrics *81*:785–788, 1988.
73. Fulginiti, V. A., Eller, J. J., Downie, A. W., et al.: Altered reactivity to measles virus: Atypical measles in children previously immunized with inactivated measles virus vaccines. J. A. M. A. *202*:1075–1080, 1967.
74. Gadomski, A. M., Lichtenstein, R., Horton, L., et al.: Efficacy of albuterol in the management of bronchiolitis. Pediatrics *43*:907–912, 1994.
75. Gagnon, S., Boota, A. M., Fischl, M. A., et al.: Corticosteroids as adjunctive therapy for severe *Pneumocystis carinii* pneumonia in the acquired immunodeficiency syndrome: A double-blind, placebo-controlled trial. N. Engl. J. Med. *323*:1444–1450, 1990.
76. Gajdusek, D. C.: *Pneumocystis carinii:* Etiologic agent of interstitial plasma cell pneumonia of premature and young infants. Pediatrics *19*:543–565, 1957.
77. Gardner, P. S.: How etiologic, pathologic, and clinical diagnoses can be made in a correlated fashion. Pediatr. Res. *11*:254–261, 1977.
78. George, R. B., and Mogabgab, W. J.: Atypical pneumonia in young men with rhinovirus infections. Ann. Intern. Med. *71*:1073–1078, 1969.
79. Gilbert, B. E., Wilson, S. Z., Knight, V., et al.: Ribavirin small-particle aerosol treatment of infections caused by influenza virus strains A/Victoria/7/83 (H1N1) and B/Texas/1/84. Antimicrob. Agents Chemother. *27*:309–313, 1985.
80. Glezen, W. P.: Acute Respiratory Disease Update. Houston, Baylor College of Medicine, 1985.
81. Glezen, W. P., Frank, A. L., Taber, L. H., et al.: Parainfluenza virus type 3: Seasonality and risk of infection and reinfection in young children. J. Infect. Dis. *150*:851–857, 1984.
82. Glezen, W. P., Loda, F. A., Clyde, W. A., et al.: Epidemiologic patterns of acute lower respiratory disease of children in a pediatric group practice. J. Pediatr. *78*:397–406, 1971.
83. Glezen, W. P., and Denny, F. W.: Epidemiology of acute lower respiratory disease in children. N. Engl. J. Med. *288*:498–505, 1973.
84. Glezen, W. P., and Denny, F. W.: Effect of passive antibody on parainfluenza virus type 3 pneumonia in hamsters. Infect. Immun. *14*:212–216, 1976.
85. Glezen, W. P., Loda, F. A., and Denny, F. W.: The parainfluenza viruses. *In* Evans, A. S. (ed.): Viral Infections of Humans: Epidemiology and Control. New York, Plenum Publishing, 1976, p. 337–349.
86. Glezen, W. P., Paredes, A., and Taber, L. H.: Influenza in children: Relationship to other respiratory agents. J. A. M. A. *243*:1345–1349, 1980.
87. Goodpasture, E. W.: The significance of certain pulmonary lesions in relation to the etiology of influenza. Am. J. Med. Sci. *158*:863–870, 1919.
88. Graham, B., Davis, T., Tang, Y., et al.: Immunoprophylaxis and immunotherapy of respiratory syncytial virus–infected mice with respiratory syncytial virus–specific immune serum. Pediatr. Res. *34*:167–172, 1993.
89. Grayston, J. T., Campbell, L. A., Kuo, C.-C., et al.: A new respiratory tract pathogen: *Chlamydia pneumoniae* strain TWAR. J. Infect. Dis. *161*:618–625, 1990.
90. Grayston, J. T., Kuo, C.-C., Wang, S. P., et al.: A new *Chlamydia psittaci* strain, TWAR, isolated in acute respiratory tract infection. N. Engl. J. Med. *315*:161–168, 1986.
91. Groothius, J. R., Simoes, E. A., Levin, M. J., et al.: Prophylactic administration of respiratory syncytial virus immune globulin to high-risk infants and young children. N. Engl. J. Med. *329*:1524–1530, 1993.
92. Grossman, L. K., Wald, E. R., Nair, P., et al.: Roentgenographic follow-up of acute pneumonia in children. Pediatrics *63*:30–31, 1979.
93. Gruber, W., Wilson, S., Throop, P., et al.: Immunoglobulin administration and ribavirus infection of the cotton rat. Pediatr. Res. 21:270–274, 1987.
94. Habib, D. M., and Perkin, R. M.: Continuous distending pressure and assisted ventilation. *In* Levin, D. L., and Morriss, F. C. (eds.): Essentials of Pediatric Intensive Care. St. Louis, Quality Medical Publishing, 1990, pp. 897–910.
95. Hable, K. A., O'Connell, E. J., and Herrmann, E. C., Jr.: Group B Coxsackieviruses as respiratory viruses. Mayo Clin. Proc. *45*:170–176, 1970.
96. Hall, C. B.: The shedding and spreading of respiratory syncytial virus. Pediatr. Res. *11*:236–239, 1977.
97. Hall, C. B.: Infectious Disease Newsletter. Rochester, NY, University of Rochester School of Medicine, 1985.
98. Hall, C. B., Douglas, R. G., Geiman, J. M., et al.: Nosocomial respiratory syncytial virus infections. N. Engl. J. Med. *293*:1343–1346, 1975.
99. Hall, C. B., Hall, W. J., and Speers, D. M.: Clinical and physiological manifestations of bronchiolitis and pneumonia: Outcome of respiratory syncytial virus. Am. J. Dis. Child. *133*:798–802, 1979.
100. Hall, C. B., McBride, J. T., Walsh, E. E., et al.: Aerosolized ribavirin treatment of infants with respiratory syncytial virus infection: A randomized double-blind study. N. Engl. J. Med. *308*:1443–1447, 1983.
101. Hall, C. B., McBride, J. T., Gala, L. L., et al.: Ribavirin treatment of respiratory syncytial viral infection in infants with underlying cardiopulmonary disease. J. A. M. A. *254*:3047–3051, 1985.
102. Hall, C. B., Powell, K. R., MacDonald, N. E., et al.: Respiratory syncytial viral infection in children with compromised immune function. N. Engl. J. Med. *315*:77–81, 1986.
103. Hammer, J., Numa, A., and Neroth, C. J.: Albuterol responsiveness in infants with respiratory failure caused by respiratory syncytial virus infection. J. Pediatr. *127*:485–490, 1995.
104. Hanshaw, J. B., and Dudgeon, J. A.: Viral Diseases of the Fetus and Newborn. Philadelphia, W. B. Saunders, 1978.
105. Harrington, R. D., Hooton, T. M., Hackman, R. C., et al.: An outbreak of respiratory syncytial virus in a bone marrow transplant center. J. Infect. Dis. *165*:987–993, 1992.
106. Harrison, H. R., English, M. G., Lee, C. K., et al.: *Chlamydia trachomatis* infant pneumonitis: Comparison with matched controls and other infant pneumonitis. N. Engl. J. Med. *298*:702–708, 1978.
107. Henderson, F. W., Clyde, W. A., Collier, A. M., et al.: The etiologic and

epidemiologic spectrum of bronchiolitis in pediatric practice. J. Pediatr. *95*:183–190, 1979.
108. Henson, D., and Mufson, M. A.: Myocarditis and pneumonitis with type 21 adenovirus infection: Association with fatal myocarditis and pneumonitis. Am. J. Dis. Child. *121*:334–336, 1971.
109. Herbert, F. A., Mahon, W. A., Wilkinson, D., et al.: Pneumonia in Indian and Eskimo infants and children. Part I. A clinical study. Can. Med. Assoc. J. *96*:257–265, 1967.
110. Herbert, F. A., Wilkinson, D., Burchak, E., et al.: Adenovirus type 3 pneumonia causing lung damage in childhood. Can. Med. Assoc. J. *116*:274–276, 1977.
111. Herrmann, E. C., Jr.: Experiences in laboratory diagnosis of adenovirus infections in routine medical practice. Mayo Clin. Proc. *43*:635–644, 1968.
112. Herrmann, E. C., Jr., and Hable, K. A.: Experiences in laboratory diagnosis of parainfluenza viruses in routine medical practice. Mayo Clin. Proc. *45*:177–188, 1970.
113. Horn, M. E. C., Brain, E., Gregg, I., et al.: Respiratory viral infection in childhood: A survey in general practice, Roehamptom, 1967–1972. J. Hyg. (Camb.) *74*:157–168, 1975.
114. Hughes, W. T., Feldman, S., and Cox, F.: Infectious diseases in children with cancer. Pediatr. Clin. North Am. *21*:583–615, 1974.
115. Hughes, W. T.: Five-year absence of *Pneumocystis carinii* pneumonitis in a pediatric oncology unit. J. Infect. Dis. *150*:305–306, 1984.
116. Institute of Medicine, National Academy of Sciences: New Vaccine Development. Establishing Priorities. Diseases of Importance in the United States. Washington, DC, National Academy Press, 1985.
117. Isaacs, D.: Problems in determining the etiology of community-acquired childhood pneumonia. Pediatr. Infect. Dis. J. *8*:143–148, 1989.
118. Jacobs, J. W., Peacock, D. B., Corner, B. D., et al.: Respiratory syncytial and other viruses associated with respiratory disease in infants. Lancet *1*:871–876, 1971.
119. Jasson, E., Wager, O., Forssell, P., et al.: Epidemic occurrence of adenovirus type 7 infection in Helsinki. Ann. Paediatr. Fenn. *8*:24–34, 1962.
120. Jarvis, W. R., Middleton, P. J.: and Gelfand, E. W.: Significance of viral infections in severe combined immunodeficiency disease. Pediatr. Infect. Dis. *2*:187–192, 1983.
121. Kattan, M., Keens, T. G., LaPierre, J. G., et al.: Pulmonary function abnormalities in symptom-free children after bronchiolitis. Pediatrics *59*:683–688, 1977.
122. Katz, B. Z., Berkman, A. B., and Shapiro, E. D.: Serologic evidence of active Epstein-Barr virus infection in Epstein-Barr virus–associated lymphoproliferative disorders of children with acquired immunodeficiency syndrome. J. Pediatr. *120*:228–232, 1992.
123. Kaye, H. S., Marsh, H. B., and Dowdle, W. R.: Seroepidemiologic survey of coronavirus (strain OC 43) related infections in a children's population. Am. J. Epidemiol. *94*:43–49, 1971.
124. Kim, H. W., Arrobio, J. O., Brandt, C. D., et al.: Epidemiology of respiratory syncytial virus infection in Washington, D.C. I. Importance of the virus in different respiratory tract disease syndromes and temporal distribution of infection. Am. J. Epidemiol. *98*:216–225, 1973.
125. Kim, H. W., Brandt, C. D., Arrobio, J. O., et al.: Influenza A and B virus infection in infants and young children during the years 1957–1976. Am. J. Epidemiol. *109*:464–479, 1979.
126. Kim, K. S., and Gohd, R. S.: Fatal pneumonia caused by adenovirus type 35. Am. J. Dis. Child. *135*:473–475, 1981.
127. Knight, V., Wilson, S. Z., Quarles, J. M., et al.: Ribavirin small-particle aerosol treatment of influenza. Lancet 2:945–950, 1981.
128. Kohn, J. L., and Koiransky, H.: Successive roentgenograms of the chest of children during measles. Am. J. Dis. Child. *38*:258–270, 1929.
129. Krasinski, K., and Borkowsky, W.: Measles and measles immunity in children infected with human immunodeficiency virus. J. A. M. A. *261*:2512–2516, 1989.
130. Lang, W. R., Howden, C. W., Laws, J., et al.: Bronchopneumonia with serious sequelae in children with evidence of adenovirus type 21 infection. Br. Med. J. *1*:73–79, 1969.
131. Laraya-Cuasay, L. R., Deforest, A., Huff, D., et al.: Chronic pulmonary complications of early influenza virus infection in children. Am. Rev. Respir. Dis. *116*:617–625, 1977.
132. Law, B. J. Wang, E. E., and Stephens, D.: Ribavirin does not reduce hospital stay in patients with respiratory syncytial virus lower respiratory tract infection. Pediatr. Res. *37*:110A, 1995.
133. Leer, J. A., Bloomfield, N. J., Green, J. L., et al.: Corticosteroid treatment in bronchiolitis: A controlled collaborative study in 297 infants and children. Am. J. Dis. Child. *117*:495–503, 1969.
134. Lepow, M. L., Balassanian, N., Emmerich, J., et al.: Interrelationships of viral, mycoplasmal, and bacterial agents in uncomplicated pneumonia. Am. Rev. Resp. Dis. *97*:533–545, 1968.
135. Lerner, A. M., Klein, J. O., Levin, H. S., et al.: Infections due to coxsackie virus group A, type 9, in Boston, 1959, with special reference to exanthems and pneumonia. N. Engl. J. Med. *263*:1265–1272, 1960.
135a. Liebovitz, E., Pollack, H., Moore, T., et al.: Comparison of PCR and standard cytological staining for detection of *Pneumocystis carinii* from respiratory specimens from patients with or at high risk for infection by human immunodeficiency virus. J. Clin. Microbiol. *33*:3004–3007, 1995.
136. Liu, C.: Diagnosis of influenzal infection by means of fluorescent antibody. Am. Rev. Respir. Dis. *83*(Suppl.):130–138, 1960.
137. Loda, F. A., Clyde, W. A., Jr., Glezen, W. P., et al.: Studies on the role of viruses, bacteria, and *M. pneumoniae* as causes of lower respiratory tract infections in children. J. Pediatr. *72*:161–176, 1968.
138. Loda, F. A., Collier, A. M., Glezen, W. P., et al.: Occurrence of *Diplococcus pneumoniae* in the upper respiratory tract of children. J. Pediatr. *87*:1087–1093, 1975.
139. Loda, F. A., Glezen, W. P., and Clyde, W. A., Jr.: Respiratory disease in group daycare. Pediatrics *49*:428–437, 1972.
140. Long, S. S.: Treatment of acute pneumonia in infants and children. Pediatr. Clin. North Am. *30*:297–321, 1983.
141. Lough, M. D., Doershuk, C. F., and Stern, R. C.: Pediatric Respiratory Therapy. 3rd ed. Chicago, Year Book Medical Publishers, 1985.
142. Louria, D. B., Blumenfield, H. L., Ellis, J. T., et al.: Studies on influenza in the pandemic of 1958–59. II. Pulmonary complications of influenza. J. Clin. Invest. *38*:213–265, 1959.
143. Macasaet, F. F., Kidd, P. A., Bolanco, C. R., et al.: The etiology of acute respiratory infections. III. The role of viruses and bacteria. J. Pediatr. *72*:829–839, 1968.
144. MacDonald, N. E., Hall, C. B., Suffin, S. D., et al.: Respiratory syncytial viral infection in infants with congenital heart disease. N. Engl. J. Med. *307*:397–400, 1982.
145. MacPherson, R. I., Cumming, G., and Chernick, V.: Unilateral hyperlucent lung in childhood: A complication of viral pneumonia. J. Can. Assoc. Radiol. *20*:225–231, 1969.
146. Maletzky, A. J., Cooney, M. K., Luce, R., et al.: Epidemiology of viral and mycoplasmal agents associated with childhood lower respiratory illness in a civilian population. J. Pediatr. *78*:407–414, 1971.
147. Markowitz, L. E., Chandler, F. W., Boldan, E. O., et al.: Fatal measles pneumonia without rash in a child with AIDS. J. Infect. Dis. *158*:480–483, 1988.
148. Martin, L. D., Rafferty, J. F., Walker, L. K., et al.: Principles of respiratory support and mechanical ventilation. *In* Rogers, M. C. (ed.): Textbook of Pediatric Intensive Care. Baltimore, Williams & Wilkins, 1992, pp. 134–203.
149. McCarthy, P. L., Frank, A. L., Ablow, R. C., et al.: Value of the C-reactive protein test in the differentiation of bacterial and viral pneumonia. J. Pediatr. *92*:454–456, 1978.
150. McCarthy, P. L., Spiesel, S. Z., Stashwick, C. A., et al.: Radiographic findings and etiologic diagnosis in ambulatory childhood pneumonias. Clin. Pediatr. *20*:686–691, 1981.
151. McCarthy, P. L., Tomasso, L., and Dolan, T. F.: Predicting fever responses of children with pneumonia treated with antibiotics. Clin. Pediatr. *19*:753–760, 1980.
152. McClelland, L., Hilleman, M. R., Hamparian, V. V., et al.: Studies of acute respiratory illnesses caused by respiratory syncytial virus. 2. Epidemiology and assessment of importance. N. Engl. J. Med. *264*:1169–1175, 1961.
153. McGowan, J. E., Bratton, L., Klein, J. D., et al.: Bacteremia in febrile children seen in a "walk-in" pediatric clinic. N. Engl. J. Med. *288*:1309–1312, 1973.
154. McIntosh, K., Chao, R. K., Krause, H. E., et al.: Coronavirus infection in acute lower respiratory tract disease of infants. J. Infect. Dis. *130*:502–507, 1974.
155. McIntosh, K., and Fishaut, J. M.: Immunopathologic mechanisms in lower respiratory tract disease in infants due to respiratory syncytial virus. Prog. Med. Virol. *26*:94–118, 1980.
156. McKinney, R. E., Maha, M. A., Connor, E. M., et al.: A multicenter trial of oral zidovudine in children with advanced human immunodeficiency virus disease. N. Engl. J. Med. *324*;1018–1025, 1991.
157. McNamara, M. J., Phillips, I. A., and Williams, O. B.: Viral and *Mycoplasma pneumoniae* infections in exacerbations of chronic lung disease. Am. Rev. Respir. Dis. *100*:19–24, 1969.
158. Meert, K. L., Sarnaik, A. P., Gelmino, M. J., et al.: Aerosolized ribavirin in mechanically ventilated children with respiratory syncytial virus lower respiratory tract disease: A prospective, double-blind, randomized trial. Crit. Care Med. *22*:566–572, 1994.
159. Menon, K., Sutcliffe, T., and Klassen, T. P.: A randomized trial comparing the efficacy of epinephrine with salbutamol in the treatment of acute bronchiolitis. J. Pediatr. *126*:1004–1007, 1995.
160. Meyers, J. D., Reed, E. C., Shepp, D. H., et al.: Acyclovir for prevention of cytomegalovirus infection and disease after allogeneic marrow transplantation. N. Engl. J. Med. *318*:70–75, 1988.
161. Mimica, L., Donoso, E., Howard, J. E., et al.: Lung puncture in the etiological diagnosis of pneumonia. Am. J. Dis. Child. *122*:278–282, 1971.
162. Minor, T. E., Dick, E. C., DeMeo, A. N., et al.: Viruses as precipitants of asthmatic attacks in children. J. A. M. A. *227*:292–298, 1974.
163. Mintz, L., Ballard, R. A., Sniderman, S. H., et al.: Nosocomial respiratory syncytial virus infections in an intensive care nursery: Rapid diagnosis by direct immunofluorescence. Pediatrics *64*:149–153, 1979.
164. Moler, F. W., Steinhart, C. M., Ohmit, S. E., et al.: Effectiveness of ribavirin in otherwise well infants with respiratory syncytial virus–associated respiratory failure. J. Pediatr. *128*:422–428, 1996.

165. Morrell, R. E., Marks, M. I., Champlin, R., et al.: An outbreak of severe pneumonia due to respiratory syncytial virus in isolated Arctic populations. Am. J. Epidemiol. *101*:231–237, 1975.
166. Mufson, M. A., Krause, H. E., Mocega, H. E., et al.: Viruses, *Mycoplasma pneumoniae*, and bacteria associated with lower respiratory tract disease among infants. Am. J. Epidemiol. *91*:912–202, 1970.
167. Murray, J. F.: The ketchup-bottle method. N. Engl. J. Med. *300*:1155–1157, 1979.
167a. Murphy, B. R., Hall, S. L., Kulkarni, A. B., et al.: An update on approaches to the development of respiratory syncytial virus and parainfluenza virus type 3 vaccines. Virus Res. *32*:13–36, 1994.
168. Murphy, S., and Florman, A. L.: Lung diseases against infection: A clinical correlation. Pediatrics *72*:1–15, 1983.
169. Murphy, T. F., Henderson, F. W., Clyde, W. A., Jr., et al.: Pneumonia: An eleven-year study in a pediatric practice. Am. J. Epidemiol. *113*:12–21, 1981.
170. Nahmias, A. J., Griffith, D., and Snitzer, J.: Fatal pneumonia associated with adenovirus type 7. Am. J. Dis. Child. *114*:36–41, 1967.
171. Nelson, K. E., Gavitt, F., Batt, M. D., et al.: The role of adenoviruses in the pertussis syndrome. J. Pediatr. *86*:335–341, 1975.
172. Nichol, K. P., and Cherry, J. D.: Bacterial-viral interrelationships in respiratory infections of children. N. Engl. J. Med. *277*:667–672, 1967.
173. Olson, L. C., Miller, G., and Hanshaw, J. B.: Acute infectious lymphocytosis presenting as a pertussis-like illness: Its association with adenovirus type 12. Lancet *1*:200–201, 1964.
174. Orenstein, D. M., Boat, T. F., Stern, R. C., et al.: The effect of early diagnosis and treatment in cystic fibrosis. Am. J. Dis. Child. *131*:973–975, 1977.
175. Osborne, D.: Radiologic appearance of viral disease of the lower respiratory tract in infants and children. A. J. R. Am. J. Roentgenol. *130*:29–33, 1978.
176. Paisley, J. W., Bruhn, F. W., Lauer, B. A., et al.: Type A_2 influenza viral infections in children. Am. J. Dis. Child. *132*:34–36, 1978.
177. Paisley, J. W., Lauer, B. A., McIntosh, K., et al.: Pathogens associated with acute lower respiratory tract infection in young children. Pediatr. Infect. Dis. *3*:14–19, 1984.
178. Parks, C. R.: Mist therapy: Rationale and practice. J. Pediatr. *76*:305–313, 1970.
179. Parrott, R. H., Vargosko, A., Luckey, A., et al.: Clinical features of infection with hemadsorption viruses. N. Engl. J. Med. *260*:731–738, 1959.
180. Parrott, R. H., Kim, H. W., Vargosko, A. J., et al.: Serious respiratory tract illness as a result of Asian influenza and influenza B infections in children. J. Pediatr. *61*:205–213, 1962.
181. Parrott, R. H.: Viral respiratory tract illness in children. Bull. N. Y. Acad. Med. *39*:629–648, 1963.
182. Person, D. A., and Herrmann, E. C., Jr.: Experiences in laboratory diagnosis of rhinovirus infections in routine medical practice. Mayo Clin. Proc. *45*:517–526, 1970.
183. Pifer, L. L: *Pneumocystis carinii*: A diagnostic dilemma. Pediatr. Infect. Dis. *2*:177–183, 1983.
184. Pifer, L. L., Hughes, W. J., Stagno, S., et al.: *Pneumocystis carinii* infection: Evidence for high prevalence in normal and immunosuppressed children. Pediatrics *61*:35–41, 1978.
185. Pinkerton, H., and Carroll, S.: Fatal adenovirus pneumonia in infants: Correlation of histologic and electron microscopic observations. Am. J. Pathol. *65*:543–548, 1971.
186. Pizzo, P.: Infectious complications in the child with cancer. J. Pediatr. *98*:341–354, 513–523, 1981.
187. Poncz, M., Kane, E., and Gill, F. M.: Acute chest syndrome in sickle cell disease: Etiology and clinical correlates. J. Pediatr. *107*:861–866, 1985.
188. Portnoy, B., Hanes, B., Salvatore, M. A., et al.: The peripheral white blood count in respirovirus infection. J. Pediatr. *68*:181–188, 1966.
189. Purtilo, D. T., Sakamoto, F., Barnabei, V., et al.: Epstein-Barr virus induced diseases in boys with x-linked lymphoproliferative syndrome. Am. J. Med. *73*:49–56, 1982.
190. Reijowen, T., Korppi, M., Pitkakangas, S., et al.: The clinical efficacy of nebulized racemic epinephrine and albuterol in acute bronchiolitis. Arch. Pediatr. Adol. Med. *149*:686–692, 1995.
191. Reilly, C. M., Hoch, S. M., Stokes, J., Jr., et al.: Clinical and laboratory findings in cases of respiratory illness caused by coryzaviruses. Ann. Intern. Med. *57*:515 525, 1962.
192. Rice, R. P., and Loda, F. A.: A roentgenographic analysis of respiratory syncytial virus pneumonia in infants. Radiology *87*:1021–1027, 1966.
193. Ross, C. A., Stott, E. J., McMichael, S., et al.: Problems of laboratory diagnosis of respiratory syncytial virus infection in childhood. Arch. Virusforsch. *14*:553–562, 1964.
194. Royall, J. A., and Levin, D. L.: Adult respiratory distress syndrome in pediatric patients. I. Clinical aspects, pathophysiology, pathology, and mechanisms of lung injury. J. Pediatr. *112*:169–180, 1988.
195. Royall, J., and Levin, D. L.: Adult respiratory distress syndrome in pediatric patients. II. Management. J. Pediatr. *112*:335–347, 1988.
196. Rubinstein, A., Morecki, R., Silverman, B., et al.: Pulmonary disease in children with acquired immune deficiency syndrome and AIDS-related complex. J. Pediatr. *108*:498–503, 1986.
197. Rusconi, F., Rancilio, L., Assael, B. M., et al.: Counter immunoelectrophoresis and latex particle agglutination in the etiologic diagnosis of presumed bacterial pneumonia in pediatric patients. Pediatr. Infect. Dis. J. *7*:781–785, 1988.
198. Saikku, P., Ruutu, P., Leinonen, M., et al.: Acute lower-respiratory-tract infection associated with chlamydial TWAR antibody in Filipino children. J. Infect. Dis. *158*:1095–1097, 1988.
199. Sanchez, I., DeKoster, J., Powell, R. E., et al.: Effect of racemic epinephrine and salbutamol on clinical score and pulmonary mechanics in infants with bronchiolitis. J. Pediatr. *122*:145–151, 1993.
200. Schmidt, G. M., Horak, D. A., Niland, J. C., et al.: A randomized, controlled trial of prophylactic ganciclovir for cytomegalovirus pulmonary infections in recipients of allogeneic bone marrow transplants. N. Engl. J. Med. *324*:1005–1011, 1991.
201. Schmidt, J. P., Metcalf, T. G., and Miltenberger, F. W.: An epidemic of Asian influenza in children at Ladd Air Force Base, Alaska, 1960. J. Pediatr. *61*:214–220, 1962.
202. Schuh, S., Canny, G., Reisman, J. J., et al.: Nebulized albuterol in acute bronchiolitis. J. Pediatr. *117*:633–637, 1990.
203. Siegel, M. M., Walter, T. K., and Ablin, A. R.: Measles pneumonia in childhood leukemia. Pediatrics *60*:38–40, 1977.
204. Siegel, S., Johnston, S., and Adair, S.: Isolation of measles virus in primary rhesus monkey cells from a child with acute interstitial pneumonia who cytologically had giant-cell pneumonia without a rash. Am. J. Clin. Pathol. *94*:464–469, 1990.
205. Siegel, W., Spencer, F. J., Smith, D. J., et al.: Two new variants of infection with coxsackie virus group B, type 5, in young children: A syndrome of lymphadenopathy, pharyngitis and hepatomegaly or splenomegaly, or both, and one of pneumonia. N. Engl. J. Med. *268*:1210–1216, 1963.
206. Simonds, R. J., Lindegren, M. L., Thomas, P., et al.: Prophylaxis against *Pneumocystis carinii* pneumonia among children with perinatally acquired human immunodeficiency virus infection in the United States. N. Engl. J. Med. *332*:786–790, 1995.
207. Simpson, W., Hacking, P. M., Court, S. D. M., et al.: The radiological findings in respiratory syncytial virus infection in children. II. The correlation of radiological categories with clinical and virological findings. Pediatr. Radiol. *2*:155–160, 1974.
208. Smith, D. W., Frankel, L. R., Mathers, L. H., et al.: A controlled trial of aerosolized ribavirin in infants receiving mechanical ventilation for severe respiratory syncytial virus infection. N. Engl. J. Med. *325*:24–29, 1991.
209. Smith, W., Andrewes, C. H., and Laidlaw, P. P.: A virus isolated from influenza patients. Lancet *2*:66–68, 1933.
210. Spence, L., and Barratt, N.: Respiratory syncytial virus associated with acute respiratory infections in Trinidadian patients. Am. J. Epidemiol. *88*:257–266, 1968.
211. Springer, C., Bar-Yishay, E., Uwayyad, K., et al.: Corticosteroids do not affect the clinical or physiological status of infants with bronchiolitis. Pediatr. Pulmonol. *9*:181–185, 1990.
212. Stagno, S., Brasfield, D. M., Brown, M. B., et al.: Infant pneumonitis associated with cytomegalovirus, *Chlamydia, Pneumocystis* and *Ureaplasma*: A prospective study. Pediatrics *68*:322–329, 1981.
213. Stagno, S., Pifer, L. L., Hughes, W. T., et al.: *Pneumocystis carinii* pneumonitis in young immunocompetent infants. Pediatrics *66*:56–62, 1980.
214. Steen-Johnsen, J., Orstavik, I., and Attramadal, A.: Severe illnesses due to adenovirus type 7 in children. Acta Paediatr. Scand. *58*:157–163, 1969.
215. Stott, E. J., Eadie, M. B., and Grist, N. R.: Rhinovirus infections of children in hospital: Isolation of three, possibly new rhinovirus serotypes. Am. J. Epidemiol. *90*:45–52, 1969.
216. Sullivan, K. M., Kopecky, K. J., and Jocom, J.: Immunomodulatory and antimicrobial efficacy of intravenous immunoglobulin in bone marrow transplantation. N. Engl. J. Med. *323*:705–712, 1990.
217. Suto, T., Yano, N., Ikeda, M., et al.: Respiratory syncytial virus infection and its serologic epidemiology. Am. J. Epidemiol. *82*:211–224, 1965.
218. Turner, R. B., Lande, A. E., Chase, P., et al.: Pneumonia in pediatric outpatients: Cause and clinical manifestations. J. Pediatr. *111*:194–200, 1987.
219. Wang, E. E., Milner, R., Allen, U., et al.: Bronchodilators for treatment of mild bronchiolitis: A factorial randomized trial. Arch. Dis. Child. *67*:289–293, 1992.
220. Wang, E. E. L., Prober, C. G., Manson, B., et al.: Association of respiratory viral infections with pulmonary deterioration in patients with cystic fibrosis. N. Engl. J. Med. *311*:1653–1658, 1984.
221. Welliver, R. C., Wong, D. T., Sun, M., et al.: The development of respiratory syncytial virus–specific IgE and the release of histamine in nasopharyngeal secretions after infection. N. Engl. J. Med. *305*:841–846, 1981.
222. Wheeler, J. G., Wofford, J., and Turner, R. B.: Historical cohort evaluation of ribavirin efficacy in respiratory syncytial virus infection. Pediatr. Infect. Dis. J. *12*:209–213, 1993.
223. Winston, D. J., Gale, R. P., Meyer, D. V., et al.: Infectious complications of human bone marrow transplantation. Medicine *58*:1–31, 1979.
224. Winternitz, M. C., Wason, I. M., and McNamara, F. P.: The Pathology of Influenza. New Haven, Yale University Press, 1920.
225. Wohl, M. E. B., and Mead, J.: Age as a factor in respiratory disease. *In* Chernick, V., and Kendig, E. L. (eds.): Disorders of the Respiratory Tract in Children. Philadelphia, W. B. Saunders, 1990, pp. 175–182.
226. Wolff, L. J., Bartlett, M. S., Baehner, R. L., et al.: The causes of interstitial

pneumonitis in immunocompromised children: An aggressive systematic approach to diagnosis. Pediatrics *60*:41–45, 1977.
227. Wright, H. T., Jr., Beckwith, J. B., and Gwinn, J. L.: A fatal case of inclusion body pneumonia in an infant infected with adenovirus type 3. J. Pediatr. *64*:528–533, 1964.
228. Wyde, P. R., Moore, D. K., Hepburn, T., et al.: Evaluation of the protective efficacy of reshaped human monoclonal antibody RSHZ19 against respiratory syncytial virus in cotton rats. Pediatr. Res. *38*:543–550, 1995.
229. Yeager, A. S.: Transfusion-acquired cytomegalovirus infection in newborn infants. Am. J. Dis. Child. *128*:478–483, 1974.
230. Yeager, A. S., Grumet, F. C., Hafleigh, E. G., et al.: Prevention of transfusion-acquired cytomegalovirus infections in newborn infants. J. Pediatr. *98*:281–287, 1981.
231. Zinserling, A.: Peculiarities of lesions in viral and *Mycoplasma* infections of the respiratory tract. Virchows Arch. Pathol. Anat. *356*:259–273, 1972.

27

BACTERIAL PNEUMONIAS

Jerome O. Klein

Bacterial pneumonia is an inflammation of the lung due to a bacterial pathogen. The pneumonias may be classified in anatomic terms, such as lobar pneumonia, bronchopneumonia, and interstitial pneumonia; however, it now is more usual to categorize this disease by the etiologic agent, as in pneumococcal or staphylococcal pneumonia.

HISTORY

Pneumonia has been a frequent and serious human illness throughout recorded history. Histologic examination of Egyptian mummies (1250 to 1000 B.C.) revealed hepatization of the lungs compatible with acute pneumococcal pneumonia. The disease was known well to the Greeks and Romans, and the symptomatology and management (including a drainage procedure for empyema) were described by Hippocrates. Laennec described the pathologic changes and physical signs of pneumonia and pleurisy in 1819, and Rokitansky distinguished lobar pneumonia from bronchopneumonia in 1842.

In 1881, Pasteur in France and Sternberg in the United States independently isolated, cultured, and described the pneumococcus. Each used inoculation of rabbits with human saliva. Pasteur used saliva from a child who had died with clinical rabies, whereas Sternberg used material from a normal subject. A fatal septicemia resulted in the rabbits, and the organisms were isolated from their blood. In 1882, Friedländer described the pneumococcus in pathologic sections of lung and pleura and in fluid obtained by lung puncture from living patients with pneumonia. In the same laboratory, Christian Gram exposed the sections to a sequence of dyes: aniline-gentian violet, a weak solution of iodine, ethanol, and Bismarck brown. Pairs of elongated cocci retained the dark aniline-gentian violet dye. The organism was referred to as "pneumococcus" by Fraenkel in 1886 because of its role as a cause of pulmonary infection.

Early methods of treatment of pneumonia included blood letting; leeching; inhalation of chloroform; subcutaneous injection of gold, silver, and platinum solutions; and oral administration of mercury, quinine, and digitalis. The investigations of the pneumococcus in the late nineteenth century led to the use in 1891 of small subcutaneous doses of rabbit serum for treatment of patients with pneumonia. These treatments usually failed, but once the many antigenically separable types of the pneumococcus were recognized, specific antisera were prepared. These materials provided prompt and striking symptomatic improvement and a marked reduction in the fatality rate for pneumococcal pneumonia. Problems arose because of hypersensitivity reactions to the animal serums and the difficulty of making type-specific diagnosis. Responses to these problems included partial elimination of some of the animal protein and adaptation of the Neufeld technique for typing of pneumococci in sputum and body fluids. Use of rabbit antisera resulted in a significant increase in survival of patients with pneumonia due to *Haemophilus influenzae*, and antistreptococcal horse serum or human serum obtained from patients convalescent from scarlet fever was used with success in patients with streptococcal pneumonia. Serotherapy was discarded after the introduction of the sulfonamides and penicillin.

Soon after the introduction of the sulfonamides for clinical use in 1935, sulfapyridine was identified as the most potent of the compounds for treatment of pneumococcal disease. By 1943, however, sulfonamide-resistant strains were reported.[71] In 1941, Abraham and colleagues[3] and in 1943, Keefer and colleagues[41] reported the efficacy of penicillin in treatment of life-threatening infections caused by gram-positive cocci, including *Streptococcus pneumoniae*. Penicillin-resistant pneumococci were identified in epidemic form in South Africa in the 1970s and now have been identified throughout the world.

A 14-valent pneumococcal polysaccharide vaccine was introduced in the United States in 1977 and a 23-valent vaccine in 1983. Most of the polysaccharides were poor immunogens for children younger than 2 years of age, and the vaccines were used only in children at risk for invasive pneumococcal infections and who were 2 years of age and older (e.g., children with sickle-cell disease, functional asplenia, or nephrosis). In October 1990, a conjugate polysaccharide vaccine for *H. influenzae* type b was approved by the Food and Drug Administration. Use of the vaccine has led to a significant decrease in the incidence of invasive disease, including pneumonia due to *H. influenzae*.

Further information about early studies of the pneumococcus and bacterial pneumonias is provided in two reference works of great value that were reprinted in 1979 by the Harvard University Press: *The Biology of the Pneumococcus* by Benjamin White and *Pneumonia* by Roderick Heffron. These works first were published in 1938 and 1939, respectively, by the Commonwealth Fund, New York. Watson and colleagues[77] have written a brief history of the pneumococcus highlighting landmarks in infectious disease discovery, including the development of Gram stain, the role of the capsule in resistance to phagocytosis, use of polysaccharides as vaccines, and evidence that DNA encodes genetic information. Symposia proceedings have focused on the pneumococcus,[61] polysaccharide pneumococcal vaccines,[40] *H. influenzae*,[23] and lower respiratory tract infections in children in developing countries.[9, 26]

MICROBIOLOGY

Because of the difficulty of documenting the microbiology of pneumonia in infants and young children, accurate data concerning the incidence and specific agents of bacterial pneumonia in children are lacking. Austrian[7] estimates that bacteria are responsible for a tenth to a third of all cases of acute pneumonias. A presumptive diagnosis of bacterial or mixed bacterial and viral infection based on antigen detection and antibody assays was made in 45 per cent of Finnish children who were hospitalized for lower respiratory tract infections.[52] Bacteriologic findings based on results of lung punctures from 1069 children in developing countries identified *S. pneumoniae*, *H. influenzae*, and *Staphylococcus aureus* as the leading pathogens.[65]

Now, as in the past, *S. pneumoniae* is the leading bacterial cause of pneumonia in all age groups except the newborn infant. *H. influenzae* type b was an important cause of pneumonia in young infants until the introduction of the conjugate polysaccharide vaccine in October 1990. In areas with high rates of immunization, pneumonia and invasive disease due to *H. influenzae* now are uncommon. Other species of bacteria are of importance in special groups: group B *Streptococcus*, *S. aureus*, and some gram-negative enteric bacilli are responsible for pneumonia in the newborn infant; group A *Streptococcus* may cause pneumonia in children with viral infections, particularly measles, chickenpox, and influenza; pneumonia caused by *S. aureus* and gram-negative enteric bacilli is a concern in children with malignancy or those who have altered host defense mechanisms. Anaerobic bacteria play a significant role in aspiration pneumonia and lung abscess. Only a few cases of pneumonia caused by *Legionella pneumophila* have been reported in children. Other species of bacteria responsible for occasional cases of pneumonia include *Neisseria meningitidis*, *Bordetella pertussis*, *Bartonella henselae*,[1] *Bacillus anthracis*, *Salmonella typhosa*, and *Francisella tularensis*.

Streptococcus pneumoniae

Although more than 80 immunologically distinct types of *S. pneumoniae* have been identified on the basis of capsular polysaccharide antigens, relatively few types are responsible for most disease in children. Types 1, 3, 6, 7, 14, 18, 19, and 23 are the types most frequently implicated in pneumonia in children; all are included in the pneumococcal vaccine introduced in the United States in 1978.

The spectrum of lower respiratory tract disease caused by *S. pneumoniae* ranges from a mild to moderate disease that can be managed without hospitalization to a severe and life-threatening disease that may be complicated by empyema or extrapulmonary manifestations, including meningitis. The usual case has sudden onset, lobar involvement, abrupt termination after appropriate chemotherapy is instituted, and rapid restoration of the involved area of the lung to normal. Although the classic pattern of pneumococcal pneumonia has a lobar distribution, bronchopneumonia and interstitial pneumonia are frequent.

Multidrug-resistant strains of pneumococci were reported from South Africa[5] in 1977. Some of the strains were highly resistant to penicillin G, requiring more than 4 μg/mL for inhibition, and were resistant to other drugs that serve as alternatives to penicillin G in pneumococcal disease, including other penicillins, cephalosporins, tetracyclines, chloramphenicol, macrolides, clindamycin, and sulfonamides. Resistance of *S. pneumoniae* to penicillin is caused by alterations in penicillin-binding proteins. Penicillin resistance is defined by the minimal inhibitory concentrations of pneumococci: less than 0.1 μg/mL = susceptible; 0.1 to 1.0 μg/mL = intermediate resistance; 2 or more μg/mL = high-level resistance. During the past few years, multidrug-resistant pneumococci have been reported from every continent.[30] High rates of resistance have been reported from Spain[56] and Papua New Guinea.[33] In Pakistan, approximately one third of pneumococci were highly resistant to trimethoprim-sulfamethoxazole, the agent used most frequently to treat children with acute lower respiratory tract infections, and one third of strains were resistant to chloramphenicol.[48]

The prevalence of resistant pneumococci in the United States varies by region, time, and culture site. A survey of hospitals by investigators at the Centers for Disease Control and Prevention identified 5 per cent of isolates with a minimal inhibitory concentration greater than 0.1 μg/mL during the period 1979 to 1987.[68] A high prevalence of multidrug-resistant pneumococci was reported during 1993 in specimens obtained from children attending a day care center in a rural Kentucky community; 53 per cent of the strains were penicillin-resistant, 33 per cent were highly resistant to penicillin, and 50 per cent were multidrug-resistant.[25] The prevalence of resistance is higher for isolates obtained from children than in isolates from adults and is higher in nasopharyngeal specimens than in specimens of blood and cerebrospinal fluid. The management issues raised by the appearance of resistant pneumococci are discussed in the section on chemotherapy for specific pathogens.

Haemophilus influenzae

Haemophilus influenzae type b accounts for most cases of pneumonia caused by this species. Pneumonia due to *H. influenzae* types a, c, or d is reported rarely. Nontypable strains are responsible for an uncertain number of cases of pneumonia and are isolated from patients with chronic bronchitis, bronchiectasis, and cystic fibrosis who have acute exacerbations of disease.

In developing countries, nontypable strains of *H. influenzae* are important causes of pneumonia. The nontypable strains gain access to the lung via spread from the upper respiratory tract but are less likely than type b strains to invade the blood stream. Of 32 isolates of *H. influenzae* obtained from blood and/or lung puncture of children with pneumonia in Papua New Guinea, 18 were nontypable, 8 were types other than b, and 6 were b; all 6 patients with type b obtained from culture of the lung aspirate also were bacteremic. Only 4 of 18 patients with nontypable *H. influenzae* in the lung puncture were bacteremic.[66] Of 105 isolates of *Haemophilus* species from cultures of blood from children with lower respiratory tract infection in Pakistan, 10 were *Haemophilus parainfluenzae*, 61 were *H. influenzae* type b, and 34 were nontypable.[78] Similar data were reported in patients with lobar pneumonia in the Gambia.[75] Thus, nontypable *H. influenzae* is unlikely to be diagnosed as the cause of pneumonia if cultures of blood alone are relied on for microbiologic diagnosis. These data also suggest that pneumonia due to nontypable *H. influenzae* probably is underdiagnosed in developed as well as developing countries.

The clinical presentation of pneumonia due to *H. influenzae* is indistinguishable from that due to *S. pneumoniae* and includes mild, moderate, and severe disease. In a series of cases in children seen at the Boston City Hospital, 17 children with pneumonia and bacteremia due to *H. influenzae* type b were identified in a 5-year period; only 4 of the children were judged to be sufficiently ill for admission to a hospital.[46] All of 13 children with mild to moderate pneumonia and bacteremia were treated successfully as outpatients. The relatively mild course of pneumonia in these patients contrasts with findings of other investigators who based their reports on the records of children admitted to the hospital.[6, 18, 38, 59] A report of 65 children with *H. influenzae* pneumonia hospitalized at Parkland Memorial Hospital in Dallas during the 14-year period beginning July 1964 included 24 children with pleural effusion, 7 with pneumothorax, and 1 who developed pneumatoceles; 10 children had associated meningitis, and 3 had purulent pericarditis.[31] Type b was the most frequent pathogen cultured from empyema fluids in children receiving care in Bethesda during the period 1974 to 1987.[18]

Beginning in the 1970s, beta-lactamase–producing strains of both nontypable and type b *H. influenzae* were reported throughout the United States.[76] The enzyme cleaves the beta-lactam ring of susceptible penicillins, rendering the antibiotic inactive against the enzyme-producing strain. During recent years in the United States, approximately 10 to 40 per cent of strains of *H. influenzae* were beta-lactamase–positive; the proportion of beta-lactamase–producing strains may vary over time in the same community.[15] Prevalence of antimicrobial resistance for a wide variety of drugs tested against isolates of *H. influenzae* was reviewed by Doern and colleagues.[24]

Staphylococcus aureus

Pneumonia and other serious infections due to *S. aureus* are of particular concern in newborn infants, patients with altered host defenses, and patients with prior viral respiratory infection (e.g., influenza). In the United States and western Europe, the most severe problem with staphylococcal disease in newborn infants occurred in the 1950s and ended around 1965. There is no satisfactory explanation for the cyclic appearance and disappearance of virulent strains of *S. aureus*. The phage type 80/81, which was so devastating in the 1950s, is no longer a major problem either in the United States or in Europe. Nevertheless, rare cases of fatal and rapidly progressive staphylococcal pneumonia still occur.[54]

In older children, staphylococcal pneumonia may not be differentiated clinically or radiologically from other bacterial pneumonias. In young infants, the course usually is severe; the onset is abrupt, with tachypnea, significant dyspnea, and restlessness. Progression of disease is rapid, and empyema, abscesses, and pneumatoceles are frequent. Although pneumatoceles are associated with staphylococcal pneumonia, they also may be seen in children with pneumonia caused by *S. pneumoniae*, group A *Streptococcus*, and *H. influenzae*. Pneumatoceles may persist for many months but are not a significant cause of morbidity, and they usually require no specific therapy.

Group B *Streptococcus*

Early-onset disease in the newborn due to group B *Streptococcus* presents as a multisystem illness during the first week of life and frequently is characterized by pneumonia, the clinical and radiologic pattern of which simulates respiratory distress syndrome.[2] The pattern of group B *Streptococcus* on chest roentgenogram includes diffuse pulmonary granularity and air bronchograms, similar to the pattern seen in infants with respiratory distress syndrome. Apnea and shock are more likely to occur in cases of pneumonia due to group B *Streptococcus*. Infants with infections caused by group B *Streptococcus* require lower respiratory pressures on mechanical ventilation than do infants with respiratory distress syndrome. At autopsy, hyaline membranes similar to those seen in infants with respiratory distress syndrome have been observed in the lungs of infants who died of pneumonia due to group B *Streptococcus*, and gram-positive cocci were present within the hyaline membranes.

Anaerobic Bacteria

Improvements in techniques for isolation and identification of the various genera and species of anaerobic bacteria have provided a better understanding of the anaerobic flora of humans and the role of these organisms in disease. Anaerobes are present on the skin, in the mouth, in the intestines, and in the genital tract. Anaerobic bacteria may be responsible for pneumonia and lung abscesses in a host who is subject to aspiration. The most common anaerobic bacteria responsible for pulmonary infection include *Fusobacterium* species, *Bacteroides melaninogenicus*, *Bacteroides fragilis*, *Peptococcus*, and *Peptostreptococcus*. The initial lesion of anaerobic infection of the lower respiratory tract is a pneumonitis with a slowly progressive clinical course. Lung abscess and necrotizing pneumonia may be a late consequence of the anaerobic pneumonitis.[11, 19]

Legionella pneumophila

In August 1976, 221 cases of respiratory illness caused by an unknown agent occurred among 4500 participants at an American Legion convention in Philadelphia. The disease was marked by high fever, recurrent chills, prominent myalgia, abnormal liver function, and a toxic encephalopathy, in addition to respiratory signs. Patients had nonproductive coughs, and their radiologic pattern showed patchy bronchopneumonia that in some cases progressed to lobar consolidation. Some patients responded promptly to therapy with erythromycin.

Investigators at the Centers for Disease Control and Prevention of the Public Health Service isolated small pleomorphic rods from lung tissues taken at autopsy. The rods were stained with silver impregnation methods and were visualized by direct immunofluorescence; however, they were seen poorly or not at all with Gram stain. The organism was designated *"Legionella pneumophila."*

The genus *Legionella* includes aerobic, fastidious, gram-negative rods that require cysteine and some form of iron for growth. Eighteen separable species have been identified. The natural habitat of *L. pneumophila* is aquatic reservoirs, including rivers, lakes, air-conditioning cooling towers, and water distribution systems. Almost all cases of respiratory infection in children have been associated with *L. pneumophila*, except for one case due to *Legionella micdadei* (the Pittsburgh pneumonia agent).[45] Diagnosis is made by culture on buffered yeast extract agar, direct fluorescent antibody staining of respiratory tract secretions, and demonstration of antibody by indirect immunofluorescence.

Seroepidemiologic studies suggest that subclinical or minor infections occur in some children.[51, 62] Prospective studies of children with lower respiratory disease, however, identified few cases due to *L. pneumophila*.[4, 55] Legionellosis in children with leukemia in relapse[45] and chronic granulomatous disease[58] indicates that the organism should be added to the list of agents that cause pneumonia in the immunocompromised child.

Group A *Streptococcus*

Pneumonia caused by group A *Streptococcus* is uncommon. Surveys of children hospitalized with pneumonia in Dallas[72] over a 9-year period and Denver[50] and Chicago[38] over a 5-year period identified only five, three, and two cases, respectively, caused by group A *Streptococcus*. Pneumonia due to group A *Streptococcus* may follow viral infection, such as influenza, measles, and chickenpox, but also occurs in children without previous illness. The disease is characterized by necrosis of respiratory tract mucosa and lung tissue with edema and localized hemorrhage. Clinical signs include chills, high and prolonged fever, dyspnea, and pleuritic chest pain. Patients remain febrile for a mean of 10 days,[72] long after the initiation of therapy with appropriate antibacterial drugs. Bacteremia and pleural effusion are frequent, and pneumatoceles may occur. The typical pleural effusion begins as a serous fluid, progresses to be serosanguineous, and may become fibrinopurulent.

Neisseria meningitidis

N. meningitidis usually is associated with asymptomatic carriage in the upper respiratory tract, but pneumonia is relatively uncommon. When pneumonia due to *N. meningitidis* does occur, it usually is due to group Y and is accompanied in some cases by bacteremia.[37] There is no distinctive clinical pattern in children, and the diagnosis usually is made by culture of blood.[10, 32]

Gram-Negative Enteric Bacilli

Pneumonia caused by gram-negative enteric bacilli occurs in newborn infants and children with altered host defense mechanisms but is seen rarely in normal infants and children. Pneumonia caused by *Pseudomonas aeruginosa* and, to a lesser extent, by *Pseudomonas cepacia* is a particular problem in children with cystic fibrosis and may occur as a severe, progressive disease leading to a fatal, necrotizing bronchopneumonia. Pneumonia caused by *Klebsiella pneumoniae* is severe, with fever, chills, and a pattern of necrosis and destruction of lung tissue.

EPIDEMIOLOGY

The respiratory pathogens *S. pneumoniae, H. influenzae*, group A *Streptococcus*, and *S. aureus* are common inhabitants of the upper respiratory tract. These organisms may be isolated from many healthy children, and it is important to differentiate the many children who are colonized (multiplication of microorganisms without signs or symptoms of disease and without immune response), children who have asymptomatic or inapparent infection (multiplication of organisms without signs or symptoms of disease but with immune response), and children with disease (clinical signs or symptoms that result from multiplication of microorganisms). Colonization may persist for periods as long as several months. The reason for colonization in some individuals and inapparent infection or disease in others is unknown. Current theories are considered in the section on pathogenesis.

Humans are the only known source for the common bacterial pathogens responsible for respiratory disease. Transmission occurs in most cases by droplet spread: the brief passage of the infectious agent through the air when the source and the patient are near each other (usually within several feet); spread occurs also during talking or sneezing. Airborne spread occurs in some cases of staphylococcal infection; organisms within droplet nuclei, dust particles, or skin squames are carried through the air for distances of more than several feet.

The incubation period of bacterial pneumonia is difficult to determine, probably because of factors, such as viral infection, that play a role in development of disease. Similarly, the period of communicability is not known accurately but probably is about 24 hours after effective antimicrobial therapy for *S. pneumoniae* and *H. influenzae*.

Bacterial pneumonia may occur during all seasons but is most prevalent during the winter and spring months, presumably because crowding in indoor spaces during these seasons favors direct transmission of infected droplets.

The highest incidence of pneumonia is in the very young and the very old. Passively acquired antibody to *S. pneumoniae* and *H. influenzae* type b is protective during the first few months of life. After the first months, if infected, the infant is susceptible to the disease until active immunity is induced as a response to inapparent infection or overt disease.

An overall male predominance is found in almost all series of bacterial pneumonia in children. Series of cases of *H. influenzae* pneumonia showed the male predominance to be 2:1 or greater.[6, 38, 59] More cases of pneumococcal pneumonia occur in males than in females in all pediatric age groups.[36]

Nosocomial pneumonia occurs in children at risk for aspiration, ventilated patients, and children with underlying pulmonary and cardiac disease and immunodeficiencies. Gram-negative bacillary organisms are responsible for a majority of bacterial pneumonias acquired in the hospital, followed in importance by gram-positive organisms. Compliance with infection control measures in intensive care units is critical to prevention of nosocomial pneumonias.[39]

Although Heffron[36] cites several studies suggesting that blacks are peculiarly susceptible to pneumonia and to pneumococcus infections in general, no studies of the incidence of disease in different racial groups that are controlled adequately for socioeconomic factors, access to medical care, and other features important in the transmission of disease have been reported.

Bacterial pneumonia uncommonly occurs in epidemic form in the community, although the incidence of disease increases during periods of epidemic viral infection, such as occurs with influenza outbreaks. Legionnaires' disease usually occurs in clusters of cases; most outbreaks have been related to airborne spread from contaminated air-conditioning cooling towers. Hospital-acquired infection may be epidemic (e.g., infections in newborn nurseries during the period of prevalence of virulent strains of *S. aureus*). Common-source outbreaks of pneumonia due to gram-negative enteric bacilli may result from contaminated aqueous solutions used in humidification equipment.

PATHOGENESIS

Most bacterial pneumonias are a result of colonization of the nasopharynx followed by aspiration or inhalation of organisms. The lung is protected from bacterial infection by a variety of mechanisms, including filtration of particles in the nares, prevention of aspiration of infected secretions by the epiglottal reflex, expulsion of aspirated materials by the cough reflex, entrapment and expulsion of organisms by mucus-secreting and ciliated cells, ingestion and killing of bacteria by alveolar macrophages, neutralization of bacteria by local and systemic nonspecific and specific immune substances (complement, opsonins, and antibodies), and transport of particles from the lung by lymphatic drainage. Pulmonary infection may occur when one or more of these barriers are altered, inhibited, or destroyed. Hematogenous spread to the lung by means of infected emboli arising from a suppurative focus, such as an abscess of the skin or soft tissue due to *S. aureus*, is infrequent.

Animal models suggest that the mechanisms of the inflammatory response in the lung are due to cell wall components of gram-positive organisms or endotoxins of gram-negative bacteria.[21, 73] An increase in cell wall components and endotoxin may follow antibiotic-caused cell death, with resulting increase in inflammation. Thus, the first stage in the healing produced by appropriate antimicrobial drugs may be accompanied by clinical deterioration due to an early increase in inflammation in the lung.

Pneumonia caused by *S. pneumoniae* begins with acute inflammation and hyperemia of the lower respiratory mucosa, exudation of edema fluid, deposition of fibrin, and infiltration of alveoli by polymorphonuclear leukocytes ("red hepatization") followed by predominance of fibrin deposition and macrophage activity ("white hepatization"). Exudate in the alveoli is digested enzymatically and absorbed or removed by coughing. Resolution then occurs, with return of lung morphology and physiology to normal. In contrast, when the pneumonia is caused by *S. aureus* or *K. pneumoniae*, destruction of tissue and formation of multiple, small abscesses are frequent.

Although clinicians have noted that symptoms and signs of minor respiratory infection caused by viruses frequently precede bacterial pneumonia, precise documentation of antecedent viral infection is scant. Studies in animal models of infection with influenza and reoviruses[42] demonstrate a limited period of vulnerability of the lung to bacterial challenge after viral infection. The effects of the viral infection appear to be mediated by alterations in the activity of the alveolar macrophage. A brief period of impaired function of these phagocytic cells results from the viral infection. Staphylococcal[27, 47] or pneumococcal pneumonias[28, 29] may occur during or shortly after infection due to influenza virus. There is no evidence that infections with other respiratory viruses precede bacterial pneumonias.[47] As an example, Hall and colleagues[34] found that the risk of secondary bacterial infection in infants hospitalized with respiratory syncytial viral infection was low (1.2 per cent of 565 children studied over 9 years).

Anatomic, physiologic, or immune defects predispose patients to lower respiratory tract infection. These include congenital anomalies (cleft palate, tracheoesophageal fistula, or sequestration of lung); congenital or acquired defects in immune function; aspiration (such as occurs in children with familial dysautonomia, in the comatose patient, in the child who has a nasogastric feeding tube in place, after seizure, or during anesthesia); and alterations in the quality of mucous secretions (as is present in patients with cystic fibrosis). Various types of pulmonary infections may develop in children who are being treated with cytotoxic and immunosuppressive drugs for malignancy, for collagen vascular disease, or as recipients of organ transplants. Patients with immune deficits may develop pneumonia due to aerobic and anaerobic gram-negative bacilli, staphylococci, *Legionella* species, *Nocardia*, various fungi (including *Aspergillus* and *Candida* species and *Pneumocystis carinii)*, and such viruses as cytomegalovirus. Some of the infections in patients with depressed immune response represent reactivation of a latent infection.

The newborn infant can acquire pneumonia by several routes, including transplacental infection, aspiration of organisms present in the birth canal during delivery, and postnatal infection in the nursery or at home from human sources or contaminated equipment or materials.

CLINICAL MANIFESTATIONS

The signs and symptoms of bacterial pneumonia vary with the bacterial pathogen, the age of the patient, and the severity of the disease. Some organisms are associated with a specific pattern of disease, such as the lobar pneumonia of *S. pneumoniae* and the empyema, abscess, and pneumatocele formation due to *S. aureus*; however, any of these manifestations may result from infection caused by any of the bacterial pathogens. In young infants, signs may be nonspecific and findings sparse on physical examination. Radiologic evidence of pneumonia may be found in infants who appear to have minimal disease or whose signs are more likely to be associated with upper respiratory tract infection. In older children, the majority of cases are mild, and undoubtedly many cases occur and remain unrecognized because signs of disease do not warrant radiography of the chest. The child with pneumonia who requires hospitalization represents a small but unknown fraction of all children with pneumonia.

Symptoms and signs of pneumonia in children may be classified for convenience into five categories: nonspecific manifestations of infection and toxicity; general signs of lower respiratory tract disease; signs of pneumonia; signs of pleural fluid; and signs of extrapulmonary disease.

Nonspecific manifestations of infection and toxicity include fever, headache, malaise, gastrointestinal complaints, restlessness, and apprehension. Rigors may occur and vary from symptoms of chilliness to a sign of teeth-chattering chills.

General signs of lower respiratory tract disease include tachypnea, dyspnea including shallow or grunting respirations, cough, expectoration of sputum, and flaring of the alae nasae. Because of the importance of tachypnea as a sign of lower respiratory tract disease, reference values for normal patients should be known.[63] Respiratory rates are correlated inversely with age during the first 3 years of life and vary between a median of 47 breaths per minute in the first months of life to 38 at the end of the first year to 28 by 3 years of age. In older children, rates vary between 15 and 25 breaths per minute. Asleep subjects have lower respiratory rates than do awake subjects. On the basis of these data, definitions of tachypnea for the purpose of diagnosing lower respiratory tract infection are 50 breaths per minute in infants 1 to 11 months of age, 40 per minute in children 1 to 4 years of age, and 30 per minute in children 5 years of age or older.[44]

Other general signs of pneumonia include a protective position and abdominal findings. The patient may lie on the affected side of the lung with legs drawn up because of chest pain. Abdominal distention may result from gastric dilatation because of swallowed air or paralytic ileus. The liver may be displaced downward by the right diaphragm or may be enlarged if congestive heart failure complicates the pneumonia.

Signs of pneumonia may be subtle in the young infant. Percussion usually is not of value in the infant or in the older child if distribution of the pneumonia is patchy. Dullness to percussion is associated more often in the young child with the presence of pleural fluid than with the involvement of the parenchyma of the lung. Auscultatory findings may include rales but are less consistent than those in the older child. Abnormal findings in the older child include dullness to percussion, decreased tactile and vocal fremitus on palpation, and decreased breath sounds and rales over involved areas on auscultation. Intercostal retraction indicates recruitment of accessory muscles that become necessary to assist respiration when significant involvement of the lung is present.

Irritation of the pleura is accompanied by chest pain that may be severe and may limit chest movement. A friction rub may be present over the involved area of pleura. As the effusion enlarges, dyspnea may increase, but pleuritic pain may diminish and become a dull ache. The pain of pleural irritation may be present at the site of inflammation. If the involved area includes the diaphragm, the pain may be referred to the posterior and lateral neck. Abdominal pain may be so severe as to suggest acute appendicitis. Pleural irritation over the right upper lobe may elicit meningismus, a sign of meningeal irritation without evidence of inflammation. Empyema may extend to involve the mediastinum or pericardium or may penetrate the chest wall to present as a soft tissue abscess (empyema necessitans). Signs of extension of empyema should be sought in the patient who does not respond appropriately to chemotherapy and surgical drainage.

Extrapulmonary infection, including abscesses of the skin and soft tissues, otitis media, sinusitis, and meningitis, may occur concomitantly with bacterial pneumonia; pericarditis and epiglottitis are particularly likely to be associated with pneumonia due to *H. influenzae* type b.

DIAGNOSIS

Microbiologic Diagnosis

Effective chemotherapy now is available for treatment of all forms of bacterial pneumonia in children. Optimal treatment, however, requires definition of the etiologic agent. The physician must differentiate viral or mycoplasmal from bacterial pneumonia; if the agent is bacterial, the probable species must be considered. An effort should be made to obtain adequate materials for bacteriologic diagnosis; these include sputum, secretions from the posterior nasopharynx, and blood. The physician also should consider the following: tracheal aspiration in young children unable to produce sputum, thoracentesis when pleural fluid is present, percutaneous lung aspiration in children who are critically ill, and lung biopsy when tissue diagnosis is important.

Methods for Obtaining Material for Examination and Culture

Sputum usually is not available from children until they are 5 years of age; younger children usually swallow their secretions. A Gram-stained smear of sputum is of value in providing immediate information about the bacterial pathogen; the presence of a significant number of organisms in association with or ingested by polymorphonuclear leukocytes suggests the likely pathogen, whereas the presence of epithelial cells indicates that the material is from the mouth and further attempts should be made to obtain sputum. The adequacy of the specimen for microbiologic evaluation may be defined by the presence of 10 or more polymorphonuclear cells per low-power field and less than 25 squamous epithelial cells per low-power field.

Secretions from the nasopharynx include organisms that may be responsible for pneumonia, but results of culture of the nasopharynx may be unrevealing or misleading because of the high rate of carriage of bacterial pathogens.

Tracheal aspiration through a catheter may be of diagnostic assistance when it is performed with direct laryngoscopy but is less valuable when the catheter is passed through the nose or mouth because of contamination with organisms present in the upper respiratory tract. Use of a double-lumen catheter ensures that the specimen will be free of contaminants.

Culture of blood provides specific bacteriologic diagnosis. Bennett and Beeson[13] suggested that most patients with pneumococcal pneumonia have bacteremia at some time during their illness. Reports of pneumococcal pneumonia in adults indicate an incidence of bacteremia of approximately 25 per cent.[8, 36] Data on the occurrence of bacteremia in children are less well documented. In a study of Boston children,[70] bacteremia occurred in 8 of 100 consecutive febrile children younger than 2 years of age who were seen in a "walk-in" clinic with radiologic evidence of pneumonia. This and other studies of febrile children seen in clinics for ambulatory children reveal many cases of unsuspected bacteremia in children with pneumonia due to *S. pneumoniae*,[16] *H. influenzae*,[46] and *N. meningitidis*.[10] Thus, the proportion of children with pneumonia who are bacteremic is uncertain, but some data are available from studies of concurrent cultures of blood and lung aspirate. Of 43 Gambian children younger than 10 years of age with pneumonia who had concurrent cultures of blood and lung aspirate, bacterial pathogens were cultured from lung aspirate only in 19 children, from blood only in 4, and from both blood and lung in 10 patients.[75]

The availability of flexible bronchoscopy and bronchoalveolar lavage has added another approach to obtain optimal specimens for microbiologic diagnosis of pneumonia.[12] The technique provides a direct view of bronchial and lung pathology, may provide evidence of endobronchial obstructions, and may identify and remove mucous or mucopurulent plugs. These techniques have been of particular value in the diagnosis of pulmonary disease in children with acquired immunodeficiency syndrome.[14]

Thoracentesis should be considered whenever fluid is present in the pleural space and microbiologic diagnosis is unrevealed by cultures of sputum, blood, or tracheal aspirate. Pleural biopsy should be performed at the time of thoracentesis if tuberculosis or tumor is included in the differential diagnosis. The area to be aspirated is defined by physical examination (the point of maximal dullness), chest radiography, and ultrasonography. Gram or acid-fast stain of the fluid may provide immediate information about the pathogen. Fluid should be sent for culture; cytology; and determination of glucose, protein, and pH.

Aspiration of pulmonary exudate (lung puncture) can provide direct, specific, and immediate information about the causative agent of pneumonia. The procedure is performed as one would carry out a thoracentesis. Lung puncture should be considered for the child who is critically ill and for whom a specific diagnosis is of immediate importance in guiding antimicrobial therapy; the child whose condition deteriorates after initial therapy and for whom an etiologic agent has not been identified; and the child who has pneumonia-complicating underlying disease or who is receiving drugs limiting normal host defense mechanisms.[43] Open or closed lung biopsy is necessary if tissue diagnosis is important.

Transtracheal percutaneous aspiration is a safe and useful method of obtaining secretions from the lower respiratory tract of adults with pneumonia who are unable to produce adequate sputum. This method bypasses the mouth flora and permits the investigator to obtain direct culture of tracheal secretions. Transtracheal aspiration has not been used in young children with pneumonia because pediatricians lack experience with the technique and are concerned about the safety of the procedure. Only one report is available: Brook and Finegold[19] used transtracheal aspiration without apparent morbidity to determine the bacteriology of lung abscesses in 10 institutionalized children 23 months to 14 years of age.

Special Methods of Isolation and Identification

Clinical microbiology laboratories have facilities for isolation and identification of aerobic bacterial pathogens associated with pneumonia, but anaerobic bacteria require special techniques. Because many anaerobic bacteria are exquisitely sensitive to oxygen, anaerobic transport media must be provided, and special methods must be used to handle materials on arrival in the laboratory.

Identification of bacterial antigens from secretions and body fluids now is possible by use of precipitin reaction, counterimmunoelectrophoresis, latex agglutination, and enzyme-linked immunosorbent assay. Identification of antigen is of particular help when prior administration of antimicrobial agents prevents successful isolation of bacteria. Counterimmunoelectrophoresis of nasopharyngeal secretions may distinguish patients with pneumococcal pneumonia from those who are carriers of this organism.[20] Detection in urine of polysaccharide antigens of *S. pneumoniae* and *H. influenzae* type b has been used for rapid diagnosis of pneumonia.[17, 74] Questions about sensitivity and specificity of the technique remain to be answered. Preliminary studies suggest value for polymerase chain reaction for detection of *S. pneumoniae* in whole blood and serum in patients with pneumonia.[64, 79]

Laboratory Tests

Elevated white blood cell counts (>15,000/mm^3) are frequent but not invariable in patients with bacterial pneumonia. A white blood cell count below 5000/mm^3 usually is associated with severe and overwhelming disease. Determinations of erythrocyte sedimentation rate and measurement of C-reactive protein did not distinguish virus from bacterial pneumonia in Finnish children.[54]

The presence of an immune response to infection may be used to document bacterial pneumonia in retrospect. At present, serologic tests for bacterial pathogens of importance in pneumonia are available only from investigative laboratories.

Chest Radiography

Although the diagnosis of pneumonia may be suggested by clinical signs, pneumonia is defined by chest radiography. In addition to plain radiography, tomography and computed tomography may be used to provide special detail about cavitation, calcification, and patency of central airways.

Roentgenographic findings may not correlate with clinical signs in young infants. Significant pneumonia may be found by roentgenography in the absence of clinical signs. Pleural effusion may be identified only with the use of a roentgenogram taken in the lateral decubitus position. The radiologic pattern may lag behind clinical improvement for weeks to months.

A chest roentgenogram should be obtained at the conclusion of the illness to determine that the pneumonia has cleared and that there is no underlying process, such as foreign body, congenital malformation, or residual atelectasis. The precise timing of such a study is uncertain, but it should be when resolution is expected, approximately 4 to 6 weeks after initial signs.

Differential Diagnosis

The differential diagnosis of bacterial pneumonia includes nonbacterial pneumonias and noninfectious causes of pulmonary disease. During each period of life, certain nonbacterial agents are prominent causes of pneumonia: pneumonia in the neonate may result from congenital infection or infection acquired at the time of delivery because of rubella, toxoplasmosis, herpes simplex infection, cytomegalovirus infection, or syphilis. From 2 weeks to 6 months of age, *Chlamydia trachomatis* is an important cause of a syndrome of afebrile pneumonia. Throughout childhood, by far the majority of pneumonias are caused by the respiratory viruses, including adenoviruses, influenza viruses, parainfluenza viruses, respiratory syncytial virus, echoviruses, and coxsackieviruses A and B. *Mycoplasma pneumoniae* is an uncommon cause of pneumonia in preschool-age children but is an important cause of pneumonia in school-age children, adolescents, and young adults. Nonbacterial pneumonias that are susceptible to available antimicrobial agents include disease caused by fungi (histoplasmosis, blastomycosis), *Rickettsia* (Q fever), and *Chlamydia* (TWAR agent and psittacosis).

It is most important to consider tuberculosis in children with persistent pulmonary disease who do not respond to penicillin or alternatives to penicillin. All children living in areas that are high risk for tuberculosis should have a tuberculin skin test if admitted to the hospital with a lower respiratory tract infection.

Noninfectious causes of pulmonary lesions include aspiration of gastric contents, aspiration of foreign body, drug reactions, sequestration of lobe, congestive heart failure, atelectasis, sarcoidosis, malignancy or tumor, alveolar proteinosis, pulmonary hemosiderosis, and desquamating interstitial pneumonia.

The bacterial causes of acute empyema include *S. aureus*, *S. pneumoniae*, *H. influenzae*, gram-negative bacilli, and anaerobic bacteria.[18] Bloody exudates (when thoracentesis occurs without trauma) suggest malignancy, infarct of the lung, connective-tissue disorder, pancreaticopleural fistula, or tuberculosis.

Clinical Guidelines in Developing Countries

Acute infections of the lower respiratory tract are the single most important cause of death in children younger than 5 years of age in developing countries. The authors of the Programme for the Control of Respiratory Infections of the World Health Organization have developed clinical guidelines for case diagnosis of pneumonia for use in developing countries. In these areas, diagnosis and management are provided for children by health care personnel who work in facilities where laboratory and radiologic tests are limited or do not exist.[60] The goals of the program are to simplify diagnosis to the smallest number of readily identifiable signs, to provide a system for classification of the illness, and to define the basis for use of antibacterial agents. The guidelines include assessment of fever, nutrition, lethargy, and color (presence or absence of cyanosis); measurement of the respiratory rate; observations of chest wall movement to detect retractions; and auscultation for stridor and wheezes.

The guidelines distinguish levels of disease for purposes of management: *very severe pneumonia* includes central cyanosis and an inability to drink; *severe pneumonia* includes chest indrawing, without cyanosis, and the ability to drink; *pneumonia* includes no chest indrawing but sustained tachypnea (>60 breaths/minute for infants younger than 2 months of age, >50 breaths/minute for children 2 to 12 months of age, >40 breaths/minute for children 12 months to 5 years of age); and *no pneumonia* includes cough in the absence of chest indrawing and tachypnea. The suggested management includes hospitalization and parenteral antibiotics for children with very severe and severe pneumonia; home care and oral antibiotics for children with pneumonia; and for children with cough but without signs of severe respiratory illness, no antibiotics but assessment and treatment of other problems.

The ability of nurses and nursing assistants in Swaziland to recognize pneumonia using the World Health Organization's protocols was evaluated by Simoes and McGrath.[67] Signs of severe disease, including stridor and abnormal sleepiness, often were overlooked, as was audible wheeze, but tachypnea and chest wall retractions were well recognized. In a study of Chinese children, tachypnea (50 cycles/minute for infants 2 to 11 months of age and 40 cycles/minute for children 1 to 5 years of age) was a good predictor of radiologically defined pneumonia and was recommended for use by village health workers in diagnosing pneumonia. Nasal flaring, retractions, stridor, and cyanosis of the tongue had high predictive values but were observed infrequently.[22] A respiratory rate of more than 50 cycles per minute or retractions were predictive of pneumonia in children with cough evaluated in Papua New Guinea.[35]

MANAGEMENT OF BACTERIAL PNEUMONIA

Therapy should be initiated promptly once bacterial pneumonia is diagnosed or strongly suspected. Initial therapy may be guided by examination of the Gram-stained smear of sputum or tracheal aspirate. If these materials are unavailable or unsatisfactory, other criteria must be used. The relative frequency of respiratory pathogens in the various age groups provides guidelines for initial therapy.

The physician must decide whether hospitalization is required for optimal management of the child. Most children with mild to moderate disease can be treated at home. Children who require hospitalization include those with severe disease, those who are toxic and have a significant degree of pulmonary dysfunction, and those whose family lack the ability to provide therapy and supportive care. Special concern is warranted for infants in the first year of life, when signs of respiratory disease are subtle and disease may progress rapidly.

Initial Choice of Antimicrobial Agents in Various Age Groups

Neonatal Pneumonia

The treatment of neonatal pneumonia is similar to that of other severe neonatal infections; initial therapy must include coverage for gram-positive cocci, particularly group B *Streptococcus*, and gram-negative bacilli.

A penicillin is the drug of choice for the gram-positive organisms. If there is reason to suspect staphylococcal infection, a penicillinase-resistant penicillin is chosen. If there is no significant risk of staphylococcal infection, penicillin G or ampicillin is used. The latter drug may provide a theoretic advantage because of greater in vitro activity against some enterococci and some gram-negative bacilli, particularly *E. coli* and *Proteus mirabilis*, when used alone or in combination with an aminoglycoside.

Choice of therapy for suspected gram-negative bacillary infection depends on the antibiotic susceptibility pattern for recent isolates obtained from newborn infants. An aminoglycoside such as gentamicin has an effective range of in vitro activity. Amikacin and tobramycin have similar activity but may be effective for strains of gram-negative enteric bacilli that are resistant to gentamicin.

Initial therapy is reevaluated when the results of cultures are available. Duration of therapy depends on the causative agent; pneumonia caused by group B *Streptococcus* or gram-negative enteric bacilli is treated for 7 to 10 days; disease caused by *S. aureus* requires 3 to 6 weeks of antimicrobial therapy, according to the severity of the disease.

Pneumonias in Children 1 Month to 10 Years of Age

The overwhelming majority of cases of bronchopneumonias at this age are caused by respiratory viruses. Therefore, if the initial clinical findings are consistent with viral infection and the child can be observed closely, antimicrobial agents may be withheld pending the results of cultures. *S. pneumoniae* and *H. influenzae* (nontypable as well as type b) are the major bacterial agents responsible for bacterial pneumonia in this age group. The rate of disease due to type b *H. influenzae* is low in children who were immunized previously with the conjugate vaccine. Although a varying proportion of pneumococci are multidrug-resistant, the prevalence of strains in most communities in the United States as of August 1996, does not warrant a change in consideration of initial management (see the section on chemotherapy for specific pathogens). Strains of beta-lactamase–producing *H. influenzae* resistant to amoxicillin and other susceptible penicillins have been isolated throughout the United States. Nevertheless, amoxicillin still is appropriate initial therapy for the young child with mild disease. If the child is moderately or seriously ill, drugs with efficacy against *S. pneumoniae* and beta-lactamase–producing *H. influenzae*, including cephalosporins (cefuroxime, ceftriaxone, cefotaxime, or ceftazidime) or chloramphenicol, should be administered by parenteral routes.

S. aureus now is an uncommon cause of pneumonia in this age group. However, if clinical signs compatible with staphylococcal disease are present, initial therapy should include a parenteral penicillinase-resistant penicillin.

Because *M. pneumoniae* is a common cause of pneumonia in school-age children and adolescents, presumptive therapy should include coverage for *S. pneumoniae* and *M. pneumoniae* in children older than 5 years of age. Erythromycin or the new macrolides, azithromycin and clarithromycin, are appropriate drugs for coverage of both pathogens.

Pneumonia in the Child 10 Years of Age or Older

S. pneumoniae and *M. pneumoniae* are the major treatable causes of pneumonia in this age group. *H. influenzae* is relatively infrequent, and initial therapy need not include coverage for this organism. Therapy outlined earlier for the school-age child continues to be appropriate for the child 10 years of age or older.

Chemotherapy for Specific Pathogens

Pneumococcal Pneumonia

Penicillin G is the drug of choice for children with pneumonia caused by *S. pneumoniae*. For most children with mild to moderately severe disease, an oral penicillin is suitable. Phenoxymethyl penicillin (penicillin V) provides significant antibacterial activity after oral administration as well as approximately twice the peak serum level provided by an equivalent dose of buffered oral penicillin G. Children who appear to be toxic, who have underlying disease, or who have complications (e.g., abscesses, empyema) require the higher serum and tissue antibacterial activity that is provided by a parenteral form. Aqueous penicillin G administered by the intravenous or intramuscular route provides high serum levels. Procaine penicillin G administered intramuscularly attains lower peak serum levels, but activity is sustained for 6 or more hours, and it is suitable for mild to moderately severe disease. A single dose of intramuscular benzathine penicillin G provides very low levels of serum antibacterial activity for periods in excess of 14 days. Although this salt has been effective in some cases of pneumococcal pneumonia, failures are frequent, and it is not recommended.

Strains of *S. pneumoniae* resistant to penicillin G (minimal inhibitory concentration 0.1 to 1.0 μg/mL = intermediately resistant and 2 μg/mL or more = highly resistant) and other effective antimicrobial agents have been identified throughout the United States. Clinical failures have occurred in some patients with meningitis due to penicillin-resistant pneumococci, but few failures have been identified in cases of sepsis or pneumonia treated with a penicillin or cephalosporin in an adequate dosage schedule. Results of a study of adults with bacteremic pneumonia caused by penicillin-resistant pneumococci suggested that patients with highly resistant strains (minimal inhibitory concentrations were 4.0 and 8.0 μg/mL) failed to respond to a penicillin, whereas patients with strains having lower minimal inhibitory concentrations did respond.[57] Susceptibility tests should be performed on all isolates of *S. pneumoniae* from sputum and body fluids (blood, cerebrospinal fluid, and pleural fluid). Presumptive therapy for mild to moderate pneumonias need not be altered because of concern for resistant pneumococci, but severe pneumonias should be treated with high-dosage parenteral therapy providing high serum and tissue concentrations and stability to beta-lactamases, such as intravenous ceftriaxone and cefotaxime. The most appropriate regimen is chosen when results of culture and susceptiblity tests are available. Vancomycin is effective uniformly against all pneumococci, including highly resistant strains, and should be considered if the susceptibility tests indicate the strain is multidrug-resistant and uniquely susceptible to vancomycin.

The dosage schedule for mild to moderate disease and severe disease is provided in Chapter 231. The duration of therapy depends on the clinical response, but therapy should be continued for at least 3 days after defervescence and significant resolution of radiologic and clinical signs; usually, a period of 5 to 7 days is sufficient.

Pneumonia Due to Haemophilus influenzae

Nontypable and type b strains of *H. influenzae* are susceptible to various antimicrobial agents, including the sulfonamides, tetracyclines, chloramphenicol, aminoglycosides, and ampicillin. All have been used with success in systemic infections (including pneumonia) due to this agent. At present, amoxicillin is considered the drug of choice in young children with mild to moderate pulmonary disease. Because of the concern for beta-lactamase–producing strains of *H. influenzae*, a second-generation (cefuroxime) or third-generation cephalosporin (ceftriaxone, cefotaxime, or ceftazidime) or intravenous chloramphenicol should be used as initial therapy of patients with severe disease when this microorganism is known or strongly suspected to be the pathogen.

The child with mild to moderate disease should be treated for a minimum of 7 days, including a period without fever of at least 3 days. The child with severe disease should be treated for 2 to 3 weeks.

Staphylococcal Pneumonia

The high incidence of staphylococci resistant to penicillin G, in the hospital and in the community, requires the use of a penicillinase-resistant penicillin whenever staphylococcal pneumonia is diagnosed or suspected. Subsequently, if the culture and sensitivity data indicate that the organism is susceptible to penicillin G, this drug should be used because of its greater efficacy and lower cost. Clinical trials indicate that all penicillinase-resistant penicillins are equally effective in treating staphylococcal pneumonia. Although the incidence of staphylococci in the community that are resistant to penicillinase-resistant penicillins is low (approximately 1 per cent in recent reports from centers in the United States), resistance should be suspected if appropriate clinical response does not occur after the use of one of these penicillins. Vancomycin has been used successfully for patients with pneumonia due to one of these resistant strains of *S. aureus*.

The rapid development of empyema, pneumatoceles, and abscesses demands close observation and meticulous nursing care. The antibiotic should be administered parenterally using a high dosage schedule for 2 to 3 weeks; an oral preparation then may be given for 1 to 3 weeks. The total duration of antibiotic therapy depends on the initial response, the presence of pulmonary and extrapulmonary complications, and the rapidity of resolution of the pneumonia.

Pneumonia Due to Anaerobic Bacteria

Most anaerobic bacteria that cause pneumonia, including strains of *B. fragilis*, are highly susceptible to penicillin G. Some strains of *B. fragilis* may be resistant to penicillin G and susceptible to chloramphenicol, clindamycin, or cefoxitin. The duration of therapy depends on the extent of the disease; pneumonia without complications clears rapidly with appropriate therapy; 7 days of therapy usually is sufficient.

Pneumonia Due to Gram-Negative Bacilli

The initial choice of therapy is guided by the following factors: the source of the infection, the disease process present (burn, cystic fibrosis), host susceptibility to infection (deficient immune mechanisms), and the antimicrobial susceptibility pattern for these organisms in the community or hospital. The basis for choice of antibiotic is similar to that outlined for neonatal pneumonia suspected to be caused by gram-negative bacilli. The duration of therapy must be tailored to the clinical course and the response to therapy. Cases of pneumonia with minimal pulmonary lesions and limited symptoms should be treated for at least 3 days after defervescence. Severe cases of pneumonia should be treated for 2 to 3 weeks.

Therapy for the Penicillin-Allergic Child

A child who has a significant history of allergic reaction to any of the penicillins must be considered sensitive to all of them, and alternative antimicrobial agents must be considered for therapy. Cephalothin and cefazolin have been used with success in the treatment of staphylococcal and pneumococcal pneumonia and may be used as alternatives to a penicillin. Erythromycin, the new macrolides, clarithromycin and azithromycin, and clindamycin are active in vitro against gram-positive cocci and are effective in the treatment of pneumococcal, staphylococcal, and anaerobic pneumonias. Because some staphylococci may be resistant to these antibiotics, it is important to test the organism for susceptibility. Vancomycin may be considered for use in the patient who is allergic to penicillin and who has severe staphylococcal disease.

Adjuncts to Chemotherapy

Antimicrobial agents are only part of the management of the child with pneumonia; close observation, nursing care (including suction of excess secretions), and the following supportive measures are of the utmost importance:

1. Maintenance of fluid and electrolyte balance
2. Humidification provided by cool mist
3. Oxygen for severe dyspnea
4. Cleansing of the mouth
5. Sparing use of antipyretics because the temperature course provides a guideline for the therapeutic response

More extensive procedures may be required under special circumstances:

1. Bronchoscopy is important in documenting the presence of a foreign body, tumor, or congenital anomaly.

2. Intubation of the trachea or tracheotomy may be considered when the patient has difficulty clearing secretions and more efficient suction of the lower respiratory tree is required.

3. Drainage of pleural effusions may be necessary when an accumulation of fluid compromises respiration. Thick, tenacious empyema may require intercostal tube drainage or closed-tube thoracostomy. Empyema due to *S. aureus* may require placement of a tube, whereas the less viscid effusion associated with *S. pneumoniae* and *S. pyogenes* rarely requires more than frequent thoracentesis. Empyema due to *H. influenzae* may be thick and viscid, requiring placement of a chest tube, or less viscid, requiring only thoracentesis. Single or multiple thoracenteses are adequate when the volume of fluid is small and the quality of the fluid allows ready drainage, as usually is true with empyema due to *S. pneumoniae* or group A *Streptococcus*. When large amounts of fluid are present or the fluid is thick and viscid, a closed drainage system with intercostal chest tube under negative pressure is placed; this frequently is necessary for empyema due to *S. aureus*. The tube should be removed as soon as its drainage function is completed because delay might result in local tissue injury, secondary infection, or sinus formation.

4. Intrapleural instillation of antibiotic should be considered in cases of empyema when the fluid is loculated because of fibrous adhesions. If a chest tube is in place, antibiotics are instilled after irrigation through the tube. In susceptible infections, aqueous penicillin G, 10,000 to 50,000 units, ampicillin, 10 to 50 mg, or a penicillinase-resistant penicillin or cephalosporin, 10 to 50 mg, may be inoculated in 10 mL of diluent (sterile water or normal saline) after the tube is clamped. The clamp is maintained for 1 hour and then released for drainage. The instillations should be repeated three to four times each day that the tube remains in place. If thoracenteses are done, antibiotic is introduced after the pleural fluid is aspirated.

PROGNOSIS

In uncomplicated cases of pneumococcal pneumonia in children in the United States, the mortality rate is very low (<1 per cent). In developing countries, pneumonia is a major cause of mortality accounting for more than one fourth of deaths in children younger than 5 years of age. Half of the pneumonia-related mortality occurs in children younger than 1 year of age. The World Health Organization estimates that about 4 million childhood deaths are caused each year by pneumonia.

Lung morphology and physiology usually return to normal after appropriate antimicrobial therapy. Fibrothorax is rare; almost all children resolve thickened pleurae with no effect on lung growth and function. Even after extensive disease associated with empyema due to *S. aureus* or *H. influenzae*, children have normal growth and development and normal pulmonary function after recovery.[49] Deaths still result from bacterial pneumonias; however, most deaths in children result from abrupt, overwhelming disease. Thus, Asmar and colleagues[6] reported 2 deaths in 43 children with pneumonia due to *H. influenzae*; both deaths occurred before antibiotics could be administered.

PREVENTION

Children who have sickle-cell anemia or who have had splenectomy are at risk for overwhelming disease due to the encapsulated organisms *S. pneumoniae* and *H. influenzae*. The most common prophylactic regimen is daily administration of oral penicillin V, which is adequate to prevent dissemination of *S. pneumoniae*.

The persistent problem of pneumococcal disease, the severe outcome in individuals with defective host defense mechanisms, and the recent reports of multiresistant strains of pneumococcus have stimulated research in usage of a pneumococcal vaccine for infants and children. The currently licensed pneumococcal vaccine contains purified polysaccharide antigens of the 23 types of pneumococcus most frequently associated with disease in adults and children. Each antigen produces a satisfactory independent antibody response in the majority of children older than 2 years of age. Protection against infection develops in about 2 weeks. Revaccination of recipients of the 23-valent vaccine after 3 to 5 years should be considered for children 10 years of age or younger who are at high risk of severe pneumococcal infection.

Children younger than 2 years of age have unsatisfactory serologic responses to a single-dose regimen. Conjugate pneumococcal vaccines utilizing the same technology used in development of the conjugate *H. influenzae* vaccines currently are in clinical trials in infants beginning at 2 months of age to determine efficacy for prevention of invasive disease and acute otitis media.

A polysaccharide vaccine for prevention of *H. influenzae* type b disease was introduced in the United States in April 1985. Antibodies to the polysaccharide antigen correlate with protection against invasive disease. Infants younger than 18 months of age have inadequate immune response to the capsular polysaccharide. The development of a new generation of vaccines prepared by coupling the capsular saccharide of *H. influenzae* type b and a protein stimulating type b–specific antibody in infants as young as 2 months of age resulted in the approval of conjugate vaccines by the Food and Drug Administration in the fall of 1990 for administration to infants in the first year of life. The subsequent experience has been a dramatic decrease in the incidence of all invasive disease due to *H. influenzae* type b in immunized infants.

References

1. Abbasi, S., and Chesney, P. J.: Pulmonary manifestations of cat-scratch disease: A case report and review of the literature. Pediatr. Infect. Dis. J. *14*:547–548, 1995.
2. Ablow, R. C., Driscoll, S. G., Effmann, E. L., et al.: A comparison of early-onset group B streptococcal neonatal infection and the respiratory distress syndrome of the newborn. N. Engl. J. Med. *294*:65–70, 1976.
3. Abraham, E. P., Gardner, A. D., Chain, E., et al.: Further observations on penicillin. Lancet *2*:177–189, 1941.
4. Anderson, R. D., Lauer, B. A., Fraser, D. W., et al.: Infections with *Legionella pneumophila* in children. J. Infect. Dis. *13*:386–390, 1981.
5. Applebaum, P. C., Bhamjee, A., Scragg, J. N., et al.: *Streptococcus pneumoniae* resistant to penicillin and chloramphenicol. Lancet *2*:995, 1977.
6. Asmar, B. I., Slovis, T. L., Reed, J. O., et al.: *Hemophilus influenzae* type b pneumonia in 43 children. J. Pediatr. *93*:389–393, 1978.
7. Austrian, R.: Treatment of pneumonia. Mod. Treat. *1*:909–923, 1964.
8. Austrian, R., and Gold, J.: Pneumococcal bacteremia with especial reference to bacteremic pneumococcal pneumonia. Ann. Intern. Med. *60*:759–776, 1964.
9. Bale, J. R.: Creation of a research program to determine the etiology and epidemiology of acute respiratory tract infection in children in developing countries. Rev. Infect. Dis. *12*(Suppl. 8):S861–S866, 1990.
10. Baltimore, R. S., and Hammerschlag, M.: Meningococcal bacteremia: Clinical and serologic studies of infants with mild illness. Am. J. Dis. Child. *131*:1001–1004, 1977.
11. Bartlett, J. G.: Anaerobic bacterial pneumonitis. Am. Rev. Respir. Dis. *119*:19–23, 1979.
12. Baselski, V. S., and Wunderink, R. G.: Bronchoscopic diagnosis of pneumonia. Clin. Microbiol. Rev. *7*:533–558, 1994.
13. Bennett, I. L., Jr., and Beeson, P. B.: Bacteremia: A consideration of some experimental and clinical aspects. Yale J. Biol. Med. *26*:241–262, 1954.
14. Birriel, J. A., Jr., Adams, J. A., Saldana, M. A., et al.: Role of flexible bronchoscopy and bronchoalveolar lavage in the diagnosis of pediatric acquired immunodeficiency syndrome–related pulmonary disease. Pediatrics *87*:897–899, 1991.
15. Bluestone, C. D., Stephenson, J. S., and Martin, L. M.: Ten-year review of otitis media pathogens. Pediatr. Infect. Dis. J. *11*(Suppl. 8):S7–S11, 1992.
16. Bratton, L., Teele, D. W., and Klein, J. O.: Outcome of unsuspected pneumococcemia in children not initially admitted to the hospital. J. Pediatr. *90*:703–706, 1977.
17. Bromberg, K., Tannis, G., and Rodgers, A.: Pneumococcal C and type polysaccharide detection in the concentrated urine of patients with bacteremia. Med. Microbiol. Immunol. *179*:335–338, 1990.
18. Brook, I.: Microbiology of empyema in children and adolescents. Pediatrics *85*:722–726, 1990.
19. Brook, I., and Finegold, S. M.: Bacteriology and therapy of lung abscess in children. J. Pediatr. *94*:10–12, 1979.
20. Congeni, B. L., and Nankervis, G. A.: Diagnosis of pneumonia by counterimmunoelectrophoresis of respiratory secretions. Am. J. Dis. Child. *1132*:684–688, 1978.
21. Cundell, D., Masure, H. R., and Tuomanen, E. I.: The molecular basis of pneumococcal infection: A hypothesis. Clin. Infect. Dis. *21*(Suppl. 3):S204–S212, 1995.
22. Dai, Y., Foy, H. M., Zonghan, Z., et al.: Respiratory rate and signs in roentgenographically confirmed pneumonia among children in China. Pediatr. Infect. Dis. J. *14*:48–50, 1995.
23. Daum, R. S., Granoff, D. M., Mäkelä, P. H., et al.: (guest eds.): Epidemiology, Pathogenesis, and Prevention of *Haemophilus influenzae* disease. J. Infect. Dis. *165*(Suppl. 1):S1–S206, 1992.
24. Doern, G. V., Jorgensen, J. H., Thornsberry, C., et al.: National collaborative study of the prevalence of antimicrobial resistance among clinical isolates of *Haemophilus influenzae*. Antimicrob. Agents Chemother. *32*:180–185, 1988.
25. Duchin, J. S., Breiman, R. F., Diamond, A., et al.: High prevalence of multidrug-resistant *Streptococcus pneumoniae* among children in a rural Kentucky community. Pediatr. Infect. Dis. J. *14*:745–750, 1995.
26. Edelstein, P. H.: Antimicrobial chemotherapy for Legionnaires' disease: A review. Clin. Infect. Dis. *21*(Suppl. 3):S265–S276, 1995.
27. Finland, M., Peterson, O. L., and Strauss, E.: Staphylococcic pneumonia occurring during an epidemic of influenzae. Arch. Intern. Med. *70*:183–205, 1942.
28. Finland, M., Ory, E. M., Meads, M., et al.: Influenza and pneumonia: Serological studies during and after an outbreak of influenza. Br. J. Lab. Clin. Med. *33*:32–46, 1948.
29. Finland, M., Barnes, M. W., and Samper, B. A.: Influenza virus isolations and serological studies made in Boston during the winter of 1943–1944. J. Clin. Invest. *24*:192–208, 1945.
30. Friedland, E. R., and McCracken, G. H., Jr.: Management of infections caused by antibiotic-resistant *Streptococcus pneumoniae.* N. Engl. J. Med. *331*:377–382, 1994.
31. Ginsburg, C. M., Howard, J. B., and Nelson, J. D.: Report of 65 cases of *Haemophilus influenzae* b pneumonia. Pediatrics *64*:283–286, 1979.
32. Goldwater, P. N., and Rice, M. S.: Primary meningococcal pneumonia in a nineteen-month-old child. Pediatr. Infect. Dis. J. *14*:155–156, 1995.
33. Gratten, M., Naraqi, S., and Hansman, D.: High prevalence of penicillin-insensitive pneumococci in Port Moresby, Papua New Guinea. Lancet *2*:192–195, 1980.
34. Hall, C. B., Powell, K. R., Schnabel, K. C., et al.: Risk of secondary bacterial infection in infants hospitalized with respiratory syncytial viral infection. J. Pediatr. *113*:266–271, 1988.
35. Harari, M., Shann, F., Spooner, V., et al.: Clinical signs of pneumonia in children. Lancet *338*:928–930, 1991.
36. Heffron, R.: Pneumonia with Special Reference to Pneumococcus Lobar Pneumonia. New York, Commonwealth Fund, 1939, pp. 308, 312, 549; reissued by Harvard University Press, Boston, 1979.
37. Hersh, J. H., Gold, R., and Lepow, M. L.: Meningococcal group Y pneumonia in an adolescent female. J. Pediatr. *64*:222–224, 1979.
38. Jacobs, N. M., and Harris, V. J.: Acute *Haemophilus* pneumonia in childhood. Am. J. Dis. Child. *133*:603–605, 1979.
39. Jacobs, R. F.: Nosocomial pneumonia in children. Infection *19*:64–72, 1991.
40. Kass, E. H. (ed.): Assessment of the pneumococcal polysaccharide vaccine. Rev. Infect. Dis. *3*(Suppl.):S1–S197, 1981.
41. Keefer, C. S., Blake, F. G., Marshall, E. K., Jr., et al.: Penicillin in the treatment of infections: A report of 500 cases. J. A. M. A. *122*:1217–1224, 1943.
42. Klein, J. O., Green, G. M., Tilles, J. G., et al.: Effect of intranasal reovirus infection on antibacterial activity of mouse lung. J. Infect. Dis. *119*:43–50, 1969.
43. Klein, J. O., and Gellis, S. S.: Diagnostic needle aspiration in pediatric practice. Pediatr. Clin. North Am. *18*:219–231, 1971.
44. Korppi, M.: Physical signs in childhood pneumonia. Pediatr. Infect. Dis. J. *14*:405–406, 1995.
45. Kovatch, A. L., Jardine, D. S., Dowling, J. N., et al.: Legionellosis in children with leukemia in relapse. Pediatrics *73*:811–815, 1984.
46. Marshall, R., Teele, D. W., and Klein, J. O.: Unsuspected bacteremia due to *Haemophilus influenzae*: Outcome in children not initially admitted to hospital. J. Pediatr. *95*:690–695, 1979.
47. Martin, C. M., Kunin, C. M., Gottlieb, L. S., et al.: Asian influenza A in Boston, 1957–1958. II. Severe staphylococcal pneumonia complicating influenza. Arch. Intern. Med. *103*:532–542, 1959.
48. Mastro, T. D., Ghafour, A., Normani, N. K., et al.: Antimicrobial resistance of pneumococci in children with acute respiratory tract infection in Pakistan. Lancet *337*:156–159, 1991.
49. McLaughlin, F. J., Goldmann, D. A., Rosenbaum, D. M., et al.: Empyema in children: Clinical course and long-term follow-up. Pediatrics *73*:587–593, 1984.
50. Molteni, R. A.: Group A β-hemolytic streptococcal pneumonia. Am. J. Dis. Child. *131*:1366–1371, 1977.
51. Muldoon, R. L., Jaecker, D. L., and Kiefer, H. K.: Legionnaires' disease in children. Pediatrics *67*:329–332, 1981.
52. Nohynek, H., Eskola, J. Laine, E., et al.: The causes of hospital-treated acute lower respiratory tract infection in children. Am. J. Dis. Child. *145*:618–622, 1991.
53. Nohynek, H., Valkeila, E., Leinonen, M., et al.: Erythrocyte sedimentation rate, white blood cell count and serum C-reactive protein in assessing etiologic diagnosis of acute lower respiratory infections in children. Pediatr. Infect. Dis. J. *14*:484–490, 1995.
54. Olcay, L., Secmeer, G., Gröğüș, S., et al.: Fatal hemorrhagic staphylococcal pneumonia. Arch. Pediatr. Adolesc. Med. *149*:925–926, 1995.
55. Orenstein, W. A., Overturf, G. D., Leedom, J. M., et al.: The frequency of *Legionella* infection prospectively determined in children hospitalized with pneumonia. J. Pediatr. *99*:403–406, 1981.
56. Pallares, R., Gudiol, F., Linares, J., et al.: Risk factors and response to antibiotic therapy in adults with bacteremic pneumonia caused by penicillin-resistant pneumococci. N. Engl. J. Med. *317*:18–22, 1987.
57. Pallares, R., Linares, J., Vadillo, M., et al.: Resistance to penicillin and cephalosporin and mortality from severe pneumococcal pneumonia in Barcelona, Spain. N. Engl. J. Med. *333*:474–480, 1995.
58. Peerless, A. G., Liebhaber, M., Anderson, S., et al.: *Legionella* pneumonia in chronic granulomatous disease. J. Pediatr. *106*:783–785, 1985.
59. Potter, A. R., and Fischer, G. W.: *Haemophilus influenzae,* the predominant cause of bacterial pneumonia in Hawaii. Pediatr. Res. *11*:504, 1977.
60. Programme for the Control of Acute Respiratory Infections: Acute respiratory infections in children: Case management in small hospitals in developing countries. Geneva, World Health Organization, 1990.
61. Quie, P. G., Giebink, G. S., and Winkelstein, J. A. (guest eds.): The pneumococcus. Rev. Infect. Dis. *3*:183–396, 1981.
62. Renner, E. D., Helms, C. M., Hierholzer, Jr., W. J., et al.: Legionnaires' disease in pneumonia patients in Iowa: A retrospective seroepidemiologic study, 1972–1977. Ann. Intern. Med. *90*:603–606, 1979.
63. Rusconi, R., Castagneto, M., Gagliardi, L., et al.: Reference values for respiratory rate in the first 3 years of life. Pediatrics *94*:350–355, 1994.
64. Salo, P., Ortqvist, A., and Leinonen, M.: Diagnosis of bacteremic pneumococcal pneumonia by amplification of pneumolysin gene fragment in serum. J. Infect. Dis. *171*:479–482, 1995.

65. Shann, F.: The management of pneumonia in children in developing countries. Clin. Infect. Dis. *21*(Suppl. 3):S218–S225, 1995.
66. Shann, F., Germer, S., Hazlett, D., et al.: Aetiology of pneumonia in children in Goroka Hospital, Papua New Guinea. Lancet *2*:537–541, 1984.
67. Simoes, E. A. F., and McGrath, E. J.: Recognition of pneumonia by primary health care workers in Swaziland with a simple clinical algorithm. Lancet *340*:1502–1503, 1992.
68. Spika, J. S., Facklam, R. R., Plikaytis, B. D., et al.: Antimicrobial resistance of *Streptococcus pneumoniae* in the United States, 1979–1987. J. Infect. Dis. *163*:1273–1278, 1991.
69. Steinhoff, M. C. (ed.): Belagio conference on the pathogenesis and prevention of pneumonia in children in developing regions. Rev. Infect. Dis. *13*(Suppl. 6), 1991.
70. Teele, D. W., Pelton, S. E., Grant, J. A., et al.: Bacteremia in febrile children under 2 years of age: Results of cultures of blood of 600 consecutive febrile children seen in a "walk-in" clinic. J. Pediatr. *87*:227–231, 1975.
71. Tillett, W. S., Cambier, M. J., Harris, W. H., Jr.: Sulfonamide-fast pneumococci: A clinical report of two cases of pneumonia together with experimental studies on the effectiveness of penicillin and tyrothricin against sulfonamide-resistant strains. J. Clin. Invest. *22*:249–255, 1943.
72. Trujillo, M., and McCracken, G. H., Jr.: Prolonged morbidity in children with group A beta-hemolytic streptococcal pneumonia. Pediatr. Infect. Dis. J. *13*:411–412, 1994.
73. Tuomanen, E. I., Austrian, R., and Masure, H. R.: Pathogenesis of pneumococcal infection. N. Engl. J. Med. *332*:1280–1284, 1995.
74. Turner, R. B., Hayden, F. G., and Hendley, J. O.: Counterimmunoelectrophoresis of urine for diagnosis of bacterial pneumonia in pediatric outpatients. Pediatrics *71*:780–783, 1983.
75. Wall, R. A., Corrah, P. T., Mabey, D. C. W., et al.: The etiology of lobar pneumonia in the Gambia. Bull. WHO *64*:553–558, 1986.
76. Ward, J. I., Tsai, T. F., Filice, G. A., et al.: Prevalence of ampicillin- and chloramphenicol-resistant strains of *Haemophilus influenzae* causing meningitis and bacteremia: National survey of hospital laboratories. J. Infect. Dis. *138*:421–424, 1978.
77. Watson, D. A., Musher, D. M., Jacobson, J. W., et al.: A brief history of the pneumococcus in biomedical research: A panoply of scientific discovery. Clin. Infect. Dis. *17*:913–924, 1993.
78. Weinberg, G. A., Ghafoor, A., Ishaq, Z., et al.: Clonal analysis of *Hemophilus influenzae* isolated from children from Pakistan with lower respiratory tract infections. J. Infect. Dis. *160*:634–643, 1989.
79. Zhang, Y., Isaacman, D. J., Wadowsky, R. M., et al.: Detection of *Streptococcus pneumoniae* in whole blood by PCR. J. Clin. Microbiol. *33*:596–601, 1995.

28

Hypersensitivity Pneumonitis and Chronic Interstitial Pneumonitis

Raymond G. Slavin

The ready access to potent antigens and the presence of large numbers of antibody-producing plasma cells, sensitized lymphocytes, and mediator substances all contribute to make the lung an important immunologic shock organ. The scope of allergic or immunologic diseases of the lung now extends far beyond classic IgE-mediated bronchial asthma.

HYPERSENSITIVITY PNEUMONITIS

Hypersensitivity pneumonitis or extrinsic allergic alveolitis is a spectrum of disorders resulting from a hypersensitivity response to inhalation of a variety of organic dusts.

Interest in these disorders began in 1932 with the first description of farmer's lung, a disease caused by exposure to moldy hay.[6] Recently, more widely available immunologic techniques have revived interest in and study of a wide variety of similar diseases associated with different antigens and different exposure situations.

Epidemiology

Several factors determine the nature of the response to organic dust inhalation.[35] First is the basic immunologic reactivity of the host. An atopic or allergic individual typically will respond to organic dust inhalation with a type 1 immune response, characterized by IgE skin-sensitizing antibody. A nonallergic or nonatopic individual will tend to respond to an organic dust challenge with a type 3 reaction, characterized by precipitating antibody. Another important host factor may be the association of human lymphocyte antigen (HLA) haplotypes with disease. In a study of pigeon breeder's disease, a common form of hypersensitivity pneumonitis, HLA-A1, B8 frequently was found, suggesting the presence of an HLA-associated immune response gene.[1]

A second factor influencing the response is the nature and source of the antigen. Perhaps most important is the particle size of the dust. The optimal size to penetrate to the alveoli is between 4 and 6 μm. Particles larger than 10 μm are trapped in the upper airway and do not reach the alveoli in amounts sufficient to cause injury.

A third factor that determines the response to an organic dust is the nature and circumstances of the exposure. An intense but intermittent exposure results in a clinical picture different from a less intense exposure of longer duration.

A variety of antigens may result in hypersensitivity pneumonitis or allergic alveolitis. As awareness of this disease process increases and other forms of environmental exposure develop, the list will continue to expand. Table 28–1 lists some general groups of organic antigens with examples of each. A significant finding is that the antigens responsible need not be related to a special exposure associated with an individual's occupation or avocation but may be found in such common areas as air conditioners or home humidifiers.

Clinical Presentation

The clinical manifestations of hypersensitivity pneumonitis essentially are the same, regardless of the offending antigen. In the acute form associated with intermittent intense antigen exposure, the main symptoms are fever, chills, cough, dyspnea, headache, body aches, and malaise developing 4 to 6 hours after inhalation of the organic dust. Remission of symptoms occurs 12 to 18 hours later in the absence of further exposure. A more insidious form associated with progressively increasing malaise, dyspnea, cough, fatigue, and weight loss is the result of constant exposure to smaller amounts of the antigen. Stiehm and associates,[44] reporting on five children with pigeon breeder's lung, commented on the insidious onset of symptoms compared with the acute onset

TABLE 28–1. Some Causes of Hypersensitivity Pneumonia

Antigens	Sources
Thermophiles	
Thermophilic actinomycetes	Moldy hay Moldy sugar cane Room humidifiers Air conditioning ducts
Fungi	
Aspergillus	Barley
Cryptostroma corticale	Maple logs
Alternaria	Wood pulp
Animal	
Avian	Pigeons, parakeets, doves
Rodent	Rats, gerbils
Amoeba	
Naegleria gruberi	Humidifiers
Chemical agents	
Trimellitic anhydride	Plastics industry

of fever and chills in 80 per cent of adult cases. They noted acute exacerbation of symptoms in three cases after heavy antigenic exposure. Physical examination is relatively unremarkable compared with the degree of cough and dyspnea. Basilar rales are present, and wheezing may be heard in atopic individuals.

Routine laboratory tests are of little diagnostic value. Leukocytosis without eosinophilia generally is present. Skin testing with the antigens responsible for extrinsic allergic alveolitis is of limited value. Extracts of thermophilic organisms are nonspecifically irritating and therefore are of no diagnostic use. When antigens such as pigeon serum or mold are used, intradermal skin testing frequently will result in a dual response, that is, an immediate wheal and erythema reaction appearing in 15 minutes followed by a late Arthus reaction because of precipitating antibody occurring 6 to 8 hours later.

The chest radiologic findings vary, depending on the type of disease. The acute form most often is associated with diffuse, finely granular infiltrates characteristic of alveolar or interstitial pneumonitis. Micronodular deposits also may be seen. In the chronic cases, the infiltrates become confluent. Radiographic changes generally resolve after 3 to 6 months but may become permanent in more severe cases.

Pulmonary function studies in hypersensitivity pneumonitis reveal a restrictive type of ventilatory impairment, usually without significant airway obstruction. Functional abnormalities include low vital capacity, decreased pulmonary compliance, diminished diffusing capacity, and a low arterial oxygen saturation, which falls further with exercise. The first pulmonary function parameter to change in hypersensitivity pneumonitis is the carbon monoxide diffusion capacity.

Pathophysiology

There is little doubt that hypersensitivity pneumonitis is mediated immunologically, but the precise mechanism presently is unclear. The type 1, IgE-mediated reaction seems to be excluded by the nonatopic status of most of the patients, the normal IgE levels, and the absence of eosinophilia and significant bronchospasm. Several features strongly suggest a type 3 immune complex–mediated disease. This hypersensitivity reaction depends on localization of antigen and precipitating antibody complexes that are slightly soluble. Complement is fixed and activated, polymorphonuclear leukocytes are attracted to the site, and lysosomal enzymes are released, resulting in extracellular digestion and tissue damage. Features of hypersensitivity pneumonitis that suggest this are precipitating antibodies in the sera of most patients against the offending organic antigen, the Arthus-like or late 6- to 8-hour skin test response to the antigen, and the interval of 4 to 6 hours between exposure and symptoms. The biopsy results, however, suggest another process.[6]

The basic pathology of the lung in hypersensitivity pneumonitis consists of small airway or alveolar involvement. There is inflammation of the alveoli and interstitial pulmonary tissue, plus some involvement of bronchioles. In the acute state, alveolar septa are thickened, with infiltrates of lymphocytes, plasma cells, and foamy histiocytes. In the chronic stage, noncaseating granulomas with epithelioid cells, Langerhans giant cells, and various degrees of fibrosis are seen. The relative absence of pulmonary vasculitis and the presence of precipitating antibody to organic dusts in a large percentage of unaffected exposed individuals[26] argue against a pure precipitating antibody/immune complex mechanism. The findings of granulomatous lesions on lung biopsy and a number of recent in vitro studies both in animals and humans support the role of cell-mediated hypersensitivity in the development of hypersensitivity pneumonitis. Symptomatic pigeon breeders with hypersensitivity pneumonitis have demonstrated production of macrophage migration inhibition factor by avian-stimulated peripheral blood and bronchoalveolar lymphocytes.[30] Animal models have been created in the guinea pig, rat, rabbit, and monkey. These studies indicate a definite cell-mediated immune response that includes macrophage migration inhibition factor production by bronchopulmonary lymphocytes, in vitro lymphocyte transformation, bronchopulmonary macrophage activation, and the ability to transfer the disease with sensitized lymphoid cells.[3] Bronchoalveolar lavage fluid from patients with chronic hypersensitivity pneumonitis contains large numbers of lymphocytes, the majority of which are T lymphocytes. Further analysis reveals that the predominant T-cell subset is the T8-positive or T-suppressor cell.[23] Lavage fluid also contains significantly increased levels of total protein, IgG, and IgM.[38] C4 and C6 levels in lavage fluid are similar to controls, indicating that there is no direct evidence of local, complement mediated reactions. One study has shown a marked increase in numbers of mast cells in lavage fluid of hypersensitivity pneumonitis,[4] which indicates that mast cell degranulation is important in regulating the number of immune and inflammatory cells in the lung and that a late-phase reaction initiated by antigen-induced mast cell degranulation may be important in the pathogenesis of hypersensitivity pneumonitis.

Differential Diagnosis

The acute presentation of chills, cough, fever, and pulmonary infiltrates frequently is mistaken for bacterial or viral pneumonia. The remission of symptoms 12 to 18 hours after admission to the hospital often is attributed to antibiotics rather than to simple avoidance of the offending organic dust.

The chronic form of hypersensitivity pneumonia may be misdiagnosed as idiopathic pulmonary fibrosis or Hamman-Rich disease.

Specific Diagnosis

The diagnosis of hypersensitivity pneumonitis should be suspected in any patient with interstitial pneumonitis or pulmonary fibrosis. A careful history usually will elicit the characteristic signs and symptoms after exposure, with remission on avoidance. The characteristic history, together with the demonstration of serum precipitins against the appropriate antigen, is presumptive evidence for hypersensitivity pneumonitis. Virtually all patients with this disease have precipitating antibody in their serum directed against the organic dust antigen, but the presence of precipitating antibody is not definite evidence that hypersensitivity pneumonitis is present. A large number of exposed but asymptomatic unaffected individuals will demonstrate precipitating antibody to the particular antigen. The serum precipitins generally are of the IgG type and can be detected by the simple Ouchterlony double-gel diffusion technique.

In some instances, aerosol challenge with the organic dust has been used as a diagnostic aid to hypersensitivity pneumonitis. Challenge with the appropriate antigen may provoke the typical findings of fever, cough, and impairment of pulmonary function within 6 to 8 hours. Inhalation must be performed with caution and should be done only under strictly controlled conditions.

Treatment

The most desirable treatment is removal of the patient from the offending environment or altering the environment to remove the offending antigen. Acute cases usually will respond to bed rest and supportive care. Corticosteroids are indicated in severe cases; generally, treatment is followed by significant improvement.

Prognosis

The prognosis of hypersensitivity pneumonitis is excellent, provided the disease is recognized in the early stage and the antigen is avoided before irreparable tissue damage has taken place. In the acute case, avoidance of the offending antigen will result in a return of pulmonary function to normal. However, in the subacute or chronic case, in which the individual is exposed to a lower antigen challenge over a long period, pulmonary fibrosis and far-advanced ventilatory insufficiency may result.

Prevention

The major preventive measures are the wearing of masks by heavily exposed individuals and altering the processing of organic antigens to prevent organism growth.

ALLERGIC BRONCHOPULMONARY ASPERGILLOSIS

Allergic bronchopulmonary aspergillosis is a hypersensitivity response to inhalation of the spores of *Aspergillus fumigatus*.[15] Pulmonary disease caused by *A. fumigatus* first was recognized in the nineteenth century when Sluyton[43] reported an aspergillus fungal mass in the lung cavity of a woman. Redon[36] later described pulmonary aspergillosis in wigmakers and pigeon breeders.

Epidemiology

The organism *Aspergillus* causes several types of diseases in humans. Invasive or septicemic aspergillosis and saprophytic or aspergilloma forms are discussed in other sections of this text. Bronchial asthma mediated by IgE may be caused by molds, including *Aspergillus*. As stated in the preceding section of this chapter, hypersensitivity pneumonitis may be caused by *Aspergillus* species.

Aspergillus is a hardy and ubiquitous organism. It thrives on a substrate with low moisture content and has been demonstrated in such diverse sources as fertile soil, air, decaying vegetation, swimming pool water, and flour. It is cultured commonly from houses and frequents basements, crawl spaces, bedding, and house dust in particular.

Allergic aspergillosis is the most common form of asthma and pulmonary eosinophilia in the United Kingdom. Initially, the incidence of the disease supposedly was greater in Great Britain than in the United States. However, more recently the disease is being reported with greater frequency in the United States because of increasing recognition by physicians whose index of suspicion is high.

Pathophysiology

Both IgE skin-sensitizing antibody and IgG precipitating antibody are thought to play major pathogenetic roles in the production of allergic aspergillosis. The presence of IgE immunoglobulin has been shown to enhance the tissue-damaging effect of IgG precipitating antibody, perhaps by stimulating the uptake of immune complexes or their products by vascular endothelial cells.[39] The importance of precipitating antibody in the pathogenesis of allergic aspergillosis is supported by a study involving serum transfer from human to monkey.[14] Transfusion of serum from a patient with allergic aspergillosis to a monkey, followed by aerosol challenge with *Aspergillus* antigen, resulted in the development of pulmonary lesions in the monkey consistent with the picture of human allergic aspergillosis. Transfusion of human serum containing only skin-sensitizing antibody caused no pulmonary lesions. In another study,[40] monkeys immunized with *A. fumigatus* to produce precipitating antibody to the organism developed marked pulmonary changes after inhalation challenge only if they also received human serum rich in IgE against *A. fumigatus*.

Study of a lung biopsy specimen from a patient with cystic fibrosis and allergic aspergillosis utilizing newly available immunohistologic techniques has provided insights into the pathogenesis of allergic aspergillosis.[41] The marked inflammatory process was largely bronchocentric. Elastin layers were intact in blood vessels and markedly disrupted in bronchioles. The paucity of vasculitis with little granulocytic infiltration argues against a precipitating antibody/immune complex pathogenesis. By immunofluorescence, major basic protein was demonstrated in eosinophils, freely deposited outside of eosinophils, and taken up by macrophages. A number of lymphocytes stained positively for IgE. Through an immunoperoxidase stain, septate hyphae of *Aspergillus* were observed clearly in the lung parenchyma. A significant increase in interleukin-2 positive-staining T cells was observed with an approximate 2:1 ratio of helper to suppressor cells.

With this information, the following pathogenesis of allergic aspergillosis could be postulated. The spores of *Aspergillus* widely are present in air, soil, and water. Ordinarily, the spores are inhaled and disposed of by expectoration or macrophage uptake in most individuals. However, in the narrowed airway and viscid secretions of the patient with asthma or cystic fibrosis, the organisms are trapped. A cardinal feature of allergic aspergillosis is that the organism actively is growing in the respiratory tract. The size of the spores and the broad temperature range at which *Aspergillus* grows make this ideally suited for colonization of the human bronchial tree. Most other fungal spores will not survive at human body temperature, but *Aspergillus* germinates, forms mycelia, and sheds antigens, both soluble and particulate in the large subsegmental bronchi. The marked inflammatory reaction occurring in the airway wall enables soluble *Aspergillus* antigen and mycelial fragments to penetrate and deposit in the lung parenchyma. Here, IgE *Aspergillus* antibody and *Aspergillus* antigen bind to cause mast cell degranulation. Among the mast cell products is eosinophil chemotactic factor of anaphylaxis, the release of which results in tissue infiltration of eosinophils. Major basic protein from the eosinophils causes marked tissue damage. Finally, the presence of a marked increase of activated T cells, particularly helper T cells, explains the presence of such cell-mediated immune tissue responses as granuloma formation.

Clinical Presentation

Patients with allergic aspergillosis complain of anorexia, headache, general aches and pains, loss of energy, temperature elevation, and acute attacks of wheezing dyspnea. They almost always are atopic and have a history of bronchial asthma. The disease tends to affect the younger age group, with most cases occurring in those younger than 40 years of age. Several children have developed the disease before 2 years of age.[17] Production of solid sputum plugs is frequent. Often, no clear relationship can be established between a history of exposure to moldy vegetable material and the onset of symptoms.

Most patients with allergic bronchopulmonary aspergillosis have general signs of airway obstruction. FEV_1 is reduced, and in most instances carbon monoxide diffusion is decreased. Therefore, although the obstructive component predominates, there also is a restrictive element.

Direct examination of sputum plugs often reveals fungal mycelium with large numbers of eosinophils in a majority of patients. Good preservation of cytoplasm indicates active growth of the fungus, in contrast to the dead mycelia devoid of cytoplasmic content seen in patients with aspergilloma. Because *Aspergillus* commonly is inhaled and expectorated by the population at large, a positive sputum culture is not diagnostic of aspergillosis. Indeed, patients with allergic aspergillosis frequently have negative cultures during episodes of pulmonary infiltration and positive cultures at other times.

Peripheral blood eosinophils generally are more than $1000/mm^3$. Significant elevation of total serum IgE is seen in most cases.[33] The majority of the total serum IgE is not specific for *A. fumigatus,* and it appears that the increase in nonspecific IgE production results from either specific inhibition of suppressor T cells or stimulation of helper T cells by factors produced by the organism.[34] It has been suggested that serial determinations of IgE may be of value in monitoring the onset of the acute phase of allergic aspergillosis.[46]

IgE and IgG antibody levels against *A. fumigatus*, as determined by either radioimmunoassay or enzyme-linked immunosorbent assay techniques, have been shown to be significantly higher in allergic aspergillosis than in uncomplicated allergic asthma. They particularly may be important in differentiating patients with allergic bronchopulmonary aspergillosis from asthmatics who have positive skin tests and positive precipitins to *A. fumigatus.*[33]

The presence of a positive immediate wheal and erythema reaction to an *Aspergillus* skin test, indicative of the presence of skin-sensitizing antibody to *Aspergillus,* is a necessary finding in allergic aspergillosis. However, a positive skin test is not diagnostic of allergic aspergillosis because 25 per cent of bronchial asthmatics are skin-test–positive to *A. fumigatus.*[31] In a high percentage of patients, the immediate wheal and erythema reaction subsides, and in 3 to 4 hours erythema and poorly defined edema begin at the skin-test site, reaching a peak at 8 hours and resolving by 24 hours. This "late" or Arthus skin reaction indicates precipitating antibody to *Aspergillus.*

Serum precipitating antibody to *A. fumigatus* is present in most patients with allergic aspergillosis. The antibody generally is of the IgG type and reflects recent or continued growth of the fungus in body tissues or within bronchi of patients with allergic aspergillosis. As in the case of immediate skin reactivity, the presence of precipitating antibody to *A. fumigatus* is not diagnostic of allergic aspergillosis because it has been demonstrated in significant numbers of patients with allergic asthma and with farmer's lung.

The patient with allergic aspergillosis will respond to bronchial challenge of an aerosol of *A. fumigatus* in the following way. An immediate fall in FEV_1 is noted, with associated wheezing. This clears shortly, to be followed in 4 to 6 hours by asthma and a fall in FEV_1. This dual bronchial response is reminiscent of the dual skin-test response and is elicited more easily with the protein fraction of *A. fumigatus.*

A variety of radiographic shadows may be seen in allergic bronchopulmonary aspergillosis.[29] The most common abnormality is a massive homogeneous shadow without fissure displacement. A rather inconspicuous radiographic appearance can represent extensive tissue damage. Thus, hairline shadows extending out from the hilum in the direction of the bronchi, called *tramlines,* represent edema of a normal bronchial wall. Ring shadows indicate cavities. A common complication of allergic aspergillosis is atelectasis of a segment or a lobe or total collapse of the whole lung. Permanent shrinkage, particularly of the upper lobes, may be seen in the later stages with hilar elevation.

A most distinctive type of bronchiectasis is seen in the patient with allergic aspergillosis. It generally is a saccular type with marked proximal involvement and peripheral or distal sparing. This suggests a localized toxic reaction in the bronchial wall resulting from the presence of the fungus, rather than the usual sequence of events leading to bronchiectasis—that is, bronchial obstruction, atelectasis, and infection. Bronchography can be quite toxic in patients with allergic bronchopulmonary aspergillosis. Computed tomography of the chest is the technique of choice in demonstrating bronchiectasis.

Differential Diagnosis

In the patient who has asthma and pulmonary shadows, the main diagnostic considerations are bacterial pneumonia, carcinoma, and tuberculosis. The frequently seen radiographic findings in allergic aspergillosis of upper lobe shrinkage and cavitation particularly are suggestive of tuberculosis.

Mucoid impaction of bronchi is defined as obstruction of proximal bronchi by plugs of inspissated mucus and exudate. The plugs usually are larger than those in allergic aspergillosis, prompting some physicians to consider the latter a condition of "microimpaction." Fungal hyphae generally are not identified in mucous plugs without other evidence of allergy to *Aspergillus*. When hypersensitivity to *Aspergillus* is well documented, the syndrome may be called *allergic aspergillosis* rather than *mucoid impaction.*[20]

Bronchocentric granulomatosis is a condition often associated with asthma, noninvasive fungi, and mucoid impaction. The lesions are quite distinctive, consisting of replacement of bronchial epithelium by granulation tissue.[20]

Specific Diagnosis

A practical approach to the diagnosis of allergic aspergillosis would be first to evaluate any patient with a history of pulmonary infiltrates and asthma with an *Aspergillus* skin test. If this is positive, then serum should be checked for a total IgE level and precipitins to *A. fumigatus*. In questionable cases, a computed tomograph of the chest can be obtained.

Asthmatics who require corticosteroids for management might well be a group with underlying allergic aspergillosis. In a study of 42 such patients, 12 were found who were suspect. Of these, three had definite and three had probable allergic aspergillosis. This subgroup is more likely to be younger, to require large corticosteroid doses, to have a higher incidence of positive skin tests to *A. fumigatus* and other antigens, and to have elevated serum IgE levels.[2] It is realized now that species of *Aspergillus* other than *A. fumigatus* may be responsible for allergic aspergillosis. In patients who are suspected of having infection due to *A. fumigatus* but whose serum is negative to a battery of *A. fumigatus* antigens, it may be necessary to isolate and extract the strain or species of *Aspergillus* in the patients' sputum to elicit precipitin reactivity. Both *A. ochraceus*[32] and *A. terreus*[21] have been shown to cause allergic aspergillosis.

Association with Cystic Fibrosis

The incidence of allergic aspergillosis appears to be increased markedly in patients with cystic fibrosis.[17, 18, 47] Making the diagnosis of allergic aspergillosis in these patients particularly is difficult because of the similarities of the two diseases. In cystic fibrosis, there is an increased frequency of atopy, positive skin tests to *A. fumigatus*, positive sputum culture, and precipitins to *A. fumigatus* and increased IgE.[22] In addition, the radiographic findings are similar, with hyperinflation, peribronchial inflammatory changes, nodular and branching densities of mucous impaction, atelectasis, predominant upper lobe infiltrates, and bronchiectasis being common to both. The diagnosis of allergic aspergillosis may be suggested if peripheral blood eosinophils are increased markedly; if the serum IgE is elevated greatly to concentrations above 1000 IU/mL; if the IgE and IgG antibodies to *Aspergillus* are elevated significantly; and if pulmonary infiltrates do not respond to antibiotics, are transient, and resolve with corticosteroids.

Treatment

The most important drugs in the treatment of allergic aspergillosis are corticosteroids. In terms of the interruption of the pathogenetic circle, corticosteroids decrease the allergic inflammatory response, decrease the viscid secretions, and relieve airway obstruction. All these factors lead to more effective removal of the fungus. Corticosteroids must be given in large enough doses over a sufficient period to accomplish these aims.[42]

A large daily dose of prednisone, 2 to 3 mg/kg or more in children, is required to clear the chest radiograph completely. The pulmonary infiltrates of allergic aspergillosis ordinarily remarkably are responsive to corticosteroids. After radiographic clearing, a daily dose of approximately 0.5 mg/kg body weight is continued for 2 weeks and then given every other day for 3 months. This alternate-day dosage then is tapered and discontinued over another 3-month period.[48] Throughout this period, bronchodilator therapy should be continued, and, particularly in the acute phase, efforts should be made to remove viscid secretions with physiotherapy and postural drainage. In stubborn cases, bronchial lavage may have to be used. Although the use of inhaled corticosteroids clearly is helpful in bronchial asthma, there is no evidence that it is beneficial in allergic aspergillosis.[48] Even when the symptoms are minimal because of the localized nature of the disease, early and strenuous treatment is important to prevent the inexorable consequence of bronchiectasis, pulmonary fibrosis, and cor pulmonale. Promising reports have described the effectiveness of itraconazole, an oral antifungal agent, in decreasing the fungal burden in allergic aspergillosis.[9]

It is imperative to monitor the patient with allergic aspergillosis carefully for disease activity. First, we have noted already that the majority of patients are young and the prospect of long-term and possibly lifelong steroid therapy is a serious possibility. It is highly desirable to discontinue corticosteroids eventually, but this can be done safely only if one has a good picture of disease activity. Second, as many as one third of acute exacerbations of allergic aspergillosis are asymptomatic. Therefore, because one cannot depend on clinical signs and symptoms, monitoring disease activity and predicting exacerbations of disease are vital. A rising serum concentration of IgE is predictive of a clinical flare, and stable or declining values imply remission. Serial chest radiographs as well as IgE measurements are extremely useful. It has been suggested that chest radiographs be obtained every 4 months for 2 years, then every 6 months for 2 years, then once a year.[48] Serial IgE levels should be obtained monthly for 2 years and then every 2 months thereafter. A rise in the concentration of IgE should prompt the institution of systemic corticosteroid therapy.

Prognosis

A long-term follow-up study of 50 patients with untreated allergic bronchopulmonary aspergillosis has been reported.[37] All followed a chronic course with airway obstruction, recurrent pulmonary consolidation, and, in many instances, severe lung destruction. One third of the patients with recurrent pulmonary consolidations were asymptomatic; that is, episodes could recur without gross functional deterioration. Therefore, the use of symptoms as a guide to therapy bears no relationship to the activity of the disease. Patients with allergic aspergillosis can continue to have clinically unrecognized pulmonary consolidations capable of progressing insidiously and causing severe lung damage. Total serum IgE levels, levels of specific IgE to *A. fumigatus*, pulmonary function measurements, and regular chest radiographs all may be helpful in monitoring the disease course.[13]

EOSINOPHILIC PNEUMONIA

Eosinophilic pneumonia refers to a poorly understood and ill-defined group of disorders that are marked by infiltrations of the lung by eosinophils with and without an excess of these cells in the peripheral blood.[25, 27]

Epidemiology

The eosinophilic pneumonias were classified by Crofton and associates[8] into five major groups on the basis of clinical criteria:

1. Loeffler syndrome or simple pulmonary eosinophilia is marked by fleeting pulmonary infiltrates and blood eosinophilia in patients who are only mildly ill or asymptomatic. Recovery occurs within a month.

2. Prolonged or chronic pulmonary eosinophilia extends considerably longer than simple pulmonary eosinophilia and is accompanied by high fever, malaise, productive cough, chest pain, weight loss, and night sweats. It can occur without blood eosinophilia. Eosinophilia associated with pulmonary infiltrates, asthma, and vasculitis now is considered to be a separate entity known as *Churg-Strauss syndrome*. This is defined as the presence of four of the following six signs or symptoms in a patient with vasculitis: asthma, eosinophilia greater than 10 per cent, migratory pulmonary infiltrates, neuropathy, sinusitis, and extravascular eosinophilia.[28]

3. Pulmonary eosinophilia with asthma is characterized by infiltrations of the lung occurring in the course of chronic asthma. The infiltrates may be transient or prolonged.

4. Tropical eosinophilia is a symptom complex of fever, dyspnea, weight loss, nocturnal bronchospasm, and marked eosinophilic leukocytosis. The term now is synonymous with pulmonary eosinophilia in the tropics.

5. Periarteritis nodosa can include lung involvement, and both eosinophils and pulmonary infiltrations are present. Chronic eosinophilic pneumonia first was described by Carrington and associates[7] in middle-aged women, 50 per cent of whom had a history of asthma. A more recent review[19] reported similar findings to those of Carrington and associates. Six per cent of patients were younger than 20 years of age. There generally is an excellent response to corticosteroids, with prolonged treatment being required to keep the illness quiescent.

Much confusion existed with regard to this classification scheme, largely because of considerable overlap. It now generally is agreed that the term *pulmonary eosinophilia* or *eosinophilic pneumonia* should be used for this entire group. *Cryptogenic pulmonary eosinophilia* refers to those instances when an etiologic diagnosis is not possible. A single etiologic agent can be associated with a number of the syndromes of pulmonary eosinophilia.

One of the most common etiologic factors in pulmonary eosinophilia is helminthic infections.[16] A major diagnostic difficulty is that the infections often are multiple. Organisms that have been implicated include *Ancylostoma, Trichinella, Ascaris, Strongyloides, Toxocara, Schistosoma,* and *Wuchereria*. In certain parts of the tropics, filariasis is an important cause of eosinophilia, asthma, and pulmonary infiltrates. Microfilariae may be found in eosinophilic abscesses in the lung and in the sputum. In *Strongyloides* infection, the pulmonary phase with the larvae tends to be much more prolonged than that of most helminths, and larvae can be found in the sputum. The pulmonary lesions in helminthic infections associated with eosinophilic pneumonia could represent foci of direct response to the parasites themselves or a response to parasites residing elsewhere.

Both cutaneous and visceral larva migrans can cause pulmonary infiltrates and eosinophilia. The cutaneous form, also called *creeping eruption*, is caused by the burrowing of the filariform larva of *Ancylostoma braziliense*, a hookworm naturally infecting dogs and cats. Pulmonary infiltrates are thought to be allergic because no larvae are present in the sputum. It is, however, possible that larvae may reach the lung and die. Visceral larva migrans may occur in children with pica who eat soil that has been contaminated by dogs. *Toxocara canis* larvae may result in systemic findings of hepatomegaly, urticaria, joint pain, pulmonary infiltrates, and wheezing.[49]

Ascaris eggs hatch in the intestine, liberating minute larvae that penetrate blood or lymph vessels in the intestinal wall. The larvae eventually reach the lungs, where they are filtered out of the blood stream. In a few days, many perforate the alveoli. Later, they migrate up the respiratory passages to the epiglottis and then down to the esophagus and small intestine, where maturation and copulation occur. If a large number of infective eggs are ingested by a child, there may be marked temperature elevation with cough, rales, hemoptysis, and lobar consolidation. During the phase of larval migration, eosinophilia is prominent.[16] *Paragonimus westermani,* the lung fluke, migrates through the peritoneal cavity and penetrates the diaphragm to reach the lungs. In the lung, the parasites produce a marked inflammatory reaction with a resultant cyst. The encapsulated parasite starts producing eggs, and, eventually, the capsule swells and ruptures, usually into a bronchiole. The clinical picture is one of chronic bronchitis with morning cough productive of a gelatinous sputum consisting of eggs, inflammatory cells, and blood.[16]

Schistosomiasis may involve the lung through embolic passage from the intestines or bladder. The eggs produce abscesses in the lung and reside therein. With healing, scarring in the lung may lead to obstruction of the pulmonary circulation, resulting in cor pulmonale.[16]

As stated in the previous section, allergic bronchopulmonary aspergillosis is one cause of eosinophilic pneumonia that can be separated from those which the etiology still is obscure. Other fungi that may be involved are *Candida* and *Helminthosporium*.

A variety of chemical agents have been associated with eosinophilic pneumonia. Either a transient Loeffler syndrome or a more prolonged form can result. The substance can be a simple heavy metal, such as nickel,[45] or more complex chemicals, such as penicillin, para-aminosalicylic acid, hydralazine, nitrofurantoin, mecamylamine, mephenesin, and chlorpropamide.[25]

An acute form of eosinophilic pneumonia has been described in children.[5] The acute onset of respiratory distress is seen with hypoxemia and diffuse pulmonary infiltrates. Many have peripheral blood eosinophilia and fever. Eosinophils are prominent in lung biopsy and bronchoalveolar lavage.

Pathophysiology

The characteristic histologic picture is the filling of alveoli with eosinophils and large mononuclear cells and by an interstitial infiltrate of eosinophils, lymphocytes, and plasma cells. Eosinophilic granules can be engulfed by the mononuclear cells. In some distal air spaces, the eosinophils accumulate in masses with central necrosis and are designated as eosinophilic abscesses. Fibrous exudates are common, and granulomatous reactions can occur. Certain histologic features have been associated with particular clinical syndromes.[25] In some cases of eosinophilic pneumonia, polypoid masses of granulation tissue containing large numbers of eosinophils protruded into bronchioles. This was felt to be reminiscent of nasal polyps found in allergic rhinitis. In patients with symptoms of 2 or more years' duration attributable to pneumonic lesions, there was evidence of severe damage to small bronchi or bronchioles.

Clinical Presentation

As stated earlier, pulmonary eosinophilia can present in a variety of ways. The patient may be asymptomatic or have symptoms ranging from low-grade fever and slight asthma for a few weeks to a severe life-threatening picture of high fever, weight loss, and severe dyspnea for several months or years. Physical examination may be normal or may reveal wheezes, rales, or changes in breath sounds. Roentgenograms may range from fleeting patchy infiltrates to massive chronic infiltrates. A peripheral density adjacent to the pleura with a central clear zone is quite characteristic in chronic pulmonary eosinophilia and has been described as a photographic negative of pulmonary edema.[7] Peripheral blood eosinophilia may or may not be present. Pulmonary function may be normal or may show obstruction to air flow and decrease in lung volume and breathing capacity indicative of an alveolar-capillary block. Thus, there may be evidence of both obstructive and restrictive disease.

Differential Diagnosis

The presence of pulmonary infiltrates is, of course, suggestive of acute bacterial or viral infection. If peripheral blood eosinophilia is absent, the differential diagnosis especially is difficult.

Specific Diagnosis

The diagnosis of eosinophilic pneumonia strongly can be suggested by the presence of pulmonary infiltrates and peripheral blood eosinophilia. Specific diagnosis, especially in instances in which blood eosinophilia is absent, can be made only by finding the characteristic histologic picture on lung biopsy specimens.

Treatment

In parasitic infections, the parasite should be identified so that specific antiparasitic agents can be administered. For specific therapy, see Chapter 223. When the causative agent is a drug or chemical, this of course must be avoided. In the majority of cases in which the causative agent is obscure, prompt and complete remission can be achieved by means of corticosteroids. In many patients, treatment may be necessary for only a few weeks, whereas in others, continuing treatment over several years may be required to maintain remission.

Prognosis

A poor prognosis is associated with severe histologic changes, including the presence of granulomatous reactions centered upon elastic tissue of bronchi or vessels, necrotizing pulmonary angiitis, or extravascular angiitis or granulomatosis. Certainly the failure of prompt clinical remission upon institution of corticosteroids indicates a poor prognosis.

Prevention

Prompt institution of appropriate therapy is vital in preventing the severe sequelae of eosinophilic pneumonia. A careful diagnostic search for helminthic infection or a possible chemical substance may uncover the offending substance. When the offending agent is unknown, prompt and vigorous corticosteroid therapy may be instituted.

CHRONIC INTERSTITIAL PNEUMONITIS

This group of conditions in children, although rare, is associated with considerable morbidity and mortality. They are characterized by derangement of the alveolar walls frequently with adjacent air spaces and distal airway involvement. They are restrictive lung diseases and generally manifest disordered pulmonary gas exchange.

Classification

Liebow and Carrington first classified chronic interstitial pneumonitis many years ago,[24] and the following varieties have been described in children.[11]

Classical or Usual Interstitial Pneumonitis

The basic pathology consists of diffuse alveolar damage with necrosis of the alveolar lining cells, exudation of fluid into the alveoli, and formation of a hyaline membrane. There is interstitial infiltration of mononuclear cells. This condition may be due to infection with viruses or *Mycoplasma* or from irritants such as hot metal fumes. Most cases heal after acute injury, but some progress to a subacute or chronic stage with interstitial fibrosis and proliferation of alveolar lining cells. The term *Hamman-Rich syndrome* has been applied to patients with the subacute course. The etiology of the subacute and chronic types is unknown, but an autosomal dominant genetic factor has been implicated in many affected children. The age of onset may be in early infancy.

Desquamative Interstitial Pneumonitis

This condition is characterized by desquamation of the type II alveolar lining cells. They can be seen to be multiplying in the lining of the alveolar walls and in the intra-alveolar exudate. Multinucleated giant cells are present, and alveolar macrophages are increased in number. There is only a minor interstitial infiltrate. The etiology is unknown.

Lymphocytic Interstitial Pneumonitis

As is evident by the name, this condition is marked by the infiltration of mature lymphocytes into the interalveolar septa and the loose connective tissue surrounding the bronchioles and arteries. Small germinal centers are present. A relentless progressive course is seen.

Bronchiolitis Obliterans

In addition to the signs of classical interstitial pneumonitis, this condition is associated with damage to the bronchioles and formation of polypoid masses of exudate. The etiology is obscure, and most children die within 2 months of the onset of symptoms.

Posttransplantation Pneumonitis

This condition is seen in the first 3 to 5 months after bone marrow and some organ transplantations. It appears to be due to a combination of infection with cytomegalovirus in particular and noninfectious factors, most notably radiation used before transplantation. It is associated with a high mortality rate.

Diagnosis

Patients with chronic interstitial pneumonitis generally have cough, tachypnea, and exercise intolerance. Physical findings include rales, chest retraction, and clubbing.[12]

As an interstitial, restrictive disease, the typical laboratory findings include hypoxemia, decrease in carbon monoxide diffusion, and decrease in vital capacity. Newer diagnostic modalities have improved the ability to diagnose chronic interstitial pneumonias. These include high-resolution computed tomography and bronchoalveolar lavage. Open lung biopsy remains the most useful diagnostic test. In one study, 80 per cent of children with chronic interstitial pneumonitis were diagnosed on open lung biopsy.[10]

Treatment

Pharmacologic treatment of pediatric interstitial lung disease largely is empirical because there are no controlled clinical trials. Agents that have been utilized are corticosteroids; hydroxychloroquine; and cytotoxic agents, such as cyclophosphamide and azathioprine. Corticosteroids are the therapy of choice for most cases of pediatric interstitial lung disease.

Lung transplantation is being performed more often, even in infants and in patients with end-stage disease.

References

1. Allen, D. H., Basten, S., and Woolcock, A. H.: Family studies in hypersensitivity pneumonitis. Chest *70*:283–284, 1976.
2. Basich, J. E., Graves, T. S., Boz, M. N., et al.: Allergic bronchopulmonary aspergillosis in corticosteroid dependent asthmatics. J. Allergy Clin. Immunol. *68*:98–102, 1981.
3. Bice, D., Salvaggio, J., and Hoffman, E.: Passive transfer of experimental hypersensitivity pneumonitis with lymphoid cells. J. Allergy Clin. Immunol. *55*:71, 1975.
4. Bjermer, L., Engstrom-Laurent, A., Lundgren, R., et al.: Bronchoalveolar mastocytosis in farmer's lung is related to the disease activity. Arch. Int. Med. *148*:1362–1365, 1988.
5. Buchheit, J., Eid, N., Rodgers, G., Jr., et al.: Acute eosinophilic pneumonia with respiratory failure: A new syndrome? Am. Rev. Respir. Dis. *145*:716–718, 1992.
6. Campbell, J. M.: Acute symptoms following work with hay. Br. Med. J. *2*:1143–1147, 1932.
7. Carrington, C. B., Addington, W. W., Goff, A. M., et al.: Chronic eosinophilic pneumonia. N. Engl. J. Med. *280*:787–798, 1969.
8. Crofton, J. W., Livingston, J. L., Oswald, N. C., et al.: Pulmonary eosinophilia. Thorax *7*:1–35, 1952.
9. Denning, D. W., Van Nye, J. E., Lewiston, N. J., et al.: Adjunctive therapy of allergic bronchopulmonary aspergillosis with itraconazole. Chest *100*:813–819, 1991.
10. Fan, L. L., Mullen, A. L. W., Brugman, S. M., et al.: Clinical spectrum of chronic interstitial lung disease in children. J. Pediatr. *121*:867–872, 1992.
11. Fan, L. L., and Langston, C. Chronic interstitial lung disease in children. Pediatr. Pulmonol. *16*:184–196, 1993.
12. Fan, L. L.: Evaluation and therapy of chronic interstitial pneumonitis in children. Curr. Opin. Pediatr. *6*:248–254, 1994.
13. Ghory, A. C., Patterson, R., Greenberger, P., et al.: Extended evaluation of allergic bronchopulmonary aspergillosis. Int. Arch. Allergy Appl. Immunol. *62*:285–291, 1980.
14. Golbert, T. M., and Patterson, R.: Pulmonary allergic aspergillosis. Ann. Intern. Med. *72*:395–403, 1970.
15. Hinson, K. F. W., Moon, A. J., and Plummer, N. S.: Bronchopulmonary aspergillosis: A review and a report of eight new cases. Thorax *7*:317–333, 1952.
16. Hunter, G. W., Swartzwelder, J. C., and Clyde, D. F.: Tropical Medicine. 5th ed. Philadelphia, W. B. Saunders, 1976, Chap. 47.
17. Imbeau, S. A., Cohen, M., and Reed, C. E.: Allergic bronchopulmonary aspergillosis in infants. Am. J. Dis. Child. *131*:1127–1130, 1977.
18. Jarmoc, L. M., and Slavin, R. G.: Hypersensitivity responses in cystic fibrosis. Immunol. Allerg. Clin. North Am. *7*:393–402, 1987.
19. Jederlinic, J. J., Sicilian, L., and Goensler, E. A.: Chronic eosinophilic pneumonia: A report of 19 cases and a review of the literature. Medicine *67*:154–162, 1988.
20. Katzenstein, A., Liebow, A. A., and Friedman, P. J.: Bronchocentric granulomatosis, mucoid impaction and hypersensitivity reactions to fungi. Am. Rev. Respir. Dis. *111*:497–537, 1975.
21. Laham, M. N., Allen, R. C., and Greene, J. C.: Allergic bronchopulmonary aspergillosis caused by *A. terreus*: Specific lymphocyte sensitivity and antigen directed serum opsonic activity. Ann. Allergy *46*:74–88, 1981.
22. Laufer, P. O., Fink, J. N., Bruns, W. T., et al.: Allergic bronchopulmonary aspergillosis and cystic fibrosis. J. Allergy Clin. Immunol. *73*:44–48, 1984.
23. Leatherman, J. W., Michael, A. F., Schwartz, B. A., et al.: Lung T cells in hypersensitivity pneumonitis. Ann. Int. Med. *100*:390–392, 1984.
24. Liebow, A. A.: New concepts and entities in pulmonary disease. *In* Liebow, A. A. and Smith, D. E. (eds.): The Lung. Baltimore, Williams and Wilkins, 1968, p. 332.
25. Liebow, A. A., and Carrington, C. B.: The eosinophilic pneumonias. Medicine *48*:251–285, 1969.
26. Lopez, M., and Salvaggio, J.: Hypersensitivity pneumonitis: Current concepts of etiology and pathogenesis. Ann. Rev. Med. *27*:453–463, 1976.
27. Lynch, J. P., and Flint, A.: Sorting out the pulmonary eosinophilic syndromes. J. Resp. Dis. *5*:61–78, 1984.
28. Masi, A. T., Hunder, G. G., Lie, J. T., et al.: The American College of Rheumatology 1990 criteria for the classification of Churg-Strauss syndrome (allergic granulomatosis and angiitis). Arth. Rheum. *33*:1094–1100, 1990.
29. McCarthy, D. S., Simon, G., and Hargreave, F. E.: The radiological appearances in allergic bronchopulmonary aspergillosis. Clin. Radiol. *21*:366–375, 1970.
30. Moore, V. L., Fink, J. N., and Barboriak, J. J.: Immunologic events in pigeon breeder's disease. J. Allergy Clin. Immunol. *53*:319–328, 1974.
31. Nelson, L. A., Callerame, M. L., and Schwartz, R. H.: Aspergillosis and atopy in cystic fibrosis. Am. Rev. Respir. Dis. *120*:863–873, 1979.
32. Novey, H. S., and Wells, I. D.: Allergic bronchopulmonary aspergillosis caused by *Aspergillus ochraceus*. Am. J. Clin. Pathol. *70*:840–843, 1978.
33. Patterson, R., and Roberts, M.: IgE and IgG antibodies against *Aspergillus fumigatus* in sera of patients with bronchopulmonary aspergillosis. Int. Arch. Allergy Appl. Immunol. *46*:150–160, 1974.
34. Patterson, R., Rosenberg, M., and Roberts, M.: Evidence that *Aspergillus fumigatus* growing in the airway of man can be a potent stimulus of specific and nonspecific IgE formation. Am. J. Med. *63*:257–262, 1977.
35. Pepys, J.: Hypersensitivity diseases of the lungs due to fungi and organic dusts. Monogr. Allergy *4*:1–147, 1969.
36. Redon, L.: Etude sur l'aspergillose chez les animaux et chez l'homme. Paris, Masson et Cie, 1897.
37. Safirstein, B. H., D'Souza, M., Simon, G., et al.: Five-year follow-up of allergic bronchopulmonary aspergillosis. Am. Rev. Respir. Dis. *108*:450–459, 1973.
38. Salvaggio, J. E.: Hypersensitivity pneumonitis. J. Allergy Clin. Immunol. *79*:448–471, 1987.
39. Siqueira, M., and Bier, O. G.: Hemorrhagic reactions at sites of passive cutaneous anaphylaxis in guinea pigs after I.V. inoculation of unrelated immune complexes. Proc. Soc. Exp. Biol. Med. *107*:779–784, 1961.
40. Slavin, R. G., Fischer, V. W., Levine, E. A., et al.: A primate model of allergic bronchopulmonary aspergillosis. Int. Arch. Allergy Appl. Immunol. *56*:325–333, 1978.
41. Slavin, R. G., Bedrossian, C. W., and Hutcheson, P. S.: A pathologic study of allergic bronchopulmonary aspergillosis. J. Allergy Clin. Immunol. *81*:718–725, 1988.
42. Slavin, R. G.: Allergic bronchopulmonary aspergillosis. *In* Cherniack, R. (ed.): Current Therapy of Respiratory Disease. 3rd ed. Philadelphia, B. C. Decker, 1989, pp. 147–150.
43. Sluyton, T.: De vegetalibus organismii animalis parasitis. Dis. Imoug. Berolini, 1847, p. 14.
44. Stiehm, E. R., Reed, C. E., and Tooley, W. H.: Pigeon breeder's lung in children. Pediatrics *39*:904–915, 1967.
45. Sunderman, F. W., and Sunderman, F. W., Jr.: Loefflers syndrome associated with nickel sensitivity. Arch. Intern. Med. *107*:405–408, 1961.
46. Turner, K. J., Elder, J. L., O'Mahony, J., et al.: The association of lung shadowing with hypersensitivity responses in patients with allergic bronchopulmonary aspergillosis. Clin. Allergy *4*:149–160, 1974.
47. Voss, M. J., Bush, R. K., Mischler, E. H., et al.: Association of allergic bronchopulmonary aspergillosis and cystic fibrosis. J. Allergy Clin. Immunol. *69*:539–546, 1982.
48. Wang, J. L., Patterson, R., Robert, M., et al.: The management of allergic bronchopulmonary aspergillosis. Am. Rev. Respir. Dis. *120*:87–92, 1979.
49. Zuelzer, W. W., and Apt, L.: Disseminated visceral lesions associated with extreme eosinophilia. Am. J. Dis. Child. *78*:153–181, 1949.

29

PLEURAL EFFUSIONS AND EMPYEMA

J. Gary Wheeler and Richard F. Jacobs

Collections of fluid in the pleural space have been described in the literature as transudates, pleural effusions, exudates, purulent pleurisy, parapneumonic effusions, empyema, and complicated empyema. Unfortunately, there is a great deal of inexactitude in the use of these terms, and, therefore, it is difficult to compare methods of diagnosis and management from one study to another. The definitions used in this chapter to describe pleural fluid collections appear immediately below.

The term transudative pleural effusion will refer to fluid in the pleural space that is a nonpurulent effusion and typically nonpneumonic in origin. The term purulent effusions will refer to those effusions that are more cellular (exudative) and typically pneumonic in origin. The term empyema will be used to describe purulent effusions with chemical or microbial evidence of a more severe process requiring drainage. Complicated empyema will describe those processes associated with loculations or a fibropurulent rind requiring more aggressive manipulations for cure. Parapneumonic effusion is a general term referring to any pleural exudative process occurring secondary to an inflammatory process in the lung.

Although the above definitions are arbitrary and the literature is inconsistent in the use of these terms, there has evolved, nevertheless, a relatively standard approach to the classification of these four types of effusions and their management.

The first description of parapneumonic infection is attributed to Hippocrates, who in the fourth century B.C. advocated incision and drainage of empyema 2 weeks after the onset of symptoms. Since then, the physiology and microbiology of effusions have been described and parapneumonic diseases and the management of fluid collections of the pleural space have been defined. In most cases, the directions of Hippocrates still are relevant: "... set him upon a stool, which is not wobbly, someone should hold his hands, then shake him by the shoulders and listen to see on which side a noise is heard. And right at this place—preferably on the left—make an incision, then it produces death more rarely."[41] This description of open drainage to normal atmospheric pressures was recognized to be associated with significant mortality from hemodynamic instability in 1918, when the Empyema Commission of the United States Army recommended that the practice be abandoned.[40] Thereafter, closed-tube drainage was introduced and mortality fell. Developments in the areas of radiology, antimicrobials, and vaccines have resulted in further improvements in care. Today, the major cause of mortality is related to the underlying disease because the management of parapneumonic effusions in children is largely successful and without residual morbidity. The physician must understand the risks of pleural effusion and empyema as well as indications for thoracentesis, implications of the results of pleural fluid studies, and the optimal management of the effusions and empyema.

EPIDEMIOLOGY

Parapneumonic effusions are known and expected complications in children with respiratory tract infections. The frequency of effusions can be as high as 20 per cent of patients with viral or mycoplasmal pneumonia[16, 21, 60] and 75 per cent of patients with proven *Staphylococcus aureus* pneumonia.[4] Empyema has been reported to occur in 6.3/1000 admissions in Israeli children[45] and as a complication of pneumonia in 1 per cent of children in the United States.[12] The most extensive study of empyema in children was from Dallas; 12 episodes per year over a 19-year period were described.[18] In adults, empyema follows a primary pulmonary process in 55 to 60 per cent of cases; surgery, 20 per cent; trauma, 6 per cent; spontaneous pneumothorax, 35 per cent; and other causes, 2 per cent.[40, 58] In children, Hoff and associates[28] found that 11 per cent of cases had an underlying illness, including hyperimmunoglobulin E syndrome, hypogammaglobulinemia, acute lymphocytic leukemia, cerebral palsy, Down syndrome, and postsurgical and congenital thrombocytopenia. The remainder were related to a primary pulmonic process. Freij and associates[18] found a rate of 8.3 per cent with similar risk factors. The mortality is highest in the first 2 years of life. After 2 years of age, children have better outcomes than adults; generally, they have less intrinsic lung disease, have greater elasticity of their chest wall, and heal more quickly than do older individuals.[10, 22]

PATHOPHYSIOLOGY

The pleurae are mesodermally derived tissues, approximately 30 to 40 μm in thickness and permeable to liquid and gas.[6, 34] The parietal pleurae, which adhere to the chest wall, are fed from the intrathoracic and superior phrenic arteries and have sensory enervation. The visceral pleurae are splanchnic in origin, with blood flow from the pulmonic and pericardiophrenic arteries and no sensory enervation. The lymphatic structures of the visceral pleurae are microscopic vessels called lacunae. They are denser in the lower lobes to accommodate greater venous pressure. Parietal structures called stomata are 4- to 10-μm pores that connect the pleurae to lymphatics. These stomata have valvular function during expiration and inspiration and can filter large structures, such as red blood cells and macrophages.[34] The venous drainage of visceral pleura is into the pulmonic veins and from the parietal pleura into intercostal and bronchial veins. Lymphatic structures are woven below and around the mesothelial cells and ultimately drain into mediastinal, intercostal, and mammary nodes. The structure of the pleura is a surface of mesothelial cells and layers of lymphatic sinuses and pores, elastic fibers, and loose vascular connective tissue and a fibroelastic layer covering the lungs and chest wall.[34]

The precise flow and distribution of pleural fluid have been debated for some time. Because of the differences in venous pressure in the intercostal and pulmonary veins, it is believed that fluid flows from the parietal venous system to the visceral system by drifting from the high pressure in parietal tissues into the negative-pressure pleural space with reabsorption on the visceral side. The latter is caused by a relatively low venous pressure system on the parietal side and the relatively high oncotic pressure of the pulmonic venous system compared with the pleural space.

The dynamics of this process are described in Starling's equation:

$$\text{Fluid movement} = k * [\{HPc\text{-}HPip\} - \{COPc\text{-}COPip\}]$$

where k is the filtration coefficient (a measure of the permeability of capillaries to fluid), HP is the hydrostatic pressure, and COP is the colloid osmotic pressure of capillaries (c) and the intrapleural compartment (ip).[9]

It now is believed that whereas the impact of Starling forces on venous flow may play a role in the normal situation, parietal lymphatics absorb most of the excess fluids in pathologic situations and play an important role in normal physiology as well, removing up to 250 to 500 mL/day in adults.[63] In addition, they are the only mechanism for absorbing cells and other debris from the pleura.

A few studies in the past have shown that up to 20 mL of pleural fluid is found normally in 30 per cent of resting adults, 70 per cent of exercising adults,[4] and 46 to 67 per cent of postpartum women.[29] It also is possible for some fluid to be transported from the peritoneum to the pleura through small communications.[4] This hypothesis is supported by reports of patients with infected abdominal fluid and pleural effusions in whom the same organisms are recovered in both sites.[8]

The raison d'être of the pleural space is not known. It has been pointed out that some mammals, such as elephants, do not have a pleural space.[71] This has served as the rationale for some methods of management of pleural disease that have included chemical obliteration of the pleural space. In the normal situation, pleural fluid in small amounts is a necessary requirement for optimal lubrication of the pleural space and for mechanical coupling of the lung and chest wall.[34] The accumulation of excess fluid (effusion) occurs in a limited set of circumstances, through either excess production or deficient absorption. Increased production occurs when vessels are leaky (septic shock) or there is active secretion of fluid with mesothelial inflammation (pleural infection). Decreased absorption occurs with lowered oncotic pressure (nephrosis), increased pulmonary hydrostatic pressure (congestive heart failure), or lymphatic obstruction (malignancy).

The mechanisms behind pleural effusions may vary among different infectious diseases. Effusion can be a "sympathetic" pleural response to a bacterial infection in the lung associated with inflammatory cytokines and altered venous/lymphatic drainage secondary to local edema. In addition, direct or hematogenous extension of a bacterial process can occur in the pleura. *Mycoplasma* particularly is pathogenic in patients with sickle-cell disease, presumably because of pulmonary sludging, which raises pulmonic venous drainage pressures and results in accumulation of effusions. In pneumococcal disease, effusions often develop several days after the acute infection, when bacteria no longer can be recovered. It is thought that these effusions may be related to immune complex disease.[9] In patients with tuberculosis, the most common cause of pleural effusions is thought to be the rupture of an old granuloma into the pleural space, with a hypersensitivity response not unlike the skin test response.[57] This, in part, explains the low yield in cultures.

Once an inflammatory process is initiated, it tends to progress through three classic stages.[2] The first is the acute exudative stage, with a thin pleural exudate characterized by normal glucose, lactate dehydrogenase, and pH, and is defined as a purulent effusion. The transitional fibropurulent stage is characterized by turbid fluid, decreased glucose concentration (<60 mg/dL) and pH (7.2 to 7.35), and elevated lactate dehydrogenase (>200 U/L) and is categorized as empyema. The chronic organizing stage is notable for a very low pH (<7.2) and glucose (<40 mg/dL), lactate dehydrogenase greater than 1000 U/L, and development of loculations and peel. This fluid is found in patients with "complicated empyema."

It often is possible to predict the pleural fluid quality based on the clinical course of the patient without actually sampling the fluid. A patient with anasarca due to heart failure or nephrosis with bilateral effusions may not need to have an effusion analyzed if otherwise stable. However, if the same patient has fever, examination of the fluid is necessary to exclude a secondary bacterial infection. Pleural fluid analysis is most helpful when the underlying disease is not known or when a primary pulmonic process is suspected. When patients have effusions caused by hydrostatic imbalance, the effusion is a transudate. Its protein and cell count do not exceed the range of normal pleural fluid (5000 cells/mL and <2 g of protein).[4, 63] Patients who have an active inflammatory process may have an exudate (defined by excess protein and cells). In children, the most common cause of exudative pleural processes is pneumonia. In adults, the majority of pleural effusions are related to congestive heart failure or malignancy,[39] but pneumonia is the most common cause of empyema.[50] Table 29–1 summarizes the general differences among pleural effusions.

A list of causes of effusions is found in Table 29–2. Some of these are important to consider in the differential diagnosis of a difficult patient, particularly iatrogenic causes, such as invasive procedures and drugs. Others are associated with specific syndromes, such as adult respiratory distress syndrome[65] and yellow nail lymphedema syndrome.[66] Motor vehicle accidents also have been noted as a common cause of serosanguineous effusions where there is disruption of normal mechanical lung function and hematoma.[57]

TABLE 29–1. Characteristics of Pleural Efflusions

	Transudative	Purulent Effusion	Empyema	Complicated Empyema
Appearance	Serous	Thin exudate	Turbid	Thick pus
Mean WBC	1000	5300	25,500	55,000
PMN%	50%	>90%	>95%	>95%
Protein (fluid/serum ratio)	<0.5	>0.5	>0.5	>0.5
LDH (fluid/serum ratio)	<0.6	>0.6	>0.6	>0.6
LDH (IU/L)		>200	>200	>1000
Glucose mg/dL	>60	<60	<60	<40
pH*	7.4–7.5	7.35–7.45	7.2–7.35	<7.2
Imaging	Fluid	Fluid	Fluid	Loculations, thick peel, scoliosis

*Should be examined immediately or stored at 0° C.

LDH, lactate dehydrogenase; PMN, polymorphonuclear neutrophils; WBC, white blood cell count.

TABLE 29–2. Causes of Pleural Effusion

Capillary leak
- Sepsis syndrome
- Vasculitis associated with immune complex disease
  - Connective tissue diseases
  - Inflammatory bowel disease
- Malignancy (lymphoreticular, sarcoma, neuroblastoma)
- Toxins (TSST-1)*
- Drugs (phenytoin, isoniazid, nitrofurantoin, amiodarone, methotrexate, bleomycin)
- Myxedema
- Trauma

Increased hydrostatic pressure
- Congestive heart failure
- Sickle-cell disease
- Pulmonary venous hypertension
- Superior vena cava syndrome
- Pregnancy

Decreased oncotic pressure
- Nephrosis
- Cirrhosis
- Protein malnutrition

Obstructed lymphatics
- Congenital lymphangiectasia
- Yellow nail syndrome
- Radiation injury
- Neoplasia (metastatic disease)
- Pneumonia

Pleural inflammation
- Pneumonia
- Lung abscess with pleural fistula
- Pleural infection (e.g., tuberculosis)
- Esophageal rupture
- Pancreatitis

Iatrogenic
- Drugs
- Central-line misplacement

*Toxic shock syndrome toxin-1.

MICROBIOLOGY

Among children with parapneumonic effusions, there has been no prospective study to establish firmly the frequency with which effusions occur and how many are associated with particular microbes. It is likely that although respiratory viruses infrequently cause symptomatic effusions, the sheer number of cases and the presence of asymptomatic cases would make viral infection the most common cause. Definite viral disease has been associated with cytomegalovirus, Epstein-Barr virus, measles, and adenovirus.[18, 20, 31, 44] Other pathogens, such as *Mycoplasma* and *Chlamydia*, are difficult to diagnose but may account for a significant number of pneumonic infections in older children and adolescents that may be associated with effusions in up to 20 per cent of cases.[16, 20, 60] Viral, chlamydial, and mycoplasmal organisms rarely are isolated in patients with effusions requiring intervention.

Several papers have established the role of different bacterial pathogens in childhood effusions. A study of 227 children by Freij and colleagues[18] found *S. aureus* (29 per cent), *Streptococcus pneumoniae* (22 per cent), and *Haemophilus influenzae* (18 per cent) as the three most frequent causes of parapneumonic effusions (Table 29–3). Other studies have verified the relative frequency of these pathogens and are listed in Table 29–4. However, the incidence of *H. influenzae* has fallen dramatically with the universal vaccination of infants using conjugate *H. influenzae* type b vaccines.[1] Certain groups of children are at higher risk for gram-negative infections (neonates,[18] immunocompromised hosts, patients with preexisting chest tubes that become infected with nosocomial pathogens, patients with a ruptured viscus, and patients with foreign body aspiration).

The administration of antibiotics prior to the diagnosis of empyema influences the recovery of organisms. In one report, the incidence of prethoracentesis antibiotics was 71 per cent in culture-negative effusions and only 41 per cent in culture-positive effusions.[28] Pretreatment with antibiotics may be associated with a decrease in the number of positive blood cultures and in the number of patients from whom *S. pneumoniae* are recovered.[50] Freij and associates[18] have reported the frequency of parapneumonic effusions occurring in children with pneumonia caused by specific pathogens. The rates of effusion by organism were as follows: group A *Streptococcus*, 86 to 91 per cent; *S. aureus*, 72 to 76 per cent; *S. pneumoniae*, 57 per cent; *H. influenzae*, 49 to 75 per cent; *Mycoplasma*, 21 per cent; and adenoviruses, 11 to 33 per cent. Anaerobes were sought carefully by Brook and Frazier,[8] who found them infrequently in patients younger than 6 years of age. They rarely were found in patients with primary pneumonia, occurring most often in patients with lung abscess and aspiration pneumonia.[8] In older patients (7 to 17 years of age), anaerobes were recovered as isolated pathogens in 44 per cent of cases.[8] Virtually every bacterial organism has been associated with pleural effusion at one time or another. *Brucella*[32] and *Yersinia*[30] both may be associated with

TABLE 29–3. Distribution of Pathogens by Ages

	No. of Cases					
Pathogen	*0–6 months*	*7–12 months*	*13–24 months*	*25 months–5 years*	*6–15 years*	*Total*
Staphylococcus aureus	27 (41)[a]	11 (17)	10 (15)	6 (9)	12 (18)	66 (100)
Streptococcus pneumoniae	7 (14)	13 (27)	16 (33)	8 (16)	5 (10)	49 (100)
Haemophilus	4 (10)	15 (38)	18 (45)	3 (7)	0	40 (100)
Sterile	3 (6)	9 (17)	17 (31)	11 (20)	14 (26)	54 (100)
Mixed bacteria	6 (60)	1 (10)	0	1 (10)	2 (20)	10 (100)
Streptococci	1 (20)	0	1 (20)	2 (40)	1 (20)	5 (100)
Gram-negative rods	2 (67)	0	1 (33)	0	0	3 (100)
All cases	50 (22)	49 (21)	63 (28)	31 (14)	34 (15)	227 (100)

[a]Numbers in parentheses, percentage of cases.

From Freij, B. J., Kusmiesz, H., Nelson, J. D., et al.: Parapneumonic effusions and empyema in hospitalized children: A retrospective review of 227 cases. Pediatr. Infect. Dis. J. *3*:578–591, 1984.

TABLE 29–4. Percentage of Pathogens Recovered in Purulent Effusions from Children

Site/Year (No. of Patients)	*Staphylococcus aureus*	*Streptococcus pneumoniae*	*Haemophilus influenzae*	Other Pathogens	Sterile	Reference
Dallas/64–82 (227)	29	22	18	8	24	18
Nashville/77–89 (61)	11	34	3	11	39	27
Washington, D.C./73–85 (33)	15	12	21	52	NR	8
Nigeria/89–91 (57)	63	NR	NR	37	NR	41
Israel/72–81 (37)	14	41	NR	35	11	44

NR, not reported.

the development of pleural effusions. The diagnosis in such cases often is suggested by a unique history in the patient.

Mycobacterial and fungal effusions are rare in children but well described. In four published reviews, only two patients (from Nigeria) were reported to have *Mycobacterium tuberculosis*.[18, 28, 42, 44] In a series of 303 children with tuberculosis younger than 2 years of age, 3.3 per cent of patients had an effusion.[27] In adolescents with tuberculosis, the incidence of effusion with tuberculosis likely approximates that of adult disease. In one series of adult patients with primary tuberculous disease, pleural effusion occurred in 29 per cent of cases.[13] In another adult series, primarily of reactivation disease, pleural effusion occurred in only 1 per cent of the patients.[22] Histoplasmosis has been associated with pleural effusion in 0 to 6 per cent of childhood histoplasmosis cases.[52] Blastomycosis has been associated with pleural effusions in 0 to 40 per cent of cases.[51, 61] Effusions secondary to other fungi (*Coccidioides, Aspergillus*) also have been described.[40] Parasitic diseases presenting with effusions are uncommon but found in patients with *Entamoeba histolytica* disease, most often from rupture of a hepatic abscess into the pleural space.[40] Echinococcal disease also has been reported.[17]

CLINICAL PRESENTATION

The clinical presentation of transudative effusions compared with purulent effusions ordinarily is distinctive, but a continuum of symptoms is shared by both. Many of the symptoms associated with pleural processes are due to the underlying disease that precipitated the effusion, making a distinct syndrome difficult to recognize in patients. Disease due to some pathogens (anaerobes, fungi, mycobacteria) also may follow a more insidious course, obscuring the symptoms of effusion. A history always should be obtained to identify systemic diseases, such as immunodeficiency diseases, cancer, and rheumatic diseases, or medications that might be associated with effusions.

Symptoms most specific for parapneumonic processes are dyspnea and pleuritic pain. Dyspnea occurs when the volume of the effusion mechanically interferes with breathing or when pain prevents adequate gas exchange. Pain occurs with irritation of the parietal pleura and upon inspiration (pleurisy). Fever is generated by the inflammatory response and pathogen-specific components (lipopolysaccharide, other toxins). With an acute bacterial process, the fever can be high and hectic, mimicking an abscess. Patients in the chronic organizational phase generally have less fever. Cough and malaise are secondary symptoms. Hemoptysis and purulent sputum also may occur. The onset of symptoms of a purulent effusion may be delayed in time and distinct from the symptoms found at the onset of the pneumonia in older children; infants, however, usually have no symptom-free period.[10] In the early phases of effusions, no symptoms may be present.

The physical examination usually is revealing. The child is tachypneic in greater than 70 per cent of cases, but breathing is shallow as a result of the child's attempt to mimimize pain. Fever and cough usually are present in more than 90 per cent of patients with purulent effusions.[42] The patient may appear toxic, with acute infection. There often is posturing toward the affected side. On auscultation, there classically is a decrease in breath sounds and occasionally a pleural rub. These often are absent in the very young child. Rales from an associated pneumonia may be heard. Depending on the stage of the process, percussion may reveal a level of dullness associated with free-flowing effusion. As the process organizes, this may be less evident. Empyemas can erode through the chest wall into the subcutaneous tissue (empyema necessitatis) or into a bronchus (bronchopleural fistula).

IMAGING

The diagnosis most often is made by radiographic examination of the chest. There is consolidation of a lobe of the lung, with an effusion obscuring the diaphragm (Fig. 29–1). A standard posterior- and anterior-standing view reveals blunting of the costal diaphragmatic gutter. As fluid tracks along the lateral and posterior chest wall, a meniscus configuration is seen. It may be difficult to distinguish this from pleural thickening, and, in such cases, a decubitus or cross-table view of the chest will allow free-flowing fluid to layer out on the dependent chest wall. In older children and adults, it is argued that a decubitus layer of fluid of more than 10 mm is a sufficient volume of fluid to attempt to extract by thoracentesis.[37] With large volumes of fluid (>1000 mL),[59] there may be compression of the lung and shift of the trachea away from the effusion (Fig. 29–2). As an empyema develops and organizes, discrete pockets of fluid (loculations) may form within the pleural cavity (Fig. 29–2). These occasionally are confused with lung abscess. Scoliosis is well defined by the chest radiograph as well and occasionally is used as an indication for surgery.[28] The observation of an air-fluid level in the pleural space signifies that air has been generated in the pleural space (gas-forming organisms) or has entered via a pneumothorax, perforated viscus, or bronchopleural fistula.

Ultrasonography has demonstrated great utility in providing better guidance for thoracentesis of pleural fluid. It is noninvasive and allows definition of empyema by showing internal echoes and septations (Fig. 29–2).[61, 73] Transudates uniformly are anechoic, although about one-third of exudates also are anechoic.[73] Ultrasonography is not as precise as computed tomography in differentiating lung abscess from an empyema. Computed tomography and magnetic resonance imaging occasionally are required to distinguish parenchymal from pleural disease or to locate a fistula.[63] Computed tomography particularly is useful in the chest radiograph that shows total opacification of the lung, and such tomo-

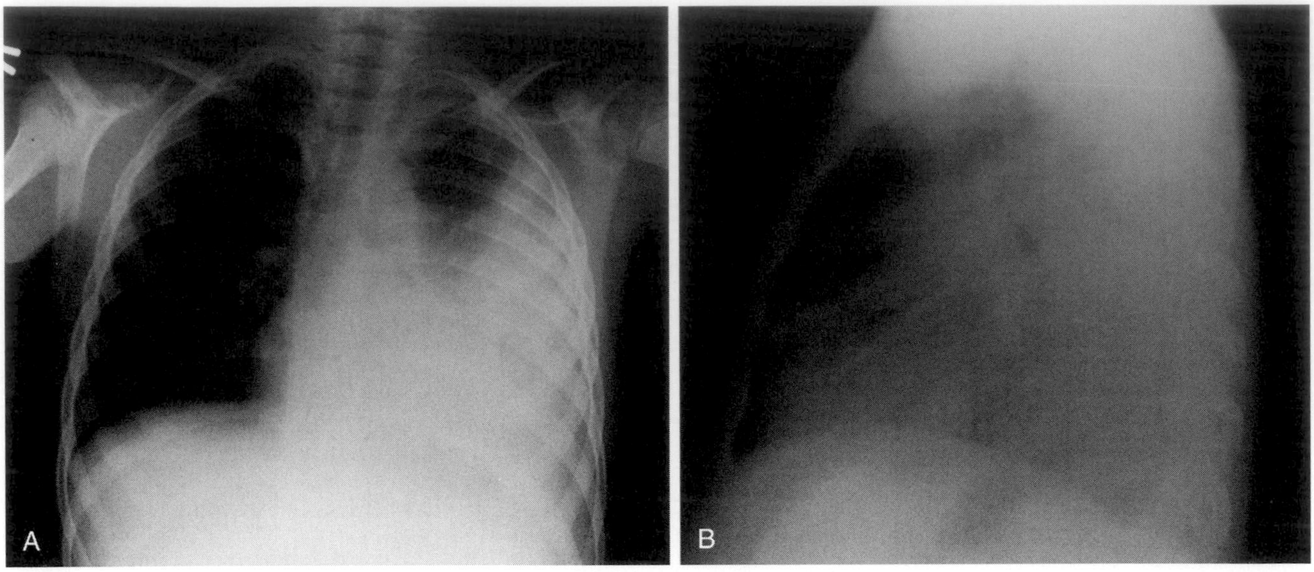

FIGURE 29–1. *Posterior* (A) *and lateral* (B) *chest radiographs demonstrate a left pleural effusion in a 9-year-old girl who had symptoms of chest wall pain, fever, and vomiting. After 1 week, her chest wall pain and shortness of breath continued and she was admitted to the hospital and treated with cefuroxime and erythromycin for pneumonia. An ultrasound examination performed 2 days later showed a large pleural effusion that was drained, with a glucose level less than 20 mg/dL, lactate dehydrogenase level greater than 99,000 U/L, protein level of 4.5 g/dL, and white blood cell count of 51,000 mm³. Gram stain of the fluid showed gram-positive cocci. Culture was negative. After failure to respond to intravenous antibiotics alone, the patient was taken to the operating room, and drainage of an empyema and several small abscesses, as well as decortication and repair of multiple bronchopleural fistulas, was performed. She was discharged 9 days later and received an additional 10 days of intravenous imipenem-cilastatin. She was well 1 month after hospital discharge.*

graphic scanning is considered to be the study of choice in this situation by some authors.[28]

THORACENTESIS

Thoracentesis plays a critical role in the management of parapneumonic effusions and in 90 per cent of adult cases yields useful information.[14] The decision to obtain fluid from the pleural cavity should be made (1) if fluid is adequate in volume and anatomically accessible and (2) if a microbial diagnosis has not been made or presumed and antibiotic therapy is intended or (3) when pulmonary function is compromised by the effusion.

The volume and location of the fluid can be determined precisely by ultrasound examination if the physical examination does not allow localization of the fluid. When a healthy child with apparent or culture-proven pneumococcal pneumonia that is community acquired has a small pleural effusion, paracentesis generally is not required. Small effusions generally can resorb, and there is a 50 per cent chance of recovering the etiologic organism from blood cultures.[18] We believe, however, that when the clinical presentation is atypical or a moderately sized effusion is present, thoracentesis almost always is indicated to define the microbial process. Atypical situations include a history of trauma, foreign body aspiration, prolonged or chronic disease, and underlying systemic diseases (congestive heart failure, malignancy).

In 1972, Light and associates,[39] in a classic paper, established the methodology by which transudates could be differentiated from exudates. Such criteria are valuable in determining if antibiotic treatment is indicated, particularly in patients with underlying diseases that predispose them to sterile effusions but who might have a comorbid infectious condition. An exudate was defined by any of the following criteria: a fluid to serum protein ratio of greater than 0.5, a lactate dehydrogenase fluid to serum ratio of greater than 0.6, a glucose less than 50 mg/dL, and a pH less than 7.2. This study was based on the results from 150 adult patients, 103 of whom had exudates.[39]

The criteria of Light and associates have been embraced and currently are used in adults and children as guidelines in the management of parapneumonic effusions. In 1984, Peterman and Speicher,[49] using adult data, recommended a two-step process to separate transudates from exudates using only the protein and lactate dehydrogenase serum to pleural fluid ratios in the initial evaluation. If a patient had an apparent exudate, additional studies were indicated, including cultures, stains, pH, and glucose. Another study in 297 adults compared several criteria for separating transudates and exudates and concluded that the criteria of Light and associates still yielded a high sensitivity (98 per cent) and a specificity of 77 per cent. A pleural fluid cholesterol concentration greater than 60 mg/dL also was used and had a sensitivity of 88 per cent and specificity of 91 per cent for exudates.[55] Although the cholesterol was not recommended for routine use, it was suggested as an extra screening test in patients with congestive heart failure in whom diuretic therapy might lead to increased pleural fluid protein concentration.[12, 55]

Once an exudate is verified, it also is necessary to determine if chest-tube drainage is needed. This is accomplished by examining several aspects of the pleural fluid. In 1980, Light and associates[38] described pleural fluid findings in adults with exudates in an attempt to determine which patients needed early chest-tube drainage of their effusions. Thirty-seven adults with acute pneumonia and parapneumonic effusions were studied. Ten patients were considered to have complicated cases if they required chest tubes or had positive cultures at time of thoracentesis. Of note, there were no clinical differences in the complicated and uncomplicated cases. Patients who required chest tubes had a pleural fluid pH of less than 7 and a glucose less than 40 mg/dL. All patients with uncomplicated effusions had a pH greater than

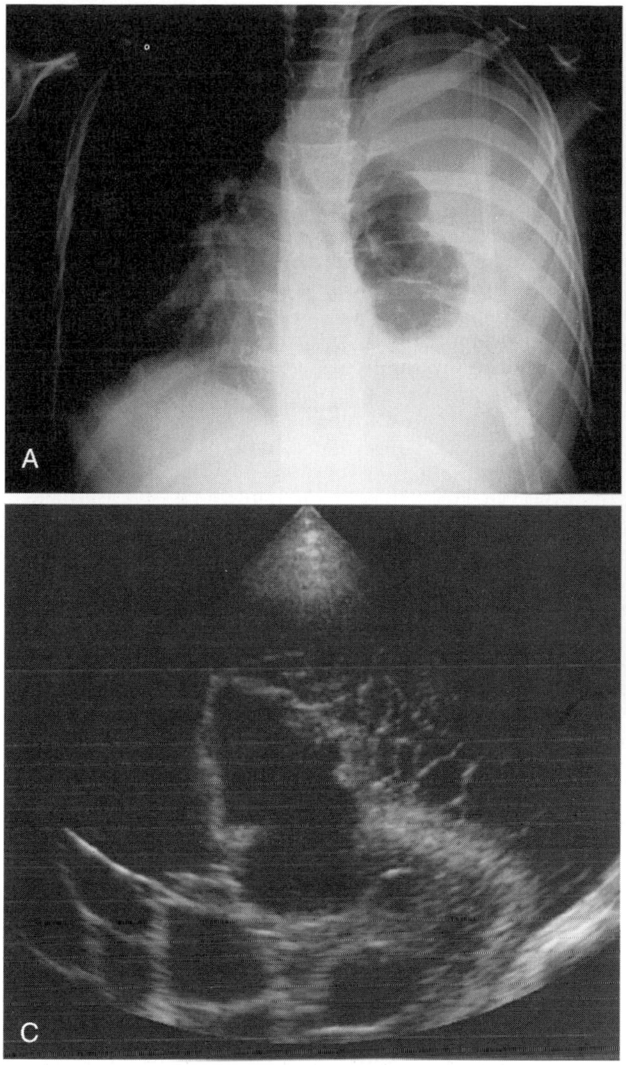

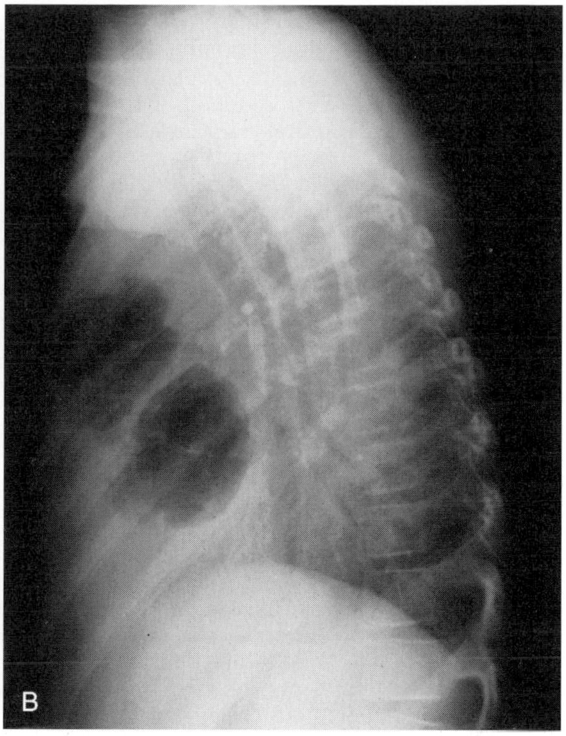

FIGURE 29–2. A *to* C, *Chest radiograph and ultrasound examination images from a 7-year-old boy with a 5-day history of vomiting, diarrhea, and low-grade fever. He had varicella 2 weeks prior. The patient was hospitalized for dehydration and developed left-sided chest pain and mild cough. Intravenous nafcillin was begun, but his condition deteriorated over the next 4 days, with an enlarging effusion and tracheal shift. Loculations were found on ultrasound examination images shown. He had a thoracotomy performed on day 6 with decortication and removal of a fibrinous rind. He was afebrile within 24 hours and received 1 week of intravenous antibiotics and 1 week of oral antibiotics. Patient was well on follow-up examination after discharge.*

7.2 and lactate dehydrogenase less than 1000 mL. Patients with a pH between 7.0 and 7.2 fell into both categories. Anaerobes were recovered from 6 of 10 complicated cases, and *S. pneumoniae* was recovered from 15 of 27 uncomplicated cases. Cell count and protein were not helpful in separating complicated from uncomplicated cases.

The application of these criteria has received limited study in children. In one series of 61 children, patients who required chest tubes or decortication had a mean pleural fluid pH of 7.24 and 7.10, respectively, compared with those who were treated with antibiotics only (pH, 7.35). The mean pleural fluid glucose was 74 g/L in the antibiotic-treated group, 10 g/L in the group treated with chest tubes, and 24 g/L in the group treated by decortication.[28] These data suggest that the criteria of Light and associates for glucose are appropriate in children but that the pH at which chest tubes are indicated may be higher in children than in adults. Additional studies are needed to confirm these observations.

Standard Gram stain and bacterial culture (aerobic and anerobic) are indicated whenever thoracentesis is carried out in patients in whom diagnosis of infection is entertained. The Gram stain usually is positive in patients with bacterial infections; when such infections are present, Gram stain may be used to direct empiric therapy until culture results are known. In one study of children, 12 of 54 sterile effusions from patients with negative blood cultures had a positive Gram stain.[18] Some experts believe that a positive Gram stain is indicative of a more severe process and that such patients are more likely to require more invasive surgical procedures.[10]

When the total white blood cell count and differential are performed, supportive information may be gained. Rarely do the results of a peripheral white blood cell count change the clinical management of the patient. The total white blood cell count in empyema fluid can vary from 5000 to 625,000/mm^3, with median values ranging from 5000 to 55,000.[18, 28] Virtually all cells are neutrophils in bacterial infections. Marked eosinophilia may be seen in parasitic, fungal, tuberculous, or hypersensitivity disease and when blood is found in the pleural space.[10] A large number of small lymphocytes are suggestive of malignancy or tuberculosis.[15, 24, 72] Other studies are required when the history suggests another underlying process. When tuberculosis is suspected by history, specific mycobacterial stains and cultures should be obtained. Identification of mycobacteria by stain and culture may be equivalent to the rate of identification of the disease process by pleural biopsy (~25 per cent).[47] Specific mycobacterial and fungal stains also should be obtained using a Ziehl-Neelsen/auramine stain and potassium hydroxide. Application of newer methods for diagnosis, such as polymerase chain reaction and tuberculosteric acid by mass spectroscopy, may be indicated.

When malignancy or metastases are suspected, cytology is necessary.[24] Most effusions in children that prove to be malignant are of lymphoreticular origin. Amylase sometimes is measured and is elevated when esophogeal rupture, acute hemorrhagic peritonitis, or pulmonary infarction is present.[36, 59] Countercurrent immunoelectropheresis and other antigen detection systems occasionally are used for diagnosis and are useful in pretreated individuals. They are only widely available for disease caused by *S. pneumoniae* and *H. influenzae* type b and not for disease caused by *S. aureus* or anaerobes. Samples for antigen detection require special preparation before analysis due to increased pleural fluid protein, which can create false-positive test results. The tests add expense and rarely, of themselves, influence management decisions.

ADDITIONAL DIAGNOSTIC STUDIES

An intradermal skin test should be applied on any child with a parapneumonic effusion to evaluate tuberculosis as a possible etiology. One-third of patients with tuberculous effusions will have a negative purified protein derivative skin test.[5] Early morning gastric aspirates also are recommended if tuberculosis is suspected.[67] Blood cultures also are indicated because up to one-third of patients will have a positive blood culture and negative pleural fluid Gram stain and culture.[18] Sputum is a less reliable source from which to determine the microbial etiology of an effusion but may be helpful in a patient with purulent sputum and a single predominant organism. It can be diagnostic in older children with reactivation or cavitary tuberculosis and also in blastomycosis and histoplasmosis. Cold agglutinins or *Mycoplasma* serology may confirm the etiology of a pleural effusion, although the nonspecificity of cold agglutinins and the delay in the rise in antibody titers make these data of marginal use in the acute management of the patient. Viral cultures are useful in only the more unusual cases and generally provide information that is not helpful in the initial management of the patient. Rapid diagnostic antigen assays, such as the rapid tests for influenza A, may be of use in defining the primary cause of respiratory disease but do not help exclude secondary bacterial pathogens causative of pneumonia and a parapneumonic effusion. When other disease, such as Wegener granulomatosis[3] and lupus erythematosus, are suspected, disease-specific tests are indicated, such as antineutrophil cytoplasmic antibody and antinucleic acid antibody.

MANAGEMENT

If a patient has an underlying disease process associated with pleural effusion and a thoracentesis has excluded bacterial infection (e.g., normal protein and lactate dehydrogenase fluid to serum ratio, normal glucose, negative cultures and Gram stain), no further treatment is indicated other than treatment of the underlying disease. These patients continue to be at risk for developing infection of the effusion and may require repeat pleural fluid examination at a later period if infection is suggested clinically.

If empyema is suggested by thoracentesis, empiric antibiotic therapy is indicated. Therapy always should include antimicrobials that are effective against *S. aureus* and *S. pneumoniae*. Acceptible regimens include nafcillin, clindamycin, first-generation cephalosporins, and cefuroxime. In patients who are vaccinated fully against *H. influenzae* (primary series and booster) and in whom the Gram stain is negative, empiric coverage against *H. influenzae* is not required. If *H. influenzae* is suspected, addition of a third-generation cephalosporin (ceftriaxone or cefotaxime) or single-drug use of cefuroxime or ampicillin-sulbactam would be effective. Ticarcillin-clavulanate, imipenem-cilastatin, and piperacillin-tazobactam would be more costly alternatives.

In patients at risk for gram-negative disease (neonates, postsurgical patients), the addition of an aminoglycoside or a third-generation cephalosporin (ceftriaxone or cefotaxime) is required. Extended-spectrum semisynthetic penicillins also would be effective (ticarcillin, mezlocillin, or piperacillin). In patients with renal failure or cephalosporin hypersensitivity, aztreonam is effective therapy for gram-negative infections. Ceftazidime, broad-spectrum β-lactams with or without a lactamase inhibitor (ticarcillin–clavulanic acid, imipenem-cilastatin, mezlocillin, or piperacillin-tazobactam), or aminoglycosides are indicated when *Pseudomonas* infection is suspected.

Anaerobic infections often are present, and in such situations, surgical drainage is believed to be a critical factor in resolving infection. Clindamycin and metronidazole are both effective, particularly when postsurgical infection or a ruptured gastrointestinal viscus is present. Upper respiratory tract anaerobes may be resistant to penicillins due to β-lactamase–producing oral flora (particularly the *Prevotella* and *Porphyromonas* species).[8] In these situations, penicillin sensitivity should be documented before using penicillin as primary therapy. For patients who have drug-resistant *S. pneumoniae*, most lung infections without associated central nervous system disease will respond to high-dose penicillin or cephalosporins.[35, 48] When the pneumococcus is highly resistant to both penicillin and cephalosporins and the patient's disease fails to improve, therapy with vancomycin and/or clindamycin may be required. Recovery of methicillin-resistant *S. aureus* requires vancomycin therapy.

With appropriate antibiotic therapy, the duration of fever in uncomplicated cases of purulent effusions usually is less than 48 to 72 hours.[46] When fever persists beyond 72 hours, surgical drainage may be required. The duration of antibiotic therapy is based on the response of the patient to the medical and/or surgical therapy provided. In one series of pediatric patients, the length of antibiotic therapy in patients who did not have surgical drainage was 10.4 days and for those with chest-tube drainage or decortication the length of intravenous therapy was 15.7 and 13.4 days, respectively.[28] The duration of combined intravenous and oral therapy was 12 to 24 days in the study reported by Freij and associates,[18] patients with *S. pneumoniae* infection receiving the shortest courses of antibiotic therapy and those infected with *S. aureus* treated for longer periods.[18] A prudent standard is to treat a minimum of 1 week beyond the last febrile day.

Closed-chest-tube drainage is the standard treatment of parapneumonic effusions in four classes of patients: those in whom (1) thick purulent material is found at thoracentesis; (2) pleural fluid pH is less than 7.35 and glucose is less than 60 mg/dL; (3) antibiotic therapy has not been associated with a timely clinical response (72 hours); and (4) pulmonary function is compromised, as demonstrated by severe hypoxemia or hypercapnia. There are no uniformly accepted criteria for suggesting the use of thoracoscopy, minithoracotomy, or urokinase therapy or decortication for individual patients.

When closed-chest-tube drainage is not associated with clinical improvement and defervescence of disease or if the lung parenchyma is trapped by the fibrinopurulent peel or fever persists, decortication often is required. If the pleural involvement is limited, a small incision (minithoracotomy) can be employed.[53] Ultrasonography and computed tomography are required to define these conditions.

Decortication has been advocated as a more expedient way

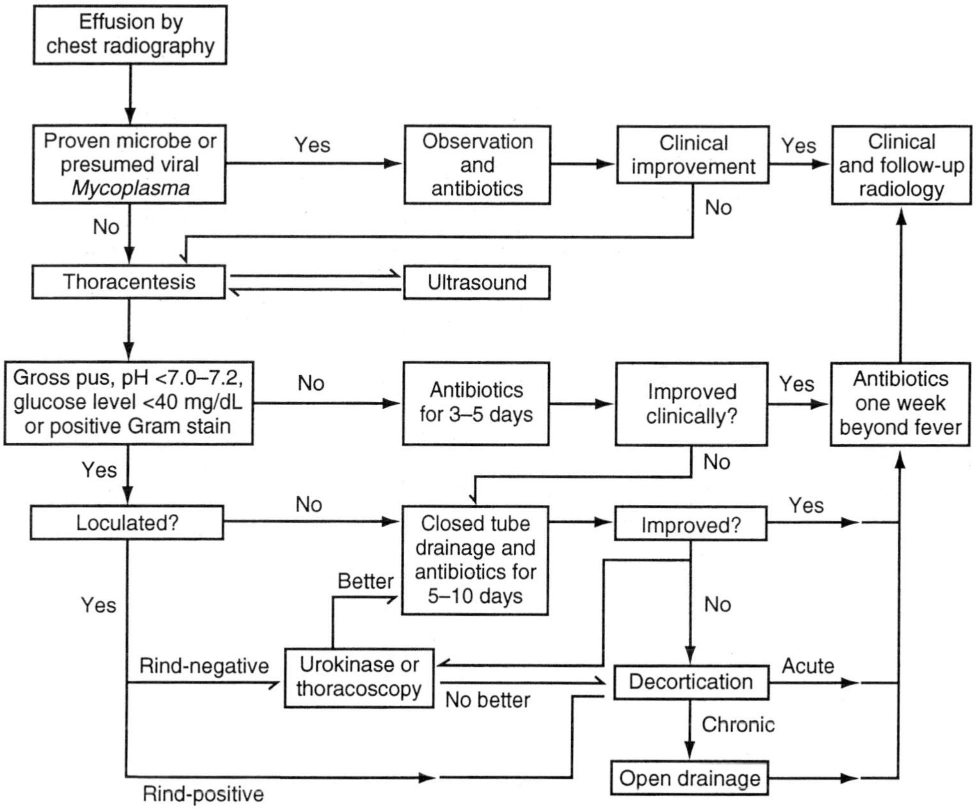

FIGURE 29–3. *Algorithm for the management of pleural fluid collections.*

to manage patients. One study reported that patients who had decortication had shorter hospital stays (11.6 days) compared with patients with thoracentesis or tube thoracostomy (28.3 days).[19] Total hospital days also were reduced in another study when patients treated with decortication (16.6 days) were compared with those treated by chest-tube drainage (21.4 days).[28] Morbidity in both cases from the operative procedure was minimal. Decortication appears to have some advantages in advanced disease in which fibrosis in the pleural cavity has resulted in a large peel. Hoff and associates[28] have used an empyema scoring system to assess the need for decortication. Any two of the following are considered indicative of severe disease and need for decortication: anaerobic infection, a pH less than 7.2, glucose less than 40 mg/dL, scoliosis, and lung entrapment.[28]

Other surgical techniques to reduce operative mortality

TABLE 29–5. Summary of Surgical Management

Procedures	Staphylococcus aureus	Streptococcus pneumoniae	Haemophilus	*Sterile*	*Mixed*	Streptococcus	*GNR*
	No. of Cases						
DT only	5 (7.5)[a]	15 (31)	16 (40)	25 (46)	0	1 (20)	0
MT	5 (7.5)	5 (10)	5 (12)	2 (4)	0	0	0
D ± T	56 (85)	29 (59)	19 (48)	27 (50)	10 (100)	4 (80)	3 (100)
Thoracotomy	1 (2)	0	1 (3)	1 (2)	0	1 (20)	0
Open drainage	1 (2)	2 (4)	0	0	1 (10)	1 (20)	0
Decortication	2 (3)	0	0	3 (6)	0	0	0
	Duration of Drainage (Days)[b]						
	n = 39	*n* = 24	*n* = 15	*n* = 22	*n* = 7	*n* = 4	*n* = 2
Range	1–43	2–12	3–41	1–20	4–54	3–6	3
Median	7	4.5	6	4.5	7	5.5	3
Mean	11.8	5.5	9.4	6.4	15.4	5	3
SD	11.1	3.0	9.6	4.7	18.5	1.4	0

[a]Numbers in parentheses, percentage of cases.
[b]Includes only surviving children who required closed-chest-tube drainage only and in whom the exact duration of drainage was known.
GNR, gram-negative rods; DT, diagnostic thoracentesis; MT, multiple thoracenteses; D ± T = closed drainage with or without initial thoracentesis.
From Freij, B. J., Kusmiesz, H., Nelson, J. D., et al.: Parapneumonic effusions and empyema in hospitalized children: A retrospective review of 227 cases. Pediatr. Infect. Dis. J. *3*:578–591, 1984.

and promote earlier hospital discharge have been proposed.[33] Although general anesthesia is required for thoracoscopy, only two small incisions are needed: one through the existing chest-tube tract for a telescope and the second through which operating instruments are passed. This allows adhesiolysis and débridement and should be done before a thick peel develops.

In chronic empyema, other approaches are used. A closed tube can be converted into an open-drainage tube. This is accomplished safely a minimum of 10 to 14 days into the course of an empyema when the visceral and parietal pleurae fuse and a pneumothorax can be avoided safely.[40] Other options include open drainage by rib resection and creation of a pleural window. The window ultimately closes with lung expansion and granulation, with disappearance of the pleural space.

The use of streptokinase in children with pleural effusion was reported in 1993.[56] The investigators utilized 12,000 to 91,000 U/kg of streptokinase over 5 days in five children with persistent empyema that had been unresponsive to chest-tube drainage and antibiotics; they reported that the treatment had immediate beneficial effects. The occasional side effects due to streptokinase reported in adults have generated concern over its safety.[7, 54] In addition, the cost of urokinase is less than that of streptokinase. Urokinase has been used in children with minimal adverse effects.[26, 54, 64] This therapy may have value in patients with organizing pleural inflammation and inadequate drainage due to loculations of pleural fluid without a peel, but at this time (1997), its use is not widespread.

Rarely are full thoracotomy and pneumonectomy required for severe pneumonic and parapneumonic disease. An occasional complication of empyema is persistent organized fluid or air collections in the pleural space, particularly in adults. A high rate of success has been reported using talc pleurodesis in these situations as well as in patients with noninfectious persistent effusions.[68, 71] Long-term complications of this therapy include development of bronchogenic carcinoma and mesothelioma (asbestos-free preparations presumably are not associated with the development of these neoplastic conditions).

One frequent cause of bloody pleural effusions is motor vehicle accidents.[40] In one series of 100 children, 56 per cent had pleural effusions associated with pulmonary contusions. These were treated with closed-chest-tube drainage; no antibiotics were used, and no infectious complications occurred.[57] Management of pleural hematoma secondary to trauma occasionally is complicated by infection because the bloody pleural fluid is an excellent growth medium. One study has suggested that empyema is less common in posttraumatic effusion with closed-chest-tube drainage than is repeated thoracentesis.[40, 69]

Complications from closed-chest-tube drainage include bleeding, exit wound infection, bronchopleural fistula, and lung laceration. Because of these rare complications, chest-tube placement, performed in the past by the pediatrician, now is delegated more frequently to the surgeon. A suggested algorithm for the management of pleural collections is shown in Figure 29–3.

PROGNOSIS AND LONG-TERM OUTCOME

The long-term outcome of patients with effusions is dependent upon the underlying cause of the effusion. Patients with empyema who previously have been well recover satisfactorily in most cases. Occasional rare complications have been reported, such as temporary paralysis of the diaphragm.[43] In three retrospective reviews, the percentage of patients who required closed-chest-tube drainage or other surgical procedures ranged from 62 to 80 per cent.[18, 28, 45] The rate of decortication ranged from 4[18] to 43 per cent.[28] The relationship of surgical management to the pathogen causing the infection is shown in Table 29–5. The immediate mortality rate for children in recent years has been reported to be from 0 to 10.8 per cent.[18, 28, 42, 45] In one of these studies, the mortality was noted to be highest in children younger than 1 year of age.[18] Studies conducted to evaluate long-term specific pulmonary disability using pulmonary function tests and lung volumes have shown normalization of these studies over time.[46]

References

1. Adams, W. G., Deaver, K. A., Cochi, S. L., et al.: Decline of childhood *Haemophilus influenzae* type b (Hib) disease in the HIB vaccine era. J. A. M. A. *269*:221–226, 1993.
2. Andrews, N. C., Parker, E. F., Shaw, R. R., et al.: Management of nontuberculous empyema. Am. Rev. Respir. Dis. *85*:935, 1962.
3. Bambery, P., Sakhuja, V., Behera, D., et al.: Pleural effusions in Wegener's granulomatosis: Report of five patients and a brief review of the literature. Scand. J. Rheumatol. *20*:445–447, 1991.
4. Baum, G. L.: Diseases of the pleura. Hosp. Med. *5*:6–25, 1969.
5. Berger, H. W., and Mejia, E.: Tuberculous pleurisy. Chest *63*:43–50, 1973.
6. Black, L. F.: The pleural space and pleural fluid. Mayo Clin. Proc. *47*:494–506, 1972.
7. Bouros, D., Schiza, S., Panagou, P., et al.: Role of streptokinase in the treatment of acute loculated parapneumonic pleural effusions and empyema. Thorax *49*:852–855, 1994.
8. Brook, I., and Frazier, E. H.: Aerobic and anaerobic microbiology of empyema. Chest *103*:1502–1507, 1993.
9. Brown, R. B., and Weinstein, L.: Pleural effusions. *In* Feigin, R. D. and Cherry, J. D. (eds.): Textbook of Pediatric Infectious Diseases. 3rd ed. Philadelphia, W. B. Saunders, 1992, pp. 309–315.
10. Brusch, J. L., and Weinstein, L.: Pleural empyema. *In* Feigin, R. D., and Cherry, J. D. (eds.): Textbook of Pediatric Infectious Diseases. 3rd ed. Philadelphia, W. B. Saunders, 1992, pp. 315–320.
11. Chartraud, S. A., and McCracken, G. H., Jr.: Staphylococcal pneumonia in infants and children. Pediatr. Infect. Dis. *1*:19–23, 1982.
12. Chonmaitree, T., and Powell, K. R.: Parapneumonic pleural effusion and empyema in children. Clin. Pediatr. *22*:414–419, 1983.
13. Choyke, P. L., Sostman, H. D., Curtis, A. M., et al.: Adult onset of pulmonary tuberculosis. Radiology *148*:357, 1983.
14. Collins, T. R., and Dahn, S. A.: Thoracentesis: Clinical value, complications, technical problems and patient experience. Chest *91*:817–822, 1987.
15. Epstein, D. M., Kline, L. R., Albeida, S. M., et al.: Tuberculous pleural effusions. Chest *91*:106–109, 1987.
16. Fine, N. L., Smith, L. R., and Sheedy, P. E.: Frequency of pleural effusions in mycoplasma and viral pneumonias. N. Engl. J. Med. *283*:790–793, 1970.
17. Fitzgerald, D., Harvey, J., Isaacs, D., et al.: The case of the persistent pleural effusions. Pediatr. Infect. Dis. J. *10*:475, 479–480, 1991.
18. Freij, B. J., Kusmiesz, H., Nelson, J. D., et al.: Parapneumonic effusions and empyema in hospitalized children: A retrospective review of 227 cases. Pediatr. Infect. Dis. J. *3*:578–591, 1984.
19. Golladay, E. S., and Wagner, C. W.: Management of empyema in children. Am. J. Surg. *158*:618–621, 1989.
20. Gothof, B. S., Kamilli, I., Keller, C., et al.: Pleural effusions in acute mononucleosis. Bildgebung *58*:218–220, 1991.
21. Grix, A., and Giammona, J. T.: Pneumonitis with pleural effusion in children due to *Mycoplasma pneumoniae*. Am. Rev. Respir. Dis. *109*:665–671, 1974.
22. Groff, D. B., Randolph, J. G., and Blader, B.: Empyema in childhood. J. A. M. A. *195*:572–574, 1966.
23. Hadlock, F. P., Park, S. K., Awe, R. J., et al.: Unusual findings in adult pulmonary tuberculosis. AJR Am. J. Roentgenol. *134*:1015, 1980.
24. Hallman, J. R., and Geisinger, K. R.: Cytology of fluids from pleural, peritoneal and pricardial cavities in children. Cytol. Fluids *38*:209–217, 1994.
25. Hamm, H., Brohan, U., Bohmer, R., et al.: Cholesterol in pleural effusions: A diagnostic aid. Chest *92*:296–302, 1987.
26. Handman, H. P., and Reuman, P. D.: The use of urokinase for loculated thoracic empyema in children: A case report and review of the literature. Pediatr. Infect. Dis. J. *12*:958–959, 1993.
27. Hardy, J. B., and Kendy, E. L., Jr.: Tuberculous pleurisy with effusion in infancy. J. Pediatr. *26*:138, 1945.
28. Hoff, S. J., Neblett, W. W., Edwards, K. M., et al.: Parapneumonic empyema

in children: Decortication hastens recovery in patients with severe pleural infections. Pediatr. Infect. Dis. J. *10*:194–199, 1990.
29. Hughson, W. G., Friedman, P., Feigin, D. S., et al.: Postpartum pleural effusion: A common radiographic finding. Ann. Intern. Med. *97*:856–858, 1982.
30. Kane, D. R., and Reuman, P. D.: *Yersinia enterocolitica* causing pneumonia and empyema in a child and a review of the literature. Pediatr. Infect. Dis. J. *11*:591–593, 1992.
31. Kato, Y., Miyata, I., Sakuma, S., et al.: A case of cytomegalovirus mononucleosis associated with pleural effusion. Acta Paediatr. Jpn. *36*:280–283, 1994.
32. Kerem, E., Diav, O., Navon, P., et al.: Pleural fluid characteristics in pulmonary brucellosis. Thorax *49*:89–90, 1994.
33. Kern, J. A. and Rodgers, B. M.: Thoracoscopy in the management of empyema in children. J. Pediatr. Surg. *28*:1128–1132, 1993.
34. Lee, K. F., and Olak, J.: Anatomy and physiology of the pleural space. Chest Surg. Clin. North Am. *4*:391–403, 1994.
35. Leggiadro, R. J., Davis, Y., and Tenover, F. C.: Outpatient drug-resistant penumococcal bacteremia. Pediatr. Infect. Dis. J. *13*:1144–1145, 1995.
36. Light, R. W.: Pleural effusions. Med. Clin. North Am. *61*:1339–1351, 1977.
37. Light, R. W.: Pleural Diseases. Philadelphia, Lea & Febiger, 1983.
38. Light, R. W., Girard, W. M., Jenkinson, S. G., et al.: Parapneumonic effusions. Am. J. Med. *69*:507–512, 1980.
39. Light, R. W., Macgregor, M. I., Luchsinger, P. C., et al.: Pleural effusions: The diagnostic separation of transudates and exudates. Ann. Intern. Med. *77*:507–513, 1972.
40. Magovern, C. J., and Rusch, V. W.: Parapneumonic and post-traumatic pleural space infections. Chest Surg. Clin. North Am. *4*:561–582, 1994.
41. Major, R. H.: Classic Descriptions of Disease. 2nd ed. Springfield, IL, Charles C Thomas, 1939, p. 620.
42. Mangete, E. D. O., Kombo, B. B., and Legg-Jack T. E.: Thoracic empyema: A study of 56 patients. Arch. Dis. Child. *69*:587–588, 1993.
43. Mazzare, M. A., and Park, M. K.: Empyema causing paralysis of hemidiaphragm. Arch. Pediatr. Adolesc. *149*:342–343, 1995.
44. Meyer, K., Girgis, N., and McGravey, V.: Adenovirus associated with con genital pleural effusion. Clin. Lab. Observations *107*:433, 1985.
45. Meyerovitch, J., Shohet, I., and Rubinstein, E.: Analysis of thirty-seven cases of pleural empyema. Eur. J. Clin. Microbiol. *4*:337–339, 1985.
46. Murphy, D., Lockhart, C. H., and Todd, J. K.: Pneumococcal empyema. Am. J. Dis. Child. *134*:659–662, 1980.
47. Nance, K. V., Shermer, R. W,. and Askin, F. B.: Diagnostic efficacy of pleural biopsy as compared with that of pleural fluid examination. Modern Pathol. *4*:320–324, 1991.
48. Pallares, R., Linares, J., Vadillo, M., et al.: Resistance to penicillin and cephalosporin and mortality from severe pneumococcal pneumonia in Barcelona, Spain. N. Engl. J. Med. *333*:474–480, 1995.
49. Peterman, T. A., and Speicher, C. E.: Evaluating pleural effusions: A two-stage laboratory approach. J. A. M. A. *252*:1051–1053, 1984.
50. Pothula, V., and Krellenstein, D. J.: Early aggressive surgical management of papapneumonic empyemas. Chest *105*:832–836, 1994.
51. Powell, D. A., and Schult, K. F.: Acute pulmonary blastomycosis in children: Clinical course and follow-up. Pediatrics *63*:736–40, 1979.
52. Quasney, M. W., and Leggiadro, R. J.: Pleural effusion associated with histoplasmosis. Pediatr. Infect. Dis. J. *12*: 415–418, 1993.
53. Raffensperger, J. G., Luck, S. R., Shkolnik, A., et al.: Mini-thoracotomy and chest tube insertion for children with empyema. J. Thorac. Cardiovasc. Surg. *84*:497–504, 1982.
54. Robinson, L. A., Moulton, A. L., Fleming, W. H., et al.: Intrapleural fibrinolytic treatment of multiloculated thoracic empyemas. Ann. Thorac. Surg. *57*:803–814, 1994.
55. Romero, S., Candela, A., Martin, C., et al.: Evaluation of different criteria for the separation of pleural transudate from exudates. Chest *104*:399–404, 1993.
56. Rosen, H., Nadkarni, V., Therous, M., et al.: Intrapleural streptokinase as adjunctive treatment for persistent empyema in pediatric patients. Chest *103*:1190–1192, 1993.
57. Roux, P., and Fisher, R. M.: Chest injuries in children: An analysis of 100 cases of blunt chest trauma from motor vehicle accidents. J. Pediatr. Surg. *27*:551–555, 1992.
58. Sahn, S. A.: Pleural manifestations of pulmonary disease. Hosp. Pract. *16*:73–89, 1981.
59. Sahn, S. A.: The differential diagnosis of pleural effusions. West. J. Med. *137*: 99–108, 1982.
60. Sahn, S. A.: Pleural effusions in the atypical pneumonias. Semin. Respir. Infect. *3*:322–334, 1988.
61. Schutze, G. S.: Blastomycosis. Clin. Infect. Dis. *22*:496–502, 1996.
62. Sherman, M. M., Subramanian, V., and Berger, R. L.: Management of thoracic empyema. Am. J. Surg. *133*:474–479, 1977.
63. Stewart, P. B.: The rate of formation and lymphatic removal of fluid in pleural effusions. J. Clin. Invest. *42*:258–262, 1963.
64. Stringel, G., and Hartman A. R.: Intrapleural instillation of urokinase in the treatment of loculated pleural effusions in children. J. Pediatr. Surg. *29*:1539–1540, 1994.
65. Tagliabue, M., Casella, T. C., Zincone G. E., et al.: CT and chest radiography in the evaluation of adult respiratory distress syndrome. Acta Radiol. *35*:230–234, 1994.
66. Tita, J. A., Wiedemann, H. P. and Weinstein, C. E.: Pleural effusions and abnormal nails. Hosp. Pract. *21*:65–68, 1986.
67. Vallejo, J. T., Ong, L. T., and Starke, J. R.: Clinical features, diagnosis and treatment of tuberculosis in infants. Pediatrics *94*:1–7, 1994.
68. Vargas, F. S., Milanez, J. R., Filomeno, L. T., et al.: Intrapleural talc for the prevention of recurrence in benign or undiagnosed pleural effusions. Chest *106*:1771–1775, 1994.
69. Varkey, B., Rose, H. D., Kutty, C. P. K., et al.: Empyema thoracis during a ten-year period: Analysis of 72 cases and comparison to a previous study (1952–1967). Arch. Intern. Med. *141*:1771–1776, 1981.
70. Weiner-Kronish, J. P.: Interrelationship of pleural and pulmonary interstitial liquid. Ann. Rev. Physiol. *55*:209–226, 1993.
71. Weissberg, D., and Ben-Zeev, I.: Talc pleurodesis. J. Thorac. Cardiovasc. Surg. *106*:689–695, 1993.
72. Yam, L. T.: Diagnostic significance of lymphocytes in pleural effusions. Ann. Intern. Med. *66*:972–982, 1967.
73. Yang, P. C., Luh, K. T., Chang, D. B., et al.: Value of sonography in determining the nature of pleural effusion: Analysis of 320 cases. Am. J. Radiol. *159*:29–33, 1992.

30

LUNG ABSCESS

J. Gary Wheeler and Richard F. Jacobs

A lung abscess is an area of necrotic material in the parenchyma of the lung initiated or complicated by infectious organisms. Although possibly originating from a pneumonia, it is distinguished by the destruction of parenchymal tissue, the presence of organization, and cavitation. Often, a lung abscess may erupt and form an adjacent empyema. Strictly, however, empyema is defined by involvement of the pleural tissues.

Lung abscess has been stereotyped in the past as a disease of male alcoholics managed with surgery.[46] Descriptions of pediatric patients have helped characterize this process and distinguish it from the presentation found in older reviews of adult patients. Notably, the incidence of lung abscess has dropped precipitously in the modern era. Smith[41] reported lung abscesses in 0.33 per cent of pediatric admissions in 1934, and Emanuel and Schulman[12] reported a rate of 0.012 per cent from 1985 to 1990. In major pediatric referral centers in Chicago, Houston, Dallas, and Montreal, the number of lung abscesses have ranged in the last two decades from 1.5 to 4.7 cases per year.[3, 12, 24, 42] Many of these cases developed in the compromised host, whereas, in the preantibiotic era, the normal host was affected more frequently. This downward trend also has been noted in adults.[34]

Improvements in pediatric diagnosis and care have resulted in a decrease in the relative numbers of cases related to underlying diseases. The morbidity and mortality rates also have fallen with the employment of antibiotic therapy and modern critical care. In 1920, Wessler and Schwarz[47] reported a 33 per cent mortality rate, with "invalidism" and hemiplegia occurring in another 27 per cent.[47] The mortality rates in the two most recent reports of lung abscess were 11 per cent and 4 per cent, respectively.[12, 42]

Although lung abscesses occur in all ages of children, two studies have suggested that there is a trend away from children younger than 5 years of age to an older population.[12, 30] In four studies, the median age ranged from 8 to 9.3 years.[3, 6, 12, 42] There does not seem to be a consistent racial or sexual predisposition to this condition in children at this time. In the 1950s, one series found boys more at risk than girls.[22] In adults, there is a twofold greater risk for males.[28, 34] Specific risk factors for lung abscess are found in Table 30–1. Most are related to some predisposition to aspiration, hematogenous spread, or compromised immunity.

PATHOPHYSIOLOGY

There are two main mechanisms to explain formation of a lung abscess. The first mechanism is by the introduction of pathogens directly into the air spaces, which typically results in solitary abscesses. This most commonly follows aspiration, with a resultant neutrophilic reaction and necrosis. Aspiration is thought to be the prevalent precipitating factor in adults, particularly in individuals with significant dental disease.[5] Most lung abscesses related to aspiration are polymicrobial and include anaerobes. The prevalence of fluoride and the relatively low incidence of dental disease in children may be additional factors for the reduced incidence of lung abscess in children, although aspiration pneumonia does occur in the absence of dental disease.

The second mechanism of lung abscess is hematogenous spread. Hematogenous seeding of the lung can lead to an initial pneumonia that develops into an abscess with further organization and cavitation. Primary pneumonia rarely progresses to necrosis and abscess in modern times; this phenomenon is explained in large part by the ready accessibility of antibiotics. Emboli from the venous circulation (septic thrombophlebitis) and right side of the heart (endocarditis) can cause single or multiple lung abscesses, often subpleural. Infection in the head and neck area also is a risk factor for vascular spread to the lung with resultant lung abscess.[38] This was a very common complication in past eras. Lung abscess complicated tonsillectomy in up to a third of cases in a 1920 report.[47] This was theorized to be secondary to aspiration during the operative procedure[41] and characteristically developed 13 to 14 days after the procedure.[47] Great improvements in modern pediatric anaesthesia with careful efforts to prevent aspiration have made this an uncommon event today.

TABLE 30–1. Underlying Risks for 46 Secondary Lung Abscesses in Pediatric Patients

Risk	No.
Neuropsychiatric causes	16
Hematologic/oncologic disorders	11
Primary pulmonary disease	8
Immunodeficiency	4
Congenital heart disease	2
Solvent aspiration	1
Foreign body aspiration	1
Prematurity	1
Chromosomal disorder	1
Endocrinopathy	1

From Tan et al.,[42] Emanuel and Shulman,[12] and unpublished data from Little Rock, Arkansas, 1989 to 1994.

A lung abscess tends to have irregular margins, with occasional bullae, and can dissect into adjacent tissues, such as the mediastinum, bronchi, and pleural space. If the abscess ruptures into a bronchus, air will enter and an air-fluid level will be noted radiographically. Dissection into the pleural space creates a purulent effusion, with air noted only if an anaerobic process is present. Dissection into the mediastinum causes a widening of the mediastinum. Air is noted if there is communication with a bronchus or in the presence of anaerobes. Multiple lung abscesses are more frequent in hematogenous or embolic disease and are found more often with more sensitive tools, such as computed tomography. Modern reviews of children have suggested that single abscesses are found more frequently than multiple abscesses.[6, 12, 42]

Microscopically, a lung abscess is definable by a collection of necrotic material: highly neutrophilic inflammation; a surrounding irregular, fibrotic wall; and microvascular infarcts. Lymphocytes often are present and seem to play a regulatory role in the formation of the abscess.[39] The infrequency of lung abscesses in patients with human immunodeficiency virus infection may be explained by this observation.

The role of preceding viral infection in undermining phagocytic host defenses is supported by the observations of preceding respiratory symptoms in patients with lung abscesses.[1] They present primarily in the cold weather[3, 12] and typically after well-defined viral illnesses, such as varicella, measles, and influenza.[20, 22, 45] The impact of chemotherapy on phagocytes also may explain the increased numbers of lung abscesses in patients with leukemia and other cancers.

On a macroscopic scale, lung abscesses do have a tendency to develop in all parts of the lung. If associated with aspiration, the anatomic site will depend on whether the subject was supine or erect at the time of aspiration. Supine patients develop abscesses in the posterior upper and lower lobes, and erect patients develop infection in the middle and basilar lower lobes. In general, there is a tendency for aspiration-related abscesses to develop more on the right than the left due presumably to the more vertical anatomy of the right stem bronchus.[12, 19]

Physicians have grouped lung abscesses into primary and secondary categories, presuming that primary versus secondary abscesses have a different microbiology, management, and outcome. The arbitrary nature of this distinction is apparent when it is appreciated how much the microbiology, clinical course, management, and outcome of both conditions overlap.[28] Primary abscesses occur in previously normal hosts without history of trauma or foreign body aspiration. Secondary abscesses are those occurring in the setting of underlying medical illnesses predisposing to infection, airway obstruction, embolization, or aspiration. In an earlier series, secondary abscesses were found more often in children younger than 1 year of age,[22] but this difference has not been corroborated in a more recent study.[12] Primary abscesses were found in 64 per cent of patients in Chicago,[12] 33 per cent in Houston,[42] and 45 per cent in Little Rock (1989 to 1994, unpublished data). A large study in Toronto from 1956 to 1965 described only 30 per cent as primary.[22]

In the modern era, lung abscess should trigger a search to exclude underlying factors that might have prognostic value and lead to treatment of underlying disease. The classic lung abscess syndrome in adults is the alcoholic who aspirates during an alcoholic binge. In children, a classic presentation would be any child with altered mental status and/or associated swallowing dysfunction. Foreign bodies can obstruct normal clearance of pathogens and precipitate a lung abscess. However, they are a surprisingly rare cause in some reports.[12, 23] Obstruction also predisposes to lung abscess in adults who have carcinoma of the lung and rarely in children with metastatic disorders. Ineffective cough in patients with neurodegenerative or myopathic disorders would be another risk factor for lung abscess, similar to that in the adult alcoholic. Patients with leukemia or who are receiving chemotherapy also are at increased risk. Occasionally, a bronchogenic cyst can become infected and mimic a lung abscess. Tricuspid or pulmonary valve endocarditis in children with complicated congenital heart disease places them at risk for lung abscess.

Immunodeficiency is another risk factor for lung abscess. Patients with chronic granulomatous disease and hyper-IgE syndrome typically are found to have lung abscesses. Patients with hypogammaglobulinemia also may develop abscesses, although bronchiectasis is the more characteristic finding. The same is true for patients with immotile cilia syndromes and cystic fibrosis, although in the latter disease abscesses surprisingly are uncommon.[8] Among pediatric patients, HIV-1 infection has not been reported as a risk factor in series from Chicago and Houston.[12, 42] Additional causes are listed in Table 30–1.

TABLE 30–2. Microbiology of Pediatric Lung Abscess

Organism	No.
Staphylococcus aureus	15
Staphylococcus coagulase-negative	2
Streptococcus pyogenes	5
Streptococcus pneumoniae	8
Alpha-hemolytic *Streptococcus*	13
Other aerobic *Streptococcus*	7
Enterococci	2
Branhamella catarrhalis	3
Escherichia coli	9
Klebsiella	8
Pseudomonas species	10
Serratia	1
Haemophilus species	7
Other gram-negative organisms	2
Bacteroides species	19
Peptostreptococcus	12
Other anaerobes	26
Candida species	3
Aspergillus	2
Mucor	1
Mycobacterium tuberculosis	1
Total	156

The information above was reported in the literature from 1976 to 1995. The isolates were recovered by direct aspiration of abscess contents, bronchoscopic aspiration, transtracheal aspiration, blood culture, or culture of surgical specimens. Data from case reports focused on procedures are included, whereas data from those focused on the organism recovered are not.[3, 6, 10, 12, 17, 18, 20, 21, 23, 24, 30, 32, 40, 42, 45]

MICROBIOLOGY

The microbiology of lung abscesses appears to be in evolution as patients and antibiotics change.[34] In the preantibiotic era, streptococci and *Mycobacterium tuberculosis* were the most common reported causes of lung abscess. After penicillin use began and tuberculosis screening and treatment became widespread, staphylococci most frequently were recovered from lung abscesses.[35] The development of better culture techniques also has increased the identification of anaerobes in lung abscess material; in past eras, these organisms probably were present but not recovered. Anaerobes clearly were suspected, though, by the fetid odor of abscesses, the time course of postoperative aspiration infections, and Gram stains of tissue and pus, which showed fusobacteria and spirochetes.[41, 47] Table 30–2 shows the microbiology of pediatric lung abscesses reported since 1975.

The primary role of anaerobes in lung abscesses has been assumed in aspiration pneumonias. Anaerobes are prominent in the oral cavity and have been recovered from the abscesses of patients with dental disease.[5] However, in many past studies, lung abscess materials have not been transported and cultured for optimal anaerobic growth. Successful growth has been described when specimens are transported in a closed syringe with culture innoculation beginning in less than 10 minutes.[6] More recent studies in which optimal culture methods were employed have corroborated the role of anaerobes in lung abscesses in children.[6, 42] In one study of mentally retarded children with seizure disorders, poor dental care, and suspected aspiration, transtracheal polymicrobial infections with aerobes were found in 9 of 10 isolates.[6] An average of 6.2 isolates were recovered per patient. *Peptostreptococcus* and *Bacteroides* species were the anaerobes recovered most frequently.[6] In a larger group of 45 children, 15 of whom had primary abscesses, 14 had polymicrobial infections.[42] Older children with neurologic disorders were the primary patients with anaerobes in both studies. Anaerobes have been recovered from normal patients along with *Streptococcus pneumoniae,* nontypable *Haemophilus influenzae,* and *Staphylococcus aureus.*[42]

The role of tissue lysins and toxins is pathogen-dependent and is felt to be critical for the development of lung abscesses. In mixed infections, there likely is synergy among the pathogens, which leads to maximally destructive qualities, as proposed by Smith in 1934.[41]

Nosocomial pathogens are becoming more frequent causes of lung abscesses as a result of the increased numbers of patients with extended hospitalizations and advanced-generation antibiotics. The wide use of third-generation antibiotics has resulted in resistant *Enterobacter* species and other gram-negative organisms' being recovered in secondary lung abscesses. In the report by Tan and associates,[42] fungal abscesses always were associated with debilitated, chronically hospitalized patients. Immunosuppression also no doubt contributes to the recovery of other unsuspected organisms (*Legionella, Neisseria mucosa, S. pneumoniae, Citrobacter*)[11, 16, 36, 37] and underscores the value of obtaining specimens in chronically hospitalized patients, atypical cases, and patients not responding to empiric treatment.

Among otherwise normal hosts, it should not be forgotten that tuberculosis can be a cause of both single and multiple abscesses. There has been a dramatic increase in the number of tuberculosis cases in the last decade. Thus, it is to be anticipated that tuberculosis will be associated more frequently with lung abscesses in the future. In patients with an international travel history, unusual pathogens should be considered, such as parasites (e.g., hydatid cysts)[13] and regional bacteria (e.g., *Pseudomonas pseudomallei*).

An important lesson for the physician is the relevance of various respiratory cultures to the microbiology of lung abscesses. Rarely is sputum of use in defining the pathogens in a lung abscess because of three factors. First, it typically is contaminated with abundant mouth flora. Second, if the lung abscess is not ruptured, there is no direct communication of the pathogens in the abscess with the airway. Third, sputum is difficult to obtain in preadolescent children. Cough cultures, performed by gagging a young child and culturing the coughed sputum on a swab before it can be swallowed, frequently is unsuccessful. However, useful information occasionally is acquired by the skilled clinician.

Bronchoscopy is very effective in recovering relevant organisms if the abscess has ruptured and has therapeutic value because it may assist in clearing secretions from the airway. This is performed infrequently in pediatric practice. Bronchoscopy is used rarely to drain the abscess. When performed, however, highly informative microbiologic information may be obtained. Transtracheal aspirates, also performed in few pediatric patients, have similar value. The upper airway frequently is colonized in debilitated patients, and thus microbiologic information so obtained must be interpreted with care. Direct aspiration of the abscess, typically under computed tomographic or ultrasound guidance, is an ideal way to provide microbiologic data and plan antimicrobial therapy. Furthermore, aspiration may have therapeutic value in decompressing the abscess.

CLINICAL FEATURES

Most patients with lung abscess have had symptoms 1 to 3 weeks before hospitalization.[12] Fever is reported to be present in 100 per cent of primary abscesses,[12, 22] and in 84 per cent of a mixed group of primary and secondary abscesses.[42] A small series of patients with secondary abscesses all had fever.[6] Cough is present in 53 to 67 per cent of cases.[22, 42] Initially, it may be nonproductive, becoming purulent when rupture into a bronchus occurs. With necrosis, hemoptysis can occur. Ipsilateral chest or shoulder pain also has been described in some patients, particularly older children.[12, 23] Weight loss may be present if the abscess is of more than a few days' duration. Other symptoms are listed in Table 30–3.[42]

There are some differences in presentation by age. Neonates and young infants typically are febrile, without localizing symptoms. Older children also are febrile but may have more cough or tachypnea and focal pain.

TABLE 30–3. Symptoms and Signs of Patients with Lung Abscess

Symptom	No. of Cases	%
Fever	38	84
Cough	24	53
Dyspnea	17	38
Chest pain	11	24
Anorexia	9	20
Purulent sputum	8	18
Rhinorrhea	7	16
Malaise/lethargy	5	11
Hemoptysis	4	9
Diarrhea	4	9
Nausea/vomiting	3	7
Irritability	3	7
Otitis media	2	4
Convulsions	2	4
Weight loss	1	2
Sore throat	1	2
Lymphadenopathy	1	2

From Tan, T. Q., Seilheimer, D. K., and Kaplan, S. L.: Pediatric lung abscess: Clinical management and outcome. Pediatr. Infect. Dis. J. *14*:51–55, 1995.

The clinical features of a lung abscess vary with the causative organisms and patient risk factors. Patients with bacterial pneumonia can present with dramatic onset of fever and overwhelming respiratory failure, such as in staphylococcal pneumonia. In these cases, there often is a recent history of influenza or varicella infection. Staphylococcal abscesses may not be noted on chest radiographs until the patient already is on ventilatory support due to the time required for an abscess to organize. Similar presentations are typical of group A beta-hemolytic *Streptococcus* and *S. pneumoniae* infections. Often, a patient has received antibiotics and there is a temporary defervescence in symptoms before the hectic fevers of an abscess re-emerge. In the latter situation, the respiratory symptoms may be less notable but virtually always are present.[12] This biphasic presentation was described more than 60 years ago in postoperative aspiration[41] and continues to be typical of many lung abscesses.

Subacute presentations are typical of patients with tuberculosis or fungal abscesses and typically are associated with other chronic systemic symptoms, such as anorexia, weight loss, and malaise. Here, the symptoms of cough may be prominent. Aspiration pneumonia may take either an indolent or acute course, depending primarily on the organisms in the abscess, the volume of aspirated material, and the status of the host.

The physical findings in lung abscess are limited. Fever almost always is present in children,[22, 42] whereas adults present with fever less frequently (19 per cent).[34] Tachypnea is a variable finding. Typically, auscultation is unrevealing, except in very large abscesses where loss of normal breath sounds is noted. Adults and older children seem to have more discrete physical findings, with rales and decreased breath sounds in about one-third of adult cases,[34] but these are infrequent in young children.[2]

An abscess can rupture into the bronchus, the mediastinum, or the pleura. In all cases, these are significant complications. In children, all organisms seem capable of these complications, but polymicrobial and anaerobic infections are suspected most frequently. Rupture into the bronchus may not be harmful if the volume of the abscess cavity does not overwhelm the host's ability to cough and clear the material. In the immunocompromised host, it may lead to disseminated pneumonia and further abscesses or death. Among adult patients who died of lung abscess, 22 per cent were found to have died of aspiration of the abscess contents.[15] In the otherwise healthy individual, rupture into the bronchus can be beneficial because it decompresses the abscess and allows for more rapid healing of the affected tissues. It is associated with the sudden production of foul-smelling, abundant, and, sometimes, blood-stained sputum. Frank hemoptysis is uncommon. Rupture into the mediastinum can be life-threatening, can be associated with chest pain and cardiac compromise, and requires surgery to drain the resulting mediastinitis. Rupture into the pleural space will result in pleuritic pain, enhancement of symptoms on inspiration, and, often, a more toxic presentation.

Routine laboratory information is of limited help. The white blood cell count and erythrocyte sedimentation rate are elevated nonspecifically, and there typically is a left shift on the white blood cell differential.[12] Certain laboratory tests may be helpful in revealing an underlying cause, such as the purified protein derivative skin test, HIV serology, or sweat chloride test. Such studies should not be routine (except the purified protein derivative skin test) and should be directed by a family history or other findings, such as chronic diarrhea or lymphadenopathy. Blood cultures are helpful, if present, but are positive in less than 10 per cent of cases.[12, 42]

DIFFERENTIAL DIAGNOSIS

The major differential diagnoses in the management of a lung abscess are anatomic. A lung abscess must be differentiated from pneumonia, from loculated empyema, and from a purulent pleural effusion with a bronchopleural fistula. Computed tomography or ultrasonography may confirm an abscess by documenting central cavitation and resolving pleural from parenchymal tissues. An abscess may be confused with a congenital cyst, pseudocyst, hydatid cyst, saccular bronchiectasis, pneumatoceole, or sequestration. Again, the chest computed tomogram allows one to define these entities in many cases by resolving the associated structures, such as the vascular supply and pleural borders.

Apart from these anatomic and infectious causes of lung abscess, the other very rare cause is cancer. Unrecognized metastatic disease from Ewing sarcoma or osteosarcomas with associated central necrosis could mimic an abscess or, by obstructing a bronchus, could promote abscess formation.

DIAGNOSIS

Currently, the diagnosis of lung abscess almost always is made by imaging the lung. In most cases, the plain film is adequate to define a lung abscess (Fig. 30–1). One visualizes a thickened cavity with an air-fluid level that can be accentuated by placing the patient in the lateral decubitus or erect position. Often, there is atelectasis as an expanding abscess compresses adjacent tissues. Pleural thickening may occur if the abscess is subpleural. Hilar adenopathy occurs in subacute situations. Visualization can be performed with bronchoscopy if the abscess ruptures into the bronchus. This is limited by the location of the abscess and skill of the bronchoscopist. The procedure usually is not performed for anatomic diagnosis but rather to obtain microbiologic specimens or exclude a foreign body.

Computed tomography is optimal in its ability to (1) identify smaller or multiple abscesses, (2) document the impact of the abscess on adjacent tissues, (3) identify cystic processes mimicing an abscess, and (4) define an abscess where an organized pneumonia obscures an air-fluid level on plain film.[17] Nuclear imaging is described[9] but used rarely and adds little to the information obtained by computed tomography.

Once a presumed abscess is defined by imaging, needle aspiration of the abscess or bronchoscopic recovery of abscess fluid should allow confirmation and identification of the infectious etiology of the process. Based on available pediatric studies, it cannot be predicted whether either procedure hastens recovery or reveals the microbiologic etiology in pretreated individuals. In an interesting case report in which an infant had abscesses in both lungs, the time to recovery was equal in the abscess that was drained and the other abscesses that were treated medically.[25] An adult study using thin-needle aspiration showed positive cultures in 92 per cent of patients not pretreated with antibiotics and in 70 per cent of those pretreated.[33]

Direct aspiration of a lung abscess may be difficult or unsuccessful if the abscess is not large or peripheral, and such complications as lung laceration are a real risk. However, Tan and associates[14] have had a satisfactory experience using direct aspiration under computed tomographic guidance (Fig. 30–2). Bronchoscopy particularly is valuable if foreign bodies are suspected or pus can be recovered. When material is obtained, a putrid quality is a clue that anaerobic organisms are present. Typically, the abscess will contain pure neutrophils. Occasionally, counterimmune electrophoresis or other antigen detection systems may assist in the microbiologic diagnosis when cultures are negative.[14] Because of the special handling required, these latter technologies usually are employed only after standard cultures have failed.

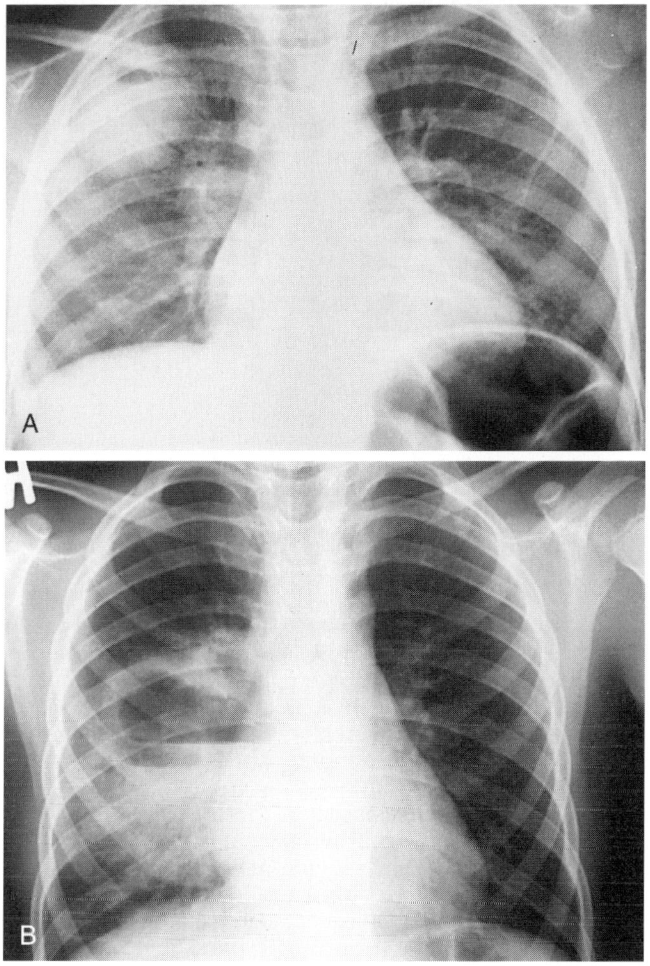

FIGURE 30–1. A, *Plain chest film of a 4-year-old black male with symptoms, including cough and fever of 104° F for 4 days. He was treated initially with oral cefaclor and re-presented with this x-ray demonstrating an air-fluid level in the right upper lobe. On intravenous cefuroxime, he was afebrile in 48 hours and went home on oral cefuroxime axetil after 4 days.* B, *Plain chest film of a 6-year-old black male who presented after 5 days of symptoms with high fevers, productive cough, dyspnea, and abdominal pain. The plain chest film reveals multiple air-fluid levels. Nafcillin and cefotaxime were begun. On day 4, an ultrasound-guided diagnostic aspiration recovered thick purulent material, but Gram stain and all cultures, including anaerobic and fungal, were negative. He was afebrile in 7 days and went home on amoxicillin–clavulanic acid at 10 days.*

TREATMENT

Although surgery clearly has a role in specific situations, the treatment of lung abscess in children often is successful when antibiotics alone are used.[35] In most cases, the need for surgery is limited to cases of failed antibiotic therapy or to an abscess complicated by rupture into adjacent tissues. New therapies such as hyperbaric oxygen[7] or papain injection[43] into the abscess have been proposed as adjuvant therapies in Russia.

The initial choice of antibiotics almost always is presump-

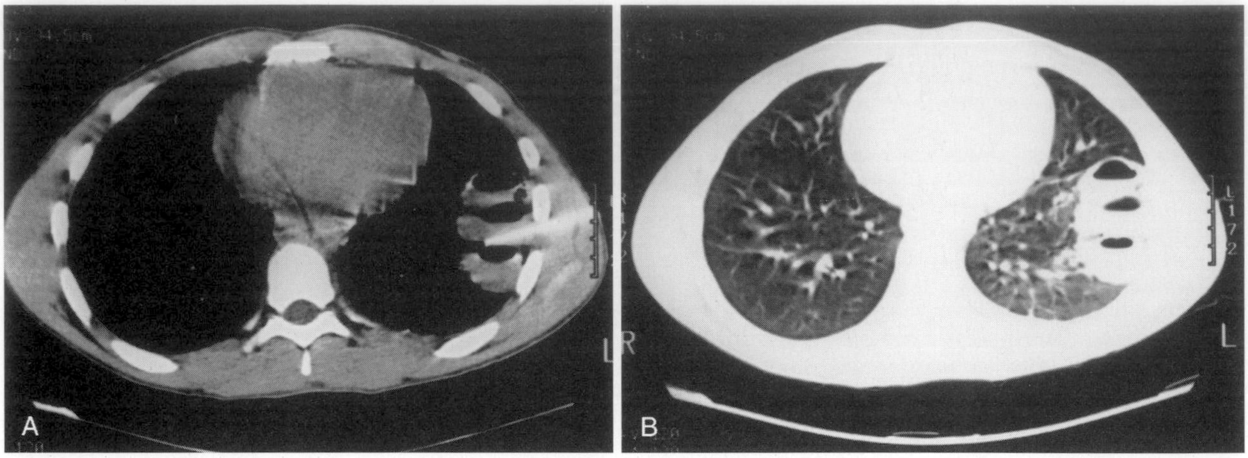

FIGURE 30–2. *This patient is a 15-year-old white male who 4 days prior to admission reported a mild aspiration during fresh-water swimming. He awoke the next day with chest and back pain. He then developed low-grade fever. His plain chest film showed a large, thick-walled abscess in the left lower lobe. The computed tomographs show* (A) *insertion of a 20-gauge needle into the abscess on the first day of admission and* (B) *detail of the wall thickness and cavitation.* Haemophilus influenzae *grew from the aspirate. Ampicillin-sulbactam was initiated and continued for 14 days.*

tive because abscess material may not be available. For primary lung abscesses in which no risk factors are identified and in the absence of positive blood cultures, it is recommended to begin therapy with a regimen that covers *S. aureus, S. pneumoniae,* and those anaerobe microorganisms that normally are found in the upper respiratory tract. Clindamycin, ampicillin plus sulbactam, or ticarcillin plus clavulanate frequently are used in this setting.

For patients at risk for aspiration or who are immunocompromised, gram-negative pathogens additionally must be considered. This spectrum of pathogens can be addressed with one of several drug regimens: (1) clindamycin and cefotaxime (or an aminoglycoside); (2) ticarcillin plus clavulanate or piperacillin plus tazobactam; or (3) nafcillin (or cefazolin), gentamicin, and metronidazole. Patients with cystic fibrosis particularly are vulnerable to *Pseudomonas* species and should receive an aminoglycoside plus an additional antipseudomonal penicillin or cephalosporin. When endocarditis is present, coverage (e.g., vancomycin, gentamicin) should be provided for staphylococci, streptococci, and enterococci while awaiting blood culture results.

It is hoped that the special problem of drug-resistant *S. pneumoniae* will remain limited due to the rarity of the isolation of this pathogen in lung abscesses. However, without effective outpatient therapy, more cases of pneumonia may progress to necrosis and abscess. As a result, there may be a resurgence of this disease. Reports from Spain suggest that most patients with resistant organisms (penicillin G, minimum inhibitory concentrations of 0.12 to 2.0) still are sensitive clinically to achievable doses of penicillins.[31]

With culture information available, therapy is directed specifically at the pathogens isolated. However, in most patients, oral or intravenous antibiotic therapy has been administered prior to aspiration of a lung abscess and, thus, may affect what organisms are recovered.[12] For this reason, coverage should be extended to include organisms that are likely but that are not recovered (such as anaerobes in a setting of aspiration).

All bacterial lung abscesses should be treated with intravenous therapy until the patient is stabile and no longer toxic. In about two-thirds to four-fifths of patients, this occurs within 3 to 7 days of instituting intravenous therapy.[12, 24] After being afebrile 48 to 72 hours, oral therapy may be considered. Certain oral drugs, such as amoxicillin plus clavulanate and clindamycin, achieve therapeutic serum levels and are effective against the spectrum of organisms in lung abscesses.

The length of total therapy for a lung abscess should be 2 to 3 weeks. Complicated infections should be treated intravenously until fever has disappeared and no evidence of continuing inflammation exists. An additional 2 to 3 weeks of oral treatment should follow. Radiographic resolution of a lung abscess that is not drained occurs over weeks. Even with drainage, the resolution may not occur more rapidly. Chest radiography should be repeated every 1 to 2 weeks, until complete resolution is documented.

Tuberculous lung abscesses spontaneously may rupture into the pleura. Treatment is not directed so much at the immediate abscess or pleuritis but at preventing spread if it erupts into a bronchus. Preventing reactivation several years later is another goal of therapy.

Clinical failure is defined by persistent fever and toxicity. Not clearly defined is the length of time one should continue treatment with intraveous antibiotics before declaring therapy a failure. Suggestions in the literature range from 1 to 3 weeks.[3, 35] When clinical failure is noted, several options are available, including physical drainage of the abscess, which permits identification of the organisms causing the disease process. Bronchoscopy may allow direct perforation of the abscess and evacuation of its contents. However, there exists a risk of fatality from aspiration of abscess contents.[16] Catheter drainage or needle aspiration (once or more) also is possible under fluoroscopy, ultrasonography, or computed tomography.[10, 20, 21, 23, 32, 44] Chest tube thoracostomy once was the standard therapy of lung abscesses.[27, 29] It now is recommended when conservative therapy fails. It may play a role in patients with large abscesses, provided the abscess abuts the parietal pleura and provides a direct path from the exterior surface to the abscess.[26] There are significant complications to tube thoracostomy, such as hemothorax, bronchopleural fistula, and empyema, which occur in a few cases.[26]

Another possible surgical indication is proximity of a lung abscess to the mediastinum. In the face of antibiotic failure, an open lung procedure and wedge resection may be required, depending on the location of the abscess.[4] The procedure typically is successful and often allows one to avoid lobectomy.[18, 46] In the complicated case, such as with a gangrenous lung, lobar resection may be necessary. Although the management of the infant with a lung abscess has been addressed with similar approaches, it has required surgery somewhat more commonly than in older children.[40, 45]

PROGNOSIS

The outcome for pediatric patients usually is very good when lung abscesses are uncomplicated, and recovery is more rapid than in adults.[28] Most patients have complete symptomatic and radiographic resolution in 3 to 6 weeks, with normal pulmonary function tests at follow-up.[3, 12] Complicated disease associated with thoracostomy tubes and empyema more likely leads to residual symptoms (pleurisy) and persistent effusions or pleural thickening on radiographs. In reports since 1982, half of the patients with lung abscess have required surgical intervention, such as thoracentesis to drain an empyema, lobectomy, or decortication, and 20 per cent have required either lobectomy or decortication.[3, 6, 12, 42] If patients require lung resection, they may experience immediate surgical complications; long-term exercise tolerance may be limited; and other problems, such as scoliosis, may develop. One study, however, found normal pulmonary functions in patients studied post lobectomy.[30] Rarely, a residual cavity may develop and become superinfected. The current mortality rate is 4 to 11 per cent[12, 42] of patients with primary and secondary lung abscesses.[12, 42] Higher risk of morbidity and mortality occurs in patients with secondary abscesses who have complications due to either a decrease in host resistance or underlying disease.[12, 34, 42]

References

1. Abramson, J. S., and Mills, E. L.: Depression of neutrophil function induced by viruses and its role in secondary microbial infections. Rev. Infect. Dis. *10*:326–341, 1988.
2. Asher, M. I., and Beaudry, P. H.: Lung abscess. *In* Chernick, V., and Kendig, E. L. (eds.): Disorders of the Respiratory Tract in Children. 5th ed. Philadelphia, W. B. Saunders, 1990, pp. 429–435.
3. Asher, M. I., Spier, S., Beland, M., et al.: Primary lung abscess in childhood: The long-term outcome of conservative management. Am. J. Dis. Child. *136*:491–494, 1982.
4. Ball, W. S., Jr., Bisset, G. S., III, and Towbin, R. B.: Percutaneous drainage of chest abscesses in children. Radiology *171*:431–434, 1989.
5. Bartlett, J. G., Gorbach, S. L., Tally, F. P., et al.: Bacteriology and treatment of primary lung abscess. Am. Rev. Respir. Dis. *109*:510–516, 1974.
6. Brook, I., and Finegold, S. M.: Bacteriology and therapy of lung abscess in children. J. Pediatr. *94*:10–12, 1979.
7. Bulynin, V. I., Koshelev, P. I. and Barsukov, V. A.: Treatment of acute lung abscess using hyperbaric oxygenation. Grudnaia i Serdechno-Sosudistaia Khirurgiia *5*:37–41, 1990.
8. Canny, G. J., Marcotte, J. E., and Levison, H.: Lung abscess in cystic fibrosis. Thorax *41*:221–222, 1985.
9. Cook, P. S., Datz, F. L., Disbro, M. A., et al.: Pulmonary uptake in indium-111 leukocyte imaging: Clinical significance in patients with suspected occult infections. Radiology *150*:557–561, 1984.
10. Cuestas, R. A., Kienzle, G. D. and Armstrong, J. D., II: Percutaneous drainage of lung abscesses in infants. Pediatr. Infect. Dis. J. *8*:390–392, 1989.
11. Dobranowski, J., and Stringer, D. A.: Diagnosis of *Legionella* lung abscess by percutaneous needle aspiration. J. Can. Assoc. Radiol. *40*:43–44, 1989.
12. Emanuel, B., and Shulman S. T.: Lung abscess in infants and children. Clin. Pediatr. *34*:2–6, 1995.
13. Fitzgerald, D., Harvey, J., Issacs, D., et al.: The case of the persistent pleural effusion. Pediatr. Infect. Dis. J. *10*:475–477, 1991.
14. Hanukoglu, A., Gutman, R., Fried, D., et al.: Lung abscess caused by *Streptococcus pneumoniae* type 3: The importance of counterimmunoelectrophoresis in laboratory diagnosis. Infection *12*:39–40, 1984.
15. Harper, P., and Terry, P. B.: Fatal lung abscesses: Review of 11 years experience. South. Med. J. *74*:281–283, 1981.
16. Hussain, Z., Lannigan, R., and Austin, T. W.: Pulmonary cavitation due to *Neisseria mucosa* in a child with chronic neutropenia. Eur. J. Clin. Microbiol. Infect. Dis. *7*:175–176, 1988.
17. Johnson, J. F., Shiels, W. E., White, C. B., et al.: Concealed pulmonary abscess: Diagnosis by computed tomography. Pediatrics *78*:283–286, 1986.
18. Kosloske, A. M., Ball, W. S., Jr., Butler, C., et al.: Drainage of pediatric lung abscess by cough, catheter, or complete resection. J. Pediatr. Surg. *21*:596–600, 1986.
19. Kuhn, C.: Bacterial infections. *In* Thurlbeck, W. M., and Churg, A. M. (eds.): Pathology of the Lung. 2nd ed. New York, Thieme Medical Publishers, 1995, p. 285.
20. Levine, M. M., Ashman, R., and Heald, F.: Anaerobic (putrid) lung abscess in adolescence. Am. J. Dis. Child. *130*:77–81, 1976.
21. Lorenzo, R. L., Bradford, G. F., Black, J., et al.: Lung abscesses in children: Diagnostic and therapeutic needle aspiration. Radiology *157*:79–80, 1985.
22. Mark, P. H., and Turner, J. A.: Lung abscess in childhood. Thorax *23*:216, 1968.
23. Mayer, T., Matlak, M. E., Condon, V., et al.: Computed tomographic findings of neonatal lung abscess. Am. J. Dis. Child. *136*:39, 1982.
24. McCracken, G. H.: Lung abscess in childhood. Hosp. Pract. *13*:35–36, 1978.
25. Melhem, R. E.: Percutaneous drainage of chest abscesses in children. Radiology *173*:575–576.
26. Mengoli, L.: Giant lung abscess treated by tube thoracostomy. J. Thorac. Cardiovasc. Surg. *90*:186–194, 1985.
27. Monaldi, V.: Endocavitary aspiration in the treatment of lung abscess. Chest *29*:193–201, 1956.
28. Neild, J. E., Eykyn, S. J., and Phillips, I.: Lung abscess and empyema. J. Med. *57*:875–882, 1985.
29. Neuhof, H., and Touroff, A. S. W.: Acute putrid abscess of the lung: Hyperacute variety. J. Thorac. Surg. *12*:98–106.
30. Nonoyama, A., Tanaka, K., Osako, T., et al.: Surgical treatment of pulmonary abscess in children under ten years of age. Chest *85*:358–362, 1984.
31. Pallares, R., Linares, J., Vadillo, M., et al.: Resistance to penicillin and cephalosporin and mortality from severe pneumococcal pneumonia in Barcelona, Spain. N. Engl. J. Med. 333:474–480, 1995.
32. Parker, L. A., Melton, J. W., Delany, D. J., et al.: Percutaneous small bore catheter drainage in the management of lung abscesses. Chest *92*:213–218, 1987.
33. Pena Grinan, N., Munoz Lucena, F, Vargas Romero, J., et al.: Yield of percutaneous needle lung aspiration in lung abscess. Chest *97*:69–74, 1990.
34. Pohlson, E. C., McNamara, J. J., Char, C., et al.: Lung abscess: A changing pattern of the disease. Am. J. Surg. *150*:97–101, 1985.
35. Powell, K.: Primary pulmonary abscess. Am. J. Dis. Child. *136*:489–490, 1982.
36. Purdy, G. D., Cullen, M., Yedlin, S., et al.: An unusual neonatal case presentation: *Streptococcus pneumoniae* pneumonia with abscess and pneumatocoele formation. J. Perinatol. *8*:378–381, 1987.
37. Shamir, R., Horev, G., Merlob, P., et al.: *Citrobacter diversus* lung abscess in a preterm infant. Pediatr. Infect. Dis. J. *9*:221–222, 1990.
38. Shanks, G. D., and Berman, J. D.: Anaerobic pulmonary abscesses: Hematogenous spread from head and neck infections. Clin. Pediatr. *25*:520–522, 1986.
39. Shapiro, M. E., Kasper, D. L., Zaleznik, D. F., et al.: Cellular control of abscess formation: Role of T cells in the regulation of abscesses formed in response to *Bacteroides fragilis*. J. Immunol. *137*:341–345, 1986.
40. Siegel, D., and McCracken, G. H., Jr.: Neonatal lung abscess. Am. J. Dis. Child. *133*:947–949, 1979.
41. Smith, D. T.: The diagnosis and treatment of pulmonary abscess in children. J. A. M. A. *103*:971–974, 1934.
42. Tan, T. Q., Seilheimer, D. K., and Kaplan, S. L.: Pediatric lung abscess: Clinical management and outcome. Pediatr. Infect. Dis. J. *14*:51–55, 1995.
43. Udod, V. M., Kolos, A. I., and Gritsuliak, Z. N.: Treatment of patients with lung abscess by local administration of papain. Vestnik. Khirurgii Imeni i Grekova *142*:24–27, 1989.
44. vanSonnenberg, E., D'Agostino, H. B., Casola, G., et al.: Lung abscess: CT-guided drainage. Radiology *178*:347–351, 1991.
45. Weber, T. R., Vane, D. W., Krishna, G., et al.: Neonatal lung abscess: Resection using one-lung anethesia. Ann. Thorac. Surg. *36*:464–467, 1983.
46. Weissberg, D.: Percutaneous drainage of lung abscess. J. Thorac. Cardiovasc. Surg. *87*:308–312, 1984.
47. Wessler, H., and Schwarz, H.: Abscess of the lung in infants and children. Am. J. Dis. Child. *19*:137–140, 1920.

31

Cystic Fibrosis

Peter W. Hiatt and Mark W. Kline

Cystic fibrosis (CF) is the most common inherited lethal disease of Caucasians. It occurs primarily among individuals of central and western European origin and affects more than 30,000 Americans. The estimated incidence in the United States is 1:2000 to 1:2600 live Caucasian births,[80] 1 in 19,000 live black births, 1 in 11,500 live Hispanic births, and 1 in 25,000 live Asian American births.[53] CF has an autosomal recessive mode of inheritance. Affected individuals are phenotypic homozygotes, and both parents usually are heterozygotes or carriers. The carrier frequency in Caucasians in the United States is approximately 1 in 25, with full siblings of children with CF having a 1 in 4 chance of being affected.

Mutations in a single gene located on the long arm of chromosome 7 account for the defective protein product in CF.[50] A range of different mutations at the DNA level account for the defective protein product in CF. The most common mutation ($_{\Delta}$F508) is the absence of three sequential nucleotides, which leads to the deletion ($_{\Delta}$) of phenylalanine (F) at the 508 position on the CF transmembrane conductance regulator protein (CFTR). About 70 per cent of individuals with CF have this mutation. More than 450 different mutations of the CF gene have been identified. Certain populations, including Ashkenazi Jews, have a relatively low incidence of the deletion of phenylalanine at the 508 position.[53]

CF transmembrane conductance regulator protein is a glycoprotein expressed at relatively low levels by surface epithelial cells in the lung, sweat glands, pancreas, liver, large intestine, and testes.[65] Higher level expression has been reported in submucosal glands. CF transmembrane conductance regulator protein appears to be very similar to a group of membrane transport proteins known as the ABC-transporter superfamily.[34] It has been confirmed that CFTR functions as an apical chloride channel mediated by cAMP. CF transmembrane conductance regulator protein appears to regulate the activity of a separate chloride channel and sodium channel balancing the rates of chloride secretion and sodium absorption.[24] CF transmembrane conductance regulator protein therefore appears to be responsible for the proper hydration of secretions in the airway, pancreas, and other tissues of patients with CF. Thus, an inability to secrete chloride and excessive sodium and water absorption contribute to altered luminal secretions. In the lung, this leads to decreased mucociliary clearance and a predisposition to chronic bacterial infections.

CLINICAL MANIFESTATIONS

Individuals with CF have exocrine gland dysfunction, which results in progressive suppurative obstructive lung disease, pancreatic insufficiency (85 to 90 per cent), elevated sweat electrolytes, male infertility (>95 per cent), and a female fertility rate of 20 to 30 per cent. Less common manifestations include hepatobiliary disease, osteoarthropathy, diabetes mellitus, nasal polyposis, and meconium ileus (Table 31–1).[11]

The potential relationship between genotype (the genetic constitution of an individual) and phenotype (the physical expression of that genotype) in CF is an active area of clinical investigation. The correlation of genotype to phenotype, to date, has not led to many clear associations between severity or course of pulmonary disease and type of genetic mutations.[9, 39] The influence of environmental factors, such as infection with respiratory tract viruses, colonization with bacterial pathogens, nutrition, passive smoke exposure, and changing medical therapy, has complicated the analysis. Multiple mutations and lack of complete understanding of the physiologic function of CFTR have delayed our understanding of the genotypic influence on phenotype in CF.

A strong association between pancreatic function and genotype has been reported for individuals homozygous for the deletion of phenylalanine at the 508 position.[8] The majority of subjects homozygous for the deletion of phenylalanine at the 508 position are pancreatic-insufficient.[13] Obstruction of the pancreatic duct begins in utero, resulting in fibrosis and loss of exocrine pancreatic function. Pancreatic fluid from patients with CF is low in enzyme and bicarbonate concentrations, resulting in maldigestion of both fat and protein. Clinically, children commonly present with steatorrhea, protein-calorie malnutrition, muscle wasting, and progressive failure to

TABLE 31–1. Clinical Features of Cystic Fibrosis at Diagnosis

Age and Clinical Feature	Approximate Prevalence (%)
0–2 Years	
Meconium ileus	10–15
Obstructive jaundice	
Hypoproteinemia/anemia	
Bleeding diathesis	
Heat prostration/hyponatremia	
Failure to thrive	
Steatorrhea	85
Rectal prolapse	20
Bronchitis/bronchiolitis	
Staphylococcal pneumonia	
2–12 Years	
Malabsorption	85
Recurrent pneumonia/bronchitis	60
Nasal polyps	6–36
Intussusception	1–5
13 Years or Older	
Chronic pulmonary disease	70
Clubbing	
Abnormal glucose tolerance	20–30
Diabetes mellitus	7
Chronic intestinal obstruction	10–20
Recurrent pancreatitis	
Focal biliary cirrhosis	15–25
Portal hypertension	2–5
Gallstones	4–14
Aspermia	98

From Chernick, V. C., and Kendig, E. L., Jr. (eds.): Kendig's Disorders of the Respiratory Tract in Children. 5th ed. Philadelphia, W. B. Saunders, 1990, p. 701.

thrive. A voracious appetite is characteristic, and stools are described as bulky, greasy, and foul smelling. Approximately 10 to 15 per cent of patients have enough preservation of pancreatic function to allow normal digestion of food (pancreatic-sufficient).[17] At least five mutations are associated with pancreatic sufficiency, whereas almost all patients homozygous for the deletion of phenylalanine at the 508 position are pancreatic-insufficient.[13]

Liver disease in CF is associated with pancreatic insufficiency.[55] Roughly 25 per cent of CF patients develop focal biliary cirrhosis, but less than 5 per cent progress to multilobar biliary cirrhosis and portal hypertension. Meconium ileus, the thick inspissated meconium that mechanically obstructs the distal ileum, occurs in 8 to 15 per cent of newborns with CF. It also is associated with pancreatic insufficiency.[40] A similar syndrome (distal intestinal obstructive syndrome) mimicking meconium ileus can occur in older children and young adults with CF.

Pulmonary disease is the primary cause of morbidity and mortality in patients with CF.[81] The lungs are morphologically normal at birth; however, within weeks they begin showing evidence of small airway abnormalities and inflammation. Progressive bronchiectasis develops with time, leading to advanced destruction of the airways and parenchyma (Figs. 31–1 and 31–2). Bronchiectatic cysts are prominent, especially in the upper lobes. Death eventually occurs from respiratory tract failure. Progressive deterioration of pulmonary function occurs, despite the routine use of antimicrobial agents. A pathogenic role for bacteria is suggested by the presence of immune complexes in the lungs, improvement clinically after treatment with antibiotics, and the improved survival observed since introduction of therapy with antipseudomonal agents.

Many children with CF present during infancy with recurrent wheezing or persistent bronchiolitis. These findings often resolve with therapy. As mucopurulent secretions increase, chronic cough develops.[11] Digital clubbing occurs gradually and correlates with severity of lung disease. On examination, there is evidence of crackles and decreased breath sounds secondary to mucopurulent secretions. Acute exacerbations may develop, requiring intravenous antibiotic therapy and frequent hospitalization. As lung disease progresses, exercise tolerance is decreased, dyspnea increases, and respiratory tract failure develops. There is marked heterogeneity in the rate of progression of pulmonary disease. Some patients live to the fifth decade of life, whereas others succumb to respiratory tract failure before their tenth birthday.

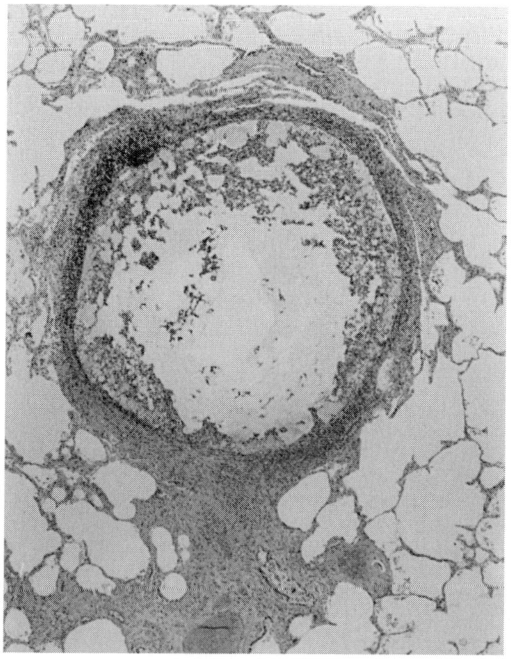

FIGURE 31–1. *Early stages of lung disease in cystic fibrosis are demonstrated in this lung specimen. Airway inflammation and bronchiectasis are present. The surrounding lung parenchyma is normal.*

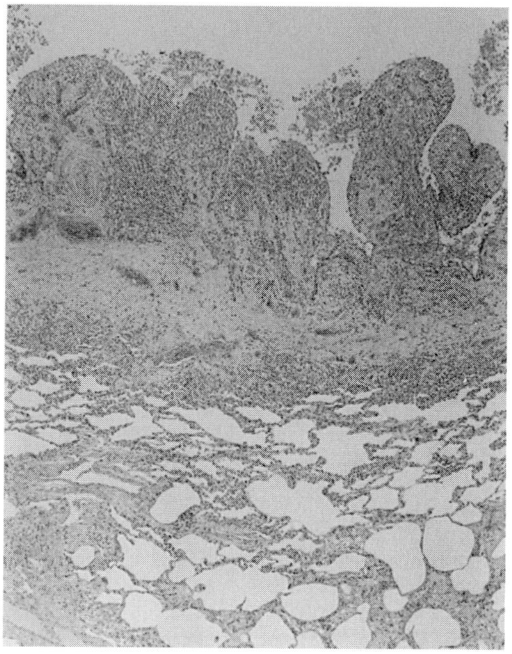

FIGURE 31–2. *Late stages of pulmonary disease are illustrated. Epithelial ulceration of the airway, loss of smooth muscle from the airway wall, inflammation, and bronchiectasis are present in the large airway at the top of the photomicrograph. Compression of the surrounding lung parenchyma occurs as bronchiectasis increases.*

DIAGNOSIS

A strong clinical suspicion is required for early recognition of CF. Most children present with a history of recurrent lower respiratory tract disease and symptoms secondary to malabsorption. Approximately 10 per cent of children will have meconium ileus at birth and/or have a family history of CF. Once the index of suspicion is raised, a quantitative pilocarpine iontophoresis sweat test[26] should be performed. Normal sweat chloride concentrations are less than 30 mEq/L, whereas the majority of individuals with CF have concentrations greater than 80 mEq/L. A sweat chloride concentration greater than 60 mEq/L is consistent with a diagnosis of CF. A minimum of 75 mg of sweat is required for accurate analysis. A positive test should be confirmed with a second sweat test on a different day. Generally, the test can be performed at any age; however, infants younger than 2 months of age frequently do not produce an adequate amount of sweat.[53] The sweat test continues to be the standard by which a diagnosis of CF is made. DNA analysis will identify approximately 70 per cent of cases as homozygous for the deletion of phenylalanine at the 508 position, with the remainder being $_{\Delta}$F508/non-$_{\Delta}$F508 or non-$_{\Delta}$F508/non-$_{\Delta}$F508. More than 450 non-$_{\Delta}$F508 mutations have been identified, but many of these have not been characterized.

PATHOGENESIS

Current knowledge of the cell biology, biochemistry, and physiology of CF is incomplete. The pathogenesis, as suggested previously, is initiated by a defect in the gene responsible for production of a transporter protein, CFTR.[50] Altered salt and water transport leads to abnormal secretions in the respiratory tract, pancreas, gastrointestinal tract, sweat glands, and other exocrine glands. In the lung, abnormal respiratory tract secretions appear to decrease mucociliary clearance and impair defenses to inhaled particulate matter and various microbial agents. These features lead to bacterial colonization and infection, inflammation, airway obstruction, and progressive lung destruction. Although the clinical features of CF are well described, the exact process by which alterations in CFTR lead to disease is unknown.

Altered chloride channel function helps to explain disease in the sweat gland, intestine, pancreas, and male genital tract. Loss of chloride from sweat can alter intestinal fluid secretion and potentially yield a dehydrated pancreatic fluid. Plugging of pancreatic ducts leads to pancreatic atrophy and loss of digestive enzymes and islet cells. The same ductular plugging and atrophy may occur in the male genital tract. Although understanding of disease pathogenesis is far from complete, better elucidation of the biology of CFTR should result in the development and institution of new therapeutic modalities.

Chronic bacterial infection of the airway is the central inciting event ultimately leading to respiratory tract impairment and death in most patients with CF. In a mouse model of CF, mucus retention and frank lung disease developed in response to recurrent bacterial infection.[14] Bacterial colonization and infection of the lower respiratory tract occur early in human infants with CF, and airway inflammation often is established already at the time the disease becomes clinically manifest.[6]

Bacterial adherence to respiratory tract epithelial cells is a necessary antecedent to infection and inflammation-induced airway damage in CF.[21, 83] Nonmucoid *Pseudomonas aeruginosa* isolates appear to adhere via pili, whereas the exopolysaccharide alginate mediates adherence of mucoid strains of the organism. Local production of cytokines and other proteins in response to bacterial infection may play an important role in modulating chronic airway inflammation.[68] Airway inflammation in CF is characterized by marked neutrophilic infiltration, with release of bioactive lipids, oxygen metabolites, myeloperoxidase, and lysozyme.[21] Proteases (e.g., elastase) derived from both neutrophils and bacteria directly damage respiratory tract epithelium and cleave proteins important in host defense.[76, 77] Chronic infection, with retention of the byproducts of inflammation, ultimately leads to the severe bronchiectatic changes and derangements of gas exchange characteristic of end-stage CF.

MICROBIOLOGY AND EPIDEMIOLOGY

Only a few etiologic agents are implicated commonly in the pulmonary infections associated with CF. Colonization of the respiratory tract with *Staphylococcus aureus* often occurs during the first 2 years of life.[27] In the preantibiotic era, 90 per cent of infection-associated deaths in patients with CF were caused by *S. aureus*. A high percentage of *S. aureus* isolates from patients receiving long-term prophylactic trimethoprim-sulfamethoxazole are thymidine-dependent.[28] These organisms grow poorly on isolation media employed commonly. In addition, mucoid colonies of *P. aeruginosa* may obscure growth of *S. aureus*, leading to an underrecognition of the true prevalence of the latter organism.

Up to 80 per cent of patients with CF develop chronic infection with *P. aeruginosa* by adolescence.[23] As infection evolves, mucoid strains of the organism predominate. The term *mucoid* describes the particular morphologic appearance of bacterial colonies on agar. Mucoidy is a result of production by the organism of large quantities of an exopolysaccharide called *alginate*.[47] Alginate synthesis by *P. aeruginosa* may be switched on by environmental stresses (e.g., high salt concentration and dehydration) in the CF patient's airway.[16] Mucoid isolates of *P. aeruginosa* appear to be more resistant to mechanical and immunologic clearance from the airway than are nonmucoid isolates. In addition, intense host immunologic responses to mucoid *P. aeruginosa* can accelerate airway injury and respiratory tract dysfunction in patients with CF.[21] Mucoid *P. aeruginosa* rarely is isolated from individuals with chronic airway diseases other than CF.

Burkholderia (*Pseudomonas*) *cepacia* has emerged as an important pathogen in CF, particularly among adolescents and young adults. Compared with colonization by *P. aeruginosa*, colonization with *B. cepacia* in CF is associated with increased morbidity and risk of early demise.[37] The so-called cepacia syndrome occurs when an adolescent or young adult with CF and relatively mild pulmonary disease becomes infected with *B. cepacia* and suffers rapid deterioration in pulmonary function, often over a period of a few months. Bacteremia also may be present. *B. cepacia*–colonized patients who undergo lung transplantation generally remain colonized and are at high risk for disseminated infection and death.[72, 74]

B. cepacia is a relatively uncommon environmental isolate.[49] Molecular epidemiologic studies suggest that the organism is transmitted person to person, either by direct physical contact or by aerosolization.[37, 43] Several studies have found an association between attendance of patients at CF summer camps and risk of *B. cepacia* colonization.[37, 57] This is in contrast to the apparently negligible risk of *P. aeruginosa* transmission in the same setting.[32] Segregation of *B. cepacia*–colonized patients is practiced in some CF centers for infection control purposes.

Selective media generally are employed for isolation of *B. cepacia* from respiratory tract secretions of patients with CF. Nevertheless, colonization is difficult to detect,[43] in part because of slow growth of the organism and overgrowth by mucoid *P. aeruginosa*.

Nontuberculous mycobacteria, especially *Mycobacterium avium-intracellulare*, can be isolated from the respiratory tract secretions of many older patients with CF.[4, 5] Recovery of these organisms sometimes is associated with exacerbation of pulmonary disease. As with *B. cepacia*, special culture techniques are required to prevent overgrowth of *P. aeruginosa* and permit isolation of nontuberculous mycobacteria.[79]

A variety of other bacteria, including *Haemophilus influenzae*, *Moraxella catarrhalis*, *Xanthomonas maltophilia*, *Alcaligenes xylosoxidans*, and Enterobacteriaceae, occasionally are isolated from the respiratory tracts of patients with CF. These organisms appear to have roles less important than those discussed earlier for *S. aureus*, *P. aeruginosa*, and *B. cepacia*. Among the fungi, *Aspergillus fumigatus* is the organism of principal interest.[27] Both allergic bronchopulmonary aspergillosis[52] and chronic necrotizing pulmonary aspergillosis[29] have been described in this population.

Bacteria play an important role in producing airway damage and altered pulmonary function, although the mechanisms by which bacteria precipitate airway disease in CF remain controversial.[7] During some pulmonary exacerbations, lack of systemic toxicity, absence of fever, and lack of an elevated white blood cell count suggest a role for nonbacterial infectious agents in initiating pulmonary disease.

A number of studies have evaluated the role of nonbacte-

TABLE 31–2. Studies Addressing the Impact of Respiratory Tract Viral Infection in Patients with Cystic Fibrosis

Authors	Number of Patients	Number of Controls	Study Duration (mo)	Age Range (yr)	Diagnostic Methods: *Serology*	Diagnostic Methods: *Cultures*	PFT Reported	Number of Culture- and Seropositive Infections in Patients	Illness per 100 Child Years	Percentage of Exacerbations Attributed to Respiratory Tract Viral Infection
Wright et al.[82]	153	0	2	1–32	+	–	–	13	47.1	39
Petersen et al.[58]	116	0	8	0.5–29	+	–	–	65	84.1	20
Wang et al.[78]	49	19	24	NR	+	+	+	105	107.1	39
Efthimiou et al.[19]	46	30	4	16–41	+	+	+	6	32.6	See text
Stroobant[75]	30	0	12	5–16	+	+	–	24	80.0	See text
Abman et al.[3]	48	0	28	0.5–5	–	+	–	21	18.8	See text
Przyklenk et al.[60]	75	0	30	4–28	+	–	–	29	15.5	78
Ong et al.[54]	36	0	12	17–32	+	+	+	12	33.3	See text
Ramsey et al.[64]	19	19	24	5–22	+	+	+	41	107.9	See text
Hordvik et al.[33]	10	0	20	5–32	+	+	+	13	78.0	See text

NR, not reported; PFT, pulmonary function tests.
From Dodge, J. A., Brock, D. J. H., and Widdicombe, J. H (eds.): Cystic Fibrosis: Current Topics. Vol. 2, New York, John Wiley & Sons, 1994, p. 219.

rial infections with pulmonary exacerbations in CF (Table 31–2). A clear correlation between respiratory tract viral infection and exacerbations of lung disease has been demonstrated in the majority of these reports.[3, 19, 33, 54, 58, 60, 64, 75, 78, 82] Most studies have focused on school age and adult CF patients. Few studies were controlled, and many failed to use active viral surveillance. Most infections were identified by a fourfold rise in antibody titer. Abman and associates,[1] assessing the effects of respiratory tract viral infections in infants with CF, found that hospitalization with respiratory syncytial virus correlated with a poor early clinical course.

Three potential mechanisms proposed for viral-induced lower airway obstruction are (1) increased thickness of the tracheobronchial wall, (2) obstruction of the airway lumen from secretions or cellular debris, and (3) altered airway smooth muscle tone.[69] Increased thickness of the airway wall can result from altered vascular permeability, inflammation, and mucosal edema. Injury to lining epithelial and mucus-secreting cells alters the consistency of mucus, affects ciliokinesis, and reduces mucociliary clearance.[10, 46] Airway smooth muscle tone is mediated by both the adrenergic and cholinergic limbs of the autonomic nervous system. There is evidence that both the afferent and efferent branches of the cholinergic reflex may be altered after viral infection, thereby increasing airway tone. Airway epithelial cells produce substances, including neutral endopeptidase and cyclooxygenase, that modulate airway hyperreactivity and smooth muscle tone. Several studies using animal models have demonstrated diminished neutral endopeptidase activity, epithelial cell damage, and greater airway responsiveness to substance P after viral infection.[18, 35, 66]

Chronic cough, pneumonia, and wheezing are early pulmonary findings in infants with CF. Two studies have reported prolonged bronchiolitis-like syndromes in infants younger than 6 months of age.[25, 45] These infants required intensive respiratory tract therapy, including bronchodilators, chest physiotherapy, and mechanical ventilation, in selected infants. Abman and associates,[2] in a prospective study, identified viral pathogens in 12 hospitalized infants with CF. Seven of the 12 isolates were respiratory syncytial virus. Infants infected with respiratory syncytial virus experienced prolonged hospitalizations, half required mechanical ventilation, and 75 per cent required supplemental oxygen at hospital discharge. When evaluated at a mean of 28 months after hospitalization, infants hospitalized with respiratory syncytial virus had developed chronic respiratory tract symptoms and worse radiograph scores. Hiatt and associates,[30, 31] assessing the effects of respiratory tract viral infection in infants with CF, found that one-half of the CF infants infected with respiratory syncytial virus required hospitalization. Although severe sequelae were not observed, pulmonary function was markedly worse after hospitalization. These studies suggest that viral respiratory tract infection, especially respiratory syncytial virus infection, has a significant detrimental impact on the early respiratory course of infants with CF.

Increased bacterial adherence to pharyngeal cells occurs during acute respiratory tract viral infections. Fainstein and associates[20] found increased adherence for *S. aureus*, *H. influenzae*, and *S. pneumoniae* after both live attenuated influenza vaccine administration and natural influenza infection. Similar findings have been reported after respiratory tract viral infection in adults with chronic bronchitis.[61, 70] *P. aeruginosa* usually does not adhere to respiratory tract epithelium unless the normal cell membrane is altered. Increased adherence of *P. aeruginosa* to epithelial cells in vitro is observed if cells first are pretreated with mild acid or trypsin or infected with influenza virus.[21] The clinical significance of these observations is not defined well. However, Johansen and Hoiby[36] reported that three-fourths of their patients developed chronic colonization with *P. aeruginosa* during the season of respiratory tract viral infection. From their observations, these investigators suggested that "respiratory [tract] viral infection paves the way for *P. aeruginosa* infection."

The interrelationship between the acquisition of *Pseudomonas* and viral respiratory tract infection remains clouded. Ong and associates[54] and Petersen and colleagues[58] reported more severe pulmonary disease with viral infection in the presence of *Pseudomonas* colonization, yet Przyklenk and coworkers[60] found no correlation. Synergism between bacteria and respiratory tract virus infection was suggested by Przyklenk and associates[60] after an increase in bacterial colony-forming units was found in the sputum of CF subjects. Hordvik and colleagues[33] and Efthimiou and associates[19] noted that CF patients with severe pulmonary disease recovered slowly from viral infection. The underlying severity of lung disease was critical in response to viral respiratory tract infection.

Malnutrition may exacerbate viral respiratory tract infection in patients with CF. Severe respiratory tract disease is reported in infants with CF and protein-calorie deficiency, compared with their well-nourished counterparts. Abman and associates[1, 2] reported that infants with CF and early hypoalbuminemia identified by newborn screening experienced higher rates of hospitalization for respiratory tract distress, a persistent need for supplemental oxygen, and chronic pulmonary symptoms. In a prospective study of infants with CF, viral lower respiratory tract infection occurred predominantly among malnourished infants.[30, 31] Both infection with respiratory syncytial virus and lower weight for height percentiles were associated with a decrease in lung function at the conclusion of the study. The incidence of viral infection in infants with CF was less than in normal controls; however, the severity of lower airway disease was dramatically worse among the CF children.

Virtually all patients with CF have radiographic evidence of sinusitis.[63] Symptomatic chronic sinusitis is common. Etiologic considerations in sinusitis and lower respiratory tract infections are similar.[67]

Infectious complications outside the respiratory tract are relatively uncommon in patients with CF. Dissemination of infection is unusual, except in the case of the cepacia syndrome. A few patients have been described with CF and brain abscess,[12, 41] probably as a consequence of sinusitis or intrapulmonic right-to-left shunting.

TREATMENT

Fundamental management of children with CF involves active bronchial clearance, control of repeated pulmonary infection, enzyme supplementation, and nutritional support. As with any chronic illness, treatment is multidisciplinary.

Antibiotics are used to control respiratory tract and serious infections. Treatment is aimed at improvement in respiratory symptoms rather than eradication of bacteria that colonize the respiratory tract. There is no consensus as to the appropriate uses of chronic and acute antibiotic therapy in CF. Continuous suppressive antibiotic therapy is employed in some centers. Other centers use antibiotics only during acute pulmonary exacerbations. Sputum culture and susceptibility test results are used to guide specific selection of antibiotics for individual subjects. The route of antibiotic administration can be oral, inhaled, or intravenous.

Despite the presence of *P. aeruginosa*, broad-spectrum oral antimicrobial therapy lacking in vitro activity against the organism often is helpful in the management of acute exacerbations of pulmonary infection. Clinical benefit may be derived from the activity of these agents against other pathogens (e.g., *S. aureus, H. influenzae*) or through a mechanism independent of bacterial killing. Prolonged courses (3 to 4 weeks) of therapy usually are prescribed. Long-term prophylactic use of oral agents also may be of benefit in some cases.

Parenteral antimicrobial therapy is indicated for clinical exacerbations that fail to respond to the use of oral agents. The goals of therapy are to reduce the burden of bacterial infection in the airway and slow infection and inflammation-associated injury to respiratory tract epithelium. Whenever possible, selection of specific therapeutic agents should be directed by the results of sputum cultures and antimicrobial susceptibility test results. Combinations of agents usually are employed to enhance antimicrobial activity in purulent respiratory tract secretions and protect against the emergence of resistant bacterial isolates. Aminoglycosides, in particular, exhibit suboptimal activity in the respiratory tract secretions of patients with CF.[48] Therapy usually includes an aminoglycoside and an antipseudomonal penicillin or cephalosporin (e.g., ceftazidime). Inclusion of an antistaphylococcal agent should be considered if *S. aureus* is suspected clinically or cultured from sputum.

Over time, with repeated courses of antimicrobial therapy, *P. aeruginosa* isolates resistant to commonly used aminoglycosides, antipseudomonal penicillins and cephalosporins, and aztreonam emerge in many patients with CF. Similarly, under pressure of therapy with quinolone antibiotics, *P. aeruginosa* may become resistant to these agents as well. As a consequence, therapeutic options frequently are limited for older patients with CF and advanced pulmonary disease.

B. cepacia inherently is resistant to aminoglycosides. Resistance to trimethoprim-sulfamethoxazole and antipseudomonal β-lactam agents frequently emerges during therapy. Some *B. cepacia* isolates are resistant to all available antimicrobial agents. Nevertheless, many patients with resistant *B. cepacia* infection respond well to treatment with antimicrobial agents to which the organism is resistant.[56]

There is enhanced clearance of most antimicrobial agents in patients with CF, necessitating the use of unusually large and frequent drug doses.[42, 73] The precise mechanisms of enhanced drug clearance are poorly understood. In the liver, both hepatic biotransformation and biliary excretion appear to be increased.[38] There is enhanced clearance of acidic drugs by the kidney.[73]

Certain antimicrobial agents, especially piperacillin and other β-lactam antibiotics, are associated with a high incidence of allergic reactions in patients with CF.[59] These reactions can limit severely options for treatment of respiratory tract infections. Useful alternatives include substitution of an agent for which there is no cross-sensitization with penicillins or cephalosporins (e.g., colistin, aztreonam) and drug desensitization.

Aerosol administration of antimicrobial agents in CF is controversial. Penicillins, cephalosporins, aminoglycosides, and colistin all have been administered by aerosolization.[22, 44, 71] One study demonstrated improved pulmonary function with aerosolized tobramycin in clinically stable CF patients.[62] The efficacy of aerosol antimicrobial therapy may be influenced by a variety of factors, including the delivery system, the physical properties of the drug, the concentration of the drug in the aerosol, particle size, and patient variables. At present, precise indications for use of aerosol antibiotics in CF are unclear.

A combined medical and surgical approach usually is indicated for the management of chronic sinusitis in CF patients.[15, 51] Other localized infections, including brain abscess, are managed similarly in patients with or without CF.

PROGNOSIS

With the current standard of care, it is anticipated that children born in the 1990s should live into the fourth or fifth decade of life. New advances in DNA technology, anti-inflammation agents, pharmocologically active compounds that alter ion transport, and gene therapy should improve further the long-term survival. The current goal of therapy is to maintain the lungs in an optimal state of health and delay the onset of deterioration in lung function for as long as possible. The future for patients born with CF should improve with the introduction of new treatments.

References

1. Abman, S. H., Reardon, M. C., Accurso, F. J., et al.: Hypoalbuminemia at diagnosis as a marker for severe respiratory course in infants with cystic fibrosis identified by newborn screening. J. Pediatr. *107*:933–935, 1985.
2. Abman, S. H., Accurso, F. J., and Sokol, R. J.: Hypoalbuminemia in young infants with cystic fibrosis. J. Pediatr. *116*:840–841, 1990.

3. Abman, S. H., Ogle, J. W., Butler, S. N., et al.: Role of respiratory syncytial virus in early hospitalizations for respiratory distress of young infants with cystic fibrosis. J. Pediatr. *113*:826–830, 1988.
4. Aitken, M. L., Burke, W., McDonald, G., et al.: Nontuberculous mycobacterial disease in adult cystic fibrosis patients. Chest *103*:1096–1099, 1993.
5. Aitken, M. L.: The role of mycobacterial infections in cystic fibrosis pulmonary disease. Pediatr. Pulmonol. *6*(Suppl.):160, 1991.
6. Armstrong, D. S., Grimwood, K., Carzino, R., et al.: Lower respiratory infection and inflammation in infants with newly diagnosed cystic fibrosis. B. M. J. *310*:1571–1572, 1995.
7. Beaudry, P. H., Marks, M. I., McDougall, D., et al.: Is anti-*Pseudomonas* therapy warranted in acute respiratory exacerbation in children with cystic fibrosis? J. Pediatr. *97*:144–147, 1980.
8. Borgo, G., Mastella, G., Gasparini, P., et al.: Pancreatic function and gene deletion F508 in cystic fibrosis. J. Med. Genet. *27*:665–669, 1990.
9. Campbell, P. W., Phillips, J. A., Krishnamani, M. R. S., et al.: Cystic fibrosis: Relationship between clinical status and F508 deletion. J. Pediatr. *118*:239–241, 1991.
10. Carson, J. L., Collier, A. M., and Hu, S. S.: Acquired ciliary defects in nasal epithelium with acute viral respiratory infections. N. Engl. J. Med. *312*:463–468, 1985.
11. Chernick, V. C., and Kendig, E. L., Jr. (eds.).: Kendig's Disorders of the Respiratory Tract in Children. 5th ed. Philadelphia, W. B. Saunders, 1990, pp. 692–730.
12. Cooper, D. M., Russell, L. E., and Henry, R. L.: Cerebral abscess as a complication of cystic fibrosis. Pediatr. Pulmonol. *17*:390–392, 1994.
13. Cutting, G. R.: Genotype defect: Its effect on cellular function and phenotypic expression. Semin. Respir. Crit. Care Med. *15*:356, 1994.
14. Davidson, D. J., Dorin, J. R., McLachlan, G., et al.: Lung disease in the cystic fibrosis mouse exposed to bacterial pathogens. Nature Genet. *9*:351–357, 1995
15. Davidson, T. M., Murphy, C., Mitchell, M., et al.: Management of chronic sinusitis in cystic fibrosis. Laryngoscope *105*:354–358, 1995.
16. Deretic, V., Schurr, M. J., Boucher, J. C., et al.: Conversion of *Pseudomonas aeruginosa* to mucoidy in cystic fibrosis: Environmental stress and regulation of bacterial virulence by alternative sigma factors. J. Bacteriol. *176*:2773–2780, 1994.
17. Di Sant'Agnese, P. A.: Fibrocystic disease of the pancreas with normal or partial pancreatic function. Pediatrics *15*:683, 1955.
17a. Dodge, J. A., Brock, D. J. H., and Widdicombe, J. H. (eds.): Cystic Fibrosis: Current Topics. Vol. 2. New York, John Wiley & Sons, 1994, p. 219.
18. Drusser, D. J., Jacoby, D. B., Djokic, T. D., et al.: Virus induces airway hyperresponsiveness to tachykinins: Role of neutral endopeptidase. J. Appl. Physiol. *67*:1504–1511, 1989.
19. Efthimiou, J., Hodson, M. E., Taylor, P., et al.: Importance of viruses and *Legionella pneumonphila* in respiratory exacerbations of young adults with cystic fibrosis. Thorax *39*:150–154, 1984.
20. Fainstein, V., Musher, D. M., and Cate, T. R.: Bacterial adherences to pharyngeal cells during viral infection. J. Infect. Dis. *141*:172–176, 1980.
21. Fick, R. B., Jr., Sonoda, F., and Hornick, D. B.: Emergence and persistence of *Pseudomonas aeruginosa* in the cystic fibrosis airway. Semin. Respir. Infect. *7*:168–178, 1992.
22. Fiel, S. B.: Aerosol delivery of antibiotics to the lower airways of patients with cystic fibrosis. Chest *107*(Suppl.):61S–64S, 1995.
23. Fitzsimmons, S. C.: The changing epidemiology of cystic fibrosis. J. Pediatr. *122*:1–9, 1993.
24. Gabriel, S. E., Clarke, L. L., Boucher, R. C., et al.: CFTR and outward rectifying chloride channels are distinct proteins with a regulatory relationship. Nature *363*:263–268, 1993.
25. Garland, J. S., Chan, Y. M., Kelly, K. J., et al.: Outcome of infants with cystic fibrosis requiring mechanical ventilation for respiratory failure. Chest *96*:136–138, 1989.
26. Gibson, L. E., and Cooke, R. E.: A test for concentration of electrolytes in sweat in cystic fibrosis of the pancreas utilizing pilocarpine by iontophoresis. Pediatrics *23*:545, 1959.
27. Gilligan, P. H., Cage, P. A., Welch, D. F., et al.: Prevalence of thymidine-dependent *Staphylococcus aureus* in patients with cystic fibrosis. J. Clin. Microbiol. *25*:1258–1261, 1987.
28. Gilligan, P. H.: Microbiology of airway disease in patients with cystic fibrosis. Clin. Microbiol. Rev. *4*:35–51, 1991.
29. Grahame-Clarke, C. N., Roberts, C. M., and Empey, D. W.: Chronic necrotizing pulmonary aspergillosis and pulmonary phycomycosis in cystic fibrosis Respir. Med. *88*:465–468, 1994.
30. Hiatt, P. W., Piedra, P., Raboudi, S., et al.: Respiratory viral infection in infants with cystic fibrosis. Am. Rev. Respir. Dis. *147*:A464, 1993.
31. Hiatt, P. W., Taber, L., Raboud, S., et al.: Respiratory viral infection and pulmonary function in infants with cystic fibrosis. Am. Rev. Respir. Dis. *145*:A115, 1992.
32. Hoogkamp-Korstanje, J. A., Meis, J. F., Kissing, J., et al.: Risk of cross-colonization and infection by *Pseudomonas aeruginosa* in a holiday camp for cystic fibrosis patients. J. Clin. Microbiol. 33:572–575, 1995.
33. Hordvik, N. L., Konig, P., Hamory, B., et al.: Effects of acute viral respiratory tract infections in patients with cystic fibrosis. Pediatr. Pulmonol. *7*:217–222, 1989.
34. Hyde, S. C., Emsley, P., Hartshorn, M. J., et al.: Structural model of ATP-binding proteins associated with cystic fibrosis, multi-drug resistance and bacterial support. Nature *346*:362–265, 1990.
35. Jacoby, D. B., Tamaoki, J., Borson, D. B., et al.: Influenza infection causes airway hyperresponsiveness by decreasing enkephalinase. J. Appl. Physiol. *64*:2653–2658, 1988.
36. Johansen, H. K., and Hoiby, N: Seasonal onset of initial colonisation and chronic infection with *Pseudomonas aeruginosa* in patients with cystic fibrosis in Denmark. Thorax *47*:109–111, 1992.
37. John, M., Ecclestone, E., Hunter, E., et al.: Epidemiology of *Pseudomonas cepacia* colonization among patients with cystic fibrosis. Pediatr. Pulmonol. *18*:108–113, 1994.
38. Kearns, G. L.: Hepatic drug metabolism in cystic fibrosis: Recent developments and future directions. Ann. Pharmacother. *27*:74–79, 1993.
39. Kerem, E., Corey, M., Kerem, B., et al.: Clinical and genetic comparisons of patients with cystic fibrosis with and without meconium ileus. J. Pediatr. *114*:767–773, 1989.
40. Kerem, E., Corey, M., Kerem, B.-S., et al.: The relationship between genotype and phenotype in cystic fibrosis: Analysis of the most common mutation (F508). N. Engl. J. Med. *323*:1517–1522, 1990.
41. Kline, M. W.: Brain abscess in a patient with cystic fibrosis. Pediatr. Infect. Dis. *4*:72–73, 1985.
42. Lindsay, C. A., and Bosso, J. A.: Optimization of antibiotic therapy in cystic fibrosis patients: Pharmacokinetic considerations. Clin. Pharmacokinet. *24*:496–506, 1993.
43. LiPuma, J. J., Marks-Austin, K. A., Holsclaw, D. S., Jr., et al.: Inapparent transmission of *Pseudomonas* (*Burkholderia*) *cepacia* among patients with cystic fibrosis. Pediatr. Infect. Dis. J. *13*:716–719, 1994.
44. Littlewood, J. M., Smye, S. W., and Cunliffe, H.: Aerosol antibiotic treatment in cystic fibrosis. Arch. Dis. Child. *68*:788–792, 1993.
45. Lloyd-Still, J. D., Kahw, K. T., and Shwachman, H.: Severe respiratory disease in infants with cystic fibrosis. Pediatrics *53*:678–682, 1974.
46. Lourenco, R. V., Stanley, E. D., Gatmaitan, B., et al.: Abnormal deposition and clearance of inhaled particles during upper respiratory viral infections. J. Clin. Invest. *50*:62A, 1971.
47. May, T. B., Shinabarger, D., Maharaj, R., et al.: Alginate synthesis by *Pseudomonas aeruginosa*: A key pathogenic factor in chronic pulmonary infections of cystic fibrosis patients. Clin. Microbiol. Rev. *4*:191–206, 1991.
48. Mendelman, P. M., Smith, A. L., Levy, J., et al.: Aminoglycoside penetration, inactivation, and efficacy in cystic fibrosis sputum. Am. Rev. Respir. Dis. *132*:761–765, 1985.
49. Mortensen, J. E., Fisher, M. C., and LiPuma, J. J.: Recovery of *Pseudomonas cepacia* and other *Pseudomonas* species from the environment. Infect. Control Hosp. Epidemiol. *16*:30–32, 1995.
50. Moss, R. B., and King, V. V.: Management of sinusitis in cystic fibrosis by endoscopic surgery and serial antimicrobial lavage: Reduction in recurrence requiring surgery. Arch. Otolaryngol. *121*:566–572, 1995.
51. Moss, R. B.: Cystic fibrosis: Pathogenesis, pulmonary infection, and treatment. Clin. Infect. Dis. *21*:839, 1995.
52. Mroueh, S., and Spock, A.: Allergic bronchopulmonary aspergillosis in patients with cystic fibrosis. Chest *105*:32–36, 1994.
53. Murphy, T. M., and Rosenstein, B. J.: Cystic Fibrosis Lung Disease: Approaching the 21st Century. University of Chicago, Pritzker School of Medicine. Published by Gardiner-Caldwell SynerMed, 1995.
54. Ong, E. L., Ellis, M. E., Webb, A. K., et al.: Infective respiratory exacerbations in young adults with cystic fibrosis: Role of viruses and atypical microorganisms. Thorax *44*:739–742, 1989.
55. Parks, R. W., and Grand, R. J.: Gastrointestinal manifestations of cystic fibrosis: A review. Gastroenterology *81*:1143–1161, 1981.
56. Peckham, D., Crouch, S., Humphreys, H., et al.: Effect of antibiotic treatment on inflammatory markers and lung function in cystic fibrosis patients with *Pseudomonas cepacia*. Thorax *49*:803–807, 1994.
57. Pegues, D. A., Carson, L. A., Tablan, O. C., et al.: Acquisition of *Pseudomonas cepacia* at summer camps for patients with cystic fibrosis: Summer camp study group. J. Pediatr. *124*:694–702, 1994.
58. Petersen, N. T., Hoiby, N., Mordhorst, C.H., et al.: Respiratory infections in cystic fibrosis patients caused by virus, *Chlamydia* and *Mycoplasma*: Possible synergism with *Pseudomonas aeruginosa*. Acta Paediatr. Scand. *70*:623–628, 1981.
59. Pleasants, R. A., Walker, T. R., and Samuelson, W. M.: Allergic reactions to parenteral beta-lactam antibiotics in patients with cystic fibrosis. Chest *106*:1124–1128, 1994.
60. Przyklenk, B., Bauernfeind, A., Bertele, R. M., et al.: Viral infections of the respiratory tract in patients with cystic fibrosis. Serodiagn. Immunother. Infect. Dis. *2*:217, 1988.
61. Ramirez-Ronda, C. H., Fuxench-Lopez, Z., and Nevarez, M.: Increased pharyngeal bacterial colonization during viral illness. Arch. Intern. Med. *141*:1599–1603, 1981.
62. Ramsey, B., and Richardson, M. A.: Impact of sinusitis in cystic fibrosis. J. Allergy Clin. Immunol. *90*:547–552, 1992.
63. Ramsey, B. W., Dorkin, H. L., Eisenberg, J. D., et al.: Efficacy of aerosolized tobramycin in patients with cystic fibrosis. N. Engl. J. Med. *328*:1740–1746, 1993.
64. Ramsey, B. W., Gore, E. J., Smith, A. L., et al.: The effect of respiratory viral infections on patients with cystic fibrosis. Am. J. Dis. Child. *143*:662–668, 1989.

65. Riordan, J. R., Rommens, J. M., Kerem, B. S., et al.: Identification of the cystic fibrosis gene: Cloning and characterization of the complementary DNA. Science *245*:1066–1073, 1989.
66. Saban, R., Dick, E. C., Fishleder, R. I., et al.: Enhancement by parainfluenza 3 infection of contractile responses to substance P and capsaicin in airway smooth muscle from the guinea pig. Am. Rev. Respir. Dis. *136*:586–591, 1987.
67. Shapiro, E. D., Milmoe, G. J., Wald, E. R., et al.: Bacteriology of the maxillary sinuses in patients with cystic fibrosis. J. Infect. Dis. *146*:589–593, 1982.
68. Shelhamer, J. H., Levine, S. J., Wu, T., et al.: NIH conference: Airway inflammation. Ann. Intern. Med. *123*:288–304, 1995.
69. Smith, A. L., and Ramsey, B.: Aerosol administration of antibiotics. Respiration *62*(Suppl. 1):19–24, 1995.
70. Smith, C. B., Golden, C., Kaluber, M. R., et al.: Interactions between viruses and bacteria in patients with chronic bronchitis. J. Infect. Dis. *134*:552–561, 1976.
71. Smith, J. J., Leme, R. J., and Taussig, L. M.: Mechanisms of viral-induced lower airway obstruction. Pediatr. Infect. Dis. *6*:837–842, 1987.
72. Snell, G. I., de Hoyos, A., Krajden, M., et al.: *Pseudomonas cepacia* in lung transplant recipients with cystic fibrosis. Chest *103*:466–71, 1993.
73. Spino, M.: Pharmacokinetics of drugs in cystic fibrosis. Clin. Rev. Allergy Immunol. 9:169–210, 1991.
74. Steinbach, S., Sun, L., Jiang, R. Z., et al.: Transmissibility of *Pseudomonas cepacia* infection in clinic patients and lung-transplant recipients with cystic fibrosis. N. Engl. J. Med. *331*:981–987, 1994.
75. Stroobant, J.: Viral infection in cystic fibrosis. J. R. Soc. Med. *79*:19–22, 1986.
76. Suter, S.: The role of bacterial proteases in the pathogenesis of cystic fibrosis. Am. J. Respir. Crit. Care Med. *150*:S118–S122, 1994.
77. Tosi, M. F., Zakem, H., and Berger, M.: Neutrophil elastase cleaves C3bi on opsonized *Pseudomonas* as well as CR1 on neutrophils to create a functionally important opsonin receptor mismatch. J. Clin. Invest. *86*:300–308, 1990.
78. Wang, E. E., Prober, C. G., Manson, B., et al.: Association of respiratory viral infections with pulmonary deterioration in patients with cystic fibrosis. N. Engl. J. Med. *311*:1653–1658, 1984.
79. Whittier, S., Hopfer, R. L., Knowles, M. R., et al.: Improved recovery of mycobacteria from respiratory secretions of patients with cystic fibrosis. J. Clin. Microbiol. *31*:861–864, 1993.
80. Wood, R. E., Board, T. F., and Doershuk, C. F.: Cystic fibrosis. Am. Rev. Respir. Dis. *113*:841, 1976.
81. Wood. R. E., Boat, T. F., and Doershuk C. F.: State of the art: Cystic fibrosis. Am. Rev. Respir. Dis. *113*:833–878, 1976.
82. Wright, P. F., Khaw, K. T., Oxman, M. N., et al.: Evaluation of the safety of amantadine-HCl and the role of respiratory viral infections in children with cystic fibrosis. J. Infect. Dis. *134*:144–149, 1976.
83. Zar, H., Saiman, L., Quittell, L., et al.: Binding of *Pseudomonas aeruginosa* to respiratory epithelial cells from patients with various mutations in the cystic fibrosis transmembrane regulator. J. Pediatr. *126*:230–233, 1995.

SECTION THREE

INFECTIONS OF THE HEART

32

INFECTIVE ENDOCARDITIS

Jeffrey R. Starke

Infective endocarditis results when microorganisms adhere to the endocardial surface of the heart. This process usually occurs on heart valves, although septal defects and mural surfaces can be affected. Most episodes of endocarditis begin on endocardium that has been altered by congenital defects, previous disease, surgery, or trauma. The clinical manifestations depend on the degree of compromise of cardiac function and the occurrence of embolic phenomena. Although bacteria are responsible for most cases, instances of infective endocarditis caused by fungi, chlamydiae, rickettsiae, and, perhaps, viruses have been described. Advances in the practice of general pediatrics and cardiology over the past three decades have contributed to changes in the predisposing conditions and etiologic agents of "modern" infective endocarditis. Prior to the 1950s, rheumatic fever was the major underlying condition, but its incidence has declined greatly since then.[243] Concurrently, improvements in the medical and surgical management of children with congenital heart disease have increased survival rates. At present, approximately 80 to 90 per cent of children with infective endocarditis have congenital heart disease.[15, 60, 211, 277, 334, 367, 412] Many cases follow cardiac surgery, especially that for replacement of valves and creation of shunts with prosthetic materials. The reported incidence of infective endocarditis in neonates is increasing, probably owing to use of sophisticated and highly invasive techniques in neonatal intensive care nurseries.[75, 259, 317]

Historically, infective endocarditis has been classified as acute or subacute, based on the progression of untreated disease.[349] The acute form has a fulminant course with high fever, systemic toxicity, and death from sepsis in several days to 6 weeks. The most common etiologic agents are *Staphylococcus aureus*, *Streptococcus pyogenes*, and *Streptococcus pneumoniae*. Children with the acute form often have no underlying cardiac lesion. Subacute disease usually occurs in patients with prior valvular disease or cardiac surgical intervention. It is characterized by a more indolent course (6 weeks to several months) with low-grade fever, vague systemic complaints, and various embolic phenomena. Viridans streptococci are the most common etiologic agents. This classification ignores the frequent overlap in clinical manifestations caused by various organisms,[349] especially the staphylococci and fungi, which are the cause of an increasing number of subacute cases in the postcardiac surgical setting. Classification based on specific etiologic agent is preferable because it has implications for the usual clinical course, predisposing factors, and appropriate medical and surgical management.

EPIDEMIOLOGY

The incidence of infective endocarditis in adults has been difficult to determine because the methods of study and criteria for diagnosis vary among series.[99, 414, 419] Accurate figures on the incidence of infective endocarditis in children are difficult to obtain. The most common method of reporting incidence in the pediatric series expresses the number of cases of infective endocarditis as the numerator and the total number of hospital admissions during the analyzed period of time as the denominator. Zakrzewski and Keith[437] reported an incidence of endocarditis of 1 in 4500 pediatric admissions at the Hospital for Sick Children in Toronto from 1952 to 1962, whereas Van Hare and colleagues[412] at Case Western Reserve found an incidence of 1 in 1280 in the period from 1972 to 1982. In a large series from Boston Children's Hospital spanning the period between 1933 and 1972, the incidence before 1963 was 1 in 4500 pediatric admissions, whereas that for 1963 to 1972 was 1 in 1800 admissions.[181] A study from a children's hospital in Australia reported an incidence of 1 in 4500 hospital admissions between 1971 and 1983.[360] More recently, one Japanese center reported an annual incidence of 0.9 cases per 1000 children seen at the cardiology clinic.[174] Although differences in referral patterns at these centers may have introduced bias into these figures, it appears that the incidence of infective endocarditis in children is rising. This might be explained by the increased survival of children with all forms of cardiovascular disease and the increase in the percentage of cases following cardiac surgery and related to intravascular catheters.[117, 189, 334] Early surgical correction of many types of congenital heart disease using effective perioperative antibiotic prophylaxis regimens ultimately may lower the incidence of postoperative infective endocarditis. However, the increasing use of invasive therapeutic modalities, especially intravenous catheters and pacemakers, may lead to an increased incidence of so-called nosocomial endocarditis.[117, 247]

The average age of children with infective endocarditis is increasing, a phenomenon that may reflect the longer life expectancy created by improved therapy for children at risk. From 1930 to 1950, the mean age for children with infective endocarditis was close to 5 years.[181] Between 1960 and the present, it has increased to 8.5 and then to 13 years.[124, 133, 181, 211, 334, 367] The number of reports of infective endocarditis in children younger than 2 years of age had been small but has increased significantly over the past decade.[29, 133, 259] The clinical course of infective endocarditis in these young children often is atypical, and some cases are diagnosed at autopsy.[180] Before the 1950s, this disease was rare in neonates, with only eight autopsy cases reported.[235] Several reports suggest a rapidly increasing rate associated with the development of intensive supportive care in neonates.[35, 75, 101, 252, 259, 264, 289, 290, 317] Symchych and colleagues[386] found a 3 per cent incidence of bacterial endocarditis among all neonatal autopsies. Endocarditis in neonates frequently occurs on the tricuspid valve when associated with an indwelling central venous catheter.[399] Congenital heart defects also predispose neonates to infectious endocarditis.[75]

Any form of structural cardiac disease may predispose to infective endocarditis, especially when turbulence of blood flow occurs.[370] In autopsy and clinical series, children with ventricular septal defect, tetralogy of Fallot, left-sided valvular disease, and systemic-pulmonary arterial communications were at highest risk, whereas those with pulmonary stenosis, coarctation of the aorta, and secundum atrial septal defect were at low risk.[47, 132, 328, 334] Hypertrophic obstructive cardiomyopathy rarely is associated with infective endocarditis.[62] Isolated pulmonic or tricuspid valve endocarditis can occur in "otherwise normal" children and adolescents with sepsis or focal bacterial infection[278] but usually is associated with congenital heart disease, intravenous catheters, or intravenous drug abuse.[55, 275] Bicuspid aortic valve is recognized as an important risk factor for infective endocarditis, especially in elderly men.[253] The underlying heart diseases in 266 pediatric cases of infective endocarditis are listed in Table 32–1.[189] A cooperative study on the Natural History of Aortic Stenosis, Pulmonary Stenosis and Ventricular Septal Defect has reported data from a controlled pediatric population collected over a period of 4 to 15 years.[130] In patients not undergoing surgical correction, the risk of acquiring endocarditis by age 30 years in those with ventricular septal defect was 9.7 per cent, compared with 1.4 per cent for aortic stenosis and 0.9 per cent for pulmonic stenosis. Aortic valvotomy in children with aortic stenosis actually increases the relative risk, whereas successful repair of ventricular septal defect significantly decreases the long-term susceptibility to infective endocarditis.[131] Similarly, endocarditis is extremely rare after ligation of patent ductus arteriosis. At present, palliative systemic-to-pulmonary shunting is the surgical procedure most often complicated by infective endocarditis.[334] In a review of 115 patients with tetralogy of Fallot, Kaplan and colleagues[191] reported an 8 per cent incidence of infective endocarditis after placement of a Pott shunt.

The increasing use of prosthetic valves and valved conduit repairs in children with complex heart disease may lead to a larger number of cases of infective endocarditis in the future.[190, 196, 367] Most medical centers report an incidence of prosthetic valve endocarditis of 2 to 4 per cent after surgery.[45, 134, 331, 370] Aortic and mitral valves most frequently are affected.[169, 237] Older studies arbitrarily divided prosthetic valve endocarditis into two categories—early and late—based on whether the infection occurred within 60 days of valve placement or later.[22] The rationale for time categorization was because of apparent differences in bacteriologic, pathogenetic, and prognostic associations. So-called early cases most often were caused by coagulase-negative staphylococci, gram-negative bacilli, and fungi, whereas oral and enterococcal streptococci, along with staphylococci, predominated in the late cases.[193] These older reports suggested that early cases were acquired via intraoperative valve contamination or secondary to postoperative extracardiac infections, whereas late cases were acquired by the same mechanisms as native valve endocarditis. Nosocomial bacteremia at any time after valve placement is a significant risk factor for endocarditis.[108] Finally, the mortality rate was thought to be higher in early versus late infection. However, more recent studies have blurred this arbitrary time distinction between early and late prosthetic valve endocarditis.[45, 169, 331] The risk probably is highest in the first 6 to 12 months and decreases to its lowest beyond 1 year after valve replacement. Coagulase-negative staphylococci are the dominant organisms both before and after the sixtieth postoperative day.[45, 195] Clinical and epidemiologic data also suggest that prosthetic valve infection caused by staphylococci occurring within the first year after placement probably is acquired at the time of surgery.[22] Identified risk factors for developing prosthetic valve endocarditis in adults include native valve endocarditis, black race, male sex, mechanical (versus biologic) prosthesis, and prolonged cardiopulmonary bypass time[169]; no comparable information is available for children.

Mitral valve endocarditis occurs frequently on an anatomically normal valve in patients with other predisposing factors.[118] An association between mitral valve prolapse and infective endocarditis has been recognized in adults and children. This heart lesion is being detected with increasing frequency in adolescent girls and may be only one component of a developmental syndrome.[354] In adults, 40 to 50 per cent of cases of infective endocarditis associated with isolated insufficient mitral valves occur in patients with mitral prolapse.[71] In some series of native valve endocarditis, mitral valve prolapse has been the most common underlying lesion.[253] The reported incidence of infective endocarditis in patients with mitral valve prolapse has varied markedly among studies, from low rates of 14 per 100,000 per year to 5 of 58 patients followed prospectively over 9 to 22 years.[159, 176] A retrospective epidemiologic analysis using matched case controls yielded an odds ratio of 8.2, indicating a substantially higher risk of endocarditis in patients with mitral valve prolapse than in normal controls.[66] It has become apparent that the risk of infective endocarditis is not uniform for all patients with mitral valve prolapse. The risk is increased in patients with a preexisting systolic murmur (but not for patients with an isolated click without a murmur), regurgitation by echocardiography, and valvular redundancy.[77, 159, 236, 245] The signs and symptoms of endocarditis associated with mitral valve prolapse may be more subtle when compared with those of other types of left-sided endocarditis.[118, 286] However, significant complications are relatively common, sometimes requiring valve replacement during the acute illness or during convalescence.[10]

Fungal endocarditis is a rare disorder in children but should be suspected in certain clinical and epidemiologic settings. It is more likely after cardiac surgery and rarely occurs on native heart valves. It is more common in neonates being cared for in intensive care settings than in older children.[75] Other predisposing factors include (1) the presence of an indwelling vascular catheter, (2) prolonged use of antibiotics, (3) intrinsic (immunodeficiency diseases, malignancy, malnutrition) or extrinsic (corticosteroids, cytotoxic drugs) immunosuppression, (4) bowel surgery resulting in transient fungemia, (5) intravenous drug abuse, and (6) preexisting or concomitant bacterial endocarditis.

Many conditions other than structural heart disease predis-

TABLE 32–1. Underlying Heart Disease in 266 Children with Infective Endocarditis

Congenital heart disease		78%
Tetralogy of Fallot	24%	
Ventricular septal defect	16%	
Congenital aortic stenosis	8%	
Patent ductus arteriosus	7%	
Transposition of the great vessels	4%	
Others	19%	
Rheumatic heart disease		14%
No heart disease		8%

From Kaplan, E. L.: Infective endocarditis in the pediatric age group: An overview. *In* Kaplan, E. L., and Taranta, A. V. (eds.): Infective Endocarditis: An American Heart Association Symposium. Dallas, American Heart Association, 1977, pp. 51–54.

pose children to infective endocarditis. The most important is the presence of an indwelling central venous catheter, especially in patients who are seriously ill or immunocompromised.[133, 225, 402, 425] The catheter acts as a foreign body and presumably causes microscopic damage by abrading endocardial and valve surfaces, resulting in a nonbacterial thrombotic vegetation.[15] Intracardiac pacemaker wires may become infected, leading to endocarditis.[8] The most common sources of organisms are infection acquired during the placement procedure and infection of the pacemaker pouch. Children with ventriculoatrial shunts placed for treatment of hydrocephalus have developed infective endocarditis, usually of the tricuspid valve.[189] In patients with arteriovenous fistulas created for hemodialysis, bacterial vegetations may develop in the fistula and on heart valves.[219, 320] Rarely, penetrating wounds or foreign bodies can initiate endocarditis.[244] One important group of patients with an increased risk for infective endocarditis is intravenous drug abusers.[249] In this group of patients, two-thirds have no evidence of underlying heart disease. There is a predilection for involvement of the tricuspid valve, followed by the mitral valve and aortic valve. Roentgenographic evidence of septic pulmonary emboli and signs of tricuspid insufficiency dominate the clinical presentation.[349] Within this group of patients, increased rates of infective endocarditis and mortality are associated with infection by the human immunodeficiency virus, particularly as CD4 cell counts fall below 200/mm^3.[313]

Although the incidence of infective endocarditis in children may be rising, the prognosis has improved dramatically over the past several decades. Current mortality rates usually are close to 10 per cent.[268, 334, 353, 360] Most survivors remain hemodynamically stable at long-term follow-up.[120, 353] However, patients who experience infective endocarditis appear to be at higher risk of recurrent endocarditis than are patients with similar cardiac abnormalities who have not had prior endocarditis.[370] The patient's functional class prior to treatment appears to be most predictive of long-term functional status. In one study, 22 per cent of children surviving infective endocarditis required surgery related to the infection, including vegetectomy, evacuation of a hematoma, atrioventricular valve replacement, and placement or replacement of a graft or intracardiac shunt.[334]

PATHOPHYSIOLOGY

Clinical observations, autopsy studies, and work with experimental animal models have demonstrated that the occurrence of several independent events is required for the development of subacute infectious endocarditis. The endocardial surface usually is disrupted by stress or injury commonly caused by turbulence of blood. This surface damage results in deposition of fibrin and platelets, which form nonbacterial thrombotic vegetations. If bacteria adhere to these deposits, infective endocarditis results. The surface of the infected vegetation becomes protected by a cover of fibrin and platelets. A tremendous proliferation of organisms may ensue (up to 10^9 colony-forming units/g).[95] The protective sheath isolates the organisms from the action of host neutrophils and antibiotics. The clinical manifestations and complications of infective endocarditis are related to both the hemodynamic changes caused by local infection and the occurrence of embolization and metastatic infection.

In experimental animals, the valvular surface must be damaged, usually by an intravenous catheter, to produce infective endocarditis.[11] The first step in the pathogenesis of subacute infective endocarditis in humans is development of hemodynamic factors that favor endocardial damage. In an autopsy study of 1024 patients with infective endocarditis, Lepeschkin[220] showed that the location of the endocardial lesions correlates with the impact of pressure, making a strong argument for the role of mechanical stress as a critical factor in the evolution of the lesions. When associated with valvular insufficiency, infective endocarditis usually occurs on the atrial surface of the mitral valve and the ventricular surface of the aortic valve. Injection of a bacterial aerosol into the air stream passing through a Venturi tube demonstrates how high pressure drives an infected fluid into a low-pressure sink.[326] This establishes a maximal deposition of bacteria in the low-pressure sink immediately beyond the orifice. Mitral insufficiency creates a Venturi effect when blood is driven from the high-pressure left ventricle into a low-pressure atrium; maximal deposition occurs around the mitral annulus on the atrial side. Similarly, with aortic valve insufficiency, the high-pressure source is the aorta and the low-pressure sink is the left ventricle, which leads to deposition on the ventricular surface of the valve. Lesions also are created more directly by a jet stream causing endocardial damage. For example, in a small, restrictive ventricular septal defect with a left-to-right shunt, a Venturi effect leads to development of lesions on the right ventricular septal side of the defect, whereas secondary lesions created by the jet effect are located on the right ventricular wall opposite the defect.[421] Heart defects with a surface area large enough to prevent a significant pressure gradient and those in which smaller volumes minimize the gradient do not create the jet and Venturi effects. This helps explain the rarity of endocarditis in atrial septal defects and the increased risk of infection complicating small but not large ventricular septal defects.

Once endocardial damage has occurred, collagen is exposed, and platelet and fibrin deposition ensues in a manner analogous to the formation of the primary plug of normal hemostasis after vascular injury.[178, 422] The subsequent sterile platelet-fibrin thrombus formed is referred to as a nonbacterial thrombotic vegetation. In experimental animals, many exogenous stresses lead to the formation of this lesion, including exposure to cold, high altitude, high cardiac output states, hormonal manipulations, and passage of a sterile catheter across a heart valve.[338] Formation of the vegetation reflects two pathogenic mechanisms: hypercoagulability and endothelial damage.[349] It nearly is impossible to establish experimental infective endocarditis without initial formation of the vegetation. Microscopic examination demonstrates that it is this lesion to which microorganisms attach during the early stages of experimental endocarditis. Nonbacterial thrombotic vegetations have been found in both adults and children with malignancy, chronic wasting diseases, uremia, connective tissue diseases, and congenital heart disease and after the placement of intracardiac catheters[229, 293] and have been associated with embolism and infarction in distant organs.[32]

Once a nonbacterial thrombotic vegetation has been established, transient bacteremia or fungemia may result in colonization of the lesion. Transient bacteremias are common, especially with traumatization of a mucosal surface. Table 32–2 lists the incidence of bacteremia in adults and children after various procedures.[107, 324] The bacteremia usually is of low grade and is proportional to the amount of trauma produced by the procedure and to the number of organisms inhabiting the surface. In addition, "silent" bacteremia probably occurs frequently. Many persons have circulating antibodies to their own oral flora as well as an increase in peripheral T cells sensitized to the flora of their dental plaque.[349]

The ability of microorganisms to adhere to the platelet-fibrin thrombus is a critical factor in the development of infective endocarditis.[148, 178] In a canine model, *S. aureus* and

TABLE 32–2. Bacteremia with Various Procedures in Adults and Children

Initiating Event	Percentage of Positive Blood Cultures	Predominant Organisms
Dental extraction (children)	30–65	*Streptococcus,* diphtheroids
Chewing gum, candy, paraffin	0–51	*Streptococcus, Staphylococcus epidermidis*
Tooth brushing	0–26	*Streptococcus*
Tonsillectomy	28–38	*Streptococcus, Haemophilus,* diphtheroids
Bronchoscopy (rigid scope)	15	*Streptococcus, Staphylococcus epidermidis*
Bronchoscopy (fiberoptic)	0	
Orotracheal intubation	0	
Nasotracheal intubation/ suctioning	16	*Streptococcus,* aerobic gram-negative rods
Sigmoidoscopy/colonoscopy	0–9.5	*Enterococcus,* aerobic gram-negative rods
Upper gastrointestinal endoscopy	8–12	*Streptococcus, Neisseria, Staphylococcus epidermidis,* diphtheroids, other
Percutaneous liver biopsy	3–14	Pneumococcus, aerobic gram-negative rods, *Staphylococcus aureus,* other
Urethral catheterization	8	Not stated
Manipulation of *Staphylococcus aureus* suppurative foci	54	

From Everett, E. D., and Hirschmann, J. U.: Transient bacteremia and endocarditis prophylaxis: A review. Medicine *56*:61–77, 1977.

the viridans streptococci, which frequently cause infective endocarditis, adhere more readily to normal aortic leaflets than do organisms uncommon in endocarditis.[141] Within isolates of *S. aureus*, strains devoid of microencapsulation are less capable of inducing endocarditis in an experimental model than are encapsulated strains.[14] Specific products, including dextran, mannan, teichoic acid, and slime, released by these organisms may enhance their ability to colonize the vegetation.[178, 204] The adherence of oral streptococci depends on the production of a complex extracellular polysaccharide: dextran. The amount of dextran produced by various viridans streptococci in broth correlates with both their adherence and their ability to produce endocarditis in the rabbit model.[346] *Candida albicans* readily is adherent and produces infective endocarditis in rabbits more easily than does *Candida krusei*, a nonadherent yeast rarely implicated in human infective endocarditis.[347] In addition, endocarditis-producing strains of streptococci and staphylococci are more potent stimulators of platelet aggregation than are other bacteria that do not produce infective endocarditis.[65, 157] This action may accelerate formation of an infected vegetation or increase removal of organisms from the circulation. The importance of adherence by organisms has been studied using preincubation of organisms with many classes of antibiotics. After incubation at subinhibitory concentrations, there is a decrease in the adhesion of streptococcal species to fibrin-platelet matrices and damaged canine valves.[351] Antibiotics may prevent infective endocarditis by both bacterial killing and inhibition of adherence to the vegetation.[137]

Host tissue factors undoubtedly play an important role in adherence of bacteria to the developing thrombus. Once bacteria become adherent to the nonbacterial thrombus, activation of the coagulation system ensues. Some organisms that produce endocarditis may be able to initiate procoagulant activity via microbial enzymes.[155] Activation of the intrinsic coagulation pathway is triggered by exposed connective tissue components and platelet aggregation.[204] However, activation of the extrinsic coagulation pathway probably is the major stimulus for growth of vegetations. Elements of the extracellular matrix, including fibronectin, laminin, and collagen, have been shown to facilitate the adherence of bacteria on fibrin-platelet matrices.[383, 401] Fibronectin may be the host receptor for organisms within the nonbacterial thrombotic vegetation.[212, 231] Laminin-binding proteins have been found on the cell walls of organisms recovered from patients with endocarditis.[365]

The platelet-organism interaction is complex and not understood completely. *Streptococcus sanguis* produces two cell-surface antigens that promote platelet aggregation: a class I antigen promotes adhesion of *S. sanguis* to platelets, while coexpression of a class II antigen promotes platelet adhesion or aggregation.[158] The induced platelet aggregation appears to be an important determinant of further vegetation development and disease progression in experimental endocarditis. In addition, streptococcal exopolysaccharide production inversely correlates with platelet adhesion while inhibiting aggregation, indicating that surface molecules may enhance endocarditis at only certain pathogenic steps.[380] Platelets also may be involved with host defense within the vegetation. After exposure to thrombin, platelets may release microbicidal proteins with bactericidal activity against some gram-positive cocci; resistance to these proteins may be a virulence factor for *S. aureus* in the development of endocarditis.[284, 435]

As bacterial colonization of a nonbacterial thrombotic vegetation progresses, it enlarges by further bacterial proliferation and platelet-fibrin deposition (Fig. 32–1). Kissane[209] describes three histologic zones: (1) necrotic endocardium; (2) a broad zone of bacterial colonies, pyknotic nuclear debris, and fibrin; and (3) a thin coating on the surface of fibrin and leukocytes. The location of the bacterial colonies below the surface and the minimal infiltration by phagocytic cells create an environment of impaired host resistance resulting in extreme bacterial proliferation. The structure of the vegetation diminishes penetration of antibiotics into the bacterial layer. In addition, the metabolic activity of bacteria within this lesion is slowed, rendering antibiotics less effective. The formation of vegetations and erosion of heart valves may cause valvular incompetence, resulting in cardiac failure.

Immunopathologic factors may have important roles in both the development and sequelae of infective endocarditis.[23] The susceptibility of a gram-negative bacillus to complement-mediated bactericidal activity is critical to its potential to create endocarditis; only "serum-resistant" organisms produce infective endocarditis in humans and experimental animals.[94] Gram-positive cocci are a more frequent cause of infective endocarditis than gram-negative bacilli. Gram-posi-

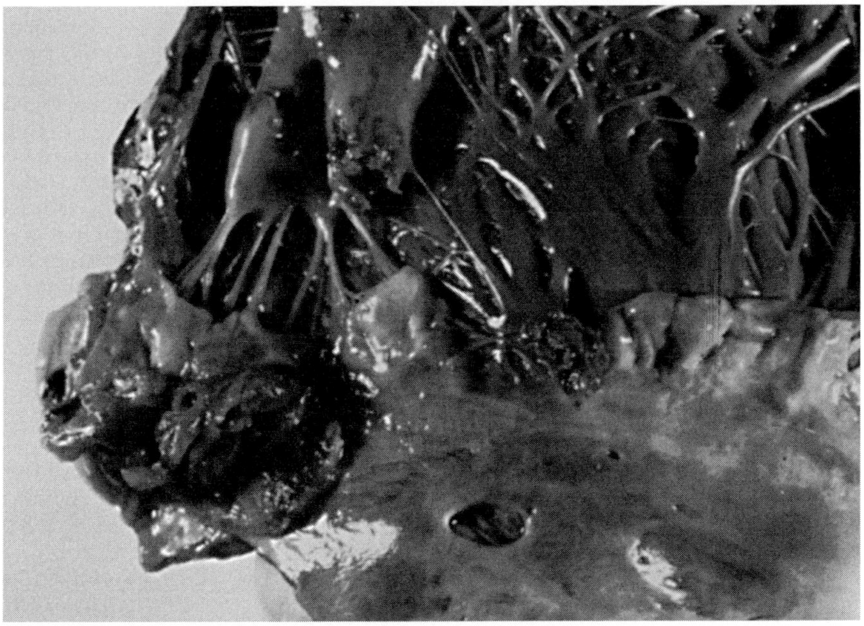

FIGURE 32–1. *Subacute endocarditis of mitral valve with vegetation and rupture of the papillary muscle, caused by* Staphylococcus aureus. *(Courtesy of Dr. Edith P. Hawkins, Texas Children's Hospital, Houston, TX.)*

tive organisms are resistant to this bactericidal activity; phagocytosis is required for killing.

The frequent presence of hypergammaglobulinemia, splenomegaly, and monocytes in the blood of patients with infective endocarditis indicates stimulation of the humoral and cellular immune systems. Macroglobulins, cryoglobulins, and agglutinating, opsonic, and complement-fixing antibodies have been associated with infective endocarditis.[163, 217] Studies in animals preimmunized with heat-killed streptococci before inducing aortic valve trauma and infection suggest that circulating antibody has a protective role.[350, 408] However, antibody to *S. aureus* and *Staphylococcus epidermidis* does not prevent the development of endocarditis in immunized animals, perhaps because this antibody does not enhance opsonophagocytosis.[349] The continuous antigenic challenge created by intravascular organisms leads to increased production of specific antibody (including opsonic, agglutinating, and complement-fixing antibodies), cryoglobulins, macroglobulins, and antibodies to bacterial heat-shock protein[314] and subsequent formation of circulating immune complexes. These are found with increased frequency in patients with a long duration of illness, hypocomplementemia, extravalvular manifestations, and right-sided disease.[25] Quantitative levels of circulating immune complexes may be helpful in distinguishing endocarditic from nonendocarditic sepsis[26] and in monitoring anti-infective therapy. Effective treatment usually leads to a prompt decrease in these levels,[24] whereas relapses may be characterized by rising titers.[197] The diffuse glomerulonephritis occasionally seen with infective endocarditis is caused by subepithelial deposition of immune complexes and complement.[146] Immune complexes can be demonstrated in some diffuse purpuric lesions seen with endocarditis.[230] Bacterial antigens have been found within these complexes.[168]

Further evidence of the stimulation of the immune system in infective endocarditis is the development of rheumatoid factor in about 50 per cent of adults with disease of greater than 6 weeks' duration.[427] Titers of rheumatoid factor correlate with hypergammaglobulinemia and, as with immune complex levels, will decrease with therapy and increase during relapse. The role of rheumatoid factor in the disease process is unknown, but it may be involved by blocking IgG opsonic activity, stimulating phagocytosis, or accelerating microvascular damage.[349] Antinuclear, antiendocardial, antisarcolemmal, and antimyolemmal antibodies also have been identified in patients with infective endocarditis; their roles in pathogenesis are unclear.[238]

The pathologic changes that occur in the heart in association with infective endocarditis are secondary to local extension of the infection. The vegetations vary in size from a millimeter to several centimeters; they frequently are singular but may be multiple. Valvular stenosis may result from large lesions. Vegetations secondary to certain organisms, especially *Candida, Haemophilus,* and *S. aureus* in acute cases, frequently are large and friable, with a propensity for embolization.[436] Ulcerative lesions may occur, leading to perforation of the valve and subsequent congestive heart failure. Other local complications include rupture of the chordae tendineae or papillary muscle (see Fig. 32–1), valve ring abscess with subsequent fistula formation and pericardial empyema,[36, 50] aneurysms of the sinus of Valsalva or ventricle,[126, 345] myocarditis, and myocardial infarction.[112] Persistent fever during appropriate medical therapy for infective endocarditis may reflect a persistent vegetation, especially with right-sided disease, or extension of infection into a valve ring and adjacent structures.[90] In such cases, surgery often is required.

The pathologic changes in distant organs usually are secondary to embolization with subsequent infarction or metastatic infection. In many cases of infective endocarditis, the causative organism is of low pathogenicity; the infections caused by septic emboli frequently are of low grade because of the reduced propensity of these organisms to invade tissue. However, the emboli in acute *S. aureus* endocarditis frequently cause severe metastatic infections and overwhelming sepsis. Emboli from right-sided heart lesions lodge in the lungs, causing pulmonary infarcts and abscesses, which usually are small and multiple. Left-sided lesions may embolize to any organ but most commonly affect the brain, kidney, spleen, and skin.[279] Cerebral emboli have been detected in 30 per cent of cases in adults and children, causing infarction, abscess, mycotic aneurysm, subarachnoid hemorrhage, meningitis, and acute hemiplegia of childhood.[143, 151, 184, 248, 335] Kidney abscess is rare, but infarcts are noted in the majority of patients at autopsy.[221, 263] Amyloidosis involving primarily the kidneys is a rare complication of chronic infective endocarditis.[156] Splenic abscess also is rare but can be a fatal complication if undetected.[182] The most common manifestation of embolization to the skin is petechiae. Janeway lesions are septic emboli consisting of bacteria, neutrophils, necrosis, and subcutaneous hemorrhage. Osler nodes are areas of thrombosis and necrosis. They may be related to both immune complex deposition and septic emboli.[2]

CLINICAL PRESENTATION

The signs and symptoms of infective endocarditis are determined by the extent of local cardiac disease; the continuous bacteremia; and the degree of involvement of distant organs caused by embolization, metastatic infection, and circulating immune complexes. As a result, the clinical presentation is highly variable and mimics many other diseases. Unexplained embolic phenomena in any organ should suggest the diagnosis of endocarditis, especially in children with known heart disease. Patients with acute bacterial endocarditis may present with florid sepsis; the endocarditis is diagnosed at autopsy. The indolent presentation of subacute endocarditis may evolve for weeks or months before medical care is sought. Endocarditis frequently occurs in children with preexisting heart disease, so that subtle changes in cardiac function may be difficult to detect early in the course. Table 32–3 lists the frequency of major clinical manifestations of bacterial endocarditis in infants and children.

Fever is the most common symptom of infective endocarditis, but it is absent in 10 per cent of cases. It usually is of low grade and has no specific pattern. Chills may accompany fever, but these rarely are seen in children. Persistent fever during antimicrobial therapy is uncommon. Prolonged (>2 weeks) fever is associated with certain etiologic agents (*S. aureus*, gram-negative bacilli, fungi); culture-negative endocarditis; and complications such as embolization of major vessels, intracardiac or peripheral abscess, tissue infarction, the need for cardiac surgery, and a higher mortality rate.[37, 218] Nonspecific symptoms such as malaise, anorexia, weight loss, and fatigue are common. Arthralgias occur in 24 per cent of patients. The arthralgias frequently are multiple and most commonly affect the large joints. Although adults may present with synovitis,[64] this finding is rare in children. Osteoarticular infection in association with infective endocarditis in adults occurs almost exclusively in intravenous drug users[344]; it is very rare in children. Gastrointestinal complaints are noted in 16 per cent of cases and include nausea, vomiting, and abdominal pain. Chest pain occurs in about 10 per cent of older children and usually is mild and nonspecific. Although chest pain usually is related to diffuse myalgias, it may be secondary to pulmonary complications or cardiac lesions, especially if the tricuspid valve is involved.

Heart murmurs occur in more than 90 per cent of children with infective endocarditis, but the vast majority of patients have underlying heart disease with preexisting murmurs. The appearance of a new murmur or significant change in a previous one occurs in only one-fourth of cases. Significant turbulence of blood flow caused by compromised valvular function must have occurred for a murmur to be detected or change. The frequent absence of changes in the cardiac examination early in the disease contributes to the long average delay in diagnosis, especially in children with preexisting heart disease. Congestive heart failure occurs in 30 per cent of children with infective endocarditis and especially is common in those patients who develop a new murmur of valvular insufficiency. Endocarditis should be suspected in any child with rheumatic or congenital heart disease who has unexplained deterioration in cardiac function. Although valvular regurgitation is the most common hemodynamic complication of endocarditis, significant obstruction of a valve or shunt requiring rapid surgery occurs rarely.[61]

Neurologic signs and symptoms are reported in about 20 per cent of children with endocarditis. They may dominate the clinical presentation, especially in endocarditis due to *S. aureus*.[151, 335] A sudden development of cerebral lesions in an infant or child should suggest this diagnosis. The manifestations are those that commonly accompany cerebral infarct or abscess—namely, acute hemiplegia of childhood, seizures, ataxia, aphasia, sensory loss, focal neurologic deficits, and alterations in mental status. They may be the presenting feature of endocarditis or may occur years after the infection has been eradicated.[438] Mycotic aneurysms of the cerebral vessels occur rarely in cases of pediatric endocarditis.[51] They usually are single, small, and peripheral but may lead to subarachnoid hemorrhage. Whereas computed tomographic scanning of the brain is useful for delineating central nervous system involvement in patients with infective endocarditis, magnetic resonance imaging may be more sensitive for detecting small infarctions and changes secondary to cerebral edema.[30] Other neurologic manifestations associated with endocarditis include cranial nerve palsies, neuropathy, visual changes, choreoathetosis, seizures, and toxic encephalopathy.

Splenomegaly is a common manifestation of endocarditis in children, occurring in 55 per cent of cases. It is found frequently in patients with long-standing disease and other evidence of immune system activation. The spleen usually is nontender and may be associated with mild hepatomegaly. Splenic infarction and abscess are rare but should be suspected in patients who develop left upper quadrant abdominal pain that radiates to the left shoulder, a pleural friction rub, or a left pleural effusion.

TABLE 32–3. Clinical Manifestations of Bacterial Endocarditis in Children

Symptom	Average Percentage	Range Percentage	Physical Finding	Average Percentage	Range Percentage
Fever	90	56–100	Fever	90	56–100
Malaise	55	40–79	Splenomegaly	55	36–67
Anorexia/weight loss	31	8–83	Petechiae	33	10–50
Heart failure	30	9–47	Embolic phenomenon	28	14–50
Arthralgia	24	16–38	New or change in heart murmur	24	9–44
Neurologic	18	12–21	Clubbing	14	2–42
Gastrointestinal	16	9–36	Osler nodes	7	7–8
Chest pain	9	5–20	Roth spots	5	0–6
			Janeway lesion	5	0–10
			Splinter hemorrhages	5	0–10

Data from references 38, 73, 124, 181, 211, 360, 367, 393, 412.

Skin manifestations are less common in children than in adults. Clubbing is found in 10 to 20 per cent of children with endocarditis but frequently is related to underlying heart disease. Petechiae are found in about one-third of patients, especially those with long-standing disease. They are most common on the extremities, oral mucosa, and conjunctivae. Splinter hemorrhages are linear red or brown streaks seen in the nailbeds. They are present in only 5 per cent of children with endocarditis and are associated with other conditions.[206] Three other types of lesions are more specific for infective endocarditis but occur in only 5 to 7 per cent of patients: Osler nodes, small (2 to 10 mm), painful nodular lesions found in the pads of fingers or toes; Janeway lesions, usually painless hemorrhagic macular plaques that frequently occur on the palms and soles[109]; and Roth spots, small pale retinal lesions associated with areas of hemorrhage located near the optic disk.

Other than fever and, perhaps, splenomegaly, no single sign or symptom occurs in greater than 50 per cent of children with endocarditis. It is obvious that there is no classic clinical presentation for this disease because the chance that even three or more signs will be present is extremely low. The appearance of any one of these clinical features in a child with predisposing heart disease should raise the suspicion of infective endocarditis, leading to an appropriate diagnostic evaluation.

The clinical presentation of infective endocarditis in infants and neonates is less specific than that in older children. The onset more often is acute and related to overwhelming infection.[180, 255] In the pre-antibiotic era, these children often presented with other foci of infection, such as osteomyelitis, meningitis, and pneumonia, which dominated the clinical picture. The widespread use of antibiotics since 1941 has caused a decrease in the number of cases of infective endocarditis occurring secondarily to other suppurative infections.[255] Although early studies concluded that congenital heart disease was not an important predisposing factor to endocarditis in infants,[128, 426] more recent reports suggest that it is.[75, 180] At present, infants with heart defects undergo corrective and palliative surgery at younger ages than in the past. Those infants who develop postoperative endocarditis likely will have clinical presentations more similar to those in older children.

Infective endocarditis is rare in the neonate and frequently is associated with indwelling vascular catheters. It may affect the tricuspid valve and have a fairly "silent" clinical presentation. Persistent bacteremia or fungemia should lead to a search for a cardiac focus of infection. Neonates frequently develop deterioration of pulmonary function, coagulopathies, thrombocytopenia, and low-grade murmurs. Skin abscesses and hepatomegaly also are common. The prognosis of neonatal intensive care–associated infective endocarditis usually is favorable, perhaps because the diagnosis often is established relatively early and antibiotics are given rapidly.[334]

Reported series of infective endocarditis in children with prosthetic valves are scarce. In early disease, fever may be the only finding because the other signs of endocarditis are masked by the medical and surgical complications occurring in the immediate postoperative period. Late infections usually produce a clinical presentation similar to that in native valve endocarditis. Clinical evidence of systemic embolization occurs in up to 40 per cent of patients. Neurologic complications carry a particularly poor prognosis for survival.[202] A new or changing murmur often indicates valvular insufficiency caused by a paravalvular leak. Florid cardiac failure is the major manifestation if local infection or abscess creates valve instability and acute, severe regurgitation.

The signs and symptoms of infective endocarditis in intravenous drug abusers may be similar, but there are several more distinctive features of their illness. Two-thirds of these patients have no predisposing heart disease. The most commonly affected valve is the tricuspid, leading to a predominance of pulmonary signs and symptoms resulting from pleural effusion, pulmonary infarction, and lung abscesses. Signs of tricuspid insufficiency (gallop rhythm, pulsatile liver, regurgitant murmur) are found in one-third of cases.[349] A large number of patients have extracardiac sites of infection that are helpful in diagnosis.[391]

LABORATORY FINDINGS

The most important diagnostic procedure is the blood culture. Because many bacteria that usually are not pathogenic cause infective endocarditis, scrupulous aseptic technique must be used to distinguish causative agents from contaminants. The yield of organisms is not increased by obtaining blood from arterial puncture or cardiac catheterization.[27] The bacteremia usually is of low grade and continuous. The first two cultures will yield the organism 90 per cent of the time; in two-thirds of cases, all blood cultures will be positive.[424] Therefore, isolated positive cultures usually are not significant. Previous outpatient antibiotic therapy may change the yield significantly. In one study, culture positivity in cases of proven endocarditis was 64 per cent in patients receiving antibiotics before cultures were drawn, compared with 100 per cent in patients without exposure to antibiotics.[297] Blood should be injected into hypertonic media if the patient has been exposed to antibiotics.

When *Candida* endocarditis is suspected, several additional points should be considered. Isolation of *Candida* species may require incubation of 1 week or longer. All blood cultures from a patient with *Candida* endocarditis may not be positive, in contrast to the usual situation with bacterial endocarditis; several positive cultures may be interspersed among negative cultures. *Candida* is isolated commonly from other infected sites, such as urine, sputum, synovial fluid, cerebrospinal fluid, lymph nodes, and bone marrow, in patients with fungal endocarditis.[337]

It is recommended that three to five sets of blood cultures be obtained from different sites within the first 24 hours in children with suspected endocarditis. Although difficult in smaller children, obtaining 3 to 5 mL of blood per culture is desirable for optimal yield. The samples should be injected into thioglycolate and trypticase soy (or brain-heart infusion) broth and held for at least 3 weeks to detect slow-growing organisms. If gram-positive cocci grow in the broth but fail to grow upon subculture, nutritionally variant streptococci should be suspected and subculture should be made onto media with either L-cysteine or pyridoxal phosphate.[48, 372] Poured plates may be made to estimate the degree of bacteremia.

Negative blood cultures are noted in 10 to 15 per cent of cases of clinically diagnosed endocarditis.[404] However, if patients did not receive prior antibiotic therapy and blood cultures were obtained properly, these cases have been less than 5 per cent of the total. Potential reasons for negative cultures include (1) right-sided endocarditis; (2) prior administration of antibiotics; (3) fungal (especially *Aspergillus*) endocarditis; (4) endocarditis caused by *Bartonella* species, rickettsiae, chlamydiae, or viruses; (5) mural endocarditis; (6) slow growth of organisms (*Candida, Haemophilus, Brucella,* nutritionally variant streptococci); (7) anaerobic infection; and (8) nonbacterial thrombotic endocarditis or an incorrect diagnosis.[147, 150, 303, 404] In some instances, intraleukocytic organisms may be seen in layered peripheral blood, even when cultures are negative.[310] If surgical resection of vegetations or valve replacement is performed, an etiology may be demonstrated by appropriate histologic examination and stains for bacteria and fungi. Organisms also may be isolated from extracardiac sites (bone marrow, urine).

Many nonspecific laboratory findings are abnormal in patients with infective endocarditis (Table 32–4). The erythrocyte sedimentation rate is elevated in 80 to 90 per cent of cases. However, it frequently is normal or low when congestive heart failure or renal failure is present. Serum C-reactive protein usually is elevated initially and returns to normal during successful therapy.[251] An increase during therapy may be caused by treatment failure but also can be caused by drug allergy or intercurrent infection. Rheumatoid factor rarely has been measured in a series of pediatric patients, but when measurements have been made, they have been positive in 25 to 50 per cent of children with endocarditis. A positive test may be a diagnostic aid in cases of culture-negative endocarditis, when other causes are excluded. Serial measurements may provide evidence of efficacy of therapy, although a fall in the titer of rheumatoid factor may lag behind the clinical and bacteriologic response.[416] Hypocomplementemia is seen in association with glomerulonephritis. Anemia is present in about 40 per cent of patients, especially in those with long-standing disease. Although hemolysis may occur in the areas of turbulence in the heart, more often it is an anemia of chronic disease. Because many patients with cyanotic heart disease normally have a compensatory polycythemia, a serial drop in hematocrit is of more significance than a single measurement. Leukocytosis occurs in a few patients, but leukopenia is rare in the absence of acute endocarditis with overwhelming sepsis. Hematuria and proteinuria, present in 25 to 50 per cent of cases, usually are secondary to microemboli in the kidneys and may be accompanied by "pyuria," casts, and bacteriuria.

Circulating immune complexes are present in the majority of adult cases of subacute endocarditis, as measured by the Raji-cell radioimmune assay[394] or the ^{125}I-Clq binding assay.[439] They frequently are absent in acute endocarditis.[197] Low levels of immune complexes have been found in 32 per cent of adults with septicemia but not endocarditis, 10 per cent of normal controls, and 40 per cent of noninfected intravenous drug abusers.[25] However, detection of levels greater than 100 μg/mL is correlated highly with the presence of endocarditis.[26] Serial measurements of immune complex levels may aid in monitoring therapeutic efficacy.[24] Systematic investigation of immune complexes has been reported infrequently in children with endocarditis. When immune complexes have been sought, the majority of patients have had significant levels,[412]

TABLE 32–4. Selected Laboratory Findings of Bacterial Endocarditis in Children

Laboratory Finding	Average Percentage	Range Percentage
Positive blood culture	87	68–98
Elevated erythrocyte sedimentation rate	80	71–96
Low hemoglobin (anemia)	44	19–79
Positive rheumatoid factor	38	25–55
Hematuria	35	28–47

Data from references 38, 73, 124, 181, 211, 360, 367, 393, 412.

including two of three children with culture-negative endocarditis.[416]

In cases in which infective endocarditis is suspected but blood cultures remain negative, serologic testing for specific organisms may prove helpful. Several techniques measure antibody to teichoic acids, which are major components of the cell wall of *S. aureus*. These antibodies are present in greater than 85 per cent of adults with staphylococcal endocarditis, but the false-positive rate is as high as 10 per cent.[19, 276] False-negative results correlate with a short (<2 weeks) duration of illness. Specific information about the accuracy of this test in children is lacking, and the tests are not readily available. Serologic testing is available or under investigation for a number of other organisms that cause infective endocarditis, including *Bartonella, Brucella, Candida, Aspergillus, Histoplasma, Cryptococcus, Chlamydia,* and *Coxiella*.[185, 207] In general, the usefulness of these tests in children with endocarditis is unproven. Some patients with nonspirochetal bacterial endocarditis who reside in locales endemic for Lyme disease will have significantly elevated levels of antibodies reactive to *Borrelia burgdorferi*.[188] Diagnostic confusion may occur because the signs and symptoms of infective endocarditis and Lyme disease can be quite similar.

Radiographic techniques have not been a great aid in the diagnosis of infective endocarditis. The findings on plain chest roentgenograms are nonspecific, but evidence of complications, such as septic pulmonary emboli or congestive heart failure, may be helpful. Computed tomography may help in the diagnosis of an infected shunt.[405] Immunoscintigraphy using technetium-labeled antigranulocyte antibodies may yield useful information when the echocardiographic findings are equivocal.[265] Cineangiography is the definitive method to determine the anatomic alterations in the heart resulting from infective endocarditis but rarely is necessary in children.

The electrocardiogram also is useful in the evaluation of patients with endocarditis because it will detect arrhythmias and conduction disturbances that complicate the disease.[57, 69] Ventricular ectopy may be related to myocardial ischemia, myocarditis, or myocardial abscess. New conduction defects imply extension of infection beyond the valve ring into the myocardium. Any degree of atrioventricular block, new left bundle branch block, or new right bundle branch block with left anterior hemiblock may represent extension of infection from the aortic valve into the ventricular septum. Junctional tachycardia, Wenckebach atrioventricular block, or complete heart block may be produced by extension of the infection from the mitral valve annulus into the atrioventricular node or proximal His bundle.[69] In general, unstable conduction block is more likely to develop in patients with aortic valve endocarditis than in those with mitral infection.[88]

Echocardiography has become a valuable adjunct to the diagnosis and treatment of endocarditis in children.[87, 138, 213, 322, 332, 355] Echocardiography can be performed via the traditional transthoracic or the transesophageal approach.[307] The sensitivity and specificity of transthoracic echocardiography still are being defined, with positive results in from 36 to 100 per cent of children in various series of pediatric patients.[40, 87, 198, 334] In general, two-dimensional echocardiography is more sensitive than the M-mode technique, especially in cases of right-sided endocarditis,[292] and is superior in diagnosing complications of the destructive process.[261] The smallest size vegetation detectable is approximately 2 mm, but the acoustic impedance of the mass relative to the surrounding structures is a more important factor than is size in identifying the vegetation. Echocardiography has identified vegetations in culture-negative cases. Its accuracy in prosthetic valve endocarditis is diminished by the difficulty in resolution around the prosthetic device.[272, 373] The serial evaluation of valvular vegetations generally does not assist in assessing the efficacy of antibiotic therapy because the diminution or disappearance of vegetations may take place long after the completion of successful medical treatment.[208] The use of transthoracic echocardiography to predict the clinical course and need for operative intervention in patients with endocarditis is controversial. A synopsis of many reports that have assessed the role of transthoracic echocardiography in the diagnosis and management of infective endocarditis suggests the following[212]: (1) because of variable sensitivity among studies for detection of vegetations, a negative study does not rule out endocarditis, especially when foreign material is present within the heart; (2) false-positive studies are quite rare (the specificity is high); (3) the reliability of transthoracic echocardiography depends on the experience of the examiner and the technical adequacy of the study; (4) transthoracic echocardiography is valuable in assessing local complications of endocarditis on native valves; and (5) in most but not all studies, patients with a vegetation identified by transthoracic echocardiography are at increased risk for systemic emboli and congestive heart failure.[44, 173, 198, 233, 323, 343, 374] Although some investigators believe that the presence of a vegetation should hasten early surgery,[84] most feel that a positive echocardiogram is adjunctive evidence that should be considered along with other clinical parameters when considering surgical intervention.[212] One study suggested that the relative risk for embolic events associated with echocardiographically visualized lesions is microorganism-dependent, with a significant attributable risk seen only in patients with viridans streptococcal infection.[368] Absence of a vegetation on transthoracic echocardiography may define the subset of patients at low risk for embolic complications.[288]

Transesophageal echocardiography is a newer technique that has been studied extensively in adults with infective endocarditis.[81] It utilizes a 5-mHz phased array transducer with Doppler and color flow encoding capabilities mounted on the tip of a flexible endoscope.[349] Biplane transesophageal echocardiography is considered the standard technique and is superior to transthoracic echocardiography because of improved spatial resolution, lack of acoustic interference from the lungs and chest wall, and closer proximity to posterior structures, such as the mitral valve and left atrium.[80] Multiplane transesophageal echocardiography facilitates and abbreviates the examination procedure and may be more accurate in providing dimensions of a vegetation associated with infective endocarditis.[80, 177] Transesophageal echocardiography generally is well tolerated by children, even with the use of an adult probe (when the child's weight is >7 kg),[355] and rarely is associated with bacteremia.[79, 215, 306] Transesophageal echocardiography generally is more sensitive than transthoracic echocardiography in the detection of intracardiac vegetations, being positive in 70 to 95 per cent of adults with strongly suspected endocarditis.[269, 359] It is significantly more sensitive in the detection of vegetations and complications in infected prosthetic values.[203, 298, 327, 373, 387] It appears to be less helpful for detection of vegetations in right-sided endocarditis.[336] Although a negative transesophageal echocardiographic study does not exclude endocarditis,[364] the procedure should be considered for patients with suspected endocarditis and a negative transthoracic echocardiograph and when perivalvular extension of infection is suspected.

To aid in the diagnosis of infective endocarditis, various sets of clinical criteria have been suggested. The von Reyn criteria were described in 1982, but echocardiographic findings were not included in the case definitions.[414] Also, the isolation of a typical infective endocarditis pathogen from blood cultures was not considered. A new set of case definitions and diagnostic criteria was proposed by investigators from Duke[97] (Tables 32–5 and 32–6). These new criteria include echocardiographic and blood culture results, resulting in more flexibility, a higher proportion of "definite" cases, and a more accurate reflection of current clinical practice. These criteria have been validated in large series of infective endocarditis in adults and children.[85, 97, 160, 342] In one pediatric series of clinically defined cases of endocarditis, no cases were rejected by the Duke criteria, whereas 25 per cent were rejected by the von Reyn criteria.[85] Three of six pathologically confirmed cases were rated as only probable or rejected by the von Reyn criteria, whereas all were definite by the Duke criteria.

MICROBIOLOGY

A wide variety of microorganisms are capable of causing infective endocarditis in humans. Table 32–7 lists those organisms isolated from patients in the major pediatric series. Gram-positive cocci are the etiologic agents in 90 per cent of

TABLE 32–5. Definition of Terms Used in the Duke Criteria for Infective Endocarditis (IE)

Major Criteria

1. Positive blood culture
   a. Typical microorganisms for IE from ≥2 blood cultures
      (1) Viridans streptococci,* *Streptococcus bovis, or* HACEK group *or*
      (2) Community-acquired *Staphylococcus aureus* or enterococci, in the absence of another primary focus, *or*
   b. Persistently positive blood cultures, with recovery of a microorganism consistent with IE from
      (1) Blood cultures drawn ≥12 hours apart *or*
      (2) All of 3 or a majority of 4 or more separate blood cultures, with first and last drawn ≥1 hour apart
2. Evidence of endocardial involvement
   a. Positive echocardiogram for IE
      (1) Oscillating intracardiac mass on valve or supporting structures, in the path of regurgitant jets, or on implanted material, in the absence of an alternative anatomic explanation, *or*
      (2) Abscess *or*
      (3) New partial dehiscence of a prosthetic valve *or*
   b. New valvular regurgitation (increase or change in preexisting murmur is not sufficient)

Minor Criteria

1. Predisposing heart condition or intravenous drug use
2. Fever ≥38° C
3. Vascular phenomena: major arterial emboli, septic pulmonary infarcts, mycotic aneurysm, intracranial hemorrhage, conjunctival hemorrhages, Janeway lesions
4. Immunologic phenomena: glomerulonephritis, Osler nodes, Roth spots, rheumatoid factor
5. Microbiologic evidence: positive blood culture but not meeting major criterion as noted previously† or serologic evidence of active infection with organism consistent with IE
6. Echocardiogram: consistent with IE but not meeting major criteria as noted previously

*Including nutritionally variant strains.

†Excluding single positive cultures for coagulase-negative staphylococci and organisms that do not cause IE.

Reprinted by permission of the publisher from Durack, D. T., Lukes, A. S., Bright, D. K., et al.: New criteria for diagnosis of infective endocarditis: Utilization of specific echocardiographic findings. Am. J. Med. *96*:200–209, 1994. Copyright 1994 by Excerpta Medica Inc.

TABLE 32–6. Duke Criteria for the Diagnosis of Infective Endocarditis (IE)

Definite

1. Pathologic criteria
   a. Microorganisms: demonstrated by culture or histology in a vegetation, in a vegetation that has embolized, or in an intracardiac abscess *or*
   b. Pathologic lesions: vegetation or intracardiac abscess present, confirmed by histology, showing endocarditis
2. Clinical criteria
   a. 2 major criteria *or*
   b. 1 major and 3 minor criteria *or*
   c. 5 minor criteria

Possible

1. Findings consistent with IE that fall short of "definite" but not "rejected"

Rejected

1. Firm alternate diagnosis explaining evidence of IE *or*
2. Resolution of IE syndrome, with antimicrobial therapy for ≤4 days, *or*
3. No pathologic evidence of IE at surgery or autopsy, with antibiotic therapy for ≤4 days

Reprinted by permission of the publisher from Durack, D. T., Lukes, A. S., Bright, D. K., et al.: New criteria for diagnosis of infective endocarditis: Utilization of specific echocardiographic findings. Am. J. Med. *96*:200–209, 1994. Copyright 1994 by Excerpta Medica Inc.

the cases in which an organism is isolated. Streptococci remain the bacteria isolated most frequently, although the percentages of cases caused by staphylococci and fungi have been increasing over the past two decades.[181, 255–334, 367, 393, 412, 436] Polymicrobial infective endocarditis, especially in nosocomial settings, appears to be increasing in incidence.[13] Characteristics of selected organisms and the type of disease they produce are considered in the following subsections.

Streptococci

Several terminologies have been used to classify streptococci. The Lancefield system defines groups (A, B, C, D, E, F, G, H) by serologic reactions. The viridans streptococci are alpha-hemolytic or nonhemolytic, may be Lancefield nontypable (*Streptococcus milleri, S. mitior, S. salivarius,* most *S. mutans,* and *S. sanguis*) or typable (*S. bovis*–group D, some *S. sanguis*–group H, some *S. milleri*–group F), and display similar characteristics in vivo. They are the most frequent etiologic agents in subacute infective endocarditis, causing 40 per cent of cases in children. They may cause rapidly progressive invasive disease.[164, 381] They are common pathogens in patients with underlying heart disease but less common in postoperative patients. They are part of the indigenous flora of the human mouth and gastrointestinal tract; procedures that disrupt the mucosal integrity in these areas predispose to viridans streptococcal bacteremia. In the pediatric population, most blood and cerebrospinal fluid isolates of viridans and nonhemolytic streptococci are not from patients with infective endocarditis.[149] Most strains are exquisitely susceptible to penicillin, although prior antibiotic administration may promote infection with resistant strains.[222] Nutritionally variant viridans streptococci are recognized with increasing frequency as a cause of culture-negative endocarditis in children.[111, 280, 375] Bacteriologic failure has occurred in up to 41 per cent of cases of endocarditis caused by nutritionally deficient streptococci despite susceptibility of the organisms to the antibiotics used.[372] Most viridans streptococci have low pathogenicity; however, *S. milleri* has a predilection for suppurative complications.[274] The prognosis of endocarditis due to nonenterococcal streptococci is excellent with good medical and surgical management; the cure rate is more than 90 per cent, although complications (emboli, congestive heart failure) occur in up to 30 per cent of cases.

TABLE 32–7. Etiologic Agents of Bacterial Endocarditis in Children

Organism	Average Percentage	Range Percentage
Streptococci		
Viridans	40.3	17–72
Enterococci	4.0	0–12
Pneumococci	3.3	0–21
Beta-hemolytic	2.7	0–8
Other	1.1	0–16
Staphylococci		
S. aureus	23.8	5–40
S. epidermidis	4.7	0–15
Gram-negative aerobic bacilli	4.0	0–15
Fungi	1.1	0–12
Miscellaneous bacteria	2.4	0–10
Culture negative	12.6	2–32

Data from references 38, 46, 73, 179–181, 211, 255, 334, 367, 393, 412, 436, 437.

Enterococcal endocarditis is much less common in children than adults,[256, 390] accounting for only 4 per cent of pediatric cases. The organism normally inhabits the gastrointestinal and genitourinary tracts; instrumentation of these areas may cause enterococcal bacteremia. More than 40 per cent of adult patients have no underlying heart disease.[321] Endocarditis should be considered in all infants and children with unexplained enterococcal bacteremia. Although the incidence of enterococcal bacteremia appears to be increasing in some neonatal intensive care units, the incidence of associated endocarditis appears to be very low. Factors that may suggest endocarditis in patients with enterococcal bacteremia include (1) preexisting heart disease, (2) community acquisition, (3) a cryptogenic source, and (4) the absence of polymicrobial bacteremia.[239] Differentiation of enterococci from other group D streptococci (*S. bovis*) is important because their respective therapeutic approaches are different.

Endocarditis caused by beta-hemolytic streptococci was more common in the pre-antibiotic era than today. Most cases are caused by Lancefield group B or G organisms,[1, 9, 125, 420] whereas group C and A streptococci rarely cause endocarditis.[34, 91, 139, 228, 295, 316] Group B streptococcal infection may lead to large, bulky vegetations, easily seen by echocardiography. Even though group B streptococcal bacteremia is common in newborn infants, endocarditis caused by this organism is rare in this age group. Similarly, *S. pneumoniae* accounted for 10 to 15 per cent of endocarditis cases in the pre-antibiotic era but currently causes less than 1 per cent.[127, 172, 291] Pneumococcal endocarditis may involve either the aortic or the mitral valve,[103, 397] and less than one-half of affected children have underlying heart disease. The clinical course frequently is fulminant.[100, 308] Concurrent meningitis and/or pneumonia occurs frequently. Valvular dysfunction and cardiac decompensation are common.[42, 315] Early surgical intervention may be required because the mortality rate is 75 per cent when medical management alone is utilized.[172]

Staphylococci

Staphylococci cause 20 to 30 per cent of cases of infective endocarditis in children. *S. aureus* is the etiologic agent in most cases of acute endocarditis and frequently infects normal heart valves.[267] The course often is fulminant when the mitral or aortic valve is involved, with frequent suppurative complications both in the heart (myocardial abscess, pericarditis, valve ring abscess) and in other organs.[106, 186, 417] *S. aureus* is responsible for more than 50 per cent of cases of endocarditis in intravenous drug abusers, but their disease tends to be less severe.[58, 59] The origin of the infecting organism is the addict's own nose or skin, not the injection paraphernalia.[403] Endocarditis associated with indwelling vascular catheters or prosthetic valves frequently is caused by *S. aureus*. Endocarditis must be suspected in any patient with *S. aureus* bacteremia, even when a peripheral focus of infection is present.[262] However, the majority of patients with *S. aureus* bacteremia do not have endocarditis.

The incidence of *S. epidermidis* endocarditis is rising rapidly.[7] Although a rare cause of endocarditis in patients without underlying heart disease,[28] it is a common etiologic agent of endocarditis after cardiac surgery.[201] This organism is the leading agent in prosthetic valve endocarditis, causing 25 to 67 per cent of early cases and 25 to 33 per cent of late cases.[134, 169, 195] Coagulase-negative staphylococcal endocarditis also has been associated with mitral valve prolapse and use of intravascular catheters in premature neonates.[12, 285] Although metastatic infection rarely occurs, *S. epidermidis* can be locally invasive; the mortality rate of *S. epidermidis* prosthetic valve endocarditis approaches 75 per cent when valve replacement is not performed. Cases of infective endocarditis caused by other species of coagulase-negative staphylococci, such as *S. capitis*, appear to be rare.[226]

Gram-Negative Organisms

Whereas gram-negative bacteria cause 4 to 5 per cent of the cases of infective endocarditis in children, the percentage of children with gram-negative enteric bacteremia who develop endocarditis is extremely low. Endocarditis should be suspected in patients with gram-negative infection when bacteremia persists despite usually appropriate antibiotic therapy.[53] Burn patients,[166] immunosuppressed hosts, narcotic addicts, and prosthetic valve recipients are at an increased risk for gram-negative endocarditis. However, in the early postoperative period after cardiac surgery, sustained gram-negative bacillary bacteremia commonly is caused by other foci of infection and does not imply the presence of endocarditis.[340] Many species of gram-negative enteric organisms have caused infective endocarditis in children, but no clear pattern has emerged. Among the more commonly reported gram-negative organisms are *Brucella, Escherichia coli, Serratia, Klebsiella-Enterobacter, Salmonella,* and *Pseudomonas*.[86, 210, 232, 384] Endocarditis due to *Salmonella* has been reported in patients with HIV infection.[116] It most often affects previously abnormal heart valves. Information is limited to case reports and general medicine reviews; discussion of individual organisms is beyond the scope of this review. Cure of left-sided endocarditis caused by the Enterobacteriaceae is uncommon with medical therapy alone.[349]

Other gram-negative organisms associated with infective endocarditis are the so-called HACEK coccobacilli (*Haemophilus, Actinobacillus, Cardiobacterium, Eikenella,* and *Kingella*). These organisms caused 57 per cent of the cases of gram-negative endocarditis seen at the Mayo Clinic from 1958 to 1979.[129] Endocarditis caused by *Haemophilus influenzae* has been reported in only four children.[78, 242] Cases due to *Haemophilus parainfluenzae* and *Haemophilus aphrophilus* are slightly more common.[31, 63, 175, 234] They usually occur in the setting of preexisting valvular disease and run a subacute course. However, central nervous system complications and emboli to major peripheral arteries are frequent.[63] Infective endocarditis in children caused by other organisms of the HACEK group is extremely rare.[6, 113, 266, 294, 315] All organisms in this group are fastidious, may require 2 to 3 weeks for primary isolation, and need subculturing onto chocolate agar in an atmosphere of 5 to 10 per cent carbon dioxide for optimal growth. These procedures should be carried out in all cases of culture-negative endocarditis.

Neisseria gonorrhoeae was responsible for 10 per cent of cases in the pre-antibiotic era, but fewer than 40 episodes have been reported since 1942.[115, 170] It frequently attacks previously normal heart valves and presents as an acute illness.[388] Valvular destruction with need for valve replacement is common. At present, nonpathogenic *Neisseria* species are isolated more frequently in endocarditis than gonococci, but they usually attack abnormal or prosthetic valves.[41, 153, 167, 305, 356]

Although 1 per cent of cases of infective endocarditis in adults is caused by anaerobic bacteria,[114] reports of anaerobic endocarditis in children are exceedingly rare.[67, 281, 367, 378]

Gram-Positive Bacilli

Infective endocarditis due to *Corynebacterium* species is unusual but may occur on normal or previously abnormal valves.[257] Both toxigenic[83] and nontoxigenic[145, 363, 395] strains of *Corynebacterium diphtheriae* cause endocarditis in children, demonstrating that the toxigenic and invasive properties of the organism are independent. Infection occurs most often on native valves and may be quite aggressive, leading to major vascular complications. *Listeria monocytogenes* endocarditis is rare, has a high mortality, and, unlike other forms of listeriosis, usually is not associated with the immunocompromised host.[21, 54] It has not been associated with listeriosis in neonates. Fewer than 40 cases of endocarditis caused by *Lactobacillus* have been reported.[144, 382] Endocarditis caused by *Erysipelothrix rhusiopathiae* is found predominately in adults who are farmers or are exposed to farm animals or products.[140, 152] Most cases of *Bacillus* endocarditis involve the tricuspid valve in intravenous drug users, but other patients, including those with prosthetic valves, have been affected.[371]

Other Organisms

A number of different bacteria rarely have been associated with endocarditis, including *Acinetobacter*,[142] *Actinomyces*,[214] *Streptobacillus*,[330] and *Rothia*.[379]

Infective endocarditis due to *Coxiella burnetii*, the causative agent of Q fever, is well documented in Northern Africa, Europe, and Australia.[216, 224] Most cases are chronic (occurring over 6 to 12 months) and involve the aortic valve. Clues to diagnosis include exposure to parturient cats or rabbits, massive splenomegaly, hypergammaglobulinemia, and thrombocytopenia.[304] The diagnosis usually is confirmed via measurement of antibodies against phase I and phase II antigens, but the organism has been isolated from leukocytes in a shell vial assay.[135] At least 20 well-documented cases of infective endocarditis caused by *Chlamydia psittaci* and *Chlamydia pneumoniae* have been reported.[161, 185, 246, 358] Most patients have had preexisting heart disease and a subacute course.[241] *Legionella* has been implicated in several cases of prosthetic valve endocarditis.[398] *Bartonella quintana* and *Bartonella henselae* have been identified as the cause of endocarditis in "culture-negative" cases.[92, 162, 174, 366] Most described cases have been in immunocompetent individuals. Diagnosis was established by serology, polymerase chain reaction, or special culture techniques.

Fungi

Most cases of fungal endocarditis in children have been described as occurring after cardiovascular surgery and prolonged intravenous and antibiotic therapy. More recently, cases have been described in neonates[250] and after prosthetic valve placement.[283] The most common causative organism is *Candida albicans,* although disease caused by other *Candida* species, including *C. krusei, C. parapsilosis, C. stellatoidea, C. tropicalis,* and *C. guilliermondi,* has been described.[312, 337, 357] Among intravenous drug abusers, *Candida* species other than *C. albicans* are more common causes of endocarditis.[329] The clinical presentation usually is indolent and not specific, with symptoms occurring from weeks to months before diagnosis. Signs and symptoms caused by emboli to large vessels, especially those supplying the brain, kidney, spleen, and extremities, should alert the physician to the possibility of fungal endocarditis.[5] Large, friable vegetations occur frequently and can be detected by echocardiography.[376] Cutaneous and ocular manifestations of systemic *Candida* infection may be present.[39] The prognosis of *Candida* endocarditis is poor and is related to the propensity for septic emboli, the tendency for invasion into the myocardium, and the poor penetration of antifungal agents into the bulky vegetation. Diagnosis frequently is delayed by the tendency for negative or intermittently positive blood cultures to occur in this disease.[183] Surgical intervention usually is required.

Aspergillus species, including *A. flavis, A. fumigatus, A. terreus,* and *A. niger,* are the second most frequent causes of fungal endocarditis, having been reported in 16 children.[16, 17] Two-thirds of these patients have underlying heart disease. *Aspergillus* endocarditis has been found in immunocompromised hosts with no prior cardiac problems.[434] The most common presenting manifestations are fever and embolic phenomena, especially to the central nervous system.[415] Fewer than 15 cases have been diagnosed ante mortem, 3 by culture of peripheral emboli. In none of the patients was antemortem blood culture-positive. Most cases occur after open-heart surgery; the most likely source of the organism is airborne inoculation of the heart during the operation.[16] Surgical removal of all infected material is recommended, although only one child has been treated successfully.

Other fungi that rarely cause endocarditis include *Histoplasma capsulatum, Coccidioides immitis, Cryptococcus neoformans, Torulopsis glabrata, Trichosporon beigelii,*[200] and *Fusarium* species.[165]

TREATMENT

In the preantibiotic era, infective endocarditis was a uniformly fatal disease. With current improved methods of diagnosis and therapy, 80 to 90 per cent of children with this disease can be expected to survive. The mortality rates are higher for acute staphylococcal infection, fungal endocarditis, and prosthetic valve endocarditis, although the tendency toward earlier surgical intervention in these entities may improve survival. The cornerstone of successful therapy is selection of antibiotics with specific activity against the causative organism. Better analysis of pharmacodynamic variables, such as bactericidal activity and postantibiotic effects of various drugs, may assist in the selection of optimal therapeutic regimens.[72, 205, 429] Although persistent infection occasionally complicates treated endocarditis,[319] deterioration of cardiac function is the major cause of morbidity and mortality.

Several general principles provide the basis for the current recommendations for treatment of endocarditis. Parenteral administration of antibiotics is preferred because the erratic absorption of oral antibiotics, especially in infants, can lead to therapeutic failure. Prolonged treatment, usually 4 to 6 weeks or longer, is necessary to sterilize the vegetations and prevent relapse. Bacteriostatic antibiotics are not effective, leading to frequent relapses and/or failure to eradicate the infection. Antibiotic combinations may produce a rapid bactericidal effect through synergistic mechanisms of action. When synergy exists, smaller doses of each drug may be used, thereby reducing toxic side effects. However, certain drug combinations (penicillin and chloramphenicol, for example) can be antagonistic and should be avoided.

Blood cultures should be obtained for several days to evaluate the effect of the antibiotics. Negative follow-up cultures do not guarantee the success of therapy, but persistent positive cultures usually require that a change of or addition to the antibiotic regimen be made. Observation of the patient's clinical course is extremely important. When fever is present initially, the temperature often returns to normal within a few days after therapy is started. However, fever can persist for weeks in patients whose eventual outcome is good. The patient must be monitored closely for cardiac arrhythmias and congestive heart failure. This may require intensive care observation and electrocardiographic monitoring. Evidence of major embolic phenomena must be sought diligently by physical examination.

Several laboratory tests may aid in monitoring therapy. In all cases of bacterial endocarditis, minimum inhibitory concentration (MIC) and minimum bactericidal concentration (MBC) must be determined for the antibiotics being used because disk susceptibility testing is unreliable and not quantitative. When combinations of antibiotics are employed, tests for bactericidal synergy, such as broth dilution, "checkerboards," or time-kill curves, may give additional information. The role of monitoring the inhibitory and bactericidal activity of the patient's serum is highly controversial. The Schlichter test determines the maximal dilutions of a patient's serum that inhibit and kill in vitro an inoculum of the organism causing the endocarditis.[318, 352] Standardization of this test is poor, with laboratories using variations in inoculum size, composition of broth, timing of samples (at expected peak or trough antibiotic concentrations in the serum), methods of dilution, and determination of bactericidal end-point.[43] In the rabbit endocarditis model, peak serum bactericidal titers greater than 1:8 correlate with therapeutic success.[52] A retrospective review of 17 reports of serum bactericidal activity in patients with endocarditis failed to show any correlation between titers greater than 1:8 and therapeutic success.[68] A prospective study suggested adjusting antibiotic doses to achieve peak titers equal to or greater than 1:64 and trough titers equal to or greater than 1:32.[423] At present, no generally accepted recommendation can be made. In general, it seems reasonable to attempt to achieve a peak serum bactericidal titer of at least 1:8 or greater if serious drug toxicity is not encountered. However, this level may not be attainable with certain organisms such as the enterococcus and gram-negative bacilli. Serum bactericidal testing particularly may be useful when synergistic combinations or less well-established antibiotic regimens are used or when response to therapy is suboptimal.[433]

Little information is available concerning optimal antibiotic therapy of infective endocarditis in children; most treatment regimens are adapted from studies of adults with endocarditis.[430] In general, these regimens have been equally successful (and generally less toxic) in children. Table 32–8 lists recommended doses of the commonly used antibiotics.

After initial evaluation of a patient with suspected infective endocarditis, the physician must make a clinical judgment about when to initiate therapy. If the findings are strongly

TABLE 32–8. Suggested Intravenous Antibiotic Doses and Schedules for Infective Endocarditis in Children

Antibiotic	Daily Dose/kg	Divided Doses Every
Aqueous crystalline penicillin G sodium	200,000–300,000 units	4 hr
Ampicillin sodium	200–300 mg	4–6 hr
Cefazolin	100 mg	6–8 hr
Ceftriaxone	75–100 mg	12–24 hr
Gentamicin sulfate	3.0–7.5 mg	8 hr
Nafcillin sodium	100–200 mg (max., 12 g)	4–6 hr
Oxacillin sodium	100–200 mg (max., 12 g)	4–6 hr
Rifampin	10–20 mg	8–12 hr
Vancomycin hydrochloride	30–60 mg	6–12 hr

indicative of the diagnosis or the child is very ill, treatment should be started as soon as the blood specimens for culture have been drawn. Initial empiric therapy depends on the clinical setting in which the tentative diagnosis is made. If the presentation is subacute, a combination of penicillin G and an aminoglycoside usually is recommended for its activity against viridans streptococci, enterococci, and most gram-negative organisms. If *S. aureus* endocarditis is a strong consideration (acute presentation, narcotic addicts), a penicillinase-resistant penicillin should be added to this regimen. Patients who recently have undergone cardiac surgery, especially prosthetic valve placement, are treated best with an aminoglycoside and vancomycin to "cover" for hospital-acquired infection caused by resistant *S. epidermidis*; some physicians would add penicillin G to this regimen to improve activity against streptococci. When culture and susceptibility data are known, antibiotic therapy can be changed as needed.

Most strains of viridans streptococci, *S. pyogenes*, *S. pneumoniae*, and nonenterococcal group D streptococci are exquisitely susceptible to penicillin, with an MIC of less than 0.2 μg/mL. However, 15 to 20 per cent of viridans streptococci have an MIC equal to or greater than 0.2 μg/mL and are defined arbitrarily as relatively resistant. In addition, some strains (particularly *S. mutans* and *S. mitior*) demonstrate tolerance, that is, an MIC to penicillin of less than 0.1 μg/mL but an MBC that is more than 10-fold higher (1.25 to 50 μg/mL). Most strains of nutritionally dependent streptococci are tolerant to penicillin.[349] Clinical failures may occur in endocarditis caused by these tolerant organisms when penicillin alone is used for treatment,[4] but, except for nutritionally dependent streptococci, therapy of tolerant viridans streptococci generally should be the same as for susceptible strains. Although most experts recommend that endocarditis caused by relatively resistant streptococci be treated with high doses of penicillin combined with 2 to 4 weeks of an aminoglycoside, some authorities feel that penicillin alone usually is adequate therapy.[33, 89] Synergy in vitro between penicillin or vancomycin and streptomycin, gentamicin, or kanamycin can be demonstrated against virtually all penicillin-susceptible streptococci.[418] This observation correlates with a more rapid rate of eradication of bacteria from cardiac vegetations in the rabbit endocarditis model when synergistic combinations of antibiotics are used.[95, 98] However, streptomycin is not synergistic for strains with high-level streptomycin resistance; gentamicin is the preferred second drug for these rare isolates.[104] In pediatric patients, gentamicin usually is substituted for streptomycin because of its lower toxicity.

Several regimens have been examined in adults with penicillin-susceptible viridans streptococcal endocarditis (Table 32–9). A 2-week course of penicillin alone leads to an unacceptable relapse rate. However, a 2-week course of intramuscular procaine penicillin and streptomycin cured 99 per cent of adults with penicillin-susceptible streptococcal endocarditis.[428] These results are similar to those obtained with β-lactams alone for 4 weeks[194] or penicillin for 4 weeks combined with streptomycin for the first 2 weeks.[432] The 2-week penicillin-gentamicin regimen is the most cost-effective and is the preferred therapy in uncomplicated cases in penicillin-susceptible streptococcal endocarditis in young adults.[349] In general, the regimen of 4 weeks of penicillin alone is preferred for patients with renal failure or at high risk from aminoglycoside-induced ototoxicity. Vancomycin or ceftriaxone for 4 weeks can be used in patients with penicillin-susceptible viridans streptococcal endocarditis who have penicillin allergy.[121, 122, 377] The regimen of 4 weeks of penicillin plus an initial 2 weeks of gentamicin is recommended in adults with a complicated course (symptoms for >3 months)[240] or with infection caused by relatively penicillin-resistant organisms (Table 32–10). Most nutritionally deficient streptococci are tolerant to penicillin. For patients with endocarditis due to these organisms, 4 to 6 weeks of penicillin with the addition of an aminoglycoside is recommended (Table 32–11).[33, 430] In patients with streptococcal infection of prosthetic valves or other prosthetic materials, a 6-week regimen of penicillin, supplemented with an aminoglycoside, is recommended. It must be emphasized that none of the regimens discussed has been evaluated specifically in children with endocarditis.

TABLE 32–9. Suggested Regimens for Therapy of Native Valve Endocarditis Due to Penicillin-Susceptible Viridans Streptococci and *Streptococcus bovis* (MIC ≤0.1 μg/mL) in Adults

Antibiotic(s)	Duration (wk)	Comments
Aqueous crystalline penicillin G sodium	4	Preferred for patients with impairment of the eighth cranial nerve or renal function
or		
Ceftriaxone sodium	4	
Aqueous crystalline penicillin G sodium	2	Gentamicin peak serum concentration of approximately 3 μg/mL is desirable
plus		
Gentamicin sulfate	2	
Vancomycin hydrochloride	4	Recommended for patients allergic to β-lactam antibiotics

From Wilson, W. R., Karchmer, A. W., Dajani, A. S., et al.: Antibiotic treatment of adults with infective endocarditis due to streptococci, enterococci, staphylococci, and HACEK microorganisms. J. A. M. A. *274*:1706–1713, 1995.

TABLE 32–10. Suggested Therapy for Native Valve Endocarditis Due to Strains of Viridans Streptococci and *Streptococcus bovis* Relatively Resistant to Penicillin G (MIC 0.1 μg/mL and 0.5 μg/mL) in Adults

Antibiotic(s)	Duration (wk)	Comments
Aqueous crystalline penicillin G sodium *plus*	4	Cefazolin or other first-generation cephalosporins may be substituted for penicillin in patients whose penicillin hypersensitivity is not of the immediate type
Gentamicin sulfate	2	
Vancomycin hydrochloride	4	Recommended for patients allergic to β-lactam antibiotics

From Wilson, W. R., Karchmer, A. W., Dajani, A. S., et al.: Antibiotic treatment of adults with infective endocarditis due to streptococci, enterococci, staphylococci, and HACEK microorganisms. J. A. M. A. *274*:1706–1713, 1995. Copyright 1990, American Medical Association.

The majority of strains of enterococci have an MIC to penicillin equal to or greater than 0.4 μg/mL and an MBC equal to or greater than 6.25 μg/mL.[273] All β-lactam antibiotics are bacteriostatic against enterococci and cannot be used alone. However, plasmid-mediated β-lactamase production has been found in rare strains of *Enterococcus faecalis*. Ampicillin-sulbactam overcomes the enzyme production and is effective in therapy.[392] Although therapy with penicillin alone is ineffective, the combination of penicillin and an aminoglycoside is synergistic and produces a bactericidal effect for most enterococcal strains.[256] Unfortunately, 20 to 50 per cent of enterococcal strains demonstrate very high resistance (MIC > 2000 μg/mL) to streptomycin, and synergy between penicillin and streptomycin does not occur.[154, 348] High-level resistance to gentamicin has been found in some isolates, and the incidence is increasing in some locales.[102, 227, 296] When these isolates are encountered, all aminoglycosides should be tested because the organism may be susceptible to one while resistant to others.[421] Fortunately, these strains rarely cause endocarditis.[273] Although vancomycin-resistant enterococci have emerged as important nosocomial pathogens,[123] they rarely cause endocarditis. Optimal therapy for these strains is not established, but a combination of high-dose penicillin plus vancomycin plus gentamicin may be effective in some cases.[49] The usual regimens for enterococcal endocarditis are listed in Table 32–11.

Most isolates of *S. aureus* are resistant to penicillin, but endocarditis due to penicillin-susceptible (MIC < 0.1 μg/mL) isolates should be treated with this agent. In general, a semisynthetic penicillinase-resistant penicillin given for 4 to 6 weeks is the drug of choice (Table 32–12). The addition of gentamicin to nafcillin produces an enhanced bactericidal effect in vitro and in experimental staphylococcal endocarditis in rabbits.[57, 339] However, the value of this combination in patients has not been proved,[341] and generally it is reserved for children with overwhelming infection. In penicillin-allergic patients or if the *S. aureus* is methicillin-resistant, vancomycin alone is recommended, although treatment failures in children with endocarditis have been reported.[110, 171, 223] Addition of rifampin or use of β-lactam drugs after desensitization is necessary in some cases.[20, 267] Ciprofloxacin has been used, but treatment failures have occurred due to emergence of resistance.[271, 389] Hospital-acquired infections with *S. epidermidis* usually are treated with vancomycin because of the high incidence of methicillin resistance among these isolates. The addition of rifampin and gentamicin to either nafcillin or vancomycin may increase bactericidal activity and is recommended in cases of prosthetic valve endocarditis secondary to staphylococci (Table 32–13).[33, 341, 430]

Therapy for endocarditis caused by gram-negative organisms must be individualized, based on in vitro susceptibility and synergy studies. Six to eight weeks of combination ther-

TABLE 32–11. Suggested Therapy for Endocarditis Due to Enterococci and Other Selected Streptococci* in Adults

Antibiotic(s)	Duration (wk)	Comments
Aqueous crystalline penicillin G sodium *plus*	4–6	Four-week therapy recommended for patients with symptoms <3 months in duration. Six-week therapy recommended for patients with symptoms >3 months in duration
Gentamicin sulfate	4–6	
Ampicillin sodium *plus*	4–6	
Gentamicin sulfate	4–6	
Vancomycin hydrochloride *plus*	4–6	Recommended for patients allergic to β-lactam antibiotics
Gentamicin sulfate	4–6	

*This table is for endocarditis due to gentamicin- or vancomycin-susceptible enterococci, viridans streptococci with an MIC >0.5 μg/mL, nutritionally variant viridans streptococci, or prosthetic valve endocarditis caused by viridans streptococci or *Streptococcus bovis*.

From Wilson, W. R., Karchmer, A. W., Dajani, A. S., et al.: Antibiotic treatment of adults with infective endocarditis due to streptococci, enterococci, staphylococci, and HACEK microorganisms. J. A. M. A. *274*:1706–1713, 1995. Copyright 1990, American Medical Association.

TABLE 32–12. Suggested Therapy for Endocarditis Due to Staphylococci in the Absence of Prosthetic Material in Adults

Antibiotic(s)	Duration	Comments
	*Methicillin-Susceptible Staphylococci**	
Nafcillin sodium or oxacillin sodium	4–6 wk	Benefit of additional aminoglycoside has not been established
Optional addition of Gentamicin sulfate	3–5 d	
Cefazolin or other first-generation cephalosporin	4–6 wk	For patients with nonimmediate type hypersensitivity to penicillin
Optional addition of Gentamicin sulfate	3–5 d	
Vancomycin hydrochloride	4–6 wk	Recommended for patients allergic to penicillin
	Methicillin-Resistant Staphylococci	
Vancomycin hydrochloride	4–6 wk	Addition of aminoglycoside or rifampin not recommended for routine use

*If *Staphylococcus* is penicillin-susceptible (MIC ≤0.1 μg/mL), aqueous crystalline penicillin G sodium can be used for 4 to 6 weeks instead of nafcillin or oxacillin.

From Wilson, W. R., Karchmer, A. W., Dajani, A. S., et al.: Antibiotic treatment of adults with infective endocarditis due to streptococci, enterococci, staphylococci, and HACEK microorganisms. J. A. M. A. *274*:1706–1713, 1995. Copyright 1990, American Medical Association.

apy with two or more drugs may be required, especially with endocarditis caused by *Klebsiella* or *Pseudomonas*.[119, 299] Surgical intervention frequently is necessary, especially for infection of the mitral or aortic valves. Endocarditis due to *Haemophilus* and other fastidious gram-negative organisms usually is responsive to ampicillin alone, but addition of an aminoglycoside may improve the outcome (Table 32–14).[63, 430] Anaerobic bacilli generally are susceptible to penicillin, but infection due to resistant *Bacillus fragilis* is treated best by combinations employing metronidazole, ticarcillin-clavulanate, or imipenem.

Survival rates of only 10 to 20 per cent in patients with fungal endocarditis are related to the poor ability of presently available antifungal agents to sterilize the vegetations. Only rare cures with medical therapy alone have been reported.[337] Most investigators believe that early surgical intervention is mandatory in every patient in whom there is conclusive evidence of intracardiac fungal infection.[406, 407] Only 33 cases of successful treatment of fungal prosthetic valve endocarditis have been reported, even when surgery was performed.[136] Whereas a prolonged course of antifungal therapy prior to operation does not improve outcome, chemotherapy should be given in conjunction with operative treatment. The drug of choice is amphotericin B at a dose of 0.5 to 1.0 mg/kg/day. This antibiotic may be either fungistatic or fungicidal, depending on the infecting organism. Although the toxicity of amphotericin B appears to be less severe in children than adults, side effects that may necessitate alterations in the usual regimen may occur. These include fever, chills, phlebitis, anemia, hypocalcemia, renal tubular acidosis, nephrotoxicity, and thrombocytopenia. The optimal dosage of amphotericin B is unknown; total doses of 20 to 50 mg/kg commonly are employed. 5-Fluorocytosine[254] and rifampin may act synergistically with amphotericin B against many strains of fungi, but their roles in fungal endocarditis are unproven. Fluconazole is less effective than amphotericin B

TABLE 32–13. Suggested Therapy for Endocarditis Due to Staphylococci in the Presence of Prosthetic Valve or Other Prosthetic Material in Adults

Antibiotic(s)	Duration (wk)	Comments
	Methicillin-Susceptible Staphylococci	
Nafcillin sodium or oxacillin sodium	≥6	First-generation cephalosporins or vancomycin should be used in patients allergic to β-lactam antibiotics
plus Rifampin	≥6	Rifampin plays a unique role in the eradication of staphylococci from prosthetic material
plus Gentamicin sulfate	2	
	Methicillin-Resistant Staphylococci	
Vancomycin hydrochloride	≥6	
plus Rifampin	≥6	
plus Gentamicin sulfate	2	

From Wilson, W. R., Karchmer, A. W., Dajani, A. S., et al.: Antibiotic treatment of adults with infective endocarditis due to streptococci, enterococci, staphylococci, and HACEK microorganisms. J. A. M. A. *274*:1706–1713, 1995. Copyright 1990, American Medical Association.

TABLE 32–14. Suggested Therapy for Endocarditis Due to HACEK* Organisms in Adults

Antibiotic(s)	Duration (wk)	Comments
Ceftriaxone sodium	4	Cefotaxime sodium or other third-generation cephalosporins may be substituted
Ampicillin sodium *plus*	4	
Gentamicin sulfate	4	

**Haemophilus* species, *Actinobacillus actinomycetemcomitans, Cardiobacterium hominis, Eikenella corrodens, Kingella kingae.*
From Wilson, W. R., Karchmer, A. W., Dajani, A. S., et al.: Antibiotic treatment of adults with infective endocarditis due to streptococci, enterococci, staphylococci, and HACEK microorganisms. J. A. M. A. *274*:1706–1713, 1995.

for the prophylaxis or treatment of experimental *Candida* endocarditis[431] but has been used successfully in a few patients.[74, 413]

Treatment for culture-negative endocarditis is problematic. In general, the same criteria used to choose empiric therapy for infective endocarditis can be employed. Antibiotics usually are continued for 6 weeks, and ongoing surveillance for an etiologic agent must be performed. In 52 adults with culture-negative endocarditis, survival correlated with initial clinical response to antibiotics; most deaths were caused by systemic emboli or congestive heart failure.[303]

Surgery has become a valuable adjunct to medical therapy in the management of infective endocarditis.[70, 260, 302, 309, 375] The generally accepted indications for surgical intervention during active endocarditis are as follows: (1) refractory congestive heart failure[258, 396]; (2) uncontrolled infection[241]; (3) more than one serious embolic episode; (4) fungal endocarditis; (5) most cases of prosthetic valve endocarditis[3, 18, 82, 105, 333]; and (6) local suppurative complications, including perivalvular or myocardial abscess with conduction system abnormalities.[385] The usual indication for surgical intervention is congestive heart failure in left-sided lesions and persistent infection in right-sided disease. Among children with endocarditis after a previous cardiac surgery, repair or takedown of infected graft material commonly is the reason for surgery.[287] In general, operative mortality is low even if surgery is performed during the active infection.[252, 270, 282] The hemodynamic status of the patient, rather than the activity of the infection, is the critical factor in determining the timing of cardiac surgery or valve replacement.[192] The aortic valve is the site most often requiring surgical intervention.[187, 311, 400]

PREVENTION

It is accepted medical practice to give prophylactic antibiotics to susceptible patients in an attempt to prevent infective endocarditis.[93, 199, 361] The rationale for such treatment is based on studies indicating that antibiotics can reduce the incidence of bacteremia after various procedures in humans[107] and can prevent experimental endocarditis in animals.[301] However, there have been no controlled trials to document the efficacy of endocarditis prophylaxis in humans.[411] Prevention of bacterial infection is most likely to be effective and cost-effective when a single antibiotic is directed against a single pathogen and when the disease occurs with high frequency in the absence of prophylaxis. Prevention of endocarditis does not meet these ideals because a variety of drugs are used against a variety of organisms, and the disease rarely occurs even if prophylaxis is not given.[93] Less than 10 per cent of all endo-

TABLE 32–15. Conditions and Procedures Related to Endocarditis Prophylaxis

Cardiac Conditions for Which Endocarditis Prophylaxis Is Recommended	Procedures for Which Endocarditis Prophylaxis Is Recommended
Prosthetic cardiac valves (mechanical and biosynthetic)	All dental procedures likely to induce gingival bleeding
Most congenital cardiac malformations	Tonsillectomy and/or adenoidectomy
Surgically constructed systemic-pulmonary shunts	Surgical procedures or biopsy involving respiratory mucosa
Rheumatic and other acquired valvular disease	Bronchoscopy, especially with a rigid scope
Idiopathic hypertrophic subaortic stenosis	Incision and drainage of infected tissue
History of bacterial endocarditis	Selected genitourinary and gastrointestinal procedures (cystoscopy, urethral catheterization, urinary tract surgery, gallbladder or colonic surgery, esophageal or anal dilatation, colonoscopy, upper gastrointestinal tract endoscopy with biopsy, proctosigmoidoscopic biopsy)
Mitral valve prolapse with valvular regurgitation	Cardiac surgery
Foreign material in the heart	*Not* routinely recommended for the following:
Not recommended for the following:	Orotracheal intubation
Isolated secundum atrial septal defect	Cardiac catheterization
Secundum atrial septal defect repaired without a patch 6 or more months earlier	Cesarean section
Patent ductus arteriosis ligated and divided 6 or more months earlier	Therapeutic abortion
Cardiac pacemaker	Intrauterine device insertion or removal
	Tympanostomy tube insertion
	Shedding of primary teeth

From Dajani, A. S., Bisno, A. L., Chung, K. J., et al.: Prevention of bacterial endocarditis: Recommendations by the American Heart Association. J. A. M. A. *264*:2919–2922, 1990.

TABLE 32–16. Recommended Antibiotic Regimens for Endocarditis Prophylaxis in Children

For Dental/Respiratory Tract Procedures			For Gastrointestinal/Genitourinary Procedures		
Regimen	***Condition***	***Dosage***	***Regimen***	***Condition***	***Dosage***
Standard	For dental procedures that cause gingival bleeding and oral/ respiratory tract surgery	Amoxicillin (<15 kg, 750 mg; 15–30 kg, 1500 mg; >30 kg, 3000 mg) one weight-appropriate dose 1 hr before the procedure, then one-half dose 6 hr later; for patients unable to take oral medications, ampicillin (50 mg/kg) IV or IM 30 min before the procedure, then 25 mg/kg 6 hr later	Standard	For genitourinary/ gastrointestinal tract procedures indicated	Ampicillin (50 mg/kg IM or IV) plus gentamicin (2.0 mg/kg IM or IV) given 30 min to 1 hr before procedure followed by amoxicillin (25 mg/kg) 6 hr later; alternatively, parenteral regimen may be given 8 hr later
Special	Parenteral regimen for use when maximal protection desired, e.g., for patients with prosthetic valves	Ampicillin (50 mg/kg IM or IV) plus gentamicin (2.0 mg/kg IM or IV) one-half hour before the procedure, followed by amoxicillin (25 mg/kg) 6 hr later; alternatively, parenteral regimen may be repeated once 8 hr later	Special	Oral regimen for minor or repetitive procedures in low-risk patients	Amoxicillin (50 mg/kg) orally 1 hr before procedure and 25 mg/ kg 6 hr later
	Oral regimen for penicillin-allergic patients and those receiving rheumatic fever prophylaxis	Erythromycin (20 mg/ kg) orally 2 hr before, then 10 mg/kg 6 hr later or clindamycin (10 mg/kg) orally 1 hr before, then 5 mg/kg 6 hr later		Penicillin-allergic patients	Vancomycin (15–20 mg/ kg IV) plus gentamicin (2 mg/kg IM or IV) 1 hr before procedure; may be repeated once 8 hr later
	Parenteral regimen for penicillin-allergic patients and those receiving rheumatic fever prophylaxis	Vancomycin (15–20 mg/ kg IV) 1 hr before; no repeated dose is necessary			

*From Dajani, A. S., Bisno, A. L., Chung, K. J., et al.: Prevention of bacterial endocarditis: Recommendations by the American Heart Association. J. A. M. A. *264*:2919–2922, 1990. Copyright 1990, American Medical Association.

carditis cases can be attributed to bacteremias caused by previous medical, surgical, or dental procedures.[409] A number of cases of prophylaxis failure have been reported,[96] but only 12 per cent of those patients received antibiotic regimens recommended by the American Heart Association. For reasons that are not clear, mitral valve prolapse was the condition most frequently associated with prophylaxis failure. The most common errors in attempted endocarditis prevention include inadequate medical histories by dentists and other health professionals to identify high-risk patients, starting prophylactic antibiotics too early, continuing preventive therapy too long, use of low-dose antibiotics, lack of prophylaxis for minor dental procedures, and confusion between prevention of rheumatic fever and prevention of infective endocarditis. Several studies have shown that adult patients at risk for infective endocarditis often have inadequate knowledge of their cardiac lesion, endocarditis, and recommended prophylaxis.[56, 410]

The Committee on Rheumatic Fever, Endocarditis and Kawasaki Disease of the Council on Cardiovascular Diseases in the Young of the American Heart Association has published recommendations for bacterial endocarditis prophylaxis.[76] The cardiac conditions and procedures for which endocarditis prophylaxis is indicated are listed in Table 32–15. The recommended antibiotic regimens are shown in Table 32–16. The major change in the most recent recommendations is the suggested use of amoxicillin—instead of penicillin V—for standard oral prophylaxis. Amoxicillin is recommended because it is absorbed better from the gastrointestinal tract and provides higher and more sustained serum levels. Endocarditis prophylaxis also is recommended for patients with indwelling transvenous cardiac pacemakers, ventriculoatrial shunts for hydrocephalus, and arteriovenous shunts for renal dialysis.[76]

References

1. Agarwala, B. N.: Group B streptococcal endocarditis in a neonate. Pediatr. Cardiol. *9*:51–53, 1988.
2. Alpert, J. S., Krous, H. F., Dalen, J. E., et al.: Pathogenesis of Osler's nodes. Ann. Intern. Med. *85*:471–476, 1976.
3. Alsip, S. G., Blackstone, E. H., Kirklin, J. W., et al.: Indications for cardiac

surgery in patients with infective endocarditis. Am. J. Med. 78:138–142, 1985.
4. Anderson, A. W., and Cruickshank, J. G.: Endocarditis due to viridans-type streptococci tolerant to beta-lactam antibiotics: Therapeutic problems. Br. Med. J. 285:85, 1982.
5. Andriole, V. T., Kravetz, H. M., Roberts, W. C., et al.: *Candida* endocarditis: Clinical and pathologic studies. Am. J. Med. 32:251–284, 1962.
6. Anolik, R., Berkowitz, R. J., Campos, J. M., et al.: *Actinobacillus* endocarditis associated with peridontal disease. Clin. Pediatr. 20:633–655, 1981.
7. Arber, N., Militano, A., Ben-Yehuda, A., et al.: Native valve *Staphylococcus epidermidis* endocarditis: Report of seven cases and review of the literature. Am. J. Med. 90:758, 1991.
8. Arber, N., Pras, E., Copperman, Y., et al.: Pacemaker endocarditis: Report of 44 cases and review of the literature. Medicine 73:299–305, 1994.
9. Backes, R. J., Wilson, W. R., and Geraci, J. E.: Group B streptococcal infective endocarditis. Arch. Intern. Med. 145:693–696, 1985.
10. Baddour, L. M., and Bisno, A. L.: Infective endocarditis complicating mitral valve prolapse: Epidemiologic, clinical and microbiological aspects. Rev. Infect. Dis. 8:117–137, 1986.
11. Baddour, L. M., Christensen, G. D., Lowrance, J. H., et al.: Pathogenesis of experimental endocarditis. Rev. Infect. Dis. 11:452–463, 1989.
12. Baddour, L. M., Phillips, T. N., and Bisno, A. L.: Coagulase-negative staphylococcal endocarditis: Occurrence in patients with mitral valve prolapse. Arch. Intern. Med. 146:119–121, 1986.
13. Baddour, L. M., Meyer, J., and Henry, B.: Polymicrobial infective endocarditis in the 1980's. Rev. Infect. Dis. 13:963–970, 1991.
14. Baddour, L. M., Lowrance, C., Albus, A., et al.: *Staphylococcus aureus* microcapsule expression attenuates bacterial virulence in a rat model of experimental endocarditis. J. Infect. Dis. 165:749–753, 1992.
15. Baltimore, R. S.: Infective endocarditis in children. Pediatr. Infect. Dis. J. 11:907–912, 1992.
16. Barst, R. J., Prince, A. S., and Neu, H. C.: *Aspergillus* endocarditis: Case report and review of the literature. Pediatrics 68:73–78, 1981.
17. Barst, R. J., Prince, A. S., and Neu, H. C.: Echocardiography in *Aspergillus* endocarditis. Pediatrics 69:252–253, 1982.
18. Baumgartner, W. A., Miller, D. C., Reitz, B. A., et al.: Surgical treatment of prosthetic valve endocarditis. Ann. Thorac. Surg. 35:87–104, 1983.
19. Bayer, A. S.: Staphylococcal bacteremia and endocarditis: State of the art. Arch. Intern. Med. 142:1169–1177, 1982.
20. Bayer, A. S.: Infective endocarditis. Clin. Infect. Dis. 17:313–332, 1993.
21. Bayer, A. S., Chow, A. W., and Guze, L. B.: *Listeria monocytogenes* endocarditis: Report of a case and review of the literature. Am. J. Med. Sci. 273:319–323, 1977.
22. Bayer, A. S., Nelson, R. J., and Slama, T. G.: Current concepts in prevention of prosthetic valve endocarditis. Chest 97:1203–1207, 1990.
23. Bayer, A. S., and Theofilopoulos, A. N.: Immunopathogenetic aspects of infective endocarditis. Chest 97:204–212, 1990.
24. Bayer, A. S., Theofilopoulos, A. N., Dixon, F. J., et al.: Circulating immune complexes in experimental streptococcal endocarditis: A monitor of therapeutic efficacy. J. Infect. Dis. 139:1–8, 1979.
25. Bayer, A. S., Theofilopoulos, A. N., Eisenberg, R., et al.: Circulating immune complexes in infective endocarditis. N. Engl. J. Med. 295:1500–1505, 1976.
26. Bayer, A. S., Theofilopoulos, A. N., Tillman, D. B., et al.: Use of circulating immune complex levels in the serodifferentiation of endocarditic and nonendocarditic septicemias. Am. J. Med. 66:58–62, 1979.
27. Beeson, P. B., Brannon, E. S., and Warren, J. V.: Observations on the sites of removal of bacteria from the blood in patients with bacterial endocarditis. J. Exp. Med. 81:9–23, 1945.
28. Belik, J., Flinn, G., Rivera, G., et al.: Successful management of bacterial endocarditis of the mitral valve due to *Staphylococcus epidermidis* in an immunosuppressed host. Acta Paediatr. Scand. 69:731–734, 1980.
29. Berkowitz, F. E., and Dansky, R.: Infective endocarditis in black South African children: Report of 10 cases with some unusual features. Pediatr. Infect. Dis. 8:787–791, 1989.
30. Bertorini, T. E., Laster, R. E., Thompson, B. F., et al.: Magnetic resonance imaging of the brain in bacterial endocarditis. Arch. Intern. Med. 149:815–817, 1989.
31. Bieger, R. C., Brewer, N. S., and Washington, J. A.: *Haemophilus aphrophilus*: A microbiological and clinical review and report of 42 cases. Medicine 57:345–355, 1978.
32. Biller, J., Challa, V. R., Toole, J. F., et al.: Nonbacterial thrombotic endocarditis: A neurologic perspective of clinicopathologic correlations of 99 patients. Arch. Neurol. 39:95–98, 1982.
33. Bisno, A. L., Dismukes, W. E., Durack, D. T., et al.: Antimicrobial treatment of infective endocarditis due to viridans streptococci, enterococci and staphylococci. J. A. M. A. 261:1471–1477, 1989.
34. Blair, D. C., and Martin, D. B.: Beta hemolytic streptococcal endocarditis: Predominance of non–group A organisms. Am. J. Med. Sci. 276:269–277, 1978.
35. Blieden, L. C., Morehead, R. R., Burke, B., et al.: Bacterial endocarditis in the neonate. Am. J. Dis. Child. 124:747–749, 1972.
36. Blumberg, E. A., Karlis, D. A., Chandrasekaran, K., et al.: Endocarditis-associated paravalvular abscesses. Chest 107:898–903, 1995.
37. Blumberg, E. A., Robbins, N., Adimora, A., et al.: Persistent fever in association with infective endocarditis. Clin. Infect. Dis. 15:983–990, 1992.
38. Blumenthal, S., Griffiths, S. P., and Morgan, B. C.: Bacterial endocarditis in children with heart disease: A review based on the literature and experience with 58 cases. Pediatrics 26:993–1017, 1960.
39. Bodey, G. P., and Luna, M.: Skin lesions associated with disseminated Candidiasis. J. A. M. A. 229:1466–1468, 1974.
40. Bricker, J., Latson, L., Huhta, J., et al.: Echocardiographic evaluation of infective endocarditis in children. Clin. Pediatr. 24:312–319, 1985.
41. Brodie, E., Adler, J. L., and Daly, A. K.: Bacterial endocarditis due to an unusual species of encapsulated *Neisseria*. Am. J. Dis. Child. 122:433–437, 1972.
42. Bruyn, G. A. W., Thompson, J., and Van Der Meer, J. W. M.: Pneumococcal endocarditis in adult patients: A report of five cases and review of the literature. Q. J. Med. 74:33–40, 1990.
43. Bryan, C. S., Marney, S. R., Alford, R. H., et al.: Gram-negative bacillary endocarditis: Interpretation of the serum bactericidal test. Am. J. Med. 58:204–215, 1975.
44. Buda, A. J., Zotz, R. J., Le Mire, M. S., et al.: Prognostic significance of vegetations detected by two-dimensional echocardiography in infective endocarditis. Am. Heart J. 112:1291–1296, 1986.
45. Calderwood, S., Swinski, L., Waternaux, C., et al.: Risk factors for the development of prosthetic valve endocarditis. Circulation 72:31–37, 1985.
46. Caldwell, R. L., Hurwitz, R. A., and Girod, D. A.: Subacute bacterial endocarditis in children. Am. J. Dis. Child. 122:312–315, 1971.
47. Canter, M. C., and Hart, R. G.: Neurologic complications of infective endocarditis. Neurology 41:1015, 1991.
48. Carey, R. B., Gross, K. C., and Roberts, R. B.: Vitamin B_6–dependent *Streptococcus mitior (mitis)* isolated from patients with systemic infections. J. Infect. Dis. 131:722–725, 1975.
49. Caron, F., Carbon, C., and Gutmann, L.: Triple-combination penicillin-vancomycin-gentamicin for experimental endocarditis caused by a moderately penicillin- and highly glycopeptide-resistant isolate of *Enterococcus faecium*. J. Infect. Dis. 164:888–893, 1991.
50. Carpenter, J. L.: Perivalvular extension of infection in patients with infectious endocarditis. Rev. Infect. Dis. 13:127–138, 1991.
51. Carr, P., Wright, M., and Handler, L. C.: Endocarditis-related cerebral aneurysms: Radiologic changes with treatment. Am. J. Neuroradiol. 16:745, 1995.
52. Carrizosa, J., and Kaye, D.: Antibiotic concentrations in serum, serum bactericidal activity, and results of therapy of streptococcal endocarditis in rabbits. Antimicrob. Agents Chemother. 12:479–483, 1977.
53. Carruthers, M.: Endocarditis due to enteric bacilli other than salmonellae: Case reports and literature review. Am. J. Med. Sci. 273:203, 1977.
54. Carvajal, A., and Frederiksen, W.: Fatal endocarditis due to *Listeria monocytogenes*. Rev. Infect. Dis. 10:616–623, 1988.
55. Cassling, R. S., Rogler, W. C., and McManus, B. M.: Isolated pulmonic valve infective endocarditis: A diagnostically elusive entity. Am. Heart J. 109:558–567, 1985.
56. Cetta, F., and Warnes, C. A.: Adults with congenital heart disease: Patient knowledge of endocarditis prophylaxis. Mayo Clin. Proc. 70:50–54, 1995.
57. Chambers, H. F.: Short-course combination and oral therapies of *Staphylococcus aureus* endocarditis. Infect. Dis. Clin. North Am. 7:69–80, 1993.
58. Chambers, H. F., Korzeniowski, O. M., Sande, M. A., et al.: *Staphylococcus aureus* endocarditis: Clinical manifestation in addicts and non-addicts. Medicine 62:170–174, 1983.
59. Chambers, H. F., Miller, R. T., and Newman, M. D.: Right-sided *Staphylococcus aureus* endocarditis in intravenous drug abusers: Two-week combination therapy. Ann. Intern. Med. 109:619–624, 1988.
60. Channer, K. S., Joffe, H. S., and Jordan, S. C.: Presentation of infective endocarditis in childhood and adolescence. J. R. Coll. Physicians Lond. 23:152–155, 1989.
61. Charney, R., Keltz, T. N., Attai, L., et al.: Acute valvular obstruction from streptococcal endocarditis. Am. Heart J. 125:544, 1993.
62. Chen, M.-R.: Infective endocarditis in hypertrophic obstructive cardiomyopathy. J. Clin. Ultrasound 20:612–614, 1992.
63. Chunn, C. J., Jones, S. R., McCutchan, J. A., et al.: *Haemophilus parainfluenzae* infective endocarditis. Medicine 56:99–113, 1977.
64. Churchill, M. A., Geraci, J. E., and Hunder, G. G.: Musculoskeletal manifestations of bacterial endocarditis. Ann. Intern. Med. 87:754–759, 1977.
65. Clawson, C. C., Rao Gunda, H. R., and White, J. G.: Platelet interaction with bacteria. IV. Stimulation of the release reaction. Am. J. Pathol. 81:411–417, 1975.
66. Clemens, J. O., Horwitz, R. I., Jaffee, C. C., et al.: A controlled evaluation of the risk of bacterial endocarditis in persons with mitral-valve prolapse. N. Engl. J. Med. 307:776–781, 1982.
67. Cofsky, R. D., and Seligman, S. J.: *Peptococcus magnus* endocarditis. South. Med. J. 78:361–362, 1985.
68. Coleman, D. L., Horwitz, R. I., and Andriole, V. T.: Association between serum inhibitory and bactericidal concentrations and therapeutic outcome in bacterial endocarditis. Am. J. Med. 73:260–267, 1982.
69. Come, P.: Infective endocarditis: Current perspectives. Compr. Ther. 8:57–70, 1982.
70. Cooley, D. A.: Surgical considerations in infective endocarditis. Tex. Heart Inst. J. 16:263–269, 1989.

71. Corrigan, D., Bolen, J., Hancock, E. W., et al.: Mitral valve prolapse and endocarditis. Am. J. Med. *63*:315–318, 1977.
72. Cremieux, A.-C., and Carbon, C.: Pharmacokinetics and pharmacodynamic requirements for antibiotic therapy of experimental endocarditis. Antimicrob. Agents Chemother. *36*:2069–2074, 1992.
73. Cutler, J. G., Ongley, P. A., Schwachman, H., et al.: Bacterial endocarditis in children with heart disease. Pediatrics *22*:706–714, 1958.
74. Czwerwiec, F. S., Bilsker, M. S., Kamerman, M. L., et al.: Long-term survival after fluconazole therapy of candidal prosthetic valve endocarditis. Am. J. Med. *94*:545–546, 1993.
75. Daher, A. H., and Berkowitz, F. E.: Infective endocarditis in neonates. Clin. Pediatr. *20*:198–206, 1995.
76. Dajani, A. S., Bisno, A. L., Chung, K. J., et al.: Prevention of bacterial endocarditis: Recommendations by the American Heart Association. J. A. M. A. *264*:2919–2922, 1990.
77. Danchin, N., Voiriot, P., Briancon, S., et al.: Mitral valve prolapse as a risk factor for infective endocarditis. Lancet *1*:743–745, 1989.
78. Danford, D. A., Kugler, J. D., Cheatham, J. P., et al.: *Hemophilus influenzae* endocarditis: Successful treatment with ampicillin and early valve replacement. Neb. Med. J. *38*:88–91, 1984.
79. Daniel, W. G., Erbel, R., Kasper, W., et al.: Safety of transesophageal echocardiography: A multicenter survey of 10,419 examinations. Circulation *83*:817–821, 1991.
80. Daniel, W. G., Mugge, A., Grote, J., et al.: Evaluation of endocarditis and its complications by biplane and multiplane transesophageal echocardiography. Am. J. Cardiac Imag. *9*:100–105, 1995.
81. Daniel, W. G., Mugge, A., Martin, R. P., et al.: Improvement in the diagnosis of abscesses associated with endocarditis by transesophageal echocardiography. N. Engl. J. Med. *324*:795–800, 1991.
82. David, T. E.: The surgical treatment of patients with prosthetic valve endocarditis. Semin. Thorac. Cardiovasc. Surg. *7*:47–53, 1995.
83. Davidson, S., Rotem, Y., Bogkowski, B., et al.: *Corynebacterium diphtheriae* endocarditis. Am. J. Med. Sci. *271*:351–353, 1976.
84. Davis, R. S., Strom, J. A., Frishman, W., et al.: The demonstration of vegetations by echocardiography in bacterial endocarditis: An indication for early surgical intervention. Am. J. Med. *57*:69, 1980.
85. Del Pont, J. M., DeCicco, L. T., Vartalitis, C., et al.: Infective endocarditis in children: Clinical analyses and evaluation of two diagnostic criteria. Pediatr. Infect. Dis. J. *14*:1079–1086, 1995.
86. Delvecchio, G., Fracassetti, O., and Lorenzi, N.: *Brucella* endocarditis. Int. J. Cardiol. *33*:328–329, 1991.
87. Dillon, T., Meyer, R. A., Korfhagen, J. C., et al.: Management of infective endocarditis using echocardiography. J. Pediatr. *96*:552–558, 1980.
88. DiNubile, M. J., Calderwood, S. B., Steinhaus, D. M., et al.: Cardiac conduction abnormalities complicating native valve active infective endocarditis. Am. J. Cardiol. *58*:1213–1217, 1986.
89. DiNubile, M. J.: Treatment of endocarditis caused by relatively resistant nonenterococcal streptococci: Is penicillin enough? Rev. Infect. Dis. *12*:112–117, 1990.
90. Douglas, A., Moore-Gillon, J., and Eykyn, S.: Fever during treatment of infective endocarditis. Lancet *1*:1341–1343, 1986.
91. Downing, G. J., and Spirazza, C.: Group C beta-hemolytic streptococcal endocarditis. Pediatr. Infect. Dis. *5*:703–704, 1986.
92. Drancourt, M., Mainardi, J. L., Brouqui, P., et al.: *Bartonella (Rochalimaea) quintana* endocarditis in three homeless men. N. Engl. J. Med. *332*:419–423, 1995.
93. Durack, D. T.: Prevention of infective endocarditis. N. Engl. J. Med. *332*:38–44, 1995.
94. Durack, D. T., and Beeson, P. B.: Protective role of complement in experimental *Escherichia coli* endocarditis. Infect. Immun. *16*:213–214, 1977.
95. Durack, D. T., Beeson, P. B., and Petersdorf, R. G.: Experimental bacterial endocarditis. III. Production and progress of the disease in rabbits. Br. J. Exp. Pathol. *54*:142–151, 1973.
96. Durack, D. T., Kaplan, E. L., and Bisno, A. L.: Apparent failure of endocarditis prophylaxis: Analysis of 52 cases submitted to a national registry. J. A. M. A. *250*:2318–2322, 1983.
97. Durack, D. T., Lukes, A. S., Bright, D. K., et al.: New criteria for diagnosis of infective endocarditis: Utilization of specific echocardiographic findings. Am. J. Med. *96*:200–209, 1994.
98. Durack, D. T., Pelletier, L. L., and Petersdorf, R. G.: Chemotherapy of experimental streptococcal endocarditis. II. Synergism between penicillin and streptomycin against penicillin-sensitive streptococci. J. Clin. Invest. *53*:829–836, 1974.
99. Durack, D. T., and Petersdorf, R. G.: Changes in the epidemiology of endocarditis. *In* Kaplan, E. L., and Taranta, A. V. (eds.): Infective Endocarditis: An American Heart Association Symposium. Dallas, American Heart Association, 1977, p. 3.
100. Edwards, K., Hruby, N., and Christy, C.: Pneumococcal endocarditis in infants and children: Report of a case and review of the literature. Pediatr. Infect. Dis. *9*:652–657, 1990.
101. Edwards, K., Ingall, D., Czapek, E., et al.: Bacterial endocarditis in 4 young infants: Is this complication on the increase? Clin. Pediatr. *16*:607–609, 1977.
102. Eliopoulos, G. M., Thauvin-Elioposlos, C., and Moellering, R. C., Jr.: Contribution of animal models in the search for effective therapy for endocarditis due to enterococci with high-level resistance to gentamicin. Clin. Infect. Dis. *15*:58–62, 1992.
103. Elward, K., Hruby, N., and Christy, C.: Pneumococcal endocarditis in infants and children: Report of a case and review of the literature. Pediatr. Infect. Dis. J. *9*:652–657, 1990.
104. Enzler, M. J., Rouse, M. S., Henry, N. K., et al.: In vitro and in vivo studies of streptomycin-resistant, penicillin-susceptible streptococci from patients with infective endocarditis. J. Infect. Dis. *155*:954–958, 1987.
105. Ergin, M. A.: Surgical techniques in prosthetic valve endocarditis. Semin. Thorac. Cardiovasc. Surg. *7*:54–56, 1995.
106. Esperson, F., and Frimodt-Moller, N.: *Staphylococcus aureus* endocarditis: A review of 119 cases. Arch. Intern. Med. *146*:1118–1121, 1986.
107. Everett, E. D., and Hirschmann, J. U.: Transient bacteremia and endocarditis prophylaxis: A review. Medicine *56*:61–77, 1977.
108. Fang, G., Keys, T. F., Gentry, L. O., et al: Prosthetic valve endocarditis resulting from nosocomial bacteremia. Ann. Intern. Med. *119*:560, 1993.
109. Farrior, J. B., and Silverman, M. E.: A consideration of the differences between a Janeway lesion and an Osler's node in infectious endocarditis. Chest *70*:239–243, 1976.
110. Faville, R. J., Zaska, D. E., Kaplan, E. L., et al.: *Staphylococcus aureus* endocarditis: Combined therapy with vancomycin and rifampin. J. A. M. A. *240*:1963–1965, 1978.
111. Feder, H. M., Olsen, N., McLaughlin, J. C., et al.: Bacterial endocarditis caused by vitamin B_6-dependent viridans group *Streptococcus*. Pediatrics *66*:309–312, 1980.
112. Feder, H. M., Chameides, L., and Diana, D. J.: Bacterial endocarditis complicated by myocardial infarction in a pediatric patient. J. A. M. A. *247*:1315–1316, 1982.
113. Felius, A., Fleer, A., and Mouloert, A.: *Actinobacillus actinomycetemcomitans* endocarditis in a child with a prosthetic heart valve. Infection *12*:260–261, 1984.
114. Felmer, J. M., and Dowell, V. R.: Anaerobic bacterial endocarditis. N. Engl. J. Med. *283*:1188–1192, 1970.
115. Fernandez, G. C., Chapman, A. J., Bolli, R., et al.: Gonococcal endocarditis: A case series demonstrating modern presentation of an old disease. Am. Heart J. *108*:1326–1334, 1984.
116. Fernandez-Guerrero, M. L., Torres-Perea, R., Gomez-Rodrigo, J., et al.: Infectious endocarditis due to non-typhi *Salmonella* in patients infected with human immunodeficiency virus: Report of two cases and review. Clin. Infect. Dis. *22*:853–855, 1996.
117. Fernandez-Guerrero, M. L., Verdejo, C., Azofra, J., et al.: Hospital-acquired infectious endocarditis not associated with cardiac survey: An emerging problem. Clin. Infect. Dis. *20*:16–23, 1995.
118. Fernicola, D. J., and Roberts, W. C.: Clinicopathologic features of active infective endocarditis isolated to the native mitral valve. Am. J. Cardiol. *71*:1186–1197, 1993.
119. Fichtenbaum, C. H., and Smith, M. J.: Treatment of endocarditis due to *Pseudomonas aeruginosa* with imipenem. Clin. Infect. Dis. *14*:353–354, 1992.
120. Fisher, R. G., Moodie, D. S., and Rice, R.: Pediatric bacterial endocarditis: Long-term follow-up. Cleve. Clin. Q. *52*:41–45, 1985.
121. Francioli, P., Etienne, J., Hoigue, R., et al.: Treatment of streptococcal endocarditis with a single daily dose of ceftriaxone sodium for 4 weeks: Efficacy and outpatient treatment feasibility. J. A. M. A. *267*:264–267, 1992.
122. Francioli, P., Ruch, W., Stamboulian, D., et al.: Treatment of streptococcal endocarditis with a single daily dose of ceftriaxone and netilmicin for 14 days: A prospective multicenter study. Clin. Infect. Dis. *21*:1406–1410, 1995.
123. Frieden, T. R., Munsiff, S. S., Low, D. E., et al.: Emergence of vancomycin-resistant enterococci in New York City. Lancet *342*:76–78, 1993.
124. Fukushige, J., Igarashi, H., and Veda, K.: Spectrum of infective endocarditis during infancy and childhood: 20-year review. Pediatr. Cardiol. *15*:127–131, 1994.
125. Gallagher, P. G., and Watanakunakorn, C.: Group B streptococcal endocarditis: Report of seven cases and review of the literature. Rev. Infect. Dis. *8*:175–188, 1986.
126. Garty, B., Berant, M., Weinhouse, E., et al.: False aneurysm of the right ventricle due to endocarditis in a child. Pediatr. Cardiol. *8*:275–277, 1987.
127. Gelfand, M. S., and Threlkeld, M. G.: Subacute bacterial endocarditis secondary to *Streptococcus pneumoniae*. Am. J. Med. *93*:91, 1992.
128. Gelfman, R., and Levine, S. A.: The incidence of acute and subacute bacterial endocarditis in congenital heart disease. Am. J. Med. Sci. *204*:324–333, 1942.
129. Geraci, J. E., and Wilson, W. R.: Endocarditis due to gram-negative bacteria. Mayo Clin. Proc. *57*:145–148, 1982.
130. Gersony, W. M., and Hayes, C. J.: Bacterial endocarditis in patients with pulmonary stenosis, aortic stenosis or ventricular septal defect. Circulation *56*:84–89, 1977.
131. Gersony, W. M., Hayes, C. J., Driscoll, D. J., et al.: Bacterial endocarditis in patients with aortic stenosis, pulmonary stenosis, or ventricular septal defect. Circulation *87*(Suppl. 1):121–126, 1993.
132. Gersony, W. M., and Hordof, A. J.: Infective endocarditis and diseases of the pericardium. Pediatr. Clin. North Am. *25*:831–846, 1978.
133. Geva, T., and Frand, M.: Infective endocarditis in children with congenital heart disease: The changing spectrum, 1965–85. Eur. Heart J. *9*:1244–1249, 1988.

134. Ghann, J. W., and Dismukes, W. E.: Prosthetic valve endocarditis: An overview. Kardiovaskulare Erkrankungan *8*:320–331, 1983.
135. Gil-Grande, R., Aguado, J. M., Pastor, C., et al.: Conventional viral cultures and shell vial assay for diagnosis of apparently culture-negative *Coxiella burnetii* endocarditis. Eur. J. Clin. Microbiol. Infect. Dis. *14*:64–67, 1995.
136. Gilbert, H. M., Peters, E. D., Lang, S. J., et al.: Successful treatment of fungal prosthetic valve endocarditis: Case report and review. Clin. Infect. Dis. *22*:348–354, 1996.
137. Glauser, M.P., Bernard, J. P., Moreillon, P., et al.: Successful single-dose amoxicillin prophylaxis against experimental streptococcal endocarditis: Evidence for two mechanisms of protection. J. Infect. Dis. *147*:568–575, 1983.
138. Goessler, M. C., Riggs, T. W., DeLeon, S., et al.: Echocardiographic diagnosis of tricuspid valve endocarditis in a child with a normal heart. Pediatr. Cardiol. *2*:141–143, 1982.
139. Goldberg, P., Shulman, S. T., and Yogev, R.: Group C streptococcal endocarditis. Pediatrics *75*:114–116, 1985.
140. Gorby, G. L., and Peacock, J. E.: *Erysipelothrix rhusiopathiae* endocarditis: Microbiologic, epidemiologic and clinical features of an occupational disease. Rev. Infect. Dis. *10*:317–325, 1988.
141. Gould, K., Ramirez-Ronda, C. H., Holmes, R. K., et al.: Adherence of bacteria to heart valves in vitro. J. Clin. Invest. *56*:1364–1370, 1975.
142. Gradon, J. D., Chapnick, E. K., and Lutwick, L. I.: Infective endocarditis of a native valve due to *Acinetobacter*: Case report and review. Clin. Infect. Dis. *14*:1145–1148, 1992.
143. Gransden, W. R., Eykyn, S. J., and Leach, R. M.: Neurologic presentations of native valve endocarditis. Q. J. Med. *73*:1135–1142, 1989.
144. Griffiths, J. K., Daly, J. S., and Dodge, R. A.: Two cases of endocarditis due to *Lactobacillus* species: Antimicrobial susceptibility, review and discussion of therapy. Clin. Infect. Dis. *15*:250–255, 1992.
145. Guard, R. W.: Non-toxigenic *Corynebacterium diphtheriae* causing subacute bacterial endocarditis: Case report. Pathology *11*:533–535, 1979.
146. Gutman, R. A., Striker, G. E., Gilliland, B. C., et al.: The immune complex glomerulonephritis of bacterial endocarditis. Medicine *51*:1–5, 1972.
147. Hall, B., and Dowling, H. F.: Negative blood cultures in bacterial endocarditis: A decade's experience. Med. Clin. North Am. *50*:159–170, 1966.
148. Hall, L. H., and Herndon, B. L.: Association of cell adherent glycocalyx and endocarditis production by viridans group streptococci. J. Clin. Microbiol. *28*:1698–1700, 1990.
149. Hamoudi, A. C., Hriban, M. M., Marcon, M. J., et al.: Clinical relevance of viridans and nonhemolytic streptococci isolated from blood and cerebrospinal fluid in a pediatric population. Am. J. Clin. Pathol. *93*:270, 1990.
150. Hampton, J. R., and Harrison, M. J.: Sterile blood cultures in bacterial endocarditis. Q. J. Med. *36*:167–174, 1967.
151. Hart, R. G., Foster, J. W., Luther, M. F., et al.: Stroke in infective endocarditis. Stroke *21*:695–700, 1990.
152. Hayek, L. J. H. E.: *Erysipelothrix* endocarditis affecting a porcine xenograft heart valve. J. Infect. *27*:203, 1993.
153. Heiddal, S., Sverrisson, J. T., Ynguason, E. E., et al.: Native-valve endocarditis due to *Neisseria sicca*: Case report and review. Clin. Infect. Dis. *16*:667–670, 1993.
154. Hellinger, W. C., Rouse, M. S., Robadan, P. M., et al.: Continuous intravenous versus intermittent ampicillin therapy of experimental endocarditis caused by aminoglycoside-resistant enterococci. Antimicrob. Agents Chemother. *36*:1272–1275, 1992.
155. Hendrix, H., Lindhout, T., Mertens, K., et al.: Activation of human prothrombin by stoichiometric levels of staphylocoagulase. J. Biol. Chem. *258*:3637–3644, 1983.
156. Herbert, M. A., Milford, D. V., Silove, E. D., et al.: Secondary amyloidosis from long-standing bacterial endocarditis. Pediatr. Nephrol. 9:33–35, 1995.
157. Herzberg, M. C., Brintzenhote, K. C., and Clawson, C. C.: Aggregation of human platelets and adhesion of *Streptococcus sanguis*. Infect. Immun. *39*:1457–1469, 1983.
158. Herzberg, M. C., MacFarlane, G. D., Gong, K., et al.: The platelet interactivity phenotype of *Streptococcus sanguis* influences the course of experimental endocarditis. Infect. Immun. *60*:4809–4818, 1992.
159. Hickey, A. J., MacMahon, S. W., and Wilcken, D. E. L.: Mitral valve prolapse and bacterial endocarditis: When is antibiotic prophylaxis necessary? Am. Heart J. *109*:431–435, 1985.
160. Hoen, B., Selton-Suty, C., Danchin, N., et al.: Evaluation of the Duke criteria versus the Beth Israel criteria for the diagnosis of infective endocarditis. Clin. Infect. Dis. *21*:905, 1995.
161. Hoen, B., Selton-Suty, C., Lacassin, F., et al.: Infective endocarditis in patients with negative blood cultures: Analysis of 88 cases from a one-year nationwide survey in France. Clin. Infect. Dis. *20*:501–506, 1995.
162. Holmes, A. H., Greenough, T. C., Balady, G. L., et al.: *Bartonella henselae* endocarditis in an immunocompetent adult. Clin. Infect. Dis. *21*:1004–1007, 1995.
163. Horwitz, D., Quismorio, F. P., and Friou, G. J.: Cryoglobulinemia in patients with infective endocarditis. Clin. Exp. Immunol. *19*:131–137, 1975.
164. Hosea, S. W.: Virulent *Streptococcus viridans* bacterial endocarditis. Am. Heart J. *101*:174–176, 1981.
165. Hsu, C.-M., Lee, P.-I., Chen, J.-M., et al.: Fatal *Fusarium* endocarditis complicated by hemolytic anemia and thrombocytopenia in an infant. Pediatr. Infect. Dis. J. *13*:1146–1148, 1994.
166. Hyams, K. C., Mader, J. T., Pollard, R. B., et al.: *Serratia* endocarditis in a pediatric burn patient. J. A. M. A. *246*:983–984, 1981.
167. Ingram, R. J. H., Cornere, B., and Ellis-Pegler, R. B.: Endocarditis due to *Neisseria mucosa*: Two case reports and review. Clin. Infect. Dis. *15*:321–324, 1992.
168. Inman, R. D., Redecha, P. B., Knechtle, S. J., et al.: Identification of bacterial antigens in circulating immune complexes of infective endocarditis. J. Clin. Invest. *70*:271–280, 1982.
169. Ivert, T. S., Dismukes, W. E., Cobbs, C. G., et al.: Prosthetic valve endocarditis. Circulation *69*:223–232, 1984.
170. Jackman, J. D., Jr., and Glamann, D. B.: Gonococcal endocarditis: Twenty-five year experience. Am. J. Med. Sci. *301*:221, 1991.
171. Jackson, M. A., and Hicks, R. A.: Vancomycin failure in staphylococcal endocarditis. Pediatr. Infect. Dis. *6*:750–752, 1987.
172. Jackson, M. J., and Rutledge, J.: Pneumococcal endocarditis in children. Pediatr. Infect. Dis. *1*:120–122, 1982.
173. Jaffe, W. M., Morgan, D. E., Pearlman, A. S., et al.: Infective endocarditis, 1983–1988: Echocardiographic findings and factors influencing morbidity and mortality. J. Am. Coll. Cardiol. *15*:1227–1233, 1990.
174. Jalava, J., Kotilainen, P., Nikkari, S., et al.: Use of the polymerase chain reaction and DNA sequencing for detection of *Bartonella quintana* in the aortic valve of a patient with culture-negative infective endocarditis. Clin. Infect. Dis. *21*:891–896, 1995.
175. Jemsek, J. G., Greenberg, S. B., Gentry, L. O., et al.: *Haemophilus parainfluenzae* endocarditis: Two cases and review of the literature in the past decade. Am. J. Med. *66*:51–57, 1979.
176. Jeresaty, R. M.: Mitral valve prolapse: Click syndrome. Prog. Cardiovasc. Dis. *15*:623–629, 1973.
177. Job, F. P., Franke, S., Lethen, H., et al.: Incremental valve of biplane and multiplane transesophageal echocardiography for the assessment of active infective endocarditis. Am. J. Cardiol. *75*:1033–1037, 1995.
178. Johnson, C. M.: Adherence events in the pathogenesis of infective endocarditis. Infect. Dis. Clin. North Am. 7:21–36, 1993.
179. Johnson, C. M., and Rhodes, K. H.: Pediatric endocarditis. Mayo Clin. Proc. *57*:86–94, 1982.
180. Johnson, D. H., Rosenthal, A., and Nadas, A.: Bacterial endocarditis in children under 2 years of age. Am. J. Dis. Child. *129*:183–186, 1975.
181. Johnson, D. H., Rosenthal, A., and Nadas, A.: A forty-year review of bacterial endocarditis in infancy and childhood. Circulation *51*:581–588, 1975.
182. Johnson, J. D., Raff, M. J., Barnwell, P. A., et al.: Splenic abscess complicating infectious endocarditis. Arch. Intern. Med. *143*:906–912, 1983.
183. Johnson, P. G., Lee, J., Domanski, M., et al.: Late recurrent *Candida* endocarditis. Chest *99*:1531–1533, 1991.
184. Jones, H. K., and Siekert, R. G.: Neurologic manifestations of infective endocarditis. Brain *112*:1295–1315, 1989.
185. Jones, R. B., Priest, J. B., and Kuo, C.: Subacute chlamydial endocarditis. J. A. M. A. *247*:655–658, 1982.
186. Julander, I.: Unfavourable prognostic factors in *Staphylococcus aureus* septicemia and endocarditis. Scand. J. Infect. Dis. *17*:179–187, 1985.
187. Jung, J. Y., Saab, S. B., and Almond, C. H.: The case for early surgical treatment of left-sided primary infective endocarditis: A collective review. J. Thorac. Cardiovasc. Surg. *70*:509–518, 1975.
188. Kaell, A. T., Volkman, D. J., Gorevic, P. D., et al.: Positive Lyme serology in subacute bacterial endocarditis: A study of four patients. J. A. M. A. *264*:2916–2918, 1990.
189. Kaplan, E. L.: Infective endocarditis in the pediatric age group: An overview. *In* Kaplan, E. L., and Taranta, A. V. (eds.): Infective Endocarditis: An American Heart Association Symposium. Dallas, American Heart Association, 1977, pp. 51–54.
190. Kaplan, E. L., Rich, H., Gersony, W., et al.: A collaborative study of infective endocarditis in the 1970's: Emphasis on infections in patients who have undergone cardiovascular surgery. Circulation *59*:327–335, 1979.
191. Kaplan, S., Helmworth, J. A., Ahern, E. N., et al.: Results of palliative procedures for tetralogy of Fallot in infants and young children. Ann. Thorac. Surg. *5*:489–495, 1968.
192. Karalis, D. G., Blumberg, A. E., Vilaro, J. F., et al.: Prognostic significance of valvular regurgitation in patients with infective endocarditis. Am. J. Med. 90:193–197, 1991.
193. Karchmer, A. W., Dismukes, W. E., Buckley, M. J., et al.: Late prosthetic valve endocarditis: Clinical features influencing therapy. Am. J. Med. *64*:199–206, 1978.
194. Karchmer, A. W., Moellering, R. C., Maki, D. G., et al.: Single-antibiotic therapy for streptococcal endocarditis. J. A. M. A. *241*:1801–1806, 1979.
195. Karchmer, A. W., Archer, G. L., and Dismukes, W. E.: *Staphylococcus epidermidis* causing prosthetic valve endocarditis: Microbiologic and clinical observations as guides to therapy. Ann. Intern. Med. *98*:447–455, 1983.
196. Karl, T., Wensley, D., Stark, J., et al.: Infective endocarditis in children with congenital heart disease: Comparison of selected features in patients with surgical correction or palliation and those without. Br. Heart J. *58*:57–65, 1987.
197. Kauffman, R. H., Thompson, J., Valentijn, R. M., et al.: The clinical impli-

cations and the pathogenetic significance of circulating immune complexes in infective endocarditis. Am. J. Med. *71*:17–25, 1981.
198. Kavey, R. W., Frank, D. M., Byrum, C. J., et al.: Two-dimensional echocardiographic assessment of infective endocarditis in children. Am. J. Dis. Child. *137*:851–856, 1983.
199. Kaye, D.: Prevention of bacterial endocarditis: 1991. Ann. Intern. Med. *114*:803–804, 1991.
200. Keay, S., Denning, D. W., and Stevens, D. A.: Endocarditis due to *Trichosporon beigelii:* In vitro susceptibility of isolates and review. Rev. Infect. Dis. *13*:383–386, 1991.
201. Keys, T. F., and Hewitt, W. L.: Endocarditis due to micrococci and *Staphylococcus epidermidis.* Arch. Intern. Med. *132*:216–220, 1973.
202. Keyser, D. L., Biller, J., Coffman, T. T., et al.: Neurologic complications of late prosthetic valve endocarditis. Stroke *21*:472, 1990.
203. Khandheria, B. K.: Transesophageal echocardiography in the evaluation of prosthetic valves. Am. J. Cardiac Imag. *9*:106–114, 1995.
204. Kielhofner, M. A., and Hamill, R. J.: Role of adherence in infective endocarditis. Tex. Heart J. *16*:239–249, 1989.
205. Kihuchi, K., Enari, T., Minami, S., et al.: Postantibiotic effects and postantibiotic sub-MIC effects of benzyl penicillin on viridans streptococci isolated from patients with infective endocarditis. J. Antimicrob. Chemother. *34*:687–696, 1994.
206. Kilpatrick, Z. M., Greenberg, P. A., and Sanford, J. P.: Splinter hemorrhages: Their clinical significance. Arch. Intern. Med. *115*:730–735, 1965.
207. Kimbrough, R. C., Ormsbee, R. A., Peacock, M., et al.: Q Fever endocarditis in the United States. Ann. Intern. Med. *91*:400–402, 1979.
208. King, M. E., and Weyman, A. E.: Echocardiographic findings in infective endocarditis. Cardiovasc. Clin. *13*:147–165, 1983.
209. Kissane, J. M.: Pathology of Infancy and Childhood. 2nd ed. St. Louis, C. V. Mosby, 1975, pp. 417–418.
210. Komshian, S. V., Tablan, O. C., Palutke, W., et al.: Characteristics of left-sided endocarditis due to *Pseudomonas aeruginosa* in the Detroit Medical Center. Rev. Infect. Dis. *12*:693–702, 1990.
211. Kramer, H., Bourgeois, M., Liersch, R., et al.: Current clinical aspects of bacterial endocarditis in infancy, childhood and adolescence. Eur. J. Pediatr. *140*:253–259, 1983.
212. Kuypers, J. M., and Proctor, R. A.: Reduced adherence to traumatized rat heart valves by a low-fibronectin-binding mutant of *Staphylococcus aureus.* Infect. Immun. *57*:2306–2312, 1989.
213. Laird, W. P., Nelson, J. D., Weinberg, A. G., et al.: Fatal *Hemophilus influenzae* endocarditis diagnosed by echocardiography in an infant. Pediatrics *64*:292–295, 1979.
214. Lam, S., Samraj, J., Rahman, S., et al.: Primary actinomycotic endocarditis: Case report and review. Clin. Infect. Dis. *16*:481–485, 1993.
215. Lamich, R., Alonso, C., Guma, J. R., et al.: Prospective study of bacteremia during transesophageal echocardiography. Am. Heart J. *125*:1454, 1993.
216. Laufer, D., Lew, P. D., Obertiansli, I., et al.: Chronic Q fever endocarditis with massive splenomegaly in childhood. J. Pediatr. *108*:535–539, 1986.
217. Laxdal, T., Messner, R. P., and Williams, R. S.: Opsonic, agglutinating and complement-fixing antibodies in patients with subacute bacterial endocarditis. J. Lab. Clin. Med. *71*:638–675, 1968.
218. Lederman, M. M., Sprague, L., Wallis, R. S., et al.: Duration of fever during treatment of infective endocarditis. Medicine *71*:52, 1992.
219. Leonard, A., Raij, L., and Shapiro, F. C.: Bacterial endocarditis in regularly dialyzed patients. Kidney Int. *4*:407–422, 1973.
220. Lepeschkin, E.: On the relation between the side of valvular involvement in endocarditis and the blood pressure resting on the valve. Am. J. Med. Sci. *224*:318–319, 1952.
221. Lerner, P. I., and Weinstein, L.: Infective endocarditis in the antibiotic era. N. Engl. J. Med. *274*:199–206, 259–266, 388–393, 1966.
222. Levin, R. M., Pulliam, L., Mondry, C., et al.: Penicillin-resistant *Streptococcus constellatus* as a cause of endocarditis. Am. J. Dis. Child. *136*:42–45, 1982.
223. Levine, D. P., Fromm, B. S., and Reddy, B. R.: Slow response to vancomycin or vancomycin plus rifampin in methicillin-resistant *Staphylococcus aureus* endocarditis. Ann. Intern. Med. *115*:674–680, 1991.
224. Levy, P. Y., Drancourt, M., Etienne, J., et al.: Comparison of different antibiotic regimens for therapy of 32 cases of Q fever endocarditis. Antimicrob. Agents Chemother. *35*:533–537, 1991.
225. Liepman, M. K., Jones, P. G., and Kauffman, C. A.: Endocarditis as a complication of indwelling right atrial catheters in leukemic patients. Cancer *54*:804–807, 1984.
226. Lina, B., Celard, M., Vandenesch, F., et al.: Infective endocarditis due to *Staphylococcus capitis.* Clin. Infect. Dis. *15*:173–174, 1992.
227. Lipman, M. L., and Silva, J.: Endocarditis due to *Streptococcus faecalis* with high-level resistance to gentamicin. Rev. Infect. Dis. *11*:325–328, 1989.
228. Liu, V. C., Stevenson, J. G., and Smith, A. L.: Group A *Streptococcus* mural endocarditis. Pediatr. Infect. Dis. J. *11*:1060–1062, 1992.
229. Liwnicz, B. H., and Lepow, H.: Nonbacterial thrombotic endocarditis in a premature child: Clinical significance and possible relationships to subvalvular hematoma. N. Y. State J. Med. *76*:912–916, 1976.
230. Lowenstein, M. B., Urman, J. D., Abeles, M., et al.: Skin immunofluorescence in infective endocarditis. J. A. M. A. *238*:1163–1165, 1977.
231. Lowrance, J. H., Baddour, L. M., and Simpson, W. A.: The role of fibronectin binding in a rat model of experimental endocarditis caused by *Streptococcus sanguis.* J. Clin. Invest. *86*:7, 1990.
232. Lubani, M., Sharda, D., and Helin, I.: Cardiac manifestations in brucellosis. Arch. Dis. Child. *61*:569–572, 1986.
233. Lutas, E. M., Roberts, R. B., Devereux, R. B., et al.: Relation between the presence of echocardiographic vegetations and the complication rate in infective endocarditis. Am. Heart J. *112*:107–113, 1986.
234. Lynn, D. C., Kane, J. G., and Parker, R. H.: *Haemophilus parainfluenzae* endocarditis: A review of forty cases. Medicine *56*:115–128, 1977.
235. Macauley, D.: Acute endocarditis in infancy and early childhood. Am. J. Dis. Child. *88*:715–721, 1954.
236. MacMahon, S. W., Hickey, A. J., Wilcken, D. E. L., et al.: Risk of infective endocarditis in mitral valve prolapse with and without precordial systolic murmurs. Am. J. Cardiol. *58*:105–108, 1986.
237. Madison, J., Wang, K., Gobel, F. L., et al.: Prosthetic aortic valve endocarditis. Circulation *51*:940–949, 1975.
238. Maisch, B., Eichstadt, H., and Kochsiek, K.: Immune reactions in infective endocarditis. I. Clinical data and diagnostic relevance of antimyocardial antibodies. Am. Heart J. *106*:329–344, 1983.
239. Maki, D. G., and Agger, W. A.: Enterococcal bacteremia: Clinical features, the risk of endocarditis and management. Medicine *67*:248–269, 1988.
240. Malacoff, R. F., Frank, E., and Andriole, V. T.: Streptococcal endocarditis (non-enterococcal, non-group A): Single vs. combination therapy. J. A. M. A. *241*:1807–1810, 1979.
241. Mansur, A. J., Grinberg, M., Lemosdaluz, P., et al.: The complications of infective endocarditis. Arch. Intern. Med. *152*:2428, 1992.
242. Marinell, P. V., Diana, D. J., and Todd, W. A.: Survival of a child after *Hemophilus influenzae* b endocarditis. Pediatr. Infect. Dis. *2*:46–47, 1983.
243. Markowitz, M.: The decline of rheumatic fever: Role of medical intervention. Lewis W. Wannamaker Memorial Lecture. J. Pediatr. *106*:545–550, 1985.
244. Markowitz, S. M., Szentpetery, S., Lower, R. R., et al.: Endocarditis due to accidental penetrating foreign bodies. Am. J. Med. *60*:571–576, 1976.
245. Marks, A. R., Choong, C. Y., Sanfilippo, A. J., et al.: Identification of high-risk and low-risk subgroups of patients with mitral-valve prolapse. N. Engl. J. Med. *370*:1031–1036, 1989.
246. Marrie, T. J., Harczy, M., Mann, O. E., et al.: Culture-negative endocarditis probably due to *Chlamydia pneumoniae.* J. Infect. Dis. *161*:127–129, 1990.
247. Martino, P., Micozzi, A., Venditti, M., et al.: Catheter-related right-sided endocarditis in bone marrow transplant recipients. Rev. Infect. Dis. *12*:250–257, 1990.
248. Masuda, J., Yutani, C., Waki, R., et al.: Histopathologic analysis of the mechanisms of intracranial hemorrhage complicating infective endocarditis. Stroke *23*:843, 1992.
249. Mathew, J., Addai, T., Anand, A., et al.: Clinical features, site of involvement, bacteriologic findings and outcome of infective endocarditis in intravenous drug users. Arch. Intern. Med. *155*:1641–1648, 1995.
250. Mayayo, E., Moralejo, J., Camps, J., et al.: Fungal endocarditis in premature infants: Case report and review. Clin. Infect. Dis. *22*:366–368, 1996.
251. McCartney, A. C., Orange, G. U., Pringle, S. D., et al.: Serum C reactive protein in infective endocarditis. J. Clin. Pathol. *41*:44–48, 1988.
252. McGuinness, G. A., Schieken, R. M., and Maquire, G. F.: Endocarditis in the newborn. Am. J. Dis. Child. *134*:577–580, 1980.
253. McKinsey, D. S., Ratts, T. E., and Bisno, A. L.: Underlying cardiac lesions in adults with infective endocarditis: The changing spectrum. Am. J. Med. *82*:681–688, 1987.
254. Medoff, G., Comfort, M., and Kabayashi, G.: Synergistic action of amphotericin B and 5-fluorocytosine against yeast-like organisms. Proc. Soc. Exp. Biol. Med. *138*:571–574, 1971.
255. Mendelsohn, G., and Hutchins, G. M.: Infective endocarditis during the first decade of life. Am. J. Dis. Child. *133*:619–622, 1979.
256. Megran, D. W.: Enterococcal endocarditis. Clin. Infect. Dis. *15*:63–71, 1992.
257. Merzbach, D., Freundlich, E., Metzker, A., et al.: Endocarditis due to *Corynebacterium.* J. Pediatr. *67*:792–796, 1965.
258. Middlemost, S., Wisenbaugh, T., Meyerowitz, C., et al.: A case for early surgery in native left-sided endocarditis complicated by heart failure: Results in 203 patients. J. Am. Coll. Cardiol. *18*:663–667, 1991.
259. Millard, D. D., and Shulman, S. T.: The changing spectrum of neonatal endocarditis. Clin. Perinatol. *15*:587–608, 1988.
260. Mills, S. A.: Surgical progress: Surgical management of infective endocarditis. Ann. Surg. *195*:367–383, 1982.
261. Mintz, G. S., Kotler, M. N., Segal, B. L., et al.: Comparison of two-dimensional and M-mode echocardiography in the evaluation of patients with infective endocarditis. Am. J. Cardiol. *43*:738–745, 1979.
262. Mirimanoff, R. O., and Glauser, M. P.: Endocarditis during *Staphylococcus aureus* septicemia in a population of non–drug addicts. Arch. Intern. Med. *142*:1311–1313, 1982.
263. Mittal, B. V.: Renal lesions in infective endocarditis. J. Postgrad. Med. *33*:193–197, 1987.
264. Moodie, D. S., and Gallen, W. J.: Pneumococcal endocarditis in a 7 week old infant. Am. J. Dis. Child. *129*:980–983, 1975.
265. Morguet, A. J., Munz, D. L., Ivancevic, V., et al.: Immunoscintigraphy using technetium-99m–labeled anti-NCA-95 antigranulocyte antibodies as an adjunct to echocardiography in subacute infective endocarditis. J. Am. Coll. Cardiol. *23*:1171–1188, 1994.

266. Morrison, V. A., and Wagner, K. F.: Clinical manifestations of *Kingella kingae* infections: Case report and review. Rev. Infect. Dis. *11*:776–782, 1989.
267. Mortara, L. A., and Bayer, A. S.: *Staphylococcus* bacteremia and endocarditis: New diagnostic and therapeutic concepts. Infect. Dis. Clin. North Am. *7*:53–67, 1993.
268. Moy, R. J. D., George, R. H., DeGiovanni, J. V., et al.: Improving survival in bacterial endocarditis. Arch. Dis. Child. *61*:394–399, 1986.
269. Mugge, A., Daniel, W. G., Frank, G., et al.: Echocardiography in infective endocarditis: Reassessment of prognostic implications of vegetation size determined by the transthoracic and transesophageal approach. J. Am. Coll. Cardiol. *14*:631–638, 1989.
270. Mullany, C. J., Chau, Y. L., Schaff, H. V., et al.: Early and late survival after surgical treatment of culture-positive active endocarditis. Mayo Clin. Proc. *70*:517–525, 1995.
271. Munoz, P., Berenguer, J., Rodriguez-Greixems, M., et al.: Ciprofloxacin and infective endocarditis. Infect. Dis. Clin. Pract. *2*:119, 1993.
272. Murphy, J. G., and Foster-Smith, K.: Management of complications of infective endocarditis with emphasis on echocardiographic findings. Infect. Dis. Clin. North Am. *7*:153–165, 1993.
273. Murray, B. E.: The life and times of the *Enterococcus*. Clin. Microbiol. Rev. *3*:46–65, 1990.
274. Murray, H. W., Gross, K. C., Masur, H., et al.: Serious infections caused by *Streptococcus milleri*. Am. J. Med. *64*:759–765, 1978.
275. Musewe, N. N., Hecht, B. M., Hesslein, P. S., et al.: Tricuspid valve endocarditis in two children with normal hearts: Diagnosis and therapy of an unusual clinical entity. J. Pediatr. *110*:735–738, 1987.
276. Nagel, J. G., Tuazon, C. V., Cardella, T. A., et al.: Teichoic acid serologic diagnosis of staphylococcal endocarditis. Ann. Intern. Med. *82*:13–18, 1975.
277. Nagunuma, M.: Infective endocarditis in children. Jpn. Circ. J. *49*:545–552, 1985.
278. Naidoo, D. P.: Right-sided endocarditis in the non–drug addict. Postgrad. Med. J. *69*:615–620, 1993.
279. Nakayama, D. K., O'Neill, J. A., Wagner, H., et al.: Management of vascular complications of bacterial endocarditis. J. Pediatr. Surg. *21*:636–639, 1986.
280. Narasimhan, S. L., and Weinstein, A. J.: Infective endocarditis due to a nutritionally deficient *Streptococcus*. J. Pediatr. *96*:61–62, 1980.
281. Nastro, L. J., and Finegold, S. M.: Endocarditis due to anaerobic gram-negative bacilli. Am. J. Med. *54*:482–496, 1973.
282. Nelson, R. J., Harley, D. P., French, W. J., et al.: Favorable ten-year experience with valve procedures for active infective endocarditis. J. Thorac. Cardiovasc. Surg. *87*:493–502, 1984.
283. Nguyen, M. H., Nguyen, M. L., Yu, V. L., et al.: *Candida* prosthetic valve endocarditis: Prospective study of six cases and review of the literature. Clin. Infect. Dis. *22*:262–267, 1996.
284. Nicolau, D. P., Freeman, C. D., Nightingale, C. H., et al.: Reduction of bacterial titers by low-dose aspirin in experimental aortic valve endocarditis. Infect. Immun. *61*:1593–1595, 1993.
285. Noel, G. J., O'Loughlin, J. E., and Edelson, P. J.: Neonatal *Staphylococcus epidermidis* right-sided endocarditis: Description of five catheterized infants. Pediatrics *82*:234–239, 1988.
286. Nolan, C. M., Kane, J. J., and Grunow, W. A.: Infective endocarditis and mitral prolapse: A comparison with other types of endocarditis. Arch. Intern. Med. *141*:447–450, 1981.
287. Nomura, F., Penny, D. J., Menahem, S., et al.: Surgical intervention for infective endocarditis in infancy and childhood. Ann. Thorac. Surg. *60*:90–95, 1995.
288. O'Brien, J. T., and Geiser, E. A.: Infective endocarditis and echocardiography. Am. Heart J. *108*:386–394, 1984.
289. O'Callaghan, C., and McDougall, P.: Infective endocarditis in neonates. Arch. Dis. Child. *63*:53–57, 1988.
290. Oelberg, D. G., Fisher, D. J., Gross, D. M., et al.: Endocarditis in high-risk neonates. Pediatrics *71*:392–397, 1983.
291. Okumura, A., Ito, K., Kondo, M., et al.: Infective endocarditis caused by highly penicillin-resistant *Streptococcus pneumoniae*: Successful treatment with cefuzonam, ampicillin and imipenem. Pediatr. Infect. Dis. J. *14*:327–329, 1995.
292. Panidis, I. P., Kotler, M. N., Mintz, G. S., et al.: Right heart endocarditis: Clinical and echocardiographic features. Am. Heart J. *107*:759–764, 1984.
293. Patchell, R. A., White, C. L., Clark, A. W., et al.: Nonbacterial thrombotic endocarditis in bone marrow transplant patients. Cancer *55*:631–635, 1985.
294. Patrick, W. D., Brown, W. D., Bowmer, M. I., et al.: Infective endocarditis due to *Eikenella corrodens*: Case report and review of the literature. Can. J. Infect. Dis. *1*:139, 1990.
295. Patterson, H. S., and Weir, M. R.: GABHS infective endocarditis: Case report. Milit. Med. *149*:92–94, 1984.
296. Patterson, J. E., and Zervos, M. J.: High-level gentamicin resistance in *Enterococcus*: Microbiology, genetic basis and epidemiology. Rev. Infect. Dis. *12*:644–652, 1990.
297. Pazin, G. J., Saul, S., and Thompson, M. E.: Blood culture positivity: Suppression by out-patient antibiotic therapy in patients with bacterial endocarditis. Arch. Intern. Med. *142*:263–269, 1982.
298. Pedersen, W. R., Walker, M., Olson, J. D., et al.: Value of transesophageal echocardiography as an adjunct to transthoracic echocardiography in evaluation of native and prosthetic valve endocarditis. Chest *100*:351–356, 1991.
299. Pefanis, A., Giamarellou, H., Karayiannakos, P., et al.: Efficacy of ceftazidime and aztreonam alone or in combination with amikacin in experimental left-sided *Pseudomonas aeruginosa* endocarditis. Antimicrob. Agents Chemother. *37*:308–313, 1993.
300. Pefanis, A., Thauvin-Eliopoulos, C., Eliopoulos, G. M., et al.: Activity of ampicillin-sulbactam and oxacillin in experimental endocarditis caused by beta-lactamase hyperproducing *Staphylococcus aureus*. Antimicrob. Agents Chemother. *37*:507–511, 1993.
301. Pelletier, L. L., Durack, D. T., and Petersdorf, R. G.: Chemotherapy of experimental streptococcal endocarditis. IV. Further observations on prophylaxis. J. Clin. Invest. *56*:319–330, 1975.
302. Perry, K. S., Tresch, D. D., Brooks, H. L., et al.: Operative approach to endocarditis. Am. Heart J. *108*:561–566, 1984.
303. Pesanti, E. L., and Smith, I. M.: Infective endocarditis with negative blood cultures: An analysis of 52 cases. Am. J. Med. *66*:43–50, 1979.
304. Peter, O., Flepp, M., Bestetti, G., et al.: Q fever endocarditis: Diagnostic approaches and monitoring of therapeutic effects. Clin. Invest. *70*:932, 1992.
305. Pollack, S., Mogtader, A., and Lange, M.: *Neisseria subflava* endocarditis: Case report and review of the literature. Am. J. Med. *76*:752–758, 1984.
306. Pongratz, G., Henneke, K. H., von der Grun, M., et al.: Risk of endocarditis in transesophageal echocardiography. Am. Heart J. *125*:190–193, 1993.
307. Popp, R. L.: Echocardiography. N. Engl. J. Med. *323*:165, 1990.
308. Powderly, W. G., Stanley, S. L., and Medoff, G.: Pneumococcal endocarditis: Report of a series and review of the literature. Rev. Infect. Dis. *8*:786–791, 1986.
309. Powell, D. C., Bivens, B. A., Bell, R. M., et al.: Endocarditis: Increasingly a surgical disease. Am. Surg. *48*:5–10, 1982.
310. Powers, D. L., and Mandell, G. L.: Intraleucocytic bacteria in endocarditis patients. J. A. M. A. *227*:313–315, 1974.
311. Prager, R. L., Maples, M. D., Hammon, J. W., et al.: Early operative intervention in aortic bacterial endocarditis. Ann. Thorac. Surg. *32*:347–350, 1981.
312. Prinsloo, J. G., and Pretorius, P. J.: *Candida albicans* endocarditis. Am. J. Dis. Child. *111*:446–447, 1966.
313. Pulvirenti, J. J., Kerns, E., Benson, C., et al.: Infective endocarditis in injection drug users: Importance of human immunodeficiency virus serostatus and degree of immunosuppression. Clin. Infect. Dis. *22*:40–45, 1996.
314. Qoronfleh, M. W., Weraarchakul, W., and Wilkinson, B. S.: Antibodies to a range of *Staphylococcus aureus* and *Escherichia coli* heat shock proteins in sera from patients with *S. aureus* endocarditis. Infect. Immun. *61*:1567–1570, 1993.
315. Rabin, R. L., Wong, P., Noonan, J. A., et al.: *Kingella kingae* endocarditis in a child with a prosthetic aortic valve and bifurcation graft. Am. J. Dis. Child. *137*:403–404, 1983.
316. Ramirez, C. A., Naragi, S., and McCulley, D. J.: Group A beta-hemolytic streptococcus endocarditis. Am. Heart J. *108*:1383–1386, 1984.
317. Rastogi, A., Luken, J. A., Pildes, R. S., et al.: Endocarditis in the neonatal intensive care unit. Pediatr. Cardiol. *14*:183–186, 1993.
318. Reller, L. B.: The serum bactericidal test. Rev. Infect. Dis. *8*:803–807, 1986.
319. Reymann, M. T., Holley, H. P., and Cobbs, C. G.: Persistent bacteremia in staphylococcal endocarditis. Am. J. Med. *65*:729–739, 1978.
320. Ribot, S., Rothfeld, D., and Frankel, H. J.: Infectious endocarditis in maintenance hemodialysis patients. Am. J. Med. Sci. *264*:183–188, 1972.
321. Rice, L. B., Calderwood, S. B., Elipoulos, G. M., et al.: Enterococcal endocarditis: A comparison of prosthetic and native valve disease. Rev. Infect. Dis. *13*:1–7, 1991.
322. Rice, M. J., McDonald, R. W., Reller, M. D., et al.: Pediatric echocardiography: Current role and a review of technical advances. J. Pediatr. 128:1–14, 1996.
323. Robbins, M. J., Frater, R. W. M., Soeiro, R., et al.: Influence of vegetation size on clinical outcome of right-sided infective endocarditis. Am. J. Med. *80*:165–171, 1986.
324. Roberts, G. J., Gardner, P., and Simmons, N. A.: Optimum sampling time for detection of dental bacteremia in children. Int. J. Cardiol. *35*:311–315, 1992.
325. Roberts, K. B., and Sidlak, M. J.: Satellite streptococci: A major cause of "negative" blood cultures in bacterial endocarditis? J. A. M. A. *241*:2293–2294, 1979.
326. Rodbard, S.: Blood velocity and endocarditis. Circulation *27*:18–28, 1963.
327. Rogers, J., Walker, M., Olson, J. D., et al.: Value of transesophageal echocardiography as an adjunct to transthoracic echocardiography in evaluation of native and prosthetic valve endocarditis. Chest *100*:351–355, 1991.
328. Rose, A. G.: Infective endocarditis complicating congenital heart disease. S. Afr. Med. J. *53*:739–743, 1978.
329. Rubinstein, E., Noreiga, E. R., Simberkoff, M. S., et al.: Fungal endocarditis: Analysis of 24 cases and review of the literature. Medicine *54*:331–344, 1975.
330. Rupp, M. E.: *Streptobacillus moniliformis* endocarditis: Case report and review. Clin. Infect. Dis. *14*:769–772.
331. Rutledge, R., Kim, B. J., and Applebaum, R. E.: Actuarial analysis of the

risk of prosthetic valve endocarditis in 1,598 patients with mechanical and bioprosthetic valves. Arch. Surg. *120*:469–472, 1985.

332. Sable, C. A., Rome, J. J., Martin, G. R., et al.: Indications for echocardiography in the diagnosis of infective endocarditis in children. Am. J. Cardiol. *75*:801–804, 1995.
333. Saffle, J. R., Gardner, P., Schoenbaum, S. C., et al.: Prosthetic valve endocarditis: The case for prompt valve replacement. J. Thorac. Cardiovasc. Surg. *73*:416–420, 1977.
334. Saiman, L., Prince, A., and Gersony, W. M.: Pediatric infective endocarditis in the modern era. J. Pediatr. *122*:847–853, 1993.
335. Salgado, A. V., Furlan, A. J., Keys, T. F., et al.: Neurologic complications of endocarditis: A 12-year experience. Neurology *39*:173–178, 1989.
336. San Roman, J. A., Vilacosta, I., Zamorano, J. L., et al.: Transesophageal echocardiography in right-sided endocarditis. J. Am. Coll. Cardiol. *21*:1226–1230, 1993.
337. Sanchez, P. J., Siegel, J. D., and Fishbein, J.: *Candida* endocarditis: Successful medical management in three preterm infants and review of the literature. Pediatr. Infect. Dis. *10*:239–243, 1991.
338. Sande, M. A.: Experimental endocarditis. *In* Kaye, D. (ed.): Infective Endocarditis. Baltimore, University Park Press, 1976, p. 11.
339. Sande, M. A., and Courtney, K. B.: Nafcillin-gentamicin synergism in experimental *Staphylococcus* endocarditis. J. Lab. Clin. Med. *88*:118–124, 1976.
340. Sande, M. A., Johnson, W. B., Hook, E. W., et al.: Sustained bacteremia in patients with prosthetic cardiac valves. N. Engl. J. Med. *286*:1067–1070, 1972.
341. Sande, M. A., and Scheld, W. M.: Combination antibiotic therapy of bacterial endocarditis. Ann. Intern. Med. *92*:390–395, 1980.
342. Sandre, R. M., and Shatran, S. D.: Infective endocarditis: Review of 135 cases over 9 years. Clin. Infect. Dis. *22*:276–286, 1996.
343. Sanfilippo, A. J., Picard, M. H., Newell, J. B., et al.: Echocardiographic assessment of patients with infectious endocarditis: Prediction or risk for complications. J. Am. Coll. Cardiol. *18*:1191–1199, 1991.
344. Sapico, F. L., Liquete, J. A., and Sarma, R. J.: Bone and joint infections in patients with infective endocarditis: Review of a 4-year experience. Clin. Infect. Dis. *22*:783–787, 1996.
345. Sapsford, R. N., Fitchett, D. H., Tarin, D., et al.: Aneurysm of left ventricle secondary to bacterial endocarditis. J. Thorac. Cardiovasc. Surg. *78*:79–86, 1979.
346. Scheld, W. M., Valone, J. A., and Sande, M. A.: Bacterial adherence in the pathogenesis of endocarditis: Interaction of bacterial dextran, platelets and fibrin. J. Clin. Invest. *61*:1394–1398, 1978.
347. Scheld, W. M., Calderone, R. A., Alliegro, G. M., et al.: Yeast adherence in the pathogenesis of *Candida* endocarditis. Proc. Soc. Exp. Biol. Med. *168*:208–217, 1981.
348. Scheld, W. M., and Mandell, G. L.: Enigmatic enterococcal endocarditis. Ann. Intern. Med. *100*:904–905, 1984.
349. Scheld, W. M., and Sande, M. A.: Endocarditis and intravascular infections. *In* Mandell, G., Bennett, J. E., and Dolin, R. (eds.): Principles and Practices of Infectious Diseases. 4th ed. New York, Churchill Livingstone, 1995, pp. 740–782.
350. Scheld, W. M., Thomas, J. H., and Sande, M. A.: Influence of preformed antibody on experimental *Streptococcus sanguis* endocarditis. Infect. Immun. *25*:781–785, 1979.
351. Scheld, W. M., Zak, O., Vosbeck, K., et al.: Bacterial adhesion in the pathogenesis of endocarditis: Effect of subinhibitory antibiotic concentrations on streptococcal adhesion in vitro and the development of endocarditis in rabbits. J. Clin. Invest. *68*:1381, 1981.
352. Schlicter, J. G., and Maclean, H.: A method of determining the effective therapeutic level in the treatment of subacute bacterial endocarditis with penicillin. Am. Heart J. *34*:209–215, 1947.
353. Schollin, J., Bjarke, B., and Wesstrom, G.: Follow-up study on children with infective endocarditis. Acta Paediatr. Scand. *78*:615–619, 1989.
354. Schulte, J. E., Gaffney, F. A., Bland, L., et al.: Distinctive anthropometric characteristics of women with mitral valve prolapse. Am. J. Med. *71*:553–558, 1981.
355. Scott, P. J., Blackburn, M. E., Wharton, G. A., et al.: Transesophageal echocardiograph in neonates, infants and children: Applicability and diagnostic value in everyday practice of a cardiothoracic unit. Br. Heart J. *68*:488–492, 1992.
356. Scott, R. M.: Bacterial endocarditis due to *Neisseria flava*. J. Pediatr. *78*:673–675, 1971.
357. Seeling, M. S., Speth, C. P., Kozinn, P. J., et al.: Patterns of *Candida* endocarditis following cardiac surgery: Importance of early diagnosis and therapy (an analysis of 91 cases). Prog. Cardiovasc. Dis. *17*:125–160, 1974.
358. Shapiro, D. S., Kenney, S. C., Johnson, M., et al.: *Chlamydia psittaci* endocarditis diagnosed by blood culture. N. Engl. J. Med. *326*:1192–1195, 1992.
359. Shively, B. K., Gurule, F. T., Roldan, C. A., et al.: Diagnostic valve of transesophageal compared with transthoracic echocardiography in infective endocarditis. J. Am. Coll. Cardiol. *18*:391–397, 1991.
360. Sholler, G. F., Hawker, R. E., and Celermajer, J. M.: Infective endocarditis in childhood. Pediatr. Cardiol. *6*:183–186, 1986.
361. Simmons, N. A.: Recommendations for endocarditis prophylaxis. J. Antimicrob. Chemother. *31*:437–438, 1993.
362. Singhi, S. C., Singh, S., and Bidwai, P. S.: *Peptococcus* endocarditis. Indian. J. Pediatr. *25*:876–878, 1988.
363. Sirisanthana, V., and Sirisanthana, T.: *Corynebacterium diphtheriae* endocarditis. Pediatr. Infect. Dis. *2*:470–471, 1983.
364. Sochowski, R. A., and Chan, K.-L.: Implication of negative results on a monoplane transesophageal echocardiographic study in patients with suspected infective endocarditis. J. Am. Coll. Cardiol. *21*:216, 1993.
365. Sommer, P., Gleyzal, C., Guerret, S., et al.: Induction of a putative laminin-binding protein of *Streptococcus gordonii* in human infective endocarditis. Infect. Immun. *60*:360–365, 1992.
366. Spach, D. H., Kanter, A. S., Daniels, N. A., et al.: *Bartonella (Rochalimaea)* species as a cause of apparent "culture-negative" endocarditis. Clin. Infect. Dis. *20*:1044–1047, 1995.
367. Stanton, B. F., Baltimore, R. S., and Clemens, J. D.: Changing spectrum of infective endocarditis in children. Am. J. Dis. Child. *138*:720–725, 1984.
368. Steckelberg, J. M., Murphy, J. G., Ballard, D., et al.: Emboli in infective endocarditis: The prognostic value of echocardiography. Ann. Intern. Med. *114*:635–640, 1991.
369. Steckelberg, M. M., Rouse, M. S., Tallan, B. M., et al.: Relative efficacies of broad-spectrum cephalosporins for treatment of methicillin-susceptible *Staphylococcus aureus* experimental infective endocarditis. Antimicrob. Agents Chemother. *37*:554–558, 1993.
370. Steckelberg, J. M., and Wilson, W. R.: Risk factors for infective endocarditis. Infect. Dis. Clin. North Am. *7*:9–19, 1993.
371. Steen, M. K., Bruno-Murtha, L. A., Chaux, G., et al.: *Bacillus cereus* endocarditis: Report of a case and review. Clin. Infect. Dis. *14*:945–946, 1992.
372. Stein, D. S., and Nelson, K. E.: Endocarditis due to nutritionally deficient streptococci: Therapeutic dilemma. Rev. Infect. Dis. *9*:908–916, 1987.
373. Stewart, W. J., and Shan, K.: The diagnosis of prosthetic valve endocarditis by echocardiography. Semin. Thorac. Cardiovasc. Surg. *7*:7–12, 1995.
374. Stewart, J. A., Silamperi, D., Harris, P., et al.: Echocardiographic documentation of vegetative lesions in infective endocarditis: Clinical implications. Circulation *61*:374–380, 1980.
375. Stinson, E. B.: Surgical treatment of infective endocarditis. Prog. Cardiovasc. Dis. *22*:145–167, 1979.
376. Stopfuchen, H., Benzing, F., Jungst, B., et al.: Echocardiographic diagnosis of *Candida* endocarditis of the tricuspid valve and of the right atrium in a young infant. Pediatr. Cardiol. *4*:49–51, 1983.
377. Stramboulian, D., Bonvehi, P., Arevalo, C., et al.: Antibiotic management of outpatients with endocarditis due to penicillin-susceptible streptococci. Rev. Infect. Dis. *13*(Suppl. 2):160–163, 1991.
378. Stuart, G., and Wren, C.: Endocarditis with acute mitral regurgitation caused by *Fusobacterium necrophorum*. Pediatr. Cardiol. 13:230–232, 1992.
379. Sudduth, E. J., Rozich, J. D., and Farrar, W. E.: *Rothia dentocariosa* endocarditis complicated by perivalvular abscess. Clin. Infect. Dis. *17*:772–775, 1993.
380. Sullam, P. M., Costerton, J. W., Yamasaki, R., et al.: Inhibition of platelet binding and aggregation by streptococcal exopolysaccharide. J. Infect. Dis. *167*:1123–1130, 1993.
381. Sussman, J. I., Baron, E. J., Tenenbaum, M. J., et al.: Viridans streptococcal endocarditis: Clinical, microbiological and echocardiographic correlations. J. Infect. Dis. *154*:597–603, 1986.
382. Sussman, J. I., Baron, E. J., Goldberg, S. M., et al.: Clinical manifestations and therapy of *Lactobacillus* endocarditis: Report of a case and review of the literature. Rev. Infect. Dis. *8*:771–776, 1986.
383. Switalski, L. M., Murchison, H., Timpl, R., et al.: Binding of laminin to oral and endocarditis strains of viridans streptococci. J. Bacteriol. *169*:1095–1101, 1987.
384. Sykes, R. M.: *Salmonella* endocarditis in a Nigerian child. East Afr. Med. J. *61*:326–327, 1984.
385. Symbas, P. N., Vlasis, S. E., Zacharupoulos, L., et al.: Immediate and long-term outlook for valve replacement in acute bacterial endocarditis. Ann. Surg. *195*:721–724, 1982.
386. Symchych, P. S., Krauss, A. W., and Winchester, P.: Endocarditis following intracardiac placement of umbilical venous catheters in neonates. J. Pediatr. *90*:287–289, 1977.
387. Taams, M. A., Gussenhoven, E. J., Bos, E., et al.: Enhanced morphological diagnosis in infective endocarditis by transesophageal echocardiography. Br. Heart J. *63*:109–113, 1990.
388. Tanowitz, H. B., Alder, J. J., and Chirito, E.: Gonococcal endocarditis. N. Y. State J. Med. *42*:2782–2783, 1972.
389. Tebas, P., Martinez, R., Roman, F., et al.: Early resistance to rifampin and ciprofloxacin in the treatment of right-sided *Staphylococcus aureus* endocarditis. J. Infect. Dis. *163*:204–205, 1991.
390. Teixeira, O. H., Carpenter, B., and Vlad, P.: Enterococcal endocarditis in early infancy. Can. Med. Assoc. J. *127*:612–613, 1982.
391. Thadelpall, H., and Francis, C. K.: Diagnostic clues in metastatic lesions of endocarditis in addicts. West. J. Med. *128*:1–7, 1978.
392. Thal, L. A., Vazquez, J., Perri, M. B., et al.: Activity of ampicillin plus sulbactam against β-lactamase producing enterococci in experimental endocarditis. J. Antimicrob. Chemother. *31*:182, 1993.
393. Thapar, M. K., Rao, P. S., Feldman, D., et al.: Infective endocarditis: A review. Paediatrician *7*:65–84, 1978.
394. Theofilopoulos, A. N., Wilson, C. B., and Dixon, F. J.: The Raji cell radioimmune assay for detecting immune complexes in human sera. J. Clin. Invest. *57*:169–182, 1976.

395. Tiley, S. M., Kociuba, K. R., Heron, L. G., et al.: Infective endocarditis due to nontoxigenic *Corynebacterium diptheriae:* Report of seven cases and review. Clin. Infect. Dis. *16*:271–275, 1993.
396. Tolan, R. W., Jr., Kleiman, M. B., Frank, M., et al.: Operative intervention in active endocarditis in children: Report of a series of cases and review. Clin. Infect. Dis. *14*:852–862, 1992.
397. Tolaymat, A., Rhatigan, R. M., and Levin, S.: Pneumococcal endocarditis in infants. South. Med. J. *72*:448–451, 1979.
398. Tompkins, L. S., Roessler, B. J., Redd, S. C., et al.: *Legionella* prosthetic-valve endocarditis. N. Engl. J. Med. *318*:530–535, 1988.
399. Tornos, M. P., Castro, A., Toran, N., et al.: Tricuspid valve endocarditis in children with normal valves. Am. Heart J. *118*:624–625, 1989.
400. Tornos, M. P., Permanyer-Miralda, G., Olona, M., et al.: Long-term complications of native valve infective endocarditis in non-addicts: A 15-year follow-up study. Ann. Intern. Med. *117*:567–572, 1992.
401. Toy, P. T. C. Y., Lai, W., Drake, T. A., et al.: Effect of fibronectin on adherence of *Staphylococcus aureus* to fibrin thrombi in vitro. Infect. Immun. *48*:83–86, 1985.
402. Tsao, M. M., and Katz, D.: Central venous catheter–induced endocarditis: Human correlate of the animal experimental model of endocarditis. Rev. Infect. Dis. *6*:783–790, 1984.
403. Tuazon, C. V., and Sheagren, J. W.: Staphylococcal endocarditis in parenteral drug abusers: Source of the organism. Ann. Intern. Med. *82*:788–790, 1975.
404. Tunkel, A. R., and Kaye, D.: Endocarditis with negative blood cultures. N. Engl. J. Med. *326*:1215–1217, 1992.
405. Turner, S. W., Wyllie, J. P., Hamilton, J. R. L., et al.: Diagnosis of infected modified Blalock-Taussig shunt by computed tomography. Ann. Thorac. Surg. *59*:1216–1217, 1995.
406. Turnier, E., Kay, J. H., Bernstein, S., et al.: Surgical treatment of *Candida* endocarditis. Chest *67*:262–268, 1975.
407. Utley, J. R., Mills, J., and Roe, B. B.: The role of valve replacement in the treatment of fungal endocarditis. J. Thorac. Cardiovasc. Surg. *69*:255–258, 1975.
408. van de Rijn, I.: Analysis of cross-protection between serotypes and passively transferred immune globulin in experimental nutritionally variant streptococcal endocarditis. Infect. Immun. *56*:117–121, 1988.
409. van der Meer, J. T. M., Thompson, J., Valkenburg, H. A., et al.: Epidemiology of bacterial endocarditis in the Netherlands. II. Antecedent procedures and use of prophylaxis. Arch. Intern. Med. *152*:1869–1873, 1992.
410. van der Meer, J. T. M., van Wijk, W., Thompson, J., et al.: Awareness of need and actual use of prophylaxis: Lack of patient compliance in the prevention of bacterial endocarditis. J. Antimicrob. Chemother. *29*:187–194, 1992.
411. van der Meer, J. T. M., van Wijk, W., Thompson, J., et al.: Efficacy of antibiotic prophylaxis for prevention of native valve endocarditis. Lancet *339*:135, 1992.
412. Van Hare, G. F., Ben-Shacher, G., Liebman, J., et al.: Infective endocarditis in infants and children during the past 10 years: A decade of change. Am. Heart J. *107*:1235–1240, 1984.
413. Venditti, M., De Bernardis, F., Micozzi, A., et al.: Fluconazole treatment of catheter-related right-sided endocarditis caused by *Candida albicans* and associated with endophthalmitis and folliculitis. Clin. Infect. Dis. *14*:422–426, 1992.
414. Von Reyn, C. F., Levy, B. S., Arbert, R. D., et al.: Infective endocarditis: An analysis based on strict case definitions. Ann. Intern. Med. *94*:505–517, 1982.
415. Walsh, T. J., and Hutchins, G. M.: *Aspergillus* mural endocarditis. Am. J. Clin. Pathol. *71*:640–644, 1979.
416. Walterspiel, J. N., and Kaplan, S. L.: Incidence and clinical characteristics of "culture negative" infective endocarditis in a pediatric population. Pediatr. Infect. Dis. *5*:328–332, 1986.
417. Watanakunakorn, C., Tan, J. S., and Phair, J. P.: Some salient features of *Staphylococcus aureus* endocarditis. Am. J. Med. *54*:473–481, 1973.
418. Watanakunakorn, C., and Glotzbecker, C.: Synergism with aminoglycosides of penicillin, ampicillin and vancomycin against nonenterococcal group D streptococci and viridans streptococci. J. Med. Microbiol. *10*:133–137, 1977.
419. Watanakunakorn, C., and Burkert, T.: Infective endocarditis at a large community teaching hospital, 1980–1990. Medicine *72*:90–102, 1993.
420. Weinberg, A. G.: Group B streptococcal endocarditis detected by echocardiography. J. Pediatr. *92*:335–336, 1978.
421. Weinstein, A. J., and Moellering, R. C.: Penicillin and gentamicin therapy for enterococcal infections. J. A. M. A. *223*:1030–1032, 1973.
422. Weinstein, L., and Schlesinger, J. J.: Pathoanatomic, pathophysiologic and clinical correlations in endocarditis. N. Engl. J. Med. *291*:832–837, 1122–1126, 1974.
423. Weinstein, M. P., Stratton, C. W., Ackley, A., et al.: Multicenter collaborative evaluation of a standardized bactericidal test as a prognostic indicator in infective endocarditis. Am. J. Med. *78*:262–269, 1985.
424. Werner, A. S., Cobbs, C. G., Kaye, D., et al.: Studies on the bacteremia of bacterial endocarditis. J. A. M. A. *202*:199–203, 1967.
425. Wheeler, J. G., and Weesner, K. M.: *Staphylococcus aureus* endocarditis and pericarditis in an infant with a central venous catheter. Clin. Pediatr. *23*:46–47, 1984.
426. White, P. D.: The incidence of endocarditis in earliest childhood. Am. J. Dis. Child. *32*:536–549, 1926.
427. Williams, R. C., and Kunkel, H. G.: Rheumatoid factor, complement and conglutinin aberrations in patients with subacute bacterial endocarditis. J. Clin. Invest. *41*:666–675, 1962.
428. Wilson, W. R., Thompson, R. L., Wilkowske, C. J., et al.: Short-term therapy for streptococcal infective endocarditis. J. A. M. A. *245*:360–363, 1981.
429. Wilson, W. R., Gilbert, D. N., Bisno, A. L., et al.: Evaluation of new anti-infective drugs for the treatment of infective endocarditis. Clin. Infect. Dis. *15*(Suppl. 1):89–95, 1992.
430. Wilson, W. R., Karchmer, A. W., Dajani, A. S., et al.: Antibiotic treatment of adults with infective endocarditis due to streptococci, enterococci, staphylococci, and HACEK microorganisms. J. A. M. A. *274*:1706–1713, 1995.
431. Witt, M. D., and Bayer, A. S.: Comparison of fluconazole and amphotericin B for prevention and treatment of experimental *Candida* endocarditis. Antimicrob. Agents Chemother. *35*:2481–2485, 1991.
432. Wolfe, J. C., and Johnson, W. D.: Penicillin-sensitive streptococcal endocarditis. Ann. Intern. Med. *81*:178–181, 1974.
433. Wolfson, J. S., and Swartz, M. N.: Serum bactericidal activity as a monitor of antibiotic therapy. N. Engl. J. Med. *312*:968–975, 1985.
434. Woods, G. L., Wood, R. P., and Shaw, B. W.: *Aspergillus* endocarditis in patients without prior cardiovascular surgery: Report of a case in a liver transplant recipient and review. Rev. Infect. Dis. *11*:263–272, 1989.
435. Yeaman, M. R., Norman, D. C., and Bayer, A. S.: *Staphylococcus aureus* susceptibility to thrombin-induced platelet microbicidal protein is independent of platelet adherence and aggregation in vitro. Infect. Immun. *60*:2368–2374, 1992.
436. Yokochi, K., Sakamato, H., Mikajima, T., et al.: Infective endocarditis in children: A current diagnostic trend and the embolic complications. Jpn. Circ. J. *50*:1294–1297, 1986.
437. Zakrzewski, T., and Keith, J. D.: Bacterial endocarditis in infants and children. J. Pediatr. *67*:1179–1193, 1965.
438. Ziment, I.: Nervous system complications in bacterial endocarditis. Am. J. Med. *47*:593–607, 1969.
439. Zubler, R. H., Lange, G., Lambert, P. H., et al.: Detection of immune complexes in unheated sera by a modified ^{125}I-Clq binding test. J. Immunol. *116*:232–239, 1976.

33

INFECTIOUS PERICARDITIS

William W. Pinsky, Richard A. Friedman, David P. Jubelirer, and Michael R. Nihill

Purulent pericarditis generally refers to bacterial infection of the pericardium. Inflammation of the pericardium, however, may result from a number of nonbacterial microorganisms or may occur with a variety of noninfectious illnesses (Table 33–1). Regardless of the cause of pericarditis, the responses of the pericardium are limited to (1) acute inflammation, (2) effusion with or without tamponade, and (3) fibrosis with or without constriction.[12] Because untreated purulent pericarditis is rapidly fatal, it is important to suspect the disease early and to approach the diagnosis aggressively.

ANATOMY AND FUNCTION

The pericardium is composed of two loosely approximated layers: the visceral and the parietal. The visceral pericardium is composed of mesothelial tissue, which closely follows the contour of the heart and extends for a short distance beyond the atria and ventricles on to the great vessels. The outer parietal pericardium is a more fibrous structure, composed of layers of collagen interlaced with elastic fibers. The pericardial sac is attached to the diaphragm below, to the sternum in front, and to the thoracic vertebrae, esophagus, and aorta posteriorly. It is surrounded by the lungs on either side and is related closely to the main bronchi and the mediastinal lymph nodes. The phrenic and vagus nerves supply a network of pain fibers to the parietal pericardium.

The dynamics of the pericardial fluid are poorly understood. The pericardial membrane is active in the transfer of water, electrolytes, and relatively small molecules. Molecules of large molecular weight, however, are absorbed poorly from the pericardial space because lymphatic channels are sparse and drainage must occur primarily through the epicardial capillaries.[50]

The function of the pericardium has been summarized by Ainger[1]: (1) prevention of overdistention of the heart, (2) protection of the heart from infection and adhesions, (3) maintenance of the heart within a fixed geometric position within the chest, and (4) regulation of the interaction between the stroke volumes of the two ventricles.

POPULATION AND INCIDENCE

In an extensive literature review of purulent pericarditis, Boyle and associates[5] reported that half of 425 cases occurred in children younger than 13 years of age. Nonetheless, acute purulent pericarditis is diagnosed infrequently. Pericardial disease of all etiologies occurs approximately once per 850 hospital admissions.[66] From 1962 to 1974, 67 cases were recognized at St. Louis Children's Hospital (Table 33–2).[66] Twelve of these children (18 per cent) had purulent pericarditis. There appears to be a predominance of cases in children younger than 2 years of age. Keith and associates[40] observed that 90 per cent of acute pericarditis in these infants is purulent. A marked male predominance (77 per cent) at all ages was reported by Boyle and coworkers[5]; however, the review by Gersony and McCracken[23] of 50 infants with purulent pericarditis indicated nearly equal sex distribution (56 per cent males). Feldman[19] showed a 57/43 distribution of males/females.

ETIOLOGY

Primary purulent pericarditis is rare and accounted for only 7 of 50 cases reported by Gersony and McCracken.[23] The disease is associated most often with infection from another site, with hematogenous or direct spread to the pericardium. Feldman[19] reviewed all cases of bacterial pericardi-

TABLE 33–1. Causes of Pericarditis

Idiopathic
- Benign
- Recurrent

Infectious
- Purulent
  1. Bacterial: *Staphylococcus aureus, Haemophilus influenzae,* streptococci, *Neisseria meningitidis, Streptococcus pneumoniae,* anaerobes, *Francisella tularensis, Salmonella,* enteric bacilli, *Pseudomonas, Listeria, Neisseria gonorrhoeae, Actinomyces,* nocardiosis
  2. Tuberculosis
  3. Fungal: histoplasmosis, coccidioidomycosis, aspergillosis, candidiasis, blastomycosis, cryptococcosis
- Viral
  1. Coxsackieviruses B
  2. Other: influenza A and B, mumps, echoviruses, adenoviruses, infectious mononucleosis, hepatitis, measles, cytomegalovirus
- Other
  1. Rickettsial: typhus, Q fever
  2. Mycoplasmal: *Mycoplasma pneumoniae*
  3. Parasitic: *Entamoeba histolytica, Echinococcus*
  4. Spirochetal: syphilis, leptospirosis
  5. Chlamydial: psitticosis
  6. Protozoal: toxoplasmosis

Noninfectious
- Postpericardiotomy syndrome
- Rheumatic fever
- Connective tissue disorders: JRA, SLE, dermatomyositis, periarteritis nodosa
- Trauma: blunt or penetrating
- Metabolic: uremia, myxedema
- Hypersensitivity: serum sickness, pulmonary infiltrates with eosinophilia, Stevens-Johnson syndrome, drugs (hydralazine, procainamide, chemotherapy)
- Neoplasm: leukemia, metastatic
- Postirradiation

JRA, juvenile rheumatoid arthritis; SLE, systemic lupus erythematosus.

TABLE 33–2. Pericarditis in Children, 1962–1974 (St. Louis Children's Hospital)*

Etiology	Number of Patients
Unknown	28
Purulent	12
Juvenile rheumatoid arthritis	9
Acute rheumatic fever	8
Uremia	5
Viral	2
Blunt chest trauma	2
Dermatomyositis	1

*Patients with postpericardiotomy pericarditis and those with small effusions at autopsy were excluded from consideration.

From Strauss, A. W., Santa Maria, M., and Goldring, D.: Constrictive pericarditis in children. Am. J. Dis. Child. *129*:822–826, 1975. Copyright 1975, American Medical Association.

tis reported in the English language literature from 1950 to 1977. Including his six cases, there were 162 reports cited. Bacteria were isolated in 146 of 162 cases (90 per cent). No other infection was found in 10 patients. The most common concomitant site involved was the lung, especially for *Staphylococcus aureus, Haemophilus influenzae,* and *Streptococcus pneumoniae.* When septic arthritis, osteomyelitis, or skin infections were found, *S. aureus* most often was the cause of pericarditis. *Neisseria meningitidis* and *H. influenzae* most often were responsible for concomitant meningitis and pericarditis.

Prior to the introduction of antibiotics, pneumococcal and streptococcal organisms were the most frequent causes of purulent pericarditis in children. The majority of cases were associated with pulmonary infections. Nearly half the patients with streptococcal pericarditis had associated postinfluenza pneumonia. Hemolytic streptococci were isolated most often; 10 per cent were nonhemolytic streptococci, and 5 per cent were viridans streptococci. Kauffman and colleagues[39] reviewed 113 cases of pneumococcal pericarditis reported since 1900. Preceding pneumonia was present in 93 per cent and empyema in 66 per cent. Pericarditis was felt to be a late event resulting from delay in appropriate therapy for pneumonia.

S. aureus is the most common organism responsible for purulent pericarditis in children.[3, 5, 19, 23, 34] Before the antibiotic era, it was responsible for only 17 per cent of cases.[5] Most cases are the result of hematogenous seeding of the pericardium from staphylococcal pneumonia with empyema, acute osteomyelitis, or soft tissue abscesses. Occasionally, the pericardium is infected during the course of staphylococcal endocarditis. *S. aureus* is the organism recovered most frequently when purulent pericarditis develops within 3 months of open heart surgery. The clinical course of acute staphylococcal pericarditis is dominated by severe toxemia. In addition to the necrotizing infection produced by *S. aureus,* the organism often releases a potent exotoxin, which produces shock and contributes to the high mortality. *S. aureus* was isolated from 73 per cent of infants who died of purulent pericarditis in the series reported by Gersony and McCracken.[23] It was responsible for 50 per cent of cases in children between 1 and 4 years of age in the review by Feldman.[19] In seven patients younger than 1 month of age, *S. aureus* was isolated from four. This finding is corroborated in literature from other countries. A review of 53 cases in Nigerian children found *S. aureus* and *Mycobacterium tuberculosis* to be equally common.[37] In New Guinea, 100 per cent of patients younger than 18 years of age between 1979 and 1982 had *S. aureus* isolated as the causative agent.[14] In both reviews, coincident lung infection was found most commonly.

The second most frequently encountered organism is *H. influenzae,* usually type b. It was responsible for 22 per cent (35 of 163) of the cases in Feldman's review.[19] Of the 18 isolates that were typed, all were type b. A single site of coexisting infection, the lung, was seen in 16 of 35 cases. Meningitis, as a single other site, was found in 5 of 35, and multiple involvement was found in 7 of 35 patients.[19] Cheatham and colleagues[10] reviewed nine cases of children with pericarditis due to *H. influenzae* between 1975 and 1979. Seven of the nine patients were younger than 1 year of age, and seven of nine had either an upper respiratory tract infection or pneumonia diagnosed 6 weeks to 2 days before the onset of illness. Two patients had coexisting meningitis. Interestingly, in the reviews from New Guinea and Nigeria, *H. influenzae* was not found as a cause of pericarditis in children.[13, 37]

Dajani and associates[14] reported that in 292 cases of *H. influenzae* disease there were no cases of pericarditis found, and other authors have reported only 3 cases of pericarditis in 83 consecutive cases of *H. influenzae* disease. Leggiadro and Balsam[46] reported two cases of *H. influenzae* pericarditis developing in children while they were receiving intravenous ampicillin for suspected sepsis. Thus, it is apparent that *H. influenzae* has become an increasingly more common agent responsible for pericarditis in the 1980s and 1990s than in previous decades. Echeverria and colleagues[17] summarized 33 cases from the literature. Pulmonary infiltrates and empyema were seen in 64 per cent of patients. Nearly 85 per cent had symptoms of an upper respiratory tract infection in the preceding 5 to 12 days.

Pneumococcal, streptococcal, and meningococcal pericarditis have diminished in frequency since the introduction of penicillin.[5] Pericardial involvement occurs in about 5 per cent of young adults with meningococcemia.[16, 31] The clinical course generally is milder than that observed with other types of purulent pericarditis. Pericardial involvement rarely is present at the time of hospital admission. Pericarditis became apparent by the third day in 13 of 17 patients reported by Dixon and Sanford.[16] In some, it did not occur until late in the course of therapy. Whether this late-onset pericardial effusion is a part of the meningococcal infection or is related to penicillin hypersensitivity has been debated in the literature.[11, 16, 52, 60]

Occasionally, other microorganisms may cause acute purulent pericarditis. Feldman[19] reported that 11 of 146 cases (8 per cent) of pericarditis in children were due to *Pseudomonas aeruginosa.* It can occur with pneumonic tularemia, salmonellosis, sepsis from enteric bacilli, listeriosis, and disseminated gonococcal disease.[5] Anaerobic bacteria also should be suspected when pericarditis develops in association with lung abscess, intra-abdominal infection, or a penetrating wound. Callanan and colleagues[7] reported the rapid development of constrictive pericarditis after purulent pericarditis due to anaerobic streptococcal infection. The child had a history of blunt trauma to the chest with no evidence of a penetrating wound 3 weeks before cardiac tamponade developed. The incidence of anaerobic infection may be underestimated because of improper handling of specimens for culture.[19]

M. tuberculosis, once a common cause of acute pericarditis in the United States,[4] now is responsible more often for chronic pericardial disease. This infection is a complication of miliary tuberculosis and rarely a primary infection. In the series of 2500 children with tuberculosis reported by Lincoln and Savell,[47] pericarditis was diagnosed in 0.4 per cent and found at necropsy in 5 per cent of patients. A review of 100 cases of tuberculous pericarditis in South African blacks by Desai[15] revealed a marked male predominance (72 per cent).

The duration of symptoms, consisting of cough and peripheral edema, in the vast majority of patients was from 0 to 120 days. Most patients were febrile and in congestive heart failure. Generalized lymphadenopathy was seen in nearly 30 per cent of patients and pulsus paradoxus in half, and a friction rub was audible in 25 per cent. Of the 52 patients who had pericardiocentesis, 40 per cent yielded fluid but none was positive for acid-fast bacilli. Pericardial effusion was demonstrated in 82 patients, 16 of whom died of tamponade and another 16 of whom went on to develop constricting pericarditis.

Orbtals and Avioli[54] describe the four stages of tuberculous pericarditis as (1) dry, (2) effusive, (3) absorptive, and (4) constrictive. Granulomata usually are found in the dry stage and heal with no sequelae. The effusive stage is common with tuberculous lymphadenitis, and usually 15 to 200 mL of fluid accumulates in the pericardial space. The absorptive stage is characterized by thickening of the pericardium with fibrin deposition. Further fibrin deposition plus calcification occurs during the constrictive phase. The disease may progress through all stages or remain in one stage alone.

Latent infection in the mediastinal lymph nodes with spread directly into the pericardium is believed to be the mode of involvement with *M. tuberculosis.*[54] The lymph nodes at the tracheal bifurcation often are the source.

Histoplasma pericarditis generally occurs with pulmonary, rather than disseminated, disease.[56] Coccidioidomycosis[9] and, rarely, blastomycosis[30] also may cause pericardial disease. Other pathogenic fungi include *Aspergillus* and *Candida.* These are more serious considerations in patients who are immunosuppressed or receiving long-term broad-spectrum antibiotics after cardiac surgery.

PATHOLOGY AND PATHOGENESIS

Pericarditis begins with fine deposits of fibrin adjacent to the great vessels; this causes the pericardial membrane to lose its smoothness and translucency. Numerous granulocytes may extend into the myocardium.[26]

Bacterial pericarditis most commonly results from direct extension of infection from involved lung and pleura. Pulmonary infections may spread to the pericardium via the bronchial circulation.[29] Pericarditis frequently arises, however, from infection elsewhere that is transmitted hematogenously. It also may be the result of an immunologically induced antibody response to a primary infection.

As pericardial fluid accumulates, intrapericardial pressure rises. The rate of rise is a function of both the speed of accumulation and the compliance of the pericardium. With slow accumulation of fluid, large volumes can be accommodated because of the gradual expansion of the parietal pericardium. As the compliance of the pericardium reaches its maximum, however, further accumulation of even small volumes of fluid results in an abrupt increase in intrapericardial pressure. If pericardial fluid accumulates at a rapid rate, marked elevation in intrapericardial pressure may occur with much smaller volumes of fluid. As little as 100 mL can cause severe tamponade in a small child, whereas up to 3 L may accumulate slowly in an older child and not result in tamponade.[1]

The most significant hemodynamic effect of pericardial effusion is restriction of ventricular filling. Ventricular end-diastolic, atrial, and venous pressures rise on the right and left sides of the heart equally. When restriction to ventricular filling becomes more pronounced, there is a fall in ventricular stroke volume and cardiac output. In an attempt to maintain cardiac output, tachycardia and peripheral vasoconstriction are seen. In addition, systemic arterial blood pressure and pulse pressure are reduced markedly.

Tamponade occurs when these compensatory mechanisms fail to maintain adequate cardiac output.

CLINICAL MANIFESTATIONS

A diagnosis of purulent pericarditis should be suspected in any patient with septicemia in whom cardiomegaly develops. The classic signs and symptoms of pericarditis are (1) precordial pain, (2) pericardial friction rub, (3) evidence of cardiac fluid, and (4) muffled heart sounds.[8] Chest pain is not a frequent symptom, especially in small children; the reported percentages vary from 15 to 80.[2, 5, 23, 34, 40, 50, 53, 72]

The most common symptoms and signs of pericarditis are fever, tachypnea, and tachycardia. These also are presenting features of associated systemic infection. However, if there is enlargement of the cardiac shadow radiographically, with or without a friction rub, and the tachypnea and tachycardia are out of proportion to the fever, either myocardial dysfunction or pericarditis should be suspected. An evanescent or ubiquitous rub may be present. The typical sound of a rub is that of a high-frequency murmur,[55] which may be to-and-fro or triphasic but may not have any correlation with the cardiac cycle.[20] Frequently, the rub is heard better with the patient leaning forward or kneeling.[20] A rub may be differentiated from a murmur by pressing the diaphragm of the stethoscope firmly against the chest wall; this amplifies the rub, and the typical scratchy quality becomes more apparent, as one opposes the visceral and parietal pericardium by compression of the chest. Rubs have been known to increase with inspiration.[62] Although it generally is true that a rub is less likely to be heard when there is a large effusion, it still may be present.[20] The heart sounds usually are muffled, and the palpable ventricular impulse generally is diminished. Both of these findings, however, may be found in congestive heart failure; they may be absent with tamponade.

Signs of cardiac tamponade may be an early complication of pericarditis in association with a systemic infection. Cardiac tamponade means that there is compression of the heart by a tense pericardial sac, usually full of fluid, resulting in a decrease in venous return to the cardiac chambers and a decrease in cardiac output. During inspiration, intrathoracic pressure falls, and there is an increase in venous return to the cavae. The tense pericardial sac limits the amount of blood that can enter the right atrium because of diastolic compression; therefore, there is a paradoxic rise in jugular venous pressure during inspiration (Kussmaul sign)[41] (Fig. 33–1).

During inspiration, there normally is a small drop in systolic blood pressure and cardiac output due to an increase in pulmonary venous capacitance. This is exaggerated with pericardial tamponade (>10 mm Hg drop in blood pressure) because of the restricted inflow into the cardiac chambers. This clinical sign has been called "paradoxic pulse," but it actually is an exaggeration of the normal respiratory cycle[25] (Fig. 33–2).

DIAGNOSIS

Radiographic appearance of a rapidly increasing cardiothoracic ratio without increasing pulmonary vascular markings is more suggestive of pericardial effusion than congestive heart failure secondary to myocardial dysfunction (Fig. 33–3). Fluoroscopy alone generally is of little value; both myocardial dysfunction and pericarditis can impair cardiac contractility.

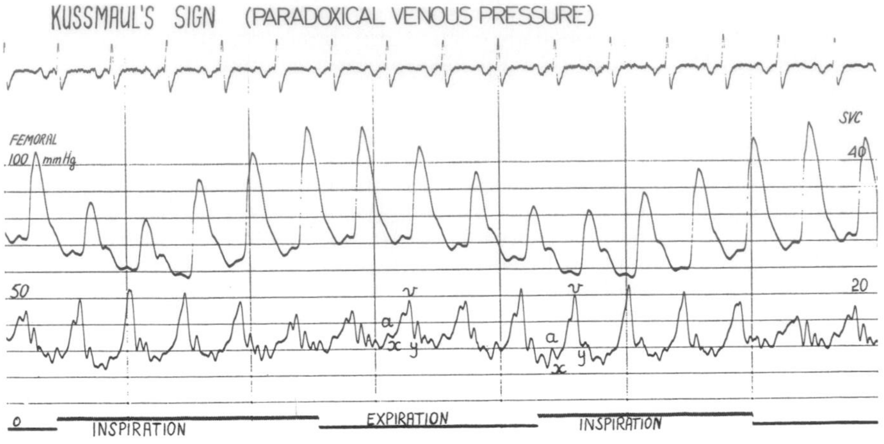

FIGURE 33–1. *Simultaneous recording of right atrial and femoral artery pressures. Note the increased V wave and exaggerated decrease in femoral artery pulse with inspiration.*

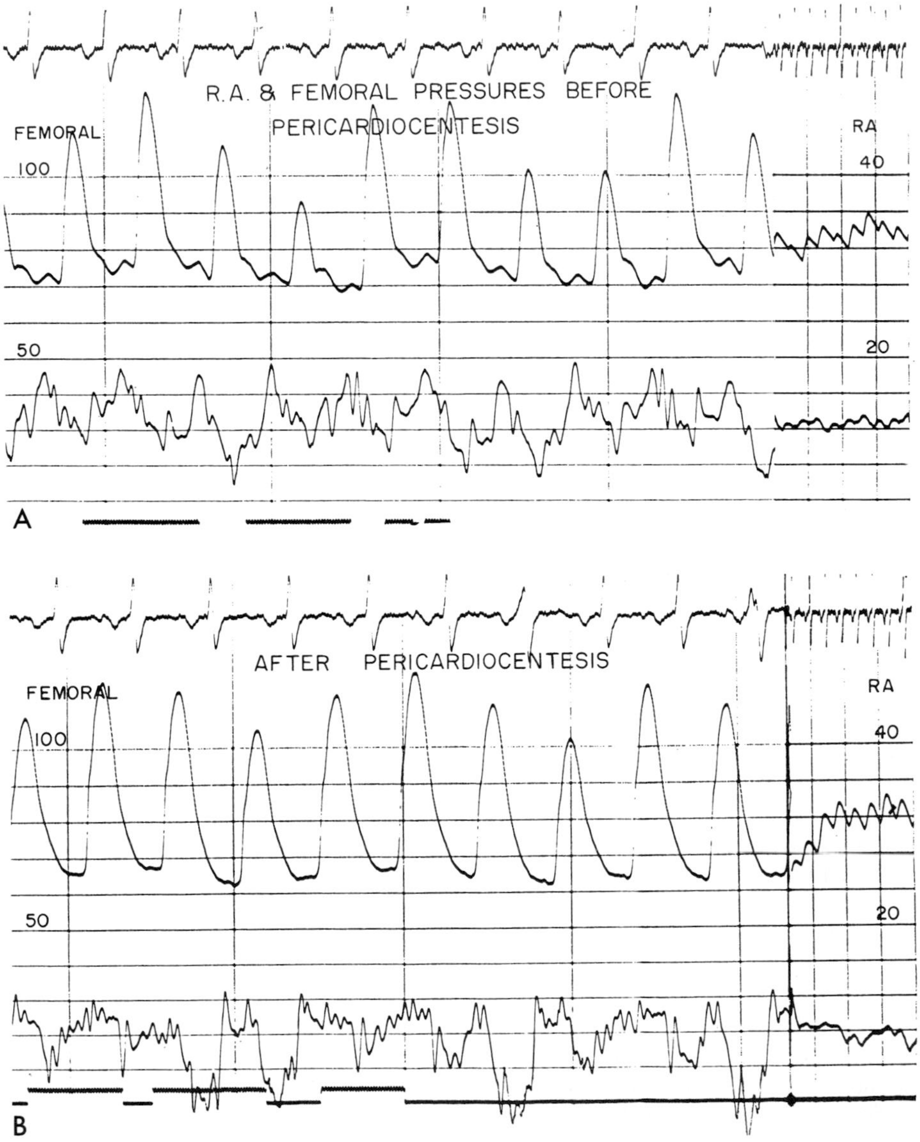

FIGURE 33–2. *Recordings of femoral artery and right atrial pressures* (A) *prior to and* (B) *after pericardiocentesis. In* A, *there is an exaggerated decrease in fall of femoral artery pressure with inspiration as well as a sustained increase in right atrial pressure.* B *demonstrates a more normal variation of femoral pressure and a lower right atrial pressure.*

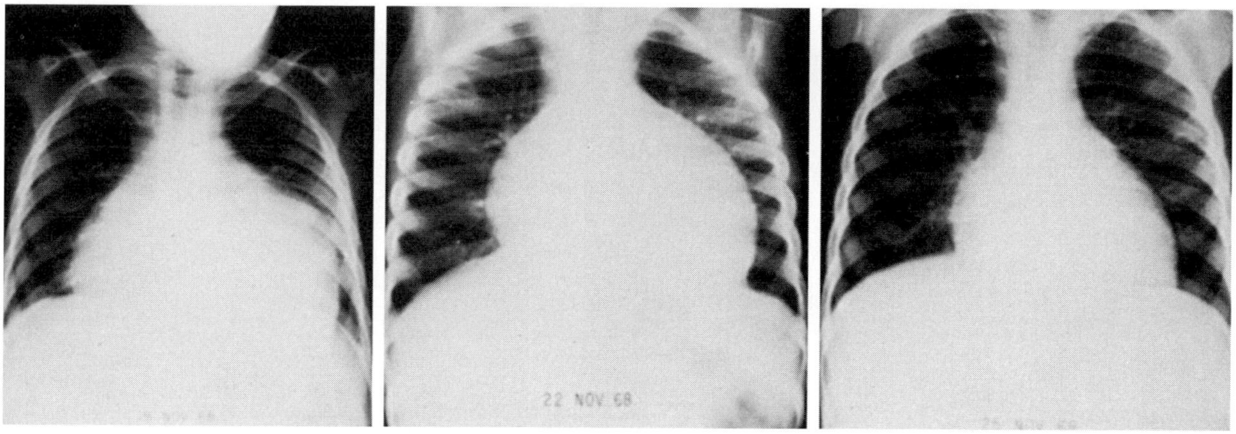

FIGURE 33–3. *A patient with pericarditis. The first two radiographs demonstrate an enlarged cardiac shadow without an increase in pulmonary vascular markings. The last shows a marked decrease in apparent heart size after pericardiocentesis.*

It is important to remember that the size of the pericardial shadow does not indicate necessarily the severity of hemodynamic effects. This is a function of the rapidity of accumulation and the volume of pericardial fluid. Thus, when acute infection results in sudden cardiac tamponade, the heart size may be normal. A large globular heart shadow with no evidence of increased pulmonary vasculature, particularly in a patient who has signs of right-sided heart failure, is strong evidence for pericardial disease. The lack of pulmonary over circulation will help to distinguish this from myocarditis; however, it may be difficult to determine whether there also are pulmonic infiltrates.

Lane and Carsky[44] demonstrated the potential of a plain lateral chest film to demonstrate pericardial effusion. The anterior mediastinal and subepicardial "fat stripes" were separated by more than 2 mm in 27 of 42 cases of proven effusion. However, 5 of 15 "negative" films and none of the "positive" films were seen in patients with purulent pericarditis. Obliteration of the retrosternal space without evidence of thymic or right ventricular enlargement also is suggestive of pericarditis. The extent of electrocardiographic abnormalities may be explained by the amount of pericardial effusion and the presence of superficial myocardial injury or myocarditis. Pericardial effusion gives rise to low-voltage QRS complexes. This is the result of the damping effect of pericardial fluid between the chest wall and the myocardium. Accumulation of fluid and fibrin under pressure also may produce an injury pattern manifested by ST-segment deviation. More than 90 per cent of patients have elevation of the ST segment, which occurs most frequently in leads I, II, V_5, and V_6. Widespread T-wave inversion indicative of epicarditis may be seen in the same leads in which ST-segment elevation occurs.

Spodick[63] has described four stages of electrocardiographic changes in acute pericarditis. In stage I, pronounced ST-segment elevation is present and depression of the PR segment may be noted. In stage II, the ST segment begins to return toward the isoelectric line, the amplitude of the T wave diminishes, and the PR segment is depressed. By stage III, the ST segment has returned to the isoelectric line and the T-wave inversion occurs. An incompletely inverted T wave (a diphasic wave or an upright T wave with a notched summit) sometimes is observed. In stage IV, these changes may resolve completely. T-wave abnormalities, however, may persist for life and do not indicate active disease necessarily.

Gintzon and Laks[24] compared the electrocardiograms of 19 patients with acute pericarditis with those of 20 healthy patients. By forming a ratio of the amplitude of the ST-segment and T-wave height in all patients, a value of 0.25 or greater in lead V_6 had a positive and negative predictive value of 1.0 for determining the presence of pericarditis. This also was true in leads I, V_4, and V_5, although the predictive values were not as high as in lead V_6. Using Spodick's criteria in their patients, Gintzon and Laks[24] were unable to distinguish healthy normal individuals from acute pericarditis patients. Their method may, therefore, prove to be more reliable, although a large study in children has not been performed.

The presence of electrical alternans is seen in a large pericardial effusion. This refers to the alternation in electrical amplitude of the T wave and the QRS complex with each cardiac cycle. Electrical alternans is thought to result from the rotational and pendular motion of the heart suspended in pericardial fluid.

Deviations from classic patterns occasionally occur, but it is not uncommon to have single electrocardiographic changes. For example, all 12 children reported by Okoroma and colleagues[53] had ST-segment elevation, whereas only 3 had concomitant low voltage.

Spodick[64] has pointed out that although many textbooks cite the frequent occurrence of dysrhythmias with pericarditis, they are an unusual occurrence in the absence of coexisting heart disease. Twenty of 49 patients with acute pericarditis had no underlying heart disease. Seven had no dysrhythmias documented on 24-hour Holter monitoring, and 10 of 20 had infrequent single ectopic beats. Only three patients had supraventricular tachycardia.

M-mode echocardiography is the most sensitive method for diagnosis of significant pericardial effusion.[28, 35] With a small to moderate effusion, only a "fluid space" is noted posteriorly (Fig. 33–4*B*). However, with a greater effusion, fluid is seen anteriorly and posteriorly and the septal motion becomes grossly abnormal. The heart may give the appearance of freely swinging (see Fig. 33–4*A*). Newer echocardiographic techniques, such as two-dimensional sector scanning, are no more useful than the conventional M-mode.

Laird and colleagues[42] found pericardial effusions on M-mode echocardiograms in 20 per cent of patients with *H. influenzae* meningitis. Counterimmunoelectrophoresis usually was positive for antigen of *H. influenzae,* and the amount usually was 20 mL or less. However, the majority of cases were asymptomatic and resolved spontaneously with resolution of the meningitis. Thus, the clinical significance of this

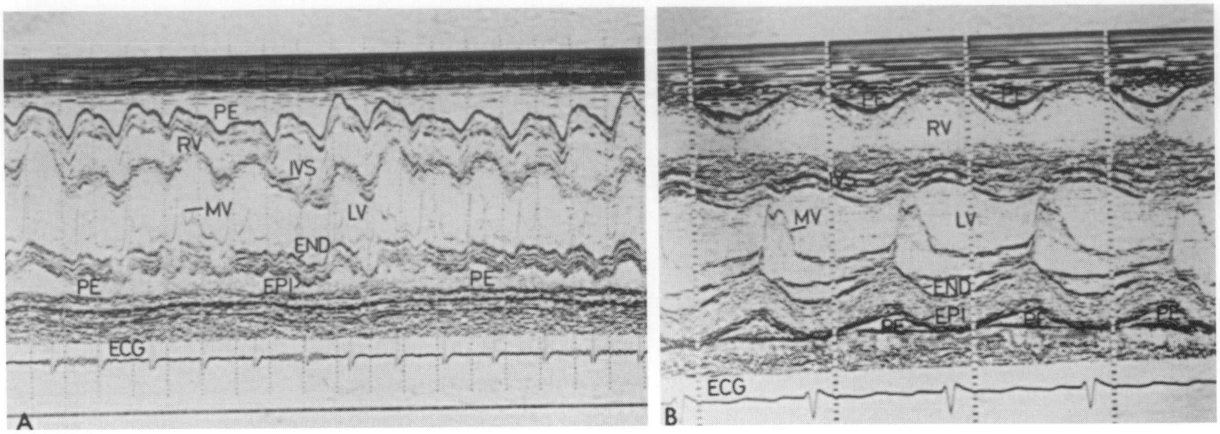

FIGURE 33–4. *Serial echocardiograms of a child prior to pericardiocentesis* (A) *and after pericardiocentesis* (B). *In* A, *note the large effusion both anterior and posterior with the "swinging" movement of the septum and anterior and posterior walls. In* B, *the heart movement is normal and there remains only a small effusion anteriorly and posteriorly. END, endocardium; EPI, epicardium; IVS, interventricular septum; LV, left ventricle; MV, mitral valve; PE, pericardial effusion; RV, right ventricle.*

pericarditis may be minimal, and these investigators felt that this technique was of limited value in patients without evidence of cardiac involvement.

Occult or unsuspected pericarditis also has been discerned with the use of radionuclide techniques. Greenberg and colleagues,[27] using iridium 111, and Shreiner and colleagues,[59] using gallium 67, demonstrated the presence of purulent pericarditis in an immunocompromised host and posttraumatic patients, respectively.

A pericardial effusion also may be diagnosed by noting a discrepancy between the position of a catheter placed adjacent to the lateral wall of the right atrium and the right cardiac border. An injection of radiopaque contrast material into the right atrium may delineate these findings further. Pressure measurements at the time of cardiac catheterization reveal the elevated right atrial pressure and further emphasize the exaggeration of venous, systemic, and left ventricular pressures imposed by inspiration (see Fig. 33–2). Injection of carbon dioxide or air into the pericardium percutaneously may delineate further the pericardial effusion fluoroscopically and differentiate freely moving fluid from loculated areas (Fig. 33–5). Radionuclide imaging also has been helpful in establishing a diagnosis of pericardial effusion.[73, 79]

The diagnosis of purulent pericarditis is established definitively only by direct examination of pericardial fluid. Purulent fluid is characterized by a predominance of polymorphonuclear leukocytes; however, this also may occur early in the course of viral and tuberculous pericarditis. Proper handling of pericardial fluid is crucial to recovery and identification of the etiologic agent: (1) Place fluid directly into broth capable of supporting aerobic and anaerobic microorganisms. Fluid also should be plated directly onto agar media, such as blood agar, chocolate agar, or MacConkey agar. (2) In addition, cultures should be submitted for *M. tuberculosis*, fungi, and viruses. (3) Several slides should be prepared for immediate examination by Gram stain and stain for acid-fast bacilli. Unstained slides should be stored in case of controversy or the need for special histochemical stains. A sample of pericardial fluid may be submitted for detection of bacterial antigens by latex agglutination or counterimmunoelectrophoresis or for detection of staphylococcal techoic acid antibodies. These techniques are useful, particularly when the patient has re-

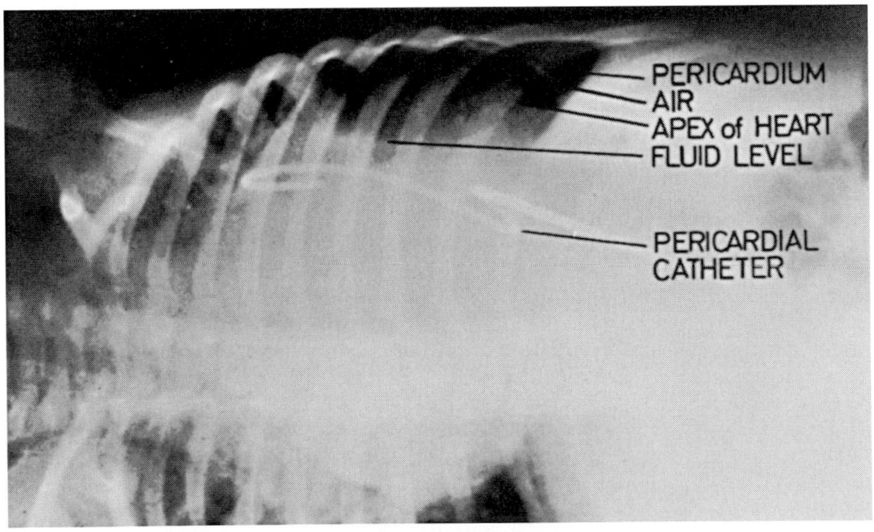

FIGURE 33–5. *Chest radiograph of a patient lying on right side with a catheter in the pericardium. Air has been injected through the catheter, outlining the pericardium and fluid within the sac.*

ceived prior antimicrobial therapy. The yield from these procedures may be increased by concomitant examination of the serum and urine of the patient.

The causative microorganism is isolated from blood cultures in the majority of patients. When indicated, cerebrospinal fluid also should be cultured. Because purulent pericarditis often follows infections of the lung or pleural space, thoracentesis or direct lung aspirate will reveal the etiologic agent in many cases. Documentation of empyema together with evidence of pericardial disease correlates highly with purulent pericarditis. Van Reken and associates,[69] however, have reported an interesting case of *H. influenzae* type b pneumonia and empyema in a patient from whom only coxsackievirus A9 was isolated from nonpurulent pericardial fluid.

Acid-fast bacilli are present on stained smears of pericardial fluid in 15 to 42 per cent of patients with tuberculous pericarditis.[4] Examination of pericardial biopsy will increase the frequency of identification of *M. tuberculosis*. Not all patients will react to intermediate-strength purified protein derivative (67 per cent), and second-strength skin tests might be necessary. The anergic state seen with miliary disease must be excluded.

Grossly bloody pericardial fluid is noted frequently in patients with *Histoplasma* pericarditis, and an aspirate of the effusion reveals a predominance of mononuclear leukocytes. Growth of *Histoplasma capsulatum* from pericardial fluid rarely is successful. Elevation of the yeast phase of the complement-fixation titer in pericardial fluid allows a more rapid diagnosis.[56] Serum precipitin antibodies to *H. capsulatum* also indicate acute histoplasmosis.

DIFFERENTIAL DIAGNOSIS

Any patient with a rapidly increasing heart size in the absence of increasing pulmonary vascular markings should be suspected of having a pericardial effusion. Purulent pericarditis must be differentiated from pericardial effusion due to collagen diseases, other infectious agents (viral, tuberculous, rickettsial, protozoan), neoplastic disorders, metabolic disorders, and congestive heart failure.[8] In addition, glycogen storage disease, congenital heart disease, primary myocardial disease, cardiac tumors, and coronary artery aberrations (anomalous origin from the pulmonary artery, medial wall necrosis, and Kawasaki disease) may be confused with pericardial effusion.[8] Appropriate analysis of pericardial fluid, as described, generally permits differentiation of purulent pericarditis from pericarditis caused by other disorders.

TREATMENT

Purulent pericarditis is a potentially life-threatening illness that requires (1) pericardial decompression and open drainage, (2) appropriate antimicrobial therapy, and (3) intense supportive therapy.

Ainger[1] stated that more than half the children with purulent pericarditis require early or emergency drainage of the pericardium for relief of critical tamponade. Although bedside needle pericardiocentesis may be lifesaving or necessary for rapid diagnosis, Fowler and Manitasas[20] reported three deaths related to pericardiocentesis performed by inexperienced physicians. Complications include arrhythmias resulting from myocardial injury, laceration of the coronary arteries leading to hemopericardium and tamponade, and pneumothorax. Ledbetter[45] described a 10-year-old girl with staphylococcal pericarditis who developed an aortic aneurysm after multiple pericardiocentesis procedures for recurrent tamponade. The subxiphoid approach is recommended, and Hoffman and Stanger[33] have described the proper technique.

Decompression and drainage of the pericardium are safest in a controlled environment, such as in an operating room or under fluoroscopy in the catheterization laboratory. If the patient is awake and agitated, premedication with intravenous diazepam (1 mg per year of age) or ketamine (0.5 to 1 mg/kg) may be given.

If pericardiocentesis is not successful in relieving symptoms and evidence of tamponade continues, immediate surgical drainage is necessary. Multiple attempts may prove unsuccessful and can lead to serious complications. The pus surrounding the heart may be too thick to be aspirated, as has been seen especially with *H. influenzae* infection.[48] A surgically created pericardial window with a drain sometimes is necessary for complete removal of fluid, which accumulates rapidly. In preparation for evacuation of the pericardial fluid during tamponade, adequate cardiac output can be maintained by stimulating the heart with pharmacologic agents that cause both a chronotropic and an inotropic effect. Isoproterenol administered intravenously at a rate of 0.05 to 0.10 μg/kg/minute is our drug of choice. This does not replace evacuating the fluid, but it gains time until the aspiration or drainage can be performed. Medications that tend to decrease heart rate and intravascular volume are contraindicated because they further compromise the patient. Wyler and colleagues[71] warn against the use of halothane anesthesia because of its known depressant effect on myocardial function. They described two patients who had reversible cardiac arrest when this agent was used during surgery to relieve tamponade.

Controversy exists regarding the approach and extent of surgery.[18, 20, 21, 43, 49, 58] Either a left anterolateral thoracotomy through the fifth intercostal space or a subxiphoid approach with removal of the xiphoid process appears best. Most surgeons favor the creation of a pericardial "window"; however, some favor more extensive removal of pericardial tissue. This decision may be influenced by the severity of pericardial inflammation or the presence of bloody pericardial fluid because these have greater potential for producing acute or chronic constriction. Care must be taken during the procedure not to injure the phrenic nerves. Morgan and colleagues[48] reviewed 15 children with purulent pericarditis between 1971 and 1981. *H. influenzae* occurred in 7 of 15 patients. Most patients had pericardiocentesis followed by an anterior interphrenic pericardiectomy and recovered completely. In a series of nine children with *H. influenzae* pericarditis, all received a limited left thoracotomy with subxiphoid approach for pericardiostomy and there were no deaths.[10]

It must be emphasized that antimicrobial therapy alone is insufficient for the successful treatment of purulent pericarditis. The survival of patients with purulent pericarditis is improved significantly when early pericardial drainage is performed (Table 33–3). In the preantibiotic era, draining the pericardium improved the mortality from nearly 100 to 45

TABLE 33–3. Influence of Pericardial Drainage on Survival in Purulent Pericarditis in Children

Treatment	Survived	Died
Antibiotics alone	5	28
Antibiotics and pericardial drainage	45	10

Data from references 2, 21, 39, 51.

per cent.[5] Occasional patients with meningococcal pericarditis have been managed successfully without pericardial drainage.[12] Fyfe and colleagues[22] described 73 of 79 patients with *H. influenzae* pericarditis seen between 1928 and 1984. The mortality before 1960 was 64 per cent (7 of 11 patients), although the majority of deaths (5 of 7) were reported prior to the antibiotic era. From 1960 to 1969, the mortality rate was 36 per cent, and from 1970 to 1979, it dropped to 11.5 per cent. From 1980 to 1984, there were 25 reported cases with no mortality. The investigators noted that when surgical drainage techniques were used with antibiotic therapy, there was no difference in mortality between patients receiving ampicillin and chloramphenicol versus ampicillin alone. This reflects the absence of ampicillin-resistant organisms in these patients.

When the etiologic agent cannot be detected rapidly, the initial antibiotic regimen should consist of two or more drugs. Because *S. aureus* is a major pathogen, a penicillinase-resistant penicillin, such as methicillin, nafcillin, or oxacillin, must be included in a dose of 200 mg/kg/24 hours (maximum, 8 g). Vancomycin may be used in a dose of 60 mg/kg/day in four divided doses (maximum, 4 g). In addition, ampicillin should be administered (300 mg/kg/24 hours) to provide protection against streptococci, pneumococci, meningococci, and *H. influenzae.* Chloramphenicol can be used when disease due to *H. influenzae* is suspected, until the sensitivity of this organism to ampicillin can be confirmed. Another equally acceptable and widely used combination for initial empiric therapy is oxacillin (150 to 200 mg/kg/day) plus cefotaxime (200 mg/kg/day), each provided every 6 hours intravenously. An aminoglycoside antibiotic should be added to this combined drug therapy when purulent pericarditis occurs after cardiac surgery, in association with genitourinary infections, or in the immunocompromised host. For the patient who is allergic to penicillin, vancomycin, clindamycin, or cefazolin is substituted for the treatment of *S. aureus;* some patients who are allergic to penicillin will be sensitive to cephalosporins. If methicillin-resistant *S. aureus* strains or penicillin and third-generation cephalosporin-resistant pneumococci are prevalent in a given locale, vancomycin should be substituted for the semisynthetic penicillin in patients who may have acquired infection nosocomially. Duration of therapy is empiric and in part determined by the nature of concomitant infection. Generally, once a pathogenic microorganism has been isolated, the most specific antimicrobial agent is continued intravenously for 3 to 4 weeks.

Using chemotherapy to treat tuberculous pericarditis has had a major impact on mortality. Prior to its use, there was an 80 to 90 per cent mortality rate in the acute phase. The other 10 to 20 per cent of patients died of constrictive pericarditis or miliary tuberculosis.[54] At present, the use of three or four drugs, including isoniazid, pyrazinamide, rifampin, and possibly streptomycin, for a period of 9 to 18 months is recommended. Corticosteroids seem to be helpful in reducing the inflammatory response to infection and enhancing the resorption of pericardial fluid.[54] Prednisone (1 mg/kg/24 hours) or an equivalent dose of other preparations over 6 to 8 weeks also is recommended. In selected cases, pericardiectomy may be indicated to prevent constrictive pericarditis.

Amphotericin B alone or with other systemic agents is indicated for treatment of fungal pericarditis; however, it rarely is required for successful therapy of *Histoplasma* pericarditis.

General supportive therapy in the acute stage of infection may include the administration of oxygen, volume expansion to increase ventricular filling pressure, and isoproterenol to facilitate systolic emptying. Digitalis and diuretics should be used cautiously and only when indicated by decreased myocardial function. Serial electrocardiograms may indicate the presence of occult arrhythmias and alert the physician to the degree of myocardial involvement. The patient must be monitored carefully for signs of reaccumulation of pericardial fluid and for the development of acute constrictive pericarditis. Strauss and colleagues[66] reported this complication in 2 of 12 children with purulent pericarditis. Acute constriction may develop within weeks of the initial pericardial infection[2, 6] and has been reported as early as the eighth day.[57] Constrictive pericarditis may be suspected by increasing jugular and central venous pressure, weight gain, enlarging liver, worsening dyspnea, and decreased urinary output. The persistence of heart failure when the cardiac silhouette is becoming smaller also suggests the development of constrictive pericarditis. Complete pericardiectomy should be performed promptly when constriction is suspected.

PROGNOSIS

The current mortality of acute purulent pericarditis ranges from 25 to 75 per cent. Accurate statistics, however, are difficult to compute from the literature because the nature and severity of underlying disease have not been considered. Factors that contribute to mortality are (1) the delay in recognition, (2) the absence of early surgical drainage, (3) the presence of cardiac tamponade, (4) the degree of myocardial involvement, (5) the etiologic agent (particularly *S. aureus*), and (6) the age of the patient. Long-term follow-up of children with purulent pericarditis is recommended. They should be followed carefully for the presence of a constrictive component as a sequela to the acute infection. Most children, however, recover fully with a return to normal activity.

VIRAL PERICARDITIS

In 1951, Christian[11] suggested that viral infections were responsible for cases of idiopathic or benign pericarditis. A viral etiology, however, has not been substantiated in many patients.

Etiology

The principal viruses implicated in pericarditis are the coxsackieviruses.[51] Adenoviruses have been recovered less frequently.[38] Previous associations with chickenpox, smallpox vaccinations, influenza,[32] influenza vaccinations,[67] and even infectious mononucleosis[36, 61] have been reported.

Clinical Manifestations

Generally, there is a history of upper respiratory tract infections 10 days to 2 weeks preceding the onset of symptoms in about 40 to 75 per cent of cases. Fever and chest and abdominal pain are the most common symptoms.[3, 11] A friction rub may be heard in 50 to 80 per cent of cases.[72] Children with viral pericarditis generally are less toxic and experience smaller elevations in body temperature than do those with purulent pericarditis. Some, however, appear acutely ill. Large amounts of pericardial fluid accumulation and tamponade are rare.

Investigative Techniques

The electrocardiographic, radiographic, echocardiographic, and nuclear scanning findings described in patients with

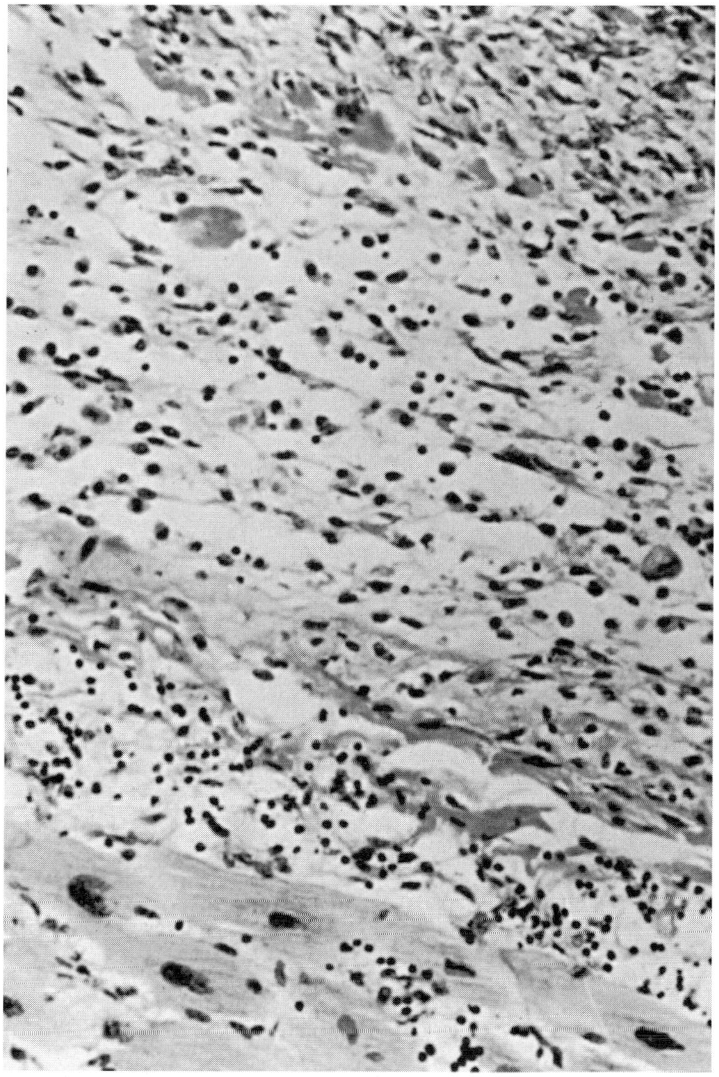

FIGURE 33–6. *Viral pericarditis showing a layer of fibrin and fibroblasts along the pericardial surface. A mononuclear cell infiltrate is in the epicardium and extends into the outer myocardium. (H and E × 400.) (Courtesy of Dr. Edith Hawkins.)*

purulent pericarditis also are observed in patients with viral pericarditis. The peripheral leukocyte count, however, may reveal fewer polymorphonuclear leukocytes than in patients with bacterial pericarditis. Mononuclear cell infiltrates in the pericardium with extension into the myocardium may be seen (Fig. 33–6).

If obtained, pericardial fluid should be sent for cell count and viral culture. Nasopharyngeal and rectal culture also should be obtained and cultured for viruses. Acute and convalescent sera should be obtained so that appropriate titers can be measured if a virus is isolated.

Course and Prognosis

Viral pericarditis generally resolves spontaneously over a 3- to 4-week period.[51] Large pericardial effusions and tamponade are rare.[8] Generally, bed rest for about 1 week and analgesics for pain are the only therapy that is required. Constrictive pericarditis is a rare occurrence. Recurrent pericarditis may develop.[51]

References

1. Ainger, L. E.: Diseases of the pericardium. *In* Kelley, V. C. (ed.): Practice of Pediatrics. Looseleaf Reference Services. Vol. III. New York, Harper Medical, 1969.
2. Benzing, G., III, and Kaplan, S.: Purulent pericarditis. Am. J. Dis. Child. *106:*287–294, 1963.
3. Boles, E. T., and Hosier, D. M.: Abdominal pain in acute myocarditis and pericarditis. Br. Heart J. *2:*165, 1940.
4. Boyd, G. L.: Tuberculous pericarditis in children. Am. J. Dis. Child. *86:*293–300, 1953.
5. Boyle, J. D., Pearce, M. L., and Guze, L. B.: Purulent pericarditis: Review of literature and report of eleven cases. Medicine *40:*119–144, 1961.
6. Caird, R., Conway, N., and McMillan, I. K. R.: Purulent pericarditis followed by early constriction in young children. Br. Heart J. *35:*201–203, 1973.
7. Callanan, D. L., Morriss, M. J., Kaplan, S. L., et al.: Constrictive pericarditis due to *Streptococcus sanguis*. South. Med. J. *74:*377–378, 1981.
8. Cayler, G. G., and Riley, H. D.: Non-rheumatic inflammatory cardiovascular diseases. *In* Moss, A. J., and Adams, F. H. (eds.): Heart Disease in Infants, Children and Adolescents. Baltimore, Williams & Wilkins, 1968, p. 851.
9. Chapman, M. G., and Kaplan, L.: Cardiac involvement in coccidioidomycosis. Am. J. Med. *23:*87–98, 1957.
10. Cheatham, J. E., Grantham, R. N., Peyton, M. D., et al.: *Haemophilus influenzae* purulent pericarditis in children. J. Thorac. Cardiovasc. Surg. *79:*933–936, 1980.
11. Christian, H. A.: Nearly ten decades of interest in idiopathic pericarditis. Am. Heart J. *42:*645, 1951.
12. Connolly, D. C., and Burchell, H. B.: Pericarditis: A ten-year survey. Am. J. Cardiol. *7:*7–13, 1961.
13. Corachan, M., Poore, P., Hadley, G. P., et al.: Purulent pericarditis in Papua, New Guinea: Report of 12 cases and review of the literature in a tropical environment. Trans. R. Soc. Trop. Med. Hyg. *77:*341–343, 1983.
14. Dajani, A. S., Asmar, B. I., and Thirumoorthi, M.: Systemic *Haemophilus influenzae* disease: An overview. J. Pediatr. *94:*355–364, 1979.
15. Desai, H. N.: Tuberculous pericarditis. A review of 100 cases. S. Afr. Med. J. *55:*877–880, 1979.

16. Dixon, L. M., and Sanford, H. S.: Meningococcal pericarditis in the antibiotic era. Milit. Med. *136:*433–438, 1971.
17. Echeverria, P., Smith, E. W. P., Ingram, D., et al.: *Haemophilus influenzae* b pericarditis in children. Pediatrics *56:*808–818, 1975.
18. Farrow, C. D., Jr., Brom, A. G., and Nauta, J.: The surgical treatment of pericarditis: A follow-up study. Dis. Chest *48:*478–483, 1965.
19. Feldman, W. E.: Bacterial etiology and mortality of purulent pericarditis in pediatric patients: Review of 162 cases. Am. J. Dis. Child. *133:*641–644, 1979.
20. Fowler, N. O., and Manitasas, G. T.: Infectious pericarditis. Prog. Cardiovasc. Dis. *16:*323–336, 1973.
21. Fredriksen, R. T., Cohen, L., and Mullins, C. B.: Pericardial window or pericardiocentesis for pericardial effusions. Am. Heart J. *82:*158–162, 1971.
22. Fyfe, D. A., Hagler, D. J., Puga, F. J., et al.: Clinical and therapeutic aspects of *Haemophilus influenzae* pericarditis in pediatric patients. Mayo Clin. Proc. *59:*415–422, 1984.
23. Gersony, W. M., and McCracken, G. H.: Purulent pericarditis in infancy. Pediatrics *40:*224–232, 1967.
24. Ginzton, L. E., and Laks, M. M.: The differential diagnosis of acute pericarditis from the normal variant: New electrocardiographic criteria. Circulation *65:*1004–1009, 1982.
25. Golinko, R. V., Kaplan, N., and Rudolph, A. M.: The mechanism of pulsus paradoxus during acute pericardial tamponade. J. Clin. Invest. *42:*229, 1963.
26. Gore, I., and Kline, I. K.: Pericarditis and myocarditis. A. Pericarditis. *In* Gould, S. E. (ed.): Pathology of the Heart and Great Vessels. 3rd ed. Springfield, IL, Charles C Thomas, 1968, p. 724.
27. Greenberg, M. L., Niebulski, H. I. J., Uretsky, B. F., et al.: Occult purulent pericarditis detected by iridium-111 leukocyte imaging. Chest *85:*701–703, 1984.
28. Gutgesell, H. P., and Paquet, M.: Atlas of Pediatric Echocardiography. Hagerstown, MD, Harper and Row, 1978, p. 161.
29. Hahn, R. S., Holman, E., and Fuerichs, J. B.: The role of the bronchial artery circulation in the etiology of pulmonary and pericardial suppuration. J. Thorac. Surg. *27:*121, 1954.
30. Herman, G. R., Marchand, E. J., and Grur, G. H.: Pericarditis: Clinical and laboratory data of 130 cases. Am. Heart J. *43:*641–652, 1952.
31. Herrick, W. W.: Meningococcal pericarditis. Med. Clin. North Am. *2:*411, 1918.
32. Hildebrandt, H. M., Maassab, H. F., and Willis, P. W.: Influenza virus pericarditis. Am. J. Dis. Child. *104:*579, 1962.
33. Hoffman, J. I. E., and Stanger, P.: Diseases of the pericardium. *In* Rudolph, A. (ed.): Pediatrics. New York, Appleton-Century-Crofts, 1977, pp. 1474–1477.
34. Horan, J. M.: Acute staphylococcal pericarditis. Pediatrics *19:*36–43, 1957.
35. Horowitz, M. S., Schultz, C. S., Stinson, E. B., et al.: Sensitivity and specificity of echocardiography diagnosis of pericardial effusion. Circulation *50:*239, 1974.
36. Hudgins, J. M.: Infectious mononucleosis complicated by myocarditis and pericarditis. J. A. M. A. *235:*262, 1976.
37. Jaiyesimi, F., Abioye, A. A., and Antia, A. U.: Infective pericarditis in Nigerian children. Arch. Dis. Child. *54:*384–390, 1979.
38. Johnson, R. T., Portnoy, B., Rodgers, N. G., et al.: Acute benign pericarditis: Virologic study of 34 patients. Arch. Intern. Med. *108:*823, 1961.
39. Kauffman, C. A., Watanakunakorn, C., and Phair, J. P.: Purulent pneumococcal pericarditis: A continuing problem in the antibiotic era. Am. J. Med. *54:*743–750, 1973.
40. Keith, J. D., Rower, R. D., and Vlad, P.: Pericarditis. *In* Dow, J. (ed.): Heart Disease in Infancy and Childhood. 2nd ed. New York, Macmillan, 1967, p. 970.
41. Kussmaul, A.: Ueber schwieglige mediastino-perikarditis und der paradoxen puls. Klin. Wochenschr. *10:*443, 1873.
42. Laird, W. P., Nelson, J. D., and Huffines, F. D.: The frequency of pericardial effusion in bacterial meningitis. Pediatrics *63:*764–770, 1979.
43. Lajos, T. Z., Black, H. E., Cooper, R. G., et al.: Pericardial decompression. Ann. Thorac. Surg. *19:*47–53, 1975.
44. Lane, E. J., and Carsky, E. W.: Epicardial fat: Lateral plain film analysis in normals and in pericardial effusion. Radiology *91:*1–5, 1968.
45. Ledbetter, M. K.: Aortic aneurysm complicating staphylococcal pericarditis. Okla. State Med. Assoc. *74:*222–225, 1981.
46. Leggiadro, R. J., and Balsam, D.: *Haemophilus influenzae* sepsis leading to pericarditis despite antimicrobial therapy. Johns Hopkins Med. J. *146:*133–136, 1980.
47. Lincoln, E. M., and Savell, E. M.: Tuberculosis in Children. New York, McGraw-Hill, 1963.
48. Morgan, R. J., Stephenson, L. W., Woolf, P. K., et al.: Surgical treatment of purulent pericarditis in children. J. Thorac. Cardiovasc. Surg. *85:*527–531, 1983.
49. Mullen, D. C., Dillon, M. L., Young, W. G., Jr., et al.: Pericardiectomy in non-tuberculous pericarditis. J. Thorac. Cardiovasc. Surg. *58:*517–529, 1969.
50. Nadas, A. S., and Levy, J. M.: Pericarditis in children. Am. J. Cardiol. *7:*109–117, 1961.
51. Neill, C. A., and Harouturuan, L. M.: Diseases of the pericardium. *In* Watson, H. (ed.): Paediatric Cardiology. London, Lloyd-Luke, 1968, p. 703.
52. O'Connell, B.: Pericarditis following meningococcal meningitis. Am. J. Dis. Child. *126:*265–267, 1973.
53. Okoroma, E., Perry, L. W., and Scott, L. P.: Acute bacterial pericarditis in children: Report of 25 cases. Am. Heart J. *90:*709–713, 1975.
54. Orbtals, D. W., and Avioli, L. V.: Tuberculous pericarditis. Arch. Intern. Med. *139:*231–234, 1979.
55. Phillips, J. H., and Burch, G. E.: Selected clues in cardiac auscultation. Am. Heart J. *63:*1, 1962.
56. Picardi, J. L., Kaufmann, C. A., Schwarz, J., et al.: Pericarditis caused by histoplasma capsulatum. Am. J. Cardiol. *37:*82–88, 1976.
57. Rubenstein, J. J., Goldblatt, A., and Daggett, W. M.: Acute constriction complicating purulent pericarditis in infancy. Am. J. Dis. Child. *124:*591–594, 1972.
58. Sethi, G. K., Nelson, R. M., and Jenson, C. B.: Surgical management of acute septic pericarditis. Chest *63:*732–735, 1973.
59. Shreiner, D. P., Krishnaswami, V., and Murphy, J. H.: Unsuspected purulent pericarditis detected by gallium-67 scanning. Clin. Nucl. Med. *6:*411–412, 1981.
60. Simon, H. B., Tarr, P. I., Hutter, A. M., et al.: Primary meningococcal pericarditis: Diagnosis by countercurrent immunoelectrophoresis. J. A. M. A. *235:*278–280, 1976.
61. Smith, J. N., Jr.: Complications of infectious mononucleosis. Ann. Intern. Med. *44:*861, 1956.
62. Spodick, D. H.: Pericardial rub: Prospective multiple observer investigation of pericardial friction in 100 patients. Am. J. Cardiol. *35:*357, 1975.
63. Spodick, D. H.: Acute Pericarditis. New York, Grune & Stratton, 1959, p. 17.
64. Spodick, D. H.: Frequency of arrhythmias in acute pericarditis determined by Holter monitoring. Am. J. Cardiol. *53:*842–845, 1984.
65. Stewart, H. J., Crane, N. F., and Deitrick, A.: Absorption from the pericardial cavity in man. Am. Heart J. *16:*198–202, 1938.
66. Strauss, A. W., Santa-Maria, M., and Goldring, D.: Constrictive pericarditis in children. Am. J. Dis. Child. *129:*822–826, 1975.
67. Streifler, J. J., Dux, S., Garty, M., et al.: Recurrent pericarditis: A rare complication of influenza vaccination. Br. Med. J. *283:*526–527, 1981.
68. Tatter, D., Gerard, P. W., and Silverman, A. H.: Fatal varicella pericarditis in a child. Am. J. Dis. Child. *108:*88, 1964.
69. Van Reken, D., Strauss, A., Hernandez, A., et al.: Infectious pericarditis in children. J. Pediatr. *85:*165–169, 1974.
70. Wagner, H. N., Jr.: An outline of the use of radioisotope techniques in medical diagnosis. Am. J. Med. Sci. *247:*601, 1964.
71. Wyler, F., Knulsi, D., Rutishauser, M., et al.: Pericarditis purulenta in children. Helv. Paediatr. Acta. *32:*135–140, 1977.
72. Weir, E. K., and Joffe, H. S.: Purulent pericarditis in children: An analysis of 28 cases. Thorax *32:*438, 1977.
73. Weiss, E. R., Blahd, W. H., Winston, M. A., et al.: Rapid diagnosis of pericardial effusion utilizing the scintillation camera. Am. J. Cardiol. *30:*258, 1972.
74. Zinssen, H. F.: Idiopathic pericarditis. Mod. Concepts Cardiovasc. Dis. *29:*611, 1960.

34

MYOCARDITIS

Richard A. Friedman, Desmond F. Duff,
Kenneth O. Schowengerdt, Jesus G. Vallejo,
and Jeffrey A. Towbin

Myocarditis refers to "inflammation of muscular walls of the heart."[218] The clinical presentation and etiology may be quite varied. In this chapter, we concentrate on proven or presumed infectious causes for myocarditis. This entity may go unrecognized in a large number of patients whose illness may resolve spontaneously, or it may lead to significant morbidity and/or mortality.

In recent years, it has become apparent that myocarditis may occur with many, if not all, of the common infectious illnesses that afflict infants and children (Table 34–1). Myocarditis also may occur as a manifestation of hypersensitivity or toxic reaction to certain drugs (Table 34–1).

In the early part of the twentieth century, most cases were classified as idiopathic, and a diffuse or focal interstitial inflammation was described on histologic examination. Fiedler[56] was the first to document the pathologic changes in an adult, and the entity of diffuse or focal idiopathic or isolated interstitial myocarditis often carries the eponym of *Fiedler myocarditis*. Rheumatic fever, diphtheria, and other bacterial infections were the only disease entities recognized as being associated with myocarditis, although some experts suspected that viruses might play a significant role in the etiology of many cases.[203]

After the discovery of the coxsackievirus group by Dalldorf and Sickles[37] in 1947 and the subsequent isolation and identification of many viruses, the number of cases of myocarditis classified as idiopathic diminished rapidly.

As a clinical entity, myocarditis is uncommon in children, representing 0.3 per cent of the 14,322 patients seen by the Cardiology Service at Texas Children's Hospital between 1954 and 1977. This experience is similar to that reported by Toronto Children's Hospital for the years 1951 to 1964.[116] It also is apparent, however, that not all cases of myocarditis are recognized clinically, and a much higher incidence is recorded in autopsy series. At Texas Children's Hospital, there is an autopsy incidence of 1.15 per cent from 4343 studies performed between 1954 and 1977. This is considerably lower than the incidence of 6.83 per cent reported by Saphir and colleagues[203] in 1944 among 1420 autopsies on children. In Saphir's series, 32 of the 97 cases had, or probably had, rheumatic carditis, whereas there were only 2 cases in the Texas Children's Hospital series. The discrepancy is even more alarming when these observations are compared with the observations of Burch and colleagues,[26] who demonstrated evidence of interstitial myocarditis in the hearts of 29 of 50 infants and young children undergoing routine postmortem studies. Zee-Cheng and associates[256] and Parrillo and coworkers[179] found that a substantial number of patients undergoing endomyocardial biopsy for unexplained myocardial dysfunction had histologic findings suggestive of myocarditis. Other investigators[222, 223] have discovered evidence of myocarditis in patients presenting with ventricular dysrhythmias. Pomerance[183] has cautioned pathologists against the overdiagnosis of myocarditis, indicating that minor foci of inflammatory cells are present in about 5 per cent of "normal" hearts. He feels that the term "myocarditis" should be used only when the pathologist is convinced that the lesion is of a magnitude to be of clinical significance. However, as pointed out by Gore and Saphir[73] and Saphir and associates,[203] unless a thorough study of the myocardium is made, focal inflammation may be missed, and if strategically placed, a small inflammatory lesion may lead to significant disease, for example, a life-threatening arrhythmia such as complete heart block.

Some of the discrepancies between the clinical and autopsy series may be explained by the fact that in a significant number of cases the manifestations of myocarditis are subclinical and may be recognized only by electrocardiographic changes or perhaps not at all. In addition, in many instances myocarditis is but one component of a generalized illness, and the cardiac dysfunction, if mild, may be overlooked.

EPIDEMIOLOGY

Whereas myocarditis generally is a sporadic disease, epidemics have been reported. Most of the epidemics have been caused by coxsackievirus group B and have affected infants in the newborn period. Gear and Measroch[68] were the first to identify coxsackievirus B in association with myocarditis, after a nursery epidemic in a maternity home in what was southern Rhodesia. Subsequent reports of nursery epidemics have appeared from what was Rhodesia,[154] South Africa,[110] the Netherlands,[234] the United States,[119] and Singapore.[106]

Infections with coxsackieviruses and echoviruses are common in the general population. Illnesses caused by these viruses include upper respiratory tract infections, gastroenteritis, orchitis, infectious mononucleosis–like syndromes, pleurodynia, meningoencephalitis, hepatitis, pneumonia, hemolytic uremic syndrome, and carditis.[44, 99, 132] Lerner and colleagues[132] state that by adult life most people in the United States have significant titers of type-specific protective antibodies. As the risk of infection in childhood is reduced because of generally improved socioeconomic conditions, a susceptible adult population will be created.[80] This concept has important ramifications for pregnant women. Infection in the mother late in pregnancy may lead to either intrauterine fetal infection or early postnatal infection of the newborn infant. Spread after birth predominantly occurs by the fecal-oral route or by the airborne route. Coxsackievirus B attaches to target cells by receptors that are not shared with other members of the enterovirus group. These receptors are thought to be an essential element in viral replication and may determine tissue tropism.[250] Approximately 50 per cent of infections with both groups of viruses are subclinical.[132] In the 1965 outbreak of coxsackievirus B infection in Europe, 5 per cent of the infected patients had cardiac manifestations.[57, 64] That same year, outbreaks in Scotland, Finland, and Austria occurred and a higher incidence of myocarditis was noted. Approximately 12 per cent of those affected presented with some cardiac dysfunction.[79, 250] Myocarditis has been described in association with coxsackievirus B serotypes 1

TABLE 34–1. Causes of Myocarditis

Agent	Reference	Agent	Reference
Viral		***Protozoa***	
Coxsackieviruses A	71, 92	*Trypanosoma cruzi*	61, 104
Coxsackieviruses B	11, 18, 44, 71, 92, 101, 112, 119, 124, 133, 153, 188, 192, 200, 237	African trypanosomiasis	158
		Toxoplasmosis	104
Echoviruses	18, 33, 46, 86, 238	Amebiasis	141
Polio viruses	59, 61, 204	***Other Parasites***	
Rubella virus	5, 71, 140	*Toxocara canis*	239
Measles virus	196	Trichinosis	35, 75, 97, 216
Adenoviruses	21, 91	***Fungi and Yeasts***	
Vaccinia virus	69, 158	Actinomycosis	104
Mumps virus	69, 130, 194, 204	Coccidioidomycosis	104
Herpes simplex virus	252	Histoplasmosis	36
Epstein-Barr virus (infectious mononucleosis)	69, 94, 103, 104	*Candida*	195
		Toxic	
Cytomegalovirus	58, 223, 234	Diphtheria	16, 131, 227, 256
Rhinoviruses	215	Scorpion	126
Hepatitis viruses	104, 163	***Drugs***	
Arboviruses	167	Sulfonamides	59, 249
Influenza viruses	46, 134, 240	Phenylbutazone	96
Varicella virus	58, 62, 154	Cyclophosphamide	8
Rickettsial		Neomercazole	104
Rickettsia rickettsii	104	***Hypersensitivity/Autoimmune***	
Rickettsia tsutsugamushi	169	Rheumatoid arthritis	152
Bacterial		Rheumatic fever	195, 204
Meningococcus	77, 195	Ulcerative colitis	160
Klebsiella	195	Systemic lupus erythematosus	87
Leptospira	104	***Other***	
Staphylococcus	69, 195	Sarcoidosis	104
Syphilis	104	Scleroderma	256
Haemophilus influenzae	69	Idiopathic	47, 56, 135, 171, 184, 224, 246, 247
Hemolytic streptococci	69, 104	Cornstarch	25
Tuberculosis	104		
Typhoid	104		
Mycoplasmal			
Mycoplasma pneumoniae	60, 69, 202		
Chlamydia psittaci	104		

through 6, and the most severe disease has occurred with types 3 and 4.[99, 118, 119] Some appreciation of the frequency also may be gained from the observations of Burch and colleagues,[26] who demonstrated coxsackievirus B antigens using an immunofluorescent technique in 41 per cent of 29 infants and children who had evidence of interstitial myocarditis at routine autopsy. Wentworth and colleagues[246] reviewed the autopsies of 2427 patients in southern Ontario, Canada. There were 1299 cases of unexpected death. Of these, 20 cases were thought to be due to viral myocarditis. Nine of the 20 had positive serologic evidence for coxsackievirus B infection. Less frequently, coxsackievirus A virus and echoviruses have been implicated as causes of myocarditis (see Table 34–1).

It is of interest that cases of idiopathic myocarditis peak during the summer months, a period corresponding to the peak fecal excretion of the enteroviruses.

Karjalainen and colleagues[114] prospectively examined 104 conscripts during a 1978 influenza A virus (H1N1) epidemic in Sweden. The incidence of myocarditis was 9 per cent of the 67 verified cases of influenza virus infection.

In 1965 in the United States, 260,222 cases of measles were reported; this number declined to 24,031 in 1975. Cardiac involvement in measles usually occurs after the onset of the illness, although at least one case has been described during the prodromal phase.[34]

The teratogenicity of the rubella virus in the first 4 months of pregnancy is well known. Ainger and colleagues,[5] however, clearly demonstrated that because of the persistence of the virus in the fetus, extensive involvement of the myocardium may lead to severe myocarditis. Of 47 infants with congenital rubella, 10 had myocarditis: 7 of these 10 had active disease, and 4 died. Morbidity in the survivors was severe. Rubella immunization programs have succeeded in reducing the number of congenital cases, so that only 28 cases of congenital rubella were recorded in the mortality and morbidity statistics of the United States in 1975.[156]

Infection of the newborn with herpes simplex virus occurs in approximately 1 of 7500 deliveries.[17] Most infections are due to type 2 virus, which is acquired from the genital tract in 95 per cent of cases. Approximately 1 per cent of pregnant women in the lowest socioeconomic groups have evidence of herpes. The spectrum of disease ranges from inapparent infection to a fatal encephalopathy. Myocardial involvement has been described, and herpesvirus has been isolated from the myocardium at autopsy.[251] Recognition of genital herpes and delivery of the infant by cesarean section would reduce the incidence of myocarditis caused by this agent.

Osama and colleagues[175] prospectively investigated 312 cases of varicella over a 1-year period. Eighteen of the 312 cases (5.8 per cent) showed evidence of myocarditis. Interestingly, there was a statistically significant increase of myocarditis in those patients who complained of skeletal myalgia.

Although diphtheria now is rare, 285 cases were reported in the United States in 1975,[156] compared with 160 cases in 1965.[155] The median for the years 1960 through 1964 was 463 cases, and the median for the years 1970 through 1974 was 224 cases. About one-third of the cases have electrocardiographic findings suggesting myocardial involvement,[61] although myocardial involvement may be as high as 84 per cent with severe infections.[16] The heart is involved only when the fauces are infected, but cardiac complications are the most common cause of death.

PATHOLOGY

Immunologic Aspects

The histologic and gross anatomic changes seen in patients with viral myocarditis have been examined extensively with the use of animal models. An understanding of the immunologic response to viral infection in these models is essential in trying to explain the spectrum of injuries seen in the hearts of patients with myocarditis.

The group B coxsackieviruses have been studied the most extensively for their ability to induce myocarditis. Rabin and associates[185] showed that after parenteral injection of coxsackievirus B in mice, viremia was detected from 24 to 72 hours and that maximum growth in tissue occurred at 72 to 96 hours. After that time, virus titers declined and could not be found at 7 to 10 days after inoculation.[250] An inverse relationship exists between virus and antibody concentrations, implying that the latter at least partially is responsible for viral clearance.[8] In addition, there also is evidence that macrophages are active in viral clearance.[172] The appearance of macrophages in coxsackievirus B myocarditis is typical for this disease at 5 to 10 days after infection.[131, 250]

Two mechanisms, probably in combination, account for the injuries seen in myocarditis from coxsackievirus B. Direct myofiber destruction by the viral particle has been demonstrated.[12, 72, 101] A second mechanism cited is cell-mediated destruction of myofibers, and it is responsible for the greatest damage to the myocardium. Mice that are pretreated with antithymocyte serum lack a normal immunologic response to infection and develop a significantly less extensive necrosis of myocardial tissue than do similarly infected animals that are treated with normal rabbit serum.[250] Also, T-cell–deficient animals clear viremia normally but do not develop a significant amount of myocarditis. This implies that the T cells are not required in elimination of virus but do play a key role in the major inflammatory response to infection.[101, 250] On the other hand, mice treated within 24 hours of or before infection with neutralizing antibody failed to develop myocarditis.[147, 148, 186, 251] Thus, the combination of macrophages and antibody suppresses viral infection, and T lymphocytes participate in the injury of myocytes.

Woodruff[250] points out that T cells can cause injury through a number of mechanisms: through accumulation of activated macrophages, through production of antibody and antibody-dependent cell-mediated cytoxicity or lysis by antibody and complement, and through direct action of cytotoxic T cells. Huber and associates,[101] using BALB/c mice infected with coxsackievirus B3, showed that cytolytic T cells were the agents responsible for the major part of myocardial cell injury. These cells damaged both virus-infected and noninfected myocytes in T-cell–deficient animals. In addition, generation of the cytotoxic T cells is thought to be stimulated by infected host cells and not by the virus. The effector cells then recognize virus-specific and major histocompatibility antigens (modified H-2 antigens) on the cell surface and act to destroy them through that recognition. The ongoing injury then may be considered an autoimmune process.[101, 250] Support for this concept is provided by Pacque and colleagues.[176] Using CD-1 mice infected with coxsackievirus B3, they found a KC1 extractable antigen present in the hearts of mice previously infected with a group B coxsackievirus that specifically was immunoreactive with immune mouse peritoneal exudate cells (i.e., stimulated production of a migration inhibitory factor). No viral activity was present in the animals that had this extractable antigen. Similar experiments in the primate model confirmed earlier findings in mice and lend further support to similar circumstances in humans.[177] Experimental evidence also has showed that the antigen responsible for cytotoxic T-cell activity is not detectable by antiserum containing antibodies directed at structural components of the viral capsid. Likewise, antiviral serum has been ineffective in preventing injury.[249] Natural killer cells have been implicated in the destruction of noninfected myocardial cells.[250] The exact mechanism of their activity currently is unknown.

Other viral agents have been used to produce myocarditis in animals. Sakamoto and colleagues,[201] using influenza A virus (H2N2), produced myocarditis in mice. However, mice pretreated with irradiation or athymic mice did not develop myocarditis. Matsumori and Kawai[147, 149] produced a model of acute and chronic myocarditis in mice using encephalomyocarditis virus, which is a picornavirus similar to the coxsackieviruses. Their model showed that acute myocarditis could progress and produce a picture of dilated cardiomyopathy similar to that seen in humans after recovery from an acute episode of myocarditis.

Studies in humans with myocarditis also have been performed. Maisch and colleagues[140] demonstrated antibody-mediated cytolysis in 30 per cent of 144 patients with myocarditis of unknown etiology as well as in 18 of 19 patients with proven viral infection (coxsackievirus B, influenza A, or mumps). The titer of a muscle-specific antimyolemmal antibody found in these patients was correlated closely to the degree of cytolysis induced in vitro with rat cardiocytes. Examining the number of positive and negative responses of neutralizing antibody to coxsackieviruses B1 to B6, Hori and colleagues[96] found that adult patients with myocarditis had been exposed to a greater number of groups than had normal control subjects. These investigators believe that an essential step in the development of myocarditis is the infection of one group by coxsackievirus B and immunization against that type plus other types of coxsackievirus B from previous exposure. However, a few cases of myocarditis in that group showed evidence of exposure to only one type of coxsackievirus B, shedding some doubt on this hypothesis.

A defect in cell-mediated immunity also has been found in patients with myocarditis. Eckstein and colleagues[52] showed a significant reduction in suppressor cell (concanavalin A–induced) activity in patients with myocarditis and congestive cardiomyopathy, compared with healthy controls.

Studies also have pointed to the effect of humoral effectors in promoting autoimmune myocarditis after viral clearance has occurred. Autoantibodies to various cellular components (antimyosin, adenine nucleotide translocator protein) have been described.[15] Inflammatory cytokines, including tumor necrosis factor and interleukin-1, have been shown in a rat model possibly to amplify injury by reducing catecholamine-induced ventricular contractility.[81] Antitumor necrosis factor antibodies administered to mice prior to inoculation with encephalomyocarditis virus improved survival and demonstrated less necrosis and inflammatory cellular infiltrate by day 14 after introduction of the virus.[253]

Specific molecules known as cell adhesion molecules also may be involved with the progression of the inflammatory response in myocarditis. One such molecule is intercellular adhesion molecule–1 (ICAM-1). ICAM-1 appears after inflammatory injury, and the expression of this molecule is up-regulated by cytokines such as interleukin-1 and tumor necrosis factor–α.[50, 95, 181] The expression of ICAM-1 has been shown to be increased in mice infected with coxsackievirus B3.[211] Treatment with anti–ICAM-1 monoclonal antibody reduced the myocardial inflammation seen with the same virus.[210]

Thus, although unequivocal proof of direct viral and humoral damage to myocytes in humans is lacking, animal models strongly suggest that this is a contributing factor. The immune response to viral infection certainly plays a major role in the damage seen long after viral clearance and may be the key element in terms of therapy for preventing further injury (Fig. 34–1).

Gross and Microscopic Features

Isolated or idiopathic myocarditis probably is a rare pathologic entity. The pathologic cardiac findings usually are nonspecific; similar gross and microscopic changes are noted, irrespective of the causative agent.[56, 73, 103, 171, 183, 195, 203] There are, however, occasions when the histology may suggest a specific etiology.

Grossly, all four chambers of the heart are enlarged and the cardiac weight is increased. The heart usually is flabby and pale. In some instances, especially with coxsackievirus B infections, petechial hemorrhages may be seen on the epicardial surfaces; pericardial fluid may be tinged with blood. On cut section, the ventricular muscle walls may be thinned. Occasionally, the ventricles are hypertrophied or increased in thickness because of edema. The valves are spared. The endocardial surface usually is unaffected but occasionally may be thickened and appear glistening white. This important observation suggests to some investigators that endocardial fibroelastosis, which presents as a congestive cardiomyopathy, represents a progression from acute viral myocarditis.[84, 105] In an elegant study of 64 hearts of children who had myocarditis or endocardial fibroelastosis, Hutchins and Vie[105] found 18 with endocardial fibroelastosis only, 5 with myocarditis only, and 41 with features of both diseases. When the history disclosed that the time from onset of illness to death was 2 weeks or less, only myocarditis was evident. When the time interval was between 2 weeks and 4 months, a combined picture was seen, whereas only endocardial fibroelastosis with occasional trivial myocarditis was evident when the time from onset of disease to death was more than 4 months. These findings are supported by Hastreiter and Miller,[84] who found microscopic evidence of myocarditis after transthoracic needle biopsy of the myocardium in a child who had the classic clinical picture of endocardial fibroelastosis, including left ventricular hypertrophy on electrocardiography.

Fruhling and associates[65] were able to extend these observations by demonstrating coxsackievirus B3 in the myocardium of 13 of 28 infants with endocardial fibroelastosis. Van Reken and associates[235] described a 5-month-old infant who died after the sudden onset of congestive cardiac failure and who had both endocardial fibroelastosis and an echovirus 9 myocarditis documented at autopsy. The virus was isolated from the heart as well as the lungs, liver, and lymph nodes.

Saphir and Field[204] observed mural thrombi in the left ventricular cavity in some patients with myocarditis and minute emboli in both coronary and cerebral vessels. Coronary emboli, although rare, may play a role in the causation of cardiac dysrhythmias, which sometimes accompany myocarditis.

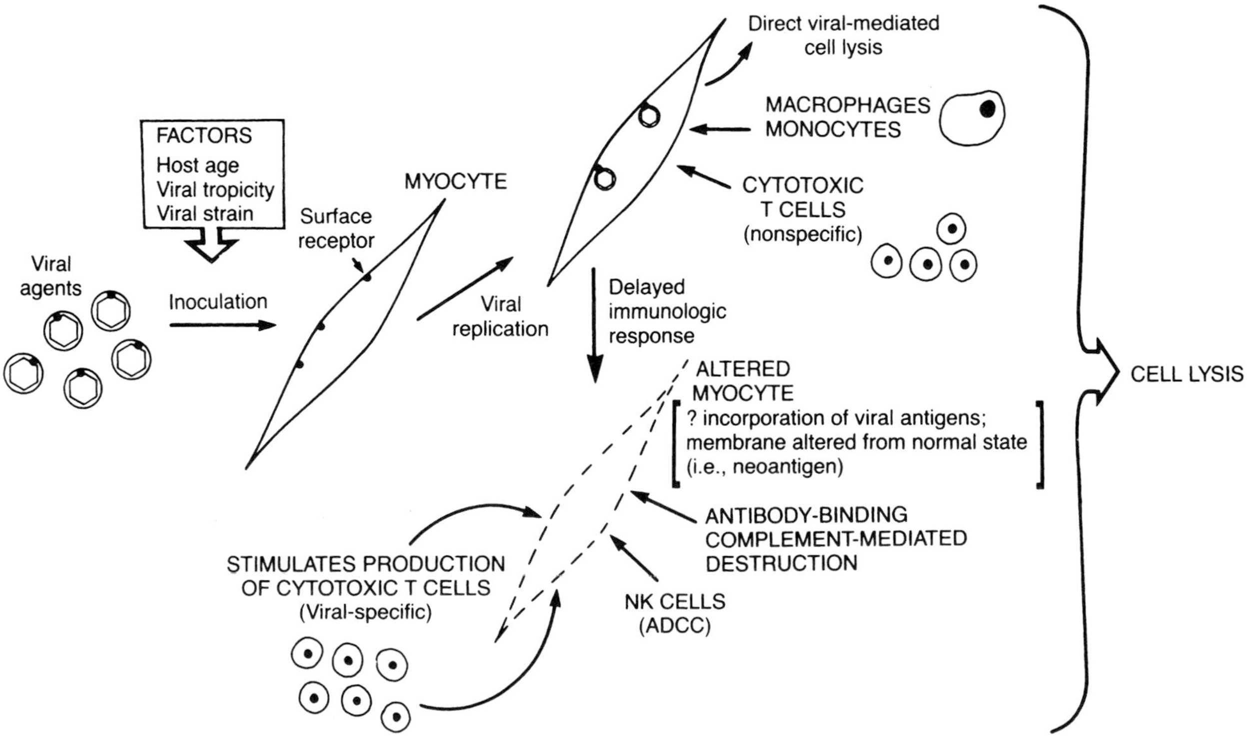

FIGURE 34–1. *Schema for pathogenesis of myocarditis. Viral agents attach to cells via surface receptors. Once a cell is infected, the cell cycle is changed. Direct virus-mediated cytolysis occurs. Cellular effectors of injury (i.e., macrophages, monocytes, and nonspecific cytotoxic T cells) are involved in the primary reaction. Myocytes that survive are altered in their structure. Cytotoxic T cells specifically targeted against the altered myocyte, natural killer (NK) cells, and complement-activated antibody–mediated cardiocytolysis or antibody-dependent cellular cytotoxicity (ADCC) take part in the secondary reaction. (Partially adapted from Maisch, B., Trostel-Soeder, R., Stechemesser, E., et al.: Diagnostic relevance of humoral and cell-mediated immune reaction in patients with acute viral myocarditis. Clin. Exp. Immunol. 48:533, 1982. Blackwell Scientific Publications Limited.)*

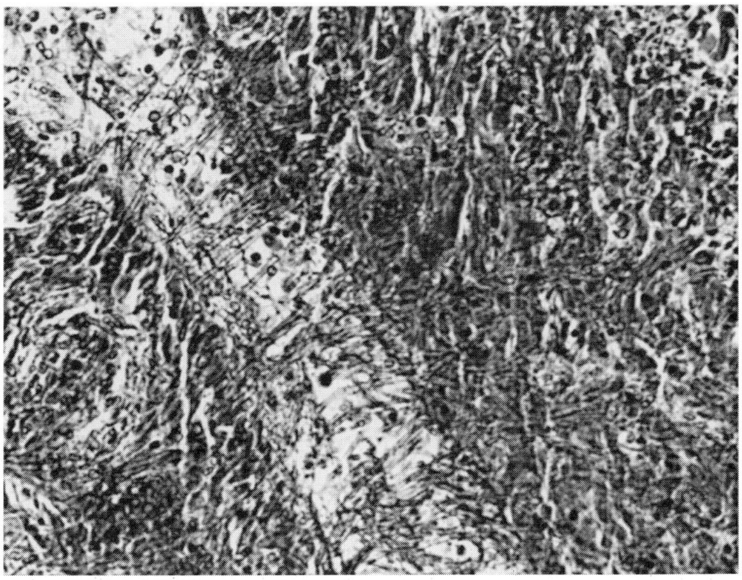

FIGURE 34–2. Candida albicans *myocarditis. Note focal necrosis of myocardium with central masses of hyphae and necrotic debris surrounded by mononuclear cell infiltrate. (H and E × 160.) (Courtesy of Dr. Edith Hawkins.)*

The microscopic picture of acute myocarditis typically shows a focal or diffuse interstitial collection predominantly of mononuclear cells—lymphocytes, plasma cells, and eosinophils. Polymorphonuclear leukocytes rarely are noted unless the cause of the carditis is bacterial. Virus particles and inclusion bodies are recognized only rarely.[187, 195]

In severe infections with any agent, but especially with coxsackieviruses and diphtheria exotoxin, there is a loss of cross-striation in the muscle fibers, edema, and, at times, extensive necrosis of the myocardium. The diphtheria exotoxin has a particular affinity also for the conductive tissue; dysrhythmias, including complete heart block, are relatively common in this form of myocarditis. The exotoxin interferes with protein synthesis by inhibition of a translocating enzyme in the delivery of amino acids. Carnitine metabolism also is affected, which results in triglyceride accumulation and a typical picture of fatty changes seen in myofibers.[192]

Although the perivascular accumulation of lymphocytes and plasma cells is described in coxsackievirus B myocarditis, it is a minor finding. When myocarditis is due to rickettsiae,[105] varicella,[58, 154] trypanosomes,[61, 182] or other parasites[59, 237] or when it occurs as a reaction to sulfonamide,[59, 237] this pattern dominates.

Myocarditis seen with bacterial infections usually differs from that of presumed viral origin (Figs. 34–2 to 34–5). The myocardial changes seen are similar to the extracardiac findings. Microabscesses and patchy focal suppurative changes may be noted.[192] Frequently, a perimyocarditis may be seen with concomitant bacterial infection of pericardium and myocardium.

Trichinella species usually cause a focal infiltrate consisting of lymphocytes and eosinophils. Larvae usually cannot be identified.

Chagas disease (see later for more in-depth discussion), which may affect 50 per cent of a population in an endemic area, is the most common causative agent of myocarditis

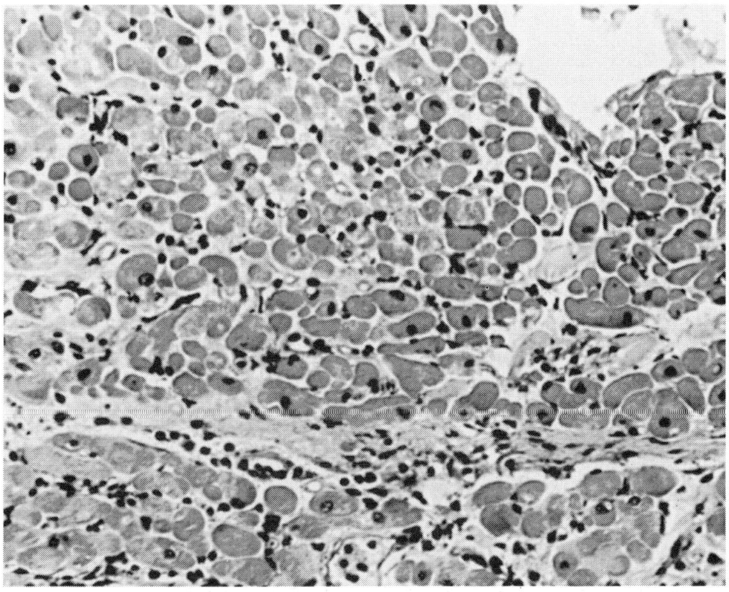

FIGURE 34–3. *Right ventricular biopsy. Presumed viral myocarditis characterized by focal mononuclear cell infiltrates. (H and E × 160.) (Courtesy of Dr. Edith Hawkins.)*

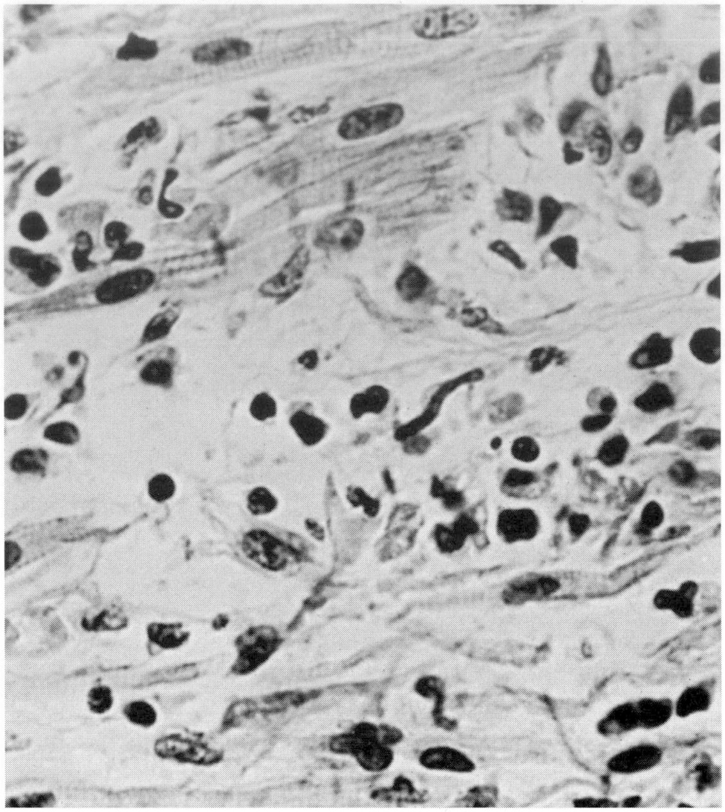

FIGURE 34–4. *Section of myocardium. Picornavirus myocarditis characterized by interstitial edema, mononuclear cell infiltrates, and focal myofiber disruption. (H and E × 400.) (Courtesy of Dr. Edith Hawkins.)*

in South America. Survivors of acute infection may suffer significant long-term morbidity, and the clinical course may result in protracted heart failure and death. Trypanosomes usually are visible, with neutrophils, lymphocytes, macrophages, and eosinophils all present in the same lesion.[192]

Some cases of myocarditis present only as disturbances in electrical conduction within the heart. Fortunately, in most instances, arrhythmias are transitory. Instances of sudden death associated with myocarditis are well documented, but the mode of death often is obscure or unclear.

It has been suggested that sudden infant death syndrome, a distressingly common entity that occurs in 1 of every 500 infants, might be due to cardiac arrhythmias in some cases.[64] James[108] found a resorptive degenerative process in the bundle of His and the left margin of the atrioventricular node but no inflammatory cells in the cases he studied of infants who died in Northern Ireland. He concluded, however, that lethal arrhythmias of conduction disturbances may be due to a developmental histologic change in these critical regions of the heart. Jankus,[109] on the other hand, demonstrated lymphocytic infiltrates in the region of the main bundle and left fascicle in a 3-month-old patient who died suddenly.

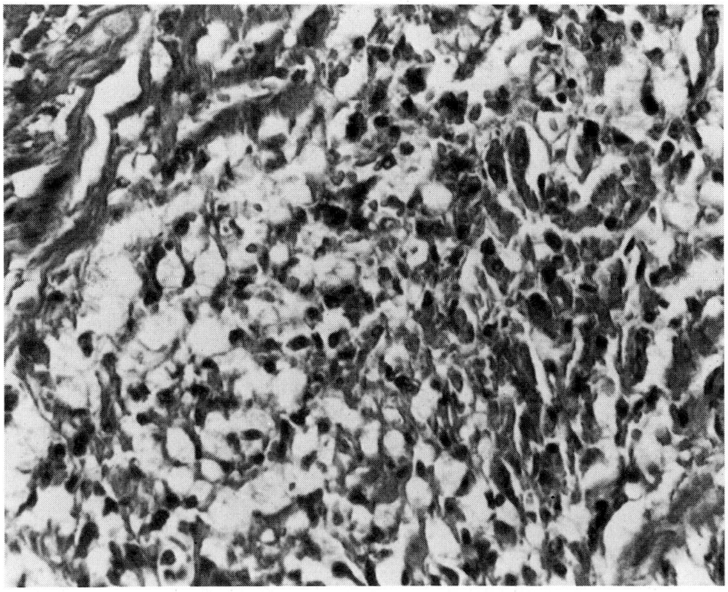

FIGURE 34–5. *Section of myocardium. Vaccinia (smallpox vaccine) myocarditis. Note mononuclear cell infiltrates and fatty degenerative changes. (H and E × 400.) (Courtesy of Dr. Edith Hawkins.)*

There were, however, no degenerative changes; again, the significance of these findings remains speculative.

Giant cells with or without granulomata are markers for the diagnosis of giant-cell myocarditis.[103] Granulomata have been observed in the myocardium in patients with tuberculosis, syphilis, rheumatoid arthritis, rheumatic heart disease, sarcoidosis, and certain fungal and parasitic infestations. Occasional giant cells have been seen in interstitial myocarditis (idiopathic or Fiedler). A significant number of cases exist, however, in which there is giant-cell myocarditis but no cause is found. Two types of giant cells are recognized, one of which appears to be myogenic in origin and is thought to represent transitional forms of myocardial fibers. This type of cell has been found without granulomata. The second and more characteristic giant cell probably is derived from interstitial histiocytes. The latter type typically is seen in patients with myocarditis of nonviral etiology, whereas the former represents a response to viral infection. Hudson[103] noted similar cells in an adult who had received neo-mercazole (carbimazole) therapy, and Hodge and Lawrence[94] reported two cases of granulomatous myocarditis associated with phenylbutazone therapy.

PATHOPHYSIOLOGY

With extensive interstitial inflammation, muscle-cell injury, or both, there is a reduction in myocardial contractility. As a consequence, the heart enlarges and the end-diastolic volume of the ventricle increases. In the normal heart, an increase in filling volume leads, by the Starling mechanism, to an increased force of contraction, ejection fraction, and cardiac output. In the presence of myocarditis, the myocardium is unable to respond in this manner, and cardiac output is reduced. Systemic blood flow may, however, be maintained by utilization of the cardiac reserve, mediated by the sympathetic nervous system and leading to vasoconstriction of the skin vessels and an increase in heart rate. With progressive disease or any stress (e.g., infection, anemia, fever), the heart may be unable to meet the oxygen demands of the tissues and the clinical picture of congestive cardiac failure may become evident. Increase in the end-diastolic volume leads to progressive increase in ventricular end-diastolic pressure. This, in turn, leads to an increased filling pressure, so that left atrial and, therefore, pulmonary venous hydrostatic pressure may be elevated above the colloid osmotic pressure, which normally prevents transudation of fluid across the capillary membranes. Pulmonary congestion and edema, as well as systemic venous engorgement—manifested in infants primarily as hepatic enlargement—are common findings in the more acute forms of myocarditis. In some infants and young children, the presentation predominantly is that of right-sided heart failure.[193]

An appreciation of the disturbance of myocardial function may be gained from the angiographic frames in Figure 34–6. The left ventricle is dilated considerably, and the outline is irregular in both diastole and systole. The ejection fraction is reduced significantly at 35 per cent instead of the normal 60 to 75 per cent.

Another means of evaluating left ventricular function is by the noninvasive technique of cardiac ultrasound. Normal standards have been established for children by Gutgesell and colleagues[82]; an example is shown in Figure 34–7*A* (a recording from a 4-year-old child). The normal shortening fraction—that is, the percentage change in ventricular dimensions between end-diastole and end-systole—is 35 ± 4 per cent, irrespective of age (range, 28 to 44 per cent). Figure 34–7*B* is from a 4-year-old child with idiopathic myocarditis and demonstrates ventricular dilatation with markedly reduced motion of the left ventricular posterior wall and septum, leading to a shortening fraction of only 12 per cent. Further assessment of ventricular function also can be achieved by measurement of systolic time intervals obtained from simultaneous recording of the electrocardiogram and the semilunar valve opening and closing points on the echocardiogram.[82]

CLINICAL PRESENTATION

The clinical presentation of myocarditis varies considerably with the age of the patient and the virulence of the organism. At one end of the spectrum, there is a fulminant and rapidly fatal illness; at the other, no apparent clinical disturbance at all. The newborn infant especially is susceptible to the severe form of myocarditis usually caused by the coxsackieviruses

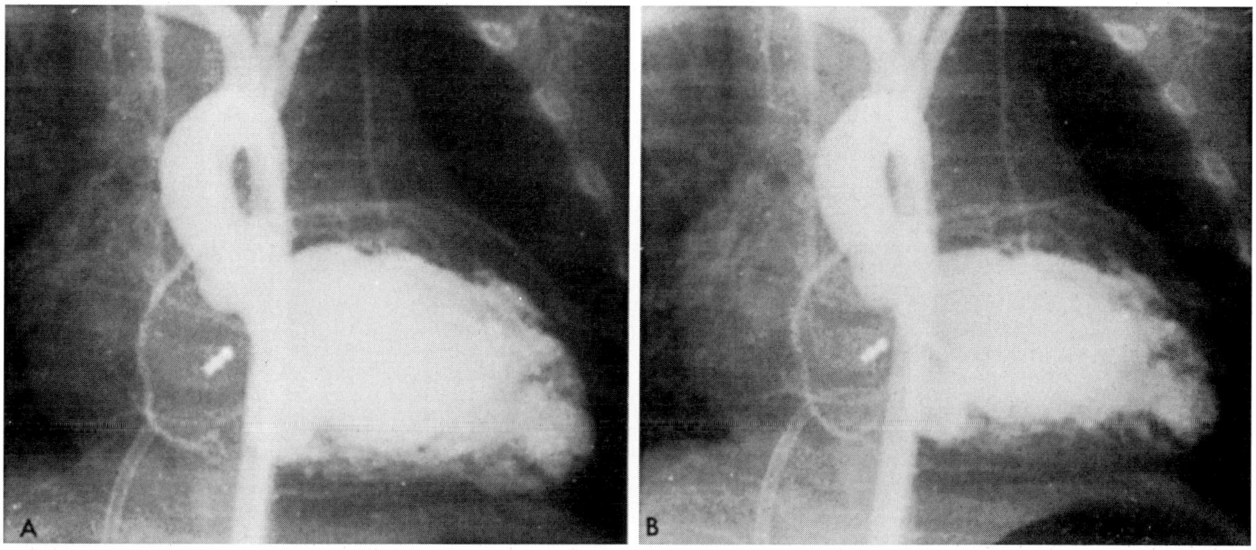

FIGURE 34–6. *The end-diastolic* (A) *and end-systolic* (B) *frames from a left ventriculogram of a patient with idiopathic myocarditis show irregularity of the wall and poor contractility.*

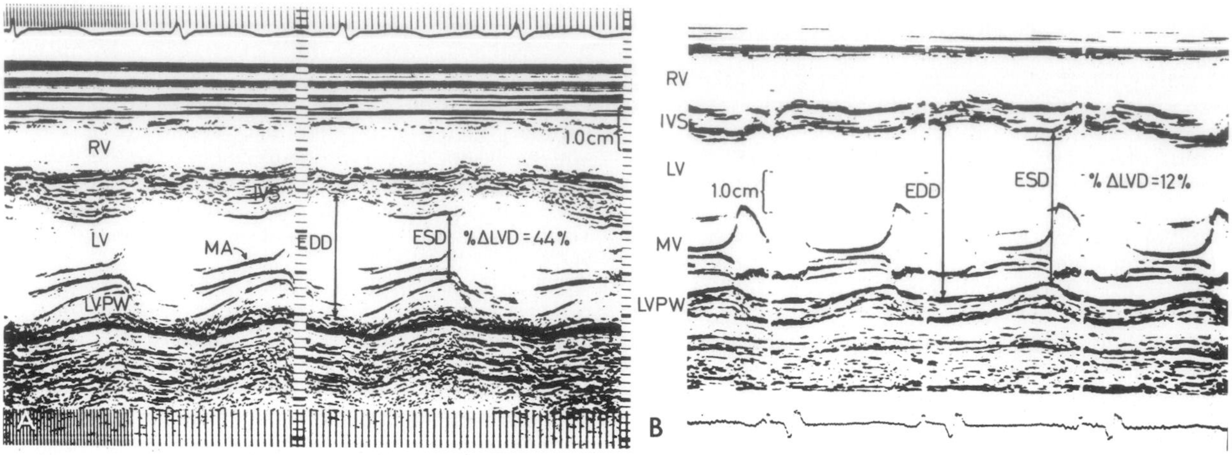

FIGURE 34–7. A, *Normal echocardiogram of a 4-year-old child. LVPW, left ventricular posterior wall; MA, mitral apparatus; EDD, end-diastolic dimension; ESD, end-systolic dimension; %ΔLVD, per cent change in left ventricular dimension (shortening fraction).* B, *Echocardiogram of a 4-year-old child with idiopathic myocarditis shows left ventricular dilatation and severely reduced shortening fraction. IVS, interventricular septum; MV, mitral valve.*

B,[119, 234] but it also is recognized with rubella[5] and herpes simplex[252] viruses as well as in association with toxoplasmosis.[61, 103]

In many of these infections, myocarditis is but one component of a generalized illness, often with severe hepatitis and encephalitis.[118, 119] In some instances, however, infections with these organisms may produce only mild clinical disturbance.[24, 107] In the report by Brightman and colleagues,[24] a nursery epidemic of coxsackievirus B5 infection in preterm infants was recognized only by chance because a virologic survey was in progress at the time at their institution. Sporadic cases also occurred among full-term infants. There were no instances of myocarditis, and all the infants recovered. Findings were lethargy, failure to gain weight, and, in some, evidence of aseptic meningitis. As noted in the review by Kibrick and Benirschke[119] of 25 infants with coxsackievirus B myocarditis, vague symptoms, such as lethargy and anorexia, may herald the onset of the severe disease, which emphasizes that close attention should be paid to all symptoms, especially in the newborn, no matter how nonspecific. Vomiting was noted in four infants. Fever was recorded in more than half of the cases; occasionally, the temperature was subnormal. Cyanosis; respiratory distress; and/or tachycardia, cardiomegaly, or electrocardiographic changes were present in 19 of 23 infants. Tachypnea, a respiratory rate higher than 60 per minute in the newborn, is an early sign of heart failure in the young infant and should alert the clinician to this diagnosis.

In older infants and children, the manifestations of myocarditis generally are less fulminant than in the newborn.[116, 193, 199, 241, 248] However, a fatal and acute illness has been reported in association with idiopathic myocarditis[135] and the myocarditis associated with enteroviruses,[119] adenoviruses,[88] mumps,[126] chickenpox,[58] diphtheria,[16] cytomegalovirus,[228] and many of the other causes listed in Table 34–1. Some older children have been reported with acute, substernal chest pain consistent with angina and have electrocardiographic changes of acute myocardial infarction.[100, 151] The usual clinical picture is that of either an acute or a subacute illness, which often begins with a mild upper respiratory infection and a low-grade fever.[9] In some infants, there are only vague, nonspecific suggestions of disease (e.g., irritability, periodic episodes of pallor) before the onset of cardiorespiratory symptoms, which begin a few days to a week or two after the onset of the initial symptoms. Abdominal pain may be a prominent complaint in some children.[241]

On examination, these infants and children often are anxious and apprehensive, but some appear apathetic and listless. Pallor may be striking, and mild cyanosis may be present. The skin may be cold and mottled. Respirations are rapid and labored, and grunting may be prominent. The pulse is thready, and blood pressure usually is normal or slightly reduced unless the infant is in profound shock. The precordium is quiet, without a prominent cardiac impulse. Tachycardia, sometimes of a marked degree, is present. The heart sounds are muffled, and a prominent gallop rhythm nearly always is heard. Fine and colleagues[57] found the most sensitive clinical sign of myocarditis to be a soft first sound at the apex. It should be noted, however, that a prolonged PR interval, which may be a nonspecific finding in many febrile illnesses,[209] also will cause a soft first sound without any other evidence of myocarditis. A high-pitched systolic murmur of mitral insufficiency is heard in some cases. The breath sounds are harsh. There may be scattered ronchi and, occasionally, fine crepitations in the lung bases. Almost uniformly, the liver is enlarged; edema is rare. Some infants are less distressed and have signs of only mild congestive cardiac failure, without the signs of peripheral circulatory failure. Others have no signs of cardiac compromise, and myocarditis is recognized only as part of a generalized illness by a disturbance in the electrocardiographic pattern.

Myocarditis in HIV Infection

Infection with HIV may affect the heart adversely. Cardiac dysfunction, including congestive heart failure, may occur; many patients who have died and undergone autopsy demonstrate myocarditis. Anderson and associates[7] retrospectively analyzed 71 consecutive necropsy patients who died of AIDS and found that 52 per cent had evidence of myocarditis. Opportunistic agents could account only for a few of the cases, and most were considered "idiopathic." Another study[14] examined autopsy specimens of 26 consecutive cases. Lymphocytic myocarditis was seen in nine patients (35 per cent), and another seven patients had lymphocytic infiltrates without myocytolysis. Acierno[3] correctly points out that a distinction must be made between "AIDS-associated myocarditis versus secondary myocarditis due to known pathogens as well as idiopathic myocarditis." Hypersensitivity or allergic-type vasculitis may occur in this disease state, with an uncontrolled hypergammaglobulinemia inducing a type I hypersensitivity reaction. Reilly and colleagues[190] found a 45 per cent incidence of myocarditis in 58 consecutive autopsy cases. Congestive heart failure, ventricular tachycardia, and other electrocardiographic abnormalities were seen in nearly 60 per cent of those patients. Two patients died suddenly, both of them with myocarditis. One study of eight children who died of noncardiac causes demonstrated myocarditis in two of four patients who underwent autopsy examination. One of those patients had disseminated cytomegalovirus infection, including numerous inclusions on microscopic examination of the heart.[221]

Thus, myocardial inflammation, with or without cell destruction, is a frequent finding in patients infected with HIV. The exact mechanism of this response, whether to the virus itself or to opportunistic agents or other toxic reactions, is not clear. Specific therapy of myocarditis in these patients has not been elucidated; therefore, no recommendations, other than inotropic support with anticongestive and afterload-reducing agents, can be made at this time.

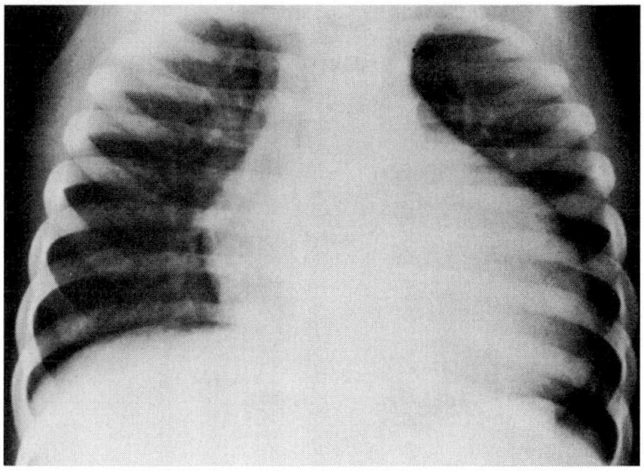

FIGURE 34–8. *Marked cardiomegaly with a mild increase in the pulmonary venous pattern in the upper lobes.*

DIAGNOSIS

The diagnosis of myocarditis often is difficult but should be suspected in any infant or child who presents in congestive heart failure and who at present has or recently had a febrile illness. The history should include information regarding travel, exposure to tuberculosis, recent drug ingestion, and illnesses in other family members or schoolmates.

A quiet precordium in the presence of a gallop rhythm and decreased intensity or muffling of the heart sounds are findings that strongly suggest the diagnosis. A tachycardia out of proportion to the level of fever also should be viewed with suspicion. A physiologic third heart sound is common in normal healthy children as well as in those with anemia and fever. At times, as with fever and associated tachycardia, the cardiac rhythm may have a gallop cadence. In association with this, however, the precordium is hyperactive and the heart sounds are increased in intensity and crisp. An unusually prominent third heart sound suggests a disturbance of ventricular compliance without other evidence of compromised cardiac function and should be investigated further with an echocardiogram, a chest radiograph, and an electrocardiogram.

The chest roentgenogram in infants and children who have signs of congestive cardiac failure invariably shows cardiomegaly, usually of a severe degree (Fig. 34–8). All four chambers may be enlarged, and there often is evidence of pulmonary venous congestion.

At times, especially in newborn infants, the first sign of illness is acute circulatory collapse; under these circumstances, the cardiac size may be normal. The same is true of children who have an arrhythmia rather than congestive heart failure. Other patients may present Stokes-Adams attacks caused by complete heart block.[134]

The occurrence of an arrhythmia, especially after a febrile illness, should alert the clinician to look for other signs of myocarditis.[33, 215] Lind and Hulquist[135] noted significant dysrhythmias in five infants with isolated myocarditis: four of the five infants died, and three of these had paroxysmal atrial tachycardia. Paroxysmal atrial tachycardia has been reported in patients with viral myocarditis[33, 215] and also has been described in patients with diphtheritic myocarditis.[16] However, atrial ectopic tachycardia may mimic sinus tachycardia and if not carefully evaluated may be the primary cause for significant myocardial dysfunction. Complete heart block has been described in children in association with acute idiopathic myocarditis,[112, 134] rubella,[72, 136] coxsackievirus,[205] and respiratory syncytial virus[13, 70] infections. In some instances, it is permanent,[13, 71, 205] and in others, temporary.[70, 112] The electrocardiogram, therefore, is an essential diagnostic tool in all patients with suspected myocarditis.

The classic electrocardiographic pattern in myocarditis is one of diffuse low-voltage QRS complexes (<5 mm total amplitude) with low amplitude or slightly inverted T waves and a small or absent Q wave in leads V_5 and V_6 (Fig. 34–9). The low voltage may be present in the standard leads and the precordial leads. Figure 34–10 depicts the electrocardiogram of an infant with acute myocarditis and shows a pattern of acute myocardial ischemia. Figure 34–11*A* is of a patient with diptheritic myocarditis, showing multifocal extrasystoles and severe intraventricular conduction delay; the electrocardiogram of this child returned to normal over a period of 3 months (Fig. 34–11*B*). The electrocardiogram from a 5-month-old infant who had mild fever, diarrhea, and vomiting for 3 to 4 days prior to admission is shown in Figure 34–12. A 2:1 atrioventricular block with normal QRS complexes is noted. This abnormality persisted in the absence of clinical symptoms for 1 year. Figure 34–13 shows a left bundle branch block noted in a 10-month-old infant with acute idiopathic myocarditis. Anomalous origin of the left coronary artery from the pulmonary artery was suspected but was excluded by catheterization. This electrocardiographic pattern persisted for at least 6 months.

Karjalainen[115] studied the electrocardiograms of 87 conscripts between 18 and 30 years of age, 28 of whom had myocarditis. The most frequent finding was T-wave changes of either reduced amplitude or inversion in the left chest leads. Sinus tachycardia followed by premature ventricular depolarizations was the most common dysrhythmia noted. Take and colleagues[225] examined serial electrocardiograms in 16 patients with proven viral myocarditis. They found the following four patterns: (1) complete normalization even in the presence of severe myocardial damage in the acute stage; (2) "pseudoinfarction" patterns with Q waves and poor R-wave progression; (3) permanent conduction disturbances that might require pacemaker support; and (4) chronic dysrhythmias, predominantly ventricular tachycardia and supraventricular tachycardia. Hoshino and colleagues[98] induced coxsackievirus B3 myocarditis in Syrian golden hamsters and

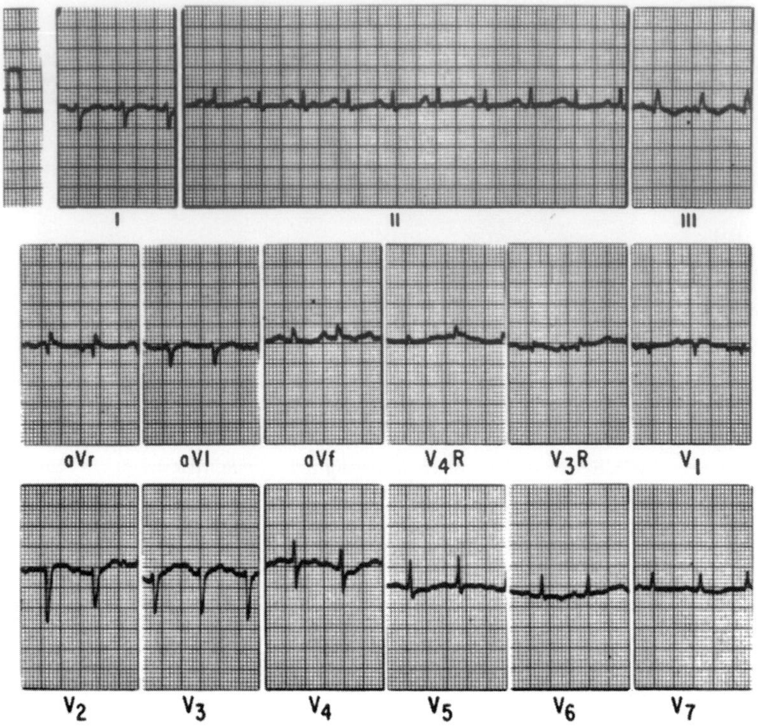

FIGURE 34–9. *Diffuse low voltage or QRS complexes with T-wave flattening and 1-mm Q waves in the lateral precordial leads—the classic pattern in myocarditis.*

found that 80 per cent of them had ST- and/or T-wave changes in their surface electrocardiogram. Most of the changes were seen between days 2 and 4, when mortality was the highest. The endocardial third of the myocardium was most involved histologically, which suggested that the subendocardial myocardial injury corresponded to the observed ST- and T-wave changes. Kishimoto and coworkers,[124] using DBA/2 mice, induced myocarditis with encephalomyocarditis virus. Acute changes were correlated with advanced atrioventricular block and both atrial and ventricular premature depolarizations. Sinus tachycardia and low voltage were seen in the late stages in the animals that survived. Chronically, the QRS voltages recovered toward normal, possibly reflecting loss of myocardial edema and/or development of ventricular hypertrophy as a compensatory mechanism for poor ventricular function.

Although T-wave and ST-segment changes are the most sensitive indices of myocardial ischemia, they also appear to

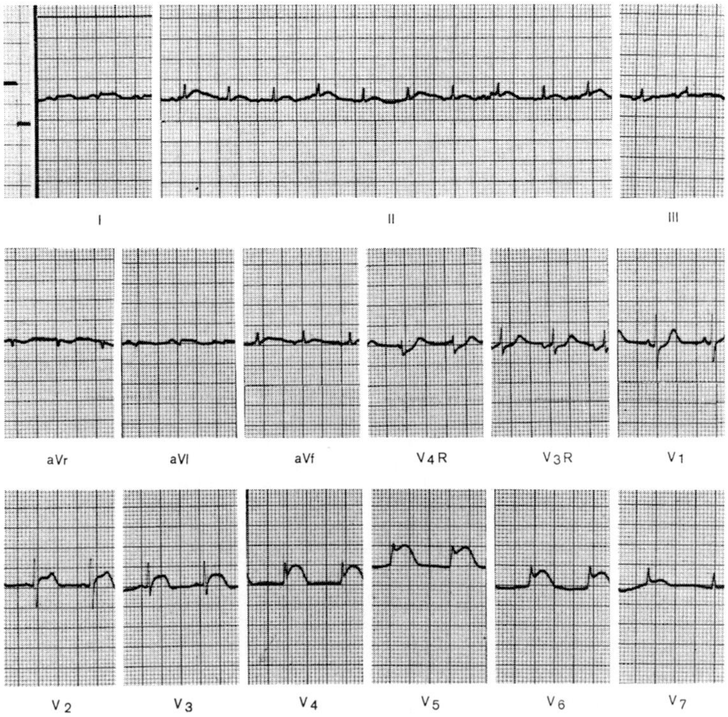

FIGURE 34–10. *In addition to low voltage, there is evidence of acute myocardial ischemia with 4- to 5-mm ST-segment elevation dominantly in the mid and lateral precordial leads.*

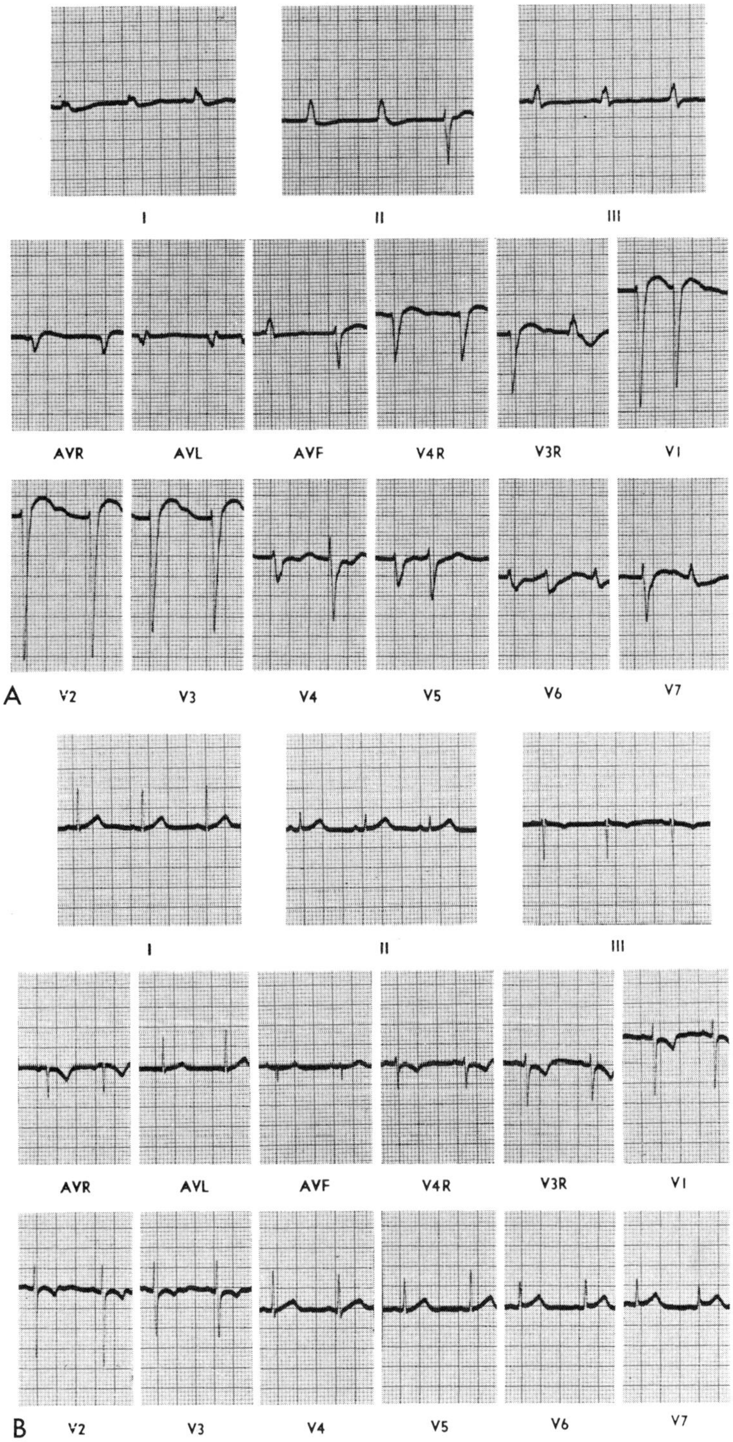

FIGURE 34–11. A, *Multifocal premature beats—atrioventricular dissociation and left bundle branch block secondary to diphtheritic myocarditis.* B, *Normal electrocardiogram 3 months after an episode of myocarditis in patient whose tracing is shown in* A.

be rather nonspecific. Prolongation of the PR interval is another nonspecific electrocardiographic finding frequently noted in patients with febrile illnesses. Scott and colleagues[209] demonstrated a 1.49 per cent prevalence of these findings among a group of 737 infants and children with respiratory tract infections but also found a similar incidence among 108 control children without respiratory infection or other febrile illness. Abt and Vinnecour[2] recorded PR prolongation and T-wave changes in infants and children who were suffering from pneumonia without other signs of myocarditis. Prolongation of the QT interval has been noted in acute myocarditis but also appears to be a rather nonspecific finding in association with certain infectious diseases, such as measles[196] and poliomyelitis.[113] Thus, a diagnosis of myocarditis cannot be established with certainty on the basis of these nonspecific changes.

The echocardiogram is useful in assessing ventricular function and helps to exclude pericardial effusion as the cause of the cardiomegaly. This ultrasound technique is an invaluable aid in the assessment of patients with suspected myocarditis.[198]

Nuclear imaging has been advocated as a potentially help-

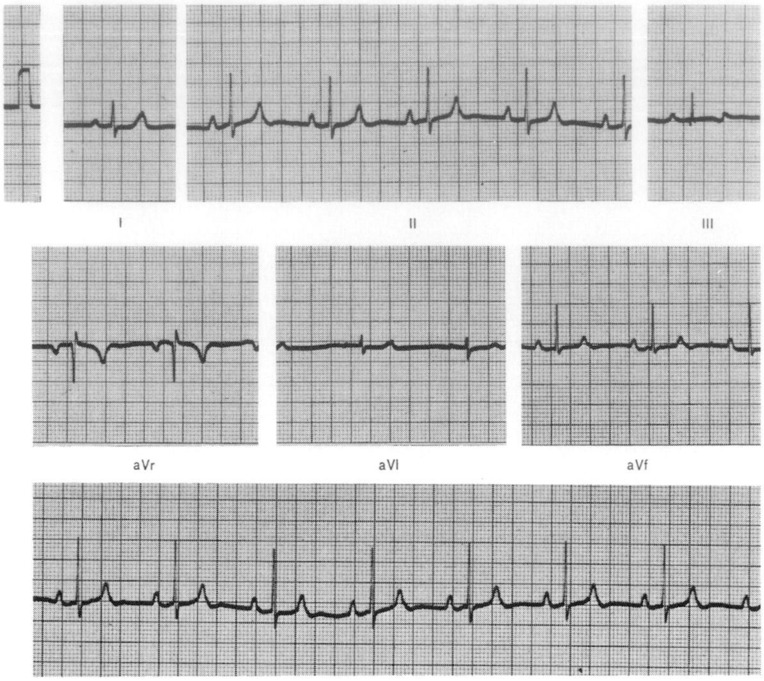

FIGURE 34–12. *Second-degree atrioventricular block with an effective ventricular rate of 60 beats/minute. The blocked P wave is placed on top of the T wave in each cycle.*

ful laboratory screening test. There is some evidence that screening patients with idiopathic-dilated cardiomyopathy with gallium-67 may select a subgroup of patients who would benefit from endomyocardial biopsy. The biopsy specimen then could be used to attempt to confirm the presence of active inflammation. O'Connell and colleagues[168] studied 68 patients with dilated cardiomyopathy who underwent 71 parallel studies with endomyocardial biopsy and gallium scanning. Five of six patients with biopsy samples that showed myocarditis also showed dense gallium uptake, and only 9 of 65 negative biopsies had "equivocally positive" gallium scans. There was a 36 per cent incidence of myocarditis on biopsy with a positive scan and only a 1.8 per cent incidence of myocarditis on biopsy with a negative scan. No large studies have been performed in children, but this technique may prove to be a safe and relatively effective method not only for selecting children for biopsy but also for following the effects of immunosuppressive therapy on the inflammatory response to the viral infection.

Techniques for examining heart muscle biopsy specimens

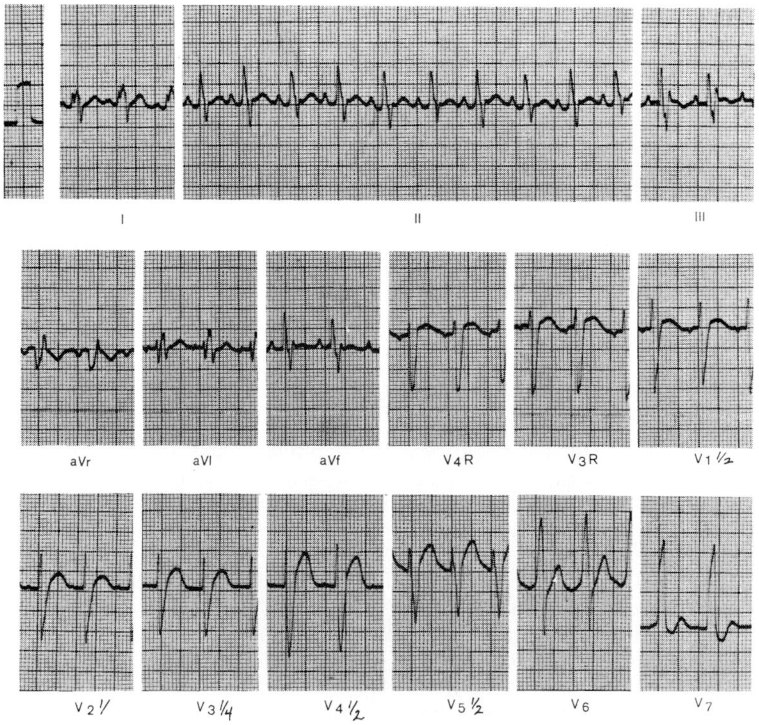

FIGURE 34–13. *Sinus tachycardia (rate, 150/minute) and left bundle branch block.*

promise to help us diagnose and plan therapy more accurately. These techniques (see later) include nucleic acid hybridization and enzymatic amplification,[231] which can be utilized to clone viral RNA or DNA. The offending virus, whose "fingerprint" is present, can be identified, yielding important epidemiologic information and possibly therapeutic guidance.

Indium-111 antimyosin imaging[43] and the presence of major histocompatibility complex class I and II antigens measured by radioimmunoassay utilizing monoclonal antibodies[89] can detect patients with active myocarditis. High titers ($\geq$1:20) of an IgG antibody (heart-reactive antibodies) measured by indirect immunofluorescence have been reported in patients with biopsy-proven myocarditis.[165]

Although none of these methods at present are applicable clinically to all patients, these noninvasive tests offer some hope that the diagnosis of inflammatory heart disease will become safer.

It is unnecessary and potentially dangerous to undertake a hemodynamic study in patients with a classic picture of acute myocarditis, including an electrocardiogram that reveals low voltage. If the clinical or electrocardiographic presentation is atypical (e.g., left ventricular hypertrophy with left axis deviation, infarction pattern, or left bundle branch block), the infant should be studied for exclusion of anomalous origin of the left coronary artery or another unsuspected anomaly.

Endomyocardial biopsy has become a relatively safe and effective means for sampling heart muscle. The technique originally was introduced in 1962 in Japan by Sakakibara and Konno[200] but did not gain wide acceptance in the United States for 10 or more years thereafter. Its widest application has been in monitoring the effectiveness of immunosuppressive therapy in heart transplant patients who may undergo the procedure multiple times.

The importance of endomyocardial biopsy in establishing the diagnosis of myocarditis and possibly classifying the phase (i.e., active, healing, healed) of the infection in the case of viral disease may have a direct impact on the type of therapy employed. Classification of myocarditis based on histologic evidence found on biopsy specimens has proved to be a difficult and at times controversial task. There is at present no widespread agreement on the criteria for establishing the diagnosis of myocarditis from biopsy samples. Sampling error due to the small amounts of tissue obtained and the focal nature of sampling and the disease process may lead to misdiagnosis. Samples usually are obtained from the right ventricular septum and/or apex and should contain at least three, and optimally five, pieces of tissue. Some investigators[232] have found sampling from other areas of the heart (e.g., the left ventricle) to be more sensitive, but these techniques have not been applied widely.

Cases of "borderline myocarditis" (specimens containing increased numbers of inflammatory cells but without evidence of myocyte necrosis) may require a repeat biopsy to confirm the diagnosis. Dec and colleagues[40] confirmed the diagnosis of myocarditis in four of six patients with an initial diagnosis of borderline myocarditis. In addition, they did not demonstrate any significant advantage to sampling the left ventricle during the repeat study. Overinterpretation or misinterpretation has been cited as a major problem in the reading of biopsy specimens. Some studies[222, 223, 240] have utilized this technique to establish a diagnosis of myocarditis in patients presenting with idiopathic congestive cardiomyopathy and in patients with serious ventricular dysrhythmias with otherwise structurally normal hearts. Edwards and associates[53] looked at endomyocardial biopsy samples from 170 biopsies and found that more than five lymphocytes per high-power field was consistent with a diagnosis of active lymphocytic myocarditis. Using endomyocardial biopsy, Fenoglio and coworkers[55] diagnosed myocarditis in 34 patients presenting with congestive heart failure of unknown etiology. They classified these patients on the basis of clinical and histologic findings. This was done in an attempt to establish subgroups of patients who might benefit from immunosuppressive therapy. Three groups were established—acute, rapidly progressive, and chronic. Immunosuppressive therapy was believed to be significantly beneficial only to the latter group in terms of clinical improvement. Dec and colleagues[42] studied 27 patients referred for endomyocardial biopsy because of the presence of congestive heart failure of unknown etiology. Two-thirds of the patients had biopsy samples read as positive for the presence of myocarditis, but unlike the study of Fenoglio and colleagues,[55] in which the histologic grouping was slightly different, there seemed to be no correlation between histologic classification and outcome. Moreover, outcome did not differ between the group receiving immunosuppressives and the group not receiving immunosuppressives. Furthermore, the biopsy was negative in 30 per cent of the patients who already had all the clinical criteria of myocarditis and was positive in two of five patients without any clinical evidence of myocarditis (viral-like illness, pericarditis, or laboratory evidence of viral infection).

Olsen[174] reviewed 1200 biopsy specimens from patients with a clinical diagnosis of idiopathic dilated congestive cardiomyopathy and found that just more than 25 per cent had a diagnosis of myocarditis established on the basis of critical evaluation of their tissue specimens. At present, there are no large series of pediatric patients in whom this technique has been used for diagnosis in therapy in myocarditis.

Most authors would agree that many cases of idiopathic dilated cardiomyopathy probably are the sequelae of unrecognized acute viral myocarditis. Thus, the role of endomyocardial biopsy in attempting to salvage patients by selecting them for specific therapy has some validity. It is hoped that early intervention in some patients guided by this technique will prevent them from progressing to transplantation or death from intractable heart failure.

Molecular Diagnostic Studies

IN SITU HYBRIDIZATION. In 1986, Bowles and colleagues[22] demonstrated the utility of molecular biologic analysis of tissue samples in the diagnosis of myocarditis. Using in situ hybridization, the authors were able to demonstrate enteroviral RNA in the myocardium of patients suspected of having myocarditis. Interestingly, these authors also were able to show that enteroviral RNA could be identified in the myocardial tissue samples obtained from patients with end-stage dilated cardiomyopathy. Hence, the belief that some cases of dilated cardiomyopathy were due to a previous episode of subclinical myocarditis gained scientific support. The ability to diagnose enteroviral myocarditis and the finding of enteroviral RNA in patients with dilated cardiomyopathy later were confirmed by other authors.[9, 10, 23] Unfortunately, because of questions of excessive false-positive results, variation between laboratories, and the difficulty in performing the test routinely in hospital laboratories, this method never gained practical popularity.

POLYMERASE CHAIN REACTION. Initially described and perfected by Mullis and Faldona,[162] polymerase chain reaction (PCR) has been utilized extensively in molecular biology. Jin and associates[111] first described the usefulness of PCR in the identification of viral genome in myocardial samples obtained from patients with suspected myocarditis. Using reverse-transcriptase PCR, which uses RNA to amplify the corresponding complementary DNA prior to final DNA amplification, the authors were able to identify enteroviral genome from cardiac tissue samples. In addition, patients with dilated cardiomyopathy were shown again to harbor enteroviral genome within myocardial specimens. Confirmation of the utility of PCR in the etiologic diagnosis of viral genome in patients with clinical myocarditis and idiopathic dilated cardiomyopathy quickly followed.[32, 51, 74, 90, 161, 180, 189, 242, 243] However, controversy existed because reports of high levels of false-positives,[51] contamination,[32] and low sensitivity[242] were published. The beauty of this method—that is, the rapid (<5 hours) and powerful amplification of specific viral genome—also is its problem because contamination may be commonplace in some laboratories. Furthermore, the method depends on the quality and quantity of nucleic acid extraction. Should any of these requirements be altered, amplification will not occur and lead to false-negative results or false-positive (i.e., contamination) results will occur.

More recently, a number of publications have demonstrated that PCR is not only a rapid and sensitive method for the diagnosis of enteroviral myocarditis but also probably the test of choice in the diagnosis of all viral-induced cardiac disease. For instance, Towbin and colleagues[229] successfully diagnosed adenoviral myocarditis in a fetus with nonimmune hydrops fetalis using PCR. In this case, adenoviral genome was amplified from fetal blood and maternal blood at 29 weeks' gestation and again at delivery at 34 weeks' gestation using blood from baby and mother, as well as placental specimens. Treatment with digoxin in utero helped the fetus improve clinically, and at delivery the newborn had normal cardiac function. Martin and associates[142] reported 34 patients with suspected acute myocarditis in which 68 per cent of samples analyzed were PCR-positive using viral primers designed to amplify enterovirus, adenovirus, cytomegalovirus, and herpes simplex virus nucleic acid. In this report, 17 control patients were PCR-negative. Interestingly, adenovirus was the most common viral genome identified (58 per cent), with enteroviruses being second most common (29 per cent). A small number of cases PCR-positive for herpes simplex virus and cytomegalovirus also were reported.

Griffin and colleagues[76] studied 58 patients with myocarditis and 28 patients with dilated cardiomyopathy due to endocardial fibroelastosis. All tissue samples were obtained at autopsy, with 79 per cent of the samples being formalin fixed and 21 per cent being fresh-frozen with liquid nitrogen. The authors demonstrated that 59 per cent of the autopsy-proven cases of myocarditis were PCR-positive, with 53 per cent of the positive samples being adenovirus and 32 per cent enterovirus; the remainder of PCR-positive cases again amplified herpes simplex virus and cytomegalovirus. Of note, the authors convincingly showed that fixed tissue samples were useful for PCR analysis, with essentially no differences in the percentage of samples amplified using either method. Particularly important was the finding that the enterovirus, an RNA virus, effectively could be identified using fixed specimens. This, therefore, suggests that previous or current cases of myocarditis in which no etiology could be identified by culture, serology, or microscopy can be studied by PCR of autopsy samples with the etiology identified retrospectively or prospectively. In addition, the authors identified adenoviral genome in 21 per cent of the cases of endocardial fibroelastosis, with no other viral genome being identified. This study, coupled with the report by Martin and associates,[142] suggested adenovirus to be a major cause of myocarditis. Although previous reports of adenoviral myocarditis had been published,[21, 31, 66, 76, 88, 212, 219, 236] this virus was considered a minor and unimportant cause of disease by most experts. Closer evaluation of these reports, however, demonstrates that a relatively high percentage of cases identified by culture and serology were adenovirus, second only to the enteroviruses coxsackieviruses and echoviruses. Lozinski and coworkers[137] confirmed the importance of adenovirus in their study of cases of myocarditis in which no etiology had been found previously; here, 66 per cent of the previously unidentified cases were identified as adenovirus.

Finally, Schowengerdt and colleagues[207] have shown that a variety of viruses may be the inciting cause of rejection in patients after heart transplantation. Using PCR of endomyocardial biopsy specimens, the authors demonstrated that a direct correlation existed between histologic rejection and PCR-positive viral studies. Studying patients undergoing serial endomyocardial biopsies, they found that viral genome could be amplified in transplant-rejecting patients who previously had negative PCR analyses. In these cases, as the rejection grade improved, PCR again became negative. The most common viruses leading to rejection were adenoviruses, cytomegalovirus, and parvovirus. The authors postulated that this form of rejection is likely to be another form of myocarditis per se. Support for this hypothesis has been presented by other clinical studies.[244]

FUTURE DIRECTIONS. The current diagnostic methods are clearly an improvement over past methods. However, these methods lack the sensitivity to identify all cases of myocarditis and are not able to pinpoint the areas of myocardium hardest hit by the viral infection. In addition, the role of inflammatory mediators is not well studied by these methods. In order to help to rectify these inadequacies, several new approaches are likely to help. These include the following:

1. *In situ PCR.* This method combines the PCR method and in situ hybridization in order to identify where in the affected tissue the viral genome resides. Hence, a sample of myocardium can be shown to have viral genome within certain myocytes but not in others. This knowledge potentially could help to understand the patchy nature of the infiltrate and the selective areas of dysfunction.
2. *Inflammatory mediators.* Using PCR and other methods, a variety of inflammatory mediators, such as cytokines and adhesion molecules, can be analyzed. In certain cases of clinical myocarditis, for instance, histology appears "negative for myocarditis." Martin and colleagues[142] have shown that in some of these cases viral genome may be amplified, particularly adenovirus. In these cases, as well as those in which the causative agent is not identified, it is likely that a cascade of inflammatory mediators is up-regulated.[127, 166, 230] Therefore, identification of this response indeed could help to diagnose inflammatory heart disease.

These methods and others are likely to continue to improve the diagnostic armamentarium in myocarditis and help to improve our understanding of this heterogeneous disease. Once understood, specific therapy is more likely to become available.

Virologic and Bacteriologic Studies[21, 85, 91, 206, 239]

In each infant or child with a diagnosis of acute myocarditis, an attempt should be made to identify the offending organism. If the patient is seen early in the illness, it may be possible to isolate the virus from throat washings, stool, blood, or the myocardium. Support for an active infection then is obtained by demonstrating a fourfold rise in antibody titer to the virus that has been isolated.

Lerner and Wilson[131] suggested criteria that would help define an etiologic association between a coxsackievirus infection and myocarditis. High-order associations included (1) isolation of the virus from the myocardium, the endocardium, or pericardial fluid and (2) localization of type-specific virus in myocardium, endocardium, or pericardium at sites of pathologic change. Moderate-order associations are present (1) when virus is isolated from pharynx or feces and a fourfold increase in type-specific, neutralizing, hemagglutination-inhibiting, or complement-fixing antibodies are demonstrated or (2) when virus is isolated from pharynx or feces with a concurrent serum titer of 1:32 or greater of type-specific IgM-neutralizing or hemagglutination-inhibiting antibodies.

Schmidt and colleagues[206] stress the usefulness of the IgM-specific antibody titer. Coxsackieviruses B1, B3, B4, B5, and B6 are identifiable with this method. Immunofluorescent methods may be used during histologic analysis to identify specific antigens in the myocardium.[26] In chronic illness, attempts at virologic identification are less fruitful.[79]

Blood for aerobic and anaerobic cultures also should be obtained in any infant with fever and signs of compromised cardiovascular function. The erythrocyte sedimentation rate and white blood cell count usually are elevated in acute myocarditis; occasionally, a leukemoid reaction may be noted.[4] A normal value for these tests does not exclude myocarditis. Elevation of serum glutamic oxaloacetic and glutamic pyruvic transaminase levels has been noted, especially in diphtheritic myocarditis,[224] but they may be elevated any time there is acute myocardial damage. Although a high level of serum transaminase activity generally is an ominous prognostic sign, Tahernia[224] found the electrocardiogram to be a more sensitive indicator of the ultimate outcome in children with diphtheritic myocarditis. Creatinine phosphokinase and lactate dehydrogenase enzymes also should be measured. Okuni and coworkers[170] noted that elevation of isoenzyme 1 of lactate dehydrogenase appeared to be very specific in their patients with idiopathic myocarditis.

DIFFERENTIAL DIAGNOSIS

Any cause of circulatory failure may mimic myocarditis, especially when acute in onset. Heart failure is well recognized in newborn infants in association with hypoxia, hypoglycemia, and hypocalcemia, whereas circulatory collapse may occur with any infection and without direct involvement of the myocardium. A careful history may help to elucidate possible precipitating factors. Biochemical investigations to exclude hypoglycemia and hypocalcemia always should be conducted in any newborn infant who has signs of heart failure. Blood cultures should be obtained when infection is suspected.

Many infants with structural cardiac defects (e.g., hypoplastic left heart syndrome or aortic valve stenosis) may not have audible murmurs when severely ill. Murmurs, however, usually appear with treatment and improvement in cardiac function. In addition, the precordium usually is hyperactive, rather than quiet, and the heart sounds are clear and increased in intensity, rather than muffled. The electrocardiogram usually shows severe right ventricular hypertrophy in the former condition and either right ventricular or left ventricular hypertrophy in the latter; thus, the electrocardiogram is useful in the differential diagnosis. The findings on an echocardiogram often are diagnostic.

Beyond the immediate neonatal period, endocardial fibroelastosis, anomalous left coronary artery arising from the pulmonary artery, Cori type II glycogen storage disease (Pompe disease), medial necrosis of the coronary arteries, left atrial myxoma,[164] and other congestive cardiomyopathies of undetermined etiology are the major disease entities that require differentiation from myocarditis.[61, 116] Common to all of these disorders is moderate to severe cardiomegaly, usually associated with congestive cardiac failure, gallop rhythm, and the infrequent occurrence or absence of murmurs. The murmurs occur primarily in association with anomalous left coronary artery and endocardial fibroelastosis. They are not more than grade 3/6 in intensity, are high pitched and apical in location, and represent some degree of mitral insufficiency.

Idiopathic myocarditis primarily occurs after 6 months of age,[193] whereas most of the conditions described earlier present before 6 months of age.

Endocardial fibroelastosis, a relatively common cause of congestive cardiac failure in infants, is impossible to differentiate from acute myocarditis on the basis of clinical examination alone.

Anomalous origin of the left coronary artery should be identified. The electrocardiogram usually shows left axis deviation of the QRS complex in the frontal plane, left ventricular hypertrophy, and a pattern of anterolateral myocardial infarction. This is recognized as a QR pattern with inverted T waves in standard leads I and AVL, as well as a broad Q wave with inverted T waves in precordial leads V_5 and V_6 and loss of anterior forces in the midprecordial leads. For definitive diagnosis, cardiac catheterization is essential.

Pericarditis, frequently caused by viruses, usually occurs in children rather than in infants. The clinical history may be identical to that of patients with myocarditis; however, considering the degree of cardiomegaly present, cardiovascular function is compromised less than in patients with myocarditis, although this is not always true because cardiac tamponade may occur in some cases. The differentiation from myocarditis may be made clinically if there is a friction rub, no gallop rhythm, and a typical pattern of chest pain. However, further studies may be required for conclusive diagnosis. The echocardiogram is invaluable in establishing this diagnosis. It is the most sensitive and least traumatic technique available and easily identifies an effusion. Myocarditis and pericarditis may occur together. This is seen most frequently in the pancarditis of rheumatic fever but may occur also in coxsackievirus B infections and in many of the collagen vascular and autoimmune diseases. Myocarditis has been described in association with rheumatoid arthritis,[152] systemic lupus erythematosus,[86] and ulcerative colitis.[160]

TREATMENT

Intensive medical care is required during the acute stage of the illness. Heart rate, respiratory rate, and blood pressure should be monitored frequently, and a careful assessment of urine output and fluid intake is mandatory. All patients require bed rest. It has been shown experimentally in mice that exercise increases virus replication in the myocardium and increases the mortality from myocarditis by 100 per cent.[67, 132] Although it always is dangerous to extrapolate directly from experimental studies in animals to the human situation, it appears prudent to suggest strict bed rest during the early stages of acute myocarditis. For infants or children with signs of congestive cardiac failure or shock, oxygen should be administered to maintain a normal arterial blood oxygen tension.

No specific therapeutic modality is known that will reverse the myocardial injury directly, but much can be done to maintain adequate tissue perfusion, prevent metabolic disturbances, and support myocardial function. When congestive cardiac failure is noted, digitalis should be administered. Because of the apparent increased sensitivity of the inflamed myocardium to digitalis, rapid digitalization in less than 24 hours should be avoided. The oral route is preferred over the intravenous route, although the latter may be required when shock is present. A dose of 0.03 mg/kg, rather than 0.04 mg/kg, should be used as a total digitalizing dose. Half the total dose is given initially, and the remainder is divided equally and administered at 8-hour intervals. Digitalization may effect dramatic improvement.[192]

Diuretics also are used frequently to treat cardiac failure. Diuretics have no direct beneficial effect on the myocardium; therefore, they should be used cautiously because rapid reduction in extracellular fluid volume may lead to shock, and the loss of potassium associated with vigorous diuresis may precipitate digitalis toxicity. When used, we prefer furosemide (Lasix) in a dosage of 1 mg/kg per dose. The frequency of administration depends on the clinical state of the patient.

In some instances, especially in the newborn infant, the primary presentation may be that of shock. The blood pressure usually is maintained close to normal levels until late in the course of disease; therefore, it cannot be a reliable index of the severity of the patient's condition. Cold extremities, increasing heart rate, and low urine output are much more sensitive indicators of a reduction in effective circulating blood volume. Although the hearts of these infants and children respond poorly to volume loading, a colloid transfusion may help in selected patients. Albumin, as a 5 per cent solution in Ringer lactate, or whole blood may be given in an initial dose of 5 mL/kg. The total amount administered should be guided by the response of the patient in terms of perfusion, urine output, heart rate, and central venous pressure. These patients may require a high filling pressure, e.g., 12 to 18 mm Hg, to achieve any cardiac output, compared with 5 mm Hg, which would achieve sufficient filling in the normal heart. If the patient remains in shock despite these high filling pressures, a positive inotropic agent is required. We prefer dopamine because it exerts an inotropic effect on the heart and concomitantly dilates the renal vessels, thereby improving urine output. The usual dosage is 2 to 10 μg/kg/minute. As the dose increases to 20 μg/kg/minute, dopamine has a more dominant alpha-adrenergic effect and may increase systemic peripheral resistance; therefore, we usually avoid doses above 15 μg/kg/minute. Dobutamine, which is a sympathomimetic amine that stimulates $beta_1$ and $beta_2$ as well as alpha-adrenergic receptors, may be quite useful when used in combination with dopamine. It has significant inotropic activity while decreasing left ventricular filling pressure. Dobutamine does not induce the positive chronotropic effect and increased ventricular irritability that is seen with dopamine. Used in combination with low doses of dopamine ($<$10 μg/kg/minute), dobutamine, in doses up to 10 μg/kg/minute, may result in significant positive inotropism while preventing a sinus tachycardia that may compromise cardiac output further. Isoproterenol, a commonly used inotropic agent, should be avoided because it causes a significant increase in heart rate and may affect cardiac function adversely. When these drugs are used, it is important to ensure normal acid-base balance because the action of these agents is decreased significantly by acidosis.

Agents such as sodium nitroprusside, phentolamine, and the nitrates have been used in adults. They have been used less extensively in children, primarily in the early postoperative period after open heart surgery, to improve cardiac function. They improve cardiac output by indirectly reducing systemic arterial resistance or venous filling pressure, or both. One study[191] demonstrated a marked improvement in the reduction of inflammation, necrosis, and dystrophic calcification in mice infected with coxsackievirus B3 when they were treated early after infection with captopril, an angiotensin-converting enzyme. Besides its known afterload-reducing effects, this agent, which contains sulfhydryl groups in its chemical structure, is capable of scavenging oxygen-free radicals in vitro. This ability may enable the drug to reduce myocyte damage by free radicals during the acute phase of the infection.

Another study failed to demonstrate any significant correlation between improved ventricular function and histologic improvement in patients with myocarditis treated with immunosuppressive therapy. Rather, a rise in the ejection fraction during the first 3 months of therapy seemed predictive of a good outcome.[41] Intravenously administered afterload-reducing agents should not be used unless facilities are available for constantly monitoring the left ventricular filling pressure (i.e., mean wedge pressure) and unless that pressure is elevated.

Arrhythmias should be recognized and treated vigorously. Digitalis should be used with caution, and intravenous administration of this drug should be performed only if the oral route is not possible. Rather than used as inotropic support, digitalis can be used to help control supraventricular arrhythmias. Levels must be monitored, especially when renal function is suspect. Lidocaine should be administered intravenously in a dose of 1 mg/kg for the acute treatment of complex ventricular arrhythmias, such as couplets and ventricular tachycardia. In cases of intractable ventricular arrhythmias, intravenously administered procainamide, 10 to 15 mg/kg as a loading dose followed by a drip of 40 to 70 μg/kg/minute, can be used. It is essential to monitor the serum level on a daily basis beginning several hours after the drip is started to prevent toxic side effects. Measures of contractility using echocardiographic techniques also are vital because procainamide is a negative inotrope. The use of intravenously administered amiodarone has been approved by the Food and Drug Administration and should be considered if the more standard therapy outlined earlier fails. However, despite aggressive management of ventricular tachycardia in the acute setting, this may prove to be a terminal event in many cases.

A temporary pacing catheter should be inserted when complete heart block occurs; in many instances, this is sufficient to allow time for spontaneous recovery of atrioventricular conduction. A permanent pacemaker may be required; if so, it should be inserted as an elective, rather than emergency, procedure. A demand pacemaker only should be used because in most instances a return to normal rhythm is expected; use of this type of pacemaker avoids the risk of competition between the patient's inherent rhythm and the pacemaker, as would occur with a fixed-rate device. If infants or children experience Stokes-Adams attacks, a transthoracic pacing wire may have to be inserted as an emergency procedure.

Antibiotics should not be given routinely unless a bacterial infection is suspected and appropriate cultures have been obtained before their use.

Immunosuppressive Agents

The use of immunosuppressive agents in the treatment of viral or suspected viral myocarditis still is controversial. Early animal studies suggested an exacerbation of virus-induced cytotoxicity when such agents were given in the acute setting and possible interference with the production of interferon.[120, 121, 197] A report[30] of 13 children with biopsy-proven myocarditis treated with prednisone approximately 3 weeks after symptoms occurred demonstrated a marked reduction in inflammation at the follow-up biopsy. However, this was an uncontrolled study and thus may not truly represent an accurate account of the role of immunosuppressive therapy. Mason and colleagues[144] used endomyocardial biopsy as a means of diagnosing and following the effects of immunosuppressive therapy in 10 patients. Eight patients received a combination of prednisone and azathioprine, and two patients received prednisone alone. Four patients improved clinically and histologically while on therapy. Two patients who had their medications discontinued suffered relapses, which were reversed with reinstitution of therapy. Only one patient worsened while on therapy, and that patient died. Although the study by Mason and associates was uncontrolled, the reversal of congestive heart failure seen in the two patients who were restarted on therapy is quite suggestive of the beneficial effect of these agents.

Daly and colleagues[38] treated nine patients using combined immunosuppressive therapy with prednisolone and azothioprine. Seven of the nine patients showed definite hemodynamic and histologic improvement after 2 months of therapy. However, after 4 months off therapy, only four of the seven patients still showed significant improvement. One patient improved with reinstitution of therapy, and two patients deteriorated. Dec and colleagues[42] treated nine patients in their study with single or combined immunosuppressive therapy. They saw improvement in 4 of 9; however, 6 of 18 patients not receiving immunosuppressive agents also improved, nullifying any statistically significant difference between the two groups. Lymphocytic myocarditis was found in 6 of 12 patients with no obvious cardiac disease but with high-grade ventricular dysrhythmias and who had undergone right ventricular endomyocardial biopsy.[240] All six patients received combined immunosuppressive therapy with prednisone and azothioprine. At follow-up, five of six patients had been cured of the dysrhythmia, and active myocardial inflammation had disappeared as proved by repeat biopsy. Although this was an uncontrolled study, the fact that none of the patients progressed to a cardiomyopathic state or died of their illness is highly suggestive of a beneficial effect.

Kereiakes and Parmley[117] have tabulated most of the studies to date showing the effects of immunosuppressive therapy in patients with myocarditis. Sixty per cent of 82 biopsy-proven cases of mycarditis showed improvement with steroids alone or in combination with azothioprine. It appears that those patients with lower-grade inflammatory changes do better than those patients showing higher-grade changes. Complications of immunosuppressive therapy, including opportunistic infections[144, 222] and a cushingoid state,[197] have been reported and may limit the amount and type of therapy. Hobbs and associates[93] treated 34 adults with biopsy-proven myocarditis with combined prednisone and azothioprine. Survival was no better in patients with histologic improvement than in those with persistent infiltrates. Most patients experienced side effects from the corticosteroids, some of them lethal. Thus, the potential benefits of this type of therapy must be weighed against the risks of immunosuppression in each patient. Steroids also have been used in diphtheritic myocarditis[227] but apparently do not prevent the observed electrocardiographic changes seen in untreated patients or the associated neuritis.

The long-awaited results of the Myocarditis Treatment Trial Investigators have been published.[145] The study was performed in adult patients, but the results nonetheless probably are applicable to the vast majority of children with this disease. Random assignment was made of 111 patients with a histopathologic diagnosis of myocarditis to one of three treatment groups. The first group received azothioprine and prednisone, the second group received cyclosporine and prednisone, and the third group did not receive any immunosuppressive therapy (i.e., they received conventional supportive therapy). Patients were treated for 24 weeks. Although three different indices of left ventricular function were studied, there was no difference between the groups treated with immunosuppressive agents and the control (conventional therapy) group. More importantly, survival was no different between the groups. It was concluded that immunosuppressive therapy was not beneficial in most patients with histologically confirmed myocarditis.

At present, there is an ongoing multicenter study of the use of intravenous gamma-globulin in children with myocarditis. This study is based on the early results of Drucker and associates,[49] who investigated the use of this agent in 21 of 46 children with myocarditis. Patients who received this drug had better left ventricular function at follow-up. In addition, survival *tended* to be higher at 1 year, although the data did not reach statistical significance because of the small number of patients in the study. Whether this proves to be beneficial or whether these early results mirror the early published experience with corticosteroids remains to be seen.

PROGNOSIS

The prognosis of acute myocarditis caused by coxsackievirus B infection in the newborn infant is poor. Kibrick and Benirschke[119] reported a 75 per cent mortality rate among 25 infants with coxsackievirus B myocarditis. The greatest number of deaths occurred in the first week of the illness. There were no apparent sequelae in the six infants who survived, although no long-term follow-up data were available. The outlook in other infants and children with clinically recognized myocarditis is somewhat better, but mortality is still significant (10 to 25 per cent). Hastreiter and Miller[84] noted complete recovery in 50 per cent of patients. A further 25 per cent became asymptomatic, but abnormal electrocardiograms and/or chest radiographs persisted. An abnormality may not be evident on the electrocardiogram unless the patients are exercised.[19] Despite lack of symptoms, many adult patients have a reduced working capacity associated with exercise stress testing.[20]

The outcome of myocarditis also is related, in part, to the etiology. Patients with diphtheritic myocarditis who have arrhythmias or conduction abnormalities have a very poor prognosis. Tahernia[224] noted in his study that all patients with disturbances of conduction died. Begg[16] also reported a 100 per cent mortality rate in patients with diphtheritic myocarditis who developed supraventricular tachycardia.

Chronic arrhythmias may persist long after the acute disease has passed. Friedman and colleagues[62] performed a retrospective analysis of 12 patients with biopsy-confirmed myocarditis and complex ventricular arrhythmias at the time of presentation (11 with ventricular tachycardia). Five of the 12 patients still were receiving antiarrhythmic therapy at a median follow-up of 50 months. Complex venticular arrhythmias still were present in these patients (three with ventricular tachycardia and two with couplets or multiforms), requiring ongoing therapy. The authors concluded that although the arrhythmias were controlled more easily than at presentation, ongoing surveillance of these patients was essential in ensuring the suppression of these potentially life-threatening arrhythmias. Thus, children who recover from myocarditis, regardless of etiology, should be followed indefinitely.

PREVENTION

Because enteroviruses may be spread by the airborne route, any newborn infant with myocarditis should be isolated with his or her mother. Individuals employed in newborn nurseries who develop signs or symptoms of enteroviral infection should be excluded from the nursery until they have recovered.

Immunization programs help to reduce the incidence of myocarditis associated with diphtheria and many of the other common infectious agents.[254]

Matsumori and colleagues[146] induced myocarditis with encephalomyocarditis virus in mice. Using ribavirin early after inoculation, they were able to show a significant reduction in myocardial injury and inflammation, presumably due to inhibition of viral replication. No studies have been conducted in humans, but this model is a promising first step in possible prevention and/or therapy of virus-induced myocarditis.

The use of myocardial biopsy techniques may help to define further the etiology of idiopathic cardiomyopathies, and with the probable availability of specific antiviral agents in the future, prevention of viral myocarditis may become a reality.

Parasitic Myocarditis

Parasitic myocarditis is an uncommon form of heart disease in the United States. In contrast, in Central and South America, infection with the protozoan *Trypanosoma cruzi* (American trypanosomiasis or Chagas disease) is a prominent cause of myocarditis.[128] Myocardial disease due to infection with other parasites, including *Trichinella, Toxoplasma,* and *Toxocara,* has been reported in the literature.

The major cardiovascular manifestation of Chagas disease is an extensive myocarditis that typically becomes evident years or even decades after the initial infection. The disease is transmitted to humans by various species of bloodsucking reduviid insects. After inoculation, the protozoa multiply and then migrate widely throughout the body. Acute Chagas disease usually is an illness of children but can occur at any age.[122] Histologic examination of the heart during the acute phase reveals intracellular parasites with a marked cellular infiltrate, particularly around myocytes that have ruptured and released the parasites.[178] It is well established that intracellular parasites are found in cardiac myocytes only during the acute phase of illness. Severe myocarditis develops in only a small proportion of acute cases, and most deaths are due to the resultant congestive heart failure and pericardial effusion. Nonspecific electrocardiographic changes are seen, but the life-threatening arrhythmias that are frequent in chronic Chagas disease generally do not occur. In the majority of patients with more acute disease (90 per cent of cases), symptoms resolve gradually over a period of weeks to months.

Chronic progressive Chagas develops in 10 to 20 per cent of previously asymptomatically infected individuals.[138] It is manifested by a chronic, diffuse, progressive fibrosing myocarditis that involves not only the myocytes but also the atrioventricular conduction system.[157, 159] On gross examination, the heart usually is enlarged and flaccid. Thrombus formation is frequent, and in some cases thrombus may fill much of the apex of the left ventricle. Histologic examination reveals focal but widespread areas of cellular infiltrates composed of plasma cells, eosinophils, mast cells, and macrophages.[157] Extensive fibrosis occurs, replacing previously damaged myocardial tissue. In contrast to the situation observed in acute disease, the presence of parasites (a rare finding) in tissue has little correlation with myocardial pathology. Inflammatory changes in the right bundle branch and the anterior fascicle of the left bundle branch explain the frequent occurrence of right bundle branch and left anterior fascicular block.[159] The clinical manifestations of chronic Chagas disease range from isolated rhythm disturbances to advanced disease characterized by cardiomegaly, chronic congestive heart failure, and arrhythmias. Syncope also is a frequent problem of the disease. In one series of 53 patients with chronic Chagas, the most frequent causes of recurrent syncope were ventricular tachycardia (43 per cent) with a poor prognosis and paroxysmal atrioventricular block (21 per cent) with a favorable prognosis.[143] Sudden death due to ventricular fibrillation is a constant threat and may develop before cardiomegaly or heart failure is diagnosed.[28, 143]

The diagnosis of chronic Chagas cannot be made only on the basis of histologic examination of the heart. Serologic testing is the method of choice for establishing the diagnosis of chronic Chagas disease. A number of highly sensitive serologic tests for the detection of anti–*T. cruzi* antibodies are available, such as indirect hemagglutination, complement fixation, indirect immunofluorescence, and enzyme-linked immunosorbent assay.[123, 214] Unfortunately, these assays lack specificity, and false-positive results have been reported in patients with other infectious diseases, such as malaria, leishmaniasis, and syphilis.[122] The current emphasis on the management of Chagas disease is on prevention because a chemotherapeutic agent that eradicates the parasite in the chronic stage of the disease is not available.

Myocarditis is one of the most serious complications of trichinosis. The disease develops when undercooked meat contaminated with infective larvae of *Trichinella* is eaten. Myocardial invasion by *Trichinella spiralis* has been well described,[216] but encystment within the myocardium has been reported only rarely.[97] At autopsy, the heart may be dilated and a pericardial effusion may be present. Histologically, a prominent focal infiltrate composed of lymphocytes and eosinophils with interstitial edema and scattered hemorrhages commonly is found.[216] Myocarditis usually is mild with few clinical signs and symptoms. However, this myocarditis may range from chest pain to fatal congestive heart failure and may mimic acute myocardial infarction.[35, 75] In one series of 114 patients with trichinosis, 21 per cent had abnormal electrocardiograms.[213] Abnormalities included prolongation of the PR interval, low voltage and/or prolongation of the QRS complex, and flattened T waves. Despite electrocardiographic evidence of myocardial involvement, less than 0.1 per cent of patients with trichinosis die of this complication.[75] The definitive diagnosis of trichinosis is based on demonstration of the larval forms in tissue biopsy samples, usually from a large tender area such as the gastrocnemius muscle. Serologic testing is available through state laboratories and the Centers for Disease Control and Prevention. Typically, serum antibody titers become positive during or after the third week of illness. The efficacy of mebendazole or albendazole in the treatment of myocarditis due to *Trichinella* infection has not been evaluated adequately.

Toxocara canis, the principal cause of visceral larva migrans, is a rare cause of myocarditis. Most reported cases have occurred in children younger than 3 years of age.[39, 63, 237] Children especially are susceptible to infection with *Toxocara* because of their habit of crawling on the ground and putting various objects into their mouths. The myocardial lesions noted on histologic examination have included granulomata and extensive eosinophilic infiltrates with foci of muscle necrosis.[39, 237] The clinical presentation may be that of acute respiratory distress due to congestive heart failure requiring administration of oxygen and diuretic therapy. However, asymptomatic infection involving the heart also has been reported.[39] The definitive diagnosis requires microscopic identification of the larvae in biopsy specimens of the liver or heart, but this finding is infrequent. An enzyme immunoassay for *Toxacara* serum antibodies, which is available at the Centers for Disease Control and Prevention, can provide presumptive evidence of toxocariasis.

Toxoplasma gondii may cause myocarditis as part of disseminated infection or less frequently an isolated cardiac infection. In infants with congenital toxoplasmosis, the clinical manifestations usually are those of meningoencephalitis, but at autopsy extensive myocardial involvement has been documented.[257] Outside the newborn period, infection with this intracellular parasite most commonly occurs in immunosuppressed individuals with malignant diseases, patients with AIDS,[27] and in patients after cardiac or bone marrow transplantation.[138] Histologic examination of the heart reveals focal interstitial infiltrates consisting of histiocytes, lymphocytes, plasma cells, eosinophils, and very few polymorphonuclear cells.[226] Toxoplasma are seen as basophilic masses within a pseudocyst in normal or damaged myocardial fibers. Clinical manifestations may include arrhythmias (atrial and ventricular), atrioventricular block, atypical chest pain, pericarditis, and heart failure.[128, 226] The diagnosis of toxoplasmic myocarditis requires the exclusion of other specific forms of heart disease and the establishment of evidence of toxoplasmosis with serologic testing. In addition, diagnosis may be aided by endomyocardial biopsy.[138] Treatment with pyrimethamine and sulfonamides (especially sulfadiazine) has been reported in patients with isolated toxoplasmic myocarditis, but the response to therapy has been variable. In one series of toxoplasmic myocarditis, relapses occurred in 17 per cent of cases after therapy.[129]

Myocardial disease also has been reported after infection with *Echinococcus granulosus* and *Plasmodium falciparum*. It is estimated that cardiac involvement occurs in less than 2 per cent of cases of echinococcosis.[45] When this occurs, the cysts usually are located in the intramyocardial region and protrude into the adjacent cardiac chambers. The clinical manifestations primarily depend on the location and size of the cyst. Rupture of the cyst is the most dreaded complication because this may lead to pericarditis, anaphylactic shock, or pulmonary emboli. Two-dimensional echocardiography is the preferred imaging study to detect and localize cysts.[173] Myocardial changes also have been documented in fatal malaria, particularly when caused by *P. falciparum*. Histologically, there is blocking of the coronary arteries and capillaries with parasites, local hemorrhage, and deposit of pigment.[143, 217] However, clinical findings suggestive of cardiac involvement are rare. In a series of 49 patients with falciparum malaria, no electrocardioigraphic evidence of cardiac involvement was noted.[217]

Myocarditis also has occurred in association with primary amebic meningoencephalitis due to *Naegleria*. In a retrospective study, focal or diffuse myocarditis was documented in more than 40 per cent of cases.[141] However, myocardial involvement is not a clinically significant manifestation of this uniformly fatal central nervous system infection.

References

1. Abelmann, W. H.: Virus and the heart. Circulation *44*:950–956, 1971.
2. Abt, A. F., and Vinnecour, M. I.: Electrocardiographic studies during pneumonia in infants and children. Am. J. Dis. Child. *47*:737, 1934.
3. Acierno, L. J.: Cardiac complications in acquired immunodeficiency syndrome (AIDS): A review. J. Am. Coll. Cardiol. *13*:1144, 1989.
4. Ainger, L. E.: Acute aseptic myocarditis: Corticosteroid therapy. J. Pediatr. *64*:716–723, 1964.
5. Ainger, L. E., Lawyer, N. G., and Fitch, C. W.: Neonatal rubella myocarditis. Br. Heart J. *28*:691, 1966.
6. Ali, N., Ferrans, V. J., Roberts, W. C., et al.: Clinical evaluation of transvenous catheter technique for endomyocardial biopsy. Chest *63*:399–402, 1973.
7. Anderson, D. W., Virmani, R., Reilly, J. M., et al.: Prevalent myocarditis at necropsy in acquired immunodeficiency syndrome. J. Am. Coll. Cardiol. *11*:792, 1988.
8. Appelbaum, F., Stranchen, J. A., Graw, R. G., Jr., et al.: Acute lethal carditis caused by high-dose combination chemotherapy: A unique clinical and pathological entity. Lancet *1*:58–62, 1976.
9. Archard, L. C., Bowles, N. E., Olsen, E. G. J., et al.: Detection of persistent coxsackievirus in dilated cardiomyopathy and myocarditis. Eur. Heart J. *8*:437–440, 1987.
10. Archard, L. C., Greeke, C. A., Richardson, P. J., et al.: Persistence of enteroviral RNA in dilated cardiomyopathy: A progression from myocarditis. *In* Schultheiss, H. E. (ed.): New Concepts in Viral Heart Disease. Berlin/Heidelberg/New York, Springer-Verlag, 1988, pp. 349–362.
11. Babb, J. M., Stoneman, M. E. R., and Stern, H.: Myocarditis and croup caused by coxsackie virus type B5. Arch. Dis. Child. *36*:551–556, 1961.
12. Bablanian, R.: Structure and functional alterations in cultured cells infected with cytocidal viruses. Prog. Med. Virol. *19*:40–83, 1975.
13. Bairan, A. C., Cherry, J. D., Fagan, L. F., et al.: Complete heart block and respiratory syncytial virus. Am. J. Dis. Child. *127*:264–265, 1974.
14. Baroldi, G., Corallo, S., Moroni, M., et al.: Focal lymphocytic myocarditis in acquired immunodeficiency syndrome (AIDS): A correlative morphologic and clinical study in 26 consecutive fatal cases. J. Am. Coll. Cardiol. *12*:463, 1988.
15. Barry, W. H.: Mechanisms of immune-mediated myocyte injury. Circulation *5*:2421–2432, 1994.
16. Begg, M. D.: Diphtheritic myocarditis: EKG study. Lancet *1*:857, 1937.
17. Behrman, R. E.: Neonatology: Diseases of the Fetus and Infant. St. Louis, C. V. Mosby, 1973.
18. Bell, E. J., and Grist, N. R.: Echo viruses, carditis and acute pleurodynia. Am. Heart J. *82*:133, 1971.
19. Bengtssen, E., and Lamberger, B.: Five-year follow-up study of cases suggestive of acute myocarditis. Am. Heart J. *72*:751, 1966.
20. Bergstrom, K., Erikson, U., Nordbring, F., et al.: Acute non-rheumatic myopericarditis: A follow-up study. Scand. J. Infect. Dis. *2*:7–16, 1970.
21. Berkovich, S., Rodriguez-Torres, R., and Lin, J. S.: Virologic studies in children with acute myocarditis. Am. J. Dis. Child. *115*:207, 1968.
22. Bowles, N. E., Richardson, P. J., Olsen, E. G. J., et al.: Detection of coxsackie-B–virus specific RNA sequences in myocardial biopsy samples from patients with myocarditis and dilated cardiomyopathy. Lancet *1*:1120–1123, 1986.
23. Bowles, N. E., Rose, M. L., Taylor, P., et al.: End-stage dilated cardiomyopathy: Persistence of enterovirus RNA in myocardium at cardiac transplantation and lack of immune response. Circulation *80*:1128–1136, 1989.
24. Brightman, V. J., McNair Scott, T. F., Westphal, M., et al.: An outbreak of coxsackie B5 virus infection in a newborn nursery. J. Pediatr. *69*:179, 1966.
25. Brynjolfsson, G., Eshaghy, B., Talano, J. V., et al.: Granulomatous myocarditis secondary to cornstarch. Am. Heart J. *94*:353–358, 1977.
26. Burch, G. E., Sun, S. C., Chu, K. C., et al.: Interstitial and coxsackie virus B myocarditis in infants and children: A comparative histologic and immunofluorescent study of 50 autopsied hearts. J. A. M. A. *203*:1–8, 1968.
27. Cappel, M. S., Mikhail, N., and Ortega, A., et al.: Toxoplasma myocarditis in AIDS. Am. Heart J. *123*:1728–1729, 1992.
28. Carrasco, H. A., Guerrero, L., Parada., H., et al.: Ventricular arrhythmias and left ventricular myocardial function in chronic chagasic patients. Int. J. Cardiol. *28*:35–41, 1980.
29. Carrasco, H. A., Parada, H., Guerrero, L., et al.: Prognostic implications of clinical, electrocardiographic and hemodynamic findings in chronic Chagas disease. Int. J. Cardiol. *43*:27–38, 1994.
30. Chan, K. Y., Iwahara, M., Benson, L. N., et al.: Immunosuppresive therapy in the management of acute myocarditis in children: A clinical trial. J. Am. Coll. Cardiol. *17*:458, 1991.
31. Chany, C., Lepine, P., Lelong, M., et al.: Severe and fatal pneumonia in infants and young children associated with adenovirus infections. Am. J. Hyg. *67*:367–378, 1958.
32. Chapman, N. M., Tracy, S., Gauntt, C. J., et al.: Molecular detection and identification of enteroviruses using enzymatic amplification and nucleic acid hybridization. J. Clin. Microbiol. *28*:843–850, 1990.
33. Cherry, J. D., Jahn, C. L., and Meyer, T. C.: Paroxysmal atrial tachycardia associated with echo 9 virus infection. Am. Heart J. *73*:681, 1967.
34. Cohen, N. A.: Myocarditis in prodromal measles. Am. J. Clin. Pathol. *40*:50–53, 1963.
35. Compton, S. J., Celeum, C. L., Lee, C., et al.: Trichinosis with ventilatory failure and persistent myocarditis. Clin. Infect. Dis. *16*:500–504, 1993.
36. Crawford, S. E., Crook, W. G., Harrison, W. W., et al.: Histoplasmosis as a cause of acute myocarditis and pericarditis: Report of occurrence in siblings and review of the literature. Pediatrics *29*:92, 1961.
37. Dalldorf, G., and Sickles, G. M.: An unidentified filterable agent isolated from the faeces of children with paralysis. Science *108*:61–62, 1984.

38. Daly, K., Richardson, P. J., Olsen, E. G. J., et al.: Acute myocarditis: Role of histological and virological examination in the diagnosis and assessment of immunosuppressive treatment. Br. Heart J. *51*:30–35, 1984.
39. Dao, A. H., and Viromani, R.: Visceral larva migrans involving the myocardium: Report of 2 cases and review of the literature. Pediatr. Pathol. *6*:449–456, 1986.
40. Dec, G. W., Fallon, J. T., Southern, J. F., et al.: "Borderline myocarditis": An indication for repeat endomyocardial biopsy. J. Am. Coll. Cardiol. *15*:283, 1990.
41. Dec, G. W., Fallon, J. T., Southern, J. F., et al.: Relation between histological findings on early repeat right ventricular biopsy and ventricular function in patients with myocarditis. Br. Heart J. *60*:332, 1988.
42. Dec, G. W., Palacios, I. F., Fallon, J. T., et al.: Acute myocarditis in the spectrum of acute dilated cardiomyopathy. N. Engl. J. Med. *312*:885–890, 1985.
43. Dec, G. W., Palacios, I., Yasuda, T., et al.: Antimyosin antibody cardiac imaging: Its role in the diagnosis of myocarditis. J. Am. Coll. Cardiol. *16*:97, 1990.
44. Dery, P., Marks, M. I., and Shapera, R.: Clinical manifestations of coxsackievirus infections in children. Am. J. Dis. Child. *128*:464–468, 1974.
45. Dighiero, J., Canabal, E. J., Aguiree, C. V., et al.: *Echinococcus* disease of the heart. Circulation *17*:127–132, 1958.
46. Downham, M. A. P. S., Gardner, P. S., McQuillin, J., et al.: Role of respiratory viruses in childhood mortality. Br. Med. J. *1*:235–239, 1975.
47. Drennan, J. M.: Acute isolated myocarditis in newborn infants. Arch. Dis. Child. *28*:288–291, 1953.
48. Drew, J. H.: Echo 11 outbreak in a nursery associated with myocarditis. Aust. Paediatr. J. *9*:90–95, 1973.
49. Drucker, N. A., Colan, S. D., Lewis, A. B., et al.: Gamma globulin treatment of acute myocarditis in the pediatric population. Circulation *89*:252–257, 1994.
50. Dustin, M. L., Staunton, D. E., and Springer, T. A.: Supergene families in the immune system. Immunol. Today *9*:213–215, 1988.
51. Easton, A., and Eglin, R. P.: The detection of coxsackievirus RNA in cardiac tissue by in situ hybridization. J. Gen. Virol. *69*:285–291, 1988.
52. Eckstein, R., Mempel, W., and Bolte, H. D.: Reduced suppressor cell activity in congestive cardiomyopathy and in myocarditis. Circulation *65*:1224–1229, 1982.
53. Edwards, W. D., Holmes, D. R., and Reeder, G. S.: Diagnosis of active lymphocytic myocarditis by endomyocardial biopsy: Quantitative criteria for light microscopy. Mayo Clin. Proc. *57*:419–425, 1982.
54. Eichenwald, H. F., and Shinefield, H. R.: Viral infections of the fetus and of the premature and newborn infant. Adv. Pediatr. *12*:249, 1962.
55. Fenoglio, J. J., Ursell, P. C., Kellogg, C. F., et al.: Diagnosis and classification of myocarditis by endomyocardial biopsy. N. Engl. J. Med. *308*:12–18, 1983.
56. Fiedler, A.: Ueber akute interstitielle myokarditis. *In* Festschrift zur Feier des funfzigjahrigen Besteheen des Strastkrankenhauses zu Dresden-Friedrichstadt. Dresden, Baensch., 1899, p. 3.
57. Fine, I., Brainerd, H., and Sokolow, M.: Myocarditis in acute infectious diseases: A clinical and electrocardiographic study. Circulation *2*:859, 1950.
58. Fowler, O. N.: Myocardial Diseases. New York, Grune & Stratton, 1973, pp. 253–279.
59. French, A. J., and Weller, C. J.: Interstitial myocarditis following the clinical and experimental use of sulfonamide drugs. Am. J. Pathol. *18*:109, 1942.
60. Friedli, B., Renevey, F., and Rouge, J. C.: Complete heart block in a young child presumably due to mycoplasma pneumonial myocarditis. Acta Paediatr. Scand. *66*:385–388, 1977.
61. Friedman, F. W., Lesch, M., and Sonnenblick, H. E.: Neonatal Heart Disease. New York, Grune & Stratton, 1973, p. 210.
62. Friedman, R. A., Kearney, D. L., Moak, J. P., et al.: Persistence of ventricular arrhythmia after resolution of occult myocarditis in children and young adults. J. Am. Coll. Cardiol. *24*:780–783, 1994.
63. Friedman, S., and Hervada, A.: Severe myocarditis with recovery in a child with visceral larva migrans. J. Pediatr. *90*:322–323, 1977.
64. Froggatt, P., Lynas, M. A., and Marshall, T. K.: Sudden death in babies: Epidemiology. Am. J. Cardiol. *22*:457–468, 1968.
65. Fruhling, L., Koru, R., Lavillaureix, J., et al.: Chronic fibroelastic myoendocarditis of the newborn and the infant (fibroelastosis). New morphological, etiological and pathogenic data. Relation to certain cardiac abnormalities. Ann. Anat. Pathol. *7*:227, 1962.
66. Gardiner, A. J. S., and Short, D.: Four faces of acute myopericarditis. Br. Heart. J. *35*:433–442, 1973.
67. Gatmaitan, B. G., Chason, J. L., and Lerner, A. M.: Augmentation of the virulence of murine coxsackie B3 myocardiopathy by exercise. J. Exp. Med. *131*:1132–1136, 1970.
68. Gear, J. H., and Measroch, V.: South African Institute for Medical Research Annual Report for 1952. 1953, pp. 38–39.
69. Gerzen, P., Granath, A., Holmgren, B., et al.: Acute myocarditis: A follow-up study. Br. Heart J. *34*:575–583, 1972.
70. Giles, T. D., and Gohd, R. S.: Respiratory syncytial virus and heart disease: A report of two cases. J. A. M. A. *236*:1128–1130, 1976.
71. Goldfinger, D., Schreiber, W., and Wosika, P. H.: Permanent heart block following German measles. Am. J. Med. *2*:320, 1947.
72. Goodman, G. C.: The cytopathology of enteroviral infection. Int. Rev. Exp. Pathol. *5*:67–110, 1966.
73. Gore, I., and Saphir, O.: Myocarditis: A classification of 1402 cases. Am. Heart J. *34*:827, 1947.
74. Grasso, M., Arbustini, E., Silini, E., et al.: Search for coxsackievirus B_3 RNA in idiopathic dilated cardiomyopathy using gene amplification by polymerase chain reaction. Am. J. Cardiol. *69*:658–664, 1992.
75. Gray, D. F., Morse, B. S., and Phillips, W. F.: Trichinosis with neurologic and cardiac involvement. Ann. Intern. Med. *57*:230–244, 1962.
76. Griffin, L. D., Kearney, D., Ni., J., et al.: Analysis of formalin-fixed and frozen myocardial autopsy samples for viral genome in childhood myocarditis and dilated cardiomyopathy with endocardial fibroelastosis using polymerase chain reaction (PCR). Cardiovasc. Pathol. *4*:3–11, 1995.
77. Grist, N. R., and Bell, E. J.: Enteroviruses and cardiac disease. Lancet *2*:1188, 1970.
78. Grist, N. R., and Bell, E. J.: Coxsackie viruses and the heart. Am. Heart J. *77*:295–300, 1969.
79. Grist, N. R.: Viruses and myocarditis. Postgrad. Med. J. *48*:746–749, 1972.
80. Grist, N. R., and Bell, E. J.: A six-year study of coxsackievirus B infections in heart disease. J. Hyg. (Camb.) *73*:165–172, 1974.
81. Gulick, T., Chung, M. L., Pieper, S. J., et al.: Interleukin-1 and tumor necrosis factor inhibit cardiac myocyte beta-adrenergic responsiveness. Proc. Natl. Acad. Sci. U. S. A. *86*:6753–6757, 1989.
82. Gutgesell, H. P., Paquet, M., Duff, D. F., et al.: Evaluation of left ventricular size and function by echocardiography: Results in normal children. Circulation *56*:457–462, 1977.
83. Harris, M. J.: Letter: Sudden infant death syndrome. Med. J. Aust. *2*:190, 1975.
84. Hastreiter, A. R., and Miller, R. A.: Management of primary endomyocardial disease: The myocarditis-endocardial fibroelastosis syndrome. Pediatr. Clin. North Am. *11*:401–430, 1964.
85. Haynes, R. E., Cramblett, H. G., Hilty, M. D., et al.: Echo virus type 3 infections in children: Clinical and laboratory studies. J. Pediatr. *80*:589–595, 1972.
86. Hejtmanick, R. M., Wright, C. J., Quint, R., et al.: The cardiovascular manifestations of systemic lupus erythematosus. Am. Heart J. *68*:119–130, 1964.
87. Helin, M., Sarola, J., and Lapinleimu, K.: Cardiac manifestations during a coxsackie B5 epidemic. Br. Med. J. *3*:97, 1968.
88. Henson, D., and Mufson, M. A.: Myocarditis and pneumonitis with type 21 adenovirus infection: Association with fatal myocarditis and pneumonitis. Am. J. Dis. Child. *121*:334–336, 1971.
89. Herskowitz, A., Ahmed-Ansari, A., Neumann, D. A., et al.: Induction of major histocompatability complex antigens within the myocardium of patients with active myocarditis: A non-histologic marker of myocarditis. J. Am. Coll. Cardiol. *15*:624, 1990.
90. Hilton, D. A., Variend, S. and Pringle, J. H.: Demonstration of coxsackievirus RNA in formalin-fixed tissue sections from childhood myocarditis by in situ hybridization and the polymerase chain reaction. J. Pathol. *170*:45–51, 1993.
91. Hirschman, Z. S., and Hammer, S. G.: Coxsackie virus myopericarditis: A microbiological and clinical review. Am. J. Cardiol. *34*:224–232, 1974.
92. Hoagland, R. J.: Cardiac involvement in infectious mononucleosis. Am. J. Med. Sci. *232*:252, 1956.
93. Hobbs, R. E., Pelegrin, D., Ratliff, N. B., et al.: Lymphocytic myocarditis and dilated cardiomyopathy: Treatment with immunosuppressive agents. Cleve. Clin. J. Med. *56*:628, 1989.
94. Hodge, P. R., and Lawrence, J. R.: Two cases of myocarditis associated with phenylbutazone therapy. Med. J. Aust. *1*:640, 1957.
95. Hogg, N., Bates, P. A., and Harvey, J.: Structure and function of intercellular adhesion molecule 1. Chem. Immunol. *50*:98–115, 1991.
96. Hori, H., Matoba, T., Shingu, M., et al.: The role of cell mediated immunity in coxsackie B viral myocarditis. Jpn. Circ. J. *45*:1409, 1981.
97. Horlich, S. S., and Bichnell, R. E.: Trichiniasis with widespread infestation of many tissues. N. Engl. J. Med. *201*:816–819, 1929.
98. Hoshino, T., Matsumori, A., Kawai, C., et al.: Electrocardiographic abnormalities in Syrian golden hamsters with coxsackievirus B1 myocarditis. Jpn. Circ. J. *46*:1305–1312, 1982.
99. Hosier, D. M., and Newton, W. A., Jr.: Serious coxsackie infection in infants and children. Am. J. Dis. Child. *96*:251–267, 1958.
100. Hoyer, M. H., and Fischer, D. R.: Acute myocarditis simulating myocardial infarction in a child. Pediatrics *87*:250, 1991.
101. Huber, S. A., Job, L. P., and Woodruff, J. F.: Lysis of infected myofibers by coxsackie virus B-3 immune T-lymphocytes. Am. J. Pathol. *98*:681, 1980.
102. Hudgins, J. M.: Infectious mononucleosis complicated by myo- and pericarditis. J. A. M. A. *235*:2626–2627, 1976.
103. Hudson, R. E. B.: Myocardial involvement (myocarditis) in infections, infestation and drug therapy. Cardiovasc. Pathol. *1*:782–854, 1965.
104. Hughes, W. T., and Rathauser, V.: Rocky Mountain spotted fever in children. Pediatr. Dig., 1970, pp. 29–34.
105. Hutchins, G. H., and Vie, S. A.: The progression of interstitial myocarditis to idiopathic endocardial fibro-elastosis. Am. J. Pathol. *66*:483–496, 1972.

106. Hwang, W. S., Chan, M. C., Wong, H. B., et al.: Fatal coxsackie virus infections of the newborn. Singapore Med. J. *16*:244–248, 1975.
107. Jahn, C. L., and Cherry, J. D.: Mild neonatal illness associated with heavy enterovirus infection. N. Engl. J. Med. *274*:394, 1966.
108. James, T. N.: Sudden death in babies: New observations on the heart. Am. J. Cardiol. *22*:479, 1968.
109. Jankus, A.: Inflammatory changes in the cardiac conducting system in sudden infant death syndrome. Med. J. Aust. *1*:594–595, 1975.
110. Javett, S. N., Heymann, S., Mundel, B., et al.: Myocarditis in the newborn infant: A study of an outbreak associated with coxsackie group B virus infection in a maternity home in Johannesburg. J. Pediatr. *48*:1–22, 1956.
111. Jin, O., Sole, M. J., and Butany, J. W.: Detection of enterovirus RNA in myocardial biopsies from patients with myocarditis and cardiomyopathy using gene amplification by polymerase chain reaction. Circulation *82*:8–16, 1990.
112. Johnson, J. L., and Lee, L. P.: Complete atrioventricular heart block secondary to acute myocarditis requiring intracardiac pacing. J. Pediatr. *78*:312–316, 1971.
113. Joos, H. A., and Yu, P. N. G.: Electrocardiographic observations in poliomyelitis: Changes of the Q-T interval in twenty-three cases. Am. J. Dis. Child. *80*:22, 1950.
114. Karjalainen, J., Nieminen, M. S., and Heikkila, J.: Influenza A1 myocarditis in conscripts. Acta. Med. Scand. *20*:27–30, 1980.
115. Karjalainen, J.: Functional and myocarditis induced T wave abnormalities. Chest *83*:6, 1983.
116. Keith, J. D., Rowe, R. D., and Vlad, P.: Heart Disease in Infancy and Childhood. 2nd ed. New York, Macmillan, 1967, pp. 996–1019.
117. Kereiakes, D. J., and Parmley, W. W.: Myocarditis and cardiomyopathy. Am. Heart J. *108*:1318–1325, 1984.
118. Kibrick, S., and Benirschke, K.: Acute aseptic myocarditis and meningoencephalitis in the newborn child infected with coxsackie virus group B3. N. Engl. J. Med. *255*:883, 1956.
119. Kibrick, S., and Benirschke, K.: Severe generalized disease (encephalohepatomyocarditis) occurring in the newborn period and due to infection with coxsackievirus group B: Evidence of intrauterine infection with this agent. Pediatrics *22*:857–874, 1958.
120. Kilbourne, E. D., Smart, K. M., and Pokorny, B. A.: Inhibition by cortisone of the synthesis and action of interferon. Nature *190*:650–651, 1961.
121. Kilbourne, E. D., Wilson, C. B., and Perrier, D.: The induction of gross myocardial lesions by a coxsackie (pleurodynic) virus and cortisone. J. Clin. Invest. *35*:362, 1956.
122. Kirchhoff, L. V.: *Trypanosoma* species (American trypanosomiasis, Chagas disease): Biology of trypanosomes. *In* Mandell, G. L., Bennett, J. E., and Dolin, R. (eds.): Mandell, Douglas and Bennett's Principles and Practices of Infectious Diseases. 4th ed. New York, Churchill Livingstone, 1995, pp. 2442–2450.
123. Kirchhoff, L. V., Gam, A. A., Gusmao, R., et al.: Increased specificity of serodiagnosis of Chagas disease by detection of antibody to the 72- and 90-kDa glycoproteins of *Trypanosoma cruzi*. J. Infect. Dis. *155*:561–564, 1987.
124. Kishimoto, C., Matsumori, A., Ohmae, M., et al.: Electrocardiographic findings in experimental myocarditis in DBA/2 mice. J. Am. Coll. Cardiol. *3*:1461–1468, 1984.
125. Kothari, U. R., Shah, S. S., Doshi, H. V., et al.: Myocarditis from scorpion sting: A clinical and electrocardiographic study of 50 cases. Indian Heart J. *28*:88–92, 1976.
126. Kussy, J. C.: Fatal mumps myocarditis. Minn. Med. *57*:285–286, 1974.
127. Lane, J. R., Neuman, D. A., Lafond-Walker, A., et al.: Role of IL-1 and tumor necrosis factor in coxsackie virus–induced autoimmune myocarditis. J. Immunol. *151*:1682–1690, 1993.
128. Laranja, F. S., Dias, E., Nobrega, G., et al.: Chagas disease: A clinical, epidemiologic and pathologic study. Circulation *14*:1035–1060, 1956.
129. Leak, D., and Meghji, M.: Toxoplasmic infection in cardiac disease. Am. J. Cardiol. *43*:841–849, 1979.
130. Ledbetter, M. K., Cannon, A. B., and Costa, A. F.: The electrocardiogram in diphtheritic myocarditis. Am. Heart J. *68*:599, 1964.
131. Lerner, A. M., and Wilson, M. F.: Virus myocardiopathy. Progr. Med. Virol. *15*:63–91, 1973.
132. Lerner, A. M., Wilson, F. M., and Reyes, M. P.: Enteroviruses and the heart (with special emphasis on the probable role of coxsackieviruses, group B, types 1–5). Mod. Concepts Cardiovasc. Dis. *64*:7–10, 1975.
133. Lewes, D., Rainford, D. J., and Lane, W. F.: Symptomless myocarditis and myalgia in viral and *Mycoplasma pneumoniae* infections. Br. Heart J. *36*:924–932, 1974.
134. Lim, C. H., Toh, C. C., Chia, B. L., et al.: Stokes-Adams attacks due to acute nonspecific myocarditis. Am. Heart J. *38*:123, 1949.
135. Lind, J., and Hulquist, G. T.: Isolated myocarditis in newborn and young infants. Am. Heart J. *38*:123, 1949.
136. Logue, B. L., and Hanson, J. L.: Complete heart block in German measles. Am. Heart J. *30*:205, 1945.
137. Lozinski, G. M., Davis G. G., Krous, H. F., et al.: Adenovirus myocarditis: Retrospective diagnosis by gene amplification from formalin-fixed, paraffin-embedded tissues. Hum. Pathol. *25*:831–834, 1994.
138. Luft, B. J., Billingham, M., and Remington, J. S.: Endomyocardial biopsy in the diagnosis of toxoplasmic myocarditis. Transplant. Proc. *6*:1871–1873, 1986.
139. Magure, J. H., Hoff, R., Sherlock, I., et al.: Cardiac morbidity and mortality due to Chagas disease: Prospective electrocardiographic study of a Brazilian community. Circulation *75*:1140–1145, 1987.
140. Maisch, B., Trostel-Soeder, R., Stechemesser, E., et al.: Diagnostic relevance of humoral and cell-mediated immune reactions in patients with acute viral myocarditis. Clin. Exp. Immunol. *48*:533, 1982.
141. Markowitz, S. M., Martinez, A. J., Duna, R. J., et al.: Myocarditis associated with primary amebic *(Naegleria)* meningoencephalitis. Am. J. Clin. Pathol. *62*:619–628, 1974.
142. Martin, A. B., Webber, S., Fricker, F. J., et al.: Acute myocarditis: Rapid diagnosis by PCR in children. Circulation *90*:330–339, 1994.
143. Martinez, M. F., Sosa, E., Nishioka, S., et al.: Clinical and electrophysiologic features of syncope in chronic chagasic heart disease. J. Cardiovasc. Electrophysiol. *5*:563–570, 1994.
144. Mason, J. W., Billingham, M. E., and Ricci, D. R.: Treatment of acute inflammatory myocarditis assisted by endomyocardial biopsy. Am. J. Cardiol. *45*:1037–1044, 1980.
145. Mason, J. W., O'Connell, J. B., Herskowitz, A., et al.: A clinical trial of immunosuppressive therapy for myocarditis: The Myocarditis Treatment Trial Investigators. N. Engl. J. Med. *333*:269–275, 1995.
146. Matsumori, A., Wang, H., Abelman, W. H., et al.: Treatment of viral myocarditis with ribavirin in an animal preparation. Circulation *71*:834–839, 1985.
147. Matsumori, A., and Kawai, C.: An experimental model for congestive heart failure after encephalomyocarditis virus myocarditis in mice. Circulation *65*:1230–1235, 1982.
148. Matsumori, A., Crumpacker, C., Abelmann, W. H., et al.: Virus vaccine and passive immunization for the prevention of viral myocarditis in mice. Circulation *68*(Suppl. III):338, 1983.
149. Matsumori, A., and Kawai, C.: An experimental model of congestive (dilated) cardiomyopathy: Dilation and hypertrophy of the heart in the chronic stage in DBA/2 mice with myocarditis caused by encephalomyocarditis virus. Circulation *66*:355–360, 1982.
150. Merkel, W. C.: *Plasmodium falciparum* malaria: The coronary and myocardial lesion observed at autopsy in two cases of acute fulminating *Plasmodium falciparum* infection. Arch. Pathol. *41*:290–298, 1946.
151. Miklozek, C. L., Crumpacker, C. S., Royal, H. D., et al.: Myocarditis presenting as acute myocardial infarction. Am. Heart. J. *115*:768, 1988.
152. Miller, J. J., and French, J. W.: Myocarditis in juvenile rheumatoid arthritis. Am. J. Dis. Child. *131*:205–209, 1977.
153. Montgomery, J., Gear, J., Prinsloo, F. R., et al.: Myocarditis of the newborn: Outbreak in maternity home in southern Rhodesia associated with coxsackie group B virus infection. S. Afr. Med. J. *29*:608–612, 1955.
154. Moore, C. M., Henry, J., Benzing, G., III, et al.: Varicella myocarditis. Am. J. Dis. Child. *118*:899–902, 1969.
155. Morbidity and Mortality Weekly Report. U.S. Department of Health, Education and Welfare. *14(1)*, 1965.
156. Morbidity and Mortality Weekly Report. U.S. Department of Health, Education and Welfare. *24(19)*, 1975
157. Morris, S. A., Tanowitz, H. B., Wittner, M., et al.: Pathophysiological insights into the cardiomyopathy of Chagas disease. Circulation *82*:1900–1909, 1990.
158. Moschos, A., Papaioannou, A. C., Nicolopoulos, D., et al.: Cardiac complications after vaccination for smallpox. Helvet. Paediatr. Acta *31*:257–260, 1976.
159. Mott, K. E., and Hagstrom, J. W. C.: The pathologic lesions of the cardiac autonomic system in chronic Chagas myocarditis. Circulation *31*:273–286, 1965.
160. Mowat, N. A., Bennett, P. N., Finlayson, J. K., et al.: Myopericarditis complicating ulcerative colitis. Br. Heart J. *36*:724–727, 1974.
161. Muir, P., Nicholson, F., Jhetan, M., et al.: Rapid diagnosis of enterovirus infection by magnetic bead extraction and polymerase chain reaction detection of enterovirus RNA in clinical specimens. J. Clin. Microbiol. *31*:31–38, 1993.
162. Mullis, K. B., and Faldona, F. A.: Specific synthesis of DNA in vitro via a polymerase catalyzed chain reaction. Methods Enzymol. *155*:335–350, 1988.
163. Nagaratnam, N., Gunawardene, K. R., and DeSilva, D. P.: Myocardial involvement in infectious hepatitis. Postgrad. Med. J. *47*:785–788, 1971.
164. Neches, W. H., Park, S. C., Lenox, C. C., et al.: Left atrial myxoma: Clinical presentation suggesting acute myocarditis. J. A. M. A. *229*:1906–1907, 1974.
165. Neumann, D. A., Burek, C. L., Baughman, K. L, et al.: Circulating heart-reactive antibodies in patients with myocarditis or cardiomyopathy. J. Am. Coll. Cardiol. *16*:839, 1990.
166. Neuman, D. A., Lane, J. R., Allen, G. S., et al.: Viral myocarditis leading to cardiomyopathy: Do cytokines contribute to pathogenesis? Clin. Immunol. Pathol. *68*:181–190, 1993.
167. Obeyesekere, I., and Hermon, Y.: Myocarditis and cardiomyopathy after arbovirus infections (dengue and chikungunya fever). Br. Heart J. *34*:821–827, 1972.
168. O'Connell, J. B., Henken, R., Robinson, J., et al.: Gallium-67 imaging in

patients with dilated cardiomyopathy and biopsy proven myocarditis. Circulation *70*:58–62, 1984.

169. Ognibene, A. J., O'Leary, D. S., Czarnecki, S. W., et al.: Myocarditis and disseminated intravascular coagulation in scrub types. Am. J. Med. Sci. *262*:233–239, 1971.
170. Okuni, M., Yamada, T., Mochizuki, S., et al.: Studies on myocarditis in childhood with special reference to the possible role of immunological process and the thymus in the chronicity of the disease. Jpn. Circ. J. *39*:463–470, 1975.
171. Okuni, M., and Takamiya, Y.: Primary myocardial disease in children, with special references to idiopathic myocarditis. Jpn. Circ. J. *35*:771–776, 1971.
172. Oldstone, M. B. A.: Virus neutralization and virus induced immune complex disease. Prog. Med. Virol. *19*:84–119, 1975.
173. Oliver, J. M., Sotillo, J. F., Dominguez, F. J., et al.: Two-dimensional echocardiographic features of *Echinococcus* of the heart and blood vessels. Circulation *78*:327–337, 1988.
174. Olsen, E. G. J.: The role of biopsy in the diagnosis of myocarditis. Herz *10*:21–25, 1985.
175. Osama, S. M., Krishnamurti, S., and Gupta, D. N.: Incidence of myocarditis in varicella. Ind. Heart J. *31*:315–320, 1979.
176. Pacque, R. E., Strauss, D. C., Nealon, T. J., et al.: Fractionation and immunologic assessment of KC1-extractable cardiac antigens in coxsackievirus B3 virus induced myocarditis. J. Immunol. *123*:358–364, 1979.
177. Pacque, R. E., Gauntt, C. J., and Nealon, T. J.: Assessment of cell mediated immunity against coxsackie B3 induced myocarditis in a primate model (*Papio papio*). Infect. Immunol. *31*:470–479, 1981.
178. Palacios-Pru, E., Carrasco, H., Scoraza, C., et al.: Ultrastructural characteristics of different stages of human Chagas myocarditis. Am. J. Trop. Med. Hyg. *41*:29-40, 1989.
179. Parrillo, J. E., Aretz, H. T., Palacios, I., et al.: The results of transvenous endomyocardial biopsy can frequently be used to diagnose myocardial disease in patients with idiopathic heart failure. Circulation *69*:93–101, 1984.
180. Petitjean, J., Kopecka, H., Freymuth, F., et al.: Detection of enteroviruses in endomyocardial biopsy by molecular approach. J. Med. Virol. *37*:76–82, 1992.
181. Pober, J. S., Gimbrone, M. A., Lapierre, L. A., et al.: Overlapping patterns of activation of human endothelial cells by interleukin 1, tumor necrosis factor, and immune interferon. J. Immunol. *137*:1893–1896, 1986.
182. Poltera, A. A., Cox, J. N., and Owor, R.: Pancarditis affecting the conducting system and all valves in human African trypanosomiasis. Br. Heart J. *38*:827–837, 1976.
183. Pomerance, A.: Classification of the secondary cardiomyopathies: The pathologist's view. Postgrad. Med. J. *48*:714–721, 1972.
184. Pomerance, A., and Davies, M. J. (eds.): The Pathology of the Heart. Philadelphia, J. B. Lippincott, 1975.
185. Rabin, E. R., Hassan, S. A., Jenson, A. B., et al.: Coxsackie virus B3 myocarditis in mice. Am. J. Pathol. *44*:775–797, 1964.
186. Rager-Zisman, B., and Allison, A. C.: Effects of immunosuppression on coxsackie B3 virus infection in mice and passive protection by circulating antibody. J. Gen. Virol. *19*:339, 1973.
187. Rantakallio, P., Saukronen, A. L., Krause, U., et al.: Follow-up study of 17 cases of neonatal coxsackie B5 meningitis and one with suspected myocarditis. Scand. J. Infect. Dis. *2*:25–28, 1970.
188. Ray, C. G., Portman, J. N., Stamm, S. J., et al.: Hemolyticuremic syndrome and myocarditis: Association with coxsackievirus B infection. Am. J. Dis. Child. *122*:418–420, 1971.
189. Redline, R. W., Genest, D. R. and Tycko, B.: Detection of enteroviral infection in paraffin-embedded tissue by the RNA polymerase chain reaction technique. Am. J. Clin. Pathol. *96*:568–571, 1991.
190. Reilly, J. M., Cunnion, R. E., Anderson, D. W., et al.: Frequency of myocarditis, left ventricular dysfunction and ventricular tachycardia in the acquired immune deficiency syndrome. Am. J. Cardiol. *62*:789, 1988.
191. Rezkalla, S., Kloner, R. A., Khatib, G., et al.: Beneficial effects of captopril in acute coxsackievirus B3 murine myocarditis. Circulation *81*:1039, 1990.
192. Robbins, S. L., and Cotran, R. S.: Pathologic Basis of Disease. 2nd ed. Philadelphia, W. B. Saunders, 1979, p. 694.
193. Rosenbaum, H. D., Nadas, A. S., and Neuhauser, E. B. D.: Primary myocardial disease in infancy and childhood. Am. J. Dis. Child. *86*:28–44, 1953.
194. Rosenberg, E. H.: Acute myocarditis in mumps (epidemic parotitis). Arch. Intern. Med. *76*:257, 1945.
195. Rosenberg, H. S., and McNamara, D. G.: Acute myocarditis in infancy and childhood. Prog. Cardiovasc. Dis. *7*:179–197, 1964.
196. Ross, L. J.: Electrocardiographic findings in measles. Am. J. Dis. Child. *83*:282–291, 1952.
197. Rytel, M. W., and Kilbourne, E. D.: Differing susceptibility of adolescent and adult mice to non-lethal infection with coxsackie virus B3. (S5596) Proc. Soc. Exp. Biol. Med. *137*:443–448, 1971.
198. Sahn, D. J., Vaucher, Y., Williams, D. E., et al.: Echocardiographic detection of large left-to-right shunts and cardiomyopathies in infants and children. Am. J. Cardiol. *38*:73–79, 1976.
199. Sainani, G. S., Dekate, M. P., and Rao, C. P.: Heart disease caused by coxsackie virus B infection. Br. Heart J. *37*:819–823, 1975.
200. Sakakibara, S., and Konno, S.: Endomyocardial biopsy. Jpn. Heart J. *3*:537, 1962.
201. Sakamoto, M., Suzuki, F., Arai, S., et al.: Experimental myocarditis induced in mice by infection with influenza A2 virus. Microbiol. Immunol. *25*:173–181, 1981.
202. Sands, M. J., Jr., Satz, J. E., Turner, W. E., Jr., et al.: Pericarditis and perimyocarditis associated with active *Mycoplasma pneumoniae* infection. Ann. Intern. Med. *86*:544–548, 1977.
203. Saphir, O., Simon, W. A., and Reingold, M. I.: Myocarditis in children. Am. J. Dis. Child. *67*:294–312, 1944.
204. Saphir, O., and Field, M.: Complications of myocarditis in children. J. Pediatr. *45*:457–463, 1954.
205. Schieken, R. M., and Myers, M. G.: Complete heart block in viral myocarditis. J. Pediatr. *87*:831–832, 1975.
206. Schmidt, N. J., Magoffin, R. L., and Lennette, E. H.: Association of group B coxsackieviruses with cases of pericarditis, myocarditis or pleurodynia by demonstration of immunoglobulin M antibody. Infect. Immunol. *8*:341–348, 1973.
207. Schowengerdt, K. O., Ni, J., Denfield, S. W., et al.: Diagnosis, surveillance, and epidemiologic evaluation of viral infection in pediatric cardiac transplant recipients using the polymerase chain reaction (PCR). J. Heart Lung Transplant. In press.
208. Schryer, M. J., and Karnauchow, P. N.: Endocardial fibroelastosis: Etiologic and pathogenetic considerations in children. Am. Heart J. *88*:557–565, 1974.
209. Scott, L. P., III, Gutelius, M. F., and Parrott, R. H.: Children with acute respiratory tract infections: An electrocardiographic survey. Am. J. Dis. Child. *119*:111–113, 1970.
210. Seko, Y., Matsuda, H., Kato, K., et al.: Expression of intercellular adhesion molecule–1 in murine hearts with acute myocarditis caused by coxsackievirus B3. J. Clin. Invest. *91*:1327–1336, 1993.
211. Seko Y., Yamazaki, T., Shinkai, Y., et al.: Cellular and molecular bases for the immunopathology of the myocardial cell damage involved in acute viral myocarditis with special reference to dilated cardiomyopathy. Jpn. Circ. J. *56*:1062–1072, 1992.
212. Shingu, M.: Laboratory diagnosis of viral myocarditis: A review. Jpn. Circ. J. *53*:87–93, 1989.
213. Solarz, S.: An electrocardiographic study on one-hundred fourteen consecutive cases of trichinosis. Am. Heart J. *34*:230–240, 1947.
214. Spencer, H. C., Allain, D. S., Sulzer, A. J., et al.: Evaluation of the micro enzyme–labeled immunosorbent assay for antibodies to *Trypanosoma cruzi*. Am. J. Trop. Med. Hyg. *29*:179–182, 1980.
215. Spencer, M. J., Cherry, J. D., Adams, F. H., et al.: Letter: Supraventricular tachycardia in an infant associated with a rhinoviral infection. J. Pediatr. *86*:811–812, 1975.
216. Spink, W. W.: Cardiovascular complications of trichinosis. Arch. Intern. Med. *56*:238–245, 1935.
217. Sprague, H. B.: The effects of malaria on the heart. Am. Heart J. *31*:426–430, 1946.
218. Stedman's Medical Dictionary. 2nd ed. Baltimore, Williams & Wilkins, 1966.
219. Sterner, G.: Adenovirus infections in childhood: An epidemiological and clinical survey among Swedish children. Acta Paediatr. *142*:1–30, 1962.
220. Sterner, G., Agell, B. O., Wahren, B., et al.: Acquired cytomegalovirus infection in older children and adults: A clinical study of hospitalized patients. Scand. J. Infect. Dis. *2*:95–103, 1970.
221. Stewart, J. M., Kaul, A., Gromisch, D. S., et al.: Symptomatic cardiac dysfunction in children with human immunodeficiency virus infection. Am. Heart J. *117*:140, 1989.
222. Strain, J. E., Grose, R. M., Factor, S. M., et al.: Results of endomyocardial biopsy in patients with spontaneous ventricular tachycardia but without apparent structural heart disease. Circulation *68*:1171–1181, 1983.
223. Sugrue, D. D., Holmes, D. R., Gersh, B. J., et al.: Cardiac histologic findings in patients with life threatening ventricular arrhythmias of unknown origin. J. Am. Coll. Cardiol. *4*:952–957, 1984.
224. Tahernia, A. C.: Electrocardiographic abnormalities and transaminase levels in diphtheritic myocarditis. J. Pediatr. *75*:1008–1014, 1969.
225. Take, M., Sekiguchi, M., Hiroe, M., et al.: Long-term follow-up of electrocardiographic findings in patients with acute myocarditis proven by endomyocardial biopsy. Jpn. Circ. J. *46*:1227–1234, 1982.
226. Theologides, A., and Kennedy, B. J.: Toxoplasmic myocarditis and pericarditis. Am. J. Med. *47*:169–173, 1969.
227. Thisyakorn, U. S. A., Wongvanich, J., and Kumpeng, V.: Failure of corticosteroid therapy to prevent diphtheritic myocarditis or neuritis. Pediatr. Infect. Dis. *3*:126–128, 1984.
228. Tiula, E., and Leinikki, P.: Fatal cytomegalovirus infection in a previously healthy boy, with myocarditis and consumption coagulopathy as presenting signs. Scand. J. Infect. Dis. *4*:57–60, 1972.
229. Towbin, J. A., Griffin, L. D., Martin, A. B., et al.: Intrauterine adenoviral myocarditis presenting as non-immune hydrops fetalis: Diagnosis by polymerase chain reaction. Pediatr. Infect. Dis. J. *13*:144–150, 1994.
230. Toyozaki, T., Saito, T., Takano, H., et al.: Expression of intercellular adhesion molecule–1 on cardiac myocytes for myocarditis before and during immunosuppressive therapy. Am. J. Cardiol. *72*:441–444, 1993.
231. Tracy, S., Wiegand, V., McManus, B., et al.: Molecular approaches to

enteroviral diagnosis in idiopathic cardiomyopathy and myocarditis. J. Am. Coll. Cardiol. *15*:1688, 1990.
232. Unverferth, D. V., Fetters, J. K., Uretsky, B., et al.: Right versus left heart biopsies: Different information. Circulation *70*(Suppl. II):402, 1984.
233. Van Creveld, S., de Groot, J. W., Hartog, H. A. P., et al.: Diagnosis and treatment of acute interstitial myocarditis in infancy. Am. Paediatr. *183*:193–202, 1954.
234. Van Creveld, S., and de Jager, H.: Myocarditis in newborns caused by coxsackie virus: Clinical and pathological data. Ann. Paediatr. *187*:100, 1956.
235. Van Reken, D. E., Geffen, W. A., and Cramer, S. F.: Clinical conference: Sudden congestive heart failure in a 5-month-old infant. J. Pediatr. *85*:724–729, 1974.
236. Van Zaane, K. D., and Van der Veen, J.: Quelques symtomes cliniques particuliers chez les enfants attenints d'ure infection a' adenovirus. Presse Med. *70*:1021–1022, 1962.
237. Vargo, T. A., Singer, D. B., Gillette, P. C., et al.: Myocarditis due to visceral larva migrans. J. Pediatr. *90*:322–323, 1977.
238. Verel, D., Warrack, A. J., Potter, C. W., et al.: Observations on the A2 England influenza epidemic: A clinicopathological study. Am. Heart J. *92*:290–296, 1976.
239. Verlinde, J. D., Van Tongeren, H. A. E., and Kret, A.: Myocarditis in newborns due to coxsackie B virus: Virus studies. Ann. Paediatr. *187*:113, 1956.
240. Vignola, P. A., Aonuma, K., Swage, P., et al.: Lymphocytic myocarditis presenting as unexplained ventricular arrhythmias: Diagnosis with endomyocardial biopsy and response to immunosuppression. J. Am. Coll. Cardiol. *4*:812–819, 1984.
241. Weber, M. W., Baldwin, J. S., and Hall, J. W.: Acute isolated myocarditis: Review of the literature and a report of a case in a 10-year-old child. Pediatrics *3*:829–835, 1949.
242. Weiss, L. M., Movahed, L. A., Billingham, M. E., et al.: Detection of coxsackievirus, B_3 RNA in myocardial tissue by the polymerase chain reaction. Am. J. Pathol. *138*:497–503, 1991.
243. Weiss, L. M., Liu, X.-F., Chang, K. L., et al.: Detection of enteroviral RNA idiopathic dilated cardiomyopathy and other human cardiac tissues. J. Clin. Invest. *90*:156–159, 1992.
244. Weiss, L. M., Movahed, L. A., Berry, G. J., et al.: In situ hybridization studies for viral nucleic acids in heart and lung allograft biopsies. Am. J. Clin. Pathol. *93*:675–679, 1990.
245. Wells, A. H., and Sax, S. G.: Isolated myocarditis, probably of sulfonamide origin. Am. Heart J. *30*:522, 1945.
246. Wentworth, P., Jentz, L. A., and Croal, A. E.: Analysis of sudden unexpected death in southern Ontario, with emphasis on myocarditis. Can. Med. Assoc. J. *120*:676–706, 1979.
247. Whitehead, J. E.: Silent infections and the epidemiology of viral carditis. Am. Heart J. *85*:711–713, 1973.
248. Williams, H., O'Reilly, R. N., and Williams, A.: Fourteen cases of idiopathic myocarditis in infants and children. Arch. Dis. Child. *28*:271–283, 1953.
249. Wong, C. Y., Woodruff, J. J., and Woodruff, J. F.: Generation of cytotoxic T lymphocytes during coxsackie B-3 infection. II. Characterization of effector cells and demonstration of cytotoxicity against viral infected fibers. J. Immunol. *118*:1165–1169, 1977.
250. Woodruff, J. F.: Viral myocarditis: A review. Am. J. Pathol. *101*:427–484, 1980.
251. Woodruff, J. F.: The influence of quantitated post-weaning undernutrition on coxsackie virus B3 infection of adult mice. II. Alteration of host defense mechanisms. J. Infect. Dis. *121*:164, 1970.
252. Wright, H. T., Jr.: Fatal infection in a newborn infant due to herpes simplex virus. J. Pediatr. *67*:130–132, 1965.
253. Yamada, T., Matsumori, A., and Sasayama, S.: Therapeutic efect of anti-tumor necrosis factor–alpha antibody on the murine model of viral myocarditis induced by encephalomyocarditis virus. Circulation *89*:846–851, 1994.
254. Yogman, M., and Echeverria, P.: Scleredema and carditis: Report of a case and review of the literature. Pediatrics *54*:108–110, 1974.
255. Zalma, V. M., Older, J. J., and Brooks, G. F.: The Austin, Texas, diphtheria outbreak: Clinical and epidemiological aspects. J. A. M. A. *211*:2125, 1970.
256. Zee-Cheng, C. S., Tsai, C. C., Palmer, D. C., et al.: High incidence of myocarditis by endomyocardial biopsy in patients with idiopathic congestive cardiomyopathy. J. Am. Coll. Cardiol. *3*:63–70, 1984.
257. Zwelzer, W. M.: Infantile toxoplasmosis. Arch. Pathol. *38*:1–19, 1944.

35

ACUTE RHEUMATIC FEVER

Diana Lennon

Acute rheumatic fever is an inflammatory disease of the heart, joints, central nervous system, and subcutaneous tissues that develops after a nasopharyngeal infection by one of the group A beta-hemolytic streptococci. The pathogenesis of this disease, a clinical syndrome without a specific diagnostic test, remains an enigma, and specific treatment is not available. Yet prevention of initial and recurrent attacks is possible by penicillin prophylaxis. Rheumatic fever especially is important because of the heart disease that often ensues and that may lead to chronic progressive damage and premature death. As succinctly stated by Lasègue many years ago, "Rheumatic fever licks the joints and bites the heart,"[123] a statement that holds true today. The unexpected upsurge in this disease in the United States in the late 1980s and into the 1990s and reports of increasing numbers of invasive group A streptococcal infections have renewed interest in group A streptococci and their abilities.

EPIDEMIOLOGY

The overall incidence and severity of acute rheumatic fever have decreased in recent years in developed areas of Western countries and in prosperous countries of Asia.[2] Reliable morbidity data on the occurrence of acute rheumatic fever in total populations are lacking because studies often consider only a segment of a population. However, the trend seems clear. Some of the best long-term data come from Denmark, where rheumatic fever has been a reportable disease for many years,[134] with a steady decline since 1900, except for a peak during World War II (Fig. 35–1). In the United States, rheumatic fever is not a reportable disease, but mortality rates (Fig. 35–2) and hospital discharge rates (Fig. 35–3) (Table 35–1) have shown a steady decline. Although this decline already was underway, it appears to have been accelerated by the introduction of penicillin.[88]

The really dramatic decline in incidence of rheumatic fever began in the United States in the late 1940s (Fig. 35–2). During the late 1950s, the 1960s, and the early 1970s, studies in the United States showed annual rates of between 13.5 and 62.5 first attacks per 100,000 children 5 to 14 years of age; however, these studies are not strictly comparable in design.[22, 32, 55, 113] Some were conducted in low-income urban areas, locations in which the incidence of rheumatic fever was believed to be higher. Secondary prevention of rheumatic fever with penicillin prophylaxis to prevent recurrent attacks probably became widespread in the 1960s. Denny and colleagues[42] showed the possibility of preventing initial attacks with injectable penicillin in 1950 in military camps. Similar controlled studies were not repeated for the general population or using oral penicillin.

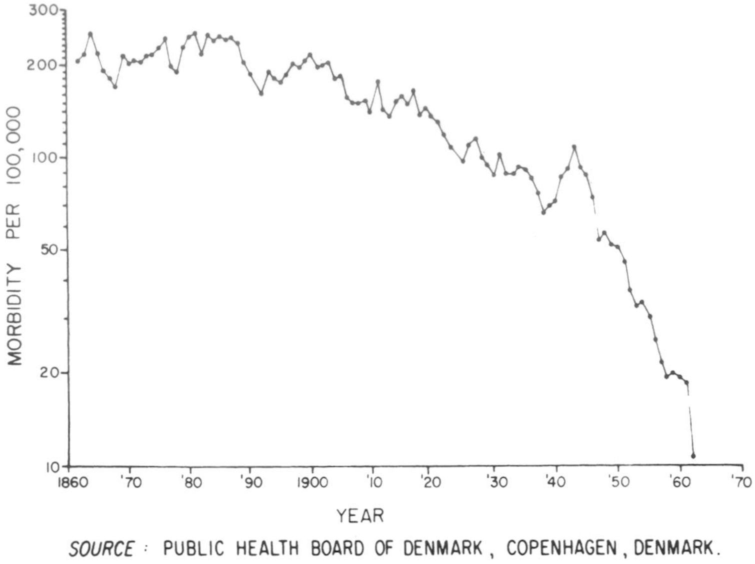

FIGURE 35–1. *Reported annual incidence of acute rheumatic fever in Denmark, 1862 to 1962. (Adapted from Public Health Board of Denmark: Reported rheumatic fever incidence in Denmark, 1862–1962. In Vensborg, P., et al.: Decreasing incidence of a history of acute rheumatic fever in chronic rheumatic heart disease. Cardiologica 53:332, 1968. Used with permission of S Karger AG, Basel.)*

The most compelling evidence that appropriate medical intervention helps to reduce initial attacks of rheumatic fever comes from a study by Gordis of health care availability in an inner-city Baltimore population at risk.[55] The rate of acute rheumatic fever was reduced by 60 per cent over a decade only in the census tracts receiving a comprehensive care program, with that reduction only occurring in patients with an identifiable preceding clinical respiratory infection. A similar trend with small numbers of patients was seen in the Navajo and Papago Native American populations using school-based intervention programs[8, 32] and in an Alaskan program.[19] Other school-based interventions[101] have reduced streptococcal prevalence rates but have not gone the necessary further step to show a reduction in rheumatic fever morbidity in a controlled, carefully demarcated population.

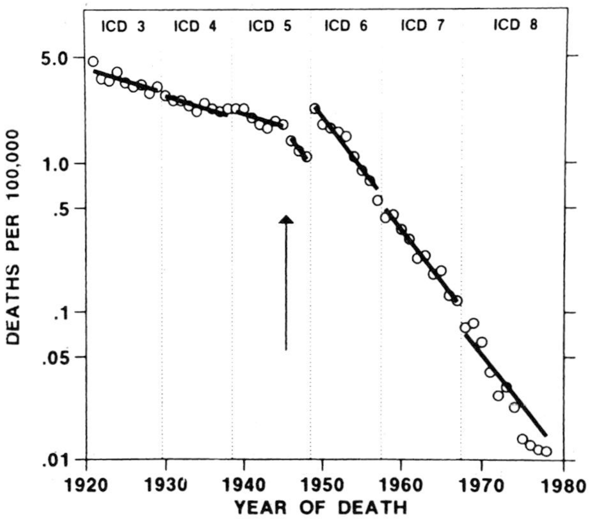

FIGURE 35–2. *United States national mortality due to rheumatic fever in persons 5 to 19 years of age, 1921 through 1978. Values are age-adjusted to the 1950 United States population. Trend lines are fitted for each era (1921 through 1945 and 1946 through 1978) separately and take International Classification of Diseases (ICD) revisions into account. The arrow separates the two eras. (From Massell, B., et al.: Penicillin and the marked decrease in morbidity and mortality from rheumatic fever in the United States. N. Engl. J. Med. 318:280–286, 1988.)*

An unexplained high incidence of acute rheumatic fever persists in Hawaii, especially in Polynesian and part-Polynesian children.[29] Similarly, rates are inexplicably higher in larger populations of Polynesian children in New Zealand.[73] Furthermore, in some areas of the continental United States, the rate of endemic rheumatic fever continues to exceed that of the general population in some children considered traditionally to be at risk (urban blacks), although not in others (recent Hispanic immigrants).[47] In contrast, in a hospital-based study in another urban area, Hispanic children, reflecting the pediatric population being served, were the most affected.[56a]

However, since the beginning of 1985, the number of acute rheumatic fever patients in several centers on the United States mainland has increased.[30, 43, 59, 72, 132, 133, 136, 137, 148] Although these numbers are not large, they represent a definite increase, although this may reflect focal outbreaks rather than increased activity nationwide[128] (Table 35–2). In fact, nationally the number of diagnoses of acute rheumatic fever may have continued to decline gradually from 1984 through 1990.[128] The populations (aside from the clusters in military populations)[26, 137] generally do not seem to be those considered to have been at risk in the past: the patients mostly are white, are middle class, and live in suburban or rural communities with ready access to medical care. In the Utah and Tennessee outbreaks,[132, 142] the families were larger than the state average. The military outbreaks[26, 137] were the first in two decades among United States military personnel. Factors other than widespread use of antibiotics and improved availability of health care may be important. Overcrowded living circumstances long have been considered to be a risk factor,[100] although this hypothesis has failed to be substantiated as an important risk factor using conditional logistic regression in modern-day studies.[135]

The disquieting feature in these recent outbreaks was the severity of the illness, especially in the Salt Lake City, Utah, outbreak: 68 per cent of patients had carditis (Table 35–3), 19 per cent had severe carditis with or without congestive heart failure, and three patients required mitral valve replacement. Earlier United States reports documented carditis in initial attacks of rheumatic fever in 40 to 51 per cent of presenting patients (1951 through 1965).[78] Longitudinal observations at the same institution suggest decreasing frequency of carditis (73 per cent from 1921 to 1930, 51 per cent from 1951 to 1960).[18, 89] Rheumatic fever in its milder form with arthritis

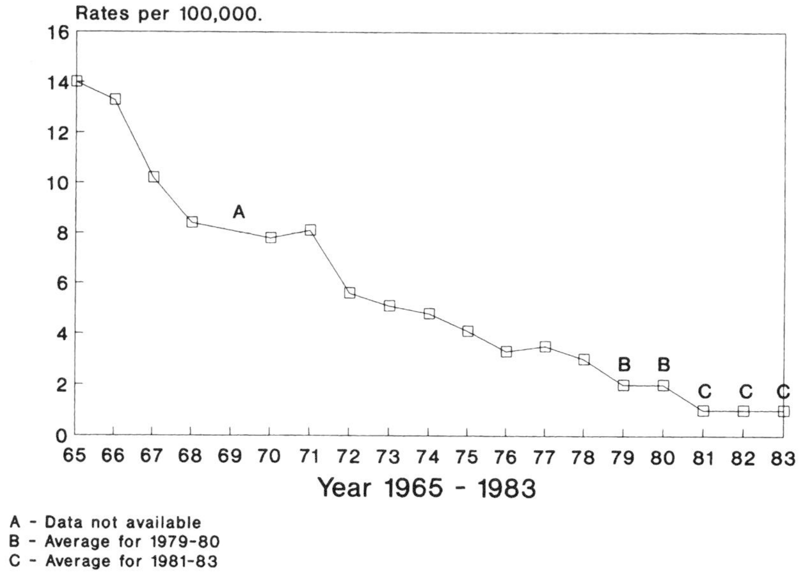

FIGURE 35–3. *Annual rates (per 100,000) of discharge of patients with rheumatic fever from short-stay nonfederal hospitals in the United States, 1965 to 1983. (From National Hospital Discharge Survey, NCHS. Adapted from Gordis, L.: The virtual disappearance of rheumatic fever in the United States: Lessons in the rise and fall of disease. Circulation 72:1155–1162, 1985.)*

as the sole major manifestation may cause difficulty in diagnosis,[57] and the patient may not be admitted to the hospital. This could affect estimates of rates of carditis in studies that are not population-based. With the use of Doppler echocardiography, carditis rates in the Utah patients rose to 85 per cent (Table 35–3). A reappraisal of diagnostic and descriptive data on rheumatic fever and its outcomes may be needed. Length of secondary penicillin prophylaxis and endocarditis prophylaxis is an important consideration for the patient with nonclinical carditis. However, the place of this new technology should be assessed carefully by longitudinal studies (see Laboratory Findings).

The prevalence of rheumatic heart disease, representing the harvest of many years of exposure to the risks of acute rheumatic fever, appears to have declined in the United States over many years.[95]

Many different racial and ethnic groups have been deemed unusually susceptible to rheumatic fever. These usually have been minority groups within a given area who are of lower socioeconomic status than the general population (e.g., Malays in Singapore, Arabs in Israel, Bantus in South Africa, Maoris in New Zealand, blacks in the United States, aborigines in Australia).[2, 20] In the United States, when differences in socioeconomic status or degree of crowding are taken into account,[52] the greater differences in the incidence of rheumatic fever,[53] prevalence of rheumatic heart disease,[95] and

TABLE 35–1. Reported Incidence of Acute Rheumatic Fever in Studies in the United States, 1970–1980

Location	Years of Study	Rate/ 100,000	Age Range in Years
Fairfax, Va.	1970–1980	1.14	0–18
Rhode Island	1976–1980	0.23	5–17
Memphis, Tenn.	1977–1981	1.88	5–17
Baltimore, Md.	1977–1981	0.50	5–19
San Fernando, Calif.	1971–1980	0.63	5–17

Adapted from Veasy, L. G., Wiedmeier, S. E., Orsmond, G. S., et al.: Resurgence of acute rheumatic fever in the intermountain area of the United States. N. Engl. J. Med. *316*:421–427, 1987. In Markowitz, M., and Kaplan, E. L.: Reappearance of rheumatic fever. Adv. Pediatr. *36*:44, 1989.

mortality from acute rheumatic fever and rheumatic heart disease,[105] at least in the population studied, disappear. Rates in blacks were slower to decline. They became very low in the 1970s, at least in some areas.[71] However, Gordis and associates[54] caution that some other socioeconomically determined factor closely paralleling crowding could be the actual determinant of rheumatic fever. Most authorities agree that the reduction in both the incidence and the severity of rheumatic fever that has been noted in the United States and in Western Europe might be due in part to a higher standard of living and less crowding. In a case-control study in the former Yugoslavia, home dampness, change of place of residence during the last 5 years, low maternal education, body weight below normal, frequent sore throat, and positive family history of rheumatic fever were found to be significant risk factors.[135]

The relationship of group A streptococcal throat infections and rheumatic fever grew out of observations of the latter occurring after outbreaks of scarlet fever.[99] The attack rate noted after group A streptococcal throat infections varied widely (from 3 per cent at Warren Air Force Base[107] to 0.39 per cent in Chicago children[118]). Further observations in the latter study reveal that exudative pharyngitis, a positive throat culture with persistence of group A streptococci beyond 21 days, and the development of significant antibody (antistreptolysin O [ASO]) responses influenced a higher attack rate, approaching 3 per cent, in the children studied.

Rheumatic fever, like streptococcal infections, is most common in children 5 to 15 years of age. First attacks of rheumatic fever are rare in children younger than 3 years of age or in adults older than 40 years of age because of the relative infrequency of streptococcal infections at those ages.

The incidence of acute rheumatic fever is highest in the spring and winter months and coincides with the seasonal variation in streptococcal pharyngitis. This may be related to the greater tendency for spread of streptococcal infections by closer contact during the colder and damper months,[123, 135] at least in some climates.

PATHOGENESIS

Evidence points toward every episode of acute rheumatic fever being preceded by a group A streptococcal upper respi-

TABLE 35–2. Reported Outbreaks in the United States of Acute Rheumatic Fever: Selected Epidemiologic Features

	Salt Lake City, Utah[132, 133]*	Columbus, Ohio[59]	Akron, Ohio[30]	Pittsburgh, Pennsylvania[136, 148]	San Diego, California[137]	Tennessee[142]*
Time	1985–1992	6/84–9/86	1986	1987–6/90	12/86–7/87	1/87–7/88
Number of cases	274	40	23	60	50	26
White %	93	80	96	97	50	80
Family Income	80% middle	73% middle	$20,000–$40,000	3 of 17 on assistance[136]	NA	$18,000
Suburban-rural residents	Majority[132]	85%	Many	75%[136]	NA	20%
History of sore throat (no.)††	77 (46)	22 (NA)	18 (NA)	4/17 (3/17)[136] 28/43 (11/43)[148]†	6 (3)	15 (7)
Family history of rheumatic fever (%)	NA	5	16	64[136]	NA	NA
Recurrences	27	1	0	2	1	0
M types of group A streptococci isolated from:						
Patients	1 × M-1; 1 × M-5	NA	M-1,-5,-18	NA	§	Mucoid M-18/T-1 Mucoid nontypable
Families	3 × M-3; 1 × M-1; 1 × M-18; 1 × M-78	NA	M-6	NA	NA	NA
Community	9 × M-18 (8/9 mucoid); 1 × M-4, M-5, M-6, M-9, M-11, M-12, 6 nontypable	Mucoid M-18	NA	NA	NA	Mucoid M-18

*Family size greater than state average.

†Respiratory illness.

††Number who sought treatment.

§San Diego: 5/7 available sera positive for antibodies to M-18, 3/7 positive for M-1 antibodies, 2/7 positive for M-5 and M-6 antibodies, 1/7 positive for M-24 antibodies.

Adapted from Veasy, L. G., Wiedmeier, S. E., Orsmond, G. S., et al.: Resurgence of acute rheumatic fever in the intermountain area of the United States. N. Engl. J. Med. *316*:421–427, 1987. Adapted from Markowitz, M., and Kaplan, E. L.: Reappearance of rheumatic fever. Adv. Pediatr. *36*:39–68, 1989. (See Table 35–1.)

TABLE 35–3. Clinical Manifestations in Four Outbreaks of Acute Rheumatic Fever

Manifestation	Salt Lake City, Utah 1985–1992 (274 patients)(%)	Columbus, Ohio 1984–1986 (40 patients)(%)	Northeastern Ohio 1986 (23 patients)(%)	Pittsburgh, Pennsylvania 1985–6/90 (60 patients)(%)	San Diego, California, Naval 1986–1987 (10 patients)(%)	Tennessee 1987–1988 (26 patients)(%)
Arthritis	36	62	78	43	100	58
Carditis	68*	50	30	52	30	73
Chorea	37	17	9	37	0	31
Erythema marginatum	4	12	1	0	0	4
Subcutaneous nodules	3	0	0	0	10	0

*85% with Doppler ultrasound examination.
Adapted from Markowitz, M., and Kaplan, E. L.: Reappearance of rheumatic fever. Adv. Pediatr. *36*:39–68, 1989.

ratory tract infection. The events that follow such infection and that culminate in rheumatic fever remain poorly defined, suggesting a complex interaction of a number of factors. With a resurgence of interest in this disease after recent outbreaks, laboratory data with the use of modern technologies carefully must be married to the epidemiology of the disease.[65] Pathogenesis involves the host, the environment (see Epidemiology), and group A *Streptococcus*, individually and collectively.

So-called rheumatogenic strains of group A streptococci have been discussed much, most recently in relation to the most recent focal upsurges of rheumatic fever.[63] However, because no factor has been described or isolated, such strains remain a hypothesis.[15] To date, rheumatic fever has been shown to occur only after nasopharyngeal infections.[140] Why the site of infection appears to predispose to the development of rheumatic fever remains an enigma, perhaps related to skin lipids.[68] Acute glomerulonephritis develops after skin or throat infections with a nephritogenic type of group A streptococci (e.g., 49, 12).[140] Certain streptococcal M-protein serotypes strongly and repetitively are implicated in epidemics of acute rheumatic fever. Serotypes M-3, -5, -14, -18, and -24 have been reported more than once in outbreaks, and M-1, -6, -19, -27, and -29 have been reported once only.[15] Other equally prevalent M types rarely, if ever, have been associated with epidemics of the disease[15] or failed to recur in susceptible patients.[16] The current resurgence lends limited support for this concept: no predominance of a single serotype within a specific geographic zone was identified in any of the published outbreaks (see Tables 35–2 and 35–4). Specific M types and their production of mucoidal colonies (see Table 35–4), considered to be related to the amount of M protein and virulence,[141] may be more relevant to epidemic rheumatic fever than to endemic rheumatic fever. In Auckland, New Zealand, an average of 45 new cases of acute rheumatic fever occur annually in children (annual age-specific rate 20/100,000/year). Nine years (1984 to 1992) of surveillance of group A streptococcal isolates from hospitalized pediatric patients (one centralized children's facility for 8 of the 9 years in question) yielded 2410 isolates. Only 3 of 38 throat isolates (32 from well-documented cases of rheumatic fever, 6 from siblings) were strains described as possibly rheumatogenic (one each of M-1, -3, and -6).[85] None was described as mucoidal.[66] In that series, M types 6, 53, 55, and 66 (and NZ 1437 when siblings were included as cases) statistically were more likely to be associated with a case of acute rheumatic fever. Both streptococcal collections[87] (see Table 35–4) are limited samples and may not be representative. In addition, as in most series, group A streptococcal isolates are isolated from a minority of cases and are not supported by streptococcal or type-specific antibody data. Strain selectivity is a further consideration: no documented evidence shows that all members of an M type equally may be able to elicit acute rheumatic fever. Some streptococci from a particular serotype may be associated with both acute rheumatic fever and acute poststreptococcal glomerulonephritis, although the two sequelae rarely occur simultaneously.[77, 86] M types have been shown to be composed of genetically diverse streptococci, not all of which may be established within a community.[86] It is possible that the M type denotes nothing more than a shared type-specific marker, leaving the property of rheumatogenicity as yet elusive. Streptococcal strains that are opacity factor–negative (a lipoprotein lipase) are unlikely to be rheumatogenic, according to earlier data (see Table 35–4).[143] This may be the case in areas where M types reflecting endemic streptococcal skin disease are more common and associated with rheumatic fever.[67, 86, 119] Surveillance of group A streptococci in different geographic zones must be encouraged to guide vaccine development.

Although current evidence strongly implicates an immunologic mechanism in the pathophysiology of rheumatic fever, the details of how the disease develops are by no means clear.[23, 122] Evidence to date strongly suggests an abnormal

TABLE 35–4. Group A Streptococci Isolated from Patients with Rheumatic Fever and from Their Siblings (1986 to May 1988)

Serotype	No. of *Cases*	No. of *Siblings*	No. of *Total*	No. (%) Mucoidal
OF-negative				
M-1, T-1	6	2	8	7 (88)
M-3, T-3	3	6	9	1 (11)
M-18, T-18	6	2	8	7 (88)
M-5, T-5/27/44	1	3	4	1 (25)
M-6, T-6	3	0	3	2 (67)
M-41, T-13	1	0	1	0 (0)
Subtotal	20	13	33	18 (55)
OF-positive				
OF-75, T-25	2	0	2	0 (0)
OF-77, T-13	2	0	2	0 (0)
OF-78, T-11	0	2	2	0 (0)
OF-48, T-28	1	0	1	1 (100)
M-2, T-2	1	0	1	0 (0)
M-4, T-4	1	0	1	0 (0)
Subtotal	7	2	9	1 (11)
Total	27	15	42	19 (45)

OF, opacity factor.
From Kaplan, E. L., Johnson, D. R., and Cleary, P. P.: Group A streptococcal serotypes isolated from patients and sibling contacts during the resurgence of rheumatic fever in the United States in the mid-1980s. J. Infect. Dis. *159*:101–103, 1989.

cell-mediated and humoral immune response to cell-membrane streptococcal antigens, which, because of molecular mimicry of human tissues, may result in continued damage to the cardiovascular and nervous systems.[23, 122] The findings of circulating immune complexes in a majority of patients[33] and the deposition of C3 and immunoglobulin in the myocardium of patients dying of acute rheumatic fever support an abnormal immune response in rheumatic fever.[66]

M proteins from highly rheumatogenic group A streptococcal types share antigenic determinants with myosin and with sarcolemma of cardiac muscle[37, 38] and with antigens of articular cartilage and synovium.[9] Thus, the immune response to streptococci may mistake the host antigens as foreign, causing tissue damage. Other streptococcal antigens, such as the group A carbohydrate component, are candidates for mistaken cross-reaction with a glycoprotein in human heart valves.[51] The group A *Streptococcus* has components that can amplify or down-regulate the immune response.[23]

The site of the initial streptococcal infection may be important: lymphatic channels have been demonstrated between the tonsils and the heart.[23] Unusual compartmentalization of rheumatic antigen-positive non–T cells in patients with acute rheumatic fever has been shown, with no positive cells detected in rheumatic tonsils but with increased numbers in peripheral blood.[56]

Cell-mediated immunity to streptococcal antigens also is enhanced in patients with rheumatic fever.[122] Lymphocytic infiltrate of heart valves was found to be composed predominantly of CD4+ helper cells.[106] Increased expression of HLA-DR on fibroblasts, which can present antigens to CD4+ lymphocytes (cytotoxic/suppressor T cells), has been observed on the heart valves of patients with acute carditis.[4] Cytotoxicity induced in normal human helper and suppressor cells in vitro by purified protein from a type M-5 group A *Streptococcus* organism has been shown to destroy several human cell types, including cultured myocardial cells.[36] T-cell subset study results are conflicting,[93, 122] but production of interleukins is reported to be enhanced.[94, 149] The role of M-protein and streptococcal pyrogenic exotoxins as superantigens, perhaps explaining the exaggeration of the streptococcal immune response, is being explored.[84, 129]

The genetic background of the human host appears to influence susceptibility to rheumatic fever. Aggregation of rheumatic fever cases in families long has been recognized.[102] However, low concordance for inheritance has been reported in monozygotic twins,[127] although affected siblings have significant concordance for arthritis, residual rheumatic heart disease, and chorea.[120] Pataroyo and associates[98] found that the B lymphocytes of patients with rheumatic fever have a specific marker (883 alloantigen) associated with host rheumatic susceptibility.[146, 147] This appears to transcend ethnicity[98] and may be similar to an immune response gene.[122] This work has been extended to family members of rheumatic fever patients using monoclonal antibodies.[46, 112] The approach promises the ability to identify those with altered risk for rheumatic fever or heart disease, which could allow targeted primary prevention. Class 1 HLAs have not been associated with acute rheumatic fever. Many studies in different populations have shown an association with HLA-DR but without a single HLA marker for susceptibility.[122] Genetic factors alone seem highly unlikely to be responsible for susceptibility to rheumatic fever.[79]

Immunity to group A streptococci, and so to rheumatic fever, depends on antibodies to the M protein; such antibodies can opsonize the bacteria in the presence of neutrophils.[12] Until lately, immunity was thought to be strain-specific and dependent on the antibodies to the variable serotype-specific regions of the protein, and vaccine development has followed this pathway.[13] Antibodies against the variable amino-terminal end of the M protein opsonize streptococci in a type-specific way, but results of experiments in animals suggest that the conserved carboxyl-terminal end also may be an immune target. There is some human evidence that this conserved epitope acts as a subunit vaccine.[104] Complexities in this area include the risk of inducing cross-reacting antibodies that could injure rather than protect.[90] Separation of the peptide fragments of M proteins (epitopes) that evoke type-specific and not cross-reacting antibodies is an important step.[21, 33] Identifying which of the 80 or so M types of the group A streptococci are likely to be rheumatogenic requires more work.

RHEUMATIC FEVER IN DEVELOPING COUNTRIES

Rheumatic heart disease is considered by some to be one of the few preventable chronic diseases.[6] In spite of impressive declines in developed countries (see Figs. 35–1, 35–2, and 35–3), rheumatic heart disease globally remains the most common form of acquired heart disease.[69] Four-fifths of the world's population live in developing countries, where the prevalence of rheumatic heart disease suggests that the incidence of acute rheumatic fever remains at high levels in areas characterized by crowded living quarters and lower socioeconomic conditions. In Soweto, South Africa, the prevalence of rheumatic heart disease has been estimated at 7.1 per 1000 schoolchildren.[91] Given the difference in medical care delivery, estimates of incidence of acute rheumatic fever must be viewed with caution. However, estimates suggest an annual incidence of 200 to 400 cases per 100,000 population in Soweto.[69] In India, the prevalence of rheumatic heart disease in schoolchildren has been estimated to be between 1.5 and 5.65 cases per 1000. The incidence of rheumatic fever (as judged by hospital admissions for rheumatic heart disease between 1966 and 1980) has remained stable in India during this period of rapid decline in the United States and the West.[2] Community-based secondary penicillin prophylaxis programs in developing countries are considered cost-effective and more achievable than primary prevention.[69]

PATHOLOGY[114]

The unique pathologic lesion of rheumatic fever is the Aschoff body, generally considered a granuloma that results from injury to collagen fibers. These classically are found in the heart, usually in the left atrial appendage, but similar foci can be found in the synovia of the joints and in and about joint capsules, tendons, and fascia.

The early pathologic response to rheumatic fever may be an exudative reaction with Aschoff-like bodies as an inflammatory focus. These are cardiac or extra-cardiac, with a central area of fibrinoid necrosis surrounded mostly by polymorphs. Clinically, this may present as arthritis and subside spontaneously in 2 to 4 weeks. No residual joint damage results. The proliferative phase of classic Aschoff nodules, with central necrosis surrounded by a rosette of large mononuclear cells, giant multinuclear cells, and other cell types, is confined to the heart, usually causing pancarditis and involving all three layers simultaneously (the pericardium, the myocardium, and the endocardium). This may result in permanent valvular damage in the following order of frequency: the mitral valve, the aortic valve, the tricuspid valve, and rarely the pulmonary valve. Therefore, the heart disease encountered clinically usually is mitral regurgitation, aortic regurgitation, or both. Scarring that leads to valvular stenoses (mitral or aortic) usually takes decades to develop but may develop much faster in hyperendemic areas. However, this is not the full story because although rheumatic mitral valve stenosis is somewhat more common in India[116] and occasionally occurs in other less advantaged populations, it was never common in the United States or the United Kingdom at the height of rheumatic fever incidence.[113]

The presence of the Aschoff body is not evidence of rheumatic activity because these lesions are found in biopsy specimens of the left atrial appendage many years after an acute attack of rheumatic fever. Little is known about the pathology of Sydenham chorea, and the pathologic changes cannot be related to the clinical manifestations. Patients rarely die of this form of rheumatic fever.

CLINICAL COURSE

The stage is set for the development of rheumatic fever in a susceptible host after a pharyngeal infection by one of the types of the group A beta-hemolytic streptococci. If the infection is not treated, most persons recover from the acute effects of the disease. About 1 to 3 per cent of children with known epidemic untreated exudative pharyngitis and a culture positive for group A streptococci develop acute rheumatic fever. The frequency drops to less than 1 per cent, as shown in the one controlled study of children,[118] when patients with less severe or less precisely diagnosed streptococcal infections are included. The preceding pharyngitis is not recognized as an illness by the patient or parent in about 10 to 33 per cent of cases of acute rheumatic fever, although 50 to 60 per cent remember having a sore throat.[55] In some series, this figure was lower (see Table 35–2). The infection is followed by a latent period that averages 19 days,[108] during which time the patient seems well. The range appears to be between 1 and 5 weeks but has been difficult to establish.[25] The average latent period is the same for recurrent attacks as for initial episodes.[25]

Acute rheumatic fever then begins. Table 35–3 suggests a clinical profile in the United States, although recurrent cases with their increased risk of carditis are included. In a prospective study in India, 67 per cent of initial episodes presented with migrating arthritis involving one or more of the large joints[115] accompanied by a fever of 38° to 39° C, malaise, and anorexia. Just as the redness, swelling, and pain in a knee subside, the whole process may start again in the ankle. Elbows and wrists also are likely to be involved. Multiple joints usually are involved, in tandem with overlap over time, when symptoms are not suppressed by anti-inflammatory therapy. The whole polyarthritic episode usually subsides over 4 weeks, leaving no residua. Carditis appears early in the illness (first 2 weeks) if it is going to occur.[1] The joint inflammation may be low-grade in some persons, without limitation of motion or outward manifestations of redness and swelling (arthralgia).

At examination, the striking findings are the patient's pallor and discomfort, especially upon movement of the affected joints. The pulse is rapid. Examination of the heart may reveal, in at least half of patients, a grade II/IV apical pansystolic murmur that is transmitted to the axilla (mitral insufficiency) with or without an apical mid-diastolic flow murmur (Carey-Coombs murmur); half of these patients also may experience an early diastolic grade II/IV murmur at the left sternal edge (aortic insufficiency). The child also can present less commonly with congestive heart failure or with cardiac enlargement, denoting active carditis. Carditis is more likely in younger children. Pericarditis may be suspected with muffled heart sounds, a frictional rub, or chest pain. It becomes less common as acute rheumatic fever in a population becomes less severe. Death is a rare but well-described sequela of the acute phase of the disease. Murmurs of mitral and aortic stenosis are associated with chronic, but not with acute, rheumatic valve disease. The distinctive skin rash, erythema marginatum, is observed in about 10 per cent of patients (Fig. 35–4). It is nonpruritic and nonpainful. The pink, slightly raised macules initially seen fuse centrally and coalesce to form a serpiginous pattern. The lesions may disappear after a few hours or may reappear intermittently over a period of weeks. Subcutaneous nodules, usually associated with severe carditis, also are uncommon (less than 10 per cent of patients). They are firm and painless and found over bony surfaces or prominences and over tendons. Acute rheumatic fever is unlikely to be diagnosed on the basis of the latter two major criteria without another major criterion.

Sydenham chorea or St. Vitus dance may be the only manifestation of rheumatic fever, or it may be associated with other disease manifestations. It becomes less common as acute rheumatic fever in a population becomes less severe. Chorea is characterized by purposeless (most often bilateral, uncoordinated, involuntary) movements, mostly of the hands, feet, and face, that develop over a period of weeks and are accentuated by excitement and emotional stress. They disappear during sleep. Sensation remains intact. The speech can be explosive and indistinct and the handwriting clumsy. Handwriting is a useful objective means of following the course of the disease. The child has difficulty in counting rapidly and in holding the protruded tongue still. The fingers

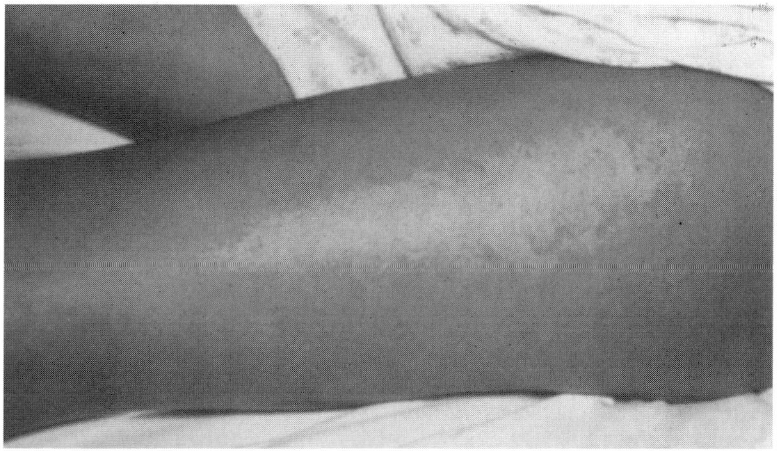

FIGURE 35–4. *Erythema marginatum in an 8-year-old girl with acute rheumatic fever.*

and wrists are hyperextended when fingers are outstretched, and the palms usually are turned outward when the arms are held above the head. The hand grip usually is weak and may consist of spasmodic contractions followed by rapid relaxation. The patient may be irritated easily and quarrelsome. Chorea typically is a delayed manifestation of rheumatic fever and may develop after other signs of the disease have subsided. It is not uncommon for chorea to appear 2 to 6 months after the streptococcal infection. Most observers think that residual heart disease is less common when chorea is the only manifestation of rheumatic fever, but the importance of prophylaxis to prevent recurrent attacks and possible subsequent carditis was reaffirmed in Kuwait.[76] Permanent serious residual neurologic deficits have not been observed. A 25-year review found the duration of chorea to be 1 to 22 weeks, with a median of 12 weeks.[96] Recurrent attacks are not uncommon.

The average duration of attack of acute rheumatic fever is approximately 3 months when unaltered by anti-inflammatory therapy.[78] Less than 5 per cent of cases persist longer than 6 months with active symptoms, so-called chronic rheumatic fever.[126]

LABORATORY FINDINGS[81, 121]

The degree of inflammation in patients with acute rheumatic fever is measured by nonspecific indicators, such as the erythrocyte sedimentation rate (ESR) and the C-reactive protein (CRP). Unless the patient has had corticosteroids or salicylates, these test results almost always are positive in patients who present with polyarthritis or acute carditis, whereas they often are normal in patients presenting with chorea. The magnitude of the ESR is proportional to the intensity of the inflammatory reaction but is not site-specific (i.e., it can be high in polyarthritis or carditis). The ESR may be decreased in congestive heart failure, whereas the CRP may be elevated in congestive heart failure due to any cause. The ESR may remain elevated for 6 weeks to 3 months in an untreated attack of acute rheumatic fever. Anti-inflammatory agents may damp down the ESR, but it will rebound if they are stopped before the rheumatic process has run its course. Chronic elevation of the ESR (more than 6 months) is not understood but is not sufficient reason on its own to limit a patient's activities.[126] The CRP may reflect the patient's rheumatic activity more precisely than may the ESR.[81]

Chest radiographs are useful in detecting cardiomegaly, which may be due to dilatation, preexisting heart disease, or pericardial effusion. The degree of enlargement is useful in judging severity. The electrocardiogram may show prolonged atrioventricular conduction time, usually evidenced by a prolonged PR interval or even greater degrees of heart block.[111] In general, an increase in the PR interval in tracings with comparable rates is considered significant.[81] Atrioventricular conduction abnormalities of themselves bear no relationship to the ultimate prognosis of patients. Changes of myocarditis and pericarditis also are seen. The role of two-dimensional and Doppler echocardiography in the diagnosis and determination of prognosis of acute rheumatic fever needs ongoing clarification.[1, 121, 132, 133, 144] In a prospective blinded study using febrile controls and strict color and pulsed Doppler criteria, pathologic left-sided heart regurgitation could be differentiated from physiologic regurgitation.[1] Several centers have observed subclinical carditis in acute rheumatic fever using similar strict criteria.[48, 49, 132, 133] The status of echocardiographic evidence as a major or minor criterion remains to be settled. It has important implications for the patient with polyarthritis as a sole major criterion[133] or the patient without major criteria and with only echocardiographic evidence of mitral or aortic regurgitation.

A positive throat culture for group A beta-hemolytic *Streptococcus* as evidence of a recent streptococcal infection is unusual, and up to 50 per cent of such patients could be carriers of the organism.[61] A positive culture may be helpful if it can be related to the time of the acute infection.

Corroboration of a previous streptococcal infection may be documented by a number of streptococcal antibody tests. The antibody titers may be elevated in the absence of clinical or bacteriologic evidence of streptococcal pharyngitis. The ASO titer is the most popular antibody test and measures the inhibition of rabbit red blood cells by specific antibody to streptolysin O, an extracellular product of beta-hemolytic streptococci that, in its reduced form, hemolyzes red blood cells. The "normal" level for an ASO titer usually is defined as the highest titer exceeded by only 20 per cent of a population but is influenced importantly by age, geography, season, and other factors. ASO titers of 500 Todd units or greater are rare in normal schoolchildren and are good evidence of a recent streptococcal infection. ASO titers below 250 Todd units could be considered normal; titers of 250 to 320 should be considered borderline elevated. About 50 per cent of patients with acute rheumatic fever have ASO titers in this range, and about 60 per cent have titers of 500 or greater.[121] Conversely, ASO titers can be normal in up to 20 per cent of acute rheumatic patients.[124] A recent streptococcal infection is more likely to be demonstrated if more than one antibody titer is measured (e.g., antistreptokinase and antihyaluronidase).[124] Another specific antibody test is antideoxyribonuclease B, which is the most favored because of better reproducibility. The Jones criteria[121] (see Table 35–5) call for an elevated or rising titer of an antistreptococcal antibody. The onset of clinical acute rheumatic fever usually coincides with the peak of the streptococcal antibody response. This may stay elevated for many weeks. However, the absence of an elevated antistreptococcal titer, if three different antibodies are measured, means the clinician can be 95 per cent certain that the patient has not had a streptococcal infection within the recent past. In patients with pure chorea, however, antibody levels may have declined to normal because of the length of the latent period between the streptococcal infection and this symptom. A slide agglutination test is available (Streptozyme antibody test, Wampole Laboratories, Stanford, CT). This test cannot be recommended at this time because of inconsistencies in results due to variations in different lots of test material.[5]

The synovial fluid in joints affected by acute rheumatic fever contains 10,000 to 100,000 white blood cells/mm^3, which mostly are neutrophils. The protein concentration is about 4 g/dL, the glucose is normal, and there is a good mucin clot.[58]

DIAGNOSIS

The signs and symptoms of rheumatic fever vary greatly, depending on the stage of the disease, the epidemiology of the rheumatic fever in that place at that time, the severity of the disease, and the sites of involvement. In the absence of a diagnostic test or pathognomonic sign, Jones suggested a series of criteria (major and minor) (Table 35–5) that has stood the test of time with ongoing modifications.[80]

The keystone on which the Jones criteria (1992 update)[121] rest is the demonstration of a recent streptococcal infection. Because relatively few acute rheumatics have positive throat cultures, the demonstration of a previous streptococcal infection by a rising titer of one or more of the extracellular

TABLE 35–5. Guidelines for the Diagnosis of Initial Attack of Rheumatic Fever (Jones Criteria 1992 Update)*

Major Manifestations†
Carditis
Polyarthritis
Chorea
Erythema marginatum
Subcutaneous nodules
Minor Manifestations†
Clinical findings
Arthralgia
Fever
Laboratory findings
Elevated acute-phase reactants
Erythrocyte sedimentation rate
C-reactive protein
Prolonged PR interval
Supporting Evidence of Antecedent Group A Streptococcal Infection
Positive throat culture or rapid streptococcal antigen test
Elevated or rising streptococcal antibody titer

*If supported by evidence of preceding group A streptococcal infection, the presence of two major manifestations or of one major and two minor manifestations indicates a high probability of acute rheumatic fever.

†See text for details.

Guidelines for the diagnosis of initial attack of rheumatic fever (Jones criteria 1992 update). J. A. M. A. *268*:2069–2073, 1992. Copyright 1992, American Medical Association.

streptococcal antibodies is critical confirmatory evidence for the establishment of a recent streptococcal infection. It must be emphasized that the mere presence of an elevated titer to one or more of the streptococcal antibodies (see Laboratory Findings) means only that the subject has had a recent group A beta-hemolytic streptococcal infection.

Clinical manifestations in recent outbreaks are summarized in Table 35–3. Prior to this, during the period of declining incidence in the United States, carditis was found in less than half of the rheumatic patients and generally was less severe.[89] Joint involvement alone therefore was the most common manifestation, making diagnostic certainty difficult.[57] A common avoidable error is the premature administration of salicylates or corticosteroids before the signs and symptoms become distinct, leaving the necessity for secondary prophylaxis, without a firm diagnosis, in doubt.

The updated criteria (1992)[121] are designed, in contrast with the revised Jones criteria (1965), to establish the diagnosis of the initial attack of acute rheumatic fever; therefore, a previous attack of rheumatic fever or rheumatic heart disease is no longer a minor manifestation. Echocardiography is not a stand-alone criterion for the diagnosis of acute rheumatic fever (see Laboratory Findings). Chorea and indolent carditis are considered as stand-alone criteria for the diagnosis of rheumatic fever. Rheumatic fever recurrences in patients with a reliable past history of rheumatic fever or clear-cut rheumatic heart disease can be diagnosed using a single major or several minor criteria if there is supporting evidence of a recent group A streptococcal infection.

So-called poststreptococcal arthritis has been discussed as a possible entity when the presenting symptoms and signs are atypical of acute rheumatic fever, fail to respond to salicylate therapy, or both. In some cases, rheumatic heart disease has ensued.[40] All such cases that fulfill the Jones criteria should be considered for a diagnosis of rheumatic fever, particularly for the purposes of secondary penicillin prophylaxis. The role of echocardiography in this diagnostic situation has yet to be clarified.

DIFFERENTIAL DIAGNOSIS

A number of other diseases might be confused with acute rheumatic fever: rheumatoid arthritis; suppurative bacterial arthritis, especially gonococcal arthritis in adolescents; reactive arthritis (e.g., after *Yersinia*[70] or *Mycoplasma*[92] infection); infective endocarditis; sickle-cell anemia; leukemia; and Lyme disease.[103]

With the help of the Jones criteria and time, these diseases usually can be excluded. For example, heart involvement with rheumatoid arthritis is rare. In suppurative arthritis, demonstration by smear and recovery by culture of the infecting bacteria provide the answer. With sickle-cell disease, the bone is affected and not the joint, and a sickle-cell preparation helps establish the diagnosis. A blood smear usually establishes the diagnosis of leukemia.

Common errors include diagnosing acute rheumatic fever when a single joint is involved, when an innocent murmur is present, when a nonspecific rash (especially an urticarial or an erythema multiforme rash) erroneously is called erythema marginatum, and when other symptoms similar to chorea (e.g., tics, phenothiazine-induced extrapyramidal syndrome) are misinterpreted.[62] Committing a child to many years of penicillin prophylaxis means careful decisionmaking at the time of diagnosis.

TREATMENT[34, 127a]

Therapy in acute rheumatic fever is symptomatic, to control inflammation, decrease fever, and control cardiac failure. Neither salicylates nor corticosteroids are considered to affect severity or outcome.[131] If the physician feels that a patient has acute rheumatic fever, a trial with salicylate is indicated as symptomatic therapy. Characteristically, the joint inflammation and fever subside in 24 to 48 hours with salicylate treatment if the serum level is 10 to 20 mg/dL, which usually is achieved by a dose of 100 mg/kg/24 hours (not exceeding 6 g/day in divided doses). This dose may be increased, but it is advisable to measure serum salicylate levels and thus adjust the dosage regimen. Higher dosage may result in the undesirable development of salicylism (tinnitus and hyperpnea). Except for the occasional patient with rheumatoid arthritis, no other forms of arthritis respond in this dramatic way to aspirin. Salicylate therapy is recommended for 1 to 2 weeks and then can be reduced gradually. There is no evidence that steroid therapy is superior, nor is there any evidence that treatment with steroid or aspirin decreases the severity or prevents the development of residual heart disease.[3, 131] Both are palliative and not curative. They are, however, effective anti-inflammatory agents for controlling the acute exudative manifestations of rheumatic fever. Steroids are more likely to reduce acute symptoms promptly and therefore may be indicated in severely ill patients in whom inflammatory edema of the myocardium may be life-threatening during the acute stage of the illness.[44] The effect of nonsteroidal anti-inflammatory drugs has not been evaluated adequately. Acetaminophen, also not critically evaluated, is used by some clinicians to provide some symptomatic relief as the signs and symptoms evolve into a diagnosable picture of acute rheumatic fever.

Bed rest has not been studied critically.[82] Restriction of physical activity until the rheumatic process has become quiescent is a time-honored method of treatment. It has been based on the assumption that the workload of the inflamed heart is related to the degree of residual scarring. Guidelines are suggested for up to 6 weeks of bed rest, depending on whether carditis is present, followed by gradual ambulation indoors over an equally long period before outside activity, in a modified fashion, takes place. The patient with severe carditis who has congestive heart failure is managed more conservatively.

It is recommended that all patients receive intramuscular benzathine penicillin, even if the throat culture does not reveal group A beta-hemolytic streptococci. The patient then can be placed on the secondary prevention treatment regimen, which may be either oral penicillin V, 250 mg twice a day, or injections of benzathine penicillin, 1.2 million units, every 4 weeks. The parenteral route has been shown to be more effective by the author's group (Fig. 35–5)[123] and others.[145] In high-risk situations, administration of benzathine penicillin every 3 weeks has been advised.[75]

Rarely, a patient has profound myocarditis and is in congestive heart failure. Under these circumstances, the patient should have the benefit of the usual measures for the treatment of congestive heart failure with bed rest, diuretics, and, if needed, oxygen and digoxin. Feinstein and Arerralo[45] did not find a higher incidence of digoxin toxicity in patients with active carditis, compared with patients with inactive rheumatic heart disease.

Cardiac Surgery in Active Rheumatic Heart Disease

Aggressive surgical therapy—with increasing acceptance that mitral repair, rather than replacement, is the treatment of choice for mitral regurgitation[7]—also may be indicated in the patient with severe active rheumatic heart disease. Strauss and associates[125] proposed that a child with rheumatic heart disease be catheterized and considered as a candidate for operation in the presence of any one of the following criteria:

1. Congestive heart failure and true chronic rheumatic fever
2. Congestive heart failure and a cardiothoracic ratio greater than 0.6
3. Functional class IV
4. Atrial fibrillation

They suggested that the decision to operate should be based on the severity of the disability and of the hemodynamic disturbance rather than on the activity or inactivity of the rheumatic process. Two-dimensional or Doppler echocardiography may spare the patient cardiac catheterization. Extensive published experience in South Africa[10] and France[28] with excellent results challenges the concept that congestive heart failure and death during active carditis are due to myocarditis rather than to incompetence of the valve. Careful postoperative management, including at least 4 months of physical rest, diuretics, and vasodilatation with angiotensin-converting enzyme inhibitors, is believed to improve the long-term outcome by avoiding enhanced blood pressure and myocardial contractility before the repair has consolidated. The acute rheumatic activity usually subsides within 2 to 3 weeks of obtaining valve competence.[10]

PROGNOSIS

The prognosis for patients with acute rheumatic fever depends on the presenting manifestations. This clearly was shown in the 20-year follow-up study from the pre-penicillin era by Bland and Jones.[18] A patient with marked cardiomegaly, congestive heart failure, or pericarditis had about a 70 to 80 per cent chance of dying in 10 years before the advent of secondary prevention programs, open heart surgery, and prosthetic valves. The prognosis today is not as ominous, although recurrence rates (with the attendant increased risk of carditis in individual patients) reported after some outbreaks[133, 148] suggest a careful look at secondary prevention and its delivery. Patients presenting with cardiomegaly or heart failure indicative of the severity of their myocarditis and who survive have up to about a 70 per cent chance of residual rheumatic heart disease at 1-year[131] and at 10-year follow-up.[31] Most have mitral insufficiency, and approximately half of these patients also have aortic insufficiency. About 50 per cent of patients are left initially with residual heart disease after an attack of rheumatic fever. This is about the same as was the case 25 to 30 years ago. However, about 25 per cent of these patients return to normal cardiac status, with a higher chance if the cardiac involvement is mild. Of patients presenting with no or questionable carditis[131] during their attack of rheumatic fever, only 6 per cent were found to have heart murmurs when re-examined 10 years later. Heart disease was present at follow-up in 30 per cent of the

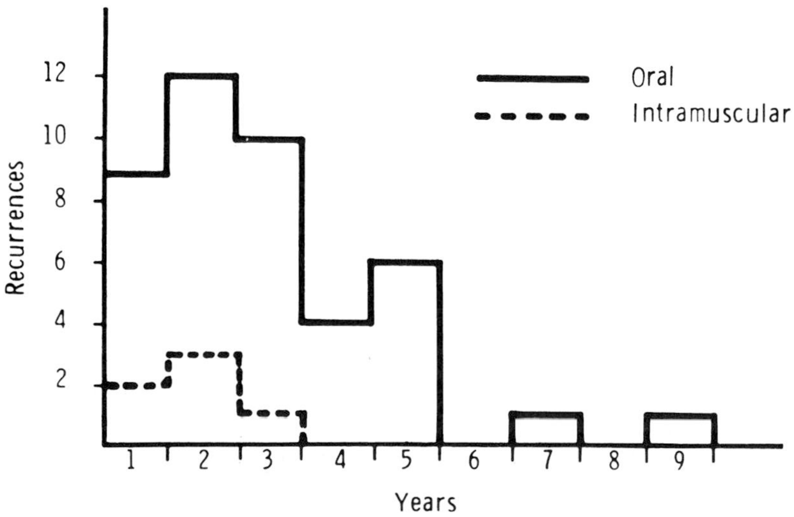

FIGURE 35–5. *Influence of oral and intramuscular penicillin prophylaxis on the recurrence of rheumatic fever. Time is between the last attack and recurrence (years). (From Newman, J. E., et al.: Patients with rheumatic fever recurrences. N. Z. Med. J. 97:678–680, 1984.)*

patients initially found to have only apical systolic murmurs and in 40 per cent of those with basal diastolic murmurs during the acute phase. Patients with chorea may have a slightly lower incidence of residual heart disease.[76]

PREVENTION[34]

Denny and associates[42, 139] made one of the most important research contributions in the last 50 years when they showed that rheumatic fever can be prevented in most susceptible subjects if the preceding pharyngeal infection by one of the group A beta-hemolytic streptococci is treated adequately. These studies used depot penicillin G. The effectiveness of other antimicrobial agents (benzathine penicillin, chlortetracycline [Aureomycin], sulfadiazine, oxytetracycline) in the prevention of rheumatic fever also was studied.[41] Eradication of the streptococcus was shown to be essential,[25] and a 10-day course of penicillin treatment was found to be more effective than a 5-day course.[138] From these studies, penicillin, a bactericidal agent against the streptococcus, became the drug of choice. Efficacy studies against rheumatic fever per se were carried out only in military populations with injectable penicillin. The ability of oral penicillin to eradicate streptococci in throats is not equal to the ability of injectable penicillin to do so.[11] The complete explanation for the decline of rheumatic fever remains unclear.

Streptococcal pharyngeal infection should be identified before treatment is started. Such an infection can be identified by throat culture or by using a rapid diagnostic antigen detection kit.[34, 39, 74, 110] The true place of these kits in the clinical setting still is evolving. Most tests have a high specificity, and so a patient with acute pharyngitis with a positive test result should be treated. Many of the tests have a less than desirable sensitivity and should be backed up by a throat culture. One study found that in a third of persons with false-negative rapid antigen detection test results, streptococcal antibody titers rose subsequently, suggesting infection.[50] Military studies showed that penicillin primary prevention treatment is effective even if started as long as 9 days after the infection,[24] so the physician may wait 24 to 48 hours for verification of infection by recovery of the group A beta-hemolytic streptococci. A dose of 1.2 million units of benzathine penicillin intramuscularly (0.6 million units if ≤27 kg) usually is adequate treatment. Because of the discomfort and a possible but small risk associated with intramuscular penicillin,[60] oral penicillin V (250 mg two or three times a day for children; 500 mg two or three times a day for adolescents and adults) may be preferred in areas in which the incidence of rheumatic fever is low. Erythromycin estolate (20 to 40 mg/kg/day in two to four divided doses; maximum, 1 g/day) may be used in patients who are allergic to penicillin. Erythromycin ethylsuccinate (40 mg/kg/day two to four times daily; maximum, 1 g/day) is an alternative. All oral treatments should be given for 10 days.

Reappearance of acute rheumatic fever in a specific geographic region should draw attention to therapeutic, preventative, and epidemiologic measures for the control of the disease. A targeted approach to particularly high-risk population groups in schools may be cost-effective and efficacious.[6, 19, 32, 101, 113, 130] Because treatment of pharyngitis seems likely to have contributed to the declining incidence of rheumatic fever, throat cultures (or a rapid antigen test) and penicillin treatment, if positive for group A streptococci, still are recommended in low-risk populations. In addition, a negative culture avoids the unnecessary prescribing of antibiotics in the 70 to 80 per cent of children with a sore throat secondary to viral pharyngitis.[117] Prompt antibiotic therapy may shorten the duration of symptoms in patients with group A beta-hemolytic streptococcal pharyngitis.[109] Cultures should be used selectively in age groups in which rheumatic fever in that population becomes rare (e.g., younger than 4 years or older than 20 years). Signs and symptoms usually not associated with streptococcal infection, such as simple coryza, hoarseness, cough, conjunctivitis, anterior stomatitis, and diarrhea,[34] may help to target the approach in a low-risk population.

A follow-up throat culture after a course of treatment for streptococcal pharyngitis is not recommended routinely unless the patient remains symptomatic or is from a family with a rheumatic person. Such follow-up cultures probably identify long-term carriers for whom repeated courses of antibiotics generally are not indicated.[117] Streptococcal carriers appear to pose little threat to themselves in the development sequelae of streptococcal infection or disseminating the organism to those around them. However, when such a carrier develops a symptomatic viral upper respiratory tract infection, it frequently is not possible to distinguish whether the group A streptococci isolated indicate current streptococcal infection or identify that individual as a chronic carrier. In one study, only 43 per cent of children with paired sera from whom group A streptococci were recovered showed a significant antibody response to one of two different streptococcal antibodies.[61] It often is reasonable to administer a single course of therapy. Indications for culturing household contacts vary according to circumstances.[34] Family contacts of high-risk patients should have a culture performed and receive treatment if the culture is positive.

Recurrent attacks of rheumatic fever can be prevented by continuous penicillin prophylaxis, either orally or parenterally.[34] The parenteral route has been shown to be more effective (1.2 million units of benzathine penicillin intramuscularly at 28-day intervals).[145] In this comprehensive study, children experienced a recurrence rate of only 0.4 per 100 patient-years of observation (Table 35–6). An international study of allergic reactions to long-term benzathine penicillin prophylaxis found that the benefits of recurrence prevention far outweighed the risks of a serious allergic reaction.[60] In areas of particularly high risk, benzathine penicillin every 21 days may be more efficacious[75] because serum levels of penicillin toward the end of the time can be unreliable,[64]

TABLE 35–6. Prophylaxis and Attack Rates of Streptococcal Infection and Rheumatic Fever Recurrences

	Parenteral Benzathine Penicillin	Oral Penicillin	Oral Sulfadiazine
Number of years	560	545	576
Number and rate of all streptococcal infections, exclusive of carrier state	24/4.3	101/18.5	102/17.7
Number and rate of rheumatic recurrences	2/0.4	30/5.5	16/2.8

Adapted from Wood, H. F., Feinstein, A. R., Taranta, A., et al.: Rheumatic fever in children and adolescents: A long-term epidemiologic study of subsequent prophylaxis, streptococcal infections, and clinical sequelae. III. Comparative effectiveness of three prophylaxis regimens in preventing streptococcal infections and rheumatic recurrences. Ann. Intern. Med. *60*(Suppl. 5), 1964, with permission.

although this should be offset against practicability and likely compliance.

Patients allergic to penicillin may be given erythromycin (250 mg twice a day). Oral regimens that have been studied for efficacy are penicillin and sulfadiazine (see Table 35–6). Sulfadiazine is not commercially available in the United States.[27] The lesser efficacy of oral regimens is related at least in part to compliance difficulties.

The risk of rheumatic fever occurring after a group A streptococcal infection rises from an attack rate of 1 to 3 per cent with the first attack of streptococcal pharyngitis to 25 to 75 per cent in subsequent attacks.[42] Those who have had carditis are at an increased risk of further carditis. Those who have not had clinical carditis are at considerably less risk of cardiac involvement with a recurrence.[76]

The risk of recurrence depends on several other factors, such as length of time since the most recent attack and the risk of acquiring streptococcal throat infections according to occupation or living circumstances. If possible, the length of prophylaxis should be individualized. The suggested length is a minimum of 5 years' prophylaxis and a maximum of lifelong prophylaxis. This approach has been validated in a study from Chile.[14]

Of equal importance is the prevention of infective endocarditis in patients with rheumatic heart disease or in those who have had rheumatic fever by administration of antimicrobial drugs before and after surgical procedures on the eyes, ears, mouth (dental extractions), nose, throat, and gastrointestinal and genitourinary tracts.[34, 35]

CONCLUSION

Although it is gratifying to have effective prophylaxis against a disease of which the pathophysiology is understood incompletely and for which there is no pharmacologic cure, rheumatic fever and its sequelae still occur in an appreciable number of young people. This is, in large part, a reflection of complacency about rheumatic fever and rheumatic heart disease among doctors and patients. Renewed educational efforts concerning this preventable disorder, among both physicians and the public, are needed. The available preventive methods should be applied vigorously.

References

1. Abernathy, M., Bass, N., Sharpe, N., et al.: Doppler echocardiography and the early diagnosis of carditis in acute rheumatic fever. Aust. N. Z. J. Med. *24*:530–535, 1994.
2. Agarwal, B. L.: Rheumatic Fever and Rheumatic Heart Disease in Developing Countries. India, Arnold Publishers, 1988, pp. 24–25.
3. Albert, D. A., Hafel, L., and Karrison, T.: The treatment of rheumatic carditis: A review and meta-analysis. Medicine *74*:1–12, 1995.
4. Amoils, B., Morrison, R. C., Wadee, A. A., et al.: Aberrant expression of HLA-DR antigen on valvular fibroblasts from patients with active rheumatic carditis. Clin. Exp. Immunol. *66*:88–94, 1986.
5. Anonymous: WHO evaluation of the streptozyme test for streptococcal antibodies. Bull. W. H. O. *64*:504, 1986.
6. Anonymous: Rheumatic fever and rheumatic heart disease. Lancet *1*:143–144, 1982.
7. Antunes, M. J.: Mitral valvuloplasty, a better alternative: Comparative study between valve reconstruction and replacement for rheumatic mitral valve disease. Eur. J. Cardiothorac. Surg. *4*:257–264, 1990.
8. Atha, M., Enos, E., Frank, C., et al.: How an American Indian tribe controlled the streptococcus. World Health Forum *3*:423–428, 1982.
9. Baird, R. W., Bronze, M. S., Kraus, W., et al.: Epitopes of group A streptococcal M protein shared with antigens of articular cartilage and synovium. J. Immunol. *146*:31–3137, 1991.
10. Barlow, J. B.: Aspects of active rheumatic carditis. Aust. N. Z. J. Med. *22*:592–600, 1992.
11. Bass, J. W.: Streptococcal pharyngitis in children: A comparison of four treatment schedules with intramuscular benzathine penicillin. J. A. M. A. *235*:1112, 1976.
12. Beachey, E. H., Seyer, J. M., Dale, J. B., et al.: Type-specific protective immunity evoked by synthetic peptide of *Streptococcus pyogenes* M protein. Nature *292*:457–459, 1981.
13. Beachey, E. H., Bronze, M., Dale, K. B., et al.: Protective and autoimmune epitopes of streptococcal M proteins. Vaccine *6*:192–196, 1988.
14. Berrios, X., del Campo, E., Guzman, B., et al.: Discontinuing rheumatic fever prophylaxis in selected adolescents and young adults: A prospective study. Ann. Intern. Med. *118*:401–406, 1993.
15. Bisno, A. L.: The concept of rheumatogenic and nephritogenic group A streptococci. *In* Read, S. E., and Zabriskie, J. B. (eds.): Streptococcal Diseases and the Immune Response. New York, Academic, 1980, pp. 789–804.
16. Bisno, A. L., Pearce, I. A., and Stollerman, G. H.: Streptococcal infections that fail to cause recurrences of rheumatic fever. J. Infect. Dis. *136*:278–285, 1977.
17. Bisno, A. L., and Land, M. A.: Incidence of acute rheumatic fever in Memphis and Shelby County, Tennessee, 1977–1981. *In* Shulman, A. (ed.): Management of Pharyngitis in an Era of Declining Rheumatic Fever. Columbus, Ross Laboratories, 1984, pp. 13–24.
18. Bland, E. F., and Jones, T. D: Rheumatic fever and rheumatic heart disease: A twenty-year report on 1,000 patients followed since childhood. Circulation *4*:836–843, 1951.
19. Brant, L. J., Bender, T. R., and Bross, D. S.: Evaluation of an Alaskan streptococcal control program: Importance of the program's intensity and duration. Prev. Med. *15*:632–642, 1986.
20. Brennan, R. E., and Patel, M. S.: Acute rheumatic fever and rheumatic heart disease in a rural central Australian aboriginal community. Med. J. Aust. *153*:335–339, 1990.
21. Bronze, M. S., Beachey, E. H., and Dale, J. B.: Protective and heart-crossreactive epitopes located within the NH_2 terminus of type 19 streptococcal M protein. J. Exp. Med. *167*:1849–1859, 1988.
22. Brownell, K. D., and Baileu-Rose, F.: Acute rheumatic fever in children. J. A. M. A. *224*:1593–1597, 1973.
23. Cairns, L. M.: Immunological studies in rheumatic fever: The immunology of rheumatic fever. N. Z. Med. J. *101*:388–391, 1988.
24. Catanzaro, F. J., Stetson, C. A., Morris, A. J., et al.: The role of the streptococcus in the pathogenesis of rheumatic fever. Am. J. Med. *17*:749–756, 1954.
25. Catanzaro, F. J., Rammelkamp, C. H., Jr., and Chamovitz, R.: Prevention of rheumatic fever by treatment of streptococcal infections. II. Factors responsible for failures. N. Engl. J. Med. *259*:51–57, 1958.
26. Centers for Disease Control and Prevention: Acute rheumatic fever among army trainees: Fort Leonard Wood, Missouri, 1987–88. M. M. W. R. *37*:519–522, 1988.
27. Centers for Disease Control and Prevention: Availability of sulfadiazine—United States. M. M. W. R. *41*:950–951, 1992.
28. Chauvaud, S., Perier, P., Touati, G., et al.: Long-term results of valve repair in children with acquired mitral valve incompetence. Circulation *74*(Suppl. 1):104–109, 1986.
29. Chun, L. T., Reddy, D. V., and Yamamoto, L. G.: Rheumatic fever in children and adolescents in Hawaii. Pediatrics *79*:549–552, 1987.
30. Congeni, B., Rizzo, C., Congeni, J., et al.: Outbreak of acute rheumatic fever in northeast Ohio. J. Pediatr. *111*:176–179, 1987.
31. Combined Rheumatic Fever Study Group, 1965: A comparison of short-term, intensive prednisone and acetylsalicylic acid therapy in the treatment of acute rheumatic fever. N. Engl. J. Med. *272*:63–70, 1965.
32. Coulehan, J., Grant, S., Reisinger, K., et al.: Acute rheumatic fever and rheumatic heart disease on the Navajo Reservation, 1962–77. Public Health Rep. *95*:62–68, 1980.
33. Cunningham, M., and Russell, M.: Study of heart-reactive antibody in antisera and hybridoma culture fluids against group A streptococci. Infect. Immun. *42*:531–538, 1983.
34. Dajani, A., Taubert, K., Ferrieri, P., et al.: Treatment of acute streptococcal pharyngitis and prevention of rheumatic fever: A statement for health professionals. Pediatrics *96*:758–764, 1995.
35. Dajani, A. S., Bisno, A. L., Chung, K., et al.: Prevention of bacterial endocarditis. Recommendations by the American Heart Association. J. A. M. A. *264*:2919–2922, 1990.
36. Dale, J. B., and Beachey, E. H.: Human cytotoxic T lymphocytes evoked by group A streptococcal M proteins. J. Exp. Med. *166*:1825–1837, 1987.
37. Dale, J. B., and Beachey, E. H.: Epitopes of streptococcal M proteins shared with cardiac myosin. J. Exp. Med. *162*:583–591, 1985.
38. Dale, J. B., and Beachey, E. H.: Protective antigenic determinant of streptococcal M protein shared with sarcolemmal membrane protein of human heart. J. Exp. Med. *156*:1165–1176, 1982.
39. Daly, J. A., Korgenski, E. K., Munson, A. C., et al.: Optical immunoassay for streptococcal pharyngitis: Evaluation of accuracy with routine and mucoid strains associated with acute rheumatic fever outbreak in the intermountain area of the United States. J. Clin. Microbiol. *32*:531–532, 1994.
40. de Cunto, C. L., Giannini, E. H., Fink, C. W., et al.: Prognosis of children with post-streptococcal reactive arthritis. Pediatr. Infect. Dis. J. *7*:683–686, 1988.
41. Denny, F. W.: A 45-year perspective on the streptococcus and rheumatic fever: The Edward H. Kass lecture in infectious disease history. Clin. Infect. Dis. *19*:1110–1122, 1994.

42. Denny, F. W., Wannamaker, L. W., Brink, W. R., et al.: Prevention of rheumatic fever: Treatment of the preceding streptococcic infection. J. A. M. A. *143*:151–153, 1950.
43. Eckerd, J. M., and McJunkin, J. E.: Recent increase in incidence of acute rheumatic fever in southern West Virginia. Scientific Newsfront *85*:279–281, 1989.
44. Editorial: Treatment of rheumatic fever. N. Engl. J. Med. *272*:101–102, 1965.
45. Feinstein, A. R., and Areralo, A. C.: Manifestations and treatment of congestive heart failure in young patients with rheumatic heart disease. Pediatrics *33*:661, 1964.
46. Feldman, B. M., Zabriskie, J. B., Silverman, E. D., et al.: Diagnostic use of B-cell alloantigen D8/17 in rheumatic chorea. J. Pediatr. *123*:84–86, 1993.
47. Ferguson, G. W., Shultz, J. M., and Bisno, A. L.: Epidemiology of acute rheumatic fever in a multiethnic multiracial urban community: The Miami-Dade County experience. J. Infect. Dis. *164*:720–725, 1991.
48. Folger, G. M., Jr., Hajar, R., Robida, A., et al.: Occurrence of valvular heart disease in acute rheumatic fever without evident carditis: Colour flow Doppler identification. Br. Heart. J. *67*:434–438, 1992.
49. Folger, G. M., Jr., and Hajar, R.: Doppler echocardiographic findings of mitral and aortic valve regurgitation in children manifesting only rheumatic arthritis. Am. J. Cardiol. *63*:1278–1280, 1989.
50. Gerber, M. A., Randolph, M. A., Chanatry, J., et al.: Antigen detection test for streptococcal pharyngitis: Evaluation of sensitivity with respect to true infections. J. Pediatr. *108*:654–658, 1986.
51. Goldstein, I., Halpern, B., and Robert, L.: Immunologic relationship between streptococcal A polysaccharide and structural glycoproteins of heart valve. Nature *213*:44–47, 1967.
52. Gordis, L.: Studies in the epidemiology and preventability of rheumatic fever. II. Socio-economic factors and the incidence of acute attacks. J. Chron. Dis. *21*:655–666, 1969.
53. Gordis, L.: Studies in the epidemiology and preventability of rheumatic fever. I. Demographic factors and the incidence of acute attacks. J. Chron. Dis. *21*:645–654, 1969.
54. Gordis, L., Lilienfeld, A., and Rodriguez, R.: A community-wide study of acute rheumatic fever in adults: Epidemiologic and preventive factors. J. A. M. A. *210*.862–865, 1969.
55. Gordis, L.: Effectiveness of comprehensive-care programs in preventing rheumatic fever. N. Engl. J. Med. *289*:331–335, 1973.
56. Gray, E. D., Regelmann, W. E., Abdin, Z., et al.: Compartmentalization of cells bearing "rheumatic" cell surface anitgens in peripheral blood and tonsils in rheumatic heart disease. J. Infect. Dis. *155*:247–252, 1987.
56a. Griffiths, S. P., and Gersony, W. M.: Acute rheumatic fever in New York City (1969–1988): A comparative study of two decades. J. Pediatr. *116*:882–887, 1990.
57. Herold, B. C., and Shulman, S. T.: Poststreptococcal arthritis. Pediatr. Infect. Dis. *7*:681–682, 1988.
58. Homer, C., and Shulman, S. T.: Clinical aspects of acute rheumatic fever. J. Rheumatol. *18*(Suppl. 29):2–13, 1991.
59. Hosier, D. M., Graenen, J., Teske, D. W., et al.: Resurgence of rheumatic fever. Am. J. Dis. Child. *141*:730–733, 1987.
60. International Rheumatic Fever Study Group: Allergic reactions to long-term benzathine penicillin prophylaxis for rheumatic fever. Lancet *337*:1308–1310, 1990.
61. Kaplan, E. L., Top, F. H., Dudding, B. A., et al.: Diagnosis of streptococcal pharyngitis: Differentiation of acute infection from the carrier state in the symptomatic child. J. Infect. Dis. *123*:490–501, 1971.
62. Kaplan, E. L.: Acute rheumatic fever. Pediatr. Clin. North Am. *25*:817–829, 1978.
63. Kaplan, E. L., Johnson, D. R., and Cleary, P. P.: Group A streptococcal serotypes isolated from patients and sibling contacts during the resurgence of rheumatic fever in the United States in the mid-1980s. J. Infect. Dis. *159*:101–103, 1989.
64. Kaplan, E. L., Berrios, X., Speth, J., et al.: Pharmacokinetics of benzathine penicillin G: Serum levels during the 28 days after intramuscular injection of 1,200,000 units. J. Pediatr. *115*:146–150, 1989.
65. Kaplan, E. L.: Epidemiological approaches to understanding the pathogenesis of rheumatic fever. Int. J. Epidemiol. *14*:499–501, 1985.
66. Kaplan, M. H., Bolande, R., Rakaita, L., et al.: Presence of bound immunoglobulins and complement in the myocardium in acute rheumatic fever. N. Engl. J. Med. *271*:637–645, 1964.
67. Kaplan, E. L., Johnson, D. R., Nanthapisud, P., et al.: A comparison of group A streptococcal serotypes isolated from the upper respiratory tract in the USA and Thailand: Implications. Bull. W. H. O. *70*:433–437, 1992.
68. Kaplan, E. L., and Wannamaker, L. W.: Streptolysin O: Suppression of its antigenicity by lipids extracted from skin. Proc. Soc. Exp. Med. *146*:205–208, 1974.
69. Kumar, R.: Controlling rheumatic heart disease in developing countries. World Health Forum *16*:47–51, 1995.
70. Laitinen, O., Leirisalo, M., and Allander, E.: Rheumatic fever and *Yersinia* arthritis: Criteria and diagnostic problems in a changing disease pattern. Scand. J. Rheumatol. *4*:145–157, 1975.
71. Land, M. A., and Bisno, A. L.: Acute rheumatic fever: A vanishing disease in suburbia. J. A. M. A. *249*:895–898, 1983.
72. Leggiadro, R. J., Birnbaum, S. E., Chase, N. A., et al.: A resurgence of acute rheumatic fever in a mid-south children's hospital. South. Med. J. *83*:1418–1420, 1990.
73. Lennon, D., Martin, D., Wong, E., et al.: Longitudinal study of poststreptococcal disease in Auckland: Rheumatic fever, glomerulonephritis, epidemiology and M typing 1981–86. N. Z. Med. J. *101*:396–398, 1988.
74. Lieu, T. A., Fleisher, G. R., and Schwartz, J. S.: Cost-effectiveness of rapid latex agglutination and throat culture for streptococcal pharyngitis. Pediatrics *85*:246–256, 1990.
75. Lue, H. C., Wu, M. H., Wang, J. K., et al.: Long-term outcome of patients with rheumatic fever receiving benzathine penicillin G prophylaxis every three weeks versus every four weeks. J. Pediatr. *125*:812–816, 1994.
76. Majeed, H. A., Yousof, A. M., Khuffash, F. A., et al.: The natural history of acute rheumatic fever in Kuwait: A prospective 6-year follow-up report. J. Chron. Dis. *39*:361–369, 1986.
77. Majeed, H. A., Yousof, A. M., Rotta, J., et al.: Group A streptococcal strains in Kuwait: A nine-year prospective study of prevalence and associations. Pediatr. Infect. Dis. J. *11*:295–300, 1992.
78. Markowitz, M., and Gordis, L.: Rheumatic Fever. Philadelphia, W. B. Saunders, 1972, pp. 62–63.
79. Markowitz, M., and Kaplan, E. L.: Reappearance of rheumatic fever. Adv. Pediatr. *36*:39–68, 1989.
80. Markowitz, M.: Evolution and critique of changes in the Jones criteria for diagnosis of rheumatic fever. N. Z. Med. J. *101*:392–394, 1988.
81. Markowitz, M., and Gordis, L.: Rheumatic Fever. Philadelphia, W. B. Saunders, 1972, pp. 80–102.
82. Markowitz, M., and Gordis, L.: Rheumatic Fever. Philadelphia, W. B. Saunders, 1972, pp. 133–136.
83. Markowitz, M.: Streptococcal disease in developing countries. Pediatr. Infect. Dis. J. *10*:S11–S38, 1991.
84. Marrack, P., and Kappler, J.: The staphylococcal enterotoxins and their relatives. Science *248*:705–711, 1990.
85. Martin, D. R., Voss, L. M., Walker, S. J., et al.: Acute rheumatic fever in Auckland, New Zealand: Spectrum of associated group A streptococci different from expected. Pediatr. Infect. Dis. J. *13*:264–269, 1994.
86. Martin, D. R., and Single, L. A.: Molecular epidemiology of group A *Streptococcus* M type 1 infections. J. Infect. Dis. *167*:1112–1117, 1993.
87. Martin, D. R.: Rheumatogenic streptococci reconsidered. N. Z. Med. J. *101*:394–396, 1988.
88. Massell, B. F., Chute, C. G., Walker, A. M., et al.: Penicillin and the marked decrease in morbidity and mortality from rheumatic fever in the United States. N. Engl. J. Med. *318*:280–286, 1988.
89. Massell, B., Amezcuac, F., and Pelargonio, S.: Evolving picture of rheumatic fever: Data from 40 years at the House of the Good Samaritan. J. A. M. A. *188*:287–294, 1964.
90. Massell, B. F., Honikman, L. H., and Amezcua, F. J.: Rheumatic fever following streptococcal vaccine: Report of 3 cases. J. A. M. A. *207*.1115–1119, 1969.
91. McLaren, M. J., Hawkins, D. M., Koornhof, H. J., et al.: Epidemiology of rheumatic heart disease in black school children of Soweto, Johannesburg. Br. Med. J. *3*:474–477, 1975.
92. Moore, P., and Mortland, T.: *Mycoplasma pneumoniae* infection mimicking acute rheumatic fever. Pediatr. Infect. Dis. J. *13*:81–82, 1994.
93. Morris, K., Mohan, C., Wahi, P. L., et al.: Increased inactivated T cells and reduction in suppressor/cytotoxic T cells in acute rheumatic fever and active heart disease: A longitudinal study. J. Infect. Dis. *167*:3979–3983, 1993.
94. Morris, K., Mohan, C., Wahi, P., et al.: Enhancement of IL-1, IL-2 production and IL-2 receptor generation in patients with acute rheumatic fever and active rheumatic heart disease: A prospective study. Clin. Exp. Immunol. *91*:429–436, 1993.
95. Morton, W. E., Huhn, L. A., and Litchy, J. A.: Rheumatic heart disease epidemiology: Observations on 17,366 Denver schoolchildren. J. A. M. A. *199*:879–884, 1967.
96. Nausieda, P. A., Grossman, B. J., Koller, W. C., et al.: Sydenham chorea: An update. Neurology *30*:331–334, 1980.
97. Newman, J. E., Lennon, D. R., and Wong-Toi, W.: Patients with rheumatic fever recurrences. N. Z. Med. J. *97*:678–680, 1984.
98. Pataroyo, M. E., Winchester, R. J., Vejerano, A., et al.: Association of a B cell alloantigen with susceptibility to rheumatic fever. Nature *278*:173–174, 1979.
99. Paul, J. R.: Epidemiology of Rheumatic Fever. 3rd ed. New York, American Heart Association, 1957, pp. 46–56.
100. Perry, C. B., and Roberts, J. A. F.: A study on the variability in the incidence of rheumatic heart disease within the city of Bristol. Br. Med. J. *193*(Suppl.):154–158, 1937.
101. Phibbs, B., Lundin, S. R., Watson, W. B., et al.: Experience of a Wyoming county streptococcal control project. West. J. Med. *148*:546–550, 1988.
102. Pickles, W. N.: A rheumatic family. Lancet *2*:241, 1943.
103. Pinals, R.: Polyarthritis and fever. N. Engl. J. Med. *330*:769–774, 1994.
104. Pruksakorn, S., Currie, B., Brandt, E., et al.: Towards a vaccine for rheumatic fever: Identification of a conserved target epitope on M protein of group A streptococci. Lancet *344*:639–642, 1994.
105. Quinn, R. W., and Federspiel, C. F.: The incidence of rheumatic fever in metropolitan Nashville, 1963–1969. Am. J. Epidemiol. *99*:273–280, 1974.
106. Raizada, V., Williams, R. C., Chopra, P., et al.: Tissue distribution of

lymphocytes in rheumatic heart valves as defined by monoclonal anti-T cell antibodies. Am. J. Med. 74:90–96, 1983.
107. Rammelkamp, C. H., Denny, F. W., and Wannamaker, L. W.: Studies on the epidemiology of rheumatic fever in the armed services. *In* Thomas, L. (ed.): Rheumatic Fever. Minneapolis, University of Minnesota Press, 1972, p. 72.
108. Rammelkamp, C. H., Jr., and Stolzer, B. L.: The latent period before the onset of acute rheumatic fever. Yale J. Biol. Med. *34*:386–398, 1961.
109. Randolph, M. F., Gerber, M. A., De Meo, K. K., et al.: Effect of antibiotic therapy on the clinical course of streptococcal pharyngitis. J. Pediatr. *106*:870–875, 1985.
110. Redd, S. C., Facklam, R. R., Collin, S., et al.: Rapid group A streptococcal antigen detection kit: Effect on antimicrobial therapy for acute pharyngitis. Pediatrics *82*:576–581, 1988.
111. Reddy, D. V., Chun, L. T., and Yamamoto, L. G.: Acute rheumatic fever with advanced degree AV block. Clin. Pediatr. *28*:326–328, 1989.
112. Regelmann, W. E., Talbot, R., Cairns, L., et al.: Distribution of cells bearing "rheumatic" antigens in peripheral blood of patients with rheumatic fever/rheumatic heart disease. J. Rheumatol. *16*:931–935, 1989.
113. Rhodes, P., and Jackson, H.: Rheumatic fever in Colorado: A conquered disease? J. A. M. A. *234*:157–158, 1975.
114. Robbins, S. L.: The heart: Rheumatic fever and rheumatic heart disease. *In* Cotran, R. S., Kumar, V., and Robbins, S. L. (eds.): Robbins Pathologic Basis of Disease. 4th ed. Philadelphia, W. B. Saunders, 1994, pp. 547–550.
115. Sanyal, S. K., Thapar, M. K., Ahmed, S. H., et al.: The initial attack of acute rheumatic fever during childhood in north India: A prospective study of the clinical profile. Circulation *49*:7–12, 1974.
116. Sanyal, S. K., Berry, A. M., Duggal, S., et al.: Sequelae of the initial attack of acute rheumatic fever in children from north India. Circulation *65*:375–379, 1982.
117. Shulman, S. T.: The decline of rheumatic fever: What impact on our management of pharyngitis? Am. J. Dis. Child. *128*:426–427, 1984.
118. Siegal, A. C., Johnson, E. E., and Stollerman, G. H.: Controlled studies of streptococcal pharyngitis in a pediatric population. N. Engl. J. Med. *265*:559–566, 1961.
119. Single, L. A., and Martin, D. R.: Clonal differences within M-types of the group A streptococci revealed by pulsed field gel electrophoresis. FEMS Microbiol. Lett. *91*:85–90, 1992.
120. Spagnuolo, M., and Taranta, M.: Rheumatic fever in siblings: Similarity of its clinical manifestations. N. Engl. J. Med. *278*:183–188, 1968.
121. Special Writing Group of the Committee on Rheumatic Fever, Endocarditis and Kawasaki Disease of the Council on Cardiovascular Disease in the Young of the American Heart Association: Jones criteria, 1992 update. J. A. M. A. *268*:2069–2073, 1992.
122. Stollerman, G. H.: Rheumatogenic streptococci and autoimmunity. Clin. Immunol. Immunopathol. *61*:131–142, 1991.
123. Stollerman, G. H.: Rheumatic Fever and Streptococcal Infection. New York, Grune & Stratton, 1975, pp. 79–86.
124. Stollerman, G. H., Lewis, A. J., Schultz, I., et al.: Relationship of immune response to group A streptococci to the course of acute, chronic and recurrent rheumatic fever. Am. J. Med. *20*:163–169, 1956.
125. Strauss, A. W., Goldring, D., Kissane, J., et al.: Valve replacement in acute rheumatic heart disease. J. Thorac. Cardiovasc. Surg. *67*:659–670, 1974.
126. Taranta, A., Spagnuolo, M., and Feinstein, A. R.: "Chronic" rheumatic fever. Ann. Intern. Med. *56*:367–388, 1962.
127. Taranta, A., Torosdag, S., Metrakos, J. D., et al.: Rheumatic fever in monozygotic and dizygotic twins. Circulation *20*:778, 1959.
127a. Taranta, A., and Markowitz, M.: Rheumatic Fever. 2nd ed. Dordrecht, Kluwer Academic Publishers, 1989, pp. 61–65.
128. Taubert, K. A., Rowley, A. H., and Shulman, S. T.: Seven-year national survey of Kawasaki disease and acute rheumatic fever. Pediatr. Infect. Dis. J. *13*:704–708, 1994.
129. Tomai, M., Kotb, M., Majumdar, G., et al.: Superantigenicity of streptococcal M protein. J. Exp. Med. *172*:359–362, 1990.
130. Tompkins, R. K., Burnes, D. C., and Cable, W. E.: An analysis of the cost-effectiveness of pharyngitis management and acute rheumatic fever prevention. Ann. Intern. Med. *86*:481–492, 1977.
131. U. K. and U. S. Joint Report: The natural history of rheumatic fever and rheumatic heart disease: Cooperative clinical trial of ACTH, cortisone and aspirin. Circulation *32*:457–476, 1965.
132. Veasy, L. G., Wiedmeier, S. E., Orsmond, G. S., et al.: Resurgence of acute rheumatic fever in the intermountain area of the United States. N. Engl. J. Med. *316*:421–427, 1987.
133. Veasy, L. G., Tani, L. Y., and Hill, H. R.: Persistence of acute rheumatic fever in the intermountain area of the United States. J. Pediatr. *124*:9–11, 1994.
134. Vendsborg, P., Fauerholdt, L., and Olsen, K. H.: Decreasing incidence of a history of acute rheumatic fever in chronic rheumatic heart disease. Cardiologica *53*:332–340, 1968.
135. Vlajinac, H., Adanja, B., Marinkovic, J., et al.: Influence of socio-economic and other factors on rheumatic fever occurrence. Eur. J. Epidemiol. *7*:702–704, 1991.
136. Wald, E. R., Dashefsky, B., Feidt, C., et al.: Acute rheumatic fever in western Pennsylvania and the Tri-State Area. Pediatrics *80*:371–374, 1987.
137. Wallace, M. R., Garst, P. D., Papadimos, T. J., et al.: The return of acute rheumatic fever in young adults. J. A. M. A. *262*:2557–2561, 1989.
138. Wannamaker, L. W., Denny, F. W., Perry, W. D., et al.: The effect of penicillin prophylaxis on streptococcal disease rates and the carrier state. N. Engl. J. Med. *249*:1–7, 1953.
139. Wannamaker, L. W., Rammelkamp, C. H., Jr., Denny, F. W., et al.: Prophylaxis of acute rheumatic fever by treatment of the preceding streptococcal infection with various amounts of depot penicillin. Am. J. Med. *10*:673–695, 1951.
140. Wannamaker, L. W.: Differences between streptococcal infections of the skin and of the throat. N. Engl. J. Med. *282*:23–30, 78–85, 1970.
141. Wannamaker, L. W.: Virulence factors in streptococci. Scand. J. Infect. Dis. *31*(Suppl.):22–27, 1982.
142. Westlake, R. M., Graham, T. A., and Edwards, K. M.: An outbreak of acute rheumatic fever in Tennessee. Pediatr. Infect. Dis. J. *9*:97–100, 1990.
143. Widdowson, J. P., Maxted, W. R., Notley, C. M., et al.: The antibody responses in man to infection with different serotypes of group A streptococci. J. Med. Microbiol. *7*:483, 1974.
144. Wilson, N. J., and Neutze, J. M.: Echocardiographic diagnosis of subclinical carditis in acute rheumatic fever. Int. J. Cardiol. *50*:1–6, 1995.
145. Wood, H. F., Feinstein, A. R., Taranta, A., et al.: Rheumatic fever in adolescents: A long-term epidemiologic study of subsequent prophylaxis, streptococcal infections, and clinical sequelae. III. Comparative effectiveness of three prophylaxis regimens in preventing streptococcal infections and rheumatic recurrences. Ann. Intern. Med. *60*(Suppl.):31–45, 1964.
146. Zabriskie, J. B.: Rheumatic fever: A model for the pathological consequences of microbial-host mimicry. Clin. Exp. Rheum. *4*:65–73, 1986.
147. Zabriskie, J. B., Lavench, D., Williams, R. C., et al.: Rheumatic fever–associated B cell alloantigens as identified by monoclonal antibodies. Arth. Rheum. *28*:1047–1051, 1985.
148. Zangwill, K. M., Wald, E. M., and Londino, A. V.: Acute rheumatic fever in western Pennsylvania: A persistent problem into the 1990's. J. Pediatr. *118*:561–563, 1991.
149. Zedan, M. M., El-Shennawy, F. A., Abou-Bakr, H. M., et al.: Interleukin-2 in relation to T cell subpopulations in rheumatic heart disease. Arch. Dis. Child. *67*:1373–1375, 1992.

36

NONINFECTIOUS CARDITIS

David R. Fulton and Jane G. Schaller

A number of diseases, primarily of the rheumatic disease category, are associated with carditis that presumably is noninfectious in nature. Rheumatic fever, the principal rheumatic disease affecting the heart, is presented in Chapter 35. Cardiac manifestations of other rheumatic diseases, including juvenile rheumatoid arthritis (JRA), ankylosing spondylitis, Reiter disease, systemic lupus erythematosus (SLE), the various vasculitis syndromes, scleroderma, dermatomyositis, and miscellaneous other diseases, are discussed here. All at times may mimic infectious diseases.

The etiologies and pathogenetic mechanisms of the rheumatic diseases are poorly understood. All are associated with chronic inflammation of various connective tissues throughout the body. Heart disease results when cardiac connective tissue is affected by such inflammation. Various regions of the heart can be involved, including the pericardium, myocardium, endocardium, coronary blood vessels, and conduction system. In some diseases, notably SLE, immune complex disease appears to be responsible for much of the inflammation and tissue damage[30, 84]; however, the primary causes of lupus itself and of the associated immune complex formation remain obscure. Immune complex mechanisms also have been shown in seropositive rheumatoid arthritis and certain forms of vasculitis.[18, 54] The finding of hepatitis antigen as the causal agent in some instances of polyarteritis,[54] presumably by an immune complex mechanism, suggests that infectious agents in fact may play a role in some rheumatic disease syndromes. However, the mechanisms of inflammation observed in most rheumatic diseases remain unknown; for example, although beta-hemolytic streptococcal infections long have been a known antecedent event for rheumatic fever, the ways in which such infections cause disease have yet to be elucidated.

Diagnoses of the various rheumatic diseases rest largely on the clinical appearances of patients; certain laboratory tests and radiographs also may be helpful. Each rheumatic disease presents a reasonably characteristic type and pattern of tissue involvement; for example, rheumatoid arthritis is characterized by chronic synovitis, dermatomyositis by inflammation of muscle and skin, and scleroderma by hardening of skin and subcutaneous tissues. There currently is no explanation for the varying and distinctive patterns of tissue involvement in these diseases. Although there are no diagnostic laboratory tests, investigations such as antinuclear antibodies, rheumatoid factors, histocompatibility antigens, radiographs, and tissue histology may be useful in classifying patients (Table 36–1).

Types of cardiac involvement that have been observed in the various rheumatic diseases are summarized in Table 36–2. Cardiac involvement, particularly pericarditis and myocarditis, can occur as isolated events without proven infectious or rheumatic etiology. Rheumatic diseases (other than rheumatic fever) most frequently associated with cardiac involvement include systemic-onset JRA (pericarditis affects 25 to 50 per cent of patients), SLE (various heart lesions affect 20 to 40 per cent of patients), and infantile polyarteritis (coronary vasculitis is found in nearly all reported patients).

PERICARDITIS

In pericarditis, the pericardium, or outer layer of the heart, is the site of inflammation. The pericardium may become thickened as a result of inflammation or fibrosis. Excessive production of pericardial fluid may give rise to pericardial effusions. If the pericardium merely is inflamed, no cardiac enlargement may be apparent but friction rubs may be heard; these often are transient and changeable. If the pericardium becomes chronically fibrotic, signs of constrictive pericarditis may ensue. If enough excess pericardial fluid is produced, signs of pericardial effusion will result. If cardiac output is compromised by pericardial constriction, from either pericardial thickening or pressure from pericardial effusion, physical signs of cardiac tamponade or cardiac failure may occur.

The pericarditis associated with rheumatic diseases may be entirely asymptomatic. The most common symptom is pain, generally substernal or anterior precordial, often exacerbated by lying flat, and sometimes referred to the left shoulder or arm. Dyspnea or tachypneas also may be present. With large pericardial effusions or with constrictive pericarditis, signs of heart failure may be present. Physical findings of pericarditis include pericardial friction rubs, tachypnea, cardiac enlargement, and congestive heart failure. With constrictive pericarditis, hepatomegaly is a cardinal sign.

TABLE 36–1. Clinical and Laboratory Features of the Rheumatic Diseases

	Characteristic Clinical Features	Laboratory Characteristics
Juvenile rheumatoid arthritis	Chronic synovitis Several subgroups Systemic-onset RF-negative polyarthritis RF-positive polyarthritis Pauciarthritis—chronic iridocyclitis Pauciarthritis—sacroiliitis	Radiographic evidence of destructive arthritis—10–30% RF—10% (RF-positive polyarthritis subgroup) ANA—25% (associated with chronic iridocyclitis)
Ankylosing spondylitis	Sacroiliitis Spinal arthritis	HL-A B27—95% Radiographic sacroiliitis—100% Radiographic spinal arthritis—late
Systemic lupus erythematosus	Multisystem disease Facial rash—50%	ANA—100% Other "autoantibodies" and lowered levels of serum hemolytic complement DNA antibodies—50% Histology: hematoxylin bodies
Dermatomyositis	Myositis, rash	Elevated serum levels of "muscle" enzymes Abnormal electromyogram Histologic myositis
Scleroderma	Cutaneous involvement	Histology of lesions ANA, RF common
Vasculitis	Multisystem disease Several distinct syndromes Henoch-Schönlein vasculitis Polyarteritis nodosa Infantile polyarteritis and mucocutaneous lymph node syndrome	Histologic vasculitis Arteriography

RF, rheumatoid factors; ANA, antinuclear antibodies.

TABLE 36–2. Cardiac Manifestations of Rheumatic Diseases

	Pericarditis	Myocarditis	Endocarditis	Coronary Vasculitis
Juvenile rheumatoid arthritis	Systemic onset + RF*-positive +	Systemic onset ± RF-positive ±	RF-positive ±	–
Ankylosing spondylitis	±	±	+ (Aortitis)	–
Systemic lupus erythematosus	+	+	+	+
Dermatomyositis	±	±	–	–
Scleroderma	+	+	±	–
Vasculitis	+	±	+	+

*RF, rheumatoid factors; ±, <5% of patients; +, ≥5% of patients; –, not associated.

Diagnosis of pericarditis rests first on suspicion of its presence. The possibility of pericarditis should be considered in any rheumatic disease patient with chest pain or dyspnea. Diagnosis depends on the demonstration of a pericardial friction rub or of pericardial fluid or thickening. The latter may be suspected on the basis of physical findings or chest radiograph and confirmed by echocardiography. Echocardiography can detect small effusions not sufficient to suggest cardiac enlargement by radiograph.[137] Electrocardiographic changes of pericarditis are not specific and may be lacking. In many instances, the pericarditis of rheumatic diseases entirely is subclinical and may be found only with incidental echocardiography[9, 16] or at autopsy.[94] On the other hand, some individuals with symptoms suggestive of pericarditis may have entirely normal findings, including echocardiography.

In the rheumatic diseases, pericarditis generally is serofibrinous in nature. Similar pleuritis, with or without pleural effusion, often also is present. This type of pericarditis resembles viral rather than bacterial pericarditis. The course generally is benign, although congestive heart failure sometimes occurs. Attacks often are self-limited but may recur. In a few rheumatic diseases, notably seropositive rheumatoid arthritis, subsequent chronic constrictive pericarditis has been reported. Pericardiocentesis to determine rheumatic etiology usually is not diagnostic.[113]

Juvenile Rheumatoid Arthritis

Significant pericarditis[9, 16, 55, 94] is associated with two subgroups of JRA: systemic-onset and seropositive disease; it occurs rarely in other patients.

In systemic-onset JRA, from 25 to 50 per cent of patients have clinical signs of pericarditis[122, 125] and higher percentages can be found by echocardiography to have pericardial effusions.[9 16] This pericarditis is serofibrinous in nature and often is associated with a similar pleuritis. Pericarditis generally occurs during febrile periods of active systemic JRA and diminishes with remission of the other systemic manifestations, generally within a period of about 6 months. Symptoms include chest pain, dyspnea, tachypnea, and pain on lying flat. Friction rubs, often transient, may be heard, and heart sounds may be muffled. Radiographic evidence of cardiac enlargement and electrocardiographic changes suggestive of pericarditis may be present. Rarely, congestive heart failure ensues. Diagnosis of pericarditis is made on the basis of history and physical and laboratory findings. Infectious pericarditis must be considered in the differential diagnosis, particularly if patients are receiving corticosteroids. Pain also must be differentiated from inflammation of costosternal junctions and other small joints of the anterior chest wall.

Therapy is geared to the underlying systemic JRA. Nonsteroidal agents or salicylates may be effective in children with only mild pericarditis. Maximum therapeutic effect may require several weeks. Congestive heart failure from the pericarditis of systemic-onset JRA is unusual; most pericarditis is relatively benign. Chest pain and dyspnea may be troublesome and may require analgesics or codeine for their relief; narcotics should be avoided for long periods, however. If pericardial effusions are very large or in the presence of congestive heart failure, corticosteroid therapy in doses of 1 to 2 mg/kg body weight of prednisone per 24 hours (40 to 60 mg/24 hours for a teenager) should result in rapid resolution of the pericarditis. Pericardiocentesis is necessary rarely, although tamponade has been reported.[155]

Prognosis for the pericarditis of systemic-onset JRA is excellent,[16, 94, 122, 139] although rare deaths have been reported.[55] Subsequent chronic constrictive pericarditis is not associated. Bouts of pericarditis generally subside within weeks to months. Some patients have recurrent pericarditis associated with subsequent attacks of systemic manifestations in future years.

Pericarditis also occurs in seropositive JRA, a subgroup similar to classic adult-onset rheumatoid arthritis.[125] This pericarditis generally is serofibrinous in nature, although granulomatous lesions resembling rheumatoid nodules sometimes are found in affected pericardium, and occasionally chronic fibrosis with subsequent constriction occurs.[5, 25, 49, 81, 111, 143] Pericarditis diagnosed by physical or electrocardiographic changes has been found in 10 per cent of adult rheumatoid patients,[81] by echocardiographic changes in 50 per cent of adult rheumatoid patients with nodules,[5] and in 40 per cent of adult rheumatoid patients at autopsy.[143] Such pericarditis often occurs years after the onset of disease and thus rarely is recognized during the childhood years. Few other extra-articular manifestations are associated, although affected patients often have severe joint disease. The course of the pericarditis generally is benign, except for those patients with chronic fibrosis and pericardial constriction. Pericardiectomy in those with seropositive disease has been successful in relieving symptoms.[37] Therapy is that of the underlying disease; occasionally, corticosteroids are needed. Distinction must be made from infectious pericarditis occurring as an independent event and from inflammation of chest wall joints.

Systemic Lupus Erythematosus

Serofibrinous pericarditis occurs in 20 to 50 per cent of patients with SLE.[6, 17, 40, 41, 59, 80, 129, 131] The histology of affected pericardium may show hematoxylin bodies, fairly characteristic of SLE, and pericardial fluid may contain typical lupus erythematosus cells, which are formed in vitro.[59] Deposits of immunoglobulins and complement have been identified in the pericardium.[67]

Clinical manifestations and diagnostic tests for pericarditis are similar to those described for systemic-onset JRA: chest pain, dyspnea, friction rub, tachycardia, distant heart sounds, congestive heart failure, cardiac enlargement, nonspecific electrocardiographic changes, and evidence of pericardial effusion on echocardiography. Pericarditis may occur as an isolated event in SLE and even may be the presenting manifestation of disease; it also may occur as a part of multisystem disease at any time during the course of disease. The use of procainamide has led to a drug-induced SLE that has been associated with constrictive pericarditis.[19, 137] Infectious pericarditis must be differentiated from SLE, particularly in patients receiving corticosteroids. Other cardiac manifestations of lupus (coronary vasculitis, myocardial infarction, and endocarditis) also must be differentiated, as must pleural or pulmonary disease of lupus or inflammation of anterior chest wall joints.

The pericarditis of lupus generally is benign and responds well to therapy of the underlying disease. Occasionally, large pericardial effusions or congestive heart failure may demand immediate therapy with corticosteroids.[4] Pericardial thickening can be assessed by echocardiography.[35] Pericardiocentesis rarely is required in younger patients.[1, 38, 73] Pain may respond to aspirin, nonsteroidal anti-inflammatory drugs, or codeine. Prognosis for the pericarditis of SLE is excellent; although bouts may be chronic or recurrent, they rarely interfere with cardiac function and rarely, if ever, result in chronic constriction.[67]

Mixed Connective Tissue Disease

Mixed connective tissue disease is a rheumatic disease syndrome that combines clinical and laboratory features of SLE, rheumatoid arthritis, dermatomyositis, and scleroderma; it is characterized by the presence of high titers of a specific antinuclear antibody reactive with ribonucleoprotein.[130, 132] Pericarditis similar to that of SLE occurs in some patients.

OTHER RHEUMATIC DISEASES OCCASIONALLY ASSOCIATED WITH PERICARDITIS

These include polyarteritis and other vasculitis syndromes,[116] scleroderma,[14, 20, 101, 134, 146] and dermatomyositis.[142, 149] Findings are similar to those described earlier. Chronic fibrosis and constriction occur rarely, if ever.

ISOLATED IDIOPATHIC PERICARDITIS

Pericarditis occurs in a number of individuals with no stigmata of either infectious or rheumatic disease.[36, 71, 154] This pericarditis may occur as a single event or may recur; pleuritis may be associated. High fevers and elevated sedimentation rates may be associated, but there are no clinical or laboratory findings diagnostic of any rheumatic or infectious disease. Although the etiology of this type of pericarditis is unknown, undiagnosed viral pericarditis may be the cause in some cases; the predilection for viral pericarditis to recur is well known. Chest trauma also may be followed by pericarditis. It also is possible that some "isolated pericarditis" represents undiagnosed rheumatic disease with pericarditis as the sole manifestation. Long-term observations are required to sort out the natural history and ultimate outcome. Patients generally respond to salicylates; sometimes corticosteroids are required.

MYOCARDITIS

Myocardial inflammation may be entirely subclinical or may cause significant cardiac dysfunction. Myocardial dysfunction results in loss of normal myocardial contractility with subsequent cardiac dilatation, decreased cardiac output, congestive heart failure, and cardiac arrhythmias. Pathologic changes include collections of inflammatory cells or deposition of fibrinoid in the myocardium, with varying degrees of damage and loss of myocardial fibers. Symptoms of myocarditis are those referable to compromised cardiac function or arrhythmias; generally, pain is not associated. Physical findings may include hypotension, tachycardia, tachypnea, diminished intensity of heart sounds, narrow pulse pressure, hepatomegaly, and rhythm disturbances. Chest radiographs may show increased cardiac size that is not attributable to pericardial fluid. However, early in the course of acute myocarditis, the heart may appear small despite significant cardiac decompensation. Electrocardiographic changes may include low voltages, left ventricular hypertrophy, nonspecific ST- and T-wave changes, and various abnormalities of cardiac rhythm.[89] Echocardiography may be helpful in excluding pericardial effusion as a component of cardiac enlargement and in identifying an enlarged, poorly contractile left ventricle. Serum levels of enzymes found in cardiac muscle may be elevated. Diagnosis of myocarditis is made on the basis of clinical and laboratory findings. Pericarditis often is associated.

Subclinical myocarditis, defined by only electrocardiographic changes or as an incidental autopsy finding, may be found in a number of rheumatic diseases but apparently is of little clinical consequence. Clinically significant myocarditis is quite rare in rheumatic diseases other than rheumatic fever but has been noted in SLE, various vasculitis syndromes, systemic-onset JRA, dermatomyositis, and scleroderma. The differential diagnosis of myocarditis associated with rheumatic diseases includes viral and other infectious myocarditis, various other known familial or metabolic cardiomyopathies, and cardiac amyloidosis.

The treatment of myocarditis is multifaceted. Digitalis should be used cautiously because many of these patients are sensitive to dosages in the therapeutic range. Diuretic therapy should be considered to decrease preload to the myocardium; however, many individuals require an elevated central venous pressure to maintain adequate cardiac output. Afterload reduction therapy using nitroprusside has been a major contribution to management but is dependent on accurate determination of underlying hemodynamics. For the patient with hemodynamic embarrassment, a pulmonary artery wedge catheter should be placed and should be equipped, preferably with a thermistor, for thermodilution determination of cardiac output. Patients with high-degree A-V block and congestive heart failure may require temporary cardiac pacing.

Juvenile Rheumatoid Arthritis

Myocarditis is rare but occurs occasionally[9, 99, 104] in systemic JRA patients who also have pericarditis. Congestive heart failure may be severe, but it generally responds to corticosteroids and diuresis. Patients may be extremely sensitive to digitalis preparations. Episodes of myocarditis may be self-limited or may become chronic.

Myocarditis also has been reported in seropositive rheumatoid arthritis, although it is rarely of clinical significance[90, 135, 151] and often is an incidental postmortem finding. Granulomatous lesions resembling rheumatoid nodules may be found in the myocardium and rarely may cause heart block.[62] Diffuse myocarditis also may be present.

Systemic Lupus Erythematosus

Myocarditis occurs in some lupus patients, as witnessed by electrocardiographic changes and autopsy findings.[17, 40, 41, 131] However, this type of heart involvement is less common in the disease than either pericarditis or endocarditis. Patients with active myositis appear more likely to manifest myocarditis. High titers of anti-RNP antibody also are found in this subset of patients.[13] Pathologic changes include fibrinoid deposition in the myocardium, myocardial inflammation, and inflammation of coronary blood vessels. Myocarditis generally is mild; subsequent congestive heart failure and cardiac arrhythmias are unusual, but the development of complete heart block with death has been reported more frequently, with early onset of atherosclerotic vascular disease and myocardial infarction.[10, 50, 153] Therapy is directed toward the underlying disease.

Dermatomyositis and Polymyositis

Although skeletal muscle involvement is, by definition, present in all patients, recognized involvement of heart muscle occurs only rarely in dermatomyositis and polymyositis. Myocardial involvement may, however, be a rare cause of cardiac arrhythmia, heart block, or congestive heart failure.[61, 96, 126, 133] Reviews of autopsy material suggest that subclinical myocardial inflammation may not be a rare event.[133]

Scleroderma

Myocardial involvement, a potentially fatal event in scleroderma, occurs in a significant number of patients with systemic scleroderma (progressive systemic sclerosis)[68, 112, 118] but rarely, if ever, in association with morphea or linear scleroderma.[85] A strong association has been found between the presence of myositis and myocarditis.[46, 152] The myocardial involvement of scleroderma is characterized histologically by collections of inflammatory cells in the myocardium, myocardial fibrosis, degeneration of myocardial fibers, and thickening of coronary blood vessels, although in one series of patients the coronary blood vessels were reported to be normal.[20] Symptoms include cardiac arrhythmias, cardiac enlargement, or congestive heart failure; some patients have precordial pain suggestive of angina. Laboratory findings include electrocardiographic changes[47] and cardiac enlargement on chest radiograph. Abnormalities of cardiac function indicated by exercise testing and thallium scanning may predate clinical evidence of myocarditis.[45] Cardiac conditions to be differentiated include hypertensive cardiac disease secondary to associated renal hypertension and cor pulmonale resulting from the pulmonary hypertension of scleroderma lung disease. There is no specific therapy for the heart disease of scleroderma; drugs such as corticosteroids, anticancer agents, and penicillamine may be warranted in life-threatening disease.[106] Conventional therapy for heart failure is indicated if present. Regular follow-up with electrocardiogram and Holter monitoring is indicated because of the likelihood for developing serious rhythm disturbances.[152] Scleroderma heart disease generally is slowly and relentlessly progressive and may be fatal.

Polyarteritis and Vasculitis

Myocardial involvement occurs at times in polyarteritis nodosa, sometimes as the result of multiple small cardiac infarcts secondary to vasculitis of the coronary blood vessels.[64] Inflammatory myocarditis of clinical significance is unusual, but electrocardiographic changes suggestive of myocarditis at times are seen in Henoch-Schönlein vasculitis, and it may be that subclinical myocarditis is not a rare event.[2, 66, 97]

ENDOCARDITIS

In endocarditis, inflammation of the inner layer of the heart causes either diffuse thickening of the endocardium (as in endocardial fibroelastosis) or valvular disease. Valvulitis is the identifying sign of acute rheumatic fever but occurs relatively rarely in other rheumatic disease syndromes. In endocarditis, the endocardium, particularly that part constituting the valve leaflets, becomes inflamed, thickened, and fibrotic, with possible resultant compromise of cardiac contractility (as in endocardial fibroelastosis) or valve function. Pathologic changes of valve leaflets similar to those of mild rheumatic fever have been described in a number of rheumatic diseases but usually are of little clinical significance. SLE, ankylosing spondylitis, some of the vasculitis syndromes, and seropositive rheumatoid arthritis at times are associated with clinically significant endocarditis. Heart valves damaged by endocarditis may function poorly, compromise cardiac function, or act as foci for bacterial endocarditis.

Clinical manifestations of endocarditis are few unless cardiac compromise is present or unless there are symptoms of coexisting pericarditis or of coronary vascular disease. Signs include valvular heart murmurs, thickened valve leaflets seen on echocardiography, selective cardiac enlargement on chest radiograph, certain electrocardiographic changes, and abnormal findings on cardiac catheterization. Diagnosis rests on one or more of such findings. Distinction must be made from bacterial endocarditis, not always an easy task in a febrile rheumatic disease patient with a heart murmur. In rheumatic diseases other than rheumatic fever, distinction also must be made between coexisting rheumatic fever and valvular heart disease caused by the particular rheumatic disease present in the patient. Congenital heart disease also must be differentiated.

Juvenile Rheumatoid Arthritis

Significant valvular heart disease rarely, if ever, occurs in the seronegative JRA subgroups.[16, 125] JRA patients with pathologic heart murmurs should be suspected of having coexisting congenital heart disease or bacterial endocarditis. Mitral regurgitation may be present in severe myocarditis resulting from ventricular dilatation or papillary muscle dysfunction.

Significant valvular heart disease does occur occasionally in patients with seropositive rheumatoid arthritis.[23, 151] In one instance, in a child with seropositive JRA, severe aortic regurgitation necessitated replacement of the aortic root with a pulmonary autograft, but the patient later died of congestive heart and allograft failure.[127] At autopsy, the pulmonary allograft showed a thickened annulus with retracted valve cusps and with histologic evidence of a rheumatic process.[138] Rheumatoid granulomatous lesions have been found in affected valve leaflets. Autopsy series have reported a high incidence of valvular lesions resembling those of chronic rheumatic fever in adult rheumatoid patients; however, few of these patients have had clinically significant heart disease,[139] and similar lesions also have been described in "normal" nonrheumatoid adults.[8, 11, 135]

Ankylosing Spondylitis

Ankylosing spondylitis is associated with aortitis and aortic valvular disease with resulting aortic insufficiency.[15, 36, 56, 141] This type of endocarditis occurs in about 5 per cent of spondylitis patients, generally some years after the onset of disease; hence it rarely is seen in children. A similar type of heart disease has been noted occasionally in Reiter disease.[108] Pathologic changes include an inflammatory process of the proximal aorta and aortic valve; the histology is reminiscent of luetic aortitis. Myocarditis, heart block, and cardiac arrhythmias may be associated. The only associated symptoms are those of cardiac decompensation or arrhythmia. Signs include the murmur of aortic insufficiency and characteristic findings of aortic insufficiency on echocardiography and cardiac catheterization.[144] Advances in the use of Doppler echocardiography permit sensitive identification of aortic regurgitation prior to auscultatory findings. There is no known form of prevention or specific therapy for this type of heart disease. Aortic valve replacement may be required. Bacterial endocarditis must be differentiated from ankylosing spondylitis.

Systemic Lupus Erythematosus

Verrucous endocarditis, or Libman-Sacks endocarditis, is a frequent autopsy finding in SLE.[40, 41, 131] One or more heart valves may be affected. Vegetations are present on one or both surfaces of the valve leaflets; they also may spread to the chordae, papillary muscles, and mural endocardium. Histologic changes include fibrinoid deposition with an accompanying inflammatory response but with minimal fibrosis and scarring. In distinction to the endocarditis of rheumatic fever, valve leaflets rarely are destroyed or seriously deformed in SLE; hence, cardiac function rarely is affected. Affected valve leaflets may be predisposed to subsequent bacterial endocarditis, however. No clinical symptoms are associated with Libman-Sacks endocarditis. Signs include cardiac murmurs, which may be quite changeable; attempts to correlate murmurs in lupus patients with the valve changes found at autopsy have not been uniformly successful, however, and it is not certain that the murmurs so common in SLE patients always are related to the observed endocarditis. Diagnosis of Libman-Sacks endocarditis is difficult to make in the living patient, although valvular murmurs certainly suggest its presence. Echocardiography occasionally may be helpful in demonstrating thickened valve leaflets.[35, 43, 53]

Differential diagnosis must include bacterial endocarditis; this distinction may be difficult in the febrile patient with SLE and a heart murmur. A thorough search for possible infectious agents should be made in such patients. The frequent treatment of lupus patients with medications, such as corticosteroids and anticancer drugs, that interfere with host inflammatory and immune responses compounds the problem. Myocarditis, pericarditis, and pulmonary disease of lupus also must be differentiated from endocarditis in SLE.

No therapy is indicated for Libman-Sacks endocarditis per se; it rarely interferes significantly with cardiac function, nor does it cause significant chronic valvular damage. If there is a possibility of bacterial endocarditis, appropriate evaluation and antibiotic therapy should be instituted.

A few patients with SLE incur significant damage to either the mitral or aortic valve, particularly the aortic valve, with resulting clinical heart disease.[8, 42] In such patients, vigorous anti-inflammatory therapy might be indicated in an attempt to stop valve destruction, but the possibility of bacterial endocarditis always must be considered.

CARDIAC DISEASE IN INFANTS OF MOTHERS WITH SYSTEMIC LUPUS ERYTHEMATOSUS

Infants of mothers with SLE usually are not affected with SLE but may show transient manifestations of the disease, presumably transplacentally passed[72, 124, 147]; these include discoid lupus, thrombocytopenia, hemolytic anemia, leukopenia, and positive tests for antinuclear antibodies. Such infants also may be affected by cardiac diseases that are not always transient. Fatal endocardial fibroelastosis has been reported in three infants of mothers with connective tissue disease.[63, 65, 95] Congenital complete heart block is a permanent sequelae of maternal SLE,[3, 26, 100] with an approximate frequency of 50 per cent of infants with neonatal lupus.[150] Antibodies to soluble tissue ribonucleoprotein antigens SSA/Ro and/or SSB/La are found in the serum of infants with neonatal lupus as well as in maternal serum.[128] Many of these mothers do not have clinical manifestations of lupus, although some eventually progress to overt expression of the disease; others have clinical manifestations of Sjögren syndrome. The development of congenital complete heart block correlates with the presence of anti–SSA/Ro and/or –SSB/La antibodies[115]; however, whether these antibodies are responsible for the conduction system damage still is uncertain. Serum from infants younger than 3 months of age has been found to contain antibody; however, none has been identified in infants older than 6 months of age, suggesting transplacental transfer of this antibody. The presence of fetal bradycardia resulting from complete heart block should suggest fetal SLE and prompt investigation of the disease in the mother. When hemodynamically significant, the bradycardia may cause fetal hydrops with ascites and pleural and pericardial effusions necessitating close serial assessment. Maternal treatment with steroids or plasmapheresis is of unclear benefit.[22, 24, 31] Postmortem immunofluorescent studies demonstrated antibody throughout the heart of an infant with congenital complete heart block and positive serology for anti-Ro (SSA).[95] The mother was clinically well and had a high serum antinuclear antibody titer. The cardiac examination was marked by elements of fibroelastosis, dystrophic calcification, and sparse inflammation, findings suggesting that intrauterine cardiac damage may result from maternally transferred autoantibody.

Reports in adults have demonstrated a high frequency of aortic and mitral regurgitation in individuals with the presence of anticardiolipin antibodies. A fetal death followed by a maternal death 28 hours later has been reported in a woman with elevated titers of anticardiolipin antibody. The fetal postmortem examination showed placental infarction and multiorgan infarction from intravascular thrombosis of small vessels.[7] Further investigation is necessary to determine if the presence of these antiphospholipid antibodies can be used as a marker in children for those at risk of developing valvulitis.[27, 48]

VASCULITIS

Endocarditis and valvulitis have been reported rarely in polyarteritis, Henoch-Schönlein vasculitis, and other vasculitis syndromes. Symptoms, signs, and diagnostic measures are similar to those described earlier. Aschoff bodies, thought by some to be pathognomonic of rheumatic fever, have been described in vasculitis.[44]

Aortic valvular disease, with resultant aortic insufficiency, is one of the cardinal findings in Cogan syndrome,[28, 34] an unusual vasculitis variant characterized also by interstitial keratitis and nerve deafness. Histology of affected valve leaflets has shown nonspecific acute and chronic inflammation with areas of fibrinoid necrosis but no demonstrable immunoglobulin or complement deposits. Therapy with corticosteroids has been considered helpful in some patients.

Takayasu aortitis, another vasculitis variant characterized by inflammation of the aorta and its major branches, also has been associated at times with endocarditis and valvular disease.[29]

CORONARY VASCULITIS

Coronary vasculitis, characterized by inflammation of coronary blood vessels, occurs in several rheumatic disease syndromes, including SLE, polyarteritis nodosa, infantile polyarteritis, and Kawasaki disease. Inflamed vessels may become weakened, leading to aneurysm formation or rupture, or narrowed, producing coronary insufficiency or myocardial infarction. Coronary vasculitis may be entirely silent or may be associated with subacute anginal symptoms of chest pain or with sudden catastrophic symptoms of massive myocardial infarction or ruptured coronary aneurysm (severe chest pain, tachycardia, vascular collapse, sudden heart failure). The diagnosis of coronary vasculitis is difficult to make ante mortem. Electrocardiographic changes suggestive of myocardial ischemia or myocardial infarction, echocardiograms showing coronary aneurysms, and increased serum levels of enzymes found in myocardial muscle may be helpful. Coronary arteriography, if necessary, may be diagnostic.

Systemic Lupus Erythematosus

Coronary vasculitis probably occurs in a significant number of SLE patients as part of a systemic vasculitis.[12, 40, 69, 129] Such coronary vasculitis is largely subclinical; any symptoms of chest pain may be difficult to differentiate from those of the pericarditis that is so common in SLE patients.

Myocardial infarction is emerging as a cause of death in relatively young SLE patients,[50, 70, 103, 145] including children.[123] Histologic changes post mortem may show accelerated atherosclerosis of coronary vessels, indistinguishable from the atherosclerotic heart disease of older patients. The role of SLE coronary vasculitis in initiating or accelerating this process is not known; other possible risk factors include the nephrotic syndrome, prolonged corticosteroid therapy, hypertension, familial atherosclerosis, and diabetes.

Polyarteritis Nodosa

Coronary vasculitis is a known concomitant of polyarteritis nodosa.[64, 114, 116] Massive myocardial infarction or ruptured aneurysms have been reported; smaller foci of myocardial damage may contribute to the "myocarditis" damage occasionally seen in polyarteritis nodosa. Symptoms, signs, and diagnostic measures are similar to those described earlier. Coronary arteriography might be diagnostic in some patients. Therapy with corticosteroids and perhaps with some of the anticancer agents is warranted, although not uniformly successful, in severe polyarteritis nodosa.

Infantile Polyarteritis Nodosa

Infantile polyarteritis nodosa has been considered a rare variant of polyarteritis nodosa, seen almost exclusively in infants and young children. Coronary vasculitis is the cardinal manifestation, and, indeed, sometimes the coronary vessels are the sole site of vasculitis.[77, 107, 117] The distribution of vascular involvement is peculiar; relatively large coronary vessels and other visceral vessels (such as the mesenteric arteries) are affected, but smaller vessels (such as those of muscle and skin) generally are spared. This condition now generally is considered to be very similar, if not identical, to Kawasaki disease.

KAWASAKI DISEASE (MUCOCUTANEOUS LYMPH NODE SYNDROME)

(See also Chapter 82.)

A fascinating constellation of signs designated as Kawasaki disease was noted initially in Japan and later in many other countries[75, 78]; more than 100,000 cases have been recognized in Japanese children. The disease has been noted with increasing frequency in the United States for the past 20 years.[88, 102] This disease affects children primarily in the first 5 years of life, although cases also occur in older children. The diagnosis rests entirely on clinical grounds: a characteristic combination of prolonged high fevers, multiform rashes, stomatitis, conjunctivitis, erythema of the hands and feet with characteristic late peeling of the digits, and lymphadenopathy. It is estimated that 0.5 to 1.0 per cent of children with Kawasaki disease die of coronary vasculitis and are found at autopsy to have changes indistinguishable from those of infantile polyarteritis nodosa. There are no specific laboratory tests diagnostic of the disease, but supportive evidence includes marked thrombocytosis. In addition, two-dimensional echocardiography accurately has demonstrated dilatation and aneurysms of the proximal coronary arteries (Fig. 36–1) as well as less specific signs of cardiac inflammation, including abnormal ventricular wall motion, pericardial effusion, mitral regurgitation, and diminished cardiac function.[32, 57, 98, 121, 156] Arteriography has confirmed coronary abnormalities in 15 to 20 per cent of all children with Kawasaki disease (Figs. 36–2 and 36–3), and of those affected, approximately 50 per cent will undergo regression of lesions by echo and/or arteriography (Fig. 36–4).[76, 120] After the clinical diagnosis in the acute stage of the illness, the treatment of choice is high-dose intravenous gamma-globulin. Efficacy has been demonstrated in several studies using total doses between 1 and 2 g/kg given as a course either in a single dose or divided over as many as 4 days.[109, 110] Our preference is to treat with 2 g/kg as a single dose administered over 8 to 10 hours. Complications associated with intravenous immunoglobulin treatment are uncommon and usually minor (rash, fever, edema), although in some children congestive heart failure may be precipitated or exacerbated. Preparations currently in use have not resulted in documented transmission of either hepatitis or HIV infection. Salicylates are used as adjunctive therapy at 100 mg/kg/day in four divided doses during the early acute phase because coagulation activation has been shown to occur in the first 3 weeks

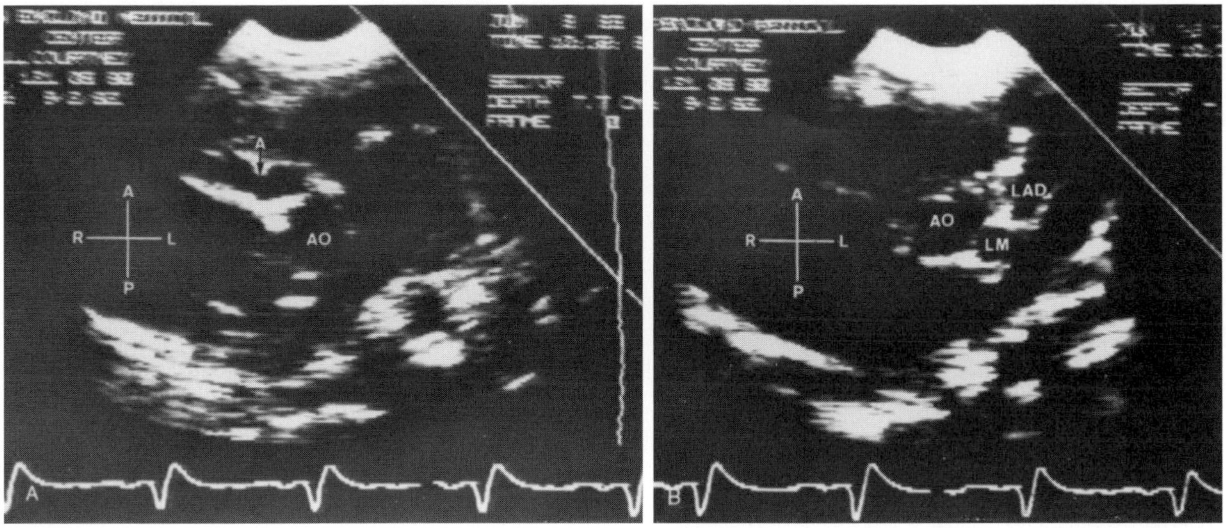

FIGURE 36–1. *Two-dimensional echocardiogram* (A) *showing a cross-sectional short axis view of the heart. The proximal right coronary artery* (A) *is dilated markedly after takeoff from the aortic root* (AO). B, *Two-dimensional echocardiogram of the aorta* (AO) *and left coronary artery in the same patient, depicting aneurysm formation of the left main coronary artery* (LM) *and the left anterior descending coronary artery* (LAD).

of the illness.[21] Elevation in beta-thromboglobulin, thromboxane A_2, and thromboxane B_2 supports the theory of platelet activation in this illness, suggesting the need for antiplatelet therapy.[21, 60] Simultaneously, we have found that low plasma prostacyclin levels are present in the first week of the illness, suggesting endothelial cell dysfunction related to the vasculitis. These levels remain low through the first 2 months of illness. The relationship of high thromboxane and low prostacyclin levels in this disease may predispose to coronary vasoconstriction and platelet aggregation potentiating ischemia. Studies of treatment with corticosteroids are inconclusive, and so this therapy has been omitted in general because it may be detrimental.[76, 79]

Once symptoms of acute inflammation have subsided (fever, rash, conjunctivitis, mucositis), single daily doses of aspirin 3 to 5 mg/kg are used until echocardiography has confirmed the absence of dilated or aneurysmal coronary arteries approximately 4 to 8 weeks after the onset of illness. In the presence of persistent coronary abnormalities, low-dose aspirin is continued indefinitely. Giant aneurysms defined as lesions exceeding 8 mm in diameter are associated more frequently with myocardial ischemia infarction and/or death. Although more aggressive therapy would seem indicated, no single approach has been accepted universally. Our preference is to add warfarin therapy to low-dose aspirin until aneurysms become less than 8 mm in diameter. Others advocate using dipyridamole to achieve coronary dilatation with aspirin therapy, and some would treat with warfarin and omit aspirin. The surgical experience involving aortocoronary bypass grafting for symptomatic patients or for critically

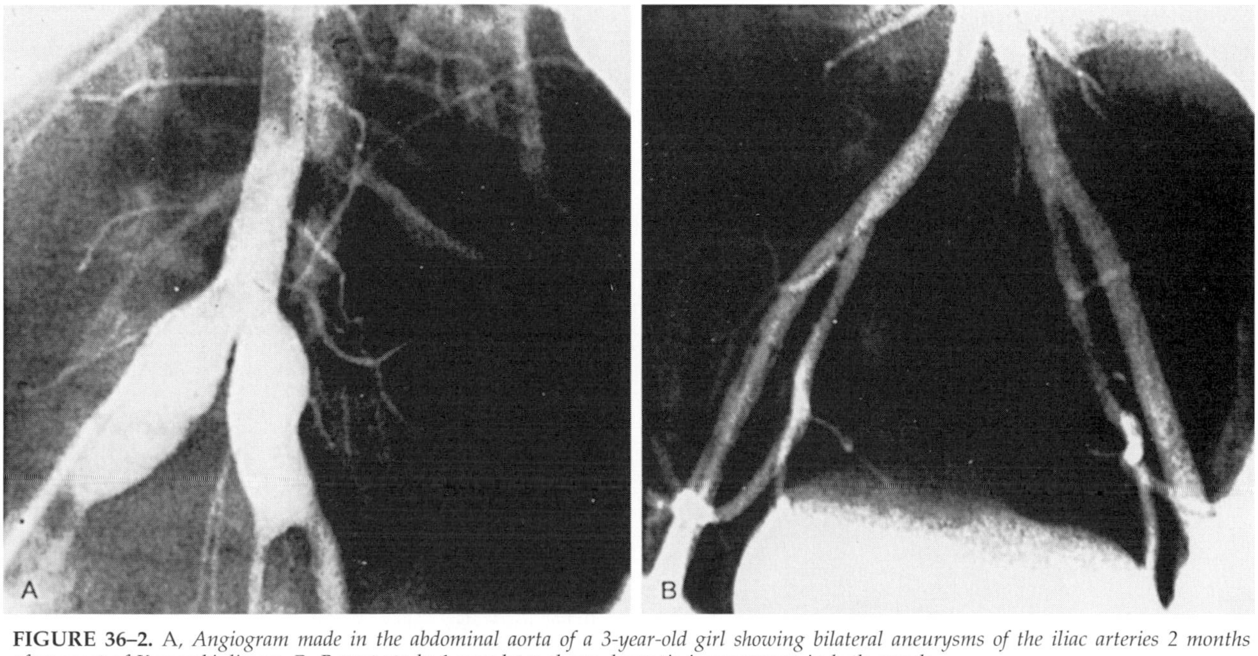

FIGURE 36–2. A, *Angiogram made in the abdominal aorta of a 3-year-old girl showing bilateral aneurysms of the iliac arteries 2 months after onset of Kawasaki disease.* B, *Repeat study 1 year later shows dramatic improvement in both vessels.*

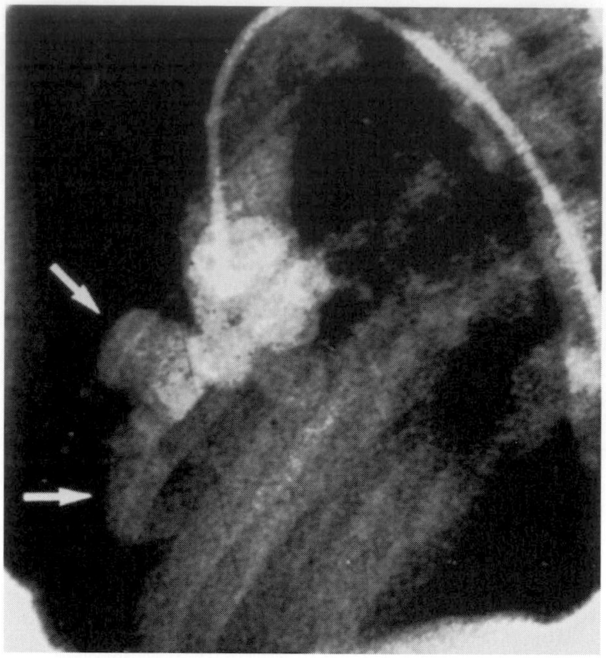

FIGURE 36–3. *Multiple aneurysms of the right coronary artery* (arrows) *delineated by an aortic root angiogram in a 3-year-old girl 2 months after the onset of Kawasaki disease.*

narrowed vessels in the absence of symptoms has improved greatly.[82, 119, 136, 148] Balloon angioplasty has not been widely successful and may predispose to rupture of calcified vessels. Early experience with rotablator therapy is promising but requires further assessment. Prevalence of this disease and the uncertain impact on the expected acquired atherosclerotic lesions of the population necessitate continued follow-up by cardiologists.

The finding of this syndrome in such widespread form in Japan is of obvious interest and raises the possibility of an infectious or environmental cause. One report suggested that rickettsiae were present in tissues[58]; this has not been confirmed. Elevated levels of serum IgE have been reported.[87] The association of this syndrome with coronary vasculitis in a minority of patients also is of great interest and suggests that some infectious or environmental agents may cause blood vessel inflammation in some patients. However, the agent(s) responsible for mucocutaneous lymph node syndrome and the mechanisms by which such agents lead to coronary vasculitis in a minority of affected patients remain to be elucidated. Investigations have demonstrated immunologic derangements in the sera of these children, including abnormalities in T-cell populations, an increase in circulating activated B cells, and cytotoxicity against skin fibroblasts by circulating mononuclear cells. In addition, T cells exhibit a decrease in suppressor-cell activity for immunoglobulin production.[91, 92] One theory suggests that Kawasaki disease may be the result of the activation of V-beta-2^+ T cells by bacterial superantigens.[93] The equivalent of the mucocutaneous lymph node syndrome is not recognized in adults.

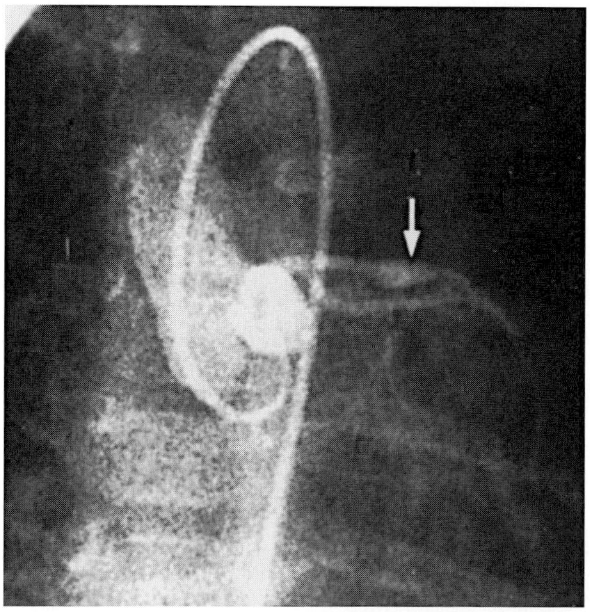

FIGURE 36–4. *Aortic root cineangiogram of an isolated aneurysm of the left coronary artery system in a 2-year-old boy.*

References

1. Aiuto, L. T., Stambouly, J. J., and Boxer, P. A.: Cardiac tamponade in an adolescent female: An unusual manifestation of systemic lupus erythematosus. Clin. Pediatr. *32*:500–567, 1993.
2. Allen, D. M., Diamond, L. K., and Howell, D. A.: Anaphylactoid purpura in children (Henoch-Schönlein syndrome). Am. J. Dis. Child. *99*:833–854, 1960.
3. Alterburger, K. M., Jedziniak, M., Roper, W. L., et al.: Congenital complete heart block associated with hydrops fetalis. J. Pediatr. *91*:618–620, 1977.
4. Auerbuch, M., Bojko, A., and Levo, Y.: Cardiac tamponade in the early postpartum period as the presenting and predominant manifestation of systemic lupus erythematosus. J. Rheumatol. *13*:444–445, 1986.
5. Bacon, P. A., and Gibson, D. G.: Cardiac involvement in rheumatoid arthritis. Ann. Rheum. Dis. *33*:20–24, 1974.
6. Bastos C. J., Queiroz, A. C., and Martinelli, R.: Cardiac involvement in systemic lupus erythematosus: Anatomopathological study. Rev. Assoc. Med. Bras. *39*:161–164, 1993.
7. Bendon, R. W., Wilson, J., Getahun, B., et al.: A maternal death due to thrombotic disease associated with anticardiolipin antibody. Arch. Pathol. Lab. Med. *111*:370–372, 1987.
8. Bernhard, G. C., Lange, R. L., and Hensly, G. T.: Aortic disease with valvular insufficiency as the principal manifestation of systemic lupus erythematosus. Ann. Intern. Med. *71*:81–87, 1969.
9. Bernstein, B., Takahashi, M., and Hanson, V.: Cardiac involvement in juvenile rheumatoid arthritis. J. Pediatr. *85*:313–317, 1974.
10. Bilazarian, S. D., Taylor, A. J., Brezinski, D., et al.: High-grade atrioventricular heart block in an adult with systemic lupus erythematosus: The association of nuclear RNP (U1 RNP) antibodies, a case report, and review of the literature. Arthritis Rheum. *32*:1170–1174, 1989.
11. Bonfiglio, T., and Atwater, E. C.: Heart disease in patients with seropositive rheumatoid arthritis: A controlled autopsy study and review. Arch. Intern. Med. *124*:714–719, 1969.
12. Bonfiglio, T., Botti, R., and Hagstrom, J.: Coronary arthritis, occlusion, and myocardial infarction due to lupus erythematosus. Am. Heart J. *83*:153–158, 1972.
13. Borenstein, D. G., Fye, W. B., Arnett, F. C., et al.: The myocarditis of systemic lupus erythematosus: Association with myocarditis. Ann. Intern. Med. *89*:619–624, 1978.
14. Botstein, G. R., and LeRoy, E. C.: Primary heart disease in systemic sclerosis (scleroderma): Advances in clinical and pathologic features, pathogenesis, and new therapeutic approaches. Am. Heart J. *102*:913–919, 1981.
15. Bottiger, L. E., and Edhag, O.: Heart block in ankylosing spondylitis and uropolyarthritis. Br. Heart J. *34*:487–492, 1972.
16. Brewer, E., Jr.: Juvenile rheumatoid arthritis: Cardiac involvement. Arthritis Rheum. *20*:231–236, 1977.
17. Brigden, W., Bywaters, E., Leffos, M., et al.: The heart in systemic lupus erythematosus. Br. Heart J. *22*:1–16, 1960.
18. Britton, M. C., and Schur, P. H.: The complement system in rheumatoid synovitis. II. Intracytoplasmic inclusions of immunoglobulins and complement. Arthritis Rheum. *14*:87–95, 1971.
19. Browning, C. A., Bishop, R. L., Heilpern, R. J., et al.: Accelerated constrictive pericarditis in procainamide-induced systemic lupus erythematosus. Am. J. Cardiol. *53*:376–377, 1984.
20. Bulkley, B. H., Ridolfi, R., Salyer, W. R., et al.: Myocardial lesions of progressive systemic sclerosis: A cause of cardiac dysfunction. Circulation *53*:483–490, 1976.

21. Burns, J. C., Glode, M. P., Clarke, S. H., et al.: Coagulopathy and platelet activation in Kawasaki syndrome: Identification of patients with high risk for development of coronary artery aneurysms. J. Pediatr. *105*:206–211, 1984.
22. Buyon, J., Roubey, R., Swersky, S., et al.: Complete congenital heart block: Risk of occurrence and therapeutic approach to prevention. J. Rheumatol. *15*:1104–1108, 1988.
23. Carpenter, D. F., Golden, A., and Roberts, W. C.: Quadrivalvular rheumatoid heart disease associated with left bundle branch block. Am. J. Med. *43*:922–929, 1967.
24. Carreira, P. E., Guiterrez-Larraya, F., and Gomez-Reino, J. J.: Successful intrauterine therapy with dexamethasone for fetal myocarditis and heart block in a woman with systemic lupus erythematosus. J. Rheumatol. *20*:1204–1207, 1993.
25. Cathcart, E. S., and Spodick, D.: Rheumatoid heart disease: A study of the incidence and nature of cardiac lesions in rheumatoid arthritis. N. Engl. J. Med. *266*:959–964, 1962.
26. Chameides, L., Truex, R. C., Vetter, V., et al.: Association of maternal systemic lupus erythematosus with congenital complete heart block. N. Engl. J. Med. *297*:1204–1207, 1977.
27. Chartash, E., Lang, D. M., Paget, S. A., et al.: Aortic insufficiency and mitral regurgitation in patients with systemic lupus erythematosus and the antiphospholipid syndrome. Am. J. Med. *86*:407–412, 1989.
28. Cheson, B. D., Bluming, A. Z., and Alroy, J.: Cogan's syndrome: A systemic vasculitis. Am. J. Med. *60*:549–555, 1976.
29. Chhetri, M. K., Pal, N. C., Neelakantan, C., et al.: Endocardial lesion in a case of Takayasu's arteriopathy. Br. Heart J. *32*:859–862, 1970.
30. Christian, C. L.: Immune complex disease. N. Engl. J. Med. *280*:878–884, 1969.
31. Chua, S., Ostman-Smith, I., Sellers, S., et al.: Congenital heart block with hydrops fetalis treated with high-dose dexamethasone: A case report. Eur. J. Obstet. Gynecol. Reprod. Biol. *42*:155–158, 1991.
32. Chung, K. J., Brandt, L., Fulton, D. R., et al.: Cardiac and coronary arterial involvement in infants and children from New England with mucocutaneous lymph node syndrome (Kawasaki disease): Angiocardiographic-echocardiographic correlations. Am. J. Cardiol. *50*:136–142, 1982.
33. Clark, W. S., Lulka, J. P., and Bauer, W.: Rheumatic aortitis with aortic regurgitation: An unusual manifestation of rheumatoid arthritis (rheumatoid spondylitis). Am. J. Med. *22*:580–592, 1957.
34. Cogan, D. G., and Dickersin, G. R.: Nonsyphilitic interstitial keratitis with vestibuloauditory symptoms. Arch. Ophthalmol. *71*:172–175, 1964.
35. Collins, R. L., Turner, R. A., Nomeir, A. M., et al.: Cardiopulmonary manifestations of systemic lupus erythematosus. J. Rheumatol. *5*:299–306, 1978.
36. Connolly, D. C., and Burchell, N. B.: Pericarditis: A ten-year survey. Am. J. Cardiol. *7*:7–14, 1961.
37. Cooper, D. K. C., Cleland, W. P., and Bentall, H. H.: Collagen diseases as a cause of constrictive pericarditis. Thorax *33*:368–371, 1978.
38. Costallat, L. T., and Coimbra, A. M.: Systemic lupus erythematosus: Clinical and laboratory aspects related to age at disease onset. Clin. Exp. Rheum. *12*:603–607, 1994.
39. Denbow, C. E., Lie, J. T., Tancredi, R. G., et al.: Cardiac involvement in polymyositis: A clinicopathologic study of 20 autopsied patients. Arthritis Rheum. *22*:1088–1092, 1979.
40. Doherty, N. E., and Siegel, R. J.: Cardiovascular manifestations of systemic lupus erythematosus. Am. Heart J. *110*:1257–1265, 1985.
41. Dubois, E. L.: Lupus Erythematosus. 2nd ed. Los Angeles, University of Southern California Press, 1976.
42. Durand, I., Blaysat, G., Chauvaud, S., et al.: Extensive fibrous endocarditis as first manifestation of systemic lupus erythematosus. Arch. Fracaises de Pediatric *50*:685–688, 1993.
43. Elkayam, V., Weiss, S., and Laniado, S.: Pericardial effusion and mitral valve involvement in systemic lupus erythematosus. Ann. Rheum. Dis. *36*:349–353, 1977.
44. Fogel, B. J., Weinberg, T., and Markowitz, M.: A fatal connective tissue disease following a wasp sting. Am. J. Dis. Child. *114*:325–329, 1967.
45. Follansbee, W. P., Curtiss, E. I., Medoger, T. A., et al.: Physiologic abnormalities of cardiac function in progressive systemic sclerosis with diffuse scleroderma. N. Engl. J. Med. *310*:142–148, 1984.
46. Follansbee, W. P., Zerbe, T. R., and Medsger, T.A.: Cardiac and skeletal muscle disease in systemic sclerosis (scleroderma): A high-risk association. Am. Heart J. *125*:194–203, 1993.
47. Follansbee, W. P., Curtiss, E. I., and Ranko, P. S.: The electocardiogram in systemic sclerosis (scleroderma): Study of 102 consecutive cases with functional correlations and review of the literature. Am. J. Med. *79*:183–192, 1985.
48. Ford, P. M., Ford, S. E., and Lillicrap, D. P.: Association of lupus anticoagulant with severe valvar heart disease in systemic lupus erythematosus. J. Rheumatol. *15*:597–600, 1988.
49. Franco, A. E., Levine, H. D., and Hall, A. P.: Rheumatoid pericarditis: Report of 17 cases diagnosed clinically. Ann. Intern. Med. *77*:837–844, 1972.
50. Friedman, D. M., Lazanas, H. M., and Fierman, A. H.: Acute myocardial infarction in pediatric systemic lupus erythematosus. J. Pediatr. *117*:263–266, 1990.
51. Fulton, D. R., Meissner, H. C., and Peterson, M. B.: Effects of current therapy of Kawasaki disease on eicosanoid metabolism. Am. J. Cardiol. *61*:1323–1327, 1988.
52. Furusho, K., Sato, K., Soeda, T., et al.: High-dose intravenous gammaglobulin for Kawasaki disease. Lancet *2*:1359, 1983.
53. Galve, E., Candell-Riera, J., Pierau, C., et al.: Prevalence, morphologic types, and evolution of cardiac valvular disease in systemic lupus erythematosus. N. Engl. J. Med. *319*:817–823, 1988.
54. Gocke, D. J., Hsu, K., Morgan, C., et al.: Association between polyarteritis and Australian antigen. Lancet *2*:1149–1153, 1970.
55. Goldenberg, J., Ferraz, M. B., Pessoa, A. P., et al.: Symptomatic cardiac involvement in juvenile rheumatoid arthritis. Int. J. Cardiol. *34*:57–62, 1992.
56. Graham, D. C., and Smythe, H. A.: The carditis and aortitis of ankylosing spondylitis. Bull. Rheum. Dis. *9*:171–174, 1958.
57. Grenadier, E., Allen, H. D., Goldberg, S. J., et al.: Left ventricular wall motion abnormalities in Kawasaki's disease. Am. Heart J. *107*:966–973, 1984.
58. Hamashima, Y., Kishi, K., and Tasaka, K.: Rickettsia-like bodies in infantile acute febrile mucocutaneous lymph node syndrome. Lancet *2*:42, 1973.
59. Harvey, A., Shulman, L., Tumulty, P., et al.: Systemic lupus erythematosus: A review of the literature and clinical analysis of 138 cases. Medicine *33*:291–437, 1954.
60. Hidaka, T., Nakano, M., Ueta, T., et al.: Increased synthesis of thromboxane A2 by platelets from patients with Kawasaki disease. J. Pediatr. *102*:94–96, 1983.
61. Hill, D. L., and Barrows, H. S.: Identical skeletal and cardiac muscle involvement in a case of fatal polymyositis. Arch. Neurol. *19*:545–551, 1968.
62. Hoffman, F. G., and Leight, L.: Complete atrioventricular block associated with rheumatoid disease. Am. J. Cardiol. *16*:585–592, 1965.
63. Hogg, G. R.: Congenital acute lupus erythematosus associated with subendocardial fibroelastosis. Am. J. Clin. Pathol. *28*:648–654, 1957.
64. Holsinger, D. R., Osmundson, P. J., and Edwards, J. E.: The heart in periarteritis nodosa. Circulation *25*:610–618, 1962.
65. Hull, D., Binns, B. A. O., and Joyce, D.: Congenital heart block and widespread fibrosis due to maternal lupus erythematosus. Arch. Dis. Child. *41*:688–690, 1966.
66. Imai, T., and Matsumoto, S.: Anaphlyactoid purpura with cardiac involvement. Arch. Dis. Child. *45*:727–729, 1970.
67. Jacobson, E. J., and Reza, M. L.: Constrictive pericarditis in systemic lupus erythematosus: Demonstration of immunoglobulins in the pericardium. Arthritis Rheum. *21*:972–974, 1978.
68. James, T. N.: De subitaneis mortibus. VIII. Coronary arteries and conduction system in scleroderma heart disease. Circulation *50*:844–856, 1974.
69. James, T., Rupe, C., and Monto, R.: Pathology of the cardiac conduction system in systemic lupus erythematosus. Ann. Intern. Med. *63*:402–410, 1965.
70. Jensen, G., and Sigurd, B.: Systemic lupus erythematosus and acute myocardial infarction. Chest *64*:653–654, 1973.
71. Johnson, R. T., Portnoy, B., Rogers, N. G., et al.: Acute benign pericarditis: Virologic study of 34 patients. Arch. Intern. Med. *108*:823–832, 1961.
72. Jordan, J. M., Valenstein, P., and Kredich, D. W.: Systemic lupus erythematosus with Libman-Sachs endocarditis in a 9-month-old infant with neonatal lupus erythematosus and congenital heart block. Pediatrics *84*:574–578, 1989.
73. Kahl, L. E.: The spectrum of pericardial tamponade in systemic lupus erythematosus. Arthritis Rheum. *35*:1343–1349, 1992.
74. Kato, H., Koike, S., and Yokoyama, T.: Kawasaki disease: Effect of treatment on coronary artery involvement. Pediatrics *63*:175–179, 1979.
75. Kato, H., Koike, S., Yamamoto, M., et al.: Coronary aneurysms in infants and young children with acute febrile mucocutaneous lymph node syndrome. J. Pediatr. *86*:892–898, 1975.
76. Kato, H., Ichinose, E., Yoshioaka, F., et al.: Fate of coronary aneurysms in Kawasaki disease: Serial coronary angiography and long-term follow-up study. Am. J. Cardiol. *49*:1758–1766, 1982.
77. Kawai, S., Okada, R., Sigimoto, H., et al.: An autopsied case of a 2-month-old infant with granulomatous pancarditis having severe vasculitis and valvulitis. Jpn. Circ. J. *47*:1325–1330, 1983.
78. Kawasaki, T., Kasaki, T., Kosaki, F., et al.: A new infantile acute febrile mucocutaneous lymph node syndrome (MLNS) prevailing in Japan. Pediatrics *54*:271–276, 1974.
79. Kijima, Y., Kamiya, T., Suzuki, A., et al.: A trial procedure to prevent aneurysm formation of the coronary arteries by steroid pulse therapy in Kawasaki disease. Jpn. Circ. J. *46*:1239–1242, 1982.
80. King, K. K., Kornreich, H. K., Bernstein, B. H., et al.: The clinical spectrum of systemic lupus erythematosus in childhood. Arthritis Rheum. *20*:287–294, 1977.
81. Kirk, J., and Cosh, J.: The pericarditis of rheumatoid arthritis. Q. J. Med. *38*:397–423, 1969.
82. Kitamura, S., Kawachi, K., Harima, R., et al.: Surgery for coronary heart disease due to mucocutaneous lymph node syndrome (Kawasaki disease): Report of six patients. Am. J. Cardiol. *51*:444–448, 1983.
83. Kitamura, S., Kawashima, Y., Fujita, T., et al.: Aortocoronary bypass grafting in a child with coronary artery obstruction due to mucocutane-

ous lymph node syndrome: Report of a case. Circulation *53*:1035–1040, 1975.
84. Koffler, D., and Kunkel, H. G.: Mechanisms of renal injury in systemic lupus erythematosus. Am. J. Med. *45*:165–169, 1968.
85. Kornreich, H. K., King, K. K., Bernstein, B. H., et al.: Scleroderma in childhood. Arthritis Rheum. *20*:343–350, 1977.
86. Krous, H. F., Clausen, C. R., and Ray, C. G.: Elevated immunoglobin E in infantile polyarteritis nodosa. J. Pediatr. *84*:841–845, 1974.
87. Kusakawa, S., and Heiner, D. C.: Elevated level of immunoglobin E in the acute febrile mucocutaneous lymph node syndrome. Pediatr. Res. *10*:108–111, 1976.
88. Landing, B. H., and Larson, E. J.: Are infantile periarteritis nodosa with coronary artery involvement and fatal mucocutaneous lymph node syndrome the same? Comparison of 20 patients from North America with patients from Hawaii and Japan. Pediatrics *59*:651–662, 1977.
89. Latinen, O., Kentala, E., and Leirisalo, M.: Electrocardiographic findings in patients with connective heart disease. Scand. J. Rheumatol. *7*:193–198, 1978.
90. Lebowitz, W. B.: The heart in rheumatoid arthritis (rheumatoid disease): A clinical and pathological study of 62 cases. Ann. Intern. Med. *58*:102–123, 1963.
91. Leung, D. Y. M., Chu, E. T., Wood, N., et al.: Immunoregulatory T cell abnormalities in mucocutaneous lymph node syndrome. J. Immunol. *130*:2002–2004, 1983.
92. Leung, D. Y. M., Seigel, L., Grady, S., et al.: Immunoregulatory abnormalities in mucocutaneous lymph node syndrome. Clin. Immunol. Immunopathol. *23*:100–112, 1982.
93. Leung, D. Y. M., Meissner, H. C., Fulton, D. R., et al.: Toxic shock syndrome toxin-secreting *Staphylococcus aureus* in Kawasaki syndrome. Lancet *342*:1385–1388, 1993.
94. Lietman, P. S., and Bywaters, E. G. L.: Pericarditis in juvenile rheumatoid arthritis. Pediatrics *32*:855–860, 1963.
95. Litsey, S. E., Noonan, J. A., O'Connor, W. N., et al.: Maternal connective tissue disease and congenital heart block: Demonstration of immunoglobulin in cardiac tissue. N. Engl. J. Med. *312*:98–100, 1985.
96. Lynch, P. G.: Cardiac involvement in chronic polymyositis. Br. Heart J. *33*:416–419, 1971.
97. MacGregor, G. A., and Vallance-Owen, J.: Cardiac involvement in anaphylactoid purpura. Lancet *2*:572–575, 1957.
98. Maeda, T., Yoshida, H., Funabashki, T., et al.: Subcostal 2-dimensional echocardiographic imaging of peripheral left coronary artery aneurysms in Kawasaki disease. Am. J. Cardiol. *52*:48–52, 1983.
99. Marin-Garcia, J., Sheridan, R., and Hanissian, A. S.: Echocardiographic detection of early cardiac involvement in juvenile rheumatoid arthritis. Pediatrics *73*:394–397, 1984.
100. McCue, C. M., Mantakas, M. E., Tingelstad, J. B., et al.: Congenital heart block in newborns of mothers with connective tissue disease. Circulation *56*:82–90, 1977.
101. McWhorter, J. E., IV, and LeRoy, E. C.: Pericardial disease in scleroderma (systemic sclerosis). Am. J. Med. *56*:566–575, 1974.
102. Melish, M. E., Hicks, R. M., and Larson, E. J.: Mucocutaneous lymph node syndrome in the United States. Am. J. Dis. Child. *130*:599–607, 1976.
103. Meller, J., Conde, C. A., Deppisch, L. M., et al.: Myocardial infarction due to coronary atherosclerosis in three young adults with systemic lupus erythematosus. Am. J. Cardiol. *35*:309–314, 1975.
104. Miller, J. J., III: Carditis in juvenile rheumatoid arthritis. Arthritis Rheum. *20*:243, 1977.
105. Miller, J. J., and French, J. W.: Myocarditis in juvenile rheumatoid arthritis. Am. J. Dis. Child. *131*:205–209, 1977.
106. Muers, M., and Stokes, W.: Treatment of scleroderma heart by D-penicillamine. Br. Heart J. *38*:864–867, 1976.
107. Munro-Faure, H.: Necrotizing arteritis of the coronary vessels in infancy: Case report and review of the literature. Pediatrics *23*:914–926, 1959.
108. Neu, L. T., Jr., Reider, R. A., and Mack, R. E.: Cardiac involvement in Reiter's disease: Report of a case with review of the literature. Ann. Intern. Med. *53*:215–220, 1960.
109. Newburger, J. W., Takahashi, M., Burns, J. C., et al.: The treatment of Kawasaki syndrome with intravenous gamma globulin. N. Engl. J. Med. *315*:341–347, 1986.
110. Newburger, J. W., Takahashi, M., Beiser, A. S., et al.: A single intravenous infusion of gammaglobulin as compared with four infusions in the treatment of acute Kawasaki syndrome. N. Engl. J. Med. *324*:1633–1639, 1991.
111. Nomeir, A. M., Turner, R., and Watts, E.: Cardiac involvement in rheumatoid arthritis. Ann. Intern. Med. *79*:800–806, 1973.
112. Oram, S., and Stokes, W.: The heart in scleroderma. Br. Heart J. *23*:243–259, 1961.
113. Permanyer-Miralda, G., Sagristá-Sauleda, J., and Soler-Soler, J.: Primary acute pericardial disease: A prospective series of 231 consecutive patients. Am. J. Cardiol. *56*:623–630, 1985.
114. Przybojewski, J. K.: Polyarteritis nodosa in the adult. S. Afr. Med. J. *60*:512–518, 1984.
115. Ramsey-Goldman, R., Hom, D., Deng, J. S., et al.: Anti SS-A antibodies and fetal outcome in maternal systemic lupus erythematosus. Arthritis Rheum. *29*:1269–1273, 1986.
116. Reidbord, H. E., McCormack, L. J., and O'Duffy, J. D.: Necrotizing angiitis. II. Findings at autopsy in twenty-seven cases. Cleve. Clin. Q. *32*:191–204, 1965.
117. Roberts, F. B., and Fetterman, G. H.: Polyarteritis nodosa in infancy. J. Pediatr. *63*:519–529, 1963.
118. Sackner, M., Heinz, E., and Steinberg, A.: The heart in scleroderma. Am. J. Cardiol. *17*:542–559, 1966.
119. Sandiford, F. M., Vargo, T. A., Shih, J., et al.: Successful triple coronary artery bypass in a child with multiple coronary aneurysms due to Kawasaki's disease. J. Thorac. Cardiovasc. Surg. *79*:283–287, 1980.
120. Sasaguri, Y., and Kato, H.: Regression of aneurysms in Kawasaki disease: A pathological study. J. Pediatr. *100*:225–231, 1982.
121. Satomi, G., Nakamura, K., Narai, S., et al.: Systemic visualization of coronary arteries by two-dimensional echocardiography in children and infants: Evaluation in Kawasaki's disease and coronary arteriovenous fistulas. Am. Heart J. *107*:497–505, 1984.
122. Schaller, J. G.: The diversity of JRA: A 1976 look at the subgroups of chronic childhood arthritis. Arthritis Rheum. *20*(Suppl.):S52–S61, 1977.
123. Schaller, J. G., and Hollister, R.: Unpublished observations.
124. Schaller, J. G.: Lupus phenomena in the newborn. Arthritis Rheum. *20*:312–314, 1977.
125. Schaller, J., and Wedgwood, R. J.: Is juvenile rheumatoid arthritis a single disease? A review. Pediatrics *50*:940–953, 1972.
126. Schaumberg, H. H., Nielsen, S. L., and Yurchak, P. M.: Heart block in polymyositis. N. Engl. J. Med. *284*:480–481, 1971.
127. Schoof, P. H., Cromme-Digkhuis, A. H., Bogers, A. J. J. C., et al.: Aortic root replacement with pulmonary autograft in children. J. Thorac. Cardiovasc. Surg. *107*:367–373, 1994.
128. Scott, J. S., Maddison, P. J., Taylor, P. V., et al.: Connective tissue disease, antibodies to ribonucleoprotein, and congenital heart block. N. Engl. J. Med. *309*:209–212, 1983.
129. Seaman, A. J., and Christerson, J. W.: Demonstration of L. E. cells in pericardial fluid: Report of a case. J. A. M. A. *149*:145–147, 1952.
130. Sharp, G. C., Irvin, W. S., Tan, E. M., et al.: Mixed connective tissue disease: An apparently distinct rheumatic disease syndrome associated with a specific antibody to an extractable nuclear antigen (ENA). Am. J. Med. *52*:148–159, 1972.
131. Shearn, M.: The heart in systemic lupus erythematosus. Am. Heart J. *58*:452–466, 1959.
132. Singsen, B. H., Bernstein, B. H., Kornreich, H. K., et al.: Mixed connective tissue disease in childhood: A clinical and serologic survey. J. Pediatr. *90*:893–900, 1977.
133. Singsen, B. H., Goldreyer, B., Stanton, R., et al.: Childhood polymyositis with cardiac conduction defects. Am. J. Dis. Child. *130*:72–74, 1976.
134. Smith, J. W., Clements, P. J., Levismen, J., et al.: Echocardiographic features of progressive systemic sclerosis (PSS): Correlation with hemodynamic and post mortem studies. Am. J. Med. *66*:28–33, 1979.
135. Sokoloff, L.: Cardiac involvement in rheumatoid arthritis and allied disorders: current concepts. Mod. Concepts Cardiovasc. Dis. *33*:847–850, 1964.
136. Suma, K., Takeuchi, Y., Shiroma, K., et al.: Early and late postoperative studies in coronary arterial lesions resulting from Kawasaki's disease in children. J. Thorac. Cardiovasc. Surg. *84*:224–229, 1983.
137. Sunder, S. K., and Shah, A.: Constrictive pericarditis in procainamide-induced lupus erythematosus syndrome. Am. J. Cardiol. *36*:960–962, 1975.
138. Suylen van, R. J., Schoof, P. H., Zoo, E., et al.: Pulmonary autograft failure after aortic root replacement in a patient with juvenile rheumatoid arthritis. Eur. J. Cardiothorac. Surg. *6*:571–572, 1992.
139. Svantesson, H., Bjorkhem, G., and Elborough, R.: Cardiac involvement in juvenile rheumatoid arthritis: A follow-up study. Acta Paediatr. Scand. *72*:345–350, 1983.
140. Tajik, A. J.: Echocardiography in pericardial effusion. Am. J. Med. *63*:29–40, 1977.
141. Takkunen, J., Vuopala, V., and Isomaki, H.: Cardiomyopathy in ankylosing spondylitis. I. Medical history and results of clinical examination in a series of 55 patients. Ann. Clin. Res. *2*:106–112, 1970.
142. Tami, L. F., and Bhasin, S.: Polymorphism of the cardiac manifestations in dermatomyositis. Clin. Cardiol. *16*:260–264, 1993.
143. Thadani, U., Iveson, J. M. I., and Wright, V.: Cardiac tamponade, constrictive pericarditis and pericardial resection in rheumatoid arthritis. Medicine *54*:261–270, 1975.
144. Thomas, D., Hill, W., Geddes, R., et al.: Early detection of aortic dilatation in ankylosing spondylitis using echocardiography. Aust. N. Z. J. Med. *12*:10–13, 1982.
145. Tsakraklides, V. G., Bleiden, L. C., and Edwards, J. E.: Coronary atherosclerosis and myocardial infarction associated with systemic lupus erythematosus. Am. Heart J. *87*:637–641, 1974.
146. Uhl, G. S., and Koppes, G. M.: Pericardial tamponade in systemic sclerosis (scleroderma). Br. Heart J. *42*:345–348, 1979.
147. Vonderheid, E. C., Koblenzer, P. J., Ming, P. M. L., et al.: Neonatal lupus erythematosus. Arch. Dermatol. *112*:698–705, 1976.
148. Wada, J., Endo, M., Takao, A., et al.: Mucocutaneous lymph node syndrome: Successful aortocoronary bypass homograft in a four-year-old boy. Chest *77*:443–446, 1980.
149. Walton, J., and Adams, R. D.: Polymyositis. Edinburgh, E. & H. Livingston, 1958.

150. Watson, R. M., Lane, A. T., Barnett, N. K., et al.: Neonatal lupus erythematosus: A clinical, serological and immunogenetic study with review of literature. Medicine *63*:362–378, 1984.
151. Weintraub, A. M., and Zvaifler, N. J.: The occurrence of valvular and myocardial disease in patients with chronic joint deformity: A spectrum. Am. J. Med. *35*:145–162, 1963.
152. West, S. G., Killian, P. J., and Lawless, O. J.: Association of myositis and myocarditis in progressive systemic sclerosis. Arthritis Rheum. *22*:1088–1092, 1979.
153. White, P. H.: Pediatric systemic lupus erythematosus and neonatal lupus. Rheum. Dis. Clin. North Am. *20*:119–127, 1994.
154. Wolff, L., and Grunfeld, O.: Pericarditis. N. Engl. J. Med. *268*:419–426, 1963.
155. Yancy, C. L., Doughty, R. A., Cohlan, B. A., et al.: Pericarditis and cardiac tamponade in juvenile rheumatoid arthritis. Pediatrics *68*:369–373, 1981.
156. Yoshikawa, J., Yanagihara, K., Owaki, T., et al.: Cross-sectional echocardiographic diagnosis of coronary artery aneurysms in patients with the mucocutaneous lymph node syndrome. Circulation *59*:133–139, 1979.

37

MEDIASTINITIS

John G. Bartlett

The mediastinum includes the extrapleural portion of the thoracic cavity situated between the two pleural sacs. The superior and inferior portions are separated arbitrarily by a line extending from the lower manubrium to the fourth thoracic vertebra. The superior mediastinum contains the thymus gland, trachea, esophagus, and aortic arch. The inferior mediastinum is divided into the anterior compartment, containing lymphatic tissue and fat; the middle compartment, containing the heart, pericardium, aorta, bifurcation of the trachea, main bronchi, and numerous lymph nodes; and the posterior compartment, containing the esophagus, thoracic duct, descending aorta, and vagus nerve. Infections of the mediastinum are relatively uncommon, but they often pose a serious threat to the vital structures in the vicinity and may prove extremely difficult to diagnose. Two forms are recognized: acute mediastinitis, which is a fulminant, septic process; and chronic mediastinitis, which is an indolent infection that produces late symptomatology due to compression of adjacent structures.

ACUTE MEDIASTINITIS

The major causes of acute mediastinitis are classified etiologically as traumatic perforation of the esophagus, nontraumatic extension from extramediastinal infections, and postoperative median sternotomy wound infections (Table 37–1).

Table 37–1. Acute Mediastinitis

1. Perforated esophagus
   - Spontaneous or postemetic
   - Foreign body
   - Instrumentation, e.g., esophagoscopy or instrumental dilatation
   - Postoperative, e.g., esophageal, proximal stomach, or thoracic surgery
   - Blunt or penetrating trauma
2. Extension of infections from adjacent structures
   - "Space Infections" of the head and neck
   - Lungs, pleura, lymph nodes, pericardium, tracheostomy
   - Subphrenic infection
   - Osteomyelitis of vertebrae
   - Hematogenous dissemination of infection from a remote site
3. Postoperative median sternotomy wound infection

Esophageal Perforation

The most common cause of acute mediastinitis is esophageal perforation.[25, 29] The stomach and duodenum represent far more frequent sites of alimentary tract perforation, and usually this is due to intrinsic diseases of these organs. In contrast, the esophagus has a thin, vulnerable wall and is perforated more easily. The most common causes of acute purulent mediastinitis, in rank order, are esophageal dilatation, foreign body extraction, chemical injury of the esophagus (lye ingestion), esophagoscopy, and ingestion of a sharp foreign body.[5] Intrinsic diseases such as strictures, carcinoma, and diverticula are associated conditions in a relatively small portion of cases.

Perforations secondary to instrumentation may produce precipitous symptoms during the procedure from transmural laceration.[29] Alternatively, there may be a superficial tear, which becomes the site of suppurative infection that subsequently extends through remaining layers. In the latter instance, several hours or days may elapse between instrumentation and the onset of symptoms. Foreign bodies that cause esophageal perforation present analogous variations in the time course from the initial injury. Sharp objects such as pins and bone fragments may cause immediate transmural penetration. More commonly, and especially with blunt objects such as coins, teeth, and food particles (e.g., corn chips), the foreign body becomes impacted in the esophagus.[28] Eventually, there is suppurative necrosis of the wall, with the onset of symptoms several days after ingestion.

Another common cause of esophageal perforation is "spontaneous" or "atraumatic" panmural rupture.[1, 9] These terms are not entirely appropriate because most cases are associated with overwhelming distention and pressure secondary to vomiting or retching. Occasional cases have been reported from air blast injuries; these indicate that 25 to 30 pounds of air pressure applied to the oropharynx will cause esophageal rupture. Neurologic diseases, possibly related to disturbances in esophageal innervation by the autonomic nervous system, appear to play a role in some atraumatic cases as well. Postoperative esophageal perforations usually represent infectious complications of anastomotic leaks occurring after esophageal resection or esophageal-pleural fistulas after thoracic surgery. The majority of these infections do not become apparent until weeks or months after surgery.

Esophageal perforations usually occur at a site of normal or pathologic narrowing, and there is a high correlation between the location of the lesion and the cause of rupture.

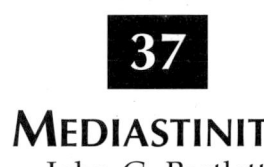

The normal esophagus has three narrow sites: the esophageal introitus, located at the level of the cricopharyngeal muscle; the midthoracic segment, where the aortic arch and left main stem bronchus indent the esophagus; and the transdiaphragmatic segment. Most perforations due to instrumentation and to foreign bodies involve the introitus, which is the narrowest segment. Perforations at this level usually are located in the posterior wall, giving egress to the prevertebral or retrovisceral space. (These spaces represent pathways for the spread of infections from the neck or mandible to the thorax, to be discussed subsequently.) Perforations at the level of the aortic arch are relatively uncommon and usually are due to ingested foreign bodies. The usual location of "spontaneous" perforations is the esophageal segment immediately above the diaphragm. In most such cases, there is a longitudinal tear on the left posterolateral wall just above the cardia, where the esophagus has little connective tissue support and its intrinsic musculature is relatively weak. Thus, the most common sites for esophageal perforation are at the proximal and distal ends, with occasional cases involving the midthoracic region. The presenting findings, as well as the underlying condition, vary with these different sites of rupture.

The predominant symptoms of acute mediastinitis developing after esophageal perforation are neck and chest pain, respiratory distress, and dysphagia. Chills, fever of 37.8° to 39° C (100° to 102° F), and leukocytosis also are common. Infants may show a staccato breathing pattern characterized by an inspiratory halt with resumption of inspiration after a brief rest.[10] The onset of symptoms usually is abrupt, and the disease tends to follow a fulminant course. Approximately 20 to 30 per cent of patients are comatose or hypotensive when first seen.[1] Mortality rates are 15 to 40 per cent and especially are high if the patient is not seen and properly treated in the early stages of the disease.[1, 5, 9, 29] An exception to this is postoperative esophageal perforation, which tends to follow a somewhat more indolent course.

Pain at the site of the lesion is a prominent complaint in about 80 per cent of patients. Perforations of the cervical esophagus are associated with pain in the neck and upper anterior chest, whereas perforations of the lower esophagus tend to cause pain in the epigastric region or precordium, which may radiate to the back, shoulder, or arm. Dyspnea usually reflects pleural involvement and is most common with lower esophageal perforations. Severe dyspnea or cyanosis suggests massive pleural effusion, pneumothorax, or a low cardiac output. Dysphagia almost invariably is present, but it may be of relatively little value in localizing the site of perforation. Physical examination often shows cervical tenderness and subcutaneous emphysema in patients with proximal perforations, whereas patients with lower esophageal perforations are more likely to have signs suggesting an acute abdominal catastrophe. Examination of the lung fields often is abnormal, but the findings are nonspecific. The Hamman sign consists of "crunching" sounds heard in synchrony with the heartbeat along the left sternal border or cardiac apex. This finding is observed in about 50 per cent of cases of mediastinal emphysema, but it also is noted with left pneumothorax, dilated esophagus, gastric dilatation, bullous emphysema, and pneumoperitoneum. The diagnosis of mediastinal emphysema also is nonspecific, as noted later.

Routine laboratory tests other than the chest radiograph generally are of little value. Pleural fluid analysis generally shows a sterile exudate early in the disease course. Pleural fluid amylase levels often are abnormal, but this varies with the time-frame of the disease course. During the first 24 hours after perforation, generally these levels are normal, i.e., 30 to 50 units/mL. After 24 hours, the pleural fluid amylase level is elevated disproportionately, compared with serum levels, to 200 to 2000 units/mL.

The principal findings on chest radiographs are a widened mediastinum, subcutaneous and mediastinal emphysema, and pleural effusions. Pleural effusions are more common with lower esophageal perforations and usually involve the left side. There also may be basilar or retrocardiac infiltrates ascribed to chemical pneumonitis in the pulmonary segment adjacent to the site of perforation. Additional changes often include basilar atelectasis, a pneumothorax, or a hydropneumothorax. Radiopaque foreign bodies may be detected with plain films, but these often are demonstrated better with mediastinal tomography or fluoroscopy.

Roentgenographic demonstration of gas in the soft tissue is highly suggestive of esophageal perforation if interpreted in the context of a compatible clinical presentation. Gas in the prevertebral tissue or superior mediastinum is most common with perforation of the upper esophagus. However, it should be noted that several other conditions also may cause mediastinal emphysema, including air entry from the retroperitoneal space along the esophagus or aorta due to a perforated stomach, perforated intestine, or perirenal insufflation; perforation of the trachea, bronchi, or marginal alveoli; air entry via cervical fascial planes after thyroidectomy, tonsillectomy, deep neck wounds, and infections of perimandibular spaces; chest wall trauma, especially with closed chest massage; and "spontaneous pneumomediastinum," an idiopathic benign condition that some authorities ascribe to ruptured blebs, bullae, or alveoli.

The diagnosis of acute mediastinitis due to esophageal perforation often can be made on the basis of a typical clinical setting coupled with the previously noted abnormalities of routine chest radiographs, mediastinal tomography, fluoroscopy (during ingestion of nonirritating water-soluble contrast media), computed tomography with contrast, or spiral computed tomography.[32] These procedures also serve to localize the site of esophageal perforation and to detect any intrinsic esophageal disease. Perforations of the intrathoracic esophagus are detected readily with these contrast studies, but perforations at the level of the introitus often give false-negative results. Esophagoscopy is considered unnecessary and, in fact, is contraindicated except for purposes of removing a foreign body.

The treatment of esophageal perforations consists of supportive measures, antimicrobials, and, in most patients, surgical intervention. Supportive measures imply several obvious considerations, such as intravenous fluid support, maintenance of an adequate airway, esophageal rest (i.e., no food), and careful monitoring of vital functions. Many patients are critically ill when seen and require intensive treatment to achieve stabilization before diagnostic tests or surgery is feasible. Others are less seriously ill initially, but the infection may progress to fulminant sepsis, serious pleural or pulmonary involvement, cardiac perforation, or aortic perforation. Vena caval obstruction is uncommon with acute mediastinitis.

Antimicrobial selection optimally is determined by bacteriologic studies. Unfortunately, valid specimens for meaningful culture seldom are obtained, and there is a paucity of reported data concerning documented pathogens. Blood and pleural fluid cultures should be obtained, but these usually are negative, except late in the course. As a consequence, antimicrobial decisions necessarily are empiric and should be directed against oral anaerobic bacteria and streptococci.[2, 4, 6, 17]

The most important component of treatment usually is surgery. Cervical perforations may respond to temporary avoidance of swallowing, antimicrobials, and endoscopic removal of any foreign body. Nevertheless, the convalescence may be protracted unnecessarily, and many authorities recommend surgical intervention. Drainage of the pretracheal space and superior mediastinum may be accomplished through a low cervical incision. Postemetic ruptures usually involve the distal esophagus; transthoracic surgical débridement with closure of the laceration strongly is recommended if the patient is seen within 12 to 24 hours of perforation. Delayed surgical intervention or extensive suppuration often precludes primary closure. An alternative approach with these "late cases" is a wide mediastinotomy with débridement and tube drainage with or without extirpation of the thoracic esophagus.[27, 29]

Extension from Adjacent Structure Infections

The mediastinum would appear to be a prime location for the spread of infections from contiguous structures. Anatomically, it is a central focus of lymph drainage, fascial planes from the abdomen and supraclavicular region transgress the mediastinum, and the adjacent pulmonary system is one of the most frequent sites of serious infection. Nevertheless, the mediastinum rarely is involved secondarily in suppurative infections.

In the preantimicrobial era, peritonsillar abscess, Ludwig angina, and other infections of the head and neck were relatively common causes of acute mediastinitis.[6, 13, 25, 34] Since the availability of penicillin, these infections have been less frequent. When they do occur, the usual initial focus is pharyngitis or a dental infection. These infections spread beyond the usual anatomic barriers to involve spaces of the neck or perimandibular area. The term *space infection* refers to suppurative involvement of potential spaces formed by fascial planes that extend from the head to the thorax.[4] The principal spaces that serve as conduits to the mediastinum are (1) the visceral division of the deep cervical fascia that envelops the esophagus, trachea, larynx, and thyroid gland and (2) the carotid sheath, which extends from the base of the skull, passes through the posterior pharyngomaxillary space along the prevertebral fascia, and enters the chest. Conditions other than pharyngitis and dental infections that may lead to suppurative involvement of these spaces include mastoiditis, laryngectomy, mediastinotomy, tracheostomy, and surgery or trauma of the oral airways. Antecedent injury in children younger than 4 years of age often is a penetrating wound to the oropharynx due to falling on a sharp or pointed object, i.e., the "pencil injury." Suppurative pleuropulmonary infections rarely are complicated by mediastinal involvement, except for loculated paramediastinal empyemas or actinomycosis. Extension of infection from vertebrae, ribs, or sternum also is unusual.

The major bacteria responsible for suppurative infections that originate in the oral cavity and extend to the mediastinum are group A beta-hemolytic streptococci and the anaerobic bacteria that are considered normal oral flora.[4, 6, 18, 24, 25] The former is the most frequent pathogen when the pharynx is the original portal of entry. Anaerobic bacteria, principally *Prevotella* species, *Bacteroides* species, fusobacteria, and peptostreptococci, are the major pathogens in spreading infections of dental origin. Clindamycin often is regarded as the agent of choice for both streptococci and anaerobes, although some authorities prefer other regimens likely to be effective, including penicillin plus metronidazole, cefoxitin, cefotetan, imipenem, or a β-lactam–β-lactamase inhibitor.[2, 6, 12, 17]

Surgical drainage is the cornerstone of treatment in "space infections." Transcervical incisions usually are employed when there is spread to the superior mediastinum. Extension of the infection below the level of the fourth thoracic vertebrae requires a parasternal or paravertebral approach, depending on whether the anterior or posterior mediastinum is involved.

MEDIASTINITIS DUE TO MEDIAN STERNOTOMY WOUND INFECTIONS

Wound infections complicate 0.5 to 2.2 per cent of median sternotomy incisions for cardiac surgery. The incidence is similar for the three major categories of thoracic surgery: repair of congenital anomalies, valve replacement, and coronary bypass surgery.[7, 10, 14, 19, 20, 22 26, 30, 33] The rate is somewhat higher after cardiac transplantation.[19, 33] Mediastinitis is considered a major complication, with potential involvement of contiguous structures, including prosthetic valves, grafts, pericardium, lung, and chest wall. The associated mortality rate is reported at 9 to 77 per cent but usually is 10 to 25 per cent.[30] Older reports showed that up to one-third of surviving patients had osteomyelitis or costochondritis that continued for months or even years and often required repeated surgical procedures. The incidence of these infections is higher with patients who have prolonged procedures, postoperative closed chest massage, infected tracheostomy stomas, reoperation in the postoperative period, and wound hematomas.[26, 30] Patient risk factors include age older than 65 years, functional cardiac status, and associated medical conditions. The role of prophylactic antibiotics in preventing mediastinitis is not established, although these drugs clearly influence bacteriologic findings, because the isolates recovered usually are resistant to the agent used. Outbreaks of mediastinitis and endocarditis have been reported with *Mycobacterium chelonei* or *Mycobacterium fortuitum*, presumably reflecting contact with nonsterile water.[20] Epidemics also have been traced to operating room personnel, who may serve as the source of *Staphylococcus aureus* or other bacteria.[14]

The clinical features of these wound infections include local pain and tenderness, erythema, purulent drainage, wound dehiscence, persistent or recurrent postoperative fever, and leukocytosis. Less frequently, there is sternal instability with a rocking motion, although this simply may indicate nonunion without necessarily implicating infection. The signs of mediastinitis usually become apparent within a few days to 3 weeks after surgery. The most common sequence is fever and systemic toxicity followed by signs of a sternal wound infection with cellulitis or purulent drainage. Computed tomography, often with aspiration, is an important adjunct in the diagnosis.[19]

The treatment of median sternotomy infections includes prolonged courses of antibiotics and surgical débridement. Antimicrobial selection optimally is based on culture results of blood, needle aspirates, or tissue specimens obtained from the infected site. The most frequent pathogens in an era when there is almost universal antimicrobial prophylaxis are *S. aureus* (including methicillin-resistant *S. aureus)* and *Staphylococcus epidermidis*; less common are coliforms, *Pseudomonas*, and *Candida albicans*. Antibiotic selection is based on sensitivity test results. *S. aureus* and *S. epidermidis* usually are treated with vancomycin due to resistance to β-lactams; rifampin or gentamicin sometimes is added to enhance antimicrobial activity. Systemic antibiotics should be given for at least 3 to 6 weeks.

Adequate surgical débridement is the most important facet of treatment. This usually will reveal gross pus and often show sternal osteomyelitis. The wound should be reopened and débrided for removal of all infected tissue. A distinction needs to be made between superficial and deep infections. Superficial infections can be treated simply with incision, packing, and a short course of antibiotics. With deep involvement, it is necessary to débride devitalized bone and irrigate the mediastinum. The wound may be managed with closed irrigation, open-wound packing, a muscle flap procedure, or an omental flap procedure.[3, 14, 16, 26, 33]

CHRONIC MEDIASTINITIS

Chronic mediastinitis is an indolent infection involving the paratracheal region, carina, and hilum. Two histologic forms are recognized: granulomatous and fibrotic. The clinical presentation and location of lesions for these two forms are identical, and there may be considerable overlap in histologic findings. Consequently, many authorities consider that common etiologic mechanisms are responsible and that the fibrotic form represents the end stage of granulomatous mediastinitis.[31] Nevertheless, one type of fibrotic mediastinitis stands apart in being associated with a fibrotic process at another anatomic site such as retroperitoneal fibrosis, orbital pseudotumor, Riedel struma, or perityphlitis of the cecum. The term *multifocal fibrosclerosis* has been used for such cases. Additional distinctive features of fibrotic mediastinitis are that symptomatic disease is more common and an etiologic organism rarely is demonstrated.

Chronic mediastinitis occurs in virtually any age group. Many patients are asymptomatic, and the lesion initially is detected by routine chest radiographs showing a widened superior mediastinum near the tracheal bifurcation or the hilum with a lobulated configuration.[11] There also may be mediastinal calcifications. Concomitant changes in the pulmonary parenchyma demonstrable by chest radiograph are variable. Symptoms, when present, usually reflect compression of adjacent structures such as the superior vena cava, esophagus, and tracheobronchial tree. There also may be low-grade fever, anemia, and weight loss. A review of 180 reported cases showed that 26 per cent of 103 patients with granulomatous mediastinitis were symptomatic, compared with 83 per cent of 77 individuals with fibrotic mediastinitis.[31] The most common signs and symptoms are those ascribed to superior vena caval obstruction.

Histoplasmosis is the most common identifiable cause of chronic mediastinitis; less common causes are tuberculosis, blastomycosis, sarcoidosis, nocardiosis, actinomycosis, and lymphomas.[8, 11, 15, 21, 22] A review of 180 cases of histoplasmosis and tuberculosis accounted for 27 per cent of cases of granulomatous mediastinitis and 4 per cent with fibrotic mediastinitis. The majority were enigmatic (31), but many investigators believe that histoplasmosis accounts for most of the "idiopathic" cases. This impression is supported by a substantially higher yield of *Histoplasma capsulatum* yeast forms in previously negative sections when a diligent search is made using periodic acid–Schiff or methenamine silver stains.[23]

Two types of mediastinal fibrosis due to histoplasmosis are recognized. The most common type, mediastinal granuloma, is caused by a cluster of nodes that coalesce and form an encapsulated mass that may be large and compress adjacent structures, especially the superior vena cava or esophagus. Surgical resection often is feasible but advocated only when there is significant obstruction. The second type is healed histoplasmosis with sclerosis. The thick fibrotic capsule may invade contiguous structures, causing stenosis of pulmonary arteries, pulmonary veins, superior vena cava, or bronchi. These lesions may require resectional surgery: resection of a subcranial mass, lobectomy, pneumonectomy, bronchoplasty, esophagoplasty, etc. Indications for surgery are arbitrary and include dyspnea, postobstructive pneumonia, and superior vena caval syndrome.[22] Surgical mortality rates may be high and the outcome variable.

The diagnostic evaluation of patients with possible chronic mediastinitis should include chest radiograph, fluoroscopy or mediastinal tomograms, tuberculin skin test, and histoplasmosis serology. Cultures of sputum for *Mycobacterium tuberculosis* and pathogenic fungi rarely are positive. The antigen assay for *H. capsulatum* using blood and urine usually is negative. Skin tests for this fungus also are not helpful. Complement-fixation titers usually exceed 1:8 in patients with chronic histoplasmosis. Venography is indicated if there is evidence of venous or vena caval obstruction, and arteriography is indicated if there is evidence of arterial involvement.

Calcifications or roentgenographic stability over a prolonged period suggests a benign condition, and if obstructive symptoms are not present, surgery often can be deferred.[23] Caution in this approach is necessary because thymomas and teratomas may cause calcified masses in the superior mediastinum and both require surgical resection. Resected tissue should be cultured and studied extensively on histologic sections for evidence of *M. tuberculosis* and fungi. When *H. capsulatum* is responsible, it usually is detected histologically; fungal cultures rarely are positive.[22, 23] The role of amphotericin B when surgically excised tissue shows *H. capsulatum* is controversial, but most authorities believe that drug treatment is unnecessary if cultures are negative.[23] Newer agents used for histoplasmosis, such as ketoconazole, fluconazole, and itraconazole, also play an uncertain role in therapy.

References

1. Abbott, O. A., Mansour, K. A., Logan, W. D., Jr., et al.: A traumatic so-called "spontaneous" rupture of the esophagus. J. Thorac. Cardiovasc. Surg. *59*:67–83, 1970.
2. Applebaum, P. C., Spangler, S. K., and Jacobs, M. R.: Beta-lactamase production and susceptibilities to amoxicillin, amoxicillin-clavulanate, ticarcillin, ticarcillin-clavulanate, cefoxitin, imipenem, and metronidazole of 320 non–*Bacteroides fragilis Bacteroides* isolates and 129 fusobacteria from 28 U.S. centers. Antimicrob. Agents Chemother. *34*:1546–1550, 1990.
3. Backer, C. L., Pensler, J. M., Tobin, G. R., et al.: Vascularized muscle flaps for life-threatening mediastinal wounds in children. Ann. Thorac. Surg. *57*:797–801, 1994.
4. Bartlett, J. G., and Gorbach, S. L.: Anaerobic infections of the head and neck. Otolaryngol. Clin. North Am. *9*:655–678, 1976.
5. Cherveniakov, A., and Cherveniakov P.: Surgical treatment of acute purulent mediastinitis. Eur. J. Cardiovasc. Thorac. Surg. *6*:407–410, 1992.
6. Civen, R., Vaisanen, M. L., and Finegold, S. M.: Peritonsillar abscess, retropharyngeal abscess, mediastinitis and nonclostridial anaerobic myonecrosis: A case report. Clin. Infect. Dis. *16*(Suppl. 4):S299–S303, 1992.
7. Curtis, J. J., Boley, T. M., Walls, J. T., et al.: Randomized prospective comparison of first- and second-generation cephalosporins as infection prophylaxis for cardiac surgery. Am. J. Surg. *166*:734–737, 1993.
8. Dukes, R. J., Strimlan, C. V., Dines, D. E., et al.: Esophageal involvement of mediastinal granuloma. J. A. M. A. *236*:2313–2315, 1976.
9. Enquist, R. W., Blanck, R. R., and Butler, R. H.: Nontraumatic mediastinitis. J. A. M. A. *236*:1048–1049, 1976.
10. Feldman, R., and Gromisch, D. S.: Acute suppurative mediastinitis. Am. J. Dis. Child. *121*:79–81, 1971.
11. Ferguson, T. B., and Burford, T. H.: Mediastinal granuloma. Ann. Thorac. Surg. *1*:125–141, 1965.
12. Finegold, S. M., and Wexler, H. M.: Therapeutic implications of bacteriologic findings in mixed aerobic-anaerobic infections. Antimicrob. Agents Chemother. *32*:611–616, 1988.
13. Garatea-Crelgo, J., and Gay-Escoda, C.: Mediastinitis from odontogenic infection: Report of three cases and review of the literature. Int. J. Oral Maxillofac. Surg. *20*:65–68, 1991.
14. Gaynes, R., Marosok, R., Mowry-Hanley, J., et al.: Mediastinitis following coronary artery bypass surgery: A 3-year review. J. Infect. Dis. *163*:117–121, 1991.
15. Goodwin, R. A., Nickell, J. A., and Des Prez, R. M.: Mediastinal fibrosis complicating healed primary histoplasmosis and tuberculosis. Medicine *51*:227–246, 1972.

16. Gottlieb, L. J., Pielet, R. W., Karp, R. B., et al.: Rigid internal fixation of the sternum in postoperative mediastinitis. Arch. Surg. *129*:489–493, 1994.
17. Gudiol, F., Manresa, F., Pallares, R., et al.: Clindamycin vs. penicillin for anaerobic lung infections. Arch. Intern. Med. *150*:2525–2531, 1990.
18. Howell, H. S., Prinz, R. A., and Pickleman, J. R.: Anaerobic mediastinitis. Surg. Gynecol. Obstet. *143*:353–359, 1976.
19. Karwande, S. V., Renlund, D. G., Olsen, S. L., et al.: Mediastinitis in heart transplantation. Ann. Thorac. Surg. *54*:1039–1045, 1992.
20. Kuritsky, J. N., Bullen, M. G., Broome, C. V., et al.: Sternal wound infections and endocarditis due to organisms of the *Mycobacterium fortuitum* complex. Ann. Intern. Med. *98*:938–939, 1983.
21. Langerstrom, C. F., Mitchell, H. G., Graham, B. S., et al.: Chronic fibrosing mediastinitis and superior vena caval obstruction from blastomycosis. Ann. Thorac. Surg. *54*:764–765, 1992.
22. Mathisen, D. J., and Grillo, H. C.: Clinical manifestations of mediastinal fibrosis and histoplasmosis. Ann. Thorac. Surg. *54*:1053–1057, 1992.
23. Medeiros, A. A.: Case records of the Massachusetts General Hospital (chronic mediastinitis due to histoplasmosis). N. Engl. J. Med. *295*:381–388, 1976.
24. Murray, P. M., and Finegold, S. M.: Anaerobic mediastinitis. Rev. Infect. Dis. *6*:5123–5127, 1984.
25. Neuhof, H.: Acute infections of the mediastinum with special reference to mediastinal suppuration. J. Thorac. Surg. *6*:194–195, 1936.
26. Newman, L. S., Szczukowski, L. C., Bain, R. P., et al.: Suppurative mediastinitis after open heart surgery. Chest *94*:546–553, 1988.
27. Payne, W. S., and Larson, R. H.: Acute mediastinitis. Surg. Clin. North Am. *49*:999–1009, 1969.
28. Reino, A. J., Jahn, A. F., Parsons, J., et al.: Traumatic pneumomediastinum in a child secondary to corn chip perforation of the esophagus. Pediatr. Emerg. Care *9*:211–215, 1993.
29. Salo, J. A., Isolauri, J. O., Heikkila, L. J., et al.: Management of delayed esophageal perforation with mediastinal sepsis. J. Thorac. Cardiovasc. Surg. *106*:1088–1091, 1993.
30. Sarr, M. G., Gott, V. L., and Townsend, T. R.: Mediastinal infection after cardiac surgery. Ann. Thorac. Surg. *38*:415–423, 1984.
31. Schowengerdt, C. G., Suyemoto, R., and Main, F. B.: Granulomatous and fibrous mediastinitis. J. Thorac. Cardiovasc. Surg. *57*:365–379, 1969.
32. Tecce, P. M., Fishman, E. K., and Kuhlman, J. E.: CT evaluation of the anterior mediastinum: Spectrum of disease. Radiographics *14*:973–990, 1994.
33. Whitehead, B., Helms, P., Goodwin, M., et al.: Heart-lung transplantation for cystic fibrosis. Arch. Dis. Child. *66*:1022–1026, 1991.
34. Zeitoun, I. M., and Dhanarajani, P. J.: Cervical cellulitis and mediastinitis caused by odontogenic infections: Report of two cases and review of the literature. J. Oral Maxillofac. Surg. *53*:203–208, 1995.

SECTION FOUR

CENTRAL NERVOUS SYSTEM INFECTIONS

❑ ❑ ❑

38

BACTERIAL MENINGITIS BEYOND THE NEONATAL PERIOD

Ralph D. Feigin and Eric Pearlman

Bacterial meningitis indicates inflammation of the meninges as a result of bacterial infection. The term *leptomeningitis* denotes inflammation of the arachnoid and pia mater, the usual distribution of meningitis. Infections of the neonate, including bacterial meningitis, are presented in Chapter 77, and central nervous system (CNS) infections caused by mycobacteria are discussed in Chapter 101.

INCIDENCE AND EPIDEMIOLOGY

Before the discovery and use of antibiotics, bacterial meningitis generally was fatal. Although antibiotic therapy has improved the prognosis in patients afflicted with bacterial meningitis dramatically, bacterial meningitis continues to be a significant cause of morbidity and mortality in children. Whereas the number of deaths attributed to many different infectious diseases in the United States decreased by 10- to 200-fold between 1935 and 1968, the number of reported deaths caused by bacterial meningitis decreased by only half during the same period.[297, 298] In 1972, the Centers for Disease Control and Prevention estimated that in the United States there were 29,000 cases of meningitis caused by *Haemophilus influenzae* type b, 4800 cases caused by *Streptococcus pneumoniae*, and 4600 cases caused by *Neisseria meningitidis*.

Population-based studies in South Carolina, Minnesota, Vermont, and New Mexico suggest that the actual incidence of bacterial meningitis ranges between 5.4 and 7.3 cases per 100,000 population.[44, 99–102]

Two hundred thirty-five patients were enrolled in a prospective study (initiated at Washington University School of Medicine and continued at the Baylor College of Medicine) of bacterial meningitis in children who were between 1 month and 15 years of age.[66, 78, 82] The organisms responsible for these infections were *H. influenzae* type b in 151 (64 per cent) patients, *S. pneumoniae* in 35 (15 per cent), and *N. meningitidis* in 26 (11 per cent). Twenty-three children[148] had meningitis caused by other organisms.

Although *H. influenzae* type b was the most common cause of bacterial meningitis in children in the United States, Canada, and Scandinavia, this pattern was not universal.[126] Davey and associates[57] reported that between 1968 and 1977, *N. meningitidis* was the most common and *H. influenzae* type b the second most common cause of bacterial meningitis in children and young adults in Great Britain. Mortality rates in this group of patients were 3.5 per cent for those with meningococcal meningitis, 7.7 per cent in children with *H. influenzae* meningitis, and 30 per cent in patients with pneumococcal meningitis.

The child between 6 and 12 months of age appears to be at greatest risk for bacterial meningitis; 90 per cent of reported cases occur between 1 month and 5 years of age.[61, 99] The age distribution of patients with bacterial meningitis has not changed appreciably during the past 40 years.[216, 270]

Annual age-specific attack rates for meningitis are shown in Table 38–1.[170] The Centers for Disease Control and Prevention found differences in attack rates for meningitis in nine reporting areas throughout the United States, although the relative frequencies of causative organisms were similar except for one region.[252] *H. influenzae* type b was the most common cause of bacterial meningitis in all regions with the exception of the west south-central region, where attack rates for meningococcal meningitis were higher than for meningitis caused by *H. influenzae* type b (1.1 compared with 0.7 cases/100,000 population/year).

The number of cases of *H. influenzae* meningitis reported through the National Bacterial Meningitis Reporting System was by far the greatest until introduction of the *H. influenzae* type b vaccine in the late 1980s. The incidence thereafter began to drop, and since 1991, meningococcal meningitis has been the most reported, followed by *S. pneumoniae* meningitis and *H. influenzae* meningitis (Fig. 38–1). Group B *Streptococcus* has been noted as the most common cause of meningitis in children 2 to 6 weeks of age, followed by *Escherichia coli, Listeria monocytogenes, H. influenzae,* and *S. pneumoniae.*[25]

Epidemiology of *Haemophilus influenzae* Meningitis

The most dramatic change in the epidemiology of bacterial meningitis since the advent of antibiotics has occurred in the past 5 years because of licensure of conjugate vaccines against *H. influenzae* type b. The first vaccines available were *H. influenzae* type b capsular polysaccharide (polyribosylribitol phosphate [PRP]) and were licensed for use in children 18 to 59 months of age in April 1985. Newer vaccines with improved immunogenicity at younger ages were developed by covalently linking the capsular polysaccharide with protein antigens. The first of these, diphtheria toxoid conjugate (PRP-D), was licensed in December 1987 for use in children 18 to 59 months of age. In October 1990, the first conjugate, PRP diphtheria CRM_{197} protein conjugate (HbOC), was approved for infant use, and in 1991, the Advisory Committee on Immunization Practices and the American Academy of Pediatrics recommended universal infant immunization at 2,

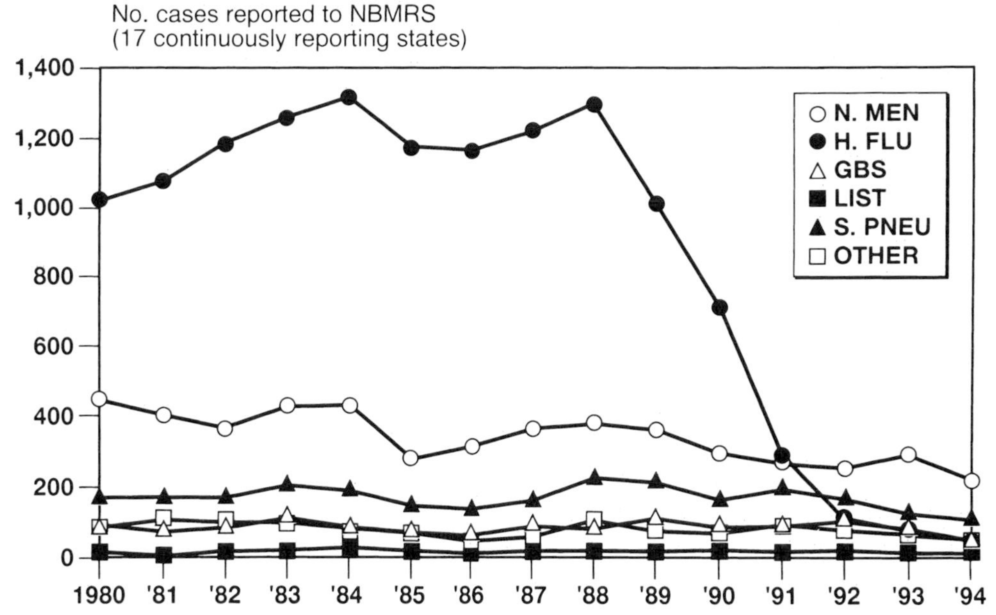

FIGURE 38–1. *Incidence of bacterial meningitis in individuals from birth to 19 years of age. A marked decline in the incidence of* Haemophilus influenzae *type b meningitis is noted over the period between 1988 and 1994. NBMRS, National Bacterial Meningitis Reporting System; N. MEN,* Neisseria meningitidis; *H. FLU,* Haemophilus influenzae *type b; GBS, group B* Streptococcus; *LIST,* Listeria monocytogenes; *S. PNEU,* Streptococcus pneumoniae.

4, and 6 months of age with either HbOC or PRP-meningococcal protein conjugate (PRP-OMP) vaccines.[8, 45]

The *Haemophilus influenzae* Study Group[5] noted that the number of cases of *H. influenzae* meningitis in children younger than 5 years of age reported through the National Bacterial Meningitis Reporting System began declining rapidly in 1988. There were 1334 cases (19.4/100,000) reported in 1980 from 20 continuously reporting states and 1451 cases (19.3/100,000) in 1988, declining to 1163 cases (15.3/100,000) in 1989, 745 cases (9.8/100,000) in 1990, and 283 cases (3.7/100,000) in 1991. In those older than 12 years of age, however, the incidence of *H. influenzae* meningitis remained relatively stable (0.06/100,000 population). Over the same period, meningococcal meningitis and pneumococcal meningitis in children younger than 5 years of age decreased from a reported 394 cases (5.7/100,000) and 190 cases (2.8/100,000) in 1980 to 194 cases (2.6/100,000) and 166 cases (2.2/100,000) in 1991, respectively.

The trend for *H. influenzae* appears to be continuing, with an incidence of 2 cases per 100,000 children younger than 5 years of age in 1993, down from 41 per 100,000 in 1987, based on reporting through the National Notifiable Diseases Surveillance System.[9]

Schoendorf and colleagues[253] evaluated national trends in mortality from meningitis from 1980 to 1991. From 1980 through 1987, mortality from *H. influenzae* meningitis decreased an average of 8.5 per cent a year from 1.72 per 100,000 children in 1980 to 0.94 per 100,000 children in 1987. From 1988 to 1991, however, mortality decreased an average of 48 per cent a year, with a death rate of 0.11 per 100,000 children in 1991. The estimated case-fatality rate for *H. influenzae* meningitis was 3.3 per cent from 1980 to 1987 and 2.3 per cent from 1988 to 1991. In comparison, mortality from *S. pneumoniae* decreased 10 per cent annually from 1980 to 1987 and 3 per cent annually from 1988 to 1991. Similarly, mortality from meningococcal meningitis decreased by 13 per cent annually from 1980 to 1987 and 12 per cent annually from 1988 to 1991.

In the United States, the mortality rate from *H. influenzae* meningitis varied by region, ranging from approximately 0.075 deaths per 100,000 population in the Northeast to 1.5 per 100,000 in the South in 1991, down from 0.7 per 100,000 and 1.8 per 100,000 in 1980, respectively. The average annual declines were similar in all four regions, ranging from 7 to 10 per cent from 1980 through 1987, increasing significantly to 42 to 46 per cent from 1988 to 1991. Other studies have demonstrated a similar decline.[40]

The dramatic decrease in the incidence of *H. influenzae*

TABLE 38–1. Annual Age-Specific Incidence of Meningitis Beyond the Neonatal Period, United States, 1978 to 1981*

Age	*Neisseria meningitidis*	*Haemophilus influenzae*	*Streptococcus pneumoniae*	Group B *Streptococcus*	*Listeria monocytogenes*	Total Meningitis
1–2 mo	9.1	18.6	5.7	10.0	1.3	56.7
3–5 mo	11.5	52.0	11.6	1.4	0.1	83.3
6–8 mo	10.6	65.1	8.0	0.3	0	88.4
9–11 mo	7.9	48.1	4.7	0	0.1	63.3
1–2 yr	3.8	19.0	1.5	0	0	25.3
3–4 yr	1.8	3.9	0.5	0	0	6.8
5–9 yr	0.7	0.7	0.3	0	0	2.0
10–19 yr	0.6	0.1	0.1	0	0	1.0

*Results are reported as number of children with meningitis per 100,000 population (before routine immunization with *H. influenzae* type b vaccines).
Adapted from Report of the Task Force on Diagnosis and Management of Meningitis. Pediatrics *78:*S959–S982, 1986.

meningitis probably has been affected by several factors. The precipitous drop that occurred shortly after universal immunization of infants strongly suggests that this practice has affected the epidemiology of this disease. Conjugate vaccination protects against nasopharyngeal colonization,[205] thus decreasing the carriage rate of *H. influenzae* type b and diminishing the reservoir for transmission, as well as providing immunity from infection. This would lessen the likelihood of infection in underimmunized children as well. Other changes in medical practice, such as the widespread use of outpatient antibiotics and improvements in supportive care, may have some effect, as demonstrated by the decrease in case-fatality rates for *H. influenzae* meningitis and the steady decrease in mortality rates before vaccination and as seen in meningococcal and pneumococcal disease.

Before universal vaccination, the incidence of *H. influenzae* meningitis varied worldwide. The incidence of *H. influenzae* meningitis in Scandinavian children younger than 5 years of age averaged from 16 to 28 cases per 100,000 children from 1975 to 1984.[219] The incidence of *H. influenzae* meningitis in the Netherlands was 22 cases per 100,000 children younger than 5 years of age.[299] A universal vaccination program in that country appears to have led to a marked decrease in the incidence, with 6 reported cases of meningitis caused by *H. influenzae* in a 1-year period after implementation of universal vaccination of infants, compared with 34 cases per 100,000 children in a 1-year period before vaccination.

The incidence of *H. influenzae* meningitis is markedly higher in nonindustrialized populations. Alaskan Eskimos had an annual incidence before the vaccination era of 282 cases per 100,000 children younger than 5 years of age.[309] The Navaho and White Mountain Apache Native Americans had a much higher incidence compared with that of Native Americans in other regions of the United States,[53, 186] and the incidence among Australian aboriginals and among certain African populations, such as those in Gambia and Senegal, was 3 to 10 times higher than that of populations in the United States and Europe.[30, 119, 141]

Nonencapsulated strains of *H. influenzae* may be found in the throat or nasopharynx of up to 80 per cent of children or adults at various periods. In contrast, only a small percentage of individuals carry *H. influenzae* type b. Turk[295] reported that when serial throat cultures were obtained in families, 0.4 per cent of adults, 0.8 per cent of children older than 5 years of age, and 3.2 per cent of children younger than 5 years of age carried *H. influenzae* type b at any one time. In a nursery of children younger than 1 year of age in the British West Indies, 45 per cent of children carried *H. influenzae* type b for several months without any evidence of clinical disease.[295] Good and associates,[127] in a study of three families, reported that four of five siblings of a child with meningitis carried *H. influenzae* type b but that this organism was not recovered from any of the parents. These and other similar data suggest that carriage of *H. influenzae* type b predominantly occurs in children of the same age, at which the frequency of disease is greatest.

In one study, the incidence of *H. influenzae* meningitis was 3.5-fold higher in blacks than in whites, but this distribution of cases appeared to be related more closely to poverty than to race.[99] In whites, there was no increase in incidence in overcrowded households, but the incidence was higher in rural than in urban areas. Fraser and his associates[99] postulated that the increased incidence in rural whites and in blacks was related to lack of access to early medical care.

Ward and colleagues[307] studied prospective data obtained in 19 states to determine the risk of spread of severe *H. influenzae* illness among household contacts of patients with *H. influenzae* meningitis. The risk in children younger than 1 year of age was 6 per cent; in children younger than 4 years of age, 2.1 per cent; and in children younger than 6 years of age, 0.5 per cent. The risk of *H. influenzae* disease in household contacts younger than 6 years of age is similar to the risk of secondary meningococcal disease in all household contacts, indicating a need for effective antimicrobial prophylaxis. The frequency with which strains of *H. influenzae* are recovered from individuals in homes of patients with *H. influenzae* disease suggests either that affected children are potent sources of infection for others in the household or that a high concentration of carriers of the type b organism precedes and predisposes to cases of *H. influenzae* meningitis.[290]

Spread of *H. influenzae* disease outside the family also has been described. Melish and associates[193] and Ginsburg and coworkers[121] described four and seven cases, respectively, among children in day care centers. Barenkamp and colleagues[23] suggested that, in addition to close contact between young children who may be carrying *H. influenzae* type b, the specific outer-membrane protein subtype may contribute to the risk of spread of invasive disease in the day care center. In one study involving 18 day care centers, the secondary attack rate in contacts younger than 4 years of age was 16 per 1000 for those who had been exposed to subtype 1H, compared with 1.6 per 1000 after exposure to other subtypes of *H. influenzae* type b. The precise risk of secondary *H. influenzae* type b infection in day care centers remains unclear.

An outbreak of *H. influenzae* type b meningitis also has been described in an enclosed hospital population.[125] Five cases were reported over a 6-month period in an enclosed population of 28 to 32 chronically ill children.

Inadequate treatment of otitis caused by *H. influenzae* type b appears to influence directly the likelihood of the development of meningitis. In one study, only 4 per cent of otitis media was caused by *H. influenzae* type b, but of patients with otitis media caused by this organism, 14 per cent developed *H. influenzae* meningitis.[142]

Recurrent invasive *H. influenzae* type b disease has been reported. Detailed studies suggest that age and high incidence of disease alone are not the only factors contributing to the recurrent disease.[38] Patients who develop recurrent disease caused by *H. influenzae* type b may represent a subset of a population with unusual disease susceptibility.

Epidemiology of Meningitis Caused by *Streptococcus pneumoniae*

The risk of developing sepsis or meningitis caused by pneumococcus depends to some extent upon the serotype with which the child is infected. Although there are 83 pneumococcal serotypes, in our experience, sepsis and meningitis most commonly are associated with serotypes 14, 6, 19, 18, 23, 4, 9, 3, and 1. These data are consistent with those of Austrian and associates,[16] who reported that pneumococcal otitis media and sepsis in children were caused most commonly by serotypes 1, 6, 14, 18, 19, and 23 and with other more recent data of Butler and colleagues.[40a] The risk of pneumococcal meningitis is 5- to 36-fold greater in blacks than in whites and is independent of income or population density.[99] In one study, 11 per cent of the black population with pneumococcal pneumonia had sickle-cell disease, a factor known to predispose the individual to pneumococcal disease.[99] Based on these data, Fraser and associates[99] suggested that 1 in every 24 children with sickle-cell disease may develop pneumococcal meningitis by 4 years of age. This incidence is 36-fold greater than the incidence of pneumococcal meningitis in a normal black population and 314-fold greater than that in white children. The greatest mortality occurs in very old and very young patients and has been estimated to be 20 to 60 per cent.[93, 101, 102, 114]

Pneumococcal infections generally occur sporadically. Household contacts of a patient with pneumococcal disease are not considered to be at increased risk of acquiring secondary infection. Concurrent pneumococcal disease (meningitis and bacteremia) has been reported, however, in the household setting.[15, 266]

The incidence of systemic infection with penicillin-resistant *S. pneumoniae* has been increasing steadily worldwide since first reported in Australia in the 1960s.[140] It has become an increasing problem in the United States since the mid-1980s[231, 277, 283, 284]; a nationwide survey documented that 6.6 per cent of isolates were resistant to penicillin (minimal inhibitory concentration [MIC] > 0.1 μg/mL). In certain areas, resistance rates are much higher. Investigations by the Centers for Disease Control and Prevention and state health departments discovered penicillin resistance in 61 per cent of nasopharyngeal cultures from children in a large day care center and in 33 per cent of isolates from children visiting a county health department in rural Kentucky. In Memphis, Tennessee, nasopharyngeal swabs from children with otitis media showed that 29 per cent of pneumococcal isolates were resistant to penicillin.[33]

The first report of meningitis caused by resistant pneumococci was published in 1974[211]; numerous case reports have appeared subsequently. Tan and colleagues[283] found that patients with systemic infections caused by penicillin-resistant pneumococci were more likely to have received a course of antibiotics within a month before their infection than were matched controls who had infections caused by pneumococci but whose isolates were susceptible to penicillin.

More recently, there has been an increase in the number of cases of systemic infection and meningitis caused by *S. pneumoniae* organisms resistant to penicillin and third-generation cephalosporins. In Kentucky and in Memphis, 27 per cent and 25 per cent of penicillin-resistant isolates, respectively, were resistant to cefotaxime (MIC > 2 μg/mL).[33] In Dallas, Texas, from 1981 to 1983, 8 per cent of *S. pneumoniae* strains isolated from children with meningitis were resistant to penicillin, but none were resistant to cephalosporins.[150] From 1991 to 1992, however, 11.6 per cent and 8 per cent of isolates were resistant to penicillin and third-generation cephalosporins, respectively, and in 1993, resistance had increased to 18.5 per cent and 12.9 per cent, respectively.[106] A prospective study involving nine children's hospitals nationwide, which identified patients with systemic infections caused by *S. pneumoniae*, found the following preliminary data: 14 per cent of isolates (ranging from 0 to 35 per cent among hospitals) were resistant to penicillin, and 4.2 per cent were resistant to third-generation cephalosporins (MIC > 1 μg/mL).[163] Isolates of penicillin-resistant and third-generation cephalosporin-resistant *S. pneumoniae* have been recovered in other regions of the world as well.[104, 106, 233] Treatment failures in patients with *S. pneumoniae* meningitis resistant to penicillin and third-generation cephalosporins also have been reported.[13, 35, 106, 167, 268]

The definition of cephalosporin resistance currently is undergoing reevaluation and change. The National Committee for Clinical Laboratory Standards has amended the definition of resistance to cefotaxime and ceftriaxone so that strains with an MIC of 2 μg/mL or greater are defined as resistant, whereas those with an MIC of 0.5 μg/mL or less are defined as fully susceptible. Strains with an MIC of 1 μg/mL are intermediate.[152] Tan and coworkers[285] reported a retrospective analysis of five children who had pneumococcal meningitis caused by strains that were penicillin-resistant and that had intermediate resistance (MIC, 0.5 to 2 μg/mL) to cefotaxime or ceftriaxone compared with strains that were penicillin-resistant but susceptible to cefotaxime or ceftriaxone (MIC, ≤0.25 μg/mL) and found no difference in clinical outcome at the time of discharge.

Epidemiology of Meningococcal Meningitis

The carriage rate for *N. meningitidis* in the civilian population has been estimated at various times to be between 1 and 15 per cent. Carriage rates in military personnel during epidemic periods have been considerably greater. Meningococcal carriers generally are adults (older than 21 years of age) who harbor the organism for months.

Greenfield and Feldman[131] studied an extended family because of an outbreak of group B meningococcal meningitis in three first cousins during a 5-month period. They found a carriage rate of 44 per cent in the members of the extended family, 50 per cent in family members who had been in direct contact with patients, 29 per cent in friends and neighbors, and 3 per cent in individuals within the community who had not been in any contact with the patients or family members. The estimated likelihood of severe meningococcal disease in family contacts usually occurring simultaneously with the first case is 1 per cent.[178] The rate is 1000-fold greater than the risk in the community. The risk of meningitis in day care center contacts of children with meningococcal disease is 1 per 1000.

No correlation has been noted between meningococcal meningitis and crowding within households, but disease appears to be more prevalent in urban than in rural areas. In a civilian population, meningococcal meningitis generally is a disease of children and young adults who have been exposed to an adult carrier, usually in the same family, or to individuals with disease or who are carrying the organism in a day care center setting. Most cases of meningococcal disease in children in recent years have been caused by group B or C meningococci; however, any known serogroup may be found in a particular individual. An association between serogroup B, serotype 2b, and a propensity for septicemia and increased fatality rates has been documented.[275]

Meningococcal diseases most frequently occur in children younger than 5 years of age, with a peak attack rate in the 6- to 12-month-old age group. A second and much larger peak occurs in adolescents.

One otherwise unprecedented outbreak occurred in a sixth grade elementary school classroom.[77] Five children from a class of 24 developed meningococcal meningitis. In addition, two siblings of one of the index cases also developed meningococcal infection. Detailed epidemiologic investigation suggested that close contact in the classroom (nose-to-nose distances of 34 inches or less) correlated with an increased rate of carriage of *N. meningitidis* and with an increased risk of developing invasive meningococcal disease.

Major outbreaks of meningococcal meningitis have occurred worldwide. In the late 1980s and early 1990s, major epidemics of *N. meningitidis* occurred throughout sub-Saharan Africa caused by a specific clone (III-1) of serogroup A *N. meningitidis*.[2, 133, 137, 223, 241] The origins of a pandemic spread of clone III-1 were traced to epidemics in Asia in the early 1980s, with spread through the Near East.[1] An outbreak occurred during the annual pilgrimage to Mecca in 1987,[198, 199] with pilgrims carrying clones back to their countries of origin, including the United States and the United Kingdom. Epidemics of closely related strains of clone III-1 serogroup A meningococcal meningitis occurred in the Sudan,[241] Ethiopia,[137] and Chad in 1988[199] and in Kenya[223] in 1989. A report in 1992 described an epidemic of clone III-1 in the Central African Republic in an area traditionally outside the "meningitis belt."[133] These epidemics generally begin during the dry season and decline at onset of the rainy season. Major outbreaks have occurred in Brazil, in Finland, and at multiple sites in Africa.[63, 218, 313] Shifts within a given community or within a country as a whole from one serogroup to another also are associated with an increased incidence of disease for several years after the new serogroup is introduced into the community.[108] The mechanisms underlying the changing patterns of meningococcal serogroups that cause disease are unknown.

Meningococcal infections also occur more frequently in patients with a deficiency of the terminal components (C5–C8) of the complement system.[72] More recently, an increased risk for meningococcal meningitis has been reported in individuals with an inherited deficiency of C9[210] and with properdin deficiency.[274] Individuals with a complement-depleting underlying illness also are at particular risk for invasive disease.[220] Screening for complement deficiency in pediatric patients with meningococcal disease has been suggested.[179]

PATHOPHYSIOLOGY

Organisms Encountered

Any organism may produce meningitis in a susceptible individual. *H. influenzae* type b, *S. pneumoniae*, and *N. meningitidis* are the responsible agents in about 95 per cent of healthy children older than 2 months of age. In compromised hosts, infection with other organisms may occur more frequently. The specific organism sometimes may be predicted based on the type of host deficit that is present.

Routes of Infection

Bacterial infection of the normally sterile leptomeningeal spaces can occur from a distant focus via the blood stream or via direct invasion from a contiguous focus. Meningitis most commonly is the result of hematogenous dissemination of organisms from a distant site of infection,[270] often from the respiratory tract. The meninges thus are seeded with microorganisms during a bacteremic period. Bacterial meningitis in children with otitis media generally follows bacteremia, although direct invasion of the meninges may occur as a complication of otitis media.

The route of infection in bacterial meningitis has been studied using a variety of animal models, but in most cases the experimental infection was initiated in a manner that did not mimic human disease. Bacterial meningitis has been induced in rats[200] and monkeys[248] after intranasal inoculation of *H. influenzae* type b. Bacteremia developed hours before meningitis could be detected histologically, a finding that supports the concept that meningitis follows hematogenous dissemination from nasopharyngeal colonization or infection. Marginating bacteria could be detected by fluorescent staining initially in the lateral and dorsal longitudinal (sagittal) sinuses and subsequently spread to the leptomeninges. In the rat model, otitis media appeared to develop by spread of infection from the subarachnoid space to the inner ear and then to the middle ear.

Meningitis may follow bacterial invasion from a contiguous focus of infection, as in infection of the mastoid or paranasal sinuses or as a complication of otitis media. Fracture through the paranasal sinuses as a result of head trauma may precede meningitis caused by *S. pneumoniae* and *H. influenzae*, which may be recurrent. Direct invasion also may occur in individuals with dermoid sinus tracts or meningomyeloceles, where a direct communication between the skin and the meninges is present. In this setting, infection most commonly is produced by organisms found on the skin. Recurrent meningitis has been reported in patients with basiethmoidal encephaloceles[280] as well as a congenital defect in the stapedial footplate.[146] Surgical obliteration of the fistula with temporal muscle and fascia prevented the recurrence of meningitis. Meningitis also may develop subsequent to osteomyelitis of the skull or vertebral column.

Neurosurgical procedures, particularly those designed for diversion of cerebrospinal fluid (CSF) in children who have hydrocephalus, may lead to subsequent development of meningitis.

Infection of the CNS may occur as the result of environmental contamination or manipulation. Meningeal infection may be acquired in utero transplacentally or during delivery via contact with the cervix or vaginal canal, which may be colonized with a variety of organisms, particularly group B streptococci and *L. monocytogenes*.[6, 17] The newborn infant, the patient with cystic fibrosis, or the burned child may develop septicemia and meningitis as a result of persistent heavy colonization with *Staphylococcus aureus*. A humidified atmosphere promotes the colonization and growth of such organisms as *Serratia marcescens* and *Pseudomonas aeruginosa*. Placing a patient in this setting leads to an increased frequency of infection with these organisms. Repeated venipuncture with contaminated equipment, such as what intravenous drug abusers experience, as well as indwelling catheters used for administration of parenteral nutrition or blood products can predispose a person to infection by bacterial (and fungal) organisms that generally are of low virulence in the normal host.

FACTORS PREDISPOSING THE HOST TO BACTERIAL MENINGITIS

Those factors that predispose the host to infection in other sites also predispose the host to bacterial infection of the CNS. There is a strong interrelationship of factors relating to the host, the organism, and environment in regard to the pathogenesis and outcome of meningitis. Although presented separately, they must be considered as a complex interplay of factors that leads to infection.

Host Factors

An increased incidence of bacterial meningitis is observed in the very young. Males are affected more frequently than females, and the severity of disease also is increased in these groups. Fraser and associates[102] reported that the greatest morbidity after bacterial meningitis occurred in individuals affected between birth and 4 years of age. The newborn infant is predisposed to septicemia and meningitis by factors that reflect physiologic deficiencies or immaturity of host defense mechanisms. These include the following: (1) decreased phagocytic and bactericidal activity of polymorphonuclear leukocytes, (2) defects in the response of neonatal leukocytes to chemotactic factors, (3) a deficiency in the capacity to support opsonization, and (4) defects in microtubular length and number that decrease the motility of the neonatal leukocyte when compared with those from older children. Deficiencies in serum complement components Clq, C3, and C5; low levels of serum properdin; and low concentrations of serum IgM and IgA have been documented repeatedly. Despite transplacental acquisition of IgG, antibodies against specific infective agents may be lacking. The precise age at which each of these factors reaches the concentration and functional activity noted in older children and adults is unclear and undoubtedly varies somewhat from individual to individual. In part, meningitis in children between 1 month and 1 year of age may reflect qualitative or quantitative differences between the inflammatory and immunologic responses seen in older children compared with infants.

The increased risk of meningitis in the normal host with less than completely mature immunologic and inflammatory responses to infection may be attributable to age alone. This is exemplified in the report of Cole and associates,[49] who studied the risk of recurrent bacteremia in young children. Within 18 months of the bacteremic illness, none of 42 children older than 24 months of age had a documented additional episode of bacteremia or systemic infection. However, 15 of 135 children (11 per cent) younger than 24 months of age at the time of the initial bacteremic disease had at least one additional documented bacteremic illness. Fourteen of these 15 children contracted both infections while younger than 2 years of age. Seven of these 15 children had meningitis. Only two patients had documented congenital or hereditary disorders of immunoglobulin or complement concentration or function.

It has been suggested that the predilection of some normal children for the development of bacteremia and meningitis may be determined genetically. Tejani and associates[292] studied 50 Caucasian children younger than 7 years of age with *H. influenzae* disease. Half of the patients had invasive disease (positive blood or CSF). The other half had fever, nasopharyngitis, and positive throat cultures for *H. influenzae* type b. The two groups of patients did not differ significantly with regard to age, number of siblings in the household younger than 12 years of age, or immunologic responses to infection. Significant differences between the two groups were seen in their genetic markers. HLA-B12 was found in 52 per cent of children with invasive disease, compared with only 16 per cent in the other group ($p < .01$). HLA-Bw40 was present in 24 per cent of children without invasive disease but was absent in children with bacteremia or meningitis caused by *H. influenzae* type b ($p < .01$).

Congenital or acquired abnormalities of the immune system may predispose the host to bacterial infections. Congenital deficiency of the three major immunoglobulin classes may predispose the host to severe bacterial infection. Congenital defects of thymic-dependent, small lymphocyte function or combined T and B defects are detrimental to host defense. A deficiency of CD4+ helper-inducer T cells in patients with bacterial meningitis has been reported and may contribute to the impaired antibody synthesis to bacterial capsular polysaccharides seen in this disease.[232] Multiple studies have demonstrated that deficiencies of various components of the complement system or increased consumption or loss of complement has been associated with increased risk of bacterial meningitis caused by encapsulated organisms.[69, 72, 111, 147, 181, 183, 210, 220, 232, 239, 242, 300]

An increased incidence of overwhelming infection, including meningitis, has been reported after splenectomy, but the likelihood of such infection depends upon the age of the child at the time of splenectomy, time since splenectomy, and the original indication for splenectomy.[73] Congenital asplenia or polysplenia also has been associated with an increased incidence of septicemia and meningitis caused by *S. pneumoniae*,[73] *H. influenzae* type b, and gram-negative enteric microorganisms.

Children with sickle-cell disease and other hemoglobinopathies experience meningitis caused by *S. pneumoniae, H. influenzae,* and *Salmonella* species more frequently than do normal children.

Children with malignancies, particularly those involving the reticuloendothelial system, appear to be prone to meningitis caused by organisms of low virulence that pose a minimal threat to normal children, presumably because of abnormalities in immunologic function. A decreased production of normal immunoglobulins, delayed and defective antibody responses to antigenic stimuli, production of abnormal immunoglobulins, depression in the clearance mechanisms of the reticuloendothelial system, and depression of cellular immunity all have been documented in children with malignancies involving the reticuloendothelial system. In addition, the use of irradiation or immunosuppressive agents and antimetabolites also predisposes the host to CNS infection. It may be difficult to attribute the occurrence of bacterial meningitis in this population directly to these agents rather than to the disease for which this therapy has been provided.

Malnutrition also predisposes children and adults to infectious disease. Impaired cellular immune responses, low levels of serum complement, impaired phagocytic activity of neutrophils, and decreased serum concentrations of transferrin have been documented in malnourished children.[84]

Systemic diseases, such as diabetes mellitus, renal insufficiency, adrenal insufficiency, cystic fibrosis, hypoparathyroidism, and exudative enteropathy, have an increased frequency and severity of CNS infections.[32] Children with diabetes mellitus, coma due to drug overdose, and Cushing syndrome have been shown to be at increased risk of bacteremia or meningitis caused by *H. influenzae* type b.[181] Defective chemotaxis, phagocytosis, and bactericidal function accompany these disorders and may explain, in part, the increased susceptibility of these individuals to infection.[84, 85]

In the normal host, bacterial infections at sites other than the leptomeninges are associated with an increased incidence of CNS infection. Infection may spread hematogenously to the meninges in children with endocarditis, pneumonia, or thrombophlebitis or by direct extension from sinusitis, mastoiditis, or osteomyelitis of the skull. Meningitis developing subsequent to performance of lumbar puncture in children younger than 1 year of age has been described.[95, 289]

PATHOLOGY

The most detailed account in English of the pathologic changes occurring with meningitis was written in 1948 by Adams, Kubik, and Bonner,[4] who described the meningeal, cerebral, and vascular changes found post mortem in 14 patients who succumbed to *H. influenzae* 14 hours to 76 days after the onset of disease. Although most in their series received inadequate treatment (effective antibiotic therapy was not available), the pathologic findings they describe differ little from subsequent reports of Smith and Landing,[271] Rorke and Pitts,[237] and Dodge and Swartz,[67] whose patients died despite administration of antibiotics. These descriptions are summarized later.

A meningeal exudate varying in thickness may be found (Fig. 38–2). Purulent material is distributed widely but may accumulate about the veins and venous sinuses, over the convexity of the brain, in the depths of the sulci, in the sylvian fissures, within the basal cisterns, and around the cerebellum. The spinal cord may be encased in pus. Ventriculitis (purulent material within the ventricles) has been

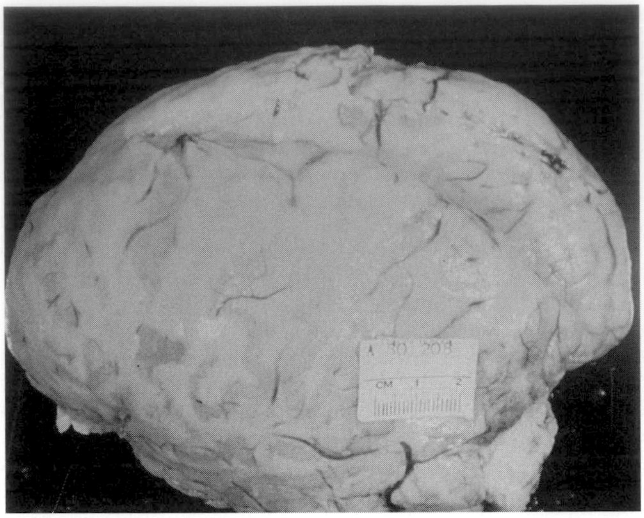

FIGURE 38–2. *Note extensive purulent exudate over entire cerebral cortex in a patient who died as a result of bacterial meningitis.*

noted repeatedly in children who died of their disease. Subsequent experience suggests that ventriculitis may be a relatively common finding in children with bacterial meningitis who survive, particularly in neonates. Invasion of the ventricular wall with perivascular collections of purulent material has been noted. Loss of ependymal lining and subependymal gliosis may be seen. In some studies, purulent exudate tended to be thicker over the convexity of the brain in pneumococcal than in other forms of meningitis.[67, 237]

Vascular and parenchymatous changes have been demonstrated at necropsy. Polymorphonuclear infiltrates extending to the subintimal region of small arteries and veins have been associated with the exudative meningeal process. Thrombosis of small cortical veins associated with necrosis of the cerebral cortex may be noted. Occlusion of one of the major venous sinuses, subarachnoid hemorrhage secondary to a necrotizing arteritis, and necrosis of the cerebral cortex in the absence of identifiable thrombosis of small vessels rarely may be observed. Reactive microglia and astrocytes may be identified in the cerebral cortex, particularly subadjacent to regions of heavy subarachnoid exudate. Because no bacteria are found in the cerebral cortex, these pathologic changes should be viewed as a noninfectious encephalopathy. "Toxic or circulatory factors" were suggested as possible causes by Adams and associates.[5] Dodge and Swartz[67] suggested systemic hypoxia and fever as additional possible causes. They also noted that an increase in intracranial pressure may interfere with cerebral circulation.

Damage to the cerebral cortex, reflecting the effects of vascular occlusion, hypoxia, bacterial invasion, toxic encephalopathy, or some combination of these factors, provides an adequate explanation for impaired consciousness, deficits in motor and sensory function, seizures, and retardation that may be observed.

Hydrocephalus is an uncommon complication of meningitis that develops beyond the newborn period. Most often, hydrocephalus is communicating and is the result of adhesive thickening of the arachnoid about the cisterns at the base of the brain. Less frequently, the aqueduct of Sylvius or the foramina of Magendie and Luschka are obstructed by fibrosis and reactive gliosis. The ensuing ventricular dilatation may be coupled with coexistent necrosis of nervous tissue because of the meningitis itself or because of occlusion of cerebral veins and, rarely, arteries. Cerebral necrosis plus increased intraventricular pressure may result in total dissolution of the cerebrum.

Subdural effusions occur frequently during the course of meningitis. The exact pathogenesis is not known. However, the high incidence of effusion and the fact that subdural fluid collections may be found early in the course of bacterial meningitis in children suggest that subdural effusions should be considered a concomitant of meningeal inflammation rather than a complication of the disease. Numerous veins traverse the subdural space, and inflammation of these and of the dural capillaries could produce an increase in vascular permeability and loss of albumin-rich fluid into the subdural space.[63] The ratio of albumin to gamma-globulin is higher in the subdural fluid of children with meningitis than it is in serum.[124] When the inflammatory process subsides, fluid formation generally ceases, but fluid may persist because of a continued transudation through newly formed vessels in the subdural membrane.

Subdural empyema, as opposed to subdural effusion, occurs rarely. It was observed in only two of the cases reported by Adams and associates,[5] in 1 of 34 patients examined by Smith and Landing,[271] and in none of the patients studied by Dodge and Swartz.[67]

Many factors contribute to the increase in intracranial pressure in patients with meningitis. Endotoxin and fragments of the cell wall of gram-positive organisms are capable of inducing the release of interleukin-1 (IL-1) and tumor necrosis factor (TNF) (cachectin) from macrophages and other sources.[65, 196] These substances, in addition to other interleukins and arachidonic acid metabolites, affect many systems, including endothelial cells, and affect profoundly the function of the vasculature and its interaction with neutrophils and other inflammatory cells. These substances play an important role in the pathogenesis of increased intracranial pressure and cerebral edema in patients with meningitis by altering cerebral blood flow, intracranial blood volume, and the permeability of the cerebral vasculature.[214] Intercellular junctions, which normally are tight, are open in experimental meningitis; this is associated with an increased permeability to circulating albumin.[229] Pinocytotic vesicles also are noted within the cytoplasm of endothelial cells. Swelling of cellular elements (cytotoxic edema) also has been noted.

Alterations in CSF resorption further exacerbate cerebral edema and increased intracranial pressure. In experimental meningitis, resorption of CSF is diminished as an accumulation of proteins, leukocytes, and other materials interfere with the function of the arachnoid villus.[251]

During the course of meningitis, excess secretion of antidiuretic hormone (ADH) occurs, which induces water retention and exacerbates electrolyte abnormalities already created secondary to the inflammatory processes occurring in the CNS. Cellular electrolyte disturbances may depolarize neuronal membranes, predisposing the host to seizure activity. Increased oxidation of glucose and increased lactate production as well as depletion of high-energy compounds, such as adenosine 5′-triphosphate and phosphocreatinine, are observed. Hypoglycorrhachia results primarily from decreased transport of glucose across the inflamed choroid plexus and from increased utilization of glucose by host tissues. Utilization of glucose by bacteria and polymorphonuclear leukocytes is of less relative importance.[67, 250]

Pathogenesis

Most cases of bacterial meningitis progress through four steps: (1) infection or colonization of the upper respiratory tract, (2) invasion of the blood from a respiratory focus, (3) seeding of the meninges by a blood-borne organism, and (4) inflammation of the meninges and brain. Less commonly, infection of the leptomeninges also can occur via contiguous spread or hematogenous dissemination from another remote site. The nasopharyngeal mucosa is colonized with *H. influenzae*, *N. meningitidis*, and *S. pneumoniae*, resulting most commonly in an asymptomatic carrier state or minor upper respiratory tract illness. This attachment is mediated by specific microbial cell surface components. *N. meningitidis* strains possess fimbriae that bind to cell surface receptors on nasopharyngeal mucosal cells[64] and appear to be transported across specialized cells within phagocytic vacuoles.[281] Once in the blood stream, the common pathogenic organisms—*H. influenzae*, *N. meningitidis*, *S. pneumoniae*, *E. coli* K1, and group B *Streptococcus*—all are capable of evading host defense mechanisms via capsular polysaccharides, which inhibit neutrophil phagocytosis and classic complement-mediated bactericidal activity. These bacteria then traverse the blood-brain barrier most likely at the cerebral capillaries and choroid plexus. Fimbriae of *E. coli* have been shown to facilitate attachment in these regions.[217] Once in the CSF, organisms multiply rapidly, liberating cell wall or membrane components (endotoxin, teichoic acid) because of insufficient opsonic and phagocytic activity.

Host defenses within the CSF before and after bacterial invasion seem to rely on two important mechanisms available to the host to clear bacteria.[265] One clearance system requires a type-specific antibody, a functional classic complement system for opsonization, and the presence of competent polymorphonuclear leukocytes for phagocytosis. The second system is dependent on the interaction of nonspecific or low-affinity antibody and the alternative complement pathway for opsonization of the organism. Clearance by this system occurs in the absence of polymorphonuclear leukocytes.

Complement and opsonic proteins either are found at very low concentrations or are absent entirely within normal CSF.[97, 265] Thus, the CSF is devoid of those factors required for bacterial clearance. When bacteria first invade the meninges, the lack of complement and opsonic proteins within the sanctuary of the CNS may permit the bacteria to multiply unrestrained for some time. The slow response of polymorphonuclear leukocytes and the lack of serum-specific antibody available during the initial inflammatory response enhance the probability that bacterial infection will be established.[29, 117, 305, 322]

The specific pathophysiologic changes in bacterial meningitis are the result of the bacterial products and the inflammatory response of the host to those products. Initial bactericidal antibiotic therapy results in a rapid release of these bacterial products such as endotoxins, teichoic acid, and peptidoglycans. Augmented permeability of the blood-brain barrier can be induced by bacterial products alone, which cause disruption of the tight junctions between capillary endothelial cells and marked increase in pinocytotic activity within endothelial cells. An influx of serum albumin into the CSF is accompanied by other low-molecular-weight proteins, including components of the complement cascade.[153]

TNF-α (cachectin) and IL-1 appear to be key mediators in initiating meningeal inflammation. Both proteins stimulate vascular endothelial cells to induce adhesion and passage of neutrophils into the CNS and trigger inflammatory processes. Astrocytes and microglia are capable of producing TNF-α.[230] TNF-α concentrations are elevated in CSF but not in serum; in animal models of bacterial meningitis; and in patients with bacterial meningitis caused by *H. influenzae*, *N. meningitidis*, *S. pneumoniae*, and *Streptococcus agalactiae*[206] but not in patients with culture-proven viral meningitis.[230] IL-1 activity can be detected in infants and children with bacterial meningitis, and its presence is correlated significantly with CSF inflammatory abnormalities, TNF-α concentrations, and adverse outcome.[206] TNF-α and IL-1 are capable of inducing phospholipase A_2 activity, triggering the production of platelet-activating factor and activation of the arachidonic acid pathway leading to the generation of prostaglandins, thromboxanes, and leukotrienes from membrane phospholipids of endothelial and polymorphonuclear cells, which modulate multiple aspects of the inflammatory process.

These cytokines activate adhesion-promoting receptors on cerebral vascular endothelial cells, resulting in attraction and attachment of leukocytes to sites of stimuli. These leukocytes release proteolytic compounds that make it possible to traverse the intercellular junctions. These enzymes in conjunction with platelet-activating factor and the arachidonic acid metabolites injure the vascular endothelium, resulting in increased blood-brain barrier permeability and activation of the coagulation cascade.

The presence of increasing amounts of chemotactic factors into the subarachnoid space leads to accumulation of large numbers of neutrophils in the CSF. The growth of bacteria is not slowed significantly by this response,[75] and the large number of neutrophils actually may have a deleterious effect on tissue damage and disease outcome.[79, 86] Poor phagocytosis by neutrophils in the meningeal spaces may be related to weak activity in fluid medium, lack of complement activity and opsonization, and poor penetration of IgM and IgG through the blood-brain barrier, even during acute *H. influenzae* and *S. pneumoniae* meningitis.[118]

Bacterial cell wall fragments, endotoxin, or both also contribute to vascular permeability. In experimental *E. coli* meningitis, the CSF endotoxin concentration increased markedly after treatment with β-lactam antibiotics. This was associated with an increase in brain water content. This effect could be blocked by polymyxin or a monoclonal antibody, both of which inactivate endotoxin.[286]

The inflammatory and vascular events described earlier act synergistically to produce the clinical symptoms and long-term sequelae that are noted in patients with bacterial meningitis. Vascular permeability leads to vasogenic edema. Inflammatory and electrolyte changes lead to cytotoxic edema. Alterations in CSF production and absorption lead to interstitial edema. The cytokines also trigger increased cerebral blood flow and further edema formation, resulting in increased intracranial pressure.[14] The increased intracranial pressure and vasculitis lead to a subsequent decrease in cerebral blood flow, which does not appear to be caused by loss of autoregulation.[14] Activation of the coagulation cascade predisposes the patient to venous, microvascular, and, rarely, arterial thrombosis. Direct neurotoxic damage by inflammatory cells also may contribute to the neuropathologic changes seen in bacterial meningitis. Superoxide and hydrogen peroxide are secreted by TNF-α–stimulated macrophages, including brain microglia, and leukocytes[227, 232]; hydrogen peroxide induces extensive neuronal damage.[215] In addition, macrophages secrete excitatory amino acids, such as glutamate, which potentially kill *N*-methyl-D-aspartate receptor–positive cells.[174]

CLINICAL MANIFESTATIONS AND PATHOPHYSIOLOGIC RELATIONSHIPS

Inflammation of the meninges generally is associated with nausea, vomiting, irritability, anorexia, headache, confusion, back pain, and nuchal rigidity. In many cases, positive Kernig and Brudzinski signs will be noted. Kernig sign is present when the leg is flexed 90 degrees at the hips and cannot be extended more than 135 degrees. Brudzinski sign is present if the thighs and legs are flexed involuntarily when the neck is flexed. All of these findings suggest irritation of inflamed sensory nerves, which in turn produce a reflex contraction of certain muscles in an attempt to minimize pain. These findings also can be the result of increased intracranial pressure and an associated distortion of nerve roots. These signs can be accompanied by hyperesthesia and photophobia. Currently, there is no satisfactory pathophysiologic explanation for photophobia. Signs of meningeal inflammation may be minimal in the infant, but irritability, restlessness, and poor feeding may be noted. Nuchal rigidity and positive Kernig and Brudzinski signs may occur late in the young child. Nuchal rigidity may not be elicited in comatose patients or when signs of focal or diffuse neurologic impairment are present. A review of 1064 cases of bacterial meningitis in children beyond the neonatal period revealed that 16 (1.5 per cent) had no meningeal signs during their entire period of hospitalization, despite the presence of CSF pleocytosis.[113] Fever, a hallmark of infection, generally is present; its absence in a patient with signs of meningeal inflammation, although infrequent, is far from unusual.

Increased intracranial pressure is the rule; this may be reflected by complaints of headache in older children and by a bulging fontanelle and diastasis of sutures in the infant. Papilledema is an uncommon finding in acute meningitis, presumably because of the relatively brief duration of increased pressure at the time of diagnosis. When papilledema is observed, venous sinus occlusion, subdural empyema, or brain abscess should be sought.

Signs of cerebral edema may be present. Vasogenic edema occurs as a consequence of increased permeability of the blood-brain barrier. Interstitial edema may occur secondary to decreased clearance of CSF at the arachnoid villae and subsequent obstructive hydrocephalus. Cytotoxic cerebral edema mediated by the release of toxic factors from neutrophils and bacteria leads to increased intracellular water and sodium concentration and loss of intracellular potassium. In many cases (88 per cent in one prospective study[78]), meningitis is associated with the release of ADH, causing water retention and a relative dumping of sodium by the kidney. If the patient then is given excessive free water during therapy, a further increase in intracranial pressure may be noted.

Transient or permanent paralysis of cranial nerves may be noted. Deafness or disturbances in vestibular function are relatively common; optic nerve involvement with blindness is rare. Involvement of the eighth cranial nerve may reflect disease at the level of the cochlear and vestibular end-organs, which may be related to concomitant infection of the inner ear. Paralysis of extraocular and facial nerves may be noted. Torticollis has been reported in two children with partially treated meningitis.[192] Obtundation, stupor, coma, and focal neurologic signs may be seen in children with bacterial meningitis. The relative frequency with which these findings are noted may be seen in Table 38–2, in which data for 235 children with bacterial meningitis who were enrolled prospectively have been analyzed according to the type of organism responsible for their meningitis. Overall, 14.9 per cent of children were semicomatose or comatose at the time of admission; rates for children with pneumococcal or meningococcal meningitis were higher than for those with *H. influenzae* disease. Focal neurologic signs were present at the time of admission in 16.5 per cent of the total group (34.3 per cent of children with pneumococcal meningitis). The presence of focal neurologic signs at the time of admission indicated poor prognosis and could be correlated with persistent abnormal neurologic examinations at 1, 3, and 6 months ($p < .01$) and at 1 year after discharge ($p < .03$). The presence of focal signs at the time of admission also correlated with the presence of retardation ($p < .001$), as determined by detailed psychometric testing after discharge. Generally, when focal signs are noted in the absence of seizures, cortical necrosis, occlusive vasculitis, or thrombosis of cortical veins has occurred. Thrombosis of meningeal vessels or cortical necrosis may be associated with hemiparesis or quadriparesis as well as with focal seizures. These signs may appear during the first 3 to 4 days of illness or, less commonly, may be noted after the first or second week of infection. A highly significant association ($p < .001$) between neurologic signs indicative of cerebral injury and late (1 to 15 years after the acute infection) afebrile seizures has been noted.[224] Ataxia has been a presenting sign of meningitis in a number of children and adults. Schwartz[255] described four children who presented with ataxia as an initial symptom. Adolescents with meningitis may present with behavioral abnormalities that may be confused with drug abuse or psychiatric disorders.[20]

Seizures before admission occur in about 20 per cent of children with bacterial meningitis and during the first or second day in the hospital in about 26 per cent. Green and colleagues[129] retrospectively examined the frequency of seizures before or at the time of presentation in children with meningitis. They found that 111 of 410 (27 per cent) children with bacterial meningitis had seizures at or before the time of diagnosis. Eighty-eight of these children had complex seizures (focal, prolonged, or more than one in a 24-hour period). They found that all children with bacterial meningitis who presented with seizures had other signs or symptoms of meningitis, such as altered level of consciousness, nuchal rigidity, or complex seizures and petechial rash. One caveat may be the child pretreated with antibiotics. One small study found that of 25 children with bacterial meningitis who presented with seizures, 4 of 7 pretreated with oral antibiotics did not have any additional signs or symptoms. Overall, seizures are noted in about 30 per cent of children with bacterial meningitis. Seizures noted before or during the first several days of hospitalization are of no particular prognostic significance. In particular, their occurrence does not herald the development of a permanent seizure disorder. Seizures that are difficult to control or that persist beyond the fourth hospital day, as well as seizures that occur for the first time late in the hospital course, may be of greater significance and have been associated with permanent sequelae of meningitis. Children with focal seizures have a greater likelihood of developing sequelae of meningitis than do those with generalized seizure activity. Focal or prolonged seizures probably are indicative of serious cerebral vascular disturbances or cerebral infarction. Seizures before admission have correlated positively with abnormal audiometric studies and permanent hearing handicaps. The frequency of seizure activity is similar for children with *H. influenzae* type b or pneumococcal meningitis; seizures occur in children with meningitis caused by these organisms approximately twice as frequently as in children with meningococcal meningitis. Seven per cent of patients with bacterial meningitis have focal or generalized seizures 3 months to 15 years after recovery from bacterial meningitis.[224]

Collections of fluid in the subdural space can be demonstrated in up to 50 per cent of infants and children during acute illness.[67] In a prospective study of infants 1 to 18 months of age with bacterial meningitis, subdural effusions were noted in 43 per cent of those with *H. influenzae* meningitis, 30 per cent of those with pneumococcal meningitis, and 22 per cent of those with meningococcal meningitis. There was no greater incidence of neurologic sequelae or developmental delay on long-term follow-up in patients with effu-

TABLE 38–2. Frequency of Selected Findings in Children with Bacterial Meningitis

	Total Group	*Haemophilus influenzae*	*Streptococcus pneumoniae*	*Neisseria meningitidis*	Others
Number of patients	235	151	35	26	23
Level of consciousness (%)					
Irritable or lethargic	184 (78.3)	117 (77.5)	24 (68.6)	21 (80.8)	22 (95.7)
Somnolent	16 (6.8)	13 (8.6)	1 (2.8)	1 (3.8)	1 (4.3)
Obtunded-semicomatose	27 (11.5)	15 (9.9)	8 (22.9)	4 (15.4)	0 (0)
Comatose	8 (3.4)	6 (4.0)	2 (5.7)	0 (0)	0 (0)
Focal neurologic signs on admission (%)	37 (16.5)	22 (14.6)	12 (34.3)	2 (7.7)	1 (4.3)
Seizures prior to admission (%)	48 (20.4)	35 (23.2)	8 (23)	3 (11.5)	2 (8.7)
Seizures in hospital (%)	61 (26)	43 (28)	12 (34)	5 (19)	1 (4.5)

sion, compared with those with bacterial meningitis who did not develop effusion.[269, 272]

Subdural effusions may cause enlargement in head circumference or may be responsible for abnormal transillumination of the skull. Vomiting, seizures, a full fontanelle, focal neurologic signs, or persistent fever may be noted at times, but these signs occur with such frequency in children with bacterial meningitis who do not have subdural effusions that it is difficult to attribute their occurrence to the subdural effusion per se.[80]

Blindness and optic atrophy may be related to optic arachnoiditis. Spastic paraparesis with sensory loss in the lower extremities may be secondary to meningomyelitis, spinal cord infarction, or both.

Arthralgia and myalgia are noted in many patients with bacterial meningitis, reflecting the systemic nature of the disease. Arthritis also may occur and does so most commonly during the course of meningococcal disease; generally it is transient. Early findings of arthritis may be related to direct invasion of the joint by the meningococcus. Arthritis that develops late in the course of meningococcal or *H. influenzae* meningitis may be an immune complex–mediated event. Petechial or purpuric lesions may be seen in 50 per cent of patients with meningococcal meningitis[67] but also may accompany any infectious or noninfectious disease process in which vasculitis occurs. Purpura, shock, and hypothermia indicate a poor prognosis.

Pericardial effusions may be present; they generally resolve during the course of antibiotic therapy. In some cases, they are the cause of persistent fever, and pericardiocentesis or an open drainage procedure may be required.

Shock may be associated with any form of overwhelming bacteremia but occurs most often in patients with fulminant meningococcemia. In a prospective study, 3.8 per cent of children with meningococcal meningitis developed profound hypotension. In the same study, shock occurred in 5.5 per cent of children with *H. influenzae* meningitis. Endotoxin has been detected by limulus lysate assay in the blood and CSF of children with meningococcal and *H. influenzae* meningitis.[16, 238] Signs of disseminated intravascular coagulation may accompany hypotension in these patients.

Facial cellulitis, including buccal and periorbital cellulitis, pneumonia, epiglottitis, endophthalmitis, and other suppurative manifestations, can present at the time of admission in any patient with bacterial meningitis. In one study of children with buccal cellulitis, more than 10 per cent (7 of 73) had concomitant bacterial meningitis documented by lumbar puncture as part of their initial evaluation.[18] Five of the seven children had no clinical evidence of meningeal irritation. *H. influenzae* and *S. pneumoniae* were cultured from two patients with periorbital cellulitis and no clinical evidence of meningeal irritation or abnormal CSF cell counts or chemistries.[243]

DIFFERENTIAL DIAGNOSIS

The signs and symptoms described earlier suggest meningeal or intracranial pathology but are not pathognomonic of acute bacterial infection. Tuberculous meningitis, fungal meningitis, aseptic meningitis, brain abscess, intracranial or spinal epidural abscesses, bacterial endocarditis with embolism, subdural empyema with or without thrombophlebitis, ruptured dermoid cysts, ruptured spinal ependymomas, and brain tumors may show similar signs and symptoms. Differentiation of these disorders depends upon careful examination of CSF obtained by lumbar puncture and additional immunologic, roentgenographic, and isotopic studies as delineated later.

DIAGNOSIS

Early diagnosis and treatment of bacterial meningitis are imperative in reducing mortality and morbidity. *Physicians must perform a lumbar puncture on any child in whom they suspect the diagnosis, unless there are specific contraindications to this procedure* (e.g., clinical signs of increased intracranial pressure in a patient with a closed fontanelle and closed sutures).

An association between performance of a lumbar puncture during bacteremia and the later development of meningitis has been reported.[95] This association was evident only in children younger than 1 year of age.[276] It seems likely that the perceptive physician selects children for lumbar puncture in whom clinical signs suggest developing meningitis before the CSF findings are diagnostic. These data suggest a need for careful observation and, if appropriate, hospitalization and antimicrobial therapy for infants younger than 1 year of age who undergo lumbar puncture and who concomitantly have risk factors (e.g., concurrent high temperature and white blood cell counts) for bacteremia.

CSF findings characteristic of various inflammatory diseases of the CNS are shown in Table 38–3.

Measurement of pressure, often neglected in infants and young children, is an important component of each CSF examination. When the pressure is very high, just enough fluid should be removed to permit a careful examination. Compression of the jugular vein should be avoided unless compression of the spinal cord is suspected. Xanthochromic CSF derives its color primarily from bilirubin pigment. Hemorrhage, bilirubin staining in icteric patients who have meningitis (i.e., neonates, leptospirosis), or an elevated protein concentration of CSF may be associated with xanthochromia.

CSF should be examined immediately. The total number of white blood cells should be counted in a counting chamber, and, after centrifugation, a differential cell count should

TABLE 38–3. Cerebrospinal Fluid Findings in Suppurative Diseases of the Central Nervous System and Meninges

Condition	Pressure (mm H_2O)	Leukocytes/mm^3	Protein (mg/dL)	Sugar (mg/dL)	Specific Findings
Acute bacterial meningitis	Usually elevated; average, 300	Several hundred to more than 60,000; usually a few thousand; occasionally less than 100 (especially meningococcal or early in disease); polymorphonuclears predominate	Usually 100 to 500, occasionally more than 1000	Less than 40 in more than half the cases	Organism usually seen on smear or recovered on culture in more than 90% of cases
Subdural empyema	Usually elevated; average, 300	Less than 100 to a few thousand; polymorphonuclears predominate	Usually 100 to 500	Normal	No organisms on smear or by culture unless concurrent meningitis
Brain abscess	Usually elevated	Usually 10 to 200; fluid is rarely acellular; lymphocytes predominate	Usually 75 to 400	Normal	No organisms on smear or by culture
Ventricular empyema (rupture of brain abscess)	Considerably elevated	Several thousand to 100,000; usually more than 90% polymorphonuclears	Usually several hundred	Usually less than 40	Organism may be cultured or seen on smear
Cerebral epidural abscess	Slight to modest elevation	Few to several hundred or more cells; lymphocytes predominate	Usually 50 to 200	Normal	No organisms on smear or by culture
Spinal epidural abscess	Usually reduced with spinal block	Usually 10 to 100; lymphocytes predominate	Usually several hundred	Normal	No organisms on smear or by culture
Thrombophlebitis (often associated with subdural empyema)	Often elevated	Few to several hundred; polymorphonuclears and lymphocytes	Slightly to moderately elevated	Normal	No organisms on smear or by culture
Bacterial endocarditis (with embolism)	Normal or slightly elevated	Few to less than 100; lymphocytes and polymorphonuclears	Slightly elevated	Normal	No organisms on smear or by culture
Acute hemorrhagic encephalitis	Usually elevated	Few to more than 1000; polymorphonuclears predominate	Moderately elevated	Normal	No organisms on smear or by culture
Tuberculous infection	Usually elevated; may be low with dynamic block in advanced stages	Usually 25 to 100, rarely more than 500; lymphocytes predominate, except in early stages when polymorphonuclears may account for 80% of cells	Nearly always elevated, usually 100 to 200; may be much higher if dynamic block	Usually reduced; less than 50 in 75% of cases	Acid-fast organisms may be seen on smear of protein coagulum (pellicle) or recovered from inoculated guinea pig or by culture
Cryptococcal infection	Usually elevated; average, 225	Average, 50 (0 to 800); lymphocytes predominate	Average, 100; usually 20 to 500	Reduced in more than half of cases; average, 30; often higher in patients with concomitant diabetes mellitus	Organisms may be seen in India ink preparation and on culture (Sabouraud medium); will usually grow on blood agar; may produce alcohol in cerebrospinal fluid from fermentation of glucose
Syphilis (acute)	Usually elevated	Average, 500; usually lymphocytes; rarely polymorphonuclears	Average, 100; gamma globulin often high, with abnormal colloidal gold curve	Normal (rarely reduced)	Positive reagin test for syphilis; spirochete not demonstrable by usual techniques of smear or by culture
Sarcoidosis	Normal to considerably elevated	0 to less than 100 mononuclear cells	Slight to moderate elevation	Normal	No specific findings

be performed on a Wright-stained smear of the sediment. The normal CSF of children 3 months of age or older contains fewer than 6 white blood cells per mm³. Ninety-five per cent of children older than 3 months of age have no polymorphonuclear leukocytes in the CSF; thus, the presence of a polymorphonuclear leukocyte in the CSF may be regarded as abnormal. When a lumbar puncture has been performed in a febrile child and a single polymorphonuclear leukocyte has been noted, careful clinical observation is imperative, and treatment should be considered until the results of the culture of the CSF are known.

If the lumbar puncture has been traumatic, a total cell count can be performed in a counting chamber. The red blood cells then can be lysed by acetic acid and a repeat cell count performed. If the total number of white blood cells compared with the number of red blood cells is in excess of that in whole blood, one can assume the presence of CSF pleocytosis. CSF protein should be measured (usually elevated in bacterial meningitis), and the CSF glucose should be compared with the blood glucose concentration that has been obtained concomitantly. In patients with bacterial meningitis, depression of CSF glucose and of the CSF to blood glucose ratio (normally about 66 per cent) is the rule.

Separate smears should be made, and these should be Gram stained for bacteria and Kinyoun stained for mycobacteria. The probability of visualizing bacteria on a Gram stain of CSF depends upon the number of organisms present. The percentage of positive smears is 25 per cent with less than 10^3 colony-forming units (CFU)/mL, 60 per cent in the range of 10^3 to 10^5 CFU/mL, and 97 per cent with greater than 10^5 CFU/mL.[173] Quellung and agglutination reactions can provide immediate identification of various organisms if the appropriate type of specific antisera is available. Treatment of the child with bacterial meningitis with an antibiotic before initial lumbar puncture usually does not alter markedly the morphologic or chemical results obtained (Table 38–4). In patients with *H. influenzae* meningitis (Table 38–5) who were pretreated, CSF cultures frequently grew *H. influenzae*; there is a tendency for pretreatment to render sterile the CSF of children with pneumococcal or meningococcal disease (see Table 38–4). Even when children received appropriate antibiotics for their meningitis intravenously for 44 to 68 hours, the bacterial character of the chemical and morphologic findings could be discerned in most cases.[31]

TABLE 38–4. Comparison of Cerebrospinal Fluid (CSF) Findings in Patients with Untreated and Pretreated Meningitis

	Untreated	Pretreated
Number of patients	143	91
Total white blood cell count × 10^3		
Mean ± 1 SD	4.9 ± 6.5	4.1 ± 5.0
Range	0–55	0.006–25.5
Per cent polys		
Mean ± 1 SD	84 ± 21	81 ± 25
Range	0–100	0–100
Glucose (mg/dL)		
Mean ± 1 SD	35 ± 28	32 ± 25
Range	0–109	0–100
CSF/blood glucose (%)		
Mean ± 1 SD	29 ± 21	29 ± 21
Range	0–78	0–94
Protein (mg/dL)		
Mean ± 1 SD	226 ± 228	174 ± 193
Range	13–2290	10–1640
Culture-positive	135	71
Gram stain–positive	114	62

TABLE 38–5. Cerebrospinal Fluid (CSF) Findings in Untreated and Pretreated Patients with *Haemophilus influenzae* Meningitis

	Untreated	Pretreated
Number of patients	92	57
Total white blood cell count × 10^3		
Mean ± 1 SD	5.6 ± 7.6	4.0 ± 4.8
Range	0.001–55	0.094–25.0
Per cent polys		
Mean ± 1 SD	91 ± 15	83 ± 22
Range	0–108	0–99
Glucose (mg/dL)		
Mean ± 1 SD	34 ± 27.5	29 ± 26
Range	0–109	0–99
Glucose CSF/blood		
Mean ± 1 SD	29 ± 21	24 ± 20
Range	0–78	0–82
Protein (mg/dL)		
Mean ± 1 SD	214 ± 129	187 ± 227
Range	25–752	29–1640
Counterimmunoelectrophoresis (CIE) (μg/mL)		
Mean ± 1 SD	1.83 ± 2.63	2.36 ± 4.73
Range	0–10.24	0.0–20.48
Culture-positive	91	51
Gram stain–positive	81	45
CIE-positive	77/88	50/55

The CSF should be cultured on a blood agar plate and a chocolate agar plate. The CSF specimens always should be cultured, even when the fluid appears to be crystal-clear and acellular or nearly so.

Countercurrent immunoelectrophoresis (CIE) has been shown to be a useful technique for rapid diagnosis (within 1 hour) and management of bacterial meningitis caused by *H. influenzae* type b; *S. pneumoniae; N. meningitidis* groups A, C, W135, and D; and group B *Streptococcus*. It also is possible to detect antigens from K1 strains of *E. coli, L. monocytogenes, Klebsiella pneumoniae,* and *P. aeruginosa*.[87, 190, 191] The methodology employed is sensitive and can detect nonviable bacteria, thus permitting the detection of bacterial antigen, even in patients who have been pretreated with appropriate antibiotics. It is imperative to use antisera that have the greatest possible sensitivity and specificity.[148, 260] Group B meningococcal antiserum, which is commercially available, is unreliable. When pneumococcal antisera are utilized, material obtained from the State Serum Institute in Copenhagen, Denmark, has proved to be highly efficacious; sensitivity is enhanced by using the various pools of pneumococcal antisera in addition to the omniserum. CIE is most effective when CSF, serum, and urine are screened concomitantly.[80] Evaluation of urine by CIE is enhanced by concentration of urine using either a Minicon B15 filter system or an ethanol precipitin technique. A negative CIE result does not exclude the diagnosis of bacterial meningitis.

Latex particle agglutination (LPA) commercial kits are available for detecting the polysaccharide antigens of *H. influenzae* type b, *S. pneumoniae, N. meningitidis,* and group B *Streptococcus*. LPA is superior to CIE in detecting PRP antigen of *H. influenzae* type b in CSF and serum. However, nonspecific agglutination of latex particles in serum, urine, and other body fluids may result in an indeterminate test. LPA detected PRP antigen in the CSF of 95 to 100 per cent of patients;

antigen was detected by CIE in only 80 to 85 per cent of the same patients.[56, 149, 249, 310] A commercial LPA kit containing antibody-coated latex particles for *H. influenzae* type b, *S. pneumoniae,* and *N. meningitidis* serogroups is available. The latex agglutination kit (Wellcogen), which contains serogroup B *N. meningitidis* antibody, detected only 27 per cent of cases of serogroup B *N. meningitidis* meningitis[202]; interaction between capsular polysaccharides of group B *N. meningitidis* and brain tissue antigens occurs.[94] A false-positive result in a latex agglutination test using the *N. meningitidis* ACYW135 kit has been reported in a patient with a ruptured dermoid tumor.[74]

Staphylococcal coagglutination also may be used to detect *H. influenzae* types a, b, c, d, e, and f; *N. meningitidis* groups A, B, C, Y, and W135; *S. pneumoniae* (83 serotypes); and group B *Streptococcus*.[68, 70]

Enzyme-linked immunosorbent assays (ELISAs) have been developed for the detection of bacterial antigen within CSF.[38] The major disadvantage of the ELISA technique described to date is the time required to perform the procedure. LPA tests or CIE can be performed within 30 to 60 minutes, whereas ELISA techniques require from 3 to 6 hours to complete. The development of homogeneous assays (enzyme-multipled immunoassay test) may permit the application of ELISA for rapid identification of microorganisms because time-consuming incubation and separation steps are eliminated.

An enzyme radioisotope assay has been developed to measure the activity of β-lactamase, an enzyme produced by many bacteria.[319] This assay offers the potential for rapid diagnosis of β-lactamase–producing bacteria.

Gas chromatography can be used to distinguish bacteria on the basis of cell components, bacterial metabolites, and products of pyrolysis.[172]

The rapidity with which results of bacterial antigen tests are obtained makes them tempting as a means to establish an early diagnosis. The degree to which they affect clinical decisions is not clear.[188] These tests are not necessary for every patient suspected of having bacterial meningitis, but they could play a role under certain circumstances, such as in those patients with a clinical presentation suspicious for bacterial meningitis and pretreatment with antibiotics or with a traumatic lumbar puncture. Antigen detection is useful in developing countries, where CSF culture yields are lower.[60]

More detailed information concerning tests that can be used for the rapid diagnosis of bacterial meningitis and other infections, including the use of the acridine orange stain and C-reactive protein, is provided in Chapter 243.

When available, evaluation of the CSF by the limulus lysate assay is a valuable adjunct to diagnosis, permitting the identification of endotoxin in CSF. A positive test, when appropriately performed, indicates infection with gram-negative organisms.[27, 238]

A number of metabolic changes have been reported in the CSF and blood of patients with meningitis (Table 38–6).

CSF lactate has been noted to be elevated significantly in patients with bacterial meningitis. The increase in CSF lactate apparently is related to decreased cerebral blood flow, cerebral hypoxia, and a change to anaerobic metabolism by the brain. CSF lactate concentration tends to parallel the CSF cellular response.[240] Although the concentration of CSF lactate in patients with bacterial meningitis generally is greater than in patients with aseptic meningitis, this is not always the case. In some patients with aseptic meningitis, CSF lactate has been in the range generally observed in patients with bacterial infections. Conversely, in patients who proved to have bacterial meningitis but who had equivocal clinical and CSF findings, measurement of CSF lactate failed to differentiate bacterial from nonbacterial infection.[240] Thus, determination of CSF lactate cannot be used reliably to differentiate viral from bacterial meningitis in the individual patient.[171]

Depression of the pH of CSF also has been described in patients with bacterial meningitis. The depression in CSF pH is more transient than the elevation of CSF lactic acid and, therefore, is of even less value in differential diagnosis.[312]

Lactic dehydrogenase, creatine phosphokinase, and glutamic oxaloacetic transaminase may be elevated in patients with bacterial meningitis. In some cases, total lactic dehydrogenase activity within CSF may be similar in patients with bacterial and aseptic meningitis, but lactic dehydrogenase isoenzymic analysis may permit differentiation of bacterial from nonbacterial infection. This procedure is time consuming and cumbersome and does not permit a specific etiologic diagnosis in any patient.[157, 212]

Speer and associates[276] found consistently elevated concentrations of elastase-α-proteinase inhibitor in the blood and CSF of children between 1 month and 12 years of age who had bacteremia, meningitis, or both. These data suggest that measurement of this enzyme inhibitor complex may be a sensitive indicator of bacterial meningitis. The study population was small (26); thus, more extensive studies will be required to ascertain the value of this test in differentiating viral, bacterial, and fungal disease early in the meningeal inflammatory process.

Despite the application of impeccable clinical judgment, examination of CSF, and use of one or more of the rapid diagnostic techniques, situations arise in which differentiation of bacterial from aseptic meningitis remains problematic. In these cases, a predominance of polymorphonuclear leukocytes generally is found in CSF, the CSF cell count is less than 100 cells/mm^3, the CSF glucose is normal or nearly so, and the Gram stain result is negative. In addition, although the patients exhibit signs and symptoms suggestive of meningitis, they do not appear acutely ill. Some investigators have advocated withholding antibiotic therapy in these individuals and repeating the lumbar puncture after 6 to 12 hours of close observation.[3, 83] Usually, the repeated examination of CSF either will substantiate the impression of aseptic meningitis (a shift to a lymphocytic differential will be noted) or will point more conclusively to a bacterial process. This course of action is not recommended if the patient has been pretreated with antibiotics or is younger than 1 year of age.

Additional laboratory data are helpful and should be obtained. Blood cultures should be obtained in every patient suspected of having bacterial meningitis. In one prospective study in which blood was obtained for culture from every patient, the cultures were positive in 80 per cent of children with *H. influenzae* meningitis, in 52 per cent of children with pneumococcal meningitis, and in 33 per cent of children with meningococcal meningitis.[81] Forty-four per cent of the entire group had received some form of antibiotic therapy before admission to hospital and before these blood cultures were obtained. If these individuals were excluded, positive blood cultures were obtained from 90 per cent, 80 per cent, and 91

TABLE 38–6. Metabolic Changes Reported in Patients with Bacterial Meningitis

Cerebrospinal fluid (CSF) lactate increased
CSF pH decreased
CSF lactic dehydrogenase increased
Creatine phosphokinase increased
Glutamine oxaloacetic transaminase increased
CSF and blood elastase-α-proteinase inhibitor increased

per cent of children with meningitis caused by *H. influenzae, S. pneumoniae,* and *N. meningitidis*, respectively.

A thorough search for foci of infection adjacent to or remote from the meninges should be performed. Repetitive neurologic evaluation also should be performed and appropriate laboratory studies undertaken to define the extent of neurologic dysfunction.

In our experience, cultures of the throat and nasopharynx have not been particularly rewarding. In most cases, no pathogen has been recovered from these sites. In some cases in which a pathogen was identified, the organism recovered was not the same as the one found in the CSF or blood.

When the concentration of bacteria within the blood is high, a Gram-stained smear of a buffy coat obtained from the blood may reveal the presence of microorganisms. If petechial lesions are present, a smear of the lesions after puncture with a small lancet may reveal microorganisms on Gram stain.

Radiographs of the chest, sinuses, skull, or spine may be helpful in disclosing a focus of infection.

Radioisotope scanning may be helpful in selected patients such as those with a leak of CSF. The pattern of distribution of radioactivity recorded by gamma camera coincides with the accumulation of purulent material. Increased concentration of isotope may relate to the inflammatory response within the meninges or in the periventricular region or to alteration in the blood-brain barrier.[120] Subdural effusions also may be recognized as crescentic accumulations of isotope over the convexities of the cerebral hemisphere.[120] Localized concentrations of radionuclide may be seen in children with meningitis, most likely as a result of cerebral vasculitis or infarction.[67] Confirmation of impaired cerebral circulation, including occlusion and narrowing of arteries, sluggish circulation, and retrograde flow, has been provided by the studies of Gado and associates.[108] In these studies, resolution of the arterial lesions was demonstrated in subsequent angiograms in two patients, despite the persistence of neurologic deficits; these findings prompted the authors to suspect vascular spasm at the earlier stage of disease. Hydrocephalus contributed to sluggish circulation through intracerebral vessels in two patients. Tyson and colleagues[296] demonstrated at least transient disturbance in the circulation of CSF in 45 per cent of patients with meningitis, but persistent hydrocephalus is a rare complication of purulent meningitis.

Computed tomography (CT), a noninvasive technique, permits the prospective and repetitive assessment of children with meningitis. This technique permits detection of ventricular dilatation, subdural effusion, decrease in brain mass, and presence of vascular lesions or of brain infarcts (Fig. 38–3). With this procedure, ventricular dilatation may be noted acutely in many children who never develop hydrocephalus after recovery from their disease.[81]

Recurrent bacterial meningitis may be the result of a communication between the nasal passage or ear and the meninges. If rhinorrhea or otorrhea is present, a leak may be suspected, but documenting that CSF is present and locating the site of leakage are difficult when the sample is small or contaminated. Sectional (2 mm) coronal cranial CT has been reported to be a relatively easy, noninvasive method for delineating anatomic abnormalities in children with recurrent meningitis.[280]

Meurman and associates[195] demonstrated that an extra band of transferrin is located in the B_2-fraction after protein electrophoresis of CSF. This extra B_2-transferrin band could not be demonstrated in serum, nasal secretions, saliva, tears, or perilymph and endolymph. The amount of sample required is small (<50 μL). We have applied this immunochemical method successfully in documenting that fluid found

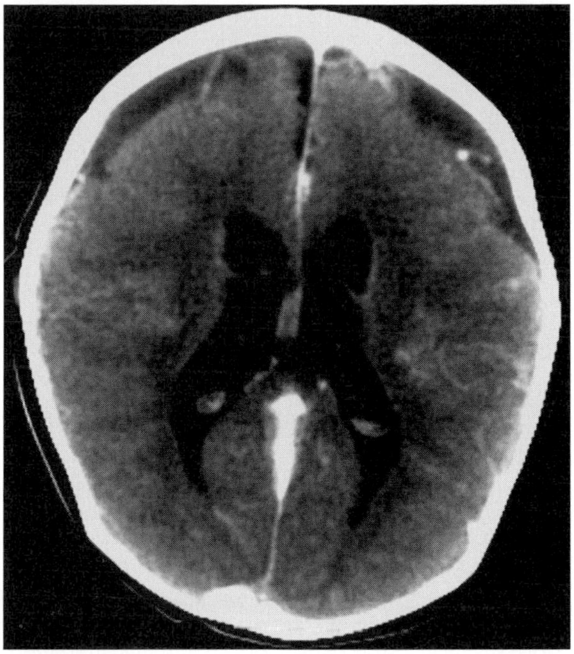

FIGURE 38–3. *Computed tomographic scan of a 2-year-old child with bacterial meningitis. Moderately severe ventricular dilatation and the presence of bilateral extracerebral fluid collections overlying the convexities of the brain (subdural effusions) are noted. Note the several prominent vessels that run through the subdural space.*

draining from the nose or ear was CSF. Differential suction may permit demonstration of the site of the anatomic communication between the nose, the ear, and the meninges. Moderate contamination with other body fluids does not invalidate the method. The method also is noninvasive and safe for the patient.

TREATMENT

Antimicrobial Therapy

Prompt treatment of bacterial meningitis with an appropriate antibiotic is essential. The initial selection always should be made before definitive cultures are available and ideally should be based on incidence and susceptibility patterns in the local community.

For many years, ampicillin and chloramphenicol were preferred as the initial empiric therapy for children older than 3 months of age and suspected of having bacterial meningitis. The development of newer cephalosporins and other antibiotics that have excellent bactericidal activity against *H. influenzae* type b, *N. meningitidis*, and *S. pneumoniae* within the CSF has led to several possible alternative approaches to the initial therapy of childhood meningitis. As experience with cefotaxime and ceftriaxone continues to amass, these drugs have become the treatment of choice in most centers. A survey of directors of programs of pediatric infectious diseases in 1992[166] indicated that 92 per cent used cefotaxime or ceftriaxone, compared with 2 per cent who continued to use ampicillin and chloramphenicol. This is a dramatic change from a 1988 survey in which ampicillin and chloramphenicol still were found to be used most frequently for initial empiric therapy.[317]

Cefotaxime sodium is a third-generation cephalosporin that has a broad spectrum of activity against both gram-positive and gram-negative organisms. It possesses a high level of resistance to hydrolysis by β-lactamase. Cefotaxime, unlike other third-generation cephalosporins, is metabolized to a fourfold or eightfold less active desacetyl derivative. Desacetyl cefotaxime, however, is a potent antibiotic itself. Moreover, the combination of cefotaxime and desacetyl cefotaxime is synergistic against 75 per cent of clinical isolates. It penetrates the blood-brain barrier and provides bactericidal activity in the CSF equivalent to or greater than that of antibiotics that have been used conventionally for treatment of bacterial meningitis in children.[201] It is an excellent choice for empiric therapy in children 3 months of age or older but must be used with ampicillin for initial therapy in children 1 to 3 months of age because *L. monocytogenes* and enterococci generally can not be treated with cefotaxime but will be sensitive to ampicillin. Cefotaxime is given as a daily dose of 200 to 300 mg/kg/day in three or four divided doses intravenously. The higher dosage is preferred by some experts because the higher CSF concentrations achieved by high-dose therapy may be beneficial for patients whose disease may be caused by *S. pneumoniae* when the organisms are of intermediate sensitivity to third-generation cephalosporins.[50a]

Ceftriaxone is another third-generation cephalosporin that possesses broad antimicrobial activity against the organisms that cause bacterial meningitis. Ceftriaxone readily penetrates the CSF of patients with inflamed meninges. In patients who receive adjunctive therapy with dexamethasone, meningeal inflammation may be reduced, possibly decreasing the penetration of antibiotics into the CSF. Gaillard and colleagues[109] found that CSF concentration of ceftriaxone in children with bacterial meningitis treated with dexamethasone was similar to that found in those not treated with steroids. The half-life of ceftriaxone in serum is approximately 4 hours; a twice-daily dose regimen provides both serum and CSF concentrations far in excess of the minimal bactericidal concentrations of most organisms that cause bacterial meningitis. Several prospective randomized studies have demonstrated that ceftriaxone is comparable to ampicillin plus chloramphenicol for the treatment of bacterial meningitis in children.[11, 24, 39, 52, 61, 123, 279]

Ceftriaxone therapy has been associated with an increased incidence of diarrhea, which is mild and self-limiting. There also is an increased incidence of "gallbladder sludge," or precipitation of ceftriaxone salts in the gallbladder, diagnosed ultrasonographically, which generally is asymptomatic but occasionally is associated with clinical symptoms of cholecystitis.[11, 247] Ceftriaxone also has a high protein-binding capacity and can displace bilirubin from albumin in vitro[134] and therefore needs to be used cautiously in neonates.

When ceftriaxone is used for the treatment of bacterial meningitis, it can be administered in a dose of 100 mg/kg/24 hours in two divided doses or one daily dose intravenously. Although a once-daily dose has proved to be effective,[34, 103, 132] is convenient, and lends itself particularly to home therapy for selected patients (after an initial period of hospitalization), we do not advocate single daily dosing; dosing errors, delayed doses, or missed doses undoubtedly will occur, and inadequate treatment could result. Moreover, although ceftriaxone can be given intramuscularly, a single dose by this route may be impractical.[34] The solution used for intramuscular administration should contain no more than 250 mg/mL. A 15-kg child receiving an 80-mg/kg daily dose would require 4.8 mL of fluid, a volume too large for injection in a single site in an infant. In addition, for non–penicillin-susceptible but ceftriaxone-susceptible organisms, administration twice a day also may be preferred.[50a]

Ampicillin and chloramphenicol have been and continue to be effective as initial treatment of bacterial meningitis, although they are used infrequently. Ampicillin is provided intravenously in a dose of 200 to 300 mg/kg/24 hours in six divided doses. An initial bolus of 100 mg/kg is given. Chloramphenicol is administered intravenously in a dose of 100 mg/kg/24 hours in four divided doses. No loading dose of chloramphenicol is required. If *N. meningitidis, S. pneumoniae,* or *H. influenzae* sensitive to ampicillin is identified, chloramphenicol is discontinued. If an ampicillin-resistant strain of *H. influenzae* is identified, chloramphenicol is continued.

Strains of *H. influenzae* type b that are resistant to ampicillin by a standardized disk susceptibility method should be reassessed using tube dilution sensitivity tests. Ampicillin resistance may be mediated by a plasmid that does not affect β-lactamase activity. Thus, rapid tests of β-lactamase activity need to be interpreted using caution, and antibiotics should not be discontinued based on these results alone. On some occasions, both β-lactamase–negative and β-lactamase–positive organisms can be isolated from the same site[282] or from different sites (blood and CSF) of the same patient (personal experience, R. D. F.).

An increasing number of strains of *S. pneumoniae* that are relatively or completely resistant to penicillin and third-generation cephalosporins have been identified.[37] Vancomycin has been used successfully in the treatment of penicillin-resistant pneumococcal meningitis[35, 106] and in experimental models of cephalosporin-resistant pneumococcal meningitis.[105] In eight reports of treatment failures with third-generation cephalosporins, a variety of treatment regimens were reported, all with success. Vancomycin, alone or in combination with rifampin, chloramphenicol, or both, was used most frequently. We have changed the recommendations for empiric therapy at our hospital to include vancomycin in addition to a third-generation cephalosporin in patients 3 months of age or older or with ampicillin and cefotaxime in patients between 1 and 3 months of age. If resistance to penicillin and cephalosporins is documented, then treatment is continued with vancomycin alone or with rifampin to complete an appropriate course. Vancomycin should be given at a dose of 60 mg/kg/24 hours in four divided doses. Peak serum concentrations in children whose renal function is normal should be between 30 and 40 μg/mL. Chloramphenicol also may be a suitable alternative for the treatment of these organisms if the pneumococcus proves to be sensitive to this antibiotic.

Cefuroxime is a second-generation cephalosporin that has been shown to be effective in vitro against *H. influenzae* type b, *S. pneumoniae,* and *N. meningitidis*. Initial clinical studies found that cefuroxime had equivalent effectiveness compared with ampicillin plus chloramphenicol. However, subsequent studies demonstrated delayed sterilization of the CSF; relapse during or after treatment was higher, and more frequent sensorineural hearing loss occurred when compared with results obtained using ampicillin, chloramphenicol, cefotaxime, and ceftriaxone.[10, 62, 174, 175, 177, 246] Therefore, cefuroxime *should not be used* to treat bacterial meningitis in children.

Other extended-spectrum cephalosporins at present being evaluated as single-drug regimens for the therapy of bacterial meningitis are ceftazidime and ceftizoxime.[41, 143, 197, 234, 235, 316] Ceftazidime has been efficacious in the treatment of meningitis caused by *P. aeruginosa.*

Concentrations of cefoperazone and cefoxitin within CSF have been assessed in patients with bacterial meningitis. Both agents may fail to reach concentrations within CSF required to kill all susceptible strains of *H. influenzae* and *S. pneumoniae* and cannot be recommended for the treatment of bacterial meningitis in children.[42, 91] Cefpirome concentrations in CSF of patients with bacterial meningitis were found to be significantly higher than the minimum bactericidal concentrations for *N. meningitidis, H. influenzae,* and *S. pneumoniae,*[316] but studies documenting its effectiveness in large numbers of children have not been performed.

Aztreonam is an antimicrobial agent that belongs to the monobactam family of antibiotics. It is effective against most gram-negative organisms, including *P. aeruginosa*. Limited data suggest its efficacy in the treatment of *Pseudomonas* and *H. influenzae* meningitis, suggesting a potential role for this agent in the treatment of patients who are allergic to penicillin and who are infected with these or other gram-negative organisms.[165, 176, 294]

Tetracycline also has proved to be effective in the treatment of *H. influenzae* meningitis when employed in a dose of 50 mg/kg/24 hours intravenously in four divided doses.[213] The adverse effects of tetracycline in children make this an unattractive alternative, to be reserved for highly selected patients.

If a history of *significant* allergy to penicillin or cephalosporin (anaphylaxis, urticaria, exfoliative dermatitis) is documented, vancomycin or chloramphenicol may be used. A cross-reactivity of approximately 10 to 15 per cent has been noted for cephalosporins in penicillin-allergic patients.

When meningitis is caused by *Streptococcus pyogenes*, ampicillin or penicillin provides effective therapy. If meningitis is caused by infection with a penicillin-resistant strain of *S. aureus*, oxacillin, methicillin, or nafcillin should be employed, using 200 mg/kg/24 hours intravenously in six divided doses. Vancomycin is effective against *S. aureus* strains resistant to penicillin and to semisynthetic penicillin derivatives[135] or in patients with *S. aureus* meningitis who are penicillin-allergic. Vancomycin also may be useful in the treatment of meningitis caused by *Flavobacterium meningosepticum*.[135] Oral metronidazole is effective in treating anaerobic infection of the CNS when response to conventional therapy has been suboptimal. A dose of 40 mg/kg/24 hours in three or four divided doses results in CSF concentrations of greater than 10 μg/mL.[26]

Imipenem and meropenem have been evaluated for the treatment of meningitis. These carbapenems are active against the bacteria that cause meningitis, but the use of imipenem cilastatins has been associated with drug-induced seizures.

The safety and efficacy of meropenem and cefotaxime were compared in a prospective randomized trial of 190 children with bacterial meningitis.[170a] Seizures occurred within 24 hours prior to antibiotic therapy in 16 per cent of patients randomized to receive meropenem and in 7 per cent of patients randomized to receive cefotaxime.

Seizures occurred in patients after therapy in 6 per cent of children receiving meropenem and in 1 per cent of those receiving cefotaxime. None of these seizures could be attributed to drug therapy. All patients responded to therapy with clinical improvement, and bacterial eradication was proved by repeat lumbar puncture in 100 per cent of patients in both groups. There was no significant difference in short-term outcomes between the two groups. These data suggest that meropenem may be effective in the treatment of bacterial meningitis in children. These data also suggest that this agent should be studied further in children who may have meningitis that is caused by organisms resistant to extended-spectrum cephalosporins. For meropenem-susceptible isolates, meropenem alone or in combination with other drugs may provide a satisfactory alternative for patients who do not tolerate vancomycin.[51a]

Current recommendations for antibiotic treatment of various microorganisms are provided in Table 38–7. An appropriate antibiotic should be continued until the patient is afebrile for 5 days but at least for 7 to 10 days in every patient. Although there are data to support a shorter course of therapy, we continue to recommend 10 days of treatment for pneumococcal and *H. influenzae* type b meningitis and 7 days for *N. meningitidis* meningitis.[151, 184, 187] If clinical improvement is noted within 24 hours, a repeat lumbar puncture is not necessary during the course of treatment or after treatment has been completed. If clinical improvement is slower than anticipated or is not noted, a repeat examination of CSF is indicated at any time. In the 1970s, lumbar puncture frequently was performed at the conclusion of therapy. Data from studies performed at that time (Table 38–8) reveal that white blood cell counts within CSF and CSF protein concentration generally had not returned completely to normal and that the CSF to blood glucose ratio may have remained depressed. In every case, CSF Gram stain should reveal no organisms and cultures should be sterile. If a lumbar puncture is performed at the conclusion of therapy, we believe retreatment to be mandatory if organisms are seen or grown. It also may be considered if more than 30 per cent of the cells are polymorphonuclear leukocytes or if the CSF glucose and the CSF to blood glucose ratio are less than 20 mg/dL and 20 per cent, respectively.

Some physicians have discharged children with meningitis from the hospital before the conclusion of a course of therapy using home management. Benefits of home therapy include a decreased risk of nosocomial infection, a return of the child to his or her normal environment sooner, and a decrease in the total cost of therapy. Financial savings of outpatient, once-daily ceftriaxone for pediatric meningitis have been estimated to be $200 per day.[225] Bradley and colleagues[34] reported the results of 54 children with bacterial meningitis treated as outpatients from 1 to 8 days (mean, 4.6 days) with intramuscular ceftriaxone given once daily. Each dose was given in conjunction with a physician's examination. Each child had to be afebrile for 24 to 48 hours before initiation of home therapy, free of neurologic dysfunction except for auditory or vestibular dysfunction, and without evidence of inappropriate secretion of ADH before being considered for outpatient therapy. No child required readmission or developed neurologic sequelae or relapse. Powell and Mawhorter[226] reported a retrospective review of 26 patients with meningitis or other serious bacterial infections who received some portion of their therapy as an outpatient with ceftriaxone without any relapse or recurrence.

Waler and Rathore[306] suggest 10 criteria for considering outpatient therapy for children with bacterial meningitis: (1) inpatient therapy for at least 6 days, (2) afebrile for at least 24 to 48 hours before outpatient therapy, (3) no significant neurologic dysfunction or focal findings, (4) no seizure activity, (5) clinically stable, (6) taking all fluids by mouth, (7) receives the first dose of outpatient antibiotic in the hospital, (8) administration of the antibiotic in the office or emergency room setting or by qualified home health nursing, (9) daily examination by a physician, and (10) reliable parents who have transportation and a telephone. We concur with the recommendations of the Committee on Infectious Diseases of the American Academy of Pediatrics,[51] which does not recommend this course of action but does recognize that it is a therapeutic option for certain patients. The dose of ceftriaxone of 80 to 100 mg/kg/24 hours intramuscularly may need to be aliquoted to account for the necessary volume of diluent to achieve a concentration of no greater than 250 mg/mL. If oral chloramphenicol is used, therapeutic serum concentrations of 15 to 25 μg/mL must be documented before discharge and maintained.

H. influenzae type b organisms have been recovered from the throats of patients after completion of a course of treatment for *H. influenzae* type b meningitis. Therefore, when members of a household to which the patient will return include children 4 years of age or younger, the patient should

TABLE 38–7. Recommendations for Antibiotic Therapy

Organism	Antibiotics	Recommended Dosages IV
Bacteroides fragilis	Chloramphenicol Metronidazole	100 mg/kg/d in 4 dd 30 mg/kg/d in 4 dd
Bacteroides other than *B. fragilis*	Penicillin G	300,000 units/kg/d in 6 dd
Clostridium	Penicillin G	300,000 units/kg/d in 6 dd
Corynebacterium	Penicillin G Erythromyin	300,000 units/kg/d in 6 dd 50 mg/kg/d in 4 dd
*Enterobacter, Klebsiella, Escherichia coli**	Ampicillin Gentamicin Amikacin Cefotaxime Ceftriaxone Ticarcillin	300 mg/kg/d in 6 dd 7.5 mg/kg/d in 3 dd 15 mg/kg/d in 3 dd 200 mg/kg/d in 4 dd 100 mg/kg/d in 2 dd 300 mg/kg/d in 4 dd
Haemophilus influenzae	Ampicillin Cefotaxime Ceftriaxone Chloramphenicol	300 mg/kg/d in 6 dd 200 mg/kg/d in 4 dd 100 mg/kg/d in 1 or 2 dd 100 mg/kg/d in 4 dd
Listeria monocytogenes	Ampicillin Gentamicin Trimethoprim-sulfamethoxazole	300 mg/kg/d in 6 dd 7.5 mg/kg/d in 3 dd 20 mg/kg/d in 4 dd (TMP component)
Neisseria meningitidis	Penicillin G	300,000 units/kg/d in 6 dd
Neisseria gonorrhoeae	Penicillin G (if sensitive to penicillin) Ceftriaxone	300,000 units/kg/d in 6 dd 100 mg/kg/d in 1–2 dd
Proteus mirabilis (indole-negative)	Ampicillin	300 mg/kg/d in 6 dd
Proteus mirabilis (indole-positive)	Cefotaxime Gentamicin Amikacin Ticarcillin	200 mg/kg/d in 4 dd 7.5 mg/kg/d in 3 dd 22.5 mg/kg/d in 3 dd 300 mg/kg/d in 4–6 dd
Pseudomonas	Gentamicin Ticarcillin Piperacillin Amikacin Ceftazidime	7.5 mg/kg/d in 3 dd 450 mg/kg/d in 4 or 6 dd 300 mg/kg/d in 4 or 6 dd 15–20 mg/kg/d in 3 dd 150–200 mg/kg/d in 3 dd
Salmonella	Ampicillin Cefotaxime Gentamicin Chloramphenicol	300 mg/kg/d in 6 dd 200 mg/kg/d in 4 dd 7.5 mg/kg/d in 3 dd 100 mg/kg/d in 4 dd
Staphylococcus aureus (penicillinase-negative)†	Penicillin G	300,000 units/kg/d in 6 dd
Staphylococcus aureus (penicillinase-positive)†	Methicillin, oxacillin or nafcillin	200 mg/kg/d in 6 dd
Staphylococcus aureus (resistant to semisynthetic penicillins)	Vancomycin	60 mg/kg/d in 4 dd
Staphylococcus (coagulase-negative)	Vancomycin	60 mg/kg/d in 4 dd
Streptococcus pneumoniae†	Penicillin G Chloramphenicol Vancomycin Cefotaxime/ceftriaxone Rifampin‡	300,000 units/kg/d in 6 dd 100 mg/kg/d in 4 dd 60 mg/kg/d in 4 dd 200–300 mg/kg/d in 3 or 4 dd/100 mg/kg/d in 1 or 2 dd 20 mg/kg/d in 2 dd
Unknown (1–3 mo of age)	Ampicillin plus Cefotaxime plus Vancomycin	300 mg/kg/d in 6 dd 200 mg/kg/d in 4 dd 60 mg/kg/d in 4 dd
Unknown (>3 mo of age)	Cefotaxime or Ceftriaxone plus Vancomycin Methicillin (or nafcillin) if question of staphylococcal infection Gentamicin (if question of *Pseudomonas*)	200 mg/kg/d in 4 dd 100 mg/kg/d in 1 or 2 dd 60 mg/kg/d in 4 dd 200 mg/kg/d in 6 dd 7.5 mg/kg/d in 3 dd

*Trimethoprim-sulfamethoxazole has been used successfully in selected patients with gram-negative enteric meningitis in a dose of 20 mg (trimethoprim) and 100 mg (sulfamethoxazole) kg/day IV in 4 divided doses (dd).

†Vancomycin may be provided in a dose of 60 mg/kg/day in 4 dd IV if patients are allergic to penicillin or penicillin derivatives or in the case of *Streptococcus pneumoniae* for multidrug-resistant pneumococci or pneumococci that are highly resistant to penicillin. In these cases, addition of rifampin also may be considered.

‡Should never be used alone.

TABLE 38–8. Cerebrospinal Fluid Findings at Conclusion of Antibiotic Treatment

	Total White Blood Cell Count		Polymorphonuclear Leukocytes (%)		Protein (mg/dL)		Glucose (mg/dL)		CSF:Blood Glucose	
	Mean + 1 SD	*Range*	*Mean + 1 SD*	*Range*	*Mean + 1 SD*	*Range*	*Mean + 1 SD*	*Range*	*Mean + 1 SD*	*Range*
Total group	41 ± 80	0–850	5.5 ± 12	0–90	46 ± 72	7–970	47 ± 12.7	21–91	55.7 ± 17	23–156
Haemophilus influenzae	53 ± 98	0–850	5.5 ± 11	0–90	43 ± 37	10–334	47 ± 13	31–100	55 ± 17	31–100
Ampicillin	56 ± 107	0–850	5.9 ± 12	0–90	44 ± 43	13–334	46 ± 14	21–91	53 ± 17	33–89
Chloramphenicol	49 ± 83	0–325	5.1 ± 10.7	0–50	41 ± 26	7–127	48 ± 11	27–90	57 ± 13	30–100
Streptococcus pneumoniae	29 ± 30	0–110	5.5 ± 11.5	0–45	42 ± 39	7–211	48 ± 9	22–68	57 ± 13	22–91
Neisseria meningitidis	16 ± 27	0–132	3.4 ± 7.9	0–27	39 ± 46	7–188	47 ± 11	29–77	47 ± 19	23–100
Others	11 ± 18	0–77	7.3 ± 19	0–75	70 ± 197	10–970	48 ± 18	37–73	70 ± 28	44–156

be given rifampin, 20 mg/kg once daily for 4 days, to prevent the occurrence of secondary cases.

Adjunctive Therapy

As described earlier, the pathogenesis and subsequent sequelae of bacterial meningitis are as much a consequence of the host response to infection as the bacterial organisms themselves. It has been hypothesized that anti-inflammatory agents as adjuncts to antimicrobial therapy may decrease the degree of tissue injury during the course of the disease.

Corticosteroids have been suggested as an adjunct to therapy of bacterial meningitis because they may (1) decrease intracranial pressure by decreasing meningeal inflammation and brain water content; (2) modulate the production of cytokines, which, in turn, lessens the meningeal inflammatory response; and (3) decrease the incidence of sensorineural hearing loss or other neurologic complications of meningitis.[174, 215]

Corticosteroids may play a role in acute management of increased intracranial pressure and cerebral herniation, although there are no data specifically indicating that corticosteroids decrease cerebral edema caused by bacterial meningitis. Odio and colleagues[215] found that dexamethasone therapy in children with bacterial meningitis decreased opening lumbar CSF pressure 12 hours after administration of the first dose, but this effect was lost by 24 hours of treatment. The significance of these findings is unclear because the steroids were not given as specific therapy for increased intracranial pressure and the majority of the subjects were not demonstrating signs of impending herniation.

Dexamethasone given 1 hour before or simultaneously with *H. influenzae* type b lipooligosaccharide significantly reduced TNF activity and meningeal inflammation in rabbits.[315] In experimental *H. influenzae* meningitis, administration of dexamethasone 1 hour before but not 1 hour after ceftriaxone was associated with significantly reduced TNF-α concentration and indices of inflammation in the CSF.[207] Dexamethasone administration has been associated with decreased concentration in CSF of prostaglandin E_2 and decreased leakage of some proteins from serum into CSF in rabbits with experimental pneumococcal meningitis.[154] In patients with bacterial meningitis, steroid-treated patients had significantly lower CSF concentrations of IL-1β, TNF-α, platelet-activating factor, and prostaglandin E_2 than those who received antibiotics alone.[194, 208, 215] Patients tend to become afebrile sooner but have an increased incidence of secondary fevers.[304]

Although our understanding of the pathophysiologic events associated with initiation of the acute inflammatory response has been enhanced by recent data, the ability of dexamethasone to reduce long-term complications of bacterial meningitis remains controversial. None of the pediatric studies of dexamethasone use in bacterial meningitis have demonstrated an overall change in mortality.

In randomized, placebo-controlled trials of dexamethasone as adjunctive therapy in bacterial meningitis[174, 215, 245, 304] and in retrospective studies[123, 164] published since 1988, 68 per cent (227 of 333) of steroid recipients in the six randomized trials had meningitis caused by *H. influenzae* type b; the remaining 32 per cent had meningitis caused by *S. pneumoniae* (38) or *N. meningitidis* (41).[228] A meta-analysis of nine controlled trials published before 1991 failed to document a reduced risk of neurologic abnormality at hospital discharge or follow-up examination.[144]

Odio and associates[215] found that the administration of dexamethasone immediately before the initiation of cefotaxime therapy was associated with a lower incidence of neurologic sequelae (14 per cent compared with 38 per cent in patients receiving cefotaxime alone). They found no significant difference in auditory sequelae, compared with those of controls. The frequency of neurologic sequelae in placebo-treated patients was significantly higher than that noted in other studies.[245, 288, 304]

Studies by Lebel and associates[174] and Schaad and colleagues[245] failed to demonstrate a significant reduction in the incidence of neurologic sequelae in steroid- compared with placebo-treated patients. A prospective, multicentered, placebo-controlled study evaluated 143 children with bacterial meningitis caused by *H. influenzae* type b (58 per cent), *S. pneumoniae* (23 per cent), and *N. meningitidis* (17 per cent).[304] Patients were treated with ceftriaxone and placebo or ceftriaxone and dexamethasone administered within 4 hours of the first dose of antibiotics. No significant difference in neurologic or developmental outcome between patients who received steroids or placebo was found.

Sensorineural hearing loss is a significant sequela of bacterial meningitis. In the two randomized studies performed by Lebel and associates,[174] dexamethasone-treated patients were significantly less likely to have moderate or severe bilateral sensorineural hearing loss; however, in one study, patients were treated with cefuroxime, which has been shown to result in delayed sterilization of the CSF and a higher rate of hearing loss, compared with treatment with ceftriaxone.[246] An additional 100 infants and children with bacterial meningitis were treated with ceftriaxone for 10 days and either dexamethasone or placebo for 4 days. A significant reduction in moderate to severe hearing loss in children with *H. influenzae* type b meningitis ($p < .001$) was reported. There were no significant differences between the two groups in other neurologic sequelae. In addition, two patients receiving dexamethasone developed gastrointestinal bleeding severe enough to require transfusion, and two others developed heme-positive stools. Odio and associates[215] found no significant difference in the incidence of moderate or severe hearing impairment between placebo and steroid groups (16 and 6 per cent, respectively).

The Swiss Meningitis Group[245] found that treating children with dexamethasone 10 minutes before ceftriaxone and then for 2 days subsequently resulted in persistent hearing loss in 5 per cent (3) of children who had received dexamethasone and in 15 per cent (8) of those who received placebo, a difference that was not significant. One of the steroid-treated and five of the placebo-treated children had unilateral hearing loss only. The group also documented a transient mild to moderate hearing impairment in five dexamethasone-treated and four placebo-treated children; in six of the nine, the impairment was shown to be caused by a conductive disturbance. Dexamethasone did not alter the incidence or natural history of the transient hearing impairment.

In the most recently published multicenter study,[304] audiologic measurements were made early in the course of the disease (within 24 hours of admission), as well as 6 weeks to 12 months after recovery from disease. The authors found no significant difference in the incidence of persistent moderate or severe hearing loss between children who received dexamethasone within 4 hours of antibiotics and those who received placebo, with the exception of bilateral deafness in children with *H. influenzae* type b meningitis (5 of 72 in placebo group vs. 0 of 67 in dexamethasone group) (p = .02). The overall incidence of moderate to severe hearing loss was 14.7 per cent (10.3 per cent unilateral and 4.4 per cent bilateral) in the dexamethasone-treated group and 22.9 per cent (13.5 per cent unilateral and 9.4 per cent bilateral; p = .33 for bilateral loss) in the placebo-treated group. Of note, these authors found that 22 children (8 in the dexamethasone group and 14 in the placebo group) had bilateral moderate or severe hearing loss at the initial evaluation. Only one child with *H. influenzae* meningitis and unilateral deafness at initial examination progressed to bilateral deafness. At follow-up, the resolution of hearing loss was nearly identical for each group, with 8 of the 22 children having normal hearing at follow-up, 5 having unilateral deafness, and 9 having bilateral deafness. These results suggest that hearing loss occurs early in the course of meningitis and that early auditory brain stem response results need to be interpreted cautiously with regard to long-term audiologic sequelae. There was a very strong relationship between hearing loss early in the disease and a low concentration of CSF glucose at presentation of meningitis, a finding that has been reported previously.[66]

The Infectious Disease Committee of the American Academy of Pediatrics (Red Book, 1994) states that "dexamethasone therapy should be considered when bacterial meningitis in infants and children 6 weeks and older is diagnosed or strongly suspected on the basis of CSF tests, including Gram-stained smears, after the physician has weighed the benefits and possible risks and before the etiology has been established." The committee recognizes that some experts continue not to recommend its use. Although recommended for treatment of *H. influenzae* type b meningitis, dexamethasone has not been supported to be of benefit for pneumococcal or meningococcal meningitis. Dexamethasone should not be used if aseptic or nonbacterial meningitis is suspected, and if it is started before the diagnosis of nonbacterial meningitis is made, it should be discontinued immediately. It should not be used in "partially treated" meningitis. No data exist on which to base a recommendation to use dexamethasone for the treatment of bacterial meningitis in infants younger than 6 weeks of age or in those with congenital or acquired abnormalities of the CNS, with or without a prosthetic device. It also should be noted that use of dexamethasone plus vancomycin may decrease the transport of vancomycin into the CSF. It is not advisable to use dexamethasone when vancomycin is used to treat meningitis caused by *S. pneumoniae* that may be resistant to penicillin, third-generation cephalosporins, or both.[36]

If dexamethasone is used, it should be used in all patients, regardless of disease severity, and should be administered as early as possible in the course of treatment in a dose of 0.15 mg/kg/dose intravenously every 6 hours for no more than 4 days. One study[245] found no difference in children treated for 2 days instead of 4 using 0.4 mg/kg/dose every 12 hours.

There is no clear evidence that dexamethasone dramatically alters the long-term sequelae of meningitis, and its use is not without risk of adverse advents. The markedly decreased frequency of meningitis caused by *H. influenzae* type b and the increased frequency of meningitis caused by *S. pneumoniae* (for which therapy with vancomycin may be necessary) suggest that initiation of dexamethasone should not be considered as a routine form of adjunctive therapy in every patient.

SUPPORTIVE CARE

In addition to antibiotic therapy, management of bacterial meningitis includes measures that apply generally to the critically ill child. Careful monitoring and attention to detail are essential. Pulse rate, blood pressure, and respiratory rate should be measured carefully every 15 minutes until stable and then every hour for the first several days. Temperature should be measured rectally every 4 hours. A thorough neurologic examination should be performed at the time of admission and at least daily thereafter. A rapid assessment of neurologic function should be performed 6 to 12 times a day for the first several days of treatment. Body weight should be measured daily for at least the first 3 to 4 days.

Head circumference should be measured and in children younger than 18 months of age at the time of admission and daily thereafter. Transillumination of the head also may be performed at the time of admission and subsequently, if indicated by the clinical course of the patient.

The following laboratory data are suggested if results of lumbar puncture indicate bacterial meningitis: (1) total peripheral white blood cell count and differential, (2) hemoglobin concentration, (3) hematocrit, (4) platelet count, (5) serum electrolytes, and (6) serum and urine osmolalities. Urine volume and specific gravity should be monitored.

A low white blood cell count may suggest a poor prognosis. Anemia associated with *H. influenzae* type b septicemia has been reported[263, 264] and has been attributed to immune hemolysis of red blood cells that are coated with soluble bacterial antigens. Shurin and Anderson[263] reported an abrupt decline in hemoglobin concentration in 17 of 19 children within 3 days of admission for *H. influenzae* type b septicemia. They concluded that the anemia related to *H. influenzae* type b septicemia was the result of injury to red blood cells by interaction of adsorbed soluble bacterial antigens with host immune mechanisms whose function is to ensure clearance of bacteria.

Every child with meningitis should be evaluated carefully in a manner that will permit identification of inappropriate secretion of ADH, recognition of seizure activity, and detection of the development of subdural effusions. Body weight, serum electrolytes, serum and urine osmolalities, urine volume, and specific gravity determinations should be made at the time of admission and followed closely (every 6 to 12 hours) for the first 24 to 36 hours in the hospital and daily for several days thereafter. Initially, the child should receive nothing by mouth because of the risk of vomiting and aspiration. In addition, delivery of all fluid intravenously ensures greater accuracy in measuring intake and output during the critical early days of therapy. Inappropriate secretion of ADH has been documented in 88 per cent of children enrolled in a prospective study of bacterial meningitis.[78] Elevated serum concentrations of ADH in the presence of hyponatremia have been documented by direct measurement of ADH concentration in serum obtained from the same children.[82]

An electrolyte solution containing approximately 40 mEq/L of sodium and chloride, 35 mEq/L of potassium, and 20 mEq/L of acetate or lactate should be administered at a rate of 1000 mL/m^2/24 hours. Fluid restriction is continued until it can be documented (frequently within 2 hours), on the basis of objective measures, that ADH secretion is not a factor or has resolved. The best indicators of retention of fluid in excess of solute are the body weight and serum sodium concentration. As serum sodium approaches normal (140 mEq/L), fluid administration may be liberalized progressively to normal maintenance levels of 1500 to 1700 mL/m^2/24 hours.

Powell and associates[227] found that elevated concentrations of arginine vasopressin in patients with bacterial meningitis who clinically were dehydrated responded to maintenance fluids plus deficit replacement with 0.9 per cent saline. This study confirms that the syndrome of inappropriate secretion of ADH should not be diagnosed in the presence of dehydration. Decreased intravascular volume is a physiologic stimulus for the release of ADH, and therefore its release is not inappropriate. Fluid restriction is not advocated for patients who are dehydrated; rehydration should be carried out with careful and frequent assessment of fluid and electrolyte status.

Singhi and colleagues[267] examined the effect of fluid restriction on body water and outcome of 50 consecutive children who had been hospitalized with acute meningitis. These children were divided into two groups—those with hyponatremia and those without hyponatremia. Patients in both groups then were assigned randomly to receive either normal maintenance or restricted fluids (65 to 70 per cent of the volume of that received by the maintenance subgroup). Thus, as few as 11 and no more than 15 patients were randomized to any of the four subgroups in the study. The authors state that there was no significant difference in overall outcome or intact survival when comparisons were made between fluid-restricted and non–fluid-restricted groups or within each group between the subgroups who received restricted fluids or maintenance fluids. However, after combining the subgroups who received restricted fluids with those on maintenance fluids, there was a trend toward higher intact survival and lower mortality in the non–fluid-restricted groups. Nevertheless, children who had an extracellular water reduction of 10 mL/kg or greater in 48 hours had a significantly lower intact survival (10 of 28, 36 per cent) than those with less than 10 mL/kg or no reduction of extracellular water (15 of 22, 64 per cent). The mortality rate also was higher in the former group (7 of 28, 25 per cent) than in the latter group (2 of 22, 9 per cent). The authors concluded that fluid restriction did not improve the outcome of acute meningitis and that a decrease in extracellular water volume at 48 hours may increase the likelihood of adverse outcome.

This study particularly is difficult to interpret within the context of previous information in the literature. In studies of large numbers of children with bacterial meningitis, evidence of inappropriate secretion of ADH correlated significantly ($p < .01$) with abnormal neurologic findings, even 3 months after discharge and with low IQ scores.[86] The original studies were carried out in patients who were *not* fluid restricted.[80] As a result of these findings, coupled with documentation of inappropriate secretion of ADH, a recommendation to fluid restrict patients who are hyponatremic at admission was made. Fluids are restricted only until evidence for inappropriate secretion of ADH can be excluded (usually within 2 hours). The average patient in subsequent studies reported by Kaplan and Feigin[158] was fluid restricted for only 0.75 days. The mortality rate in the largest single study reported by Feigin[76] of individuals who were fluid restricted was 0.5 per cent compared with 9 and 25 per cent in the groups reported in the studies by Singhi and associates.[267] Moreover, Singhi and associates did not assess other important outcome variables, such as the number of patients with hearing loss or those whose psychometric performance might or might not have been impaired. The total number of patients in any of their study groups was relatively small. Although their data are intriguing, other differences either in the population studied or in the management of the patients may have accounted for these differences. In addition to the increased mortality in the patients studied by Singhi and associates noted earlier, there also was an extraordinarily high frequency of hydrocephalus and a very high frequency of seizures and status epilepticus noted, compared with groups of patients who have been studied in the United States. Because cerebral edema and increased intracranial pressure have been noted as major disturbances in seriously ill patients with meningitis and because many of the deaths and some of the sequelae have been related to the effects of cerebral edema and intracranial hypertension, we continue to recommend fluid restriction in patients with hyponatremia and liberalization of fluids as soon as the effects of excess ADH secretion have been dissipated (usually less than 1 day).

Meningitis complicated by shock creates a complex fluid management problem. Shock associated with meningitis is secondary to septicemia and generally is treated with large quantities of intravenous fluid to maintain blood pressure and adequate tissue perfusion (see Chapter 72). Patients with meningitis without shock benefit from initial fluid restriction to avoid worsening of cerebral edema and severe hyponatremia with subsequent seizures. Children with meningitis and shock should receive sufficient quantities of isotonic fluid to maintain a systolic blood pressure of 80 to 90 mm Hg, a urine output equal to or greater than 500 mL/m^2/24 hours, and adequate cerebral perfusion, as indicated by mental status. Central venous pressure monitoring is useful to guide fluid resuscitation and prevent fluid overload. The addition of albumin (1 g/kg) to intravenous fluids may decrease the total volume of fluid needed to maintain adequate perfusion. Vasopressors, such as dopamine, dobutamine, and isoproterenol, also may provide support of blood pressure and perfusion and reduce intravenous fluid requirements.

When increased intracranial pressure is suggested by such signs as progressive lethargy, increased muscle tone, or bulging anterior fontanelle, elevation of the head approximately 30 degrees may be helpful. Increased intracranial pressure associated with deterioration in mental status or signs of cerebral herniation (Fig. 38–4) may be treated more vigorously with mannitol administered intravenously (0.5 g/kg) infused over 30 minutes and repeated as necessary. If steroids are used for this purpose, the recommended steroid is dexamethasone in a dose of 10 to 12 mg/m^2/day in four divided doses for no more than 4 or 5 days.[159]

Head circumference measurement and transillumination permit assessment of the development of subdural effusions or may suggest other causes for an enlarging head. CT may be helpful in detecting large subdural effusions or hydrocephalus. Because effusions can be considered as part of the pathophysiologic changes that occur with bacterial meningitis, CT to evaluate effusions does not need to be part of the routine evaluation of a child with meningitis. CT should be

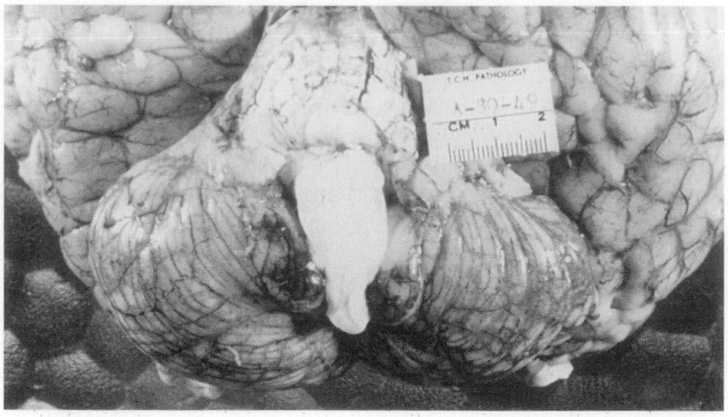

FIGURE 38–4. *Inflammation and hemorrhage of cerebellar tonsils from child with cerebellar herniation through foramen magnum due to bacterial meningitis. (From Kaplan, S. Current management of common bacterial meningitides. Reproduced with permission of Pediatrics in Review 7:77, copyright 1985.)*

performed in children with focal neurologic signs. In children with hemiparesis or quadriparesis, CT may document cerebrovascular abnormalities. CT also should be performed in children with papilledema on an emergency basis before proceeding with the initial lumbar puncture. *Administration of antibiotics should not be delayed for diagnostic imaging in patients in whom bacterial meningitis is suspected.*

Treatment of subdural effusions, consisting of subdural paracentesis, should take place only when one suspects that the effusions are responsible for seizures or for prolonged fever as a result of subdural empyema. Paracentesis also may be useful if the effusion is responsible for symptoms of increased intracranial pressure or is the cause of focal neurologic signs.[78, 86] In most cases, subdural taps are not required.

Seizures, when noted, should be treated expeditiously. A patent airway must be maintained and appropriate anticonvulsants administered. Sodium phenobarbital (7 mg/kg loading dose) may be administered parenterally followed by a maintenance dose of 5 mg/kg/day in two divided doses. If necessary, diazepam (up to 0.2 mg/kg) or lorazepam (0.05 mg/kg/dose up to 4 mg maximum) infused intravenously over 1 to 2 minutes may be used. If prolonged seizure control is needed, phenytoin (5 mg/kg/day) in two divided doses may be used. Phenytoin generally does not depress the respiratory center to the same extent that phenobarbital does, and it also may benefit the patient by inhibiting the secretion of ADH. If the seizure activity no longer is apparent after the second hospital day and there are no focal neurologic signs at the time of discharge from the hospital, anticonvulsants may be discontinued. Phenytoin and phenobarbital can induce hepatic microsomal enzymes; their use may increase the rate of metabolism of chloramphenicol and possibly cause a significant decrease in the serum concentration of this antibiotic.[226]

An electroencephalogram is indicated in patients with meningitis and seizures when focal seizures are noted, seizures persist after more than 72 hours after presentation, seizures occur after the third day of hospitalization, a subdural effusion is noted, or prolonged alteration in sensorium is present. An electroencephalogram may be of value in distinguishing abnormal intermittent posturing from movements associated with seizure activity.

Patients with disseminated intravascular coagulation syndrome may benefit from heparin therapy, although there are no controlled studies that document unequivocally the efficacy of this form of therapy. Heparin may be given in a dose of 1 mg/kg intravenously and repeated every 4 hours as needed.

Persistent fever (lasting longer than 8 or 9 days) has been noted.[19] Suppurative complications, however, including subdural or pleural empyema, septic arthritis, and pericarditis, should be sought carefully. The rare occurrence of brain abscess in association with bacterial meningitis may lead to persistent fever as well. Furthermore, nosocomial intercurrent infection, usually viral, may cause prolonged fever in a child with meningitis. Persistent fever may be related to the severity of the infection. Poor therapeutic response (especially in multidrug-resistant organisms) occurs, and repeated lumbar puncture must be considered on an individual basis. Drug fever often is cited but rarely is the cause of persistent fever and remains a diagnosis of exclusion.

PROGNOSIS AND SEQUELAE

The prognosis in individual patients with bacterial meningitis depends upon many factors, including the following: (1) the age of the patient, (2) the time course or progression of illness before effective antibiotic therapy, (3) the specific microorganism causing the disease, (4) the number of organisms[89] or the quantity of capsular polysaccharide material present in the meninges and CSF at the time of diagnosis, (5) the rapidity with which CSF is sterilized after initiation of antibiotic therapy, and (6) the presence of disorders that may compromise host response to infection.[177]

The younger the patient and the greater the antigenic load at the time of admission, the worse the prognosis. Bacterial colony counts appear to be a more reliable indication of sequelae than does antigen concentration. Seizures, subdural effusions, bacteremia, and a more prolonged period of fever are more frequent in children who have more than 10^7 CFU/mL of a particular organism in CSF at the time of admission.[90] Children with colony counts equal to or greater than 10^7 CFU/mL also are significantly more likely to experience hearing loss and speech disturbance than are children with meningitis but lower concentrations of bacteria within CSF specimens.[90] The presence of TNF in serum has been associated with a fatal outcome in patients with meningococcal meningitis.[302] Elevated concentrations of IL-1β and TNF within the CSF of patients with bacterial meningitis also have been correlated significantly ($p < .002$) with a higher incidence of neurologic sequelae of disease.[206]

The mortality rate for bacterial meningitis in children who are beyond the neonatal period has been reduced to between 1 and 5 per cent. Although antibiotic therapy has reduced the mortality rate, as many as 50 per cent of the survivors of meningitis have some sequelae of their disease.[67, 86, 257, 278] Most studies from which estimates of sequelae have been derived have been retrospective, and the patients were enrolled over a period of many years (1951–1968). Although antibiotic treatment of these individuals may have been relatively standardized during this period, ancillary methods employed in their care were not controlled.

Sell and associates,[257] in a retrospective study of *H. influenzae* meningitis, reported that 11 of 86 children died and that 29 per cent of the survivors had severe or significant handicaps. Included in the group classified as severely handicapped were those whose IQ was 70 or less. These investigators also noted that 14 per cent of survivors had possible residual abnormalities; included in this group were children who scored 70 to 80 on intelligence tests. In addition, postmeningitic children functioned at significantly lower levels than did their age-matched peers.[258] Thus, minor residual deficits appear to be a frequent concomitant of bacterial meningitis.

The frequency of complications of meningitis can be assessed most appropriately by prospective evaluation.

In 1975, Sell[256] began a prospective study of 50 infants and children who recovered from *H. influenzae* meningitis. Fifty per cent of this group were entirely normal, 9 per cent were normal except for behavioral problems, and 28 per cent had significant handicaps. The major handicaps noted included hearing loss (10 to 11 per cent), language disorders or delayed language development (15 per cent), impaired vision (2 to 4 per cent), mental retardation (10 to 11 per cent), motor abnormalities (3 to 7 per cent), and seizures (2 to 8 per cent). Twenty-one postmeningitic children were paired with a sibling and tested by the Wechsler Intelligence Scale for Children. The mean IQ of the postmeningitic children was 86 and that of control children 97 ($p < .05$). Comparison of results for individual pairs revealed that 29 per cent of postmeningitic children scored one full standard deviation below their siblings; no survivor had a score one standard deviation higher than his or her sibling.

The most recent results of our own large prospective study of bacterial meningitis in children revealed that 32.8 per cent of children had abnormalities detectable on neurologic examination at the time of discharge, but by 5 years after discharge, specific deficits were noted in only 11.1 per cent of the total group.[79] As a result of the onset of late seizures in some of these patients, the frequency of neurologic sequelae 15 years after discharge was 14 per cent.[224] Specific complications or sequelae of meningitis in these patients are shown in Table 38–9. Shortly after discharge, hemiparesis or quadriparesis was noted in 30 patients (12.4 per cent of the total group), but at 1 year after discharge, paralysis was noted in only 5. These data reflect the tendency for even major neurologic defects to clear unpredictably with time. This important observation suggests the need to maintain cautious optimism in discussing long-term complications of meningitis with parents.

A study by Taylor and associates[288] attempted to gain additional insight into the sequelae of *H. influenzae* meningitis, with particular emphasis on neuropsychologic function. Although the study was retrospective, it permitted a more detailed neuropsychologic assessment made at an earlier age than that reported by investigators in previous studies. In addition, the index patients were compared with their siblings who were closest in age and the same sex, and the study was controlled for occupational and educational status. Only 14 per cent of children who had been afflicted with *H. influenzae* meningitis had any residual neurologic sequelae. Mean full-scale IQ was 102 for the index children and 109 for the control children.

In 1995, Grimwood and colleagues[131a] reported the results of a prospective cohort study of 158 meningitis survivors, ages 3 months to 14 years, who were treated in a single center between 1983 and 1986. Between 1991 and 1993, 130 children (82 per cent of the original cohort) were evaluated at a mean age of 8.4 years and a mean of 6.7 years after their meningitis. Blended, audiologic, behavior, neurologic, neuropsychologic, and sociodemographic assessments were compared with those of sex- and grade-matched control children.

There was a systematic increase in the risk of abnormality or for poorer functioning for children with meningitis versus control children across all categories tested. The differences reached statistical significance for tests of fine motor function, intelligence, neuropsychologic function, school behavior, and auditory figure-ground differentiation.

Eleven children who had experienced meningitis (85 per cent of the cohort studied) had major deficits (hydrocephalus, persistent seizures, spasticity, blindness, IQ < 70, or profound hearing loss). Twenty-four (18.5 per cent) of the survivors of meningitis and 14 (10.8 per cent) of the control children had minor deficits (IQ, 70 to 80; inability to read; abnormalities in speech discrimination, possibly referable to mild to moderate hearing loss; or school behavior problems).

Overall, one in four of the children in this study had either a serious disabling sequela or a functionally important behavior disorder or neuropsychologic or auditory dysfunction that adversely affected academic performance.

Meta-analysis of 19 reports of prospectively enrolled and evaluated cohorts from developing countries published between 1980 and 1990[22] determined the mean probability of mortality to be 3.8 per cent for *H. influenzae* type b, 7.5 per cent for *N. meningitidis*, and 15.3 per cent for *S. pneumoniae*, with an overall probability of 4.8 per cent. The mean probabilities of sequelae in the survivors were deafness, 10.5 per cent; mental retardation, 4.2 per cent; spasticity, paresis, or both, 3.5 per cent; and seizure disorder, 4.2 per cent. The mean probability of no detectable sequelae was 83.6 per cent.

Other specific sequelae or complications of bacterial meningitis that have been observed include cranial nerve involvement, hemiparesis or quadriparesis, muscular hypertonia, ataxia, permanent seizure disorders, and the development of obstructive hydrocephalus. Subdural effusions (as noted earlier) are so frequent in young children that they can be considered a part of the general disease process rather than as a persistent or troublesome complication of the meningeal infection. Brain abscess after bacterial meningitis is exceed-

TABLE 38–9. Complications or Sequelae of Meningitis

	Total	*Haemophilus influenzae*	*H. influenzae* (Ampicillin)	*H. influenzae* (Chloramphenicol)	*Streptococcus pneumoniae*	*Neisseria meningitidis*	Others
Number	235	151	90	61	35	26	23
Deaths <12 hr in hospital	4	4	3	1	0	0	0
Deaths >12 hr in hospital	1	0	0	0	0	1	0
Shock	8	6	5	1	1	1	0
Paralysis							
Early	30	18	7	11	7	3	2
Persistent	5	4	1	3	4	0	0
Persistent tone	5	4	1	3	1	2	0
Ataxia							
Early	7	5	2	3	2	0	0
Persistent	1	1	0	1	0	0	0
Visual problems	7	4	2	2	3	0	0
Clinically significant hearing deficit	25	17	6	11	5	2	1
Hydrocephalus	1	1	1	0	0	0	0

ingly rare[92]; when found, the possibility that it preceded the development of meningeal infection must be entertained, and a careful search for other sites of such infections as endocarditis should be initiated.

Bacteriologic relapse after treatment of meningitis (particularly that caused by *H. influenzae* and treated with ampicillin) has been highlighted in a number of reports.[19, 48, 50, 130, 138, 139, 251, 320] Relapse of *H. influenzae* meningitis after chloramphenicol treatment also has been reported, but, in all except three cases, treatment failure occurred in patients who received a portion of chloramphenicol intramuscularly, a route now known to be unreliable and one no longer sanctioned.[59, 180, 222] It has been difficult to assess precisely the frequency of relapse in children who have received an appropriate antibiotic to which the organism is sensitive or an appropriate dose intravenously and for an extended period. In one retrospective study in which these criteria were fulfilled, the relapse rate after treatment of *H. influenzae* meningitis with ampicillin was 4 per cent.[259] Currently, the relapse rate is less than 1 per cent.

Evoked response audiometry was used to detect hearing deficits in the patients described by Feigin and Dodge.[79] Some deficit in auditory nerve function was documented by this sensitive technique in 6 per cent of children with *H. influenzae* meningitis, in 31 per cent of children with pneumococcal meningitis, and in 10.5 per cent of children with meningococcal disease.

Significant hearing loss after bacterial meningitis has been reported frequently. The mechanisms responsible for hearing deficits include spread of infection along the auditory canal and cochlear aqueduct, serous or purulent labyrinthitis, and, with time, replacement of the membranous labyrinth with fibrous tissue and new bone.[27, 155, 182, 185, 236] Deafness generally is noted early in the course of bacterial meningitis and is independent of the therapy provided.[66, 156, 161, 204, 256, 301] Ataxia has been reported as a presenting sign of bacterial meningitis in children with hearing loss noted in the same individuals at a later date.[160, 255] Presumably, the insult to the vestibular and auditory systems occurred concomitantly in these children. The early loss of hearing noted by several investigators suggests that hearing loss is *not* associated specifically with the use of a particular antimicrobial agent. It is apparent that early diagnosis and treatment will not prevent the development of deafness in many children who develop loss of hearing as a consequence of bacterial meningitis.

Estimates of the frequency of hearing loss in retrospective studies vary from 2.4 to 29 per cent.[41, 48, 92, 209] In our own prospective studies, 7 per cent of children have experienced marked to extensive (75-db loss or greater) hearing losses.[156, 161] Occasionally, hearing loss noted early may improve over a period of weeks to months.[236]

In our own studies, there has been no correlation between loss of hearing and either the age of the patient at the onset of meningitis or duration of illness before admission.[66, 161] There was a significant correlation between hearing loss and the presence of seizures before admission, the duration of fever in the hospital after therapy had been initiated (which presumably reflects more severe disease), treatment with antibiotics administered orally before a definitive diagnosis of bacterial meningitis, and a depressed CSF to blood glucose ratio at the time of admission.[66, 161, 162]

Because hearing deficits are so common in patients with bacterial meningitis, hearing evaluation using evoked response audiometry in young, uncooperative children is recommended routinely at the time of or shortly after discharge from the hospital. Repeated audiometric evaluation is recommended after discharge if the results of initial examination are abnormal. Pure tone audiometry can be used for older, cooperative children. It is important to differentiate hearing deficits because of conductive disturbances from those related to damage to the eighth cranial nerve. Some children who have repetitive episodes of otitis media may experience conductive loss that is unrelated to the meningitis.

In our own studies, the mean IQ ($\pm$1 SD) of the entire group of patients (235) after recovery was 94 ($\pm$23), with a range of 33 to 150. Twenty-nine children (17.3 per cent) had IQs less than 80, and 22 (11.6 per cent) had IQs less than 70. A comparison of these patients with their own siblings and other control children revealed no significant difference in mean IQ. A significantly greater proportion ($p < .01$) of children who recovered from meningitis had IQs less than 80 than did children from control groups. These results differ from those of Sell,[256] which were noted previously. Tejani and associates[291] also prospectively evaluated children who had recovered from bacterial meningitis using siblings as controls. They reported no significant differences in the verbal performances or full-scale IQs between meningitis patients and the sibling control population.

Feldman and Michaels[88] more recently reported that children who recovered from meningitis caused by *H. influenzae* and who were evaluated 10 to 12 years later maintained grades and scores comparable with those of their siblings as they progressed to middle school. Their academic success may require more school and family support to compensate for minor differences in IQs that had been noted.

The prospective nature of these studies has permitted an assessment of factors that herald a poor prognosis and that may be discernible at or near the time of admission. Evidence of inappropriate secretion of ADH was correlated significantly ($p < .01$) with abnormal neurologic examinations at 3 months after discharge and with low IQs. The age of the child correlated inversely with the development of subdural effusion ($p < .01$), the occurrence of hearing deficits ($p < .02$), and low IQ ($p < .05$). Thus, the significantly increased impact of the disease upon young children could be documented conclusively. The presence of focal neurologic findings in patients who were not postictal at the time of admission correlated significantly ($p < .001$) with abnormal neurologic examination, which was noted previously. Focal deficits indicative of cerebral injury noted at admission or during the course of hospitalization were associated significantly ($p < .001$) with the development of late (1 to 15 years after discharge) afebrile seizures.[224] Thus, focal neurologic findings at the time of admission proved to be a most reliable predictor of permanent sequelae of bacterial meningitis. Focal deficits at admission also correlated significantly with low IQs ($p < .001$), even at 2 and 3 years after discharge from hospital. The quantity of antigen in the initial CSF specimen and the number of organisms present also correlated significantly ($p < .01$) with sequelae of meningitis.[86]

CT has revealed evidence of cerebral infarction in children who had a diagnosis of bacterial meningitis established within 1 or 2 days of the onset of symptoms of a febrile illness.[273] In most of these cases, evidence of abnormalities in cerebrovascular dynamics (arteritis, thrombosis, thrombophlebitis), ventricular dilatation, or both have been observed. In some of these cases, infarction has been associated with profound hypotension related to endotoxemia (personal experience). It is apparent that brain infarction is *not* related causally to a delay in diagnosis and therapy in many cases.

PREVENTION

Haemophilus influenzae Meningitis

In the past 10 years, methods of preventing meningitis caused by *H. influenzae* type b have improved. The dramatic decrease in the incidence of *H. influenzae* type b invasive disease and meningitis has been attributed to the introduction of vaccines that initially were found to be effective at 15 months of age[4] and then later were found to be effective as early as 2 months of age.[253] There currently are three conjugate vaccines approved for infants beginning at 2 months of age: HbOC, PRP-OMP, and PRP conjugated to tetanus toxoid (PRP-T). In December 1990, the Advisory Committee on Immunization Practices and the American Academy of Pediatrics recommended universal infant immunization at 2, 4, and 6 months of age with HbOC or at 2 and 4 months of age with PRP-OMP.[8, 45]

Passive immunization against *H. influenzae* type b also is under investigation. One such approach involves an attempt to extend the period of passive immunity in the infant by immunizing pregnant women with an appropriate vaccine. Researchers at the University of Rochester have performed two studies of this type. Results obtained suggest that the concentrations of antibody to *H. influenzae* in the infants of immunized mothers should protect all of the children studied for 6 months and about half of them for up to 12 months.[145]

Passive immunization of infants also has been studied using bacterial polysaccharide immunoglobulin.[7, 244] This preparation given in a single intramuscular dose of 0.5 mL/kg provides significant protection for infants from *H. influenzae* type b disease for 3 or 4 months.

Children studied for the acquisition of secretory antibody developed antibody to the capsule in nasal secretions after infection, and this mucosal antibody persisted in some children for up to 2 years.[221] Children with high levels of mucosal antibody developed only low concentrations of serum antibody. These data suggest a potential for an early IgA response in young infants; the functional maturation of the mucosal immune system may precede that of the serum immune system with respect to antibodies to the capsule of *H. influenzae* type b.[145]

The single most comprehensive study concerning the spread of *H. influenzae* type b infection among household contacts was coordinated by the Centers for Disease Control and Prevention.[307] Data collected from 19 states were analyzed prospectively. *H. influenzae* meningitis was reported in 1403 patients. Eighty-two per cent of exposed families were investigated for the occurrence of *H. influenzae* disease within 30 days of its onset in the index patient. Systemic disease caused by *H. influenzae* type b developed in 9 of 1687 contacts (0.5 per cent) who were younger than 6 years of age. The risk in patients younger than 4 years of age was 2.1 per cent; the risk in children younger than 1 year of age was 6 per cent. The risk of secondary infection of household contacts in the 30 days after onset of meningitis in the index case was 585 times greater than the age-adjusted risk in the general population and was similar to the risk of secondary meningococcal disease in household contacts. This nationwide study provided an important impetus for finding a chemoprophylactic regimen that could prevent secondary infection in household contacts.

A number of antibiotic regimens were studied between 1978 and 1984 to determine whether they could eliminate nasopharyngeal carriage of *H. influenzae* and prevent invasive disease. Antibiotics effective in treating local or invasive disease often were ineffective in eliminating the carrier state. Ampicillin, erythromycin-sulfisoxazole, cefaclor, and trimethoprim-sulfamethoxazole all have been ineffective in reliably eliminating *H. influenzae* from the nasopharynx.[261]

A number of studies have appeared between 1978 and 1984 in which investigators utilized rifampin to determine whether it was efficacious in eradicating nasopharyngeal carriage of *H. influenzae* type b organisms.[43, 54, 55, 116, 128, 262, 308, 318] Some of these studies were retrospective, some prospective; some randomized, and others nonrandomized. Regardless of study design, rifampin administered in a 20 mg/kg dose provided once each day for 4 days proved to be superior in eradicating nasopharyngeal carriage of *H. influenzae* to a 10 mg/kg dose once a day or a 10 mg/kg dose twice a day.

On the basis of an analysis of these data, the Infectious Disease Committee of the American Academy of Pediatrics recommended that rifampin be provided orally once each day for 4 days in a 20 mg/kg dose (maximum dose, 600 mg/day) to all household contacts (children and adults), irrespective of age in those households with at least one unvaccinated contact younger than 4 years of age.[168] However, rifampin prophylaxis is not required when all of the household contacts younger than 4 years of age have been immunized fully. Children within the household who have been exposed to the index case and develop a febrile illness should receive prompt medical evaluation and, if indicated, antimicrobial therapy appropriate for *H. influenzae* invasive disease, whether or not they already are receiving rifampin prophylaxis.

Although the Infectious Disease Committee of the American Academy of Pediatrics also made a similar recommendation for day care center and nursery school contacts, the committee has reconsidered this recommendation and no longer insists upon rifampin prophylaxis when only a single case has been reported in a day care center.

There is no information to document the safety of rifampin administered during pregnancy. Therefore, prophylaxis with rifampin is not recommended for pregnant women who are contacts of infected infants. The recommendations that have been made were espoused after careful consideration of the cost of the drug, of the possibility that resistance to rifampin might develop among selected isolates of *H. influenzae* type b, of the difficulties encountered because rifampin is formulated only as a capsule, and of the possibility that prophylaxis may eradicate carriage from some children in whom carriage of *H. influenzae* might elicit an antibody response that could protect them from invasive disease.[107]

The more crucial issue is to ascertain whether rifampin prophylaxis not only is effective in eliminating nasopharyngeal carriage but also actually can prevent secondary disease. A nationwide, collaborative, placebo-controlled trial was conducted among household (children younger than 6 years of age) and day care center contacts of people with invasive *H. influenzae* type b disease.[21] Four of 765 placebo-treated contacts experienced secondary disease versus none of 1112 rifampin-treated contacts. This difference was statistically significant ($p = .027$). Rifampin was provided during this study either in a 10 mg/kg dose or a 20 mg/kg dose, or a placebo was provided. The 20 mg/kg dose for 4 days was provided after previous studies (see earlier) documented the superiority of that regimen to the 10 mg/kg dose. If one patient from the placebo-treated group is moved to the rifampin-treated group, the difference is not statistically significant. Household and day care center contacts were pooled before the data were analyzed. When a separate analysis of the data is made for each of the groups of contacts, no statistically significant difference is achieved for day care center contacts of children with *H. influenzae* infection.

Patients receiving rifampin should be advised routinely that their urine, sweat, and tears will be stained orange. Individuals should be advised to refrain from the use of contact lenses during rifampin therapy because the lenses may be stained permanently.

Meningococcal Infection

We advocate the use of chemoprophylaxis in all household members of a patient with meningococcal meningitis and in day care nursery contacts, preferably within 24 hours of the diagnosis of the primary case.[131, 169] Schoolroom classmates and hospital contacts of patients usually are not given prophylactic treatment. Meningococcal infections caused by sulfonamide-sensitive bacteria may be prevented by prophylaxis with sulfonamides, using sulfadiazine in a dose of 0.5 to 1.0 g twice daily for 3 to 5 days.

Minocycline and rifampin have proved to be 80 to 90 per cent effective in eradicating carriage of meningococci.[136, 138] Both drugs are secreted in the saliva in concentrations greater than the MICs for meningococci. The use of minocycline has been accompanied by frequent and significant vestibular reactions, even after a single dose of 100 mg and, in our opinion, generally should not be used.[44, 46, 47, 314]

Rifampin can be utilized in a dose of 600 mg twice daily for four doses in adults and in doses of 10 mg/kg/dose for four doses in children between 1 and 12 years of age. A dose of 5 mg/kg every 12 hours for four doses can be used in children between 3 months and 1 year of age.[203] The emergence of rifampin-resistant strains in treated meningococcal carriers has been reported to occur with a frequency of 0 to 27 per cent.[58, 71, 311] No rifampin-resistant isolates from cases have been reported among those submitted to the Centers for Disease Control and Prevention in Atlanta, Georgia, since 1970.

A short course of low-dose penicillin V has not proved to be effective prophylaxis for meningococcal disease. A 10-day course of penicillin G in therapeutic dosage has not been evaluated critically as a means of meningococcal prophylaxis in a civilian population. In our own limited trials, we have been impressed with the value of this approach; further studies appear to be warranted.

A single intramuscular dose of ceftriaxone has proved to be an effective alternative to rifampin for prophylaxis in meningococcal contacts.[254] This approach to prophylaxis particularly may be useful in circumstances in which compliance with the use of oral rifampin is considered to be questionable.

Four meningococcal polysaccharide vaccines are licensed in the United States for selective use: (1) monovalent A, (2) monovalent C, (3) bivalent groups A and C, and (4) quadrivalent groups A, C, Y, and W-135. The use of these vaccines in military recruits in the United States has produced a significant reduction in epidemics of meningococcal disease.[12]

A single dose of serogroup C vaccine seems to be about 70 per cent effective, for a period of 6 to 9 months, in preventing meningococcal disease in children who are older than 2 years of age.[287] Single 50-μg injections in children younger than 2 years of age do not produce adequate antibody responses.[287] A serogroup A polysaccharide vaccine has been field tested by the World Health Organization and is effective in children 3 months of age or older.[303, 305] Serogroup-specific monovalent vaccines may be used to control outbreaks of disease caused by either type A or type C meningococci and may be of value for travelers to countries with epidemic disease.[76, 169] Bivalent A/C vaccine or quadrivalent A/C/Y/W-135 vaccine currently is given to all American military personnel. The vaccine is administered as a single dose parenterally in the volume specified by the package insert. Reactions noted after immunizations previously have been mild and infrequent; localized erythema of 1 or 2 days' duration is not unusual.

The safety of the vaccine in pregnant women has not been established.

An effective serogroup B meningococcal vaccine has not been produced to date. In an effort to enhance the immunologic activity of meningococcal serogroup B polysaccharide, it has been complexed noncovalently with serotype 2 outer-membrane proteins. Use of the product has been shown to be safe and immunogenic in humans.[321] This preparation offers the hope that an appropriately immunogenic serogroup B meningococcal vaccine may be available in the near future.[98]

References

1. Achtman, M.: Molecular epidemiology of epidemic bacterial meningitis. Rev. Med. Microbiol. *1*:29–38, 1990.
2. Achtman, M.: Clonal properties of meningococci from epidemic meningitis. Trans. Royal Soc. Trop. Med. Hyg. *85*(Suppl.):24–31, 1991.
3. Adair, C. V., Gould, R. L., and Smadel, J. E.: Aseptic meningitis, a disease of diverse etiology: Clinical and etiologic studies on 854 cases. Ann. Intern. Med. *39*:675–704, 1953.
4. Adams, R. D., Kubik, C. S., and Bonner, F. J.: The clinical and pathological aspects of influenzal meningitis. Arch. Pediatr. *65*:354–376, 1948.
5. Adams, W. G., Deaver, K. A., Cochi, S. L., et al.: Decline of childhood *Haemophilus influenzae* type b (Hib) disease in the Hib vaccine era. J. A. M. A. *269*:221–226, 1993.
6. Allbritton, W. L., Wiggins, G. L., and Feeley, J. C.: Neonatal listerioses: Distribution of serotypes in relation to age at onset of disease. J. Pediatr. *88*:481–483, 1976.
7. Ambrosino, D. M., Landesman, S. H., Gorham, C. C., et al.: Passive immunization against disease due to *Haemophilus influenzae* type b: Concentrations of antibody to capsular polysaccharide in high-risk children. J. Infect. Dis. *153*:1–7, 1986.
8. American Academy of Pediatrics, Committee on Infectious Disease: *Haemophilus influenzae* type b conjugate vaccines: Recommendations for immunization of infants and children 2 months of age and older: Update. Pediatrics *88*:169–172, 1991.
9. Anderson, G., Smithee, L., Rados, M., et al.: Progress toward elimination of *Haemophilus influenzae* type b disease among infants and children—United States, 1987–1993. M. M. W. R. *43*:144–148, 1994.
10. Arditi, M., Herold, B. C., and Yogev, R.: Cefuroxime treatment failure and *Haemophilus influenzae* meningitis: Case report and review of the literature. Pediatrics *84*:132–135, 1989.
11. Aronoff, S. C., Reed, M. O., O'Brien, C. A., et al.: Comparison of the efficacy and safety of cetriaxone to ampicillin/chloramphenicol in the treatment of childhood meningitis. Antimicrob. Agents Chemother. *13*:143–151, 1984.
12. Artenstein, M. S., Gold, R., Zimmerly, J. D., et al.: Prevention of meningococcal disease by group C polysaccharide vaccine. N. Engl. J. Med. *282*:417–420, 1970.
13. Asensi, F., Otero, M. C., Perez-Tamarit, D., et al.: Risk/benefit in the treatment of children with imipenem-cilastatin for meningitis caused by penicillin-resistant pneumococcus. J. Chemother. 5:133–134, 1993.
14. Ashwal, S., Tomasi, L., Schneider, S., et al.: Bacterial meningitis in children: Pathophysiology and treatment. Neurology *42*:739–748, 1992.
15. Asmar, B. I., and Dajani, A. S.: Concurrent pneumococcal disease in two siblings. Am. J. Dis. Child. *136*:946–947, 1982.
16. Austrian, R., Lukens, J., and Seeler, R. A.: Pneumococcal infections in sickle cell anemia. Am. J. Dis. Child. *123*:614–615, 1972.
17. Baker, C. J., and Barrett, F. F.: Transmission of group B streptococci among parturient women and their neonates. J. Pediatr. *83*:919–925, 1973.
18. Baker, R. C., and Bausher, J. C.: Meningitis complicating acute bacteremic facial cellulitis. Pediatr. Infect. Dis. *5*:421–423, 1986.
19. Balagtas, R. C., Levin, S., Nelson, K. E., et al.: Secondary and prolonged fevers in bacterial meningitis. J. Pediatr. *77*:957–964, 1970.
20. Baldwin, L. N., Henderson, A., Thomas, P., et al.: Acute bacterial meningitis in young adults mistaken for substance abuse. BMJ *306*:775–776, 1993.
21. Band, J., Fraser, D. W., and Ajello, G.: Prevention of *Hemophilus influenzae* type b disease. J. A. M. A. *25*:2381–2386, 1984.
22. Baraff, L. J., Lee, S., and Schriger, D. L.: Outcomes of bacterial meningitis in children: A meta-analysis. Pediatr. Infect. Dis. J. *12*:389–394, 1993.
23. Barenkamp, S. J., Granoff, D. M., and Munson, R. S., Jr.: Outer-membrane protein subtypes of *Haemophilus influenzae* type b and spread of disease in day-care centers. J. Infect. Dis. *144*:210–217, 1981.
24. Barson, W. J., Miller, M. A., Brady, M. T., et al.: Prospective comparative trial of ceftriaxone versus conventional therapy for treatment of bacterial meningitis in children. Pediatr. Infect. Dis. *4*:362–368, 1985.
25. Baumgartner, E. T., Augustine, A., and Steele, R. W.: Bacterial meningitis in older neonates. Am. J. Dis. Child. *137*:1052–1054, 1983.
26. Berlow, S. J., Caldarelli, D. D., Matz, G. J., et al.: Bacterial meningitis: A prospective investigation. Laryngoscope *90*:1445–1452, 1980.
27. Berman, B. W., King, F. H., Jr., Rubenstein, D. S., et al.: *Bacteroides fragilis* meningitis in a neonate successfully treated with metronidazole. J. Pediatr. *93*:793–795, 1978.
28. Berman, N. S., Siegel, S. E., Nachum, A., et al.: Cerebrospinal fluid endotoxin concentrations in gram-negative bacterial meningitis. J. Pediatr. *88*:553–556, 1976.
29. Bernhardt, L. L., Semberkoff, M. S., and Rahal, J. J., Jr.: Deficient cerebrospinal fluid opsonization in experimental *Escherichia coli* meningitis. Infect. Immun. *32*:411–413, 1981.

30. Bijlmer, H. A.: World-wide epidemiology of *Haemophilus influenzae* meningitis: Industrialized versus non-industrialized countries. Vaccine *9*(Suppl.*)*:S5–s9, 1991.
31. Blazer, S., Berant, M., and Alon, U.: Bacterial meningitis: Effect of antibiotic treatment on cerebrospinal fluid. Am. J. Clin. Pathol. *80*:386–387, 1983.
32. Bohr, V., Hansen, B., Jessen, O., et al.: Eight hundred and seventy-five cases of bacterial meningitis. Part I of a three-part series: Clinical data, prognosis, and the role of specialized hospital departments. J. Infect. *7*:21–30, 1983.
33. Block, S., Hedrick, J., Wright, P., et al.: Drug-resistant *Streptococcus pneumoniae*—Kentucky and Tennessee, 1993. M. M. W. R. *43*:23–25, 1994.
34. Bradley, J. S., Ching, D. K., and Phillips, S. E.: Outpatient therapy of serious pediatric infections with ceftriaxone. Pediatr. Infect. Dis. J. *7*:160–164, 1988.
35. Bradley, J. S., and Conner, J. D.: Ceftriaxone failure in meningitis caused by *Streptococcus pneumoniae* with reduced susceptiblity to beta-lactam antibiotics. Pediatr. Infect. Dis. J. *10*:871–873, 1991.
36. Brady, M. T., Kaplan, S. L., and Taber, L. H.: Association between persistence of pneumococcal meningitis and dexamethasone administration. J. Pediatr. *99*:924–926, 1981.
37. Breiman, R. F., Butler, J. C., Tenover, F. C., et al.: Emergence of drug-resistant pneumococcal infections in the United States. J. A. M. A. *271*:1831–1835, 1994.
38. Brenneman, G., Silimperi, D., and Ward, J.: Recurrent invasive *Haemophilus influenzae* type b disease in Alaskan natives. Pediatr. Infect. Dis. J. *6*:388–392, 1987.
39. Bryan, J. P., Rocha, H., da Silva, H. R., et al.: Comparison of ceftriaxone and ampicillin plus chloramphenicol for the therapy of acute bacterial meningitis. Antimicrob. Agents Chemother. *28*:361–368, 1985.
40. Buchanan, G. A., and Darville, T.: Impact of immunization against *Haemophilus influenzae* type b (HIB) on the incidence of HIB meningitis treated at Arkansas Children's Hospital. South. Med. J. *87*:38–40, 1994.
40a. Butler, J. C., Breiman, R. F., and Lipman, H. B.: Serotype distribution of *Streptococcus pneumoniae* infections among preschool children in the United States, 1978–1994: Implications for development of conjugate vaccine. J. Infect. Dis. *171*:885–889, 1995.
41. Cable, D., Edralin, G., and Overturf, G. D.: Human cerebrospinal fluid pharmacokinetics and treatment of bacterial meningitis with ceftizoxime. Antimicrob. Agents Chemother. *10*:C121–c127, 1982.
42. Cable, D., Overturf, G., and Edralin, G.: Concentrations of cefoperazone in cerebrospinal fluid during bacterial meningitis. Antimicrob. Agents Chemother. *23*:688–691, 1983.
43. Campbell, L. R., Zedd, A. J., and Michaels, R. H.: Household spread of infection due to *Haemophilus influenzae* type b. Pediatrics *66*:115–117, 1980.
44. Centers for Disease Control: Bacterial meningitis and meningococcemia: United States—1978. M. M. W. R. *28*:277–278, 1979.
45. Centers for Disease Control: *Haemophilus* b conjugate vaccines for prevention of *Haemophilus influenzae* type b disease among infants and children two months of age and older. Recommendations of the Immunization Practices Advisory Committee (ACIP). M. M. W. R. *40*:1–7, 1991.
46. Centers for Disease Control: Vestibular reactions to minocycline after meningococcal prophylaxis—New Jersey. M. M. W. R. *24*:9–11, 1975.
47. Centers for Disease Control: Vestibular reactions to minocycline followup—Georgia, New York, Vermont. M. M. W. R. *24*:55–56, 1975.
48. Cherry, J. D., and Sheenan, C. P.: Bacteriologic relapse in *Haemophilus influenzae* meningitis: Inadequate ampicillin therapy. N. Engl. J. Med. *278*:1001–1003, 1968.
49. Cole, F. S., Saryan, J. A., and Smith, A. L.: The risk of additional systemic bacterial illness in infants with systemic *Streptococcus pneumoniae* disease. J. Pediatr. *99*:91–94, 1981.
50. Coleman, S. J., Auld, E. B., Connor, J. D., et al.: Relapse of *Hemophilus influenzae* type b meningitis during intravenous therapy with ampicillin. J. Pediatr. *74*:781–784, 1969.
50a. Committee on Infectious Diseases of the American Academy of Pediatrics: Therapy for children with invasive pneumococcal infections. Pediatrics *99*:289–299, 1997.
51. Committee on Infectious Diseases of the American Academy of Pediatrics: Treatment of bacterial meningitis. Pediatrics *81*:904–907, 1988.
52. Congeni, B. L.: Comparison of ceftriaxone and traditional therapy of bacterial meningitis. Antimicrob. Agents Chemother. *25*:40–44, 1984.
53. Cox, F., Trincher, R., Rissing, J. P., et al.: Rifampin prophylaxis for contacts of *Haemophilus influenzae* type b disease. J. A. M. A. *245*:1043–1045, 1981.
54. Coulehan, J. L., Michaels, R. H., Hallowel, C., et al.: Epidemiology of *Haemophilus influenzae* type b disease among Navajo Indians. Public Health Rep. *99*:404–409, 1984.
55. Daum, R. S., Glode, M. P., Goldmann, D. A., et al.: Rifampin chemoprophylaxis for household contacts of patients with invasive infections due to *Haemophilus influenzae* type b. J. Pediatr. *98*:485–491, 1981.
56. Daum, R. S., Silber, G. R., Kamon, J. S., et al.: Evaluation of a commercial latex particle agglutination test for rapid diagnosis of *Haemophilus influenzae* type b infection. Pediatrics *69*:466–471, 1982.
57. Davey, P. G., Cruikshank, J. K., McManus, I. C., et al: Bacterial meningitis—Ten years' experience. J. Hyg. *88*:383–401, 1982.
58. Deal, W. B., and Sanders, E.: Efficacy of rifampin in treatment of meningococcal carriers. N. Engl. J. Med. *281*:641–645, 1969.
59. Deane, G. E., Furman, J. E., Bentz, A. R., et al.: Treatment of meningitis with chloromycetin palmitate: Results of therapy in twenty-three cases. Pediatrics *11*:368–380, 1953.
60. Deivanayagam, N., Ashaok, T. P., Nedunchelian, K., et al.: Evaluation of CSF variables as a diagnostic test for bacterial meningitis. J. Trop. Pediatr. *39*:284–287, 1993.
61. Del Rio, M., Chrane, D., Shelton, S., et al.: Ceftriaxone versus ampicillin and chloramphenicol for treatment of bacterial meningitis in children. Lancet *1*:1241–1244, 1983.
62. Del Rio, M. D. A., Chrane, D. F., Shelton, S., et al.: Pharmacokinetics of cefuroxime in infants and children with bacterial meningitis. Antimicrob. Agents Chemother. *22*:990–994, 1982.
63. de Morais, J. S., Munford, R. S., Rise, J. N., et al.: Epidemic disease due to serogroup L *Neisseria meningitidis* in São Paulo, Brazil. J. Infect. Dis. *129*:568–571, 1974.
64. Devoe, I. W., and Gilchrist, J. E.: Pili on meningococci from primary cultures of nasophopharyngeal carriers and cerebrospinal fluid of infants with acute disease. J. Exp. Med. *141*:297–305, 1975.
65. Dinarello, C. A., and Mier, J. W.: Lymphokines. N. Engl. J. Med. *317*:940–945, 1987.
66. Dodge, P. R., Davis, H., Feigin, R. D., et al.: Prospective evaluation of hearing impairment as a sequela of acute bacterial meningitis. N. Engl. J. Med. *311*:869–874, 1984.
67. Dodge, P. R., and Swartz, M. N.: Bacterial meningitis: A review of selected aspects. II. Special neurologic problems, postmeningitic complications and clinicopathological correlations. N. Engl. J. Med. *272*:1003–1010, 1965.
68. Drow, D. L., Welch, D. F., Hensel, D., et al.: Evaluation of Phadebact CSF test for detection of the four most common causes of bacterial meningitis. J. Clin. Microbiol. *18*:1358–1361, 1983.
69. Edwards, K. M., Alford, R., Gewurz, H., et al.: Recurrent bacterial infections associated with C^3 nephritic factor and hypocomplementemia. N. Engl. J. Med. *308*:1138–1141, 1983.
70. Edwards, M. S., Kasper, D. L., and Baker, C. J.: Rapid diagnosis of type III group B streptococcal meningitis by latex particle agglutination. J. Pediatr. *95*:202–205, 1979.
71. Eickhoff, T. C.: In-vitro and in-vivo studies of resistance to rifampin in meningococci. J. Infect. Dis. *123*:414–420, 1971.
72. Ellison, R. T., III, Kohler, P. F., Curd, J. G., et al.: Prevalence of congenital or acquired complement deficiency in patients with sporadic meningococcal disease. N. Engl. J. Med. *308*:913–916, 1983.
73. Eraklis, A. J., Kevy, S. V., Diamond, L. K., et al.: Hazard of overwhelming infection after splenectomy in childhood. N. Engl. J. Med. *276*:1225–1229, 1967.
74. Erdem, G., Kanra, G., Topcu, M., et al.: False-positive latex agglutination test with *Neisseria meningitidis* ACTW135 in a patient with intracranial dermoid tumor. Pediatr. Infect. Dis. J. *13*:550–551, 1994.
75. Ernst, J. D., Decazes, J. M., and Sande, M. A.: Experimental pneumococcal meningitis: The role of leukocytes in pathogenesis. Infect. Immun. *41*:275–279, 1983.
76. Feigin, R. D.: Bacterial meningitis beyond the newborn period. *In* Feigin, R. D., and Cherry, J. D. (eds.): Textbook of Pediatric Infectious Diseases. 2nd ed. Philadelphia, W. B. Saunders, 1987, pp. 439–465.
77. Feigin, R. D., Baker, C. J., Herwaldt, L. A., et al.: Epidemic meningococcal disease in an elementary-school classroom. N. Engl. J. Med. *307*:1255–1257, 1982.
78. Feigin, R. D., and Dodge, P. R.: Bacterial meningitis: Newer concepts of pathophysiology and neurologic sequelae. Pediatr. Clin. North Am. *23*:541–556, 1976.
79. Feigin, R. D., and Dodge, P. R.: Personal communications, 1974–1991.
80. Feigin, R. D., and Dodge, P. R.: Personal data.
81. Feigin, R. D., and Dodge, P. R.: Personal experience: Unpublished data for prospective studies of bacterial meningitis, 1974–1979.
82. Feigin, R. D., and Kaplan, S.: Inappropriate secretion of antidiuretic hormone (ADH) in children with bacterial meningitis. Am. J. Clin. Nutr. *30*:1482–1484, 1977.
83. Feigin, R. D., and Shackelford, P. G.: Sequential lumbar puncture as a diagnostic aid in aseptic meningitis. N. Engl. J. Med. *289*:571–574, 1973.
84. Feigin, R. D., and Shearer, W. T.: Opportunistic infection in children. Part I. In the compromised host. J. Pediatr. *87*:507–514, 1975.
85. Feigin, R. D., and Shearer, W. T.: Opportunistic infection in children. Part II. In the compromised host. J. Pediatr. *87*:677–694, 1975.
86. Feigin, R. D., Stechenberg, B. W., Chang, M. J., et al.: Prospective evaluation of treatment of *Hemophilus influenzae* meningitis. J. Pediatr. *88*:773–775, 1976.
87. Feigin, R. D., Wong, M., Shackelford, P. G., et al.: Countercurrent immunoelectrophoresis of urine as well as CSF and blood for the diagnosis of bacterial meningitis. J. Pediatr. *89*:773–773, 1976.
88. Feldman, H. M., and Michaels, R. H.: Academic achievement in children ten to 12 years after *Haemophilus influenzae* meningitis. Pediatrics *81*:339–344, 1988.
89. Feldman, W. E.: Concentrations of bacteria in cerebrospinal fluid of patients with bacterial meningitis. J. Pediatr. *88*:549–552, 1976.
90. Feldman, W. E., Ginsburg, C. B., McCracken, G. H., et al.: Relation of concentrations of *Haemophilus influenzae* type b in cerebrospinal fluid to late sequelae of patients with meningitis. J. Pediatr. *100*:209–218, 1982.

91. Feldman, W. E., Moffitt, S., and Manning, N. S.: Penetration of cefoxitin into cerebrospinal fluid of infants and children with bacterial meningitis. Antimicrob. Agents Chemother. *21*:468–471, 1982.
92. Feldman, W. E., and Schwartz, J.: *Haemophilus influenzae* type b brain abscess complicating meningitis: Case report. Pediatrics *72*:473–475, 1983.
93. Finland, M., and Barnes, M. W.: Acute bacterial meningitis at Boston City Hospital during 12 selected years, 1935–1972. J. Infect. Dis. *136*:400–415, 1977.
94. Finne, J., Bitter Suermann, D., Goridis, C., et al.: An IgG monoclonal antibody to group B meningococci cross-reacts with developmentally regulated polysialic acid units of glycoproteins in neural and extraneural tissues. J. Immunol. *138*:4402–4407, 1987.
95. Fischer, G. W., Brenz, R. W., Alden, E. R., et al.: Lumbar puncture and meningitis. Am. J. Dis. Child. *129*:590–592, 1975.
96. Fothergill, L. D., and Wright, J.: Influenzal meningitis: The relation of age incidence to the bactericidal power of blood against the causal organism. J. Immunol. *24*:273–284, 1933.
97. Franciosi, R. A., Knostman, J. D., and Zimmerman, R. A.: Group B streptococcal neonatal and infant infections. J. Pediatr. *82*:707–718, 1973.
98. Frasch, C. E., Pepple, B. S., Cate, T. R., et al.: Immunogenicity and clinical evaluation of group B *Neisseria meningitidis* outer membrane protein vaccines. *In* Weinstein, L., and Fields, B. N. (eds.): Seminar in Infectious Diseases. Vol. 4. Bacterial Vaccines. New York, Thieme-Stratton, 1982, pp. 263–267.
99. Fraser, D. W., Darby, C. P., Koehler, R. E., et al.: Risk factors in bacterial meningitis: Charleston County, South Carolina. J. Infect. Dis. *127*:271–277, 1973.
100. Fraser, D. W., Geil, C. C., and Feldman, R. A.: Bacterial meningitis in Bernalilla County, New Mexico: A comparison with three other American populations. Am. J. Epidemiol. *100*:29–34, 1974.
101. Fraser, D. W., Henke, C. E., and Feldman, R. A.: Changing patterns of bacterial meningitis in Olmstead County, Minnesota, 1935–1970. J. Infect. Dis. *128*:300–307, 1973.
102. Fraser, D. W., Mitchell, J. E., Silverman, L. P., et al.: Undiagnosed bacterial meningitis in Vermont children. Ann. J. Epidemiol. *102*:394–399, 1975.
103. Frenkel, L. D., and the Multicenter Ceftriaxone Pediatric Study Group: Once-daily administration of ceftriaxone for the treatment of selected serious bacterial infections in children. Pediatrics *82*:486–491, 1988.
104. Friedland, I. R., and Klugman, K. P.: Antibiotic-resistant pneumococcal disease in South African children. Am. J. Dis. Child. 146:920–923, 1992.
105. Friedland, I. R., Paris, M., Ehrett, S., et al.: Evaluation of antimicrobial regimens for treatment of experimental penicillin- and cephalosporin-resistant pneumococcal meningitis. Antimicrob. Agents Chemother. *37*:1630–1636, 1993.
106. Friedland, I. R., Shelton, S., Paris, M., et al.: Dilemmas in diagnosis and management of cephalosporin-resistant *Streptococcus pneumoniae* meningitis. Pediatr. Infect. Dis. J. *12*:196–200, 1993.
107. Fulginiti, V. A.: Recommendations for rifampin prophylaxis of *Haemophilus* infections by the Committee on Infectious Diseases of the American Academy of Pediatrics. Pediatr. Infect. Dis. *1*:377–378, 1982.
108. Gado, M., Axley, J., Appleton, D. B., et al.: Angiography in the acute and post-treatment phases of *Haemophilus influenzae* meningitis. Radiology *110*:439–444, 1974.
109. Gaillard, J. L., Abadie, G., Cheron, J., et al.: Concentrations of ceftriaxone in cerebrospinal fluid of children with meningitis receiving dexamethasone therapy. Antimcrob. Agents Chemother. *38*:1209–1210, 1994.
110. Garcia, H., Kaplan, S. L., and Feigin, R. D.: Cerebrospinal fluid concentration of arginine vasopressin in children with bacterial meningitis. J. Pediatr. *98*:67–70, 1981.
111. Garred, P., Michaelsen, T. E., Bjune, G., et al.: A low serum concentration of mannan-binding protein is not associated with serogroup B or C meningococcal disease. Scand. J. Immunol. *37*:468–470, 1993.
112. Gary, N., Powers, N., and Todd, J. K.: Clinical identification and comparative prognosis of high-risk patients with *Haemophilus influenzae* meningitis. Am. J. Dis. Child. *143*:307–311, 1989.
113. Geiseler, P. J., and Nelson, K. E.: Bacterial meningitis without clinical signs of meningeal irritation. South. Med. J. *75*:448–450, 1982.
114. Geiseler, P. J., Nelson, K. E., and Levin, S.: Community-acquired purulent meningitis: A review of 1,316 cases during the antibiotic era, 1954–1976. Rev. Infect. Dis. *2*:725–744, 1980.
115. General recommendations on immunization: Recommendations of the Advisory Committee on Immunization Practices (ACIP). M. M. W. R. *43*(RR-1):1–38, 1994.
116. Gessert, C., Granoff, D. M., and Gilsdorf, J.: Comparison of rifampin and ampicillin in day care center contacts of *Haemophilis influenzae* type b disease. Pediatrics *66*:1–4, 1980.
117. Giampaolo, C., Scheld, W. M., Boyd, J., et al.: Leukocyte and bacterial interrelationships in experimental meningitis. Ann. Neurol. *9*:328–333, 1982.
118. Gigliotti, F., Lee, D., Insel, R. A., et al.: IgG penetration into the cerebrospinal fluid in a rabbit model of meningitis. J. Infect. Dis. *156*:394–398, 1987.
119. Gilbert, G.: Epidemiology of *Haemophilus influenzae* type b disease in Australia and New Zealand. Vaccine *9*(Suppl.):S10–S13, 1991.
120. Gilday, D. L.: Various radionuclide patterns of cerebral inflammation in infants and children. A. J. R. Am. J. Roentgenol. *120*:247–253, 1974.
121. Ginsburg, C. M., McCracken, G. H., Jr., and Parke, J. J.: *Haemophilus influenzae* type b disease in a day-care center. Pediatr. Res. *11*:435, 1977.
122. Girgis, N. I., Abu El Ella, A. H., Farid, Z., et al.: Intramuscular ceftriaxone versus ampicillin-chloramphenicol in childhood bacterial meningitis. Scand. J. Infect. Dis. *20*:613–617, 1988.
123. Girgis, N. I., Farid, Z., Mikhail, I. A., et al.: Dexamethasone treatment for bacterial meningitis in children and adults. Pediatr. Infect. Dis. J. *5*:210–215, 1989.
124. Gitlin, D.: Pathogenesis of subdural collections of fluid. Pediatrics *16*:345–351, 1955.
125. Glode, M. N. P., Schiffer, M. S., Robbins, J. B., et al.: An outbreak of *Hemophilus influenzae* type b meningitis in an enclosed hospital population. J. Pediatr. *88*:36–40, 1976.
126. Gold, R.: Bacterial meningitis—1982. Am. J. Med. *75*:98–101, 1983.
127. Good, P. G., Fousek, M. D., Grossman, M. F., et al.: A study of the familial spread of *Hemophilus influenzae*, type b. Yale J. Biol. Med. *15*:913–918, 1943.
128. Granoff, D. M., Gilsdorf, J., Gessert, C., et al.: *Haemophilus influenzae* type b disease in a day care center: Eradication of carrier state by rifampin. Pediatrics *63*:397–401, 1979.
129. Green, S. M., Rothrock, S. G., Clem, K. J., et al.: Can seizures be the sole manifestation of meningitis in febrile children? Pediatrics *92*:527–534, 1993.
130. Greene, H. L.: Failure of ampicillin in meningitis. Lancet *1*:861, 1968.
131. Greenfield, S., and Feldman, H. A.: Familial carriers and meningococcal meningitis. N. Engl. J. Med. *277*:487–502, 1967.
131a. Grimwood, K., Anderson, V. A., Bond, L., et al.: Adverse outcomes of bacterial meningitis in school-age survivors. Pediatrics *95*:646–656, 1995.
132. Grubbauer, H. M., Dornbusch, H. J., Dittrich, P., et al.: Ceftriaxone monotherapy for bacterial meningitis in children. Chemotherapy *36*:441–447, 1990.
133. Guibourdenche, M., Caugant, D. A., Hervé, V., et al.: Characteristics of serogroup A *Neisseria meningitidis* strains isolated in the Central African Republic in February 1992. Eur. J. Clin. Microbiol. Infect. Dis. *13*:174–177, 1994.
134. Gulian, J.-M., Gonard, V., Dalmasso, C., et al.: Bilirubin displacement by ceftriaxone in neonates: Evaluation by determination of "free" bilirubin and erythrocyte-bound bilirubin. J. Antimicrob. Chemother. *19*:823–829, 1987.
135. Gump, D. W.: Vancomycin for treatment of bacterial meningitis. Rev. Infect. Dis. *3*:S289–s292, 1981.
136. Guttler, R. B., Counts, G. W., Avent, C. K., et al.: Effect of rifampin and minocycline on meningococcal carrier rates. J. Infect. Dis. *124*:199–205, 1971.
137. Haimanot, R. T., Caugant, D. A., Fekadu, D., et al.: Characteristics of serogroup A *Neisseria meningitidis* responsible for an epidemic in Ethiopia, 1988–89. Scand. J. Infect. Dis. *22*:171–174, 1990.
138. Hall, B. D.: Failure of ampicillin in meningitis. Lancet *1*:1033, 1968.
139. Haltalin, K. C., and Smith, J. B.: Reevaluation of ampicillin therapy for *Haemophilus influenzae* meningitis: An appraisal based on a review of cases of persistent or recurrent infection. Am. J. Dis. Child. *122*:328–336, 1971.
140. Hansman, D., and Andrews, G. A.: A resistant pneumococcus. Lancet *2*:264–265, 1967.
141. Hansman, D., Hanna, J., and Morey, F.: High prevalence of invasive *Haemophilus influenzae* disease in central Australia, 1986. Lancet *2*:927, 1986.
142. Harding, A. L., Anderson, P., Howie, V. M., et al.: *Hemophilus influenzae* isolated from children with otitis media. *In* Sell, S. H., and Karzon, D. T. (eds.): *Haemophilis influenzae*. Nashville, Vanderbilt University Press, 1973.
143. Hatch, D., Overturf, G. D., Kovacs, A., et al.: Treatment of bacterial meningitis with ceftazidime. Pediatr. Infect. Dis. *5*:416–420, 1986.
144. Haven, P. L., Wendelgerger, K. J., Hoffman, G. M., et al.: Corticosteroids as adjunctive therapy in bacterial meningitis. Am. J. Dis. Child. *143*:1051–1055, 1989.
145. Hill, J. C.: Summary of a workshop on *Haemophilus influenzae* type b vaccines. J. Infect. Dis. *148*:167–175, 1983.
146. Hirakawa, K., Kurokawa, M., Yajin, K., et al.: Recurrent meningitis due to a congenital fistula in the stapedial footplate. Arch. Otolaryngol. *109*:697–700, 1983.
147. Hogasen K., Michaelsen, T., Mellbye, O. J., et al.: Low prevalence of complement deficiencies among patients with meningococcal disease in Norway. Scand. J. Immunol. *37*:487–489, 1993.
148. Ingram, D. L., Anderson, P., and Smith, D. H.: Counter-current immunoelectrophoresis in the diagnosis of systemic disease caused by *Hemophilus influenzae*, type b. J. Pediatr. *81*:1156–1159, 1972.
149. Ingram, D. L., Pearson, A. W., and Occhiuti, A. R.: Detection of bacterial antigens in body fluids with the Wellcogen *Haemophilus influenzae* b, *Streptococcus pneumoniae*, and *Neisseria meningitidis* (ACYW135) latex agglutination tests. J. Clin. Microbiol. *18*:1119–1121, 1983.
150. Jackson, M. A., Shelton, S., Nelson, J. D., et al.: Relatively penicillin-resistant pneumococcal infections in pediatric patients. Pediatr. Infect. Dis. J. *3*:129–132, 1984.
151. Jadavji, T., Biggar, W. D., Gold, R., et al.: Sequelae of acute bacterial meningitis in children treated for seven days. Pediatrics *78*:21–25, 1985.
152. Jorgensen, J. H., Swenson, J. M., Tenover, F. C., et al.: Development of quality control interpretive criteria of antimicrobial susceptibility testing

of *Streptococcus pneumoniae*. *In* Program and Abstracts of the 33rd Interscience Conference on Antimicrobial Agents and Chemotherapy, New Orleans. American Society for Microbiology, 1993, p. 167.

153. Kadurugamuwa, J. L., Hengstler, B., and Zak, O.: Cerebrospinal fluid protein profile in experimental pneumococcal meningitis and its alteration by ampicillin and anti-inflammatory agents. J. Infect. Dis. *159*:26–34, 1989.
154. Kadurugamuwa, J. L., Hengstler, B., and Zak, O.: Effects of antiinflammatory drugs on arachidonic-acid metabolites and cerebrospinal fluid (CSF) proteins during infectious pneumococcal meningitis in rabbits. Pediatr. Infect. Dis. *6*(Suppl.):1153–1154, 1987.
155. Kaene, W. M., Postic, W. P., Rowe, L. D., et al.: Meningitis and hearing loss in children. Otolaryngology *105*:39–44, 1979.
156. Kaplan, S. L., Catlin, F. I., Weaver, T., et al.: Onset of hearing loss in children with bacterial meningitis. Pediatrics *73*:575–578, 1984.
157. Kaplan, S. L., and Feigin, R. D.: Rapid identification of the invading microorganism. Pediatr. Clin. North Am. *27*:783–803, 1980.
158. Kaplan, S. L., and Feigin, R. D.: The syndrome of inappropriate secretion of antidiuretic hormone in children with bacterial meningitis. J. Pediatr. *92*:758–61, 1978.
159. Kaplan, S. L., and Fishman, M. A.: Supportive therapy for bacterial meningitis. Pediatr. Infect. Dis. J. *6*:670–677, 1987.
160. Kaplan, S. L., Goddard, J., VanKleeck, M., et al.: Ataxia and deafness in children due to bacterial meningitis. Pediatrics *68*:8–13, 1981.
161. Kaplan, S. L., Mason, E. O., Jr., Mason, S. K., et al.: Prospective comparative trial of moxalactam versus ampicillin or chloramphenicol for treatment of *Haemophilus influenzae* type b meningitis. J. Pediatr. *104*:447–453, 1984.
162. Kaplan, S. L., Smith, E. O., Wills, C., et al.: Association between preadmission oral antibiotic therapy and cerebrospinal fluid findings and sequelae caused by *Haemophilus influenzae* type b meningitis. Pediatr. Infect. Dis. *5*:626–632, 1986.
163. Kaplan, S. L., and the U.S. Pediatric Multicenter Pneumococcal Surveillance Group: One-year surveillance of systemic pneumococcal infections in children. Pediatr. Res. *37*:197A, 1995.
164. Kennedy, W. A., Hoyt, M. J., and McCracken, G. H.: The role of corticosteroids in children with penumococcal meningitis. Am. J. Dis. Child. *145*:1374–1478, 1991.
165. Kilpatrick, M., Girgis, N., Farid, Z., et al.: Aztreonam for treating meningitis caused by gram-negative rods. Scand. J. Infect. Dis. *23*:125–126, 1991.
166. Klass, P. E., Klein, J. O.: Therapy of bacterial sepsis, meningitis and otitis media in infants and children: 1992 poll of directors of programs in pediatric infectious diseases. Pediatr. Infect. Dis. J. *11*:702–705, 1992.
167. Kleiman, M. D., Weinberg, G. A., Reynolds, J. K., et al.: Meningitis with beta-lactam–resistant *Streptococcus pneumoniae*: The need for early repeat lumbar puncture. Pediatr. Infect. Dis. J. *12*:782–784, 1993.
168. Klein, J. O. (ed.): *Haemophilus influenzae* infections. *In* Report of the Committee on Infectious Diseases. 19th ed. Evanston, IL, American Academy of Pediatrics, 1982, pp. 105–107.
169. Klein, J. O. (ed.): Meningococcal Infections. *In* Report of the Committee on Infectious Diseases. 19th ed. Evanston, IL, American Academy of Pediatrics, 1982, pp. 139–141.
170. Klein, J. O., Feigin, R. D., and McCracken, G. H., Jr.: Report of the Task Force on Diagnosis and Management of Meningitis. Pediatrics *78*:S959–s982, 1986.
170a. Klugman, K. P., Dagan, R., and The Meropenem Meningitis Study Group: Randomized comparison of meropenem with cefotaxime for treatment of bacterial meningitis. Antimicrob. Agents Chemother. *39*:1140–1146, 1995.
171. Komorowski, R. N., Farmer, S. G., and Hause, L. L.: Cerebrospinal fluid lactic acid in diagnosis of meningitis. J. Clin. Microbiol. *8*:89–92, 1978.
172. LaForce, F. M., Brice, J. L., and Tornabene, T. G.: Diagnosis of bacterial meningitis by gas-liquid chromatography. II. Analysis of spinal fluid. J. Infect. Dis. *140*:453–464, 1979.
173. LaScolea, L. J., Jr., and Dryja, D.: Quantitation of bacteria in cerebrospinal fluid and blood of children with meningitis and its diagnostic significance. J. Clin. Microbiol. *19*:187–190, 1984.
174. Lebel, M. H., Freij, B. J., Syrogiannopoulos, G. A., et al.: Dexamethasone therapy for bacterial meningitis: Results of two double-blind, placebo-controlled trials. N. Engl. J. Med. *319*:964–971, 1988.
175. Lebel, M. H., Hoyt, M. J., and McCracken, G. H.: Comparative efficacy of ceftriaxone and cefuroxime for treatment of bacterial meningitis. J. Pediatr. *114*:1049–1054, 1989.
176. Lebel, M. H., and McCracken, G. H., Jr.: Aztreonam: Review of the clinical experience and potential uses in pediatrics. Pediatr. Infect. Dis. J. *7*:331–339, 1988.
177. Lebel, M. H., and McCracken, G. H., Jr.: Delayed cerebrospinal fluid sterilization and adverse outcome of bacterial meningitis in infants and children. Pediatrics *83*:161–167, 1989.
178. Leedom, J. M., Ivler, D., Mathies, A. W., et al.: The problem of sulfadiazine-resistant meningococci. Antimicrob. Agents Chemother. *6*:281–292, 1966.
179. Leggiadro, R. J., and Winkelstein, J. A.: Prevalence of complement deficiencies in children with systemic meningococcal disease. Pediatr. Infect. Dis. J. *6*:75–76, 1987.
180. Lepper, M. H., and Spies, H. W.: Nontuberculous bacterial infections of the nervous system. Gen. Pharmacol. *25*:83–93, 1962.
181. Lerman, S. J.: Systemic *Hemophilus influenzae* infection: A study of risk factors. Clin. Pediatr. *21*:360–364, 1982.
182. Liebman, E. P., Ronis, M. L., Loyrinic, J. H., et al.: Hearing improvement following meningitis deafness. Arch. Otolaryngol. *90*:470–473, 1969.
183. Lim, D., Gerurz, A., Lint, T. F., et al.: Absence of the sixth component of complement in a patient with repeated episodes of meningococcal meningitis. J. Pediatr. *89*:42–47, 1976.
184. Lin, T. Y., Chrane, D. F., Nelson, J. D., et al.: Seven days of ceftriaxone therapy is as effective as ten days' treatment for bacterial meningitis. J. A. M. A. *253*:3559–3563, 1985.
185. Lindsay, J.: Profound childhood deafness: Inner ear pathology. Assn. Otol. Rhinol. Laryngol. *82*(Suppl. 5):88–102, 1973.
186. Losonsky, G. A., Santosham, M., Sehgal, V. M., et al.: *Haemophilus influenzae* disease in the White Mountain Apaches: Molecular epidemiology of a high risk population. Pediatr. Infect. Dis. *3*:539–547, 1984.
187. Marks, W. A., Stutman, H. R., Marks, M. I., et al.: Cefuroxime versus ampicillin plus chloramphenicol in childhood bacterial meningitis: A multicenter randomized controlled trial. J. Pediatr. *109*:123–130, 1986.
188. Maxson, S., Lewno, M. J., and Schutze, G. E.: Clinical usefulness of cerebrospinal fluid bacterial antigen studies. J. Pediatr. *125*:235–238, 1994.
189. McCracken, G. J., Jr., and Lebel, M. H.: Dexamethasone therapy for bacterial meningitis in infants and children. Am. J. Dis. Child. *143*:287–289, 1989.
190. McCracken, G. H., Jr., and Sarff, L. D.: Current status and therapy of neonatal *E. coli* meningitis. Hosp. Pract. *9*:57–64, 1974.
191. McCracken, G. H., Sarff, L. D., Glode, M. P., et al.: Relation between *Escherichia coli* K1 capsular polysaccharide antigen and clinical outcome in neonatal meningitis. Lancet *2*:246–250, 1974.
192. McIntosh, D., Brown, J., Hanson, R., et al.: Torticollis and bacterial meningitis. Pediatr. Infect. Dis. J. *12*:160–161, 1993.
193. Melish, M. E., Nelson, A. J., Martin, T. E., et al.: Epidemic spread of *Hemophilus influenzae* type b disease in a day care center. Pediatr. Res. *10*:348, 1976.
194. Mertsola, J., Kennedy, W. A., Waagner, D., et al.: Endotoxin concentrations in cerebrospinal fluid correlate with clinical severity and neurologic outcome of *Haemophilus influenzae* type b meningitis. Am. J. Dis. Child. *145*:1099–1103, 1991.
195. Meurman, O. H., Irjala, K., Suonpaa, J., et al.: A new method for the identification of cerebrospinal fluid leakage. Acta Otolaryngol. *87*:366–369, 1979.
196. Michie, H. R., Manogue, K. R., Spriggs, D. R., et al.: Detection of circulation tumor necrosis factor after endotoxin administration. N. Engl. J. Med. *318*:1481–1486, 1988.
197. Modai, J., Vittecoq, D., Decazes, J. M., et al.: Penetration of ceftazidime into cerebrospinal fluid of patients with bacterial meningitis. Antimicrob. Agents Chemother. *24*:126–128, 1983.
198. Moore, P. S., Harrison, L. H., Telzak, E. E., et al.: Group A meningococcal carriage in travelers returning from Saudi Arabia. J. A. M. A. *260*:2686–2689, 1988.
199. Moore, P. S., Reeves, M. W., Schwartz, B., et al.: Intercontinental spread of an epidemic group A *Neisseria meningitidis* strain. Lancet *2*:260–263, 1989.
200. Moxon, E. R., Smith, A. L., Averill, D. R., et al.: *Hemophilus influenzae* meningitis in infant rats after intranasal inoculation. J. Infect. Dis. *129*:154–162, 1974.
201. Mullaney, D. T., and John, J. F.: Cefotaxime therapy: Evaluation of its effect of bacterial meningitis, CSF drug levels, and bactericidal activity. Arch. Intern. Med. *143*:1705–1708, 1983.
202. Muller, P. D., Donald, P. R., Burger, R. J., et al.: Detection of bacterial antigens in cerebrospinal fluid by a latex agglutination test in "septic unknown" meningitis and serogroup B meningococcal meningitis. South Afr. Med. J. *76*:214–215, 1989.
203. Mumford, R. J., deVasconelas, Z. J. S., Phillips, C. J., et al.: Eradication of carriage of *Neisseria meningitidis* in families: A study in Brazil. J. Infect. Dis. *129*:644–649, 1974.
204. Munoz, O., Benitez-Diaz, L., Martinez, M. C., et al.: Hearing loss after *Hemophilus influenzae* meningitis: Follow-up study with auditory brainstem potentials. Ann. Otol. Rhinol. Laryngol. *92*:272–275, 1983.
205. Murphy, T. V., Pastor, P., Medley, F., et al.: Decreased *Haemophilus* colonization in children vaccinated with *Haemophilus influenzae* type b conjugate vaccine. J. Pediatr. *122*:517–523, 1993.
206. Mustafa, M. M., Lebel, M. H., Ramilo, O., et al.: Correlation of interleukin 1β and cachectin concentrations in cerebrospinal fluid and outcome from bacterial meningitis. J. Pediatr. *115*:208–213, 1989.
207. Mustafa, M. M., Ramilo, O., Mertsola, J., et al.: Modulation of inflammation and cachectin activity in relation to treatment of experimental *Haemophilus influenzae* type b meningitis. J. Infect. Dis. *160*:818–825, 1989.
208. Mustafa, M. M., Ramilo, O., Saez-Llorens, X., et al.: Cerebrospinal fluid prostaglandins, interleukin 1β, and tumor necrosis factor in bacterial meningitis: Clinical and laboratory correlations in placebo and dexamethasone-treated patients. Am. J. Dis. Child. *144*:883–887, 1990.
209. Nadol, J. B., Jr.: Hearing loss as a sequela of meningitis. Laryngoscope *88*:739–755, 1978.
210. Nagata, M., Hara, T., Aoki, T., et al.: Inherited deficiency of ninth component of complement: An increased risk of meningococcal meningitis. J. Pediatr. *114*:260–264, 1989.

211. Naraqui, S., Kirkpatrick, G. P., and Kabins, S.: Relapsing pneumococcal meningitis: Isolation of an organism with decreased susceptibility to penicillin G. J. Pediatr. *85*:671–673, 1974.
212. Neches, W., and Platt, M.: Cerebrospinal fluid LDH in 287 children including 53 cases of meningitis of bacterial and non-bacterial etiology. Pediatrics *41*:1097–1103, 1968.
213. Nelson, K. E., Levin, S., Spies, H. W., et al.: Treatment of *Hemophilus influenzae* meningitis: A comparison of chloramphenicol and tetracycline. J. Infect. Dis. *125*:459–465, 1972.
214. Niemoller, U. M., and Tauber, M. G.: Brain edema and increased intracranial pressure in the pathophysiology of bacterial meningitis. Eur. J. Clin. Microbiol. Infect. Dis. *8*:109–117, 1989.
215. Odio, C. M., Faingezicht, I., and Paris, M.: The beneficial effects of early dexamethasone administration in infants and children with bacterial meningitis. N. Engl. J. Med. *324*:1515–1531, 1991.
216. Parke, J. C., Jr., Schneerson, R., and Robbins, J. B.: The attack rate, age, incidence, racial distribution and case fatality rate of *Hemophilus influenzae*, type b meningitis in Mecklenburg County, North Carolina. J. Pediatr. *81*:765–769, 1972.
217. Parkkinen, J., Korhonen, T. K., Pere, A., et al.: Binding sites in the rat brain for *Escherichia coli S. fimbriae* associated with neonatal meningitis. J. Clin. Invest. 81:860–865, 1988.
218. Peltola, H., Makela, P. H., Kayhty, H., et al.: Clinical efficacy of meningococcus group A capsular polysaccharide vaccine in children three months to five years of age. N. Engl. J. Med. *297*:686–691, 1977.
219. Peltola, H., Rod, T. O., Jonsdottir, K., et al.: Life-threatening *Haemophilus influenzae* infections in Scandinavia: A five-country analysis of the incidence and the main clinical and bacteriologic characteristics. Rev. Infect. Dis. *12*:708–715, 1990.
220. Peter, G., Weigart, M. B., Bissel, A. R., et al.: Meningococcal meningitis in familial deficiency of the fifth component of complement. Pediatrics *67*:882–886, 1981.
221. Pichichero, M. E., Hall, C. B., and Insel, R. A.: A mucosal antibody response following systemic *Haemophilus influenzae* type b infection in children. J. Clin. Invest. *67*:1482–1489, 1981.
222. Pickup, J. D., and Mathur, B. S.: *Haemophilus influenzae* meningitis treated with parenteral and intrathecal Penbritin. Postgrad. Med. J. *40*:204–207, 1964.
223. Pinner, R. W., Onyango, F., Perkins, B. A., et al.: Epidemic meningococcal disease in Nairobi, Kenya, 1989. J. Infect. Dis. *166*:359–364, 1992.
224. Pomeroy, S. L., Holmes, S. J., Dodge, P. R., et al.: A prospective evaluation of the neurologic sequelae of bacterial meningitis in children with special emphasis on late seizures. N. Engl. J. Med. *323*:1651–1657, 1990.
225. Powell, D. A., Nahata, M. C., Durrell, D. C., et al.: Interactions among chloramphenicol, phenytoin and phenobarbital in a pediatric patient. J. Pediatr. *98*:1001–1003, 1981.
226. Powell, K. R., and Mawhorter, S.: Outpatient treatment of serious infections in infants and children with ceftriaxone. J. Pediatr. *110*:889–901, 1987.
227. Powell, K. R., Sugarman, L. I., Eskenazi, A. I., et al.: Normalization of plasma arginine vasopressin concentrations when children with meningitis are given maintenance plus replacement fluid therapy. J. Pediatr. *117*:515–522, 1990.
228. Prober, C. G.: The role of steroids in the management of children with bacterial meningitis. Pediatrics *95*:29–31, 1995.
229. Quagliarello, V. J., Long, W. J., and Scheld, W. M.: Morphologic alterations of the blood brain barrier with experimental meningitis in the rat: Temporal sequence and role of encapsulation. J. Clin. Invest. *77*:1084–1095, 1986.
230. Ramilo, O., Mustafa, M. M., Porter J., et al.: Detection of interleukin-1 β but not tumor necrosis factor–alpha in cerebrospinal fluid of children with aseptic meningitis. Am. J. Dis. Child. *144*:349–352, 1990.
231. Rauch, A. M., O'Ryan, M., Van, R., et al.: Invasive disease due to multiply resistant *Streptococcus pneumoniae* in a Houston, Texas, day-care center. Am. J. Dis. Child. *144*:923–927, 1990.
232. Raziuddin, S., El-Awad, M. E., Mir, N. A.: Bacterial meningitis: T cell activation and immunoregulatory CD4+ T cell subset alteration. J. Allergy Clin. Immunol. *87*:1115–1120, 1991.
233. Ridgway, E. J., Allen, K. D., Neal, T. J., et al.: Penicillin-resistant pneumococcal meningitis. Lancet *339*:931, 1992.
234. Rodriguez, W. J., Khan, W. N., Gold, B., et al.: Ceftazidime in the treatment of meningitis in infants and children over one month of age. Am. J. Med. *79*(Suppl. 2A):52–55, 1985.
235. Rodriguez, W. J., Puig, J. R., Khan, W. N., et al.: Ceftazidime vs. standard therapy for pediatric meningitis: Therapeutic, pharmacologic and epidemiologic observations. Pediatr. Infect. Dis. *5*:408–415, 1986.
236. Roeses, R. J., and Campbell, J. C.: Recovery of auditory function following meningitis deafness. J. Speech Hear. Dis. *40*:405–411, 1975.
237. Rorke, L. B., and Pitts, F. W.: Purulent meningitis: The pathological basis of clinical manifestations. Clin. Pediatr. 2:64–71, 1963.
238. Ross, S., Rodriguez, W., Controni, G., et al.: Limulus lysate test for gram-negative bacterial meningitis: Bedside application. J. A. M. A. *233*:1366–1369, 1975.
239. Rowe, P. C., McLean, R. H., Wood, R. A., et al.: Association of homozygous C4B deficiency with bacterial meningitis. J. Infect. Dis. *160*:448–451, 1989.
240. Rutledge, J., Benjamin, D., Hood, L., et al.: Is the CSF lactate measurement useful in the management of children with suspected bacterial meningitis? J. Pediatr. *98*:20–24, 1981.
241. Salih, M. A., Ahmed, H. S., Karrar, Z. A., et al.: Features of a large epidemic of group A meningococcal meningitis in Khartoum, Sudan, in 1988. Scand. J. Infect. Dis. *22*:161–170, 1990.
242. Sanal, O., Loos, M., Ersoy, F., et al.: Complement component deficiencies and infection C_5, C_8, C_3. Eur. J. Pediatr. *151*:676–679, 1992.
243. Sankrithi, U. M., and Lipuma, J. J.: Clinically inapparent meningitis complicating periorbital cellulitis. Pediatr. Emerg. Care *7*:28–29, 1991.
244. Santhosham, M., Reid, R., and Ambrosino, D. M.: Prevention of *Haemophilus influenzae* type b infections in high-risk infants treated with bacterial polysaccharide immune globulin. N. Engl. J. Med. *317*:923–929, 1987.
245. Schaad, U. B., Lips, U., Gnehm, H. E., et al.: Dexamethasone therapy for bacterial meningitis in children. Lancet *342*:457–461, 1993.
246. Schaad, U. B., Suter, S., and Gianella-Borradori, A., et al.: A comparison of ceftriaxone and cefuroxime for the treatment of bacterial meningitis in children. N. Engl. J. Med. *322*:141–147, 1990.
247. Schaad, U. B., Wedgwood-Krucko, J., and Tschaeppeler, H.: Reversible ceftriaxone-associated biliary pseudolithiasis in children. Lancet *2*:1411–1413, 1988.
248. Scheifele, D., Daum, R., Syriopoulou, V., et al.: A primate model of *Hemophilus influenzae*, type b meningitis. 16th Interscience Conference on Antimicrobial Agents and Chemotherapy, Chicago. October 27–29, 1976. Abstract 238.
249. Scheifele, D. W., Ward, J. I., and Siber, G. R.: Advantage of latex agglutination over countercurrent immunoelectrophoresis in the detection of *Haemophilus influenzae* type b antigen in serum. Pediatrics *68*:888–891, 1981.
250. Scheld, W. M.: Pathophysiological correlates in bacterial meningitis. J. Infect. *3*(Suppl. 1):5–18, 1981.
251. Scheld, W. M.: Pathogenesis and pathophysiology of pneumococcal meningitis. *In* Sande, M. A., Smith, A. L., and Root, R. K. (eds.): Bacterial Meningitis. New York, Churchill Livingstone, 1985, pp. 37–69.
252. Schlech, W. F., Ward, J. L., Band, J. D., et al.: Bacterial meningitis in the United States, 1978–1981: The National Bacterial Meningitis Surveillance Study. J. A. M. A. *253*:1749–1954, 1985.
253. Schoendorf, K. C., Adams, W. G., Kiely, J. L., et al.: National trends in *Haemophilus influenzae* meningitis mortality and hospitalization among children, 1980 through 1991. Pediatrics *93*:663–668, 1994.
254. Schwartz, B., Al-Tobaiqi, A., Al-Ruwais, A., et al.: Comparative efficacy of ceftriaxone and rifampin in eradicating pharyngeal carriage of group A *Neisseria meningitidis*. Lancet *1*:1239–1242, 1988.
255. Schwartz, J. F.: Ataxia in bacterial meningitis. Neurology *22*:1071–1074, 1972.
256. Sell, S. H.: Long-term sequelae of bacterial meningitis in children. Pediatr. Infect. Dis. *2*:90–93, 1983.
257. Sell, S. H. W., Merrill, R. E., Doyne, E. D., et al.: Long-term sequelae of *Hemophilus influenzae* meningitis. Pediatrics *49*:206–211, 1972.
258. Sell, S. H. W., Webb, W. W., Pate, J. E., et al.: Psychological sequelae to bacterial meningitis: Two controlled studies. Pediatrics *49*:212–217, 1972.
259. Shackelford, P. G., Bobinski, J. E., Feigin, R. D., et al.: Therapy of *Haemophilus influenzae* meningitis reconsidered. N. Engl. J. Med. *287*:634–638, 1972.
260. Shackelford, P. G., Campbell, J., and Feigin, R. D.: Countercurrent immunoelectrophoresis in the evaluation of childhood infection. J. Pediatr. *85*:478–481, 1974.
261. Shapiro, E. D.: Prophylaxis for contacts of patients with meningococcal or *Haemophilus influenzae* type b disease. Pediatr. Infect. Dis. *1*:132–138, 1982.
262. Shapiro, E. D., and Ward, E. R.: Efficacy of rifampin in eliminating pharyngeal carriage of *Haemophilus influenzae* type b. Pediatrics *66*:5–8, 1980.
263. Shurin, S. B., and Anderson, P.: Anemia associated with *H. influenzae* b (Hib) septicemia is due to immune *Hemophilus* of RBC coated with soluble bacterial antigens. Pediatr. Res. *17*:932, 1983.
264. Sills, R. H., Caserta, M. T., and Landaw, S. A.: Decreased erythrocyte deformability in the anemia of bacterial meningitis. J. Pediatr. *101*:395–398, 1982.
265. Simberkoff, M. D., Moldovec, N. H., and Rahal, J. J., Jr.: Absence of detectable bactericidal and opsonic activities in normal and infected human cerebrospinal fluids: A regional host defense deficiency. J. Lab. Clin. Med. *95*:362–372, 1980.
266. Singer, J. I., and Berger, O. G.: Simultaneous occult pneumococcal bacteremia in identical twins. J. Pediatr. *98*:250–251, 1981.
267. Singhi, S. C., Singhi, P. D., Srinivas, B., et al.: Fluid restriction does not improve the outcome of acute meningitis. Pediatr. Infect. Dis. J. *14*:495–503, 1995.
268. Sloas, M. M., Barrett, F. F., Chesney, P. J., et al.: Cephalosporin treatment failure in penicillin- and cephalosporin-resistant *Streptococcus pneumoniae* meningitis. Pediatr. Infect. Dis. J. *11*:662–666, 1992.
269. Smith, A. L.: Neurologic sequelae of meningitis. N. Engl. J. Med. *319*:1012–1014, 1988.
270. Smith, D. H., Ingram, D. L., Smith, A. L., et al.: Bacterial meningitis. Pediatrics *52*:586–600, 1973.
271. Smith, J. F., and Landing, B. H.: Mechanisms of brain damage in *H. influenzae* meningitis. J. Neuropathol. Exp. Neurol. *19*:248–265, 1960.

272. Snedeker, J. D., Kaplan, S. L., Dodge, P. R., et al.: Subdural effusion and its relationship with neurologic sequelae of bacterial meningitis in infancy: A prospective study. Pediatrics *86*:163–170, 1990.
273. Snyder, R. D., Stovring, J., Cushing, A. H., et al.: Cerebral infarction in childhood bacterial meningitis. J. Neurol. Neurosurg. Psych. *44*:581–585, 1981.
274. Soderstrom, C., Sjoholm, A. G., Svensson, R., et al.: Another Swedish family with complete properdin deficiency: Association with fulminant meningococcal disease in one male family member. Scand. J. Infect. Dis. *21*:259–265, 1989.
275. Spanjaard, L., Bol, P., de Marie, S., et al.: Association of meningococcal serotypes with the course of disease: Serotypes 2a and 2b in the Netherlands, 1959–1981. J. Infect. Dis. *155*:277–282, 1987.
276. Speer, C. P., Rethwilm, M., and Gahr, M.: Elastase-alpha 1-proteinase inhibitor: An early indicator of septicemia and bacterial meningitis in children. J. Pediatr. *111*:667–671, 1987.
277. Spika, J. S., Facklam, R. R., Plikaytis, B. D., et al. (The Pneumococcal Surveillance Working Group): Antimicrobial resistance of *Streptococcus pneumoniae* in the United States, 1979–1987. J. Infect. Dis. *163*:1273–1278, 1991.
278. Sproles, E. T., III, Azerrad, J., Williamson, C., et al.: Meningitis due to *Hemophilus influenzae*: Long-term sequelae. J. Pediatr. *75*:782–788, 1969.
279. Steele, R. W., and Bradsher, R. W.: Comparison of ceftriaxone with standard therapy for bacterial meningitis. J. Pediatr. *103*:138–141, 1983.
280. Steele, R. W., McConnell, J. R., Jacobs, R. F., et al.: Recurrent bacterial meningitis: Coronal thin-section cranial computed tomography to delineate anatomic defects. Pediatrics *76*:950–953, 1985.
281. Stephen, D. S., and McGee, Z. A.: Attachment of *Neisseria meningitidis* to human mucosal surfaces: Influence of pili and type of receptor cell. J. Infect. Dis. *143*:525–532, 1981.
282. Stewardson-Krieger, S., and Naidu, S.: Simultaneous recovery of β-lactamase–negative and β-lactamase–positive *Haemophilus influenzae* type b from cerebrospinal fluid of a neonate. Pediatrics *68*:253–254, 1981.
283. Tan, T. Q., Mason, E. O., Jr., and Kaplan, S. L.: Penicillin-resistant systemic pneumococcal infections in children: A retrospective case-control study. Pediatrics *92*:761–767, 1993.
284. Tan, T. Q., Mason, E. O., Jr., and Kaplan, S. L.: Systemic infections due to *Streptococcus pneumoniae* relatively resistant to penicillin in a children's hospital: Clinical management and outcome. Pediatrics *90*:928–933, 1992.
285. Tan, T. Q., Schutze, G. E., Mason, E. O., Jr., et al.: Antibiotic therapy and acute outcome of meningitis due to *Streptococcus pneumoniae* considered intermediately susceptible to broad-spectrum cephalosporins. Antimicrob. Agents Chemother. *38*:918–923, 1994.
286. Tauber, M. G., Shibl, A. M., Hackbarth, C. J., et al.: Antibiotic therapy endotoxin concentration in cerebrospinal fluid and brain edema in experimental *Escherichia coli* meningitis in rabbits. J. Infect. Dis. *156*:456–462, 1987.
287. Tauney, A. E., Galvao, P. A., DeMorais, J. S., et al.: Disease prevention by meningococcal serogroup C polysaccharide vaccine in pre-school children—São Paulo, Brazil. Unpublished.
288. Taylor, H. G., Mills, E. L., Ciampi, A., et al.: The sequelae of *Haemophilus influenzae* meningitis in school-age children. N. Engl. J. Med. *323*:1657–1663, 1990.
289. Teele, D. W., Dashefsky, B., Rakusan, T., et al.: Meningitis after lumbar puncture in children with bacteremia. N. Engl. J. Med. *305*:1079–1081, 1981.
290. Tejani, A., Dobias, B., Nangia, B. S., et al.: Intra-family spread of *Haemophilus influenzae* type b infection. Am. J. Dis. Child. *131*:778–781, 1977.
291. Tejani, A., Dobias, B., and Sambursky, J.: Long-term prognosis after *H. influenzae* meningitis: Prospective evaluation. Dev. Med. Child. Neurol. *24*:338–343, 1982.
292. Tejani, A., Mahadevan, R., and Dobias, B.: Occurrence of HLA types in *H. influenzae* type b disease. Tissue Antigens *17*:205–211, 1981.
293. Tracey, K. J., Vlassara, J., and Cerami, A.: Cachectin/tumor necrosis factor. Lancet *1*:1122–1125, 1989.
294. Trujillo, H., Harry, N., Arango, A., et al.: Aztreonam in the treatment of aerobic, gram-negative bacillary infections in pediatric patients. Chemotherapy *35*(Suppl.):25–30, 1989.
295. Turk, D. C.: Distribution of *Hemophilus influenzae* in healthy human communities. *In* Turk, D. C., and May, J. R. (eds.): *Hemophilus influenzae*: Its Clinical Importance. London, English University Press, 1965.
296. Tyson, J. E., Gilmartin, R. C., Jr., Friedman, B. I., et al.: ^{131}I-HSA cisternography in children with meningitis. *In* Harbert, J. C. (ed.): Cisternography and Hydrocephalus. Springfield, IL, Charles C Thomas, 1972, pp. 413–432.
297. U.S. Department of Commerce, Bureau of the Census: Mortality Statistics, 1935. Washington, D.C., Government Printing Office, 1937.
298. U.S. Department of Health, Education and Welfare, Public Health Service: Vital Statistics of the United States, 1968. Vol. II. Mortality. Washington, D.C., Government Printing Office, 1970.
299. van Alphen, L., Spanjaard, L., van der Ende, A., et al.: Predicted disappearance of *Haemophilus influenzae* type b meningitis in Netherlands. Lancet *344*:195, 1994.
300. Veeder, M. H., Folds, J. D., Yount, W. J., et al.: Recurrent bacterial meningitis associated with C8 and IgA deficiency. J. Infect. Dis. *144*:399–402, 1981.
301. Vienny, H., Despland, P. A., Lutschg, J., et al.: Early diagnosis and evolution of deafness in childhood bacterial meningitis: A study using brainstem auditory evoked potentials. Pediatrics *73*:579–586, 1984.
302. Waage, A., Halstensen, A., and Espevik, T.: Association between tumour necrosis factor in serum and fatal outcome in patients with meningococcal disease. Lancet *1*:355–357, 1987.
303. Wahden, M. H., Rizk, F., and El-Akkad, A. M.: A controlled field trial of a serogroup A meningococcal polysaccharide vaccine. Bull. W. H. O. *48*:667–673, 1973.
304. Wald, E. R., Kaplan, S. L., Mason, E. O., Jr., et al.: Dexamethasone therapy for children with bacterial meningitis. Pediatrics *95*:21–28, 1995.
305. Waldvogel, F. A.: Pathophysiological mechanisms in psycogenic infection: Two examples—pleural empyema and acute bacterial meningitis. *In* Majno, G., Cotran, R. S., and Kaufman, N. (eds.): Current Topics in Inflammation and Infection. Baltimore and London, Williams & Wilkins, 1982, pp. 115–122.
306. Waler, J. A., and Rathore, M. H.: Outpatient management of pediatric bacterial meningitis. Pediatr. Infect. Dis. J. *14*:89–92, 1995.
307. Ward, J. I., Fraser, D. W., Baraff, L. J., et al.: *Hemophilus influenzae* meningitis: A national study of secondary spread in household contacts. N. Engl. J. Med. *19*:122–126, 1979.
308. Ward, J. I., Gorman, C., Philips, C., et. al.: *Haemophilus influenzae* type b disease in a day care center. J. Pediatr. *92*:713–717, 1978.
309. Ward, J. I., Lum, M. K. W., Hall, D. B., et al.: Invasive *Haemophilus influenzae* type b disease in Alaska: Background epidemiology for a vaccine efficacy trial. J. Infect. Dis. *153*:17–26, 1986.
310. Ward, J. I., Siber, G. I., Scheifele, D. W., et al.: Rapid diagnosis of *Hemophilus influenzae* type b infections by latex particle agglutination and counterimmunoelectrophoresis. J. Pediatr. *93*:37–42, 1978.
311. Weidmer, C. E., Dunkel, T. B., Pettyjohn, F. S., et al.: Effectiveness of rifampin in eradicating the meningococcal carrier state in a relatively closed population: Emergence of resistant strains. J. Infect. Dis. *24*:172–178, 1971.
312. Weil, M. L.: Infections of the nervous system. *In* Menkes, J. H. (ed.): Textbook of Child Neurology. Philadelphia, Lea & Febiger, 1980, pp. 276–304.
313. Whittle, H. C., and Greenwood, B. M.: Meningococcal meningitis in the northern savanna of Africa. Trop. Doct. *6*:99–104, 1976.
314. Williams, D. N., Laughlin, L. W., and Lee, Y. H.: Minocycline: Possible vestibular side-effects. Lancet *2*:744–746, 1974.
315. Wispelway, B., Long, J. M., Castracene, J. M., et al.: Cerebrospinal fluid interleukin-1 activity following intracisternal inoculation of *Haemophilus influenzae* lipooligosaccharide. Presented at the 28th Interscience Conference on Antimicrobial Agents and Chemotherapy. Los Angeles, October 26, 1988.
316. Wolff, M., Chavanet, P., Kazmierczak, A., et al.: Diffusion of cefpirome into the cerebrospinal fluid of patients with purulent meningitis. J. Antimicrob. Chemother. *29A*:59–62, 1992.
317. Word, B. M., and Klein, J. O.: Current therapy of bacterial sepsis and meningitis in infants and children: A poll of directors of programs in pediatric infectious diseases. Pediatr. Infect. Dis. J. *7*:267–270, 1988.
318. Yogev, R., Melick, C., and Kabat, K.: Nasopharyngeal colonization with *Haemophilus influenzae* type b: Attempted eradication by cefaclor or rifampin. Pediatrics *67*:430–433, 1981.
319. Yolken, R. H., and Hughes, W. T.: Rapid diagnosis of infections caused by β-lactamase–producing bacteria by means of an enzyme radioisotopic assay. J. Pediatr. *97*:715–720, 1980.
320. Young, L. M., Haddow, J. E., and Klein, J. O.: Relapse following ampicillin treatment of acute *Haemophilus influenzae* meningitis. Pediatrics *41*:516–518, 1968.
321. Zollinger, W. D., Mandrell, R. E., Guffiss, J. M., et al.: Complex of meningococcal group B polysaccharide and type 2 outer membrane protein immunogenic in man. J. Clin. Invest. *63*:836–848, 1979.
322. Zwahlen, A., Nydegger, U. E., Vaudaux, P., et al.: Complement-mediated opsonic activity in normal and infected human cerebrospinal fluid: Early response during bacterial meningitis. J. Infect. Dis. *145*:635–646, 1982.

39

PARAMENINGEAL INFECTIONS

Scott L. Pomeroy, Mary E. Sutton, and Philip R. Dodge

Abscess formation may occur in the parenchyma of the central nervous system or in the epidural or subdural spaces, altering neurologic function by direct destruction of nervous tissue, by infarction after inflammatory occlusion of veins and arteries, or by compression due to mass effect.

Although brain abscess, subdural empyema, cranial epidural abscess, and spinal epidural infections are discussed as separate entities, more than one condition may coexist in a patient.

BRAIN ABSCESS

Brain abscess is uncommon in children. On the basis of the experience at St. Louis Children's Hospital, a physician can expect to see 40 or more cases of bacterial meningitis for each case of brain abscess (Table 39–1). In children, as in adults, brain abscess hardly ever is secondary to bacterial meningitis, although an abscess may give rise to meningitis as a consequence of rupture into the ventricle or rarely into the subarachnoid space. In infants, especially in neonates, it often is uncertain which came first, and it seems probable that it could occur either way. In this very young group, the abscess may be enormous before the lesion is recognized clinically.[26]

Sources of Infection, Pathogenesis, and Pathology

Organisms invade the parenchyma of the brain usually as a consequence of a contiguous infection of nonneural tissues or as the result of hematogenous spread from a remote site. Initially, a rather diffuse inflammatory response in the brain occurs, polymorphonuclear leukocytes predominating. Over a period of many days to weeks, necrosis and liquefaction occur in the center of the lesion. Reactive astroglia, fibroblasts, and macrophages surround this nidus of tissue destruction. Both mononuclear and polymorphonuclear leukocytes may be seen scattered throughout this zone. The resulting capsule may, in chronic abscesses, be several millimeters to centimeters in thickness. Especially in the early stages of the process, there may be widespread cerebral edema of the white matter around the abscess cavity. Figure 39–1 shows the gross appearance of a well-defined abscess of hematogenous origin; in Figures 39–2, 39–3, and 39–4, various microscopic features are illustrated. Britt and Enzmann[6] reported a correlation between the histopathologic stages of abscess formation and clinical and computed tomographic (CT) findings in both experimental animals and humans.

Whenever symptoms and signs of intracranial disease develop in a patient with infection of the middle ear; mastoids; paranasal sinuses; or soft tissues of the face, orbit, or scalp, brain abscess should be considered in the differential diagnosis. The infection most often is subacute or chronic and spreads intracranially by infected veins or, less commonly, by osteomyelitis. Abscess also may complicate comminuted fractures of the skull and develop after intracranial surgery, including the insertion of shunts to divert cerebrospinal fluid (CSF) from a lateral ventricle to another compartment of the body (e.g., right atrium, peritoneal cavity). In infants and young children, a sharp object may penetrate the skull, leaving minimal external evidence of trauma. This especially is so with orbital trauma because the posterior wall of the orbit is so thin that a pencil point, as well as a sharp stick, has been incriminated as the mode for introducing the infective agent in frontal lobe abscess[2, 14] and even rarely in cerebellar abscess.[1] Congenital lesions, including dermal sinuses, usually over the posterior fossa, and various forms of ruptured anterior (nasal) and posterior encephaloceles may provide direct access for microorganisms to brain tissue.

Patients with congenital cyanotic heart disease in whom venous blood is shunted into the systemic circulation, bypassing the lungs, are prone to develop brain abscess. Curiously, this rarely occurs before the age of 2 years, and the abscess or abscesses usually are in areas of brain perfused by the middle cerebral arteries. Evidence of associated endocarditis is rare in these cases, although acute bacterial endocarditis may be complicated by septic infarction of brain and abscess formation.[25] Peripheral arteriovenous shunts, lung abscess, pulmonary thrombophlebitis, and collections of purulent material elsewhere in the body may provide an infective source for a cerebral abscess. Patients with either congen-

TABLE 39–1. Number of Patients with Bacterial Meningitis, Subdural Empyema, and Brain Abscess (St. Louis Children's Hospital)

	1974	1975	1976	1977	Total
Bacterial meningitis	36	25	47	14	122
Subdural empyema	0	0	0	1	1
Brain abscess	0	0	2	1	3
Epidural abscess	0	0	0	0	0

The 1994 distribution of intracranial suppurative disease essentially remains unchanged.

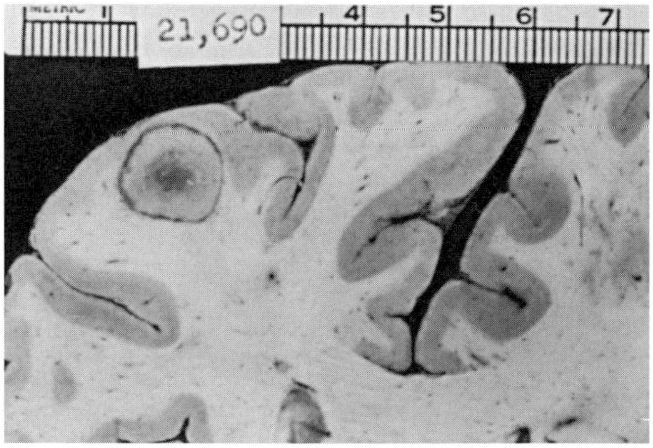

FIGURE 39–1. *Circumscribed cerebral abscess of hematogenous origin.*

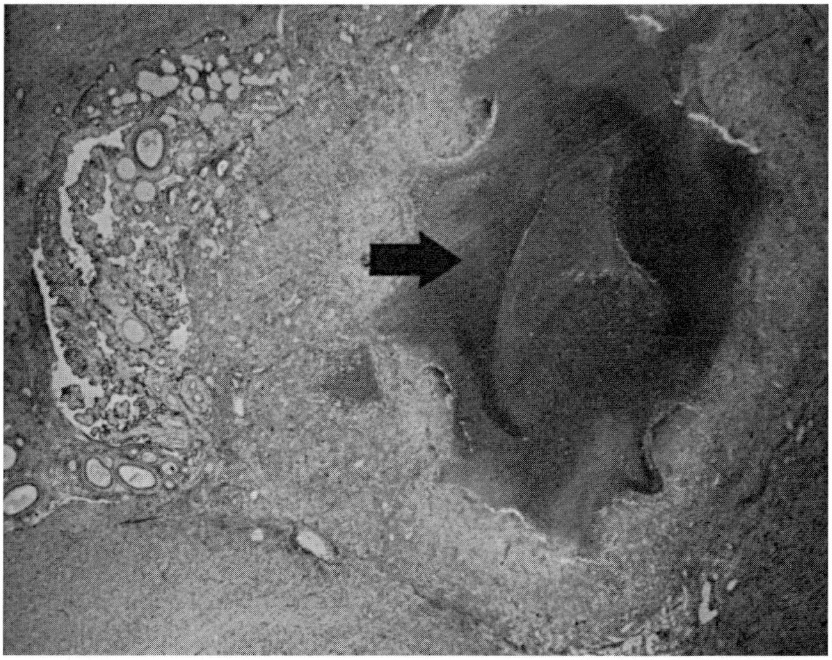

FIGURE 39–2. *Area of necrosis and liquefaction in a cerebral abscess (arrow).*

ital or acquired immune suppression also are at increased risk for brain abscess. Esophageal dilation has been associated with brain abscess, but this must be a rare entity in which the pathogenesis is unknown.[22] In some cases, no source can be found.

A wide range of microorganisms can be recovered from brain abscesses, including most bacteria and certain fungi and parasites. It is imperative that one considers this fact when the pus is subjected to laboratory investigation. Smears of the sample should be examined microscopically after Gram staining and after staining for acid-fast bacilli and fungi. Cultures should be incubated under appropriate conditions for aerobic and anaerobic bacteria, for mycobacteria, and for fungi. Unless this is appreciated, it may be concluded inappropriately that the pus is sterile. Sterile pus has been reported in about 25 per cent of abscesses, but the techniques used in attempting recovery of an agent rarely were detailed enough to afford reasonable assurance that no viable microorganisms were present. More than one organism—in fact, several—may be recovered from an abscess, especially in patients in whom there is direct access to the intracranial cavity from a contiguous extracerebral infection.

Among the aerobic species frequently seen are strains of streptococci, staphylococci, *Escherichia coli, Proteus, Nocardia,* and *Haemophilus influenzae*. Anaerobic bacteria, including various species of streptococci and *Bacteroides*, have been cul-

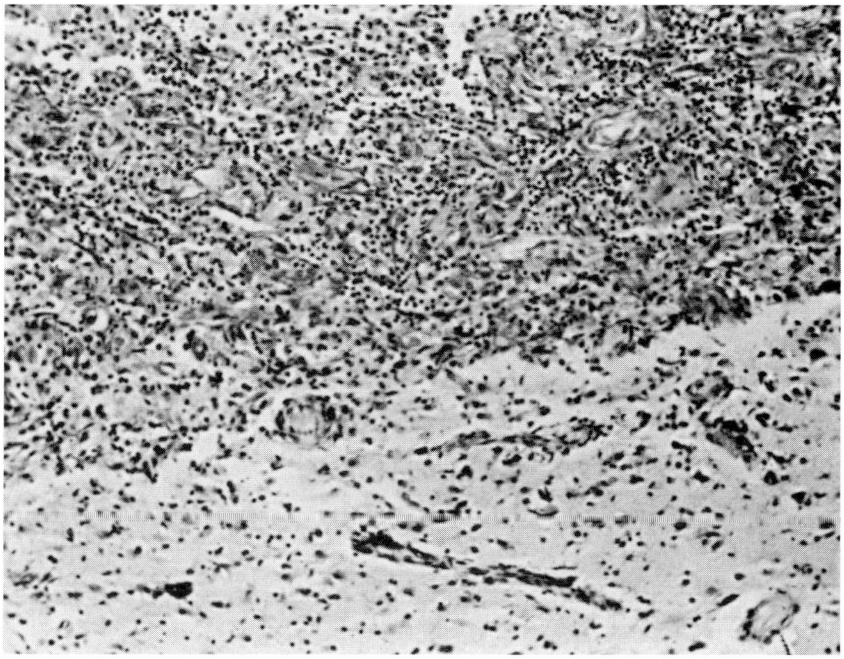

FIGURE 39–3. *Astroglia and fibroblasts forming the capsule of a cerebral abscess.*

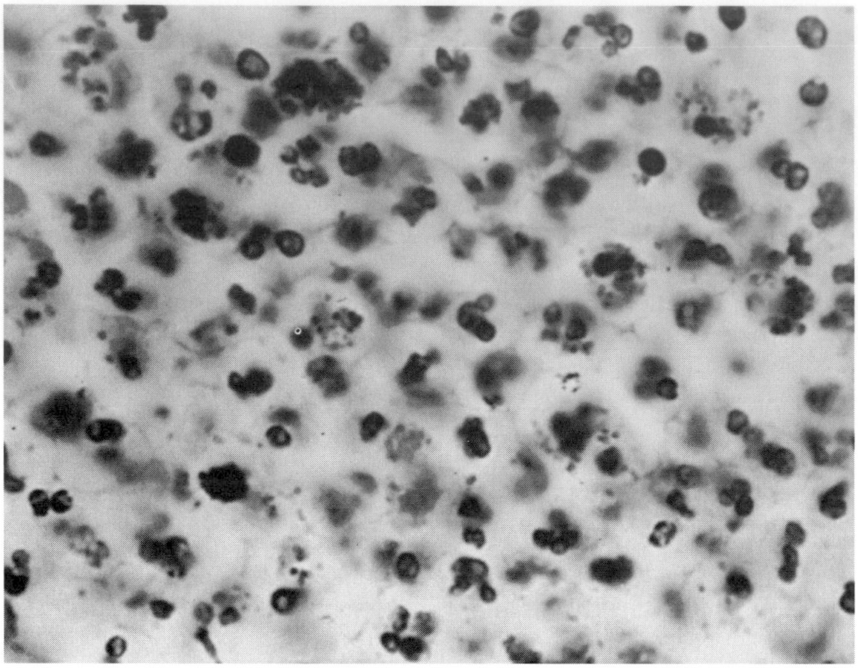

FIGURE 39–4. *Mononuclear and polymorphonuclear leukocytes in the center of a cerebral abscess.*

tured most commonly. *Haemophilus aphrophilus*, which thrives in an environment rich in carbon dioxide, has been recovered rarely from brain abscesses in children. Pneumococci have been cultured infrequently in recent years, which contrasts with past years. *Salmonella* organisms may be recovered.[18, 20] Gram-negative organisms, such as *Proteus* and *Citrobacter*[26] but not *E. coli*, are recovered commonly from abscesses in neonates. Offending fungi include *Cladosporium trichoides* and species of *Candida* and *Aspergillus*, but these are uncommon, as are amebic abscesses, at least in the United States. However, opportunistic infections have become increasingly important with induced immunosuppression and with the advent of AIDS. Fungal abscesses, in particular, may occur in immunosuppressed patients, although abscesses due to many other organisms, including *Toxoplasma gondii*, are becoming more common as well.[12, 24]

Clinical Manifestations

The clinical course in patients with brain abscess is protean. During the initial stages of disease, there may be fever, generalized malaise, vomiting, and headache, which often is localized to the region of the infection. In infants and young children, the presence of headache is difficult to document, although in the former the anterior fontanelle may bulge, which reflects increased intracranial pressure. Focal neurologic signs depend upon the site of the lesion or lesions and may be prominent or inconspicuous and either sudden or slow in their development. Thus, for example, a patient with a frontal abscess may exhibit few symptoms and signs except for raised intracranial pressure for weeks or months, whereas abscesses involving regions of the central nervous system concerned with motor, sensory, language, or visual functions usually will cause deficits relatively early in the course of the disease.

Leukocytosis and an elevated sedimentation rate may or may not be present, and recovery of a microorganism from the blood would be exceptional except when septicemia related to an acute endocarditis is present. The CSF characteristically is sterile, although inflammatory cells (a few to 400 polymorphonuclear cells and lymphocytes) and a modest elevation in protein with a normal concentration of glucose often can be found. The CSF pressure usually is elevated. Because of this, caution must be exercised lest a disturbance in intracranial dynamics precipitate herniation of cerebral tissue at either the tentorium or foramen magnum, a complication occurring all too frequently, even in the absence of lumbar puncture. Whenever brain abscess is a serious diagnostic consideration, especially in the presence of signs of increased intracranial pressure, a CT or other scan should be obtained before performing a lumbar puncture. If evidence of a probable abscess is demonstrated by imaging, lumbar puncture should be avoided.

Chronic abscesses are accompanied less frequently by systemic symptoms and laboratory evidence of infection. Rather, they produce symptoms and signs of an intracranial mass lesion and may be confused with neoplastic disease. An exception exists when rupture of the abscess into the ventricular system evokes a catastrophic complication, which is discussed later.

FRONTAL LOBE ABSCESS. In infants and children, infection of facial tissues or ethmoidal sinuses, often with orbital cellulitis, leads most frequently to intracranial infection by way of veins that drain into the cavernous sinus, which may itself become infected and thrombosed.[30] Amputation of a nasal meningoencephalocele leading to a cerebrospinal rhinorrhea predisposes to intracranial spread of infection, including abscess. Apical dental abscesses in older children are a potential source.[21] In neonates, abscesses frequently are multiple and involve the frontal lobes most commonly, although the source of the infection leading to abscess formation frequently is obscure.[26]

In older children, papilledema frequently is seen, and disturbed behavior of the child may lead to the incorrect diagnosis of a primary psychiatric disorder. Forced grasping and sucking may be prominent, and later a hemiparesis evolves. Because frontal lobe lesions remain relatively silent, rather massive abscess cavities can develop before focal neurologic signs appear. Frequently, depressed consciousness and signs of temporal lobe herniation, often with rupture into the lateral ventricle, preclude effective treatment before death.

TEMPORAL LOBE ABSCESS. Most temporal lobe abscesses are of otogenic origin. Developing as they do because of mastoiditis and phlebitis, associated infection within the epidural and subdural space is common, and lateral sinus and cortical vein thromboses also occur. Although it has been reported that the abscess may develop on the side opposite to the ear disease, we have not observed this. Nonfluent or fluent dysphasia can be witnessed when the dominant hemisphere is involved, and a contralateral upper quadrant field defect or complete homonymous hemianopsia may be demonstrated. Extension anteriorly can interfere with motor function, affecting the face and arm most conspicuously. Herniation of the mesial temporal lobe through the incisura of the tentorium usually produces an ipsilateral third nerve palsy and upper brain stem dysfunction. Prognosis is poor when the diagnosis is delayed until this stage.

PARIETAL LOBE ABSCESS. Usually of hematogenous origin, a parietal lobe abscess often is relatively asymptomatic with regard to focal neurologic features, until it encroaches upon the sensorimotor cortex. Extension posteriorly and inferiorly may cause an inferior quadrant field defect and homonymous hemianopsia or dysphasia when the dominant hemisphere is involved. Dyspraxia and spatial neglect contralaterally suggest dysfunction of the nondominant hemisphere.

CEREBELLAR ABSCESS. As with temporal lobe abscesses, cerebellar abscesses usually are of otogenic origin. The same pathogenic factors prevail as in temporal lobe abscesses, but the infection simply extends below the tentorium. On occasion, an infection of the soft tissues of the neck, such as a carbuncle, leads to development of a cerebellar abscess.

Most cerebellar abscesses develop in the hemispheres so that the neurologic syndrome is lateralized, with ataxia and tremor being ipsilateral to the lesion. Dizziness and nystagmus (most prominent on gaze to the side of the lesion) may be discerned if the lesion extends close to the midline, in which case ataxia of gait also is to be expected. Skew deviation of the eyes and abducens nerve palsy may be seen. Vomiting is prominent and papilledema is present in about half the cases; these findings relate primarily to increased intracranial pressure from the mass itself or from swelling of surrounding uninfected tissue, either of which may impair circulation of CSF. Sudden death results from apnea associated with herniation of cerebellar tissue through the foramen magnum. Upward herniation through the incisura of the tentorium can produce symptoms and signs similar to those observed in downward herniation from supratentorial lesions.

BRAIN STEM ABSCESS. Brain stem abscesses are very rare and infrequently diagnosed during life. Otogenic or hematogenous sources have been reported. Most often, the lesion is confused clinically with a primary glioma because of multiple cranial nerve palsies and signs of involvement of ascending and descending tracts.

Rupture of Brain Abscess into the Ventricular System

Rupture of an abscess into the ventricle with consequent ventricular empyema is a dreaded complication because the mortality rate exceeds 50 per cent, and residual neurologic deficits, including hydrocephalus, are the rule in those who survive. Frequently, rupture occurs before the diagnosis of abscess has been established and surgical removal can be accomplished. A sudden worsening in the patient's clinical state heralds this event. High fever, shock, meningismus, and altered consciousness are prominent among the clinical signs. Whereas a modest pleocytosis and elevated protein concentration in CSF may have been noted earlier, the findings of 50,000 to 100,000 polymorphonuclear leukocytes and markedly reduced sugar concentration in the CSF are usual. Organisms may be demonstrated on smear of the CSF and cultured from the fluid. In other words, the patient has, in fact, developed purulent meningitis, and treatment for this must include high doses of antibiotics as well as surgery (see Treatment). The concurrence of abscess and meningitis in the past has led to the assumption that brain abscess can be a complication of meningitis, but this is rarely, if ever, the case, although meningitis may develop during the incipient stages of abscess formation after intracranial invasion of organisms from a contiguous extracranial source. In such circumstances, it may appear that the abscess is consequent upon the leptomeningitis. Given a potential source of infection in the ear or paranasal sinuses, the clinician must be wary and appreciate the possibility of this sequence of events. Abscess has been reported to complicate *Citrobacter* meningitis in premature infants, but careful pathologic study has demonstrated vasculitis and liquefaction necrosis of the white matter without capsule formation.[11]

Diagnosis

Magnetic resonance imaging (MRI) currently is the diagnostic procedure of choice for the diagnosis and localization of cerebral abscesses, although CT scanning is an excellent alternative if MRI is not available. Administration of contrast material intravenously is advised because the abscess otherwise may be missed.[17, 28] Figure 39–5 illustrates the appearance on CT scan of a left frontal cerebral abscess in a neonate. The presence of gas within the abscess cavity on MRI/CT scanning should suggest communication of the abscess with air outside the skull, although gas-forming bacteria in the abscess cavity may be responsible on rare occasions.[32] Abnormalities on electroencephalography may be localized and of help in excluding a more generalized, bilateral, intracranial disease, such as encephalitis. Unilateral slow waves (delta, 1–3/sec) characterize the usual electroencephalography findings in cerebral abscesses.

Once the diagnosis of brain abscess has been established, a careful search should be made for a source of infection serving as a site of origin for either hematogenous spread or direct inoculation of organisms into the central nervous system. In addition to data obtained from the history and physical examination, the MRI/CT evaluation should be extended to include the mastoids and paranasal sinuses. An echocardiogram should be obtained to assess for concurrent endocarditis. Other testing should be guided by the history and findings on physical examination.

Treatment

Surgery remains the definitive treatment for cerebral abscess, but controversy continues as to whether excision of the abscess is preferable to single or multiple aspirations of the cavity. Experience indicates that aspiration of abscess contents for diagnostic or therapeutic purposes can be accomplished through precise CT scan–guided stereotactic needle placement. After aspiration alone, a cure can be achieved in many cases by prolonged therapy with antibiotics while monitoring the size of the abscess with serial CT scans or in

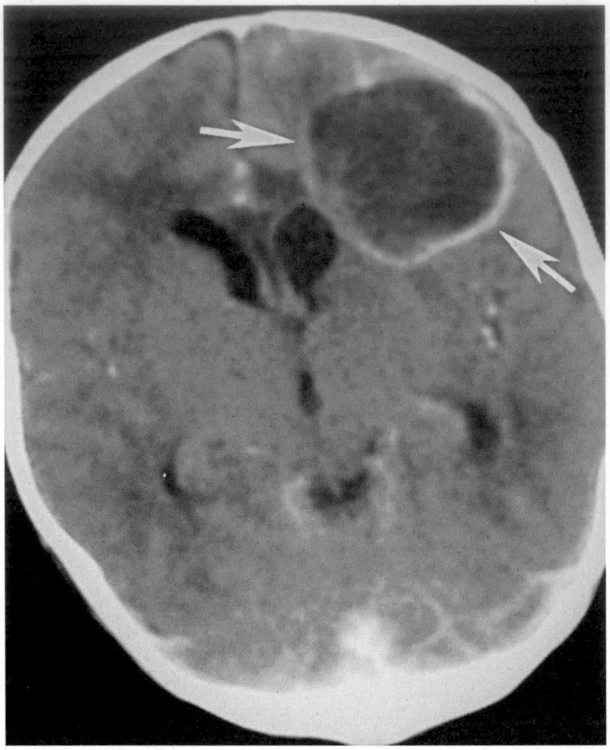

FIGURE 39–5. *Contrast-enhanced computed tomographic scan shows a ring-enhancing left frontal cerebral abscess (arrows) in a 3-week-old male infant with concurrent* Enterobacter *meningitis (courtesy of Drs. C. D. Robson and P. D. Barnes).*

young infants by real-time ultrasonography[4, 10, 20, 26] (Fig. 39–6). In some cases, repeated aspiration of the abscess contents may be necessary. Surgical excision may be associated with increased risk of neurologic sequelae and should be reserved for those not responding to antibiotics with or without aspiration and for those patients in whom increased intracranial pressure threatens life.[16, 23] While cultures are pending, the selection of antibiotics should be guided by the primary source of infection, pertinent patient history, and the results of microscopic examination of the pus (Table 39–2). The duration of therapy varies according to the individual but ranges from 2 to 8 weeks, with shorter duration therapy reserved

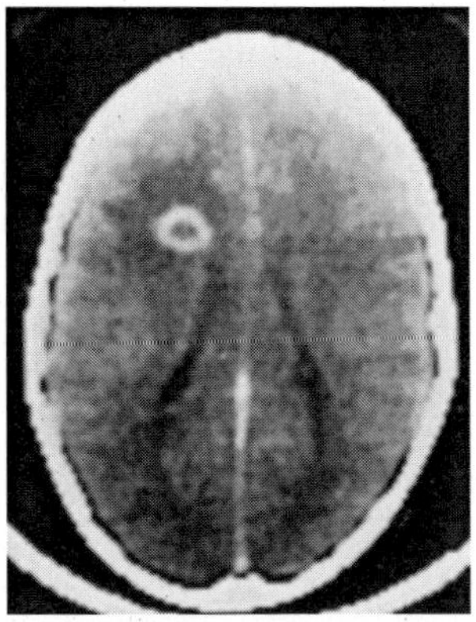

FIGURE 39–6. *Frontal lobe abscess adjacent to the lateral ventricle into which the abscess had ruptured. The patient had purulent meningitis. Note edema (lucent area) surrounding the abscess. The abscess cavity was evacuated by needle aspiration subsequent to computed tomographic scanning.*

TABLE 39–2. Suggested Initial Empiric Antibiotic Therapy for Brain Abscess in Children*

Primary Source	Antibiotic Regimen
Cyanotic heart disease	Penicillin and chloramphenicol
Meningitis	Third-generation cephalosporin with or without an aminoglycoside
Ventriculo-peritoneal shunt infection	Vancomycin and ceftazidime
Otitis/mastoiditis	Nafcillin or vancomycin, ceftazidime, and metronidazole
Sinusitis	Nafcillin or vancomycin and chloramphenicol
Head trauma	Nafcillin or vancomycin and chloramphenicol
Unknown	Nafcillin or vancomycin, third-generation cephalosporin, and metronidazole

*Immunosuppressed children should be treated with broad coverage and with consideration of amphotericin B therapy. Antituberculous therapy should be considered for children with exposure to tuberculosis.

From Sáez-Llorens, X. J., Umana, M. A., Odio, C. M., et al.: Brain abscess in infants and children. Pediatr. Infect. Dis. *8*:449–458, 1989.

only for those patients with complete surgical excision of the abscess.

Regardless of the therapeutic modalities employed, neurologic deficits after treatment remain disappointingly high, about 50 per cent in some series, although widespread availability of CT scanning has allowed for a reduction in mortality of from 30 to about 10 per cent.[16, 23, 27] Eradication of potential sources of infection before the abscess has developed is logical preventive medicine, and the fewer cases of parameningeal sepsis, including cerebral abscess, in recent years are encouraging. Early diagnosis and treatment are imperative and can be facilitated by the liberal use of MRI/CT scanning when this diagnosis is even a remote consideration.

SUBDURAL EMPYEMA

Pyogenic infection in the subdural space is designated as subdural empyema or sometimes, but less correctly, as subdural abscess. The sources of infection and microorganisms responsible are the same as those encountered in brain abscess. It is a relatively rare disease; only one case was seen at St. Louis Children's Hospital during a period when 122 patients with bacterial meningitis and 3 patients with cerebral abscess were treated (see Table 39–1). The primary source of subdural empyema in this single case was not found, which increasingly is true in pediatric experience. Farmer, Wise, and Jacobson[9, 15] found associated meningitis in six of eight infants with subdural empyema (seen over a 16-year period), suggesting that the latter was a complication of the former. We, too, have encountered this situation, albeit rarely, and more often than not the subdural fluid is turbid rather than frankly purulent.

In older children, the infection appears not to follow leptomeningitis. Although leptomeningitis may complicate subdural empyema, infections of the paranasal sinuses and mastoid region, usually chronic, spread to the subdural space directly because of osteomyelitis or by way of infected veins that penetrate the skull. Understandably, extension to cortical veins and to major venous sinuses occurs frequently in association with subdural empyema, as discussed elsewhere in this section. Why in some cases the infection is restricted to one or another anatomic site or sites (e.g., epidural space, subdural space, parenchyma of the brain or blood vessels) is unknown. Subdural empyema may be hematogenous in origin. It is an infrequent but recognized complication of intracranial surgery.

The anatomy of the subdural space is such that the infection often extends widely over one or both cerebral hemispheres, and accumulation of pus in the parafalcine region is well known.

Clinical Manifestations

The symptoms and signs of the primary source of infection may be prominent, subtle, or absent. Increasingly severe headache, high fever, signs of meningeal irritation, and progressive neurologic deficits referable to the site of the lesion are reported in the typical untreated case. Seizures, focal or generalized, are prominent, especially when cortical injury from associated vasculitis is present. Signs of increased intracranial pressure become prominent as the mass of pus enlarges. In infants, a fullness of fontanelle, vomiting, and depressed responsiveness are seen. Transillumination of the skull can be positive. Older children may, in addition, develop papilledema. As the intracranial pressure rises, symptoms and signs progress, ultimately leading to temporal lobe or cerebellar herniation and the characteristic syndromes of these complications.

Diagnosis

The laboratory findings reflect the active infectious process; peripheral leukocytosis and a predominance of polymorphonuclear leukocytes with immature cells are seen.

The CSF in infants reflects the common association with leptomeningitis, and the findings depend upon when the fluid is examined. Before the meningitis has been treated adequately, organisms may be cultured; the glucose concentration may be low and the protein concentration high in the CSF. Later, the CSF findings are those of treated meningitis, yet viable organisms can be recovered from the subdural collections when the CSF is sterile. Also, specific antigen may be demonstrated in subdural collections by tests such as countercurrent immunoelectrophoresis in the absence of viable organisms. In older children, the characteristic CSF findings include elevated pressure with a few to a few hundred or more leukocytes, polymorphonuclear leukocytes predominating. The protein concentration frequently is elevated, the glucose concentration normal, and the fluid sterile.

In the past two or more decades, subdural empyema in children has become more difficult to diagnose clinically because of antimicrobial therapy, which, when initiated early, may attenuate the dramatic nature of the disease, especially those symptoms and signs of acute infection. Because the diagnosis of subdural empyema often is confused with that of brain abscess, radiographic studies are necessary to establish the correct diagnosis. The CT scan (Fig. 39–7) and MRI are effective noninvasive techniques, as discussed in relation to brain abscess. Cerebral angiography can demonstrate a failure of the cerebral vessels to approximate the inner surface of the skull. These studies reveal the extent of subdural disease and may define an epidural abscess or other infectious exudate collection concurrent with subdural empyema (Fig. 39–8).

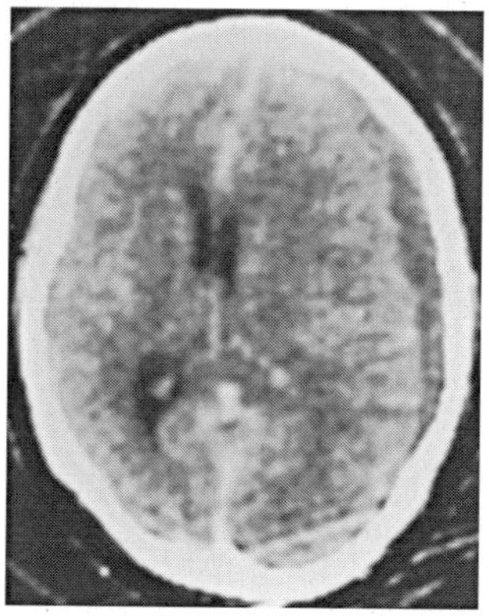

FIGURE 39–7. *Computed tomographic scan showing subdural empyema with marked displacement of the ventricular system.*

Treatment

Until a causative organism (or organisms) is identified, the patient should receive broad-spectrum antibiotics intravenously in dosages appropriate for bacterial meningitis. Once the offending organism is known, the sensitivities of that organism to specific medications will dictate more precise antibiotic therapy.

In infants, antibiotic therapy may be sufficient when the fluid is cloudy only, but if thick purulent material is obtained by subdural paracentesis or, in older children, if the clinical and radiographic evidence indicates a subdural empyema, then surgery is requisite. Depending upon individual circumstances, craniotomy or multiple burr holes with irrigation of the subdural space should be accomplished.

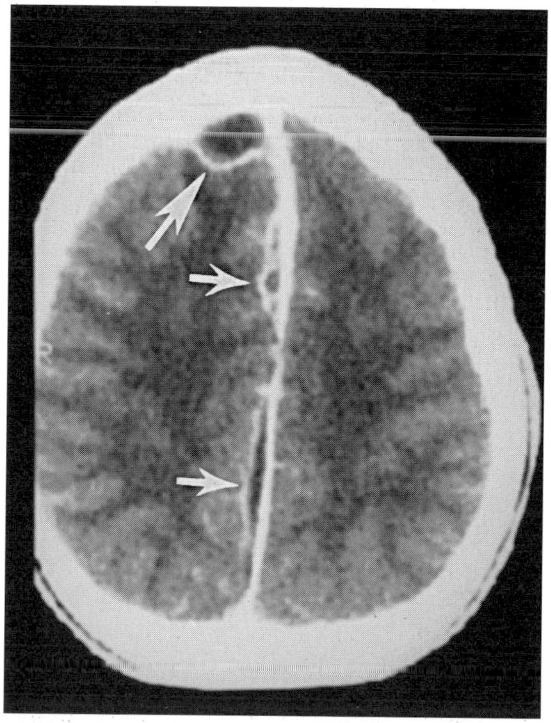

FIGURE 39–8. *Contrast-enhanced computed tomographic scan demonstrates a right frontal epidural abscess (large arrow) concurrent with an interhemispheric subdural abscess (small arrows) in a 13-year-old male who developed headache, fever, and vomiting after fracture of the right frontal sinus (courtesy of Drs. C. D. Robson and P. D. Barnes).*

Unfortunately, as with brain abscess, the mortality and morbidity rates are high (20 to 40 per cent) in most series but lower in some.[8, 29, 33] Early diagnosis and treatment are imperative, and it would appear that the early use of CT scanning is responsible for improved therapeutic results.[33]

CRANIAL EPIDURAL ABSCESS

Because the dura closely is adherent to the inner aspect of the cranium, epidural abscesses rarely attain a large size and consequently do not exert significant pressure on the brain. Their importance lies in their serving as a focus for spread of infection into the subdural space, leptomeninges, or brain. In addition, the infection may involve local penetrating vessels and lead to occlusion of these with extension to venous sinuses and other vessels. Infection of the middle ear, mastoid bone, or ancillary air sinuses may lead to epidural abscess, as in the case of subdural empyema and brain abscess. Often, epidural abscess coexists with the other lesions and presumably develops first. Osteomyelitis may be evident. This usually is the case with mastoiditis and often is evident after head injury with comminuted fracture of the skull or after intracranial surgery. An adolescent boy with osteomyelitis and epidural abscess complicating a wrestling injury has been reported.[31] Local pain, tenderness, and fever may be the only signs. Treatment usually includes antibiotic drugs and surgery in the presence of osteomyelitis. Exclusion of associated intracranial infections is mandatory; the epidural infection serves to raise these diagnostic possibilities.

SPINAL EPIDURAL INFECTIONS

Spinal epidural infections may be acute or chronic, and they may be restricted in their extent or extend longitudinally over many segments of the spinal cord because the epidural space offers no resisting structures. Most often, the process affects the posterior region of the spine, with maximal pus or granulomatous tissue being found over the dorsal aspect of the cord or spinal roots. However, in Danner and Hartman's[7] series from the New York Hospital, in about half of the patients the pus primarily was anterior to the cord. In the case of spinal osteomyelitis, the pus may be more viscous ventrally. Occasionally, the purulent material may encircle the neural elements. In infants and children, this is a rare condition; no case was encountered at the St. Louis Children's Hospital during the 39 months in which 122 cases of bacterial meningitis were seen. In an extensive report by Baker and colleagues[3] covering a 27-year period at the Massachusetts General Hospital, only 6 of 39 patients were younger than 20 years of age, and the youngest was 11. The incidence ranged from 0.2 to 1.2 hospital admissions a year. In approximately half the patients in this series, acute purulent material was discovered at operation or autopsy, with *Staphylococcus aureus* being incriminated in more than half the cases. In the remainder, a granulomatous process was found, associated with a wide variety of bacteria. There was no instance of tuberculous infection, although in many regions of the world this organism remains an important consideration. Nonbacterial infective agents may include fungi or parasites.

The neural dysfunction results, in all probability, from direct compression of the spinal cord and/or roots and nerves, but impaired circulation from associated inflammation and occlusion of vessels is at least a contributory factor in some cases. It often is difficult to determine with certainty the extent to which each of the above mechanisms contributes to neural dysfunction. Extensive necrosis of the cord may result in advanced cases in which a prompt diagnosis has not been made.

Sources of Infection

In tuberculous and other chronic infections, osteomyelitis and intervertebral disk infection are common, but those afflicted primarily are adults.[18] Acute spinal epidural infections usually follow hematogenous spread from furuncles, pharyngitis, dental abscesses, decubitus ulcers, and urinary tract and wound infections. They may complicate spinal surgery, and, rarely, lumbar puncture has been implicated as a source.[5] Osteomyelitis is uncommon. A history of minor trauma to the back may be reported. Presumably, trauma results in local tissue injury or hemorrhage, forming a nidus for the developing infection.

Clinical Manifestations

Fever is the rule, the temperature being higher in patients with acute infections. Such patients appear septic, and toxic delirium occurs frequently. Heusner,[13] in his classic paper dealing primarily with acute epidural abscesses, divided the clinical phases as follows: (1) spinal ache, (2) root pain, (3) weakness, and (4) paralysis. Although because of certain therapeutic implications this separation is a useful way to consider the disorder, phases 3 and 4 are combined in the following discussion. It is axiomatic that the various stages often overlap.

PHASE 1: SPINAL ACHE. This was a universal finding in Heusner's experience. In a report from Baker and associates,[3] all 39 patients had backache of varying degrees of severity. Local tenderness was absent in only two of their patients and should be searched for by carefully tapping over the spine.

PHASE 2: ROOT PAIN. Root pain is characteristic and also is an early symptom that may assist in localization of the pathologic process. Root pain especially is prominent with lumbosacral disease in which roots are implicated without involvement of spinal cord. The diagnosis is suspected infrequently until functional motor and sensory loss occurs, which is unfortunate because therapy is most effective during the early stages. Progression to symptoms and signs of spinal cord involvement usually occurs within a few days, except when the process is granulomatous, in which case the time course tends to be prolonged, extending over several or more weeks.

PHASES 3 AND 4: WEAKNESS AND PARALYSIS. Once weakness and impaired sensation referable to disease of the spinal cord appear, the progression to paralysis can be rapid, and immediate surgical treatment is imperative to maximize the likelihood of reasonable functional recovery. However, as stated earlier, even appropriate therapy at this stage often is ineffective in restoring normal neurologic functions. Death occurs in at least 20 per cent of cases; this rate has not changed significantly since 1948, in spite of the availability of a wide range of antibiotic agents.

Diagnosis

The diagnosis of spinal epidural infection is established by MRI of the spine (Fig. 39–9). This also may reveal evidence for concurrent osteomyelitis of the spine, which is present in about 20 per cent of chronic lesions. Once discovered, immediate neurosurgical intervention is necessary to prevent long-

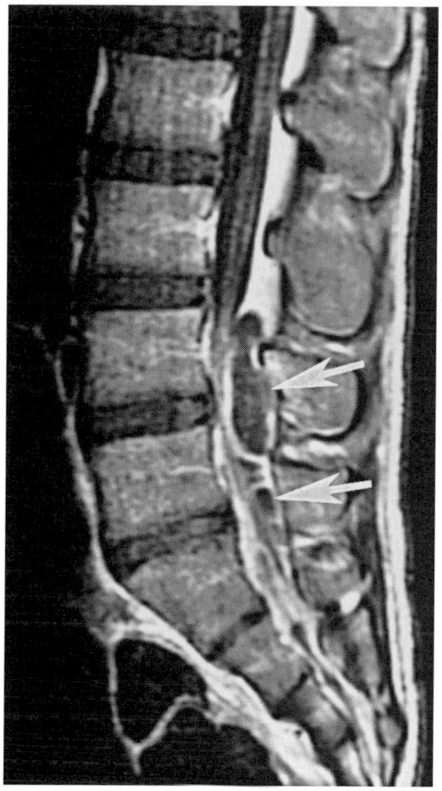

FIGURE 39–9. *Gadolinium-enhanced sagittal T1-weighted magnetic resonance image shows a rim-enhancing lumbar spinal epidural abscess (arrows) in a 15-year-old male with a 3-week history of lower back pain, followed by rapidly progressive left leg numbness with decreased bowel and bladder function.* Staphylococcus aureus *was cultured from purulent fluid removed after L4/5 laminectomy (courtesy of Drs. C. D. Robson and P. D. Barnes).*

term neurologic sequelae. At the time of surgery, stains and cultures for aerobic and anaerobic bacteria, mycobacteria, and fungi should be obtained. If lumbar puncture is attempted when epidural abscess is suspected, the spinal needle (with stylet) is advanced slowly in the lumbar region, with periodic removal of the stylet and with suction being applied gently *before* the thecal sac is entered. If purulent material is obtained, the diagnosis is established, and the pus must be examined by a Gram-stained smear and cultured on various media under aerobic and anaerobic conditions. The leptomeninges should not be penetrated if purulent material is encountered; otherwise, CSF should be obtained. Characteristically, the CSF is clear or slightly opalescent and yellow in the presence of a block. Pleocytosis with a few to many hundred cells (lymphocytes predominating) reflects a contiguous infectious process, but in the absence of meningitis, there will be no organisms, and the CSF glucose concentration should be normal. The protein concentration always is elevated, and the level may be very high (several hundred to 2000 mg/dL) in the presence of a partial or total manometric block.

The differential diagnosis includes myelitis due to bacterial meningitis, syphilis, viruses, and a parainfectious process, as well as to the syndrome of acute transverse myelopathy of unknown cause. Spinal ache is most prominent in acute transverse myelopathy, but as a general rule, the entire illness is compressed in time, with paresis or paralysis evolving over hours or a few days from the outset of the disease. Impaired circulation of CSF does not occur in this or the aforementioned disorders. Rarely, a lymphoma may mimic a spinal epidural abscess. Spinal cord tumors, vascular malformations, and arachnoiditis are considerations when the course of disease is prolonged and evidence of sepsis is either minimal or absent, as occurs with chronic epidural infections.

Treatment

Prompt surgical removal of purulent or granulomatous material is essential. This should be combined with the intravenous administration of an appropriate antibiotic. Initial empiric antibiotic coverage is similar to that for brain abscess, although antifungal therapy need not be included unless cultures or stains are positive for fungi. Treatment typically should be continued for 3 to 4 weeks but continued for twice this period if there is osteomyelitis. Despite advances, the morbidity and mortality of spinal epidural abscess remain distressingly high. Up to one third of children with the disease die, and another third are left with permanent neurologic sequelae, including weakness, incontinence, and sensory abnormalities. Rapid diagnosis and treatment are essential to ensure a successful outcome.

References

1. Amano, K., and Kamano, S.: Cerebellar abscess due to penetrating orbital wound. J. Comput. Assist. Tomogr. *6*:1163–1166, 1982.
2. Anonymous: Case records of the Massachusetts General Hospital: Weekly clinicopathological exercises: Case 13-1973. N. Engl. J. Med. *288*:674–679, 1973.
3. Baker, A. S., Ojemann, R. G., Swartz, M. N., et al.: Spinal epidural abscess. N. Engl. J. Med. *293*:464–468, 1975.
4. Berg, B., Franklin, G., Cuneo, R., et al.: Nonsurgical cure of brain abscess: Early diagnosis and follow-up with computerized tomography. Ann. Neurol. *3*:474–478, 1978.
5. Bergman, I., Wald, E. R., Meyer, J. D., et al.: Epidural abscess and vertebral osteomyelitis following serial lumbar punctures. Pediatrics *72*:476–480, 1983.
6. Britt, R. H., and Enzmann, D. R.: Clinical stages of human brain abscesses on serial CT scans after contrast infusion. J. Neurosurg. *59*:972–989, 1983.
7. Danner, R. L., and Hartman, B. J.: Update of spinal epidural abscess: 35 cases and review of the literature. Rev. Infect. Dis. *9*:265–274, 1987.
8. Dill, S. R., Cobbs, C. G., and McDonald, C. K.: Subdural empyema: Analysis of 32 cases and review. Clin. Infect. Dis. *20*:372–386, 1995.
9. Farmer, T. W., and Wise, G. R.: Subdural empyema in infants, children and adults. Neurology *23*:254–261, 1973.
10. Ferriero, D. M., Derechin, M., Edwards, B. S. B., et al.: Outcome of brain abscess treatment in children: Reduced morbidity with neuroimaging. Pediatr. Neurol. *3*:148–152, 1987.
11. Foreman, S. D., Smith, E. E., Ryan, N. J., et al.: Neonatal *Citrobacter* meningitis: Pathogenesis of cerebral abscess formation. Ann. Neurol. *16*:655–659, 1984.
12. Hagensee, M. E., Bauwens, J. E., Kjos, B., et al.: Brain abscess following marrow transplantation: Experience at the Fred Hutchinson Cancer Research Center, 1984–1992. Clin. Infect. Dis. *19*:402–408, 1994.
13. Heusner, A. P.: Nontuberculous spinal epidural infections. N. Engl. J. Med. *239*:845–854, 1948.
14. Horner, F. A., Berry, R. G., and Frantz, M.: Broken pencil points as a cause of brain abscess. N. Engl. J. Med. *271*:342–345, 1964.
15. Jacobson, P. E., and Farmer, T. W.: Subdural empyema complicating meningitis in infants: Improved prognosis. Neurology *31*:190–193, 1981.
16. Jadavji, T., Humphreys, R. P., and Prober, C. G.: Brain abscesses in infants and children. Pediatr. Infect. Dis. *4*:394–398, 1985.
17. Joubert, M. J., and Stephanov, S.: Computerized tomography and surgical treatment in intracranial suppuration. J. Neurosurg. *47*:73–78, 1977.
18. Kaufman, D. M., Kaplan, J. G., and Litman, N.: Infectious agents in spinal epidural abscesses. Neurology *30*:844–850, 1980.
19. Kinsella, T. R., Yogev, R., Shulman, S. T., et al.: Treatment of *Salmonella* meningitis and brain abscess with the new cephalosporins: Two case reports and a review of the literature. Pediatr. Infect. Dis. *6*:476–480, 1987.
20. Kondziolka, D., Duma, C. M., and Lunsford, L. D.: Factors that enhance the likelihood of successful stereotactic treatment of brain abscesses. Acta Neurochir. *127*:85–90, 1994.
21. Lampe, R. M., Cheldelin, L. V., and Brown, J., III: Brain abscess following dental extraction in a child with cyanotic congenital heart disease. Pediatrics *61*:659–660, 1978.

22. Leahy, W. R., Toyka, K. V., and Fischbeck, K. H., Jr.: Cerebral abscess in children secondary to esophageal dilatation. Pediatrics *59*:300–301, 1977.
23. Mampalam, T. J., and Rosenblum, M. L.: Trends in the management of bacterial brain abscesses: A review of 102 cases over 17 years. Neurosurgery *23*:451–458, 1988.
24. Piazza, E., Condorelli, A., Arcidiacono, R., et al.: Intracerebral mass lesions in patients affected by AIDS. Acta Neurochir. *83*:116–120, 1986.
25. Pruitt, A. A., Rubin, R. H., Karchmer, A. W., et al.: Neurologic complications of bacterial endocarditis. Medicine *57*:329–343, 1977.
26. Renier, D. R., Flandin, C., Hirsch, E., et al.: Brain abscesses in neonates: A study of 30 cases. J. Neurosurg. *69*:877–882, 1988.
27. Sáez-Llorens, X. J., Umana, M. A., Odio, C. M., et al.: Brain abscess in infants and children. Pediatr. Infect. Dis. *8*:449–458, 1989.
28. Shaw, M. D. M., and Russell, J. A.: Value of computed tomography in the diagnosis of intracranial abscess. J. Neurol. Neurosurg. Psychiatr. *40*:214–220, 1977.
29. Smith, H. P., and Hendrick, E. B.: Subdural empyema and epidural abscess in children. J. Neurosurg. *58*:392–397, 1983.
30. Sutton, D. L., and Ouvrier, R. A.: Cerebral abscess in the under 6 month age group. Arch. Dis. Child. *58*:901–905, 1983.
31. Tudor, R. B., Carson, J. P., Pulliam, M. W., et al.: Pott's puffy tumor, frontal sinusitis, frontal bone osteomyelitis, and epidural abscess secondary to a wrestling injury. Am. J. Sports Med. *9*:390–391, 1981.
32. Young, R. F., and Frazee, J.: Gas within intracranial abscess cavities: An indication for surgical excision. Ann. Neurol. *16*:35–39, 1984.
33. Zimmerman, R. D., Leeds, N. E., and Danziger, A.: Subdural empyema: CT findings. Radiology *150*:417–422, 1984.

Additional Reading

Bell, W. E., and McCormick, W. F.: Focal suppurative infections of the nervous system. *In* Neurologic Infections in Children. Major Probl. Clin. Pediatr. *12*:90–123, 1975.
Dodge, P. R., and Swartz, M. N.: Infections and inflammatory diseases of the central nervous system and its coverings. *In* Beeson, P. R., and McDermott, W. (eds.): Textbook of Medicine. 14th ed. Philadelphia, W. B. Saunders, 1975, pp. 670–683.

40

FUNGAL MENINGITIS

J. Thomas Cross, Jr., and Richard F. Jacobs

Fungi are rare causes of meningitis in children. *Candida albicans*, *Cryptococcus neoformans*, and *Coccidioides immitis* are the most common isolates in the pediatric age group. Diagnosis can be difficult. Fungal meningitis frequently is chronic in nature, and, thus, patients may have few symptoms. The lack of obvious meningeal signs and symptoms and the relative uncommonness of a fungal etiology often delay diagnosis. Inherent problems with the diagnosis of fungal central nervous system infections begin with the basic microbiology of the organisms. Their fastidious growth, prolonged time for culture, and requirement of special media can make diagnosis difficult in meningitis.

Because it frequently is difficult to cultivate many fungi from the cerebrospinal fluid (CSF), the use of serologic tests for antibodies and antigens will help define the infection quicker and with more sensitivity. These tests can be done on CSF, serum, and in some instances urine.[149] For most infections, amphotericin B is the drug of choice, although its supremacy is being tested by some of the newer azoles in recent and current clinical trials. Central nervous system (CNS) disease due to fungi generally has a high morbidity and mortality.

EPIDEMIOLOGY

The epidemiology of fungal meningitis depends upon many factors. The geographic location of the patient or travel to an endemic area can be an important clue to defining the etiology of the infection. The geographic distribution of fungal meningitis varies in the United States and worldwide. Histoplasmosis generally occurs in endemic areas of the Mississippi River Valley.[148] Coccidioidomycosis occurs in the San Joaquin Valley as well as in Mexico and the desert Southwest.[3, 97] Cryptococcosis has worldwide distribution rather than discrete endemic areas but seems to be associated with pigeon droppings and nesting areas of other birds.[81] Blastomycosis has a sporadic pattern of infectivity but generally occurs in states bordering the Mississippi and Ohio river basins, with occasional outbreaks occurring in the Great Lakes region and Canada.[41, 67, 117] *Candida* species, *Aspergillus* species, *Sporothrix schenckii*, and other fungal pathogens generally are not defined by geographic boundaries but depend more on environmental exposures and the immunocompetence of the individual patient.

Many fungal infections (particularly those due to *Candida* species and *Histoplasma*) generally are not responsible for meningitis, unless the host is immunocompromised. Cases of cryptococcal meningitis have increased dramatically in association with the AIDS epidemic. A review from the mid-1980s by the Centers for Disease Control and Prevention showed an incidence rate of 6.8 per cent for cryptococcal meningitis in patients with AIDS; however, the rate in pediatric AIDS patients was 10 times lower (0.6 per cent).[118] In the pre-AIDS era, patients known to be at risk for disseminated cryptococcosis included patients with lymphoma, patients on high-dose corticosteroid therapy, and patients with underlying cellular immune dysfunction.[22] Risk factors for *Candida* species meningitis are very similar to those for candidemia: prolonged antimicrobial therapy, indwelling venous catheters, hyperalimentation, corticosteroid use, recent intra-abdominal surgery, and intravenous drug abuse.[113, 131] Pediatric cases are most common in the neonate, particularly in the very low birth weight infant.[8, 46, 58, 61, 123] In the early 1980s, 3.8 per cent of infants weighing less than 1500 g in a large pediatric teaching hospital developed systemic fungal infections, mostly due to *Candida* species. The mean birth weight was 809 g, with 86 per cent of the infants weighing less than 1000 g.

Inhalation is the most common means by which many fungi infect the host. Other fungi can be inoculated directly into the skin; this can occur in the outdoor environment or in the hospital setting (intravenous catheters, etc.), especially in very low birth weight infants.[8]

CLINICAL MANIFESTATIONS

Candida species infection in very low birth weight newborns can be particularly difficult to diagnose because of the broad range of symptoms. Most infants with disseminated candidiasis with meningitis present with respiratory distress and a supplemental oxygen requirement, with most progressing to require mechanical ventilation.[8] *Candida* usually is identified in endotracheal washings, urine, and blood in patients with *Candida* meningitis, but the infants have symptoms on average 11 days before the diagnosis is made. Ophthalmologic examinations may be very important in disseminated *Candida* infections.[26] A careful funduscopic examination also can help determine if increased intracranial pressure is present with the presence of papilledema. Marked abdominal distention also is common in disseminated *Candida* infections in low birth weight infants and frequently is associated with guaiac-positive stools. Temperature instability, elevated white blood cell counts, and feeding intolerance also are present in a majority of cases. Hepatomegaly may indicate the presence of systemic infection.

Physical findings that are diagnostic for other causes of fungal meningitis (*Cryptococcus, Blastomyces, Histoplasma*, etc.) are rare because they usually are chronic infections. However, it is very important to look carefully for other manifestations of fungal infections, especially the presence of skin lesions. All superficial lesions, nodules, and draining abscesses should be investigated because they may give a clue to the etiology of subacute and chronic infections (*Coccidioides, Blastomyces, Cryptococcus*, etc.).[52] Fungal stains, including India ink, should be performed on all biopsy specimens and drainage material, and all specimens should be processed for culture. Bone involvement is common with certain fungal infections (*Cryptococcus* and *Blastomyces*).

The significance of isolating a fungus from CSF cannot be overemphasized. The finding of fungal organisms should be considered a true infection and appropriate antifungal therapy initiated. However, the significance of a single CSF culture for *Candida* or an unlikely meningeal pathogen (*Paecilomyces*) with an otherwise normal CSF should lead the physician to consider the possibility of contamination.[5] Repeat CSF cultures should be sought in such patients.

Infection with Specific Organisms

Candidal Meningitis

Candidal meningitis remains relatively rare in children. Arisoy and associates[5] reported that 2 per cent of all positive CSF cultures were fungal organisms. *Candida* species accounted for 94.5 per cent of the fungal isolates. Nine of 23 patients were newborns, eight of whom were very low birth weight infants. Risk factors for positive CSF fungal cultures from neonates included antimicrobial therapy, umbilical catheterization, total parenteral nutrition, intubation, and prematurity.[35, 36] Risk factors in children beyond the neonatal period included concurrent bacterial infection, chronic systemic or CNS disease, and the presence of central venous catheters. Histopathology models in animals have revealed hyphal invasion, vasculitis, abscesses, and acute and chronic inflammatory infiltration of meninges and brain parenchyma.[60]

Children with HIV infection are at risk for disseminated *Candida* infections, including meningitis. In one study, 27 per cent of HIV-infected patients with disseminated *Candida* infections had CNS involvement.[79] Nearly all HIV-infected patients who develop *Candida* infection do so as a result of hospital-acquired infection. Predisposing factors include oral candidiasis, central venous catheters, prolonged antibiotic therapy, and total parenteral nutrition. In HIV-infected patients, neutropenia, surprisingly, is not a major risk factor. However, simultaneous pulmonary disease, particularly viral, bacterial, or *Pneumocystis carinii* pneumonias, is present in a majority of HIV-infected patients with disseminated *Candida* infection. A majority of patients are febrile more than 14 days, with peak temperatures of more than 39° C before the diagnosis is made.

Recently, the incidence of infection with *Candida* species other than *C. albicans* has increased dramatically in immunocompromised children, particularly those with malignancies. *C. tropicalis* meningitis in a recent case series was uniformly fatal.[38] In addition to patients with malignancies and HIV infections, other children at risk for infection have been reported, including a child with myeloperoxidase deficiency.[83]

Candida species have become another concern because of the development of resistance. *C. lusitaniae* resistance to amphotericin B has been noted, and meningitis in an adult patient with a resistant strain has been reported.[114] *C. krusei* recently has been noted to have azole resistance, particularly in immunocompromised patients receiving suppressive azole therapy. These fungal infections already are difficult to treat without the added burden of drug resistance.

Candida meningitis usually responds to therapy with intravenous amphotericin B alone or in combination with oral flucytosine. The use of flucytosine is controversial; however, most reports support its use in meningitis. Flucytosine has been difficult to use in low birth weight infants because of the immaturity of their gastrointestinal tracts and the risks of necrotizing enterocolitis. The use of amphotericin alone for systemic candidiasis including meningitis in neonates has been used successfully in patients who could not tolerate oral medication.[21] The *most* important factor in successful treatment was the initiation of therapy quickly, once systemic *Candida* infection was suspected, frequently before the organism was isolated. Prolonged delays in initiating therapy results in high mortality. Amphotericin B initiated at a dose of 0.25 mg/kg of body weight diluted in 5 or 10 per cent dextrose-water can be infused over 2 to 4 hours. In most neonates, the drug dosage can be increased in 0.25 mg/kg increments at 6- to 12-hour intervals until the desired 1 mg/kg daily dose is attained. In older children and adolescents, a test dose usually is given, with an initial dose of 0.1 mg/kg (1 mg maximum). If this is tolerated, the initial dose of therapy (0.25 mg/kg) is given. In severely ill patients, the dose can be increased rapidly in 6- to 12-hour intervals to 1 mg/kg/dose. Flucytosine generally is recommended in a dose of 150 mg/kg/day divided every 6 hours. The use of flucytosine often requires monitoring and adjustment of dosage based on serum determinations.

Cryptococcosis

Cryptococcal meningitis was relatively rare in the United States in the pre-HIV era. However, with the growth of the AIDS epidemic, this infection has become a common cause of meningitis in adults in certain areas of the United States and infects 2 to 9 per cent of adult AIDS patients.[27, 32, 69, 153] However, it remains relatively uncommon in pediatric patients.[94, 110] Cryptococcosis is a systemic fungal infection, and meningitis is its most serious manifestation. Patients with initial pulmonary involvement may have very few symptoms but can present with fever, cough, weight loss, and dyspnea on exertion.[87] In adult studies, progressively severe headaches without the presence of fever were noted commonly.[133] Patients with cryptococcal meningitis frequently have few symptoms but can present with nausea, dizziness, and irritability. Nuchal rigidity usually is absent. Careful examination for cranial nerve palsies, which in adults are found in about one-fifth of patients, should be performed.

Diplopia, in particular, is one of the most common manifestations of cryptococcal meningitis. Papilledema is seen in nearly a third of patients with cryptococcal meningitis.[31] Patients with coexistent AIDS frequently have very few symptoms.[32] In adults, prognostic factors that may indicate a poor outcome include altered mental status, a CSF cryptococcal antigen titer greater than 1:1024, and a CSF white blood cell count less than 20/mm^3.[107, 112]

Pediatric patients with cryptococcal meningitis usually present with signs and symptoms not referable to the CNS.[122] Leggiadro and associates[78] reported on 13 children with AIDS compiled from 11 institutions who were diagnosed with extrapulmonary cryptococcosis. Meningitis was diagnosed in 62 per cent of these patients and was the most common clinical manifestation of extrapulmonary disease. Patients who initially responded to antifungal therapy did not die of the fungal infection but succumbed to other illnesses related to their immunodeficiency.

Leggiadro and associates[77] also reported on eight children with acute lymphoblastic leukemia who developed extrapulmonary cryptococcosis. Of these immunocompromised children, 63 per cent had meningitis. Fever was the most common symptom, occurring in 60 per cent of the children with meningitis. Headache was present in only 40 per cent. A significant number of the children were completely asymptomatic (40 per cent) and had lumbar punctures performed as routine management of their acute lymphoblastic leukemia, with the subsequent unexpected growth of *C. neoformans* on culture. One child had cutaneous lesions and another had ptosis and unsteady gait. Treatment in this series of patients included amphotericin B (intravenous and/or intrathecal) alone or combined with oral flucytosine. In these patients with acute lymphoblastic leukemia, relapse was a major complication, occurring in 60 per cent of patients thought to have been treated successfully. The relapses occurred within 2 to 6 months of completing therapy. Treatment of the relapses generally included combination therapy of amphotericin B and flucytosine with the occasional use of intrathecal amphotericin B.

Other illnesses that may lead to cryptococcal meningitis include systemic lupus erythematosus being treated with corticosteroids alone or in combination with azathioprine,[2, 77, 80, 108] chronic mucocutaneous candidiasis,[57, 144] and hyper-IgE syndrome.[128]

Direct examination of the CSF using the India ink test can provide an immediate presumptive diagnosis of cryptococcal meningitis. The sensitivity of this test is variable, but in recent studies in adult AIDS patients, the stain approached 75 per cent positivity.[27] Other useful stains include silver, periodic acid–Schiff, and mucicarmine. Gram stain of CSF is insensitive and unreliable.

Diagnosis of cryptococcal meningitis is aided today by the use of serologic tests. The most common test is the cryptococcal capsular polysaccharide antigen test, which can be performed on serum, CSF, or other sterile body fluids. The sensitivity of this test is nearly 100 per cent in the serum of HIV-positive patients.[28, 69, 153] The CSF antigen test appears in some studies to be less sensitive, with a 91 per cent sensitivity.[27] False-positive results have been reported due to cross-reactions of antigens in disseminated infections with *Trichosporon beigelii*.[89] Culture still is the gold standard for diagnosis and monitoring the success of therapy.

Treatment of cryptococcal meningitis is prolonged and in immunocompromised patients frequently requires lifelong maintenance therapy. In adults with HIV infection, multiple regimens have been suggested. Based on a comparison study between amphotericin B and fluconazole therapy for the initial treatment of cryptococcal meningitis, Saag and associates[112] demonstrated that patients with any of three poor prognostic signs (change in mental status, CSF cryptococcal antigen >1:1024, or white blood count <20/mm^3) should have initial therapy with amphotericin B. In patients with "mild" disease, the use of fluconazole therapy alone had an efficacy similar to that of amphotericin B, but the time to negative cultures using fluconazole alone was more prolonged. There was no difference in overall survival between the two groups, but patients who received fluconazole had an increased frequency of early death compared with the amphotericin B group. Treatment recommendations are variable. Recent reports support the use of 0.5 to 0.7 mg/kg/day of amphotericin B with or without flucytosine in a dose of 75 to 100 mg/kg/day in four divided doses.[106] Recent data suggest that amphotericin B in a dose of 0.7 mg/kg/day plus flucytosine in a dose of 100 mg/kg/day for 14 days followed by fluconazole at a dose of 400 mg/day had a trend toward superiority compared with amphotericin B alone at the same dose.[141] Larsen and associates[74] have recommended that amphotericin B in combination with flucytosine be used for therapy in AIDS patients. After the initial symptoms have resolved and the patient is afebrile, many physicians recommend switching to fluconazole at a dose of 400 mg/day to complete an 8- to 10-week course, followed by fluconazole 200 mg/day indefinitely.[107, 112] Recently, Larsen and associates[73] have noted similar good results with the use of fluconazole (400 mg/day) combined with flucytosine (150 mg/kg divided daily).

In nonimmunocompromised patients, the use of amphotericin B in a dose of 0.3 mg/kg/day and 150 mg of flucytosine in four divided oral doses daily for a 6-week course has shown efficacy in clinical trials.[11] In patients with renal compromise associated with amphotericin B, flucytosine levels must be monitored carefully. It is recommended that the dose of flucytosine be reduced to 75 to 100 mg/kg/day and continuing doses be adjusted to maintain serum flucytosine levels between 25 and 60 μg/mL.[6, 39] Serum cryptococcal antigens are not useful in monitoring response to therapy, and the use of CSF cryptococcal antigens to monitor response to therapy also is controversial. The best method to judge successful therapy is by the demonstration of sterility of CSF fungal cultures.

In pediatrics, a combination of amphotericin B and flucytosine has been used most frequently. In children with AIDS, amphotericin B in a dose of 0.5 to 1.0 mg/kg/day with or without flucytosine (150 mg/kg/day divided into four doses) is recommended for 4 to 8 weeks, followed by maintenance therapy with fluconazole of 3 to 6 mg/kg/day indefinitely.[147]

Histoplasmosis

Infection with *Histoplasma capsulatum*, usually a benign and self-limited disease, is endemic in many parts of the United States. Disseminated disease including meningitis is very rare in children.[65] Case reports in adults generally involve immunocompromised individuals.[44, 138] Clinical presentations reported in the literature show a wide variability in presentation of meningitis. In these cases, 39 per cent presented with meningitis associated with acute dissemination, 25 per cent with single histoplasmoma that presented as symptomatic mass lesions alone or with dissemination, 25 per cent with chronic meningitis without evidence of dissemination, and the remainder with meningitis as a manifestation of recurrent disease. Rarely, embolization to the brain due to *Histoplasma* endocarditis has been associated with meningitis.[148]

Meningitis occurring in AIDS patients has become relatively common in endemic areas. In one report, 8 per cent of the AIDS-defining illnesses in children were due to disseminated histoplasmosis.[115] The duration of symptoms is quite variable. In non-AIDS patients, the symptoms generally last more than 6 months but can last as long as 7 years.[33, 44, 101, 145] In the AIDS patient, symptoms usually present more acutely in a much shorter time frame.[148] In a recent series, neurologic findings occurred in all but 6 per cent of the patients.[148] The most common signs and symptoms include depressed consciousness (29 per cent), headaches (24 per cent), confusion (22 per cent), cranial nerve deficits (19 per cent), other focal deficits (16 per cent), seizures (14 per cent), personality changes (12 per cent), and ataxia (11 per cent). Findings more commonly observed with acute bacterial meningitis, such as meningismus, a present Babinski sign, or papilledema, were seen in less than 8 per cent of the cases. In adult non-AIDS patients, the death rate is about 12 per cent with a relapse rate of 44 per cent. In adult AIDS patients, the death rate is as high as 100 per cent in some series.[4, 148]

Diagnosis can be aided by serologic testing. High levels of anti-*H. capsulatum* antibodies were detected in the serum of 70 per cent of patients tested. Cerebrospinal fluid serology was helpful in 75 per cent of patients who were tested. Culture of the CSF was positive in less than half of the cases in one review.[65] However, in a second series in AIDS patients, blood cultures were positive in 49 per cent, bone marrow in 53 per cent, respiratory secretions in 58 per cent, and brain/meninges cultures in 75 per cent of those individuals tested. Serologic testing can be negative because 10 to 25 per cent of patients with disseminated disease lack a positive antibody response. The serology also can be falsely positive in patients with other fungal diseases or tuberculosis. Additionally, the antibody response to acute *Histoplasma* infection may remain elevated for years, without evidence of dissemination or meningeal disease. The use of *Histoplasma* antigen has become widely held as a useful test in the immunocompromised patient with disseminated *Histoplasma*. Recent data from Wheat and associates[148] showed that in AIDS patients with meningitis, antigen was found in the urine of six of seven patients.

Treatment with amphotericin B is considered standard therapy. A total dose of at least 30 mg/kg is felt by many to be necessary to ensure a cure. Children with meningitis due to *H. capsulatum* should have the amphotericin B dose advanced rapidly to 1 mg/kg/day. The use of intrathecal amphotericin B is not recommended for *H. capsulatum* meningitis. Additionally, AIDS patients whose induction therapy was successful must remain on an anti-*Histoplasma* agent indefinitely. There are a few case reports of children with disseminated histoplasmosis and AIDS but none with meningitis, and in these children, it is necessary to continue antifungal therapy indefinitely.[24, 115] The case report by Schutze and associates[115] demonstrated that ketoconazole was ineffective for preventing recurrence of nonmeningeal disseminated disease, and, with ketoconazole's poor CNS penetration, it is likely to be ineffective for prophylaxis of meningitis. In patients with AIDS, some success has occurred with the use of itraconazole for suppressive therapy in disseminated disease. However, few data exist on the use of itraconazole for suppressive therapy for meningitis or other CNS lesions due to *Histoplasma*. Based on the present data available, amphotericin B in a weekly dose of 1 mg/kg intravenous is the best agent for maintenance therapy in patients with meningitis. Fluconazole in one case report was effective in an adult with *Histoplasma* meningitis refractory to amphotericin B therapy.[132]

Coccidioidomycosis

C. immitis meningitis is more common than *Histoplasma* as a cause of chronic meningitis. Approximately 1 per cent of children with symptomatic pulmonary disease develop disseminated disease.[62] From 15 to 20 per cent of patients with disseminated coccidioidomycosis develop meningitis.[62, 66] Exposure history is very important in this disease and relies on careful questioning of the patient about travel to or residence in an endemic area.[129, 130] Additionally, exposure of wounds by colonized soil has been implicated in at least one pediatric case.[93]

CSF shows a mononuclear pleocytosis with an elevated protein and decreased glucose concentration. Diagnosis of coccidioidal meningitis is made easier by the availability of reliable serologic tests. Smith and associates[124] showed that complement-fixing antibodies appeared in the CSF only in patients with meningitis and provided a sensitivity of 76 per cent. Ninety-six per cent sensitivity was seen when the complement-fixation test was incubated at 4° C.[98] McGinnis,[88] in his review of the literature based on pooling five studies, showed that *Coccidioides* could be cultured from the CSF in 76 per cent of patients with meningitis and was seen on direct examination of the CSF in only 8 per cent of the cases. He concluded that these values were too high and were likely skewed because of reporting bias. Other experts in the field also believe that the rate of positive CSF cultures is much lower (approximately 33 per cent) and that finding the organism in the CSF by direct examination is very rare.[127]

Coccidioidomycosis in infancy was described more than 40 years ago and continues to be a problem today.[134] Infants usually have severe disease with high mortality and morbidity. In the 1980s, two studies reported on children with *Coccidioides* species meningitis who were treated with oral, intravenous, or intrathecal imidazoles.[54, 119] The authors noted promising results with the use of ketoconazole and imidazole therapy when compared with standard intravenous or intrathecal amphotericin B.

If untreated, *Coccidioides* meningitis is uniformly fatal. Therapy with amphotericin B both intravenous and intrathecal reduced the mortality rate to 30 per cent.[98] The use of fluconazole has been found in adult studies to have a success rate as high as 79 per cent.[12] It appears safe in clinical use, although there has been a case report of a pregnant woman with *Coccidioides* meningitis treated with fluconazole who delivered a child with congenital malformations. However, the child was felt to have an autosomal recessive disorder (Antley-Bixler syndrome) and not teratogenic malformations due to fluconazole.[76] It appears that fluconazole may be the superior agent for sustaining remission of meningitis due to *Coccidioides* because of its oral bioavailability, the toxicity associated with amphotericin B, and the elimination of the need for intrathecal administration.[104]

Itraconazole has proven efficacy in nonmeningeal coccidioidomycosis, with 63 per cent of adult patients treated showing a complete response.[137] The use of itraconazole for meningeal involvement led to great hope for the use of an oral agent in this disease.[135] Unfortunately, adult patients with *Coccidioides* meningitis had high relapse rates (40 to 50 per cent), which made them dependent on lifelong therapy with itraconazole.[50] However, the alternative of continued intrathecal amphotericin B makes this treatment much more appealing.

At present, intravenous and intrathecal amphotericin B still is standard therapy for coccidioidal meningitis. Amphotericin B intrathecally can be administered into the lumbar area, into the cisterna magna or by using an Ommaya reservoir.[30, 43, 71, 152] In younger children, intraventricular or intracisternal therapy using the Ommaya reservoir allows ease of administration but has the disadvantage of increased susceptibility to secondary bacterial infection. The initial dose of amphotericin B into the CSF is 0.025 mg. This then is increased by doubling the dose until a maintenance dose of 0.1 to 0.5 mg is attained. Once this dose has been achieved, therapy can be given every other day, alternating with the intravenous administration of amphotericin B. Therapy is continued until the child's condition has stabilized, and at this point intrathecal therapy gradually can be stretched out to every 3 weeks. This is continued until the CSF indices are normal and cultures have been negative for at least 1 year. Miconazole, an imidazole compound, also has been used in the treatment of *Coccidioides* meningitis and, in combination with oral ketoconazole, has had good results in nine children.[119] Fluconazole in a dose of 400 to 600 mg/day for 9 to 12 months has been shown to be effective in adults.[42, 136] A corresponding dose of 6 mg/kg/day in pediatric patients also has been used, but no controlled studies using this agent in pediatric patients have been published to date.

Blastomycosis

Blastomyces dermatitidis is an uncommon cause of chronic meningitis, which is difficult to diagnose premortem unless the patient has other signs of systemic blastomycosis. However, when systemic blastomycosis occurs, it is not uncommon for it to involve the CNS in up to 5 per cent of cases.[18] Common sites for this organism include bone, genitourinary tract, and skin.[9, 19] Although examination of CSF obtained by lumbar puncture usually is negative (9 per cent sensitivity), ventricular fluid (four of four patients tested) appears to have a higher yield.[70] Typically, fungal meningitis is associated with a lymphocytic pleocytosis; however, meningitis due to *B. dermatitidis* frequently has a neutrophilic predominance.[53] Previously, blastomycosis most often affected patients who were immunocompetent. Recent reports indicate that patients with AIDS are at a high risk of chronic infection.[53] Because of the difficulty in diagnosing meningitis due to *B. dermatitidis* and the similarities to tuberculous meningitis, patients usually are treated for presumptive tuberculous meningitis.[47, 92] Although meningitis is the most common form of CNS blastomycosis, solitary mass lesions also can occur.[111]

Diagnosis relies on the characteristic histopathologic appearance in tissues and occasionally culture of CSF obtained from the ventricles. However, if the difficulty in performing these procedures is prohibitive, looking for other sources of blastomycosis is indicated, including sputum and urine. A study in AIDS patients showed that sputum examination was useful for the diagnosis of disseminated blastomycosis.[99]

Treatment of systemic blastomycosis including meningitis relies on amphotericin B in a dose of 1 mg/kg/day.[126] Duration of therapy is unknown, but adults with systemic disease usually require a minimum of 2 g to prevent relapse of nonmeningeal disease.[100] In adult patients who have been "cured" of their meningitis, doses between 2400 and 3150 mg were required. This would correspond to a total dose of 35 to 45 mg/kg in a child.

Aspergillosis

Central nervous system *Aspergillus fumigatus* infections as well as infections with other *Aspergillus* species in immunocompromised patients usually are fatal. Conditions that place the patient at risk include organ transplantation, malignancies, and neutropenia. In most reported cases, patients were receiving high-dose corticosteroid therapy in addition to broad-spectrum antibiotics.[10, 72] In many cases, fever was present and pulmonary findings preceded neurologic manifestations. *Aspergillus* infection of the CNS usually is acquired by hematogenous spread from the lungs. Other modes of acquisition include extension from a contiguous focus (sinuses) and intravenous drug abuse.[91]

Brain abscesses are the most typical manifestation of *Aspergillus* species infection in the CNS, but meningoencephalitis, isolated spinal cord lesions, and mycotic aneurysms also have been described.[25, 37, 146, 151] The use of magnetic resonance imaging has been suggested to be superior to computed tomography for the delineation of lesions in the CNS in patients with bone marrow transplantation.[90] The lesions are consistent with acute infarcts.

Some of the early reports of CNS aspergillosis occurred in infants who appeared to be normal.[1, 84] The diagnosis of meningitis relies on CSF cultures, but frequently the results of a bronchoscopy or biopsy will be more helpful and provide a more expedient diagnosis. Because the disease is uniformly fatal, the importance of treating pulmonary aspergillosis before the development of meningeal involvement cannot be overemphasized. Amphotericin B in doses of 1 to 1.5 mg/kg/day is recommended with or without the addition of flucytosine and/or rifampin.[48, 142]

Sporotrichosis

Sporothrix schenckii, although a primarily lymphocutaneous disease, has been reported to cause meningitis.[34, 40, 68, 102, 121] It is suggested that meningeal seeding occurs via hematogenous spread from the lungs, as is seen in most other fungal infections.[34] Meningeal involvement with sporotrichosis produces similar CSF indices and abnormalities as seen with the other fungal meningitides.[33] The use of CSF fungal culture is insensitive for the diagnosis of meningitis due to sporotrichosis. The use of *S. schenckii* antibody in the CSF has been shown to be effective in diagnosing meningitis in patients without other overt signs of this infection.[116]

Treatment of this infection is very difficult. Amphotericin B alone has been successful on occasion. Some experts recommend the addition of flucytosine, but no studies have evaluated the efficacy of this combination. The azoles, particularly itraconazole, had excellent results in nonmeningeal disease, but successful treatment of meningitis with this agent has not been proved.

Mucormycosis

Meningitis due to *Mucor* species as well as other zygomycetes usually occurs as a result of direct extension from paranasal sinus disease. Infection with these organisms most commonly is seen in the immunocompromised host and particularly in patients with diabetes mellitus or those receiving high doses of corticosteroids. Patients (particularly dialysis patients) undergoing chelation therapy with deferoxamine have been found to be at risk for infection.[16, 17, 64, 150] The association with deferoxamine therapy is seen with *Cunninghamella*.[109] *Mucor* causing CNS disease has been reported in children but is very rare.[51, 59] Treatment employs amphotericin B in doses of 1 to 1.5 mg/kg/day but usually is unsuccessful. Surgical excision of rhinocerebral infection is recommended along with antifungal therapy.

Other Fungal Infections

Acremonium species are common soil fungi that may cause chronic meningitis in humans.[96] *Xylohypha bantiana*, an uncommon dematiaceous fungus, has been reported to have caused a fungal brain abscess in an adolescent girl; this report increases the number of cases reported in the literature to nearly 40.[95] Cerebral chromoblastomycosis also has been reported.[120] Other fungal organisms causing CNS infection include *Paracoccidioides brasiliensis* (South American blastomycosis),[103] *Prototheca wickerhamii*,[63] *B. capitatus*,[45] *Rhodotorula* species,[86, 105] and *Pseudoallescheria boydii*.[13]

DIAGNOSIS

Specific information about each organism's diagnosis is discussed in previous sections. Table 40–1 provides specific data for some of the fungal meningitides. Overall, the problem with diagnosing many of these infections is that most have nonspecific signs and symptoms without reference to the CNS. Also, standard culture media may not be useful for these organisms, and cultures can take weeks before an organism is identified. The use of antigen and antibody testing has proved quite useful for the diagnosis of *Cryptococcus*, *Coccidioides*, and *Histoplasma* infections. It is hoped that polymerase chain reaction technology may be helpful in the future as it has been for bacterial and mycobacterial diagnoses.

CSF may be helpful in some instances. As much CSF as can be removed safely should be obtained, especially at the time of ventriculography or pneumoencephalography.[33] A minimum of 5 mL of spinal fluid has been suggested, based on experimental work.[82] Repeated cultures of large volumes of CSF may be helpful.[33] The fluid obtained should be centrifuged and the sediment saved for culture and India ink preparation, while the supernatant is sent for serologic tests. Use of the India ink should be interpreted with caution and must be followed up with cultures because artifacts frequently can cause misinterpretation.[33] The cumulative efficacy of repeated lumbar punctures for cryptococcal meningitis improved the sensitivity of the India ink smear from 26 per cent in one lumbar puncture to 52.6 per cent with the second.[88] If large volumes are available, membrane filtration may be used to concentrate the fungal elements. The membrane containing the fungi is placed aseptically on isolation media and incubated at 30° C for up to 4 weeks. The CSF that passes through the membrane then can be used for serology or chemistry determinations.[88] The remaining CSF can be inoculated onto Sabouraud glucose agar, blood agar, and brain-heart infusion agar or into broth media or into both types of media. CSF cultures for *Histoplasma*, *Blastomyces*, and other dimorphic fungi generally are unhelpful.

Serologic techniques are extremely useful for *Cryptococcus* and *Coccidioides*. Approximately 100 per cent sensitivity is seen with serum cryptococcal antigen tests in HIV-positive patients.[28, 69, 153] The CSF antigen test in HIV-positive patients appears in some studies to be less sensitive (91 per cent).[27] In patients not HIV-infected, the sensitivity of the serologic test in the CSF approaches 90 per cent.[55] For coccidioidal meningitis, the sensitivity rate is more than 76 per cent.[98, 124]

Candida can be cultured but may require a prolonged incubation period, necessitating empiric therapy while awaiting cultures. For other organisms, such as *Histoplasma*, *Blastomyces*, and *Coccidioides*, it can be helpful to culture other body fluids, such as blood, urine, sputum, or draining wounds.

ANTIFUNGAL AGENTS AND TREATMENT GUIDELINES

Amphotericin B remains the treatment of choice for most CNS fungal infections. Amphotericin B has less than 5 per cent oral bioavailability and is more than 90 per cent protein bound.[14] It has a very prolonged terminal elimination half-life of 15 days, with only about 3 per cent of the parent compound found unchanged in the urine.[7] CSF concentrations are about 2 to 4 per cent of those found in serum.[43, 140] The dose recommended varies, depending upon the organism and the severity of the illness. However, in most children and infants, a dose of 1 mg/kg/day appears to be satisfactory, particularly in view of the increased clearance of the drug compared with that in adults.[12, 125] Table 40–2 gives guidelines for initiating therapy in infants and children with fungal meningitis.

Toxicity and adverse effects are universal with the use of amphotericin B. Acetaminophen and diphenhydramine may be helpful in reducing the incidence of fever, nausea, and chills. The use of hydrocortisone to reduce febrile reactions has been documented to be effective.[139] However, great variability of patient responses to this treatment occurs. Addi-

TABLE 40–1. Fungal Cerebrospinal Fluid Characteristics[47, 54, 88, 148]

Organism	WBCs	Protein	Glucose	Smears	Serology	Cultures
Blastomyces	Variable up to 15,000 cells/mm³ with PMNs or lymphocytes	Elevated up to 300 mg/dL	Normal or low	Rare on smear	No good serology	CSF cultures rarely +; increased yield with ventricular taps
Candida	Mean = 600 cells/mm³ up to 1900 cells/mm³ with lymphocytes or PMNs	Elevated	Low or normal	40% + on smears	Serology not helpful	CSF cultures useful
Coccidioides	100–750 WBCs mostly lymphocytes	150–2000 mg/dL	21–62% serum	Rare on smear	CSF CF Ab + in 75–95%	CSF cultures + in 33–60%
Cryptococcus	40–400 WBCs mostly lymphocytes	High	Low	India ink + in 25–50%	CSF and serum cryptococcal Ag + in 85–90%	CSF cultures + in 75%
Histoplasma	0–300 WBCs lymphocytes or PMNs; most 11–101/mm³	Usually elevated but can be normal	Usually low (<40 mg/dL) to normal	Rare on smear	Polysaccharide Ag in urine, blood, CSF + in 61%	CSF cultures + in 27–65%

+, positive; Ab, antibody; Ag, antigen; CF, complement fixation; CSF, cerebrospinal fluid; PMNs, polymorphonuclear leukocytes; WBCs, white blood cells

TABLE 40–2. Guidelines for Administration of Amphotericin B

Administer a test dose of 1 mg (0.1 mg/kg for infants weighing less than 10 kg) by mixing in 25–50 mL dextrose 5% in water infused over 20–30 minutes.
If the patient develops a reaction to the test dose or develops cardiopulmonary impairment, cautiously try a second dose of 50–100 μg.
If this is tolerated, the drug should be prepared in a concentration of 0.1 mg/mL of 5% dextrose with phosphate buffers. DO NOT USE 0.9% NaCl solution, which will precipitate the drug.
For uncomplicated infections, institute therapy with 0.25 mg/kg administered over 2–6 hours after the test dose is complete.
Increase the daily dose on subsequent days to the maximum dose for the specific infection being treated (up to 1.5 mg/kg/day for *Aspergillus*).
If the patient is critically ill or immunocompromised, the physician can proceed directly to the full therapeutic dose after the test dose by increasing the dose in increments of 0.25 mg/kg every 6 to 12 hours.

tionally, the use of corticosteroids can potentiate water retention and amphotericin B–induced hypokalemia; thus, the dosage of corticosteroids should be kept to a minimum.[43] If chills occur, they can be terminated with the use of meperidine.[20]

Amphotericin B induces reversible impairment of renal function in 80 per cent of patients during the first 2 weeks of therapy.[23] In most cases, renal function returns to normal after cessation of the drug. The manifestations of its toxicity include renal tubular acidosis, azotemia, oliguria, and potassium/magnesium wasting. Other nephrotoxic drugs worsen the azotemia. Renal failure in adult studies has been shown to be ameliorated by the use of salt loading.[56] The adult studies used 500 cc of 0.9 per cent sodium chloride solution as pre- and posthydration; in children, 10 mL/kg appears to work as well. Hypokalemia along with hypomagnesemia occurs frequently and may require supplementation. A normocytic, normochromic anemia occurs in many patients who receive amphotericin B, with an 18 to 35 per cent decrease in hemoglobin seen after 10 weeks of therapy; this anemia appears partially related to changes in erythropoietin levels.[85]

Collaborative studies in adult patients with CNS cryptococcosis without HIV have shown that initial therapy with amphotericin B (0.3 mg/kg/day) and flucytosine (150 mg/kg/day) results in better outcomes than amphotericin B alone (0.6 mg/kg/day).[11] Because amphotericin B induces azotemia and thus can result in the accumulation of toxic levels of flucytosine, most authorities have recommended reducing the dose of flucytosine to 75 to 100 mg/kg/day and maintaining serum flucytosine levels between 25 and 60 μg/mL.[6, 39] The importance of repeated CSF cultures is the cornerstone of therapy and must be emphasized. Although cryptococcal antigen is extremely useful as a diagnostic aid, the conversion of CSF cultures to negative is the critical feature for clinical success. Lifetime maintenance with fluconazole is the standard of care for cryptococcal meningitis in patients with AIDS. If amphotericin B must be used as maintenance therapy, a dose of 1 mg/kg intravenous once to twice weekly is given for the rest of the patient's life.

Intravenous amphotericin B, in combination with intrathecal therapy, is for severe, coccidioidal CNS infections. The total duration of therapy is variable and sometimes requires treatment for several years. As in cryptococcal disease, patients with AIDS require lifetime suppressive therapy.

Candidal meningitis usually responds to therapy with intravenous amphotericin B alone or in combination with oral flucytosine. *Histoplasma* meningitis generally is treated with amphotericin B alone, without intrathecal therapy. In the rare cases of CNS infections due to *B. dermatitides, S. schenckii,* and *Aspergillus* species, intravenous amphotericin B is considered to be the drug of choice. CNS *Aspergillus* infection should be treated with 1 to 1.5 mg/kg/day; therapy is quite prolonged, sometimes for several months.

Ketoconazole has not been an effective agent for most fungal CNS disease processes. It has been supplanted by the newer azoles, fluconazole and itraconazole, because of their better bioavailability and more favorable results in recent clinical trials.

Fluconazole is a very effective agent for the suppression of cryptococcal meningitis in AIDS as well as immunocompetent patients and appears in fact to be superior to amphotericin B in AIDS patients for prolonged maintenance therapy. Fluconazole absorption by the gastrointestinal tract is not affected by the presence of food or gastric acidity.[15] Fluconazole is highly water-soluble and minimally bound to plasma proteins.[75] The terminal elimination half-life of fluconazole is 22 to 31 hours, with 80 per cent of the drug excreted unchanged in the urine.[29] Fluconazole readily penetrates into CSF in inflamed or noninflamed meninges, achieving levels that are 60 to 80 per cent of serum levels. Rifampin, cyclosporin A, and phenytoin have significant interactions with fluconazole. Adverse effects are relatively uncommon, especially when compared with those associated with amphotericin B. Nausea and vomiting occur in less than 5 per cent of patients. Asymptomatic elevations of plasma aminotransferases occur in less than 1 to 7 per cent of patients.[29] In children with cryptococcal meningitis, a dose comparable to the adult loading dose of 8 mg/kg/day (400 mg daily, maximum dose) is used, followed by 4 to 6 mg/kg/day (200 mg daily, maximum dose) for 10 to 12 weeks after sterilization of the CSF. Maintenance therapy for cryptococcal meningitis in patients with AIDS is 4 to 6 mg/kg/day (200 mg daily, maximum dose).

Data for itraconazole use in pediatrics are very limited, and itraconazole is not recommended at this time for CNS fungal infections in children. Itraconazole has increased absorption when taken with food.[143] Itraconazole is highly protein-bound (>99 per cent); less than 1 per cent is excreted unchanged in urine.[49] CSF concentrations are relatively low compared with those of fluconazole; however, itraconazole is much more lipophilic, allowing it to show efficacy in treatment of some fungal meningitides. Additional data should be forthcoming in the next several years on this and the other azoles, particularly for treatment of coccidioidal meningitis in children. Promising results in an adult study have been published.[135]

CONCLUSION

With the large increase of immunocompromised children in the last 10 years due to the epidemic of HIV, the advent of new antineoplastic agents, the growth of organ transplantation, and the increased use of corticosteroids, the relative rarity of fungal meningitides has been replaced by a burgeoning upswing in the incidence and prevalence of these infections. New modalities for diagnosis are needed because many of these fungal infections still require weeks for identification. We expect that trials in progress will help determine and differentiate which azole is comparable or superior to amphotericin B for the treatment of many fungal meningitides.

References

1. Allan, G. W., and Anderson, D. H.: Generalized aspergillosis in an infant 18 days of age. Pediatrics *26*:432–440, 1960.
2. al-Rasheed, S. A., and al-Fawaz, I. M.: Cryptococcal meningitis in a child with systemic lupus erythematosus. Ann. Trop. Paediatr. *10*:323–326, 1990.
3. Ampel, N. M., Wieden, M. A., and Galgiani, J. N.: Coccidioidomycosis: Clinical update. Rev. Infect. Dis. *11*:897, 1989.
4. Anaissie, E., Fainstein, V., Samo, T., et al.: Central nervous system histoplasmosis: An unappreciated complication of the acquired immunodeficiency syndrome. Am. J. Med. *84*:215–217, 1988.
5. Arisoy, E. S., Arisoy, A. E., Dunne, W. M., Jr.: Clinical significance of fungi isolated from cerebrospinal fluid in children. Pediatr. Infect. Dis. J. *13*:128–133, 1994.
6. Armstrong, D.: Treatment of opportunistic fungal infections. Clin. Infect. Dis. *16*:1–9, 1993.
7. Atkinson, A. J., and Bennett, J. E.: Amphotericin B pharmacokinetics in humans. Antimicrob. Agents Chemother. *13*:271, 1978.
8. Baley, J. E., Kliegman, R. M., and Fanaroff, A. A.: Disseminated fungal infections in very low-birth-weight infants: Clinical manifestations and epidemiology. Pediatrics *73*:144–152, 1984.
9. Baumgardner, D. J., Buggy, B. P., Mattson, B. J., et al.: Epidemiology of blastomycosis in a region of high endemicity in north central Wisconsin. Clin. Infect. Dis. *15*:629–635, 1992.
10. Beal, M. F., O'Carroll, C. P., Kleinman, G. M., et al.: Aspergillosis of the central nervous system. Neurology *32*:473–479, 1982.
11. Bennett, J. E., Dismukes, W. E., Duma, R. J., et al.: A comparison of amphotericin B alone and combined with flucytosine in the treatment of cryptococcal meningitis. N. Engl. J. Med. *301*:126–131, 1979.
12. Benson, J. M., and Nahata, M. C.: Pharmacokinetics of amphotericin B in children. Antimicrob. Agents Chemother. *33*:1989–1993, 1989.
13. Berenguer, J., Diaz-Mediavilla, J., Urra, D., et al.: Central nervous system infection caused by *Pseudoallescheria boydii*: Case report and review. Rev. Infect. Dis. *11*:890–896, 1989.
14. Block, E. R., Bennett, J. E., Livoti, L. G., et al.: Flucytosine and amphotericin B: Hemodialysis effects on the plasma concentration and clearance. Ann. Intern. Med. *80*:613–617, 1974.
15. Blum, R., A., D'Andrea, D. T., Florentino, B. M., et al.: Increased gastric pH and the bioavailability of fluconazole and ketoconazole. Ann. Intern. Med. *114*:755–757, 1991.
16. Boelaert, J. R., de Locht, M., Van Cutsem, J., et al.: Mucormycosis during deferoxamine therapy is a siderophore-mediated infection: In vitro and in vivo animal studies. J. Clin. Invest. *91*:1979–1986, 1993.
17. Boelaert, J. R., Vergauwe, P. L., and Vandepitte, J. M.: Mucormycosis infection in dialysis patients. Ann. Intern. Med. *107*:782–783, 1987.
18. Bradsher, R. W.: Blastomycosis. Clin. Infect. Dis. *14*(Suppl. 1):S582–S590, 1992.
19. Bradsher, R. W., Rice, D. C., and Abernathy, R. S.: Ketoconazole therapy for endemic blastomycosis. Ann. Intern. Med. *103*:872–879, 1985.
20. Burks, L. C., Aisner, J., Fortner, C. L., et al.: Meperidine for the treatment of shaking chills and fever. Arch. Intern. Med. *140*:483–484, 1980.
21. Butler, K. M., Rench, M. A., and Baker, C. J.: Amphotericin B as a single agent in the treatment of systemic candidiasis in neonates. Pediatr. Infect. Dis. J. *9*:51–56, 1990.
22. Butler, W. T., Alling, D. W., Spickard, A., et al.: Diagnostic and prognostic value of clinical and laboratory findings in cryptococcal meningitis: A follow-up study of forty patients. N. Engl. J. Med. *270*:59–66, 1964.
23. Butler, W. T., Bennett, J. E., Alling, D. W., et al.: Nephrotoxicity of amphotericin B: Early and late effects in 81 patients. Ann. Intern. Med. *61*:175–187, 1964.
24. Byers, M., Feldman, S., and Edwards, J.: Disseminated histoplasmosis as the acquired immunodeficiency syndrome-defining illness in an infant. Pediatr. Infect. Dis. J. *11*:127–128, 1992.
25. Casey, A. T., Wilkins, P., and Uttley, D.: Aspergillosis infection in neurosurgical practice. Br. J. Neurosurg. *8*:31–39, 1994.
26. Chen, J. Y.: Neonatal candidiasis associated with meningitis and endophthalmitis. Acta Pediatr. Jpn. *36*:261–265, 1994.
27. Chuck, S. L., and Sande, M. A.: Infections with *Cryptococcus neoformans* in the acquired immunodeficiency syndrome. N. Engl. J. Med. *321*:794–799, 1989.
28. Clark, R. A., Greer, D., Atkinson, W., et al.: Spectrum of *Cryptococcus neoformans* infection in 68 patients infected with human immunodeficiency virus. Rev. Infect. Dis. *12*:768–777, 1990.
29. Como, J. A., and Dismukes, W. E.: Oral azole drugs as systemic antifungal therapy. N. Engl. J. Med. *330*:263–272, 1994.
30. Dennis, M., and Rusch, J. R.: The Ommaya Reservoir in fungal meningitis: A case report. *In* Ajello, L. (ed.): Coccidioidomycosis. Tucson, University of Arizona Press, 1967, pp. 119–122.
31. Diamond, R. D.: *Cryptococcus neoformans. In* Mandell, G. L., Bennett, J. E., and Dolin, R. (eds.): Principles and Practice of Infectious Diseases. 4th ed. New York, Churchill Livingstone, 1995, pp. 2331–2340.
32. Dismukes, W. E.: Cryptococcal meningitis in patients with AIDS. J. Infect. Dis. *157*:624–628, 1988.
33. Ellner, J. J., and Bennett, J. E.: Chronic meningitis. Medicine *55*:341–396, 1976.
34. Ewing, G. E., Bosl, G. J., and Peterson, P. K.: *Sporothrix schenckii* meningitis in a farmer with Hodgkin's disease. Am. J. Med. *68*:455–457, 1980.
35. Faix, R. G.: Systemic *Candida* infections in infants in intensive care nurseries: High incidence of central nervous system involvement. J. Pediatr. *105*:616–622, 1984.
36. Faix, R. G., Kovarik, S. M., Shaw, T. R., et al.: Mucocutaneous and invasive candidiasis among very low birth weight (<1500 grams) infants in intensive care nurseries: A prospective study. Pediatrics *83*:101–107, 1989.
37. Feely, M., and Steinberg, M.: *Aspergillus* infection complicating transsphenoidal yttrium-90 pituitary implant. J. Neurosurg. *46*:530–532, 1977.
38. Flynn, P. M., Marina, N. M., Rivera, G. K., et al.: *Candida tropicalis* infections in children with leukemia. Leuk. Lymphoma *10*:369–376, 1993.
39. Francis, P., and Walsh, T. J.: Evolving role of flucytosine in immunocompromised patients: New insights into safety, pharmacokinetics, and antifungal therapy. Clin. Infect. Dis. *15*:1003–1008, 1992.
40. Freeman, J. W., and Ziegler, D. K.: Chronic meningitis caused by *Sporotrichum schenckii*. Neurology *27*:989–992, 1977.
41. Furcolow, M. L., Chick, E. W., Busey, J. F., et al.: Prevalence and incidence studies of human and canine blastomycosis. I. Cases in the United States, 1885–1968. Am. Rev. Respir. Dis. *102*:60–67, 1970.
42. Galgiani, J., N., Catanzaro, A., Cloud, G. A., et al.: Fluconazole therapy for coccidioidal meningitis: The NIAID-Mycoses Study Group. Ann. Intern. Med. *119*:28–35, 1993.
43. Gallis, H. A., Drew, R. H., and Pickard, W. W.: Amphotericin B: 30 years of clinical experience. Rev. Infect. Dis. *12*:308–329, 1990.
44. Gelfand, J. A., and Bennett, J. E.: Active *Histoplasma* meningitis of 22 years duration. J. A. M. A. *233*:1294–1295, 1975.
45. Girmenia, C., Micozzi, A., Venditti, M., et al.: Fluconazole treatment of *Blastoschizomyces capitatus* meningitis in an allogeneic bone marrow recipient. Eur. J. Clin. Microbiol. Infect. Dis. *10*:752–756, 1991.
46. Glick, C., Graves, C. R., and Feldman, S.: Neonatal fungemia and amphotericin B. South. Med. J. *86*:1368–1371, 1993.
47. Gonyea, E. F.: The spectrum of primary blastomycotic meningitis: A review of central nervous system blastomycosis. Ann. Neurol. *3*:26–39, 1978.
48. Gordon, M. A., Holzman, R. S., Senter, H., et al.: *Aspergillus oryzae* meningitis. J. A. M. A. *235*:2122–2123, 1976.
49. Grant, S. M., and Clissold, S. P.: Itraconazole: A review of its pharmacodynamic and pharmacokinetic properties and therapeutic use in superficial and systemic mycoses. Drugs *37*:310–344, 1989.
50. Graybill, J. R.: Future directions of antifungal chemotherapy. Clin. Infect. Dis. *14*(Suppl. 1):S170–S181, 1992.
51. Hale, L. M.: Orbital cerebral phycomycosis: Report of a case and a review of the disease in infants. Arch. Ophthalmol. *86*:39–43, 1971.
52. Hamner, R. W., Baum, E. W., and Pritchett, P. S.: Coccidioidal meningitis diagnosed by skin biopsy. Cutis *29*:603–610, 1982.
53. Harley, W. B., Lomis, M., and Haas, D. W.: Marked polymorphonuclear pleocytosis due to blastomycotic meningitis: Case report and review. Clin. Infect. Dis. *18*:816–818, 1994.
54. Harrison, H. R., Galgiani, J. N., Reynolds, A. F., Jr., et al.: Amphotericin B and imidazole therapy for coccidioidal meningitis in children. Pediatr. Infect. Dis. *2*:216–221, 1983.
55. Hay, R. J., Mackenzie, D. W. R., Campbell, C. K., et al.: Cryptococcosis in the United Kingdom and the Irish Republic: An analysis of 69 cases. J. Infect. *2*:13–22, 1980.
56. Heidemann, H. T., Gerkens, J. F., Spickard, W. A., et al.: Amphotericin B nephrotoxicity in humans decreased by salt repletion. Am. J. Med. *75*:476–481, 1983.
57. Imperato, P. J., Buckley, C. E., and Callaway, J. L.: *Candida* granuloma. Arch. Dermatol. *97*:139–146, 1968.
58. Isaacs, D., Barfield, C. P., Grimwood, K., et al.: Systemic bacterial and fungal infections in infants in Australian neonatal units: Australian Study Group for Neonatal Infections. Med. J. Aust. *162*:198–201, 1995.
59. Isaacson, C., and Levin, S. E.: Gastrointestinal mucormycosis in infancy. S. Afr. Med. J. *35*:581–584, 1961.
60. Jafari, H. S., Saez-Llorens, X., Grimprel, E., et al.: Characteristics of experimental *Candida albicans* infection of the central nervous system in rabbits. J. Infect. Dis. *164*:389–395, 1991.
61. Johnson, D. E., Thompson, T. R., Green, T. P., et al.: Systemic candidiasis in very low-birth-weight infants (<1500 grams). Pediatrics *73*:138–143, 1984.
62. Kafka, J. A., and Catanzaro, A.: Disseminated coccidioidomycosis in children. J. Pediatr. *98*:355–361, 1981.
63. Kaminski, Z. C., Kapila, R., Sharer, L. R., et al.: Meningitis due to *Prototheca wickerhamii* in a patient with AIDS. Clin. Infect. Dis. *15*:704–706, 1992.
64. Kaneko, T., Abe, F., Ito, M., et al.: Intestinal mucormycosis in a hemodialysis patient treated with desferrioxamine. Acta. Pathol. Jpn. *41*:561–566, 1991.
65. Karalakulasingam, R., Arora, K. K., and Adams, G.: Meningoencephalitis caused by *Histoplasma capsulatum*: Occurrence in a renal transplant and review of the literature. Arch. Intern. Med. *136*:217–220, 1976.
66. Kelly, P. C.: Coccidioidal meningitis. *In* Stevens, D. A. (ed.): Coccidioidomycosis: A Text. New York, Plenum Medical Book Co., 1980, pp. 163–194.
67. Klein, B. S., Vergeront, J. M., Weeks, R. J., et al.: Isolation of *Blastomyces dermatitidis* in soil associated with a large outbreak of blastomycosis in Wisconsin. N. Engl. J. Med. *314*:529–534, 1986.

68. Klein, R. C., Ivens, M. S., Seabury, J. H., et al.: Meningitis due to *Sporotrichum schenckii.* Arch. Intern. Med. *118*:145–149, 1966.
69. Kovacs, J. A., Kovacs, A. A., Polis, M., et al.: Cryptococcosis in the acquired immunodeficiency syndrome. Ann. Intern. Med. *103*:533–538, 1985.
70. Kravitz, G. R., Davies, S. F., Eckman, M. R., et al.: Chronic blastomycotic meningitis. Am. J. Med. *71*:501–505, 1981.
71. Kucers, A., and Bennett, N. McK.: Amphotericin B. *In* Kucers, A., and Bennett, N. McK. (eds.): The Use of Antibiotics. 4th ed. Philadelphia, J. B. Lippincott, 1987, pp. 1441–1477.
72. Lammens, M., Robberecht, W., Waer, M., et al.: Purulent meningitis due to aspergillosis in a patient with systemic lupus erythematosus. Clin. Neurol. Neurosurg. *94*:39–43, 1992.
73. Larsen, R. A., Bozzette, S. A., Jones, B. E., et al.: Fluconazole combined with flucytosine for treatment of cryptococcal meningitis in patients with AIDS. Clin. Infect. Dis. *19*:741–745, 1994.
74. Larsen, R. A., Leal, M. A. E., and Chan, L. S.: Fluconazole compared with amphotericin B plus flucytosine for cryptococcal meningitis in AIDS: A randomized trial. Ann. Intern. Med. *113*:183–187, 1990.
75. Lazar, J. D., and Hilligoss, D. M.: The clinical pharmacology of fluconazole. Semin. Oncol. *17*(Suppl. 6):14–18, 1990.
76. Lee, B. E., Feinberg, M., Abraham, J. J., et al.: Congenital malformations in an infant born to a woman treated with fluconazole. Pediatr. Infect. Dis. J. *11*:1062–1064, 1992.
77. Leggiadro, R. J., Barrett, F. F., and Hughes, W. T.: Extrapulmonary cryptococcosis in immunocompromised infants and children. Pediatr. Infect. Dis. J. *11*:43–47, 1992.
78. Leggiadro, R. J., Kline, M. W., and Hughes, W. T.: Extrapulmonary cryptococcosis in children with acquired immunodeficiency syndrome. Pediatr. Infect. Dis. J. *10*:658–662, 1991.
79. Leibovitz, E., Rigaud, M., Chandwani, S., et al.: Disseminated fungal infections in children infected with human immunodeficiency virus. Pediatr. Infect. Dis. J. *10*:888–894, 1991.
80. Lesser, R. L., Simon, R. M., Leon, H., et al.: Cryptococcal meningitis and internal ophthalmoplegia. Am. J. Ophthalmol. *87*:682–687, 1979.
81. Littman, M. L., and Walter, J. E.: Cryptococcosis: Current status. Am. J. Med. *45*:922–932, 1968.
82. Louria, D. B., Feder, N., Mitchell, W., et al.: Influence of fungus strain and lapse on time in experimental histoplasmosis and of volume of inoculum in cryptococcosis upon recovery of the fungi. J. Lab. Clin. Med. *53*:311–317, 1959.
83. Ludviksson, B. R., Thorarensen, O., Gudnason, T., et al.: *Candida albicans* meningitis in a child with myeloperoxidase deficiency. Pediatr. Infect. Dis. J. *12*:162–164, 1993.
84. Luke, J. L., Bolande, R. P., and Gross, S.: Generalized aspergillosis and *Aspergillus endocarditis* in infancy. Pediatrics *31*:115–122, 1963.
85. MacGregor, R. R., Bennett, J. E., and Erslev, A. J.: Erythropoietin concentration in amphotericin B-induced anemia. Antimicrob. Agents Chemother. *14*:270–273, 1978.
86. Marinova, I., Szabadosova, V., Brandeburova, O., et al.: *Rhodotorula* spp. fungemia in an immunocompromised boy after neurosurgery successfully treated with miconazole and 5-flucytosine: case report and review of the literature. Chemotherapy *40*:287–289, 1994.
87. McDonald, R., Greenberg, E. N., and Kramer, R.: Cryptococcal meningitis. Arch. Dis. Child. *45*:417–420, 1970.
88. McGinnis, M. R.: Detection of fungi in cerebrospinal fluid. Am. J. Med. *75*:129–138, 1983.
89. McManus, E. J., and Jones, J. M.: Detection of a *Trichosporon beigelii* antigen cross-reactive with *Cryptococcus neoformans* capsular polysaccharide in serum from a patient with disseminated *Trichosporon* infection. J. Clin. Microbiol. *21*:681–685, 1985.
90. Miaux, Y., Ribaud, P., Williams, M, et al.: MR of cerebral aspergillosis in patients who have had bone marrow transplantation. Am. J. Neuroradiol. *16*:555–562, 1995.
91. Morrow, R., Wong, B., Finkelstein, W. E., et al.: Aspergillosis of the cerebral ventricles in a heroin abuser: Case report and review of the literature. Arch. Intern. Med. *143*:161–164, 1983.
92. Morse, H. G., Nichol, W. P., Cook, D. M., et al.: Central nervous system and genitourinary blastomycosis: Confusion with tuberculosis. West. J. Med. *139*:99–103, 1983.
93. Morwood, D. T., Nichter, L. S., and Wong, V.: An unusual complication of an open-head injury: Coccidioidal meningitis. Ann. Plast. Surg. *23*:437–441, 1989.
94. Nicholas, S. W., Dondheimer, D. L., Willoughby, A. D., et al.: Human immunodeficiency virus infection in childhood, adolescence, and pregnancy: A status report and national research agenda. Pediatrics *83*:293–308, 1989.
95. Palaoglu, S., Sav, A., Basak, T., et al.: Cerebral phaeohyphomycosis. Neurosurgery *33*:894–897, 1993.
96. Papadatos, C., Pavatou, M., and Alexiou, D.: *Cephalosporium* meningitis. Pediatrics *44*:749–751, 1969.
97. Pappagianis, D: Epidemiology of coccidioidomycosis. *In* Stevens D. A. (ed.): Coccidioidomycosis: A Text. New York, Plenum Medical, 1980, p. 63.
98. Pappagianis, D., and Crane, R.: Survival in coccidioidal meningitis since introduction of amphotericin B. *In* Ajello, L. (ed.): Coccidioidomycosis: Current Clinical and Diagnostic Status. Miami, Symposia Specialists Medical Books, 1977, pp. 223–237.
99. Pappas, P. G., Pottage, J. C., Powderly, W. G., et al.: Blastomycosis in patients with the acquired immunodeficiency syndrome. Ann. Intern. Med. *116*:847–853, 1992.
100. Parker, J. D., Doto, I. L., and Tosh, F. E.: A decade of experience with blastomycosis and its treatment with amphotericin B. Am. Rev. Respir. Dis. *99*:895–902, 1969.
101. Parsons, R. J., and Zarafonetis, C. J. D.: Histoplasmosis in man: Report of seven cases and a review of seventy-one cases. Arch. Intern. Med. *75*:1–23, 1945.
102. Penn, C. C., Goldstein, E., and Bartholomew, M. R.: *Sporothrix schenckii* meningitis in a patient with AIDS. Clin. Infect. Dis. *15*:741–743, 1992.
103. Pereira, W. C., Tenuto, R. A., Raphael, A., et al.: Localizacaco encefalica da blastomicose Sul-Americana, Arq. Neuro-Psiquiat. (Sao Paulo) *23*:113–126, 1965.
104. Perez, J. A., Jr., Johnson, R. A., Caldwell, J. W., et al.: Fluconazole therapy in coccidioidal meningitis maintained with intrathecal amphotericin B. Arch. Intern. Med. *155*:1665–1668, 1995.
105. Pore, R. S., and Chen, J.: Meningitis caused by *Rhodotorula*. Sabouoraudia *14*:331–335, 1976.
106. Powderly, W. G.: Therapy for cryptococcal meningitis in patients with AIDS. Clin. Infect. Dis. *14*(Suppl. 1):S54–S59, 1992.
107. Powderly, W. G., Saag, M. S., Cloud, G. A., et al.: A controlled trial of fluconazole or amphotericin B to prevent relapse of cryptococcal meningitis in patients with the acquired immunodeficiency syndrome. N. Engl. J. Med. *326*:793–798, 1992.
108. Rapaport, S. I., Ames, S. B., and Duvall, B. J.: A plasma coagulation defect in systemic lupus erythematosus arising from hypoprothrombinemia combined with antiprothrombinase activity. Blood *15*:212–227, 1960.
109. Rex, J. H., Ginsberg, A. M., Fries, L. F., et al.: *Cunninghamella bertholletiae* infection associated with deferoxamine therapy. Rev. Infect. Dis. *10*:1187–1194, 1988.
110. Rogers, M. F., Thomas, P. A., Starcher, E. T., et al.: Acquired immunodeficiency syndrome in children: Report of the Centers for Disease Control national surveillance, 1982–1985. Pediatrics *79*:1008–1014, 1987.
111. Ross, K. L., Bryan, J. P., Maggio, W. W., et al.: Intracranial blastomycoma. Medicine (Baltimore) *66*:224–235, 1987.
112. Saag, M. S., Powderly, W. G., Cloud, G. A., et al.: Comparison of amphotericin B with fluconazole in the treatment of acute AIDS-associated cryptococcal meningitis. N. Engl. J. Med. *326*:83–89, 1992.
113. Salaki, J. S., Louria, D. B., and Chmel, H.: Fungal and yeast infections of the central nervous system: A clinical review. Medicine (Baltimore) *63*:108–132, 1984.
114. Sarma, P. S., Durairaj, P., and Padhye, A. A.: *Candida lusitaniae* causing fatal meningitis. Postgrad. Med. J. *69*:878–880, 1993.
115. Schutze, G. E., Tucker, N. C., and Jacobs, R. F.: Histoplasmosis and perinatal human immunodeficiency virus. Pediatr. Infect. Dis. J. *11*:501–502, 1992.
116. Scott, E. N., Kaufman, L., Brown, A. C., et al.: Serologic studies in the diagnosis and management of meningitis due to *Sporothrix schenckii*. N. Engl. J. Med. *317*:935–940, 1987.
117. Sekshon, A. S., Borgorus, M. S., and Sims, H. V.: Blastomycosis: Report of three cases from Alberta with a review of Canadian cases. Mycopathologia *1*:53–63, 1979.
118. Selik, R., Starcher, E., and Curran J.: Opportunistic diseases reported in AIDS patients: Frequencies, associations, and trends. AIDS *1*:175–182, 1987.
119. Shehab, Z. M., Britton, H., and Dunn, J. H.: Imidazole therapy of coccidioidal meningitis in children. Pediatr. Infect. Dis. J. *7*:40–44, 1988.
120. Shimosaka, S., and Waga, S.: Cerebral chromoblastomycosis complicated by meningitis and multiple fungal aneurysms after resection of a granuloma: Case report. J. Neurosurg. *59*:158–161, 1983.
121. Shoemaker, E. H., Bennett, H. D., Fields, W. S., et al.: Leptomeningitis due to *Sporotrichum schenckii*. Arch. Pathol. *64*:222, 1957.
122. Siewers, C. M. F., and Cramblett, H. G.: Cryptococcosis (torulosis) in children: A report of four cases. Pediatrics *34*:393–400, 1964.
123. Smego, R. A., Perfect, J. R., and Durack, D. T.: Combined therapy with amphotericin B and 5-fluorocytosine for candida meningitis. Rev. Infect. Dis. *6*:791–801, 1984.
124. Smith, C. E., Saito, M. T., and Simons, S. A.: Pattern of 39,500 serologic tests in coccidioidomycosis. J. A. M. A. *160*:546–552, 1956.
125. Starke, J. R., Mason, E. O., Jr., Kramer, W. G., et al.: Pharmacokinetics of amphotericin B in infants and children. J. Infect. Dis. *155*:766–774, 1987.
126. Steele, R. W., and Abernathy, R. S.: Systemic blastomycosis in children. Pediatr. Infect. Dis. J. *2*:304–307, 1983.
127. Stevens, D.: *Coccidioides immitis. In* Mandell, G. L., Bennett, J. E., and Dolin, R. (eds.): Principles and Practice of Infectious Diseases. 4th ed. New York, Churchill Livingstone, 1995, pp. 2365–2375.
128. Stone, B. D., and Wheeler, J. G.: Disseminated cryptococcal infection in a patient with hyperimmunoglobinemia E syndrome. J. Pediatr. *117*:92–95, 1990.
129. Takeda, K., Oritsu, M., and Sakuta, M.: A case of coccidioidomycosis with central nervous system involvement. Rinsho Shinkeigaku *33*:1184–1187, 1993.

130. Taylor, G. D., Boettger, D. W., Miedzinski, L. J., et al.: Coccidioidal meningitis acquired during holidays in Arizona. Can. Med. Assoc. J. *142*:1388–1390, 1990.
131. Taylor, G. D., Buchanan-Chell, M., Kirkland, T., et al.: Trends and sources of nosocomial fungaemia. Mycoses *37*:187–190, 1994.
132. Tiraboschi, I., Parera, I. C., Pikielny, R., et al.: Chronic *Histoplasma capsulatum* infection of the central nervous system successfully treated with fluconazole. Eur. Neurol. *32*:70–73, 1992.
133. Tjia, T. L., Yeow, Y. K., and Tan, C. B.: Cryptococcal meningitis. J. Neurol. Neurosurg. Psychiatry *48*:853–858, 1985.
134. Townsend, T. E., and McKay, R. W.: Coccidioidomycosis in infants. Am. J. Dis. Child. *86*:51–53, 1953.
135. Tucker, R. M., Denning, D. W., Dupont, B., et al.: Itraconazole therapy for chronic coccidioidal meningitis. Ann. Intern. Med. *112*:108–112, 1990.
136. Tucker, R. M., Galgiani, J. N., Denning, D. W., et al.: Treatment of coccidioidal meningitis with fluconazole. Rev. Infect. Dis. *12*(Suppl. 3):S390–S399, 1990.
137. Tucker, R. M., Williams, P. L., Arathoon, E. G., et al.: Treatment of mycoses with itraconazole. Ann. N. Y. Acad. Sci. *544*:451–470, 1988.
138. Tynes, B. S., Crutcher, J. C., and Utz, J. P.: Histoplasma meningitis. Ann. Intern. Med. *59*:615–621, 1963.
139. Tynes, B. S., Utz, J. P, Bennett, J. E., et al.: Reducing amphotericin B reactions: A double-blind study. Am. Rev. Respir. Dis. *87*:264–268, 1963.
140. Utz, J. P., Garriques, I. L., Sande, M. A., et al: Therapy of cryptococcosis with a combination of flucytosine and amphotericin B. J. Infect. Dis. *132*:368–373, 1975.
141. Van der Horst, C., Saag, M., Cloud, G., et al.: Part 1. Randomized double-blind comparison of amphotericin B plus flucytosine (AMB + FC) to AMB alone (Step 1) followed by a comparison of fluconazole to itraconazole (Step 2) in the treatment of acute cryptococcal meningitis in patients with AIDS. Abstract #I216. Presented at 35th Interscience Conference on Antimicrobial Agents and Chemotherapy. San Francisco, September 20, 1995.
142. Van de Wyngaert, F. A., Sindic, C. J., Rousseau, J. J., et al.: Spinal arachnoiditis due to *Aspergillus meningitis* in a previously healthy patient. J. Neurol. *233*:41–43, 1986.
143. Van Peer, A., Woestenborghs, R., Heykants, J., et al.: The effects of food and dose on the oral systemic availability of itraconazole in healthy subjects. Eur J. Clin. Pharmacol. *36*:423–426, 1989.
144. Van'T Wout, J. W., DeGraeff-Meeder, E. R., Paul, L. C., et al.: Treatment of two cases of cryptococcal meningitis with fluconazole. Scand. J. Infect. Dis. *20*:193–198, 1988.
145. Venger, B. H., Landon, G., and Rose, J. E.: Solitary histoplasmoma of the thalamus: Case report and literature review. Neurosurgery *20*:784–787, 1987.
146. Venugopal, P. V., Venugopal, T. V., Thiruneelakantan, D., et al.: Cerebral aspergillosis: Report of two cases. Sabouraudia *15*:225–230, 1977.
147. Walsh, T. J.: Fungal infections complicating pediatric HIV infection. *In* Pizzo, P. A., and Wilfert, C. M. (eds.): Pediatric AIDS: The Challenge of HIV Infection in Infants, Children, and Adolescents. 2nd ed. Baltimore, Williams and Wilkins, 1994, pp. 321–343.
148. Wheat, L. J., Batteiger, B. E., and Sathapatayavongs, B.: *Histoplasma capsulatum* infections of the central nervous system: A clinical review. Medicine *69*:244–260, 1990.
149. Wheat, L. J., Connolly-Stringfield, P. A., Baker, R. L., et al.: Disseminated histoplasmosis in the acquired immune deficiency syndrome: Clinical findings, diagnosis and treatment and review of the literature. Medicine (Baltimore) *69*:361–374, 1990.
150. Windus, D. W., Stokes, J. J., Julian, B. A., et al.: Fatal *Rhizopus* infections in hemodialysis patients receiving deferoxamine. Ann. Intern. Med. *107*:678–680, 1987.
151. Young, R. C., Bennett, J. E., Vogel C. L., et al. Aspergillosis: The spectrum of the disease in 98 patients. Medicine *49*:147–173, 1970.
152. Zealear, D. S., and Winn, W. A.: The neurosurgical approach in the treatment of coccidioidal meningitis: Report of ten cases. *In* Ajello, L. (ed.): Coccidioidomycosis. Tucson, University of Arizona Press, 1967, pp. 43–53.
153. Zuger, A., Louie, E., Holzman, R. S., et al.: Cryptococcal disease in patients with the acquired immunodeficiency syndrome: Diagnostic features and outcome of treatment. Ann. Intern. Med. *104*:234–240, 1986.

41

EOSINOPHILIC MENINGITIS

Barbara W. Stechenberg

The term *eosinophilic meningitis* may include any meningitis, infectious or noninfectious, in which one finds a cerebrospinal fluid pleocytosis with a significant percentage of eosinophils. Such a finding strongly suggests invasion of the central nervous system by a helminthic parasite. In the last 20 years, the term *eosinophilic meningitis* has been applied more specifically to a typical form of meningitis caused by *Angiostrongylus cantonensis* (Chen), a rat lungworm found primarily in the Pacific Islands and Southeast Asia.

The first documented case of eosinophilic meningitis was reported from Taiwan in 1945.[1] The patient was a 15-year-old boy who developed severe headache and vomiting. Examination of the cerebrospinal fluid revealed 528 leukocytes, of which 50 per cent were eosinophils. Ten actively moving nematodes also were recovered from the specimen. Since the early 1960s, many new cases have been reported, with particularly large numbers from Thailand,[18, 19] Tahiti,[23] and Taiwan,[33] as well as Hawaii.[10]

ETIOLOGIC AGENTS

The organism that presumably is involved in the majority of cases is the rodent lungworm. *A. cantonensis,* which as an adult is 17 to 25 mm long and 0.25 to 0.36 mm at its maximum width, has a smooth cuticle and three minute lips at the cephalic end. The male has a copulatory bursa supported by bursal rays.

In its life cycle, rodents such as *Rattus rattus* are the principal hosts. These rodents ingest mollusks containing third-stage larvae, which travel from the liver and lung into the general circulation. The larvae selectively leave the circulation to enter the central nervous system within the first 48 hours. There they develop into young adults in about 2 weeks.[30] From the brain, they then travel to the pulmonary arteries, where their eggs are laid. These hatch in the pulmonary capillaries; the first-stage forms then travel from the alveolar spaces up the rat trachea to the gastrointestinal tract, from which they are eliminated in the feces. The larvae can survive for about 2 weeks under humid conditions. The third-stage larvae develop in the intermediate hosts in about 2 weeks.

More recently, another form of eosinophilic meningitis has been attributed to another nematode, *Gnathostoma spinigerum.* The adult *G. spinigerum* is stout and reddish and has a globose cephalic bulb that is separated from the body by a slight constriction. The head and anterior part of the body have spines. Males and females may be 11 to 25 mm and 25 to 54 mm in length, respectively. The adults lie coiled in lesions along the alimentary canal, from which they release eggs into the feces, where they become embryonated. The eggs hatch upon reaching water, releasing a larva that is ingested by a copepod (*Cyclops*) and continues to develop. When the infected copepod is eaten by a fish, frog, snake, or bird, a third-stage larva develops and becomes encapsulated in the intermediate host. When ingested by the definitive host (cats, dogs, hogs, mink, humans), the parasite localizes in the stomach wall.[24]

EPIDEMIOLOGY

The geographic distribution of eosinophilic meningitis depends on the distribution of *A. cantonensis.* A large number of cases have been reported from Taiwan and Thailand. Other areas include Vietnam, the Society Islands, especially Tahiti, Hawaii, the Marshall Islands, and Ponape. Rodents infected with the worm have been documented in other areas of the Pacific Islands and Asia. Disease has been reported from Cuba, Egypt, and many other countries. As infected rodents are carried to other countries on cargo ships, spread of these organisms will continue to increase. Two cases have been diagnosed in the continental United States in travelers from endemic regions.[6, 14]

The seasonal incidence of the disease varies in different areas, but the months of highest prevalence usually correspond with the more humid periods in each country.

Patients with eosinophilic meningitis have eaten terrestrial snails, slugs, fish, or freshwater shrimp, all of which can serve as intermediate hosts for the parasites.[27, 28, 29] In Thailand, the most common source is the *Pila* snails, which are eaten raw or pickled.[16] They may be served as an appetizer with alcoholic beverages; this may explain, in part, the increased incidence of the disease in males.[18] The giant African snail, *Achatina fulica,* is very common in Taiwan and may carry thousands of roundworm larvae, thus explaining the higher incidence of recovery of organisms from the patients on Taiwan.[29] The larvae also may remain infective in water for about 60 hours. Cases have been associated with the ingestion of leafy vegetables, presumed to be contaminated by slugs or snails.[10]

The distribution of disease among age groups is variable. In Thailand, most of the cases occur in the third to fourth decade of life, but in Taiwan and Hawaii, most cases occur in children younger than 15 years of age.[18, 33] Although eosinophilic meningitis has been rare in very young children, one report documented disease in five children younger than 2 years of age.[26]

PATHOGENESIS

The pathogenesis of this disease in humans has not been studied rigorously but is presumed to parallel that in the rodent host. The larvae are ingested, make their way into the general circulation, and selectively enter the central nervous system. The number of nematodes found on autopsy specimens has been varied. In a Taiwanese 5-year-old girl, 150 nematodes were found on the surface of the cerebrum and cerebellum and in the subarachnoid spaces and more than 500 were recovered from the normal saline in which the spinal cord and meninges were placed. *A. cantonensis* also were found in the pulmonary arteries.[33]

Pathologic specimens have demonstrated a leptomeningitis in which plasma cells and eosinophils predominate. There may be tortuous tracts of variable size in the brain and spinal cord parenchyma surrounded by variable reaction and degenerating neurons. Granuloma may form around dead *A. cantonensis.*[15, 22]

Hemorrhagic, necrotic tracts caused by the organisms have been associated more commonly with *G. spinigerum* infection,[4] but even *Angiostrongylus* is capable of causing a vascular reaction, including thrombosis and rupture of vessels and arteritis, leading to aneurysm formation.[15] The tracts caused by *G. spinigerum* may be larger and more necrotic.

CLINICAL MANIFESTATIONS

On the basis of information obtained from patients with a history of ingestion of the intermediate hosts, the incubation period is between 7 and 30 days. Most patients with typical eosinophilic meningitis have an abrupt onset of their disease; a more insidious onset may be noted in 20 per cent of cases. Headache is the most common and distressing symptom. It usually is intermittent but is frequent and severe. Other common symptoms are nausea; vomiting, often projectile; intermittent somnolence; malaise; anorexia; constipation; and fever with temperatures usually reaching a maximum of 38° to 39° C in the early phase of the disease, although many patients have no documented fever. Nuchal rigidity is seen more commonly in the older patients, often in association with severe headache. Paresthesias occur in a large variety of locations and are expressed as pain, numbness, itching, or a sense of worms crawling on the skin. Some patients also note diplopia with or without strabismus. Convulsions are unusual.

Physical examination is normal in half the patients. Positive physical findings may include mild hepatomegaly, mild changes in deep tendon reflexes (usually decreased), nuchal rigidity, absent abdominal wall reflexes, and, less commonly, ophthalmoplegia or facial paralysis. Twelve per cent of Thai patients had abnormal funduscopic examinations.[9]

Cerebrospinal fluid examination reveals grossly turbid or opalescent fluid in the majority of patients, with leukocyte counts usually between 100 and 5000 per mm^3. All counts usually reach their maximum in the first 3 weeks of disease, dropping sharply thereafter. In general, the percentage of eosinophils in the cerebrospinal fluid is high, often greater than 50 per cent. Fluids with higher cell counts tend to have a higher percentage of eosinophils.[19, 33] The proportion of eosinophils may decrease after the first 4 weeks. Cerebrospinal fluid protein is moderately high (often 50 to 200 mg/dL), but the glucose concentration usually is normal.

Peripheral white blood cell count is variable, but the differential cell count often shows striking eosinophilia. Examination of the feces may reveal concurrent infestation with other parasites, such as *Ascaris* or *Trichuris.*

The clinical manifestations of the eosinophilic radiculomyeloencephalitis thought to be associated with *G. spinigerum* overlap to some degree with those of typical eosinophilic meningitis. Headache, however, is less prominent. Many of the patients report sharp, shooting pains of the trunk or limbs, flaccid paralyses, and impairment of superficial sensation.[17] Impairment of the sensorium may be very sudden in association with cerebral hemorrhage. Grossly bloody spinal fluid is common when myeloencephalitis is present, but it is extremely rare in typical eosinophilic meningitis.

DIFFERENTIAL DIAGNOSIS

The diagnosis of eosinophilic meningitis caused by *A. cantonensis* can be made definitively only by isolation of the parasite from the cerebrospinal fluid. In regions where the nematodes are endemic, many cases are diagnosed only on the basis of the typical clinical manifestations and the markedly reduced probability of other causes. Serology and intradermal skin testing have been unreliable in the past, although the enzyme-linked immunosorbent assay appears to show more promise for diagnosis.[2]

Other helminths may invade the central nervous system of humans and may be associated with an eosinophilic pleocytosis.[31] These include *Taenia solium,* the pork tapeworm causing cerebrospinal cysticercosis; *Schistosoma* species; *Paragonimus westermani;* and *Echinococcus.* The diseases produced generally have a chronic and intermittent course. Signs of a space-occupying lesion and convulsions are frequent. Visceral myiasis with central nervous system invasion of the botfly larvae may cause cerebrospinal fluid eosinophilia.[3] Two cases of eosinophilic meningitis associated with the raccoon ascarid, *Baylisascaris procyonis,* have been reported, both in children.[7, 8] The larvae of *Trichinella spiralis* and *Toxocara canis* can invade the central nervous system, but pleocytosis appears to be unusual[3, 33]; the evidence for an association of eosinophilic meningitis with these parasites often is circumstantial.[11]

Neurosyphilis and tuberculous meningitis rarely have been associated with eosinophils in the cerebrospinal fluid as have several malignancies, particularly lymphomas, involving the central nervous system.[11, 13] Other known causes of significant eosinophilic pleocytosis include intrathecal injection of various foreign proteins, rabies vaccination, the insertion of rubber tubing into the central nervous system during neurosurgery, lymphocytic choriomeningitis,[11] coccidioidomycosis,[21, 25] and Rocky Mountain spotted fever.[5] Eosinophilic pleocytosis has been documented in infants with congenital toxoplasmosis and late-onset group B streptococcal meningitis.[12, 32] Eosinophilia in the cerebrospinal fluid indicating hypersensitivity has been hard to document, although one case report described the association of eosinophilic meningitis and ibuprofen therapy.[20]

TREATMENT

In a study in Thailand in which the disappearance of headache was used as the criterion for improvement, no significant differences were noted among groups when 284 patients were treated with analgesics alone, 96 patients were treated with analgesics and steroids (30 to 60 mg of prednisone daily for 5 days), and 56 patients were treated with analgesics and antibiotics (penicillin or tetracycline).[14] Treatment with thiabendazole also has been tried without significant benefit.

COURSE AND PROGNOSIS

In most patients, eosinophilic meningitis is a self-limited disease characterized by repeated attacks of severe headache, vomiting, intermittent fever, and somnolence. Many patients experience a dramatic improvement soon after a lumbar puncture, so repeated lumbar punctures may be performed at weekly intervals to relieve the headache. In the majority of patients, most symptoms disappear within 4 weeks of onset, often within a few days after the first lumbar puncture, leaving no sequelae. The mortality rate in large series from Thailand and Taiwan has been less than 5 per cent; the incidence of permanent sequelae also has been less than 5 per cent for *Angiostrongylus* infection.[19, 32] The mortality in gnathostomiasis is higher, ranging from 7.7 to 25 per cent.[24] There is no evidence that immunity develops after recovery from infection; many recurrences have been reported.[19, 23, 33]

PREVENTION

Prevention of the disease can be effected only by rodent control and proper cooking of mollusks, shrimp, fish, and other intermediate hosts. Careful washing of fruits and vegetables that may be contaminated by rodent feces also is important. The larvae may remain infective in water for as long as 60 hours, so protection of the water supply should be attempted.

References

1. Beaver, P. C., and Rosen, L.: Memorandum on the first report of *Angiostrongylus* in man by Nomura and Lin, 1945. Am. J. Trop. Med. Hyg. *13*:589–590, 1964.
2. Bhopale, M. K., Limaye, L. S., Pradhan, V. R., et al.: Studies on suspected clinical and experimental angiostrongyliasis: Serological responses. J. Hyg. Epidemiol. Microbiol. Immunol. *29*:283–288, 1985.
3. Char, D. F. B., and Rosen, L.: Eosinophilic meningitis among children in Hawaii. J. Pediatr. *70*:28–35, 1967.
4. Chitanondh, H., and Rosen, L.: Fatal eosinophilic encephalomyelitis caused by the nematode *Gnathostoma spinigerum.* Am. J. Trop. Med. Hyg. *16*:638–645, 1967.
5. Crennan, J. M., and VanScoy, R. E.: Eosinophilic meningitis caused by Rocky Mountain spotted fever. Am. J. Med. *80*:288–289, 1986.
6. Fischer, P. R.: Eosinophilic meningitis. West. J. Med. *139*:372–373, 1983.
7. Fox, A. S., Kazacos, K. R., Gould, N. S., et al.: Fatal eosinophilic meningoencephalitis and visceral larva migrans caused by the raccoon ascarid *Baylisascaris procyonis.* N. Engl. J. Med. *312*:1619–1623, 1985.
8. Huff, D. S., Neatie, R. C., Binder, M. J., et al.: Case 4: The first fatal *Baylisascaris* infection in humans: An infant with eosinophilic meningoencephalitis. Pediatr. Pathol. *2*:345–352, 1984.
9. Kanchanaranya, C., and Punyagupta, S.: Case of ocular angiostrongyliasis associated with eosinophilic meningitis. Am. J. Ophthalmol. *71*:931–934, 1971.
10. Koo, J., Pien, F., and Kliks, M. M.: *Angiostrongylus* (parastrongylus) eosinophilic meningitis. Rev. Infect. Dis. *10*:1155–1162, 1988.
11. Kuberski, T.: Eosinophils in the cerebrospinal fluid. Ann. Intern. Med. *91*:70–75, 1979.
12. Miron, D., Snelling, L. K., Josephson, S. L., et al.: Eosinophilic meningitis in a newborn with group B streptococcal infection. Pediatr. Infect. Dis. J. *12*:966–967, 1993.
13. Mulligan, M. J., Vasu, R., Grossi, C. E., et al.: Case report: Neoplastic meningitis with eosinophilic pleocytosis in Hodgkin's disease: A case with cerebellar dysfunction and a review of the literature. Am. J. Med. Sci. *296*:322–326, 1988.
14. Noskin, G. A., McMenamin, M. B., and Grohmann, S. M.: Eosinophilic meningitis due to *Angiostrongylus cantonensis.* Neurology *42*:1423–1424, 1992.
15. Nye, S. W., Tangchai, P., and Sundarakiti, S.: Lesion of the brain in eosinophilic meningitis. Arch. Pathol. *89*:9–19, 1970.
16. Punyagupta, S.: Eosinophilic meningoencephalitis in Thailand: Summary of nine cases and observations on *Angiostrongylus cantonensis* as a causative agent and *Pila ampullacea* as a new intermediate host. Am. J. Trop. Med. Hyg. *14*:370–374, 1965.
17. Punyagupta, S., Limtrakul, C., Vichipanthu, P., et al.: Radiculomyeloencephalitis associated with eosinophilic pleocytosis: Report of nine cases. Am. J. Trop. Med. Hyg. *17*:551–560, 1968.
18. Punyagupta, S., Bunnag, T., Juttijudata, P., et al.: Eosinophilic meningitis in Thailand: Epidemiologic studies of 484 typical cases and the etiologic role of *Angiostrongylus cantonensis.* Am. J. Trop. Med. Hyg. *19*:950–958, 1970.
19. Punyagupta, S., Juttijudata, P., and Bunnag, T.: Eosinophilic meningitis in Thailand: Clinical studies of 484 typical cases probably caused by *Angiostrongylus cantonensis.* Am. J. Trop. Med. Hyg. *24*:921–931, 1975.
20. Quinn, J. P., Weinstein, R. A., and Caplan, L. R.: Eosinophilic meningitis and ibuprofen therapy. Neurology *34*:108–109, 1984.
21. Ragland, A. S., Arsura, E., Ismail, Y., et al.: Eosinophilic pleocytosis in coccidioidal meningitis: frequency and significance. Am. J. Med. *95*:254–256, 1993.
22. Rosen, L., Chappel, R., Laqueur, G. L., et al.: Eosinophilic meningoencephalitis caused by a metastrongylid lungworm of rats. J. A. M. A. *179*:620–624, 1962.
23. Rosen, L., Loison, G., Laigret, J., et al.: Studies on eosinophilic meningitis. 3. Epidemiologic and clinical observations on Pacific Islands and the possible etiologic role of *Angiostrongylus cantonensis.* Am. J. Epidemiol. *85*:17–44, 1967.
24. Rusnak, J. M., and Lucey, D. R.: Clinical gnathostomiasis: Case report and review of the English language literature. Clin. Infect. Dis. *16*:33–50, 1993.
25. Schermoly, M. J., and Hinthorn, D. R.: Eosinophilia in coccidioidomycosis. Arch. Intern. Med. *148*:895–896, 1988.
26. Shih, S.-L., Hsu, C.-H., Huanig, F.-Y., et al.: *Angiostrongylus cantonensis* infection in infants and young children. Pediatr. Infect. Dis. J. *11*:1064–1065, 1992.

27. Wallace, G. D., and Rosen, L.: Studies on eosinophilic meningitis. 2. Experimental infection of shrimp and crabs with *Angiostrongylus cantonensis.* Am. J. Epidemiol. *84*:120–131, 1966.
28. Wallace, G. D., and Rosen, L.: Studies on eosinophilic meningitis. 4. Experimental infection of freshwater and marine fish with *Angiostrongylus cantonensis.* Am. J. Epidemiol. *85*:395–402, 1967.
29. Wallace, G. D., and Rosen, L.: Studies on eosinophilic meningitis. V. Molluscan hosts of *Angiostrongylus cantonensis* on Pacific Islands. Am. J. Trop. Med. Hyg. *18*:206–216, 1969.
30. Wallace, G. D., and Rosen, L.: Studies on eosinophilic meningitis. VI. Experimental infection of rats and other homoiothermic vertebrates with *Angiostrongylus cantonensis.* Am. J. Epidemiol. *89*:331–344, 1969.
31. Weller, P. F., Eosinophilic meningitis. Am. J. Med. *95*:250–253, 1993.
32. Woods, C. R., and Englund, J.: Congenital toxoplasmosis presenting with eosinophilic meningitis. Pediatr. Infect. Dis. J. *12*:347–348, 1993.
33. Yii, C.: Clinical observations on eosinophilic meningitis and meningoencephalitis caused by *Angiostrongylus cantonensis* on Taiwan. Am. J. Trop. Med. Hyg. *25*:233–249, 1976.

42

Aseptic Meningitis and Viral Meningitis

James D. Cherry

Aseptic meningitis is an inflammatory process of the meninges. It is relatively common and is caused by many different etiologic factors. The cerebrospinal fluid (CSF) is characterized by pleocytosis, increased protein, and the absence of microorganisms on Gram stain and on routine culture. Usually, the illnesses are self-limited; with some etiologies, however, the resulting diseases may be severe, protracted, recurrent, or progressive and lead to disability and death.

"Serous meningitis," "lymphocytic meningitis," and "nonparalytic poliomyelitis" are terms that were used in the past to denote aseptic meningitis. Viral meningitis is an inflammation of the leptomeninges caused by infections with many different viruses. Viruses are the cause of most cases of aseptic meningitis.

HISTORY

Aseptic meningitis is a syndrome that first was described by Wallgren in 1925.[148] Wallgren's criteria for this diagnosis included (1) an acute onset with obvious signs and symptoms of meningeal involvement; (2) alteration of CSF typical of meningitis, which may show a small or large number of cells; (3) absence of bacteria in the CSF, as demonstrated by appropriate culture; (4) a relatively short, benign course of illness; (5) absence of local parameningeal infection (e.g., otitis, sinusitis, trauma) or a general disease that might have meningitis as a secondary manifestation; and (6) absence from the community of epidemic disease, of which meningitis is a feature. In 1951, Wallgren[147] redefined aseptic meningitis as a syndrome likely to be encountered in a large number of different infectious diseases.

The clinical occurrence of aseptic meningitis first was recognized in epidemic poliomyelitis and in mumps at the beginning of the 20th century.[51, 152] Rivers and Scott[113] reported the recovery of lymphocytic choriomeningitis (LCM) virus from the CSF of several patients with aseptic meningitis in 1935, and in 1934 Johnson and Goodpasture[75] proved that mumps was caused by a virus.

The discovery of coxsackieviruses in 1948 by Dalldorf and Sickles[39] and the introduction of tissue culture in 1949 by Enders, Weller, and Robbins,[52] which resulted in the discovery of echoviruses, paved the way for the widespread investigation into the etiology of aseptic meningitis.

Rasmussen[109] reported on 374 cases evaluated at the Walter Reed Army Institute of Research laboratory between 1941 and 1946 and found the probable or definite etiology in 26 per cent of "viral" disease of the central nervous system (CNS). Mumps and LCM viruses were the two etiologic agents identified in his study.

In 1953, Adair and associates[4] reviewed 480 additional cases of aseptic meningitis occurring in military personnel and their dependents from 1947 through 1952 and were able to confirm the etiology in 25 per cent of those patients. Herpes simplex virus and *Leptospira* species were added to the previously identified mumps and LCM viruses as causes of aseptic meningitis. Meyer and associates[92] extended these studies to include 713 more children and adults with acute CNS syndromes of "viral" etiology admitted to military and Veterans Administration hospitals between 1953 and 1958. Of these 713 patients, 430 had the clinical syndrome of aseptic meningitis. Approximately 80 per cent of these patients were hospitalized in the United States. An etiologic diagnosis was determined in 71 per cent of patients with aseptic meningitis. In addition to the agents identified earlier, poliovirus, coxsackieviruses of groups A and B, and echoviruses and arthropod-borne viruses were identified as causes of aseptic meningitis. Lepow and colleagues[86, 87] reported the probable viral etiology in 54 per cent of the 407 patients they studied in Cleveland between 1955 and 1958. Lennette and associates[85] in 1958 determined a viral etiology in 65 per cent of 511 children and adults with presumed viral CNS disease in Los Angeles; 368 of these patients were diagnosed as having aseptic meningitis. Sköldenberg[128] analyzed 3117 patients admitted to the Hospital for Infectious Diseases in Stockholm between 1955 and 1964 with the diagnosis of aseptic meningitis with or without encephalitis or myelitis, and a virologic or clinical diagnosis (or both) of an associated virus infection was established in 72.6 per cent. More recently, Berlin and associates[13] carried out an aseptic meningitis surveillance study in pediatric ambulatory clinics and emergency rooms of three Baltimore hospitals between July 1986 and December 1990. They identified a single viral agent in 169 (62 per cent) of the 274 cases with laboratory study; there were 168 enteroviruses and 1 adenovirus.

ETIOLOGY

Etiologic agents and factors in aseptic meningitis are listed in Table 42–1. At present, the diagnostic work-up of aseptic meningitis usually is not undertaken vigorously, and therefore the etiologic agent is identified in only about 10 per cent of all cases. However, epidemiologic study and intensive investigations at some centers indicate that the vast majority of cases result from viral infections. Enteroviruses account

TABLE 42–1. Etiologic Agents, Factors, and Diseases Associated with Aseptic Meningitis

Viruses
- Enteroviruses (echoviruses, coxsackieviruses A and B, polioviruses, and enteroviruses)
- Arboviruses (in the United States: Eastern equine, Western equine, Venezuelan equine, St. Louis, Powassan, California, Colorado tick fever. In other areas of the world, many other arboviruses are important.)
- Mumps
- Herpes simplex type 2
- Human herpesvirus type 6
- HIV-1
- Adenoviruses
- Varicella-zoster
- Epstein-Barr
- Lymphocytic choriomeningitis
- Encephalomyocarditis
- Cytomegalovirus
- Rhinoviruses
- Measles
- Rubella
- Influenza A and B
- Parainfluenza
- Parvovirus B19
- Rotaviruses
- Coronaviruses
- Variola

Postvaccine
- Measles
- Vaccinia
- Polio
- Rabies

Bacteria
- *Mycobacterium tuberculosis*
- Pyogenic—partially treated
- *Leptospira* species (leptospirosis)
- *Treponema pallidum* (syphilis)
- *Borrelia* species (relapsing fever)
- *Borrelia burgdorferi* (Lyme disease)
- *Nocardia* species (noncardiosis)
- *Bartonella henselae*

Fungi
- *Blastomyces dermatitidis*
- *Coccidioides immitis*
- *Cryptococcus neoformans*
- *Histoplasma capsulatum*
- *Candida* species
- Other: *Alternaria* species, *Aspergillus* species, *Cephalosporium* species, *Cladosporium trichoides, Dreschslera hawaiiensis, Paracoccidioides brasiliensis, Petriellidium boydii, Sporotrichum schenckii, Ustilago* species, *Zygomycete* species

Chlamydia
- *C. psittaci*
- *C. pneumoniae*

Rickettsia
- *R. rickettsii* (Rocky Mountain spotted fever)
- *R. prowazekii* (typhus)
- *Coxiella burnetii*
- *Ehrlichia canis*

Mycoplasma
- *M. pneumoniae*
- *M. hominis*

Parasites (eosinophilic meningitis)
- Roundworms: *Angiostrongylus cantonensis, Gnathostoma spinigerum, Baylisascaris procyonis, Strongyloides stercoralis, Trichinella spiralis, Toxocara canis*
- Tapeworms: Cysticorosis
- Flukes: *Paragonimus westermani,* schistosomiasis, fascioliasis

Parasites (noneosinophilic meningitis)
- *Toxoplasma gondii* (toxoplasmosis)
- *Naegleria fowleri*
- *Acanthamoeba*

Parameningeal Infections

Malignancy
- Leukemia
- Central nervous system tumor

Immune Diseases
- Behçet syndrome
- Lupus erythematosus
- Sarcoidosis

Miscellaneous
- Kawasaki disease
- Heavy metal poisoning
- Intrathecal injections (contrast media, antibiotics, etc.)
- Foreign bodies (shunt, reservoir)
- Antimicrobial agents
- Other drugs
- Epidermoid, dermoid, other cysts

for approximately 85 per cent of all cases of aseptic meningitis.[27, 42–44, 65, 98] The following enteroviruses have been associated with aseptic meningitis: polioviruses 1 to 3; coxsackieviruses A 1 to 14, 16 to 18, 21, 22, and 24; coxsackieviruses B 1 to 6; echoviruses 1 to 9, 11 to 27, and 29 to 33; and enterovirus 71. The most common specific types in the vaccine era in the United States are coxsackievirus B5 and echoviruses 4, 6, 9, and 11. Arboviruses account for about 5 per cent of cases of aseptic meningitis in North America, St. Louis encephalitis virus being the most common.[19, 23, 25, 30] In the prevaccine era, mumps virus was the agent responsible for the greatest number of cases of aseptic meningitis; today in the United States, use of vaccine has made mumps meningitis rare.[24]

Aseptic meningitis is an occasional manifestation of acute and recurrent genital infections with herpes simplex virus type 2.[8, 12, 37, 48, 129, 141] In contrast with herpes simplex virus type 1 CNS infections, which without treatment usually are fatal, type 2 aseptic meningitis in otherwise immunocompetent persons is a benign, self-limited illness. Adenoviral types 1, 2, 3, 5, 6, 7, 12, 14, and 32 have been associated with meningitis and meningoencephalitis.[13, 35, 42–44, 54, 80, 103, 126, 131] Although rare, adenoviral CNS infections tend to be more severe than enteroviral infections. Pleocytosis is noted occasionally in herpes zoster, but neurologic involvement in primary varicella-zoster viral infections usually is an encephalitis rather than a benign meningitis.[42, 107, 111, 151] Echevarria and colleagues[50] detected DNA sequences specific for varicella-zoster virus in the CSF of six patients with acute aseptic meningitis who had no cutaneous lesions. Meningoencephalitis with sequelae in an infant with human herpesvirus type 6 has been reported.[159] A variety of neurologic disorders, including aseptic meningitis, are rare complications of Epstein-Barr virus infection.[53, 64, 135, 143]

On occasion, meningitis or meningoencephalitis occurs as a manifestation of acute illness with HIV-1 infection.[9, 67] Neurologic manifestations develop 3 to 6 weeks after primary infection at the same time as an infectious mononucleosis-like illness.

Although LCM virus was an important historical cause of aseptic meningitis, it rarely is recognized today as a cause of meningitis, except in animal exposure outbreak situations.[14, 45, 92] In 1974, eight cases of aseptic meningitis caused by LCM virus were found in New York State.[45] Many sporadic instances of LCM virus infection probably go unrecognized. Physicians should be alert to the possibility in all situations of rodent (pet or wild) exposure. Encephalomyocarditis virus is another rodent virus that rarely is recognized in humans.[149] It is associated with a variety of neurologic manifestations, including aseptic meningitis.[57]

Most noncongenital infections with cytomegalovirus in nonimmunocompromised persons are unrecognized. However, occasional instances of aseptic meningitis have been noted.[42–44] Rarely, aseptic meningitis has been noted during illnesses caused by rhinoviruses, influenza A and B viruses, parainfluenza viruses, parvovirus B19 virus, rotaviruses, and coronaviruses.[7, 22, 38, 42–44, 74, 99, 100, 112, 144, 156] Most infections with measles, rubella, and variola viruses that involve the CNS are encephalitic.[26, 28, 95]

Neurologic illness is a rare complication of measles, smallpox, polio, and rabies viral vaccines. In most instances, the illnesses are complex and severe, but on occasion, aseptic meningitis is the only manifestation.[13, 26, 30, 96, 133] Aseptic meningitis and encephalitis resulting from mumps vaccine administration have been noted in Canada and Europe.[6, 33, 91, 94] The Leningrad 3 and Urabe Am 9 strains of vaccine viruses have been implicated. In the United States, where the Jeryl Lynn vaccine strain has been used exclusively, the rate of encephalitis in vaccinees is no higher than the observed background incidence of similar illness in the population.[24]

Certain bacteria are important to recognize as etiologic agents in aseptic meningitis because the illnesses are treatable and early therapy is crucial. Of most importance is tuberculous meningitis. Early treatment of this illness nearly always results in complete cure, whereas diagnostic delay or inadequate treatment frequently results in permanent neurologic sequelae. Lyme disease, relapsing fever, brucellosis, and leptospirosis are illnesses, acquired either directly or indirectly from animals, in which aseptic meningitis may be a part of the disease process.[15, 17, 76, 84, 104, 132, 155, 158, 161] Partially treated common bacterial meningitides are a relatively common cause of meningitis in which cultures of CSF fail to grow organisms. Fortunately, antigen detection systems, such as latex agglutination, can be useful in identifying the causative agents in some of these cases.

A large number of fungi and yeasts cause meningitis.[120] Many fungal meningitides only occur in immunocompromised persons. The following agents are the most common causes of meningitis in children and adults with normal immunologic status: *Blastomyces dermatitidis, Coccidioides immitis, Cryptococcus neoformans, Cladosporium* species, *Histoplasma capsulatum,* and *Paracoccidioides brasiliensis.*

Mycoplasma pneumoniae is an important cause of neurologic illness.[21, 106] Pönkä[106] noted that 8 of 560 hospitalized patients with *M. pneumoniae* infections had aseptic meningitis and 18 had encephalitis or meningoencephalitis. *Mycoplasma hominis* and *Ureaplasma urealyticum* are rare causes of neonatal meningitis.[58, 89, 145, 146] Meningitis and meningoencephalitis have been associated with *Chlamydia pneumoniae* infections.[130, 137]

Parasites are an occasional cause of aseptic meningitis. Of much interest is eosinophilic meningitis, which is caused by *Angiostrongylus cantonensis*, a rat lungworm.[31, 67, 114, 150] Aseptic meningitis due to *A. cantonensis* has been observed on several islands in the Pacific, and the infection may be acquired by the consumption of freshwater shrimp. A number of drugs and biologics have been implicated in aseptic meningitis.[10, 20, 46, 63, 90, 93, 108, 157] Of most importance in pediatrics are trimethoprim-sulfamethoxazole and intravenous immunoglobulin. Other causes of aseptic meningitis are listed in Table 42–1.[47, 56, 62, 63, 69, 73, 81, 82, 90, 93, 125]

EPIDEMIOLOGY

Because many different types of organisms cause aseptic meningitis, there is no unified epidemiologic pattern. The epidemiology of the specific individual infectious agents or diseases is presented in detail in the various respective chapters of this book, and only a brief overview is presented here.

Approximately 85 per cent of all cases of aseptic meningitis are caused by enteroviral infections. Because of this, the basic epidemiologic pattern of aseptic meningitis reflects these agents. In temperate climates, most cases occur in the summer and fall; infection with enteroviruses is spread directly from person to person, and the incubation period usually is 4 to 6 days. Epidemiologic considerations in aseptic meningitis caused by agents other than enteroviruses depend markedly on season, geography, climatic conditions, animal exposures, and many other factors related to the specific pathogens.

CLINICAL MANIFESTATIONS

Aseptic meningitis has many different causes (Table 42–1), and clinical manifestations vary somewhat with the different diseases. In some instances, the signs and symptoms resulting from meningeal inflammation dominate the clinical illness, whereas in other instances, the main signs and symptoms reflect other organ system involvement. Clinical manifestations in aseptic meningitis, regardless of etiology, also vary markedly by patient age.

Enteroviruses[2, 16, 40, 55, 59, 66, 68, 70, 71, 78, 79, 83, 110, 115, 117–119, 121, 127, 136, 139, 153]

Enteroviruses are the most common cause of aseptic meningitis, and they can be considered the prototype for a description of general clinical manifestations of aseptic meningitis. However, even among the enteroviruses there are significant differences in clinical manifestations among the different viral types. Some general aspects of epidemic enteroviral aseptic meningitis are presented by viral type in Chapter 170.

The onset of illness generally is acute, although it may be insidious over a week or so or may be preceded by a nonspecific acute febrile illness of a few days' duration. Almost all children have fever, and most older children have headache, which most often is retro-orbital or frontal in location. Photophobia is common. Temperature elevation is variable, ranging from 38° to 40.5° C (100.4° to 105° F), and usually lasts about 5 days. Occasionally, fever is biphasic, with the initial elevation occurring before the onset of neurologic signs and symptoms. Anorexia, nausea, and vomiting are common complaints, and abdominal pain and diarrhea also frequently are reported.

Meningeal signs (stiff neck and back, tightness of the hamstring muscles, Brudzinski and Kernig signs) usually are present, but deep tendon reflexes usually are normal or hyperactive. Seizures occur occasionally, usually when there is concomitant high fever. Muscle weakness rarely is reported, but myalgia occasionally is noted. In young children, fever, irritability, and lethargy are the most common findings. Infants may be irritable and show resentment to handling, and the fontanelle may be tense.

Other manifestations of enteroviral infections also occur in children with aseptic meningitis. Most common is pharyngitis, which occurs during infection with all of the neurotropic enteroviral types. Rash is common but varies by viral type. With echovirus 9 meningitis, 30 to 50 per cent of children have rashes, whereas with echovirus 6, exanthem is rare. Enanthem, pleurodynia, pericarditis, myocarditis, and conjunctivitis are other findings noted in children with enteroviral aseptic meningitis.

CSF leukocyte counts vary from a few cells to a few thousand/mm^3; the median is in the range of 100 to 500 cells/mm^3. The percentage of neutrophils also varies greatly. Initially, a predominance of neutrophils is common, but later CSF examinations show a decline in the percentage of neutrophils. The CSF protein usually is elevated mildly, and the glucose concentration most often is normal; rarely, hypoglycorrhachia is noted.

The duration of illness is variable. Usually, disability because of neurologic involvement lasts 1 to 2 weeks.

Aseptic Meningitis Caused by Other Agents

In meningitis caused by arboviruses, there usually is brain involvement as well (meningoencephalitis). However, with both St. Louis and California viral infections in children, the illness commonly is benign without changes in sensorium or other findings indicative of brain involvement. Seizures are more common in arboviral meningitides than in enteroviral illnesses of otherwise comparable severity. When neurologic disease due to mumps is recognized, there usually is evidence of brain involvement. However, CSF examination in mild cases of mumps often reveals pleocytosis.

Tuberculous meningitis usually has a gradual onset over a period of 2 to 3 weeks. Initially, there may be personality change, irritability, anorexia, listlessness, and low-grade fever. This is followed by signs of increased intracranial pressure, such as drowsiness, stiff neck, cranial nerve palsies, inequality of the pupils, vomiting, and convulsions. Finally, coma, irregular pulse and respirations, and high fever occur. In fungal diseases, the course of meningitis is similar to that in tuberculosis. In both tuberculosis and several fungal meningitides, such as those due to *C. immitis, H. capsulatum,* and *C. neoformans*, there may be historical and radiographic evidence of pulmonary disease.

Aseptic meningitis due to *M. pneumoniae* is unique in that it frequently follows a respiratory illness (pharyngitis, bronchitis, or pneumonia) by a few days to 3 weeks. In nonenteroviral aseptic meningitides, the CSF findings generally are similar to those in enteroviral disease. In general, the likelihood of a predominance of neutrophils is less in other aseptic meningitides, and low glucose levels are likely in parameningeal bacterial infections, partially treated bacterial meningitides, brain tumors, leukemic infiltration, *M. pneumoniae* infections, fungal infections, and tuberculosis.

Recurrent Aseptic Meningitis (Mollaret Meningitis)

In 1944, Mollaret[97] described three patients with recurrent aseptic meningitis whom he had observed over a period of 15 years. Subsequently, many other cases have been reported, and some cases have been noted in children.[18, 33, 34, 72, 105, 134, 140] The illness is characterized by recurrent attacks of fever with meningeal signs and symptoms. The attacks last several days and are separated by symptom-free periods of weeks or months. During attacks, there is CSF pleocytosis, which in addition to neutrophils and lymphocytes contains endothelial cells (Mollaret cells). The disease remits spontaneously. The disease has been considered of unknown etiology, but Steel and colleagues[134] recovered herpes simplex virus type 1 from the CSF of a patient during a recurrence. Epstein-Barr virus infection has been associated with recurrent meningitis, and recurrent meningitis has been found to be an early manifestation of systemic lupus erythematosus.[64, 122] Studies using the polymerase chain reaction or DNA probes suggest that herpes simplex virus type 2 is the major cause of recurrent aseptic meningitis.[33, 105, 140] Recurrent aseptic meningitis in an 8-year-old girl secondary to an intracranial cyst has been reported.[81]

DIFFERENTIAL DIAGNOSIS

Careful analysis of the history and epidemiologic circumstances may point toward one of the specific causes listed in Table 42–1. During the summer and autumn, the presence of pleurodynia, herpangina, or unexplained febrile eruptions in the community suggests the possibility of enteroviral infections; the coexistence of acute paralytic disorders in other patients suggests poliomyelitis; encephalitis in horses points to the possibility of an arbovirus infection; a history of swimming in waters contaminated by urine from infected animals suggests leptospiral infection. Exposure to ticks might suggest Lyme disease, relapsing fever, or rickettsial disease, depending on the geographic location and other symptoms of the illness. Knowledge of clear-cut exposure to or concurrent evidence of mumps or of one of the common exanthems is helpful in the differential diagnosis.

The association of pneumonia or other respiratory illness preceding aseptic meningitis strongly suggests the possibility of *M. pneumoniae* as the etiologic agent.

Most difficult from the diagnostic, therapeutic, and prognostic points of view are instances of incipient or partially treated bacterial (especially when due to *Haemophilus influenzae*) or mycobacterial meningitis. The clinical findings, the dosage of antibiotic previously used, and the spinal fluid smear, latex agglutination, or other rapid antigen identification test, culture, and glucose level may be helpful in bacterial meningitis. The quantitative determination of C-reactive protein in the CSF also may be useful in differentiating bacterial from viral meningitis.[1, 36, 41, 101, 102] Lindquist and associates[88] found that the determination of CSF concentrations of lactate was the most useful test in differentiating bacterial from nonbacterial causes of meningitis. Studies suggest that the presence of tumor necrosis factor–α in the CSF is rare in viral infections but common in bacterial disease.[5, 49, 60] When tuberculous meningitis is suspected, a careful evaluation of contacts, a careful examination of an appropriately stained smear from the pellicle of the CSF that was allowed to settle, and a positive tuberculin reaction may confirm the diagnosis. Because combined bacterial and viral infection has occurred, examinations of cerebrospinal fluid should be repeated if there is the slightest doubt. The possibility that the observed meningeal reaction is of neither viral nor bacterial origin must be considered. Finally, CNS tumor must be considered in the differential diagnosis, particularly if there is hypoglycorrhachia and prominent signs of increased intracranial pressure.

SPECIFIC DIAGNOSIS

A meticulous history is essential and must evaluate exposure in the past 2 to 3 weeks to illness in contacts; exposure to mosquitoes, ticks, and animals during recent vacations, picnics, and so on; awareness of illness in animals, especially horses and other Equidae, in the patient's environment; recent travel from the home area; recent injections or medications of any kind; and the possibility of accidental exposure to heavy metals.

The CSF must be examined carefully to exclude disorders that respond to specific therapy. Smears for bacteria, appropriate rapid antigen identification tests, and cultures of the CSF are mandatory; the history and clinical findings may indicate the need for acid-fast stain and culture of the sediment for mycobacteria. Other circumstances may indicate the need for excluding fungal or protozoal infection; atypical cells may require cytopathologic study to exclude neural neoplasms, which may present acutely.

In any patient suspected of having viral meningitis, spinal fluid, blood, feces, and throat swabs should be collected and sent to a laboratory offering viral diagnostic services. An additional serum specimen should be collected 10 to 21 days later so that paired serums can be examined for antibody titer rises. This particularly is useful in arboviral, LCM viral, encephalomyocarditis viral, leptospiral, borrelial, rickettsial, mycoplasmal, and toxoplasmal infections. Although these studies may not provide an immediate diagnosis, they may give early warning of a specific epidemic, and they are useful for prognostication, particularly in very young infants.

Several studies indicate that an enteroviral etiology of aseptic meningitis can be diagnosed by the demonstration of enteroviral RNA by polymerase chain reaction assay.[3, 61, 77, 116, 123, 124, 142]

TREATMENT

Hospitalization usually is necessary because of the possibility of treatable bacterial disease and the frequent need of fluid therapy for dehydration. Treatment is symptomatic. Headache and hyperesthesia are treated with rest, analgesics, and a reduction in room light, noise, and visitors. Antipyretics are recommended for fever. It is prudent to use acetaminophen rather than aspirin because of the associated risk of Reye syndrome with the latter antipyretic. Codeine, morphine, and the phenothiazine derivatives often are used for pain and vomiting, but they rarely are necessary in children, and they should be avoided because they may induce misleading signs and symptoms.

Several weeks after apparent recovery, careful neuromuscular assessment should be conducted to ensure that muscular weakness is not a sequel. Bilateral audiometry is recommended, especially when mumps virus was involved.

Treatment for such illnesses as tuberculous meningitis, fungal meningitides, and other illnesses for which specific therapies are available is covered in specific chapters of this book.

PROGNOSIS

The prognosis in aseptic meningitis depends on the etiology. Some illnesses have an ominous prognosis (tuberculous meningitis, parameningeal infections, rickettsial infections), but the patients usually do well if appropriate specific therapy is instituted early in the course of the illness. In *C. immitis* meningitis, the prognosis for cure is guarded even with early optimal therapy.

In enteroviral and other viral meningitides, children usually recover completely. Some patients complain of fatigue, irritability, decreased ability to concentrate, muscle pain, muscle weakness and spasm, and incoordination for several weeks after an acute illness. Although the outcome of enteroviral meningitis most often is without residual, some infants who have enteroviral meningitis in the first few months of life have an increased risk for altered language development.[11, 154] It therefore is important formally to evaluate such children from ages 3 to 6 years.

PREVENTION

The universal use of polio and mumps vaccines in children clearly is effective in controlling these two diseases. Control of insect vectors by suitable spraying methods and eradication of insect breeding sites is important in the control of many arboviruses. The control of animal vectors such as mice and rats alters the incidence of infections with LCM and encephalomyocarditis viruses.

References

1. Abramson, J. S., Hampton, K. D., Babu, S., et al.: The use of C-reactive protein from cerebrospinal fluid for differentiating meningitis from other central nervous system diseases. J. Infect. Dis. *151*:854–858, 1985.
2. Abzug, M. J., Levin, M. J., and Rotbart, H. A.: Profile of enterovirus disease in the first two weeks of life. Pediatr. Infect. Dis. J. *12*:820–824, 1993.
3. Abzug, M. J., Loeffelholz, M., and Rotbart, H. A.: Clinical and laboratory observations: Diagnosis of neonatal enterovirus infection by polymerase chain reaction. J. Pediatr. *126*:447–450, 1995.
4. Adair, C. V., Gauld, R. L., and Smadel, J. E.: Aseptic meningitis, a disease of diverse etiology: Clinical and etiologic studies on 854 cases. Ann. Intern. Med. *39*:675–704, 1953.
5. Akalin, H., Akdis, A. C., Mistik, R., et al.: Cerebrospinal fluid interleukin-1 beta/interleukin-1 receptor antagonist balance and tumor necrosis factor concentrations in tuberculous, viral and acute bacterial meningitis. Scand. J. Infect. Dis. *26*:667–674, 1994.
6. Anonymous: Mumps meningitis and MMR vaccination. Lancet *2*:1015–1016, 1989.
7. Arisoy, E. S., Demmler, G. J., Thakar, S., et al.: Meningitis due to parainfluenza virus type 3: Report of two cases and review. Clin. Infect. Dis. *17*:995–997, 1993.
8. Atia, W. A., Ratnatunga, C. S., Greenfield, C., et al.: Aseptic meningitis and herpes simplex proctitis: A case report. Br. J. Vener. Dis. *58*:53–58, 1982.
9. Atwood, W. J., Berger, J. R., Kaderman, R., et al.: Human immunodeficiency virus type 1 infection of the brain. Clin. Microbiol. Rev. *6*:339–366, 1993.
10. Auxier, G. G.: Aseptic meningitis associated with administration of trimethoprim and sulfamethoxazole. Am. J. Dis. Child. *144*:144–145, 1990.
11. Bergman, I., Painter, M. J., Wald, E. R., et al.: Outcome in children with enteroviral meningitis during the first year of life. J. Pediatr. *110*:705–709, 1987.
12. Bergstrom, T., Vahlne, A., Alestig, K., et al.: Primary and recurrent herpes simplex virus type 2–induced meningitis. J. Infect. Dis. *162*:322–330, 1990.
13. Berlin, L. E., Rorabaugh, M. L., Heldrich, F., et al.: Aseptic meningitis in infants <2 years of age: Diagnosis and etiology. J. Infect. Dis. *168*:888–892, 1993.
14. Biggar, R. J., Woodall, J. P., Walter, P. D., et al.: Lymphocytic choriomeningitis outbreak associated with pet hamsters: Fifty-seven cases from New York State. J. A. M. A. *232*:494–500, 1975.
15. Bingham, P. M., Galetta, S. L., Athreya, B., et al.: Neurologic manifestations in children with Lyme disease. Pediatrics *96*:1053–1056, 1995.
16. Bowen, G. S., Fisher, M. C., DeForest, A., et al.: Epidemic of meningitis and febrile illness in neonates caused by echo type 11 virus in Philadelphia. Pediatr. Infect. Dis. *2*:359–363, 1983.
17. Bruhn, F. W.: Lyme disease. Am. J. Dis. Child. *138*:467–470, 1984.
18. Bruyn, G. W., Straathof, L. J. A., and Raymakers, G. M. J.: Mollaret's

meningitis: Differential diagnosis and diagnostic pitfalls. Neurology *12*:745–753, 1962.
19. Calisher, C. H.: Medically important arboviruses of the United States and Canada. Clin. Microbiol. Rev. *7*:89–116, 1994.
20. Carlson, J., and Wiholm, B. E.: Trimethoprim-associated aseptic meningitis. Scand. J. Infect. Dis. *19*:687–691, 1987.
21. Cassell, G. H., and Cole, B. C.: Mycoplasmas as agents of human disease. N. Engl. J. Med. *304*:80–89, 1981.
22. Cassinotti, P., Schultze, D., Schlageter, P., et al.: Persistent human parvovirus B19 infection following an acute infection with meningitis in an immunocompetent patient. Eur. J. Clin. Microbiol. Infect. Dis. *12*:701–704, 1993.
23. Centers for Disease Control: Arboviral Surveillance: United States, 1990. M. M. W. R. *39*:593–598, 1990.
24. Centers for Disease Control: ACIP: Mumps prevention. M. M. W. R. *38*:388–400, 1989.
25. Centers for Disease Control: Arboviral infections of the central nervous system: United States, 1985. M. M. W. R. *35*:341–350, 1986.
26. Centers for Disease Control: Measles surveillance, 1977–1981. Issued September 1982.
27. Centers for Disease Control: Enterovirus surveillance, summary 1970–1979. Issued November 1981.
28. Centers for Disease Control: Encephalitis surveillance, annual summary 1978. Issued May 1981.
29. Centers for Disease Control: Neurotropic diseases surveillance, summary 1974–1976. Issued October 1977.
30. Centers for Disease Control: Neurotropic viral diseases surveillance: Aseptic meningitis, annual summary 1975. Issued July 1977.
31. Char, D. F. B., and Rosen, L.: Eosinophilic meningitis among children in Hawaii. J. Pediatr. *70*:28–35, 1967.
32. Cizman, M., Mozetic, M., Radescek-Rakar, R., et al.: Aseptic meningitis after vaccination against measles and mumps. Pediatr. Infect. Dis. *8*:302–308, 1989.
33. Cohen, B. A., Rowley, A. H., and Long, C. M.: Herpes simplex type 2 in a patient with Mollaret's meningitis: Demonstration by polymerase chain reaction. Ann. Neurol. *35*:112–116, 1994.
34. Coleman, W. S., Lischner, H. W., and Grover, W. D.: Recurrent aseptic meningitis without sequelae. J. Pediatr. *87*:89–91, 1975.
35. Connor, J. D., Buchta, R. M., DeGenaro, F., Jr., et al.: Potpourri of adenoviral infections. West. J. Med. *120*:55–61, 1974.
36. Corrall, C. J., Pepple, J. M., Moxon, E. R., et al.: C-reactive protein in spinal fluid of children with meningitis. J. Pediatr. *99*:365–369, 1981.
37. Craig, C. P., and Nahmias, A. J.: Different patterns of neurologic involvement with herpes simplex virus types 1 and 2: Isolation of herpes simplex virus type 2 from the buffy coat of two adults with meningitis. J. Infect. Dis. *127*:365–372, 1973.
38. Craver, R. D., Gohd, R. S., Sundin, D. R., et al.: Isolation of parainfluenza virus type 3 from cerebrospinal fluid associated with aseptic meningitis. Clin. Microbiol. Infect. Dis. *99*:705–707, 1993.
39. Dalldorf, G., and Sickles, G. M.: An unidentified, filtrable agent isolated from the feces of children with paralysis. Science *108*:61–62, 1948.
40. Davies, J. W., McDermott, A., and Severs, D.: Epidemic virus meningitis due to echo 9 virus in Newfoundland. Can. Med. Assoc. J. *79*:162–167, 1958.
41. DeBeer, F. C., Kirsten, G. F., Gie, R. P., et al.: Value of C reactive protein measurement in tuberculous, bacterial, and viral meningitis. Arch. Dis. Child. *59*:653–656, 1984.
42. Deibel, R., and Flanagan, T. D.: Central nervous system infections: Etiologic and epidemiologic observations in New York State, 1976–1977. N. Y. State J. Med. *79*:689–695, 1979.
43. Deibel, R., Flanagan, T. D., and Smith, V.: Central nervous system infections: Etiologic and epidemiologic observations in New York State, 1975. N. Y. State J. Med. *77*:1398–1404, 1977.
44. Deibel, R., Flanagan, T. D., and Smith, V.: Central nervous system infections in New York State: Etiologic and epidemiologic observations, 1974. N. Y. State J. Med. *75*:2337–2342, 1975.
45. Deibel, R., Woodall, J. P., Decher, W. J., et al.: Lymphocytic choriomeningitis virus in man: Serologic evidence of association with pet hamsters. J. A. M. A. *232*:501–504, 1975.
46. Derbes, S. J.: Trimethoprim-induced aseptic meningitis. J. A. M. A. *252*:2865–2866, 1984.
47. Dimmitt, D. C., Fishbein, D. B., and Dawson, J. E.: Human ehrlichiosis associated with cerebrospinal fluid pleocytosis: A case report. Am. J. Med. *87*:677–678, 1989.
48. Do, A. N., Green, P. A., and Demmler, G. J.: Herpes simplex virus type 2 meningitis and associated genital lesions in a three year-old child. Pediatr. Infect. Dis. J. *13*:1014–1016, 1994.
49. Dulkerian, S. J., Kilpatrick, L., Costarino, A. T., Jr., et al.: Cytokine elevations in infants with bacterial and aseptic meningitis. J. Pediatr. *126*:872–876, 1995.
50. Echevarria, J. M., Casas, I., Tenorio, A., et al.: Detection of varicella-zoster virus-specific DNA sequences in cerebrospinal fluid from patients with acute aseptic meningitis and no cutaneous lesions. J. Med. Virol. *43*:331–335, 1994.
51. Enders, J. F.: Mumps. *In* Rivers, T. M., and Horsfall, F. L. (eds.): Viral and Rickettsial Infections of Man. Philadelphia, J. B. Lippincott, 1959, pp. 780–789.
52. Enders, J. R., Weller, T. H., and Robbins, F. C.: Cultivation of the Lansing strain of poliomyelitis virus in cultures of various human embryonic tissues. Science *109*:85–87, 1949.
53. Evans, A. S., and Niederman, J. C.: Epstein-Barr virus. *In* Evans, A. S. (ed.): Viral Infections of Humans. Epidemiology and Control. 2nd ed. New York, Plenum Medical, 1982, pp. 253–281.
54. Faulkner, R., and Van Rooyen, C. E.: Adenoviruses types 3 and 5 isolated from the cerebrospinal fluid of children. Can. Med. Assoc. J. *87*:1123–1125, 1962.
55. Forbes, J. A.: Meningitis in Melbourne due to ECHO virus. Part I. Clinical aspects. Med. J. Aust. *1*:246–248, 1958.
56. Fryden, A., Kihlstrom, E., Maller, R., et al.: A clinical and epidemiological study of "ornithosis" caused by *Chlamydia psittaci* and *Chlamydia pneumoniae* (strain TWAR). Scand. J. Infect. Dis. *21*:681–691, 1989.
57. Gajdusek, D. C.: Review article: Encephalomyocarditis virus infection in childhood. Pediatrics *16*:902–906, 1955.
58. Garland, S. M., and Murton, L. J.: Neonatal meningitis caused by *Ureaplasma urealyticum*. Pediatr. Infect. Dis. *6*:868–870, 1987.
59. Gilbert, G. L., Dickson, K. E., Waters, M. J., et al.: Outbreak of enterovirus 71 infection in Victoria, Australia, with a high incidence of neurologic involvement. Pediatr. Infect. Dis. *7*:484–488, 1988.
60. Glimaker, M., Kragsbjerg, P., Forsgren, M., et al.: Tumor necrosis factor–alpha in cerebrospinal fluid from patients with meningitis of different etiologies: High levels of TNF-alpha indicate bacterial meningitis. J. Infect. Dis. *167*:882–889, 1993.
61. Glimaker, M., Johansson, B., Olcen, P., et al.: Detection of enteroviral RNA by polymerase chain reaction in cerebrospinal fluid from patients with aseptic meningitis. Scand. J. Infect. Dis. *25*:547–557, 1993.
62. Golden, S. E.: Aseptic meningitis associated with *Ehrlichia canis* infection. Pediatr. Infect. Dis. *8*:335–337, 1989.
63. Gordon, M. F., Allon, M., and Coyle, P. K.: Drug-induced meningitis. Neurology *40*:163–164, 1990.
64. Graman, P. S.: Mollaret's meningitis associated with acute Epstein-Barr virus mononucleosis. Arch. Neurol. *44*:1204–1205, 1987.
65. Grist, N. R., Bell, E. J., and Assaad, F.: Enteroviruses in human disease. Prog. Med. Virol. *24*:114–157, 1978.
66. Guthrie, N.: Coxsackie B5 meningitis: Report of an outbreak in a high school football squad. J. Tenn. State Med. Assoc. *55*:355–356, 1962.
67. Hammer, S. M., and Connolly, K. J.: Viral aseptic meningitis in the United States: Clinical features, viral etiologies, and differential diagnosis. Curr. Clin. Top. Infect. Dis. *12*:1–25, 1992.
68. Hanninen, P., and Pohjonen, R.: Echovirus type 6 meningitis: Clinical and virological observations during an epidemic in Turku in 1968. Scand. J. Infect. Dis. *3*:121–125, 1971.
69. Haynes, R. E., Sanders, D. Y., and Cramblett, H. G.: Rocky Mountain spotted fever in children. J. Pediatr. *76*:685–693, 1970.
70. Haynes, R. E., Cramblett, H. G., and Kronfol, H. J.: Echovirus 9 meningoencephalitis in infants and children. J. A. M. A. *208*:1657–1660, 1969.
71. Helin, I., Widell, A., Borulf, S., et al.: Outbreak of coxsackievirus A-14 meningitis among newborns in a maternity hospital ward. Acta Paediatr. Scand. *76*:234–238, 1987.
72. Hermans, P. E., Goldstein, N. P., and Wellman, W. E.: Mollaret's meningitis and differential diagnosis of recurrent meningitis. Am. J. Med. *52*:128–140, 1972.
73. Heusner, A. P.: Nontuberculous spinal epidural infections. N. Engl. J. Med. *239*:845–854, 1948.
74. Holzel, A., Smith, P. A., and Tobin, J. O. H.: A new type of meningoencephalitis associated with a rhinovirus. Acta Paediatr. Scand. *54*:168–174, 1965.
75. Johnson, C. D., and Goodpasture, E. W.: An investigation of the etiology of mumps. J. Exp. Med. *59*:1–20, 1934.
76. Jorbeck, H. J. A., Guftafsson, P. M., Lind, H. C. F., et al.: Tick-borne *Borrelia* meningitis in children. Acta Paediatr. Scand. *76*:228–233, 1987.
77. Kammerer, U., Kunkel, B., and Korn, K.: Nested PCR for specific detection and rapid identification of human picornaviruses. J. Clin. Microbiol. *32*:285–291, 1994.
78. Karzon, D. T., and Barron, A. L.: An epidemic of aseptic meningitis syndrome due to echo virus type 6. I. Correlation of enterovirus isolation with illness. II. Clinical study. III. Sequelae. Pediatrics *29*:409–417, 418–431, 432–437, 1962.
79. Karzon, D. T., Eckert, G. L., Barron, A. L., et al.: Aseptic meningitis epidemic due to echo 4 virus. Am. J. Dis. Child. *101*:610–622, 1961.
80. Kelsey, D. S.: Adenovirus meningoencephalitis. Pediatrics *61*:291–293, 1978.
81. Kitai, I., Navas, L., Rohlicke, C., et al.: Recurrent aseptic meningitis secondary to an intracranial cyst: A case report and review of clinical features and imaging modalities. Pediatr. Infect. Dis. J. *11*:671–675, 1992.
82. Kriss, T. C., Kriss, V. M., and Warf, B. C.: Recurrent meningitis: The search for the dermoid or epidermoid tumor. Pediatr. Infect. Dis. J. *14*:697–700, 1995.
83. LaForest, R. A., McNaughton, G. A., Beale, A. J., et al.: Outbreak of aseptic meningitis (meningoencephalitis) with rubelliform rash: Toronto, 1956. Can. Med. Assoc. J. *77*:1–4, 1957.

84. Lecour, H., Miranda, M., Magro, C., et al.: Human leptospirosis: A review of 50 cases. Infection *16*:8–12, 1989.
85. Lennette, E. H., Magoffin, R. L., and Knouf, E. G.: Viral central nervous system disease: An etiologic study conducted at the Los Angeles County General Hospital. J. A. M. A. *179*:687–695, 1962.
86. Lepow, M. L., Carver, D. H., Wright, H. T., Jr., et al.: A clinical, epidemiologic and laboratory investigation of aseptic meningitis during the four-year period 1955–1958. I. Observations concerning etiology and epidemiology. N. Engl. J. Med. *266*:1181–1187, 1962.
87. Lepow, M. L., Coyne, N., Thompson, L. B., et al.: A clinical, epidemiologic and laboratory investigation of aseptic meningitis during the four-year period 1955–1958. II. The clinical disease and its sequelae. N. Engl. J. Med. *266*:1188–1193, 1962.
88. Lindquist, L., Linne, T., Hansson, L. O., et al.: Value of cerebrospinal fluid analysis in the differential diagnosis of meningitis: A study in 710 patients with suspected central nervous system infection. Eur. J. Clin. Microbiol. Infect. Dis. *7*:374–380, 1988.
89. Mardh, P. A.: *Mycoplasma hominis* infection of the central nervous system in newborn infants. Sex. Transm. Dis. *10*:331–334, 1983.
90. Martin, M. A., Massanari, R. M., Nghiem, D. D., et al.: Nosocomial aseptic meningitis associated with administration of OKT3. J. A. M. A. *259*:2002–2005, 1988.
91. McDonald, J. C., Moore, D. L., and Quennec, P.: Clinical and epidemiologic features of mumps meningoencephalitis and possible vaccine-related disease. Pediatr. Infect. Dis. *8*:751–755, 1989.
92. Meyer, H. M., Jr., Johnson, R. T., Crawford, I. P., et al.: Central nervous system syndromes of "viral" etiology: A study of 713 cases. Am. J. Med. *29*:334–347, 1960.
93. Mifsud, A. J.: Drug-related recurrent meningitis. J. Infect. *17*:151–153, 1988.
94. Miller, E., Goldacre, M., Pugh, S., et al.: Risk of aseptic meningitis after measles, mumps, and rubella vaccine in UK children. Lancet *341*:979–982, 1993.
95. Miller, H. G., Stanton, J. B., and Gibbons, J. L.: Parainfectious encephalomyelitis and related syndromes: A critical review of the neurological complications of certain specific fevers. Q. J. Med. *100*:427–505, 1956.
96. Miller, H. G., and Stanton, J. B.: Neurological sequelae of prophylactic inoculation. Q. J. Med. *89*:1–27, 1954.
97. Mollaret, P.: La meningite endothelio-leukocytaire multirecurrente benigne: Syndrome nouveau ou maladie nouvelle? Rev. Neurol. *72*:57–76, 1944.
98. Moore, M.: Enteroviral disease in the United States, 1970–1979. J. Infect. Dis. *146*:103–108, 1982.
99. Okumura, A., and Ichikawa, T.: Aseptic meningitis caused by human parvovirus B19. Arch. Dis. Child. *68*:784–785, 1993.
100. Paisley, J. W., Bruhn, F. W., Lauer, B. A., et al.: Type A2 influenza viral infections in children. Am. J. Dis. Child. *132*:34–36, 1978.
101. Peltola, H., and Valmari, P.: Serum C-reactive protein as detector of pretreated childhood bacterial meningitis. Neurology *35*:251–253, 1985.
102. Peltola, H. O.: C-reactive protein for rapid monitoring of infections of the central nervous system. Lancet *1*:980–983, 1982.
103. Pereira, M. S., and MacCallum, F. O.: Infection with adenovirus type 12. Lancet *1*:198–199, 1964.
104. Peter, G.: Leptospirosis: A zoonosis of protean manifestations. Pediatr. Infect. Dis. *1*:282–288, 1982.
105. Picard, F. J., Dekaban, G. A., Silva, J., et al.: Mollaret's meningitis associated with herpes simplex type 2 infection. Neurology *43*:1722–1727, 1993.
106. Pönkä, A.: Central nervous system manifestations associated with serologically verified *Mycoplasma pneumoniae* infection. Scand. J. Infect. Dis. *12*:175–184, 1980.
107. Preblud, S. R.: Age-specific risks of varicella complications. Pediatrics *68*:14–17, 1981.
108. Rao, S. P., Teitlebaum, J., and Miller, S. T.: Intravenous immune globulin and aseptic meningitis. Am. J. Dis. Child. *146*:539–540, 1992.
109. Rasmussen, A. F.: The laboratory diagnosis of lymphocytic choriomeningitis and mumps. *In* Rocky Mountain Conference on Infantile Paralysis. Denver, University of Colorado School of Medicine, 1946, p. 45.
110. Reeves, W. C., Quiroz, E., Brenes, M. M., et al.: Aseptic meningitis due to echovirus 4 in Panama City, Republic of Panama. Am. J. Epidemiol. *125*:562–575, 1987.
111. Reimer, L. G., and Reller, L. B.: CSF in herpes zoster meningoencephalitis. Arch. Neurol. *38*:668, 1981.
112. Riski, H., and Hovi, T.: Coronavirus infections of man associated with diseases other than the common cold. J. Med. Virol. *6*:259–265, 1980.
113. Rivers, T. M., and Scott, T. F. M.: Meningitis in man caused by a filterable virus. Science *81*:439–440, 1935.
114. Rosen, L., Loison, G., Laigret, J., et al.: Studies on eosinophilic meningitis. 3. Epidemiologic and clinical observations on Pacific islands and the possible etiologic role of *Angiostrongylus cantonensis*. Am. J. Epidemiol. *85*:17–44, 1967.
115. Rotbart, H. A.: Enteroviral infections of the central nervous system. Clin. Infect. Dis. *20*:971–981, 1995.
116. Rotbart, H. A., Sawyer, M. H., Fast, S., et al.: Diagnosis of enteroviral meningitis by using PCR with a colorimetric microwell detection assay. J. Clin. Microbiol. *32*:2590–2592, 1994.
117. Rotem, C. E.: Meningitis of virus origin. Lancet *1*:502–504, 1957.
118. Rothenberg, R., Murphy, W., O'Brien, C. L., et al.: Aseptic meningitis associated with ECHO virus type 9: An outbreak in Norfolk, Va. South. Med. J. *63*:280–285, 1970.
119. Sabin, A. B., Krumbiegel, E. R., and Wigand, R.: ECHO type 9 virus disease: Virologically controlled clinical and epidemiologic observations during a 1957 epidemic in Milwaukee with notes on concurrent similar diseases associated with coxsackie and other ECHO viruses. Prog. Pediatr. *96*:197–219, 1958.
120. Salaki, J. S., Louria, D. B., and Chmel, H.: Fungal and yeast infections of the central nervous system: A clinical review. Medicine *63*:108–132, 1984.
121. Samuda, G. M., Chang, W. K., Yeung, C. Y., et al.: Monoplegia caused by enterovirus 71: An outbreak in Hong Kong. Pediatr. Infect. Dis. *6*:206–208, 1987.
122. Sands, M. L., Ryczak, M., and Brown, R. B.: Recurrent aseptic meningitis followed by transverse myelitis as a presentation of systemic lupus erythematosus. J. Rheumatol. *15*:862–864, 1988.
123. Sawyer, M. H., Holland, D., Aintablian, N., et al.: Diagnosis of enteroviral central nervous system infection by polymerase chain reaction during a large community outbreak. Pediatr. Infect. Dis. J. *13*:177–182, 1994.
124. Schlesinger, Y., Sawyer, M. H., and Storch, G. A.: Enteroviral meningitis in infancy: Potential role for polymerase chain reaction in patient management. Pediatrics *94*:157–162, 1994.
125. Shaked, Y., and Samra, Y.: Q fever meningoencephalitis associated with bilateral abducens nerve paralysis, bilateral optic neuritis and abnormal cerebrospinal fluid findings. Infection *17*:394–396, 1989.
126. Simila, S., Jouppila, R., Salmi, A., et al.: Encephalomeningitis in children associated with an adenovirus type 7 epidemic. Acta Paediatr. Scand. *59*:310–316, 1970.
127. Singer, J. I., Maur, P. R., Riley, J. P., et al.: Management of central nervous system infections during an epidemic of enteroviral aseptic meningitis. J. Pediatr. *96*:559–563, 1980.
128. Sköldenberg, B.: On the role of viruses in acute infectious diseases of the central nervous system: Clinical and laboratory studies on hospitalized patients. Scand. J. Infect. Dis. *3*(Suppl.):5–95, 1975.
129. Sköldenberg, B., Jeansson, S., and Wolontis, S.: Herpes simplex virus type 2 and acute aseptic meningitis. Scand. J. Infect. Dis. *7*:227–232, 1975.
130. Socan, M., Beovic, B., and Kese, D.: *Chlamydia* pneumonia and meningoencephalitis. N. Engl. J. Med. *331*:406, 1994.
131. Sohier, R., Chardonnet, Y., and Prunieras, M.: Adenoviruses: Status of current knowledge. Prog. Med. Virol. *7*:253–325, 1965.
132. Southern, P. M., Jr.: Relapsing fever. *In* Tice, F. (ed.): Practice of Medicine. Vol. 3. Scranton, Hoeber Medical Div., Harper & Row, 1969, pp. 1–19.
133. Spillane, J. D., and Wells, C. E. C.: The neurology of Jennerian vaccination: A clinical account of the neurological complications which occurred during the smallpox epidemic in South Wales in 1962. Brain *87*:1–44, 1964.
134. Steel, J. G., Dix, R. D., and Baringer, J. R.: Isolation of herpes simplex virus type 1 in recurrent (Mollaret) meningitis. Ann. Neurol. *11*:17–21, 1982.
135. Sumaya, C. V., and Ench, Y.: Epstein-Barr virus infectious mononucleosis in children. I. Clinical and general laboratory findings. Pediatrics *75*:1003–1010, 1985.
136. Sumaya, C. V., and Corman, L. I.: Enteroviral meningitis in early infancy: Significance in community outbreaks. Pediatr. Infect. Dis. *1*:151–154, 1982.
137. Sundelof, B., Gnarpe, H., and Gnarpe, J.: An unusual manifestation of *Chlamydia pneumoniae* infection: Meningitis, hepatitis, iritis and atypical erythema nodosum. Scand. J. Infect. Dis. *25*:259–261, 1993.
138. Suzuki, N., Terada, S., and Inoue, M.: Neonatal meningitis with human parvovirus B19 infection. Arch. Dis. Child. Fetal Neonatal Ed. *73*:F196–F197, 1995.
139. Syverton, J. T., McLean, D. M., daSilva, M. M., et al.: Outbreak of aseptic meningitis caused by coxsackie B5 virus: Laboratory, clinical and epidemiologic study. J. A. M. A. *164*:2015–2019, 1957.
140. Tedder, D. G., Ashley, R., Tyler, K. L., et al.: Herpes simplex virus infection as a cause of benign recurrent lymphocytic meningitis. Ann. Intern. Med. *121*:334–338, 1994.
141. Terni, M., Caccialanza, P., Cassai, E., et al.: Aseptic meningitis in association with herpes progenitalis. N. Engl. J. Med. *285*:503–504, 1971.
142. Thoren, A., and Widell, A.: PCR for the diagnosis of enteroviral meningitis. Scand. J. Infect. Dis. *26*:249–254, 1994.
143. Tsutsumi, H., Kamazaki, H., and Nakata, S.: Sequential development of acute meningoencephalitis and transverse myelitis caused by Epstein-Barr virus during infectious mononucleosis. Pediatr. Infect. Dis. J. *13*:665–667, 1994.
144. Vreede, R. W., Schellekens, H., and Zuijderwijk, M.: Isolation of parainfluenza virus type 3 from cerebrospinal fluid. J. Infect. Dis. *165*:1166, 1992.
145. Waites, K. B., Duffy, L. B., Crouse, D. T., et al.: Mycoplasmal infections of cerebrospinal fluid in newborn infants from a community hospital population. Pediatr. Infect. Dis. *9*:241–245, 1990.
146. Waites, K. B., Rudd, P. T., Crouse, D. T., et al.: Chronic *Ureaplasma urealyticum* and *Mycoplasma hominis* infections of central nervous system in preterm infants. Lancet *1*:17–21, 1988.
147. Wallgren, A.: Die ätiologie der enzephalomeningitis bei kindern, besonders des syndromes der akuten abakteriellen (aseptichen) meningitis. Acta Paediatr. Scand. *40*:541–565, 1951.

148. Wallgren, A.: Une nouvelle maladie infectieuse du systeme nerveus central? Acta Paediatr. Scand. *4*(Suppl.):158–182, 1925.
149. Warren, J.: Encephalomyocarditis viruses. *In* Horsfall, F. L., and Tamm, I. (eds.): Viral and Rickettsial Infections of Man. Philadelphia, J. B. Lippincott, 1965, pp. 562–568.
150. Weller, P. F.: Eosinophilic meningitis. Am. J. Med. *95*:250–253, 1993.
151. Weller, T. H.: Varicella-Herpes zoster virus. *In* Evans, A. S. (ed.): Viral Infections of Humans: Epidemiology and Control. 2nd ed. New York, Plenum Medical, 1982, pp. 569–595.
152. Wickman, I.: Studien über poliomyelitis acuta: Zugleich ein beitrag zur kenntnis der myelitis acuta. Berlin, S. Karger, Engl. Trans. Nev. and Ment. Dis. Monog. Ser. No. 16, p. 1913, 1905.
153. Wilfert, C. M., Lehrman, S. N., and Katz, S. L.: Enteroviruses and meningitis. Pediatr. Infect. Dis. *2*:333–341, 1983.
154. Wilfert, C. M., Thompson, R. J., Jr., Sunder, T. R., et al.: Longitudinal assessment of children with enteroviral meningitis during the first three months of life. Pediatrics *67*:811–815, 1981.
155. Williams, C. L., Strobino, B., Lee, A., et al.: Lyme disease in childhood: Clinical and epidemiologic features of ninety cases. Pediatr. Infect. Dis. *9*:10–14, 1990.
156. Wong, C. J., Price, Z., and Bruckner, D. A.: Aseptic meningitis in an infant with rotavirus gastroenteritis. Pediatr. Infect. Dis. *3*:244–246, 1984.
157. Wong, J. G., Hathaway, S. C., Paat, J. J., et al.: Drug-induced meningitis: A case involving trimethoprim-sulfamethoxazole. Postgrad. Med. *96*:117–124, 1994.
158. Wong, M. L., Kaplan, S., Dunkle, L. M., et al.: Leptospirosis: A childhood disease. J. Pediatr. *90*:532–537, 1977.
159. Yanagihara, K., Tanaka-Taya, K., Itagaki, Y., et al.: Human herpesvirus 6 meningoencephalitis with sequelae. Pediatr. Infect. Dis. J. *14*:240–242, 1995.
160. Yerly, S., Gervaix, A., Simonet, V., et al.: Rapid and sensitive detection of enteroviruses in specimens from patients with aseptic meningitis. J. Clin. Microbiol. *34*:199–201, 1996.
161. Young, E. J.: Human brucellosis. Rev. Infect. Dis. *5*:821–842, 1983.

43

ENCEPHALITIS AND MENINGOENCEPHALITIS

James D. Cherry and W. Donald Shields

Encephalitis is an inflammation of the brain, and meningoencephalitis is a similar inflammatory illness in which both the brain and meninges are involved. The diagnosis of encephalitis can be established with absolute certainty only by the microscopic examination of brain tissue, and similarly the etiology is established only by the recovery from or the demonstration in brain tissue of an infectious agent. In clinical practice, the diagnosis frequently is based on neurologic manifestations, the recovery of infectious agents from other sites in the body, the serologic evidence of a specific infection, and relevant epidemiologic findings.

Encephalitis frequently is classified as primary or postinfectious or parainfectious.[26] Primary encephalitis is an illness in which encephalitis is the major manifestation. Symptoms are caused by direct invasion and replication of an infectious agent in the central nervous system, resulting in objective clinical evidence of cerebral or cerebellar dysfunction. Postinfectious or parainfectious encephalitis follows or occurs in combination with other illnesses that are not central nervous system illnesses or after a vaccine or other product has been administered. Manifestations may be mediated immunologically.

When neurologic clinical findings suggest encephalitis but inflammation of the brain has not occurred (such as in Reye syndrome), the condition is identified by the less specific term "encephalopathy." Frequently, when encephalitis or meningoencephalitis occurs, other areas of the nervous system also are involved, such as the spinal cord (myelitis), nerve roots (radiculitis), and nerves (neuritis).

HISTORY

Rabies encephalitis was recognized in ancient times in Europe and Asia.[95] In 100 A.D., Celsus noted the relationship of animal rabies to human disease. "Sleeping sickness" associated with epidemic influenza was noted early in the eighteenth century.[187] For the last 100 years, epizootics of encephalitis in equine animals have been observed in the United States, and in 1933, St. Louis encephalitis virus was isolated from the brains of humans dying of epidemic encephalitis.[132, 144] Meningoencephalitis was recognized as a complication of mumps at the beginning of the twentieth century.[56] Nonpolio enteroviruses have been known as a cause of encephalitis for the last 40 years; during the same period, more than 400 zoonotic arthropod-borne viruses have been discovered, and of these, 100 or more cause encephalitis in humans.[12]

ETIOLOGY

Etiologic agents in acute encephalitis, meningoencephalitis, and acute illnesses with an encephalitic component are presented in Table 43–1. All of the infectious agents or diseases are presented more fully and are referenced more completely in other areas of this book (see Index).

Viruses

Adenoviruses are an uncommon but not rare cause of encephalitis and meningoencephalitis.[31, 45, 46, 50, 108, 140, 145] Adenoviral types 1, 2, 3, 5, 6, 7, 11, 12, and 32 have been recovered from either the brain or cerebrospinal fluid in afflicted patients. Herpes simplex virus type 2 is a leading cause of severe and frequently fatal encephalitis in neonates.[192] In older children, the usual cause is herpes simplex virus type 1.[49, 113, 166, 184, 192] Recurrent genital infection with herpes simplex virus type 2 occasionally is associated with an aseptic meningitis, but this type 2 virus almost never causes encephalitis outside of the newborn period.

Encephalitis can occur in association with primary infection with varicella-zoster virus (chickenpox) and with endogenous recurrent disease (herpes zoster).[22, 39, 44, 54, 93, 109, 111, 154, 176] In chickenpox, the rate of encephalitis is about 0.3 per 1000 cases,[32] and the case-fatality rate is about 17 per cent.[149] Between 0.5 and 5 per cent of patients with herpes zoster have encephalitis.[94] This complication is more common in immunocompromised patients.

In infectious mononucleosis, encephalitis occurs in less than 1 per cent of cases; in addition, encephalitis rarely is the

TABLE 43–1. Etiologic Agents in Acute Encephalitis and Acute Meningoencephalitis

Etiologic Agents	Frequency*
Viruses	
Spread person to person only	
Adenoviruses	+ +
Herpes simplex types 1 and 2	+ + +
Varicella-zoster	+ +
Epstein-Barr	+
Cytomegalovirus	+ +
Variola	+
Enteroviruses	+ +
Reoviruses	+
Rubella	+ +
Influenza A and B	+ +
Respiratory syncytial	+
Parainfluenza 1–3	+
Mumps	+ + +
Measles	+ +
Hepatitis B	+
Human parvovirus	+
Hepatitis A	+
Rotavirus	+
Reovirus	+
Human herpes type 6	+ +
Spread to people by mosquitoes or ticks	
Arboviruses†—those that occur in the United States are the following: St. Louis, eastern equine, western equine, Venezuelan equine, California, Powassan, and Colorado tick fever	+ + +
Spread by warm-blooded mammals	
Rabies	+ + +
Herpesvirus simiae (herpes B)	+
Lymphocytic choriomeningitis	+ +
Encephalomyocarditis	+
Vesicular stomatitis	+
Bacteria	
Haemophilus influenzae, Neisseria meningitidis, Streptococcus pneumoniae, Mycobacterium tuberculosis, and other bacterial meningitides often have an encephalitic component.	+ + +
Spirochetal infections: *Treponema pallidum, Leptospira, Borrelia burgdorferi,* and other *Borrelia* species infections	+ + +
Brucella species	+
Actinomyces and *Nocardia*	+
Bartonella henselae	+
Other	
Chlamydia psittaci, Chlamydia pneumoniae	+
Rickettsial infections: Rocky Mountain spotted fever, ehrlichiosis, Q fever, and typhus	+ + +
Mycoplasma infections: *Mycoplasma pneumoniae* and *Mycoplasma hominis*	+ +
Fungal: *Coccidioides immitis, Cryptococcus neoformans,* and other fungal meningitides often have an encephalitic component.	+ +
Protozoal: *Plasmodium* species, *Trypanosoma* species, *Naegleria* species, *Acanthamoeba, Balamuthia mandrillaris,* and *Toxoplasma gondii*	+ + +
Helminths: *Trichinella spiralis, Schistosoma* species, *Strongyloides stercoralis*	+ +
Drug: trimethoprim	+

*Frequency refers to the rate of occurrence of encephalitis or encephalitis component in the particular disease cited and not its relative overall occurrence; + + + = frequent, + + = infrequent; + = rare.
†See Chapters 175, 178, 179, 190, and 191 for viral diseases in other countries transmitted by arthropods.

sole manifestation of Epstein-Barr virus infection.[41, 43, 87, 183] Severe chronic involvement of the brain is common in congenital cytomegalovirus infection.[83] Encephalitis due to acquired cytomegalovirus infection is relatively uncommon and usually occurs in immunocompromised children.[87, 175] Several cases have been described in previously healthy persons, however. Human herpesvirus 6 is an important cause of acute febrile illness, as well as roseola infantum, in young children.[81] Febrile convulsions are common in human herpesvirus 6 infections, and encephalitis is a rare complication of roseola. Studies indicate that human herpesvirus 6 is an infrequent cause of encephalitis in children.[91, 92, 125, 195] Smallpox (variola virus infection) prior to its world eradication was a rare cause of encephalitis.

Enteroviruses now are the leading viral cause of neurologic disease in children in the United States, and they are a major cause of encephalitis.[11, 31, 37, 45–47, 50, 76, 87, 101, 104, 108, 115, 132, 136, 138, 140] The following viral types have been associated with encephalitis: coxsackieviruses A2, 4–7, 9, 10, 16, and B1–5; echoviruses 1–9, 11–25, 27, 30, and 33; and enterovirus 71. A variety of neurologic illnesses, including encephalitis, have occurred rarely in reoviral infections.[55, 99, 109, 112, 197]

Neurologic involvement is a common manifestation of congenital rubella virus infection,[83] and encephalitis is a rare complication of noncongenital disease.[133] Some data suggest a rate of encephalitis in rubella between 1 per 5000 and 1 per 10,000 cases.[31] In the prevaccine era, the encephalitis rate in one epidemic in 1964 was 1 per 5000 cases, and in another epidemic in 1942 it was 1 per 6000 cases.[122, 172] In addition to Reye syndrome (see Chapter 59), which is an uncommon but important neurologic disease associated with influenza viral infections, encephalitis also occurs with some regularity as a manifestation of influenza viral infection.[11, 31, 39, 45–47, 59, 65, 66, 109, 140, 146, 154] During every influenza epidemic, university hospital pediatric services see one or two cases of encephalitis in children with influenza. On rare occasions, encephalitis occurs during the course of respiratory infections with respiratory syncytial virus and parainfluenza virus infections.[6, 15, 32, 45, 47, 109, 186]

Prior to the widespread use of mumps vaccine, this virus was the leading cause of meningoencephalitis in the United States. Today mumps is rare. The rate of encephalitis in mumps is about 3 episodes per 1000 cases.[27] The death-to-case rate is 1.4 per cent. In the prevaccine era, measles was an important cause of severe encephalitis in children.[30, 32] Measles is relatively rare in the United States, and therefore encephalitis is uncommon. Encephalitis occurs at a rate of 0.74 per 1000 cases of measles. The death-to-case rate is 14 per cent.

Hepatitis B virus is a rare cause of encephalitis, and encephalitis has been reported as a complication of erythema infectiosum on two occasions (human parvovirus infection).[6, 7, 80] A case of encephalitis in a 3-year-old boy caused by vesicular stomatitis virus has been presented.[153] This virus can be spread by direct contact with infected animals or by insects.

Arboviruses are the most important worldwide cause of severe encephalitis. The occurrence of specific arboviruses is both seasonal and highly geographic. There are more than 400 different arboviruses, and information about illnesses caused by specific types in various areas of the world is detailed in Chapters 175, 178, 179, 190, and 191.[12, 87] In the United States, seven arboviruses (eastern equine, western equine, Venezuelan equine, St. Louis, Powassan, California, and Colorado tick fever) that cause encephalitis have been isolated. Illness due to St. Louis virus has been the most common arboviral disease in the United States.

Each year in the United States, the causative agent is not determined in about 75 per cent of the cases of encephalitis. However, the season of occurrence (summer and fall) of these cases of undetermined etiology suggests that these cases most likely are caused by enteroviruses and arboviruses.

Human rabies is uncommon in the United States, but more than 20,000 cases and deaths occur worldwide every year.[194] Since the early 1970s, there have been about two cases of rabies per year in the United States, and about 50 per cent of the cases have occurred in children and teenagers.[3, 29] Encephalitis due to herpes B virus is rare and occurs predominantly in monkey handlers and usually after monkey bites.[90] Except in outbreak situations, lymphocytic choriomeningitis virus rarely is recognized as a cause of encephalitis.[14] However, serologic surveys have indicated that neurologic disease due to this virus is not rare in the United States.[46–48, 96, 132] Rare cases of encephalitis are caused by encephalomyocarditis virus; infection of humans with this virus is fairly common, but most infections go unrecognized.[180]

Bacteria

Signs and symptoms of acute encephalitis (drowsiness, coma, convulsions, mental confusion) are common in *Haemophilus influenzae, Neisseria meningitidis,* and *Streptococcus pneumoniae* bacterial meningitides, but the true etiology usually is established easily by the examination of the cerebrospinal fluid. Spirochetal infections are a more common cause of nervous system disease, and specifically encephalitis, than generally is appreciated. Encephalitis is a recognized complication of leptospirosis, Lyme disease, and relapsing fever.[15, 20, 147, 177] *Brucella* species are an infrequent cause of meningoencephalitis.[196] Encephalitis due to *Bartonella henselae* is an uncommon complication of cat-scratch disease.[23, 130, 141, 179]

Neurologic disease is a relatively common complication of pertussis. A 10-year study in the United States indicated a rate of neurologic disease in infants of about 9 per 1000 cases.[57] An extensive review by Miller and associates[133] suggested that the neurologic disease occurring with pertussis rarely, if ever, is inflammatory, and therefore it is better classified as an encephalopathy.

Other Agents

Encephalitis is an uncommon event in psittacosis, occurring in 1 to 3 per cent of cases.[24, 62] It can be caused by both *Chlamydia psittaci* and *Chlamydia pneumoniae.* Neurologic involvement is common in Rocky Mountain spotted fever.[85, 103] In one study, two-thirds of the ill children had evidence of encephalitis. Neurologic sequelae are common.[68] Neurologic involvement also occurs in nonspotted fever rickettsial infections.[51, 67, 120, 155, 170] *Coxiella burnetii, Ehrlichia canis, Rickettsia typhi,* and *Rickettsia canada* all have been implicated.

Mycoplasma pneumoniae is an important cause of encephalitis.[25, 40, 110, 148, 173] Pönkä[148] noted that 4.8 per cent of hospitalized patients with *M. pneumoniae* infections had central nervous system manifestations, and the majority had encephalitis or meningoencephalitis. *Mycoplasma hominis* is a rare cause of neonatal meningoencephalitis.[121]

A large number of fungi cause neurologic illness.[165] These illnesses are most common in immunocompromised persons, but some infections occur in apparently normal persons. Meningitis and brain abscess are the most common pathologic events, but encephalitis is associated commonly with meningitis. The following fungal agents are the most common causes of meningoencephalitis in children and adults with normal immunologic status: *Blastomyces dermatitidis, Coccidioides immitis, Cryptococcus neoformans, Cladosporium* species, *Histoplasma capsulatum,* and *Paracoccidioides brasiliensis.*

Involvement of the brain in parasitic infections is common, and the reader is referred to Section 22 for a complete review. Cerebral malaria is a common complication of *Plasmodium falciparum* infection. Meningoencephalitis and enlarging cerebral mass lesions rarely occur in acute acquired toxoplasmosis.[182] The free-living amoeba *Naegleria fowleri* is a rare cause of encephalitis, but infection with this agent usually is fatal.[168, 181] Most cases occur in children and young adults and are caused by swimming or playing in contaminated water. Fatal encephalitis also has resulted from infection with *Balamuthia mandrillaris,* a soil ameba formerly thought to be innocuous.[73, 185] A recurrent encephalitis due to trimethoprim administration has been reported.[86]

Postimmunization

Neurologic disease, including encephalitis and meningoencephalitis, has occurred after immunization with a variety of prophylactic and therapeutic preparations. Depending on the type of immunizing agent, the encephalitis can be the result of an immunologic reaction, a central nervous system infection with the vaccine virus, or a combination of infection and immunologic reaction. Historically, many of the observed neurologic reactions occurred after the administration of antiserums prepared in animals in the treatment of specific diseases. Antiserums to the following diseases or infectious agents have been noted in association with neurologic illness: tetanus, diphtheria, scarlet fever, tuberculosis, gas gangrene, pneumococcus, gonococcus, meningococcus, and streptococci.[2, 89, 105, 134, 159] Of 100 neurologic syndromes complicating serum administration reviewed by Miller and Stanton,[134] only 10 per cent were of a cerebral or meningeal type.

Neurologic disease was a common complication of rabies vaccine derived from animal nervous tissue.[134] The incidence of complication was between 3 per 1000 and 1 per 6000 cases.[16, 134] About 10 per cent of the neurologic disease attributed to this rabies vaccine was meningoencephalitic or encephalomyelitic. Encephalitis has not been observed after the use of the presently available human diploid-cell rabies vaccine.[28]

Encephalitis was an important complication of smallpox vaccination.[4, 19, 60, 71, 101, 117, 139, 178] The rate of encephalitis varied markedly from one study to another, from 1 in 4000 primary vaccinations in the Netherlands[139] to about 1 in 80,000 primary vaccinations in the United States.[116]

Neurologic disease, including encephalitis, occurs rarely after the administration of typhoid-paratyphoid vaccine.[134] Neurologic disease also rarely has been attributed to tetanus toxoid and diphtheria toxoid administration, but the manifestations rarely are central.

Encephalitis and encephalopathy have been observed after influenza immunization.[64, 72, 160, 193] However, in the extensive surveillance that occurred in the United States during the period October 1, 1976, to December 16, 1976, when 45,651,113 persons received the A/New Jersey/76 influenza vaccine, no epidemiologic evidence of an association between vaccine and encephalitis was noted.[79] Two children with acute disseminated encephalomyelitis after Japanese B encephalitis vaccination have been reported.[142]

Neurologic disease after pertussis immunization is a well-known event.[34–36] Pathologic evidence in fatal cases suggests encephalopathy rather than encephalitis.[42] Because neurologic illness similar to that which follows pertussis vaccination is not infrequent in infants who have not been vaccinated, it has been difficult to establish a true rate of pertussis vaccine encephalopathy or to establish with certainty that there is such an entity at all. The analysis of studies suggests that encephalopathy caused by pertussis vaccine does not occur.[35, 36, 75]

Neurologic disease, including encephalitis, is a rare complication of measles immunization.[30, 33, 61, 114] The rate in vaccines in the United States is less than 1 per million. In contrast, the finding in the National Childhood Encephalopathy Study in England, Scotland, and Wales indicated a rate of 1 per 87,000 immunizations.[1] This high rate of encephalopathy may be an artifact due to the misclassification of complicated febrile convulsions as encephalopathy. Meningoencephalitis is a rare complication of mumps immunization with some vaccine virus strains.[126] This has not been a problem in the United States, however.

A fatal encephalitis occurred in a 3-year-old child after 17D yellow fever vaccination.[151]

Postinfectious Encephalitis

Postinfectious or parainfectious encephalitis is an illness that follows a demonstrated or presumed viral infection and is thought to be immune-mediated rather than due to a direct effect of the virus in nerve cells.[74, 96, 97, 98, 163] This has been studied extensively by Johnson and Griffin[74, 97, 98] in encephalitis associated with measles. They have described a periventricular demyelinating disease and have not been able to isolate measles virus or identify measles antigens in nervous tissue. However, others, including one of us (J. D. C.), have recovered measles virus from the cerebrospinal fluid and brain of affected patients.[61, 129, 131, 152, 169] We believe that immune mechanisms may play a role in the pathogenesis of measles and perhaps other postinfectious neurologic illnesses, but the process is stimulated by the direct presence of the antigen in the nervous system. The mechanism of disease is important regarding possible treatment: steroids might be useful in immune-mediated disease but could be detrimental in an acute viral infection.

In contrast with measles, other apparent postinfectious encephalitides that usually have a subacute onset are immune-mediated and have multifocal white matter lesions.[18, 78, 106, 128] Specifically, acute disseminated encephalomyelitis usually is subacute in onset and is characterized by optic neuritis, myelitis, ataxia, hemiparesis, cranial nerve palsies, and multifocal white matter lesions that are indistinguishable on magnetic resonance imaging (MRI) from those seen in multiple sclerosis. Patients with this illness respond dramatically to treatment with steroids.

Chronic Encephalitic or Encephalopathic Illnesses

"Slow infections" that cause encephalitic and encephalopathic illness in humans have been recognized for many years. Many of these illnesses now are recognized as viral infections or due to prions. Viral illnesses include progressive multifocal leukoencephalopathy (JC, SV40, and BK viruses), subacute sclerosing panencephalitis (measles virus), and AIDS (HIV-1 and HIV-2). Prion diseases, called transmissible spongiform encephalopathies, include kuru, Jakob-Creutzfeldt disease, and Gerstamann-Straussler-Scheinke disease.[150] They are related to scrapie of sheep and bovine spongiform encephalopathy (mad cow disease), which are prion diseases of animals. These chronic illnesses are presented in Chapter 160.

EPIDEMIOLOGY

Because encephalitis has many different causes, there is not a unified epidemiologic pattern. The specific epidemiology of each individual infectious agent or disease is presented in detail in the various respective chapters of this book; only a brief overview is presented here. The vast majority of cases occur in the summer and fall, reflecting arboviral and enteroviral etiologies. Encephalitis due to arboviruses occurs in localized outbreaks and epidemics with boundaries determined by the range of particular mosquito vectors and the prevalence of natural reservoir animals.

Arboviruses are zoonoses in which humans are infected accidentally by an arthropod vector, humans not being essential in the life cycle of arboviruses. Most commonly, mosquitoes or other insects acquire arboviruses by biting infected birds, which often have prolonged viremia without illness. The insect vectors, although preferring birds, bite other vertebrates, including humans and horses. Encephalitis in horses and mules may be the first indication of incipient trouble in an area; veterinarians often are the first to detect an impending epidemic. Rural exposure is not a sine qua non; urban and suburban outbreaks are frequent.

Although enteroviral disease, including aseptic meningitis, occurs in epidemics, severe encephalitis caused by these agents usually is a sporadic event.

Sporadic cases of encephalitis occur in any season; epidemiologic considerations that must be reviewed in a search for the causative agent include geographic area; climatic conditions; animal, water, food, soil, and personal exposures; and host factors.

PATHOGENESIS[4, 13, 25, 40, 52, 58, 61, 68, 74, 77, 83, 87, 94, 96, 132–134, 137, 190]

Because there are multiple causes of encephalitis and meningoencephalitis, the lack of a unified pathogenesis is not surprising. Clinical manifestations of encephalitis can result from either a direct or an indirect effect of an infectious agent on the brain. Rabies, arbovirus infection, herpes simplex, and enteroviral encephalitides are examples in which the viral infections directly involve tissue cells within the brain. In contrast, encephalitic symptoms in bacterial meningitides and in rickettsial infections may be caused by the vasculitis and liberated toxins of the surrounding infection. In addition, in many postinfectious or parainfectious encephalitides, it is clear that immunologic events are important in the pathogenesis. In this category are measles and *M. pneumoniae* infections.

Postinfectious or parainfectious encephalitis is an acute demyelinating disease of the brain in which the findings suggest an autoimmune process. Usually, there is little evidence of an active infectious process when symptoms occur. However, it is probable that viral or other agents initially invaded the central nervous system and then were cleared but were a trigger for the subsequent disease. An immune (T-cell) response to myelin basic protein occurs.

In the majority of encephalitides, such as those due to arboviruses, mumps, and enteroviruses, the central nervous system infection is secondary to a primary viral infection elsewhere in the body. In general, the infectious agents, whether from ingestion, as in enteroviral infections, or from the bite of a mosquito, as in an arboviral infection, enter the lymphatic system. In the lymphatics, viral multiplication occurs, which results in seeding of the blood stream and then infection of other organs in the body. Viral multiplication then occurs at these secondary infection sites; extensive secondary viremia occurs; and then the central nervous system becomes infected. Actual involvement of nervous tissue may result from growth across or passive diffusion through brain capillaries or centripetal axonal transport of virus from the olfactory neuroepithelium to the olfactory bulb.[137]

Infection of the brain also may occur via the peripheral nerves. This retrograde spread of virus is important in rabies and herpes simplex virus encephalitis.

PATHOLOGY[42, 96, 133, 134, 178]

It is difficult to determine the etiology of encephalitis at autopsy, although morphologic identification of falciparum malaria, trypanosomiasis, and fungal encephalitis is possible. In viral encephalitides, the histopathologist may recognize rabies (Negri bodies) or an agent of the herpesvirus group (intranuclear inclusion bodies).

Tissue sections of the brain generally reveal meningeal congestion and mononuclear infiltration, perivascular cuffs of lymphocytes and plasma cells, some perivascular tissue necrosis with myelin breakdown, neuronal disruption in various stages (including ultimately neuronophagia), and endothelial proliferation or necrosis. A marked degree of demyelination with preservation of neurons and their axons is considered to be predominantly postinfectious or parainfectious (autoimmune) encephalitis. The severity and the extent of observed lesions vary with the infectious agent as well as with the degree of reaction of the host. The cerebral cortex, especially the temporal lobe, often is affected severely by herpes simplex virus; the arboviruses tend to affect the entire brain; and rabies has a predilection for the basal structures. Involvement of the spinal cord, nerve roots, and peripheral nerves is variable.

CLINICAL MANIFESTATIONS

The clinical findings in encephalitis are determined by (1) the severity of involvement and anatomic localization of the affected portions of the nervous system, (2) the inherent pathogenicity of the offending agent, and (3) the immune and other reactive mechanisms of the patient ("host factors"). There is, accordingly, a wide range of severity of clinical manifestations even with the same etiologic agent. Evidence of brain parenchymal involvement is the hallmark of encephalitis. Children with encephalitis may demonstrate evidence of diffuse disease, such as behavioral or personality changes; decreased consciousness; and generalized seizures or localized changes, such as focal seizures, hemiparesis, movement disorders, cranial nerve defects, and ataxia. Some children may appear to be mildly affected initially only to lapse into coma and sudden death. In others, the illness is ushered in by high fever, violent convulsions interspersed with bizarre movements, and hallucinations alternating with brief periods of clarity, and the children emerge with relatively few sequelae.

Most commonly, the initial manifestations resemble an undifferentiated acute systemic illness with fever, headache, or, in infants, screaming spells, abdominal distress, nausea, and vomiting. Signs of an associated mild nasopharyngitis may suggest a respiratory infection. As the temperature rises, new findings direct attention to the nervous system: mental dullness eventuating in stupor; bizarre movements; convulsions; nuchal rigidity, often not as pronounced as in purely meningitic illness; and focal neurologic signs, which may be stationary, progress, or fluctuate. Loss of bowel and bladder control and unprovoked emotional outbursts may occur.

Specific Forms of Encephalitis

Specific forms of encephalitis or complicating manifestations of encephalitis include Guillain-Barré syndrome, acute transverse myelitis, acute hemiplegia, brain stem encephalitis, and acute cerebellar ataxia. Acute cerebellar ataxia is characterized by an abrupt onset of truncal ataxia resulting in varying degrees of gait disturbance. Children with this illness have tremulousness of the head and trunk when in the upright position and of the extremities when attempting to move them against gravity. The duration of illness varies from 3 to 4 days to several weeks, and up to 30 per cent of those affected have minimal to moderate permanent residual ataxia.

Brain stem encephalitis is a rare disorder but is important because clinical signs appear much like those of a brain stem glioma. The differentiation is made by the time of onset of symptoms. Brain stem glioma usually has slowly progressive symptoms over several weeks or months. Brain stem encephalitis evolves over as few as 1 to 7 days. Both disorders may be associated with radiographic evidence of brain stem enlargement. Brain stem encephalitis resolves after 1 to 4 weeks' duration, whereas glioma continues to progress until radiation therapy is given.

Most cases of brain stem encephalitis appear to be postinfectious and thus are similar to postinfectious cerebellar ataxia or Guillain-Barré syndrome. Indeed, the conditions often overlap (i.e., there may be evidence of peripheral nerve involvement or cerebellar ataxia in a patient with brain stem encephalitis). In postinfectious cases, the onset of brain stem encephalitis begins 1 to 3 weeks after a nonspecific viral infection. Brain stem encephalitis has been reported to occur as a result of specific, identifiable, and possibly treatable infectious agents, including herpes simplex virus,[158, 167] varicella-zoster virus,[161] and cytomegalovirus,[63, 100] as well as *Listeria monocytogenes*[5, 9] and *Propionibacterium acnes*.[21] Brain stem encephalitis may arise in HIV-infected patients and may be due to one of the treatable causes, such as herpes simplex virus.[63, 82, 160]

DIFFERENTIAL DIAGNOSIS

The evaluation of the patient with an acute central nervous system illness (encephalopathy) must be considered carefully, and the sequence of tests should be dictated by the specific circumstances of the individual patient. Several disease processes may have a presentation similar to that of encephalitis or meningoencephalitis. The differential diagnosis of acute encephalopathy includes the following:

1. Metabolic diseases, such as hypoglycemia, uremic encephalopathy, hepatic encephalopathy, and rare genetic inborn errors of metabolism, including disorders of glucose or ammonia metabolism
2. Toxic disorders, such as drug ingestion or Reye syndrome
3. Mass lesions, such as tumor or abscess
4. Subarachnoid hemorrhage from arteriovenous malformation or aneurysm
5. Embolic lesions due to bacterial endocarditis
6. Acute demyelinating disorders, including acute multiple sclerosis and acute hemorrhagic leukoencephalitis
7. Status epilepticus, especially nonconvulsive status epilepticus, such as complex-partial status or absence status
8. Infectious diseases, including viral, bacterial, fungal, chlamydial, mycoplasmal, and parasitic
9. Postinfectious diseases, including Guillain-Barré syndrome, brain stem encephalitis, Miller-Fisher syndrome, and acute cerebellar ataxia
10. Acute confusional migraine

In some of these disorders, a lumbar puncture (LP) is unnecessary and may even be contraindicated; in others, an immediate LP is essential. For example, a patient who has a cerebellar tumor with acute obstruction of the fourth ventricle may present with a decreasing level of consciousness due to the rapidly rising intracranial pressure. Nuchal rigidity may be present. The family may not have recognized the more subtle changes in cerebellar functions for the months before the acute obstruction and may give a history only of acute encephalopathy. In that case, an LP could be followed by serious sequelae. Thus, before an LP is performed, the patient should be assessed for the possibility of increased intracranial pressure and the potential for herniation. The history should be reviewed carefully, questioning specifically for symptoms of neurologic problems in the days or weeks prior to the acute disorder. The physical examination must be performed, particularly looking for focal neurologic abnormalities, cerebellar signs, and evidence of increased intracranial pressure. A careful funduscopic examination is essential. The presence of papilledema would indicate that computed tomography (CT) should be considered prior to the LP. If on funduscopic examination spontaneous venous pulsations are noted, intracranial pressure is not increased, and the LP can be performed. Rarely, a specific etiologic diagnosis is necessary for immediate institution of appropriate antimicrobial therapy. In such circumstances, an LP may be necessary even with clear evidence of increased intracranial pressure, but it should be performed by an experienced physician using a small-gauge needle, with only enough cerebrospinal fluid removed to make the diagnosis.

Most patients with encephalitis should undergo neuroimaging to aid diagnosis of treatable conditions, such as herpes simplex virus encephalitis. As a general principle, MRI is more sensitive than is CT[119, 171] in detecting the often subtle changes associated with encephalitis. Thus, MRI should be the imaging technique of choice if it is readily available. In most cases of viral encephalitis, CT and MRI yield normal results, but there may be nonspecific swelling[189] or edema.[119] One important exception to this is herpes simplex encephalitis. As previously noted, MRI is more sensitive than is CT and may identify temporal lobe abnormalities earlier than CT can. MRI usually shows increased signal on T2-weighted images in one or both temporal lobes. Similarly, CT usually shows a low-density lesion in one or both temporal lobes, there often is a mass effect, and contrast infusion enhances the lesions. Although MRI may demonstrate abnormalities earlier in the disease process than may CT, normal neuroimaging cannot be relied on to exclude the diagnosis of herpes simplex encephalitis. Electroencephalography (EEG) often is the most dependable test early in its course. In one study of five biopsy-proven cases, the CT results were normal in the first 1 to 7 days, but the EEG results were abnormal in all five cases.[72] In another study, 11 patients had CT; 5 were normal, 6 abnormal.[52] All five patients with normal scans had grossly abnormal EEG results and ultimately died of the herpes simplex virus encephalitis. Of the six with abnormal CT results, only two had grossly abnormal EEG results, whereas four had just focal slowing. Only two of the six died.

In addition to herpes, other encephalitides may yield abnormal neuroimaging. CT and MRI results often are abnormal with disorders due to arbovirus or enterovirus infections. When imaging is abnormal, it usually is nonspecific, demonstrating areas of decreased density (with CT) or increased signal intensity (with MRI) in the gray or white matter. These findings are thought to represent edema or necrosis. Postinfectious disorders most often are associated with selective oligodendrocyte involvement.[10] Imaging thus shows increased signal in white matter with T2-weighted MRI or low-density white matter with CT.[8, 18, 84, 106, 143] Patients with acute hemorrhagic leukoencephalitis, a rare disease that is rapidly progressive and often fatal, may present with a clinical picture similar to that of herpes simplex encephalitis. In contradistinction to herpes simplex virus infection, however, the CT results often are abnormal within the first day or two.[162, 188] Thus, if a patient with suspected herpes simplex encephalitis has abnormal CT results early in the course, acute hemorrhagic leukoencephalitis should be considered.

EEG results generally are normal or nonspecifically abnormal in encephalitis, showing diffuse slowing. In the setting of acute encephalopathy, the presence of periodic lateralized epileptiform discharges (PLEDs) in the EEG results strongly suggests the possibility of herpes simplex virus encephalitis. Early in the course, there may be generalized slowing of the background frequencies and focal slowing over the affected temporal lobe. Within a few days, the characteristic PLEDs pattern develops in most cases. Later in the course, the background activity between the bursts of PLEDs gradually may flatten. Occasionally, other areas of the brain appear to be involved primarily with herpes simplex virus. In one reported case, the EEG results showed a right occipital slow-wave focus, but the presence of PLEDs suggested the possibility of herpes encephalitis. The CT results were normal, but a radioisotope scan also showed right occipital uptake. A biopsy specimen of the right temporal lobe grew herpes simplex virus.[13] PLEDs, although strongly suggestive of herpes simplex virus encephalitis, are not diagnostic. PLEDs have been reported with infectious mononucleosis encephalitis,[70] and periodic complexes are characteristic of the "slow virus" and prion disorders, including Jakob-Creutzfeldt disease and subacute sclerosing panencephalitis. The EEG abnormalities in neonatal herpes encephalitis are similar. The characteristic EEG results yield periodic or pseudoperiodic complexes, usually triangular or sharp waves, occurring in a multifocal pattern.[135] In one study of 34 infants with herpes encephalitis, 21 underwent EEG; the results of 19 of the 21 were abnormal. The results of 3 showed only focal slowing, but those of 16 showed the characteristic periodic or pseudoperiodic complexes.[164] The authors then reviewed 500 other neonatal EEG records and found 20 with similar complexes. Eleven patients had meningoencephalitis of unknown etiology, three had hemorrhage, and two suffered asphyxia. Four were placed in a "miscellaneous" category. Thus, periodic or pseudoperiodic complexes in neonatal EEG results strongly suggest herpes simplex virus encephalitis, but they are not diagnostic.

Single photon emission computed tomography (SPECT) has not been studied well yet, but there are reports of SPECT use in the early identification of herpes simplex encephalitis. The results suggest that SPECT may be more sensitive in the early diagnosis of herpes simplex virus encephalitis than CT. Ackerman and colleagues[1] found that SPECT demonstrated greater sensitivity and more precise localization than did conventional radionuclide scanning and CT. Launes and associates[118] studied 14 encephalitis patients and found that SPECT detected temporal lobe abnormalities in all 6 with herpes simplex virus encephalitis and yielded normal results in the remaining 8 who had other etiologies.

The modalities used to study the patient with suspected herpes simplex virus encephalitis depend on availability in an individual hospital. EEG and MRI are more sensitive than CT and should be performed preferentially. If these studies do not support the diagnosis in a patient in whom herpes simplex virus infection is strongly suspected, SPECT should be performed if available. Identification of a localized temporal lobe abnormality only suggests a probable diagnosis of herpes simplex; absolute diagnosis depends on identification of the virus by brain biopsy.[191] However, in many cases, the clinical course coupled with the cerebrospinal fluid studies and identification of a localized abnormality is enough to warrant treatment with antiviral agents without a brain biopsy. Intracranial ultrasonography in the neonate has been shown to be helpful in the diagnosis and follow-up of infants with herpes simplex virus or cytomegalovirus infections.[123]

SPECIFIC DIAGNOSIS

A meticulous history is essential and must evaluate exposure in the past 2 to 3 weeks to illness in contacts; exposure to mosquitoes, ticks, and animals during recent vacations, picnics, and so on; awareness of illness in animals, especially horses and other equidae, in the patient's environment; recent travel from the home area; recent injections of any kind; and the possibility of accidental exposure to heavy metals, pesticides, or other questionable substances.

The cerebrospinal fluid must be examined carefully to exclude other disorders that respond to specific therapy. Smears for bacteria, appropriate rapid antigen identification tests, and cultures of the cerebrospinal fluid are mandatory; the history and clinical findings may indicate the need for acid-fast stain and culture of the sediment for mycobacteria. Other circumstances may indicate the need for excluding fungal or protozoal infection; atypical cells may require cytopathologic study to exclude neural neoplasms that may present acutely.

The availability of polymerase chain reaction has allowed the definitive and rapid diagnosis of herpes simplex virus encephalitis, thus eliminating the need for brain biopsy.[49, 113, 166, 192] Herpes simplex virus DNA was detected in the cerebrospinal fluid of 53 of 54 patients with biopsy-proven herpes simplex virus encephalitis.[113] The etiology of encephalitis due to other herpes group viruses also has been determined by polymerase chain reaction assay of cerebrospinal fluid.[44, 125, 183] In the future, routine polymerase chain reaction assay is likely to become available for the diagnosis of *M. pneumoniae* infection, enterovirus infections, and other encephalitides.

In viral encephalitis, the cerebrospinal fluid frequently is clear; the leukocyte count ranges from none to several thousand, often with a significant percentage of polymorphonuclear cells initially, moderate or no elevation of protein, and an initially normal level of glucose relative to the simultaneously determined blood glucose level. In any patient suspected of having viral meningoencephalitis, spinal fluid, blood, feces, and throat swabs should be collected and sent to a laboratory offering viral diagnostic services. An additional serum specimen should be collected 10 to 21 days later. Although these studies may not provide an immediate diagnosis, they may give early warning of a specific epidemic, and the use of specific antiviral chemotherapy may be indicated by the preliminary culture results.

Inquiry regarding recent illness, recent injections, and especially recent exposures away from the home environment sometimes is helpful. The incubation periods of some arboviruses are such that mosquito bites acquired at least 1 week earlier or insect bites now healed may give a clue. Occasionally, patients who have traveled to Africa or Asia in preceding weeks present with encephalitis due to viruses, trypanosomiasis, or falciparum malaria with bizarre systemic and central nervous system signs and symptoms.

TREATMENT

With the exception of the use of acyclovir for herpes simplex virus and varicella-zoster encephalitis, the use of ganciclovir for cytomegalovirus encephalitis, and the antimicrobial treatment of spirochetal, chlamydial, mycoplasmal, fungal, and parasitic infections, treatment is nonspecific and empirical, aimed at maintaining life and supporting each involved organ system. The effectiveness of various recommended regimens in most instances has not been evaluated objectively.

Until a bacterial etiology and, in particular, a brain abscess are excluded substantially, parenteral antibiotic therapy should be administered.

It is crucial to anticipate and be prepared for convulsions, cerebral edema, hyperpyrexia, inadequate respiratory exchange, disturbed fluid and electrolyte balance, aspiration and asphyxia, abrupt cardiac and respiratory arrest of central origin, cardiac decompensation, and gastrointestinal bleeding. The syndrome of disseminated intravascular coagulation may be an additional complication. For these reasons, all patients with severe encephalitis should be cared for in intensive care units. Cardiac monitoring should be maintained. Repeat CT and MRI are helpful in following comatose patients and often show signs of brain swelling before the patient has the typical clinical indicators of increased intracranial pressure, such as Cushing triad (systolic hypertension, bradycardia, and slowing of respirations), dilated pupils, and decorticate or decerebrate posturing. The Cushing triad is an unreliable indicator of increased pressure, and, when the other signs of increased intracranial pressure occur, it often is late in the course and the patient's cerebral perfusion already is at risk.[127] If brain swelling becomes a problem, it may be necessary to place an intracranial pressure monitor. The intracranial pressure then should be maintained below 15 mm Hg if at all possible using the standard techniques for reduction of intracranial pressure, including hyperventilation, osmotic diuretics, and cerebrospinal fluid removal. As a last resort, barbiturate coma may be necessary. A related consequence of increased pressure is the syndrome of inappropriate antidiuretic hormone secretion. Careful monitoring of the fluid and electrolyte balance is essential in all seriously ill encephalitis patients.

All fluids, electrolytes, and medications initially are given parenterally. In prolonged states of coma, parenteral hyperalimentation is indicated. Normal blood levels of glucose, magnesium, and calcium must be maintained in order to minimize the threat of convulsions.

Status epilepticus caused by encephalitis should be treated vigorously using a structured protocol to ensure optimal control.[174] Most epileptologists now recommend intravenous lorazepam, 0.1 to 0.2 mg/kg, up to 4 mg maximum, as the initial therapy. Seizures due to encephalitis may be difficult to control, and other anticonvulsant medications may be required to achieve and maintain seizure control. If after a second attempt lorazepam fails to control the seizures, intravenous phenytoin is the next drug of choice. The dose is 18 to 20 mg/kg, maximum 1000 mg, given over 20 minutes with careful monitoring of vital signs because phenytoin can cause cardiac arrhythmias. If the seizures still persist, phenobarbital, 20 to 25 mg/kg, should be administered. Patients receiving large amounts of anticonvulsant medications are at risk of respiratory arrest, and the treating physician must be prepared to support the respiratory system at any time. If seizures persist after all three medications, pentobarbital coma can be considered.

A number of methods have been proposed to minimize cerebral edema and to diminish the consequences of cerebral anoxia; these measures are difficult to evaluate and generally are reserved for patients with severe illness whose condition appears to be desperate.

1. Dexamethasone, 0.1 to 0.2 mg/kg intravenously in an initial dose followed by 0.05 to 0.1 mg/kg intravenously every 4 to 6 hours, is given. This large dose should be reduced gradually after a few days if recovery or improvement is evident. Dexamethasone probably should not be used in acute viral diseases because steroids may potentiate the viral infection.
2. Other substances employed in an effort to reduce elevated intracranial pressure include (a) mannitol, given intravenously, as a 20 per cent solution in a dose of 0.25 to 1 g/kg over a 30- to 60-minute period (this may be repeated every 8 to 12 hours), and (b) glycerol, by nasogastric tube, using 0.5 to 1.0 mL/kg diluted with twice that volume of orange juice. This is nontoxic and may be repeated every 6 hours for an extended period.

For more than 40 years, steroids and adrenocorticotropic hormone frequently have been used as empiric therapy for encephalitis. However, no controlled studies have demonstrated any efficacy. In two comparative studies of measles encephalitis, steroids were found to offer no benefit, and in both studies the steroid recipients appeared to have had worse outcomes.[17, 198] More recently, in a carefully controlled study, no benefit of high-dose dexamethasone was found in the treatment of acute encephalitis due to Japanese encephalitis virus.[88]

In contrast with these investigations are more recent clinical experiences in the treatment of acute disseminated encephalomyelitis, in which MRI studies have indicated multifocal white matter lesions.[18, 78, 106, 128] Steroid-treated patients have responded dramatically with clinical improvement and resolution of the lesions as demonstrated by MRI. Steroids along with specific antibiotic therapy also may offer benefit in the treatment of encephalitis due to *M. pneumoniae* infection.[110, 173]

It is our opinion that steroids should not be used to treat encephalitis if there is an active infection unless the infection can be treated concomitantly with an effective antimicrobial agent. Plasmapheresis and intravenous immunoglobulin have been used empirically to treat brain stem encephalitis as well as other encephalitides, but no studies have been done that indicate that such therapies are helpful.

Equipment and personnel for handling such emergencies as cardiac and respiratory arrest constantly must be on hand. Early consultation with an anesthesiologist or intensive care specialist is useful in anticipation of the need for artificially assisted respiration.

Supportive and rehabilitative efforts are important after the patient recovers. Motor incoordination, convulsive disorders, squint, total or partial deafness, or behavioral disturbances may appear only after some time. Visual disturbances due to chorioretinopathy and perceptual amblyopia also may make a delayed appearance. Special facilities and, at times, institutional placement may become necessary.

PROGNOSIS

The prognosis in all encephalitides is guarded with respect to both immediate outcome and sequelae. Sequelae involving the central nervous system may be intellectual, motor, psychiatric, epileptic, visual, or auditory. Cardiovascular, intraocular, pulmonary, hepatic, and other systems sometimes are affected permanently. The short-term and long-term prognoses depend to some extent on etiology and age. Young infants usually have severe disease and sequelae. In general, herpes simplex viruses carry a worse prognosis for survival and residual disability than do the enteroviruses.

Rautonen and associates[156] examined prognostic factors in childhood acute encephalitis at the Children's Hospital, University of Helsinki, during a 20-year period from 1968 to 1987. In this study were 462 cases with the following etiologies: mumps virus, measles virus, rubella virus, varicella-zoster virus, herpes simplex virus, enteroviruses, respiratory viruses, *M. pneumoniae,* other agents, and cause undetermined. They found that mortality was fivefold greater in infants compared with older children. Children who were disorientated or unconscious before admission had fourfold and 25-fold greater risks of death and severe damage, respectively, than had children whose level of consciousness had been normal. Patients with herpes simplex virus or *M. pneumoniae* infection had the greatest risks of death or serious residual damage when compared with children with encephalitis of other etiologies.

California encephalitis has a low mortality rate but occurs most frequently in the pediatric age group. Of those patients who experience seizures in the acute phase of their disease,

25 per cent have a permanent seizure disorder.[69] Psychologic sequelae were present in 15 per cent in one series but were not found to be significant in several series if the children were evaluated several years after their illness.[38, 124, 157]

Prognosis in encephalitis due to western equine virus is guarded; 56 per cent of infants younger than 1 month of age have had recurring seizures with marked motor and behavioral changes. After 1 year of age, the sequelae appear to diminish; only 5 per cent of adults have neurologic sequelae. Fifty-seven per cent of infants who survived western equine virus infection and who were younger than 1 year of age at the time of infection had major neurologic sequelae requiring either a special school or institutionalization late in life. Severe retardation, paralysis, spasticity, recurrent convulsions, hearing deficits, and speech difficulties all were reported as complications.[53, 58]

Eastern equine encephalitis has a high mortality rate. Infants and children younger than 5 years of age who survive usually have severe sequelae consisting of mental retardation, convulsions, and paralysis. This is in contradistinction to adults older than 40 years of age who survive, who recover completely or have only slight damage.

St. Louis encephalitis has a low mortality rate. Although neurologic sequelae are reported, their incidence is low in the pediatric age group.

PREVENTION

The widespread use of effective attenuated viral vaccines for measles, mumps, and rubella almost has eliminated central nervous system complications from these diseases in the United States. The control of encephalitis due to arboviruses has been less successful because specific vaccines for the arbovirus diseases that occur in North America are not available. Control of insect vectors by suitable spraying methods and eradication of insect breeding sites is useful.

References

1. Ackerman, E. S., Tumeh, S. S., Charron, M., et al.: Viral encephalitis: Imaging with SPECT. Clin. Nucl. Med. *13*:640–643, 1988.
2. Allen, I. M.: The neurological complications of serum treatment: With report of a case. Lancet 2:1128–1131, 1931.
3. Anderson, L. J., Nicholson, K. G., Tauxe, R. V., et al.: Human rabies in the United States, 1960 to 1979: Epidemiology, diagnosis and prevention. Ann. Intern. Med. *100*:728–735, 1984.
4. Angulo, J. J., Pimenta-de-Campos, E., and de Salles-Gomes, L. F.: Postvaccinial meningo-encephalitis: Isolation of the virus from the brain. J. A. M. A. *187*:151–153, 1964.
5. Armstrong, R. W., and Fung, P. C.: Brainstem encephalitis (Rhombencephalitis) due to *Listeria monocytogenes*. Case report and review. Clin. Infect. Dis. *16*:1089–1093, 1993.
6. Assaad, F., and Borecka, I.: Nine-year study of WHO virus reports on fatal viral infections. Bull. W. H. O. *55*:445–453, 1977.
7. Balfour, H. H., Jr., Schiff, G. M., and Bloom, J. E.: Encephalitis associated with erythema infectiosum. J. Pediatr. *77*:133–136, 1970.
8. Barnes, P. D., Poussaint, T. Y., and Burrows, P. E.: Imaging of pediatric central nervous system infections. Neuroimaging Clin. North Am. *4*:367–391, 1994.
9. Barontini, F., and Leoncini, F.: Brainstem encephalitis due to *Listeria monocytogenes*: Favourable outcome after early antibiotic therapy. Ital. J. Neurol. Sci. *10*:85–87, 1989.
10. Becker, L. E.: Infections of the developing brain. Am. J. Neuroradiol. *13*:537–550, 1992.
11. Beghi, E., Nicolosi, A., Kurland, L. T., et al.: Encephalitis and aseptic meningitis, Olmsted County, Minnesota, 1950–1981. I. Epidemiology. Ann. Neurol. *16*:283–294, 1984.
12. Berge, T. O. (ed.): International Catalogue of Arboviruses including Certain Other Viruses of Vertebrates. 2nd ed. U.S. Dept. of Health, Education and Welfare, Public Health Service, No. (CDC) 75–8301, 1975.
13. Bergey, G. K., Coyle, P. K., Kromholz, A., et al.: Herpes simplex encephalitis with occipital localization. Arch. Neurol. *39*:312–313, 1982.
14. Biggar, R. J., Woodall, J. P., Walter, P. D., et al.: Lymphocytic choriomeningitis outbreak associated with pet hamsters: Fifty-seven cases from New York State. J. A. M. A. *232*:494–500, 1975.
15. Bingham, P. M., Galetta, S. L., Athreya, B., et al: Neurologic manifestations in children with Lyme disease. Pediatrics *96*:1053–1056, 1995.
16. Blatt, N. H., and Lepper, M. H.: Reactions following antirabies prophylaxis: Report on sixteen patients. Am. J. Dis. Child. *86*:395–402, 1953.
17. Boe, J., Solberg, C. O., and Saeter, T.: Corticosteroid treatment for acute meningoencephalitis: A retrospective study of 346 cases. Br. Med. J. *1*:1094–1095, 1965.
18. Boulloche, J., Parain, D., Mallet, E., et al.: Postinfectious encephalitis with multifocal white matter lesions. Neuropediatrics *20*:173–175, 1989.
19. Brown, E. H.: Complications of smallpox vaccination. Postgrad. Med. J. *41*:634–635, 1965.
20. Bruhn, F. W.: Lyme disease. Am. J. Dis. Child. *138*:467–470, 1984.
21. Camarata, P. J., McGeachie, R. E., and Haines, S. J.: Dorsal midbrain encephalitis caused by *Propionibacterium acnes*. Report of two cases. J. Neurosurg. *72*:654–659, 1990.
22. Carithers, H. A., and Margileth, A. M.: Cat-scratch disease: Acute encephalopathy and other neurologic manifestations. Am. J. Dis. Child. *145*:98–101, 1991.
23. Carmack, M. A., Twiss, J., Enzmann, D. R., et al.: Multifocal leukoencephalitis caused by varicella-zoster virus in a child with leukemia: Successful treatment with acyclovir. Pediatr. Infect. Dis. J. *12*:402–406, 1993.
24. Carr-Locke, D. L., and Mair, H. J.: Neurological presentation of psittacosis during a small outbreak in Leicestershire. Br. Med. J. *3*:853–854, 1976.
25. Cassell, G. H., and Cole, B. C.: Mycoplasmas as agents of human disease. N. Engl. J. Med. *304*:80–89, 1981.
26. Centers for Disease Control: Case definitions for public health surveillance. M. M. W. R. *39*:1–43, 1990.
27. Centers for Disease Control: Mumps surveillance, January 1977–December 1982. Issued September 1984.
28. Centers for Disease Control: Rabies prevention: United States, 1984. M. M. W. R. *33*:393–408, 1984.
29. Centers for Disease Control: Rabies surveillance: Annual summary 1980–1982. Issued August 1983.
30. Centers for Disease Control: Measles surveillance: Annual report 1977–1981. Issued September 1982.
31. Centers for Disease Control: Encephalitis surveillance: Annual summary 1978. Issued May 1981.
32. Centers for Disease Control: Encephalitis surveillance: Annual summary 1977. Issued December 1979.
33. Centers for Disease Control: Measles surveillance: 1973–1976. Issued July 1977.
34. Cherry, J. D.: The epidemiology of pertussis and pertussis immunization in the United Kingdom and the United States: A comparative study. Curr. Probl. Pediatr. *14*:1–78, 1984.
35. Cherry, J. D.: "Pertussis vaccine encephalopathy": It is time to recognize it as the myth that it is. J. A. M. A. *263*:1679–1680, 1990.
36. Cherry, J. D., Brunell, P. A., Golden, G. S., et al.: Report of the Task Force on Pertussis and Pertussis Immunization—1988. Pediatrics *81*:939–984, 1988.
37. Chonmaitree, T., Menegus, M. A., Schervish-Swierkosz, E. M., et al.: Enterovirus 71 infection: Report of an outbreak with two cases of paralysis and a review of the literature. Pediatrics *67*:489–493, 1981.
38. Chun, R. W. M., Thompson, W. H., Grabow, J. D., et al.: California arbovirus encephalitis in children. Am. J. Dis. Child. *124*:530–533, 1968.
39. Cizman, M., and Jazbec, J.: Etiology of acute encephalitis in childhood in Slovenia. Pediatr. Infect. Dis. J. *12*:903–908, 1993.
40. Clyde, W. A., Jr.: Neurological syndromes and mycoplasmal infections. Arch. Neurol. *37*:65–66, 1980.
41. Connelly, K. P., and DeWitt, L. D.: Neurologic complications of infectious mononucleosis. Pediatr. Neurol. *10*:181–184, 1994.
42. Corsellis, J. A. N., Janota, I., and Marshall, A. K.: Immunization against whooping cough: A neuropathological review. Neuropathol. Appl. Neurobiol. *9*:261–270, 1983.
43. Dagan, R., and Shahak, E.: Prolonged meningoencephalitis due to Epstein-Barr virus with favorable outcome in a young infant. Infection *21*:400–402, 1993.
44. Dangond, F., Engle, E., Yesseyan, L., et al.: Pre-eruptive varicella cerebellitis confirmed by PCR. Pediatr. Neurol. *9*:491–493, 1993.
45. Deibel, R., and Flanagan, T. D.: Central nervous system infections: Etiologic and epidemiologic observations in New York State, 1976–1977. N. Y. State J. Med. *79*:689–695, 1979.
46. Deibel, R., Flanagan, T. D., and Smith, V.: Central nervous system infections: Etiologic and epidemiologic observations in New York State, 1975. N. Y. State J. Med. *77*:1398–1404, 1977.
47. Deibel, R., Woodall, J. P., Decher, W. J., et al.: Lymphocytic choriomeningitis virus in man: Serologic evidence of association with pet hamsters. J. A. M. A. *232*:501–504, 1975.
48. Deibel, R., Flanagan, T. D., and Smith, V.: Central nervous system infections in New York State: Etiologic and epidemiologic observations, 1974. N. Y. State J. Med. *75*:2337–2342, 1975.
49. DeVincenzo, J. P., and Thorne, G.: Mild herpes simplex encephalitis diagnosed by polymerase chain reaction: A case report and review. Pediatr. Infect. Dis. J. *13*:662–664, 1994.

50. Donat, J. F., Rhodes, K. H., Groover, R. V., et al.: Etiology and outcome in 42 children with acute nonbacterial meningoencephalitis. Mayo Clin. Proc. *55*:156–160, 1980.
51. Drancourt, M., Raoult, D., Xeridat, B., et al.: Q fever meningoencephalitis in five patients. Eur. J. Epidemiol. *7*:134–138, 1991.
52. Dutt, M. K., and Johnston, I. D. A.: Computed tomography and EEG in herpes simplex encephalitis. Arch. Neurol. *39*:99–102, 1982.
53. Earnest, M. P., Goolishian, H. A., Calverley, J. R., et al.: Neurologic, intellectual, and psychologic sequelae following western equine encephalitis: A study of 35 cases. Neurology *21*:969–974, 1971.
54. Elliott, K. J.: Other neurological complications of herpes zoster and their management. Ann. Neurol. *35*:S57–S61, 1994.
55. El-Rai, F. M., and Evans, A. S.: Reovirus infections in children and young adults. Arch. Environ. Health *7*:700–704, 1963.
56. Enders, J. F.: Mumps. *In* Rivers, T. M., and Horsfall, F. L., Jr. (eds.): Viral and Rickettsial Infections of Man. Philadelphia, J. B. Lippincott, 1959, pp. 780–789.
57. Farizo, K. M., Cochi, S. L., Zell, E. R., et al.: Epidemiological features of pertussis in the United States, 1980–1989. Clin. Infect. Dis. *14*:708–719, 1992.
58. Finlay, K. H., Fitzgerald, L. H., Richter, R. W., et al.: Western encephalitis and cerebral ontogenesis. Arch. Neurol. *16*:140–167, 1967.
59. Flewett, T. H., and Hoult, J. G.: Influenzal encephalopathy and postinfluenzal encephalitis. Lancet *2*:11–15, 1958.
60. Flexner, S.: Postvaccinal encephalitis and allied conditions. J. A. M. A. *94*:305–311, 1930.
61. Forman, M. L., and Cherry, J. D.: Isolation of measles virus from the cerebrospinal fluid of a child with encephalitis following measles vaccination. The program for the American Pediatric Society, 1967.
62. Fryden, A., Kihlstrom, E., Maller, R., et al.: A clinical and epidemiological study of "ornithosis" caused by *Chlamydia psittaci* and *Chlamydia pneumoniae* (strain TWAR). Scand. J. Infect. Dis. *21*:681–691, 1989.
63. Fuller, G. N., Guiloff, R. J., Scaravilli, F., et al.: Combined HIV-CMV encephalitis presenting with brainstem signs. J. Neurol. Neurosurg. Psychiatry *52*:975–979, 1989.
64. Genz, R. D., and Beecham, H. J.: Meningoencephalitis after influenza inoculation. N. Engl. J. Med. *299*:721–722, 1978.
65. Glezen W. P., Paredes, A., and Taber, L. H.: Influenza in children: Relationship to other respiratory agents. J. A. M. A. *243*:1345–1349, 1980.
66. Glezen, W. P.: Consideration of the risk of influenza in children and indications for prophylaxis. Rev. Infect. Dis. *2*:408–420, 1980.
67. Golden, S. E.: Aseptic meningitis associated with *Ehrlichiae canis* infection. Pediatr. Infect. Dis. *8*:335–337, 1989.
68. Gorman, R. J., Saxon, S., and Snead, O. C.: Neurologic sequelae of Rocky Mountain spotted fever. Pediatrics *67*:354–357, 1981.
69. Grabow, J. D., Matthews, G. G., Chun, R. W. M., et al.: The electroencephalogram and clinical sequelae of California arbovirus encephalitis. Neurology *19*:394–404, 1969.
70. Greenberg, D. A., Weinkle, D. J., and Aminoff, M. J.: Periodic EEG complexes in infectious mononucleosis encephalitis. J. Neurol. Neurosurg. Psychiatry *45*:648–651, 1982.
71. Greenberg, M.: Complications of vaccination against smallpox. Am. J. Dis. Child. *76*:492–502, 1948.
72. Greenberg, S. B., Taber, L., Septimus, E., et al.: Computerized tomography in brain biopsy proven herpes simplex encephalitis. Arch. Neurol. *38*:58–59, 1981.
73. Griesemer, D. A., Barton, L. L., Reese, C. M., et al.: Amebic meningoencephalitis caused by *Balamuthia mandrillaris*. Pediatr. Neurol. *10*:249–254, 1994.
74. Griffin, D. E.: Post-infectious and post-vaccinal disorders of the central nervous system. Immunol. Allergy Clin. North Am. *8*:239–249, 1988.
75. Griffith, A. H.: Permanent brain damage and pertussis vaccination: Is the end of the saga in sight? Vaccine *7*:199–210, 1989.
76. Grist, N. R., Bell, E. J., and Assaad, F.: Enteroviruses in human disease. Prog. Med. Virol. *4*:114–157, 1978.
77. Gross, W. L., Ravens, K. G., and Hansen, H. W.: Meningoencephalitic syndrome following influenza vaccination. J. Neurol. *217*:219–222, 1978.
78. Grossman, M., and Azimi, P. H.: An encephalitis syndrome in a seven-year-old. Pediatr. Infect. Dis. J. *14*:550–555, 1995.
79. Guerrero, I. C., Retailliau, H. F., Brandling-Bennett, A. D., et al.: No increased meningoencephalitis after influenza vaccine. N. Engl. J. Med. *300*:565, 1979.
80. Hall, C. B., and Horner, F. A.: Encephalopathy with erythema infectiosum. Am. J. Dis. Child. *131*:65–67, 1977.
81. Hall, C. B., Long, C. E., Schnabel, K. C., et al: Human herpesvirus-6 infection in children: A prospective study of complications and reactivation. N. Engl. J. Med. *331*:432–438, 1994.
82. Hamilton, R. L., Achim, C., Grafe, M. R., et al.: Herpes simplex virus brainstem encephalitis in an AIDS patient. Clin. Neuropathol. *14*:45–50, 1995.
83. Hanshaw, J. B., Dudgeon, J. A., and Marshall, W. C.: Congenital cytomegalovirus. *In* Hanshaw, J. B., Dudgeon, J. A., and Marshall, W. C. (eds.): Viral Diseases of the Fetus and Newborn. 2nd ed. Philadelphia, W. B. Saunders, 1985, pp. 92–131.
84. Hattori, H., Kawamori, J., Takao, T., et al.: Computed tomography in postinfluenzal encephalitis. Brain Dev. *5*:564–567, 1983.
85. Haynes, R. E., Sanders, D. Y., and Cramblett, H. G.: Rocky Mountain spotted fever in children. J. Pediatr. *76*:685–693, 1970.
86. Hedlund, J., Aurelius, E., and Andersson, J.: Recurrent encephalitis due to trimethoprim intake. Scand. J. Infect. Dis. *22*:109–112, 1990.
87. Ho, D. D., and Hirsch, M. S.: Acute viral encephalitis. Med. Clin. North Am. *69*:415–429, 1985.
88. Hoke, C. H., Jr., Vaughn, D. W., Nisalak, A., et al.: Effect of high-dose dexamethasone on the outcome of acute encephalitis due to Japanese encephalitis virus. J. Infect. Dis. *165*:631–637, 1992.
89. Hughes, R. R.: Neurological complications of serum and vaccine therapy. Lancet *2*:464–467, 1944.
90. Hummeler, K., Davidson, W. L., Henle, W., et al.: Encephalomyelitis due to infection with *Herpesvirus simiae* (herpes B virus): A report of two fatal, laboratory-acquired cases. N. Engl. J. Med. *261*:64–67, 1959.
91. Irving, W. L., Chang, J., Raymond, D. R., et al.: Roseola infantum and other syndromes associated with acute HHV-6 infection. Arch. Dis. Child. *65*:297–300, 1990.
92. Ishiguro, N., Yamada, S., Takahashi, T., et al.: Meningoencephalitis associated with HHV-6 related exanthem subitum. Acta Paediatr. Scand. *79*:987–989, 1990.
93. Jackson, M. A., Burry, V. F., and Olson, L. C.: Complications of varicella requiring hospitalization in previously healthy children. Pediatr. Infect. Dis. J. *11*:441–445, 1992.
94. Jemsek, H., Greenberg, S. B., Taber, L., et al.: Herpes zoster-associated encephalitis: Clinicopathologic report of 12 cases and review of the literature. Medicine *62*:81–97, 1983.
95. Johnson, H. N.: Rabies. *In* Rivers, T. M., and Horsfall, F. J., Jr. (eds.): Viral and Rickettsial Infections of Man. 3rd ed. Philadelphia, J. B. Lippincott, 1959, pp. 405–431.
96. Johnson, R. T.: Viral Infections of the Nervous System. New York, Raven Press, 1982, pp. 87–128.
97. Johnson, R. T.: The pathogenesis of acute viral encephalitis and postinfectious encephalomyelitis. J. Infect. Dis. *155*:359–364, 1987.
98. Johnson, R. T.: The virology of demyelinating diseases. Ann. Neurol. *36*:S54–S60, 1994.
99. Joske, R. A., Keall, D. D., Leak, P. J., et al.: Hepatitis-encephalitis in humans with reovirus infection. Arch. Intern. Med. *113*:811–816, 1964.
100. Kanzaki, A., Yubuki, S., and Yuki, N.: Bickerstaff's brainstem encephalitis associated with cytomegalovirus infection. J. Neurol. Neurosurg. Psychiatry *58*:260–261, 1993.
101. Kaplan, M. H., Klein, S. W., McPhee, J., et al.: Group B coxsackievirus infections in infants younger than three months of age: A serious childhood illness. Rev. Infect. Dis. *5*:1019–1032, 1983.
102. Kappus, K. D., Sather, G. E., Kaplan, J. E., et al.: Human arboviral infections in the United States in 1980. J. Infect. Dis. *145*:283–286, 1982.
103. Katz, D. A., Dworzack, D. L., Horowitz, E. A., et al.: Encephalitis associated with Rocky Mountain spotted fever. Arch. Pathol. Lab. Med. *109*:771–773, 1985.
104. Kennedy, C.: Acute viral encephalitis in childhood. Br. Med. J. *310*:139–140, 1995.
105. Kennedy, F.: Certain nervous complications following the use of therapeutic and prophylactic sera. Am. J. Med. Sci. *177*:555–559, 1929.
106. Kesselring, J., Miller, D. H., Robb, S. A., et al.: Acute disseminated encephalomyelitis: MRI findings and the distinction from multiple sclerosis. Brain *113*:291–302, 1990.
107. Kohl, S., and James, A. R.: Herpes simplex virus encephalitis during childhood: Importance of brain biopsy diagnosis. J. Pediatr. *107*:212–215, 1985.
108. Koskiniemi, M., Manninen, V., Vaheri, A., et al.: Acute encephalitis: A survey of epidemiological, clinical and microbiological features covering a twelve-year period. Acta Med. Scand. *209*:115–120, 1981.
109. Koskiniemi, M., and Vaheri, A.: Effect of measles, mumps, rubella vaccination on pattern of encephalitis in children. Lancet *1*:31–34, 1989.
110. Koskiniemi, M.: CNS manifestations associated with *Mycoplasma pneumoniae* infections: Summary of cases at the University of Helsinki and review. Clin. Infect. Dis. *17*:S52–S57, 1993.
111. Kovacs, S. O., Kuban, K., and Strand, R.: Lateral medullary syndrome following varicella infection. Am. J. Dis. Child. *147*:823–825, 1993.
112. Krainer, L., and Aronson, B. E.: Disseminated encephalomyelitis in humans with recovery of hepato-encephalitis virus (HEV). J. Neuropathol. Exp. Neurol. *18*:339–342, 1969.
113. Lakeman, F. D., Whitley, R. J., and the NIAID Collaborative Antiviral Study Group: Diagnosis of herpes simplex encephalitis: Application of polymerase chain reaction to cerebrospinal fluid from brain-biopsied patients and correlation with disease. J. Infect. Dis. *171*:857–863, 1995.
114. Landrigan, P. J., and Witte, J. J.: Neurologic disorders following live measles virus vaccination. J. A. M. A. *223*:1459–1462, 1973.
115. Landry, M. L., Ponseca, S. S., Cohen, S., et al.: Fatal enterovirus type 71 infection: Rapid detection and diagnostic pitfalls. Pediatr. Infect. Dis. J. *14*:1095–1100, 1995.
116. Lane, J. M., Ruben, F. L., Neff, J. M., et al.: Complications of smallpox vaccination, 1968: Results of ten statewide surveys. J. Infect. Dis. *122*:303–309, 1970.

117. Lane, J. M., Ruben, R. L., Neff, J. M., et al.: Complications of smallpox vaccination, 1968: National surveillance in the United States. N. Engl. J. Med. *281*:1201–1208, 1969.
118. Launes, J., Nikkinen, P., Lindroth, L., et al.: Diagnosis of acute herpes simplex encephalitis by brain perfusion single photon emission computed tomography. Lancet *1*:1188–1191, 1988.
119. Lester, J. W., Carter, M. P., and Reynolds, T. L.: Herpes encephalitis: MR monitoring of response to acyclovir therapy. J. Comput. Assist. Tomogr. *12*:941–943, 1988.
120. Linnemann, C. C., Jr., Pretzman, C. I., and Peterson, E. D.: Acute febrile cerebrovasculitis: A non-spotted fever group rickettsial disease. Arch. Intern. Med. *149*:1682–1684, 1989.
121. Mardh, P. A.: *Mycoplasma hominis* infection of the central nervous system in newborn infants. Sex. Transm. Dis. *10*:331–334, 1983.
122. Margolis, F. J., Wilson, J. L., and Top, F. H.: Postrubella encephalomyelitis: Report of cases in Detroit and review of literature. J. Pediatr. *23*:158–165, 1943.
123. Matsumoto, N., Yano, S., Miyao, M., et al.: Two-dimensional ultrasonography of the brain: Its diagnostic usefulness in herpes simplex encephalitis and cytomegalic inclusion disease. Brain Dev. *5*:327–333, 1983.
124. Matthews, C. G., Chun, R. W. M., Grabow, J. D., et al.: Psychological sequelae in children following California arbovirus encephalitis. Neurology *18*:1023–1030, 1968.
125. McCullers, J. A., Lakeman, F. D., and Whitley, R. J.: Human herpesvirus 6 is associated with focal encephalitis. Clin. Infect. Dis. *21*:571–576, 1995.
126. McDonald, J. C., Moore, D. L., and Quennec, P.: Clinical and epidemiologic features of mumps meningoencephalitis and possible vaccine-related disease. Pediatr. Infect. Dis. *8*:751–755, 1989.
127. McDowall, D. G.: Monitoring the brain. Anesthesiology *45*:117–134, 1976.
128. McHugh, K., and McMenamin, J. B.: Acute disseminated encephalomyelitis in childhood. Irish Med. J. *80*:412–414, 1987.
129. McLean, D. M., Best, J. M., Smith, P. A., et al.: Viral infections of Toronto children during 1965. II. Measles encephalitis and other complications. Can. Med. Assoc. J. *94*:905–910, 1966.
130. Melis, K., Bochner, A., Vandenberghe, P., et al.: Cat-scratch disease with reversible encephalopathy. Eur. J. Pediatr. *149*:2–25, 1989.
131. Meulin, V. T., Kackell, Y., Muller, D., et al.: Isolation of infectious measles virus in measles encephalitis. Lancet *2*:1172–1175, 1972.
132. Meyer, H. M., Jr., Johnson, R. T., Crawford, I. P., et al.: Central nervous system syndromes of "viral" etiology: A study of 713 cases. Am. J. Med. *2*:334–347, 1960.
133. Miller, H. G., Stanton, J. B., and Gibbons, J. L.: Parainfectious encephalomyelitis and related syndromes. Q. J. Med. *100*:427–505, 1956.
134. Miller, H. G., and Stanton, J. B.: Neurological sequelae of prophylactic inoculation. Q. J. Med. *89*:1–27, 1954.
135. Mizrahi, E. M., and Tharp, B. R.: A characteristic EEG pattern in neonatal herpes simplex encephalitis. Neurology *32*:1215–1220, 1982.
136. Modlin, J. F., Dagan, R., Berlin, L. E., et al.: Focal encephalitis with enterovirus infections. Pediatrics *88*:841–845, 1991.
137. Monath, T. P., Cropp, C. B., and Harrison, A. K.: Mode of entry of a neurotropic arbovirus into the central nervous system: Reinvestigation of an old controversy. Lab. Invest. *48*:399–410, 1983.
138. Moore, M.: Enteroviral disease in the United States, 1970–1979. J. Infect. Dis. *146*:103–108, 1982.
139. Nanning, W.: Prophylactic effect of antivaccinia gammaglobulin against post-vaccinal encephalitis. Bull. W. H. O. *27*:317–324, 1962.
140. Noah, N. D., and Urquhart, A. M.: Virus meningitis and encephalitis in 1979. J. Infect. *2*:379–383, 1980.
141. Noah, R. L., Bresee, J. S., Gorensek, M. J., et al.: Cluster of five children with acute encephalopathy associated with cat-scratch disease in South Florida. Pediatr. Infect. Dis. J. *14*:866–869, 1995.
142. Ohtaki, E., Murakami, Y., Komori, H., et al.: Acute disseminated encephalomyelitis after Japanese B encephalitis vaccination. Pediatr. Neurol. *8*:137–139, 1992.
143. Okuno, T., Takao, T., Ito, M., et al.: Contrast-enhanced hypodense areas in a case of acute disseminated encephalitis following influenza A virus. Comput. Radiol. *6*:215–217, 1982.
144. Olitsky, P. K., and Casals, J.: Arthropod-borne group A virus infections of man. *In* Rivers, R. M., and Horsfall, F. L., Jr. (eds.): Viral and Rickettsial Infections of Man. Philadelphia, J. B. Lippincott, 1959, pp. 286–304.
145. Osamura, T., Mizuta, R., Yoshioka, H., et al.: Isolation of adenovirus type 11 from the brain of a neonate with pneumonia and encephalitis. Eur. J. Pediatr. *152*:496–499, 1993.
146. Paisley, J. W., Bruhn, F. W., Lauer, B. A., et al.: Type A2 influenza viral infections in children. Am. J. Dis. Child. *132*:34–36, 1978.
147. Peter, G.: Leptospirosis: A zoonosis of protean manifestations. Pediatr. Infect. Dis. *1*:282–288, 1982.
148. Ponka, A.: Central nervous system manifestations associated with serologically verified *Mycoplasma pneumoniae* infection. Scand. J. Infect. Dis. *12*:175–184, 1980.
149. Preblud, S. R.: Age-specific risks of varicella complications. Pediatrics *68*:14–17, 1981.
150. Prusiner, S. B., and Hsiao, K. K.: Human prion diseases. Ann. Neurol. *35*:385–395, 1994.
151. Public Health Service, U.S. Dept. Health, Education and Welfare, joint statement: Fatal viral encephalitis following 17D yellow fever vaccine inoculation: Report of a case in a 3-year-old child. J. A. M. A. *198*:203–204, 1966.
152. Purdham, D. R., and Batty, P. F.: A case of acute measles meningoencephalitis with virus isolation. J. Clin. Pathol. *27*:994–996, 1974.
153. Quiroz, E., Moreno, N., Peralta, P. H., et al.: A human case of encephalitis associated with vesicular stomatitis virus (Indiana serotype) infection. Am. J. Trop. Med. Hyg. *39*:312–314, 1988.
154. Rantala, H., and Uhari, M.: Occurrence of childhood encephalitis: A population-based study. Pediatr. Infect. Dis. J. *8*:426–430, 1989.
155. Raoult, D., and Marrie, T.: Q fever. Clin. Infect. Dis. *20*:489–496, 1995.
156. Rautonen, J., Koskiniemi, M., and Vaheri, A.: Prognostic factors in childhood acute encephalitis. Pediatr. Infect. Dis. J. *10*:441–446, 1991.
157. Rie, H. E., Hilty, M. D., and Cramblatt, H. G.: Intelligence and coordination following California encephalitis. Am. J. Dis. Child. *125*:824–827, 1973.
158. Robb, L., and Butt, W.: Brain stem encephalitis due to herpes simplex virus. Aust. Paediatr. J. *25*:246–247, 1989.
159. Robinson, L. J.: Neurologic complications following the administration of vaccines and serums: Report of a case of peripheral paralysis following the injection of typhoid vaccine. N. Engl. J. Med. *216*:831–837, 1937.
160. Rosenberg, G. A.: Meningoencephalitis following an influenza vaccination. N. Engl. J. Med. *283*:1209–1210, 1970.
161. Rosenblum, M. K.: Bulbar encephalitis complicating trigeminal zoster in the acquired immune deficiency syndrome. Hum. Pathol. *20*:292–295, 1989.
162. Rothstein, T., and Shaw, C. M.: Computerized tomography as a diagnostic aid in acute hemorrhagic leukoencephalitis. Ann. Neurol. *13*:331–333, 1983.
163. Rubeiz, H., and Roos, R. P.: Viral meningitis and encephalitis. Semin. Neurol. *12*:165–177, 1992.
164. Sainio, K., Granstrom, M. L., Pettay, O., et al.: EEG in neonatal herpes simplex encephalitis. Electroencephalogr. Clin. Neurophysiol. *56*:556–561, 1983.
165. Salaki, J. S., Louria, D. B., and Chmel, H.: Fungal and yeast infections of the central nervous system: A clinical review. Medicine *63*:108–132, 1984.
166. Schlesinger, Y., Butler, R. S., and Brunstrom, J. E.: Expanded spectrum of herpes simplex encephalitis in childhood. J. Pediatr. *126*:234–241, 1995.
167. Schmidbauer, M., Budka, H., and Ambros, P.: Herpes simplex virus (HSV) DNA in microglial nodular brainstem encephalitis. J. Neuropathol. Exp. Neurol. *48*:645–652, 1989.
168. Seidel, J. S., Harmatz, P., Visvesvara, G. S., et al.: Successful treatment of primary amebic meningoencephalitis. N. Engl. J. Med. *306*:346–348, 1982.
169. Shaffer, M. F., Rake, G., Hodes, H. L.: Isolation of virus from a patient with fatal encephalitis complicating measles. Am. J. Dis. Child. *64*:815–819, 1942.
170. Shaked, Y., and Samra, Y.: Q fever meningoencephalitis associated with bilateral abducens nerve paralysis, bilateral optic neuritis and abnormal cerebrospinal fluid findings. Infection *17*:394–395, 1989.
171. Shaw, D. W. W., and Cohen, W. A.: Viral infections of the CNA in children: Imaging features. A. J. R. Am. J. Roentgenol. *160*:125–133, 1993.
172. Sherman, F. E., Michaels, R. H., and Kenny, F. M.: Acute encephalopathy (encephalitis) complicating rubella. J. A. M. A. *192*:675–681, 1965.
173. Sheth, R. D., Goulden, K. J., and Pryse-Phillips, W. E.: The focal encephalopathies associated with *Mycoplasma pneumoniae*. Can. J. Neurol. Sci. *20*:319–323, 1993.
174. Shields, W. D.: Status epilepticus. Pediatr. Clin. North Am. *36*:383–393, 1989.
175. Siegman-Igra, Y., Michaeli, D., Doron, A., et al.: Cytomegalovirus encephalitis in a noncompromised host. Isr. J. Med. Sci. *20*:163–166, 1984.
176. Sillimsan, C. C., Tedder, D., Ogle, J. W., et al.: Unsuspected varicella-zoster virus encephalitis in a child with acquired immunodeficiency syndrome. J. Pediatr. *123*:418–422, 1993.
177. Southern, P. M., Jr.: Relapsing fever. *In* Tice, F. (ed.): Practice of Medicine. Vol. 3. Scranton, Hoeber Medical Division, Harper & Row, 1969, pp. 1–19.
178. Spillane, J. D., and Wells, C. E. C.: The neurology of Jennerian vaccination: A clinical account of the neurological complications which occurred during the smallpox epidemic in South Wales in 1962. Brain *87*:1–44, 1964.
179. Steiner, M. M., Vuckovitch, D., and Hadawi, S. A.: Cat-scratch disease with encephalopathy: Case report and review of the literature. J. Pediatr. *62*:514–520, 1963.
180. Tesh, R. B.: The prevalence of encephalomyocarditis virus neutralizing antibodies among various human populations. Am. J. Trop. Med. Hyg. *27*:144–149, 1978.
181. Thong, T. H.: Primary amoebic meningoencephalitis. Fifteen years later. Med. J. Aust. *1*:352–354, 1980.
182. Townsend, J. J., Wolinsky, J. S., Baringer, J. R., et al.: Acquired toxoplasmosis: A neglected cause of treatable nervous system disease. Arch. Neurol. *32*:335–343, 1975.
183. Tsutsumi, H., Kamazaki, H., Nakata, S., et al: Sequential development of acute meningoencephalitis and transverse myelitis caused by Epstein-Barr virus during infectious mononucleosis. Pediatr. Infect. Dis. J. *13*:665–667, 1994.

184. Uren, E. C., Johnson, P. D. R., Montanaro, J., et al.: Herpes simplex virus encephalitis in pediatrics: Diagnosis by detection of antibodies and DNA in cerebrospinal fluid. Pediatr. Infect. Dis. J. *12*:1001–1006, 1993.
185. Visvesvara, G. S., Martinez, A. J., Schuster, F. L., et al.: *Leptomyxid ameba*, a new agent of amebic meningoencephalitis in humans and animals. J. Clin. Microbiol. *28*:2750–2756, 1990.
186. Wallace, S. J., and Zealley, H.: Neurological, electroencephalographic, and virological findings in febrile children. Arch. Dis. Child. *45*:611–623, 1970.
187. Warren, J.: Encephalitis lethargica. *In* Rivers, T. M., and Horsfall, F. L., Jr. (eds.): Viral and Rickettsial Infections of Man. Philadelphia, J. B. Lippincott, 1959, pp. 914–915.
188. Watson, R. T., Ballinger, W. E., and Quisling, R. G.: Acute hemorrhagic leukoencephalitis: Diagnosis by computed tomography. Ann. Neurol. *15*:611–612, 1984.
189. Weisberg, L. A.: The role of CT in the evaluation of patients with intracranial CNS infectious-inflammatory disorders. Comput. Radiol. *8*:29–36, 1984.
190. Whitley, R. J.: Viral encephalitis. N. Engl. J. Med. *323*:242–250, 1990.
191. Whitley, R. J., Cobbs, C. G., Alford, C. A., Jr., et al.: Diseases that mimic herpes simplex encephalitis: Diagnosis, presentation and outcome. J. A. M. A. *262*:234–239, 1989.
192. Whitley, R. J., and Lakeman, F.: Herpes simplex virus infections of the central nervous system: Therapeutic and diagnostic considerations. Clin. Infect Dis. *20*:414–420, 1995.
193. Woods, C. A., and Ellison, G. W.: Encephalopathy following influenza immunization. J. Pediatr. *65*:745–748, 1964.
194. World Health Organization: World Health Statistics Annual. Vol. 11, Infectious Diseases: Cases and Deaths. Geneva, World Health Organization, 1978.
195. Yoshikawa, T., Nakashima, T., Suga, S., et al.: Human herpesvirus-6 DNA in cerebrospinal fluid of a child with exanthem subitum and meningoencephalitis. Pediatrics *89*:888–890, 1992.
196. Young, E. J.: Human brucellosis. Rev. Infect. Dis. *5*:821–842, 1983.
197. Zalan, E., Leers, W. D., and Labzoffsky, N. A.: Occurrence of reovirus infection in Ontario. Can. Med. Assoc. J. *87*:714–715, 1962.
198. Ziegra, S. R.: Corticosteroid treatment for measles encephalitis. J. Pediatr. *39*:322–323, 1961.
199. Zinserling, A. V., Aksenov, O. A., Melnikova, V. F., et al.: Extrapulmonary lesions in influenza. Tohoku J. Exp. Med. *140*:259–272, 1983.

44

TRANSVERSE MYELITIS OR MYELOPATHY

Scott L. Pomeroy, Mary E. Sutton, and Philip R. Dodge

Transverse myelitis is a clinical syndrome with complete or partial loss of neurologic functions as a result of an intrinsic spinal cord lesion of unclear etiology. Most often, the lesion involves a limited number of segments, usually in the cervical or thoracic cord. Although inflammation is implied and at times present on pathologic examination, it is an inconsistent finding. For this reason, the term *transverse myelopathy* is preferred by many neurologists.

ETIOLOGY AND PATHOGENESIS

As a syndrome rather than a disease, the spectrum of probable causes is broad. However, the cause remains unknown in the majority of patients who have the typical clinical findings.

Abramsky and Teitelbaum[1] studied 10 patients with idiopathic myelitis, one of whom was a 14-year-old male. They presented immunologic evidence suggesting that cell-mediated autoimmune mechanisms may be an important factor in the pathogenesis of acute transverse myelitis. Antecedent infection is noted more often in children than in older persons.[3] A variety of organisms have been identified in association with transverse myelitis, including *Borrelia burgdorferi* (Lyme disease), Epstein-Barr virus, and *Mycoplasma pneumoniae*.[8, 11, 14] Transverse myelitis also has been described in association with systemic lupus erythematosus and as a rare complication of acute bacterial meningitis.[5, 13] McCarthy and Amer[7] reported that the ages ranged from 3 years to 30 years, although the exact number of children was not cited.

PREVALENCE

During a 20-year period, 62 Jewish patients in Israel were reported to have transverse myelitis, for an average incidence rate of 1.3 per million population.[3] The syndrome is encountered more commonly in adults than in children. Altrocchi[2] reviewed the 67 patients (44 adults and 23 children) who were encountered over a 25-year period at the Columbia Presbyterian Medical Center in New York. Males and females were affected about equally. Cases associated with compressive lesions, serious trauma, and radiation myelopathy; patients with evidence of concomitant cerebral involvement; and patients thought to have multiple sclerosis were excluded.

PATHOLOGY

The pathology of myelitis or myelopathy includes varying degrees of destruction affecting either white or gray matter or often both, usually in an asymmetric fashion, with this irregular pattern of involvement persisting over the longitudinal extent of the lesion. Patchy destruction frequently involves several segments of the spinal cord but may be even more extensive. Demyelination, neuronal injury, and incomplete or complete necrosis of neural tissue have been described and may, at times, be associated with inflammatory cells, macrophages, or proliferation of astroglia. The form of the reaction probably is related to the duration of the disease and its cause. Thickening of small arteries and veins within or adjacent to the parenchyma of the spinal cord has been prominent in only a few of the recorded cases.

Because death rarely occurs in the acute state of the illness today, recent reports characteristically lack postmortem studies employing modern histochemical and cytologic techniques.

CLINICAL MANIFESTATIONS

The onset usually is abrupt, with the neurologic deficit evolving from the initial symptoms to maximal disability within hours to a few days or occasionally a few weeks. A premonitory history of an upper respiratory tract or other infection or minor trauma is reported in about 25 per cent of patients. The earliest symptoms are (1) muscle weakness, usually involving the lower limbs, (2) sensory aberrations, (3) back discomfort, and (4) root pain, all occurring with about equal frequency. Signs may be asymmetric, but bilateral involvement of the spinal cord is invariable at some time in the course of the disorder. Bladder and bowel dysfunction are nearly universal as paresis of the limbs and sensory disturbances progress.

The degree of paraparesis is variable, but moderate to severe weakness of the legs occurs in about two thirds of patients. Weakness may affect the arms in as many as one quarter of patients. Sensory loss also is seen in approximately two thirds of reported cases, pain and temperature being affected more often than position and vibratory sensation. Segmental paresthesias and dysesthesias may occur. Stretch reflexes often are lost in the acute stage of the disease but become exaggerated later. Babinski signs are usual. Meningeal signs are encountered in up to one-third of patients. There is fever in about one half of patients, although this may be referable to complicating infections of the lung or urinary tract.

The cerebrospinal fluid findings are extremely variable, even during the acute stage of the disease. In some patients, the cerebrospinal fluid may be acellular with only a slight rise in the protein concentration, but there may be several hundred or a thousand or more leukocytes, often with a predominant polymorphonuclear reaction in the acute state. The protein concentration may be elevated to several hundred milligrams per deciliter, and the percentage of gamma globulin can be increased significantly. The sugar content typically is normal. Gadolinium-enhanced magnetic resonance imaging may demonstrate increased T2 signal and spinal cord enlargement at the site of the lesion (Fig. 44–1).[12]

DIAGNOSIS

Although the diagnosis of transverse myelitis or myelopathy can be suspected on clinical grounds, the physician should consider first those diseases that demand specific and prompt treatment. Spinal epidural abscess can mimic transverse myelitis closely, although the course of the latter condition usually is more rapid. Magnetic resonance imaging or contrast myelography should be performed to establish the diagnosis. The risk of these procedures is minimal, and the danger of missing a compressive suppurative lesion that should be treated by surgery is of overriding concern. Intraspinal neoplasms and other compressive tumors also will be excluded by magnetic resonance imaging or myelography, except in those rare instances in which an acutely inflamed, swollen cord may mimic an intra-axial mass.[10]

Syphilis, especially the meningovascular form, may mimic nonspecific myelitis and deserves immediate treatment. The treatable nutritional myelopathies evolve more slowly and have a pattern of spinal cord involvement that is more diffuse. Other evidence of vitamin B_{12} deficiency or of pellagra should make exclusion of these disorders relatively easy. A vascular nevus at the segmental level of the spinal cord lesion should signal the possibility of an intraspinal vascular malformation that can be defined by selective spinal cord angiography.

Every effort should be made to establish the diagnosis of specific viral infections by the appropriate cultures and serologic tests. Appropriate serologic tests (complement fixation or enzyme-linked immunosorbent assay) and cultures should be obtained to exclude disease due to *Mycoplasma*. A diagnosis of multiple sclerosis may become obvious only when lesions of the central nervous system disseminated in time and space appear. Transverse myelitis has been described after the inadvertent intra-arterial injection of benzathine penicillin and after intrathecal administration of chemotherapeutic agents.[15]

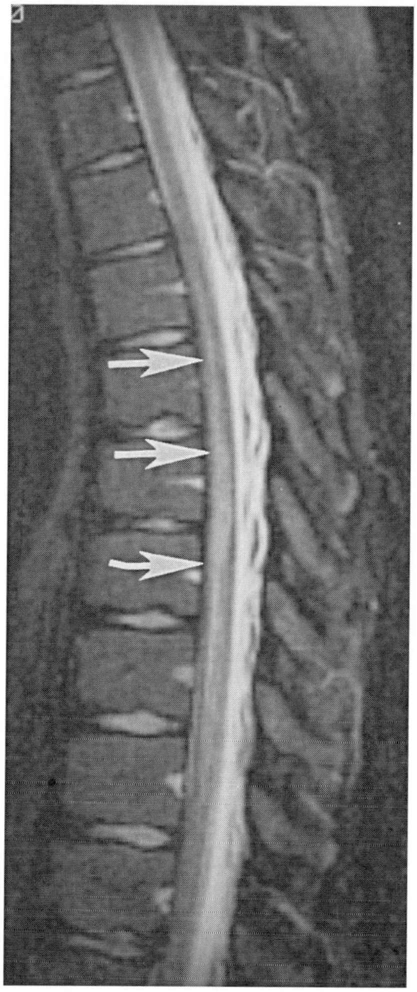

Figure 44–1. *Sagittal T2-weighted magnetic resonance image reveals increased signal and expansion of the midthoracic spinal cord in a 14-year-old female who presented with subacute onset paraplegia after an Epstein-Barr virus infection. (Courtesy of Drs. C. D. Robson and P. D. Barnes.)*

TREATMENT

There is no specific treatment for transverse myelitis or myelopathy of unknown cause. The efficacy of pharmacologic doses of the glucocorticoids is unproved but might be considered, particularly if there is evidence of swelling of the spinal cord.[9] Prevention or appropriate treatment for the complications of paraplegia is critical.

PROGNOSIS

Proper supportive care, including therapy for complicating infection, prevention of pressure sores, and attention to urinary tract function, renders the prognosis for survival excellent. According to Altrocchi,[2] one-third of patients make a good or complete recovery, one-third do moderately well, and one-third have a poor recovery. Lipton and Teasdall[6] found similar results in adults. Children tend to do better; more than 50 per cent recover completely or have a good outcome.[4] Recurrent neurologic problems are rare among the survivors.

References

1. Abramsky, O., and Teitelbaum, D.: The autoimmune features of acute transverse myelopathy. Ann. Neurol. 2:36–40, 1977.
2. Altrocchi, P. H.: Acute transverse myelopathy. Arch. Neurol. *9*:111–119, 1963.
3. Berman, M., Feldman, S., Alter, M., et al.: Acute transverse myelitis: Incidence and etiologic considerations. Neurology *31*:966–971, 1981.
4. Dunne, K., Hopkins, I. J., and Shield, L. K.: Acute transverse myelopathy in childhood. Dev. Med. Child Neurol. *28*:198–204, 1986.
5. Linssen, W. H. J. P., Fiselier, T. J. W., Gabreëls, G. J. M., et al.: Acute transverse myelopathy as the initial manifestation of probably systematic lupus erythematosus in a child. Neuropediatrics *19*:212–215, 1988.
6. Lipton, H. L., and Teasdall, R. D.: Acute transverse myelopathy in adults. Arch. Neurol. *28*:252–257, 1973.
7. McCarthy, J. T., and Amer, J.: Postvaricella acute transverse myelitis: A case presentation and review of the literature. Pediatrics *62*:202–204, 1978.
8. Mills, R. W., and Schoolfield, L.: Acute transverse myelitis associated with *Mycoplasma pneumoniae* infection: A case report and review of the literature. Pediatr. Infect. Dis. J. *11*:228–231, 1992.
9. Paine, R. S., and Byers, R. K.: Transverse myelopathy in childhood. Am. J. Dis. Child. *85*:151–163, 1953.
10. Ropper, A. H., and Poskanzer, D. C.: The prognosis of acute and subacute transverse myelopathy based on early signs and symptoms. Ann. Neurol. *4*:51–59, 1978.
11. Rousseau, J. J., Lust, C., Bangerle, P. F., et al.: Acute transverse myelitis as presenting neurological feature of Lyme disease. Lancet *2*:1222–1223, 1986.
12. Sanders, K. A., Khandji, A. G., and Mohr, J. P.: Gadolinium-MRI in acute transverse myelopathy. Neurology *40*:1614–1616, 1990.
13. Seay, A. R.: Spinal cord dysfunction complicating bacterial meningitis. Arch. Neurol. *41*:545–546, 1984.
14. Tsutsumi, H., Kamazaki, H., Nakata, S., et al.: Sequential development of acute meningoencephalitis and transverse myelitis caused by Epstein-Barr virus during infectious mononucleosis. Pediatr. Infect. Dis. *13*:665–667, 1994.
15. Weir, M. R., and Fearnow, R. G.: Transverse myelitis and penicillin. Pediatrics *71*:988, 1983.

Additional Reading

Dodge, P. R.: Transverse myelitis or myelopathy. *In* Beeson, P. B., McDermott, W., and Wyngaarden, J. B. (eds.): Textbook of Medicine. 15th ed. Philadelphia, W. B. Saunders, 1979, pp. 811–812.

Greenfield, J. G., and Turner, J. W. A.: Acute and subacute necrotic myelitis. Brain *62*:227–252, 1939.

Hoffman, H. L.: Acute necrotic myelopathy. Brain *78*:377–393, 1955.

45

GUILLAIN-BARRÉ SYNDROME

Daniel G. Glaze

The Guillain-Barré syndrome (GBS) is an acute, demyelinating disease of the peripheral nervous system. With the decline in the incidence of poliomyelitis, GBS has emerged as the most frequent cause of acute, severe generalized human paralytic disease.[180, 189] This disorder typically occurs several weeks after an upper respiratory or gastrointestinal tract illness, but it has been associated with other factors, including immunization and surgery. It is characterized by progressive motor weakness, hyporeflexia, and minor sensory disturbances. An elevated protein concentration contrasts with a relatively normal cell count in the cerebrospinal fluid (CSF). There is no diagnostic test for GBS; the diagnosis is based on the clinical features supported by other data, including CSF protein elevation, electrophysiologic changes, and pathologic changes of the peripheral nerves. The precise diagnostic limits of GBS remain uncertain.[8] It generally is accepted that GBS is mediated immunologically. However, the specific immunologic alterations necessary to initiate the events that result in demyelinization of human peripheral nerve are unclear. The primary treatment modality is supportive care, but the efficacy of other therapies, such as plasma exchange transfusion and intravenous immunoglobulin (IVIG) therapy, in shortening the duration of the illness and decreasing the need for mechanical ventilation has been demonstrated.[50, 89, 196, 197] This chapter presents an overview of GBS, including diagnostic inclusion and exclusion criteria, the role of preceding viral infection and immunization, immunologic aspects, and treatment modalities.

HISTORY

Although bearing the names of Guillain and Barré, this disorder first was recognized by Landry in 1859.[106] He reported 10 patients who usually first had generalized weakness, then paresthesia and transitory muscle cramps, and then rapidly ascending paralysis that involved the respiratory muscles last. He named this disorder *acute ascending paralysis*, postulated that it occurred after another illness, and considered it to be a severe disease because 2 of the 10 patients died. Other reports of this disorder appeared, but, in 1916, Guillain, Barré, and Strohl[73] clearly characterized this disorder and first called attention to the "albuminocytologic dissociation" (increased CSF protein with absence of cells). Barré and Guillain favored an infectious cause; in 1955, Waksman and Adams[202] pointed out the similarity in the clinical and pathologic picture between GBS and experimental allergic neuritis in rabbits. Melnick,[125] in 1963, found antibodies to nervous tissue in 19 of 38 GBS patients. In 1960, Osler and Sidell[141] indicated the need for exact diagnostic criteria for GBS and presented 12 diagnostic criteria restricting the definition of the disorder. Most subsequent studies arrived at a broader concept of the disorder.[5, 9, 53] After the reports of significant increase of GBS in association with the 1976 inoculation program for swine flu and sponsored by the National Institute of Neurological and Communicative Disorders and Stroke (NINCDS), inclusion and exclusion diagnostic criteria were proposed.[8–10]

DIAGNOSTIC CRITERIA

The diagnosis of GBS is based on the clinical history and examination and supported by clinical laboratory (i.e., CSF) and electrodiagnostic (i.e., nerve conduction velocities) evaluations. The "typical" case of GBS often follows a recognizable nonspecific infection, more often viral than bacterial, after a period of a few days or weeks. The paralytic stage usually begins with pain or paresthesia, followed by hypotonic, ascending paralysis without pyramidal tract involvement—loss of deep tendon reflexes rather than hyperreflexia or pathologic reflexes. Initial weakness usually is noted in the lower extremities and less commonly in the upper extremities or the face. A significant number of patients experience minimal to moderate sensory loss in a glove-stocking distribution. Maximum paralysis is reached in about 3 weeks, with more acute than chronic courses occurring. In 46 to 75 per cent of persons, cranial nerves may be affected, including VII, IX/X, or both, giving rise to facial weakness and difficulties in swallowing. Respiratory weakness occurs in 12 to 20 per cent of patients, and some may require mechanical ventilation. Pain, usually described as similar to muscular discomfort after exercise, has been reported to occur in 55 per cent of GBS patients, and it may precede weakness in a few patients.[161] Routine laboratory findings are unremarkable, except for characteristic elevation of CSF protein (typical values of 50 to 200 mg/dL) without appearances of cells. CSF protein usually peaks during the second to eighth weeks, with a slow decline thereafter. Although most patients experience "complete" recovery, some (20 per cent) have permanent residual disease (weakness, muscle atrophy) or rarely (1 to 4 per cent) die of respiratory failure.[14, 121]

As has been emphasized by Asbury,[8] the problem is not with recognition of a typical case but with knowing the delimiting boundaries of the disorder. To define those limits, criteria have been reported and are presented in Table 45–1.[10, 11] These criteria include features required for diagnosis: progressive motor weakness of more than one limb and areflexia.

Clinical features supporting the diagnosis include the following: progression of symptoms with signs of motor weakness ceasing to progress by 4 weeks into the illness; symmetry of symptoms; sensory, cranial nerve, and autonomic dysfunction; recovery; and absence of fever.

Laboratory features supporting diagnosis include CSF protein elevation after the first week of symptoms or rise on serial lumbar punctures and fewer than 10 mononuclear leukocytes/mm³.

The major features of physiologic studies of GBS include early conduction block, early reduction in distal evoked compound muscle action potential amplitude, and a later reduction in motor conduction velocity.[35] Electrodiagnostic features supporting diagnosis include evidence of nerve conduction slowing in about 80 per cent of cases characterized by conduction velocity usually less than 60 per cent of normal, patchy distribution, and some unaffected nerves; conduction studies yield normal results in the other 20 per cent.[8, 9]

Certain features cast doubt on the diagnosis or rule out the diagnosis. The latter include a purely sensory syndrome, a current history of hexacarbon abuse, abnormal porphyrin metabolism (increased excretion of porphobilinogen and δ-aminolevulinic acid in the urine), evidence of recent diphtheric infection or lead neuropathy and intoxication, or a definite diagnosis of a condition such as poliomyelitis, botulism, hysterical paralysis, or toxic neuropathy (nitrofurantoin, dapsone, or organophosphorus).[8, 9]

A diagnostic process has been suggested.[8] If the clinical features and temporal evolution are typical and without variant features or features that rule out GBS, the diagnosis may be made on clinical grounds alone. Laboratory findings, such as CSF protein elevation, may not appear until after a week, whereas electrodiagnostic findings may never appear. However, if clinical features are unusual, laboratory studies may provide important supportive information, and a diagnosis of GBS may have to be delayed to evaluate fully these tests. Asbury and Cornblath[11] reported that certain variant features are seen on occasion in otherwise typical cases of GBS. These variant features include the following:

1. Fever at onset of neuritic symptoms
2. Severe sensory loss with pain
3. Progression beyond 4 weeks
4. Cessation of progression without recovery or with major permanent residual deficit
5. Sphincter dysfunction
6. CNS involvement
7. No rise in CSF protein in the period of 1 to 10 weeks after onset of symptoms
8. Counts of 11 to 50 mononuclear leukocytes/mm³ in CSF

These authors suggested that the presence of one of these symptoms, signs, or laboratory results should raise doubt about the validity of the diagnosis and that the presence of two or more suggest that the diagnosis of GBS is incorrect. Also, manifestations of systemic illness or constitutional symptoms or both preceding or coinciding with signs and symptoms of involvement of peripheral nervous system should suggest a diagnosis of a systemic illness or intoxication and not GBS. In HIV-seropositive patients with features consistent with GBS, CSF cell counts frequently are elevated.[11]

TABLE 45–1. Criteria for Diagnosis of Guillain-Barré Syndrome[8, 9]

Required

Progressive motor weakness in more than one extremity
Areflexia (at least distal with hyporeflexia of the biceps and knee jerks)

Strongly Supportive

Clinical features (in order of importance)
- Progression: ceases by 4 weeks
- Relative symmetry
- Mild sensory symptoms or signs
- Cranial nerve involvement
- Recovery: usually 2–4 weeks after progression ceases
- Autonomic dysfunction
- Absence of fever at onset of neurologic symptoms

Cerebrospinal Fluid Features

- Protein: elevated after first week of symptoms, or rising on serial lumbar punctures
- Cells: 10 or fewer mononuclear leukocytes/mm³

Electrodiagnostic features
- Nerve conduction slowing

Casting Doubt

Marked, persistent asymmetry of weakness
Persistent bladder or bowel dysfunction
Bowel or bladder dysfunction at onset
More than 50 mononuclear leukocytes/mm³ in cerebrospinal fluid
Presence of polymorphonuclear leukocytes in cerebrospinal fluid
Sharp sensory level

Rule Out the Diagnosis

Current history of hexacarbon abuse
Abnormal porphyrin metabolism
Recent diphtheria infection
Evidence of lead neuropathy or intoxication
Purely sensory syndrome
Definite diagnosis of poliomyelitis, botulism, hysterical paralysis, or toxic neuropathy

CLINICAL VARIANTS

Typically, GBS has an acute onset followed by rapidly ascending weakness. In some patients, onset is stuttering with periods of progression and plateaus before reaching the nadir of involvement. Onset is subacute in some patients, with a slow progression that can take place over a few weeks.[123] In addition to weakness and areflexia, other individual features may be observed in patients with GBS. These include total and incomplete external ophthalmoplegia[65, 70]; papilledema[38]; and autonomic dysfunction, including hypertension, postural hypotension, and cardiovascular disturbances.[38, 39, 184, 192] Hypertension may be a consequence of sympathetic nervous system hypersensitivity and increased excretion of catecholamines[38, 73, 192] but has been associated with increased renin-angiotensin activity.[169] Cardiovascular disturbances have been reported to be more prevalent in GBS patients who are severely paralyzed and require mechanical ventilation.[39] Autonomic dysfunction in GBS, including tachycardia and other arrhythmias, may contribute to morbidity.[39, 192]

One criticism of the NINCDS Ad Hoc Committee criteria is that they are too restrictive.[8, 10] The criteria initially were designed for use during field studies of GBS. Certain variants are allowed: fever at onset of neuritic symptoms; severe sensory loss with pain; occasional progression beyond 4 weeks; major permanent residual deficits; transient bladder paralysis; and, possibly, CNS involvement such as ataxia (cerebellar), dysarthria, extensor plantar responses, and ill-defined sensory levels. These features need not exclude the diagnosis of GBS.[8, 9]

Specific variants in which the clinical features are atypical but may fall in the spectrum of GBS have been described.[8, 9] Findings of ophthalmoplegia, ataxia, and areflexia have been designated as Miller Fisher syndrome.[60, 158] The rapid onset of these symptoms usually indicates a benign course with fairly complete recovery within weeks to months.[8, 9] Sensory loss and areflexia without motor weakness or simultaneous onset of symmetric cranial nerve dysfunction may be accepted as variants of GBS if characterized by rapid onset and recovery, elevation of CSF protein, and the typical electrodiagnostic pattern of demyelination.[8, 9]

EPIDEMIOLOGY

Since the decline in the incidence of poliomyelitis, GBS has been reported to be the most frequent cause of acute, generalized human paralytic disease.[180] However, trends in the incidence of GBS are difficult to assess because earlier epidemiologic studies[14, 21, 109, 180] were based on small numbers of cases and lacked common and well-defined diagnostic criteria for GBS. The results of these studies may not be comparable because of diagnostic and methodologic differences.[14] Schonberger and associates[173] have reviewed these epidemiologic data for GBS.

Case Reports

Leneman[108] reported an extensive list of 1100 cases. Of these cases, 638 were associated with a variety of infectious diseases, 150 cases with allergic phenomenon or immune responses, 96 cases with metabolic or endocrine disturbances, 14 cases with toxic agents, 33 cases with neoplasms, 1 case with an influenza vaccination, and 365 cases with no known antecedent or underlying disease. However, as has been emphasized,[173] it is difficult to determine whether reported associations are etiologic or merely coincidental.

Case Control Studies

Five studies[4, 47, 95, 126, 184] that compared the frequency of suspected etiologic factors in a group of GBS patients and a selected group without GBS were reviewed. These studies provided evidence that important risk factors for GBS include recent nonspecific antecedent respiratory infection (48 per cent[126]; 43 to 65 per cent of GBS cases in other reports[94, 109]), recent gastrointestinal infection (32 per cent),[95] or recent cytomegalovirus (CMV) infection (32.6 per cent).[47] Three studies[4, 107, 184] found no association of human leukocyte antigen type and GBS.

Incidence Rates in Well-Defined Populations

Ten studies were reviewed,[14, 21, 25, 72, 82, 94, 95, 104, 109, 136] and the crude average annual incidence rate of GBS per 100,000 population ranged from 0.6 to 1.9. It has been suggested that the similarities of these incidence rates are consistent with a hypothesis that the triggering agents responsible for GBS are widespread and multiple and that susceptibility to GBS in geographically scattered populations is similarly low.[173] However, higher incidences have been reported, including an increased risk within a 5-week period after A/New Jersey influenza vaccine was administered during 1976.[172] Also, for a large, well-defined Colorado population, an incidence of 4 cases per 100,000 per year for 1981 to 1983 was reported, which contrasted with an incidence of 1.2 cases per 100,000 per year for 1975 to 1980.[94] The increased incidence could not be accounted for on the basis of patient characteristics or predisposing factors. These studies of incidence rates have indicated a higher incidence for males and, in one study, for whites compared with blacks.[173] Peak incidences in the first decade of life,[162] in the fifth and sixth decades,[119, 155, 180] or in both younger and older patients[180] have been observed. These findings may be due to socioeconomic factors, which might influence the age at which viral infections were acquired, or due to age-dependent immune system peculiarities.[180] No clear seasonal or geographic clustering of GBS has been observed.

One study[14] has presented an updated evaluation of GBS using more rigid criteria proposed by the NINCDS Ad Hoc Committee (Table 45–2). The incidence of GBS from 1935 to 1980 in Olmsted County, Minnesota, was 1.8 per 100,000 person-years (age- and sex-adjusted). The rate increased from 1.2 (1935 to 1956) to 2.4 (1970 to 1980). Males were affected more than females (2.3 vs. 1.2). The incidence rate increased with age from 0.8 in those younger than 18 years of age to 3.2 for those 60 years of age or older. In the 4 weeks preceding the onset of neurologic symptoms, 65 per cent of the 48 patients had an antecedent infection, including 21 patients with upper respiratory tract illnesses, 10 with gastrointestinal tract illnesses, and 9 with nonspecific febrile illnesses. A nadir was reached after onset at an average of 8 days. Illness duration was an average of 12 weeks. Two (4 per cent) of the 48 patients died as a result of GBS; minimal residua were observed in about 20 per cent, whereas no patient had severe residua.

SENTINEL NEUROLOGISTS' SURVEILLANCE OF GUILLAIN-BARRÉ SYNDROME IN THE UNITED STATES

Between January 1, 1978, and March 31, 1979, neurologists who were members of the American Association of Neuropa-

TABLE 45–2. Antecedent Factors

Strongly Suggestive Evidence
- Cytomegalovirus
- Epstein-Barr virus
- Coxsackieviruses A
- *Campylobacter jejuni*
- *Mycoplasma pneumoniae*

Suggestive Evidence
- A/New Jersey 1976 influenza immunization

Survey Study or Anecdotal Reports
- Viral Agents:
  - Echoviruses
  - Coxsackieviruses A and B
  - Influenza viruses A and B
  - Measles
  - Varicella virus
  - Rubella
  - Mumps
  - Hepatitis viruses
  - Herpes simplex viruses
  - Rabies
  - HIV
- Nonviral Agents:
  - *Francisella (Pasteurella) tularensis* (tularemia)
  - *Chlamydia*
  - *Plasmodium* (malaria)
  - *Toxoplasma gondii*
  - *Mycobacterium tuberculosis*
- Noninfectious Agents:
  - Immunizations
    - Trivalent oral poliovirus
    - Diphtheria-tetanus-pertussis
    - Measles-mumps-rubella
    - Rabies
    - Influenza, other than A/New Jersey
    - Polyvalent pneumococcal
    - Hepatitis
    - *Haemophilus influenzae* type b
  - Surgery
  - Trauma
  - Epidural anesthesia
  - Neoplasm (Hodgkin)
  - Vasculitides (systemic lupus erythematosus)
  - Drug hypersensitivities
  - Heroin addiction
  - Drug (zimeldine)

thologists (AAN) were surveyed by the Centers for Disease Control and Prevention (CDC).[173] This survey indicated that the incidence rate for males was 39 per cent higher than for females and 50 to 60 per cent higher for whites than for blacks. The incidence rates were highest for persons 50 to 74 years of age. Sixty-seven per cent of the patients for whom information was available indicated that they had had an antecedent illness within 8 weeks before the onset of GBS: 58 per cent primarily respiratory, 22 per cent gastrointestinal, and 10 per cent both respiratory and gastrointestinal. The peak interval between the antecedent respiratory or gastrointestinal tract illness and the onset of GBS was 2 weeks. Five per cent of GBS patients had undergone surgery within 8 weeks prior to the onset of GBS; the significance of this in comparison with the general population has not been confirmed.

A report based on a retrospective epidemiologic survey carried out in southern California found the mean annual incidence of GBS to be 0.60 (95 per cent confidence intervals, 0.48 to 0.73) per 100,000 children younger than 15 years of age.[154] This study was based on the review of medical records of all children discharged from 22 hospitals caring for children in Los Angeles and Orange counties with the diagnosis of any kind of neuropathy. The criteria proposed by the GBS study group were used to identify the children with GBS and excluded those with a history or evidence of poliomyelitis, diphtheria, botulism, hexacarbon abuse, porphyria, lead intoxication, toxic neuropathy, exposure to organophosphates, or tic paralysis.[68] From 1980 to 1986, 93 affected children younger than 15 years of age living in the study area were identified. Eighty-eight had progressive motor weakness of more than one limb; five had Miller Fisher variant with ataxia, areflexia, and ophthalmoplegia. Ninety-two had an initial lumbar puncture, and all of these had CSF cell counts of no more than 50 monocytes or 2 polymorphonuclear leukocytes; 79 had a repeat lumbar puncture, and all of these had elevated CSF protein after 1 week of symptoms. In all patients, disease progressed for days to a few weeks and recovery ensued 2 to 4 weeks after progression of symptoms was halted. Eighty-eight had relative symmetry of weakness, and 22 had autonomic dysfunction. In seventy-one patients (76 per cent), the onset of GBS was preceded by an infection. There was no significant difference in the incidence of GBS between boys and girls, among ethnic groups, or in the annual and monthly occurrence. The incidence was significantly higher in 2-year-old children than in any other group.[154]

Age-related differences in the expression of GBS in children have been observed.[169] In children younger than 5 years of age, there was a greater incidence of bulbar nerve (cranial nerves IX, X, XII) dysfunction. In children younger than 5 years of age, muscle weakness was the most frequent initial symptom, occurring in 72 per cent. In children older than 5 years of age, limb pain was the most frequent initial symptom (53.4 per cent). The interval between previous illness and onset of GBS was shorter for children older than 5 years of age and typically was 2 to 14 days. There were no statistically significant differences in respiratory complications or fatal outcome between the groups of older and younger children with GBS.

PATHOLOGY AND PATHOGENESIS

GBS has been described as a distinctive neuropathy characterized pathologically by the presence of inflammatory lesions scattered throughout the peripheral nervous system.[138, 150] Asbury and associates[9, 10] studied 19 fatal cases and observed that the pathologic hallmark of this disorder is a perivenular mononuclear inflammatory infiltrate, which was observed throughout the peripheral nervous system, even in the cases of shortest clinical course (1 to 4 days). They observed that the lesions were predominantly lymphocytic and that the inflammatory infiltrate tended to cluster about small endoneural and epineural vessels, particularly veins, in a seemingly random, multifocal manner. All levels appeared vulnerable to attack, including anterior and posterior roots, ganglia, proximal and distal nerve trunks, terminal twigs, cranial nerves, and sympathetic chains and ganglia. The site of maximal involvement correlated with the degree of premorbid clinical findings. Segmented demyelination was the predominant form of nerve fiber damage, and myelin destruction was restricted to these regions of nerve trunks that were infiltrated by inflammatory cells. Subsequent reports have confirmed the observation that primary demyelination occurs only in tissue infiltrated by inflammatory cells. These studies have shown that the destructive process is affected by macrophages in the presence of lymphocytes and only directed at that part of the Schwann cell plasma membrane forming the myelin sheath.[23, 149, 150, 205, 210] However, Kanda and associates[92] reported the findings of a necropsy of early fulminant GBS in an adult. Using semi-thin sections, they observed less extensive mononuclear infiltrates and found nerve fibers with myelin splitting, even in regions where inflammatory cell reaction was not conspicuous. Small myelinated fibers preferentially were involved, and there were no abnormalities of unmyelinated fibers. Sensory roots were involved as severely as motor roots. These authors concluded that the underlying pathology of GBS is heterogeneous. They suggested that some cases involve only perivascular infiltration and are cell-mediated. Other cases may involve demyelination without lymphocytic infiltration and are mediated primarily humorally.

Motor nerve biopsy in one patient with severe GBS showed pronounced subperineural edema, macrophage infiltration, and axons that had been demyelinated completely and some associated with intratubal macrophages. This biopsy indicated primary demyelination as the pathologic process.[76]

Role of Infection

The onset of GBS frequently follows an acute febrile infectious illness. GBS has been reported to occur after childhood illnesses, such as mumps,[28, 45] varicella,[19, 40, 203] measles,[45, 48, 110, 145] or rubella.[45, 166] However, the association of these childhood illnesses with GBS is rare.[45] Epidemiologic studies have indicated the significant occurrence of upper respiratory or gastrointestinal tract illnesses prior to the onset of GBS and support the concept that both these categories of illness constitute important risk factors for GBS.[58, 95, 126] One case-control study[126] reported a higher incidence of elevated specific complement-fixation antibody titers in GBS cases compared with controls for infectious mononucleosis and parainfluenza. Although influenza A and B infections have been observed in GBS patients,[17, 134, 135, 204] this case-control study found no significantly higher incidence of elevated complement-fixation titers in GBS patients compared with controls for influenza A or B.[126] Additionally, during outbreaks of influenza A2 in 1960 to 1961 and influenza B in 1961 to 1962, the incidence of GBS was high; however, the largest number of cases occurred from November 1959 to October 1960, when the prevalence of influenza was comparatively low.[126] Infectious hepatitis has been reported in association with GBS,[143, 147] and four case reports have observed hepatitis B antigenemia in GBS patients.[59, 120, 132, 133] Acute viral hepatitis rarely is complicated by GBS. GBS has been associated with serologically documented cases of acute A, B, non-A/non-B, and delta hepatitis.[111, 186, 191] Immune complexes containing hepatitis B surface antigen in the serum and CSF were found in patients with GBS. These complexes were present with acute hepatitis B during the acute phase of GBS and disappeared when the neurologic symptoms resolved.[186, 191] However, a causal association has not been established, and it has been emphasized that many of the populations at risk for hepatitis B and A also are at risk for infections with other viruses, such as Epstein-Barr virus and CMV.[186] Echoviruses and various serotypes of coxsackieviruses A and B viral isolates have been described in GBS patients.[54, 56, 61, 87, 90, 96, 99, 117, 126, 142, 194] Most isolates were obtained from stool, although in a few cases isolates were obtained from CSF.[45] Recovery of virus does not prove causation; some isolates were recovered when enterovirus was prevalent in the community and in one instance equaled the frequency from controls.[45, 117] Direct isolation of coxsackievirus A4 from nerve roots and dorsal root ganglia has been reported.[56] GBS also has been reported after herpes simplex type 2 encephalitis[128, 179] and during the course of rabies infection.[199]

Laboratory research has suggested an important association of herpesviruses and GBS. Dowling and Cook[45] reported that 15 per cent of GBS patients tested had IgM antibody in high titer against CMV antigen in tissue culture cells. Other studies also have observed an association between CMV and GBS.[7, 30, 47, 91, 129, 146, 171] Dowling and Cook[45] reported a wide spectrum of antecedent illness in CMV-positive patients, ranging from asymptomatic infection to typical respiratory tract and gastrointestinal tract symptoms. There was a predilection for CMV-positive GBS to occur in patients younger than 30 years of age, corresponding to the age incidence described in heterophil-negative, CMV-induced, mononucleosis-like illness.[45] Time clustering of cases was observed, with CMV antibody–positive cases appearing in 10- to 16-week clusters. Dowling and Cook[45] suggest that in cases associated with preceding surgery, GBS may be consequent to CMV, either acquired during transfusion or caused by activation of latent virus or occurrence of nontransfusion, non-A/non-B hepatitis.[45] Dowling and Cook[44] also observed the frequent (8 per cent) occurrence of positive IgM antibodies to Epstein-Barr virus in GBS. In contrast, less than 2 per cent (1 of 75) of GBS patients demonstrated IgM herpes simplex virus–specific antibody.[16] These studies indicate that two herpesviruses are common antecedents of the syndrome, but the precise mechanism by which these initiate destruction of myelin is not known. However, Hart and Kennedy[77] emphasized the difficulty of establishing CMV as a cause of GBS. Utilizing serologic tests, they confirmed active CMV infection in three patients with GBS. They reported that CMV can be isolated in up to 1 per cent of asymptomatic persons and in up to 10 per cent of pregnant women. Isolation may be coincidental. These authors suggested that latent CMV may be activated by other viruses, and isolation may reflect such a nonspecific phenomenon. GBS has been observed in association with human immunodeficiency virus infection.[37] Elevated levels of circulating antibody to Epstein-Barr virus, CMV, and other infectious agents are common in these patients and may be responsible directly for some cases of GBS occurring in association with human immunodeficiency virus infection.[122]

Nonviral infectious agents may precede GBS. Indeed, a preceding infection with *Campylobacter jejuni* associated with a diarrheal illness commonly precedes GBS.[157] After two case reports,[29, 152] a retrospective study was conducted to determine serologic evidence of recent *C. jejuni* infection in GBS.[91] Thirty-eight per cent (20) of 56 GBS patients were found to have serum evidence, CSF serologic evidence (including documentation of rise in titer, two or more elevated antibody titers, or positive CSF titer), or both. Twenty per cent of these GBS patients had preceding diarrheal illnesses. Groups of normal controls and those with other neurologic disorders had no evidence of recent *C. jejuni* infection. IgA- and IgM-specific antibody was found only in the CSF of patients with recent *C. jejuni* infection, suggesting production of specific antibodies in the nervous system because it is unlikely that these are diffused passively into the CSF. GBS patients with serologic evidence of *C. jejuni* appeared to have a significantly more severe illness; 90 per cent of *C. jejuni* GBS patients required mechanical ventilation. A report noted mild illness in GBS patients with positive serology and stool culture for *C. jejuni*.[151] During a more recent prospective, case-controlled study in a cohort of patients with GBS (96 patients) or Miller Fisher syndrome (7 patients) who were admitted to hospitals throughout England and Wales between November 1992 and April 1994, Rees and associates[156a] found evidence of recent *C. jejuni* infection in 26 per cent of the patients with

GBS or Miller Fisher syndrome, compared with 16 per cent of household controls and 1 per cent of age-matched hospital controls. No specific serotypes were associated with GBS. Seventy per cent of the patients with *C. jejuni* infection reported having had a diarrheal illness within 12 weeks before the onset of the neurologic illness. *C. jejuni* was associated with axonal degeneration, slow recovery, and greater disability after 1 year. The median interval from onset of diarrhea to the onset of symptoms for all *C. jejuni*–positive patients was 9 days, suggesting that GBS is a consequence of an immune response to *C. jejuni* rather than a direct effect of the organism or one of its toxins.[88]

Mycoplasma pneumoniae is the second most prominent nonviral agent reported in association with GBS. One report observed that 5 per cent of GBS patients had serologic evidence of active *Mycoplasma* infection.[66] GBS has been reported rarely after infection with *Francisella tularensis* (tularemia), *Chlamydia* (psittacosis), *Plasmodium* (malaria), *Mycobacterium tuberculosis,* and *Toxoplasma gondii.*[20, 69, 126, 130, 170, 201]

In summary, patients with GBS frequently give a history of prodromal symptoms. An association between GBS and an infectious agent long has been considered. McFarlin[119] has suggested that demyelination of peripheral nerve results from direct infection of Schwann cells by the infectious agent, producing prodromal symptoms, or from immunologic mechanisms triggered by the infection. McFarlin[119] favors the second possibility because epidemiologic and virologic surveys of patients with GBS have failed to identify reactivity with a single infectious agent and because the disorder can be triggered by other events, including surgery and immunizations. In addition, the clinical course may be shortened by plasmapheresis.

Role of Immunization

Infrequently, GBS occurs after immunization, including smallpox, diphtheria, tetanus, pertussis, combined mumps-rubella, hepatitis B, rabies, *Haemophilus influenzae* type b, and polyvalent-pneumococcal vaccines.[41, 63, 75, 85, 98] However, a nationwide GBS surveillance conducted from December 16, 1976, until January 31, 1977, suggested an excess risk of GBS related to A/New Jersey influenza vaccine for persons 18 years of age or older.[24] The peak time of onset of GBS was 2 to 3 weeks after receiving the vaccine.[118] For the 10 weeks after vaccination with A/New Jersey vaccine, the risk was approximately 13.3 cases per 100,000 for vaccine recipients, which was five to six times higher than that in unvaccinated persons (2.6/100,000).[118, 172, 173]

A subsequent survey of persons older than 18 years of age vaccinated in the 1978 to 1979 influenza campaign revealed that the relative risk of vaccine-associated GBS (those vaccinated within 8 weeks before the onset of GBS) was 1.4, which was significantly below the risk, 6.2, associated with A/New Jersey vaccine for the equivalent 8-week period.[24, 86, 173] The survey of 1979 to 1980 also did not reveal an increased incidence of GBS for vaccinated versus nonvaccinated persons.[86, 93, 173] The clustering of GBS onset in the second and third weeks after the influenza vaccinations administered in 1976 was not observed after vaccinations administered in either 1978 to 1979 or 1979 to 1980.[173] These results suggested that A/New Jersey influenza vaccine differed from subsequent influenza vaccines in its ability to trigger GBS.[173] The neurotigenic P2 protein of peripheral nerve myelin has been shown to have been present in the 1976 influenza vaccine and to have been biologically active.[179] P2 may have been a factor in the production of GBS after the A/New Jersey influenza vaccination in susceptible persons.[178] Subsequently, the CDC report forms have been reviewed by Kurland and associates.[105] They have expressed concern that (1) the CDC did not establish diagnostic criteria for GBS, (2) records were abstracted by health workers with varying qualifications, and no copies of clinical records were made for subsequent review, (3) cases had not been followed up systematically, and (4) the clinical records never underwent standardized neurologic assessment.

To deal with these concerns and criticisms, the CDC systematically reanalyzed all known and suspected cases of GBS in the states of Michigan and Minnesota for the 4 months in question. Nearly all hospital records were reviewed blindly to identify all cases of GBS. References to prior vaccination, prior viral illnesses, and triggering events were masked. After breaking the code, it was observed that the ratio of vaccinated to unvaccinated cases was as initially reported. The relative risk of GBS developing in the vaccinated population in those two states was 7.10, roughly comparable with prior estimates, whereas the risk of GBS developing more than 6 weeks after vaccination was no different than the background rate of cases in the community. Asbury[8] concluded that an "epidemic" of GBS actually took place, but the precise cause of the illness remains undetermined. It is not clear whether there was a special antigenic site on the A/New Jersey viral product. Patients with GBS who were vaccinated were spread throughout all 141 lots, and the problem could not be traced to individual lots or a single manufacturer. Subsequent surveillance for GBS in the subsequent (1979) influenza programs did not show any excess cases of GBS.[8]

GBS has occurred after the administration of rabies vaccine prepared in suckling mouse brain.[22, 81] A severe protracted course with involvement of cranial nerves, increased mortality rate (20 per cent), and increased long-term sequelae were observed. GBS less commonly occurs after immunization with Sample-type vaccine prepared in brain/spinal cord of mature animals.

The number of GBS cases was increased in both children and adults in Finland in 1985 after a mass vaccination program with oral polio vaccine.[97, 193] This was a one-time campaign involving the entire Finnish population, and further study of the association between oral polio vaccine and GBS in Finland was not possible. This relationship was examined further during a retrospective epidemiologic survey in southern California.[154] No apparent temporal association between GBS and oral polio vaccine was noted. The frequency of GBS was low in the age groups during which children usually are immunized (before 2 years of age and 5 years of age). It was concluded that the failure to find a correlation between the usual age of oral polio vaccine immunization and the incidence of GBS by age coupled with the failure to find any children with GBS with onset within 1 month of oral polio vaccine immunization provided strong evidence against a causal relationship between oral polio vaccine administration and GBS. It was suggested that the differences noted in the outcomes of these studies may be related to the fact that, in the former study, the entire population of Finland already was vaccinated with inactivated polio vaccine and because different types of oral polio vaccine were used in Finland and California.

Immunologic Factors

Current opinion strongly favors the hypothesis that GBS is an autoimmune disease. There is much evidence that GBS represents an aberrant immune response to peripheral nerve components.[5] McFarlin[119] suggested that the following support an autoimmune mechanism in GBS: (1) plasmapheresis shortens the clinical course of GBS, (2) sera from patients with GBS contain IgM antibodies against a component of peripheral nerve myelin, (3) lipid antigen reacts with these antibodies, and (4) at least one lipid, sulfate-3-glucoronyl paragloboside, can produce an experimental disease similar to GBS. This hypothesis is supported by the similarities of GBS, experimental allergic neuritis, and Marek disease.[188, 202] Serum antibodies or antibody-like factors have been demonstrated in peripheral nervous system tissues in experimental allergic neuritis and in GBS.[32, 42, 112, 115, 137, 164, 165, 188, 190, 198] P2, a neurotigenic component of peripheral nervous system myelin administered in complete Freund adjuvant, has been shown to induce experimental allergic neuritis[202]; sensitization to P2 has been reported in GBS.[1, 3, 178] Sensitized lymphocytes capable of producing demyelination have been found in experimental allergic neuritis and GBS.[6, 58, 68, 208] Evidence of hypersensitization to peripheral nervous system antigens utilizing the technique of macrophage migration inhibition factor assay has been reported in experimental allergic neuritis[176] and GBS.[68, 101, 113, 159] However, the cause of GBS and the nature of the antigen or antigens against which the immune response is directed are not known precisely. There is evidence that an intense immunologic response is an invariable accompaniment of the disease.[3, 31, 86, 164, 167] Both cell-mediated immunity and humoral immunity have been found to be altered in GBS and may contribute to the pathogenesis and pathology of GBS.

Several lines of investigation have implicated a cell-mediated immunologic reaction to the constituent of myelin as being of primary importance in the pathogenesis of GBS.[2, 3, 5, 68, 86, 101, 167] Activated lymphocytes can be identified in early phases of GBS.[43] Secretion of mediators, such as macrophage migration inhibitory factor (a measure of T-cell sensitization), in the presence of P2 protein has been demonstrated during the acute phase of GBS.[15, 68, 101, 159, 177] By means of in vitro lymphocytic transformation technique, lymphocytes sensitized to P2 were found in GBS[3]; others have not confirmed these results and suggest that P2 may not be the antigen in GBS.[86] Goust and associates[68] have reported circulating immune complexes in GBS and an association between increased immune complex and decreased suppressor cell function. Abnormal T-cell subsets have been reported,[114] but other investigators did not reproduce this finding.[83, 86] Additional evidence of cell-mediated immunity in GBS is suggested by studies observing demyelinization of rat peripheral nerves in tissue culture by circulating immunocytes from GBS patients or lymph node cells from animals with experimental allergic neuritis.[6, 65, 86, 168]

Activation of T cells has been reported in GBS.[79, 80, 187] Taylor and Hughes[187] observed an increase in the levels of T cells bearing activator markers (interleukin-2 receptor and transferrin receptor) in the serum of GBS patients compared with normal controls. Hartung and associates[79, 80] have demonstrated T-cell activation in the acute phase of GBS, as evidenced by increased interleukin-2 receptor expression on T cells, increased serum concentrations of interleukin-2 and soluble interleukin-2 receptor, and increased numbers of DR-positive circulating T cells. They reported that increased soluble interleukin-2 receptor concentrations that were found in several samples decreased with clinical improvement. The suggested role of activated T cells in GBS could include cytotoxic effect on Schwann cells, myelinotoxic effects, recruitment of macrophages in a delayed hypersensitivity reaction, or helping B cells to produce antibody against myelin. Activated T cells also may play a role in recovery.[79, 80]

Both protective and destructive roles have been ascribed to antibodies in GBS.[6, 209] It has been suggested that the destructive effects of antibodies are mediated either directly by lysis of peripheral myelin with or without a requirement for complement or indirectly by opsonizing myelin, which then is attacked by macrophages.[86] Serum and CSF immunoglobulins of restricted electrophoretic heterogenicity have been reported to be increased in GBS, and these increased levels return toward normal with clinical improvement.[31, 33, 112] Autoantibodies to erythrocytes and circulating antigen-antibody complexes have been found in GBS.[32, 33, 43, 46, 68] Antineural antibody in GBS sera was demonstrated first by Melnick[125]; antineural antibodies also have been reported in the CSF of GBS patients.[164] The cytotoxic effect of GBS serum in vitro has been reported.[31, 34, 49] Several studies have suggested the presence of antineuronal antibodies in GBS patients. Indirect immunofluorescence has been used to demonstrate that sera of GBS patients have IgG antibody to monkey dorsal root ganglia.[44] Tissue studies have demonstrated the presence of immunoglobulins in peripheral nerves of GBS patients.[174]

Some findings indicate that sera from GBS patients react with multiple antigens in peripheral nerve myelin.[46, 103, 152, 211] Complement-fixing antibodies to peripheral nerve myelin have been detected in the serum of GBS patients.[100, 125] Rising titers of complement-fixing anti–peripheral nerve myelin antibodies (IgM) were found during the acute phase of GBS, and decreasing titers were observed during convalescence.[102] Koski and associates[102, 103] found that some of the anti–peripheral nerve myelin antibody in all serum from patients with GBS that was tested binds a neutral glycolipid of human peripheral nerve myelin and cross-reacts with Forssman antigen, a cross-species antigen found in many infectious diseases. These investigators suggested that IgM antibodies, triggered by multiple infectious agents in patients with GBS, can bind to a glycolipid surface determinant of human peripheral nerve myelin and, after penetration of the damaged blood-nerve barrier, participate in the demyelination of peripheral nerve through activation of complement. Yu and associates[211] found that sera from GBS patients reacted with antigens in peripheral nerve myelin, including one lipid, SGPG; in rabbits, immunization with SGPG produced weakness and physiologic abnormalities consistent with a demyelinating neuropathy.[211]

In summary, GBS is regarded as an autoimmune disorder involving both cellular and humoral immune mechanisms.[196] Immunologic studies have not resulted in a simple concept of the pathogenesis of GBS. The animal model of GBS, experimental allergic neuritis, has allowed analysis of the pathogenetic mechanisms involved in the demyelinating process.[196] In the Lewis rat, the disease can be transferred by $CD4^+$ T cells reactive to neuroautoantigens P2 and P0. In the rabbit, experimental allergic neuritis serum injected intraneurally demyelinates rat nerve largely because of antigalactocerebroside antibody.[148] In humans, no peripheral nerve antigen has been identified as the responsible target.[197] Involvement of the cellular immune system has been implicated. T and B cells become activated at the onset of GBS, as indicated by an increase of activation markers, including interleukin-2, soluble interleukin-2 receptor, and tumor necrosis factor–α in serum and CSF.[13, 78, 175, 196] The serum levels of these decrease with recovery.[13, 175] Disruption of myelin has been reported secondary to increased serum concentrations of the cytokine tumor necrosis factor–α.[175] Increased serum concentrations of tumor necrosis factor–α are detected in 50 per cent of patients with GBS as well as in 26 per cent of patients with unrelated neuropathies and other neurologic disorders. Increased serum concentrations of tumor necrosis factor–α are not specific for GBS. Tumor necrosis factor–α serum concentrations correlate with clinical severity and decrease as patients recover[175] and are similar in patients with GBS, whether or not preceding infections were noted. Thus, it is unlikely that these elevations are merely secondary to the antecedent infection. In contrast, soluble concentrations of interleukin-2 receptor are elevated in healthy relatives of GBS patients, as well as in GBS patients. These data suggest that these concentrations may be secondary to environmental or infectious factors rather than related to the pathogenic mechanism responsible for GBS.[175] The involvement of complement is suggested by findings that include increased concentrations of the soluble terminal complement in serum and CSF and increases of C3a and C5a in CSF alone.[78, 148, 196] One study demonstrated a breakdown of the blood-nerve barrier by activated T cells, allowing the development of focal conduction block and demyelinization in the presence of circulating antimyelin antibodies.[148] Elevated serum concentrations of endothelial leukocyte adhesion molecule-1 have been demonstrated in GBS during the acute phase, with serum concentrations returning to normal by 14 days. Endothelial leukocyte adhesion molecule-1 may be important by virtue of breakdown of the blood-nerve barrier.[140] Serum antibodies against such major glycolipids as GM1, GD1b, and LN1 have been reported in the acute phase of GBS.[55, 139, 200, 212] In GBS, the specificity of antiganglioside antibodies is variable.[26, 206] The presence of anti-GM1 ganglioside IgG antibodies may be associated with a more severe and predominantly motor form of GBS. Serum anti-GQ1b ganglioside antibodies have been observed in the Miller Fisher variant of GBS.[26, 88, 139, 206] These findings suggest some association between antigenic specificities of antiglycolipid antibodies and clinical forms of GBS. However, the exact role of these antibodies—neurotoxic, directly responsible for the symptoms, or as incidental byproducts—is not established clearly.[26, 197, 206]

Although studies confirm the activation of the immune system in GBS, it is unknown whether the increase in activation markers is caused by preceding infection; why they are only found in some, but not all, GBS patients; and what their role is in destruction of myelin.

Pathogenesis

The diversity of preceding infectious factors and the observation that GBS may occur after noninfectious factors, such as surgery, trauma, epidural anesthesia, drug administration, and immunizations[5, 24, 57, 183] (see Table 45–2), have suggested that infection is not a necessary precondition for the development of GBS.[45] A single factor such as the release of antigen may be common to the mechanism leading to nerve damage, the peripheral nervous system may possess a limited repertoire of pathologic responses and may react to diverse insults in a restricted fashion, or both may be true.[177] As noted, a number of reports have indicated alterations of both cell-mediated immunity and humoral immunity in GBS and have suggested an immunologic basis for the demyelinization in GBS. However, the exact mechanism and precise interaction of a preceding event and the patient's cell-mediated and humoral immune responses in causing demyelinization are not known. It is not clear whether GBS is the result of an autoimmune process or represents neural injury from an immune response to viral antigen that might be present in neural tissue.[31] Proposed mechanisms for the immunopathogenesis of GBS lesions have included (1) antibody or cell-mediated immunity to an infectious agent with secondary neural injury, (2) autoantibody or cell-mediated immunity to peripheral nerve system tissue, and (3) demyelinization due to deposition of circulatory antigen-antibody complexes in blood vessels of peripheral nerves.[31] It has been suggested that GBS is a syndrome and not a disease and that it may have several different causes.[182]

It has become increasingly evident that the expression of GBS varies considerably.[51, 196] Although the NINCDS Ad Hoc Committee proposed criteria for the research diagnosis of GBS, this committee recognized the occurrence of heterogeneous clinical presentations with fever, severe sensory loss or pain, and progression beyond 4 weeks as variants.[68] Ataxic (Miller Fisher syndrome) and autonomic variants also have been described. In view of these findings, it may be difficult to set minimal criteria for the diagnosis of GBS. For example, insistence on areflexia is too restrictive; pain may occur in one-half of patients and should not be an exclusion criterion. GBS could be viewed as a family of closely related diseases that can be categorized by class of axon (motor, sensory, autonomic, or mixtures), pathologic process (inflammatory-demyelinating, antibody attack), preceding infection, associated antibody, underlying disease mechanism, or response to treatment.[196]

The clinical variability of GBS may reflect different pathogenetic mechanisms. Pathologic studies suggest the heterogeneity of GBS. Studies by Asbury and coworkers[8–11] indicated the early occurrence of inflammatory cells as the primary mechanism resulting in demyelination. The lesions were found along all of the nerve but with variable expression among patients corresponding to their clinical deficits. The role of lymphocytic infiltration has been reappraised. Lymphocytic infiltration varies widely among persons with GBS. It has been shown that severe demyelination can occur without lymphocytic infiltration. Heterogeneity is suggested further by the experimental allergic neuritis models.[148, 196] The rat experimental allergic neuritis model is a T-cell–dependent response to the antigen P2. In the rabbit model, demyelination results from a B-cell–dependent response to galactocerebroside. These models suggest that the variability of GBS may depend on the relative contribution of T-cell and B-cell responses.[148, 196]

The association of *C. jejuni* infection preceding GBS and the occurrence of antiganglioside antibodies may contribute to an understanding of pathogenesis of GBS. *C. jejuni* remains an important candidate as an infectious agent promoting an immune reaction in GBS.[55, 71, 91, 156, 196] Only certain *C. jejuni* strains appear to be associated with GBS. The features of GBS that have been linked with antecedent *C. jejuni* infection include more severe disease, a greater degree of axonal degeneration, a poorer prognosis, a higher proportion of children, and a higher association with anti-GM1 and -GO1a antibodies. However, other reports indicate that "typical" GBS with demyelination of moderate severity can be associated with recent *C. jejuni* infection.[55, 91] There is evidence for shared antigenic determinants among certain infective agents associated with GBS and various antigens within peripheral nerve: (1) shared antigenic determinants between herpes simplex ribonucleotide reductase and peripheral nerve P0 glycoprotein have been demonstrated, (2) amino acid sequence homology between CMV and varicella-zoster virus and P0 glycoprotein has been observed, and (3) antibodies to ganglioside have been detected in patients with GBS after *C. jejuni* and *M. pneumoniae* infection.[148] Some studies indicate that molecular mimicry may contribute to the presence of antiganglioside antibodies after *C. jejuni* infection.[55, 139, 212] It is suggested that humoral immune mechanisms directed at an infectious agent cross-react with antigens of the peripheral nervous system and cause an immunopathologic disease. The family of glycoconjugates, including gangliosides, is one candidate of the myelin antigenic groups with which antibodies have been identified in GBS. The frequency of these antibodies may be as high as 35 per cent of patients with

GBS. Nevertheless, the presence of high titers of antiglycoconjugate antibodies is not correlated necessarily with the more severe course of this disease.[55, 71, 91, 200]

C. jejuni has a lipopolysaccharide capsule that is rich in glycoconjugates containing sialic acid and that resemble human glycoconjugates.[71] A terminal tetrasaccharide immunogenically identical to the ganglioside GM1 present in human peripheral nerve has been demonstrated on the outer membrane of a *Campylobacter* strain cultured from a GBS patient.[12] Serologic evidence of an antecedent *C. jejuni* infection has been shown to correlate with the presence of anti-GM1 antibodies.[55, 88, 200, 212] Anti-GM1 IgG antibodies in GBS sera recognize surface epitopes on whole *Campylobacter* bacteria, and this recognition is strain-specific.

C. jejuni but not *Escherichia coli* bacteria can absorb GM1 antibodies of the IgG class.[139] Studies suggest that molecular mimicry might play a role in the pathogenesis of GBS. Molecular mimicry is suggested further by the observation that the GQ1b epitope is present in the lipopolysaccharide fractions of *C. jejuni* isolated from patients with the Miller Fisher variant.[206, 212] Direct infection of cells of the peripheral nervous system leading to an immune attack seems unlikely in the case of *C. jejuni* because extraintestinal infection and especially peripheral nervous system infection probably are not relevant. *C. jejuni* may generate toxins that directly damage peripheral nerves. Although strain-specific toxins may play a role in post–*C. jejuni* GBS, an immune mechanism remains most likely.[71] Especially appealing is that the association with *C. jejuni* provides indirect support for the "shared epitope" or "molecular mimicry" model of the immunopathogenesis of GBS. It is hypothesized that an infectious agent with a specific antigenetic repertoire induces an immune response involving T-cell activation and antibodies that cross-react with gangliosides present in peripheral nerves.[55]

OUTCOME

Most patients with GBS recover spontaneously. However, epidemiologic studies have indicated that 10 to 23 per cent of patients may require mechanical ventilation, 7 to 22 per cent have some disability, 3 to 10 per cent relapse, and 2 to 5 per cent die.[8, 14, 64, 84, 116, 124, 153, 207] Patients may be left with residual symptoms, such as facial weakness, weakness in the lower extremities with foot drop, weakness and atrophy of hands, and autonomic dysfunction (impotence and urinary retention).[123] In the North American study of the effect of plasmapheresis,[74] the median time to recovery of independent walking was 85 days for controls compared with 169 days for patients who were on a respirator. This same study indicated that children walked at 52 days. Five prognostic factors were identified: age, requirement for respiratory support, rate of progress, abnormal physiologic characteristics of peripheral nerve function, and plasmapheresis.[123]

In children, complete recovery from motor or sensory deficit after an episode of GBS has been reported in 70 per cent of cases after 12 months and in 82 per cent after 15 years.[163] Kleyweg and associates[100] compared the outcome of GBS in groups of children and adults. They observed that 22 per cent of the children compared with 30 per cent of adults required mechanical ventilation, with a median duration of 21.5 days in the children and 32 days in the adults. Mean duration of hospitalization for the children was 84 days and in the adult group 86 days. Two of 18 children died. At 1 year, 77 per cent of the children had a good outcome, and at 2 years, 83 per cent had a good outcome; for the adults, good outcomes at 1 and 2 years were observed in 86 and 92 per cent, respectively. Significant slowing of motor and sensory nerve conduction or electromyographic abnormalities may persist for weeks to years after recovery.[153, 163] Reported unfavorable signs for complete recovery in children included a period longer than 18 days of plateau between greatest weakness and beginning weakness, weakness and maximum motor deficit of greater than 3 weeks, or marked paralysis alone (need for assisted ventilation).[53, 163, 207]

TREATMENT

There is no specific treatment for GBS. Intensive nursing and medical care are essential for proper management. Most deaths are related to respiratory failure, pulmonary embolism, and autonomic dysfunction.[84] Respiratory function must be monitored closely, especially during the acutely progressive phase. The need for endotracheal intubation and mechanical ventilation has been suggested if vital capacity falls below 12 to 15 mL/kg, arterial Po_2 falls below 70 mm Hg, or clinical signs of fatigue develop; tracheostomy may be indicated if paralysis is prolonged.[160] Physiotherapy and preventive measures for pulmonary embolism are indicated. Because of autonomic dysfunction, the electrocardiogram and blood pressure must be monitored. Hyponatremia is a reported complication and probably is caused by inappropriate secretion of antidiuretic hormone[144]; fluid and sodium balance and adequate nourishment must be maintained. Reassurance and attention to anxiety, anger, and depression are important during the progressive phase of GBS, especially for patients being ventilated.[84]

Other treatment modalities have been utilized in an attempt to hasten recovery, shorten ventilatory and intensive care unit time, and decrease the incidence of residual neurologic deficits. Adrenocorticotropic hormone, prednisone, and prednisolone have been used in GBS with varying results. In one controlled study, in eight patients with mild or moderate GBS, adrenocorticotropic hormone shortened the duration of GBS but not the hospital stay.[185] The opposite conclusion was reached from a larger, randomized trial of prednisolone in severely affected patients requiring ventilation.[67] Improvement was less in the prednisolone group than in the controls. A controlled, randomized trial of plasma exchange combined with prednisone was compared with supportive care alone in GBS patients.[127] Improvement in the treated group over the controls was not significant; the investigators suggested that the potential beneficial effect of plasma exchange (discussed later) may have been affected adversely by prednisone.[127] It appears that steroids have little effect on GBS. A beneficial effect of steroids on chronic or subacute demyelinating polyradiculoneuropathy has been reported.[27, 52, 131] Also, steroids have hastened improvement in experimental allergic neuritis when begun before or at the time of onset of neurologic signs; such an effect would be difficult to demonstrate in GBS, in which it rarely is possible to make the diagnosis and initiate treatment within 24 hours from the onset of symptoms.[84] McKhann[120] suggested that assessment of steroids in GBS may have been complicated because of relative late administration of steroids in GBS. A controlled study of the use of steroids early in the course of the disease has been undertaken.[120]

The efficacy of plasmapheresis has been demonstrated in two large clinical trials in adults involving 245 patients in the North American trial and 220 patients in the French trial.[62, 74] In the North American trial, a total of 200 to 500 mL/kg of plasma were exchanged on three to five occasions.[74] In the French study, two plasma volumes were exchanged on 4 alternative days.[62] In the patients treated by plasmapheresis in both studies, improvement started earlier, the need for artificial respiration was reduced significantly, and the median time until independent locomotion was decreased by 32 and 41 days, respectively, compared with the control group. Studies in children also have demonstrated the efficacy of plasmapheresis for treatment of GBS. In children, the benefits have included decrease in the number of days of mechanical ventilation and time until motor recovery, as well as a decrease in the overall cost of care.[89, 197] Although plasmapheresis can be a cumbersome procedure with many technical difficulties, it has been used safely in critically ill children as young as 8 months of age. Mild hypotension related to rapid fluid removal has been reported, but no major complications or deaths related to plasmapheresis have been reported in pediatric patients with GBS. Reported complications in adults include hypotension, transfusion reactions, hypocalcemia, arrhythmias, cardiopulmonary arrest, and infection due to transmitted blood products or sepsis secondary to indwelling catheters.

In children, a short intensive course of plasmapheresis has been recommended for those with significant motor weakness, rapid progress of symptoms, impending respiratory failure, or bulbar insufficiency. Significant motor weakness includes having a limited ability to walk, being bed-bound, or needing ventilatory assistance. Plasmapheresis should be initiated within the first 7 days of the onset of disease symptoms.[89, 196]

Contraindication to the use of plasmapheresis in some patients with GBS and complications and lack of universal ability of plasmapheresis led to a study of IVIG as an alternative to plasmapheresis therapy. A multicentered study conducted in the Netherlands compared IVIG with plasmapheresis.[195, 196] A dose of 0.4 g/kg/day of IVIG was administered on 5 consecutive days. Significantly more patients (53 per cent) treated with IVIG improved over the first 4 weeks when compared with the group treated by plasmapheresis (34 per cent). Other outcome variables, including time until functional improvement, the proportion of patients with multiple complications, and the proportion of patients needing artificial ventilation in the second week, favored therapy with IVIG. It was concluded that IVIG is at least as effective as treatment by plasmapheresis. Ongoing studies are comparing the efficacy of plasmapheresis therapy with that of IVIG. These include administration of IVIG after completion of a course of plasmapheresis and the efficacy of high-dose methylprednisolone coupled with IVIG.[50, 195, 196] Treatment with plasmapheresis or IVIG should start as soon as possible, at least before the end of the second week of illness. It also may be used in patients whose disease still is progressing in the third or fourth week of illness. Mildly affected patients also may benefit from therapy with IVIG. No large trials of IVIG therapy have been performed exclusively in children. Small studies indicate similar improvement in children as in adults when plasmapheresis or IVIG therapy is used. A retrospective review of children receiving plasmapheresis compared with children treated with IVIG revealed a shorter time for improvement and fewer days of mechanical ventilation in the group treated by IVIG.[197]

Advantages of IVIG therapy for GBS include its wide availability, ease of administration, safety, and absence of serious complications. Therapy with IVIG generally is less expensive than plasmapheresis.[197]

In children, reported complications of plasmapheresis or IVIG therapy have included headache (aseptic meningitis), hypotension, dyspnea, diuresis, fever, and transient microscopic hematuria.[89, 197]

In adults, high-dose IVIG has been observed to increase blood viscosity. This appears to occur immediately after completion of the IVIG infusion, and the effect decreases over the next month. It has been speculated that such an effect could impair blood flow and trigger a cardiovascular or cerebrovascular embolus and ischemic event.[36] Other reported adverse reactions have included pain at the site of infusion, flushing, chest tightness, chills, fever, dizziness, and nausea. An uncontrolled study reported symptomatic relapse of GBS.[18] It was suggested that antibody specificities of different immunoglobulin preparations vary considerably, which may yield different therapeutic results. Further deterioration during IVIG or plasmapheresis treatment may occur. About 10 per cent of patients with GBS treated with either IVIG or plasmapheresis may improve initially and deteriorate subsequently. Re-treatment is not associated with a further improvement. It has been shown that more than one-third of patients start to improve during the second week of treatment.[195, 196] Thus, it has been suggested that the chosen therapy should be continued at least until the second week after its initiation. Subsequently, a change in therapy may be appropriate. In most cases, a subsequent change in therapy has been of little benefit because the majority of patients are at the end of their third or beginning of their fourth week of disease; any treatment then is unlikely to be beneficial.[195, 196]

In summary, controlled studies in adults and a retrospective study in children suggest that therapy with IVIG is at least as effective as plasmapheresis.[195–197] The mode action of IVIG therapy is not known. Potential suggested mechanisms have included provision of a source of anti-idiotypic antibodies with selective reduction or suppression of antimyelin antibodies, provision of neutralizing or antitoxin antibodies, and enhancement of competitive macrophage inhibition.[123, 174]

References

1. Abramsky, O., and Korn-Luhetzky, I.: Association with auto-immune diseases and cellular immune response to the neurotigenic protein in Guillain-Barré syndrome. Trans. Am. Neurol. Assoc. *105*:350–354, 1980.
2. Abramsky, O., Teitelbaum, D., and Arnon, R.: Experimental allergic neuritis induced by a basic neurotigenic protein (P_1L) of human peripheral nerve origin. Eur. J. Immunol. *7*:213–217, 1977.
3. Abramsky, O., Webb, C., Teitelbaum, D., et al.: Cell mediated immunity to neural antigens in idiopathic polyneuritis and myeloradiculitis. Neurology *25*:1154–1159, 1975.
4. Adams, D., Gibson, J. D., Thomas, P. K., et al.: HLA antigens in Guillain-Barré syndrome. Lancet 2:504–505, 1977.
5. Arnason, B. G. W.: Inflammatory polyradiculoneuropathies. *In* Dyck, P. J., Thomas, P. K., and Lambert E. H. (eds.): Peripheral Neuropathy. Vol. 2. Philadelphia, W. B. Saunders, 1975, pp. 1110–1148.
6. Arnason, B. G. W., Winkler, G. F., and Hadler, N. M.: Cell mediated demyelination of peripheral nerve in tissue culture. Lab. Invest. *21*:1–10, 1969.
7. Arnold, A. G., Lawrence, D. S., and Corbitt, G.: Cytomegalovirus infection and the Guillain-Barré syndrome. Postgrad. Med. J. *54*:112–114, 1978.
8. Asbury, A. K.: Diagnostic considerations in Guillain-Barré syndrome. Ann. Neurol. *9*(Suppl.):1–5, 1981.
9. Asbury, A. K.: Guillain-Barré syndrome: Historical aspects. Ann. Neurol. *27*(Suppl.):S2–S6, 1990.
10. Asbury, A. K., Arnason, B. G., Karp, H. R., et al.: Criteria for diagnosis of Guillain-Barré syndrome. Ann. Neurol. *3*:565–566, 1978.
11. Asbury, A. K., and Cornblath, D. R.: Assessment of current diagnostic criteria for Guillain-Barré syndrome. Ann. Neurol. *27*(Suppl.):S21–S24, 1990.
12. Banerjii, N. K., and Miller, J. H. D.: Guillain-Barré syndrome in children with special reference to serial nerve conduction studies. Dev. Med. Child Neurol. *14*:56–63, 1972.
13. Bansil, S., Mithen, F. A., Cook, S. D., et al.: Clinical correlation with serum-soluble interleukin-2 receptor levels in Guillain-Barré syndrome. Neurology *41*:1302–1305, 1991.
14. Beghi, E., Kurland, L. T., Mulder, D. W., et al.: Guillain-Barré syndrome: Clinicoepidemiologic features and effect of influenza vaccine. Arch. Neurol. *42*:1053–1057, 1985.
15. Behan, P. O., Lamarche, J. B., Feldman, R. G., et al.: Lymphocyte transformation in the Guillain-Barré syndrome. Lancet *1*:421, 1970.
16. Bernsen, H. J., Van-Loon, A. M., Poels, R. F., et al.: Herpes simplex virus specific antibody determined by immunoblotting in cerebrospinal fluid of a patient with the Guillain-Barré syndrome. J. Neurol. Neurosurg. Psychiatry *52*:788–791, 1989.

17. Bertrand, A., Janbon, F., Clot, J., et al.: Guillain-Barré polyradiculoneuritis and influenza virus. Presse Med. 79:2328, 1971.
18. Bleck, T. P.: IVIG for GBS: Potential problems in the alphabet soup. Neurology 43:857–858, 1993.
19. Boucharlat, J., Groslambert, R., and Chateau, R.: Polyradiculoneuritis as a symptom of varicella (a case report). J. Med. Lyon 49:1443–1445, 1968.
20. Bouchez, B., Poirriez, J., Arnott, G. E., et al.: Acute polyradiculoneuritis during toxoplasmosis. J. Neurol. 231:347, 1985.
21. Brewis, M., Poskanzer, D. C., Rolland, C., et al.: Neurological diseases in an English city. Acta Neurol. Scand. 42(Suppl. 24):1–89, 1966.
22. Cabrera, J., Griffin, D. E., and Johnson, R. T.: Unusual features of the Guillain-Barré syndrome after rabies vaccine prepared in suckling mouse brains. J. Neurol. Sci. 81:239–245, 1987.
23. Carpenter, S.: An ultrastructural study of an acute fatal case of the Guillain-Barré syndrome. J. Neurol. Sci. 15:125–140, 1972.
24. Centers for Disease Control: National surveillance for Guillain-Barré syndrome January 1978–March 1979. M. M. W. R. 28:547–548, 1979.
25. Chen, K. M., Brody, J. A., and Kurland, L. T.: Patterns of neurologic disease on Guam. I. Epidemiologic aspects. Arch. Neurol. 19:573–578, 1968.
26. Chiba, A., Kusunoki, S., Shimizu, T., et al.: Serum IgG antibody to ganglioside GQ1b is a possible marker of Miller Fisher syndrome. Ann. Neurol. 31:677–679, 1992.
27. Colan, R. V., Snead, O. C., Oh, S. S., et al.: Steroid-responsive polyneuropathy with subacute onset in childhood. J. Pediatr. 97:374–377, 1980.
28. Collens, W. S., and Rabinowitz, M. A.: Mumps polyneuritis: Quadriplegia with bilateral facial paralysis. Arch. Intern. Med. 41:61–65, 1928.
29. Constant, O. C., Bentley, C. C., Denman, A. M., et al.: The Guillain-Barré syndrome following *Campylobacter enteritis* with recovery after plasmapheresis. J. Infect. 6:89–91, 1983.
30. Constantino, T., and Weintraub, A.: The Guillain-Barré syndrome as a complication of the postperfusion syndrome. Am. Heart J. 84:678–680, 1972.
31. Cook, S. D., and Dowling, P. C.: The role of autoantibody and immune complexes in the pathogenesis of Guillain-Barré syndrome. Ann. Neurol. 9(Suppl.):70–79, 1981.
32. Cook, S. D., Dowling, P. C., Murray, M. R., et al.: Circulating demyelinating factors in acute idiopathic polyneuropathy. Arch. Neurol. 24:136–144, 1971.
33. Cook, S. D., Dowling, P. C., and Whitaker, J. N.: Serum immunoglobulins in the Guillain-Barré syndrome. Neurology 20:403, 1970.
34. Cook, S., Murray, M. R., Whitaker, J. N., et al.: Myelinotoxic antibody in the Guillain-Barré syndrome. Neurology 19:284, 1969.
35. Cornblath, D. R.: Electrophysiology in Guillain-Barré syndrome. Ann. Neurol. 27(Suppl.):S17–S20, 1990.
36. Dalakas, M. C.: High-dose intravenous immunoglobulin and serum viscosity: A risk of precipitating thromboembolic events. Neurology 44:223–226, 1994.
37. Dalakas, M. C., and Pezeshkpour, G. H.: Neuromuscular disease associated with human immunodeficiency virus infection. Ann. Neurol. 23(Suppl.):S38–S48, 1988.
38. Davidson, D. L. W., and Jellinek, E. H.: Hypertension and papilloedema in the Guillain-Barré syndrome. J. Neurol. Neurosurg. Psychiatry 40:144–148, 1977.
39. Davies, A. G., and Dingle, H. R.: Observations on cardiovascular and neuroendocrine disturbance in the Guillain-Barré syndrome. J. Neurol. Neurosurg. Psychiatry 35:176–179, 1972.
40. Davis, J., and Rowlatt, R. J.: Transient severe hypertension and polyradiculitis after chickenpox. Br. Med. J. 2:1608, 1978.
41. D'Cruz, O. F., Shapiro, E. D., Spiegelman, K. N., et al.: Acute inflammatory demyelinating polyradiculoneuropathy (Guillain-Barré syndrome) after immunization with *Haemophilus influenzae* type b conjugate vaccine. J. Pediatr. 115:743–746, 1989.
42. Dowling, P. C., Bosch, V. V., Cook, S. D., et al.: Serum immunoglobulins in Guillain-Barré syndrome. J. Neurol. Sci. 57:435–440, 1982.
43. Dowling, P. C., and Cook, S. D.: Circulating complexes in neurologic disease. J. Neuropathol. Exp. Neurol. 1:161, 1972.
44. Dowling, P. C., and Cook, S. D.: Antibodies to dorsal root ganglia in Guillain-Barré syndrome. Neurology 23:423, 1973.
45. Dowling, P. C., and Cook, S. D.: Role of infection in Guillain-Barré syndrome: Laboratory confirmation of herpesviruses in 41 cases. Ann. Neurol. 9(Suppl.):44–55, 1981.
46. Dowling, P. C., Cook, S. D., and Whitaker, J. N.: Cold agglutinin in positive Guillain-Barré syndrome. Trans. Am. Neurol. Assoc. 95:234–235, 1970.
47. Dowling, P., Menonna, J., and Cook, S.: Cytomegalovirus complement fixation antibody in Guillain-Barré syndrome. Neurology 27:1153–1156, 1977.
48. Drueke, T. B., Pujade-Lauraine, E., Poisson, M., et al.: Measles virus and Guillain-Barré syndrome during long-term hemodialysis. Am. J. Med. 60:444–446, 1976.
49. Dubois-Dalcq, M., Buyse, M., Buyse, G., et al.: The action of Guillain-Barré syndrome serum on myelin: A tissue culture and electronmicroscopic analysis. J. Neurol. Sci. 13:67–83, 1971.
50. The Dutch Guillain-Barré Study Group: Treatment of Guillain-Barré syndrome with high dose immune globulin combined with methylprednisone: A pilot study. Ann. Neurol. 35:749–752, 1994.
51. Dyck, P. J.: Is there an axonal variety of GBS? Neurology 43:1277–1280, 1993.
52. Dyck, P. J., O'Brien, P. C., Oviatt, K. F., et al.: Prednisone improves chronic inflammatory demyelinating polyradiculoneuropathy more than no treatment. Ann. Neurol. 11:136–141, 1982.
53. Eberle, E., Brink, S., Azen, S., et al.: Early predictors of incomplete recovery in children with Guillain-Barré polyneuritis. J. Pediatr. 86:356–359, 1975.
54. Eiben, R. M., and Gersiny, W. M.: Recognition, prognosis and treatment of the Guillain-Barré syndrome (acute idiopathic polyneuritis). Med. Clin. North Am. 47:1371–1380, 1963.
55. Enders, U., Karch, H., Toyka, K. V., et al.: The spectrum of immune responses to *Campylobacter jejuni* and glycoconjugates in Guillain-Barré syndrome and in other neuroimmunological disorders. Ann. Neurol. 34:136–144, 1993.
56. Estrada-Gonzales, R., and Mas, P.: Virological studies in acute polyradiculoneuritis—Landry-Guillain-Barré syndrome: Various findings in relation to coxsackie A4 virus. Neurol. Neurocir. Psiquiatr. 18(Suppl. 2–3):527–531, 1977.
57. Fagius, J., Osterman, P. O., and Siden, A.: Guillain-Barré syndrome following zimeldine treatment. J. Neurol. Neurosurg. Psychiatry 48:65–69, 1985.
58. Feasby, T. E., Hahn, A. F., and Gilber, J. J.: Passive transfer of demyelinating activity in Guillain-Barré polyneuropathy. Neurology 30:363, 1980.
59. Feutren, G., Gerbal, J.-L., Allinquant, B., et al.: Association of Guillain-Barré syndrome and B-virus hepatitis: Simultaneous presence of anti-DS-DNA antibodies and HBs antigen in cerebrospinal fluid. J. Clin. Lab. Immunol. 11:161–164, 1983.
60. Fisher, M.: An unusual variant of acute idiopathic polyneuritis syndrome of ophthalmoplegia, ataxia and areflexia. N. Engl. J. Med. 255:57–65, 1956.
61. Forbes, F. J., Brumlik, J., and Harding, H. B.: Acute ascending polyradiculomyelitis associated with Echo 9 virus. Dis. Nerv. Syst. 28:537–540, 1967.
62. French Cooperative Group of Plasma Exchange in Guillain-Barré Syndrome: Efficiency of plasma exchange in Guillain-Barré syndrome: Role of replacement fluids. Ann. Neurol. 22:753–761, 1987.
63. Friedland, M. L., and Wittels, E. G.: An unusual neurologic reaction following polyvalent pneumococcal vaccine in a patient with hairy cell leukemia. Am. J. Hematol. 14:189, 1983.
64. Gashi, F., and Kenrick, M. M.: Guillain-Barré syndrome: Review of the literature, case presentation, and psychiatric management. South. Med. J. 68:1524–1528, 1975.
65. Gibberd, F. B.: Ophthalmoplegia in acute polyneuritis. Arch. Neurol. 23:161–164, 1970.
66. Goldschmidt, B., Menonna, J., Fortunato, T., et al.: Mycoplasma antibody in Guillain-Barré syndrome and other neurological disorders. Ann. Neurol. 7:108–112, 1980.
67. Goodall, J. A. D., Kosmidis, J. C., and Geddes, A. M.: Effect of corticosteroids on course of Guillain-Barré syndrome. Lancet 1:524–526, 1974.
68. Goust, J. M., Chenais, F., Carnes, J. E., et al.: Abnormal T cell subpopulations and circulating immune complexes in the Guillain-Barré syndrome and multiple sclerosis. Neurology 28:421–425, 1978.
69. Grattan, C. E. H., and Berman, P.: Chlamydial infection as a possible aetiological factor in the Guillain-Barré syndrome. Postgrad. Med. J. 58:776–777, 1982.
70. Green, S. H.: Polyradiculitis (Landry-Guillain-Barré syndrome) with total external ophthalmoplegia: Encephalomyelo-radiculo-neuropathy. Develop. Med. Clin. Neurol. 13:369–373, 1976.
71. Griffin, J. W., and Ho, T. W. H.: The Guillain-Barré syndrome at 75: The *Campylobacter* connection. Ann. Neurol. 34:125–127, 1993.
72. Gudmundsson, K. R.: Prevalence and occurrence of some rare neurological diseases in Iceland. Acta Neurol. Scand. 45:114–118, 1969.
73. Guillain, G., Barré, J. A., and Strohl, A.: Sur un syndrome de radiculonevrite avec hyperalbuminose du liquide cephalo-rachidien sans regraphiques des reflexes tendineux. Bull. Soc. Med. Hop. Paris 40:1462–1470, 1916.
74. The Guillain-Barré Syndrome Study Group: Plasmapheresis and acute Guillain-Barré syndrome. Neurology 35:1096–1104, 1985.
75. Gunderman, J. R.: Guillain-Barré syndrome: Occurrence following combined mumps-rubella vaccine. Am. J. Dis. Child. 125:834–835, 1973.
76. Hall, S. M., Hughes, R. A. C., Atkinson, P. F., et al.: Motor nerve biopsy in severe Guillain-Barré syndrome. Ann. Neurol. 31:441–444, 1992.
77. Hart, I. K., and Kennedy, P. G.: Guillain-Barré syndrome associated with cytomegalovirus infection. Q. J. Med. 67:425–430, 1988.
78. Hartung, H. P.: Immune-mediated demyelination. Ann. Neurol. 33:563–567, 1993.
79. Hartung, H. P., Hughes, R. A., Taylor, W. A., et al.: T-cell activation in Guillain-Barré syndrome and in MS: Elevated serum levels of soluble IL-2 receptors. Neurology 40:215–218, 1990.
80. Hartung, H. P., and Toyka, K. V.: T-cell and macrophage activation in experimental autoimmune neuritis and Guillain-Barré syndrome. Ann. Neurol. 27(Suppl.):S57–S63, 1990.
81. Hemachudha, T., Griffin, D. E., Chen, W. W., et al.: Immunologic studies of rabies vaccination-induced Guillain-Barré syndrome. Neurology 38:375–378, 1988.

82. Hogg, J. E., Kobrin, D. E., and Schoenberg, B. S.: The Guillain-Barré syndrome, epidemiologic and clinical features. J. Chronic Dis. *32*:227–231, 1974.
83. Hughes, R. A. C., Aslan, S., and Gray, I. A.: Lymphocyte subpopulations and suppression cell activity in acute polyradiculoneuritis (Guillain-Barré syndrome). Clin. Exp. Immunol. *51*:448–454, 1983.
84. Hughes, R. A. C., Kadlubowski, M., and Hufschmidt, A.: Treatment of acute inflammatory polyneuropathy. Ann. Neurol. *9*(Suppl.):125–133, 1981.
85. Hurwitz, E. S., Schonberger, L. B., Nelson, D. B., et al.: Guillain-Barré syndrome and the 1978–1979 influenza vaccine. N. Engl. J. Med. *304*:1557–1561, 1981.
86. Iqbal, A., Oger, J. J.-F., and Arnason, B. G.: Cell-mediated immunity in idiopathic polyneuritis. Ann. Neurol. *9*(Suppl.):65–68, 1981.
87. Jackson, A. L.: A clinical study of the Landry-Guillain-Barré syndrome with reference to aetiology, including the role of coxsackie virus infections. S. Afr. J. Lab. Clin. Med. *7*:121–137, 1961.
88. Jacobs, B. C., Endtz, H., van der Meche, F. G., et al: Serum anti-GQ1b IgG antibodies recognize surface epitopes on *Campylobacter jejuni* from patients with Miller Fisher syndrome. Ann. Neurol. *37*:260–264, 1995.
89. Jansen, P. W., Perkin, R. M., and Ashwal, S.: Guillain-Barré syndrome in childhood: Natural course and efficacy of plasmapheresis. Pediatr. Neurol. *9*:16–20, 1993.
90. Kabins, S., Keller, R., Peitchel, R., et al.: Acute idiopathic polyneuritis caused by cytomegalovirus. Arch. Intern. Med. *136*:100–101, 1976.
91. Kaldor, J., and Speed, B. R.: Guillain-Barré syndrome and *Campylobacter jejuni*: A serological study. Br. Med. J. *288*:1867–1870, 1984.
92. Kanda, T., Hayashi, H., Tanabe, H., et al.: A fulminant case of Guillain-Barré syndrome: Topographic and fibre size related analysis of demyelinating changes. J. Neurol. Neurosurg. Psychiatry *52*:857–564, 1989.
93. Kaplan, J. E., Katona, P., Hurwitz, E. S., et al.: Guillain-Barré syndrome in the United States, 1979–1980 and 1980–1981: Lack of an association with influenza vaccination. J. A. M. A. *248*:696–700, 1982.
94. Kaplan, J. E., Poduska, P. J., McIntosh, G. C., et al.: Guillain-Barré syndrome in Larimer County, Colorado: A high incidence area. Neurology *35*:581–584, 1985.
95. Kennedy, R. H., Danielson, M. A., Mulder, D. W., et al.: Guillain-Barré syndrome: A 42 year epidemiologic and clinical study. Mayo Clin. Proc. *53*:93–99, 1978.
96. Kibrich, S.: Current status of coxsackie and Echo viruses in human disease. Prog. Med. Virol. *6*:27–70, 1964.
97. Kinnunen, E., Färkkilä, M., Hovi, T., et al.: Incidence of Guillain-Barré syndrome during a nationwide oral poliovirus vaccine campaign. Neurology *39*:1034–1036, 1989.
98. Kisch, A. L.: Guillain-Barré syndrome following smallpox vaccination: Report of a case. N. Engl. J. Med. *258*:83, 1958.
99. Kleinman, H., Ramras, K. G., Cooney, M. K., et al.: Aseptic meningitis due to Echo virus type 7. N. Engl. J. Med. *267*:1116–1121, 1962.
100. Kleyweg, R. P., Van-der-Meche, F. G., Loonen, M. C., et al.: The natural history of the Guillain-Barré syndrome in 18 children and 50 adults. J. Neurol. Neurosurg. Psychiatry *52*:853–856, 1989.
101. Knowles, M., Saunders, M., Currie, S., et al.: Lymphocyte transformation in the Guillain-Barré syndrome. Lancet *2*:1168–1170, 1969.
102. Koski, C. L.: Characterization of complement-fixing antibodies to peripheral nerve myelin in Guillain-Barré syndrome. Ann. Neurol. 27(Suppl.): S44–S47, 1990.
103. Koski, C. L., Chou, D. K., and Jungalwala, F. B.: Anti-peripheral nerve myelin antibodies in Guillain-Barré syndrome bind a neutral glycolipid of peripheral myelin and cross-react with Forssman antigen. J. Clin. Invest. *84*:280–287, 1989.
104. Kurland, L. T.: Descriptive epidemiology of selected neurologic and myopathic disorders with particular reference to a survey in Rochester, Minnesota. J. Chronic. Dis. *8*:378–418, 1958.
105. Kurland, L. T., Wiederholt, W. C., Kirkpatrick, J. W., et al.: Swine influenza vaccine and Guillain-Barré syndrome: Epidemic or artifact? Arch. Neurol. *42*:1089–1090, 1985.
106. Landry, O.: Note sur la paralysis ascendante aique. Gaz. Hebdom. Med. Chir. *6*:472–474, 486–488, 1859.
107. Latovitzki, N., Suciu-Foca, N., Penn, A. S., et al.: HLA typing and Guillain-Barré syndrome. Neurology *29*:743–745, 1979.
108. Leneman, F.: The Guillain-Barré syndrome. Arch. Intern. Med. *118*:139–144, 1966.
109. Lesser, R. P., Hauser, W. A., Kurland, L. T., et al.: Epidemiologic features of the Guillain-Barré syndrome. Neurology *23*:1269–1272, 1973.
110. Lidin-Janson, G., and Strannegard, O.: Two cases of Guillain-Barré syndrome and encephalitis after measles. Br. Med. J. *2*:572, 1972.
111. Lin, S. M., Ryu, S. T., and Liaw, Y. F.: Guillain-Barré syndrome associated with acute delta-hepatitis virus superinfection. J. Med. Virol. *28*:144–145, 1989.
112. Link, H.: Immunoglobulin abnormalities in Guillain-Barré syndrome. J. Neurol. Sci. *18*:11–23, 1973.
113. Lisak, R. P., Kuchmy, D., Armati-Gulsin, P. J., et al.: Serum-mediated Schwann cell cytotoxicity in the Guillain-Barré syndrome. Neurology *34*:1240–1243, 1984.
114. Lisak, R. P., Zweiman, B., Guerrero, F., et al.: Circulating T-cell subsets in Guillain-Barré syndrome. J. Neuroimmunol. *8*:93–101, 1985.
115. Lisak, R. P., Zweiman, B., and Norman, M.: Antimyelin antibodies in neurologic diseases: Immunofluorescent demonstration. Arch. Neurol. *32*:163–167, 1975.
116. Loffel, N. B., Rossi, L. W., Mumenthaler, M., et al.: The Landry-Guillain-Barré syndrome: Complications, prognosis, and natural history in 123 cases. J. Neurol. Sci. *33*:71–79, 1977.
117. Lopez, F., Lopez, J. H., Holquin, H., et al.: An outbreak of acute polyradiculoneuropathy in Columbia in 1968. Am. J. Epidemiol. *98*:226–230, 1973.
118. McFarland, H. R., and Heller, G. L.: Guillain-Barré disease complex: A statement of diagnostic criteria and analysis of 100 cases. Arch. Neurol. *14*:196–201, 1966.
119. McFarlin, D. E.: Immunological parameters in Guillain-Barré syndrome. Ann. Neurol. *27*(Suppl.):S25–S29, 1990.
120. McKhann, G. M.: Guillain-Barré syndrome: Clinical and therapeutic observations. Ann. Neurol. *27*(Suppl.):S13–S16, 1990.
121. McLeod, J. G., Walsh, J. C., Prineas, J. W., et al.: Acute idiopathic polyneuritis: A clinical and electrophysiological follow-up study. J. Neurol. Sci. *27*:145–162, 1976.
122. Marks, J. S., and Halpin, T. J.: Guillain-Barré syndrome in recipients of A/New Jersey influenza vaccine. J. A. M. A. *243*:2490–2494, 1980.
123. Marshall, J.: The Landry-Guillain-Barré syndrome. Brain *86*:55–66, 1963.
124. Marti-Masso, J. F., Obeso, J. A., Cosme, A., et al.: Guillain-Barré syndrome associated with a type B acute hepatitis. Med. Clin. (Barc.) *73*:447–450, 1979.
125. Melnick, S. C.: Thirty-eight cases of the Guillain-Barré syndrome: An immunological study. Br. Med. J. *1*:368–373, 1963.
126. Melnick, S. C., and Flewelt, T. H.: Role of infection in the Guillain-Barré syndrome. J. Neurol. Neurosurg. Psychiatry *27*:385–407, 1964.
127. Mendell, J. R., Kissel, J. T., Kennedy, M. S., et al.: Plasma exchange and prednisone in Guillain-Barré syndrome: A controlled randomized trial. Neurology *35*:1551–1555, 1985.
128. Menonna, J., Goldschmidt, B., Haidri, N., et al.: Herpes simplex virus IgM specific antibodies in Guillain-Barré syndrome and encephalitis. Acta Neurol. Scand. *56*:223–231, 1977.
129. Mozes, B., Pines, A., Sayar, Y., et al.: Guillain-Barré syndrome associated with acute cytomegalovirus mononucleosis syndrome. Eur. Neurol. *23*:237–239, 1984.
130. Mushinski, J. F., Taniguchi, R. M., and Stiefel, J. W.: Guillain-Barré syndrome associated with ulceroglandular tularemia. Neurology *14*:877–879, 1964.
131. Newman, M. J., and Nelson, N.: Treatment of subacute polyneuritis with corticosteroids. Can. J. Neurol. Sci. *1*:180–184, 1974.
132. Ng, P. L., Powell, I. W., and Campbell, C. P.: Guillain-Barré syndrome during the pre-icteric phase of acute type B viral hepatitis. Aust. N. Z. J. Med. *5*:367–369, 1975.
133. Niermeyer, P., and Girs, C. H.: Guillain-Barré syndrome in acute HBS Ag-positive hepatitis. Br. Med. J. *4*:732–733, 1975.
134. Novak, M.: Guillain-Barré syndrome as a sequela of influenza. Cesk. Neurol. Neurochir. *38*:314–316, 1975.
135. Nowicki, J.: Neurological syndromes occurring in the course of influenza. Neurol. Neurochir. Pol. *7*:695–699, 1973.
136. Nyland, H.: Epidemiology of Guillain-Barré syndrome in mid-western Norway. Acta. Neurol. Scand. *57*(Suppl. 67):223, 1978.
137. Nyland, H., and Aarli, J. A.: Guillain-Barré syndrome: Demonstration of antibodies to peripheral nerve tissue. Acta Neurol. Scand. *58*:35–43, 1978.
138. Nyland, H., Matre, R., and Mork, S.: Immunological characterization of sural nerve biopsies from patients with Guillain-Barré syndrome. Ann. Neurol. *9*(Suppl.):80–86, 1981.
139. Oames, P. G., Jacobs, B. C., Hazenberg, M. P. H., et al.: Anti-GM_1 IgG antibodies and *Campylobacter* bacteria in Guillain-Barré syndrome: Evidence of molecular mimicry. Ann. Neurol. *38*:170, 1995.
140. Oka, N., Akiguchi, I., Kawasaki, T., et al.: Elevated serum levels of endothelial leukocyte adhesion molecules in Guillain-Barré syndrome and chronic inflammatory demyelinating polyneuropathy. Ann. Neurol. *35*:621–624, 1994.
141. Osler, L. D., and Sidell, A. D.: The Guillain-Barré syndrome: The need for exact diagnostic criteria. N. Engl. J. Med. *262*:964–969, 1960.
142. Parker, W., Witt, J. C., Dawson, J. W., et al.: Landry-Guillain-Barré syndrome: The isolation of an Echovirus type 6. Can. Med. Assoc. J. *82*:813–815, 1960.
143. Partnow, M. J., Devereaux, M. W., and Humphries, T. S.: Infectious hepatitis and the Guillain-Barré syndrome. J. Med. Soc. N. J. *77*:118–120, 1980.
144. Penney, M. D., Murphy, D., and Walters, G.: Resetting of osmoreceptor response as cause of hyponatremia in acute idiopathic polyneuritis. Br. Med. J. 2:1474–1476, 1979.
145. Phillips, P. E.: Guillain-Barré syndrome after measles. Br. Med. J. *4*:50–57, 1972.
146. Plachy, U., Lichy, J., Horacek, J., et al.: Polyradiculoneuritis syndrome in cytomegalovirus infection. Cesk. Neurol. Neurochir. *42*:396–401, 1979.
147. Plough, J. C., and Ayerle, R. S.: The Guillain-Barré syndrome associated with acute hepatitis. N. Engl. J. Med. *249*:61–62, 1953.
148. Pollard, J. D., Westland, K. W., Harvey, G. K., et al.: Activated T cells of non-neural specificity open the blood-nerve barrier to circulating antibody. Ann. Neurol. *37*:467–475, 1995.

149. Prineas, J. W.: Acute idiopathic polyneuritis: An electron microscopic study. Lab. Invest. *26*:133–146, 1972.
150. Prineas, J. W.: Pathology of the Guillain-Barré syndrome. Ann. Neurol. *9*(Suppl.):6–19, 1981.
151. Pryor, W. M., Freiman, J. S., Gillies, M. A., et al.: Guillain-Barré syndrome associated with *Campylobacter* infection. Aust. N. Z. J. Med. *14*:687, 1984.
152. Quarles, R. H., Ilyas, A. A., and Willison, H. J.: Antibodies to gangliosides and myelin proteins in Guillain-Barré syndrome. Ann. Neurol. *27*(Suppl.):S48–S52, 1990.
153. Raman, P. T., and Taori, G. M.: Prognostic significance of electrodiagnostic studies in the Guillain-Barré syndrome. J. Neurol. Neurosurg. Psychiatry *39*:163–170, 1976.
154. Rantala, H., Cherry, J. D., Shields, W. D., et al.: Epidemiology of Guillain-Barré syndrome in children: Relationship of oral polio vaccine administration to occurrence. J. Pediatr. *124*:220–223, 1994.
155. Ravin, H.: The Landry-Guillain-Barré syndrome: A survey and a clinical report of 127 cases. Acta Neurol. Scand. *43*(Suppl. 30):1–64, 1967.
156. Rees, J. H., and Hughes, R. A. C.: *Campylobacter jejuni* and Guillain-Barré syndrome. Ann. Neurol. *35*:248–249, 1994.
156a. Rees, J. H., Soudain, S. E., Gregson, N. A., et al.: *Campylobacter jejuni* infection and Guillain Barré syndrome. N. Engl. J. Med *333*:1374–1379, 1995.
157. Rhodes, K. M., and Tattersfield, A. E.: Guillain-Barré syndrome associated with *Campylobacter* infection. Br. Med. J. *285*:173–174, 1982.
158. Richter, R. B.: The ataxic form of polyradiculoneuritis (Landry-Guillain-Barré syndrome). J. Neuropathol. Exp. Neurol. *21*:171–184, 1962.
159. Rocklin, R. E., Sheremata, W. A., Feldman, R. G., et al.: The Guillain-Barré syndrome and multiple sclerosis: In vitro cellular responses to nervous tissue antigens. N. Engl. J. Med. *284*:803–808, 1971.
160. Ropper, A. H., and Kehne, S. M.: Guillain-Barré syndrome: Management of respiratory failure. Neurology *35*:1662–1665, 1985.
161. Ropper, A. H., and Shahani, B. T.: Pain in Guillain-Barré syndrome. Arch. Neurol. *41*:511–514, 1984.
162. Rosenberg, R. N., and Mendoza, G.: Idiopathic acute symmetrical polyradiculoneuritis: The Landry-Guillain-Barré-Strohl syndrome. West. J. Med. *120*:124–130, 1974.
163. Rossi, L. N., Mumenthaler, M., Lutschg, J., et al.: Guillain-Barré syndrome in children with special reference to the natural history of 38 personal cases. Neuropadiatrie *7*:42–51, 1976.
164. Ryberg, B.: Extra- and intrathecal production of antinerve and antibrain antibodies in Guillain-Barré syndrome: Evaluation by an antibody index. Neurology *34*:1378–1381, 1984.
165. Ryberg, B., Hindfelt, B., Nilsson, B., et al.: Antineural antibodies in Guillain-Barré syndrome and lymphocytic meningoradiculitis (Bannwarth's syndrome). Arch. Neurol. *41*:1277–1281, 1984.
166. Saeed, A. A., and Lange, L. S.: Guillain-Barré syndrome after rubella. Postgrad. Med. J. *54*:333–334, 1978.
167. Saida, T., Saida, K., Lisak, R. P., et al.: In vivo demyelinating activity of sera from patients with Guillain-Barré syndrome. Ann. Neurol. *11*:69–75, 1982.
168. Saida, T., Saida, K., Silbergerg, D. H., et al.: Transfer of demyelination by intraneural injection of experimental allergic neuritis serum. Nature *272*:639–641, 1978.
169. Sakakihara, Y., Kamoshita, S.: Age-associated changes in the symptomatology of Guillain-Barré syndrome in children. Dev. Med. Child Neurol. *31*:611–616, 1991.
170. Samantray, S. K., Johnson, S. C., Mathai, K. V., et al.: Landry-Guillain-Barré-Strohl syndrome: A study of 302 cases. Med. J. Aust. *2*:84–91, 1977.
171. Schmitz, H., and Enders, G.: Cytomegalovirus as a frequent cause of Guillain-Barré syndrome. J. Med. Virol. *1*:21–27, 1977.
172. Schonberger, L. B., Bergman, D. J., Sullivan-Bolyai, J. Z., et al.: Guillain-Barré syndrome following vaccination in the national influenza immunization program, United States, 1976–1977. Am. J. Epidemiol. *110*:105–123, 1979.
173. Schonberger, L. B., Hurwitz, E. S., Katona, P., et al.: Guillain-Barré syndrome: Its epidemiology and associations with influenza vaccination. Ann. Neurol. *9*(Suppl.):31–38, 1981.
174. Shahar, E., Murphy, E. G., and Roifman, C. M.: Benefit of intravenously administered immune serum globulin in patients with Guillain-Barré syndrome. J. Pediatr. *116*:141–144, 1990.
175. Sharief, M. K., McLean, B., Thompson, E. J.: Elevated serum levels of tumor necrosis factor in Guillain-Barré syndrome. Ann. Neurol. 33:591–596, 1993.
176. Siebert, D. G., and Seals, J. E.: Polyneuropathy after herpes simplex type 2 meningitis. South. Med. J. *77*:1476, 1984.
177. Shermata, W., and Behan, P. O.: Experimental allergic neuritis: A new experimental approach. J. Neurol. Neurosurg. Psychiatry *36*:139–145, 1973.
178. Sheremata, W., Colby, S., Lusky, G., et al.: Cellular hypersensitization to peripheral nervous antigens in the Guillain-Barré syndrome. Neurology *25*:833–839, 1975.
179. Sheremata, W., Eylar, E. H., Szymanska, I., et al.: Peripheral nerve myelin P2 protein in influenza vaccine. Ann. Neurol. *10*:91–92, 1981.
180. Soffer, D., Feldman, S., and Alter, M.: Epidemiology of Guillain-Barré syndrome. Neurology *28*:686–690, 1978.
181. Stapleton, F. D., Skoglund, R. R., and Daggett, R. B.: Hypertension associated with the Guillain-Barré syndrome. Pediatrics *62*:588–590, 1978.
182. Steinberg, A. D.: Modulation of a complex immune system. Ann. Neurol. *9*(Suppl.):117–124, 1981.
183. Steiner, I., Argov, Z., Cahan, C., et al.: Guillain-Barré syndrome after epidural anesthesia: Direct nerve root damage may trigger disease. Neurology *35*:1473–1475, 1985.
184. Stewart, G. J., Pollard, J. D., McLeod, J. G., et al.: HLA antigens in the Landry-Guillain-Barré syndrome and chronic relapsing polyneuritis. Ann. Neurol. *4*:285–289, 1975.
185. Swick, H. M., and McQuillen, M. P.: The use of steroids in the treatment of idiopathic polyneuritis. Neurology *26*:205–212, 1976.
186. Tabor, E.: Guillain-Barré syndrome and other neurologic syndromes in hepatitis A, B, and non-A, non-B. J. Med. Virol. *21*:207–216, 1987.
187. Taylor, W. A., and Hughes, R. A.: T lymphocyte activation antigens in Guillain-Barré syndrome and chronic idiopathic demyelinating polyradiculoneuropathy. J. Neuroimmunol. *24*:33–39, 1989.
188. Tindall, R. S. A., Zinn, P., and Rosenberg, R. N.: Humoral immunity in the Guillain-Barré syndrome: Evidence for circulating IgG and IgM. Neurology *30*:362–363, 1980.
189. Toyka, K. V., Augspach, R., Paulus, W., et al.: Plasma exchange in polyradiculoneuropathy. Ann. Neurol. *8*:205–206, 1980.
190. Tse, K. S., Arbesman, C. E., Tomasi, et al.: Demonstration of antimyelin antibodies by immunofluorescence in Guillain-Barré syndrome. Clin. Exp. Immunol. *8*:881–887, 1971.
191. Tsukada, N., Koh, C. S., Inoue, A., et al.: Demyelinating neuropathy associated with hepatitis B virus infection: Detection of immune complexes composed of hepatitis B virus surface antigen. J. Neurol. Sci. *77*:203–216, 1987.
192. Tuck, R. R., and McLeod, J. G.: Autoimmune dysfunction in Guillain-Barré syndrome. J. Neurol. Neurosurg. Psychiatry *44*:983–990, 1981.
193. Uhari, M., Rantala, H., and Niemela, M.: Cluster of childhood Guillain-Barré cases after an oral polio vaccine campaign. Lancet *2*:440–441, 1989.
194. Usui, T., Hammada, Y., and Anta, M.: A case of Guillain-Barré associated with coxsackie. Tokushima J. Exp. Med. *21*:17–19, 1974.
195. Van der Meche, F. G.: The Guillain-Barré syndrome: Plasma exchange or immunoglobulins intravenously. J. Neurol. Neurosurg. Psych. *57*(Suppl.): 33–34, 1995.
196. Van der Meche, F. G., and Van Doorn, P. A.: Guillain-Barré syndrome and chronic inflammatory demyelinating polyneuropathy: Immune mechanisms and update on current therapies. Ann. Neurol. *37*(Suppl. 1):S14–S31, 1995.
197. Vajsar, J., Sloane, A., Wood, E., et al.: Plasmapheresis vs. intravenous immunoglobulin treatment in childhood Guillain-Barré syndrome. Arch. Pediatr. Adolesc. Med. *148*:1210–1212, 1994.
198. Vedeler, C. A., Nyland, H., and Matre, R.: Antibodies to peripheral nerve tissue in sera from patients with acute Guillain-Barré syndrome demonstrated by a mixed hemagglutination technique. J. Neuroimmunol. *2*:209–214, 1982.
199. Verma, A. K., Maheshwari, M. C., Chardhary, C., et al.: Acute ascending motor paralysis due to rabies: A clinicopathological report. Eur. Neurol. *24*:160–162, 1985.
200. Vriesendrop, F. J., Mishu, B., Blasher, M. J., et al.: Serum antibodies to GM1, GD1b, peripheral nerve myelin, and *Campylobacter jejuni* in patients with Guillain-Barré syndrome and controls: Correlation and prognosis. Ann. Neurol. *34*:130–135, 1993.
201. Vyravanathan, S., and Senanayake, N.: Guillain-Barré syndrome associated with tuberculosis. Postgrad. Med. J. *59*:516–517, 1983.
202. Waksman, B. H., and Adams, R. D.: Allergic neuritis: An experimental disease of rabbits induced by the injection of peripheral nervous tissue and adjuvants. J. Exp. Med. *102*:213–235, 1955.
203. Welch, R. G.: Chickenpox and the Guillain-Barré syndrome. Arch. Dis. Child. *37*:557–559, 1962.
204. Wells, C. E. C., James, W. R. I., and Evans, A. D.: Guillain-Barré syndrome and virus of influenza A (Asian strain): Report of two fatal cases during the 1957 epidemic in Wales. Arch. Neurol. Psych. *81*:699–705, 1959.
205. Whitaker, J. N., Hirano, A., Cook, S. D., et al.: The ultrastructure of circulating immunocytes in Guillain-Barré syndrome. Neurology *20*:765–770, 1970.
206. Willison, H. J., Veitch, J., Paterson, G., et al.: Miller Fisher syndrome is associated with serum antibodies to GQ1b ganglioside. J. Neurol. Neurosurg. Psychiatry *56*:204–206, 1993.
207. Winer, J. B., Hughes, R. A. C., Greenwood, R. J., et al.: Prognosis in Guillain-Barré syndrome. Lancet *1*:1202–1203, 1985.
208. Winkler, G. F.: In vitro demyelination of peripheral nerve induced with sensitized cells. Ann. N. Y. Acad. Sci. *122*:287–296, 1965.
209. Winkler, G. F., and Arnason, B. G. W.: Antiserum to immunoglobulin A: Inhibition of cell mediated demyelination in tissue culture. Science *153*:75–76, 1966.
210. Wisniewki, H., Terry, R. D., Whitaker, J. N., et al.: The Landry-Guillain-Barré syndrome: A primary demyelinating disease. Arch. Neurol. *21*:269–276, 1969.
211. Yu, R. K., Ariga, T., Kobriyama, T., et al.: Autoimmune mechanisms in peripheral neuropathies. Ann. Neurol. *27*(Suppl.):S30–S35, 1990.
212. Yuki, N., Taki, T., Takahasi, M., et al.: Molecular mimicry between GQ1b ganglioside and lipopolysaccharides of *Campylobacter jejuni* isolated from patients with Fisher's syndrome. Ann. Neurol. *36*:791–793, 1994.

SECTION FIVE

GENITOURINARY TRACT INFECTIONS

❑ ❑ ❑

46

URINARY TRACT INFECTIONS

Melvin I. Marks and Antonio C. Arrieta

Urethritis refers to inflammation of the urethra and periurethral tissues in males and females and may be associated with a variety of infectious and noninfectious disorders. Cystitis is an inflammatory condition of the bladder that may occur as an infection localized to this site or as part of a more generalized urinary tract infection, including urethritis, pyelonephritis, or both. Pyelonephritis refers to inflammation of the kidney parenchyma, calyces, or pelvis. These disorders are discussed individually in three consecutive sections of this chapter.

URETHRITIS

Epidemiology

The cause of urethritis varies with age of the patient, sexual practices, and hygienic standards.[12, 45] *Chlamydia* infections and gonorrhea are common in adolescents; fecal contamination or irritation due to physical or chemical substances is more usual in the preschooler. Transmission during sexual activity is the usual means of spread of *Neisseria gonorrhoeae* and *Chlamydia trachomatis* in teenagers and in sexually abused patients[24, 40]; nonvenereal transmission also has been described in prepubertal children.[46] Manifestations after nonvenereal spread may include vaginitis, balanitis, and conjunctivitis in addition to urethritis.[46] The home and social environments of the prepubertal child must be examined to identify fully the pattern of spread and infection in the patient and contacts because complex psychosocial diagnoses and therapies often are involved.[33] Concentrations of children with gonorrhea and chlamydial infections occur in large urban centers, usually in poor socioeconomic environments.

Gonococcal infections in children 4 to 10 years of age should be considered evidence of possible sexual abuse. Household contacts have been found to have positive cultures in 27 to 63 per cent of such cases. Prepubertal females infected with *N. gonorrhoeae* as a result of sexual abuse outnumber males by a ratio of at least 3:1 and in one report 8:1.[14, 17]

Pathophysiology

Infection due to *N. gonorrhoeae* usually is localized to the urethra in males and to the vagina in young females; however, rectal carriage sometimes occurs in the absence of urethral colonization. Serum and local antibody, urine bactericidal antibody,[31] phagocytosis, and other host-defense mechanisms are involved. Gonococcal virulence factors include pili,[50] the ability to attach to urethral epithelial cells,[52] and production of extracellular proteases that cleave IgA.[37]

Chlamydia infections are the most frequent cause of sexually transmitted disease in the United States.[11] Chlamydiae are structurally complex organisms that are obligate intracellular parasites and contain both DNA and RNA. Attachment, which is not understood completely, is the first step in the infectious process of the susceptible host cell. This is followed by phagocytosis and then the failure of cellular lysosomes to fuse with the phagosome containing the elementary body. The latter may be mediated in part by macromolecules in the chlamydial cell envelope. After these two crucial events, the elementary bodies undergo biologic changes and, after approximately 72 hours, they are released from the host cell as new infective elementary bodies.

Urethritis in younger children also may be caused by the introduction of fecal bacteria contaminants or pinworms into the urethra during the early years of toilet training, particularly in young girls. Inflammation may be related to bubble bath and other chemical and physical irritants. Edema of the mucosa and the presence of inflammation and red blood cells are common features of the histopathology of urethritis that lead to dysuria, hematuria, and microscopic pyuria.

Clinical Presentation

Gonococcal urethritis is characterized by a 2- to 8-day incubation period after sexual intercourse. The onset often is sudden, with dysuria and profuse urethral discharge in the male and leukorrhea in the female. The urethral discharge often is thick, profuse, and yellow. The patient usually has no fever. In prepubertal females, leukorrhea is more prominent as a sign of gonococcal infections, and urethritis is less common. This may be related to the method of infection or to the different sensitivity of the vaginal epithelial surface to infection in the prepubertal child. Leukorrhea may be minimal in the female, and dysuria may be absent.[43] Septic arthritis (secondary to gonococcemia) occurs in less than 1 per cent of adolescent girls and less frequently in boys.[43] Diagnosis often is made earlier in adolescent boys than in girls, perhaps because of the prominence of urethral discharge in boys and misinterpretation of the significance of leukorrhea in females. Gonococcal urethritis also may cause asymptomatic pyuria in boys.[15] Occasionally, prepubertal patients have conjunctivitis or balanitis without significant urethritis. Clinical presentations also may include systemic illness with fever, arthritis, and skin lesions secondary to bacteremia. These lesions often begin on the extremities as small erythematous macules, which progress to circular papules with an area of central necrosis.

The clinical presentation of nongonococcal urethritis may

be similar to that described earlier for gonorrhea, but more commonly there is a longer incubation period (often 8 to 14 days after sexual intercourse) and a scanty exudate, which may be clear in character and intermittent. This condition also is called *nonspecific urethritis* and may be present in association with, or subsequent to, gonococcal urethritis. In the latter case, the scant urethral discharge may persist after the patient has been treated for gonorrhea. Asymptomatic urethral colonization with *C. trachomatis* also is reported in males.[49]

An equivalent syndrome, acute urethral syndrome, has been described in sexually active females. The patient experiences an acute onset of dysuria and increased frequency, and pyuria (eight or more white blood cells/mm^3 of midstream urine) is common. Bacterial cultures of the urine often are sterile or demonstrate less than 10^5 bacteria/mL; coliform bacteria, *Staphylococcus saprophyticus*, and *C. trachomatis* are the most common causes. Although *C. trachomatis* usually causes nonspecific urethritis in males, mucopurulent (yellowish secretion) cervicitis often is the female counterpart[8]; these infections frequently are asymptomatic in both sexes, an important consideration in designing strategies for diagnosis and management of contacts. For example, asymptomatic chlamydial infection may be the forerunner of pelvic inflammatory disease or infertility.

The patient with urethritis due to trauma may have hematuria and dysuria without fever. The trauma may be obvious or related to masturbation or introduction of foreign bodies into the urethra. Patients with urethritis secondary to bubble bath or soap usually have transient dysuria and no systemic signs. Fecal contamination of the urethra may be accompanied by hematuria, dysuria, and pyuria. Cystitis or vaginitis may be apparent, and fever is variable or absent.

Differential Diagnosis (Table 46–1)

Noninfectious

Trauma, soap, bubble bath, masturbation, radiation, and caustic substances may lead to urethritis. Urethritis also may be a component of several systemic syndromes, including erythema multiforme (Stevens-Johnson syndrome) and, occasionally, other forms of allergy. The term *Reiter syndrome* denotes the association of nongonococcal urethritis with conjunctivitis and arthritis.

Infectious

The most common forms of urethritis in sexually active adolescents and young adults are gonococcal and so-called nongonococcal urethritis. These may occur together or sequentially. Nongonococcal urethritis causally has been related to infections with *C. trachomatis* in approximately 30 to 50 per cent of cases,[23, 42] with *Ureaplasma urealyticum* (T-strain mycoplasma) in up to 70 per cent[9] and with a combination of these agents in 23 per cent. The remainder of cases of infectious urethritis in postpubescent, sexually active patients may be due to a variety of pathogenic microorganisms, including *Gardnerella vaginalis, Mycoplasma hominis, Trichomonas vaginalis, Candida albicans,* herpes simplex type 2, *Treponema pallidum* (syphilis), and other bacteria, such as staphylococci, Enterobacteriaceae, and, occasionally, streptococci, including group B.[18, 51]

Mycoplasma genitalium is a newly identified species, first isolated from males with urethritis.[10, 55] Studies also have implicated a causative role in *Chlamydia*-negative nongonococcal urethritis to anaerobic organisms of the *Bacteroides* species, in particular, *Bacteroides ureolyticus*.[3]

In younger children, urethritis usually has noninfectious causes as outlined earlier, although gonorrhea, *Chlamydia*, and fecal bacteria may be important as well.

TABLE 46–1. Etiology of Urethritis

Infectious	Noninfectious
Gonococcus	Reiter syndrome
Chlamydia	Erythema multiforme
Ureaplasma	Allergy
Trichomonas	Masturbation
Candida	Trauma
Herpes simplex virus type 2	Soap
Syphilis	Drugs
Enteric bacteria	
Staphylococcus	
Enterobius	
Gardnerella	
Streptococcus	
Mycoplasma	

Specific Diagnosis

The best method for diagnosis of gonorrhea in the sexually active male is to obtain urethral discharge by manually stripping the urethra or, if that is unproductive, by gently inserting a swab into the distal urethra. The best culture technique for isolating *N. gonorrhoeae,* a fastidious organism, is immediate inoculation of this material onto a selective growth medium, such as modified Thayer-Martin agar.[27] Chocolate agar also may be used because of the occasional strain of gonococcus that is susceptible to the vancomycin in modified Thayer-Martin medium. Any delay in inoculation of the plates necessitates the use of a transport method using growth media in a carbon dioxide environment that will support the gonococcus at ambient temperatures; JEMBEC and Transgrow are examples of these.[27] Also useful, but not as satisfactory, are transport-holding media, such as the Amies modification of Stuart medium. The principle involved in these techniques takes advantage of the growth requirements of *N. gonorrhoeae* as well as its marked susceptibility to the effects of drying, cold, and overgrowth by other bacteria. The male patient should undergo Gram staining of the urethral exudate at the same time; demonstration of kidney-shaped, gram-negative, intracellular diplococci is presumptively diagnostic (Fig. 46–1). Reliance on Gram stain, however, can lead to errors, particularly in smears characterized by a predominance of extracellular diplococci.[3] A rapid method (approximately 3 hours) has been devised that detects gonococcal antigen in urethral exudate with a high degree of accuracy.[15]

Sexually active females with urethritis also should undergo urethral culture. Gram stain is not reliable for the diagnosis of gonorrhea in females of this age. Vaginal, cervical, and rectal swabs are recommended. Asymptomatic colonization with gonococci seems to be more common in females, although it has been described in adolescent males.[22] It should be remembered that pharyngitis, conjunctivitis, balanitis, and other less common manifestations of gonorrhea may coexist with urethritis. Samples obtained from these sites should be handled as described earlier. Blood agar and other specialized media may be indicated to identify nongonococcal causes of urethritis.

Prepubescent gonococcal urethritis is diagnosed in males as described earlier. Vaginal swabs are most useful in females, even though leukorrhea may not be prominent. Endo-

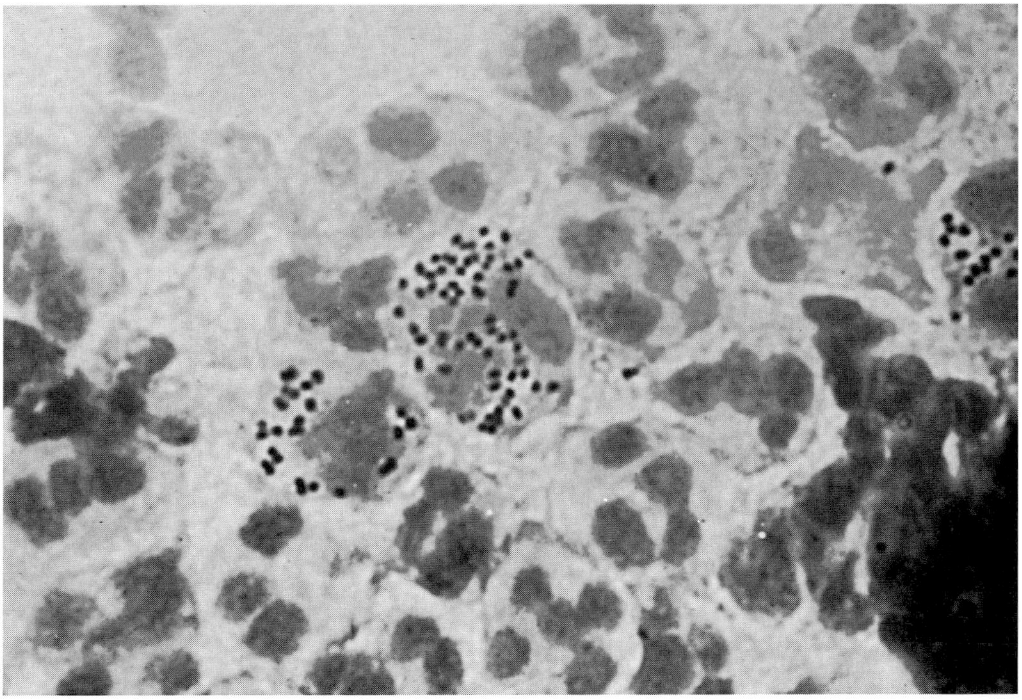

FIGURE 46–1. *Gram-stained smear of urethral discharge from a teenage boy with gonorrhea.*

cervical cultures are not recommended for the diagnosis of gonorrhea in prepubescent females. The yield of vaginal swabs appears adequate for most diagnostic purposes; however, rectal swabs also may be useful in females. Demonstration of kidney-shaped, gram-negative, intracellular diplococci in the prepubescent male and female is useful for a presumptive diagnosis and institution of therapy. Confirmation of diagnosis requires growth of *N. gonorrhoeae* identified by Gram stain characteristics, a positive oxidase reaction, and carbohydrate utilization (acid production from glucose degradation but none from sucrose, maltose, or lactose).[77]

The emergence of penicillin-resistant strains of *N. gonorrhoeae* has increased. These isolates make up approximately 1 per cent of the cases in the United States, with the highest percentage (71 per cent) in New York City, Los Angeles, and Florida. It is remarkable that one-third of the cases in Dade County, Florida, are caused by penicillin-resistant strains of *N. gonorrhoeae*.

Antimicrobial resistance by *N. gonorrhoeae* may be mediated by different mechanisms:

1. *Plasmid-mediated*: Two plasmids are recognized—β-lactamase and tet-M. The former is responsible for β-lactamase production and confers resistance to β-lactam antibiotics. It can be detected by several methods, including tests performed directly on urethral exudates. Penicillinase-producing *N. gonorrhoeae* accounts for approximately 1 per cent of the isolates in the United States. The tet-M plasmid confers resistance to tetracyclines, and disk sensitivity testing is required.
2. *Chromosomal-mediated*: This is a cumulative effect of many chromosomal mutations. It may confer resistance to multiple antibiotics, including β-lactams, tetracyclines, spectinomycin, and erythromycin.[14, 23, 41]

Other infectious causes of urethritis may be defined by specific techniques in the patients and their contacts, including "wet mount" for *Trichomonas*, Gram stain and culture on Sabouraud dextrose agar for *C. albicans*, and culture for herpes simplex virus type 2.

New culture techniques for *Chlamydia*, such as the use of microtiter cell monolayers, have increased the recovery rates, decreased the cost, and shortened the turnaround time, making cultures practical from a clinical point of view (Fig. 46–2).[6] Still, the rigorous transport conditions and the small number of laboratories with cell culture techniques have limited the availability of *Chlamydia* cultures. Fortunately, noncultural methods are available. These include direct immunofluorescence staining of smears using monoclonal antibodies and enzyme immunoassay techniques. The sensitivity of the direct fluorescent antibody test for symptomatic men is 92 per cent, and the specificity is 97 per cent. In the case of women from high-prevalence populations, the sensitivity is 90 per cent and the specificity is 95 per cent. The sensitivity of enzyme-linked immunosorbent assay, on the other hand, is 79 per cent in asymptomatic men, and the specificity is 97 per cent. In women in high-prevalence populations, the sensitivity and specificity are 89 and 95 per cent, respectively.[6, 19, 25, 29, 47] Several studies have explored the use of first-void urine samples for the detection of *C. trachomatis* infections. The leukocyte esterase dipstick test of first-void urine in men yielded conflicting results, but it may lack sensitivity, particularly in asymptomatic men.[16, 36] The detection of *C. trachomatis* by enzyme immunoassay (Chlamydiazyme) in the sediment of first-void urine has a sensitivity of 55 to 87 per cent in men and 61 per cent in women. In both sexes, it was highly specific (98 per cent).[2, 5] DNA amplification by polymerase chain reaction in first-void urine in men proved to be highly sensitive and specific (100 per cent). The possibility of contamination may hinder the use of polymerase chain reaction techniques for large-scale screening.[7, 35, 39]

Ureaplasma and other genital mycoplasmas only can be identified by culture at this time. This test should be reserved for recurrent cases with poor response to treatment.[3, 10, 25, 55] Selection of patients for these procedures can be facilitated by microscopic examination of urethral secretions (more than four polymorphonuclear leukocytes/high-power field

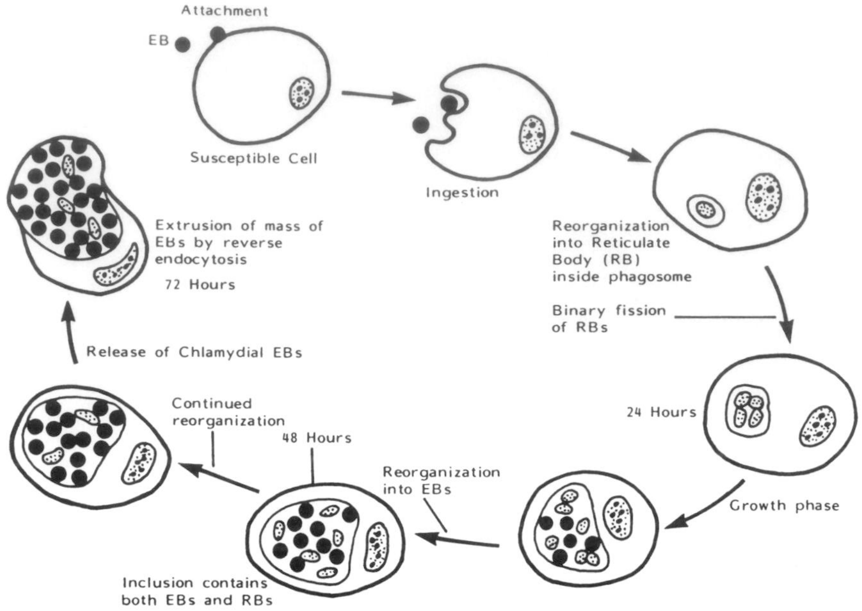

FIGURE 46–2. *Schematic description of the growth cycle of* Chlamydia trachomatis. *(From Batteiger, B. E., and Jones, R. B.: Chlamydial infections. Infect. Dis. Clin. North Am. 1:55–81, 1987.)*

[hpf])[51] and urine (more than 10 white blood cells/hpf in sediment from the initial 20 mL of void)[1] for purulence, even in asymptomatic subjects. Specimens of urethral and vaginal discharge secondary to fecal contamination, foreign bodies, and so on can be examined by conventional diagnostic bacterial techniques.

Treatment (Table 46–2)

The treatment of urethritis should include treatment of the sexual partners of the index case to avoid reinfection as well as further spread of infection. Frequently, patients with urethritis have mixed infections with *N. gonorrhoeae* and the pathogens linked with nongonococcal urethritis, such as *C. trachomatis* and *U. urealyticum*. Also, patients with gonococcal urethritis are at risk for early incubating syphilis. One must consider these factors, as well as the possibility of systemic infection, when choosing a treatment regimen for urethritis.[32]

After the neonatal period, sexual abuse is the most common cause of gonococcal infection among preadolescent children. Anorectal and pharyngeal infections with *N. gonorrhoeae* are common and frequently asymptomatic among these patients.[22]

In September 1994, the Centers for Disease Control and Prevention published treatment guidelines for sexually transmitted diseases, including urethritis (see Table 46–2). Every attempt should be made to ascertain the specific diagnosis. If this is not possible, the treatment regimen chosen always should be appropriate for both nongonococcal urethritis and gonococcal infection. Follow-up generally is not needed unless symptoms recur or persist.[56] Single-dose azithromycin for nongonococcal urethritis (as well as for gonococcal urethritis) and either intramuscular or oral single-dose regimens for uncomplicated genital infections are likely to increase compliance.[20, 21, 28, 30, 34, 38, 48, 53] If these regimens fail, infections with other pathogens, such as herpes simplex virus or *T. vaginalis*, or bacterial urethritis should be considered. Appropriate testing and specific treatment should be provided when indicated.[56]

Prognosis

Gonococcal urethritis may subside and lead to asymptomatic carriage in females. Such carriage may last for weeks to months in adults; however, this period is undefined in children. Untreated gonococcal urethritis also may lead to prostatitis and epididymitis in the male, as well as urethral stricture. Systemic complications of gonorrheal infections can include arthritis, endocarditis, and necrotic skin lesions.

Chlamydia infections frequently have been associated with pelvic inflammatory disease in women, resulting sometimes in infertility or ectopic pregnancy. Chlamydiae can be transmitted to the newborn in the birth canal, which can produce conjunctivitis or pneumonia.[44]

The frequency of *U. urealyticum* is higher in sperm samples from men of infertile couples.[40] It also has been associated in women with premature delivery and postpartum fever. In the newborn, this organism might be linked with the development of bronchopulmonary dysplasia.[55] *Ureaplasma* central nervous system infection occasionally is reported in newborns.[54, 55]

Prevention

An effective, specific gonococcal vaccine has yet to be developed. The mainstays of prevention continue to be education and hygiene, for which case finding and reporting are essential. Prepubescent gonorrhea can be prevented from recurring only by careful family counseling and psychosocial therapy; at times, court intervention may be necessary. Although postexposure antibiotic prophylaxis effectively prevents gonorrhea in most cases, this and the use of a condom (a less effective method of prevention) are not amenable to widespread public health application. Early reporting and therapy are necessary for prevention, but control is not always successful.

Prevention of noninfectious causes of urethritis usually depends on education and specific counseling of the family. Offending physical agents and allergens, if these are implicated, must be removed.

TABLE 46–2. Antibiotic Regimen for Urethritis

Nongonococcal Urethritis	
Recommended regimen	Doxycycline 100 mg b.i.d. × 7 days
Alternative regimen	Erythromycin base 500 mg q.i.d. × 7 days *or* Erythromycin ethyl succinate 800 mg q.i.d. × 7 days If patient cannot tolerate high-dose erythromycin, erythromycin base 250 mg q.i.d. × 14 days *or* erythromycin ethyl succinate 400 mg q.i.d. × 14 days
Chlamydial Infection	
Recommended regimen (adults and adolescents)	Doxycycline 100 mg b.i.d. × 7 days *or* Azithromycin 1 g PO single dose
Alternative regimens	Ofloxacin 300 mg b.i.d. × 7 days Erythromycin base 500 mg q.i.d. × 7 days Erythromycin ethyl succinate 800 mg q.i.d. × 7 days Sulfisoxazole 500 mg q.i.d. × 10 days
Children	
<45 kg	Erythromycin 50 mg/kg/day q.i.d. × 10–14 days
≥45 kg <8 years of age	Use adult regimen of erythromycin
>8 years of age	Use same regimen of doxycyline (consider adult regimen of azithromycin)
Gonococcal Infection	
Recommended regimen (adults and adolescents)	Ceftriaxone 125 mg IM single dose *or* Cefixime 400 mg PO single dose *or* Ciprofloxacin 500 mg PO single dose *or* Ofloxacin 400 mg PO single dose *plus* Regimen effective for *Chlamydia*
Children	
≥45 kg	Use adult regimen
<45 kg	Ceftriaxone 125 mg IM single dose If bacteremia, arthritis, or meningitis, ceftriaxone 50–100 mg/kg/day (max. 2 g/day) IV × 7–14 days

CYSTITIS

This section discusses infections in which the major inflammation is localized to the bladder and conditions in which infections of the upper tract and lower tract cannot be distinguished clearly, such as asymptomatic bacteriuria.

Many criteria—clinical, cystoscopic, radiologic, immunologic, and histopathologic—can be used to define cystitis. In general, the condition refers to the presence of significant inflammatory changes in the bladder clinically manifested as dysuria, increased frequency, and, occasionally, hematuria and urinary retention. Suprapubic pain, urgency, pruritus, and incontinence also may be present. Criteria for bacterial cystitis include significant bacteriuria with dysuria and increased frequency but no back or renal pain. For investigative purposes, additional criteria to distinguish cystitis from disease involving the upper urinary tract have been employed. These include low-grade temperature elevation (lower than 38.5° C, or 101.3° F), urinary concentrating capacity of greater than 800 mOsm/L after 14 hours of fluid deprivation, and an erythrocyte sedimentation rate of less than 25 mm/hr.[30] Serum C–reactive protein correlates well with clinical, but not occult, pyelonephritis.[15]

Pathophysiology and Epidemiology

Cystitis generally is unassociated with any discernible uropathy. When predisposing factors are present, they usually are conditions that disturb flow or allow residual urine to remain in the bladder. Such conditions are found in children with indwelling urinary catheters, neurogenic bladder syndromes, and congenital and acquired obstructions.[36] The gastrointestinal tract is the major reservoir for bacteria infecting the urinary tract. This particularly is true for *Escherichia coli,* in which the same serotype of infecting bacteria often is in the feces of the patient before urinary tract infection (UTI) develops. The distal urethra normally is colonized by enteric and perineal bacteria, which subsequently enter the bladder by several mechanisms. Urethral trauma, retrograde "milking" during intercourse or masturbation, and turbulent flow in the short urethra of the female[8] are common examples. The long male urethra and bactericidal prostatic secretions may be contributing factors to the relative infrequency of cystitis in boys.[16] The protective role of prostatic secretions in the prepubescent male is unclear.

UTI is more common in uncircumcised infants than in age-matched female and circumcised male infants. The presence of a foreskin is associated with a greater quantity of periurethral and urethral bacteria and a greater likelihood of the presence of, as well as a higher concentration of, potentially uropathogenic organisms. This difference persists until about 12 months of age, when the foreskin is more easily retractable and hygiene is easier.[4, 74]

Bacteria that enter the bladder normally are cleared by urine flow, and subsequent infection does not occur. Local bladder defense mechanisms include urinary bactericidal substances, inhibitory pH, and complete emptying; polymorphonuclear and mononuclear leukocytes and local secretion of IgA and IgG antibodies also appear to be important.[28, 69] Local immunoglobulin defenses in the bladder and vagina[68] probably are more important in chronic and recurrent cystitis and may contribute to the increasing resistance of girls to repeated infections in later life.

Unfortunately, urine also may be a good culture medium, and bacteria may grow to significant numbers in residual urine, leading to inflammatory changes in the bladder. Mucosal edema and leukocytic infiltration are prominent histopathologic features (Fig. 46–3). Cystitis often is associated with proximal urethritis, and the two inflamed areas are responsible for the clinical symptoms and signs of this condition.

Transient reflux often occurs secondary to inflammatory edema of the ureterovesical junction, which may interfere with the normal sphincter-like action of the area.[17] Subsequent radiographic and clinical studies of such patients demonstrate spontaneous resolution of reflux in about half the children. Moreover, surgical therapy seldom has improved the prognosis in the remainder.[2, 73] This has led to a much more conservative estimate of the incidence of congenital obstructions. Normal bladder neck diameters vary from 3 to 19 mm, distal urethral segments from 2 to 8 mm, and meatal diameters from 2 to 7 mm.[63] These wide variations, as well as the frequent presence of transient reflux on voiding cystourethrography during infections, should caution the physician and radiologist against making a diagnosis of obstruction or significant reflux in such patients. The incidence of other congenital obstructions, such as those due to diverticula, duplications, exstrophy, and stenoses, is low. Acquired obstruction and stasis may be subsequent to repeated bladder and urethral infections, trauma, indwelling catheters, and surgical procedures. Neuromuscular abnormalities, such as meningomyelocele with neurogenic bladder, also are important causes of stasis and subsequent cystitis. Extragenital causes of urinary obstruction include fecal impaction because of constipation and Hirschsprung disease with megacolon.

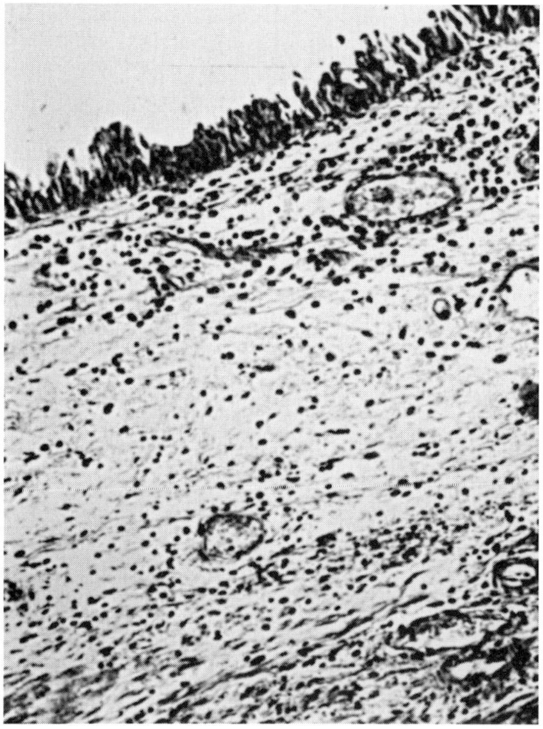

FIGURE 46-3. *Bladder mucosa in recurrent cystitis, showing marked submucosal edema with infiltration of tissues by mononuclear and neutrophilic cells. (H and E × 135) (Courtesy of R. Bolande, M.D.)*

Clinical Presentation

The symptoms and signs of cystitis include daytime dribbling, nocturnal enuresis, abdominal and suprapubic pain, dysuria, low-grade fever, altered frequency, urgency, pyuria, and hematuria.[72]

Dribbling or foul-smelling urine may be the only complaint in girls with otherwise asymptomatic bacteriuria and normal genitourinary tracts. Onset of pain with or without fever suggests accompanying urethritis. The sudden onset of painful hematuria suggests infection of the lower urinary tract, including acute hemorrhagic cystitis of viral origin. School age males outnumber females 3:1 in this condition.[49] Rare presentations of cystitis include parasites or gas (pneumaturia) in the urine.[45]

Screening programs have detected bacteriuria in 1 to 2 per cent of preschool and school age girls and 0.03 per cent of boys; about two-thirds of the girls are asymptomatic.[13] One of the difficulties of anatomically classifying these patients with regard to UTI is the lack of tests that are readily available and that can differentiate reliably. Many of the patients probably have infections of both the upper and the lower urinary tract. Several investigators have attempted to estimate the contribution of lower tract disease to the "asymptomatic bacteriuria" syndrome. On the basis of normal results of six tests designed to segregate patients into those with upper or lower tract disease, 48 per cent of 60 schoolgirls with asymptomatic bacteriuria had cystitis only.[40] These tests were normal renal concentrating capacity, fewer than 50 white blood cells/mm^3 in the urine, fewer than 1000 bacteria/mL in all of three final urine specimens taken every 20 minutes after a bladder washout, erythrocyte sedimentation rate of less than 20 mm/hour, C-reactive protein of less than 10 μg/mL, and the absence of antibodies in the patient's serum against her own strain of bacteria (usually *E. coli*). Intravenous pyelography and voiding cystourethrography also were used. Twelve per cent of the patients in this cohort had disease of the upper tract, and the remaining percentage could not be classified. Thus, asymptomatic bacteriuria may be one of the clinical presentations of cystitis, pyelonephritis, or infections of the upper and lower urinary tract.

In the neonate, nonspecific systemic symptoms may predominate and include fever, poor feedings, and lethargy. It has been observed that 31 per cent of neonates with UTI developed bacteremia, compared with 18 per cent of infants 1 to 3 months of age and 6 per cent of infants 4 to 8 months of age. Bacteremia in infants may lead to life-threatening sepsis and meningitis. In children younger than 2 years of age, fever alone is an unusual presentation of UTI, more so in boys. If abdominal pain also is present, UTI can be diagnosed in almost one-third of patients.[9, 14, 24]

Differential Diagnosis

Infectious

E. coli is responsible for more than 90 per cent of first episodes of acute bacterial cystitis in children[72] and causes about 75 per cent of recurrent infections. Specific O-antigen serotypes of *E. coli,* resistance to serum killing, hemolysin production, and adhesiveness to uroepithelium characterize strains associated most frequently with acute and recurrent UTIs.[41] In young women, *S. saprophyticus* is second only to *E. coli* as a cause of cystitis.[32] Enteric bacteria, including *Enterobacter, Klebsiella,* and *Proteus,* are common in the group of patients in which infection is not caused by *E. coli* or *S. saprophyticus.*

Other causes of acute cystitis include *Pseudomonas,* other staphylococci, and yeasts, such as *Candida* species and *Torulopsis glabrata.*[44] Often these organisms become pathogenic secondary to the use of intraurethral catheters or in immunosuppressed and immunoincompetent hosts. *Gardnerella vaginalis,*[59] *Haemophilus influenzae,*[19, 26] and *Streptococcus pneumoniae* all have been reported to cause UTI as well. These bacteria, anaerobes,[53] and the more fastidious aerobes, such as *N. gonorrhoeae, Neisseria meningitidis,* cell wall–defective bacteria, *M. hominis,*[29] and *U. urealyticum*, may require special techniques for culture and identification.

The presence of gas-forming microorganisms, including bacteria *(E. coli)* and fungi *(C. albicans, T. glabrata),* may lead to symptoms of pneumaturia and the diagnosis of emphysematous cystitis.[44]

The most important causes of viral cystitis demonstrated to date are adenoviruses.[50] Type 11 has been the most common cause of acute hemorrhagic cystitis in school age boys. Occasionally, type 21 has been demonstrated in these patients as well.

Granulomatous cystitis is the histopathologic description of cystitis due to *Mycobacterium tuberculosis,* as well as schistosomiasis and other parasitic infections. Certain parasitic granulomas, such as *Toxocara* and microfilariae, also may contain numerous eosinophils.[35] *Enterobius vermicularis* infestation occasionally leads to signs and symptoms of cystitis and inflammatory changes of the bladder wall.

Chronic interstitial cystitis (discussed later) may be caused by *M. hominis, U. urealyticum,* or both in sexually active females.[29]

Noninfectious

Cyclophosphamide and methenamine mandelate are two drugs that may lead to hematuria and inflammatory changes in the urinary bladder.[56] Trauma, foreign bodies, the presence of catheters, and surgical procedures all may predispose to nonbacteriuric cystitis.

Several poorly characterized conditions have been proposed in the surgical literature to account for cases of cystitis without demonstrable infectious, traumatic, or drug-induced causes. For example, interstitial cystitis is a diagnosis suggested by symptoms of diurnal frequency, sterile urine, and cystoscopic appearance of petechiae on the bladder mucosa. The pathology of this condition is not well described, and its clinical diagnosis often is controversial.[21] Distention of the bladder by hydrostatic pressure is a suggested form of therapy for this condition. This approach should be reserved for patients in whom all of the causes listed earlier have been ruled out carefully. It also is important to rule out neuropsychiatric disorders, including syndromes of hyperkinesis and neuroses, that may give signs of diurnal frequency and symptoms of abdominal and suprapubic pain, dysuria, and urgency.[21]

Specific Diagnosis

A careful history should be obtained with particular attention to previous UTIs, trauma, foreign bodies, sexual activity, urethritis, and neuropsychiatric conditions. Urinalysis and culture performed on a bagged specimen of urine seldom are useful in patients who have diarrhea, incontinence, or poor hygiene. These tests also are of little value in females during menstruation or when the bag is permitted to remain attached for a considerable length of time. In these situations, or if the initiation of therapy is urgent, a suprapubic bladder aspiration is recommended, despite the minimally increased risks of this invasive technique.[47] In other patients and when therapy can be withheld temporarily, a midstream clean-catch technique is used.

A standard technique for the examination of urine is recommended. Centrifuging approximately 5 mL of urine at 3000 rpm for 3 minutes permits a consistent interpretation of the sediment. The presence of more than 20 white blood cells/hpf of the sediment correlates with a significant bacterial colony count of more than 100,000 colonies/mL in most cases. Pyuria also has been demonstrated in states of extreme dehydration along with foreign bodies and calculi in certain cases of drug-induced chemical cystitis and after the administration of oral poliovirus vaccine.[54] Cellular staining methods may be necessary to differentiate renal epithelial cells from leukocytes, particularly when malignancy or parasitic or other diseases are suspected.[37]

The presence of more than three bacteria (3+) in the unstained sediment (3+ or 4+ usually refers to more than 100 bacteria/hpf) correlates with significant bacteriuria in more than 90 per cent of cases.[54] A Gram stain of uncentrifuged urine that demonstrates the presence of bacteria correlates with the presence of significant bacteriuria in approximately 95 per cent of cases (Fig. 46–4). A negative urinalysis, however, does not rule out necessarily the presence of significant bacteriuria. A positive finding of bacteriuria (or funguria), pyuria, and hematuria on urinalysis necessitates careful evaluation of the patient.

Urine culture is essential to diagnosis of UTI. The diagnosis should be documented accurately because it may suggest the need for careful ultrasonography and/or radiologic examination and follow-up evaluation that is expensive, is stressful for the patient and family, and may lead to exposure to a variety of therapeutic drugs and procedures. Alternatively, it is not in the best interest of the patient to permit the persistence of disease in severely distressed patients pending satisfaction of the rigid criteria for laboratory confirmation of this diagnosis.

The diagnosis of bacterial UTI is based on the presence of more than 100,000 colonies/mL urine of a single type of bacteria in pure culture. The accuracy of a single culture of urine that has been obtained by midstream clean-catch technique in predicting UTI is 80 per cent. The accuracy of two consecutive positive cultures is 95 per cent, and with three the accuracy is almost 100 per cent.[7] Colony counts of 10,000 to 100,000 colonies/mL associated with clinical signs and symptoms of cystitis suggest the need for additional cultures (perhaps by suprapubic aspiration) and an evaluation of the factors that may have contributed to these equivocal results. Increased urine excretion rates (as with excessive fluid intake), the presence of bacteriostatic agents in the urine, an extremely acid urine (pH less than 5), highly diluted urine with a specific gravity of less than 1.003, the presence of fastidious organisms (including anaerobes), and other conditions (including recurrent obstruction and the presence of foreign bodies) may be responsible.[6, 54] Colony counts of less than 10^5/mL also may be noted in urine from patients with

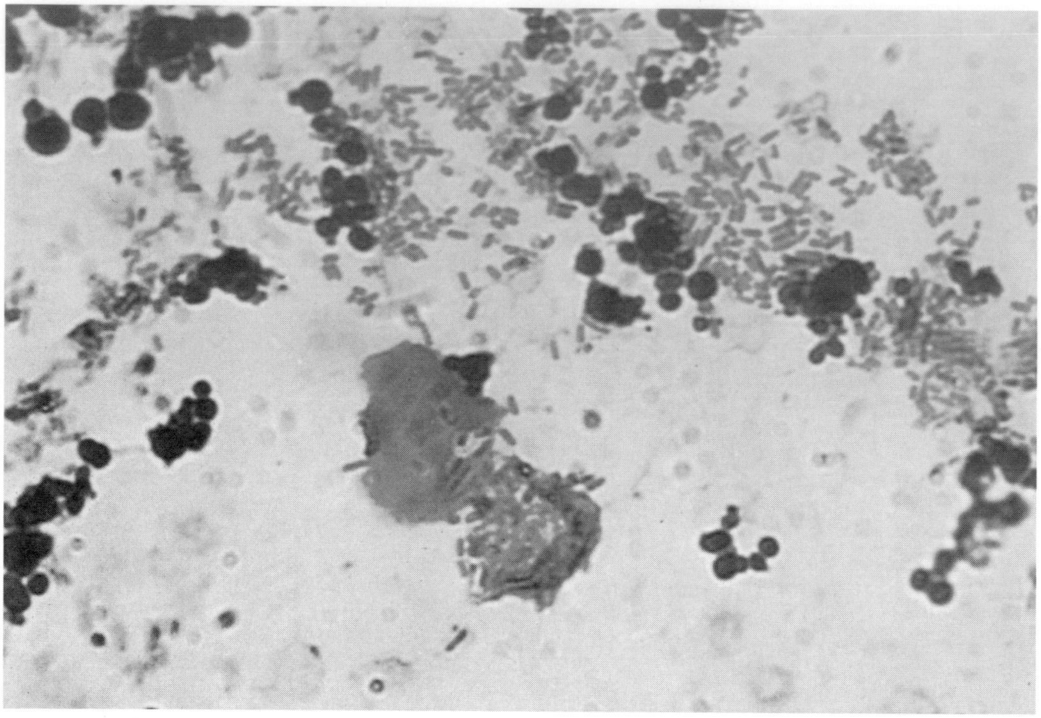

FIGURE 46–4. *Gram stain of uncentrifuged urine demonstrating many leukocytes and gram-negative rods* (Escherichia coli) *(× 400). (Courtesy of G. Ahronheim, M.D.)*

staphylococcal[32] or fungal cystitis and in patients with indwelling urinary catheters.[67]

The isolation of any bacteria from a suprapubic aspirate of the bladder is significant. A skin culture after cleansing the suprapubic area with povidone-iodine may help distinguish contamination by skin organisms, such as *S. epidermidis* and diphtheroids, from true cystitis. Specimens from patients with indwelling urinary catheters are obtained best by direct puncture of the catheter and aspiration with a sterile needle. Opening the closed drainage system or culturing the catheter tip or urine from the bag rarely is a useful technique.[7]

All urine samples should be plated immediately on blood agar and MacConkey or a similar medium that supports the growth of gram-negative organisms. Other media are appropriate in specific situations (e.g., chocolate agar for *H. influenzae,* a Sabouraud dextrose agar for fungi). A predetermined standardized inoculum of urine (e.g., 0.001 mL using a calibrated loop) is spread over the surface of the plate. After overnight incubation at 37° C (98.6° F), the number of colonies spread over the plate is counted and multiplied by 1000. When urine has been obtained directly from the bladder by suprapubic aspiration, 0.1 mL of urine should be spread evenly over the plate; any growth at all is considered significant. Specimens obtained directly by catheterization of the bladder usually should be processed in the same manner as urine obtained by suprapubic bladder aspiration, but the presence of urethritis, traumatic catheterization, and chronic indwelling catheters may hinder the interpretation of results.

If any of these specimens cannot be inoculated and incubated immediately, the urine should be placed in the refrigerator at 4° C (39.2° F) until it can be processed.[7]

Chemical or microbiologic screening techniques are available commercially for the screening of asymptomatic patients in the office of the physician.[67, 72] The frequency of false-negative and false-positive results encountered with most of these techniques is such that they are not recommended for application to the symptomatic patient with cystitis or to persons with infection of the upper tracts.[7, 23] They may be useful and economical for screening asymptomatic female infants and children (Table 46–3).[9]

Specimens obtained from patients with clinical signs of acute hemorrhagic cystitis may be processed by inoculation of tissue cultures (e.g., HEK, HeLa, HEp-2 cell lines) appropriate for growing adenoviruses. Infection also may be documented by adenovirus serology (e.g., complement fixation). It probably is best to reserve these studies for cases in which bacterial culture results have been negative.

Although radiographic examination and/or ultrasonography of the urinary tract is not necessarily indicated in patients with cystitis, examinations often are performed because

TABLE 46–3. Screening Tests for Urinary Tract Infections

Chemical

Nitrite: Produced from dietary nitrates by bacteria, notably *Escherichia coli, Klebsiella,* and *Proteus* species. *Enterococcus,* mycobacteria, and fungi do not reduce nitrates. Can be coupled to urine dip-tests; however, few hours can be required for the color change. Hence, false-negative results may be related to the type and concentration of microorganisms or to the short time of urine in the bladder.

Esterases: Depends on the presence of leukocyte esterases in the urine. Hence, sensitivity depends on the degree of pyuria, and specificity is related to the cause of pyuria.

Microbiologic

Bac T screen: This inexpensive and simple colorimetric test detects bacteriuria. Bacteria are trapped in the filter and then stained with safranine dye. Pink to red indicates more than 100,000 bacteria/mL. Does not require bacterial growth. Can differentiate gram-positive and gram-negative bacteria by repeating the procedure with violet dye, iodine, and alcohol wash. Is 93 to 97 per cent sensitive.

of the difficulty in differentiating this condition from upper tract disease. The chances of detecting significant developmental and obstructive abnormalities in the urinary tract are lowest in patients with cystitis associated with obvious urethritis, in those with hemorrhagic cystitis, and in girls with their first episode of asymptomatic bacteriuria. If radiographic examination is performed, an intravenous pyelogram and voiding cystourethrogram (VCUG) may demonstrate a thickened bladder wall with irregular mucosal contours and, occasionally, vesicoureteral reflux and the presence of residual urine.[72] Many of these findings are transient; reflux and residual urine may be present only during the 2 or 3 weeks of active cystitis.

These radiographic bladder changes are described most frequently in patients with chronic recurrent UTI. The child with a single episode of cystitis or with asymptomatic bacteriuria detected in mass screening programs usually has no abnormalities of the bladder on radiographic examination. Criteria used to diagnose bladder neck obstruction and urethral or meatal stenosis should be strict.[63] Radiographic studies should be delayed whenever possible for at least 6 weeks after bacteriologic and clinical resolution of the infection. This minimizes transient reflux and radiographic signs of obstruction secondary to acute inflammation.

In a representative study of children with UTI, intravenous pyelogram results were normal in 73 of 90 patients.[62] Duplication of the renal pelvis or ureter was the most common abnormality detected. VCUG results were normal in 42 of 65 patients; however, most abnormalities reported were reflux. Many of these radiographs presumably were taken during periods of active inflammation, and criteria for patient selection were not defined carefully. The presence of reflux into the bladder from the urethra or the ureters from the bladder should not be perceived as an indication for surgical intervention or cystoscopy until further studies provide additional support. Ultrasound and radioisotopic techniques have become more significant in the imaging evaluation of children with UTI (see pyelonephritis section).[3, 52, 75] The role of cystoscopy in the diagnosis of cystitis is limited. Most patients with bacterial and viral inflammatory disease of the bladder do not require this procedure. If cystoscopy is performed in children with recurrent cystitis, an increase in trabeculation of the bladder wall, erythema, and, occasionally, cysts or ulcerations are seen. None of these findings suggests an etiologic diagnosis.

Differentiation between disease of the upper and lower urinary tract is difficult. Two fluorescent antibody–coated bacteria techniques were used to evaluate this test in children in a Scandinavian study.[18] Fluorescence was negative in 27 of 28 children with cystitis. Positive fluorescence indicating the presence of pyelonephritis was found in only 7 of 20 children. The tests included a sheep antihuman IgG fluorescent-conjugated preparation, as well as a *Staphylococcus* protein A fluorescent conjugate. The technical complexity of the fluorescent method to detect antibody coating of bacteria, the problem of nonspecific reactions, and the specificity of the reagents used are confounding factors.[42, 46] C-reactive protein concentrations[30] and urinary lactic dehydrogenase isoenzymes[43] also have been studied in an attempt to localize accurately the site of UTIs, but neither has gained wide acceptance. C-reactive protein correlates with the presence of symptomatic pyelonephritis.[67] Lactic dehydrogenase isoenzyme 1 is found more frequently in the urine of patients with cystitis.[75]

Treatment (Table 46–4)

The specific treatment of acute bacterial cystitis requires a consideration of the pharmacokinetics of the drugs used, the site of infection, the interactions of the drugs and bacteria (or fungi), and the natural history of the disease. Most antimicrobials are excreted by glomerular filtration or tubular secretion and therefore are highly concentrated in the urine.[66] The usual drugs employed in the treatment of acute bacterial cystitis are sulfonamides, ampicillin, and nitrofurantoins. All are absorbed adequately from the gastrointestinal tract, are concentrated greatly in the urine, are of low toxicity, and are inexpensive. Oral penicillin has been shown to be useful clinically in the treatment of cystitis; urinary concentrations of this drug often approach 300 to 500 μg/mL, whereas the usual minimum inhibitory concentrations for *E. coli* range from 12.5 to 50 μg/mL. These in vitro data have been correlated with successful clinical outcomes.[33] Because of the variable oral absorption and a relative degree of resistance, the margin of safety probably is greater for agents other than penicillin in such infections. Cefixime, an orally absorbed third-generation cephalosporin, has been evaluated for the treatment of UTIs in children in a once-a-day regimen. Its in vitro activity against clinical isolates and clinical cure rate are excellent. Cefixime should be reserved for the treatment of infections due to bacteria resistant to other antibiotics that are less expensive and equally effective.[11] The quinolones, norfloxacin and ciprofloxacin in particular, are being evaluated extensively for use in children. These drugs are well absorbed from the gastrointestinal tract and have excellent activity against staphylococci and gram-negative enteric bacteria, including *Pseudomonas aeruginosa.* They may prove a useful alternative in the treatment of children with chronic or recurrent infections, particularly if *P. aeruginosa* or multiresistant *E. coli* is involved.[61] Norfloxacin also has been evaluated in a prophylaxis regimen at a dose of 2 to 6 mg/kg/day with good results, although breakthrough infections with enterococci and quinolone-resistant *Pseudomonas* do occur.[70]

TABLE 46–4. Antimicrobial Agents for Acute Bacterial Cystitis

	Dose (mg/kg/24 hr)	Frequency (dose/24 hr)	Route
Sulfisoxazole	120–150	4	Oral or parenteral
Ampicillin	50–100	4	Oral or parenteral
Amoxicillin	25	3	Oral
Cephalexin	50	4	Oral
Cefixime	8	1–2	Oral
Nitrofurantoin	5	4	Oral
Piperacillin	200	4	Parenteral
Gentamicin	3–5	3	Parenteral
Ciprofloxacin*	10–20	2	Oral
Norfloxacin*	10	2	Oral

*Use with caution in patients younger than 18 years of age.

The quinolones should be reserved for when other antibiotics with a better-documented safety profile are not useful. Quinolones always should be used with caution in children younger than 18 years of age.

The interaction of the antibiotic with the environment at the site of infection also is important. This is illustrated best by the enhancement of antimicrobial activity at various pHs. For example, erythromycin is extremely active against enteric bacteria and *Pseudomonas* at an alkaline pH.[76] An oral program employing erythromycin and bicarbonate, therefore, may be used for episodes of recurrent cystitis due to susceptible bacteria, without the hospitalization often required for the use of parenteral drugs. The anticoliform activity of polymyxin B is increased at an alkaline pH, whereas its anti-*Pseudomonas* activity is increased at an acid pH.[48] Penicillins and nitrofurantoins are more active in an acid environment, whereas methenamine-containing drugs require an acid medium for any significant activity.[48]

After institution of therapy in a patient with bacterial cystitis, a repeat clinical and microbiologic examination is recommended after 48 to 72 hours. At this time, the results of in vitro susceptibility studies usually are available, and they can be correlated with the clinical and bacteriologic progress of the disease. Lack of bacteriologic cure (growth in the urine) at 48 to 72 hours suggests in vivo resistance. If this is correlated with in vitro resistance, a more appropriate alternative drug should be prescribed on the basis of susceptibility testing.

Bacterial cystitis can be treated effectively with as little as one dose of antibiotic[8, 71]; however, regimens of 1 to 3 days are common.[57] Whatever regimen is selected, follow-up is critical because a variable percentage of patients (5 to 30 per cent) continue to have bacteriuria or become reinfected.[62] Because differentiation of simple bladder infection (with or without urethritis) from cystitis with upper tract involvement often is not possible, therapy frequently lasts 1 to 2 weeks. The advantages of increasing urine flow with increased fluid intake seem to outweigh the disadvantages of dilution of the antimicrobial effect of the drugs administered.

A culture obtained within a week after cessation of therapy also is important in documenting bacteriologic cure. The recurrence rate of UTI in children is sufficient to warrant cultures at monthly intervals for 3 months, then at 3-month intervals for a subsequent 6-month period, then twice yearly.[38] Many variations of this program are acceptable, as long as the patient is followed for at least 2 years and undergoes bacteriologic and clinical examinations.

The prophylaxis and treatment of recurrent UTI are intended to maintain the patient as symptom-free as possible and to prevent progressive renal damage.[31] The use of co-trimoxazole (trimethoprim-sulfamethoxazole),[9, 64] methenamine mandelate,[22] and nitrofurantoins is well accepted as a long-term prophylactic regimen.[38] Sulfonamides alone may be less useful because of the development of bacterial resistance. Both nitrofurantoin macrocrystals and co-trimoxazole are associated with negligible recurrence rates during long-term prophylactic administration to adults and children with chronic recurrent UTI.[64, 66] Nitrofurantoin may cause peripheral neuropathy in the presence of renal failure; overt disease that reappears despite continuous therapy also may be noted. Some children also may experience nausea and vomiting with this drug. Reappearance of symptoms during the course of continuous administration is less common with co-trimoxazole, but use of this drug is associated with a slightly increased rate of colonization of the gastrointestinal tract of patients with coliforms that are resistant to this fixed combination of drugs.[39, 65] The emergence of plasmid-mediated resistance is a potential, but as yet unrealized, risk of long-term use of these agents.[39] Dosages are given in Table 46–5.

Once UTI recurs, two courses of treatment may be warranted. One is to institute therapy with one of the agents listed earlier (after effective treatment of the acute infection as described) for 3 to 6 months and to continue to follow the patient clinically and bacteriologically. A single bedtime dose of co-trimoxazole or nitrofurantoin is an effective regimen. The other is to treat intercurrent infections as soon as they are detected. The former technique is preferred because secondary changes, such as bladder mucosal thickening, reflux, and numbers of recurrences, are decreased by this method. In using this technique, the additional risks of adverse reactions from the agents used, their expense, and the induction of resistance should be recognized, but these generally are acceptable.[27]

Long-term prophylaxis (at least 1 year) is essential in patients with demonstrable underlying genitourinary abnormalities leading to obstruction or abnormal voiding, which are documented by clinical or radiologic means. Patients with calculi, duplications, and obstructive uropathy and some with neurogenic bladder fall into this category. Surgical correction of these conditions should be followed by long-term chemoprophylaxis until urine flow pattern has returned to normal,[43] after which a trial without chemoprophylaxis is warranted. Intermittent urethral catheterization has been highly successful in managing many children with a neurogenic bladder.[10, 51] Surgical procedures for urinary diversion, such as bladder reconstruction and ileal conduits, often are associated with an extremely high risk of recurrent infection, obstruction, and subsequent loss of renal function.[37, 43] These procedures rarely are indicated, because most patients should respond to intermittent catheterization and chemoprophylaxis.[25] If urinary diversion is required, colonic conduit with antiperistaltic ureteral implantation or ureterosigmoid diversion can be attempted.[55] Vesicostomy also may be used to provide continuous drainage in cases with obstruction or extensive intrarenal reflux.[25]

Patients with indwelling urinary catheters frequently develop cystitis. Catheterization for as short a term as possible is recommended. When prolonged catheterization is necessary, systemic antimicrobials or continuous bladder irrigation has been used. In such situations, systemic antimicrobials have been shown to be effective only for about 4 days, after which the infection rate in these patients is the same as that in untreated controls. The risk of development of resistant organisms is enhanced considerably.[20] Careful use of closed systems and aseptic techniques are the most important aspects of indwelling bladder catheterization. The use of local antimicrobial irrigations instilled via the catheter is acceptable, provided it does not detract from the aseptic technique used; when available, triple-lumen catheters permit continuous irrigation with solutions containing, for example, polymyxin-neomycin-bacitracin.

Prognosis

The natural history of disease in patients with cystitis as distinct from upper tract infection is not defined clearly. Many patients with acute urethritis and cystitis appear to have single episodes of infection without any evidence of

TABLE 46–5. Antimicrobial Agents for Prophylaxis of Recurrent Cystitis

	Dose (mg/kg/24 hr)	Frequency (dose/24 hr)	Route
Co-trimoxazole (trimethroprim-sulfamethoxazole)	2/10	1–2	Oral
Nitrofurantoin	2	1	Oral
Sulfisoxazole	100	4	Oral
Methenamine mandelate	50	3	Oral

recurrence, even after short-term antibiotic therapy. When an underlying cause of obstruction and infection can be defined, such as fecal contamination, foreign body, pinworms, or detergent irritation, removal or avoidance of these factors influences prognosis.

One group of investigators followed 40 girls with recurrent attacks of cystitis (defined by clinical and radiographic criteria). No evidence of renal damage, retardation of physical growth, or the development of hypertension was obtained.[72] A similar study in 61 children describes two patients in each of a control (no antibiotic) and a treated (antibiotic therapy) group who developed radiographic signs of pyelonephritis during a 2-year follow-up.[58] Children with asymptomatic bacteriuria are more likely to develop glycosuria in pregnancy, but they otherwise retain good renal function to 18 years of age, even without antibacterial prophylaxis (they did receive treatment for symptomatic episodes).[12] A study in Göteborg, Sweden, evaluated screening for bacteriuria and symptomatic UTI in the first year of life. It showed that radiologic abnormalities in the screening group were remarkably few. No major abnormalities were found, and only 11 per cent of patients had reflux, none with dilatation. Asymptomatic bacteriuria cleared spontaneously in the vast majority of cases or after antibiotic treatment for other infections in a few cases. A patient detected during screening rarely developed symptomatic UTI. With this in mind, infants with asymptomatic bacteriuria detected during screening constitute a very low-risk group.[34] With careful attention to clinical and bacteriologic surveillance, as well as judicious use of antimicrobial therapy, the outlook for children with recurrent cystitis appears to be excellent.

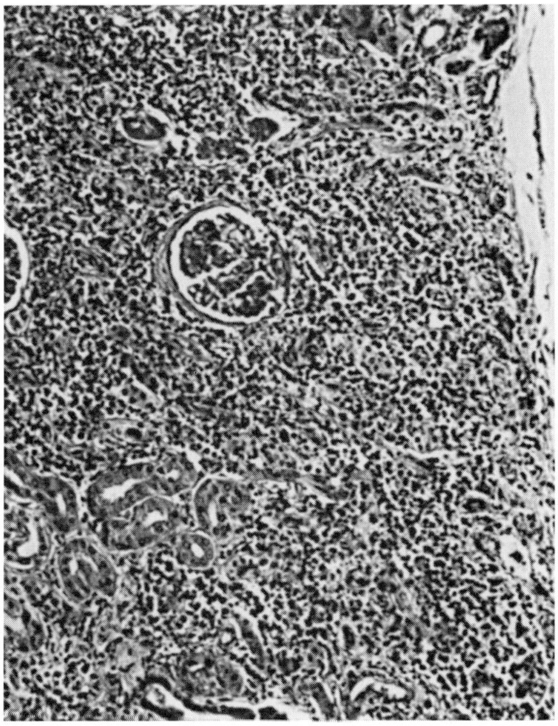

FIGURE 46–5. *Chronic active interstitial pyelonephritis. Interstitial infiltration of subcapsular renal parenchyma by mononuclear cells. Beginning periglomerular fibrosis with atrophy and degeneration of tubules is shown. (H and E × 135) (Courtesy of R. Bolande, M.D.)*

PYELONEPHRITIS

Pyelonephritis usually is due to bacterial infection. Some prefer the term "upper urinary tract infection" when the kidney, renal pelvis, or ureters are involved. In fact, the abbreviation *UTI* is used here when referring to infections of the urinary tract, including the kidney parenchyma and other portions. Histopathologic features of acute pyelonephritis include the presence of polymorphonuclear and mononuclear leukocytes, edema, and parenchymal necrosis, often of a focal nature. Renal atrophy, calyceal destruction, and distortion and fibrosis also may be present in chronic cases (Fig. 46–5). Many characteristics of these microscopic lesions are common to other clinicopathologic entities, including focal and generalized glomerulonephritides. This probably has led to a considerable overestimate of the frequency of bacterial pyelonephritis in the past.

Clinical and radiographic criteria also are used to define pyelonephritis. Thus, chills, high fever, flank pain, and costovertebral angle tenderness (the latter two being difficult to elicit in children younger than 4 years of age) are considered to be characteristic of pyelonephritis, whereas suprapubic pain, dysuria, frequency, and dribbling are more common with cystitis. The presence of radiographic abnormalities above the ureterovesical junction usually is accepted as evidence of pyelonephritis or upper urinary tract disease as well. Kunin[34] prefers more careful descriptive clinicoradiologic terms—that is, "recurrent urinary tract infections (symptomatic or not) associated with reflux (or not) with the development of cortical scars."

When histopathologic or radiologic evidence of kidney involvement is demonstrated, the diagnosis of pyelonephritis is irrefutable; however, cases without these features often are difficult to categorize. Cystitis (with or without urethritis), ureteritis, pyelitis, pyelonephritis, or combinations of these are all possible.

Studies of urinary enzymes or of antibody labeling of bacteria have been used in an attempt to localize infection to the bladder or kidney but have met with only limited success, particularly in the pediatric age group.[51] Because of this overlap, see also the section on cystitis for a more complete view of the pathophysiology, diagnosis, and therapy of UTIs.

Epidemiology

There are marked age and sex differences in the incidence, pathogenesis, clinical presentation, and prognosis of pyelonephritis in children. Newborns most often acquire their infection via the hematogenous route, and signs of pyelonephritis are difficult to discern clinically at this age. Edelmann and associates[17] surveyed 836 full-term infants, using suprapubic aspiration to confirm the diagnosis in each case, and described a 0.7 per cent occurrence of UTI. As with other infections of newborns, boys were infected more commonly, and premature infants seemed more susceptible (2.9 per cent incidence) than full-term babies.

Randolph and associates[59] diagnosed UTI in 3.6 per cent of 800 infants in a private practice survey. The technique used (urine bag) almost certainly overestimates the incidence of infection in this age group. Bacterial recurrences occurred up to 3 years after the initial infection in 9 of 25 infants followed.

The most comprehensive surveys of UTI have been performed in school age children. With careful diagnostic criteria, the prevalence of urinary infection was about 1 per cent in schoolgirls and 0.03 per cent in boys.[34–36] Approximately 5 per cent of schoolgirls have UTIs during their school years. Sexual activity may increase the risk of infection.[55] Prognosis

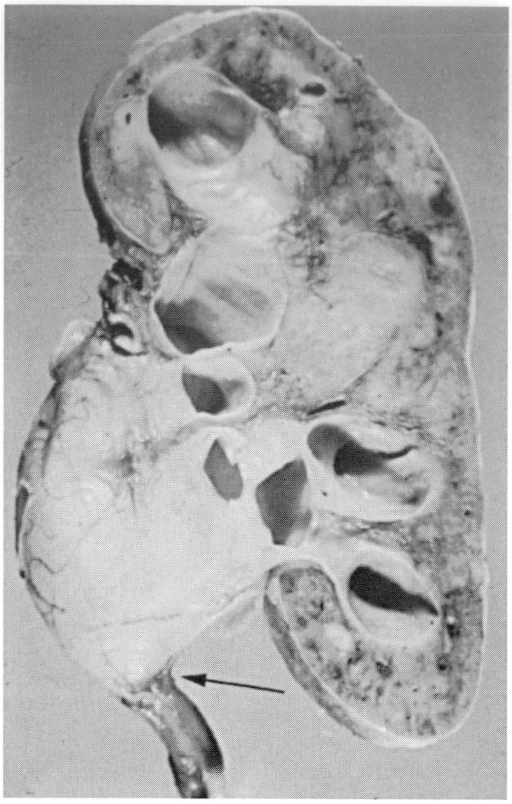

FIGURE 46–6. *Marked hydronephrosis, pyelectasis, and caliectasis due to congenital ureteropelvic obstruction* (arrow). *The renal parenchyma is compressed; corticomedullary demarcation is observed. (Courtesy of R. Bolande, M.D.)*

seems good in these patients, although recurrence in later life (often associated with pregnancy) may be anticipated in some patients.

The route of infection in girls is usually ascending, and the reservoir for infecting bacteria is in the gastrointestinal tract.[76] Urethral and preputial colonization with potential urinary tract pathogens has been observed in infants less than 1 year of age, allowing for the presence of the prepuce to be a risk factor for the development of UTI in young infant boys, in particular those younger than 6 months (see cystitis section).[1, 83] UTI in boys is associated more often with underlying renal structural abnormalities than in girls.[11, 21]

Nosocomial UTIs, including pyelonephritis, may occur in any age group.[76] The epidemiology of these infections is complex, but the most common predisposing factors include indwelling urinary catheters, surgery, or debilitating conditions. The spread of infection to these patients often can be traced to contaminated catheters or collecting equipment. Careful epidemiologic monitoring for nosocomial UTIs is important in intensive care units and particularly when indwelling catheters and genitourinary surgery are involved. The usual route of hospital-acquired infection is by direct ascending contamination of the urinary tract. Patients receiving intravenous hyperalimentation and others with bacteremia may acquire their UTIs after hematogenous spread. Bacteriologic markers, such as pyocin, O antigen, P antigen (fimbria), phage, or antibiotic typing of bacterial isolates, may be used in hospital epidemiologic surveillance.[76]

Pathophysiology

Residual urine, obstruction, other abnormalities of flow, and renal parenchymal injury are important predisposing factors to development of pyelonephritis. Hence, congenital abnormalities of the drainage system (Fig. 46–6) and acquired obstruction secondary to recurrent infection, nephrolithiasis, neurogenic bladder, surgery, and even constipation may be present.[54] It often is necessary to obstruct the outflow system or to traumatize the kidney to cause pyelonephritis in animal models.[67] Experimental studies in animals also have elucidated some of the virulence factors of the infecting bacteria that are critical in the development of UTIs. The presence of pili may be essential for adherence of bacteria to renal epithelial cells, penetration of these cells, and development of pyelonephritis.[18, 67] Adherence can be inhibited by IgA antibody, which is produced locally in association with infection of the urinary tract.

Because *E. coli* is the most common pathogen found in patients with UTI, several experimental efforts have concentrated on the identification of virulence factors and their role in the pathogenesis of UTI. The clonotyping of *E. coli* based on its O:K:H antigens has identified a few combinations more frequently associated with pyelonephritis.[7, 48] A study by Marild and associates[48] showed an increased frequency of eight O groups (1, 2, 4, 6, 7, 16, 18, and 75) in association with acute pyelonephritis, confirming previous reports. They also found that the K1 antigen occurred in 38 per cent of the isolates, with K1, K2, K5, and K12 found in 60 of 84 strains (71 per cent); antigens H1, H4, H5, H6, and H7 were expressed in 53 per cent of the isolates. The O1:K1:H7 clone was most common, accounting for 17 per cent of all *E. coli* isolates from 84 patients with pyelonephritis (Table 46–6).

Certain virulence factors may enhance bacterial colonization and subsequent invasion of the urinary tract. Bacteria possessing these properties have been called uropathogens. Enhanced ability to attach to mucosal surfaces is the best-understood virulence factor in uropathogenic *E. coli*. This property has been related to the presence of structures, called adhesins, found on bacterial pili. Three types of adhesins have been characterized: (1) type 1 pili, (2) *P. fimbriae*, and (3) x-binding adhesins.[7]

TABLE 46–6. O:K:H Serotypes Associated with Pyelonephritis in 84 Patients

	O:K:H	n	%
Multiple			
	1:1:0	5	6
	1:1:7	14	17
	2:7:0	2	2
	4:0:5	2	2
	4:12:5	5	6
	6:5:1	4	5
	7:1:0	3	4
	15:52:1	2	2
	16:1:0	4	5
	16:1:6	3	4
	18:5:0	6	7
	75:5:0	5	6
	Total	55	66
Single			
	2:0:4, 2:0:6, 2:1:0, 2:1:4, 2:5:4, 3:2:2, 4:0:0, 4:2:5, 4:6:5, 6:2:1, 6:13:1, 6:N:31, 7:N:16, 15:N:1, 16:2:6, 21:2:2, 21:0:5, 21:N:0, 25:7:1, 37:0:4, 44:2:18, 78:0:0, 83:1:4, 88:7:8, 153:0:0, N:13:0, R:2:2, R:14:0, R:1:6.		
	Total	29	34

From Marild, S., Jodal, U., Orskov, I., et al.: Special virulence of the *Escherichia coli* O1:K1:H7 clone in acute pyelonephritis. J. Pediatr. *115*:40–45, 1989.

Epithelial cell receptors may have specific biochemical sequences to which the adhesins of certain uropathogens may attach. The active component of the cellular receptor to which *P. fimbriae* adheres was identified as the globo series of glycolipids (globo$^+$), which include the disaccharide galactose α 1→4 galactose β (gal-gal$^+$). This disaccharide apparently is necessary for attachment of uropathogens.[7, 73]

The presence of gal-gal$^+$ isolates frequently has been associated with intense inflammatory responses, severe reflux, and renal abnormalities. The clone O1:K1:H7 expresses globo$^+$ adhesins frequently, which may account for its increasing role in the pathogenesis of pyelonephritis.[13, 14, 48, 49]

Bacterial interference (that is, the ability of one strain of bacteria to inhibit the growth of other bacteria) also may play a role in the development of UTIs, particularly those that develop by the ascending route.[22] Bacteriocins, interference, environmental factors, tropism, and other virulence factors mentioned earlier may explain the rarity of polymicrobial UTI. Genetic predilection of the host, including gender and anatomic features, also may determine the expression of infection.

Pyelonephritis has several effects on the host in addition to the stimulation of immune responses and severe inflammatory changes. A decrease in renal concentrating ability is a fairly consistent finding in patients with pyelonephritis.[41, 63] Because a prolonged period of fluid deprivation often is necessary to demonstrate this effect, its clinical usefulness is limited in children and infants. Antibodies coating bacteria in upper tract disease usually are of the IgG class and are directed against the O antigen. IgG, IgA, and IgM antibodies are produced in kidney tissue during pyelonephritis.[68] The biologic significance of local antibody production in the kidney is uncertain, although it has been postulated that this may prevent reinfection or mediate cytotoxicity by sensitized lymphocytes. Persistence of *E. coli* antigen in the renal parenchyma long after pyelonephritis has cleared may contribute to this defense mechanism.

Other immunologic effects observed in experimental pyelonephritis include the migration of large numbers of polymorphonuclear leukocytes to the kidney parenchyma. These cells may contribute to renal injury directly by means of release of proteolytic enzymes or through cytotoxic mediators.[81] The role of T cells in the pathogenesis and immunity of pyelonephritis is unclear. Although T lymphocytes may be present in the kidney during infection, their function may be inhibited, rather than stimulated, by the inflammatory response.[12, 80] Antibody to kidney and bacterial antigens commonly is present in the urine of patients with chronic pyelonephritis, implicating roles for both host immune factors and bacteria in tissue injury.[62] The presence of cytokines (IL-6, IL-1β, IL-8) in the urine of children with UTI, independent from serum concentrations, clearly documents a local inflammatory response. This may open new ways to diagnose complicated UTIs as well as therapeutic approaches to decrease inflammation, which may result in lowering the risk of scarring.[2, 3, 75]

Clinical Presentation

The classic symptoms and signs of pyelonephritis (chills, fever, flank pain, and costovertebral angle tenderness) are more obvious in older than in younger patients but are not a constant finding at any age. As many as two-thirds of preschool and school age girls may be asymptomatic with their first UTI. Renal parenchymal infection can be demonstrated in 10 per cent of those patients and reflux in an additional 20 per cent.[41] Although renal findings usually are associated with fever, a decrease in renal concentrating ability, an elevated erythrocyte sedimentation rate, and increased concentrations of C-reactive protein, this is not always the case.[41] Fever is an important sign of pyelonephritis and, although more common in patients with upper tract disease, also may be prominent in children with bladder infection.[84] Rare presentations include encephalopathy secondary to increased ammonia production by *Proteus* species.[64]

Age may be an important determinant of the clinical syndrome associated with UTI. Although infants with pyelonephritis may have colic, newborns have accelerated weight loss, poor feeding, or jaundice in the first few days of life as their only presenting sign, or they may be completely asymptomatic.[16, 50] The jaundice may be secondary to immaturity of hepatic enzymes as well as to bacterial hepatitis, endotoxic liver damage, red cell hemolysis, or a combination of these.[50] A review of 80 newborns with symptomatic UTIs revealed the following features: many of these infections were associated with bacteremia; boys were infected more frequently than girls; weight loss was common; and a history of maternal UTIs was common. *E. coli* was the most common infecting organism; 5 per cent of the infected patients had radiographic signs of obstructive uropathy; and 25 per cent of the patients had recurrent infection within 3 months after treatment was completed.[4]

Differential Diagnosis

E. coli accounts for approximately 90 per cent of pyelonephritis in girls and 65 per cent in boys.[11] Other major causative bacteria usually are derived from enteric flora and include *Proteus* in boys and a variety of Enterobacteriaceae in both sexes. Coagulase-negative staphylococci may be important in patients with underlying renal abnormalities and in sexually active subjects.[30, 45] A retrospective study of children with UTIs from the Children's Hospital in Boston found that gram-positive cocci were the organisms found most frequently in boys with pyelonephritis. *E. coli* was responsible for 21 per cent of the infections and *Staphylococcus albus* for 23 per cent. Moreover, 75 per cent of the boys had an anatomic abnormality (more than 25 per cent had obstructive lesions), and half had renal scarring.[6] These bacteria are less virulent, and infection often is confined to the bladder. Occasionally, staphylococci are associated with severe pyelonephritis.[45]

Fungi are a much less common cause of UTI, although *C. albicans* may invade the kidneys via the hematogenous or ascending route. Renal candidiasis rarely is proved in vivo but should be suspected in patients with underlying renal abnormalities, after surgery, and in severely debilitated hosts. Cultures of *Candida* directly from the kidney or the upper tract collecting system, the presence of kidney lesions suggestive of abscess on radiograph or scan, and persistent candiduria despite removal of predisposing factors are important clues to this diagnosis. The treatment of this condition should be aggressive because the prognosis may be grave.[23]

Anaerobic bacteria rarely cause UTI but should be suspected in patients with underlying renal disease, pyuria, and negative aerobic bacterial cultures.[65] Suprapubic aspiration and careful anaerobic culture may be necessary to confirm this diagnosis. Renal tuberculosis, although extremely rare now in North America, should be ruled out in these cases as well.

Patients with nephrolithiasis may have more complicated infections and may be more difficult to treat because of obstruction by the calculi and bacterial colonization of the stones. Struvite stones are infected more commonly than calcium oxalate ones, and *Proteus mirabilis* or other urea-splitting bacteria often are present.[74] Xanthogranulomatous pyelonephritis is a rare, chronic, suppurative renal infection characterized by the presence of granulomas, abscesses, and lipid-laden foam cells. Nephrectomy may be necessary to eradicate infection.[19] The clinical or radiologic presentation often is a mass lesion, and the differential diagnosis includes Wilms tumor, neuroblastoma, tuberculosis, and renal carcinoma.[19] A staghorn calculus may be present, and radiologic diagnosis occasionally indicates an obstructed, nonfunctioning kidney.[21, 32] *Proteus* and *Staphylococcus* species frequently are cultured from these lesions; however, antibiotic treatment rarely is successful without surgery.[61]

Viruses rarely have been demonstrated to cause clinical or pathologic lesions compatible with pyelonephritis. Viruria, hematuria, and proteinuria have been associated with mumps, coxsackievirus, echovirus, adenovirus, and hepatitis virus.[71] In general, illness associated with these and other viral infections behaves more like glomerulonephritis than pyelonephritis.

Specific Diagnosis

Pyuria, proteinuria, hematuria, and white blood cell casts in the urine often are noted in patients with pyelonephritis. Pyuria can be used to discriminate pyelonephritis from cystitis or asymptomatic bacteriuria. In young (<16 weeks), febrile infants, the presence of five or more white blood cells/hpf in the sediment correlated with pyelonephritis as documented with a positive TC-DSMA scan. In older children, Hoberman and associates noted a high correlation between a white blood cell count greater than or equal to 10/mm^3 with significant bacteriuria (>50,000 colony-forming units/mL in culture) and evidence of renal involvement on TC-DSMA scan.[27, 38] Details of collection and interpretation of the urinalysis and urine culture are discussed in the cystitis section.

Specimens obtained by adhesive bags are least useful in confirming the diagnosis of pyelonephritis and are most inaccurate in very young patients and in those with diarrhea, poor hygiene, neurogenic bladder, and underlying surgical conditions.[17, 37] Nevertheless, bagged specimens often can be used effectively in screening for UTIs and for follow-up. Two consecutive, midstream, clean-catch specimens containing more than 100,000 colonies/mL of a single bacterial isolate should be used whenever possible as a criterion to confirm the clinical diagnosis of UTI. When this is not possible, suprapubic bladder aspiration is the method of choice for confirming the diagnosis. Suprapubic aspiration should be carried out with sterile technique and with sufficient precautions to avoid trauma to the patient. The use of catheterized specimens rarely is necessary in children and requires extremely careful technique and skill. The catheter may introduce infection into the bladder, and interpretation of quantitative bacteriology after catheterization in children may be difficult.

Patients with ileal conduits present specific problems because the distal 4 cm of the conduit usually are colonized heavily. A double-lumen catheter has been recommended for obtaining urine samples from such patients. With such a catheter, counts of more than 1000 colonies/mL usually are significant.[72]

Gram stain of the urine, quantitative bacteriology, and the fluorescent antibody technique are discussed in the cystitis section. Urinary lactic dehydrogenase isoenzyme assays may be useful in defining kidney involvement. Although total urinary lactic dehydrogenase may be elevated in both cystitis and pyelonephritis, isoenzyme 5 appears to predominate in the urine of patients with kidney infection.[8] Experience in performing the assay, enzyme elevations due to other nephropathies, interfering effects of drugs such as nitrofurantoin, and the lability of the enzyme at room and freezer temperatures are limiting factors.

Radiographic and ultrasonographic studies are recommended in all patients with suspected pyelonephritis. This is performed best 6 or more weeks after complete resolution of clinical and bacterial signs of infection. Voiding cystourethrograms probably are unnecessary in most of these patients, unless a specific obstructive lesion of the lower urinary tract is suspected. Plain radiographs and ultrasonography can be used to rule out stones and major urinary tract malformations during the acute stages of infection.[66] These studies often are indicated in newborns and in patients with UTI associated with abdominal pain, hypertension, masses, or azotemia. Estimates of the frequency of radiographic abnormalities of the renal tract in children with UTI vary widely. This is caused partly by the difficulty of differentiating upper and lower tract infection as well as by the various definitions used for radiologic abnormalities.

In a study of children with first UTIs, Forbes and associates[20] defined parenchymal changes (renal atrophy, calyceal damage), gross structural abnormalities (of which duplications of the collecting system account for about a third), or both in 18 per cent of children (Fig. 46–7) and minor radiologic abnormalities (meatal or distal urethral narrowing, reflux, and bladder abnormalities) in 53 per cent. One-half of these radiologic changes reverted to normal within the follow-up period. Surgical attempts to improve function usually were not successful. A study carried out exclusively in boys described a 76 per cent frequency of upper tract renal abnormalities on intravenous pyelogram.[11] When patients with urethritis, transient cystitis, and nosocomial disease are excluded, as many as one-half of boys and one-third of girls probably have reflux, significant renal abnormalities, or both detected by radiology after their first UTI.

Hayden and associates[26] from the University of Texas, Galveston, recommend a stepwise approach to imaging evaluations of UTI in children (Fig. 46–8).

Step 1. Real-time ultrasonography should be the initial imaging technique. It identifies significant congenital anomalies, provides accurate measurements of the kidney for assessment of present and future growth, and demonstrates the presence of hydronephrosis and provides information regarding anatomy of the bladder, vesicourethral junction, and proximal urethra.

Step 2. If the sonographic examination is abnormal, radionuclide scintigraphy using ^{99}Tc-DTPA is indicated to evaluate renal function and urodynamics.

Step 3. If sonography is normal and differentiation of upper from lower tract infection is important, renal radionuclide cortical imaging with ^{99}Tc-glucoheptonate should be performed.

Step 4. A VCUG is performed on all boys with UTI, regardless of the findings of ultrasonography or cortical imaging scintigraphy. The VCUG is the best examination for the evaluation of vesicourethral reflux and the anatomy and physiology of the bladder and urethra. For follow-up evaluation of vesicourethral reflux, radionuclide cystography is indicated. Radionuclide cystography instead of VCUG also can be used satisfactorily as the first study in girls, in whom detailed anatomic definition of the bladder and urethra is not needed.

Computed tomography provides the most complete anatomic definition of the kidneys and adjacent retroperitoneum. The use of contrast also can yield some functional information. The disadvantages of this test include cost and the need

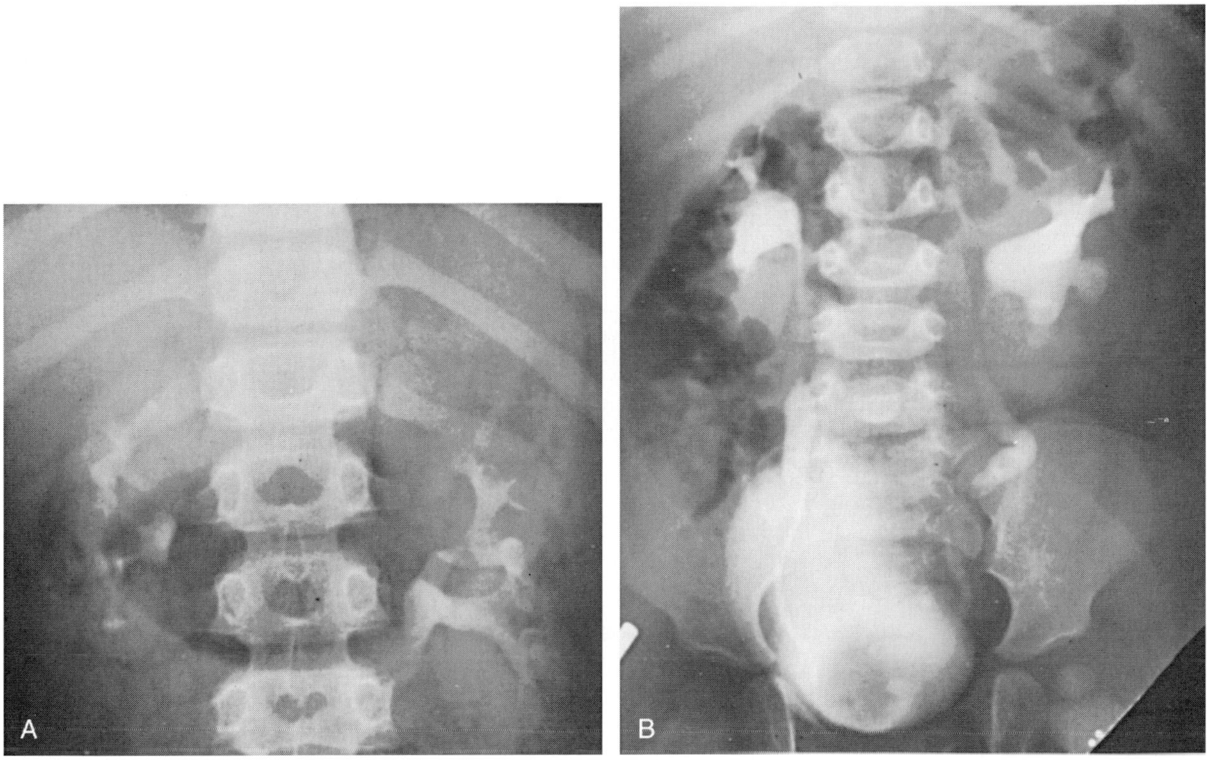

FIGURE 46–7. A, *Intravenous pyelogram demonstrating chronic pyelonephritis in an 8-year-old girl with a 5-year history of recurrent urinary tract infection. Note the small size and irregular contour of the right kidney and the calyceal distortion. There is compensatory hypertrophy of the normal left kidney.* B, *Ureterocele presenting a filling defect in the bladder of a 1.5-year-old girl. Note the displacement of the inferior pole of the left kidney, tortuosity of the left ureter, and left hydronephrosis. (Courtesy of B. Nogrady, M.D.)*

of sedation for young children. Magnetic resonance imaging for the evaluation of UTI is experimental at this time.[26, 46]

Retrograde cystourethrography is indicated in the preoperative and postoperative evaluation of patients with severe reflux. The amount of residual urine (normal <10 mL) can be estimated and the degree of reflux carefully measured. Unilateral obstruction and reflux also can be defined better by this procedure than by intravenous pyelography or voiding cystourethrography.

Cystoscopy rarely is indicated in children with pyelonephritis. It may be used for selected cases in which ureteral catheterization may be necessary, as with unilateral obstructive lesions and in cases that are resistant to conventional therapy.[33]

Radioisotope scanning and computed tomography are useful for identification of renal abscesses and for the diagnosis of anatomic abnormalities, cystic lesions, and hydronephrosis.

Treatment

There are several acceptable treatment programs for acute and chronic UTIs in infants and children. Specific dosages and drugs are outlined in the cystitis section. Principles of treatment of pyelonephritis include accurate diagnosis and monitoring of therapy by clinical, microscopic, and bacteriologic means. Careful follow-up, radiologic examination, and attention to hygiene and other predisposing conditions are important. A minimum duration of therapy of 2 weeks is important for the treatment of pyelonephritis.[10]

Drugs that are well concentrated in the urine and excreted by glomerular filtration or tubular secretion are most useful, and knowledge of the activities of these agents in urine at various pHs may be useful to the clinician. Amoxicillin, ampicillin, sulfonamides, cephalosporins, and aminoglycosides are all effective when the bacteria are susceptible. Because of the more limited activity of penicillins and the combination of erythromycin plus bicarbonate against certain gram-negative bacteria, these agents probably should be reserved for patients with cystitis or urethritis.[31] Co-trimoxazole (sulfamethoxazole-trimethoprim) offers little advantage over sulfisoxazole or amoxicillin alone in the treatment of acute pyelonephritis.[28, 47]

Experimental evidence in animal models has demonstrated excellent penetration of most antibiotics into the papillary and medullary regions of the kidney, which are the initial sites of infection in many cases of pyelonephritis. Hydration may decrease the concentration of some drugs in these sites, although this has little effect on ampicillin.[79] Studies in rats have indicated that diuresis plus ampicillin gave better bacteriologic results than either ampicillin or diuresis alone.[39] The clinical significance of these experimental animal studies is not clear, although logic would support the use of moderate diuresis and appropriate antimicrobial therapy. Drugs should be selected on the basis of in vitro susceptibility data whenever possible, and this selection should be confirmed by the clinical and microbiologic response during therapy, as well as the persistence of this response thereafter.

Recurrent pyelonephritis effectively may be prevented by several regimens, although none can be relied on to cure the condition completely. Certain agents, such as nalidixic and oxolinic acid, should not be used in children because of the high incidence of side effects and the rapid development of bacterial resistance in vivo. Several drugs, alone and in combination, may be chosen for long-term treatment of UTIs. Co-trimoxazole, nitrofurantoin, and methenamine compounds are all useful. The duration of such therapy is arbi-

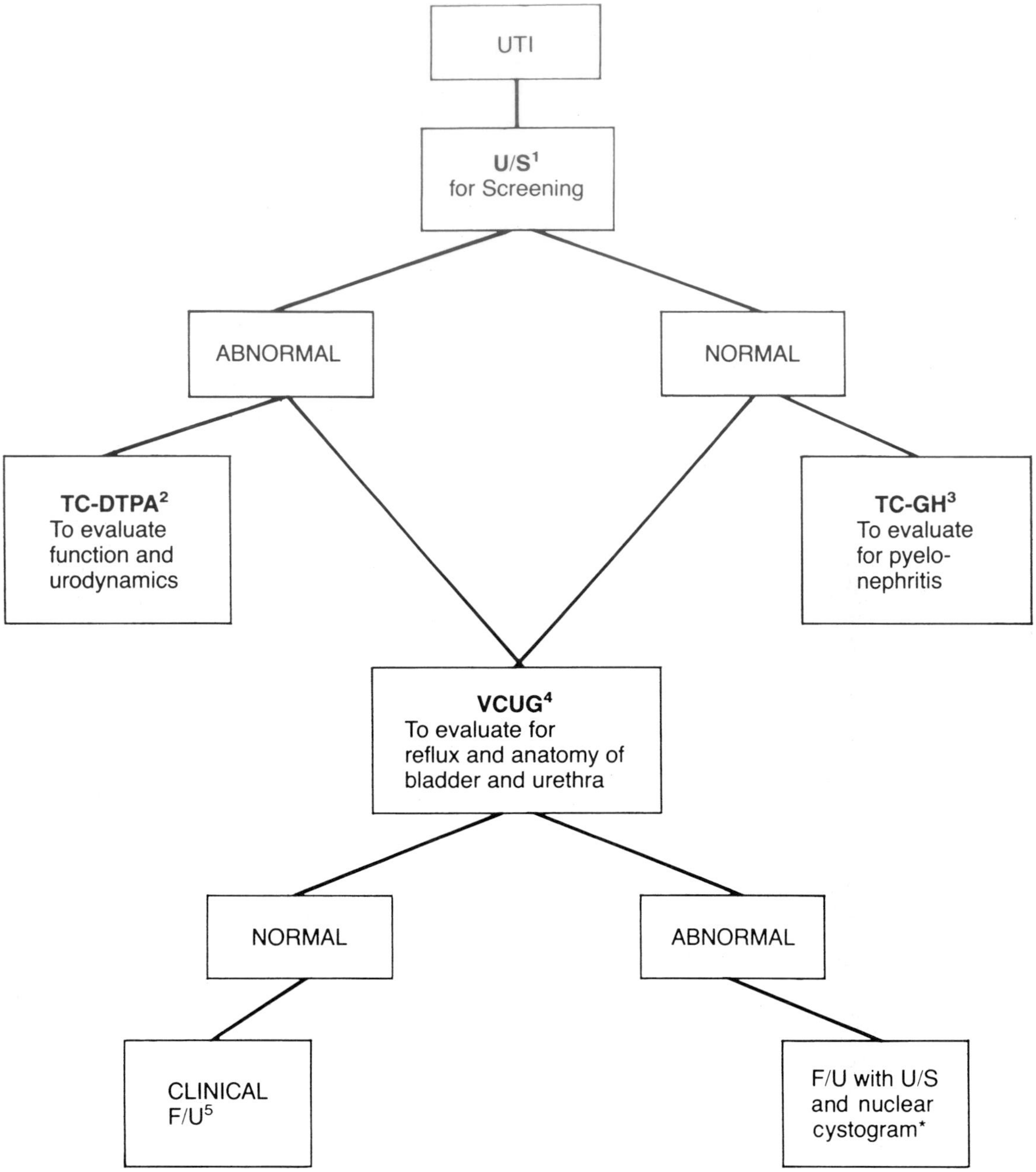

*Nuclear cystogram may replace voiding cystourethrogram in girls
[1]Ultrasonography
[2]Radionuclide scintigraphy with Tc-99-DTPA
[3]Radionuclide scintigraphy with Tc-99-glucoheptonate
[4]Voiding cystourethrogram
[5]Follow-up

FIGURE 46–8. *Diagnostic imaging approach for the patient with initial urinary tract infection. VCUG, voiding cystourethrogram.*

trary. Long durations (1 to 2 years) should be used in patients with renal abnormalities or frequent recurrent infections in the past and in whom compliance can be ensured.

Some patients with gross structural abnormalities, duplications, valves, ureteroceles, diverticula, and bladder exstrophies require a combination of surgical and medical therapy. Duplication of the collecting system with persistent reflux to the lower pole segment also may require surgical intervention. Colonic diversions or bladder reimplantation[58] may be useful in some patients formerly treated by ileal conduit; the long-term results of the latter procedure have been poor because of repeated infections and obstruction.[52] Urinary diversion should be reserved for patients in whom frequent catheterization, manual techniques for expression of the bladder, and antiseptic therapy have failed to prevent recurrent infection or loss of renal function.

The role of surgical repair is less clear in the treatment of patients with reflux.[60] Surgical repair of vesicoureteral reflux (usually ureteral reimplantation) may be useful in patients selected because of frequent recurrences or persistence of reflux despite antibiotic therapy or because of severe reflux with pyelonephritis.[82] In one such treatment group, however, postoperative ureteral dysfunction and obstruction occurred in 2 per cent of the patients and recurrent infection in 21 per cent. Prospective evaluation of patients with reflux by means of retrograde cystourethrography during a period of medical therapy seems reasonable. Persistence of reflux that is difficult to control with medical therapy and that is associated with progressive upper urinary tract damage justifies a surgical approach. Careful follow-up data have suggested that meatotomy seldom has a therapeutic or prophylactic effect on UTIs.[20]

Prognosis

Patients with major radiologic abnormalities and renal damage at the time of initial infection generally do poorly, as do patients with persistent intrarenal reflux, who have many infection recurrences. These patients and those with severe abnormalities of flow due to neurogenic and neuromuscular disorders or secondary to trauma or surgery may progress to severe renal failure on the basis of recurrent infection and obstruction.[77] Nephrolithiasis and stricture are grave complications in children with frequent recurrences and reflux. In addition, adverse effects of long-term antibiotic prophylaxis may include nephrotoxicity and superinfection with a variety of microorganisms, including *C. albicans*. Reflux nephropathy is responsible for a significant percentage of end-stage renal disease in late childhood and for 5 to 15 per cent of end-stage disease in white adults younger than 50 years of age. It also is the most common cause of severe hypertension in children. Renal parenchymal injury occurs early, usually before the age of 3 years. Most renal scars are present when reflux initially is discovered and usually are detected during evaluation after a UTI. Although the etiology and pathogenesis of reflux nephropathy are not clear yet, there is general consensus that early detection of reflux and prevention of infection can reduce the amount of damage to the kidney.

Because reflux occurs in less than 1 per cent of the general population, universal screening would not be a cost-effective strategy for prevention of renal disease. Identifying groups at risk is critical for this purpose. Siblings of children found to have reflux during evaluation after a UTI were found to have reflux themselves in 34 to 46 per cent of cases evaluated. The reflux was grade IV to V in approximately 60 per cent of the patients. The incidence of reflux in siblings was not related to previous history of UTI.[56, 57] Furthermore, scarring was detected in 38 per cent of asymptomatic patients with reflux. The best method of screening is debatable. VCUGs offer detail imaging of the urethra and allow for standardized grading of reflux; nuclear cystograms expose the patient to less radiation, and there have been some attempts to correlate findings with the currently accepted grading score. Renal damage is assessed better by cortical scintigraphy with TC-DSMA scan.[5]

Despite these dismal notes, it should be appreciated that most young infants and children with a first UTI do well. The capacity for compensatory renal growth in infants and children often is remarkable.[9] Patients with isolated lower tract signs and symptoms do best. Patients who contract their first UTI as newborns and those with renal damage or structural abnormalities of the kidney or collecting system at the time of their first infection do less well.[78]

The recurrence rate after first infection is approximately 30 to 40 per cent for children without demonstrable renal abnormalities. These recurrences usually happen within 6 months; however, 1 per cent of patients may have recurrences up to 6 years after the first infection. Follow-up for pyelonephritis should include urine cultures at least four times a year for the first 2 years and probably yearly up to 6 years.[10, 20, 24] Approximately 60 per cent of patients with one recurrence have a second recurrence.[10] The prognosis in patients with multiple recurrences and no underlying structural abnormalities is unclear. Most long-term studies indicate that it is rare for these children to develop renal abnormalities. Most patients have less severe clinical presentations with their recurrences than with their first infection. It is suggested that girls in particular may maintain their predisposition for UTIs into adulthood and that these may be manifested most commonly during pregnancy.[43]

Prevention

Chemoprophylaxis has been discussed under treatment in both this section and the one on cystitis. Several approaches are useful and should be guided by the individual's compliance and response to this therapy. A single dose of nitrofurantoin administered at bedtime (2.5 mg/kg) is useful for the prevention of recurrences. A double-blind crossover study compared nitrofurantoin with placebo in children without any major urinary tract abnormalities. Patients receiving the drug had 0.2 episodes per patient year, and patients receiving placebo had 4.2 episodes per patient year.[44] Clinical experience with co-trimoxazole (sulfamethoxazole-trimethoprim) has been equally favorable. Patients with clear evidence of upper tract disease and those with structural abnormalities may respond to long-term chemoprophylaxis as well.

Efforts at immunoprophylaxis are under investigation. The evidence that five K antigen types of *E. coli* are responsible for the majority of cases of acute pyelonephritis in children offers additional rationale for these studies.[29] Preliminary investigations in rabbits indicated that active immunization with "common antigen" derived from *Salmonella* could prevent pyelonephritis by both the ascending and the hematogenous routes.[15] Subsequent studies confirmed the ability of subcutaneous immunization with *E. coli* to prevent hematogenous pyelonephritis but could not confirm the prevention of infection due to the ascending route by either subcutaneous or intravesical immunization.[53] Continued investigations into the pathogenesis and immunology of experimental UTI may provide better approaches in the future.

References

URETHRITIS

1. Adger, H., Shafer, M.-A., Sweet, R. L., et al.: Screening for *Chlamydia trachomatis* and *Neisseria gonorrhoeae* in adolescent males: Value of first-catch urine examination. Lancet *2*:944–945, 1984.
2. Adjei, O., and Lal, V.: Non-invasive detection of *Chlamydia trachomatis* genital infections in asymptomatic males and females by enzyme immunoassay (Chlamydiazyme). J. Trop. Med. Hyg. *98*:51–54, 1994
3. Ahmed-Jushuf, I. H., Pratt, B. C., and Parya, O.: Incidence of *Ureaplasma urealyticum* in endourethral swabs compared with first voided urine from men. Genitourin. Med. *64*:78–80, 1988.
4. Arnold, A. J., and Kleris, G. S.: The "borderline" smear in men with urethritis. J. A. M. A. *244*:157–159, 1980.
5. Backman, M., Ruden, A. K., Ringertz, O., et al.: Detection of *Chlamydia trachomatis* in urine from men with urethritis. Eur. J. Clin. Microbiol. Infect. Dis. *12*:447-449, 1993.

6. Batteiger, B. E., and Jones, R. B.: Chlamydial infections. Infect. Dis. Clin. North Am. *1*:55–81, 1987.
7. Bauwens, J. E., Clark, A. M., Loeffelholz, M. J., et al.: Diagnosis of *Chlamydia trachomatis* urethritis in men by polymerase chain reaction assay of first-catch urine. J. Clin. Microb. *31*:3013–3016, 1993.
8. Bowie, W. R., Alexander, E. R., Floyd, J. F., et al.: Differential responses of chlamydial and ureaplasma-associated urethritis to sulfafurazole (sulfisoxazole) and aminocyclitols. Lancet 2:1276–1278, 1976.
9. Brunham, R. C., Paavonen, J., Stevens, C. E., et al.: Mucopurulent cervicitis: The ignored counterpart in women of urethritis in men. N. Engl. J. Med. *311*:1–6, 1984.
10. Cassell, G. H., Davis, J. K., Waites, K. B., et al.: Pathogenesis and significance of urogenital mycoplasmal infections. Adv. Exp. Med. Biol. *224*:93–115, 1987.
11. Centers for Disease Control: *Chlamydia trachomatis* infections: Policy guidelines for prevention and control. M. M. W. R. *34*(Suppl. 3S):53S, 1985.
12. Chacko, M. R., and Lovchik, J. C.: *Chlamydia trachomatis* infection in sexually active adolescents: Prevalence and risk factors. Pediatrics *73*:836–840, 1984.
13. Dallabetta, G., and Hook, E. W., III: Gonococcal infections. Infect. Dis. Clin. North Am. *1*:25–54, 1987.
14. Dawar, S., and Hellerstein, S.: Gonorrhea as a cause of asymptomatic pyuria in adolescent boys. J. Pediatr. *81*:357–358, 1972.
15. Demetriou, E., Sackett, R., Welch, D. F., et al.: Evaluation of an enzyme immunoassay for detection of *Neisseria gonorrhoeae* in an adolescent population. J. A. M. A. *252*:247–250, 1984.
16. Domeika, M. A., Bassiri, M., and Mardh, P. A.: Non-invasive sampling for detection of genital infection with *Chlamydia trachomatis* in males utilizing urinary leukocyte esterese tests and immunoassays. Infection *22*:65–68, 1994.
17. Folland, D. S., Burke, R. E., Hinman, A. R., et al.: Gonorrhea in preadolescent children: An inquiry into source of infection and mode of transmission. Pediatrics *60*:153, 1977.
18. Greenberg, R. N., Rein, M. F., Sanders, C. V., et al.: Urethral syndrome in women. J. A. M. A. *245*:923, 1981.
19. Hagay, Z. J., Sarov, B., and Sachs, J.: Detecting *Chlamydia trachomatis* in men with urethritis: Serology v isolation in cell culture. Genitourin. Med. *65*:166–170, 1988.
20. Handsfield, H. H., McCormack, W. M., Hook, E. W., et al.: A comparison of single-dose cefixime with ceftriaxone as treatment for uncomplicated gonorrhea. N. Engl. J. Med. *325*:1337–1340, 1991.
21. Hammerschlag, M. R., Golden, N. H., Oh, M. K., et al.: Single dose of azithromycin for the treatment of genital chlamydial infections in adolescents. J. Pediatr. *122*:961–965, 1993.
22. Hein, K., Marks, A., and Cohen, M.: Asymptomatic gonorrhea: Prevalence in a population of urban adolescents. J. Pediatr. *90*:634–635, 1977.
23. Herve, V. M. A., Georges, A. J., Massanga, M., et al.: Evaluation of a method for rapid detection of penicillinase-producing *Neisseria gonorrhoeae* in urethral exudates. J. Clin. Microbiol. *27*:227–228, 1989.
24. Holmes, K. K., Handsfield, H. H., Wang, S. P., et al.: Etiology of nongonococcal urethritis. N. Engl. J. Med. *292*:1199–1205, 1975.
25. Hooton, T. M., and Barnes, R. C.: Urethritis in men. Infect. Dis. Clin. North Am. *1*:165–178, 1987.
26. Ingram, D. L., Runyan, D. K., Collins, A. D., et al.: Vaginal *Chlamydia trachomatis* infection in children with sexual contact. Pediatr. Infect. Dis. *3*:97–99, 1984.
27. Kellog, D. S., Jr., Holmes, K. K., and Hill, G. A.: Laboratory diagnosis of gonorrhea. Cumitech *4*:1–10, 1976.
28. Lauharanta, J., Saarinen, K., Mustonen, M. T., et al.: Single-dose oral azithromycin versus seven-day doxycycline in treatment of non-gonococcal urethritis and cervicitis. J. Antimicrob. Chemother. *31*(Suppl.):177–183, 1993.
29. Mahony, J., Castriciano, S., Sellors, J., et al.: Diagnosis of *Chlamydia trachomatis* genital infections by cell culture and two enzyme immunoassays detecting different chlamydial antigens. J. Clin. Microbiol. *27*:1934–1938, 1989.
30. Martin, D. H., Mroczkowski, T. F., Dalu, Z. A., et al.: A controlled trial of single dose of azithromycin for the treatment of chlamydial urethritis and cervicitis. N. Engl. J. Med. *327*:921–925, 1992.
31. McCutchan, J. A., Wunderlich, A., and Braude, A. I.: Role of urinary solutes in natural immunity to gonorrhea. Infect. Immunol. *15*:149–155, 1977.
32. Moran, J. S., and Levine, W. C.: Drugs of choice for the treatment of uncomplicated gonococcal infections. Clin. Infect. Dis. *20*(Suppl.):S47-S65, 1995.
33. Neinstein, L. S., Goldenring, J., and Carpenter, S.: Non-sexual transmission of sexually transmitted diseases: An infrequent occurrence. Pediatrics *74*:67–76, 1984.
34. Odugbemi, T., Oyewold, F., Isichei, C. S., et al.: Single oral dose of azithromycin for therapy of susceptible sexually transmitted diseases: A multicenter open evaluation. W. Afr. J. Med. *12*:136–140, 1993.
35. Palmer, H. M., Gilroy, C. B., Thomas, B. J., et al.: Detection of *Chlamydia trachomatis* by the polymerase chain reaction in swabs and urine from men with non-gonococcal urethritis. J. Clin. Pathol. *44*:321–325, 1991.
36. Patrick, D. M., Rekart, M. L., Knowles, L.: Unsatisfactory performance of the leukocyte esterase test of first voided urine for rapid diagnosis of urethritis. Genitourin. Med. *70*:187–190, 1994.
37. Plaut, A. G., Gilbert, J. V., Artenstein, M. S., et al.: *Neisseria gonorrhoeae* and *Neisseria meningitidis*: Extracellular enzyme cleaves human immunoglobulin A. Science *190*:1103–1105, 1975.
38. Plourde, P. J., Tyndall, M., Agoki, E., et al.: Single-dose cefixime versus single-dose ceftriaxone in the treatment of antimicrobial-resistant *Neisseria gonorrhoeae* infection. J. Infect. Dis. *166*:919–922, 1992.
39. Rasmussen, S. J., Smith-Vaughan, H., Nelson, M., et al.: Detection of *Chlamydia trachomatis* in urine using enzyme immunoassay and DNA amplification. Mol. Cell. Probes 7:425–430, 1993.
40. Rettig, P. J.: Pediatric genital infection with *Chlamydia trachomatis*: Statistically nonsignificant, but clinically important. Pediatr. Infect. Dis. *3*:95–96, 1984.
41. Rice, R. J., Biddle, J. W., JeanLouis, Y. A., et al.: Chromosomally mediated resistance in *Neisseria gonorrhoeae* in the United States: Results of surveillance and reporting, 1983–1984. J. Infect. Dis. *153*:340–345, 1986.
42. Richmond, S. J., and Sparling, P. F.: Genital chlamydial infections. Am. J. Epidemiol. *103*:428–435, 1976.
43. Ris, H. W., and Dodge, R. W.: Gonorrhea in adolescent girls in a closed population. Am. J. Dis. Child. *123*:185–189, 1972.
44. Robertson, J. A.: Alternative therapy for genital mycoplasma infections. Eur. J. Clin. Microbiol. Infect. Dis. *7*:603–605, 1988.
45. Shafer, M.-A., Beck, A., Blain, B., et al.: *Chlamydia trachomatis*: Important relationships to race, contraception, lower genital tract infection, and Papanicolaou smear. J. Pediatr. *104*:141–146, 1984.
46. Shore, W. B., and Winkelstein, J. A.: Nonvenereal transmission of gonococcal infections to children. J. Pediatr. *79*:661–663, 1971.
47. Stamm, W. E.: Diagnosis of *Chlamydia trachomatis* genitourinary infections. Ann. Intern. Med. *108*:710–717, 1988.
48. Stamm, W. E.: Azithromycin in the treatment of uncomplicated genital chlamydial urethritis and cervicitis. Am. J. Med. *9*:195–225, 1991.
49. Stamm, W. E., Koutsky, L. A., Benedetti, J. K., et al.: *Chlamydia trachomatis* urethral infections in men. Prevalence, risk factors, and clinical manifestations. Ann. Intern. Med. *100*:47–51, 1984.
50. Swanson, J., Sparks, E., Young, D., et al.: Studies on *Gonococcus* infection. X. Pili and leukocyte association factor as mediators of interactions between gonococci and eukaryotic cells in vitro. Infect. Immunol. *11*:1352–1361, 1975.
51. Swartz, S. L., Kraus, S. J., Herrmann, K. L., et al.: Diagnosis and etiology of nongonococcal urethritis. J. Infect. Dis. *138*:445–454, 1978.
52. Tramont, E. C.: Inhibition of adherence of *Neisseria gonorrhoeae* by human genital secretions. J. Clin. Invest. *59*:117–124, 1977.
53. Weber, J. T., and Johnson, R. E.: New treatments for *Chlamydia trachomatis* genital infection. Clin. Infect. Dis. *20*(Suppl.):S66–S71, 1995.
54. Wilkinson, A. E., Seth, A. D., and Rodin, P.: Infection with penicillinase-producing gonococcus. Br. Med. J. *2*:1233–1235, 1976.
55. Wong, E. S., Hooton, T. M., Hill, C. C., et al.: Clinical and microbiological features of persistent or recurrent nongonococcal urethritis in men. J. Infect. Dis. *158*:1098–1101, 1988.

CYSTITIS

1. Adam, D.: Use of quinolones in pediatric patients. Rev. Infect. Dis. *11*:S1113–S1116, 1989.
2. Aladjem, M., Boichis, H., Hertz, M., et al.: The conservative management of vesicoureteric reflux: A review of 121 children. Pediatrics *65*:78–80, 1980.
3. Alon, U., Berant, M., and Pery, M.: Intravenous pyelography in children with urinary tract infection and vesicourethral reflux. Pediatrics *83*:332–336, 1989.
4. Amir, J., Varsano, I., and Mimouni, M.: Circumcision and urinary tract infection in infants. Am. J. Dis. Child. *140*:1092, 1986.
5. Avner, E. D., Ingelfinger, J. R., Herrin, J. T., et al.: Single-dose amoxicillin therapy of uncomplicated pediatric urinary tract infections. J. Pediatr. *102*:623–626, 1983.
6. Bailey, R. R.: Urinary infection and bacterial excretion-rates in urine. Lancet *1*:187–188, 1971.
7. Barry, A. L., Smith, P. B., and Turck, M.: Laboratory diagnosis of urinary tract infection. Cumitech *2*:1–11, 1975.
8. Bran, J. L., Levison, M. E., and Kaye, D.: Entrance of bacteria into the female urinary bladder. N. Engl. J. Med. *286*:626–629, 1972.
9. Burns, M. W., Burns, J. L., and Krieger, J. N.: Pediatric urinary tract infection. Pediatr. Clin. North Am. *34*:1111–1120, 1987.
10. Crooks, K. K., and Enrile, B. G.: Comparison of the ileal conduit and clean intermittent catheterization for myelomeningocele. Pediatrics *72*:203–206, 1983.
11. Dagan, R., Einhorn, M., Lang, R., et al.: Once-daily cefixime compared with twice-daily trimethoprim-sulfamethoxazole for treatment of urinary tract infection in infants and children. Pediatr. Infect. Dis. J. *11*:198–203, 1992.
12. Davison, J. M., Sprott, M. S., and Selkon, J. B.: The effect of covert bacteriuria in schoolgirls on renal function at 18 years and during pregnancy. Lancet *2*:651–655, 1984.
13. Dodge, W. F., West, E. F., and Travis, L. B.: Bacteriuria in school children. Am. J. Dis. Child. *127*:364–370, 1974.

14. Durbin, W. A., Jr., and Georges, P.: Management of urinary tract infections in infants and children. Pediatr. Infect. Dis. *3*:564–574, 1984.
15. Eichenwald, H. F.: Some aspects of the diagnosis and management of urinary tract infection in children and adolescents. Pediatr. Infect. Dis. *5*:760–765, 1986.
16. Fair, W. R., and Wehner, N.: Further observations on the antibacterial nature of prostatic fluid. Infect. Immunol. *3*:494–495, 1971.
17. Forbes, P. A., Drummond, K. N., and Nogrady, M. B.: Initial urinary tract infections: Observations in children without major radiologic abnormalities. J. Pediatr. *75*:187–192, 1969.
18. Forsum, U., Hjelm, E., and Jonsell, G.: Antibody-coated bacteria in the urine of children with urinary tract infections. Acta Pediatr. Scand. *65*:639–642, 1976.
19. Gabre-Kidan, T., Lipsky, B. A., and Plorde, J. J.: *Hemophilus influenzae* as a cause of urinary tract infections in men. Arch. Intern. Med. *144*:1623–1627, 1984.
20. Garibaldi, R. A., Burke, J. P., Dickman, M. L., et al.: Factors predisposing to bacteriuria during indwelling urethral catheterization. N. Engl. J. Med. *291*:215–219, 1974.
21. Geist, R. W., and Antolak, S. J.: Interstitial cystitis in children. J. Urol. *104*:922–925, 1970.
22. Gerstein, A. R., Okun, R., Gonick, H. C., et al.: The prolonged use of methenamine hippurate in the treatment of chronic urinary tract infection. J. Urol. *100*:767–771, 1968.
23. Gillenwater, J. Y., Gleason, C. H., Lohr, J. A., et al.: Home urine cultures by the dip-strip method: Results in 289 cultures. Pediatrics *58*:508–512, 1976.
24. Ginsburg, C. M., and McCracken, G. H.: Urinary tract infections in young infants. Pediatrics *69*:409–412, 1982.
25. Gonzales, E. T.: Annual meeting of the section on pediatric urology. Pediatrics *74*:893–897, 1984.
26. Granoff, D. M., and Roskes, S.: Urinary tract infection due to *Hemophilus influenzae*, type b. J. Pediatr. *84*:414–416, 1974.
27. Gruneberg, R. N., Smellie, J. M., Leakey, A., et al.: Long-term low-dose co-trimoxazole in prophylaxis of childhood urinary tract infection: Bacteriological aspects. Br. Med. J. *2*:206–208, 1976.
28. Hand, W. L., Smith, J. W., Miller, T. E., et al.: Immunoglobulin synthesis in lower urinary tract infection. J. Lab. Clin. Med. *75*:19–29, 1970.
29. Hedelin, H. H., Mardh, P. A., Brorson, J. E., et al.: *Mycoplasma hominis* and interstitial cystitis. Sex. Transm. Dis. *10*:327–330, 1983.
30. Hellerstein, S.: Recurrent urinary tract infections in children. Pediatr. Infect. Dis. *1*:271–281, 1982.
31. Hellerstein, S., Duggan, E., Welchert, E., et al.: Serum C-reactive protein and the site of urinary tract infections. J. Pediatr. *100*:21–25, 1982.
32. Hovelius, B., and Mardh, P. A.: *Staphylococcus saprophyticus* as a common cause of urinary tract infections. Rev. Infect. Dis. *6*:328–337, 1984.
33. Hulbert, J.: Gram-negative urinary infection treated with oral penicillin G. Lancet *2*:1216–1219, 1972.
34. Jodal, U.: The natural history of bacteriuria in childhood. Infect. Dis. Clin. North Am. *1*:713–729, 1987.
35. Johnson, H. W., Elliott, G. B., Israels, S., et al.: Granulomatous cystitis of children, bilharzia-like, occurring in British Columbia. Pediatrics *40*:808–815, 1967.
36. Kamhi, B., Horowitz, M. I., and Kovetz, A.: Isolated neurogenic dysfunction of the bladder in children with urinary tract infection. J. Urol. *106*:151–153, 1971.
37. Kern, W. H.: Epithelial cells in urine sediments. Am. J. Clin. Pathol. *56*:67–72, 1971.
38. Kunin, C.: Urinary tract infections in children. Hosp. Pract. *11*:91–98, 1976.
39. Levy, S. B.: Fecal flora in recurrent urinary-tract infection. N. Engl. J. Med. *296*:813–814, 1977.
40. Lindberg, U., Jodal, U., Hanson, L. A., et al.: Asymptomatic bacteriuria in school girls. Acta Paediatr. Scand. *64*:432–440, 1975.
41. Lomberg, H., Hellstrom, M., Jodal, U., et al.: Virulence-associated traits in *Escherichia coli* causing first and recurrent episodes of urinary tract infection in children with or without vesicoureteral reflux. J. Infect. Dis. *150*:561–569, 1984.
42. Lorentz, W. B., and Resnick, M. I.: Comparison of urinary lactic dehydrogenase with antibody-coated bacteria in the urine sediment as means of localizing the site of urinary tract infection. Pediatrics *64*:672–677, 1979.
43. Lyon, R. P., Scott, M. P., and Marshall, S.: Intermittent catheterization rather than urinary diversion in children with meningomyelocele. J. Urol. *113*:409–417, 1975.
44. Marks, M. I.: Iatrogenic pneumaturia. J. Urol. *106*:407–408, 1971.
45. Marks, M. I., Langston, C., and Eickhoff, T. C.: *Torulopsis glabrata*: An opportunistic pathogen in man. N. Engl. J. Med. *283*:1131–1134, 1970.
46. Montplaisir, S., Courteau, C., Martineau, B., et al.: Limitations of the direct immunofluorescence test for antibody-coated bacteria in determining the site of urinary tract infections in children. Can. Med. Assoc. J. *125*:993–1002, 1981.
47. Morrell, R. E., Duritz, G., and Oltorf, C.: Suprapubic aspiration associated with hematoma. Pediatrics *69*:455–457, 1982.
48. Mou, T. W.: Effect of urine pH on the antibacterial activity of antibiotics and chemotherapeutic agents. J. Urol. *87*:978–987, 1962.
49. Mufson, M. A., and Belshe, R. B.: A review of adenoviruses in the etiology of acute hemorrhagic cystitis. J. Urol. *115*:191–194, 1976.
50. Numazaki, Y., Kumasaka, T., Yano, N., et al.: Further study on acute hemorrhagic cystitis due to adenovirus type 11. N. Engl. J. Med. *289*:344–347, 1973.
51. Orikasa, S., Koyanagi, T., Motomura, M., et al.: Experience with non-sterile, intermittent self-catheterization. J. Urol. *115*:141–142, 1976.
52. Parrott, T. S.: Cystitis and urethritis. Pediatr. Rev. *10*:217–222, 1989.
53. Pass, R. F., and Waldo, F. B.: Anaerobic bacteremia following suprapubic bladder aspiration. J. Pediatr. *94*:748–750, 1979.
54. Pryles, C. V., and Lustik, B.: Laboratory diagnosis of urinary tract infection. Pediatr. Clin. North Am. *18*:233–244, 1971.
55. Rabinovitch, H.: Personal communications, 1977.
56. Ross, R. R., and Conway, G. F.: Hemorrhagic cystitis following accidental overdose of methenamine mandelate. Am. J. Dis. Child. *119*:86–87, 1970.
57. Ruberto, U., D'Eufemia, P., Ferretti, L., et al.: Effect of 3- vs. 10-day treatment of urinary tract infections. J. Pediatr. *104*:483–484, 1984.
58. Savage, D. C. L., Adler, K., Howie, G., et al.: Controlled trial of therapy in covert bacteriuria of childhood. Lancet *1*:358–361, 1975.
59. Savige, J. A., Gilbert, G. L., Fairley, K. F., et al.: Bacteriuria due to *Ureaplasma urealyticum* and *Gardnerella vaginalis* in women with preeclampsia. J. Infect. Dis. *148*:605, 1983.
60. Saxena, S. R., Laurance, B. M., and Shaw, D. G.: The justification for early radiological investigations of urinary-tract infection in children. Lancet *2*:403–404, 1975.
61. Schaad, U., Salam, M. A., Augard, Y., et al.: Use of fluoroquinolones in pediatrics: Consensus report of an International Society of Chemotherapy commission. Pediatr. Infect. Dis. J. *14*:1–9, 1995.
62. Shapiro, E. D.: Short course antimicrobial treatment of urinary tract infections in children: A critical analysis. Pediatr. Infect. Dis. *1*:294–297, 1982.
63. Shopfner, C. E.: Modern concepts of lower urinary tract obstruction in pediatric patients. Pediatrics *45*:194–196, 1970.
64. Smellie, J. M., Gruneberg, R. N., Leakey, A., et al.: Long-term low-dose co-trimoxazole in prophylaxis of childhood urinary tract infection: Clinical aspects. Br. Med. J. *2*:203–206, 1976.
65. Stamey, T. A., Condy, M., and Mihara, G.: Prophylactic efficacy of nitrofurantoin macrocrystals and trimethoprim-sulfamethoxazole in urinary infections. N. Engl. J. Med. *296*:780–783, 1977.
66. Stamey, T. A., Fair, W. R., Timothy, M. M., et al.: Serum versus urinary antimicrobial concentrations in cure of urinary-tract infections. N. Engl. J. Med. *291*:1159–1163, 1974.
67. Stark, R. P., and Maki, D. G.: Bacteriuria in the catheterized patient: What quantitative level of bacteriuria is relevant? N. Engl. J. Med. *311*:560–564, 1984.
68. Tuttle, J. P., Jr., Sarvas, H., and Koistinen, J.: The role of vaginal immunoglobulin A in girls with recurrent urinary tract infections. J. Urol. *120*:742–744, 1978.
69. Uehling, D. T., and Stiehm, E. R.: Elevated urinary secretory IgA in children with urinary tract infection. Pediatrics *47*:40–46, 1971.
70. Van Wijk, J. A. E., de Jong, T. P. V. M., Van Gool, J. D., et al.: Using quinolones in urinary tract infections in children. Adv. Antimicrob. Antineopl. Chemother. *11*(Suppl.):157–161, 1992.
71. Wallen, L., Zeller, W. P., Goessler, M., et al.: Single-dose amikacin treatment of first childhood *E. coli* lower urinary tract infections. J. Pediatr. *103*:316–319, 1983.
72. Welch, T. R., Forbes, P. A., Drummond, K. N., et al.: Recurrent urinary tract infection in girls. Arch. Dis. Child. *51*:114–119, 1976.
73. White, R. H. R., and Taylor, C. M.: Prospective trial of operative versus non-operative treatment of severe vesicoureteric reflux: Two years' observation in 96 children. Br. Med. J. *287*:171–174, 1983.
74. Wiswell, T. E., and Roscelli, J. D.: Corroborative evidence for the decreased incidence of urinary tract infections in circumcised male infants. Pediatrics *78*:96–99, 1986.
75. Zaloga, G. P., and Hill, T.: Advances in diagnostic testing for urinary tract infection. Infect. Urol. 2:117–125, 1989.
76. Zinner, S. H., Sabath, L. D., Casey, J. I., et al.: Erythromycin and alkalinisation of the urine in the treatment of urinary-tract infections due to Gram-negative bacilli. Lancet *1*:1267–1268, 1971.

PYELONEPHRITIS

1. Amir, J., Varsano, I., and Mimouni, M.: Circumcision and urinary tract infection in infants. Am. J. Dis. Child. *140*:1092, 1986.
2. Arrieta, A., Sequeira, A., Vargas-Shiraishi, O. M., et al.: Interleukin (IL) 1 αβ and IL-6 in urine and serum of children with urinary tract infections (UTI). Pediatr. Res. *37*:4, 1995.
3. Benson, M., Jodal, U., Andreasson, A., et al.: Interleukin 6 response to urinary tract infection in childhood. Pediatr. Infect. Dis. J. *13*:612–616, 1994.
4. Bergstrom, T., Larson, H., Lincoln, K., et al.: Studies of urinary tract infections in infancy and childhood. J. Pediatr. *80*:858–866, 1972.
5. Buonomo, C., Treves, S. T., Jones, B., et al.: Silent renal damage in symptom-free siblings of children with vesicoureteral reflux: Assessment with technetium 99m dimercaptosuccinic acid scintigraphy. J. Pediatr. *122*:721–723, 1993.
6. Burbige, K. A., Retik, A. B., Colodny, A. H., et al.: Urinary tract infection in boys. J. Urol. *132*:541–542, 1984.

7. Burns, M. W., Burns, J. L., and Krieger, J. N.: Pediatric urinary tract infection. Pediatr. Clin. North Am. *34*:1111–1120, 1987.
8. Carvajal, H. F., Passey, R. B., Berger, M., et al.: Urinary lactic dehydrogenase isoenzyme 5 in the differential diagnosis of kidney and bladder infection. Kidney Int. *8*:176–184, 1975.
9. Claësson, I., Jacobsson, B., Jodal, U., et al.: Compensatory kidney growth in children with urinary tract infection and unilateral renal scarring: An epidemiologic study. Kidney Int. *20*:759–764, 1981.
10. Cohen, M.: Urinary tract infections in children. I. Females aged 2 through 14, first two infections. Pediatrics *50*:271–276, 1972.
11. Cohen, M.: The first urinary tract infection in male children. Am. J. Dis. Child. *130*:810–813, 1976.
12. Coles, G. A., Chick, S., Hopkins, M., et al.: The role of the T cell in experimental pyelonephritis. Clin. Exp. Immunol. *16*:629–636, 1974.
13. De Man, P., Claeson, I., and Johanson, I.: Bacterial attachment as a predictor of renal abnormalities in boys with urinary tract infection. J. Pediatr. *115*:915–921, 1989.
14. De Man, P., Jodal, U., Lincoln, K., et al.: Bacterial attachment and inflammation in the urinary tract. J. Infect. Dis. *158*:29–35, 1988.
15. Dominique, G., Salhi, A., Rountree, C., et al.: Prevention of experimental hematogenous and retrograde pyelonephritis by antibodies against enterobacterial common antigen. Infect. Immun. *2*:175–182, 1970.
16. Du, J. N.: Colic as the sole symptom of urinary tract infection in infants. Can. Med. Assoc. J. *115*:334–337, 1976.
17. Edelmann, C. M., Ogwo, J. E., Fine, B. P., et al.: The prevalence of bacteriuria in full-term and premature newborn infants. J. Pediatr. *82*:125–132, 1973.
18. Eden, C. S., Hanson, L. A., Jodal, U., et al.: Variable adherence to normal human urinary tract epithelial cells of *Escherichia coli* strains associated with various forms of urinary tract infection. Lancet *2*:490–492, 1976.
19. Elder, J. S., and Vaughan, E. D.: Xanthogranulomatous pyelonephritis: The great imitator. Infect. Surg. February, 145–158, 1984.
20. Forbes, P. A., Drummond, K. N., and Nogrady, M. B.: Initial urinary tract infections. J. Pediatr. *75*:187–192, 1969.
21. Graivier, L., and Vargas, M. A.: Xanthogranulomatous pyelonephritis in childhood. Am. J. Dis. Child. *123*:156–158, 1972.
22. Guze, L. B., Hubert, E. G., and Kalmanson, G. M.: Pyelonephritis. X. Microbial interference in streptococcal infections in the rat kidney. J. Lab. Clin. Med. *74*:274–287, 1969.
23. Guziel, L. P., Stone, W. J., Schaffner, W., et al.: Primary renal candidiasis with renal granulomata and salt-losing nephropathy. Am. J. Med. Sci. *269*:123–130, 1975.
24. Hallett, R. J., Pead, L., and Maskell, R.: Urinary infections in boys: A three-year prospective study. Lancet *2*:1107–1110, 1976.
25. Harles, E. M. J., Bullen, J. J., and Thompson, D. A.: Influence of estrogen on experimental pyelonephritis caused by *Escherichia coli*. Lancet *2*:283–286, 1975.
26. Hayden, C. K., Swischuk, L. E., Fawcett, H. D., et al.: Urinary tract infections in childhood: A current imaging approach. Radiographics *6*:1023–1037, 1986.
27. Hoberman, A., Wald, E., Reynolds, E., et al.: Pyuria and bacteriuria in urine specimens obtained by catheter from young children with fever. J. Pediatr. *124*:513–519, 1994.
28. Howard, J. B., and Howard, J. E., Sr.: Double-blind comparison of trimethoprim-sulfamethoxazole (TMP/SMX) and sulfamethoxazole (SMX) in the treatment of acute urinary tract infections in infants and children. Abstract Z41, Proceedings of the 15th Interscience Conference on Antimicrobial Agents and Chemotherapy, 1975.
29. Kaijser, B., Hanson, L. A., Jodal, U., et al.: Frequency of *E. coli* K antigens in urinary tract infections in children. Lancet *1*:663–666, 1977.
30. Khan, A. J., Evans, H. E., Bombach, E., et al.: Coagulase-negative staphylococcal bacteriuria: A rarity in infants and children. J. Pediatr. *86*:309–311, 1975.
31. Klastersky, J., Debusscher, L., and Daneau, D.: Effectiveness of erythromycin plus alkalinization and of nitrofurantoin in the treatment of urinary tract infections. Curr. Therap. Res. *13*:427–433, 1971.
32. Klugo, R. C., Anderson, J. A., Reid, R., et al.: Xanthogranulomatous pyelonephritis in children. J. Urol. *117*:350–352, 1977.
33. Koutsaimanis, K. G., and Roberts, A. P.: Infection of each side of upper urinary tract with a different organism in a case of bilateral chronic pyelonephritis. Lancet *1*:471–472, 1971.
34. Kunin, C. M., Deutscher, R., and Paquin, A.: Urinary tract infections in school children: An epidemiologic, clinical and laboratory study. Medicine *43*:91–130, 1964.
35. Kunin, C. M.: The natural history of recurrent bacteriuria in schoolgirls. N. Engl. J. Med. *282*:1443–1448, 1970.
36. Kunin, C. M.: A ten-year study of bacteriuria in schoolgirls: Final report of bacteriologic, urologic and epidemiologic findings. J. Infect. Dis. *122*:382–393, 1970.
37. Kunin, C. M.: Urinary tract infections in infancy. J. Pediatr. *86*:483–484, 1975.
38. Landau, D., Turner, M. E., Brennan, J., et al.: The value of urinalysis in differentiating acute pyelonephritis from lower urinary tract infection in febrile infants. Pediatr. Infect. Dis. J. *13*:777–781, 1994.
39. Levison, S. P., and Kaye, D.: Influence of water diuresis on antimicrobial treatment of enterococcal pyelonephritis. J. Clin. Invest. *51*:2408–2413, 1972.
40. Lidefelt, K. J., Bollgren, I., Kallenius, G., et al.: P-fimbriated *Escherichia coli* in children with acute cystitis. Acta Paediatr. Scand. *76*:775–780, 1987.
41. Lindberg, U., Claesson, I., Hanson, L. A., et al.: Asymptomatic bacteriuria in schoolgirls. I. Clinical and laboratory findings. Acta Paediatr. Scand. *64*:425–431, 1975.
42. Lindberg, U., Hanson, L. A., Jodal, U., et al.: Asymptomatic bacteriuria in schoolgirls. II. Differences in *Escherichia coli* causing asymptomatic and symptomatic bacteriuria. Acta Paediatr. Scand. *64*:432–436, 1975.
43. Lindblad, B. S., and Ekengren, K.: The long-term prognosis is of non-obstructive urinary tract infection in infancy and childhood after the advent of sulphonamides. Acta Paediatr. Scand. *58*:25–32, 1969.
44. Lohr, J. A., Nunley, D. H., Howards, S. S., et al.: Prevention of recurrent urinary tract infections in girls. Pediatrics *59*:562–565, 1977.
45. Mabeck, C. E.: Significance of coagulase-negative staphylococcal bacteriuria. Lancet *2*:1150–1152, 1969.
46. Magill, H. L., Riggs, W., Boulden, T. F., et al.: Diagnostic imaging in children with urinary tract infection: Review of current concepts and suggested guidelines. South. Med. J. *80*:1557–1565, 1987.
47. Mannisto, P. T.: Comparison of oxolinic acid, trimethoprim, and trimethoprim-sulfamethoxazole in the treatment and long-term control of urinary tract infection. Curr. Ther. Res. *20*:645–654, 1976.
48. Marild, S., Jodal, U., Orskov, I., et al.: Special virulence of the *Escherichia coli* O1:K1:H7 clone in acute pyelonephritis. J. Pediatr. *115*:40–45, 1989.
49. Marild, S., Wettergren, B., Hellstrom, M., et al.: Bacterial virulence and inflammatory response in infants with febrile urinary tract infection or screening bacteriuria. J. Pediatr. *112*:348–354, 1988.
50. McNicholl, B.: Urinary tract infection and jaundice. Am. J. Dis. Child. *120*:89–91, 1970.
51. Merritt, J. L., and Keys, T. F.: Limitations of the antibody-coated bacteria test in patients with neurogenic bladders. J. A. M. A. *247*:1723–1725, 1982.
52. Middleton, A. W., Jr., and Hendren, W. H.: Ileal conduits in children at the Massachusetts General Hospital from 1955 to 1970. J. Urol. *115*:591–595, 1976.
53. Montgomerie, J. Z., Kalmanson, G. M., Hubert, E. G., et al.: Pyelonephritis. XIV. Effect of immunization on experimental *Escherichia coli* pyelonephritis. Infect. Immun. *6*:330–334, 1972.
54. Neumann, P. Z., deDomenico, I. J., and Nogrady, M. B.: Constipation and urinary tract infection. Pediatrics *52*:241–245, 1973.
55. Nicolle, L. E., Harding, G. K. M., Preiksaitis, J., et al.: The association of urinary tract infection with sexual intercourse. J. Infect. Dis. *146*:579–583, 1982.
56. Noe, H. N.: The long-term results of prospective sibling reflux screening. J. Urol. *148*:1739–1742, 1992.
57. Peeden, J. N., Jr., and Noe, H. N.: Is it practical to screen for familial vesicoureteral reflux within a private pediatric practice? Pediatrics *89*:4, 1992.
58. Perlmutter, A. D.: Experiences with urinary undiversion in children with neurogenic bladder. J. Urol. *123*:402–406, 1980.
59. Randolph, M. F., Morris, K. E., and Gould, E. B.: The first urinary tract infection in the female infant. J. Pediatr. *86*:342–348, 1975.
60. Ransley, P. G.: Vesicoureteric reflux: Continuing surgical dilemma. Urology *22*:246–255, 1978.
61. Rasoulpour, M., Banco, L., Mackay, I. M., et al.: Treatment of focal xanthogranulomatous pyelonephritis with antibiotics. J. Pediatr. *105*:423–425, 1984.
62. Ratner, J. J., Thomas, V. L., Sanford, B. A., et al.: Antibody to kidney antigen in the urine of patients with urinary tract infections. J. Infect. Dis. *147*:434–444, 1983.
63. Ronald, A. R., Cutler, R. E., and Turck, M.: Effect of bacteriuria on renal concentrating mechanisms. Ann. Intern. Med. *70*:723–733, 1969.
64. Samtoy, B., and DeBeukelaer, M. M.: Ammonia encephalopathy secondary to urinary tract infection with *Proteus mirabilis*. Pediatrics *65*:294–297, 1980.
65. Segura, J. W., Kelalis, P. P., Martin, W. J., et al.: Anaerobic bacteria in the urinary tract. Mayo Clin. Proc. *47*:30–33, 1972.
66. Sherwood, T., and Whitaker, R. H.: Initial screening of children with urinary tract infections: Is plain film radiography and ultrasonography enough? Br. Med. J. *288*:827, 1984.
67. Silverblatt, F. J.: Host-parasite interaction in the rat renal pelvis. A possible role for pili in the pathogenesis of pyelonephritis. J. Exp. Med. *140*:1696–1711, 1974.
68. Smith, J., Holmgren, J., Ahlstedt, S., et al.: Local antibody production in experimental pyelonephritis: Amount, avidity, and immunoglobulin class. Infect. Immun. *10*:411–415, 1974.
69. Smith, J. W., and Kaijser, B.: The local immune response to *Escherichia coli* O and K antigens in experimental pyelonephritis. J. Clin. Invest. *58*:276–281, 1976.
70. Smith, J. W., Jones, S. R., and Kaijser, B.: Significance of antibody-coated bacteria in urinary sediment in experimental pyelonephritis. J. Infect. Dis. *135*:577–581, 1977.
71. Smith, R. D., and Aquino, J.: Viruses and the kidney. Med. Clin. North Am. *55*:89–106, 1971.
72. Spence, B., Stewart, W., and Cass, A. S.: Use of a double-lumen catheter to

determine bacteriuria in intestinal loop diversions in children. J. Urol. *108*:800–801, 1972.
73. Svanborg Eden, C., and De Man, P.: Bacterial virulence in urinary tract infection. Infect. Dis. Clin. North Am. *1*:731–750, 1987.
74. Thompson, R. B., and Stamey, T. A.: Bacteriology of infected stones. Urology *11*:627–633, 1973.
75. Tullus, K., Fituri, O., Burman, L. G., et al.: Interleukin 6 and 8 in the urine of infants and children with acute pyelonephritis. ICAAC Abstract, 1992.
76. Tullus, K., Horlin, K., Svenson, S. B., et al.: Epidemic outbreaks of acute pyelonephritis caused by nosocomial spread of P fimbriated *Escherichia coli* in children. J. Infect. Dis. *150*:728–736, 1984.
77. Warshaw, B. L., Edelbrock, H. H., Ettenger, R. B., et al.: Progression to end-stage renal disease in children with obstructive uropathy. J. Pediatr. *100*:183–187, 1982.
78. Wein, A. J., and Schoenberg, H. W.: A review of 402 girls with recurrent urinary tract infection. J. Urol. *107*:329–331, 1972.
79. Whelton, A., Sapir, D. G., Carter, G. C., et al.: Intrarenal distribution of penicillin, cephalothin, ampicillin and oxytetracycline during varied states of hydration. J. Pharmacol. Exp. Ther. *179*:419–428, 1971.
80. Williams, T. W., Friedlander, A. M., Lyons, J. M., et al.: Cellular immunity in pyelonephritis: Identification of suppressor cell activity of spleen cells in response to concanavalin A and inhibition of lymphocyte-mediated L cell cytotoxicity. J. Immunol. *116*:778–781, 1976.
81. Williams, T. W., Lyons, J. M., and Braude, A. I.: In vitro lysis of target cells by rat polymorphonuclear leukocytes isolated from acute pyelonephritic exudates. J. Immunol. *119*:671–674, 1977.
82. Willscher, M. K., Bauer, S. B., Zammuto, P. J., et al.: Infection of the urinary tract after anti-reflux surgery. J. Pediatr. *89*:743–746, 1976.
83. Wiswell, T. E., and Roscelli, J. D.: Corroborative evidence for the decreased incidence of urinary tract infections in circumcised male infants. Pediatrics *78*:96–99, 1986.
84. Woodward, J. R., and Holden, S.: The prognostic significance of fever in childhood urinary infections. Clin. Pediatr. *15*:1051–1054, 1976.

47

RENAL ABSCESS

Edmond T. Gonzales, Jr.

Although acute pyelonephritis is a relatively common infection in children, the primary development of a renal abscess or progression of pyelonephritis to a renal or perinephric abscess is a distinctly uncommon situation. Renal abscess may be a primary problem—that is, one that develops in a kidney without an antecedent infection or underlying anatomical abnormality—or it may occur secondarily in a patient with previously recognized acute pyelonephritis or in a child with congenital urologic abnormalities known to predispose to the development of pyelonephritis.

A primary renal abscess is thought to develop most often after an episode of bacteremia and frequently occurs in younger children. The most common organisms involved in these abscesses are gram-positive cocci—primarily *Staphylococcus aureus* and less often a streptococcus. In some cases, a cutaneous infection might have been present prior to the development of the renal abscess, and this infection is thought to be the primary source for the bacteremia.[8] In older children and teenagers, tuberculous abscess and caseous necrosis of the renal parenchyma also should be included in this primary classification. However, these tend to be indolent infections, although renal tuberculosis may be complicated by bacterial infection because of associated ureteral strictures and severe tuberculous cystitis. Pediatricians, though, should become familiar with this "adult" malady because of the resurgence of tuberculosis and the generally older age group that many pediatricians are caring for now.

When a renal abscess occurs in association with a recognized urologic disorder, the responsible organism most often is a gram-negative bacillus or an enterococcus—bacteria usually seen in simple urinary tract infections and pyelonephritis.[11] Examples of urologic disorders one might encounter with these infections include congenital and acquired obstructions (ureteropelvic and ureterovesical obstruction, retrocaval ureter, ureteral stricture after surgical intervention), calculous disease (obstructing and nonobstructing), infundibular stenosis, and renal dysplasia with cystic changes.

Anaerobic organisms also have been implicated as a cause of renal abscess. They often are present simultaneously with the more usual aerobic bacteria, but they can cause infections and abscesses alone. These anaerobic renal infections develop most commonly in association with infections complicating bowel injury or surgery, renal transplant, malignancy, and orodental infections.[1]

Children with HIV infection seem to have an increased risk of developing renal abscesses, both from the more common traditional organisms[3] and from unusual opportunistic fungal organisms—especially *Aspergillus*.[6] As expected, these children also tend to have a more fulminate course that often requires extensive surgical intervention and drainage.

The presence of a renal abscess implies the destruction and liquefaction of tissue in a confined space. Two other infectious disorders of the kidney frequently are included in this general category, although technically they do not always develop true abscess formation. These two processes are xanthogranulomatous pyelonephritis and acute lobar nephronia.

Xanthogranulomatous pyelonephritis describes a more chronic form of severe renal parenchymal destruction that often is associated with chronic stone disease. The process may involve the whole kidney or may be focal. In children, the focal form is more common. The pathognomonic histologic finding is an accumulation of lipid-laden macrophages that coalesce into discrete yellow nodules. Small abscess cavities often are studded throughout the kidney. The most common organism recovered from the kidney is *Proteus*, and urinary calculi are common. Although these patients often present with acute symptoms, these symptoms frequently are superimposed on more chronic symptoms, such as weight loss, failure to thrive, and anemia. Treatment is complete or partial nephrectomy because the renal destruction generally is severe.[6]

Acute lobar nephronia describes a focal area of intense edema at the site of infection in acute pyelonephritis.[2] This usually is recognized as a mass effect on an initial screening renal ultrasonogram. Computed tomography (CT) of the kidney demonstrates poor uptake in the involved segment but no well-defined liquefaction (Fig. 47–1). Whether this is just an exaggerated response to infection or actually represents a preabscess change remains unknown. However, in my expe-

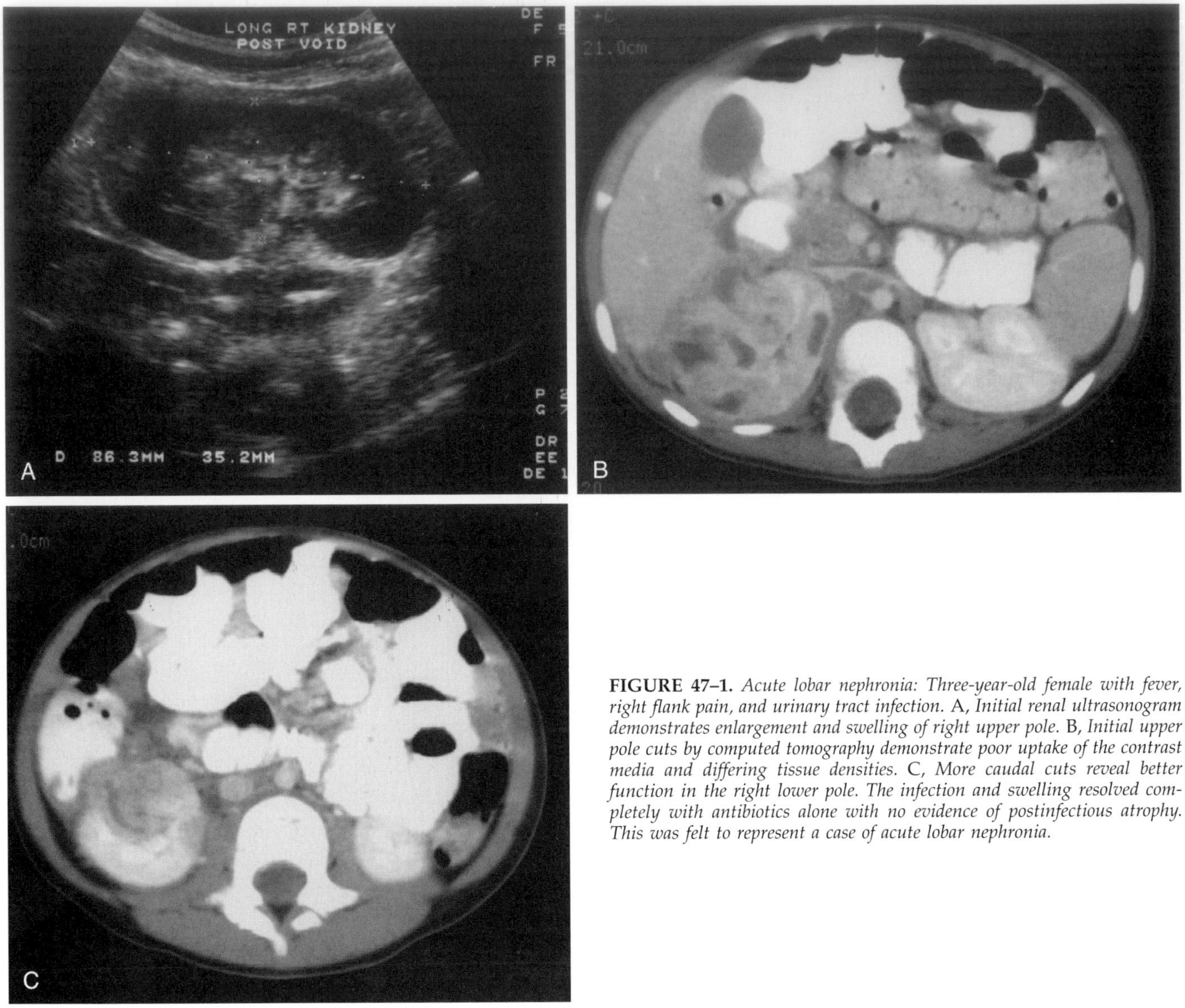

FIGURE 47–1. *Acute lobar nephronia: Three-year-old female with fever, right flank pain, and urinary tract infection.* A, *Initial renal ultrasonogram demonstrates enlargement and swelling of right upper pole.* B, *Initial upper pole cuts by computed tomography demonstrate poor uptake of the contrast media and differing tissue densities.* C, *More caudal cuts reveal better function in the right lower pole. The infection and swelling resolved completely with antibiotics alone with no evidence of postinfectious atrophy. This was felt to represent a case of acute lobar nephronia.*

rience, these lesions generally go on to satisfactory healing with antibiotics alone. The development of an abscess is unlikely.

If a somewhat more indolent process is encountered, one should consider obtaining appropriate stains and cultures for tuberculosis.

CLINICAL PRESENTATION

Children with acute renal abscess present with fever and localized pain in the costovertebral location. However, the initial findings generally do not differentiate between acute pyelonephritis with or without an abscess. If the abscess has spread into the perinephric region, one might be able to recognize psoas muscle irritation in the patient—that is, the patient is more comfortable with the ipsilateral leg in a position of flexion and experiences pain with full extension. A large abscess may be palpable as a flank mass. Findings on urinalysis can be confusing. In a primary (hematogenous) abscess, the urine may be deceptively benign and the culture generally is negative.[12] Abscesses associated with underlying urologic disorders can be expected to contain organisms. Generally, severe leukocytosis is present. All of these findings, though, are nonspecific, and the diagnosis often must await further diagnostic studies.

DIAGNOSTIC EVALUATION

All children admitted with a febrile urinary tract infection should undergo renal ultrasonography as soon as it is reasonable after admission. The findings on this initial study can direct significantly the choice of therapeutic options. If both kidneys are normal and unobstructed, organism-specific therapy is satisfactory in the overwhelming majority of patients. If significant obstruction or stones are present, antibiotic therapy may not be as effective, and interventional drainage may become necessary if the response to antibiotics is inadequate. At the time of this initial screening study, findings may suggest the presence of a renal abscess. These findings would include a mass effect within the margins of the kidney with a thickened wall and material within the mass of varying sonographic density (Fig. 47–2). Similar findings can be seen in cases of infection involving severe ureteropelvic junction obstruction or infundibular stenosis with isolated caliceal

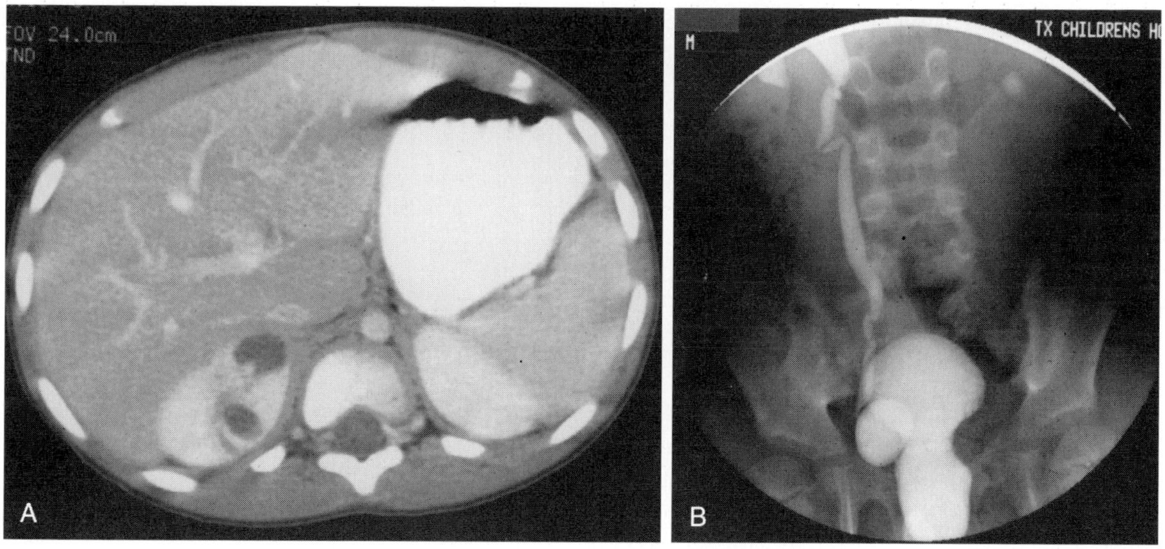

FIGURE 47–2. *Renal abscess (secondary): Six-month-old male with urinary tract infection. Screening renal ultrasonogram demonstrated a small mass in the right kidney.* A, *Computed tomography shows two clearly defined cystic areas consistent with small parenchymal abscesses. Treatment consisted of intravenous antibiotics only.* B, *A voiding cystogram revealed the presence of vesicoureteral reflux.*

dilatation, in which purulent material within the dilated collecting system layers out and can mimic a renal abscess (Figs. 47–3 and 47–4).

Once the diagnosis of an abscess is suspected on ultrasonography, CT of the involved kidney is in order.[5] CT defines more clearly the margins of the abscess, assesses whether loss of function is significant, and can screen the rest of the kidney for small satellite abscesses.[10] If loss of function in the affected kidney appears to be significant, a dimercaptosuccinic acid renal scan should be included because this is an even more sensitive test to quantitate overall renal function. Currently, gallium-67 scintigraphy is not used frequently to diagnose an obscure inflammatory mass. Today, improved computed tomographic technology strongly suggests the diagnosis, and, when necessary, percutaneous aspiration can confirm clearly whether an abscess is present without additional studies and at the same time that material for culture is being obtained.

If a child with a urinary tract infection and a previously normal renal ultrasonogram is on culture-specific antibiotics and subsequently develops a new fever, ultrasonography should be repeated. A previously small, unrecognized abscess may have been treated inadequately and now may be more obvious.

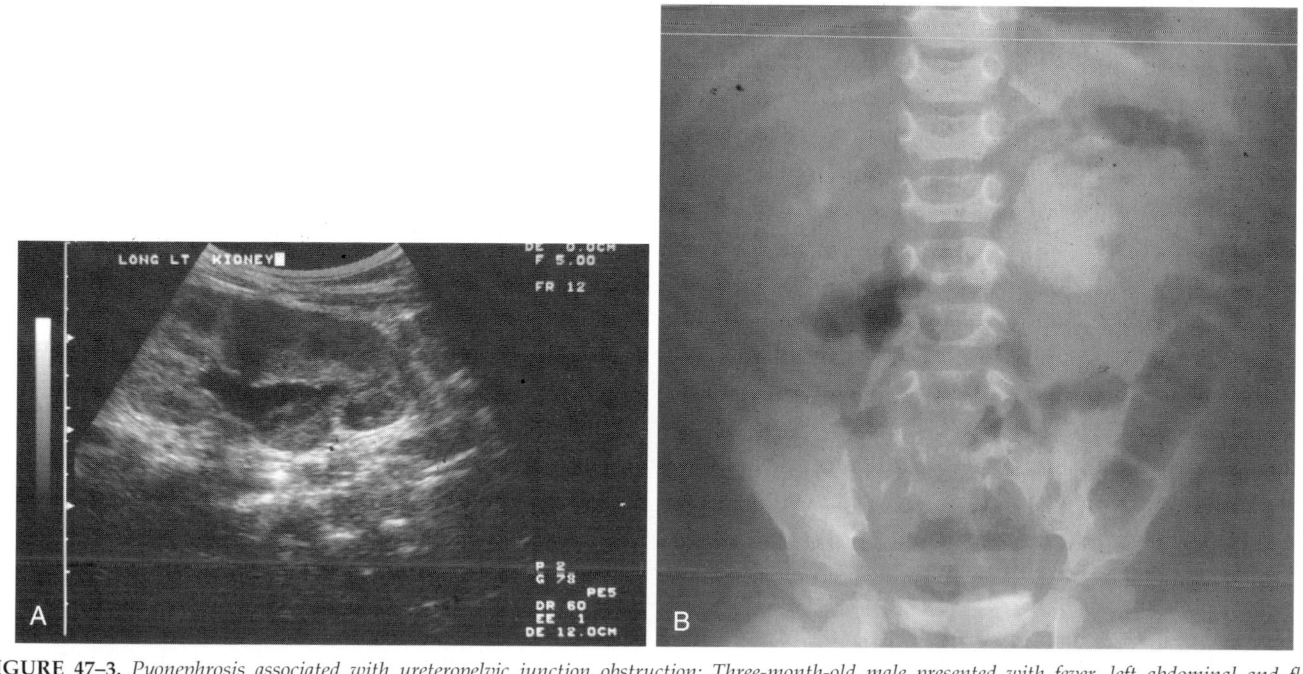

FIGURE 47–3. *Pyonephrosis associated with ureteropelvic junction obstruction: Three-month-old male presented with fever, left abdominal and flank tenderness, and urinary tract infection.* A, *Renal ultrasonogram demonstrates a medially placed cystic mass with layered fluids of different density consistent with purulent material. The position of the mass is most consistent with the renal pelvis.* B, *An intravenous pyelogram confirms a ureteropelvic junction obstruction. This infant was treated initially with percutaneous nephrostomy drainage in addition to appropriate antibiotics.*

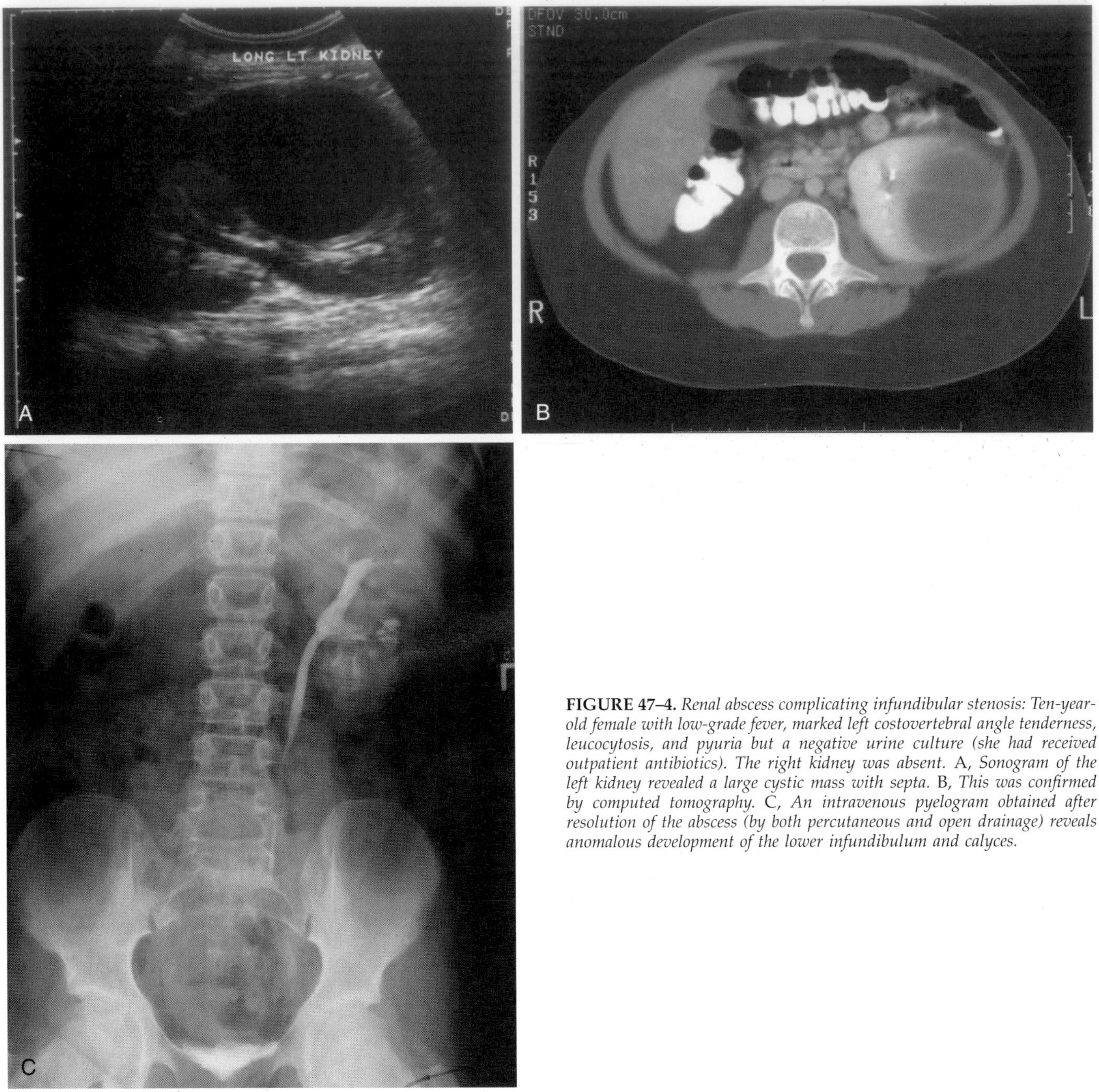

FIGURE 47–4. *Renal abscess complicating infundibular stenosis: Ten-year-old female with low-grade fever, marked left costovertebral angle tenderness, leucocytosis, and pyuria but a negative urine culture (she had received outpatient antibiotics). The right kidney was absent.* A, *Sonogram of the left kidney revealed a large cystic mass with septa.* B, *This was confirmed by computed tomography.* C, *An intravenous pyelogram obtained after resolution of the abscess (by both percutaneous and open drainage) reveals anomalous development of the lower infundibulum and calyces.*

Occasionally, imaging studies cannot distinguish between a renal abscess and severe acute lobar nephronia. The latter condition also may demonstrate tissues of differing density by ultrasonography or CT. In these situations, ultrasonography- or CT-guided percutaneous aspiration of the lesion may be necessary to see if purulent material can be obtained.

THERAPEUTIC CONSIDERATIONS

Once the diagnosis of an abscess is confirmed, several factors dictate the choice of therapeutic options. These factors include the overall status of the patient, size and number of abscesses, whether the abscess appears to be unilocular or septate, associated uropathies, and the extent of renal function in the involved kidney. Included in these considerations is some insight into the responsible organism. If this is a solitary abscess in a child with an unimpressive urinalysis and an otherwise normal kidney, one should suspect a staphylococcal abscess. This can be confirmed by percutaneous aspiration, Gram stain, and culture. If the urinalysis reveals an obvious infection, one can assume that the urine culture reflects the organism responsible for the abscess. The only caution here is if the abscess is complicated by significant stone disease. In this situation, there may be more than one organism in the urinary tract, and the urine culture alone may be misleading. Again, percutaneous aspiration accurately can identify the organism responsible for the abscess.

Renal abscesses traditionally have been managed by open surgical drainage. With the introduction of safe percutaneous access, particularly when used with ultrasonography or CT guidance, single, unilocular lesions now can be managed effectively with percutaneous placement of an indwelling catheter that allows not only for primary drainage but also for irrigation of the cavity with appropriate antibiotic solution.[1, 7] Small renal abscesses have been treated successfully with antibiotics alone.[9, 14]

When function is insufficient to justify renal salvage and ultimate nephrectomy is planned, a short course of specific antibiotics and percutaneous drainage, if the abscess is large, is initiated in order to decrease the inflammation in the perinephric tissues and reduce the possibility of causing bacteremia at the time of surgery.

When required, surgical repair of associated congenital anomalies of the urinary tract generally is performed at a separate session after the abscess has resolved. Reconstructive surgery in the presence of active infection increases significantly the risk of surgical complications and the possibility of additional surgical procedures.

CONCLUSIONS

The treatment of renal abscess today is multifaceted, and each case must be individualized. In addition to culture-specific antibiotics, treatment may include observation only, percutaneous drainage, or open surgical drainage. The diagnostic evaluation, including renal ultrasonography, CT, and percutaneous aspiration, generally can confirm that an abscess is present and assist in the decision regarding the therapeutic options.

References

1. Barker, A. P., and Ahmed, S.: Renal abscess in childhood. Aust. N. Z. J. Surg. *61*:217–221, 1991.
2. Boam, W. D., and Miser, W. F.: Acute focal bacterial pyelonephritis. Am. Fam. Phys. *52*:919–924, 1995.
3. Brandels, J. M., Baskin, L. S., Kogan, B. A., et al.: Recurrent *Staphylococcus aureus* renal abscess in a child positive for the human immunodeficiency virus. Urology *46*:246–248, 1995.
4. Brook, I.: The role of anaerobic bacteria in perinephric and renal abscesses in children. Pediatrics *92*:261–264, 1994.
5. Gerzof, S. G., and Gale, M. E.: Computer tomography and ultrasonography for diagnosis and treatment of renal and retroperitoneal abscesses. Urol. Clin. North Am. *9*:185–193, 1982.
6. Martinez-Jabalonas, J., Osca, J. M., Ruiz, J. L., et al.: Renal aspergillosis and AIDS. Eur. Urol. *27*:167–169, 1995.
7. Pedersen, J. F., Hancke, S., and Kristensen, J. V.: Renal carbuncle: Antibiotic therapy governed by ultrasonically guided aspiration. J. Urol. *109*:777–778, 1973.
8. Rote, A. R., Bauer, S. B., and Retik, A. B.: Renal abscess in children. J. Urol. *119*:254–258, 1978.
9. Schiff, M., Glickman, M., Weiss, R. M., et al.: Antibiotic treatment of renal carbuncle. Ann. Intern. Med. *8*:305, 1977.
10. Thornbury, J. R.: Acute renal infections. Urol. Radiol. *12*:209–213, 1991.
11. Timmons, J. W., and Perlmutter, A. D.: Renal abscess: A changing concept. J. Urol. *115*:299–301, 1976.
12. Vachvanichsanong, P., Dissaneewate, P., Patrapinyokul, S., et al.: Renal abscess in healthy children: Report of three cases. Pediatr. Nephrol. *6*:273–275, 1992.
13. Watson, A. R., Marsden, H. B., Cendon, M., et al.: Renal pseudotumors caused by xanthogranulomatous pyelonephritis. Arch. Dis. Child. *57*:635, 1982.
14. Wipplemann, C. F., Schafer, O., Baetz, R., et al.: Renal abscess in childhood: Diagnostic and therapeutic program. Pediatr. Infect. Dis. J. *10*:446–450, 1991.

48

PROSTATITIS

Edmond T. Gonzales, Jr.

Prostatitis, a major source of chronic infection and symptoms in adult males, is rare in prepubertal children. Although postpubertal teenagers may develop prostatitis, even in this age group the diagnosis is recognized infrequently. The disorder commonly called prostatitis generally is divided into three separate clinical problems: acute prostatitis, chronic prostatitis, and prostatodynia.

Acute prostatitis is a severe infection generally associated with significant toxicity (high fever, elevated white blood cell count, systemic symptoms). There may be marked urinary symptoms, such as frequency, dysuria, and urinary retention. The urine usually is infected. On rectal examination, the prostate is enlarged, boggy (edematous), and exquisitely tender. Care must be taken in performing the rectal examination or in placing a transurethral catheter because bacteremia can result. The responsible organism usually is one of the gram-negative pathogens responsible for common cases of urinary tract infection. Treatment generally is begun with broad-spectrum parenteral antibiotics, pending the availability of culture-proven sensitivities and a satisfactory clinical response.

Chronic prostatitis is a more indolent infection associated with intermittent urinary tract infection, bladder irritative symptoms, and perineal discomfort. Ejaculation may be painful. Expressed prostatic secretions usually show an increase in white blood cells. Chronic prostatitis generally is recognized to occur in two different patterns: bacterial and nonbacterial. The clinical features of the two disorders are remarkably similar, including an increase in the white blood cells in expressed prostatic secretions, but patients with chronic bacterial prostatitis generally also have recurring episodes of urinary tract infection with the same organism, most often one of the gram-negative pathogens. In most studies, chronic nonbacterial prostatitis is more common than chronic bacterial prostatitis.

The cause for nonbacterial prostatitis remains enigmatic. Prostatic secretions do not show a common organism consistently, and urinary tract infection does not recur. However, culture of prostatic secretions notoriously is unreliable because of the means by which this material is collected; these secretions are contaminated easily as they pass through the urethra.[8] A specific causative relationship has not been found for either *Ureaplasma urealyticum* or *Chlamydia trachomatis* in nonbacterial prostatitis, two organisms commonly implicated in urethritis.[11]

The treatment of chronic bacterial prostatitis is frustrating because few patients truly are cured and relapse is common after antibiotics are discontinued. Several studies have confirmed satisfactory concentration of most common antibiotics in the prostatic tissues,[3–5] but no study has explained convincingly the high treatment failure rate. It is postulated that antibiotic levels may be inadequate within the acini of the prostatic glands and their secretions, but this has not been proved.[9] Normal prostatic secretions exhibit an antibacterial effect that is not present in men with chronic bacterial prostatitis. Several investigators have shown this factor to be free zinc or a zinc-based compound.[10] This antibacterial factor is depressed or absent in men with chronic prostatitis, but whether this causes or results from prostatitis remains unknown. The most successful antibiotic therapy has been with trimethoprim-sulfamethoxazole or one of the fluoroquinalones.[6] In many instances, though, low-dose maintenance chemoprophylaxis with trimethoprim-sulfamethoxazole or nitrofurantoin remains the most effective means to control symptoms.

A final population of patients has all the symptoms described for patients with chronic (bacterial) prostatitis but no history of urinary tract infection and microscopically normal prostatic secretions. To distinguish this group of patients from those with prostatic infection, the term "prostatodynia" is used. The etiology of prostatodynia is unknown, but most investigators feel that the disorder is a form of perineal and urethral muscle dysfunction with sphincter spasm, high voiding pressures within the prostatic urethra, reflux of urine into the prostatic ducts, and ultimately development of a chemical prostatitis.[2, 7] Treatment generally consists of the use of alpha-adrenergic blocking agents to relax the bladder neck and proximal prostatic urethra and diazepam to relax the striated muscle of the perineum. Although most patients seem to experience some benefit, the results of therapy are difficult to quantitate, and underlying psychosocial issues are thought to be responsible for the symptoms of many patients. Psychologic assessment and indicated treatment are an essential part of total management of these patients.

In the older age group still seen within a pediatric practice, symptoms similar to those of the chronic form of prostatitis also might occur with urethritis. As noted earlier, *Chlamydia* and *Ureaplasma* commonly are found in the urethral discharge in these patients[1] and are believed to be responsible for these specific symptoms. These organisms also have been implicated as a cause of epididymitis in young men. These organisms are transmitted sexually and are treated effectively with a tetracycline (minocycline or doxycycline) or erythromycin. Therefore, it seems reasonable to prescribe these drugs empirically for sexually active young adults with lower tract irritative symptoms and symptoms consistent with urethritis while awaiting cultures.

"Nonspecific urethritis" is the term commonly used for the infection in men with irritative voiding symptoms and a clear mucoid discharge in whom the culture of the discharge reveals a mixture of common perineal and gram-negative organisms but without a predominant organism felt to be responsible for the infection. Undoubtedly, some of these patients have undiagnosed chlamydial or ureaplasmal infection. Although specific treatment is empiric, a tetracycline or erythromycin seems to be a prudent first choice in most cases. Finally, one must not overlook the possibility of gonococcal urethritis.

In the male, ectopic ureters can drain into the prostatic urethra or the seminal vesicle. With this anomaly, the ipsilateral renal parenchyma generally is dysplastic, the ureter is highly dilated, and the seminal vesicle may be markedly distended, forming a large cyst-like structure behind the prostate, the bladder neck, and the trigone. If this anomaly becomes infected, pain in the perineum and on rectal examination generally is significant. Occasionally, frankly purulent material is passed at the urethral meatus or expressed from the urethra after rectal examination.

In most cases, the kidney drained by the ectopic ureter is highly dysplastic and shows little or no function. Ultimate management usually consists of a nephroureterectomy (ureteroneocystostomy if the kidney works) and, if the seminal vesicle is unusually large, partial excision and decompression of the seminal vesicle. Even though these abnormalities are congenital and are recognized easily by fetal ultrasonography, they can present at almost any age if not identified prior to birth. Unless a palpable flank or lower abdominal mass is felt, infection generally is the presenting symptom. Despite the severe degree of abnormality and ureteral and seminal vesicle dilation, development of infection can be delayed well into the adult years. Infrequently, distortion at the bladder neck can result in obstruction to urinary flow.

In summary, prostatitis as it is seen and described in the adult is rare in the population likely to be seen by a pediatrician. When it does occur, it affects the pubertal adolescent, and even here it may be difficult to distinguish true prostatitis from simple urethritis.

The appropriate evaluation of the adolescent male who presents with a lower tract urinary infection generally begins with renal ultrasonography. Special attention should be directed to the region of the bladder and prostate. With this imaging modality, one can assess the presence and normalcy of both kidneys, the degree of bladder wall thickening, the ability of the bladder to empty, and whether any cystic masses are behind the bladder or prostate. Any obvious abnormality justifies obtaining a voiding cystourethrogram. A thickened detrusor or a recurrence of infection suggests the possibility of urethral obstruction. Although properly performed voiding cystourethrography does image the entire urethra, other diagnostic tests might include retrograde urethrography or determination of the urinary flow rate, especially if one suspects a urethral stricture. Cystoscopy usually is not necessary if all imaging study results are normal, although cystoscopy may be used to confirm, and at times manage, obvious urethral obstruction.

References

1. Bowie, W. R., Wang, S. P., Alexander, E. R., et al.: Etiology of non-gonococcal urethritis: Evidence for *C. trachomatis* and *U. urealyticum*. J. Clin. Invest. *59*:735–742, 1977.
2. Hellstrom, W. J., Schmidt, R. A., Lue, T. F., et al.: Neuromuscular dysfunction in non-bacterial prostatitis. Urology *30*:183–188, 1987.
3. Hensle, T. W., Prout, G. R., Jr., and Griffin, P.: Minocycline diffusion into benign prostatic hyperplasia. J. Urol. *118*:609–611, 1977.
4. Larsen, E. H., Grasser, T. C., Dorflinger, T., et al.: The concentration of various quinolone derivatives in the human prostate. *In* Weidner, W., Brunner, H., Krause, W., et al. (eds.): Therapy of Prostatitis. Munich, W. Zucksweidt Verlag, 1986, pp. 40–44.
5. Meares, E. M., Jr.: Prostatitis: Review of pharmacokinetics and therapy. Rev. Infect. Dis. *4*:475–483, 1982.
6. Meares, E. M., Jr.: Prostatitis syndromes: New perspectives about old woes. J. Urol. *123*:141–147, 1980.
7. Meares, E. M., Jr.: Prostatodynia: Clinical findings and rationale for treatment. *In* Weidner, W., Brunner, H., Krause, W., et al. (eds.): Therapy of Prostatitis. Munich, W. Zucksweidt Verlag, 1986, pp. 207–212.
8. Meares, E. M., Jr., and Stamey, T. A.: Bacteriologic localization patterns in bacterial prostatitis and urethritis. Invest. Urol. *5*:492–518, 1968.
9. Nielsen, O. S., Frimodt-Moeller, N., Maiqaard, S., et al.: Penicillanic acid derivatives in the canine prostate. Prostate *1*:79–85, 1980.
10. Parrish, R. F., Perinette, E. P., and Fair, W. R.: Evidence against a zinc binding peptide in pilocarpine-stimulated canine prostatic secretions. Prostate *4*:189–193, 1983.
11. Shortliffe, L. M., and Wehner, N.: The characterization of bacterial and non-bacterial prostatitis by prostatic immunoglobulins. Medicine *65*:399–414, 1986.

49

Gynecologic Infections in Childhood and Adolescence

Mariam R. Chacko and Charles R. Woods, Jr.*

Gynecologic infections in premenarcheal girls are, for the most part, limited to the vulva and vagina. Their clinical picture and management differ somewhat from those of similar infections in older patients. Gynecologic infections in postmenarcheal girls, however, include all of the infections found in adult women; the symptoms accompanying them are like those in the adult, and their treatment essentially is the same.

This section reviews the clinical aspects of gynecologic infections in the pre- and postmenarcheal female, with the exception of those associated with pregnancy. The normal vaginal microenvironment is presented, followed by sections on premenarcheal vulvovaginitis; other infections of the premenarcheal genital tract; issues of sexual abuse in children with genital tract infections; postmenarcheal lower genital tract infections, including infectious causes of vulvovaginitis, infections of the Bartholin ducts and glands, and vulvovaginal ulcerative disorders; infections of the cervix and uterus; infections of the uterine tubes, including pelvic inflammatory disease, salpingitis, and tubo-ovarian abscess; and ovaritis.

Information is provided regarding trichomoniasis, candidiasis, gonorrhea, syphilis, chlamydial infections, bacterial vaginosis, herpes genitalis, condyloma acuminata, molluscum contagiosum, lymphogranuloma venereum, granuloma inguinale, chancroid, tuberculosis, Behçet syndrome, and vulvar vestibulitis, as well as group A streptococci, *Shigella,* and other agents that occasionally cause genital tract disease.

Additional information concerning principles of gynecologic infections in children and young adults can be found in referenced sources.[40, 58, 114, 187, 190, 214] Although the infectious complications of pregnancy are not included, physicians concerned with adolescent patients will bear in mind that pregnancy among young teenage girls is not uncommon and that there is a high incidence of abortion in this age group. Physicians must be on the alert, therefore, for signs of a pregnancy-related infection when confronted with a septic state in an adolescent female.

NORMAL VAGINAL FLORA

The vagina is inhabited by nonpathogenic bacteria from birth. A wide range of aerobic and anaerobic species have been cultured from asymptomatic girls. The results of several modern series[61, 82, 88, 94, 106, 185] are summarized in Table 49–1.

Most girls harbor several organisms in the vagina at any given time. Vaginal cultures obtained during anesthesia for elective surgery from 19 healthy girls 3 months to 5.7 years of age yielded a mean of 12 bacterial species.[112] Anaerobes predominated, with a mean of 8.7 species versus 3.4 aerobic species. Another series of 25 asymptomatic girls 2 months to 15 years of age found a mean of 8.7 different species per patient vaginal specimen.[95] The mean number of aerobes was approximately four and of anaerobes approximately five. Another series of adolescents 13 to 21 years of age noted a mean of about three aerobic organisms in non–sexually active subjects versus six in sexually active patients. Anaerobic flora were not evaluated in this study.[204] This heterogeneity of the vaginal microflora during childhood and adolescence is similar to that found in adult women.[137]

There are differences in the types of bacteria isolated at various ages, however. The vagina and its microbial flora form an ecosystem that changes over time from infancy to childhood to adolescence and adulthood.[111] The major forces that influence these changes are fluctuations in estrogen levels and advent of sexual activity. Hygienic practices and medications, including oral contraceptives and antimicrobial agents, also affect the complex interactions between the vari-

TABLE 49–1. Vaginal Organisms Isolated from Asymptomatic Girls, 2 Months to 16 Years of Age[61, 82, 88, 94, 106, 186]

Coagulase-negative staphylococci (35–73)*	*Mycoplasma hominis*
Diphtheroids (14–78)	*Ureaplasma urealyticum*
Streptococcus viridans (13–39)	*Gardnerella vaginalis*‡
Enterococci (29–62)	*Peptostreptococcus* species (29–56)
Group B *Streptococcus* (5–11)	*Peptococcus* species (39–76)
Group D *Streptococcus*	*Veillonella* species
Staphylococcus epidermidis	*Eubacterium* species
Staphylococcus aureus	*Propionobacterium acnes*
Streptococcus pneumoniae	*Bacteroides fragilis*
Micrococcus species	*Bacteroides melaninogenicus*
Lactobacillus species (10–39)†	Other *Bacteroides* species
Escherichia coli (12–67)	*Prevotella* species
Klebsiella species (15–52)	*Bifidobacterium* species
Enterobacter species	*Clostridium perfringens*
Proteus species (3–5)	Other *Clostridium* species
Pseudomonas aeruginosa (5–6.5)	*Fusobacterium* species
Citrobacter species	*Candida* species (3–18)
Haemophilus influenzae	Other yeasts
Neisseria species other than gonococci	*Actinomyces* species
Moraxella (Branhamella) catarrhalis	
Flavobacterium species	
Alcaligenes species	
Acinetobacter species	

*Percentage range when the organism was isolated from patients in at least two studies. If no range is present, the organism was isolated from 3 to 33 per cent of patients in a single study.
†Eighty-eight per cent of girls were older than 11 years of age in one series.
‡Isolated in a number of cases without discharge.

*Parts of this chapter were revised from material written previously by John W. Huffman, who is deceased.

ous flora present in the vagina in terms of persistence, predominance, and overgrowth.

Gram-negative enteric bacteria and enterococci commonly are encountered in infants and toddlers prior to completion of toilet training but less frequently thereafter.[96, 112] Lactobacilli are the predominant flora in most females by the end of adolescence and may play a protective role in limiting overgrowth of other flora.[111] In childhood, lactobacilli are present more often in girls younger than 2 years of age than in older prepubertal girls. The incidence of colonization increases from puberty. The presence of yeasts and *Gardnerella vaginalis,* although much less common in all ages, parallels that of lactobacilli.[96]

Colonization with lactobacilli and *G. vaginalis* also increases with onset of sexual activity. *Mycoplasma hominis* and *Ureaplasma urealyticum* are more common in sexually active adolescents and in girls of any age who have been sexually abused than in non–sexually active girls. However, genital mycoplasmas were found in 17 per cent of one series of young girls who had not suffered any sexual abuse.[99, 204]

Several of these organisms also are associated with cases of vulvovaginitis. Alteration of the vaginal microenvironment by factors such as poor hygiene, foreign bodies, and hormonal fluctuations allows overgrowth by these part-time commensals and part-time pathogens, with resultant vulvovaginitis.

PREMENARCHEAL VULVOVAGINITIS[12, 46, 50, 78, 106, 115, 183]

Infections and inflammation of the vulva and vagina account for 85 to 90 per cent of all genital problems in premenarcheal girls. These are encountered most commonly in children between 2 and 7 years of age.[170] Infections of the vulva and vagina usually occur together and generally are discussed as one entity—vulvovaginitis. The various types of vulvovaginitis are differentiated by determining the agent causing the inflammation in a particular case or group of cases.

Genital discharge and perineal or vulvar discomfort are the most common symptoms that bring a child with vulvovaginitis to the physician.[115, 170] The discomfort may be only minor pain or soreness, or it may be intense perineal burning or pruritus. The discharge may be scanty serous fluid, bloody, or profuse and purulent. Infections of the vulva and vagina, however, can cause neither discomfort nor discharge. Genital erythema is the most common sign in girls with vulvovaginitis and is present in more than 80 per cent of cases. Visible discharge is present in one-third of cases.[170]

In several situations, a child may have a genital discharge and yet not have a vulvovaginal infection. For example, most female babies have a rather profuse discharge from the vagina during the newborn period. The grayish-white, somewhat mucoid material that covers the baby's vulva and fills the vagina consists of desquamated vaginal mucosa and cervical epithelium that has undergone hypertrophy because of prenatal stimulation by the placental and maternal hormones. Microscopic examination of the material reveals masses of large, superficial vaginal epithelial cells (Fig. 49–1). The condition lasts for up to several weeks, is not pathogenic, and does not require treatment. Another example of a genital discharge without infection is the urinary leakage from an ectopic ureter opening into the genital tract.

A pubertal girl nearing her menarche may have a copious viscous, transparent secretion that fills her vagina, bathes the vulvar tissues, and soils her underclothing. Parents of such a girl may be concerned that she has a vaginal infection. Inspection discovers no signs of infection; instead, the vulvar and vaginal tissues are thick and moist—a sign of increased estrogen stimulation. Microscopic examination of the vaginal fluid reveals masses of estrogenized superficial vaginal epithelial cells and few leukocytes (Fig. 49–2). Test results for pathogenic bacteria are negative. The family should be reassured that the girl does not have an infection. Frequent bathing and frequent changes of underclothing are all that need be prescribed.

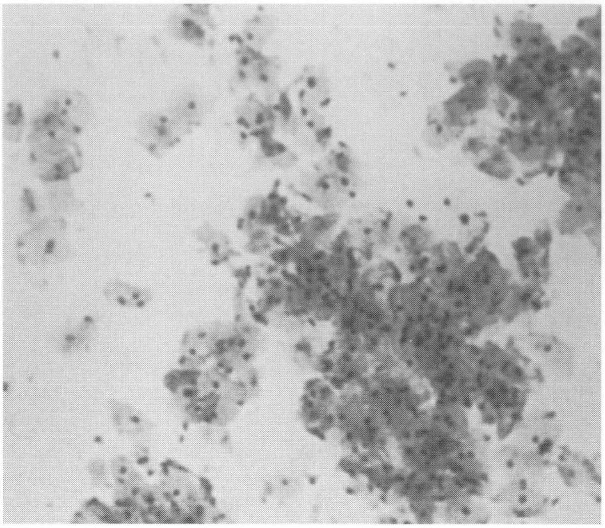

FIGURE 49–1. *Cytosmear from the vaginal discharge of a newborn infant.*

Poor hygiene with subsequent overgrowth of a mixed aerobic and anaerobic bacterial flora is the most common cause of premenarcheal vulvovaginitis.[166] However, inflammation of the lower genitourinary tract also may be caused by a variety of specific microorganisms, chemicals, and other physical agents. Contact irritation and allergic reactions induced by soaps, detergents, and medications are frequent causes of vulvovaginitis. Some systemic diseases and focal skin disorders may mimic vulvovaginitis or allow it to de-

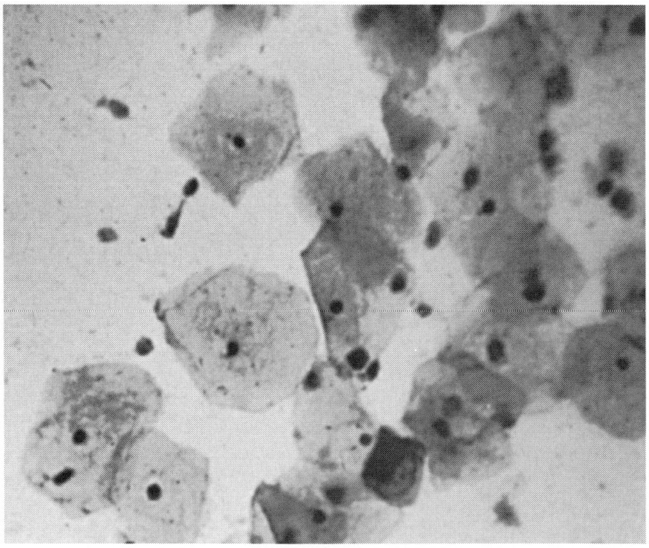

FIGURE 49–2. *Cytosmear from the vaginal secretion of a pubertal girl. Masses of epithelial cells and few bacteria or leukocytes attest to its nonpathologic character.*

velop as a secondary process when they involve the vulvar or perineal tissues.[68] Anatomic abnormalities may be associated with vulvovaginitis. An increased incidence of vulvovaginitis and urinary tract infections has been reported in girls with high posterior commissures.[234] Drainage from an ectopic ureter into the vagina can cause chronic vulvovaginitis and lead to vaginal calculus formation.[31] Labial adhesions were present in 7 per cent of girls with vulvovaginitis in one recent series.[170] Table 49–2 gives an outline of the causes of vulvovaginitis in premenarcheal girls. This chapter primarily addresses vulvovaginitis that results from infection.

The child's history may not be helpful in some cases of vulvovaginitis. It is necessary to determine whether other children in the family or the patient's playmates are affected similarly and whether other family members have any genital infection as evidenced by vaginal or penile discharge, genital pain, or pruritus. The history should include information as to the manner of and circumstances surrounding onset of the disorder, its duration, whether it is recurrent, and the nature of any preceding treatment. The possibility that the child may have had or has a systemic disorder affecting the genitalia should be explored.

Sexual abuse is a possible factor that must be considered when a child has a genital infection, regardless of the nature of the infection or the socioeconomic status of the family. This particularly is true when the child has a sexually transmissible disease, but any infectious organism can be transmitted to a child's genitalia by the fingers of a person fondling her vulva. Sexual abuse does not necessarily require penile vaginal penetration.

The type of discharge is seldom significant. At the onset of an infection, the discharge is likely to be thick, purulent,

TABLE 49–2. Etiologic Factors in Premenarcheal Vulvovaginitis[8, 115, 136, 148, 165]

Bacterial Infections

- Nonspecific mixed infections secondary to
  - Poor perineal hygiene
  - Foreign body in vagina
  - Respiratory tract infections
  - Skin infections (impetigo)
  - Urinary tract infection
- Specific nonvenereal infection
  - Hemolytic streptococci (group A streptococci)
  - *Shigella flexneri, sonnei*
  - *Neisseria meningitidis, sicca*
  - *Haemophilus influenzae* type b
  - *Streptococcus pneumoniae*
  - *Corynebacterium diphtheriae*
  - *Yersinia enterocolitica*
  - *Mycobacterium tuberculosis*
  - *Moraxella (Branhamella) catarrhalis*
  - *Staphylococcus aureus*
- Specific venereal infections
  - *Neisseria gonorrhoeae*
  - *Treponema pallidum*
  - *Chlamydia trachomatis*
  - Chancroid *(Haemophilus ducreyi)*
  - Granuloma inguinale
- Bacterial vaginosis
  - *Gardnerella vaginalis*
  - *Mobiluncus curtisii*
  - *Mobiluncus mulieris*

Fungal Infections

- *Candida albicans*
- Other yeasts
- Dermatophytes

Protozoan and Parasitic Infections

- Trichomoniasis
- Amebiasis
- *Enterobius vermicularis*
- Hirudiniasis
- Schistosomiasis
- Other parasites (ascariasis, trichuriasis)

Viral Infections

- Venereal
  - Herpes simplex
  - Condyloma accuminatum (papillomavirus)
  - Molluscum contagiosum
- Involvement as part of systemic infection
  - Measles
  - Chickenpox
  - Mononucleosis
  - Coxsackievirus
  - Smallpox

Infestations

- Pediculosis
- Scabies

Contact Irritation or Allergic Reactions

- Bubble bath preparations
- Hair shampoos
- Vulvar deodorant sprays
- Soaps, laundry detergents
- Nylon, rayon underclothing
- Other medications

Vulvar or Perineal Skin Diseases

- Local
  - Seborrhea
  - Lichen sclerosus et atrophicus
  - Lichen planus
  - Lichen simplex chronicus
  - Premalignant leukoplakia
  - Erythrasma *(Corynebacterium minutissimum)*
  - Bartholinitis
  - Skenitis
- Involvement as part of a systemic disorder
  - Psoriasis
  - Atopic dermatitis
  - Drug eruption
  - Generalized pruritus with excoriation
    - Chronic liver disease
    - Chronic renal disease
    - Metabolic errors
    - Psychosomatic
  - Crohn disease
  - Sjögren syndrome
  - Kawasaki disease
  - Stevens-Johnson syndrome
  - Typhoid

Physical Factors

- Sand (sandbox)
- Chemical or thermal trauma
- Physical trauma (accidents, abuse, masturbation)
- Tight garments (maceration in warm climates)
- Anatomic abnormalities
  - Neoplasms (sarcoma botryoides)
  - Polyps
  - Labial agglutination, adhesion
  - Prolapsed urethra
  - Ectopic ureter
  - Rectal fistula
  - Draining pelvic abscess via fistula

and profuse. It may become scanty and seropurulent in later chronic stages of infection.[115] Discharges that are odorless and bloody or serosanguineous may result from noninfectious conditions, such as vulvar irritation, trauma, precocious puberty, foreign body, urethral prolapse, or a tumor; vulvovaginitis caused by *Shigella* or group A streptococci also can cause bleeding. Foul-smelling discharge suggests a foreign body but also may result from a necrotic tumor. Specific diagnoses are made more often when symptoms have been present for less than 1 month.[227]

A general physical examination should precede that of the genital tract. Gynecologic examination begins with abdominal inspection and palpation followed by external examination of the perineum and genitalia, including the vulva, urethral meatus, clitoris, hymen, and anus. This should be done with the child in a supine, frog-leg position.[227] The labia can be retracted gently to visualize the anterior vagina. Speculum and bimanual examinations generally are inappropriate in prepubertal children.[173] Note should be made of structural abnormalities, inflammation, sores and ulcerations, and excoriations.

Visualization of the vagina and cervix without instrumentation is possible with the child in the prone knee-chest position.[61] This method is useful in children older than 2 years of age. In this position, with labial traction, the vaginal muscles relax and stretch open the hymenal membrane. An otoscope head or a magnifying lens with a good wall light is used to visualize the cervix. Because the vagina of the prepubertal child is short, the presence of a foreign body or a lesion may be visualized.[59]

If visualization with instrumentation is required, vaginoscopy may be performed using a pediatric cystoscope or a hysteroscope (Fig. 49–3). Alternatively, the Cameron-Myers vaginoscope may be used. However, visualization of the vagina with this instrument often is inadequate because of its small distal portal.[173] General anesthesia may be required for vaginoscopy for children who are small or unable to cooperate during the procedure.

When a vaginal discharge is present, samples should be obtained for culture, Gram stain, saline, and potassium hydroxide preparations. A urine analysis with microscopic examination should be performed. A complete blood cell count

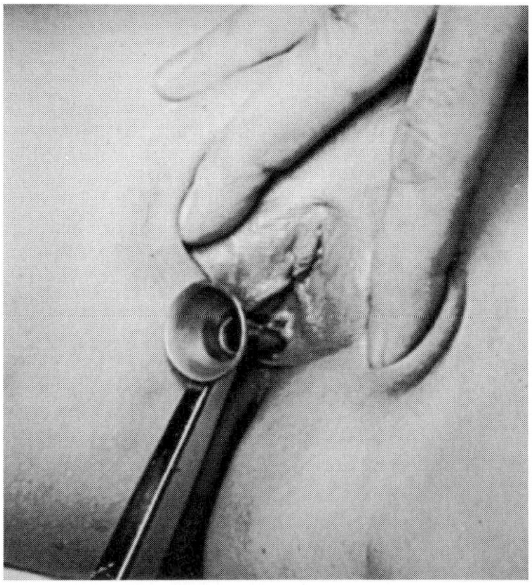

FIGURE 49–3. *Vaginoscopy is performed to exclude foreign bodies and tumors when a child has a vaginal discharge.*

TABLE 49–3. Tests Using Vaginal Discharge or Aspirate

Gram stain for bacteria and polymorphonuclear cells
Bacterial cultures (aerobic and anaerobic)
Cultures for gonococci and chlamydiae (no rapid tests)
Cultures for yeast and fungi (Nickerson medium)
Wet preparation for fungal elements (10% potassium hydroxide); white and red blood cells; vaginal epithelium (clue cells, estrogenic effect); flagellates (trichomonas); parasitic ova (pinworms)

may be useful when pyogenic infection is suspected or bleeding has occurred.

Separate vulvar and vaginal cultures are necessary in all cases of vulvovaginitis, and material for culture from the vagina should be obtained without vulvar contamination (Table 49–3).

A nasopharyngeal Calgiswab or wire Dacron swab moistened in nonbacterocidal saline can be inserted easily into the vagina through the hymenal opening with minimal pain. A dry swab can be painful. The swab may be used to obtain specimens to test for gonorrhea, *Chlamydia* infection, and other nonspecific bacterial infections; it is the preferred method to test for *Chlamydia trachomatis.* When multiple samples are needed, it has been suggested that vaginal secretions be obtained using a catheter-within-a-catheter technique or an eye dropper with tubing (Fig. 49–4).[172, 173] However, these aspiration methods have not been tested for their ability to obtain adequate vaginal epithelial cells, which is an important factor in the isolation of *C. trachomatis.* The distal 4 inches of a soft, size-12 bladder catheter and the proximal 4 inches of butterfly needle intravenous tubing are excised from their parent devices using a sterile technique. The latter is attached to a tuberculin syringe that has been filled with 0.5 to 1.0 mL of sterile fluid and then is inserted into the bladder catheter. The catheter-within-a-catheter is inserted into the vagina. The fluid is flushed in and out of the upper vagina several times before final aspiration into the syringe and removal of the device. Alternatively, a plastic or glass eyedropper or syringe with 4 to 5 cm of intravenous tubing attached can be used to aspirate secretions. The specimens obtained generally are adequate for wet mount, stains, cultures, and any required forensic studies.[173]

Nonspecific Vulvovaginitis

Nonspecific vulvovaginitis is identified by vaginal cultures that yield a growth of mixed bacteria not related etiologically to a specific disease. It is the most frequently encountered premenarcheal genital disorder.[115] It accounts for 25 to 75 per cent of cases of vulvovaginitis diagnosed in this age group in referral centers.[227] In most cases, as noted in Table 49–2, identifiable secondary factors contribute to nonspecific vulvovaginitis.

Several factors other than those listed in Table 49–2 contribute to the occurrence of vulvovaginal infections in young children. The developing immature labia minora and majora flare outward as a little girl squats or sits. As a result, they do not protect the vestibular and vulvar mucosas from contamination as they do later in life. The nonestrogenized prepubertal vulvar and vaginal epithelium, consisting as it does of only a few layers of cells, is traumatized easily and infected readily; there is, however, no evidence that an estrogen deficiency is a causative factor in premenarcheal vulvovaginitis. The alkaline vaginal reaction during childhood is not as

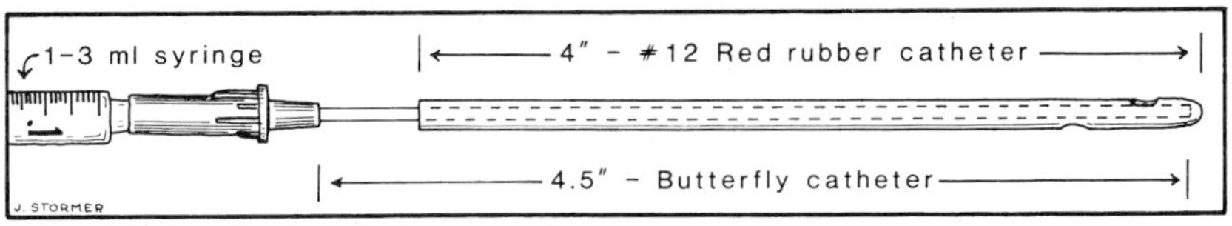

FIGURE 49–4. *Assembled catheter-within-a-catheter for obtaining specimens from a prepubertal child. (From Pokorny, S. F., and Stormer, L. V. N.: Atraumatic removal of secretions from the prepubertal vagina. Am. J. Obstet. Gynecol. 156:581, 1987.)*

resistant to infection as is the acid vaginal secretion of the postmenarcheal female. Because children frequently do not cleanse themselves properly after defecation, the perineum and vulva are contaminated more often by feces than in the older patient. The child is more likely than an older person to touch her vulva with unclean hands; this is augmented by a child's interest in her own and other children's genitalia. Infected adults, in caring for a child, may transmit their infection to her.

Vulvovaginitis Secondary to Poor Perineal Hygiene

A vulvovaginal infection is considered to be secondary to poor perineal hygiene when bacteria native to the lower gastrointestinal tract are found on properly obtained cultures from the vagina. In a large series of cases of vulvovaginitis subjected to culture, *Escherichia coli* or other coliform organisms were found in 70 per cent of patients in the series.[106] It is believed that the infection is caused by vulvar and vaginal contamination with feces as the result of improper cleansing after defecation. This is supported by the fact that the infection is resolved in many cases when proper perineal hygiene is the only treatment recommended. Symptoms reappear when the child's genitalia are not kept clean. Reappearance and disappearance of premenarcheal vulvovaginitis secondary to poor perineal hygiene are related directly to the appearance and disappearance of coliform organisms in the child's vagina.

Children with nonspecific vulvovaginitis secondary to poor perineal hygiene do not have any uniform historic findings. If asked, the parent may be able to describe the way the child cleanses herself after defecation. Many children wipe themselves from back to front after defecation. In girls, this easily results in fecal contamination of the vulvar area.

On examination, the vulvar mucosa and outer third of the vagina usually are hyperemic and covered with a scant, light gray, mucoid discharge. Frequently, a clue to the cause of the infection is fecal soiling about the anus or on the perineum. Inspection of the child's underpants shows fecal material in the area that comes in contact with the vulva unless, as often is the case, the girl has been bathed and dressed in clean clothes before visiting the physician.

Treatment is prophylactic, hygienic, and therapeutic. Instructions to the parents of little girls regarding perineal and vulvar cleansing when the children are bathed decreases the likelihood that their daughters will develop nonspecific vulvovaginitis. Little girls should be taught that the genitalia should be kept clean and that they should wash their hands both before and after urination and defecation. Routine inspection of the perineum, vulva, hymen, and clitoris should be a part of every general examination, including well-child checkups.[115]

Proper cleansing of the perineum and anus after defecation and sitz baths relieves this type of infection in many cases. Sitz baths (warm water with or without Aveeno colloidal oatmeal or baking soda) of a 10- to 15-minute duration should be taken two to six times per day, depending on the severity of the vulvovaginal inflammation.[60] For intense, oozing inflammation, wet compresses with Burow solution (1:40) or plain water may be applied as often as every 3 to 4 hours instead of sitz baths.[8] In mild cases, the vulva may be washed twice a day with water or a mild, unscented, nonmedicated soap (Basis, unscented Dove, Neutrogena). The perineum should be patted dry gently after baths or treatments. Complete drying may be facilitated by sitting for 10 minutes with legs spread apart or by a hair dryer on low or cool setting. Hair dryers should be used cautiously, however, because inadvertent use of high or hot settings could result in burns. The girl should be instructed to urinate with the labia and legs spread apart in order to minimize urinary reflux into the vagina. Witch hazel pads (Tucks) may be used to provide mild analgesia and to wipe after defecation.[60]

White cotton underpants, with frequent changes to absorb discharge, and loose-fitting clothing should be worn for several days to a few weeks after symptoms resolve. Continued wearing of these also may be helpful in preventing recurrences of vulvovaginitis, especially in girls who live in warmer climates.

As the inflammation and exudate subside over 1 to 2 days, sitz baths may be reduced in frequency and alternated two to four times a day, with application of either calamine lotion or protective ointments, such as zinc oxide, Desitin, Vaseline, and A&D ointment.

If pruritus is a significant symptom, an oral agent, such as hydroxyzine hydrochloride (Atarax) or diphenhydramine hydrochloride (Benadryl), may be used. Topical applications of 1 per cent hydrocortisone cream or triamcinolone acetonide (Mycolog) cream may be utilized as inflammation resolves but should be avoided in the acute phase.[60]

Shampooing the hair while sitting in a bathtub and using harsh soaps, bubble baths, or other preparations that might lead to chemical irritation of the vulvar skin and vaginal mucosa should be avoided throughout the course of vulvovaginitis.[16, 26] Application of powders should be avoided, at least until acute symptoms have resolved.

Between 15 and 20 per cent of the children have recurrences at some time, usually a month or more after resolution of the initial episode. In most instances, recurrences can be attributed to poor perineal hygiene. The parents must understand the need for perineal cleanliness. Older girls are warned that discharge and pruritus will continue if they do not cleanse themselves properly.[115]

Patients who do not improve after 2 to 3 days on the aforementioned regimen should be re-evaluated. Specimens taken from the vagina should be sent for aerobic and anaerobic bacterial cultures, if not done initially. An intravaginal medication, such as Sultrin vaginal cream, which consists of sulfathiazole, sulfacetamide, and sulfabenzamide, may be given.[2, 77] Approximately 1.0 mL is inserted into the vagina with a 5-mL Luer syringe each night for 7 nights (the applicator that comes with the tube of cream is too large to insert into the immature vagina). A 5-cm piece of 12- or 14-French urethral catheter attached to the syringe facilitates the application of the cream, if the patient is cooperative (Fig. 49–5). Warning against and instruction on how to avoid inserting the cream into the child's urethra and bladder must be given.[115] Alternatively, the vagina may be irrigated with a

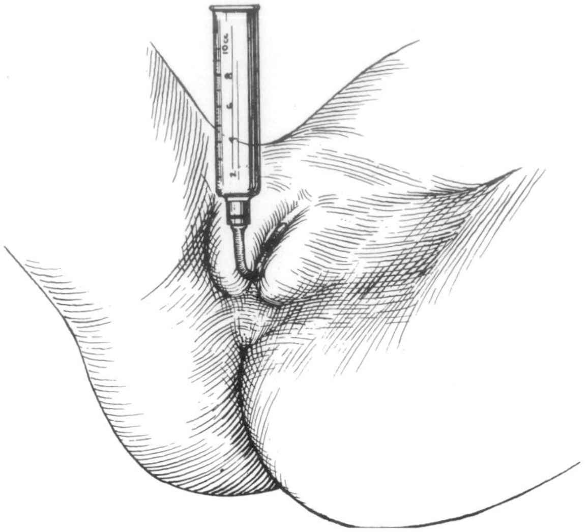

FIGURE 49–5. *The barrel of a Luer-type syringe and attached piece of urethra catheter are used for vaginal lavage when the patient with a vaginal infection is an older child.*

1 per cent povidone-iodine (Betadine) solution with this same method and caveat.[60]

Intractable nonspecific vulvovaginal infections that are not caused by foreign bodies, intestinal parasites, or poor perineal hygiene are encountered occasionally. They are resistant not only to the regimens described earlier but also to antibiotics. Lowering the vaginal pH from an alkaline or neutral to an acid reaction often helps in these difficult cases. This may be achieved either by the local use of estrogen or by the daily flushing into the child's vagina of a solution of 1 mL of lactic acid, USP, in 250 mL of tap water by employing a 10-mL Luer-type syringe and a section of a rubber or plastic urethral catheter, as shown in Figure 49–5.[115]

Estrogens cause thickening of the thin prepubertal vaginal mucosa, which lowers the vaginal pH. These events generally are therapeutic. Estrogens are not recommended for treatment of routine cases of premenarcheal vulvovaginitis for two reasons: results do not appear superior to nonhormonal therapies in these cases,[115] and prolonged administration of topical estrogens may cause isosexual pseudoprecocity. For intractable cases, estrogen should be applied topically and not orally. A globule of estrogen cream (Premarin vaginal cream), measuring not more than 5 mm in diameter, should be rubbed gently onto the inner surfaces of the labia minora and external surface of the hymen. This procedure is repeated daily for 2 to 4 weeks. After 7 to 10 days, the vulvar and vaginal tissues usually thicken, and a mucoid vaginal secretion may appear. The family must understand clearly that the cream must be used for no longer than instructed. The cream should be discontinued if thelarche occurs.

Oral or parenteral antibiotics may be indicated if symptoms persist for 2 to 3 weeks or if a specific pathogen that requires antibiotic treatment is isolated. When possible, selection of antibiotic agents and route of administration should be based on susceptibility testing of organisms isolated from vaginal cultures. Nonspecific vulvovaginal infections are relatively benign, superficial, mucosal inflammations that do not affect the child's general health. They usually respond to less potent chemotherapeutic agents when these are needed. Many antibiotics are absorbed through the vaginal mucosa. Indiscriminate use of vaginal, oral, or parenteral antibiotics may result in the child's becoming sensitized to them.

Nonspecific Vulvovaginitis Secondary to Intestinal Parasites[60]

Pinworms (*Enterobius vermicularis*) are the causative factor in many cases of recurrent or intractable nonspecific vulvovaginitis in children. Infection occurs when the worms in the lower bowel crawl out of the anus onto the perineum and migrate into the vagina, where they deposit ova. They carry *E. coli* and other coliform bacteria. Vulvovaginitis develops when these organisms are introduced into the vagina.

Other intestinal parasites seldom invade the vagina, although Huffman[115] knew of one case in which a specimen of *Ascaris lumbricoides* was discovered in a child's vagina.[85]

Infestation with pinworms is relatively common and is not associated necessarily with poor hygiene. Although it is more common in children from families in lower socioeconomic groups, children from affluent homes are not free from it. Pinworm ova may be deposited in playground soil, on toys or books, and on the hands of infected persons. Infection frequently is asymptomatic.

A child with a pinworm infection and vulvovaginitis usually has a history of a chronic vaginal discharge that has recurred, despite repeated efforts to eradicate it. Parents may say that they have seen worms on the child's perineum and that the youngster awakens at night because of perineal itching. Other children in the family or the girl herself may have had pinworms previously.

Examination reveals a low-grade inflammation of the vulva and vagina. There may be excoriations from scratching about the perineum. Vaginoscopy shows an inflammatory reaction extending to, but not including, the cervix. Vaginal cultures produce a mixed growth of nonpathogenic bacteria, with *E. coli* and other coliform bacteria generally predominating.

The diagnosis depends on finding pinworm ova on smears from the child's perineum or in the vaginal discharge or a report from parents that worms are visible on the child's perianal skin. As a rule, the perineal smear is most likely to demonstrate the presence of pinworms, but pinworm ova may be discovered in a wet smear of the vaginal secretions (Fig. 49–6).

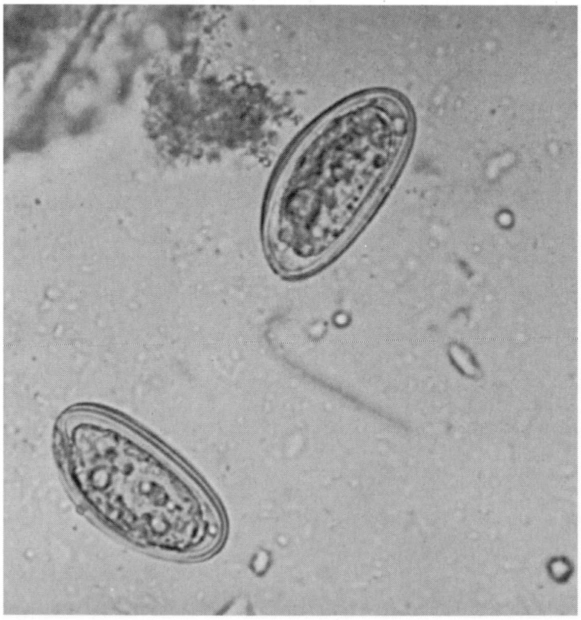

FIGURE 49–6. *Pinworm ova discovered in a vaginal smear from a child with intractable vulvovaginitis.*

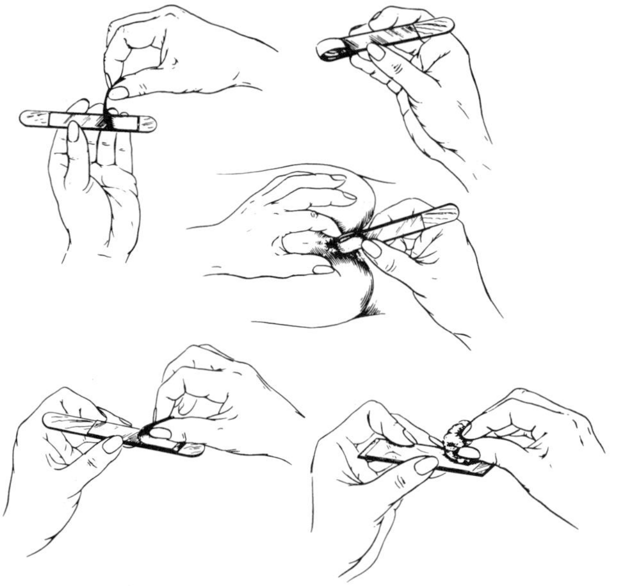

FIGURE 49–7. *Technique for obtaining a perianal smear for the detection of pinworm ova. Scotch tape and a tongue depressor are used.*

When a perineal smear for the ova of *E. vermicularis* is to be obtained, the parent is given a wooden tongue blade, a piece of Scotch tape, and a glass microscopic slide. The tape is attached, adhesive side out (Fig. 49–7), to the tongue blade. The tape is applied firmly to several areas about the child's anus. The tape then is removed and applied, adhesive side down, to the glass slide. It then is sent to the laboratory for examination.

The type of discharge, the appearance of the vaginal mucosa, or the presence or absence of pruritus does not aid diagnosis. A history of a previous infection with pinworms in the patient, a member of the family, or a playmate is significant. Pinworms should be suspected when a child has bouts of recurrent intractable nonspecific vulvovaginitis.

Treatment consists of eradicating the pinworms. All members of the family are presumed to be infected and also must be treated. There are several highly effective drugs for this purpose, among which are pyrantel pamoate, given as a single dose of 11 mg/kg not to exceed 1 g, and mebendazole, 100 mg orally as a single dose. Either treatment should be repeated after 2 weeks. Three negative perianal smears, taken at weekly intervals, should be obtained before it can be assumed that the worms have been eradicated.

The vulvovaginitis caused by coliform organisms carried on pinworms is treated as are other cases of nonspecific vulvovaginitis caused by poor perineal hygiene (discussed earlier).

Nonspecific Vulvovaginitis Secondary to Vaginal Foreign Bodies

Foreign bodies account for about 4 per cent of cases of vaginal discharge in premenarcheal girls.[8] When a foreign body remains in the vagina for some time, it inevitably causes nonspecific vulvovaginitis.

Usually, the parent is unaware of the fact that the child has inserted something into her vagina. The youngster is brought to a physician because of the child's profuse, foul-smelling, sometimes blood-tinged discharge. The presence of such a discharge is almost pathognomonic of the presence of a foreign body.

All sorts of objects have been found in children's vaginas, including safety pins, glass beads, coins, beans, bits of crayon, and parts of toys. By far the most common objects are bits of toilet paper or shreds of cloth from nightclothes or bedding (Fig. 49–8).[108, 116]

The history does not contribute to the diagnosis unless the child has a record of having put objects in her vagina previously; "repeaters" are common. Even without a profuse discharge or bleeding, a foul odor from the vagina strongly suggests a foreign body. Examination reveals inflammation of the vulvar and vaginal mucosa. Although foreign material may be seen when the labia are separated, vaginoscopy is necessary to explore the full length of the vagina. Rarely, a metallic object that has been in the vagina for some time erodes the mucosa and becomes hidden in granulation tissue. When such a condition is suspected, a radiograph should be obtained. However, most foreign bodies, such as glass, plastics, paper, or cloth, are not radiopaque, and radiographic examination fails to detect the foreign material. Soft foreign bodies, such as toilet paper, can be flushed out of the vaginal canal. Vaginoscopy should be performed when a hard foreign body is suspected or when the flushing technique fails.

Extraction of a foreign body usually is a simple office procedure, but, in older girls particularly, large objects (light bulbs, perfume bottles, flashlights) may be forced into the vagina. The size of the object and edema of the vaginal mucosa from pressure may make removal a difficult task, even when the patient is anesthetized.

The nonspecific vulvovaginitis caused by a foreign body disappears gradually after removal. Recovery can be hastened by using the treatments previously described. The child should be re-examined periodically to guard against repetition of the problem.

Specific Vulvovaginal Infections

Included in this group are those infections of the premenarcheal vulva and vagina due to bacteria that cause specific diseases in other sites.

Gonorrheal Vulvovaginitis[30, 60, 107, 202, 226, 239]

Gonococcal infections of the prepubertal genital tract manifest as vulvovaginitis and not the endocervicitis seen in post-

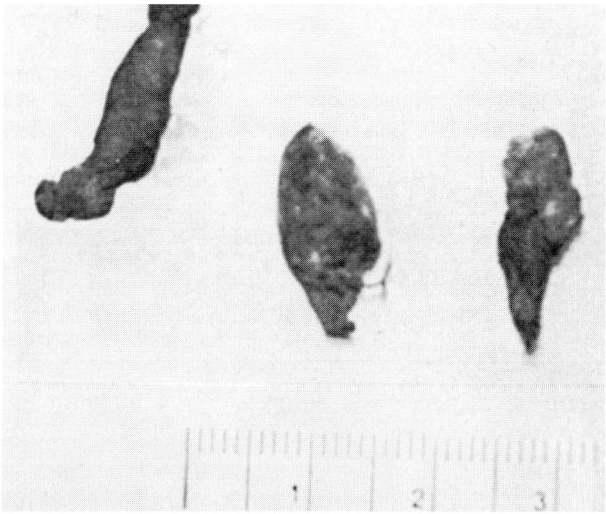

FIGURE 49–8. *Bits of paper or cloth are, by far, the most frequently found vaginal foreign bodies in children.*

menarcheal females. The alkaline environment of the unestrogenized vaginal tissues of the young girl appears to limit spread of infection to the upper genital tract. Gonorrhea is less common in children now than in the past but must be considered whenever a girl has vulvovaginitis.

Sexual contact should be suspected strongly and is almost always the source when a child has a gonococcal infection. Whether gonococcal infection is transmitted through nonsexual contact is controversial. It has been suggested that transmission may occur from freshly infected bedding, towels, a toilet seat, or digital transmission from an infected adult. There is, however, no absolute evidence for this source of infection.

Neisseria gonorrhoeae was the most common cause of vulvovaginal discharge among prepubertal girls in Rwanda in the late 1980s. Sexual contact was considered likely in all cases because of existence of a cultural belief that a man with a purulent urethral discharge could be cured by rubbing his penis on the external genitalia of a prepubertal girl.[21]

Gonorrheal infections in nurseries have been traced to rectal thermometers, other instruments, fomites, and attendants. However, before attributing a gonococcal infection to an environmental source, the possibility of sexual abuse must be considered strongly and investigated, and supportive epidemiologic evidence should be sought (e.g., cultures of potential reservoirs).

The acute stage of gonorrheal vulvovaginitis is characterized by inflammation and a purulent discharge. The child may complain of vulvar discomfort, dysuria, frequent urination, and pain on walking. The mother may have noted vulvar redness, swelling, or discharge. The child usually is otherwise well. Asymptomatic vaginal infection is rare.

An acute inflammatory reaction is the first indication of infection. The vulvar tissues are edematous and hyperemic. They are covered by a profuse, thick, yellowish discharge that exudes from the vagina. The entire vaginal mucosa is inflamed acutely.

The urethra, paraurethral glands, and the major vestibular (Bartholin) glands are involved rarely in a premenarcheal gonorrheal infection. Vulvovaginal infections, including gonorrhea, in prepubertal children rarely, if ever, affect the upper genitalia (uterus, uterine tubes, ovaries, or pelvic peritoneum). Symptoms suggestive of pelvic peritonitis have been reported in premenarcheal children who had gonorrheal vulvovaginitis; all of the patients recovered promptly after the administration of penicillin.[30, 75]

The acute phase lasts for a few weeks, after which most of the symptoms, except the discharge, disappear. The vulvar and vaginal tissues may, in some cases, remain hyperemic and macerated. The discharge becomes scanty and seropurulent. The disease pursues a chronic course if it is not treated.

The diagnosis of gonorrheal vulvovaginitis and its differentiation from other types of vulvovaginitis are established by vaginal smears and cultures. Specimens from the pharynx and rectum to test for *N. gonorrhoeae* also should be obtained. Because of the potential medicolegal use of the test results for *N. gonorrhoeae* among children, only standard culture systems should be used for the diagnosis of *N. gonorrhoeae* in children.[32] At this time, DNA probes and enzyme immunoassay for the gonococcus are neither recommended nor approved for use in children. Gram-negative intracellular diplococci in vaginal smears from a child with a history of exposure or typical clinical findings are a sufficient reason to start treatment, but they do not establish a definitive diagnosis. Other forms of *Neisseria*, particularly *Moraxella (Branhamella) catarrhalis* and *Neisseria sicca*, may be present in association with vulvovaginitis. A definitive diagnosis of gonorrhea is made only when *N. gonorrhoeae* is differentiated from other *Neisseria* species based on glucose utilization. Additional confirmation of *N. gonorrhoeae* is recommended in children. Monoclonal fluorescent-antibody tests or DNA probe confirmation tests currently are available. Isolates should be preserved to permit repeated or additional analyses.

Children weighing less than 45 kg with uncomplicated gonococcal vulvovaginitis, urethritis, pharyngitis, or proctitis are treated with a single dose of 125 mg of intramuscular ceftriaxone. A single dose of intramuscular spectinomycin 40 mg/kg may be given if ceftriaxone is not tolerated. Treatment of children 9 years of age or older weighing more than 45 kg follows the guidelines for postmenarcheal females.[32] Cefotaxime is approved only for treatment of gonococcal ophthalmia. Oral cephalosporins, such as cefixime and cefpodoxime, have not received adequate evaluation in the treatment of gonococcal infections in children to permit recommendation.[32] Ciprofloxacin or other quinolones may be considered in children who are allergic to cephalosporins and spectinomycin. Local treatment is limited to gentle cleansing of the vulva and perineum. For hospitalized children, contact isolation precautions are recommended until 24 hours after administration of effective parenteral therapy.

Follow-up cultures should be obtained from all infected sites 2 weeks after treatment to ensure that it has been effective. All children with gonorrhea should be evaluated for coinfection with *C. trachomatis* and syphilis.

Premenarcheal Chlamydial Vaginitis

Until the diagnosis of *C. trachomatis* infection could be confirmed by tissue-culture isolation, *C. trachomatis* vaginal infection in children rarely was reported. Rectovaginal infection has been suspected because of its association with other sexually transmitted diseases. Rettig and Nelson[182] reported *C. trachomatis* in 27 per cent of children with *N. gonorrhoeae.* Although sexual abuse must be suspected strongly when a child has vaginal *C. trachomatis*, persistence of perinatal infection for 2 to 3 years and sometimes longer has been reported. Subclinical rectal and vaginal *C. trachomatis* infection has been reported in 15 per cent of infants of mothers with active *C. trachomatis* infection.[93, 101, 125]

Unlike premenarcheal gonorrhea infections, chlamydial vaginitis primarily is an asymptomatic condition. When children with *C. trachomatis* vaginal infections have symptoms, 25 per cent have a vaginal discharge and 12 per cent have vaginal bleeding.

Direct tissue culture isolation of *C. trachomatis* remains the most reliable diagnostic test available. *Chlamydia* culture requires isolation of the organism in tissue culture and confirmation of the characteristic intracytoplasmic inclusions by fluorescent monoclonal-antibody staining.[32] Nonculture *Chlamydia* tests, such as enzyme immunoassay or DNA probes, are not approved for use with vaginal specimens from children. False-positive results have been reported with these tests in children suspected of having been sexually abused.[4] This probably results from cross-reactivity with common anogenital organisms: *Streptococcus*, groups A and B; *Acinetobacter* species; *N. gonorrhoeae; G. vaginalis; E. coli;* and *Proteus* species. A polymerase chain reaction assay has been approved for genital specimens in adults but has not been evaluated yet in children.[100, 101]

The treatment of choice for children with chlamydial infection is erythromycin, 50 mg/kg/day in four divided doses for 7 to 14 days. A single course is effective in approximately 80 per cent of cases; a second course may be required. Children who are 8 years of age or older should be treated with doxycycline, 100 mg twice a day for 7 days.[100] Azithromycin has been approved as a single-dose therapy for urethral and cervical infections in adults. Studies of this agent in children are under way, but it is not recommended for chlamydial infections in children.[101]

Premenarcheal Vaginal Trichomoniasis[42]

Although vaginal trichomoniasis seldom is encountered in prepubertal children, a number of reports in the literature confirm its occurrence in infants and children. Trichomoniasis in newborn infants has been described by Worwag.[240] Huffman[115] observed *Trichomonas vaginalis* in 3 per cent of cases of premenarcheal vulvovaginitis.

The absence of glycogen in the anestrogenic prepubertal vagina presumably is the reason why the infection is found infrequently in little girls. The incidence of trichomoniasis rises with the increasing amounts of glycogen in the vaginal mucosa, which estrogen induces during the several years preceding the menarche. There is a marked increase in the incidence of the infection after the menarche. All of the patients Huffman observed were near menarche and had clearly defined signs of estrogen stimulation.

Infection acquired from the mother's vagina during delivery explains vaginal trichomoniasis in newborn infants.[42] Although the source of the infection in many older children is not known, sexual transmission must be considered and further medical and social evaluation for sexual abuse performed.

The symptoms of trichomoniasis in children are similar to those in postmenarcheal girls. The child has more or less vulvar pruritus; an acrid, grayish-white, frothy discharge; and dysuria. Diffuse vaginal inflammation rather than the punctate vaginitis is seen in young patients. The condition is chronic, with frequent exacerbations. The child's general health is not affected.

The diagnosis is made by finding the trichomonads in the vaginal secretions and urine. Culture media for trichomonads are available. The more practical diagnostic test is a wet preparation for motile, triflagellated organisms. Trichomonads sometimes are found on stained smears of the discharge.

An oral trichomonacide, metronidazole (Flagyl), is effective in the treatment of vaginal trichomoniasis not only in adults but also in premenarcheal children. The dose for children between 8 and 12 years of age is 125 mg (15 mg/kg/day) three times daily for 7 to 10 days. Metronidazole has a low level of toxicity. Possible side reactions are described in the discussion of trichomoniasis in adolescent girls.[60] The nonspecific vulvovaginitis present when a patient suffers from trichomoniasis is treated in the same way as that secondary to poor perineal hygiene (see earlier).

Recurrences of the infection are a common problem. They are encountered less frequently if a search, both through interrogation and examination, is made for similar infections in other members of the family. Sexual contact as a source of reinfection ought to be considered.

Bacterial Vaginosis

Platt[171] described two cases of infection with *G. vaginalis* in newborn infants, one of whom died; he also found a generalized infection with the same organism in seven fetuses. He noted that the organism is sensitive to penicillin, tetracycline, chloramphenicol, erythromycin, kanamycin, and bacitracin but recommended that antimicrobial sensitivity tests precede treatment.

Bacterial vaginosis as defined in adolescents and adults (see Postmenarcheal Bacterial Vaginosis) has not been well defined in premenarcheal girls. Hammerschlag and associates[95] reported the presence of a vaginal odor in girls after sexual abuse who also had laboratory results consistent with *G. vaginalis,* namely a positive amine test result (characteristic amine or fishy odor when vaginal secretions are mixed with 10 per cent potassium hydroxide) and clue cells. The entity bacterial vaginosis is characterized by an overgrowth of *G. vaginalis* and anaerobes. Therefore, a diagnosis of bacterial vaginosis in premenarcheal girls should not be made solely on a positive culture for *G. vaginalis.* Whether the presence of *G. vaginalis* in the premenarcheal vagina indicates sexual transmission is controversial.[15, 93] *G. vaginalis* has been isolated from children with a history of sexual abuse and children without a history of sexual abuse. In children with a history of sexual abuse, its presence in the prepubertal vagina is not associated with vaginal discharge, odor, or erythema.[15] Huffman[115] reported encountering this organism in eight children between 8 and 11 years of age. Each of them had a profuse mucopurulent discharge and some vulvar irritation. Until the relationship between *G. vaginalis,* bacterial vaginosis, and sexual abuse in children can be clarified further, the presence of bacterial vaginosis with a vaginal discharge should prompt the physician to elicit the possibility of sexual abuse by history and examination. However, the presence of *G. vaginalis* is not diagnostic of sexual abuse.

The treatment of bacterial vaginosis in children older than 8 years of age is metronidazole, 125 mg (15 mg/kg/day), orally three times daily for 10 days. Girls weighing more than 45.4 kg (100 lb) are treated as adolescents (see later). A gentle vaginal lavage using a dilute lactic acid solution may be performed nightly.

Mycotic (Fungal) Vulvovaginitis[199]

Mycotic infections with *Candida albicans* constitute a considerable proportion of the cases of vulvovaginitis occurring in infants and children. A history of moniliasis in another member of the family, particularly the mother, explains some cases. In most instances, however, the child received antibiotic therapy shortly before the onset of her genital symptoms. Uncontrolled diabetes mellitus in either children or adults frequently is associated with mycotic vulvitis.[209] Immunosuppression (diabetes, HIV infection) should be considered in a child with recurrent or persistent infections. Most mycotic infections are acquired nonsexually during childhood, and sexual transmission is unlikely.

The child suffering from mycotic vulvovaginitis usually complains of vulvar pruritus and burning, a result of urine coming in contact with desquamated or excoriated areas on the vulva. Vulvar redness and some vaginal discharge may have been observed.

Examination reveals a diffuse hyperemia of the vulvar mucosa, and this often extends onto the perineal skin. The involved areas are red and shiny and may be edematous. Excoriated areas are caused by scratching. If the condition has existed for some time, the edema, secondary infection, and repeated scratching may produce thickened and fissured lesions closely resembling chronic eczema or lichen sclerosis et atrophicus (Fig. 49–9).

The vaginal mucosa is dusky red. There may be small, whitish plaques on the vulvar or vaginal surface or white curdled material in the rather scanty discharge. Microscopic examination shows that the plaques and curds are composed of masses of mycotic mycelia.

The diagnosis is established by finding hyphae and spores on wet preparations of the discharge or of material scraped from the vulvar skin (Fig. 49–10). It can be confirmed further by identifying *C. albicans* in cultures of material from the vagina or vulva on Sabouraud or Nickerson media.

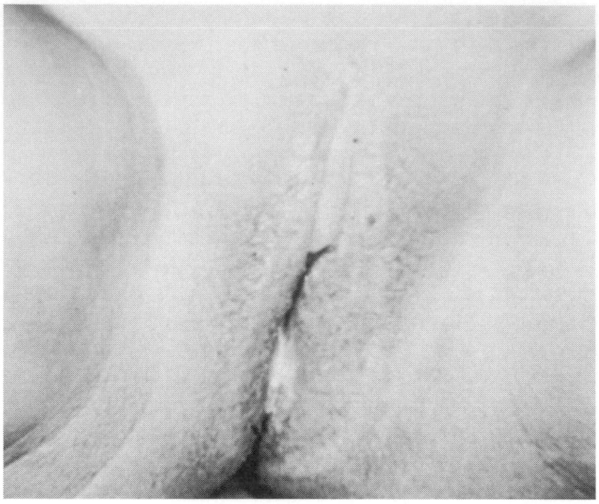

FIGURE 49–9. *Mycotic vulvovaginitis. The child is a diabetic.*

Local treatment consists of cleansing the child's perineum and vulva four times daily with soap and warm water. A cream containing nystatin (Mycostatin) is applied to the affected area after cleansing and at each diaper change.

Mycotic infections are difficult to cure in children who are taking antibiotics or who receive repeated courses of antibiotic therapy. In such cases, if the patient is an infant or small child, 1 mL of nystatin suspension (Mycostatin), 100,000 units/mL, is injected into the vagina three times a day for 10 days. One milliliter of the same suspension is administered orally four times daily. Treatment is continued if a culture still reveals the presence of *C. albicans* after 10 days of therapy.

Intravaginal therapy may be used in recurrent infection.

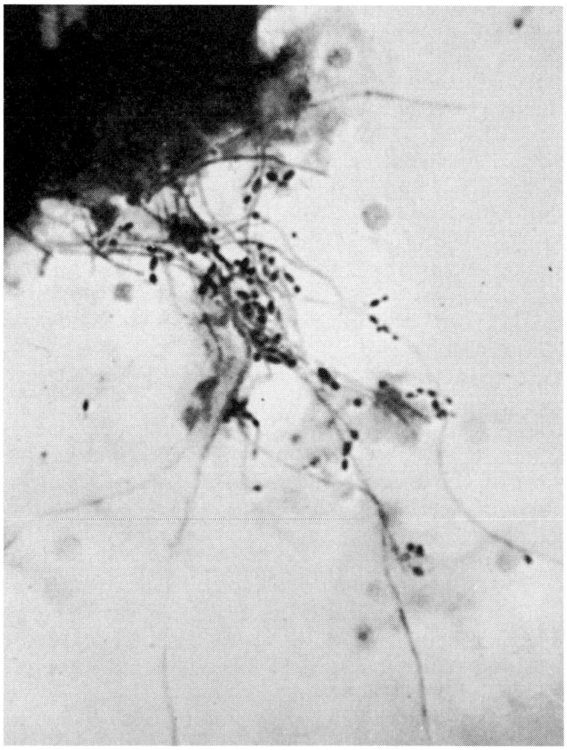

FIGURE 49–10. *Hyphae of* Candida albicans *discovered on wet smear of vaginal discharge.*

One milliliter of 0.5 per cent aqueous solution of gentian violet is injected into the vagina with a sterile eyedropper each night for 10 nights. Some children are sensitive to gentian violet and develop herpes-like lesions on the vulva after its application; its use should be discontinued if there is evidence of sensitization.[115]

Vulvovaginal infections with *C. albicans* in older girls are treated with fungicidal vaginal creams or suppositories as described in the section on vaginal infections in adolescent girls.

Nongonorrheal Neisserial Vulvovaginitis

Occasionally, other forms of *Neisseria* are the causative agents in cases of premenarcheal vulvovaginitis. These gram-negative, intra- and extracellular diplococci resemble *N. gonorrhoeae* on stained smears. *M. catarrhalis* also is identical on Gram stain. Gram-negative diplococci should be speciated completely by the microbiology laboratory to avoid misidentification of nongonococcal diplococci as gonococci and vice versa. Especially for pediatric patients, misidentification can result in serious medicolegal consequences for the family when unwarranted intervention is initiated or in failure to protect the child's welfare when appropriate measures are deemed unnecessary.[6]

N. sicca, generally considered nonpathogenic, has been isolated from children with vulvovaginal infections that clinically resembled gonorrhea.[237] *Neisseria meningitidis* also has been reported as the cause of vulvovaginitis.[64, 88] Nongonococcal *Neisseria* species may be considered the cause of vulvovaginal infections when isolated as the predominant flora in the setting of vaginal inflammation and discharge.

Treatment of vulvovaginitis due to nongonococcal *Neisseria* species or *M. catarrhalis* is the same as for *N. gonorrhoeae.* Most nongonococcal *Neisseria* species are not resistant to penicillin, but the need for therapy generally is based on the Gram stain finding of gram-negative diplococci, which for therapeutic purposes should be considered gonococci pending culture results. Data are not available, but a single dose of ceftriaxone likely should be as effective for these noninvasive *Neisseria* infections as it is for gonorrhea.

Chemoprophylaxis, generally with rifampin, should be considered for family members and other contacts in cases of meningococcal vulvovaginitis.

Group A Streptococcal Vulvovaginitis

Group A *Streptococcus* is a frequent cause of vulvovaginitis in premenarcheal girls, accounting for 9 to 20 per cent of cases in several series.[52, 58, 60, 106, 215] Most cases occur among girls 2 to 7 years of age, but cases among infants and teenagers have been reported.[22, 52, 84, 198, 215] A marked seasonal variation in incidence in some geographic regions, with peak rates in late fall and winter, may explain the low numbers of cases of vulvovaginitis caused by group A streptococci in some series.[147] The nasopharynx appears to be the primary reservoir for group A streptococci in these girls. Infection occurs from self-inoculation by hand to nose to vulvovaginal area.[198] The skin also may serve as the source of group A streptococcal vulvovaginitis.[147, 215] Preceding or concurrent symptoms of upper respiratory tract infection are uncommon, but many girls with group A streptococcal vulvovaginitis have throat cultures positive for *Streptococcus pyogenes.*[84, 215] Group A streptococcal vulvovaginitis may occur during the course of scarlet fever.[22, 105, 106] Concomitant streptococcal proctitis and perianal skin infections have been reported.[67, 131, 210]

The signs and symptoms of group A streptococcal vulvovaginitis often overlap with those caused by other bacterial infections, but symptoms usually are abrupt in onset.[215] Most patients present within 1 week of onset. Vaginal discharge and dysuria are the most common complaints. The girls usually are afebrile. Localized tenderness and an intense, fiery-red erythema of the vulvar tissues are frequent findings. Pruritus and excoriation may be present. The discharge usually is seropurulent but may be serosanguineous. The color may be white or green. Petechiae may be present on the vaginal mucosa.[84, 198, 215] The diagnosis of *S. pyogenes* infection may be missed if vaginal secretions are not plated onto sheep blood agar or other media that readily support the growth of streptococci.[215]

The vulvovaginitis caused by group A streptococci usually responds to oral antimicrobial therapy within 24 hours. A 10-day course of oral penicillin or erythromycin usually is sufficient. A second course sometimes is necessary when perianal disease is present.[210] Adjunctive use of the hygienic measures for nonspecific vulvovaginitis hastens clinical improvement.

Vulvovaginitis Secondary to Bacteria that Colonize the Nasopharynx

It is not uncommon to obtain the history that an upper respiratory tract infection preceded the onset of vulvovaginitis by a few days. The suspicion that the two conditions are related is strengthened when vaginal cultures yield organisms that commonly colonize the nasopharynx. It is assumed that vulvovaginitis results from autoinoculation of the microbes from the nasopharynx to the genitalia. The onset of vulvovaginal symptoms in these infections tends to be more acute, the inflammation and discomfort more marked, and the discharge less profuse and less purulent than in nonspecific vulvovaginitis.[115]

Haemophilus influenzae and *Staphylococcus aureus* are the species isolated most commonly from cultures in this setting. *Streptococcus pneumoniae* occasionally is seen. *H. influenzae* was the organism isolated most frequently in a recent series of 200 girls with vulvovaginitis.[170] Acute and chronic cases of *H. influenzae* vulvovaginitis occur, and the discharge usually is mucoid or mucopurulent, yellow, and odorless. Vulvovaginitis can be caused by serotypes a, b, and c and nontypable strains.[106, 144] Concurrent otitis media or urinary tract infection may be present. All three of these species occasionally are found in vaginal cultures from asymptomatic children. It is their isolation in pure culture from symptomatic girls that leads to the clinical conclusion of cause and effect.

Vulvovaginitis caused by these organisms often responds to the treatments described earlier for nonspecific vulvovaginitis due to poor perineal hygiene. Systemic antibiotics may be required for persistent cases or may be helpful early in severely symptomatic cases. The choice of agent depends on the anticipated or known antimicrobial susceptibilities of the specific organism.

The vagina is a well-recognized source of *S. aureus* colonization in cases of toxic shock syndrome associated with this organism. Such cases generally have occurred in adolescent and adult females in association with tampon use. Vulvovaginitis due to *S. aureus* in prepubertal girls has not been reported in association with toxic shock syndrome.

Vulvovaginitis Secondary to Skin Infections

Like the child with an upper respiratory tract infection, one with impetigo or an infected superficial wound may transmit bacteria from the wound to her genitalia through handling. Cultures in such cases usually yield hemolytic streptococci or *S. aureus*. Treatment is like that described for nonspecific vulvovaginitis secondary to respiratory tract infections.

Shigella *Vulvovaginitis*

Vulvovaginitis may be caused by infection with pathogens from the intestinal tract, especially when the organisms are endemic in a community. *Shigella* species, mainly *S. flexneri* and *S. sonnei*, appear to account for the majority of these cases.[21, 47, 152] A vaginal discharge without pain, pruritus, or dysuria is the most frequent presentation of *Shigella* vulvovaginitis.[152] The course can be acute, but discharge that persists for 4 weeks to several months before diagnosis is common. Bloody discharge has been observed in about half of the cases reported from developed countries[108] but was not seen among 27 girls with *Shigella* vulvovaginitis in Rwanda between 1988 and 1991.[21] Discharge may be purulent and heavy; it occasionally is absent. The vulvar tissues usually appear inflamed.

In most instances, *Shigella* vulvovaginitis is not associated with current or recent diarrhea.[21, 152] A vaginal foreign body, which may present with similar symptoms and course, was considered likely in a number of patients prior to diagnosis of *Shigella* infection.[152]

Local application of triple-sulfa cream (Sultrin) may clear the infection in some cases. However, refractory cases were noted in two series.[47, 152] Systemic treatment with an antibiotic to which the *Shigella* isolate is susceptible is recommended. Single-dose therapy with third-generation cephalosporins is not effective; 5- to 7-day courses of oral agents generally are required.[21] Amoxicillin, trimethoprim-sulfamethoxazole, and cefixime are reasonable choices for susceptible isolates. A growing number of *Shigella* isolates are resistant to ampicillin and trimethoprim-sulfamethoxazole. As with other causes of vulvovaginitis, adjunctive use of hygienic measures may help resolve the process and prevent recurrence.

Other Specific Causes of Premenarcheal Vulvovaginitis[71, 136, 169]

Diphtheritic, amebic, and other types of specific vulvovaginitis in children have been reported in the literature. Most of them are associated with primary disease elsewhere. When present in vaginal specimens, the bacterial pathogens discussed earlier usually are isolated in pure or nearly pure culture.

Diphtheritic vulvovaginitis may be primary in the genitalia, but most of the cases reported in the literature have been secondary to a nasopharyngeal infection. Although diphtheria is uncommon today, sporadic cases occasionally appear in areas where immunization is not practiced regularly.

The vulva is the most common genital site involved in diphtheria,[169] but diphtheritic lesions may occur in the vagina without vulvar involvement. The diagnosis is suspected when a child has the severe systemic symptoms produced by upper respiratory tract diphtheria and a local ulceration covered by a gray adherent membrane; it is confirmed by finding *Corynebacterium diphtheriae* in the discharge from the lesion.[57] The treatment of diphtheria is the same regardless of the site of the infection; it is discussed elsewhere in this book (see Chapter 95).

One case of vulvovaginitis with *Yersinia enterocolitica* isolated as the predominant organism has been reported.[230] This 4-year-old girl also had a positive stool culture and associated fever and abdominal pain but no diarrhea. Other members of the community in which she lived developed diarrhea with cultures positive for *Y. enterocolitica*. The outbreak was linked to contaminated food. Infections with this organism may be missed because special culture techniques are required for its isolation.

Rarely, ulcerative vulvovaginitis due to *Entamoeba histolytica* or related to typhoid fever has been reported. As a rule, specific genital infections with pathogenic organisms usually found in the gastrointestinal tract are the result of fecal contamination of the vulva and vagina. The treatment of infections caused by *E. histolytica* is described in Chapter 208.

Other Infections of the Premenarcheal Female Genitalia

Other specific and nonspecific infections of the premenarcheal female genitalia, including herpes genitalis, condylomata acuminata, molluscum contagiosum, lymphogranuloma venereum, cervicitis, and salpingitis, are discussed in the part of this chapter devoted to genital infections in the adolescent.

Pelvic inflammatory disease (i.e., infection of the uterine tubes, ovaries, and pelvic peritoneum) is extremely rare in premenarcheal girls. With the exceptions of gonorrhea and the inflammation caused by a foreign body, most vulvar and vaginal infections do not involve the upper third of the vagina and do not approach the cervix of premenarcheal patients. The premenarcheal cervix and endometrium apparently are barriers rather than passageways for bacteria causing all types of vulvovaginitis in children.

Reported cases of ascending pelvic infection, including gonorrhea, are most unusual; this is true of case reports in the literature before the advent of antibiotics as well as those of more recent times. Girls have been described who had lower abdominal symptoms after having presented with nonspecific or gonorrheal vulvovaginitis, but, almost without exception, a causal relation between the lower genital tract infection and that in the pelvis was not confirmed by surgical inspection or culture of the pelvic exudate.

When intrapelvic infection has been reported in premenarcheal girls, it usually has been part of either generalized primary peritonitis or of peritonitis secondary to a ruptured appendix or some other intra-abdominal infection.[195]

Pelvic infection that is part of an intra-abdominal infection characteristically affects the surfaces of the uterine tubes, uterus, and ovaries, producing a perisalpingitis and periovaritis; periappendicitis also is present even if the infection did not begin as appendicitis. An ascending infection from the lower genital tract, such as that caused by gonorrhea, involves the tubal mucosa, producing endosalpingitis and pyosalpingitis.

Identical bacteria should be identified in cultures from the lower genitalia and from the pelvic exudate before an ascending infection is considered the cause of a pelvic infection in a specific case in which the patient is a premenarcheal child.

Peritonitis in a child usually is an acute disease. Its diagnosis and treatment are considered in Chapter 62.

Occasionally, an abscess forms in the lowermost part of the pelvis of a patient who has purulent peritonitis. Pelvic abscesses are drained surgically after they have localized; their diagnosis and surgical treatment are considered in more detail in the discussion of pelvic inflammatory disease in adolescents (see later).

SEXUALLY TRANSMITTED DISEASES IN SEXUALLY ABUSED CHILDREN

Isolation of a sexually transmitted disease in a child places a health care provider in an awkward position of having to report the case to a children's protective service agency for investigation of sexual abuse. The possibility of nonsexual transmission of these diseases often is raised, particularly when a preliminary investigation cannot elicit a history of sexual abuse. The challenges involved in eliciting and validating sexual abuse in children are many. Verbal communication in children younger than 2 to 3 years of age is impossible or difficult to interpret. Fear of disclosure by children or family members, due to threats of violence, may be a major barrier to validating a case in an older child.[145]

The first step to managing such situations is for a physician to perform a genital examination on the child, looking for evidence of vulvar and hymenal trauma. A brief interview of the child in a nondirected way with open-ended questions also should be performed. Regardless of whether the child divulges any information, the case should be reported to the local children's protective service agency. The objective is for an agency caseworker also to interview the child in a nonthreatening manner. The caseworker also should request that all household members be tested for sexually transmitted diseases. More than one visit and interview by the caseworker may be necessary to accomplish this. Based on a review of the literature, common sexually transmitted diseases in prepubertal children and their potential mode of transmission are presented in Table 49–4.

Gonococcal Infection

In infants, perinatal nonsexual transmission is considered the most likely cause for gonococcal infection. Branch and Paxton[23] found that in 1- to 11-month-old children, all the mothers were found to have gonococcal infection, and no history of sexual contact could be elicited. The authors concluded that transmission of the gonorrhea was perinatal, from freshly contaminated hands, or through fomites.

Children with gonococcal infection frequently are found to have a history of sexual contact. Branch and Paxton[23] found that 93 per cent of children 1 to 9 years of age with gonorrhea had sexual contact with relatives in the household. Ingram and colleagues[118] found that 35 per cent of 1- to 4-year-old children and 100 per cent of children older than 4 years of age with gonorrhea reported sexual contact with an extended older male family member. Folland and colleagues[70] elicited a history of sexual contact from 34 per cent of children with gonococcal urethritis and vaginitis.

Other infected adults and children often are found in an infected child's environment.[174] Testing of household members can detect infected adults at a rate of 18 to 29 per cent.[5, 155] In a retrospective study of 14 Native Alaskan children with gonococcal infection, 3 reported sexual contact. Seven children slept with their parents, one or both of whom had gonorrhea; the authors assumed that these children acquired the infection by nonsexual means.[206]

N. gonorrhoeae has been shown to survive for 20 to 24 hours in infected secretions on towels and handkerchiefs.[212] However, *N. gonorrhoeae* from toilet seats has survived up to 2 hours after inoculation, but no gonococcus was recovered from toilet seats in public restrooms or a clinic for sexually transmitted diseases.[83, 173] Nonsexual transmission to adults is rare.

It is conceivable that nonsexual transmission occurs among children who sleep and bathe with their parents. However,

TABLE 49–4. Common Sexually Transmitted Diseases (STDs) in Prepubertal Children and Their Possible Mode of Transmission

	Perinatal	STD Rate in Alleged Sexual Abuse Cases	Alleged Sexual Abuse Rate in STD Cases	Infected Household Members	Survival on Fomites	Other
Neisseria gonorrhoeae	Up to 1 year of age[23]	5%–7%[47a, 197a]	35%, 1–4 years of age[118] 100%, older than 4 years of age[118] 93%, 1–9 years of age[23]	18%–29%, no history of sexual abuse elicited[5, 155]	24 hours on wet fomites; 2 hours on dry fomites. None from public toilet seats[83, 173]	None
Chlamydia trachomatis	Up to 3 years of age[193]	6%–8%[119, 120] 4% cases vs. 7% controls[98]	75%	No data	No data	None
Trichomonas vaginalis	Up to 1 year of age	No data	Case report[122] History of sexual abuse not obtained in Polish studies[133]	43% fathers, 72% mothers, no history of sexual abuse elicited (Poland)[133]	Up to 6 hours on wood surface and discharge.[128] Isolated from bathing implements[157]	Bathing tanks (India).[157] Mud baths, warm mineral waters (Poland).[133] Water from toilets[29]
Syphilis	Congenital	0%–5%[47a, 197a]	Case reports	No data	No data	None
Bacterial vaginosis/ nonspecific vaginitis	No data	13% cases vs. 4% controls[97]	Case reports	No data	No data	None
Herpes simplex virus	Period unknown	No data	Case reports	Case report (mother with infected finger)[126]	2 hours on latex gloves, toilet seat[138] 24 72 hours on speculum and gauze[138]	Auto inoculation from oral lesions[154]
Human papilloma virus	Up to 3 years of age[45]	No data	27%–90%[37]	No data	No data	None

sexual transmission is the more common and most likely mode of transmission. An investigation for sexual abuse must be pursued in a child with gonorrhea.

Chlamydial Infection

C. trachomatis can be transmitted to an infant from the infected mother during the perinatal period. *C. trachomatis* has been isolated from the conjunctiva, nasopharynx, vagina, and rectum of infants born to infected mothers.[193] Perinatally acquired rectal and vaginal chlamydial infection in infants can persist for up to 372 and 383 days, respectively. Persistent chlamydial infection of the pharynx in infants can persist for up to 2 years.[19]

Sexual abuse as a potential mode of transmission of *C. trachomatis* infection should be considered in children older than 1 year of age.[76, 98] Ingram and associates[119] found that 6 per cent of girls who allegedly were sexually abused and no girls who denied sexual abuse had *C. trachomatis* infection. Except for one child, all the children in the control group were determined later to have been sexually abused. In a prospective study, Ingram and associates[120] found *C. trachomatis* in 8 per cent of girls with a history of sexual abuse, compared with 0 per cent in girls with no history of sexual abuse. In the former group, three girls were found also to have rectal and one pharyngeal infection.

In conclusion, perinatally acquired genital chlamydial infection is a strong possibility in children younger than 1 year of age. Perinatal transmission is possible in children as old as 3 years of age. After 1 year of age, however, sexual transmission should be a strong consideration in children with genital chlamydial infection. Therefore, an investigation for sexual abuse must be pursued in a child diagnosed with genital chlamydial infection. No studies have evaluated the presence of *C. trachomatis* on fomites and its coexistence in family members of infected children.

Syphilis

Syphilis infections not found to be acquired congenitally should be considered sexually transmitted.[85] Sexually acquired infection is a strong possibility in all prepubertal children with syphilis. Syphilitic lesions and positive serologic results have been detected in alleged sexual abusers of children with syphilis.[1] There are no data on the survival of *Treponema pallidum* on fomites. An investigation for sexual abuse must be pursued in a child diagnosed with syphilis.

Trichomonas vaginalis Infection

T. vaginalis has been found in the nasopharynx and vagina of newborns born to infected mothers. Therefore, transmission of *T. vaginalis* in infants as old as 1 year of age probably is perinatal. The mode of transmission in children after 1 year of age is controversial. There is a report of two cases of *T. vaginalis* in premenarcheal girls who were sexually abused.[122] Prevalence studies either do not address the mode of transmission at all or, if they do, do not address the possibility of sexual abuse.[66, 133] In addition, a vaginal wet mount for trichomonads is not done routinely in children assessed for possible sexual abuse. A survey from Poland found one case of *T. vaginalis* in children 2 to 7 years of age and a significantly higher number of cases in 8- to 10-year-old girls. The numbers increased even further after 10 years of age. This suggests a strong association between *T. vaginalis* and the presence of an estrogenic environment, which promotes glycogen production and decreases vaginal pH.[133]

The Polish survey tested families of women infected with *T. vaginalis* and found that almost a third of their sexual partners and 8 per cent of the children (mostly girls) had *T. vaginalis.* When families of men infected with *T. vaginalis* were tested, 91 per cent of their sexual partners and 13 per cent of the children had *T. vaginalis.* When families of children (mostly girls) infected with *T. vaginalis* were tested, 72 per cent of their mothers and 43 per cent of their fathers had the infection. The investigators thought the infection in the latter group originated from mothers and the primary mode of transmission to be nonsexual (beds, sponges, towels, overcrowding). Information regarding sharing of potentially infected fomites, sexual abuse, or physically intimate behavior between parents and children was not gathered in these cases.[133]

Although *T. vaginalis* has been known to survive on fomites in controlled experiments, its ability to spread by these means is not known. There are no documented cases of adults being infected by fomites. *T. vaginalis* has been found to survive for up to 6 hours on droplets of discharge and enameled surfaces of wood blocks.[128] It has been isolated from droplets of water splashed from toilets containing urine of an infected person.[29] *T. vaginalis* also has been found to survive in mudbaths, bathing waters, warm mineral waters, and moist bathing implements.[133, 157] In rural India, a survey found that young girls who bathed in tanks or rivers had a significantly higher risk of acquiring *T. vaginalis* compared with those who used pipe or well water.[36]

In conclusion, it is conceivable that *T. vaginalis* is transmitted to children nonsexually. The likelihood of perinatal transmission is probable in infants younger than 1 year of age. However, it also is possible that a child or an infant younger than 1 year of age with *T. vaginalis* may have been sexually abused. In a child older than 1 year of age, the probability of sexual abuse must be considered and the case must be investigated. Perinatal transmission and transmission of infection through fomites should not be assumed without an investigation for sexual abuse.

Bacterial Vaginosis

The significance of bacterial vaginosis and *G. vaginalis* and their relationship to sexual abuse in prepubertal girls are unclear. Based on the presence of clue cells and a positive amine test result in vaginal secretions, bacterial vaginosis has been diagnosed in 13 per cent of sexually abused children, compared with 4 per cent of girls who denied sexual abuse.[97] Similar prevalence rates for *G. vaginalis* have been reported in children who have and have not been sexually abused.[15] There are no data regarding the survival of *G. vaginalis* on fomites.

In conclusion, although the prevalence of *G. vaginalis* and bacterial vaginosis is higher in sexually abused children than in nonabused children, their significance as a marker for sexual abuse is unclear. It therefore is recommended that the child be questioned for sexual abuse. However, an investigation by a children's protective service agency is not necessary.

Herpes Genitalis

Perinatal transmission of herpes simplex virus types 1 and 2 in the form of stomatitis occurs in infants. Herpes simplex virus type 2 is not common. Types 1 and 2 have been isolated in the genital area in children alleging sexual abuse.[81, 126] However, there are no studies reporting the coexistence of herpes simplex virus genital infection in household members and infected children. Physical contact by a mother's infected finger has been reported.[126] Autoinoculation from the mouth to the genitals as a mode of transmission is possible, especially when oral herpes simplex virus infection precedes herpes simplex virus genital lesions.[154] Herpes simplex virus has been known to survive for 2 hours on latex gloves and toilet seats, 24 hours on a speculum, and 72 hours on gauze.[138] However, transmission of herpes simplex virus from fomites requires direct contact of viable virus with either mucous membrane or a break in the skin, making fomite transmission unlikely. It is recommended that the child with herpes simplex virus genital infection be evaluated for sexual abuse and the case be reported to the authorities.

Venereal Warts

Perinatal transmission of human papilloma virus from an infected mother to her baby is well documented. The incubation period after exposure to the virus may range from 1 to 20 months.[45] Because the exact incubation period for development of genital lesions is not known, perinatal transmission has been found to be the most likely cause for genital warts in almost 96 per cent of patients younger than 3 years of age.[45] In children 3 years of age or older, a history of sexual abuse has been elicited in 27 to 90 per cent with venereal warts.[37, 109] Based on failure to identify sexual abuse, a report from a dermatology clinic concludes that transmission of human papilloma virus possibly occurs by fomites.[37] No reports in the literature address survival of the virus on fomites or in infected household members.

In conclusion, sexual abuse is the most common means of acquiring human papilloma virus infection and should be suspected in all prepubertal children older than 3 years of age who are infected. In children younger than 3 years of age, sexual abuse should be suspected and investigated as well, even though perinatal transmission is a strong possibility.

POSTMENARCHEAL LOWER GENITAL TRACT INFECTIONS

Infections of the postmenarcheal female clitoris, urinary tract, vulva, vagina, and cervix produce a variety of overlapping symptoms, including vulvar pruritus, dysuria, and increased or altered vaginal discharge and spotting. As a result, it is difficult to distinguish among various lower genital tract infections based solely on symptoms. History, physical examination, and laboratory tests play an important role in assisting the clinician in diagnosing urethritis, vaginitis, or cervicitis.

Pruritus and Dysuria

Pruritus of the genitalia or perineal skin is a common complaint. This should be approached as a symptom and not as a disease in itself. Itching may be associated with vulvovaginitis of many causes and with local and systemic skin disorders that involve the genital region[148] (see Table 49–2). The underlying process should be treated in addition to providing symptomatic relief of pruritus.[73]

The complaint of dysuria generally leads to evaluation for possible urinary tract infection. However, in adolescent girls, dysuria frequently is associated with vulvitis, vaginitis, or another manifestation of sexually transmitted disease without evidence of a concurrent urinary tract infection. In one series, almost 60 per cent of patients whose chief complaint was dysuria fell into this category.[48] Dysuria in these cases probably is secondary to irritation of ulcerated areas by urine flow.

Disorders of the Clitoris

The clitoral hood occasionally develops cellulitis with induration, edema, and erythema, analogous to posthitis in the male. Staphylococci or streptococci are the most common etiologies. Oral antibiotics with efficacy against these organisms usually are effective. Warm soaks or sitz baths also may provide symptomatic relief.[58]

Clitorimegaly with erythema can occur with vulvovaginitis of any etiology but most often is associated with herpes simplex virus infections.[49] Edematous enlargement of the clitoris, as well as labia, without erythema has been reported in patients with Crohn disease.[151]

Postmenarcheal Urethritis

Dysuria is classified into external dysuria and internal dysuria. External dysuria is pain from urine flowing over the vulva. This history suggests vulvitis and vaginitis. Internal dysuria is pain with initiation of urination and is not associated with urine flowing over the vulva. This indicates urethritis or a urinary tract infection. Careful history and examination assists the physician in differentiating urethritis from vaginitis.

Urethritis in postmenarcheal females is common, particularly when they are sexually active. *T. vaginalis* may cause urethritis with internal dysuria. A teenager with an acute gonococcal cervical infection may have associated urethritis due to *C. trachomatis* infection of the urethra. This has been implicated as an important cause of dysuria in sexually active females. This is called the acute urethral syndrome, and the clinical presentation includes dysuria, frequency, and pyuria with significant bacteriurea.[213] Urethral infection may occur with or without cervical infection. Stamm and colleagues[213] noted that 50 per cent of females with acute-onset dysuria and frequency had sterile pyuria; *C. trachomatis* was isolated in 31 per cent of these cases.

Thus, when a sexually active adolescent female presents with internal dysuria, in addition to being tested for conventional uropathogens, she should be screened for common sexually transmitted diseases, such as gonorrhea and *Chlamydia* and *Trichomonas* infection of the vagina, cervix, and urethra. A urine analysis and microscopy for presence of leukocytes and bacteria should be performed in these patients as well. For treatment of urethritis caused by sexually transmitted organisms, the sections in this chapter on trichomoniasis, gonorrhea, and chlamydial infections should be reviewed.

Paraurethral Duct Abscess, Bartholinitis, and Bartholin Abscess

The paraurethral ducts lie on each side of the urethral meatus. The Bartholin glands are small, bean-shaped glands that lie on each side of the vaginal opening, behind the hymen. Each gland opens by means of a long single duct immediately external to the hymen. Infections of the paraurethral and Bartholin ducts are more common in adult women but occasionally occur in the adolescent female.

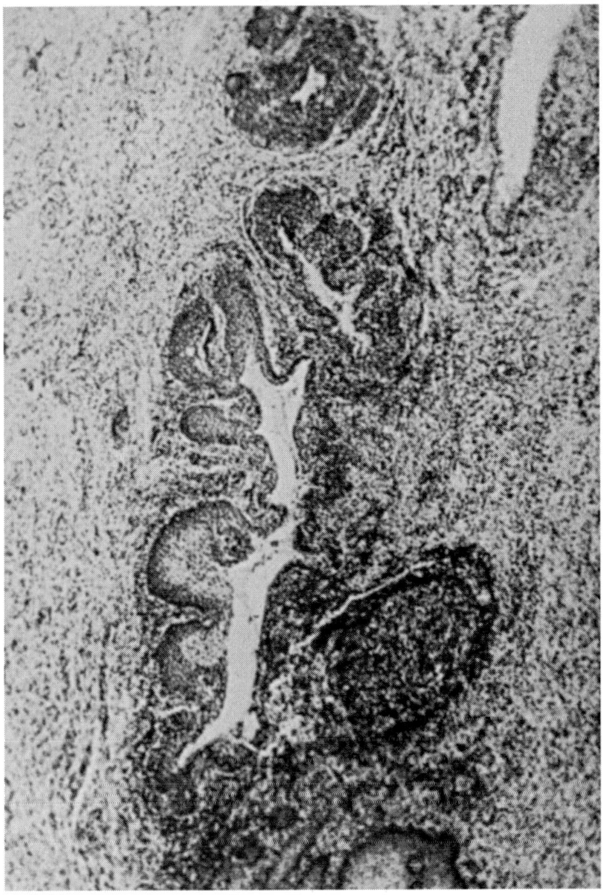

FIGURE 49–11. *Acute gonorrheal major vestibular (Bartholin) gland duct abscess.*

A paraurethral duct abscess (Fig. 49–11) creates a small, exquisitely painful swelling in the urethrovaginal septum. If the abscess is not incised and drained, it may rupture into the urethra, creating a urethral diverticulum. Discharge for a Gram stain should be obtained from the urethral lumen and the paraurethral ducts by downward and outward pressure on the urethrovaginal septum (Fig 49–12).

Bartholinitis, or inflammation of the Bartholin ducts, causes pain, tenderness, and a linear ropey-shaped swelling, best palpated by holding the vulvar mucosa and labia majora between the fingers. Purulent or mucoid exudate can be expressed occasionally from the Bartholin duct.

N. gonorrhoeae and *C. trachomatis* have been isolated from ductal exudate in women with bartholinitis.[44, 179] Bartholinitis should be treated with antibiotics that provide coverage for *N. gonorrhoeae, C. trachomatis,* and anaerobes. Sitz baths provide symptomatic relief.

A Bartholin abscess is seen most often in women 20 to 29 years of age and is the second most common urogenital complication of gonorrhea after pelvic inflammatory disease in women. Risk factors for Bartholin abscess are similar to risk factors for sexually transmitted diseases.[3]

Infection of a Bartholin cyst results in a markedly tender abscess (Fig. 49–13). The abscess can rupture spontaneously and drain foul-smelling, purulent material externally through the skin. Multiple organisms tend to be isolated from Bartholin abscesses. An early study using percutaneous aspirates from abscesses predominantly demonstrated anaerobes and facultative organisms. *N. gonorrhoeae* was isolated in 8 per cent of cases and gram-negative bacilli in 16 per cent of cases.

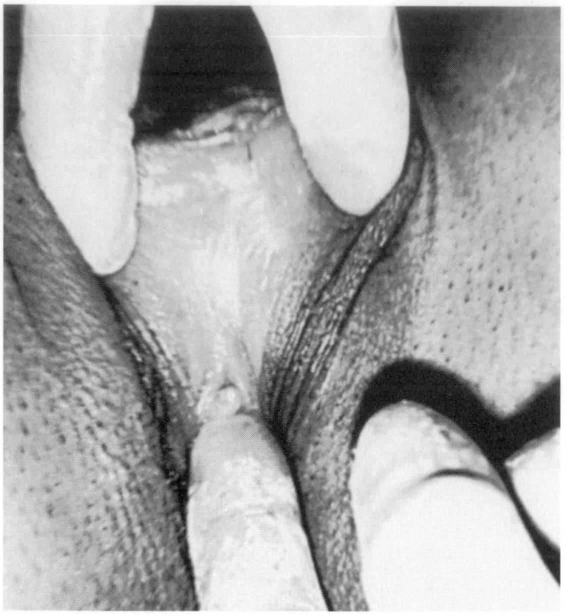

FIGURE 49–12. *Urethral and paraurethral duct discharge is obtained by downward and outward digital pressure on the distal urethrovaginal septum.*

Although genital Mycoplasmataceae were isolated from the duct secretions, they were not isolated directly from abscesses.[139] More recently, *Porphyromonas asaccharolyticus* (a black-pigmented, gram-negative anaerobe), *Salmonella panama* (after an attack of *Salmonella* enteritis), and tuberculosis have been associated with Bartholin abscess.[43, 51, 56] Huffman[115] encountered tuberculosis of the Bartholin gland in a 14-year-old sexually inactive female with pulmonary tuberculosis. She had painless, unilateral swelling of the left labia majora with a brown discharge exuding from a small sinus. *Mycobacterium tuberculosis* was isolated in the discharge.

A Bartholin abscess should be incised and drained by applying a surface anesthetic, ethyl chloride, making a 1- to 1½-cm, full-thickness incision on the medial aspect of the labia majora. The cavity should be probed with a sterile cotton-tipped swab to break up loculations within the abscess. To allow for further drainage, one should pack the abscess cavity with sterile gauze. Alternatively, a Word catheter can be inserted into the cavity and the balloon inflated. Clinical experience indicates that the packing method is far more painful to the patient and healing takes longer.

Antibiotic coverage for anaerobes, *N. gonorrhoeae,* and *C. trachomatis* should be provided for at least 2 weeks, and a nonsteroidal medication is recommended for inflammation and pain. Frequent sitz baths further help with drainage and healing. Close follow-up during the first week is advised. The packing or the catheter may be removed after 4 days of antibiotics. Although marsupialization frequently was used to treat recurrent Bartholin abscesses, incision with drainage and primary suture of the abscess cavity under an antibiotic (clindamycin) now have been found to cause more rapid healing and significantly decrease the incidence of recurrent abscesses.[10]

Postmenarcheal Vulvovaginitis

The most common types of vulvovaginitis in postmenarcheal females are *T. vaginalis* vaginitis, vulvovaginal candidiasis, and bacterial vaginosis. Although gonococcal infection most frequently is manifested by cervicitis, the vulvovaginal manifestations of gonococcal infection are discussed separately from gonococcal cervicitis. *C. trachomatis* does not infect the postmenarcheal vulvar mucosa but infects the urethra and endocervix.

Postmenarcheal Vaginal Trichomoniasis

Vaginal trichomoniasis in the postmenarcheal girl is characterized by vaginal inflammation, leukorrhea, vulvovaginal pruritus, and the presence of *T. vaginalis* in the vaginal fluid.

T. vaginalis is a triflagellated protozoan (Fig. 49–14). The organism, somewhat larger than a polymorphonuclear leukocyte, has a distinctive vibrating or whip-like movement when seen microscopically in fresh wet smears taken from the vagina. It quickly succumbs to a lowering of the pH, drying, cooling, and changing osmotic pressure of the fluid surrounding it.

Most infections are encountered in sexually active young women; the incidence increases during the early reproductive years. Trichomoniasis is found only rarely in premenarcheal girls, sexually inactive adolescents, and postmenopausal women. Generally, it is accepted that, in the great majority of cases, trichomoniasis is a sexually transmitted disease. However, Huffman[115] has seen trichomoniasis in patients who had not had coitus. *T. vaginalis* has been shown to survive in chlorinated swimming pools, bathing tanks, mud baths, and warm mineral waters.[134, 157]

Trichomoniasis frequently is asymptomatic. When symptomatic, patients complain of a profuse, irritating discharge. Both discharge and pruritus tend to be more severe just before and immediately after a menstrual period. Recurrent exacerbations of the infection are common. Patients occasionally report dysuria and abdominal pain.

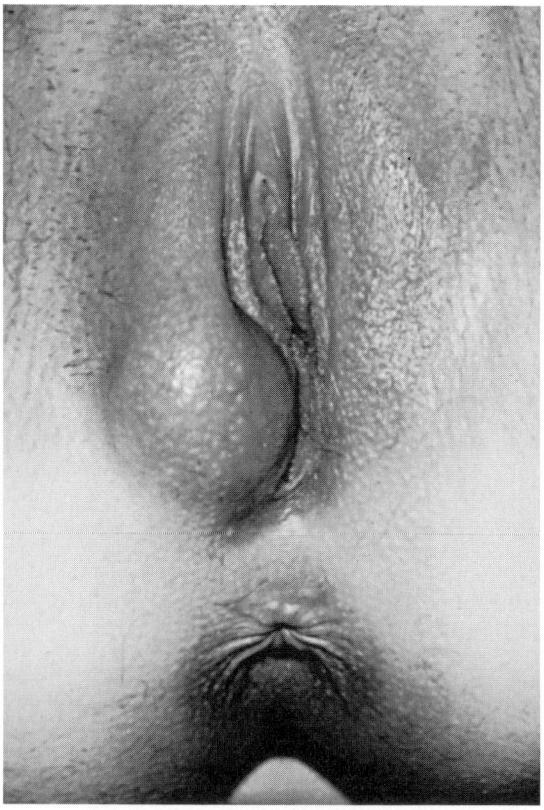

FIGURE 49–13. *Paraurethral duct abscess.*

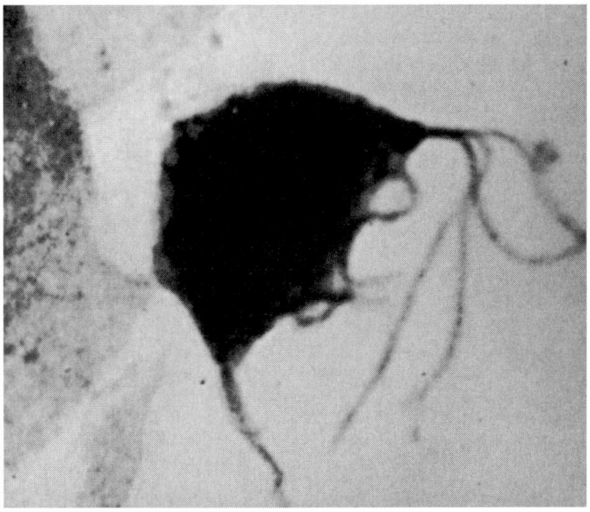

FIGURE 49–14. Trichomonas vaginalis *is a triflagellated protozoan that, when motile, is identified easily in wet smears of the vaginal discharge.*

Examination reveals diffuse vulvitis with erythema and excoriations and copious leukorrhea that covers the vulvar tissues. The discharge typically is frothy or bubbly, grayish-yellow, and watery or mucopurulent. It has a pH of between 5 and 7 and an acrid or musty odor. A "strawberry" or punctate vaginal eruption with hemorrhagic spots has been described as typical of trichomoniasis. Such eruptions frequently are not present, even in severe cases. More often, diffuse inflammation causes the vaginal mucosa to be brilliant red.

The diagnosis of trichomoniasis is confirmed by finding trichomonads in a wet smear of the vaginal fluid. It is important that the slide be viewed promptly because the organisms do not remain viable for long outside the vagina and are difficult to detect once they cease to be motile. The observer sees numerous ovoid-shaped, motile organisms. The sensitivity of this test ranges from 40 to 75 per cent. A vaginal cytosmear to detect trichomoniasis is not recommended because of the high rate of error in identifying trichomonads in stained smears. Other methods used to diagnose trichomoniasis include the Papanicolaou smear, isolation by special culture medium, and direct fluorescent immunoassay. The last two methods are the most sensitive but are not used routinely in clinical settings.[187]

Treatment[32]

A single 2-g oral dose of metronidazole (Flagyl) is the recommended treatment of choice. An alternative regimen is metronidazole 500 mg orally twice daily for 7 days. The cure rate is 95 per cent in females. If symptoms persist and the wet smears from her vagina still show trichomonads, the course of treatment is repeated. Only in unusually persistent cases is a third course necessary. The patient is warned of possible gastrointestinal side effects (nausea, diarrhea). Alcohol sometimes aggravates the side effects of metronidazole therapy; the patient should be instructed not to consume alcoholic beverages when under treatment. She should be told that trichomoniasis is a sexually transmitted disease and that her partner should be treated and use a condom.

Metronidazole is not recommended during the first trimester of pregnancy because of reports of spontaneous abortion, developmental anomalies, and perinatal deaths. Clotrimazole vaginal suppositories, one a day for 6 days, cures two-thirds of patients. Gentle vaginal douching with vinegar and water may relieve symptoms somewhat. Metronidazole gel has not been studied for the treatment of trichomoniasis and therefore should not be used.

Postmenarcheal Mycotic Vulvovaginitis

Several factors play a role in causing the increased incidence of vaginal candidiasis that occurs after the menarche and continues during the reproductive years. Menstruation, by altering the vaginal pH, may offer a favorable medium for the growth of mycotic organisms. Sexual contact undoubtedly explains some cases. In view of their widespread distribution, *Candida* species not surprisingly are common in the intestinal tract and frequently are found in stool cultures. Fecal contamination of the vulva during cleansing after defecation at a time when the normal vulvar and vaginal flora are depleted and not able to inhibit fungal growth would permit the development of symptomatic vulvovaginal candidiasis. Uncleanliness, the ingestion of large quantities of carbohydrates, and tight-fitting underclothes (which keep the perineum warm and moist) are factors that contribute to the growth of mycotic organisms. The widespread use of antibiotics that disturb the vaginal flora and of oral contraceptives are additional factors that increase the incidence of candidal infections. Other predisposing factors include pregnancy, obesity, immunosuppressive therapy, and heroin or other drug addiction. The frequent association of vulvar and vaginal candidiasis with uncontrolled diabetes mellitus suggests that any patient suffering from recurrent *Candida* infection be examined for diabetes mellitus. If a patient has a recurrent unexplainable or resistant infection, a glucose tolerance test should be performed.

C. albicans and *Torulopsis glabrata* are the yeast-like fungi most often found in the vagina. *C. albicans* is responsible for 80 to 95 per cent and *T. glabrata* for 3 to 16 per cent of fungal infections. Other *Candida* species are found less often in the vagina but can be pathogenic. *Candida tropicalis,* like *C. albicans,* produces systemic infections in immunosuppressed hosts. Mycotic vulvovaginitis causes severe vulvar and vaginal itching; usually, the patient does not have an excessive discharge. The discharge that is present is white, thick, and curdled and has a yeasty sour odor. There may be pain during and after voiding or external dysuria as a result of urine coming in contact with excoriated areas on the urethra and vulva.

Examination in the acute stage reveals intense inflammation of the vulva and vagina, and this may extend to the perineal skin. The involved areas are shiny, beefy red with linear excoriations, and edematous. *C. albicans* typically forms patches of mycelia that create adherent white plaques scattered over the inflamed surfaces. Superficial, red, weeping areas remain after the plaques are pulled away. Other *Candida* species, notably *C. tropicalis,* do not form adherent plaques but produce a cottage cheese–like discharge similar to that found with *C. albicans.* The vaginal pH usually is within a normal range (below 4.5).

The diagnosis is established by finding hyphae and buds of the fungus in the vaginal fluid (see Fig. 49–11), in the curdled discharge, in material scraped from the vulvar mucosa, or on the perineal skin. A wet smear in normal saline may suffice, but debris and cellular material may make it difficult to identify the fungus. If so, a smear using 10 per cent potassium hydroxide solution is helpful. The slide is heated gently until bubbles appear under the coverslip. The potassium hydroxide solution dissolves other extraneous material without affecting the fungus. With an experienced microscopist, this method yields a sensitivity of 86 per cent in symptomatic females. The diagnosis is confirmed by culture on Nickerson or Sabouraud medium.

Treatment[32]

Several vaginal preparations can be used. The commonly used antifungal creams are imidazoles (clotrimazole and miconazole) and polyenes (nystatin). The polyenes are not used now because of increasing resistance of fungi to this compound. The imidazoles are available as creams, tablets, and coated tampons. Intravaginal treatment with 100-mg vaginal tablets clotrimazole every night for 7 days produces a cure rate of 90 per cent. Comparable cure rates are observed with 100 to 200 mg of clotrimazole or miconazole (two tablets) for 3 days. The shorter regimen may result in better compliance. Creams and tablets are equally effective.

Gentian violet, which has been used for many years, still is the most effective treatment for vulvovaginal candidiasis.[115] A 1 per cent aqueous solution is painted on the cervix and the vaginal and vulvar mucosa. Care is taken to rotate the speculum so that the anterior and posterior vaginal walls are treated. Likewise, the creases between the folds of the vulvar mucosa are covered with the dye. The speculum is reinserted, opened, and left in place for 5 minutes so that all painted surfaces will become dry.

Gentian violet has two disadvantages: it causes herpes-like lesions on the vulvas of a few patients, and it is messy. Many adolescents refuse this treatment. The patient is advised not to have intercourse until the infection is eradicated, but if she chooses to do so anyway, her partner should be told to wear a condom, not only to prevent getting the dye on his penis but to avoid being a carrier of the fungus.

Treatment with gentian violet is repeated once weekly for 3 weeks and should include one treatment during a menstrual period. The patient is instructed to use a fungicidal vaginal cream nightly between office visits. Creams and suppositories containing gentian violet are less effective and are not recommended. Oral nystatin (two Mycostatin oral tablets, each containing 500,000 units of nystatin, three times daily) should be taken concurrently with local treatment to reduce the mycotic population in the gastrointestinal tract.

Oral ketoconazole is an effective preparation for treatment of difficult relapsing vulvovaginal candidiasis. The oral regimen is 200 mg twice daily for 5 days, and the cure rate is 90 per cent.[32] Low-dose prophylactic treatment also may be used in these cases. Oral ketoconazole should not be used for uncomplicated vulvovaginal candidiasis.

Postmenarcheal Bacterial Vaginosis

Bacterial vaginosis is a noninflammatory polymicrobial condition caused by an ecologic change in the vagina; an overgrowth of anaerobes, especially *Bacteroides* and *Mobiluncus* species, *G. vaginalis,* and *M. hominis*; and a decrease in the concentration of lactobacilli.[9, 77–79, 164]

Bacterial vaginosis is considered a sexually transmitted disease based on the occurrence of bacterial vaginosis with other sexually transmitted diseases and in male partners of females with this condition. However, bacterial vaginosis has been described in non–sexually active adolescent girls.[28]

As a rule, the patient's primary complaint is an offensive odor with moderately profuse, gray-colored leukorrhea that stains her underwear. She may have mild pruritus or dyspareunia.

A clinician often is able to identify this condition simply by the odor of the discharge. Examination shows little or no vulvar or vaginal erythema. The urethral and vulvar glands are not involved. The vagina contains a thick, homogeneous, grayish-white discharge. The pH of vaginal secretions in bacterial vaginosis is between 5 and 6. A pH greater than 5 also is noted when blood, cervical secretions, and *T. vaginalis* are present in vaginal secretions. Therefore, taking care to obtain nonbloody vaginal secretions uncontaminated by cervical secretions is important. *T. vaginalis* tends to be associated with a vaginal pH between 6 and 8.

Microscopic examination of some of the discharge mixed with normal saline solution in a wet preparation shows masses of desquamated vaginal epithelial cells and cellular debris. Clusters of bacteria adhere to the surface of many of the vaginal cells; these "clue cells" (Fig. 49–15) are characteristic of the condition. Absence of erythrocytes and leukocytes in the discharge is another characteristic finding. The clinical diagnosis is made by the presence of any three of the following four criteria: (1) a homogenous gray malodorous discharge, (2) a pH of vaginal secretions greater than 4.5, (3) a fishy odor elicited with release of amines when 10 per cent potassium hydroxide is added to vaginal secretion (whiff test), and (4) the presence of clue cells.[9]

The most reliable diagnostic test for bacterial vaginosis is a Gram stain of vaginal secretions. A predominance of gram-variable cocci and curved rods (anaerobes) and occasional long gram-positive rods (lactobacilli) are seen. A wet mount, however, is a rapid and helpful test for clue cells in a busy clinical setting. Cultures for *G. vaginalis* and anaerobes are not useful clinically in nonpregnant females.

In most cases, bacterial vaginosis responds to metronidazole, 500 mg orally twice daily for 7 days, or a 2-g oral dose repeated once at 48 hours.[32] Alternative regimens include clindamycin cream 2 per cent intravaginally every night for

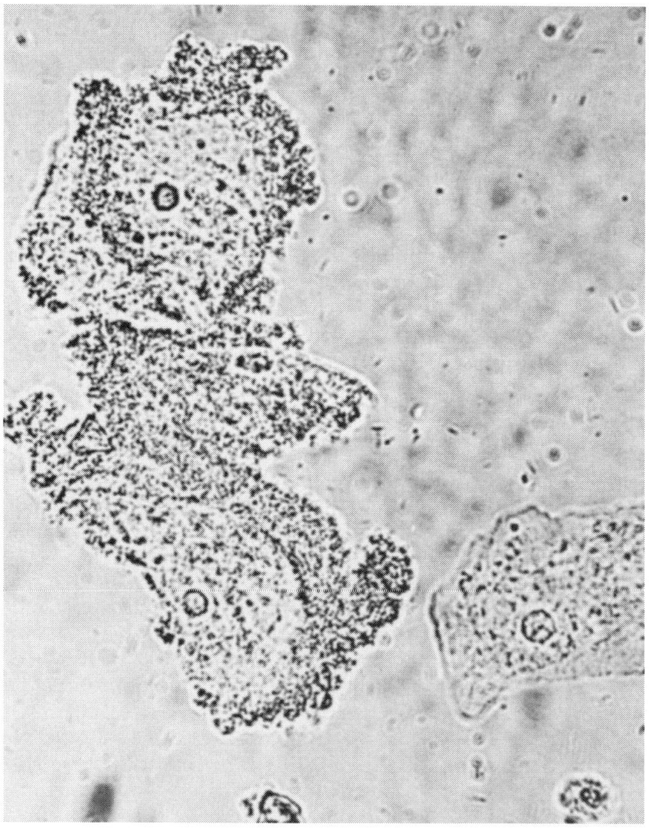

FIGURE 49–15. *Bacteria clinging to the sides of a vaginal epithelial cell ("clue cell") is significant in bacterial vaginosis. (Courtesy of Dr. Herman L. Gardner.)*

7 days and metronidazole gel 0.75 per cent intravaginally twice a day for 5 days. These regimens provide effective coverage of anaerobes and *G. vaginalis.* Treatment of the sexual partner has not proved to be beneficial.[32]

Postmenarcheal Vulvovaginal Gonorrhea

The endocervical canal is the primary site of gonococcal infection in adolescent females. Structures in the external genitalia, urethra, vulvar mucosa, and vestibular glands also may be infected.[143]

Symptoms usually begin 3 to 5 days after exposure to an infected partner. The associated vaginal (endocervical) discharge is profuse and purulent. The urethral discharge is much less evident in females than in males. Inflammation of the vulvar tissues often causes pruritus and burning.

The urethral and vulvar symptoms resolve after a few weeks without treatment. The vaginal discharge continues as a result of persisting endocervical infection. This profuse leukorrhea leads to irritation of the vaginal tissues, and this may allow secondary nonspecific vaginitis to develop.

Postmenarcheal girls suspected of having acute gonorrhea should be evaluated before urination in order to detect a urethral discharge, which may be the only evidence of acute infection. The perimeatal tissues and urethral labia are edematous and hyperemic during the acute stage of infection. The urethral mucosa often is everted. A purulent discharge similar to that from the endocervix may exude from the urethra, paraurethral ducts, and the major and minor vestibular glands.

Untreated acute gonorrhea in the female often leaves residual lesions that include chronic urethritis, Bartholinitis, thickenings of Bartholin ducts, thickening of Bartholin glands, and chronic cervicitis. Discharge from the urethral lumen and paraurethral ducts is obtained by downward and outward pressure on the urethrovaginal septum (see Fig. 49–14). Smears for Gram stain and material for cultures are taken from the urethra and endocervix. Treatment of gonococcal infection is discussed in the section on gonococcal cervicitis.

Postmenarcheal Nonspecific Vulvitis[74, 77]

Nonspecific vulvitis in postmenarcheal patients is related closely to intertrigo. Bacterial invasion of the vulvar mucosa is incited by local uncleanliness and by warmth and maceration of the tissues. Chronic, profuse leukorrhea is a common cause. Secondary pyogenic infections frequently are superimposed on vulvar mycotic dermatitis or other skin disorders.

The patient suffering from a nonspecific vulvitis complains of vulvar burning and pruritus. Acid urine flowing over the inflamed surface often causes acute distress. The patient frequently describes this as dysuria. In adolescent females, dysuria represents a genital tract infection more often than a urinary tract infection.[48] In vulvitis, a discharge usually is present as well, either from a preexisting vaginitis or from vulvar lesions. She frequently complains of distress when walking or sitting.

The vulvar tissues are red, glazed, edematous, and sodden. There may be fissured, excoriated, or desquamated areas. If the condition has persisted for some time, the mucosa tends to be dry and scaly.

The role of leukorrhea in causing vulvitis merits special mention. The maceration, constant moisture, and low-grade infection caused by a vaginal discharge and the constant irritation of a discharge-soaked perineal pad all contribute to the development of vulvar inflammation.

At first sight, acute nonspecific vulvitis may resemble the erythema caused by contact with any one of a variety of physical or chemical agents. Among the latter are rayon and nylon underclothing; rubberized girdles; soaps and detergents used for bathing or washing clothing; bubble-bath preparations and other bathing aids; perfumed or medicated douches; "hygienic" vulvar sprays; locally applied medications; condom lubricants; and contraceptive suppositories, foams, and jellies. As a rule, contact vulvitis causes little discharge and a more intense erythema than nonspecific vulvitis, from which it must be differentiated.

Treatment

The first step in the treatment of nonspecific vulvitis is the eradication of any cervical or vaginal disorder causing chronic leukorrhea. Mycotic infections superimposed on nonspecific vulvitis require candidacidal therapy. Patients with acute vulvitis recover more promptly if they are put at bed rest so that friction of the parts is avoided. The vulva is kept dry and exposed to the air as much as possible. Air drying with an electric hair dryer (warm, not hot, air) is soothing and promotes healing. The tissues are cleansed gently with a mild soap and warm water twice daily. Many patients find ice-cold witch hazel compresses (Tucks) soothing. Acute nonspecific inflammations of the vulva usually respond to the local application of bacitracin ointment.

Nonspecific vulvar irritation may be caused by warm weather, nylon underpants, obesity, poor hygiene, or sitting on sand. Adolescents complain of pruritus, dysuria, and discomfort. Treatment includes applying 1 per cent hydrocortisone cream three times a day to the vulva, wearing cotton underpants, and avoiding precipitating factors.[55]

Postmenarcheal Nonspecific Vulvovaginitis[58, 115]

Nonspecific vulvovaginitis is characterized by leukorrhea, inflammation of the vulvovaginal mucosa, and vaginal cultures that reveal a mixed growth of common pathogenic organisms. The diagnosis is made less frequently because bacterial vaginosis and other specific organisms have been identified as specific causes of vulvovaginitis that formerly were considered to be nonspecific. A diagnosis of nonspecific vulvovaginitis is not made in a specific case until a thorough study has ruled out other agents as causes of a patient's symptoms.

Leukorrhea is the primary symptom. An offensive odor and pruritus usually are not complaints. Dyspareunia may be reported by sexually active adolescents.

The vaginal mucosa shows varying degrees of hyperemia and edema. The discharge is not distinctive. Frequently, a discharge is not noted on examination. The normally acid vaginal fluid is neutral or alkaline. Wet-smear preparations do not reveal clue cells, trichomonads, or mycotic hyphae; lactobacilli are absent. The smear reveals masses of leukocytes, erythrocytes, and cellular debris. Cultures, which are negative for organisms causing specific disease entities, commonly yield *E. coli,* other coliform bacteria, and nonspecific pathogens. In addition to aerobic and anaerobic cultures, chlamydial, mycoplasmal, and viral specimens should be taken if laboratory facilities are available for processing them.

Nonspecific vulvovaginitis has several contributory factors. Vaginal foreign bodies cause discharges that are profuse, extremely malodorous, and sometimes bloody. The most frequent offender is a forgotten menstrual tampon or toilet paper. Improper or inadequate cleansing of the perineum after defecation also is responsible for many cases of chronic nonspecific vulvovaginitis, especially in mentally handicapped adolescent girls. Inquiry regarding perineal cleansing should be a part of the examination in such cases. If a male partner inserts his penis into the rectum first and then into the vagina or inadvertently touches the anal area before vaginal intercourse, coliform organisms are carried into the vagina.

The possibility that a vaginal discharge is caused by a tumor always should be remembered. A discharge, with or without bleeding, may be one of the first symptoms of adenosis or adenocarcinoma of the vagina and cervix. These neoplasms are associated with prenatal exposure to diethylstilbestrol and related synthetic estrogens.

Treatment[115]

The treatment of nonspecific vulvovaginitis in the postmenarcheal patient can be frustrating when no causative agent is found. Often, it is impossible to identify the causative agent.

Instruction in proper perineal cleansing after defecation eradicates a major source of nonspecific vaginal infections in teenagers just as it does in children. Advice regarding sexual habits is necessary in some cases if coital-related infections are to be avoided. Leukorrhea associated with oral contraceptives must be tolerated by the patient, or her method of contraception must be changed. Noninfectious cervical hypersecretion during the early postmenarcheal period can be controlled by frequent bathing and frequent changes of underclothing.

In the majority of cases, nonspecific vulvovaginitis unassociated with a chronic cervicitis responds to sulfonamide (Sultrin vaginal cream) or antimicrobial creams (AVC vaginal cream) inserted at bedtime for 14 days. As a general rule, creams are preferable because they spread over a larger area of the vaginal mucosa than do suppositories. Acidification of the vagina by the nightly insertion of an acetic acid preparation, pH 4.0 (Aci-Jel cream), for a few weeks may be all that is necessary; it hastens the return of a normal vaginal flora and creates an unfriendly environment for nonspecific pathogens.

Vaginal douching sometimes is considered helpful in the treatment of nonspecific vulvovaginitis. Recent data, however, suggest a causative relationship between vaginal douching and pelvic inflammatory disease in inner-city populations at high risk for acquiring sexually transmitted diseases.[237] Therefore, vaginal douching strongly should be discouraged.

TOXIC SHOCK SYNDROME

First recognized in the late 1970s, toxic shock syndrome is a relatively uncommon, serious, sometimes fatal, acute infection most often encountered in otherwise healthy adolescent girls and young women who use menstrual tampons. It also has been reported, however, in men, children, women who do not use tampons, and nonmenstruating women. All types of tampons have been associated with it. Its incidence has decreased since women have become aware of the hazards associated with the improper use of menstrual tampons. This entity is discussed fully in Chapter 74.

VULVOVAGINAL VIRAL INFECTIONS

Herpes Genitalis

The Premenarcheal Patient[102]

Herpes simplex virus infections of the genitalia are rare in children. The mode of acquisition of the infection is not known always, but case reports describe the possibility of autoinoculation from oral lesions, physical contact by a mother's infected finger, and sexual abuse.[126] Therefore, the presence of herpes simplex virus genital lesions in a child or any disease that is known to be sexually transmitted in an adult should raise a question about whether she has been subjected to some type of sexual molestation. It is known that the virus can be isolated from the pharynx or vagina of about 5 per cent of asymptomatic adults. Such persons are carriers and may transmit the infection to susceptible contacts. It is not surprising, therefore, that children would have either herpes simplex virus type 1 or 2 genital lesions.

Herpetic lesions on the vulva begin as small, erythematous spots. Papules quickly develop on the inflamed areas. The papules, in turn, become serum-filled vesicles that rupture, leaving slightly eroded red areas. The latter become covered with crusts, which remain for a few days.

The lesions typically cause pruritus and burning. If they do not become secondarily infected, they heal within 2 weeks.

Herpes limited to the genitalia of a healthy child is a painful but relatively benign disease. An infection in a poorly nourished child may spread beyond the vulva and become a serious, life-endangering matter.

The treatment of genital herpes is discussed later.

The Adolescent Patient[153]

Herpes simplex virus is the most common cause of vesiculoulcerative disease of the adult genitalia. It is sexually transmitted, and its increasing frequency in teenage girls is related to their sexual activity.

As noted in Chapter 163, there are two types of herpes simplex virus, which can be antigenically and culturally distinguished from each other. Type 1 is the causative agent in oronasal cold sores. Type 2 is responsible for 90 per cent of genital herpes, but as Chang[35] has pointed out, genital infections with type 1 have become more common; he relates their increasing incidence to the more frequent engagement in genital-oral sex play.

Seroprevalence studies show that type 2 antibodies do not begin to appear until the early teens. The frequency gradually rises through late adulthood and is related to sexual activity, especially with multiple partners. Type 2 infections are highly contagious and may be transmitted by carriers who are asymptomatic. Approximately 9 per cent of private patients and 22 per cent of public clinic patients have serologic evidence of prior type 2 infection.[26, 208] Because of its frequency and its diverse clinical appearance, it should be considered in the differential diagnosis of all vulvar vesiculoulcerative lesions. It may, because of its acute symptoms, mask the presence of concurrently acquired other venereal disease; the patient with herpes genitalis always should be examined for gonorrhea and syphilis.

Three presentations of genital disease are recognized: primary initial, nonprimary initial, and recurrent infection. Primary initial genital herpes infection develops with no preexisting herpes antibody. A nonprimary initial infection develops in a person for the first time with preexisting herpes antibody. Recurrent infection is diagnosed when a person has a history of prior similar genital infection. Patients with nonprimary initial infection have fewer lesions, less pain, fewer constitutional symptoms, shorter duration of viral shedding, and an overall shorter course of illness.[187]

A primary infection begins with sexual contact with an infected person 2 to 8 days preceding the onset of symptoms. There is likely to be a prodromal episode of fever, malaise, and myalgias, often accompanied by vulvar paresthesia and burning; dysuria; and tender, nonsuppurative inguinal lymphadenopathy.

The primary lesions, often involving all of the vulvar tissues, the vaginal mucosa, and the cervix, occur over a 2-week period. They first appear as papules surrounded by an erythematous zone, and these subsequently become vesiculopustular lesions. The vesicles enlarge and rupture, exposing shallow ulcerations. During the acute phase of a severe infection, there is more or less edema and generalized erythema of the vulvar mucosa (Fig. 49–16).

As a rule, the ulcers become covered with a firm yellow crust that drops off after a week or so, leaving a smooth, red area that eventually disappears. The lesions usually are asymptomatic in from 10 to 21 days, depending on the severity of the infection. Secondary bacterial infection and a coexisting immunodeficiency state, such as HIV infection, delay healing. Urethral and vesical involvement may cause severe dysuria, leading to retention of urine. Proctitis may occur in females who engage in anal intercourse, although perianal ulcers also may occur without anal intercourse.

Herpes simplex virus can be cultured from the cervix in 90 per cent of females with primary type 2 infection. The cervix appears abnormal in almost 90 per cent of cases with positive cultures. The cervical lesions are ulcerations on the exocervix and may range from erythema to severe necrotic cervicitis. Acute cervicitis may be the only manifestation of primary herpes simplex virus infection.

Inguinal lymphadenopathy and moderate lower abdominal pain may be present, but, if they are, they usually occur only with the more severe first eruption. Tender inguinal lymphadenopathy is the last to resolve. If the urethra is involved, dysuria may be severe enough to cause urinary retention. The insertion of a vaginal speculum may be exquisitely painful. Extension to the perianal area may cause severe discomfort on defecation. Complete healing of lesions at all sites occurs in about 3 weeks. Once healed, herpetic lesions rarely leave scars.

The diagnosis of herpes genitalis usually is not difficult. The intense pain and the superficial vesiculoulcerative lesions with their irregular margins and red areolae sufficiently are characteristic to make clinical identification easy in a typical case. A laboratory confirmation should be attempted in all children and adolescents. Direct isolation of herpes simplex virus by tissue culture is the most reliable method and is best when the specimen is taken from a lesion within the first 48 hours of onset of symptoms. The presence of multinucleated giant cells in a cervicovaginal smear (Papanicolaou smear) (Fig. 49–17) or in the herpetic fluid smear with Tzanck preparation confirms the diagnosis for practical purposes. These tests, however, are only 40 to 50 per cent sensitive compared with culture. Serodiagnosis with type-specific antisera by Western blot assay showing a rise in anti–herpes simplex virus titer may be useful in documenting a primary type 2 infection but has limited usefulness in secondary infection.

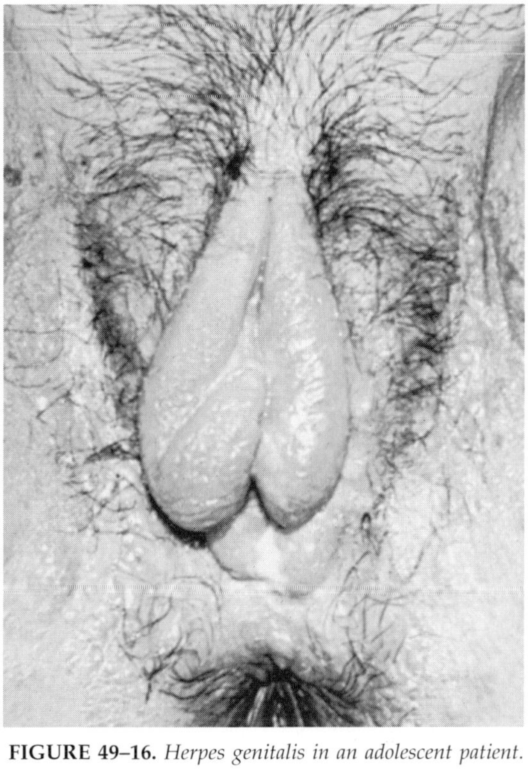

FIGURE 49–16. *Herpes genitalis in an adolescent patient.*

For many weeks after the infection has subsided clinically and the patient appears to be cured, type 2 virus can be recovered from her cervix and vagina. The latent virus may infect others or cause recurrent infections in its host. Although the recurrence rate of herpes genitalis is unknown, as many as 80 per cent of patients with type 2 infection develop recurrent episodes. Factors influencing recurrence rates are severity of the initial episode and host immune response to the disease. Emotional stress, heat, moisture, climate change, menstruation, pregnancy, oral contraceptive use, anesthesia, and trauma appear to be triggering factors. The median time from a primary infection to a secondary or recurrent infection is about 120 days.[40, 208, 232] Such recurrent episodes, although painful, usually are less severe than primary infections. Some patients have recurrences immediately preceding or at the time of each menstrual period. It has been suggested that genital herpes and squamous cell carcinoma of the cervix are related. Most of the evidence favoring this association originally came from seroepidemiologic studies. A much stronger association now has been observed between human papilloma virus DNA and cervical cancer. At most, herpes simplex virus may be causative or may be a cofactor in some cases of cervical cancer.[40, 65]

Treatment[32]

Acyclovir is the current drug of choice for genital herpes simplex virus infection. For the treatment of initial genital herpes, acyclovir orally, one 200-mg capsule five times a day, is administered for 7 to 10 days until clinical resolution occurs. Its use is reported to shorten the time the patient has pain, decrease the number of new lesions, hasten crusting, and reduce the time the virus can be found in the lesions. The earlier the treatment is started after the initial lesions appear, the sooner the patients obtain relief. In severe primary herpes infection with marked systemic symptoms, intravenous acyclovir, 15 to 30 mg/kg/day every 8 hours for 5 to 7 days or until clinical resolution occurs, is recommended. Frequent or severe recurrent disease may benefit from acyclovir if started within 2 days of onset of lesions or at the beginning of the prodrome. Oral acyclovir may be given at 200 mg five times a day for 5 days or 800 mg twice a day for 5 days. Daily suppressive treatment reduces recurrences by at least 75 per cent among patients with frequent recurrences. Oral acyclovir may be given at 200 mg two to five times a day or 400 mg twice a day for 1 year. Acyclovir should be discontinued after 1 year to reassess the recurrence rate.[32] The dosage regimen of oral acyclovir in treating prepubertal herpes genitalis is not known and, therefore, is not used commonly in this age group for mild cases. In moderate to severe cases, clinicians have prescribed approximately 50 per cent of the adult dose.

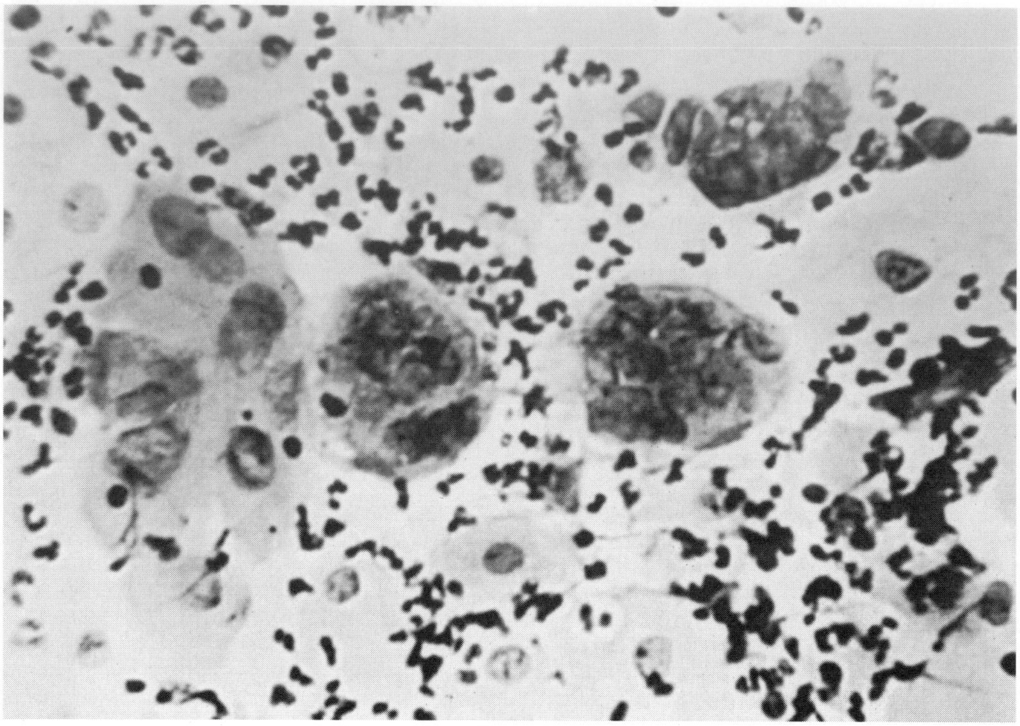

FIGURE 49–17. *Multinucleated giant cells in the vaginal smear are characteristic of herpes genitalis. (Courtesy of Dr. Herman L. Gardner.)*

Recurrences can be reduced in frequency in some cases if the patients can avoid stress-inducing situations. Topical anesthetics; cold, wet compresses; and sitz baths with 1:40 Burow solution frequently lessen local discomfort. Severe dysuria may be relieved by urinating when sitting in water. Local therapies used in the past, such as povidone-iodine solutions, photodynamic-dye light therapy, and topical surfactant, have not been found to be beneficial, but messy and potentially toxic.

Lesions caused by herpes simplex virus are relatively common among patients with HIV infection. Immunocompromised patients benefit from increased dosage of acyclovir; 400 mg orally three to five times a day has been found to be effective. For severe disease, hospitalization may be required for intravenous acyclovir treatment.[32]

Condylomata Acuminata[38, 58, 163]

Condylomata acuminata (venereal warts) are encountered in both premenarcheal children and teenage girls. The agent causing them is the human papilloma virus, a small, slow-growing virus of the papovavirus group. Several types of human papilloma virus cause exophytic genital warts and subclinical infection of the vagina and cervix. These include types 6, 11, 16, 18, and 31. Types 16, 18, and 31 have been associated with premalignant and malignant cervical carcinoma in females.

The Premenarcheal Patient[45, 87]

Perinatal transmission of the human papilloma virus to an infant is a recognized mode of infection. The incubation period can range from 2 months to 20 months or more. Therefore, initial onset of genital warts in a child older than 3 years of age is less likely to result from perinatal transmission. Condylomata acuminata are acquired by children as a result of close physical contact with an infected person, by digital infection of a child's genitalia by such a person, or by sexual contact with a person with the disease.[200] A history of condylomata in other members of the family, particularly the mother or older sisters who care for the child, sometimes may be elicited. Perinatal exposure, poor hygiene, and shared bathing have been suggested sources of infection.[216, 217] In one study, up to 91 per cent of cases were reported to be sexually transmitted.[109] However, types 6, 11, 16, and 18 are seen in adults with anogenital warts and are the most common genital types seen in children. This finding has raised questions about warts in children resulting from sexual abuse. In a number of cases, however, the mode of transmission is not known.[46]

Warts may cover the entire vulva. Most often, however, those in premenarcheal girls are single or scattered cauliflower-like lesions (Fig. 49–18) that have a predilection for the smooth, moist mucosa covering the inner surfaces of the labia minora, for the mucosa about the urethral meatus, and for the lining of the fossa navicularis. The vestibular mucosa may be studded with innumerable minute excrescences.

Condylomata in children seldom become ulcerative, but sessile condylomata arising within the vagina may become necrotic, produce a bloody vaginal discharge, and resemble, on cursory examination, a mixed mesodermal tumor (sarcoma botryoides) of the vagina. Although not tumors, condylomata acuminata should be considered in the differential diagnosis of vaginal neoplasms. As DNA typing becomes more widely available, a biopsy of the warts should be performed for diagnosis and to assess prognosis. HIV infection should be considered in infants and children with severe, extensive warts.

The Adolescent Patient[45, 187]

Condylomata acuminata develop in adolescent girls by sexual transmission. In support of the contention that the

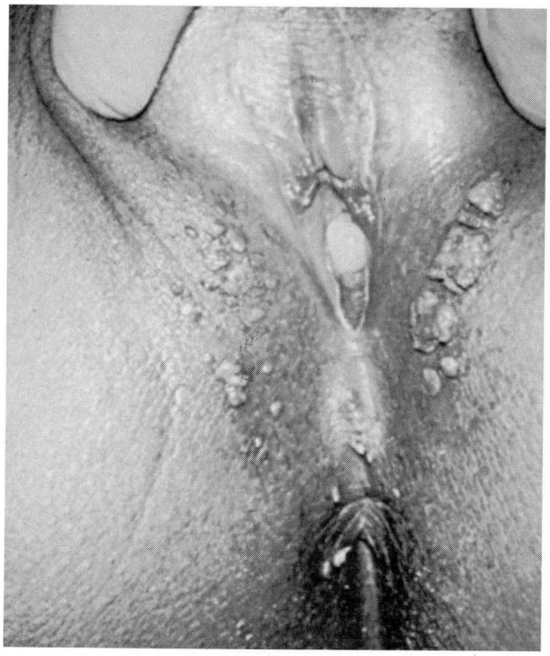

FIGURE 49–18. *Condylomata acuminata usually are single or scattered relatively small warts in premenarcheal children.*

infection is venereal is Teokharov's[224] observation that approximately 65 per cent of the sexual partners of persons with condylomata developed the disease within 3 to 4 months after contact. The prevalence of human papilloma virus in adolescent and young adult females ranges from 11 to 46 per cent, depending on the method of human papilloma virus DNA detection used. The polymerase chain reaction technique is more sensitive than the dot-blot hybridization method (ViraPap; Life Technologies, Gaithersburg, MD). As seen in adult women, the prevalence of human papilloma virus in adolescents as detected by DNA isolation techniques is far higher than the prevalence of active disease. The cell mediated or T-cell immune system appears to play an important role in whether the presence of virus results in clinically manifested disease. Cofactors of human papilloma virus infection are herpes, cervicitis, and tobacco use. Immunosuppression from a variety of conditions is associated with a greater likelihood of human papilloma virus disease in patients. These include renal transplant, Hodgkin disease, and HIV infection patients.[186, 187]

In the teenage postmenarcheal girl, condylomata usually form discrete, sessile, vegetative, wart-like growths covered with folded grayish-pink epithelium. They are found most frequently on the smooth mucosa of the vulvar vestibule. Usually, they are accompanied by more or less vaginal discharge, which is increased by moisture that exudes from between the leaf-like folds of the warty masses. Most often there is associated pruritus and secondary infection. Warts are more likely to become necrotic in adults than in children. Contact lesions frequently appear on contiguous surfaces. Huge condylomatous masses (Fig. 49–19) that completely hide the introitus are not uncommon in adolescent patients; if not treated, these huge growths may invade the rectum. Vaginal and cervical lesions commonly accompany those on the vulva.

Vulvar condylomata have a 50 to 60 per cent incidence of cervical disease detected by the presence of koilocytotic cells on Papanicolaou smears from the cervix. Therefore, a Papanicolaou smear is recommended twice a year in adolescents with vulvar and vaginal warts. Application of 3 to 5 per cent acetic acid to suspicious areas on the cervix reveals tiny white "acetowhite" flecks. In cases with cervical human papilloma virus infection without dysplasia, approximately 15 per cent progress to cervical intraepithelial neoplasm during a 2-year period.

Treatment

The goal of treatment is removal of warts and the amelioration of symptoms—not the eradication of human papilloma virus. No therapy has been shown to eradicate human papilloma virus. Cryotherapy is the most effective method of treating single or multiple small condylomata in infants and children.[115] General anesthesia usually is required. Emans and Goldstein[60] recommend carbon dioxide laser under general anesthesia. This may be done in an outpatient surgery setting when few lesions are present. Electrocautery, electrocoagulation, or laser treatment may result in deep scarring after use and distort the vulva. Hospitalization is necessary for more extensive lesions. The older child usually tolerates cryotherapy without general anesthesia if she knows that there will be some tingling or burning sensation with it. Liquid nitrogen may be used in the same manner as solid carbon dioxide. Podophyllin ointment (see later) should not be used for the eradication of condylomata acuminata in young children because a child may digitally transfer some of the ointment to other body areas.

Warts occasionally disappear after application of 3 per cent iodochlorhydroxyquin (Vioform) with 1 per cent hydrocortisone. This preparation or other ointments containing bacitracin or polymyxin B may be worth trying before cryotherapy is used.

Currently available therapeutic methods are 22 to 94 per cent effective in clearing exophytic genital warts, and recurrence rates are high—at least 25 per cent within 3 months. Treatment appears to be more successful for genital warts

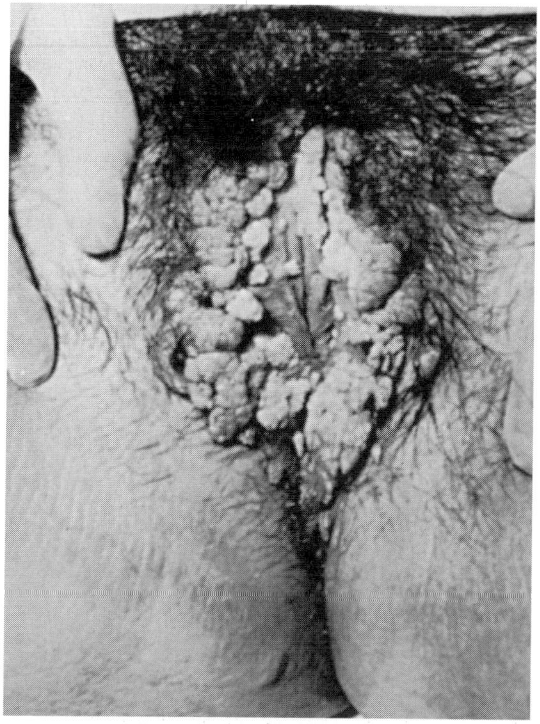

FIGURE 49–19. *Condylomata acuminata may form large masses covering the vulva in postmenarcheal patients.*

that are small and present for less than 1 year.[32] Condylomata acuminata can be treated with 25 per cent podophyllin in compound tincture of benzoin or a solution of 85 per cent trichloroacetic acid. The lesions that are treated so should be less than a centimeter in diameter and should not be in a confluent mass. The solution is applied to the wart only (not to the surrounding skin) for a period of 1 to 4 hours and then is removed with soap and water; treatment is repeated once weekly until the lesions have disappeared (usually 3 or 4 weeks). Urethral, anal, vaginal, and cervical lesions should not be treated with podophyllin. Normal skin is irritated by the ointment, and there is danger of injury to delicate tissues, particularly the eyes, if the patient inadvertently carries the medication to areas other than the point of application. Electrocautery, electrocoagulation, or laser treatment often is used for larger or resistant lesions (Fig. 49–20). These procedures are not recommended for lesions proximal to the anal range. Huge masses must be excised.

Alternative treatments for adolescents are topical 5-fluorouracil in 5 per cent creams and local interferon. 5-Fluorouracil is preferable for vaginal and intraurethral warts because it causes erosive dermatitis of normal surrounding skin. Use of 5-fluorouracil appears to be more effective than use of the laser for exophytic warts in the vagina.[45]

All adolescents with condylomatous changes noted on the Papanicolaou smear or with cervical warts should undergo colposcopy with biopsies of suspicious areas.

Molluscum Contagiosum[140]

Molluscum contagiosum is a viral infection of the skin characterized by small, discrete, translucent, grayish-pink, umbilicated, wart-like papules that sometimes are surrounded by a narrow ring of erythema. The lesions, which are asymptomatic, usually are less than 5 mm in diameter and may be missed by both the patient and an examiner. The disease, transmitted by close physical contact, is encountered most often in postmenarcheal patients on the inner surfaces of the thighs and perineum. Although lesions on the lower abdomen and thighs have caused it to be classed with the venereal diseases, coitus is not necessary for its transmission. Pediatricians frequently encounter it on the nongenital skin of children. It can be contracted from contaminated towels, bedding, garments, and so on. Lesions of molluscum contagiosum on the lower abdomen, pubis, thighs, or perineum of a child are tacit evidence of sexual contact.

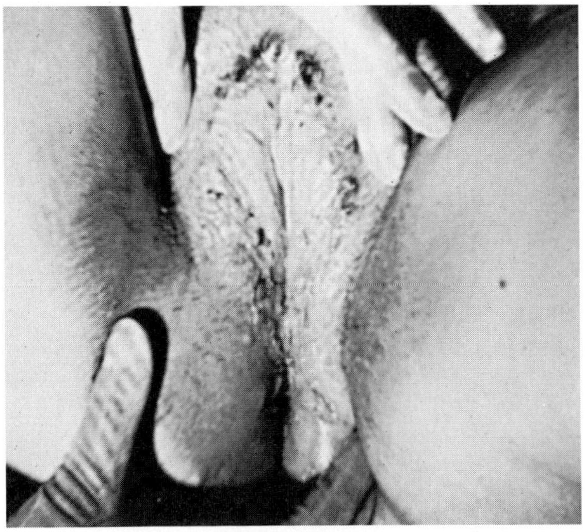

FIGURE 49–20. *The appearance of the vulva 10 days after electrocoagulation and surgical excision of the condylomatous mass shown in Figure 49–19.*

The appearance of the lesions usually is sufficient to establish the diagnosis. It can be confirmed by finding large, intracytoplasmic inclusion bodies in a smear or biopsy from a lesion.

Treatment consists of lifting off the roof of each lesion and lightly curetting its base. Cryotherapy also gives good results.

VULVOVAGINAL GRANULOMATOUS AND ULCERATIVE DISORDERS

Sexually transmitted genital ulcerative diseases occur throughout the world but are found most frequently in tropical countries. Genital ulcers are a relatively common finding on evaluation of adolescent and adult patients with genital symptoms. They are less common in young children. Ulcers usually are secondary lesions that result from breakdown of vesicles, papules, or pustules. By the time many patients with genital infections seek medical attention for their symptoms, the primary lesion has proceeded to ulceration.[207] Microbial causes vary by geographic region and socioeconomic status: herpes simplex is the most common cause in Western Europe and North America, whereas chancroid is most common in the tropics; in the United States, syphilis and chancroid are more common among urban minority groups, whereas herpes simplex is more common among more affluent groups. Complications of sexually transmitted genital ulcerative diseases also are more common in developing countries. The complication often is the reason for presentation.[150]

Herpes simplex virus infection, syphilis, chancroid, lymphogranuloma venereum, granuloma inguinale, and tuberculosis all may present with genital ulcers as a major clinical finding (Table 49–5). Although each of these diseases has a characteristic lesion and course, there is considerable overlap, so diagnosis based on history and physical appearance alone often is inaccurate. Herpetic ulcers, contrary to classic presentations, can be painless, and syphilis chancres can be painful at times. Secondary infection of an ulcerated area may cause pain in lesions that are characteristically painless. Also, more than one sexually transmitted disease may be present among at least 3 to 10 per cent of patients with genital ulcers.

Genital ulcers also may result from infestation, fixed drug eruption, mechanical or chemical trauma, autoimmune processes (such as Behçet syndrome and Crohn disease), and neoplasia. Presence of ulcers in sites other than the genital regions or oropharynx suggests a noninfectious etiology.

In the United States, most patients with genital ulcers have herpes genitalis, syphilis, chancroid, or a combination thereof. Empiric treatment often must be given before diagnostic test results are available, and laboratory confirmation of a specific diagnosis is lacking in at least one-quarter of patients with genital ulcer disease. Treatment for syphilis and chancroid should be considered in such circumstances, especially in geographic regions where chancroid morbidity is notable (see later).[32, 161] The diagnosis and treatment of the listed infectious etiologies of genital ulcers and Behçet syndrome are discussed in this chapter and elsewhere in this text.

Genital ulcers of any etiology, but especially those caused by herpes, syphilis, chancroid, and granuloma inguinale, are associated with an increased risk of HIV infection. Serologic testing for HIV infection therefore should be considered in the management of patients with genital ulcers.[32, 150] Improved treatment of sexually transmitted diseases can affect

TABLE 49–5. Diagnostic Features of Genital Ulcerations Caused by Sexually Transmitted Diseases

Feature	Primary Syphilis	Genital Herpes	Chancroid	Lymphogranuloma Venereum	Granuloma Inguinale
Incubation period	9–90 days, avg. 2–4 weeks	2–7 days	Range 1–35 days, avg. 3–7 days	3 days to 3 weeks, avg. 10–14 days	Precise data unavailable; probably from a few days to several months
Number of lesions	Usually one, may be multiple	Multiple; may coalesce, more with primary episodes than with recurrences	Usually 1–3, may be multiple	Usually single	Single or multiple
Description of genital ulcers	Sharply demarcated round or oval ulcer with slightly elevated edges; may be irregular, symmetric "kissing chancre"	Small, superficial, grouped vesicles, erosions, or both; lesions may coalesce, forming bullae or large areas of ulcerations; lesions have irregular borders	Superficial, shallow, sharply demarcated ulcer; irregular, ragged, undermined edge; size from a few millimeters to 2 cm in diameter	Papule, pustule, vesicle, or ulcer discrete and transient; frequently overlooked	Sharply defined, irregular ulcerations or hypertrophic, verrucous, necrotic, or cicatricial granulomas
Base	Red, smooth, and shiny or crusty; oozing serous exudate when squeezed	Bright red and smooth	Rough, uneven, yellow to gray	Variable	Usually friable, rough, beefy granulations; can be necrotic, verrucous, or cicatricial
Induration	Firm; does not change shape with pressure	None	Soft; changes shape with pressure	None	Firm granulation tissue
Pain	Painless; may become tender if secondarily infected	Common; more prominent with initial infection than recurrences	Common	Variable	Rare
Inguinal lymphadenopathy	Unilateral or bilateral, firm, movable, and nontender; does not suppurate	Usually bilateral, firm, and tender; more common in primary episodes than in recurrences	Unilateral, bilateral rarely occurs; overlying erythema; matted, fixed, and tender; suppuration may occur	Unilateral or bilateral; initially movable, firm, and tender; later indolent; fixed and matted; "sign of groove" may suppurate; fistulae	Pseudobuboes; subcutaneous perilymphatic granulomatous lesions that produce inguinal swellings
Constitutional symptoms	Rare	Common in primary episode; less likely in recurrences	Rare	Frequent	Rare
Course of untreated disease	Slowly (2–6 weeks) resolves to latency	Recurrence is the rule	May progress to erosive lesions	Local lesions heal; systemic disease may progress; disfiguring; late complications	Worsens slowly
Diagnostic tests	Dark-field examination, direct immunofluorescence, FTA-ABS, VDRL	Tzanck smear, culture, Pap smear, direct immunofluorescence, electron microscopy, direct immunoperoxidase staining, serology	Culture, biopsy (rarely used), Gram-stained smears have low specificity	Complement fixation, isolation of the microorganism by culture	"Donovan bodies" in tissue smears; biopsy

From Mroczkowski, T. R., and Martin, D. H.: Genital ulcer disease. Dermatol. Clin. North Am. *12*:753–764, 1994.

the rate of HIV seroconversion in a population: HIV seroconversion was reduced by 40 per cent over a 2-year follow-up period in rural communities in Tanzania where treatment programs were instituted, compared with control communities with no programs.[89]

Lymphogranuloma Venereum

Lymphogranuloma venereum is a sexually transmitted disease characterized by chronicity, indolent inflammatory infiltration, granulomatous ulceration, abscess formation, and fibrotic cicatrization of the inguinal, perineal, and rectal lymphatics. The infecting agent is *C. trachomatis* subtypes L1 to L3. It occurs more often in tropical than in temperate climates.

The Premenarcheal Patient

Lymphogranuloma venereum has been reported in children.[14, 86, 233] The disease usually is acquired in childhood as a result of sexual contact. Transmission also may occur by accidental inoculation of infected material from family members, such as by handling of garments or towels that have been contaminated by drainage from ulcerative lesions or buboes. However, sexual abuse always should be considered. There is little evidence of transplacental or perinatal transmission of the lymphogranuloma venereum serovars of *C. trachomatis*.[86]

The primary lesion, a small papule or superficial and relatively asymptomatic ulcer, seldom is seen in either children or older patients. A prodromal episode of fever, malaise, and joint pain accompanied by leukocytosis, anemia, and an increased sedimentation rate may precede local signs. These symptoms often are mild and not diagnostically significant.

The most common presentations in prepubertal children are inguinal lymphadenopathy and proctitis. The glands may be swollen and tender for a time and then regress spontaneously. More often, if treatment is not initiated, they progress to abscess formation and then rupture, developing draining sinuses. Rectal, anal, and deep pelvic tissue infiltration with rectal and colonic strictures is not common in children. Arthritis, usually of the knees and erythema nodosum, occasionally occurs in children, as it does in older patients.[86]

The Adolescent Patient

Adolescents usually acquire lymphogranuloma venereum through sexual activity. The primary lesion, a small papule, vesicle, or shallow ulcer on the vulva (Fig. 49–21), vaginal wall, or cervix, seldom is seen. Cervicitis is a more common presentation of primary lymphogranuloma venereum, and the primary lesion often is asymptomatic, heals rapidly, and leaves no scar. The incubation period usually is 2 to 5 days after exposure, but several weeks may elapse before the primary lesion appears.[86, 115]

Painful enlargement of the inguinal lymph nodes generally occurs after the initial lesions. Inguinal adenitis usually is unilateral in the early stages of infection. The perirectal lymph nodes occasionally are the first to be involved; pain on defecation is an early symptom when this occurs. The rectovaginal septum may become involved when the posterior vagina is a primary site of infection.

If the disease goes untreated, it may enter a secondary stage called the inguinal syndrome, in which the inguinal glands and the surrounding subcutaneous tissues become a brawny mass that adheres to the indurated, purplish-red overlying skin. The nodes increase in size and form abscesses

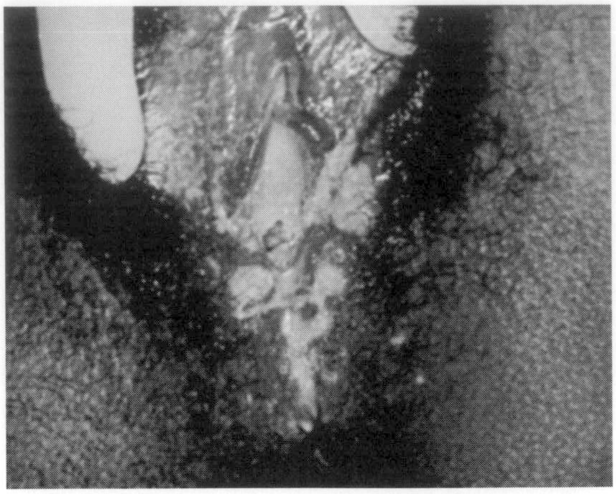

FIGURE 49–21. *Early lesions of lymphogranuloma venereum in the form of herpetic-like ulcers in an adolescent. The diagnosis was confirmed serologically.*

(buboes). Unless aspirated, the buboes rupture and create chronically draining sinuses.[115] Enlargement of lymph nodes above and below the inguinal ligament may lead to the "groove" sign.[86] Complaints of lower abdominal pain and backache may indicate concurrent proctitis. The deep iliac nodes may be enlarged in 75 per cent of cases; rupture of these may cause large pelvic abscesses.

Healing of draining buboes is slow, and severe scarring occurs. In the vast majority of cases, healing of buboes indicates the end of the disease. Relapses have been reported in 20 per cent of untreated cases. Disseminated disease, hepatitis, pneumonia, arthritis, erythema nodosum, erythema multiforme, and ocular infection can occur in association with the inguinal syndrome.

The anogenitorectal syndrome is a subacute manifestation of lymphogranuloma venereum. It includes proctocolitis and hyperplasia of intestinal and perirectal lymphatic tissue. Perirectal abscesses often develop and lead to ischiorectal and rectovaginal fistulas, anal fistulas, and rectal stricture or stenosis. The clinical presentation consists of fever, rectal pain, and abdominal cramping. Progression of the disease causes rectal bleeding and purulent rectal discharge. Rectal strictures lead to constipation and "pencil stools." Weight loss, bowel perforation, and peritonitis may occur. Genital elephantiasis (esthiomene) may occur with chronic infection.

The diagnosis of lymphogranuloma venereum is considered whenever a patient has a tender, enlarged inguinal gland or an ulcerative or granulomatous lesion of the vulva, perineum, vagina, or cervix. Acutely painful, unilateral inguinal lymphadenitis strongly suggests lymphogranuloma venereum. A definitive diagnosis is made by identification of *C. trachomatis* serotypes L1, L2, or L3 in tissue cultures of material from buboes or ulcerative lesions. Sensitivity of culture for lymphogranuloma venereum is only about 50 per cent, however.[124] Serologic tests may be used when cultures are negative or buboes are not present. Complement fixation has been available since the 1930s and 1940s. In clinical settings suggestive of lymphogranuloma venereum, a complement fixation antibody titer of 1:64 or higher is considered diagnostic. Most patients with lymphogranuloma venereum have titers of 1:128 or higher. Titers between acute and convalescent specimens may not rise because most patients present for care well after the acute phase of the infection. Cross-reaction with other chlamydial serotypes occurs, but titers higher than 1:16 are rare with chlamydial urethritis. Microimmunofluorescence is more specific than complement fixation and can detect IgM and IgG titers. This test is not widely available, however.[124]

Complement fixation remains the recommended test for diagnosis when the clinical presentation leads to a presumptive diagnosis of lymphogranuloma venereum. If complement fixation titers are negative, repeat testing in a few weeks may be helpful in patients who happen to present relatively early in the course of illness. DNA probes or monoclonal antibodies specific for lymphogranuloma venereum serovars may become available in the near future.

Lymphogranuloma venereum must be differentiated from syphilis, with which it may coexist. False-positive venereal disease research laboratories results may occur with 20 per cent of patients with lymphogranuloma venereum. When the diagnosis is in doubt, specific tests for antitreponemal antibodies must be used to rule out syphilis. The disease is differentiated from other granulomatous and ulcerative disorders by specific tests for each, by biopsy, and by the clinical appearance of the lesions (see Table 49–4).

Treatment[32]

The earlier the diagnosis is made and treatment started, the better the response to therapy and the less serious the tissue destruction. Fluctuant buboes are aspirated, not incised, before they rupture. The discharge from the ulcerated areas and buboes is infectious, so precautions against transmission of the disease must be taken. The patient will be more comfortable if kept in bed. Ice cold compresses may be applied to the inguinal areas. The vulva is cleansed gently twice daily.

The preferred treatment for lymphogranuloma venereum is doxycycline, 100 mg orally twice a day for 21 days.[32] Alternatives, which are preferred in pediatric patients younger than 8 years of age, are erythromycin and sulfisoxazole. Either of these also should be given for 21 days. Because of the potential for shorter treatment courses and improved compliance, azithromycin may become a treatment option for lymphogranuloma venereum in the future. It cannot be recommended now because data are insufficient.

After treatment is initiated, patients should be followed clinically until signs and symptoms have resolved. Persons who have had sexual contact with a patient with lymphogranuloma venereum during the 30 days before the onset of symptoms should be examined, tested for chlamydial infection, and treated.[32]

Adolescents are likely to be treated before they develop the extensive anal and rectal strictures and distorting vulvar cicatrizations for which extensive surgery sometimes is necessary in older patients.

Granuloma Inguinale[24, 54, 103, 134, 159]

Granuloma inguinale is a chronic disease characterized by ulcerative granulomatous lesions of the skin and subcutaneous tissues (Fig. 49–22) (see Table 49–5). Common synonyms for the infection include granuloma venereum and donovanosis. The disease most often affects the external genitalia, perineum, and inguinal regions, but the vagina, cervix, and, rarely, distant extragenital sites may be involved. The disease is caused by *Calymmatobacterium granulomatis* (*Donovania granulomatis,* Donovan bodies), an encapsulated, gram-negative bacillus.

Granuloma inguinale is common in the tropical and subtropical regions of the world.[160] It is relatively rare in developed countries. In the United States, 19 cases were reported in 1993, of whom 4 involved female patients who were suspected to have been seen as a result of international travel and immigration.[53] A case in a white adolescent female in California was reported in 1985.[90] The male-to-female ratio appears to be at least 2:1. The disease is rare in premenarcheal children, but it should be considered in the differential diagnosis of granulomatous lesions of the genitalia in adolescents.

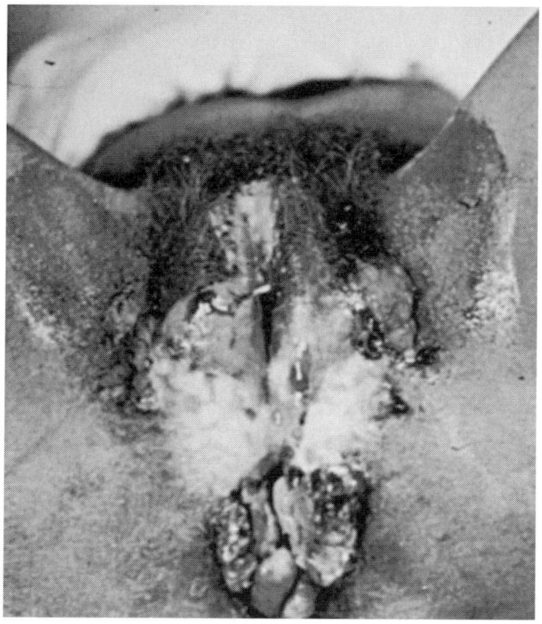

FIGURE 49–22. *Granuloma inguinale.*

The disease clearly is transmitted during sexual intercourse among adolescents and adults. However, the close physical contact of the inguinal, perineal, and genital regions that occurs during sexual activity, and not intercourse per se, probably is more important for transmission of the infection. The organism is not highly contagious; sexual partners of patients with granuloma inguinale often do not become infected. Breaches in the integrity of the skin or mucous membranes, such as with minor trauma, may be required for an inoculum to establish a successful infection.[103] The disease apparently can be transmitted to young children by contaminated clothing or towels. Close physical contact, such as sitting on the lap of an infected parent, also has been reported as a mode of transmission to young children.[241]

The incubation period usually is less than 2 weeks but may be as long as 3 months.[103] The first manifestation of infection usually is single or multiple small, relatively painless hard nodules on the vulva or perineum that erode the skin and form ulcers. Genital tract bleeding is the next most common presentation. Ulcers are shallow and have a beefy, granular base that is friable and bleeds easily. The edges are nodular, raised, and undermined. They usually are painless, unless they become infected secondarily.[159]

If left untreated, lesions progress slowly outward by eccentric expansion of the leading edge. Over time, this ulcerative stage involves large areas of the perineum, external genitalia, and surrounding skin surfaces. The central areas usually remain ulcerative but may become hypertrophic. Hypertrophic lesions consist of large, vegetating masses with overgrowth of granulation tissue. Less frequently, lesions develop extensive, destructive necrosis or are dry with sclerotic scarring, which distorts the tissues. Lymphedema of distal tissues is common during the course of the disease. Lymphatic obstruction or elephantiasis occasionally results in enlargement of the clitoris or labia.[103, 159] Subcutaneous granulation tissue occurs in about 5 per cent of cases and may mimic the appearance of bubo formation, called pseudobuboes. When true regional adenopathy occurs in the course of granuloma inguinale, it generally represents a response to a secondary infection and may be painful.

Extragenital disease may occur in up to 6 per cent of cases and usually involves the head and neck. Autoinoculation is postulated as the source of infection of these sites.[73] Occasional involvement of the liver, thorax, and bones remote from the primary genital site suggests that hematogenous spread can occur. Systemic disease is encountered more frequently in females with cervical lesions and is associated with prolonged spiking fever, anemia, and weight loss.[25, 130, 176]

Successful isolation of *C. granulomatis* rarely has proved feasible. Reliable culture techniques are not available yet. Therefore, the diagnosis of granuloma inguinale is based on the presence of Donovan bodies in large, histiocytic cells on crush preparations from lesions (Fig. 49–23). A portion of granulation tissue is removed and pressed onto a clean slide, which is allowed to air-dry. The slide then is stained with Giemsa, Wright, or Warthin-Starry stain. Donovan bodies, which are pathognomonic for granuloma inguinale, are vacuolar compartments within the cytoplasm, which contain up to 20 to 30 viable organisms.[54] Histopathologic study of biopsy specimens sometimes is required for diagnosis. Biopsy should be performed in very early, very sclerotic, or heavily superinfected specimens. Organisms that are more scarce or smear or crush specimens are likely to fail in such circumstances. Biopsy also should be performed when malignancy is thought possible or when antibiotic therapy does not lead to improvement.[124]

Complement fixation and indirect immunofluorescence have been developed but have limited specificities. A more recently developed serologic test using indirect immunofluorescence may be helpful in the future for epidemiologic studies.[124]

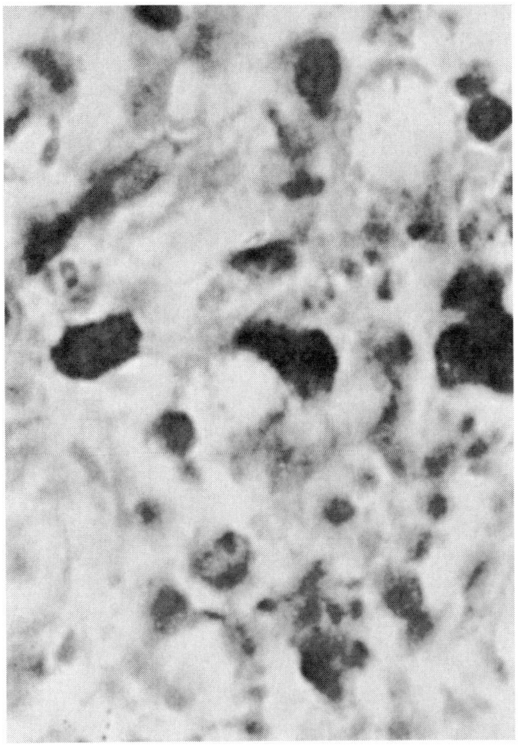

FIGURE 49–23. *Donovan bodies.*

The differential diagnosis of granuloma inguinale includes carcinoma, syphilis, tuberculosis, chancroid, lymphogranuloma venereum, condyloma acuminata, blastomycosis, schistosomiasis, and other granulomatous diseases.[17, 103, 159] Sexually transmitted diseases, such as syphilis, may coexist with granuloma inguinale. Darkfield examination of tissue specimens and serologic tests for syphilis should be performed. Biopsy may be required to rule out neoplasia or tuberculosis.[73] Chancroid ulcers tend to be deeper and more ragged and often have associated bubo formation. Physical examination alone, however, often is not sufficient to distinguish any one of these processes from the others (see Table 49–5). Granuloma inguinale also is associated with the development of carcinoma within areas that have been involved in the ulcerative process.

Treatment

Tetracycline probably is the drug of choice for treatment of granuloma inguinale. Doxycycline is likely as effective and may result in improved compliance. Alternatives include trimethoprim-sulfamethoxazole and erythromycin, either of which could be used in a young child. Chloramphenicol and gentamicin also may be used.[184]

Treatment should be continued for at least 2 to 3 weeks and until ulcerative lesions have re-epithelialized. Vulvar lesions usually heal within 2 weeks of therapy, but cervical and pelvic lesions may require greater than 3 months of therapy. Incomplete treatment may result in recurrence with extensive fibrosis and scarring.[17] The disease recurs in about 10 per cent of cases. Surgery may be required for complications of granuloma inguinale, such as elephantiasis, strictures, and pelvic abscesses.[184]

Precautions regarding infections should be taken in the home or hospital until the lesions are healed. Sexual contacts of persons with donovanosis should be traced and examined but treated only if lesions are found.[184] Adolescent girls who have had granuloma inguinale should be kept under clinical surveillance for many years for potential development of carcinomas in the perineum and genital tract.

Chancroid[4, 236]

Chancroid is an acute, ulcerative disease that primarily involves the external genitalia. The causative agent, *Haemophilus ducreyi,* is a fastidious, gram-negative coccobacillus that is transmitted by physical contact, usually during sexual intercourse with an infected person. The incubation period usually is 3 to 7 days but may be longer.

Chancroid is well established as a co-factor for transmission of HIV infection.[32, 33] It is more common in tropical and subtropical regions than in developed countries. Its frequency is increasing in many parts of the world.[162] Chancroid is endemic in the United States, and discrete outbreaks occasionally are seen. The disease is underrecognized and underreported.[33]

Chancroid rarely is encountered in young children but occasionally is seen in sexually active adolescents.[101, 162] It is far more common in males than females for reasons that are unclear, although asymptomatic carriage in females has been hypothesized.[20, 101, 162]

The first sign of infection is a small, hyperemic macule. The macule becomes a papule and then a pustule before ulceration. The ulcer is painful and usually deep, with irregular borders and undermined edges. The base is gray and covered with purulent exudate laden with the ducreyi bacillus. Ulcers may occur on the vulva, vaginal mucosa, cervix, or anus but usually are found on the labia minora. Dysuria is a frequent complaint. Tenesmus and rectal bleeding may be associated with anal lesions. Single ulcers are common, but multiple ulcers occur more often. These may become contiguous to form large, eroded areas. Phagedenic destruction of the external genitalia may occur when treatment is not sought early in the course or a secondary infection develops in the ulcers. In such cases, scarring persists, despite successful eradication of the microbe.

Associated, painful inguinal adenitis occurs in one-quarter to one-half of cases. Adenitis is more common when genital ulcers have been present for more than 10 days. The skin overlying the nodes frequently is erythematous.

Many patients with chancroid have concurrent infections with other sexually transmitted diseases. Patients should be tested for HIV infection and syphilis when chancroid is diagnosed. Repeat testing should be performed in 3 months if initial results are negative.[32]

In the United States, a probable diagnosis of chancroid is made clinically if (1) the person has one or more painful genital ulcers and has no evidence of *T. pallidum* infection by either darkfield examination of ulcer exudate of a serologic test for syphilis performed at least 7 days after the onset of ulcers and (2) the clinical presentation of the ulcers is not typical of herpes genitalis or tests for herpes simplex virus are negative. When present, the combination of a painful ulcer with tender inguinal adenopathy suggests chancroid. A painful genital ulcer accompanied by suppurative inguinal adenopathy almost is pathognomonic for chancroid.[32]

Definitive diagnosis of chancroid requires isolation of *H. ducreyi* on special culture media that are not commercially available. Even when available, the sensitivity of culture usually is less than 80 per cent.[32] When culture is performed, exudate from the purulent base of the ulcer or material aspirated from buboes should be inoculated on medium that consists of chocolate agar with vancomycin, 3 μg/mL, and Isovitalex, 1 per cent. Gram-negative coccobacilli in a "school-of-fish" grouping on Gram stain suggests *H. ducreyi,* but this pattern often is not present. Diagnosis also can be based on the histologic appearance of tissue obtained by biopsy.

Rapid diagnostic tests using enzyme immunoassays and the polymerase chain reaction are under development but are not available for clinical use.[33, 197]

Treatment

Azithromycin (1 g orally in a single dose in adolescents and adults), ceftriaxone (250 mg intramuscularly in a single dose), and erythromycin base (500 mg orally four times a day for 7 days in adolescents and adults) are effective agents for the treatment of chancroid among patients without HIV infection. Trimethoprim-sulfamethoxazole no longer is recommended because of the frequency of resistant isolates of *H. ducreyi.* Amoxicillin plus clavulanic acid may be effective and requires a 7-day course. Quinolones, such as ciprofloxacin, also may be effective but are not approved for use in pediatric patients.[32]

Patients should be re-examined 3 to 7 days after initiation of therapy. Ulcers should improve symptomatically within 3 days and show objective improvement within 7 days if treatment is effective. If no clinical improvement occurs, the diagnosis may be incorrect, there may be co-infection with another sexually transmitted agent, the infecting strain may be resistant to the prescribed antimicrobial agent, compliance with multiple-dose regimens may have been poor, the patient may have HIV infection, or there may be some combination of these explanations. The time required for complete healing of ulcers is related to their size. Large ulcers may require 2 or more weeks.[32]

Resolution of fluctuant lymphadenopathy (buboes) is slower than that of ulcers. Drainage of buboes, when they occur, usually is required for resolution of the infection. Needle aspiration, if adequate drainage can be accomplished, is preferred over surgical incision because it results in less cicatricial scarring. Discharge from buboes and vulvar lesions is highly infectious; patient care should include precautions regarding infections. Healed ulcers frequently leave significant scarring.

Persons who have had sexual contact with a patient who has chancroid during the 10 days before onset of symptoms and thereafter should be examined and treated for chancroid, even in the absence of symptoms.[32] Patients co-infected with HIV should be followed closely. Longer courses of therapy may be required, and healing may be slower. Optimal duration of therapy in these patients is unknown.

Tuberculosis[104, 194, 218]

Even before the advent of chemotherapy for the treatment of tuberculosis, tuberculous disease of the lower genital tract was uncommon. Today, the scrofulous type is rare, and primary tuberculosis of the vulva and vagina is rarer still.

The primary lesions of vulvar tuberculosis are described as a relatively painless, slowly developing, localized, nodular thickening of the skin and subcutaneous tissues or as ulcerative "sores" that are rather firm, slightly raised, reddish areas. The ulcers are demarcated sharply, with undermined edges and granular, grayish-brown bases with tubercles and areas of caseation studding their bases.

The scrofulous type is characterized by fistulous tracts and burrowing sinuses that extend from underlying tuberculous infection in the bowel, bladder, or pelvic viscera. Drainage from the ulcers and sinuses keeps the surrounding skin macerated and leads to extension of the disease.

The diagnosis is not a problem if the patient is known to have visceral tuberculosis, as most often is the case. Isolation of *M. tuberculosis* from the discharge or lesions or examination of the biopsy specimen from the base of an ulcer is confirmatory. Primary tuberculosis of the vulva must be differentiated from other granulomatous diseases, and the scrofulous type must be distinguished from syphilis, lymphogranuloma inguinale, and Crohn disease.

Tuberculosis of the upper genital tract also is uncommon but frequently leads to infertility when it occurs, likely due to scarring of the uterine tubes.[191]

Treatment

The chemotherapeutic agents used in the treatment of pulmonary and other types of systemic tuberculosis also are effective in the treatment of the disease when it affects the genitalia. The treatment of tuberculosis is described in Chapter 101.

VULVOVAGINAL ULCERATIVE INFECTIONS

Behçet Syndrome[110, 129, 146, 158, 177]

In 1937, Behçet described a syndrome characterized by recurrent genital ulcers, aphthous stomatitis, and ocular inflammation. Arthritis, abnormalities of the central nervous system, a variety of skin lesions, and other systemic symptoms also may be associated with the disease. The cause of

Behçet syndrome is not known, but an autoimmune basis has been suggested. Onset usually occurs between 20 and 30 years of age. It is rare in children and occurs more often in girls than boys.[129]

The vulvar lesions take the form of destructive, deep ulcerations that, as they recur, result in marked scarring and distortion with a progressive loss of vulvar tissue (Fig. 49–24). In spite of their destructiveness, the lesions are relatively painless. The oral lesions resemble common aphthous ulcers and may precede all other manifestations of Behçet syndrome by 5 to 10 years or longer. Ocular inflammation may present as iridocyclitis or chorioretinitis or other posterior segment lesions. Hypopyon may be seen in some cases.

The vulvar lesions of Behçet syndrome are nonspecific in character. The diagnosis is based on the associated findings and negative test results for diseases that might resemble the vulvar ulcers, notably syphilis, herpes, the granulomatous disorders, and Crohn disease. Histologic study of biopsied material from an ulcer shows only vasculitis and chronic inflammation.

Many agents, including streptococcal vaccine, chloroquine, and estrogen preparations, have been used to treat Behçet syndrome in the past. Modern treatment regimens most commonly have used systemic corticosteroids, with or without chlorambucil; colchicine; azathioprine; or thalidomide. Recent studies have suggested that cyclosporin[167] and interferon-α[7] may be effective. Plastic surgery for the correction of vaginal distortions is contraindicated because trauma may be followed by an exacerbation of the disease.

Vulvar Vestibulitis

A syndrome of severe and persistent superficial dyspareunia has been recognized as a distinct clinical entity for many years. Vulvar vestibulitis is the term most commonly used for this syndrome,[18, 138, 175] although other terms, such as focal vulvitis, have been used.[168] The syndrome consists of the triad of severe pain on vestibular touch on attempted vaginal entry, tenderness to pressure localized within the vulvar vestibule, and physical findings limited to vulvar erythema of varying degrees.[142] Areas of focal, tender inflammation or ulceration on the vestibular mucosa that are 3 to 10 mm in size also have been described.[168]

Chronic inflammation in the squamous mucosa and in the periglandular and periductal connective tissue is the typical histopathologic finding. The infiltrate consists predominantly of T lymphocytes and plasma cells with a smaller number of B lymphocytes.[142, 175]

The etiology is unknown and likely multifactorial. Subclinical infection with human papillomavirus has been suspected in some cases.[142] In situ hybridization studies for human papilloma virus types 6, 11, 16, 18, 31, and 35 were all negative in a recent series of 36 cases, casting doubt on an etiologic role, at least for these human papilloma virus types.[175] Chronic recurrent infections (e.g., candidiasis, bacterial vaginosis), chronic alteration of vaginal pH, and use of chemical and destructive therapeutic agents have been associated with the syndrome.[142] A recent case control study suggested an increased risk of developing vulvar vestibulitis among women who used oral contraceptives, especially if use began before 17 years of age, compared with those who never used them.[18] First intercourse at 15 years of age or younger also increased risk relative to first intercourse at 16 years of age or older.

Patients with acute vulvar vestibulitis should be evaluated and treated for any sexually transmitted diseases that are found. A history of all medicinal agents or other treatment modalities used by the patient should be obtained. Any agent that might be contributing to the problem should be discontinued if possible. Topical steroids may be effective once any infections have been controlled. If the condition is chronic and no specific etiology can be found, surgical excision may be the only way to provide relief. Antimicrobial agents and steroids are of no benefit in such cases.[142]

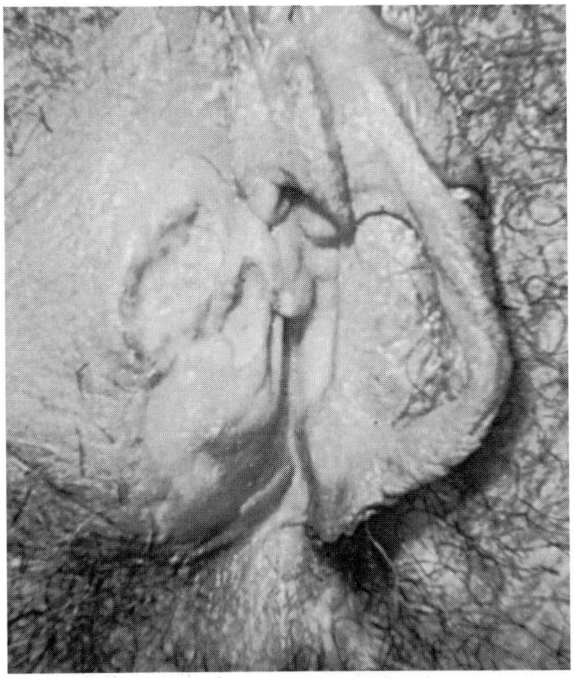

FIGURE 49–24. *Vulvar lesions in Behçet syndrome. (From Friedrich, E. G., Jr.: Vulvar Disease. Philadelphia, W. B. Saunders, 1976. Reproduced by permission of the author.)*

CERVICITIS

Premenarcheal

As a rule, the cervix is not involved when a premenarcheal child has vaginitis because most vaginal infections affect only the distal half of the vagina in children; the exception is gonococcal vaginitis, which usually also involves the squamous epithelium over the external cervix. Cervicitis also may occur when there is a vaginal foreign body.

Endocervicitis is unusual in premenarcheal females because the endocervical glands and mucosa are developed poorly prior to menarche, thus providing a poor environment for invading organisms.

Erosions of the cervix seldom are seen in children older than 1 year of age. So-called "congenital ectopy" is not the result of infection. It is a persistence of the fetal paramesonephric (müllerian) glandular epithelium on the outer cervix. That epithelium normally recedes into the endocervical canal as the cervix develops postnatally.

Inflammation of the external cervix, which occasionally occurs with vaginitis in a premenarcheal child, need not be treated; it heals as the vaginitis improves. Electrocauterization, chemical cauterization, or cryotherapy of the immature cervix rarely, if ever, is necessary. It carries with it the very real danger of causing stenosis of the endocervical canal, leading to serious problems when the child is older.

Postmenarcheal[113, 185]

The structure of the cervix during the reproductive years makes it vulnerable to infections induced by a number of factors. The long, narrow, deeply pocketed cervical canal, lined by open cryptic glands bathed in alkaline secretion and washed periodically by menstrual blood, is an excellent nidus for bacterial growth. Pathogenic bacteria in the vagina find ready access to the cervical canal. Use of oral contraceptive pills promotes cervical ectopy, thus increasing the vulnerability of the endocervical cells to chlamydial infection.

Early recognition and aggressive treatment of cervicitis in sexually active adolescents is an important way to prevent the serious complications of pelvic inflammatory disease and tubo-ovarian abscess. Clinical recognition of infections of the cervix was difficult in the past because of the lack of objective diagnostic criteria for cervical inflammation.

There also was confusion over normal cervical changes that occur during the reproductive period, such as the difficulty in differentiating normal ectopic columnar epithelium on the exocervix (ectopy) from cervicitis. When the squamocolumnar junction is exposed on the exocervix, it is called ectopy. It appears bright shiny red in contrast with the dull pearly pink appearance of the exocervix. This area does not bleed easily when touched with a swab. Ectopy is not an abnormal finding. During adolescence, the normal cervix may exhibit no ectopy, a small area of ectopy, or at times up to 50 per cent ectopy. When ectopy appears edematous, raised, and friable (often with marked bleeding when touched lightly with a swab), cervicitis should be suspected.

Nabothian inclusion cysts, shiny grayish transparent cysts on the cervix, are normal. Diethylstilbestrol exposure should be suspected in a female born before 1974 with cervical changes, such as fibrous ridges, a circular fold covering the cervix, and a cockscomb appearance on the anterior aspect of the cervix.

Mucopurulent cervicitis primarily is endocervicitis associated with *C. trachomatis, M. hominis, U. urealyticum, N. gonorrhoeae, G. vaginalis,* and group B *Streptococcus.* In contrast, *T. vaginalis* causes an exocervicitis by an extension of vaginitis. Because of the high prevalence of coexisting infections of the cervix, it often is difficult to associate any one organism with clinical signs and symptoms of cervicitis. Studies, however, have noted a strong association between mucopurulent cervicitis and *C. trachomatis.* This organism is isolated in almost 50 per cent of cases of cervicitis.[113]

The criteria for diagnosis of mucopurulent cervicitis include the presence of mucopurulent secretion from the endocervix, erythema of the cervix, and friable ectopy. The mucopurulent secretion in chlamydial cervicitis is tenacious mucoid material mixed with yellow exudate and is difficult to remove from the endocervix. The ectopic area on the cervix may appear erythematous and friable. In chronic chlamydial cervicitis, the ectopic area may be swollen and irregular with a cobblestone appearance. This is called hypertrophic cervicitis. In gonococcal cervicitis, the endocervical mucosa is swollen, intensely inflamed, and often friable as well. In contrast with a mucopurulent discharge in chlamydia cervicitis, there is a profuse, yellowish-green acrid discharge in gonococcal cervicitis.

Cervical erosions occur in sexually active adolescents. Infections other than those listed earlier as causing mucopurulent cervicitis also can involve the vulva, vagina, and cervix. A chancre, the primary lesion of syphilis, may appear on the cervix, where it forms an irregularly shaped ulcer that only remotely resembles a chancre on the vulva. Tuberculosis, herpes simplex virus, granuloma inguinale, lymphogranuloma venereum, chancroid, schistosomiasis, and actinomycosis also may affect the cervix. The cervical lesions of most of these infections are altered by the warmth and moisture of the vagina and are atypical in appearance. None of them is common, but all of them should be considered in the differential diagnosis when a patient has an unusual ulcerative or fungating lesion of the cervix.[115]

Treatment

The first step in the clinical management of cervicitis is to wipe the cervix with a large swab to remove vaginal secretions. Endocervical specimens then are obtained for a Gram stain and tests for *C. trachomatis* and *N. gonorrhoeae.* Cervicitis is suspected when an adequate endocervical Gram stain has more than 5 to 10 polymorphonuclear cells per field under oil immersion. The presence of at least eight pairs of gram-negative intracellular diplococci in at least three polymorphonuclear cells strongly suggests gonococcal cervicitis. The absence of gram-negative intracellular diplococci but the presence of more than 5 to 10 polymorphonuclear cells per oil immersion field suggests nongonococcal cervicitis.[27, 149] When cervical erosions or ulcers are seen, a specimen for herpes simplex virus culture should be obtained. *T. vaginalis* is identified by microscopic examination of vaginal secretions in saline.

Treatment of cervicitis follows the same guidelines provided for treatment of gonococcal and chlamydial cervicitis: 125 mg of intramuscular ceftriaxone in a single dose along with 100 mg of doxycycline orally twice a day or 500 mg of tetracycline four times a day orally for 10 days. When *T. vaginalis* vaginitis is diagnosed or herpes simplex virus strongly suspected, the appropriate treatment for these infections should be given (see the sections on trichomoniasis and herpes genitalis).

Integral to treating the patient is notification, examination, and treatment of the patient's sexual partners if gonococcal and/or chlamydial infection is found. The partners should be treated with the same regimen, and written information should be provided with names of diseases and medications. A follow-up examination of the patient is recommended in 14 days. In cases with minimal or no improvement, medication compliance problems and untreated sexual partners should be considered. Another course of doxycycline or tetracycline is prescribed and treatment of partners encouraged. This management approach causes resolution of signs and symptoms in most cases. When signs of cervicitis persist, despite this treatment approach, a Papanicolaou smear should be obtained for evidence of dysplasia. Erosions heal spontaneously after the irritating discharge ceases. Nabothian follicle cysts are innocent structures that should be left alone unless they interfere with cervical drainage. The management of specific cervical infections is part of the treatment of the disease causing them.

Chlamydial

Some of the highest rates of chlamydial infection (8 to 25 per cent) have been reported in adolescents.[34, 69, 72, 189] It is three to four times more common than gonococcal cervicitis. *C. trachomatis* causes cervicitis by infecting columnar and transitional epithelium of the cervix. Cervical ectopy appears to be a predisposing factor for *C. trachomatis* infection.[13]

C. trachomatis predominantly is an asymptomatic disease in adolescent girls.[34] A clinical diagnosis is made when friable ectopy with a mucopurulent cervical discharge (mucopus) is noted. Chlamydial cervicitis is suspected when a Gram stain of an adequate endocervical smear demonstrates more than 5 to 10 polymorphonuclear cells per field with oil immersion in the absence of gram-negative intracellular diplococci.[27, 149]

C. trachomatis is diagnosed by identifying intracellular inclusion bodies in tissue culture. The tissue-culture method is considered the gold standard.[192] Because of the high cost of this technique, it is not widely available. Serologic tests are not helpful for the diagnosis of chlamydial genital infections, except in pelvic inflammatory disease.

Three rapid tests for detecting *C. trachomatis* currently are being used predominantly: the direct fluorescent antibody test or Micro Trak (Abbott), the Chlamydiazyme (Syva) test, and the DNA probe assay or Gen-Probe (Gen-Probe). Other rapid tests, including polymerase chain reaction and enhanced optical immunoassays, now are available. The Micro Trak test detects *Chlamydia* elementary bodies in a cervical specimen using a direct fluorescent-antibody method. This method takes 15 to 20 minutes to perform and has a sensitivity of 61 to 90 per cent and specificity of 95 to 97 per cent when compared with the culture method. The Chlamydiazyme test is an enzyme-linked immunosorbent assay and takes 4 to 5 hours to perform. It has a sensitivity of 85 to 100 per cent and specificity of 88 to 97 per cent. The Gen-Probe is 80 per cent sensitive and 100 per cent specific in detecting *Chlamydia* infection in females.[196] Overall, the rapid antigen-detection tests perform best in adolescent populations with high prevalence rates of *C. trachomatis* infection.[132, 205] Treatment was discussed earlier in this section.

Gonococcal

Gonococcal cervicitis may be symptomatic or asymptomatic. The risk of infection varies with the population. Adolescents seen in private practices in the suburbs have a significantly lower rate of gonococcal cervicitis than do adolescents seen in large outpatient hospital clinics or community clinics serving inner-city populations. Although it has been estimated that gonococcal cervicitis predominantly is an asymptomatic condition in females, many patients, after careful questioning, in fact do have symptoms. Asymptomatic endocervical infection among adolescent females seen in urban settings ranges from 3 to 12 per cent. Anal gonorrhea usually is secondary to the discharge from gonococcal cervicitis infecting the anus. Primary anal gonorrhea as a result of anal intercourse should be suspected in a sexually active adolescent with anal discomfort. In addition, gonococcal infection should be considered in the differential diagnosis of pharyngitis in sexually active adolescents.[228] Gonococcal endocarditis, arthritis, and dermal abscesses occur but are beyond the scope of this chapter.

The presenting complaints in gonococcal cervicitis include vaginal discharge, dysuria, urinary frequency, and dyspareunia. On examination, the patient has a normal-appearing cervix or the cervix appears erythematous and friable, with a foul-smelling purulent discharge draining from the cervical os. Laboratory diagnosis is made by detecting gram-negative intracellular diplococci on Gram stain and detecting *N. gonorrhoeae* by culture or a rapid test.

Material for cultures is obtained from the endocervix using sterile cotton-tipped applicators and either placed in transport medium (Amies charcoal transport medium) or, preferably, streaked on Thayer-Martin or Martin-Lewis culture plates, which are sent promptly to the laboratory (in a carbon dioxide environment) for incubation and bacterial identification.

Alternatively, the candle jar method can be used or plates containing carbon dioxide–generating tablets can be placed in a plastic bag to provide a carbon dioxide environment. When using screw-cap bottles containing Stuart medium and carbon dioxide, the bottle must be held upright when inoculated to prevent escape of carbon dioxide. An enzyme immunoassay for the detection of *N. gonorrhoeae* (Gonozyme) is available. Field testing has indicated so far that this test is more sensitive in males than in females in clinics with a high prevalence rate of gonorrhea and is less sensitive than culture. A major drawback is the inability to test *N. gonorrhoeae* for antibiotic resistance. The DNA hybridization technique to detect *N. gonorrhoeae* also has low sensitivity in infected females, compared with culture.[142a] It is recommended, therefore, that gonorrhea infection in females be confirmed by culture.

Current treatment of gonococcal infection has been influenced by the emergence of antibiotic-resistant strains, including penicillinase-producing *N. gonorrhoeae,* tetracycline-resistant strains, and chromosomally resistant strains. The high frequency of chlamydial infection in persons with gonorrhea (as high as 45 per cent in certain populations), the lack of a rapid on-site diagnostic test for chlamydial infection, and the serious complications resulting from untreated gonorrhea and chlamydial infections also have influenced the treatment approach.

Nonpregnant females with genital and pharyngeal gonorrhea are treated for gonococcal and chlamydial infections with a single dose of intramuscular ceftriaxone (125 mg) or a single dose of oral cefixime (400 mg) plus doxycycline (100 mg) orally twice a day for 7 days. An alternative to doxycycline is 500 mg of tetracycline orally four times a day for 7 days. Compliance with doxycycline may be better. An alternative to cephalosporins is a single dose of intramuscular spectinomycin (2 g) followed by the doxycycline regimen. A single oral dose of ciprofloxacin (500 mg) or ofloxacin (400 mg) may be used only in nonpregnant teenagers older than 16 years of age. Pregnant females with genital and pharyngeal gonorrhea are treated with ceftriaxone plus 500 mg of erythromycin (base or stearate) orally four times a day for 7 days. A single oral dose of amoxicillin (3 g) or intramuscular procaine penicillin (4.8 million units), with probenecid (1 g) plus doxycycline (100 mg) twice a day for 7 days orally, is an acceptable regimen for proven cases of non–penicillinase-producing *N. gonorrhoeae* strains in endemic areas and in areas where penicillinase-producing *N. gonorrhoeae* strains are not endemic.

A test-of-cure visit after ceftriaxone and cefixime treatment to ensure cure is not necessary. Other treatment regimens, however, require a test-of-cure visit 4 to 7 days after completion of treatment. Sexual partners should be notified, examined, tested, and treated.[32]

UPPER GENITAL TRACT INFECTIONS

Pelvic Inflammatory Disease

Pelvic inflammatory disease in postmenarcheal girls is a common problem (Fig. 49–25). Although salpingitis has been reported in virgins, this condition primarily occurs in sexually active adolescents at risk for acquiring sexually transmitted diseases.[115]

Pelvic inflammatory disease is defined as an acute clinical syndrome (unrelated to pregnancy or surgery) attributed to the ascent of microorganisms from the vagina and endocervix to the endometrium, fallopian tubes, or contiguous structures, resulting in pelvic and generalized peritonitis. Use of terms specifically describing anatomic sites involved is preferable (e.g., endometritis, salpingitis, salpingo-oophoritis). However, in most adolescents with acute severe infec-

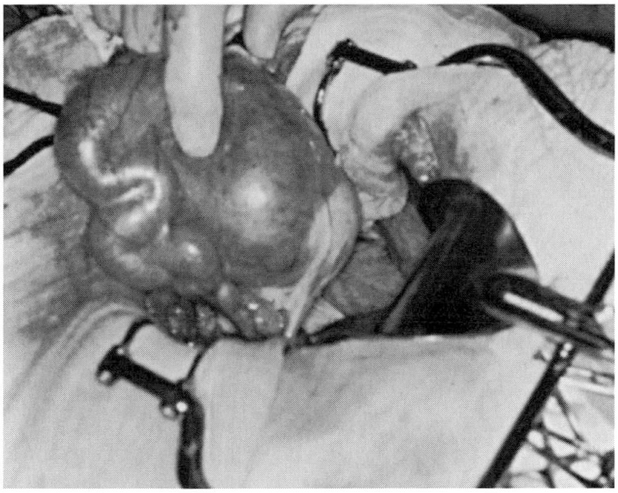

FIGURE 49–25. *Large hydrosalpinx, the result of gonorrheal salpingitis in an older teenage girl who had repeated gonorrheal infections. The other tube also was diseased.*

tion, it is difficult to differentiate these entities; thus, use of the term pelvic inflammatory disease is common.

Epidemiologic investigation on the risk of developing pelvic inflammatory disease has demonstrated a calculated annual risk of 1:8 in sexually active adolescents versus 1:80 in women who are 24 years of age or older. Reasons hypothesized for this age-related difference are physiologic and social. The former includes alterations in cervical mucus due to immature and anovulatory menstrual cycles, early onset of sexual activity, and multiple sexual partners. Besides age, other factors influencing the risk of pelvic inflammatory disease are method of contraception, history of gonococcal or chlamydial lower genital tract infection, and uterine instrumentation such as with use of an intrauterine device or during dilatation and curettage. The insertion of an intrauterine device and dilatation and curettage are performed rarely in adolescents.

Oral contraceptives are used commonly by adolescents. Their possible protective effect on the development of pelvic inflammatory disease has been reported. Compared with other methods of contraception, oral contraceptive users have a lower risk of pelvic inflammatory disease.[201] Laparoscopic studies also have shown that women with pelvic inflammatory disease who were using oral contraceptive pills have significantly milder degrees of fallopian tube inflammation compared with non–pill users. This suggests that the pill may reduce potential tubal damage. Another study, however, reports that by promoting cervical ectopy, oral contraceptives potentially are a risk factor for chlamydial pelvic inflammatory disease.[203, 223, 238]

Women who have had one episode of pelvic inflammatory disease have a 20 to 25 per cent chance of developing subsequent ones. Reasons for this may be reinfection from untreated sexual partners, an inadequately treated first infection, or increased susceptibility of the tubal epithelium to infection.[62, 235]

Pathogenic bacteria reach the endometrium and fallopian tubes by one of three routes: hematogenous, direct from a contagious site of infection, or ascending infection from the lower genital tract. The first two routes are uncommon.[235]

The mechanism for ascending infection from the vagina and cervix to the endometrium and fallopian tubes is thought to be multifactorial. During menses and midcycle, cervical mucus is less viscous and more permeable to ascending infection. In vitro experiments show that *N. gonorrhoeae, C. trachomatis, U. urealyticum,* and other aerobic and anaerobic agents can adhere to spermatozoa and migrate with them.[225] Whether this can occur in vivo is not known. The majority of organisms found in nongonococcal and nonchlamydial pelvic inflammatory disease also are found in bacterial vaginosis. This suggests that bacterial vaginosis may be a predisposing or a precipitating factor for pelvic inflammatory disease. It also has been suggested that *T. vaginalis* can act as a vector for transporting bacteria.[127] Another possible factor is upward transport of bacteria from orgasmic myometrial contractions.[235] Vaginal douching also has been reported to be a risk factor in promoting ascending infection.[237]

Endometritis

Premenarcheal girls rarely, if ever, suffer from endometrial infections. Infections of the endometrium in postmenarcheal females are considered rare clinical entities, except for postabortive and puerperal endometritis. Poor compliance with prophylactic antibiotics places an adolescent at an increased risk for endometritis after an abortion. Recent evidence suggests that endometritis occurs in up to 40 per cent of patients with asymptomatic endocervical chlamydial infection.[123] The gonococcus, on its way upward to the uterine tubes, produces a fleeting infection of the endometrium, but the symptoms produced are overshadowed by those of the vulvar and cervical infections. Young women who wear intrauterine devices are likely to have asymptomatic, low-grade, chronic endometritis.

Endometrial tuberculosis, rare in the United States, Australia, and several other countries, but relatively common in Scotland and elsewhere, is encountered most often in patients with pulmonary tuberculosis. In older patients, the infection reaches the uterus via the gastrointestinal tract and by lymphatic spread. It is not acquired as a result of an ascending infection or through coitus with an infected male. The symptoms of endometrial tuberculosis vary from none at all to amenorrhea, pelvic pain, dysmenorrhea, and abnormal uterine bleeding. It may be an incidental finding in a patient without discoverable tuberculosis in other organs who is subjected to curettage for menstrual irregularity or infertility. Often, there is a history of healed or active pulmonary disease. Ninety per cent of patients with pelvic tuberculosis have tuberculous endometritis.

Endometrial tuberculosis is diagnosed by histologic study of curetted tissue or by demonstrating acid-fast *M. tuberculosis* in cultures of curettings or menstrual blood.

Additional information on endometrial tuberculosis and the management of tuberculosis is described elsewhere in this book (see Chapter 101).

Salpingitis

The pathogenesis of salpingitis has been studied best with *N. gonorrhoeae* and *C. trachomatis.* In the fallopian tube, gonococci attach to nonciliated epithelial cells and induce sloughing of the ciliated epithelial cells into the lumen. Gonococci also enter the subepithelial space, where a local inflammatory response is produced, and may reach the blood stream. A purulent exudate is produced within the tube and may cause pelvic peritonitis. Chlamydial infection produces a similar picture, except that it causes a predominantly lymphocytic infiltrate in the submucosa compared with gonococcal pelvic inflammatory disease, in which a predominantly polymorphonuclear leukocytic infiltrate occurs in the submucosa.[167, 221, 235]

Salpingitis also is caused by several microbial agents that

have been isolated directly from the fallopian tubes. The current classification categorizes salpingitis into gonococcal; chlamydial; and nongonococcal, nonchlamydial salpingitis. The most commonly recovered organisms from the upper tract in salpingitis are mixed anaerobes (25 to 84 per cent), followed by *N. gonorrhoeae* (25 to 50 per cent), *C. trachomatis* (25 to 43 per cent), facultative bacteria *(G. vaginalis, E. coli,* group B *Streptococcus),* and genital tract mycoplasmas.[62] The mixed anaerobes include *Bacteroides* species and *Peptostreptococcus* species. Nongonococcal and nonchlamydial pelvic inflammatory disease is more common in females with severe pelvic inflammatory disease, chronic pelvic inflammatory disease, and recurrent pelvic inflammatory disease. Approximately 10 to 17 per cent of females with endocervical *N. gonorrhoeae* and 10 to 30 per cent with endocervical *C. trachomatis* develop pelvic inflammatory disease. Initially, it was thought that *N. gonorrhoeae* initiated the infection and superinfection with anaerobes followed. It now is apparent that both anaerobes and aerobes can initiate pelvic inflammatory disease without *C. trachomatis* or *N. gonorrhoeae.*

It often is difficult clinically to differentiate gonococcal; chlamydial; and nongonococcal, nonchlamydial salpingitis. Gonococcal and chlamydial salpingitis seem to occur most often within a week of menstruation.[222] The onset of nongonococcal, nonchlamydial salpingitis does not seem related to menses. The course of chlamydial salpingitis may be slow, with mild symptoms initially. As a result, patients delay seeking treatment. The erythrocyte sedimentation rate is elevated and tubal damage significant at the time of presentation in the case of chlamydial salpingitis. In contrast, gonococcal salpingitis usually has an acute presentation with a dramatic onset of symptoms and earlier presentation to the clinic. Fever is more common in females with gonococcal salpingitis and pelvic peritonitis than in females with chlamydial salpingitis. A recent report showed that compared with adults, adolescents with salpingitis tend to seek health care later in the course of their illness.[211]

The classic presentation of acute pelvic inflammatory disease is lower abdominal pain, which usually is bilateral and continuous and may worsen with movement. After the onset of abdominal pain is the onset of fever, nausea, and vomiting. The temperature may reach 39° to 39.5° C (102° to 103° F). It is unusual for a chill to precede the fever. Other common presenting symptoms include vaginal discharge, irregular vaginal bleeding, and urinary symptoms.

On physical examination, the patient usually looks sick and uncomfortable. Tachycardia is present in proportion to the fever, if present. Abdominal examination reveals a markedly tender and often tense lower abdomen. Rebound tenderness indicates generalized peritonitis. The genital examination may show a purulent vaginal discharge in the vaginal vault. Even gentle bimanual rectovaginal abdominal palpation causes great distress. Attempted mobilization of the cervix is extremely painful. The uterus is tense and tender. The adnexa may not be outlined because of discomfort produced by the examination. Palpation of the adnexa unilaterally or bilaterally may be extremely painful. An adnexal swelling may be palpated, but this finding is not reliable in diagnosing an adnexal mass. In the less acutely tender patient, the examination may reveal a thickened, tender tube.

Common laboratory findings in patients with pelvic inflammatory disease include a peripheral white blood cell count greater than 10,000/mm^3 and an erythrocyte sedimentation rate greater than 15 mm/hour. In addition, endocervical gonorrhea and chlamydial infection may be present simultaneously in 10 to 30 per cent of cases. Ultrasonography of the pelvic cavity helps to exclude adnexal masses and detection of a pelvic abscess. A study in the use of pelvic ultrasonography in adolescents with pelvic inflammatory disease showed that the presence of fluid in the cul-de-sac was not helpful in differentiating patients with and without pelvic inflammatory disease.[86a] However, almost 20 per cent of patients with pelvic inflammatory disease had a tubo-ovarian abscess; in the absence of a tubo-ovarian abscess, adnexal volume was significantly larger in patients with pelvic inflammatory disease compared with patients without it.[86a]

The clinical diagnosis of pelvic inflammatory disease is made by having a high index of suspicion of this entity. Many of the classic symptoms seen with this condition are similar to those seen in other gynecologic, urinary, and gastrointestinal tract conditions. Although these diagnoses need to be considered in a case of acute onset of abdominal pain, over the years clinical criteria for the diagnosis of pelvic inflammatory disease have been developed (Table 49–6). Jacobson and Westrom[121] were the first investigators to use clinical criteria to differentiate pelvic inflammatory disease from other acute clinical conditions, such as appendicitis, ovarian cysts, and ectopic pregnancy. The clinical diagnosis was confirmed by laparoscopy. Only 65 per cent of cases with clinical diagnosis of pelvic inflammatory disease were confirmed by laparoscopy. No symptoms and signs were specific for pelvic inflammatory disease. Laparoscopy is the only means of making a definitive diagnosis. The benefits of using laparoscopy are to make an accurate diagnosis rapidly by direct visualization of the fallopian tubes and adjacent structures, to obtain cultures of tubal exudate, and to evaluate outcome of therapy. This diagnostic method, however, is not without risks and adds to the cost of care.[220] Therefore, for practical reasons, the clinical criteria developed by Jacobson and Westrom have been expanded to aid in the diagnosis and increase the index of suspicion of pelvic inflammatory disease. These are listed in Table 49–6. The more criteria that can be met, the more likely that a tubal infection is present. However, those who use strict criteria will miss patients with mild disease.[92, 121, 198, 229]

The differential diagnosis of pelvic inflammatory disease is that of the acute abdomen. Conditions of the urinary tract that should be considered include cystitis, pyelonephritis, and urethritis. Gastrointestinal tract conditions include appendicitis, constipation, diverticulitis, gastroenteritis, in

TABLE 49–6. Clinical Criteria for the Diagnosis of Acute Pelvic Inflammatory Disease

All three of the following must be present:

- History of lower abdominal pain and the presence of abdominal tenderness, with or without rebound tenderness
- Tenderness with motion of the cervix and uterus
- Adnexal tenderness

Plus one or more of the following:

- Temperature ≥38° C
- White blood cell count ≥ 10,500 mm/hr
- Elevated sedimentation rate > 15 mm/hr
- Evidence of *Neisseria gonorrhoeae* and/or *Chlamydia trachomatis* in the endocervix; Gram stain from the endocervix positive for gram-negative intracellular diplococci or a monoclonal-directed smear positive for *Chlamydia* (or similar rapid tests) or >5 white blood cells per oil immersion field on Gram stain of endocervical discharge
- Pelvic abscess or inflammatory complex on bimanual examination or by sonography
- Purulent material (white blood cells present) from peritoneal cavity by culdocentesis or laparoscopy

flammatory bowel disease, and irritable bowel syndrome. Gynecologic conditions include dysmenorrhea, ectopic pregnancy, endometriosis, endometritis, mittelschmerz, torsion or rupture of ovarian cyst, ruptured follicle, septic abortion, and threatened abortion.

As in pelvic inflammatory disease, early diagnosis of acute appendicitis and ectopic pregnancy is important. In acute appendicitis, an adolescent is more likely to have nausea, vomiting, a short history of right lower quadrant abdominal pain, lower grade fever, higher leukocyte count in relation to the fever, and relatively little discomfort with the pelvic examination than in pelvic inflammatory disease. Occasionally, however, the appendix hangs over the pelvic brim, resulting in pelvic tenderness. A ruptured appendix and peritonitis may simulate pelvic inflammatory disease closely. Differentiating pelvic inflammatory disease from ectopic pregnancy is less difficult if the history suggests pregnancy. It should be remembered that pelvic inflammatory disease can occur during the first trimester of pregnancy. In ectopic pregnancy, the patient does not have fever or leukocytosis. The symptoms almost always are unilateral. There are signs of hematoperitoneum if the tube is ruptured. A serum pregnancy test and pelvic ultrasonography for a gestational sac should be performed immediately when an ectopic pregnancy is suspected.

Treatment[32]

The major goals of treatment of pelvic inflammatory disease are preservation of fertility and prevention of other long-term sequelae, including ectopic pregnancy. Females with a history of one or more episodes of pelvic inflammatory disease have an infertility rate of 21 per cent, compared with 3 per cent in controls, and a sixfold increase in ectopic pregnancy, even with antibiotic treatment.[235] Therefore, to reduce sequelae of this condition, there must be early recognition of pelvic inflammatory disease, use of broad-spectrum antibiotics to treat a polymicrobial disease, careful clinical re-evaluation 48 hours after initiating antibiotic treatment to assess antibiotic response, and evaluation and treatment of sexual partners. Screening the patient for other sexually transmitted diseases, such as trichomoniasis, bacterial vaginosis, and syphilis, also is important.

Although 75 per cent of females with pelvic inflammatory disease are treated on an ambulatory basis, no empirical studies show the value of ambulatory versus inpatient treatment in terms of either short-term goals of improvement of acute symptoms and elimination of bacterial infection or long-term goals of preventing ectopic pregnancy and infertility. Because of the seriousness of the sequelae and problems with compliance among this age group, most adolescents should be hospitalized for treatment to ensure compliance with medication. Other reasons for hospitalization are uncertain diagnosis, presence of tubo-ovarian abscess, pregnancy, temperature above 38.5° C, nausea and vomiting that preclude the use of oral medications, and lack of improvement after 48 hours of oral antibiotic treatment.

The current Centers for Disease Control and Prevention recommendations for treatment of pelvic inflammatory disease in both ambulatory and hospitalized patients address antibiotic coverage for the polymicrobial etiology of this condition (Tables 49–7 and 49–8).[32] Other second- and third-generation cephalosporins may be used as alternatives to cefoxitin and cefotetan in the inpatient treatment of pelvic inflammatory disease. However, they are less active against anaerobic bacteria. For outpatient treatment of pelvic inflammatory disease, oral ofloxacin with clindamycin is an alternative regimen for adolescents older than 16 years of age. Ofloxacin is effective against *N. gonorrhoeae* and *C. trachomatis.* In addition to antibiotic treatment, bed rest is recommended with elevation of the back and knees. Warm, moist packs to the lower abdomen sometimes are soothing.[115] Intravenous fluids are administered for hydration when necessary. When the diagnosis of pelvic inflammatory disease is certain, oral analgesic agents may be prescribed. Until nausea and vomiting are controlled, a liquid diet is prescribed.

Complications associated with pelvic inflammatory disease are perihepatitis (14 per cent), tubo-ovarian abscess (up to 20 per cent), chronic abdominal pain from adhesions surrounding fallopian tubes and ovaries (18 per cent), and recurrent pelvic inflammatory disease (20 to 25 per cent).

The classic presentation of perihepatitis or Fitz-Hugh–Curtis syndrome[63] is severe right upper abdominal pain, which often radiates to the shoulder. Concurrent left upper abdominal pain also may be present. Lower abdominal pain and evidence of acute or subacute pelvic inflammatory disease is common. The right upper quadrant pain lasts about 48 hours. Nausea, fever, and leukocytosis are common features. There may be elevation of the erythrocyte sedimentation rate and liver enzymes. The pathogenesis of perihepatitis is thought

TABLE 49–7. Ambulatory Management of Pelvic Inflammatory Disease[32]

Regimen A

Cefoxitin 2 g IM plus probenecid, 1 g PO concurrently or ceftriaxone 250 mg IM, or equivalent cephalosporin

plus

Doxycycline 100 mg PO two times a day for 10 to 14 days

Regimen B (>16 Years of Age)

Ofloxacin 400 mg PO two times a day for 14 days

plus

Either clindamycin 450 mg PO four times a day or metronidazole 500 mg PO two times a day for 14 days

Alternative for patients who do not tolerate doxycycline or who are pregnant:

Erythromycin, 500 mg PO four times a day for 10 to 14 days may be substituted for doxycycline. This regimen, however, is based on limited clinical data.

TABLE 49–8. Inpatient Treatment of Pelvic Inflammatory Disease[32]

Regimen A

Cefoxitin 2 g IV every 6 hours or cefotetan IV 2 g every 12 hours

plus

Doxycycline 100 mg every 12 hours PO or IV

The above regimen is given for at least 48 hours after the patient clinically improves. After discharge from hospital, doxycycline is continued 100 mg PO two times a day for a total of 10 to 14 days.

Regimen B

Clindamycin IV 900 mg every 8 hours

plus

Gentamicin loading dose IV or IM (2 mg/kg) followed by a maintenance dose (1.5 mg/kg) every 8 hours

The above regimen is given for at least 48 hours after the patient improves. After discharge from hospital, doxycycline is continued 100 mg PO two times a day for a total of 10 to 14 days.

to be from direct spread of *N. gonorrhoeae* and *C. trachomatis* from the fallopian tubes into the peritoneal cavity, along the paracolic sulci. From there, they reach the subphrenic space and hepatic surface. However, spread from the reproductive tract also is possible via retroperitoneal lymphatics.[63]

The diagnosis is made by having a high index of suspicion. Perihepatitis frequently mimics cholelithiasis, hepatitis, pleuritis, subphrenic abscess, perforated peptic ulcer, nephrolithiasis, appendicitis, ectopic pregnancy, abdominal trauma, and pancreatitis. Treatment of this condition is similar to that of pelvic inflammatory disease.

Tubo-ovarian Abscess[41, 178]

The incidence of tubo-ovarian abscess ranges from 14 to 38 per cent in hospital-based adolescents and adults with salpingitis.[86a, 91, 135, 156] This is the most frequent complication of pelvic inflammatory disease and may lead to irreversible tubal and ovarian damage. Infected exudate spreading over the surface of the ovary as a result of acute peritonitis or a tubal infection produces an inflammatory reaction in the ovarian epithelium, periovaritis, that is followed by residual thickening of the ovarian capsule; periovarian adhesions to the omentum, bowel, and tube; and firm fixation of the ovary to the undersurface of the broad ligament and the lateral pelvic wall. Periovaritis frequently accompanies both primary and secondary peritonitis and is common after suppurative appendicitis with rupture. Involvement of the ovarian substance, usually created by infection entering the ovary through a ruptured follicle at ovulation, leads to ovaritis and ovarian abscess.

Intraovarian infections and ovarian abscesses are unusual in premenarcheal children because there are no ruptured follicles to act as a gateway for infection.[188] They are, however, rather common in adolescents. The ovary rarely escapes an infection that involves the tube. The two organs may form a tubo-ovarian abscess, which ruptures spontaneously and spills its infectious and irritating contents into the peritoneal cavity. The most common organisms recovered from tubo-ovarian abscesses are *E. coli, Bacteroides fragilis,* other *Bacteroides* species, *Peptostreptococcus, Peptococcus,* and aerobic streptococci.[178] It usually is difficult to diagnose the presence of a tubo-ovarian abscess clinically. Bimanual examination frequently does not demonstrate a pelvic mass.[41] Four potentially useful clinical features that suggest the presence of a pelvic abscess are pain, persistent fever, adnexal tenderness (for more than 7 days), and an erythrocyte sedimentation rate of greater than 30 mm/hour.[41] Ultrasonography of the pelvis is valuable to confirm the presence of an abscess.[86a]

The prompt administration of antibiotics greatly has reduced the incidence of pelvic abscess. Most of those encountered today are in patients who have not had adequate care and delay seeking treatment. Adolescents are far more likely to delay seeking treatment than young adult females.[211]

A conservative approach is favored for the treatment of a developed tubo-ovarian or ovarian abscess (i.e., bed rest, supportive care, intravenous antibiotics). The choice of antibiotics for treatment of tubo-ovarian abscess should include the following considerations: effectiveness against β-lactamase–producing anaerobes, adequate coverage against resistant bacteroides species, penetration into the abscess, and ability to remain stable in an abscess environment. The antibiotics regimens for inpatient treatment of pelvic inflammatory disease fulfill these considerations and therefore are appropriate for the treatment of tubo-ovarian abscess (see Table 49–8). In addition to cefoxitin, cefotetan, and clindamycin, metronidazole provides good activity against anaerobes.[178] Many hospitals prefer the use of triple antibiotics, cefoxitin, and gentamicin plus clindamycin or metronidazole. Clinical response to treatment should be noted in 72 hours, with decrease in pain, fever, and total leukocyte count. Pelvic ultrasonography should be repeated at this time to note any further increase in abscess size. The duration of intravenous antibiotic therapy for tubo-ovarian abscess has not been standardized and may range from 7 to 14 days. The patient may be placed on oral antibiotics once she is afebrile and asymptomatic and the abscess size has stabilized. Oral antibiotics are provided to complete 3 weeks of treatment. The abscess either resolves without drainage or becomes an encapsulated pool of pus. The latter eventually "points" either in the cul-de-sac or anteriorly in the abdominal wall.

Surgical intervention may be needed in up to 25 per cent of cases either during the initial period or within a year, usually depending on the size of the abscess. An abscess larger than 10 cm has a 60 per cent chance, an abscess of 7 to 9 cm has a 35 per cent chance, and an abscess of 4 to 6 cm has a 20 per cent chance of requiring surgical intervention.[178] As a rule, vaginal drainage of a pelvic abscess in a small child is ill-advised because of the restricted surgical field and because the pelvic tissues are thick and unyielding. Instead, suprapubic drainage is preferable in a premenarcheal child. Vaginal incision and drainage in the adolescent, however, are performed simply and quickly if the abscess has been allowed to reach the floor of the pelvic basin.

Occasionally, an abscess that has been present for some time has a thick, granulation tissue wall, or much of its wall is composed of stretched-out ovarian tissue. In such cases, drainage is followed by a chronically discharging sinus. It persists until the walls of the abscess are excised. Such a procedure is performed abdominally. It may be exceedingly difficult because of adhesions. The patient frequently has a stormy, febrile postoperative course.

Ovaritis

A massive inflammatory swelling of the ovary may be secondary to an acute systemic disease. It must be differentiated from an ovarian tumor. The acute exanthemas and mumps are complicated most frequently by ovaritis. The presence of an enlarged, tender, boggy, smooth, mobile ovary in a child with mumps or one of the exanthemas is an indication for repeated examination and watchfulness. If the swelling is ovaritis, the ovary becomes less tender and gradually shrinks. Mumps ovaritis, particularly, may convert one or both ovaries into swellings 6 to 8 cm in diameter. The enlargement may persist for several months. Treatment is palliative. Analgesics are given for discomfort and fever.[11]

References

1. Ackerman, A. B., Goldfaden, G., and Cosmides, J. C.: Acquired syphilis in prepubertal children. Arch. Dermatol. *106*:92–93, 1972.
2. Adams, R.: Topical therapy: A formulary for pediatric skin disease. *In* Gellis, S., and Kagan, B. (eds.): Current Pediatric Therapy 3. Philadelphia, W. B. Saunders, 1976, pp. 446–454.
3. Aghajanian, A., Bernstein, L., and Grimes, D. A.: Bartholin's duct abscess and cyst: A case-control study. South. Med. J. *87*:26–29, 1994.
4. Alergant, C.: Chancroid. Practitioner *209*:624–627, 1972.
5. Alexander, E. R.: Misidentification of sexually transmitted organisms in children: Medicolegal implications. Pediatr. Infect. Dis. J. *7*:1–2, 1988.
6. Alexander, W. J., Griffith, H., Housch, J. G., et al.: Infections in sexual contacts and associates of children with gonorrhea. Sex. Transm. Dis. *11*:156–158, 1983.
7. Alpsoy, E., Yilmaz, E., and Basaran, E.: Interferon therapy for Behçet disease. J. Am. Acad. Dermatol. *31*:617–619, 1994.
8. Altchek, A.: Vulvovaginitis, vulvar skin disease, and pelvic inflammatory disease. Pediatr. Clin. North Am. *28*:397–432, 1981.

9. Amsel, R., Totten, P. A., Speigel, C. A., et al.: Nonspecific vaginitis: Diagnostic criteria, microbial and epidemiologic associations. Am. J. Med. *74*:14–22, 1983.
10. Andersen, P. G., Christensen, S., Detlefsen, G. U., et al.: Treatment of Bartholin's abscess: Marsupialization versus incision, curettage and suture under antibiotic cover: A randomised study with 6 months' follow up. Acta Obstet. Gynecol. Scand. *71*:59–62, 1992.
11. Andreoli, C., and Vischi, F.: Parotitis and ovaritis. Panminerva Med. *3*:358–361, 1961.
12. Andrew, D., and Bumstead, E.: The role of fomites in the transmission of vaginitis. Can. Med. Assoc. J. *112*:1181–1183, 1975.
13. Arya, O. P., Mallinson, H., and Goddard, A. D.: Epidemiological and clinical correlates of chlamydial infection of the cervix. Br. J. Vener. Dis. *57*:118–124, 1981.
14. Banov, L., Jr.: Rectal lesions of lymphogranuloma venereum in childhood. Am. J. Dis. Child. *83*:660–662, 1952.
15. Bartley, D. L., Morgan, L., and Rimsza, M. E.: *Gardnerella vaginalis* in prepubertal girls. Am. J. Dis. Child. *141*:1014–1017, 1987.
16. Bass, H. N.: "Bubble bath" as an irritant to the urinary tract of children. Clin. Pediatr. *7*:174, 1968.
17. Bassa, A. G. H., Hoosen, A. A., Moodley, J., et al.: Granuloma inguinale (Donovanosis) in women: An analysis of 60 cases from Durban, South Africa. Sex. Transm. Dis. *20*:164–167, 1993.
18. Bazin, S., Bouchard, C., Brisson, J., et al.: Vulvar vestibulitis syndrome: An exploratory case-control study. Obstet. Gynecol. *83*:47–50, 1994.
19. Bell, T. A., Stamm, W. E., Wang, S. P., et al.: Chronic *Chlamydia trachomatis* infections in infants. J. A. M. A. *267*:400–402, 1992.
20. Blackmore, C. A., Limpakarnjanarat, K., Rigau-Perez, J. G., et al.: An outbreak of chancroid in Orange County, California: Descriptive epidemiology and disease-control measures. J. Infect. Dis. *151*:840–844, 1985.
21. Bogaerts, Lepage, P., De Clercq, A., et al.: *Shigella* and gonococcal vulvovaginitis in prepubertal Central African girls. Pediatr. Infect. Dis. J. *11*:890–892.
22. Boisvert, P., and Walcher, D.: Hemolytic streptococcal vaginitis in children. Pediatrics *2*:24–29, 1948.
23. Branch, G., and Paxton, R.: A study of gonococcal infections among infants and children. Public Heath Rep. *80*:347–352, 1965.
24. Breschi, L. C., Goldman, G., and Shapiro, S. R.: Granuloma inguinale in Vietnam. J. Am. Vener. Dis. Assoc. *1*:118–120, 1975.
25. Brigden, M., and Guard, R.: Extragenital granuloma inguinale in North Queensland. Med. J. Aust. *2*:565–567, 1980.
26. Brown, J. L.: Hair shampooing technique and pediatric vulvovaginitis. Pediatrics *83*:146, 1989.
27. Brunham, R. C., Paavonen, J., Stevens, C. E., et al.: Mucopurulent cervicitis: The ignored counterpart in women of urethritis in men. N. Engl. J. Med. *311*:1–6, 1984.
28. Bump, R. C., and Buesching, W. J.: Bacterial vaginosis in virginal and sexually active adolescent females: Evidence against exclusive sexual transmission. Am. J. Obstet. Gynecol. *158*:935–939, 1988.
29. Burgess, J. A.: *Trichomonas vaginalis* infection from splashing in water closets. Br. J. Vener. Dis. *39*:248–250, 1963.
30. Burry, V.: Gonococcal vulvovaginitis and possible peritonitis in prepubertal girls. Am. J. Dis. Child. *121*:536–537, 1971.
31. Capraro, V., and Capraro, E.: Infections of the genital organs in children and adolescent girls. Gynecol. Prat. *22*:179–190, 1971.
32. Centers for Disease Control and Prevention: 1993 sexually transmitted diseases treatment guidelines. M. M. W. R. *42*(RR-14), 1993.
33. Centers for Disease Control and Prevention: Chancroid detected by polymerase chain reaction: Jackson, Mississippi, 1994–1995. M. M. W. R. *44*:567–574, 1995.
34. Chacko, M. R., and Lovchick, J. C.: *Chlamydia trachomatis* infection in sexually active adolescents: Prevalence and risk factors. Pediatrics *73*:836–840, 1984.
35. Chang, T.: Genital herpes, the source of infection. Int. J. Dermatol. *14*:201–202, 1975.
36. Charles, S. X.: Epidemiology of *Trichomonas vaginalis* in rural adolescent and juvenile children. J. Trop. Pediatr. *37*:90, 1991.
37. Cohen, B. A., Honig, P., and Androphy, E.: Anogenital warts in children. Arch. Dermatol. *126*:1575–1580, 1990.
38. Cohen, M. S., Hook, P., and Androphy, E.: Anogenital warts in children. Arch. Dermatol. *126*:1575–1580, 1990.
39. Cohen, M. S., Hook, E. W., and Hitchcock, P. J.: Sexually transmitted diseases in the AIDS era: Part I. Infect. Dis. Clin. North Am. *7*:739–914, 1993.
40. Corey, L.: Genital herpes. *In* Holmes, K. K., Mårdh, P.-A., Sparling, P. F., et al. (eds.): Sexually Transmitted Diseases. New York, McGraw-Hill, 1984, pp. 449–474.
41. Cromer, B. A., Brandstaetter, L. A., Fischer, R. A., et al.: Tubo-ovarian abscess in adolescents. Adolesc. Pediatr. Gynecol. *3*:21–24, 1990.
42. Crowther, I.: *Trichomonas* vaginitis in infancy. Lancet *1*:1074, 1962.
43. Cummins, A. J., and Atia, W. A.: Bartholin's abscess complicating food poisoning with *Salmonella panama*: A case report. Genitourin. Med. *70*:46–48, 1994.
44. Davies, J. A., Res, E., and Hobson, D.: Isolation of *Chlamydia trachomatis* from Bartholin's ducts. Br. J. Vener. Dis. *54*:409–413, 1978.
45. Davis, A. J., and Emans, S. J.: Human papilloma virus in the pediatric and adolescent patients. J. Pediatr. *115*:1–9, 1989.
46. Davis, B.: Deodorant vulvitis. Obstet. Gynecol. *36*:812, 1970.
47. Davis, T.: Chronic vulvovaginitis in children due to *Shigella flexneri*. Pediatrics *56*:41–44, 1975.
47a. DeJong, A. R.: Sexually transmitted diseases in sexually abused children. Sex. Transm. Dis. *13*:123–126, 1986.
48. Demetriou, E., Emans, S. J., and Masland, R. P.: Dysuria in adolescent girls: Urinary tract infection or vaginitis? Pediatrics *70*:299–301, 1982.
49. Dershewitz, R. A., and Levitsky, L. L.: Vulvovaginitis: A cause of clitorimegaly. Am. J. Dis. Child. *138*:887–888, 1984.
50. Dewhurst, C. J.: Practical Pediatric and Adolescent Gynecology. New York, Marcel Dekker, 1980, pp. 83–92.
51. Dhall, K., Das, S. S., and Dey, P.: Tuberculosis of Bartholin's gland. Int. J. Gynaecol. Obstet. *48*:223–224, 1995.
52. Dhar, V., Roker, K., Adhami, Z., et al.: Streptococcal vulvovaginitis in girls. Pediatr. Dermatol. *10*:366, 1993.
53. Division of STD/HIV Prevention: Sexually Transmitted Disease Surveillance, 1993. U.S. Department of Health and Human Services, Public Health Service. Atlanta, Centers for Disease Control and Prevention, 1994, pp. 55–57.
54. Dodson, R. F., Fritz, G. S., Hubler, W. R., et al.: Donovanosis: A morphologic study. J. Invest. Dermatol. *62*:611–614, 1974.
55. Donald, F. E., Slack, D. B., and Colman, G.: *Streptococcus pyogenes* vulvovaginitis in children in Nottingham. Epidemiol. Infect. *106*:459–465, 1991.
56. Duerden, B. I.: Black-pigmented gram-negative anaerobes in genito-urinary tract and pelvic infections. FEMS Immunol. Med. Microbiol. *6*:223–227, 1993.
57. Eigen, L.: Vaginal diphtheria. J. Med. Assoc. N. J. *29*:778–780, 1932.
58. Emans, S. J., and Goldstein, D. P. (eds.): Pediatric and Adolescent Gynecology. 3rd ed. Boston, Little Brown, 1990.
59. Emans, S. J. H., and Goldstein, D. P.: Office evaluation of the child and adolescent. *In* Emans, S. J. H., and Goldstein, D. P. (eds.): Pediatric and Adolescent Gynecology. 3rd ed. Boston, Little Brown, 1990, pp. 1–45.
60. Emans, S. J. H., and Goldstein, D. P.: Vulvovaginal problems in the prepubertal child. *In* Emans, S. J., and Goldstein, D. P. (eds.): Pediatric and Adolescent Gynecology. 3rd ed. Boston, Little Brown, 1990, pp. 67–93.
61. Emans, S. J. H., and Goldstein, D. P.: The gynecologic examination of the prepubertal child with vulvovaginitis: Use of the knee-chest position. Pediatrics *65*:758–760, 1980.
62. Eschenbach, D. A.: Acute pelvic inflammatory disease. Urol. Clin. North Am. *11*:65–81, 1984.
63. Eschenbach, D.: Fitz-Hugh-Curtis syndrome. *In* Holmes, K. K., Mårdh, P.-A., Sparling, P. F., et al. (eds.): Sexually Transmitted Diseases. New York, McGraw-Hill, 1984, pp. 633–638.
64. Fallon, P., and Robinson, E. T.: Meningococcal vulvovaginitis. Scand. J. Infect. Dis. *6*:295–296, 1974.
65. FDA Drug Bulletin: Oncogenic potential of new herpes simplex therapy. FDA Drug Bull. *5*:3, 1975.
66. Feo, L. G.: The incidence of *Trichomonas vaginalis* in various age groups. Am. J. Trop. Med. Hyg. *5*:786 790, 1956.
67. Figueroa-Colón, R., Grunow, J. E., Torres-Pinedo, R., et al.: Group A streptococcal proctitis and vulvovaginitis in a prepubertal girl. Pediatr. Infect. Dis. J. *3*:439–442, 1984.
68. Fink, C. W.: A perineal rash in Kawasaki disease. Pediatr. Infect. Dis. *2*:140–141, 1983.
69. Fisher, M., Swenson, P. D., Risucci, D., et al.: *Chlamydia trachomatis* in suburban adolescents. J. Pediatr. *111*:617–620, 1987.
70. Folland, D. S., Burke, R. E., Hinman, A. R., et al.: Gonorrhea in preadolescent children: An inquiry into source of infection and mode of transmission. Pediatrics *60*:153–156, 1977.
71. Forssner, H.: Vaginaltresia mit diphtherischer pathogenese. Acta Med. Scand. *59*:690–695, 1923.
72. Frazer, J. J., Rettig, P. J., and Kaplan, D. W.: Prevalence of cervical *Chlamydia trachomatis* and *Neisseria gonorrhoeae* in female adolescents. Pediatrics *71*:333–336, 1983.
73. Freinkel, A. L.: Granuloma inguinale of cervical lymph nodes simulating tuberculous lymphadenitis: Two case reports and review of published reports. Genitourin. Med. *64*:339–343, 1988.
74. Friedrich, E.: Vulvar Disease. Philadelphia, W. B. Saunders, 1976.
75. Fuld, G.: Gonococcal peritonitis in a prepubertal child. Am. J. Dis. Child. *115*:621–622, 1968.
76. Fuster, C. D., and Neinstein, L. S.: Vaginal *Chlamydia trachomatis*: Prevalence in sexually abused pubertal girls. Pediatrics *79*:235–238, 1987.
77. Gardner, H.: The vulvovaginitides (new interpretation and treatment methods). *In* Traymor, M., and Green, T., Jr. (eds.): Progress in Gynecology. Vol. 6. New York, Grune & Stratton, 1975, p. 307.
78. Gardner, H., and Dukes, C.: *Haemophilus vaginalis* vaginitis: A newly defined specific infection previously classified "non-specific" vaginitis. Am. J. Obstet. Gynecol. *69*:962–976, 1955.
79. Gardner, H. L.: *Hemophilus vaginalis* after twenty five years. Am. J. Obstet. Gynecol. *137*:385–391, 1980.
80. Gardner, J. J.: Comparison of the vaginal flora in sexually abused and nonabused girls. J. Pediatr. *120*:872–877, 1992.

81. Gardner, M., and Jones, J. G.: Genital herpes acquired by sexual abuse of children. J. Pediatr. *104*:243–244, 1984.
82. Gerstner, G. J., Grünberger, W., Boschitsch, E., et al.: Vaginal organisms in prepubertal children with and without vulvovaginitis. Arch. Gynecol. *231*:247–252, 1982.
83. Gilbaugh, J. H., and Fuchs, P. C.: The gonococcus and the toilet seat. N. Engl. J. Med. *301*:91–93, 1979.
84. Ginsberg, C. M.: Group A streptococcal vaginitis in children. Pediatr. Infect. Dis. J. *1*:36–37, 1982.
85. Ginsburg, C. M.: Acquired syphilis in prepubertal children. Pediatr. Infect. Dis. J. *2*:232–234, 1983.
86. Goh, B. T., and Forster, G. E.: Sexually transmitted diseases in children: Chlamydial oculo-genital infection. Genitourin. Med. *69*:213–221, 1993.
86a. Golden, N., Cohen, H., Gennari, G., et al.: The use of pelvic ultrasonography in evaluation of adolescents with pelvic inflammatory disease. Am. J. Dis. Child. *141*:1235–1238, 1987.
87. Grace, D. A., Ochsner, J. A., McLain, C. R., et al.: Vulvar condylomata acuminata in prepubertal females. J. A. M. A. *201*:151–152, 1967.
88. Gregory, J. E., and Abramson, E.: Meningococci in vaginitis. Am. J. Dis. Child. *121*:423, 1971.
89. Grosskurth, H., Mosha, F., Todd, J., et al.: Impact of improved treatment of sexually transmitted diseases on HIV infection in rural Tanzania: Randomised controlled trial. Lancet *346*:530–536, 1995.
90. Growdon, W. A., Lebherz, T. B., Moore, J. G., et al.: Granuloma inguinale in a white teenager: A diagnosis easily forgotten, poorly pursued. West. J. Med. *143*:105–108, 1985.
91. Hager, W. D.: Followup of patients with tubo-ovarian abscess(es) in association with salpingitis. Obstet. Gynecol. *61*:680–684, 1983.
92. Hager, W. D., Eschenbach, D. A., Spence, M. R., et al.: Criteria for diagnosis and grading of salpingitis. Obstet. Gynecol. *61*:113, 1983.
93. Hammerschlag, M. R.: Chlamydial infections. J. Pediatr. *114*:727–734, 1989.
94. Hammerschlag, M. R.: *Chlamydia trachomatis* in children. Paediatr. Ann. *23*:349–353, 1994.
95. Hammerschlag, M. R., Alpert, S., Onderdonk, A. B., et al.: Anaerobic microflora of the vagina in children. Am. J. Obstet. Gynecol. *131*:853–856, 1978.
96. Hammerschlag, M. R., Alpert, S., Rosner, I., et al.: Microbiology of the vagina in children: Normal and potentially pathogenic organisms. Pediatrics *62*:57–62, 1978.
97. Hammerschlag, M. R., Cummings, M., Doraiswamy, B., et al.: Nonspecific vaginitis following sexual abuse in children. Pediatrics *75*:1028–1031, 1985.
98. Hammerschlag, M. R., Doraiswamy, B., Alexander E. R., et al.: Are rectogenital chlamydial infections a marker of sexual abuse in children? Pediatr. Infect. Dis. J. *3*:100–104, 1984.
99. Hammerschlag, M. R., Doraiswamy, B., Cox, P., et al.: Colonization of sexually abused children with genital mycoplasmas. Sex. Transm. Dis. *14*:23–25, 1987.
100. Hammerschlag, M. R., Rettig, P. J., and Shields, W. E.: False-positive results with the use of chlamydial antigen detection tests in the evaluation of suspected sexual abuse in children. Pediatr. Infect. Dis. J. *7*:11–14, 1988.
101. Hammond, G. W., Slutchuk, M., Scatliff, J., et al.: Epidemiologic, clinical, laboratory, and therapeutic features of an urban outbreak of chancroid in North America. Rev. Infect. Dis. *2*:867–878, 1980.
102. Hare, M., and Mowla, A.: Genital herpesvirus infection in a prepubertal girl. Br. J. Obstet. Gynaecol. *84*:141–142, 1977.
103. Hart, G.: Donovanosis. *In* Holmes, K. K., Mårdh, P.-A., Sparling, P. F., et al. (eds.): Sexually Transmitted Diseases. New York, McGraw-Hill, 1990, pp. 273–277.
104. Hay, D., and Cole, F.: Postgranulomatous epidermoid carcinoma of the vulva. Am. J. Obstet. Gynecol. *108*:479–484, 1970.
105. Hedlund, P.: Acute vulvovaginitis in patients with streptococcal infections. Nord. Med. *49*:566–567, 1953.
106. Heller, R. H., Joseph, J. M., and Davis, H. J.: Vulvovaginitis in the premenarcheal child. J. Pediatr. *74*:370–377, 1969.
107. Hellgren, L.: Gonorre-tonsillit efter genitooral kontakt. Lakartidningen *68*:569–571, 1971.
108. Henderson, P., and Scott, R.: Foreign body vaginitis caused by toilet tissue. Am. J. Dis. Child. *111*:529–532, 1966.
109. Herman-Giddens, M. E., Gutman, L. T., and Berson, N. L.: Association of coexisting vaginal infections and multiple abusers in female children with genital warts. Sex. Transm. Dis. *1*:63–67, 1987.
110. Hewitt, A. B.: Behçet's disease. Br. J. Vener. Dis. *47*:52–53, 1971.
111. Hill, G. B., Eschenbach, D. A., and Holmes, K. K.: Bacteriology of the vagina. Scand. J. Urol. Nephrol. *86*(Suppl.):23–39, 1984.
112. Hill, G. B., St. Claire, K. K., and Gutman, L. T.: Anaerobes predominate among the vaginal microflora of prepubertal girls. Clin. Infect. Dis. *20*(Suppl. 2):S269–S270, 1995.
113. Holmes, K. K.: Lower genital tract infections in women: Cystitis/urethritis, vulvovaginitis and cervicitis. *In* Holmes, K. K., Mårdh, P.-A., Sparling, P. F., et al. (eds.): Sexually Transmitted Diseases. New York, McGraw-Hill, 1990, pp. 527–545.
114. Holmes, K. K., Mårdh, P.-A., Sparling, P. F., et al. (eds.): Sexually Transmitted Diseases. New York, McGraw-Hill, 1990.
115. Huffman, J. W.: Gynecologic infections in childhood and adolescence. *In* Feigin, R. D., and Cherry, J. D. (eds.): Textbook of Pediatric Infectious Diseases. 2nd ed. Philadelphia, W. B. Saunders, 1987, pp. 555–587.
116. Huffman, J. W., Dewhurst, C. J., and Capraro, V. J.: The Gynecology of Childhood and Adolescence. 2nd ed. Philadelphia, W. B. Saunders, 1981.
117. Ingram, D. L.: *Neisseria gonorrhoeae* in children. Pediatr. Ann. *23*:341–345, 1994.
118. Ingram, D. L., White, S. T., Durfee, M. F., et al.: Sexual contact in children with gonorrhea. Am. J. Dis. Child. *136*:994–996, 1982.
119. Ingram, D. L., Runyan, D. K., Collins, A. D., et al.: Vaginal *Chlamydia trachomatis* infection in children with sexual contact. Pedatr. Infect. Dis. J. *3*:97–99, 1984.
120. Ingram, D. L., White, S. T., Occhiuti, A. R., et al.: Childhood vaginal infections: Association of *Chlamydia trachomatis* with sexual contact. Pediatr. Infect. Dis. J. *5*:226–229, 1986.
121. Jacobson, L., and Westrom, L.: Objectivized diagnosis of acute pelvic inflammatory disease. Am. J. Obstet. Gynecol. *105*:1088–1098, 1969.
122. Jones, J. G., Yamauchi, T., and Lambert, B.: *Trichomonas vaginalis* infestation in sexually abused girls. Am. J. Dis. Child. *139*:846–847, 1985.
123. Jones, R. B., Mammel, J. B., Shepard, M. K., et al.: Recovery of *Chlamydia trachomatis* from the endometrium of women at risk for chlamydial infection. Am. J. Obstet. Gynecol. *155*:35–39, 1986.
124. Joseph, A. K., and Rosen, T.: Laboratory techniques used in the diagnosis of chancroid, granuloma inguinale, and lymphogranuloma venereum. Dermatol. Clin. *12*:1–8, 1994.
125. Judson, F. N., and Ehret, J.: Laboratory diagnosis of sexually transmitted infections. Pediatr. Ann. *23*:361–369, 1994.
126. Kaplan, K. M., Fleisher, G. R., Paradise, J. E., et al.: Social relevance of genital herpes simplex in children. Am. J. Dis. Child. *138*:872–874, 1984.
127. Keith, L. G., Berger, G. S., Edelman, D. A., et al.: On the causation of pelvic inflammatory disease. Am. J. Obstet. Gynecol. *149*:215–224, 1984.
128. Kessel, J. F., and Thompson, C. F.: Survival of *Trichomonas vaginalis* infestation in vaginal discharge. Proc. Soc. Exp. Biol. Med. *74*:755–758, 1950.
129. Kim, D.-K., Chang, S. N., Bang, D., et al.: Clinical analysis of 40 cases of childhood-onset Behçet's disease. Pediatr. Dermatol. *11*:95–101, 1994.
130. Kirkpatrick, D. J.: Donovanosis (granuloma inguinale): A rare cause of osteolytic bone lesions. Clin. Radiol. *21*:101–105, 1970.
131. Kokx, N. P., Comstock, J. A., and Facklam, R. R.: Streptococcal perianal disease in children. Pediatrics *80*:659–663, 1987.
132. Krowchuk, D. P., Anglin, T. M., Lembo, R. M., et al.: Use of enzyme immunoassay for the rapid diagnosis of *Chlamydia trachomatis* endocervical infection in female adolescents. J. Adolesc. Health Care *9*:296–300, 1988.
133. Kurnatowska, A., and Komorowska, A.: Urogenital trichomoniasis in children. *In* Honigsberg, B. M. (ed.): Trichomonads: Parasites in Humans. New York, Springer-Verlag, 1989, pp. 246–273.
134. Lal, S., and Nicholas, C.: Epidemiological and clinical features in 165 cases of granuloma inguinale. Br. J. Vener. Dis. *465*:461–463, 1970.
135. Landers, D. V., and Sweet, R. L.: Tubo-ovarian abscess: Contemporary approach to management. Rev. Infect. Dis. *5*:876–884, 1983.
136. Lang, W. R.: Pediatric vaginitis. N. Engl. J. Med. *253*:1153–1160, 1955.
137. Larsen, B., and Galask, R. P.: Vaginal microbial flora: Composition and influences of host physiology. Ann. Intern. Med. *96*(Part 2):926–930, 1982.
138. Larson, T., and Bryson, Y. J.: Fomites and herpes simplex virus. J. Infect. Dis. *151*:746–747, 1985.
139. Lee, Y.-H., Rankin, J. S., Alpert, S., et al.: Microbiological investigation of Bartholin's gland abscesses and cysts. Am. J. Obstet. Gynecol. *129*:150–153, 1977.
140. Lynch, P.: Molluscum contagiosum venereum. Clin. Obstet. Gynecol. *15*:966–975, 1972.
141. Marinoff, S. C., and Turner, M. L. C.: Vulvar vestibulitis syndrome: An overview. Am. J. Obstet. Gynecol. *165*:1228–1233, 1991.
142. Mårdh, P.-A., and Danielson, D.: *Neisseria gonorrhoea*. *In* Holmes, K. K., Mårdh, P.-A., Sparling, P. F., et al. (eds.): Sexually Transmitted Diseases. New York, McGraw-Hill, 1990, pp. 903–916.
143. McCormack, W. M.: Clinical spectrum of gonococcal infection in women. Lancet 2:1182–1185, 1977.
144. Mcfarlane, D. E., and Sharma, D. P.: *Haemophilus influenzae* and genital tract infections in children. Acta Paediatr. Scand. *76*:363–364, 1987.
145. Mishaw, C. O.: Sexual abuse and sexually transmitted diseases in prepubertal children. Semin. Pediatr. Infect. Dis. *4*:131–138, 1993.
146. Monacelli, M., and Nazzaro, P.: Behçet's Disease. Basel/New York, S. Karger, 1966.
147. Morris, C. A.: Seasonal variation of streptococcal vulvo-vaginitis in an urban community. J. Clin. Pathol. 24:805–807, 1971.
148. Morrison, J. C., and Fish, S. A.: Adolescent genital dermatoses. South. Med. J. *69*:1136–1140, 1976.
149. Moscicki, B., Shafer, M. A., Millstein, S. G., et al.: The use and limitations of endocervical gram stains and mucopurulent cervicitis as predictors for *Chlamydia trachomatis* in female adolescents. Am. J. Obstet. Gynecol. *157*:65–71, 1987.
150. Mroczkowski, T. F., and Martin, D. H.: Genital ulcer disease. Dermatol. Clin. *12*:753–764, 1994.
151. Muram, D., Savage, M. O., Harries, J. T., et al.: Crohn's disease of the vulva in a prepubertal girl. Pediatr. Adolesc. Gynecol. *1*:189–195, 1983.

152. Murphy, T. V., and Nelson, J. D.: *Shigella* vaginitis: Report of 38 patients and review of the literature. Pediatrics *63*:511–516, 1979.
153. Nahmias, A.: Herpes simplex infection. *In* Gellis, S., and Kagan, B. (eds.): Current Pediatric Therapy 7. Philadelphia, W. B. Saunders, 1976, pp. 599–603.
154. Nahamias, A. J., Dowdle, W. R., Naib, Z. M., et al.: Genital infection with herpes virus hominis types 1 and 2 in children. Pediatrics *42*:659–666, 1968.
155. Nair, P., Glazer-Semmel, E., Gould, C., et al.: *Neisseria gonorrhoeae* in asymptomatic prepubertal household contacts of children with gonococcal infection. Clin. Pediatr. *25*:160–163, 1986.
156. Nebel, W. A., and Lucas, W. E.: Management of tubo-ovarian abscess. Obstet. Gynecol. *32*:382–386, 1968.
157. Neinstein, L. S., Goldenring, J., and Carpenter, S.: Nonsexual transmission of sexually transmitted diseases: An infrequent occurrence. Pediatrics *74*:67–76, 1984.
158. O'Duffy, J. D., Carney, J. A., and Deodhar, S.: Behçet's disease. Ann. Intern. Med. *75*:561–570, 1971.
159. O'Farrell, N.: Clinico-epidemiological study of donovanosis in Durban, South Africa. Genitourin. Med. *69*:108–111, 1993.
160. O'Farrell, N.: Global eradication of donovanosis: An opportunity for limiting the spread of HIV-1. Genitourin. Med. *71*:27–31, 1995.
161. O'Farrell, N., Hoosen, A. A., Coetzee, K. D., et al.: Genital ulcer disease: Accuracy of clinical diagnosis and strategies to improve control in Durban, South Africa. Genitourin. Med. *70*:7–11, 1994.
162. Orellana-Diaz, O., and Hernandez-Perez, E.: Chancroid in El Salvador. Int. J. Dermatol. *27*:243–245, 1988.
163. Oriel, J.: Natural history of genital warts. Br. J. Vener. Dis. *47*:1–13, 1971.
164. Owen, R., Christiansen, G., Hansen, E., et al.: Reports from the working groups at the Symposium on Bacterial Vaginosis: Taxonomy of anaerobic curved rods. Scand. J. Urol. Nephrol. *86*(Suppl.):259–266, 1984.
165. Pacor, M. L., Biasi, D., Lunardi, C., et al.: Cyclosporin in Behçet's disease: Results in 16 patients after 24 months of therapy. Clin. Rheumatol. *13*:224–227, 1994.
166. Paradise, J. E., Campos, J. M., Friedman, H. M., et al.: Vulvovaginitis in premenarcheal girls: Clinical features and diagnostic evaluation. Pediatrics *70*:193–198, 1982.
167. Patton, D. C.: Immunopathology and histopathology of experimental chlamydial salpingitis. Rev. Infect. Dis. *7*:746–753, 1985.
168. Peckham, B. M., Maki, D. G., Patterson, J. J., et al.: Focal vulvitis: A characteristic syndrome and cause of dyspareunia. Am. J. Obstet. Gynecol. *154*:855–864, 1986.
169. Peter, R., and Vesely, K.: Kindergynakologie. Leipzig, Georg Thieme, 1966.
170. Pierce, A. M., and Hart, C. A.: Vulvovaginitis: Causes and management. Arch. Dis. Child. *67*:509–512, 1992.
171. Platt, M.: Neonatal *Hemophilus vaginalis (Corynebacterium vaginalis)* infection. Clin. Pediatr. *10*:513–516, 1971.
172. Pokorny, S. F., and Stormer, J.: Atraumatic removal of secretions from prepubertal vagina. Am. J. Obstet. Gynecol. *156*:581–582, 1987.
173. Pokorny, S. F.: Prepubertal vulvovaginopathies. Obstet. Gynecol. Clin. North Am. *19*:39–58, 1992.
174. Potterat, J. J., Markewich, G. S., King, R. D., et al.: Child-to-child transmission of gonorrhea: Report of asymptomatic genital infection in a boy Pediatrics *60*:153–156, 1977.
175. Prayson, R. A., Stoler, M. H., and Hart, W. R.: Vulvar vestibulitis: A histopathologic study of 36 cases, including human papillomavirus in situ hybridization analysis. Am. J. Surg. Pathol. *19*:154–160, 1995.
176. Rajam, R. V., Rangiah, P. N., and Anguli, V. C.: Systemic donovaniasis. Br. J. Vener. Dis. *30*:73, 1954.
177. Rakover, Y., Adar, H., Tal, I., et al.: Behçet disease: Long-term follow-up of three children and review of the literature. Pediatrics *83*:986–992, 1989.
178. Reed, S. D., Landers, D. V., and Sweet, R. L.: Antibiotic treatment of tubo-ovarian abscess: Comparison of broad-spectrum β-lactam agents versus clindamycin-containing regimens. Am. J. Obstet. Gynecol. *164*:1556–1561, 1991.
179. Rees, E.: Gonococcal bartholinitis. Br. J. Vener. Dis. *43*:150–156, 1967.
180. Regard, M. M., Chacko, M. R., Kozinetz, C. A., et al.: Reliability of cervical findings and endocervical polymorphonuclear cells in detecting chlamydial and gonococcal cervicitis in young women receiving contraceptive services. Adolesc. Pediatr. Gynecol. *6*:129–134, 1993.
181. Rein, M. F.: Survival of gonococci outside the body. N. Engl. J. Med. *301*:1347, 1979.
182. Rettig, P. J., and Nelson, J. D.: Genital tract infection with *Chlamydia trachomatis* in prepubertal children. J. Pediatr. *99*:206–210, 1981.
183. Rey-Stocker, I.: Vulvitis and vaginitis in the infant. Gynaecologia *168*:413–415, 1969.
184. Richens, J.: The diagnosis and treatment of donovanosis (granuloma inguinale). Genitourin. Med. *67*:441–452, 1991.
185. Rosenfeld, W. D., and Clark, J.: Vulvovaginitis and cervicitis. Pediatr. Clin. North Am. *36*:489–511, 1989.
186. Rosenfeld, W., Vermund, S., Wentz, S., et al.: High prevalence rate of human papilloma virus infection and association with abnormal Papanicolaou smears in sexually active adolescents. Am. J. Dis. Child. *143*:1443–1447, 1989.
187. Rosenfeld, W. D., and Litman, N.: Sexually transmitted diseases. *In* Friedman, S. B., Fisher, M., and Schonberg, S. K. (eds.): Comprehensive Adolescent Health Care. St. Louis, Quality Medical Publishing, 1992, pp. 995–1015.
188. Roth, R.: Acute abdomen in infancy and childhood: Case report of acute gonorrheal tubo-ovarian abscess in infant of 2 months. Mississippi Doctor *24*:159–161, 1946.
189. Saltz, G. R., Linneman, C. C., Brookman, R. R., et al.: *Chlamydia trachomatis* cervical infections in female adolescent. J. Pediatr. *98*:981–985, 1981.
190. Sanfilippo, J. S.: Pediatric and adolescent gynecology. Obstet. Gynecol. Clin. North Am. *19*:1–239, 1992.
191. Saracoglu, O. F., Mungan, T., and Tanzer, F.: Pelvic tuberculosis. Int. J. Gynecol. Obstet. *37*:115–120, 1992.
192. Schachter, J.: Biology of *Chlamydia trachomatis*. *In* Holmes, K. K., Mårdh, P.-A., Sparling, P. F., et al. (eds.): Sexually Transmitted Diseases. New York, McGraw-Hill, 1984, pp. 243–257.
193. Schachter, J., Grossman, M., Sweet, R. L., et al.: Prospective study of perinatal transmission of *Chlamydia trachomatis*. J. A. M. A. *255*:3374–3377, 1986.
194. Schaefer, G.: Tuberculosis of the female genital tract. Clin. Obstet. Gynecol. *13*:965–998, 1970.
195. Scheid, F.: Diseases of adnexa in children and their differentiation from appendicitis. Med. Klin. *18*:1277–1279, 1922.
196. Schubiner, H. H., Lebar, W., Jemal, C., et al.: Comparison of three new non-culture tests in the diagnosis of *Chlamydia* genital infections. J. Adolesc. Health Care *11*:505–509, 1990.
197. Schulte, J. M., and Schmid, G. P.: Recommendations for treatment of chancroid, 1993. Clin. Infect. Dis. *20*(Suppl. 1):S39–S46, 1995.
197a. Schwarcz, S. K., and Whittington, W. L.: Sexual assault and sexually transmitted diseases: Detection and management in adults and children. Rev. Infect. Dis. *12*(Suppl. 6):S682–S690, 1990.
198. Schwartz, R. H., Wientzen, R. L., and Barsanti, R. G.: Vulvovaginitis in prepubertal girls: The importance of group A *Streptococcus*. South. Med. J. *75*:446–447, 1982.
199. Seelig, M.: The role of antibiotics in the pathogenesis of *Candida* infections. Am. J. Med. *40*:887–917, 1966.
200. Seidel, J., Zonang, J., and Totten, E.: Condylomata acuminata as a sign of sexual abuse in children. J. Pediatr. *95*:553–554, 1979.
201. Senanayake, P., and Kramer, D. G.: Contraception and the etiology of pelvic inflammatory disease: New perspectives. Am. J. Obstet. Gynecol. *138*:852–860, 1980.
202. Sgroi, S.: Pediatric gonorrhea beyond infancy. Pediatr. Ann. *8*:326–336, 1979.
203. Shafer, M. A., Beck, A., Blain, B., et al.: *Chlamydia trachomatis*: Important relationships to race, contraception, lower genital tract infection, and Papanicolaou smear. J. Pediatr. *104*:141–146, 1984.
204. Shafer, M. A., Sweet, R. L., Ohm-Smith, M. J., et al.: Microbiology of the lower genital tract in postmenarcheal adolescent girls: Differences by sexual activity, contraception, and presence of nonspecific vaginitis. J. Pediatr. *107*:974–981, 1985.
205. Shafer, M.-A., Vaughn, E., Lipkin, E. S., et al.: Evaluation of fluorescein conjugated monoclonal antibody test to detect *Chlamydia trachomatis* in adolescent girls. J. Pediatr. *108*:779–783, 1986.
206. Shore, W. B., and Winkelstein, J. A.: Nonvenereal transmission of gonococcal infections to children. J. Pediatr. *79*:661–663, 1971.
207. Silber, T. J.: Genital ulcer syndrome. Semin. Adolesc. Med. *2*:155–162, 1986.
208. Smith, E. W., Peutherer, J. F., Robertson, D. H., et al.: Virological studies in genital herpes. Lancet *2*:1089–1090, 1976.
209. Sonck, C., and Somersalo, O.: The yeast flora of the anogenital region in diabetic girls. Arch. Dermatol. *88*:846–852, 1963.
210. Spear, R. M., Rothbaum, R. J., Keating, J. P., et al.: Perianal streptococcal cellulitis. J. Pediatr. *107*:557–559, 1985.
211. Spence, M. R., Adler, J., and McLellan, R.: Pelvic inflammatory disease. J. Adolesc. Health Care *11*:304–309, 1990.
212. Srivastava, A. C.: Survival of gonococci in urethral secretions with reference to the nonsexual transmission of gonococcal infection. J. Med. Microbiol. *13*:593–596, 1980.
213. Stamm, W. E., Wagner, K. F., Amsel, R., et al.: Causes of acute urethral syndrome in women. N. Engl. J. Med. *303*:409–415, 1980.
214. Strasburger, V. C.: Adolescent gynecology. Pediatr. Clin. North Am. *36*:471–478, 1989.
215. Straumanis, J. P., and Bocchini, J. A.: Group A beta-hemolytic streptococcal vulvovaginitis in prepubertal girls: A case report and review of the past twenty years. Pediatr. Infect. Dis. J. *9*:845–848, 1990.
216. Stringel, G., Spence, J., and Corsini, L.: Genital warts in children. Can. Med. Assoc. J. *132*:1397–1398, 1985.
217. Stumph, P. G.: Increasing occurrence of condyloma acuminata in premenarcheal children. Obstet. Gynecol. *56*:262–264, 1980.
218. Swain, V.: Tuberculous vulvovaginitis: Report of a case in infancy. Lancet *1*:868–869, 1937.
219. Sweet, R. L.: Pelvic inflammatory disease and infertility in women. Infect. Dis. Clin. North Am. *1*:199, 1987.
220. Sweet, R. L.: Use of laparoscopy to determine microbiologic etiology of acute salpingitis. Am. J. Obstet. Gynecol. *134*:68–74, 1979.

221. Sweet, R. L., Banks, J., Sung, M., et al.: Experimental chlamydial salpingitis in the guinea pig. Am. J. Obstet. Gynecol. *138*:952–956, 1980.
222. Sweet, R. L., Blankfort-Doyle, M., Robbie, M. O., et al.: The occurrence of chlamydial and gonococcal salpingitis during the menstrual cycle. J. A. M. A. *255*:2062–2064, 1986.
223. Swensson, L., Westrom, T., and Mårdh, P.-A.: Contraceptives and acute salpingitis. J. A. M. A. *251*:2553–2555, 1984.
224. Teokharov, B. A.: Non-gonococcal infections in the female genitalia. Br. J. Vener. Dis. *45*:334–340, 1969.
225. Toth, A., O'Leary, W. M., and Ledger, W.: Evidence for microbial transfer by spermatozoa. Obstet. Gynecol. *59*:556–559, 1982.
226. Tunnessen, W. W., Jr., and Jastremski, M.: Prepubescent gonococcal vulvovaginitis. Clin. Pediatr. *13*:675–676, 1974.
227. Vandeven, A. M., and Emans, J.: Vulvovaginitis in the child and adolescent. Pediatr. Rev. *14*:141–147, 1993.
228. Van Overbeek, J.: Gonorrheal infections in the oropharynx. Arch. Otolaryngol. *102*:94–96, 1976.
229. Washington, A. E., Sweet, R. L., and Shafer, M. B.: Pelvic inflammatory disease and its sequelae in adolescents. J. Adolesc. Health Care *6*:298, 1985.
230. Watkins, S., and Quan, L.: Vulvovaginitis caused by *Yersinia enterocolitica*. Pediatr. Infect. Dis. J. *3*:444–445, 1984.
231. Weaver, J.: Non-gonorrheal vulvovaginitis due to gram-negative intracellular diplococci. Am. J. Obstet. Gynecol. *60*:257–260, 1950.
232. Webb, D. H., and Fife, K. H.: Genital herpes simplex virus infection. Infect. Dis. Clin. North Am. *1*:97–122, 1987.
233. Weinstock, H., and Keesol, S.: Lymphogranuloma venereum: Report of 24 cases in children. Urol. Cutan. Rev. *50*:520–522, 1946.
234. Weisserbacher, G., and Wiltschke, H.: Chronic urinary tract infections and vulvitis in girls with high posterior commissures. Pediatr. Padol. *9*:60–65, 1974.
235. Westrom, L., and Mårdh, P.-A.: Acute pelvic inflammatory disease (PID). *In* Holmes, K. K., Mårdh, P.-A., Sparling, P. F., et al. (eds.): Sexually Transmitted Diseases. New York, McGraw-Hill, 1990, pp. 593–613.
236. Willcox, R.: Chancroid. *In* Morton, R. S., and Harris, J. R. (eds.): Recent Advances in Sexually Transmitted Diseases. New York, Longman, 1975.
237. Wolner-Hanssen, P., Eschenbach, D. A., Paavonen, J., et al.: Association between vaginal douching and acute pelvic inflammatory disease. J. A. M. A. *263*:1936–1941, 1990.
238. Wolner-Hanssen, P., Svensson, L., and Mårdh, P.-A.: Laparoscopic findings and contraceptive use in women with signs and symptoms suggestive of acute salpingitis. Obstet. Gynecol. *66*:233–238, 1985.
239. Woods, C. R.: Gonococcal infections in children and adolescents. Semin. Pediatr. Rev. *14*:141–147, 1993.
240. Worwag, Z.: Trichomoniasis in newborn infants. Ginekol. Pol. *43*:57–63, 1971.
241. Zigas, V.: Medicine from the past: Donovanosis project in Goilala (1951–1954). Papua New Guinea Med. J. *14*:148, 1971.

50

SEXUALLY TRANSMITTED DISEASES

Laura T. Gutman

Chlamydia Infections

THE ORGANISM

Chlamydiaceae is a family of obligate intracellular bacterial parasites. There is one genus—*Chlamydia*—which contains three distinct species. *Chlamydia trachomatis* is inhibited by sulfonamides and produces iodine-staining cytoplasmic inclusions. *Chlamydia psittaci* is not inhibited by sulfonamides and does not produce iodine-staining inclusions in cytoplasmic vesicles. *Chlamydia pneumoniae* is the species identified most recently (Table 50–1).

Although *Chlamydia* organisms are found in a variety of vertebrates, they infect primarily birds, humans, and other mammals. Trachoma, genital trachoma, inclusion conjunctivitis, and lymphogranuloma venereum (LGV) are the most common human diseases caused by these organisms. Humans may be infected with *Chlamydia* species that normally are associated with disease of other animals, such as those causing psittacosis. *C. pneumoniae* has characteristics differentiating it from the other human chlamydial strains (see Chapter 193).

A unique developmental cycle characterizes *Chlamydia.* It consists of three major stages:[1] Attachment is followed by organism-induced phagocytosis by the host cell. The elementary body, the infective form of *Chlamydia,* is a small, dense, spherical body 0.2 to 0.4 μm in diameter with a rigid envelope.[2] This elementary body then enlarges to 0.7 to 1 μm in diameter; this is the noninfective initial body, a granular and reticulated form of the organism with a flexible envelope. The initial bodies are within the phagocytic vacuole and direct the cell's synthetic functions to their own metabolic needs.[3] The initial bodies multiply by binary fission; the daughter organisms reorganize into infective elementary bodies with the characteristic dense appearance.

The phagocytized elementary body with the surrounding invaginated host-cell membrane becomes the inclusion body as replication of the organism proceeds. Intracellular inclu-

TABLE 50–1. Characteristics Distinguishing *Chlamydia* Species

C. trachomatis	*C. psittaci*	*C. pneumoniae*
Iodine-staining glycogen produced by microcolony	Microcolony does not produce glycogen	Microcolony does not produce glycogen
Round elementary body	Round elementary body	Pear-shaped elementary body
Folate biosynthesis	No folate biosynthesis	No folate biosynthesis
Restriction endonuclease pattern distinguishes species	Restriction endonuclease pattern distinguishes species	Restriction endonuclease pattern distinguishes species
16 serovars determined by immunofluorescence	Uncertain number of serovars	1 serovar

sion bodies contain large, noninfectious initial bodies and elementary bodies that are capable of initiating infection. These large inclusion bodies are intracellular bacterial microcolonies. About 48 to 72 hours after infection, the host cell ruptures and the elementary bodies are released to begin a new infectious cycle. Thus, *Chlamydia* is adapted uniquely to survival in the host. The elementary body survives adverse environmental features, is infectious, and induces its own phagocytosis. Inside the phagocytic vacuole, the elementary body prevents fusion of the phagosome and lysosomes, protecting itself from enzymatic destruction. The reticular bodies are the metabolic, multiplying form of the organism and successfully parasitize the host cell's production of energy.

In *C. trachomatis,* the maturation of initial bodies into elementary bodies is accompanied by a rapid increase in the synthesis of DNA. The elementary body has an electron-dense eccentrically located nucleoid. The molecular weight of the *C. trachomatis* double-stranded DNA is approximately 600×10^6 daltons and is among the smallest of the prokaryotic genomes. Only that of *Mycoplasma* species is smaller. This DNA is approximately one-quarter the size of that of *Escherichia coli.* The elementary body is limited by a discrete cell wall, which stains gram-negative. The envelope of *Chlamydia* reticulate bodies consists of inner and outer cytoplasmic membranes, like other gram-negative bacteria. The envelope has a major outer-membrane protein, but unlike other gram-negative bacteria, no peptidoglycan layer is interposed. The rigidity of the elementary body envelope may be due to disulfide cross-linkage because elementary bodies differ from reticulate bodies in the extent of complexing of the outer membrane proteins by disulfide bonding. The outer membrane has a unique patch of projections made up of approximately 18 hexagonally arrayed cylindrical projections that extend through the outer membrane and are located on the far side of the cell away from the nucleoid. The *Chlamydia* organisms are unable to synthesize their own high-energy compounds, including adenosine 5′-triphosphate, and utilize energy-rich host-cell metabolites for macromolecular synthesis.

Antigenic Structure

The antigens to which the host develops antibodies and immunity also provide the serologic identification of *Chlamydia* and are located in the cell envelope. All *Chlamydia* possess a common heat-stable antigen present at all times during the developmental cycle. This antigen is associated with the cell wall and resembles polysaccharides of other gram-negative bacteria containing 2-keto-3-deoxyoctanoic acid. Because it is genus-specific, its presence can be used only for detection, not for identification of chlamydial strains.

The major outer-membrane protein is the predominant site of immunoreactive groups defining species specificity (i.e., differentiating *C. trachomatis* from *C. psittaci*) and serovar specificity. There are 16 serovars (strain variations) of *C. trachomatis.* These specificities were detected by microimmunofluorescence and confirmed by peptide mapping of major outer-membrane proteins. The immune response to these proteins is somewhat protective against reinfection by the same strain but also may contribute to the adverse consequences of chlamydial infection.[65]

Microimmunofluorescence Typing

Antigenic subdivision of *C. trachomatis* serovars may be based on immunofluorescent techniques (Table 50–2). Studies of strains isolated from the eyes and the genital tract have revealed 14 or more distinguishable types: A through L. Types A, B, and C have been isolated primarily from the eyes of persons with trachoma in trachoma-endemic areas. The types appear to correlate with the site of isolation of organisms and the epidemiology of infection. Isolation of these types from genital sites is rare. Types D through L usually are isolated from the eyes of persons in areas where trachoma is nonendemic and most frequently from the genital tracts of adults. Included among strains D through L are isolates from infants who were born to mothers with cervical infection and developed inclusion conjunctivitis. However, genital types also occasionally may be isolated from ocular sites in areas of endemic ocular trachoma.[47]

TABLE 50–2. Human Diseases Caused by *Chlamydia trachomatis*

Serovar	Major Diseases
A, B, C	Endemic trachoma of the eye
D–M	Inclusion conjunctivitis of newborn and adult
	Nongonococcal urethritis
	Cervicitis
	Salpingitis
	Pneumonitis of newborn
	Proctitis
L_1, L_2, L_3	Lymphogranuloma venereum

With the immunofluorescent test, lymphogranuloma strains may be immunotyped into one of three subtypes—L_1, L_2, or L_3—and usually are isolated from patients with clinically characteristic LGV. Using these methods to explore the serologic response to proven LGV, researchers have found that persons infected with any of the LGV strains characteristically demonstrate a very high antibody titer to the isolated strains and to the antigenically related strains. In addition, there is antibody to a broad range of other *C. trachomatis* antigenic types in patients with LGV. This is in marked contrast to the moderate and specific immune response of persons with ocular trachoma and the slightly more vigorous and widely reactive response of persons with chlamydial urethritis. These findings probably reflect the marked increase in biologic capacity for invasion and virulence shown by LGV strains, compared with other *C. trachomatis* strains in humans. Trachoma-like strains seldom invade beyond mucous membranes, whereas LGV strains frequently are isolated from regional lymph nodes and may cause systemic disease.

LABORATORY DIAGNOSIS

Culture and Antigen Detection

Isolation of *Chlamydia* may be accomplished by inoculation of infected material into embryonated eggs, selected tissue culture cell lines, or experimental animals.

Tissue cell culture methods for isolating *Chlamydia* may include use of centrifugation for enhancing absorption of *Chlamydia* to cells; use of susceptible cell lines; the pretreatment of cells to increase detection of inclusions; and use of commercially available fluorescein-conjugated monoclonal antibody, which allows species-specific immunofluorescent detection of infected cells.[22, 71] Cell lines commonly used to isolate *Chlamydia* include irradiated McCoy and HeLa cells. Use of *Chlamydia* transport media enhances the survival of organisms from clinical specimens. Specimens must be placed on ice immediately after collection and never stored at -20° C.

Chlamydial antigen detection tests have been developed and are commercially available. Direct fluorescent antibody tests and enzyme immunoassay systems have been developed. More recently, amplified DNA assays have been developed.[61, 83] The tests have been evaluated extensively in adults who are at high risk for sexually transmitted diseases, and the results of the assay of urethral and cervical specimens often have been comparable with culture results.[25, 91] These assay methods also are highly sensitive and specific in the diagnosis of neonatal inclusion conjunctivitis,[11, 44, 69, 75] but the evaluation of other pediatric specimens usually requires culture for adequate diagnosis.

Cytopathologic examination of infected specimens may provide an adequate diagnosis. *C. trachomatis* develops compact, clearly defined, glycogen-containing intracellular microcolonies or inclusions. These are found in infected yolk sac preparations, infected animal tissue, inoculated tissue culture cells, and conjunctival scrapings of persons with active trachoma or inclusion conjunctivitis. Demonstration of the causative agent in ocular diseases may be made by everting the tarsal plate, removing the exudate, and gently scraping epithelial cells from the surface. The inclusions in scrapings are basophilic and stain a mahogany color with iodine, are gram-negative, and may stain with fluorescent antibody or Giemsa stain.

Serologic Tests

The microimmunofluorescent technique provided the initial means for measuring type-specific antibody response to *C. trachomatis*. In the majority of patients for whom the identity of the infecting strain is known, type-specific antibody develops. Exceptions include patients with LGV, in whom antibody frequently is reactive with more than one type. Early antibody formation is of the IgM class and persists for approximately 1 month before being succeeded by IgG. In the few instances in which serial antibody determinations have been made, type-specific antibody has been observed to decrease fairly rapidly after primary infection, often within 1 or 2 months. Unfortunately, such antibody tests are not available for many clinical services.

Frei Test

The Frei test is only of historic interest and was an intradermal skin test used primarily for the diagnosis of LGV. The test initially used boiled lymph node material excised from a patient with LGV; a later reagent was lymphogranuloma antigen, a crude protein antigen prepared from infected chick embryo yolk sac material by acid extraction. The site of the skin test injection was examined at 48 and 72 hours for the formation of a subcutaneous nodule. The Frei test was much less sensitive than antibody determination as measured by complement fixation in the diagnosis of infections due to *C. trachomatis*.

EPIDEMIOLOGY

The basic epidemiologic characteristics of genital trachoma were appreciated very early in the twentieth century. The most comprehensive early review in English was in 1942 by Thygeson and Stone,[94] in which the association between disease of the eye of the infant, the maternal cervix, and other siblings was described, suggesting transmission by mucous membrane to mucous membrane. Thirteen mothers of infants with inclusion conjunctivitis had cervical material examined, and 10 of these specimens were positive. Ocular disease typical of inclusion conjunctivitis had occurred in 17 of 37 siblings of infants with inclusion conjunctivitis, and unexplained postpartum fever occurred in 9 of 38 infected women. In a study of nonpregnant women, chronic pelvic inflammatory disease, cervicitis, and vaginal discharge affected the *Chlamydia*-positive women. A proportion of male patients with nongonococcal or postgonococcal urethritis are infected with *Chlamydia* and are consorts of women whose infants have inclusion conjunctivitis. Finally, accidental inoculation of infected genital secretions into the eyes of adults with resulting inclusion conjunctivitis has been reported.[84] The constellation of disease, which includes inclusion conjunctivitis of the newborn, cervical disease of the adult female, and urethritis and ophthalmitis of adults, was described fully in the pre-antibiotic era and while the causative agent was believed to be a virus.

Chlamydia may be isolated from approximately 40 per cent of men with nongonococcal or postgonococcal urethritis.[51, 79] Approximately 35 per cent of female contacts of men with chlamydial urethritis themselves have cervical or urethral disease due to *Chlamydia*. Conversely, the majority of fathers of infants with inclusion conjunctivitis also harbored urethral *Chlamydia*. Finally, multiple sites of disease in adults are common; most persons who have chlamydial disease of the eye also have genital infection and/or pharyngeal colonization or disease.

Prevalence rates of chlamydial infections in sexually active female adolescents vary from 8 per cent in asymptomatic women to more than 20 per cent (Table 50–3). *C. trachomatis* now is the most prevalent sexually transmitted pathogen in the United States.

In contrast to the responses to the epidemic of gonorrhea from the 1970s and 1980s, which included national programs for screening and ascertainment of disease, there has not been a major initiative for the control of chlamydial disease. It appears that localized programs have had notable successes,[2] but widespread implementation has not occurred in spite of recommendations to do so.[21] Genital disease continues therefore to occur on a widespread basis, and children and adolescents who are abused or assaulted are at risk.[35]

Adolescents

The following conditions are associated with an increased rate of chlamydial infection in female adolescents:

1. The majority of female adolescents infected with *Chlamydia* are unaware of symptomatic disease.

TABLE 50–3. Prevalence of Cervical *Chlamydia trachomatis* Infections in Sexually Active Female Adolescents

Author, Date, Place	Number (% Infected)	Population
Golden,[36] 1984, New York	19/186 (10.2%)	Sexually active
Fraser,[32] 1978, Oklahoma	10/125 (8%)	Sexually active
Saltz,[81] 1981, Ohio	22/100 (22%)	Sexually active
Fisher,[30] 1987, New York	29/200 (14.5%)	Sexually active
Mulcahy,[67] 1987, Leeds	49/307 (16.2%)	Residential care
Biro,[16] 1994, Ohio	20/228 (8.7%)	Asymptomatic
	39/251 (15.5%)	Symptomatic

2. Laboratory findings that are correlated with chlamydial endocervicitis in female adolescents include the presence of polymorphonuclear cells on endocervical Gram stains.[66, 85] Populations of adolescents with a high rate of disease due to *Chlamydia* also have a high rate of other sexually transmitted diseases, such as gonorrhea and *Trichomonas* infections.[27, 39, 67] The infections often are polymicrobial.[39]

3. Behavioral risk factors for infection with *Chlamydia* in adolescents include multiple sexual partners, sexual contact with men with urethritis, omission of the use of condoms, and history of infection with a sexually transmitted disease.[23, 74, 77, 89] Use of oral contraception may be a risk factor for the acquisition of chlamydial endocervicitis.[85]

4. Genital infection with *Chlamydia* in women is asymptomatic in approximately a third of infections.[16] Infection also may be associated with cervical erosions and bleeding, pelvic inflammatory disease, proctitis, salpingitis, vaginal discharge, and urethritis.

5. Female adolescents often experience repeated chlamydial disease. Factors leading to recurrences include problems with completion of planned therapy, low rates of partner notification, and low rates of treatment of partners.[18]

Children

C. trachomatis is a sexually transmissible disease that may affect children. The infant may be infected during passage through an infected birth canal. When that happens, there may be delay before cultures are positive,[13] and the child subsequently may shed the organism for a relatively prolonged period, sometimes as long as 3 years.[14, 15] However, when children who are older than about 3 years of age are shown to be infected with *C. trachomatis* at vaginal, rectal, or pharyngeal sites, they should be assumed to have been the probable victim of sexual abuse (see later).[5] Studies have documented the association of *C. trachomatis* infections in children with sexual exposure.[52, 53] Conversely, children who are undergoing a medical evaluation for sexual abuse or rape should have cultures taken from vaginal, rectal, and pharyngeal sites for *C. trachomatis*. Table 50–4 tabulates the rates of vaginal, rectal, or pharyngeal *Chlamydia* from five studies of prepubertal children who were evaluated for sexual abuse. Rates of *C. trachomatis* from vaginal cultures of these girls ranged from 1 to 17 per cent.

EFFECT ON PREGNANCY

The possibility of an adverse effect on a pregnancy by chlamydial infection of the cervix must be considered before the risk to a newborn infant is examined. Studies of pregnant women have indicated that approximately 7 to 12 per cent of women in the United States harbor *Chlamydia* in the cervix during pregnancy. Some studies have shown a significantly increased incidence of premature delivery, low birth weight, and perinatal death for infected women, compared with controls.[34, 62] Other studies have indicated that only women with recent and active chlamydial infection may be at particular risk of fetal loss.[4] The added risk to the pregnancy for women with recent or invasive chlamydial disease has been confirmed by the demonstration of significantly increased rates of prolonged rupture of the membranes and preterm deliveries in infected mothers.[90]

Other serious complications of reproduction appear to be associated highly with chlamydial disease, including pelvic inflammatory disease, ectopic pregnancy, and infertility.[97] These complications follow asymptomatic disease and are the cause of considerable disability, absenteeism, and medical expense. These complications appear to be especially prevalent in infected female adolescents, compared with infected women.

CLINICAL MANIFESTATIONS

Inclusion Conjunctivitis in Infants

"Inclusion conjunctivitis" usually is a disease of the newborn eye that is contracted during delivery through an infected birth canal. It is caused by *C. trachomatis,* which also is the cause of adult ocular trachoma. The term "TRIC agent" historically encompassed both diseases.

Attempts to establish an experimental animal model for ocular *C. trachomatis* infection have been made by infecting the cervices of pregnant Taiwan monkeys. Conjunctival challenge of the infants at approximately 7 months of age resulted in severe pannus formation, identical with that shown by animals who had previous *Chlamydia* ocular infections. These findings suggested that an infection of the infant had sensitized the infant to subsequent challenge.[3] The disease was similar to trachoma, which suggested that prior sensitization and the host response had contributed to the observed pathogenesis.

Inclusion conjunctivitis was recognized to be a separate disease of the newborn period very early in the twentieth century, and accurate clinical descriptions have been widely available for more than 60 years. Table 50–5 shows results of four studies of infants who were born to mothers who had *Chlamydia* isolated from cervical cultures during pregnancy and one study of randomized therapy. The rate of conjunctivitis in these studies was 15 to 37 per cent of exposed infants. The randomized therapy study indicated that topical prophylaxis was not efficacious.

TABLE 50–4. Prevalence of Genital *Chlamydia* Infections in Sexually Abused Prepubertal Girls

Author, Date, Place	Number Positive/Number Evaluated (%) *Vagina*	*Rectum*	*Pharynx*	Population
Bump,[20] 1987, Ohio	4/29 (14%)	ND	ND	Symptomatic
Ingram,[53] 1986, North Carolina	10/124 (8%)	3/124 (2%)	2/124 (2%)	Children evaluated for abuse
Fuster,[33] 1987, California	8/147 (17%)	ND	ND	Children evaluated for abuse
Hauger,[48] 1988, New York	4/93 (4%)	1/81 (1%)	0/76 (0%)	Children evaluated for abuse
Shapiro,[86] 1993, Ohio	8/615 (1.3%)	1/490 (0.2%)	ND	Children evaluated for abuse
Siegel,[87] 1995, Ohio	2/242 (0.8%)	1/242 (0.4%)	ND	Children evaluated for abuse
Ingram,[54] 1992, North Carolina	17/1473 (1.2%)	6/1473 (0.4%)	—	Children evaluated for abuse

ND, No data.

TABLE 50–5. Incidence of Conjunctivitis and of Pneumonia in Infants Born to Mothers with Cervical *Chlamydia trachomatis* Infection

Author, Date	Conjunctivitis (Patients Infected/Studied)	Pneumonia (Patients Infected/Studied)
Heggie,[50] 1981	20/95 (21%)	3/95 (3%)
Schachter,[82] 1986	23/131 (18%)	21/131 (16%)
Datta,[26] 1988	18/49 (37%)	6/49 (12%)
Hammerschlag,[41] 1989	35/230 (15%)	2/230 (1%)

A preponderance of premature infants appears among children in whom the diagnosis is made.[37] This may be attributable to a longer hospitalization and consequent recognition of the disease or to increased susceptibility to the infection in premature infants.

The presentation of neonatal inclusion conjunctivitis usually begins a few days after birth, although it may present on the day of birth. Onset as late as the second week after birth is not rare. The child usually is in good general health, and there are few if any signs of systemic disease. Unilateral involvement is common. The discharge may be mucopurulent but often is very minimal, with crusting and slight edema of the lids as the only signs of disease. Other bacteria often infect the eye concomitantly, and culture may yield *Staphylococcus epidermidis* and *Neisseria, Corynebacterium,* and *Streptococcus* species. Findings during examination of the eye often include edema of both upper and lower lids, diffuse injection of the palpebral conjunctiva, and prominence of small blood vessels. The exudate contains mainly polymorphonuclear leukocytes, and examination of the exudate usually will not reveal the inclusions that are to be found in the epithelial cells. Direct immunofluorescent staining of exudate obtained on a small swab will reveal elementary bodies.

Inclusion conjunctivitis of the newborn has a clinical spectrum, which may include scarring.[40] Early studies showed that the majority of untreated children who had inclusion conjunctivitis as infants developed sequelae of some form, although it usually was mild and did not compromise vision.[31, 38, 63] In Goscienski's series,[37, 38] all children had received therapy at the time the disease was recognized, and the proportion of children who developed sequelae was minimal.

Attempts to provide prophylaxis for chlamydial disease of the newborn by topical treatment of the eye, analogous to gonococcal prophylaxis, generally have been unsuccessful. Table 50–6 summarizes four studies on the efficacy of silver nitrate, erythromycin, and tetracycline used as topical therapy for exposed infants. The efficacy of each was only moderate at best, and it is apparent that exposed infants require systemic therapy.

Ocular trachoma is not discussed in any detail in this chapter. The staging of disease has been well described.[93] In 1966, Jones and associates[55] provided a comparison of the stages of adult trachoma with those of inclusion conjunctivitis in infants. The stages are summarized in Table 50–7.

The diagnosis of chlamydial ophthalmia in the newborn period may be made by tissue culture, direct fluorescent antibody, or enzyme immunoassay methods. For ocular disease, the last two methods provide results that are similar in sensitivity and specificity to results from culture.[43, 75]

Respiratory Tract Disease in Infants

Infections of other mucous membranes are recognized commonly in children who are born to mothers who have genital *Chlamydia* infection or who have neonatal ocular disease. Periauricular adenopathy is an accompanying physical finding. Otitis media, laryngitis, and rhinopharyngitis are concomitant events that are reported frequently, and a decrease in the number of upper respiratory diseases may occur after treatment of trachoma in children. A preceding nasal discharge and vulvovaginitis of female infants commonly accompany inclusion conjunctivitis.

Although lower respiratory tract disease has been recognized for many years in infants born to mothers with genital *Chlamydia* infection, interest in chlamydial disease of the respiratory tract was stimulated by several studies in the 1970s. In 1977, Beem and Saxon[9] reported 18 infants with chlamydial pneumonia who shed *Chlamydia* from the upper respiratory tract. Half of these infants had not had conjunctivitis.

Chlamydial pneumonia in infancy usually presents between 3 and 11 weeks of age with a persistent, staccato cough, rales, and wheezing, but without fever.[95] Otitis media is present in more than half the cases.[45] Laboratory findings have been few and include a mild peripheral eosinophilia and elevated IgG and IgM. The elevation of the serologic titer to the infecting strain, measured by microimmunofluorescence, usually is greater than 1:32 acutely.[73] Tracheal secre-

TABLE 50–6. Chlamydial Ophthalmia Neonatorum: Efficacy of Prophylaxis

Author, Date, Place, Method	Mothers Infected (%)	Study Drug	Number of Exposed Babies	Number Infected/1000 Exposed Infants	Reduction (%)
Bell et al.,[12] 1987, Washington; prospective, nonrandom	100%	Silver nitrate	93	230	?
	100%	Erythromycin	27	150	?
Laga,[56] 1986, Kenya; alternate patients	100%	Silver nitrate	81	111	66%
	100%	Tetracycline	95	63	80%
	100%	None	—	304	—
Hammerschlag et al.,[41] 1989, New York; randomized	100%	Silver nitrate	76	200	?
	100%	Erythromycin	92	140	?
Chen,[24] 1992, Taiwan; randomized	Unknown	Tetracycline	Unknown	13	None
		Erythromycin	Unknown	15	None
		Silver nitrate	Unknown	17	None
		None	—	16	None
		Erythromycin x2	Unknown	14	None

TABLE 50–7. Comparison of Stages of Ocular Trachoma with Those of Inclusion Conjunctivitis in the Adult

Inclusion Conjunctivitis	Trachoma
Stage 1	
No corneal involvement No follicles in upper tarsus	Follicles developed among papillae in upper tarsal plate Corneal epithelium hazy Infiltrating periphery of cornea Edema of limbus Micropannus develops
Stage II	
Follicular disease in lower lid and fornix Upper tarsus and cornea not involved	Increasing development of follicles and papillary hypertrophy Follicles become yellowish, soft Pannus extends into marginal infiltration of cornea Limbal follicles may develop
Stage III	
Healing without scarring Cornea unaffected	Healing by resolution of follicles with scarring Limbal follicles resolve to leave Herbert pits Pannus and keratitis gradually subside
Stage IV	
Conjunctiva returns to normal No scars	Conjunctival scarring remains Trichiasis or entropion may occur Inactive pannus persists, often with corneal opacity and Herbert pits

Data from Jones, B. R., Al-Hussaini, M. K., Dunlop, E. M. C., et al.: Infection by TRIC agent and other members of the Bedsonia group; with a note on Reiter's disease. I. Ocular disease in the adult. Trans. Ophthalmol. Soc. U. K. *86*:291–312, 1966.

tions reveal a pronounced eosinophilic exudate. The course often is protracted over several weeks, and fatalities may occur.

Chronic pulmonary disease may persist long after the acute phase has ended.[46] Initial studies of infants with pneumonitis have demonstrated that the acute clinical syndromes due to *Pneumocystis, Ureaplasma,* cytomegalovirus, and *Chlamydia* are indistinguishable.[19] Follow-up studies on infants who had clinically apparent chlamydial pneumonia in the neonatal period have shown that the majority had obstructive airway disease and physician-diagnosed asthma at 7 or more years of age.[99] In addition, there is a significant mortality rate in the first years of life due to chronic obstructive pulmonary disease in premature infants who are infected with *C. trachomatis.*[68] These studies demonstrate the importance of the prevention of infection in the newborn, preferably by screening and treating women of child-bearing age.

Genital Tract Disease in Prepubertal Children

Although infection with *Chlamydia* is recognized to cause approximately 40 per cent of nongonococcal urethritis in adult men and is associated with mucopurulent cervicitis and sterile pyuria in women, the pediatric role of chlamydial infections in symptomatic disease has been described less well. Pediatric studies of chlamydial disease have emphasized perinatal diseases and genital tract disease of sexually active teenagers resembling those of adults.[32] However, there are indications that chlamydial disease frequently accompanies gonococcal infection in prepubertal girls as well as in adults. Rettig and Nelson[78] demonstrated that 27 per cent of children with genital tract gonorrhea had accompanying infection with *Chlamydia.* In this and other reports, children presented with postgonococcal urethritis, vulvovaginitis, and asymptomatic infection. A persistent discharge after therapy for gonorrhea has been a major finding in dually infected children.[53]

The diagnosis of rectal or vaginal chlamydial infection in a prepubertal child should be based on a culture result because indirect methods are insufficiently sensitive or specific in this setting.[42, 48, 72, 101]

Although indirect methods for identifying genital chlamydial infection and disease have been successful for adult patients, the only acceptable techniques for identifying genital *Chlamydia* in prepubertal children use cell culture systems. Indirect methods are both insensitive and nonspecific in young children.[21, 42, 48, 72] Because anal or genital chlamydial infection in a child older than 3 years of age is confirming evidence of sexual abuse, the diagnosis of infection must be secure. Only cell culture systems offer adequate specificity. In addition, children often harbor sparse numbers of infecting organisms, and in that setting, the culture systems also may have greater sensitivity than alternative techniques.[58] For these reasons, the clinician who is caring for a child who requires an evaluation for chlamydial infection must be informed of the availability of culture services and ensure optimal handling and transport of specimens. Issues specific for chlamydial diagnosis in children include the following:

1. The clinician should have appropriate transport media.
2. The clinician should be prepared to place the specimen on ice immediately after collection and ensure that it remains at 4° C until processed.
3. The clinician should ensure that the specimen has been identified and labeled and the chain of custody maintained.
4. The clinician should ensure that the receiving laboratory is competent to identify *C. trachomatis.*
5. When evaluating pharyngeal specimens from children suspected of having been orally abused, the laboratory may need to distinguish between *C. trachomatis* and *C. pneumoniae.* The species may be distinguished through the use of species-specific antibody reagents.[8]
6. The clinician must be prepared to address the social and legal implications of the diagnosis of anal or genital chlamydial infection in a postnatal, prepubertal child (Table 50–8).

Salpingitis and Pelvic Inflammatory Disease

Salpingitis and pelvic inflammatory disease of female adolescents and women have been associated with genital tract infections with *Chlamydia* and gonococci. Teenagers especially are likely to experience severe and fibrosing disease of the fallopian tubes when they contract either of these infections.[36] Treatment of these diseases in this age range therefore especially is important. For a discussion of pelvic inflammatory disease in relation to gonococcal disease, see Chapter 49; for medications for hospitalization of children

TABLE 50–8. Special Significance of Genital Pediatric Sexually Transmitted Diseases and Recommendations Regarding Reporting for Suspected Abuse to the Relevant Community Agency

Infection	Evidence of Abuse	Recommended Action
Neisseria gonorrhoeae	Certain	Report
Acquired syphilis	Certain	Report
Chlamydia trachomatis	Probable (age restrictions)	Report
Trichomonas vaginalis	Probable	Report
Genital warts	Probable (age restrictions)	Report
Bacterial vaginosis	Uncertain	Evaluate for abuse
Herpes simplex virus type 2	Probable	Report
Herpes simplex virus type 1 (genital)	Possible	Report

Data from American Academy of Pediatrics: Guidelines for the evaluation of sexual abuse of children. Pediatrics *87*:254–260, 1991.

and adolescents for treatment of pelvic inflammatory disease, see Table 49–5.

Lymphogranuloma Venereum

Lymphogranuloma inguinale, climatic bubo, tropical bubo, and esthiomene are synonyms for a venereal disease that appeared from time to time throughout the eighteenth century. The distribution of this disease caused by the LGV biovar of *C. trachomatis* now is worldwide. It occurs more commonly in blacks than in whites and is recognized more frequently in males than in females. Humans are the sole natural host. LGV should not be confused with granuloma inguinale, which is caused by *Calymmatobacterium granulomatis*.

Autopsies of and biopsy specimens from patients with chronic LGV infection have revealed lesions of the lymph nodes, composed of aggregations of large mononuclear cells, forming abscesses surrounded by epithelioid cells. A few giant cells of the Langhans type may be found. Numerous plasma cells may invade the granuloma formation. Occasionally, necrotic lesions with few or no granulocytes but also surrounded by giant cells are present, usually in disease of long duration. Varying degrees of fibrosis occur, with bands of granulation and connective tissue and a thickened capsule.

Several biologic characteristics differentiate strains of *Chlamydia* that are LGV-like from those of patients with oculogenital trachoma. Animal pathogenicity of LGV-like strains shows virulence for mouse brain and failure to cause disease in monkey eye. The reverse is true for most strains from patients with oculogenital diseases. Most LGV strains rapidly are lethal for embryonated eggs at low inocula, which is not true for other *C. trachomatis*.

It should be noted that the definition of LGV-like strains usually implies that the strain was isolated from a patient with LGV-like disease. However, strains from such patients occasionally most closely have resembled trachoma-like strains or *C. psittaci* strains. There is, therefore, a general but not altogether specific relationship between biologic characteristics of a given strain and the clinical syndrome of the patient from whom it was isolated.

The incidence and epidemiology of LGV have received little attention; the limited information pertains almost exclusively to adults. Fewer than 1000 cases are reported yearly in the United States, and cases in children are recognized rarely. Table 50–9 contains brief sketches of pediatric patients reported in English publications since 1935. It is notable that the majority are females between the ages of 3 and 12 years. Notable also is the frequent occurrence of LGV in adult family members, especially the mothers of infected girls. In the five male patients, no family members or other source was noted.

LGV in adults in the past has been recognized most commonly in tropical countries, in persons who are promiscuous, in male homosexuals, and in persons of low socioeconomic positions. During the Vietnam War, numerous Americans returning from a tour of duty in the Far East were found to be infected.[1] Reports of disease in middle-class individuals have been more frequent.[60]

Clinical aspects of LGV in children appear to be similar to those of adults. The primary lesions seldom are recognized but may be apparent as small, multiple, slightly tender lesions on the genitalia. The onset after known sexual assault indicates an incubation period as short as 1 week, but delay in onset of clinical signs apparently may be many months. Inguinal adenopathy and rectal disease are equally common presentations in males and females; rectal involvement was

TABLE 50–9. Case Reports of Children with Lymphogranuloma Venereum (LGV)

Source	Sex	Age	Clinical Presentation and Source
Elitzak and Kornblith,[29] 1935	F	8	Rectal bleeding and ulceration; both parents had LGV
Levy,[57] 1937	F	6	Inguinal adenopathy; both parents had LGV
Sonck,[88] 1939	F	9	Rectal bleeding and stricture; both parents had LGV
	F	4	Rectal bleeding and stricture; mother had LGV
Sisters	F	5	Rectal stricture and arthritis
Sisters	F	7	Rectal stricture and arthritis
Sisters	F	6	Minimal rectal findings
			Mother of these 3 girls grossly infected with LGV
Weinstock and Keesal,[98] 1946	M	3	Inguinal adenopathy; no source noted
Roth and Schulick,[80] 1951	M	6	Cervical adenopathy; no source noted
Banov,[7] 1952	M	10	Rectal strictures; no source
Annamunthodo and Stewart,[6] 1962	F	11	Inguinal adenopathy; sexual assault 6 days previously
	F	12	Rectal bleeding and stricture; no source noted
	F		Unspecified 4 girls with inguinal adenopathy
	M		Unspecified 2 males with inguinal adenopathy
Tomeh and Wilfert,[96] 1973	F	4	Inguinal adenopathy; teenage male presumed source

noted in 7 of the 11 girls referred to in Table 50–9. Late follow-up studies on involved children are very rare; consequently, the course of disease is not described well. Inguinal nodes frequently suppurate, drain, and presumably eventually heal. Proctitis and rectal strictures appear to have a worse prognosis, and many of the involved children are noted to have become wasted, anemic, and chronically ill. Several clinical findings may accompany the primary complaints. Eosinophilia, erythema nodosum, arthritis, leukocytosis, and elevated erythrocyte sedimentation rates are common in children.[88]

Descriptions of the presentation of LGV proctitis in children have been similar to those of adults. Tenesmus, blood per rectum, purulent rectal discharge, and abdominal pain predominate. Stools become loose and frequent, and rectal strictures progress slowly. Therapy of rectal strictures has not been entirely satisfactory because recurrent fibrosing disease tends to lead to relapses.

Extragenital disease rarely is reported in children, but the diagnosis is not sought commonly. Cervical adenopathy has been reported.[80] Other findings from adult experience that may be expected to occur in children include meningoencephalitis,[100] hepatitis,[1] various forms of rash, and other oral and cervical lesions.[92]

Reiter Syndrome

Reiter syndrome is characterized by urethritis, arthritis, and conjunctivitis. Other common manifestations include dermal disease (keratoderma blennorrhagicum), cardiac disease, additional ulcerative lesions of mucous membranes, and development of brittle nails. It is a syndrome of uncertain etiology in which a role for *Chlamydia* has been suggested.[28]

Reiter syndrome occurs in epidemic forms and also sporadically. Epidemic forms frequently accompany outbreaks of diarrheal diseases, such as shigellosis. Sporadic cases of Reiter syndrome frequently follow venereal diseases in the adult, particularly an episode of gonococcal or nongonococcal urethritis. Evidence that Reiter syndrome may represent an unusual host response to a rather common pathogen is provided by the observation that the vast majority of patients with Reiter syndrome have the second segregant series histocompatibility antigen, W27. This antigen also is common in persons with ankylosing spondylitis and suggests that the cellular response may participate in disease pathogenesis.[64]

Epidemiologic aspects of Reiter syndrome in children differ only slightly from those in adults. Gastrointestinal disease is the most frequent predisposing event. Furthermore, it is common for other family members also to have Reiter syndrome when children are involved.[59] There appears to be a male predominance, and children of any age may acquire the syndrome.

In children, conjunctivitis has been the most common initial complaint of Reiter syndrome, followed by urethritis and arthritis. Major symptoms usually develop within 2 weeks and last for approximately 2 to 3 months. The joint disease usually involves large joints of the lower extremities and is asymmetric in distribution; purulent fluid may be obtained. Heel pain is a common complaint of children and adults. Residual functional damage appears to be very rare in children. Antimicrobial therapy has been of no proven benefit in children and adults.

PREVENTION AND TREATMENT

Prevention of Ophthalmia Neonatorum

Instillation of a prophylactic agent into the eyes of all newborn infants is recommended to prevent gonococcal ophthalmia neonatorum and is required by law in most states. Although all regimens listed effectively prevent gonococcal eye disease, their efficacy in preventing *Chlamydia* eye disease is not clear.[17, 24] Furthermore, they do not eliminate nasopharyngeal colonization with *C. trachomatis*.[49] Treatment of gonococcal and chlamydial infections in pregnant women is the best method for preventing neonatal gonococcal and chlamydial disease.[70]

TABLE 50–10. Dose of Erythromycin in the Newborn Period

	Body Weight <2000 g	Body Weight >2000 g
Age 0–7 days	20 mg/kg/day q 12 hr	20 mg/kg/day q 8 hr
Age >7 days	30 mg/kg/day q 8 hr	40 mg/kg/day q 8 hr

The recommended regimen is as follows: erythromycin (0.5 per cent) ophthalmic ointment, once; tetracycline (1 per cent) ophthalmic ointment, once; or silver nitrate (1 per cent) aqueous solution, once. One of these should be instilled into the eyes of every neonate as soon as possible after delivery and definitely within 1 hour after birth. Single-use tubes or ampules are preferable to multiple-use tubes.

The efficacy of tetracycline and erythromycin in the prevention of tetracycline-resistant *Neisseria gonorrhoeae* and penicillinase-producing *N. gonorrhoeae* ophthalmia is unknown, although both probably are effective because of the high concentration of drug in these preparations. Bacitracin is not recommended.

Treatment

CHLAMYDIAL CONJUNCTIVITIS OF THE NEWBORN. Erythromycin estolate or erythromycin ethylsuccinate orally for 10 to 14 days is recommended[10] (Table 50–10).

***CHLAMYDIA TRACHOMATIS* PNEUMONIA.** Erythromycin estolate or erythromycin ethylsuccinate orally for 14 to 21 days is recommended. The dosage is 20 to 50 mg/kg/day, every 6 hours.

CHLAMYDIAL SALPINGITIS, VAGINITIS, CERVICITIS, AND URETHRITIS IN PREPUBERTAL CHILDREN. The recommended regimen is as follows: erythromycin, 40 mg/kg/day orally, divided every 6 hours for 14 days, or (children 9 years of age or older) doxycycline, 4 mg/kg/day, given twice daily for 14 days. Azithromycin has become a first-choice therapy for adults, but pediatric studies for its use have not been completed.

LYMPHOGRANULOMA VENEREUM IN CHILDREN. Optimal therapy has not been established. Because of the long duration and chronic nature of LGV, therapy appropriately may be longer than for other chlamydial infections. Six weeks or more of sulfonamide or erythromycin therapy is standard. Povidone-iodine has been shown to be an adequate skin antiseptic for *C. trachomatis*.[76]

References

1. Abrams, A. J.: Lymphogranuloma venereum. J. A. M. A. *205:*199–202, 1968.
2. Addiss, D. G., Vaughn, M. L., Ludka, D., et al.: Decreased prevalence of *Chlamydia trachomatis* infection associated with a selective screening program in family planning clinics in Wisconsin. Sex. Transm. Dis. *20:*28–35, 1993.

3. Alexander, E. R., and Chiang, W.-T.: Infection of pregnant monkeys and their offspring with TRIC agents. Am. J. Ophthalmol. *63*:1145–1153, 1967.
4. Alexander, E. R., and Harrison, H. R.: Role of *Chlamydia trachomatis* in perinatal infection. Rev. Infect. Dis. *5*:713–719, 1983.
5. American Academy of Pediatrics: Guidelines for the evaluation of sexual abuse of children. Pediatrics *87*:254–260, 1991.
6. Annamunthodo, H., and Stewart, D. B.: Lymphogranuloma venereum in children. *In* Sigel, M. M. (ed.): Lymphogranuloma Venereum. Coral Gables, University of Miami Press, 1962, pp. 169–171.
7. Banov, L.: Rectal lesions of lymphogranuloma venereum in childhood: Review of the literature and report of a case in a ten-year-old boy with rectal strictures. Am. J. Dis. Child. *83*:660–662, 1952.
8. Bauwens, T. E., Gibbons, M. S., Hubbard, M. M., et al.: *Chlamydia pneumoniae* (strain TWAR) isolated from two symptom-free children during evaluation for possible sexual assault. J. Pediatr. *119*:591–593, 1991.
9. Beem, M. O., and Saxon, E. M.: Respiratory-tract colonization and a distinctive pneumonia syndrome in infants infected with *Chlamydia trachomatis*. N. Engl. J. Med. *296*:306–319, 1977.
10. Beem, M. O., Saxon, E., and Tipple, M. A.: Treatment of chlamydial pneumonia in infancy. Pediatrics *63*:198, 1979.
11. Bell, T. A., Quo, C. C., Stamm, W. E., et al.: Direct fluorescent monoclonal stain for rapid diagnosis of infant *Chlamydia trachomatis* infections. Pediatrics *74*:224–228, 1984.
12. Bell, T. A., Sandstrom, K. I., Gravett, M. G., et al.: Comparison of ophthalmic silver nitrate solution and erythromycin ointment for prevention of naturally acquired *Chlamydia trachomatis*. Sex. Transm. Dis. *14*:195–200, 1987.
13. Bell, T. A., Stamm, W. E., Kuo, C. C., et al.: Delayed appearance of *Chlamydia trachomatis* infections acquired at birth. Pediatr. Infect. Dis. J. *6*:928–931, 1987.
14. Bell, T. A., Stamm, W. E., Wang, S. P., et al.: Chronic *Chlamydia trachomatis* infections in infants. J. A. M. A. *267*:400–402, 1992.
15. Bell, T. A.: *Chlamydia trachomatis* infections in infants: Perinatal or sexual transmission? Infect. Med. *10*:32–36, 1993.
16. Biro, F. M., Reising, S. F., Doughman, J. A., et al.: A comparison of diagnostic methods in adolescent girls with and without symptoms of *Chlamydia* urogenital infection. Pediatrics *93*:476–480, 1994.
17. Black-Payne, C., Bocchini, J. A., and Cedotal, C.: Failure of erythromycin ointment for postnatal ocular prophylaxis of chlamydial conjunctivitis. Pediatr. Infect. Dis. J. *8*:491–498, 1989.
18. Blythe, M. J., Katz, B. P., Batteiger, B. E., et al.: Recurrent genitourinary chlamydial infections in sexually active female adolescents. J. Pediatr. *121*:487–493, 1992.
19. Brasfield, D. M., Stagno, S., Whitley, R. J., et al.: Infant pneumonitis associated with cytomegalovirus, *Chlamydia, Pneumocystis,* and *Ureaplasma:* Follow-up. Pediatrics *79*:76–83, 1987.
20. Bump, R. C.: *Chlamydia trachomatis* as a cause of prepubertal vaginitis. Obstet. Gynecol. *65*:384–388, 1987.
21. Centers for Disease Control: False-positive results with the use of chlamydial tests in the evaluation of suspected sexual abuse. M. M. W. R. *39*:932–935, 1991.
22. Centers for Disease Control and Prevention: Recommendations for laboratory testing for *Chlamydia trachomatis*. Lab. Med. *25*:168–175, 1994.
23. Chacko, M. R., and Lovchik, J. C.: *C. trachomatis* infection in sexually active adolescents: Prevalence and risk factors. Pediatrics *73*:836–840, 1984.
24. Chen, J.-Y.: Prophylaxis of ophthalmia neonatorum: Comparison of silver nitrate, tetracycline, erythromycin and no prophylaxis. Pediatr. Infect. Dis. J. *11*:1026–1030, 1992.
25. Chernesky, M. A., Mahoney, J. B., Castriciano, S., et al.: Detection of *Chlamydia trachomatis* antigens by enzyme immunoassay and immunofluorescence in genital specimens from symptomatic and asymptomatic men and women. J. Infect. Dis. *154*:141–148, 1986.
26. Datta, P., Laga, M., Plummer, F. A., et al.: Infection and disease after perinatal exposure to *Chlamydia trachomatis* in Nairobi, Kenya. J. Infect. Dis. *158*:524–528, 1988.
27. Dattel, B. J., Landers, D. V., Coulter, K., et al.: Isolation of *Chlamydia trachomatis* and *Neisseria gonorrhoeae* from the genital tract of sexually abused prepubertal females. Adolesc. Pediatr. Gynecol. *2*:217–220, 1989.
28. Dawson, C. R., Schachter, J., Ostler, H. B., et al.: Inclusion conjunctivitis and Reiter's syndrome in a married couple. Arch. Ophthalmol. *83*:300–306, 1970.
29. Elitzak, J., and Kornblith, B. A.: Lymphogranuloma inguinale: With rectal manifestations in a child. Am. J. Dis. Child. *49*:703–709, 1935.
30. Fisher, M., Swenson, P. D., Risucci, D., et al.: *Chlamydia trachomatis* in suburban adolescents. J. Pediatr. *111*:617–620, 1987.
31. Forster, R. K., Dawson, C. R., and Schachter, J.: Late follow-up of patients with neonatal inclusion conjunctivitis. Am. J. Ophthalmol. *69*:467–472, 1970.
32. Fraser, J. J., Rettig, P. G., and Kaplan, D. W.: Prevalence of cervical *Chlamydia trachomatis* and *Neisseria gonorrhoeae* in female adolescents. Pediatrics *71*:333–336, 1978.
33. Fuster, C. D., and Neinstein, L. S.: Vaginal *Chlamydia trachomatis* prevalence in sexually abused prepubertal girls. Pediatrics *79*:235–238, 1987.
34. Gencay, M., Koskiniemi, M., Saikku, P., et al.: *Chlamydia trachomatis* seropositivity during pregnancy is associated with perinatal complications. Clin. Infect. Dis. *21*:424–426, 1995.
35. Glaser, J. B., Schachter, J., Benes, S., et al.: Sexually transmitted diseases in post pubertal rape victims. J. Infect. Dis. *164*:726–730, 1991.
36. Golden, N., Hammerschlag, M., Neuhoff, S., et al.: Prevalence of *Chlamydia trachomatis* cervical infection in female adolescents. Am. J. Dis. Child. *138*:562–564, 1984.
37. Goscienski, P. J.: Inclusion conjunctivitis in the newborn infant. J. Pediatr. *77*:19–26, 1970.
38. Goscienski, P. J., and Sexton, R. R.: Follow-up studies in neonatal inclusion conjunctivitis. Am. J. Dis. Child. *124*:180–182, 1972.
39. Gutman, L. T., Weisner, P. J., Holmes, K. K., et al.: Microbiologic correlates of cervicitis. Clin. Res. *20*:529, 1972.
40. Gutman, L. T., and Wilfert, C. M.: Chlamydial infections. *In* Feigin, R. D., and Cherry, J. D. (eds.): Textbook of Pediatric Infectious Diseases. 2nd ed. Philadelphia, W. B. Saunders, 1987, pp. 1867–1877.
41. Hammerschlag, M. R., Cummings, C., Roblin, P. M., et al.: Efficacy of neonatal ocular prophylaxis for the prevention of chlamydial and gonococcal conjunctivitis. N. Engl. J. Med. *320*:769–772, 1989.
42. Hammerschlag, M. R., Rettig, P. J., and Sheilds, M. E.: False positive results with the use of chlamydial antigen detection tests in the evaluation of suspected sexual abuse in children. Pediatr. Infect. Dis. J. *7*:11–14, 1988.
43. Hammerschlag, M. R., Roblin, P. M., Cummings, C., et al.: Comparison of enzyme immunoassay and culture for diagnosing chlamydial conjunctivitis and respiratory infections in infants. J. Clin. Microbiol. *25*:2306–2308, 1987.
44. Hammerschlag, M. R., Gelling, M., Dumornay, W., et al.: Office diagnosis of neonatal chlamydial conjunctivitis. Pediatr. Infect. Dis. J. *10*:540–541, 1991.
45. Harrison, H. R., English, M. G., Lee, C. K., et al.: *Chlamydia trachomatis* infant pneumonitis. N. Engl. J. Med. *298*:702–708, 1978.
46. Harrison, H. R., Taussig, L. M., and Fulginiti, V.: *Chlamydia trachomatis* and chronic respiratory disease in children. Pediatr. Infect. Dis. *1*:29–33, 1982.
47. Harrison, H. R., Boyce, W. T., Wang, S.-P., et al.: Infection with *Chlamydia trachomatis* immunotype J associated with trachoma in children in an area previously endemic for trachoma. J. Infect. Dis. *151*:1034–1036, 1985.
48. Hauger, S. B., Brown, J., Agre, F., et al.: Failure of direct fluorescent antibody staining to detect *Chlamydia trachomatis* from genital tract sites of prepubertal children at risk for sexual abuse. Pediatr. Infect. Dis. J. *7*:660–662, 1988.
49. Heggie, A. D., Jaffe, A. C., Stuart, L. A., et al.: Topical sulfacetamide vs. oral erythromycin for neonatal chlamydial conjunctivitis. Am. J. Dis. Child. *139*:564–566, 1985.
50. Heggie, A. D., Lumicao, G. G., Stuart, L. E., et al.: *Chlamydia trachomatis* infection in mothers and infants: A prospective study. Am. J. Dis. Child. *135*:507–511, 1981.
51. Holmes, K. K., Handsfield, H. H., Wang, S.-P., et al.: Etiology of nongonococcal urethritis. N. Engl. J. Med. *29*:1199–1205, 1975.
52. Ingram, D. L., Runjan, D. K., Collins, A. D., et al.: Vaginal *Chlamydia trachomatis* infection in children with sexual contact. Pediatr. Infect. Dis. *3*:97–99, 1984.
53. Ingram, D. L., White, S. T., Occhiuti, A. R., et al.: Childhood vaginal infections: Association of *Chlamydia trachomatis* with sexual contact. Pediatr. Infect. Dis. J. *5*:226–229, 1986.
54. Ingram, D. L., Everett, V. D., Lyna, P. R., et al.: Epidemiology of adult sexually transmitted disease agents in children being evaluated for sexual abuse. Pediatr. Infect. Dis. J. *11*:945–950, 1992.
55. Jones, B. R., Al-Hussaini, M. K., Dunlop, E. M. C., et al.: Infection by TRIC agent and other members of the Bedsonia group; with a note on Reiter's disease. I. Ocular disease in the adult. Trans. Ophthalmol. Soc. U.K. *86*:291–312, 1966.
56. Laga, M., Nsanze, H., Plummer, F. A., et al.: Comparison of tetracycline and silver nitrate for the prophylaxis of chlamydial and gonococcal ophthalmia neonatorum. *In* Oriel, D., et al. (eds.): Chlamydial Infections. Cambridge, Cambridge University Press, 1986, pp. 301–304.
57. Levy, H.: Lymphogranuloma venereum in childhood: Review of the literature with report of a case. J. Pediatr. *11*:812–823, 1937.
58. Lin, J. S., Jones, W. E., Yan, L., et al.: Underdiagnosis of *Chlamydia trachomatis* infection: Diagnostic limitations in patients with low-level infection. Sex. Transm. Dis. *19*:259–265, 1992.
59. Lockie, G. N., and Hunder, G. G.: Reiter's syndrome in children: A case report and review. Arthritis Rheum. *14*:767–772, 1971.
60. McLelland, B. A., and Anderson, P. C.: Lymphogranuloma venereum: Outbreak in a university community. J. A. M. A. *235*:56–57, 1976.
61. Mahony, J. B., Luinstra, K. E., Tyndall, M., et al.: Multiplex PCR detection of *Chlamydia trachomatis* and *Neisseria gonorrhoeae* in genitourinary specimens. J. Clin. Microbiol. *33*:3049–3053, 1995.
62. Martin, D. H., Koutsky, L., Eschenbach, D. A., et al.: Prematurity and perinatal mortality in pregnancies complicated by maternal *Chlamydia trachomatis* infections. J. A. M. A. *247*:1585–1588, 1982.
63. Mordhorst, C. H., and Dawson, C.: Sequelae of neonatal inclusion conjunctivitis and associated disease in parents. Am. J. Ophthalmol. *71*:861–867, 1971.
64. Morris, R., Metzger, A. L., Bluestone, R., et al.: HL-A W27: A clue to the diagnosis and pathogenesis of Reiter's syndrome. N. Engl. J. Med. *290*:554–556, 1974.
65. Morrison, R. P.: Immune responses to *Chlamydia trachomatis* are protective

and pathogenic. *In* Bowie, W. R., et al. (eds.): Chlamydial Infections. Cambridge, Cambridge University Press, 1990, pp. 163–172.
66. Moscicki, B., Shafer, M.-A., Millstein, S. G., et al.: The use and limitations of endocervical Gram stains and mucopurulent cervicitis as predictors for *Chlamydia trachomatis* in female adolescents. Am. J. Obstet. Gynecol. *157*:65–71, 1987.
67. Mulcahy, F. M., and Lacey, C. J. N.: Sexually transmitted infections in adolescent girls. Genitourin. Med. *63*:119–121, 1987.
68. Numazaki, K., Chiba, S., Kogawa, K., et al.: Chronic respiratory disease in premature infants caused by *Chlamydia trachomatis*. J. Clin. Pathol. *39*:84–88, 1986.
69. Numazaki, K., and Chiba, S.: Diagnostic value of rapid detection of *Chlamydia trachomatis* by using amplified enzyme immunoassay in infants with respiratory infections. Diagn. Microbiol. Infect. Dis. *17*:233–234, 1993.
70. Patamasucon, P., Rettig, P. J., and Nelson, J. D.: Cefuroxime therapy of gonorrhea and coinfection with *Chlamydia trachomatis* in children. Pediatrics *68*:534–538, 1981.
71. Pate, M. S., and Hook, E. W.: Laboratory to laboratory variation in *Chlamydia trachomatis* culture practices. Sex. Transm. Dis. *22*:322–326, 1995.
72. Porder, K., Sanchez, N., Roblin, P. M., et al.: Lack of specificity of chlamydiazyme for detection of vaginal chlamydial infection in prepubertal girls. Pediatr. Infect. Dis. J. *8*:358–360, 1989.
73. Poulakkainen, M., Saikku, P., Leinonen, M., et al.: Chlamydial pneumonitis and its serodiagnosis in infants. J. Infect. Dis. *149*:598–604, 1984.
74. Rahm, V. A., Odlind, V., and Pettersson, R.: *Chlamydia trachomatis* in sexually active teenage girls. Factors related to genital chlamydial infection: A prospective study. Genitourin. Med. *67*:317–321, 1991.
75. Rapoza, P. A., Quinn, T. C., Kiessling, L. A., et al.: Assessment of neonatal conjunctivitis with a direct immunofluorescence monoclonal antibody stain for *Chlamydia*. J. A. M. A. *255*:3369–3373, 1986.
76. Reeve, P.: The inactivation of *Chlamydia trachomatis* by povidone-iodine. J. Antimicrob. Chemother. *2*:77–80, 1976.
77. Remapedi, G., and Abdalian, S. E.: Clinical predictors of *Chlamydia trachomatis* endocervicitis in adolescent women. Am. J. Dis. Child. *143*:1437–1442, 1989.
78. Rettig, P. J., and Nelson, J. D.: Genital tract infection with *Chlamydia trachomatis* in prepubertal children. J. Pediatr. *99*:206–210, 1981.
79. Richmond, S. J., and Sparling, P. F.: Genital chlamydial infections. Am. J. Epidemiol. *103*:428–435, 1976.
80. Roth, D., and Schulick, R.: Isolated cervical lymphogranuloma venereum in a child. Pediatrics *8*:489–493, 1951.
81. Saltz, G. R., Linnemann, C. C., Brookman, R. R., et al. *Chlamydia trachomatis* cervical infection in female adolescents. J. Pediatr. *98*:981–985, 1981.
82. Schachter, J., Grossman, M., Sweet, R. L., et al.: Prospective study of prenatal transmission of *Chlamydia trachomatis*. J. A. M. A. *255*:3374–3377, 1986.
83. Schachter, J., Moncada, J., and Whidden, R.: Noninvasive tests for diagnosis of *Chlamydia trachomatis* infection. Application of ligase chain reaction to first-catch urine specimens of women. J. Infect. Dis. *172*:1411–1414, 1995.
84. Scott, B. D., and Fortenberry, J. D.: Postgonococcal conjunctivitis due to *Chlamydia trachomatis*. Sex. Transm. Dis. *13*:172–173, 1986.
85. Shafer, M. A., Beck, A., Blain, B., et al.: *Chlamydia trachomatis:* Important relationships to race, contraception, lower genital tract infection, and Papanicolaou smear. J. Pediatr. *104*:141–146, 1984.
86. Shapiro, R. A., Schubert, C. J., and Myers, P. A.: Vaginal discharge as an indicator of gonorrhea and *Chlamydia* infection in girls under 12 years old. Pediatr. Emerg. Care *9*:341–345, 1993.
87. Siegel, R. M., Schubert, C. S., Myers, P. A., et al.: The prevalence of sexually transmitted diseases in children and adolescents evaluated for sexual abuse in Cincinnati: Rationale for limited STD testing in prepubertal girls. Pediatrics *96*:1090–1094, 1995.
88. Sonck, C. E.: Five cases of lymphogranuloma inguinale in children (with rectal manifestations and arthropathies). Acta Dermato-vener. *20*:171–190, 1939.
89. Stergachis, A., Scholes, D., Heidrich, F. E., et al.: Selective screening for *Chlamydia trachomatis* infection in a primary care population of women. Am. J. Epidemiol. *138*:143–153, 1993.
90. Sweet, R. L., Landers, D. V., Walker, C., et al.: *Chlamydia trachomatis* infection and pregnancy outcome. Am. J. Obstet. Gynecol. *156*:824–831, 1987.
91. Tam, M. R., Stamm, W. E., Handsfield, H. H., et al.: Culture-independent diagnosis of *Chlamydia trachomatis* using monoclonal antibodies. N. Engl. J. Med. *310*:1146–1150, 1984.
92. Thorsteinsson, S. B., Musher, D. M., Min, K.-W., et al.: Lymphogranuloma venereum: A course of cervical lymphadenopathy. J. A. M. A. *235*:1882, 1976.
93. Thygeson, P.: Trachoma Manual and Atlas. Washington, D.C., Public Health Service Publication No. 541, 1958.
94. Thygeson, P., and Stone, W.: Epidemiology of inclusion conjunctivitis. Arch. Ophthalmol. *27*:91–122, 1942.
95. Tipple, M. A., Beem, M. O., and Saxon, E. M.: Clinical characteristics of the afebrile pneumonia associated with *Chlamydia trachomatis* infection in infants less than 6 months of age. Pediatrics *63*:192–197, 1979.
96. Tomeh, M. O., and Wilfert, C. M.: Venereal diseases of infants and children at Duke University Medical Center. N. Carolina Med. J. *34*:109–113, 1973.
97. Washington, A. E., Johnson, R. E., and Sanders, L. L.: *Chlamydia trachomatis* infections in the United States: What are they costing us? J. A. M. A. *257*:2070–2072, 1987.
98. Weinstock, H. L., and Keesal, S.: Lymphogranuloma venereum: Report of a case in a child. Urol. Cutaneous Rev. *50*:520–522, 1946.
99. Weiss, S. G., Newcomb, R. W., and Beem, M. O.: Pulmonary assessment of children after chlamydial pneumonia of infancy. J. Pediatr. *108*:659–664, 1986.
100. Zarafonetis, C. J. D.: Meningoencephalitis in lymphogranuloma venereum: A report of two cases. N. Engl. J. Med. *230*:567–573, 1944.
101. Zeeberg, B., Thelin, I., and Schalen, C.: *Chlamydia trachomatis* antigen detection by chlamydiazyme combined with *Chlamydia* blocking reagent verification. Int. J. Sex. Transm. Dis. AIDS *3*:355–359, 1992.

Trichomonas vaginalis Infection

Trichomonas vaginalis is a flagellated protozoal pathogen of the human urogenital tract. It is recognized to be one of the more common causes of sexually transmitted diseases, but because cases are not reportable, incidence data are weak or unavailable. Disease in adults has been reviewed.[7]

Recognized *T. vaginalis* disease occurs in populations that are sexually active or in children who are sexually abused or assaulted. The infection appears to be symptomatic in females more commonly than in males. Asymptomatic male carriers provide an important source of disease that may be unrecognized and untreated. Some males have urethral symptoms with a minor discharge,[13] but more are asymptomatic. In adult males, the rate of identification of infection decreases rapidly after last contact.[14]

Identification of *T. vaginalis* infection in women usually is achieved through the direct examination of urine or wet mount of secretions (vaginal or urethral). Diagnosis requires the recognition of motile protozoa of characteristic morphology. The organisms are larger than polymorphonuclear leukocytes, which often accompany an infection.

A wet mount is an insensitive method of identifying *T. vaginalis* disease, even for patients with florid disease, and will reveal only approximately 40 to 80 per cent of cases.[22] Several culture systems are available, and all are much more sensitive than direct examination.[11] Diamond medium is one such method.[12] For circumstances in which a definitive diagnosis is sought and a wet mount has been negative, a culture may yield a diagnosis.[16, 18] When the patient is infected with low concentrations of organisms, a wet mount is unlikely to be effective and a culture then is essential for diagnosis.[10, 11] However, culture methods are expensive and labor-intensive. A probe technique is available and appears to provide identification of infections that is more sensitive than a direct wet mount but less sensitive than a culture.[3]

Laboratory assays for the diagnosis of *T. vaginalis* infection have not been evaluated in pediatric populations. Virtually all reports of genital *T. vaginalis* infection in children have resulted from recognition of disease using a wet-mount technique. Because this technique is insensitive, it is presumed that the infection is underrecognized in children. Reported rates of recognized *T. vaginalis* infection in populations of children being examined for possible sexual abuse have been 0 to 4 per cent (Table 50–11).

In infants who are born to mothers infected with *T. vaginalis*, infection or disease may occur occasionally, but it appears to be a rare event. In two studies of exposed infants evaluated by repeated perinatal culture, none of 14 and none of 430 were infected.[4, 23] Another study yielded rates of infant infection of 0.6 per cent when assessed by culture and 0.1 per cent by wet mount.[1] *T. vaginalis* also has been isolated from infant respiratory tracts.[17] The infections of infants, when recognized, appear to be of relatively short duration and remit spontaneously.

TABLE 50–11. Prevalence of Genital *Trichomonas vaginalis* in Populations of Prepubertal Girls*

Author(s), Date, Location	Population	Rate
Lang,[15] 1959	Girls with vaginitis	4/110 (3.6%)
Yordan and Yordan,[27] 1992, Connecticut	Evaluation for sexual abuse	3/288 (1%)
Feo,[5] 1956, Philadelphia	Pediatric clinic patients 1–9 years of age	3/84 (3.6%)
White et al.,[26] 1983, Raleigh	Children <13 years of age Sexual abuse evaluation	4/409 (1%)
Gray and Kotcher,[6] 1960	Girls with vaginitis	4/92 (4%)
Siegel et al.,[25] 1995, Cincinnati	Prepubertal girls Sexual abuse evaluation	0/119 (0%)
Ingram et al.,[8] 1992, Raleigh	Girls with discharge evaluated for sexual abuse	3/141 (2%)

*Diagnosis by wet-mount observation.

Reports of how *T. vaginalis* is transmitted to children are very sparse. *T. vaginalis* infection is a sexually transmitted disease among adults, and there is no evidence that, beyond the newborn period, transmission to children occurs by any other means. The organism has site specificity for the urethra and vagina and is very sensitive to desiccation. No cases of fomite transmission have been documented.[21]

T. vaginalis infection is accepted to be a sexually transmitted disease in children, as in adults.[20, 24] However, because of the paucity of study data and because most experience is derived from case reports,[2, 9] the American Academy of Pediatrics has categorized *T. vaginalis* infection as one that is "probable" evidence of sexual abuse (see Table 50–8). As in other instances of children with sexually transmitted diseases, the child with *T. vaginalis* infection should be reported to the agency constituted by that community to receive reports of child sexual abuse. The child should receive a complete evaluation for suspected sexual abuse.[19]

In adults, there is a low diagnostic yield of specimens from male partners of infected women. Nevertheless, asymptomatic men are a major source of disease and of recurrent disease in their partners if untreated. For children with *T. vaginalis* infection, the failure to identify the organism in a given person should not be used as evidence that that person was not a perpetrator or assailant of the child. Similarly, recurrent disease in a child is likely to occur because the child's perpetrator has not been identified and/or treated and the child is experiencing reabuse.

The therapy of choice is metronidazole administered as 15 mg/kg/day orally divided into three doses per day for 7 days. Identified perpetrators or contacts also should be treated.

Additional information regarding *Trichomonas* infection can be found in Chapter 213.

References

1. Al-Sahili, F. L., Curran, J. P., and Wang, J.-S.: Neonatal *Trichomonas vaginalis*. Pediatrics *53*:196–200, 1974.
2. Altchek, A.: Pediatric vulvovaginitis. J. Reprod. Med. *29*:359–375, 1984.
3. Biselden, A. M., and Hinier, S. L.: Evaluation of Affirm VP Microbial identification test of *Gardnerella vaginalis* and *Trichomonas vaginalis*. J. Clin. Microbiol. *32*:148–152, 1994.
4. Bramley, M.: Study of female babies within entering confinement with vaginal trichomoniasis. Br. J. Vener. Dis. *52*:58–62, 1976.
5. Feo, L. G.: The incidence of *Trichomonas vaginalis* in the various age groups. Am. J. Trop. Med. Hyg. *5*:786–790, 1956.
6. Gray, L., and Kotcher, E.: Vulvovaginitis in childhood. Clin. Obstet. Gyncol. *3*:165–174, 1960.
7. Heine, P., and McGregor, J. A.: *Trichomonas vaginalis*: A reemerging pathogen. Clin. Obstet. Gyncol. *36*:137–144, 1993.
8. Ingram, D. L., Everett, V. D., Lyna, P. R., et al.: Epidemiology of adult sexually transmitted disease agents in children being evaluated for sexual abuse. Pediatr. Infect. Dis. J. *11*:945–950, 1992.
9. Jones, J. G., Yamauchi, T., and Lambert, B.: *Trichomas vaginalis* infestation in sexually abused girls. Am. J. Dis. Child. *139*:846–847, 1985.
10. Judson, F. N., and Ehret, J.: Laboratory diagnosis of sexually transmitted infections. Pediatr. Ann. *23*:361–369, 1994.
11. Krieger, J. N., Tam, M. R., Stevens, C. E., et al.: Diagnosis of trichomoniasis: Comparison of conventional wet-mount examination with cytologic studies, cultures, and monoclonal antibody staining of direct specimens. J. A. M. A. *259*:1223–1227, 1988.
12. Krieger, J. N., Jenny, C., Verdon, M., et al.: Clinical manifestations of trichomoniasis in men. Ann. Intern. Med. *118*:844–849, 1993.
13. Krieger, J. N.: *Trichomonas* in men: Old issues and new data. Sex. Transm. Dis. *22*:83–96, 1995.
14. Krieger, J. N., and Rein, M. F.: Trichomoniasis. *In* Mandell, G. L. (ed.): Atlas of Infectious Diseases. Philadelphia, Churchill Livingstone, 1996, pp. 6.2–6.11.
15. Lang, W.: Premenarchal vaginitis. Obstet. Gynecol. *13*:723–729, 1959.
16. Linstead, D. J.: Cultivation of *Trichomonas* parasitic in humans. *In* Honigberg, B. M. (ed.): Trichomonads Parasitic in Humans. New York, Springer-Verlag, 1989, p. 91.
17. McLaren, L. C., Davis, L. E., Healy, G. R., et al.: Isolation of *Trichomonas vaginalis* from the respiratory tract of infants with respiratory disease. Pediatrics *71*:888–890, 1983.
18. McMillan, A.: Laboratory diagnostic methods and cryopreservation of *Trichomonas*. *In* Honigberg, B. M. (ed.): Trichomonads Parasitic in Humans. New York, Springer-Verlag, 1989, p. 299.
19. Matson, N., and Gutman, L. T.: Child sexual abuse and sexually transmitted diseases. *In* Holmes, K. K., Cates, W., Jr., Lemon, S. M., et al. (eds.): Sexually Transmitted Diseases. 3rd ed. New York, McGraw-Hill, 1996.
20. Mishaw, C. O.: Sexual abuse and sexually transmitted diseases in prepubertal children. Semin. Pediatr. Infect. Dis. *4*:131–138, 1993.
21. Neinstein, L. S., Goldenring, J., and Carpenter, S.: Nonsexual transmission of sexually transmitted diseases: An infrequent occurrence. Pediatrics *74*:67–76, 1984.
22. Rein, M. F., and Muller, M.: *Trichomonas vaginalis* and trichomoniasis. *In* Holmes, K. K., Cates, W., Jr., Lemon, S. M., et al. (eds.): Sexually Transmitted Diseases. 2nd ed. New York, McGraw-Hill, 1990, p. 481.
23. Robinson, S. C., and Halifax, N. S.: Observations on vaginal *Trichomonas*. 1. In pregnancy. J. Can. Med. Assoc. *84*:948–949, 1961.
24. Ross, J. D. C., Scott, G. R., and Busuttil, A.: *Trichomonas vaginalis* infection in prepubertal girls. Med. Sci. Law *33*:82–85, 1993.
25. Siegel, R. M., Schubert, C. J., Myers, P. A., et al.: The prevalence of sexually transmitted diseases in children and adolescents evaluated for sexual abuse in Cincinnati: Rationale for limited STD testing in prepubertal girls. Pediatrics *96*:1090–1094, 1995.
26. White, S., Loda, F., Ingram, D., et al.: Sexually transmitted diseases in sexually abused children. Pediatrics *72*:16–21, 1983.
27. Yordan, E. E., and Yordan, R. A.: Sexually transmitted diseases and human immunodeficiency virus screening in a population of sexually abused girls. Adolesc. Pediatr. Gynecol. *5*:187–191, 1992.

Herpes Simplex Virus Infections of the Genital Tract

Herpes simplex virus (HSV) infections of the genital tract in adults most commonly (>80 per cent) are caused by HSV-2, whereas HSV-1 more commonly is found in oral infections and disease. In newborn HSV disease, HSV-2 predominates.

Beyond the newborn period, the large majority of HSV disease in children is caused by HSV-1. This virus infects the mucosa of the mouth (herpes stomatitis, cold sores) and is transmitted through direct contact of infected secretions, such as by hand-to-mouth contact and kisses.[14] A large proportion of infected children experience only subclinical infection. Group day care facilities probably have enhanced the rate at which young children are experiencing HSV-1 infection.[20]

HSV infection of the adult genital tract is a sexually transmitted disease, and nonsexual transmission is a rarity. Fomite transmission has not been documented.[15] Studies of children with genital HSV disease indicate that the majority fulfill accepted criteria for a diagnosis of sexual abuse. However, the numbers of reported cases are small, and even large studies of children evaluated for abuse usually include only a few children with recognized genital HSV infection (Table 50–12).

Sexual abuse of children may involve acts during which adults have oral contact with the child's genitals, may include finger contact, and may include genital contact with the child's genitalia. Consequently, either HSV-1 or HSV-2 may be isolated from children who are confirmed to have been sexually abused. As an example, a report of six children with genital HSV disease included five cases of HSV-1 and one of HSV-2.[12] Sexual abuse was confirmed in four of the six. The type of HSV isolated from a child's genitalia does not provide evidence that the infection was or was not transmitted during an abusive encounter.

In spite of the fact that the HSV type does not indicate the likelihood that the infection was or was not the result of abuse, the two types have been used to indicate different levels of concern regarding sexual abuse of the child. All children with genital HSV infection should be reported for suspected abuse to the agency constituted in the community to receive such reports. The child then should receive a complete medical and social evaluation for possible abuse. Regarding the interpretation of an HSV-2 genital infection, the American Academy of Pediatrics recommends that it be regarded as probable evidence of abuse (see Table 50–8). In contrast, HSV-1 infection should be regarded as possible evidence of abuse. It appears from adult studies that genital HSV disease is only moderately contagious among sexual couples who are practicing barrier protection. Bryson and associates[1] found a yearly transmission rate of 10 per cent from infected partners to noninfected partners. It also appears that abusive transmission to children is a relatively rare event (Table 50–12). Supporting these expectations are seroepidemiologic studies of the prevalence of type-specific antibody to HSV-2 in pediatric populations. In the United States, a study of 785 children younger than 10 years of age revealed only one with HSV-2 antibody.[10] A Swedish study of children somewhat older (14 to 15 years of age) showed that 0.4 per cent had HSV-2 antibodies.[3] In accordance with the infrequency of recognition of genital HSV disease are the individual published case reports. These reports usually also note that the child has been recognized to have been sexually abused.[6–8, 12]

Diagnosis of HSV infection or disease of the genital tract of children may be clinically difficult. Although some children present with typical clusters of painful bullous lesions, others will have a diffuse, denuded, erythematous mucosal epithelium. Some children have very slow healing of untreated lesions and also may have frequent recurrences. It should be remembered that anal abuse of children is common and perianal HSV disease may result. Children with painful and persistent mucosal lesions should be evaluated for possible HIV infection.

Growth of HSV using tissue culture methods is the standard means for diagnosing HSV disease of children.[11] This method has the advantage of allowing typing of an isolate, and a full range of confirming methods may be used on the isolate. As with other pediatric sexually transmitted diseases, the diagnosis has major social implications, and therefore a standard test should be used. Other diagnostic methods for mucosal lesions include rapid assays that may assist in an immediate diagnosis but, if used, also should be followed by a culture.

There are no studies of the efficacy of genital HSV disease treatment in children. Consequently, recommendations may omit the mention of children or rely on extrapolations from adult data. It is apparent from numerous studies of adults that persons with genital HSV disease may benefit from therapy during several clinical settings, and it is presumed that children will experience similar benefits.[2]

When considering therapy for children with HSV infection at any body site, a dominant consideration is the age of the child. Infants who are infected with HSV have very high rates of dissemination from cutaneous sites to the central nervous system. Consequently, it is recommended that all infected infants be evaluated for extent of disease and receive a full course of parenteral antiviral chemotherapy.[23]

The requirement that infants who are in the newborn period receive parenteral therapy is based on extensive study and experience. Beyond the newborn period, there is relatively little information regarding the risk that an untreated skin or mucosal infection will disseminate the disease; the risk appears to decrease with increasing age. I treat all HSV-infected infants who are younger than 1 year of age with either parenteral therapy or high-dose oral therapy.

The situations in which oral therapy for genital HSV disease is most likely to benefit the child who is beyond early infancy are discussed next.

The first clinically apparent episode of genital HSV disease in children is likely to be true primary disease. Because primary disease is characterized by a relatively frequent occurrence of both local and systemic symptoms and may have a long duration, such children are likely to benefit from antiviral chemotherapy. Oral acyclovir is the drug of choice.[4] The recommended dosing schedule is 400 mg orally three times daily for 10 days. The dosing often is not based on weight because of extremely low rates of toxicity and because of the relatively poor absorption.

Because a majority of children infected with HSV-2 have genital recurrences of disease, a decision should be made

TABLE 50–12. Prevalence of Genital Herpes Simplex Virus Disease in Populations of Prepubertal Girls

Author(s), Date, Location	Population	Rate
Ingram et al.,[9] 1992, Raleigh	Sexual abuse evaluation	2/1500 (0.1%)
Siegel et al.,[21] 1995, Cincinnati	Sexual abuse evaluation	0/704 (0%)
DeJong,[5] 1986, Philadelphia	Abused girls 1–13 years of age	1/532 (0.2%)
Yordan and Yordan,[24] 1992, Connecticut	Abused girls	1/288 (0.2%)

about the treatment of recurrences.[18] Adult studies indicate that treatment will shorten the duration of lesions.[17] A regimen that is effective in adults and suitable for children is acyclovir, 400 mg orally three times daily for 5 days. Therapy for recurrent disease is most effective if started at first signs of recurrent symptoms, and patient-initiated therapy may improve the results.

Children who have frequent recurrences of genital disease may be treated best with a regimen of prolonged continuous suppressive therapy. Acyclovir has been tolerated well in large numbers of adults for a year, with no significant laboratory or clinical adverse reactions.[16] In two studies, small numbers of children have received acyclovir for prolonged periods. One report indicated that children on suppressive regimens should be evaluated periodically for neutropenia,[13] although the other report described no adverse reactions.[19]

Adults receiving continuous suppressive therapy have had excellent control of recurrences.[22] It is recommended that therapy be suspended at least yearly to determine if disease still is recurring. A dose schedule is acyclovir, 400 mg orally twice daily.

More detailed information concerning postnatal HSV infection is found in Chapter 163.

References

1. Bryson, Y., Dillon, M., Bernstein, D. I., et al.: Risk of acquisition of genital herpes simplex virus type 2 in sex partners of persons with genital herpes: A prospective couple study. J. Infect. Dis. *167*:942–946, 1993.
2. Centers for Disease Control: 1993 Sexually Transmitted Diseases Treatment Guidelines. M. M. W. R. *42*(Suppl. RR-14):1–102, 1993.
3. Christenson, B., Bottiger, M., Svensson, A., et al.: A 15-year surveillance study of antibodies to herpes simplex virus type 1 and 2 in a cohort of young girls. J. Infect. Dis. *25*:147–154, 1992.
4. Corey, L., Benedetti, J., Critchlow, C., et al.: Treatment of primary first-episode genital herpes simplex virus infections with acyclovir. J. Antimicrob. Chemother. *12*:79–88, 1983.
5. DeJong, A. R.: Sexually transmitted disease in sexually abused children. Sex. Transm. Dis. *13*:123–126, 1986.
6. Do, A. N., Green, P. A., and Demmier, G. J.: Herpes simplex virus type 2 meningitis and associated genital lesions in a three-year-old child. Pediatr. Infect. Dis. J. *13*:1014–1016, 1994.
7. Gardner, M., and Jones, J. G.: Genital herpes acquired by sexual abuse of children. J Pediatr. *101*:243–422, 1984.
8. Hare, M. J., and Mowla, G.: Genital herpes virus infection in a prepubertal girl. Br. J. Obstet. Gynaecol. *84*:141–142, 1977.
9. Ingram, D. L., Everett, V. D., and Lyna, P. R.: Epidemiology of adult sexually transmitted disease agents in children being evaluated for sexual abuse. Pediatr. Infect. Dis. J. *11*:945–950, 1992.
10. Johnson, R. E., Nahmias, A. J., Magder, L. S., et al.: A seroepidemiologic survey of the prevalence of herpes simplex virus type 2 infection in the United States. N. Engl. J. Med. *321*:7–12, 1989.
11. Judson, F. N., and Ehret, J.: Laboratory diagnosis of sexually transmitted infections. Pediatr. Ann. *23*:361–369, 1994.
12. Kaplan, K. M., Fleisher, G. R., Paradies, J. E., et al.: Social relevance of genital herpes simplex to children. Am. J. Dis. Child. *138*:872–874, 1984.
13. Kimberlin, D., Powell, D., Gruber, W., et al.: Administration of oral acyclovir suppressive therapy after neonatal herpes simplex virus disease limited to the skin, eyes, and mouth: Results of a phase I/II trial. Pediatr. Infect. Dis. J. *15*:247–254, 1996.
14. Kohl, S.: Herpes simplex virus infection: The neonate to the adolescent. Israeli J. Med. Sci. *30*:392–398, 1994.
15. Larson, T., and Bryson, Y. J.: Fomites and herpes simplex virus infection: A multicenter double blind trial. J. A. M. A. *260*:201–206, 1994.
16. Mertz, G. J., Jones, C. C., Mills, J., et al.: Long-term acyclovir suppression of frequently recurring genital herpes simplex virus infection: A multicenter double-blind trial. J. A. M. A. *260*:201–206, 1988.
17. Reichman, R. C., Badger, G. J., Mertz, G. J., et al.: Treatment of recurrent genital herpes simplex infections with oral acyclovir: A controlled study. J. A. M. A. *251*:2103–2107, 1984.
18. Reeves, W. C., Corey, L., Adams, H. G., et al.: Risk of recurrence after first episodes of genital herpes: Relation to HSV type and antibody response. N. Engl. J. Med. *305*:315–319, 1981.
19. Rudd, C., Rivadeneira, E. D., and Gutman, L. T.: Dosing considerations for oral acyclovir following neonatal herpes disease. Acta Paediatr. *83*:1237–1243, 1994.
20. Schmitt, D. C., Johnson, D. W., and Henderson, F. W.: Herpes simplex type I infections in group day care. Pediatr. Infect. Dis. J. *10*:729–734, 1991.
21. Siegel, R. M., Schubert, C. J., Myers, P. A., et al.: The prevalence of sexually transmitted diseases in children and adolescents evaluated for sexual abuse in Cincinnati: Rationale for limited STD testing in prepubertal girls. Pediatrics *96*:1090–1094, 1995.
22. Strauss, S. E., Takiff, H. E., Seidlin, M., et al.: Suppressing of frequently recurring genital herpes: A placebo-controlled double-blind trial of oral acyclovir. N. Engl. J. Med. *310*:1545–1550, 1984.
23. Whitley, R., Arvin, A., Prober, C., et al.: Predictors of morbidity and mortality in neonates with herpes simplex virus disease. N. Engl. J. Med. *324*:450–454, 1991.
24. Yordan, E. E., and Yordan, R. A.: Sexually transmitted diseases and human immunodeficiency virus screening in a population of sexually abused girls. Adolesc. Pediatr. Gyneol. *5*:187–191, 1992.

Donovanosis (Granuloma Inguinale)

Donovanosis is a genital ulcer disease that is recognized very rarely in children and may or may not be transmitted sexually. The causative agent is a pleomorphic gram-negative rod that multiplies within host cells and is named *Calymmatobacterium granulomatis*. The intracellular microcolonies may be seen in Giemsa stain and are named Donovan bodies.

The disease is very rare in the United States, with fewer than 100 cases reported annually. The disease has not been recognized in young children in the United States.

In adults, the infection is recognized to cause a slowly progressing ulcerative disease, usually of the genital and perineal areas and with exuberant granulation tissue. The disease may progress to involve bones and other adjacent structures and may disseminate.

Clinicians who are concerned that a child may suffer from this disease should refer to the adult experiences in the diagnosis and treatment of donovanosis.[1, 2]

Doxycycline or tetracycline is the antibiotic used most frequently. Doxycycline is provided in a dose of 100 mg twice a day, and tetracycline is provided in a dose of 500 mg orally four times each day until the lesions heal completely (usually 21 days).

More detailed information concerning *C. granulomatis* may be found in Chapter 135.

References

1. Holmes, K. K., Cates, W., Jr., Lemon, S. M., et al. (eds.): Sexually Transmitted Diseases. 3rd ed. New York, McGraw-Hill, 1996.
2. Richens, J.: The diagnosis and treatment of donovanosis (granuloma inguinale). Genitourn. Med. *67*:441–452, 1991.

Chancroid

Chancroid is a bacterial infection that causes genital ulcer disease. It virtually never has been recognized in prepubertal children in the United States, although it is seen occasionally in adolescents. The disease typically causes deep genital ulcers with irregular borders and undermined edges.[1] There may be a gray coating of the lesion. Lesions typically are quite painful and start with a macule that progresses to one or more related ulcers.

Chancroid in adults is transmitted sexually and is seen commonly in developing countries.[2] Chancroid has received a great deal of attention because the rapidly increasing numbers of cases in the United States have occurred in populations in which sex is exchanged for drugs.[3] Chancroid breaches mucosal barriers and plays a major role in facilitating sexual transmission of HIV.[4] For these reasons, vigorous attempts are being made to control the spread of chancroid.

The causative agent is *Haemophilus ducreyi*, which is a small gram-negative coccobacillus that stains poorly with Gram iodine and is facultatively anaerobic.[5] Culture techniques require the services of a laboratory that is capable of processing such specimens. Media, atmospheric conditions, moisture, and rapid processing influence the outcome of culture results. Clinicians who suspect this disease should consult their available laboratory for advice and assistance.

Advances have been made in the identification of *H. ducreyi* genome through polymerase chain reaction methods.[6] As with all other diagnostic techniques for chancroid, there is no pediatric experience with the use of polymerase chain reaction for diagnosis of disease. There is no reliable serologic diagnosis.

Treatment regimens in children are not established and may be based on extrapolations from adult experiences. Single-dose therapy with parenteral ceftriaxone at 250 mg intramuscularly has led to very acceptable results in adults. Alternatively, erythromycin at 30 mg/kg/24 hours in four divided doses for 7 days may be used. The total daily dose should not exceed 2 g. Azithromycin in a single oral dose of 1 g has been used in adults.

References

1. Chacko, M. R.: Diagnosis and management of genital ulcers. Semin. Pediatr. Infect. Dis. *4*:182–190, 1993.
2. Martin, D. H., and DiCarlo, R. P.: Recent changes in epidemiology of genital ulcer disease in the United States: The crack cocaine connection. Sex. Transm. Dis. *21*:S76–S80, 1994.
3. Schmid, G. P., Saunders, L. L., Blount, J. H., et al.: Chancroid in the United States: Re-establishment of an old disease. J. A. M. A. *258*:3265–3268, 1987.
4. Trees, D. L., and Morse, S. H.: Chancroid and *Haemophilus ducreyi*: An update. Clin. Microbiol. Rev. *8*:357–375, 1995.
5. Wasserheit, J. N.: Epidemiologic synergy: Interrelationships between human immunodeficiency virus infection and other sexually transmitted diseases. Sex. Transm. Dis. *19*:61–77, 1992.
6. West, B., Wilson, S. M., Changalucha, J., et al.: Simplified PCR for detection of *Haemophilus ducreyi* and diagnosis of chancroid. J. Clin. Microbiol. *33*:787–790, 1995.

Other Sexually Transmitted Diseases

The clinical presentation, diagnosis, and treatment of gonorrhea and syphilis are presented in Chapters 94 and 150, respectively. These disorders also are discussed in detail in Chapter 49.

SECTION SIX

GASTROINTESTINAL TRACT INFECTIONS

❑ ❑ ❑

51

ESOPHAGITIS

Sudipta Misra and Marvin E. Ament

Infectious esophagitis is distinct from other gastrointestinal infections because it is rare in previously healthy persons, predominantly of fungal and viral etiologies, and usually a harbinger of immunodeficiency due to acquired, drug-induced, or congenital causes. Infection by multiple organisms is common in these patients. Even in normal children, infectious esophagitis is associated commonly with conditions that compromise esophageal defense mechanisms.[39] The incidence of infectious esophagitis in children is unknown. Among patients with AIDS, as many as 10 per cent can have *Candida* infection.[6, 29] Seventy-one to 100 per cent of AIDS patients presenting with both oral candidiasis and odynophagia had endoscopic evidence of esophageal candidiasis.[7, 27, 32]

PATHOPHYSIOLOGY AND CAUSATIVE ORGANISMS

The defense mechanisms of the esophagus against infection include a mucosal lining of stratified squamous epithelium that is resistant to microbial invasion, motility (continuous flow of luminal contents that discourages colonization by microbes), and the general immune mechanism of the body. Compromise in any one or more of these factors leads to esophageal infections. Immunosuppression (as seen in AIDS), chronic mucocutaneous candidiasis (a lymphocyte function defect), post–organ transplant immunosuppression, chemotherapy, malignancy, and prolonged steroid treatment are the most common underlying etiologic factors for fungal and viral infections of the esophagus.[3, 8, 17, 23, 29] Dysmotility of the esophagus, in addition to mucosal injury secondary to gastroesophageal reflux, can make the esophagus vulnerable to infections in immunocompetent children. The esophagus can be infected by local invasion (*Candida*, herpes simplex virus [HSV], bacterial), as a result of systemic infection (cytomegalovirus [CMV], *Candida*, *Pneumocystis*), or by contiguous spread from the mediastinum or neck (tuberculosis, retropharyngeal abscess).

Most of the esophageal infections are caused by fungi and viruses. However, esophagitis in immunocompromised patients can be polymicrobial in origin. *Candida albicans*, HSV, and CMV are the major pathogens.[6, 29, 38, 39] Other less common pathogens include fungi, such as *Aspergillus* and *Histoplasma* species[19, 25]; viruses, such as varicella-zoster, Epstein-Barr, HIV, and papilloma viruses[14, 15, 28, 34]; and protozoas, such as *Cryptosporidium*, *Pneumocystis carinii*, and *Leishmania donovani*.[9, 13, 16] Bacterial infections of the esophagus probably are underreported. As much as 10 to 16 per cent of esophageal infections can have a bacterial etiology, mostly in granulocytopenic patients and as secondary infection in fungal or viral esophagitis. Gram-positive and gram-negative oropharyngeal bacterial flora and *Mycobacterium tuberculosis* are the common pathogens.[11, 37] Tubercular esophagitis, caused by both typical and atypical mycobacteria, is found mainly in immunocompromised patients in the United States. *Helicobacter pylori* has been isolated from Barrett esophagitis. However, this "infection" appears to be related to the gastroesophageal reflux disease rather than direct invasion of the esophagus by *H. pylori*.[26]

CLINICAL PRESENTATION

Infectious esophagitis can present with esophageal, abdominal, or systemic symptoms (Table 51–1). Dysphagia (difficulty in swallowing) and odynophagia (painful swallowing) are the most common symptoms of esophagitis. Complaints also may include a sensation of food "sticking" behind the sternum or a feeling of food or liquid bolus passing through the chest. Drooling is unusual in esophagitis per se but may be present with pharyngeal involvement. Dysphagia and odynophagia may not be apparent in small children, and esophageal involvement may be overlooked. Even in adults, only 59 to 79 per cent of patients with documented esophageal infections had these symptoms. About a quarter of the patients with esophageal candidiasis were asymptomatic.[5] Oral lesions may be present in 27 to 37 per cent of the patients with *Candida*, HSV, or HIV esophagitis and are rare with CMV infection and tuberculosis.[5] Oral thrush, however, is common in infants and immunocompromised patients. The frequency of *Candida* esophagitis in infants with oral thrush is not known. The presence of oral thrush and esophageal symptoms does not exclude concomitant esophageal infection with pathogens other than *Candida* or idiopathic esophageal ulcerations associated with HIV. Oropharyngeal lesions are less common in HSV esophagitis than in *Candida* esophagitis. A history of recurrent cold sores, vesicular lesions on the nasolabial folds, and esophageal symptoms are the typical presenting features of HSV esophagitis in an immunocompetent host. Nausea and vomiting are associated

TABLE 51–1. Signs and Symptoms of Infectious Esophagitis

Dysphagia	Fever
Odynophagia	Diarrhea
Oral lesions	Cough
Nausea/vomiting	Skin rash
Abdominal pain	Hematemesis

more commonly with CMV esophagitis, reflecting the systemic nature of the illness. Abdominal pain in esophagitis may be due to referred pain from the distal esophagus, associated gastritis (as in CMV infection), or concomitant intra-abdominal infections in the immunocompromised host (advanced stage of HIV infection). Fever mostly is due to systemic infection (CMV) or secondary infections (mediastinal abscess or pneumonia in tuberculosis). Fever is not common in bacterial esophagitis. Cough is characteristic of tubercular infection, tracheobronchial fistulae, or high-grade esophageal obstruction. A maculopapular truncal skin rash and fever may be present in patients with idiopathic esophageal ulceration during acute HIV seroconversion.[28] Diarrhea can be present in CMV infection (diffuse involvement of the gastrointestinal tract) or HIV infection (opportunistic enteral infections, HIV enteropathy). It must be emphasized that most of the reported studies are from adult subjects. Symptoms may differ in children, especially with subjective complaints, such as dysphagia and odynophagia. Because esophagitis is not looked for commonly in the absence of dysphagia or odynophagia, infectious esophagitis may be underdiagnosed in infants and children. In one report of fungal esophagitis in children, hematemesis was the most common presenting symptom.[39]

DIFFERENTIAL DIAGNOSIS

Gastroesophageal reflux is the most common cause of esophagitis in children. In previously healthy children, esophageal symptoms are likely to be due to reflux esophagitis, whereas in immunocompromised patients, infectious esophagitis needs to be ruled out. Secondary bacterial or fungal infections can be present in reflux esophagitis, especially with severe inflammation and obstruction. Absence of reflux symptoms, such as long-standing heartburn, brash taste in the mouth, vomiting, spitting up (in infants), pillow wetting, and coughing, does not rule out reflux esophagitis entirely. Immunodeficiency, systemic signs, and oral lesions suggest infectious esophagitis. Endoscopy, biopsies, and endoscopic brush specimens may be required for diagnosis. Achalasia, diffuse esophageal spasm, foreign-body impaction, and mediastinal or retropharyngeal abscesses can present with esophageal symptoms and may be secondarily infected.

Specific diagnosis is essential for management of infectious esophagitis. Although clinical profile, barium esophagogram, and endoscopic appearances can provide some clue, histopathology, immunohistochemistry, and cultures of endoscopic biopsies and brush specimens are essential for confirmation. Viral serology may offer indirect evidence of infection in difficult cases.

Barium Esophagography

The usefulness of an esophagogram in infectious esophagitis is limited by the fact that it does not provide an etiologic diagnosis and some patients have normal or nonspecific findings. These studies are useful for assessing motility and for excluding obstruction, perforation, and fistulas of the esophagus. Barium studies are not indicated if endoscopy is planned. Double-contrast barium esophagography with air and barium, which details the mucosal lining, is the radiologic investigation of choice. However, children may not tolerate this procedure well.[21]

Candida esophagitis generally is diffuse, whereas HSV or CMV lesions are more frequent in the mid to distal esophagus. Discrete longitudinal plaques, grossly irregular or "shaggy" appearance, or tiny nodular lesions with granular appearance are characteristic of *Candida* esophagitis (Fig. 51–1). Discrete superficial stellate ulcers in the mid-esophagus with normal-appearing surrounding mucosa are characteristic of HSV esophagitis. CMV lesions may mimic HSV lesions on barium esophagography. However, oval or elongated large ulcers are found mostly in CMV and idiopathic esophageal ulceration with HIV infection.[20, 36] Esophagograms in tuberculosis can show intramural pseudodiverticula, extrinsic compression, or esophageal displacement by mediastinal lymph nodes and sinus tracts.[10]

Esophagoscopy

Characteristic macroscopic lesions are associated with some of the infectious agents. However, macroscopic appear-

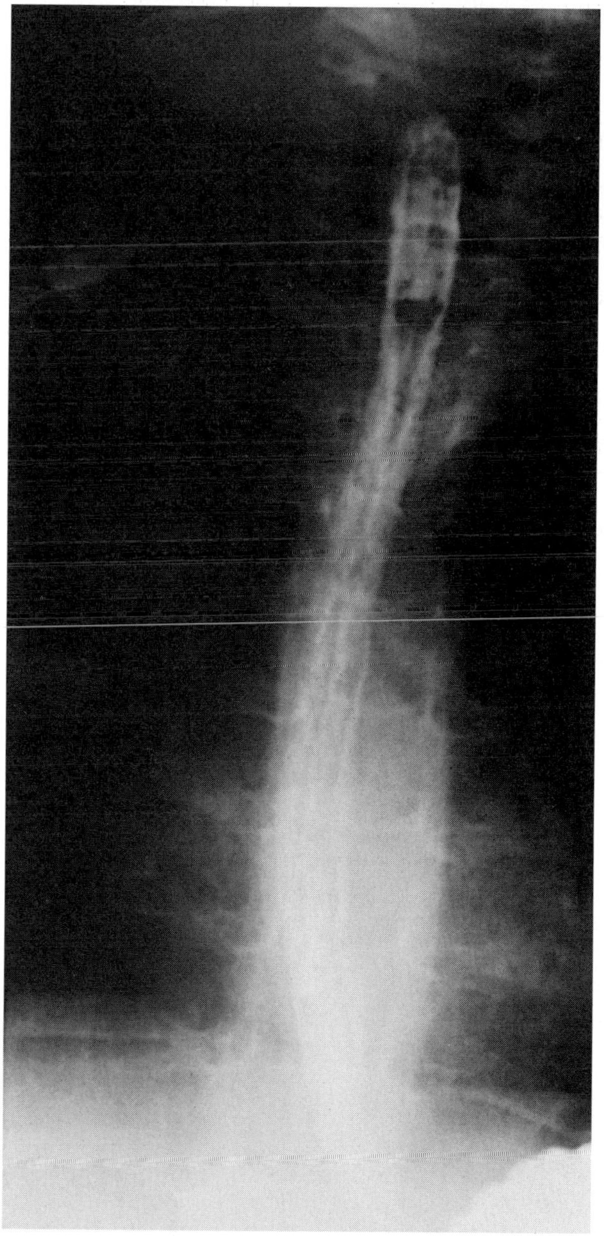

FIGURE 51–1. *Barium esophagogram in* Candida *esophagitis. Note the diffuse mucosal irregularity suggestive of inflammation and longitudinal filling defects suggestive of plaques. (Courtesy of Sjirk Westra, M.D., Division of Pediatric Radiology, UCLA Medical Center, Los Angeles, CA.)*

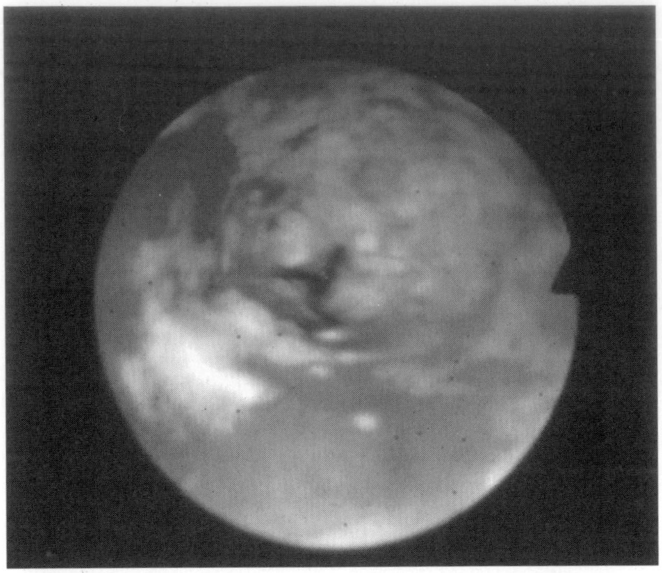

FIGURE 51–2. *Endoscopic appearance of* Candida *esophagitis. Note the diffuse inflammation and whitish longitudinal plaques. (Courtesy of George Gershman, M.D., Division of Pediatric Gastroenterology and Nutrition, UCLA Medical Center, Los Angeles, CA.)*

ances overlap considerably, and histopathology or immunohistochemistries (or both) of endoscopic biopsies and brush specimens are essential for diagnosis. A diffuse esophageal lesion is characteristic of *Candida* infection, whereas CMV and HSV infections mainly involve the distal esophagus. Whitish, longitudinal plaques adhering to the mucosa are characteristic of *Candida* infection (Fig. 51–2).[18] Plaques swallowed from oral thrush, common in infants and immunocompromised children, can be washed away, revealing a nonulcerated underlying mucosa. Similar-appearing plaques, however, also may be seen in CMV, HSV, and bacterial esophagitis, in "pill" esophagitis, and after sucralfate ingestion. Small, 1- to 3-mm vesicles are characteristic of HSV esophagitis, but by the time endoscopy is performed, these vesicles usually slough off to sharply demarcated ulcers with a raised edge, necrotic base, and normal-appearing surrounding mucosa. In progressive disease, these ulcers may coalesce to resemble *Candida* esophagitis.[1] Multiple superficial ulcers in the distal esophagus are common in CMV esophagitis. However, large elongated ulcers also are typical of CMV infection but may occur in idiopathic esophageal ulcerations in HIV infection as well.[20] Complete denudation of the mucosa is unusual with CMV infection.[33] Endoscopy in varicella-zoster virus esophagitis can show vesicles, discrete ulcers, or necrotizing esophagitis, depending on the stage of the disease. Tubercular ulcers of the esophagus usually are of varying size, distinct, and shallow with a necrotic base.

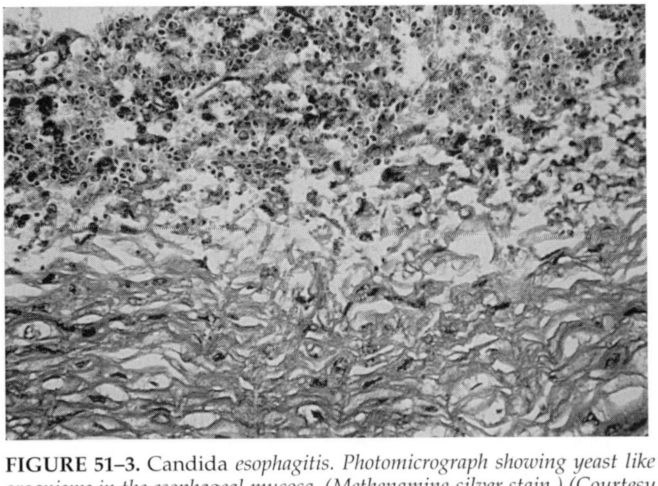

FIGURE 51–3. Candida *esophagitis. Photomicrograph showing yeast like organisms in the esophageal mucosa. (Methenamine-silver stain.) (Courtesy of Klaus Lewin, M.D., Department of Pathology, UCLA Medical Center, Los Angeles, CA.)*

Biopsies and Brushings

Endoscopic biopsies should be obtained from the edge as well as the base of the lesions. In CMV infection, biopsies from the edge do not yield diagnostic information.[33] The pathologist should be alerted to the possibility of fungal and viral as well as polymicrobial infections. Appropriate fixatives should be used for routine hematoxylin and eosin stain, Gram stain, and special stains for fungi and bacteria, such as *Mycobacterium*. *Candida* and *Aspergillus* can be demonstrated by silver stain, periodic acid–Schiff stain, or Gram stain (Fig. 51–3). Diagnostic histopathologic changes, such as multinucleated giant cells, ballooning degeneration, intranuclear Cowdry type A inclusion bodies and margination of chromatin in HSV (Fig. 51–4), and amphophilic intranuclear inclusions and small multiple cytoplasmic inclusion bodies in CMV infection (Fig. 51–5), can be diagnostic. However, immunohistochemical studies and DNA hybridization techniques often are required for diagnosis. Viral cultures with or without immunohistochemical techniques may aid confirmation. Materials obtained by endoscopy-guided brushings can reveal features of *Candida* or viral infection described earlier. Blind brushings of the esophagus may be useful for *Candida* infection when endoscopy is not possible or is not available.[7]

If abdominal pain, fever, or other unusual symptoms are present, the possibility of disseminated or abdominal infections should be excluded by appropriate investigations.

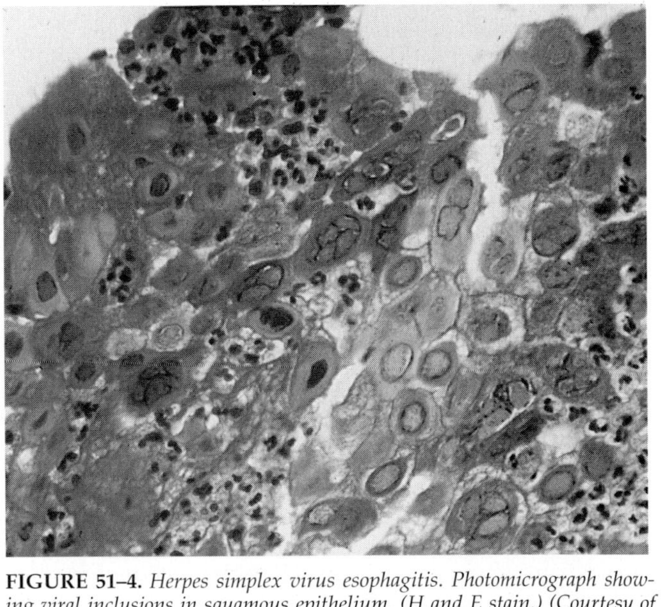

FIGURE 51–4. *Herpes simplex virus esophagitis. Photomicrograph showing viral inclusions in squamous epithelium. (H and E stain.) (Courtesy of Klaus Lewin, M.D., Department of Pathology, UCLA Medical Center, Los Angeles, CA.)*

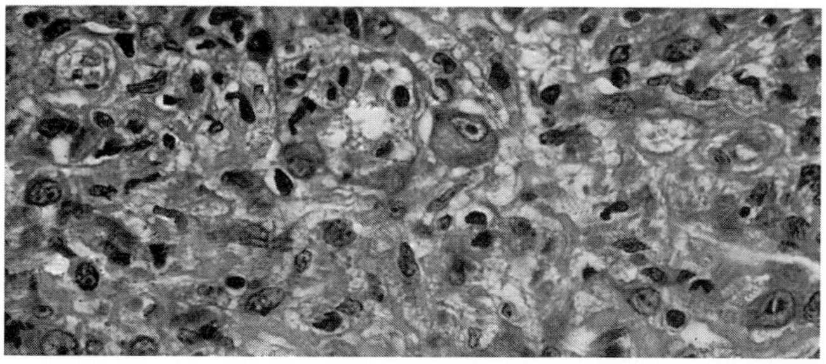

FIGURE 51–5. *Cytomegalovirus esophagitis. Photomicrograph showing intracytoplasmic inclusion bodies in the lamina propria. (H and E stain.) (Courtesy of Klaus Lewin, M.D., Department of Pathology, UCLA Medical Center, Los Angeles, CA.)*

TREATMENT

Candida Esophagitis

Treatment depends on the severity of infection as well as the degree of immunocompetency. Normal children and children in the early stages of HIV infection who have minimal lymphocyte dysfunction and normal granulocyte function can be treated with topical or oral antifungal agents (Table 51–2). Nystatin and ketoconazole are the agents used commonly.[39] For patients with severe infection or granulocyte dysfunction, intravenous amphotericin B is used. In infection confined to the esophagus, a 10- to 14-day course often suffices (see Table 51–2). In disseminated infection, a total dose of 30 to 50 mg/kg may be required. Nephrotoxicity is the major toxic effect of amphotericin B. Coadministering amphotericin B with lipid emulsions or using newer microsomal preparations may reduce this toxic effect.[24, 35] Intravenous fluconazole is an alternative to amphotericin B. Oral nystatin, oral amphotericin B, and fluconazole have been used with success for prophylaxis against esophageal candidiasis in AIDS patients and after organ transplantation.

Other Fungal Esophagitis

Amphotericin B given intravenously is the treatment of choice in aspergillosis and histoplasmosis.

Viral Esophagitis

Immunocompetent children with HSV need only supportive care. However, in immunocompromised patients, intravenous acyclovir is indicated (see Table 51–2). Foscarnet and vidarabine are the other alternatives. HSV prophylaxis with oral acyclovir has been successful in solid-organ and bone marrow transplantation patients, as well as in patients with AIDS. Ganciclovir and foscarnet are used for CMV infection (see Table 51–2). Ganciclovir, although effective, causes granulocytopenia. Foscarnet is less toxic but can only suppress CMV and does not eradicate it. Organ transplant recipients who are seropositive for CMV or receive the graft from a CMV-seropositive donor should receive prophylaxis with intravenous acyclovir or ganciclovir (see Table 51–2).[31] Oral acyclovir is only partially effective in this situation. Acyclovir is the treatment of choice for varicella-zoster virus. Prophylaxis effectively has reduced the rate of varicella-zoster virus infections in post-transplantation patients. HIV-associated idiopathic ulcers do not respond to empiric antiviral or antifungal therapy. Systemic steroid therapy may improve the symptoms and the ulcers in these cases.[4] However, the healing is slow, treatment for more than 1 month may be required, and symptoms recur if the therapy is interrupted. Topical therapy with a slurry of sucralfate and dexamethasone may be a useful alternative.[30]

Bacterial Esophagitis

Bacterial esophagitis should be treated with appropriate broad-spectrum antibiotics. Blood cultures always should be obtained to exclude septicemia. Tuberculosis is treated with

TABLE 51–2. Treatment of Fungal and Viral Esophagitis

Drug	Route	Dose	Duration	Limiting Toxic Effect
Antifungal				
Nystatin	Oral	5–10 × 10^6 units q 3 hours	2–6 weeks	Unpleasant taste
Amphotericin B	Oral	10–100 mg q 4 hours	2–6 weeks	Unpleasant taste
Clotrimazole (oral troches)	Oral	10 mg q 4–6 hours	2 weeks	Nausea, vomiting, resistance
Ketoconazole	Oral	3.3–6.6 mg/kg/day	10–14 days	Resistance, hepatotoxicity (rare)
Fluconazole*	Intravenous	3–6 mg/kg/day	10–14 days	Resistance
Amphotericin B*	Intravenous	0.5–1.0 mg/kg/day	10–14 days	Nephrotoxicity
Flucytocine*	Oral	50–100 mg/kg q 6 hours (with amphotericin B)	Complicated *Candida* infection	Bone marrow suppression, resistance with monotherapy
Nystatin	Oral	2–5 × 10^6 units q 6–8 hours	Prophylaxis	Unpleasant taste
Antiviral				
Acyclovir*	Intravenous	250 mg/m² q 8 hours	2–3 weeks	Neuropathy, encephalopathy
Ganciclovir*	Intravenous	10 mg/kg q 12 hours	2–3 weeks	Granulocytopenia
Foscarnet*	Intravenous	60 mg/kg q 8 hours 90 mg/kg/day maintenance	2–3 weeks	
Acyclovir*	Oral	10 mg/kg q 6 hours	Prophylaxis	Gastrointestinal disturbance, headache
Acyclovir*	Intravenous	250 mg/m² q 8 hours	Prophylaxis	Neuropathy, encephalopathy
Ganciclovir*	Intravenous	5 mg/kg/day	Prophylaxis	Granulocytopenia

*Dose should be adjusted for renal function.

standard antitubercular drugs. Patients with AIDS respond more poorly to the drug therapy than do immunocompetent patients. Surgery is required for fistulas, obstruction, and perforations.

Lack of response to appropriate therapy may indicate concomitant superinfection by other organisms or resistance to the drugs used. Fungal and bacterial superinfections are common in viral esophagitis. Repeat endoscopy is indicated for documenting eradication of infection.

PROGNOSIS

Candida esophagitis carries a poor prognosis for AIDS patients. The survival is about 1 year after an episode of *Candida* esophagitis in children with AIDS.[6, 29] *Candida* esophagitis, if not successfully treated, can lead to strictures, obstruction, and perforation of the esophagus. Viral esophagitis usually does not have long-term sequelae.

Acknowledgment

We are grateful to John Tse, Pharm. D., Department of Pharmacology, UCLA Medical Center, Los Angeles, California, for reviewing the drugs and dosages (see Table 51–2).

References

1. Agha, F. P., Lee, H. H., and Nostrand, T. T.: Herpetic esophagitis: A diagnostic challenge in the immunocompromised patient. Am. J. Gastroenterol. *81*:246–253, 1986.
2. Alexander, J. A., Brouillette, E. D., Chien, M. C., et al.: Infectious esophagitis following liver and renal transplantation. Dig. Dis. Sci. *33*:1121–1126, 1988.
3. Ammann, J., and Hong, R.: Disorders of the T cell system. *In* Stein, E. R. (ed.): Immunologic Disorders in Infants and Children. Philadelphia, W. B. Saunders, 1989, p. 286.
4. Bach, M. C., Valenti, A. J., Howell, D. A., et al.: Odynophagia from aphthous ulcers of the pharynx esophagus in the acquired immunodeficiency syndrome. Ann. Intern. Med. *109*:338–339, 1988.
5. Baehr, P. H., and McDonald, G. B.: Esophageal infections: Risk factors, presentation, diagnosis and treatment. Gastroenterology *106*:509–532, 1994.
6. Blanche, S., Tardieu, M., Duliege, M., et al.: Longitudinal study of 94 symptomatic infants with perinatally transmitted human immunodeficiency virus infection. Am. J. Dis. Child. *144*:1210–1215, 1990.
7. Bonacini, M., Laine, L., Gal, A. A., et al.: Prospective evaluation of blind brushings in the esophagus for *Candida* esophagitis in patients with human immunodeficiency virus infection. Am. J. Gastroenterol. *85*:385–389, 1990.
8. Brouillette, D. E., Alexander, J., Yoo, Y. K., et al.: T-cell population in liver transplant recipients with infectious esophagitis. Dig. Dis. Sci. *34*:92–96, 1989.
9. Datry, A., Similowski, T., Jais, P., et al.: AIDS-associated leishmaniasis: An unusual gastro-duodenal presentation. Trans. R. Soc. Trop. Med. Hyg. *84*:239–240, 1990.
10. DeSilva, R., Stoopak, P. M., and Raufman, J. P.: Esophageal fistulas associated with mycobacterial infections in patients at risk for AIDS. Radiology *175*:449–453, 1990.
11. Eng, J., and Sabanathan, S.: Tuberculosis of the esophagus. Dig. Dis. Sci. *36*:536–540, 1991.
12. Ginsburg, C. H., Braden, G. L., Tauber, A. I., et al.: Oral clotrimazole in the treatment of esophageal candidiasis. Am. J. Med. *71*:891–895, 1981.
13. Grimes, M. M., LaPook, J. D., and Bar, M. H.: Disseminated *Pneumocystis carinii* in a patient with acquired immunodeficiency syndrome. Hum. Pathol. *18*:307–308, 1987.
14. Hirsch, M. S.: Herpes group virus infections in the compromised host. *In* Rubin, R. H., and Young, L. S. (eds.): Clinical Approach to Infection in the Compromised Host. 2nd ed. New York, Plenum, 1988, pp. 347–366.
15. Javdan, P., and Pitman, E. R.: Squamous papilloma of esophagus. Dig. Dis. Sci. *29*:317–320, 1984.
16. Kazlow, P. G., Shah, K., Benkov, K. J., et al.: Esophageal cryptosporidiosis in a child with acquired immune deficiency syndrome. Gastroenterology *91*:1301–1303, 1986.
17. Kesten, S., Hyland, R. H., Pruzanski, W. R., et al.: Esophageal candidiasis associated with beclomethasone dipropionate aerosal therapy. Drug Intell. Clin. Pharm. *22*:568–569, 1988.
18. Kodsi, B. E., Wickremesinghe, C., Kozinn, P. J., et al.: *Candida* esophagitis: A prospective study of 27 cases. Gastroenterology *71*:715–719, 1976.
19. Lee, J. H., Neumann, D. A., and Welsh, J. D.: Disseminated histoplasmosis presenting with esophageal symptomatology. Dig. Dis. Sci. *22*:831–834, 1977.
20. Levine, M. S., Loerscher, G., Katzka, D. A., et al.: Giant human immunodeficiency virus related ulcers in the esophagus. Radiology *180*:323, 1991.
21. Levine, M. S., Macones, A. J., Jr., and Laufer, I.: *Candida* esophagitis: Accuracy of radiographic diagnosis. Radiology *154*:581–587, 1985.
22. Mathieson, R., and Dutta, S. K.: *Candida* esophagitis. Dis. Dig. Sci. *28*:365–370, 1983.
23. Naito, Y., Yoshikawa, T., Oyamada, H., et al.: Esophageal candidiasis. Gastroenterol. Jpn. *23*:363–370, 1988.
24. Ng, T. T., and Denning, D. W.: Liposomal amphotericin B (AmBisone) therapy in invasive fungal infections: Evaluation of United Kingdom compassionate data. Arch. Intern. Med. *155*:1093–1098, 1995.
25. Obrecht, W. F., Jr., Richter, J. E., Olympio, G. A., et al.: Tracheoesophageal fistula: A serious complication of infectious esophagitis. Gastroenterology *87*:1174–1179, 1984.
26. O'Connor, H. J., and Cunnane, K.: *Helicobacter pylori* and gastroesophageal reflux disease: A prospective study. Irish J. Med. Sci. *163*:369–373, 1994.
27. Porro, G. B., Parente, F., and Cernuschi, M.: The diagnosis of esophageal candidiasis in patients with acquired immunodeficiency syndrome: Is endoscopy always necessary? Am. J. Gastroenterol. *84*:143–146, 1989.
28. Rabeneck, L., Popovic, M., Gartner, S., et al.: Acute HIV infection presenting with painful swallowing and painful ulcers. J. A. M. A. *263*:2318–2322, 1990.
29. Scott, G. B., Hutto, C., Makuch, R. W., et al.: Survival in children with perinatally acquired immunodeficiency virus type I infection. N. Engl. J. Med. *321*:1791–1796, 1989.
30. Sokol-Anderson, M. L., Prelutsky, D. J., and Westblom, T. U.: Giant esophageal aphthous ulcers in AIDS patients: Treatment with low dose corticosteroids. AIDS *5*:1537–1538, 1991.
31. Stratta, R. J., Schaeffer, M. S., Cushing, K. A., et al.: Successful prophylaxis of cytomegalovirus disease after primary CMV exposure in liver transplant recipients. Transplantation *51*:90–97, 1991.
32. Tavitian, A., Raufman, J. P., and Rosenthal, L. E.: Oral candidiasis as a marker for esophageal candidiasis in acquired immunodeficiency syndrome. Ann. Intern. Med. *104*:54–55, 1986.
33. Theise, N. D., Rotterdam, H., and Dieterich, D.: Cytomegalovirus esophagitis in AIDS: Diagnosis by endoscopic biopsy. Am. J. Gastroenterol. *86*:1123–1126, 1991.
34. Tilbe, K. S., and Lloyd, D. A.: A case of viral esophagitis. J. Clin. Gastroenterol. *8*:494–495, 1986.
35. Vita, E., and Schroeder, D. J.: Intralipid in prophylaxis of amphotericin B nephrotoxicity. Ann. Pharmacol. *28*:1182–1183, 1994.
36. Wall, S. D., and Jones, B.: Gastrointestinal tract in immunocompromised host, opportunistic infections and other complications. Radiology *185*:327–335, 1992.
37. Walsh, T. J., Belitsos, N. J., and Hamilton, S. R.: Bacterial esophagitis in immunocompromised patient. Arch. Intern. Med. *146*:1345–1348, 1986.
38. Yolkin, R. H., Hart, W., and Berman, J.: Viral infection and gastrointestinal dysfunction in children with HIV infection. *In* Bizzo, B. A., and Wilford, C. M. (eds.): Pediatric AIDS: The Challenge of HIV in Infants, Children and Adolescents. Baltimore, Williams & Wilkins, 1991, pp. 277–287.
39. Young, C., Chang, M. H., and Chang, M. H.: Fungal esophagitis in children. Acta Paediatr. Sin. *34*:436–442, 1993.

52

APPROACH TO PATIENTS WITH GASTROINTESTINAL TRACT INFECTIONS AND FOOD POISONING

Larry K. Pickering and Thomas G. Cleary

The approach to patients with gastrointestinal tract infections begins with a thorough medical history, including information about epidemiologic factors, a physical examination, and knowledge of the pathophysiology of various enteropathogens. Gastrointestinal tract infections include a wide range of symptom complexes and can be produced by a variety of enteropathogens. Most infectious diarrheal illness can be classified into one of several categories based on the causative agent, its pathophysiologic mechanism, and the clinical response. This information then can be used to determine the appropriate use of laboratory facilities and to determine therapy. All patients with diarrhea require some degree of fluid and electrolyte therapy, a few need other nonspecific support, and for some, specific antimicrobial therapy is indicated to shorten the illness and eradicate fecal excretion of the organism.

EPIDEMIOLOGY AND ETIOLOGY

Establishing the cause of diarrhea often is difficult because of variations in host susceptibility and response to infection, geographic location, season, and complexity of laboratory techniques necessary to identify fully the causative agents. In the United States and other parts of the world, acute infectious diarrhea is caused by many enteropathogens, but on the basis of epidemiologic and etiologic considerations, a number of major categories can be listed (Table 52–1): (1) outbreaks of diarrhea in child care centers and hospitals, (2) food-borne or water-borne diarrhea, (3) antimicrobial-associated diarrhea, (4) diarrhea of travelers, (5) diarrhea in immunosuppressed hosts, including persons with AIDS, and (6) others, which include sporadic episodes in which an epidemiologic factor cannot be identified. Answers to the following questions should be obtained from all patients with diarrhea: Does the patient attend or work in a child care center? Do other family members or acquaintances also have diarrhea? Is the patient taking or has the patient recently taken an antimicrobial agent? Has the patient traveled to or returned from a developing country within the previous week? Is the patient immunosuppressed or taking immunosuppressive agents? Is the patient infected with HIV?

When a patient complains of moderate or severe diarrhea, a decision should be made as to whether he or she should be hospitalized or treated as an outpatient. The following patients with diarrhea should be considered for hospitalization: (1) infants and elderly persons who appear "toxic" or have high temperatures, (2) patients with excessive loss of fluid and electrolytes through stools, especially when associated with vomiting, (3) persons with grossly bloody stools, and (4) persons who are immunosuppressed, including those with AIDS. Once the decision has been made either to hospitalize or to treat on an outpatient basis, appropriate diagnostic procedures and therapy can be instituted.

Outbreaks in Child Care Centers or Hospitals

The risk of an individual acquiring a gastrointestinal tract infection varies with age, environment, season, exposure, and immune status. Clinical and epidemiologic data often guide classification of an episode of acute infectious diarrhea into one of the categories mentioned earlier. If predisposing factors are not present, the episode can be classified as sporadic. Most cases of sporadic diarrhea occur in children younger than 5 years of age, although all age groups are affected. Infants who are breastfed are relatively protected from con-

TABLE 52–1. Major Categories of Acute Infectious Diarrhea

Category of Diarrhea	Epidemiologic Considerations	Most Commonly Involved Enteropathogens
Outbreaks	Child care centers Hospitals	Enteric viruses *Giardia lamblia*
Food-borne or water-borne	Other people involved after common food or water exposure	See Tables 52–2 and 52–3
Antimicrobial-associated colitis	Recent administration of an antimicrobial agent	*Clostridium difficile*
Travelers	Recent travel to a developing country	Enterotoxigenic *Escherichia coli* *Campylobacter* *Shigella* *Salmonella*
Immunosuppressed hosts	Underlying disease, including HIV infection; recent administration of an immunosuppressive drug	See Table 52–4

taminated food and water. Some protection also is afforded by factors present in human milk.[292] At weaning, the risk of diarrhea increases. When an episode of acute infectious diarrhea occurs, an association with other cases should be sought, especially when highly contagious organisms, such as *Shigella, Escherichia coli* O157:H7, *Giardia lamblia*, rotavirus, astrovirus, or enteric adenovirus, are isolated and in conditions in which close contact is facilitated, such as institutions for mentally retarded persons or child care centers.[162, 244, 245, 269, 270, 285, 286, 290, 364] Following respiratory tract illness, diarrhea is the second most common disease among children in child care facilities,[162] occurring most frequently in children younger than 3 years of age.

The National Nosocomial Infectious Surveillance (NNIS) system of the Centers for Disease Control and Prevention (CDC) reported that from 1985 to 1991, nosocomial diarrhea occurred in general pediatric care units at a rate of 11 per 10,000 discharges, in newborn nurseries at a rate of 11 per 10,000 discharges, and in high-risk nurseries at a rate of 20 per 10,000 discharges.[243] Studies of these pediatric populations have identified viral enteropathogens as the most frequent nosocomial agents, with rotavirus being the most frequently identified.[123]

Food-Borne or Water-Borne Diarrhea

Reporting of food-borne and water-borne diseases in the United States began in 1923 because of concern about typhoid fever and infantile diarrhea.[22] In 1978, food-borne and water-borne outbreaks first were published in separate annual summaries. These reported outbreaks account for a small fraction of the outbreaks that occur.

An outbreak of food-borne or water-borne disease is defined as an incident in which two or more persons experience a similar illness, usually involving the gastrointestinal tract, after ingesting common food or water intended for drinking.[22, 197] The CDC criteria state that a single case of botulism or chemical poisoning constitutes an outbreak if laboratory studies indicate that the food or water was contaminated by *Clostridium botulinum* or a chemical. Food-borne or water-borne disease can be produced by food or water contaminated with bacteria or bacterial toxin, a chemical, virus, or parasite.[8, 146, 147, 188] Table 52–2 outlines the various characteristics of food-borne or water-borne outbreaks, including those not characterized by diarrhea. Although most enteropathogens are spread by food or water, the epidemiology of outbreaks often suggests specific etiologic agents. A determination of the incubation period and the presence or absence of selected clinical findings (especially fever, vomiting, and bloody diarrhea) often leads the physician toward the correct diagnosis in outbreaks of food-borne or water-borne disease. As a general rule, when outbreaks are divided by incubation period of the illness, those less than 1 hour usually are caused by chemical poisoning; those of 1 to 7 hours, either by *Staphylococcus aureus* or *Bacillus cereus* emetic toxins; those of 8 to 14 hours, *Clostridium perfringens* or *B. cereus* enterotoxins; and those more than 14 hours, other infectious or toxic agents.

During the period from 1988 to 1992, a total of 2423 confirmed outbreaks of food-borne disease comprising 77,373 cases were reported to the CDC in Atlanta from various regions of the United States.[22] Among outbreaks in which the etiology was determined, bacterial pathogens caused the largest number of outbreaks (79 per cent) and cases (90 per cent), with *Salmonella, S. aureus,* and *C. botulism* isolated most frequently. Chemical agents caused 14 per cent of outbreaks and 2 per cent of cases, with ciguatoxin, heavy metals, mushrooms, paralytic shellfish, and scombrotoxin accounting for the outbreaks due to chemical agents (Table 52–3). Parasites caused 2 per cent of outbreaks and 1 per cent of cases and viruses 4 per cent of outbreaks and 6 per cent of cases. Hepatitis A and Norwalk-like viruses accounted for the outbreaks due to viruses. The etiologic agent was not detected in 59 per cent of outbreaks, indicating the need for improved investigative techniques. Food was eaten in a delicatessen, cafeteria, or restaurant in 37 per cent of the outbreaks, with the most common contributing factor being improper storage or inadequate holding temperature, followed by poor personal hygiene of the food handler. Outbreaks of gastroenteritis due to caliciviruses (CVs) have been associated with consumption of contaminated oysters, salad, and bakery products, and the virus has been transmitted by food handlers.[146, 200, 250, 310]

The ingestion of raw fish (sushi or sashimi) has led to infection with *Vibrio parahaemolyticus* and various parasites from infected fish. Parasites acquired through ingestion of raw fish include larval nematodes of the family Anisakidae, fish tapeworm of the species *Diphyllobothrium*, the fluke *Nanophyetus salmincola* from salmon, and many other helminths.[329, 387] The majority of worm infections acquired from raw fish in the United States have been acquired from dishes prepared at home and not from sushi restaurants.

Symptoms in patients with chemical poisoning generally begin within 1 to 2 hours after ingestion, although certain mushroom toxins may produce symptoms for up to 24 hours (see Table 52–3). Heavy metals, such as cadmium, iron, and tin, cause irritation of the gastric mucosa, with nausea, vomiting, and abdominal cramps, which usually resolve 2 to 3 hours after the offending agent has been removed.

The toxic syndromes acquired from fish and shellfish can be grouped clinically into two categories: the histamine-like syndrome of scombroid poisoning and the neurotoxic syndrome, including ciguatera, paralytic shellfish poisoning, and neurotoxic shellfish poisoning, and puffer fish poisoning due to tetrodotoxin.[106] The neurologic symptoms produced by fish, shellfish, and the Chinese restaurant syndrome agent include paresthesia, reversal of hot-cold sensations, loss of proprioception, flushing, weakness, and burning sensations. Chinese restaurant syndrome appears to be caused by excessive amounts of monosodium glutamate in foods. Fish poisoning may be caused by scombrotoxin, ciguatoxin, or tetrodotoxin. Scombroid fish poisoning is characterized by symptoms resembling those of histamine release. Shellfish poisoning can be of two types: paralytic, due to neurotoxins, including saxitoxin, and neurotoxic, due to several poorly characterized neurotoxins. Domoic acid from contaminated mussels causes acute widespread neurologic dysfunction and gastrointestinal tract manifestations followed by chronic residual memory deficits and motor neuropathy or axonopathy.[280, 352]

Infectious diseases associated with consumption of raw and lightly cooked shellfish (mussels, clams, oysters, lobsters, and other mollusks) are caused by bacterial agents that are native to the marine environment and by viral and bacterial agents from sewage effluents and other sources that contaminate environmental waters. As filter-feeding organisms, shellfish amplify public health problems associated with environmental contamination because they accumulate microbial pathogens at densities many times those found in overlying waters.[310]

The current public health problems of greatest concern to consumers of molluscan shellfish are associated with viral pathogens. The numbers of cases and outbreaks caused by these pathogens far exceed those of all other infectious diseases. The *Vibrio* genus (specifically *Vibrio vulnificus*) presents the most serious problem in terms of the severity of human illness and death, especially in persons with liver disease.[155]

TABLE 52–2. Characteristics of Food-Borne or Water-Borne Outbreaks of Diarrhea

Usual Incubation Periods	Clinical Illness		Causative Agent	Epidemiologic and Laboratory Diagnosis
	Fever	*Vomiting*		
5 minutes–6 hours (usually <3 hours)	Rare	Common	Chemical	Demonstration of toxin or chemical from food or epidemiologic incrimination of food
1–6 hours (usually <1 hour)	Rare	Profuse	*Staphylococcus aureus* enterotoxin *Bacillus cereus* emetic toxin	Detection of toxin in food, isolation of organisms in food (>10^5/g) or in vomitus or stool
8–14 hours	Rare	Occasional	*Clostridium perfringens* enterotoxin *Bacillus cereus* enterotoxin	Isolation of organisms or toxin from food (>10^5g) or stools of ill persons, epidemiologic incrimination of food
16–96 hours	Common	Occasional	*Shigella* *Salmonella* *Vibrio parahaemolyticus* Invasive *Escherichia coli* *Yersinia enterocolitica*	Isolation of organisms from food or stools of ill persons
12–36 hours	Clinical syndrome compatible with botulism		*Clostridium botulinum*	Isolation of organism or toxin from food (10^5/g) or stools, demonstration of toxin in serum or food
16–96 hours	Occasional	Occasional	*E. coli* enterotoxin *V. parahaemolyticus* enterotoxin *Vibrio cholerae* enterotoxin *Y. enterocolitica* enterotoxin	Isolation of organism from food and stools of ill persons, identification of toxin, epidemiologic incrimination of food
3–5 days	Uncommon	Frequent	*E. coli* O157:H7 and other enterohemorrhagic *E. coli*	Isolation of organism from food or identification of toxin in stools of ill persons, epidemiologic incrimination of food
1–3 days	Occasional	Common	Caliciviruses	Antigen detection (enzyme immunoassay) in stool, immune electron microscopy of stool, serology
1–7 days	Occasional	Occasional	*Campylobacter jejuni*	Isolation of organisms from food or stools of ill persons, epidemiologic incrimination of food

TABLE 52–3. Chemical Causes of Food Poisoning

Type of Chemical or Poison	Food	Clinical Symptoms	Onset of Symptoms (Hours)
Heavy metals such as, cadmium, copper, iron, tin	Water, less often food	Gastrointestinal	1
Scombrotoxin	Fish (tuna, mackerel, bonito, mahi-mahi, bluefish)	*Due to histamine:* flushing, headache, burning of mouth and throat, urticaria, gastrointestinal	1
Ciguatoxin	Fish (barracuda, amberjack, snapper, grouper)	*Neurologic:* paresthesia, reversal of cold-hot sensations, gastrointestinal	1–6
Tetrodotoxin	Puffer fish	*Neurologic:* paresthesia, numbness, loss of proprioception	1
Paralytic or neurotoxic compounds	Shellfish (clams, oysters, scallops, mussels, other mollusks)	Paresthesia, weakness, respiratory difficulties, gastrointestinal	1–4
Domoic acid	Mussels	Gastrointestinal; *acute CNS:* headache, seizures, hemiparesis, ophthalmoplegia, abnormalities of arousal; *chronic CNS:* memory deficits, motor neuropathy or axonopathy	Within 24
Monosodium glutamate	Chinese food	Burning sensation, heavy feeling in chest, pressure over face, flushing, gastrointestinal	1
Ibotenic acid, muscimol	Mushroom	*CNS:* confusion, delirium, visual disturbances, lethargy	2
Coprine	Mushroom	*Disulfiram-like effect:* nausea, vomiting, headache, hypotension, flushing, paresthesia and tachycardia	2
Muscarine	Mushroom	*Parasympathetic:* sweating, salivation, lacrimation, blurred vision, diarrhea, bradycardia, hypotension	2
Psilocybin, psilocin	Mushroom	*CNS:* hallucinations, anxiety, mood elevation, weakness	2
Diverse, mostly unknown	Mushroom	Gastrointestinal	2
Monomethylhydrazine, gyromitrin	Mushroom	Cellular destruction, gastrointestinal, loss of coordination, convulsion, coma, death	6–12
Amatoxins, phallotoxins	Mushroom	Cellular destruction, gastrointestinal, hepatic, and/or renal necrosis	6–24

CNS, central nervous system.

Mushrooms produce seven clinical syndromes, generally within 2 hours of ingestion[142] (see Table 52–3), except for poisoning due to amatoxins, phallotoxins, amantin, monomethylhydrazine, and gyromitrin, which may produce symptoms, including death, up to 24 hours after ingestion.[142] Mushrooms also can be contaminated with other agents, including *S. aureus* enterotoxin A.[209]

Bacterial diseases associated with ingestion of unpasteurized milk include salmonellosis and campylobacteriosis and, less frequently, infection with *Brucella, E. coli, Listeria monocytogenes, Mycobacterium, S. aureus, Streptococcus* species, *Streptobacillus moniliformis,* and *Yersinia enterocolitica.*[300] A nationwide outbreak of *Salmonella enteritidis* gastroenteritis involved 224,000 persons in the United States and was associated with ingestion of contaminated ice cream. The origin of the contamination was pasteurized ice cream premix that was contaminated in tanker trailers that previously had carried nonpasteurized liquid eggs containing *S. enteritidis.*[149] Consumption of raw milk has been associated with a chronic diarrhea syndrome of unknown cause,[272] initially identified in Minnesota. It is characterized by acute onset with marked urgency and a lack of systemic symptoms. The duration of illness is at least 9 months and generally has involved adults. Clinical and laboratory data indicate that diarrhea is caused by a secretory mechanism. There is no evidence of secondary transmission. Antimicrobial therapy has not been successful.[272] In addition, an outbreak of chronic diarrhea involving 72 people who ingested untreated drinking water was reported.[277] The cause and pathophysiologic mechanism of the illness remain unknown.

Since 1971, the number of reported water-borne outbreaks in the United States has averaged 30 per year (range, 13 to 53), involving approximately 7600 people per year (range, 1569 to 21,149).[197] During the 2-year period from 1993 to 1994, 17 states and one territory reported a total of 30 outbreaks associated with drinking water. These outbreaks caused an estimated 405,366 persons to become ill, including 403,000 from an outbreak of cryptosporidiosis in Milwaukee, the largest water-borne outbreak ever documented in the United States,[220] and 2366 from the other 29 outbreaks. This probably represents only a small fraction of the total number of outbreaks that occurred. Ingestion of pathogens during swimming has been associated with outbreaks.[140, 299, 345] Pathogens incriminated in water-borne outbreaks are different from those most often responsible for food poisoning. *G. lamblia* has been the most common pathogen documented to be spread by water, and *Cryptosporidium* has produced the largest outbreak; *Shigella,* hepatitis A virus, *Salmonella,* CVs, *Campylobacter,* and chemicals occasionally produce disease.[33, 140, 145, 186, 220, 299, 345] The cryptosporidiosis outbreak that occurred in Milwaukee in 1993 dramatically demonstrated the potential of this organism to cause water-borne disease.[220] Large outbreaks aboard passenger cruise ships continue to occur,[193] with a mean of 323 passengers involved in the 10 outbreaks investigated from 1986 to 1988.[197]

The main therapeutic modality in most patients with food

poisoning is supportive care because the majority of these illnesses are self-limited. Exceptions include botulism, paralytic shellfish poisoning, long-acting mushroom poisoning, and enterohemorrhagic *E. coli* (EHEC) infection, all of which may be fatal in previously healthy people. Food-borne disease due to any agent can produce fatalities in infants, the elderly, debilitated people, or persons with immune deficiencies.

Antimicrobial-Associated Diarrhea

Diarrhea is common after the use of an antimicrobial agent. Changes in bowel flora may result in abnormal stools in the absence of a documented enteropathogen, and discontinuation of the medication may be sufficient to eliminate symptoms. In a small number of patients with antibiotic-induced diarrhea, a severe and potentially fatal form of colitis may develop.[218]

Pseudomembranous or antimicrobial-associated colitis (AAC) refers to the presence of a pseudomembrane or of multiple plaque-like lesions in the colon induced by administration of an antimicrobial agent within the preceding 8 weeks. Pseudomembranous colitis not associated with antibiotic use occurs with *Shigella dysenteriae* serotype 1 and EHEC.[185, 294] The specific cause of essentially all cases of AAC are toxins produced by *Clostridium difficile*.[331] Intestinal flora generally can prevent proliferation and toxin production by *C. difficile;* however, administration of antibiotics to some persons allows *C. difficile* to proliferate and produce sufficient toxin to cause mucosal damage. Many antimicrobial agents have been reported to cause this condition; ampicillin, the cephalosporins, clindamycin, lincomycin, erythromycin, and trimethoprim-sulfamethoxazole (TMP-SMX) have been implicated most frequently.[19] Tetracycline, metronidazole, miconazole, and chloramphenicol are rare causes of AAC, whereas vancomycin has not been reported to cause the condition. Cancer chemotherapeutic agents also have been associated with AAC. In addition, nosocomial infection with *C. difficile* occurs and can result in asymptomatic carriage or diarrhea.[234, 235]

Patients with AAC present with watery diarrhea that often contains blood and mucus. Diarrhea may be the only manifestation of disease or may occur in association with nausea, vomiting, abdominal pain or cramps, fever, or leukocytosis. Extraintestinal *C. difficile* infections, including bacteremia, are uncommon.[117] If not treated appropriately, gastrointestinal tract symptoms may progress to toxic megacolon, colonic perforation, shock, and death. The diagnosis of AAC in a patient with diarrhea is supported by the following:[222, 330]

1. A history of ongoing or recent antimicrobial therapy. Twenty to 40 per cent of episodes occur after the drug has been discontinued.
2. Finding leukocytes on a stain of fecal material.
3. Exclusion of other agents known to cause fecal leukocytes.
4. Identification of *C. difficile* toxins in stool specimens.
5. Sigmoidoscopy with rectal biopsy to identify pseudomembrane or plaques that contain mucin, fibrin, leukocytes, and sloughed epithelial cells.

Plaques or pseudomembrane are not always present in patients with AAC, but when they are, *C. difficile* usually can be presumed to be the cause of disease. Proctoscopy, with or without mucosal biopsy, is the quickest way to establish the diagnosis. The finding of *C. difficile* in feces suggests but does not confirm that *C. difficile* is the cause of the diarrhea. The finding of fecal toxin is a more useful method of diagnosing *C. difficile*–induced disease than is bacterial culture.[241] *C. difficile* and its toxins can be detected by employing a variety of tissue culture assays, enzyme immunoassays, latex agglutination, and molecular techniques.[68, 199, 218, 241] The toxic effect in tissue culture should be neutralized by antitoxin. This organism and the toxins may be found in the gastrointestinal tract of some healthy persons,[235, 246] particularly infants.[92]

The most important aspect of therapy in patients with AAC is discontinuation of the antimicrobial agent. If this is done, symptoms usually resolve within 1 to 2 weeks; however, if symptoms persist or worsen or if the patient has severe diarrhea, specific therapy with metronidazole,[238, 351] vancomycin,[97, 392] or bacitracin[97, 392] should be instituted. To decrease the emergence of vancomycin-resistant enterococci in hospitals, many experts recommend metronidazole first in treatment of most patients with *C. difficile* colitis.[381] Oral vancomycin should be reserved for seriously ill patients or for those who do not respond to metronidazole. Resistance to metronidazole and bacitracin has been reported. The response rate to bacitracin is slower and less certain than that to vancomycin[97, 392] and potentially toxic if absorbed from an inflamed intestine. Teicoplanin, a glycopeptide antibiotic, has been used to treat patients with *C. difficile* disease.[81] Patients who are unable to take oral therapy should be treated with both intravenous vancomycin and metronidazole as well as oral vancomycin delivered through a nasogastric tube, if possible, or an ostomy tube, if present. After initiation of therapy, symptoms generally resolve within several days, and titer decreases and fecal toxin disappears eventually. Recurrence of colitis after discontinuation of metronidazole or vancomycin has been documented in 10 to 20 per cent of patients.[18] Relapses are treated with a second course of either metronidazole or vancomycin. The combination of recommended antibiotics and *Saccharomyces boulardii* administered orally was effective and safe therapy for patients with recurrent disease due to *C. difficile*.[236] No benefit of *S. boulardii* was demonstrated for patients during their initial episodes.

Travelers' Diarrhea

Travelers' diarrhea is the most common health problem encountered by persons from the United States, Northern Europe, Canada, or Australia who travel to Latin America, Asia, the Middle East, or Africa, where diarrhea is hyperendemic.[99–102, 135, 219] Half of these travelers experience diarrhea within the first few weeks after arrival. Enterotoxigenic *E. coli* (ETEC) is the most commonly identified cause of travelers' diarrhea, but the illness can be caused by a variety of bacteria, viruses, and parasites,[36, 99–102, 228] including *Shigella* species, *Campylobacter jejuni, Aeromonas* species, *Plesiomonas shigelloides, Salmonella* species, *V. parahaemolyticus* (in Asia), *G. lamblia,* enteroaggregative *E. coli* (EAEC), and rotavirus. There is limited information from existing studies concerning pathogens associated with diarrhea among children or the elderly who travel. Studies of diarrhea of travelers visiting the United States and Great Britain from developed and developing countries showed attack rates of 2 and 0.6 per cent, respectively.[124, 319]

The clinical illness varies, reflecting the diversity of causative agents. Typically, illness occurs within several weeks of arrival in a foreign country and is defined as the passage of at least three unformed stools in a 24-hour period, together with cramps, nausea, fecal urgency, tenesmus, or a combination thereof. Bloody diarrhea, vomiting, and documented temperature elevation are less frequent. About 50 per cent of persons who become ill have mild disease, 15 to 40 per cent are forced to alter their scheduled activities, and 15 to 30 per cent are confined to bed.[219] Travelers may experience more than one episode. Because travelers' diarrhea is caused by a variety of enteropathogens, it is likely to be spread by many fecally contaminated vehicles. Most studies implicate food, particularly uncooked food,[111, 356] and untreated water and ice. Careful attention to food consumption with avoidance of foods that are not steaming hot, raw vegetables, fruit not peeled by the traveler, and tap water, including ice, is critical to disease prevention.[111, 239] Predisposing factors and host factors that increase susceptibility to travelers' diarrhea or complicate its course include young age, short duration of travel, eating in restaurants, season, reduced gastric acidity, chronic and active gastrointestinal tract disease, and immunodeficiency disorders.[103, 111, 159]

Several studies have evaluated prevention and treatment of travelers' diarrhea in adults using either antidiarrheal compounds or antibiotic compounds.[239] Compounds that have been shown to be effective chemoprophylactic agents include doxycycline, bismuth subsalicylate,[101] TMP-SMX, and fluoroquinolones.[112] These compounds have been shown to offer 50 to 100 per cent protection against travelers' diarrhea.[321] Potential problems with antibiotic regimens include resistance of bacteria, such as ETEC, *Salmonella* species, and *Shigella* species, and side effects, such as nausea, diarrhea, and photosensitivity reactions. Large doses of bismuth subsalicylate can result in significant serum salicylate concentrations.[118, 287] The bioavailability of salicylate in one ounce of Pepto-Bismol is equivalent to that of one 325-mg adult aspirin tablet.[118]

Because of the uncertain risk of widespread prophylactic administration of these antimicrobial agents, including development of resistance among enteric bacteria[253] and the mildness of most cases of travelers' diarrhea, prophylactic use of antimicrobial agents generally is not recommended.[135] Instruction of travelers in regard to appropriate dietary practices as a prophylactic measure is recommended.[111, 356]

If a person becomes ill in a locale where laboratory facilities are inadequate, the choice of a therapeutic agent must be made on an empiric basis.[239] Antidiarrheal compounds as therapy for travelers' diarrhea have been used in persons with nondysenteric disease. Bismuth subsalicylate has been shown to be effective in decreasing the incidence of diarrhea by up to 60 per cent.[100] Loperamide should not be used in infants or older children with bloody diarrhea or fever, although older children and adults with watery diarrhea may benefit. Other nonantimicrobial compounds have been shown to be ineffective or dangerous or have not been evaluated.[301]

Because many episodes of travelers' diarrhea are caused by bacteria that are susceptible to TMP-SMX, a 3- to 5-day course of this antibiotic may help travelers who develop diarrhea with three or more loose stools in an 8-hour period, especially if associated with symptoms such as nausea, vomiting, abdominal cramps, fever, or blood in stools.[102] In areas where *C. jejuni* is common or where resistance to TMP-SMX by other enteropathogens is high, ciprofloxacin or ofloxacin may be a better choice for treatment of adults. Ciprofloxacin is equivalent to TMP-SMX in therapy of diarrhea due to susceptible organisms and expands the coverage to resistant organisms and *C. jejuni,* which generally is resistant to TMP-SMX.[103, 112, 238, 253] In a study of 227 U.S. adults with acute diarrhea in Mexico, the combination of loperamide and TMP-SMX for 3 days provided the most rapid relief of travelers' diarrhea when compared with the placebo group.[113] A single dose of TMP-SMX also was efficacious, but loperamide alone was not.

If a person develops chronic diarrhea after an episode of travelers' diarrhea, the differential diagnosis should include persistent infection, particularly with *Giardia, Cryptosporidium, Cyclospora,* or *Isospora;* antibiotic-associated colitis; small intestinal bacterial overgrowth; transient disaccharidase deficiency; initial manifestation of ulcerative colitis or regional enteritis; postdysenteric colitis; irritable bowel syndrome; or tropical sprue.[105] An underlying immune system defect such as occurs with AIDS also should be considered.

Immunocompromised Hosts, Including Persons with AIDS

Causes of gastrointestinal tract disease in children with AIDS can be grouped under the major headings of infection, malignancy, and HIV enteropathy. The location of involvement of the gastrointestinal tract by infectious agents determines the clinical symptoms and the ease with which these organisms can be diagnosed and treated (Table 52–4). Organisms and diseases of the gastrointestinal tract that fulfill the CDC surveillance case definition of AIDS[55] are candidiasis, cryptosporidiosis, cytomegalovirus, herpes simplex, *Mycobacterium avium* complex, *Microsporidium,* isosporiasis, and *Salmonella.*[7, 95, 170, 194, 293, 383] In addition, the AIDS wasting syndrome (HIV infection without superimposed opportunistic enteric infection of known cause) is part of the CDC case definition for AIDS.[55] Patients with AIDS have been shown to have D-xylose malabsorption and steatorrhea, and, on jejunal and rectal biopsies, a specific pathologic process can be demonstrated in the lamina propria of the small intestine and colon.[194] A significant proportion of patients with AIDS and severe small intestinal injury have enterocyte infection, often with *Cryptosporidium* or various *Microsporidium* organisms.[134, 195] Infections with several enteropathogens in persons with AIDS are more frequent and more likely to be severe, recurrent, persistent, or associated with extraintestinal disease. Diarrhea also is common in bone marrow transplant

TABLE 52–4. Organisms that Cause Gastrointestinal Tract Infections in Patients with AIDS

Area	Organisms
Esophagus	*Candida albicans**
	Cytomegalovirus (CMV)*
	Herpes simplex virus (HSV)*
Hepatobiliary	CMV
	*Cryptosporidium**
	Hepatotropic viruses
	Mycobacterium avium complex (MAC)*
Small intestine	*Campylobacter* species
	CMV*
	*Cryptosporidium**
	Giardia lamblia
	*Isospora belli**
	MAC*
	*Microsporidium** (*Enterocytozoon bieneusi* and *Septata intestinalis*)
	Salmonella species*
	Strongyloides stercoralis
Large intestine	*Campylobacter* species
	Clostridium difficile
	CMV*
	Entamoeba histolytica
	HSV*
	Salmonella species*
	Shigella species

*Indicator diseases of the gastrointestinal tract that fulfill the Centers for Disease Control and Prevention surveillance case definition of AIDS.[55]

TABLE 52–5. Pathogenic Bacteria Associated with Acute Infectious Diarrhea

Agent	Frequency (%)	Country or Area	Epidemiologic Considerations
Aeromonas hydrophila	<1	United States	Water, food, or animal exposure
	5–27	India, Australia, Great Britain, Thailand	
Bacillus cereus	<1	Worldwide	Food exposure
Campylobacter jejuni	1–5	United States, Finland, Canada, Indonesia, Belgium	Animal or food exposure
	5–14	Great Britain, Switzerland, Australia, France, Brazil, Zaire, Bangladesh, Gambia	
	35	South Africa	
Clostridium difficile	Unknown	United States	Exposure to antimicrobial agents
Clostridium perfringens	<1	United States, New Guinea	Food exposure
Plesiomonas shigelloides	Unknown	Tropical and subtropical	Water, fish, or animal exposure
Salmonella species	<1–6	Bangladesh, Finland, Canada, United States, Japan, Australia	Travel, exposure to carrier, food exposure
	10–12	Brazil, Mexico	
Shigella species	1–8	Australia, United States, Canada, Brazil	Exposure to an infected person or to contaminated food
	5–14	Bangladesh, Mexico	
Staphylococcus aureus	<1	United States	Food exposure
Vibrio cholerae O1	<1	United States	Travel, food, or water exposure
	4	Philippines	
	12–14	Bangladesh	
V. cholerae O139	1	Southeast Asia	Food or water
Vibrio parahaemolyticus	<1	United States, Japan, Bangladesh	Seafood exposure
Yersinia enterocolitica	<1–3	United States, Brazil, Finland, Canada	Food or animal exposure

recipients[390] and may be caused by any of the earlier-mentioned organisms. Guidelines for prevention of opportunistic infections, including those involving the gastrointestinal tract, have been published.[59]

ORGANISMS THAT CAUSE ACUTE GASTROENTERITIS

Bacteria

Many bacterial, viral, and parasitic organisms produce diarrhea in humans. Tables 52–5 and 52–6 show the major bacterial enteric pathogens associated with acute infectious diarrhea and their relative frequencies in various parts of the world. Each organism is discussed here in alphabetical order for ease of reference. The relative importance of each organism as a cause of diarrhea varies in different populations.

Aeromonas hydrophila

Aeromonas species are gram-negative bacteria found in soil and fresh and brackish water worldwide; they are recognized as colonizers and pathogens of cold-blooded animals, including fish, reptiles, and amphibians.[5] *Aeromonas* species have been associated with a wide spectrum of human disease, most frequently gastroenteritis, soft tissue infection, and bacteremia, especially in immunocompromised hosts.[5] Three species, *A. hydrophila, A. sobria,* and *A. caviae,* have been associated with human disease, but DNA hybridization studies indicate that there are more genotypes.[173] Because many clinical laboratories cannot perform precise identification, most species isolated are reported as *A. hydrophila.* The role of *A. hydrophila* in human diarrhea remains uncertain. Despite the association of this organism with acute gastroenteritis and its more frequent isolation from patients with diarrhea than from healthy controls,[171] volunteers who have been fed

TABLE 52–6. Pathogenic *Escherichia coli* Associated with Acute Infectious Diarrhea

Class of *E. coli*	Frequency (%)	Country	Usual Presentation of Disease
Enterohemorrhagic	1–4	United States, Great Britain, Canada	Bloody diarrhea and hemorrhagic colitis, water- and food-borne outbreaks, associated with hemolytic uremic syndrome
Enterotoxigenic	1–4	Finland, Australia, United States, Canada	Watery diarrhea in children living in and travelers visiting developing countries
	6–16	Brazil, Mexico, Philippines	
	18–20	El Salvador, Bangladesh	
Enteroinvasive	<1–1	United States, Finland, Mexico	Dysentery in adults and watery diarrhea, occasionally food-borne outbreaks
	1–20	Brazil	
Enteropathogenic	4–8	Finland, Japan, Canada,	Acute and chronic diarrhea in infants in nurseries, diarrhea in children <1 year of age in developing countries
	18–28	El Salvador	
	43–50	Mexico, Brazil	
		India, South Africa	
Enteroaggregative	12–34	India, Mexico	Chronic watery diarrhea in children in developing countries

the organism have not become ill.[249] *A. hydrophila* has been isolated from stools of less than 3 per cent of healthy humans[5]; however, in Thailand, the isolation rate from healthy controls increased with age, up to 27 per cent in adults.[5] *A. hydrophila* strains have been shown to produce both cytotoxin and enterotoxin, including heat-labile (cholera-like) enterotoxin and heat-stable enterotoxins.[12] Enterotoxin-producing strains were identified with 97 per cent accuracy using a hemolysin assay.[47] Other toxic or invasive properties may be important in disease production because one-quarter of patients have a dysentery-like illness.[171]

Bacillus cereus

B. cereus is an aerobic, spore-forming, gram-positive bacillus that is a rare cause of food poisoning in the United States.[57, 217, 354] Although frequently present in food, it should be suspected as the cause of gastrointestinal tract illness only if appropriate symptoms are present and if incriminated food, particularly fried rice, contains 10^5 or more *B. cereus* organisms per gram.[354] Two distinct forms of gastrointestinal tract illness can be produced by this organism. One is caused by production of a low-molecular-weight (<10,000 Da) preformed emetic toxin that survives high temperatures, exposure to trypsin, and pH extremes. The other is caused by a high-molecular-weight (48,000 Da) heat-labile enterotoxin that is sensitive to high temperatures, proteolytic enzymes, and acids and is formed in vivo.[359] If the strain causing illness produces the emetic toxin, a syndrome occurs that resembles illness produced by staphylococcal enterotoxin with nausea, vomiting, and abdominal cramps that begin within several hours of ingestion. The diagnosis may be difficult to confirm because heating may kill the organism but leave the toxin intact. If the strain produces enterotoxin, profuse watery diarrhea and abdominal pain begin within 12 hours, with minimal or no vomiting. Some strains produce both toxins, whereas others produce only enterotoxin. Symptoms due to either toxin resolve in less than 24 hours, and fever is rare. Spores of *B. cereus* are resistant to heat and therefore may withstand a brief period of cooking or boiling. *B. cereus* can grow in temperatures ranging from 25° C to 40° C.

Campylobacter

Campylobacter species are recognized as one of the most important causes of acute diarrheal disease in humans throughout the world.[50, 131] The taxonomy of the genus *Campylobacter* has been revised extensively. Currently, 15 *Campylobacter* species and 6 subspecies are recognized.[267] Most *Campylobacter* and *Campylobacter*-like organisms have been assigned to rRNA super-family VI, which includes the genus *Helicobacter,* the family Campylobacteraceae, and a number of other taxa. *C. jejuni, C. coli, C. concisus, C. fetus, C. lari, C. hyointestinalis, C. sputorum,* and *C. upsaliensis* have been incriminated as enteropathogens for humans; *C. jejuni* and *C. coli* are the two predominant species, although the use of certain selective media may preclude isolation of others.[266, 267] *C. fetus,* recognized as a cause of fever, bacteremia, and meningitis in immunocompromised hosts and abortion, rarely causes diarrhea. *C. jejuni* typically produces illness in previously healthy persons. In many parts of the United States and Canada, *C. jejuni* is the most commonly documented bacterial cause of diarrhea.[39] Infected persons complain of diarrhea, cramping abdominal pain, chills, and fever. Gross rectal bleeding and mucus and the presence of fecal leukocytes may occur, resembling the illness produced by *Shigella.*[39] The clinical presentation also may mimic that of inflammatory bowel disease. Both a heat-labile enterotoxin and mucosal invasion have been incriminated in the pathogenesis.[315] *C. jejuni* also has been associated with septicemia, abortion, and Guillain-Barré syndrome.[306] Many clinical microbiology laboratories do not differentiate *C. jejuni* and *C. coli.* Both produce diarrhea, and differences with regard to susceptibility patterns and clinical illness are minimal.

A thermophilic strain of *Campylobacter* has been distinguished from *C. jejuni* by its nalidixic acid resistance and halotolerance. The species name *C. lari* was proposed because the great majority of isolates were from sea gulls (genus *Larus).*[28] This organism has been shown to produce diarrhea and rarely septicemia in humans. The significance of *C. lari, C. sputorum, C. hyointestinalis,* and *C. upsaliensis* as causes of diarrhea in humans has not been defined fully. *C. sputorum* and *C. upsaliensis* have been associated with abscesses in humans.[267]

Helicobacter pylori (formerly *C. pylori)* has been isolated from the stomach and duodenum of patients with histologically confirmed type B antral gastritis, peptic ulcer disease, duodenal ulcers, and gastric lymphoma.[40, 267, 376] Data from human volunteer studies, therapeutic trials with antimicrobial agents, and studies in animal models indicate that *H. pylori* is the cause of these syndromes.[38, 40, 267, 376] It is not associated with diarrhea.

Clostridium difficile

C. difficile and its toxins have been shown to be the cause of pseudomembranous colitis or AAC.[19, 20, 218] Interpretation of the finding of *C. difficile* or its toxins in stools from infants presents a special problem because both may be found without illness.[92, 246] Colitis results from toxin production within the intestinal lumen. The toxins produced by *C. difficile* lead to progression of disease, but the manner in which disease occurs appears to be more complex than just direct action of the toxin on gut mucosa. The initial reaction appears to involve the binding of toxin A to its receptor in the brush border membrane, but the mechanism by which the toxin kills mucosal cells and causes the enterotoxic response is not known. The extensive damage that occurs from the action of toxin A and the intense inflammatory infiltrate probably result in dissemination of both toxins A and B into the systemic circulation. Toxin A, which no longer is enterotoxic (i.e., neutralized with monoclonal antibody that neutralizes the enterotoxic activity), still is lethal when injected. This raises the possibility that toxin A acts by a different mechanism once it leaves the intestine. Toxin B also acts on tissues outside of the intestine, but the receptor for the toxin and the target tissues have not been identified. Because these toxins cause inflammation and sometimes mucosal necrosis without bacterial invasion, there may be watery diarrhea with or without blood in the feces.

Clostridium perfringens

C. perfringens types A, C, and D produce an enterotoxin that is implicated in the pathogenesis of disease caused by this organism.[233, 331] Most food-borne outbreaks are caused by type A. *C. perfringens* causes a short-duration food poisoning syndrome.[141] After ingestion of contaminated meat or poultry products, in vivo sporulation occurs in the small intestine with release of a structural spore protein that has enterotoxic and cytotoxic properties. The heat-labile, 35-kDa, single-polypeptide enterotoxin induces fluid accumulation in ileal loops in animals and produces diarrhea in humans. Within 14 hours after the meal, watery diarrhea and abdominal pain with minimal nausea, vomiting, or fever ensue.[141] Illness resolves in less than 24 hours. Less than 5 per cent of

C. perfringens isolates contain the chromosomal *cpe* gene encoding this toxin. *C. perfringens* type C also is associated with a rare destructive intestinal disease called enteritis necroticans or pig-bel. These strains produce three toxins (alpha-toxin, beta-toxin, and an enterotoxin) of potential pathogenetic significance.[331] This illness occurs after ingestion of undercooked pig at pork feasts in Papua, New Guinea. It is characterized by vomiting, abdominal pain, bloody diarrhea, and small bowel necrosis, with peritonitis, shock, and death.[254]

Escherichia coli

There are several recognized categories of *E. coli* that produce diarrhea: EHEC, ETEC, enteroinvasive *E. coli* (EIEC), enteropathogenic *E. coli* (EPEC), and EAEC (see Table 52–6).[208, 331] *E. coli* is among the most common causes of bacterial diarrhea in humans worldwide.

EHEC produces bloody diarrhea, usually without fever. This hemorrhagic colitis syndrome has been recognized to be caused most often by *E. coli* O157:H7 and other EHEC strains, which produce large quantities of a potent cytotoxin[168, 184, 224, 264, 309, 331] similar or identical to the cytotoxin produced by *S. dysenteriae* serotype 1.[184, 264, 265] Several closely related toxins are recognized. The cytotoxin that essentially is identical to shigatoxin is called Shiga toxin I (or verotoxin 1) when produced by *E. coli.* A structurally and functionally related toxin that is distinct immunologically is called Shiga toxin II (or verotoxin 2). Both toxins are encoded by bacteriophages. Multiple additional variants exist that are more closely related to the second toxin.[65] EHEC lacks the 140-MDa plasmid that is associated with the invasiveness characteristic of EIEC, but it does possess a 60-MDa plasmid.[309] *E. coli* organisms that produce high levels of cytotoxin are clinically important because, like *S. dysenteriae* 1,[265] they have been incriminated as etiologic agents of hemolytic uremic syndrome.[64, 183, 294] These pathogens often possess adherence genes related to those of EPEC.[25]

E. coli disease may be caused by heat-stable and heat-labile enterotoxins, which are among the best characterized of all enterotoxins.[79, 93, 214, 331, 350] Heat-stable enterotoxin a and heat-labile enterotoxin I are associated with disease in humans and other animals, whereas heat-stable enterotoxin b is associated primarily with disease in piglets and heat-labile enterotoxin II has been associated only with animal disease. ETEC strains from humans with diarrhea produce heat-stable enterotoxin a only, heat-labile enterotoxin I only, or both together. These toxins often are produced by strains that have colonization factor antigens, which are important in adherence of the organism to the gastrointestinal tract.[214] ETEC belongs to many different serogroups and causes disease in patients of all ages, especially infants and children living in developing countries and travelers from developed to developing countries.

EIEC is related antigenically and biochemically to *Shigella*[61] and causes either a dysentery-like illness or watery diarrhea. EIEC possesses a 140-MDa plasmid, which encodes for invasiveness and which probably contributes to dysenteric illness. This plasmid is related closely to the plasmids that are associated with *Shigella* virulence.[325] The watery diarrhea may be due to an enterotoxin referred to as EIEC enterotoxin.[331] Infections generally occur in adults; food-borne outbreaks have been reported.

EPEC have been incriminated as causing both sporadic and epidemic diarrhea in infants, especially in developing countries.[89, 208, 358] Originally, EPEC was a term used to describe all *E. coli* organisms associated with diarrheal syndromes. Currently, the term EPEC is defined more narrowly. Volunteer studies[89] and studies comparing rates of isolation from sick and healthy infants[208] have demonstrated that EPEC organisms are pathogens, although these strains rarely cause diarrhea in older children and adults. The specific mechanisms of disease production may be related to adherence, which can be demonstrated in HEp-2 cells.[21, 228] EPEC adherence to microvilli is known to be encoded by a gene, *bfp*A, which has homology to the pilin gene of *V. cholerae* and two genes, *eae*A and *esp*B (formerly *eae*B).[90, 91, 130, 342] Some strains currently classified as EPEC have an adhesin (AIDA-I) that causes the organisms to adhere to tissue culture cells in a diffuse pattern.[30] EPEC causes a distinctive histopathologic lesion in the human intestine that involves destruction of microvilli and close adherence of bacteria to the membrane of the enterocyte with cap-like pedestals on which each bacterium rests. The classic histopathologic lesion is called the attacking/effacing lesion. F actin, myosin, and other cytoskeletal elements are clustered beneath the attached bacteria.[331]

EAEC[371] have been associated with acute[227] and chronic[32, 202] diarrhea in developing countries and in adults with travelers' diarrhea in whom no other mechanism for their diarrhea could be defined.[226] These *E. coli* organisms are detected in the HEp-2 cell assay in which three distinct patterns of adherence can be observed: localized, diffuse, and aggregative.[228] The localized phenotype is characteristic of some EPEC strains. In contrast, *E. coli* organisms that exhibit the diffuse or aggregative patterns represent two categories associated with diarrhea (EAEC). The aggregating phenotype is due to a protein called aggregative adherence fimbria I.[257] EAEC strains have been reported to produce three toxins that potentially are able to stimulate intestinal secretion and are called EAEC heat-stable enterotoxin 1, a 120-kDa heat-labile protein, and a 108- to 116-kDa protein.[256, 328, 331] The extent of disease caused by EAEC strains and the relation to EPEC strains are being investigated.[73]

Plesiomonas shigelloides

P. shigelloides is a gram-negative bacillus that has been associated with opportunistic infections in immunocompromised hosts and with sporadic cases of diarrhea in immunocompetent hosts in a variety of countries.[43, 161, 179] Organisms produce heat-stable and heat-labile enterotoxins, but their association with disease is unknown.[331] The organism has been isolated from surface water and the intestines of freshwater fish and many animals, including dogs and cats.[355] It is common in tropical and subtropical areas from which most stool isolates have been reported.[161] Persons with *P. shigelloides* infection describe self-limited diarrhea, occasionally characterized by blood and mucus. The organism is a rare cause of extraintestinal illness, such as meningitis or bacteremia.[43] Appropriate antimicrobial therapy appears to shorten the duration of diarrheal illness.[161, 179] The organism has failed to produce illness when fed to volunteers, and its role as an enteric pathogen remains unproven.[151]

Salmonella

Most hospital laboratories biochemically differentiate three species of *Salmonella: S. cholerae-suis, S. typhi,* and *S. enteritidis.* Most of the 1700 serotypes of *Salmonella* now are grouped together as *S. enteritidis.* Several clinical syndromes are due to *Salmonella*: (1) the carrier state, (2) acute gastroenteritis, (3) bacteremia, enteric fever, or both, and (4) dissemination with localized suppuration, such as abscess, osteomyelitis, or meningitis. Although *S. typhi* is the prototype of *Salmonella* able to penetrate intestinal mucosa, reach intestinal lymphatic tissue, and disseminate, other *Salmonella* organisms only occasionally behave in this manner.[67] Invasion of intestinal epithelium by *S. typhi* and occasionally by nontyphoidal *Salmonella* strains is a well-known virulence trait of *Salmonella* species. Most nontyphoidal *Salmonella* serotypes are associated with watery diarrhea; the pathogenesis of the secretory response to *Salmonella* is not understood completely.[12, 331] *Salmonella* rarely causes an illness similar to pseudomembranous colitis.[164] *Salmonella* gastroenteritis occurs throughout life but is most common in the first year, decreases during early childhood, and remains relatively constant throughout the adult years.[58] Reptiles, including turtles, snakes, lizards, and iguanas, are vectors for certain serotypes of *Salmonella* and have been associated with episodes of salmonellosis.[1] Numerous outbreaks of disease due to *Salmonella* have been reported after ingestion of contaminated food products, including eggs and ice cream.[149, 353]

Shigella

There are four serogroups of *Shigella* containing more than 40 serotypes and subtypes.[133, 187] *S. sonnei* currently is a more common cause of bacillary dysentery in the United States and Europe than is *S. flexneri,* whereas *S. boydii* and *S. dysenteriae* are uncommon causes of diarrhea in the United States. Patients with *Shigella* isolated from stool may present with several clinical patterns: (1) asymptomatic excretion,[283] (2) enterotoxin-like diarrhea, (3) bacillary dysentery,[346] (4) an arthritis similar to that seen in Reiter syndrome,[3] and (5) hemolytic-uremic syndrome occurring after infection with *S. dysenteriae* 1. The arthritis occurs 2 to 5 weeks after the dysenteric illness, characteristically in patients with histocompatibility antigen HLA-B27. Postinfectious arthritis also occurs in patients after *Salmonella, Campylobacter,* and *Y. enterocolitica* infections. The molecular mechanisms by which *Shigella* organisms invade epithelial cells have been defined.[133] *S. dysenteriae* 1 produces Shiga toxin in high levels.[265] Infection by *Shigella* species is rare in the first few months of life but is common between 6 months and 10 years of age.

Staphylococcus aureus

Two enteric syndromes have been associated with *S. aureus*. Although previously considered a cause of AAC, it currently is unclear whether antibiotic-associated staphylococcal enteritis actually exists as a disease entity, because most antibiotic-associated diarrhea is associated with *C. difficile*.[20] The existence of the other major staphylococcal enteric syndrome is well established. Staphylococcal food poisoning is caused by ingestion of food contaminated with preformed *S. aureus* heat-stable enterotoxin.[108, 209] Although multiple enterotoxins (A to F) have been described, only enterotoxin types A to E cause enteric disease. Type A has been responsible for more than half of the reported outbreaks of staphylococcal food poisoning in the United States.[160, 209] All toxins are antigenically related, low-molecular-weight proteins. Illness due to these preformed toxins begins within 1 to 6 hours after ingestion and lasts less than 12 hours. Nausea, vomiting, abdominal pain, and diarrhea without fever occur.

Vibrio cholerae

Strains of *V. cholerae* are classified according to somatic or O groups. *V. cholerae* strains are separated further into two main serotypes (Ogawa and Inaba) and two biotypes (classic and El Tor).[180] *V. cholerae* responsible for epidemic cholera belong to serogroups O1 and O139; all other *V. cholerae* strains belonging to serogroups other than O1 and O139 occasionally cause diarrhea or extraintestinal infections.[172] Cholera affects persons of all ages, but children are involved disproportionately. *V. cholerae* O1 primarily is a problem in Asia, Africa, and South America, although a focus is present in the Gulf Coast of the United States.[180, 216] *V. cholerae* O139 primarily is a problem in Southeast Asia. Most clinical isolates of *V. cholerae* O1 in the United States are travel-associated, and many are resistant to antimicrobial agents.[221] Epidemic cholera appeared in Peru in January 1991 and subsequently spread throughout the Americas, including the United States.[54, 221] The epidemic strain is biotype El Tor, serotype Inaba. It can be differentiated from the strain of *V. cholerae* that is endemic to the U.S. Gulf Coast by hemolysin production and by molecular subtyping techniques.

V. cholerae O1 adheres to and multiplies on small intestinal mucosa. Diarrhea occurs after elaboration of several toxins, the most important of which is cholera toxin, a heat-labile enterotoxin composed of one A and five B subunits.[331] The B subunits bind the toxin to the terminal galactose of the G_{M1} ganglioside receptors present on intestinal mucosal cells. The A subunit adenosine 5′-diphosphate ribosylates the guanosine 5′-triphosphate–binding regulatory protein of adenylate cyclase in gut epithelium.[331] The resulting intracellular increase in cyclic adenosine monophosphate causes inhibition of sodium absorption and causes chloride and fluid secretion in the small intestine. Most non-O1 strains isolated from ill persons in the United States lack cholera toxin–like activity[172] and, when tested with gene probes, are found not to possess gene sequences homologous to those of cholera toxin.[180] Two additional toxins are produced by *V. cholerae,* Zot (zonula occludens toxin) and Ace (accessory cholera enterotoxin). Strains of *V. cholerae* belonging to serotypes other than O1 and O139 are much less significant pathogens, although they can cause mild and occasionally profuse, watery diarrhea. Other *Vibrio* species, including *V. fluvialis, V. mimicus, V. hollisae,* and *V. furnissii,* have been shown occasionally to cause gastrointestinal tract disease.[172]

Vibrio parahaemolyticus

V. parahaemolyticus, a common marine isolate, has been found in water, shellfish, fish, and plankton.[155] Although widely distributed in coastal waters, *V. parahaemolyticus* is an uncommon cause of diarrhea, except in Japan, where consumption of raw seafood is common. Clinical manifestations of infection include diarrhea, abdominal cramps, nausea, and less frequently vomiting, headache, low-grade fever, and chills.[172] A dysentery-like syndrome has been described in India and Bangladesh.[166] Preexisting liver disease predisposes infected persons to septicemia and death.[155] A selective culture medium is required for isolation of the organism from stool cultures. The pathophysiology of illness is uncertain, although a 23-kDa protein called thermostable direct hemolysin either is responsible for the disease or is linked closely to the virulence genes.[262]

Yersinia enterocolitica

Y. enterocolitica is a gram-negative bacillus that appears to be a common cause of gastroenteritis among children in Europe and Canada but is a relatively uncommon cause of enteritis in the United States,[72] where *Y. enterocolitica* O8 has been the predominant clinical serotype.[205] The ingestion of contaminated milk or food such as chitterlings[205] has been implicated as the mode of transmission in reported outbreaks. The clinical manifestations vary depending on the age of the person involved.[163] Illness in children younger than 5 years of age usually is self-limited gastroenteritis. Stools may contain blood and mucus or be watery. Associated symptoms consist of fever, vomiting, and abdominal pain. Older children may present with abdominal pain associated with mesenteric adenitis that mimics acute appendicitis. Adults develop diarrhea and abdominal pain less frequently than do children but may present with polyarthritis, arthralgia, or erythema nodosum. Disease is caused at least in part by production of a heat-stable enterotoxin[72, 82, 331] and by a 42- to 44-MDa plasmid encoding for invasiveness.

The role of other bacteria in enteric infection remains speculative. Although enterotoxin production and other potential virulence properties have been described, *Klebsiella, Citrobacter, Bacteroides fragilis,* and *Enterobacter* have not been proved to be diarrheal pathogens.

Viruses

Acute infectious diarrhea of viral origin generally is a self-limited disease characterized by various combinations of diarrhea, nausea, vomiting, abdominal cramps, headaches, myalgias, and low-grade fever.[114, 197, 229, 231, 232, 245, 269, 365, 391] Bowel movements are watery and generally do not contain mucus or blood. Vomiting is the most common manifestation of this condition. Rotavirus, enteric adenovirus, astrovirus, and calicivirus are common causes of viral gastroenteritis (Table 52–7). Some caliciviruses characteristically produce epidemics of illness in adults and children,[177] whereas rotavirus, astroviruses, and enteric adenovirus generally cause endemic illness in infants and young children.

Rotaviruses

Rotavirus is a 70-nm particle that on electron microscopy resembles a wheel with radiating spokes (Fig. 52–1). Rotavirus first was associated with diarrhea in children by Bishop and associates in 1973.[34] Since then, human rotavirus has been established as a major cause of acute gastroenteritis in infants, children, and various animal species worldwide.[230] Six antigenically distinct groups of rotavirus (A through F) have been recognized. Three of these groups (A, B, and C) have been identified in humans. The group A rotaviruses are those associated with infantile diarrhea.[114] Group B rotaviruses have caused epidemics of cholera-like illness in China and sporadic cases elsewhere.[114, 255] Outside Southeast Asia, few humans have antibody to group B rotaviruses. Group C rotaviruses have caused outbreaks of diarrhea in children in many countries.[44]

Group A rotaviruses have two outer capsid proteins, a hemagglutinin (VP4) and a glycoprotein (VP7), each of which induces neutralizing antibodies.[114] There are 14 different antigenic types of VP7 (which define serotype) and seven human serotypes of VP4 (also designated P serotypes because VP4 is protease-sensitive), including two subtypes. This number, combined with the ability of the gene segments to reassort independently, indicates that rotaviruses are complex antigenically.[114] Although 10 human rotavirus serotypes are known, VP7 (also designated G serotype) serotypes 1, 2, 3, and 4 appear to be of epidemiologic importance. Epidemiologic studies indicate that the four widespread serotypes are endemic in most regions, that one serotype tends to be predominant at any particular time, that predominant serotypes differ between regions in the same country, and that predictable cycles of change of the predominant serotype may occur.[231]

TABLE 52–7. Viruses Associated with Gastroenteritis

Virus	Approximate Size (nm)
Rotavirus	70
Enteric adenovirus (types 40 and 41)	70–80
Astrovirus	20–30
Calicivirus	35–39
Parvovirus	20–30
Coronavirus	80–180
Pestivirus	40–60
Breda virus	100

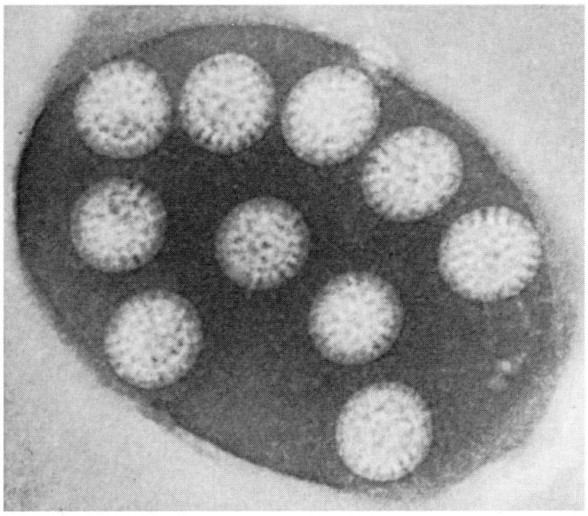

FIGURE 52–1. *Electron micrograph of virus particles in a fecal specimen from an infant with diarrhea. (Phosphotungstic acid × 238,000.)*

Rotavirus gastroenteritis affects more than 90 per cent of children by 3 years of age and may cause moderate to severe vomiting that precedes diarrhea. It accounts for 10 to 50 per cent of the cases of diarrhea in children and is the most common cause of diarrhea in infants and children during winter months in colder climates. Rotavirus accounts for 35 to 50 per cent of infants and young children hospitalized for acute diarrhea. In the United States, rotavirus accounts for 82,000 hospitalizations per year and 150 deaths.[230] Stools usually are watery or soft, and the presence of blood or leukocytes is rare. Asymptomatic rotavirus infections are frequent,[269, 288] and reinfection has been reported.[369, 370] The mechanism of spread is fecal-oral; whether respiratory transmission occurs is uncertain. Shedding of virus most frequently occurs from a few days before to 10 days after the onset of illness.[288] Rotavirus outbreaks in child care centers are common; they usually occur in the colder months, are caused by a single serotype,[269] and are manifested by the fact that half the infected children are asymptomatic.[17]

The incubation period of human rotavirus infection ranges from 2 to 4 days. Animal models suggest that whereas morphologic changes in the villous tip cells contribute to malabsorption and diarrhea, altered cell function, resulting in enzyme deficiencies, results from enterocyte immaturity and may account for the major part of the disordered physiologic findings. Although there is no specific therapy for children with rotavirus infection, immunizations are being evaluated.[242]

Astroviruses

Astroviruses, identified in 1975, are 20 to 30 nm in diameter and have a characteristic five- to six-pointed star. The virus genome is a positive-strand RNA of approximately

7500 nucleotides that encodes four structural proteins.[132] Eight different antigenic types have been described. Astrovirus gastroenteritis occurs worldwide and has been associated with outbreaks of mild gastroenteritis in schools, child care centers, pediatric wards, and nursing homes.[132, 192, 201, 244, 245] Illness is restricted primarily to children and the elderly; 80 per cent or more of adults have antibodies against the virus.[201] The incubation period is 3 to 4 days.[192] Symptoms include fever and malaise, followed by watery diarrhea that may last approximately 3 days. Vomiting is uncommon. Short-term monosaccharide intolerance and more prolonged cow's milk protein intolerance have been reported after astrovirus infection.[258]

Caliciviruses

CVs include morphologically "typical" and "atypical" small round structural viruses that cause illness in both animals (AnCVs) and humans (HuCVs). HuCVs mainly cause acute gastroenteritis, except for hepatitis E virus (HEV), which causes hepatitis. Multiple syndromes such as hemorrhagic pneumonia, hepatitis, abortion, mucosal infection, and gastroenteritis have been associated with AnCVs. Many HuCV strains have been described, including Norwalk virus, the prototype HuCV[37, 138, 139, 174, 175, 181]; Snow Mountain agent[88]; Hawaii agent; Taunton agent; Montgomery County agent; "minireovirus"; Sapporo virus; and many recently characterized strains.[176, 247] Because HuCVs, except for HEV, can not be passed in cell culture or animal models, HuCVs were poorly classified in the premolecular phase of HuCV research and generally were called Norwalk virus–related or Norwalk virus–like viruses. The classification of small round structural viruses as CVs has been confirmed, and three HuCV genogroups have been described: Snow Mountain–like, Norwalk virus–like, and Sapporo-like.

The major public health concern about HuCVs has been their ability to cause large outbreaks of gastroenteritis. Such outbreaks usually have high attack rates and have occurred in schools, restaurants, summer camps, hospitals, nursing homes, and cruise ships.[88, 139, 156, 176, 177, 182, 307] Exposure to a common source of the virus, such as contaminated food or water, usually can be identified. Outbreaks resulting from consumption of uncooked shellfish is common. HuCVs also can be spread by person-to-person transmission. The syndrome of HuCV-associated gastroenteritis includes diarrhea, vomiting, nausea, abdominal cramps, fever, and malaise; diarrhea and vomiting are most common. The recognition of HEV as a CV further highlights the importance of HuCV as a cause of human illness. HEV also causes large outbreaks with a transmission pattern similar to that of HuCV-associated gastroenteritis.

Enteric Adenoviruses

Human adenoviruses of subgroups A to F have been identified as etiologic agents in a wide range of human diseases, including conjunctivitis, upper respiratory tract infections, and pneumonia. A subgroup of fastidious adenoviruses (group F) with a distinct set of antigenic determinants and specific tissue culture growth characteristics have been shown to be associated with acute gastroenteritis and are called enteric adenoviruses.[42, 365] These agents fail to propagate in conventional cell lines used to grow adenoviruses but grow readily in 293 cells, an adenovirus type 5 transformed line.

The enteric adenoviruses in group F include serotypes 40 and 41.[196] Types 40 and 41 both appear to be widespread and endemic causes of diarrhea in children. Antibody prevalence to enteric adenovirus increases from 20 per cent during the first 6 months of life to a maximum of 50 per cent or greater by the third or fourth year of life.[336] Seasonal shifts in the predominance of types 40 and 41, similar to those described for rotavirus, may occur. A 9-year study in Washington, D.C., found that enteric adenovirus types 40 and 41 circulate simultaneously all year.[42] Infection with enteric adenovirus appears to increase in the summer, although with a less marked seasonal variation than that exhibited by rotavirus, which peaks in the winter.[42] Outbreaks of enteric adenovirus diarrhea have been described in child care centers where asymptomatic excretion is common.[365]

Pestivirus antigen was detected by monoclonal antibody enzyme immunoassay in the stools of 30 of 128 children with diarrhea of unknown cause, in 1 of 28 children without diarrhea, and 1 of 31 children with rotavirus infection.[391] The diarrhea was mild and accompanied by respiratory tract symptoms. In 1984, a virus resembling the Breda virus of calf diarrhea was detected in stools of 20 persons with gastroenteritis.[23] Additional studies are required to determine the etiologic role of these and other viruses, including parvovirus and coronavirus, in human disease.

Parasites

The most important protozoa known to cause diarrhea in various populations in the United States are *Entamoeba histolytica, G. lamblia,* and four spore-forming protozoa: *Cryptosporidium parvum, Isospora belli, Microsporidium* species, and *Cyclospora cayetanensis.* Among helminths, *Strongyloides stercoralis* and occasionally *Trichuris trichiura* may produce diarrhea. Data are lacking associating *Ascaris* or hookworm with diarrhea, but both cause abdominal pain. HIV infections have stimulated renewed interest in several of these organisms, including various *Microsporidium* species, *C. parvum,* and *I. belli*[95, 134]; the latter two are part of the CDC surveillance definition for AIDS.[55] The role of *Blastocystis hominis, Balantidium coli,* and *Dientamoeba fragilis* as a cause of diarrhea is not known. With the onset of AIDS and further development of diagnostic techniques, four intestinal protozoa have emerged as major pathogens of the intestinal tract: cryptosporidia, microsporidia, *Isospora,* and *Cyclospora.*[134]

Cryptosporidium

Cryptosporidium organisms are coccidian protozoa that invade and replicate within the microvillous region of epithelial cells lining the digestive and respiratory tracts of vertebrates.[76] *Cryptosporidium* organisms are related taxonomically to *Toxoplasma, Sarcocystis, Isospora,* and *Plasmodium* species. A review of 38 studies that evaluated persons with diarrhea reported an overall *Cryptosporidium* prevalence of 2.1 per cent in industrialized nations and 8.5 per cent in developing nations.[74] Children 6 to 24 months of age seem to be at a particularly high risk for acquiring this organism. Cryptosporidia have been implicated as a cause of diarrhea in travelers and of epidemics in hospitals, child care centers, and other institutions worldwide.[75, 191, 225] Other groups at risk include animal handlers, travelers to foreign countries with a high prevalence of *Cryptosporidium,* and hospital personnel.[75, 96, 191, 225] Person-to-person transmission probably is the principal route of infection, although water also is important in transmission. The largest water-borne outbreak of diarrhea documented in the United States was due to *Cryptosporidium.*[220] Volunteer studies in adults showed that 132 oocysts cause disease.[104] The incubation period in humans has been estimated to be 2 to 14 days.[74]

Cryptosporidiosis can present with a wide spectrum of symptoms, including asymptomatic excretion, acute diarrhea, chronic diarrhea, epidemic diarrhea, severe life-threatening, watery diarrhea, and biliary tract disease.[51] Watery diarrhea is the hallmark of symptomatic infections, but there are few, if any, features that distinguish gastroenteritis due to *Cryptosporidium* in the immunocompetent patient from other enteric infections. Stools do not contain blood or leukocytes. Vomiting, flatulence, abdominal pain, and low-grade fever routinely accompany diarrhea.[144] Symptoms usually subside in an average of 9 days. Patients with T-cell immunodeficiencies also are at a high risk of acquiring this infection and of having a protracted clinical course with unremitting, profuse diarrhea lasting for months accompanied by profound malabsorption and weight loss. The prevalence of enteritis due to *Cryptosporidium* in patients with AIDS is reported to be 3 to 4 per cent in the United States, and approximately 15 per cent of patients with AIDS and diarrhea harbor the parasite.[203, 340] The frequency with which *Cryptosporidium* and microsporidia are identified in stools of patients with AIDS reflects the CD4 count, with identification of the organisms and symptoms being more frequent when the count is less than 100 cells/μL.[122] Biliary tract infection with *Cryptosporidium* produces two syndromes: sclerosing cholangitis-type lesions that cause progressive, irregular obstruction and dilation of the intra- and extrahepatic bile ducts[27] and acalculous cholecystitis caused by infection of the wall of the gall bladder.[153] Symptoms have been characterized by right upper quadrant pain, nausea, and vomiting. Pancreatitis and appendicitis also have been reported in association with *Cryptosporidium* infection.[95, 293]

Entamoeba histolytica

The life cycle of *E. histolytica* involves encystment of a trophozoite, followed by release of the trophozoite from the cyst under appropriate conditions in the gastrointestinal tract[305] (Fig. 52–2). The trophozoites vary in size and are found in stools of patients with dysentery or diarrhea. The cyst is more resistant to environmental stresses and is the infective stage. Cysts are found more frequently in formed stools. The minimum period between the ingestion of cysts and development of symptoms is 8 days. The incubation period ranges up to 95 days.

There are distinct species of *Entamoeba* that morphologically are identical. *E. dispar* is the more prevalent species and is associated solely with an asymptomatic carrier state. The pathogenic species, now called *E. histolytica*, can invade tissue and cause symptomatic disease.[305] Species can be differentiated by zymodemes (patterns of electrophoretic mobility of certain parasitic isoenzymes), RNA and DNA probes, and antigen detection tests such as enzyme immunoassay.[143]

The clinical patterns that occur in patients with amebiasis consist of (1) intestinal amebiasis, with the gradual onset of colicky abdominal pain and frequent bowel movements, tenesmus, and little or no constitutional disturbance, (2) amebic dysentery characterized by profuse diarrhea containing blood and mucus and the presence of constitutional signs, such as fever, dehydration, and electrolyte alterations, (3) hepatic amebiasis, which usually presents as abscess formation without gastrointestinal symptoms,[2, 305] and (4) asymptomatic excretion. Patients may experience tender hepatomegaly, jaundice, weight loss, fever, and anorexia. The frequency of liver abscess development in patients with amebiasis is between 1 and 5 per cent. The complications of intestinal amebiasis include perforation, ameboma, stricture, hemorrhage secondary to erosion into a blood vessel, intussusception, ischiorectal abscess, fistulas, and rectal prolapse. Persons in the third through fifth decades of life have the highest incidence of infection and clinical symptoms, although persons of all ages are susceptible.

Giardia lamblia

G. lamblia is a flagellated protozoan that is an important cause of diarrhea, particularly in certain high-risk populations and in persons who travel to hyperendemic areas. Children appear to be more susceptible to *Giardia* than are adults. Conditions other than age that predispose to giardiasis are hypogammaglobulinemia, secretory IgA deficiency, peptic ulcer disease, biliary tract disease, and pancreatitis. The parasite may exist in two forms: cyst and trophozoite (Fig. 52–3). After being ingested, each cyst divides into two trophozoites, which subsequently mature. The trophozoites usually are seen in duodenal aspirates and loose stools, whereas the cysts can be found in formed stools. The cysts can remain viable and infectious in water for more than 3 months.

Individuals vary in their response to infection with *Giardia*, with the following clinical manifestations: (1) asymptomatic, (2) an acute illness with a sudden onset of explosive, watery, foul-smelling stools, flatulence, abdominal distention, nausea, anorexia, and the absence of blood and mucus, and (3) chronic diarrhea and malabsorption with exacerbations and remissions of flatulence, abdominal distention, and abdominal pain often lasting for months.[289]

Strongyloides stercoralis

S. stercoralis is a nematode that infects humans via the intestinal tract or through skin if either comes in contact

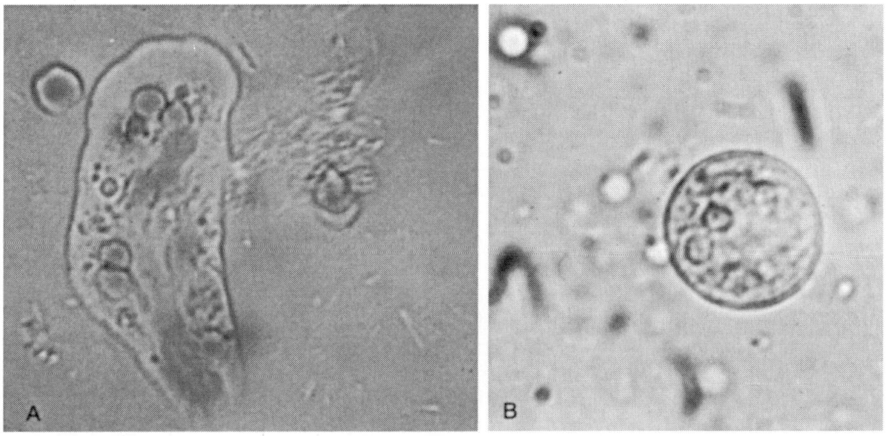

FIGURE 52–2. A, *Trophozoite of* Entamoeba histolytica *with ingested material in the cytoplasm.* B, *Cyst of* E. histolytica *seen in a merthiolate-iodine-formalin–stained preparation from a stool specimen. Note two visible nuclei. (× 1000.) (From DuPont, H. L., and Pickering, L. K.: Infections of the Gastrointestinal Tract. New York, Plenum Publishing, 1980.)*

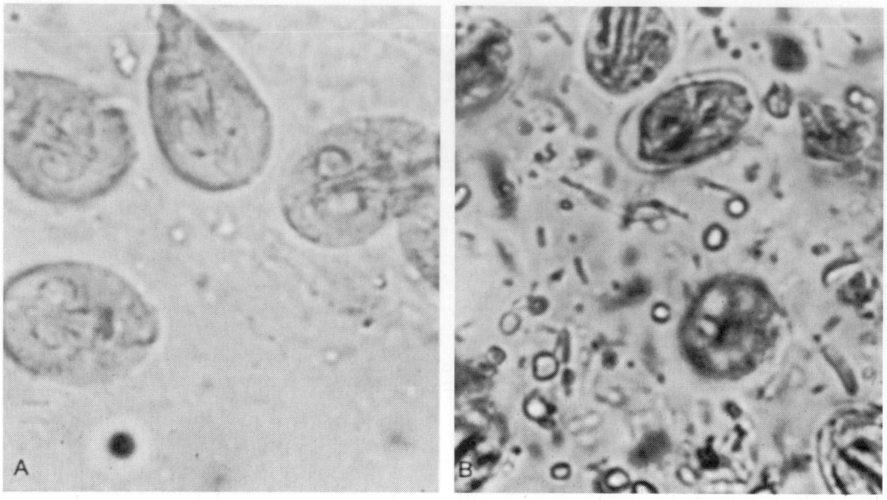

FIGURE 52–3. A, *Trophozoites of* Giardia lamblia *seen in a merthiolate-iodine-formalin–stained preparation of stool from a patient with diarrhea.* (× *1000.)* B, *Cysts of* G. lamblia *seen in a merthiolate-iodine-formalin–stained preparation of stool from a patient without diarrhea.* (× *1000.)*

with soil that contains the larvae. Approximately one-third of people with strongyloidiasis are asymptomatic, and the remainder may have skin, pulmonary, or, more frequently, gastrointestinal tract involvement. People at risk include residents and travelers to endemic areas; natives and residents of the Appalachian region in the United States; institutionalized persons; and those treated with corticosteroids, cimetidine, and antacids.[31, 127] Epigastric abdominal pain occurs and is associated with diarrhea that contains mucus and blood.[31] Some patients may complain of nausea, vomiting, and weight loss with evidence of malabsorption. Eosinophilia and an urticarial rash are prominent features of infection. People infected with *S. stercoralis* should be treated with thiabendazole in an attempt to eradicate the infection.[237]

Isospora belli

Isospora was established as a cause of diarrhea in humans in the early 1900s, when sporadic cases of isosporiasis and a few clinical series were reported in the medical literature.[87] *I. belli* has gained importance with the advent of AIDS, where it has been shown to be an important cause of severe and prolonged gastroenteritis.[275] Humans are the only known host for *I. belli,* but the actual prevalence of this parasite is unknown. Infection can occur in adults and children and has been reported in infants with severe diarrhea.[115, 211, 271] *Isospora* has been encountered in 15 per cent of patients with AIDS in Haiti and in 0.2 per cent in the United States, although the true prevalence in this population is unknown. This organism also has been implicated as a cause of travelers' diarrhea.[129]

Transmission is fecal-oral from one human to another, but the infective dose in humans is unknown. Oocysts may be present in stools for as long as 120 days after infection. No animal reservoir of *I. belli* has been documented. Transmission is believed to occur by ingestion of oocysts contaminating food, water, or environmental surfaces.[273] *I. belli* oocysts are resistant to commonly used disinfectants and may remain viable for months in a cool, moist environment.

The clinical spectrum of disease caused by *Isospora* is indistinguishable from that described for *Cryptosporidium.* The spectrum includes asymptomatic infection, acute diarrhea in children in developing countries, and chronic diarrhea or severe protracted life-threatening diarrhea in persons with AIDS. Infection of the biliary tract in persons with AIDS by *Isospora* has been associated with acalculous cholecystitis.[26] The incubation period was 8 to 14 days in four persons who had been exposed to the organism in the laboratory.[148] Fever, malaise, abdominal pain, and headache all have been reported. Stools are watery and do not contain blood or leukocytes. Malabsorption, steatorrhea, severe weight loss, and chronic diarrhea lasting months to years are most likely in immunocompromised hosts.[80, 383]

Microsporidia

Microsporidia are ubiquitous, spore-forming, intracellular protozoal parasites that cause disease in a wide range of vertebrate and invertebrate hosts. There are more than 100 genera of microsporidia. The nontaxonomic term human microsporidia can refer to any of the five microsporidia known to cause disease in humans: *Enterocytozoon, Septata, Encephalitozoon* species, *Pleistophora* species, and *Nosema* species. Of these, *Enterocytozoon bieneusi* and *Septata intestinalis* are the most important in gastrointestinal tract disease of humans.[13, 377] Most cases of microsporidia-related infections reported have occurred in patients with AIDS.[53] Information about the epidemiology, mode of transmission, and clinical features of microsporidia are limited. Infections with these organisms have been documented in immunocompetent and immunosuppressed persons from Africa, Asia, Europe, and North and South America.[53, 333, 334]

Sources of infection for humans are unknown. In animals, transmission occurs by ingestion of spores shed into the environment. Human-to-human fecal-oral route may play a role in transmission. The clinical spectrum appears to depend on the immune status of the host. *E. bieneusi* and *S. intestinalis* have been detected in intestinal biopsy specimens of patients with AIDS with a clinical picture of prolonged diarrhea and weight loss.[48, 84, 308] The primary location of all intestinal spore-forming protozoal infection is the small intestine, but colonic infection has been reported with *E. bieneusi.*[134] Infection of the biliary tract with *E. bieneusi* and *S. intestinalis* in patients with AIDS can cause sclerosing cholangitis-type lesions[297, 385] and acalculous cholecystitis caused by infection of the wall of the gall bladder.[49] *S. intestinalis* can infect lamina propria macrophages, fibroblasts, and endothelial cells and can disseminate to other organs, including liver, respiratory tract, and kidney.[134, 385]

Extraintestinal infection occurs after infection with other species of microsporidia. Microsporidial keratoconjunctivitis has been documented in patients with AIDS.[53] One patient had a corneal perforation requiring emergency corneal grafting; two recovered spontaneously, and the other two died of AIDS-related complications without improvement of the ocular infection.

Cyclospora

Cyclospora cayetonensis (formerly cyanobacteria or blue-green algae-like bodies) is a coccidian protozoa that first was diagnosed as causing infection in humans in 1977.[271] *Cyclospora* is transmitted by the fecal-oral route; direct person-to-person transmission is unlikely because excreted oocysts require days to weeks under favorable environmental conditions to sporulate and become infectious. An animal reservoir has not been described. Outbreaks of diarrhea due to consumption of water and fresh fruits contaminated with *Cyclospora* have been described,[60, 165] and travelers to developing countries are at increased risk for contacting diarrhea due to *Cyclospora*.[268, 276] Most of the reported cases have occurred during the spring and summer. The mean incubation period appears to be 7 days. Clinical manifestations include asymptomatic excretion, acute watery diarrhea, and diarrhea that may be protracted from days to weeks with frequent, watery stools, which may remit and relapse.

DIAGNOSIS

The diagnosis of the cause of an episode of acute infectious diarrhea depends on epidemiologic information, the clinical syndrome, laboratory tests, and knowledge or assessment of an organism for virulence factors. Because virulence properties determine clinical manifestations of disease, an understanding of pathophysiologic mechanisms guides the laboratory evaluation and empiric therapy. The major virulence properties of enteropathogens include adherence; production of enterotoxin, cytoskeleton-altering toxin, cytotoxin, and toxins with neural activity; and epithelial cell invasion.[331] Certain enteropathogens may produce diarrhea by other mechanisms, and enteric pathogens may possess one or several of these virulence properties (Table 52–8).

Enterotoxins are bacterial products that act on the mucosal epithelium of the small intestine, causing fluid secretion and profuse watery diarrhea without intestinal damage so that stools are devoid of blood and leukocytes. Fluid secretion is related to enzymatic effect on intestinal cells, often through specific receptors, and increased cyclic nucleotide levels.[251] The prototype is the heat-labile cholera toxin produced by *V. cholerae*, which causes adenosine diphosphate ribosylation of an adenylate cyclase regulatory protein, leading to an increase in intracellular cyclic adenosine monophosphate. This causes active fluid secretion and inhibition of reabsorption of salt and water. Immunologically and functionally similar heat-labile enterotoxins are produced by *E. coli* and other enteric pathogens (see Table 52–8). Other enterotoxins produced by *E. coli*, *Y. enterocolitica*, and other enteric pathogens are called heat-stable enterotoxins. These heat-stable enterotoxins activate guanylate cyclase. Other enterotoxins act by independent mechanisms that have not been characterized.[331] Bacterial toxins are the sole cause of disease only occasion-

TABLE 52–8. Virulence Characteristics of Enteropathogens

Organisms	Virulence Properties
Bacteria	
Aeromonas	Entertoxin (aerolysin)
Bacillus cereus	Emetic toxin, diarrhea-associated enterotoxin
Campylobacter jejuni	Invasion, heat-labile enterotoxin (LT), cytotoxin, cytolethal distending toxin (CLDT)
Clostridium difficile	Cytotoxin and enterotoxin
Clostridium perfringens type A	Cytotoxin
Clostridium perfringens type C	Cytotoxins (beta, alpha)
Escherichia coli	
Enterohemorrhagic	Shiga toxins I and II (or verotoxins I and II)
Enteropathogenic	Adherence and production of attaching and effacing lesion
Enterotoxigenic	LT, stable toxin (ST), adherence
Invasive	Invasion
Enteroadherent	Adherence, heat-stable and heat-labile toxins
Plesiomonas shigelloides	LT
Salmonella	Invasion, LT, complement resistance
Shigella dysenteriae 1	Invasion, shiga toxin
Other *Shigella*	Invasion, shigella enterotoxin *(S. flexneri)*, CLDT
Staphylococcus aureus	Enterotoxins A to E, delta toxin
Vibrio cholerae	Cholera toxin, hemolysin, adherence, zona occludens toxin, accessory cholera enterotoxin
Vibrio parahaemolyticus	Thermostable direct hemolysin
Yersinia enterocolitica	ST, invasion
Parasites	
Cryptosporidium	Invade intestinal epithelial cells
Cyclospora cayetanensis	Invade intestinal epithelial cells
Entamoeba histolytica	Invasion, enzyme and cytotoxin production
Enterocytozoon bieneusi	Invade intestinal epithelial cells
Giardia lamblia	Adheres to mucosa by ventral suckers
Isospora belli	Invades intestinal epithelial cells
Septata intestinalis	Invades intestinal epithelial and subepithelial cells
Stronglyloides stercoralis	Invasion of intestinal epithelium with inflammatory reaction
Viruses	
Rotavirus, astrovirus, calicivirus, enteric adenovirus	Mucosal lesion, destruction of absorptive cells (villus tip cells)

ally; more frequently, they must act in concert with other virulence factors of bacteria, such as adherence mechanisms.[12]

Cytotoxins are defined by their ability to produce cell or tissue damage, usually resulting in cell death, by inhibition of protein synthesis. Cytotoxic activity is demonstrated in vitro by its effects on cells in tissue culture.[65] In vivo cytotoxins cause damage to intestinal epithelial cells and destruction of normal absorptive mechanisms, which result in intestinal hemorrhage and diarrhea containing blood. Fluid loss probably is related to impaired absorption. Unlike enterotoxins, cytotoxins do not cause active fluid secretion by the gut, nor do they leave the gut undamaged. The prototype of this group of toxins is Shiga toxin, which is produced mainly by *S. dysenteriae* serotype 1.[16, 261, 265] Functionally, immunologically, and structurally, closely related toxins (Shiga-like toxins or verotoxins) are produced by certain serotypes of *E. coli.* This group of toxins has been implicated in hemorrhagic colitis and plays a role in the pathogenesis of the hemolytic uremic syndrome.[65, 183] Cytotoxin production has been demonstrated in other pathogens, but most of them are not well characterized, and their role in human disease needs to be clarified (see Table 52–8).[331]

Another class of enteric toxins is the cytoskeleton-altering toxins, which produce an alteration in cell shape without inducing significant cell injury, most often because of rearrangement of F actin. This toxin may be associated with evidence of net secretion in in vitro or in vivo intestinal cell models of disease.[331] Many organisms, including *Aeromonas, C. jejuni, C. difficile,* EPEC, ETEC, *P. shigelloides, Salmonella* species, *Shigella* species, and *V. cholerae,* produce toxins with cytoskeleton-altering properties.[331]

Enteric bacteria also may produce toxins with neural activity. At least part of the secretory activity of these toxins is attributable to the release of one or more neurotransmitters from the enteric nervous system, or the toxin alters smooth muscle activity in the intestine.[137] No enteric toxin has been shown to stimulate secretion only through neural mechanisms. Organisms shown to have neural activity include *C. difficile,* ETEC, *S. aureus,* and *V. cholerae.*[331]

Invasiveness is another virulence trait of some bacteria. Bacterial invasion of gastrointestinal tract epithelium is characterized clinically by fever, abdominal pain, tenesmus, and stools containing blood, mucus, and fecal leukocytes.[284] *Shigella* species invade and destroy epithelial cells of the gastrointestinal tract, causing diffuse or focal colitis. This invasion is demonstrated in the laboratory by the guinea pig keratoconjunctivitis test (Sereny test).[332] The invasiveness of *Shigella* and EIEC is encoded by 120- to 140-MDa plasmids. *Salmonella* species pass through gut epithelium, often with little mucosal damage to the lamina propria, where they elicit a chemotactic response resulting in an influx of polymorphonuclear leukocytes. Further invasion, resulting in systemic infection, is infrequent, except in immunocompromised hosts and in infections due to *S. typhi, S. paratyphi,* and *S. cholerae-suis*. These organisms reach the lamina propria and elicit an influx of macrophages, which ingest the *Salmonella* organisms, drain into the mesenteric lymph nodes, and reach the blood stream via the lymphatic system.[347] *V. parahaemolyticus* also is thought to be invasive.[172] The pathology of *Campylobacter* colitis suggests invasiveness as well as enterotoxin production as a mechanism of disease. The fact that pathogenic *Y. enterocolitica* organisms are Sereny test–positive and may cause a dysentery-like illness suggests invasiveness as a virulence mechanism.

Adherence, the ability of organisms to attach and colonize gut epithelium, is the least specific virulence property in terms of associated clinical findings. The ability of ETEC to adhere to and colonize the upper small intestine in order to cause disease by production of enterotoxin has been described.[107, 125, 214] This adherence capacity has been related to fimbria such as K88, K99, or multiple colonization-factor antigens for piglet, calf, and human strains, respectively. The production of these adherence antigens appears to be coded genetically by transmissible plasmids.[388] These fimbriated colonization-factor antigen adhesins are distinct from type 1 pili and cause mannose-resistant hemagglutination in the laboratory. *V. cholerae* organisms adhere to intestinal mucosa in the same manner. EPEC are examples of organisms in which adherence appears to be a major pathogenic mechanism. EPEC colonize the small intestine and cause a diarrheal syndrome that tends to be chronic.[62, 312] The loss of absorptive microvillous surface that occurs with adherence of EPEC partially may explain the resulting diarrhea[313] (Fig. 52–4). EAEC also adhere and cause diarrhea without enteroinvasion. The enteric protozoal pathogens adhere to and invade enterocytes and may cause symptoms of chronic malabsorption.

Many enteric pathogens produce diarrhea by several mechanisms. For example, enterotoxin and cytotoxin production is common among organisms that are invasive. Thus, shigellosis may have an early secretory diarrheal phase and a late dysenteric phase. Both host and microbiologic factors ultimately determine clinical expression in the individual patient. Not all of the recognized virulence properties of a given species are obvious clinically in each episode of disease. *Salmonella* infection, for example, may manifest clinically as mild or severe watery diarrhea with or without dysenteric symptoms.

LABORATORY EVALUATION

Proper identification of the causative agent of an episode of acute infectious diarrhea may facilitate appropriate ther-

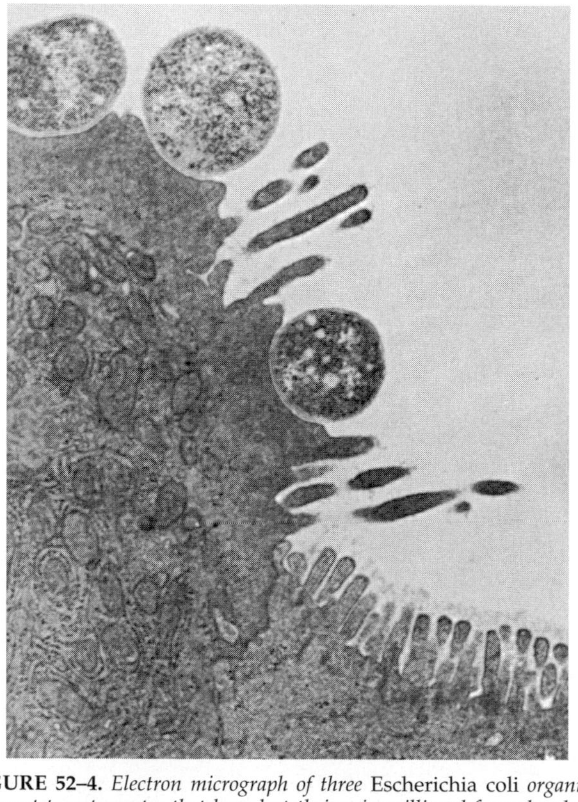

FIGURE 52–4. *Electron micrograph of three* Escherichia coli *organisms adherent to enterocytes that have lost their microvilli and formed pedestals on which the bacteria lie. (× 25,000.) (Courtesy of Dr. R. J. Rothbaum.)*

apy. A gross examination of the stool specimen should be routine in all patients with diarrhea, even if no laboratory studies are performed. Diarrheal stool that is watery and without mucus or blood usually is caused by an enterotoxin, virus, or protozoan organism, or it may be caused by infection outside the gastrointestinal tract. The color of stools generally conveys little information if the stool does not contain blood. Infectious causes to be considered when stools contain blood or mucus include a cytotoxin-producing bacteria; an enteroinvasive bacteria causing mucosal inflammation; or an enteric parasite associated with blood in stools such as *E. histolytica, B. coli,* and *T. trichiura.* When present, blood usually is mixed evenly into the stool, except in the case of *E. histolytica* infections, in which blood often is on the surface of the stool, and some EHEC infections, in which the stool may be blood-streaked. Stools that particularly are foul-smelling are consistent with *Salmonella* and other bacteria, as well as *Giardia, Cryptosporidium,* and *Strongyloides.* Stools with little odor suggest an enterotoxin, such as cholera toxin or heat-stable/heat-labile *E. coli* or viral enteropathogen. Laboratory tests used to detect enteropathogens are listed in Tables 52–9 and 52–10.

Microscopic Examination

Microscopic examination of stool specimens for evidence of fecal leukocytes provides information concerning the cause of diarrhea in addition to determining the anatomic location and presence of mucosal inflammation. Fecal leukocytes are produced in response to bacteria that diffusely invade the colonic mucosa and indicate that the patient has colitis. There is no inflammatory bacterial enteritis in which the results of the fecal leukocyte examination are positive in all cases. Thus, the examination results are more helpful when positive than when negative. When the results are positive, the patient likely has an invasive or cytotoxin-producing organism, such as *Shigella, Salmonella, Campylobacter,* invasive *E. coli, C. difficile,* or *Y. enterocolitica,* although ulcerative colitis and Crohn disease also are associated with fecal leukocytes. Fecal leukocytes generally are not present in stools from patients with diarrhea secondary to viruses, enterotoxin-producing bacteria, or parasites. The leukocytes seen in cytotoxin-associated and invasive bacterial diarrhea syndromes are polymorphonuclear leukocytes. The exception to this is infection by *S. typhi,* in which the leukocytes are mononuclear. If the fecal leukocyte examination shows evidence of inflammatory enteritis, further laboratory evaluation is indicated. The fecal lactoferrin assay has been shown to be a more accurate test than fecal leukocytes or occult blood in patients with inflammatory diarrhea.[167]

Parasites that cause diarrhea usually do not produce numerous fecal leukocytes. Normally, it is unnecessary to examine stools for ova and parasites unless there is a history of recent travel to high-risk areas, stool cultures are negative for other enteropathogens, the patients are involved in an outbreak of diarrhea, diarrhea persists for longer than 1 week, or the patients are immunosuppressed. *G. lamblia* and *S. stercoralis* can be visualized in stools, duodenal fluid, and small intestinal biopsy material. Both trophozoites and cysts of *G. lamblia* and larvae of *Strongyloides* can be identified on direct smears of stool specimens (see Fig. 52–3); however, the sensitivity of stool examination for most parasites can be improved by using a concentration technique[273] and by placing stools in vials containing polyvinyl alcohol or 10 per cent formalin (Para Pak, Meridian Diagnostics, Cincinnati, OH). Trichrome and iron hematoxylin both are useful as permanent stains for *Giardia.* An advantage of trichrome is that it may be used in polyvinyl alcohol-preserved specimens. Pooling of preserved fecal samples is an efficient and economical procedure for detection of ova and parasites.[4]

In patients in whom giardiasis, cryptosporidiosis, isosporiasis, or strongyloidiasis is considered and in whom stools are negative, aspiration or biopsy of the duodenum or upper jejunum may be indicated. Because these organisms live in the upper intestine, this procedure is more reliable than is examination of stool specimens.[311] Duodenal biopsy is a sensitive and specific method of diagnosing giardiasis, strongyloidiasis, and spore-forming protozoa. Small intestinal biopsy should be considered in patients with characteristic clinical symptoms, negative stool and duodenal fluid specimens, and one of the following: abnormal radiographic findings such as edema and segmentation in the small intestine, abnormal lactose tolerance test results, absent secretory IgA, hypogammaglobulinemia, achlorhydria, AIDS, and severe malabsorptive diarrhea with weight loss. Electron microscopic examination of tissue sections may be useful in identifying fine structures of a parasite (Fig. 52–5).

TABLE 52–9. Laboratory Tests Used to Detect Enteropathogens

Laboratory Tests	Organisms Suggested or Identified
Microscopic examination of stool	
Fecal leukocytes	Invasive or cytotoxin-producing bacteria
Trophozoites, cysts, oocysts, or spores	*Giardia lamblia, Entamoeba histolytica, Cryptosporidium, Isospora belli, Cyclospora, Enterocytozoon bieneusi, Septata intestinalis*
Rhabditiform larva	*Strongyloides*
Spiral or S-shaped gram-negative bacilli	*Campylobacter jejuni*
Stool culture	
Standard	*Escherichia coli, Shigella, Salmonella, Campylobacter jejuni*
Special	*Yersinia enterocolitica, Vibrio cholerae, Vibrio parahaemolyticus, Clostridium difficile, E. coli* O157:H7
Enzyme immunoassay or latex agglutination	Rotavirus, *G. lamblia,* enteric adenovirus, *C. difficile*
Serotyping	*E. coli* O157:H7 and other enterohemorrhagic *E. coli,* enteropathogenic *E. coli*
Latex agglutination after broth enrichment	*Salmonella, Shigella*
Tests performed in research laboratories	Toxin-producing bacteria, small round viruses, invasive *E. coli,* enteroadherent *E. coli,* gene probe or polymerase chain reaction for virulence genes

TABLE 52–10. Laboratory Evaluation of Patients with Presumed Bacterial Diarrhea

Organism	Tests
Aeromonas hydrophila	Screen colonies grown on MacConkey agar for positive oxidase test
	Culture on modified blood agar
Bacillus cereus	Culture food (>10^5 organisms/g), demonstrate enterotoxin by enzyme immunoassay
Campylobacter jejuni	Stool culture using Skirrows, Campy-BAP, or Butzler's media incubated at 42° C with 5% O_2 and 10% CO_2
	Gram stain for "gull wing," *Vibrio*-like organisms, and fecal leukocytes; darkfield or phase contrast of stool for organisms with darting motility
	Nucleic acid probe
	Serology
Clostridium difficile	Culture feces anaerobically on cycloserine, cefoxitin, fructose agar
	Demonstrate cytotoxin in stool by enzyme immunoassay or tissue culture cytotoxicity and neutralization with antitoxin
Clostridium perfringens	Culture food (>10^5 organisms/g) and feces
	Serotype organism
Escherichia coli	Standard stool culture for initial isolation
ETEC	
Stable toxin	Suckling mouse assay
	Gene probe hybridization assay
Labile toxin	Rabbit ileal loop
	Y-1 adrenal or Chinese hamster ovary cell assay
	Gene probe hybridization assay
	GM, enzyme immunoassay
EPEC	Serogroup, gene probe assay
	Small bowel biopsy for routine microscopy and electron microscopy
EIEC	Gene probe assay
	Biologic assays for invasiveness (Serény or HeLa cell)
EHEC	MacConkey sorbitol agar for O157:H7
	Gene probe or polymerase chain reaction to detect toxin gene sequences
	Serotyping
	Free/cytotoxin in stool by enzyme immunoassay or tissue culture
	Serologic responses to verotoxins or lipopolysaccharide of *E. coli* O157
EAEC	HEp-2 adherence assay, DNA probes
Plesiomonas shigelloides	Culture
Salmonella species	Standard stool culture; blood, bone marrow, and urine cultures if disseminated
	Serotype by Kaufman-White classification
Shigella species	Examine stool for fecal leukocytes
	Standard stool culture
Staphylococcus aureus	Culture food and skin lesions of food handlers
	Phage type
	Demonstrate enterotoxin in food
Vibrio cholerae	Culture feces on thiosulfate citrate bile salt agar
	Serotype
Vibrio parahaemolyticus	Culture feces on thiosulfate citrate bile salt agar
	Test for Kanagawa reaction (beta hemolysis on Wagatsuma agar), which is a marker for pathogencity
Yersinia enterocolitica	Standard stool culture with cold enrichment; blood culture if disseminated
	Serology
	Lack of rhamnose fermentation by toxin-producing strains
	Suckling mouse assay for stable toxin

EAEC, enteroaggregative *E. coli*; EHEC, enterohemorrhagic *E. coli*; EIEC, enteroinvasive *E. coli*; EPEC, enteropathogenic *E. coli*; ETEC, enterotoxigenic *E. coli*.

Medications, including antibiotics, antacids, antidiarrheal compounds, and certain enema and laxative preparations, as well as contrast material for radiographic studies, can interfere with identification of the organism by altering morphology or causing a temporary disappearance of parasites from stool specimens. Patients should not receive these compounds for 48 to 72 hours prior to collection of stool for testing. Detection of antigen to *G. lamblia* in feces is a rapid and sensitive diagnostic test.[190, 361]

E. histolytica can be diagnosed by microscopic examination of fresh stool specimens or bowel wall scrapings for cysts or trophozoites (see Fig. 52–2). Trophozoites generally are found in liquid stools, whereas cysts are detected in formed stools. A concentration technique may be helpful in the demonstration of amebic cysts. Examination of several stool samples by an experienced technician may be necessary because excretion of cysts often is intermittent and interpretation is difficult. Confusion in differentiating amebic cysts from fecal leukocytes may occur. A number of serologic tests for amebiasis to detect different types and concentrations of antibodies are available.[375] Serologic test results for amebas almost always are positive in acute amebic dysentery and hepatic amebiasis. A liver scan may indicate the presence of a liver abscess.

Diagnosis of *Cryptosporidium, Isospora, Cyclospora,* and microsporidia is based on morphology and staining of stool or by histologic examination of tissue sections.[134] Among the most widely used stains to visualize oocysts of *Cryptosporidium, Isospora,* and *Cyclospora* are standard acid-fast or modified acid-fast stains, which are based on the use of reagents

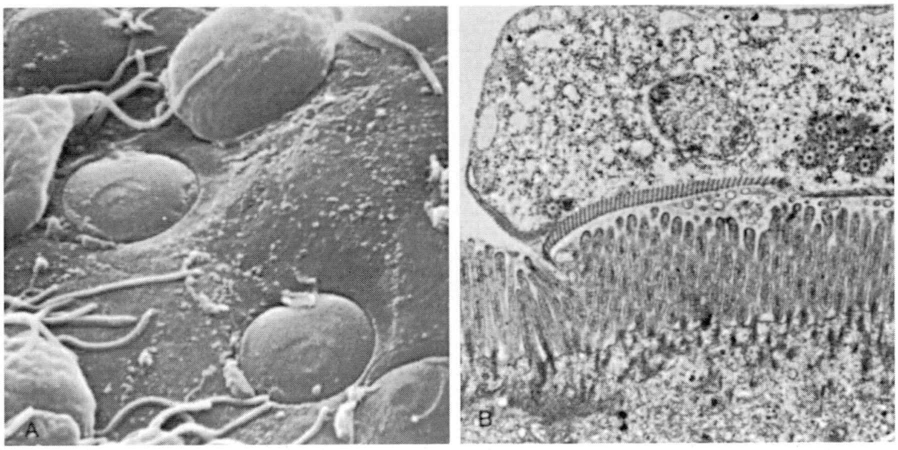

FIGURE 52–5. A, *Scanning electron micrograph of an intestinal villus revealing firm attachment of* Giardia muris *trophozoites to the microvillous border (MVB). Circular dome-shaped lesions in the MVB are produced by attachment of the adhesive disk of trophozoite. (× 4600.) (Courtesy of Dr. S. L. Erlandsen.)* B, *Transmission electron micrograph of a* G. muris *trophozoite illustrating how lesions in the MVB are produced. Note that the edges of the adhesive disk penetrate the MVB and compress the microvilli centrally. The microvilli also show some vesiculation under the adhesive disk. (× 20,000.) (Courtesy of Dr. S. L. Erlandsen.)*

that enhance the penetration of fuchsin into the organism without the need for heating (modified Kinyoun acid-fast stain). Using a modified acid-fast stain, *Cryptosporidium* oocysts, which are 4 to 6 μm in size with four crescentic sporozoites, stain red and can be differentiated readily from yeasts that stain green.[150] Easy-to-use enzyme immunoassays[362] and fluorescent monoclonal antibody-based assays[126, 317] for detection of *Cryptosporidium* antigen in stool specimens have been developed. A fluorescent assay is commercially available (MerFluor, *Cryptosporidium,* Meridian Diagnostics, Cincinnati, OH). In a study of seven microscopy-based *Cryptosporidium* oocyst detection methods, false-positive results were detected by acid-fast and auramine-rhodamine stains but not by monoclonal antibody-based methods.[9] Oocysts of *I. belli* often are visualized by wet-mount preparations because of their size, which is 20 to 30 microns with four sporozoites in two sporocysts. *Cyclospora* oocysts are 8 to 10 μm in diameter and are nonrefractile spherical organisms containing two sporozoites in two sporocysts that are seen easily on wet-mount preparations and exhibit variable acid-fastness. An acid-fast stain is commercially available (VOLU-SOL, Medical Industries, Las Vegas, NV).

Microsporidia are difficult to differentiate from bacteria and debris because of the small size of the spores, which measure 1 to 2 μm. Formalin-fixed stool or duodenal fluid is stained using a calcofluor stain, a modified trichrome stain, or a fluorescent stain.[85, 378] Gram, acid-fast, periodic acid–Schiff, and Giemsa stains also have been used to stain the organism.[308, 333] A nonspecific fluorescence method or enzyme immunoassay may enhance speed and sensitivity[366] and may become more useful as specific antibodies become widely available. Small bowel biopsy may be more sensitive than stool examination for diagnosis of intestinal microsporidiosis.[24] Spores are gram-positive, and parts of the internal structure are positive for acid-fast or periodic acid–Schiff stains. After preliminary identification by these stains, further examination by electron microscopy is needed to classify adequately the microsporidia into an appropriate genus. Routine histopathologic studies can provide presumptive identification in infected biopsy tissue; diagnostic confirmation requires electron microscopy. Reliable serologic tests are not available. Sensitive polymerase chain reaction assays are being evaluated for *E. bieneusi* and *S. intestinalis.*[77, 116]

Standard Diagnostic Stool Cultures

Stool cultures cannot be justified in all patients with acute diarrhea. Patients with mild, self-limited illness do not need to have stool specimens cultured. When culture is indicated, the specimen should be inoculated onto culture plate media adequate to isolate *E. coli, Shigella, Salmonella,* and *C. jejuni.* Standard stool culture media should include differential, mildly selective media, such as MacConkey or eosin methylene blue agar; selective media, such as *Salmonella-Shigella* agar, xylose-lysine-deoxycholate, or Hektoen Enteric medium; a less inhibitory medium to increase the recovery of *Shigella,* such as Tergitol 7 with 1 per cent triphenyltetrazolium chloride; and an enrichment broth (selenite F or GN broth) to increase the yield of *Salmonella.* For isolation of *Campylobacter,* Skirrow, Campy-BAP, or Butzler medium also should be routine. Several *Campylobacter* species, such as *C. upsaliensis, C. hyointestinalis,* and *C. laris,* require use of selective medium for identification.[267, 374] The Association of State and Territorial Public Health Laboratory Directors and Epidemiologists recommends that clinical laboratories screen all bloody stool specimens for *E. coli* O157:H7 with sorbitol MacConkey medium.[41] Fecal specimens can be transported to the laboratory in a non–nutrient-holding medium, such as Cary-Blair, when immediate culture is not possible. This medium prevents drying or overgrowth of specific organisms.

E. coli grown in a hospital microbiology laboratory usually is considered to be normal flora. Proving pathogenicity is difficult because tissue culture and animal assays used to document pathogenicity are expensive and time-consuming and require special expertise. These assays currently are available only in reference or research laboratories. Enzyme immunoassays and gene probe hybridization assays are available in research laboratories for diagnosis of ETEC, EIEC, EAEC, and EPEC infections. *Shigella* organisms are identified in the standard evaluation of stool cultures. Unfortunately, it has been shown in volunteer studies that these organisms are not isolated always in culture from patients ill with shigellosis.

Salmonella organisms routinely are isolated by clinical microbiology laboratories. Speciation is important in salmonellosis because *S. cholerae-suis* and *S. typhi* cause more severe disease than do other *Salmonella* species. *S. enteritidis,* the third major species, is more variable in severity. Serotyping of *S. enteritidis* usually is not helpful in the individual case, although it is crucial in evaluation of an outbreak. Because there are so many *Salmonella* serotypes, isolation of an unusual serotype can be of use in the investigation of a food-borne epidemic. As with *Shigella,* isolation of a *Salmonella* species, even without demonstration of virulence properties, is considered adequate to make an etiologic diagnosis. Serologic studies are of no value in the individual patient. DNA probes can be used to detect *S. typhi*.[314]

Special Diagnostic Cultures

Other bacterial enteropathogens require modified laboratory procedures for identification. If these agents are suspected, the laboratory should be notified so that appropriate culture methods can be used. *Y. enterocolitica* can be isolated from routine media, but a differential selective medium, such as cefsulodin-triclosan (Irgasan)-novobiocin agar is more effective. If routine enteric media are inoculated, recovery of organisms is optimized by plating them onto MacConkey agar, followed by incubation at 25° C for 48 hours. Cold enrichment techniques may increase the yield of the organism from contaminated specimens such as feces. Stool cultures positive for *Y. enterocolitica* only after prolonged cold enrichment may represent environmental strains of low virulence, unrelated to human disease. Biotyping and serotyping for 0:3, 0:8, and 0:9 are helpful in determining the clinical relevance of such isolates.

V. cholerae strains can be isolated from stool using thiosulfate-citrate-bile-salt-sucrose agar, which is the most convenient and frequently used selective media. This media is suitable for most enteropathogenic *Vibrio* species, except *V. hollisae*. Placing the specimen into an enrichment broth, such as alkaline peptone water with 1 per cent sodium chloride (pH 8.5) for 5 hours before placing on thiosulfate-citrate-bile-salt-sucrose agar, enhances the isolation of vibrios. Serotyping is necessary to classify organisms into those that cause typical epidemic cholera (O1 and O139 serotypes) and those that cause less severe disease (non-O1, or nonagglutinating vibrios). The assays for cholera toxin are the same as those for heat-labile *E. coli* but routinely are not indicated. *V. parahaemolyticus*, like other vibrios, can be cultured on thiosulfate-citrate-bile-salt-sucrose agar. Strains associated with diarrhea are Kanagawa-positive on Wagatsuma agar (i.e., show hemodigestion resembling beta-hemolysis), which is a marker for pathogenicity. *V. parahaemolyticus* can be serotyped based on the O and K antigens.

A. hydrophila can be overlooked easily on standard stool cultures. A specialized blood agar has been suggested for isolation.[5] Oxidase testing of organisms that resemble *E. coli* can select organisms as possible *Aeromonas* species.[5] If oxidase-positive colonies are found, they can be evaluated biochemically to determine species.

C. difficile can be isolated by anaerobic stool culture on agar containing cycloserine, cefoxitin, and fructose. For definitive diagnosis, it is necessary to demonstrate the presence of toxin in stool specimens and its neutralization with antitoxin or by use of enzyme immunoassay.

C. perfringens is isolated commonly from feces of well persons. Diagnosis of *C. perfringens* food poisoning requires isolation of the organisms from incriminated food in a significant quantity ($>10^5$ organisms/g), demonstration of the same serotype of *C. perfringens* from food and feces of ill persons, or demonstration of a serotype of *C. perfringens* in feces of sick but not healthy controls.

S. aureus may be isolated from food and may not be the cause of illness because not all strains of *Staphylococcus* produce enterotoxin. Conversely, the absence of *S. aureus* from food that has been reheated just prior to being eaten does not exclude staphylococcal food poisoning because heating may destroy the organism without inactivating the toxin. Thus, isolation of *S. aureus* from food is only suggestive evidence of etiology. Isolation of the same phage type *S. aureus* from a skin lesion on the hands of a food handler and the food or feces of ill persons can confirm the diagnosis. Although staphylococcal enterotoxins can be demonstrated by their ability to cause emesis after intragastric inoculation of monkeys, they are identified most conveniently using immunologic techniques available in reference laboratories.

B. cereus can be diagnosed by demonstration of greater than 10^5 organisms/g in the incriminated food. Stool culture is unreliable in the individual patient because *B. cereus* may be isolated from feces of well persons. An enzyme immunoassay to demonstrate the diarrheogenic enterotoxin has been developed.

Serotyping and Toxin Detection

Certain serotypes have been associated with ETEC, EIEC, EPEC, and EHEC. Studies of somatic *E. coli* antigens are not helpful in establishing the diagnosis of ETEC because more than 50 different serogroups of *E. coli* have been shown to produce heat-stabile enterotoxins, heat-labile enterotoxins, or both.

Serogroup determination is required for definition of EPEC. Currently, 170 distinct O and 56 H antigens are recognized. The EPEC organisms belong primarily to serogroups O26, O55, O86, O111, O114, O119, O125, O126, O127, O128, and O142.[208] Serogrouping has a role in definition of outbreaks of enteritis among infants but currently is not recommended in sporadic diarrheal disease. Persistent diarrhea in an infant associated with an EPEC serogroup may warrant small bowel biopsy. Changes typical of EPEC on light microscopy of small intestine are flattening and loss of villi with chronic inflammatory changes in the lamina propria. On electron microscopy, bacteria can be seen adherent to epithelial cells that have lost their microvilli and formed "pedestals" with bacteria attached (see Fig. 52–4).[62, 312, 313]

EIEC organisms are identified by demonstration of invasiveness in tissue culture (HeLa cells), by their ability to produce keratoconjunctivitis when inoculated into eyes of guinea pigs or rabbits (Sereny test),[332] or by demonstration of the genes encoding invasiveness. These dysentery-producing EIEC belong to a small number of serogroups: O28, O112, O124, O136, O143, O144, O152, O164, and O167.[61] The O antigens of EIEC are related closely to various *Shigella* O antigens. EIEC may be suspected when a nonmotile, lysine decarboxylase–negative *E. coli* strain is isolated from a patient thought clinically to have shigellosis.[357]

EHEC are noninvasive organisms that produce Shiga-like cytotoxin (also called verotoxin). Although *E. coli* O157:H7 is the most commonly recognized strain causing this disease,[309] more than 50 serotypes have been recognized as pathogens. *E. coli* O157:H7 should be suspected when an *E. coli* strain that does not ferment sorbitol is isolated from a patient with the syndrome[380] and may be identified definitively by serotyping and quantitation of toxin. The other EHEC serotypes are not distinctive biochemically and can be identified only by demonstration of production of Shiga toxin I, II, or I/II or by demonstration of the genes responsible for toxin production.[98] EAEC organisms can be defined by their adherence to HEp-2 cells in tissue culture or by DNA probes.[21, 228]

Virus Detection

Rotavirus has been identified by examination of stool specimens for 70-nm particles by electron microscopy (see Fig. 52–1). Commercially available enzyme immunoassay and latex agglutination kits are available to detect rotavirus antigen in stool specimens.[83, 210] Assay procedures using monoclonal antibodies have improved the sensitivity and specificity to greater than 95 per cent.[83, 189] Other diagnostic methods less suitable for routine use include gel electrophoresis, polymerase chain reaction, and viral culture. To detect non–group A rotaviruses, gel electrophoresis and electron microscopy are required because they are not detected by the commercially available assays.

Attempts at in vitro propagation of the CV agents by routine techniques have been unsuccessful, and no readily available animal model has been developed for study of these viruses. This has made it difficult to study these agents by conventional neutralization test methods. The technique of immune electron microscopy has proved useful in the study of volunteers with experimentally induced Norwalk virus gastroenteritis and in the diagnosis of naturally occurring Norwalk-like agent gastroenteritis.[181] The cloning of Norwalk virus led to the development of several new diagnostic assays, including enzyme immunoassay based on baculovirus-expressed viral capsid proteins and reverse transcriptase polymerase chain reaction to detect viral RNA.[174–177] The antigen enzyme immunoassays are highly specific and detect closely related strains within the same genogroup. The antibody enzyme immunoassays are relatively type-specific with low levels of cross-reaction among strains that are distinct in the antigen enzyme immunoassays. Monoclonal antibodies against the recombinant capsids have been generated and are useful for the development of type-specific assays. Reverse transcriptase polymerase chain reaction more broadly is reactive and useful for genetic classification of the family.[174–177] These assays are available only in research laboratories.

Diagnosis of enteric adenovirus can be established by immune electron microscopy of stool specimens, enzyme immunoassay of stool specimens, or propagation in a line of human embryonic kidney cells transformed by adenovirus type 5 (293 cells).[42, 270] Restriction enzyme analysis is the definitive method for classifying individual enteric adenovirus isolates. Commercially available assays for detection of enteric adenovirus currently are available.[365]

Astroviruses grow well in human embryo kidney cells in the presence of trypsin. Electron microscopy, immune electron microscopy, immunofluorescence on cell culture, enzyme immunoassay, and polymerase chain reaction can be used as detection methods but are available only in reference or research laboratories.[132]

Proctosigmoidoscopy

When symptoms of colitis are severe or the etiology of an inflammatory enteritis syndrome remains obscure after laboratory evaluation, proctoscopic examination may help to establish the diagnosis. Table 52–11 shows the usual proctoscopic findings in the various enteric syndromes that are characterized by fever, abdominal pain, and diarrhea with mucus and blood. Noninfectious diseases, such as Crohn disease and ulcerative colitis, enter the differential diagnosis when symptoms of inflammatory enteritis become chronic. Proctitis with or without diarrhea may be related to child abuse or to sexual practices. The causes of proctitis include all of the aforementioned etiologies as well as *N. gonorrhoeae,* herpes simplex virus, lymphogranuloma venereum, and *Chlamydia trachomatis.*

TREATMENT

Enteric infections generally are self-limited conditions, but nonspecific therapy can provide relief for some patients, and

TABLE 52–11. Proctoscopic Findings of Persistent Inflammatory Colitis

Organism or Disease	Gross Findings	Microscopic Findings
Shigella species	Diffuse erythema with loss of vascular pattern, mucocpurulence, mild friability, occasional aphthoid ulcers	Edema, capillary congestion, focal hemorrhages, crypt hyperplasia, goblet cell depletion, mononuclear and polymorphonuclear leukoycte infiltrate, loss of epithelial cells with microulcerations
Salmonella species	Hyperemic, friable mucosa with petechiae and ulcerations, occasional pseudomembranous changes	Edema, inflammation, microabscesses, ulcerations
Campylobacter jejuni	Diffuse exudative edema	Inflammatory infiltrate with polymorphonuclear leukocytes, eosinophils, mononuclear cells, degeneration, loss of mucus, crypt abscesses, ulcerations
Clostridium difficile	Pseudomembranous colitis with 1- to 5-mm white-yellow nodules or plaques, minimal friability, sometimes nonspecific colitis	Fibrin, mucus, necrotic epithelial cells, leukocytes adherent to the underlying inflamed tissues
Clostridium perfringens	Rarely pseudomembranous colitis	Findings similar to those produced by *C. difficile*
Entamoeba histolytica	Discrete ulcers (mm to cm in diameter) with undermined edges amid normal mucosa	Trophozoites in flask-shaped ulcers that extend into submucosa, inflammatory cells near periphery but not near trophozoites; wet mount shows motile amoeba containing erythrocytes
Ulcerative colitis	Friability, inflammatory polyps on heaped up granulation tissue, deep linear ulcers	Mucosal ulceration extending to lamina propria, diffuse inflammation, vascular engagement, microabscesses in crypts
Crohn colitis	Hyperemic mucosa with linear ulcers	Inflammation involving all layers of bowel with lymphocytes, histiocytes, and plasma cells forming granulomas

specific therapy may shorten the illness and eradicate fecal shedding of the organism. In caring for patients with diarrhea and dehydration, there are several major therapeutic considerations: (1) fluid and electrolyte therapy, (2) dietary manipulation, (3) nonspecific therapy with antidiarrheal compounds, and (4) specific therapy with antimicrobial agents.

Fluid and Electrolyte Therapy

Patients who develop diarrhea lose fluid and electrolytes via the gastrointestinal tract by several mechanisms: vomiting, loss of fecal fluid caused by the infecting enteropathogen, and fecal water loss in excess of sodium due to the intraluminal osmotic effect of unabsorbed nutrients.[154] The composition and amount of lost fluid depend on the rate of stool loss and the causative agent. The higher the rate of stool loss, the greater the sodium loss, probably as a result of rapid passage of intestinal contents through the colon, where sodium/potassium exchange occurs. Stools from patients with cholera or ETEC infection contain sodium in a concentration of 80 to 120 mEq/L, whereas stools from patients with rotavirus infection have sodium concentrations of less than 50 mEq/L.[327] In secretory diarrheal disorders, fluid loss generally is derived from the small intestine and colonic reabsorption is overwhelmed. In viral gastroenteritis, small bowel absorptive capacity primarily is impaired, and in dysenteric or invasive diarrhea, reabsorptive capacity of the large intestine is reduced. If vomiting also is a manifestation, this loss is compounded. Continued loss of fluid or electrolytes may lead to dehydration with potentially severe sequelae. Children, especially infants, are more susceptible to dehydration because of the greater basal fluid and electrolyte requirements per kilogram and because they depend on others to meet these needs.

Important factors to be considered in evaluating patients with diarrhea and possible dehydration include (1) an estimation of deficiency, (2) ongoing daily requirements, (3) continued losses and their replacement, and (4) correction of the underlying cause.[154, 301] The clinical signs and symptoms that may help in estimating deficiencies and determining the severity of dehydration include thirst, dryness of the mucous membranes, decrease in urinary output, tachycardia, loss of skin elasticity and turgor, and mottling and coolness of the skin. These signs may be misleading in patients who are malnourished or in those with hypertonic dehydration.

Fluids should not be withheld in the treatment of any patient with diarrheal disease. Oral therapy should consist of rapid rehydration with replacement of ongoing losses during the first 6 to 12 hours of therapy with a glucose electrolyte solution,[327] followed by early initiation of a modified diet.[223] If fluid and electrolyte deficits are significant, priority should be given to rehydration as rapidly as possible with oral electrolyte solutions containing 90 mEq/L of sodium, 20 mEq/L of potassium, and 2 to 2.5 per cent glucose concentration. Additional free water is given as desired. If the patient is too young to ask for or obtain free water, two parts of this electrolyte solution should be alternated with one part water without added electrolytes.[63] This is the content of the World Health Organization solution used for rehydration in developing parts of the world.[327] Intravenous therapy is required only if the patient is in shock, is obtunded, or has ileus or if vomiting precludes intake; otherwise, fluid and electrolyte therapy should be administered orally. Once the patient is rehydrated, an orally administered maintenance solution containing approximately 50 mEq/L of sodium should be used. Patients with mild diarrhea without clinical dehydration (less than 3 per cent weight loss) can be managed at home by supplementing their diet with oral electrolyte solutions containing glucose. The glucose in these solutions is necessary to promote intestinal absorption of sodium and water in the small intestine.[335]

Commercial preparations of ready-to-feed glucose electrolyte solutions are available in the United States and should be used in preference to homemade solutions for fluid maintenance. The sodium and potassium content of various commercially available preparations is outlined in Table 52–12. Gatorade and other sports drinks do not supply the quantity of electrolytes necessary to replace the continued stool losses of severe diarrhea. They are high in carbohydrate content. A concentration of 2 per cent glucose is recommended for optimal absorption of the salt and water solution. Higher concentrations of sugar are not tolerated well because of high osmotic activity that may exacerbate diarrhea. The carbohydrate concentration, in millimolar units, should not exceed the sodium concentration by more than 2:1. If this occurs, the excess carbohydrate produces osmotic retention of water in the intestine with subsequent loss in stool.[301] The preparation of glucose and salt solutions at home is not recommended because errors in preparing the solutions may result in hypertonic dehydration in infants.[207] The use of rice-based oral rehydration solutions that contain glucose polymers and amino acids has been shown to increase the absorption of salt, water, and glucose from the intestine and may be more beneficial than glucose-based oral rehydration solutions.[326, 337]

Other fluids that may be consumed at home include decarbonated soda beverages, fruit juices, and Jell-O. All contain small amounts of sodium and potassium and carbohydrate concentrations of 10 to 15 per cent, which may exceed the absorptive capacity of the intestine.[335] These solutions should not be used if rehydration requires more than one or two feedings. Kool-Aid and tea are not recommended because

TABLE 52–12. Content of Solutions Used for Oral Rehydration

Solution	Sodium (mmol/L)	Potassium (mmol/L)	Carbohydrate (mmol/L)	Osmolarity (mOsm/L)
Rehydration				
World Health Organization solution*	90	20	111	310
Rehydralyte (Ross)	75	20	140	310
Maintenance Prevention				
Infalyte (Mead Johnson)	50	25	70	200
Naturalyte (Unlimited Beverage)	45	20	140	265
Pedialyte (Ross)	45	20	140	250
Pediatric electrolyte (NutraMax)	45	20	140	250

*Packets of oral rehydration salts are available in the United States from Cera Products, Columbia, MD, (410) 997-2334 and Jianas Brothers, Kansas City, MO, (816) 421-2880.

they are low in both sodium and potassium and thus have little advantage over sugar and water. Six hours after the child has begun drinking a fluid and electrolyte solution, feeding should be restarted.[45, 301]

Dietary Manipulation

Of all common childhood illnesses, diarrhea has the most significant adverse nutritional effect. Restoration of feeding is important to reduce the nutritional defects caused by diarrhea. However, optimal conditions have not been defined in nutrient management of different diarrheal states.[45] Once rehydration is complete, food may be reintroduced while the oral electrolyte solution is continued to replace ongoing losses from stools and for maintenance. Breast feeding in infants should be resumed as soon as possible, preferably immediately after rehydration. Some infants experience temporary lactose intolerance after diarrheal illness,[15] although the vast majority of young children with acute diarrhea can be managed successfully with continued feeding of undiluted nonhuman milk.[46, 223, 301] Routine dilution of milk and routine use of lactose-free milk formula are not necessary, especially when oral rehydration therapy and early feeding are part of the approach to the clinical management of acute diarrhea.

In some children and infants, the carbohydrate fraction of milk may exacerbate diarrhea because of disaccharidase deficiency acquired as a result of diarrhea.[15] The development of lactase deficiency during a diarrheal illness may require some alteration in diet. In children with moderate or severe acute diarrhea, it may be necessary to reduce or eliminate lactose from the diet early in the illness to minimize the effects of lactose intolerance. Relative lactose tolerance has been shown to persist for 2 to 6 weeks after some episodes of diarrhea. Other disaccharidases may be reduced during infection, influencing the absorption of other sugars. Soy-based, lactose-free formulas can be used safely during the acute phase of diarrheal illness in infants.[326] If diarrhea persists for more than 3 weeks, conditions that should be considered include not only disaccharidase deficiency but also celiac disease, cystic fibrosis, parasitic disease, allergic gastroenteropathy, bacterial overgrowth syndrome, EPEC disease, and chronic nonspecific diarrhea.[213]

Nonspecific Therapy with Antidiarrheal Compounds

Many compounds are available for symptomatic treatment of patients with diarrhea. These substances are prescribed by physicians, administered by parents, or taken by patients who are eager to relieve the symptoms of acute diarrheal disease. Their purpose is to decrease the volume of diarrhea by increasing absorption of water and electrolytes, decrease intestinal secretion, or decrease intestinal motility. These over-the-counter and prescription preparations act on the gastrointestinal tract by one or more of these mechanisms. Table 52–13 lists some commercially available antidiarrheal agents and their mechanism of action, major value, and toxicity. Most of these compounds are not approved for children younger than 2 to 3 years of age.

Drugs that alter intestinal motility can be classified into antimuscarinics and synthetic or natural opium alkaloids.[71, 98, 296] These compounds usually have a rapid onset of action (see Table 52–13). They decrease the volume of stool output and relieve abdominal cramps and pain, probably by producing segmental contractions of the intestine, which retard movement of intestinal contents responsible for diarrhea and restrict the intestinal distention that normally causes abdominal pain. Drugs that affect intestinal motility may worsen the symptoms of *Shigella* or other invasive bacteria by inhibiting intestinal transit and allowing the enteropathogen to be in contact with the intestinal mucosa for a longer period.[98] These agents may accelerate the development of AAC.[263] Drugs that have central opiate-like effects can lead to overdose; fatalities in children have occurred.[128, 296, 316] Two to four doses of these compounds over a 24-hour period may be used in adolescents or adults to treat severe cramps, but prolonged therapy is not advised, and use in children is not recommended. The combination of TMP-SMX plus loperamide was effective in the treatment of adults with travelers' diarrhea,[113] which resulted in the shortest mean duration of diarrhea when compared with that in patients taking placebo or TMP-SMX alone. In infants, loperamide can cause ileus, emesis, and drowsiness.[252] The practice parameter of the American Academy of Pediatrics does not recommend this class of compounds to treat diarrhea in children.[301]

A number of chemically inert agents are used internally as adsorbents to bind toxins and water to reduce the number and improve consistency of bowel movements. When these substances are given by mouth, they can adsorb not only bacteria and toxins but also drugs, nutrients, and enzymes. The only agents currently used widely are compounds containing activated attapulgite, which have been shown to be effective in animals by reducing diarrhea and producing formed stools,[121, 301] but studies in humans are lacking. Disadvantages include nonspecific changes in adsorption of nutrients, enzymes, and antibiotics, particularly if the absorbent is used for a prolonged period.

Lactobacillus preparations have been given to recolonize the intestine with saccharolytic flora and alter the intestinal pH as a way of deterring potential pathogens.[66, 279] Ingesting lactulose, lactobacilli, and yogurt results in an increased production of short-chain fatty acids and a decrease in pH in the intestine, which may inhibit the growth of *Salmonella* and *Shigella*; however, there is no evidence of the effectiveness of these compounds in the symptomatic treatment of diarrhea. Feeding selected microorganisms, including *Bifidobacterium bifidum, Saccharomyces boulardii, Lactobacillus acidophilus,* and *Streptococcus thermophilus,* to children and adults has been shown to be effective in prevention and treatment against intestinal disease.[109, 320]

Indomethacin, aspirin, chlorpromazine, and imidazole decrease the intestinal secretion of fluid and electrolytes. Indomethacin has been shown to be effective in radiation-induced diarrhea, and chlorpromazine is effective in diarrhea caused by *V. cholerae*; however, the usefulness of these compounds in patients with various forms of acute infectious diarrhea is unknown. Laboratory studies showed that bismuth subsalicylate (Pepto-Bismol) inhibited intestinal secretion caused by *E. coli* and cholera enterotoxins,[110] reduced diarrhea in adult students who became ill in Mexico,[100] and prevented diarrhea among U. S. students traveling to Mexico.[101] Studies supporting its use in children are limited.[343, 344] Potential problems with this compound relate to the absorption of salicylate[118, 287] and bismuth.[240] Octreotide (Sandostatin) is a long-acting octapeptide with pharmacologic actions mimicking those of the natural hormone somatostatin. It has been used in patients with AIDS who have severe refractory secretory diarrhea[52] but is not approved by the Food and Drug Administration for this purpose.

Specific Therapy with Antimicrobial Agents

Antimicrobial therapy is administered to selected patients with gastroenteritis to abbreviate the clinical course and de-

TABLE 52–13. Antidiarrheal Compounds Used as Nonspecific Therapy for Patients with Acute Diarrhea

Mechanism of Action	Generic Name	Trade Name	Value	Comments
Alteration of intestinal motility	Loperamide	Imodium, Imodium A-D, Maalox Antidiarrheal, Pepto Diarrhea Control		
			Decreases diarrhea, rapid onset action	Numerous side effects and contraindications, not recommended or approved for use in infants and young children, may potentiate *Shigella* or *Salmonella* infections or accelerate the course of antimicrobial associated colitis
	Difenoxin and atropine	Motofen*		
	Diphenoxylate and atropine	Lomotil*		
	Tincture of opium	Paregoric*		
Alteration of secretion	Bismuth subsalicylate	Pepto-Bismol	Decreases diarrhea and cramps of travelers	Potential for salicylate and/or bismuth overdose, darkens stool
	Octreotide	Sandostatin	Decreases diarrhea in patients with vasoactive intestinal peptide secreting and metastatic carcinoid tumors	Used for relief of refractory AIDS-associated diarrhea; not approved by the Food and Drug Administration for this condition
Adsorption of toxins and water	Attapulgite	Diasorb, Donnagel, Kaopectate, Rheaban	Increases form of stool	Safe, minimally effective, decreases absorption of nutrients and drugs, causes abdominal fullness
Alteration of intestinal microflora	Lactobacillus	Pro-Bionate, Superdophilus	Value unproven	Safe, contraindicated in those with lactose tolerance

* Requires a prescription.

crease excretion of the causative organisms.[291] A stool culture should be obtained when antibiotic treatment is anticipated, and antibiotic susceptibility testing of any suspected pathogen should be performed to ensure optimal therapy. Changing susceptibility patterns makes the initial selection of an antimicrobial agent difficult. Antimicrobial agents should not be used routinely or liberally for gastroenteritis of unknown etiology.

Shigella

Several antibiotics have been used successfully in eradicating clinical symptoms and fecal shedding of *Shigella.* Table 52–14 outlines suggested antimicrobial therapy for children and adults who are presumed to have shigellosis or from whom *Shigella* organisms are isolated from stool. TMP-SMX is the treatment of choice for susceptible *Shigella* organisms,[260] although TMP-SMX resistance appears to be increasing, especially in isolates associated with foreign travel.[348] The history of resistance among *Shigella* strains has shown progressive acquisition of multiresistance, first to sulfonamides, shortly after their commercial availability; then to tetracycline, chloramphenicol, and streptomycin less than 10 years after they were introduced; and subsequently to ampicillin, kanamycin, and TMP-SMX.[253, 295] In children with known ampicillin-susceptible strains, ampicillin can be given. Amoxicillin is not as effective as ampicillin in the treatment of shigellosis and should not be used.[259] Ciprofloxacin, ofloxacin, and ceftriaxone have been used successfully to treat adults with shigellosis[29, 178]; in adults, fluoroquinolones are the first drug of choice.[238] Intramuscular ceftriaxone[178, 368] or oral cefixime[11] is effective therapy and is preferable empiric therapy wherever TMP-SMX resistance is common. Although at present not recommended for use in children in the United States, nalidixic acid can be used as an alternative drug in children[323] for resistant strains, keeping in mind that *Shigella* resistance has been described.[253] Patients who are transient asymptomatic carriers may be managed without antimicrobial therapy if they understand and employ excellent standards of personal hygiene. Treatment of these patients, however, reduces fecal shedding of the organism and prevents spread of infection.

Salmonella

Table 52–15 shows antimicrobial therapy of patients with the various clinical manifestations of *Salmonella.* The type of syndrome produced by *Salmonella* influences the selection and duration of antimicrobial therapy. Antibiotics should not be used in the treatment of persons who are nontyphoid *Salmonella* carriers or in the vast majority of patients with mild gastroenteritis. Antimicrobial therapy may, on occasion, convert intestinal carriage into systemic disease with bacteremia, prolong excretion of *Salmonella,*[10] or encourage development or selection of resistant strains. Antimicrobial agents should be considered in patients with enterocolitis if the disease appears to be evolving into one of the systemic syndromes and in patients with a major disease or condition that impairs host resistance to infection, including neonates, young infants, and patients with hemoglobinopathies, including sickle-cell anemia, AIDS, leukemia, or lymphoma. Antibiotic treatment of *Salmonella* infection should be given for all patients with (1) typhoid fever, (2) bacteremia caused by nontyphoidal strains, and (3) dissemination with localized suppuration.

Despite excellent in vitro activity, several antibiotics, including first- and second-generation cephalosporins, have been ineffective in the therapy of patients with *Salmonella* infection. Selection of antimicrobial agents for therapy is complicated by the emergence of *Salmonella* strains that are resistant to multiple antibiotics[206, 295] and by increased risk of *Salmonella* infection associated with prior antimicrobial exposure.[278] Antibiotics of first choice for the treatment of patients with various *Salmonella* syndromes include ceftriaxone, cefotaxime, ciprofloxacin, and ofloxacin.[238] The fluoroquinolones are approved by the Food and Drug Administration only for persons older than 17 years of age. Alternative drugs include chloramphenicol, ampicillin or amoxicillin, and TMP-SMX. Response is gradual, with temperatures returning to normal within 3 to 5 days in most patients.

In the United States, *S. typhi* generally has remained susceptible, but resistance is increasing because of importation of resistant strains.[206, 295, 318] Resistance is common in nontyphoidal *Salmonella* strains, which have their major reservoirs in animals. Third-generation cephalosporins such as cefotaxime and ceftriaxone are effective against *S. typhi* and nontyphoidal *Salmonella,* which are resistant to ampicillin, chloramphenicol, and TMP-SMX.[169, 248, 338, 341] Ciprofloxacin and ofloxacin are active in vitro against *Salmonella* organisms, including *S. typhi,*[303, 338, 372] and have been used clinically with success.[14, 69, 212, 372] With an intravascular localized infection, such as endocarditis or aneurysmal infection, chloramphenicol should be avoided because it is not a cidal drug. Patients who have defects in host defense mechanisms, such as those with AIDS, should be treated with ampicillin or a third-generation cephalosporin antibiotic, depending on suscepti-

TABLE 52–14. Antimicrobial Therapy of Patients with Shigellosis

	Antimicrobial Agent	Children	Adults
Strain of unknown susceptibility	Ceftriaxone	50 mg/kg IM as a single dose daily for 5 days	1.5 g/day as a single daily dose for 5 days
	Cefixime	8 mg/kg/day in 2 oral doses for 5 days	—
	Nalidixic acid*	55 mg/kg/day in 4 oral doses for 5 days	—
Trimethoprim-sulfamethoxazole (TMP-SMX)–susceptible strains	TMP-SMX	TMP 10 mg/kg/day plus SMX 50 mg/kg/day orally divided twice daily for 5 days	TMP (160 mg) plus SMX (800 mg) orally twice daily for 5 days
Ampicillin-susceptible strain	Ampicillin	50–75 mg/kg/day orally divided four times daily for 5 days	500 mg orally four times for 5 days
Suspected or proven multidrug-resistant strain	Ciprofloxacin	Not recommended	500 mg orally two times daily for 3–5 days
	Ofloxacin	Not recommended	400 mg orally two times daily for 3–5 days

*Not recommended for use in children in the United States.

TABLE 52–15. Antimicrobial Therapy of Patients with *Salmonella* Infections

Clinical Manifestation	Antimicrobial Agent	Dosage	
		Children	*Adults*
Carrier state	None	None	None
Acute gastroenteritis*	None	None	None
Bacteremia and/or enteric fever†	Ampicillin	200 mg/kg/day IV divided every 4 hours for 2 weeks	6 g/day IV divided every 4 hours for 2 weeks
	or		
	Chloramphenicol	75 mg/kg/day orally or IV divided every 6 hours for 2 weeks	3 g/day IV or orally divided every 6 hours for 2 weeks
	or		
	Trimethoprim-sulfamethoxazole (TMP-SMX)	TMP 10 mg/kg/day plus SMX 50 mg/kg/day divided every 12 hours for 2 weeks	TMP 160 mg plus SMX 800 mg every 12 hours for 2 weeks
Dissemination with localized suppuration (osteomyelitis)† or bacteremia in patients with AIDS	Ampicillin or Chloramphenicol or TMP-SMX	Administer for 4–6 weeks	
Meningitis or ampicillin-chloramphenicol and TMP-SMX–resistant organisms	Cefotaxime	200 mg/kg/day IV divided every 6 hours for 2 weeks (at least 4 weeks for meningitis)	12 g/day IV divided every 6 hours for 2 weeks
	or		
	Ceftriaxone	100 mg/kg/day IV every 12 hours for 2 weeks (at least 4 weeks for meningitis)	4 g/day IV divided every 12 hours or once per day for 2 weeks

*Patients with hyperpyrexia and systemic signs or symptoms should be treated empirically until bacteremia is excluded. Although of unproven efficacy, antibiotic therapy for children in the first 3 months of life also is recommended by most authorities; a 7- to 10-day course of therapy probably is sufficient.

†Ciprofloxacin or ofloxacin can be used to treat resistant organisms in persons older than 17 years of age. Both are available for intravenous as well as oral use. Neither is recommended for pregnant women.

bility.[170, 339] Corticosteroids can be beneficial in patients with severe typhoid fever, in whom prompt relief of manifestations of toxemia might be life-saving,[157] although they may increase the relapse rate.[70]

Ampicillin or amoxicillin combined with probenecid is the treatment of choice for chronic enteric carriers who have normally functioning gall bladders without cholelithiasis.[282] When gallbladder disease is present, the failure of ampicillin is common. Ciprofloxacin[119] has been shown to be successful in the eradication of *S. typhi* in chronic carriers in adults. Three typhoid fever vaccines are commercially available in the United States for specific situations.[56]

Campylobacter

Several studies have evaluated the susceptibility of *Campylobacter* species to antimicrobial agents.[349] Furazolidone and the aminoglycosides showed a high degree of in vitro susceptibility; tetracycline, erythromycin, and chloramphenicol were active against most strains tested, whereas penicillin, ampicillin, the cephalosporins, and TMP-SMX were relatively inactive. Clindamycin, metronidazole, ticarcillin, and carbenicillin also showed activity against *Campylobacter* isolates. Isolation of *Campylobacter* from stool does not imply the need for antibiotics. The decision concerning therapy should be individualized, but therapy probably should be used in patients with high temperatures, bloody diarrhea, or severe diarrhea. In patients with *Campylobacter* enteritis, erythromycin and a fluoroquinolone are the agents of choice when a decision has been made to initiate therapy.[238] Gentamicin and a tetracycline are alternative drugs. In double-blind, placebo-controlled trials of erythromycin for the treatment of patients with enteritis due to *C. jejuni*, erythromycin was shown promptly to eradicate *C. jejuni* from the feces but did not alter the clinical course when begun 4 or more days after the onset of symptoms.[6] Studies in which therapy was started early showed that *C. jejuni* rapidly was eliminated from stools, but they gave conflicting results with regard to resolution of clinical illness.[324, 384] The treatment of choice for patients with *C. fetus* infection is gentamicin or imipenem.[238]

Other Bacterial Agents (Table 52–16)

Antimicrobial agents have been employed frequently in attempts to treat infantile gastroenteritis caused by EPEC and as a means of controlling the spread of EPEC strains in hospital nurseries. Although no definitive studies support the effectiveness of these drugs, they may be useful in certain situations, particularly when life-threatening infection occurs or when epidemic spread of the strains continues, despite the use of strict hand washing and appropriate isolation. Agents used in the treatment of mild EPEC diarrhea include oral nonabsorbable antibiotics, such as neomycin and gentamicin. TMP-SMX may be useful in the treatment of patients with diarrhea due to EPEC. If systemic infection is suspected, parenteral therapy should be started and modified according to antimicrobial susceptibility of the organism isolated.

Diarrhea due to ETEC usually is limited, but studies in adults have shown that antimicrobial agents such as TMP-SMX and ciprofloxacin are effective.[112] The treatment of patients with diarrhea due to EIEC is similar to that for patients with shigellosis (see Table 52–14). Antimicrobial treatment of patients infected with EHEC is controversial; controlled studies are needed.

Antimicrobial agents decrease the diarrhea associated with cholera by eradicating the vibrios from the gastrointestinal tract[373] and thus reducing the volume of fluid loss. Doxycycline or tetracycline is the drug of choice in most instances for O1 and O39 infection, including children in whom the benefits of a 1- to 2-day course outweigh the risks of dental staining.[54, 302, 389] TMP-SMX can be used in children younger than 8 years of age for *V. cholerae* O1, but O139 strains often are resistant. Ampicillin probably is the safest agent for use during pregnancy. Other effective antimicrobial agents are the fluoroquinolones, azithromycin, cephems, and penems.[136, 389] Diarrhea due to *V. parahaemolyticus* is self-limited, so that antimicrobial therapy shortens neither the clinical course nor the duration of excretion. Antimicrobial therapy has not been proved efficacious in the treatment of uncomplicated enterocolitis caused by *Y. enterocolitica*.[72] Patients with *Y. enterocolitica*–induced septicemia or extraintestinal focal infection or compromised hosts with enterocolitis should receive antibiotic therapy. The drug of choice is TMP-SMX, and alternative drugs are a fluoroquinolone, an aminoglycoside, cefotaxime, or ceftizoxime. Table 52–16 outlines the antimicrobial therapy of these bacterial pathogens.

Protozoal Agents

Several drugs available in the United States have been shown to be effective in the treatment of patients with giardiasis (e.g., metronidazole, furazolidone, paromomycin).[78, 237] Metronidazole is not approved for the treatment of patients with giardiasis in the United States and is carcinogenic in animals. Tinidazole and ornidazole are nitroimidazole drugs similar to metronidazole but are not marketed in the United States. Paromomycin is not absorbed and not highly effective but has been proposed for use during pregnancy.[198]

In a review of comparative drug trials for the treatment of giardiasis, Davidson[78] reported that metronidazole cured 92 per cent of 219 patients and furazolidone cured 84 per cent of 150 patients. Approximately 7 per cent of the metronidazole-treated patients and 10 per cent of the furazolidone-treated patients had side effects that were serious enough to report. The only drug available in a liquid preparation is furazolidone. The dosage schedule for the treatment of patients with giardiasis is shown in Table 52–17.

In treating patients with amebiasis, iodoquinol is the best luminal amebicide presently available in the United States.[237] This drug is effective against both cysts and trophozoites in the lumen of the gut but is ineffective against tissue forms of the disease. Invasive amebiasis of the intestine, liver, or other organs necessitates the additional use of tissue amebicides, such as metronidazole. Liver abscess or other extraintestinal forms of disease should be treated with metronidazole in the dose recommended for intestinal disease. Table 52–18 lists the recommended drugs for the treatment of children and adults with various forms of amebiasis.

Patients with intestinal strongyloidiasis should receive thiabendazole (25 mg/kg/dose) every 12 hours for four doses (50 mg/kg/day; maximum, 3 g/day) or ivermectin (200 μg/kg/day) for 1 to 2 days. Immunosuppressed patients with disseminated disease may require continued therapy

Table 52–16. Antimicrobial Therapy of Bacterial Pathogens Causing Gastroenteritis

Organism	Antibiotic Therapy: *Children*	Antibiotic Therapy: *Adults*
Campylobacter jejuni		
Gastroenteritis	None, or if colitis is present, erythromycin 30 mg/kg/day orally divided 4 times daily for 5–7 days	None or erythromycin 250 mg orally 4 times daily for 5–7 days or ciprofloxacin or ofloxacin
Sepsis	Aminoglycoside	Aminoglycoside
Clostridium difficile (antimicrobial-associated colitis)	Metronidazole 35 mg/kg/day orally divided 3 times daily for 7 days or Vancomycin 40 mg/kg/day orally divided 4 times daily for 7 days	Metronidazole 250 mg orally 4 times daily for 7 days or Vancomycin 125 mg orally 4 times daily for 7 days
Escherichia coli		
Enteropathogenic	None or trimethoprim-sulfamethoxazole (TMP-SMX)	None or TMP-SMX
Enterotoxigenic	None or TMP-SMX	None, TMP-SMX, or fluoroquinolone
Invasive	Same as for shigellosis (see Table 63–14)	Same as for shigellosis
Vibrio cholerae	Tetracycline 12.5 mg/kg every 6 hours for 2 days or doxycycline 6 mg/kg once TMP 10 mg/kg/day plus SMX 50 mg/kg/day divided every 12 hours for 2 days	Tetracycline 500 mg every 6 hours for 2 days or doxycycline 300 mg once or Ciprofloxacin or ofloxacin
Vibrio parahaemolyticus	None	None
Yersinia enterocolitica		
Gastroenteritis	Probably none	Probably none
Sepsis	TMP-SMX or An aminoglycoside or Cefotaxime or Ceftizoxime	TMP-SMX or An aminoglycoside or A fluoroquinolone or Cefotaxime or Ceftizoxime

TABLE 52–17. Antimicrobial Therapy of Patients with Giardiasis

Antimicrobial Agent	Dose: Children	Dose: Adults	Comments
Metronidazole (Flagyl)	15 mg/kg/day orally three times daily for 7 days (maximum, 750 mg/day)	250 mg orally three times daily for 7 days	Metallic taste, nausea, headache, dry mouth, mutagenic in bacteria, carcinogenic in animals, disulfiram-like reaction with alcohol
Furazolidone (Furoxone)	6 mg/kg/day orally four times daily for 10 days (maximum, 400 mg/day)	100 mg orally four times daily for 10 days	Nausea, vomiting, disulfiram-like reaction with alcohol, mild hemolysis in G6P-D–deficient individuals, hypoglycemia, allergic reactions
Paromomycin	Not recommended	30 mg/kg/day orally three times per day for 7 days	Not highly effective, proposed for use in pregnancy

for 2 to 3 weeks, but mortality is high despite therapy. A thorough examination should be performed before giving immunosuppressive therapy to a patient with a past history of infection with *S. stercoralis.*

There is no therapeutic agent proved to be beneficial consistently for the treatment of patients with cryptosporidiosis. More than 80 different drugs, including antibiotics, antiparasitic agents, antidiarrheal medications, anti-inflammatory drugs, and inflammatory mediators, have been tried in animals and humans without conclusive results.[322, 386] Infection is self-limited in immunocompetent patients. Paromomycin and azithromycin both have shown promise in small numbers of immunosuppressed patients.[35, 120, 152, 367, 382] Immune therapy using transfer factor, a dialyzable extract from bovine leukocytes, was beneficial in five of eight patients with cryptosporidiosis.[215] Hyperimmune bovine colostrum has been used with some success in a child with agammaglobulinemia[360] and in a patient with AIDS.[363] Immune bovine colostrum has been shown to neutralize *C. parvum* sporozoites and partially to protect mice against oral challenge with *C. parvum* oocysts.[281] Nonspecific therapy with octreotide may control the severe diarrhea that occurs in patients with AIDS but has no effect on the infection[52] and is not approved for this use by the Food and Drug Administration.

In contrast to *Cryptosporidium,* for which no effective drug treatment has been effective consistently, for isosporiasis, TMP-SMX is effective and is the drug of choice.[237] TMP-SMX at a dose of 160 mg TMP and 800 mg SMX four times a day for 10 days followed by the same dose twice a day for 3 weeks is recommended for adults. Other drugs, including pyrimethamine-sulfadoxine (Fansidar), metronidazole, and furazolidone, have been reported to be successful for the treatment of patients with isosporiasis.[274, 379] Pyrimethamine probably is an effective alternative in patients allergic to sulfa drugs.[274] Problems in the treatment of isosporiasis have been encountered in patients with AIDS, in whom a high incidence of recurrence has been reported after treatment has been stopped. Continuation of therapy indefinitely in adults with either pyrimethamine-sulfadoxine or TMP-SMX has been shown to be effective in preventing recurrence of disease,[274] although further studies are necessary to determine the adequacy of this approach. All of these drugs are considered investigational for isosporiasis by the Food and Drug Administration.

There is no recommended therapy for infections due to *E. bieneusi* or *S. intestinalis,* although albendazole (400 mg twice a day in adults) may be effective.[86, 94, 204] Patients with *Cyclospora* infection respond to TMP-SMX (TMP 5 mg/kg and SMX 25 mg/kg four times daily for 10 days, then twice a day for 7 days; maximum, 160 mg/800 mg per dose), but relapses are common.[158] HIV-infected patients may need higher doses and long-term maintenance.[276]

TABLE 52–18. Antimicrobial Therapy of Patients with Amebiasis

Asymptomatic amebic cyst	Iodoquinol (Yodoxin) or	30 mg/kg/day divided three times daily for 20 days (not to exceed 2 g/day)	650 mg three times daily for 20 days
	Paromomycin (Humatin) or	25–30 mg/kg/day divided three times daily for 7 days	25–30 mg/kg/day three times daily for 7 days
	Diloxanide furoate*	20 mg/kg/day divided three times daily for 10 days	500 mg three times daily for 10 days
Mild to moderate intestinal disease	Metronidazole (Flagyl) followed by	35–50 mg/kg/day divided three times daily for 10 days (maximum, 2250 mg/day)	750 mg three times daily for 10 days
	Iodoquinol	See above	See above
Severe intestinal disease, liver abscess, or other extraintestinal disease	Metronidazole followed by Iodoquinol	See above See above	See above See above

*Available in the United States from the CDC Drug Service, Centers for Disease Control and Prevention, Atlanta, GA 30333; (404) 639-2888.

References

1. Ackman, D. M., Drabkin, P., Birkhead, G., et al.: Reptile-associated salmonellosis in New York State. Pediatr. Infect. Dis. J. *14*:955–959, 1995.
2. Ahmed, L., El Rooby, A., Kassem, M. I., et al.: Ultrasonography in the diagnosis and management of 52 patients with amebic liver abscess in Cairo. Rev. Infect. Dis. *12*:330, 1990.
3. Aho, K., Ahvonen, P., Alkio, P., et al.: HLA-27 in reactive arthritis following infection. Ann. Rheum. Dis. *34*(Suppl.):29–30, 1975.
4. Aldeen, W. E., Whisenant, J., Hale, D., et al.: Comparison of pooled formalin-preserved fecal specimens with three individual samples for detection of intestinal parasites. J. Clin. Microbiol. *31*:144–145, 1993.
5. Altwegg, M., and Geiss, H. K.: *Aeromonas* as a human pathogen. CRC Crit. Rev. Microbiol. *16*:253, 1989.
6. Anders, B. J., Paisley, J. W., Lauer, B. A., et al.: Double-blind placebo controlled trial of erythromycin for treatment of *Campylobacter* enteritis. Lancet *1*:131–132, 1982.
7. Angulo, F. J., and Swerdlow, D. L.: Bacterial enteric infections in persons infected with human immunodeficiency virus. Clin. Infect. Dis. *21*(Suppl. 1):S84–S93, 1995.
8. Archer, D. L., and Young, F. E.: Contemporary issues: Diseases with a food vector. Clin. Microbiol. Rev. *1*:377, 1988.
9. Arrowood, M. J., and Sterling, C. R.: Comparison of conventional staining methods and monoclonal antibody-based methods for *Cryptosporidium* oocyst detection. J. Clin. Microbiol. *27*:1490, 1989.
10. Aserkoff, B., and Bennett, J. V.: Effect of antibiotic therapy in acute salmonellosis on the fecal excretion of salmonellae. N. Engl. J. Med. *281*:636–640, 1969.
11. Ashkenazi, S., Amir, J., Waisman, Y., et al.: A randomized, double-blind study comparing cefixime and TMP/SMX in the treatment of childhood shigellosis. J. Pediatr. *123*:817–821, 1993.
12. Ashkenazi, S., Cleary, T. G., and Pickering, L. K.: Bacterial toxins associated with diarrheal disease. *In* Lebenthal, E., and Duffy, M. (eds.): Textbook of Secretory Diarrhea. Vol. 18. New York: Raven Press, 1990, p. 255.
13. Asmuth, D. M., DeGirolami, P. C., Federman, M., et al.: Clinical features of microsporidiosis in patients with AIDS. Clin. Infect. Dis. *18*:819–825, 1994.
14. Asperilla, M. O., Smego, R. A., Jr., and Scott, L. K.: Quinolone antibiotics in the treatment of *Salmonella* infections. Rev. Infect. Dis. *12*:873, 1990.
15. Avery, G. B., Villavicencio, O., Lilly, J. R., et al.: Intractable diarrhea in early infancy. Pediatrics *41*:712–722, 1968.
16. Bartlett, A. V., Prado, D., Cleary, T. G., et al.: Production of Shigatoxin and other cytotoxins by serogroups of *Shigella*. J. Infect. Dis. *154*:996, 1986.
17. Bartlett, A. V., Reves, R. R., and Pickering, L. K.: Rotavirus in infant toddler day care centers: Epidemiology relevant to disease control strategies. J. Pediatr. *113*:435, 1988.
18. Bartlett, J. G., Tedesdo, F. J., Shull, S., et al.: Symptomatic relapse after oral vancomycin therapy of antibiotic-associated pseudomembranous colitis. Gastroenterology *78*:431–434, 1980.
19. Bartlett, J. G.: Antimicrobial agents implicated in *Clostridium difficile* toxin-associated diarrhea or colitis. Johns Hopkins Med. J. *149*:6–9, 1981.
20. Bartlett, J. G.: *Clostridium difficile:* History of its role as an enteric pathogen and the current state of knowledge about the organism. Clin. Infect. Dis. *18*(Suppl. 4):S265–S272, 1994.
21. Baudry, B., Savarino, S. J., Vial, P., et al.: A sensitive and specific DNA probe to identify enteroaggregative *Escherichia coli*, a recently discovered diarrheal pathogen. J. Infect. Dis. *161*:1249, 1990.
22. Bean, N. H., Goulding, J. S., Lao, C., et al.: Foodborne disease outbreaks in the United States 1988–1992. M. M. W. R. *45*:1–66, 1996.
23. Beards, G. M., Green, J. G., Hall, C., et al.: An enveloped virus in stools of children and adults with gastroenteritis that resembles the Breda virus of calves. Lancet *1*:1050, 1984.
24. Beauvais, B., Sarfati, C., Molina, J. M., et al.: Comparative evaluation of five diagnostic methods for demonstrating microsporidia in stool and intestinal biopsy specimens. Ann. Trop. Med. Parasitol. *87*:99–102, 1993.
25. Beebakhee, G., Louie, M., De-Azavedo, J., et al.: Cloning and nucleotide sequence of the *eae* gene homologue from enterohemorrhagic *Escherichia coli* serotype 0157:H7. FEMS Microbiol. Lett. *70*:63–68, 1992.
26. Benator, D. A., French, A. L., Beaudet, L. M., et al.: *Isospori belli* infection associated with acalculous cholecystitis in a patient with AIDS. Ann. Intern. Med. *121*:663–664, 1994.
27. Benhamou, Y., Caumes, E., Gerosa, Y., et al.: AIDS-related cholangiopathy: Critical analysis of a prospective series of 26 patients. Dig. Dis. Sci. *38*:1113–1118, 1993.
28. Benjamin, J., Leaper, S., Owen, R. J., et al.: Description of *Campylobacter laridis,* a new species comprising the nalidixic acid resistant thermophilic *Campylobacter* (NARTC) group. Curr. Microbiol. *8*:231–238, 1983.
29. Bennish, M. L., Salam, M. A., Haider, R., et al.: Therapy for shigellosis. II. Randomized, double-blind comparison of ciprofloxacin and ampicillin. J. Infect. Dis. *162*:711, 1990.
30. Benz, I., and Schmidt, M. A.: AIDA-I, the adhesin involved in diffuse adherence of the diarrhoeagenic *Escherichia coli* strain 2787 (0126:H27), is synthesized via a precursor molecule. Mol. Microbiol. *6*:1539–1546, 1992.
31. Berk, S. L., Verghese, A., Alvarez, S., et al.: Clinical and epidemiologic features of strongyloidiasis: A prospective study in rural Tennessee. Arch. Intern. Med. *147*:1257, 1987.
32. Bhan, M. K., Raj, P., Levine, M. M., et al.: Enteroaggregative *E. coli* associated with persistent diarrhea in a cohort of rural children in India. J. Infect. Dis. *159*:1061, 1989.
33. Birkhead, G., and Vogt, R. L.: Epidemiologic surveillance for endemic *Giardia lamblia* infection in Vermont: The roles of waterborne and person-to-person transmission. Am. J. Epidemiol. *129*:762, 1989.
34. Bishop, R. F., Davidson, G. P., Holmes, I. H., et al.: Virus particles in epithelial cells of duodenal mucosa from children with acute nonbacterial gastroenteritis. Lancet *2*:1281–1283, 1973.
35. Bissuel, F., Cotte, L., and Rabondonirina, M.: Paromomycin: An effective treatment for cryptosporidial diarrhea in patients with AIDS. Clin. Infect. Dis. *18*:447–449, 1994.
36. Black, R. E.: Pathogens that cause travelers' diarrhea in Latin America and Africa. Rev. Infect. Dis. *8*:131S, 1986.
37. Blacklow, N. R., Cukor, G., Bedigian, M. K., et al.: Immune response and prevalence of antibody to Norwalk enteritis virus as determined by radioimmunoassay. J. Clin. Microbiol. *10*:903, 1979.
38. Blaser, M. J.: *Helicobacter pylori* and the pathogenesis of gastroduodenal inflammation. J. Infect. Dis. *161*:626, 1990.
39. Blaser, M. J., Wells, J. G., Feldman, R. A., et al.: *Campylobacter* enteritis in the United States. Ann. Intern. Med. *98*:360–365, 1983.
40. Bourke, B., Jones, N., and Sherman, P.: *Helicobacter pylori* infection and peptic ulcer disease in children. Pediatr. Infect. Dis. J. *15*:1–13, 1996.
41. Boyle, T. G., Pemberton, A. G., Wells, J. G., et al.: Screening for *Escherichia coli* 0157:H7: A nationwide survey of clinical laboratories. J. Clin. Microbiol. *33*:3275–3277, 1995.
42. Brandt, C. D., Kim, H. W., Rodriguez, W. J., et al.: Adenoviruses and pediatric gastroenteritis. J. Infect. Dis. *151*:437–443, 1985.
43. Brenden, R. A., Miller, M. A., and Janda, J. M.: Clinical disease spectrum and pathogenic factors associated with *Plesiomonas shigelloides* infections in humans. Rev. Infect. Dis. *10*:303, 1988.
44. Bridges, J. C., Pedley, S., and McCrae, M. A.: Group C rotaviruses in humans. J. Clin. Microbiol. *23*:760, 1986.
45. Brown, K. H., and McClean, W. C.: Nutritional management of acute diarrhea: An appraisal of the alternatives. Pediatrics *73*:119–125, 1984.
46. Brown, K. H., Peerson, J. M., and Fontaine, O.: Use of nonhuman milks in the dietary management of young children with acute diarrhea. A meta-analysis of clinical trials. Pediatrics *93*:17–27, 1994.
47. Burke, V., Robinson, J., Beaman, J., et al.: Correlation of enterotoxicity with biotype in *Aeromonas* spp. J. Clin. Microbiol. *18*:1196–1200, 1983.
48. Cali, A., and Owen, R. L.: Intracellular development of *Enterocytozoon:* A unique microsporidian found in the intestine of AIDS patients. J. Protozool. *37*:145, 1990.
49. Cali, A., Kotler, D. P., and Orenstein, J. M.: *Septata intestinalis* N. G., N. Sp., an intestinal microsporidian associated with chronic diarrhea and dissemination in AIDS patients. J. Eukaryot. Microbiol. *40*:101–112, 1993.
50. Calva, J. J., Ruiz-Palacios, G. M., Lopez-Vidal, A. B., et al.: Cohort study of intestinal infection with *Campylobacter* in Mexican children. Lancet *1*:503, 1988.
51. Carter, M. J., and Anzimlt, T.: *Cryptosporidium:* An important cause of gastrointestinal disease in immunocompetent patients. N. Z. Med. J. *99*:101, 1986.
52. Cello, J. P., Grendell, J. H., Basuk, P., et al.: Effect of octreotide on refractory AIDS-associated diarrhea: A prospective, multicenter trial. Ann. Intern. Med. *115*:705–710, 1991.
53. Centers for Disease Control: Microsporidian keratoconjunctivitis in patients with AIDS. M. M. W. R. *39*:188, 1990.
54. Centers for Disease Control: Update: Cholera—Western Hemisphere, and recommendations for treatment of cholera. M. M. W. R. *40*:562–566, 1991.
55. Centers for Disease Control and Prevention: 1993 revised classification system for HIV infection and expanded surveillance case definition for AIDS among adolescents and adults. M. M. W. R. *41*(RR-17):1–19, 1992.
56. Centers for Disease Control and Prevention: Typhoid immunization. M. M. W. R. *43*:1–7, 1994.
57. Centers for Disease Control and Prevention: *Bacillus cereus* food poisoning associated with fried rice at two child care centers: Virginia, 1993. M. M. W. R. *43*:177–178, 1994.
58. Centers for Disease Control and Prevention: Summary of notifiable diseases, United States, 1994. M. M. W. R. *43*:1–81, 1995.
59. Centers for Disease Control and Prevention: USPHS/IDSA guidelines for the prevention of opportunistic infections in persons infected with human immunodeficiency virus: A summary. M. M. W. R. *44*:1–34, 1995.
60. Centers for Disease Control and Prevention: Outbreaks of *Cyclospora cayetanensis* infection: United States, 1996. M. M. W. R. *45*:549–551, 1996.
61. Cheasty, T., and Rowe, B.: Antigenic relationships between the enteroinvasive *Escherichia coli* O antigens O28ac, O112ac, O124, O136, O143, O144, O152, and O164 and *Shigella* O antigens. J. Clin. Microbiol. *17*:681–684, 1983.
62. Clausen, C. R., and Christie, D. L.: Chronic diarrhea in infants caused by adherent enteropathogenic *Escherichia coli.* J. Pediatr. *100*:358–361, 1982.
63. Cleary, T. G., Cleary, K. R., DuPont, H. L., et al.: The relationship of oral rehydration solution to hypernatremia in infantile diarrhea. J. Pediatr. *99*:739, 1981.
64. Cleary, T. G.: Cytotoxin-producing *Escherichia coli* and hemolytic uremic syndrome. Pediatr. Clin. North Am. *35*:485, 1988.

65. Cleary, T. G., and Lopez, E. L.: The Shiga-like toxin producing *E. coli* and hemolytic uremic syndrome. Pediatr. Infect. Dis. *8*:720, 1989.
66. Clements, M. L., Levine, M. M., Black, R. E., et al.: *Lactobacillus* prophylaxis for diarrhea due to enterotoxigenic *Escherichia coli*. Antimicrob. Agents Chemother. *20*:104–8, 1981.
67. Cohen, M. L., and Gangarosa, E. J.: Nontyphoid salmonellosis. South. Med. J. *71*:1540–1545, 1978.
68. Collier, M. C., Stock, F., DeGirolami, P. C., et al.: Comparison of PCR-based approaches to molecular epidemiologic analysis of *Clostridium difficile*. J. Clin. Microbiol. *34*:1153–1157, 1996.
69. Connolly, M. J., Snow, M. H., and Ingham, H. R.: Ciprofloxacin treatment of recurrent *Salmonella* septicaemia in a patient with acquired immune deficiency syndrome. J. Antimicrob. Chemother. *18*:647, 1986.
70. Cooles, P.: Adjuvant steroids and relapse of typhoid fever. J. Trop. Med. Hyg. *89*:229, 1986.
71. Cornett, J. W. D., Aspeling, R. L., and Mallegol, D.: A double-blind comparative evaluation of loperamide versus diphenoxylate with atropine in acute diarrhea. Curr. Ther. Res. Clin. Exp. *21*:629–637, 1977.
72. Cover, T. L., and Aber, R. C.: *Yersinia enterocolitica*. N. Engl. J. Med. *321*:16, 1989.
73. Cravioto, A., Gross, R. J., Scotland, S. M., et al.: An adhesin factor found in strains of *Escherichia coli* belonging to traditional infantile enteropathogenic *Escherichia coli* serotypes. Curr. Microbiol. *3*:95–99, 1979.
74. Crawford, F. G., and Vermund, S. H.: Human cryptosporidiosis. CRC Crit. Rev. Microbiol. *16*:113, 1988.
75. Current, W. L., Reese, N. C., Ernst, J. V., et al.: Human cryptosporidiosis in immunocompetent and immunodeficient persons: Studies of an outbreak and experimental transmission. N. Engl. J. Med. *308*:1252–1257, 1983.
76. Current, W. L.: *Cryptosporidium:* Its biology and potential for environmental transmission. CRC Crit. Rev. Environ. Control *17*:21, 1986.
77. DaSilva, A. J., Schwartz, D. A., Visvesvara, G. S., et al.: Sensitive PCR diagnosis of infections by *Enterocytozoon bieneusi* (microsporidia) using primers based on the region coding for small-subunit rRNA. J. Clin. Microbiol. *34*:986–987, 1996.
78. Davidson, R. A.: Issues in clinical parasitology: The treatment of giardiasis. Am. J. Gastroenterol. *79*:256–261, 1984.
79. Dean, A. G., Ching, Y. C., Williams, R. G., et al.: Test for *Escherichia coli* enterotoxin using infant mice: Application in a study of diarrhea in children in Honolulu. J. Infect. Dis. *125*:407–411, 1972.
80. DeHovitz, J. A., Pape, J. W., Boncy, M., et al.: Clinical manifestations and therapy of *Isospora belli* infection in patients with the acquired immunodeficiency syndrome. N. Engl. J. Med. *315*:87, 1986.
81. DeLalla, F., Privitera, G., Rinaldi, E., et al.: Treatment of *Clostridium difficile*–associated disease with teicoplanin. Antimicrob. Agents Chemother. *33*:1125, 1989.
82. Delor, I., Kaeckenbeeck, A., Wauters, G., et al.: Nucleotide sequence of *yst*, the *Yersinia enterocolitica* gene encoding the heat-stable enterotoxin, and prevalence of the gene among pathogenic and nonpathogenic yersiniae. Infect. Immun. *58*:2983, 1990.
83. Dennehey, P. H., Gauntlett, D. R., and Tente, W.: Comparison of nine commercial immunoassays for the detection of rotavirus in fecal samples. J. Clin. Microbiol. *26*:1630, 1988.
84. Desportes, I., Le Charpentier, Y., Galian, A., et al.: Occurrence of a new microsporidian: *Enterocytozoon bienusi* n.g., N.sp., in the enterocytes of human patients with AIDS. J. Protozool. *32*:250, 1985.
85. Didier, E. S., Orenstein, J. M., Aldras, A., et al.: Comparison of three staining methods for detecting microsporidia in fluids. J. Clin. Microbiol. *33*:3138–3145, 1995.
86. Dietrich, D. T., Lew, E. A., Kotler, D. P., et al.: Treatment with albendazole for intestinal disease due to *Enterocytozoon bieneusi* in patients with AIDS. J. Infect. Dis. *169*:178–183, 1994.
87. Dobell, C.: A revision of the coccidia parasitic in man. Parasitology *11*:147, 1919.
88. Dolin, R., Reichman, R. C., Roessner, K. D., et al.: Detection by immune electron microscopy of the Snow Mountain agent of acute viral gastroenteritis. J. Infect. Dis. *146*:184–189, 1982.
89. Donnenberg, M. D., and Kaper, J. B.: Enteropathogenic *Escherichia coli*. Infect. Immun. *60*:3953–3961, 1992.
90. Donnenberg, M. S., Yu, J., and Kaper, J. B.: A second chromosomal gene necessary for intimate attachment of enteropathogenic *E. coli* to epithelial cells. J. Bacteriol. *175*:4670–4680, 1993.
91. Donnenberg, M. S., Giron, J. A., Nataro, J. P., et al.: A plasmid-encoded type IV fimbrial gene of enteropathogenic *Escherichia coli* associated with localized ahderence. Mol. Microbiol. *6*:3427–3437, 1992.
92. Donta, S. T., and Myers, M. G.: *Clostridium difficile* toxin in asymptomatic neonates. J. Pediatr. *100*:431–434, 1982.
93. Donta, S. T., Wallace, R. B., Whipp, S. C., et al.: Enterotoxigenic *Escherichia coli* and diarrhea disease in Mexican children. J. Infect. Dis. *135*:482–485, 1977.
94. Dore, G. J., Marriott, D. J., Hing, M. C., et al.: Disseminated microsporidiosis due to *Septata intestinalis* in nine patients infected with the human immunodeficiency virus: Response to therapy with ablendazole. Clin. Infect. Dis. *21*:70–76, 1995.
95. Doyle, M. G., and Pickering, L. K.: Gastrointestinal tract infections in children with AIDS. Semin. Pediatr. Infect. Dis. *1*:64, 1990.
96. Dryjanski, J., Gold, J. W., Ritchie, M. T., et al.: Cryptosporidiosis: Case report in a health team worker. Am. J. Med. *80*:751, 1986.
97. Dudley, M. N., McLaughlin, J. C., Carrington, G., et al.: Oral bacitracin vs. vancomycin therapy for *Clostridium difficile*--induced diarrhea: A randomized double-blind trial. Arch. Intern. Med. *146*:1101, 1986.
98. DuPont, H. L., and Hornick, R. B.: Adverse effects of Lomotil therapy in shigellosis. J. A. M. A. *226*:1525–1528, 1973.
99. DuPont, H. L., Olarte, J., Evans, D. G., et al.: Comparative susceptibility of Latin American and United States students to enteric pathogens. N. Engl. J. Med. *295*:1520–1521, 1976.
100. DuPont, H. L., Sullivan, P., Pickering, L. K., et al.: Symptomatic treatment of diarrhea with bismuth subsalicylate among students attending a Mexican university. Gastroenterology *73*:715–718, 1977.
101. DuPont, H. L., Evans, D. G., Sullivan, P., et al.: Prevention of travelers' diarrhea (emporiatric enteritis) by prophylactic administration of bismuth subsalicylate. J. A. M. A. *243*:237–241, 1980.
102. DuPont, H. L., Reves, R. R., Galindo, E., et al.: Treatment of travelers' diarrhea with trimethoprim/sulfamethoxazole and with trimethoprim alone. N. Engl. J. Med. *307*:841–844, 1982.
103. DuPont, H. L., Ericsson, C. D., Robinson, A., et al.: Current problems in antimicrobial therapy for bacterial enteric infection. Am. J. Med. *82*(Suppl.):324, 1987.
104. Dupont, H. L., Chappell, C. L., Sterling, C. R., et al.: The ineffectivity of *Cryptosporidium parvum* in healthy volunteers. N. Engl. J. Med. *332*:855–859, 1995.
105. Dupont, H. L., and Capsuto, E. G.: Persistent diarrhea in travelers. Clin. Infect. Dis. *22*:124–128, 1996.
106. Eastaugh, J., and Shepherd, S.: Infectious and toxic syndromes from fish and shellfish consumption: A review. Arch. Intern. Med. *149*:1735, 1989.
107. Eidels, L., Proia, R., and Hart, D. A.: Membrane receptors for bacterial toxins. Microbiol. Rev. *47*:596–620, 1983.
108. Eisenberg, M. S., Gaarslev, K., Brown, W., et al.: Staphylococcal food poisoning aboard a commercial aircraft. Lancet *2*:595–599, 1975.
109. Elmer, G. W., Surawicz, C. M., and McFarland, L. V.: Biotherapeutic agents: A neglected modality for the treatment and prevention of selected intestinal and vaginal infections. J. A. M. A. *275*:870–876, 1996.
110. Ericsson, C. D., DuPont, H. L., Evans, D. G., et al.: Bismuth subsalicylate inhibits activity of crude toxins of *Escherichia coli* and *Vibrio cholerae*. J. Infect. Dis. *136*:693–696, 1977.
111. Ericsson, C. D., Pickering, L. K., Sullivan, P., et al.: The role of location of food consumption in the prevention of travelers' diarrhea in Mexico. Gastroenterology *79*:812–816, 1980.
112. Ericsson, C. D., Johnson, P. C., DuPont, H. L., et al.: Ciprofloxacin or trimethoprim/sulfamethoxazole as initial therapy for travelers' diarrhea. Ann. Intern. Med. *106*:216, 1987.
113. Ericsson, C. D., DuPont, H. L., Mathewson, J. J., et al.: Treatment of travelers' diarrhea with sulfamethoxazole and trimethoprim and loperamide. J. A. M. A. *263*:257, 1990.
114. Estes, M. K., and Cohen, J.: Rotavirus gene structure and function. Microbiol. Rev. *53*:410, 1989.
115. Faust, E. C., Giraldo, L. E., Caicedo, G., et al.: Human isosporosis in the Western Hemisphere. Am. J. Med. *10*:343, 1983.
116. Fedorko, D. P., Nelson, N. A., and Cartwright, C. P.: Identification of microsporidia in stool specimens by using PCR and restrition endonucleases. J. Clin. Microbiol. *33*:1739–1741, 1995.
117. Feldman, R. J., Kallich, M., and Weinstein, M. P.: Bacteremia due to *Clostridium difficile*: Case report and review of extraintestinal *C. difficile* infections. Clin. Infect. Dis. *20*:1560–1562, 1995.
118. Feldman, S., Chen, S. L., Pickering, L. K., et al.: Salicylate absorption from a bismuth subsalicylate antidiarrheal preparation. Clin. Pharmacol. Therapeut. *29*:788–792, 1981.
119. Ferreccio, C., Morriss, G., Valdivieso, C., et al.: Efficacy of ciprofloxacin in the treatment of chronic typhoid carriers. J. Infect. Dis. *157*:1235, 1988.
120. Fichtenbaum, C. J., Ritchie, D. J., and Powderly, W. G.: Use of paromomycin for treatment of cryptosporidiosis in AIDS. Clin. Infect. Dis. *16*:298–300, 1993.
121. Fioramonti, J., Droy-Lefaix, M. T., and Bueno, L.: Changes in gastrointestinal motility induced by cholera toxin and experimental osmotic diarrhoea in dogs: Effects of treatment with an argillaceous compound. Digestion *36*:230, 1987.
122. Flanigan, T., Whalen, C., and Turner, J.: *Cryptosporidium* infection and CD4 counts. Ann. Intern. Med. *116*:840–842, 1992.
123. Ford-Jones, E. L., Mindorff, C. M., Gold, R., et. al.: The incidence of viral-associated diarrhea after admission to a pediatric hospital. Am. J. Epidemiol. *131*:711–718, 1990.
124. Freedman, B. J.: Travelers' diarrhoea: Does it occur in the United Kingdom? J. Hyg. (Camb.) *79*:73–75, 1979.
125. Gaastra, W., and deGraaf, F. K.: Host-specific fimbiral adhesions of noninvasive enterotoxigenic *Escherichia coli* strains. Microbiol. Rev. *46*:129–161, 1982.
126. Garcia, L. S., Brewer, T. C., and Bruckner, D. A.: Incidence of *Cryptosporidium* in all patients submitting stool specimens for ova and parasites

examination: Monoclonal antibody IFA method. Diagn. Microbiol. Infect. Dis. *11*:25, 1988.
127. Genta, R. M.: Global prevalence of strongyloidiasis: Critical review with epidemiologic insights into the prevention of disseminated disease. Rev. Infect. Dis. *11*:755, 1989.
128. Ginsburg, C. M.: Lomotil (diphenoxylate and atropine) intoxication. Am. J. Dis. Child. *125*:241, 1973.
129. Girard, D. E., and Keefe, E. B.: *Isospora* and travelers' diarrhea. Ann. Intern. Med. *106*:908, 1987.
130. Giron, J. A., Ho, A. S., and Schoolnik, G. K.: An inducible bundle-forming pilus of enteropathogenic *Escherichia coli*. Science *254*:710–713, 1991.
131. Glass, R. I., Stoll, B. J., Hug, M. I., et al.: Epidemiologic and clinical features of endemic *Campylobacter jejuni* infection in Bangladesh. J. Infect. Dis. 148:292–96, 1983.
132. Glass, R. I., Noel, J., Mitchell, D., et al: The changing epidemiology of astrovirus-associated gastroenteritis. Arch. Virol. In press.
133. Goldberg, M. B., and Sansonetti, P. J.: *Shigella* subversion of the cellular cytoskelton: A strategy for epithelial colonization. Infect. Immun. *61*:4941–4946, 1993.
134. Goodgame, R. W.: Understanding intestinal spore-forming protozoa: Cryptosporidia, microsporidia, isospora, and cyclospora. Ann. Intern. Med. *124*:429–441, 1996.
135. Gorbach, S. L., Carpenter, C. C. J., Grayson, R., et al.: Travelers' diarrhea: Consensus conference. J. A. M. A. *253*:2700–2704, 1985.
136. Gotuzzo, E., Seas, C., Echevarria, J., et al.: Ciprofloxacin for the treatment of cholera: A randomized, double-blind controlled clinical trial of a single dose in Peruvian adults. Clin. Infect. Dis. *20*:1485–1490, 1995.
137. Goyal, R. K., and Hirando, I.: The enteric nervous system. N. Engl. J. Med. *334*:1106–1115, 1996.
138. Greenberg, H. B., Valdesuso, J. R., Kapikian, A. Z., et al.: Prevalence of antibody to the Norwalk virus in various countries. Infect. Immun. *26*:270, 1979.
139. Greenberg, H. B., Valdesuso, J., Yolken, R. H., et al.: Role of Norwalk virus in outbreaks of non-bacterial gastroenteritis. J. Infect. Dis. *139*:564, 1979.
140. Greensmith, C. T., Stanwick, R. S., Elliot, B. E., et al.: Giardiasis associated with the use of a water slide. Pediatr. Infect. Dis. *7*:91, 1988.
141. Gross, T. P., Kamara, L. B., Hatheway, C. L., et al.: *Clostridium perfringens* food poisoning: Use of serotyping in an outbreak setting. J. Clin. Microbiol. *27*:660, 1989.
142. Hanrahan, J. P., and Gordon, M. A.: Mushroom poisoning: Case reports and a review of therapy. J. A. M. A. *251*:1057–1061, 1984.
143. Haque, R., Neville, L. M., Hahn, P., et al.: Rapid diagnosis of *Entamoebla* infection by using *Entamoeba* and *Entamoeba histolytica* stool antigen detection kits. J. Clin. Microbiol. *33*:2558–2561, 1995.
144. Hart, C. A., Baxby, D., and Blundell, N.: Gastroenteritis due to *Cryptosporidium:* A prospective survey in a children's hospital. J. Infect. *9*:264, 1984.
145. Hayes, E. B., Matte, T. D., O'Brien, T. R., et al.: Large community outbreak of cryptosporidiosis due to contamination of a filtered public water supply. N. Engl. J. Med. *320*:1376, 1989.
146. Hedberg, C. W., and Osterholm, M. T.: Outbreaks of food-borne and waterborne viral gastroenteritis. Clin. Microbiol. Rev. *6*:199–210, 1993.
147. Hedberg, C. W., MacDonald, K. L., and Osterholm, M. T.: Changing epidemiology of food-borne disease: A Minnesota prospective. Clin. Infect. Dis. *18*:671–682, 1994.
148. Henderson, A. E., Gillespie, G. W., Kaplan, P., et al.: The human *Isospora*. Am. J. Hyg. *78*:302, 1963.
149. Hennessy, T. W., Hedberg, C. W., Slutsker, L., et al.: A national outbreak of *Salmonella enteritidis* infections from ice cream. N. Engl. J. Med. *334*:1281–1286, 1996.
150. Henricksen, S. A., and Pohlenz, J. F. L.: Staining of cryptosporidia by a modified Ziehl-Neelsen technique. Acta Vet. Scand. *22*:594, 1981.
151. Herrington, D. A., Tzipori, S., Robins-Browne, R. M., et al.: In vitro and in vivo pathogenicity of *Plesiomonas shigelloides*. Infect. Immun. *55*:979, 1987.
152. Hicks, P., Zwiener, J., Squires, J., et al.: Azithromycin therapy for *Cryptosporidium parvum* infection in four children infected with human immunodeficiency virus. J. Infect. Dis. *129*:297–300, 1996.
153. Hinnant, K., Schwartz, A., Rotterdam, H., et al.: Cytomegaloviral and cryptosporidial cholecystitis in two patients with AIDS. Am. J. Surg. Pathol. *13*:57–60, 1989.
154. Hirschhorn, N.: Treatment of acute diarrhea in children: Historical and physiological perspective. J. Clin. Nutr. *33*:637–663, 1980.
155. Hlady, W. G., and Klontz, K. C.: The epidemiology of *Vibrio* infections in Florida, 1981–1993. J. Infect. Dis. *173*:1176–1183, 1996.
156. Ho, M., Glass, R. I., Monroe, S. S., et al.: Viral gastroenteritis aboard a cruise ship. Lancet 2:961, 1989.
157. Hoffman, S. L., Punjabi, N. H., Kumala, S., et al.: Reduction of mortality in chloramphenicol-treated severe typhoid fever by high-dose dexamethasone. N. Engl. J. Med. *310*:82, 1984.
158. Hoge, C. W., Shlim, D. R., Ghimire, M., et al.: Placebo-controlled trial of co-trimoxazole for cyclospora infections among travellers and foreign residents in Nepal. Lancet *345*:691–693, 1995.
159. Hoge, C. W., Shlim, D. R., Echeverria, P., et al.: Epidemiology of diarrhea among expatriate residents living in a highly endemic environment. J. A. M. A. *275*:533–538, 1996.
160. Holmberg, S. D., and Blake, P. A.: Staphylococcal food poisoning in the United States: New facts and old misconceptions. J. A. M. A. *251*:487–489, 1984.
161. Holmberg, S. D., Wachsmuth, I. K., Hickman-Brenner, F. W., et al.: *Plesiomonas* enteric infections in the United States. Ann. Intern. Med. *105*:690, 1986.
162. Holmes, S. J., Morrow, A. L., and Pickering, L. K.: Child care practices: Effects of social changes on epidemiology of infectious diseases and antibiotic resistance. Epidemiol. Rev. *18*:10–28, 1996.
163. Hoogkamp-Korstanje, J. A. A., and Stolk-Engelaar, V. M. M.: *Yersinia enterocolitica* infection in children. Pediatr. Infect. Dis. J. *14*:771–775, 1995.
164. Hovius, S. E. R., and Rietra, P. J.: *Salmonella* colitis clinically presenting as pseudomembranous colitis. Neth. J. Surg. *34*:81–82, 1982.
165. Huang, P., Weber, J. T., Sosin, D. M., et al.: The first reported outreak of diarrheal illness associated with *Cyclospora* in the United States. Ann. Intern. Med. *123*:409–414, 1995.
166. Hughes, J. M., Boyce, J. M., Aleem, A. R. M. A., et al.: *Vibrio parahaemolyticus* enterocolitis in Bangladesh: Report of an outbreak. Am. J. Trop. Med. Hyg. *27*:106–112, 1978.
167. Huicho, L., Campos, M., Rivera, J., et al.: Fecal screening tests in the approach to acute infectious diarrhea: A scientific overview. Pediatr. Infect. Dis. J. *15*:486–494, 1996.
168. Hunt, C. M., Harvey, J. A., Youngs, E. R., et al.: Clinical and pathological variability of infection by enterohaemorrhagic (verocytotoxin producing) *E. coli*. J. Clin. Pathol. *42*:847, 1989.
169. Islam, A., Butler, T., Nath, S. K., et al.: Randomized treatment of patients with typhoid fever by using ceftriaxone or chloramphenicol. J. Infect. Dis. *158*:742, 1988.
170. Jacobs, J. L., Gold, J. W. M., Murray, H. W., et al.: *Salmonella* infections in patients with the acquired immunodeficiency syndrome. Ann. Intern. Med. *102*:186–188, 1985.
171. Janda, J. M., and Duffey, P. S.: Mesophilic aeromonads in human disease: Current toxonomy, laboratory identification and infectious disease spectrum. Rev. Infect. Dis. *10*:980, 1988.
172. Janda, J. M., Powers, C., Bryant, R. G., et al.: Current perspectives on the epidemiology and pathogenesis of clinically significant *Vibrio* spp. Clin. Microbiol. Rev. *1*:245, 1988.
173. Janda, J. M., Abbott, S. L., Khashe, S., et al.: Further studies on biochemical characteristics and serologic properties of the genus *Aeromonas*. J. Clin. Microbiol. *34*:1930–1933, 1996.
174. Jiang, X., Graham, D. Y., Wang, K., et al.: Norwalk virus genome cloning and characterization. Science *250*:1580–1583, 1991.
175. Jiang, X., Wang, M., Graham, D. Y., et al.: Expression, self-assembly and antigenicity of the Norwalk virus capsid protein. J. Virol. *66*:6527–6532, 1992.
176. Jiang, X., Matson, D. O., Velazquez, F. R., et al.: A study of Norwalk-related viruses in Mexican children. J. Med. Virol. *47*:309–316, 1995.
177. Jiang, X., Turf, E., Hu, J., et al.: Outbreaks of gastroenteritis in elderly nursing homes and retirement facilities associated with human caliciviruses. J. Med. Virol. *50*:335–341, 1996.
178. Kabir, I., Butler, T., and Khanam, A.: Comparative efficacies of single intravenous doses of ceftriaxone and ampicillin for shigellosis in a placebo-controlled trial. Antimicrob. Agents Chemother. *29*:645, 1986.
179. Kain, K. C., and Kelly, M. T.: Clinical features, epidemiology, and treatment of *Plesiomonas shigelloides* diarrhea. J. Clin. Microbiol. *27*:998, 1989.
180. Kaper, J. B., Morris, J. G., Jr., and Levine, M. M.: Cholera. Clin. Microbiol. Rev. *8*:48–86, 1995.
181. Kapikian, A. Z., Wyatt, R. G., Dolin, R., et al.: Visualization by immune electron microscopy of a 27-nm particle associated with acute infectious nonbacterial gastroenteritis. J. Virol. *10*:1075–1081, 1972.
182. Kaplan, J. E., Gary, G. W., Baron, R. C., et al.: Epidemiology of Norwalk gastroenteritis and the role of Norwalk virus in outbreaks of acute nonbacterial gastroenteritis. Ann. Intern. Med. *96*:756–761, 1982.
183. Karmali, M. A., Petric, M., Lim, C., et al.: The association between idiopathic hemolytic uremic syndrome and infection by verotoxin-producing *Escherichia coli*. J. Infect. Dis. *151*:775–782, 1985.
184. Karmali, M. A.: Infection by verocytotoxin-producing *Escherichia coli*. Clin. Microbiol. Rev. 2:15, 1989.
185. Kelber, M., and Ament, M. E.: *Shigella dysenteriae* I: A forgotton cause of pseudomembranous colitis. J. Pediatr. *89*:595, 1976.
186. Kent, G. P., Greenspan, J. R., Herndon, J. L., et al.: Epidemic giardiasis caused by a contaminated public water supply. Am. J. Public Health *78*:139, 1988.
187. Keusch, G. T., and Bennish, M. L.: Shigellosis: Recent progress, persisting problems and research issues. Pediatr. Infect. Dis. *8*:713, 1989.
188. Kluytmans, J., van Leeuwen, W., Goessens, W., et al.: Food-initiated outbreak of methicillin-resistant *Staphylococcus aureus* analyzed by pheno- and genotyping. J. Clin. Microbiol. *33*:1121–1128, 1995.
189. Knisley, C. V., Bednarz-Prashad, A. J., and Pickering, L. K.: Detection of rotavirus in stool specimens with monoclonal and polyclonal antibody-based assay systems. J. Clin. Microbiol. *23*:897–900, 1986.
190. Knisley, C. V., Englekirk, P. G., Pickering, L. K., et al.: Rapid detection of *Giardia* antigen in stool using enzyme immunoassays. Am. J. Clin. Pathol. *91*:704, 1989.
191. Koch, K. L., Phillips, D. J., Aber, R. C., et al.: Cryptosporidiosis in hospital

personnel: Evidence for person-to-person transmission. Ann. Intern. Med. *102*:593, 1985.
192. Konno, T., Suzuki, H., Ishida, M., et al.: Astrovirus-associated epidemic gastroenteritis in Japan. J. Med. Virol. *9*:1, 1982.
193. Koo, D., Maloney, K., and Tauxe, R.: Epidemiology of diarrheal disease outbreaks on cruise ships, 1986 through 1993. J. A. M. A. *275*:545–547, 1996.
194. Kotler, D. P., Gaetz, H. P., Lange, M., et al.: Enteropathy associated with acquired immunodeficiency syndrome. Ann. Intern. Med. *101*:421–428, 1984.
195. Kotler, D. P., Francisco, A., Clayton, F., et al.: Small intestinal injury and parasitic diseases in AIDS. Ann. Intern. Med. *113*:444, 1990.
196. Kotloff, K. L., Losonsky, G. A., Morris, J. G., et al.: Enteric adenovirus infection and childhood diarrhea: An epidemiologic study in three clinical settings. Pediatrics *84*:219, 1989.
197. Kramer, M. N., Herwaldt, B. L., Craun, G. F., et al.: Surveillance for waterborne-disease outbreaks: United States 1993–1994. M. M. W. R. *45*(SS-1):1, 1996.
198. Kreutner, A. K., Del Bene, V. E., and Amstey, M. S.: Giardiasis in pregnancy. Am. J. Obstet. Gynecol. *140*:895–901, 1981.
199. Kristjansson, M., Samore M. H., Gerding, D. N., et al.: Comparison of restriction endonuclease analysis, ribotyping, and pulsed-field gel electrophoresis for molecular differentiation of *Clostridium difficile* strains. J. Clin. Microbiol. *32*:1963–1969, 1994.
200. Kuritsky, J. N., Osterholm, M. T., Greenberg, H. B., et al.: Norwalk gastroenteritis: A community outbreak associated with bakery product consumption. Ann. Intern. Med. *201:519–521,* 1984.
201. Kurtz, J., and Lee, T.: Astrovirus gastroenteritis: Age distribution of antibody. Med. Microbiol. Immunol. *177*:227, 1978.
202. Lacroix, J., Delage, G., Gosselin, F., et al.: Severe protracted diarrhea due to multiresistant adherent *Escherichia coli.* Am. J. Dis. Child. *138*:693–696, 1984.
203. Laughon, B. E., Druckman, D. A., Vernon, A., et al.: Prevalence of enteric pathogens in homosexual men with and without acquired immunodeficiency syndrome. Gastroenterology *94*:984, 1988.
204. Lecuit, M., Oksenhendler, E., and Sarfati, C.: Use of albendazole for disseminated microsporidian infection in a patient with AIDS. Clin. Infect. Dis. *19*:332–333, 1994.
205. Lee, L. A., Gerber, A. R., Lonsway, D. R., et al.: *Yersinia enterocolitica* 0:3 infections in infants and children, associated with the household preparation of chitterlings. N. Engl. J. Med. *322*:984, 1990.
206. Lee, L. A., Puhr, N. D., Maloney, K., et al.: Increase in antimicrobial-resistant *Salmonella* infections in the United States. J. Infect. Dis. *170*:128–134, 1994.
207. Levine, M. M., Hughes, T. P., Black, R. E., et al.: Variability of sodium and sucrose levels of simple sugar/salt oral rehydration solutions prepared under optimal and field conditions. J. Pediatr. *97*:324–327, 1980.
208. Levine, M. M., and Edelman, R.: Enteropathogenic *Escherichia coli* of classic serotypes associated with infant diarrhea: Epidemiology and pathogenesis. Epidemiol. Rev. *6*:31–51, 1984.
209. Levine, W. C., Bennett, R. W., Choi, Y., et al.: Staphylococcal food poisoning caused by imported canned mushrooms. J. Infect. Dis. *173*:1263–1267, 1996.
210. Lew, J. F., LeBaron, C. W., Glass, R. I., et al.: Recommendations for collection of laboratory specimens associated with outbreaks of gastroenteritis. M. M. W. R. *39*(RR-14):1–13, 1990.
211. Liebman, W. M., Thaler, M. M., DeLorimier, A., et al.: Intractable diarrhea of infancy due to intestinal coccidiosis. Gastroenterology *78*:579, 1980.
212. Limson, B. M., and Littana, R. T.: Ciprofloxacin vs. co-trimoxazole in *Salmonella* enteric fever. Infection *17*:105, 1989.
213. Lo, C. W., and Walker, W. A.: Chronic protracted diarrhea of infancy: A nutritional disease. Pediatrics *72*:786–800, 1983.
214. Lopez-Vidal, Y., Calva, J. J., Trujillo, A., et al.: Enterotoxins and adhesions of enterotoxigenic *Escherichia coli:* Are they risk factors for acute diarrhea in the community? J. Infect. Dis. *162*:442, 1990.
215. Louie, E., Barkowsky, W., and Klesius, P. H.: Treatment of cryptosporidiosis with oral bovine transfer factor. Clin. Immunol. Immunopathol. *44*:329, 1987.
216. Lowry, P. W., Pavia, A. T., McFarland, L. M., et al.: Cholera in Louisiana: Widening spectrum of seafood vehicles. Arch. Intern. Med. *149*:2079, 1989.
217. Luby, S., Jones, J., Dowda, H., et al.: A large outbreak of gastroenteritis caused by diarrheal toxin-producing *Bacillus cereus.* J. Infect. Dis. *167*:1452–1455, 1993.
218. Lyerly, D. M., Krivan, H. C., and Wilkins, T. D.: *Clostridium difficile:* Its diseases and toxins. Clin. Microbiol. Rev. *1*:1, 1988.
219. MacDonald, K. L., and Cohen, M. L.: Epidemiology of travelers' diarrhea: Current perspectives. Rev. Infect. Dis. *8*:117S, 1986.
220. MacKenzie, W. R., Hoxie, N. J., Proctor, M. E., et al.: A massive outbreak in Milwaukee of *Cryptosporidium* infection transmitted through the public water supply. N. Engl. J. Med. *331*:161–167, 1994.
221. Mahon, B. E., Mintz, E. D., Greene, K. D., et al.: Reported cholera in the United States, 1992–1994: A reflection of global changes in cholera epidemiology. J. A. M. A. *276*:307–312, 1996.
222. Manabe, Y. C., Vinetz, J. M., Moore, R. D., et. al.: *Clostridium difficile* colitis: An efficient clinical approach to diagnosis. Ann. Intern. Med. *123*:835–840, 1995.
223. Margolis, P. A., Litteer, T., Hare, N., et al.: Effects of unrestricted diet on mild infantile diarrhea. Am. J. Dis. Child. *144*:162, 1990.
224. Martin, D. L., MacDonald, K. L., White, K. E., et al.: The epidemiology and clinical aspects of the hemolytic uremic syndrome in Minnesota. N. Engl. J. Med. *323*:1161, 1990.
225. Martino, P., Gentile, G., Caprioli, A., et al.: Hospital acquired cryptosporidiosis in a bone marrow transplantation unit. J. Infect. Dis. *158*:647, 1988.
226. Mathewson, J. J., Johnson, P. C., DuPont, H. L., et al.: A newly recognized cause of travelers' diarrhea: Enteroadherent *Escherichia coli.* J. Infect. Dis. *151*:471–475, 1985.
227. Mathewson, J. J., Oberhelman, R. A., DuPont, H. L., et al.: Enteroadherent *E. coli* as a cause of diarrhea among children in Mexico. J. Clin. Microbiol. *25*:1917, 1987.
228. Mathewson, J. J., and Cravioto, A.: HEp-2 cell adherence as an assay for virulence among diarrheagenic *Escherichia coli.* J. Infect. Dis. *159*:1057, 1989.
229. Matson, D. O., Estes, M. K., Glass, R. I., et al.: Human calicivirus-associated diarrhea in children attending day care centers. J. Infect. Dis. *159*:71, 1989.
230. Matson, D. O., and Estes, M. K.: Impact of rotavirus infection at a large pediatric hospital. J. Infect. Dis. *162*:598, 1990.
231. Matson, D. O., Estes, M. K., Burns, J. W., et al.: Serotype variation of human group A rotaviruses in two regions of the United States. J. Infect. Dis. *162*:605, 1990.
232. Matson, D. O., Estes, M. K., Tanaka, T., et al.: Asymptomatic human calicivirus infection in a day care center. Pediatr. Infect. Dis. *9*:190, 1990.
233. McClane, B. A., and Wnek, A. P.: Studies of *Clostridium perfringens* enterotoxin action at different temperatures demonstrate a correlation between complex formation and cytotoxicity. Infect. Immun. *58*:3109, 1990.
234. McFarland, L. V., Mulligan, M. E., Kwok, R. Y. Y., et al.: Nosocomial acquisition of *Clostridium difficile* infection. N. Engl. J. Med. *320*:204, 1989.
235. McFarland, L. V., Surawicz, C. M., and Stamm, W. E.: Risk factors for *Clostridium difficile* carriage and *C. difficile*-associated diarrhea in a cohort of hospitalized patients. J. Infect. Dis. *162*:678, 1990.
236. McFarland, L. V., Surawicz, C. M., Greenberg, R. N., et al.: A randomized placebo-controlled trial of *Saccharomyces boulardii* in combination with standard antibiotics for *Clostridium difficile* disease. J. A. M. A. *271*:1913–1918, 1994.
237. Medical Letter: Drugs for parasitic infections. Med. Lett. *37*:99–108, 1995.
238. Medical Letter: The choice of antibacterial drugs. Med. Lett. *38*:25–34, 1996.
239. Medical Letter: Advice for travelers. Med. Lett. *38*:17–20, 1996.
240. Mendelowitz, P. C., Hoffman, R. S., and Weber, S.: Bismuth absorption and myoclonic encephalopathy during bismuth subsalicylate therapy. Ann. Intern. Med. *112*:140, 1990.
241. Merz, C. S, Kramer, C., Forman, M., et al.: Comparison of four commercially available rapid enzyme immunoassays with cytotoxin assay for detection of *Clostridium difficile* toxin(s) from stool specimens. J. Clin. Microbiol. *32*:1142–1147, 1994.
242. Midthun, K., and Kapikian, A. Z.: Rotavirus vaccines: An overview. Clin. Microbiol. Rev. *9*:423–434, 1996.
243. Mitchell, D. K., and Pickering, L. K.: Nosocomial gastrointestinal tract infections in pediatric patients. *In* Mayhall, C. G. (ed.): Hospital Epidemiology and Infection Control. Baltimore, Williams & Wilkins, 1995, pp. 506–523.
244. Mitchell, D. K., Van, R., Morrow, A. L., et al.: Outbreaks of astrovirus gastroenteritis in day care centers. J. Pediatr. *123*:725–732, 1993.
245. Mitchell, D. K., Monroe, S. S., Jiang, X., et al.: Virologic features of an astrovirus diarrhea outbreak in a day care center revealed by reverse transcriptase-polymerase chain reaction. J. Infect. Dis. *172*:1437–1444, 1995.
246. Mitchell, D. K., Van, R., Mason, E. H., et al.: Prospective study of toxigenic *Clostridium difficile* in children given amoxicillin/clavulanate for otitis media. Pediatr. Infect. Dis. J. *15*:514–519, 1996.
247. Moe, C. L., Gentsch, J., Grohmann, G., et al.: Application of PCR to detection of Norwalk virus in fecal specimens from outbreaks of gastroenteritis. J. Clin. Microbiol. *32*:642–648, 1994.
248. Moosa, A., and Rubidge, C. J.: Once daily ceftriaxone vs. chloramphenicol for treatment of typhoid fever in children. Pediatr. Infect. Dis. *8*:696, 1989.
249. Morgan, D. R., Johnson, P. C., DuPont, H. L., et al.: Lack of correlation between known virulence properties of *Aeromonas hydrophila* and enteropathogenicity for humans. Infect. Immun. *50*:62, 1985.
250. Morse, D. L., Guzewich, J. J., Hanrahan, J. P., et al.: Widespread outbreaks of clam- and oyster-associated gastroenteritis: Role of Norwalk virus. N. Engl. J. Med. *314*:678–681, 1986.
251. Moss, J., Burns, D. L., Hsia, J. A., et al.: Cyclic nucleotides: Mediators of bacterial toxin action in diseases. Ann. Intern. Med. *101*:653, 1984.
252. Motala, C., Hill, I. D., Mann, M. D., et al.: Effect of loperamide on stool output and duration of acute infectious diarrhea in infants. J. Pediatr. *117*:467, 1990.
253. Murray, B. E.: Problems and mechanisms of antimicrobial resistance. Infect. Dis. Clin. North Am. *3*:423, 1990.
254. Murrell, T. G. C., Egerton, J. R., Rampling, A., et al.: The ecology and

epidemiology of the pig-bel syndrome in man in New Guinea. J. Hyg. *64*:375–396, 1966.
255. Nakata, S., Estes, M. K., Graham, D. Y., et al.: Detection of antibodies to group B adult diarrhea rotaviruses in humans. J. Clin. Microbiol. *25*:812, 1987.
256. Nalin, D. R., Harland, E., Ramlal, A., et al.: Comparison of low and high sodium and potassium content in oral rehydration solution. J. Pediatr. *97*:848–853, 1980.
257. Nataro, J. P., Yikang, D., Giron, J. A., et al.: Aggregative adherence fimbria I expression in enteroaggregative *Escherichia coli* requires two unlinked plasmid regions. Infect. Immun. *61*:1126–1131, 1993.
258. Nazer, H., Rice, S., and Walker-Smith, J. A.: Clinical associations of stool astrovirus in childhood. J. Pediatr. Gastroenterol. Nutr. *1*:555, 1982.
259. Nelson, J. D., and Haltalin, K. C.: Amoxicillin less effective than ampicillin against *Shigella* in vitro and in vivo: Relationship of efficacy to activity in serum. J. Infect. Dis. *129*(Suppl.):222–227, 1974.
260. Nelson, J. D., Kusmiesz, H., and Jackson, L. H.: Comparison of trimethoprim-sulfamethoxazole and ampicillin therapy for shigellosis in ambulatory patients. J. Pediatr. *89*:491–493, 1976.
261. Newland, J. W., and Neill, R. J.: DNA probes for Shiga-like toxins I and II and for toxin-converting bacteriophages. J. Clin. Microbiol. *26*:1292, 1988.
262. Nishibuchi, M., Fasano, A., Russell, R. G., et al.: Enterotoxigenicity of *V. parahaemolyticus* with and without genes encoding thermostable direct hemolysin. Infect. Immun. *60*:3539–3545, 1992.
263. Novak, E., Lee, J. G., Seckman, C. E., et al.: Unfavorable effect of atropine-diphenoxylate (Lomotil) therapy in lincomycin-caused diarrhea. J. A. M. A. *235*:1451, 1976.
264. O'Brien, A. D., Lively, T. A., Chang, T. W., et al.: Purification of *Shigella dysenteriae* 1 (Shiga)-like toxin from *Escherichia coli* O157:H7 strain associated with haemorrhagic colitis. Lancet *2*:573, 1983.
265. O'Brien, A. D., and Holmes, R. K.: Shiga and Shiga-like toxins. Microbiol. Rev. *51*:206, 1987.
266. Olive, D. M., Johny, M., and Sethi, S. K.: Use of an alkaline phosphatase-labeled synthetic oligonucleotide probe for detection of *Campylobacter jejuni* and *Campylobacter coli*. J. Clin. Microbiol. *28*:1565, 1990.
267. On, S. L. W.: Identification methods for campylobacters, helicobacters, and related organisms. Clin. Microbiol. Rev. *9*:405–422, 1996.
268. Ooi, W. W., Zimmerman, S. K., and Needham, C. A.: *Cyclospora* species as a gastrointestinal pathogen in immunocompetent hosts. J. Clin. Microbiol. *33*:1267–1269, 1995.
269. O'Ryan, M., Matson, D. O., Estes, M. K., et al.: Molecular epidemiology of rotaviruses in children attending day care centers in Houston. J. Infect. Dis. *162*:810, 1990.
270. O'Ryan, M., and Matson, D. O.: Viral gastroenteritis pathogens in the day care center setting. Semin. Pediatr. Infect. Dis. *1*:252, 1990.
271. Ortega, Y. R., Sterling, C. R., Gilman R. H., et al.: *Cyclospora* species: A new protozoan pathogen of humans. N. Engl. J. Med. *328*:1308–1312, 1993.
272. Osterholm, M. T., MacDonald, K. L., White, K. E., et al.: An outbreak of brainerdiasis: An outbreak of a newly recognized chronic diarrhea syndrome associated with raw milk consumption. J. A. M. A. *256*:484–490, 1986.
273. Panosian, C. B.: Parasitic diarrhea. Infect. Dis. Clin. North Am. *2*:685, 1988.
274. Pape, J. W., Verdier, R., Johnson, W. D., et al.: Treatment and prophylaxis of *Isospora belli* infection in patients with the acquired immunodeficiency syndrome. N. Engl. J. Med. *320*:1044, 1989.
275. Pape, J. W., and Johnson, W. D., Jr.: *Isospora belli* infection. Prog. Clin. Parasitol. *2*:119–127, 1991.
276. Pape, J. W., Verdier, R. I., Boncy, M., et al.: *Cyclospora* infection in adults infected with HIV: Clinical manifestations, treatment and prophylaxis. Ann. Intern. Med. *121*:654–657, 1994.
277. Parsonnet, J., Trock, S. C., Bopp, C. A., et al.: Chronic diarrhea associated with drinking untreated water. Ann. Intern. Med. *110*:985, 1989.
278. Pavia, A. T., Shipman, L. D., Wells, J. G., et al.: Epidemiologic evidence that prior antimicrobial exposure decreases resistance to infection by antimicrobial-sensitive *Salmonella*. J. Infect. Dis. *161*:255, 1990.
279. Pearce, J. L., and Hamilton, J. R.: Controlled trial of orally administered lactobacilli in acute infantile diarrhea. J. Pediatr. *84*:261–262, 1974.
280. Perl, T. M., Bédard, L., Kosatsky, T., et al.: An outbreak of toxic encephalopathy caused by eating mussels contaminated with domoic acid. N. Engl. J. Med. *322*:1775, 1990.
281. Perryman, L. E., Riggs, M. W., Mason, P. H., et al.: Kinetics of *Cryptosporidium parvum* sporozoite neutralization by monoclonal antibodies, immune bovine serum, and immune bovine colostrum. Infect. Immun. *58*:157, 1990.
282. Phillips, W. E.: Treatment of chronic carriers with ampicillin. J. A. M. A. *217*:913–915, 1971.
283. Pickering, L. K., DuPont, H. L., Evans, D. G., et al.: Isolation of enteric pathogens in asymptomatic students from the United States and Latin America. J. Infect. Dis. *135*:1003–1005, 1977.
284. Pickering, L. K., DuPont, H. L., Olarte, J., et al.: Fecal leukocytes in enteric infections. Am. J. Clin. Pathol. *68*:562–565, 1977.
285. Pickering, L. K., Evans, D. G., Munoz, O., et al.: Prospective evaluation of enteropathogens in children with diarrhea in Houston and Mexico. J. Pediatr. *93*:383–388, 1978.
286. Pickering, L. K., Evans, D. G., DuPont, H. L., et al.: Diarrhea caused by *Shigella*, *Rotavirus*, and *Giardia* in day care centers: Prospective study. J. Pediatr. *99*:51–56, 1981.
287. Pickering, L. K., Feldman, S., Ericsson, C. D., et al.: Absorption of salicylate and bismuth from a bismuth subsalicylate containing compound (Pepto-Bismol). J. Pediatr. *99*:654–656, 1981.
288. Pickering, L. K., Bartlett, A. V., Reves, R. R., et al.: Asymptomatic excretion of rotavirus before and after rotavirus diarrhea in children in day care centers. J. Pediatr. *112*:361, 1988.
289. Pickering, L. K., and Engelkirk, P. G.: *Giardia lamblia*. Pediatr. Clin. North Am. *35*:565, 1988.
290. Pickering, L. K.: Bacterial and parasitic enteropathogens in day care. Semin. Pediatr. Infect. Dis. *1*:263, 1990.
291. Pickering, L. K., and Matson, D. O.: Therapy for diarrheal disease in children. *In* Blaser, M. J., Smith, P. D., Ravdin, J. I., et al. (eds.): Infections of the Gastrointestinal Tract. New York, Raven Press, 1995, pp. 1401–1415.
292. Pickering, L. K., and Morrow, A. L.: Factors in human milk that protect against diarrhea disease. Infection *21*:355–357, 1993.
293. Pickering, L. K.: Infections of the gastrointestinal tract. *In* Pizzo, P. A., and Wilfert, C. M. (eds.): Pediatric AIDS. The Challenge of HIV Infection in Infants, Children and Adolescents. 2nd ed. Baltimore, Williams & Wilkins, 1994, pp. 377–404.
294. Pickering, L. K., Obrig, T. G., and Stapleton, F. B.: Hemolytic uremic syndrome and enterohemorrhagic *Escherichia coli*. Pediatr. Infect. Dis. J. *13*:459–475, 1994.
295. Pickering, L K.: Emerging antibiotic resistance in enteric bacterial pathogens. Semin. Pediatr. Infect. Dis. In press.
296. Pitman, F. E.: Adverse effects of Lomotil. Gastroenterology *67*:408–410, 1974.
297. Pol, S., Romana, C. A., Richard, S., et al.: Microsporidia infection in patients with the human immunodeficiency virus and unexplained cholangitis. N. Engl. J. Med. *328*:95–99, 1993.
298. Pollard, D. R., Johnson, W. M., Lior, H., et al.: Rapid and specific detection of verotoxin genes in *Escherichia coli* by the polymerase chain reaction. J. Clin. Microbiol. *28*:540, 1990.
299. Porter, J. D., Ragazzoni, H. P., Buchanon, J. D., et al.: *Giardia* transmission in a swimming pool. Am. J. Public Health *78*:659, 1988.
300. Potter, M. E., Kaufmann, A. F., Blake, P. A., et al.: Unpasteurized milk. The hazards of a health fetish. J. A. M. A. *252*:2048–2054, 1984.
301. Provisional Committee on Quality Improvement, Subcommittee on Acute Gastroenteritis, American Academy of Pediatrics: Practice parameter: The management of acute gastroenteritis in young children. Pediatrics *97*:424–436, 1996.
302. Rabbani, G. H., Islam, M. R., Butler, T., et al.: Single-dose treatment of cholera with furazolidone or tetracycline in a double-blind randomized trial. Antimicrob. Agents Chemother. *33*:1447, 1989.
303. Ramirez, C. A., Bran, J. L., Mejia, C. R., et al.: Open, prospective study of the clinical efficacy of ciprofloxacin. Antimicrob. Agents Chemother. *28*:128, 1985.
304. Rateau, J. G., Morgant, G., Droy-Priot, M. T., et al.: A histological, enzymatic and water-electrolyte study of the action of smectite, a mucoprotective clay, on experimental infectious diarrhoea in the rabbit. Curr. Med. Res. Opin. *8*:233, 1982.
305. Ravdin, J. I.: Amebiasis. Clin. Infect. Dis. *20*.1453–1466, 1995.
306. Rees, J. H., Soudain, S. E., Gregson, N. A., et al.: *Campylobacter jejuni* infection and Guillain-Barré syndrome. N. Engl. J. Med. *333*:1374–1379, 1995.
307. Reid, J. A., White, D. G., Caul, E. O., et al.: Role of infected food handler in hotel outbreak of Norwalk-like viral gastroenteritis: Implications for control. Lancet *2*:321, 1988.
308. Rijpstra, A. C., Canning, E. U., van Ketel, R. J., et al.: Use of light microscopy to diagnose small intestinal microsporidiosis in patients with AIDS. J. Infect. Dis. *157*:827, 1988.
309. Riley, L. W., Remis, R. S., Helgerson, S. D., et al.: Hemorrhagic colitis associated with a rare *Escherichia coli* serotype. N. Engl. J. Med. *308*:681–685, 1983.
310. Rippey, S. R.: Infectious diseases associated with molluscan shellfish consumption. Clin. Microbiol. Rev. *7*:419–425, 1994.
311. Rosenthal, P., and Liebman, W. M.: Comparative study of stool examination, duodenal aspiration and pediatric Entero-test for giardiasis in children. J. Pediatr. *96*:278–279, 1980.
312. Rothbaum, R., McAdams, A. J., Giannella, R., et al.: A clinicopathologic study of enterocyte-adherent *Escherichia coli*: A cause of protracted diarrhea in infants. Gastroenterology *83*:441–454, 1982.
313. Rothbaum, R. J., Partin, J. C., Saalfield, K., et al.: An ultrastructural study of enteropathogenic *Escherichia coli* infection in human infants. Ultrastruct. Pathol. *4*:291–301, 1983.
314. Rubin, F. A., McWhirter, P. D., Punjabi, N. H., et al.: Use of a DNA probe to detect *Salmonella typhi* in the blood of patients with typhoid fever. J. Clin. Microbiol. *27*:1112, 1989.
315. Ruiz-Palacios, G. M., Torres, J., Torres, N. I., et al.: Cholera-like enterotoxin produced by *Campylobacter jejuni*: Characterization and significance. Lancet *2*:250–252, 1983.
316. Rumack, B. H., and Temple, A. R.: Lomotil poisoning. Pediatrics *53*:495, 1974.
317. Rusmak, J., Hadfield, T. L., Rhodes, M., et al.: Detection of *Cryptosporidium*

oocysts in human fecal specimens by an indirect immunofluorescence assay with monoclonal antibodies. J. Clin. Microbiol. *27*:1135, 1989.

318. Ryan, C. A., Hargrett-Bean, N. T., and Blake, P. A.: *Salmonella typhi* infections in the United States, 1975–1984: Increasing role of foreign travel. J. Infect. Dis. *11*:1, 1989.
319. Ryder, R. W., Wells, J. G., and Gangarosa, E. J.: A study of travelers' diarrhea in foreign visitors to the United States. J. Infect. Dis. *136*:605–607, 1977.
320. Saavedra, J. M., Bauman, N. A., Oung, I., et al.: Feeding of *Bifidobacterium bifidum* and *Streptococcus thermophilus* to infants in hospital for prevention of diarrhoea and shedding of rotavirus. Lancet *344*:1046–1049, 1994.
321. Sack, R. B.: Antimicrobial prophylaxis of travelers diarrhea: A selected summary. Rev. Infect. Dis. *2*(Suppl.):160, 1986.
322. Saez-Llorens, X., Odio, C. M., Umaña, M. A., et al.: Spiramycin vs. placebo for treatment of acute diarrhea caused by *Cryptosporidium*. Pediatr. Infect. Dis. *8*:136, 1989.
323. Salam, M. A., and Bennish, M. L.: Therapy for shigellosis. I. Randomized, double-blind trial of nalidixic acid in childhood shigellosis. J. Pediatr. *113*:901, 1988.
324. Salazar-Lindo, E., Sack, B., Chea-Woo, E., et al.: Early treatment with erythromycin of *Campylobacter jejuni* associated dysentery in children. J. Pediatr. *109*:355, 1986.
325. Sansonetti, P. J., Kopecko, D. J., and Formal, S. B.: Involvement of a plasmid in the invasive ability of *Shigella flexneri*. Infect. Immun. *35*:852–860, 1982.
326. Santosham, M., Foster, S., Reid, R., et al.: Role of soy-based, lactose-free formula during treatment of acute diarrhea. Pediatrics *76*:292–298, 1985.
327. Santosham, M., and Greenough, W. B., III: Oral rehydration therapy: Global prospective. J. Pediatr. *118*:44–51, 1991.
328. Savarino, S. J., Fasano, A., Watson, J., et al.: Enteroaggregative *Escherichia coli* heat-stable enterotoxin 1 represents another subfamily of *E. coli* heat-stable toxin. Proc. Natl. Acad. Sci. U. S. A. *90*:3093–3097, 1993.
329. Schantz, P. M.: The dangers of eating raw fish. N. Engl. J. Med. *320*:1143, 1989.
330. Schleupner, M. A., Garner, D. C., Sosnowski, K. M., et al.: Concurrence of *Clostridium difficile* toxin A enzyme-linked immunosorbent assay, fecal lactoferrin assay, and clinical criteria with *C. difficile* cytotoxin titer in two patient cohorts. J. Clin. Microbiol. *33*:1755–1759, 1995.
331. Sears, C. L., and Kaper, J. B.: Enteric bacterial toxins: Mechanisms of action and linkage to intestinal secretion. Microbiol. Rev. *60*:167–215, 1996.
332. Serény, B.: Experimental *Shigella* keratoconjunctivitis: A preliminary report. Acta Microbiol. Acad. Sci. *2*:293–296, 1955.
333. Shadduck, J. A., and Greeley, E.: *Microsporidia* and human infections. Clin. Microbiol. Rev. *2*:158, 1989.
334. Shadduck, J. A., Meccoli, R. A., Davis, R., et al.: Isolation of a microsporidian from a human patient. J. Infect. Dis. *162*:773, 1990.
335. Shedl, H. P., and Clifton, J. A.: Solute and water absorption by the human small intestine. Nature *199*:1264–1267, 1963.
336. Shinozaki, T., Araki, K., Ushijima, H., et al.: Antibody response to enteric adenovirus types 40 and 41 in sera from people in various age groups. J. Clin. Microbiol. *25*:1679, 1987.
337. Sloven, D. G., Jirapinyo, P., and Lebenthal, E.: Hydrolysis and absorption of glucose polymers from rice compared with corn in chronic diarrhea in infancy. J. Pediatr. *116*:876, 1990.
338. Smith, M. D., Duong, N. M., Hoa, N. T. T., et al.: Comparison of ofloxacin and ceftriaxone for short-course treatment of enteric fever. Antimicrob. Agents Chemother. *38*:1716–1720, 1994.
339. Smith, P. D., Macher, A. M., Bookman, M. A., et al.: *Salmonella typhimurium* enteritis and bacteremia in the acquired immunodeficiency syndrome. Ann. Intern. Med. *102*:207, 1985.
340. Smith, P. D., Lane, H. C., Gill, V. J., et al.: Intestinal infections in patients with the acquired immunodeficiency syndrome (AIDS). Ann. Intern. Med. *108*:328, 1988.
341. Soe, G. B., and Overturf, G. D.: Treatment of typhoid fever and other systemic salmonelloses with cefotaxime, ceftriaxone, cefoperazone, and other newer cephalosporins. Rev. Infect. Dis. *9*:719, 1987.
342. Sohel, I., Puente, J. L., Murray, W. J., et al.: Cloning and characterization of the bundle-forming pilin gene of enteropathogenic *Escherichia coli* and its distribution in *Salmonella* serotypes. Mol. Microbiol. *7*:563–575, 1993.
343. Soriano-Brücher, H. E., Avendaño, P., O'Ryan, M., et al.: Use of bismuth subsalicylate in acute diarrhea in children. Rev. Infect. Dis. *12*:S51, 1990.
344. Soriano-Brücher, H., Avendaño, P., O'Ryan, M., et al.: Bismuth subsalicylate in the treatment of acute diarrhea in children: A clinical study. Pediatrics *87*:18–27, 1991.
345. Sorvillo, F. J., Waterman, S. H., Vogt, J. K., et al.: Shigellosis associated with recreational water contact in Los Angeles County. Am. J. Trop. Med. Hyg. *38*:613, 1988.
346. Speelman, P., Kabir, I., and Islam, M.: Distribution and spread of colonic lesions in shigellosis: A colonoscopic study. J. Infect. Dis. *150*:899–903, 1984.
347. Sprinz, H. E., Gangarosa, E. J., Williams, M., et al.: Histopathology of the upper small intestine in typhoid fever: Biopsy study of experimental disease in man. Am. J. Dig. Dis. *11*:615–624, 1966.
348. Tauxe, R. V., Puhr, N. D., Wells, J. G., et al.: Antimicrobial resistance of *Shigella* isolates in the U.S.A.: The importance of international travel. J. Infect. Dis. *162*:1107, 1990.
349. Taylor, D. E., and Courvalin, P.: Mechanisms of antibiotic resistance in *Campylobacter* species. Antimicrob. Agents Chemother. *32*:1107, 1988.
350. Taylor, W. R., Schell, W. L., Wells, J. G., et al.: A foodborne outbreak of enterotoxigenic *Escherichia coli* diarrhea. N. Engl. J. Med. *306*:1093–1095, 1982.
351. Teasley, D. G., Gerding, D. N., Olson, M. M., et al.: Prospective randomized trial of metronidazole versus vancomycin for *Clostridium difficile*-associated diarrhea and colitis. Lancet *2*:1043–1046, 1983.
352. Teitelbaum, J. S., Zatorre, R. J., Carpenter, S., et al.: Neurologic sequelae of domoic acid intoxication due to the ingestion of contaminated mussels. N. Engl. J. Med. *322*:1781, 1990.
353. Telzak, E. E., Budnick, L. D., Greenberg, M. S. Z., et al.: A nosocomial outbreak of *Salmonella enteritis* infection due to the consumption of raw eggs. N. Engl. J. Med. *323*:394, 1990.
354. Terranova, W., and Blake, P. A.: Current concepts: *Bacillus cereus* food poisoning. N. Engl. J. Med. *298*:143–144, 1978.
355. Tippen, P. S., Meyer, A., Blank, E. C., et al.: Aquariam-associated *Plesiomonas shigelloides* infection: Missouri. M. M. W. R. *38*:617, 1989.
356. Tjoa, W. S., DuPont, H. L., Sullivan, P., et al.: Location of food consumption and travelers' diarrhea. Am. J. Epidemiol. *106*:61–66, 1977.
357. Toledo, M. R. F., and Trabulsi, L. R.: Correlation between biochemical and serological characteristics of *Escherichia coli* and results of the Sereny test. J. Clin. Microbiol. *17*:419–421, 1983.
358. Toledo, M. R. F., Alvariza, M. C. B., Murahovschi, J., et al.: Enteropathogenic *Escherichia coli* serotypes and endemic diarrhea in infants. Infect. Immun. *39*:586–589, 1983.
359. Turnbill, P. C. B.: Studies on the production of enterotoxins by *Bacillus cereus*. J. Clin. Pathol. *29*:941–948, 1976.
360. Tzipori, S., Roberton, D., and Chapman, C.: Remission of cryptosporidiosis in an immunodeficient child with hyperimmune bovine colostrum. B. M. J. *293*:1276, 1986.
361. Ungar, B. L. P., Yolken, R. H., Nash, T. E., et al.: Enzyme-linked immunosorbent assay for the detection of *Giardia lamblia* in fecal specimens. J. Infect. Dis. *149*:90–97, 1984.
362. Ungar, B. L.: Enzyme-linked immunoassay for detection of *Cryptosporidium* antigens in fecal specimens. J. Clin. Microbiol. *28*:2491, 1990.
363. Ungar, B. L. P., Ward, D. S., Fayer, R., et al.: Cessation of *Cryptosporidium*-associated diarrhea in an acquired immunodeficiency syndrome patient after treatment with hyperimmune bovine colostrum. Gastroenterology *98*:486, 1990.
364. Van, R., Wun, C.-C., Morrow, A. L., et al.: The effect of diaper type and overclothing on fecal contamination in day care centers. J. A. M. A. *265*:1840–1844, 1991.
365. Van, R., Wun, C. C., O'Ryan, M. L., et al.: Outbreaks of human enteric adenovirus types 40 and 41 in Houston day care centers. J. Pediatr. *120*:516–521, 1992.
366. van Gool, T., Snijders, F., Reiss, P., et al.: Diagnosis of intestinal and disseminated microsporidial infections in patients with HIV by a new rapid fluorescence technique. J. Clin. Pathol. *46*:694–6949, 1993.
367. Vargas, S. L., Shenep, J. L., Flynn, P. M., et al.: Azithromycin for treatment of severe *Cryptosporidium* diarrhea in children with cancer. J. Pediatr. *123*:154–156, 1993.
368. Varsano, I., Eidlitz-Marcus, T., Nassinovitch, M., et al.: Comparative efficacy of ceftriaxone and ampicillin for treatment of severe shigellosis in children. J. Pediatr. *118*:627–632, 1991.
369. Velazquez, F. R., Calva, J. J., Guerrero, M. L., et al.: Cohort study of rotavirus serotype patterns in symptomatic and asymptomatic infections in Mexican children. Pediatr. Infect. Dis. J. *12*:56–61, 1993.
370. Velazquez, F. R., Matson, D. O., Calva, J. J., et al.: Natural protection conferred by rotavirus infections: Implications for vaccine strategies. N. Engl. J. Med. *335*:1022–1028, 1996.
371. Vial, P. A., Robins-Browne, R., Lior, H., et al.: Characterization of enteroadherent-aggregative *E. coli,* a putative agent of diarrheal disease. J. Infect. Dis. *158*:70, 1988.
372. Vinh, H., Wain, J., Hanh, V. T. N., et al.: Two or three days of ofloxacin treatment for uncomplicated multidrug-resistant typhoid fever in children. Antimicrob. Agents Chemother. *40*:958–961, 1996.
373. Wallace, C. K., Anderson, P. N., Brown, T. C., et al.: Optimal antibiotic therapy in cholera. Bull. W. H. O. *39*:239–245, 1968.
374. Walmsley, S. L., and Karmali, M. A.: Direct isolation of atypical thermophilic species from human feces on selective agar medium. J. Clin. Microbiol. *27*:668, 1989.
375. Walsh, J. A.: Problems in recognition and diagnosis of amebiasis: Estimation of the global magnitude of morbidity and mortality. Rev. Infect. Dis. *8*:228–238, 1986.
376. Walsh, J. H., and Peterson, W. L.: The treatment of *Helicobacter pylori* infection in the management of peptic ulcer disease. N. Engl. J. Med. *333*:984–989, 1995.
377. Webber, R., Bryan, R. T., Schwartz, D. A., et al.: Human microsporidial infections. Clin. Microbiol. Rev. 7:426–61, 1994.
378. Webber, R., Bryan, R. T., Owen, R. L., et al.: Improved light microscopial detection of microsporidia spores in stool and duodenal aspirates. N. Engl. J. Med. *326*:161–166, 1992.

379. Weiss, L. M., Perlman, D. C., Sherman, J., et al.: *Isospora belli* infection: Treatment with pyrimethamine. Ann. Intern. Med. *109*:474, 1988.
380. Wells, J. G., Davis, B. R., Wachsmuth, K., et al.: Laboratory investigation of hemorrhagic colitis outbreaks associated with a rare *Escherichia coli* serotype. J. Clin. Microbiol. *18*:512–520, 1983.
381. Wenisch, C., Parschalk, B., Masenhundl, M., et al.: Comparison of vancomycin, teicoplanin, metronidazole, and fusidic acid for the treatment of *Clostridium difficile*–associated diarrhea. Clin. Infect. Dis. *22*:813–818, 1996.
382. White, A. C., Chappell, C. L., Hayat, C. S., et al.: Paromomycin for cryptosporidiosis in AIDS: A prospective, double-blind trial. J. Infect. Dis. *170*:19–24, 1994.
383. Whiteside, M. E., Barkin, J. S., May, R. G., et al.: Enteric coccidiosis among patients with the acquired immunodeficiency syndrome. Am. J. Trop. Med. Hyg. *33*:1065–1072, 1984.
384. Williams, D., Schorling, J., Barrett, L. J., et al.: Early treatment of *jejuni* enteritis. Antimicrob. Agents Chemother. *33*:248, 1989.
385. Willson, R., Harrington, R., and Stewart, B.: Human immunodeficiency virus 1-associated necrotizing cholangitis caused by infection with *Septata intestinalis*. Gastroenterology *108*:247–251, 1995.
386. Wittenberg, D. F., Miller, N. M., and Vanden Ende, J.: Spiramycin is not effective in treating *Cryptosporidium* diarrhea in infants: Results of a double-blind randomized trial. J. Infect. Dis. *159*:131, 1989.
387. Wittner, M., Turner, J. W., Jacquette, G., et al.: Eustrongylidiasis: A parasitic infection acquired by eating sushi. N. Engl. J. Med. *320*:1124, 1989.
388. Yamamoto, T., Honda, T., Miwatani, T., et al.: A virulence plasmid in *Escherichia coli* enterotoxigenic for humans: Intergenetic transfer and expression. J. Infect. Dis. *150*:688–698, 1984.
389. Yamamoto, T., Nair, G. B., Albert, M. J., et al.: Survey of in vitro susceptibilities of *Vibrio cholerae* 01 and 0139 to antimicrobial agents. Antimicrob. Agents Chemother. *39*:241–244, 1995.
390. Yolken, R. H., Bishop, C. A., Townsend, T. R., et al.: Infectious gastroenteritis in bone-marrow transplant recipients. N. Engl. J. Med. *306*:1009–1012, 1982.
391. Yolken, R., Leister, F., Dubovi, E., et al.: Infantile gastroenteritis associated with excretion of pestivirus antigens. Lancet *1*:517, 1989.
392. Young, G. P., Ward, P. B., Bayley, N., et al.: Antibiotic-associated colitis due to *Clostridium difficile:* Double-blind comparison of vancomycin with bacitracin. Gastroenterology *89*:1038, 1985.

53

ANTIBIOTIC-ASSOCIATED COLITIS

George D. Ferry

Clostridium difficile colonization and infection accounts for 10 to 25 per cent of antibiotic-associated diarrhea and is the major cause of antibiotic-associated pseudomembranous colitis.[8] Diarrhea and colitis develop when antibiotics, especially those with a broad spectrum of activity, disturb the bowel flora and allow overgrowth of *C. difficile*. Toxin production then leads to inflammation and secretion of fluids from the colon, resulting in watery diarrhea. If inflammation progresses and pseudomembranous colitis develops, the diarrhea becomes bloody. Colitis induced by *C. difficile* has been reported without prior antibiotics, but this is uncommon.

HISTORY

Pseudomembranous colitis was recognized as early as 1893[22] and derives its name from the numerous plaque-like lesions in the colon. The plaques are membranes of epithelial debris containing fibrin, mucus, and polymorphonuclear leukocytes overlying necrotic glands.[55] It was not until the early 1950s that an association with antibiotics was suggested. The organism that initially received the most attention as a possible cause was *Staphylococcus aureus*.[58] Stool cultures frequently were positive for *S. aureus* after antibiotic use, and autopsies showed enterocolitis with ulcers and pseudomembranes in both the small and the large bowel. The association with *C. difficile*, a gram-positive anaerobic bacillus, was shown in 1977 and 1978 with the report of toxin production related to pseudomembranous changes in the colon.[9, 10, 40] *C. difficile* can colonize the intestine without causing diarrhea and was identified as part of the normal flora of infants and newborns in 1935.[29] Early studies suggested that *Clostridium sordellii* might be related to pseudomembranous colitis, but subsequent investigation has shown that *C. sordellii* antitoxin neutralizes *C. difficile* cytotoxicity but is not a cause of colitis.[10]

ETIOLOGY AND PATHOGENESIS

C. difficile can be cultured in low numbers in 5 per cent of healthy adults,[20] but in hospitalized patients, the incidence of colonization and positive cultures reaches 20 per cent or more.[44] *C. difficile* spores are viable for long periods, up to 5 months,[35] and can be cultured from flooring, toilets, and bedding, as well as from the stool and hands of carriers[19, 35] (Table 53–1). A number of studies have shown that neonates frequently are colonized with *C. difficile*.[29, 31, 70] In a London study, 2 to 52 per cent of infants in three postnatal wards had positive cultures, but none developed diarrhea or colitis.[39] There was no evidence that infants were colonized from their mothers. The rate of colonization appears to be related to the length of time infants are hospitalized.[57] After 1 year of age, colonization decreases significantly.[28] *C. difficile* is not only a common contaminant in hospitals[19, 35]; person-to-person transmission between children in day care centers also has been reported.[34]

Infection with *C. difficile* is common and accounts for 10 to 25 per cent of cases of uncomplicated antibiotic-associated diarrhea.[8, 63] Most infections cause watery diarrhea, but 5 to 10 per cent progress to pseudomembranous colitis.[36] In day care centers, the incidence of *C. difficile* infection not related to antibiotics may be as high as 50 per cent.[34] Community-acquired diarrhea due to *C. difficile* studied in a health maintenance organization population identified 51 cases, with an incidence of 7.7 cases/100,000 person-years.[30] Half of these cases occurred after antibiotic use. Increased age and exposure to more than one antibiotic within a 42-day period increased the risk.[30] *C. difficile* diarrhea was uncommon in patients younger than 20 years of age. Risk factors included inflammatory bowel disease, HIV infection, and chronic antibiotic treatment. Pseudomembranous colitis can occur sporadically or in epidemics.[48, 51]

Virulence may differ among strains of *C. difficile*, some being highly toxigenic and others having low virulence.[37] Toxin production by the organism and clinical illness are absent in 25 per cent of patients with positive cultures.[20] Two toxins are produced by *C. difficile*. Toxin B is a cytotoxin that produces cytopathic effects in tissue culture but appears to have little effect in vivo.[43, 53] Toxin A is an enterotoxin that binds to receptors on the enterocyte and stimulates salt and water secretion. This secretory effect does not occur via the

TABLE 53–1. Distribution of *Clostridium difficile* Isolates Taken from the Environment of Two Pediatric Units

Sites Cultured	No. Positive/No. Sampled (%) Pediatric Ward (case-associated)	Newborn Intensive Care Unit (control)
Surfaces		
Bedpan hoppers	0/25	0/15
Chart covers	0/30 (3.3)	0/20
Cribs (occupied)	2/45 (4.4)	1/20 (5)
Dust mops, dust pans on cleaning carts	2/6 (33.3)	0/4
Floors		
Bathroom	4/40 (10)	NA
Clean storage room	2/30 (6.7)	0/20
Patient's room	6/50 (12)	1/30 (3.3)
Soiled room	2/30 (6.7)	0/20
Hospital garments	0/20	0/11
Linens, blankets (clean)	0/20	0/8
Linens, blankets (in use)	5/50 (10)	3/37 (8.1)
Medical devices (e.g., stethoscopes)	0/25	0/20
Mobiles, toys	1/20 (5)	0/12
Scales	8/40 (20)	1/30 (3.3)
Washbasins, sinks, tubs	4/40 (10)	1/30 (3.3)
Air (30 cu. ft. per sample)	0/7	0/2
TOTAL	37/478 (7.7)*	7/279 (2.5)*

*$p < .005$.

From Kim, K.-H., Fekety, R., Batts, D. H., et al.: Isolation of *Clostridium difficile* from the environment and contacts of patients with antibiotic-associated colitis. J. Infect. Dis. *143*:44–50, 1981.

adenylate or guanylate cyclase cycle, as is the case with cholera toxin and *Escherichia coli* heat-stable enterotoxin. Toxin A has a significant chemotactic effect on neutrophils, leading to local inflammation and release of inflammatory mediators.[53] In experimental models, injection of toxin A into rabbit ileal loops results in increased fluid secretion, inflammation and necrosis of epithelial cells, and a release of prostaglandin E2 and leukotriene B4 into the lumen.[67] Superoxide anion generation from granulocytes has not been found with either toxin A or toxin B.[53]

Serum antibodies to *C. difficile* toxins A and B are common, being found in 60 to 70 per cent of patients older than 3 years of age.[69] In adults, specific serum IgA and IgG antibodies to toxin A have been detected in 57 to 60 per cent of patients.[52] Antibodies have been found in colonic mucosa and duodenal aspirates in 10 per cent of patients. Binding of toxin A significantly was inhibited by colonic aspirates with high-IgA antitoxin-A antibody. These antibodies appear to persist throughout life, but it is not clear that they protect against diarrhea or colitis.[33] Protection against diarrhea and pseudomembranous colitis in newborns may be due to a lack of the intestinal receptor for toxin A.[17] Although breast milk contains antibody against *C. difficile*, it is unclear whether this influences disease activity.[71]

In the normal host, many bacteria inhibit growth of *C. difficile*, especially lactobacilli, *Bacteroides*, group D enterococci, and *E. coli*.[56] Treatment with any antibiotic can result in overgrowth of *C. difficile* and lead to pseudomembranous colitis. Oral antibiotics are associated with colitis more often than are parenteral antibiotics, and broad-spectrum antibiotics are responsible for most cases. Multiple antibiotics have been implicated in antibiotic-associated diarrhea in children, including clindamycin, ampicillin, cephalosporin, penicillin, chloramphenicol, gentamicin, and trimethoprim-sulfamethoxazole.[1, 65] Cefixime also has been associated with pediatric pseudomembranous colitis.[27] Long-term antibiotic treatment of acne has been complicated rarely by diarrhea or colitis.[18]

C. difficile infection has been reported during chemotherapy, methotrexate being the most common precipitating agent.[3] The spectrum of illness has been mild to fulminant colitis, just as in antibiotic-associated disease. *C. difficile* also has occurred as an outbreak with associated diarrhea in AIDS patients who were admitted to the same hospital ward.[4]

CLINICAL MANIFESTATIONS

The spectrum of clinical signs and symptoms related to *C. difficile* infection ranges from the asymptomatic carrier state to a fulminant colitis and toxic megacolon.[66] Most have watery diarrhea, but 10 to 15 per cent have bloody stools.[36] Diarrhea most often begins 3 to 21 days after the use of antibiotics. Most children with diarrhea have a self-limited illness with watery stools, fever, and abdominal pain.[59, 65] Patients with pseudomembranous colitis present with cramping abdominal pain, fever, and watery, green, foul stools progressing to bloody diarrhea.[16] Colitis often is a mild, self-limited illness once antibiotics are stopped, but it may be severe and require intensive antibiotic and supportive therapy.

Toxic megacolon, or toxic dilatation of the small bowel, may develop without preceding diarrhea. In these critically ill patients, colitis may lead to perforation and peritonitis. In a series of 201 surgical patients, 5 developed toxic megacolon and 4 of the 5 died.[54] Confirmation of the diagnosis may depend on finding the typical pseudomembranous ulcers on colonoscopy. Response to treatment generally is rapid: symptoms clear in 50 per cent of patients within 6 to 14 days and in 100 per cent by 1 month.

The role of *C. difficile* infection in inflammatory bowel disease has been controversial. Some studies have shown no significant association,[45] whereas others have implicated *C. difficile* in the relapse of Crohn disease and ulcerative colitis.[13, 38] The organism has been found in 8 per cent of patients in remission,[15] the same as in the general population. The presence of toxin seems to correlate with the degree of bleeding and disease activity.[26] In one study of 59 patients, toxin was found in 11 (19 per cent). Four of the 11 had received no prior antibiotics. These patients responded promptly to vancomycin, suggesting that the flare of colitis was related to *C. difficile*.[68]

LABORATORY STUDIES

Stool examination often shows blood and mucus, and fecal leukocytes are present in 50 per cent of patients.[20] *C. difficile* can be cultured on selective media, such as cycloserine-cefoxitin-fructose agar.[24] Stool culture is the most sensitive diagnostic tool, but it is not as specific as assaying for *C. difficile* toxin.[25] Because not all organisms produce toxin, a causative role for *C. difficile* in diarrhea and colitis generally is based on detecting toxin in the stool rather than on a positive culture.[25, 41] *C. difficile* toxin production can be diagnosed by a variety of techniques. The most accurate is the assay for toxin B demonstrating its cytopathic effect on cell-culture monolayers.[20] The sensitivity of enzyme-linked immunosorbent assay screening tests for toxins A and B generally is in the range of 80 to 90 per cent.[20] Newer enzyme immunoassay kits are reported to have a sensitivity of 93 to 99 per cent and a specificity of 93 to 100 per cent.[2] Polymerase chain reaction amplification of a segment of the toxin A gene also has been used to identify *C. difficile* from stool specimens in patients with antibiotic-associated diarrhea.[32] This test appears to be highly accurate when compared with a stool culture and toxin assay. Latex agglutination for *C. difficile* antigen is less sensitive than culture and not as specific as toxin assay.[25, 50]

Endoscopic diagnosis of *C. difficile* is useful when urgent diagnosis is needed prior to laboratory confirmation of a positive assay for toxin (Fig. 53–1). Flexible sigmoidoscopy is a rapid diagnostic tool, but in one study of 29 patients with a positive toxin assay, only 55 per cent had typical pseudomembranous colitis, 14 per cent had nonspecific colitis, and 31 per cent were normal.[11] In cases with a typical endoscopic appearance, *C. difficile* toxin is positive in 95 per cent.[23] Flexible sigmoidoscopy will detect 90 per cent of patients with colitis.[11, 63]

The colon typically appears red with raised, circular, yellow plaques.[23, 62] These pseudomembranous plaques vary from 2 to 5 mm in diameter and are scattered throughout the involved area. In the earliest stage, 1- to 2-mm ulcers may be seen but may not have an obvious membrane. Biopsies of these small lesions show the same endothelial degeneration and pseudomembrane as do larger lesions.[23]

Plain radiography of the abdomen in patients with colitis may show a variety of abnormalities, including colonic ileus, small bowel ileus, ascites, and nodular haustral thickening.[12] In severely ill patients with pseudomembranous colitis, leukocyte scintigraphy has demonstrated a constant and diffuse pattern of intense radio tracer.[47] Although not specific, this test may be useful whenever endoscopy can not be performed.

DIFFERENTIAL DIAGNOSIS

Bloody diarrhea occurring after recent use of antibiotics should suggest the possibility of pseudomembranous colitis.

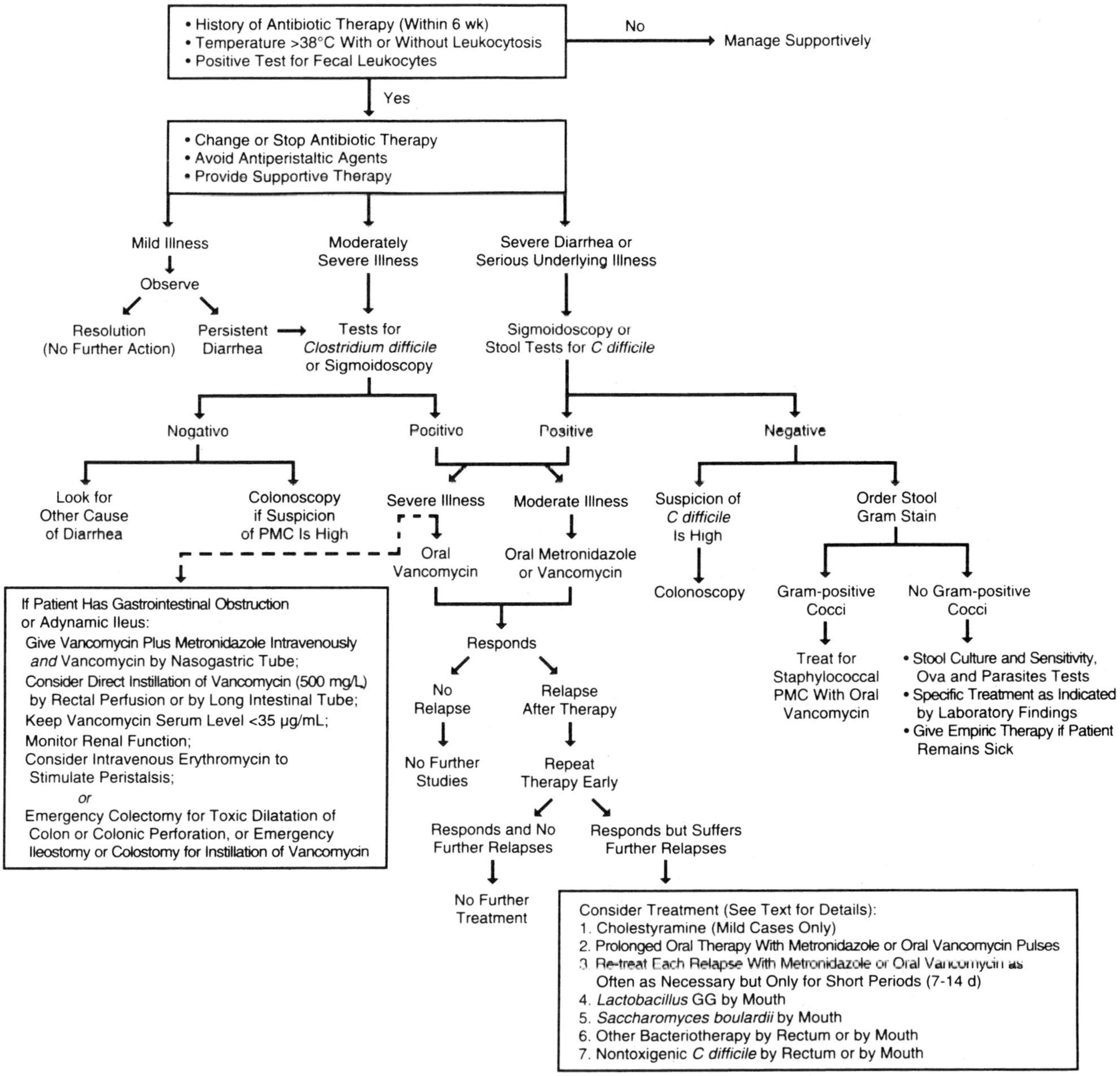

FIGURE 53–1. *Algorithm for management of antibiotic-associated diarrhea and colitis. PMC, pseudomembranous colitis. (From Fekety, R., and Shah, A. B.: Diagnosis and treatment of* Clostridium difficile *colitis. J. A. M. A. 269:72, 1993.)*

TABLE 53–2. Comparison of Results of Treatment with Various Regimens for *Clostridium difficile*–Associated Diarrhea and Colitis

Author	Regimen	No. Responding/Total	No. Relapsing/Total
Gerding and Brazier[25]	Metronidazole	37/39 (95%)	2/39 (5%)
	Vancomycin	45/45 (100%)	6/45 (13%)
Greenfield et al.[26]	Metrondiazole	19/19 (100%)	6/19 (32%)
	Fusidic acid	20/20 (100%)	5/20 (25%)
George et al.[24]	Vancomycin	21/21 (100%)	6/18 (33%)
	Bacitracin	21/21 (100%)	5/12 (42%)
Gremse et al.[27]	Vancomycin	15/15 (100%)	3/15 (20%)
	Bacitracin	12/15 (80%)	5/15 (33%)

From Bartlett, J. G.: *Clostridium difficile:* Clinical considerations. Rev. Infect. Dis. *12*:S243–S251, 1990.

Stool specimens should be obtained for *C. difficile* toxin, along with routine cultures for *Salmonella, Shigella, Campylobacter,* and type-specific *E. coli.* The possibility of inflammatory bowel disease, either ulcerative colitis or Crohn disease of the colon, always should be considered, especially if treatment fails to resolve the colitis. A hemorrhagic colitis related to penicillin has been described, but no pseudomembranes are seen on colonoscopy, and studies for *C. difficile* yield negative results.[46]

TREATMENT

In mild cases, discontinuing antibiotics and implementing supportive measures alone lead to gradual resolution of symptoms.[62] Antiperistaltic agents should be avoided because they may cause toxin retention and complications.[14] Vancomycin is the accepted treatment of choice for pseudomembranous colitis, but both vancomycin and metronidazole clear 80 to 100 per cent of infections (Table 53–2).[5, 7, 72] The effective oral dose of vancomycin is 40 to 50 mg/kg/day. The adult dose is 125 mg four times daily for mild cases and up to 500 mg/dose for severe cases.[7, 21] Intravenous vancomycin is not effective. Metronidazole is effective in doses of 15 to 20 mg/kg/day, with adult doses ranging from 250 mg four times daily up to 500 mg three times a day. Oral bacitracin, 25,000 units four times daily, has been used in some adult patients. Systemic signs of infection generally clear within 24 to 48 hours, and diarrhea gradually subsides over 7 to 10 days.

Relapse is a major problem and occurs in 5 to 33 per cent of patients treated with either vancomycin or metronidazole (see Table 53–2).[6–8, 60, 61] If a relapse produces severe symptoms, re-treatment generally is required.[61] In mild relapse, patients may be watched to see whether they clear the infection spontaneously. Other therapeutic regimens to treat relapse have included weaning to the point at which vancomycin or metronidazole is administered every other or every third day.[64] In some patients, cholestyramine has helped to clear recurrent diarrhea.[20] One study in children showed an excellent response to gamma-globulin given intravenously.[42]

Response to treatment is poor with ileus, toxic megacolon, or colonic perforation. In these cases, installation of vancomycin by clamped nasogastric tube or direct colonic instillation can be tried. The colonic dose for adults is 2000 mg initially followed by 100 mg every 6 hours.[49]

PREVENTION

To date, no good mechanism has evolved to prevent the spread of and colonization with *C. difficile* or to prevent antibiotic-related pseudomembranous colitis. Private rooms and enteric precautions are used commonly, but their efficacy is unknown.

References

1. Ahmad, S. H., Kumar, P., Fakhir, S., et al.: Antibiotic associated colitis. Indian J. Pediatr. *60*:591–4, 1993.
2. Altaie, S. S., Meyer, P., and Dryja, D.: Comparison of two commercially available enzyme immunoassays for detection of *Clostridium difficile* in stool specimens [published erratum appears in J. Clin. Microbiol. *32*:1623, 1994]. J. Clin. Microbiol. *32*:51–53, 1994.
3. Anand, A., and Glatt, A. E.: *Clostridium difficile* infection associated with antineoplastic chemotherapy: A review. Clin. Infect. Dis. *17*:109–113, 1993.
4. Barbut, F., Mario, N., Meyohas, M. C., et al.: Investigation of a nosocomial outbreak of Clostridium difficile–associated diarrhoea among AIDS patients by random amplified polymorphic DNA (RAPD) assay. J. Hosp. Infect. *26*:181–189, 1994.
5. Bartlett, J. G.: Treatment of antibiotic-associated pseudomembranous colitis. Rev. Infect. Dis. *6*(Suppl. 1):S235–S241, 1984.
6. Bartlett, J. G.: Treatment of *Clostridium difficile* colitis. Gastroenterology *89*:1192–1195, 1985.
7. Bartlett, J. G.: *Clostridium difficile:* Clinical considerations. Rev. Infect. Dis. *12*(Suppl. 2):S243–S251, 1990.
8. Bartlett, J. G.: *Clostridium difficile*: History of its role as an enteric pathogen and the current state of knowledge about the organism. Clin. Infect. Dis. *18*(Suppl. 4):S265–S264, 1994.
9. Bartlett, J. G., Chang, T. W., Gurwith, M., et al.: Antibiotic-associated pseudomembranous colitis due to toxin-producing clostridia. N. Engl. J. Med. *298*:531–534, 1978.
10. Bartlett, J. G., Moon, I. V., Chang, T. W., et al.: Role of *Clostridium difficile* in antibiotic-associated pseudomembranous colitis. Gastroenterology *75*:778–782, 1978.
11. Bergstein, J. M., Kramer, A., Wittman, D. H., et al.: Pseudomembranous colitis: How useful is endoscopy? Surg. Endosc. *4*:217–219, 1990.
12. Boland, G. W., Lee, M. J., Cats, A., et al.: Pseudomembranous colitis: Diagnostic sensitivity of the abdominal plain radiograph. Clin. Radiol. *49*:473–475, 1994.
13. Bolton, R. P., Sherriff, R. J., and Read, A. E.: *Clostridium difficile*–associated diarrhea: A role in inflammatory bowel disease? Lancet *1*:383–384, 1980.
14. Church, J. M., and Fazio, V. W.: A role for colonic stasis in the pathogenesis of disease related to *Clostridium difficile.* Dis. Colon Rectum *29*:804–809, 1986.
15. Dorman, S. A., Liggoria, E., Winn, W. C., et al.: Isolation of *Clostridium difficile* toxin from patients with inactive Crohn's disease. Gastroenterology *82*:1348–1351, 1982.
16. Drapkin, M. S., Worthington, M. G., Chang, T-W., et al.: *Clostridium difficile* colitis mimicking acute peritonitis. Arch. Surg. *120*:1321–1322, 1985.
17. Eglow, R., Pothoulakis, C., Israel, E., et al.: Age-related increase in receptor binding for *Clostridium difficile* toxin A (TxA) in rabbit intestine. Gastroenterology *96*:A136, 1989.
18. Facklam, D. P., Gardner, J. S., Neidert, G. L., et al.: An epidemiologic postmarketing surveillance study of prescription acne medications. Am. J. Public Health *80*:50–53, 1990.
19. Fekety, R., Kim, K.-H., Brown, D., et al.: Epidemiology of antibiotic-associated colitis: Isolation of *Clostridium difficile* from the hospital environment. Am. J. Med. *70*:906–908, 1981.
20. Fekety, R., and Shah, A. B.: Diagnosis and treatment of *Clostridium difficile* colitis. J. A. M. A. *269*:71–75, 1993.
21. Fekety, R., Silva, J., Kaufman, C., et al.: Treatment of antibiotic-associated *Clostridium difficile* colitis with oral vancomycin: Comparison of two dosage regimens. Am. J. Med. *86*:15–19, 1989.

22. Finney, J. M. T.: Gastroenterostomy for cicatrizing ulcer of the pylorus. Bull. Johns Hopkins Hosp. *4*:53, 1893.
23. Gebhard, R. L., Gerding, D. N., Olson, M. M., et al.: Clinical and endoscopic findings in patients early in the course of *Clostridium difficile*–associated pseudomembranous colitis. Am. J. Med. *78*:45–48, 1985.
24. George, W. L., Sutter, V. L., Citron, D. M., et al.: Selective and differential medium for isolation of *Clostridium difficile*. J. Clin. Microbiol. *9*:214–219, 1979.
25. Gerding, D. N., and Brazier, J. S.: Optimal methods for identifying *Clostridium difficile* infections. Clin. Infect. Dis. *16*(Suppl. 4):S439–S442, 1993.
26. Greenfield, C., Ramierex, J. R. A., Pounder, R. E., et al.: *Clostridium difficile* and inflammatory bowel disease. Gut *24*:713–717, 1983.
27. Gremse, D. A., Dean, P. C., Farquhar, D. S.: Cefixime and antibiotic-associated colitis. Pediatr. Infect. Dis. J. *13*:331–333, 1994.
28. Hafiz, S. L., and Oakley, C. L.: *Clostridium difficile*: Isolation and characteristics. J. Med. Microbiol. *9*:129–136, 1976.
29. Hall, I. C., and O'Toole, E: Intestinal flora in newborn infants. Am. J. Dis. Child. *49*:390, 1935.
30. Hirschhorn, L. R., Trnka, Y., Onderdonk, A., et al.: Epidemiology of community-acquired *Clostridium difficile*–associated diarrhea. J. Infect. Dis. *169*:127–133, 1994.
31. Holst, E., Helin, I., and Mårdh, P.-H.: Recovery of *Clostridium difficile* from children. Scand. J. Infect. Dis. *13*:41–45, 1981.
32. Kato, N., Ou, C. Y., Kato, H., et al.: Detection of toxigenic *Clostridium difficile* in stool specimens by the polymerase chain reaction. J. Infect. Dis. *167*:455–458, 1993.
33. Kelly, C. P., Pothoulakis, C., Orellana, J., et al.: Human colonic aspirates containing immunoglobulin A antibody to *Clostridium difficile* toxin A inhibit toxin A–receptor binding. Gastroenterology *102*:35–40, 1992.
34. Kim, K., DuPont, H. L., and Pickering, L. K.: Outbreaks of diarrhea associated with *Clostridium difficile* and its toxin in day care centers: Evidence of person-to-person spread. J. Pediatr. *102*:376–382, 1983.
35. Kim, K.-H., Fekety, R., Batts, D. H., et al.: Isolation of *Clostridium difficile* from the environment and contacts of patients with antibiotic-associated colitis. J. Infect. Dis. *143*:42–50, 1981.
36. Knoop, F. C., Owens, M., and Crocker, I. C.: *Clostridium difficile*: Clinical disease and diagnosis. Clin. Microbiol. Rev. *6*:251–265, 1993.
37. Kuijpor, E. J., Oudbier, J. H., Stuifbergen, W. N., et al.: Application of whole-cell DNA restriction endonuclease profiles to the epidemiology of *Clostridium difficile*--induced diarrheas. J. Clin. Microbiol. *25*:751–753, 1987.
38. LaMont, J. T., and Trnka, Y.: Therapeutic implications of *Clostridium difficile* toxin during relapse of inflammatory bowel disease. Lancet *1*:381–383, 1980.
39. Larson, H. E., Barclay, F. E., Honour, P., et al.: Epidemiology of *Clostridium difficile* in infants. J. Infect. Dis. *146*:727–733, 1982.
40. Larson, H. E., and Price, A. B.: Pseudomembranous colitis: Presence of clostridial toxin. Lancet 2:1312–1314, 1977.
41. Lashner, B. A., Todorczuk, J., Salum, D. F., et al.: *Clostridium difficile* culture-positive toxin-negative diarrhea. Am. J. Gastroenterol. *81*:940–943, 1986.
42. Leung, D. Y., Kelly, C. P., Boguniewicz, M., et al.: Treatment with intravenously administered gamma globulin of chronic relapsing colitis induced by *Clostridium difficile* toxin. J. Pediatr. 118:633–637, 1991.
43. Lyerly, D. M., Lockwood, D. E., Richardson, S. H., et al.: *Clostridium difficile*: Its disease and toxins. Clin. Microbiol. Rev. *1*:1–18, 1988.
44. McFarland, L. V., Mulligan, M. E., Kwok, R. Y., et al.: Nosocomial acquisition of *Clostridium difficile* infection. N. Engl. J. Med. *320*:204–210, 1989.
45. Meyers, S., Mayer, L., Bottone, E., et al.: Occurrence of *Clostridium difficile* toxin during the course of inflammatory bowel disease. Gastroenterology *80*:697, 1981.
46. Moulis, H., and Vender, R. J.: Antibiotic-associated hemorrhagic colitis. J. Clin. Gastroenterol. *18*:227–231, 1994.
47. Nathan, M. A., Seabold, J. E., Brown, B. P., et al.: Colonic localization of labeled leukocytes in critically ill patients: Scintigraphic detection of pseudomembranous colitis. Clin. Nuclear Med. *20*:99–106, 1995.
48. Nolan, N. P. N.: An epidemic of pseudomembranous colitis: Importance of person to person spread. Gut *28*:1467–1473, 1987.
49. Pasic, M., Jost, R., Carrel, T., et al.: Intracolonic vancomycin for pseudomembranous colitis. N. Engl. J. Med. *329*:583, 1993.
50. Peterson, L. R., and Kelly, P. J.: The role of the clinical microbiology laboratory in the management of *Clostridium difficile* associated diarrhea. Infect. Dis. Clin. North Am. *7*:277–293, 1993.
51. Pierce, P. F., Jr., Wilson, R., and Silva, J. J., et al.: Antibiotic associated pseudomembranous colitis: An epidemiologic investigation of a cluster of cases. J. Infect. Dis. *145*:269–274, 1982.
52. Pothoulakis, C.: Human colonic aspirates containing immunoglobulin A antibody to *Clostridium difficile* toxin A inhibit toxin A–receptor binding. Gastroenterology *102*:35–40, 1992.
53. Pothoulakis, C., Sullivan, R., Melnick, D. A., et al: *Clostridium difficile* toxin A stimulates intracellular calcium release and chemotactic response in human granulocytes. J. Clin. Invest. *81*:1741–1745, 1988.
54. Prendergast, T. M., Marini, C. P., D'Angelo, A. J., et al.: Surgical patients with pseudomembranous colitis: Factors affecting prognosis. Surgery *116*:768–774, 1994.
55. Price, A. B., and Davies, D. R.: Pseudomembranous colitis. J. Clin. Pathol. *30*:1–12, 1977.
56. Rolfe, R. D., Helebian, S., and Finefold, S. M.: Bacterial interference between *Clostridium difficile* and normal fecal flora. J. Infect. Dis. *143*:470–475, 1981.
57. Sheretz, R. J., and Sarubbi, F. A.: The prevalence of *Clostridium difficile* and toxin in a nursery population: A comparison with patients with necrotizing enterocolitis and an asymptomatic group. J. Pediatr. *100*:435–439, 1982.
58. Speare, G. S.: *Staphylococcus* pseudomembranous enterocolitis, a complication of antibiotic therapy. Am. J. Surg. *88*:523, 1954.
59. Sutphen, J. L., Grand, R. J., Flores, A., et al.: Chronic diarrhea associated with *Clostridium difficile* in children. Am. J. Dis. Child. *137*:275–278, 1983.
60. Teasley, D. G., Gerding, D. N., Olson, M. M., et al.: Prospective randomized trial of metronidazole versus vancomycin for *Clostridium difficile*–associated diarrhea and colitis. Lancet *2*:1043–1046, 1983.
61. Tedesco, F. J.: Pseudomembranous colitis: Pathogenesis and therapy. Med. Clin. North Am. *66*:655–664, 1982.
62. Tedesco, F. J., Barton, R. W., and Alpers, D. H.: Clindamycin-associated colitis: A prospective study. Ann. Intern. Med. *81*:429–433, 1974.
63. Tedesco, F. J., Corless, J. K., and Brownstein, R. E.: Rectal sparing in the antibiotic-associated pseudomembranous colitis: A prospective study. Gastroenterology *83*:1259–1260, 1982.
64. Tedesco, F. J., Gordon, D., and Fortson, W. C.: Approach to patients with multiple relapses of antibiotic-associated pseudomembranous colitis. Am. J. Gastroenterol. *80*:867–868, 1985.
65. Thompson, C. M., Gilligan, P. H., Fisher, M. C., et al.: *Clostridium difficile* cytotoxin in a pediatric population. Am. J. Dis. Child. *137*:271–274, 1983.
66. Triadafilopoulos, G., and Hallstone, A. E.: Acute abdomen as the first presentation of pseudomembranous colitis. Gastroenterology *101*:685–691, 1991.
67. Triadafilopoulos, G., Pothoulakis, C., Weiss, R., et al.: Comparative study of *Clostridium difficile* toxin A and cholera toxin in rabbit ileum. Gastroenterology *97*:1186-1892, 1989.
68. Trnka, Y. M., and LaMont, J. T.: Association of *Clostridium difficile* toxin with symptomatic relapse of chronic inflammatory bowel disease. Gastroenterology *80*:693–6966, 1981.
69. Viscidi, R., Laughon, B. E., and Yoken, R.: Serum antibody response to toxins A and B of *Clostridium difficile*. J. Infect. Dis. *148*:93–100, 1983.
70. Viscidi, R., Willey, S., and Bartlett, J. G.: Isolation rates and toxigenic potential of *Clostridium difficile* isolates from various patient populations. Gastroenterology *81*:5–9, 1981.
71. Wada, N., Nishida, N., Iwaki, S., et al.: Neutralizing activity against *Clostridium difficile* toxin in the supernatant of cultured colostral cells. Infect. Immun. *29*:545–550, 1980.
72. Young, G. P., Ward, P. B., Bayley, N., et al.: Antibiotic colitis due to *Clostridium difficile*: Double-blind comparison of vancomycin with bacitracin. Gastroenterology *89*:1038–1045, 1985.

54

WHIPPLE DISEASE

Roberto A. Guerrero and Mark A. Gilger

Whipple disease is a rare, systemic bacterial infection that until recently was uniformly fatal. In its most common form, Whipple disease affects white, middle-aged men with diarrhea, weight loss, abdominal pain, arthralgias, and fever. Although it is extraordinarily rare in children, its recognition may be critical. Simple treatment with appropriate antibiotics may be both curative and lifesaving.[21]

HISTORY

Whipple disease was described in 1907 by Dr. George Hoyt Whipple,[59] at that time an Instructor in Pathology at The Johns Hopkins University.[6] Curiously, Whipple's description probably was not the first. Allchin and Webb appear to have described a patient with "Whipple's disease" in 1895.[38] Nonetheless, in Whipple's account, a 37-year-old medical missionary was admitted to the Johns Hopkins Hospital with low-grade fever, steatorrhea, and an abdominal mass. The patient had a 5-year history of sporadic migratory polyarthritis. These attacks of arthritis were associated with a gradual loss of both weight and strength. His skin was pigmented with a brownish hue. Laboratory evaluation found severe anemia and an enormous number of fatty acid crystals in the stool. Explorative laparotomy revealed large, firm mesenteric lymph nodes, and a diagnosis of either Hodgkin disease or tuberculosis was made. The patient died 1 week later, and autopsy revealed marked fatty deposition within intestinal mucosa and the mesenteric and retroperitoneal lymph nodes. Other findings included polyserositis (peritonitis, pleuritis, and pericarditis) and endocarditis. Histology revealed infiltration of the lamina propria of the small intestine by large, foamy mononuclear cells that did not stain for fat. Fatty acids and triglycerides were found in dilated lymph channels. Silver stains of the mesenteric lymph nodes showed "great numbers of rod-shaped organisms" that resembled the tubercle bacillus. Whipple suggested that these bacillus-like organisms in the nodes could be the cause. Whipple reported "a hitherto undescribed disease characterized anatomically by deposits of fat and fatty acids in the intestinal and mesenteric lymphatic tissues."[59] He concluded that the patient suffered from "an obscure disease of fat metabolism" and proposed the term "intestinal lipodystrophy."[12] Whipple recognized the most important features of this disease except for the involvement of the central nervous system. In 1949, Black-Schaffer demonstrated that macrophages within the intestinal mucosa of patients with Whipple disease are stained intensely by the periodic acid–Schiff method,[27] proving that the macrophages contained glycoprotein or mucopolysaccharide, not fat, as Whipple suggested. In 1961, Yardley and associates took tissue samples from Whipple's original patient and found them to be strongly periodic acid–Schiff positive,[50] thus confirming the diagnosis of "Whipple disease."

In 1992, Relman and colleagues[45] identified a gram-positive bacillus to be associated with Whipple disease using polymerase chain reaction. They reported a unique 1321–base pair, 16s ribosomal RNA sequence amplified by polymerase chain reaction on intestinal and lymph node tissue from five unrelated patients with Whipple disease. They suggested that the responsible bacillus is a member of the actinomycetes. The actinomycetes are gram-positive bacteria with DNA rich in guanine and cytosine.[60] The genus consists of Actinomycetaceae, Streptomycetaceae, and the Nocardioform group.[9] The Whipple disease bacillus appears most closely related to four actinobacteria: *Dermatophilus congolensis*, *Arthrobacter globiformis*, *Terrabacter tumescenes*, and *Micrococcus luteus*.[45] Relman concluded that, with the phylogenetic relations of the Whipple disease bacillus, the features of the illness, and its distinct morphologic characteristics, there were sufficient grounds to propose a new genus and species name: *Tropheryma whippelii* (from the Greek *trophe*, or nourishment; *eryma*, or barrier, due to the malabsorption it causes; and *whippelii*, in honor of George Whipple). Wilson and associates argued that by using "bootstrap" analysis (a measure of statistical confidence), the Whipple bacillus is only 67 per cent associated with actinobacteria, which is far from the 95 per cent confidence level needed for a scientific conclusion.[52] They suggested that the Whipple bacillus may represent yet another, separate, fourth line of descent within the actinomycetes.

EPIDEMIOLOGY

Whipple disease characteristically occurs in white, middle-aged males. Its true incidence and prevalence are unknown because fewer than 1000 cases have been reported worldwide. It is extremely rare in children,[1, 2, 4, 7, 26] with fewer than 10 reported cases. The youngest case was in a newborn,[13] and the oldest case was in a person 83 years of age.[33] The peak age of presentation is 40 to 49 years.[17] In a literature review of 114 patients,[33] 88 per cent were males and 12 per cent were females. Most of these patients were white. The vast majority of patients reported as having Whipple disease are from continental Europe or the United States.[8] In an extensive review of 741 cases,[11] Dobbins found that most academic centers in the United States had records of three or four unreported individuals. He estimated that for every published report there were at least two to three unpublished cases, and, therefore, some 1500 to 2000 individuals probably have had Whipple disease.[12]

ETIOLOGY AND PATHOGENESIS

Despite Whipple's account of "great numbers of rod-shaped organisms,"[59] all attempts to culture the organism have been unsuccessful. It is, however, widely accepted that the disease is caused by an organism known as Whipple bacillus.[17, 33, 59] However, such a bacterial etiology of Whipple disease should be confirmed by fulfilling Koch's postulates of pathogenicity, which thus far has not been possible. Many other organisms have been isolated from patients with Whipple disease, such as *Corynebacterium* (anaerobic and aerobic), *Haemophilus* species, *Brucella*, and atypical *Streptococcus* (alpha-hemolytic),[17, 33] but none of these organisms can be found consistently.

There is scant support for a primary humoral immune

deficiency in Whipple disease,[20] but there is stronger evidence for a distinct defect in the cell-mediated immune function. Dobbins[10] reviewed data on 30 patients with HLA-A and -B locus typing and 47 patients with HLA-B27 typing. He found an increased incidence of patients who were HLA-B27–positive (28 per cent), even with absence of concomitant sacroileitis. Other reports, however, have failed to confirm the increased association with the HLA-B27 antigen.[3] Marth and associates[35] studied 27 patients with Whipple disease. They found a significantly reduced number of cells expressing the complement receptor 3 L-chain (CD11B), a reduced proliferation to phytohemagglutinin and to sheep red blood cells, and a hypoergic skin reaction. These findings indicated a defect of cell-mediated immunity. In patients with active disease, there is an increase in CD8-positive cells, which results in a reduced CD4:CD8 ratio. Such defects of cellular immunity appear to persist in patients for several years, despite complete remission of the disease.

Oral acquisition of the Whipple bacillus appears most likely,[17] emphasizing greater involvement of the duodenum and proximal jejunum than the more distal small intestine. There have been only three reports of siblings with this disease; thus, contagious spread of Whipple disease seems unlikely.[21] Whipple bacillus has been identified free in the small intestine next to the glycocalyx of the enterocyte's microvilli, in epithelial cells, and in the lamina propria.[17] Even in patients with extraintestinal Whipple disease, the organism usually is identified in the small bowel.[17] The bacillus appears to spread through the lymphatics as well as through systemic circulation[17, 28, 39] and then can involve several extraintestinal organs.

Whipple bacillus can be seen faintly by light microscopy. The bacilli are seen best by transmission electron microscopy, which reveals a rod-shaped organism 0.2 μm wide and 1.5 to 2.5 μm long[21] (Fig. 54–1). The ultrastructure of the Whipple bacillus wall is similar to that of other gram-positive bacteria, with the exception of an additional surface membrane. This membrane is different from the outer membrane of gram-negative bacteria because it is thinner, has a symmetric profile, and has no periodic acid–Schiff positive components.[52] Once the bacillus has been ingested by the macrophage, the degenerative process that occurs leads to the accumulation of bacterial remnants that are resistant to degradation. The polysaccharide-containing portion of the bacillus wall correlates to these remnants, and its progressive accumulation leads to the typical intramacrophagic inclusions. These inclusions are periodic acid–Schiff positive and one of the key features in the histologic diagnosis of Whipple disease.[52]

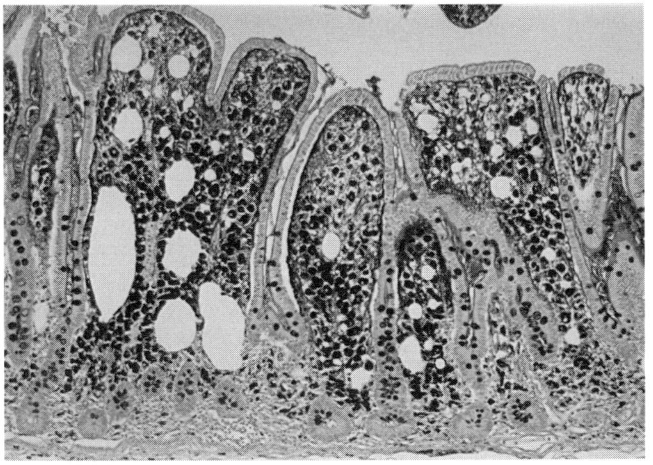

FIGURE 54–2. *Light microscopic photograph of intestinal mucosa from the proximal jejunum of a patient with untreated Whipple disease. The villi appear somewhat blunted and swollen with periodic acid–Schiff positive macrophages stuffed in the lamina propria. (Courtesy of Kenneth P. Batts, M. D., Mayo Clinic, Rochester, MN; Jeffrey Craver, M. D., Depaul Health Center, Bridgeton, MO; and Milton J. Finegold, M. D., Baylor College of Medicine, Houston, TX.)*

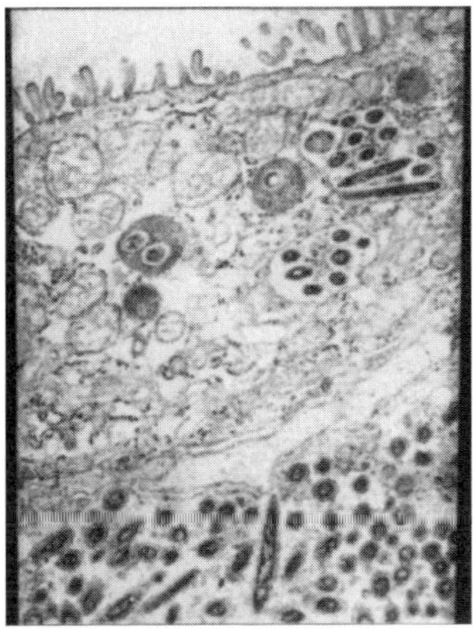

FIGURE 54–1. *Electron micrograph of the invasion of enterocytes by Whipple bacilli. There are numerous bacilli within the lamina propria. (Magnification × 25,000.) (From Tyor, M. P.: Whipple's disease: The Duke connection. N. C. Med. J. 55:237–240, 1994.)*

Biopsy specimens from the small intestine in patients with Whipple disease usually show characteristic changes. The intestinal villi are preserved,[17] but there is distortion of the architecture.[20] There usually is a clubbed appearance of the intestinal villi[33] due to the accumulation of foamy macrophages in the lamina propria.[17] The enterocytes may appear normal[15, 33] or may show flattening and vacuolization and occasionally appear cuboidal[15, 33] (Fig. 54–2). Lipid accumulation with large fat droplets within the lamina propria and smaller droplets within and in between the absorptive cells is common.[33] In some instances, there are prominent, dilated lacteals.[17] Ectors and associates[15] reported reduced and even absent lactase and major histocompatibility complex class II (HLA-DR) expression. Lactase and major histocompatibility complex class II expression normalized within 3 to 6 months of starting antibiotic therapy.

The characteristic feature of Whipple disease is the presence of periodic acid–Schiff positive, diastase-resistant macrophages.[21] These findings are not pathognomonic, however, because intestinal periodic acid–Schiff positive macrophages can be found in other conditions,[17] such as histiocytosis, melanosis coli, and *Mycobacterium avium-intracellulare* infection, and even within macrophages in healthy individuals. The macrophages in Whipple disease do not stain with Ziehl-Neelsen.[15, 21] There often is a sickle-shaped appearance of the periodic acid–Schiff positive granules in the macrophages of patients with Whipple disease.[33] Sieracki and and Fine[51] observed systemic involvement in the autopsies of five patients with Whipple disease. The sickle-shaped, periodic acid–Schiff positive macrophages were believed to be specific for Whipple disease, demonstrating involvement of the entire gastrointestinal tract and the pancreas; diffuse involvement of the retroperitoneum and lymph nodes, the adrenals, the liver with sickle-form particles in Kupffer cells and in histiocytes, the brain, the heart, and the visceral pleura of the lungs; and minimal involvement of the genitourinary tract, skeletal muscles, and bone marrow. James and associates[28] examined the vessels of the gastrointestinal system and found abundant bacilli in the arteries of the small intestinal serosa and liver. They noted focal degeneration and fibrosis in the tunica media with arteritis and intimal proliferation. Rickman and coworkers[46] reported a case that confirmed the presence of Whipple bacillus in the vitreous of the eye.

Whipple bacillus produces a predominantly histiocytic inflammatory reaction, with infiltration by macrophages.[16] Noncaseating, epithelioid cell, sarcoid-like granulomas are located preferentially in peripheral lymph nodes and the liver.[14, 16] These granulomas occasionally can be seen in different tissues, with three reports of granulomas in the intestinal tract.[16] Mesenteric lymph nodes often are strikingly enlarged.[8]

Electron microscopy can be useful, often revealing the presence of the rod-shaped bacterium[21] (see Fig. 54–1). Electron microscopy also demonstrates intestinal macrophages containing bacteria with signs of lysis.[52] Silva and associates[52] described steps of a degradative process of the bacillus that starts with disorganization of the surface membrane and the thick outer wall. With the loss of intracellular material, there are bacterial ghosts composed of the three inner layers of the envelope. The two electron-dense layers of the cytoplasmic membrane become disorganized and solubilized, leaving the inner dense layer of the cell wall as the final bacterial remnant (Fig. 54–3).

TABLE 54–1. Major Symptoms and Signs in Whipple Disease

	Percentage of Cases
Symptoms	
Weight loss	65–100
Chronic diarrhea	60–85
Arthralgia	65–80
Abdominal pain	60
Fever	10–55
Central nervous system–related complaints	10–40
Signs	
Malnutrition	90–95
Hypotension	70
Lymphadenopathy	55
Hyperpigmentation	45–55
Abdominal tenderness	50
Edema	30
Abdominal mass	20
Hepatomegaly	1–14
Splenomegaly	5–10
Ascites	8

Data from references 8, 20, 21, 31, 33.

CLINICAL MANIFESTATIONS

The clinical manifestations of Whipple disease vary, depending on the organ system involved. The disease is viewed best as a multisystemic illness, with focus on the gastrointestinal tract.[5] Malabsorption is the key feature of clinical disease, but there are no specific signs or symptoms for Whipple disease. Table 54–1 illustrates the major symptoms and signs of Whipple disease. In children, failure to thrive, malnutrition, and chronic diarrhea appear most commonly. Abdominal distention, abdominal pain, and generalized lymphadenopathy may be found.[2] Response to antibiotic treatment may be dramatic, with rapid weight gain and resolution of symptoms.[4]

GASTROINTESTINAL TRACT. One of the most common symptoms is weight loss, being found in 65 to 100 per cent of cases.[8, 17, 21, 33] Indeed, weight loss may be the only symptom.[7] Diarrhea is reported in 60 to 85 per cent of patients.[8, 17, 21, 33] The diarrhea usually is watery or fatty in nature.[33] Several mechanisms have been proposed to explain the malabsorption and steatorrhea in Whipple disease.[17] Direct infection and secondary enterocyte dysfunction may prevent the esterification of fatty acids to triglycerides, as well as inhibit the uptake of carbohydrates and amino acids. Blockage of transport of triglyceride-rich chylomicrons into lacteals may occur due to the deposition of foamy macrophages in the lamina propria. Lymphatic obstruction may occur due to involvement of the mesenteric lymph nodes. Malabsorption and diarrhea tend to resolve within a few days after antibiotic treatment, whereas the lacteal dilatation and periodic acid–Schiff positive macrophages can remain for months to years. Occult gastrointestinal bleeding frequently is found, but melena and gross gastrointestinal bleeding are rare.[17, 21, 33]

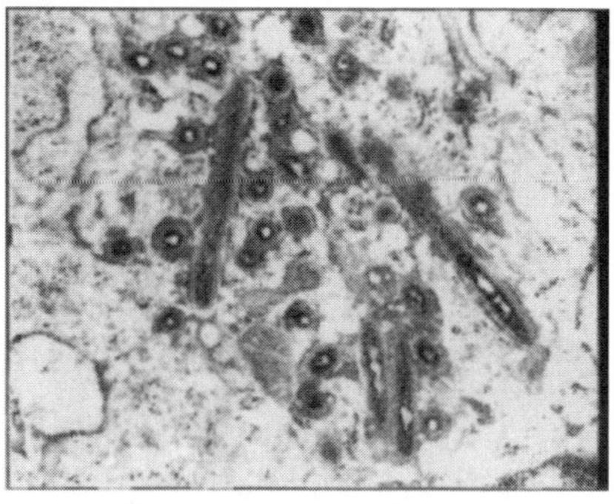

FIGURE 54–3. *Electron micrograph illustrating numerous rod-shaped bacilliform bodies within the cytoplasm of a macrophage. (Magnification × 13,750.) (From Tyor, M. P.: Whipple's disease: The Duke connection. N. C. Med. J. 55:237–240, 1994.)*

Abdominal pain is found in up to 60 per cent of patients.[8, 17, 21, 33] The pain is nonspecific, generally is epigastric in location, and may be worse after meals.[33] Such pain and anorexia may lead to reduced caloric intake and further weight loss.[17] Abdominal distention is common and may be secondary to intra-abdominal lymphadenopathy or to thickening of loops of diseased intestine.[17, 33] Ascites occasionally is seen and may be chylous, secondary to lymphatic obstruction.[7, 21]

JOINTS. Arthralgia is the most frequent nongastrointestinal symptom in Whipple disease,[17, 33] presenting in 65 per cent of adult cases.[33] Arthralgia may precede gastrointestinal symptoms by a number of years or even decades[17, 31] and is less common in children. Generally, joint symptoms continue unchanged with the onset of gastrointestinal symptoms.[17] Acute migratory arthralgia or arthritis may last for days or weeks[21, 25, 31] and may persist as the disease progresses. The involved joints, in decreasing order of frequency, are knees, ankles, hips, fingers, wrists, elbows, hands, and spine.[17] Examination may reveal joint pain, swelling, limited range of motion, and warmth.[49] Fever sometimes is present.[17] Spondylitis, with or without sacroileitis, may develop.[4] Permanent joint destruction and deformity are uncommon but can be severe.[17, 49] Arthrocentesis may reveal an inflammatory arthritis, with cell counts of 6000 to 75,000, often with a polymorphonuclear leukocyte predominance.[17] Synovial biopsy may demonstrate periodic acid–Schiff positive macrophages.[17]

CENTRAL NERVOUS SYSTEM. Whipple disease can be

confined to the brain[47] but usually is accompanied by other manifestations.[21] Central nervous system and neurologic manifestations, such as headache, diplopia, meningoencephalitis, depression, confusion, and personality changes, are uncommon[8, 17, 33] but may be significant.[8, 17, 20, 33, 41] Table 54–2 lists the spectrum of potential central nervous system involvement.

EYE. Indirect involvement of the central nervous system, as well as direct involvement of the eye, can produce visual problems.[17] Ophthalmoplegia and diplopia can occur, with involvement of cranial nerves III, IV, and VI.[17] Reduced visual acuity and papilledema can occur with compromise of the optic nerve.[17] Numerous ophthalmologic findings have been reported, including vasculitis, vitritis, optic atrophy, uveitis, chorioretinitis, vitreous opacities, glaucoma, keratitis, retinal hemorrhages, disk edema, and lacrimal duct obstruction.[17, 57] Rickman and associates[46] reported a case of ocular disease without marked central nervous system or gastrointestinal disease.

SKIN. Hyperpigmentation of the skin in sun-exposed areas occurs in roughly one half of cases.[20, 33] The mechanism of hyperpigmentation is uncertain but is not related to adrenal insufficiency.[17] Subcutaneous nodules may be found and can reveal periodic acid–Schiff positive macrophages and bacilli on electron microscopy.[24]

HEART. The heart frequently is involved in Whipple disease. Endocarditis, myocarditis, pericarditis, pancarditis, and coronary arteritis have been found.[17, 36] A blood culture–negative endocarditis may be caused by Whipple disease.[17] Chronic aortic regurgitation is the most common clinical finding of endocardial involvement.[17] Pericarditis with polyserositis (pleuritis, peritonitis) has been found.[19] The electrocardiographic abnormalities are nonspecific but include first-degree atrioventricular block, left ventricular hypertrophy, sinus tachycardia, left bundle branch block, intraventricular conduction delay, old inferior wall infarct, and short PR interval.[20] Sossai and associates[53] reported a case of regression of a right bundle branch block after treatment with antibiotics, but the block spontaneously recurred 2 years later.

SKELETAL MUSCLE. Skeletal muscle may be involved, diagnosed by electromyography or muscle biopsy.[54] Proximal muscle weakness is most common. Muscle biopsy reveals a nonspecific myopathy.

LYMPH NODES AND SPLEEN. Whipple disease may involve any lymph node in the body.[17] Mesenteric lymph nodes frequently are involved, and splenomegaly is found in 5 to 10 per cent of cases.[33]

PULMONARY. Cough, pleuritic chest pain, and dyspnea have been reported.[55] Pleural involvement may appear as a pleural rub. Pleural adhesions and granulomas have been reported at autopsy.[4, 55] Chest radiography often reveals pleural thickening, parenchymal shadowing, and elevation of the diaphragm.[55] Lung function tests may demonstrate decreased lung volumes.[55]

KIDNEY. Renal involvement in Whipple disease is rare.[17] However, granulomata have been found, as well as focal glomerulonephritis.[30]

HEMATOLOGIC. Anemia is common and usually is of a hypochromic, microcytic variety.[17, 20, 21] Macrocytic anemia also may be seen due to folate malabsorption. Leukocytosis, thrombocytosis,[40] and bone marrow involvement may be found.[43] Low serum iron concentration and an elevated erythrocyte sedimentation rate frequently are seen.[20] There is a single case report of extraintestinal lymphoma in association with Whipple disease found at autopsy.[23]

TABLE 54–2. Central Nervous System Symptoms and Signs of Whipple Disease

Headache
Incoordination
Mental and personality changes
Confusion
Lethargy, coma
Ataxia
Convulsions
Motor weakness
Dementia
Depression
Papilledema
Ophthalmoplegia
Visual difficulties (diplopia, blurring)
Nystagmus
Pupillary abnormalities
Ptosis
Hemiparesis
Polydipsia
Hyperphagia
Hearing loss
Sensory loss
Numbness
Slurred speech
Dizziness
Tinnitus
Loss of vibratory and position sense
Sleep disorders
Stiff neck
Facial pain
Muscle rigidity
Muscular jerks and twitches
Hyperreflexia (± positive Babinski)

DIAGNOSIS

There are no specific laboratory findings of Whipple disease. Anemia and low albumin probably are the most common, being found in about 90 per cent of patients. Low serum iron and folate are seen in perhaps 30 per cent of cases. Hypokalemia, hypocalcemia, low cholesterol and carotene, prolonged prothrombin time, and increased transaminases are less common. Elevated fecal fat is found in more than 90 per cent of cases. The D-xylose malabsorption test frequently is abnormal.

Barium x-ray studies of the small bowel may show marked thickening of the mucosal folds and separation of bowel loops, suggesting a malabsorptive disease. Such findings usually resolve completely with successful antibiotic therapy.

One of the key features in the histologic diagnosis of Whipple disease is the accumulation of periodic acid–Schiff positive, diastase-resistant macrophages in the lamina propria of the small intestine.[4, 20, 34] These findings are not pathognomonic, and infection with *M. avium-intracellulare* must be excluded.[34] Whipple bacillus does not stain acid-fast,[34] whereas mycobacteria readily are identified. Small bowel involvement by *M. avium* complex can have similar endoscopic, histologic, and radiographic findings to those of Whipple disease.[42] Periodic acid–Schiff positive macrophages occasionally can be seen in the mucosa of the large bowel and rectum in unrelated diseases, such as histiocytosis, and benign problems, such as melanosis coli and pneumatosis intestini.[34] Electron microscopy can confirm the diagnosis by visualization of the characteristic bacillus.[21, 52]

Endoscopy of the small bowel may be helpful because characteristic lesions may be seen and biopsy specimens obtained. There are no clear data as to where the intestinal specimens should be taken[34] because intestinal involvement

TABLE 54–3. Treatment of Whipple Disease: Initial Antibiotic Regimen and Relapse

Antibiotic(s)	Number of Patients	Total Number of Relapses	CNS Relapses
TCN[a] alone	49	21	9[b]
PCN + STM + TCN[a]	15	2	0
PCN/PCN[a]	8	3	2
PCN + STM	5	2	0
TMP-SMX[a]	3	0	0
Other	8	3	2
Total	88	31	13

CNS, central nervous system; PCN, penicillin; STM, streptomycin; TCN, tetracycline; TMP-SMX; trimethoprim-sulfamethoxazole; [a]oral therapy; [b]includes two patients treated with TCN only in whom CNS relapse was the second relapse.

Data from Keinath, R. D., Merrell, D. E., Vlietstra, R., et al.: Antibiotic treatment and relapse in Whipple's disease: Long-term follow-up of 88 patients. Gastroenterology *88*:1867–1873, 1985.

usually is patchy. Random biopsies of the small bowel are suggested, beginning at the ligament of Treitz.[37] Endoscopic findings include yellow-white plaques and an erythematous, erosive, friable mucosa.[22]

Polymerase chain reaction amplification may be used to detect and identify unculturable bacterial pathogens.[58] To set up a polymerase chain reaction, the only prerequisite information that is needed is the nucleotide sequences flanking each end of the target.[44] Specific identification of the Whipple bacillus can be achieved by amplification of the 1321–base pair bacterial, 16s ribosomal RNA gene isolated from infected tissue.[45] Muller and associates[39] applied this polymerase chain reaction technique to demonstrate *T. whippelii* in peripheral blood mononuclear cells and cells derived from pleural effusion in a patient with Whipple disease. Lowsky and colleagues[32] used similar polymerase chain reaction techniques to detect *T. whippelii* in erythrocytes.

TREATMENT

Antibiotics are the mainstay of therapy for Whipple disease.[8] However, because the Whipple bacillus has never been cultured, no actual antimicrobial sensitivities are available.[17, 21] All antibiotic treatment strategies are empiric, based only on the accumulated anecdotal experience. Table 54–3 illustrates several antibiotic treatments and the likelihood of relapse. In general, response to antibiotics is good and often dramatic. Symptoms such as diarrhea quickly resolve, and weight gain is rapid. Several antibiotics alone or in combination have been tried, including chloramphenicol, penicillin, streptomycin, ampicillin, trimethoprim-sulfamethoxazole, erythromycin, and doxycycline.[8, 17, 18, 21] Keinath and associates[29] analyzed the antibiotic response rate of 88 patients with documented Whipple disease. Thirty-one experienced relapse, with a mean time of relapse of 4.2 years after initial diagnosis. Central nervous system relapse occurred in 13 of 88, and all central nervous system and cardiac relapses were late.

All patients with Whipple disease should receive antibiotics that penetrate the blood-brain barrier.[29, 48] Tetracycline and penicillin do not penetrate the blood-brain barrier well, unless the meninges are inflamed.[48] The preferred treatment in both adults and children is trimethoprim-sulfamethoxazole given orally twice a day for 1 year.[48] If the small bowel is involved, repeat small bowel biopsy is suggested at least 6 months to 1 year after treatment to document the disappearance of the bacillus. In patients intolerant to trimethoprim-sulfamethoxazole, penicillin or ampicillin is recommended. Feurle and Marth[18] noted that trimethoprim-sulfamethoxazole was more efficacious than tetracycline in inducing clinical remission of Whipple disease. However, they observed the development of aqueductal stenosis with hydrocephalus in a patient during trimethoprim-sulfamethoxazole treatment and indicated that even trimethoprim-sulfamethoxazole is no safeguard against cerebral recurrence. Central nervous system relapse has a poor prognosis.[17, 18, 21, 29] Feurle and Marth[18] suggested an experimental therapy for central nervous system recurrence using a highly active bactericidal compound, such as a third-generation cephalosporin, a quinolone, or intrathecal antibiotic therapy, that readily crosses the blood-brain barrier. In adult patients, Keinath and associates[29] recommended treatment with parenteral penicillin (1.2 million units daily) plus streptomycin (1 g daily) for 10 to 14 days, followed by trimethoprim-sulfamethoxazole (one double-strength tablet twice daily) for 1 year. Due to the extreme rarity of Whipple disease in children, prudent management dictates long-term surveillance after resolution of symptoms.

Because Whipple disease is a malabsorptive disorder, the patient's nutritional needs must be assessed carefully. Specific attention must be paid to replace any vitamin or mineral deficiencies. Iron, folate, vitamin D, and calcium, for example, typically are given until the steatorrhea resolves.

CONCLUSIONS

Whipple disease, despite its rarity in children, deserves diagnostic consideration in any child with failure to thrive, malnutrition, and chronic diarrhea. Such findings, especially with central nervous system manifestations or arthralgias, should raise the spectre of Whipple disease. Diagnosis of Whipple disease can be made using modern molecular tests, such as polymerase chain reaction, that allow identification of previously unculturable microbial pathogens. Finally, simple antibiotic treatment with oral trimethoprin-sulfamethoxazole can result in dramatic resolution of symptoms, whereas failure to consider this rare disease can lead to catastrophic events.

References

1. Ament, M. E.: Malabsorption syndromes in infancy and childhood. J. Pediatr. *81*:867–884, 1972.
2. Aust, C. H., and Smith, E. B.: Whipple's disease in a 3-month-old infant. Am. J. Clin. Pathol. *37*:66–74, 1962.
3. Bai, J. C., Mota, A. H., Maurino, E., et al.: Class I and class II HLA antigens in a homogeneous Argentinian population with Whipple's disease: Lack of association with HLA-B27. Am. J. Gastroenterol. *86*:992–994, 1991.
4. Barakat, A. Y., Bitar, J., and Nassar, V. H.: Whipple's disease in a seven-year-old child: Report of a case. Am. J. Proctol. *24*:312–315, 1973.

5. Bayless, T. M., and Knox, D. L.: Whipple's disease: A multisystemic infection. N. Engl. J. Med. *300*:920, 1979.
6. Birch, C. A.: Whipple's disease: George Hoyt Whipple (born 1878). Practitioner *212*(1270 Spec. No.):581–582, 1974.
7. Bruni, R., and Massimo, L.: Descrizione un rarissimo caso di mallatia de Whipple nell eta pediatrica. Minerva Pediatr. *11*:935–943, 1959.
8. Comer, G. M., Brandt, L. J., and Abissi, C. J.: Whipple's disease: A review. Am. J. Gastroenterol. *78*:107–114, 1983.
9. Couper, R.: Whipple's disease: The bacillus unmasked. J. Pediatr. Gastroenterol Nutr. *17*:339–344, 1993.
10. Dobbins, W. O., III: HLA antigens in Whipple's disease. Arthritis Rheum. *30*:102–105, 1987.
11. Dobbins, W. O., III: Whipple's disease. Mayo Clin. Proc. *63*:623–624, 1988.
12. Dobbins, W. O., III: Whipple's disease: An historical perspective. Q. J. Med. *56*:523–531, 1985.
13. DePra, M., Casagrande, A., and Guarino, M.: Whipple's disease: Apropos of a case demonstrating the existence of the congenital form. Minerva Pediatr. *26*:1723–1743, 1974.
14. Desmet, V. J., and Geboes, K.: Review article: Liver lesions in inflammatory bowel disorders. J. Pathol. *151*:247–255, 1987.
15. Ectors, N. L., Geboes, K. J., DeVos, R. M., et al.: Whipple's disease: A histological, immunocytochemical and electron microscopic study of the small intestinal epithelium. J. Pathol. *172*:73–79, 1994.
16. Ectors, N., Geboes, K., Wynants, P., et al.: Granulomatous gastritis and Whipple's disease. Am. J. Gastroenterol. *87*:509–515, 1992.
17. Feldman, M.: Southern Internal Medicine Conference: Whipple's disease. Am. J. Med. Sci. *291*:56–67, 1986.
18. Feurle, G. E., and Marth, T.: An evaluation of antimicrobial treatment for Whipple's disease: Tetracycline versus trimethoprim-sulfamethoxazole. Dig. Dis. Sci. *39*:1642–1648, 1995.
19. Finch, W.: Arthritis and the gut. Postgrad. Med. *86*:229–235, 1989.
20. Flemin, J. L., Wiesner, R. H., and Shorter, R. G.: Whipple's disease: Clinical, biochemical and histopathologic features and assessment of treatment in 29 patients. Mayo Clin. Proc. *63*:539–551, 1988.
21. Gaist, D., and Ladefoged, K.: Whipple's disease. Scand. J. Gastroenterol. *29*:97–101, 1994.
22. Geboes, K., Ectors, N., Heidbuchel, H., et al.: Whipple's disease: Endoscopic aspects before and after therapy. Gastrointest. Endosc. *36*:247–252, 1990.
23. Gillen, C. D., Coddington, R., Montieth, P. G., et al.: Extraintestinal lymphoma in association with Whipple's disease. Gut *34*:1627–1629, 1993.
24. Good, A. E, Beals, T. F, Simmons, J. L., et al.: A subcutaneous nodule with Whipple's disease: Key to early diagnosis? Arthritis Rheum. *23*:856–859, 1980.
25. Gran, J. T., and Husby, G.: Joint manifestations in gastrointestinal diseases. Dig. Dis. *10*:295–312, 1992.
26. Hamilton, J. R.: Whipple disease. *In* Behrman, R. E., Vaughn, V., and Nelson, W. E. (eds.): Textbook of Pediatrics. Philadelphia, W. B. Saunders, 1983, p. 935.
27. Harvey, A. M.: Teacher and distinguished pupil: William Henry Welch and George Hoyt Whipple. Johns Hopkins Med. J. *135*:178–190, 1974.
28. James, T. N., Bulkley, B. H., and Kent, S. P.: Case report: Vascular lesions of the gastrointestinal system in Whipple's disease. Am. J. Med. Sci. *288*:125–129, 1984.
29. Keinath, R. D., Merrell, D. E., Vlietstra, R., et al.: Antibiotic treatment and relapse in Whipple's disease: Long-term follow-up of 88 patients. Gastroenterology *88*:1867–1873, 1985.
30. Kraunz, R. F.: Whipple's disease with cardiac and renal abnormalities. Arch. Intern. Med. *123*:701–706, 1969.
31. Leirisalo-Repo, M.: Enteropathic arthritis, Whipple's disease, juvenile spondyloarthropathy and uveitis. Curr. Opin. Rheumatol. *6*:385–390, 1994.
32. Lowsky, R., Archer, G. L., Fyles, G., et al.: Brief report: Diagnosis of Whipple's disease by molecular analysis of peripheral blood. N. Engl. J. Med. *331*:1343–1346, 1994.
33. Maizel, H., Ruffin, J. M., and Dobbins, W. O., III: Whipple's disease: A review of 19 patients from one hospital and a review of the literature since 1950. Medicine *49*:175–205, 1970.
34. Marbet, V. A., Stalder, G. A., and Gyr, K. E.: Whipple's disease: A multisystemic disease with changing presentation. Dig. Dis. *4*:119–128, 1986.
35. Marth, T., Roux, M., VonHerbay, A., et al.: Persistant reduction of complement receptor 3 L-chain expressing mononuclear blood cells and transient inhibitory serum factors in Whipple's disease. Clin. Immunol. Immunopathol. *72*:217–226, 1994.
36. McAllister, H. A., and Fenoglio, J. J.: Cardiac involvement in Whipple's disease. Circulation *52*:152–156, 1975.
37. Moorthy, S., Nolley, G., and Hermos, J. A.: Whipple's disease with minimal intestinal involvement. Gut *18*:152–155, 1977.
38. Morgan, A. D.: The first recorded case of Whipple's disease. Gut *2*:370–372, 1961.
39. Muller, C., Stain, C., and Burghuber, O.: *Tropheryma whippelii* in peripheral blood mononuclear cells and cells of pleural effusion. Lancet *341*:701, 1993.
40. Nuzum, C. T., Sandler, R. S., and Paulk, H. T.: Thrombocytosis in Whipple's disease. Gastroenterology *80*:1465–1467, 1981.
41. Ojeda, E., Redondo, J., Lapaza, J., et al.: Enfermedad de Whipple: Manifestaciones neurologicas y revision de los casos publicados en la literatura nacional. Rev. Clin. Esp. *183*:365–367, 1988.
42. Poorman, J. C., and Katon, R. M.: Small bowel involvement by *Mycobacterium avium* complex in a patient with AIDS: Endoscopic, histologic and radiographic similarities to Whipple's disease. Gastrointest. Endosc. *4*:753–759, 1994.
43. Rausing, A.: Bone marrow biopsy in diagnosis of Whipple's disease. Acta Med. Scand. *193*:5–8, 1973.
44. Relman, D. A.: Whipple's disease: A disorder associated with a visible but uncultured bacillus. J. Infect. Dis. *168*:1–8, 1993.
45. Relman, D. A., Schmidt, T. M., MacDermott, R. P., et al.: Identification of the uncultured bacillus of Whipple's disease. N. Engl. J. Med. *327*:293–300, 1992.
46. Rickman, L. S., Freeman, W. R., Green, W. R., et al.: Brief report: Uveitis caused by *Tropheryma whippelii* (Whipple's bacillus). N. Engl. J. Med. *332*:363–366, 1995.
47. Romanul, F. C. A., Radvany, J., and Rosales, R. K.: Whipple's disease confined to the brain: A case studied clinically and pathologically. J. Neurol. Neurosurg. Psychiatr. *40*:901–909, 1977.
48. Ryser, R. J., Locksley, R. M., Eng, S. C, et al.: Reversal of dementia associated with Whipple's disease by trimethoprim-sulfamethoxazole, drugs that penetrate the blood-brain barrier. Gastroenterology *86*:745–752, 1984.
49. Scheib, J. S., and Quinet, R. J: Whipple's disease with axial and peripheral joint destruction. South. Med. J. *83*:684–687, 1990.
50. Sharma, O. P.: Beethoven's illness: Whipple's disease rather than sarcoidosis? J. Royal Soc. Med. *87:283–285*, 1994.
51. Sieracki, J. C., and Fine, G.: Whipple's disease: Observations on systemic involvement. II. Gross and histologic observations. Arch. Pathol. *67*:81–93, 1959.
52. Silva, M. T., Macedo, P. M., and Moura Nunes, J. F.: Ultrastructure of bacilli and the bacillary origin of the macrophagic inclusions in Whipple's disease. J. Gen. Microbiol. *131*:1001–1013, 1985.
53. Sossai, P., DeBoni, M., and Cielo, R.: The heart and Whipple's disease. Int. J. Cardiol. *23:275–276*, 1989.
54. Swash, M., Schwartz, M. S., Vandenberg, M. J., et al.: Myopathy in Whipple's disease. Gut. *18*:800–804, 1977.
55. Symmons, D. P. N., Shepard, A. N., Boardman, P. L., et al.: Pulmonary manifestations of Whipple's disease. Q. J. Med. *56*:497–504, 1985.
56. Tyor, M. P.: Whipple's disease: The Duke connection. N. C. Med. J. *55*:237–240, 1994.
57. Vine, A. K.: Retinal vasculitis. Semin. Neurol. *14*:354–360, 1994.
58. von Weizsacker, F., and Blum, H. E.: Impact of molecular biology in gastroenterology. Digestion *54*:125–129, 1993.
59. Whipple, G. H.: A hitherto undescribed disease characterized anatomically by deposits of fat and fatty acids in the intestinal mesenteric lymphatic tissues. Johns Hopkins Hosp. Bull. *18*:382–391, 1907.
60. Woese, C. R.: Bacterial evolution. Microbiol. Rev. *51*:221–271, 1987.

S E C T I O N   S E V E N

LIVER DISEASES

❑ ❑ ❑

55

Viral Hepatitis Due to Hepatitis Viruses A–E and GB Virus

Richard D. Aach

Viral hepatitis is a systemic infection in which the principal clinical manifestations are caused by hepatic-cell inflammation and necrosis. Until relatively recently, it was believed that there were two different types of viral hepatitis caused by two immunologically distinct viruses. Infectious hepatitis, short-incubation hepatitis, MS-1 hepatitis, and hepatitis A were terms used for one, whereas serum hepatitis, homologous serum jaundice, long-incubation hepatitis, MS-2 hepatitis, and hepatitis B were designations for the other (Table 55–1). The current preferred designations are type A and type B, respectively. Three additional agents have been well characterized, and they have been designated as hepatitis C virus (HCV); hepatitis D virus (HDV), or delta hepatitis; and hepatitis E virus (HEV). A sixth agent, at present called the GB virus (GBV), recently has been identified.

Other viruses, such as cytomegalovirus and the Epstein-Barr virus, can give rise to an illness with chemical and laboratory derangements similar to those of viral hepatitis. However, because involvement of other organs usually is more dominant, these illnesses are discussed elsewhere in this text.

HISTORY

The first description of viral hepatitis has been attributed to the Hippocratic School in the second century B.C. Curiously, the second citing of this illness and its possible contagiousness awaited Pope Zachanas' account about a thousand years later.[49] After another hiatus of almost 800 years, reports of epidemic jaundice began to appear. In Bachman's *World Atlas of Epidemic Disease*, 80 epidemics of jaundice were listed between the early 1600s and 1874.[23] The first recorded outbreak of hepatitis in the United States occurred in Norfolk, Virginia, in 1812.

During wartime, in both the United States and other countries, epidemics of jaundice were a serious problem among the military. Thus, camp jaundice, or field jaundice, severely affected the armies fighting the Napoleonic Wars, the American Civil War, the Franco-Prussian Wars, and both World Wars. Although other causes of jaundice, such as yellow fever and leptospirosis, probably were included in these descriptions, viral hepatitis A undoubtedly was responsible for the vast majority of these epidemics.

Descriptions of sporadic (isolated) cases of hepatitis A are of more recent vintage. Case records date back more than 150 years, but the prevailing opinion for many years, championed by Virchow, was that so-called catarrhal jaundice was caused by blockage of the common bile duct or ampulla of Vater by a mucus plug.[242] In Osler's classic *Principles and Practice of Medicine*, uncertainty about the true hepatocellular origin is evidenced by his discussion: "The nature of acute catarrhal jaundice is still unknown. It may possibly be an acute infection. In favor of this view are the occurrences in epidemic form and the presence of slight fever." However, Osler's recommended therapy reflected the prevailing view, for he suggested that "...irrigation of the large bowel with cold water may be practiced. The cold is supposed to excite peristalsis of the gall-bladder and ducts, and thus aid in the expulsion of the mucus."[168] That epidemic and catarrhal

TABLE 55–1. Types of Viral Hepatitis*

	Hepatitis A	Hepatitis B	Hepatitis C	Hepatitis D	Hepatitis E	GB Hepatitis
Viral designation	HAV	HBV	HCV	HDV	HEV	GBV
Genome	HAV RNA	HBV DNA	HCV RNA	HDV RNA	HEV RNA	GBV RNA
Virus family	*Picornaviridae*	*Hepadnaviridae*	*Flaviviridae*	Unique	*Caliciviridae*	*Flaviviridae*
Primary mode of spread	Enteral	Parenteral	Parenteral	Parenteral	Enteral	?
Chronicity	No	Yes	Yes	Yes	No	?
Prophylaxis	Immunoglobulin	HBIG	No	HBIG†	No	?
Vaccine	Yes	Yes	No	Yes†	No	No

*Five types of viral hepatitis due to five distinct viral agents have been identified. The responsible viral agents have been characterized fully, as have their epidemiologic features and clinical manifestations. The causative agent for a sixth agent, the GB virus, recently has been recognized. The salient characteristics of each type of viral hepatitis are shown. HBIG, hepatitis B immunoglobulin.

†Prevention of hepatitis D virus infection is accomplished by preventing transmission of hepatitis B virus.

jaundice were the same condition, namely hepatitis A, awaited the observations of Cockayne in 1912.[49] Of note, the suggestion of a viral etiology was not made until the 1920s, approximately 20 years before experimental studies supported this view.

The earliest recognizable description of presumed viral hepatitis B dates to the 1880s. In what ranks as a classic epidemiologic study, Luerman[141] in 1883 reported an outbreak of hepatitis among shipyard and warehouse workers in Bremen, Germany, who received smallpox vaccine that contained lymph of human origin. Of the 1350 employees receiving this material, 191 became jaundiced 2 to 6 months later. Luerman noted that workers given vaccine of a different origin at the same time and workers hired after the contaminated vaccine had been administered did not develop jaundice. He also pointed out the more prolonged nature of this form of hepatitis, in contrast to epidemic jaundice. However, despite the thoroughness with which he documented the epidemiologic and clinical features, Luerman was unable to fit the pieces of the puzzle together to account for its occurrence. Indeed, that this form of hepatitis is a distinct viral disease transmitted percutaneously was not appreciated for another 50 years.

The introduction of arsphenamine for the treatment of syphilis in the early 1900s soon was followed by reports of postarsenical jaundice, almost certainly hepatitis B and/or C.[98] As new forms of percutaneous therapy were introduced for hospitalized and clinic patients in the 1920s and 1930s, jaundice was observed as a not unusual late sequela. Unaware that hepatitis could be transmitted readily by inoculation with very small amounts of contaminated blood, physicians puzzled over whether or not jaundice after malarial treatment for neurosyphilis, insulin therapy for diabetes, and intravenous gold for rheumatoid arthritis was a complication of the underlying diseases or a complication of treatment. The problem was compounded by the fact that certain forms of therapy, such as the use of heavy metals, could, on occasion, give rise to drug-induced hepatitis.

One wonders how long hepatitis B would have remained unrecognized had not large-scale inoculations with live, attenuated, yellow fever vaccine been introduced in the mid 1930s. The live vaccines were stabilized by human serum. Instances of icterus occurring after vaccination were far too numerous to explain away as fortuitous or as complications of the vaccines per se.

The most famous epidemic of postvaccine hepatitis occurred among U.S. military personnel in 1942. Anticipating that U.S. troops likely would be engaged in combat where yellow fever was endemic, a mass inoculation program was instituted early during World War II. Certain lots of vaccine were stabilized with pooled human serum contaminated with hepatitis B virus (HBV). These contaminated lots gave rise to more than 28,000 recognized cases of icteric hepatitis 2 to 6 months later.[1] In addition, several epidemics of hepatitis occurred after the use of pooled measles and pooled mumps convalescent serum of human origin. In one epidemic, 44.7 per cent of soldiers receiving one lot of mumps convalescent serum subsequently became jaundiced.[27]

Viral hepatitis was a common problem in World War II. In all, about 250,000 of American military forces acquired hepatitis, many in the Mediterranean area, where hepatitis A was endemic. The administration of pooled plasma to battle casualties also gave rise to many cases of hepatitis. Pooling of plasma circumvented the need to crossmatch the donor and recipient. As the war progressed, the need for refrigeration was obviated by the technical advance of lyophilization. Unfortunately, the hepatitis agents tolerated lyophilization, storage at room temperature, and reconstitution. Thus, plasma could be made from very large donor pools, often more than 100 donors per lot, and one or a few units harboring hepatitis virus would contaminate the entire lot. As a result, posttransfusion hepatitis was observed commonly among military casualties given pooled plasma. By June 1945, 23 per cent of all cases of viral hepatitis in army hospitals were associated with the prior use of this material.[197]

In addition, much information about viral hepatitis was gained from a limited number of well-designed experiments using conscientious objectors as volunteers.[94] These volunteer studies, like epidemiologic observations, were believed to demonstrate two forms of disease: infectious hepatitis (hepatitis A) and serum hepatitis (hepatitis B).[143, 144] Both were caused by viral agents, as evidenced by infectivity of material even after passage through filters with a mean pore diameter of 50 nm, serial transmission from one human volunteer to another, and destruction of the agents by boiling. Recovery from one type of infection was observed to confer immunity to that type of hepatitis but did not result in cross-immunity to infection by the other viral agent.[160]

In the 1950s and 1960s, better definition of the epidemiologic features of hepatitis A and B was seen.[126] The introduction of serum transaminases as routine laboratory tests led to the recognition that both hepatitis A and B more often gave rise to anicteric than icteric infection, and even subclinical illness occurred with transaminase elevations only. Nevertheless, further progress was hampered greatly by the inability to grow the viral agents in tissue culture and organ explants. Fortunately, several independent observations largely circumvented this major obstacle during the late 1960s and early 1970s.

First came the realization that viral hepatitis was not restricted to human beings, as originally believed, but was transmissible to subhuman primates.[55, 98] The ability to conduct studies in susceptible chimpanzees and marmosets has been of immense value in confirming the infectivity of materials, characterization of the viral agents, acquisition of reagents for serologic testing, and evaluation of candidate vaccines against hepatitis B.

The second observation was the serendipitous discovery by Blumberg and associates[34] of the Australian (Au) antigen in the blood of an Australian aborigine. Although first reported in 1965, it was not related specifically to viral hepatitis infection until 1968.[35, 141, 174] By the early 1970s, the Au antigen was recognized as an immunologic marker unique to hepatitis B. Over the next several years, this antigen was given a number of designations, including the SH antigen, the hepatitis-associated antigen (HAA), the hepatitis B antigen (HBAg), and, finally, the preferred designation, hepatitis B surface antigen (HBsAg). Sensitive tests (vide infra) soon were developed for detection of HBsAg and its antibody, anti-HBs.

The third major breakthrough was the identification by Feinstone and associates,[77] in 1973, of virus-like particles in the stools of patients with hepatitis A virus (HAV) infection. In short order, tests were developed to detect antigenic determinants specific in these particles, HAAg, and HAV and its antibody, anti-HAV. Thus, by 1975, specific serologic markers for type A and type B hepatitis were available for investigational, epidemiologic, and clinical studies. Based on studies using tests for these serologic markers, hepatitis not associated with either hepatitis A or hepatitis B soon was recognized and called non-A, non-B hepatitis.[15, 101, 175, 224] In 1977, another hepatitis virus agent was discovered as the result of investigations of liver biopsy samples from chronic hepatitis B carriers using immunofluorescent staining.[189] These studies demonstrated a different pattern of staining in certain carriers soon appreciated to be due to a unique viral agent, called the hepatitis delta virus. This is a defective RNA virus that can replicate only when HBV infection also is present.

Epidemiologic observations and experimental studies with nonhuman primates soon demonstrated at least two distinct non-A, non-B agents, one transmitted percutaneously and the other a water-borne non-A, non-B agent that has been responsible for several common-source epidemics: so-called enterically transmitted non-A, non-B hepatitis.[125, 226]

Efforts to isolate and characterize the etiologic agents responsible for non-A, non-B hepatitis met with frustration for more than 15 years. In 1988, a viral agent responsible for most non-A, non-B hepatitis spread percutaneously was identified successfully.[47] The viral agent identified is called HCV. In 1990, the agent responsible for enteric non-A, non-B hepatitis was characterized by the same methodologic approach.[187] It has been given the designation of HEV and the infection it produces, hepatitis E. One additional viral hepatitis agent has been isolated recently. It is called GBV at present. GB are the initials of the individual whose blood provided the source of the virus.

HEPATITIS A

Virology and Serology

During hepatitis A, HAV can be recovered in the stool in large numbers (Fig. 55–1).[63] When viewed by immune electron microscopy, HAV has a surface with cuboid symmetry. Both intact, electron-dense "full" and "empty" particles suggestive of viral capsids can be seen by immune electron microscopy. HAV particles have been detected in the liver, bile, and serum of infected subhuman primates, as well as in the feces of chimpanzees and human beings with hepatitis A.[150] During infection, HAV can be demonstrated by immunofluorescence within the cytoplasm of infected hepatocytes.

HAV is an RNA virus belonging to the family *Picornaviridae* in a newly established genus designated *Hepatovirus*.[39] The virus is nonenveloped, is 27 nm in diameter, and has four surface polypeptides. Its genome consists of positive single-stranded RNA, which contains about 8000 nucleotides and has a molecular weight of approximately 2.8 million daltons.[209] Like other members of *Picornaviridae*, it has only one open-reading frame encoding a single large polyprotein processed by a protease (3Cpro), which is included within the polyprotein. Four distinct genotypes of HAV have been identified, but all are related very closely antigenically, so all four belong to a single serotype, i.e., HAA or HAV.

The buoyant density of HAV particles recovered from acute-phase stool, determined by isopyknic binding in cesium chloride, is 1.4 g/mL.[76] A lighter population with a buoyant density of 1.32 to 1.33 g/mL also has been described.[150] Both populations of particles react with anti-HAV and produce hepatitis A when inoculated into subhuman primates. In addition, morphologically and serologically identical particles with a density of 1.34 g/mL have been recovered from the liver of experimentally infected marmosets.

Purified HAV is inactivated completely after heating at 100° C for 5 minutes, exposure to ultraviolet light, and 1:4000 formalin at 37° C for 3 days. HAV is inactivated partially by heating at 60° C for 1 hour. It is acid- and ether-stable.[180]

HAV has been cultivated in vitro in culture lines from rhesus monkey kidney and human diploid lung cells.[179] The ability to grow HAV in vitro has led to the development of both live attenuated vaccine candidates and an inactivated vaccine that was licensed recently.

Utilizing purified HAV from infected human stool and marmoset liver, researchers developed tests that detect anti-HAV in the serum. Other techniques used soon thereafter include complement fixation, immune adherence hemagglutination, radioimmunoassay, and enzyme-linked immunosorbent assay (ELISA). Radioimmunoassay also can demonstrate HAV in the serum of experimentally infected chimpanzees. Screening for HAVAg has not proved feasible for the routine diagnosis of acute hepatitis A because it only is present transiently and in low titer. However, tests for the presence of IgM anti-HAV, which appears shortly after the onset of acute type A infection, are applicable readily for clinical and epidemiologic use. They are used routinely to establish the diagnosis of acute hepatitis A.

Typical Course of Hepatitis A

The interval between exposure to HAV and the onset of clinically apparent illness (incubation period) averages about 28 to 30 days, with a range of 15 to 50 days. HAV can be demonstrated in the stool at least 5 days before the serum transaminases begin to increase, usually 1 or 2 weeks before the appearance of clinical symptoms (Fig. 55–2).[63, 64] Fecal excretion of HAV reaches maximal levels at the time of peak transaminase elevation and then decreases rapidly as jaundice appears. These findings are consistent with earlier volunteer studies and epidemiologic observations that the

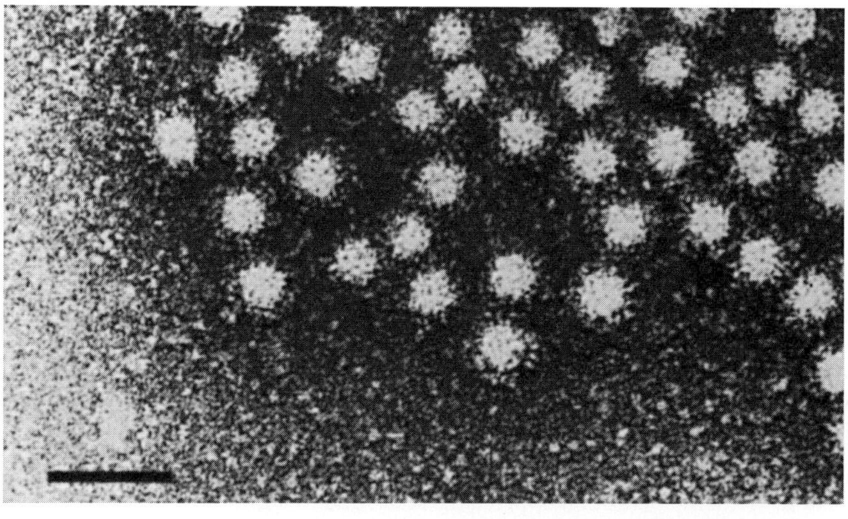

FIGURE 55–1. *Twenty-seven–nanometer hepatitis A virus (HAV) isolated from stool filtrate of a patient with acute HAV infection. The HAV particles are aggregated by convalescent serum containing anti-HAV antibodies. The line represents 100 nm. (Courtesy of Dr. Jules Dienstag, taken at the Laboratory of Infectious Diseases. NIAID, NIH, DHEW, Bethesda, MD.)*

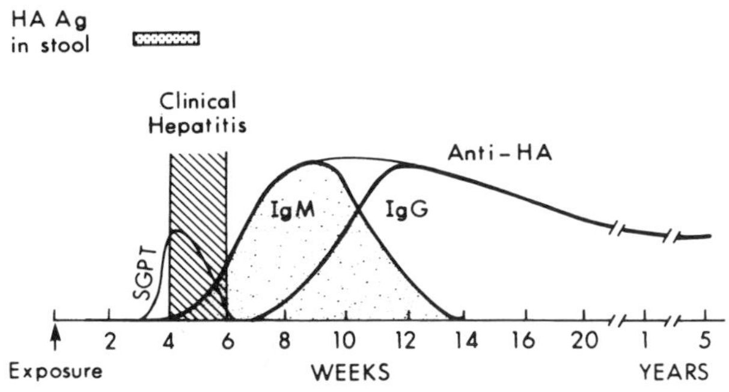

FIGURE 55–2. *Typical pattern of acute hepatitis A virus infection. Hepatitis A antigen (HAAg) fecal excretions precede serum transaminase elevations and clinical manifestations of infection by 1 to 2 weeks. Anti-HA appears in the serum early during the clinically apparent illness stage and persists thereafter. Anti-HA predominantly is IgM initially but after 2 to 3 months is detectable primarily as IgG.*

feces of hepatitis A patients are infectious for up to 3 weeks before and approximately 1 week after the appearance of jaundice.[25] Fecal shedding generally ceases within a 2- to 4-week period, but in a few patients it is prolonged, lasting up to 40 weeks.[87] Viremia is maximal during the prodromal phase of infection before there is chemical serologic or clinical evidence of hepatitis. The degree of viremia usually is 2 to 3 $\log^{10}$ less than the amount of viruses excreted in the stool but may continue throughout the period of fecal shedding.

As HAV disappears from the stool, usually while the patient is symptomatic, anti-HAV becomes detectable in the serum by complement fixation and radioimmunoassay but not by immune adherence hemagglutination. The anti-HAV titer rises rapidly, and, after several weeks, it can be demonstrated also by immune adherence hemagglutination. This pattern of detection is due to the fact that anti-HAV predominantly is IgM during the first several weeks after seroconversion. IgM anti-HAV activity peaks during the first 6 months after its appearance and then gradually declines to undetectable levels within 6 to 12 months. Thereafter, anti-HAV resides exclusively in the 7s, IgG fraction. IgG anti-HAV activity persists for years after recovery and is an indicator of prior type A infection and immunity to reinfection with HAV. Solid-phase antibody-captive immunoassays are employed routinely for the detection of IgM anti-HAV. ELISAs also are available for total anti-HAV, i.e., both IgM and IgG anti-HAV. These tests also are positive at the onset of acute hepatitis A but may remain reactive indefinitely after recovery from infection because of sustained IgG anti-HAV seropositivity. Therefore, a positive test for total anti-HAV is not diagnostic of an acute or recent infection.

To date, neither chronic hepatitis A nor an HAV carrier state has been demonstrated.

Epidemiology

Hepatitis A is worldwide in distribution. The predominant mode of transmission is by direct contact (person to person) via the fecal-oral route. Spread occurs particularly among children in the same household. As a result, hepatitis A is more widespread where there are crowding and poor sanitation, such as in underdeveloped countries, in lower social classes in urban areas of the United States, and in homes for the mentally disadvantaged. In a large-scale study of residents of the greater New York City area, anti-HAV was found in approximately 75 per cent of individuals in the lower social class, in contrast to a 20 to 30 per cent prevalence among the middle and upper-middle classes.[219] The peak rates of clinically evident hepatitis occur among children and young adolescents 5 to 15 years of age. Outbreaks of hepatitis A have occurred in a number of large cities in the United States over the past several years with epidemiologic characteristics of person-to-person spread.

The Sentinel County study by the Centers for Disease Control and Prevention has led to an estimation of the relative frequencies of the different ways HAV is transmitted in the United States. Household exposure accounts for 24 per cent, transmission in day care centers for 18 per cent, homosexual activity for 11 per cent, exposure during travel to areas endemic for hepatitis A 4 per cent, and intravenous drug abuse for 2 per cent. Of note, a risk factor cannot be identified in about 40 per cent of cases.

Approximately 50 "common-source" epidemics of hepatitis A have been ascribed to simultaneous exposure of multiple individuals to food or water contaminated by HAV.[154] Raw clams,[65] raw oysters,[149] milk,[157] potato salad,[112] and orange juice[72] are but some of the vehicles that became contaminated inadvertently by human waste harboring HAV and thus served as the common source for hepatitis A cases.

Hepatitis A also has spread from subhuman primates to animal handlers in zoos and animal colonies.[98] Typically, hepatitis A is transmitted from newly arrived animals who do not appear ill or have mild, nonspecific illness (e.g., diarrhea in the absence of jaundice). The animals are believed to have acquired hepatitis A during captivity in many instances because they often are kept and cared for shortly after capture in villages where hepatitis A is endemic.

Of note, hepatitis A is transmitted only very rarely by blood transfusion. An increased prevalence of anti-HAV has not been found in patients who have received multiple transfusions or among staff and patients in dialysis units where hepatitis is endemic. Vertical transmission does not play an important role in the spread of hepatitis A.

HEPATITIS B

Biophysiology, Serology, and Virology

HBsAg resides on the surface of HBV as spherical particles, 22 nm in diameter, and tubular structures of the same width but up to 700 nm in length.[84] HBV, originally called the Dane particle after its discoverer,[50] is 42 nm in diameter (range, 40 to 45 nm) and can be found in complete and incomplete forms. The 22-nm spheres and tubules have a buoyant density of 1.20 g/mL in cesium chloride.[86] Complete HBV has a double-layered outer coat that surrounds a discrete spherical inner core, 27 nm in diameter (Fig. 55–3). Incomplete HBV particles devoid of inner core also are observed on electron microscopy.

The inner core of HBV has two antigen determinants: the hepatitis B core antigen (HBcAg) and HBeAg.[225] HBcAg is demonstrable when the outer coat is disrupted by detergent.[10] In contrast, HBeAg can be detected readily in the serum early in the course of acute and chronic hepatitis B. After recovery (or later in the course of chronic hepatitis), anti-HBe rather than HBeAg is present.[145] HBeAg's presence correlates with the level of circulating HBV (vide infra).[167] The inner core of HBV is denser than the surface coat, with a buoyant density of 1.32 g/mL. Immunofluorescent studies employing antibodies specific for HBsAg (anti-HBs) and HBcAg (anti-HBc) demonstrate that surface antigen is made within the cytoplasm of the infected hepatocyte, whereas the core is synthesized within the nucleus.[24]

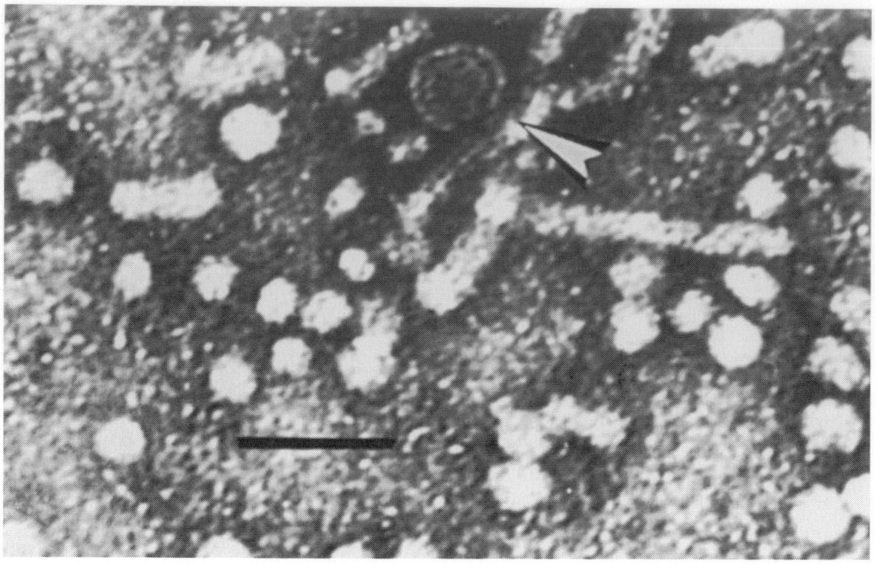

FIGURE 55–3. *Electron micrograph of hepatitis B virus particles. Most particles are 20 to 25 nm in diameter and consist of both spheres and tubules. A larger, 42-nm, Dane particle also is present (arrow). Hepatitis B surface antigen determinants are present on the surface of all three forms.*

The 22-nm particles, tubules, and outer coat of the Dane particle are composed of protein, lipid, and polysaccharide but no nucleoprotein. The surface protein is composed of two major polypeptides, both with HBsAg determinants. The larger polypeptide has a molecular weight of 28,000 daltons and is glycosylated, whereas the smaller polypeptide with a molecular weight of 23,000 daltons is not.[85] The small spheres and tubules are believed to be capsid- or surface-coat material synthesized in excess during HBV replication.

The Dane particle's inner core contains hepatitis B–specific DNA polymerase and circular DNA.[190] HBV DNA consists of 3200 nucleotides. It is circular and double-stranded, except for one small region of variable length that is single-stranded. HBV DNA is synthesized from an RNA intermediate by reverse transcription, similar to the process of replication of retroviruses.[218]

The simultaneous presence of endogenous DNA polymerase and double-stranded DNA is unique; this combination has not been found in any other known group of viruses infecting primates. However, these are characteristics of a newly identified family of HBV-like viruses that are species-specific and include agents that infect the pekin duck, Beechey ground squirrel, and woodchuck.[79, 217] These viruses have similar structural biologic features. Intact virions and smaller defective surface-antigen particles circulate in the serum of the infected host. They all infect the hepatocyte and produce both acute and chronic infection. The woodchuck hepatitis virus, like HBV in humans, has been associated with the development of hepatocellular carcinoma. These agents, including HBV, now are considered to be members of the same family of viruses, to which the term hepadnavirus group has been applied.

The DNA of HBV has been cloned in *Escherichia coli* and yeast-cell cultures. The nucleotide sequence has been determined in full, and the base pairs coding for each of the HBV determinants have been identified (Fig. 55–4).[45, 84, 169, 212] The HBV genome has four open-reading frames that code as the pre-S, S, C, X, and P genes. The S gene codes for the predominant polypeptide of HBsAg consisting of 226 amino acids. The pre-S region encodes two other proteins recognized as pre-S and pre-S2 epitopes, which are important in the attachment of HBV to the hepatocyte.[167]

Investigations have shown that HBeAg is synthesized by the C gene, the same gene that codes for HBcAg.[246] This gene has two initiation codons for protein synthesis. The first (pre-C) start codon yields HBeAg, whereas the second (C) start codon leads to synthesis of HBcAg. These two products of the gene initially reside on a single protein, which then undergoes proteolytic clearage at the C terminal and yields HBeAg, which is secreted into the circulation from the infected cell. HBcAg, on the other hand, accumulates in the hepatocyte, where it is utilized for HBV assembly. Because HBeAg is synthesized by the C gene, which is essential for HBV synthesis, HBeAg correlates with the level of HBV in the blood and, therefore, is an indirect measure of the degree of infectivity.[17]

The P gene, which overlaps the other genes, codes for HBV DNA polymerase. This enzyme has reverse transcriptase activity and functions to repair the missing nucleotides in the inner or short strand of DNA.[99] The X gene codes for a protein (HBxAg) containing 154 amino acids whose function(s) is less well understood. It appears to be involved in HBV expression, perhaps as a transcriptional activator.[205]

The relative proportion of circulating 22-nm spheres, filaments, and HBV varies considerably in different HBsAg-positive sera. However, the smaller spherical forms and tubules virtually always are present in much greater numbers than HBV. DNA polymerase activity and circulating HBV particles usually are more abundant during the first 1 to 4 weeks of acute infection and in the serum of approximately 5 to 10 per cent of HBsAg carriers. The level of circulating HBV does not appear to be correlated with the titer of HBsAg. Serum specimens strongly positive for HBsAg (i.e., detectable by agar gel diffusion) contain approximately 3×10^{15} of the 22-nm diameter particles per milliliter. Currently available assays can detect HBsAg levels less than 5 to 10 ng of protein or 10^{12} particles per milliliter.

HBsAg is ether- and acid-stable. Surface antigenicity resists exposure to formalin (1:2000) at 37° C for 96 hours and heating at 100° C for 1 minute and at 60° C for 10 hours. HBV infectivity, on the other hand, is inactivated by boiling, sodium hypochlorite, and formalin (see the section on prevention) (vide infra).

Although a single immunoprecipitation line is formed when HBsAg-positive serum is tested in agar gel diffusion with high-titer anti-HBs, the surface coat actually contains a heterogeneous group of antigens. This makes it possible to subtype HBsAg-positive material. All surface antigens are coded by the HBV and not the infected host. One antigen, a, is common to all HBsAg particles. There are, in addition, at least two pairs of subtype-specific determinants. One of each pair, d or y and w or r, also resides on the surface coat.[24, 133] Thus, four HBsAg subtypes can be identified: HBsAg/adw, HBsAg/ayw, HBsAg/adr, and HBsAg/ayr. Using monospecific antisera, researchers can accomplish subtyping by immunodiffusion, counterelectrophoresis, hemagglutination, and radioimmunassay. With use of immunodiffusion, a "spur," denoting either d or y antigen, is formed when serum containing HBsAg/adw and HBsAg/ayr is added to wells adjacent to wells containing anti-ay and anti-ad antisera, respectively (Fig. 55–5). The w and r antigens are identifiable with monospecific anti-HBs prepared in a similar fashion. There is no apparent correlation between the HBsAg subtype and the virulence of the infecting HBV or an increased risk of the development of chronic hepatitis B.[258]

On the other hand, the presence of HBeAg correlates with the degree of hepatocellular necrosis and inflammation.[17, 145, 233] By immunoelectrophoresis, HBeAg is demonstrated in the majority of patients with elevated transaminases and histologic evidence of chronic hepatitis B. However, anti-HBe is found in asymptomatic HBsAg carriers who have normal or nearly normal liver function tests and liver biopsies, a population in which HBeAg uncommonly is present. It was hoped initially that testing for HBeAg might prove useful in determining early in the course of acute illness which patients' status would progress to chronic hepatitis. Unfortunately, HBeAg has not been found to be a predictor of chronicity.[75]

Infants born of mothers who acquire anti-HB during their third trimester are at considerable risk of acquiring hepatitis.[232] The risk is much lower if hepatitis begins in the first or second trimester and there is recovery before the third trimester begins.

Transmission of hepatitis to neonates occurs with high frequency from HBsAg-carrier mothers whose blood also has HBeAg.[165] Vertical, or perinatal, transmission from mother to newborn infant is much less frequent if the HBsAg-positive mother is HBeAg-negative. Carrier mothers who are anti-HBe–positive transmit hepatitis B to their newborn but less frequently. Thus, although the presence of HBeAg in serum indicates a high degree of infectivity, its absence does not ensure an HBV-negative, noninfectious state.

Of note, variants of HBV exist. The predominant variant is the result of a mutation in the precore region of the HBV genome that affects the translation and transcription of HBeAg. Patients infected with this "HBeAg-minus" HBV phenotype have high levels of circulating HBV-DNA but are HBeAg-negative.[166] Instead of circulating HBeAg, anti-HBe is present in the blood. Individuals with chronic hepatitis B infected with these precore mutants tend to have more severe hepatitis and a more progressive course compared with patients with chronic hepatitis B due to nonmutuant HBV.[41] Fulminant hepatitis B also has been shown to be a consequence of infection due to HBV precore mutants in both children and adults.[95, 198]

Epidemiology

Hepatitis B is one of the most important causes of acute and chronic hepatitis worldwide. In the United States, there are approximately 200,000 new cases of hepatitis B each year and an estimated 1 million individuals who chronically are infected with HBV.[19] The number of HBV carriers worldwide is thought to approach 300 million.

The HBV carrier rate in the United States is estimated to be between 0.1 and 0.4 per cent.[221] Carriers are far more prevalent in Asian countries and developing nations. In Ja-

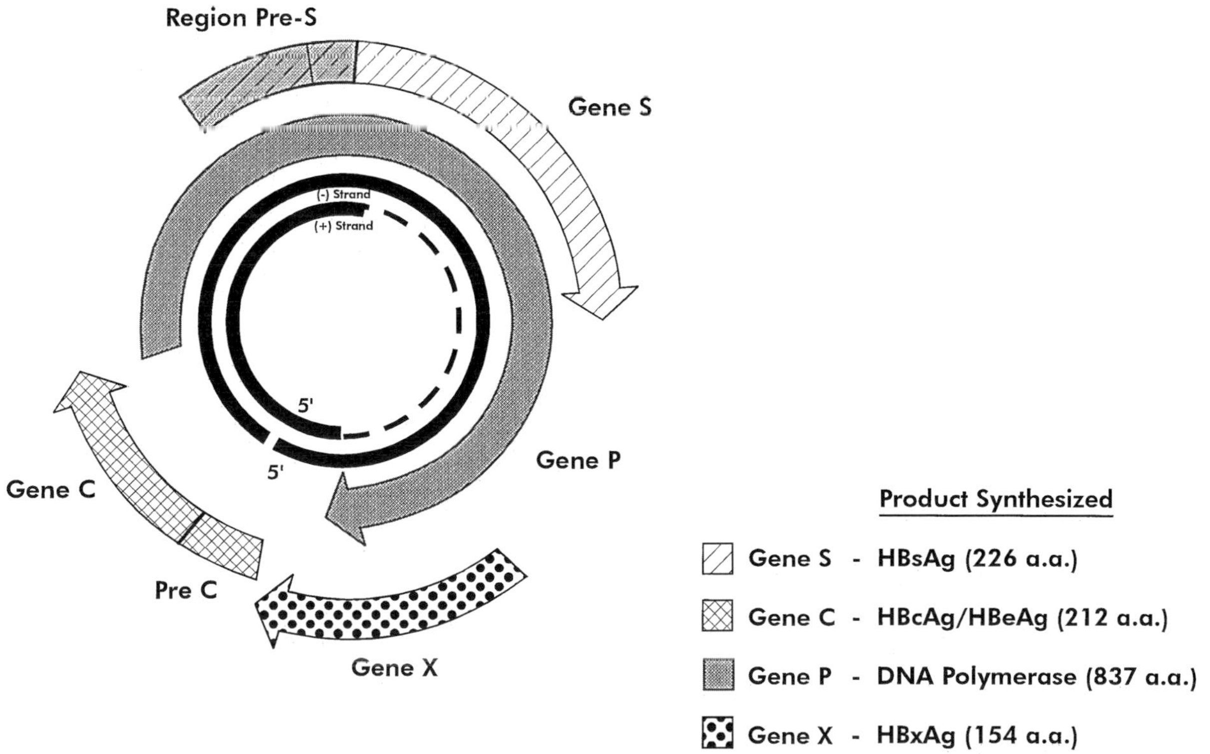

FIGURE 55–4. *Schematic representation of the hepatitis B virus genome (HBV DNA). The genome consists of double-stranded DNA with 3200 nucleotides. Functionally, it is divided into the pre-S, S, pre-C, C, P, and X domains. The products synthesized by HBV DNA are indicated in the figure.*

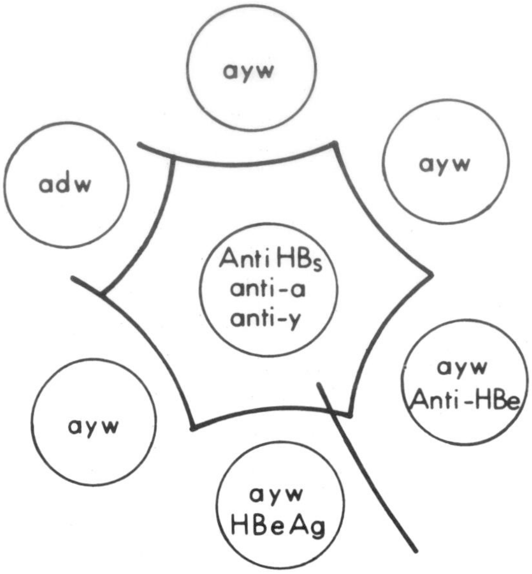

FIGURE 55–5. *Agar gel diffusion patterns of hepatitis B surface antigen (HBsAg) subdeterminants and the HBsAg/anti-HBe system. The center well contains high-titer anti-HBs with anti-a and anti-y antibodies. Outer wells contain HBsAg-positive sera. Five wells hold serum with HBsAg/ayw. The well at 10 o'clock contains HBsAg/adw. The y subdeterminant is recognizable as a spur on either side of the well containing HBsAg/adw. An HBeAg/anti-HBe immunoprecipitation band has formed at the 5 o'clock position. It crosses the HBsAg/anti-HBs line, indicating a reaction of nonidentity.*

pan, 1 per cent of the adult population harbors HBsAg; in other Asian populations, the carrier rate varies from 5 to 15 per cent.

Approximately 15 per cent of Americans are anti-HBs–positive, the vast majority without a prior illness recognizable (even in retrospect) as viral hepatitis. The prevalence of anti-HBs increases with age. In a survey of residents in the Washington, D.C., area, anti-HBs was not observed in the serum of infants younger than 1 year of age but was found in 3 per cent of children 5 to 9 years of age, 7 per cent of those 10 to 14 years of age, 24 per cent of adults between 20 and 29 years of age, and 32 per cent of adults older than 50 years of age.[138] In the drug culture, anti-HBs has been found in approximately two-thirds of those surveyed, and the HBsAg carrier rate also is increased.[204]

Hepatitis B is more common among health care professionals than in the general population because of their greater contact with patients who are infected with HBV, often with clinically silent and unrecognized infection.[211] Prevalence rates among physicians and nurses range up to 1 per cent and 25 to 50 per cent for HBsAg and anti-HBs, respectively. Nurses and physicians, particularly professional staff of renal dialysis and oncology units, where they are exposed to immunosuppressed, highly infectious individuals, are at special risk of acquiring hepatitis B.[139, 244] Hepatitis B particularly is an occupational hazard to the general surgeon, the surgical nurse, and the technician in the clinical laboratory. Dentists, especially oral surgeons, also are more likely to acquire hepatitis B.[137, 156]

Hepatitis B can be transmitted other than by percutaneous inoculation. HBsAg has been detected in saliva, semen, vaginal secretions, and even breast milk.[96, 139, 240] Thus, it is not surprising that hepatitis B occurs more frequently among patients with venereal disease, male homosexuals,[220] and spouses of patients acutely ill with hepatitis B. Once considered to be a major and frequent cause of posttransfusion hepatitis, HBV infection is seen very rarely among transfusion recipients in the United States since screening of blood donors for HBsAg, anti-HBc, and alanine aminotransferase became mandatory. The rate of posttransfusion hepatitis B among recipients in the 1970s, after HBsAg screening was initiated among voluntary donors, was 1 per cent.[3] In a series conducted from 1988 to 1992, not one case of HBV infection was detected among more than 4000 transfusion recipients.[31]

Perinatal transmission from surface-antigen–positive mothers to newborn offspring has been emphasized in the previous section in relation to HBeAg. The risk of transmission is 70 to 90 per cent if the mother is HBeAg-positive and 10 to 40 per cent if the mother is HBeAg-negative.[214, 215] Exposure usually takes place at the time of delivery rather than in utero.[200] HBsAg or signs of infection (often mild) in the neonate usually begin during the first 3 months of life and typically are asymptomatic and unrecognized. However, infection in the newborn is likely to evolve into chronic disease. In the United States, approximately 10 per cent of all acute HBV infections occur among children 10 years of age or younger but account for roughly one-third of chronic HBV infections. Perinatally acquired hepatitis B in the Far East is believed to be the basis for the high prevalence of the HBsAg carrier state and higher incidence of hepatomas in these populations (see the hepatoma section) (vide infra).

Diagnosing Acute Viral Hepatitis B

The diagnosis of acute hepatitis B usually is easy to establish. The de novo appearance of HBsAg in the blood is diagnostic of acute HBV infection. However, the time of appearance, duration, and titer of HBsAg positivity also are variable. HBsAg is not detectable always by even the most sensitive tests in patients with acute illness.[104] IgM antibody to HBcAg also is indicative of recent HBV infection, and assays for its presence are used to establish a diagnosis of acute or recent HBV infection when HBsAg is not detected.[46] A diagnosis of acute hepatitis B can be made in these patients by detecting HBV DNA by a polymerase chain reaction assay or by demonstrating the de novo appearance of anti-HBc. Seroconversion of anti-HBs after recovery is other evidence that the episode of hepatitis was due to HBV. Some patients with self-limited type B infection fail to develop detectable levels of anti-HBs or have only transiently demonstrable anti-HBs after recovery. However, these patients generally are HBsAg-positive during infection and have detectable anti-HBc.

Typical Course of Acute Hepatitis B

The severity and duration of hepatitis B infection are highly variable. As in hepatitis A, most patients have a mild, self-limited illness with nonspecific constitutional symptoms or subclinical infection without symptoms. Based on prospective studies of individuals exposed to blood known to be contaminated with HBV, serologic evidence of acute hepatitis B or serum transaminase elevation is accompanied by symptoms in only about 25 to 30 per cent.[3]

The typical sequence of events in hepatitis B is as follows. The incubation period (time of exposure to first symptoms) averages 90 days, with a range of 60 to 180 days (Fig. 55–6). HBsAg usually first appears in the serum several weeks after exposure, generally about 4 weeks before clinical evidence of infection. However, it has been detected as early as 7 days and as long as 4 months after exposure. HBsAg serum positivity soon is followed by HBV DNA, DNA polymerase, and HBeAg in the serum.

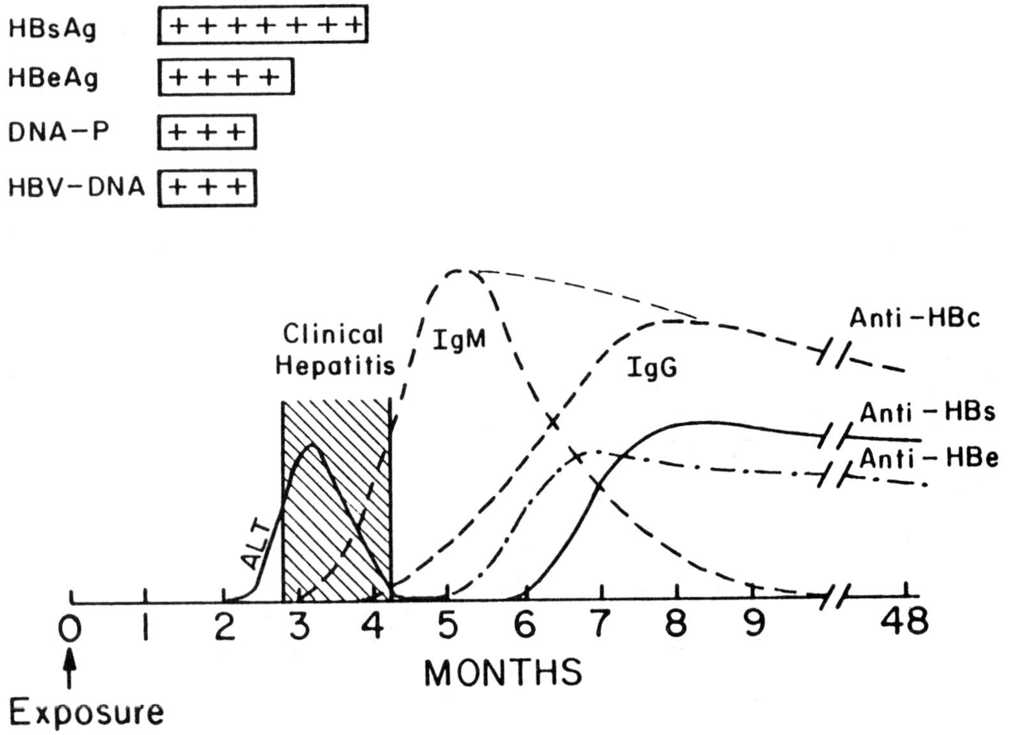

FIGURE 55–6. *Sequence of events in acute hepatitis B virus infection. Clinically evident hepatitis is preceded by hepatitis B surface antigen (HBsAg) serum positivity. Anti-HBc seroconversion occurs during the clinical phase of illness, whereas anti-HBs usually appears 1 to 3 months after recovery. Anti-HBc circulates as IgM during the first 6 to 12 months of its appearance.*

Serum transaminase levels begin to increase next, usually 1 to 4 weeks after HBsAg first appears, and reach peak levels at about the time symptoms of hepatitis begin. In the majority of patients, anti-HBc appears early during the clinical phase of illness when HBsAg still is detectable.[104] It is present predominantly in the IgM fraction during the first 4 to 6 months after its appearance.[46] At about the time of appearance of anti-HBc, DNA polymerase activity and then HBeAg disappear from the serum. However, tests for HBsAg usually do not become negative until symptoms, signs of infection, and liver function tests have become normal. Although anti-HBs seroconversion may occur at any stage of acute illness, anti-HBs usually makes its appearance during convalescence, 1 to 3 months after HBsAg has cleared.[132] Thus, the finding of HBsAg with or without anti-HBc denotes very early acute hepatitis B, whereas the finding of IgM anti-HBc alone in high titer strongly is suggestive of early convalescence, remote infection without a measurable anti-HBs response, or HBV infection with HBsAg levels too low to detect by standard assays.[103] The simultaneous presence of anti-HBc and anti-HBs suggests infection in the past (months to years) with complete resolution of infection. The finding of anti-HBs alone also implies remote infection with full recovery or may be due to hepatitis B vaccination.

Chronic Hepatitis B

Chronic HBV infection, with or without evidence of chronic hepatitis, is a well-recognized complication of type B hepatitis.[184] Chronic hepatitis B is characterized by continued HBsAg positivity of at least 6 months' duration; a high-titer anti-HBc, which is present predominantly or exclusively as an IgG fraction; and the absence of anti-HBs in the serum.[46, 105] Generally, chronic hepatitis B is most active during the first few years after its onset, during which time the virus is replicating actively. Serum levels of HBV DNA and HBeAg positivity are high. There is active hepatitis during this "replicative" stage demonstrated on liver biopsy and by an elevated alanine aminotransferase level. Over time, the degree of hepatocellular inflammation and necrosis diminishes and, later in the course, actually may disappear. HBV DNA no longer may be detected or circulates in low titer, HBeAg clears followed by the appearance of anti-HBe, and the serum alanine aminotransferase may normalize. These features are typical of the asymptomatic carrier state. HBV DNA at this stage of illness usually is integrated into the genome of infected liver cells. It is not unusual for the transition to a carrier state to be ushered in by an episode simulating acute hepatitis B.[54] In addition, some patients with quiescent infection may have one or more exacerbations easily confused with acute hepatitis B if it is not known that they are infected chronically.[54] These clinical exacerbations are indicative of a recurrence of active viral replication demonstrable by high levels of HBV DNA and the reappearance of HBeAg. In some patients, IgM anti-HBc may reappear transiently in the serum. The precipitating factors for these exacerbations are not known.

The long-term consequences of untreated chronic hepatitis B among adults understandably have been a subject of considerable interest. Although a number of articles have appeared in the literature on the subject, there still is much to be learned about the natural history of chronic HBV infection. There virtually are no natural history studies that span more than 10 to 15 years of follow-up. Furthermore, reports have demonstrated considerable variation in the severity, frequency of complications, and rate of progression of chronic HBV infection. These diverse patterns may relate to differences in the expression of HBV infection as a result of a number of modifying factors. The patient's gender as well as differences in the pattern of immune response either genetically predetermined or influenced by environmental factors, the age at onset of infection, and the presence of coexistent disease may affect the clinical manifestation and course of the disease. However, virtually all studies show that chronic

HBV infection is associated with considerable long-term morbidity and mortality.

The largest study examining this subject was conducted in Taiwan.[26] This prospective study followed 220,707 Chinese adult males, of whom 15.2 per cent had HBV infection. Among those who died, 54 per cent were HBsAg-positive individuals whose deaths were attributable to cirrhosis or a hepatoma. In contrast, only 1.5 per cent of the deaths among noninfected controls were due to these two conditions. The relative risk of hepatoma among the HBV-infected group was 223 times greater than that of the control group. In a study conducted in London, 100 consecutive HBV carriers were followed for a mean period of 44 months.[241] Seven of the patients in this series died of a hepatoma during follow-up.

Natural history studies of chronic HBV among children are just beginning to appear in the literature. They differ in their findings from a very benign course[37] to an incidence of greater than 3 per cent of cirrhosis on initial biopsy.[70, 191] Furthermore, HBV-associated hepatoma has been observed among both Asian and white children.[44, 58, 173] These findings indicate that chronic hepatitis B can be a rapidly progressive and fatal disease among children.

The risk of developing chronic HBV is correlated highly with the age of the susceptible person at the time of initial infection. Approximately 90 per cent of those infected prior to 1 year of age develop chronic HBV infection, whereas the rate decreases to approximately 40 per cent between 1 and 10 years of age and is less than 10 per cent among adults.[118, 151] Immunosuppression, either as a complication of disease (e.g., AIDS, chronic renal failure) or therapeutically induced by medications (e.g., corticosteroids), also increases the risk of chronic HBV infection.

Hepatitis D

The agent responsible for delta hepatitis (the delta agent, or HDV) is unique in that it is an incomplete virus that requires the "helper" function of HBV. It circulates in the blood stream in a subpopulation of HBsAg particles 35 to 37 nm in diameter.[188] The HDV genome consists of circular and single-stranded RNA that have approximately 1700 base pairs.[245] The genome has only one open-reading frame that codes for structured HDVAg protein. HDV's envelope of HBsAg enables the agent to bind to receptor sites on the surface of the hepatotype, which then is followed by cell entry. The replication of HDV is associated with suppression of HBV synthesis and a corresponding decrease in the production of HBV determinants. The agent is transmissible to humans and subhuman primates, but it is associated always with HBV infection.

Two patterns of infection have been described: (1) simultaneous acute "co-infection" of HBV and HDV, which usually results in overt self-limited hepatitis; and (2) HDV "superinfection" of a patient who is infected chronically with HBV.[36] Hepatitis is much more severe in HDV superinfection, with mortality rates as high as 20 per cent. Those surviving usually have continued HBV and HDV infection and a much more severe form of chronic hepatitis, which may progress rapidly to cirrhosis. Delta hepatitis should be suspected in fulminant hepatitis or when a patient with chronic hepatitis B has an acute flare-up.

Three genotypes have been identified on the basis of sequence analysis of the HDV gene.[254] The severity of infection and rate of progression of hepatitis D have been linked with the specific HDV genotype. Types I and III give rise most often to fulminant hepatitis and severe chronic hepatitis. The course of disease in patients with type II genotype generally is less severe.

The diagnosis of hepatitis D infection is made by demonstrating the anti-HD antibodies in the serum by solid-phase radioimmunoassay or ELISA. In HDV co-infection, anti-HD may be of low titer and transient. Serial testing may be required for detection. In contrast, chronic delta hepatitis is characterized by continued high titers of anti-HD. During the first several months after HDV infection, anti-HD is predominantly in the IgM fraction, but, thereafter, it is found almost exclusively as IgG. Direct assays for HDV RNA have proved to be highly sensitive and specific but are not routinely available for clinical use.

The delta agent is worldwide in distribution, with an endemic concentration in the Mediterranean, particularly in Italy. Outbreaks of hepatitis D with high mortality rates have occurred among Yucpa Indians in South America.[92] Gene-sequencing studies have implicated HDV of type III genotype as the etiologic agent.[43] It also is present in the drug culture, where it has been spreading in recent years.

HEPATITIS C

The development of serologic tests diagnostic for hepatitis A and B that were negative in most instances of posttransfusion hepatitis led to the recognition of at least one additional form of viral hepatitis spread percutaneously.[65, 78, 175] Given the name non-A, non-B hepatitis, its virologic etiology was demonstrated by transmission to chimpanzees with blood implicated in posttransfusion hepatitis.[15, 101, 224] A number of serologic tests and candidate viral agents were described, but a specific non-A, non-B hepatitis agent was not identified for almost 15 years.

In 1988, a non-A, non-B hepatitis viral agent was identified by studying the antigen expressed from a cDNA library in bacteriophage derived from the DNA and RNA of highly infectious chimp serum.[47] Using the serum of a patient with chronic non-A, non-B hepatitis as a presumed source of antibody directed against viral antigens and exhaustive methodical screening of the cDNA library of more than 1 million clones by immunoblot technique, researchers eventually found a clone that expressed an antigen agent that was encoded by a portion of a viral genome. The viral antigen originally identified was used to develop an immunologic test to detect antibody to the virus in the circulation of infected individuals.[108, 128] This discovery also led to the sequencing of the virus. The agent identified has been designated HCV. It is 30 to 50 nm in diameter and consists of an outer lipid envelope, HCV antigen, and a core containing a genome consisting of linear single-stranded RNA of approximately 9400 nucleotides (Fig. 55–7).[128]

HCV belongs to a distinct genus of the *Flaviviridae* family. It shares some characteristics with *Pestivirus* (bovine viral diarrhea and hog cholera virus), as well as with other flaviviruses (dengue viruses, yellow fever virus, and Japanese encephalitis virus).[108]

The HCV genome has been well characterized (Fig. 55–7).[108, 247] A highly conserved noncoding region at the 5′ end of the genome precedes a large sequence that codes for the structural proteins of the virus, i.e., the core protein and two envelope glycoproteins (E_1 and E_2). This region is followed by sequences that encode nonstructural (NS) proteins. These domains are designated E_2/NS_1, NS_2, NS_3, NS_4, and NS_5. Not all of the functions of the nonstructural proteins are known. It appears that NS_3 codes for a viral protease involved in the processing of polyproteins and a helicase enzyme that plays a role in the unwinding of the RNA genome necessary for

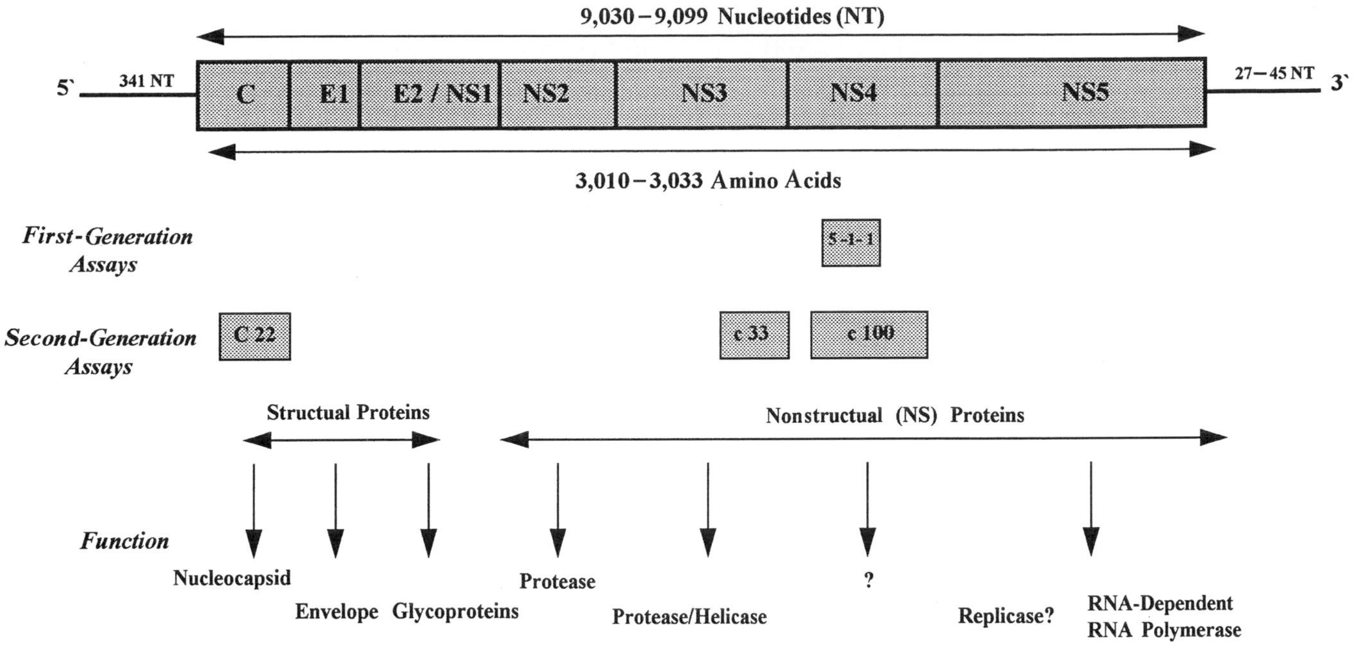

FIGURE 55–7. *Schematic representation of the hepatitis C virus (HCV) genome. The HCV genome is single stranded with approximately 9400 nucleotides. The 5′ end is highly conserved. Sequencing has demonstrated that the genome is divided into domains that encode for nucleocapsid glycoprotein and other structural proteins (C, E1, and E2) and the domains that code for nonstructural proteins (NS1, NS2, NS3, NS4, and NS5). The designations of the recombinant proteins used in the first- and second-generation assays are shown, as are the portions of the genome from which they were encoded. Not all of the specific functions of the proteins products of the HCV genome are known.*

replication to proceed. No function has been identified for the products of NS_4. The NS_5 region encodes an RNA-dependent RNA polymerase that is responsible for the replication of the RNA genome.

Of note, HCV has a propensity to mutate. Hypervariable regions exist throughout the genome, most notably in the E_1, E_2/NS_1, and NS_5 regions. As a result, mutant HCV, termed quasispecies of HCV, are produced continually during the course of infection and circulate with the dominant strain.[120, 210] Over time, owing to immune pressure, one of the HCV mutants may become the predominant strain.

Careful analyses of the HCV nucleotide sequences of many specimens worldwide have led to the identification of 6 major genotypes, which can be divided into 11 specific subtypes.[210] The major types display 60 to 65 per cent homology with one another, whereas the related subtypes show 75 to 80 per cent homology. It is very likely that additional phenotypes will be recognized. The genotypes are designated by Arabic numerals, and the subtypes are identified by lowercase letters in the order in which they were discovered. Thus, the first HCV agent cloned by Choo and associates[47] is designated type Ia, the second agent recognized (in Japan) is Ib, and so on. Genotypes 1, 2, and 3 are present worldwide. Types 1 and 2 are the primary subtypes in Western Europe and the Far East. Type 3 is common in Europe but infrequent in the Far East, except Thailand. In the United States, HCV subtypes Ia and Ib have been recognized most frequently, whereas subtypes 2a, 2b, and 3a are uncommon. Less is known about the other genotypes at present.

Clinical studies suggest that there may be an important association between the HCV genotype and the severity of hepatitis C infection, as well as the likelihood of a favorable response to interferon (IFN)–α therapy.[210] Thus, type 1 infection tends to produce more aggressive disease and is less responsive to treatment with IFN than is type 2 infection. Definitive information about the other genotypes is not available yet. It should be noted that some investigations have related the severity and response to therapy to the rate of replication of the virus and the level of viremia.[133] Thus, the more virulent genotypes may have the higher replication rates.

A number of diagnostic tests for HCV have been developed. Those approved for routine use detect anti-HCV directed toward antigenic determinants encoded by the HCV genome. The initial (first-generation) tests represented a major diagnostic breakthrough but recognized only a small amount of antigenic determinants coded by the NS_5 portion of the genome. It suffered from problems of sensitivity and particularly specificity, which resulted in a high number of false-positive results. Furthermore, there was a very long interval of several months to up to a year between the onset of infection and the first appearance of antibody.[14] To address the problems of specificity, a different anti-HCV assay was developed for supplemental testing of ELISA-positive specimens. This assay is the recombinant-strip immunoblot assay. HCV antibody is detected by different HCV antigenic determinants immobilized at distinct sites on a membrane. The determinants at each site are coded for by different regions of the genome, e.g., core, envelope, and NS domains (see Fig. 55–7). IgG also is present on the membrane to differentiate specific from nonspecific antibody binding. Depending on the determinant(s) recognized, results are given as positive (more than one reactive HCV-specific site), negative (no HCV-specific binding), or indeterminant (only one reactive HCV determinant). There is a close correlation with a positive result and HCV infection, whereas a negative recombinant-strip immunoblot assay result argues strongly for a false-positive ELISA.

First-generation ELISAs and recombinant-strip immunoblot assays have given way to second-generation test systems. These assays use the same methodologies as the first-generation tests but detect additional HCV antigenic determinants to improve on sensitivity and specificity. The test now most used for routine testing in the clinical laboratories and blood banks is an ELISA. Comparison of different second-generation assays has shown concordant results in 96 per cent of samples of hospitalized patients and healthy adults with sensitivities ranging from 94 to 100 per cent and specificities of 98 to 100 per cent.[158]

Problems still exist with some patients who are anti-HCV–positive but do not have demonstrable HCV RNA by highly sensitive polymerase chain reaction assays. This pattern is due to the persistence of antibody after infection has cleared, to a nondetectable level of viral replication in a patient with ongoing hepatitis C, or to methodologic problems. Third-generation anti-HCV assays have been developed and are in use outside the United States but as yet have not been licensed in the United States. They follow the pattern of utilizing additional HCV determinants for enhanced anti-HCV detection. In addition, a growing number of viral nucleic acid assays have been utilized in clinical studies to recognize HCV RNA in the serum. Polymerase chain reaction assays have the advantage of extreme sensitivity because they can detect only a few HCV-RNA copies per milliliter. They also have been modified to quantitate accurately the level of viremia. These assays must be performed under very strict conditions because they are contaminated easily and currently do not lend themselves for testing large numbers of specimens. However, they have proved very valuable in better understanding the different patterns of HCV infection and the genetic heterogeneity of HCV. They also have yielded important information in the evaluation of IFN in the treatment of chronic HCV infection. Polymerase chain reaction assays have demonstrated that the level of circulatory HCV is an important predictor of the response to therapy.[235] They also are the most sensitive means of identifying a relapse after IFN treatment.[208]

Clinical Features

The clinical features of hepatitis C have been characterized well from prospective studies of patients acquiring posttransfusion hepatitis in which the precise time of exposure is known (Fig. 55–8). Hepatitis C has an incubation period of approximately 45 days, with a range of 14 to 115 days.[3] HCV usually appears in the blood stream 7 to 14 days after exposure, well before the initial rise of serum transaminases and the onset of symptoms. HCV antibody seroconversion is delayed, generally not occurring until 1 to 3 months after the onset of illness. As with hepatitis A and B, anti-HCV is present as IgM and IgG early in the course of infection. However, testing for IgM anti-HCV has not proved useful for diagnostic purposes in hepatitis C because it may persist well after the acute stage of illness. HCV antibody may persist for years after recovery, or it may fall gradually in titer to nondetectable levels over time.

Like hepatitis A and B, most cases of hepatitis C are subclinical or anicteric. The mortality rate of hepatitis C is less than 1 per cent. However, at least 50 to 75 per cent of patients who acquire hepatitis C develop chronic hepatitis and become chronic HCV carriers with prolonged viremia.[12, 18, 28, 122]

Chronic hepatitis C often is asymptomatic or may be accompanied by constitutional symptoms, such as easy fatigability and malaise, particularly when there is laboratory evidence of a flare. Typically, serum enzyme levels (e.g., alanine aminotransferase) wax and wane with episodic elevations from normal or minimally increased levels to values two to five times the normal range for periods of several weeks to many months. These exacerbations can last for several weeks to many months and may relate to the emergence of a new mutant HCV strain.

HCV antibody persists in most patients who develop chronic disease. However, some patients have been observed to remain viremic after anti-HCV has disappeared.[18] This observation has two implications: (1) loss of anti-HCV does not mean necessarily that HCV infection has cleared, and (2) chronic HCV infection may be more common than previously appreciated.

Studies of the natural history of chronic HCV infection in adults are beginning to appear in the literature.[116, 121, 196] Approximately 20 to 25 per cent of individuals with chronic hepatitis C develop cirrhosis, and 10 to 15 per cent develop overt clinical evidence of hepatic dysfunction due to cirrhosis. Liver-related mortality due to cirrhosis or hepatocellular carcinoma ranges from 2 to 9 per cent. Comparable information about the natural history of chronic HCV infection in children has not accrued yet.

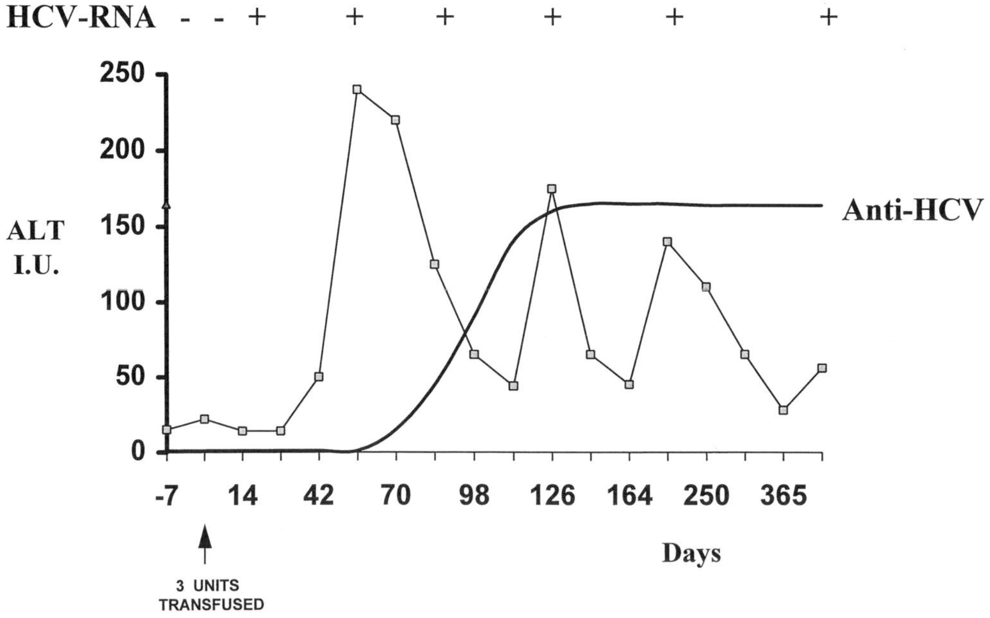

FIGURE 55–8. *Schematic representation of the course of hepatitis C virus (HCV) infection. HCV RNA can be detected in the serum within 7 to 14 days after exposure. Clinical manifestations of infection usually begin during the sixth to eighth week. Anti-HCV seroconversion often is delayed for several months. In the majority of patients, infection becomes chronic, with continued viremia and anti-HCV positivity. Repeated exacerbations are frequent in chronic HCV infection, with elevated serum transaminase levels lasting several weeks to many months.*

The consequences of chronic hepatitis C also was the subject of a large-scale study that examined the long-term results of five different prospective investigations of post-transfusion hepatitis initiated in the 1970s.[201] In this study, a small but significant excess of liver-related deaths occurred among the patients with hepatitis. However, no difference was found in the rate of mortality between patients with chronic hepatitis after transfusion and matched controls who did not acquire hepatitis. The lack of a more significant difference in the overall mortality rates may be due to the very indolent nature of chronic HCV infection and, thus, the long interval between the onset of HCV infection and the first clinical expression of complications. In a study conducted in Japan, the mean interval between acute infection and cirrhosis was 14 years, whereas clear evidence of clinical cirrhosis averaged 18 years.[116] Clinical manifestations of hepatocellular carcinoma appeared 23 years after exposure.

Epidemiology

Epidemiologic surveys conducted by the Centers for Disease Control and Prevention indicate that there are about 150,000 new cases of hepatitis C in the United States each year. The majority of patients for whom exposure is known are intravenous drug abusers who share contaminated needles and syringes. Blood transfusion, once a major source of non-A, non-B/C hepatitis transmission,[14] is estimated to account for less than 10 per cent of all cases as a result of routine donor testing for anti-HCV, "surrogate markers" (an elevated alanine aminotransferase level and anti-HBc positivity),[5] and HIV. The estimated risk of acquiring hepatitis today from transfused blood is 1 per cent or less.[4, 66, 161] With the advent of improved tests for anti-HCV, the utility of continued surrogate marker screening has been questioned.[31] Perinatal spread is infrequent, unlike that of HBV, unless the pregnant female is co-infected with HIV or has a very high level of circulating HCV.[164]

Seroprevalence studies have demonstrated a 60 to 90 per cent rate of anti-HCV among intravenous drug addicts and patients with hemophilia who had received pooled unscreened blood products.[19] Chronic hemodialysis patients have a rate of about 20 per cent. Among individuals with high-risk sexual behavior or household members exposed to a chronic HCV carrier, anti-HCV has been demonstrated in 1 to 10 per cent. The anti-HCV seroprevalence rate among health care workers is 1 to 2 per cent. Based on earlier observations of infections acquired from single-unit transfusions, the carrier HCV rate was estimated to be 1 to 2 per cent among "healthy" volunteer blood donors (R. D. Aach, personal observations). This is in accord with volunteer donor screening, which has demonstrated an anti-HCV positivity rate of 0.5 to 1.5 per cent in the United States.

HEPATITIS E

First recognized in 1977, hepatitis E originally was given the names of epidemic non-A, non-B hepatitis and enterically transmitted non-A, non-B hepatitis.

The viral agent responsible for hepatitis E (HEV) is a small, nonenveloped virus, 27 to 35 nm in diameter. It has a genome that consists of single-stranded RNA with about 6500 nucleotides.[187] It has three different open-reading frames, the first of which codes for RNA-dependent, RNA polymerase. The size and lack of an envelope feature suggest that it is a calicivirus from a recently recognized family of single-stranded RNA viruses responsible for infectious diarrhea, primarily in children. However, the genomic organization and expression strategy of HEV indicate that HEV is a unique, nonenveloped RNA virus that infects human beings.

HEV is known to be transmitted enterically by ingestion of contaminated drinking water. Spread from person to person and from contaminated food likely occurs but has not been documented yet.

There have been more than 30 well-documented waterborne epidemics of hepatitis E.[114, 226, 250] The majority have been in developing countries, primarily in India and Pakistan, but outbreaks also have occurred in Burma, China, Mexico, Russia, and South America. HEV is a common cause of acute viral hepatitis in undeveloped countries.[170] Infection also may occur sporadically not associated with an epidemic. Among healthy blood donors in Egypt and Saudi Arabia, anti-HEV indicative of prior infection was found in 4 per cent and 9 per cent, respectively.[170] The seroprevalence rate varies between 0.9 and 2.5 per cent in Western Europe and Great Britain.[170] There have been no epidemics recognized in the United States, but a few patients have been diagnosed who were exposed to HEV elsewhere before entering the country. Only one patient has been reported to date in whom exposure appeared to take place in the United States.[129]

HEV has an incubation period of 2 to 9 weeks; most people become ill around 40 days after exposure. Young adults appear to be the most at risk to clinical illness. Fatalities are uncommon, and the overall mortality rate is less than 0.5 per cent. However, pregnant women are predisposed to more severe illness, and, in some epidemics, fatality rates of approximately 20 per cent have been described.[124] Vertical transmission from mother to infant can occur, and an increase in fetal wastage has been observed.[115, 159] Infection is self-limited. Chronic hepatitis and a carrier state have not been recognized.

Early assays for diagnosing HEV infection included immune electron immunoassay and immunofluorescent probing of hepatocytes. They were important in the identification of HEV and defining the course of HEV infection but were laborious and limited in their application. With the sequencing of the HEV genome, recombinant HEV proteins have been produced that are utilized for anti-HEV detection in more clinically applicable Western blot assays and ELISAs.

The virologic and serologic course of hepatitis E is similar to that of hepatitis A. HEV can be demonstrated in the liver and then the stool for several days before the serum transaminases begin to rise. Viremia often is present. Fecal shedding of the virus peaks soon after the serum transaminases become elevated and generally disappears within 2 weeks[48] but can be prolonged.[159] IgM anti-HEV appears early during the acute phase and soon is followed by IgG anti-HEV. IgM anti-HEV disappears approximately 6 months after the beginning of infection, whereas IgG anti-HEV persists.

NON-A–E HEPATITIS

Approximately 5 to 10 per cent of patients with a clinical diagnosis of viral hepatitis are not found to have test results diagnostic of the five known agents.[4, 19, 114] Until recently, there was considerable debate as to whether this was due to another viral hepatitis agent. Some investigators believed that the tests for the known hepatitis agents were not sensitive enough, but this has not been substantiated by more recent assays that exquisitely are sensitive. Alternatively, some believed that these patients represented a "wastebasket" assortment of different conditions that give rise to a clinical picture that simulates viral hepatitis. Examples of such disorders include congestive heart failure, autoimmune hepatitis, unrecognized alcoholic liver disease, obesity, medication-associated hepatitis, and infection with such agents as cytomogalovirus and Epstein-Barr virus. However, carefully taken histories were negative for these disorders, and liver biopsy specimens of selected patients demonstrated histologic changes typical of viral hepatitis. Serologic studies excluded cytomegalovirus and Epstein-Barr virus.

There are other lines of evidence for at least one additional hepatitis agent. Epidemiologic studies of intravenous drug users have demonstrated multiple, distinct clinical episodes of viral hepatitis in the same individual, some of which were not related to the characterized agents.[155] Chimpanzees who had recovered fully from experimentally transmitted non-A, non-B hepatitis were found to develop a second discrete bout of non-A, non-B hepatitis when rechallenged with another infected blood donor source.[101] Furthermore, differences have been described in the ultrastructural and physiochemical properties of a non-A, non-B agent(s) present in the blood of known infectious blood donors and experimentally infected chimpanzees.[40] As a result of these observations, there has been a gradually increasing consensus that at least one additional hepatitis agent does exist. It variously has been termed non-A, B, C; non-A–E; and hepatitis X. Very limited demographic and epidemiologic data currently are available, and its clinical course is poorly characterized. The majority of cases have been identified among patients who have received transfusions.

Understandably, scientists at a number of laboratories have been working intensely to identify the agent(s) and develop diagnostic assays. Two independently developed prototype assays recently have identified a viral candidate. It has been given the tentative designation of GBV.[199, 257] Early assessment of the genomic characteristics of the GB agent indicate that it is a member of the *Flaviviridae* family, similar to HCV but belonging to a distinct genus.[83]

CLINICAL PATTERNS OF VIRAL HEPATITIS

The clinical and laboratory features of viral hepatitis vary considerably from one infected individual to another. The majority of individuals who acquire hepatitis have subclinical or mild illness, but a small number of patients develop a rapidly fatal illness, with death in several days to several weeks from profound hepatic failure. Although hepatitis usually is self-limited, with complete recovery, it can become chronic, with continued evidence of infection, hepatocellular necrosis, or both.

In general, the clinical manifestations, except for chronicity, are similar for all viral types. HBV, HCV, and HDV can lead to chronic hepatitis; HAV and HEV do not. Hepatitis A tends to be a mild illness in children and more often is subclinical than is infection caused by the other agents responsible for viral hepatitis. However, the severity of hepatitis A increases with age. Approximately 75 per cent of adults with acute hepatitis A have symptoms and/or jaundice. Thus, clinical manifestations of hepatitis among adults more frequently accompanies HAV infection rather than that due to HBV or HCV. HDV is the most virulent virus and almost always gives rise to clinically evident hepatitis, which is often severe. Hepatitis E particularly is severe in pregnant females. Despite these generalizations, it virtually is impossible to determine the type of acute hepatitis on clinical, biochemical, or morphologic grounds alone. Serologic testing is required for an etiologic diagnosis.

Acute infection due to viral hepatitis agents can be subdivided into the broad clinical categories described later.

Subclinical Hepatitis

The subclinical form of infection is not associated with symptoms or signs. It is recognized by the finding of transiently elevated serum transaminases or serologic evidence of viral hepatitis. Large-scale epidemiologic surveys and prospective studies of exposed patients demonstrate that this is the most common pattern of infection, particularly in childhood. Subclinical infection accounts for more than 50 per cent of all hepatitis cases.

Clinical Hepatitis

The term clinical hepatitis refers to patients who have symptomatic illness usually accompanied by abnormal physical findings during acute infection. By tradition, clinical hepatitis is divided into anicteric and icteric disease, based upon the presence or absence of jaundice. Bilirubinuria producing amber or brownish urine and a serum bilirubin greater than 2 mg/dL also have been used as criteria for icteric hepatitis. In most epidemics and prospective studies, the ratio of anicteric to icteric infection varies between 2:1 and 6:1. Like subclinical infection, anicteric hepatitis is more frequent among children and young adults than in infected individuals older than 40 years of age.

Earlier descriptions of clinically overt hepatitis based on studies of epidemics stressed a difference in the mode of onset of the classic symptoms and signs of infectious (type A) and serum (type B) hepatitis. Type A infection has a more abrupt onset with "flu-like symptoms." The patient often can recall the day or even the exact hour that symptoms first appeared. In contrast, type B infection was described as having a more insidious onset with gradually worsening symptoms over a period of 1 or 2 weeks. Unfortunately, there are so many exceptions to these patterns that this distinction is not of great value in differentiating the type of hepatitis in the individual patient.

The major symptoms experienced by 65 to 95 per cent of patients with clinical hepatitis are severe anorexia, lassitude, weakness, fever, headache, abdominal discomfort or pain, and nausea usually accompanied by vomiting. Less common complaints include rhinorrhea, sore throat, cough, diarrhea, and constipation. Patients with anicteric hepatitis have similar clinical manifestations, although they are less frequent, less intense, and of shorter duration.

The duration of the preicteric phase is approximately 7 days but can vary widely from less than 1 day to more than 2 weeks. In general, it is shorter in hepatitis A than in hepatitis B or C.

The most common sequence of events is improvement in the flu-like features of the preicteric phase coincidental with the appearance of dark urine, light stools, and jaundice. Fever, nausea, and anorexia abate over a period of several days as jaundice deepens, while malaise and easy fatigability clear more gradually. Jaundice rapidly increases in intensity over a period of several days to a week and then gradually fades. The colors of the urine and stool return to normal several days before jaundice disappears. Approximately a third of patients experience pruritus, at times intense, during the icteric phase of illness.

The total duration of illness, as defined by symptoms and abnormal liver tests, is variable. It tends to be longer in clinical hepatitis B and C than in hepatitis A. It generally is of shorter duration in children and adolescents than in adults. Thus, the mean duration of jaundice for children younger than 15 years of age with hepatitis A averages 10 days, and recovery usually is complete within 3 weeks after the onset of jaundice. Illness in adults may continue for 4 to 6 weeks. Many patients, particularly adults, have easy fatigability for months after a bout of hepatitis. Patients with icteric hepatitis often lose 5 to 10 pounds of weight while acutely ill.

Physical Findings

Patients with mild anicteric infection may have an entirely normal physical examination, although an enlarged and mildly tender liver may be palpated.

The patient examined during the preicteric phase of more clinically overt infection appears acutely ill, with fever between 37.5° and 38.5° C and occasionally as high as 39.0° C. The patient usually appears somnolent and lethargic but is oriented well. Posterior cervical adenopathy is common; general lymphadenopathy is unusual. The liver may not be enlarged until late in the preicteric phase, but pain is elicited often on palpation of the right upper quadrant or upon tapping the lower right thorax laterally (Murphy punch tenderness). A soft, nontender spleen is felt in approximately 15 per cent of patients.

Fever usually disappears during the icteric phase, and the patient appears more alert. The cervical nodes become less prominent, and splenomegaly disappears. The skin appears yellow when examined under natural light, particularly that of the face, shoulders, and arms. The conjunctivae overlaying the sclerae and the mucous membranes, especially the soft palate, appear yellow or golden. In instances of low-grade hyperbilirubinemia, these may be the only sites where jaundice can be appreciated. Palmar erythema and several spider angiomas may be found transiently and do not denote severe or chronic illness. Excoriations due to scratching are evident upon examination of a patient who develops pruritus during the icteric phase.

Laboratory Findings

Hemogram

Although red blood cell survival time is shortened during acute viral hepatitis, anemia is not a feature of self-limited, uncomplicated infection. Early in the acute phase, particularly in hepatitis A, the white blood cell count may be low,[5] usually between 3000 and 4000/mm^3. This is caused by a temporary granulocytopenia, which results in a relative lymphocytosis. Large atypical lymphocytes, like those seen in infectious mononucleosis, are present in the peripheral smear. However, they are few in number and rarely exceed 10 per cent of the total white blood cell count. A leukocytosis is unusual and when found is suggestive of impending fulminant hepatitis or another process (e.g., toxic hepatitis) simulating acute viral hepatitis.

Liver Chemistries

As has been emphasized, the total serum bilirubin need not be increased during acute viral hepatitis (i.e., anicteric infection). When it is elevated, both the indirect (unconjugated) and the direct (conjugated) fractions are increased. At plasma bilirubin values above 2 mg/dL, the urine becomes brownish or amber due to conjugated bilirubinuria. At the onset of hyperbilirubinemia, the urine urobilinogen level transiently increases because of interruption of the enterohepatic circulation, which prevents recycling of urobilinogen after absorption of this bile pigment from the colon. As the illness intensifies, little if any bilirubin is excreted into the bile, resulting in light or acholic stools and disappearance of urobilinogen in the urine. During this (acholic) phase, the clinical and chemical picture may simulate biliary tract obstruction, particularly if pruritus is a prominent complaint. As the patient begins to recover and the serum bilirubin falls, the color of the stool returns to normal. Rapid clearing of the increased bilirubin load via the bile results in increased formation of urobilinogen in the gut and therefore increased absorption and urinary excretion of urobilinogen for a short period.

In a few patients, the total serum bilirubin does not return entirely to normal after otherwise full recovery. Only the unconjugated serum bilirubin is increased, and, although it fluctuates in value, it rarely exceeds 4 mg/dL. It is not clear whether persistent unconjugated hyperbilirubinemia represents Gilbert syndrome acquired as a consequence of viral hepatitis or is Gilbert disease, first brought to light because of the close clinical and laboratory scrutiny required in the management of acute hepatitis. In either case, it is a benign condition with no sequelae.

The serum transaminases—serum glutamic oxaloacetic transaminase (or aspartate aminotransferase) and serum glutamic pyruvic transaminase (or alanine aminotransferase)—are elevated in all patients with acute viral hepatitis, except for those individuals with totally subclinical infection manifested only by serologic changes. The serum transaminases begin to increase 1 to 2 weeks before the onset of symptoms and peak about the time jaundice first appears. In approximately 80 per cent of patients, the alanine aminotransferase is higher than the aspartate aminotransferase and falls more slowly. Peak values are highly variable, but values greater than 10 times the upper limits of the normal are typical. The height of the serum elevation does not correlate closely with the extent of hepatic necrosis. However, the serum transaminases virtually are the last tests to return to normal. Serum lactic acid dehydrogenase and gamma-glutamyltranspeptidase also are elevated but offer no additional information to that provided by alanine aminotransferase or aspartate aminotransferase determinations in a patient with acute hepatitis.

The serum alkaline phosphatase also is elevated, but the level rarely exceeds two to three times the normal value. The prothrombin time and other parameters of clotting function are not deranged unless the patient has severe infection or is malnourished. In the latter instance, 5 to 10 mg of vitamin K administered parenterally rapidly corrects the prothrombin time. If the prothrombin time does not return to normal within 24 to 48 hours after parenteral vitamin K, severe (fulminant or subacute) hepatitis is suggested. Although a relatively nonspecific test of clotting function, the prothrombin time is one of the best correlates of the extent of hepatic damage.

The serum albumin and globulin concentrations are normal in self-limited viral hepatitis. Qualitative changes—namely increases in beta- and gamma-globulin levels—can be demonstrated by serum protein electrophoresis. An elevated level of IgG is seen in HBV infection, whereas a rise in the IgM level is typical of acute hepatitis A. Unfortunately, these differences usually are not marked or reproducible enough to be helpful in the differential diagnosis. A low serum albumin or elevated globulin (twofold or greater) suggests a more severe or prolonged illness, such as subacute or chronic active hepatitis (vide infra).

A small percentage of patients with benign viral hepatitis have low-titer, circulating autoantibodies during the acute phase of illness. Antinuclear, antismooth muscle, antimito-

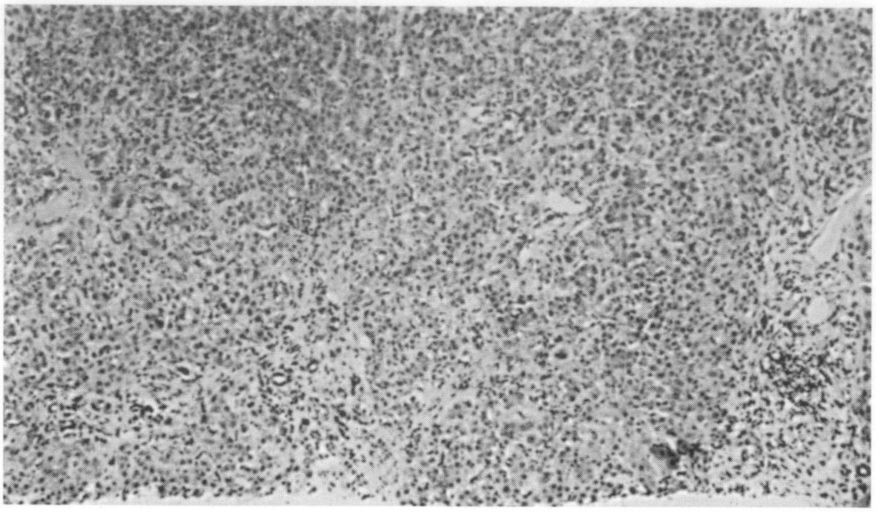

FIGURE 55–9. *Morphology of acute viral hepatitis. Focal areas of liver cell necrosis, inflammatory infiltrate, and cellular disarray are present throughout the lobule.*

chondrial, and antithyroid antibodies may be present individually or in combination. Antinuclear antibodies usually are of the homogeneous pattern. These phenomena clear with resolution of acute illness if caused by viral hepatitis.

Pathology

Acute viral hepatitis of all known etiologies gives rise to diffuse necroinflammatory changes in the liver. Evidence of liver cell damage, spotty necrosis, and an inflammatory cell infiltrate (lobular hepatitis) are the characteristic morphologic changes of acute viral hepatitis.[153] Necrotic and degenerating parenchymal cells are present throughout the liver lobule but may be concentrated more heavily in the centrilobular areas (Fig. 55–9). Parenchymal cell involvement is accompanied by lobular infiltration of inflammatory cells, predominantly mononuclear in type (Fig. 55–10). The same infiltrate is contained in portal triads. The extent of necrosis and inflammatory cell infiltration varies from lobule to lobule. Hepatocytes are pleomorphic. Degenerating cells stain less intensely. Dead or dying cells either are swollen with balloon degeneration leading to lytic necrosis or are shrunken with small, rounded, intensely red staining "acidophilic bodies" that, after death by apocytosis, are extruded into the perisinusoidal space (Fig. 55–11). Small bile ducts may undergo proliferation, and there is proliferation of Kupffer cells in the hepatic sinusoids.

Differences in the histologic features of hepatitis A, B, and C have been described.[62, 229] In hepatitis A, hepatic cell injury tends to be more heavily concentrated in the periportal region of the liver lobule where abundant plasma cells are present. In hepatitis B, infected cells may have a ground-glass appearance, best brought out by orcein or Victoria blue staining. Immunologic staining may reveal HBsAg in the cytoplasm and HBcAg in the nucleus of infected cells. In hepatitis B, there is a denser, more uniform lymphocytic infiltration in the portal triads. Lymphocytes also are distributed throughout the lobule, often adjacent to abnormal hepatocytes and acidophilic bodies. In hepatitis C, the degree of lymphocytic infiltration is relatively less but acidophilic bodies are abundant, and there may be evidence of sinusoidal cell activation. Micro- or macrovesicular steatosis may be found, particularly in chronic hepatitis C. Microvesicular steatosis also may be seen in hepatitis D along with granular eosinophilic necrosis. Otherwise, the changes of acute HDV infection are the same as those of acute hepatitis B. In hepatitis E, cholestasis, rosette formation of liver cells, and polymorphonuclear leukocytes can be distinguishing features. However, the differences, except for specific immunologic staining, generally are not so distinctive as to be diagnostic

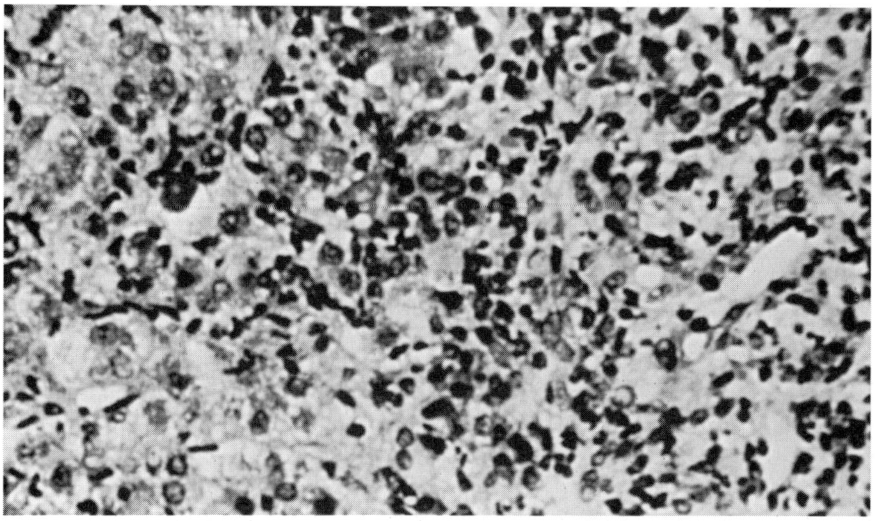

FIGURE 55–10. *Higher-power view of inflammatory infiltrate in acute viral hepatitis. Mononuclear cells, primarily lymphocytes, predominate. Some plasma cells can be found.*

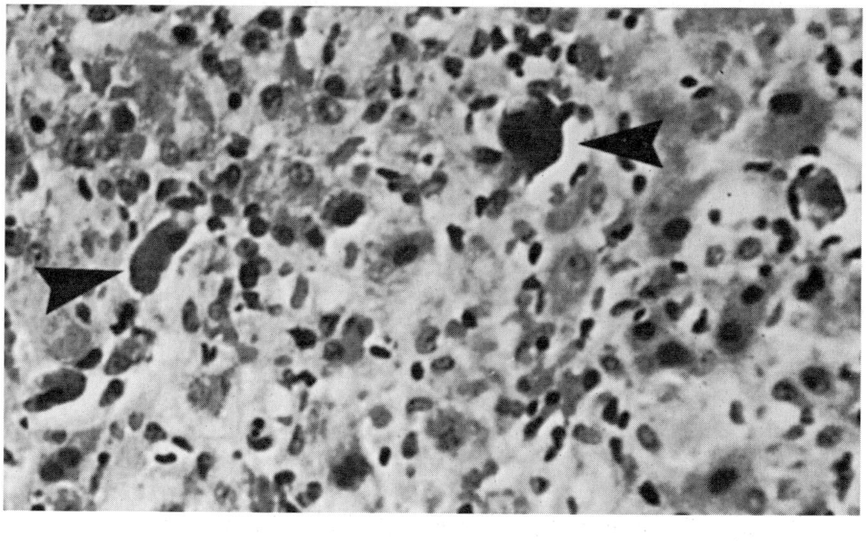

FIGURE 55–11. *Intensely staining "acidophilic bodies" (arrow) in liver biopsy, also showing hepatic cell degeneration and focal necrosis with surrounding mononuclear infiltrate. These changes are characteristic of but not specific for viral hepatitis. Similar histologic characteristics may be found in drug-induced hepatitis.*

in the individual patient and certainly are not a substitute for serologic studies.

With clinical and chemical improvement, variable degrees of lobular collapse are found with condensation of reticulum in areas where necrotic hepatic cells have "dropped out." Large phagocytic cells appear within the lobules and later the portal tracts. These scavenger macrophages contain ceroid pigment and stainable iron. Portal tracts often are expanded and at times linked together by inflammatory infiltration.

As resolution proceeds, liver cell necrosis disappears, although hepatic parenchymal cells may remain pleomorphic. Small focal collections of inflammatory cells still are present in the lobules and in most portal triads. Ceroid pigment–laden macrophages persist, and slender strands of fibrosis may extend a short distance from some portal tracts. Fibrosis is accompanied by little or no inflammatory cell component. The morphologic features at this stage of recovery often are difficult to distinguish from the pathologic changes of chronic persistent hepatitis (vide infra). These residual changes gradually resolve over 4 to 12 months in self-limited infection but continue indefinitely in chronic hepatitis.

Variants of Viral Hepatitis

A small proportion of patients with viral hepatitis run an atypical course. This may take one of three basic forms: (1) atypical self-limited infection, (2) life-threatening hepatitis (fulminant and subacute hepatitis), and (3) the development of chronic hepatitis. In addition, there is a group of miscellaneous complications that rarely are seen.

Atypical Forms of Self-Limited Hepatitis

CHOLESTATIC ACUTE VIRAL HEPATITIS. This unusual variant closely simulates extrahepatic biliary tract obstruction. In addition to acholic stools and brownish urine, there is marked jaundice and intense pruritus. The clinical course may be more prolonged, lasting a month or more.[67] Laboratory tests are typical of cholestasis. The serum bilirubin exceeds 10 mg/dL and may be greater than 20 mg/dL. The serum alkaline phosphatase is greater than three times the upper limits of normal; the serum cholesterol, beta-lipoprotein, and gamma-glutamyltranspeptidase are elevated. Features that help distinguish this hepatitis variant from biliary tract obstruction are a history of exposure to viral hepatitis, the flu-like prodrome of hepatitis, and high serum transaminase values (e.g., greater than five times normal). The liver usually is enlarged and diffusely tender, and liver biopsy reveals the characteristic changes of acute viral hepatitis. This variant resolves completely over time. Cholestasis has been a predominant feature in several outbreaks of hepatitis E and occurs as a variant of hepatitis A. Its pathogenesis is unknown, but it does not appear to be related to the viral load and does not carry a more grave prognosis.

A major problem is distinguishing cholestatic viral hepatitis from drug-induced hepatitis if the patient has been taking one of a multitude of agents that can produce cholestasis.[134, 216, 256] A carefully taken, complete history is critical, as are serologic tests for viral hepatitis. Fortunately, drug-induced hepatitis is seen infrequently in children.

RELAPSING VIRAL HEPATITIS. An exacerbation of clinical illness accompanied by a rise of serum transaminases (and less frequently of serum bilirubin) may occur in patients with acute viral hepatitis, particularly those with hepatitis C. It usually occurs within the first few months of onset, often during the recovery phase, when symptoms largely have disappeared and the laboratory test results are improving. It may coincide with resumption of more strenuous activity, although several studies have demonstrated that moderate exertion does not influence adversely the overall course in young, otherwise healthy persons.

A relapsing pattern occurs in about 20 per cent of patients with acute hepatitis A, but complete recovery is the rule. Patients with acute hepatitis C who experience relapse are more apt to develop chronic hepatitis.[227] Relapses may be evidenced only by serum transaminase elevations several weeks to months after tests indicative of acute hepatitis have returned to normal. For this reason, full recovery from acute hepatitis C should not be presumed until an interval of at least 6 months of normal values has elapsed.

In some instances, apparent relapses actually represent a second bout of acute hepatitis caused by a different viral agent, such as HCV after HBV infection. This phenomenon has been documented well among recipients of blood transfusions and illicit drug users.[152]

Life-Threatening Hepatitis

FULMINANT HEPATITIS. This grave complication is the clinical counterpart of massive hepatic necrosis.[183] Fulminant hepatitis has been defined conventionally as liver dysfunction severe enough to produce hepatic failure as shown by the presentation of hepatic encephalopathy within 8 weeks of the first symptoms of illness.[234] This definition has been modified by some workers in the field to require that the time interval between the onset of jaundice and encephalitis is no greater than 2 weeks. Subfulminant liver failure is the term used when the time interval from onset of infection to evidence of profound hepatic failure is 2 to 12 weeks.[29]

The frequency of fulminant hepatitis varies considerably with the type of infection. Fulminant hepatitis occurs rarely (<0.5 per cent of cases) in recognized HAV infection[182] and in approximately 1 per cent of individuals with documented acute HBV infection.[183] Before serologic testing was available, mortality rates of up to 30 per cent were described in a few outbreaks of serum hepatitis.[67] In retrospect, this presumably was due to HDV superinfection of chronic hepatitis B rather than HBV (or HCV) infection alone. Fulminant hepatitis is an infrequent complication of hepatitis C[253] and virtually is unknown as a sequela of HCV infection acquired from blood transfusion. It is a major complication of pregnant women who become infected with HEV.

Fulminant viral hepatitis is manifested by the development of profound hepatic failure, usually during the first week of illness. Some patients with typical benign acute hepatitis suddenly develop signs of fulminant illness. This complication should be suspected strongly whenever a patient develops hepatic encephalopathy, fluid retention, oliguria, or evidence of impaired clotting. Hyperexcitability and impaired mentation, soon followed by increasing somnolence and then deep coma, are features of hepatic encephalopathy. Some patients develop generalized convulsions. Complaints of severe abdominal pain are common, as is an unexplained increase in temperature or development of fever, protracted nausea, and vomiting accompanied by rapidly deepening jaundice.

Physical examination reveals an agitated, confused, or comatose jaundiced patient. The liver is small or rapidly decreases in size, in contrast to the hepatomegaly characteristic of benign acute viral hepatitis. Ecchymoses, gastrointestinal bleeding, and oozing at needle puncture sites represent profound disturbances in coagulation. Asterixis and hyperventilation are additional manifestations of hepatic encephalopathy, and neurologic examination may reveal spasticity, hyperreflexia, and a positive Babinski sign(s).

Laboratory derangements of fulminant viral hepatitis include a leukocytosis with an increase in the number of circulating neutrophils. The serum fibrinogen level is decreased markedly in concentration, and the prothrombin time is prolonged due to deficient synthesis of factors II, V, VII, and X. Consumption coagulopathy, the result of deposition of fibrin into areas of hepatic necrosis, also contributes to the clotting disturbance.[97] The serum electrolytes are normal, except for a low serum bicarbonate secondary to hyperventilation with resultant respiratory alkalosis. Some patients have an anion gap due to lactic acidosis. Arterial blood gases and pH as well as serum lactate and pyruvate levels should be obtained if an anion gap is present. The blood glucose concentration must be monitored carefully. Hypoglycemia can develop rapidly and be difficult to correct. It is a common cause of death, particularly in children with fulminant hepatitis, who especially are prone to develop this complication.

The blood ammonia often is elevated, but its concentration does not correlate well with the status of the patient. The same is true of conventional liver tests. If fulminant hepatitis evolves rapidly, the total serum bilirubin may be elevated only slightly when the patient first is seen. The height of the serum transaminase (alanine aminotransferase and aspartate aminotransferase) elevations do not reflect necessarily the degree of hepatic necrosis, and values of 500 to 2000 IU/mL are typical. The serum albumin usually is normal because of its long half-life, unless there is a significant extravascular leak with attendant edema and ascites. Hyponatremia may develop owing to a combination of the administration of fluids low in sodium, an increased level of antidiuretic hormone, and, perhaps, the "sick cell syndrome." Fluid retention also is common for these reasons plus hyperaldosteronism. Azotemia, oliguria, and a 24-hour urine sodium excretion of less than 5 mEq in the absence of evidence of prerenal origin are ominous indicators of the hepatorenal syndrome.

Fulminant viral hepatitis carries a high fatality rate, ranging between 75 and 95 per cent in patients who do not receive a liver transplant. Most patients die within a week, but death may occur in less than 24 hours of onset. Younger patients, particularly children and young adults, have the best prognosis.

Of note, follow-up studies of patients who survive fulminant viral hepatitis have shown complete clinical recovery, in many instances with little or no histologic residual.[107, 113]

SUBACUTE OR SEVERE VIRAL HEPATITIS. Approximately 5 per cent of patients with viral hepatitis develop hepatic failure more slowly over a period of several weeks or months. The term subacute hepatitis has been applied to this condition, although some of the most severely ill patients also fit the category of subfulminant liver failure. The pathologic counterpart of this variant is submassive hepatic necrosis. Such patients usually have a longer prodromal period than in typical viral hepatitis, with continued low-grade fever, extreme fatigue, anorexia, nausea, and vomiting lasting more than 4 weeks. Hepatomegaly and splenomegaly are frequent findings, as are ascites and peripheral edema.

Laboratory tests of special significance include a serum bilirubin usually in excess of 10 mg/dL, low serum albumin, prolonged prothrombin time not corrected by vitamin K injections, and a very high gamma-globulin level.

Older individuals, especially women older than 40 years of age, particularly are prone to develop this complication. There is some evidence that failure of hepatic regeneration, not just the extreme degree of hepatic necrosis, plays an important role in the pathogenesis of this variant.

Chronic Viral Hepatitis

The transition from acute to chronic hepatitis should be suspected strongly when biochemical evidence of infection extends beyond 4 months.[207] It is defined, however, by evidence of hepatitis and continued infection for at least 6 months.

Based largely on clinical and pathologic study of patients with chronic hepatitis of autoimmune origin, chronic hepatitis of any etiology, including chronic viral hepatitis, by convention has been subdivided into three basic groups. These are chronic persistent hepatitis, chronic active hepatitis, and lobular hepatitis. Grouping in this fashion was considered to be of value in predicting the likely course of a patient with chronic hepatitis.

Chronic persistent hepatitis is considered the form of continued process that tends not to progress, even though associated with continued pathologic changes and liver test abnormalities, namely elevated serum transaminases. Other terms used for this condition include portal hepatitis, transaminitis, triaditis, and unresolved hepatitis. Liver biopsy reveals primarily a mild to moderate portal triad mononuclear infiltrate.

Chronic active hepatitis is the designation given to the form of continued liver inflammation and necrosis that can progress and over time result in cirrhosis and its complications. The histologic counterpart consists of periportal necrosis and mononuclear infiltration, often with abundant plasma cells. The limiting plate that normally surrounds the portal triad is destroyed, a pattern called piecemeal necrosis. More extensive necrosis of entire lobules (multilobular necrosis) and "bridging" necrosis with broad areas of cell death and inflammatory infiltrates extending between adjacent portal triads or central veins are more severe forms of chronic active hepatitis.[42] In one series of 429 cases of acute hepatitis B, 10 per cent developed chronic hepatitis B.[184] Of these, approximately two-thirds had chronic persistent hepatitis on liver biopsy and one-third had histologic changes of chronic active hepatitis. In hepatitis C, there is a greater tendency toward chronic active hepatitis than chronic persistent hepatitis.

Lobular hepatitis is seen less commonly than chronic persistent and chronic active hepatitis in patients with chronic viral hepatitis. It is associated generally with few or no symptoms, minor elevation of the serum transaminase, and a benign clinical course. Liver biopsy reveals foci of liver cell necrosis and inflammatory cell infiltration in the liver cell lobules.

It is important to emphasize that more recent observations of patients with chronic viral hepatitis demonstrate that the distinction between these subgroups, particularly chronic persistent hepatitis and chronic active hepatitis, may not be clear-cut. Findings on serial biopsies of patients with chronic hepatitis B have been found to vary over time, changing from features of chronic persistent to those of chronic active hepatitis and vice versa. Thus, the predictive value of this grouping as to prognosis in patients with chronic viral hepatitis is more limited than originally was believed.

It should be noted that these same clinical and morphologic pictures are seen in patients after the administration of certain therapeutic agents (methyldopa, oxyphenisatin, isoniazid, and halothane), individuals with Wilson disease, and, of course, individuals with autoimmune chronic hepatitis.

Because of the variable morphologic features of some patients with chronic viral hepatitis over time and the increasing number of etiologies giving rise to the same patterns, the classification of chronic hepatitis has been revised.[59] It now is defined on the basis of etiology, the degree of activity, and the stage of liver disease. The necroinflammatory changes are graded semiquantitatively with the new classification as showing minimal, mild, moderate, or severe activity. The changes on biopsy then are staged as to the degree of progression relating to fibrosis (mild, moderate, or severe fibrosis) or cirrhosis.

CIRRHOSIS. Cirrhosis is a complication of chronic hepatitis B and D and of hepatitis C (see individual chapters). It most often is macronodular (postnecrotic) with regenerating nodules of different size surrounded by fibrosis. A mononuclear infiltrate frequently is present in remnants of portal triads with adjacent hepatic cell necrosis. The degree of fibrosis and infiltration is variable, depending on the duration of disease and its activity. In several surveys, up to 25 per cent of patients with macronodular cirrhosis were HBsAg-positive. Cirrhosis occurs as a late complication in approximately 20 to 25 per cent of patients with chronic hepatitis C.

HEPATOMA. Primary adenocarcinoma of the liver is a well-recognized sequela of chronic hepatitis due to HBV and HCV. In areas of the world where the HBV carrier rate is high, 50 to 70 per cent of patients who develop hepatomas are HBsAg-positive.[231] Longitudinal studies indicate that HBV is a tumor-associated virus and that hepatoma may be the ultimate "end stage" of chronic hepatitis B infection. The association of hepatoma is greatest in underdeveloped countries and the Far East. Investigators employing DNA probes have shown HBV nucleotide sequences integrated into the DNA of hepatoma cells.[206] Integration occurs after prolonged HBV infection and is an important factor in the malignant transformation of infected liver cells, although other precipitation factors, such as aflatoxin, cirrhosis, HCV, and possibly tobacco, may be important as well. Cirrhosis need not be present for a hepatoma to develop. Hepatoma occurs more frequently in males than in females, usually after an interval of 20 to 30 years after the onset of HBV infection. It rapidly is fatal in most instances.

Primary hepatocellular carcinoma is a major late complication of chronic hepatitis C as well.[60, 193] As indicated earlier, 2 to 9 per cent of patients with chronic hepatitis C die of either cirrhosis or hepatoma. Epidemiologic investigations also show a strong relationship between chronic HCV infection and the development of a hepatoma. There is a much higher prevalence of anti-HCV positivity among patients with hepatoma compared with nonhepatoma controls.[33] The relationship between HCV infection and hepatoma is increased significantly in hepatoma patients who have chronic hepatitis B as well.[33] In the United States, hepatoma is associated with anti-HCV positivity in 25 to 50 per cent of cases.

The mechanism by which HCV induces malignant transformation is unknown. Integration of viral genome sequences into the DNA of the hepatotype would not be expected to occur because HCV is an RNA virus. HCV has been found in both malignant and nonmalignant liver tissue at autopsy. Virtually all anti-HCV patients who develop a hepatoma have well-established cirrhosis. HCV indirectly could be responsible by producing cirrhosis, which carries an increased risk of malignancy. However, one report described the finding of HCV-associated hepatoma in the absence of cirrhosis, suggesting that the viral agent may be truly oncogenic.[57] This finding needs to be confirmed.

OTHER COMPLICATIONS. HBV may give rise to the serum sickness–like syndrome in patients with acute infection as well as polyarteritis nodosa and glomerulonephritis in chronic HBV infection.[11, 88, 242] The pathogenesis of these variants is believed to be the formation of soluble immune complexes of HBsAg and anti-HBs with activation of both the classic and alternate complement system. HBsAg, IgG, and complement have been demonstrated in the joint fluid and synovium of involved joints, the endothelium of affected vessels in polyarteritis nodosa, and in a subepithelial location along the glomerular basement membrane in HBV-positive patients with glomerulonephritis. The serum sickness–like syndrome can occur in either anicteric or icteric hepatitis. In patients with icteric hepatitis, the syndrome usually begins 1 to 4 weeks before other clinical features of liver cell necrosis appear. It rarely lasts more than a week. This syndrome also has been associated with acute hepatitis A, but it occurs much less frequently than in hepatitis B and its pathogenesis has not been studied comparably.

HCV infection has been associated with types II and III cryoglobulinemia.[20, 32] Among 19 patients with type II or mixed cryoglobulinemia in one series,[20] 16 had demonstrable HCV RNA in the serum. HCV antibody was detected in the serum in only 8 patients. Both HCV RNA and anti-HCV, presumably as immune complexes, were concentrated in the cryoprecipitate. These observations suggest that HCV may be a major cause of type II cryoglobulinemia and that the diagnosis of hepatitis C may be missed unless the serum is examined for HCV RNA or the cryoprecipitate also is tested for the presence of anti-HCV.

Other associations on less firm grounds include porphyria cutanea tarda, polyarteritis nodosa, Sjögren syndrome, autoimmune chronic hepatitis, and lichen planus.[119, 163]

A number of other complications of viral hepatitis are seen rarely. These include neurologic problems, such as the Guillain-Barré syndrome, encephalitis, meningitis, and a peripheral neuropathy associated with acute infection. Rapid hemolysis with bilirubin levels exceeding 20 mg/dL has been observed in hepatitis patients who also have sickle cell anemia or glucose-6-phosphatase deficiency.[194] More than 100 instances of aplastic anemia in association with acute hepatitis now have been reported in the literature.[93] This complication usually follows the acute stage of illness when the patient appears to be recovering. Children particularly are prone to develop postinfection aplastic anemia, which unfortunately often is fatal. No form of therapy has proved effective in reversing this complication. Earlier reports have linked non-A, non-B hepatitis with this complication.[255] However, hepatitis patients with aplastic anemia have not been found to have hepatitis C. Furthermore, some of these patients have received a variety of medications, including chloramphenicol, which also can produce aplastic anemia.

IMMUNOPATHOGENESIS

Hepatitis A

There are conflicting data about the mechanism(s) by which HAV infection leads to hepatocellular necrosis. HAV belongs to the *Piconaviridae* family, whose members, in general, directly are cytopathic to infected cells. Furthermore, there appears to be a correlation between the amount of HAV produced during infection and the severity of infection.[64] An argument against a cytopathic mechanism is the observation that HAV replication and fecal shedding appear to begin well before the onset of hepatocellular necrosis. Also, HAV can be grown in tissue culture, such as marmoset liver explants, without any evidence of cytotoxicity.[30] There also is evidence that lymphocytes isolated from the blood and liver during acute hepatitis A are cytotoxic to HAV-infected cells.[147, 237] This suggests that hepatocellular necrosis may be the result of HAV-specific cytotoxic lymphocytes, which mount an attack on infected liver cells. Thus, it is possible that hepatocellular necrosis is due to both direct viral cytotoxicity and cell-mediated immunity.

Hepatitis B

There is abundant evidence indicating that HBV is not directly cytopathic. Cell injury is believed to be due to the host's cell-mediated immune response to HBV infection.[69] The prevailing theory is that cytotoxic lymphocytes mount an attack on the infected hepatocytes. They specifically are directed against HBV antigens expressed on the cell surface of the infected cell and human leukocyte antigen class I determinants induced by endogenous interferon.[81] HBcAg and possibly HBeAg are the HBV antigens recognized by the cytotoxic lymphocytes.[228] There is much to support this mechanism. It would explain the different clinical patterns associated with HBV infection. It has been known for some time that the HBV titer or the rate of HBV replication does not correlate with the severity of infection. Indeed, the highest levels of circulating HBV are seen in the asymptomatic HBV carrier state and in patients who are immunosuppressed. In contrast, the amount of detectable HBV in fulminant hepatitis B is quite low. These findings are consistent with the postulation that the host's immune response determines the clinical expression of HBV infection. Thus, self-limited hepatitis B would represent an effective immune response with termination of HBV infection. Fulminant hepatitis can be explained by an exaggerated immune response to HBV infection. Chronic hepatitis would be due to an immune response insufficient to clear all infected cells. Such an inadequate immune response could result from one or more factors, including an intrinsic defect in the processing of HBV antigens by class II CD4 lymphocytes, an abnormality of expression of HBV antigens on the surface of infected hepatocytes, a suboptimal IFN augmentation in response to infection, and a defect in IFN induction of human leukocyte antigen determinants. There is evidence to support more than one of these possible abnormalities. A vigorous human leukocyte antigen class II CD4 T-cell response to HBV nucleocapsid antigenic determinants has been demonstrated in acute self-limited hepatitis B and is believed to be critical for termination of infection.[80] In chronic hepatitis B, the response by CD4 T lymphocytes to HBcAg and HBeAg is much lower.[80, 81] In addition, low levels of IFN have been found in patients with chronic hepatitis B compared with those who recover fully from infection.[53] This observation offers an explanation of why treatment with exogenous IFN may be effective in inducing a clinical response and even recovery from infection in patients with chronic hepatitis B.

Hepatitis C

The immunopathogenesis of hepatitis C is not understood well at present. There have been very limited investigations on this subject to date. The similarity of the clinical features of HCV to HBV, such as sustained infection and chronic hepatitis, which can take the form of a clinically silent carrier state, suggests at first glance that they may have the same pathogenesis. There are clear differences between the two agents, however, that make this unlikely. In contrast to that due to HBV, chronic infection due to HCV is believed to result from the virus' propensity to mutate, thereby escaping the infected host's defense mechanisms. There also is a difference in the clinical manifestations of a response to IFN therapy, which suggests a different immunopathogenesis for the two agents (see the treatment section) (vide infra). The hepatitis-like flare typically seen prior to an IFN response in chronic hepatitis B is not seen in treated patients with chronic HCV infection. There is limited indirect evidence that supports a direct cytotoxic effect of the virus. A correlation appears to exist between the extent of viral replication and the level of HCV RNA in the circulation with the severity of the infection in chronic hepatitis C.[133] Furthermore, patients with chronic hepatitis C who are immunosuppressed due to HIV co-infection have more rapid progression of hepatocellular disease. The apparent relationship between the HCV genotype and the rate of progression of hepatitis C also implies that HCV plays a major role in determining the clinical manifestations of hepatitis C. However, there are some observations suggesting that the clinical manifestations of chronic hepatitis C are due to the immune response of the host. Human leukocyte antigen class I HCV-specific T-cytotoxic lymphocytes have been isolated from the liver during HCV infection.[123] In addition, immunosuppressive agents given to HCV-infected chimpanzees decrease the necroinflammatory response, with a flare in the level of activity when the agents are discontinued.[125] An exacerbation of liver disease also has been observed in HCV-infected bone marrow transplant recipients when their immunosuppressive therapy has been completed or withdrawn. In summary, it is quite possible that the clinical manifestations of HCV infection are due to both a viral cytopathic effect and the host's immune defense.

Hepatitis D

The hepatocellular manifestations of HDV infection are believed to be due to a direct cytotoxic effect of the virus.[188] Evidence for a direct relationship between the agent and severity of expression stems from HDV gene-sequencing studies. As indicated in an earlier section of this chapter, three genotypes of HDV have been identified and cloned.[254] Types I and III genotypes have been found to be much more virulent than type II.[254]

Hepatitis E

The pathogenetic mechanism by which hepatocellular necrosis occurs in HEV infection is unknown. Of major importance is why pregnant women particularly are susceptible to severe and frequently fatal hepatitis E.[124]

DIFFERENTIAL DIAGNOSIS

Establishing the correct diagnosis on the basis of history, physical examination, and laboratory findings does not pose a problem in the typical case of acute viral hepatitis, although serologic studies are required for determining the specific type of infection. Neonatal hepatitis and biliary atresia are diagnostic considerations in the newborn infant. However, the clinical manifestations of both these conditions begin earlier than does viral hepatitis, usually during the first 3 weeks of life. In general, the serum transaminases are not as high in neonatal hepatitis as in viral hepatitis, and the clinical features are more those of obstructive jaundice, as in biliary atresia, than of hepatocellular injury. Cytomegalic inclusion disease, rubella, herpes simplex, varicella, toxoplasmosis, *Listeria* infection, and syphilis also can give rise to a clinical picture simulating neonatal hepatitis. Evidence of intrauterine infection (microcephaly, chorioretinitis, intraventricular calcification, congenital heart disease, and so on) or an associated hemolytic anemia is helpful in distinguishing these conditions from viral hepatitis. Unfortunately, liver biopsy may not be diagnostic, for even in viral hepatitis it may reveal primarily giant cell transformation and a variable degree of portal cell inflammatory cell infiltrate. These morphologic changes reflect a common pattern of injury to a wide variety of different hepatic insults in the newborn. Serologic studies should lead to the correct diagnosis.

In the older child and adult, infectious mononucleosis can simulate viral hepatitis, but the degree of hepatocellular injury, as shown by the height and duration of the serum transaminase elevations, generally is less impressive. In addition, patients with infectious mononucleosis usually have more sustained fever, more prominent pharyngitis, generalized lymphadenopathy, and a tender, enlarged spleen. The diagnosis of infectious mononucleosis can be made by finding greater than 15 per cent atypical lymphocytes on peripheral smear, a positive heterophil agglutination test, and/or the appearance of Epstein-Barr virus antibodies.

In the child and adolescent, Reye syndrome may be difficult to distinguish from fulminant viral hepatitis. Reye syndrome should be suspected when, over a matter of hours, evidence of profound hepatic failure with encephalopathy appears several days after varicella or an acute upper respiratory tract infection. This usually occurs in children who were given aspirin to treat the viral infection. Results of liver function tests may be identical to those seen in early fulminant viral hepatitis, with elevated serum transaminases, hypoprothrombinemia, hypofibrinogenemia, hypoglycemia, and an elevated blood ammonia with little or no elevation in the serum bilirubin because of the abruptness of onset of profound hepatic failure. In the absence of serologic evidence of viral hepatitis, examination of a liver biopsy specimen should help distinguish between the two conditions. In Reye syndrome, fine microdroplets of fat in hepatocytes are present in a panlobular distribution, with only minimal evidence on biopsy of hepatocellular injury and necrosis typical of viral hepatitis.

Drug-induced hepatitis can show chemical and morphologic findings indistinguishable from those of viral hepatitis. Patients with drug-induced hepatitis may have other features of hypersensitivity, including a rash, arthralgias and arthritis, and eosinophilia. A history of exposure to such agents as halothane, methyldopa, and nitrofurantoin and a history of drug allergies strongly suggest a hypersensitivity reaction. Acute hepatic failure due to hepatotoxins rarely is encountered today but should be suspected if there has been recent exposure to halogenated hydrocarbons (e.g., carbon tetrachloride) or inorganic phosphorus or ingestion of large doses of acetaminophen or the *Amanita* genus of mushroom.

Alcoholic liver disease, particularly acute alcoholic hepatitis, on occasion can be confused with viral hepatitis. Alcoholic liver disease occasionally may be seen in the adolescent and young adult. In addition, acute viral hepatitis may be contracted by the alcoholic. In acute alcoholic hepatitis, there usually is ample physical evidence of more chronic liver disease with wasting (despite its misleading terminology, implying only acute disease). Helpful laboratory clues include anemia, leukocytosis, hypoalbuminemia, and serum transaminase levels less than 300 IU/mL. When in doubt, a liver biopsy specimen examination should permit ready distinction from viral hepatitis.

TREATMENT

Acute Hepatitis

There is no specific form of therapy for acute viral hepatitis. Absolute bed rest was recommended for many years because it was felt to hasten recovery and prevent relapses. However, clinical studies have not demonstrated a beneficial effect of absolute bed rest.[186] Therefore, most hepatologists recommend limited activity in a home setting until there is a definite improvement in the clinical status of the patient and the liver function tests. Hospitalization, once standard practice for patients with icteric hepatitis, is reserved for individuals who cannot receive adequate care at home, are very symptomatic, or have evidence of severe (e.g., fulminant or subacute) hepatitis. Patients with less serious illness should eat a well-balanced diet of 40 to 50 calories/kg of body weight with about 4 to 5 g of protein/kg of body weight. Frequent small meals, four to five times a day, are desirable if nausea is a problem. Many patients are able to tolerate better a large breakfast as their major or only meal of the day, for nausea is less and the appetite is better in the morning. Supplemented high-calorie products may be tried if required. However, high-calorie, high-protein diets either high or low in fat do not accelerate the rate of recovery. If the patient is unable to eat, at least 700 calories/24 hours should be given intravenously as 10 per cent glucose and water along with intravenous multivitamins. Hyperalimentation with intravenous amino acids and possibly intralipid may be given if the patient is severely ill and unable to eat, although hepatic encephalopathy can be precipitated or aggravated by such therapy. Vegetable protein, which is rich in branched-chain amino acids, is less likely to be associated with encephalopathy than are animal proteins, which have a higher proportion of aromatic amino acids.

The patient's physical activity can be increased in graded fashion once the liver studies have improved substantially (e.g., serum bilirubin less than 2 mg/dL, alanine aminotransferase and aspartate aminotransferase less than four to five times the upper limit of normal). Children should not return to school or adults to work until jaundice has resolved and the serum enzymes are no more than twice the upper limits of normal.

Corticosteroids, standard immunoglobulin, and hepatitis B immunoglobulin* should not be used in the treatment of acute viral hepatitis. They have not been shown to be beneficial. In HBV infection, corticosteroids may be associated with a greater risk of developing chronic hepatitis. They are not beneficial in fulminant hepatitis either. Serious superimposed bacterial or fungal infections are more frequent when corticosteroids are used in high dose for fulminant hepatitis.[91]

There is preliminary information to suggest that treatment of acute hepatitis C with a 4- to 12-week course of IFN-α may reduce the risk of chronic infection and hepatitis.[131, 239] However, some patients who initially respond later have been found to be infected with HCV. Although this information is promising, more is needed.

For fulminant viral hepatitis, careful monitoring in the intensive care unit for cerebral edema (controlled with mannitol), cardiopulmonary dysfunction, and infection is the mainstay of therapy. Curiously, patients with the shortest interval between the onset of symptoms and profound liver failure appear to have a better prognosis. Emergency orthotopic liver transplantation has emerged as a lifesaving measure for an increasing number of patients who in the past would have died. The type of viral hepatitis also is important in the outcome. Patients with fulminant hepatitis A have the best prognosis, whether they have received transplants or not. Among those who received transplants, more than 60 per cent were alive after 1 year.[249] Survival rates after transplant for hepatitis B–induced fulminant hepatitis are on the order of 40 per cent, whereas non-A, non-B hepatitis 1-year survival rates are 20 to 25 per cent.[249] The proportion of cases who had HCV infection among the latter group is not known.

The selection criteria for transplantation varies from center to center and are not standardized. Criteria that have been used include a factor V level below 20 per cent in a patient who is encephalopathic, a substantially reduced liver volume on ultrasonography or computed tomography, less than 50 per cent viable hepatocytes in a transjugular liver biopsy specimen, and a combination of factors including age, rapidity of onset and course of illness, and liver volume.[249]

Chronic Viral Hepatitis

Administration of large doses of anti-HBs and transfer factor has not been successful in terminating chronic hepatitis B and the HBV carrier state. Early studies using adenine arabinoside also gave disappointing results.[90]

At present, IFN-α is the only medication approved for the treatment of chronic hepatitis B.[52, 61, 171] Among adults, the response rate to IFN is approximately 40 per cent among chronic hepatitis B patients treated with the recommended regimen of 5 million units of IFN subcutaneously daily for 16 weeks, with or without a preceding 6-week period of priming with prednisone.[171] A response is defined by the loss of circulating HBeAg and HBV DNA, normalization of the serum alanine aminotransferase activity, and improvement in the degree of necroinflammatory changes on liver biopsy. About 6 to 10 per cent of patients lose HBsAg and HBV DNA, which is indicative of the termination of HBV infection. Typically, a response is heralded with an acute flare-up, with clinical and laboratory features simulating acute viral hepatitis. INF should be used with caution and in low dose in patients with clinically overt cirrhosis due to chronic HBV infection.[101] It is contraindicated in patients with far-advanced liver disease because the flare can precipitate profound hepatic failure and death.

The best predictors of a response to IFN are a high initial serum alanine aminotransferase activity (>200 IU/L), a low blood HBV-DNA level, short duration of chronic infection, and the absence of other conditions that can alter the immune state, such as HIV infection. In general, responders maintain their response long term, and a few may even clear HBV infection over time.

Results of IFN therapy of children with chronic hepatitis B are varied. Randomized controlled trials have not shown a beneficial effect, but the majority of children in these studies had normal alanine aminotransferase values or were Asian, factors known to correlate with a poor response.[130, 171] In one series, the rate of response to IFN among European children who had increased alanine aminotransferase levels was comparable with that of the response to serum in white adults.[153] The dose used in this study was 3 million units/m^2 three times a week for 6 months.

Medical therapy for chronic hepatitis D is limited to IFN, and the results are disappointing. Although about 50 per cent of patients respond initially to therapy, more than 90 per cent experience relapse after IFN is discontinued. HDV and HDV RNA may disappear from the blood but persist in the liver. Those who have a long-term response clear HBsAg and HBV DNA from the serum and liver, but both may reappear later. A response may require a longer course of treatment with IFN therapy than for hepatitis B alone.

INF also is the only therapeutic agent shown to be effective in chronic hepatitis C.[52, 106] Licensed for use in adults, the standard protocol is a dose of 3×10^6 units given subcutaneously three times a week for 6 months. Multiple therapeutic trials have shown that approximately 40 per cent of those treated with this regimen respond with a return of the alanine aminotransferase level to normal values and an improved sense of well-being if symptomatic.[52, 61] Of those responding, about 75 per cent have evidence of morphologic improvement on liver biopsy. Unlike the acute hepatitis–like flare that typically heralds a response to therapy in chronic hepatitis B, patients with chronic hepatitis C who respond demonstrate a gradual fall in serum alanine aminotransferase levels. This virtually always occurs within the first 3 months of treatment. Patients not demonstrating clinical improvement within 3 months are unlikely to respond favorably with continued therapy. Among those who respond initially, 50 to 70 per cent experience relapse after therapy is discontinued, usually within the first 6 to 12 months. A relapse is associated with the reappearance of HCV RNA in the serum and the liver if it had cleared during therapy, followed by elevation of the serum alanine aminotransferase level. Relapses usually respond to retreatment with IFN. Predictors of a good initial response to INF include a low serum alanine aminotransferase value, a low HCV-RNA level, minimal activity on liver biopsy, absent cirrhosis, and HCV genotypes other than type 1.

Higher doses of IFN and longer duration of therapy have been examined in more recent clinical trials. Careful analysis of these clinical trials suggests that the response rate at 1 to 2 years after treatment may be 10 to 15 per cent higher among those treated when a larger total dose of IFN is used (vide infra).

Most patients treated with IFN have side effects that are

*Hepatitis B immunoglobulin prepared from recipients of multiple transfusions has an anti-HBs titer of at least 1:100,000 by passive hemagglutination, compared with titers of 1:64 to 1:128 for standard immunoglobulin.

dose related. Side effects include depression, reversible alopecia, and bone marrow depression. However, the majority of patients treated with the standard protocol are able to complete the full course of therapy. The source of IFN, whether recombinant (e.g., α2) or natural (lymphoblastoid), does not appear to influence the outcome or side effects of IFN.

Based on the finding that a greater total dose of IFN increases the probability of a sustained response rate, some hepatologists are treating chronic hepatitis C patients with 3 million units thrice weekly for 12 months or more. This regimen is preferred because a dose of 5 to 10 million units per administration is more likely to give rise to side effects that may necessitate discontinuation of therapy.

IFN should be administered under the direction of physicians familiar with chronic hepatitis and the use of this agent and only when the patient can be followed closely.

Ribavirin therapy by itself brings about a reduction in the alanine aminotransferase level but does not appear to decrease HCV replication. Early results of clinical trials suggest that it may exert a synergistic effect when given in combination with IFN. If true, combination therapy with these two agents might prove effective in treating those patients whose disease fails to respond to IFN alone.

There still are many unanswered questions about IFN treatment of chronic hepatitis C in adults. Although there are predictors of patients more likely to respond to therapy, there virtually is no way to predict early in the course of chronic infection which patients will do poorly unless treated. As a result, there is no consensus as to who should be treated with IFN, other than those patients with clear evidence of progression, incapacitating symptoms, or chronic HCV complicated with cryoglobulinemia. Furthermore, there is very limited information about the long-term outcome of those patients responding to IFN. It is not known whether a remission, once achieved, will be sustained long term and whether an IFN-induced remission favorably influences the development of cirrhosis or the risk of a hepatoma. Such information is very much needed.

To date, there are only limited data from a few pilot studies about the use of IFN in the treatment of children with chronic hepatitis C.[110, 192] Although encouraging, larger controlled trials are needed before specific recommendations can be formulated.

Liver transplantation is another mode of therapy reserved for patients with end-stage liver disease due to chronic viral hepatitis B and C. Patients with hepatitis B do poorly after orthotopic liver transplantation if their new liver is not protected against becoming infected.[230] HBV infection after transplantation usually leads to very rapid and progressive liver disease, graft failure, or the very serious complication of "fibrosing" cholestatic hepatitis.[51, 238] Candidates do best if their serum is HBV RNA–negative or in very low titer prior to transplant. Protection during and after transplant with immunoglobulin containing high-titer anti-HB has been found to reduce significantly the chances of HBV reinfection after liver transplantation.[230] Disease recurrence has been treated with IFN-α, and some patients have responded.[238] However, experience with this regimen in transplant recipients is limited. In one large multicenter study, the overall survival rate of 372 patients who received transplants for chronic hepatitis B at 1 year and 3 years was 75 per cent and 63 per cent, respectively.[195] They had received hepatitis B immunoglobulin prior to and after transplantation.

Recurrent HBV and HDV infections are frequent complications of patients who receive transplants for end-stage liver disease due to hepatitis D.[22] In general, the course after HBV and HDV graft reinfection is milder than in infections due to HBV alone. Presumably, this is due to the inhibitory effect of HDV on HBV replication. As a result, there is less risk of recurrent HBV infection in patients who receive transplants for hepatitis D than in patients who have only chronic hepatitis B.

There is a growing body of knowledge about the effectiveness of liver transplantation for chronic HCV infection. In one published series consisting of 97 patients, 1- and 3-year survival rates were 94 per cent and 87 per cent, respectively.[41] Despite these promising results, the vast majority of patients who received transplants for end-stage disease due to chronic hepatitis C became reinfected after the transplantation.[252] The presence of recurrent HCV infection may be missed because infection usually is silent or low-grade in activity and because immunosuppressive therapy may result in false-negative anti-HCV determinations. Testing for HCV RNA may be required for diagnosis. Although HCV reinfection clearly is less severe than reinfection of HBV in transplant recipients, the long-term outcome of recurrent HCV infection is not known yet.

PREVENTION

General Measures

Good personal hygiene is known to be effective in reducing the spread of hepatitis A. Disposable equipment, such as needles and syringes, should be used whenever possible and nondisposable materials, such as instruments and containers, sterilized with heat after thorough cleansing. Heat sterilization can be accomplished by boiling in water (100° C) for 10 minutes, autoclaving (steam under pressure at 121° C at 15 lb/square inch) for 15 minutes, or with dry heat (160° C) for 2 hours. When heat sterilization is not possible, one of several alternatives presumed to be viricidal should be used: (1) soaking in 0.5 to 1.0 per cent sodium hypochlorite for 30 minutes, (2) soaking in 40 per cent aqueous formalin (16 per cent formaldehyde) for 12 hours or formalin 20 per cent in 70 per cent alcohol for 18 hours, (3) soaking in 2 per cent aqueous alkalinized glutaraldehyde for 10 hours, or (4) gas sterilization with ethylene oxide.[172]

Standard precautions, which embody the major features of universal precautions, are recommended for all hospitalized patients, regardless of their diagnosis.[68] Standard precautions are designed to minimize the risk of transmission of infectious agents, including viral hepatitis, from both recognized and unrecognized sources in the hospital setting. They apply to the handling of blood, all body fluids, secretions or excretions, nonintact skin, and mucous membranes. The use of gloves, which are changed between individual patient contacts, and prompt washing of the hands are essential components of standard precautions, as is the proper disposal of potentially contaminated sharp instruments, such as needles and scalpel blades. A gown should be worn when there is a chance of splashing or spraying infectious body fluids or secretions. Contact precautions, which include private room placement, applies to patients with hepatitis A. Contact precautions are designed to prevent spread of infection by direct or indirect contact. They also apply to patients with the other types of viral hepatitis expected to contaminate the environment or who are unable to assist in maintaining appropriate hygienic control.

Staff who are acutely ill with hepatitis should not be allowed to manage patients until they have recovered fully. Based on prospective studies,[17] the current Public Health Service statement on control of hepatitis B does not recommend restriction of activity of health care individuals with chronic hepatitis B unless they clearly have been implicated in the spread of hepatitis.

Immunoprophylaxis

Hepatitis A

Conventional immunoglobulin (formally designated immune serum globulin) is 80 to 90 per cent effective in preventing clinically evident hepatitis A if given within 1 to 2 weeks of exposure. It is recommended for all household contacts who have not had hepatitis A or in special circumstances, as in a school or institution where there is clear evidence that an outbreak has occurred.[6, 19] Immunoglobulin totally may prevent infection or attenuate the infection to a subclinical level, permitting the development of naturally acquired immunity, i.e., passive-active immunization. The immunoglobulin dosage recommended by the Public Health Service for hepatitis A prophylaxis is shown in Table 55–2.

An inactivated hepatitis A vaccine (Havrix) was licensed in February 1995. The vaccine is derived from HAV grown in human diploid cells that is inactivated with formalin after purification.[178] The vaccine has been tested extensively and has been shown to be both safe and highly effective if used appropriately. Field trials demonstrated an efficacy rate of greater than 90 per cent in preventing clinical hepatitis.[109, 248] Early observations suggest that protection induced by immunization may be very long lasting. The recommended dosage schedule for vaccination is shown in Table 55–3.

The vaccine is recommended for persons older than 2 years of age who are at increased risk for hepatitis A via international travel.[7] Additional recommendations from the Advisory Committee on Immunization Practices will be forthcoming and are likely to include residents of a community experiencing an outbreak of hepatitis A, military personnel, persons engaged in high-risk sexual activity, workers in day care centers, care takers of the developmentally challenged, primate handlers, and laboratory workers handling specimens containing HAV. Primary immunization should be completed at least 2 weeks prior to exposure. The vaccine also can be given to individuals exposed to hepatitis A who require both immediate and long-term protection. In this case, the initial dose should be given concomitantly with immunoglobulin but at a different site and then repeated for the full course.

The vaccine is contraindicated in people who are hypersensitive to any of its components. Caution is urged in pregnant women and mothers who are breast feeding because of a lack of experience in these settings.

Hepatitis B

Prevention of infection after exposure to HBV by passive and active immunization, or a combination of the two, has been evaluated carefully in several large clinical trials. Initial studies examined the effect of immunoglobulin.[176, 223] These studies were followed by investigations that compared the protection afforded by immunoglobulin with that of hepatitis B immunoglobulin.[89, 176, 177, 203] Subsequently, clinical trials determined the efficacy of hepatitis B vaccine given alone[82, 127, 183, 213, 223] or in conjunction with hepatitis B immunoglobulin.[251] Based on the results of these multiple trials, specific recommendations for pre-exposure and post-exposure prophylaxis of hepatitis B have been made by the Advisory Committee on Immunization Practices.

The degree of protection offered by immunoglobulin after exposure to hepatitis B has been debated for many years. Clinical trials that compared the efficacy of immunoglobulin and hepatitis B immunoglobulin demonstrated that the latter is more effective than the former, although protection by both is only temporary, generally lasting several weeks to several months, respectively. Hepatitis B immunoglobulin is recommended for immediate prophylaxis after parenteral (e.g., needle stick) or sexual exposure.[185]

A vaccine for hepatitis B has been available since 1982. The first approved vaccine consisted of highly purified alum-absorbed HBsAg (20-nm particles) derived from the blood of chronic HBV carriers. It had been tested extensively in chimpanzees and humans and found to be highly immunogenic and noninfectious. Nonetheless, it was not received with great popularity due to its source, which raised concern (not realized) that it might transmit HIV. This fear has been allayed by the introduction of recombinant vaccine preparations.[111]

Currently, only recombinant vaccines are available for use in the United States. They are safe and effective and have a low incidence of side effects comparable with other vaccines. Approximately 20 to 35 per cent of those vaccinated develop pain at the site of injection, low-grade fever, or rash.[223] Serious side effects, such as Guillain-Barré syndrome and AIDS, have not been linked causally linked to the vaccines. They can be given to anti-HBs–positive individuals and to HBsAg carriers without adverse effects. Pregnancy is not a contraindication to the use of the vaccines for persons who otherwise are eligible.[19]

The recommended primary vaccination series, whether pre-exposure or post-exposure, consists of three intramuscular injections of the hepatitis B vaccine of the same dosage (Table 55–4). The second and third injections are given 3 and 6 months after the first dose. Specific doses vary by age group, clinical status, and vaccine manufacturer. The manufacturer's package insert should be consulted for specific dosage. The anti-HBS response rate is approximately 90 per cent after the full series among healthy individuals and about 50 per cent among immunocompromised patients.[82, 213, 223] Of note, children, including newborns, are very responsive to the vaccine; approximately 95 per cent develop anti-HBs.

TABLE 55–2. Guidelines for Conventional Immunoglobulin Prophylaxis Against Hepatitis A Virus Infection

	Body Weight (lb)	Immunoglobulin Dose (mL)
Household contacts; travelers who bypass tourist routes in countries having epidemic hepatitis	<50	0.5
	50–100	1.0
	>100	2.0
Foreign travelers staying 3 or more months in tropical areas or developing countries	<50	1.0
	50–100	2.5
	>100	5.0

TABLE 55–3. Vaccination Schedule Recommended for Prevention of Hepatitis A Virus Infection

Age Group (yr)	Dose (EL.U)*	Volume (mL)	No. Doses	Scheduled (mo)
2–18	720	0.5	2	0, 6–12
>18	1440	1.0	2	0, 6–12

The licensed inactivated vaccine (Havrix) is distributed by SmithKline Beecham Pharmaceuticals (Philadelphia). It should be administered by intramuscular injection into the deltoid muscle.

*Measure as enzyme-linked immunosorbent units.

TABLE 55–4. Postexposure Prophylaxis

	HBIG (Administered IM)		Vaccine* (Administered IM)	
Exposure	***Dose***	***Time***	***Dose***	***Time***
Perinatal	0.5 mL	Within 12 hr	0.5 mL	12 hr of birth, 1 mo, and 6 mo
Percutaneous	0.06 mL/kg BW	24 hr, repeat at 1 mo	1.0 mL	7 d, 1 mo, and 6 mo
Sexual	0.06 mL/kg BW	Within 14 d	1.0 mL	7 d of HBIG, 3 mo, and 6 mo†

*Administer in deltoid muscle, at different arm than HBIG.
†Administer at 1 mo and 6 mo if sexual partner(s) remain positive for HBsAg.
BW, body weight; HBIG, hepatitis B immunoglobulin; HBsAg, hepatitis B surface antigen; IM, intramuscularly.

PRE-EXPOSURE PROPHYLAXIS. Pre-exposure prophylaxis is accomplished by administration of the three-dose regimen described in the previous section. Immunization with hepatitis B vaccine was recommended originally for susceptible persons whose occupation or social setting puts them at special risk for acquiring hepatitis B (Table 55–5).[9] However, this policy has proved to be a failure. Although a vaccine for hepatitis B has been available for more than 35 years, less than 30 per cent of the 22 million individuals in the United States considered at high risk to hepatitis B have been vaccinated. Furthermore, as many as 40 per cent of new cases of hepatitis B do not fall within high-risk groups. For these reasons, the Advisory Committee on Immunization Practices has expanded the recommendations of vaccination to a strategy that has as its goal the ultimate elimination of HBV transmission in the United States. Recommendations include (1) infants and children at the time they receive their other routine vaccinations, (2) infants and children younger than 11 years of age who are Pacific Islanders or who live in households of first-generation immigrants from countries of high or intermediate HBV endemicity, and (3) 11- to 12-year-old children who have not been vaccinated previously.[8] For adults, the vaccine still is recommended prophylactically for high-risk groups.

Unknown is whether a booster dose should be given to those immunized during childhood when they become adolescents or adults. Approximately 40 per cent of these vaccinated lose detectable anti-HBs within 7 years of vaccination. However, protection apparently outlives anti-HBs positivity.[148] As a result, the Advisory Committee on Immunization Practices currently does not recommend a routine vaccine booster dose. It should be pointed out that some hepatologists do favor administering a routine booster dose 5 to 7 years after the primary series.

TABLE 55–5. Groups at Greater Risk for Acquiring Hepatitis B Virus Infection

1. Health care workers (medical, dental, laboratory, and support staff) in contact with patients and blood products
2. Clients and staff of institutions for mentally retarded
3. Hemodialysis patients
4. Patients who receive repeated blood transfusions and those with clotting disorders who are recipients of factor VII or IX concentrate
5. Homosexually active males
6. Users of illicit injectable drugs
7. Household sexual contacts of hepatitis B virus carriers
8. Other high-risk populations
   a. Alaskan Eskimos and immigrants from areas where hepatitis B virus is highly endemic
   b. Immigrants from eastern Asia and sub-Saharan Africa
   c. Long-term inmates of correctional facilities

Among adults, prescreening to determine susceptibility is advised on a cost-effective basis only for those individuals who fall into a particularly high-risk group, such as male homosexuals and illicit drug users. For these groups, the cost of first testing a blood sample for evidence of prior or current hepatitis B is less than the administration of the vaccine. To determine susceptibility to HBV infection, a sample of blood of the person to be vaccinated should be tested for the presence of anti-HBs or anti-HBc. In most instances, anti-HBs testing alone is adequate. An anti-HBs value of 10 mIU/mL or greater is considered evidence of naturally acquired immunity due to prior HBV infection. Uncertainty exists about the status of immunity of persons with anti-HBs levels less than 10 mIU/mL. These individuals either should be considered susceptible and vaccinated or should be tested for the presence of anti-HBc. If anti-HBc–positive, they should be considered immune. If anti-HBc–negative, they should be vaccinated.

POSTEXPOSURE PROPHYLAXIS. Hepatitis B immunoglobulin administered before, simultaneous with, or shortly after the hepatitis B vaccine does not prevent active immunization as long as hepatitis B immunoglobulin and the vaccine are administered at different sites.[222] It therefore is possible to provide immediate passive protection after exposure to HBV with hepatitis B immunoglobulin and at the same time initiate active long-standing immunity with hepatitis B vaccine. Hepatitis B immunoglobulin and hepatitis B vaccine do not interfere with oral polio or diphtheria-tetanus-pertussis vaccine administered to children at 2 months of age. Prophylaxis after exposure has occurred is recommended in the following situations: (1) perinatal exposure of an infant born to an HBsAg-positive mother; (2) accidental mucosal, ocular, or percutaneous exposure to HBsAg-positive blood and secretions; and (3) sexual exposure to an HBsAg-positive individual (see Table 55–4).[19, 185]

All pregnant women should be screened for hepatitis B, preferably during the third trimester. This is to identify the newborn who requires immunoprophylaxis shortly after delivery. Protection is maximal when administered on the day of birth.[56] If prenatal testing was not performed, the mother should be screened for HBsAg as soon as possible after delivery.

Early prophylaxis for exposed infants is important for the prevention of acute hepatitis B and the very high probability of the development of chronic hepatitis and an HBV carrier state. The administration of hepatitis B vaccine and hepatitis B immunoglobulin injected at different sites is approximately 95 per cent effective in protecting against hepatitis B. The 5 per cent of neonates not protected by this regimen are believed to have acquired hepatitis B in utero.

The regimen to be followed is shown in Table 55–4. It consists of the intramuscular administration of 0.5 mL of hepatitis B immunoglobulin after the newborn has become stable, preferably within 12 hours of delivery. This is followed by the intramuscular administration of hepatitis B vaccine in three doses. The first vaccine dose should be administered 12 hours after birth at a site different from that used for hepatitis B immunoglobulin. The second and third doses should be administered 1 month and 6 months after the first dose. Testing for anti-HBs and HBsAg at 6 months may be performed. If anti-HBs–positive, the child can be considered immune; if HBsAg-positive, it indicates a therapeutic failure and a third vaccine dose should not be given. The child then should be managed for HBV infection. If the infant is negative for both tests, he or she should be revaccinated if the mother remains HBsAg-positive.

For needle stick, mucous membrane, or ocular exposure to blood known to contain HBsAg and for human bites from HBsAg-positive individuals that penetrate the skin, hepatitis B immunoglobulin in a dose of 0.06 mL/kg of body weight should be given as soon as possible, preferably within 24 hours. The same dose of hepatitis B immunoglobulin should be repeated at 1 month. However, if repeated exposure to HBV is likely, hepatitis B vaccine should be administered intramuscularly at a separate site either concurrently or within 7 days of exposure. Second and third courses of the same dose of vaccine should be given 1 and 6 months later. Administration of hepatitis B immunoglobulin need not be repeated when active vaccination is initiated in this fashion.

Prophylaxis also is recommended for sexual contacts of persons with acute hepatitis B. Information based on limited studies suggests that hepatitis B immunoglobulin probably is effective within 14 days of exposure to HBV by this route. The exposed sexual partner should be screened for susceptibility (i.e., the absence of anti-HBS or anti-HBc) if the time required to obtain the test results does not delay the administration of hepatitis B immunoglobulin beyond 14 days of exposure. A full series of hepatitis B vaccine also should be initiated at the time hepatitis B immunoglobulin first is given if the patient is found to be susceptible. Only the initial dose of hepatitis B immunoglobulin is required if the full vaccine series is initiated simultaneously.

Of some concern are a few reports of HBV pre-S gene escape mutants that can infect individuals who have been vaccinated and had a good anti-HBs response.[42] Fortunately, the magnitude of this problem does not appear to be great.

A variety of other hepatitis B vaccine candidates currently are under evaluation. Possible future vaccines include immunogenic polypeptide components that are synthesized de novo, naked DNA, and HBV S gene inserted into the genome of live attenuated virus for delivery of childhood vaccines.[136, 236] The ability to synthesize a vaccine offers the potential for large-scale production of material that is low in cost. It then could be utilized on a worldwide basis with the goal of eradicating hepatitis B. Incorporating the pre-S gene into the vaccine could protect against mutant HBV strains as well.

Hepatitis C

Studies that have examined the efficacy of immunoglobulin in preventing hepatitis C are few in number and present conflicting results.[117, 204] Consequently, no formal recommendations have been made for the use of immunoglobulin after exposure to hepatitis C. However, some authorities recommend immunoglobulin in a dose of 0.06 mL/kg of body weight (or 5 mL for adults) after clear evidence of percutaneous, mucosal, or sexual exposure to hepatitis C blood or secretions.[202]

An effective vaccine for the prevention of hepatitis C has not been developed and may be very difficult to achieve. Chimpanzees who have recovered from HCV infection are reinfected after rechallenge with both homologous and heterologous strains of HCV.[73] Neutralizing anti-HCV antibodies are produced in response to HCV, but they are not effective in halting infection or preventing reinfection. It appears that although the anti-HCV elicited is capable of neutralizing the original infecting HCV strain, escape mutants appear that are resistant to immune attack.[74] Thus, the prosperity of HCV to mutant, like HIV, poses a serious problem in providing short-term protection by immunoglobulin and in developing an effective vaccine for long-term immunity. One approach to circumventing this problem is to identify antigens coded for by the more highly conserved regions of the HCV genome. Once identified, they can be studied to determine if they are able to elicit protective antibodies against all strains of HCV.

Hepatitis D

A vaccine to prevent hepatitis D does not exist. Recombinant HDAg has been tested in the woodchuck, and, although immunogenic, it does not prevent infection. Prevention of HDV/HBV coinfection is accomplished with hepatitis B immunoglobulin prophylaxis by preventing hepatitis B after exposure. Long-term protection is provided by vaccination against hepatitis B. However, this strategy is not effective in the prevention of HDV superinfection in patients with chronic HBV infection. Such individuals should be advised strongly against high-risk activity, such as continued intravenous drug use and promiscuous sexual activity.

Hepatitis E

No Advisory Committee on Immunization Practices recommendations have been made for prophylaxis against HEV, and a vaccine is not available. It is logical to assume that immunoglobulin given shortly after exposure could prevent HEV infection if it is obtained from individuals who have recovered from hepatitis E and, therefore, have high-titer anti-HEV. Immunoglobulin from undeveloped countries where HEV is endemic is likely to be the best source of protective immunoglobulin.

References

1. Aach, R. D., Lander, J. J., Sherman, L. A., et al.: Transfusion-transmitted viruses: Interim analysis of hepatitis among transfused and non-transfused patients. *In* Vyas, G. N., Cohen, S. N., and Schmid, R. (eds.): Viral Hepatitis. Philadelphia, Franklin Institute Press, 1978, p. 383.
2. Aach, R. D., Stevens, C. E., Hollinger, F. B., et al.: Hepatitis C virus infection in post-transfusion hepatitis: An analysis of the transfusion-transmitted viruses study with first and second generation assays. N. Engl. J. Med. *325*:1325–1329, 1991.
3. Aach, R. D., Szmuness, W., Mosley, J. W., et al.: Serum alanine aminotransferase of donors in relation to the risk of non-A, non-B hepatitis in recipients: The Transfusion-Transmitted Viruses Study. N. Engl. J. Med. *304*:989–994, 1981.
4. Advisory Committee on Immunization Practices: Immune globulins for protection against viral hepatitis. M. M. W. R. *530*:423–433, 1981.
5. Advisory Committee on Immunization Practices: Licensure of inactivated hepatitis A vaccine. M. M. W. R. *44*:559–560, 1995.
6. Advisory Committee on Immunization Practices: Update: Recommendations to prevent hepatitis B virus transmission—United States. M. M. W. R. *44*:574–575, 1995.
7. Advisory Committee on Immunization Practices: Recommendations for protection against viral hepatitis. M. M. W. R. *39*:1–26, 1990.
8. Almeida, J. D., Rubenstein, D., and Stott, E. J.: New antigen-antibody system in Australia-antigen–positive hepatitis. Lancet 2:1225–1227, 1971.
9. Alpert, E., Isselbacher, K. J., and Schur, P. H.: The pathogenesis of arthritis associated with viral hepatitis. N. Engl. J. Med. *285*:185–189, 1971.
10. Alter, M. J.: The detection, transmission and outcome of hepatitis C virus infection. Infect. Agents Dis. 2:155–166, 1993.
11. Alter, H. J., Chalmers, T. C., Freeman, B. M., et al.: Health care workers

positive for hepatitis B surface antigen: Are their contacts at risk? N. Engl. J. Med. *292*:454–457, 1975.
12. Alter, H. J., Holland, P. V., Purcell, R. H., et al.: Post-transfusion hepatitis after exclusion of commercial and hepatitis B antigen-positive donors. Ann. Intern. Med. *77*:691–699, 1972.
13. Alter, H. J., Purcell, R. H., Holland, P. V., et al.: Transmissible agent in non-A, non-B hepatitis. Lancet *1*:459–463, 1978.
14. Alter, H. J., Purcell, R. H., Shik, J. W., et al.: Detection of antibody to hepatitis C virus in prospectively followed transfusion recipient with acute and chronic non-A, non-B hepatitis. N. Engl. J. Med. *321*:1494–1500, 1989.
15. Alter, H. J., Seeff, L. B., Kaplan, P. M., et al.: Type B hepatitis: The infectivity of blood positive for e antigen and DNA polymerase after accidental needle stick exposure. N. Engl. J. Med. *295*:909–913, 1976.
16. Alter, M. J., Margolis, H. S., Krawczynski, K., et al.: The natural history of community-acquired hepatitis C in the United States. N. Engl. J. Med. *327*:1899–1905, 1992.
17. Alter, M. J., and Must, E. E.: The epidemiology of viral hepatitis in the United States. Gastroenterol. Clin. North Am. *23*:437–455, 1994.
18. Angello, V., Chung, R. T., and Kaplan, L. M.: A role of hepatitis C virus infection in type II cryoglobulinemia. N. Engl. J. Med. *327*:1490–1495, 1992.
19. Anonymous: Jaundice following yellow fever vaccination. J. A. M. A. *119*:1110, 1942.
20. Anonymous: Morphological criteria in viral hepatitis: Review by an international group. Lancet *1*:333–337, 1971.
21. Asher, M. L., Lak, J. R., Emond, J., et al.: Liver transplantation for hepatitis C virus–related cirrhosis. Hepatology *20*(Suppl.):245–275, 1994.
22. Aynes, S., Bonino, S., and Rizzetto, M.: Patterns of hepatitis delta virus reinfection and disease in liver transplantation. Gastroenterology *101*:1649–1655, 1991.
23. Bachmann, L.: Infectious hepatitis in Europe. *In* Rodenwalt, E. (ed.): World Atlas of Epidemic Diseases. Part. I. Hamburg, Falk-Verlag, 1952, p. 67.
24. Bancroft, W. H., Mundon, F. K., and Russel, P. K.: Detection of additional antigenic determinants of hepatitis B antigen. J. Immunol. *109*:842–848, 1972.
25. Batten, P. J., Runte, V. E., Skinner, H. G., et al.: Infectious hepatitis: Infectiousness during the presymptomatic phase of the disease. Am. J. Hyg. *77*:129, 1963.
26. Beasley, R. P., Hwang, L. W., Lin, C. C., et al.: Hepatocellular carcinoma and hepatitis B virus: A prospective study of 22,707 men in Tawain. Lancet 2:1129–1132, 1981
27. Beeson, P. B., Chesney, G., McFarlan, A. M., et al.: Hepatitis following injection of mumps convalescent plasma. Lancet *1*:814, 1944.
28. Berman, M., Alter, H. J., Ishak, K. G., et al.: The chronic sequelae of non-A, non-B hepatitis. Ann. Intern. Med. *91*:1–6, 1979.
29. Bernuau, J., Rueff, B., and Benhamou, J.: Fulminant and subfulminant liver failure: Definitions and causes. Semin. Liver Dis. *6*:97–106, 1986.
30. Binn, L. N., Lemon, S. M., Marchwicki, R. H., et al.: Primary isolation and serial passage of hepatitis A virus strains in primate cell cultures. J. Clin. Microbiol. *20*:28–33, 1984.
31. Blajchman, M. A., Bull, S. B., and Feinman, S. V.: Post-transfusion hepatitis: Impact on non-A, non-B hepatitis surrogate tests. Lancet *345*:21–25, 1995.
32. Bloch, K. J.: Cryoglobulinemia and hepatitis C viruses. N. Engl. J. Med. *327*:1521–1552, 1992.
33. Blum, H. E.: Does hepatitis C virus cause hepatocellular carcinoma? Hepatology *19*:251–258, 1994.
34. Blumberg, R. S., Alter, H. J., Visnich, S., et al.: A "new" antigen in leukemia sera. J. A. M. A. *191*:541, 1965.
35. Blumberg, B. S., Stunick, A. I., and London, W. T.: Hepatitis and leukemia: Their relation to Australia antigen. Bull. N. Y. Acad. Med. *44*:1566–1586, 1968.
36. Bonimo, F., and Smedile, A.: Delta agent (type D) hepatitis. Semin. Liver Dis. *6*:28–33, 1986.
37. Bortolotti, F., Cadrobbi, P., Crivellaro, C., et al.: Long-term outcome of chronic type B hepatitis in patients who have acquired hepatitis B infection in childhood. Gastroenterology *99*:805–811, 1990.
38. Boyer, J. L., and Klatskin, G.: Pattern of necrosis in acute viral hepatitis: Prognostic value of bridging (subacute hepatic necrosis). N. Engl. J. Med. *283*:1063–1071, 1970.
39. Bradley, D. W.: Introduction: The diversity of human hepatitis viruses. Semin. Virol. *4*:269–271, 1993.
40. Bradley, D. W., Maynard, J. E., Popper, H., et al.: Post-transfusion non-A, non-B hepatitis: Physiochemical properties of two distinct agents. J. Infect. Dis. *148*:254–265, 1983.
41. Brunetto, M., Stemler, M., Bonino, F., et al.: A new hepatitis B virus strain in patients with severe anti-HBe positive chronic hepatitis B. J. Hepatol. *10*:258–261, 1990.
42. Carman, W. F, Zanetti, A. R., Karayiannis, P., et al: Vaccine-induced mutant of hepatitis B virus. Lancet *336*:325–329, 1990.
43. Casey, J. L., Brown, T. L., Colan, E. J., et al.: A genotype of hepatitis D virus that occurs in northern South America. Proc. Natl. Acad. Sci. U. S. A. *90*:9016–9020, 1993.
44. Chang, M. H., Chen, P. J., Chen, J. Y., et al.: Hepatitis B virus–related hepatocellular carcinoma in childhood. Hepatology *13*:316–320, 1991.
45. Charnay, P., Pourcel, C., Louise, A., et al.: Cloning in *Escherichia coli* and physical structure of hepatitis B virion DNA. Proc. Natl. Acad. Sci. U. S. A. *76*:2222–2226, 1979.
46. Chau, K. H., Hargie, M. P., Decker, R. H., et al.: Serodiagnosis of recent hepatitis B infection by IgM class anti-HBc. Hepatology *3*:142–149, 1983.
47. Choo, Q.-L., Kuo, G., Weiner, A. J., et al.: Isolation of a cDNA clone derived from a blood-borne non-A, non-B viral hepatitis genome. Science *244*:359–362, 1989.
48. Clayson, E. T., Myint, K. S., Snitbhan, R., et al.: Viremia, fecal shedding and IgM and IgG responses in patients with hepatitis E. J. Infect. Dis. *172*:927–933, 1995.
49. Cockayne, E. A.: Catarrhal jaundice sporadic and epidemic, and its relation to acute yellow atrophy of the liver. Q. J. Med. *6*:1, 1912.
50. Dane, D. S., Cameron, C. H., and Briggs, M.: Virus-like particles in serum of patients with Australia-antigen–associated hepatitis. Lancet *1*:695–698, 1970.
51. Davies, S. E., Portmann, B. C., O'Grady, J. G., et al.: Hepatic histological findings after transplantation for chronic hepatitis B virus infection including a unique pattern of fibrosing cholestatic hepatitis. Hepatology *13*:150–157, 1991.
52. Davis, G. L., Balart, L. A., Schiff, E. R., et al.: Treatment of chronic hepatitis C with recombinant interferon alpha: A multicenter, randomized, controlled trial. N. Engl. J. Med. *321*:1501–1506, 1989.
53. Davis, G. L., and Hoofnagle, J. H.: Interferon in viral hepatitis. Hepatology *6*:1038–1041, 1986.
54. Davis G. L., and Hoofnagle, J. H.: Reactivation of chronic type B hepatitis presenting as acute viral hepatitis. Ann. Intern. Med. *102*:762–765, 1985.
55. Deinhardt, F., Holmes, A. W., Capps, R. B., et al.: Studies on the transmission of human viral hepatitis to marmoset monkeys. I. Transmission of disease, serial passages, and description of liver lesions. J. Exp. Med. *125*:673–688, 1967.
56. Delaplane, D., Yogev, R., Crussi, F., et al.: Fatal hepatitis B in early infancy: The importance of identifying HBsAg positive pregnant women and providing immunoprophylaxis to their newborns. Pediatrics *72*:176–180, 1983.
57. DeMitri, M. S., Poussin, K., Baccarini, P., et al.: HCV associated liver cancer without cirrhosis. Lancet *345*:413–415, 1995.
58. DePotter, C., Robberrecht, E., Laureys, G., et al.: Hepatitis B related childhood hepatocellular carcinoma. Cancer *60*:414–418, 1987.
59. Desmet, V. J., Gerber, M. A., Hoofnagle, J. H., et al.: Classification of chronic hepatitis: Diagnosis, grading and staging. Hepatology *19*:1513 1520, 1994.
60. DiBisceglie, A. M.: Hepatitis C and hepatocellular carcinoma. Semin. Liver Dis. *15*:64–69, 1995.
61. DiBisceglie, A. M., Martin, P., Kassianides, C., et al.: Recombinant interferon alpha therapy for chronic hepatitis C: A randomized double blind, placebo-controlled trial. N. Engl. J. Med. *321*:1506–1510, 1989.
62. Dienes, H. P., Popper, H., Arnold, W., et al.: Histologic observations in human hepatitis non-A, non-B. Hepatology 2:562–571, 1982.
63. Dienstag, J. L., Feinstone, S. M., Kapikian, A. Z., et al.: Fecal shedding of hepatitis A antigen. Lancet *1*:765–767, 1975.
64. Dienstag, J. L., Routenberg, J. A., Purcell, R. H., et al.: Foodhandler-associated outbreak of hepatitis A. Ann. Intern. Med. *83*:647–650, 1975.
65. Dienstag, J. L., Purcell, R. H., Alter, H., et al.: Non-A, non-B post-transfusion hepatitis. Lancet *1*:560–562, 1977.
66. Donahue, J. G., Munoz, A., Ness, P. M., et al.: The declining risk of post-transfusion hepatitis C virus infection. N. Engl. J. Med. *327*:369–373, 1992.
67. Dougherty, W. J., and Altman, R.: Viral hepatitis in New Jersey, 1960–1961. Am. J. Med. *32*:704, 1962.
68. Draft Guidelines for Isolation Precautions in Hospitals: Part I. "Evolution of isolation practices" and Part II. "Recommendations for isolation precautions in hospitals"; notice of comment period. Federal Register *59*(No. 214):55552–55570, 1994.
69. Dubin, I. N., Sullivan, B. H., LeGolvan, P. C., et al.: The cholestatic form of viral hepatitis: Experiences with viral hepatitis at Brooke Army Hospital during the years 1951 to 1953. Am. J. Med. *29*:55, 1960.
70. Dupuy, J. M., Kostewicz, E., and Alagille, D.: Hepatitis B in children: An analysis of 80 cases of acute and chronic hepatitis B. J. Pediatr. *92*:17–20, 1978.
71. Eddleston, A. L. W. F., and Williams, R.: Inadequate antibody response to HB Ag or suppressor T-cell defect in development of active chronic hepatitis. Lancet 2:1543–1545, 1974.
72. Eisenstein, A. B., Aach, R. D., Jacobsohn, W., et al.: An epidemic of hepatitis in general hospital: Probable transmission by contaminated orange juice. J. A. M. A. *185*:171, 1963.
73. Farci, P., Alter, H. J., Govindarajan, S., et al: Lack of protective immunity against reinfection with hepatitis C virus. Science *258*:135–140, 1992.
74. Farci, P., Alter, H. J., Wong, D. C., et al.: Prevention of HCV infection in chimpanzees following antibody-mediated in-vitro neutralization. Proc. Natl. Acad. Sci. U. S. A. *91*:7792–7796, 1994.
75. Fay, O., Tanno, H., and Roncoroni, M.: Prognostic implications of the e antigen of hepatitis B virus. J. A. M. A. *238*:2501–2503, 1977.
76. Feinstone, S. M., Kapikian, A. Z., Gerin, J. L., et al.: Buoyant density of

the hepatitis A virus–like particle in cesium chloride. J. Virol. *13*:1412–1414, 1974.
77. Feinstone, S. M., Kapikian, A. Z., and Purcell, R. H.: Hepatitis A: Detection by immune electron microscopy of a virus-like antigen associated with acute illness. Science *182*:1026–1028, 1973.
78. Feinstone, S. M., Kapikian, A. Z., Purcell, R. H., et al.: Transfusion-associated hepatitis not due to viral hepatitis A or B. N. Engl. J. Med. *292*:767–770, 1975.
79. Feitelson, M. A., Marion, P. L., and Robinson, W. S.: Antigenic and structural relationships of the surface antigen of hepatitis B virus, ground squirrel hepatitis virus, and woodchuck hepatitis virus. J. Virol. *39*:447–454, 1981.
80. Ferrari, C., Bartoletti, A., Penna, A., et al.: Identification of immunodominant T cell epitopes of the hepatitis B virus nucleocapsid antigen. J. Clin. Invest. *88*:214–222, 1991.
81. Ferrari, C., Penna, A., Bartoletti, A., et al.: Cellular immune response to hepatitis B virus (HBV) encoded antigens in acute and chronic HBV infection. J. Immunol. *145*:3442–3449, 1990.
82. Francis, C. P., Hadler, S. C., Thompson, S. E., et al.: The prevention of hepatitis B with vaccine: Report of the Centers for Disease Control multicenter efficacy trial among homosexual men. Ann. Intern. Med. *97*:362–366, 1982.
83. Fry, K. E., Linnen, J. M., Zhang-Keck, Z. Y., et al.: Sequence analysis of a new RNA virus (hepatitis G virus, HGV) reveals a unique virus in the *Flaviviridae* family. Hepatology *22*:181A, 1995.
84. Galibert, F., Mandart, E., Fitoussi, F., et al.: Nucleotide sequence of hepatitis B virus genome (sub type ayw) cloned *E. coli*. Nature *281*:646–650, 1979.
85. Gerin, J. L., Shih, J. W. K., and Hoyer, B. H.: Biology and characterization of hepatitis B virus. *In* Szmuness, W. J., Alter, H. J., and Maynard, J. E. (eds.): Viral Hepatitis, 1981 International Symposium. Philadelphia, Franklin Institute Press, 1982, p. 49.
86. Gerin, J. L., Shih, J. W. K., Kaplan, P. M., et al.: Biophysical and biochemical characterization of hepatitis B antigen. Am. J. Med. Sci. *270*:115–121, 1975.
87. Glikson, M., Galum, E., Oren, R., et al.: Relapsing hepatitis A: A review of 14 cases and a literature survey. Medicine (Baltimore) *71*:14–23, 1992.
88. Gocke, D. J.: Extrahepatic manifestations of viral hepatitis. Am. J. Med. Sci. *270*:49–206, 1975.
89. Grady, G. F., and Lee, V. A.: Hepatitis B immune globulin-prevention of hepatitis from accidental exposure among medical personnel. N. Engl. J. Med. *293*:1067–70, 1975.
90. Greenberg, H. B., Pollard, R. B., Lutwick, L. I., et al.: Effect of human leukocyte interferon on hepatitis B virus infection in patients with chronic active hepatitis. N. Engl. J. Med. *295*:517–522, 1976.
91. Gregory, P. B., Knaver, C. M., Kempson, R. L., et al.: Steroid therapy in severe viral hepatitis. N. Engl. J. Med. *294*:681–687, 1976.
92. Hadler, S. C., de Monzon, M., Ponzetto, A., et al.: An epidemic of severe hepatitis due to delta virus infection in Yucpa Indians of Venezuela. Ann. Intern. Med. *100*:339–349, 1984.
93. Hagler, L., Pastore, R. A., Bergin, J. J., et al.: Aplastic anemia following viral hepatitis: Report of two fatal cases and literature review. Medicine *54*:139–164, 1975.
94. Havens, W. P., Jr.: Infectious hepatitis. Medicine *27*:279, 1948.
95. Hawkins, A. E., Gilson, R. J., Beath, S. V., et al.: Novel application of a point mutation assay: Evidence for transmission of hepatitis B viruses with pre-core mutations and their detections in infants with fulminant hepatitis B. J. Med. Virol. *44*:13–21, 1994.
96. Heathcote, J., Cameron, C. H., and Dane, D. S.: Hepatitis-B antigen in saliva and semen. Lancet *1*:71–73, 1974.
97. Hillenbrand, P., Parbhoo, S. P., Jedrychowski, A., et al.: Significance of intravascular coagulation and fibrinolysis in acute hepatic failure. Gut *15*:83–88, 1974.
98. Hillis, W. D.: An outbreak of infectious hepatitis among chimpanzee handlers at a United States Air Force base. Am. J. Hyg. *73*:316, 1961.
99. Hindman, S. H., Gravelle C. R., Murphy, B. L., et al.: "e" antigen, Dane particles, and serum DNA polymerase activity in HBsAg carriers. Ann. Intern. Med. *85*:458–460, 1976.
100. Hofmann, A.: Ikterus mit letalem ausgang nach salvarsan. Munch. Med. Wochenschr. *58*:1773, 1911.
101. Hollinger, F. B., Gitnick, G. L., Aach, R. D., et al.: Non-A, non-B transmission in chimpanzees: A project of the transfusion-transmitted viruses study group. Intervirology *10*:60–68, 1978.
102. Hollinger, F. B., Mosley, J. W., Szmuness, W., et al.: Transfusion-transmitted virus study: Experimental evidence for two non-A, non-B hepatitis agents. J. Infect. Dis. *142*:400–407, 1980.
103. Hoofnagle, J. H., DiBisceglie, A. M., Waggoner, J. J., et al.: Interferon alpha for patients with clinically apparent cirrhosis due to chronic hepatitis B. Hepatology *104*:1116–1121, 1993.
104. Hoofnagle, J. H., Gerety, R. H., and Barker, L. F.: Antibody to hepatitis B core antigen. Amer. J. Med. Sci. *270*:179–187, 1975.
105. Hoofnagle, J. H., Gerety, R. J., Ni, L. Y., et al.: Antibody to hepatitis B core antigen: A sensitive indicator of hepatitis B virus replication. N. Engl. J. Med. *290*:1336–1340, 1974.
106. Hoofnagle, J. H., Mullen, K. D., Jones, D. B., et al.: Treatment of chronic non-A, non-B hepatitis with recombinant human alpha-interferon: A preliminary report. N. Engl. J. Med. *315*:1575–1578, 1986.
107. Horney, J. T., and Galambos, J. T.: The liver during and after fulminant hepatitis. Gastroenterology *73*:639–645, 1977.
108. Houghton, M., Weiner, A., Kuo, G., et al.: Molecular biology of hepatitis C viruses: Implications for diagnosis, development and control of viral disease. Hepatology *14*:381–388, 1991.
109. Innis, B. L., Snitbhan, R., Kunasol, P., et al: Protection against hepatitis A by an inactivated vaccine. J. A. M. A. *271*:1328–1334, 1994.
110. Iorio, R., Fariello, I., Guida, S., et al.: Alpha lymphoblastoid interferon therapy in 12 children with chronic hepatitis C. Hepatology *18*:237A, 1993.
111. Jilg, W., Lorbeer, B., Schmidt, M., et al.: Clinical evaluation of a recombinant hepatitis B vaccine. Lancet *2*:1174–1175, 1984.
112. Joseph, P. R., Millar, J. D., Henderson, D. A., et al.: An outbreak of hepatitis traced to food contamination. N. Engl. J. Med. *273*:188, 1965.
113. Karvountzis, G. G., Redeker, A. G., and Peters, R. L.: Long-term follow-up studies of patients surviving fulminant viral hepatitis. Gastroenterology *67*:870–877, 1974.
114. Khuroo, M. S.: Study of an epidemic of non-A, non-B hepatitis: Possibility of another human hepatitis virus distinct from post-transfusion non-A, non-B type. Am. J. Med. *68*:818–824, 1980.
115. Khuroo, M. S., Kamili, S., Jameel, S.: Vertical transmission of hepatitis E virus. Lancet *315*:1025–1026, 1995.
116. Kiyosawa, K., Akahane, Y., Nagata, A., et al.: Significance of blood transfusion in non-A, non-B chronic liver disease in Japan. Vox Sanguinis *43*:45–52, 1982.
117. Knodell, R. G., Conrad, M. E., Ginsberg, A. L., et al.: Efficacy of prophylactic gamma globulin in preventing non-A, non-B post-transfusion hepatitis. Lancet *1*:557–561, 1976.
118. Koff, R. S.: Management of the hepatitis B surface antigens (HBsAg) carrier. Semin. Liver Dis. *1*:33–43, 1981.
119. Koff, R. S., and Dienstag, J. L.: Extra hepatic manifestations of hepatitis C and the association with alcoholic liver disease. Semin. Liver Dis. *15*:101–109, 1995.
120. Koizumi, K., Enomoto, N., Kurosaki, M., et al.: Diversity of quasispecies in various disease stages of chronic hepatitis C virus infection and its significance in interferon treatment. Hepatology *22*:30–35, 1995.
121. Koretz, R. L., Abbey, H., Coleman, E., et al.: Non-A, non-B post-transfusion hepatitis: Looking back in the second decade. Ann. Intern. Med. *119*:110–115, 1993.
122. Koretz, R. L., Suffin, S. C., and Gitnick, G.: Post-transfusion chronic liver disease. Gastroenterology *77*:797–803, 1976.
123. Koziel, M. J., Dudley, D., Wong, J. T., et al.: Intrahepatic cytotoxic T lymphocytes specific for hepatitis C virus in persons with chronic hepatitis. J. Immunol. *149*:3339–3344, 1992.
124. Krawczynski, K.: Hepatitis E. Hepatology *17*:932–941, 1993.
125. Krawczynski, K., Beach, M., Bradley, D. W., et al.: Immunosuppression and pathogenetic studies of acute hepatitis C virus (HCV) infection in chimpanzees. Hepatology *16*:131A, 1992.
126. Krugman, S., Giles, J. P., Hammond, J., et al.: Infectious hepatitis: Evidence for two distinctive clinical, epidemiological and immunological types of infection. J. A. M. A. *200*:365–373, 1967.
127. Krugman, S., Overby, L. R., Mushabwar, I. K., et al.: Viral hepatitis type B: Studies on natural history and prevention re-examined. N. Engl. J. Med. *300*:101–106, 1979.
128. Kuo, G., Choo, Q.-L., Alter, H. J., et al.: An assay for circulating antibodies to a major etiologic virus of human non-A, non-B hepatitis. Science *244*:362–264, 1989.
129. Kwo, P. Y., Balan, V. J., Carpenter, H. A., et al.: Acute hepatitis E acquired in the U.S. Hepatology *22*(Suppl.):182A, 1995.
130. Lai, C. L., Lin, H. J., Lau, J. N., et al.: Effect of recombinant alpha 2 interferon with or without prednisone in Chinese HBsAg carrier children. Q. J. Med. *78*:155–163, 1991.
131. Lampertico, P., Rumi, M., Romeo, A., et al.: A multicenter, randomized controlled trial of recombinant interferon-alpha 2b in patients with acute transfusion-associated hepatitis C. Hepatology *19*:19–22, 1994.
132. Lander, J. J., Holland, P. V., Alter, H. J., et al.: Antibody to hepatitis-associated antigen: Frequency and pattern of response as detected by radio immunoprecipitation. J. A. M. A. *200*:1079–1082, 1972.
133. Lau, J. Y. N., Davis, G. L., Kniffen, J., et al.: Significance of serum hepatitis C virus RNA levels in chronic hepatitis C. Lancet *341*:1501–1504, 1993.
134. LeBouvier, G. L.: The heterogenicity of Australia antigen. J. Infect. Dis. *123*:671, 1971.
135. Lee, W. M.: Drug-induced hepatotoxicity. N. Engl. J. Med. *333*:1118–1127, 1995.
136. Lerner, R. A., Green, P., Alexander, H. et al.: Chemically synthesized peptides predicted from the nucleotide sequence of the hepatitis B virus genome elicit antibodies reactive with the native envelope protein of Dane particles. Proc. Natl. Acad. Sci. U. S. A. *78*:3403–3407, 1981.
137. Levin, M. L., Maddrey, W. C., Wands, J. R., et al.: Hepatitis B transmission by dentists. J. A. M. A. *228*:1139–1140, 1974.
138. Lewis, T. L., Alter, H. J., Chalmers, T. C., et al.: A comparison of the frequency of hepatitis B antigen and antibody in hospital and non-hospital personnel. N. Engl. J. Med. *289*:647–651, 1973.

139. Linnemann, C. C., and Goldberg, S.: HBAg in breast milk. Lancet *2*:155, 1974.
140. London, W. T., Di Figlia, M., Sutnick, A. I., et al.: An epidemic of hepatitis in a chronic hemodialysis unit: Australia antigen and differences in host response. N. Engl. J. Med. *281*:571–578, 1969.
141. London, W. T., Sutnick, A. I., Blumberg, B. S., et al.: Australian antigen and acute viral hepatitis. Ann. Intern. Med. *70*:55–59, 1969.
142. Luerman, A.: Eine icterusepidemie. Berl. Klin. Wochenschr. *22*:20, 1885.
143. MacCallum, F. O., and Bauer, D. J.: Homologous serum jaundice: Transmission experiments with human volunteers. Lancet *1*:622, 1944.
144. MacCallum, F. O., and Bradley, W. H.: Transmission of infective hepatitis to human volunteers. Lancet *2*:228, 1944.
145. Magnius, L. O., and Espmark, J. A.: New specificities in Australia antigen positive sera distinct from the LeBouvier determinants. J. Immunol. *109*:1017–1021, 1972.
146. Magnius, L. O., Lindholm, A., Lundin, P., et al.: A new antigen-antibody system: Clinical significance in long-term carriers of hepatitis B surface antigen. J. A. M. A. *231*:356–359, 1975.
147. Maier, K., Gabriel, P., Koscielniak, E., et al.: Human gamma interferon production by cytotoxic T lymphocytes sensitized during hepatitis A virus infection. J. Virol. *62*:3756–3763, 1988.
148. Margolis, H. S.: Prevention of acute and chronic liver disease through immunization: Hepatitis B and beyond. J. Infect. Dis. *168*:9–14, 1993.
149. Mason, J. O., and McLean, W. R.: Infectious hepatitis traced to the consumption of raw oysters: An epidemiologic study. Am. J. Hyg. *75*:90, 1962.
150. Maynard, J. E., Lorenz, D., Bradley, D. W., et al.: Review of infectivity studies in non-human primates with virus-like particles associated with MS-1 hepatitis. Am. J. Med. Sci. *270*:81–85, 1975.
151. McMahon, B. J., Alward, W. L. M., Hall, D. B., et al.: Acute hepatitis B virus infection: Relation of age to the clinical expression of disease and subsequent development of the carrier state. J. Infect. Dis. *151*:599–603, 1985.
152. Mimms, L. T., Mosley, J. W., Hollinger, B., et al.: Effect of concurrent accute infection with hepatitis C virus on acute hepatitis B infection. BMJ *307*:1095–1097, 1993.
153. Moreno, M. R., Rua, M. J., Molina, J., et al: Prospective randomized controlled trial of interferon-alpha in children with chronic hepatitis B. Hepatology *13*:1035–1039, 1991.
154. Mosley, J. W.: Transmission of viral diseases by drinking water. *In* Berg, G. (ed.): Transmission of Viruses by the Water Route. New York, Interscience, 1965, p. 5.
155. Mosley, J. W., Redeker, A. G., Feinstone, S. M., et al.: Multiple hepatitis viruses in multiple attacks of acute viral hepatitis. N. Engl. J. Med. *296*:75–78, 1977.
156. Mosley, J. W., and White, E.: Viral hepatitis as an occupational hazard of the dentist. J. Am. Dent. Assoc. *90*:992–997, 1975.
157. Murphy, W. J., Petrie, L. M., Work, S. D., Jr., et al.: Outbreak of infectious hepatitis apparently milk-borne. Am. J. Public Health *36*:169, 1946.
158. Nakagiri, I., Ichihara, K., Ohmoto, K., et al.: Analysis of discordant test results from five second-generation assays for anti-hepatitis C virus antibodies also tested by polymerase chain reaction–RNA assay and other laboratory and clinical tests for hepatitis. J. Clin. Microbiol. *31*:2974–2980, 1993.
159. Nanda, S. K., Ansari, I. H., Acharya, S. K., et al.: Protracted viremia during acute sporadic hepatitis E virus infections. Gastroenterology *108*:225–230, 1995.
160. Neefe, J. R., Gellis, S. S., Stokes, J., et al.: Homologous serum hepatitis and infectious (epidemic) hepatitis: Studies in volunteers bearing on immunological and other characteristics of the etiological agents. Am. J. Med. *1*:3, 1946.
161. Nelson, K. E., Ahmed, F., Mess, P., et al.: The incidence of post-transfusion hepatitis. N. Engl. J. Med. *328*:1280–1281, 1993.
162. Nordenfelt, E., and Kjellen, L.: Dane particles, DNA polymerase, and e-antigen in two different categories of hepatitis B antigen carriers. Intervirology *5*:225–232, 1975.
163. Nowicki, M. J., and Balistreri, W. F.: Hepatitis C virus: Identification, epidemiology and clinical controversies. J. Pediatr. Gastroenterol. Nutr. *20*:248–274, 1995.
164. Ohto, H., Terazawa, S., Sasaki, N., et al.: Transmission of hepatitis C virus from mothers to infants. N. Engl. J. Med. *330*:744–750, 1994.
165. Okada, K., Kamiyama, I., Inomata, M., et al.: e-Antigen and anti-e in the serum of asymptomatic carrier mothers as indicators of positive and negative transmission of hepatitis B virus to their infants. N. Engl. J. Med. *294*:746–749, 1976.
166. Okamoto, H., Yotsumoto, Y., Akahane, Y., et al.: Hepatitis B viruses with pre-core region defects prevail in persistently infected hosts along with sero-conversion to the antibody against e antigen. J. Virol. *64*:1298–1303, 1990.
167. Okamoto, H., Imsi, M., Usuda, S., et al.: Hemagglutination assay of polypeptide coded by the pre-S region of hepatitis B virus with monoclonal antibody: Human serum albumin in serums containing hepatitis B antigens. J. Immunol. *134*:1212–1216, 1985.
168. Osler, W.: Principles and Practice of Medicine. New York, D. Appleton, 1892.
169. Pasek, M., Gotto, T., Gilbert, W., et al.: Hepatitis B virus genes and their expression in *E. coli*. Nature *282*:575–579, 1979.
170. Paul, D. A., Knigge, M. F., Ritter, A., et al.: Determination of hepatitis E virus seroprevalence by using recombinant fusion proteins and synthetic peptides. J. Infect. Dis. *169*:801–806, 1994.
171. Perrillo, R. P., Schiff, E. R., Davis, G. L., et al.: A randomized, controlled trial of interferon alpha-2b alone and after prednisone withdrawal after the treatment of chronic hepatitis B. N. Engl. J. Med. *323*:295–301, 1990.
172. Perspectives on the control of viral hepatitis, type B. M. M. W. R. *25*(Suppl.):3, 1976.
173. Pontisso, P., Morisa, G., Ruvoletto, M. G., et al.: Latent hepatitis B virus infection in childhood hepatocellular carcinoma. Cancer *69*:2731–2735, 1992.
174. Prince, A. M.: An antigen detected in the blood during the incubation period of serum hepatitis. Proc. Natl. Acad. Sci. U. S. A. *60*:814–821, 1968.
175. Prince, A. M., Brotman, B., Grady, G. F., et al.: Long-incubation post-transfusion hepatitis without serological evidence of exposure to hepatitis B virus. Lancet *2*:241–246, 1974.
176. Prince, A. M., Szmuness, W. F., Mann, M. K., et al.: Hepatitis B immune globulin: Final report of a controlled multicenter trial of efficacy in prevention of dialysis-associated hepatitis. J. Infect. Dis. *137*:131–144, 1978.
177. Prince, A. M., Szmuness, W., Woods, K. P., et al.: Antibody against serum-hepatitis antigen: Prevalence and protective use as immune serum globulin in prevention of serum-hepatitis infections. N. Engl. J. Med. *285*:933–938, 1971.
178. Provost, P. J., Conti, P. A., Giesa, P. A., et al.: Studies in chimpanzees of live, attenuated hepatitis A vaccine candidates. Proc. Soc. Exp. Biol. Med. *172*:357–363, 1983.
179. Provost, P. J., McAleer, W. J., and Hilleman, M. R.: In-vitro cultivation of hepatitis A virus. *In* Szmuness, W. J., Alter, H. J., and Maynard, J. E. (eds.): Viral Hepatitis, 1981 International Symposium. Philadelphia, Franklin Institute Press, 1982, p. 21.
180. Provost, P. J., Wolanski, B. S., Miller, W. J., et al.: Biophysical and biochemical properties of CR 326 human hepatitis A virus. Am. J. Med. Sci. *287*:87–92, 1975.
181. Purcell, R. H., and Gerin, J. L.: Hepatitis B subunit vaccine: A preliminary report of safety and efficacy tests in chimpanzees. Am. J. Med. Sci. *270*:395–399, 1975.
182. Rakela, J., Redeker, A. G., Edwards, V. M., et al.: Hepatitis A virus infection in fulminant hepatitis and chronic active hepatitis. Gastroenterology *74*:879–882, 1978.
183. Redeker, A. G.: Fulminant hepatitis. *In* Schaffner, F., Sherlock, S., and Leevy, C. (eds.): The Liver and Its Diseases. New York, Intercontinental Medical Book Corp., 1974, p. 149.
184. Redeker, A. G.: Chronic hepatitis. Med. Clin. North Am. *59*:863–867, 1975.
185. Redeker, A. G., Mosley, M. W., Gocke, D. J., et al.: Hepatitis B immune globulin as a prophylactic measure for spouses exposed to acute type B hepatitis. N. Engl. J. Med. *293*:1055–1059, 1975.
186. Repsher, L. H., and Freebern, R. K.: Effects of early and vigorous exercise on recovery from infectious hepatitis. N. Engl. J. Med. *281*:1393–1396, 1969.
187. Reyes, G. R., Purdy, M. A., Kim, J. P., et al.: Isolation of cDNA from the virus responsible for enterically transmitted non-A, non-B hepatitis. Science *247*:1335–1339, 1990.
188. Rizzetto, M.: The Delta agent. Hepatology *3*:729–737, 1983.
189. Rizzetto, M., Canese, M. G., Avico, S., et al.: Immunofluorescence detection of a new antigen/antibody system (delta/anti-delta) associated with hepatitis B virus in liver and serum of HBsAg carriers. Gut *18*:997–1003, 1977.
190. Robinson, W. S., and Lutwick, L.: The virus of hepatitis, type B. N. Engl. J. Med. *295*:1168–1175, 1976.
191. Ruiz-Moreno, M., Camps, T., and Aquado, J. G.: A serological and histological follow-up of chronic hepatitis B infection. Arch. Dis. Child. *64*:1165–1169, 1989.
192. Ruiz-Moreno, M., Rua, M. J., Castillo, I., et al.: Treatment of children with chronic hepatitis C with recombinant interferon-alpha: A pilot study. Hepatology *16*:882–885, 1992.
193. Saito, I., Miyamura, T., Ohbayashi, A., et al.: Hepatitis C virus infection is associated with the development of hepatocellular carcinoma. Proc. Natl. Acad. Sci. U. S. A. *87*:6547–6549, 1990.
194. Salen, G., Goldstein, F., Haurani, F., et al.: Acute hemolytic anemia complicating viral hepatitis in patients with glucose-6-phosphate dehydrogenase deficiency. Ann. Intern. Med. *65*:1210–1220, 1966.
195. Sameral, D., Muller, R., Alexander, G., et al.: Liver transplantation in European patients with hepatitis B surface antigen. N. Engl. J. Med. *329*:1842–1847, 1993.
196. Sanchez-Tapias, J. M., Barrera, J., Costa, J., et al.: Hepatitis C virus infection in patients with non-alcoholic chronic liver disease. Ann. Intern. Med. *112*:921–924, 1990.
197. Sartwell, P. E.: Infectious hepatitis in relation to blood transfusion. Bull. U.S. Army Med. Dept. *7*:90, 1947.
198. Sato, S., Suzuki, K., Akahene, Y. et al.: Hepatitis B virus strains with mutations in the core promoter in patients with fulminant hepatitis. Ann. Intern. Med. *122*:241–248, 1995.
199. Schaluder, G. C., Dawson, G. J., Simons, J. N., et al.: Molecular and

serologic analysis in the transmission of the GB hepatitis agents. J. Med. Virol. *46*:81–90, 1995.
200. Schweitzer, I. L.: Vertical transmission of the hepatitis B surface antigen. Am. J. Med. Sci. *270*:287–291, 1975.
201. Seeff, L. B., Buskell-Bales, Z., Wright, E. C., et al.: Long-term mortality after transfusion-associated non-A, non-B hepatitis. N. Engl. J. Med. *327*:1906–1911, 1992.
202. Seeff, L. B., and Hoofnagle, J. H.: Immunoprophylaxis of viral hepatitis. Gastroenterology *77*:161–182, 1979.
203. Seeff, L. B., Wright, E. C., Zimmerman, H. J., et al.: Type B hepatitis after needle stick exposure: Prevention with hepatitis B immune globulin: Final report of the Veterans Administration Cooperative Study. Ann. Intern. Med. *88*:285–293, 1978.
204. Seeff, L., Zimmerman, H. J., Wright, E. C., et al.: Hepatic disease in asymptomatic parenteral narcotic drug abusers: A Veterans Administration Collaborative Study. Am. J. Med. Sci. *270*:41–47, 1975.
205. Seto, E., Yen, T. S., Peterlin, B. M., et al.: Trans-activation of the human immunodeficiency virus long terminal repeat by the hepatitis B virus X protein. Proc. Natl. Acad. Sci. U. S. A. *85*:8286–8290, 1988.
206. Shafritz, D. A., Shouval, D., Sherman, H. I., et al.: Integration of hepatitis B virus DNA into the genome of liver cells in chronic liver disease and hepatocellular carcinoma: Studies in percutaneous liver biopsies and postmortem tissue specimens. N. Engl. J. Med. *305*:1067–1073, 1981.
207. Sherlock, S.: Predicting progression of acute type B hepatitis to chronicity. Lancet *2*:354–357, 1976.
208. Shindo, M., Arai, K., Sokawa, Y., et al.: Hepatic hepatitis C virus RNA as a predictor or a long-term response to interferon-alpha therapy. Ann. Intern. Med. *122*:586–591, 1995.
209. Siegl, G.: Structure and biology of hepatitis A virus. *In* Szmuness, W. J., Alter, H. J., and Maynard, J. E. (eds.): Viral Hepatitis, 1981 International Symposium. Philadelphia, Franklin Institute Press, 1982, p. 13.
210. Simmonds, P.: Variability of hepatitis C virus. Hepatology *21*:570–583, 1995.
211. Smith, J. L., Maynard, J. E., Berquist, K. R., et al.: Comparative risk of hepatitis B among physicians and dentists. J. Infect. Dis. *133*:705–706, 1976.
212. Sninsky, J. J., Siddiqui, A., Robinson, W. S., et al.: Cloning and endonuclease mapping of the hepatitis B viral genome. Nature *279*:346–348, 1979.
213. Stevens, C. E., Alter, H. J., Taylor, P. E., et al.: Hepatitis B vaccine in patients receiving hemodialysis: Immunogenicity and efficacy. N. Engl. J. Med. *311*:496–501, 1984.
214. Stevens, C. E., Beasley, R. P., Tsui, J., et al.: Vertical transmission of hepatitis B antigen in Taiwan. N. Engl. J. Med. *292*:771–774, 1975.
215. Stevens, C. E., Neurath, R. A. Beasley, R. P., et al.: HBeAg and anti-HBe detection by radioimmunoassay: Correlation with vertical transmission of hepatitis B virus in Taiwan. J. Med. Virol. *3*:237–241, 1979.
216. A comprehensive survey of the literature on adverse drug reactions up to January 1985. *In* Stricker, B. H. C., and Spoelstra, P. (eds.): Drug-Induced Hepatic Injury. New York, Elsevier Science Publishing, 1985, pp. 45–76.
217. Summers, J.: Three recently described animal virus models for human hepatitis B virus. Hepatology *1*:179–183, 1981.
218. Summers, J., and Mason, W. S.: Replication of a genome of a hepatitis B like virus by reverse transcription of an RNA intermediate. Cell *29*:403–415, 1982.
219. Szmuness, W., Dienstag, J. L., Purcell, R. H., et al.: Distribution of antibody to hepatitis A antigen in urban adult populations. N. Engl. J. Med. *295*:755–759, 1976.
220. Szmuness, W., Much, M. I., Prince, A. M., et al.: On the role of sexual behavior in the spread of hepatitis B infection. Ann. Intern. Med. *83*:489–495, 1975.
221. Szmuness, W., Prince, A. M., Brotman, B., et al.: Hepatitis B antigen and antibody in blood donors: An epidemiologic study. J. Infect. Dis. *127*:17–25, 1973.
222. Szmuness, W., Stevens, C. E., Oleszko, W. R., et al.: Passive-active immunization against hepatitis B immunogenicity studies in adult Americans. Lancet *1*:575–577, 1981.
223. Szmuness, W., Stevens, C. E., Zang, E. A., et al.: A controlled clinical trial of the efficacy of the hepatitis B vaccine (Heptavax B): A final report. Hepatology *1*:377–381, 1981.
224. Tabor, E., Gerety, R. J., Drucker, J. A., et al.: Transmission of non-A, non-B hepatitis from man to chimpanzees. Lancet *1*:463–466, 1978.
225. Takahashi, K., Akahane, Y., Gotanda, T., et al.: Demonstration of hepatitis B e antigen in the core of Dane particles. J. Immunol. *122*:275–279, 1979.
226. Tandon, B. N., Joshi, Y. K., Jain, S. K., et al.: An epidemic of non-A, non-B hepatitis in north India. Indian J. Med. Res. *75*:739–744, 1982.
227. Tateda, A., Kikuchi, K., Numazaki, Y., et al.: Non-B hepatitis in Japanese recipients of blood transfusion: Clinical and serologic studies after the introduction of laboratory screening of donor blood for hepatitis B surface antigen. J. Infect. Dis. *139*:511–518, 1979.
228. Thomas, H. C., Meron, J., and Waters, J.: Virus-host interaction in chronic hepatitis B infection. Semin. Liver Dis. *8*:342–349, 1988.
229. Thung, S. N., Gerber, M. A., and Popper, H.: Basic morphologic patterns of viral hepatitis A, B, non-A, non-B, and delta agent in animal and man. *In* Chisari, F. V. (ed.): Advances in Hepatitis Research. New York, Masson Publishers USA, 1984, p. 293.
230. Todo, S., Demetris, A. J., Van Thiel, D. H., et al.: Orthotopic liver transplantation for patients with hepatitis B virus-related liver disease. Hepatology *13*:619–626, 1991.
231. Tong, M. J., Sun, S. L., Schaeffer, B. T., et al.: Hepatitis associated antigen and hepatocellular carcinoma in Taiwan. Ann. Intern. Med. *75*:687–691, 1971.
232. Tony, M. J., Thursby, M., Rekata, J., et al.: Studies on the maternal-infant transmission of the viruses which cause anti-hepatitis. Gastroenterology *89*:160–164, 1985.
233. Trepo, C. G., Magnius, L. O., Schaefer, R. A., et al.: Detection of e antigen and antibody: Correlations with hepatitis B surface and hepatitis B core antigens, liver disease, and outcome in hepatitis B infections. Gastroenterology *71*:804–808, 1976.
234. Trey, C., and Davidson, C: The management of fulminant hepatitis failure. *In* Popper, H., and Schaffner, F. (eds.): Progress in Liver Disease. New York, Grune & Stratton, 1970, p. 282.
235. Tsubota, A., Chayama, K., Ikeda, K., et al.: Factors predictive of response to interferon-alpha therapy in hepatitis C virus infection. Hepatology *19*:1088–1094, 1994.
236. Ulmer, J. B., Donnely, J. J., Parker, S. E., et al.: Heterologous protection against influenza by injection of DNA encoding viral protein. Science *259*:1745–1749, 1993.
237. Vallbracht, A., Maier, K., Stierhof, Y. D., et al.: Liver-derived cytotoxic T cells in hepatitis A virus infection. J. Infect. Dis. *160*:209–217, 1989.
238. Van Thiel, D. H., Wright, H. I., and Fagiuoli, S.: Liver transplantation for hepatitis B virus–associated cirrhosis: A progress report. Hepatology *20*:20s–23s, 1994.
239. Viladomi, L., Genesca, J., Estaban, J. I., et al: Interferon-alpha in acute post-transfusion hepatitis C: A randomized controlled trial. Hepatology *15*:767–769, 1992.
240. Villarejos, V. M., Visona, K. A., Gutierrez, A., et al.: Role of saliva, urine and feces in the transmission of type B hepatitis. N. Engl. J. Med. *291*:1375–1378, 1974.
241. Viola, L. A., Barrison, I. G., Coleman, J. C., et al.: Natural history of liver disease in chronic hepatitis B surface antigen carriers: Survey of 100 patients from Great Britain. Lancet *2*:1156–1159, 1981.
242. Virchow, R.: Über das vorkommen und den nachweis des hapatogenen insbesondere des katarrhabischen icterus. Virchows Arch. [Pathol. Anat.] *32*:117, 1865.
243. Wands, J. R., Mann, E., Alpert, E., et al.: The pathogenesis of arthritis associated with acute hepatitis B surface antigen-positive hepatitis: Complement activation and characterization of circulating immune complexes. J. Clin. Invest. *55*:930–936, 1975.
244. Wands, J. R., Walter, J. A., Davis, T. T., et al.: Hepatitis B in an oncology unit. N. Engl. J. Med. *291*:1371–1375, 1974.
245. Wang, K. S., Choo, Q.-L., Weiner, A. J., et al.: Structure, sequence and expression of the hepatitis delta(s) viral genome. Nature *323*:508–514, 1986.
246. Weimer, T., Salfield, J., and Will, H.: Expression of the hepatitis B virus core gene in vitro and in vivo. J. Virol. *61*:3109–3113, 1987.
247. Weiner, A. J., Kuo, G., Bradley, D. W., et al.: Detection of hepatitis C viral sequences in non-A, non-B hepatitis. Lancet *335*:1–3, 1990.
248. Werzberger, A., Mensch B., Kuter, B., et al: A controlled trial of formalin inactivated hepatitis A vaccine in healthy children. N. Engl. J. Med. *327*:453–457, 1992.
249. Williams, R., and Wendon, J.: Indications for orthotic liver transplantation in fulminant liver failure. Hepatology *20*:55–105, 1994.
250. Wong, D. C., Purcell, R. H., Sreenivasan, M. A., et al.: Epidemic and endemic hepatitis in India: Evidence for non-A, non-B hepatitis virus etiology. Lancet *2*:876–879, 1980.
251. Wong, V. C. W., Ip, H. M. H., Reesink, H. W., et al.: Prevention of the HBsAg carrier status in newborn infants in mothers who are chronic carriers of HBsAg and HBeAg by administration of hepatitis B vaccine and hepatitis B immune globulin: Double-blind randomized placebo-controlled study. Lancet *1*:921–926, 1984.
252. Wright, T. L., Donegan, E., Hsu, H. H., et al.: Recurrent and acquired hepatitis C viral infection in liver transplant recipients. Gastroenterology *103*:317–322, 1992.
253. Wright, T. L., Hsu, H., Donegan, E., et al.: Hepatitis C virus not found in fulminant non-A, non-B hepatitis. Ann. Intern. Med. *115*:111–112, 1991.
254. Wu, J. C., Choo, J. B., Chen, T. Z., et al.: Genotyping of hepatitis D virus by restriction-fragment length polymorphism and relation to outcome of hepatitis D. Lancet *346*:939–941, 1995.
255. Zeldis, J. B., Dienstag, J. L., and Gale, R. P.: Aplastic anemia and non-A, non-B hepatitis. Am. J. Med. *74*:64–68, 1983.
256. Zimmerman, H. J.: Update of hepatoxicity from drugs in common use: Nonsteroidal drugs, anti-inflammatory drugs, antibiotics, anti-hypertensives and cardiac and psychotropic agents. Semin. Liver Dis. *10*:322–338, 1990.
257. Zuckerman, A. J.: The new GB hepatitis viruses. Lancet *345*:1453–1454, 1995.
258. Zuckerman, G. R., Hacker, E. J., and Aach, R. D.: Epidemiological-clinical correlates of hepatitis B antigen subtypes. Gastroenterology *66*:408–414, 1974.

56

Viral Hepatitis Due to Viruses Other than Hepatitis Viruses A–E

Sandy T. Hwang and George D. Ferry

Hepatitis is a feature of many viral illnesses, but the clinical manifestations of liver injury vary widely, depending on the agent, patient age, or associated conditions. Liver involvement may be of no clinical significance with only minor enzyme elevations, or hepatitis may be a prominent manifestation of the illness, such as in yellow fever. In neonates, viral infections such as herpes simplex virus (HSV) infection, coxsackievirus infection, echovirus infection, cytomegalovirus (CMV) infection, and rubella virus infection may lead to serious hepatic involvement along with the generalized viral illness. Many viral infections take on a much greater clinical signficance in the presence of immunosuppression after transplantation.

CYTOMEGALOVIRUS

Infection with CMV is most common in neonates, adolescents, and the immunocompromised host. Many infections go unrecognized, but antibodies to CMV gradually increase with age. Five to 10 per cent of children have CMV antibodies by 2 years of age. This rises to 50 to 80 per cent by 30 years of age.[94, 105]

Neonatal infection with CMV presents as neonatal hepatitis in one-third of cases, with jaundice beginning in the first few days of life and progressing to an obstructive picture with elevated direct-reacting bilirubin.[105] The clinical and laboratory findings often are suggestive of biliary atresia, but needle liver biopsy will show neonatal hepatitis. CMV inclusions may be seen in both hepatocytes and biliary epithelium.[27] Patients with significant hepatitis may have no other manifestation of infection, or they may have the full-blown pattern of thrombocytopenia, bleeding, anemia, hepatosplenomegaly, and central nervous system damage with calcification and microcephaly. The course of CMV hepatitis is one of gradual resolution of inflammation, and most cases resolve without cirrhosis.[11, 69]

In young children, asymptomatic CMV infection may lead to hepatosplenomegaly and elevations of aminotransferases.[39, 93] There is no evidence that chronic liver disease develops in these children after CMV infection, but there is one report of a 4-year-old who presented with fever, jaundice, and fatal CMV hepatitis and two other young children with prolonged elevated aminotransferases after recovery from acute CMV infection.[84]

CMV infection in adolescents and young adults may be asymptomatic with only aminotransferase elevation or present with a generalized infection with fever, fatigue, malaise, jaundice, splenomegaly, and lymphocytosis.[44, 59] Fever often lasts 2 to 4 weeks. Most cases have elevated liver enzymes, but the hepatitis is subclinical.[43, 44] Peak aminotransferase levels occur during the second week of illness in patients with CMV mononucleosis.[43] Occasional patients develop significant cholestatic jaundice with pruritus; jaundice in these cases can last for 20 to 40 days.[59, 95]

Diagnosis of CMV hepatitis often is based on elevated IgM antibodies, a fourfold rise in IgG antibodies in paired sera, and negative tests for Epstein-Barr virus (EBV) infection and hepatitis A, B, and C. Viral isolation from urine and/or saliva often is used in conjunction with serology. The serum IgM level in neonates is not a reliable indicator of the presence of disease,[40] and up to 1 per cent of neonates are asymptomatic excretors.[105] Persistence of fever and atypical lymphocytes is suggestive of CMV infection.[116] Liver biopsy may be suggestive, but inconclusive, of CMV hepatitis. Indirect immunofluorescence with specific monoclonal antibodies can confirm the diagnosis.[65, 95]

Treatment of nonimmunocompromised patients is supportive. There is a case report of successful treatment of congenital CMV hepatitis with resolution of hepatomegaly and ascites and improved aminotransferases with a 21-day course of ganciclovir.[108]

EPSTEIN-BARR VIRUS

A ubiquitous agent, EBV infects approximately 80 per cent of individuals by adulthood.[66] Primarily asymptomatic in young children, EBV infection causes a wide spectrum of disease in older children and adults and may cause significant liver injury.

The classic presentation of EBV infection is infectious mononucleosis with fever, rash, tonsillopharyngitis, lymphadenopathy, and hepatosplenomegaly. Subclinical hepatitis is a common finding, with elevated aminotransferases reported in 70 to 90 per cent of patients.[43, 111] Jaundice is uncommon.[43, 66, 111] Aminotransferases usually are mild to moderately elevated during the course of acute symptoms and normalize within weeks to 3 months.[43, 84, 105, 111] Liver biopsy rarely is indicated, but histologic findings include lymphocytic portal infiltration, hepatocellular ballooning and mitosis, and mild cholestasis.[66] Chronic liver disease and liver failure are rare complications. There have been case reports of acute hepatic failure in previous healthy pediatric patients with EBV infection,[19, 20, 114] but immunodeficiency may be a factor in severity of disease. Sainsbury and associates[96] reported a case of a 17-year-old immunosuppressed male with acute hepatic failure that resolved 3 weeks after the onset of symptoms. Shaw and Evans[99] reported the discovery of C4 deficiency in an otherwise healthy 5-year-old who developed fulminant hepatic failure secondary to primary EBV infection.

Sporadic fatal infectious mononucleosis, a rare but distinct diagnosis, affects 1 in 3000 cases of EBV mononucleosis.[66] Patients present with significant lymphadenopathy, splenomegaly, and other typical symptoms of mononucleosis. The median age of patients is 10 to 11 years. The median survival time is 4 to 8 weeks, with the usual cause of death being fulminant hepatic failure.[63, 66] Hepatomegaly and jaundice usually are present.[63] Histologic features are portal infiltration with atypical lymphocytes, immunoblasts, and plasma cells with periportal necrosis.[63, 66] Iijima and colleagues[48] suggested that the mechanism of liver injury is abnormal killing activity of T cells and natural-killer cells. There was no evidence that EBV directly infects hepatocytes.

Severe or fatal infectious mononucleosis with hepatitis and liver failure as prominent features also is seen in patients with X-linked lymphoproliferative syndrome after a primary EBV infection.[63, 66] Patients have a defect in mounting a T-cell response to EBV-induced lymphoproliferation.[66] All patients are male and tend to acquire EBV infection early in life (median age, 2.4 years).[97] Clinical presentation and histologic findings are similar to those in sporadic fatal infectious mononucleosis. Approximately 60 per cent die of hepatic failure.[63] Treatment with antiviral agents, immunosuppression, interferon, and immunoglobulin has not proved to be beneficial.[97]

Diagnosis of EBV infection usually is made serologically. In acute primary infection, the presence of IgM to viral capsid antigen is sufficient. The lack of antibodies to nuclear antigen and the presence of antibodies to the early antigen support the diagnosis of primary infection.[110] Heterophil antibodies often are used to document EBV infection, but they tend to be negative in young children with infectious mononucleosis.[66] In atypical or severe infections, tissue detection of EBV DNA can be made by Southern blot hybridization, in situ hybridization, or polymerase chain reaction.[66]

Treatment of infectious mononucleosis is supportive. Studies have shown that both parenteral and peroral acyclovir inhibit oropharyngeal virus shedding during administration, but there is no significant improvement in clinical symptoms or in aminotransferase elevation.[2, 118]

VARICELLA-ZOSTER VIRUS

Elevated aminotransferases are common in uncomplicated varicella infections,[91] with persistent vomiting as the most common symptom leading to a diagnosis of hepatitis.[28] Because liver biopsies rarely are available in mild cases, whether enzyme elevations represent the mildest and early stage of Reye syndrome or mild focal hepatitis is unclear.[25]

Certainly, varicella-zoster virus may disseminate widely in immunocompromised hosts. In a review of varicella infections in immunocompromised children, 50 per cent had disseminated disease. All had hepatitis associated with fever, rash, and pneumonitis.[82] The more severe group had a typical sequence of events beginning with fever, rash, and abdominal pain followed by the elevation of aminotransferases. Autopsies in children who received chemotherapy for cancer have shown varying degrees of liver involvement from mild to severe. Lesions include large hemorrhagic, necrotic areas and eosinophilic intranuclear inclusions in peripheral hepatocytes scattered throughout the liver.[73] In immunocompromised hosts, early treatment is essential. Immunoglobulin should be given at the time of exposure, and intravenous acyclovir should be started within 2 days of the onset of the rash.[5]

HERPES SIMPLEX VIRUS

Immunocompromised individuals are more susceptible to hepatitis due to HSV, but normal individuals have been reported with herpes hepatitis.[21, 35, 126] Newborns and pregnant women also are more susceptible to infection.[103, 121] HSV-1 and HSV-2 are equally infectious.[18]

Neonatal HSV hepatitis generally is a part of disseminated infection, and 50 to 60 per cent of patients die of the infection in spite of administration of acyclovir or vidarabine.[122] Patients present with fever, lethargy, respiratory distress, central nervous system symptoms, hemorrhage, and fulminant hepatic failure.[10, 74] Hepatomegaly with or without jaundice is seen in 80 per cent of neonates with fatal HSV infection.[74] The course is rapidly progressive, and the majority die within the first 8 days of illness.[74]

Immunocompromised patients usually have HSV hepatitis associated with disseminated disease. Fever, respiratory symptoms, abdominal pain and tenderness, moderately elevated aminotransferases, an increase in band form neutrophils in the blood, and thrombocytopenia commonly are seen.[50, 54] The course usually is rapid, and the diagnosis is made at postmortem or within 48 hours before death.[54] Hypotension, metabolic acidosis, gastrointestinal hemorrhage, and coagulopathy are correlated with a poor prognosis.[54]

The diagnosis of herpes can be confirmed by cultures of vesicles, the oropharynx, conjunctivae, urine, and stool. Liver biopsy shows overwhelming necrosis with numerous intranuclear inclusions; positive immunoperoxidase staining and in situ hybridization can make an earlier diagnosis.[10, 117] Treatment with intravenous acyclovir, 30 mg/kg/day, leads to recovery in 40 to 60 per cent of patients.[117, 122]

ADENOVIRUSES

Hepatitis secondary to adenoviral infection is seen commonly in immunocompromised patients,[41, 100, 120, 124] neonates with systemic illness, and young children with disseminated disease.[85] Patients usually have high fever, malaise, cough, tachypnea, vomiting, diarrhea, and hepatomegaly.[85, 124] Infection can progress to fulminant liver failure and death. Serum aminotransferases and bilirubin levels are elevated moderately.[41, 100, 120, 124] Liver biopsies show random circumscribed lesions of monocytes and neutrophils with necrosis or confluent hepatocellular necrosis and intranuclear target inclusions.[16, 52, 124] Diagnosis is based on viral isolation from blood, urine, sputum, stool, and tissue; a fourfold rise in complement fixation antibodies or the demonstration of IgM antibody by enzyme-linked immunosorbent assay; and histology. Immunostaining with antiviral monoclonal antibody or the presence of viral particles seen on electron microscopy of liver tissue can make an early diagnosis.[16, 52] There is a high fatality rate in immunocompromised patients.[100, 124] Treatment is supportive.

PARAMYXOVIRUSES

Of all the paramyxoviruses, the measles virus is associated most often with hepatic involvement. This usually is subclinical and transient, evidenced by elevated aminotransferases during the exanthematous phase of the disease. Hepatomegaly and jaundice are uncommon findings.[31, 34, 83, 98, 101] Patients present with typical symptoms of measles—fever, cough, coryza, conjunctivitis, and a diffuse maculopapular rash. The reported incidence of hepatic involvement in adolescents and young adults varies between 30 and 80 per cent.[31, 34, 36, 83, 98] One study revealed that 16.3 per cent of pediatric patients had abnormal aminotransferases during a measles outbreak.[61]

Diagnosis of measles is made according to clinical symptoms, physical findings, and a fourfold rise in hemagglutination-inhibition antibody titer to measles virus or the demonstration of measles IgM antibody by enzyme-linked immunosorbent assay or immunofluorescence. Liver biopsy rarely is indicated. Percutaneous liver biopsy in three adults during the peak of enzyme elevation revealed nonspecific findings of minimal nuclear vacuolization and sinusoidal inflammation. Viral particles were not detected, and antimeasles antibody staining was negative, suggesting an immunologic as opposed to a direct viral insult.[75]

Prognosis is good, with normalization of aminotransferases in most cases by 2 weeks to 3 months.[31, 61, 83, 98, 101] One report described 10 patients with severe giant-cell hepatitis characterized by chronic active hepatitis or subclinical liver failure, leading to death or liver transplantation. Biopsies revealed syncytial giant cells and intracytoplasmic particles that resemble paramyxovirus nucleocapsids.[90] This may represent a subset of patients with measles or other paramyxoviral hepatitis with poor prognosis.

ENTEROVIRUSES (COXSACKIEVIRUSES/ECHOVIRUSES)

Enteroviral infections occur in all age groups, but the incidence is increased in infants, especially during the neonatal period. There is seasonal variation, with occurrences primarily between June and November, and affected neonates usually have a history of recent maternal illness prior to delivery.[55, 81] In general, neonates tend to have a more severe illness than do older children and adults. A review of 338 infants with nonpolio enteroviral infections showed that 74 per cent had "severe" disease characterized by aseptic meningitis/encephalitis, sepsis, carditis, and hepatitis.[81] Infection is acquired through vertical transmission during delivery or close human contact. Diagnosis is made by viral isolation from blood, urine, cerebrospinal fluid, stool, and tissue and confirmed by demonstrating antibody titer rise to the specific virus.

Significant liver involvement with hemorrhagic centrilobular necrosis without significant inflammation has been reported in fatal coxsackievirus B infections of neonates. Jaundice, increased aminotransferases, and hepatomegaly were common. Extensive liver dysfunction usually is seen in the setting of systemic illness manifested by high fevers, respiratory symptoms, carditis, meningoencephalitis, and disseminated intravascular coagulation with hemorrhage.[45, 123] In contrast to the neonate, only transient elevation of aminotransferases is seen during the first week of coxsackievirus B myocarditis in older children and adults.[117a]

A severe form of systemic echoviral infection in neonates is associated with massive centrilobular hepatic necrosis as well. Patients are characterized by jaundice, prolonged bleeding, moderately elevated aminotransferases, and high mortality.[76, 77] A review of 61 neonatal echoviral illnesses revealed that 70 per cent of cases were due to serotype 11 and that 68 per cent of all cases met criteria for severe hepatitis—aminotransferase levels at least three times normal, prothrombin time at least two times normal, and/or hepatic necrosis seen post mortem. This syndrome was associated with symptoms within the first week of life and a mortality of 83 per cent.[77] Other serotypes associated with hepatitis are 6, 7, 9, 14, 17, and 19.[47, 77] Multiple case reports of disseminated echovirus 11 infection show hepatic necrosis on pathology.[17, 77, 78, 92] As opposed to neonatal illness, fatal echoviral infections in older children appear to involve primarily the respiratory tract with no evidence of significant liver injury.[12]

Therapy primarily is supportive. One case report described the use of 1 g/kg intravenous immunoglobulin in a 6-day-old neonate with severe echovirus 11 infection and hepatitis. The patient had a good outcome with normalization of aminotransferases.[51] There also is one case report of a successful orthotopic liver transplantation in a 13-day-old with echovirus 11 hepatic necrosis.[17]

PARVOVIRUS B19

Human parvovirus B19 is a viral agent that produces a spectrum of illness including erythema infectiosum, hydrops fetalis, arthritis, and aplastic anemia.[115] Although the incidence is more common in children between the ages of 5 and 14 years, parvoviral infections are seen in infants and adults as well. Transmission usually is through respiratory droplets or transplacental infection, and infections occur in the winter and spring months.[115]

There are reported cases of intrauterine infection with resultant hydrops fetalis and hepatic involvement.[1, 71] Pathologic findings of two aborted fetuses with nonimmune hydrops and evidence of midtrimester infection were significant for hepatocellular necrosis, ballooning and degeneration of nuclei, excessive iron deposition, and significant hematopoeisis with eosinophilic nuclear changes.[1] Another hydropic neonate who died at 4 days of age had liver pathology revealing bile duct proliferation, cholestasis, and periportal fibrosis. Increased hematopoiesis also was seen, and the authors suggest that hepatic damage may be secondary to direct viral effects as well as the cytotoxic effects of excessive iron.[71] The diagnosis can be made by evidence of maternal seroconversion during pregnancy with the development of virus-specific IgM and IgG and the presence of virus-specific IgM and IgG in patient serum. Treatment is supportive.

Langnas and associates[56] reported that parvovirus B19 may be an etiology of non-A, non-B, non-C fulminant liver failure, especially if there is associated aplastic anemia. The presence of serum antiparvovirus B19 IgG was noted and viral DNA in liver tissue was detected by polymerase chain reaction in four of six patients with fulminant liver failure and aplastic anemia. Massive hepatic necrosis without evidence of inflammation or viral inclusions was seen on biopsies of these patients. All eventually underwent liver transplantation.

RUBELLA VIRUS

Prior to the advent of its vaccine, rubella virus infection was a common illness in children between 5 and 9 years of age.[30] Symptoms include low-grade fever, malaise, cough, conjunctivitis, and rash. Lymphadenopathy, especially in the postauricular, suboccipital, and cervical regions, usually is present. One study reported a 12 per cent incidence of subclinical hepatitis in pediatric patients during a rubella epidemic.[109] Enzyme levels peaked 3 to 10 days after the appearance of the rash and normalized within a month. Alkaline phosphatase, gamma-glutamyltransferase, and bilirubin levels were normal.[109]

Liver involvement more commonly is known to be associated with congenital rubella. Hepatomegaly and jaundice begin within the first few days of life.[53, 80, 107] Patients have elevated aminotransferases and direct hyperbilirubinemia. These findings accompany the other signs of multisystem involvement—intrauterine growth retardation, cataracts, congenital heart defects, thrombocytopenia, purpura, and deafness.[24, 53, 80, 107] Liver biopsies have shown mild periportal inflammation and cholestasis, a typical picture consistent with neonatal giant cell hepatitis with multinucleated giant cells, and mild interlobular fibrosis.[24, 80, 107] The course either can be transient with eventual normalization of liver values or can become chronic with cholestasis.[53, 80]

The diagnosis of rubella can be made serologically by the

presence of virus-specific IgM or a fourfold rise in antibody titer. A definitive diagnosis can be confirmed by the isolation of rubella virus in the urine, cerebrospinal fluid, or nasopharyngeal washings.[30] Treatment is supportive.

HEMORRHAGIC FEVER VIRUSES

Viral hemorrhagic fevers are a group of diseases caused by twelve distinct RNA viruses from four different families (Table 56–1). These hepatotropic viruses cause zoonotic infections in persons of all ages.[60] Person-to-person transmission and contact with infected animals also are important ways to acquire them.[32, 33, 60, 62]

The different diseases share many clinical manifestations. Patients usually experience a combination of the following symptoms: fever, malaise, headache, retro-orbital pain, myalgia, conjunctivitis, rash, and hemorrhage.[13, 29, 32, 33, 49, 62] Hepatitis is common during the acute phase of the illness.[13, 23, 29, 32, 33, 49, 62, 125] Moderately elevated aminotransferases (usually <500 U/L) are a consistent finding with liver involvement.[23, 32, 33, 119, 125] However, there are reports of levels reaching several thousand in severe cases.[33, 67] Levels normalize in patients who survive the acute illness.[23, 33] Jaundice is rare[9, 23, 33, 49, 67] but when seen is suggestive of severe yellow fever.[49]

Findings on liver biopsy are similar among the different viruses. There is evidence of hepatocellular acidophilic necrosis primarily in the midzonal distribution, presence of Councilman bodies, hepatocellular mitoses, insignificant inflammation, and varying amounts of steatosis.[9, 13, 23, 49, 67, 119] Cholestasis and cirrhosis typically are not present.[9, 49]

History of travel to an endemic region (especially rural areas), contact with sick animals, history of an arthropod bite, or the presence of typical symptoms should lead the clinician to suspect the diagnosis.[32] Diagnosis can be made by viral isolation from the blood and/or a greater than fourfold rise in virus-specific antibodies.[9, 32, 49]

Treatment is supportive. Ribavirin has been evaluated in animal and human studies.[46] There appears to be a benefit to the use of ribavirin in Lassa fever and hemorrhagic fever with renal syndrome. Intravenous ribavirin given to patients with Lassa fever has been shown to improve the case-fatality rate significantly, especially if it is given within 6 days of illness onset.[68]

HUMAN HERPESVIRUS 6

Human herpesvirus 6 infection commonly results in exanthem subitum in infants and young children or in an acute febrile illness without a rash.[37] There have been several case reports of liver involvement in neonates,[70] infants,[3, 112, 113] and adults[22, 102, 104] with primary human herpesvirus 6 infection. Patients can have transiently elevated aminotransferases during the acute phase of illness, presenting usually with fever, vomiting, anorexia, rash, or a mononucleosis-like illness.[22, 102, 104] A few patients have developed fulminant hepatic failure resulting in either full recovery or death.[3, 70] Diagnosis of primary infection can be made by isolation of virus in blood with confirmation by immunofluorescence, electron microscopy, or polymerase chain reaction; the presence of virus-specific IgM; or evidence of seroconversion.[3, 22, 37, 70, 102, 104] Treatment is supportive. Chronic liver disease with elevated aminotransferases has been reported in a 6-month-old infant; a trial of interferon-α given subcutaneously daily resulted in improved enzyme levels 1 month later.[113]

VIRAL HEPATITIS AFTER LIVER TRANSPLANTATION

Opportunistic viral infections are an important cause of morbidity and mortality in patients with solid organ transplants and chronic immunosuppression. Table 56–2 provides the relative frequency of the common causes of viral hepatitis in liver transplant patients.[65]

CYTOMEGALOVIRUS. CMV hepatitis is one of the most common infections in liver transplant recipients[87] and is seen

TABLE 56–1. The Hemorrhagic Fever (HF) Viruses, Their Distribution, and Their Principal Mode of Transmission

Family, Virus	Disease	Distribution	Means of Transmission
Arenaviridae			
Lassa	Lassa fever	West Africa	Rodent
Junin	Argentine HF	Argentina	Rodent
Machupo	Bolivian HF	Bolivia	Rodent
Bunyaviridae			
Rift Valley fever	Rift Valley fever	Sub-Saharan Africa	Mosquito
Crimean-Congo HF	Crimean-Congo HF	Africa, Asia, southern former Soviet Union	Tick
Hantaan and related viruses	HF with renal syndrome	Asia, Balkans, former Soviet Union, Europe	Rodent
Filoviridae			
Marburg	Marburg HF	Sub-Saharan Africa	Unknown
Ebola	Ebola HF	Sub-Saharan Africa	Unknown
Flaviviridae			
Yellow fever	Yellow fever	Tropical Americas, sub-Saharan Africa	Mosquito
Dengue	Dengue fever, dengue HF, dengue shock syndrome	Asia, Africa, Pacific, Americas	Mosquito
Kyasanur Forest disease	Kyasanur Forest disease	India	Tick
Omsk	Omsk HF	Former Soviet Union	Tick

From LeDuc, J. W.: Epidemiology of hemorrhagic fever viruses. Rev. Infect. Dis. *11*(Suppl. 4):730–735, 1989. University of Chicago, publisher.

TABLE 56–2. Spectrum of Opportunistic Viral Hepatitis in Liver Transplant Recipients

	No. of Cases	Mean Time after Transplant (days)	Mean Time after OKT3 (days)
Cytomegalovirus hepatitis			
Primary	11	7.1	26.4
Reactivation or reinfection	40	46.8	26.4
Epstein-Barr virus hepatitis	6	59.6	15.2
Herpes simplex virus hepatitis	3	14.7	5.5
Adenoviral hepatitis	2	34.5	
Total	62		

From Markin, R. S., Langnas, A. N., Donovan, J. P., et al.: Opportunistic viral hepatitis in liver transplant recipients. Transplant. Proc. *23*:1520–1521, 1991. Reprinted by permission of Appleton & Lange, Inc.

frequently on biopsy specimens obtained to rule out allograft rejection. Regardless of the status of the recipient, 19 to 23 per cent receiving a seropositive graft will develop CMV liver involvement.[6, 8, 88] If the donor is seronegative for CMV, the percentage drops to 5.

Symptoms often are compatible with either hepatitis or rejection and include fever (85 per cent), myalgia, and arthralgia (30 per cent).[88] Gamma-glutamyltransferase often is increased significantly, while aminotransferases, bilirubin, and alkaline phosphatase are elevated moderately.[88] A small per cent of patients have leukopenia and thrombocytopenia.[15] A combination of rejection and CMV hepatitis is seen in 14 to 25 per cent of cases.[15, 88] The majority of infections occur after repeat transplantation or heavy immunosuppression with repeat corticosteroid bolus therapy, the use of OKT3, or azathioprine.[15] Primary infection is followed by persistent latent infection, and reactivation and primary infection post transplantation occur with equal frequency. CMV hepatitis occurs most often within 1 month after heavy immunosuppression.[65]

Immunostaining of liver biopsy tissue with monoclonal antibody to early CMV antigen is the most sensitive technique for diagnosis.[8, 89] This immunoperoxidase stain often is positive before typical inclusions are seen. Polymerase chain reaction detection of CMV DNA also is a good technique.[7] Viral isolation from liver biopsy is good, but the technique takes too long to be useful clinically in deciding on treatment or on differentiation from acute rejection.[8] The typical pathology involves lobules and the biliary tree. Parenchymal inflammation with clusters of neutrophils is typical,[8, 65] but cholangitis also is common.

Treatment initially was to lower the dose of immunosuppression. Trials using intravenous ganciclovir at 7.5 to 10 mg/kg/day have shown good results, with decreased viremia and resolution of hepatitis.[86, 106] Immunoglobulin is recommended for rapidly progressive disease.[106] Prophylactic oral acyclovir up to 3200 mg/day for 3 months has been used.[79] Intravenous ganciclovir, 10 mg/kg/day for 2 weeks, followed by oral acyclovir, appears to be more efficacious in preventing or delaying infection.[66a]

EPSTEIN-BARR VIRUS. In several large series, EBV hepatitis has been found to occur in 2 per cent of patients after orthotopic liver transplantation.[57, 58, 65] Infection may be primary or from reactivation; pediatric patients tend to have more primary infections.[58, 65] Breinig and colleagues[14] found that about 50 per cent of pediatric recipients are seronegative for EBV prior to surgery. Patients usually develop infection within 2 months after transplantation,[14, 58, 65] and infection usually is related to a recent course of OKT3.[58, 65] Clinically, patients may present with elevated aminotransferases and/or fever of unclear etiology.[58] EBV hepatitis also is suspected if a patient originally diagnosed with allograft rejection does not improve with the usual therapy.[58, 64] Serologic evidence of either primary infection or reactivation by a fourfold rise in viral capsid antibody coupled with histologic findings is used to make the diagnosis.[14, 57, 58] Histologic findings include portal infiltration with immunoblasts, lymphocytes, and plasma cells. Helpful features are the loss of eosinophils during the transition from rejection to infection and the lack of bile duct damage.[58] The application of EBV nuclear antigen staining and polymerase chain reaction to liver tissue can help make a diagnosis quickly.[14, 57, 58] A subset of patients may have evidence of posttransplantation lymphoproliferative disorder, which necessitates more aggressive therapy due to the risk of progression to malignancy.[57, 65, 66] Therapy involves reduction of immunosuppression and the use of an antiviral agent (acyclovir, ganciclovir) and possibly an immunoglobulin adjuvant.[57, 58] Langnas and associates[58] reported patient and graft survival of 70 per cent at 1 year.

ADENOVIRUS. Adenovirus infection after liver transplantation is related most often to significant immunosuppression, especially after OKT3. In a large series, 2.2 per cent of liver recipients had adenovirus hepatitis and 40 per cent of them died of fulminant liver failure.[16] Types 1, 2, and 5 have been recovered most often, with type 5 the most common with hepatitis.[72] Infections usually occur within the first 2 months after transplantation.[16, 52, 72] Fever, enteritis, upper airway infection, and rash may occur. Aminotransferases, bilirubin, and gamma-glutamyltransferase may be elevated moderately, but aspartate aminotransferase appears to be significantly higher than alanine aminotransferase and may give an early clue to the diagnosis. The only treatment to date is to reduce immunosuppression.

HERPES SIMPLEX VIRUS. In a large series of liver transplant patients, less than 1 per cent developed HSV hepatitis[65]; however, its significance lies in its high mortality despite the use of antivirals.[38] The mean time for development of infection is 15 days after surgery.[65] This implies transmission from the donor organ or a blood transfusion, although it also may be secondary to a primary exposure.[26] Patients usually present with fulminant hepatic failure,[4, 26] developing symptoms of fever, mental status change, significantly increased transaminases, and, later, jaundice.[26] Therapy is the institution of acyclovir once the diagnosis is suspected.

References

1. Anand, A., Gray, E., Brown, T., et al.: Human parvovirus infection in pregnancy and hydrops fetalis. N. Engl. J. Med. *316*:183–186, 1987.
2. Andersson, J., Britton, S., Ernberg, I., et al.: Effect of acyclovir on infectious mononucleosis: A double-blind, placebo-controlled study. J. Infect. Dis. *153*:283–290, 1986.
3. Asano, Y., Yoshikawa, T., Suga, S., et al.: Fatal fulminant hepatitis in an infant with human herpesvirus-6 infection. Lancet *335*:862–863, 1990.
4. Awad, J., Peters, M. G., Brunt, E., et al.: Herpes viral hepatitis in liver transplant recipients. Clin. Transplant. *6*:16–20, 1992.
5. Balfour, H. H.: Intravenous acyclovir therapy for varicella in immunocompromised children. J. Pediatr. *104*:134–136, 1984.
6. Barkholt, L., Ericzon, B. G., Tollemar, J., et al.: Infections in human liver recipients: Different patterns early and late after transplantation. Transplant. Int. *6*:77–84, 1993.
7. Barkholt, L. M., Ehrnst, A., Veress, B., et al.: New criteria for diagnosing cytomegalovirus hepatitis in liver transplant patients. Transplant. Proc. *27*:1224–1225, 1995.

8. Barkholt, L. M., Ehrnst, A., Veress, B.: Clinical use of immunohistopathologic methods for the diagnosis of cytomegalovirus hepatitis in human liver allograft biopsy specimens. Scand. J. Gastroenterol. *29*:553–560, 1994.
9. Bechtelsheimer, H., Korb, G., and Gedigk, P.: The morphology and pathogenesis of "Marburg virus" hepatitis. Hum. Pathol. *3*:255–263, 1972.
10. Benador, N., Mannhardt, W., Schranz, D., et al.: Three cases of neonatal herpes simplex virus infection presenting as fulminant hepatitis. Eur. J. Pediatr. *149*:555–559, 1990.
11. Berenberg, W., and Nankervis, G.: Long-term follow-up of cytomegalic inclusion disease of infancy. Pediatrics *46*:403–410, 1970.
12. Berry, P., and Nagington, J.: Fatal infection with echovirus 11. Arch. Dis. Child. *57*:22–29, 1982.
13. Bhamarapravati, N.: Hemostatic defects in dengue hemorrhagic fever. Rev. Infect. Dis. *11*(Suppl. 4):826–829, 1989.
14. Breinig, M., Zitelli, B., Starzl, T., et al.: Epstein-Barr virus, cytomegalovirus, and other viral infections in children after liver transplantation. J. Infect. Dis. *156*:273–279, 1987.
15. Bronsther, O., Makowka, L., Jaffe, R., et al.: Occurrence of cytomegalovirus hepatitis in liver transplant patients. J. Med. Virol. *24*:423–434, 1988.
16. Cames, B., Rahier, J., Burtomboy, G., et al.: Acute adenovirus hepatitis in liver transplant recipients. J. Pediatr. *120*:33–37, 1992.
17. Chuang, E., Maller, E., Hoffman, M., et al.: Successful treatment of fulminant echovirus 11 infection in a neonate by orthotopic liver transplantation. J. Pediatr. Gastroenterol. Nutr. *17*:211–214, 1993.
18. Corey, L., and Spear, P.G.: Infections with herpes simplex viruses (1). N. Engl. J. Med. *314*:686–691, 1986.
19. Dai-ming, W., and Zheng, P.: Severe hepatitis associated with Epstein-Barr virus in childhood. Chin. Med. J. *101*:454–455, 1988.
20. Deutsch, J., Wolf, H., Becker, H., et al.: Demonstration of Epstein-Barr virus DNA in a previously healthy boy with fulminant hepatic failure. Eur. J. Pediatr. *145*:94–98, 1986.
21. Dienes, H. P., Schirmacher, P., Weise, K., et al.: Herpes simplex virus hepatitis and related problems. Int. Rev. Exp. Pathol. *35*:1–38, 1994.
22. Dubedat, S., and Kappagoda, N.: Hepatitis due to human herpesvirus-6. Lancet *2*:1463–1464, 1989.
23. Elisaf, M., Stefanaki, S., Repanti, M., et al.: Liver involvement in hemorrhagic fever with renal syndrome. J. Clin. Gastroenterol. *17*:33–37, 1993.
24. Esterly, J., Slusser, R., and Ruebner, B.: Hepatic lesions in the congenital rubella syndrome. J. Pediatr. *71*:676–685, 1967.
25. Ey, J. L., Smith, S. M., and Fulginiti, V. A.: Varicella hepatitis without neurologic symptoms or findings. Pediatrics *67*:285–287, 1981.
26. Fagiuoli, S., Shah, G., Wright, H., et al.: Types, causes, and therapies of hepatitis occurring in liver transplant recipients. Dig. Dis. Sci. *38*:449–455, 1993.
27. Ferry, G. D., Selby, M. L., Udall, J., et al.: Guide to early diagnosis of biliary obstruction in infancy: Review of 143 cases. Clin. Pediatr. *24*:305–311, 1985.
28. Fleisher, G., Henry, W., McSorley, M., et al.: Life-threatening complications of varicella. Am. J. Dis. Child. *135*:896–899, 1981.
29. Frame, J.: Clinical features of Lassa fever in Liberia. Rev. Infect. Dis. *11*:783–789, 1989.
30. Freij, B., South, M., and Sever, J.: Maternal rubella and the congenital rubella syndrome. Clin. Perinatol. 15:247–257, 1988.
31. Gavish, D., Kleinman, Y., Morag, A., et al.: Hepatitis and jaundice associated with measles in young adults. Arch. Intern. Med. *143*:674–677, 1983.
32. Gear, H. S.: Clinical aspects of African viral hemorrhagic fevers. Rev. Infect. Dis. *11*(Suppl. 4):777–782, 1989.
33. Gear, J. S. S., Cassel, G., Gear, A., et al.: Outbreak of Marburg virus disease in Johannesburg. Br. Med. J. *4*:489–493, 1975.
34. Giladi, M., Schulman, A., Kedem, R., et al.: Measles in adults: A prospective study of 291 consecutive cases. Br. Med. J. *295*:1314, 1987.
35. Goodman, Z. D., Ishak, K. G., and Sesterhenn, I. A.: Herpes simplex hepatitis in apparently immunocompetent adults. Am. J. Clin. Pathol. *85*:694–699, 1986.
36. Gremillion, D., and Crawford, G.: Measles pneumonia in young adults: An analysis of 106 cases. Am. J. Med. *71*:539–542, 1981.
37. Hall, C., Long, C., Schnabel, K., et al.: Human herpesvirus-6 infection in children: A prospective study of complications and reactivation. N. Engl. J. Med. *331*:432–438, 1994.
38. Hanley, C. J., Braun, D. K., Brown, K., et al.: Fulminant hepatic failure secondary to herpes simplex virus hepatitis: Successful outcome after orthotopic liver transplantation. Transplantation *59*:145–149, 1995.
39. Hanshaw, J. B., Betts, R. F., Simon, G., et al.: Acquired cytomegalovirus infection. N. Engl. J. Med. *272*:602–609, 1965.
40. Hanshaw, J. B.: Cytomegalovirus infections. Pediatr. Rev. *16*:43–48, 1995.
41. Hierholzer, J. C.: Adenoviruses in the immunocompromised host. Clin. Microbiol. Rev. *5*:262–274, 1992.
42. (See reference 117a.)
43. Horwitz, C. A., Burke, M. D., Grimes, P., et al.: Hepatic function in mononucleosis induced by Epstein-Barr virus and cytomegalovirus. Clin. Chem. *26*:243–246, 1980.
44. Horwitz, C. A., Henle, W., Henle, G., et al.: Clinical and laboratory evaluation of cytomegalovirus-induced mononucleosis in previously healthy individuals. Medicine *65*:124–134, 1986.
45. Hosier, D., and Newton, W.: Serious coxsackie infection in infants and children. Am. J. Dis. Child. *96*:251–267, 1958.
46. Huggins, J.: Prospects for treatment of viral hemorrhagic fevers with ribavirin, a broad-spectrum antiviral drug. Rev. Infect. Dis. *11*(Suppl. 4):750–759, 1989.
47. Hughes, J., Wilfert, C., Moore, M., et al.: Echovirus 14 infection associated with fatal neonatal hepatic necrosis. Am. J. Dis. Child. *123*:61–67, 1972.
48. Iijima, T., Sumazaki, R., Mori, N., et al.: A pathological and immunohistological case report of fatal infectious mononucleosis, Epstein-Barr virus infection, demonstrated by in situ and Southern blot hybridization. Virchows Arch. Pathol. Anat. *421*:73–78, 1992.
49. Ishak, K., Walker, D., Coetzer, J., et al.: Viral hemorrhagic fevers with hepatic involvement: Pathologic aspects with clinical correlations. Prog. Liver Dis. *7*:495–515, 1982.
50. Johnson, J., Egaas, S., Gleaves, C., et al.: Hepatitis due to herpes simplex virus in marrow-transplant recipients. Clin. Infect. Dis. *14*:38–45, 1992.
51. Johnston, J., and Overall, J.: Intravenous immunoglobulin in disseminated neonatal echovirus 11 infection. Pediatr. Infect. Dis. J. *8*:254–256, 1989.
52. Koneru, B., Jaffe, R., Esquivel, C. O., et al.: Adenoviral infections in pediatric liver transplant recipients. J. A. M. A. *258*:489–492, 1987.
53. Korones, S., Ainger, L., Monif, G., et al.: Congenital rubella syndrome: Study of 22 infants. Am. J. Dis. Child. *110*:434–440, 1965.
54. Kusne, S., Schwartz, M., Breinig, M., et al.: Herpes simplex virus hepatitis after solid organ transplantation in adults. J. Infect. Dis. *163*:1001–1007, 1991.
55. Lake, A., Lauer, B., Clark, J., et al.: Enterovirus infections in neonates. J. Pediatr. *89*:787–791, 1976.
56. Langnas, A., Markin, R., Cattral, M., et al.: Parvovirus B19 as a possible causative agent of fulminant liver failure and associated aplastic anemia. Hepatology *22*:1661–1665, 1995.
57. Langnas, A., Castaldo, P., Markin, R., et al.: The spectrum of Epstein-Barr virus infection with hepatitis following liver transplantation. Transplant. Proc. *23*:1513–1515, 1991.
58. Langnas, A., Markin, R., Inagaki, M., et al.: Epstein-Barr virus hepatitis after liver transplantation. Am. J. Gastroenterol. *89*:1066–1070, 1994.
59. Laskus, T., Lupa, E., Cianciara, J., et al.: Cytomegalovirus infection presenting as hepatitis. Digestion *47*:167–171, 1990.
60. LeDuc, J. W.: Epidemiology of hemorrhagic fever viruses. Rev. Infect. Dis. *11*(Suppl. 4):730–735, 1989.
61. Lotan, C., Matoth, I., and Korman, S.: Liver involvement in measles. Eur. J. Pediatr. *145*:160–161, 1986.
62. Malison, M. and Waterman, S.: Dengue fever in the United States. J. A. M. A. *249*:496–500, 1983.
63. Markin, R. S., Linder, J., Zuerlein, K., et al.: Hepatitis in fatal infectious mononucleosis. Gastroenterology *93*:1210–1217, 1987.
64. Markin, R. S., Wood, P. R., Shaw, B. W., et al.: Immunohistologic identification of Epstein-Barr virus–induced hepatitis reactivation after OKT3 therapy following orthotopic liver transplant. Am. J. Gastroenterol. *85*:1014–1019, 1990.
65. Markin, R. S., Langnas, A. N., Donovan, J. P., et al.: Opportunistic viral hepatitis in liver transplant recipients. Transplant. Proc. *23*:1520–1521, 1991.
66. Markin, R. S.: Manifestations of Epstein-Barr virus–associated disorders in liver. Liver *14*:1–13, 1994.
66a. Martin, M., Manez, R., Linden, P., et al.: A prospective randomized trial comparing sequential ganciclovir–high-dose acyclovir to high-dose acyclovir for prevention of cytomegalovirus disease in adult liver transplant recipients. Transplantation *59*:779–785, 1994.
67. McCormick, J. B., Walker, D. H., King, I. J., et al.: Lassa virus hepatitis: A study of fatal Lassa fever in humans. Am. J. Trop. Med. Hyg. *35*:401–407, 1986.
68. McCormick, J. B., King, I. T., Webb, P. A., et al.: Lassa fever: Effective therapy with ribavirin. N. Engl. J. Med. *314*:20–26, 1986.
69. McCracken, G. H., Jr., Shinefield, H. R., Cobb, K., et al.: Congenital cytomegalic inclusion disease: A longitudinal study of 20 patients. Am. J. Dis. Child. *117*:522–539, 1969.
70. Mendel, I., De Matteis, M., Bertin, C., et al.: Fulminant hepatitis in neonates with human herpesvirus 6 infection. Pediatr. Infect. Dis. J. *14*:993–997, 1995.
71. Metzman, R., Anand, A., DeGiulio, P., et al.: Hepatic disease associated with intrauterine parvovirus B19 infection in a newborn premature infant. J. Pediatr. Gastroenterol. Nutr. *9*:112–114, 1989.
72. Michaels, M. G., Green, M., Wald, E. R., et al.: Adenovirus infection in pediatric liver transplant recipients. J. Infect. Dis. *165*:170–174, 1992.
73. Miliauskas, J. R., and Webber, B. L.: Disseminated varicella at autopsy in children with cancer. Cancer *53*:1518–1525, 1984.
74. Miller, D., Hanshaw, J., O'Leary, D., et al.: Fatal disseminated herpes simplex virus infection and hemorrhage in the neonate. J. Pediatr. *76*:409–415, 1970.
75. Modai, D., Pik, A., Marmor, Z., et al.: Liver dysfunction in measles, liver biopsy findings. Dig. Dis. Sci. *31*:333, 1986.
76. Modlin, J.: Perinatal echovirus and group B coxsackievirus infections. Clin. Perinatol. *15*:233–245, 1988.
77. Modlin, J.: Perinatal echovirus infection: Insights from a literature review

of 61 cases of serious infection and 16 outbreaks in nurseries. Rev. Infect. Dis. *8*:918–926, 1986.
78. Modlin, J.: Fatal echovirus 11 disease in premature neonates. Pediatrics *66*:775–779, 1980.
79. Mollison, L. C., Richards, M. J., Johnson, P. D. R., et al.: High-dose oral acyclovir reduces the incidence of cytomegalovirus infection in liver transplant recipients. J. Infect. Dis. *168*:721–724, 1993.
80. Monif, G., Asofsky, R., and Sever, J.: Hepatic dysfunction in the congenital rubella syndrome. Br. Med. J. *1*:1086–1088, 1966.
81. Morens, D.: Enteroviral disease in early infancy. J. Pediatr. *92*:374–377, 1978.
82. Morgan, E., and Smalley, L.: Varicella in immunocompromised children: Incidence of abdominal pain and organ involvement. Am. J. Dis. Child. *137*:883–885, 1983.
83. Nickell, M., Cannady, P., and Schwitzer, G.: Subclinical hepatitis in rubeola infections in young adults. Ann. Intern. Med. *90*:354–355, 1979.
84. Nigro, G., Bartmann, U., Mattia, S., et al.: Acute hepatitis in childhood: Virological, immunological, and clinical aspects. Biomed. Pharmacol. *46*:155–160, 1992.
85. Odio, C., McCracken, G. H., Jr., and Nelson, J. D.: Disseminated adenovirus infection: A case report and review of the literature. Pediatr. Infect. Dis. *3*:46–49, 1984.
86. Paya, C., Hermans, P., Smith, T., et al.: Efficacy of ganciclovir in liver and kidney transplant recipients with severe cytomegalovirus infection. Transplantation *46*:229–234, 1988.
87. Paya, C. V., Hermans, P. E., Washington, J. A. II, et al.: Incidence, distribution, and outcome of episodes of infection in 100 orthotopic liver transplantations. Mayo Clin. Proc. *64*:555–564, 1989.
88. Paya, C., Hermans, P. E., Wiesner, R. H., et al.: Cytomegalovirus hepatitis in liver transplantation: Prospective analysis of 93 consecutive orthotopic liver transplantations. J. Infect. Dis. *160*:752–758, 1989.
89. Paya, C. V., Holley, K. E., Wiesner, R. H., et al.: Early diagnosis of cytomegalovirus hepatitis in liver transplant recipients: Role of immunostaining, DNA hybridization and culture of hepatic tissue. Hepatology *12*:119–126, 1990.
90. Phillips, M. J., Blendis, L. M., Poucell, S., et al.: Syncytial giant-cell hepatitis: Sporadic hepatitis with distinctive pathological features, a severe clinical course, and paramyxoviral features. N. Engl. J. Med. *324*:455–460, 1991.
91. Pitel, P. A., McCormick, K. L., Fitzgerald, E., et al.: Subclinical hepatic changes in clinical varicella infection. Pediatrics *65*:631–633, 1980.
92. Reyes, M., Ostrea, E., Roskamp, J., et al.: Disseminated neonatal echovirus 11 disease following antenatal maternal infection with a virus-positive cervix and virus-negative gastrointestinal tract. J. Med. Virol. *12*:155–159, 1983.
93. Rowe, W. P., Hartley, J. W., Cramblett, H. G., et al.: Detection of human salivary gland virus in the mouth and urine of children. Am. J. Hyg. *67*:57–65, 1958.
94. Rowe, W. P., Hartley, J. W., Waterman, S., et al.: Cytopathogenic agent resembling human salivary gland virus recovered from tissue culture of human adenoids. Proc. Soc. Exp. Biol. Med. *92*:418–424, 1956.
95. Sacks, S. L., and Freeman, H. J.: Cytomegalovirus hepatitis: evidence for direct hepatic viral infection using monoclonal antibodies. Gastroenterology *86*:346–350, 1984.
96. Sainsbury, R., Smith, P., LeQuesne, G., et al.: Gallbladder wall thickening with infectious mononucleosis hepatitis in an immunosuppressed adolescent. J. Pediatr. Gastroenterol. Nutr. *19*:123–125, 1994.
97. Seemayer, T., Grierson, H., Pirruccello, S., et al.: X-linked lymphoproliferative disease. Am. J. Dis. Child. *147*:1242–1245, 1993.
98. Shalev-Zimels, H., Weizman, Z., Lotan, C., et al.: Extent of measles hepatitis in various ages. Hepatology *8*:1138–1139, 1988.
99. Shaw, N., and Evans, J.: Liver failure and Epstein-Barr virus infection. Arch. Dis. Child. *63*:432–433, 1988.
100. Shields, A., Hackman, R., Fife, K., et al.: Adenovirus infections in patients undergoing bone marrow transplantation. N. Engl. J. Med. *312*:529–533, 1985.
101. Siegel, D., and Hirschman, S.: Hepatic dysfunction in acute measles infection of adults. Arch. Intern. Med. *137*:1178–1179, 1977.
102. Sobue, R., Miyazaki, H., Okamoto, M., et al.: Fulminant hepatitis in primary human herpesvirus-6 infection. N. Engl. J. Med. *324*:1290, 1991.
103. Stagno, S., and Whitley, R. J.: Herpesvirus infections of pregnancy. Part II. Herpes simplex virus and varicella-zoster virus infections. N. Engl. J. Med. *313*:1327–1330, 1985.
104. Steeper, T., Horwitz, C., Ablashi, D., et al.: The spectrum of clinical and laboratory findings resulting from human herpesvirus-6 (HHV-6) in patients with mononucleosis-like illnesses not resulting from Epstein-Barr virus or cytomegalovirus. Am. J. Clin. Pathol. *93*:776–783, 1990.
105. Stern, H.: Cytomegalovirus and EB virus infections of the liver. Br. Med. Bull. *28*:180–185, 1972.
106. Stratta, R., Shaeffer, M., Markin, R., et al.: Cytomegalovirus infection and disease after liver transplantation: An overview. Dig. Dis. Sci. *37*:673–685, 1992.
107. Strauss, L., and Bernstein, J.: Neonatal hepatitis in congenital rubella. Arch. Path. *86*:317–327, 1968.
108. Stronati, M., Revello, M., Cerbo, R., et al.: Ganciclovir therapy of congenital human cytomegalovirus hepatitis. Acta. Paediatr. *84*:340–341, 1995.
109. Sugaya, N., Nirasawa, M., Mitamura, K., et al.: Hepatitis in acquired rubella infection in children. Am. J. Dis. Child. *142*:817–818, 1988.
110. Sumaya, C.: Epstein-Barr virus serologic testing: Diagnostic indications and interpretations. Pediatr. Infect. Dis. *5*:337–342, 1986.
111. Sumaya, C., and Ench, Y.: Epstein-Barr virus infectious mononucleosis in children I. Clinical and general laboratory findings. Pediatrics *75*:1003–1010, 1985.
112. Tajiri, H., Nose, O., Baba, K., et al.: Human herpesvirus-6 infection with liver injury in neonatal hepatitis. Lancet *335*:863, 1990.
113. Takikawa, T., Hayashibara, H., Harada, Y., et al.: Liver dysfunction, anaemia, and granulocytopenia after exanthema subitum. Lancet *340*:1288–1289, 1992.
114. Tazawa, Y., Nishinomiya, F., Noguchi, H., et al.: A case of fatal infectious mononucleosis presenting with fulminant hepatic failure associated with an extensive CD8-positive lymphocyte infiltration in the liver. Hum. Pathol. *24*:1135–1139, 1993.
115. Thurn, J.: Human parvovirus B19: Historical and clinical review. Rev. Infect. Dis. *10*:1005–1011, 1988.
116. Toghill, P. J., Bailey, M. E., Williams, R., et al.: Cytomegalovirus hepatitis in the adult. Lancet *1*:1351–1354, 1967.
117. Tomita, T., Garcia, F., and Mowry, M.: Herpes simplex hepatitis before and after acyclovir treatment. Arch. Pathol. Lab. Med. *116*:173–177, 1992.
117a. Toshima, H., Hironori, T., Ohkita, Y., and Shingu, M.: Clinical features of acute coxsackie B viral myocarditis. Jpn. Circ. J. *43*:441–444, 1979.
118. Van der Horst, C., Joncas, J., Ahronheim, G., et al.: Lack of effect of peroral acyclovir for the treatment of acute infectious mononucleosis. J. Infect. Dis. *164*:788–792, 1991.
119. Vieira, W. T., Gayotto, L. C., de Lima, C. P., et al.: Histopathology of the human liver in yellow fever with special emphasis on the diagnostic role of the Councilman body. Histopathology *7*:195–208, 1983.
120. Washington, K., Gossage, D. L., and Gottfried, M. R.: Pathology of the liver in severe combined immundeficiency and DiGeorge syndrome. Pediatr. Pathol. *13*:485–505, 1992.
121. Whitley, R. J., Nahmias, A. J., Visintine, A. M., et al.: The natural history of herpes simplex virus infection of mother and newborn. Pediatrics *66*:489–494, 1980.
122. Whitley, R., Arvin, A., Prober, C., et al.: A controlled trial comparing vidarabine with acyclovir in neonatal herpes simplex virus infection. N. Engl. J. Med. *324*:444–449, 1991.
123. Wong, S., Tam, A., Ng, T., et al.: Fatal coxsackie B1 virus infection in neonates. Pediatr. Infect. Dis. J. *8*:638–641, 1989.
124. Zahradnik, J., Spencer, M., and Porter, D.: Adenovirus infection in the immunocompromised patient. Am. J. Med. *68*:725–732, 1980.
125. Zhang, T. M., Yang, Z. Q., Zhang, M. Y., et al.: Early analysis of viremia and clinical tests in patients with epidemic hemorrhagic fever. Chin. Med. J. *106*:608–610, 1993.
126. Zuelzer, W., and Stulberg, C.: Herpes simplex virus as the cause of fulminating visceral disease and hepatitis in infancy. Am. J. Dis. Child. *83*:421–439, 1952.

57

CHOLANGITIS AND CHOLECYSTITIS

Ann O. Scheimann, George D. Ferry, and Richard D. Aach

Cholangitis is considered a clinical diagnosis composed of signs and symptoms of biliary tract–associated sepsis. Bacterbilia, evidence of biliary colonization, increased biliary pressure, and clinical evidence of septicemia are necessary for the diagnosis.[27] Cholangitis may involve large or small ducts; pericholangitis generally refers to involvement of the small ducts of the portal triad.[99]

Cholecystitis refers to an acute or chronic inflammation of the gallbladder and cystic ducts. Pediatric patients with cholecystitis commonly exhibit classic adult signs of gallbladder inflammation—nausea, vomiting, right upper quadrant abdominal pain, and a palpable mass.

HISTORY OF CHOLANGITIS AND CHOLECYSTITIS

Biliary tract–associated infections in the pediatric patient population first were described by Joseph Gibson in 1734, when he reported a case of a 12-year-old who died after a febrile illness with right upper quadrant tenderness and jaundice. At autopsy, the gallbladder and common bile duct were distended and filled with concretions.[34] In 1877, Charcot described the classic triad associated with cholangitis—fever/chills, jaundice, and right upper quadrant pain.[18] The first cholecystectomy was performed by Howe in 1922 on a 5-year-old with cholecystitis.[79]

Both cholecystitis and cholangitis are uncommon but not rare pediatric illnesses. Inflammation of the biliary conduit system or cholangitis generally occurs in the presence of underlying ductal anomalies or immunocompromise. Acute cholecystitis requires stasis and concomitant obstruction to flow secondary to intrinsic (calculous) or extrinsic (acalculous) factors.

CHOLANGITIS

Etiology and Pathogenesis

Hematogenous colonization and abnormalities of biliary flow initiate inflammatory changes and subsequent infection. Early research conducted on patients with cholecystitis and cholangitis by Rosenow[86] in 1916 and Wilkie[117] in 1927 indicated that the most common route of infection was direct hematogenous spread into the gallbladder wall. Experiments conducted by Scott and Khan[98] in 1967 and Scott[97] in 1971 corroborated this hypothesis. Others described obstruction to flow from underlying ductal anomalies (Caroli disease, congenital hepatic fibrosis, choledochal cyst) resulting in ongoing colonization via hematogenous spread and inflammatory changes.[1, 47, 61, 92] Biliary drainage via a Roux-en-Y connection directly to the porta hepatitis—the Kasai procedure—may predispose to ascending colonization from the jejunal flora.[28, 50] The high incidence of post–Kasai procedure cholangitis correlates with decreased biliary and duodenal motility.[102] Thus, the major factors leading to cholangitis in children are the combination of bacterial colonization and relative stasis.

Escherichia coli is the most commonly isolated agent causing cholangitis, accounting for nearly one-half of initial episodes.[97] *Klebsiella, Enterococcus, Pseudomonas, Enterobacter, Serratia, Bacteroides,* and *Clostridium perfringens* account for most other infections (Table 57–1).[9, 65, 108, 119] Enterobacteriaceae and occasionally *Pseudomonas aeruginosa* are more common in cholangitis due to congenital hepatic fibrosis.[88]

Clinical Presentation

The majority of adults present with Charcot triad of fever, right upper quadrant abdominal pain, and jaundice (55 to 70 per cent); a small minority develop shock (7 per cent).[87, 90, 108] Cholangitis within the pediatric age group most often is a complication of the Kasai procedure. These children can have fever (100 per cent), acholic stools, or increase in bilirubin (68 per cent), and many present with signs of shock.[28, 88] In our experience, the majority of children with cholangitis exhibit only fever and elevation in bilirubin, gamma-glutamyltransferase, and/or aminotransferases. Septic shock has been infrequent. Cholangitis rarely occurs without an underlying predisposition but should be considered in the differential diagnosis of fever of unknown origin.[120]

Minimal information currently exists on the morbidity of cholangitis. A review of 26 cases of cholangitis in patients with congenital hepatic fibrosis reported 13 deaths due to the acute infection and 3 deaths from unrelated causes. One child had repeated cholangitis, and nine others had no further episodes of cholangitis.[88]

Laboratory Studies

Laboratory abnormalities commonly encountered with episodes of cholangitis in adults include elevated alkaline phosphatase (96 per cent) and elevated total bilirubin levels (88 per cent). Children commonly present with elevated or low white blood cell counts, an increase in serum gamma-glutamyltransferase or alkaline phosphatase levels, an increase in transaminase activity, and coagulopathy.[74, 88]

Blood cultures are positive in 50 per cent of patients. Cultures of hepatic tissue obtained via percutaneous biopsy may increase the diagnostic yield significantly.[85] In one pediatric study, hepatic cultures provided an etiologic agent in nearly 40 per cent of patients with negative blood cultures.[108] Diagnostic evaluation for cholangitis should include a complete blood cell count, liver enzyme profile including alkaline phosphatase and gamma-glutamyltransferase levels, blood culture (aerobic and anaerobic), and urine culture. An ultrasound or computed tomographic scan may be helpful in identifying abscesses, stones, ductal dilatation, or other periportal masses causing obstruction. In addition to a culture, a percutaneous liver biopsy may confirm any underlying pathology.[108]

TABLE 57–1. Biliary Tract Organisms in Adult Patients with Cholangitis

Organisms	Blood Bourgault et al., 1979[9]	Bile Wong et al., 1981[119]	Bile and Blood Marne et al., 1986[65]
Aerobes			
Escherichia coli	20%	57%	68%
Klebsiella	8%	44%	31%
Pseudomonas aeruginosa	6%	16%	1%
Serratia	2%	0	1%
Morganella morgani	3%	0	0
Aeromonas	2%	0	4%
Haemophilus influenzae	1%	0	1%
Citrobacter freundii	1%	0	1%
Proteus	1%	7%	4%
Pseudomonas maltophilia	1%	0	0
Enterobacter	1%	0	13%
Enterococcus faecalis	0	14%	25%
Viridans streptococci	0	2%	12%
Anaerobes			
Bacteroides fragilis	2%	5%	38%
Clostridium perfringens	1%	7%	38%
Fusobacterium	1%	0	5%
Peptostreptococci	0	0	9%

Differential Diagnosis

Patients exhibiting either Charcot triad or elevation of biliary tract–associated enzymes in the presence of fever of unknown origin deserve further diagnostic evaluation for biliary tract pathology via ultrasonography or scintigraphy. In some cases, an endoscopic retrograde cholangiopancreatography may be indicated for delineation of stones or obstruction.[27]

The differential diagnosis for fever, right upper quadrant abdominal pain, jaundice, and elevation in liver enzymes includes acute viral hepatitis, obstruction, and cholestasis associated with sepsis; drug-induced cholestasis; amebic abscess; and primary sclerosing cholangitis.

Acute viral hepatitis generally exhibits fever and high transaminases (aspartate aminotransferase, alanine aminotransferase) with lesser degrees of elevation in biliary tract–associated enzymes (alkaline phosphatase, gamma-glutamyltransferase). Bile flow often becomes sluggish in the presence of septicemia (especially with gram-negative organisms), but generally a thorough examination indicates a nonbiliary primary focus. Occasionally, biliary tract imaging or percutaneous liver biopsy is required to distinguish between biliary sludge and cholangitis.[27] Amebic abscesses generally present with fever, abdominal pain, and tender hepatomegaly and rarely exhibit jaundice or elevation of biliary tract enzymes.[39]

Drugs, such as chlorpromazine and erythromycin estolate, can produce idiosyncratic reactions, such as fever, nausea, vomiting, cholestatic jaundice, and right upper quadrant abdominal pain. Biliary caliber on noninvasive imaging often reveals normal biliary duct size; liver biopsy demonstrates eosinophilic and lymphocytic infiltrates with focal hepatocyte necrosis.[24]

Children with primary sclerosing cholangitis, an inflammatory condition of the biliary ductules usually associated with inflammatory bowel disease, generally present with malaise, jaundice, and weight loss and rarely present with fever, unless secondary cholangitis arises.[2, 62, 99, 100] Endoscopic retrograde cholangiopancreatography is diagnostic, with characteristic findings of irregular narrowing and stricture of the hepatic, common bile, and, often, intrahepatic ducts (Fig. 57–1). Histologic changes of pericholangiolar edema, portal edema, pericholangitis, and "onion skinning" around interlobular bile ducts may be seen in some areas.

Special Topics in Cholangitis

Cholangitis in Biliary Atresia

John Thomson first described biliary atresia in 1892 in the *Edinburgh Medical Journal*.[109] In 1928, W. E. Ladd[58] reported the first correctable biliary atresia operation, and Kasai and Suzuki[53] reported the first successful surgical correction of a previously "uncorrectable" biliary atresia in 1959. The Kasai procedure, a hepatic portojejunostomy in Roux-en-Y fashion, now is the standard operation for infants with biliary atresia.[50] The incidence of cholangitis, after the Kasai procedure, is highest in the first postoperative year. In 1973, Kobayashi and associates[56] reported a 47 per cent incidence (8 of 17) of

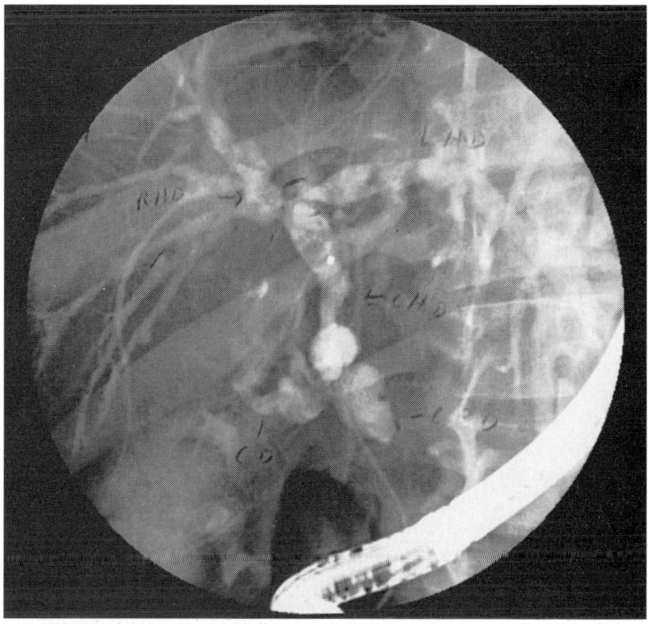

FIGURE 57–1. *An ERCP (endoscopic retrograde cholangiopancreatography) photograph of an adolescent with ulcerative colitis and recent onset of nausea and progressive jaundice demonstrating characteristic "beading" of the biliary tree reported in sclerosing cholangitis. (Courtesy of M. A. Gilger, M.D., Baylor College of Medicine.)*

cholangitis within 3 to 8 months after the initial surgery. Cholangitis appeared to compromise gains in biliary flow and resulted in three deaths. Others report a 43 to 78 per cent incidence of cholangitis after portojejunostomy, with the highest incidence (93 per cent) within the first 3 to 12 months after surgery and rare occurrences after 2 years.[28, 36, 57] The incidence of cholangitis varies in different ethnic groups. The highest incidence is in Hispanic patients (61 per cent), followed by white (54 per cent), Asian (54 per cent), and black (37 per cent) patients.[52] Cholangitis after a Kasai procedure may result from destruction of the sphincter of Oddi and ascending colonization of bile from the jejunal limb. Several modifications of the original Kasai procedure designed to minimize postoperative cholangitis gave rise to mixed results until researchers found success with an on-line Roux-en-Y intussusception valve designed to simulate the sphincter of Oddi and decrease ascending bacterial colonization.[26, 62, 103] The incidence of cholangitis declined to 13 per cent after addition of the intussusception valve at the time of the Kasai procedure.[26, 72, 103] Variability in operative success may result from differences in motility of the biliary tract and duodenum after a Kasai procedure.[102]

Both aerobic and anaerobic organisms have been retrieved from infants with post–Kasai procedure cholangitis in similar proportions to adult cholangitis series.[11, 41] *E. coli* is the most common organism, accounting for 50 per cent of the first and second episodes; 75 per cent of *E. coli* were resistant to ampicillin if treated postoperatively with ampicillin as prophylaxis.[28] Colonization of biliary cultures with *Candida albicans* without systemic involvement has been reported by Chen and associates[20] in a 1-year-old child with recurrent cholangitis after a Kasai procedure.[20]

Each episode of cholangitis carries a 1 per cent mortality rate, and continuing episodes of cholangitis can diminish biliary flow resulting in progression to cirrhosis.[28, 75] Early postoperative infections increase the mortality rate. Kobayashi and colleagues[56] reported an 88 per cent mortality rate among patients with cholangitis within 1 month of the Kasai procedure and a 16 per cent mortality rate among patients with cholangitis more than 1 month after the Kasai procedure. An episode of cholangitis diminished the 5-year survival rate from 91 to 54 per cent among Dutch patients with biliary atresia.[46]

Cholangitis After Liver Transplantation

Bacterial intra-abdominal infections are common in liver transplant patients and occur mainly in the first 2 months after transplantation. Infections are rare after 6 months.[71] Infectious complications of biliary origin are noted throughout the postoperative period; late cholangitis after transplantation occurs with biliary stricture formation.[49, 71] One early series of both adult and pediatric liver transplant recipients reported up to a 30 per cent incidence of cholangitis (some patients with bacteremia after transplant with no source identified).[78] More recent pediatric data report a 5 to 11 per cent incidence of posttransplant cholangitis in living-related and orthotopic liver transplant for biliary atresia.[47, 97, 107, 111]

Children with cholangitis after liver transplantation often present with fever, rising liver enzymes, and bacteremia.[57] Gram-negative bacilli, especially *Enterobacter* species, enterococci, and anaerobes, most frequently are isolated with polymicrobial sepsis.[64, 77] A history of broad-spectrum antibiotics and malnutrition has been associated with *C. albicans* cholangitis after transplantation.[35] Percutaneous liver biopsy is critical for culture as well as for discrimination between cholangitis and posttransplant rejection (Fig. 57–2).

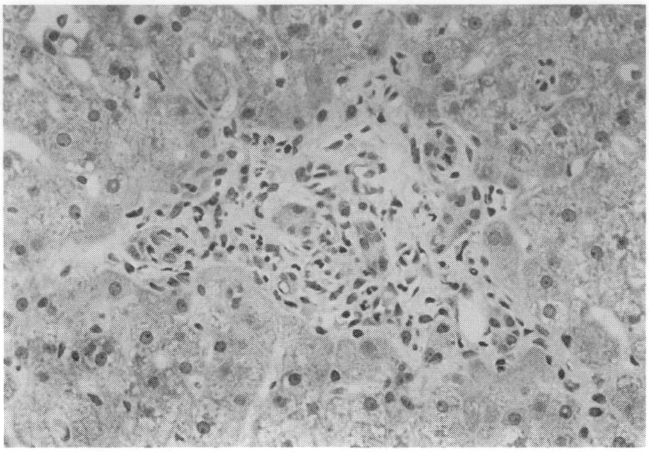

FIGURE 57–2. *Percutaneous liver biopsy from a child with fever and jaundice 6 months after orthotopic transplantation demonstrating acute ductal inflammation consistent with acute cholangitis. (Courtesy of M. Finegold, M.D., and G. S. Gopalakrishna, M.D., Baylor College of Medicine.)*

Cholangitis in the Immunocompromised

Biliary tract disease is more common in adults with HIV infection than in children. AIDS cholangiopathy associated with adult AIDS may give rise to sclerosing cholangitis, stenosis, and long-stricture formation from cytomegalovirus, *Cryptosporidium*, *Mycobacterium avium-intracellulare*, blastomycosis, and *Trichosporon*.[15, 16] AIDS cholangiopathy seriously should be considered in HIV-infected children with evidence of biliary ductal dilatation on ultrasonography. AIDS-related cholangitis has been reported in a 9-year-old girl with perinatally acquired AIDS and evidence of ductal dilatation by ultrasound, with bacterial overgrowth and abscess formation found at autopsy.[89]

Similar opportunistic biliary infections have been reported in HIV-negative children with other immunodeficiencies. Gremse and associates[38] described a similar picture of sclerosing cholangiopathy in a 10-year-old child with familial T-cell deficiency, IgA/IgG deficiencies, and chronic cryptosporidial enteritis. *C. albicans* cholangitis has been described in a leukemic child with abdominal distention and vomiting.[96]

Other Biliary Tract Pathogens in Normal Hosts

Opportunistic agents have caused biliary tract infections in normal pediatric hosts. *Cryptococcus neoformans* cholangitis was reported by Bucuvalas and colleagues[12] in a 15-year-old girl with cirrhosis who eventually succumbed to liver failure. *C. albicans* cholangitis secondary to fungus-ball formation was reported in a 3-year-old girl 2 months after abdominal surgery for blunt trauma.[13]

Parasitic infection with *Echinococcus* and *Clonorchis sinensis* rarely may result in symptomatic cholangitis in pediatric patients. An isolated case report of a 12-year-old son of a shepherd describes symptomatic echinococcal cholangitis from rupture of daughter hydatid cysts. Marsupialization of the cyst cavity was required.[63] Childhood recurrent pyogenic cholangitis is a clinical syndrome affecting Asian children after infestation with *C. sinensis*. This infection causes inflammation of the biliary ducts with consequent stricture and stone formation. *Klebsiella pneumoniae, E. coli, Proteus mirabilis,* and *Streptococcus faecalis* are the most common isolates during attacks of cholangitis.[6, 90]

TABLE 57–2. Biliary Levels of Antibiotics*

Antimicrobial Agent	Ratio of Antibiotic Level in Bile to Serum**	Antimicrobial Agent	Ratio of Antibiotic Level in Bile to Serum**
Penicillins		***Aminoglycosides***	
Penicillin G	0.5	Streptomycin	0.4–3.0
Ampicillin	1.0–2.0	Gentamicin	0.3–0.6
Mezlocillin	10	Amikacin	0.3
Nafcillin	40	Tobramycin	0.1–0.2
Oxacillin	0.2–0.4	***Tetracyclines/Macrolides/***	
Piperacillin	10–15	***Chloramphenicol***	
Cephalosporins		Tetracyclines	5.0–10.0
Cefazolin	0.7	Doxycycline	10–20
Cefmetazole	~10	Erythromycin	8.0–25.0
Cefoperazone	8–12	Clindamycin	2.5–3.0
Cefotaxime	0.1–0.5	Chloramphenicol	0.2
Cefoxitin	2.8	***Miscellaneous***	
Ceftazidime	0.3	Amphotericin B	2–7
Ceftizoxime	0.1–0.3	Aztreonam	0.6
Ceftriaxone	10	Ciprofloxacin	~2.0
Cefuroxime	0.4	Imipenem	0.04
Cephalothin	0.4–0.8	Ketoconazole	Minimal
		Metronidazole	1.0
		Rifampin	100
		Trimethoprim-sulfamethoxazole	1.0–2.0/0.4–0.7
		Vancomycin	0.5

*With obstruction, virtually none enters bile; **>1.0 indicates bile level exceeds serum.
From Sanford, J. P., Gilbert, D. N., and Sande, M. A.: Sanford Guide to Antimicrobial Therapy. Dallas, Antimicrobial Therapy, Inc., 1995.

Treatment

Treatment for cholangitis should include appropriate antibiotic coverage (based upon sensitivities) and supportive measures. A limited number of adult studies of cholangitis have evaluated antibiotic coverage, including mezlocillin, ampicillin plus gentamicin, perfloxacin, cefoperazone, piperacillin, and ampicillin plus tobramycin, noting good results with mezlocillin, piperacillin, and cefoperazone. Optimal response to antibiotic therapy occurred when the combination of sensitive organisms and adequate serum/biliary antibiotic levels was obtained with minimal nephrotoxicity. Prolonged treatment of cholangitis with ceftriaxone should be avoided because of its propensity to cause biliary sludge formation not found with cefoperazone.[17, 33, 71, 104] (See Table 57–2 for antimicrobial levels within bile according to Sanford and associates.[93]) Adequate biliary drainage is crucial to the clearance of organisms. Both endoscopic retrograde cholangiopancreatography and percutaneous transhepatic cholangiography are useful in visualization of the biliary tree to rule out obstruction and for therapeutic stent placement. Both procedures are lower in risk than open surgical manipulation (Fig. 57–3).[61]

Few reports are available in the current literature regarding therapy for post–Kasai procedure cholangitis. Rothenberg and colleagues[88] recommend early treatment for potential cholangitis (fever > 38° C, alteration in bilirubin and liver function tests) with a 7- to 10-day course of antibiotics for initial episodes of cholangitis and a 40-day course for refractory cholangitis. This group noted that third-generation cephalosporins (ceftriaxone, ceftazidime, cefotaxime) offered better efficacy than penicillins, ampicillin, or cefazolin (62.7 per cent success vs. 26 per cent). Others report increasing resistance among biliary isolates to ampicillin (from 65 to 75 per cent), trimethoprim (from 36 to >59 per cent), and gentamicin (from 12 to >36 per cent) with continued sensitivity to cephalosporins (from 9 to >13 per cent).[28] Rothenberg and associates[88] favored consideration of reoperation to augment biliary excretion and administration of oral corticosteroids to decrease ductular edema with recurrent cholangitis.[51] After an initial episode of post–Kasai procedure cholangitis, many advocate long-term prophylaxis with high-dose (20 mg/kg/day trimethoprim) trimethoprim-sulfamethoxazole for 1 year. In cases of recurrent cholangitis, prophylaxis is recommended for 18 months to 2 years, despite concerns over selection of resistant bacterial strains and lack of controlled study data.[3, 4, 19, 46, 55]

Several case reports stress the importance of a thorough evaluation for cystic collections in patients with recurrent cholangitis after biliary atresia repair.[28, 48, 116] Endoscopic retrograde cholangiopancreatography and percutaneous transhepatic cholangiography are employed to search for ductal dilatation and sludge formation, as well as potential stent placement if ductal narrowing is discovered during the procedure (Fig. 57–3). Certain patient subgroups may require surgical exploration of the biliary tree.[65, 108]

Therapy for posttransplant cholangitis is similar to that for cholangitis in biliary atresia and includes antimicrobial coverage for *Pseudomonas* species. Recurrent episodes of cholangitis require careful evaluation for cystic changes within the liver that might require drainage.[35]

CHOLECYSTITIS

Etiology and Pathogenesis

Cholecystitis in children most often is chronic in duration, and two-thirds of cases are associated with gallstones.[70] Gallstones generally arise from increased bilirubin turnover (hemoglobinopathies) or perturbation in the equilibrium between cholesterol/lecithin/bile salts.[10, 94] Elevations in cholesterol production secondary to obesity and pregnancy or depletions in the bile salt pool found in cystic fibrosis or

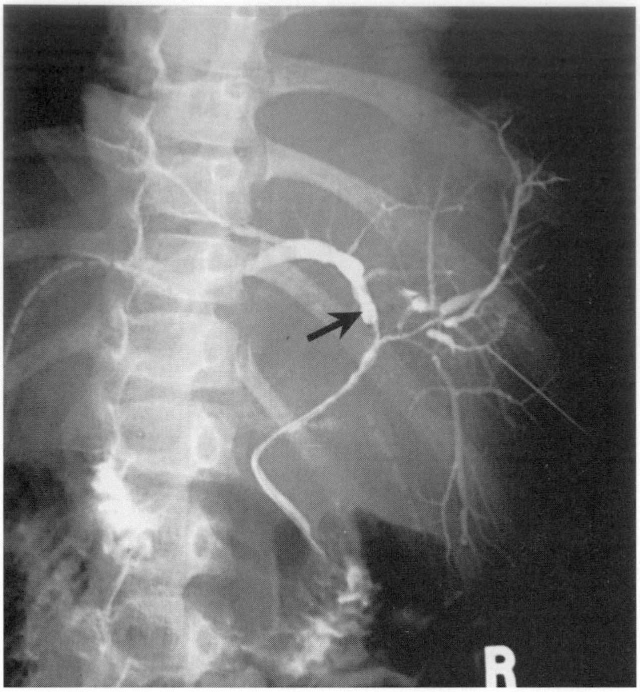

FIGURE 57–3. *Percutaneous cholangiogram from a girl with cholangitis approximately 1 year after orthotopic liver transplantation. A biliary stricture is noted (arrow). Placement of a biliary stent to improve drainage resulted in resolution of cholangitis. (Courtesy of G. S. Gopalakrishna, M.D., Baylor College of Medicine.)*

Crohn disease impair formation of micelles within the bile. Poor formation of micelles creates a nidus for stone formation.[10, 40, 42] Cholecystitis results from acute obstruction or stasis of the gallbladder. This commonly is associated with one or more predisposing conditions, including cystic duct obstruction, severe systemic infection, anesthesia/surgery, trauma, and dehydration.[105]

The mechanism for the underlying inflammation remains unclear, although ischemia, bacteria, distention, and lysolecithin are proposed factors in pathogenesis.[70] Early canine research suggested that obstruction of the cystic duct will result in acute cholecystitis only in the presence of concentrated bile.[69] More recent experimental data suggest a role for lysolecithin, generated from biliary lecithin by phospholipase A (found in the gallbladder mucosa). Lysolecithin enhances synthesis of prostaglandin E_2, which transforms the internal surface of the gallbladder into a secretory mucosa, stimulates mucus production, and increases the viscosity of bile.[60, 73, 110] Earlier bacterial culture data from Edlund and colleagues[29] suggest that bacteria play a secondary role in calculous cholecystitis.

Biliary stasis appears crucial for the development of acalculous cholecystitis. Stasis may result from sepsis, dehydration, trauma/burns, anesthesia/surgery, or total parenteral nutrition. Alterations in tone of the sphincter of Oddi (from opiates) can exacerbate stasis and impair defenses against enteric bacteria. Changes in vascular tone can hinder mucosal protection, allowing initiation of the lysolecithin cascade.[94] Various infectious agents or diseases have been associated with the development of acalculous cholecystitis, including leptospirosis,[5, 68, 105] *Salmonella typhi*,[80, 106, 118] *Salmonella paratyphi*,[80] *Mycoplasma pneumoniae*,[45] scarlet fever,[23, 95, 101] group B *Streptococcus* sepsis,[84] group A *Streptococcus* sepsis,[84] *Staphylococcus aureus* septicemia, [84] and ascariasis.[21] Other conditions associated with acalculous cholecystitis include familial Mediterranean fever,[21] Henoch-Schönlein syndrome,[8, 66] nephrotic syndrome,[21] polyarteritis nodosa,[21] leukemia,[21] Kawasaki disease,[21] and hemoglobinopathies (including sickle-cell and thalassemia major).[7, 13] Gangrenous acalculous cholecystitis has been reported in association with neonatal necrotizing enterocolitis and AIDS patients with cytomegalovirus or *Cryptosporidium* infection.[30, 94]

Clinical Presentation

Pediatric patients with cholecystitis typically present with findings similar to those of adults. Abdominal pain localized to the right upper quadrant or epigastric region is the most common symptom during an acute attack; one-third of patients will have a palpable gallbladder.[94] Poorly localized pain, periumbilical pain, right lower quadrant pain, and back pain have been reported in some pediatric patients.[105] Patients commonly complain of low-grade fever, nausea, anorexia, and vomiting. Mild jaundice develops in 20 to 30 per cent of patients, even in the absence of common bile duct stones.[94, 105] In contrast to adults, jaundice in children is hypothesized to arise generally from biliary obstruction secondary to surrounding inflammation, edema, or ductal compression via mesenteric nodes rather than directly from the presence of common duct stones.[112] Fever, abdominal tenderness, and jaundice may be minimal in the seriously ill patient, leading to a delayed diagnosis of acute cholecystitis.[94]

Laboratory Studies

The majority of patients with cholecystitis have nonspecific laboratory data. A mild leukocytosis and left shift are present in the majority of patients. Slight elevations in bilirubin and biliary tract–associated enzymes, including amylase and lipase, can be present in patients with hemoglobinopathy and choledocholithiasis without clinical evidence of acute pancreatitis.[82]

Other commonly utilized diagnostic tools include plain abdominal films, oral cholecystography, abdominal ultrasound, and cholescintigraphy. Holcomb and Robertson reported, respectively, 36 and 47 per cent incidences in children of radiopaque gallstones (generally noncholesterol stones); 15 per cent of adult gallstones are radiopaque.[43, 82, 83] Real-time ultrasound is the screening tool of choice in suspicious cases of cholecystitis.[37] Ultrasonography can image nonradiolucent calculi, ductal anomalies, and surrounding anatomy. Sonographic criteria for cholecystitis include cholelithiasis, thickening of the gallbladder wall (>3 mm in children), and nonvisualization of the gallbladder.[44] Gallbladder wall thickening is not specific for cholecystitis or always detectable; hypoalbuminemia, hepatitis, and physiologic contraction of the gallbladder also can produce wall thickening.[67] Cholescintigraphy can assist in clarifying uncertain ultrasound findings. During acute cholecystitis, the ^{99}technetium-labeled iminodiacetic acid scan will demonstrate continuity of bile flow from the extrahepatic biliary system into the intestines with nonvisualization of the gallbladder. The sensitivity and specificity of cholescintigraphy are 100 per cent and 95 per cent, respectively; occasional false-positive results occur in seriously ill fasted and total parenteral nutrition–dependent patients.[115] Employment of intravenous morphine during scintigraphy enhances sensitivity by increasing sphincter of Oddi pressure/common bile duct pressure, which increases the likelihood of gallbladder visualization.[31] Advances in ultrasound technology have resulted in infrequent utilization of oral cholecystograms, which have a significant number of false-positive results.[82]

Differential Diagnosis

The diagnosis of cholecystitis is straightforward when classic symptoms of nausea, vomiting, jaundice, and right upper quadrant pain are present. In the pediatric population, atypical symptoms often are encountered and can lead to misdiagnoses, including appendicitis (most common),[45, 105, 114] intussusception,[105] choledochal cyst,[45] viral hepatitis,[45] and peritonitis/acute abdominal process.[45] Serum transaminases (to exclude hepatitis) and ultrasonography/cholescintigraphy can help in the diagnosis. Careful resumption of feedings, serial physical examinations, and serial ultrasonography may discriminate between distention or hydrops of the gallbladder associated with scarlet fever, Kawasaki disease, and mesenteric adenitis from cholecystitis.[21, 23, 42, 43] For some pediatric patients, the diagnosis of cholecystitis only can be confirmed at exploratory laparotomy.

Treatment

Adequate treatment of acute cholecystitis requires hospitalization for analgesia, rehydration, and surgical monitoring. Thereafter, the approach to treatment differs between calculous and acalculous cholecystitis. For calculous cholecystitis, early cholecystectomy generally is the treatment of choice; for elective cholecystitis procedures, laparoscopic cholecystectomy often is utilized.[113] Antibiotics often are administered due to the high probability of biliary infection and the potential for hematogenous dissemination. However, biliary drug levels are suboptimal in the presence of obstruction.[93, 94]

The management of acalculous cholecystitis has changed radically over the past several years due to improved ultrasonographic diagnostics. Although a cholecystectomy to remove the distended gallbladder was performed in previous years,[4, 21, 68, 101, 114] acalculous cholecystitis currently is managed conservatively with hydration, appropriate antibiotic coverage, and careful monitoring of gallbladder dimensions.[25, 94, 118] Cholecystostomy or radiologic-guided drainage of the gallbladder can be employed if rupture is probable. Gangrenous cholecystitis necessitates surgical excision.[30, 32]

Complications of Cholecystitis

Cholecystitis may result in occasional complications, including perforation of the gallbladder (most frequent), gangrenous cholecystitis, cholangitis, pancreatitis, and carcinoma of the gallbladder (rare). Free perforation, associated with a 30 per cent mortality rate in adults, occurs in 1 to 2 per cent of cholecystitis patients; a few cases of gangrenous cholecystitis, associated with a mortality rate of more than 50 per cent, have been reported in the pediatric literature.[29, 32] Localized perforation can evolve into a palpable abscess, requiring drainage, or develop into a cholecystoenteric fistula. Ascending cholangitis can develop in patients with calculous cholecystitis. Pancreatitis occurs more commonly in adults with acute cholecystitis than in children.[10] Carcinoma of the gallbladder in earlier adult series had a high correlation with cholelithiasis (60 to 90 per cent). Two pediatric patients with cholelithiasis and cholecystitis have been recorded in the literature with coincidental carcinoma of the gallbladder at the time of operation.[112]

References

1. Alvarez, F., Hadchonel, M., and Bernard, O.: Latent chronic cholangitis in congenital hepatic fibrosis. Eur. J. Pediatr. *139*:203–205, 1982.
2. Barbaratis, C., Grases, P., Shepherd, H. A., et al.: Histological features of sclerosing cholangitis in patients with ulcerative colitis. J. Clin. Pathol. *38*:778–783, 1985.
3. Barkin, R. M., and Lilly, J. R.: Biliary atresia and the Kasai operation: Continuing care. J. Pediatr. *96*:1015–1019, 1980.
4. Barton, L. L., Escobedo, M. B., Keating, J. P., et al.: Leptospirosis with acalculous cholecystitis. Am. J. Dis. Child. *126*:350–351, 1973.
5. Barton, L. L., and Rathore, M. H.: Antibiotic prophylaxis of cholangitis after the Kasai procedure. J. Pediatr. Gastroenterol. Nutr. *11*:559–560, 1990.
6. Bergman, K. S., and Harris, B. H.: Oriental cholangitis. J. Pediatr. Surg. *21*:573–575, 1986.
7. Borgna-Pignatti, C., De Stefano, P., Pajno, D., et al.: Cholelithiasis in children with thalassemia major: An ultrasonographic study. J. Pediatr. *99*:243–244, 1981.
8. Bosio, M., Ravelli, A., Ruperto, N., et al.: Sindrome di Schönlein-Henoch con severo intervessamento multisistemico. Minerva Pediatr. *45*:197–201, 1993.
9. Bourgault, A. M., England, D. M., Rosenblatt, J. E., et al.: Clinical characteristics of anaerobic bactibilia. Arch. Intern. Med. *139*:1346–1349, 1979.
10. Brenner, R. W., and Stewart, C. F.: Cholecystitis in children. Rev. Surg. *21*:327, 1964.
11. Brook, I., and Altman, R. P.: The significance of anaerobic bacteria in biliary tract infection after hepatic portoenterostomy for biliary atresia. Surgery *95*:281–283, 1984.
12. Bucuvalas, J. C., Bove, K. E., Kaufman, R. A., et al.: Cholangitis associated with *Cryptococcus neoformans*. Gastroenterology *88*:1055–1059, 1985.
13. Cabrol, S., Desjardin, F., Baruchel, S., et al.: L'hydrocholecyste, cause meconnue de crises douloreuses abdominales ches le drepanocytaire. Arch. Fr. Pediatr. *42*:859–861, 1985.
14. Carstensen, H., Nilsson, K. O., Nettelblad, S. C., et al.: Common bile duct obstruction due to an intraluminal mass of candidiasis in a previously healthy child. Pediatrics *77*:858–861, 1986.
15. Cello, J. P.: Human immunodeficiency virus–associated biliary tract disease. Semin. Liver Dis. *12*:213–218, 1992.
16. Cello, J. P.: Acquired immunodeficiency syndrome cholangiopathy: Spectrum of disease. Am. J. Med. *86*:539–546, 1989.
17. Chacon, J. P., Criscuolo, P. D., Kobata, C. M., et al.: Prospective randomized comparison of pefloxacin and ampicillin plus gentamicin in the treatment of bacteriologically proven biliary tract infections. J. Antimicrob. Chemother. *26*:167–172, 1990.
18. Charcot, J. M.: Le Cons Sur Les Maladies du Fole de Voies Filiares et de Reins. Paris, Faculté de Medicine de Paris, 1877.
19. Chaudhary, S., and Turner, R. B.: Trimethoprim sulfamethoxazole for cholangitis following hepatic portoenterostomy for biliary atresia. J. Pediatr. *99*:656–658, 1981.
20. Chen, C. C., Chang, P. Y., and Chen, C. L.: Refractory cholangitis after Kasai's operation caused by candidiasis: A case report. J. Pediatr. Surg. *21*:736–737, 1986.
21. Crankson, S., Nazer, H., and Jacobsson, B.: Acute hydrops of the gallbladder in childhood. Eur. J. Pediatr. *151*:318–320, 1992.
22. Crystal, R. F., and Fink, R. L.: Acute acalculous cholecystitis in childhood. Clin. Pediatr. *10*:423–426, 1971.
23. Dickenson, S. J., Corley, G., and Santulli, T. V.: Acute cholecystitis as a sequel of scarlet fever. Am. J. Dis. Child. *121*:331–333, 1971.
24. Dienstag, J. L., Wands, J. R., and Isselbacher, K. J.: Acute hepatitis. *In* Wilson, J. D., et al. (eds.): Harrison's Principles of Internal Medicine. 12th ed. New York, McGraw-Hill, 1991, pp. 1322–1337.
25. Dinulos, J., Mitchell, D. K., Edgerton, J., et al.: Hydrops of the gallbladder associated with Epstein-Barr virus infection: A report of two cases and review of the literature. Pediatr. Infect. Dis. J. *13*:924–929, 1994.
26. Donahoe, P. K., and Hendren, W. H.: Roux-en-Y on-line intussusception to avoid ascending cholangitis in biliary atresia. Arch. Surg. *118*:1091–1094, 1983.
27. Dooley, J. S.: Cholangitis and biliary tract infections. *In* McIntyre, N., Benhamou, J., et al. (eds.): Oxford Textbook of Clinical Hepatology. Oxford, Oxford Publishing Corp., 1991, pp. 1134–1139.
28. Ecoffey, C., Rothman, E., Bernard, O., et al.: Bacterial cholangitis after surgery for biliary atresia. J. Pediatr. *111*:824–829, 1987.
29. Edlund, Y. A., Mollstedt, B. O., and Ouchterlong, O.: Bacteriological investigation of the biliary system and liver in biliary tract disease connected to clinical data and microstructure of the gallbladder and liver. Acta Chirurg. Scand. *116*:461, 1958.
30. Fernandes, E. T., Hollabaugh, R. S., Boulden, T. F., et al.: Gangrenous acalculous cholecystitis in a premature infant. J. Pediatr. Surg. *24*:608–609, 1989.
31. Flancbaum, L., and Alden, S. M.: Morphine cholescintigraphy. Surg. Gynecol. Obstet. *171*:227–232, 1990.
32. Gangopadhyay, A. N., Biswas, S. K., Arya, N. C., et al.: An unusual presentation of infantile gangrenous cholecystitis. Indian Pediatr. *30*:542–544, 1993.
33. Gerecht, W. B., Henry, N. K., Hoffman, W. W., et al.: Prospective randomized comparison of mezlocillin therapy alone with combined ampicillin and gentamicin therapy for patients with cholangitis. Arch. Intern. Med. *149*:1279–1284, 1989.

34. Gibson, J.: An extraordinarily large gallbladder and hydropick cysts. Medical Essays and Observations 2:352, 1734.
35. Gleghorn, E. E., Rosenthal, P., Vachon, L., et al.: Long-term external catheter biliary drainage for recurrent cholangitis after hepatoportoenterostomy. J. Pediatr. Gastroenterol. Nutr. *5*:485–488, 1986.
36. Gottrand, F., Bernard, O., Hadchouel, M., et al.: Late cholangitis after successful surgical repair of biliary atresia. Am. J. Dis. Child. *145*:213–215, 1991.
37. Greenburg, M., Kangarloo, H., Cochran, S. T., et al.: The ultrasonographic diagnosis of cholecystitis and cholelithiasis in children. Radiographics *137*:745–749, 1980.
38. Gremse, D. A., Bucuvalas, J. C., and Bongiovanni, G. L.: Papillary stenosis and sclerosing cholangitis in an immunodeficient child. Gastroenterology *96*:1600–1603, 1989.
39. Harrison, H. R., Crowe, C. P., and Fulginiti, V. A.: Amebic liver abscess in children: Clinical and epidemiologic features. Pediatrics *64*:923–928, 1979.
40. Heubi, J. E., O'Connell, N. C., and Setchell, K. D.: Ileal resection/dysfunction in childhood predisposes to lithogenic bile only after puberty. Gastroenterology *103*:636–640, 1992.
41. Hitch, D. C., and Lilly, J. R.: Identification, quantification, and significance of bacterial growth within the biliary tract after Kasai's operation. J. Pediatr. Surg. *13*:563–569, 1978.
42. Holcomb, G. W., Jr., and Holcomb, G. W., III: Cholelithiasis in infants, children, and adolescents. Pediatr. Rev. *11*:268–274, 1990.
43. Holcomb, G. W., Jr., O'Neill, J. A., and Holcomb, G. W., III: Cholecystitis, cholelithiasis, and common duct stenosis in children and adolescents. Ann. Surg. *191*:626–635, 1980.
44. Holt, R. W., Wagner, R., and Homa, M.: Ultrasonic diagnosis of cholelithiasis. J. Pediatr. *92*:418–419, 1978.
45. Horii, Y., Sugimoto, T., Sakamoto, I., et al.: Acute acalculous cholecystitis complicating *Mycoplasma pneumoniae* infection. Clin. Pediatr. *31*:376–377, 1992.
46. Houwen, R. H., Zwierstra, R. P., Severijnen, R. S., et al.: Prognosis of extrahepatic biliary atresia. Arch. Dis. Child. *64*:214–218, 1989.
47. Howlett, S. A., Shulman, S. T., Ayoub, E. M., et al.: Cholangitis complicating congenital hepatic fibrosis. Am. J. Dig. Dis. *20*:790–795, 1975.
48. Ishii, K., Matsuo, S., Hirayama, Y., et al.: Intrahepatic biliary cysts after hepatic portoenterostomy in four children with biliary atresia. Pediatr. Radiol. *19*:471–473, 1989.
49. Kalayoglu, M., D'Alessandro, A., M., Knechtle, S. J., et al.: Long-term results of liver transplantation for biliary atresia. Surgery *114*:711–717, 1993.
50. Karrer, F. M., Hall, R. J., Stewart, B. A., et al.: Congenital biliary tract disease. Surg. Clin. North Am. *70*:1403–1418, 1990.
51. Karrer, F. M., and Lilly, J. R.: Corticosteroid therapy in biliary atresia. J. Pediatr. Surg. *20*:693–695, 1985.
52. Karrer, F. M., Lilly, J. R., Stewart, B. A., et al.: Biliary atresia registry: 1976 to 1989. J. Pediatr. Surg. *25*:1076–1080, 1990.
53. Kasai, M., and Suzuki, S.: A new operation for noncorrectable biliary atresia: Hepatic portoenterostomy. Shujitsu *13*:733, 1959.
54. Kimura, K.: Letter to editor. J. Pediatr. Surg. *25*:376, 1990.
55. Kobayashi, A., Itabashi, F., and Ohbe, Y.: Long-term prognosis in biliary atresia after portoenterostomy: Analysis of 35 patients who survived beyond 5 years of age. J. Pediatr. *105*:243–246, 1984.
56. Kobayashi, A., Utsunomiya, T., Obe Y., et al.: Ascending cholangitis after successful repair of biliary atresia. Arch. Dis. Child. *48*:697–703, 1973.
57. Kusne, S., Dummer, J. S., Singh, N., et al.: Infections after liver transplantation: An analysis of 101 consecutive cases. Medicine *67*:132–143, 1988.
58. Ladd, W. E.: Congenital atresia and stenosis of the bile ducts. J. A. M. A. *91*:1082, 1928.
59. Lai, E. C., Mok, F. P., Tan, E. S., et al.: Endoscopic biliary drainage for severe acute cholangitis. N. Engl. J. Med. *326*:1582–1586, 1992.
60. Lee, S. P., LaMont, J. T., and Carey, M. C.: Role of gallstone mucus hypersecretion in the evolution of the cholesterol gallstones. J. Clin. Invest. *67*:1712–1723, 1981.
61. Lipsett, P. A., and Pitt, H. A.: Acute cholangitis. Surg. Clin. North Am. *70*:1297–1312, 1990.
62. Ludwig, J.: Small-duct primary sclerosing cholangitis. Semin. Liver Dis. *11*:11–17, 1991.
63. Macris, G. J., and Galanis, N. N.: Rupture of *Echinococcus* cysts of the liver: Report of nine cases. Am. Surg. *32*:36–44, 1966.
64. Markin, R. S., Stratta, R. J., and Woods, G. L.: Infection after liver transplantation. Am. J. Surg. Pathol. *14*(Suppl. 1):64–78, 1990.
65. Marne, C., Pallaves, R., Martin, R., et al.: Gangrenous cholecystitis and acute cholangitis associated with anaerobic bacteria in bile. Eur. J. Clin. Microbiol. *5*:35–39, 1986.
66. McCrindle, B. W., Wood, R. A., and Nussbaum, A. R.: Henoch-Schönlein syndrome: Unusual manifestations with hydrops of the gallbladder. Clin. Pediatr. *27*:254–256, 1988.
67. McGahan, J. P., Phillips, H. E., Stadalnik, R. C., et al.: Ultrasound and radionuclide scanning in acute pediatric abdominal pain. J. Clin. Ultrasound *11*:251–258, 1983.
68. McKiernan, J., O'Brien, D. J., and Dundon, S.: Leptospirosis and acalculous cholecystitis. Irish Med. J. *69*:71–72, 1976.
69. Morris, C. P., Hohf, R. P., and Ivy, A. C.: An experimental study of the role of stasis in the etiology of cholecystitis. Surgery *32*:673, 1952.
70. Motil, K. A.: Cholecystitis. *In* Oski, F. A., DeAngelis, C. D., Feigin, R. D., et al. (eds.): Principles and Practice of Pediatrics. 2nd ed. Philadelphia, J.B. Lippincott, 1990, pp. 1779–1783.
71. Muller, E. L., Pitt, H. A., Thompson, J. E., Jr., et al.: Antibiotics in infections of the biliary tract. Surg. Gynecol. Obstet. *165*:285–292, 1987.
72. Nakajo, T., Hashizume, K., Saeki, M., et al.: Intussusception-type antireflux valve in the Roux-en-Y loop to prevent ascending cholangitis after hepatic portoenterostomy. J. Pediatr. Surg. *25*:311–314, 1990.
73. Neiderhiser, D., Thornell, E., Bjorck, S., et al.: The effect of lysophosphatidylcholine on gallbladder function in the cat. J. Lab. Clin. Med. *101*:699–707, 1983.
74. Novak, D. A., and Dolson, D. J.: Bacterial, parasitic, and fungal infections of the liver. *In* Suchy, F. J. (ed.): Liver Disease in Children. St. Louis, Mosby–Year Book, 1994, pp. 550–568.
75. Ohuchi, N., Ohi, R., Takahashi, T., et al.: Postoperative changes of intrahepatic portal veins in biliary atresia: A 3-D reconstruction study. J. Pediatr. Surg. *21*:10–14, 1986.
76. Patriquin, H. B., DiPietro, M., Barber, F. E., et al.: Sonography of thickened gallbladder wall: Causes in children. A. J. R. Am. J. Roentgenol. *141*:57–60, 1983.
77. Paya, C. V., and Hermans, P. E.: Bacterial infections after liver transplantation. Eur. J. Clin. Microbiol. Infect. Dis. *8*:499–504, 1989.
78. Paya, C. V., Hermans, P. E., Washington, J. A., II, et al.: Incidence, distribution, and outcome of episodes of infection in 100 orthotopic liver transplantations. Mayo Clin. Proc. *64*:555–564, 1989.
79. Potter, A. H.: Gallbladder disease in young subjects. Surg. Gynecol. Obstet. *46*:795–808, 1928.
80. Rao, S. D., Lewin, S., Shetty, B., et al.: Acute acalculous cholecystitis in typhoid fever. Indian Pediatr. *29*:1431–1435, 1992.
81. Rathore, M. H.: Cholangitis after the Kasai operation for biliary atresia. J. Pediatr. Surg. *25*:376, 1990.
82. Rescorla, F. J., and Grosfeld, J. L.: Cholecystitis and cholelithiasis in children. Semin. Pediatr. Surg. *1*:94–106, 1992.
83. Robertson, J. F., Carachi, R., Sweet, E. M., et al.: Cholelithiasis in childhood: A follow-up study. J. Pediatr. Surg. *23*:246–249, 1988.
84. Robinson, A. E., Erwin, J. H., Wiseman, H. J., et al.: Cholecystitis and hydrops of the gallbladder in the newborn. Radiology *122*:749–751, 1977.
85. Rogers, C. A., Isenberg, J. N., Leonard, A. S., et al.: Ascending cholangitis diagnosed by percutaneous hepatic aspiration. J. Pediatr. *88*:83–86, 1976.
86. Rosenow, E. C.: The etiology of cholangitis and gallstones and their production by the intravenous injection of bacteria. J. Infect. Dis. *29*:527, 1916.
87. Roth, P., and Cohen, S.: Cholangitis, a review of the literature with a report of an illustrative case. Am. J. Gastroenterol. *53*:154–163, 1970.
88. Rothenberg, S. S., Schroter, G. P., Karrer, F. M., et al.: Cholangitis after the Kasai operation for biliary atresia. J. Pediatr. Surg. *24*:729–732, 1989.
89. Rusin, J. A., Sivit, C. J., Rakusan, T. A., et al.: AIDS-related cholangitis in children: Sonographic findings. A. J. R. Am. J. Radiol. *159*:626–627, 1992.
90. Saik, R. P., Greenburg, A. G., Farris, J. M., et al.: Spectrum of cholangitis. Am. J. Surg. *130*:143–150, 1975.
91. Saing, H., Tam, P. K., Choi, T. K., et al.: Childhood recurrent pyogenic cholangitis. J. Pediatr. Surg. *23*:424–429, 1988.
92. Sanchez, C., Gonzalez, E., and Garau, J.: Trimethoprim-sulfamethoxazole treatment of cholangitis complicating congenital hepatic fibrosis. Pediatr. Infect. Dis. *5*:360–363, 1986.
93. Sanford, J. P., Gilbert, D. N., and Sande, M. A.: Sanford Guide to Antimicrobial Therapy. Dallas, Antimicrobial Therapy, Inc., 1995.
94. Schaffer, E. A.: Gallbladder disease. *In* Walker, A., et al. (eds.): Pediatric Gastrointestinal Disease: Pathophysiology, Diagnosis, Management. Vol. 2, 2nd ed. Salem, Mosby, 1966, pp. 1416–1417.
95. Schottmuller, H.: Hepatitis and cholecystitis: A specific complication of scarlet fever. Klin. Wochenschr. *10*:17–20, 1931.
96. Schreiber, M., Black, L., Noah, Z., et al.: Gallbladder candidiasis in a leukemic child. Am. J. Dis. Child. *136*:462–463, 1982.
97. Scott, A. J.: Bacteria and disease of the biliary tract. Gut *12*:487–492, 1971.
98. Scott, A. J., and Khan, G. A.: Origin of bacteria in bileduct bile. Lancet *2*:790–792, 1967.
99. Sherlock, S., and Dooley, J.: Diseases of the Liver and Biliary System. 9th ed. Oxford, Blackwell Scientific Publications, 1993, pp. 249–259.
100. Sisto, A., Feldman, P., Garel, L., et al.: Primary sclerosing cholangitis in children: Study of five cases and review of the literature. Pediatrics *80*:918–923, 1987.
101. Strauss, R. G.: Scarlet fever with hydrops of the gallbladder. Pediatrics *44*:741–745, 1969.
102. Takano, K., Iwafuchi, M., Uchiyama, M., et al.: Studies on intestinal motility and mechanism of cholangitis after biliary reconstruction. J. Pediatr. Surg. *24*:1225–1231, 1989.
103. Tanaka, K., Shirahase, I., Utsunomiya, H., et al.: A valved hepatic portoduodenal intestinal conduit for biliary atresia. Ann. Surg. *213*:230–235, 1991.
104. Tanaka, K., Uemoto, S., Tokunaga, Y., et al.: Living related liver transplantation in children. Am. J. Surg. *168*:41–48, 1994.
105. Ternberg, J. L., and Keating, J. P.: Acute acalculous cholecystitis: Complication of other illnesses in childhood. Arch. Surg. *110*:543–547, 1975.
106. Thambidorai, C. R., Shyamala, J., Sarala, R., et al.: Acute acalculous cholecystitis associated with enteric fever in children. Pediatr. Infect. Dis. J. *14*:812–813, 1995.

107. Thompson, J. E., Jr., Pitt, H. A., Doty, J. E., et al.: Broad spectrum penicillin as an adequate therapy for acute cholangitis. Surg. Gynecol. Obstet. *171*:275–282, 1990.
108. Thompson, J. E., Jr., Tompkins, R. K., and Longmire, W. P., Jr.: Factors in the management of acute cholangitis. Ann. Surg. *95*:137–145, 1982.
109. Thomson, J.: On congenital obliteration of the bile ducts. Edinburgh Med. J. *37*:523, 604, 724, 1892.
110. Thornell, E., Jivegard, L., Bukhave, K., et al.: Prostaglandin E_2 formation by the gallbladder in experimental cholecystitis. Gut *27*:370–373, 1986.
111. Uemoto, S., Tanaka, K., Fujita, S., et al.: Infectious complications in living related liver transplantation. J. Pediatr. Surg. *29*:514–517, 1994.
112. Ulin, A. W., Nosal, J. L., and Martin, W. L.: Cholecystitis in childhood: Associated obstructive jaundice. Surgery *31*:312, 1952.
113. Ware, R., Filston, H. C., Schultz, W. H., et al.: Elective cholecystectomy in children with sickle hemoglobinopathies: Successful outcome using preoperative transfusion regimen. Ann. Surg. *208*:17–22, 1988.
114. Washburn, M. E., and Barcia, P. J.: Uncommon cause of right upper quadrant abdominal mass in the newborn: Acute cholecystitis. Am. J. Surg. *140*:704–705, 1980.
115. Weissman, H. S., Badia, J., Sugarman, L. A., et al.: Spectrum of 99m-Tc-IDA cholescintigraphic patterns in acute cholecystitis. Radiology *138*:167–175, 1981.
116. Werlin, S. L., Sty, J. R., Starshak, R. J., et al.: Intrahepatic biliary abnormalities in children with congenital extrahepatic biliary atresia. J. Pediatr. Gastroenterol. Nutr. *4*:537–541, 1985.
117. Wilkie, A. L.: The bacteriology of recurrent cholecystitis: A clinical and experimental study. Br. J. Surg. *15*:450, 1927.
118. Winkler, A. P., and Gleich, S.: Acute cholecystitis caused by *Salmonella typhi* in an 11-year-old. Pediatr. Infect. Dis. J. *7*:125–128, 1988.
119. Wong, W., Teoh-Chan, C. H., Huang, C. T., et al: The bacteriology of recurrent cholangitis and associated diseases. J. Hyg. *87*:407–412, 1981.
120. Wyllie, R., and Fitzgerald, J. F.: Bacterial cholangitis in a 10-week-old infant with fever of undetermined origin. Pediatrics *65*:164–167, 1980.

58

Pyogenic Liver Abscess

Sheldon L. Kaplan

Pyogenic liver abscesses are encountered infrequently in normal children and generally have been reported in the compromised pediatric host. The rarity of liver abscesses may be explained, in part, by the rich blood supply, unique architecture, and extensive reticuloendothelial system of the liver, all of which present an effective barrier against bacterial invasion.

The precise incidence of pyogenic liver abscesses in children is unknown. Adult patients with hepatic abscesses constitute approximately 6 to 10 cases per 100,000 admissions; there is a 0.29 to 0.57 per cent incidence of liver abscesses in autopsies of adult patients.[10, 41] In the only large series of liver abscesses in children in the literature, Dehner and Kissane[9] reported a 0.38 per cent incidence at autopsy in patients younger than 15 years of age. In this series, 11 of 27 (41 per cent) patients were younger than 2 years of age, and 18 of 27 (67 per cent) were younger than 6 years of age. In a review of admissions to Milwaukee Children's Hospital, Chusid[8] found five children (four of whom were younger than 6 months of age) with at least one hepatic abscess and estimated an incidence of three cases for every 100,000 admissions. Pineiro-Carrero and Andress[38] estimated an incidence of approximately 25 cases per 100,000 admissions in their pediatric population (11 cases over 14 years).

PATHOGENESIS

Bacteria can establish an inflammatory focus in the liver by four major routes. Direct extension from contiguous structures is the most common mode in adults and precedes 28 to 40 per cent of hepatic abscesses in adults.[6, 39, 41] Biliary tract infection (cholangitis, cholecystitis), pancreatitis, and penetrating gastric or duodenal ulcer are examples of diseases associated with liver abscesses due to extension from a contiguous focus of infection. In a review of this problem at St. Louis Children's Hospital, 3 of 27 children (11 per cent) were considered to have a liver abscess secondary to inflammation of contiguous organs.[9] Although biliary tract disease is relatively uncommon in children, ascending cholangitis is a particularly frequent complication of the hepatic portoenterostomy procedure for congenital biliary atresia and may lead to infections of the liver in such patients.[11, 36] Liver abscesses also may develop as a complication of liver transplantation, especially if technical problems related to vascular supply or biliary drainage develop.[13, 27]

The portal system is the second most common route by which bacteria may reach the liver in adults; 6 to 20 per cent of liver abscesses in adults derive from this source.[29, 41] In Dehner and Kissane's series,[9] hepatic infection via the portal vein was encountered in two children, both cases occurring prior to 1940. In the newborn period, solitary liver abscesses, especially due to gram-negative organisms, have complicated the use of umbilical vein catheterization or have been secondary to omphalitis.[5] Prematurity and necrotizing enterocolitis also are important predisposing conditions.[17]

Portal vein inflammation and bacteremia can be associated with infections within the abdominal cavity. Appendicitis, diverticulitis, perirectal abscesses, regional enteritis, ulcerative colitis, and omphalitis all are possible sources of portal vein sepsis.[9] A pyogenic liver abscess may be an unusual complication of an ingested foreign body with subsequent portal venous bacteremia.[34] Since antibiotics have been available, portal vein inflammation or pylephlebitis has become a less common source of hepatic infection in children.

Systemic bacteremia with hematogenous spread of bacteria to the liver via the hepatic artery appears to be the most common source of liver abscess in children but is implicated in less than 20 per cent of adult patients.

In the St. Louis series, the systemic hematogenous route was responsible for 21 of 27 (78 per cent) cases of liver abscesses.[9] In five of the patients examined prior to 1940, the bacteremia was associated with infection, which would be considered manageable today (pneumonia, cellulitis, and osteomyelitis). Seven of 13 patients encountered after 1940 had bacteremia associated with leukemia. Anaerobic bacteremia associated with retropharyngeal or peritonsillar abscesses presumably has preceded anaerobic liver abscesses in several children.[7] Likewise, liver abscesses in neonates may be preceded by a systemic bacteremia without evidence of portal or biliary tract involvement.[32]

Liver abscesses occur more frequently in compromised pediatric hosts than in normal children. Johnston and

Baehner[22] reported that hepatic or perihepatic abscesses were present in 41 of 92 (45 per cent) patients with chronic granulomatous disease. In addition to functional disorders of phagocytes, chronic neutropenia also predisposes to the development of liver abscesses.[37] Wintch and colleagues[48] noted that 5 of 10 children with hepatic abscesses in their institution had an underlying defect in host defense.

Penetrating and nonpenetrating trauma to the liver may lead to liver abscesses, presumably due to bacterial proliferation within small collections of blood and bile that result from the trauma. Hepatic abscess may be a rare complication of ventriculoperitoneal shunts following penetration of peritoneal catheter into the liver.[35] This mode of infection is uncommon in children.

Unexplained or cryptogenic hepatic abscesses are encountered in most series and accounted for nearly 20 per cent of cases in one series.[29] Lee and Block[30] have proposed that these cryptogenic liver abscesses "originate from anaerobic bacterial invasion of hepatic infarcts." This theory is supported by reports that describe pyogenic liver abscesses as a complication of hepatic infarction in patients with sickle cell anemia.[44] Normal gastrointestinal bacterial flora were isolated from 9 of 11 patients with liver abscesses at the Mayo Clinic. This finding suggested to Lazarchick and associates[29] that unrecognized intra-abdominal collections of pus were responsible. Although the reasons are unclear, diabetes mellitus also predisposes to the development of liver abscesses.[1, 20, 39]

Biliary tract disease generally predisposes to the development of multiple liver abscesses. In contrast, blunt trauma to the liver or portal system inflammation most commonly predisposes to a single abscess. In the neonate, liver abscesses may be solitary or multiple because of systemic bacteria.[32, 33] Solitary abscesses are most common in the right lobe of the liver.[29]

Hepatic and splenic abscesses due to *Candida* species are well described in patients with cancer.[45, 47] Multiple abscesses are typical. Presumably, these organs are infected hematogenously, usually at a time when the host is neutropenic.

MICROBIOLOGY

Gram-negative organisms have been the predominant isolates from liver abscesses in adults. *Escherichia coli, Klebsiella, Aerobacter, Pseudomonas,* and *Proteus* species have been implicated most frequently. Anaerobic organisms also are important; anaerobic organisms were recovered from 45 per cent of patients with liver abscesses in the UCLA series.[43] In contrast with the adult experience, Dehner and Kissane[9] reported that 33 per cent of liver abscesses in children were due to *Staphylococcus aureus*, whereas gram-negative organisms were found in only 32 per cent. Two or more organisms were recovered from liver abscesses in 52 per cent of children. In a review of 96 children (no neonates) with pyogenic liver abscesses, *S. aureus*, gram-negative enterics, and anaerobes were the most commonly isolated organisms, in that order.[25] In neonates, gram-negative enterics are isolated most commonly. Anaerobes, particularly *Fusobacterium necrophorum*, have been isolated from liver abscesses in children without underlying disease.[14] Human rotavirus–like particles were identified in the material aspirated from a liver abscess but were considered a secondary phenomenon and not the primary etiology of the liver abscess.[18] Fungi, particularly *Candida albicans,* have been associated with liver abscesses in children with leukemia who have received parenteral hyperalimentation.[2] Most of these children also have systemic *C. albicans* infection.

CLINICAL MANIFESTATIONS

The clinical manifestations of pyogenic liver abscesses are nonspecific. A high index of suspicion plus an awareness of this illness is necessary to make the diagnosis. A history of preceding abdominal surgery or trauma is helpful when present, as is the knowledge that host response to infection is compromised.

Fever, nausea, vomiting, anorexia, weakness, and malaise are prominent symptoms that may last several weeks. Abdominal or pleuritic pain, weight loss, and diarrhea are less common. A history of abdominal pain and fever of unknown origin in an otherwise healthy child suggests the diagnosis of pyogenic liver abscess.[24] In contrast, fever often is not observed in the neonate.[12] Patients with a macroscopic or single abscess frequently experience a subacute to chronic course. In contrast, patients with multiple abscesses generally experience a more acute febrile illness.

Hepatomegaly occurs in 40 to 80 per cent of patients; abdominal tenderness is less common. The presence of right upper quadrant tenderness or even a mass may be subtle and not appreciated unless the physician specifically and carefully examines this region. Other physical findings include jaundice (generally associated with biliary tract disease and not liver abscesses per se), abdominal distension, and evidence of pleuropulmonary involvement (i.e., elevated or fixed hemidiaphragm, rales, and pleural effusion).

DIAGNOSIS

Routine laboratory studies are of little help in attempting to establish a diagnosis. Anemia and leukocytosis are common. Liver function tests generally reflect underlying disease of the liver itself. These changes generally are not caused by the abscess. When abscesses are secondary to biliary tract obstruction, alkaline phosphatase and bilirubin concentrations generally are elevated. Transaminase concentrations generally are normal to mildly elevated in most cases. A rapidly enlarging, tender liver in a patient with normal transaminase concentrations should alert the clinician to the possibility of liver abscess. Lazarchick and colleagues[29] found that the serum albumin concentration was the single most important test with regard to prognosis: 14 of 16 patients with a serum albumin level of less than 2 g/dL died.

Blood cultures are positive more commonly in patients with multiple abscesses than in those with solitary abscesses.

More than 50 per cent of adult patients have abnormalities on chest radiograph. Atelectasis, pulmonary infiltrates, pleural effusion, and elevated or fixed right hemidiaphragm are the most common findings.

Currently, computed tomography (CT) provides the most accurate information concerning the size, location, and number of abscesses within the liver parenchyma (Fig. 58–1).[23, 28, 38] Lesions 1 cm in diameter can be detected by CT. Multiple small abscesses may appear in clusters in a pattern suggesting early coalescence of the abscesses.[21] Liver abscesses appear as areas of low attenuation. The "target" lesions of hepatic candidiasis are not visualized by CT when the patient is neutropenic, and repeat scans may be necessary before these characteristic lesions are observed.[47] Structures contiguous with the liver also are demonstrated by CT; this is important when a surgical approach to drainage is being planned. Magnetic resonance imaging does not have any major advantages over CT for detecting or characterizing liver abscess.[31] Ultrasonography also is a sensitive technique for detecting liver abscesses, and because it is noninvasive and does not require exposure to radiation, it is recom-

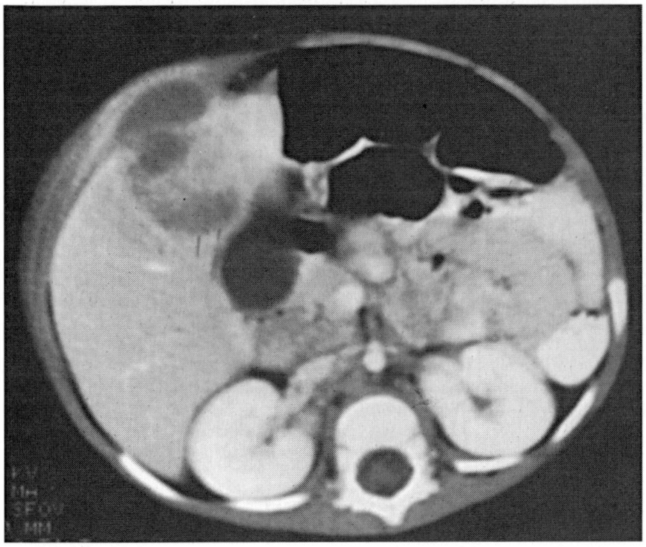

Figure 58–1. *Abdominal computed tomograph showing a 4- × 5-cm encapsulated, septate, circular mass within the liver. A low-density soft-tissue mass is noted in the abdominal wall from apparent extension from the intrahepatic mass.*

mended for initial evaluation.[26, 28] Hepatic angiography further defines the vascular anatomy in the area of the liver abscess and may provide information necessary for surgical management in selected cases. Nuclear medicine techniques rarely are indicated as a diagnostic method if liver abscess is suspected.

TREATMENT

Numerous reports have documented that patients with undiagnosed and untreated liver abscesses generally die and that surgical drainage of the solitary pyogenic liver abscess is the key to successful therapy. The choice of extraserous or transperitoneal open drainage or percutaneous closed aspiration depends on the location and size of the abscess and the experience and preference of the surgeon.[36, 41] A number of surgical investigators have reviewed the surgical management of liver abscesses.[15, 17]

Numerous groups have described percutaneous catheter drainage of liver abscesses in adults.[3, 4, 16, 26] A catheter is placed into the cavity under CT or ultrasound guidance; material is aspirated, and once an abscess is documented, a draining catheter is placed. The cavity can be irrigated with saline initially. Criteria for the selection of patients for percutaneous drainage have been established.[16] Optimally, the route of percutaneous aspiration is direct into the abscess cavity and does not involve any uninfected organs or space. Drainage may proceed for 2 or more weeks or until there is decreased drainage from the cavity, the patient is afebrile and improving, and radiography demonstrates that the cavity is becoming smaller.[19] Surgical back-up is mandatory when this drainage technique is utilized because spillage of abscess material into the peritoneal cavity, hemorrhage, and other complications may occur. Percutaneous drainage of liver abscesses in children has been performed successfully, and this technique can be considered an alternative approach to surgical drainage of such abscesses, especially in the right lobe of the liver.[11, 38]

Appropriate antibiotic therapy initially is based on knowledge of the organisms most commonly involved, Gram stain of the purulent material, and culture and susceptibility to antibiotics of the organisms that are recovered.

If a hematogenous source of infection is suspected or the host has an immune deficiency disease, *S. aureus* and streptococci are more likely. Biliary tract disease and blunt trauma more frequently are associated with gram-negative aerobic and anaerobic organisms. A logical antibiotic combination for the initial therapy of children with liver abscesses includes a penicillinase-resistant penicillin, such as nafcillin, plus an aminoglycoside. The optimal duration and route of administration of antibiotics for children with a solitary pyogenic liver abscess that has been drained have not been determined. In general, 2 to 4 weeks of antibiotic therapy administered parenterally, followed by an appropriate oral antibiotic to complete a (minimum) 4-week total course, should prove adequate.

Penicillin, clindamycin, chloramphenicol, cefoxitin, or metronidazole is administered for anaerobic isolates, depending on susceptibility.

Multiple liver abscesses are more difficult to treat because complete surgical drainage usually is not possible. Prolonged antibiotic therapy plus treatment of any underlying illnesses is the keystone to effective management. Sabbaj and associates[42, 43] recommend 4 months of therapy with appropriate antibiotics for patients with multiple hepatic abscesses.

Fungal liver abscesses are difficult to document by culture of the abscess material; thus, histologic evidence of a fungal infection of the liver must be sought.[2] Amphotericin B, with or without fluorocytosine, is administered in the treatment of fungal liver abscesses.[47] In a neutropenic rabbit model, combination therapy with amphotericin and fluorocytosine was superior to amphotericin B alone in clearing disseminated candidiasis.[46] The optimal duration of therapy is unknown, but prolonged therapy, guided by repeat CT and biopsies, should be provided until the lesions have resolved.[47]

COMPLICATIONS AND PROGNOSIS

Complications of hepatic abscesses are variable and relatively common. Twenty-eight per cent of the patients reported by Rubin and associates[41] and 44 per cent of the patients studied by Pitt and Zuidema[39] had one or more complications. Pleural and pulmonary inflammation, peritonitis, subphrenic or subhepatic abscesses, and hemobilia are just a few of the possible complications.[9, 41]

Polymicrobial bacteremia, hypoalbuminemia, multiple liver abscesses, or the presence of any complication is associated with increased mortality rates in patients with liver abscesses. The overall mortality rates largely depend on underlying pathology and therefore are difficult to interpret. Nevertheless, mortality figures from recent reports vary between 15 and 80 per cent. An increased awareness and suspicion of liver abscesses, in conjunction with newer diagnostic techniques, should reduce substantially the mortality of this disease.

References

1. Altemeier, W. A., Schowengerdt, C. G., and Whiteley, D. H.: Abscesses of the liver: Surgical considerations. Arch. Surg. *101*:258–265, 1970.
2. Bartley, D. L., Hughes, W. T., Parvey, L. S., et al.: Computed tomography of hepatic and splenic fungal abscesses in leukemic children. Pediatr. Infect. Dis. *1*:317–321, 1982.
3. Berger, L. A., and Osborne, D. R.: Treatment of pyogenic liver abscesses by percutaneous needle aspiration. Lancet *1*:132–134, 1982.
4. Bernardino, M. E., Berkman, W. A., Plemmons, M., et al.: Percutaneous drainage of multiseptated hepatic abscess. J. Comput. Assist. Tomogr. *8*:38–41, 1984.

5. Brans, Y. M., Ceballos, R., and Cassady, G.: Umbilical catheters and hepatic abscesses. Pediatrics *53*:264–265, 1974.
6. Branum, G. D., Tyson, G. S., Branum, M. A., et al.: Hepatic abscess: Changes in etiology, diagnosis, and management. Ann. Surg. *212*:655, 1990.
7. Brook, I., and Fraizer, E. H.: Role of anaerobic bacteria in liver abscesses in children. Pediatr. Infect. Dis. J. *12*:743, 1993.
8. Chusid, M. J.: Pyogenic hepatic abscess in infancy and childhood. Pediatrics *62*:554–559, 1978.
9. Dehner, L. P., and Kissane, J. M.: Pyogenic hepatic abscesses in infancy and childhood. J. Pediatr. *74*:763–773, 1969.
10. de la Maza, L. M., Faramary, N., and Berman, L. D.: The changing etiology of liver abscess. J. A. M. A. *227*:161–163, 1974.
11. Diament, M. J., Stanley, P., Kangarloo, H., et al.: Percutaneous aspiration and catheter drainage of abscesses. J. Pediatr. *108*:204–208, 1986.
12. Doerr, C. A., Demmler, G. J., Garcia-Pratts, J. A., et al.: Solitary pyogenic liver abscess in neonates: Report of three cases and review of the literature. Pediatr. Infect. Dis. J. *13*:64, 1994.
13. Ecoffey, C., Rothman, E., Bernard, O., et al.: Bacterial cholangitis after surgery for biliary atresia. J. Pediatr. *111*:824–829, 1987.
14. Embree, J. E., Williams, T., and Law, B. J.: Hepatic abscesses in a child caused by *Fusobacterium necrophorum*. Pediatr. Infect. Dis. *7*:359–360, 1988.
15. Gaisford, W. D., and Mack, J. B. D.: Surgical management of hepatic abscess. Am. J. Surg. *118*:317–326, 1969.
16. Gerzof, S. G., Robbins, A. H., Johnson, W. C., et al.: Percutaneous catheter drainage of abdominal abscesses: A five-year experience. N. Engl. J. Med. *305*:353–357, 1981.
17. Goldsmith, H. S., and Chen, W. F.: Management of a pyogenic abscess of the liver. Surg. Clin. North Am. *53*:711–715, 1973.
18. Grunow, J. E., Dunton, S. F., and Waner, J. L.: Human rotavirus-like particles in a hepatic abscess. J. Pediatr. *106*:73–76, 1985.
19. Hoffer, F. A., Fellows, K. E., Wyly, J. B., et al.: Therapeutic catheter procedures in pediatrics. Pediatr. Clin. North Am. *32*:1461, 1985.
20. Holt, J. M., and Spry, C. J. F.: Solitary pyogenic liver abscess in patients with diabetes mellitus. Lancet *2*:198–200, 1966.
21. Jeffrey, R. B., Jr., Tolentino, C. S., Chang, F. C., et al.: CT of small pyogenic hepatic abscesses: The cluster sign. A. J. R. Am. J. Roentgenol. *151*:487–489, 1988.
22. Johnston, R. B., and Baehner, R. L.: Chronic granulomatous disease: Correlation between pathogenesis and clinical findings. Pediatrics *48*:730–739, 1971.
23. Kandel, G., and Marcon, N. E.: Pyogenic liver abscess: New concepts of an old disease. Am. J. Gastroenterol. *79*:65–71, 1984.
24. Kaplan, S. L., and Feigin, R. D.: Pyogenic liver abscess in normal children with fever of unknown origin. Pediatrics *58*:614–616, 1976.
25. Kays, D.W.: Pediatric liver cysts and abscesses. Semin. Pediatr. Surg. *1*:107, 1992.
26. Kuligowska, E., Connors, S. K., and Shapiro, J. H.: Liver abscess: Sonography in diagnosis and treatment. A. J. R. Am. J. Roentgenol. *138*:253–257, 1982.
27. Kusne, S., Dummer, J. S., Singh, N., et al.: Infections after liver transplantation: An analysis of 101 consecutive cases. Medicine *67*:132–143, 1988.
28. Laurin, S., and Kaude, J. V.: Diagnosis of liver-spleen abscesses in children: With emphasis on ultrasound for the initial and follow-up examinations. Pediatr. Radiol. *14*:198–204, 1984.
29. Lazarchick, J., DeSouza, E., Silvia, N. A., et al.: Pyogenic liver abscess. Mayo Clin. Proc. *48*:349–355, 1973.
30. Lee, J. F., and Block, G. E.: The changing clinical pattern of hepatic abscesses. Arch. Surg. *104*:456–470, 1972.
31. Mendez, R. J., Schiebler, M. L., Outwater, E. K. et al.: Hepatic abscesses: MR imaging findings. Radiology *190*:431, 1994.
32. Moss, T. J., and Pysher, T. J.: Hepatic abscess in neonates. Am. J. Dis. Child. *135*:726–728, 1981.
33. Murphy, F. M., and Baker, C. J.: Solitary hepatic abscess: A delayed complication of neonatal bacteremia. Pediatr. Infect. Dis. *7*:414–416, 1988.
34. Noel, G. J., and Karasic, R. B.: Liver abscess following ingestion of a foreign body. Pediatr. Infect. Dis. *3*:342–344, 1984.
35. Paone, R. F., and Mercer, L. C.: Hepatic abscess caused by a ventriculoperitoneal shunt. Pediatr. Infect. Dis. J. *10*:338, 1991.
36. Patterson, H. C.: Open aspiration in solitary liver abscess. Am. J. Surg. *119*:326–329, 1970.
37. Pincus, S. H., Boxer, L. A., and Stossel, T. P.: Chronic neutropenia in childhood: Analysis of 16 cases and a review of the literature. Am. J. Med. *61*:849–861, 1976.
38. Pineiro-Carrero, V. M., and Andres, J. M.: Morbidity and mortality in children with pyogenic liver abscess. Am. J. Dis. Child. *143*:1424–1427, 1989.
39. Pitt, H. A., and Zuidema, G. D.: Factors influencing mortality in the treatment of pyogenic hepatic abscess. Surg. Gynecol. Obstet. *140*:228–234, 1975.
40. Rogers, C. A., Isenberg, J. N., Leonard, A. S., et al.: Ascending cholangitis diagnosed by percutaneous hepatic aspiration. J. Pediatr. *88*:83–86, 1976.
41. Rubin, R. H., Swartz, M. N., and Malt, R.: Hepatic abscess: Changes in clinical, bacteriologic and therapeutic aspects. Am. J. Med. *57*:601–610, 1974.
42. Sabbaj, J.: Anaerobes in liver abscess. Rev. Infect. Dis. *6*:S152–S156, 1984.
43. Sabbaj, J., Sutter, V. L., and Finegold, S. M.: Anaerobic pyogenic liver abscess. Ann. Intern. Med. *77*:629–638, 1972.
44. Shulman, S. T., and Beem, M. O.: A unique presentation of sickle cell disease: Pyogenic hepatic abscess. Pediatrics *47*:1019–1022, 1971.
45. Tashjian, L. S., Abramson, J. S., and Peacock, J. E., Jr.: Focal hepatic candidiasis: A distinct clinical variant of candidiasis in immunocompromised patients. Rev. Infect. Dis. *6*:689–703, 1984.
46. Thaler, M., Bacher, J., O'Leary, T., et al.: Evaluation of single-drug combination antifungal therapy in an experimental model of candidiasis in rabbits with prolonged neutropenia. J. Infect. Dis. *158*:80–88, 1988.
47. Thaler, M., Pastakia, B., Shawker, T. H., et al.: Hepatic candidiasis in cancer patients: The evolving picture of the syndrome. Ann. Intern. Med. *108*:88–100, 1988.
48. Wintch, R. W., Reines, H. D., and Rambo, W. M.: Liver abscess: A changing entity Am. J. Surg. *48*:11–15, 1982.

59

REYE SYNDROME

James P. Keating

Reye syndrome is defined as acute postinfectious encephalopathy with microvesicular fat in the liver parenchyma and elevation of serum transaminases. In fact, the clinical presentation is striking. The usual patient, recovering from a mild viral illness, develops a disturbance in consciousness heralded by persistent retching, which is followed after a few hours by confusion and delirium. Fever, hyperventilation, and leukocytosis suggest an infectious process, but spinal fluid and pathology specimens from liver and brain contain little evidence of inflammation. The stereotyped postures (decorticate, decerebrate, and opisthotonos) of deep coma and death may occur within 2 days of the onset of vomiting. The illness in its classic form is distinctive, explosive, and terrifying.

EPIDEMIOLOGY

The syndrome affects the sexes equally. It probably occurs in all countries, but most epidemiologic data are derived from observations made in Australia, the United States, the United Kingdom, South Africa, and Thailand. For reasons yet undetermined, the illness predominantly occurs in white children, is rare after 18 years of age, is more likely to attack rural and suburban children (1.8 cases per 100,000 population younger than 18 years of age) than their city-living contemporaries (0.42 per 100,000 population younger than 18 years of age), and is associated strongly with mild infectious illnesses[8] caused by the influenza B and varicella viruses.

Reye syndrome rarely attacks more than one child in a

family, but siblings appear to be affected more frequently than can be explained by chance or by a heightened awareness of the symptoms of the syndrome in the parents of an affected child.[3,9] In some families, the second sibling's illness occurred years after the first. The rarity of recurrence of the syndrome in survivors argues against persistent individual susceptibility. Episodes mimicking Reye syndrome[13] occur in youngsters with defects in ureagenesis and fatty acid metabolism, but metabolic defects have not been found in Reye syndrome survivors. A toxic cause of Reye syndrome has not been proved, despite clinical similarities to Jamaican vomiting illness (hypoglycin toxicity), aflatoxin poisoning, and salicylate toxicity.

Reye syndrome is a reportable disease in most states. Influenza B–related "clusters" of cases occurred in 1962, 1967, 1969, 1974, 1977, and 1980. In the 1973/1974 outbreak, 326 cases were recognized, with a case-fatality rate of 41 per cent.[8] In 1980, 335 cases were reported, with a fatality rate of 12 per cent.[4] Several case-control studies identified a statistical association between aspirin taken during the antecedent viral illness and the development of Reye syndrome.[16] Although the etiologic role of aspirin has not been proved, both the use of aspirin during minor childhood illness[19] and the frequency of diagnosis of Reye syndrome decreased during the 1980s (Table 59–1).[5] In 1984, the median age increased, a change that may reflect a reduction in salicylate use in young children.

CLINICAL MANIFESTATIONS

Persistent retching usually is the first symptom. It may begin within a day of the onset of the antecedent viral illness but more typically starts 4 or 5 days later, often as the child returns to his or her usual activities. The duration of vomiting usually is less than 24 hours. Confusion begins as the vomiting abates and commonly is misinterpreted as a side effect of antiemetic medications. As vomiting ceases, the child is perceived to be frightened, confused, and detached (stage I). Next, perseveration and profanity occur and, as the coma deepens, merge with unnerving screams. The pupils are large and become decreasingly reactive to light; occasional patients complain of being unable to see. Agitated delirium (stage II) can persist for 24 hours and can progress at any time to deeper coma. Decorticate and decerebrate posturing (stage III and stage IV, respectively) appears, and ultimately brain stem reflexes (pupillary and oculovestibular) are lost (stage V). The complete neurologic sequence usually is completed within 2 days of onset. Later deterioration is exceptional, and if it occurs, complicating infection should be suspected.[6] Neither papilledema nor elevation in cerebrospinal fluid pressure is found early in the illness.

Death occurs within 2 to 3 days of onset, although modern life support techniques may delay or change the outcome. Happily, deterioration may stop at any point. A child who is decerebrate one day may demand food the next (an occurrence that has great potential for reinforcement of whatever therapy was employed). A slower path to recovery is taken by many patients, and neurologic improvement may occur as late as several months after the acute episode. Full neurologic recovery is the rule, but some patients suffer severe neurologic sequelae.[2]

The syndrome has been described in children with leukemia, Kawasaki disease, juvenile rheumatoid arthritis, systemic lupus erythematosus, rheumatic fever, sickle-cell anemia, nephrotic syndrome, juvenile diabetes mellitus, seizure disorders, and mental retardation.[9] When the victim suffers from a preexisting illness, it may be difficult, even with a properly processed liver biopsy, to be certain of the diagnosis.

The signs and symptoms of pancreatitis dominate the early clinical picture in a minority of cases,[9] and several patients have undergone exploratory laparotomy. The biochemical and clinical course of Reye syndrome patients with elevated serum amylase concentrations differs little from that of the group as a whole, although extraordinary fluid needs and hypocalcemia may occur.

Azotemia and oliguria may be no more than reflections of the dehydrated state, which usually is present on admittance and is aggravated by osmotic diuresis and restricted water infusion. Fatty changes are seen in renal tubular cells, but the lesion in most patients is mild. Successful transplantation has been achieved using kidneys taken from Reye patients.[12] Hyperuricemia (serum uric acid may be as high as 15 mg/dL) is believed to be a result of increased production as well as decreased excretion.

TABLE 59–1. Reye Syndrome (RS) Incidence

Year	Total	Varicella-Associated	Incidence of RS*	Fatality Rate (%)
1974	379	—	0.6	41
1977	454	73	0.7	42
1978	236	69	0.4	29
1979	389	113	0.6	32
1980	555	103	0.9	23
1981	297	77	0.5	30
1982	213	45	0.3	35
1983	198	28	0.3	31
1984	204	26	0.3	26
1985	93	15	0.2	31
1986	101	5	0.2	27
1987	36	7	0.1	29
1988	20	4	0.0	30

*Per 100,000 United States population younger than 18 years of age.
Modified from Centers for Disease Control: Reye syndrome surveillance: United States, 1987 and 1988. M. M. W. R. *38*:325–327, 1989.

PATHOPHYSIOLOGY

The antecedent viral illnesses are, at least in retrospect, no more severe than those occurring in the general population. Even in influenza B epidemics, Reye syndrome occurs in a tiny minority of infected children (1 in 20,000). These observations have led to speculation concerning host factors (e.g., hereditary enzymatic deficiency, environmental toxins, medications) that might be necessary for the development of the syndrome. Investigation continues, but the pathophysiology of the syndrome is descriptive and speculative.

The presence of a metabolic encephalopathy combined with evidence of hepatic disturbance led some authorities to speculate that Reye syndrome was a form of hepatic coma, a belief that shaped early therapeutic efforts (e.g., neomycin, exchange transfusion, plasmapheresis). Although the neurologic and metabolic findings in Reye syndrome are similar to those that occur in acute hepatic failure, the time course is much shorter in the syndrome and jaundice is absent.

Another theory of pathogenesis centers on an early mitochondrial injury. Based on the ultrastructure of liver tissue obtained by needle biopsy, investigators in Cincinnati demonstrated morphologic changes in mitochondria early in the illness. Transient depression of mitochondrial function, reflected in the activity of the enzyme ornithine transcarbamylase,[1] corroborated the morphologic observations.

Serum enzyme abnormalities include elevations in serum

glutamic-oxaloacetic transaminase (aspartate transaminase), serum glutamic-pyruvic transaminase (alanine transaminase), L-lactate dehydrogenase, creatine kinase, and, occasionally, amylase. Transaminase values range from 2 to 200 times the normal range but usually are between 200 and 600 mIU/mL. Serum alkaline phosphatase and gamma-glutamyltranspeptidase are normal. Prothrombin time usually is prolonged by 3 to 10 seconds. Histopathologic evidence of skeletal and cardiac muscle, as well as pancreas, liver, and brain involvement, indicates that multiple organs may contribute to the serum enzyme abnormalities.[21]

Blood ammonia concentrations usually are elevated in comatose patients but may be normal. When these concentrations are measured early in the illness, a value in excess of 500 μg/dL is predictive of a severe course of illness.

Hypoglycemia, present in 13 of 19 patients in the original report,[20] is, in fact, an infrequent finding. Depletion of hepatic glycogen has been observed histologically; impaired hepatic gluconeogenesis is reflected in accumulation of precursors (lactate, pyruvate, alanine) in serum and defective pyruvate incorporation into glucose.[14, 15] The relative contributions of starvation, increased utilization, and decreased gluconeogenesis probably vary from patient to patient; normal blood glucose concentrations are maintained easily by intravenous infusion of glucose-containing fluids.

Aminoaciduria was described in the original report. Increased serum concentrations of the gluconeogenic amino acids have been documented amply[15]; the pattern of the aminogram is similar to that found in serum from patients with fulminant hepatic failure. Efforts to affect the course by infusion of amino acid solutions have not been effective.

The characteristic acid-base findings are those of a mixed disturbance.[11] Laboratory values on admittance typically indicate primary respiratory alkalosis ($P_{CO_2} \leq 25$ mm Hg) and primary metabolic acidosis ($CO_2 \leq 15$ mEq/L); pH often is in, or near, the normal range, despite significant abnormalities in the other Henderson-Hasselbalch variables. This complex disturbance, also seen in salicylism, hepatic coma, and endotoxemia, is attributed to disturbances in the brain stem respiratory control centers and in oxidative metabolism in liver and muscle. If respiratory failure does not occur, hyperventilation and hypocapnia persist for 24 to 48 hours. Extreme hypocapnia ($P_{CO_2} < 20$ mm Hg) may occur for hours in patients fated to make a complete recovery.

Controversy exists concerning hyperventilation in Reye syndrome. The reduction in cerebral blood flow that is associated with hypocapnia may be beneficial, because cerebral edema occurs in most severely ill Reye syndrome patients; conversely, reduction of blood flow to the brain may produce ischemic injury. If hyperventilation is a salutary response, the patient should be permitted to maintain his or her own respiratory pattern; if hyperventilation is viewed by the clinician as dangerous, pharmacologic paralysis and mechanical ventilation are substituted, usually maintaining a P_{CO_2} of 25 mm Hg.

Hypophosphatemia, which may disrupt the transport and utilization of oxygen, has occurred in patients with Reye syndrome receiving phosphate-free glucose solutions.[17] The reported serum inorganic phosphorus concentrations (<1.0 mg/dL [normal, 4.5 to 6.5 mg/dL]), if sustained for 24 hours, may be associated with a reduction in erythrocytic organic phosphates and a shift in the oxygen-hemoglobin dissociation curve. Although available data indicate that the hypophosphatemic period is too brief to be of major importance in most Reye syndrome patients, the use of phosphate-containing fluids and monitoring of serum concentrations of phosphate are recommended.

DIAGNOSIS AND DIFFERENTIAL DIAGNOSIS

The clinical diagnosis of Reye syndrome can be made if there is (1) acute onset of a disturbance in consciousness, (2) elevation of aspartate transaminase or alanine transaminase to twice-normal concentrations, (3) histologic changes consistent with the syndrome seen in biopsy specimens or postmortem material, and (4) absence of another reasonable explanation for the findings. When the classic temporal sequence of symptoms and signs occurs in clustered cases, diagnosis can be made with confidence on the basis of the aforementioned criteria. When the presentation is atypical, additional studies may be necessary. Both liver biopsy and lumbar puncture are diagnostic procedures that improve the accuracy of diagnosis. Unfortunately, neither is free of complications, and the risk must be weighed against the potential value for each patient. Satisfaction of the fourth criterion demands a careful history, which, in the circumstances surrounding this illness, can be a test of the physician's equanimity, experience, and breadth of knowledge. Emphasis should be placed on drug intoxication, unwitnessed head trauma, central nervous system infection, and inborn errors of metabolism.

Salicylate hepatoxicity may cause serum enzyme elevations when alteration in consciousness is due to some process other than Reye syndrome. When the serum salicylate concentration exceeds 20 mg/dL, owing to the excessive dosage or dehydration, transaminase elevations quantitatively similar to those seen in Reye syndrome may be found. Cumulative salicylism, a serious form of salicylate intoxication, shares many clinical features with Reye syndrome, including severe neurologic dysfunction and death.[18] Acetaminophen and intramuscular injections of antibiotics, anticonvulsants, or antiemetics may cause serum enzyme elevations. The combination of one or more of these medicines and a disturbance in consciousness from ingestion, trauma, vascular lesions, or infection of the central nervous system may lead to an incorrect diagnosis of Reye syndrome.

Fulminant hepatic failure causes an acute encephalopathic illness with agitation, posturing, mydriasis, hyperventilation, hypoprothrombinemia, and a mixed acid-base disturbance similar to that observed in Reye syndrome patients. Jaundice always is absent in Reye syndrome and almost always is present in fulminant hepatic failure. A history of exposure to hepatotoxins should be sought. In some patients, liver biopsy is the only means by which the two entities can be differentiated.

A delirious or confusional state may occur in acute pancreatitis, owing to pancreatic enzymes released into the circulation or central nervous system or to hypovolemia, hypocalcemia, narcotic overdose, or head trauma. Distinguishing between pancreatic encephalopathy and Reye syndrome may present difficulty in comatose children with hyperamylasemia.

In addition, those inborn errors of metabolism that are associated with hyperammonemia and neurologic disturbances, particularly ornithine transcarbamylase deficiency, carnitine deficiency,[7] glutaric aciduria, variants of the ketotic hyperglycinemia, and defects of fatty acid metabolism, are important considerations. Hypoglycemia, transaminase elevations, and hepatic steatosis are features of glycogen storage disease, fructose-1,6-diphosphatase deficiency, and fructose aldolase deficiency.

TREATMENT

Treatment consists of intensive supportive care[10] directed at airway maintenance, tissue oxygenation, and control of cerebral edema. Early diagnosis and glucose infusion may improve prognosis, if only by reducing the likelihood of inappropriate medical and surgical therapy. The prevention of coma by initiation of glucose infusion early in the illness is emphasized by some authorities. Exchange transfusion, plasmapheresis, peritoneal dialysis, hypothermic total-body washout, amino acid infusion, bowel sterilization, and barbiturate coma have been reported as helpful, but none is of proven value.

Although there is no proof of a causal role of aspirin, prudent practitioners avoid its use in children with viral illness, exceptions being made when the value of the medication outweighs the possible risk.

References

1. Brown, T., Hug, G., Lansky, L., et al.: Transiently reduced activity of carbamyl phosphate synthetase and ornithine, transcarbamylase in livers of children with Reye syndrome. N. Engl. J. Med. *294*:861–867, 1976.
2. Brunner, R. L., O'Grady, D. J., Partin, J. C., et al.: Neuropsychologic consequences of Reye syndrome. J. Pediatr. *95*:706–711, 1979.
3. Centers for Disease Control: Reye syndrome in three siblings. M. M. W. R. *28*:64–69, 1979.
4. Centers for Disease Control: Reye syndrome. M. M. W. R. *29*:112, 1980.
5. Centers for Disease Control: Reye syndrome surveillance: United States, 1987 and 1988. M. M. W. R. *38*:325–327, 1989.
6. Chalhub, E. G., DeVivo, D. C., Keating, J. P., et al.: Reye syndrome complicated by a generalized herpes simplex type I infection. J. Pediatr. *98*:73–76, 1981.
7. Chapoy, P. R., Angelini, C., Brown, W. J., et al.: Systemic carnitine deficiency: A treatable inherited lipid-storage disease presenting as Reye's syndrome. N. Engl. J. Med. *303*:1389–1394, 1980.
8. Corey, L., Rubin, R. J., Hattwick, M. A. W., et al.: A nationwide outbreak of Reye's syndrome: Its epidemiologic relationship to influenza B. Am. J. Med. *61*:615–625, 1976.
9. DeVivo, D. C., and Keating, J. P.: Reye's syndrome. Adv. Pediatr. *22*:175–229, 1975.
10. DeVivo, D. C., Keating, J. P., and Haymond, M. W.: Acute encephalopathy with fatty infiltration of the viscera. Pediatr. Clin. North Am. *23*:527–538, 1976.
11. DeVivo, D. C., Keating, J. P., and Haymond, M. W.: Reye syndrome: Results of intensive support care. J. Pediatr. *87*:875–880, 1975.
12. Firlit, C. F., Jonasson, O. J., Kahan, B. D., et al.: Reye's syndrome cadaveric kidneys: Their use in human transplantation. Arch. Surg. *109*:797, 1974.
13. Glasgow, A. M.: Reye's syndrome mimickers. J. Natl. Reye Syndrome Found. *1*:105, 1980.
14. Haymond, M. W., Karl, I. E., DeVivo, D. C., et al.: Sequential metabolic observations in Reye's syndrome. *In* Pollack, J. D. (ed.): Reye's Syndrome. New York, Grune & Stratton, 1975, pp. 215–225.
15. Haymond, M. W., Karl, I. E., Keating, J. P., et al.: Metabolic response to hypertonic glucose administration in Reye syndrome. Ann. Neurol. *3*:207–215, 1978.
16. Hurwitz, E. S., Barrett, M. J., Bregman, D., et al.: Public Health Service study on Reye's syndrome and medications. N. Engl. J. Med. *313*:849–857, 1985.
17. Keating, J. P., Karl, I. E., DeVivo, D. C., et al.: Hypophosphatemia in Reye's syndrome. *In* Pollack, J. D. (ed.): Reye's Syndrome. New York, Grune & Stratton, 1975, pp. 255–259.
18. Makela, A. L., Lang, H., and Koppella, P.: Toxic encephalopathy with hyperammonemia during high-dose salicylate therapy. Acta Neurol. Scand. *61*:146–151, 1980.
19. Remington, P. L., Rowley, D., McGee, H., et al.: Decreasing trends in Reye syndrome and aspirin use in Michigan, 1979 to 1984. Pediatrics *77*:93–98, 1986.
20. Reye, R. D. K., Morgan, G., and Baral, J.: Encephalopathy and fatty degeneration of the viscera: A disease entity in childhood. Lancet *2*:749–752, 1963.
21. Roe, C. R., Schonberger, L. B., Gelbach, S. H., et al.: Enzymatic alterations in Reye's syndrome: Prognostic implications. Pediatrics *55*:119–126, 1975.

SECTION EIGHT

OTHER INTRA-ABDOMINAL INFECTIONS

❑ ❑ ❑

60

APPENDICITIS AND PELVIC ABSCESS

Thomas L. Kuhls

The ability to diagnose appendicitis accurately in a child continues to be one of the most fundamental skills that a pediatric surgeon has to master, although the diagnosis often is difficult in young patients. The surgeon ultimately is responsible for deciding whether a child is taken to the operating room for appendectomy; however, a primary care physician often is the first person to evaluate the patient who complains of abdominal pain. Pediatricians with expertise in infectious diseases frequently are involved in the care of children who present with subtle or atypical manifestations of appendicitis, have unusual microorganisms recovered from their appendices, or have complications as a result of appendiceal rupture, such as the development of wound infections, sepsis, peritonitis, intra-abdominal abscesses, and pelvic abscesses.

HISTORY

As early as the 16th century, physicians began describing patients with clinical manifestations suggestive of perforated appendicitis. Until the late 1800s, the inflammatory process was called typhlitis or perityphlitis because it was believed that the illness originated from the cecum. In 1886, Reginald Fitz[51] recognized that the source of the inflammation was the appendix and suggested that a laparotomy be performed early in the course of the illness. Shortly afterwards, Charles McBurney[95] reported that in patients with appendicitis, tenderness is greatest 2 inches from the anterior iliac spine on a line drawn to the umbilicus. Despite intensive research and refinement of our understanding of appendicitis during the last century, the accuracy of diagnosing this inflammatory process has not improved substantially. The rates of removing nondiseased appendices or finding already perforated appendices at laparotomy both remain at approximately 20 per cent.

Despite the continued difficulties in diagnosing appendicitis, the mortality rate from appendicitis greatly has decreased since Fitz reported a 40 per cent operative mortality rate. In 1936, Bancroft and Skoluda[13] reported a mortality rate of 8 per cent and a complication rate of 11 per cent for appendicitis, most likely because of the availabilities of general anesthesia and better aseptic surgical techniques. The second major improvement in outcome occurred in the 1940s, when sulfonamides and banked blood widely became available.[93] It was not until the 1970s that anaerobes, such as *Bacteroides fragilis*, were found frequently to cause postoperative infections in patients with appendicitis and that treating these microorganisms could reduce further the rate of postoperative complications.[77] In the 1990s, death from appendicitis is rare in the United States.

PATHOPHYSIOLOGY

It is believed that the initial event in the development of most cases of appendicitis is obstruction of the appendiceal lumen.[138] Only occasionally do microorganisms invade the appendiceal mucosa and initiate the inflammatory process. Appendiceal obstruction can be caused by inspissated feces (fecalith), hypertrophied lymphoid tissue that develops during a systemic viral infection or bacterial enterocolitis, infestation by parasites, appendiceal wall hemorrhage associated with anaphylactic purpura, inspissated barium, or ingested seeds. Continued mucus production by the appendiceal mucosa distal to the obstruction causes the appendix to distend. Vascular congestion and ischemia occur as the increased intraluminal pressure of the appendix becomes greater than the venous pressure, and edema develops as lymphatic flow becomes obstructed. Stasis of intestinal flow and intestinal ischemia allow the microorganisms in the appendix to invade the tissues, and this enhances the already developing inflammatory response. Bacteria then may translocate across the appendiceal wall and reach the peritoneal cavity.[14] If the process is severe and arteriolar blood flow to the appendix is obstructed, transmural infarction occurs and the appendix ruptures. Microorganisms then are liberated into the peritoneal cavity, causing generalized peritonitis and abscess formation. Animal studies have suggested that synergism between enteric aerobes, such as *Escherichia coli*, and anaerobes, such as *B. fragilis*, is important in the development of intra-abdominal and pelvic abscesses after perforation.[57]

As the appendix distends in the early stages of appendicitis, the visceral afferent autonomic nerves that enter the spinal cord at T8 to T10 are stimulated, thus referring the pain to the epigastric and periumbilical areas of the abdomen.[138] When the inflammatory response reaches the serosal surface of the appendix, the parietal peritoneum is stimulated and the pain intensifies in the right lower quadrant. If perforation occurs, the peritoneal inflammatory response causes more generalized abdominal tenderness.

Although appendiceal obstruction may play an important role in the early stages of most cases of appendicitis, not all obstructed appendices become inflamed. Ten per cent of normal appendices removed during abdominal surgical procedures contain inspissated fecal material. Also, children may develop recurrent, crampy abdominal pain, possibly from intermittent appendiceal obstruction.[129]

The classic description of the pathophysiology of appendicitis does not explain easily many epidemiologic features of this disease, including its peak incidence during adolescence, its low incidence in newborns and infants, its higher incidence in males, and its higher incidences in certain races. It has been suggested that the amount and reactivity of the lymphoid tissue in the wall of the appendix are key determinants to the development of appendicitis.[85] The amount of lymphoid tissue in the appendix is greatest during adolescence and may be genetic. In a case-control study from Italy, prolonged breast feeding during infancy was associated with a decreased risk of developing acute appendicitis later in life.[117] The investigators hypothesized that breast feeding may have decreased the amount of stimulation to intestinal lymphocytes by microbial and food antigens early in life, so that appendiceal lymphoid tissues were less reactive to antigenic challenge during adolescence and adulthood.

MICROBIOLOGY

Numerous microorganisms have been implicated as a cause of acute appendicitis; however, there has been considerable debate as to whether or not simply isolating an organism from the appendical lumen is enough proof to define causation (Table 60–1).[1] There have been scattered reports from mostly developing countries that demonstrate parasites (*Balantidium coli, Entamoeba histolytica, Strongyloides stercoralis, Enterobius vermicularis, Schistosoma* species, *Cryptosporidium parvum*, and *Angiostrongylus costaricensis*) within inflamed appendiceal tissues, suggesting that the parasites may have initiated the inflammation.[3, 40, 83, 91, 101, 105, 123, 134] Also, it is plausible that roundworms, such as *Ascaris lumbricoides*, occasionally obstruct the appendiceal lumen and initiate the cascade of inflammatory events leading to perforated appendicitis.[89, 112] Parasites such as *E. vermicularis*, however, can be identified in the lumina of 1 to 12 per cent of surgically removed appendices obtained from persons living in highly endemic areas.[22] In some studies, pinworms were found more frequently in appendices that had no evidence of appendiceal inflammation; thus, they probably were a part of the normal appendiceal flora and were not causing the patient's abdominal pain, or they caused symptoms that mimicked acute appendicitis necessitating surgical intervention.[37, 157] Other parasites that have been identified in the lumen of appendices from patients who have undergone surgery for abdominal pain include *Taenia* species, *Anisakis* species, and *Trichuris trichiura*.[7, 44, 59]

TABLE 60–1. Microorganisms Associated with Acute Appendicitis in Children

Parasites	**Enteric Aerobes**
Balantidium coli	*Escherichia coli*
Entamoeba histolytica	*Shigella* species
Strongyloides stercoralis	*Salmonella* species
Enterobius vermicularis	*Campylobacter* species
Schistosoma species	*Yersinia* species
Cryptosporidium parvum	*Enterococcus* species
Angiostrongylus costaricensis	*Streptococcus milleri*
Ascaris lumbricoides	*Citrobacter* species
Taenia species	*Klebsiella* species
Anisakis species	*Enterobacter* species
Trichuris trichiura	*Proteus* species
Viruses	**Other Bacteria**
Coxsackieviruses B	*Streptococcus pneumoniae*
Adenoviruses	*Haemophilus influenzae*
Epstein-Barr	*Haemophilus segnis*
Measles	*Pasteurella multocida*
Cytomegalovirus (in AIDS patients)	*Pseudomonas* species
	Eikenella corrodens
	Staphylococcus species
Anaerobes	
Bacteroides species	
Bilophilia wadsworthia	
Peptostreptococcus species	
Fusobacterium species	
Clostridium species	

Bacterial pathogens, such as *Shigella* species, *Salmonella* species, *Campylobacter* species, and *Yersinia* species, have been isolated occasionally from appendiceal tissues or peritoneal fluid of persons with nonperforated and perforated appendicitis; but again, it is unknown if they played a role in the pathogenesis of disease.[19, 31, 71, 111, 152] It is much more common for these organisms, however, to cause enterocolitis or mesenteric adenitis, with symptoms mimicking appendicitis.[152] Also, enterohemorrhagic *E. coli* O157:H7 and O111:H have been isolated infrequently from the stools of children with appendicitis.[33, 149] Rarely, encapsulated organisms, such as *Streptococcus pneumoniae, Haemophilus influenzae*, and *Haemophilus segnis*, have been isolated from appendiceal tissues or peritoneal fluid of young children with appendicitis, and often these organisms were isolated in pure culture.[10, 61, 106] *Pasteurella multocida* also has been isolated occasionally from the peritoneal fluid or appendiceal lumen of patients with perforated and nonperforated appendicitis.[121]

The role of viruses in causing appendicitis is controversial, although it has been suggested that a systemic viral infection may cause hypertrophied lymphoid aggregates that obstruct the appendiceal lumen. Thirty years ago, elevated levels of antibodies against coxsackieviruses B or adenoviruses were found in the sera of some children with appendicitis.[147] A later study, however, could not confirm this finding.[102] Six adolescents with infectious mononucleosis have developed appendicitis.[82] Another child has had histologic evidence of measles virus infection in the wall of an inflamed appendix.[54] Because of the rarity of documented simultaneous viral infections and appendicitis, it is doubtful whether these viruses play a major role in the pathogenesis of acute appendicitis.

In most cases of appendicitis, infectious agents do not appear to be involved directly in the initial stages of the inflammatory process. However, microorganisms that normally inhabit the appendix are liberated into the peritoneal cavity when there is appendiceal perforation or when there is translocation through the inflamed tissues; thus, it is not surprising that polymicrobial infections develop as a complication of the disease process.[18, 146] In a study of 30 adolescents and adults with nonperforated and perforated appendicitis, 223 different anaerobes and 82 aerobes were recovered from cultures of their appendiceal tissues, peritoneal fluid, and contents of abscesses.[18] An average of 10 different organisms were isolated per specimen collected. As with previous studies, *E. coli* and *B. fragilis* were the most frequently isolated organisms, occurring in more than 70 per cent of the patients. Other anaerobes that frequently were isolated included *Bacteroides* species, *Bilophila wadsworthia*, *Peptostreptococcus* species, *Fusobacterium* species, and *Clostridium* species. Unlike other studies, group D streptococci were isolated in only 20 per cent of the patients with appendicitis, whereas viridans streptococci (including members of the *Streptococcus milleri* group[67, 87, 118]) and *Pseudomonas* species were isolated more frequently (33 per cent and >25 per cent, respectively).[18]

Other aerobes that occasionally have been isolated from appendiceal tissues or abscesses include *Citrobacter* species; *Eikenella corrodens*; *Klebsiella* species; groups C, F, and G beta-hemolytic streptococci; *Enterobacter* species; *Proteus* species; and staphylococci.[42, 68, 88, 120, 146] Only rarely are yeasts cultured from appendiceal tissues of immunocompetent patients.[42]

Adults and children with appendicitis usually are not bacteremic at the time of diagnosis, especially if the appendix is not perforated. Occasionally, *Klebsiella pneumoniae, E. coli, B. fragilis,* and *B. wadsworthia* are isolated from the blood of patients with nonperforated appendicitis.[20, 113, 116, 128] In a review of 1000 children and adults with appendicitis, 10 per cent of persons with perforation had positive blood cultures, whereas none of the patients without perforation had bacteremia.[78]

In immunocompromised patients who develop appendicitis, the microorganisms that are isolated from appendiceal tissues or peritoneal cultures usually are identical to those found in immunocompetent persons.[104] In adults infected with human immunodeficiency virus, however, appendicitis has been caused by cytomegalovirus infection and neoplastic obstruction of the base of the appendix by Kaposi sarcoma.[32, 79, 108] Patients with acquired immunodeficiency with gastrointestinal *Mycobacterium avium* complex or *Mycobacterium tuberculosis* infections may develop symptoms that mimic appendicitis.[39, 153]

EPIDEMIOLOGY

The reported incidences of acute appendicitis vary widely, depending on where the studies were performed and what methodologies were used. It generally is believed that the numbers of cases of acute appendicitis have been decreasing over the last few decades.[2, 96, 122] In the United States, 1.5 million appendectomies were performed for acute appendicitis during the years 1979 to 1984.[2] In California, 25,413 appendectomies (1 per 1000 residents) were performed for acute appendicitis in 1984.[84] Although appendicitis occurs in all age groups, the highest incidence occurs during the second decade of life.[2, 85] Appendicitis is uncommon in children younger than 5 years of age and extremely rare in infants younger than 6 months of age. It has been suggested that patients with AIDS have a higher incidence of appendicitis than the normal population.[75]

In most studies, there is a modest increase in incidence of appendicitis in males compared with females.[2, 5, 85] It has been estimated that the lifetime risk of appendicitis for males is 8.6 per cent, whereas in females it is 6.7 per cent.[2] In a study of acute appendicitis in California from 1983 to 1986, whites had twice the rate of appendicitis of blacks and Asians.[85] Other studies from the United States and South Africa have revealed similar findings.[2, 154] It is unknown whether the reported racial differences are due to errors of measurement, sociodemographic factors, environmental factors, factors related to body constitution, or genetic factors. Children with appendicitis have a more frequent history of having family members who have previously had appendicitis, suggesting that genetic background plays a role in the susceptibility to appendicitis.[15]

Numerous studies have demonstrated that the peak rates of appendicitis occur during the summer months, whereas the lowest rates occur during the winter months.[2, 26, 85, 162] The reasons for this seasonal pattern are unknown, but changes in diet and exposure to allergens have been suggested as explanations.[85] Also, enteric infections occur most commonly during the summer months and may play a role in raising the incidence of appendicitis during that particular time of the year.

CLINICAL MANIFESTATIONS

In school age children and adolescents with appendicitis, the median duration of symptoms prior to the time of hospital admission is 24 to 28 hours.[124] Pain in the right iliac fossa is the most common sign of appendicitis, occurring in 88 to 99 per cent of persons with the disease.[124, 125] Pain shifts from the periumbilical area to the right lower quadrant of the abdomen in approximately two-thirds of pediatric patients with appendicitis. In three-quarters of the children, the pain becomes worse during movement. Importantly, the characteristics of the abdominal pain do not always predict accurately which children have appendicitis. Twenty-five per cent of children found to have mesenteric adenitis at laparotomy report a shift in their abdominal pain to the right iliac fossa, and 33 per cent experience worsening of their pain during movement.[124]

Nausea and vomiting are found in 86 to 96 per cent of children with appendicitis.[124, 125] Vomiting usually occurs after the onset of abdominal pain but may precede the pain in nearly 20 per cent of cases. If only nausea or vomiting is present, it is less likely that the child has appendicitis.[124] Anorexia is less common in children than adults, occurring in 47 to 75 per cent of cases of appendicitis. Because 50 per cent of children found to have normal appendices at surgery complain of anorexia, it is not a helpful clinical finding to differentiate appendicitis from other causes of right iliac fossa pain. Similarly, complaints of diarrhea (9 to 16 per cent), constipation (5 to 28 per cent), and dysuria (7 per cent) occasionally can be elicited from children with appendicitis.[124, 127] Fever may be helpful as a clinical sign of appendicitis if it is present (>37.5° C in 68 to 96 per cent of cases), but absence of fever does not exclude the possibility of acute appendicitis. Very high temperatures (>39° C) suggest that perforation already has occurred or that another intra-abdominal process is present.[138]

During the physical examination, the child frequently lies quietly on the examination table with the right hip flexed. Tenderness in the right iliac fossa is the most sensitive sign of appendicitis, occurring in 93 to 100 per cent of cases of appendicitis.[124, 125] If the psoas muscle is irritated from the inflamed appendix, the child feels increased pain when the right hip is flexed actively. Likewise, if the obturator internus muscle is involved, pain is elicited when the flexed thigh is rotated internally.[138] Guarding is found in 80 to 91 per cent of cases of appendicitis, compared with 50 per cent of cases of mesenteric adenitis and 8 per cent of cases of nonspecific abdominal pain.[124] Similarly, rebound tenderness is found in 56 to 83 per cent of cases of appendicitis, 33 per cent of cases of acute mesenteric adenitis, and 1 per cent of cases of nonspecific abdominal pain.[124] The development of diffuse abdominal tenderness and absent bowel sounds usually indicates perforation. Extremely hyperactive bowel sounds suggest that the patient may not have appendicitis. Occasionally, a mass can be palpated in the right lower quadrant of the abdomen in children with appendicitis who are relaxed or well sedated. Rectal tenderness is more common in children with appendicitis (44 to 68 per cent) than in those with other causes of abdominal pain (12 per cent); however, findings during the rectal examination seldom alter the clinical decision of the surgeon.[124]

In preschool age children, the diagnosis of appendicitis becomes more difficult because of the relative inability of young children to express their symptoms and because they often do not cooperate during the physical examination.[159, 160] Most young children with appendicitis are seen early in the course of their symptoms and are prescribed antibiotics, antihistamines, or antipyretics. By the time it is realized that the child has appendicitis, the appendix usually is perforated (50 to 90 per cent).[159, 160] Unlike with older children, vomiting is the most frequently observed initial symptom of appendicitis, and abdominal pain may be absent or may never localize in the right iliac fossa.[124] Sleep disturbances, irritability, restlessness, and crying are common manifestations of appendicitis in this age group. The preschool age child is more likely to have a palpable inflammatory mass at presentation.[138]

During the newborn period, appendicitis is extremely uncommon.[9, 27, 135, 136] The symptoms of neonatal appendicitis include abdominal distention; vomiting; irritability; diarrhea; erythema, edema, or cellulitis of the abdominal wall; gastrointestinal hemorrhage; abdominal rigidity; lethargy; and jaundice. Usually, the symptoms of neonatal appendicitis are indistinguishable from the symptoms of necrotizing enterocolitis. Underlying conditions, such as total colonic Hirschsprung disease, meconium plugs, or hernias, may predispose the newborn to this condition.

In children who are undergoing chemotherapy for leukemia, acute appendicitis may present with only vague abdominal pain, abdominal distension, lack of abdominal guarding, fever, dehydration, diarrhea, or such unusual symptoms as gastrointestinal bleeding.[6] The symptoms of appendicitis may be identical to the symptoms of typhlitis.

The differential diagnosis of acute abdominal pain in children is extensive. Conditions that can present with symptoms suggestive of acute appendicitis are outlined in Table 60–2.

TABLE 60–2. Differential Diagnosis of Acute Appendicitis in Children

Cecal and Colonic Diseases	**Reproductive Tract Diseases**
Crohn disease	Intrauterine and ectopic pregnancy
Intestinal obstruction	Ovarian torsion
Typhlitis (leukemics)	Ovarian cysts
Infectious colitis (bacterial, parasitic)	Pelvic inflammatory disease
Necrotizing enterocolitis (newborns)	Testicular torsion
Constipation	**Urinary Tract Diseases**
Small Intestinal Diseases	Hydronephrosis
Gastroenteritis (including mesenteric adenitis)	Pyelonephritis
Duodenal ulcers (acute and perforated)	Urolithiasis
Intestinal obstruction	Wilms tumor
Intussusception	Urachal abscess
Meckel diverticulitis	**Systemic Illnesses**
Volvulus	Anaphylactoid purpura
Intestinal duplication	Lymphoma (Burkitt)
Hepatobiliary and Pancreatic Diseases	Rocky Mountain spotted fever
Cholecystitis	Tuberculosis
Hepatitis	Cytomegalovirus infection (in AIDS patients)
Hydrops of the gallbladder	Diabetic ketoacidosis
Pancreatitis	Porphyria
Other Diseases	Sickle-cell disease
Spontaneous peritonitis	
Pneumonia	
Omental torsion	
Psoas abscess	

DIAGNOSIS

The diagnosis of acute appendicitis should be established without laboratory studies when a child complains of abdominal tenderness in the right lower quadrant that initially started in the periumbilical area, develops nausea and vomiting, and has rebound tenderness in the right lower quadrant with guarding during an abdominal examination.[138] The child should be taken to the operating room for an appendectomy as soon as possible before perforation occurs. Many children, however, do not have all of the "classic" clinical manifestations of appendicitis; thus, there has been a great emphasis on using various laboratory tests to help clinicians accurately diagnose the disease.

For decades, physicians have valued peripheral blood leukocyte counts, neutrophil counts, C-reactive protein concentrations, and erythrocyte sedimentation rates to help them distinguish appendicitis from other noninflammatory causes of abdominal pain. When properly evaluated, however, these tests have been found to be too insensitive to use as reliable tools for diagnosing appendicitis.[41, 43, 47, 76, 110, 115] Although these tests help to confirm a physician's suspicions when results are positive, normal results clearly do not rule out the possibility that the child has appendicitis. Certain groups of patients commonly have normal leukocyte counts despite having acute appendicitis. Four studies have demonstrated that black persons with acute appendicitis frequently do not develop leukocytosis.[66, 78, 92, 107] Similarly, patients with acquired immunodeficiency syndrome with appendicitis often do not have elevated white blood cell counts.[104]

The role of routine radiologic studies in the diagnosis of appendicitis continues to be controversial. A chest radiograph often is obtained because right lower lobe pneumonia can cause severe abdominal pain in children. Although radiographs of the abdomen frequently are obtained in children complaining of abdominal pain, there are no sensitive or specific signs of appendicitis.[25, 58] Abnormalities described in association with acute appendicitis include an abnormal bowel gas pattern, a mass, a fecalith, and obliteration of normal fat planes in the right lower quadrant. Gas in the appendiceal lumen is thought to be diagnostic of acute appendicitis but may occur rarely in its absence.

Prior to the use of sonography to diagnose appendicitis, barium enema was used to evaluate patients with right lower quadrant abdominal pain.[49] Findings suggestive of acute appendicitis include partial or absent visualization of the appendix, pressure defects on the cecum, and irritability of the cecum or terminal ileum as demonstrated by fluoroscopy. Five to 10 per cent of normal appendices, however, can not be visualized during the procedure. Also, changes consistent with acute appendicitis have been found in patients with small bowel obstruction, acute enterocolitis, pelvic hemorrhage, pelvic inflammatory disease, hemorrhagic ovarian cysts, and torsion of the ovary. Examination results have been normal in a few patients with histologically proven acute appendicitis.

In the 1990s, graded compression sonography has become the diagnostic procedure of choice in evaluating patients with possible appendicitis.[35, 137, 141, 142, 163, 165] The transducer is used to apply gradual pressure to the abdomen. The technician must make sure that all gas and fluid contents from the loops of bowel are expressed for the examination to be adequate. A noncompressible, enlarged (>6 mm in diameter in adolescents) appendix or a fecalith is the major criterion used for diagnosing appendicitis by sonography.[164] Interruption in the continuity of the echogenic submucosa suggests necrosis of the appendiceal wall and impending perforation. An echogenic periappendiceal mass indicates inflammation of the mesenteric or omental fat. Loculated or generalized fluid collections suggest that perforation already has occurred.

Most studies of graded compression sonography have demonstrated that the procedure is 70 to 90 per cent sensitive and greater than 90 per cent specific in diagnosing acute appendicitis in adults and children.[164] False-positive sonographic results occur in obese patients who have noncompressible appendices because of overlying fat and in children who have inflamed appendices due to Crohn disease, ulcerative colitis, or adjacent salpingitis. False-negative results occur if retrocecally located appendices are not visualized properly, if the cecum is filled with gas or feces and is not compressed adequately, or if perforation has occurred, allowing the appendix to be compressible. In one study, a noncompressible appendix was identified in only 38 per cent of pediatric patients with perforated appendicitis, thus making the other sonographic findings of appendicitis important in diagnosing the disease.[119] When a normal appendix is found during the sonographic evaluation, the examination then should be turned to diagnose other causes of abdominal pain that can mimic appendicitis.

Computed tomography also has been used to diagnose appendicitis when diagnosis cannot be made on clinical grounds alone.[21] However, intravenous contrast agents and high-resolution, thin-section scanning techniques have to be utilized to visualize the appendix adequately. Usually, diluted oral barium or Gastrografin is given to the child, and small bowel opacification can be facilitated with metoclopramide. An enlarged appendix with a circumferentially and symmetrically thickened bowel wall that is enhanced with contrast is the most common computed tomographic finding in appendicitis. Periappendiceal inflammatory reaction or fluid collections may be identified. If the appendix is not well visualized, the presence of a fecalith along with pericecal inflammatory changes strongly suggests appendicitis. However, fecaliths can be visualized in normal appendices by computed tomography and are of no clinical significance unless other inflammatory changes are present. In a study comparing high-resolution computed tomography with graded compression sonography in evaluating patients with suspected appendicitis, computed tomography had higher sensitivity, accuracy, and negative predictive value than did sonography; however, the specificity and positive predictive values were similar.[12] Because sonography can be completed more rapidly, is cheaper, and does not require ionizing radiation and sedation, it remains the preferred initial imaging study in children. Radiolabeled autologous leukocyte scans have been used to diagnose appendicitis in children; however, this modality should be reserved for atypical presentations of disease when localizing signs are not present.[62]

TREATMENT

In previously healthy children with signs of acute appendicitis and no clinical evidence of perforation, nasogastric suctioning should be established and imbalances in fluid and electrolyte concentrations should be corrected quickly. The child should be taken to the operating room as soon as possible for exploratory laparotomy and appendectomy. Although some controversy still remains, most studies have demonstrated that prophylactic antibiotics given perioperatively decrease the postoperative wound infection rate, even in noncomplicated cases of childhood appendicitis.[16, 72, 109, 161] There is no general agreement concerning the appropriate antimicrobial agent or agents that should be used or the appropriate duration of treatment required after surgery to reduce the complication rate. Although most surgeons continue the antibiotics for 1 to 5 days after surgery, one prospective, randomized study demonstrated that a single perioperative dose of gentamicin or metronidazole was as effective as continuing both medications for 24 hours.[148] Few data support the routine intraoperative collection of peritoneal fluid cultures in children with nonperforated appendicitis, although 5 to 20 per cent of cultures grow enteric aerobes, anaerobes, or both.[29, 52, 97] Immunocompromised patients, however, should undergo intraoperative cultures, including cultures for mycobacteria and cytomegalovirus.

Controversy remains considerable as to whether immediate appendectomy should be performed on children in whom a palpable mass is associated with their appendicitis or who show evidence of appendiceal rupture with or without abscess formation at the time of presentation.[138] Most surgeons believe that early intervention is preferred, despite the high complication rate, to prevent severe complications such as death, fistula formation, and abscess rupture.[86] If a laparotomy is performed, there also is debate as to whether the wound should be closed primarily and whether transperitoneal drains should be placed at the time of surgery.[28, 36, 46, 86, 132] During the surgical procedure, most surgeons irrigate the peritoneal cavity with copious amounts of saline or antibiotics to lower the quantity of bacteria in the abdomen.[86] It is unclear if the addition of antibiotics to the lavage fluid further decreases the rate of postoperative complications in children with perforated appendicitis who are receiving systemic antibiotics.[94]

It has been demonstrated that more than 70 per cent of children with palpable masses respond to conservative, nonoperative management consisting of intravenous fluids and broad-spectrum antibiotics.[138] If the child does not improve or a walled-off abscess develops, drainage of the area and appendectomy should be performed. If the child responds to conservative management, an interval appendectomy should be performed 6 to 8 weeks after resolution of the symptoms. Proponents of initial conservative management believe that the complication rate after interval appendectomy is significantly lower than when the procedure is performed during the acute stage of disease.

In the 1990s, there has been increasing interest in performing laparoscopic appendectomies in children with nonperforated and perforated appendicitis.[45, 56] Although the procedure has to be performed by a surgeon experienced in laparoscopic techniques, the advantages of the procedure are a reduction in scarring, a shorter hospital stay, and an earlier return to normal activity. However, the mean total cost of a laparoscopic appendectomy is similar to that of the more commonly performed open appendectomy.

Antimicrobial agents should be administered routinely to children when perforation or appendiceal abscess is suspected or discovered during surgery. Antibiotics active against aerobes and anaerobes that normally inhabit the intestinal tract have been effective in treating children with perforated appendicitis. Treatment failures are most common when *B. fragilis* or *Pseudomonas* species are isolated from intraoperative cultures and antimicrobial agents without activity against these organisms are used.[63] The antimicrobial combination of ampicillin, gentamicin, and clindamycin has been the gold standard of therapy since the 1970s.[86, 131] The importance of including ampicillin in the regimen for adequate enterococcal coverage continues to be controversial. Animal studies and clinical trials using antibiotics with poor enterococcal activity have shown that ampicillin probably is not required in the treatment of perforated appendicitis.[57] Because of the increasing problem of ampicillin resistance in enterococcal strains, ampicillin probably should be reserved for the rare child with enterococcal bacteremia or with persistent intra-abdominal infection in which enterococci have been isolated. Some medical centers use metronidazole instead of clindamycin because of the former's broader activity against enteric anaerobes, whereas other institutions substitute cefotaxime for gentamicin.[131]

In recent years, there have been efforts to determine whether single antibiotics are effective in treating perforated appendicitis. To date, the only agents that have been shown to be effective in treating children with perforated appendicitis are cefoxitin, imipenem-cilastatin, and ticarcillin-clavulanate.[99, 139, 140, 150] Because the latter two antibiotics are more expensive, they should be reserved for special circumstances. In a few medical centers, nearly 50 per cent of *B. fragilis* isolates are resistant to cefoxitin, thus making it questionable as to whether cefoxitin should be used routinely as a single agent in these institutions.[53]

Most patients with perforated appendicitis are treated with intravenous antibiotics for 5 to 10 days. If complications occur, such as the development of an intra-abdominal abscess, phlegmon, wound infection, or enterocutaneous fistula, another surgical procedure often is performed and antibiotic treatment is prolonged. In recent years, there has been an effort to shorten the hospital stay of children with perforated appendicitis. Home antimicrobial therapy through a peripherally inserted, centrally placed catheter can reduce costs and hasten hospital discharge in selected children with this condition.[145]

PROGNOSIS AND EARLY COMPLICATIONS

Currently in the United States, the risk of dying of appendicitis is very low. It was estimated that the mortality rate for nonperforated and perforated appendicitis in California during the 1980s was 0.02 per cent.[84] In smaller series of children and adults reported in the 1990s, the mortality rate was 0 per cent.[86, 93] It has been stated that the risk of death from appendicitis should be the risk of death from general anesthesia.[93] However, the mortality rate appears higher in the rare newborn or premature infant who develops appendicitis.[136] Also, factors contributing to the death of children rarely may include delay in diagnosis, inadequate fluid replacement, immunodeficiency, and postoperative vascular or infectious complications.

The most predictive factor of postoperative morbidity from appendicitis is perforation. Age, obesity, duration of the surgical procedure, and nutritional status also are risk factors for the development of complications.[72] Wound infection rates in children who receive at least perioperative antibiotics have ranged between 0 and 7 per cent.[148] The microorganisms that cause wound infections usually are the same organisms that are isolated in cultures obtained during the appendectomy. Occasionally, children develop peritonitis, intra-abdominal abscesses, psoas abscesses, fistulas, pylephlebitis of the portal vein, scrotal abscesses, or pneumoperitoneum during the course of treatment of appendicitis.[11, 60, 64, 69, 126] The next section focuses on pelvic abscess as an early complication of appendicitis because the topic is not discussed elsewhere in this textbook.

PELVIC ABSCESS

The pelvic area is a common site for abscesses because it is the most dependent portion of the peritoneal cavity. Pelvic abscesses most commonly occur in children in whom intestinal perforations have occurred after appendicitis, who have suffered penetrating abdominal or retroperitoneal injury, or who have undergone an abdominal surgical procedure.[4, 55] Occasionally, adolescents with pelvic inflammatory disease or Crohn disease develop a pelvic abscess.[130]

In children with perforated appendicitis, a coexisting pelvic abscess often is diagnosed at the time of laparotomy. In patients who recently have had penetrating trauma to the abdomen or pelvic inflammatory disease or who have undergone gastrointestinal surgery, a pelvic abscess should be suspected when they have continued fever or complain of abdominal pain despite adequate treatment of the initial disease process. Symptoms may not develop until days to months after therapy is terminated. No characteristic physical findings are associated with a pelvic abscess, although abdominal palpation or rectal examination may elicit tenderness or there may be signs of intestinal obstruction.

If a pelvic abscess is suspected, sonographic and usually computed tomographic evaluation of the pelvis should be completed.[55] The bladder should be filled before the procedure, so that it can displace bowel loops from the pelvis, act as an anatomic marker, and act as a standard of fluidity against which an abscess cavity can be compared. "Walled-off" fluid collections in the pelvis can be identified, and sometimes the rectum, sigmoid colon, or bladder is compressed because of mass effect from the abscess cavity.[55] Because most pelvic abscesses develop as complications of intestinal or pelvic infections, enteric aerobes and anaerobes are the organisms most commonly isolated from the abscess cavity. Only rarely do yeasts cause pelvic abscesses.[151, 158] An *Actinomyces* pelvic abscess developed in an adult who had an intrauterine device.[114] Rarely, tuberculous abscesses can develop as a complication of genital tuberculosis.[156]

When a pelvic abscess is identified, antibiotics covering intestinal aerobes and anaerobes, such as clindamycin and gentamicin, should be started and the abscess contents should be drained. In most situations, it is difficult to reach the abscess cavity by an anterior approach. In recent years, there has been considerable interest in using computed tomography or sonography to guide percutaneous drainage of pelvic abscesses by transgluteal, transrectal, transparacoccygeal, or transvaginal approaches.[4, 17, 30, 48, 50, 80, 81] Although transgluteal catheter placement is easiest, the sciatic nerve and gluteal vessels must be avoided.[90] Also, there may be an increased risk of wound infection because microorganisms may track along the outside of the catheter to the skin. Many surgeons prefer the transrectal approach because it often is the most direct route to the abscess. However, transvaginal drainage has been used with good results in young women. Most often, drainage catheters can be removed after 7 to 10 days of treatment.

Abscesses also may develop within the muscles of the pelvic girdle, including the psoas and internal obturator muscles.[23, 143, 144] Similar to true pelvic abscesses, pelvic muscle abscesses usually cause fever in children, who occasionally have abdominal complaints. However, most children begin to limp, refuse to walk, or complain of pain in the buttocks, thigh, or groin.[23, 143] Often, a suppurative hip infection initially is suspected. A pelvic muscle abscess is diagnosed by sonography, computed tomography, or magnetic resonance imaging. Labeled leukocyte scans sometimes are useful in localizing the infection to within the pelvis, especially when the child has no symptoms other than fever or refusing to walk.

Pelvic muscle abscesses (psoas abscesses) usually develop as a complication of Crohn disease or appendicitis; however, they also may develop after an episode of bacteremia. *Staphylococcus aureus* is the most common cause of a primary pelvic muscle abscess.[23, 143, 144] *S. pneumoniae, H. influenzae* type b, *E.*

coli, Enterococcus faecalis, S. milleri group, *Yersinia enterocolitica, Salmonella* species, *Proteus mirabilis,* and *Actinomyces* species also have been reported to cause hematogenously acquired abscesses.[23, 24, 34, 38, 65, 70, 73, 133] Bacteremia secondary to intravenous drugs abuse or the presence of central lines occasionally predisposes persons to this type of infection.[74, 155] Rarely, tuberculous psoas abscesses develop as a complication of vertebral osteomyelitis.

Pelvic muscle abscesses usually are drained by a percutaneous or surgical approach, and antibiotic therapy is based on Gram stain and culture results. Successful therapy with antibiotics alone has been reported.[144] The duration of treatment is individualized and depends on the child's response and the drainage techniques used.

LATE COMPLICATIONS

Most children who have undergone appendectomy or drainage of a pelvic abscess do not have late complications. Occasionally, patients later develop signs of bowel obstruction from peritoneal adhesions. Some studies have suggested that the future risk of infertility is greater in women who have perforated appendices or pelvic abscesses, presumably because of adhesion formation that impairs the migration of ova in the reproductive tract.[103] Although some retrospective studies have suggested that patients with appendectomies have a higher rate of developing malignancies later in life, prospective and controlled studies have failed to demonstrate this association.[98, 100] It has been reported that patients who have had appendicitis are three times more likely to develop right inguinal hernias than are persons who have not undergone removal of the appendix.[8]

References

1. Addiss, D. G., and Juranek, D. D.: Lack of evidence for a causal association between parasitic infections and acute appendicitis. J. Infect. Dis. *164*:1036–1037, 1991.
2. Addiss, D. G., Shaffer, N., Fowler, B. S., et al.: The epidemiology of appendicitis and appendectomy in the United States. Am. J. Epidemiol. *132*:910–925, 1990.
3. Adebamowo, C. A., Akang, E. E. U., Ladipo, J. K., et al.: Schistosomiasis of the appendix. Br. J. Surg. *78*:1219–1221, 1991.
4. Alexander, A. A., Eschelman, D. J., Nazarian, L. N., et al.: Transrectal sonographically guided drainage of deep pelvic abscesses. A. J. R. Am. J. Roentgenol. *162*:1227–1230, 1994.
5. Andersson, R., Hugander, A., Thulin, A., et al.: Indications for operation in suspected appendicitis and incidence of perforation. Br. Med. J. *308*:107–110, 1994.
6. Angel, C. A., Rao, B. N., Wrenn, E., et al.: Acute appendicitis in children with leukemia and other malignancies: Still a diagnostic dilemma. J. Pediatr. Surg. *27*:476–479, 1992.
7. Arenal Vera, J. J., Marcos Rodriquez, J. L., Borrego Pintado, M. H., et al.: Anisakiasis as a cause of acute appendicitis and rheumatologic picture: The first case in medical literature. Revista Espanola de Enfermedades Digestivas *79*:355–358, 1991.
8. Arnbjornsson, E.: Development of right inguinal hernia after appendectomy. Am. J. Surg. *143*:174–175, 1982.
9. Arora, N. K., Deorari, A. K., Bhatnagar, V., et al.: Neonatal appendicitis: A rare cause of surgical emergency in preterm babies. Indian Pediatr. *28*:1330–1333, 1991.
10. Astagneau, P., Goldstein, F. W., Francoual, S., et al.: Appendicitis due to both *Streptococcus pneumoniae* and *Haemophilus influenzae*. Eur. J. Clin. Microbiol. Infect. Dis. *11*:559–560, 1992.
11. Babcock, D. S.: Ultrasound diagnosis of portal vein thrombosis as a complication of appendicitis. A. J. R. Am. J. Roentgenol. *133*:317–319, 1979.
12. Balthazar, E. J., Birnbaum, B. A., Yee, J., et al.: CT and sonography correlation in acute appendicitis: Prospective evaluation of 100 patients. Radiology *190*:31–35, 1994.
13. Bancroft, F. W., and Skoluda, E. R.: Appendicitis: A study of 596 cases. N. Y. State J. Med. *36*:507–509, 1936.
14. Baron, E. J., Bennion, R., Thompson, J., et al.: Microbiological comparison between acute and complicated appendicitis. Clin. Infect. Dis. *14*:227–231, 1992.
15. Basta, M., Morton, N. E., Mulvihill, J. J., et al.: Inheritance of acute appendicitis: Familial aggregation and evidence of polygenic transmission. Am. J. Hum. Genet. *46*:377–382, 1990.
16. Bauer, T., Vennits, B., Holm, B., et al.: Antibiotic prophylaxis in acute nonperforated appendicitis. Ann. Surg. *209*:307–311, 1989.
17. Bennett, J. D., Kozak, R. I., Taylor, B. M., et al.: Deep pelvic abscesses: Transrectal drainage with radiologic guidance. Radiology *185*:825–828, 1992.
18. Bennion, R. S., Baron, E. J., Thompson, J. E., et al.: The bacteriology of gangrenous and perforated appendicitis revisited. Ann. Surg. *211*:165–171, 1990.
19. Bennion, R. S., Thompson, J. E., Gil, J., et al.: The role of *Yersinia enterocolitica* in appendicitis in the southwestern United States. Am. Surg. *57*:766–768, 1991.
20. Bernard, D., Verschraegen, G., Claeys, G., et al.: *Bilophila wadsworthii* bacteremia in a patient with gangrenous appendicitis. Clin. Infect. Dis. *18*:1023–1024, 1994.
21. Birnbaum, B. A., and Balthazar, E. J.: CT of appendicitis and diverticulitis. Radiol. Clin. North Am. *32*:885–898, 1994.
22. Bredesen, J., Lauritzen, A. F., Kristiansen, V. B., et al.: Appendicitis and enterobiasis in children. Acta Chir. Scand. *154*:585–587, 1988.
23. Bresee, J. S., and Edwards, M. S.: Psoas abscess in children. Pediatr. Infect. Dis. J. *9*:201–206, 1990.
24. Brooks, D. J., Cant, A. J., Lambert, H. P., et al.: Recurrent *Salmonella* septicaemia with aortitis, osteomyelitis and psoas abscess. J. Infect. *7*:156–158, 1983.
25. Brooks, D. W., and Killen, D. A.: Roentgenographic findings in acute appendicitis. Surgery *57*:377–384, 1965.
26. Brumer, M.: Appendicitis: Seasonal incidence and postoperative wound infection. Br. J. Surg. *57*:93–99, 1970.
27. Buntain, W. L., Krempe, R. E., and Kraft, J. W.: Neonatal appendicitis. Ala. J. Med. Sci. *21*:295–299, 1984.
28. Burnweit, C., Bilik, R., and Shandling, B.: Primary closure of contaminated wounds in perforated appendicitis. J. Pediatr. Surg. *26*:1362–1365, 1991.
29. Busuttil, R. W., Davidson, R. K., Fine, M., et al.: Effect of prophylactic antibiotics in acute nonperforated appendicitis. Ann. Surg. *194*:502–509, 1981.
30. Butch, R. J., Mueller, P. R., Ferrucci, J. T., et al.: Drainage of pelvic abscesses through the greater sciatic foramen. Radiology *158*:487–491, 1986.
31. Chandler, N. D., and Parisi, M. T.: Radiological cases of the month: *Yersinia enterocolitica* masquerading as appendicitis. Arch. Pediatr. Adolesc. Med. *148*:527–528, 1994.
32. Chetty, R., Slavin, J. L., and Miller, R. A.: Kaposi's sarcoma presenting as acute appendicitis in an HIV-1 positive patient. Histopathology *23*:590–591, 1993.
33. Cimolai, N., Anderson, J. D., Bhanji, N. M., et al.: *Escherichia coli* 0157:H7 infections associated with perforated appendicitis and chronic diarrhoea. Eur. J. Pediatr. *149*:259–260, 1990.
34. Coakham, H. B., and Ashby, E. C.: Actinomycosis in recurrent psoas abscess. Proc. R. Soc. Med. *65*:880, 1972.
35. Crady, S. K., Jones, J. S., Wyn, T., et al.: Clinical validity of ultrasound in children with suspected appendicitis. Ann. Emerg. Med. *22*:1125–1129, 1993.
36. Curran, T. J., and Muenchow, S. K.: The treatment of complicated appendicitis in children using peritoneal drainage: Results from a public hospital. J. Pediatr. Surg. *28*:204–208, 1993.
37. Dahlstrom, J. E., and Macarthur, E. B.: *Enterobius vermicularis*: A possible cause of symptoms resembling appendicitis. Aust. N. Z. J. Surg. *64*:92–94, 1994.
38. Davies, D., King, S. M., Parekh, R. S., et al.: Psoas abscess caused by *Haemophilus influenzae*, type b. Pediatr. Infect. Dis. J. *10*:411–412, 1991.
39. Dezfuli, M. G., Oo, M. M., Jones, B. E., et al.: Tuberculosis mimicking acute appendicitis in patients with human immunodeficiency virus infection. Clin. Infect. Dis. *18*:650–651, 1994.
40. Dodd, L. G.: *Balantidium coli* infestation as a cause of acute appendicitis. J. Infect. Dis. *163*:1392, 1991.
41. Doraiswamy, N. V.: The neutrophil count in childhood acute appendicitis. Br. J. Surg. *64*:342–344, 1977.
42. Dougherty, S. H., Saltzstein, E. C., Peacock, J. B., et al.: Perforated or gangrenous appendicitis treated with aminoglycosides. Arch. Surg. *124*:1280–1283, 1989.
43. Dueholm, S., Bagi, P., and Bud, M.: Laboratory aid in the diagnosis of acute appendicitis: A blinded, prospective trial concerning diagnostic value of leukocyte count, neutrophil differential count, and C-reactive protein. Dis. Colon Rectum *32*:855–859, 1989.
44. Duong, T. H., Dumon, H., Quilici, M., et al.: Taenia et appendicite, ou appendicite a taenia. Presse Med. *15*:2020, 1986.
45. El Ghoneimi, A., Valla, J. S., Limonne, B., et al.: Laparoscopic appendectomy in children: Report of 1,379 cases. J. Pediatr. Surg. *29*:786–789, 1994.
46. Elmore, J. R., Dibbins, A. W., and Curci, M. R.: The treatment of compli-

cated appendicitis in children: What is the gold standard? Arch. Surg. *122*:424–427, 1987.

47. Eriksson, S., Granstrom, L., and Bark, S.: Laboratory tests in patients with suspected acute appendicitis. Acta Chir. Scand. *155*:117–120, 1989.
48. Eschelman, D. J., and Sullivan, K. L.: Use of a colapinto needle in US-guided transvaginal drainage of pelvic abscesses. Radiology *186*:893–894, 1993.
49. Fedyshin, P., Kelvin, F. M., and Rice, R. P.: Nonspecificity of barium enema findings in acute appendicitis. A. J. R. Am. J. Roentgenol. *143*:99–102, 1984.
50. Feld, R., Eschelman, D. J., Sagerman, J. E., et al.: Treatment of pelvic abscesses and other fluid collections: Efficacy of transvaginal sonographically guided aspiration and drainage. A. J. R. Am. J. Roentgenol. *163*:1141–1145, 1994.
51. Fitz, R. H.: Perforating inflammation of the vermiform appendix, with special reference to its early diagnosis and treatment. Am. J. Med. Sci. *92*:321–346, 1886.
52. Foster, P. D., and O'Toole, R. D.: Primary appendectomy: The effect of prophylactic cephaloridine on postoperative wound infection. J. A. M. A. *239*:1411–1412, 1981.
53. Fraulin, F. O. G., and Thurston, O. G.: Value of cultures of tissue samples taken at operation for lower intestinal perforation. Can. J. Surg. *36*:261–265, 1993.
54. Gaulier, A., Sabatier, P., Prevot, S., et al.: Do measles early giant cells result from fusion of non-infected cells? An immunohistochemical and in situ hybridization study in a case of morbillous appendicitis. Virchows Arch. [A] *419*:245–249, 1991.
55. Gazelle, G. S., and Mueller, P. R.: Abdominal abscess: Imaging and intervention. Radiol. Clin. North Am. *32*:913–932, 1994.
56. Gilchrist, B. F., Lobe, T. E., Schropp, K. P., et al.: Is there a role for laparoscopic appendectomy in pediatric surgery? J. Pediatr. Surg. *27*:209–214, 1992.
57. Gorbach, S. L.: Intraabdominal infections. Clin. Infect. Dis. *17*:961–967, 1993.
58. Graham, A. D., and Johnson, H. F.: The incidence of radiographic findings in acute appendicitis compared to 200 normal abdomens. Milit. Med. *131*:272–276, 1966.
59. Gupta, S. C., Gupta, A. K., Keswani, N. K., et al.: Pathology of tropical appendicitis. J. Clin. Pathol. *42*:1169–1172, 1989.
60. Haas, G. P., Shumaker, B. P., and Haas, P. A.: Appendicovesical fistula. Urology *24*:604–609, 1984.
61. Heltberg, O., Korner, B., and Schouenborg, P.: Six cases of acute appendicitis with secondary peritonitis caused by *Streptococcus pneumoniae*. Eur. J. Clin. Microbiol. *3*:141–143, 1984.
62. Henneman, P. L., Marcus, C. S., Inkelis, S. H., et al.: Evaluation of children with possible appendicitis using technetium 99m leukocyte scan. Pediatrics *85*:838–843, 1990.
63. Heseltine, P. N. R., Yellin, A. E., Appleman, M. D., et al.: Perforated and gangrenous appendicitis: An analysis of antibiotic failures. J. Infect. Dis. *148*:322–329, 1983.
64. Hoffer, F. A., Ablow, R. C., Gryboski, J. D., et al.: Primary appendicitis with an appendico-tuboovarian fistula. A. J. R. Am. J. Roentgenol. *138*:742–743, 1982.
65. Humphreys, H., Keane, C. T., Marron, P., et al.: Infective sacroiliac arthritis and psoas abscess caused by *Streptococcus milleri*. J. Infect. *19*:77–78, 1989.
66. Hyman, P., and Westring, D. W.: Leukocytosis in acute appendicitis: Observed racial difference. J. A. M. A. *229*:1630–1632, 1974.
67. Jackson, D. S., Welch, D. F., Pickett, D. A., et al.: Suppurative infections in children caused by non–beta-hemolytic members of the *Streptococcus milleri* group. Pediatr. Infect. Dis. J. *14*:80–82, 1995.
68. Jakobsen, J., Andersen, J. C., and Klausen, I. C.: Beta-haemolytic streptococci in acute appendicitis. Acta Chir. Scand. *154*:301–303, 1988.
69. Janik, J. S., and Firor, H. V.: Pediatric appendicitis: A 20-year study of 1,640 children at Cook County (Illinois) Hospital. Arch. Surg. *114*:717–719, 1979.
70. Kahn, F. W., Glasser, J. E., and Agger, W. A.: Psoas muscle abscess due to *Yersinia enterocolitica*. Am. J. Med. *76*:947–949, 1984.
71. Kazlow, P. G., Freed, J., Rosh, J. R., et al.: *Salmonella typhimurium* appendicitis. J. Pediatr. Gastroenterol. Nutr. *13*:101–103, 1991.
72. Kizilcan, F., Tanyel, F. C., Buyukpamukcu, N., et al.: The necessity of prophylactic antibiotics in uncomplicated appendicitis during childhood. J. Pediatr. Surg. *27*:586–588, 1992.
73. Knobel, B., Sommer, I., and Schwartz, G.: Primary psoas abscess three years after ipsilateral nephrectomy. Infection *13*:27–28, 1985.
74. Kwok, T., and Coles, J.: Psoas abscess as a complication of subclavian venous catheterization. Postgrad. Med. J. *66*:771–772, 1990.
75. LaRaja, R. D., Rothenberg, R. E., Odom, J. W., et al.: The incidence of intra-abdominal surgery in acquired immunodeficiency syndrome: A statistical review of 904 patients. Surgery *105*:175–179, 1989.
76. Lau, W. Y., Ho, Y. C., Chu, K. W., et al.: Leucocyte count and neutrophil percentage in appendectomy for suspected appendicitis. Aust. N. Z. J. Surg. *59*:395–398, 1989.
77. Leigh, D. A., Simmons, K., and Normal, E.: Bacterial flora of the appendix fossa in appendicitis and postoperative wound infection. J. Clin. Pathol. *27*:997–1000, 1974.
78. Lewis, F., Holcroft, J., Boey, J., et al.: Appendicitis in critical review of diagnosis and treatment in 1000 cases. Arch. Surg. *110*:677–684, 1975.
79. Lin, J., Bleiweiss, I. J., Mendelson, M. H., et al.: Cytomegalovirus-associated appendicitis in a patient with the acquired immunodeficiency syndrome. Am. J. Med. *89*:377–379, 1990.
80. Lomas, D. J., Dixon, A. K., Thomson, H. J., et al.: CT-guided drainage of pelvic abscesses: The peranal transrectal approach. Clin. Radiol. *45*:246–249, 1992.
81. Longo, J. M., Bilbao, J. I., deVilla, V. H., et al.: CT-guided paracoccygeal drainage of pelvic abscesses. J. Comput. Assist. Tomogr. *17*:909–914, 1993.
82. Lopez-Navidad, A., Domingo, P., and Cada Falch, G.: Acute appendicitis complicating infectious mononucleosis: Case report and review. Rev. Infect. Dis. *12*:297–302, 1990.
83. Loria-Cortes, R., and Lobo-Sanahuja, J. F.: Clinical abdominal angiostrongylosis. Am. J. Trop. Med. Hyg. *29*:538–544, 1980.
84. Luckmann, R.: Incidence and case fatality rates for acute appendicitis in California: A population-based study of the effects of age. Am. J. Epidemiol. *129*:905–918, 1989.
85. Luckmann, R., and Davis, P.: The epidemiology of acute appendicitis in California: Racial, gender, and seasonal variation. Epidemiology *2*:323–330, 1991.
86. Lund, D. P., and Murphy, E. U.: Management of perforated appendicitis in children: A decade of aggressive treatment. J. Pediatr. Surg. *29*:1130–1134, 1994.
87. Madden, N. P., and Hart, C. A.: *Streptococcus milleri* in appendicitis in children. J. Pediatr. Surg. *20*:6–7, 1985.
88. Maia, A., Goldstein, F. W., Acar, J. F., et al.: Isolation of *Eikenella corrodens* from human infections: Report of six cases. J. Infect. *2*:347–353, 1980.
89. Malde, H. M., and Chadha, D.: Roundworm obstruction: Sonographic diagnosis. Abdom. Imaging *18*:274–276, 1993.
90. Malden, E. S., and Picus, D.: Hemorrhagic complication of transgluteal pelvic abscess drainage: Successful percutaneous treatment. J. Vasc. Interv. Radiol. *3*:323–328, 1992.
91. Malik, A. K., Hanum, N., and Yip, C. H.: Acute isolated amoebic appendicitis. Histopathology *24*:87–88, 1994.
92. Marrero, R. R., Barnwell, S., and Hoover, E. L.: Appendicitis in children: A continuing clinical challenge. J. Natl. Med. Assoc. *84*:850–852, 1992.
93. Maxwell, J. M., and Ragland, J. J.: Appendicitis: Improvements in diagnosis and treatment. Am. Surg. *57*:282–285, 1991.
94. McAllister, T. A., Fyfe, A. H., Young, D. G., et al.: Cefotaxime lavage in children undergoing appendicectomy. Drugs *35*(Suppl. 2):127–132, 1988.
95. McBurney, C.: Experience with early operative interference in cases of disease of the vermiform appendix. N. Y. State Med. J. *50*:676, 1889.
96. McCahy, P.: Continuing fall in the incidence of acute appendicitis. Ann. R. Coll. Surg. Engl. *76*:282–283, 1994.
97. McNamara, M. J., Pasquale, M. D., and Evans, S. R. T.: Acute appendicitis and the use of intraperitoneal cultures. Surg. Gynecol. Obstet. *177*:393–397, 1993.
98. McVay, J. R.: The appendix in relation to neoplastic disease. Cancer *17*:929–937, 1964.
99. Meller, J. L., Reyes, H. M., Loeff, D. S., et al.: One drug versus two-drug antibiotic therapy in pediatric perforated appendicitis: A prospective randomized trial. Surgery *110*:764–768, 1991.
100. Moertel, C. G., Nobrega, F. T., Elveback, L. R., et al.: A prospective study of appendectomy and predisposition to cancer. Surg. Gynecol. Obstet. *138*:549–553, 1974.
101. Mogensen, K., Pahle, E., and Kowalski, K.: *Enterobius vermicularis* and acute appendicitis. Acta Chir. Scand. *151*:705–707, 1985.
102. Morrison, J. D.: *Yersinia* and viruses in acute non-specific abdominal pain and appendicitis. Br. J. Surg. *68*:284–286, 1981.
103. Mueller, B. A., Daling, J. R., Moore, D. E., et al.: Appendectomy and the risk of tubal infertility. N. Engl. J. Med. *315*:1506–1508, 1986.
104. Mueller, G. P., and Williams, R. A.: Surgical infections in AIDS patients. Am. J. Surg. *169*(Suppl. 5A):34S–38S, 1995.
105. Nadler, S., Cappell, M. S., Bhatt, B., et al.: Appendiceal infection by *Entamoeba histolytica* and *Strongyloides stercoralis* presenting like acute appendicitis. Dig. Dis. Sci. *35*:603–608, 1990.
106. Namnyak, S. S., Martin, D. H., Ferguson, J. D. M., et al.: *Haemophilus segnis* appendicitis. J. Infect. *23*:339–341, 1991.
107. Natesha, R., Barnwell, S., Weaver, W., et al.: Is there evidence for a racial difference in the misdiagnosis in patients explored for appendicitis? J. Natl. Med. Assoc. *81*:269–271, 1989.
108. Neumayer, L. A., Makar, R., Ampel, N. M., et al.: Cytomegalovirus appendicitis in a patient with human immunodeficiency virus infection. Arch. Surg. *128*:467–468, 1993.
109. Nguyen, B.-L., Raynor, S., and Thompson, J. S.: Selective versus routine antibiotic use in acute appendicitis. Am. Surg. *5*:280–283, 1992.
110. Nordback, I., and Harju, E.: Inflammation parameters in the diagnosis of acute appendicitis. Acta Chir. Scand. *154*:43–48, 1988.
111. Nussinovitch, M., Shapiro, R. P., Cohen, A. H., et al.: Shigellosis complicated by perforated appendix. Pediatr. Infect. Dis. J. *12*:352, 1993.
112. Ochoa, B.: Surgical complications of ascariasis. World J. Surg. *15*:222–227, 1991.

113. Park, J. W.: *Escherichia coli* septicemia associated with acute appendicitis. South. Med. J. *84*:667–668, 1991.
114. Pearlman, M., Frantz, A. C., Floyd, W. S., et al.: Abdominal wall *Actinomyces* abscess associated with an intrauterine device. J. Reprod. Med. *36*:398–402, 1991.
115. Peltola, H., Ahlqvist, J., Rapola, J., et al.: C-reactive protein compared with white blood cell count and erythrocyte sedimentation rate in the diagnosis of acute appendicitis in children. Acta Chir. Scand. *152*:55–58, 1986.
116. Peters, J., Greenberg, S., and Gentry, L.: Sepsis associated with non-perforated appendicitis. South. Med. J. *75*:75–76, 1982.
117. Pisacane, A., de Luca, U., Impagliazzo, N., et al.: Breast feeding and acute appendicitis. Br. Med. J. *310*:836–837, 1995.
118. Poole, P. M., and Wilson, G.: *Streptococcus milleri* in the appendix. J. Clin. Pathol. *30*:937–942, 1977.
119. Quillin, S. P., Siegel, M. J., and Coffin, C. M.: Acute appendicitis in children: Value of sonography in detecting perforation. A. J. R. Am. J. Roentgenol. *159*:1265–1268, 1992.
120. Raffensperger, J.: *Eikenella corrodens* infections in children. J. Pediatr. Surg. *21*:644–646, 1986.
121. Raffi, F., David, A., Mouzard, A., et al.: *Pasteurella multocida* appendiceal peritonitis: Report of three cases and review of the literature. Pediatr. Infect. Dis. *5*:695–698, 1986.
122. Raguveer-Saran, M. K., and Keddie, N. C.: The falling incidence of appendicitis. Br. J. Surg. *67*:681, 1980.
123. Ramsden, K., and Freeth, M.: Cryptosporidial infection presenting as an acute appendicitis. Histopathology *14*:209–211, 1989.
124. Rasmussen, O., and Hoffmann, J.: Assessment of the reliability of the symptoms and signs of acute appendicitis. J. R. Coll. Surg. Edinb. *36*:372–377, 1991.
125. Reynolds, S. L., and Jaffe, D. M.: Diagnosing abdominal pain in a pediatric emergency department. Pediatr. Emerg. Care *8*:126–128, 1992.
126. Robertson, F. M., Olsen, S. B., Jackson, M. R., et al.: Inguinal-scrotal suppuration following treatment of perforated appendicitis. J. Pediatr. Surg. *28*:267–268, 1993.
127. Rothrock, S. G., Skeoch, G., Rush, J. J., et al.: Clinical features of misdiagnosed appendicitis in children. Ann. Emerg. Med. *20*:45–50, 1991.
128. Ruff, M. E., Friedland, I. R., and Hickey, S. M.: *Escherichia coli* septicemia in nonperforated appendicitis. Arch. Pediatr. Adolesc. Med. *148*:853–855, 1994.
129. Schisgall, R. M.: Appendiceal colic in childhood: The role of inspissated casts of stool within the appendix. Ann. Surg. *192*:687–693, 1980.
130. Schratter-Sehn, A. U., Lochs, H., Handl-Zeller, L., et al.: Endosonographic features of the lower pelvic region in Crohn's disease. Am. J. Gastroenterol. *88*:1054–1057, 1993.
131. Schropp, K. P., Kaplan, S., Golladay, E. S., et al.: A randomized clinical trial of ampicillin, gentamicin and clindamycin versus cefotaxime and clindamycin in children with ruptured appendicitis. Surgery *172*:351–356, 1991.
132. Schwartz, M. Z., Tapper, D., and Solenberger, R. I.: Management of perforated appendicitis in children. Ann. Surg. *197*:407–411, 1983.
133. Scott, B. D., and Schmidt, J. H.: Pneumococcal meningitis due to psoas abscess. South. Med. J. *82*:1310–1311, 1989.
134. Shakir, A. F., Youngberg, G., and Alvarez, S.: Strongyloides infestation as a cause of acute appendicitis. J. Tenn. Med. Assoc. *79*:543–544, 1986.
135. Sharma, A. K., Shukla, A. K., Agarwal, L. D., et al.: Appendicitis in the newborns. Indian Pediatr. *29*:1293–1294, 1992.
136. Shaul, W. L.: Clues to the early diagnosis of neonatal appendicitis. J. Pediatr. *98*:473–476, 1981.
137. Siegel, M. J.: Acute appendicitis in childhood: The role of US. Radiology *185*:341–342, 1992.
138. Silen, M. L., and Tracy, T. F.: The right lower quadrant "revisited." Pediatr. Clin. North Am. *40*:1201–1211, 1993.
139. Sirinek, K. R., and Levine, B. A.: Antimicrobial management of surgically treated gangrenous or perforated appendicitis: Comparison of cefoxitin and clindamycin-gentamicin. Clin. Ther. *9*:420–428, 1987.
140. Sirinek, K. R., and Levine, B. A.: A randomized trial of ticarcillin and clavulanate versus gentamicin and clindamycin in patients with complicated appendicitis. Surg. Gynecol. Obstet. *172*:30–35, 1991.
141. Sivit, C. J.: Diagnosis of acute appendicitis in children: Spectrum of sonographic findings. A. J. R. Am. J. Roentgenol. *161*:147–152, 1993.
142. Sivit, C. J., Newman, K. D., Boenning, D. A., et al.: Appendicitis: Usefulness of US in diagnosis in a pediatric population. Radiology *185*:549–552, 1992.
143. Snook, M. E., and LiPuma, J. J.: Pelvic muscle abscess: An unusual cause of gait disturbance in young children. Clin. Pediatr. *32*:298–299, 1993.
144. Souid, A. K., Sadowitz, P. D., Weiner, L., et al.: Obturator internus muscle abscess: A case report and review of the literature. Am. J. Dis. Child. *147*:1278–1279, 1993.
145. Stovroff, M. C., Totten, M., and Glick, P. L.: PIC lines save money and hasten discharge in the care of children with ruptured appendicitis. J. Pediatr. Surg. *29*:245–247, 1994.
146. Thadepalli, H., Mandal, A. K., Chuah, S. K., et al.: Bacteriology of the appendix and the ileum in health and in appendicitis. Am. Surg. *57*:317–322, 1991.
147. Tobe, I.: Inapparent virus infection as a trigger of appendicitis. Lancet *1*:1343–1346, 1965.
148. Tsang, T. M., Tam, P. K. H., and Saing, H.: Antibiotic prophylaxis in acute non-perforated appendicitis in children: Single dose of metronidazole and gentamicin. J. R. Coll. Surg. Edinb. *37*:110–112, 1992.
149. Uchimura, M., Tsuruoka, Y., Hukuda, T., et al.: Isolation of vero toxin-producing *Escherichia coli* (enterohemorrhagic *E. coli*) 0111:H- from 2 cases diagnosed as appendicitis. Kansenshogaku Zasshi *65*:905–908, 1991.
150. Uhari, M., Seppanen, J., and Heikkinen, E.: Imipenem-cilastatin vs. tobramycin and metronidazole for appendicitis-related infections. Pediatr. Infect. Dis. J. *11*:445–450, 1992.
151. Urizar, R. E., Lepow, M., Neumann, M., et al.: Fungal peritonitis with splenic-pelvic abscess in a patient on continuous ambulatory peritoneal dialysis. Peritoneal Dialysis Int. *13*:162–163, 1993.
152. Van Noyen, R., Selderslaghs, R., Bekaert, J., et al.: Causative role of *Yersinia* and other enteric pathogens in the appendicular syndrome. Eur. J. Clin. Microbiol. Infect. Dis. *10*:735–741, 1991.
153. Visvanathan, K., Jones, P. D., and Truskett, P.: Abdominal mycobacterial infection mimicking acute appendicitis in an AIDS patient. Aust. N. Z. J. Surg. *63*:558–560, 1993.
154. Walker, A. R., and Walker, B. F.: Appendicitis in South Africa inter-ethnic school pupils. Am. J. Gastroenterol. *82*:219–222, 1987.
155. Walsh, T. R., Reilly, J. R., Hanley, E., et al.: Changing etiology of iliopsoas abscess. Am. J. Surg. *163*:413–416, 1992.
156. Wehner, J. H., De Bruyne, K., Kagawa, F. T., et al.: Pulmonary tuberculosis, amenorrhea, and a pelvic mass. West. J. Med. *161*:515–518, 1994.
157. Wiebe, B. M.: Appendicitis and *Enterobius vermicularis*. Scand. J. Gastroenterol. *26*:336–338, 1991.
158. Wiesenfeld, H. C., Berg, S. R., and Sweet, R. L.: *Torulopsis glabrata* pelvic abscess and fungemia. Obstet. Gynecol. *83*:887–889, 1994.
159. Williams, N., and Kapila, L.: Acute appendicitis in the preschool child. Arch. Dis. Child. *66*:1270–1272, 1991.
160. Williams, N., and Kapila, L.: Acute appendicitis in the under 5-year-old. J. R. Coll. Surg. Edinb. *39*:168–170, 1994.
161. Winslow, R. E., Dean, R. E., and Harley, J. W.: Acute nonperforating appendicitis. Arch. Surg. *118*:651–655, 1983.
162. Wolkomir, A., Kornak, P., Elsakr, M., et al.: Seasonal variation of acute appendicitis: A 56-year study. South. Med. J. *80*:958–960, 1987.
163. Wong, M. L., Casey, S. O., Leonidas, J. C., et al.: Sonographic diagnosis of acute appendicitis in children. J. Pediatr. Surg. *29*:1356–1360, 1994.
164. Yacoe, M. E., and Jeffrey, R. B.: Sonography of appendicitis and diverticulitis. Radiol. Clin. North Am. *32*:899–912, 1994.
165. Zaki, A. M., MacMahon, R. A., and Gray, A. R.: Acute appendicitis in children: When does ultrasound help? Aust. N. Z. J. Surg. *64*:695–698, 1994.

61

PANCREATITIS

Thomas L. Kuhls

Before 1980, pancreatitis was thought to be a rare cause of abdominal pain in children and a disease primarily of adults.[65] Because of better recognition of symptoms in children and the more frequent use of medications that cause pancreatic inflammation, pancreatitis currently is being diagnosed more frequently in pediatric practices. It now is estimated that 1 in 50,000 children develop pancreatitis, an estimate nearly 10 times higher than those of previous decades.[31] The mortality rate for children with pancreatitis is 14 per cent.[78]

Compared with the causes of pancreatitis in adults—primarily alcoholism, cholelithiasis, and trauma—the causes of childhood pancreatitis are more diverse. Microorganisms account for a significant proportion of cases of pancreatitis in children. Also, antimicrobial agents have been associated with severe and occasionally fatal episodes of pancreatitis, and bacterial infections may complicate the natural history of acute and chronic pancreatitis. Thus, pediatricians who care for children with pancreatitis must have expertise in the diagnosis and treatment of infectious diseases.

CLINICAL MANIFESTATIONS

More than 80 per cent of children with pancreatitis complain of abdominal pain.[56, 112, 129, 136] However, only 30 per cent of pediatric patients have epigastric pain as usually described by adults.[129] In children, other sites of tenderness or diffuse pain include the right upper quadrant of the abdomen, the periumbilical area, the entire abdomen, and less commonly the right lower quadrant of the abdomen.

The onset of pain usually is rapid and increases to a maximum intensity in a few hours. It usually is described as sharp and excruciating in nature. Only one-third of children complain of pain that radiates to other areas, including the back, lower part of the abdomen, upper abdominal quadrants, and anterior chest wall.[129] In school age children, the pain often intensifies after meals.

Most children with pancreatitis have nausea and vomiting. Children younger than 5 years of age occasionally experience vomiting without abdominal tenderness.[136] Fever is present in only 30 per cent of children with pancreatitis, but temperatures higher than 38.5° C are observed occasionally.[129]

On physical examination, children usually are found lying quietly on their sides with their knees flexed. They have epigastric tenderness to palpation and decreased or absent bowel sounds. Abdominal distention is found in 30 per cent of children with pancreatitis and is more common in the preschool-age child.[129, 136] Occasionally, rebound tenderness, guarding of the epigastrium, jaundice, an abdominal mass, or ascites is detected. Rarely, ecchymoses of the flanks (Grey Turner sign) or the umbilical area (Cullen sign) can be identified but usually only when life-threatening hemorrhagic pancreatitis is present.

LABORATORY DIAGNOSIS

The single most common useful laboratory test for the clinical diagnosis of pancreatitis in children is measurement of serum amylase, but the level correlates poorly with the severity of the disease.[31, 56, 65] The serum concentration quickly rises within hours after symptoms in more than 90 per cent of children with pancreatitis. High serum amylase concentrations can be observed in numerous other illnesses, including acute cholecystitis, intestinal obstruction, perforated abdominal organs, appendicitis, salpingitis, ruptured ectopic pregnancy, and salivary gland disease. The serum amylase concentration can return to normal in 24 to 72 hours after the onset of symptoms, and the diagnosis of pancreatitis therefore can be missed. In this situation, the urine amylase concentration can remain elevated for at least 1 week.

Rarely, serum amylase concentrations are not elevated during the course of pancreatitis in children.[104] Also, marked hyperlipidemia may interfere with the laboratory measurement of amylase.[13] Serum lipase is useful in these situations; however, high serum concentrations often are not detected until 24 hours after the beginning of the illness. Because lipase is produced only in the pancreas and intestinal cells, measurement of its serum concentration helps to distinguish children with high serum amylase concentrations of pancreatic, compared with salivary, origin. Measurement of serum trypsinogen may be the most sensitive and specific way of detecting acute pancreatitis, but it is not available currently in most clinical laboratories.[129]

Nonspecific laboratory findings in children with pancreatitis can include leukocytosis with increased immature polymorphonuclear leukocytes and an elevated erythrocyte sedimentation rate. In children with fulminant hemorrhagic pancreatitis, anemia develops quickly. Other associated findings include hyperglycemia, hypertriglyceridemia, hypoalbuminemia, and hypocalcemia. Elevated transaminases and alkaline phosphatase generally are observed only when the episode of pancreatitis is caused by biliary obstruction, such as in gallstone-related disease.

The radiographic features of childhood pancreatitis also are nonspecific. Radiographs of the abdomen may demonstrate a localized ileus of the jejunum in the midepigastric or left upper quadrant region adjacent to the pancreas (sentinel loop), distended transverse colon without visualization of the descending colon due to adjacent pancreatic inflammation (colon cutoff sign), duodenal distention with air-fluid levels, or loss of the left psoas shadow.[56] Occasionally, chest radiography reveals an elevated left hemidiaphragm or pleural effusion.

In recent years, the ability to diagnose pancreatitis in children has been improved greatly by ultrasonography.[30] Normally, echodensity of the pancreas is equal to or greater than that of the left lobe of the liver. During acute pancreatitis, edema causes the gland to enlarge and become less dense than the liver. These two findings can aid the diagnosis of pancreatitis, and such complications as abscesses and pseudocysts can be identified. Visualization of the pancreas by ultrasonography may be obscured because of overlying bowel gas. In such cases, computed tomography is useful in detecting pancreatic size and density.

Endoscopic retrograde cholangiopancreatography is a difficult procedure in children but occasionally should be considered for children with pancreatitis to exclude gallstones, pseudocysts, strictures, or ascaris infection.[93]

NONINFECTIOUS ETIOLOGIES

An etiology for childhood pancreatitis can be determined in more than 90 per cent of cases if diagnostic evaluation is thorough.[136] However, the frequency of each specific cause depends highly on the patient population of the particular medical center. For instance, 33 per cent of children with pancreatitis at Children's Hospital of Michigan have biliary tract–related disease because of their large sickle-cell anemia patient population.[136] At Yale–New Haven Hospital, on the other hand, drug-related pancreatitis accounts for 30 per cent of the total cases of childhood pancreatitis because of the frequent use of immunosuppressive and cancer chemotherapeutic agents in this hospital setting.[56]

Table 61–1 outlines the most common noninfectious causes of pancreatitis in children. In most series, trauma is the leading cause of acute pancreatitis. Because the pancreas is immobilized by the stomach, duodenum, and vertebrae and because the organ is highly vascular, it is susceptible to blunt and penetrating trauma. Less developed abdominal wall musculature in pediatric compared with adult patients may enhance the susceptibility of pancreatic injury after episodes of blunt trauma. Child abuse has been recognized increasingly as a cause of trauma-related pancreatitis since the 1980s. Postoperative pancreatitis occurs most commonly after abdominal or cardiac surgery.[39] Pancreatitis also may be associated with traumatic brain injury in children.[122]

TABLE 61–1. Noninfectious Causes of Childhood Pancreatitis

Trauma
Blunt
Penetrating
Postoperative
Brain injury
Drugs
Immunosuppressives (azathioprine, steroids, asparaginase)
Diuretics (thiazides, furosemide, ethacrynic acid)
Valproic acid
Sulfasalazine
Growth hormone
Ethyl alcohol
Antimicrobials (pentamidine, interferon-α, sulfonamides, tetracycline, rifampin, metronidazole, nitrofurantoin, erythromycin, 2′, 3′-dideoxyinosine)
Cholelithiasis
Anatomic malformations
Metabolic diseases
Hyperlipoproteinemia types I, IV, V
Cystic fibrosis
Diabetes mellitus
Hyperparathyroidism
Aminoacidurias
Glycogen storage disease type 1
Vasculitis
Kawasaki syndrome
Henoch-Schönlein purpura
Systemic lupus erythematosus
Miscellaneous
Crohn disease
Scorpions of Trinidad and Israel
Reye syndrome
Familial
Anticholinesterase insecticide intoxication

Medications used in pediatric practice increasingly are causing episodes of pancreatitis in children. Azathioprine, steroids, and L-asparaginase have been associated with cases of childhood pancreatitis, and immunosuppressive agents most likely play a role in posttransplantation pancreatitis.[8, 79, 99, 131] Valproic acid is a commonly used pediatric anticonvulsant that can cause pancreatitis.[134] Also, diuretics, including hydrochlorothiazide and furosemide, have been associated with disease.[79] Acute pancreatitis recently has been associated with growth hormone therapy and sulfasalazine treatment of inflammatory bowel disease.[44, 80] Alcohol consumption is an uncommon cause of pancreatitis in younger children; however, it can cause illness occasionally in the adolescent population.

Physicians with expertise in the management of infectious diseases are becoming more aware of drug-induced pancreatitis because many antimicrobial agents can cause pancreatic inflammation. Pentamidine isethionate is used in the treatment of *Pneumocystis carinii* pneumonia, African trypanosomiasis, and leishmaniasis. It may cause hypoglycemia due to toxicity to pancreatic islet cells[58] and is associated with severe and occasionally fatal episodes of pancreatitis.[84, 87, 137] In children and adults, aerosolized pentamidine prophylaxis for *P. carinii* pneumonia also has been associated with severe cases of pancreatitis in patients with AIDS.[50, 84] Recently, interferon-α, which is used in the treatment of malignancies and chronic hepatitis, has been associated with the development of pancreatitis.[116]

Sulfonamides, including trimethoprim-sulfamethoxazole, have been implicated on occasion as a cause of acute pancreatitis in adults.[3, 7] Symptoms have recurred when the patients have been re-exposed to the medication. The abdominal pain often is accompanied by a hypersensitivity-type skin rash. Tetracycline-induced pancreatitis has been described in children with and without overt liver disease.[37, 119] Also, metronidazole, erythromycin, rifampin, and nitrofurantoin have been added to the list of agents that can cause pancreatitis in previously healthy persons.[12, 26, 48, 90, 101, 105]

Most recently, pancreatitis has been a major dose-limiting toxic effect of the HIV-inhibiting drug 2′,3′-dideoxyinosine in adult and pediatric patients with AIDS.[22, 23, 29, 73] Most episodes of pancreatitis occur when the dose is 360 mg/m^2/day or more and usually resolve when the medication is discontinued. It is possible that the concomitant administration of pentamidine with 2′, 3′-dideoxyinosine increases the risk of developing pancreatitis. In pediatric patients with AIDS, serum amylase concentrations often are elevated in children without pancreatic symptoms, whereas children with pancreatitis can have normal serum amylase concentrations. Thus, the serum lipase concentration is useful in evaluating HIV-infected children for possible pancreatic inflammation.[23, 84] Increased liver transaminases or lipase concentrations prior to the administration of 2′,3′-dideoxyinosine may be helpful in predicting which children will develop pancreatitis.[23] In all children with symptoms consistent with pancreatitis, 2′,3′-dideoxyinosine should be withheld pending the results of a lipase concentration, and it should be discontinued if the concentration is elevated. Similarly, 2′,3′-dideoxyinosine should be discontinued during and for 1 week after pentamidine treatment for *P. carinii* pneumonia.[42]

Obstruction of the common bile duct, pancreatic duct, or sphincter of Oddi may cause pancreatitis.[4, 96] Gallstones or congenital anatomic malformations, including annular pancreas, pancreas divisum, choledochal cysts, and intrapancreatic duplication cysts, can cause pancreatitis by obstructing normal pancreatic flow. Metabolic diseases often are associated with recurrent episodes of pancreatitis. They include hyperlipoproteinemias, cystic fibrosis, diabetes mellitus, hyperparathyroidism, aminoacidurias, and glycogen storage disease type I.[56, 66, 113] Recurrent hereditary pancreatitis usually occurs in an autosomal dominant pattern, with onset occurring between infancy and adolescence.[100]

Pancreatitis also can occur in syndromes in which vasculitis is a major component of the disease process. It has been associated with common pediatric diseases, including Kawasaki syndrome, Henoch-Schönlein purpura, and systemic lupus erythematosus.[18, 56, 118] Other pediatric diseases have been associated with pancreatitis, including Crohn disease and Reye syndrome.[36, 45, 107, 108] The venom of the scorpions *Tityus trinitatis* and *Leiurus quinquestriatus* can cause pancreatitis in patients who have been stung; however, these species do not live naturally in the United States.[10, 115] The gastrointestinal symptoms that are observed in children with anticholinesterase insecticide poisoning may be caused by pancreatitis.[130]

INFECTIOUS ETIOLOGIES

Infections caused by various microorganisms have been demonstrated by culture, histologic examination, or antibody titer rise during the course of acute pancreatitis in humans (Table 61–2). However, a true causal relationship usually is not demonstrated. Although not all of the following infectious agents have been shown to be associated with cases of childhood pancreatitis, they must be considered as possible etiologic agents because adult patients with infectious pancreatitis have been described.

Viral Infections

Mumps virus and group B coxsackieviruses are the best documented causes of pancreatitis in children. Usually, mumps pancreatitis occurs in the presence of parotitis; however, abdominal pain and vomiting may occur for days before the development of salivary swelling.[127] Rarely, mumps virus can cause pancreatitis without other common clinical manifestations.[88] Because more than 80 per cent of children with mumps parotitis have elevated serum amylase concentrations, the diagnosis of pancreatitis should be aided by ultrasonography and serum lipase concentrations.[49] It has been estimated that 15 per cent of children with mumps virus infection have abdominal tenderness and vomiting suggestive of the diagnosis of pancreatitis.[56] Only in a single report has the pancreatitis been hemorrhagic and severe.[40] Occasionally, chronic or recurring pancreatitis develops after mumps infection.[133]

TABLE 61–2. Microorganisms Associated with Episodes of Acute Pancreatitis

Viruses	**Mycoplasmas and Bacteria**
Mumps virus	*Mycoplasma pneumoniae*
Group B coxsackieviruses	*Escherichia coli*
Hepatitis A virus	*Salmonella* species
Hepatitis B virus	*Campylobacter jejuni*
Epstein-Barr virus	*Yersinia* species
Varicella-zoster virus	*Legionella* species
Cytomegalovirus	*Mycobacterium tuberculosis*
Adenoviruses	*Leptospira* species
Parainfluenza viruses	*Brucella melitensis*
HIV	
Measles virus	**Fungi**
Parasites	*Aspergillus* species
Ascaris lumbricoides	*Candida* species
Clonorchis sinensis	*Cryptococcus neoformans*
Fasciola hepatica	
Taenia saginata	
Echinococcus granulosus	
Wuchereria bancrofti	
Cryptosporidium parvum	
Toxoplasma gondii	
Plasmodium falciparum	

Pancreatitis has been caused by group B coxsackieviruses in children. Associated clinical manifestations include aseptic meningitis, mild diarrhea, rash, and myocarditis.[25, 60] It is unknown how commonly these enteroviruses cause pancreatic inflammation. Thirty-one per cent of patients with aseptic meningitis during an epidemic of group B coxsackievirus infection had increased serum amylase concentrations in one epidemiologic study.[89] Multiple studies have demonstrated coxsackievirus B–induced damage to pancreatic acinar cells in mouse models of infection.[14, 114, 125] Coxsackievirus B strains recently have been isolated from biopsied pancreatic tissue of patients with chronic pancreatitis.[110]

It was thought previously that acute pancreatitis only occurred in cases of viral hepatitis when fulminant liver disease developed. In 1986, the case of a 12-year-old boy with mild hepatitis A virus infection and pancreatitis was reported.[76] Also, hepatitis B viral antigens have been detected in pancreatic glandular cells of patients with severe acute hemorrhagic pancreatitis.[124] The role of hepatitis B virus in the pathogenesis of pancreatic inflammation in these patients is unknown.

Human herpesviruses are an uncommon cause of childhood pancreatitis. Occasionally, children and adolescents with infectious mononucleosis develop pancreatitis.[71, 75, 86] There has been a single report of a case of an adult with chickenpox of 4 days' duration who developed acute pancreatitis and pseudocyst formation.[70] Also, an immunocompetent 22-year-old developed pancreatitis during a period that seroconversion to cytomegalovirus was documented.[68]

Viral pancreatitis also occurs in the immunocompromised patient. Cytomegalovirus has been identified in pancreatic specimens from autopsies of AIDS, transplant, and cancer chemotherapy patients.[61, 63, 94] Also, the symptoms of pancreatitis have resolved in a few patients with AIDS treated with ganciclovir or foscarnet.[28] Adenovirus has caused hemorrhagic pancreatitis and death in a child who received a bone marrow transplant, and varicella-zoster virus has caused pancreatitis and death in a patient with AIDS.[41, 92] The case of an infant with severe combined immunodeficiency in whom disseminated parainfluenza virus infection developed (temporally associated with the development of pancreatitis) has been reported; however, there was no attempt to culture the virus from postmortem pancreatic tissue.[43]

To date, it is unclear whether HIV directly causes pancreatitis. Laboratory-diagnosed episodes of pancreatitis in adults and children with AIDS do occur, but it is unknown whether the pancreatic inflammation is due to HIV or an unrecognized opportunistic pathogen.[19, 120, 135]

Interstitial pancreatitis also is relatively common in children with congenital rubella syndrome.[85]

Parasite Infestations and Infections

Ascaris lumbricoides can migrate in the intestines to the ampulla of Vater and subsequently to the pancreatic duct or common bile duct. Biliary or pancreatic duct obstruction can cause acute pancreatitis.[9, 24, 32, 33, 69] Ascariasis is diagnosed when adult roundworms are identified in the duodenum by radiographs of the upper gastrointestinal tract (Fig. 61–1) or more commonly by ultrasonography or retrograde cholangiopancreatography. Often, a history of seeing worms in the feces can be elicited. The flukes *Clonorchis sinensis* and *Fasciola hepatica* and the cestode *Taenia saginata* also can migrate to the pancreatic and biliary drainage systems and cause pancreatitis.[15, 111, 123] Rarely, hepatic hydatid cysts can obstruct biliary drainage and cause pancreatic inflammation.[17, 82] Recently, *Wuchereria bancrofti* has been found to be a cause of chronic pancreatitis.[62] Parasitic infestations should be considered as a cause of pancreatitis, particularly in immigrant children and patients who have traveled to developing nations.

Cryptosporidium parvum has been identified in the bile of a patient with AIDS with elevated serum amylase and right upper quadrant abdominal pain.[46] Cholangiopancreatography demonstrated biliary and pancreatic ductal disease, but no other opportunistic pathogens could be isolated. Cryptosporidia also have been observed in interlobular pancreatic ducts of experimentally infected immunocompromised mice.[121] It is unknown whether cryptosporidial infection causes pancreatitis in immunocompetent patients; however, a previously healthy adolescent developed pancreatitis after a course of cryptosporidial diarrhea.[51] *Toxoplasma gondii* cysts have been found in postmortem pancreatic tissues of patients with AIDS.[1, 57] Rarely, pancreatitis occurs during acute episodes of falciparum malaria.[64] Other systemic manifestations of malaria often are present, including high fever, hepatitis, intestinal malabsorption, encephalitis, and pulmonary insufficiency.

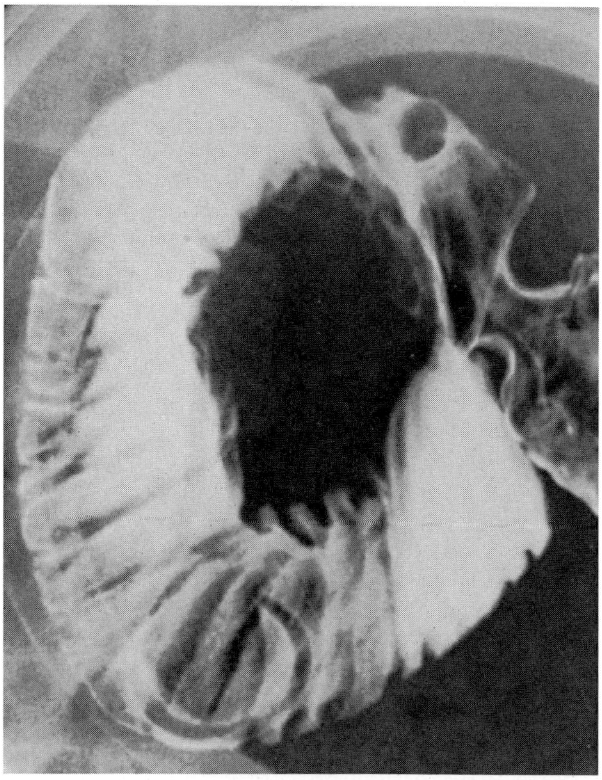

FIGURE 61–1. *An ascaris close to the ampulla of Vater, the body and tail lying in the second and third parts of the duodenum. The patient is a 9-year-old girl with acute pancreatitis.*

Mycoplasmal and Bacterial Infections

In adolescents and adults, moderately severe symptoms of pancreatitis have occurred just before or during the course of atypical pneumonia.[54, 81] In these cases, most patients have had cold agglutinins in their sera, and all have had significant changes in *Mycoplasma pneumoniae* antibody titers. There has been some controversy over whether *M. pneumoniae* can cause acute pancreatitis without evidence of pneumonia. Although complement-fixing IgM antibodies against *M. pneumoniae* often significantly increase during the course of acute pancreatitis, it has been argued that pancreatic cellular antigenic components similar to *Mycoplasma* lipid antigens are exposed during the disease process and that the elicited antibodies cross-react in *Mycoplasma* serologic assays.[74]

It generally is accepted that common pyogenic bacteria do not cause acute pancreatitis. However, secondary invasion of inflamed pancreatic tissue does occur. There is some evidence that circulating endotoxin from *Escherichia coli* can cause extrahepatic cholestasis and pancreatitis.[34] Occasionally, pancreatitis occurs during acute episodes of enteritis. *Salmonella typhimurium, Salmonella typhosa, Campylobacter jejuni, Yersinia enterocolitica,* and *Yersinia pseudotuberculosis* all have been reported to cause clinically evident and laboratory-proven cases of pancreatitis.[6, 35, 52, 55, 95, 106, 109]

Along with *M. pneumoniae* infection, legionnaires' disease must be considered when a patient develops acute pancreatitis with pneumonia.[83, 132] Also, miliary tuberculosis can present with symptoms of pancreatitis.[38, 103] The prognosis of tuberculous pancreatitis generally is poor.

Pancreatitis has been reported in children with leptospirosis.[11] Also, *Brucella melitensis* has been added to the list of uncommon causes of acute pancreatitis.[2]

Fungal Infections

Fungal infections have not been reported to cause acute pancreatitis in immunocompetent patients. However, *Aspergillus* has caused fatal hemorrhagic pancreatitis in an adult cancer patient undergoing chemotherapy.[47] *Candida* species and *Cryptococcus neoformans* have been isolated from pancreatic tissues of patients with AIDS, but whether they cause clinical symptoms of pancreatitis is unknown.[135]

PATHOGENESIS

Enzymes to polysaccharides, fats, and proteins are produced and stored in pancreatic acinar cells. They exist intracellularly in an inactive precursor form. After cholecystokinin-pancreozymin stimulation, the proenzymes are released into the pancreatic ducts and flow into the duodenum. The enzymes normally do not become enzymatically active until they reach the intestinal lumen.

Pancreatitis occurs when the proteolytic enzymes are activated within the pancreas, causing autodigestion and inflammation of the gland.[13] The specific mechanisms that activate the pancreatic enzymes during specific pathologic processes have not been elucidated. Drug-induced and infectious pancreatitis are thought to be caused by direct toxic effects on acinar cells. Gallstones, ascaris infection, and congenital abnormalities are believed to damage acinar cells by obstructing pancreatic flow. Traumatic pancreatitis probably occurs by direct injury to the glandular cells, whereas vasculitis may cause changes in pancreatic blood flow, thus eliciting premature proteolytic enzyme activation.

Autodigestion of the pancreas causes inflammation. The inflammatory response can be relatively mild, as occurs commonly in episodes of infectious pancreatitis, or more severe, with hemorrhagic necrosis, as occurs typically after alcohol consumption in adults.

TREATMENT

Despite our increasing recognition of cases of childhood pancreatitis, there have been no major advances in the treatment of the disease since the mid-1970s.[77] Animal data have demonstrated that such medications as glucagon, aprotinin, 5-fluorouracil, and somatostatin may be useful in the treatment of pancreatitis; however, trials in adults have not substantiated their efficacy.[27, 117] The continuing main objectives of treatment are to relieve abdominal pain, to reduce pancreatic exocrine secretion, and to treat aggressively systemic manifestations, such as shock, electrolyte abnormalities, and anemia.[65]

Meperidine continues to be the most common medication used for pain control. Usually, children fast, or nasogastric suction is applied to decrease duodenal acid-stimulated secretin release. Feeding with carbohydrate solutions is not restarted until all symptoms have resolved. Intravenous fluids and colloids are used during the acute episode to maintain intravascular volume. Parenteral nutrition is started if the patient has fasted for more than 5 days. During the entire course of acute pancreatitis, the hematologic and biochemical parameters of the child must be monitored closely.

If the episode of pancreatitis is drug-induced, the medication should be discontinued immediately. Often, the symptoms recur if the medication is restarted. Pancreatitis caused by *M. pneumoniae* or bacteria should be treated with proper antimicrobials. Obstructions to pancreatic flow (e.g., gallstones, roundworms, congenital abnormalities) may have to be removed or altered surgically or endoscopically.[20, 72]

COMPLICATIONS

During the acute episode of pancreatitis, renal, hematologic, central nervous system, pulmonary, and cardiovascular complications can occur, caused by shock.

In 12 per cent of children with pancreatitis, an inflammatory mass develops in the first weeks after the onset of illness.[126] Continued or increasing abdominal pain, nausea, or vomiting often accompanies the development of a phlegmon, abscess, or pseudocyst. An inflammatory phlegmon usually develops into a thin-walled pseudocyst of the lesser sac but may become secondarily infected, causing abscess formation. Patients in whom an inflammatory mass develops must be followed closely with frequent physical examinations and serial ultrasound studies. In children with pseudocysts, acute abdominal pain accompanied by hypotension often signifies bleeding into the pseudocyst or rupture of the pseudocyst into the peritoneum. Slowly leaking pseudocysts may cause pancreatic ascites. Pseudocysts either are resected surgically or are drained externally when complications occur. About 33 per cent of pseudocysts resolve spontaneously within 6 weeks.[102]

The development of fever and leukocytosis during the course of pancreatitis should suggest the development of an infected pseudocyst or pancreatic abscess. The role of prophylactic antibiotics in preventing suppurative complications of acute pancreatitis is controversial; prophylactic antibiotics should be considered only when pancreatic necrosis is severe.[16, 97, 98] Infections, when they do occur after prophylactic antimicrobials, often are caused by bacteria that are resistant to commonly used antimicrobials. In adults, infectious complications account for 80 per cent of deaths associated with acute pancreatitis.[21] Isolates from pancreatic abscesses have yielded intestinal flora in more than 90 per cent of cases, but *Candida* species are becoming more common in many medical centers.[5, 128] Even with early diagnosis and surgical intervention, deaths due to pancreatic abscesses reach 22 to 57 per cent.[56, 59] Rarely, fistulas from pseudocysts or abscesses to other abdominal organs develop.[53]

Osteolytic lesions resembling osteomyelitis may develop weeks to months after an acute episode of pancreatitis.[67, 91] It has been hypothesized that elevated serum lipase causes intramedullary fat necrosis in the bone. Usually, the lesions are asymptomatic and resolve spontaneously without therapy.

References

1. Ahuja, S. K., Ahuja, S. S., Thelmo, W., et al.: Necrotizing pancreatitis and multisystem organ failure associated with toxoplasmosis in a patient with AIDS. Clin. Infect. Dis. *16*:432–434, 1993.
2. Al-Awadhi, N. Z., Ashkenani, F., and Khalaf, E. S.: Acute pancreatitis associated with brucellosis. Am. J. Gastroenterol. *84*:1570–1574, 1989.
3. Alberti-Flor, J. J., Hernandez, M. E., Ferrer, J. P., et al.: Fulminant liver failure and pancreatitis associated with the use of sulfamethoxazole-trimethoprim. Am. J. Gastroenterol. *84*:1577–1579, 1989.
4. Albu, E., Buiumsohn, A., Lopez, R., et al.: Gallstone pancreatitis in adolescents. J. Pediatr. Surg. *22*:960–962, 1987.
5. Aloia, T., Solomkin, J., Fink, A. S., et al.: *Candida* in pancreatic infection: A clinical experience. Am. Surg. *60*:793–796, 1994.
6. Andrén-Sandberg, A., and Höjer, H.: Necrotizing acute pancreatitis induced by *Salmonella* infection. Int. J. Pancreatol. *15*:229–230, 1994.
7. Antonow, D. R.: Acute pancreatitis associated with trimethoprim sulfamethoxazole. Ann. Intern. Med. *104*:363–365, 1986.
8. Aziz, S., Bergdahl, L., Baldwin, J. C., et al.: Pancreatitis after cardiac and cardiopulmonary transplantation. Surgery *97*:653–661, 1985.
9. Baldwin, M., Eisenman, R. E., Prelipp, A. M., et al.: *Ascaris lumbricoides* resulting in acute cholecystitis and pancreatitis in the midwest. Am. J. Gastroenterol. *88*:2119–2121, 1993.
10. Bartholomew, C.: Acute scorpion pancreatitis in Trinidad. Br. Med. J. *1*:666–668, 1970.
11. Bell, M. J., Ternberg, J. L., and Feigin, R. D.: Surgical complications of leptospirosis in children. J. Pediatr. Surg. *13*:325–330, 1978.
12. Berger, T. M., Cook, W. J., O'Marcaigh, A. S., et al.: Acute pancreatitis in a 12-year-old girl after an erythromycin overdose. Pediatrics *90*:624–626, 1992.
13. Blake, R. L.: Acute pancreatitis. Primary Care *15*:187–199, 1988.
14. Blay, R., Simpson, K., Leslie, K., et al.: Coxsackie-virus-induced disease, $CD4^+$ cells initiate both myocarditis and pancreatitis in DBA/2 mice. Am. J. Pathol. *135*:899–907, 1989.
15. Bouteloup, C., Michel, P., Desechalliers, J.-P., et al.: Pancréatite aiguë récidivante a *Taenia saginata*. Gastroenterol. Clin. Biol. *16*:818–820, 1992.
16. Bradley, E. L.: Antibiotics in acute pancreatitis: Current status and future directions. Am. J. Surg. *158*:472–477, 1989.
17. Braithwaite, P. A., and Brodribb, R. K.: Hepatic hydatid disease presenting as pancreatitis. Med. J. Aust. *2*:369–370, 1983.
18. Branski, D., Gross, V., Gross-Kieselstein, E., et al.: Pancreatitis as a complication of Henoch-Schönlein purpura. J. Pediatr. Gastroenterol. Nutr. *1*:275–276, 1982.
19. Brivet, F., Coffin, B., Bedossa, P., et al.: Pancreatic lesions in AIDS. Lancet *2*:570–571, 1987.
20. Brown, C. W., Werlin, S. L., Geenen, J. E., et al.: The diagnosis and therapeutic role of endoscopic retrograde cholangiopancreatography in children. J. Pediatr. Gastroenterol. Nutr. *17*:19–23, 1993.
21. Buggy, B. P., and Nostrant, T. T.: Lethal pancreatitis. Am. J. Gastroenterol. *78*:810–814, 1983.
22. Butler, K. M., Husson, R. N., Balis, F. M., et al.: Dideoxyinosine in children with symptomatic human immunodeficiency virus infection. N. Engl. J. Med. *324*:137–144, 1991.
23. Butler, K. M., Venzon, D., Henry, N., et al.: Pancreatitis in human immunodeficiency virus–infected children receiving dideoxyinosine. Pediatrics *91*:747–751, 1993.
24. Capallo, D. V., and Gongaware, R. D.: Biliary ascariasis. South. Med. J. *77*:1201–1202, 1984.
25. Capner, P., Lendrum, R., Jeffries, D. J., et al.: Viral antibody studies in pancreatic disease. Gut *16*:866–870, 1975.
26. Celifarco, A., Warschauer, C., and Burakoff, R.: Metronidazole-induced pancreatitis. Am. J. Gastroenterol. *84*:958–964, 1989.
27. Choi, T. K., Mok, F., Zhan, W. H., et al.: Somatostatin in the treatment of acute pancreatitis: A prospective randomized controlled trial. Gut *30*:223–227, 1989.

28. Colebunders, R., Van den Abbeele, K., Fleerackers, Y., et al.: Two AIDS patients with life-threatening pancreatitis successfully treated, one with ganciclovir the other with foscarnet. Acta Clin. Belg. *49*:229–232, 1994.
29. Cooley, T. P., Kunches, L. M., Saunders, C. A., et al.: Once-daily administration of 2′, 3′-dideoxyinosine (ddI) in patients with the acquired immunodeficiency syndrome or AIDS-related complex: Results of a phase 1 trial. N. Engl. J. Med. *322*:1340–1345, 1990.
30. Cox, K. L., Ament, M. E., Sample, W. F., et al.: The ultrasonic and biochemical diagnosis of pancreatitis in children. J. Pediatr. *96*:407–411, 1980.
31. Cox, K. L.: Pancreatitis in children. Pediatric Case Reports in Gastrointestinal Diseases (Ross Laboratories) *6*:1–7, 1986.
32. Daojin, C., and Xiaorong, L.: Forty-two patients with acute ascaris pancreatitis in China. J. Gastroenterol. *29*:676–678, 1994.
33. Das, S.: Pancreatitis in children associated with round worms. Indian Pediatr. *14*:81–83, 1977.
34. Dev, G., Sikka, M., Sehgal, S., et al.: *Escherchia coli* infection producing pancreatitis and extrahepatic-cholestasis. Indian Pediatr. *24*:249–253, 1987.
35. de Bois, M. H. W., Schoemaker, M. C., van der Werf, S. D. J., et al.: Pancreatitis associated with *Campylobacter jejuni* infections: Diagnosis by ultrasonography. Br. Med. J. *298*:1004, 1989.
36. Ellis, G. H., Mirkin, L. D., and Mills, M. C.: Pancreatitis and Reye's syndrome. Am. J. Dis. Child. *133*:1014–1016, 1979.
37. Elmore, M. F., and Rogge, J. D.: Tetracycline-induced pancreatitis. Gastroenterology *81*:1134–1136, 1981.
38. Fan, S. T., Yan, K. W., Lau, W. Y., et al.: Tuberculosis of the pancreas: A rare cause of massive gastrointestinal bleeding. Br. J. Surg. *73*:373, 1986.
39. Feiner, H.: Pancreatitis after cardiac surgery: A morphologic study. Am. J. Surg. *131*:684–688, 1976.
40. Feldstein, J. D., Johnson, F. R., Kallick, C. A., et al.: Acute hemorrhagic pancreatitis and pseudocyst due to mumps. Ann. Surg. *180*:85–88, 1974.
41. Fernández, R. A., Varona, T. L., Jaquotot, J. M. K., et al.: Pancreatitis aguda asociada a infección por virus de la varicela-zoster en un paciente con síndrome de immunodeficiencia adquirida. Med. Clin. (Barc.) *98*:339–341, 1992.
42. Foisy, M. M., Slayter, K. L., Hewitt, R. G., et al.: Pancreatitis during intravenous pentamidine therapy in an AIDS patient with prior exposure to didanosine. Ann. Pharmacother. *28*:1025–1028, 1994.
43. Frank, J. A., Warren, R. W., Tucker, J. A., et al.: Disseminated parainfluenza infection in a child with severe combined immunodeficiency. Am. J. Dis. Child. *137*:1172–1174, 1983.
44. Garau, P., Orenstein, S. R., Neigut, D. A., et al.: Pancreatitis associated with olsalazine and sulfasalazine in children with ulcerative colitis. J. Pediatr. Gastroenterol. Nutr. *18*:481–485, 1994.
45. Glassman, M., Tahan, S., Hillemeier, C., et al.: Pancreatitis in patients with Reye's syndrome. J. Clin. Gastroenterol. *3*:165–169, 1981.
46. Gross, T. L., Wheat, J., Bartlett, M., et al.: AIDS and multiple system involvement with *Cryptosporidium*. Am. J. Gastroenterol. *81*:456–458, 1986.
47. Guice, K. S., Lynch, M., and Weatherbee, L.: Invasive aspergillosis: An unusual cause of hemorrhagic pancreatitis. Am. J. Gastroenterol. *82*:563–565, 1987.
48. Gumaste, V. V.: Erythromycin-induced pancreatitis. Am. J. Med. *86*:725, 1989.
49. Haddock, G., Coupar, G., Youngson, G. G., et al.: Acute pancreatitis in children: A 15-year review. J. Pediatr. Surg. *29*:719–722, 1994.
50. Hart, C. C.: Aerosolized pentamidine and pancreatitis. Ann. Intern. Med. *111*:691, 1989.
51. Hawkins, S. P., Thomas, R. P., and Teasdale, C.: Acute pancreatitis: A new finding in *Cryptosporidium* enteritis. Br. Med. J. *294*:483–484, 1987.
52. Hearne, S. E., Whigham, T. E., and Brady, C. E.: Pancreatitis and typhoid fever. Am. J. Med. *86*:471–473, 1989.
53. Henderson, J. M., and MacDonald, J. A. E.: Fistula formation complicating pancreatic abscess. Br. J. Surg. *63*:233–234, 1976.
54. Herbaut, C., Tielemans, C., Burette, A., et al.: *Mycoplasma pneumoniae* infection and acute pancreatitis. Acta. Clin. Belg. *38*:186–188, 1983.
55. Hermans, P., Gerard, M., Van Laethem, Y., et al.: Pancreatic disturbances and typhoid fever. Scand. J. Infect. Dis. *23*:201–205, 1991.
56. Hillemeier, C., and Gryboski, J. D.: Acute pancreatitis in infants and children. Yale J. Biol. Med. *57*:149–159, 1984.
57. Hofman, P., Michiels, J.-F., Mondain, V., et al.: Pancréatite aiguë toxoplasmique. Gastroenterol. Clin. Biol. *18*:895–897, 1994.
58. Hughes, W. T., Feldman, S., Chaudbary, S. C., et al.: Comparison of pentamidine isethionate and trimethoprim-sulfamethoxazole in the treatment of *Pneumocystis carinii* pneumonia. J. Pediatr. *92*:285–291, 1978.
59. Hurley, J. E., and Vargish, T.: Early diagnosis and outcome of pancreatic abscesses in pancreatitis. Am. Surg. *53*:29–33, 1987.
60. Imrie, C. W., Ferguson, J. C., and Sommerville, R. G.: Coxsackie and mumps virus infection in a prospective study of acute pancreatitis. Gut *18*:53–56, 1977.
61. Iwasaki, T., Tashiro, A., Satodate, R., et al.: Acute pancreatitis with cytomegalovirus infection. Acta Pathol. Jpn. *37*:1661–1668, 1987.
62. Jesudason, S. R. B., Mathai, V., Muthusami, J. C., et al.: *Wuchereria bancrofti* induced pancreatitis. Trop. Gastroenterol. *13*:115–118, 1992.
63. Joe, L., Ansher, A. F., and Gordin, F. M.: Severe pancreatitis in an AIDS patient in association with cytomegalovirus infection. South. Med. J. *82*:1444–1445, 1989.
64. Johnson, R. C., DeFord, J. W., and Carlton, P. K.: Pancreatitis complicating falciparum malaria. Postgrad. Med. *61*:181–183, 1977.
65. Jordan, S. C., and Ament, M. E.: Pancreatitis in children and adolescents. J. Pediatr. *91*:211–216, 1977.
66. Kahler, S. G., Sherwood, W. G., Woolf, D., et al.: Pancreatitis in patients with organic acidemias. J. Pediatr. *124*:239–243, 1994.
67. Keating, J. P., Shackelford, G. D., Shackelford, P. G., et al.: Pancreatitis and osteolytic lesions. J. Pediatr. *81*:350–353, 1972.
68. Keidar, S., Porath, E. B., Naftali, V., et al.: Acute pancreatitis associated with rising cytomegalovirus titer. Isr. J. Med. Sci. *23*:296–297, 1987.
69. Khuroo, M. S., Zargar, S. A., Yattoo, G. N., et al.: *Ascaris*-induced acute pancreatitis. Br. J. Surg. *79*:1335–1338, 1992.
70. Kirschner, S., and Raufman, J. P.: Varicella pancreatitis complicated by pancreatic pseudocyst and duodenal obstruction. Dig. Dis. Sci. *33*:1192–1195, 1988.
71. Koutras, A.: Epstein-Barr virus infection with pancreatitis, hepatitis, and proctitis. Pediatr. Infect. Dis. *2*:312–313, 1983.
72. Kozarek, R. A., Christie, D., and Barclay, G.: Endoscopic therapy of pancreatitis in the pediatric population. Gastrointest. Endoscop. *39*:665–669, 1993.
73. Lambert, J. S., Seidlin, M., Reichman, R. C., et al.: 2′, 3′-dideoxyinosine (ddI) in patients with the acquired immunodeficiency syndrome or AIDS-related complex: A phase 1 trial. N. Engl. J. Med. *322*:1333–1340, 1990.
74. Leinikki, P. O., Panzar, P., and Tykka, H.: Immunoglobulin M antibody response against *Mycoplasma pneumoniae* lipid antigen in patients with acute pancreatitis. J. Clin. Microbiol. *8*:113–118, 1978.
75. Lifschitz, C., and LaSala, S.: Pancreatitis, cholecystitis, and choledocholithiasis associated with infectious mononucleosis. Clin. Pediatr. *20*:131, 1981.
76. Lopez Morante, A., Rodriquez de Lope, C., San Miguel, G., et al.: Acute pancreatitis in hepatitis A infection. Postgrad. Med. J. *62*:407–408, 1986.
77. Löser, C., and Fölsch, U. R.: A concept of treatment in acute pancreatitis: Results of controlled trials, and future developments. Hepato-Gastroenterology *40*:569–573, 1993.
78. Mader, T. J., and McHugh, T. P.: Acute pancreatitis in children. Pediatr. Emerg. Care *8*:157–161, 1992.
79. Mallory, A., and Kern, F.: Drug-induced pancreatitis: A critical review. Gastroenterology *78*:813–820, 1980.
80. Malozowski, S., Hung, W., Scott, D. C., et al.: Acute pancreatitis associated with growth hormone therapy for short stature. N. Engl. J. Med. *332*:401–402, 1995.
81. Mardh, P. A., and Ursing, B.: The occurrence of acute pancreatitis in *Mycoplasma pneumoniae* infection. Scand. J. Infect. Dis. *6*:167–171, 1974.
82. Mathai, V., Jesudason, S. R. B., Muthusami, J. C., et al.: Chronic pancreatitis caused by intraductal hydatid cysts of the pancreas. Br. J. Surg. *81*:1029, 1994.
83. Michel, O., Naeije, N., Csoma, M., et al.: Acute pancreatitis in Legionnaires' disease. Eur. J. Respir. Dis. *66*:62–64, 1985.
84. Miller, T. L., Winter, H. S., Luginbuhl, L. M., et al.: Pancreatitis in pediatric human immunodeficiency virus infection. J. Pediatr. *120*:223–227, 1992.
85. Monif, G. R. G.: Rubella virus and the pancreas. Med. Chir. Dig. *3*:195–197, 1974.
86. Mor, R., Pitlik, S., Dux, S., et al.: Parotitis and pancreatitis complicating infectious mononucleosis. Isr. J. Med. Sci. *18*:709–710, 1982.
87. Murphey, S. A., and Josephs, A. S.: Acute pancreatitis associated with pentamidine therapy. Arch. Intern. Med. *141*:56–58, 1981.
88. Naficy, K., Nategh, R., and Ghadimi, H.: Mumps pancreatitis without parotitis. Br. Med. J. *1*:529–533, 1973.
89. Nakao, T., Nitta, T., Miura, R., et al.: Clinical and epidemiological studies on an outbreak of aseptic meningitis caused by Coxsackie B5 and A9 viruses in Aomori in 1961. Tohoku J. Exp. Med. *83*:94–102, 1964.
90. Nelis, G. F.: Nitrofurantoin-induced pancreatitis: Report of a case. Gastroenterology *84*:1032–1034, 1983.
91. Neuer, F. S., Roberts, F. F., and McCarthy, V.: Osteolytic lesions following traumatic pancreatitis. Am. J. Dis. Child. *131*:738–740, 1977.
92. Niemann, T. H., Trigg, M. E., Winick, N., et al.: Disseminated adenoviral infection presenting as acute pancreatitis. Hum. Pathol. *24*:1145–1148, 1993.
93. Novis, B. H., Narunsky, L., and Bank, S.: Endoscopic retrograde cholangiopancreatography in the evaluation of pancreatic disease. S. Afr. Med. J. *50*:1501–1505, 1976.
94. Parham, D. M.: Post-transplantation pancreatitis associated with cytomegalovirus (report of a case). Hum. Pathol. *12*:663–665, 1981.
95. Pastore, M., Pellegrino, M., Maruzzi, M., et al.: Pancreatite in corso di salmonellosi maggiore. Minerva Pediatr. *45*:471–473, 1993.
96. Patamasucon, P., Pillsbury, H. L., and Colon, A. R.: Childhood pancreatitis with biliary calcareous disease. J. Pediatr. Surg. *17*:189–190, 1982.
97. Pederzoli, P., Bassi, C., Vesentini, S., et al.: A randomized multicenter clinical trial of antibiotic prophylaxis of septic complications in acute necrotizing pancreatitis with imipenem. Surg. Gynecol. Obstet. *176*:480–483, 1993.
98. Pederzoli, P., Bassi, C., Vesentini, S., et al.: Antibiotics in acute pancreatitis: The debate revisited. Am. J. Gastroenterol. 90:666–667, 1995.

99. Penn, I., Durst, A. L., Machado, M., et al.: Acute pancreatitis and hyperamylasemia in renal homograft recipients. Arch. Surg. *105*:167–172, 1972.
100. Perrault, J.: Hereditary pancreatitis. Gastroenterol. Clin. North Am. *23*:743–752, 1994.
101. Perry, W., Jenkins, M. V., and Stamp, T. C. B.: Lysosomal enzymes and pancreatitis during rifampicin therapy. Lancet *1*:492, 1979.
102. Pollak, E. W., Michas, C. A., and Wolfman, E. F.: Pancreatic pseudocyst: Management in 54 patients. Am. J. Surg. *135*:199–201, 1978.
103. Rushing, J. L., Hanna, C. J., and Selecky, P. A.: Pancreatitis as the presenting manifestation of miliary tuberculosis. West. J. Med. *129*:432–436, 1978.
104. Ruzena, S.: Normal serum amylase in acute pancreatitis. Dig. Dis. Sci. *34*:960–961, 1989.
105. Sanford, K. A., Mayle, J. E., Dean, H. A., et al.: Metronidazole-associated pancreatitis. Ann. Intern. Med. *109*:756–757, 1988.
106. Schulz, T. B.: Association of pancreas affection and yersiniosis. Acta Med. Scand. *205*:255–256, 1979.
107. Scully, R. E., Mark, E. J., McNeely, W. F., et al.: Case records of the Massachusetts General Hospital: Case 3-1994. N. Engl. J. Med. *330*:196–200, 1994.
108. Seidman, E. G., Deckelbaum, R. J., Owen, H., et al.: Relapsing pancreatitis in association with Crohn's disease. J. Pediatr. Gastroenterol. Nutr. *2*:178–182, 1983.
109. Sherl, N. D., and Patterson, D. L. H.: Pancreatitis with *Salmonella* gastroenteritis. J. Med. Soc. N. J. *68*:129–130, 1971.
110. Shirobokov, V. P., Zhurba, T. B., and Zemlyansky, V. V.: Properties of the coxsackie viruses isolated from pancreatic tissue of patients with chronic pancreatitis. Mikrobiol. Zh. *50*:78–81, 1988.
111. Shugar, R. A., and Ryan, J. J.: *Clonorchis sinensis* and pancreatitis. Am. J. Gastroenterol. *65*:400–403, 1975.
112. Sibert, J. R.: Pancreatitis in children: A study in the north of England. Arch. Dis. Child. *50*:443–448, 1975.
113. Slyper, A. H., Wyatt, D. T., and Brown, C. W.: Clinical and/or biochemical pancreatitis in diabetic ketoacidosis. J. Pediatr. Endocrinol. *7*:261–264, 1994.
114. Smith, R., and Deibel, R.: Coxsackie virus infection in mice. Association with pancreatitis and subclinical disease. Arch. Intern. Med. *135*:238–239, 1975.
115. Sofer, S., Shalev, H., Weizman, Z., et al.: Acute pancreatitis in children following envenomation by the yellow scorpion *Leiurus quinquestriatus*. Toxicon *29*:125–128, 1991.
116. Sotomatsu, M., Shimoda, M., Ogawa, C., et al.: Acute pancreatitis associated with interferon-α therapy for chronic myelogenous leukemia. Am. J. Hematol. *48*:211–212, 1995.
117. Steinberg, W. M., and Schlesselman, S. E.: Treatment of acute pancreatitis. Comparison of animal and human studies. Gastroenterology *93*:1420–1427, 1987.
118. Stoler, J., Biller, J. A., and Grand, R. J.: Pancreatitis in Kawasaki disease. Am. J. Dis. Child. *141*:306–308, 1987.
119. Torosis, J., and Vender, R.: Tetracycline-induced pancreatitis. J. Clin. Gastroenterol. *9*:580–581, 1987.
120. Torre, D., Montanari, M., Fiori, G. P., et al.: HIV and the pancreas. Lancet *2*:1212, 1987.
121. Ungar, B. L. P., Burris, J. A., Quinn, C. A., et al.: New mouse models for chronic *Cryptosporidium* infection in immunodeficient hosts. Infect. Immun. *58*:961–969, 1990.
122. Urban, M., Splaingard, M., and Werlin, S. L.: Pancreatitis associated with remote traumatic brain injury in children. Child's Nerv. Syst. *10*:388–391, 1994.
123. Veerappan, A., Siegel, J. H., Podany, J., et al.: *Fasciola hepatica* pancreatitis: Endoscopic extraction of live parasites. Gastrointest. Endoscop. *37*:473–475, 1991.
124. Vital Durand, D., Trepo, C., Bouletreau, P., et al.: Hepatite fulminante a virus HB avec pancreatite aigue: Deux observations. Ann. Med. Interne *132*:120–123, 1981.
125. Vuorinen, T., Kallajoki, M., Hyypia, T., et al.: Coxsackie B3–induced acute pancreatitis: Analysis of histopathological and viral parameters in a mouse model. Br. J. Exp. Pathol. *70*:395–403, 1989.
126. Warner, R. L., Othersen, H. B., and Smith, C. D.: Traumatic pancreatitis and pseudocyst in children: Current management. J. Trauma *29*:597–601, 1989.
127. Warren, W. R.: Serum amylase and lipase in mumps. Am. J. Med. Sci. *230*:161–168, 1955.
128. Warshaw, A. L.: Pancreatic abscesses. N. Engl. J. Med. *287*:1234–1236, 1972.
129. Weizman, Z., and Durie, P. R.: Acute pancreatitis in childhood. J. Pediatr. *113*:24–29, 1988.
130. Weizman, Z., and Sofer, S.: Acute pancreatitis in children with anticholinesterase insecticide intoxication. Pediatrics *90*:204–206, 1992.
131. Werlin, S. L., Casper, J., Antonson, D., et al.: Pancreatitis associated with bone marrow transplantation in children. Bone Marrow Transplant. *10*:65–69, 1992.
132. Westblom, T. U., and Hamory, B. H.: Acute pancreatitis caused by *Legionella pneumophila*. South. Med. J. *81*:1200–1201, 1988.
133. Wood, C. B., Bradbrook, R. A., and Blumgart, L. H.: Chronic pancreatitis in childhood associated with mumps virus infection. Br. J. Clin. Pract. *28*:67–69, 1974.
134. Wyllie, E., Wyllie, R., Cruse, R. P., et al.: Pancreatitis associated with valproic acid therapy. Am. J. Dis. Child. *138*:912–914, 1984.
135. Zazzo, J. F., Pichon, F., and Regnier, B.: HIV and the pancreas. Lancet *2*:1212–1213, 1987.
136. Ziegler, D. W., Long, J. A., Philippart, A. I., et al.: Pancreatitis in childhood: Experience with 49 patients. Ann. Surg. *207*:257–261, 1988.
137. Zuger, A., Wolf, B. Z., El-Sadr, W., et al.: Pentamidine-associated fatal acute pancreatitis. J. A. M. A. *256*:2383–2385, 1986.

62

PERITONITIS AND INTRA-ABDOMINAL ABSCESS

W. Lance George

Intra-abdominal infection can take several forms: peritonitis, intraperitoneal abscess, visceral abscess, and retroperitoneal infection.[7] Peritonitis, intraperitoneal abscess, and certain forms of visceral abscess are reviewed in this chapter. Liver abscess is reviewed in Chapter 58. Retroperitoneal infection is covered in Chapter 63.

PERITONITIS

Peritonitis is inflammation of the serous lining of the peritoneal cavity. It may be caused by infection or chemical irritation. Peritonitis arising outside the abdominal cavity and reaching the peritoneal cavity via the blood stream or lymphatics is termed primary. Peritonitis is secondary when it arises within the abdominal cavity or is iatrogenic.

Epidemiology and Etiology

Peritonitis is a serious infection. Although relatively common in the preantibiotic era, primary peritonitis now accounts for less than 2 per cent of cases of peritonitis.[5, 8] Predisposing factors appear to be postnecrotic cirrhosis, nephrotic syndrome, and, possibly, urinary tract infection. Ascites typically is present. Primary peritonitis usually is a monomicrobial infection; the most likely organisms are *Streptococcus pneumoniae*, *Streptococcus pyogenes*, *Escherichia coli* and other enteric organisms, and *Staphylococcus aureus*.[5, 8]

The majority of cases of peritonitis are secondary and relate to such processes as rupture of an intra-abdominal viscus or extension of an abscess of one of the solid organs within the abdominal cavity.[1, 2, 4–7] This type of peritonitis usually is polymicrobial and involves 5 to 10 (or more) different species of bacteria.[7] These infecting agents usually are from the gastrointestinal flora but may be from the female genital tract flora; some infections are caused by microorganisms introduced from outside the body in the course of surgery, trauma, or peritoneal dialysis. Bacterial peritonitis secondary to appendicitis or lesions of the colon, for example, typically is a mixed infection involving a number of organisms, with anaerobes predominating numerically. Although various anaerobes may be involved, the major ones typically encountered are members of the *Bacteroides fragilis* group, other *Bacteroides* species (and anaerobic gram-negative bacilli recently renamed but previously classified in the genus *Bacteroides*), anaerobic gram-positive cocci (primarily members of the genus *Peptostreptococcus*), and clostridia.[4, 6, 7] The major nonanaerobes encountered include *E. coli, Klebsiella* species, *Enterococcus* species, and viridans streptococci.[7] Peritonitis originating from higher in the bowel will have lower numbers of anaerobes and coliforms. Recent antimicrobial therapy may alter the composition of the infecting flora. Peritonitis derived from the female genital tract may involve group A or B streptococci and *Neisseria gonorrhoeae* in addition to the aforementioned bacteria.[7] Peritonitis occurring after abdominal surgery often involves *S. aureus* and gram-negative bacilli, such as *Klebsiella, Enterobacter, Proteus,* and *Pseudomonas*, particularly when antimicrobial prophylaxis has been given.[7] Organisms most frequently involved in peritonitis due to peritoneal dialysis are *S. aureus*, coagulase-negative staphylococci, and diphtheroids.

Neonatal peritonitis may arise from a transplacental infection in utero but more commonly is acquired during or shortly after birth. Most often, it is secondary to bacteremia, direct extension from umbilical infection, or perforation of the bowel.[5] After the neonatal period, peritonitis is uncommon until later childhood, with appendicitis a common background factor.[5] Other processes that predispose to peritonitis are intussusception, volvulus, incarcerated hernia, ruptured Meckel diverticulum, and inflammatory bowel disease.[5]

Nonbacterial peritonitis[5] may result from the introduction into the peritoneal cavity of blood, bile, pancreatic juice, gastroduodenal juices, or meconium. Meconium peritonitis results from perforation of the bowel in utero or shortly after birth. This occurs most often as a complication of meconium ileus in infants with cystic fibrosis but sometimes is caused by intestinal obstruction due to other causes.

Pathophysiology

Normally, the peritoneal cavity is remarkably resistant to infection. The two major factors involved in peritonitis are a continuing source of infection in the peritoneal cavity and the presence of foreign material, such as mucus, enzymes, bile, and feces, that protects bacteria from host defense mechanisms or injures the peritoneal lining.[7] In ways that are not understood yet, free hemoglobin facilitates peritonitis.

Plaques of fibrinous material accumulate on the inflamed peritoneal surface and cause loops of bowel to adhere to one another and to the parietal peritoneum. There is an outpouring of serous fluid and leukocytes. The greater omentum adheres to areas of peritonitis. These various factors, as well as ileus, tend to localize infection to a portion of the peritoneal cavity. An important factor determining the outcome is the ratio of bacteria to available leukocytes. If peritoneal defenses and supportive measures are adequate, the process may resolve spontaneously. A second possible outcome is the development of an abscess or abscesses. If host defenses are insufficient, a diffuse, spreading peritonitis may ensue.

Clinical Presentation

The characteristic findings are pain, abdominal distention, absence of abdominal respiratory movement, diffuse abdominal muscle spasm, tenderness, rebound tenderness, decreased or absent peristalsis, rigidity of the abdominal wall, tenderness on rectal or vaginal examination, and fever.[4, 7] Toxemia and shock also may be present. The underlying process may determine the mode of onset and add other features to the presentation. In primary peritonitis, the onset varies from insidious to rapid with extreme prostration. Diarrhea is common, and vomiting may occur. The child may show restlessness, irritability, and anxiety.[4] The temperature often is 39.5° to 40.5° C (103° to 105° F) and may be accompanied by chills or convulsions. However, in extreme situations, and especially in early infancy, the temperature may be normal or even subnormal.[4] Similarly, the very young patient may not have pain and muscle spasm, and patients in shock or receiving corticosteroids may show atypical findings.[4, 7] In such patients, the most important finding usually is a completely silent abdomen on auscultation. There also may be an unexplained rise in pulse rate or drop in blood pressure.

The white blood cell count usually is 16,000 to 25,000/mm^3, with 90 per cent or more polymorphonuclear leukocytes and an increase in immature forms.[4, 7] In primary peritonitis, the white blood cell count may be as high as 35,000 cells/mm^3.

Differential Diagnosis

The differential considerations include such entities as arachnidism, porphyria, diabetic acidosis, lead poisoning, drug poisoning, pulmonary disease, and renal disease.[4, 7] In acute pancreatitis and in diabetic acidosis, there may be glycosuria and hyperglycemia, but these are not typical of peritonitis. Hematuria and pyuria usually are an indication of involvement of the genitourinary tract, but they may relate to adjacent inflammatory disease, such as appendicitis. Mild elevations of the serum amylase may be seen in peritonitis with almost any cause, but very high serum amylase levels indicate acute pancreatitis.

Specific Diagnosis

Roentgenograms of the abdomen in different planes (supine, upright, or left lateral decubitus) may reveal free air due to a ruptured viscus in the peritoneal cavity, gas within an abscess, features of ileus or obstruction, evidence of peritoneal fluid, and obliteration of the psoas shadow or other peritoneal lines.[7] Ultrasonography and computed tomographic scanning often are helpful in determining the underlying cause of the peritonitis. Radiologic examination of the intestinal tract and gallium- and indium-labeled white blood cell scans also may be useful. Obviously, these tests may suggest the presence of peritonitis; in general, though, they are more likely to reveal the primary disease process (in the case of secondary peritonitis) or complications of the illness, such as intra-abdominal abscess. Occasionally, peritoneoscopy or needle biopsy of the peritoneum may be helpful.

Needle aspiration of peritoneal fluid or peritoneal lavage may be very helpful. The presence of pus, blood, or free-floating fat globules is helpful in limiting the diagnostic possibilities. A foul odor to aspirated fluid indicates the presence of anaerobic bacteria. Gram stain and aerobic and anaerobic cultures should be performed on fluid obtained. The unique morphology of certain anaerobes on Gram stain can provide an early clue to the likely presence of these organisms. It is important that material transported to the laboratory be kept under anaerobic conditions during transport.

Treatment

Therapeutic principles include (1) improvement of vascular perfusion by correction of fluid and electrolyte deficiencies, (2) combating effects of bacteria and their toxic products, (3) reduction of paralytic ileus, (4) elimination of the underlying source of infection by excision or closure, (5) aspiration of the infected peritoneal exudate and drainage of the site of the primary lesion, and (6) treatment of local or distant complications. Most cases of peritonitis require surgical intervention, which should be undertaken at the earliest time consistent with proper preparation of the patient.[5, 7]

Antimicrobial therapy also is very important.[5, 7] Primary bacterial peritonitis due to streptococci or pneumococci is treated best with penicillin G in a daily dosage of 200,000 to 500,000 units/kg body weight, given in four to six divided doses, administered intravenously. Because of recent increases in the incidence of both relative and absolute resistance of *S. pneumoniae* to penicillin G, antimicrobial susceptibility should be determined as soon as possible. In postoperative peritonitis, one of the penicillinase-resistant penicillins, such as nafcillin, should be used when *S. aureus* is involved, and an aminoglycoside, such as gentamicin or amikacin, should be used when gram-negative aerobic or facultative bacteria are involved. The dosage of nafcillin is 100 to 200 mg/kg/24 hours, given intravenously in four to six doses. Gentamicin is given to children in a daily dosage of 6 to 7.5 mg/kg body weight administered intramuscularly or intravenously in three doses. The dosing of gentamicin and amikacin is different for infants and neonates younger than 7 days of age; consult Chapter 77 for information. For amikacin, the daily dose is 15 mg/kg body weight, intramuscularly or intravenously in two to three doses. In peritonitis involving bowel flora, an aminoglycoside should be combined with clindamycin, metronidazole, cefoxitin, chloramphenicol, or a broad-spectrum penicillin (e.g., ticarcillin) as initial therapy.[5, 7]

The combination of a β-lactam agent with a β-lactamase inhibitor (e.g., ampicillin-sulbactam, ticarcillin–clavulanic acid) may be useful for treatment of peritonitis in adults, but only limited data are available for children. Similarly, imipenem has an extremely broad spectrum of activity but has not been evaluated extensively in children.[7] Furthermore, certain broader spectrum cephalosporins (e.g., cefotaxime, ceftizoxime) may be effective for treatment of polymicrobial peritonitis in which the infecting flora are susceptible. Dosages (all daily doses based on kilograms of body weight intravenously) are the following: clindamycin, 15 to 40 mg in three to four doses; chloramphenicol, 50 to 100 mg (as 10 per cent solution) in three to four doses; cefoxitin (>3 months of age only), 80 to 160 mg in four to six doses; and ticarcillin, 50 to 300 mg in four to six doses. One of several newer agents (ampicillin/sulbactam, ticarcillin/clavulanic acid, and imipenem) or metronidazole, although not necessarily approved for use in children, might be considered in very seriously ill children. Dosages of all agents given require adjustment for children in the neonatal age group. All dosages assume normal renal and hepatic function. The duration of therapy must be individualized, but in general it should be prolonged (at least 2 to 3 weeks), particularly in cases of secondary peritonitis. In individuals who are quite ill, it would be prudent to add penicillin G to the regimen when clindamycin or metronidazole is used because penicillin is active against a number of anaerobes that may be resistant to clindamycin and against streptococci resistant to metronidazole. The regimen just described for peritonitis involving bowel microflora also is very good for infections related to the female genital tract.

Intraperitoneal administration of antimicrobial agents is neither necessary nor desirable. Modification of therapy, based on susceptibility data, particularly when an aminoglycoside is being used, is essential to lessen the risks of oto- and nephrotoxicity, colonization with antimicrobial-resistant bacteria, and potential superinfection.

Prognosis

The introduction of antimicrobial agents has resulted in a remarkable decrease in the mortality rate in diffuse peritonitis. However, there still may be significant mortality, depending on the underlying cause of the peritonitis and whether or not certain complications are present. Important complications of peritonitis are septic shock, intra-abdominal or retroperitoneal abscesses, postoperative wound infection, adhesions, fistula formation, and respiratory failure.

Prevention

Early appropriate treatment of potential causes of peritonitis may prevent its occurrence. The incidence of postoperative peritonitis may be reduced by the use of good surgical technique and careful asepsis. Preoperative bowel preparation with oral neomycin or kanamycin plus tetracycline or erythromycin lowers the incidence of peritonitis and other postoperative infections. Many surgeons prefer the use of parenteral antimicrobials (with or without oral antimicrobial bowel preparation) for prophylaxis of infection related to colonic surgery, but this does not appear to be superior to mechanical cleansing of the bowel and administration of oral medications as described earlier. When there has been contamination of the peritoneal cavity with bowel contents, such as with perforated viscus, antimicrobial agents should be given along with appropriate drainage. (This represents therapy rather than prophylaxis; see details of therapeutic regimens.)

INTRA-ABDOMINAL ABSCESS

Intra-abdominal abscess may represent abscess in a solid viscus alone (e.g., hepatic or pancreatic abscess), intraperitoneal abscess secondary to spread of an abscess from a solid viscus, or intraperitoneal abscess secondary to peritonitis.[5, 7]

Etiology and Pathogenesis

Excluding retroperitoneal infections (discussed in Chapter 63), the most common visceral abscesses involve the liver (discussed in Chapter 58), the pancreas, and the spleen.[5, 7]

Pancreatic abscess is an uncommon infection; it usually develops as a complication of pancreatitis, which, in children, is of biliary tract, postoperative, or posttraumatic origin.[5] Pancreatic necrosis, whether due to pancreatitis, surgical trauma, or accidental trauma, appears to be a key step in the pathogenesis; reflux into the pancreatic duct of bile contaminated by bowel flora results in infection of the necrotic pancreatic tissues and subsequent abscess formation. Approximately one-half of pancreatic abscesses are polymicrobial and involve Enterobacteriaceae, *Enterococcus*, viridans streptococci, and, less frequently, *S. aureus*. Anaerobic bacteria also are involved in pancreatic abscess; unfortunately, studies adequate to determine the incidence of anaerobes in this type of infection have not been conducted.[5–7] The anaerobes most likely to be present are members of the *B. fragilis* group[6]; properly collected and processed anaerobic (and aerobic) cultures of pancreatic abscess contents are mandatory, however, because of the limited data available. Pancreatic abscess due to *S. aureus* probably occurs by hematogenous infection in most instances.

Splenic abscess, like pancreatic abscess, is an uncommon infection. Although some splenic abscesses develop as a consequence of contiguous infection, the usual predisposing factors are sickle hemoglobinopathies, other causes of splenic infarct (e.g., emboli to the spleen from an infected cardiac valve), and splenic hematoma.[5] The occurrence of bacteremia or fungemia, particularly in the presence of a splenic lesion, then may result in abscess development. Organisms that have caused splenic abscess include *S. aureus;* streptococci; and Enterobacteriaceae, including *Salmonella* and fungi, particularly *Candida* species. Polymicrobial abscess usually arises from an adjacent infection and frequently involves bowel anaerobes and coliform bacteria.

Intraperitoneal abscesses are complications of either primary and secondary peritonitis or occasionally spread from infection in a solid viscus; such abscesses may be solitary or multiple. Surgical or accidental trauma may be an important antecedent event. The location of an intraperitoneal abscess generally is dependent on the site of the primary infection and on the direction in which free peritoneal fluid may flow.[7] Appendicitis is associated with right lower quadrant and pelvic abscesses, reflecting the location of the appendix.[3] More than half of subphrenic abscesses in children also are due to appendicitis, reflecting the propensity for intraperitoneal fluid to flow from the cecum to the diaphragm along the right paracolic gutter.[3, 7] In general, the bacterial flora of intraperitoneal abscesses reflects the flora of the primary infection (as reviewed earlier).

Clinical Presentation

Intraperitoneal abscess is characterized by a high intermittent fever, shaking chills, abdominal pain, and tenderness over the involved area.[5, 7] The presence (and persistence) of leukocytosis in the range of 20,000 to 50,000 cells/mm^3, even in the absence of significant fever, is highly suggestive of abscess. Intraperitoneal abscess may develop after surgery on a diseased but uninfected organ. The typical course for maturation of an abscess is approximately 5 to 10 days.[7] Therefore, the postoperative patient initially may have signs and symptoms consistent with either the postsurgical state or early infection. If significant fever and leukocytosis persist for more than 48 to 72 hours postoperatively, intraperitoneal (or visceral) abscess should be considered, assuming other infections have been excluded. Subphrenic, as opposed to subhepatic, abscesses often are accompanied by costal tenderness and pulmonary or pleural involvement.

Specific Diagnosis

A detailed knowledge of the patient's recent medical and surgical history and a high index of suspicion are essential for prompt diagnosis of intra-abdominal abscess. Routine chest and abdominal radiography may provide important clues. The presence of a pleural effusion may suggest subphrenic abscess; the presence of gas, manifested either by an air-fluid level or a mottled collection of gas bubbles (the so-called soap bubble appearance) on abdominal radiography, is strongly suggestive of abscess.

There are several other procedures that may be needed to detect or delineate an intra-abdominal abscess.[5, 7] Ultrasonographic examination of the abdomen is relatively sensitive and can be performed relatively rapidly. Radionuclide scanning also may be helpful. Gallium scanning commonly is used but has the limitation that the isotope is excreted into the bowel lumen and, therefore, may confound interpretation. Indium-labeled white cell scans also are useful for the detection of intraperitoneal abscesses. This isotope is not excreted into the bowel, and a scan is likely to be positive during the first 1 to 2 weeks of abscess formation. Thereafter, the sensitivity of indium scanning appears to decrease. At present, the most specific test for intra-abdominal abscess is computed tomography when given with intravenous and intraluminal contrast.[7] Magnetic resonance imaging offers the advantage of elimination of radiation exposure. However, it has not been evaluated extensively for diagnosis of intra-abdominal abscess and generally requires more time to perform than does computed tomography; this may be a distinct disadvantage with small children. Careful consideration should be given in each case to the benefits and risks of radiation exposure in the aforementioned tests.

Treatment

The treatment of intra-abdominal abscesses includes appropriate supportive care, institution of antimicrobial therapy after obtaining appropriate cultures, drainage of the abscess, and surgical correction of any primary intra-abdominal disease process.

After appropriate cultures, such as blood cultures, have been obtained, it is prudent to initiate antimicrobial therapy when intraperitoneal abscess is suspected; this usually occurs prior to drainage of the abscess. Obviously, such therapy is empiric and should be based on the most likely pathogens, as discussed earlier.

Early drainage is important. With certain lesions (e.g., hepatic abscess, subphrenic abscess, some postoperative abscesses), percutaneous drainage may be feasible.[7] This technique has proved quite useful in adult patients and may have limited application in older children. In general, though, laparotomy for abscess drainage, closure of associated bowel perforations, and so forth will be required.[5, 7]

Prognosis

The length of morbidity of patients with intra-abdominal abscesses is appreciable. The presence of multiple abscesses or inadequate surgical drainage is associated with significantly greater mortality.

References

1. Altemeier, W. A.: The bacterial flora of acute, perforated appendicitis with peritonitis. Ann. Surg. *107*:517–528, 1938.
2. Altemeier, W. A.: The pathogenicity of the bacteria of appendicitis and peritonitis: An experimental study. Surgery *11*:374–384, 1942.
3. Altemeier, W. A., Culbertson, W. R., Fullen, W. D., et al.: Intra-abdominal abscesses. Am. J. Surg. *125*:70–79, 1973.
4. Brook, I.: Bacterial studies of peritoneal cavity and postoperative wound infection following perforated appendix in children. Ann. Surg. *192*:208–212, 1980.
5. Brook, I.: Anaerobic Infections in Childhood. Boston, G. K. Hall, 1983.
6. Finegold, S. M.: Anaerobic Bacteria in Human Disease. New York, Academic Press, 1977.
7. Finegold, S. M., and George, W. L. (eds.): Anaerobic Infections in Humans. San Diego, Academic Press, 1989.
8. Golden, G. T., and Shaw, A.: Primary peritonitis. Surg. Gynecol. Obstet. *135*:513–516, 1973.

63

RETROPERITONEAL INFECTION

W. Lance George

Infection in the retroperitoneal space technically includes perinephric abscess and many subphrenic abscesses, but in practice, the term retroperitoneal infection or abscess usually refers to infection in the lumbar and iliac regions. Many intra-abdominal organs, such as the pancreas, the duodenum, and parts of the colon, lie posteriorly to the peritoneum and technically are retroperitoneal. Infections that involve these organs usually are manifested as disease within the affected organ and, therefore, are discussed in other chapters in this section.

EPIDEMIOLOGY AND ETIOLOGY

Retroperitoneal infection arises in a variety of ways. Most often, it is related to posterior perforations of the appendix or colon, to infections of the kidney or spine, to suppurative lymphadenitis in the iliac area, and to bacteremia (usually due to *Staphylococcus aureus*).[1, 2] Suppurative lymphadenitis of the iliac region usually is secondary to streptococcal infection of the lower extremities in children.[1, 6] Infections that result from perforation of the appendix or colon posteriorly involve bowel flora. The most common organisms involved are gram-negative anaerobic bacilli, particularly members of the *Bacteroides fragilis* group, clostridia, anaerobic cocci and streptococci, coliforms (chiefly *Escherichia coli*), and enterococci. Infections originating in the spine most often involve *S. aureus*, but a variety of gram-negative bacilli (*Klebsiella, Proteus*, and *Pseudomonas*) also may be implicated. Infections originating in the kidney may involve a variety of organisms.[5, 8]

Renal cortical abscesses almost invariably are caused by metastatic implantation of *S. aureus* from another focus.[8] Perinephric abscess also may involve *S. aureus*, but at present the most common organisms are those that are involved in acute pyelonephritis—*E. coli, Proteus, Klebsiella, Enterobacter*, and *Pseudomonas*.[5, 8] Hematogenous infection of the retroperitoneal space most often involves *S. aureus*, but streptococci also may be found. It has been appreciated that retropsoas and subgluteal abscesses may follow paracervical-pudendal infiltration anesthesia.[7] The solution used for anesthesia may become contaminated with vaginal or rectal flora during administration. The organisms most commonly encountered in these infections are *E. coli, Bacteroides*, and anaerobic streptococci. Retroperitoneal actinomycosis appears on occasion, the primary focus usually being the kidney or the spine. Tuberculosis may be involved in similar fashion.

Less commonly, infection in structures other than those just mentioned may be responsible for retroperitoneal infection. Included are the duodenum (on the right), the ureters, spermatic or ovarian vessels, and para-aortic lymph nodes. Infection in any of these structures may be responsible for retroperitoneal abscess or infection. Elective surgical procedures involving the retroperitoneum may be complicated by retroperitoneal infection. Accidental penetrating trauma to the retroperitoneum, particularly if intra-abdominal viscera also are injured, is prone to result in retroperitoneal infection; such infection most often is caused by colonic flora.

CLINICAL PRESENTATION

Typically, there is a lack of severe constitutional symptoms. Most patients have some pain in the abdomen, flank, or back; the area of pain usually is related directly to the location of the infectious process.[1, 6] Fever often is of low grade.[2]

In infection of the lumbar fossa, there is tenderness and spasm of the back muscles on the affected side, and a mass often is palpable in the lumbar region. On the other hand, there may be a prominent and tender abdominal mass without pain or spasm in the lumbar region.[6] There may be flexion of the hip (psoas sign), but this is more common with infections lower in the retroperitoneal area. There usually is low-grade fever and leukocytosis.

With infection in the iliac fossa, the pain is noted in the iliac or inguinal region; when the psoas muscle is involved, severe pain may be referred to the hip, the thigh, or the knee.[3, 4, 6] A mass usually can be felt in the lower abdomen, and rectal examination may reveal fullness and tenderness. Hip spasm (psoas sign) often is present.

SPECIFIC DIAGNOSIS

Because retroperitoneal infection is relatively rare and the presentation often is not dramatic, there may be a considerable delay in diagnosis. The possibility of retroperitoneal infection should be considered in patients with fever and low back pain. Careful physical examination may reveal the findings just described. A palpable mass is a very important finding, but it may be difficult to palpate retroperitoneal abscesses. Palpation under anesthesia may be helpful. Blood cultures may be positive. Radiographic procedures, including flat plates of the abdomen, barium contrast studies, and pyelography, are helpful. They may delineate the inflammatory mass, show displacement of the kidney or ureter in some cases, reveal an absent or fuzzy psoas shadow, or demonstrate scoliosis with concavity on the side of the infection. Ultrasonic examination of the retroperitoneum is a rapid and rather sensitive means of evaluation. Computed tomography or magnetic resonance imaging performed after injection of contrast agents provides the most precise anatomic information. Radionuclide scans (gallium- and indium-labeled white blood cell scans) may be of value in selected cases.[4]

TREATMENT

The treatment for retroperitoneal abscess is incision and drainage and antimicrobial therapy (see Chapter 62, Peritonitis and Intra-abdominal Abscess).

PROGNOSIS

The prognosis is not as good as in intra-abdominal abscess because of the difficulties in diagnosis. This leads to significant delay in diagnosis and, therefore, in institution of appropriate therapy. A significant number of retroperitoneal infections are diagnosed only at autopsy.

PREVENTION

Early detection and treatment of conditions that are complicated by retroperitoneal infection (posterior perforations of the appendix or colon, kidney and spine infections, bacteremia, and suppurative lymphadenitis in the iliac area) will prevent retroperitoneal infection.

References

1. Altemeier, W. A., and Alexander, J. W.: Retroperitoneal abscess. Arch. Surg. *83*:512–524, 1961.
2. Daviglius, G. R., and Rush, B. F.: Retroperitoneal abscess, a clinical study. Arch. Surg. *83*:322–328, 1961.
3. Firor, H. V.: Acute psoas abscess in children. Clin. Pediatr. *11*:228–231, 1972.
4. Gordin, F., Stamler, C., and Mills, J.: Pyogenic psoas abscesses: Noninvasive diagnostic techniques and review of the literature. Rev. Infect. Dis. *5*:1003–1011, 1983.
5. Malgieri, J. J., Kursh, E., and Persky, L.: The changing clinicopathological pattern of abscesses in or adjacent to the kidney. J. Urol. *118*:230–232, 1977.
6. Neuhof, H., and Arnheim, E. E.: Acute retroperitoneal abscess and phlegmon: A study of sixty-five cases. Ann. Surg. *119*:741–758, 1944.
7. Svancarek, W., Chirino, O., Schaefer, G., Jr., et al.: Retropsoas and subgluteal abscesses following paracervical and pudendal anesthesia. J. A. M. A. *237*:892–894, 1977.
8. Thorley, J. D., Jones, S. R., and Sanford, J. P.: Perinephric abscess. Medicine *53*:441–451, 1974.

S E C T I O N N I N E

MUSCULOSKELETAL INFECTIONS

❑ ❑ ❑

64

Osteomyelitis and Septic Arthritis

Paul Krogstad and Arnold L. Smith

Osteomyelitis

Osteomyelitis, in the strictest sense, means inflammation of bones. This term usually refers to an infection caused primarily by bacteria, but osteomyelitis also may be caused by fungi and viruses. Acute osteomyelitis, if not treated adequately, results in a chronic lesion.

The incidence of osteomyelitis in normal children has been examined in several populations over the last 40 years. Estimates have varied from as low as 1/20,000 adolescent females in New Zealand to as high as 1/1000 in Australian aboriginals.[20, 66] Males appear to be at greater risk, having the disease 1.2 to 3.7 times as often as do females.[66, 149] Overall, 40 per cent of the patients with osteomyelitis are younger than 20 years of age, but one-third are younger than 2 years of age, and one-half are younger than 5 years of age.[98, 121, 170] The incidence is increased in sickle-cell disease and perhaps in immunocompromised patients (see later).

The primary etiologic agent in osteomyelitis is *Staphylococcus aureus;* it is incriminated in as many as 89 per cent of cases. Other causative organisms include streptococcal species, Enterobacteriaceae, *Salmonella,* and *Haemophilus influenzae.* Rarely, viruses, rickettsia, fungi, and certain mycobacteria cause osteomyelitis.

Microorganisms can be introduced into bone in three ways: (1) by direct inoculation, primarily after trauma but also during surgery; (2) by local invasion from a contiguous focus of infection, usually cellulitis; and (3) by hematogenous implantation secondary to bacteremia. Regardless of the routes of infection, the common denominator is microscopic bone death.

HEMATOGENOUS OSTEOMYELITIS

Pathogenesis[30, 91, 176]

In long tubular bones, the infection first begins in the metaphysis, the broad cancellous end of the bone shaft adjacent to the epiphyseal growth plate. The cartilaginous epiphyseal growth plate (the physis) is nourished by diffusion of nutrients from a narrow plexus of capillaries fed by the metaphyseal branches of the nutrient artery; these capillaries drain into a large sinusoidal plexus that ultimately joins the large sinusoidal veins in the bone marrow (Fig. 64–1).[79] Thrombosis of the slow-flowing sinusoidal vessels secondary to trauma or embolization provides a nidus for infection. Blood-borne bacteria can seed the poorly perfused area and proliferate, protected from the host defense mechanisms. *S. aureus* has the ability to adhere to type I collagen of bone fibrils via a ligand that is distinct from the fibronectin receptor.[24] Once *S. aureus* binds to collagen, bacterial replication gives rise to microcolonies that are surrounded by a glycocalyx.[74] Continued injury, elicited by *S. aureus* exoproducts and the host cellular inflammatory response to the injury, causes the accumulation of exudate under pressure. The pressure compresses blood vessels of bone, producing focal bone necrosis. The low ratio of surface area to mass combined with the blood vessel anatomy described earlier is not conducive to reabsorption of necrotic cortical bone.[30, 91]

The very early stages of osteomyelitis, actually a cellulitis of the marrow, may be aborted by appropriate chemotherapy. In the absence of therapy, necrosis of cortical bone and marrow continues. The exudate under pressure is forced through the haversian systems and Volkmann canals and into the cortex (see Fig. 64–1). Given this pathogenesis, it is not surprising that osteomyelitis usually involves only a single bone; only 7 per cent in one series had more than one bone involved at the time of diagnosis.[121]

Bacterial Etiology

S. aureus is the primary pathogen, and group A streptococci are next in frequency. *H. influenzae* type B is an uncommon cause of osteomyelitis; however, in almost all reported series (Table 64–1),[98, 121, 132, 167] it has been found as the etiologic agent in 2 to 5 per cent of diagnosed cases. This incidence is likely to decrease further as immunization makes invasive disease due to *H. influenzae* a rarity. Uncommon organisms usually are suspected because of specific epidemiologic considerations, such as sickle-cell disease, or because of clinical features of the infection (e.g., indolent infection caused by *Kingella kingae*). Anaerobic microorganisms should be consid-

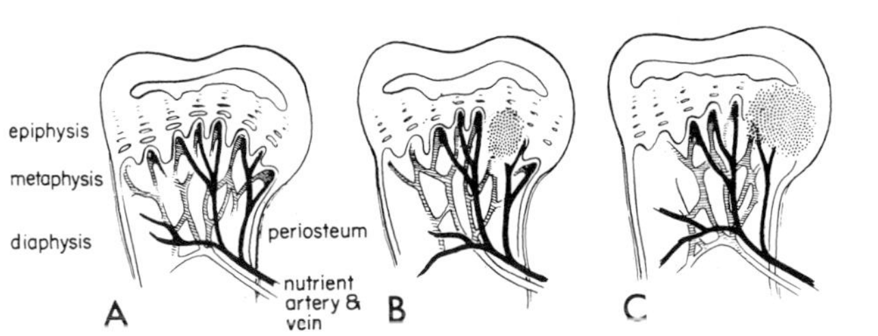

FIGURE 64–1. A, *The sluggish blood flow in the sinusoidal venous connections, located at the metaphyseal-epiphyseal junction, is thought to predispose to traumatic thrombosis and infarction.* B, *Bacteremic seeding of the relatively avascular area initiates the infection, which then spreads through the Volkmann canals and the haversian systems, causing septic thrombosis.* C, *The infection tends to spread laterally through the cortex, elevating or rupturing through the periosteum.*

TABLE 64–1. Etiology of Acute Hematogenous Osteomyelitis in Children

Organisms	Number of Bacteriologically Confirmed Cases			
	Nelson[121] *n* = *297*	*LaMont et al*[98] *n* = *90*	*Unkila-Kallio et al*[167] *n* = *44*	*Roine et al*[132] *n* = *38*
Gram-positive bacteria				
Staphylococcus aureus	67%	70%	89%	89%
Coagulase-negative staphylococci	3%	1%		
Streptococcus pneumoniae	2%	6%	2%	
Other streptococci	12%	16%	2%	3%
Gram-negative bacteria				
Haemophilus influenzae	5%	8%	7%	8%
Pseudomonas aeruginosa	3%			
Salmonella species	2%			
Escherichia coli	<1%			
Kingella kingae	<1%			
Mixed or unusual organisms	4%			

ered if there is an existing infectious focus in which these organisms commonly reside (e.g., sinusitis, mastoiditis, lung abscess).

Signs and Symptoms

The clinical presentation of osteomyelitis depends upon the age of the patient (Fig. 64–2). In the newborn infant, the relatively thin cortex and loosely applied periosteum are poor barriers to the spread of infection. Consequently, the purulence rapidly ruptures through both these structures into the contiguous muscular bed. With progression of the infection, the purulent material often dissects the muscle bundles, with the red, swollen, discolored limb taking on the appearance of a sausage. In addition, the nutrient metaphyseal capillaries perforate the epiphyseal growth plate in the newborn infant. In children in this age group, the capsule of the diarthrodial joints frequently extends to or is slightly more distal than is the epiphyseal plate. Both of these anatomic situations permit the infection to involve the epiphysis and perforate into the adjacent joint cavity. In older infants,

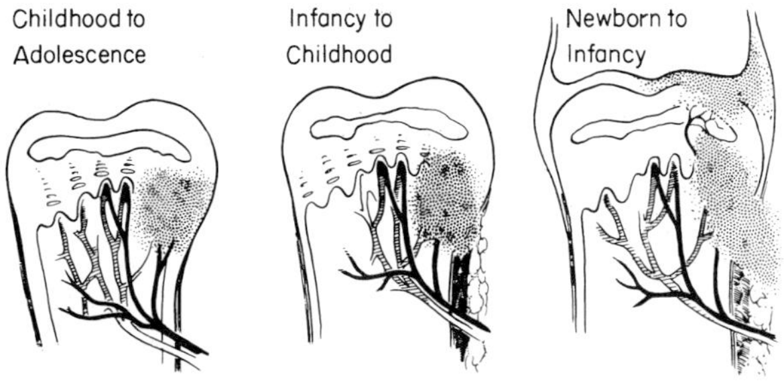

FIGURE 64–2. *In young infants and neonates, particularly in the hip where the epiphyseal growth plate is traversed by nutrient vessels terminating in the distal ossification center, septic thrombophlebitis of the nutrient vessels can lead to growth discrepancies. With the capsule of the joint extending to the metaphysis, rupture of the infection through the cortex leads to septic arthritis. Because of the thin cortex and loose periosteum, the osteomyelitis may come to medical attention as a deep soft tissue abscess. In older infants and early childhood, the thicker cortex and denser periosteum are a greater barrier to the infection. Local tenderness from subperiosteal edema or abscess is the rule. In late childhood and adolescence, the lesion is extremely well localized, rarely penetrating the bony cortex. In this age group, invasive procedures, such as windowing or drilling, are necessary for obtaining infected material.*

the cortex (see Fig. 64–2) is thicker and the periosteum slightly more dense. Both of these function more efficiently as barriers to infection, and, consequently, the infection rarely ruptures and spreads to the soft tissues of the extremity. Subperiosteal abscess and contiguous edema, however, readily develop. In children in this age group, the nutrient metaphyseal capillaries are atrophic. Thus, the avascular epiphyseal growth plate acts as a barrier for the spread of infection to the epiphysis and adjacent joint. The subperiosteal purulence almost always is at the metaphysis, the area in which the cortex is the thinnest.[71] In children and adolescents (4 to 16 years of age), the metaphyseal cortex is considerably thicker, with a dense, fibrous periosteum. The pathogenesis of the infection is the same in this age group, but the infection rarely ruptures and spreads to the outer cortical lamellae. As a result, signs and symptoms of this illness tend to be very focal.

The bacteremic phase of hematogenous osteomyelitis may be recognized by malaise and low-grade fever, may be entirely subclinical, or may be characterized by severe constitutional symptoms with a temperature as high as 40° C. There is no correlation between the magnitude of these signs and symptoms and the severity of subsequent osteomyelitis. In addition, systemic signs and symptoms are no more frequent in any one age group than in another.

The newborn infant usually is irritable when the affected extremity is touched or moved. Pseudoparalysis may occur, and if the disease remains untreated, massive swelling of the extremity may be seen. A plain radiograph is invaluable in this age group: the majority will have changes consistent with osteomyelitis on the initial radiograph.[95, 114, 174]

In infants and young children, there usually are pain and, because osteomyelitis is more common in the lower extremities, a limp. The child refuses to use the affected extremity and displays variable constitutional symptoms. The hallmark of the disease is the marked focality of symptoms; point tenderness and well-localized pain suggest the diagnosis. Percussion of the long bone away from the area of point tenderness often elicits pain at the site of osteomyelitis.

In late childhood and adolescence, there is less restriction of extremity function. The point tenderness is circumscribed more sharply and may be found only as a small area of discomfort present at rest. This disease most often affects the lower extremities, producing a mild limp. Most commonly, tubular bones are involved, but infection in other bones also occurs (Table 64–2). Deep venous thrombophlebitis also has been associated with osteomyelitis in these older patients and may be the presenting symptom. There is some suggestion that this process is associated with a contiguous periosteal abscess.[90]

Nontubular Bone Osteomyelitis

Less than 20 per cent of all cases of osteomyelitis involve nontubular bones. Infection of the calcaneus appears to be most common. In patients with hematogenous infection, there is destruction just under the epiphyseal line in the metaphysis posteriorly and medially, where the blood supply is greatest. This is present in all patients in addition to the destruction of the adjacent epiphysis, particularly in its middle to superior portion. Periosteal new bone formation occurs very late, reossification requiring 3 to 4 months. Osteomyelitis in the other cuboidal bones is rare.

Almost equal in frequency of occurrence of infection of the calcaneus is infection of the bones of the pelvis.[7, 121] Of the bones of the pelvis, the ischium is involved most commonly. The next most frequent involvement is of the ilium, followed by the sacroiliac joint. The pubis is involved only in 20 per cent of the cases of pelvic osteomyelitis.[78, 119] Pelvic osteomyelitis causes an increase in the erythrocyte sedimentation rate in nearly all patients, and two-thirds have a peripheral leukocyte count greater than 10,000 cells/mm^3.[119] The most common organism causing pelvic osteomyelitis is *S. aureus*, which is isolated from either blood or an aspirate from the bone lesions in approximately 80 per cent of the cases. The diagnosis of pelvic osteomyelitis often is difficult. Most patients are judged to have disease in the hip at the time medical attention is sought. Most often, patients with pelvic osteomyelitis have hip pain and abnormality of gait but allow their hips passively to be put through a range of motion. Point tenderness at the site of the lesion can be elicited in approximately half the patients. Sacroiliitis often is difficult to define. Compressing the pelvis, which stresses the sacroiliac joint, produces local pain. Tenderness, if present, in the buttocks or the sciatic notch is an invaluable diagnostic finding.[1, 29, 43, 115, 175] Pelvic osteomyelitis can mimic appendicitis and urinary tract infection; it is more common in individuals with inflammatory bowel disease. In the majority, the plain films of the pelvis are not rewarding, whereas the technetium 99m (Tc 99m) bone scan indicates the diagnosis in approximately 90 per cent.[108, 119] Computed tomography has revealed infection not evident by Tc 99m scanning.[96] Magnetic resonance imaging is likely to reveal abnormalities[166]; however, comparative data are not available. Antibiotic therapy alone is adequate in a majority of the cases of pelvic osteomyelitis. Only when there is a lack of response to antimicrobial therapy is surgery indicated. Osteomyelitis in the pelvic bones has a uniformly good prognosis; chronic infection or sequelae are extremely rare.

Hematogenous osteomyelitis of the flat bones is extremely rare but has been described in the skull, ribs, sternum, and scapula.[116, 121, 168]

TABLE 64–2. Site of Bone Involvement in Acute Hematogenous Osteomyelitis

Bone Type	Per Cent
Tubular	
Femur	36
Tibia	33
Humerus	10
Fibula	7
Radius	3
Ulna	2
Clavicle	1
Cuboidal	
Calcaneous	3
Patella	1
Tarsals and phalanges	0.5
Irregular	
Ilium	2.2
Pubis	0.5
Ischium	0.1
Flat	
Ribs	0.5
Skull	0.3
Sternum	0.2
Scapulae	0.1

Bone classification is according to Jaffe.[87a]

Epiphyseal Osteomyelitis[62, 107, 165]

Rarely, hematogenous osteomyelitis may arise in the epiphysis of tubular bones of young children. This may occur when microorganisms are delivered to the epiphysis by transphyseal vessels. After 15 to 18 months of age, these vessels are lost and the physis acts as a physical barrier to the spread of infection from the metaphysis. However, the vascular anatomy of the epiphysis is very similar to that of the metaphysis, and in some cases infection may occur when bacteria are delivered to venous sinusoids by terminal branches of epiphyseal arteries. Hematogenous epiphyseal osteomyelitis may be acute or subacute in presentation. In the acute presentation, septic arthritis initially may be diagnosed when joint swelling and abnormal fluid are removed by diagnostic aspiration. In cases with a more indolent presentation, pain, limp, or other symptoms prompt an evaluation for the possibility of an osteoarticular infection. The correct diagnosis is made when a radionuclide bone scan or plain radiographs taken weeks later show evidence of increased bone turnover or the lytic changes characteristic of osteomyelitis. Treatment appropriate for epiphyseal osteomyelitis has been followed by complete recovery without apparent sequelae 2 to 6 years after diagnosis.

Pseudomonas *Infections*

This organism was an infrequent cause of bone infection until the advent of antibiotics. Almost all cases of hematogenous *Pseudomonas aeruginosa* osteomyelitis occur in individuals with a history of injecting illicit drugs. The disease is characterized by some pain accompanied by very few constitutional symptoms. The spinal vertebrae and pelvic bones are involved most frequently.[81, 105, 136]

Chronic Hemodialysis Patients

These patients, with multiple invasions of their vascular compartment, appear to be at greater risk for hematogenous osteomyelitis. Their indwelling intravenous cannulas can be colonized with *Staphylococcus epidermidis* or *S. aureus*, and osteomyelitis may develop. The thoracic spine and ribs are the bones most commonly involved; other tubular and cuboidal bones that have been traumatized also can become infected. There are no specific clinical features associated with this illness.

Infection After Closed Fractures

Several groups of workers[25, 37, 172] have noted acute hematogenous osteomyelitis occurring after closed fractures of tubular bones. In all reported cases, the diagnosis was not recognized until fluctuation was apparent at the fracture site. However, there are clues to its diagnosis: after initial postfracture pain has subsided, the pain of osteomyelitis appears. It begins as early as 1 week and as late as 6 weeks after injury. The pain differs from that associated with the fracture by being progressive, and it is not relieved by immobilization. When the cast is removed, a local erythema and warmth are apparent and are increased when it would seem that these findings would be resolving if they were secondary to the fracture. Patients are febrile and may be thought to have another focus of infection before the diagnosis is realized. Anaerobic superinfection of staphylococcal osteomyelitis at the fracture site has been recognized.[160] Adequate débridement, administration of appropriate antibiotics, and external fixation have been used in such cases. The outcome, however, is variable.

Polymicrobial Osteomyelitis

Isolation of multiple bacteria from bone pus is uncommon in acute osteomyelitis.[125] In more than half the cases, it represents spread from contiguous infectious foci and most often occurs in the skull, face, hands, or feet. Distal extremities compromised by vascular insufficiency or immobile because of peripheral neuropathy often are the site of polymicrobial osteomyelitis (including paraplegia due to spina bifida). In children, *S. aureus* and streptococci are the most common isolates: in a small number of cases, gram-negative bacilli are additional organisms.[125]

Chronic Recurrent Multifocal Osteomyelitis

This illness, characterized by chronic focal, multiple inflammatory lesions in bone with periodic exacerbations and remission, moderate bone pain, and sterile lesions, first was described by Giedion and coworkers.[63] Initially, this disease is difficult to distinguish from pyogenic osteomyelitis; there seems to be no difference other than the apparent absence of an infecting agent. Repeated biopsy of lesions that prove to be sterile usually leads to the diagnosis. It is more common in girls younger than 10 years of age. At presentation, slightly more than half have fever, and virtually all have an increased erythrocyte sedimentation rate (or increased C-reactive protein). The lesions primarily are in the distal femur, the distal tibia, and the proximal tibia. Virtually all long tubular bones can be involved, the metaphysis being involved in all lesions reported to date. Patients may have from 2 to 18 lesions, which on biopsy show a nonspecific chronic inflammatory process. Occasionally, there is a predominance of plasma cells, leading to this disease erroneously being called plasma-cell osteomyelitis. In the first reported cases, the lesions were symmetric. However, this feature has not been present consistently as more cases have been described. Many of the cases are in children of northern European origin.[14, 94, 169] Approximately 20 per cent of patients have a pustular eruption of the palms and soles at the same time that they come to medical attention with bone lesions: this illness is called pustulosis palmaris et plantaris. Some patients also may have Sweet syndrome, in which painful, indurated, cutaneous plaques are found accompanied by fever and leukocytosis. It well may be that Sweet syndrome and pustulosis palmaris et plantaris are variations of the same illness. In addition, Sweet syndrome and congenital dyserythropoietic anemia also have been associated with chronic recurrent multifocal osteomyelitis.[47, 108] The long-term outlook in children with this disease is good.[14] Glucocorticoids and nonsteroidal anti-inflammatory agents have been administered to children with this disease. All appear to afford transient relief. However, there is recurrence of symptoms and lesions when these agents have been discontinued.

Osteomyelitis in the Newborn

Infection of the bones of newborns has distinct physiologic and clinical features that merit emphasis.[6] Although rare, osteomyelitis in the neonate may occur in infants with certain risk factors, such as prematurity, skin infections, and complicated delivery.[58, 95] As indicated earlier, the epiphyseal-metaphyseal junction frequently is within the joint capsule, and blood vessels that penetrate the epiphysis are common, particularly in the hip, shoulder, and knee of the newborn. In newborns, osteomyelitis in the long tubular bones frequently (50 to 70 per cent of cases) is accompanied by contiguous septic arthritis. Fever is present in a third to a half of the newborns; of these, half have a "septic" or "toxic" appearance. Half of the infants have multiple bones involved. Antecedent infections are present in half the cases and usually are nosocomial; infection of heel puncture sites, arterial cannulae, lungs, and cut-down sites and cephalhematoma all have been described.[6, 39] *S. aureus* is the etiologic agent in more than 90 per cent of cases; gram-negative bacilli cause a minority of cases.

Group B streptococci have been isolated with increasing frequency.[46] Infants with infection due to this organism are older (2 to 4 weeks of age), there is no recognized preceding infection, and a single bone is involved, often the right tibia or humerus.[6]

Osteomyelitis in the skull, an uncommon disease, can occur in the neonate. This often is associated with a cephalhematoma with or without loss of skin integrity.[100] It can be due to fetal monitoring without a cephalhematoma.[110] A variety of bacteria have been isolated from such lesions; as one might expect, most of these have been organisms present as vaginal flora. Radiographic changes (i.e., bony erosion) are a late finding, but computed tomography of the skull appears to assist in the diagnosis. Infection of a cephalhematoma should be considered if it is enlarging, if it is inflamed, or if there is laboratory evidence of infection (such as an increased C-reactive protein or leukocyte count). In most cases, the lesion is drained and treated with an antibiotic appropriate for the infecting organism.

In older series of osteomyelitis, sequelae appear to have been common. However, in more recent series,[95, 178] approximately three-fourths of all cases had a good outcome, even when the hip was involved. When seen, sequelae include avascular necrosis of the femoral head, bony deformities, and limb shortening.[124]

Osteomyelitis in Children with Hemoglobinopathies

After pneumonia, osteomyelitis is the second most common infection in children with sickle-cell disease.[9] Patients at risk are those with hemoglobin SS, hemoglobin S-Thal, or hemoglobin SO-Arab and certain children with hemoglobin SC disease.[73, 146] The disease does not differ in its initial clinical manifestations but is characterized by a propensity for simultaneous involvement of multiple sites, a tendency toward recurrence, and a greater frequency in children 18 to 48 months of age. *Salmonella* osteomyelitis occurs in less than 1 per cent of normal patients with *Salmonella* bacteremia,[176] but the frequency of *Salmonella* osteomyelitis in sickle-cell disease is several hundred times that occurring in the general population, with an incidence estimated at 0.36 per cent per annum.[9, 42, 126]

Seventy per cent of all lesions or blood cultures in children with hemoglobinopathy and presumptive osteomyelitis yield *Salmonella* microorganisms, 10 per cent contain *S. aureus*, and aerobic gram-negative rods are isolated in 7 per cent, including *Shigella sonnei*,[134] *Escherichia coli*,[72] *Serratia* species,[57] and *Arizona hinshawii*.[83]

A number of factors probably contribute to the greater incidence of osteomyelitis in patients with sickle-cell hemoglobinopathy. It has been suggested that individuals with such hemoglobinopathies are exposed more frequently to *Salmonella*, but this epidemiologic influence has not been confirmed. Injuries to the intestinal mucosa from local thrombosis during a thrombotic crisis may facilitate entrance of the organisms into the blood stream.[176] Once blood stream infection occurs, the splenic dysfunction in these patients may allow a prolonged period or greater magnitude of the bacteremia. It is not clear whether bacteria lodge in infarcted bone or whether there is a different pathogenesis. Infarction occurs in the capital femoral epiphysis, hands, feet, and vertebrae, whereas osteomyelitis involves the metaphyseal-diaphyseal junction of long tubular bones.[48, 126]

Infants with the hand and foot syndrome are not distinguished easily from those with osteomyelitis of the phalanges of the hands or tarsal bones of the feet.[12, 31, 173] Changes on plain radiographs due to osteomyelitis are more severe than are those usually found in sickle-cell disease. The most common radiographic findings are a longitudinal intracortical diaphyseal fissure and overabundant periosteal new bone formation. The cortical fissures are thought to represent a layer of purulent exudate in and between the periosteal new bone and dead bone.[42]

Radionuclide scans often are used to help differentiate osteomyelitis from bone infarction. In theory, bone infarction should have decreased uptake of Tc 99m in the early "blood pool" phase of the scan; increased uptake would be found only as the lesion healed.[92] However, in one series with 34 sites of infarction, there was increased Tc 99m uptake in 10, normal uptake in 9, and decreased uptake surrounded by zones of increased concentration in the remaining 15 sites.[65] Gallium 67 or bone marrow scans of lesions with technetium sulfur colloid may be of value in differentiating infarction from infection; increased uptake of the radionuclide is seen more frequently with infection than infarction.[128] Acute infarction and osteomyelitis cannot be differentiated by gadolinium-enhanced magnetic resonance imaging, perhaps because of preexisting abnormalities of the bone marrow. However, magnetic resonance imaging may be useful for presurgical evaluation.[17] Generally, patients with bony infarcts have had dactylitis as an infant and multiple episodes; the temperature usually is less than 39° C. Children with hemoglobinopathy and osteomyelitis lack the history and have a modest leukocytosis of immature granulocytes.[85]

If fever, leukocytosis, and local symptoms persist despite hydration and other supportive measures, needle aspiration of the area must be considered. Identification of an infectious pathogen particularly is important because there are no well-established regimens for the treatment of gram-negative osteomyelitis. Because of its tendency to recur, a balance between the potential toxicity of the drugs used and the longest possible duration of therapy is sought.

Osteomyelitis in HIV Infection[53, 84, 111, 150]

Although recurrent invasive bacterial infections often complicate HIV infection in children and adults, there are few reports of osteomyelitis in these patients. Many of the existing reports involve patients with recent intravenous drug use, which probably acted as a predisposing factor. *S. aureus* was recovered most commonly, although *E. coli*, *Salmonella enteritidis*, *Cryptococcus neoformans*, *Mycobacterium kansasii*, *Histoplasma capsulatum*, and other organisms also were seen in individual cases. To date, there is no evidence that the presenting signs and symptoms or treatment needed for recovery from osteomyelitis are affected by co-infection with HIV.

Brodie Abscess[151]

In some patients, a subacute form of osteomyelitis occurs, resulting in the formation of intraosseous abscesses. These patients most often are adolescents who present with complaints of long bone pain and tenderness. Bony defects are detected by radiography in most patients. The erythrocyte sedimentation rate usually is normal. Treatment consists of surgical drainage and curettage followed by antimicrobial therapy, as for other forms of hematogenous osteomyelitis. A variety of organisms have been isolated from these lesions, including *H. influenzae*,[97] but *S. aureus* and other gram-positive cocci are the usual pathogens involved. The prognosis generally is good, although deformities occur in some cases.

Differential Diagnosis

Osteomyelitis can be confused with a number of other diseases associated with fever, pain, and tenderness in an extremity. These diseases include rheumatic fever, septicemia, septic arthritis, cellulitis, Ewing sarcoma, leukemia, reflex neurovascular dystrophy, thrombophlebitis, bone infarction secondary to sickle-cell or Gaucher disease, and toxic synovitis.

Diagnosis

Bacteriology

The cornerstone of the diagnosis of osteomyelitis is the isolation of bacteria or other microbes from bone or from anatomic structures that are contiguous to bone. Overall, such cultures (bone, subperiosteal exudate, or joint fluid) provide a bacteriologic diagnosis in 66 to 76 per cent of cases. Blood cultures are rewarding less frequently; an organism was recovered from blood in only 36 to 76 per cent of patients in three series.[41, 121, 168]

In neonates, needle aspirations of the soft tissue or incision and drainage of bone may yield the offending organism. In infants and young children, subperiosteal needle aspirations can be used if the point tenderness is localized easily. In older children and adolescents, noninvasive culturing of the bone is less rewarding. In this age group, windowing or drilling to drain the pus from the bone yields valuable material for culture but is controversial; some orthopedic surgeons believe that the risk of epiphyseal damage and subsequent length discrepancy secondary to the procedure is too great. Thus, there is more reliance on blood cultures and noninvasive methods.

A diagnosis of osteomyelitis also should be entertained in a child with deep thrombophlebitis who has not had that extremity immobilized either in bed or with a cast.[82]

Radiology

PLAIN RADIOGRAPHS. Conventional radiographs first were used to aid in the diagnosis of osteomyelitis. Because bone density must decrease 50 per cent to be detected by x-ray,[7] the less ossified bones of neonates indicate infection more reliably than do those of older children and adults. In contrast, Waldvogel and Papageorgion[171] found in the adults that plain radiographs were of no diagnostic value in 23 per cent and were misleading in an additional 16 per cent.

Radiographic changes occur in three stages.[26] The first stage, occurring approximately 3 days after the onset of symptoms, is a small, local, deep soft tissue swelling in the region of the metaphysis (Fig. 64–3). Thus, when early diagnosis of osteomyelitis is sought, examination of the radiograph should be directed to the soft tissue rather than the bone. The second stage, occurring 3 to 7 days after the onset of symptoms, is swelling of the muscles and obliteration of the interposed translucent fat planes. This is due to continued spread of edema fluid and can progress, particularly in neonates and young infants, to superficial soft tissue edema; the skin may take on an orange-peel texture.

Third, the radiographic picture typically associated with osteomyelitis does not occur until 10 to 21 days after the onset of symptoms. The variability depends upon the specific bone involved: in general, long tubular bones tend to show bone destruction and periosteal new bone formation 2 to 3 weeks earlier than do membranous or irregular bones.

RADIONUCLIDE IMAGING. Radionuclide scanning has been found to be a valuable adjunct to the diagnosis of osteomyelitis.[44] Bone imaging using technetium 99m (Tc 99m) polyphosphate or diphosphonate compounds is based on initial flow through the bone and adsorption of covalently bonded Tc 99m phosphate adduct to the surface of the hydroxyapatite crystal in bone. With microautoradiographic techniques, it is found that Tc 99m pyrophosphate is concentrated in the cement line, located at the junction of osteoid and mineralized bone.[162]

Most institutions perform a three-phase bone scan. Shortly after injection (2 to 5 seconds), a nuclear angiogram (flow phase) image is obtained of the area of suspected osteomyelitis. The second phase (the blood pool phase) consists of a single image obtained 5 to 10 minutes after injection. The third image is obtained 2 to 4 hours after injection. In this latter phase, specificity of the diphosphonate compounds for the bone is revealed. Anything increasing local blood flow to the area, particularly if accompanied by inflammation, results in increased general uptake in the first two phases, but osteomyelitis results in focal uptake in the third phase with the intensity of the signal detected reflecting the level of osteoblastic activity.[38] The overall accuracy of a Tc 99m image revealing osteomyelitis exceeds 90 per cent (Fig. 64–4).[28, 40, 44, 64, 96, 140] It is clear that osteomyelitis can be diagnosed by Tc 99m scan and treated successfully without the development of evidence of bone changes on plain radiographs. In one study, seven children with bacteriologically proven osteomyelitis had the diagnosis suggested by a Tc 99m methylene diphosphonate scan; only three of the seven ultimately developed typical radiographic bone changes.[164] Serial bone scans have been performed in children with osteomyelitis.[142] In general, changes on the nuclide scan are more characteristic when patients have had an illness of longer duration.

However, bone scans that utilize Tc 99m may be nondiagnostic in neonates.[58] There is destruction of cortical bone, and periostial new bone formation often is present on plain film radiographs of bones with normal Tc 99m uptake. The false-negative result of bone scans probably is due to the paucity of mineralization in the neonate's bones. Ischemia of bone, probably due to infarction, also has been noted on the initial bone scan.[114] Overall, the sensitivity of bone scan in neonates is uncertain but may be as low as 30 per cent.[5]

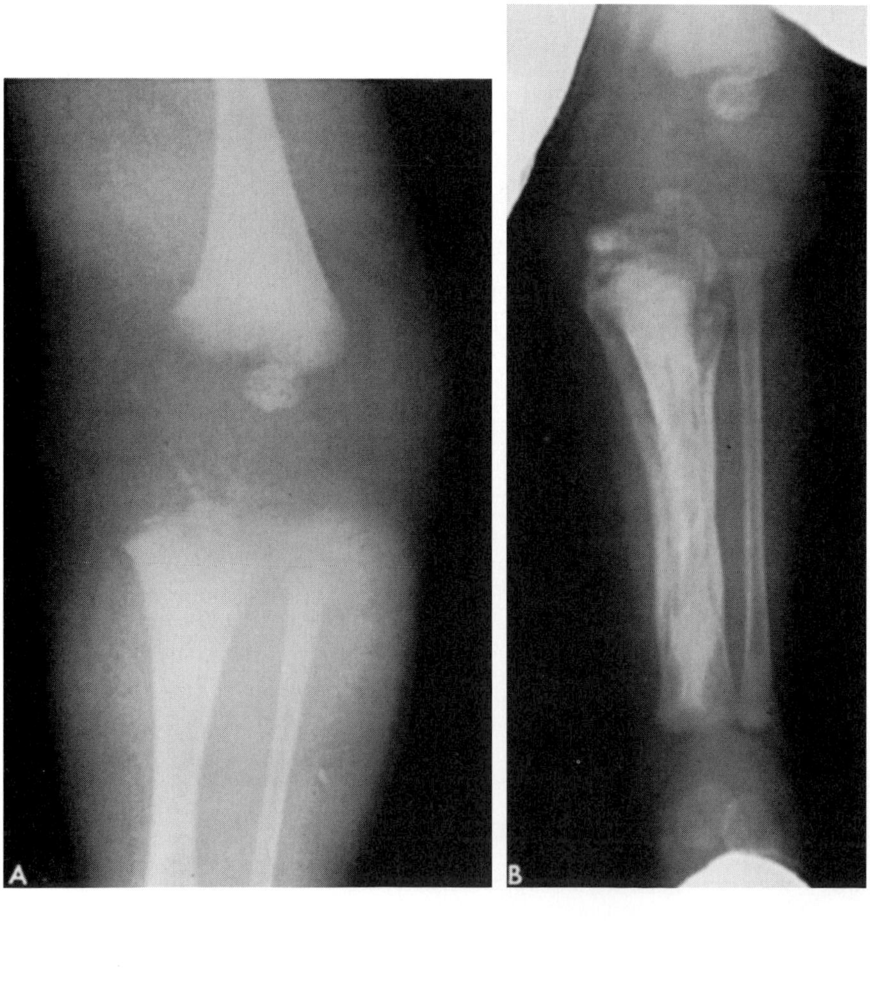

FIGURE 64–3. A, *Left knee of an infant that shows an increase in water density around the proximal tibia and fibula. No fat lines are apparent on this plain film.* B, *Two layers of subcutaneous fat lines between the muscles and the skin can be seen, as well as an exaggerated involucrum involving almost all of the tibia 6 weeks later.*

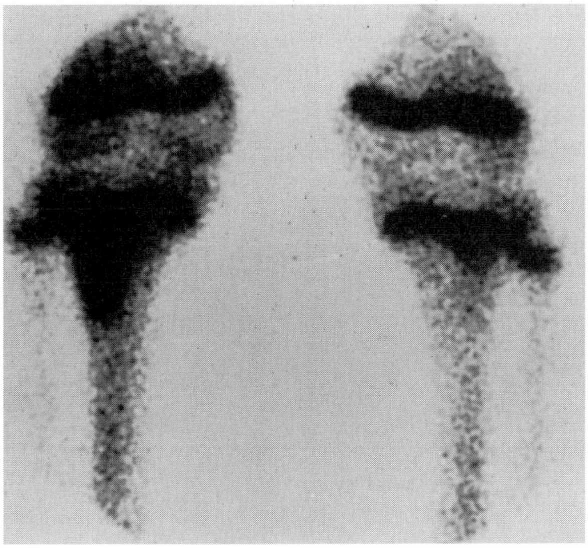

FIGURE 64–4. *A technetium pyrophosphate scan of an adolescent boy with pain and tenderness of the proximal right tibia. Exaggerated uptake of the isotope on the right metaphyseal-epiphyseal junction is seen, compared with the left. (Courtesy of Dr. Joel Blumhagen.)*

Older infants with osteomyelitis and a nondiagnostic Tc 99m bone scan also have been described.[13, 75] In such instances, the gallium 67 scan may be of value. Gallium 67 is a transition metal, which, like iron, is bound to plasma proteins; the unbound portion, 10 to 25 per cent, is excreted in the urine. It localizes in inflammatory foci because of increased capillary permeability (leaking plasma proteins), in vivo leukocyte labeling, binding to lactoferrin in the lesion, and perhaps direct bacterial uptake. Because of the slower elimination of gallium from the blood, its uptake in an inflammatory focus is less dependent on blood flow. Delayed elimination, however, often results in poor contrast of bone to soft tissue, delaying reliable interpretation for 24 to 72 hours after injection.[80] Fifteen of 16 cases of osteomyelitis with a nondiagnostic Tc 99m scan had changes on gallium 67 scan typical of osteomyelitis.[148] Combined evaluation with both gallium imaging and Tc bone scan may lead to greater diagnostic certainty when the studies are not conclusively diagnostic.[145]

A number of studies have been conducted to examine the utility of indium 111–labeled leukocyte scans for the diagnosis of osteomyelitis. This method involves removing leukocytes from the patient and injecting them back into the patient after in vitro labeling. A sensitivity of approximately 86 per cent has been ascribed to this method.[138] The sensitivity appears to be best for detection of long bone lesions. False-positive scans can result from a variety of processes, including fracture and infarction. Enthusiasm for this modality also is limited by the higher organ absorption of the radiation dose.[60] A number of other scintigraphic methods for the detection of osteomyelitis have been examined, including Tc 99m hexamethylpropyleneamine oxide–labeled leukocytes and monoclonal antibodies. At present, no distinct advantages have been ascribed to these newer methods.

MAGNETIC RESONANCE IMAGING AND COMPUTED TOMOGRAPHY. Magnetic resonance imaging can give more specific anatomic information than can computed tomography or plain radiography. The major advantage of magnetic resonance imaging is that it delineates accurately subperiosteal or soft tissue collections of pus, permitting surgical drainage, and it can identify sinus tracts for removal.[56, 157, 166] In acute osteomyelitis, bone marrow edema due to the accumulation of purulent material leads to decreased signal in T1-weighted images. In T2-weighted images of the same area, increased signal is seen. Fat-suppression sequences, including short-time inversion recovery, decrease the signal from fat. Short-time inversion recover sequences thus allow more sensitive detection of bone marrow edema, but the specificity of this method of detection of osteomyelitis probably is lower than that of conventional T1 and T2 sequences. Magnetic resonance imaging may have a particular advantage in diagnosis of spinal osteomyelitis because the distinction between the vertebral body and the adjacent disk is seen clearly. Loss of this border is one of the first abnormalities detected by magnetic resonance imaging in spinal osteomyelitis.

Computed tomography occasionally is used in the diagnosis and management of osteomyelitis because it provides excellent definition of cortical bone and high spatial resolution. Computed tomographic abnormalities commonly found in osteomyelitis include increased density of bone marrow due to accumulation of purulent material, as well as periosteal purulence. Computed tomography particularly is useful in detecting sequestra and delineation of subperiosteal abscesses. It previously has been used to define infections of the spine. However, magnetic resonance imaging by and large has replaced computed tomography for this indication.

Treatment

Acute bacterial hematogenous osteomyelitis should be treated, at least initially, with parenteral antibiotics for two reasons. First, the most common pathogen, *S. aureus*, is prone to disseminate and cause metastatic abscesses as well as primary infection of other organ systems. It should be kept in mind that in the pre-antibiotic era, the mortality rate in *S. aureus* osteomyelitis in children was 20 per cent.[71] Thus, the proliferation of this organism needs to be stopped as quickly as possible. Second, the concomitant physiologic changes resulting from bacteremia in acute osteomyelitis are not conducive to the absorption of oral antibiotics.

Initial antimicrobial therapy always should be directed against *S. aureus* and group A streptococci. In most instances, this consists of penicillinase-resistant semisynthetic penicillin, such as nafcillin or oxacillin. Cefuroxime, a second-generation cephalosporin, also has been used for empiric therapy with good results.[121] Antimicrobial coverage for *H. influenzae* also should be considered for younger children, particularly in those who have not been immunized adequately. Under these circumstances, use of cefuroxime or addition of ampicillin, chloramphenicol, or a third-generation cephalosporin (such as cefotaxime) to oxacillin or nafcillin might be warranted. Other agents may be administered in the presence of epidemiologic factors suggesting the possibility of other pathogens: ampicillin, chloramphenicol, or third-generation cephalosporins for *Salmonella* osteomyelitis; ceftazidime and aminoglycosides for *P. aeruginosa*; ampicillin and aminoglycosides for enteric gram-negative organisms; and clindamycin for suspected anaerobic infections.[51, 131] When an organism is isolated or identified by other means, antimicrobial therapy can be chosen with greater specificity. Staphylococci should be treated with penicillin G if they are susceptible to this antibiotic. In most cases, staphylococci must be treated with a penicillinase-resistant penicillin (oxacillin or nafcillin) administered parenterally in a dosage of 200 mg/kg/day in four to six divided doses.[70, 85, 132] Infection with methicillin-resistant strains of *S. aureus* should be treated with vancomycin, 40 mg/kg/day administered every 6 hours. Ceftriaxone

TABLE 64–3. Antibiotic Use and Duration Relative to Failure Rate in Acute Staphylococcal Osteomyelitis

Study	Number of Patients	Antibiotic Therapy Drug	Duration (Days)	Percentage Failure Rate
Green[70]	62	Cloxacillin	35	6
Blockey and Watson[16]	113	Cloxacillin	21	15
Feigin et al.[51]	19	Clindamycin	42	5
Rodriguez et al.[131]	25	Clindamycin	63	0
Tetzlaff et al.[161]	15	Cephalexin	19	0
Dich et al.[111]	37	Penicillin class	≤21	19
Dich et al.[41]	48	Penicillin class	21–50	2
Geddes et al.[60a]	9	Clindamycin	42–84	0
Bryson et al.[22a]	14	Dicloxacillin	≥35	0
Walker[171a]	14	Cephaloridine-cephalexin	≥28	0
Prober and Yeager[127]	22	Penicillin class	≥35	0
Nelson et al.[122]	23	Cephalosporins	≥21	1*

*Poor absorption of antibiotics administered by the oral route was documented.

should be used with great caution for the treatment of staphylococcal osteomyelitis; numerous treatment failures have been described.

The need for surgical therapy also must be evaluated. Subperiosteal and soft tissue abscesses and intramedullary purulence should be drained. Sequestra, if present, should be removed. If contiguous infectious foci are present, they should be débrided adequately and treated with effective antimicrobial therapy. Immobilization of the affected extremity or splinting may afford relief from pain and sometimes is used to prevent pathologic fractures from occurring when extensive bone involvement is detected by plain radiography.

Duration of appropriate therapy is as important a factor in outcome as is the specific antimicrobial agent chosen. In all reported series, a short duration of therapy has been associated with poor outcome. Harris[76] noted that 4 of 45 patients with acute hematogenous osteomyelitis who experienced relapse had been treated for 4 to 10 days. Likewise, Dich and colleagues[41] noted a 19 per cent failure rate in 37 patients treated for 3 weeks or less; the rate was 2 per cent in 48 patients treated for 21 to 50 days (Table 64–3). Similar data were provided by Blockey and Watson.[16] Thus, the minimum duration of treatment for hematogenous osteomyelitis appears to be 4 to 6 weeks. A conservative approach would be to administer antibiotics until the erythrocyte sedimentation rate is within the normal range.[122] During successful treatment of osteomyelitis, this rate generally increases during the first several days and then declines in the weeks that follow.[167] Failure of the erythrocyte sedimentation rate to decrease during the second week of treatment may indicate the need for surgical drainage or indicate the development of chronic osteomyelitis.[156] Measurement of C-reactive protein, another acute-phase reactant, also has been used to monitor the response to therapy for osteoarticular infections. In one study, C-reactive protein returned to normal levels more rapidly in children with an uneventful clinical course, compared with that in children whose treatment was complicated by prolonged fever, pain, or signs of inflammation or who required repeated surgical drainage.[132] In the same study, slower decline of C-reactive protein values also was associated with more extensive radiographic changes or persistent symptoms 1 to 2 months after discharge from the hospital.

Once controversial, completion of the treatment of osteomyelitis by oral administration of antibiotics has gained acceptance. Such treatment avoids the cost, pain, inconvenience, and hazards of long-term intravenous therapy. In most series in which oral therapy was employed (see Table 64–3), treatment was continued with intravenous antibiotics until the patient was afebrile, until local signs and symptoms of infection were reduced considerably, and until the patient was maintaining caloric and fluid balance by the oral route. In severe or complicated cases, it is advisable to delay switching to the oral route until after the peripheral leukocyte count has normalized and after the erythrocyte sedimentation rate has decreased by 20 per cent or more. Guidelines to indicate when oral therapy[121, 122] is an acceptable option include the following: ability to swallow and retain medication, etiologic agent established, ability of the laboratory to monitor degree of antibiotic absorption, and a clear clinical response to intravenously administered antibiotics.[122]

Antibiotics administered orally for osteomyelitis must be given in doses that often are two to three times those recommended in package inserts. Specific antibiotics and the recommended starting doses are listed in Table 64–4. The assumption implicit in successful oral therapy is that the antibiotic reaches an effective concentration at the focus of infection. Compliance with the prescribed dose and frequency and absorption into the blood stream are necessary to fulfill this assumption. Continued oral therapy on an inpatient basis facilitates management of such patients. However, most patients have their planned treatment course concluded as outpatients. Patient (or parent) education and a continuing time commitment by a physician or nurse are essential to maintain the compliance required for successful treatment.

Absorption of the antibiotic to produce effective concentrations at the site of infection is documented by measuring the concentration of the antibiotic or the antibacterial activity in serum. Advantages of measuring the peak (0.5 to 2 hours

TABLE 64–4. Initial Antibiotic Dosages for Oral Treatment of Osteomyelitis

Drug	Dosage (mg/kg/day)	Interval Between Doses (hr)
Amoxicillin	100	6
Cefaclor	150	6
Chloramphenicol	75	8
Cephalexin	150	6
Clindamycin	40	8
Cloxacillin	125	6
Dicloxacillin	100	6
Penicillin V	125	4

after administration) serum bactericidal titer include testing against the pathogen isolated from that patient and documenting the bactericidal activity of the antibiotic and specifically tailoring treatment. A peak serum bactericidal titer greater than or equal to 1:8 is sought.[127, 161] Dosages of β-lactams often can be increased to 200 mg/kg/day without serious adverse side effects. Diarrhea, a frequent complication of high-dose oral β-lactam therapy, can be mitigated by reduction in dose and the administration of probenecid (40 mg/kg/day, every 6 hours; maximum dose, 2 g/day). A disadvantage of assessing the serum bactericidal activity is the difficulty of performing the test when other antibiotics are present in the serum sample. For example, nafcillin would interfere with evaluating the bioactivity of dicloxacillin. Chemical assays of a specific agent circumvent this problem. Dicloxacillin, for example, can be administered orally and the dose adjusted based on dicloxacillin measurements before the intravenous administration of another β-lactam has been discontinued. This avoids several days of inadequate therapy, should the dosage of the oral agent need to be adjusted.

NONHEMATOGENOUS OSTEOMYELITIS

Nonhematogenous infections of the bone arise either through inoculation or from a contiguous focus of infection.

Puncture Wound Osteomyelitis

Inoculation osteomyelitis most commonly involves either the foot or the patella. Soft tissue infections occur after puncture wounds of the foot approximately 15 per cent of the time, and osteomyelitis occurs in 1.5 per cent of such cases.[55] Osteomyelitis of the foot after puncture wounds in children should be termed osteochondritis. The first report of this condition[88] pointed out that the majority of patients were between 9 and 18 years of age and that *P. aeruginosa* was the predominant organism responsible for these infections. After the initial pain of the puncture wound subsides (in 24 to 48 hours), the signs of osteochondritis appear after another 48 to 72 hours. Typically, there is point tenderness as well as localized swelling, erythema, and pain over the puncture wound entrance. In general, there are very few constitutional symptoms, with no or low-grade fever. There is no peripheral leukocytosis; the erythrocyte sedimentation rate is increased minimally. Although the offending organism most commonly is *P. aeruginosa* (90 per cent of the time), staphylococci, streptococci, and other organisms also have been isolated.[19, 55, 86, 87] In some series,[87] up to 20 per cent yielded *P. aeruginosa* and *S. aureus* on culture. The predominance of *Pseudomonas* can be explained partially on the basis of tropism of that organism for cartilage. The organism is not found commonly in surveys of the skin of the feet,[67, 112, 158] but culture of the sponge liner from sneakers often yields *P. aeruginosa*.[54] Most patients developing *P. aeruginosa* osteochondritis received prophylactic oral antibiotics active against gram-positive pathogens.

Surgical débridement of the necrotic cartilage is the mainstay of treatment. Four to 5 days after adequate débridement the local signs and symptoms of infection resolve, allowing the patient to bear weight on the foot. In contrast, antibiotic therapy alone after a diagnostic aspiration may have to be continued 6 to 8 weeks before weight bearing is possible. Prompt initiation of antibiotics active against *P. aeruginosa* generally is successful.[86, 87] Long-term follow-up of *P. aeruginosa* osteochondritis indicates that many patients have asymptomatic, radiographic abnormalities.[10] Radiographic abnormalities are more common in patients in whom an adjacent joint initially was involved.[10] It is important to emphasize that puncture wound osteochondritis cannot be assumed to be due to *P. aeruginosa*. In addition to *S. aureus* and group A streptococci, *Stenotrophomonas* (*Pseudomonas*) *maltophilia*[8] and *Serratia marcescens*[118] may cause infections of the foot after puncture wounds that are indistinguishable clinically from those due to *P. aeruginosa*. Thus, surgical exploration is imperative for obtaining an etiologic diagnosis because many gram-negative nonfermenting bacilli can infect the foot; these may vary markedly in antibiotic susceptibility. A semisynthetic penicillinase-resistant penicillin and an aminoglycoside or cetfazidime often are employed as initial therapy.[86, 87]

Osteomyelitis of the patella is a disease of children between 5 and 15 years of age, the time in life in which the patella is vascularized. By adulthood, the vessels almost completely atrophy. In almost all cases, the diagnosis is caused by inoculation, such as kneeling on a needle. The most common etiologic agent is *S. aureus*; the signs of osteomyelitis appear 1 week after the puncture. There are no constitutional symptoms, but extension of the leg produces pain over the anterior aspect of the patella. The diagnosis is made by isolation of the organism from the patella. Radiographic confirmation of the diagnosis often requires 2 to 3 weeks. Because the bone lacks periosteum, there is no periosteal elevation, but rarefaction and sclerosis may be seen on the profile view or on tomograms. The treatment of this disease is similar to that for other forms of osteomyelitis.

Contiguous Osteomyelitis

Osteomyelitis related to an infected contiguous focus rarely is seen in children. In one review, only 10 per cent of the patients with osteomyelitis due to a contiguous septic focus were younger than 20 years of age. Almost all cases of osteomyelitis from a contiguous source in childhood are nosocomial or are due to an infected burn wound. The probability of postoperative osteomyelitis is a function of the surgeon's experience, the technique, the length of time the wound was open, and whether or not prophylactic antibiotics had been administered.[152] The interval between the precipitating event and the pain and the appearance of persistent sinus drainage or ulceration is 2 to 4 weeks. The peripheral white blood cell count often is normal, as is the erythrocyte sedimentation rate. More than half of the cases are due to multiple organisms. When there are small draining sinuses, the correlation between the sinus culture and the bone biopsy is good. However, with large open areas, organisms obtained from the wound culture may not be important etiologically, and a bone biopsy is necessary for definitive bacteriologic diagnosis. Staphylococci and streptococci predominate; however, nosocomial gram-negative organisms often are seen.

Spinal Osteomyelitis

Spinal osteomyelitis can involve either the intervertebral disk or the vertebral bodies per se. It is worthwhile to conceptualize these infections as different entities because of the different pathophysiology and prognosis.

Diskitis

The intervertebral disk consists of three components: paired cartilaginous articulation, the fibrous ring (annulus fibrosus), and the nucleus pulposus. The axial vessels that parallel the fetal notocord are atrophied by birth, leaving the avascular, mucilaginous nucleus pulposus. The disk has two arterial supplies: periosteal vessels and vessels descending from the central portion of the vertebral body.[32, 52] The vessel from the central portion of the adjacent vertebra begins to atrophy in the first year and is obliterated completely by 10 years of age. This leaves only the capillary network in the annulus fibrosis, which is derived from the terminal radial ramifications of the periosteal vessels. If the loss of this vascular supply is precipitous, it leads to idiopathic disk necrosis, usually presenting as asymptomatic calcification.[139, 154] (In males, this most commonly occurs in the cervical area.) If, however, bacteremia occurs during the loss of the blood supply, intervertebral disk infection may occur.

Intervertebral disk infection does not have a sex predominance, but the majority of the children are younger than 5 years of age.[144] It occurs almost exclusively in the lumbar region (the L4 and L5 disks most frequently are involved, followed by the L3 and L4). The disease comes to medical attention with the patient's refusal to walk. There may be backache and progressive limp. Nonambulatory infants often become irritable and refuse to sit. On examination, the most striking feature is percussion tenderness over the contiguous spine; hip pain and stiffness, with loss of lordosis of the lower back, are present. On occasion, compression of the spine produces pain at the infected disk. The median duration of symptoms prior to diagnosis is approximately 10 weeks (range, 1 to 18 months). Higher lesions (T8 to L1) can mimic gastrointestinal disease with abdominal pain, ileus, and vomiting, but the most important entities in the differential diagnosis are vertebral osteomyelitis and spinal or paraspinal tumors. Most patients have a history of a recent upper respiratory infection.[18, 93, 99, 130, 135, 147] Fever generally is absent or low-grade. There is peripheral leukocytosis in a third of the patients, and virtually all have an increased erythrocyte sedimentation rate. Forty-six per cent of the patients in the series noted earlier had biopsy specimens that grew microorganisms. Most commonly, *S. aureus* is recovered, with rare isolates of pneumococci and gram-negative organisms, including *K. kingae*. Evaluation for suspected diskitis usually involves careful history taking and physical examination, a complete blood count, determination of the erythrocyte sedimentation rate, a blood culture, and plain lateral radiographs of the lumbosacral spine.

Typical radiographic findings are depicted in Figure 64–5. On lateral film, the first finding is narrowing of the disk space, usually not detectable until 2 to 4 weeks after the onset of symptoms. This narrowing often is overlooked if the loss of the normal progressive (from cephalad to caudad) increase in disk width is not appreciated. This is followed by destruction of the adjacent cartilaginous vertebral end-plates, followed by herniation of the disk into the vertebral body. Rarely, vertebral body compression or wedging is noted. In older children, anterior spontaneous fusion is common. In all individuals, reactive bone proliferation is rare, as are paravertebral soft tissue masses. Because of the overlap of this syndrome with noninfectious disk necrosis, it is not surprising to find that investigators in the earlier literature advocated treatment of this disease solely by bed rest. In view of the low yield and generally favorable prognosis of diskitis, biopsy or aspiration for culture generally is not performed. In general, however, antistaphylococcal therapy is instituted. This therapy frequently is provided orally and for a prolonged period (5 to 6 months). Others have suggested 5 to 7 days of intravenous antistaphylococal therapy, followed by 7 to 14 days of a similar oral agent.[34] Very young children do well, and the disk space will be preserved; spontaneous spinal fusion is common in older individuals.

Vertebral Osteomyelitis

The intervertebral disk loses its vascular supply with age, a process usually being completed by 30 years of age.[159] As a result, bacteremic pyogenic infections of the spine most often occur in the vertebral bodies. The venous drainage of the vertebral bodies is composed of three different freely communicating but valveless systems. Intraosseous vertebral veins drain the center of each body and form a large channel with exits through the nutrient foramen. This in turn anastomoses with the anterior and posterior internal plexus (between the dura mater and the vertebral body). The internal venous plexus has anastomotic connections through the vertebral ligaments with the external venous plexus. The external venous plexus communicates freely with the segmental veins on the ventral surface of the body wall (Batson plexus).

It is thought that reversal of blood flow or thrombosis in the sluggishly flowing vertebral veins is the first event in vertebral osteomyelitis. Because of the vascular communication, osteomyelitis usually involves two adjacent vertebral bodies, initially skipping the interposed disk. The same process of septic thrombophlebitis involving the internal venous plexus can produce epidural abscess (with cord compression) as well as infarction of the vertebral body. Spread along the external venous plexus can lead to a paraspinous mass. In the thoracic area, it may produce mediastinitis.[37] In the cervical area, retropharyngeal abscess can occur. The lumbar area is involved much more commonly than is the thoracic area, which is in turn more commonly involved than is the cervical region.[2, 89, 153]

Children with vertebral osteomyelitis usually are older than 8 years of age and seek medical attention because of dull, constant back pain. Often, the child appears toxic and febrile (>39° C) after an indolent course with low-grade fever for 3 or 4 months. Percussion of the spinal dorsal process frequently elicits exquisite tenderness. Usually, the paraspinous muscles around the involved vertebrae are in spasm, with rigidity of the area. Radiographic examination of a patient with vertebral osteomyelitis shows the earliest change to be a localized rarefaction of one vertebral plateau, followed by involvement of adjacent vertebrae. Marked destruction of the bone, usually anteriorly, is followed by abundant anterior osteophytic reactions with bridging and bone sclerosis (Fig. 64–6). Magnetic resonance imaging is useful in the diagnosis of vertebral osteomyelitis[113] because the vertebral disk and the vertebral body clearly are discernible. Most vertebral osteomyelitis begins anteriorly at the margin between the disk and the anterior part of the vertebral body. In some cases, magnetic resonance imaging has detected evidence of osteomyelitis when radionuclide imaging studies were normal.[163] It radiologically is impossible to distinguish pyogenic osteomyelitis from tuberculous lesions, but the latter usually are characterized by less bone destruction, less bone proliferation, and less sclerosis. The osteophytic bridging between adjacent vertebrae is extremely rare in spinal tuberculosis.

Both Tc 99m and gallium 67 are taken up by the lesion in vertebral osteomyelitis. An advantage of scanning with both isotopes is identification of paraspinous abscess with gallium 67.[137]

Most cases of vertebral osteomyelitis are caused by *S. aureus*. Organisms causing urinary tract infections can cause osteomyelitis, presumably by local spread through the Batson plexus.[21, 77, 101] However, urinary tract infection rarely precedes vertebral osteomyelitis; approximately 2 per cent of all

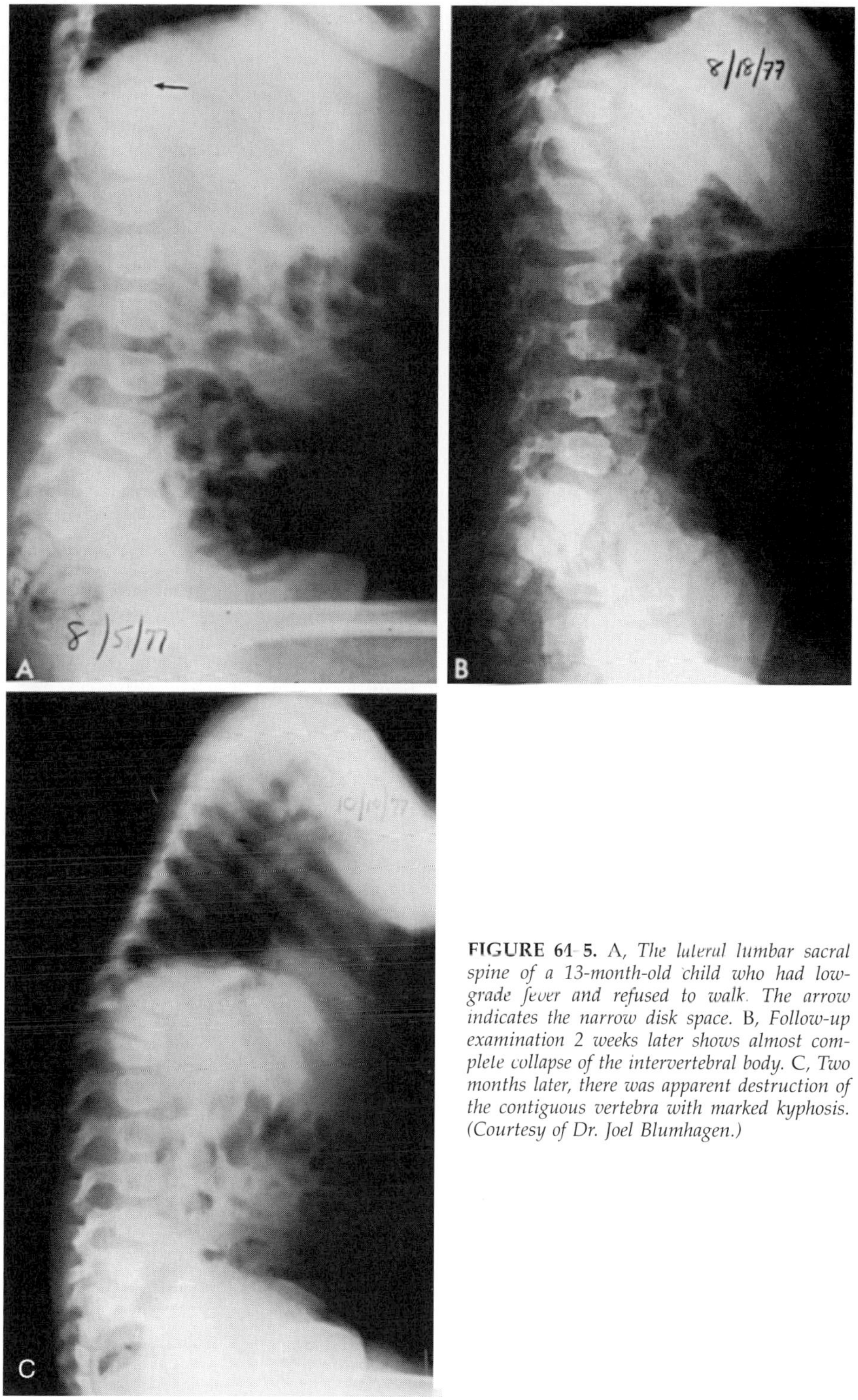

FIGURE 64-5. A, *The lateral lumbar sacral spine of a 13-month-old child who had low-grade fever and refused to walk. The arrow indicates the narrow disk space.* B, *Follow-up examination 2 weeks later shows almost complete collapse of the intervertebral body.* C, *Two months later, there was apparent destruction of the contiguous vertebra with marked kyphosis. (Courtesy of Dr. Joel Blumhagen.)*

cases can be shown to be related to infection of the urinary tract.[61] The best method of establishing the diagnosis is through examination of bone biopsy specimens and cultures.[120]

P. aeruginosa has been recognized as a pathogen in vertebral osteomyelitis.[102, 105, 177] All patients were intravenous drug abusers, and the organisms presumably were inoculated along with the illicit drug. Not surprisingly, younger heroin addicts have been found to have *P. aeruginosa* infection in their intervertebral disks.[22, 141] In the areas of the world where brucellosis is endemic, spinal osteomyelitis due to *Brucella* species needs to be considered.[104] Fungal pathogens causing vertebral osteomyelitis include *Coccidioides immitis* in endemic areas and *Candida* species (often in immunocompromised patients).

The therapy of spinal osteomyelitis includes immobilization. Whether this should be accomplished by simple bed rest or with a body cast is controversial. Antibiotic administration

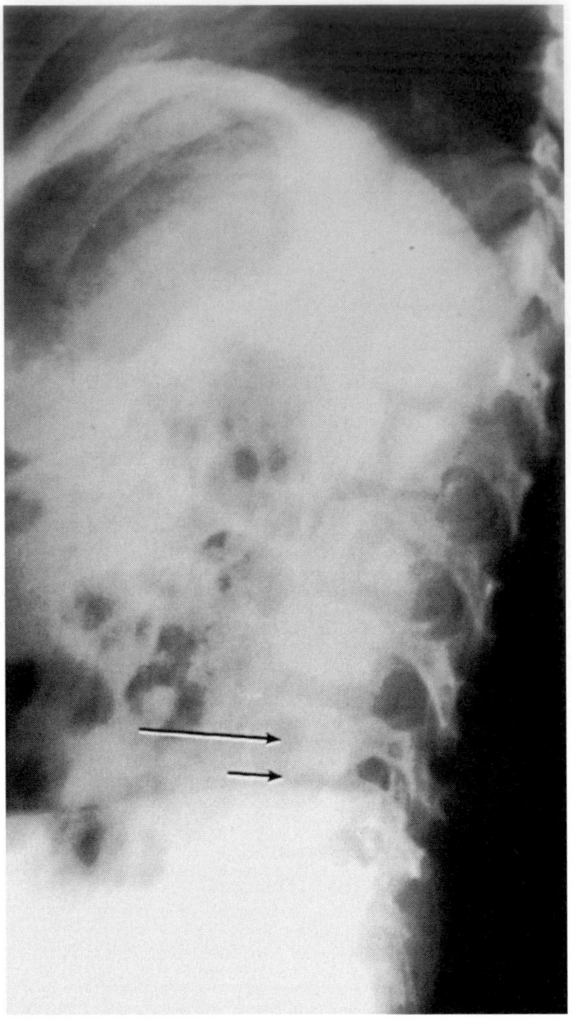

FIGURE 64–6. *The large arrow indicates the lytic lesion with some anterosclerosis in the lumbar vertebra. A small arrow indicates involvement of the adjacent lower vertebra and narrowing of the disk space. (Courtesy of Dr. Joel Blumhagen.)*

always is indicated. The average duration of treatment of bacterial vertebral osteomyelitis is 2 months. There are, however, no data available that can be used for determining the most appropriate duration of therapy. The need for surgical drainage in some cases should not be overlooked, because spinal cord compression caused by epidural or subdural abscess can lead to permanent paraplegia. A paraspinal mass may rupture into the abdominal cavity or erode the aorta; both are catastrophic complications.[59] The optimal therapy for fungal infections of the vertebra is not clear at present.

UNUSUAL MICROBIAL CAUSES OF OSTEOMYELITIS

Anaerobic Organisms

Four distinct clinical entities of infection due to anaerobic bacteria exist: bacteremic seeding of previously normal bones in children and young adults, superinfection of a fracture site already infected with *S. aureus*, an indolent (months to years after surgery) infection of a prosthetic device, and a contiguous chronic infection.[160] Of the latter type, the most common such infections occur in the skull; another 40 per cent occur in the extremities. *Bacteroides* is the most common infecting genus. *Bacteroides fragilis* is the most common *Bacteroides* species and usually is associated with paranasal, sinus, or mastoid infection. In the majority of cases, a foul odor is noted when the bone is incised or the focus opened; trauma often has been an inciting influence.[103]

Actinomyces

More than half of all such actinomycotic infections involve the facial or cervical area. The most common site of actinomycotic bone infection is the jaw, the mandible being involved more frequently than the maxilla. Local signs and symptoms of fever and discharge from a sinus indicate the presence of the disease. Radiographically, periosteal elevation is followed by lytic changes. Often, there will be several "eggshell" areas of new bone.

Forty per cent of all actinomycotic infections occur in the vertebral bodies. In this illness, the infection almost always is associated with a focus elsewhere; the condition comes to medical attention because of mild pain, tenderness, and some stiffness. It can be distinguished from tuberculosis radiographically because of the diffuse honeycombing of the vertebral bodies and the periosteal reaction; large lytic lesions usually are absent. Long-term (>3 months) penicillin G therapy is indicated at dosages of 150,000 units per kilogram of body weight per day, i.e., approximately 100 mg/kg/day.

Unusual Aerobes

Prior to the development of effective vaccines, *H. influenzae* was an unusual cause of osteomyelitis. There are no distinguishing features other than its propensity to occur in the upper extremities.[49, 50, 69, 158a] As with other *Haemophilus* infections, it usually occurs in children between 3 months and 6 years of age.

Brucella species can produce abscesses in the vertebral bodies or long bones, although these are not striking features of the disease. Malaise, headaches, nightsweats, and minimally tender cervical adenopathy, with hepatosplenomegaly, predominate.

K. kingae is a fastidious gram-negative organism that causes osteomyelitis, diskitis, and septic arthritis. These osteoarticular infections often have a particularly indolent presentation. Blood cultures are positive in few patients, and peripheral leukocytosis usually is absent. The diagnosis is established in most cases by culture of joint fluid or purulent fluid removed from focal lesions in bone identified by plain radiographs or three-phase bone scan. These organisms are susceptible to a wide variety of antimicrobial agents. Treatment with β-lactam antibiotics generally has been employed in most patients described and appears uniformly to be successful.[36, 68, 179]

Fungi

Coccidioidomycosis may be characterized by cough, chest pain, nightsweats, and anorexia and often is associated with erythema nodosum or erythema multiforme. This disease commonly is found in the southwestern United States. Extrapulmonary involvement is suggested by persistent high temperature and toxicity. *C. immitis* primarily occurs in cancellous bone, e.g., the vertebral bodies, distal tubular bones, and the skull.[129] These lesions are not distinct radiographically from those seen in osteomyelitis from other causes.[143]

Blastomycosis may mimic coccidioidomycosis, but the pulmonary involvement is much more varied, and fusion of the vertebral bodies is rare. There is a propensity to verrucous, reddened, weeping skin lesions, and prostate involvement may be seen. Bone involvement is frequent; the skull and vertebral bodies are infected most frequently. It is impossible to distinguish this from other forms of osteomyelitis on radiographic examination.

Aspergillus osteomyelitis is being recognized with increasing frequency.[27, 33, 133] Most commonly, it is a disease of the immunosuppressed with *Aspergillus* pneumonia followed by disseminated disease. However, bone disease occurring by hematogenous spread has developed in normal individuals[33, 133] without intravenous inoculation, such as that associated with drug abuse. Penetrating trauma also has produced *Aspergillus* osteomyelitis.

Rhizopus osteomyelitis of the femur without direct introduction has been reported in an immunocompromised adolescent.[45]

Disseminated *C. neoformans* may be seen in 5 to 10 per cent of patients with pulmonary disease. Slowly destructive, very discrete bone lesions may be part of the dissemination. These occur primarily in the long tubular bones without marginal sclerosis. This radiologic reaction is confused most commonly with tumor and, occasionally, with tuberculosis.[23, 106]

CHRONIC OSTEOMYELITIS

This illness is a result of infection occurring secondary to a surgical procedure or after major trauma. Inadequate treatment of acute hematogenous osteomyelitis also can lead to chronic osteomyelitis. Diagnosis of chronic osteomyelitis poses no problem; patients have a painful, nonfunctional extremity with a chronically draining sinus. Cultures of the purulent exudate or of the necrotic bone usually reveal *S. aureus*. Gram-negative bacteria, including *H. influenzae*,[97] may be isolated from the intraosseous abscess.

Treatment of chronic osteomyelitis involves the long-term administration of appropriate antibiotics and surgery, which is essential for the removal of any necrotic debris. Few controlled trials comparing different modes of therapy have been performed. Antimicrobial regimens for chronic staphylococcal osteomyelitis that have been studied include oral cloxacillin plus probenecid for 6 to 12 months; 9 of the 19 patients apparently were treated successfully.[11] In another study, the outcome of a 6-week course of nafcillin was compared with that of nafcillin and oral rifampin. No statistically significant differences were observed with the addition of rifampin, but the majority (10/17) of the patients showed no evidence of disease activity 2 years after cessation of antibiotics.[123]

The high failure rate in these and other studies have led to the study of a variety of adjunctive measures to improve the outcome of chronic osteomyelitis. Local irrigation with antibiotic solutions, with[109] or without[3] added detergents, has been examined. The use of surgically implanted polymethylmethacrylate beads impregnated with an antibiotic (usually gentamicin) has been compared with conventional antibiotic therapy and with therapy with both.[15] No differences were seen among the three groups in a preliminary analysis. Hyperbaric oxygen also has been suggested as an aid to therapy, but no comparative studies have been performed.[35, 117] Because perpetuation of chronic infection appears to be due to the presence of avascular bone and tissue, advances such as the use of laser Doppler flowmetry ultimately may improve the outcome of this disease.[155] Surgical approaches to close open wounds and improve blood flow after débridement with mobilized tissue flaps also appear to bring about prolonged remission in some patients.[4] Complications of chronic osteomyelitis include secondary amyloidosis and local sarcomatosis or carcinomatous changes at the site of infection. The high likelihood of a poor outcome in chronic osteomyelitis must be kept in mind during treatment for acute hematogenous osteomyelitis. Failure to comply with a regimen of oral therapy may result in chronic infection.[156]

References

1. Ailsby, R. L., and Staheli, L. T.: Pyogenic infections of the sacroiliac joint in children: Radioisotope bone scanning as a diagnostic tool. Clin. Orthop. *100*:96–100, 1974.
2. Ambrose, G. B., Alpert, M., and Neer, C. S.: Vertebral osteomyelitis: A diagnostic problem. J. A. M. A. *197*:619–622, 1966.
3. Anderson, L. D., and Horn, L. G.: Irrigation-suction technique in the treatment of acute hematogenous osteomyelitis, chronic osteomyelitis, and acute and chronic joint infections. South. Med. J. *63*:745–754, 1970.
4. Anthony, J. P., and Mathes, S. J.: Update on chronic osteomyelitis. Clin. Plast. Surg. *18*:515–523, 1991.
5. Ash, J. M., and Gilday, D. L.: The futility of bone scanning in neonatal osteomyelitis: Concise communication. J. Nucl. Med. *21*:417–420, 1980.
6. Asmar, B. I.: Osteomyelitis in the neonate. Infect. Dis. Clin. North Am. *6*:117–132, 1992.
7. Babaiantz, L.: Les osteopathies atrophiques. J. Radiol. Radiother. Nucl. Med. *19*:333, 1948.
8. Baltimore, R. S., and Jenson, H. B.: Puncture wound osteochondritis of the foot caused by *Pseudomonas maltophilia*. Pediatr. Infect. Dis. J. *9*:143–144, 1990.
9. Barrett-Connor, E.: Bacterial infection and sickle cell anemia: An analysis of 250 infections in 166 patients and a review of the literature. Medicine *50*:97–112, 1971.
10. Barton, L. L., Hoddy, D. M., Rathore, M. H., et al.: Long-term radiologic outcome of *Pseudomonas* osteomyelitis of the foot. Pediatr. Infect. Dis. J. *9*:476–478, 1980.
11. Bell, S. M.: Further observations on the value of oral penicillins in chronic staphylococcal osteomyelitis. Med. J. Aust. 2:591–593, 1976.
12. Bennett, O. M.: *Salmonella* osteomyelitis and the hand-foot syndrome in sickle cell disease. J. Pediatr. Orthop. *12*:534–538, 1992.
13. Berkowitz, I. D., and Wenzel, W.: "Normal" technetium bone scans in patients with acute osteomyelitis. Am. J. Dis. Child. *134*:828–830, 1980.
14. Bjorksten, B., Gustavson, K. H., Eriksson, B., et al.: Chronic recurrent multifocal osteomyelitis and pustulosis palmoplantaris. J. Pediatr. *93*:227–237, 1978.
15. Blaha, J. D., Calhoun, J. H., Nelson, C. L., et al.: Comparison of the clinical efficacy and tolerance of gentamicin PMMA beads on surgical wire versus combined and systemic therapy for osteomyelitis. Clin. Orthop. *295*:8–12, 1993.
16. Blockey, N. J., and Watson, J. T.: Acute osteomyelitis in children. J. Bone Joint Surg. *52*:77–88, 1970.
17. Bonnerot, V., Sebag, G., de Montalembert, M., et al.: Gadolinium-DOTA enhanced MRI of painful osseous crises in children with sickle cell anemia. Pediatr. Radiol. *24*:92–95, 1994.
18. Boston, H. J., Bianco, A. J., and Rhodes, K. H.: Disk space infections in children. Orthop. Clin. North Am. *6*:953–964, 1975.
19. Brand, R. A., and Black, H.: *Pseudomonas* osteomyelitis following puncture wounds in children. J. Bone Joint Surg. *56*:1637–1642, 1974.
20. Bremner, A., and Neligan, G.: Pyogenic osteitis. Recent Adv. Pediatr. 354, 1958.
21. Bruno, M. S., Silverberg, T. N., and Goldstein, D. H.: Embolic osteomyelitis of the spine as a complication of infection of the urinary tract. Am. J. Med. *19*:865–878, 1960.
22. Bryan, V., Franks, L., and Torres, H.: *Pseudomonas aeruginosa* cervical diskitis with chondro-osteomyelitis in an intravenous drug abuser. Surg. Neurol. *1*:142–144, 1973.

22a. Bryson, Y. J., Connor, J. D., LeClerc, M., et al.: High-dose oral dicloxacillin treatment of acute staphylococcal osteomyelitis in children. J. Pediatr. *94*:673–675, 1979.

23. Burch, K. H., Fine, G., Quinn, E. L., et al.: *Cryptococcus neoformans* as a cause of lytic bone lesions. J. A. M. A. *231*:1057–1059, 1975.
24. Buxton, T., Rissing, J., Horner, J., et al.: Binding of a *Staphyloccous aureus* bone pathogen to type I collagen. Microb. Pathogen. *8*:441–448, 1990.
25. Canale, S. T., Puhl, J., Watson, F. M., et al.: Acute osteomyelitis following closed fractures: Report of three cases. J. Bone Joint Surg. *57*:415–418, 1975.
26. Capitanio, M. A., and Kirkpatrick, J. A.: Early roentgen observations in acute osteomyelitis. Am. J. Roentgenol. *108*:488–496, 1970.
27. Casscells, S. W.: *Aspergillus* osteomyelitis of the tibia: A case report. J. Bone Joint Surg. *60*:994–995, 1978.
28. Charkes, N. D.: Skeletal blood flow: Implications for bone-scan interpretation. J. Nucl. Med. *21*:91, 1980.

29. Chung, S. M., and Borns, P.: Acute osteomyelitis adjacent to the sacro-iliac joint in children: Report of two cases. J. Bone Joint Surg. *55*:630–634, 1973.
30. Collin, D. H.: Pathology of Bone. London, Butterworths, 1966, pp. 209–227.
31. Constant, E., Green, R. L., and Wagner, D. K.: *Salmonella* osteomyelitis of both hands and the hand-foot syndrome. Arch. Surg. *102*:148–151, 1971.
32. Conventry, M. B., Ghormley, R. K., and Kernohan, J. W.: Intervertebral disc: Its microscopic anatomy and pathology. J. Bone Joint Surg. *27*:105–112, 1945.
33. Corrall, C. J., Merz, W. G., Rekedal, K., et al.: *Aspergillus* osteomyelitis in an immunocompetent adolescent: A case report and review of the literature. Pediatrics *70*:455–461, 1982.
34. Cushing, A. H.: Diskitis in children. Clin. Infect. Dis. *17*:1–6, 1993.
35. Davis, J. C., Heckman, J. D., DeLee, J. C., et al.: Chronic non-hematogenous osteomyelitis treated with adjuvant hyperbaric oxygen. J. Bone Joint Surg. *68*:1210–1217, 1986.
36. DeGroot, R., Glover, D., Clausen, C., et al.: Bone and joint infections caused by *Kingella kingae*: Six cases and review of the literature. Rev. Infect. Dis. *10*:998–1004, 1988.
37. Delorimier, A. A., Haskin, D., and Massie, F. S.: Mediastinal mass caused by vertebral osteomyelitis. Am. J. Dis. Child. *111*:639–643, 1966.
38. Demopulos, G. A., Bleck, E. E., and McDougall, I. R.: Role of radionuclide imaging in the diagnosis of acute osteomyelitis. J. Pediatr. Orthoped. 8:558–565, 1988.
39. Deshpande, P. G., Wagle, S. U., Mehta, S. D., et al.: Neonatal osteomyelitis and septic arthritis. Ind. Pediatr. *27*:453–457, 1990.
40. Deutsch, S. D., Gandsman, E. J., and Spraragen, S. C.: Quantitative regional blood-flow analysis and its clinical application during routine bone-scanning. J. Bone Joint Surg. *63*:295–305, 1981.
41. Dich, V. Q., Nelson, J. D., and Haltalin, K. C.: Osteomyelitis in infants and children: A review of 163 cases. Am. J. Dis. Child. *129*:1273–1278, 1975.
42. Diggs, L. W.: Bone and joint lesions in sickle-cell disease. Clin. Orthoped. *52*:119–143, 1967.
43. Dunn, E. J., Bryan, D. M., Nugent, J. T., et al.: Pyogenic infections of the sacro-iliac joint. Clin. Orthoped. *118*:113, 1976.
44. Duszynski, D. O., Kuhn, J. P., Afshani, E., et al.: Early radionuclide diagnosis of acute osteomyelitis. Radiology *117*:337–340, 1975.
45. Echols, R. M., Selinger, D. S., Hallowell, C., et al.: *Rhizopus* osteomyelitis: A case report and review. Am. J. Med. *66*:141–145, 1979.
46. Edwards, M. S., Baker, C. J., Wagner, M. L., et al.: An etiologic shift in infantile osteomyelitis: The emergence of the group B *Streptococcus*. J. Pediatr. *93*:578–583, 1978.
47. Edwards, T. C., Stapleton, F. B., Bond, M. J., et al.: Sweet's syndrome with multifocal sterile osteomyelitis. Am. J. Dis. Child. *140*:817–818, 1986.
48. Epps, C. J., Bryant, D. D., Coles, M. J., et al.: Osteomyelitis in patients who have sickle-cell disease: Diagnosis and management. J. Bone Joint Surg. *73*:1281–1294, 1991.
49. Farr, H.: Acute hematogenous osteomyelitis due to type B *Haemophilus* osteomyelitis and arthritis. Lancet *1*:517–518, 1966.
50. Farrand, R. J., Johnstone, J. M., and McCabe, A. F.: *Haemophilus* osteomyelitis and arthritis. Br. Med. J. *2*:334–336, 1968.
51. Feigin, R. D., Pickering, L. K., Anderson, D., et al.: Clindamycin treatment of osteomyelitis and septic arthritis in children. Pediatrics *55*:213–223, 1975.
52. Ferguson, W. R.: Some observations on circulation in fetal and infant spine. J. Bone Joint Surg. *32*:640–648, 1950.
53. Fernandez, M. S., Quiralte, J. del A. A., et al.: Osteoarticular infection associated with the human immunodeficiency virus. Clin. Exp. Rheumatol. *9*:489–493, 1991.
54. Fisher, M. C., Goldsmith, J. F., and Gilligan, P. H.: Sneakers as a source of *Pseudomonas aeruginosa* in children with osteomyelitis following puncture wounds. J. Pediatr. *106*:607–609, 1985.
55. Fitzgerald, R. J., and Cowan, J. D.: Puncture wounds of the foot. Orthop. Clin. North Am. *6*:965, 1975.
56. Fletcher, B. D., Scoles, P. V,. and Nelson, A. D.: Osteomyelitis in children: Detection by magnetic resonance: Work in progress. Orthoped. Clin. North Am. Radiology *150*:57–60, 1980.
57. Fonk, J., and Coonrod, J. D.: *Serratia* osteomyelitis in sickle cell disease. J. A. M. A. *217*:80–81, 1970.
58. Fox, L., and Sprunt, K.: Neonatal osteomyelitis. Pediatrics *62*:535–542, 1978.
59. Freehafer, A. A., Furey, J. G., and Pierce, D. S.: Pyogenic osteomyelitis of the spine resulting in spinal paralysis. J. Bone Joint Surg. *441*:710–716, 1962.
60. Gainey, M. A., Siegel, J. A., Smergel, E. M., et al.: Indium-111–labeled white blood cells: Dosimetry in children. J. Nucl. Med. *29*:689–694, 1988.
60a. Geddes, A. M., Finch, R. S., Goodall, A. C., et al.: The treatment of pediatric infections with clindamycin. *In* Hejzlar, M., Simonsky, M., and Masak, S. (eds.): Advances in Antimicrobial and Antineoplastic Chemotherapy. Baltimore, University Park Press, 1972, pp. 1207–1208.
61. Genster, H. G., and Andersen, J. J. F.: Spinal osteomyelitis complicating urinary tract infection. J. Urol. *107*:109–111, 1971.
62. Gibson, W. K., Bartosh, R., and Timperlake, R.: Acute hematogenous epiphyseal osteomyelitis. Orthopedics *14*:705–707, 1991.
63. Giedion, A., Holthusen, W., Masel, L. F., et al.: Subacute and chronic "symmetrical" osteomyelitis. J. Urol. *107*:109–111, 1972.
64. Gilday, D. L., Paul, D. J., and Paterson, J.: Diagnosis of osteomyelitis in children by combined blood pool and bone imaging. Radiology *117*:331–335, 1975.
65. Gilfand, M. J., and Harcke, H. T.: Skeletal imaging in sickle cell disease. J. Nucl. Med. *19*:698–709, 1978.
66. Gillespie, W. J.: Epidemiology in bone and joint infection. Infect. Dis. Clin. North Am. *4*:361–376, 1990.
67. Goldstein, E. J., Ahonkhai, V. I., Cristofaro, R. L., et al.: Source of *Pseudomonas* in osteomyelitis of heels. J. Clin. Microbiol. *12*:711–713, 1980.
68. Goutzmanis, J. J., Gonis, G., and Gilbert, G. L.: *Kingella kingae* infection in children: Ten cases and a review of the literature. Pediatr. Infect. Dis. J. *10*:677–683, 1991.
69. Granoff, D. M., Sargent, E., and Jolivette, D.: *Haemophilus influenzae* type b osteomyelitis. Am. J. Dis. Child. *132*:488–490, 1976.
70. Green, J. H.: Cloxacillin in the treatment of osteomyelitis. Br. Med. J. *2*:414–416, 1967.
71. Green, W. T.: Osteomyelitis of infants: A disease different from osteomyelitis of older children. Arch. Surg. *32*:462–493, 1936.
72. Greenberg, L. W., and Haynes, R. E.: *Escherichia coli* osteomyelitis in an infant with sickle-cell disease. Clin. Pediatr. *9*:436–438, 1990.
73. Griesemer, D. A., Winkelstein, J. A., and Luddy, R.: Pneumococcal meningitis in patients with a major sickle hemoglobinopathy. J. Pediatr. *92*:82–84, 1978.
74. Gristina, A., Oza, M., Webb, L., et al.: Adherence bacterial colonization in the pathogenesis of osteomyelitis. Science *228*:990–993, 1985.
75. Handmaker, H., and Giammona, S. T.: Improved early diagnosis of acute inflammatory skeletal-articular diseases in children: A two-radiopharmaceutical approach. Pediatrics *73*:661–669, 1984.
76. Harris, N. H.: Some problems in the diagnosis and treatment of acute osteomyelitis. J. Bone Joint Surg. *42*:535–542, 1960.
77. Henson, F. W., Jr., and Coventry, M. B.: Osteomyelitis of the vertebrae as a result of infection of the urinary tract. Surg. Gynecol. Obstet. *102*:207–214, 1956.
78. Highland, T. R., and LaMont, R. L.: Osteomyelitis of the pelvis in children. Pediatrics *73*:661–669, 1984.
79. Hobo, T.: Zúr pathogenese der vitalfarbungalehre. Acta Sch. Med. Univ. Kioto *4*:1–29, 1921.
80. Hoffer, P.: Gallium and infection. J. Nucl. Med. *21*:484, 1980.
81. Holzman, R. S., and Bishko, F.: Osteomyelitis in heroin addicts. Ann. Intern. Med. *75*:693–696, 1971.
82. Horvath, F. L., Brodeur, A. E., and Cherry, J. D.: Deep thrombophlebitis associated with acute osteomyelitis. J. Pediatr. *79*:815–818, 1971.
83. Hruby, M. A., Honig, G. R., Lolekha, S., et al.: *Arizoni hinshawii* osteomyelitis in sickle cell anemia. Am. J. Dis. Child. *125*:867–868, 1973.
84. Hughes, R. A., Rowe, I. F., Shanson, D., et al.: Septic bone, joint and muscle lesions associated with human immunodeficiency virus infection. Br. J. Rheumatol. *31*:381–388, 1992.
85. Jackson, M. A., and Nelson, J. D.: Etiology and medical management of acute suppurative bone and joint infections in pediatric patients. J. Pediatr. Orthoped. *2*:313–323, 1982.
86. Jacobs, R. F., Adelman, L., Sack, C. M., et al.: Management of *Pseudomonas* osteochondritis complicating puncture wounds of the foot. Pediatrics *69*:432–435, 1982.
87. Jacobs, R. F., McCarthy, R. E., and Elser, J. M.: *Pseudomonas* osteochondritis complicating puncture wounds of the foot in children: A 10-year evaluation. J. Infect. Dis. *160*:657–661, 1989.
87a. Jaffe, H. L.: Metabolic, Degenerative, and Inflammatory Diseases of the Bones and Joints. Philadelphia, Lea & Febiger, 1972.
88. Johanson, P. H.: *Pseudomonas* infections of the foot following puncture wounds. J. A. M. A. *204*:262–264, 1968.
89. Jordan, M. C., and Kirby, W. M.: Pyogenic vertebral osteomyelitis. Treatment with antimicrobial agents and bed rest. Arch. Intern. Med. *128*:405–410, 1971.
90. Jupiter, J. B., Ehrlich, M. G., Novelline, R. A., et al.: The association of septic thrombophlebitis with subperiosteal abscesses in children. J. Pediatr. *101*:690–695, 1982.
91. Kahn, D. S., and Pritzker, K. P.: The pathophysiology of bone infection. Clin. Orthoped. *96*:12–20, 1973.
92. Keeley, K., and Buchanan, G. R.: Acute infarction of long bones in children with sickle cell anemia. J. Pediatr. *101*:170–175, 1982.
93. Kemp, H., Jackson, J., and Jeremia, J.: Pyogenic infections occurring primarily in intervertebral discs. J. Bone Joint Surg. *55*:698–714, 1963.
94. King, S. M., Laxer, R. M., Manson, D., et al.: Chronic recurrent multifocal osteomyelitis: A noninfectious inflammatory process. Pediatr. Infect. Dis. J. *6*:907–911, 1987.
95. Knudsen, C. J., and Hoffman, E. B.: Neonatal osteomyelitis. J. Bone Joint Surg. *72*:846–851, 1990.
96. Kozin, F., Carrera, G. F., Ryan, L. M., et al.: Computed tomography in the diagnosis of sacroiliitis. Am. J. Dis. Child. *134*:828–830, 1980.
97. Kurlandsky, L. E., Quinn, P. H., and Sills, E. M.: *Haemophilus influenzae* as a cause of Brodie's abscess in an infant. Johns Hopkins Med. J. *144*:15–17, 1979.

98. LaMont, R. L., Anderson, P. A., Dajani, A. S., et al.: Acute hematogenous osteomyelitis in children. J. Pediatr. Orthoped. *7*:579–583, 1987.
99. Lascari, A. D., Graham, M. H., and MacQueen, J. C.: Intervertebral disk infection in children. J. Pediatr. *70*:751–757, 1967.
100. Lee, P. Y.: Infected cephalhaematoma and neonatal osteomyelitis. J. Infect. *21*:191–193, 1990.
101. Leigh, T. F., Kelly, R. P., and Weens, H. S.: Spinal osteomyelitis associated with urinary tract infections. Radiology *65*:334–342, 1955.
102. Lewis, R., Gorbach, S., and Altner, P.: Spinal *Pseudomonas* chondro-osteomyelitis in heroin users. N. Engl. J. Med. *286*:1303, 1972.
103. Lewis, R. P., Sutter, V. L., and Finegold, S. M.: Bone infections involving anaerobic bacteria. Medicine *57*:279–305, 1978.
104. Lifeso, R. M., Harder, E., and McCorkel, S. J.: Spinal brucellosis. Br. J. Bone Joint Surg. *67*:345–351, 1985.
105. Light, R. W., and Dunham, T. R.: Vertebral osteomyelitis due to *Pseudomonas* in the occasional heroin user. J. A. M. A. *228*:12–72, 1974.
106. Littman, M. L., and Walter, J. E.: Cryptococcosis: Current status. Am. J. Med. *45*:922–932, 1968.
107. Longjohn, D. B., Zionts, L. E., and Stott, N. S.: Acute hematogenous osteomyelitis of the epiphysis. Clin. Orthoped. *316*:227–234, 1995.
108. Majeed, H. A., Kalaawi, M., Mohanty, D., et al.: Congenital dyserythropoietic anemia and chronic recurrent multifocal osteomyelitis in three related children and the association with Sweet syndrome in two siblings. J. Pediatr. *115*:730–734, 1989.
109. Makin, M., Geller, R., Jacobs, J., et al.: Non-toxic detergent irrigation of chronic infections: An experimental evaluation. Clin. Orthoped. *92*:320–324, 1973.
110. McGregor, J. A., and McFarren, T.: Neonatal cranial osteomyelitis: A complication of fetal monitoring. Obstet. Gynecol. *73*:490–492, 1989.
111. Medina, F., Fuentes, M., Jara, L. J., et al.: *Salmonella* pyomyositis in patients with the human immunodeficiency virus. Br. J. Rheumatol. *34*:568–571, 1995.
112. Miller, E. H., and Semian, D. W.: Gram-negative osteomyelitis following puncture wounds of the foot. Medicine (Baltimore) *57*:279–305,1978.
113. Modic, M. T., Feiglin, D. H., Piraino, D. W., et al.: Vertebral osteomyelitis: Assessment using MR. Radiology *157*:157–166, 1985.
114. Mok, P. M., Reilly, B. J., and Ash, J. M.: Osteomyelitis in the neonate. Clinical aspects and the role of radiography and scintigraphy in diagnosis and management. Radiology *145*:677–682, 1982.
115. Morgan, A., and Yates, A. K.: Diagnosis of acute osteomyelitis of the pelvis. Postgrad. Med. J. *42*:74–78, 1966.
116. Morrey, B. F., Bianco, A. J., and Rhodes, K. H.: Hematogenous osteomyelitis at uncommon sites in children. Mayo Clin. Proc. *53*:707–713, 1978.
117. Morrey, B. F., Dunn, J. M., Heimbach, R. D., et al.: Hyperbaric oxygen and chronic osteomyelitis. Clin. Orthoped. *144*:121–127, 1979.
118. Murray, M. M., Welch, D. F., and Kuhls, T. L.: *Serratia* osteochondritis after puncture wounds of the foot. Pediatr. Infect. Dis. J. *9*:523–524, 1990.
119. Mustafa, M. M., Saez, L. X., McCracken, G. J., et al.: Acute hematogenous pelvic osteomyelitis in infants and children. Pediatr. Infect. Dis. *9*:416–421, 1990.
120. Nagal, D. A., Albright, J. A., Keggi, K. J.: Closer look at spinal lesions: Open biopsy of vertebral lesions. J. A. M. A. *191*:975–978, 1965.
121. Nelson, J. D.: Acute osteomyelitis in children. Infect. Dis. Clin. North Am. *4*:513–522, 1990.
122. Nelson, J. D., Bucholz, R. W., Kusmiesz, H., et al.: Benefits and risks of sequential parenteral-oral cephalosporin therapy for suppurative bone and joint infections. J. Pediatr. Orthoped. *2*:255–262, 1982.
123. Norden, C. W., Bryant, R., Palmer, D., et al.: Chronic osteomyelitis caused by *Staphylococcus aureus*: Controlled clinical trial of nafcillin therapy and nafcillin-rifampin therapy. South. Med. J. *79*:947–951, 1986.
124. Peters, W., Irving, J., and Letts, M.: Long-term effects of neonatal bone and joint infection on adjacent growth plates. J. Pediatr. Orthoped. *12*:806–810, 1992.
125. Pichichero, M. E., and Friesen, H. A.: Polymicrobial osteomyelitis: Report of three cases and review of the literature. Rev. Infect. Dis. 4:86–96, 1982.
126. Piehl, F. C., Davis, R. J., and Prugh, S. I.: Osteomyelitis in sickle cell disease. J. Pediatr. Orthoped. *13*:225–227, 1993.
127. Prober, C. G., and Yeager, A. S.: Use of the serum bactericidal titer to assess the adequacy of oral antibiotic therapy in the treatment of acute hematogenous osteomyelitis. J. Pediatr. *95*:131–135, 1979.
128. Rao, S., Solomon, N., Miller, S., et al.: Scintigraphic differentiation of bone infarction from osteomyelitis in children with sickle cell disease. J. Pediatr. *107*:685–688, 1985.
129. Rhangos, W. C., and Chick, E. W.: Mycotic infections of bone. South. Med. J. *57*:664–674, 1964.
130. Rocco, H. D., and Eyring, E. J.: Intervertebral disk infections in children. Am. J. Dis. Child. *123*:448–452, 1972.
131. Rodriguez, W., Ross, S., Khan, W., et al.: Clindamycin in the treatment of osteomyelitis in children: A report of 29 cases. Am. J. Dis. Child. *131*:1088–1093, 1977.
132. Roine, I., Faingezicht, I., Arguedas, A., et al.: Serial serum C-reactive protein to monitor recovery from acute hematogenous osteomyelitis in children. Pediatr. Infect. Dis. J. *14*:40–44, 1995.
133. Roselle, G. A., and Baird, I. M.: *Aspergillus flavipes* group osteomyelitis. Arch. Intern. Med. *139*:590–592, 1979.
134. Rubin, H. M., Eardley, W., and Nichols, B. L.: *Shigella sonnei* osteomyelitis and sickle-cell anemia. Am. J. Dis. Child. *116*:83–87, 1968.
135. Rubin, R. C., Jacobs, G. B., Cooper, P. R., et al.: Disc space infections in children. Childs Brain *3*:180–190, 1977.
136. Salahuddin, N. I., Madhavan, T., Fisher, E. J., et al.: *Pseudomonas* osteomyelitis: Radiologic features. Radiology *109*:41–47, 1973.
137. Sapico, F. L., and Montgomerie, J. Z.: Pyogenic vertebral osteomyelitis: Report of nine cases and review of the literature. Rev. Infect. Dis. *1*:754, 1979.
138. Schauwecker, D. S.: Osteomyelitis: Diagnosis with In-111–labeled leukocytes. Radiology *171*:141–146, 1989.
139. Schechter, L. S., Smith, A., and Pearl, M.: Intervertebral disk calcification in childhood. Am. J. Dis. Child. *123*:608–611, 1972.
140. Scoles, P. V., Hilty, M. D., and Sfakianakis, G. N.: Bone scan patterns in acute osteomyelitis. Clin. Orthoped. *153*:210–217, 1980.
141. Selby, R. C., and Pillay, K. V.: Osteomyelitis and disc infection secondary to *Pseudomonas aeruginosa* in heroin addiction: Case report. J. Neurosurg. *37*:463–466, 1972.
142. Sfakianakis, G. N., Scoles, P., Welch, M., et al. Evolution of bone imaging findings in osteomyelitis. J. Nucl. Med. *199*:706, 1978.
143. Smith, C. E., Beard, R. R., Whiting, E. G., et al. Varieties of coccidioidal infection in relation to epidemiology and control of the disease. Am. J. Public Health *36*:1394–1402, 1946.
144. Smith, R. F., and Taylor, T. K.: Inflammatory lesions of intervertebral discs in children. J. Bone Joint Surg. *49*:1508–1520, 1967.
145. Sorsdahl, O. A., Goodhart, G. L., Williams, H. T., et al.: Quantitative bone gallium scintigraphy in osteomyelitis. Skeletal Radiol. 22:239–242, 1993.
146. Specht, E. E.: Hemoglobinopathic *Salmonella* osteomyelitis: Orthopedic aspects. Clin. Orthoped. *79*:110–118, 1971.
147. Spiegel, P. G., Kengla, K. W., Isaacson, A. S., and Wilson, J. J.: Intervertebral disc-space inflammation in children. J. Bone Joint Surg. *54*:284–296, 1972.
148. Staab, E. V., and McCartney, W. H.: Role of gallium 67 in inflammatory disease. Semin. Nucl. Med. *8*:219–234, 1978.
149. Starr, C. L.: Acute hematogenous osteomyelitis. Arch. Surg. *4*:567–587, 1922.
150. Steinbach, L. S., Tehranzadeh, J., Fleckenstein, J. L., et al.: Human immunodeficiency virus infection: Musculoskeletal manifestations. Radiology *186*:833–838, 1993.
151. Stephens, M. M., and MacAuley, P.: Brodies abscess: A long-term review. *In* Urist, M. R. (ed.): Clinical Orthopaedics and Related Research. Philadelphia, J. B. Lippincott, 1988, pp. 211–216.
152. Stevens, J.: Post-operative orthopedic infections. J. Bone Joint Surg. *46*:96, 1964.
153. Stone, D. B, and Bonfiglio, M.: Pyogenic vertebral osteomyelitis: A diagnostic pitfall for the internists. Arch. Intern. Med. *112*:491–500, 1963.
154. Swick, H. M.: Calcification of intervertebral discs in childhood. J. Pediatr. *86*:364–369, 1975.
155. Swiontkowski, M. F.: Surgical approaches in osteomyelitis: Use of laser Doppler flowmetry to determine nonviable bone. Infect. Dis. Clin. North Am. *4*:501–512, 1990.
156. Syrogiannopoulos, G. A., and Nelson, J. D.: Duration of antimicrobial therapy for acute suppurative osteoarticular infections. Lancet *1*:37–40, 1988.
157. Tang, J. S., Gold, R. H., Bassett, L.W., et al.: Musculoskeletal infection of the extremities: Evaluation with MR imaging. Radiology *166*:205–209, 1988.
158. Taplin, D.: Environmental influences on the microbiology of the skin. Arch. Environ. Health *11*:546, 1968
158a. Taylor, J. C., and Fallon, R. J.: Osteomyelitis due to *Hemophilus influenzae*. Lancet *1*:715, 1966.
159. Taylor, J. R.: Growth of human intervertebral discs and vertebral bodies. J. Anat. *120*:49–68, 1975.
160. Templeton, W. C. I., Wawrukiewicz, A., Melo, J. C., et al.: Anaerobic osteomyelitis of long bones. Rev. Infect. Dis. *5*:692–712, 1983.
161. Tetzlaff, T. R., McCracken, G. J., and Nelson, J. D.: Oral antibiotic therapy for skeletal infections of children. II. Therapy of osteomyelitis and suppurative arthritis. J. Pediatr. *92*:485–490, 1978.
162. Tilden, R. L., Jackson, J. J., Enneking, W. F., et al.: 99m Tc–polyphosphate: Histological localization in human femurs by autoradiography. J. Nucl. Med. *14*:576–578, 1973.
163. Torda, A. J., Gottleib, T., and Bradbury, R.: Pyogenic vertebral osteomyelitis analysis of 20 cases and review. Clin. Infect. Dis. *20*:320–328, 1995.
164. Treves, S., Khettry, J., Broker, F. H., et al.: Osteomyelitis: Early scintigraphic detection in children. Pediatrics *57*:173–186, 1976.
165. Trueta, J.: The three types of acute hematogenous osteomyelitis. J. Bone Joint Surg. *41*:671–680, 1959.
166. Unger, E., Moldofsky, P., Gatenby, R., et al.: Diagnosis of osteomyelitis by MR imaging. AJR Am. J. Roentgenol. *150*:605–610, 1988.
167. Unkila-Kallio, L., Kallio, M. J., Eskola, J., et al.: Serum C-reactive protein, erythrocyte sedimentation rate, and white blood cell count in acute hematogenous osteomyelitis of children. Pediatrics *93*:59–62, 1994.
168. Unkila-Kallio, L., Kallio, M. J., and Peltola, H.: Acute haematogenous osteomyelitis in children in Finland: Finnish Study Group. Ann. Med. *25*:545–549, 1993.

169. VanHowe, R. S., Starshak, R. J., and Chusid, M. J.: Chronic, recurrent multifocal osteomyelitis: Case report and review of the literature. Clin. Pediatr. 28:54–59, 1989.
170. Vaughan, P. A., Newman, N. M., and Rosman, M. A.: Acute hematogenous osteomyelitis in children. J. Pediatr. Orthopaed. 7:652–655, 1987.
171. Waldvogel, F. A., and Papageorgiou, P. S.: Osteomyelitis: The past decade. N. Engl. J. Med. 303:360–370, 1980.
171a. Walker, S. H.: Staphylococcal osteomyelitis in children: Success with cephaloridine-cephalexin therapy. Clin. Pediatr. 12:98–100, 1973.
172. Watson, F. M., and Whitesides, T. J.: Acute hematogenous osteomyelitis complicating closed fractures. Clin. Orthoped. 117:296–302, 1976.
173. Watson, R. J., Burko, H., Megas, H., et al.: The hand-foot syndrome in sickle cell disease in young children. Pediatrics 31:775–829, 1963.
174. Weissberg, E. D., Smith, A. L., and Smith, D. H.: Clinical features of neonatal osteomyelitis. Pediatrics 53:505–509, 1974.
175. Weld, P. W.: Osteomyelitis of the ileum, masquerading as acute appendicitis. J. A. M. A. 173:634–636, 1960.
176. Widen, A. L., and Cardon, L.: *Salmonella typhimurium* osteomyelitis with sickle cell hemoglobin C disease: A review and case report. Ann. Intern. Med. 54:510–521, 1961.
177. Wiesseman, G. J., Wood, V. E., Kroll, L. L., et al.: *Pseudomonas* vertebral osteomyelitis in heroin addicts. J. Bone Joint Surg. 55A:1416–1424, 1973.
178. Williamson, J. B., Galasko, C. S., and Robinson, M. J.: Outcome after acute osteomyelitis in preterm infants. Arch. Dis. Child. 65:1060–1062, 1990.
179. Yagupsky, P., Howard, C. B., Einhorn, M., et al.: *Kingella kingae* osteomyelitis of the calcaneus in young children. Pediatr. Infect. Dis. J. 12:540–541, 1993.

Septic Arthritis

This section concerns acute bacterial infections of the joints. The terms septic arthritis, acute suppurative pyarthrosis, and infectious arthritis are used interchangeably; they refer to the presence of organisms in the joint space, not associated with contiguous osteomyelitis.

EPIDEMIOLOGY

The incidence of septic arthritis has been evaluated in several populations. It is clear that septic arthritis occurs most commonly in childhood. In a review from the preantibiotic era, half the patients were younger than 20 years of age.[35] Another series from a general hospital, collected since antibiotics became available for systemic use, revealed that 41 of 66 patients (62 per cent) were younger than 20 years of age.[6, 63] In more recent studies, the incidence of septic arthritis in children has been estimated as 5.5 to 12 cases per 100,000 individuals.[25] Describing the age distribution of septic arthritis in childhood is difficult because of varying age intervals selected by authors of different studies. In one representative study, 21 of 38 cases (55 per cent) occurred in children younger than 1 year of age; individuals older than 13 years of age were excluded from the tabulation.[64]

A history of trauma often is sought as a predisposing determinant of septic arthritis or osteomyelitis, although many investigators have questioned a relationship because of the great frequency of trauma in any normal healthy child. Other hereditary or acquired conditions also may predispose to the development of septic arthritis. Acute suppurative arthritis may follow joint surgery, joint injections, or surgery on or instrumentation of the urinary or intestinal tracts. Gram-negative organisms are the most frequent causes of disease when these predisposing factors are present. *Salmonella* septic arthritis may develop during the course of *Salmonella* bacteremia in the normal host but occurs with increased frequency in patients with sickle-cell disease or other hemoglobinopathies. Although septic arthritis occurs in HIV-infected children and adults,[46] there are as yet no data to substantiate that HIV increases the incidence of musculoskeletal infections in children.

A history of upper respiratory infection during the 2 weeks prior to the development of septic arthritis was noted by Feigin (personal communication) in 44 per cent of the patients that he reviewed over 10 years. Of particular interest, upper respiratory infection or otitis media was reported or observed in 77 per cent of those patients who developed pyarthrosis caused by *Haemophilus influenzae,* whereas it was reported in only 18 per cent of the children who developed pyarthrosis due to *Staphylococcus aureus.* In contrast, 42 per cent of children with septic arthritis due to *S. aureus* reported or were observed to have skin or soft tissue infections adjacent to the site of the pyarthrosis. Septic arthritis has been described during varicella, presumably due to bacteremia resulting from infected skin lesions. This must be differentiated from the apparent ability of varicella-zoster virus to cause joint inflammation on its own.[49, 61]

PATHOPHYSIOLOGY

Synovial joints, also termed diarthrodial joints, are composed of a movable articulation containing synovia. The latter is a transparent viscous fluid, which lubricates the joint and nourishes the avascular articular cartilage. The synovial membrane is responsible for the formation of the joint fluid. It is composed of a prominent capillary network embedded in a connective tissue network containing at least two types of cells. One morphologic type (type A) appears to be related to mononuclear phagocytes, whereas fibroblast-like type B cells appear to be responsible for the synthesis of hyaluronic acid. Joint fluid is formed by filtration through the capillary network, i.e., the net balance of back diffusion into the capillary bed and diffusion into the joint space. Diarthrodial joints normally contain small amounts of fluid (e.g., 0.5 to 3 mL in the knee)[69] with glucose and electrolyte concentrations equal to plasma. There is a partial pressure of oxygen of 60 to 70 torr, an albumin concentration of 1 to 2 g/dL, and an IgG content of 50 mg/dL.[16, 17, 23, 68, 69]

Diffusion from the joint space is increased by any mechanism that increases pressure (distention with injected solution, active or passive motion, or external massage). Particulate material is removed from the joint space by the synovial membrane macrophages and free monocytes (the latter usually are present in concentrations $<50 \times 10^6$/L). The viscosity of joint fluid is due to the hyaluronic acid: enzymatic depolymerization produces a viscosity approximately equivalent to that of water. With the loss of hyaluronidate from the synovia, the articular cartilage, with continued use, is eroded and becomes sclerotic.[8] Only the vasculature of the synovial membrane is innervated, which has two consequences: (1) joint pain is localized poorly because it results from stretching the fibrous joint capsule, and (2) inflammation within the joint cavity elicits an axon reflex leading to vasodilation and warmth over an infected joint. Lymphatic channels are present in all the joint tissues except cartilage; these drain to the regional flexor lymph nodes.

Bacteria can enter the joint space one of three ways: hematogenous spread, direct inoculation, or contiguous extension. The synovial membrane has been shown to have a high effective blood flow, approximately equal to that of the brain (if it is assumed that there is 1 g of synovial membrane in an adult knee joint). Thus, a large number of bacteria in blood may be envisioned as being delivered to the synovial membrane per unit time.

Inoculation arthritis follows the puncture of the joint by a contaminated object. In one series, 5 of 35 cases of septic arthritis were due to puncture wounds. Not surprisingly, there is a predilection for the knee; four of five cases cited in this study were secondary to kneeling on sewing needles.[64]

Generally, contiguous extension of an infection into the joint space appears to be rare, particularly in children. In one series, 10 of 77 cases of septic arthritis had disease originating from a contiguous focus.[12] Of these, none were in the joints of the foot, and eight occurred before the availability of many antibiotics (1951). This surprisingly high frequency of septic arthritis due to spread of infection from a contiguous focus has not been seen in more recent studies.

ETIOLOGY

S. aureus is the most common infecting agent causing septic arthritis. Streptococci (group A organisms and pneumococci) have been responsible for most other gram-positive infections. (Table 64–5). Although it is becoming a rare entity in areas where immunization has been extensively used, *H. influenzae* septic arthritis generally is seen only in children younger than 2 years of age.[33, 66] Arthritis due to *Streptococcus pneumoniae* also generally occurs in these younger children.[38] *Salmonella* species causes approximately 1 per cent of the total cases of septic arthritis. Enteric gram-negative organisms appear to be an increasing cause of septic arthritis. The source often is unknown in pediatric cases, except when a puncture wound is apparent. In one series, Enterobacteriaceae accounted for 13 of 76 cases of arthritis; only 1 of the 13 occurred in a child.[28] All the adults in this series had preexisting joint disease, underlying serious systemic disease (malignancy or diabetes), and a known focus of infection elsewhere in the body. *Kingella kingae* has been recognized increasingly as a cause of septic arthritis[18, 48]; in one series from Israel, it was the most common bacterial isolate (48 per cent of cases).[76]

In newborns and sexually active adolescents with suspected septic arthritis, *Neisseria gonorrhoeae* should be considered.[28, 41, 42] This disease in newborns has nonspecific prodromal symptoms: poor feeding, irritability, and fever. The portal of entry is unknown, and the joints below the hip usually are involved (knee, ankles, and metatarsal). During adolescence, gonococcal arthritis occurs as a manifestation of sepsis with fever, chills, skin rash, and multiple small joint involvement, often with tenosynovitis[22]; the illness often follows the onset of menses by a few days.

Unusual causes of septic arthritis include *Pseudomonas aeruginosa* (most commonly seen in the sternoclavicular joint of heroin addicts),[71] *Enterobacter, Bacteroides,*[1] and *Campylobacter fetus.* Other unusual causes of septic arthritis, such as *Serratia* species and *Corynebacterium pyogenes,* generally occur in patients with malignancy who are immunosuppressed.[13, 45, 56] In one series, 7 of 32 patients with gram-negative bacillary arthritis had an underlying malignancy.[28] Other rare bacterial causes of septic arthritis include *Propionibacterium acnes*[77] and *Pasteurella multocida.*[31]

Streptobacillus moniliformis infection of joints may become evident 2 to 3 days after a rat bite; a macular rash commonly is present at the time of presentation. Discussion of Lyme arthritis is beyond the scope of this chapter, but intermittent, inflammatory arthritis occurs in most patients after *Borrelia burgdorferi* is transmitted by a tick bite.[40] *Brucella* and mycobacteria (*Mycobacterium tuberculosis* and "atypical" species), as well as *Nocardia asteroides,* may cause a chronic monoarticular arthritis with a granulomatous reaction.

DIAGNOSIS

Clinical Findings

Almost all patients have fever and constitutional symptoms within the first few days of the infection.[24] The frequency of specific joint involvement in hematogenous septic arthritis of childhood is indicated in Table 64–6. Lower extremity (knee, hip, and ankle) infections account for about 80 per cent of the total number of cases.[52] Focal findings in the joint involved almost always are present. In infants, in whom the hip is one of the most common joints involved, swelling, tenderness, and heat may be absent. Most commonly, the infant lies with the involved leg abducted and externally rotated. Often, there is dislocation.[54] When the capsule of the joint can be examined, swelling is noted; effusion was present in 22 of 24 cases in one series.[73] Because pain fibers are located in the capsule, any maneuver that increases the intracapsular pressure also produces pain. In the hip, this can be elicited by compression of the head of the femur into the acetabulum. A portal of entry almost never is apparent; bilateral hip joint infection occurs in a small number of cases.[58] Pyogenic sacroiliitis often is accompanied by tenderness detected by pressure applied over the sacrum during a digital rectal examination and by pain during flexion, abduction, and external hip rotation (Faber maneuver).[2]

Radiologic Findings

The findings on plain film radiographs are due to capsular swelling. In the joints readily accessible to physical examination, radiographs add little to the diagnostic evaluation, but when septic arthritis of the hip is suspected in a child, they are a valuable adjunct and may identify other causes of hip pain, such as Legg-Calvé-Perthes disease, slipped capital femoral epiphysis, and fracture.[19] Films of the hip should be made with the child in the "frog leg position," as well as with the legs extended at the knee and slightly internally

TABLE 64–5. Bacterial Etiology of Septic Arthritis in Children

Year of Report and Reference	Gram-Positive Organisms			Gram-Negative Organisms			Total in Study
	Staphylococcus aureus	*Streptococci*	*Pneumococci*	Haemophilus influenzae	*Enterobacteriaceae*	Salmonella	
1941[35]	50	45	2	0	0	0	97
1956[74]	12	9	0	3	0	1	25
1958[64]	18	8	5	3	3	1	38
1962[58]	19	0	0	0	2	0	21
1972[50]	39	19	8	37	13	2	118
1975[47]	37	10	0	14	6	0	67
Total	175	91	15	57	24	4	366
Per cent	48	25	4	16	7	1	

TABLE 64–6. Joints Involved in Septic Arthritis of Children

Reference	Knee	Hip	Ankle	Wrist	Elbow	Shoulder	Small Diathrodial Joints
35	40	50	13	2	8	9	2
74	8	13	2	6	9	2	3
64	8	19	2	0	6	3	0
52	60	19	23	8	16	8	2
24	37	41	13	2	3	3	0
Total (=440)	153	142	53	18	42	25	7
Per cent	35	32	12	4	10	6	2

rotated. The early signs of septic arthritis are due to swelling of the capsule, which displaces the fat lines. One of the oldest signs is the obturator sign: as the tendon of the obturator internus passes over the capsule of the hip joint, the margins of this muscle are displaced medially into the pelvis[36] (Fig. 64–7). With continued swelling of the hip joint capsule, the femoral head is displaced laterally and upward.[14] One of the most consistent findings is obliteration or lateral displacement of the gluteal fat lines (see Fig. 64–7).[75] Coincident with the filling of the capsule with exudate, the femoral portion of the Shenton line is raised and its arc widened.[75] If there is a high index of suspicion of septic arthritis and if attempted arthrocentesis does not yield fluid, an arthogram should be considered. This might be of value in cases with delayed treatment, because characteristic arthrographic findings may be present that include cartilaginous abnormalities and subluxation.[27] Lacy fibrin strands with exudate may be seen. In children older than 1 year of age, subluxation of the femoral head from the hip joint is uncommon.[72] If a technetium bone scan is performed, there is increased uptake on either side of the joint during the "blood pool" phase of the scan. The utility of ultrasound in the evaluation of septic arthritis of the hip has been demonstrated. In a series of 96 patients, none of the 40 patients with normal sonographic findings had septic arthritis.[39, 78]

Bacterial infections causing pyogenic sacroiliitis particularly may be difficult to diagnose; computed tomography appears to be the diagnostic radiologic method of choice.[2]

Joint Fluid Findings

Diagnostic evaluation for suspected septic arthritis generally includes determination of the erythrocyte sedimentation rate and peripheral blood leukocyte count and differential. However, these may be only mildly elevated in cases of proven infection.[19] Blood for cultures always should be obtained. The primary criterion for the diagnosis of septic arthritis is identification of organisms in the joint fluid (Table 64–7), which should be Gram-stained and cultured aerobically and anaerobically. The need to examine a Gram-stained smear carefully must be emphasized because joint fluid exerts a bacteriostatic effect upon microorganisms and organisms that can be seen may not grow in culture. In some series, 30 per cent of joint aspirates are sterile in patients with other clinical and laboratory findings of a septic joint, including positive blood cultures. The joint fluid also should be examined for the number and type of leukocytes. The joint fluid should be collected in a heparinized syringe so that the large clot that usually forms in the fluid derived from patients with septic arthritis or juvenile rheumatoid arthritis does not preclude the enumeration of the leukocytes. The median synovial fluid leukocyte count in bacterial arthritis range in one study was 60.5×10^9 cells/L[67]; in this and other studies,[62] polymorphonuclear leukocytes accounted for 75 to 90 per cent of these cells. The cell density generally is lower in fluid obtained from patients with acute rheumatic fever, juvenile rheumatoid arthritis, or other inflammatory causes of arthritis.[67] The glucose concentration often is decreased in septic arthritis, but it also may be depressed in rheumatoid arthritis and other conditions. It should be remembered that a joint fluid leukocyte density of 5×10^9 cells/L has been found in patients ultimately proved to have septic arthritis; thus, minimally turbid fluid with a seemingly low number of cells still should be processed for bacterial culture and Gram stain. Examination of the fluid for uric acid and other types of crystals should be considered for selected children (e.g., those with hyperuricemia).

DIFFERENTIAL DIAGNOSIS

The differential diagnosis of bacterial arthritis includes epiphyseal osteomyelitis, viral arthritis (varicella-zoster, parvovirus B19, rubella, and others), mycobacterial and fungal arthritis, traumatic arthritis, bacterial endocarditis, villonodu-

TABLE 64–7. Joint Fluid Findings in Childhood Arthritides

Diagnosis	Spontaneous Clotting	Mucin Clot	Leukocytes: Cells/μL	Leukocytes: % PMN	Glucose As Percentage of Blood Value
Septic	Rapid formation of large clot	Curdled milk	73,000	90	30
Rheumatic fever	Small to absent	Tight rope	18,000	60	75
Juvenile rheumatoid arthritis	Large clot	Small, friable masses	15,000	60	75

PMN, polymorphonuclear leukocytes.

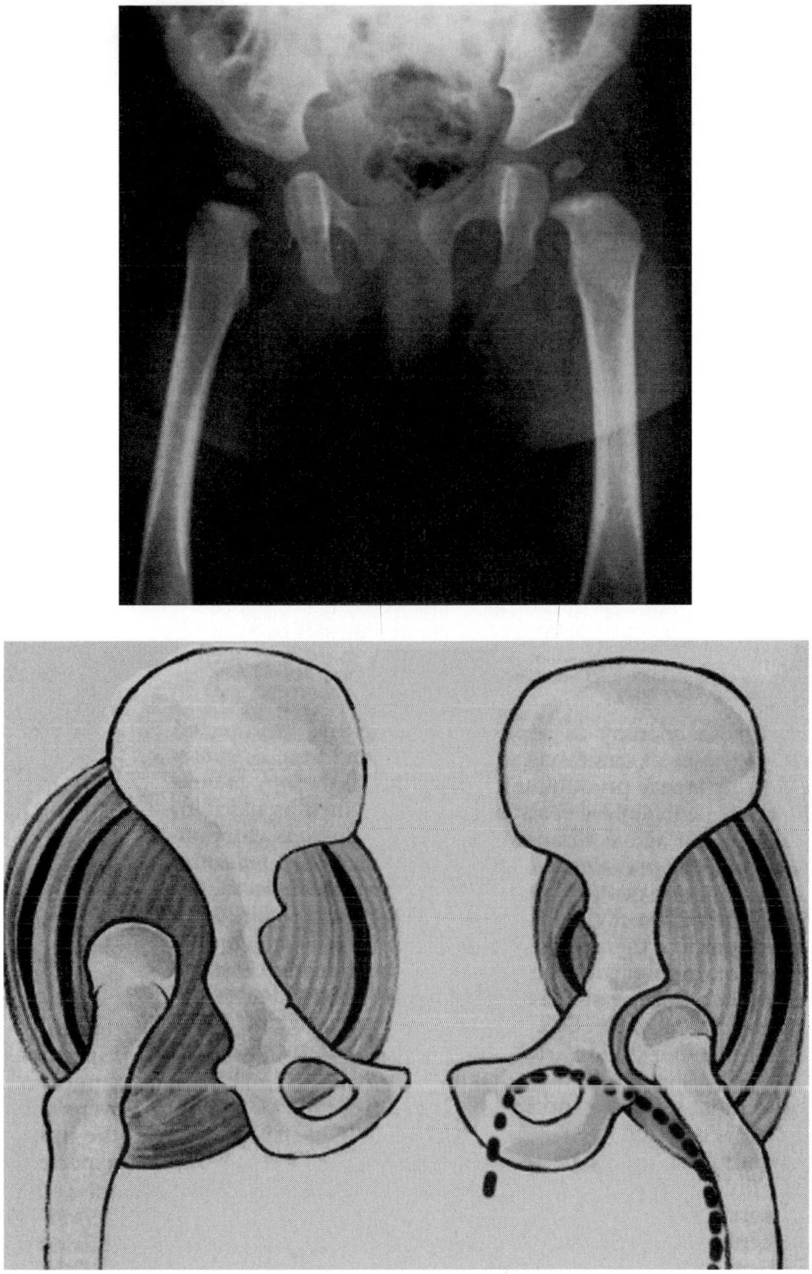

FIGURE 64–7. *The obturator sign in the hip is one of the oldest signs of septic arthritis. Another consistent finding is obliteration or lateral displacement of the gluteal fat lines and loss of continuity of the Shenton line. These findings are illustrated radiographically and schematically.*

lar synovitis, leukemia, deep cellulitis, serum sickness, ulcerative colitis, granulomatous colitis, Schönlein-Henoch purpura, traumatic arthritis, fracture, Legg-Calvé-Perthes disease, slipped femoral capital epiphysis, and metabolic diseases affecting joints (e.g., ochronosis). Toxic synovitis (also referred to as irritable hip, reactive synovitis, and transient synovitis) frequently is seen in childhood. Most patients are afebrile and have a minimally elevated or normal erythrocyte sedimentation rate.[19]

TREATMENT

Antibiotic Therapy

Antibiotic therapy of septic arthritis should be directed toward the most common pathogens. In children, *S. aureus* and other gram-positive organisms predominate.[51] Although the risk of invasive *H. influenzae* infection is low in areas of effective immunization, cases continue to be reported. Initial therapy therefore should contain a penicillinase-resistant penicillin (such as nafcillin) and an agent active against *H. influenzae* (such as cefotaxime). Cefuroxime, which is active against *S. aureus* (and other gram-positive pathogens) and *H. influenzae,* is a useful alternative. Chloramphenicol is a well-established alternative to the use of third-generation cephalosporins. After a definitive diagnosis has been established, antibiotic therapy should be changed to the most effective and least toxic drug.

All antibiotics that have been studied penetrate into the joint fluid readily; soon after administration, at the time of the serum peak, the joint fluid concentration averages 30 per cent of the serum value.[5, 7, 50, 60] However, the efflux of antibiotic from joint fluid back to serum is slow. Immediately prior to the next systemic dose, the joint fluid antibiotic concentrations frequently exceed those present in the serum. Thus, antibiotics, whether administered orally or parenterally, can achieve efficacious concentrations in joint fluid.[50, 60]

Occasionally, antibiotics have been infused directly into the joint space. This usually is unnecessary because of the excellent penetration[3] and is contraindicated with certain agents; many antibiotics (such as cephalothin) are capable of evoking an intense inflammatory reaction, much as they do if they are infiltrated beneath the skin. Tetzlaff and associates[70] have demonstrated that septic arthritis can be treated for 1 week parenterally, with the balance of the drug given orally. These investigators caution that the drug dosage should be adjusted for each patient to ensure a peak serum bactericidal titer of at least 1:8 and that the patient should remain hospitalized so that compliance can be ensured. The minimum duration of therapy was 3 weeks, the mean being 4 weeks.

The adequacy of antibiotic therapy can be assessed by serial joint fluid examinations, leukocyte density, and culture results.[73] Not surprisingly, the time required for resolution of joint symptoms and the time for the synovia to become sterile are proportional to the duration of symptoms prior to the initiation of appropriate antibiotic therapy.[37] In one study of therapy for septic arthritis, some patients still had cultures yielding their infecting bacteria after up to 1 week of therapy. In these patients, the cellular density ranged from 25×10^9 to 253×10^9 cells/L (mean, 109×10^9 cells/L) at the beginning of therapy; 92 per cent of the cells were polymorphonuclear leukocytes. By the end of 2 weeks of therapy, all cultures were sterile and the leukocyte density ranged from 4.9×10^9 to 23×10^9 cells/L, with a mean of 12.3×10^9 cells/L.[73] Similar studies of the rate of resolution of indicators of inflammation in joint fluid suggested that after 9 days of treatment, those ultimately recovering completely had a density of $\leq 5 \times 10^9$ cells/L; however, in those with recrudescent infection or poor outcome, there were 6×10^{10} cells/L.[30] When an effusion reaccumulates, one should remove it by arthrocentesis, not only to make the patient more comfortable but also so that serial assessment of therapy can be made. In general, disease due to *S. aureus* and Enterobacteriaceae is treated longer than that caused by *H. influenzae* or meningococci. Radiographs should be obtained during therapy, seeking bone changes indicative that osteomyelitis may have been present.

Surgical Treatment

In infants, septic arthritis found in the hips and shoulders is a surgical emergency; these joints should be drained as soon as the diagnosis is apparent to prevent bony destruction.[58] In a study in adults, the outcome was better in patients treated by repeated needle aspiration than by surgical drainage.[29] Eighty per cent of the patients treated by needle aspiration were thought to have a good outcome, compared with 47 per cent treated by surgical drainage. All wrist joint infections in this series were treated only by needle aspiration; in the treatment of septic arthritis of the knee, however, the outcome almost was equivalent. The investigators noted that surgical drainage should be employed in the treatment of any joint whenever the presence of large amounts of fibrin, tissue debris, or loculation prevents adequate drainage by needle aspiration. The other feature of this study, which relates surgery to a poor outcome, is that more hip joint infections were drained surgically. Because the sequelae of infection of the hip joint generally are greater, poorer results would be expected.

PROGNOSIS

The most important variables affecting adverse outcome are the duration of symptoms prior to initiation of specific therapy and the infants' being younger than 1 year of age.[44] Seven of eight patients with "permanent" hip dislocation had symptoms for 7 or more days before treatment.[74] Similarly, all patients with spontaneous ankylosis had symptoms longer than 7 days.[74] Comparable data were obtained by Samilson and colleagues:[64] 8 of 10 patients with pathologic dislocation of the hip had symptoms for more than 7 days. A detailed analysis of the factors affecting the satisfactory outcome in hematogenous septic arthritis of childhood showed no significant difference of the joint when arthrotomy, with or without irrigation, was compared with repeated aspiration.[47] Likewise, the specific antibiotic used had no effect on the outcome as long as it was effective against the infecting organism.

The literature does suggest that Enterobacteriaceae and *S. aureus* infections are associated with more sequelae than are *H. influenzae* infections.[20, 30, 53, 73]

SPECIAL PROBLEMS

Neonatal Septic Arthritis

This problem deserves special attention because of its subtle signs and symptoms,[15] the potential catastrophic consequences of untreated disease,[57] and the unusual organisms occasionally seen.

Any newborn who has swelling in the region of the thigh and the buttock and holds that leg flexed with slight abduction and external rotation at the hip should be suspected of having femoral-acetabular septic arthritis. It can occur from 1 to 28 days after a femoral venipuncture (in most newborns, 5 to 9 days) and should not be confused with femoral vein thrombosis.[4, 11] In the *majority* of the newborns, there is no toxemia, fever, or leukocytosis. More than one joint may be involved at the time of presentation. The progression of the disease in newborns can be so indolent that the hip spontaneously drains along the obturator internus and is manifested as a lower abdominal mass just above the inguinal canal.[21] Problems in recognition of the disease in newborn infants undoubtedly contribute to the poor outcome. In one series, the delay from onset to diagnosis was an average of 1 week; only two of the nine infants in this series had a normal hip examination at follow-up.[57]

In most series, the causative agents are staphylococci and streptococci,[4, 11, 15, 57] but Enterobacteriaceae have been observed.[9] More importantly, *Candida albicans* has been described, and the gonococcus[28, 41, 42] should not be forgotten. In gonococcal arthritis, the symptoms, which usually become apparent between 1 and 5 weeks of age, usually are polyarthritic (with more than one joint involved).[26] As previously noted, other symptoms of neonatal gonococcal arthritis are no different from those caused by other pathogens.

Initial antibiotic therapy for neonatal septic arthritis should be directed toward *S. aureus* and the nosocomial gram-negative bacteria that are prevalent in the nursery. Antibiotic therapy can be altered when the susceptibility of the causative bacterium is known. As noted earlier, the usual duration of therapy is 3 to 4 weeks, and radiography should be performed toward the end of treatment. Oral therapy has been used successfully to complete treatment for septic arthritis in the newborn,[59] but the absorption of antibiotics in this age range is unpredictable.[65] Consequently, either intravenous therapy or serum antibactericidal activity measurements should be used to verify absorption.[70]

Joint Infections During Rheumatoid Arthritis

This condition appears to be more frequent in adults with rheumatoid arthritis than in children. In one series, only 2 of 17 patients were younger than 10 years of age.[6] Its notable features are that the hips are not involved generally and that there is frequent infection of multiple joints (17 of 44 patients had more than one joint involved). Because of the preexisting joint disease, the diagnosis often is delayed and the outcome usually is poor. Septic arthritis should be considered if there is an unusual worsening of one joint during a flare-up of rheumatoid arthritis.

Reactive Arthritis

After certain bacterial infections, particularly with *Shigella*[10, 55] but also including *Chlamydia trachomatis*, *Salmonella*,[34] and *Yersinia*, a reactive arthritis can occur.[43] This postinfectious joint inflammation appears to occur with greater frequency in individuals who are carriers of the histocompatibility antigen HLA-B27, perhaps as a result of molecular similarities between bacterial antigens and the human protein. It also appears that during the initial infection, bacterial antigens may be deposited in the synovium and that these can persist for a long period, leading to pathogenic inflammation.[32]

In general, onset of joint symptoms takes place a few days to several weeks after the transient and often mild episode of diarrhea. The arthritis may mimic rheumatic fever and is characterized by daily low-grade fever and an increased erythrocyte sedimentation rate. This entity can be distinguished from septic arthritis by analysis of the synovial fluid. Resolution of joint symptoms in reactive cases takes 7 to 10 days, regardless of administration of broad-spectrum antibiotics.

References

1. Ament, M. E., and Gaal, S. A.: Bacteroides arthritis. Am. J. Dis. Child. *114*:427–428, 1967.
2. Aprin, H., and Turen, C.: Pyogenic sacroiliitis in children. Clin. Orthop. *287*:98–106, 1993.
3. Argen, R, J., Wilson, C. J., and Wood, P.: Suppurative arthritis. Clinical features of 42 cases. Arch. Intern. Med. *117*:661–666, 1996.
4. Asnes, R. S., and Arendar, G. M.: Septic arthritis of the hip: A complication of femoral venipuncture. Pediatrics *38*:837–841, 1966.
5. Baciocco, E. A., and Iles, R. L.: Ampicillin and kanamycin concentrations in joint fluid. Clin. Pharmacol. Ther. *12*:858–863, 1971.
6. Baitch, A.: Recent observations of acute suppurative arthritis. Clin. Orthop. *22*:153–165, 1962.
7. Balboni, V. G., Shapiro, I. M., and Kydd, D. M.: The penetration of penicillin into joint fluid following intramuscular administration. Am. J. Med. Sci. *210*:588–591, 1945.
8. Barnett, C. H., Davies, D. V., and MacConcill, M. A.: Synovial Joints. Springfield, IL, Charles C Thomas, 1961.
9. Bodganovitich, A.: Neonatal arthritis due to *Proteus vulgaris*. Arch. Dis. Child. *23*:65–66, 1948.
10. Calin, A., and Fries, J. F.: An "experimental" epidemic of Reiter's syndrome revisited: Follow-up evidence on genetic and environmental factors. Ann. Intern. Med. *84*:564–566, 1976.
11. Chacha, P. B.: Suppurative arthritis of the hip joint in infancy: A persistent diagnostic problem and possible complication of femoral venipuncture. J. Bone Joint Surg. (Am.) *53*:538–544, 1971.
12. Chartier, Y., Martin, W. J., and Kelly, P. J.: Bacterial arthritis: Experiences in the treatment of 77 patients. Ann. Intern. Med. *50*:1462–1472, 1959.
13. Chmel, H., and Armstrong, D.: Acute arthritis caused by *Aeromonas hydrophilia*: Clinical and therapeutic aspects. Arthritis Rheum. *19*:169–172, 1976.
14. Chont, L. K.: Roentgen sign of early suppurative arthritis of the hip in infancy. Radiology *38*:708–714, 1942.
15. Chung, S. M, and Pollis, R. E.: Diagnostic pitfalls in septic arthritis of the hip in infants and children. Clin. Pediatr. *14*:758–761, 1975.
16. Curtiss, P. J.: Joint infections: Pathophysiology. Clin. Orthop. *96*:129, 1973.
17. Daniel, D., Akeson, W., Amiel, D., et al.: Lavage of septic joints in rabbits: Effects of chondrolysis. J. Bone Joint Surg. (Am.) *58*:393–395, 1976.
18. de Groot, R., Glover, D., Clausen, C., et al.: Bone and joint infections caused by *Kingella kingae*: Six cases and review of the literature. Rev. Infect. Dis. *10*:998–1004, 1988.
19. Del Beccaro, M. A., Champoux, A. N., Bockers, T., et al.: Septic arthritis versus transient synovitis of the hip: The value of screening laboratory tests. Ann. Emerg. Med. *21*:1418–1422, 1992.
20. Flatauer, F. E., and Khan, M. A.: Septic arthritis caused by *Enterobacter agglomerans*. Arch. Intern. Med. *138*:788, 1978.
21. Freiberg, J. A., and Perlman, R.: Pelvic abscesses associated with acute purulent infection of the hip joint. J. Bone Joint Surg. *18*:417–427, 1936.
22. Garcia-Kutzbach, A., and Masi, A. T.: Acute infectious agent arthritis (IAA): A detailed comparison of proved gonococcal and other blood-borne bacterial arthritis. J. Rheumatol. *1*:93–101, 1974.
23. Gardner, E. D.: Physiology of joints. J. Bone Joint Surg. (Am.) *45*:152–159, 1963.
24. Gillespie, R.: Septic arthritis of childhood. Clin. Orthop. *96*:152–159, 1973.
25. Gillespie, W. J.: Epidemiology in bone and joint infection. Infect. Dis. Clin. North Am. *4*:361–376, 1990.
26. Glaser, S., Boxerbaum, B., and Kennell, J. H.: Gonococcal arthritis in the newborn: Report of a case and review of the literature. Am. J. Dis. Child. *112*:185–188, 1966.
27. Glassberg, G. B., and Ozonoff, M. B.: Arthrographic findings in septic arthritis of the hip in infants. Radiology *128*:151–155, 1978.
28. Goldenberg, D. L., Brandt, K. D., Cathcart, E. S., et al.: Acute arthritis caused by gram-negative bacilli: A clinical characterization. Medicine (Baltimore) *53*:197–208, 1974.
29. Goldenberg, D. L., Brandt, K. D., Cohen, A. S., et al.: Treatment of septic arthritis: Comparison of needle aspiration and surgery as initial modes of joint drainage. Arthritis Rheum. *18*:83–90, 1975.
30. Goldenberg, D. L., and Cohen, A. S.: Acute infectious arthritis: A review of patients with nongonococcal joint infections (with emphasis on therapy and prognosis). Am. J. Med. *60*:369–377, 1976.
31. Gomez, R. J., Shah, M., Gorevic, P., et al.: *Pasteurella multocida* arthritis: Case report. J. Bone Joint Surg. (Am.) *62*:1212–1213, 1980.
32. Granfors, K., Jalkanen, S., von Essen, R., et al.: *Yersinia* antigens in synovial-fluid cells from patients with reactive arthritis [see comments]. N. Engl. J. Med. *320*:216–221, 1989.
33. Granoff, D. M., Sargent, E., and Jolivette, D.: *Haemophilus influenzae* type b osteomyelitis. Am. J. Dis. Child. *132*:488–490, 1978.
34. Hakansson, U., Low, B., Eitrem, R., et al.: HL-A27 and reactive arthritis in an outbreak of salmonellosis. Tissue Antigens *6*:366–367, 1975.
35. Heberling, J. A.: A review of two hundred and one cases of suppurative arthritis. J. Bone Joint Surg. *23*:917–921, 1941.
36. Hefke, H. W., and Turner, V. C.: The obturator sign as the earliest roentgenographic sign in the diagnosis of septic arthritis and tuberculosis of the hip. J. Bone Joint Surg. *24*:857–869, 1942.
37. Ho, G. J., and Su, E. Y.: Therapy for septic arthritis. J. A. M. A. *247*:797–800, 1982.
38. Jacobs, N. M.: Pneumococcal osteomyelitis and arthritis in children: A hospital series and literature review. Am. J. Dis. Child. *145*:70–74, 1991.
39. Jamillo, D., Treves, S. T., Kasser, J. R., et al.: Osteomyelitis and septic arthritis in children: Appropriate use of imaging to guide treatment. A. J. R. Am. J. Roentgen. *165*:339–403, 1995.
40. Kalish, R.: Lyme disease. Rheum. Dis. Clin. North Am. *19*:399–426, 1993.
41. Kleiman, M. B., and Lamb, G. A.: Gonococcal arthritis in a newborn infant. Pediatrics *52*:285–287, 1973.
42. Kohen, D. P.: Neonatal gonococcal arthritis: Three cases and review of the literature. Pediatrics *53*:436–440, 1974.
43. Koopman, W. J.: Host factors in the pathogenesis of arthritis triggered by infectious organisms: Overview. Rheum. Dis. Clin. North Am. *19*:279–292, 1993.
44. Lunseth, P. A., and Heiple, K. G.: Prognosis in septic arthritis of the hip in children. Clin. Orthop. 81–85, 1979.
45. Martin, C. M., Merrill, R. H., and Barrett, O. J.: Arthritis due to *Serratia*. J. Bone Joint Surg. (Am.) *52*:1450–1452, 1970.
46. Merchan, E. C., Magallon, M., Manso, F., et al.: Septic arthritis in HIV positive haemophiliacs: Four cases and a literature review. Int. Orthop. *16*:302–306, 1992.
47. Morrey, B. F., Bianco, A. J., and Rhodes, K. H.: Septic arthritis in children. Orthop. Clin. North Am. *6*:923–934, 1975.
48. Morrison, V. A., and Wagner, K. F.: Clinical manifestations of *Kingella kingae* infections: Case report and review. Rev. Infect. Dis. *11*:776–782, 1989.
49. Mulhern, L. M., Friday, G. A., and Perri, J. A.: Arthritis complicating varicella infection. Pediatrics *48*:827, 1971.
50. Nelsen, J. D.: The bacterial etiology and antibiotic management of septic arthritis in infants and children. Pediatrics *50*:437–440, 1972.
51. Nelson, J. D.: Antibiotic concentrations in septic joint effusions. N. Engl. J. Med. *284*:349–353, 1971.
52. Nelson, J. D., and Koontz, W. C.: Septic arthritis in infants and children: A review of 117 cases. Pediatrics *38*:966–971, 1966.
53. Newman, J. H.: Review of septic arthritis throughout the antibiotic era. Ann. Rheum. Dis. *35*:198–205, 1976.

54. Nicholson, J. T.: Pyogenic arthritis with pathologic dislocation of the hip in infants. J. A. M. A. *141*:826–831, 1949.
55. Noer, H. R.: An "experimental" epidemic of Reiter's syndrome. J. A. M. A. *198*:693–698, 1966.
56. Norenberg, D. D., Bigley, D. V., Virata, R. L., et al.: *Corynebacterium pyogenes* septic arthritis with plasma cell synovial infiltrate and monoclonal gammopathy. Arch. Intern. Med. *138*:810–811, 1978.
57. Obletz, B.: Acute suppurative arthritis of the hip in the neonatal period. J. Bone Joint Surg. (Am.) *42*:23–30, 1960.
58. Obletz, B. E.: Suppurative arthritis of the hip joint in infants. Clin. Orthop. *22*:27–33, 1962.
59. Perkins, M. D., Edwards, K. M., Heller, R. M., et al.: Neonatal group B streptococcal osteomyelitis and suppurative arthritis: Outpatient therapy. Clin. Pediatr. *28*:229–230, 1989.
60. Plott, M. A., and Roth, H.: Penetration of clindamycin into synovial fluid. Clin. Pharmacol. Ther. *11*:577–580, 1970.
61. Priest, J. R., Urick, J. J., Groth, K. E., et al.: Varicella arthritis documented by isolation of virus from joint fluid. J. Pediatr. *93*:990, 1978.
62. Ropes, M.: Joint fluid findings in disease. Bull. Rheum. Dis *7*(Suppl.):21, 1957.
63. Russell, A. S., and Ansell, B. M.: Septic arthritis. Ann. Rheum. Dis. *31*:40–44, 1972.
64. Samilson, R. L., Bersani, F. A., and Watkins, M. B.: Acute suppurative arthritis in infants and children: The importance of early diagnosis and surgical drainage. Pediatrics *21*:798–803, 1958.
65. Schwartz, G. J., Hegyi, T., and Spitzer, A.: Subtherapeutic dicloxacillin levels in a neonate: Possible mechanisms. J. Pediatr. *89*:310–312, 1976.
66. Schwartz, R. H., and Reing, C. M.: Acute hematogenous osteomyelitis secondary to *Hemophilus influenzae*. J. Pediatr. Orthop. *1*:385–389, 1981.
67. Shmerling, R. H., Delbanco, T. L., Tosteson, A. N. A., et al.: Synovial fluid tests. J. A. M. A. *264*:1009–1014, 1990.
68. Simkin, P. A., and Pizzorno, J. E.: Transynovial exchange of small molecules in normal human subjects. J. Appl. Physiol. *36*:581–587, 1974.
69. Stravino, V. D.: The synovial system. Am. J. Phys. Med. *51*:312–320, 1972.
70. Tetzlaff, T. R., McCracken, G. J., and Nelson, J. D.: Oral antibiotic therapy for skeletal infections of children. II. Therapy of osteomyelitis and suppurative arthritis. J. Pediatr. *92*:485–490, 1978.
71. Tindel, J. R., and Crowder, J. G.: Septic arthritis due to *Pseudomonas aeruginosa*. J. A. M. A. *218*:559–561, 1971.
72. Volberg, F. M., Sumner, T. E., Abramson, J. S., et al.: Unreliability of radiographic diagnosis of septic hip in children. Pediatrics *74*:118–120, 1984.
73. Ward, J., Cohen, A. S., and Bauer, W.: The diagnosis and therapy of acute suppurative arthritis. Arthritis Rheum. *3*:522–535, 1960.
74. Watkins, M. B., Samilson, R. L., and Winter, D. M.: Acute suppurative arthritis. J. Bone Joint Surg. (Am.) *38*:1313–1320, 1956.
75. White, H.: Roentgen findings of acute infectious disease of the hip in infants and children. Clin. Orthop. *2*:34–42, 1962.
76. Yagupsky, P., Bar-Ziv, Y., Howard, C. B., et al.: Epidemiology, etiology, and clinical features of septic arthritis in children younger than 24 months. Arch. Pediatr. Adolesc. Med. *149*:537–540, 1995.
77. Yocum, R. C., McArthur, J., Petty, B. G., et al.: Septic arthritis caused by *Propionibacterium acnes*. J. A. M. A. *248*:1740–1741, 1982.
78. Zawin, J. K., Hoffer, F. A., Rand, F. F., et al.: Joint effusion in children with an irritable hip: US diagnosis and aspiration. Radiology *187*:459–463, 1993.

65

BACTERIAL MYOSITIS AND PYOMYOSITIS

Charles Grose

Myositis is not a common manifestation of bacterial infection, but when it occurs, the consequences to the patient may be severe or even fatal. *Staphylococcus aureus* and group A streptococci are the most likely causative organisms. Myositis also has been associated with several other infectious agents, including clostridia, viruses, fungi, and parasites. These pathogens have been listed in Table 65–1; they are not discussed further herein because the muscle diseases caused by these agents are described thoroughly in the individual chapters on the specific microorganisms. This discussion focuses on two forms of pyogenic myositis, designated as acute bacterial myositis and tropical pyomyositis. The former is caused primarily by group A streptococci and the latter by *Staphylococcus aureus*. Tropical (or staphylococcal) pyomyositis is by far the more common of the two bacterial diseases and should be considered a distinct nosologic entity.

PYOMYOSITIS

The pathologic entity termed spontaneous acute myositis was recognized by Virchow in the mid-nineteenth century, but the first clinical description of suppurative myositis generally is attributed to the Japanese surgeon Scriba.[20] In 1904, another Japanese surgeon, Miyake,[17] extensively reviewed the subject of skeletal muscle abscesses and added an additional 33 cases. As the British and French expanded their colonial empires at the turn of the century, the disease was recognized with increasing frequency in the native populations, as well as in the soldiers who lived in the tropical areas of Asia and Africa (reviewed by Traquair[26]). It therefore acquired the name by which it now is known widely, tropical pyomyositis.

TABLE 65–1. Infectious Causes of Myositis

Bacterial	Fungal
Tropical pyomyositis	Disseminated candidiasis
Acute bacterial myositis	**Parasitic**
Clostridial myonecrosis	Trichinosis
Viral	Toxoplasmosis
Coxsackievirus myositis	Cysticercosis
Postinfluenza myositis	

The suitability of this designation was confirmed by an epidemiologic study in East Africa, which discovered that the disease was found commonly only in regions with a truly tropical climate, i.e., a fairly constant high temperature and high relative humidity, at an altitude below 4000 ft.[15] However, it should not be forgotten that pyomyositis has been described in children from geographic regions of the United States as diverse as New England,[9] northern California,[2] Iowa,[16] and Texas.[12, 22] A large number of reported cases within the continental United States have occurred in and around San Antonio, Texas.[5] In a 10-year chart review, there were one or two cases of pyomyositis annually per 4000 pediatric admissions. All of the cases occurred during the warmest months of May through October, when San Antonio experiences a modified subtropical climate—which underscores the original appellation of *tropical* pyomyositis. In contrast, a review of consultations of pediatric infectious disease at the University of Iowa Hospital disclosed fewer cases of pyomyositis among children younger than 16 years of age.[7] Thus, pyomyositis appears to occur more commonly in children who live in the southernmost regions of the United States, e.g., San Antonio at latitude 29° N, than in those who live in the northern regions, e.g., Iowa City at latitude 41° N.

Pathophysiology

The etiologic agent of the skeletal muscle abscesses in more than 90 per cent of the cases is *S. aureus*. To date, phage-typing of many isolates in different countries has not identified a particular staphylococcal strain that is more likely to cause pyomyositis.[10] The second most common bacteriologic isolate is *Streptococcus*, including both group A and nonhemolytic strains. Whether more virulent streptococcal infections are occurring in the 1990s is an issue that remains unresolved.

The experimental conditions under which staphylococci cause muscle abscesses were studied extensively by Miyake.[17] When healthy rabbits were given boluses of staphylococci intravenously, they occasionally developed small abscesses in the kidney, liver, or spleen but never in the skeletal muscles. However, when specific muscles were damaged by mechanical pinching or electrical current 24 or 48 hours prior to the intravenous injection of bacteria, small abscesses developed at some of the injured sites in nearly half the animals within 2 to 28 days. Abscesses were not found in healthy muscle tissue.

The role of trauma received further support from a study of pyomyositis in the British Army.[3] After physicians found this disease to be a common problem in Gurkha army recruits, they investigated 32 cases and made the following observations: two-thirds of the men recalled trauma at the affected site, the incidence of abscesses increased as the severity of physical training increased, and the abscesses occurred three times more commonly on the dominant (right) side of the body. In an analysis of 78 cases in Uganda, abscesses also were found more commonly on the right side of the body.[15]

From both experimental evidence and clinical observations, it appears that two conditions are necessary for pyomyositis to occur: muscle injury and bacteremia, usually staphylococcal. A reported case is illustrative.[12] A 12-year-old girl caught her left foot in the wheel of a moving bicycle and tumbled to the ground. One week later she developed a furuncle of the foot, and within the next 2 weeks she developed painful lumps in muscles of the thigh, shoulder, and chest wall (which had been injured during the original accident). Cultures from both the furuncle and blood, as well as from the incised muscle abscesses, grew *S. aureus*. All isolates were identified as phage type 94. Thus, the initial episode of trauma resulted in a staphylococcal skin lesion and, presumably, a bacteremia that seeded sites of previously bruised muscle. Since the 1978 report, the author has cared for six additional cases of pyomyositis in children (Table 65–2). An analysis of all seven cases clearly illustrates the association of pyomyositis with trauma. The sources of muscle trauma have ranged from bicycle accidents to strenuous aerobic exercises. These cases also may explain the predilection of the disease to occur in warmer climates, viz., concomitant skin infections and muscle trauma are more likely to occur in a climate where children can play or work out-of-doors with fewer clothes for most of the year.

In a "medical progress" article on *S. aureus*, Sheagren[21] reiterated that pyomyositis in tropical countries often occurs in individuals who are malnourished and who have multiple parasitic infections. This association has not been noted in the children with pyomyositis seen in south Texas[5] or Iowa.[7] None of the children had been malnourished or vitamin-deficient, and none had parasitic infestation or marked eosinophilia. Extensive immunologic evaluations also have been normal; the tests included quantitative immunoglobulins, enumeration of T-lymphocyte subpopulations, total hemolytic complement levels, and leukocyte function as tested by reduction of nitroblue tetrazolium.

Clinical Presentation

Pyomyositis often is considered a disease of adolescents and young adults, even though it occurs in individuals of all ages, including infants and young children.[6] Boys are affected more often than girls. However, as more girls enter competitive sporting activities, pyomyositis is being reported in female athletes.[16] The majority of children with pyomyositis have a solitary lesion, but multiple lesions are not rare. The most common site of abscess formation is the thigh, followed by the calf, buttock, arm, scapula, and chest wall. The muscle lesions are firm or "woody" to palpation with a well-defined border. The sign of fluctuation may be difficult to elicit. Erythema and warmth often are not apparent because of the deep location of the masses, although diffuse tenderness is present usually. When a muscle in an extremity is involved, the entire limb may be swollen. Occasionally, none of the abscess are palpable, and the patient has only fever and vague muscle pain of a few weeks' duration.

The American children with pyomyositis ranged in age

TABLE 65–2. Pyomyositis and Trauma

Case	Sex	Age (yr)	Source of Trauma	Circumstances of Trauma	Extent of Disease
1*	F	12	Bicycle accident	Thrown from bicycle onto street after foot was caught in the wheel	Right deltoid/right chest wall/left thigh/right groin
2	M	3	Fall while running	Fell while running on street	Left calf/right scapula/right buttock
3	M	11	Hay bale accident	Struck in abdomen by bale of hay thrown from a hay baler	Abdominal wall musculature
4	M	6	Blunt trauma to abdomen	Struck in abdomen during mock fistfight with sibling	Abdominal wall musculature
5	F	17	Aerobics exercises	Injured while instructing others in aerobics exercises	Left thigh
6	M	7	Bicycle accident	Fell from fast moving bicycle onto street	Left calf
7	F	13	Volleyball accident	Fell several times diving for volleyball during training exercises	Left iliopsoas

*Cases 1 and 2 from reference 12, cases 3 and 4 from reference 5, cases 5 and 6 from reference 7, and case 7 from reference 16.

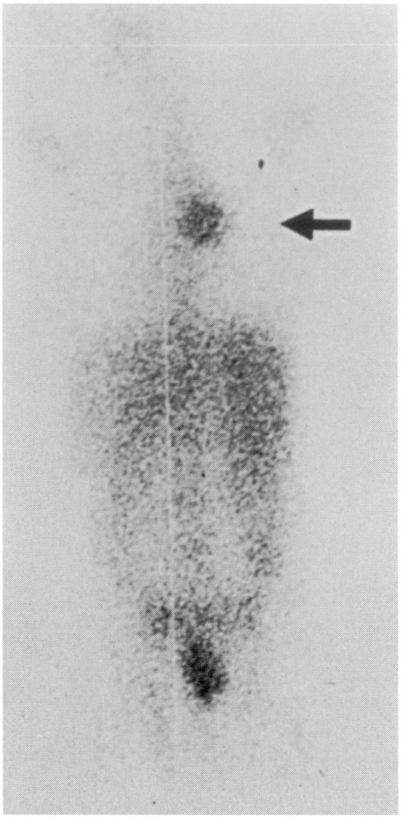

FIGURE 65–1. *Scintigram of a patient with pyomyositis. Posterior gallium-67 citrate scan shows abnormally high uptake over the right scapula (arrow), where an abscess cavity was located within the muscle. Increased radioactivity also is observed in the bladder, a normal finding.*

from 2 years of age through the teenage years and, in general, had similar presenting complaints.[7, 11] Many had incurred a recent accidental injury (often involving a leg) that usually was not considered serious. After a few days, the children developed low-grade fever (38.3° to 39.0° C), muscle pain, and, occasionally, an impaired gait. These symptoms persisted from a few days to a few weeks until a mass appeared. When first examined, many of the patients were considered to have only a contusion or a hematoma; occasionally, a child was diagnosed as having a rhabdomyosarcoma. Although the disease usually occurs in individuals who are otherwise healthy, pyomyositis has been reported in patients with malignancy. Pyomyositis also may develop in children with AIDS.[19] However, the pathophysiology of pyogenic muscle abscess may not be the same in immunodeficient individuals with increased susceptibility to bacterial infection. It should be re-emphasized that the majority of children with pyomyositis have no definable immunologic abnormalities.

An unusual clinical presentation is acute abdominal pain. Beck and Grose[5] described two children with pyomyositis whose initial complaints were confined to the abdominal wall. One of the children was a 6-year-old who had been struck in the abdomen in a mock fistfight with an older sibling. One week later, he developed a low-grade fever and began to walk with a stoop; after another week, his mother detected a "knot" in his right midabdominal wall. The second case involved the 11-year-old son of a rancher who was struck in the abdomen by a bale of hay tossed from a hay baler. When he subsequently developed symptoms of abdominal pain, the diagnosis of appendicitis was entertained. When a mass later became palpable in his abdominal wall, rhabdomyosarcoma was suspected. A correct diagnosis was made after the use of both scintigraphy and sonography and is described below.[5]

Diagnosis

The diagnosis of pyomyositis should be considered in any child with fever and muscle pain, especially if there is a recent history of trauma. When a child has visible masses at commonly involved sites, such as the thigh, the diagnosis of pyomyositis can be made by needle aspiration of a mass. If a febrile child complains of myalgia in an extremity but has no palpable masses, the differential diagnosis must include the more common inflammatory and infectious conditions of the bone or joint. A definitive diagnosis usually depends on one or more radiologic procedures. Plain films may demonstrate a soft tissue swelling or even a widened fascial plane suggestive of a mass lesion. In addition, a combination of plain roentgenography and radionuclide (^{99m}Tc phosphate) bone scintigraphy often can exclude osteomyelitis and pyoarthritis. If the diagnosis still is in question, scanning with gallium or indium can localize a muscle abscess very precisely and can visualize other intramuscular abscesses too small to palpate (Fig. 65–1). Alternatively, it has been shown that ultrasonography also can detect muscle abscesses and may be preferable as an initial procedure because it avoids the radiation exposure from computed tomography (CT) or scintigrams (Fig. 65–2). Nevertheless, gallium-67 citrate scanning remains a sensitive diagnostic procedure for detection of small muscle abscesses.[5, 14] Because of the intensity of the signal, the scan often can be completed within 1 to 4 hours after injection of the isotope.

Magnetic resonance imaging (MRI) can be very helpful in delineating the extent of a muscle abscess. In many cases, the abscess is much larger than suspected by physical symptoms and signs. The MRI scans of an illustrative case are presented in Figure 65–3. The patient was a 17-year-old girl with a swollen left lower thigh. Interestingly, she worked part-time as an attendant in an athletic club, where she participated in some of the vigorous exercise programs. Radiographs of the knee were normal, whereas a technetium bone scan showed slightly increased radionuclide uptake in the soft tissues around the distal left femur. MRI of the left and right thighs demonstrated a large fluid collection extending from the mid to distal left femur. Surgical exploration identified extensive abscess formation around the posterior aspect of the femur; the culture grew *S. aureus*. The

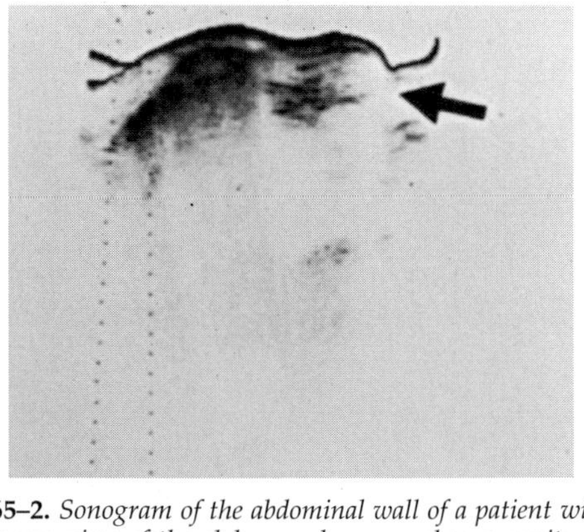

FIGURE 65–2. *Sonogram of the abdominal wall of a patient with pyomyositis. Transverse view of the abdomen shows an abscess cavity in the right belly of the rectus abdominis muscle (arrow).*

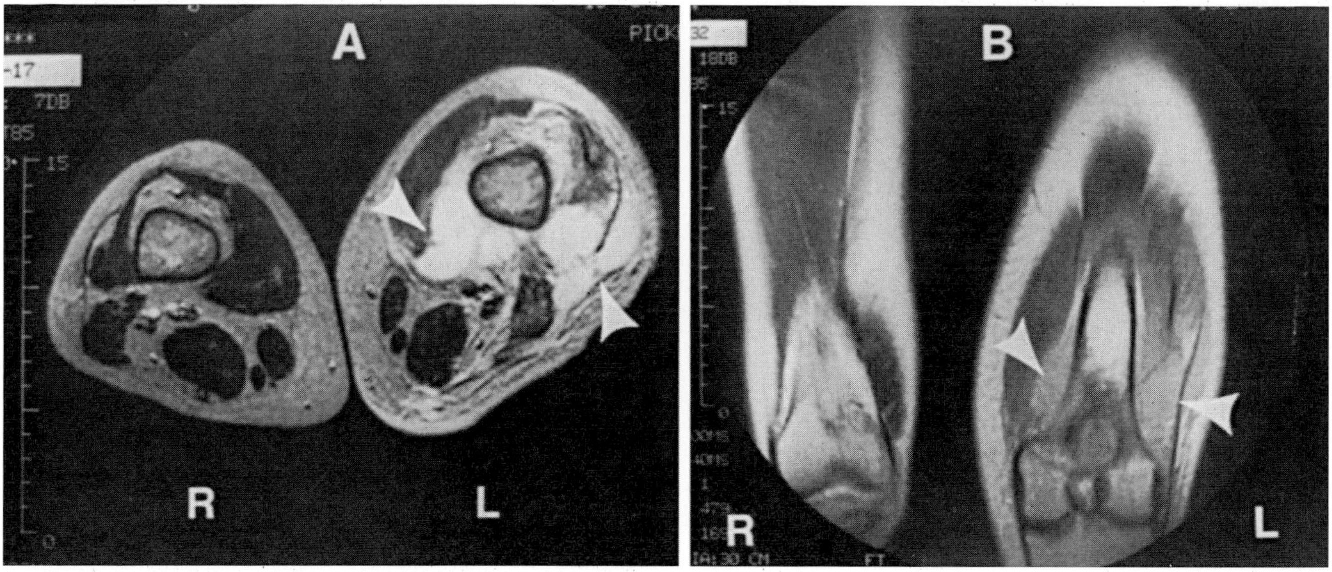

FIGURE 65–3. *Magnetic resonance imaging of the thighs of a patient with pyomyositis.* A *includes axial images of the right (R) and left (L) thighs, whereas* B *shows coronal images around the distal femoral shafts and femoral condyles. The scans demonstrate several well-defined areas of extremely high intensity in the muscle bundles and fascial planes from the mid to distal left femur (designated by arrows). The high signal intensity suggests a fluid collection (e.g., an abscess) rather than a neoplastic process. Edema of the subcutaneous tissues also is evident in the lateral aspect of the swollen left thigh. There are no abnormal signals within the bone.*

affected muscle groups included the vastus medialis, vastus intermedius, vastus lateralis, and biceps femoris. There was no involvement of the bone. CT can be substituted for MRI, but MRI is the preferred procedure if readily available.

Treatment

Because pyomyositis is an abscess of skeletal muscle, the treatment is surgical incision and drainage. However, it has been the experience of several physicians that smaller lesions resolved spontaneously, even prior to the antibiotic era. An important role for systemic antibiotics is to prevent the formation of further muscle abscesses, especially in a patient with proven bacteremia. Because *S. aureus* is the most likely agent, a semisynthetic penicillinase-resistant penicillin is the preferred antibiotic. Usually, nafcillin or oxacillin is administered intravenously every 6 hours at a total daily dosage of 150 to 200 mg/kg. When pyomyositis occurs in a patient with penicillin hypersensitivity, clindamycin (40 mg/kg/day, divided every 8 hours) can be substituted because of its excellent coverage of gram-positive cocci. Parenteral therapy is continued until clinical improvement is evident, usually within a few days after surgical drainage. Thereafter, the antibiotics can be given orally at a reduced dosage for an additional 2 to 3 weeks. Either a penicillin derivative (dicloxacillin at 25 mg/kg/day) or clindamycin (20 to 30 mg/kg/day) is acceptable.

ACUTE BACTERIAL MYOSITIS

Far less common than tropical pyomyositis is the condition of acute bacterial myositis, usually caused by group A streptococci. Often in this condition, the bacterial infection is not confined to distinct abscesses within the muscle but instead extends diffusely through one or more muscle groups. As with pyomyositis, the disease occurs more commonly in males than in females and, in general, is associated with prior physical exertion and perhaps minor trauma. Unlike pyomyositis, most published cases of acute bacterial myositis have occurred in adults and not in children.[4] The disease has been divided into the following four main types by Svane:[25] (1) a malignant form with septicemia and a uniformly fatal outcome; (2) an acute form with a more protracted clinical course, as well as other foci of suppuration such as the bones, joints, or viscera; (3) a subacute form with better clinical prognosis; and (4) a benign type associated with more distinct muscle abscesses. The benign type of acute bacterial myositis by the Svane classification is the same disease process as described in the preceding section on pyomyositis.

Clinical Presentation

The main clinical difference between the acute myositis syndrome and the pyomyositis syndrome is the virulence of the former disease, especially the malignant type. A case in a San Antonio native is illustrative. The patient was a muscular 23-year-old jackhammer operator who was admitted because of high fever, malaise, and pains in his arms. On examination, both upper extremities were tender to palpation, and faint erythema was visible over the same areas. He soon became incoherent, and his general condition quickly deteriorated. Death followed within 24 hours. Blood cultures drawn prior to death grew A streptococci, and cultures of the biceps muscles obtained at autopsy grew the same organism. This case is similar to others described in the literature.[4, 25] It also is most intriguing that the patient worked as a jackhammer operator, who presumably would incur considerable minor trauma to the muscles of the upper arms and shoulders. Two reported cases of streptococcal myositis in children involved the left thigh and the left paravertebral muscles, respectively.[18] The first child developed septic shock and required intensive care for 27 days before a definitive diagnosis was made by CT.

A case of generalized myositis with staphylococcal septicemia has been described in a 15-year-old boy.[1] The patient presented with signs of fever and very diffuse muscle swelling and tenderness. All muscle groups of the extremities appeared inflamed and markedly tender; the creatine phosphokinase enzymes were markedly elevated. Culture of a muscle biopsy grew *S. aureus*, as did previously drawn blood cultures. The patient experienced a stormy hospital course with severe hypotension and shock syndrome, requiring treatment with intravenous fluids, corticosteroids, dopamine, heparin, and assisted ventilation. He also received a total of 4 weeks of antistaphylococcal antibiotic therapy.

Diagnosis

Blood cultures are positive most often in patients with the most significant clinical symptoms. The muscle biopsy findings have been well described by Svane.[25] They include marked swelling and multiple hemorrhages with destruction of the musculature. There is abundant interfibrillar inflammatory exudate with masses of neutrophils and lymphocytes, together with large numbers of gram-positive cocci. Bacterial cultures of the affected muscle give a profuse growth of bacteria. In rare circumstances, myositis has occurred as a delayed complication of chickenpox, often together with fasciitis.[13, 17, 24] In this situation, bacteremia may not be documented because the bacterial process usually is the result of contiguous spread from a secondarily infected pock lesion. These streptococcal complications of chickenpox often occur in an extremity, which may become swollen and painful. Under these circumstances, MRI can be an extremely valuable diagnostic tool to gauge the depth and extent of inflammation.[27]

Treatment and the Eagle Effect

The treatment of acute streptococcal or staphylococcal myositis of the malignant type is a medical emergency. As soon as the diagnosis is suspected, bacteriologic cultures should be obtained and intravenous therapy with a high-dose semisynthetic penicillin should be initiated, e.g., nafcillin given at a dosage of 50 mg/kg every 6 hours. If the cultures yield group A streptococci rather than *Staphylococcus*, the antibiotic can be switched to penicillin G at an equivalent high dosage. Surgical consultation is required to evaluate the need for débridement and drainage. MRI may be advisable to document the extent of the disease and the response to antibiotic therapy. In severe cases of bacterial myositis, the total duration of hospitalization can exceed 4 weeks.[1, 18]

The apparent resurgence of serious streptococcal infection has led to an increased interest in what has been called the "Harry Eagle effect," named after the scientist who first described the failure of penicillin to eradicate group A streptococcal infection in a mouse model.[8] Eagle inoculated mice intramuscularly with group A streptococci and observed a markedly retarded bactericidal action of penicillin on organisms in the older abscesses, even though the bacteria remained highly sensitive to the antibiotic. Even massive doses of penicillin 10,000 times greater than the minimum inhibitory concentration were not effective at eradication of bacteria. Subsequent studies by other investigators confirmed the existence of the Eagle effect and, in addition, disclosed that clindamycin demonstrated superior efficacy to penicillin in treatment of streptococcal myositis in the mouse model.[23] In an editorial comment, Stevens[24] observed that penicillin most likely fails to kill stationary-phase streptococci present in muscle infections, an explanation for the Eagle effect. Thus, he suggests that streptococcal myositis or fasciitis be treated with intravenous clindamycin (40 mg/kg/day) if the condition fails to respond to penicillin therapy.

References

1. Adamski, G. B., Garin, E. H., Ballinger, W. E., et al.: Generalized nonsuppurative myositis with staphylococcal septicemia. J. Pediatr. *96*:694–697, 1980.
2. Altrocchi, P. H.: Spontaneous bacterial myositis. J. A. M. A. *217*:819–820, 1971.
3. Ashken, M. H., and Cotton, R. E.: Tropical skeletal muscle abscesses (pyomyositis tropicans). Br. J. Surg. *50*:846–852, 1963.
4. Barrett, A. M., and Gresham, G. A.: Acute streptococcal myositis. Lancet *1*:347–351, 1958.
5. Beck, W., and Grose, C.: Pyomyositis presenting as acute abdominal pain. Pediatr. Infect. Dis. *3*:445–448, 1984.
6. Chacha, P. B.: Muscle abscesses in children. Clin. Orthop. *70*:174–180, 1970.
7. Diamandakis, V., and Grose, C.: Bad consequences of bicycle accidents. Pediatr. Infect. Dis. J. *13*:422–425, 1994.
8. Eagle, H.: Experimental approach to the problem of treatment failure with penicillin. I. Group A streptococcal infection in mice. Am. J. Med. *13*:389–399, 1952.
9. Echeverria, P., and Vaughn, M. C.: Tropical pyomyositis: A diagnostic problem in temperate climates. Am. J. Dis. Child. *129*:856–857, 1975.
10. Foster, W. D.: The bacteriology of tropical pyomyositis in Uganda. J. Hyg. (Lond.) *63*:517–524, 1965.
11. Goldberg, J. S., London, W. L., and Nagel, D. M.: Tropical pyomyositis: A case report and review. Pediatrics *63*:298–300, 1979.
12. Grose, C.: Staphylococcal pyomyositis in south Texas. J. Pediatr. *93*:457–458, 1978.
13. Grose, C.: Varicella-zoster virus infections: Chickenpox, shingles, and varicella vaccine. *In* Glaser, R., and Jones, J. F. (eds.): Herpesvirus Infections. New York, Marcel Dekker, 1994, pp. 117–185.
14. Hirano, T., Srinivasan, G., Janakiraman, N., et al.: Gallium 67 citrate scintigraphy in pyomyositis. J. Pediatr. *97*:596–598, 1980.
15. Marcus, R. T., and Foster, W. D.: Observations on the clinical features, aetiology and geographic distribution of pyomyositis in East Africa. East Afr. Med. J. *45*:167–176, 1968.
16. Meehan, J., Grose, C., Soper, R. T., and Kimura, K. Pyomyositis in an adolescent female athlete. J. Pediatr. Surg. *30*:127–128, 1995.
17. Miyake, H.: Beitrage zur kenntnis der sogenannten myositis infectiosa. Mitt. Grenageb. Med. Chir. *13*:155–198, 1904.
18. Moore, D. L, Delage, G., Labelle, H., et al.: Peracute streptococcal pyomyositis: Report of two cases and review of the literature. J. Pediatr. Orthop. *6*:232–235, 1986.
19. Raphael, S. A., Wolfson, B. J., Parker, P., et al.: Pyomyositis in a child with acquired immunodeficiency syndrome. Am. J. Dis. Child. *143*:779–781, 1989.
20. Scriba, J.: Beitrag zur aetiologie der myositis acuta. Dtsch. Z. Chir. *22*:497–502, 1885.
21. Sheagren, J. N.: *Staphylococcus aureus*: The persistent pathogen. N. Engl. J. Med. *310*:1368–1373, 1984.
22. Sirinavin, S., and McCracken, G. H.: Primary suppurative myositis in children. Am. J. Dis. Child. *133*:263–265, 1979.
23. Stevens, D. L., Gibbons, A. E., Bergstrom, R., and Winn, V. The Eagle effect revisited: Efficacy of clindamycin, erythromycin, and penicillin in the treatment of streptococcal myositis. J. Infect. Dis. *158*:23–28, 1988.
24. Stevens, D. L.: Editorial response: Varicella gangrenosa with toxic shock-like syndrome. Clin. Infect. Dis. *20*:1061–1062, 1995.
25. Svane, S.: Peracute spontaneous streptococcal myositis. Acta Chir. Scand. *137*:155–163, 1971.
26. Traquair, R. N.: Pyomyositis. J. Trop. Med. Hyg. *50*:81–89, 1947.
27. Zittergruen, M., and Grose, C.: Magnetic resonance imaging for early diagnosis of necrotizing fasciitis. Pediatr. Emerg. Care *9*:26–28, 1993.

66

MISCELLANEOUS CAUSES OF MYOSITIS

Bernhard L. Wiedermann

In addition to the many gram-positive and gram-negative bacteria that may cause both pyogenic and nonpyogenic myositis, a host of other infectious agents have been implicated in acute and chronic inflammatory diseases of muscle. The pathophysiology of these disorders varies with the etiologic agent, but three basic categories exist. First, the microorganism can cause muscle injury by direct invasion of skeletal muscle. This is demonstrated most commonly for some of the parasitic causes of myositis, such as trichinosis, but it also has been seen rarely with viral etiologies. The second and probably most common mechanism of myositis is a postinfectious syndrome. Patients with this syndrome present with symptoms of muscle inflammation in the convalescent stage of a (usually) minor respiratory infection. The mechanism of this process has not been determined, but an autoimmune basis is suspected. Finally, systemic infections that result in diffuse vasculitis may present with severe myalgias; dengue, Rocky Mountain spotted fever, and leptospirosis are examples.

The major clinical syndromes encompassed by the nonbacterial causes of myositis are discussed here. The reader is referred to chapters on the specific pathogens for a more complete discussion of the etiologic agents.

CLINICAL SYNDROMES

Benign Acute Childhood Myositis

Benign acute childhood myositis originally was described in Lundberg's classic 1957 report of 74 cases of "myalgia cruris epidemica."[40] As more cases have been described, a prototype clinical picture has emerged.[2, 7, 11, 44, 45, 49, 62, 70] Typically, school age children are affected, with a male-female ratio of 2:1. There usually is an initial upper respiratory illness with resolution of symptoms over a period of days. During this resolution, there is a relatively abrupt presentation of calf pain and tenderness. The pain can be severe enough to interfere with normal ambulation. On examination, muscle tenderness is present and primarily involves the gastrocnemius and soleus muscles. Muscle swelling is uncommon, and there usually are no findings of systemic illness. Other muscle groups in the lower extremities, upper extremities, and neck also have been reported to be involved. There is marked elevation of serum creatinine phosphokinase and other muscle enzymes. Myoglobinuria usually is absent, distinguishing this entity from the more severe myositides, which cause extensive destruction of muscle tissue. Many different viruses, including influenza A and B, parainfluenza viruses, enteroviruses, adenoviruses, measles, and mumps, as well as *Mycoplasma pneumoniae*, have been implicated as etiologic agents (Table 66–1).

Histologic examination of muscle biopsy specimens generally shows edema and acute inflammatory infiltrates. Occasionally, scattered areas of necrosis are evident, with minimal perivascular inflammation. In general, examinations for viral particles by electron microscopy or indirect fluorescent antibody staining have been negative, suggesting an autoimmune mechanism for this disease.

No specific treatment for benign acute childhood myositis is needed; the illness resolves spontaneously, usually within several days.

Myositis with Myoglobinuria

Myositis with myoglobinuria probably is not distinct from benign acute childhood myositis but instead represents a more severe form of the acute myositis continuum. The presence of myoglobinuria in a child with myositis implies a more severe degree of muscle destruction than that seen with typical benign acute childhood myositis. The differences in clinical manifestations are more reflective of the host rather than the specific infectious agent, but it is useful from a clinical standpoint to discuss this group of patients separately. Influenza A virus infection seems to be the most

TABLE 66–1. Miscellaneous (Nonpyogenic) Causes of Myositis

Benign Acute Childhood Myositis/Myoglobinuric Myositis
Influenza viruses A and B[8, 11, 14–16, 25, 38, 47, 49–51, 58, 62, 66–68, 70, 78]
Parainfluenza viruses 2 and 3[72, 79]
Echoviruses 6 and 9[33, 35, 60]
Coxsackieviruses[8]
Rotavirus[28]
Measles virus[1]
Rubella virus (immunization)[27]
Adenovirus 21[48, 77]
Varicella-zoster virus[57]
Cytomegalovirus[29, 54]
Epstein-Barr virus[23, 36, 63]
Herpes simplex virus type 2[63]
Mycoplasma pneumoniae[7]
Pleurodynia
Coxsackieviruses A and B[5, 17, 34]
Many echoviruses[34]
Parasitic Myositis
Trichinella spiralis[4, 24, 52]
Cysticercus cellulosae (Taenia solium)[10, 43]
Toxoplasma gondii[26, 71]
Toxocara species[75]
Microsporidia[12, 39, 41]
Sarcocystis[6]
Wucheria bancrofti[53, 59]
Spirochetal Myositis
Borrelia burgdorferi[3, 18, 61, 64, 65]
Leptospira species[22]
Chronic Polymyositis
HIV-1[20, 31, 76]
Human T-cell lymphotrophic virus type I[19, 56]
Coxsackieviruses (?)[10]

common organism implicated in myoglobinuric myositis.[8, 13–15, 50, 51, 66, 78] In general, these patients may be more likely than those with benign acute childhood myositis to present with muscle pain during the acute phase of the precipitating infection, and their muscle pain is more severe and more generalized. The offending microorganism may be demonstrable more readily in muscle tissue. However, none of these features can distinguish these entities clearly in any individual patient, and a urinalysis is the most important test to obtain in this regard.

Patients with myoglobinuria will have positive results in tests for urinary occult blood by dipstick but have no demonstrable erythrocytes on microscopic urine examination. The diagnosis can be confirmed by specific myoglobin determination in urine. Once this diagnosis is made, it is important to monitor renal function in these individuals because of the risk of myoglobinuric renal failure. Patients with severe myoglobinuria may have an underlying disorder of muscle, such as carnitine palmityl transferase deficiency or paroxysmal rhabdomyolysis, which should be considered.[21, 37]

No specific therapy exists for this disorder. Supportive care, including that appropriate for patients with renal failure, is most important. Amantadine therapy for patients with early influenza A infection might be effective but has not been evaluated in this clinical situation.

Epidemic Pleurodynia (see also Chapter 170)

Epidemic pleurodynia (Bornholm disease) is an acute viral syndrome most commonly seen with coxsackievirus B infection in children and young adults.[5, 17, 34] The typical syndrome consists of fever and pain involving the chest and upper abdomen. Tenderness without muscle swelling is present in the affected areas, and pain may be aggravated by sudden movement with coughing or deep inspiration. The symptoms may mimic those of acute appendicitis in the younger child. Upper respiratory and gastrointestinal symptoms suggestive of viral illness often are present. A pleural friction rub may be heard on examination, but chest radiographs and routine laboratory tests generally are unrewarding. Clinical manifestations usually wane after 2 to 3 days but may reappear several days later. No specific therapy is available.

Parasitic Myositis

Myositis resulting from parasitic disease usually occurs with tissue invasion by the pathogen, and therefore most of these individuals will have significant eosinophilia as the primary diagnostic clue.

Trichinosis

Trichinella spiralis is the most common cause of this clinical entity, resulting from ingestion of the encysted larvae in undercooked meat, primarily pork and wild game.[4] Initially, patients present with fever, diarrhea, and abdominal pain during the intestinal phase of infection. In the second week of illness, this is replaced with signs and symptoms related to dissemination via the blood stream and invasion of skeletal muscle. Fever, malaise, eyelid edema, and pain, tenderness, and swelling of muscles are the predominant symptoms.[24, 52] The most frequent sites involved are in the upper body and include extraocular muscles, muscles of mastication, neck, deltoids, intercostals, and diaphragm. Untreated, the illness resolves slowly, with calcification developing in affected muscle tissue after several months. Trichinosis occurring in natives of northern Canada may present with less prominent or absent symptoms of myositis.[42]

A history of ingestion of undercooked meat or the presence of an outbreak of myositis in the community accompanied by the finding of eosinophilia in the patient strongly suggests a diagnosis of trichinosis. Muscle biopsy is the most direct and accurate method of confirming the diagnosis, but serologic tests may be helpful.[32, 74]

Mebendazole, albendazole, or flubendazole may be effective treatment for trichinosis.[46] Systemic corticosteroids have been helpful in alleviating severe symptoms.

Cysticercosis

Cysticercosis occurs with human ingestion of eggs of the pork tapeworm, *Taenia solium*, in material from a human source (feces or vomitus). Cysticercosis is not common in the United States but frequently is found in Mexico, Central and South America, and parts of Africa. After ingestion, virtually any organ system in the body can be infected, with skeletal muscle among the most common sites.[10, 43] Typically, muscular involvement is asymptomatic, although fever, myalgias, and eosinophilia can be seen. More commonly, cysticercal myositis is diagnosed incidentally in a patient with central nervous system involvement or by histologic examination of subcutaneous nodules that are present occasionally. Calcific densities in skeletal muscle, in a classic "puffed rice" appearance, are highly suggestive of the diagnosis. Granulomatous reactions commonly are seen in tissue. Treatment with praziquantel has resulted in resolution of the subcutaneous nodules; it is difficult to judge the effects of treatment on muscular involvement, which normally has a benign course.[43] Individuals with cysticercal myositis should have careful neurologic and ophthalmologic evaluations performed for detection of potentially more serious manifestations of the disease.

Other Parasites

Myalgias are a frequent complaint in acquired *Toxoplasma gondii* infection, and toxoplasmosis rarely may present with a polymyositis-like syndrome.[26, 71] *Toxocara* myositis was diagnosed in two previously healthy children by clinical and serologic means.[75] Both had resolution of symptoms within 72 hours and received no specific therapy. Microsporidiosis reportedly caused myositis in a young man with AIDS as well as in another adult patient with a nonspecific immunodeficiency.[12, 39, 41] The diagnoses were made by demonstration of microsporidia in biopsy material. *Sarcocystis* and *Wucheria bancrofti* have been reported to cause inflammatory muscle disease.[6, 53, 59]

Spirochetal Myositis

Although spirochetes are classified correctly as bacteria, the clinical presentation of myositis due to spirochetes has more similarities to viral myositis than to overt bacterial pyomyositis. Thus, these entities are discussed briefly here.

Borrelia burgdorferi

Muscular pain is not an uncommon complaint in patients with acute Lyme disease, and there are several reports of patients with Lyme disease who have myositis as a major feature at initial presentation.[3, 18, 61, 64] Lyme myositis primarily is a feature in stage II Lyme disease, appearing anywhere from 2 to 5 months after infection. Clinically, proximal muscles, particularly the thigh muscles, are involved, with a rather painful swelling that may wax and wane over several months. Orbital myositis, usually considered an idiopathic condition, has been reported in association with Lyme disease in a 5-year-old girl.[65] Typically, biopsy specimens show chronic inflammation surrounding intramuscular veins. Spirochetes can be demonstrated in tissue, and antibiotic treatment for Lyme disease appears to result in a favorable response in most individuals with Lyme myositis.[3, 61, 64]

Leptospirosis

Myalgia often is a prominent and severe component in the initial presentation of leptospirosis.[22] It is somewhat surprising, therefore, that the histologic changes in muscle are not more prominent. Most commonly, only minimal changes (of cytoplasmic vacuoles in the myofibrillar cells) are seen, with occasional acute inflammatory infiltrates. With resolution of the infection, healing of muscle occurs without fibrosis.

Retroviral Myositis

Published reports of muscle involvement related to primary infection with HIV-1 or human T-cell lymphotrophic virus type I (HTLV-I) suggest a role for these retroviruses in the production of a relatively chronic form of myositis.

HIV-1

Myalgia is a frequent finding in patients with HIV-1 infection. Generalized disease usually is present, and muscular atrophy may be prominent. It is difficult, however, to ascribe all of these changes to HIV-1 infection because these individuals usually have multiple medical problems that could contribute to muscle wasting. The p24 antigen has been demonstrated in affected muscle tissue, and viral-like particles have been seen,[19, 56] but immunohistologic studies do not suggest direct infection of muscle fibers by HIV-1. Intravenous immunoglobulin therapy may have benefited one adult with HIV-1–associated polymyositis.[73]

Human T-Cell Lymphotrophic Virus Type I

The association between HTLV-I infection and a polymyositis-like syndrome is more clear-cut than is the case with HIV-1 disease. Although more prominently a cause of tropical spastic paraparesis, a myelopathy primarily involving the lower extremities, some studies strongly suggest an etiologic role in some cases of polymyositis.[20, 31, 76] Initially, seroepidemiologic data implicated HTLV-I in this syndrome, and, more recently, specific virologic data in individual cases have strengthened this contention. One patient with combined infection with HTLV-I and HIV-1 and diffuse muscle weakness had evidence of HTLV-I in muscle biopsy specimens demonstrated by in situ hybridization and by immunocytochemistry.[20] There was no evidence of HIV-1 material in the biopsy by those methods.

Although these cases of retroviral myopathy occurred in adults, the clinical entity should be recognized so that the cases of infants and children with polymyositis-like symptoms and risk factors for either HIV-1 or HTLV-I disease can be evaluated for these infections appropriately.

Other Forms of Chronic Polymyositis

Limited data may suggest a causal role for other infectious agents, primarily enteroviruses and mumps virus, in idiopathic polymyositis. Virus-like particles have been noted in muscle tissue sections from patients with chronic myositis, and coxsackievirus A9 has been isolated from the muscle of an individual with polymyositis.[69] Coxsackievirus B antigen has been demonstrated by in situ hybridization in patients with polymyositis and with acute and chronic dermatomyositis but not in normal controls or samples from muscular dystrophy patients.[9] Mumps long has been suspected as an etiologic agent of inclusion-body myositis because the structure of abnormal muscle filaments bears some resemblance to mumps virus nucleoproteins.[55] However, no evidence of mumps antigen was detected by hybridization or immunocytochemical means in muscle tissues of 20 patients with such myositis.[55] Further studies are necessary before a true link can be established between chronic, idiopathic myositis and viral infections.

References

1. Ando, T., Suzuki, M., and Sato, T.: A case of myoglobinuria associated with measles. Shonika *15*:981, 1974.
2. Antony, J. H., Procopis, P. G., and Ouvrier, R. A.: Benign acute childhood myositis. Neurology *29*:1068, 1979.
3. Atlas, E., Novak, S. N., Duray, P. H., et al.: Lyme myositis: Muscle invasion by *Borrelia burgdorferi*. Ann. Intern. Med. *109*:245, 1988.
4. Bailey, T. M., and Schantz, P. M.: Trichinosis surveillance, United States, 1986. CDC Surveillance Summaries *37*(SS-5):1, 1988.
5. Bain, H. N., McLean, D. M., and Walker, S. J.: Epidemic pleurodynia (Bornholm disease) due to coxsackie B-5 virus: The interrelationship of pleurodynia, benign pericarditis, and aseptic meningitis. Pediatrics *27*:889, 1961.
6. Beaver, P. C., Gadgil, R. K., and Morera, P.: *Sarcocystis* in man: A review and report of five cases. Am. J. Trop. Med. Hyg. *28*:819, 1979.
7. Belardi, C., Roberge, R., Kelly, M., et al.: Myalgia cruris epidemica (benign acute childhood myositis) associated with a *Mycoplasma pneumoniae* infection. Ann. Emerg. Med. *16*:579, 1987.
8. Berlin, B. S., Simon, N. M., and Bovner, R. N.: Myoglobinuria precipitated by viral infection. J. A. M. A. *227*:1414, 1974.
9. Bowles, N. E., Sewry, C. A., Dubowitz, V., et al.: Dermatomyositis, polymyositis, and coxsackie-B-virus infection. Lancet *1*:1004, 1987.
10. Brown, W. J., and Voge, M.: Cysticercosis: A modern day plague. Pediatr. Clin. North Am. *32*:953, 1985.
11. Buchta, R. M.: Myositis and influenza. Pediatrics *60*:761, 1977.
12. Chupp, G. L., Alroy, J., Adelman, L. S., et al.: Myositis due to *Pleistophora* (Microsporidia) in a patient with AIDS. Clin. Infect. Dis. *16*:15, 1993.
13. Christenson, J. C., and San Joaquin, V. H.: Influenza-associated rhabdomyolysis in a child. Pediatr. Infect. Dis. J. *9*:60, 1990.
14. Cunningham, E., Kohli, R., and Venuto, R. C.: Influenza-associated myoglobinuric real failure. J. A. M. A. *242*:2428, 1979.
15. DiBona, F. J., and Morens, D. M.: Rhabdomyolysis associated with influenza: Report of a case with unusual fluid and electrolytes abnormalities. J. Pediatr. *91*:943, 1977.
16. Dietzman, D. E., Schaller, J. G., Ray, C. G., et al.: Acute myositis associated with influenza B infection. Pediatrics *57*:255, 1967.
17. Disney, M. E., Howard, E. M., and Wood, B. S. B.: Bornholm disease in children. Br. Med. J. *1*:1351, 1953.
18. Duray, P. H.: Clinical pathologic correlations of Lyme disease. Rev. Infect. Dis. *11*:S1487, 1989.
19. Espinoza, L. R., Aguilar, J. L., Berman, A., et al.: Rheumatic manifestations associated with human immunodeficiency virus infection. Arthritis Rheum. *32*:1615, 1989.
20. Evans, B. K., Gore, I., Harrell, L. E., et al.: HTLV-I-associated myelopathy and polymyositis in a US native. Neurol *39*:1572, 1989.
21. Favara, B. E., Vawter, G. F., and Wagner, R., et al.: Familial paroxysmal rhabdomyolysis in children: A myoglobinuric syndrome. Am. J. Med. *42*:196, 1967.
22. Feigin, R. D., and Anderson, D. C.: Human leptospirosis. CRC Crit. Rev. Clin. Lab. Sci. *5*:413, 1975.
23. Friedman, B. I., and Libby, R.: Epstein-Barr virus infection associated with rhabdomyolysis and acute renal failure. Clin. Pediatr. *25*:228, 1986.
24. Gould, S. E.: Clinical manifestations. A. Symptomatology. *In* Gould, S. E. (ed.): Trichinosis in Man and Animals. Springfield, Charles C Thomas, 1970, p. 269.
25. Greco, T. P., Askenase, P. W., and Kashgarian, M.: Postviral myositis: Myxovirus-like structures in affected muscles. Ann. Intern. Med. *86*:193, 1977.
26. Greenlee, J. E., Johnson, W. D., Campa, J. F., et al.: Adult toxoplasmosis presenting as polymyositis and cerebral ataxia. Ann. Intern. Med. *82*:367, 1975.

27. Hanissian, A. S., Martinez, A. J., Jabbour, J. T., et al.: Vasculitis and myositis secondary to rubella vaccination. Arch. Neurol. *28*:202, 1973.
28. Hattori, H., Torii, S., Nagafuji, H., et al.: Benign acute myositis associated with rotavirus gastroenteritis. J. Pediatr. *121*:748, 1992.
29. Hughes, G. S., and Hunt, R.: Cytomegalovirus infection with rhabdomyolysis and myoglobinuria. Ann. Intern. Med. *101*:276, 1984.
30. Illa, I., Nath, A., and Dalakas, M.: Immunocytochemical and virological characteristics of HIV-associated inflammatory myopathies: Similarities with seronegative polymyositis. Ann. Neurol. *29*:474, 1991.
31. Ishii, K., Yamato, K., Iwahara, Y., et al: Isolation of HTLV-1 from muscle of a patient with polymyositis. Am. J. Med. *90*:267, 1991.
32. Ivanoska, D., Cuperlović, K., Gamble, H. R., et al.: Comparative efficacy of antigen and antibody detection tests for human trichinellosis. J. Parasitol. *75*:38, 1989.
33. Jehn, U. W., and Fink, M. K.: Myositis, myoglobinemia, and myoglobinuria associated with enterovirus echo 9 infection. Arch. Neurol. *37*:457, 1980.
34. Johnson, K. M., Bloom, H. H., Forsyth, B., et al.: The role of enteroviruses in respiratory disease. Am. Rev. Respir. Dis. *88*:240, 1963.
35. Josselson, J., Pula, T., and Sadler, J. H.: Acute rhabdomyolysis associated with an echovirus 9 infection. Arch. Intern. Med. *140*:1671, 1980.
36. Kantor, R. J., Norden, C. W., and Wein, T. P.: Infectious mononucleosis associated with rhabdomyolysis and renal failure. South. Med. J. *71*:346, 1978.
37. Kelly, K. J., Garland, J. S., Tang, T. T., et al.: Fatal rhabdomyolysis following influenza infection in a girl with familial carnitine palmityl transferase deficiency. Pediatrics *84*:312, 1989.
38. Kessler, H. A., Trenholme, G. M., Harris, A. A., et al.: Acute myopathy associated with influenza A/Texas/1/77 infection. J. A. M. A. *243*:461, 1980.
39. Ledford, D. K., Overman, M. D., Gonzalvo, A., et al.: Microsporidiosis myositis in a patient with the acquired immunodeficiency syndrome. Ann. Intern. Med. *102*:628, 1985.
40. Lundberg, A.: Myalgia cruris epidemica. Acta Paediatr. *46*:18, 1957.
41. Macher, A. M., Neafie, R., Angritt, P., et al.: Microsporidial myositis and the acquired immunodeficiency syndrome (AIDS): A four-year follow-up. Ann. Intern. Med. *109*:343, 1988.
42. MacLean, J. D., Viallet, J., Law, C., et al.: Trichinosis in the Canadian Arctic: Report of five outbreaks and a new clinical syndrome. J. Infect. Dis. *160*:513, 1989.
43. Manson-Bahr, P. E. C., and Bell, D. R. (eds.): Tapeworms (cestaodes). *In* Manson's Tropical Diseases. 19th ed. Philadelphia, Bailliere Tindall, 1987, p. 521.
44. Mason, W., and Keller, E.: Acute transient myositis with influenza-like illness. J. Pediatr. *86*:813, 1975.
45. McKinlay, I. A., and Mitchell, I.: Transient acute myositis in childhood. Arch. Dis. Child. *51*:135, 1979.
46. Medical Letter on Drugs and Therapeutics: Drugs for parasitic infections. Med. Lett. *37*:99, 1995.
47. Mejlszenkier, J. D., Safran, A. P., Healy, J. J., et al.: The myositis of influenza. Arch. Neurol. *29*:441, 1973.
48. Meshkinpour, H., and Vaziri, M. D.: Acute rhabdomyolysis associated with adenovirus infection. J. Infect. Dis. *143*:133, 1981.
49. Middleton, P. J., Alexander, R. M., and Szymanski, M. T.: Severe myositis during recovery from influenza. Lancet *2*:533, 1970.
50. Minow, R. A., Gorbach, S., Johnson, B. L., et al.: Myoglobinuria associated with influenza A infection. Ann. Intern. Med. *80*:359, 1980.
51. Morgensen, J. L.: Myoglobinuria and renal failure associated with influenza. Ann. Intern. Med. *80*:362, 1974.
52. Most, H.: Trichinosis: Preventable yet still with us. N. Engl. J. Med. *298*:1178, 1978.
53. Narasimhan, C., George, T. J., Thomas George, K., et al.: *W. bancrofti* as a causal agent of polymyositis. J. Assoc. Physicians India *40*:471, 1992.
54. Naylor, C. D., Jevnikar, A. M., and Witt, N. J.: Sporadic viral myositis in two adults. Can. Med. Assoc. J. *137*:819, 1987.
55. Nishino, H., Engel, A. G., and Rima, B. K.: Inclusion body myositis: The mumps hypothesis. Ann. Neurol. *25*:260, 1989.
56. Nordstrom, D. M., Petropolis, A. A., Giorno, R., et al.: Inflammatory myopathy and acquired immunodeficiency syndrome. Arthritis Rheum. *32*:475, 1989.
57. Norris, F. H., Jr., Dramov, B., Calder, C. D., et al.: Virus-like particles in myositis accompanying herpes zoster. Arch. Neurol. *21*:25, 1969.
58. Partin, J. C., Schubert, W. K., Partin, J. S., et al.: Isolation of influenza virus from liver and muscle biopsy specimens from a surviving case of Reye's syndrome. Lancet *2*:599, 1976.
59. Poddar, S. K., Misra, S., and Singh, N. K.: Acute polymyositis associated with *W. bancrofti*. Acta Neurol. Scand. *89*:225, 1994.
60. Poels, P., Ewals, J., Joosten, E., et al.: Rhabdomyolysis associated with simultaneous Epstein-Barr virus infection and isolation of echovirus 6 from muscle: A dual infection. J. Neurol. Neurosurg. Psychiatry *52*:412, 1989.
61. Reimers, C. D., Pongratz, D. E., Neubert, U., et al.: Myositis caused by *Borrelia burgdorferi*: Report of four cases. J. Neurol. Sci. *91*:215, 1989.
62. Ruff, R. L., and Secrist, D.: Viral studies in benign acute childhood myositis. Arch. Neurol. *39*:261, 1982.
63. Schlesinger, M. J. J., Gandara, D., and Bensch, K. G.: Myoglobinuria associated with herpes-group viral infection. Arch. Intern. Med. *138*:422, 1978.
64. Schoenen, J., Sianard-Gainko, J., Carpentier, M., et al.: Myositis during *Borrelia burgdorferi* infection (Lyme disease). J. Neurol. Neurosurg. Psychiatry *52*:1002, 1989.
65. Seidenberg, K. B., and Leib, M. L.: Orbital myositis with Lyme disease. Am. J. Ophthalmol. *109*:13, 1990.
66. Simon, N. M., Rovner, R. N., and Berlin, B. S.: Acute myoglobinuria associated with type A2 (Hong Kong) influenza. J. A. M. A. *212*:1704, 1970.
67. Stang, H.: Acute transient myositis associated with influenza virus infection. Pediatr. Infect. Dis. J. *8*:257, 1989.
68. Stevens, D., Burman, D., Clarke, S. K. R., et al.: Temporary paralysis in childhood after influenza B. Lancet *2*:1354, 1974.
69. Tang, T. T., Sedmak, G. V., Siegesmund, K. A., et al.: Chronic myopathy associated with coxsackievirus type A9: A combined electron microscopical and viral isolation study. N. Engl. J. Med. *292*:608, 1975.
70. Tepperberg, J.: Transient acute myositis in children. J. A. M. A. *238*:27, 1977.
71. Teutsch, S. M., Juranek, D. D., Sulzer, A., et al.: Epidemic toxoplasmosis associated with infected cats. N. Engl. J. Med. *300*:695, 1979.
72. Ueda, K., Robbins, D. A., Itaka, K., et al.: Fatal rhabdomyolysis associated with parainfluenza type 3 infection. Hiroshima J. Med. Sci. *27*:99, 1978.
73. Viard, J.-P., Vittecoq, D., Lacroix, C., et al.: Response of HIV-1–associated polymyositis to intravenous immunoglobulin. Am. J. Med. *92*:580, 1992.
74. Walls, K. W.: Serodiagnostic tests for parasitic diseases. *In* Lennette, E. H., Balows, A., Hausler, W. J., et al. (eds.): Manual of Clinical Microbiology. 4th ed. Washington, D.C., American Society for Microbiology, 1985, p. 945.
75. Walsh, S. S., Robson, W. J., and Hart, C. A.: Acute transient myositis due to *Toxocara*. Arch. Dis. Child. *63*:1087, 1988.
76. Wiley, C. A., Nerenberg, M., Cros, D., et al.: HTLV-I polymyositis in a patient also infected with the human immunodeficiency virus. N. Engl. J. Med. *320*:992, 1989.
77. Wright, J., Couchonnal G., and Hodges, G. R.: Adenovirus type 21 infection: Occurrence with pneumonia, rhabdomyolysis, and myoglobinuria in an adult. J. A. M. A. *241*:2420, 1979.
78. Zamkoff, K., and Rosen, N.: Influenza and myoglobinuria in brothers. Neurology *29*:340, 1979.
79. Zvolanek, J. R.: Benign acute childhood myositis associated with parainfluenza type 2 infection. Pediatr. Infect. Dis. *3*:594, 1984.

S E C T I O N   T E N

SKIN INFECTIONS

❑ ❑ ❑

67

CUTANEOUS MANIFESTATIONS OF SYSTEMIC INFECTIONS

James D. Cherry

Many illnesses caused by infectious agents have associated cutaneous manifestations. In some cases, the exanthem may be the hallmark of the disease, and in others, only a vague indicator of a more significant underlying process. When an exanthem occurs, it often offers important clues to the etiology of a patient's illness. Although most exanthematous illnesses in children are benign, their differential diagnosis is critical because the early manifestations of potentially fatal bacterial and rickettsial diseases frequently have cutaneous findings.

HISTORY

Exanthematous manifestations of infectious illnesses have been important since medical antiquity. Major epidemics of both measles and smallpox occurred in the Roman Empire and in China at the beginning of the Christian era.[19, 107] Scarlet fever was recognized as a distinct entity in the 17th century, and chickenpox and rubella were identified in the 18th and 19th centuries, respectively.[12]

In the writings of the early 20th century, maculopapular exanthematous illnesses of children frequently were referred to by number. Scarlet fever and measles historically were the first two classic maculopapular exanthems of childhood. Which one had the honor of being the "first disease" is unknown today. By the beginning of the 20th century, it was clear that rubella was a distinct entity, and it was the "third disease."[57, 59, 72, 129, 147–149] In 1900, Dukes[57] described an exanthematous illness with characteristics of both rubella and scarlet fever, which he felt was a "fourth disease." It is the general opinion today that his disease was not a distinct entity. Shaw[149] suggested that Dukes' cases had mild atypical scarlet fever, and Powell[129] raised the possibility that the illness resulted from epidermolytic toxin-producing staphylococci. It seems most probable that rubella and scarlet fever were both epidemic in the student population under Dr. Dukes' care; combined infections led to the confusion.

Erythema infectiosum (see Chapter 158) commonly is referred to as fifth disease, and roseola infantum (see Chapter 68) qualifies as the sixth disease.[148]

During the last 40 years, interest in exanthematous diseases has been renewed because a large number of previously unknown viruses and other infectious agents that cause cutaneous manifestations have been discovered. In addition, the pattern of disease caused by classic exanthem-producing agents has changed; smallpox has been eradicated, the epidemiology of measles and rubella has been altered by immunization, and ecologic changes have resulted in differences in bacterially induced rashes.

ETIOLOGIC AGENTS

Many different types of viruses, chlamydiae, rickettsiae, mycoplasmas, bacteria, fungi, and protozoan and metazoan agents cause illnesses with associated cutaneous manifestations. Although this chapter is devoted to systemic infectious diseases with cutaneous manifestations, the demarcation between exanthematous disease of systemic and local origin is not always readily apparent. For example, the recurrent cold sore due to herpes simplex virus infection frequently is thought of as a local problem, although its nature and pathogenesis involve central virus latency and host systemic immune functions. Similarly, superficial fungal diseases and other local infections, such as warts, may be quite dependent upon more general immunologic functions of the host. The exanthems of enteroviral infections frequently are confused with those caused by insect bites and allergic problems.

Table 67–1 presents viruses that have cutaneous manifestations in humans. Erythema infectiosum is caused by human parvovirus B19.[3, 170] Adenovirus types 1, 2, 3, 4, 7, and 7a have been isolated from children and young adults with exanthem.[42, 91, 173, 174] The overall clinical expression rate of exanthem in adenovirus infection rarely has been studied. Fukumi and associates[67] noted that rash occurred in 2 per cent of adenoviral infections; Hope-Simpson and Higgins[81] indicated a rate of about 8 per cent.

Six species in the *Herpesvirus* genus have cutaneous manifestations associated with infection, but the clinical expression rates vary greatly. Nearly all primary varicella infections are associated with exanthem, whereas exanthem with acquired cytomegalovirus infection is rare.[14, 17, 41, 136, 155, 173] Exanthem in Epstein-Barr virus infection varies from 3 to nearly 100 per cent, depending upon the presence or absence of concomitant ampicillin administration.[11, 22, 79, 86, 92, 119, 130, 162, 163] Although firm data are lacking, probably less than 10 per cent of primary infections with herpes simplex virus type 1 are associated with cutaneous manifestations. Erythema multiforme occasionally occurs with recurrent herpes simplex virus infections.[30, 65, 88, 117] Human herpesvirus 6 is a major cause of roseola infantum.[6, 170, 180]

At present, human illnesses with cutaneous manifestations due to poxviruses are rare. Smallpox as a disease ceases to exist, and because of this, the use of vaccinia virus for immunization has decreased dramatically. Monkeypox, orf, and paravaccinia (milker's nodules) continue to occur as isolated events in exposed individuals.[140, 173, 174] Human infection with Tanapox virus is a geographically related illness occurring in limited areas of Kenya.

In the present era, enteroviruses are the leading cause of exanthematous diseases.[42, 46, 90, 173, 174] Thirty-six types have been associated with rash illnesses. The clinical expression

Text continued on page 720

TABLE 67–1. Clinical Characteristics of Viral Infections with Cutaneous Manifestations

Virus	Disease or Syndrome	Incubation Period (Days)	Main Season	Clinical Characteristics	Exanthem: Lesions	Exanthem: Distribution	Usual Duration (Days)
Parvovirus (See Figs. 67–7 and 67–8)	Erythema infectiosum	7–17	Winter and spring	Biphasic illness with mild prodromal period with headache and malaise for 2–3 days, then 7-day symptom-free period, followed by typical exanthem	Three-stage exanthem: initially, rash on cheeks (slapped-cheek appearance) and then erythematous maculopapular rash on trunk and limbs. Finally, rash develops a reticular pattern	Starts on face. More prominent on extensor surfaces of extremities	7–21
Wart	Warts		Nonseasonal	Local cutaneous disease	Papular or nodular isolated lesions	Most common on extremities	100+
Adenovirus types 1, 2, 3, 4, 7, and 7a		6–9	Winter and spring	Fever and signs and symptoms of respiratory illness. Occasionally, rash occurs after defervescence (roseola-like)	Most commonly erythematous, maculopapular, and discrete (rubelliform) but occasionally confluent (morbilliform); rarely erythema multiforme and Stevens-Johnson syndrome	Usually starts on face and spreads downward to trunk and extremities	3–5
Herpes simplex types 1 and 2 (See Fig. 67–5)	Cold sores, genital herpes, neonatal herpes, or other	2–12	Nonseasonal	Primary disease associated with fever and systemic symptoms. Recurrent disease due to exogenous and endogenous infections	Singular or grouped vesicular lesions varying in size from 2 to 10 mm, frequently on a mildly erythematous base. Occasionally erythema multiforme. Stevens-Johnson syndrome and erythema nodosum	Lesions in primary infection with type 1 virus mainly are in and around the mouth. Recurrent type 1 lesions usually perioral. Primary and recurrent type 2 lesions usually on genitals	7–14
Human herpes-virus 6	Roseola infantum		Nonseasonal	Fever 3–5 days' duration, rapid defervescence, and then the appearance of rash	Erythematous macular or maculopapular	Most prominent on neck and trunk. Face and extremities may be affected	1–2
Varicella-zoster (See Fig. 67–4)	Chickenpox (varicella)	12–20	Late fall, winter, and spring	Malaise and fever of 5–6 days' duration	Basic lesion is vesicular, but lesions go through stages: macules, papules, vesicles, and crusts. Lesions occur in crops	Lesions more profuse on trunk than on extremities. Proximal extremities are more involved than are distal	8–10
	Herpes zoster		Nonseasonal	Endogenous infection. Pain and paresthesia with dermatome distribution	Basic lesion is vesicular, but lesions go through stages: macules, papules, vesicles, and crusts	Lesions localized to the area of skin innervated by a single sensory ganglion	10–28
Epstein-Barr	Infectious mononucleosis	28–49	Nonseasonal	Fever, pharyngitis, and lymphadenopathy. Exanthem occurs in 3–13% of cases. If ampicillin administered, then exanthem in 50% of cases	Most commonly erythematous, macular, maculopapular, and discrete (rubelliform). In association with ampicillin administration, the rash may be more vivid. Erythema multiforme and urticaria may occur	Mainly on trunk and proximal extremities	2–7
Cytomegalovirus	Cytomegalovirus mononucleosis		Nonseasonal	Acquired: Mild febrile illness with lymphadenopathy Congenital: Disseminated disease	Erythematous, maculopapular, and discrete. Vesicular or petechial in congenital infection	Located mainly on trunk and proximal extremities	2–7
Vaccinia	Roseola vaccinatum, eczema vaccinatum, vaccination "take," or disseminated vaccinia		Nonseasonal	Illness due to direct exposure via vaccination or exposure to a vaccinee	Vaccination and eczema vaccinatum: Lesions go through stages: papule, vesicle, pustule, and scab. Roseola vaccinatum: erythematous maculopapular lesions. Occasionally erythema multiforme. Disseminated vaccinia: papular or vesicular lesions	Lesions in roseola vaccinatum, eczema vaccinatum, and disseminated vaccinia are generalized	7–14
Variola	Smallpox	8–17	Seasonal by geographic area	Abrupt onset of high fever, headache, and muscle and joint pains. Rash appears 2–4 days after onset	Basic lesion is vesicular, but lesions go through stages: macules, papules, vesicles, pustules, and crusts	Most prominent on exposed body surfaces. Starts on extremities and face. Spreads centripetally	12–20
Monkeypox				Similar to mild smallpox. Exposure to monkeys. No human-to-human spread	Similar to mild smallpox	Similar to mild smallpox	

Orf	Ecthyma contagiosum	4–7	Spring	Disease of sheep acquired by humans	Initially erythematous papule. Becomes umbilicated, nodular, and then vesicular. Occasionally erythema multiforme	Solitary lesion, usually on hands	30–40
Molluscum contagiosum	Molluscum contagiosum			Local cutaneous disease	Umbilicated nodular lesions: singular or clusters	Most common on face, inner thigh, breasts, and genitalia	100+
Paravaccinia	Milker's nodules	4–7		Human infection acquired from infected calves	Nodular lesion. Occasionally erythema multiforme	Solitary lesion, usually on hands	30–40
Tanapox				A virus of monkeys. Human infection associated with fever and regional lymphadenopathy	Umbilicated vesicular lesion	Upper body. Solitary lesion	35–56
Coxsackieviruses A2, 4, 5, 7, 9, 10, and 16; coxsackieviruses B1–5; echoviruses 1–7, 9, 11–14, 16–19, 22, 24, 25, 30, and 33; enterovirus 71 (See Figs. 67–9 through 67–16)		4–7	Summer and fall	Fever and mild to moderate pharyngitis. Occasionally, herpangina, meningitis, and other manifestations of systemic viral infection. Exanthem occurs in 5–50% of infections, depending on virus type. Rash may occur during fever or after defervescence. Hand, foot, and mouth syndrome	Most commonly erythematous, maculopapular, and discrete. May have macular, petechial, vesicular, and urticarial components. Rarely erythema multiforme	Usually starts on face and spreads downward to trunk and extremities. May have peripheral distribution (hand, foot, and mouth syndrome)	3–7
Rhinoviruses (many types)		2–4	Fall, winter, and spring	Mild fever and signs and symptoms of respiratory illness. Exanthem occurs in about 5% of cases	Erythematous, maculopapular, and discrete	Starts on face and spreads downward to trunk and extremities	1–4
Foot and mouth		3–4		Direct animal contact. Fever, sore mouth, and lymphadenopathy. Vesicles and ulcers within the mouth	Vesicular lesions	Hands and feet	3–6
Colorado tick fever		3–5	Summer	Fever, chills, eye pain, myalgia, and headache. Diphasic course. Rash in only about 10% of cases	Occasionally maculopapular but usually petechial	Maculopapular rash is generalized. Petechial rash most prominent on arms, legs, and trunk	2–7
Reovirus 2 and 3		4–7	Summer	Fever, mild pharyngitis, and cervical adenopathy	Erythematous or maculopapular. Discrete or confluent. Occasionally vesicular	Starts on face and spreads downward to trunk and extremities	3–9
Rotavirus		2–4	Fall, winter, and spring	Gastroenteritis	Petechial and morbilliform	Generalized	7–14
Chikungunya, O'nyong nyong, Ross River, Sindbis			During periods of arthropod prevalence	Fever, headache, eye pain, and marked myalgia, arthralgia, and arthritis. Geographically localized diseases.	Rubelliform and morbilliform. Frequently vesicular and petechial	Starts on face and spreads downward to trunk and extremities	4–7
Rubella (See Fig. 67–3)	Rubella (German measles)	15–21	Winter and spring	Mild symptoms with onset 1–5 days before rash. Fever usually <38.5° C (101.5° F). Headache, malaise, and suboccipital and postauricular lymphadenopathy	Erythematous, maculopapular, and discrete	Starts on face and spreads downward to trunk and extremities	3–5
West Nile				Sudden onset of fever, chills, and drowsiness. Rash may appear during or after fever. Geographically localized disease	Erythematous, macular, and maculopapular	Starts on trunk and spreads to extremities	3–6

Table continued on following page

TABLE 67–1. Clinical Characteristics of Viral Infections with Cutaneous Manifestations *Continued*

Virus	Disease or Syndrome	Incubation Period (Days)	Main Season	Clinical Characteristics	Exanthem: *Lesions*	Exanthem: *Distribution*	Usual Duration (Days)
Dengue and Kunjin		7	During periods of specific arthropod prevalence	Sudden onset of high fever, then severe headache, myalgia, arthralgia, abdominal pain, and marked diaphoresis. Fever lasts 5–6 days and ends by crisis. Rash appears within 48 hours of onset of fever. Geographically localized disease	Initially, macular, flushed appearance, then erythematous, maculopapular rash. May be scarlatiniform. Frequently becomes petechial and purpuric. Small vesicles occur in Kunjin virus infection	Initial macular rash is more prominent centrally. Maculopapular rash may start on hands and feet and spread to trunk	3–10
Influenza A and B		2–5	Fall, winter, and spring	Fever, cough, headache, muscle aches, and pains. Usually in young children. Rash an occasional occurrence	Erythematous, maculopapular, and discrete (rubelliform). Rarely erythema multiforme	Starts on face and trunk and spreads to extremities	1–3
Respiratory syncytial		2–5	Fall, winter, and spring	Fever, coryza, and respiratory distress (bronchitis, bronchiolitis, or pneumonia). Usually in children <2 years of age	Erythematous, maculopapular, and discrete (rubelliform)	Starts on face and trunk and spreads to extremities	1–3
Parainfluenza 1–3		2–5	Fall, winter, and spring	Fever, coryza, nasopharyngitis, croup, and bronchitis. Usually in young children	Erythematous, maculopapular, and discrete (rubelliform)	Starts on face and trunk and spreads to extremities	1–3
Mumps	Mumps	14–21	Fall, winter, and spring	Fever, headache, and salivary gland swelling	Erythematous, maculopapular, and discrete. Also, urticaria and vesicles. Rarely, erythema multiforme	Most prominent on trunk	2–5
Measles (See Figs. 67–1 and 67–2)	Measles	8–12	Winter and spring	Onset with fever, cough, coryza, and conjunctivitis. About 2 days after onset, appearance of enanthem (Koplik spots) and 2 days later, onset of exanthem	Erythematous, maculopapular, and confluent. Develops a brownish appearance, and fine desquamation occurs	Starts behind ears and on forehead. Spreads downward over body. Confluence most prominent on face, trunk, and proximal extremities	5–7
Lassa	Lassa fever			Sudden onset of fever, chills, headache, and sore throat. Progresses to pneumonia and renal failure Geographically localized outbreaks	Macular and sometimes petechial	Localized or general	
Hepatitis B	Papular acrodermatitis of childhood	50–180		Insidious onset with arthralgia, arthritis, and rash occurring prior to jaundice	Maculopapular, macular, and/or urticarial. In young children, papular (Gianotti-Crosti syndrome or papular acrodermatitis of childhood). Rarely erythema multiforme	Generalized	4–10
Marburg		5–7		Headache, conjunctivitis, photophobia, myalgia, vomiting, diarrhea, and fever (biphasic). Exposure to vervet monkeys	Initially erythematous macular, then discrete maculopapular, and finally, confluent maculopapular. Exfoliation occurs. Occasionally purpura	Generalized	2–14
HIV		14–60	Nonseasonal	Fever, pharyngitis, myalgia, arthralgias, adenopathy, and rash	Macular	Mainly chest and abdomen	7

From references 1, 3–7, 9, 11, 14, 17, 20, 30, 36, 38, 40, 42, 46, 48, 51, 65, 66, 68, 79, 88, 89, 91, 92, 96, 98, 99, 113, 114, 117, 119, 124, 130, 134, 136, 137, 140, 141, 144, 153, 154, 162–164, 166–168, 172–174, 180.

TABLE 67–2. Clinical Characteristics of Chlamydial, Rickettsial, and Mycoplasmal Infections with Cutaneous Manifestations

Agent	Disease or Syndrome	Incubation Period (Days)	Main Season	Clinical Characteristics	Exanthem: Lesions	Exanthem: Distribution	Usual Duration (Days)
Chlamydia psittaci	Psittacosis	7–14	Nonseasonal	Fever, chills, headache, and cough. Respiratory distress	Erythematous macules. Occasionally erythema multiforme or erythema nodosum	Mainly on trunk	2–7
Rickettsia akari	Rickettsialpox	7–14	Nonseasonal	Fever, chills, headache, backache, and malaise 4–7 days after onset of primary lesion at site of mite bite. Geographically localized disease	Initial lesion at site of mite bite is papular and then vesicular, and finally an eschar forms. Two days after onset of fever, erythematous maculopapular discrete rash occurs. Lesions progress to small vesicles and later to scabs	Most prominent on trunk and proximal extremities	7–10
Rickettsia typhi	Endemic, murine typhus	7–14	Nonseasonal	Fever and headache. Rash appears on 4th–7th day. Geographically localized disease	Initially discrete macules and then erythematous maculopapular. May become purpuric	Initially upper trunk and axilla. Progresses to entire body except face, palms, and soles	7–14
Rickettsia prowazekii	Epidemic typhus	10–14	Nonseasonal	Sudden onset of fever, chills, headache, and myalgias. Rash appears on 4th–7th day. Geographically localized disease	Initially discrete macules and then progresses to maculopapular and petechial lesions. Sometimes purpuric	Appears first on trunk and spreads to extremities. Spares palms and soles	7–14
Rickettsia quintana	Trench fever	8–18	Nonseasonal	Usually, mild fever, headache, chilliness, and tibial bone pain	Macular rash	Mainly on trunk	2–7
Rickettsia tsutsugamushi	Scrub typhus	7–21	Nonseasonal	Sudden onset of chills, fever, and headache	Local lesion at site of chigger bite is present at onset of symptoms, characterized by vesicle, ulcer, and eschar. Maculopapular rash occurs 5–8 days after onset of fever	Maculopapular rash first occurs on trunk and then becomes generalized	7–14
Rickettsia rickettsii	Rocky Mountain spotted fever	3–12	Summer	Abrupt onset of fever, chills, and headache. Rash appears 2–4 days after onset	Early maculopapular, then petechial, and sometimes purpuric	Rash starts on distal extremities. Rarely involves the trunk	7–14
Other tick-borne *Rickettsiae*			Tick seasons	Similar to mild Rocky Mountain spotted fever	Similar to Rocky Mountain spotted fever; eschar at site of tick bite	Similar to Rocky Mountain spotted fever	7–14
R. siberica	North Asian tick-borne rickettsiosis						
R. australis	Queensland tick typhus						
R. conorii	Boutonneuse fever						
Coxiella burnetii	Q fever	20–40	Nonseasonal	Acute febrile illness with chills, headache, and myalgia	Fine discrete macular rash occurring during febrile illness. Transient urticarial rash also noted	Mainly on trunk	2–7
Ehrlichia canis	Ehrlichiosis	14–28	Tick seasons	Similar to Rocky Mountain spotted fever, but rash usually not on palms and soles	Similar to endemic typhus	Similar to endemic typhus	7–14
Mycoplasma pneumoniae		21	All seasons	Gradual onset of fever, malaise, headache, and cough	Maculopapular rashes occur in 5–15% of cases. Vesicular and bullous lesions common (Stevens-Johnson syndrome); more common in males. Papular, petechial, and urticarial lesions also noted. Erythema multiforme common	Rash most prominent on trunk and proximal extremities	7–14

From references 8, 9, 13, 25, 29, 33–35, 43, 44, 58, 70, 76, 95, 100, 106, 112, 116, 120, 143, 152, 155, 179.

TABLE 67–3. Bacteria Associated with Cutaneous Manifestations

Agent	Disease or Syndrome	Clinical Characteristics	Exanthem: *Lesions*	Exanthem: *Distribution*
Gram-positive cocci				
Staphylococcus aureus exfoliative toxin–producing (mainly phage group 2) (See Figs. 67–17 and 67–18)	Bullous impetigo	Usually occurs in infants. May be epidemic	Rapid progression from vesicles to bullous lesions	Most common in diaper area
	Scalded-skin syndrome. Toxic epidermal necrolysis (Ritter disease in infants <4 months of age; Lyell syndrome in older children)	Usually occurs in infants and children 1 month–5 years of age. Mucopurulent nasal and eye discharge. Fever	Scarlatiniform eruption with exfoliation. Positive Nikolsky sign. Crusty appearance around eyes and under nose	Generalized. Most marked on trunk
	Staphylococcal scarlet fever or staphylococcal scarlatiniform eruption	Fever and staphylococcal infection in throat but no evidence of pharyngitis	Scarlet fever–like rash with desquamation. Pastia lines present	Generalized
Staphylococcus aureus (nonexfoliative toxin–producing)	Septicemic disease	Severe septicemia with osteomyelitis, arthritis, endocarditis, or pneumonia	Diffuse, erythematous, confluent, and macular rash (flush). With endocarditis, may have petechiae and splinter hemorrhages. Osler nodes. Janeway spots	Trunk and proximal extremities
Staphylococcus aureus (toxin-1 [TSST-1]–producing)	Toxic shock syndrome	Fever, intense myalgias, vomiting, and diarrhea. Mental confusion and hypotension	Erythematous, deep red (sunburn-like) rash. Desquamation occurs	Generalized
Staphylococcus aureus (nonexfoliative toxin–producing)	Folliculitis, furuncles, or carbuncles	See Bacterial Skin Infections, Chapter 69		
Streptococcus pyogenes	Scarlet fever	Fever, pharyngitis, and cervical lymphadenitis. Rash onset within 2 days of first symptoms. Incubation period 3–4 days	Diffuse erythematous and fine maculopapular (looks and feels like red sandpaper). Rash darker in skin folds (Pastia lines). Desquamation occurs	Circumoral pallor. Generalized rash, with trunk and proximal extremities being most involved
	Erysipelas	Fever, headache, and vomiting. Localized infection	Circumscribed area that is raised and erythematous. Advancing edge is irregular	Anywhere
	Impetigo	Localized superficial pyoderma. See Bacterial Skin Infections, Chapter 69	Discrete and coalescent lesions of a vesicular nature. Quickly becomes more pustular and then crusts over with a yellowish-brown appearance	Forearms, legs, and face
	Septicemia	Fever and systemic foci of infection	Petechiae	Diffuse
	Miscellaneous skin manifestations of *S. pyogenes* infections		Erythema multiforme, erythema nodosum, and erythema marginatum	
Streptococcus pneumoniae	Septicemia	Fever	Petechiae	Diffuse
Enterococcal and viridans group streptococci	Endocarditis	Endocarditis	Petechiae, splinter hemorrhages, Osler nodes, and Janeway spots	
Gram-negative cocci				
Neisseria gonorrhoeae	Gonococcemia	Fever and polyarthralgias	Papular, petechial, purpuric, pustular, and/or necrotic lesions	Most common on extremities. Extensor surfaces over joints
Neisseria meningitidis	Meningococcemia	Fever and pharyngitis. Sudden onset of rash	Characteristic rash is petechial or purpuric. Early lesions may be erythematous, maculopapular, or urticarial	Generalized
Moraxella catarrhalis	Bacteremia	Fever and pharyngitis	Maculopapular and petechial	Generalized
Gram-positive bacilli				
Bacillus anthracis	Anthrax	Fever, headache, malaise, and joint pains	Initially, macular, pruritic lesion. Later, a papule forms and then vesiculation. Vesicles last 2–6 days, and then eschar forms	Usually, single lesion initially at point of exposure. Secondary lesions in area develop later
Listeria monocytogenes	Listeriosis	Neonatal meningitis with hepatosplenomegaly	Maculopapular, discrete lesions. Pustules	Trunk and legs
Erysipelothrix insidiosa	Crab or fishnet dermatitis	Fever and local pain	Erysipeloid lesion (violet or red)	Hands
Corynebacterium diphtheriae	Cutaneous diphtheria	Secondary infection in cutaneous wounds	Impetigo or ecthyma-like rarely. Erythema multiforme	Exposed surfaces
Arcanobacterium hemolyticum	Scarlet fever–like illness	Fever and pharyngitis	Scarlet fever–like rash occasionally. Rubelliform	Generalized rash with peripheral predominance
Enteric gram-negative bacilli				
Salmonella typhi	Typhoid fever	Malaise, headache, and marked fever. Rash onset 10 days after onset of fever	Rose spots. 2–4 mm macular lesions	Discrete lesions on the abdomen

Other *Salmonella* species	Septicemic salmonellosis	Similar to mild typhoid fever	Similar to typhoid fever	Similar to typhoid fever
Shigella sonnei	Shigellosis	Diarrhea	Urticaria	Diffuse
Campylobacter species		Gastroenteritis	Skin pustules and erythema nodosum	Lower legs
Other gram-negative bacilli				
Francisella tularensis	Tularemia	Chills, fever, headache, and localized lymphadenopathy	Initial papule that later ulcerates	Site of inoculation
Haemophilus ducreyi	Chancroid	Local pain and tenderness	Pustular lesions that ulcerate	External genitalia
Haemophilus influenzae	Septicemia	Fever	Petechiae. Reddish-purple cellulitis	Diffuse. Cellulitis mainly on cheeks and extremities
Streptobacillus moniliformis	Rat-bite fever	Fever, chills, malaise, headache, and polyarthritis	Erythematous, maculopapular rash that may become petechial	Most prominent on extremities, including palms and soles
Yersinia pestis	Septicemic plague	Sudden onset of fever	Initial generalized erythema followed by petechiae and purpura	Generalized
Yersinia pseudotuberculosis		Mesenteric lymphadenitis	Erythema nodosum and scarlatiniform eruption	Lower legs and generalized
Yersinia enterocolitica	Yersiniosis	Enterocolitis	Erythema nodosum and urticaria	Lower legs and generalized
Bartonella bacilliformis	Bartonellosis, Carrion disease, or Oroya fever	Initially intermittent fever, malaise, and myalgias 30–60 days after initial fever, exanthem appears	Erythematous maculopapular. Later recurrent nodules	Face and extensor surface of extremities
Calymmatobacterium granulomatis	Granuloma inguinale	See *Calymmatobacterium granulomatis*, Chapter 135	Nodular, ulcerovegetative, hypertrophic, or cicatricial lesions	Genitals
Pseudomonas aeruginosa	Ecthyma gangrenosa	Septicemia (usually in immunocompromised patients)	Initially, vesicular and then hemorrhagic. Become ulcerated with central black necrotic eschar	Anywhere
	Pseudomonas folliculitis (health spa dermatitis)	Headache, malaise, and fatigue	Papular and pustular	Generalized
Pseudomonas mallei	Glanders, melioidosis	Fever, malaise, chills, arthralgia, and muscle pains	Nodule or ulcer at site of inoculation and then widespread papules, bullae, and pustules	Generalized
Brucella species	Brucellosis	Acute or subacute febrile illness. Exanthem in 8% of cases	Erythematous and maculopapular. Occasionally vesicles	Generalized
Legionella pneumophila	Legionnaires' disease	Severe pneumonia	Maculopapular	Anterior trunk
Bartonella henselae	Cat-scratch fever	Subacute regional lymphadenitis	Erythematous maculopapular, morbilliform, petechial, erythema nodosum, erythema multiforme, and erythema marginatum. May be pruritic	Generalized
Acid-fast bacilli				
Mycobacterium tuberculosis	Lupus vulgaris	Usually, associated with other manifestations of tuberculosis	Reddish-brown nodular or scaling lesions	Mainly on face and neck
	Papulonecrotic tuberculids	Associated with disseminated tuberculosis	Initially, vesicular. Become pustules, umbilical, and ulcerated and then form scabs and leave scars	Single or multiple lesions anywhere
Atypical mycobacteria			Granulomatous and ulcerative lesions at site of superficial injury	Usually on hands
Mycobacterium leprae	Erythema nodosum leprosum	General findings of lepromatous leprosy	Erythematous nodular lesions	Disseminated. Most prominent on face and extremities
Spirochetes				
Treponema pallidum	Chancre	Primary	Large ulcers with indurated edges	Genital
		Secondary syphilis	Erythematous maculopapules that frequently are scaly (psoriasiform)	Generalized, including palms and soles
Treponema pertenue	Yaws		Papular lesions at sites of inoculations. Lesions ulcerate, leaving a wart-like appearance	Anywhere
Borrelia burgdorferi	Lyme disease (erythema chronicum migrans)	Skin, cardiac, neurologic, and joint abnormalities	Expanding erythematous annular lesions	Thighs, buttocks, or axillae
Treponema carateum	Pinta		Initially, erythematous, papular lesions. Increase in size over 1-month period and become scaly	Exposed surfaces of body
Spirillum minus	Rat-bite fever	Fever and chills	Discrete, macular rash	Trunk and extremities, including palms and soles
Leptospira species	Leptospirosis	Fever, conjunctivitis, and anorexia. Rash rarely is noted	Erythematous maculopapular rash	Mainly on trunk
Borrelia species	Relapsing fever	Relapsing fever, headache, myalgia, and photophobia	Morbilliform and petechial. Erythema multiforme	Generalized

From references 2, 9, 12, 16, 18, 23, 24, 26–28, 31, 32, 35, 45, 50, 54, 56, 58, 60, 63, 71, 73, 75, 82–85, 87, 93, 94, 97, 101, 103, 105, 109, 115, 118, 122, 123, 125, 127, 128, 131, 132, 138, 142, 146, 156–161, 166, 169, 170, 171, 175, 177, 178, 184.

rate varies greatly among the different types; it is as high as 50 per cent in children with coxsackievirus A16 and echovirus 9 infections. Only about 15 per cent of those infected with echovirus 4 have exanthem, and rash is a rarity in echovirus 6 infections. Hope-Simpson and Higgins[81] noted exanthem in about 5 per cent of patients with rhinoviral respiratory illness.

Two per cent of patients with Colorado tick fever encephalitis have exanthem.[42] Although infection with reoviruses is common, exanthem has been noted on only nine occasions.[42, 99] A morbilliform rash has been observed in one adult with a rotavirus infection, and a 4-year-old boy was noted to have a petechial rash in association with a rotaviral illness.[51, 137]

Of the *Togaviridae* family of viruses, rubella virus is the most important as a worldwide cause of exanthematous disease. Several alphaviruses also frequently cause exanthems.[89, 114, 173, 174] Each of these viruses has a marked geographic distribution. Similarly, flaviviruses also have exanthem as part of their clinical presentation, and they too have specific geographic boundaries.[173, 174]

Exanthem generally is not considered to be a manifestation of influenza virus infection. However, Hope-Simpson and Higgins[81] noted it in approximately 8 per cent of patients with influenza B virus isolation and in 1 or 2 per cent of those infected with influenza A virus. Measles virus is the most notable of the *Paramyxoviridae* family with an associated exanthem. However, exanthem is rather frequent in young children with parainfluenza virus types 1, 2, and 3 infections and also in respiratory syncytial virus illnesses.[68, 77, 78, 164, 167] Hope-Simpson and Higgins[81] noted a 15 per cent occurrence of rash in respiratory syncytial virus infection and an approximate 15 per cent occurrence in parainfluenza virus infections. Exanthem also has been noted on rare occasions with mumps virus infection.[41]

Lassa fever virus, Marburg virus, and hepatitis B virus all have been associated with exanthem on occasion.[38, 53, 124, 141, 173] Hepatitis B virus is the main cause of papular acrodermatitis (Gianotti-Crosti syndrome) in children.[144] A macular rash has been noted in association with acute infection with HIV-1.[4, 113, 154]

Chlamydiae, rickettsiae, and mycoplasmas associated with cutaneous manifestations are listed in Table 67–2. Of the chlamydiae, only *Chlamydia psittaci* has been associated with exanthem. In contrast, all rickettsiae that infect humans, with the exception of *Coxiella burnetii,* usually display some cutaneous manifestations as part of their systemic disease.[139] About 4 to 7 per cent of adults with Q fever have exanthem.[33, 152] Of the mycoplasmas that infect humans, only *Mycoplasma pneumoniae* is associated with exanthem.[8, 43, 44, 47] In epidemics, exanthem occurs in about 15 per cent of persons with respiratory illness.

In Table 67–3, bacterial agents in which cutaneous manifestations are part of the clinical illness are presented (see Chapter 69). The clinical expressions of exanthem vary tremendously among the different etiologic agents, as do the conditions associated with a specific infection. For example, infections in young infants with phage group II staphylococci usually result in cutaneous disease, whereas the same organisms in adults rarely cause illness. Symptomatic infection with *Streptococcus pneumoniae* is associated with cutaneous manifestations only occasionally; on the other hand, similar systemic disease with *Neisseria meningitidis* virtually always is associated with the characteristic petechial exanthem. Of the other bacterial agents listed in Table 67–3, exanthem is most important in the following: *Neisseria gonorrhoeae, Salmonella typhi, Streptobacillus moniliformis, Spirillum minus, Pseudomonas aeruginosa,* and *Treponema pallidum.*

Fungal, protozoan, and metazoan agents associated with cutaneous manifestations in humans are listed in Tables 67–4, 67–5, and 67–6, respectively. These agents and their diseases, discussed more completely in other chapters, are included here for completeness of differential diagnosis.

EPIDEMIOLOGY

Tables 67–1 through 67–6 show clearly that there are many possible etiologic agents in exanthematous disease; because of this, there obviously is no unified epidemiology. Epidemiologic events related to specific agents are considered in appropriate sections throughout this text. Each agent with exanthem as a clinical manifestation has a unique epidemiologic pattern, which, if understood, separates it from many of the other agents that cause otherwise identical clinical illnesses. In the evaluation of all patients with rash, exposure, season, and incubation period are important aspects of the diagnostic process.

PATHOPHYSIOLOGY AND PATHOLOGY OF EXANTHEMS

Even though the skin can respond in only a limited number of ways, it is obvious from the extensive number of etiologic agents that multiple pathogenic mechanisms must occur. In many sections of this book, the pathology and pathophysiology of specific agents are presented in detail. An overview is presented here.

The cutaneous manifestations of systemic diseases can be separated into three broad categories. The first category involves the dissemination of infectious agents by the blood (viremia, bacteremia, and so on), resulting in secondary infection at the cutaneous site. The clinical cutaneous findings in this type of infection can be the direct result of infectious agents in the epidermis, dermis, or dermal capillary endothelium or can be the result of an immune response between the organism and antibody or cellular factors in the cutaneous location. The possible events in the skin of this type of infection are presented in Table 67–7. Chickenpox, many enteroviral infections, and meningococcemia are examples of diseases in which the infectious agents have reached the skin by the blood and are causing the cutaneous findings without the additional contribution of host immune factors. In illnesses such as measles, rubella, and gonococcemia, the timing, histologic picture, and difficulty of direct recovery on culture of the agent suggest both a direct effect and an immune-mediated response.

The second category of pathogenesis relates to the dissemination of known specific toxins of infectious agents. The infection is in a localized area of the body, but the toxin liberated by the infectious agents reaches the skin by bloodborne dissemination. Three examples of toxin-mediated exanthematous disease are streptococcal scarlet fever, staphylococcal scalded skin syndrome, and toxic shock syndrome.

The third category of pathogenesis in systemic disease with exanthem is poorly understood but appears to have an immunologic basis. Most important in this category are the clinical pictures of erythema multiforme exudativum (Stevens-Johnson syndrome) and erythema nodosum. In the former, in disease due to *M. pneumoniae* and herpes simplex virus, organisms have been isolated or identified at the skin site. In the majority of cases, however, neither antigen localization nor disseminated toxin has been identified.

Important clinical aspects of exanthematous diseases are the distribution and progression of the lesions, yet little is

TABLE 67–4. Fungi Associated with Cutaneous Manifestations

Agent	Disease or Syndrome	Clinical Characteristics	Exanthem	
			Lesions	*Distribution*
Dermatophytic fungi	Tinea capitis, tinea cruris, tinea pedis, or tinea circinata		Localized, brownish, maculopapular lesions that are scaly. Erythema nodosum	
Candida albicans	Congenital cutaneous candidiasis	Congenital infection	Discrete vesicular lesions	Generalized
	Chronic mucocutaneous candidiasis	Immunodeficiency disease	Confluent, erythematous, and exudative lesions	Generalized, including scalp
	Acquired candidiasis		Confluent, fiery red lesions	Most common in diaper area
	Systemic candidiasis	Severe opportunistic infection	Erythematous nodular lesions	Generalized
Histoplasma capsulatum	Histoplasmosis	Primary respiratory infection	Erythema nodosum, erythema multiforme, and erythematous maculopapular	
Cryptococcus neoformans	Cryptococcosis	Primary respiratory infection	Erythema nodosum and acneiform eruptions	
Coccidioides immitis	Coccidioidomycosis	Primary respiratory infection	Initially, erythematous, maculopapular rash. Later, erythema multiforme and erythema nodosum	Generalized maculopapular rash
Sporotrichum schenckii	Sporotrichosis	Cutaneous inoculation	Nodular lesions that ulcerate	Usually, hands, arms, and legs
Blastomyces dermatitidis	Blastomycosis	Primary respiratory infection	Nodular lesions that ulcerate. Erythema nodosum	

From references 9, 10, 21, 35, 58, 62, 69, 104, 108, 133, 151, 168, 176.

TABLE 67–5. Cutaneous Manifestations of Protozoan and Helminthic Infections

Agents	Disease or Syndrome	Cutaneous Manifestations
Plasmodium species	Malaria	Occasionally generalized urticaria in chronic infection
Toxoplasma gondii	Acquired toxoplasmosis	Occasionally generalized erythematous, maculopapular rash
	Congenital toxoplasmosis	Generalized petechial rash
Giardia lamblia	Giardiasis	Rarely urticaria
Entamoeba histolytica	Amebiasis	Rarely urticaria
Leishmania tropica	Oriental sore	Red nodular lesion that ulcerates. Lasts 2–3 months
Leishmania braziliensis and *mexicana*	American cutaneous leishmaniasis	Erythematous papular lesion that vesiculates and ulcerates
Trypanosoma gambiense	African trypanosomiasis	Red nodular lesion at site of bite, followed by generalized, pruritic, erythema multiforme-like rash
Trypanosoma cruzi	American trypanosomiasis or Chagas disease	Nodular lesion at site of bite. Generalized, recurrent, erythematous, maculopapular rash
Trichomonas vaginalis	Vulvovaginalis	Rarely urticaria and erythema multiforme
Ascaris lumbricoides	Roundworm infestation	Erythema nodosum
Enterobius vermicularis	Pinworm infestation	Rarely urticaria
Necator americanus	Hookworm disease	Papules and papulovesicles on exposed surfaces (feet). Generalized urticaria
Trichinella spiralis	Trichinosis	Urticaria common. Also, generalized maculopapular rash may occur. Petechiae frequently develop
Strongyloides stercoralis	Strongyloidiasis. Also, creeping eruption (cutaneous larva migrans)	Erythematous, maculopapular lesions on feet. Creeping eruption
Ancylostoma braziliense	Creeping eruption (cutaneous larva migrans)	Creeping eruption
Schistosoma haematobium, mansoni, and *japonicum*	Schistosomiasis	Pruritic papular eruption where exposed, generalized urticaria, and granulomatous lesions
Trichobilharzia ocellata, physellae, and *stagnicolae*	Swimmer's itch or collector's itch	Initial erythema and urticaria, followed by papules and vesiculation. Pruritic
Wuchereria bancrofti	Filariasis	Localized erythema, urticaria, and erythema nodosum
Onchocerca volvulus	Onchocerciasis	Chronic, papular, scaly rash
Echinococcus granulosus and *multilocularis*	Echinococcosis	Frequent urticaria

From references 9, 15, 35, 47, 58, 61, 74, 110.

TABLE 67–6. Cutaneous Manifestations of Arthropod Bites and Stings

Agents	Disease	Cutaneous Manifestations
Spiders		
Loxosceles reclusa	Recluse spider bite or brown spider bite	Erythema followed by blister and necrosis
Ticks	Tick bite	Initial pruritus at site; becomes ulcerated and granulomatous
Mites		
Sarcoptes scabiei	Scabies	Pruritic burrows in body creases and generalized. Become erythematous and then papular urticaria
Trombicula irritans	Chigger bite	Marked pruritus and then papular urticaria
Other mites: Food, grain, murine, and fowl		Marked pruritus and then papular urticaria
Lice		
Pediculus humanus	Body lice or pediculosis	Erythematous, maculopapular, pruritic lesions. Sometimes urticaria
Phthirus pubis	Crabs	Pruritus and erythema under pubic hair
Bedbugs and kissing bugs		
Cimex lectularius	Bedbug bite	Pruritic papular urticaria
Triatoma sanguisuga	Kissing bug bite	Papular urticaria. Occasionally hemorrhagic nodular lesions
Gypsy moth caterpillar		
Lymantria dispar	Gypsy moth rash	Pruritic blotchy erythema and maculopapular
Moths		
Hylesia alinda	Moth-associated dermatitis	Erythema and pruritis. Feeling of warmth in area of rash. May have vesicular lesions
Ants		
Solenopsis saevissima	Fire ant bite	Painful papular urticarial lesions that become pustular and then nodular
Fleas		
Pulex irritans (human flea) and fleas of many animals	Flea bite	Papular urticaria
Flies and mosquitoes	Fly and mosquito bite	Papular, nodular, and urticarial lesions in sensitive persons

From references 37, 39, 52, 58, 80, 121, 135, 145, 150.

TABLE 67–7. Aspects of Pathogenesis in Exanthems Associated with Blood-borne Dissemination of the Infectious Agent

Anatomic Location	Spread of Agent	Histology	Clinical Expressions	Pathophysiology
Blood	Free in plasma → Infection; Associated with leukocytes → Infection			
Dermal capillary endothelium	Infection → Damage to vessel; Free in plasma ↓ To dermis through breaks in basement membrane (secondary to trauma) ↓; Infection ↓ Contiguous spread ↓; Associated with leukocytes ↓ To dermis by diapedesis ↓	Damage to vessel; endothelial swelling; perivascular edema; cellular infiltration; hemorrhage	Macule; papule; petechia	Direct effect of agent or immune reaction with pathologic consequences
Dermis	Infection | Contiguous spread ↓	Edema: cellular infiltration; hemorrhage; microscopic visualization of organism	Papule; urticaria; purpura; vesicle	Direct effect of agent or immune reaction with pathologic consequences; histamine release
Epidermis	Infection	Cytopathic effects (inclusions, ballooning, vacuolation, necrosis, nuclear disruption); microscopic visualization of organism	Papule; vesicle; ulcer	Direct effect of agent

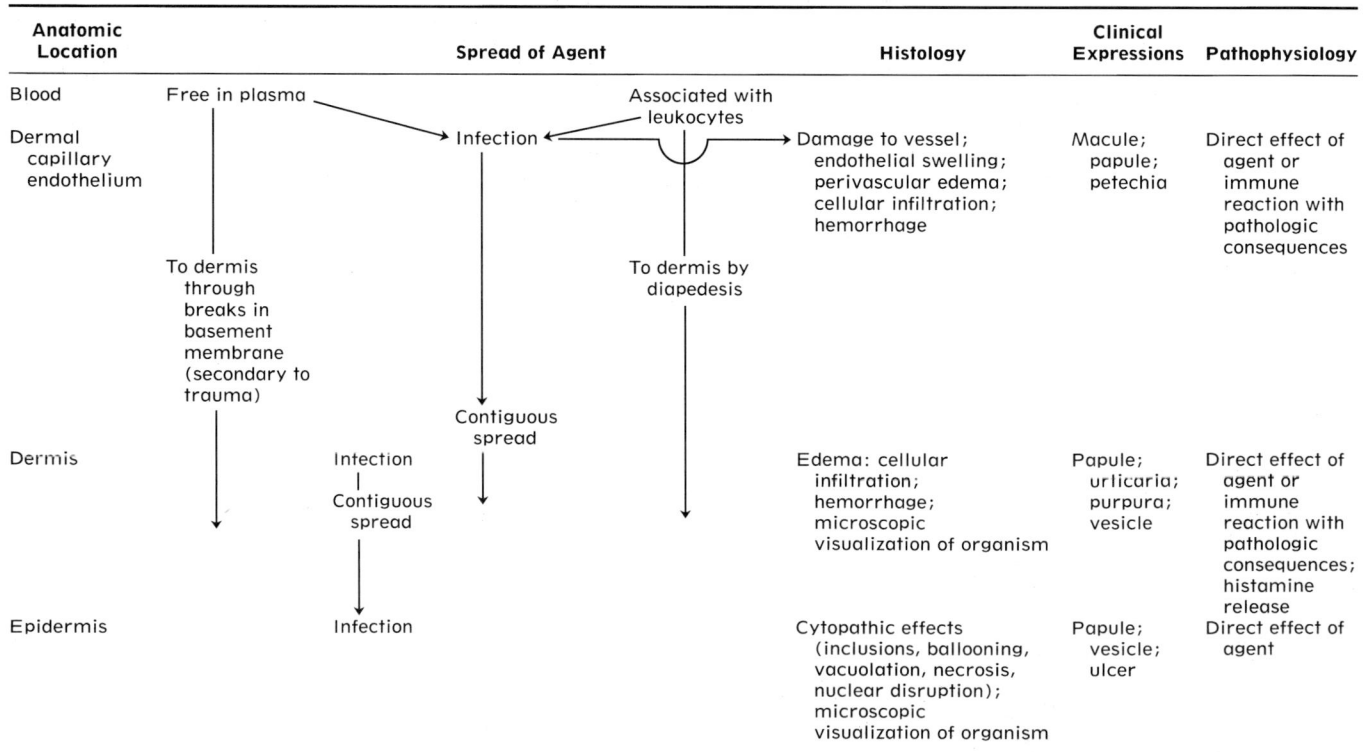

Modified from Cherry, J. D.: Newer viral exanthems. Adv. Pediatr. *16*:233–286, 1969. Used with permission.

known of the cause of these aspects. Differences in skin thickness, vascularity, proliferation rate, temperature, and metabolic activity are important in animal diseases with cutaneous manifestations.[42, 64, 102, 111, 126] In humans, similar factors must be important but obviously affect the various etiologic agents differently (e.g., the more central exanthem of chickenpox compared with that of the hand, foot, and mouth syndrome of coxsackievirus A16 infection).

CLINICAL MANIFESTATIONS

The clinical findings in exanthematous diseases resulting from systemic infections are varied and depend upon the inciting pathogens. Upon examination of the skin alone, it frequently is difficult to differentiate an exanthematous disease resulting from systemic infection (e.g., coxsackievirus A9, rubella virus infection) from primary cutaneous diseases of infectious and noninfectious origins, such as insect bites, acne, and poison ivy contact. In Tables 67–1 through 67–6, clinical characteristics of viral, chlamydial, rickettsial, bacterial, fungal, parasitic, and arthropod-induced illnesses with primary or secondary cutaneous manifestations are presented. In Tables 67–8 through 67–17, etiologic agents and clinical manifestations are presented on the basis of the more pronounced cutaneous manifestations or syndrome associations. The clinician must keep in mind that other aspects of an illness (e.g., exposure, season, incubation period, geographic location, patient age, associated signs and symptoms) may be more important in determining the underlying etiologic agent. Clinical manifestations of specific exanthematous diseases are presented in greater detail in other chapters of this book.

Erythematous Macular Exanthems

When all infectious diseases with exanthems are taken into consideration, the occurrence of illnesses in which the lesions are just macular is a rarity. However, many important, severe diseases have a transitory erythematous macular rash early in their course, and recognition of this fact can be lifesaving. Infectious agents associated with illnesses in which macular exanthems have been observed are presented in Table 67–8.

The most common rash in infectious mononucleosis is erythematous and maculopapular, but rarely (most often in association with ampicillin administration), the exanthem is generalized, confluent, fiery red, and macular. Blotchy or diffuse erythematous macular rashes have been caused specifically by 12 different enterovirus types. The majority of these descriptions are of neonates, other very young infants, and adults; children in the peak ages for enteroviral exanthematous diseases do not seem to present only with macular lesions. In neonates, enteroviral disease with a blotchy macular rash in association with fever and lethargy usually is confused with bacterial sepsis.

Patients with dengue, Lassa, and Marburg fevers frequently have a macular, flushed appearance before developing other cutaneous manifestations. Similarly, in both murine and epidemic typhus, the initial skin manifestations are macular but progress rapidly to more pronounced findings.

Bacterial septicemia with both common and exotic organisms is associated frequently with a generalized flush. In staphylococcal disease, this particularly is apparent in endocarditis and osteomyelitis. The most famous disease with a macular rash is typhoid fever. Rose spots are most common on the abdomen but also occur on the chest and back. They are erythematous, macular lesions of 2 to 4 mm. Lesions also have been noted in leptospirosis and psittacosis. Rose spots also are seen occasionally in septicemic illnesses due to other *Salmonella* species.

TABLE 67–8. Infectious Agents Associated with Illness in Which a Macular Exanthem Has Been Observed

Infectious Agent	Illness
Human herpesvirus 6	Roseola infantum
Epstein-Barr virus	Infectious mononucleosis
Coxsackieviruses B1, 2, 5	—
Echoviruses 2, 4, 5, 14, 17–19, 30	—
Enterovirus 71	—
Dengue virus	Dengue fever
Lassa virus	Lassa fever
Marburg virus	Marburg fever
Parvovirus	Erythema infectiosum
HIV-1	Manifestation of acute infection
Chlamydia psittaci	Psittacosis
Rickettsia typhi	Murine typhus
Rickettsia prowazekii	Epidemic typhus
Rickettsia quintana	Trench fever
Coxiella burnetii	Q fever
Mycoplasma pneumoniae	—
Staphylococcus aureus	Septicemia and toxic shock syndrome
Streptococcus pyogenes	Scarlatina and septicemia
Bacillus anthracis	Anthrax
Salmonella typhi	Typhoid fever
Salmonella species	Septicemic salmonellosis
Spirillum minus	Rat-bite fever
Leptospira species	Leptospirosis
Yersinia pestis	Plague

The slapped-cheek appearance in erythema infectiosum (Fig. 67–6, Color Plate II) is caused by an erythematous macular flush of the cheeks. The full-blown rash in streptococcal scarlet fever is maculopapular, but frequently in mild cases and in those altered by antibiotic therapy, the exanthem is only macular in character (scarlatina).

Erythematous Maculopapular Exanthems

(Figs. 67–2 and 67–3, Color Plate I; Fig. 67–10, Color Plate II; Fig. 67–13, Color Plate III)

The erythematous maculopapular rash is the most common cutaneous manifestation of systemic infection. It also is an exceedingly common occurrence in allergic conditions. However, all too frequently the rash of an infectious illness is ascribed to an allergy to an administered drug rather than correctly to the disease process. The converse—an allergic rash illness that is attributed mistakenly to an infectious agent—rarely is true. Infectious agents associated with illnesses in which maculopapular exanthems occur are presented in Table 67–9.

Both by number of possible etiologic agents and by total infections, viruses account for the vast majority of illnesses with maculopapular eruptions. Although the distribution and the progression of rashes are important aspects relating to differential diagnosis, the single most important point is whether the lesions are discrete (rubelliform) or confluent (morbilliform). Adenoviruses are not uncommon causes of erythematous maculopapular eruptions. In most instances, signs and symptoms of upper respiratory infection are present. Most commonly, the lesions are discrete, but, occasionally, a confluent morbilliform rash is present. A roseola infantum picture—occurrence of rash after the fever falls by crisis—is not infrequent. As a rule, the exanthem in adenoviral infections starts on the head and spreads to the trunk and extremities.

Text continued on page 730

FIGURE 67–1. *Koplik spots. Involvement of the buccal and lower labial mucosa.*

FIGURE 67–2. *Measles exanthem. Note the generalized erythematous confluent base supporting small papular and microvesicular lesions.*

FIGURE 67–3. *Rubella exanthem. Rash is erythematous, maculopapular, and discrete. (From Cherry, J. D.: Newer viral exanthems. Adv. Pediatr.* 16:233–286, *1969. Used with permission.)*

FIGURE 67–4. *Chickenpox exanthem. Typical lesions in all stages: vesicles, papulovesicles, and papules. (From Cherry, J. D.: Newer viral exanthems. Adv. Pediatr.* 16:233–286, *1969. Used with permission.)*

FIGURE 67–5. *Primary herpes simplex virus infection in an infant. Note severe stomatitis and papulovesicular and vesicular lesions under lower lip and on cheek.*

FIGURE 67–6. *Slapped-cheek appearance with relative circumoral papillor in erythema infectiosum.*

FIGURE 67–7. *Rash with lace-like, or reticular, pattern in erythema infectiosum.*

FIGURE 67–8. *Confluent exanthem in a patient with a human parvovirus infection.*

FIGURE 67–9. *Vesicular and maculopapular lesions on the foot and lower leg. Hand, foot, and mouth syndrome due to coxsackievirus A16. (From Cherry, J. D., and Jahn, C. L.: Hand, foot, and mouth syndrome: Report of six cases due to coxsackievirus, group A, type 16. Pediatrics* 37:637, *1966. Used with permission of Pediatrics.)*

FIGURE 67–10. *Erythematous maculopapular lesions on the buttocks. Hand, foot, and mouth syndrome due to coxsackievirus A16. (From Cherry, J. D., and Jahn, C. L.: Hand, foot, and mouth syndrome: Report of six cases due to coxsackievirus, group A, type 16. Pediatrics* 37:637, *1966. Used with permission of Pediatrics.)*

FIGURE 67–11. *Two large ulcerative lesions on the underside of the tongue. Hand, foot, and mouth syndrome due to coxsackievirus A16.*

FIGURE 67–12. *Papulourticarial lesions in coxsackievirus A9 infection. (From Cherry, J. D.: Newer viral exanthems. Adv. Pediatr.* 16:233–286, *1969. Used with permission.)*

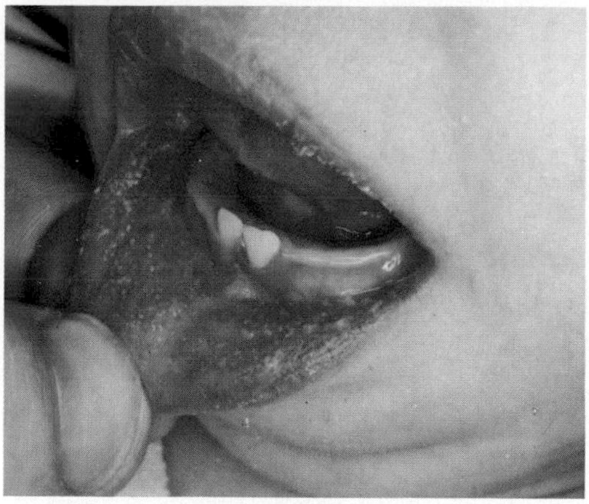

FIGURE 67–1

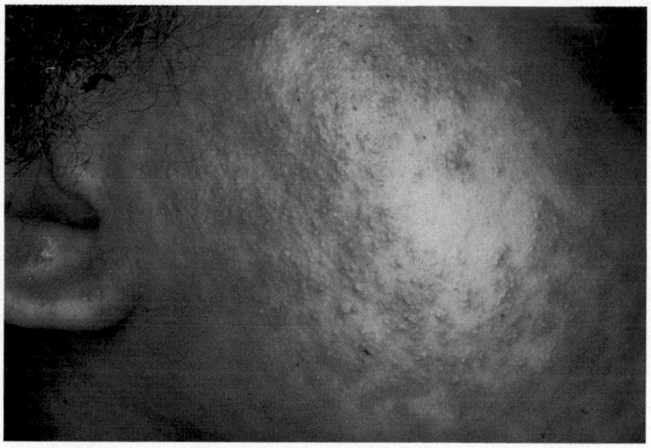

FIGURE 67–2

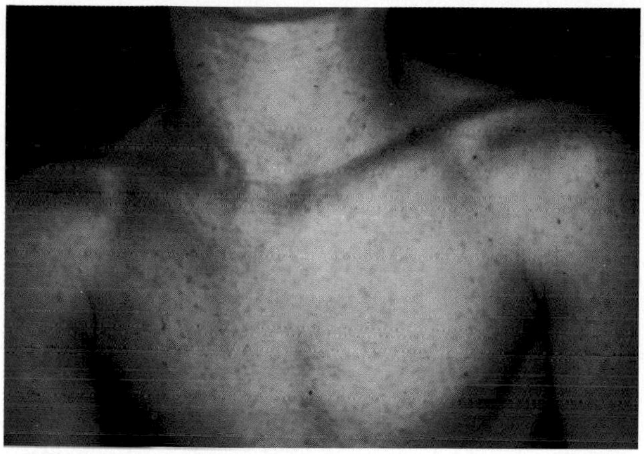

FIGURE 67–3

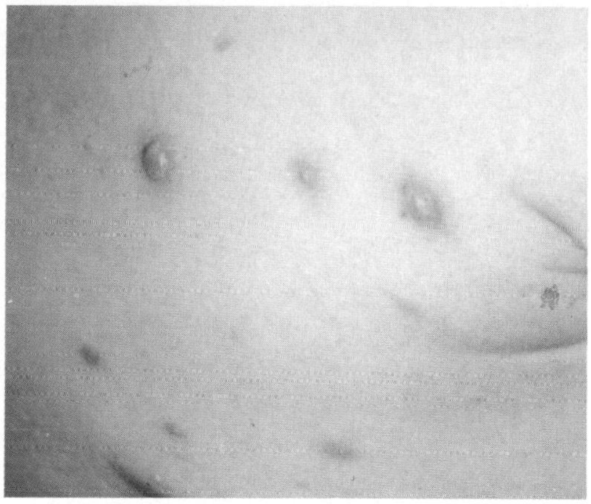

FIGURE 67–4

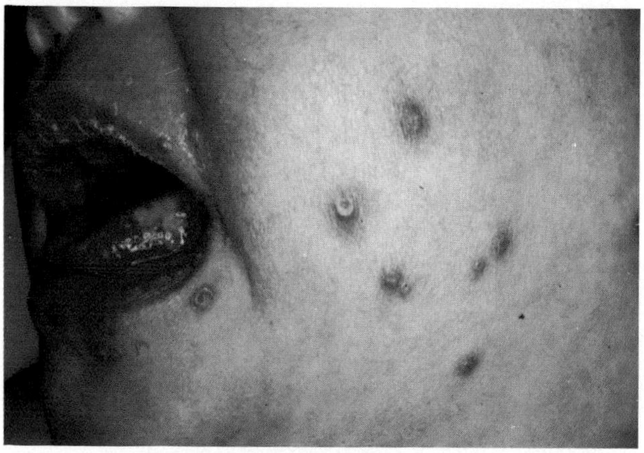

FIGURE 67–5

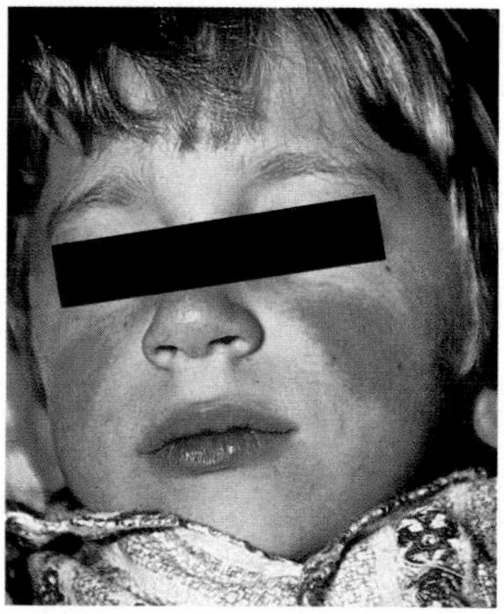

FIGURE 67–6

COLOR PLATE I. *See legends on opposite page*

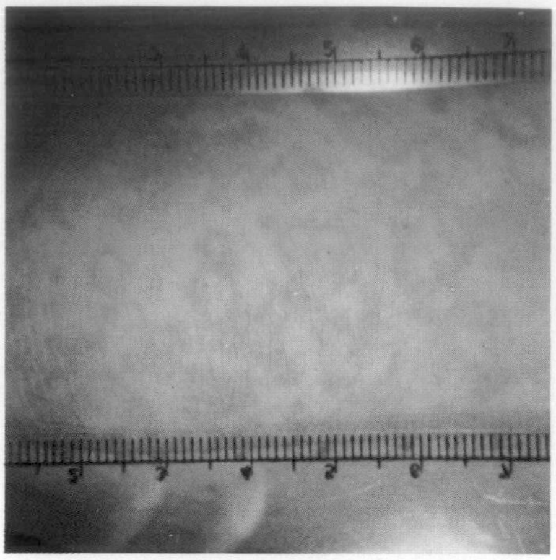

FIGURE 67–7

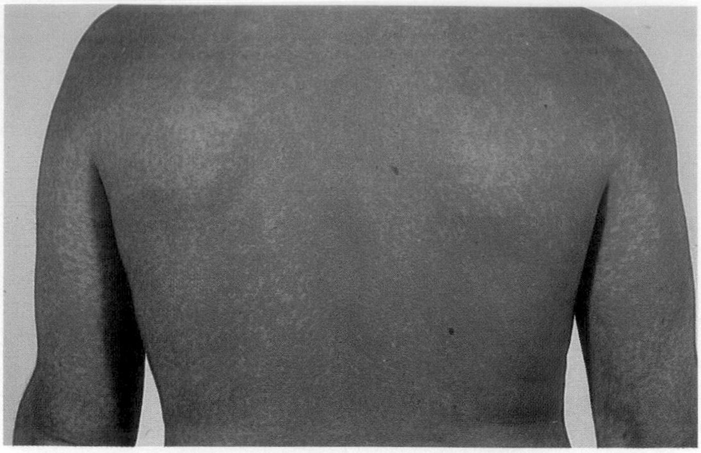

FIGURE 67–8

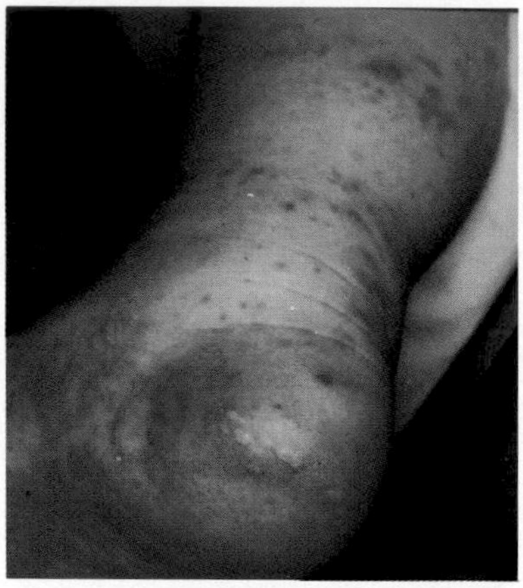

FIGURE 67–9

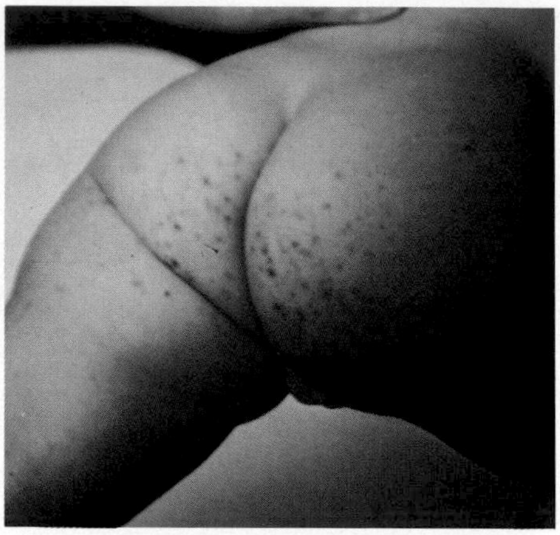

FIGURE 67–10

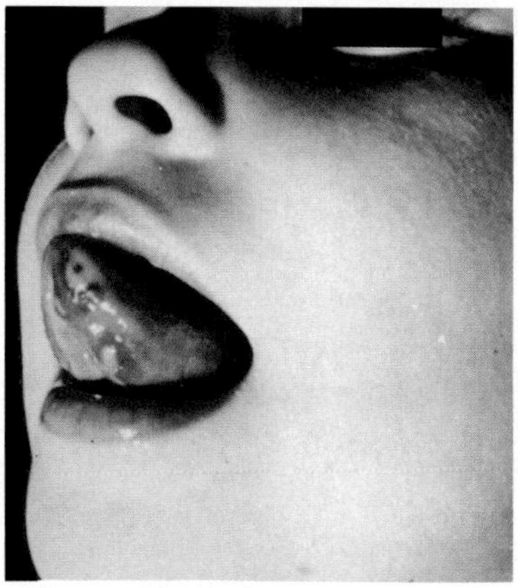

FIGURE 67–11

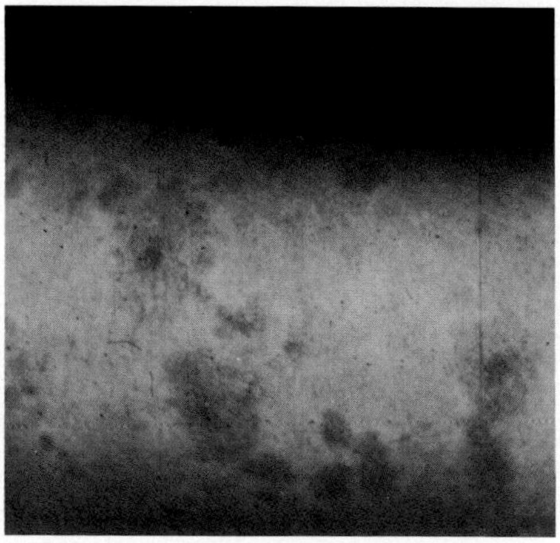

FIGURE 67–12

COLOR PLATE II. *See legends on page 724*

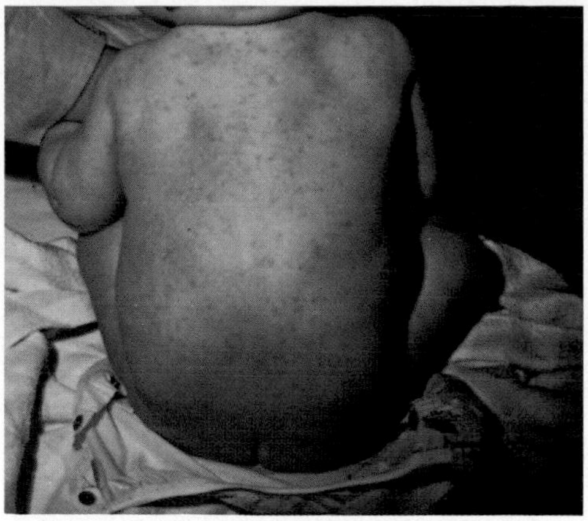

FIGURE 67–13

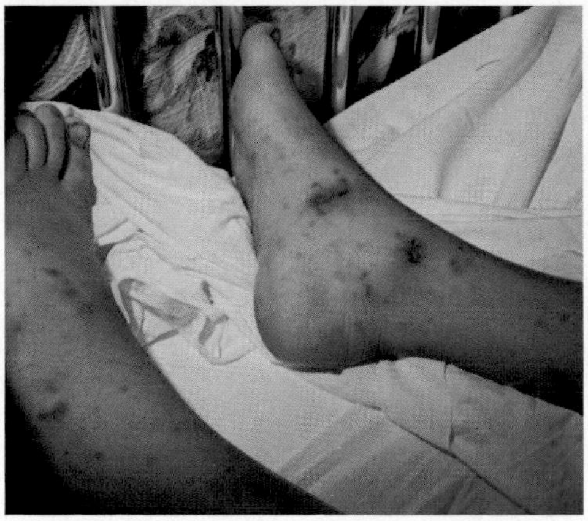

FIGURE 67–14

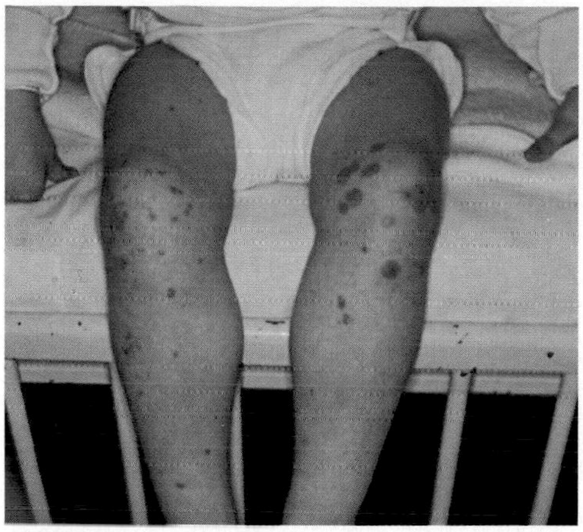

FIGURE 67–15

FIGURE 67–16

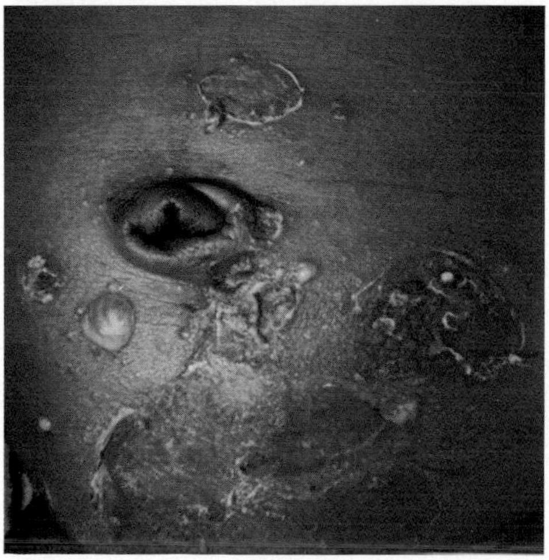

FIGURE 67–17

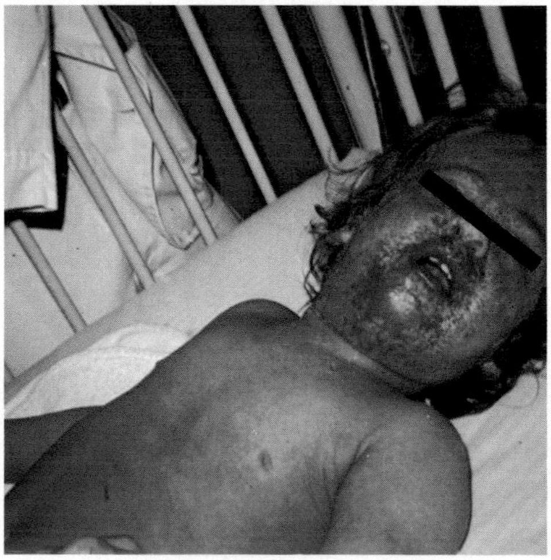

FIGURE 67–18

COLOR PLATE III. *See legends on page 729*

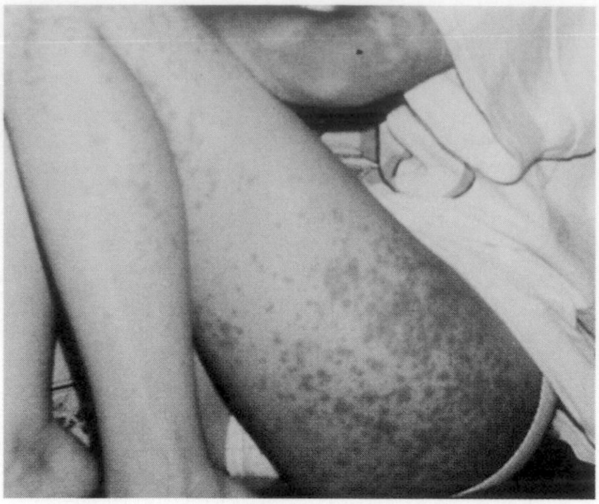

FIGURE 67–19

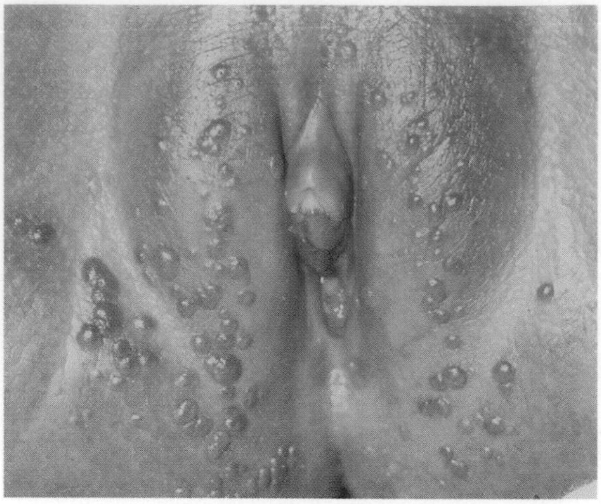

FIGURE 67–20

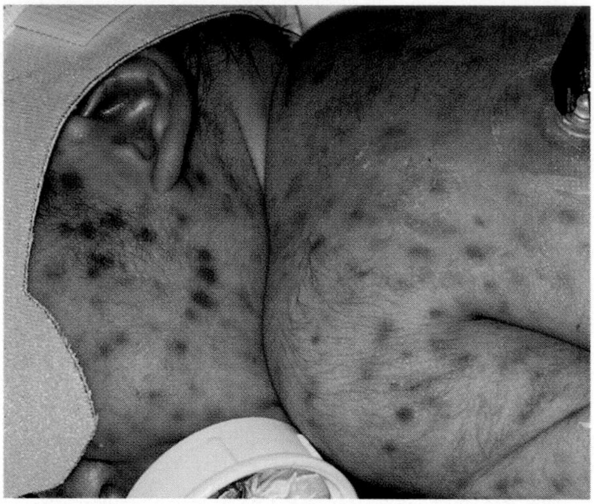

FIGURE 67–21

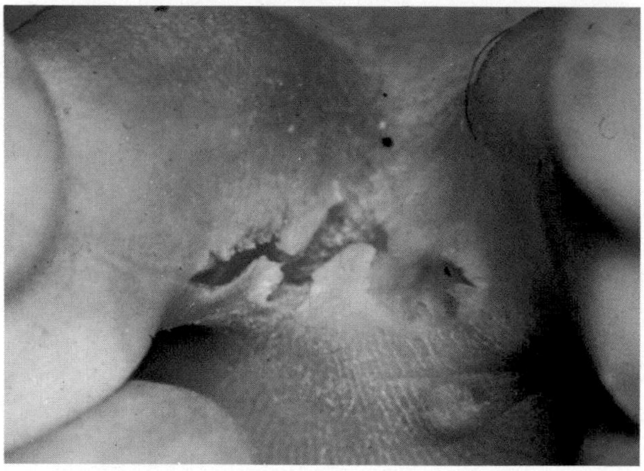

FIGURE 67–22

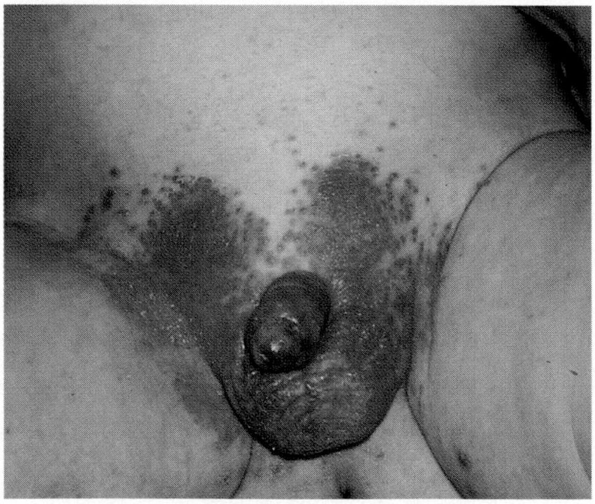

FIGURE 67–23

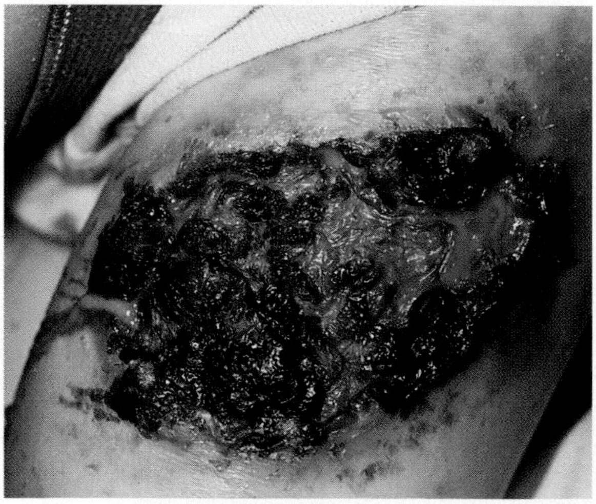

FIGURE 67–24

COLOR PLATE IV. *See legends on opposite page*

FIGURE 67–13. *Erythematous, discrete, maculopapular, and petechial rash of echovirus 9 infection. (From Cherry, J. D.: Newer viral exanthems. Adv. Pediatr. 16:233–286, 1969. Used with permission.)*

FIGURE 67–14. *Petechial and purpuric rash in a child with coxsackievirus A9 infection.*

FIGURE 67–15. *Erythematous, papular, papulovesicular, and petechial lesions suggestive of anaphylactic purpura in a child with coxsackievirus A4 infection.*

FIGURE 67–16. *Acute urticaria in a child with hand, foot, and mouth syndrome due to coxsackievirus A16 infection.*

FIGURE 67–17. *Bullous impetigo in newborn infant due to exfoliative toxin–producing* Staphylococcus aureus.

FIGURE 67–18. *Scalded skin syndrome due to exfoliative toxin producing* Staphylococcus aureus.

FIGURE 67–19. *Erythematous maculopapular discrete and confluent rash on thigh and arm in a 16-year-old girl with pharyngitis and* Arcanobacterium haemolyticum *isolated from throat. (From Mackenzie, A., Fuite, L. A., Chan, F. T. H., et al.: Clin. Infect. Dis. 21:177–181, 1995. University of Chicago, publisher.)*

FIGURE 67–20. *Numerous flat-topped and dome-shaped slightly erythematous papules over the skin of the perineum of a young girl with bowenoid papulosis.*

FIGURE 67–21. *Numerous isolated purple papules of dermal erythropoiesis overlying icteric skin of a neonate with congenital cytomegalovirus infection.*

FIGURE 67–22. *Tinea pedis, demonstrating the peeling, macerations, and fissuring in the fourth interdigital space of the foot characteristic of dermatophytic infections.*

FIGURE 67–23. *Clinical photograph of an infant with* Candida *diaper dermatitis. Confluent and discrete erythematous papules and plaque involving the scrotum, penis, and superpubic and inguinal area.*

FIGURE 67–24. *An extensive crusted erosion on the left thigh of a child with cryptococcal skin infection.*

TABLE 67–9. Infectious Agents Associated with Illnesses in Which Maculopapular Exanthems Occur

Infectious Agent	Illness	Character of Rash: Discrete	Character of Rash: Confluent
Parvovirus	Erythema infectiosum	+++	+
Adenoviruses 1, 2, 3, 4, 7, 7a		+++	+
Human herpesvirus 6	Roseola infantum	+++	+
Epstein-Barr virus	Infectious mononucleosis	+++	+
Cytomegalovirus		++++	
Vaccinia virus	Roseola vaccinatum	+++	+
Coxsackieviruses A2, 4, 5, 7, 9, 10, 16		+++	+
Coxsackieviruses B1–5		+++	+
Echoviruses 1–7, 9, 11, 13, 14, 16–19, 22, 25, 30, 33		+++	+
Enterovirus 71		++++	
Rhinoviruses (many types)		++++	
Colorado tick fever virus	Colorado tick fever	++++	
Reoviruses 2, 3		++	++
Rotavirus		++++	
Alphaviruses: Chikungunya, Sindbis, O'nyong nyong fever, Ross River		++	++
Rubella virus	Rubella (German measles)	+++	+
Flavivirus: Dengue, Kunjin	Dengue and Kunjin fever	++	++
Influenza viruses A, B		++++	
Respiratory syncytial virus		++++	
Parainfluenza viruses 1–4		++++	
Mumps virus	Mumps	++++	
Measles virus	Measles	+	+++
Hepatitis B virus		++++	
Marburg virus	Marburg fever	++	++
Rickettsia akari	Rickettsialpox	++++	
Rickettsia typhi	Murine typhus	+++	+
Rickettsia prowazekii	Epidemic typhus	+++	+
Rickettsia tsutsugamushi	Scrub typhus	+++	+
Rickettsia rickettsii	Rocky Mountain spotted fever	+	+++
Ehrlichia canis	Ehrlichiosis	+++	+
Mycoplasma pneumoniae		++	++
Staphylococcus aureus (exfoliative toxin–producing)	Staphylococcal scarlet fever		++++
Streptococcus pyogenes	Scarlet fever		++++
Corynebacterium hemolyticum		++	++
Neisseria meningitidis	Meningococcemia	++++	
Moraxella catarrhalis		++++	
Listeria monocytogenes	Listeriosis	++++	
Streptobacillus moniliformis	Rat-bite fever	+++	+
Yersinia pseudotuberculosis			++++
Bartonella bacilliformis	Bartonellosis	++++	
Brucella species	Brucellosis	++++	
Legionella pneumophila	Legionnaires disease	++++	
Bartonella henselae	Cat-scratch fever	+++	+
Treponema pallidum	Secondary syphilis	+++	+
Leptospira species	Leptospirosis	++++	
Borrelia species	Relapsing fever		++++
Coccidioides immitis	Coccidioidomycosis	+++	+
Toxoplasma gondii	Toxoplasmosis	++++	
Strongyloides stercoralis	Strongyloidiasis	++++	

Enteroviruses account for the greatest number of erythematous maculopapular rash illnesses; 36 different serologic types have been implicated. The enteroviral types most commonly associated with maculopapular exanthems are coxsackieviruses A9 and B5 and echoviruses 4, 9, and 16. Echovirus 9 has been the most common cause of enteroviral exanthem for the last 30 years (see Fig. 67–13, Color Plate III). Although morbilliform rashes do occur, the more usual cutaneous manifestation is one suggestive of rubella. The exanthem usually starts on the head and upper trunk and spreads to the extremities.

Although not common manifestations of respiratory viruses (rhinoviruses, influenza A and B viruses, respiratory syncytial virus, and parainfluenza viruses types 1 through 4), exanthems probably occur more often than generally is realized. Because children infected with these agents frequently are given antibiotics, confusion often occurs between an allergic and an infectious etiology. With all the respiratory viruses, the signs and symptoms of respiratory illness (cough, coryza, croup, bronchiolitis, and so on) are prominent. The exanthems virtually always are discrete and rubelliform in character.

In dengue, the exanthem goes through several stages. Initially, it is macular, then erythematous maculopapular, and finally hemorrhagic. Similarly, the exanthems in the rickettsial diseases go through stages that vary in relation to the specific agent (see Table 67–2). In Rocky Mountain spotted fever, the rash starts on the distal extremities. Although the hallmark of meningococcemia is a petechial or purpuric rash, in the initial stages the exanthem may be erythematous and maculopapular. Also, maculopapular eruptions are observed in chronic meningococcemia. The most notable cutaneous lesion in coccidioidomycosis is erythema nodosum, but early in infection a rubelliform rash is not unusual.

Vesicular Exanthems (Figs. 67–4 and 67–5, Color Plate I; Fig. 67–9, Color Plate II)

There are three main categories of vesicular exanthems: single or localized lesions, generalized lesions in greatest concentration on the trunk and head, and generalized lesions with the greatest concentration on the extremities. Infectious agents associated with illnesses in which vesicular rashes occur are presented in Table 67–10. The exanthem in primary or recurrent herpes simplex virus infection is localized, as it is in recurrent endogenous varicella-zoster infection (herpes zoster), ecthyma contagiosum, Tanapox, scrub typhus, anthrax, and papulonecrotic tuberculids (see Fig. 67–5, Color Plate I).

The most common vesicular exanthematous disease of children today is chickenpox (see Fig. 67–4, Color Plate I). It should be a readily recognizable disease, but all too frequently it is confused with enteroviral infections or insect bites and allergic conditions. Chickenpox has a long incubation period (16 days) and is associated with mild fever and an exanthem that starts on the head and upper trunk and spreads to the extremities. The rash always is more prominent on the trunk than on the extremities. At any time during the first few days of the rash, lesions in all stages (macules, papules, and vesicles) can be seen. Individual lesions in chickenpox form scabs that persist for about 7 days.

TABLE 67–10. Infectious Agents Associated with Illnesses in Which Vesicular Exanthems Occur

Infectious Agent	Illness
Herpes simplex virus types 1 and 2	Cold sores, genital herpes, or neonatal herpes
Varicella-zoster virus	Chickenpox (varicella) or herpes zoster
Vaccinia virus	Disseminated vaccinia or eczema vaccinatum
Variola virus	Smallpox
Monkeypox virus	
Orf virus	Ecthyma contagiosum
Tanapox virus	
Coxsackieviruses A4, 5, 8, 10, 16	
Coxsackieviruses B1–3	
Echoviruses 6, 9, 11, 17	
Enterovirus 71	
Reovirus 2	
Alphaviruses: Chikungunya, O'nyong nyong fever, Ross River, Sindbis	
Kunjin virus	
Mumps virus	Mumps
Measles virus	Atypical measles
Rickettsia akari	Rickettsialpox
Rickettsia tsutsugamushi	
Mycoplasma pneumoniae	
Streptococcus pyogenes	Impetigo
Pseudomonas aeruginosa	
Brucella species	Brucellosis
Bacillus anthracis	Anthrax
Mycobacterium tuberculosis	Papulonecrotic tuberculids
Candida albicans	Congenital cutaneous candidiasis
Leishmania braziliensis	American cutaneous leishmaniasis
Necator americanus	Hookworm disease

TABLE 67–11. Infectious Agents Associated with Illnesses in Which Petechial and/or Purpuric Exanthems Occur

Infectious Agent	Illness
Varicella-zoster virus	Hemorrhagic chickenpox
Cytomegalovirus	Congenital cytomegalovirus infection
Variola virus	Hemorrhagic smallpox
Coxsackieviruses A4, 9	
Coxsackieviruses B2–4	
Echoviruses 4, 7, 9	
Colorado tick fever virus	Colorado tick fever
Rotavirus	
Alphaviruses: Chikungunya, O'nyong nyong fever, Ross River, Sindbis	
Rubella virus	Rubella (German measles) or congenital rubella
Respiratory syncytial virus	
Measles virus	Hemorrhagic (black measles) or atypical measles
Lassa virus	Lassa fever
Marburg virus	
Rickettsia typhi	Murine typhus
Rickettsia prowazekii	Epidemic typhus
Rickettsia rickettsii and other tick-borne rickettsiae	Rocky Mountain spotted fever
Ehrlichia canis	Ehrlichiosis
Mycoplasma pneumoniae	
Streptococcus pyogenes	Scarlet fever or septicemia
Streptococcus pneumoniae	Pneumococcal septicemia
Enterococcal and viridans group streptococci	Endocarditis
Neisseria gonorrhoeae	Gonococcemia
Neisseria meningitidis	Meningococcemia
Moraxella catarrhalis	
Haemophilus influenzae	*H. influenzae* septicemia
Pseudomonas aeruginosa	Ecthyma gangrenosa
Streptobacillus moniliformis	
Yersinia pestis	Septicemic plague (Black Death)
Bartonella henselae	Cat-scratch fever
Treponema pallidum	Congenital syphilis
Borrelia species	Relapsing fever
Toxoplasma gondii	Congenital toxoplasmosis
Trichinella spiralis	Trichinosis

In contrast to that of chickenpox, the exanthem in enteroviral infections frequently is peripheral in distribution, and the lesions generally heal without scabs. The incubation period (5 days) is much shorter than that of chickenpox. The hand, foot, and mouth syndrome is a common presentation of enteroviral vesicular rash illnesses (see Figs. 67–9, 67–10, and 67–11, Color Plate II). The most common etiologic agent in the hand, foot, and mouth syndrome is coxsackievirus A16, but the syndrome also has been attributed to coxsackieviruses A5, A9, A10, B1, and B3 and enterovirus 71.

Enteroviral infections with vesicular exanthems in which the hand, foot, and mouth distribution is not present quite frequently are diagnosed erroneously as insect bites or poison ivy.

Petechial and/or Purpuric Exanthems (Figs. 67–14 and 67–15, Color Plate III)

A large number of infectious agents are associated with petechial and purpuric skin manifestations. These are listed in Table 67–11. Infectious diseases with hemorrhagic rashes can be fulminant fatal events or relatively benign illnesses. On a worldwide basis, meningococcemia perhaps is the most important and feared, although not the most prevalent of the petechial and/or purpuric exanthematous diseases. The relatively sudden onset of fever and a petechial rash must be considered and treated as meningococcemia unless another etiology can be established with absolute certainty. The most important of differential diagnostic problems is exanthem due to enteroviral infection. Many different enterovirus illnesses have sudden onsets with fever and petechial rashes. In addition, the situation frequently is complicated further by the occurrence of meningitis. The most important enterovirus in its ability to mimic meningococcemia is echovirus 9.

Purpuric and petechial lesions in infectious illnesses can result from a direct or indirect (immunologic) effect of the infectious agent at the cutaneous site or from the occurrence of thrombocytopenia. Thrombocytopenia is most common in acquired rubella virus infections.

Urticarial Exanthems (Fig. 67–12, Color Plate II; Fig. 67–16, Color Plate III)

The occurrence of urticaria all too frequently leads the physician to suspect an allergic or dermatologic condition.[164, 165] However, it has become quite evident in recent years that when urticaria occurs in association with an acute febrile illness, the cutaneous reaction is a direct effect of an infectious agent, and its mediation does not require an allergic response. Listed in Table 67–12 are infectious agents associated with urticarial exanthems.

Papular urticaria is very common in children in the summer and fall and most commonly is the result of insect bites (see Table 67–6). However, virtually identical lesions occur in infections with coxsackieviruses A as well as other enteroviruses (see Fig. 67–12, Color Plate II). The main point for differentiation is the fact that fever regularly occurs in the virus-induced exanthems but is not a characteristic associated with insect bites.

Early in meningococcemia the exanthem can be urticarial, so illness of sudden onset with fever and this cutaneous manifestation should never be taken lightly.

TABLE 67–12. Infectious Agents Associated with Illnesses in Which Urticarial Exanthems Occur

Infectious Agent	Illness
Epstein-Barr virus	Infectious mononucleosis
Coxsackieviruses A9, 16, B4, 5	
Echovirus 11	
Mumps virus	Mumps
Hepatitis B virus	
Mycoplasma pneumoniae	
Neisseria meningitidis	Meningococcemia
Shigella sonnei	Shigellosis
Yersinia enterocolitica	Yersiniosis
Plasmodium species	Malaria
Coxiella burnetii	Q fever
Giardia lamblia	Giardiasis
Entamoeba histolytica	Amebiasis
Trichomonas vaginalis	Vulvovaginalis
Enterobius vermicularis	Pinworm infestation
Necator americanus	Hookworm disease
Trichinella spiralis	Trichinosis
Schistosoma species	Schistosomiasis
Trichobilharzia species	Swimmer's itch or collector's itch
Wuchereria bancrofti	Filariasis
Echinococcus species	Echinococcosis
Sarcoptes scabiei	Scabies
Trombicula irritans	Chigger bites
Other mites	Mite bites
Pediculus humanus	Pediculosis
Bedbugs, kissing bugs, ants, fleas, flies, and mosquitoes	Bites and stings

TABLE 67–13. Infectious Agents Associated with Papular, Nodular, and Ulcerative Lesions

Agent	Illness*
Wart virus	Warts (P and N)
Orf virus	Ecthyma contagiosum (N)
Molluscum contagiosum virus	Molluscum contagiosum (P and N)
Hepatitis B virus	Gianotti-Crosti syndrome (P)
Paravaccinia virus	Milker's nodules (N)
Francisella tularensis	Tularemia (U)
Haemophilus ducreyi	Chancroid (U)
Bartonella bacilliformis	Bartonellosis (N)
Calymmatobacterium granulomatis	Granuloma inguinale (N and U)
Pseudomonas aeruginosa	Ecthyma gangrenosa (U)
Pseudomonas aeruginosa	*Pseudomonas* folliculitis (P)
Pseudomonas mallei	Glanders (N and U)
Mycobacterium tuberculosis	Lupus vulgaris (N) Papulonecrotic tuberculids (U)
Atypical mycobacteria	(U)
Mycobacterium leprae	(N)
Treponema pallidum	Chancre (U)
Treponema pertenue	Yaws (P and U)
Sporotrichum schenckii	Sporotrichosis (U)
Blastomyces dermatitidis	Blastomycosis (N and U)
Candida albicans	Systemic candidiasis (N)
Leishmania tropica	Oriental sore (N and U)
Leishmania braziliensis and *mexicana*	American cutaneous leishmaniasis (P and U)
Trypanosoma species	Trypanosomiasis (N)
Necator americanus	Hookworm disease (P)
Schistosoma species	Schistosomiasis (P)
Trichobilharzia species	Swimmer's itch or collector's itch (P)
Onchocerca volvulus	Onchocerciasis (P)
Loxosceles reclusa	Recluse spider bites (U)
Ticks	Tick bites (U)
Sarcoptes scabiei	Scabies (P)
Trombicula irritans	Chigger bites (P)
Other mites	Mite bites (P)
Cimex lectularius	Bedbug bites (P)
Triatoma sanguisuga	Kissing bug bites (P and N)
Solenopsis saevissima	Fire ant bites (P and N)
Fleas	Flea bites (P)
Flies and mosquitoes	Fly and mosquito bites (P)

*P, papular; N, nodular; U, ulcerative.

Papular, Nodular, and Ulcerative Lesions

In many instances, the lesions in this category occur as single events at the site of primary inoculation. Specific illnesses and etiologic agents are listed in Table 67–13.

Distinctive Clinical Features or Syndromes

Erythema Multiforme

Erythema multiforme is a self-limited skin eruption that is erythematous and characterized by distinctive target or iris lesions, or both. Small vesicles and urticarial areas also may develop. Occasionally, the disease is severe and associated with mucosal involvement and genital lesions. In this latter illness—the Stevens-Johnson syndrome, bullous erythema multiforme, erythema multiforme exudativum major—severe ulcerative, oral, and genital lesions occur; generalized exanthems become bullous; and conjunctivitis is present. The illness is associated with fever and general distress.

Although the pathogenesis of erythema multiforme is unknown, it is clear that multiple factors, including infectious agents, cause its occurrence. Infectious agents associated with erythema multiforme are listed in Table 67–14. The single most important infectious cause of erythema multiforme and Stevens-Johnson syndrome is *M. pneumoniae*. When *M. pneumoniae* is the instigating agent, there nearly always is a concomitant pneumonia.

Herpes simplex virus frequently has been recovered from the throats of persons with erythema multiforme, but the cause-and-effect relationship in many cases must be questioned. However, in a recent study, herpes simplex virus DNA was found in skin lesions of 11 of 31 patients with erythema multiforme.[49]

Erythema Nodosum

Erythema nodosum most commonly occurs on the anterior aspect of the lower legs but may occur anywhere on the body. The lesions are raised, erythematous, and painful to touch. Their usual size is about 2 to 4 cm, and their duration is from 2 to 6 weeks.

Erythema nodosum is less common today than three decades ago, and the frequency of specific associated infectious agents also is different. In the past, streptococcal and mycobacterial infections were the most common related agents. Now, the exanthem most often is associated with respiratory infection with *Histoplasma capsulatum*, *Cryptococcus neoformans*, and *Coccidioides immitis*. Infectious agents associated with erythema nodosum are listed in Table 67–15.

Hand, Foot, and Mouth Syndrome

The hand, foot, and mouth syndrome is a clearly recognizable viral illness characterized by vesicular lesions in the anterior mouth and on the hands and feet in association with fever. Although several enteroviruses (coxsackieviruses A5, A9, A10, A16, B1, and B3 and enterovirus 71) have been implicated, as well as herpes simplex and foot and mouth disease viruses, most of these cases are caused by coxsackievirus A16.

TABLE 67–14. Infectious Agents Associated with Erythema Multiforme

Agent	Illness
Adenovirus 7	Respiratory infection
Herpes simplex virus type 1	Perioral or respiratory infection
Epstein-Barr virus	Infectious mononucleosis
Varicella virus	Chickenpox
Coxsackieviruses A10, 16, B5	Enterovirus syndrome
Echovirus 6	Enterovirus syndrome
Poliomyelitis virus	Poliomyelitis
Vaccinia virus	Smallpox vaccination
Variola virus	Smallpox
Orf virus	Ecthyma contagiosum
Paravaccinia virus	Milker's nodules
Influenza A virus	Influenza
Mumps	Mumps
Hepatitis B virus	Serum hepatitis
Chlamydia psittaci	Psittacosis
Chlamydia trachomatis	Lymphogranuloma venereum
Mycoplasma pneumoniae	Respiratory symptoms
Staphylococcus aureus	Septicemia
Streptococcus pyogenes	Respiratory symptoms
Neisseria gonorrhoeae	Gonorrhea
Corynebacterium diphtheriae	Diphtheria
Pseudomonas aeruginosa	Septicemia
Salmonella species	Gastroenteritis
Francisella tularensis	Tularemia
Yersinia species	Gastrointestinal symptoms
Vibrio parhaemolyticus	Gastroenteritis
Treponema pallidum	Syphilis
Bartonella henselae	Cat-scratch fever
Mycobacterium tuberculosis	Tuberculosis
Mycobacterium leprae	Leprosy
Coccidioides immitis	Coccidioidomycosis
Histoplasma capsulatum	Histoplasmosis
Trichomonas vaginalis	Vulvovaginalis

TABLE 67–15. Infectious Agents Associated with Erythema Nodosum

Agent	Illness
Herpes simplex virus	Perioral or respiratory infection
Chlamydia psittaci	Psittacosis
Chlamydia trachomatis	Lymphogranuloma venereum
Streptococcus pyogenes	Respiratory infection
Neisseria meningitidis	Meningococcemia
Corynebacterium diphtheriae	Diphtheria
Campylobacter species	Gastroenteritis
Haemophilus ducreyi	Chancroid
Yersinia species	Gastrointestinal symptoms
Treponema pallidum	Syphilis
Bartonella henselae	Cat-scratch fever
Mycobacterium leprae	Leprosy
Trichophyton species	Kerion of scalp
Histoplasma capsulatum	Histoplasmosis
Cryptococcus neoformans	Cryptococcosis
Coccidioides immitis	Coccidioidomycosis
Blastomyces dermatitidis	Blastomycosis
Ascaris lumbricoides	Roundworm infestation
Wuchereria bancrofti	Filariasis

Roseola-Like Illness

Roseola infantum is a classic pediatric illness characterized by a fever of 3 to 5 days in duration, rapid defervescence, and then the appearance of an erythematous macular or maculopapular rash that persists for 1 to 2 days. Roseola is an age-related response to infection with many viruses. Recent studies suggest that a leading cause of roseola infantum is primary infection with human herpesvirus 6. The following other viruses have been noted in association with roseola: adenoviruses 1, 2, 3, and 14; coxsackieviruses A6, A9, B1, B2, B4, and B5; echoviruses 9, 11, 16, 25, 27, and 30; parainfluenza virus type 1; and measles vaccine virus.

Rocky Mountain Spotted Fever–Like Illness

Rocky Mountain spotted fever is a clinical illness characterized by fever and a petechial rash located mainly on the distal extremities. The illness is caused by *Rickettsia rickettsii* and is prevalent in many areas of North America; the infectious agent is transmitted to humans by ticks. In other areas of the world, other tick-borne *Rickettsiae* (*R. siberica, R. australis, R. conorii*) produce similar human illness. Infection with *Ehrlichia canis* also can cause an illness similar to Rocky Mountain spotted fever.

The most important illness confused with Rocky Mountain spotted fever is atypical measles (see Chapter 183). This illness, which has both the constitutional symptoms of Rocky Mountain spotted fever and a rash most prominent on the extremities, occurs almost exclusively upon exposure to measles virus in some persons previously immunized with inactivated (killed) measles vaccine.

Rat-bite fever due to *S. moniliformis* also has been misdiagnosed as Rocky Mountain spotted fever.[128]

TABLE 67–16. Infectious Agents Associated with Exanthem and Meningitis

Agent	Illness
Herpes simplex virus type 2	Recurrent genital herpes
Coxsackieviruses A2, 9, B1, 4, 5	Enterovirus syndrome
Echoviruses 4, 6, 9, 11, 14, 17, 25, 33	Enterovirus syndrome
Colorado tick fever virus	Colorado tick fever
Reovirus 2	Respiratory infection
Neisseria meningitidis	Meningococcemia
Listeria monocytogenes	Listeriosis
Toxoplasma gondii	Toxoplasmosis

Exanthem and Meningitis

Aseptic and also bacterial meningitis frequently present both exanthem and symptoms and signs of neurologic involvement. Infectious agents associated with exanthem and meningitis are presented in Table 67–16. Of most importance in this category is the differential diagnosis of enteroviral syndromes and meningococcemia.

Exanthem and Pulmonary Involvement

Infectious agents associated with exanthem and pulmonary involvement are listed in Table 67–17. In patients older than 5 years of age, the leading cause of exanthem and pneumonia is *M. pneumoniae* infection. In younger children, adenoviruses are the most important etiologic agents. With the exception of the enteroviral infections, which are more likely to involve young children, most of the illnesses listed in Table 67–17 occur in older children and young adults.

Gianotti-Crosti Syndrome (Papular Acrodermatitis)

This is a distinct clinical entity characterized by a papular (lichenoid) exanthem, generalized lymphadenopathy, hepatomegaly, and acute anicteric hepatitis.[38, 140, 143] In most instances, this illness was found to be associated with hepatitis B virus infection. The syndrome also has been noted in association with Epstein-Barr virus, cytomegalovirus, coxsackievirus B, and respiratory syncytial virus infections.[55, 92, 141, 158]

TABLE 67–17. Infectious Agents Associated with Exanthem and Pulmonary Involvement

Agent	Illness
Adenoviruses 7, 7a	Respiratory infection
Herpes simplex virus type 1	Respiratory infection
Varicella-zoster virus	Chickenpox pneumonia
Epstein-Barr virus	Infectious mononucleosis
Coxsackievirus A9	Enterovirus syndrome
Echovirus 11	Enterovirus syndrome
Reovirus 3	Respiratory infection
Measles virus	Measles pneumonia and atypical measles
Chlamydia psittaci	Psittacosis
Mycoplasma pneumoniae	*M. pneumoniae* pneumonia
Neisseria meningitidis	Meningococcal pneumonia
Mycobacterium tuberculosis	Tuberculosis
Histoplasma capsulatum	Histoplasmosis
Cryptococcus neoformans	Cryptococcosis
Coccidioides immitis	Coccidioidomycosis

DIAGNOSIS

Differential Diagnosis

The diagnosis of infectious exanthems frequently is considered an impossible task by many physicians. Other physicians glibly call the first maculopapular exanthem of childhood roseola and the first vesicular rash chickenpox without consideration of more appropriate choices. The hallmark of diagnosis in exanthematous disease is the careful elicitation of historic data. Differential diagnosis requires the consideration of noninfectious etiologies as well as different infectious agents. Listed in Table 67–18 are the major considerations in the diagnosis of diseases with cutaneous manifestations.

A history of exposure is most important in differential diagnosis. For example, was the patient exposed to poison ivy, insects, or a person ill with a specific disease? In infectious illnesses with high clinical expression rates (measles, chickenpox, rubella), it is quite unusual when proper questioning is employed not to find the contact case or at least other cases in the community. On the other hand, in illnesses with low rates of clinical expression of exanthem, such as adenoviral and some enteroviral infections, the source may not be apparent.

The consideration of the seasonal occurrence of different infectious agents as well as insects particularly is useful in the differential diagnosis. In temperate climates, enteroviral and arthropod-mediated diseases occur in the summer and fall. Exanthems with measles, varicella-zoster, and rubella viruses occur most often in the winter and spring. The diagnosis of rubella is important because of the fetal consequences. All too frequently rubella is over- and underdiagnosed; this can be avoided if its seasonal prevalence is understood.

The incubation period is important in separating exanthem due to rubella, varicella-zoster, or measles viruses from rash illnesses due to enteroviruses or common respiratory viruses. The former have long incubation periods, whereas in the others, the period from exposure to the onset of illness is less than 1 week. Age can be useful. Today in the United States, measles and rubella often are illnesses of adolescents and young adults. Enterovirus exanthem frequency is related inversely to age.

The questioning to obtain pertinent history of previous exanthems can give useful information if it is done with care. For example, if patients are asked whether they had rubella, the answer is quite unreliable. However, if the past illness is documented by year, season, and symptomatology, accurate information often is obtained. The relationship of rash to fever is most important in the diagnosis of roseola. The presence or absence of fever is important in separating exanthems of infectious and noninfectious etiologies. Frequently, insect bites are diagnosed as chickenpox by parents and physicians as well. Chickenpox rarely occurs without fever.

TABLE 67–18. Important Aspects in the Diagnosis of Exanthematous Illness

Exposure	Type of rash
Season	Distribution of rash
Incubation period	Progression of rash
Age	Exanthem
Previous exanthems	Other associated symptoms
Relation of rash to fever	Laboratory tests
Adenopathy	

From Cherry, J. D.: Newer viral exanthems. Adv. Pediatr. *16*:233–286, 1969. Used with permission.

The type and distribution of exanthem obviously are important. They virtually are diagnostic in hand, foot, and mouth syndrome, Rocky Mountain spotted fever, and atypical measles. Enanthem can lead to a specific diagnosis (Koplik spots in measles) or a category diagnosis (herpangina in enteroviral infections). Other characteristics, such as those listed in Tables 67–8 through 67–17, obviously are useful in delineating a specific illness.

Specific Diagnosis

As in other infectious diseases, specific diagnosis depends upon the acquisition of proper cultures, serologic tests, and microscopic study of secretions or histologic or cytologic preparations. These techniques are discussed in other chapters of this book.

Vesicular lesions always should be scraped for cytologic study or direct antigen identification (varicella, herpes simplex), and, frequently, petechial lesions should be scraped and stained in search of infectious agents (meningococci). The etiology of viral infections can be established by virus isolation, direct antigen detection, or serologic methods. In most instances, a virus recovered from the throat indicates acute infection and is the likely cause of a particular illness. Serologic study without culture is useful in rickettsial diseases, some viral infections, and a few illnesses of bacterial origin. Serologic study without virus isolation generally is not useful in enteroviral illnesses.

TREATMENT, PROGNOSIS, AND PREVENTION

Treatment, prognosis, and prevention of exanthematous diseases are presented in appropriate chapters throughout this text.

References

1. Africk, J. A., and Halprin, K. M.: Infectious mononucleosis presenting as urticaria. J. A. M. A. *209*:1524–1525, 1969.
2. Ahvonen, P.: Human yersiniosis in Finland. II. Clinical features. Ann. Clin. Res. *4*:39–48, 1972.
3. Anderson, M. J., Lewis, E., Kidd, I. M., et al.: An outbreak of erythema infectiosum associated with human parvovirus infection. J. Hyg. (Lond.) *93*:85–93, 1984.
4. Anonymous: Needlestick transmission of HTLV-III from a patient infected in Africa. Lancet *2*:1376–1377, 1984.
5. Arkwright, J. A.: Foot-and-mouth disease in man. Lancet *1*:1191–1192, 1928.
6. Asano, Y., Yoshikawa, T., Suga, S., et al.: Viremia and neutralizing antibody response in infants with exanthem subitum. J. Pediatr. *114*:535–539, 1989.
7. Athreya, B. H., and Coriell, L. L.: Erythema multiforme exudativum major: A review and report of four cases. Clin. Pediatr. *3*:68–74, 1964.
8. Azimi, P. H., Chase, P. A., and Petru, A. M.: Mycoplasmas: Their role in pediatric disease. Curr. Probl. Pediatr. *14*:7–46, 1984.
9. Baer, R. L.: Erythema multiforme—1976. Am. J. Med. Sci. *271*:119–120, 1976.
10. Baley, J. E., Kliegman, R. M., and Fanaroff, A. A.: Disseminated fungal infections in very low-birth weight infants: Clinical manifestations and epidemiology. Pediatrics *83*:144–152, 1984.
11. Balfour, H. H., Jr., Forte, F. A., Simpson, R. B., et al.: Penicillin-related exanthems in infectious mononucleosis identical to those associated with ampicillin. Clin. Pediatr. *11*:417–421, 1972.
12. Baron, J., and Shapiro, E. D.: Unsuspected bacteremia caused by *Branhamella catarrhalis*. Pediatr. Infect. Dis. *4*:100–101, 1985.
13. Barrett, P. K. M., and Greenberg, M. J.: Outbreak of ornithosis. Br. Med. J. *2*:206–207, 1966.
14. Baumgartner, J. D., Glauser, M. P., Burgo-Black, A. L., et al.: Severe cytomegalovirus infection in multiply transfused, splenectomised, trauma patients. Lancet *2*:63–66, 1982.
15. Beall, G. N.: Urticaria: A review of laboratory and clinical observations. Medicine *43*:131–151, 1964.
16. Benoit, F. L.: Chronic meningococcemia: Case report and review of the literature. Am. J. Med. *35*:103–112, 1963.
17. Berant, M., Naveh, Y., and Weissman, I.: Papular acrodermatitis with cytomegalovirus hepatitis. Arch. Dis. Child. *58*:1024–1025, 1983.
18. Berger, B. W.: Erythema chronicum migrans of Lyme disease. Arch. Dermatol. *120*:1017–1021, 1984.
19. Black, F. L.: Measles. *In* Evans, A. S. (ed.): Viral Infections of Humans: Epidemiology and Control. New York, Plenum, 1976, pp. 297–316.
20. Blatt, J., Kastner, O., and Hodes, D. S.: Cutaneous vesicles in congenital cytomegalovirus infection. J. Pediatr. *92*:509, 1978.
21. Bodey, G. P., and Fainstein, V.: Systemic candidiasis. *In* Bodey, G. P., and Fainstein, V. (eds.): Candidiasis. New York, Raven Press, 1985, pp. 135–168.
22. Boughton, C. R.: Glandular fever: A study of hospital series in Sydney. Med. J. Aust. *2*:529–535, 1970.
23. Bowmer, E. J., McKiel, J. A., Cockcroft, W. H., et al.: *Listeria monocytogenes* infections in Canada. Can. Med. Assoc. J. *109*:125–135, 1973.
24. Bowmer, M. I., Leggat, I., and Barrowman, J. A.: Disseminated gonococcal infection. Can. Med. Assoc. J. *126*:1188–1190, 1982.
25. Bradford, W. D., and Hawkins, H. K.: Rocky Mountain spotted fever in childhood. Am. J. Dis. Child. *131*:1228–1232, 1977.
26. Breese, B. B.: Streptococcal pharyngitis and scarlet fever. Am. J. Dis. Child. *132*:612–616, 1978.
27. Breese, B. B.: Pharyngitis and scarlet fever. *In* Breese, B. B., and Hall, C. B. (eds.): Beta Hemolytic Streptococcal Diseases. Boston, Houghton Mifflin, 1978, pp. 65–78.
28. Breese, B. B.: Streptococcal skin infections. *In* Breese, B. B., and Hall, C. B. (eds.): Beta Hemolytic Streptococcal Diseases. Boston, Houghton Mifflin, 1978, pp. 176–211.
29. Brettman, L. R., Lewin, S., Holzman, R. S., et al.: Rickettsialpox: Report of an outbreak and a contemporary review. Medicine *60*:363–372, 1981.
30. Brody, I.: Topical treatment of recurrent herpes simplex and post-herpetic erythema multiforme with low concentrations of zinc sulphate solution. Br. J. Dermatol. *104*:191–194, 1981.
31. Browne, S. G.: Mycobacterial diseases: Leprosy. *In* Fitzpatrick, T. B., Eisen, A. Z., Wolff, K., et al. (eds.): Dermatology in General Medicine. New York, McGraw Hill, 1979, pp. 1492–1505.
32. Bruhn, F. W.: Lyme disease. Am. J. Dis. Child. *138*:467–470, 1984.
33. Buckley, B.: Q fever epidemic in Victorian general practice. Med. J. Aust. *1*:593–595, 1980.
34. Burnett, J. W.: Uncommon bacterial infections of the skin. Arch. Dermatol. *86*:597–607, 1962.
35. Caputo, R. V., and Solomon, L. M.: Vascular reactive diseases. *In* Solomon, L. M., Esterly, N. B., and Loeffel, E. D. (eds.): Adolescent Dermatology. Philadelphia, W. B. Saunders, 1978, pp. 404–432.
36. Carlstrom, G., Alden, J., Belfrage, S., et al.: Acquired cytomegalovirus infection. Br. Med. J. *2*:521–525, 1968.
37. Carslaw, R. W.: Skin infestation. Practitioner *216*:154–158, 1976.
38. Castellano, A., Schweitzer, R., Tong, M. J., et al.: Papular acrodermatitis of childhood and hepatitis B infection. Arch. Dermatol. *114*:1530–1532, 1978.
39. Centers for Disease Control: Moth-associated dermatitis: Cozumel, Mexico. M. M. W. R. *39*:219–221, 1990.
40. Chanarin, I., and Walford, D. M.: Thrombocytopenic purpura in cytomegalovirus mononucleosis. Lancet *2*:238–239, 1973.
41. Cherry, J. D.: Newer viral exanthems. Adv. Pediatr. *16*:233–286, 1969.
42. Cherry, J. D., Hurwitz, E. S., and Welliver, R. C.: *Mycoplasma pneumoniae* infections and exanthems. J. Pediatr. *87*:369–373, 1975.
43. Cherry, J. D., and Jahn, C. L.: Exanthem and enanthem associated with mumps virus infection. Arch. Environ. Health *12*:518–521, 1966.
44. Cherry, J. D., and Welliver, R. C.: *Mycoplasma pneumoniae* infections of adults and children. West. J. Med. *125*:47–55, 1976.
45. Chesney, P. J., Davis, J. P., Purdy, W. K., et al.: Clinical manifestations of toxic shock syndrome. J. A. M. A. *246*:741–748, 1981.
46. Chonmaitree, T., Menegus, M. A., and Powell, K. R.: The clinical relevance of "CSF viral culture": A two-year experience with aseptic meningitis in Rochester, New York. J. A. M. A. *247*:1843–1847, 1982.
47. Clark, R. F.: Localized urticaria due to *Enterobius vermicularis*. Arch. Dermatol. *84*:1026, 1961.
48. Cowdrey, S. C., and Reynolds, J. S.: Acute urticaria in infectious mononucleosis. Ann. Allergy *27*:182–187, 1969.
49. Darragh, T. M., Egbert, B. M., Berger, T. G., et al.: Identification of herpes simplex virus DNA in lesions of erythema multiforme by the polymerase chain reaction. J. Am. Acad. Dermatol. *24*: 23–36, 1991.
50. Daye, S., McHenry, J. A., and Roscelli, J. D.: Pruritic rash associated with cat scratch disease. Pediatrics *81*:559–561, 1988.
51. Delage, G., McLaughlin, B., and Berthiaume, L.: A clinical study of rotavirus gastroenteritis. J. Pediatr. *93*:455–457, 1978.
52. Derbes, V. J.: Arthropod bites and stings. *In* Fitzpatrick, T. B., Eisen, A. Z., Wolff, K., et al. (eds.): Dermatology in General Medicine. New York, McGraw-Hill, 1979, pp. 1656–1668.
53. Dienstag, J. L., Rhodes, A. R., Bhan, A. K., et al.: Urticaria associated with acute viral hepatitis type B: Studies of pathogenesis. Ann. Intern. Med. *88*:34–40, 1978.

54. Dooley, J. R.: Haemotropic bacteria in man. Lancet 2:1237–1239, 1980.
55. Draelos, Z. K., Hansen, R. C., and James, W. D.: Gianotti-Crosti syndrome associated with infections other than hepatitis B. J. A. M. A. *256*:2386–2388, 1986.
56. Dryer, R. F., Goellner, P. G., and Carney, A. S.: Lyme arthritis in Wisconsin. J. A. M. A. *241*:498–499, 1979.
57. Dukes, C.: On the confusion of two different diseases under the name of rubella (rose-rash). Lancet 2:89–94, 1900.
58. Duncan, W. C.: Cutaneous manifestations of infectious diseases. *In* Hoeprich, P. D. (ed.): Infectious Diseases: A Modern Treatise of Infectious Processes. Hagerstown, MD, Harper & Row, 1977, pp. 68–74.
59. Editor's Reply: First, second, third, fourth and fifth diseases. Am. J. Dis. Child. *108*:440–441, 1964.
60. Ellis, M. E., Pope, J., Mokashi, A., et al.: *Campylobacter* colitis associated with erythema nodosum. Br. Med. J. *285*:937, 1982.
61. Farah, F. S.: Protozoan and helminth infections. *In* Fitzpatrick, T. B., Eisen, A. Z., Wolff, K., et al. (eds.): Dermatology in General Medicine. New York, McGraw-Hill, 1979, pp. 1635–1656.
62. Fass, R. J., and Saslaw, S.: Earth day histoplasmosis: A new type of urban pollution. Arch. Intern. Med. *128*:588–590, 1971.
63. Fell, H. W. K., Nagington, J., Naylor, G. R. E., et al.: *Corynebacterium haemolyticum* infections in Cambridgeshire. J. Hyg. (Lond.) *79*:269–275, 1977.
64. Fenner, F.: The clinical features and pathogenesis of mouse-pox (infectious ectromelia of mice). J. Pathol. Bacteriol. *60*:529–552, 1948.
65. Fiumara, N. J., and Solomon, J.: Recurrent herpes simplex virus infections and erythema multiforme: A report of three patients. Sex. Transm. Dis. *10*:144–146, 1983.
66. Flaum, A.: Foot-and-mouth disease in man. Acta Pathol. Microbiol. Scand. *16*:197–213, 1939.
67. Fukumi, H., Nishikawa, F., Kokubu, Y., et al.: Isolation of adenovirus from an exanthematous infection resembling roseola infantum. Jpn. J. Med. Sci. Biol. *10*:87–91, 1957.
68. Gardner, S. D.: The isolation of parainfluenza 4 subtypes A and B in England and serological studies of their prevalence. J. Hyg. (Camb.) *67*:545–550, 1969.
69. Goodwin, R. A., Loyd, J. E., and Des Prez, R. M.: Histoplasmosis in normal hosts. Medicine *60*:231–266, 1981.
70. Griffith, G. L., and Luce, E. A.: Massive skin necrosis in Rocky Mountain spotted fever. South. Med. J. *71*:1337–1340, 1978.
71. Gustafson, T. L., Band, J. D., Hutcheson, R. H., Jr., et al.: *Pseudomonas* folliculitis: An outbreak and review. Rev. Infect. Dis. *5*:1–8, 1983.
72. Hall, C. B.: The exanthematous family tree: Diseases one, two, three and five? Am. J. Dis. Child. *131*:816, 1977.
73. Halliday, H. L., and Hirata, T.: Perinatal listeriosis: A review of twelve patients. Am. J. Obstet. Gynecol. *133*:405–410, 1979.
74. Hamrick, H. J., and Moore, G. W.: Giardiasis causing urticaria in a child. Am. J. Dis. Child. *137*:761–763, 1983.
75. Hannuksela, M., and Ahvonen, P.: Skin manifestations in human yersiniosis. Ann. Clin. Res. *7*:368–373, 1975.
76. Harrison, D. L.: A case of human ornithosis presenting as an obscure febrile illness associated with macular rash. Practitioner *190*:245–246, 1963.
77. Herrmann, E. C., Jr., and Hable, K. A.: Experiences in laboratory diagnosis of parainfluenza viruses in routine medical practice. Mayo Clin. Proc. *45*:177–188, 1970.
78. Hilleman, M. R., Hamparian, V. V., Ketler, A., et al.: Acute respiratory illnesses among children and adults: Field study of contemporary importance of several viruses and appraisal of the literature. J. A. M. A. *180*:445–453, 1962.
79. Hoagland, R. J.: The clinical manifestations of infectious mononucleosis: A report of two hundred cases. Am. J. Med. Sci. *240*:55–62, 1960.
80. Honig, P. J.: Bites and parasites. Pediatr. Clin. North Am. *30*:563–581, 1983.
81. Hope-Simpson, R. E., and Higgins, P. G.: A respiratory virus study in Great Britain: Review and evaluation. Prog. Med. Virol. *11*:354–407, 1969.
82. Horton, J. M., and Blaser, M. J.: The spectrum of relapsing fever in the Rocky Mountains. Arch. Intern. Med. *145*:871–875, 1985.
83. Humphrey, T., Sanders, S., and Stadius, M.: Leptospirosis mimicking MLNS. J. Pediatr. *91*:853–854, 1977.
84. Jacobs, R. F., Hsi, S., Wilson, C. B., et al.: Apparent meningococcemia: Clinical features of disease due to *Haemophilus influenzae* and *Neisseria meningitidis.* Pediatrics *72*:469–472, 1983.
85. Johnson, R. A.: Atypical mycobacteria. *In* Fitzpatrick, T. B., Eisen, A. Z., Wolff, K., et al. (eds.): Dermatology in General Medicine. New York, McGraw-Hill, 1979, pp. 1505–1508.
86. Joncas, J., Chiasson, J. P., Turcotte, J., et al.: Studies on infectious mononucleosis. III. Clinical data, serologic and epidemiologic findings. Can. Med. Assoc. J. *98*:848–854, 1968.
87. Kalis, P., LeFrock, J. L., Smith, W., et al.: Listeriosis. Am. J. Med. Sci. *271*:159–169, 1976.
88. Kazmierowski, J. A., Peizner, D. S., and Wuepper, K. D.: Herpes simplex antigen in immune complexes of patients with erythema multiforme: Presence following recurrent herpes simplex infection. J. A. M. A. *247*:2547–2550, 1982.
89. Kennedy, A. C., Fleming, J., and Solomon, L.: Chikungunya viral arthropathy: A clinical description. J. Rheumatol. *7*:231–236, 1980.
90. Kennett, M. L., Birch, C. J., Lewis, F. A., et al.: Enterovirus type 71 infection in Melbourne. Bull. W. H. O. *51*:609–615, 1974.
91. Kiernan, J. P., Schanzlin, D. J., and Leveille, A. S.: Stevens-Johnson syndrome associated with adenovirus conjunctivitis. Am. J. Ophthalmol. *92*:543–545, 1981.
92. Konno, M., Kikuta, H., Ishikawa, N., et al.: A possible association between hepatitis B antigen–negative infantile papular acrodermatitis and Epstein-Barr virus infection. J. Pediatr. *101*:222–224, 1982.
93. Krause, V. W., Embree, J. E., MacDonald, S. W., et al.: Congenital listeriosis causing early neonatal death. Can. Med. Assoc. J. *127*:36–38, 1982.
94. Krober, M. S., Bass, J. W., and Barcia, P. J.: Scarlatiniform rash and pleural effusion in a patient with *Yersinia pseudotuberculosis* infection. J. Pediatr. *102*:879–881, 1983.
95. Lackman, D. B.: A review of information on rickettsialpox in the United States. Clin. Pediatr. *2*:296–301, 1963.
96. Lambie, J. A., and Gustafson, A. A.: Contagious ecthyma in man: Report of two cases with laboratory studies. Lancet *87*:400–402, 1967.
97. Le, C. T.: Tick-borne relapsing fever in children. Pediatrics *66*:963–966, 1980.
98. Leavell, U. W., Jr., McNamara, M. J., Meulling, R. J., et al.: Ecthyma contagiosum (orf). South. Med. J. *58*:239–243, 1965.
99. Lerner, A. M., Cherry, J. D., Klein, J. O., et al.: Infections with reoviruses. N. Engl. J. Med. *267*:947–952, 1962.
100. Linnemann, C. C., Jr., and Janson, P. J.: The clinical presentations of Rocky Mountain spotted fever: Comments on recognition and management based on a study of 63 patients. Clin. Pediatr. *17*:673–679, 1978.
101. Litt, I. F., Edberg, S. C., and Finberg, L.: Gonorrhea in children and adolescents: A current review. J. Pediatr. *85*:595–607, 1974.
102. Liu, C., and Coffin, D. L.: Studies on canine distemper infection by means of fluorescein-labeled antibody. I. The pathogenesis, pathology, and diagnosis of the disease in experimentally infected ferrets. Virology *3*:115–131, 1957.
103. Maki, M., Vesikari, T., Rantala, I., et al.: *Yersinia* in children. Arch. Dis. Child. *55*:861–865, 1980.
104. Martinez-Roig, A., Llorens-Terol, J., and Torres, J. M.: Erythema nodosum and kerion of the scalp. Am. J. Dis. Child. *136*:440–442, 1982.
105. Mast, W. E., and Burrows, W. M.: Erythema chronicum migrans in the United States. J. A. M. A. *236*:859–860, 1976.
106. McDade, J. E.: Ehrlichiosis: A disease of animals and humans. J. Infect. Dis. *161*:609–617, 1990.
107. McNeill, W. H.: Plagues and Peoples. Garden City, New York, Anchor Press–Doubleday, 1976, pp. 105, 119.
108. Medeiros, A. A., Marty, S. D., Tosh, F. E., et al.: Erythema nodosum and erythema multiforme as clinical manifestations of histoplasmosis in a community outbreak. N. Engl. J. Med. *274*:415–420, 1966.
109. Melish, M. E., and Glasgow, L. A.: Staphylococcal scalded skin syndrome: The expanded clinical syndrome. J. Pediatr. *78*:958–967, 1971.
110. Milder, J. E., Walzer, P. D., Kilgore, G., et al.: Clinical features of *Strongyloides stercoralis* infection in an endemic area of the United States. Gastroenterology *80*:1481–1488, 1981.
111. Mims, C. A.: Pathogenesis of rashes in virus diseases. Bacteriol. Rev. *30*:739–760, 1966.
112. Moraga, F. A., Martinez-Roig, A., Alonso, J. L., et al.: Boutonneuse fever. Arch. Dis. Child. *57*:149–151, 1982.
113. Neisson-Vernant, C., Arfi, S., Mathez, D., et al.: Needlestick HIV seroconversion in a nurse. Lancet *2*:814, 1986.
114. Niklasson, B., Espmark, A., LeDuc, J. W., et al.: Association of a Sindbis-like virus with Ockelbo disease in Sweden. Am. J. Trop. Med. Hyg. *33*:1212–1217, 1984.
115. Nussbaum, M., Scalettar, H., and Shenker, I. R.: Gonococcal arthritis-dermatitis (GADS) as a complication of gonococcemia in adolescents. Clin. Pediatr. *14*:1037–1040, 1975.
116. Older, J. J.: The epidemiology of murine typhus in Texas, 1969. J. A. M. A. *214*:2011–2017, 1970.
117. Orton, P. W., Huff, J. C., Tonnesen, M. G., et al.: Detection of a herpes simplex viral antigen in skin lesions of erythema multiforme. Ann. Intern. Med. *101*:48–50, 1984.
118. Patamasucon, P., Schaad, U. B., and Nelson, J. D.: Melioidosis. J. Pediatr. *100*:175–182, 1982.
119. Patel, B. M.: Skin rash with infectious mononucleosis and ampicillin. Pediatrics *40*:910–911, 1967.
120. Paterson, P. Y., and Taylor, W.: Rickettsialpox. Bull. N. Y. Acad. Med. *42*:579–587, 1966.
121. Perlman, F.: Arthropod sensitivity. *In* Criep, L. H. (ed.): Dermatologic Allergy. Philadelphia, W. B. Saunders, 1967, pp. 222–244.
122. Peter, G.: Leptospirosis: A zoonosis of protean manifestations. Pediatr. Infect. Dis. *1*:282–288, 1982.
123. Pfister, L. E., Gallagher, M. V., Potterfield, T. G., et al.: *Neisseria catarrhalis:* Bacteremia with meningitis. J. A. M. A. *193*:399–401, 1965.
124. Pittsley, R. A., Shearn, M. A., and Kaufman, L.: Acute hepatitis B simulating dermatomyositis. J. A. M. A. *239*:959, 1978.
125. Place, E. H., and Sutton, L. E.: Erythema arthriticum epidemicum (Haverhill fever). Arch. Intern. Med. *54*:659–684, 1934.

126. Platt, H.: The susceptibility of the skin and epidermoid mucous membranes to virus infection in man and other animals. J. Pathol. Bacteriol. *76*:479–497, 1948.
127. Pollowitz, J. A.: Acute urticaria associated with shigellosis: A case report. Ann. Allergy *45*:302–303, 1980.
128. Portnoy, B. L., Satterwhite, T. K., and Dyckman, J. D.: Rat bite fever misdiagnosed as Rocky Mountain spotted fever. J. South. Med. Assoc. *72*:607–609, 1979.
129. Powell, K. R.: Filatow-Dukes' disease: Epidermolytic toxin-producing staphylococci as the etiologic agent of the fourth childhood exanthem. Am. J. Dis. Child. *133*:88–90, 1979.
130. Pullen, H., Wright, N., and Murdoch, J. McC.: Hypersensitivity reactions to antibacterial drugs in infectious mononucleosis. Lancet *2*:1176–1178, 1967.
131. Rasmussen, J. E., and Graves, W. H.: *Pseudomonas aeruginosa*, hot tubs, and skin infections. Am. J. Dis. Child. *136*:553–554, 1982.
132. Resnick, S. D.: Toxic shock syndrome: Recent developments in pathogenesis. J. Pediatr. *116*:321–328, 1990.
133. Richter, H. S.: Coccidioidomycosis: A report of 300 new cases. G. P. *39*:89–92, 1969.
134. Robbins, F. C.: Measles: Clinical features. Am. J. Dis. Child. *103*:266–273, 1962.
135. Rook, A.: Papular urticaria. Pediatr. Clin. North Am. *8*:817–833, 1961.
136. Rustgi, V. K., Sacher, R. A., O'Brien, P., et al.: Fatal disseminated cytomegalovirus infection in an apparently normal adult. Arch. Intern. Med. *143*:372–373, 1983.
137. Ruzicka, T., Rosendahl, C., and Braun-Falco, O.: A probable case of rotavirus exanthem. Arch. Dermatol. *121*:253–254, 1985.
138. Saari, T. N., and Triplett, D. A.: *Yersinia pseudotuberculosis* mesenteric adenitis. J. Pediatr. *85*:656–659, 1974.
139. Sabin, A. B.: Research on dengue during World War II. Am. J. Trop. Med. *1*:30–50, 1952.
140. Sanchez, R. L., Hebert, A., Lucia, H., et al.: Orf: A case report with histologic, electron microscopic, and immunoperoxidase studies. Arch. Pathol. Lab. Med. *109*:166–170, 1985.
141. San Joaquin, V. H., and Marks, M. I.: Gianotti disease or Gianotti-Crosti syndrome? J. Pediatr. *101*:216–217, 1982.
142. Saslaw, S.: Chronic meningococcemia: Report of a case. N. Engl. J. Med. *266*:605–607, 1962.
143. Schaffner, W.: The rickettsioses. *In* Fitzpatrick, T. B., Eisen, A. Z., Wolff, K., et al. (eds.): Dermatology in General Medicine. New York, McGraw-Hill, 1979, pp. 1563–1570.
144. Schneider, J. A., Poley, J. R., Millunchick, E. W., et al.: Papular acrodermatitis (Gianotti-Crosti syndrome) in a child with anicteric hepatitis B, virus subtype adw. J. Pediatr. *101*:219–222, 1982.
145. Shama, S. K., Etkind, P. H., Odell, T. M., et al.: Gypsy-moth-caterpillar dermatitis. N. Engl. J. Med. *306*:1300–1301, 1982.
146. Shanson, D. C., Gazzard, B. G., Midgley, J., et al.: *Streptobacillus moniliformis* isolated from blood in four cases of Haverhill fever: First outbreak in Britain. Lancet 2:92–94, 1983.
147. Shapiro, L.: The numbered diseases. First through sixth. J. A. M. A. *194*:210, 1965.
148. Shapiro, L.: On the numbered exanthemata. Clin. Pediatr. *6*:611–612, 1967.
149. Shaw, E. B.: Fifth disease. Am. J. Dis. Child. *131*:816, 1977.
150. Shelley, E. D., Shelley, W. B., Pula, J. F., et al.: The diagnostic challenge of nonburrowing mite bites: *Cheyletiella yasguri*. J. A. M. A. *251*:2690–2691, 1984.
151. Siewers, C. M. F., and Cramblett, H. G.: Cryptococcosis (torulosis) in children: A report of four cases. Pediatrics *34*:393–400, 1964.
152. Spelman, D. W.: Q fever: A study of 111 consecutive cases. Med. J. Aust. *1*:547–553, 1982.
153. Steere, A. C., Broderick, T. F., and Malawista, S. E.: Erythema chronicum migrans and Lyme arthritis: Epidemiologic evidence for a tick vector. Am. J. Epidemiol. *108*:312–321, 1978.
154. Stricof, R. L., and Morse, D. L.: HTLV-III/LAV seroconversion following a deep intramuscular needlestick injury. N. Engl. J. Med. *314*:1115, 1986.
155. Strong, W. B.: Petechiae and streptococcal pharyngitis. Am. J. Dis. Child. *117*:156–160, 1969.
156. Swartz, M. N., and Weinberg, A. N.: Infections due to gram-positive bacteria. *In* Fitzpatrick, T. B., Eisen, A. Z., Wolff, K., et al. (eds.): Dermatology in General Medicine. New York, McGraw-Hill, 1979, pp. 1426–1445.
157. Swartz, M. N., and Weinberg, A. N.: Miscellaneous bacterial infections with cutaneous manifestations. *In* Fitzpatrick, T. B., Eisen, A. Z., Wolff, K., et al. (eds.): Dermatology in General Medicine. New York, McGraw-Hill, 1979, pp. 1459–1473.
158. Taieb, A., Plantin, P., DuPasquier, P., et al.: Gianotti-Crosti syndrome: A study of 26 cases. Br. J. Dermatol. *115*:49–59, 1986.
159. Taylor, P. R., Weinstein, W. M., and Bryner, J. H.: *Campylobacter fetus* infection in human subjects: Association with raw milk. Am. J. Med. *66*:779–783, 1979.
160. Tertti, R., Granfors, K., Lehtonen, O. P., et al.: An outbreak of *Yersinia pseudotuberculosis* infection. J. Infect. Dis. *149*:245–250, 1984.
161. Thomas, P., Moore, M., Bell, E., et al.: *Pseudomonas* dermatitis associated with a swimming pool. J. A. M. A. *253*:1156–1159, 1985.
162. Timar, L., Budai, J., Gero, A., et al.: Rare complications and unusual syndromes associated with Epstein-Barr virus. Pediatr. Infect. Dis. *4*:212–213, 1985.
163. Timar, L., Budai, J., and Koller, M.: A prospective study on infectious mononucleosis in childhood: Symptoms, serology, Epstein-Barr virus specific leukocyte migration inhibition. Infection *10*:139–143, 1982.
164. Toth, M., Barna, M., and Voltay, B.: Aetiology of acute respiratory diseases in infants and children. Acta Paediatr. Hung. *6*:367–374, 1966.
165. Tudor, R. B.: Urticaria in childhood. Lancet *82*:273–274, 1962.
166. Turner, T. W., and Wilkinson, D. S.: *Pasteurella pseudotuberculosis* as a cause of erythema nodosum. Br. J. Dermatol. *81*:823–826, 1969.
167. Unger, A., Tapia, L., Minnich, L. L., et al.: Atypical neonatal respiratory syncytial virus infection. J. Pediatr. *100*:762–764, 1982.
168. Utz, J. P., and Shadomy, H. J.: Deep fungus infections. *In* Fitzpatrick, T. B., Eisen, A. Z., Wolff, K., et al. (eds.): Dermatology in General Medicine. New York, McGraw-Hill, 1979, pp. 1533–1563.
169. Van Arsdall, J. A., Wunderlich, H. F., Melo, J. C., et al.: The protean manifestations of Legionnaires disease. J. Infect. Dis. *7*:51–62, 1983.
170. Ware, R.: Human parvovirus infection. J. Pediatr. *114*:343–348, 1989.
171. Weinberg, A. N., and Swartz, M. N.: Gram-negative coccal and bacillary infections. *In* Fitzpatrick, T. B., Eisen, A. Z., Wolff, K., et al. (eds.): Dermatology in General Medicine. New York, McGraw-Hill, 1979, pp. 1445–1459.
172. Weller, T. H.: The cytomegaloviruses: Ubiquitous agents with protean clinical manifestations. I and II. N. Engl. J. Med. *285*:203–214 and 267–274, 1971.
173. Wenner, H. A.: Virus diseases associated with cutaneous eruptions. Prog. Med. Virol. *16*:269–336, 1973.
174. Wenner, H. A., and Lou, T. Y.: Virus diseases associated with cutaneous eruptions. Prog. Med. Virol. *5*:219–294, 1963.
175. Wiesenthal, A. M., and Todd, J. K.: Toxic shock syndrome in children aged 10 years or less. Pediatrics *74*:112–117, 1984.
176. Winn, W. A., Levine, H. B., Broderick, J. E., et al.: A localized epidemic of coccidioidal infection: Primary coccidioidomycosis occurring in a group of ten children infected in a backyard playground in the San Joaquin Valley of California. N. Engl. J. Med. *268*:867–870, 1963.
177. Wolff, K.: Mycobacterial diseases: Tuberculosis. *In* Fitzpatrick, T. B., Eisen, A. Z., Wolff, K., et al. (eds.): Dermatology in General Medicine. New York, McGraw-Hill, 1979, pp. 1473–1492.
178. Wong, M. L., Kaplan, S., Dunkle, L. M., et al.: Leptospirosis: A childhood disease. J. Pediatr. *90*:532–537, 1977.
179. Woodward, T. E.: Rocky mountain spotted fever: Epidemiological and early clinical signs are keys to treatment and reduced mortality. J. Infect. Dis. *150*:465–468, 1984.
180. Yamanishi, K., Shiraki, K., Kondo T., et al.: Identification of human herpesvirus-6 as a causal agent for exanthem subitum. Lancet *1*:1065–1067, 1988.
181. Young, E. J.: Human brucellosis. Rev. Infect. Dis. *5*:821–842, 1983.

68

ROSEOLA INFANTUM (EXANTHEM SUBITUM)

James D. Cherry

Roseola infantum (exanthem subitum, pseudorubella, exanthem criticum, sixth disease, 3-day fever) is a common acute illness of young children characterized by a fever of 3 to 5 days' duration, rapid defervescence, and then the appearance of an erythematous macular or maculopapular rash that persists for 1 to 2 days.

HISTORY

Zahorsky[64] generally is given credit for the original description of roseola infantum. However, in his writings, he clearly pointed out that the syndrome was described in earlier pediatric and dermatology texts.[65–67] The descriptions in the older literature did not separate the syndrome from the known exanthematous diseases (measles, rubella, and scarlet fever), an omission that Zahorsky corrected.

In 1921, Veeder and Hempelmann[61] described the syndrome further and noted that leukopenia and relative lymphocytosis occurred. These investigators objected to the name "roseola infantum," which in the past had been used to describe a large group of diseases of indefinite causes. They suggested the term "exanthem subitum" because it was "descriptive of the most striking clinical symptom, namely, the sudden, unexpected appearance of the eruption on the fourth day." At present, the term "roseola" is used most commonly to describe the syndrome.

From 1920 through 1940, many excellent clinical descriptions of the syndrome were published.[4, 5, 8, 14, 15, 17, 21, 22, 31, 67, 68] From 1940 through 1988, papers relating to roseola were concerned with unusual manifestations and complications[6, 9–11, 19, 27, 41–43, 47, 49, 55] and attempts to recover an etiologic agent.[23, 26, 35, 40, 56] In 1988, Yamanishi and associates[63] identified human herpesvirus 6 in the blood of infants with roseola, and since then, this virus and disease association has been confirmed on many occasions.[1–3, 7, 16, 18, 24, 25, 28–30, 34, 36–39, 48, 50, 52, 57–59]

EPIDEMIOLOGY

In his original paper, Zahorsky[64] reported that roseola occurred most commonly in the fall. In his second paper, a year-round incidence was observed[65]; in 1925, he pointed out that most cases occurred in the spring, summer, and fall.[66] Breese[8] noted that the greatest number of cases occurred in the summer and early fall. In contrast, 55 per cent of Clemens' cases occurred in February, March, and April; 16 per cent were seen in October.[14] In a review of 243 cases over a 10-year period, Juretic[33] noted that the peak month was May. Juretic also reviewed the seasonal incidence in 10 other studies and found only minor variations by month. Prevalence was greatest in March, April, and October and least in December. One epidemic of roseola in a maternity hospital occurred in the summer,[31] another epidemic in an infants' home occurred in the fall,[4] and a hospital outbreak was noted in the winter.[15]

Roseola predominantly is an illness of young children. It is rare before 3 months of age or after 4 years of age. In a review of 1462 cases, the peak age range prevalence was from 7 to 13 months of age; 55 per cent of the cases occurred within the first year of life and 90 per cent within the first 2 years of life.[33] Occasional cases have been seen in older children, adolescents, and young adults, as well as in neonates and other infants younger than 6 months of age.[22, 31]

Although Faber and Dickey[17] found twice as many girls as boys with the syndrome, the sex ratio in most large studies has been equal.[5, 8, 14, 22, 40] Although three epidemics have been reported and cases frequently occur in groups by season, the majority of cases occur sporadically without known exposure. The syndrome, when seen sporadically, generally is considered to be noncontagious, but occasional secondary cases have been reported.[4, 8, 15, 31] The incubation period range in epidemics is 5 to 15 days.[4, 8, 15]

It is surprising to ascertain that the attack rate of roseola has not been well studied. Berenberg and associates[5] state that roseola is the most common exanthem encountered in children younger than 2 years of age. Breese[8] noted that 16 per cent of a group of infants that he followed for the first 12 months of life had definite roseola. He estimated that 30 per cent of children would have clinical roseola. Juretic[33] looked at the frequency of roseola in 6735 children; the yearly attack rate over a 10-year period varied from 1 to 10 per cent, with a mean of 3.3 per cent.

ETIOLOGY

In 1941, Breese[8] reported rather vigorous attempts to isolate a filterable virus from three children with pre-eruptive roseola. These studies included extensive animal inoculations, but no viral agents were uncovered. In 1950, Kempe and associates[35] reported the passage of the illness to a 6-month-old susceptible infant by the intravenous injection of serum from an 18-month-old child with pre-eruptive roseola. Febrile illnesses without exanthem also were produced in monkeys with serum and throat washings from a child with the syndrome. In similar experiments, Hellström and Vahlquist[26] produced the syndrome in three children 6 to 9 days after the intramuscular administration of blood from typical roseola cases.

In electron microscopic studies, Reagan and associates[53] noted uniform virus-like particles (100 to 110 nm) in the blood of an 18-month-old child with the syndrome. Febrile illness was produced in two monkeys after inoculation of the concentrated virus-containing material.

Since the advent of the present era of diagnostic virology in the early 1950s, numerous viral agents have been recovered from children with roseola. In 1951, Neva and associates[46] studied an epidemic exanthematous illness (Boston exanthem) due to echovirus 16, in which many of the illnesses were characteristic of roseola. In 1954, Neva[44] observed additional cases of roseola-like illness associated with echovirus 16 infection. In 1974, Hall and colleagues[24] noted four additional echovirus 16 infections with clinical manifestations of roseola. In addition, the reporting of roseola in Rochester, New York, nearly doubled during the time of echovirus 16 activity in the area. Roseola-like illnesses also have been noted in association with these enteroviruses: coxsackievirus A6 and 9 and B1, 2, 4, and 5; and echovirus 9, 11, 25, 27, and 30.[12, 13, 24, 57, 62] It seems probable that outbreaks of roseola that occur in the summer and fall are due to enteroviral infections.

In addition to enteroviruses, adenovirus types 1, 2, 3, and 14 and parainfluenza type 1 virus have been recovered from children with roseola.[20, 32, 45, 62] Saitoh and associates[56] detected rotavirus capsomeres in fecal specimens of nine children with roseola. In contrast with these findings, Gurwith and colleagues[23] studied fecal specimens from five children with roseola, and in none were viral particles identified. One of 13 children in this study did develop antibody to rotavirus around the time of illness, however.

In addition to the occurrence of roseola in association with a large number of natural viral infections, its pattern (fever and then rash with defervescence) was observed frequently in recipients of Edmonston B measles vaccine.[12]

In 1988, Yamanishi and associates[63] isolated human herpesvirus 6 from four infants with roseola, and all four had significant titer rises to this virus. Shortly after this report, several other investigators noted similar findings.[1, 2, 16, 28, 37, 59, 60] The implication from these studies, as suggested by the various authors, is that human herpesvirus 6 is the cause of roseola. This viewpoint obviously overlooks or ignores the past experience in which other viral agents have been associated with the clinical syndrome. More recent studies indicate that human herpesvirus 6 is a major cause of roseola and the cause of acute febrile illness without exanthem in infants.[3, 7, 24, 29, 36, 39, 40, 50, 52, 58]

In a study of 1653 infants and young children with acute febrile illnesses, Hall and colleagues[24] found that 160 (9.7 per cent) had primary human herpesvirus 6 infections; 27 (17 per cent) of the children infected with human herpesvirus 6 had roseola. In a study of clinical roseola, Okada and associates[48] noted that 81 per cent had serologic evidence of human herpesvirus 6 infection and that 8 per cent had an echovirus 18 infection. In a study of roseola in Italy, Braito and Uberti[7] found serologic evidence of human herpesvirus 6 infection in only 30 per cent of the cases. In 33 per cent of the remaining cases, they attributed the illnesses to another infectious agent.

At present, it seems that human herpesvirus 6 is a major but not the sole cause of roseola.

PATHOPHYSIOLOGY

The pathophysiologic process of roseola is unknown. Watson[62] has suggested that roseola is not an infection due to one particular pathogen but is the result of an immunizing reaction against many different viruses. He also suggests that the rash is due to the neutralization of virus in the skin at the end of the period of viremia.

Because viremia is common in human herpesvirus 6, enteroviral, and adenoviral infections, it is reasonable to believe that the rash in roseola is related to an immunologic event resulting from the virus that is localized in the skin. Why the pattern of fever and then rash with defervescence is so clearly age-dependent is unknown. Most of the viruses that in the past have been associated with roseola cause other exanthematous manifestations in older patients.[12]

CLINICAL PRESENTATION

The basic clinical pattern of roseola is a febrile period of 3 to 5 days, defervescence, and the appearance of a rash that persists for 1 to 2 days. Because the syndrome is due to many different viruses, it is apparent that the illness may be associated with a large number of other symptoms and signs. The major manifestations have been reviewed on several occasions.[5, 8, 14, 22, 33, 65]

Illness usually occurs with the apparent abrupt onset of fever. Slight irritability and malaise are frequent, but more commonly the child's temperature is taken because a parent notes that the child feels warm. The temperature commonly is in the range of 38.9° to 40.6° C (102° to 105° F). Despite the high fever, the child usually is active, alert, and generally unphased. The fever is either constant or intermittent, with its greatest degree in the early evening. Restlessness and irritability are noted with higher temperatures. The usual duration of fever is 3 to 5 days, but it has been noted to persist for 9 days. The temperature most often returns to normal by crisis, but in some cases, temperature "lysis" occurs over a 24- to 36-hour period.

Mild cough and coryza are noted frequently in cases occurring in the winter and spring, and headache and abdominal pain are reported in older children, mainly in the summer and fall. Vomiting and diarrhea are infrequent occurrences.

On initial physical examination during the febrile period, most children appear to be happy, alert, and playful. However, with high temperatures, some children are irritable; occasionally, a child appears to be sick, which suggests more serious illness, such as meningitis or septicemia. Examination within the oral cavity frequently reveals one or more abnormalities. Mild inflammation of the pharynx and tonsils is most common. Occasionally, small exudative follicular lesions are noted on the tonsils. In other cases, small ulcerative lesions on the soft palate, uvula, and tonsillar pillars are observed. Usually, the lesions on the soft palate consist of only erythematous macules and maculopapules presumably due to lymphoid hyperplasia.

Mild injection of the tympanic membranes is common. Enlargement of the suboccipital, posterior cervical, and postauricular lymph nodes is common, but the degree is not particularly remarkable.

Berliner[6] noted that children with roseola had palpebral edema. He felt that the "heavy eyelids" or "droopy" or "sleepy" appearance resulting from this edema was diagnostic of the syndrome before the appearance of the rash. Bulging of the anterior fontanelle also has been noted in roseola.[49]

The appearance of the rash in roseola usually coincides with the subsidence of fever, but it may occur after an afebrile interlude of several hours to 2 days. When defervescence occurs by lysis, commonly the onset of the exanthem occurs before the temperature has returned entirely to a normal level. However, by definition, it is incorrect to call an illness roseola if the fever and rash are truly concomitant.

Zahorsky[64, 65] originally described the rash as morbilliform, but it is clear that his use of "morbilliform" was not as ours is today (i.e., measles-like—erythematous maculopapular with confluence). The rash is erythematous and macular or maculopapular, and the lesions are discrete. The lesions are 2 to 5 mm in diameter, and they blanch on pressure. Frequently, individual lesions are surrounded by a whitish ring. The rash is most prominent on the neck and trunk, but the proximal extremities and the face also may be affected. Although they have been reported,[14, 21] pruritus and desquamation usually do not occur. The rash usually persists for 24 to 48 hours. In occasional cases, well-documented rashes have been observed to appear and resolve within 2 to 4 hours.

Except for the white blood cell count, routine laboratory studies are of little use in roseola. The total white blood cell count usually is low. However, early in the febrile period, high counts occasionally are found. The total count drops to its lowest level at the third to the sixth day of illness and then gradually returns to normal over the ensuing 7 to 10 days. During the same time frame, the percentage of lymphocytes increases from a normal value of about 50 per cent to 60 to 80 per cent on days 3 to 10 and then returns to normal over the next 7 days. Frequently, extreme counts in the range of 3000 cells/mm^3 with 90 per cent lymphocytes are found, which raises the consideration of a granulocytic defect.

CLINICAL COMPLICATIONS

The most important complications of roseola are convulsions and other neurologic symptoms.[2, 5, 9–11, 17, 19, 22, 27, 30, 38, 42, 51, 54, 55] The incidence of convulsions has varied widely among reports. Juretic[33] found not one instance of convulsions in the 243 cases in his study. Breese[8] did not report convulsions in any of 100 roseola attacks that he studied. In contrast, Greenthal[22] noted convulsions in 6 per cent of his cases, and Faber and Dickey[17] found seizures in 8 of 26 cases of roseola. Möller[42] noted that 8 per cent of children admitted to the hospital because of febrile convulsions eventually were diagnosed with roseola infantum.[42]

Möller[42] also reported cerebrospinal fluid evaluations in 29 cases of roseola and febrile convulsions. In six instances, the pressure was elevated; in two, there were five white blood cells/mm^3; and in another instance, there were nine white blood cells/mm^3. In most other cerebrospinal fluid examinations, the findings have been within normal limits, but occasionally mild pleocytosis with mononuclear cells has been noted.[5, 27] There have been a surprising number of reports of encephalitis in association with roseola,[11, 19, 27, 30] and residua have been common. Hemiplegia after illness has been noted,[11, 19, 51, 54] and permanent paresis and mental retardation have occurred in some affected patients.

Thrombocytopenic purpura has been noted in five children with roseola; all of these patients recovered.[47]

DIAGNOSIS

Although it is fortuitous to note leukopenia with relative lymphocytosis, the only necessity in establishing the diagnosis of a roseola is to document the fever, defervescence, and exanthem pattern. All too frequently, however, the first exanthematous illness that a child has is called roseola regardless of whether the exanthem and the fever are concomitant or whether there was no febrile period at all.

The only problem in differential diagnosis occurs when a febrile child is receiving antibiotics and a rash follows defervescence. This is a fairly frequent happening, and unfortunately the child usually is labeled allergic to the antibiotic rather than suspected to have roseola. In most instances of drug allergy, the exanthem lasts longer than roseola does, and in allergic cases, pruritus and fever may accompany the rash.

TREATMENT AND PROGNOSIS

There is no specific treatment for roseola. When fever is a problem, it may be treated with acetaminophen. Note that acetaminophen can alter the temperature curve, so the correct diagnosis may be obscured. Febrile seizures and other neurologic complications should, of course, be treated vigorously.

In the vast majority of cases, the outlook is excellent. When encephalitis occurs, the prognosis must be guarded.

Because roseola is the result of infection with multiple different viruses, there currently is no practical way to prevent it.

References

1. Asano, Y., Yoshikawa, T., Suga, S., et al.: Viremia and neutralizing antibody response in infants with exanthem subitum. J. Pediatr. *114*:535–539, 1989.
2. Asano, Y., Nakashima, T., Yoshikawa, T., et al.: Severity of human herpesvirus-6 viremia and clinical findings in infants with exanthem subitum. J. Pediatr. *118*:891–895, 1991.
3. Asano, Y., Yoshikawa, T., Suga, S., et al.: Clinical features of infants with primary human herpesvirus 6 infection (exanthem subitum, roseola infantum). Pediatrics *93*:104–108, 1994.
4. Barenberg, L. H., and Greenspan, L.: Exanthema subitum (roseola infantum). Am. J. Dis. Child. *58*:983–993, 1939.
5. Berenberg, W., Wright, S., and Janeway, C. A.: Roseola infantum (exanthem subitum). N. Engl. J. Med. *241*:253–259, 1949.
6. Berliner, B. C.: A physical sign useful in diagnosis of roseola infantum before the rash. Pediatrics *25*:1034, 1960.
7. Braito, A., and Uberti, M.: Roseola infantum and its correlation with HHV6. Eur. J. Pediatr. *153*:209, 1994.
8. Breese, B. B., Jr.: Roseola infantum (exanthem subitum). N. Y. State J. Med. *41*:1854–1859, 1941.
9. Broberger, A. O.: Exanthema subitum och feberkramper. Nord. Med. *59*:523–525, 1958.
10. Brunner, V. N.: 172 Fälle von exanthema subitum aus praxis und klinik. Helv. Paediatr. Acta *14*:408–425, 1959.
11. Burnstine, R. C., and Paine, R. S.: Residual encephalopathy following roseola infantum. Am. J. Dis. Child. *98*:144–152, 1959.
12. Cherry, J. D.: Newer viral exanthems. Adv. Pediatr. *16*:233, 1969.
13. Cherry, J. D., Lerner, A. M., Klein, J. O., et al.: Coxsackie B5 infections with exanthems. Pediatrics *31*:455–462, 1963.
14. Clemens, H. H.: Exanthem subitum (roseola infantum): Report of eighty cases. J. Pediatr. *26*:66–77, 1945.
15. Cushing, H. B.: An epidemic of roseola infantum. Can. Med. Assoc. J. *17*:905–906, 1927.
16. Enders, G., Biber, M., Meyer, G., et al.: Prevalence of antibodies to human herpesvirus 6 in different age groups, in children with exanthema subitum, other acute exanthematous childhood diseases, Kawasaki syndrome, and acute infections with other herpesviruses and HIV. Infection *18*:12–15, 1990.
17. Faber, H. K., and Dickey, L. B.: The symptomatology of exanthem subitum. Arch. Pediatr. *44*:491–496, 1927.
18. Fox, J. D., Ward, P., Briggs, M., et al.: Production of IgM antibody to HHV6 in reactivation and primary infection. Epidemiol. Infect. *104*:289–296, 1990.
19. Friedman, J. H., Golomb, J., and Aronson, L.: Hemiplegia associated with roseola infantum (exanthem subitum). N. Y. State J. Med. *50*:1749–1750, 1950.
20. Fukumi, H., Nishikawa, F., Kokubu, Y., et al.: Isolation of adenovirus from an exanthematous infection resembling roseola infantum. Jpn. J. Med. Sci. Biol. *10*:87–91, 1957.
21. Greenthal, R. M.: An unusual exanthem occurring in infants. Am. J. Dis. Child. *23*:63–65, 1922.
22. Greenthal, R. M.: Roseola infantum (exanthem subitum). Wis. Med. J. *40*:25–27, 1941.
23. Gurwith, M., Gurwith, D., Wenman, W., et al.: Exanthem subitum not associated with rotavirus. N. Engl. J. Med. *305*:174–175, 1981.
24. Hall, C. B., Cherry, J. D., Hatch, M. H., et al.: The return of Boston exanthem: Echovirus 16 infections in 1974. Am. J. Dis. Child. *131*:323–326, 1977.
25. Hall, C. B., Long, C. E., Schnabel, K. C., et al.: Human herpesvirus-6 infection in children: A prospective study of complications and reactivation. N. Engl. J. Med. *331*:432–438, 1994.
26. Hellström, B., and Vahlquist, B.: Experimental inoculation of roseola infantum. Acta Paediatr. *40*:189–197, 1951.
27. Holliday, P. B., Jr.: Pre-eruptive neurological complications of the common contagious diseases: Rubella, rubeola, roseola, and varicella. J. Pediatr. *36*:185–198, 1950.
28. Huang, L. M., Lee, C. Y., Chen, J. Y., et al.: Primary human herpesvirus 6 infections in children: A prospective serologic study. J. Infect. Dis. *165*:1163–1164, 1992.
29. Irving, W. L., Chang, J., Raymond, D. R., et al.: Roseola infantum and other syndromes associated with acute HHV6 infection. Arch. Dis. Child. *65*:1297–1300, 1990.
30. Ishiguro, N., Yamada, S., Takahashi, T., et al.: Meningoencephalitis associated with HHV-6-related exanthem subitum. Acta Paediatr. Scand. *79*:987–989, 1990.
31. James, U., and Freier, A.: Roseola infantum: An outbreak in a maternity hospital. Arch. Dis. Child. *23–24*:54–58, 1948–1949.
32. Jansson, E., Wager, O., Forssell, P., et al.: An exanthema subitumlike rash in patients with adenovirus infection. Ann. Paediatr. Fenn. *7*:3–11, 1961.
33. Juretic, M.: Exanthema subitum: A review of 243 cases. Helv. Paediatr. Acta *18*:80–95, 1963.
34. Kawaguchi, S., Suga, S., Kozawa, T., et al.: Primary human herpesvirus-6 infection (exanthem subitum) in the newborn. Pediatrics *90*:628–630, 1992.
35. Kempe, C. H., Shaw, E. B., Jackson, J. R., et al.: Studies on the etiology of exanthema subitum (roseola infantum). J. Pediatr. *37*:561–568, 1950.
36. Knowles, W., and Gardner, S.: High prevalence of antibody to human

herpesvirus 6 and seroconversion associated with rash in 2 infants. Lancet 2:912–913, 1988.
37. Kodo, S., Kondo, K., Kondo, T., et al.: Detection of human herpesvirus 6 DNA in throat swabs by polymerase chain reaction. J. Med. Virol. *32*:139–142, 1990.
38. Kondo, K., Nagafuji, H., Hata, A., et al.: Association of human herpesvirus 6 infection of the central nervous system with recurrence of febrile convulsions. J. Infect. Dis. *167*:1197–1200, 1993.
39. Kusuhara, K., Ueda, K., Okada, K., et al.: Do second attacks of exanthema subitum result from human herpesvirus-6 reactivation or reinfection? Pediatr. Infect. Dis. J. *10*:468–469, 1991.
40. Letchner, A.: Roseola infantum: A review of fifty cases. Lancet *2*:1163–1165, 1955.
41. McEnery, J. T.: Postoccipital lymphadenopathy as a diagnostic sign in roseola infantum (exanthem subitum). Clin. Pediatr. *9*:512–514, 1970.
42. Möller, K. L.: Exanthema subitum and febrile convulsions. Acta Paediatr. *45*:534–540, 1956.
43. Moore, W. F., Jr.: Roseola infantum. Hawaii Med. J. *22*:431–434, 1963.
44. Neva, F. A.: A second outbreak of Boston exanthem disease in Pittsburgh during 1954. N. Engl. Med. J. *254*:838, 1956.
45. Neva, F. A., and Enders, J. F.: Isolation of a cytopathogenic agent from an infant with a disease in certain respects resembling roseola infantum. J. Immunol. *72*:315–321, 1954.
46. Neva, F. A., Feemster, R. F., and Gorback, I. J.: Clinical and epidemiological features of an unusual epidemic exanthem. J. A. M. A. *155*:544, 1954.
47. Nishimura, K., and Igarashi, M.: Thrombocytopenic purpura associated with exanthem subitum. Pediatrics *60*:260, 1977.
48. Okada, K., Ueda, K., Kusuhara, K., et al.: Exanthema subitum and human herpesvirus 6 infection: Clinical observations in fifty-seven cases. Pediatr. Infect. Dis. J. *12*:204–208, 1993.
49. Oski, F. A.: Roseola infantum: Another case of bulging fontanel. Am. J. Dis. Child. *101*:376–378, 1961.
50. Portolani, M., Cermelli, C., Moroni, A., et al.: Human herpesvirus-6 infections in infants admitted to hospital. J. Med. Virol. *39*:146–151, 1993.
51. Posson, D. D.: Exanthem subitum (roseola infantum) complicated by prolonged convulsions and hemiplegia. J. Pediatr. *35*:235–236, 1949.
52. Pruksananonda, P., Hall, C. B., Insel, R. A., et al.: Primary human herpesvirus 6 infection in young children. N. Engl. J. Med. *326*:1445–1450, 1992.
53. Reagan, R. L., Chang, S. C., Moolten, S. E., et al.: Electron microscopic studies of the roseola infantum (exanthem subitum) virus. Tex. Rep. Biol. Med. *13*:929–933, 1955.
54. Rosenblum, J.: Roseola infantum (exanthem subitum) complicated by hemiplegia. Am. J. Dis. Child. *69*:234–236, 1945.
55. Rothman, P. E., and Naiditch, M. J.: Nervous complications of exanthem subitum. Calif. Med. J. *88*:39–44, 1958.
56. Saitoh, Y., Matsuno, S., and Mukoyama, A.: Exanthem subitum and rotavirus. N. Engl. J. Med. *304*:845, 1981.
57. St. Geme, J. W., Jr., Prince, J. T., Scherer, W. F., et al.: A clinical study of an exanthem due to ECHO virus type 9. J. Pediatr. *54*:459–467, 1959.
58. Suga, S., Yazaki, T., Kajita, Y., et al.: Detection of human herpesvirus 6 DNAs in samples from several body sites of patients with exanthem subitum and their mothers by polymerase chain reaction assay. J. Med. Virol. *46*:52–55, 1995.
59. Takahashi, K., Sonoda, S., Kawakami, K., et al.: Human herpesvirus 6 and exanthem subitum. Lancet *1*:1463, 1988.
60. Ueda, K., Kusuhara, K., Hirose, M., et al.: Exanthem subitum and antibody to human herpesvirus-6. J. Infect. Dis. *159*:750–752, 1989.
61. Veeder, B. S., and Hempelmann, T. C.: A febrile exanthem occurring in childhood (exanthem subitum). J. A. M. A. *77*:1787–1789, 1921.
62. Watson, G. I.: The roseolar reaction. Br. Med. J. *4*:719–720, 1974.
63. Yamanishi, K., Okuno, T., Shiraki, K., et al.: Identification of human herpesvirus-6 as a causal agent for exanthem subitum. Lancet *1*:1065–1067, 1988.
64. Zahorsky, J.: Roseola infantilis. Pediatrics *22*:60–64, 1910.
65. Zahorsky, J.: Roseola infantum. J. A. M. A. *61*:1446–1450, 1913.
66. Zahorsky, J.: Roseola infantum: The rose rash of infants. Arch. Pediatr. *42*:610–613, 1925.
67. Zahorsky, J.: Roseola infantum: A critical survey of some recent literature. Arch. Pediatr. *57*:405–409, 1940.
68. Zahorsky, J.: Roseola infantum, a critical survey of recent literature. Arch. Pediatr. *64*:579–583, 1947.

69

BACTERIAL SKIN INFECTIONS

Marian E. Melish and Alison A. Bertuch

The skin frequently is involved during the course of a multitude of infectious diseases. At least three pathogenetic patterns in which infection leads to skin disease can be identified:

1. The infection does not involve the skin directly, but skin lesions develop as a result of toxic or immunologic mechanisms. Examples of toxin-mediated skin disease are provided by the two generalized forms of the staphylococcal scalded skin syndrome. In these diseases, toxin is elaborated by the infecting organism at a local site of infection, is disseminated by the hematogenous route, and acts in the skin to produce the characteristic skin lesions. An example of immunologically mediated skin disease is the appearance of sterile skin lesions associated with disseminated gonococcal septicemia.
2. The skin is infected as part of a generalized illness. Examples are multiple viral diseases, including measles, varicella, and smallpox; certain bacterial infections, such as *Neisseria meningitidis* meningitis and *Pseudomonas aeruginosa* septicemia; and septic emboli, which develop in the course of endocarditis. Skin lesions also occur as an integral part of systemic mycobacterial infections, such as leprosy and tuberculosis.
3. The skin itself is infected primarily. The disease may be self-limited, or infection may spread to other contiguous sites or initiate disseminated disease.

Only primary skin infections are discussed in this chapter. Skin infections may arise on previously normal skin or, more frequently, in skin that has been injured either acutely or chronically.

NORMAL SKIN FLORA

The skin is a dynamic environment that is host to a variety of microorganisms. As a habitat, the skin has various "climatic" zones, which support different types and densities of organisms. Moist intertriginous zones support larger bacterial populations than does exposed, dry skin, such as forearm skin. Areas rich in sebaceous secretions, such as scalp and face, also carry large numbers of organisms. Personal hygiene and the presence of skin disease have a profound effect on skin flora.

The skin flora can be subdivided into resident and transient flora. The resident flora consists of organisms that are present regularly on the skin, predominantly the nonpathogenic *Staphylococcus epidermidis*, micrococci, and anaerobic and aerobic diphtheroids, particularly *Propionibacterium acnes*. The transient flora consist of a wide variety of organisms occasionally resident on the skin. These transient organisms may be pathogens that colonize the skin temporarily. Transient flora usually are removed easily from normal skin by scrubbing but may be difficult to remove from diseased skin.

Transient flora may be pathogens or nonpathogens. Streptococci, *Staphylococcus aureus*, enteric organisms, and *Candida* species frequently are found on the skin but do not become established permanently.

In determining whether an organism isolated at or near a skin lesion is pathogenic, the normal flora and the site of isolation must be considered. Both *S. epidermidis* and diphtheroids, such as *P. acnes*, occasionally may cause pyogenic disease but almost certainly would be recovered from any skin site sampled. *S. aureus* and beta-hemolytic streptococci rarely are recovered from scrubbed normal skin and are likely pathogens when recovered from skin lesions.

SUPERFICIAL SKIN INFECTIONS

Many clinical disorders with differing courses and etiologies are subsumed under the term pyoderma, which broadly means "purulent skin infection." Common bacterial infections include two clinically and bacteriologically distinct forms of impetigo, folliculitis, furunculosis, hidradenitis, erysipelas, and cellulitis. The most superficial of skin infections generally are termed, imprecisely, impetigo. Considerable confusion and idle argument can be avoided if the two entities, which clinically, bacteriologically, and histologically are diverse, are considered separately. The two basic forms of disease generally called impetigo are the thick-crusted variety, which may be caused by streptococci or staphylococci, and bullous impetigo, which is of staphylococcal origin. In the United States, the thick-crusted variety generally is implied by the term impetigo or impetigo contagiosa, whereas the British literature tends to combine both varieties under this term without clear separation. Further confusing the issue are textbooks of pediatrics, medicine, dermatology, and dermatopathology, which either lump these two forms together or split them into numerous, generally meaningless subcategories.

Impetigo

Clinical Features

Simple superficial impetigo is the most common skin infection encountered in children. Generally, it is diagnosed and treated on clinical grounds alone (Fig. 69–1). The typical lesion begins as an erythematous papule in a traumatized area, such as an abrasion or insect bite. There may be small transient vesicles, but the lesion rapidly evolves to its clinically recognizable crusted form. The lesion itself is of varying size, ranging from a few millimeters to 1 to 2 cm, and consists of a central crusted plaque surrounded by a discrete erythematous margin. Minimal edema can be appreciated within the erythematous margin. The crust is thick and of an amber or honey color. The lesions are not excessively purulent; when the crust is removed, a cloudy, amber serous fluid exudes from the moist erythematous base. In general, the lesions are discrete and limited initially, although with time they may become quite large and coalescent. Scalp impetigo particularly is likely to become coalescent and be extensive by the time the patient seeks care.

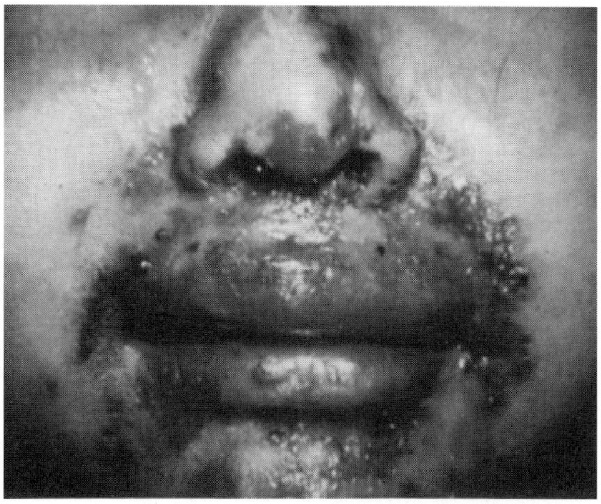

FIGURE 69–1. *Common impetigo. This lesion is characterized by the presence of a thick honey-colored crust made up of dried exudate. Lesions are seen commonly about the nose and mouth or on extremities.*

Impetigo is an indolent, well-tolerated infection. An average delay of 2 to 3 weeks in seeking medical attention has been noted in several studies.[15, 24] In one study, concern about regional adenitis rather than skin lesions prompted most visits. Among certain groups, such as Polynesians living in Hawaii and Samoa, the rural poor in the humid climate of the southern United States, and children on a Minnesota Indian reservation in the summer, skin infections nearly are universal. In these groups, "sores" are considered a normal attribute of childhood and cause concern only when cellulitis, painful adenopathy, or other complications occur. Patients with impetigo seek medical attention late because the skin lesions are not painful and only moderately are tender to the touch; tenderness does not extend beyond the margin of the lesion. Generally, lesions are slowly progressive. Fever and systemic signs are not encountered, even with extensive superficial impetigo. Regional adenopathy does appear in a considerable proportion of patients.[24] The majority of lesions are found on exposed areas, particularly the extremities.

The clinical condition tends to remain stable for considerable periods, and many lesions heal spontaneously, particularly in people with good personal hygiene. Other lesions may become chronic and form stable ulcers with erosion through the dermis.

Epidemiology

Impetigo primarily is a disease of children, occurring both endemically and in epidemics. Both sporadic cases and epidemic outbreaks have occurred in adolescents and adults, particularly among servicemen and among players on athletic teams. Although certain investigators have declared impetigo to be a problem primarily of preschool children,[64] multiple series have shown the entire range of the pediatric age group to be affected, with a mean age of patients of 5 years.[15, 24] In Hawaii, impetigo is as prevalent among schoolchildren as preschool children, although younger children tend to be seen for treatment earlier. Impetigo is spread within families and among those in close physical contact, as in schools and camps.

Climate dramatically affects the prevalence of impetigo. Reports from widely diverse geographic areas confirm that it is more prevalent during warm, humid weather. It is extremely prevalent and seen year-round in tropical areas. In the southern United States (e.g., Alabama), it is endemic but more prevalent in the summer, [24] whereas in northern latitudes (e.g., Minnesota), it is seen primarily during the warm, humid months.[3] It is strikingly less prevalent in dry climates. A warm, humid atmosphere promotes the development of impetigo by providing maximum opportunities for insect bites and cutaneous trauma on uncovered limbs and also may enhance bacterial multiplication.

Etiology

For many years, group A beta-hemolytic streptococci were considered to be the primary etiologic agent, with staphylococci, when present, thought to be a secondary invader.[22, 24, 34, 63, 64] In the 1980s, however, a reversal was observed, with the majority of the lesions yielding *S. aureus*, often as the sole pathogen.[6, 7, 9, 23, 75] Furthermore, studies demonstrated that therapies directed at streptococci alone were significantly less effective than were those regimens that employed antistaphylococcal agents.[6, 20, 23]

During the late 1960s, elegant studies on the natural history of impetigo tracing skin and respiratory tract colonization through the development of overt impetiginous lesions were carried out at the Red Lake Indian Reservation in Minnesota among 31 children in families at high risk for the development of impetigo. During the study period (summer and fall), all children developed impetigo. Group A streptococci were found on normal skin a mean of 10 days before the development of impetigo in 74 per cent of episodes. Colonization of nose and throat followed skin acquisition of streptococci in 97 per cent. The index streptococcal strain was seen to spread among families, other members acquiring skin streptococci a mean of 5 days after its acquisition by the index family member. A longer interval, 21 days, separated the appearance of overt skin disease among family members.[22, 34] Although streptococci were isolated from skin sites all over the body, impetigo lesions generally appeared on the exposed portions of the extremities, suggesting that cutaneous trauma is important in the development of skin lesions. In contrast to streptococcal colonization, staphylococcal colonization of the nose was found a mean of 13 days before the development of skin lesions in 65 per cent of episodes.[22]

Diagnosis and Treatment

The diagnosis of impetigo can be made by the clinical appearance of the lesions, their superficial nature, and the absence of systemic toxicity. Bacterial culture usually is unnecessary except when the presentation is atypical or when the patient has failed to respond to initial therapy. Therapy must be directed at both staphylococci and streptococci. For superficial, localized infections not involving the mouth, the recommended treatment is the topical antibiotic agent mupirocin, applied three times per day for 7 to 10 days. In controlled clinical trials, mupirocin was demonstrated to be as effective as erythromycin given by mouth in three or four divided doses and was associated with a lower incidence of adverse effects.[7, 9, 52, 57] For widespread infection or infection surrounding the mouth, an oral agent is indicated. Appropriate oral agents used generally for 10 days include erythromycin, clindamycin, dicloxacillin, and cephalexin.[6, 7, 9, 15, 23, 24, 26, 28, 44] The emergence of erythromycin-resistant *S. aureus* from impetigo lesions has resulted in a re-evaluation of the efficacy of erythromycin in this setting. The results have been conflicting, with some, but not all, groups concluding that in vitro resistance correlates with treatment failure.[21, 57, 59] Effective therapy for patients with impetigo can be expected to result in rapid healing of lesions and to prevent secondary cases in contacts and may prevent deep suppurative disease. If no response is observed within 7 days of treatment, antibiotic resistance or noncompliance should be suspected and a lesion should be cultured.

Prophylaxis

Simple cleanliness and prompt attention to minor wounds will do much to prevent impetigo. It is our practice to spend time teaching patients with established impetigo and their parents to bathe regularly and to apply antibiotic ointment to insect bites and early infected lesions as soon as they are noted, in hopes of preventing future overt disease. In a specific epidemic situation in which patients had poor hygiene and a high attack rate of streptococcal impetigo, prophylactic long-acting benzathine penicillin given intramuscularly was found to reduce the frequency of new impetigo lesions in treated children.[33] Although capable of reducing epidemic spread of impetigo under certain conditions, the prophylactic administration of benzathine penicillin generally is not indicated.

Patients with recurrent staphylococcal impetigo should be evaluated for nasal carriage of *S. aureus*. Application of mupirocin to the anterior nares four times daily has been shown to eliminate nasal carriage in the majority of patients within 2 to 4 days, although in many patients the nares become recolonized with the same phage type within months.[16, 31] To date, clinical trials evaluating the impact of elimination of *S. aureus* nasal carriage on recurrent impetigo have not been performed.

Prognosis

Superficial impetigo generally has a good outcome. Severe local and distant metastatic suppurative complications are quite rare but do occur. The nonsuppurative complication of acute poststreptococcal glomerulonephritis occurs more commonly and is of considerable importance. Streptococcal skin infections play the major etiologic role in the high seasonal occurrence of acute glomerulonephritis in the southeastern United States,[27, 28] in the recurrent outbreaks of nephritis at the Red Lake Indian Reservation,[3] in epidemic outbreaks in Trinidad,[65, 68] and in the high endemic prevalence of glomerulonephritis in children in tropical areas such as Hawaii. Certain types of streptococci, particularly the Red Lake strain, type 49, and types 2, 55, 56, and 31,[2, 88] have been demonstrated repeatedly to be more prevalent in impetigo resulting in nephritis, compared with uncomplicated impetigo. After infection with a nephritogenic strain of streptococci, the magnitude of the antistreptococcal antibody response measured by anti-DNAase B is significantly greater in those developing nephritis than in controls. This suggests that a hyperimmune mechanism is of central importance in the pathogenesis of glomerulonephritis.[29, 41] Treatment of established impetigo does not prevent the complication of acute poststreptococcal glomerulonephritis, at least in part because so much antigenic exposure has occurred before the patient presents for treatment.[22, 27, 29, 33, 41, 65, 88]

The pattern of antibody response is different after skin infection compared with throat infection. Elevated anti-DNAase B levels are seen after skin infection, with lesser or no elevation in antistreptolysin O titers; both antibodies tend to be elevated after throat infection. The Streptozyme test, which incorporates several antistreptococcal antibodies, should be positive after significant streptococcal skin infection and occasionally may be useful in retrospective diagnosis. This subject has been reviewed extensively.[88]

Bullous Impetigo

Clinical Features (see Fig. 67–17)

In the United States, bullous impetigo is considerably less common than is the thick-crusted variety and easily is differentiated by the characteristic superficial thin-walled bullae, ranging from 0.5 to 3 cm in diameter (Fig. 69–2). Although

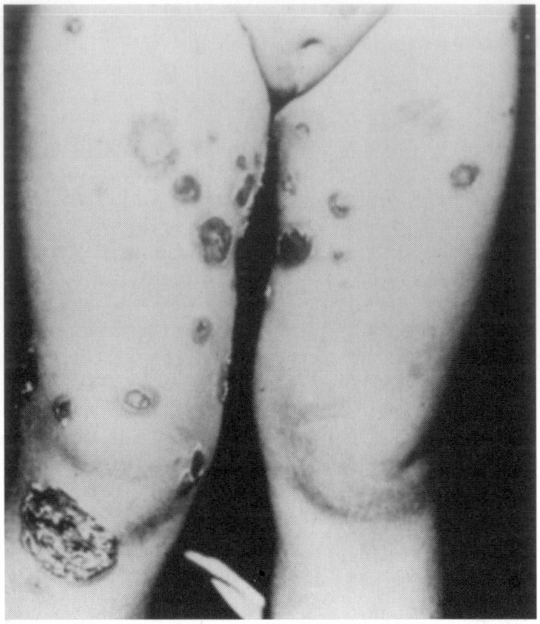

FIGURE 69–2. *Bullous impetigo is composed of superficial thin-walled bullae that spontaneously rupture to form circular plaques.*

there may be a thin ring of erythema surrounding the base of the individual lesion, the bullae usually arise from normal-appearing skin. Lesions are found most often in small groups of three to six bullae confined to a single area. In neonates, lesions are found most often on the perineum, periumbilical area, or both. In older children, the extremities are involved most frequently. Occasionally, extensive areas of skin are involved with extremely large numbers of bullae. Bullae may be either flaccid or tense but always appear to have thin, delicate walls. Fluid within bullae varies from clear to cloudy to frankly purulent. After the fragile bullae rupture, a thin, flat, clear varnish-like coating quickly forms over the denuded area (Fig. 69–3). This crust differs markedly from the thick "stuck-on" crusts associated with the more common form of impetigo. Also, in contrast to streptococcal impetigo, regional lymphadenopathy usually is absent.

Etiology

The etiology of bullous impetigo is exclusively staphylococcal. Staphylococci can be recovered in pure culture from aspirated bullous fluid.[23, 25, 54] Multiple studies of staphylococci isolated from bullous impetigo at first suggested that these staphylococci were limited to phage group II strains, most notably phage type 71.[14, 25, 63] The discovery of the staphylococcal epidermolytic toxins demonstrated the mechanism by which these particular staphylococci cause the characteristic bullae.[54] Epidermolytic toxins A and B, elaborated by many phage group II strains (3A, 3C, 55, and 71), also are elaborated by occasional strains of staphylococci belonging to other phage groups. Therefore, any staphylococci elaborating epidermolytic toxin may be responsible, whatever the phage type. No organisms other than staphylococci have been demonstrated to make these products. The toxins are low-molecular-weight proteins capable of disrupting the intercellular attachments of epidermal cells of the stratum granulosum.[50, 55] Epidermolytic toxin separates the upper layers of epidermis of both adult and infant human skin, other primate skin, and mouse skin. It is inactive in many other mammalian species. The genes encoding both toxin proteins have been cloned.[47, 62] Sequence analysis suggests that the toxins act as proteases. However, the specific skin substrate has not been identified.[4] Antibody to the form of epidermolytic toxin most common in the United States develops with age; it is found in the majority of adults and in children older than 5 years of age.[56]

Antitoxin antibody may be protective against the generalized forms of the staphylococcal scalded skin syndrome (Ritter disease, toxic epidermal necrolysis, staphylococcal scarlet fever) by preventing the hematogenous dissemination of epidermolytic toxin. In the localized lesions of bullous impetigo, antitoxin antibody does not appear to prevent the development of new lesions or to promote faster healing. In this situation, epidermolytic toxin is produced locally and acts locally; although antibody is able to neutralize toxin in the blood stream, it may be unable to neutralize toxin at the site of its action.

Histologic examination of skin lesions of bullous impetigo shows the development of a cleavage plane high in the epidermis at the stratum granulosum immediately below the cornified layer. Organisms and polymorphonuclear leukocytes may be seen within the bullae. Epidermolytic toxin also is present within the fluid of the bullae (Fig. 69–4).

Epidemiology

Bullous impetigo occurs in both endemic and epidemic patterns. Common-source, nursery-associated epidemics have

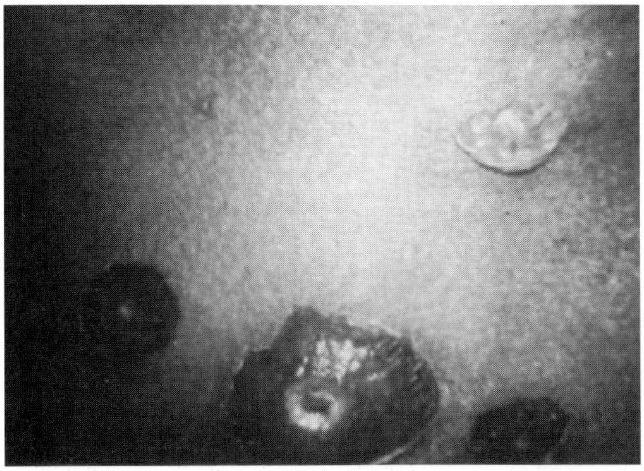

FIGURE 69–3. *The plaques of bullous impetigo dry to a thin, shiny, varnish-like veneer.*

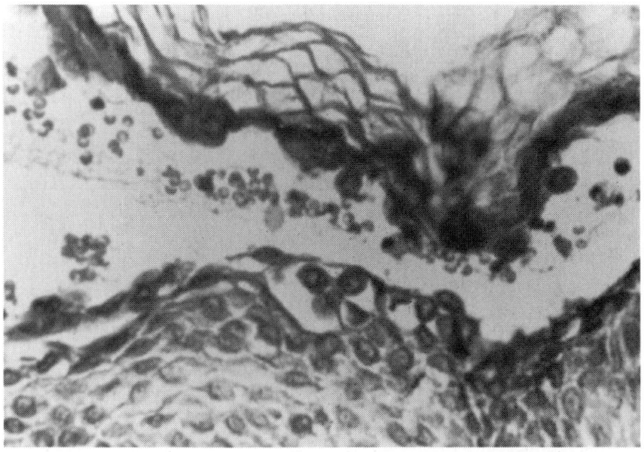

FIGURE 69–4. *The bullae in bullous impetigo are formed after cleavage of the superficial epidermis at the granular cell layer. Staphylococci, leukocytes, and epidermolytic toxin all are found within the bulla fluid.*

been noted repeatedly among neonates exposed to high rates of staphylococcal colonization. Staphylococcal skin disease rarely is manifested during the short neonatal hospital stay but becomes apparent within a month after discharge. If infection surveillance practices do not recognize that this nosocomial infection generally is manifested after hospital discharge, outbreaks of considerable size can be overlooked. In the United States since 1972, bullous impetigo appears to have been the most common manifestation of nursery-associated staphylococcal disease. A few more severely involved infants with generalized epidermolytic toxin–mediated skin disease (Ritter disease) are seen frequently in these outbreaks. Among older children in the United States, bullous impetigo generally has a sporadic incidence pattern. Small outbreaks may occur among family members or close contacts. Larger outbreaks have been reported, particularly in Britain,[63] but in the United States, bullous impetigo decidedly is less common than is the thick-crusted variety, accounting for only 7 per cent of 500 patients in Dillon's series from Alabama[25] and 8 per cent in a smaller, more recent study.[23] It is unclear whether abrasions or insect bites play as important a role in the initiation of bullous impetigo as they do in the thick-crusted variety.

Differential Diagnosis

When present in small groups in a single area, the lesions of bullous impetigo usually are recognized correctly, but confusion arises, particularly when single lesions or extensive involvement is present. Frequently, single lesions are mistaken for thermal burns; we have seen two cases in which child abuse mistakenly was alleged—the single bulla observed was thought to have resulted from a cigarette burn. Extensive lesions are likely to be confused with other bullous dermatoses of childhood, including dermatitis herpetiformis, bullous pemphigoid, pemphigus, and Stevens-Johnson syndrome. Firm diagnosis can be made by aspirating bullae, demonstrating polymorphonuclear leukocytes and gram-positive cocci in the aspirate, and culturing staphylococci from this material. Skin biopsy occasionally is necessary to secure diagnosis of extensive cases; the specimen will show a cleavage plane high in the epidermis. Organisms and polymorphonuclear leukocytes are found within the cleft. Examination of the biopsy specimen is definitive and rules out other bullous diseases.

Treatment

Systemic antistaphylococcal antibiotics, usually administered orally, are effective in eradicating the infection, which frequently progresses rapidly if untreated. Epidermolytic toxin–producing staphylococci overwhelmingly are penicillin-resistant. The semisynthetic β-lactamase–resistant penicillins, cephalosporins, erythromycin, or lincomycin-clindamycin antibiotics should be used for a 10-day course. Patients with bullous impetigo have been included in some of the clinical trials comparing oral antistaphylococcal antibiotics with mupirocin. Whether they were over- or under-represented in the relatively small group of patients whose mupirocin treatment failed was not reported.[7, 21, 52, 72] When effective systemic antibiotic therapy is employed, topical therapy is unnecessary.

Perianal Streptococcal Dermatitis

Perianal cellulitis secondary to group A beta-hemolytic streptococci first was described in 1966 in 10 patients who had marked perirectal erythema with moderate edema and tenderness.[1] This condition was recognized and further defined in the past decade. Kokx and associates[45] reported 31 patients encountered over a 9-month period in a single pediatric practice, suggesting that the infection is common. Signs and symptoms include superficial, sharply marginated perineal erythema with local tenderness and pruritus. Rectal pain usually on defecation occurs in one-half and blood in stools in one-third of patients seen. Fever and other signs of systemic illness were not seen. Regional lymphadenopathy was not recognized in any series. Group A beta-hemolytic streptococci in heavy growth were recovered from perianal surface cultures in all patients, and direct antigen tests on swabs were positive in more than 85 per cent tested. More than half of the patients had the same T type of *Streptococcus* in pharyngeal cultures.[1, 45, 46, 51, 78] In two studies, control groups of asymptomatic children were tested for the presence of perianal streptococci. Six per cent were found to have streptococci, usually with sparse growth of organisms in contrast to the heavy growth found in patients.[1, 45] Intrafamilial spread of perianal dermatitis was common.[1, 45] Treatment with systemic antistreptococcal agents results in prompt eradication of symptoms in most cases, but recurrences were seen in more than one-third in the largest series.[45] In patients with recurrent or persistent disease, repeat courses of penicillin were not always successful, and treatment with clindamycin or penicillin plus rifampin ultimately was required for the eradication of symptoms. Successful treatment with topical mupirocin has been reported.[53]

Although this condition originally was termed perianal streptococcal cellulitis and bears a superficial resemblance to erysipelas with the intense, sharply marginated erythema, the absence of systemic symptoms and progressive disease is evidence that this is a superficial lesion and not a true cellulitis.[45, 46]

Folliculitis, Furunculosis, and Carbuncles

This group of infections is characterized by a common origin in hair follicles, abscess formation with central purulence, and a common etiology, nearly always coagulase-positive staphylococci. Folliculitis, the most limited of these infections, refers to small abscesses, each involving only a single follicle, with very limited surrounding tissue reaction. Furuncles also develop about hair follicles but become deeper inflammatory nodules surrounded by a zone of intense tissue reaction (Fig. 69–5). Carbuncles are considerably more extensive, with wider and deeper tissue infiltration, and generally are made up of several interconnecting furuncles or abscesses.

Epidemiology

These infections are fairly common among children of all age groups. Widespread folliculitis and furunculosis were seen commonly among neonates and their families in the nursery-associated staphylococcal outbreaks of the 1950s. Recently, more of these outbreaks have taken the form of bullous impetigo. Beyond infancy, late school age and adolescent children appear somewhat more prone to these pyodermas. Clusters of infection involving multiple family members are seen frequently, and conventional wisdom suggests that towels, washcloths, and shared items of clothing and bedding may be involved in transmission. Poor hygiene appears to be a powerful contributing force, but some persons with meticulous hygiene are subject to recurrent disease.

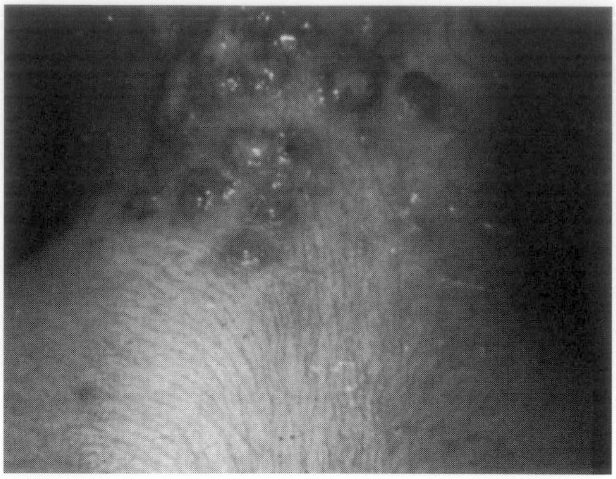

FIGURE 69–5. *Furunculosis. All stages in the formation of superficial staphylococcal abscesses are represented here, from early folliculitis, to the older nodular inflammatory furuncles, to the small carbuncle made up of multiple interconnecting furuncles.*

Pathophysiology and Clinical Presentation

Lesions are limited to hair-bearing areas and are most prevalent in the axilla, breast area, perineum, extremities, and neck. In most cases, lesions appear to arise de novo with no preexisting focus implicated. Small lesions of folliculitis frequently are self-limited, responding to scrubbing and soaks, whereas larger lesions tend to persist, progressing to a firm, painful, erythematous nodule. With time, a thick-walled abscess becomes established with a purulent necrotic center that may rupture spontaneously. The duration of untreated lesions is extremely variable. Although most infections are contained well by an intense local inflammatory reaction, spread to surrounding tissues—manifested as extensive cellulitis—may occur at any time, even in the normal host. Metastatic dissemination of organisms or direct extension to deeper tissues, such as underlying bone, also may be noted. The likelihood of extension is much greater in patients whose inflammatory reaction is compromised by corticosteroid therapy or neutropenia.

Coagulase-positive staphylococci nearly always are the cause of this group of pyodermas, particularly in the absence of trauma to the skin. Infections that begin in contaminated wounds may appear later as abscesses that look like staphylococcal furuncles. In these cases, a wide variety of organisms may be responsible.

Outbreaks of hot tub–, swimming pool–, and whirlpool-associated folliculitis due to *P. aeruginosa* have been described in several epidemiologic reports. Pruritus, malaise, and low-grade fever are associated features. The infection is self-limited, generally resolving without treatment within 7 to 14 days.[17, 40, 89] Recurrent eruptions may occur if the recreational or nonrecreational source is not identified and exposures recur.[84]

Certain patients are subject to recurrent staphylococcal abscesses. Although impaired circulation and diabetes mellitus have been cited as predisposing causes, the majority of patients with this problem have neither condition. Hill and colleagues[42, 43] have reported abnormal neutrophil chemotaxis in various groups of patients subject to recurrent staphylococcal abscesses, including patients with atopy, elevated IgE, and chronic eczema.

In our experience with patients with recurrent abscesses, no abnormality has been found in white blood cell function when phagocytosis, nitroblue tetrazolium dye reduction, ability to respond to phagocytosis with a metabolic burst, and in vitro chemotaxis were studied. The reasons for predilection to recurrent staphylococcal infection remain obscure for most patients.

Diagnosis and Management

The diagnosis of furunculosis can be made by inspection. Early lesions can be treated with warm soaks to encourage spontaneous drainage. Larger localized lesions should be incised and drained. Gram stain of pus recovered should be performed if the lesions are atypical or if the history suggests that organisms other than *S. aureus* may be involved, particularly when infection occurs secondary to trauma. If organisms other than gram-positive cocci are seen, culture should be done. Patients with an extensive carbuncle or a carbuncle or furuncle associated with cellulitis or fever should be treated with systemic antistaphylococcal antibiotics for 7 to 10 days. Application of bacitracin ointment around the lesion after drainage protects the surrounding skin. Patients should be cautioned that draining lesions are a potential source of infection to others and that they should not be allowed to work as food handlers or to have direct contact with hospitalized patients until the lesion has healed. After drainage has occurred, erythema and edema subside, but a dense scar is a frequent sequel to all but very small lesions.

The most serious problem associated with these pyodermas is local or metastatic spread of infection. This can be minimized by prompt therapy. Febrile, systemically ill patients always should be evaluated by cultures of blood and lesions and have a careful search for metastatic foci that may be present in the heart, bones, joints, deep tissues, or brain.

Evaluation and treatment of the child with recurrent furunculosis pose a challenge. Careful history and physical examination should be performed, looking for evidence of breaks in the skin barrier. Chronic dermatoses, such as eczema, ichthyosis, and seborrhea, may be predisposing factors. In adults, diabetes mellitus is mentioned frequently as a predisposing factor to recurrent furunculosis. The reason for the association noted in adults is unclear. It may be secondary to poor perfusion, to depressed granulocytic chemotactic function noted in diabetic ketoacidosis, or to some undefined host factors. As discussed earlier, tests of white blood cell function, including qualitative nitroblue tetrazolium dye reduction, phagocytosis, and chemotaxis, may be indicated. Except for nitroblue tetrazolium dye reduction, these tests are not widely available. It is unclear whether diabetes itself predisposes to recurrence of staphylococcal infections in children.

Prophylaxis against recurrent disease should be attempted. The patient should be instructed in a strict regimen of personal hygiene, including hexachlorophene soap,[74] showers rather than baths, and one-time-only use of washcloths and towels. Skin trauma and irritants such as deodorants should be avoided. The patient should have antibiotic ointment to apply to small wounds and should not share bed linens or clothes with other family members. Dressings from draining skin lesions should be changed frequently.

At present, there are no other safe and effective prophylactic measures for patients with recurrent staphylococcal infection. Many of these patients continue to develop infections despite meticulous hygiene, good diet, and good general health. Some have periods of recurrent infection followed by long periods with no problems. Patients with these problems are easy prey for those who claim great benefits from dietary measures, megavitamins, and so on, and they should be given anticipatory guidance to help them evaluate these claims. The therapies offered by medical practitioners also should be scrutinized carefully. Various staphylococcal vaccines have been used but have not been evaluated well, and no benefit has been demonstrated. A careful search for nasal colonization and its elimination by bacitracin or mupirocin ointment or by the brief administration of systemic antibiotics are of unproven worth but are relatively innocuous.

CONTAMINATED WOUNDS

A list of all the circumstances under which skin injury occurs and the organisms that may cause infection in these wounds would be very long. Infections of the greatest clinical importance in pediatrics are those arising in human and animal bites, soil-contaminated wounds, water-contaminated wounds, thermal burns, and surgical wounds. Staphylococci and streptococci, being ubiquitous and frequently found on the normal skin, may be involved in any of these infections. This fact is so well known that there is an assumption widely acted on that these organisms are the likely cause of infection in nearly all skin wounds. Failure to consider the pathogenic potential of other organisms as well as failure to provide adequate drainage often leads to inadequate therapy. Management of infected wounds requires careful collection of the exudate from deep within the wound, Gram stain of the exudate, and careful culture and identification of all organisms present. Multiple agents are involved frequently.

Human Bites

Human bites, particularly those involving the hand, may result in rapidly progressive and extremely destructive infections of the soft tissues, tendons, joints, and bone. Bite injuries are sustained frequently by a fist blow to the mouth, which results in an apparently trivial laceration by a tooth over the metacarpophalangeal joint, as well as by full-mouth bites to the hand or fingers. Infections nearly always are polymicrobial and involve staphylococci, anaerobic gram-positive mouth flora, aerobic streptococci, and mouth spirochetes. Infections typically develop rapidly, within 24 hours of injury, and the pus is foul-smelling.

Because only those patients receiving treatment are included, the exact proportion of human bites that do become infected is unknown, although it is believed to be high.[5, 8, 77] Disturbed by a retrospective study of human bite–associated hand infections, which showed that two-thirds of the infections developed despite early medical attention to the bite, Chuinard and D'Ambrosia[19] developed a protocol that apparently reduced the incidence of serious complications in a group of patients studied prospectively. They stressed careful examination of the wound after tourniquet application to allow a bloodless field, excisional débridement, copious irrigation, and provision for adequate external drainage by means of a wick. Antibiotics (cephalosporins or antistaphylococcal penicillin) were given to all patients, and the wound was followed carefully with daily dressing changes. Human bites should never be sutured or closed early. Analysis of the organisms involved demonstrates that antibiotic therapy should be directed at staphylococci and mouth anaerobes that are sensitive to penicillin. High oral doses of penicillinase-resistant penicillins or cephalosporins will cover these organisms. Alternatively, clindamycin or erythromycin may be used in the penicillin-allergic patient. Infections frequently develop despite antibiotic coverage if débridement is not performed or if the wound is closed. For severe infection requiring parenteral antibiotics, cefoxitin, a first-generation cephalosporin plus a penicillinase-resistant penicillin, or ticarcillin–clavulanate potassium generally will provide the coverage needed.

Many patients seek treatment with established infection. For any but minor infections, and particularly when the hand is involved, these patients need radical débridement, deep wound culture, and a period of intravenous antibiotic treatment.

Animal Bites

Animal bites apparently are somewhat less likely to become infected than are human bites. When infection occurs, it most often is polymicrobial, with the most frequent isolates being *S. aureus*, anaerobic cocci, and *Pasteurella multocida*, a short gram-negative rod.[11, 48] In the clinical laboratory, *P. multocida* has been confused with *Neisseria, Haemophilus influenzae,* and *Mima polymorpha* by colony characteristics, but it can be distinguished readily by its growth and biochemical characteristics. Principles of preventive management of animal bites include careful inspection, débridement, and irrigation. Primary suturing of the wound increases infection risks, so that if suturing of the wound is performed, prophylatic antibiotic therapy should be given and daily follow-up examinations of the wound should be performed. Penicillin provides coverage against *P. multocida,* streptococci, and most anaerobes. If staphylococci are suspected, a first-generation cephalosporin or a pencillinase-resistant penicillin should be added. It should be recognized that infection may develop despite early antibiotic treatment.[83] The characteristics of the infection are the rapid development and progression to cellulitis or abscess formation, marked local tenderness, and pain. Resolution is slow, despite débridement, drainage, and appropriate antibiotic therapy. Lymphadenopathy, systemic toxicity, and osteomyelitis may occur. Tenosynovitis and osteomyelitis are associated particularly with cat bites, apparently because the sharp teeth of a cat are more likely to penetrate and inoculate tendons, joint spaces, and the periosteum.[82, 83]

Soil-Contaminated Wounds

A wide variety of organisms, including gram-negative enterics and gas-forming anaerobes, such as those responsible for gas gangrene and tetanus, may contaminate and cause infection in dirty wounds. Prevention of infection should be practiced by complete exploration, adequate débridement, copious irrigation, and avoidance of early closure. Gas gangrene (clostridial cellulitis or myositis), the most dreaded complication of contaminated wounds, can be prevented only by making the local environment unsatisfactory for the growth of clostridia. To do this, foreign bodies must be removed, devitalized tissue excised, and drainage promoted.

The same principles apply in the management of the obviously infected wound. The wound area should be inspected carefully for signs of rapidly progressive extension or for characteristics of clostridial cellulitis. Rapid progression, bullae, crepitation of surrounding tissues, or evidence of gas in the subcutaneous tissue seen by radiograph suggests this diagnosis. Gram stain of the exudate may show gram-positive rods. Clostridial cellulitis requires extensive surgical débridement with multiple incisions into the involved tissue. Large intravenous doses of penicillin (300,000 units/kg/day) should be given. Less extensive wound infections or abscesses also should be managed by débridement, by obtaining exudate from deep in the wound for Gram stain and culture, and by provision for drainage. Pending culture results, combinations of an antistaphylococcal penicillin and an aminoglycoside, such as gentamicin, or a third-generation cephalosporin should be given for all but the most trivial infections.

Water-Contaminated Wounds

Infection arising in wounds sustained in or contaminated by stagnant fresh water may become infected with organisms found in stagnant water, particularly *Aeromonas hydrophila* or pseudomonads and coliforms. *Aeromonas* inoculated in this manner may cause extensive necrotizing wound infections characterized by rapid progression, even in healthy hosts. *Aeromonas* and pseudomonads are resistant to penicillin and ampicillin but sensitive to chloramphenicol, third-generation cephalosporins, trimethoprim-sulfamethoxazole, and some aminoglycosides, such as gentamicin and tobramycin.[38, 66, 76, 85]

Surgical Wounds

Surgical wound infections continue to be caused predominantly by coagulase-positive staphylococci and by group A beta-hemolytic streptococci. In abdominal wounds with peritonitis, anaerobic and aerobic enteric floras may be etiologic agents.

The responsible organisms are inoculated into the wound at the time of surgery. The size of the inoculum capable of causing infection varies with the organisms. Under experimental conditions, as few as 10^2 group A beta-hemolytic streptococci may cause infection, whereas wound tissue may resist more than 10^7 coagulase-positive staphylococci. The condition of the wound plays a major role in resistance to infection; the presence of hematoma, necrotic tissue, diminished blood supply, or foreign bodies decreases the innate local resistance to infection. For example, a braided suture alone has been demonstrated to alter resistance such that an inoculum of 10^4 staphylococci easily initiates infection.

The clinical manifestations of wound infection vary with the infecting organism. For staphylococcal and enteric organisms, the onset usually is insidious and delayed until 4 to 6 days after surgery. Generally, low-grade fever or mild systemic signs, such as increased anorexia or lethargy, are noted first, signs difficult to evaluate in postoperative patients. The wound itself may not show edema, erythema, and tenderness for 1 to 2 days after the onset of fever. Daily inspection, gentle probing, and removal of a stitch are indicated and frequently reveal exudate deep within the wound. When surgery is performed for peritonitis secondary to a ruptured viscus, it should be remembered that gram-negative enterics, particularly the anaerobe *Bacteroides fragilis,* may cause infection. Gram stain of the exudate distinguishes between the gram-positive staphylococci and the gram-negative enterics.

The wound should be opened sufficiently to allow drainage and to demonstrate the extent of involvement. Antibiotics should be given to prevent dissemination of infection but are less important than is provision for surgical drainage. Staphylococcal infections should be treated with an antistaphylococcal penicillin. Postoperative wound infections often are treated with ampicillin or a cephalosporin prior to culture results or in the absence of culture. This is a particularly ill-advised strategy. Neither antibiotic provides broad gram-negative coverage, and, most importantly, *B. fragilis* usually is resistant to both. Chloramphenicol, clindamycin, and cefoxitin are the agents most effective against *B. fragilis;* aminoglycosides, particularly gentamicin, provide the most complete coverage against gram-negative aerobes.

Fortunately, group A beta-hemolytic streptococcal wound infections are less common, accounting for only 3 per cent of wound infections encountered in one large series from a general surgical service.[30] These infections occur earlier, usually within 1 to 2 days of the operation, and are characterized by high fever, leukocytosis, and tachycardia. The wound may appear normal, but deep aspiration may reveal gram-positive cocci on Gram stain and streptococci on culture. Because postoperative streptococcal infections may be severe and fulminant, a high degree of suspicion, careful wound evaluation and aspiration, and prompt antibiotic therapy when gram-positive cocci are found are essential. In overwhelming streptococcal disease, clindamycin should be used rather than penicillin because of the decreased efficacy of penicillin against streptococci at the stationary growth phase.[80] If Gram stain clearly does not show the cocci to be in chains, differentiating them from staphylococci, methicillin or oxacillin may be used instead of penicillin, at doses of 100 to 200 mg/kg/day.

ERYSIPELAS

Erysipelas (Fig. 69–6) refers to a specific form of superficial cellulitis that is caused by group A beta-hemolytic streptococci and that involves the dermis and uppermost portions of the subcutaneous tissue layer. There is marked involvement of the superficial lymphatics. The characteristic appearance consists of a rapidly enlarging, deeply erythematous plaque with a sharply demarcated, slightly elevated, advancing margin. The involved skin is painful to the touch and indurated and frequently has a peau d'orange appearance. Occasionally, large tension bullae develop in the erythematous zone. The lesion advances rapidly and may involve large areas of skin (the entire trunk or extremities) within a 12-hour period. Patients generally have fever and chills and appear quite toxic. The leukocyte count is elevated, with a polymorphonuclear predominance.

The portal of entry of streptococci may be a surgical wound, the umbilicus in a newborn, or any break in the skin. However, the initiating lesion frequently is trivial or inapparent. In nonsurgical erysipelas, the older literature indicates that the face is involved most commonly and that the rash frequently shows a butterfly distribution over the nose and cheeks. It also is stated that the neonate and the elderly are most likely to be affected. This is at variance with our own experience, as we have encountered erysipelas most frequently as a circumferential, rapidly progressive lesion of the extremities, particularly the legs, in preschool children or schoolchildren. In a retrospective study including 535 patients, Chartier and Grosshans[18] found the lower extremities involved in 85 per cent of the cases. We also have encountered it in association with surgical wounds in children and young adults on several occasions.

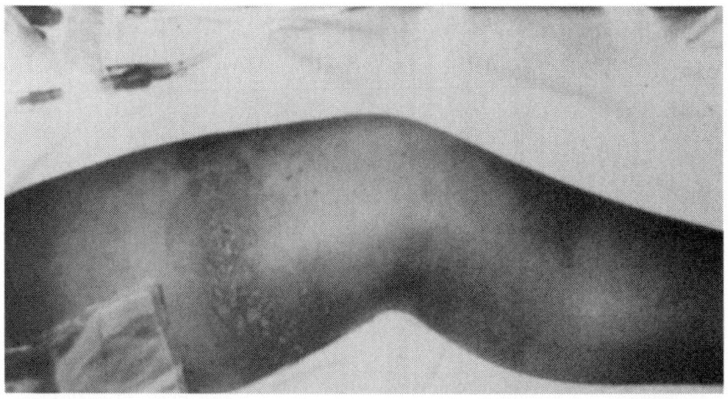

FIGURE 69–6. *Erysipelas. A sharply demarcated, tender band of indurated erythema surrounds the leg. A collection of small bullae is seen at the upper border.*

Histologically, the dermis and uppermost subcutaneous tissue show intense edema with vascular dilatation. The lymphatic channels and tissue spaces are infiltrated heavily with streptococci and polymorphonuclear leukocytes.

Streptococci can be recovered by aspiration of the superficial tissue of the lesion, particularly at the advancing margin. Whenever there is a central or initiation wound, this often is found to be infected with streptococci and also is a good source for culture. Frequently, streptococci are present in the throat, and an antistreptolysin O titer rise can be demonstrated in convalescence.

Because of the acute toxicity of patients and because of the rapidity of spread of this lesion, we take an aggressive approach to its management. With the intense, superficial, sharply demarcated erythema and edema, the diagnosis is recognizable immediately on clinical grounds alone. We prefer intravenous antibiotic therapy (preferably penicillin) for an initial period of 24 to 48 hours, followed by oral therapy. Fever subsides within 24 hours of the initiation of therapy, and the progression of the lesion rapidly halts, but erythema and edema in the tissues already involved may persist for 2 to 5 days. After a clinical response is obtained, oral antibiotic therapy may be given to complete a 10-day course.

Erysipelas, more colorfully and descriptively called St. Anthony's fire in the Middle Ages, is treated frequently as a historic curiosity rarely encountered in the antibiotic era. This is at variance with our experience, as we have encountered it frequently in such diverse locales as upper New York State, Southern California, and Hawaii.

CELLULITIS

Cellulitis refers to a group of infections in which the subcutaneous tissue primarily is involved with an additional involvement of the dermis. Usually, the epidermis itself is not affected. Cellulitis is manifested by an area of edema, erythema, warmth, and tenderness. Erysipelas is a distinctive and superficial member of the cellulitis group and one whose etiology can be diagnosed reliably on clinical grounds alone. Because the cellulitis infections other than erysipelas involve deeper layers of the subcutaneous tissue, the lateral margin of involvement is indistinct, with erythema and edema gradually merging with the surrounding unaffected area.

A wide variety of organisms may cause cellulitis, particularly after trauma or in immunocompromised hosts, but the most common organisms implicated are coagulase-positive staphylococci, group A beta-hemolytic streptococci, and, until recently, *H. influenzae* type b. Staphylococcal infections tend to be more localized and more likely to have a purulent center; streptococcal infections tend to spread more rapidly, and *H. influenzae* type b infections may have a peculiar, deep blue-red coloration. None of these features is pathognomonic, and a careful search for the responsible organism must be undertaken. Streptococcal and staphylococcal cellulitis may occur at any site and among persons of any age. These infections generally are associated with previous trauma or infection in the area involved, although the site of inoculation may be trivial or overlooked. Because of the association with previous trauma, most cellulitis occurs on the extremities. Cellulitis may extend to involve deeper underlying tissues and is associated particularly with osteomyelitis and septic arthritis.

Haemophilus influenzae Type B Cellulitis

H. influenzae type b cellulitis has some unique characteristics. Although not limited to young children, generally it occurs at the age of greatest risk for disease due to *H. influenzae* type b (from 3 months to 4 years, with the peak at approximately 9 months). Fortunately, the incidence of *H. influenzae* type b cellulitis has declined dramatically since the initiation of routine immunization. Unlike other forms of cellulitis, it is associated nearly always with systemic disease because most patients are bacteremic. Although it may occur on the extremities, most often it has been described as a unilateral infection of the cheek. The reason for the observed affinity to the cheek has not been explained. An association of cheek cellulitis with ipsilateral otitis media has been noted, and the hypothesis has been advanced that the cheek infection results from extension of middle ear infection through lymphatic channels to the buccinator nodes. Many patients with *H. influenzae* type b cellulitis manifest a recognizable deep blue-red or purple discoloration, which has been reported by many to be pathognomonic for this condition. This feature is not universal by any means, nor is a dusty purple hue limited to this form of cellulitis.[37, 58, 70]

Diagnosis

The presence of cellulitis is recognized easily. Fever is nearly universal with *H. influenzae* type b infections and is found in most patients with other forms of cellulitis, unless the area of involvement is very limited. Blood culture should be performed; it is likely to be positive in patients with *H. influenzae* type b disease but generally is negative in streptococcal and staphylococcal infections. Aspiration of the infected area may yield the etiologic agent and should be attempted in all cases. The technique and site of aspiration have not been evaluated formally, but empirically it would seem that the most inflamed central portion and not the advancing margin would be the most appropriate place to sample. In erysipelas, the advancing margin is most likely to contain the organism, but in other types of cellulitis, the advancing margin is indistinct and probably represents only the edema, which extends from the site of more active infection. We employ a No. 22 needle on a 3-mL syringe. We inject 0.1 mL of sterile water or sterile saline (without preservative) into the subcutaneous tissue and then exert negative pressure on the syringe to recover fluid. If no fluid returns, we send the syringe and needle directly to the laboratory to be rinsed with culture medium.

Treatment

Although Gram stains of aspirates may allow an early presumptive diagnosis of the offending agent, in many cases therapy necessarily will be started on empiric grounds before the culture results are known. If the aspirate Gram stain is negative, coverage for both streptococci and staphylococci should be provided for most cases of cellulitis. An antistaphylococcal penicillin or first-generation cephalosporin given intravenously is sufficient coverage for both organisms. In underimmunized children younger than 4 years of age, coverage for *H. influenzae* type b should be provided for facial cellulitis. If the cellulitis is located on the extremities, it is less likely to be due to *H. influenzae* type b, but coverage still should be provided if the child has high fever and significant toxicity, if the child has evidence of infection elsewhere (such as meningitis, septic arthritis, or pneumonia), or if the lesion has a peculiar blue-purple discoloration. Adequate coverage for streptococci, staphylococci, *Streptococcus pneumoniae*, and *H. influenzae* can be provided by cefotaxime or ceftriaxone.

In dealing with cellulitis in an immunocompromised patient, maximum efforts should be made to identify an etiologic agent because a wide variety of organisms may be involved. Empiric therapy in the compromised host should include coverage for *Pseudomonas* and gram-negative enterics as well as more common etiologic agents. This can be achieved by using an aminoglycoside in combination with a systemic antistaphylococcal penicillin or third-generation cephalosporin, such as ceftazidime.

Once antibiotics have been started, therapy should be given for a total of at least 10 days, but intravenous administration may be discontinued whenever erythema, warmth, and edema have shown marked reduction. Application of warm compresses to the affected area may promote suppuration and drainage and increase patient comfort. If abscess formation occurs within the lesion, it should be drained surgically.

NECROTIZING CELLULITIS AND NECROTIZING FASCIITIS

A confusing terminology has arisen around a group of infections characterized by involvement of cutaneous and subcutaneous tissues, together with some degree of involvement of deeper underlying tissues of the fascia and muscle. Precision in terminology is hampered by difficulty in determining the exact tissue planes involved in each case. Additional confusion is provided because different etiologic agents, often acting synergistically, may be responsible for infections with similar clinical manifestations. Terms that have been used for infections that overlap in their clinical manifestations include the following:

Necrotizing fasciitis
Acute streptococcal hemolytic gangrene
Synergistic necrotizing cellulitis
Progressive synergistic gangrene
Meleney synergistic gangrene
Bacterial synergistic gangrene
Gangrenous erysipelas
Necrotizing erysipelas

All these terms refer to extensive cellulitis with severe involvement of subcutaneous tissue, including fascia, muscle, or both. Necrosis of underlying tissue and a need for surgical débridement are characteristic of these infections.

Microbiology

Most often, more than one etiologic agent is found.[12, 36] A synergistic relationship between an aerobe (such as *S. aureus*, group A beta-hemolytic *Streptococcus*, or a gram-negative enteric organism) and one or more anaerobes (such as *Peptostreptococcus, Prevotella*, and *Porphyromonas* species and *B. fragilis* group) is encountered frequently. *Pseudomonas* species and gram-negative enteric organisms often are isolated in neutropenic patients.[61] Synergistic infection is not essential to the pathogenesis: single organisms may be equally destructive.

Clinical Manifestations

Initially, infections in this group appear much like ordinary cellulitis, with erythema, edema, and tenderness. The severity of pain, however, often is out of proportion to the physical findings. The area of involvement rapidly becomes extensive. The induration is marked, frequently extending beyond the area of erythema. A dusky area indicating poor perfusion of tissue frequently appears. Blebs and bullae often occur, and areas of skin necrosis become apparent, generally in the center of the involved area. Infections in the necrotizing fasciitis/necrotizing cellulitis group can be separated from gas gangrene clinically by the absence of gas or crepitance in the tissues. Many patients with necrotizing fasciitis develop severe systemic illness and remarkable general debilitation. Edema, hypoproteinemia, and proteinuria may develop before the process is halted. Hypocalcemia, related to deposition of calcium in necrotic tissue, is seen in a considerable number of patients.

Suspicion of necrotizing fasciitis warrants immediate surgical consultation because both definitive diagnosis and therapy are made surgically. The most characteristic aspect of the clinical course of these infections is their relentless progress, despite administration of antibiotic therapy effective against the responsible agent (even in large doses by parenteral routes).

Risk factors for the development of necrotizing fasciitis include congenital and acquired immunodeficiencies, varicella, trauma, and surgery.[10, 32, 61] In neonates, omphalitis and circumcision are predisposing conditions.[39] The use of nonsteroidal anti-inflammatory agents may contribute to progression by impairing granulocytic function.[73]

Diagnosis

A microbiologic diagnosis may be made by the isolation of bacteria from blood, tissue aspirate, or wounds. A laboratory search for anaerobic organisms should be made. Smears or biopsied specimens of affected tissue should be examined for the presence of organisms, particularly because previous antibiotic therapy may have rendered cultures sterile without halting the clinical progression.

Diagnosis of the tissue plane involved is more important than microbiologic diagnosis is because it leads to effective surgical débridement. An incision extending to the fascia should be made with an attempt to pass a probe laterally along the fascial plane. If necrotic fascia or subcutaneous tissue is present, the probe will move easily through the tissues. A thin, serous, frequently malodorous liquid may run from the wound. Material removed from necrotic areas should be cultured and Gram stained.

Delays in diagnosis and proper surgical treatment are associated with significantly higher morbidity and mortality.[49] In children, the severity of extremity pain may make an adequate physical examination difficult. The use of magnetic resonance imaging may facilitate early diagnosis.[69, 91] Definitive diagnosis, however, requires surgical exploration.

Treatment

Surgical débridement of necrotic tissue is the sine qua non of effective therapy. After confirmation of subcutaneous, fascial, or muscle necrosis, extensive incision and débridement of fat, fascia, and any involved muscle to the limits of the involved area must be carried out. It has been a common experience that unless débridement extending to healthy tissue is made, the surgery will have to be repeated (Fig. 69–7).[8, 71, 81, 90] The adequacy of resection may be established by frozen biopsy or by resection to freely bleeding margins. Postoperatively, frequent dressing changes are necessary to débride remaining devitalized tissue.

Antibiotic therapy and meticulous supportive care should be seen as adjuncts to surgery that may be necessary for resolution of infection and very frequently for survival. Whereas Gram staining provides important information re-

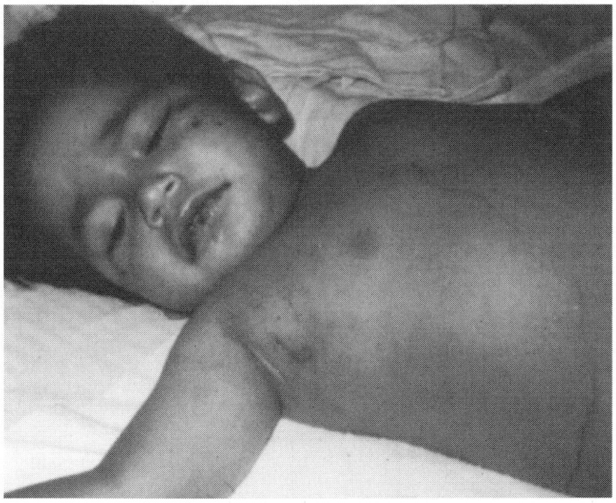

FIGURE 69–7. *Necrotizing fasciitis. The patient had fever and a large area of erythema surrounding a central necrotic lesion under the axilla. The area of erythema is outlined in ink on the chest; it extended to the midline in back. At surgery, extensive necrosis of the fascia of the pectoralis major and latissimus dorsi muscles was present.*

garding the relative significance of organisms cultured, initial empiric therapy should provide coverage for mixed aerobic and anaerobic infection. Combinations of a penicillinase-resistant penicillin, such as nafcillin, and an aminoglycoside, such as gentamicin, or a third-generation cephalosporin should be used until culture results are available. Antibiotics of the penicillin group cover anaerobes, with the exception of *B. fragilis* found in the bowel. Clindamycin, chloramphenicol, or cefoxitin is the drug of choice when *B. fragilis* is encountered. Clindamycin also is recommended in situations in which specimens yield only group A beta-hemolytic *Streptococcus* because penicillin has inferior efficacy in this clinical setting.[79]

Prognosis

Patients with infections of the necrotizing fasciitis/cellulitis group tend to become seriously ill and may die if not treated promptly. Supportive care should include careful fluid therapy, evaluation for hypocalcemia, and adequate nutritional support. The extensive surgical débridement often needed may require a prolonged convalescence and rehabilitation for the patient, including skin grafting and physical therapy.

MYCOBACTERIAL SKIN INFECTION

Mycobacterial skin infections are encountered occasionally in children, most often in the form of chronic granulomatous lesions in traumatized sites. Swimming pool granuloma, caused by *Mycobacterium marinum,* arises most frequently in abrasions sustained in swimming pools or from fish tanks.[67] Histologically, noncaseating granuloma extending to the dermis or subcutaneous tissues may be seen. The Langerhans giant cells are present, whereas the organisms may or may not be seen.

Clinically, the infection is indolent, with no systemic manifestations. Solitary bluish-red nodular lesions appear at a site of previous trauma and enlarge over a 2- to 3-week period. They may break down and crust. Lymphangitis and lymphadenopathy are very rare.[35, 60]

The organisms generally are resistant to most antituberculous drugs. Minocycline, trimethoprim-sulfamethoxazole, and clarithromycin may be effective.[13, 87] The lesions tend to heal spontaneously within a few months. Surgical excision has been attempted, but local recurrence may be observed.

Mycobacterium chelonea, a rapid-growing atypical mycobacterium, characteristically produces multiple, minimally tender, subcutaneous nodules, which may or may not drain. Similar to *M. marinum,* it is resistant to most available antimicrobials with the exception of clarithromycin.[86]

References

1. Amron, D. P., Anderson, A. S., and Wannamaker, L. W.: Perianal cellulitis associated with group A streptococci. Am. J. Dis. Child. *112*:546–552, 1966.
2. Anthony, B. B., Kaplan, E. L., Chapman, S. S., et al.: Epidemic acute nephritis with reappearance of type 49 *Streptococcus*. Lancet 2:787–790, 1967.
3. Anthony, B. F., Perlman, L. V., and Wannamaker, L. W.: Skin infections and acute nephritis in American Indian children. Pediatrics *39*:263–269, 1967.
4. Bailey, C. J., Lockhart, B. P., Redpath, M. B., et al.: The epidermolytic (exfoliative) toxins of *Staphylococcus aureus*. Med. Microbiol. Immunol. *184*:53–61, 1995.
5. Baker, M. D., and Moore, S. E.: Human bites in children: A six-year experience. Am. J. Dis. Child. *141*:1285–1290, 1987.
6. Barton, L. L., and Friedman, A. D.: Impetigo: A reassessment of etiology and therapy. Pediatr. Dermatol. *4*:185–188, 1987.
7. Barton, L. L., Friedman, A. D., Sharkey, A. M., et al.: Impetigo contagiosa. III. Compartive efficacy of oral erythromycin and topical mupirocin. Pediatr. Dermatol. *6*:134–138, 1989.
8. Baxter, C. R.: Surgical management of soft tissue infections. Surg. Clin. North Am. *52*:1483–1499, 1972.
9. Britton, J. W., Fajardo, J. E., and Krafte-Jacobs, B.: Comparison of mupirocin and erythromycin in the treatment of impetigo. J. Pediatr. *117*:827–829, 1990.
10. Brogan, T. V., Nizet, V., Waldhausen, J. H. T., et al.: Group A streptococcal necrotizing fasciitis complicating primary varicella: A series of fourteen patients. Pediatr. Infect. Dis. J. *14*:588–594, 1995.
11. Brook, I.: Microbiology of human and animal bite wounds in children. Pediatr. Infect. Dis. J. *6*:29–32, 1987.
12. Brook, I., and Frazier, E. H.: Clinical and microbiological features of necrotizing fasciitis. J. Clin. Microbiol. *33*:2382–2386, 1995.
13. Brown, B. A., Wallace, R. J., Jr., and Onyi, G. O.: Activities of clarithromycin against eight slowly growing species of nontuberculous mycobacteria, determined by using broth microdilution MIC system. Antimicrob. Agents Chemother. *36*:1987–1990, 1992.
14. Brudin, G., and Laurell, G.: Phagetyping in staphylodermia. Acta Derm. Venereol. (Stockholm) *43*:25–28, 1963.
15. Burnett, J. W.: The route of antibiotic administration in superficial impetigo. N. Engl. J. Med. *268*:72–75, 1963.
16. Casewell, M. W., and Hill, R. L. R.: Elimination of nasal carriage of *Staphylococcus aureus* with mupirocin ("pseudomonic acid"): A controlled trial. J. Antimicrob. Chemother. *17*:365–372, 1986.
17. Chandrasekar, P. H., Rolston, K. V. I., Kannangara, W. et al.: Hot tub–associated dermatitis due to *Pseudomonas aeruginosa*. Arch. Dermatol. *120*:1337–1340, 1984.
18. Chartier, C., and Grosshans, E.: Erysipelas. Int. J. Dermatol. *29*:459–467, 1990.
19. Chuinard, R. G., and D'Ambrosia, R. D.: Human bite infection of the hand. Am. J. Bone Joint Surg. *59*:416–418, 1977.
20. Dagan, R., and Bar-David, Y.: Comparison of amoxicillin and clavulanic acid (Augmentin) for the treatment of non-bullous impetigo. Am. J. Dis. Child. *143*:916–918, 1989.
21. Dagan, R., and Bar-David, Y.: Double-blind study comparing erythromycin and mupirocin for treatment of impetigo in children: Implications of a high prevalence of erythromycin-resistant *Staphylococcus aureus* strains. Antimicrob. Agents Chemother. *36*:287–290, 1992.
22. Dajani, A. S., Ferrieri, P., and Wannamaker, L. W.: Natural history of impetigo. II. Etiologic agents and bacterial interactions. J. Clin. Invest. *51*:2863–2871, 1972.
23. Demidovich, C. W., Wittler, R. R., Ruff, M. E., et al.: Impetigo: Current etiology and comparison of penicillin, erythromycin and cephaloxin therapies. Am. J. Dis. Child. *144*:1313–1315, 1990.
24. Derrick, C. W., and Dillon, H. C.: Further studies on the treatment of streptococcal skin infection. J. Pediatr. *77*:696–700, 1970.
25. Dillon, H. C.: Bullous impetigo: Clinical and bacteriologic aspects. Clin. Res. *15*:39, 1967.
26. Dillon, H. C.: The treatment of streptococcal skin infections. J. Pediatr. *76*:676–684, 1970.
27. Dillon, H. C.: Streptococcal infections of the skin and their complications:

Impetigo and nephritis. *In* Wannamaker, L. W., and Matson, E. (eds.): Streptococci and Streptococcal Diseases. New York, Academic Press, 1972.
28. Dillon, H. C., and Derrick, C. W.: Clinical experience with clindamycin hydrochloride. I. Treatment of streptococcal and mixed streptococcal-staphylococcal skin infections. Pediatrics *55*:205–212, 1975.
29. Dillon, H. C., and Reeves, M. S. A.: Streptococcal immune responses in nephritis after skin infection. Pediatrics *56*:333–346, 1974.
30. Dineen, P.: Infections following surgical operation. *In* Hoeprich, P. D. (ed.): Infectious Diseases. Hagerstown, MD, Harper & Row, 1972.
31. Doebbeling, B. N., Breneman, D. L., Neu, H. C., et al.: Elimination of *Staphylococcus aureus* nasal carriage in health care workers: Analysis of six clinical trials with calcium mupirocin ointment. Clin. Infect. Dis. *1993*:466–474, 1993.
32. Farrell, L. D., Karl, S. R., Davis, P. K., et al.: Postoperative necrotizing fasciitis in children. Pediatrics *82*:874–879, 1988.
33. Ferrieri, P., Dajani, A. S., and Wannamaker, L. W.: A controlled study of penicillin prophylaxis against streptococcal impetigo. J. Infect. Dis. *129*: 429–438, 1974.
34. Ferrieri, P., Dajani, A. S., Wannamaker, L. W., et al.: Natural history of impetigo. I. Site sequence of acquisition and familial patterns of spread of cutaneous streptococci. J. Clin. Invest. *51*:2851–2862, 1972.
35. Ginsburg, C. M.: Superficial fungal and mycobacterial infections of the skin. Pediatr. Infect. Dis. *4*(Suppl.):519–523, 1965.
36. Giuliano, A., Lewis, F., Hadley, K., et al.: Bacteriology of necrotizing fasciitis. Am. J. Surg. *134*:52–57, 1977.
37. Goetz, J. P., Tafari, N., and Boxerbaum, B.: Needle aspiration in *Haemophilus influenzae* type b cellulitis. Pediatrics *54*:504–506, 1974.
38. Gold, W. L., and Salit, I. E.: *Aeromonas hydrophila* infections of skin and soft tissue: Report of 11 cases and review. Clin. Infect. Dis. *16*:69–74, 1993.
39. Goldberg, G. N., Hansen, R. C., and Lynch, P. J.: Necrotizing fasciitis in infancy: Report of three cases and review of the literature. Pediatr. Dermatol. 2:55–63, 1984.
40. Gustafson, T. L., Band, J. D., Hutcheson, R. H., Jr., et al.: *Pseudomonas* folliculitis: An outbreak and review. Rev. Infect. Dis. *5*:1–8, 1983.
41. Hall, W. D., Blumberg, R. W., and Moody, M. D.: Studies in children with impetigo: Bacteriology, serology and incidence of glomerulonephritis. Am. J. Dis. Child. *125*:800–806, 1973.
42. Hill, H. E., and Quie, P. G.: Raised serum IgE levels and defective neutrophil chemotaxis in three children with eczema and recurrent bacterial infections. Lancet *1*:183–187, 1974.
43. Hill, H. R., Williams, P. B., Kruger, G. G., et al.: Recurrent staphylococcal abscesses associated with defective neutrophil chemotaxis and allergic rhinitis. Ann. Intern. Med. *85*:39–43, 1976.
44. Hughes, W. T., and Wan, R. T.: Impetigo contagiosa: Etiology, complications and comparison of therapeutic effectiveness of erythromycin and antibiotic ointment. Am. J. Dis. Child. *113*:449–453, 1967.
45. Kokx, N. P., Comstock, J. A., and Facklam, R. R.: Streptococcal perianal disease in children. Pediatrics *80*:659–663, 1987.
46. Krol, A. L.: Perianal streptococcal dermatitis. Pediatr. Dermatol. *7*:97–100, 1990.
47. Lee, C. Y., Schmidt, J. J., Johnson-Winegar, A. D., et al.: Sequence determination and comparison of the exfoliative toxin A and toxin B genes from *Staphylococcus aureus*. J. Bacteriol. *169*:3904–3909, 1987.
48. Lee, M. L. H., and Behr, A. J.: Dog bites and local infection with *Pasteurella septica*. Br. J. Med. *2*:169–171, 1960.
49. Lille, S. T., Sato, T. T., Engrav, L. H., et al.: Necrotizing soft tissue infections: Obstacles in diagnosis. J. Am. Coll. Surg. *182*:7–11, 1996.
50. Lillibridge, C. L.: Site of action of exfoliative toxin in the staphylococcal scalded skin syndrome. J. Pediatr. *50*:728–738, 1972.
51. Marks, V. J., and Maksimak, M. J.: Perianal cellulitis. J. Am. Acad. Dermatol. *18*:587–588, 1988.
52. McLinn, S.: A bacteriologically controlled, randomized study comparing the efficacy of 2% mupirocin ointment (Bactroban) with oral erythromycin in the treatment of patients with impetigo. J. Am. Acad. Dermatol. *22*:883–885, 1990.
53. Medina, S., Gomez, M. I., de Misa, R. F., et al.: Perianal streptococcal cellulitis: Treatment with topical mupirocin. Dermatology *185*:219, 1992.
54. Melish, M. E.: The staphylococcal scalded skin syndrome: The expanded clinical syndrome. J. Pediatr. *78*:959–966, 1971.
55. Melish, M. E., Glasgow, L. A., and Turner, M. D.: The staphylococcal scalded skin syndrome: Isolation and partial characterization of the exfoliative toxin. J. Infect. Dis. *125*:129–140, 1972.
56. Melish, M. E., Stuckey, M., and Sprouse, S.: Development of antibody to *Staphylococcus* epidermolytic toxin. Pediatr. Res. *12*(Part II):496, 1978.
57. Mertz, P. M., Marshall, D. A., Eaglestein, W. H., et al.: Topical mupirocin treatment of impetigo is equal to oral erythromycin therapy. Arch. Dermatol. 125:1069–1073, 1989.
58. Minnefor, A. B., Murray, J. J., and Davis, P. H.: *Hemophilus influenzae* cellulitis of the lower extremity. Am. J. Dis. Child. *124*:920–921, 1972.
59. Misko, M. L., Terracina, J. R., and Diven, D. G.: The frequency of erythromycin-resistant *Staphylococcus aureus* in impetiginized dermatoses. Pediatr. Dermatol. *12*:12–15, 1995.
60. Mollohan, C. S., and Romer, M. S.: Public health significances of swimming pool granuloma. Am. J. Public Health *51*:883–891, 1961.
61. Murphy, J. J., Granger, R., Blair, G. K., et al.: Necrotizing fasciitis in childhood. J. Pediatr. Surg. *30*:1131–1134, 1995.
62. O'Toole, P. W., and Foster, T. J.: Nucleotide sequence of the epidermolytic toxin A gene of *Staphylococcus aureus*. J. Bacteriol. *169*:3910–3915, 1987.
63. Parker, M. T., Tomlinson, A. J. H., and Williams, R. E. O.: Impetigo contagiosa: The association of certain types of *Staphylococcus aureus* and *Streptococcus pyogenes* with superficial skin infections. J. Hyg. (Cambridge) *53*:458–473, 1955.
64. Parker, M. T., and Williams, R. E. O.: Further observations on the bacteriology of impetigo and pemphigus neonatorum. Acta. Pediatr. Scand. *50*:101–112, 1961.
65. Peter, G., and Smith, A. L.: Group A streptococcal infections of the skin and pharynx. N. Engl. J. Med. *297*:311–317, 1977.
66. Phillips, J. A., Bernhardt, H. E., and Rosenthal, S. G.: *Aeromonas hydrophilia* infections. Pediatrics *53*:110–112, 1974.
67. Philpott, J. D., Woodburne, A. R., and Philpott, O. S.: Swimming pool granuloma: A study of 290 cases. Arch. Dermatol. *88*:158–162, 1963.
68. Potter, E. V., Siegel, A. C., Simon, N. M., et al.: Streptococcal infections and epidemic acute glomerulonephritis in south Trinidad. J. Pediatr. *72*:871–876, 1968.
69. Rahmouni, A., Chosidow, O., Mathieu, D., et al.: MR imaging in acute infectious cellulitis. Radiology *192*:493–496, 1994.
70. Rasmussen, J. E.: *Haemophilus influenzae* cellulitis. Br. J. Dermatol. *88*:547–550, 1973.
71. Rea, W. J., and Wyrick, J. J.: Necrotizing fasciitis. Ann. Surg. *172*:957–963, 1970.
72. Rice, T. D., Duggan, A. K., and DeAngelis, C.: Cost-effectiveness of erythromycin versus mupirocin for the treatment of impetigo in children. Pediatrics *89*:210–214, 1992.
73. Rimailho, A., Riou, B., Richard, C., et al.: Fulminant necrotizing fasciitis and nonsteroidal anti-inflammatory drugs. J. Infect. Dis. *155*:143–146, 1987.
74. Ruby, R. J., and Nelson, J. D.: The influence of hexachlorophene scrubs on the response to placebo or penicillin therapy in impetigo. Pediatrics *52*:854–859, 1973.
75. Schachner, L., Taplin, D., Scott, G. B., et al.: A therapeutic update of superficial skin infections. Pediatr. Clin. North Am. *30*:397–404, 1983.
76. Semel, J. D., and Trenholme, G.: *Aeromonas hydrophila* water-associated traumatic wound infections. J. Trauma *30*:324–327, 1990.
77. Shields, C., Patzakis, M. S., Meyers, M. H., et al.: Hand infections secondary to human bites. J. Trauma *15*:235–236, 1975.
78. Spear, R. M., Rothbaum, R. J., Keating, J. P., et al.: Perianal streptococcal cellulitis. J. Pediatr. *107*:557–559, 1985.
79. Stevens, D. L., Gibbons, A. E., Bergstrom, R., et al.: The Eagle effect revisted: Efficacy of clindamycin, erythromycin and penicillin in the treatment of streptococcal myositis. J. Infect. Dis. *158*:23–28, 1988.
80. Stevens, D. L., Yan, S., and Bryant, A. E.: Penicillin-binding protein expression at different growth stages determines penicillin efficacy in vitro and in vivo: An explanation for the inoculum effect. J. Infect. Dis. *167*:1401–1405, 1993.
81. Stone, H. H., and Martin, J. D.: Synergistic necrotizing cellulitis. Ann. Surg. *175*:702–711, 1972.
82. Szaley, C.: Osteomyelitis secondary to animal bites. Clin. Pediatr. *11*:687–689, 1972.
83. Tindall, J. P., and Harrison, C. M.: *Pasteurella multocida* infections following animal injuries, especially cat bites. Arch. Dermatol. *105*:412–416, 1972.
84. Trueb, R. M., Gloor, M., and Wuthrich, B.: Recurrent *Pseudomonas* folliculitis. Pediatr. Dermatol. *11*:35–38, 1994.
85. Von Graevenitz, A., and Mensca, A. H.: The genus *Aeromonas* in human bacteriology. N. Engl. J. Med. *278*:245, 1968.
86. Wallace, R. J., Jr., Brown, B. A., and Onyi, G. O.: Skin, soft tissue, and bone infections due to *Mycobacterium chelonae chelonae*: Importance of prior corticosteroid therapy, frequency of disseminated infections, and resistance to oral antimicrobials other than clarithromycin. J. Infect. Dis. *166*:405–412, 1992.
87. Wallace, R. J., Jr., O'Brien, R., Glassroth, J., et al.: Diagnosis and treatment of disease caused by nontuberculous mycobacteria. Am. Rev. Respir. Dis. *142*:940–953, 1990.
88. Wannamaker, L. W.: Differences between streptococcal infections of the throat and of the skin. N. Engl. J. Med. *282*:23–29, 78–85, 1970.
89. Washburn, J., Jacobson, J. A., Marston, E., et al.: *Pseudomonas aeruginosa* rash associated with a whirlpool. J. A. M. A. *235*:2205, 1976.
90. Wilson, H. E., and Haltalin, K. C.: Acute necrotizing fasciitis in childhood. Am. J. Dis. Child. *125*:591–595, 1973.
91. Zittergruen, M., and Grose, C.: Magnetic resonance imaging for early diagnosis of necrotizing fasciitis. Pediatr. Emerg. Care *9*:26–28, 1993.

70

VIRAL AND FUNGAL SKIN INFECTIONS

Stacey E. Gallas and Moise L. Levy

VIRAL INFECTIONS

Viral infections, especially in children, often have cutaneous manifestations. Primary viral skin infections and viral exanthems are discussed in this chapter. Viral exanthems are cutaneous eruptions that accompany an acute viral infection.[211] Primary viral skin infections and exanthematous diseases long have been recognized, are prominent in medical history, and, in the case of afflictions such as warts, also have a role in folklore.[28] Perhaps the best known historical classification of exanthems is Dukes' numbering system of six exanthematous diseases (Table 70–1). Because of the myriad of viruses, bacteria, and other agents known to be capable of producing cutaneous manifestations, such a numbering system is impractical, if not impossible. There are a large number of viruses that have been reported to have cutaneous manifestations, and as many new viruses are isolated, the number continues to grow. This chapter focuses on the cutaneous manifestations of the more common, recently reported, and some historically significant viral diseases. Further details on the viruses and the illnesses they cause can be found in the chapters of this text devoted to specific viral agents.

The pathophysiologic mechanism producing a viral eruption varies, depending on the virus. One of four different mechanisms usually is responsible. The first of these is direct invasion of the skin secondary to viremia.[79] Similarly, a virus primarily may infect the skin and lead to a virally induced skin tumor, such as a wart.[211] The third and probably most common mechanism is when a virus present in the skin reacts with circulating or cell-mediated immune factors manifesting as an exanthem.[79] Fourth, a systemic immunologic response involving the presence of circulating immune factors may lead to a cutaneous reaction without the presence of virus or deposition of viral antigen in the skin.[79]

The type of exanthem produced depends on the virus itself, the pathophysiologic mechanisms involved, the location of the eruption, and local and systemic immune factors. One virus may produce a variety of manifestations, even within the same host. When presented with an exanthem, the physician is faced with the frequently difficult challenge of determining a cause. Viral infections and their exanthems often are benign and self-limited, but recognition of etiologic agents that might prove dangerous to an immunocompromised host or a developing fetus or differentiation from a bacterial cause or drug eruption often is important. Although certain exanthems, such as those caused by varicella or classic measles, may be obvious based on the morphology of the rash and associated signs and symptoms, others, such as enteroviral exanthems, may be very difficult to diagnose accurately and many times are given a final diagnosis of rash associated with viral illness. There are certain factors that can be helpful in determining the cause of the exanthem. Useful historical data include awareness of viral infections currently prevalent in the community, any available information on exposure to known illnesses, a history of previous viral illnesses, and any associated symptoms (e.g., enanthems).[69] When presented with an unusual pattern of exanthem, a history of previous trauma, sunburn, or other cause of skin damage is important because clustering of lesions in areas of altered skin integrity is a common phenomenon.[69] In addition, medical history, especially any history of primary or secondary immunodeficiencies or skin diseases, is necessary. Apart from careful examination of the rash itself, fever and physical signs of rhinitis, pharyngitis, conjunctivitis, lymphadenopathy, and hepatosplenomegaly are signs that are indicative of, but not specific for, the presence of a systemic viral illness.[69] A few laboratory studies, other than specific viral detection methods, can be helpful in diagnosing the cause of an exanthem. A complete blood cell count and differential can provide further support to a suspected diagnosis of a viral versus a bacterial exanthem, or, if eosinophilia is seen, the diagnosis of a drug eruption may become more likely.[69] In patients with purpura or cutaneous vasculitis, a platelet count and possibly coagulation studies should be done to exclude a primary hematologic abnormality.[69]

In a prospective study of 100 children with fever and widespread erythematous rashes, it was found that not all illnesses presumed to be viral were, and because of the frequency and variable presentation of group A beta hemolytic streptococcal infection, a throat swab was a very useful routine study in their population.[84] Further laboratory analysis should be undertaken after the previously mentioned factors are explored and the need for a specific diagnosis is established. Specific viral detection methods include culture, acute and convalescent serum antibody titers, antigen detection methods (e.g., immunofluorescence, enzyme-linked immunosorbent assay), and histopathology. The use of these tests in detecting certain viruses is more extensively discussed in this chapter under the sections on specific viral infections.

Molluscum Contagiosum

Molluscum contagiosum virus (MCV) is a poxvirus and is the largest true virus causing disease in humans.[79, 120] The molluscum virus has not been grown in tissue or egg culture.[86, 110, 120] MCV has been divided into two subtypes based on DNA analysis: MCV-1 and MCV-2.[86, 110] MCV-1 is much more common and accounts for 66 to more than 90 per cent of isolates.[68, 86, 164] Unlike herpesviruses, the subtypes do not have a proclivity for genital versus nongenital areas.[68, 86, 110] However, in one study, MCV-2 was not isolated from any patient younger than 15 years of age[164]; another study found

TABLE 70–1. Dukes' Classification of Exanthems

First disease*	Measles
Second disease	Scarlet fever
Third disease	Rubella
Fourth disease†	Dukes' disease
Fifth disease	Erythema infectiosum
Sixth disease	Roseola infantum

*It is not known definitively if measles or scarlet fever was the first disease.

†This disorder had characteristics of many infections and today is not believed to represent a distinct entity.

Data from references 36, 79, 106.

MCV-2 more commonly in HIV-infected patients and localized to genital areas.[68]

Epidemiology

Molluscum contagiosum is a common viral skin disease in children. The disease now is being seen with increasing frequency in sexually active and immunodeficient individuals.[68, 86] The infection may occur at any age, with the highest incidence reported to be in patients younger than 5 years of age[79, 120] in some studies and at school age in others.[98, 110] The infection is two to three times more common in school age and sexually active males than in females.[79, 86, 120] Transmission is via close contact, including routine play, sports, sexual activity, and breast feeding.[86, 98, 110, 120] Spread by fomites also is possible.[68, 79, 110] The incidence of disease is highest in warm climates and in areas of overcrowding.[79, 86, 110, 120]

Clinical Manifestations

The incubation period for molluscum is between 2 and 7 weeks; however, there has been a report of an infant presenting with molluscum contagiosum at 1 week of age.[86, 120] The typical lesions of molluscum contagiosum are 1 to 5 mm; dome-shaped, white, skin-colored, or pink papules with a distinctive central umbilication (Fig. 70–1). Giant molluscum up to 1 to 2 cm can be seen.[79, 107, 110] Usually, 2 to 30 lesions are present.[86, 120] In children, molluscum most commonly is seen on the face, neck, trunk, and extremities but may be seen on any part of the body, including the mucous membranes.[86] Periocular molluscum may lead to a secondary keratoconjunctivitis or trachoma.[86, 173] Molluscum least commonly is seen on the palms and soles.[86, 98] In some cases, molluscum contagiosum is a sexually transmitted disease, raising the issue of sexual abuse when infection is seen in the genital area. The most common etiology of genital molluscum is autoinoculation; however, if the lesions occur solely in the genital area or there is a question about the patient's social situation, the possibility of abuse should be explored.[110, 120]

Atypical molluscum lesions are being seen more commonly, especially with the improved survival of patients with AIDS and other immunocompromised patients. The incidence of molluscum contagiosum in HIV infection is 5 to 18 per cent,[86, 107, 180] with the highest incidence in individuals with CD4 counts of less than 100 cells/mm^3.[86]

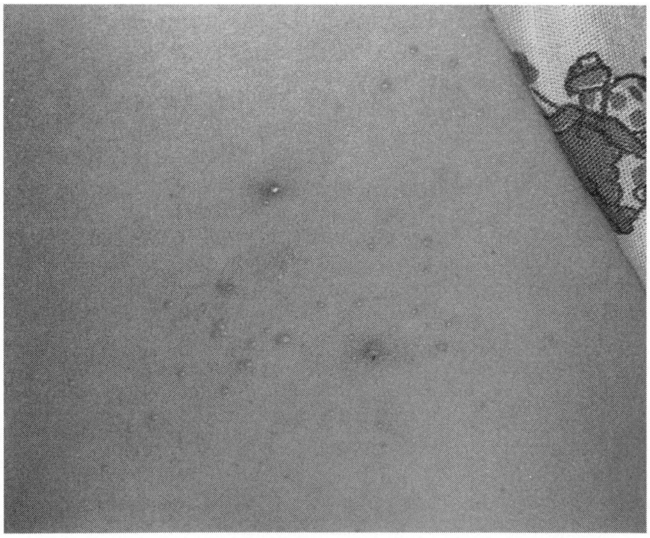

FIGURE 70–1. *Skin-colored, dome-shaped papules characteristic of molluscum contagiosum on the skin of the thigh. Some papules demonstrate mild erythema at their bases.*

Molluscum lesions in immunocompromised patients often are large, are situated more deeply in the epidermis, and may number in the hundreds.[107, 180] HIV-positive adults usually have molluscum contagiosum lesions on the face, neck, and trunk, as opposed to the genital area in immunocompetent adults.[86] There is one case report of molluscum contagiosum presenting as a large facial tumor in a man with AIDS.[107] There has been only one study in which molluscum contagiosum was evaluated in immunocompromised children. In this study, molluscum contagiosum was not felt to be more common or more severe in this population.[105] However, this study included only six patients (five with various cancers and one with AIDS), and two of the patients were described as being disease-free and immunocompetent at the time of onset of molluscum contagiosum. This and other studies suggest that the presence and degree of cellular immunodeficiency may be important in the presentation of molluscum contagiosum.[105, 180]

Patients with atopic dermatitis also may be predisposed to more severe MCV infection.[98, 105] There is not enough available information to know if this is related to the eczema itself, which may alter the skin barrier, or to the use of corticosteroids. The term molluscum dermatitis, more commonly seen in patients with atopic dermatitis, is used to describe an eczematous reaction that may occur around molluscum contagiosum lesions and is felt to represent a delayed type hypersensitivity reaction to viral antigens in the dermis.[79, 216]

Diagnosis

The diagnosis of molluscum contagiosum almost always is clinical. However, there are situations in which the virus presents atypically and microscopic diagnosis is useful. Structurally, the molluscum lesion is formed by one or more epidermal lobules extending into the dermis with an opening onto the surface.[86] The basement membrane is intact, and dermal inflammation is rare.[79, 86] The central umbilication is filled with molluscum bodies and keratin fragments.[86] The characteristic microscopic finding is a lobular collection of large, round keratinocytes with characteristic intracytoplasmic inclusion bodies, termed molluscum bodies.[110, 120, 216] The contents of a papule can be expressed and smeared on a slide and then stained with Wright, Giemsa, Gram, or Papanicolaou stains to illustrate these structures (Fig. 70–2).[79, 120, 216] The molluscum bodies (also called Henderson-Patterson bodies) are spherical, eosinophilic hyaline masses, which become more basophilic in the upper epidermis and contain viral colonies.[79, 110, 216]

Antibodies to molluscum are produced in most immunocompetent patients with MCV infection.[86] These antibodies have been identified in various studies by immunofluorescence, gel filtration, and other techniques.[86] Antibody detection currently is not a clinically relevant method of diagnosis.

Differential Diagnosis

Molluscum contagiosum, especially atypical forms, can be difficult to differentiate from many other disorders. Molluscum may be confused with verrucae, furuncles, juvenile xanthogranulomas, syringomas, and hidrocystomas.[79, 110, 120] Large lesions may mimic basal cell carcinoma or keratoacanthomas.[110, 120, 216] Lesions around the eye may be mistaken for chalazion, granulomata, adnexal tumors, and lid abscesses.[110, 120] Cryptococcosis and other deep fungal infections

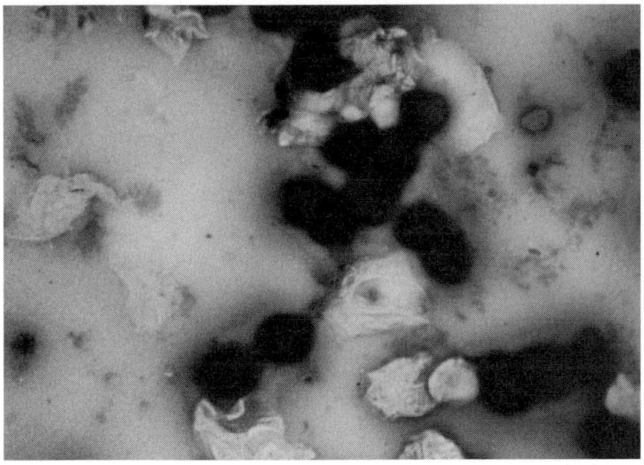

FIGURE 70–2. *Multiple basophilic molluscum bodies from a crush preparation of the contents of a papule of molluscum contagiosum. (×400.) (Courtesy of Sue Baer, M.D.)*

are important clinical considerations, especially in the immunocompromised patient.[110, 140]

Treatment

Many different modalities, including benign neglect, ultimately will result in the resolution of molluscum contagiosum in the immunocompetent patient. Treatment may be undertaken to avoid autoinoculation and spread to others and for cosmetic reasons. Superficial curettage or expression of the plug after a superficial incision is made is an effective but often frightening method of treatment in young children. In some cases, application of a topical local anesthetic, such as EMLA (eutectic mixture of lidocaine-prilocaine), may be necessary prior to treatment. Cryotherapy using liquid nitrogen also is effective.[68, 79, 110, 120] Application of local irritants, such as cantharidin 0.7 to 0.9 per cent in flexible collodion, podophyllin in tincture of benzoin, 0.05 to 0.1 per cent tretinoin, trichloracetic acid, or 10 per cent benzoyl peroxide, also can be used either alone or after superficial incision.[79, 86, 110, 120, 216] These treatments can be dangerous around the eye, and, in many cases, lesions in this location should be allowed to resolve spontaneously. Systemic treatment of molluscum contagiosum has been tried with griseofulvin and methisazone (a compound with activity against variola and vaccinia), but neither has shown definitive or consistent effectiveness.[86] In the vast majority of cases, molluscum contagiosum will resolve without treatment in 4 weeks to several months.

Treatment of molluscum in the immunocompromised patient can be problematic. No one treatment has been shown to be effective or has prevented recurrences universally. Trichloracetic acid peels were shown to be helpful in reducing lesion counts in one study of HIV-positive patients.[86] Combination therapy using cantharidin, tretinoin, and curettage controlled MCV infection in about 50 per cent of HIV-positive patients with CD4 counts less than 200 cells/mm^3.[86] The use of interferon-α was unsuccessful in another study.[86, 180] There has been one report of zidovudine leading to resolution of molluscum contagiosum in an HIV-positive patient with a CD4 count of 115 cells/mm^3.[86, 180] However, zidovudine has not been helpful in controlling molluscum contagiosum in other HIV-positive patients.[180]

Prevention

Because of the generally benign nature of infection, no specific isolation is needed for individuals with molluscum contagiosum. Spread of infection can be decreased by treatment and by avoidance of close contact with infected individuals.

Herpes Simplex Virus Infection

Herpes simplex virus (HSV) types 1 and 2 are members of the herpesvirus family, which includes varicella-zoster virus (VZV), cytomegalovirus (CMV), Epstein-Barr virus (EBV), and human herpesviruses (HHVs). The word herpes is derived from the Greek word *herpein,* meaning "to creep," and first was used to describe herpes facialis.[116, 140] Infection with HSV-1 and -2 may be asymptomatic or produce a variety of different clinical manifestations (see Chapter 163). HSV-1 has a predilection for the oral mucosa, whereas HSV-2 is more common in genital infection, although both viruses can infect any site. This section concentrates on aspects of infection directly relevant to cutaneous and mucous membrane infection.

Epidemiology

HSV infections occur worldwide and have no seasonal variation. Humans are the only reservoir of disease. HSV is transmitted via direct contact with body fluids and secretions of infected individuals or of asymptomatic carriers. The prevalence of HSV infection varies in different populations. Seroprevalence is highest in lower socioeconomic groups and in underdeveloped countries. The seroprevalence of HSV-2 is higher in women than in men.[184] Antibody to HSV-1 is acquired most commonly during childhood, whereas HSV-2 seroconversion occurs after adolescence.

Pathogenesis

Other than in the fetal and the immediate perinatal period, initial infection with HSV occurs at the mucous membranes or less commonly at the skin surface. Once HSV has entered the epidermis, it replicates locally and then travels to the regional nerve ganglia where it remains for the host's lifetime.[79, 145] The incubation period for primary infection varies from 2 to 20 days,[116, 145] and infection may be asymptomatic. After the initial infection, the virus remains latent in the sensory neural ganglia and may cause recurrent infection via intra-axonal transmission to the same area as the original infection.[28, 116] Recurrent infection almost always is less severe than initial infection, and the host often sheds virus while asymptomatic.[116, 207] In the immunocompetent host, herpes simplex usually begins as and remains a localized infection.

Clinical Manifestations

The manifestations of cutaneous and mucocutaneous HSV vary depending on the site of infection. Each of the herpetic disease manifestations will be considered separately.

Oral or perioral HSV is the most frequent form of primary infection seen in children.[79, 116] The disease is seen most commonly between 1 and 5 years of age.[116, 145] Initial infection may manifest as gingivostomatitis. Recurrent gingivostomatitis may occur in the immunocompromised host. This illness often is preceded by fever, mouth and throat soreness, and refusal to eat or drink.[79, 116, 145] Painful vesicles then appear on the lips, gingiva, buccal mucosa, and anterior portions of the tongue and hard palate (Fig. 70–3; see also Fig. 67–5, Color Plate I). The lesions are friable and may bleed easily. The breath often is foul smelling, and there may be accompanying cervical or submental adenopathy. In the normal host, the

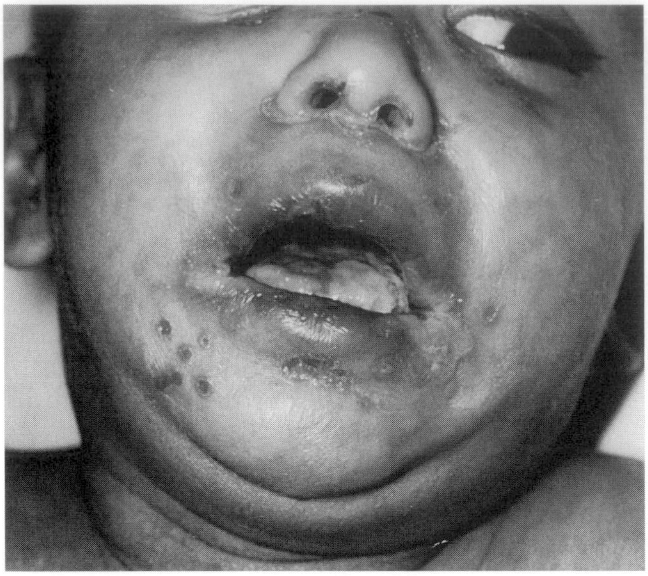

FIGURE 70–3. *Punched-out superficial erosions around the mouth and erosions on the tongue of a child with herpetic gingivostomatitis.*

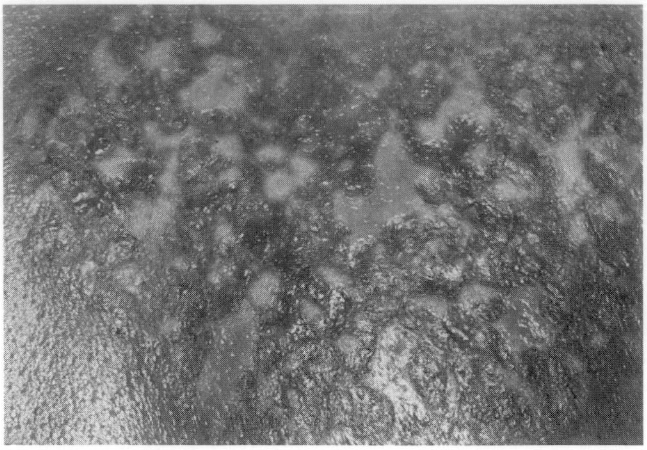

FIGURE 70–4. *Confluent erosions and exudate involving the perianal skin of a male with herpes simplex virus infection.*

entire illness usually lasts from 10 to 14 days. Herpetic pharyngitis more often is seen in older adolescents and, in increasing numbers of cases, is secondary to HSV-2 infection.[116]

It has been estimated that one-third to one-half of all adults experience recurrent oral-facial herpes infections.[140, 145, 207] Recurrences more often are seen after primary infection with HSV-1 rather than with HSV-2.[116] Herpes labialis is the most common form of recurrent oral infection. Most patients experience a prodrome of local pain, burning, or tingling sensations for 6 hours to several days before the appearance of lesions in the same area. Recurrences often are precipitated by emotional or physical factors, such as stress, sunlight, local trauma, or illness. The lesions begin as a papule, then form a vesicle that ulcerates and crusts with resolution of the lesion usually within a week. Most lesions are located on the vermilion border and affect the lower lip more frequently than the upper lip. Herpes facialis is a less common form of recurrent disease. Lesions may be seen on the chin, cheeks, or nose. The disease follows a pattern similar to that of herpes labialis.

Genital HSV may represent either primary or recurrent infection. The incidence of this infection is rising in the adult population.[116, 184] HSV-2 causes 75 to 95 per cent of infections in the United States, but infection with HSV-1 is increasing.[116, 140] Initial HSV-2 infection may be less severe if the patient previously has been infected with HSV-1.[79] HSV-2 infection recurs more commonly than does HSV-1.[79, 116, 207] The lesions present as painful, grouped vesicles, often on an erythematous base, and progress to ulceration. The lesion is located most commonly on the penile shaft, prepuce, and glans in males and on the vulva, vagina, and cervix in females. In homosexual males, erosive anal and perianal lesions may be seen (Fig. 70–4). Infection in females may be accompanied by cervicitis, urethritis, and cystitis with dysuria. Painful inguinal lymphadenopathy and systemic symptoms of fever, malaise, myalgias, and headache often accompany infection. Aseptic meningitis also can complicate primary disease.[116, 140] Duration of primary disease is 2 to 3 weeks, and recurrent disease lasts 1 to 2 weeks. Genital HSV infection is seen infrequently in children. Rarely, it can be introduced by a caregiver with contaminated hands or by autoinoculation. Whenever this disease is seen in the child, the possibility of sexual abuse should be explored carefully.

Herpetic ocular infections may present as primary or recurrent infection. This infection usually is due to HSV-1 and may present as keratitis, conjunctivitis, or blepharitis. Typical herpetic vesicles can be seen around the eye and on the lid. Unilateral keratoconjunctivitis with pain, photophobia, chemosis, excessive tearing, and blurred vision is the typical presentation. Preauricular lymphadenopathy may be present. Dendritic ulcers are seen on examination. If there is deeper corneal involvement, stromal keratitis, uveitis, and chorioretinitis can occur.[79, 116, 140, 145] Deterioration in vision and possibly blindness are serious sequelae of this disease.

Although mucocutaneous infection is more common, primary or recurrent HSV infection can affect any part of the skin. In children, herpetic whitlow is the most common cutaneous HSV infection. Herpetic whitlow often occurs when virus is inoculated into the skin by finger or thumb sucking at the time of oral HSV infection. There has been one report of herpetic whitlow occurring in a 12-day-old as a result of the mother biting the infant's nails for fear of hurting the child by clipping them.[113] Similarly, herpetic whitlow was seen in the great toe of a 3-year-old whose mother bit the toenails.[73] In adults, herpetic whitlow often occurs secondary to autoinoculation from genital herpes or due to occupational exposure in health care workers. The finger or toe is painful, erythematous, and edematous, with vesicles or pustules present (Fig. 70–5). Fever and regional lymphadenopathy often

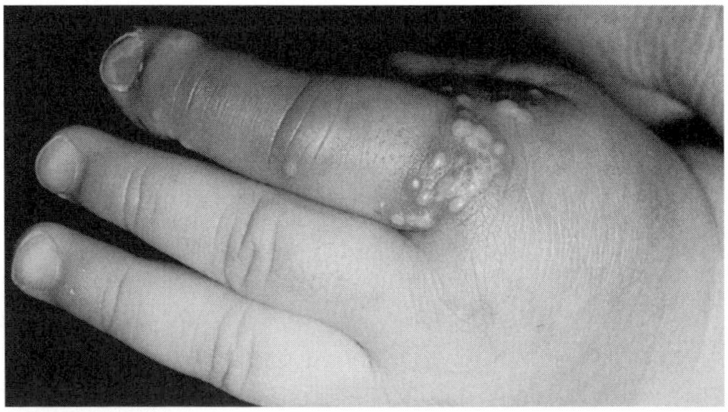

FIGURE 70–5. *Photograph of the left hand of a young child demonstrating grouped tense vesicles typical of a herpetic whitlow.*

accompany primary infection but are less common in recurrent infection. Cutaneous HSV infection also may occur in athletes involved in contact sports. The most commonly described syndromes are herpes gladiatorum in wrestlers and scrum-pox in rugby players. The lesions appear as the typical grouped vesicles, usually on an erythematous base in areas of contact.

Neonatal HSV is discussed extensively in Chapter 76. The cutaneous manifestations only will be discussed here. As genital HSV infection becomes more common, so does neonatal infection. The majority of neonatal HSV is acquired during the birth process.[79, 145, 152] Less commonly, infection is acquired postnatally from an infected caregiver, and least commonly seen is infection transmitted in utero.[79, 145, 152] Perinatally acquired infection may be localized and present with skin, oral, or eye infection only; it may involve only the central nervous system or may be disseminated with or without central nervous system involvement.[145, 152] Cutaneous or mucocutaneous lesions usually are present in infants with perinatal acquisition of HSV but may not be apparent at birth.[79] Almost all infants with HSV acquired in utero have skin lesions.[152] Skin lesions may reoccur later in infancy in infants with neonatal HSV.[145, 152] The cutaneous lesions are vesicular or sometimes bullous and appear similar to the lesions in older children (Figs. 70–6 and 70–7).

Eczema herpeticum is a cutaneous disorder due to primary or recurrent HSV infection of skin affected by another primary dermatologic disorder. This disorder also is called Kaposi varicelliform eruption, but the term eczema herpeticum will be used here because Kaposi varicelliform eruption can refer to similar infections caused by vaccinia virus types 1 and 2 and coxsackievirus A16.[141] Eczema herpeticum originally was thought to affect only infants, but it now is known to occur in children and adults of any age and is being seen with increasing frequency, which may be due to the increasing frequency of HSV infections.[141] The disorder is seen most often in patients with atopic dermatitis but has been reported to complicate a number of other primary and acquired dermatologic disorders, including seborrheic dermatitis, neurodermatitis, benign familial pemphigus, pemphigus foliaceus, mycosis fungoides, Darier disease, Sézary syndrome, pityriasis rubra pilaris, ichthyosis vulgaris, congenital ichthyosiform erythroderma, Wiskott-Aldrich syndrome, irritant contact dermatitis, burns, and skin grafts.[141] The reason for more

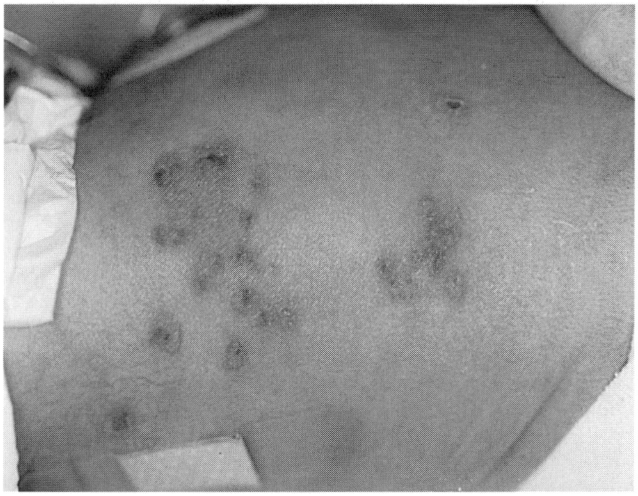

FIGURE 70–7. *Congenital crusted erosions on the skin of the left flank and abdomen of a newborn with herpes simplex virus infection.*

severe herpetic infection in these skin disorders is unknown, but it may be related to the abnormal skin itself or an underlying cellular immunologic defect.[57] In a study of 179 patients with atopic dermatitis, the extent of eczema was unrelated to the occurrence of eczema herpeticum.[57] The eruption begins as clusters of vesicles in areas of abnormal skin and rapidly may become very widespread (Fig. 70–8). Systemic symptoms of fever, malaise, and lymphadenopathy may be present.[141] The lesions usually spread for 7 to 10 days and may become hemorrhagic and crusted and evolve into ulcerations.[79, 141] Varying stages of disease may be seen in the same patient.[79] In primary infection, the process generally resolves in 2 to 6 weeks.[141] Recurrent infection resolves more quickly.[141] Failure of infected-appearing eczema to respond to appropriate antibiotic therapy may indicate superinfection with HSV and a need for acyclovir therapy.[57] Complications of eczema herpeticum include secondary bacterial infection and scarring.[141]

Erythema multiforme (EM) minor and Stevens-Johnson syndrome (EM major) can be precipitated by HSV infection. HSV now is known to be the most frequent precipitating factor in EM minor.[125, 139, 207, 210] In a study by Weston and

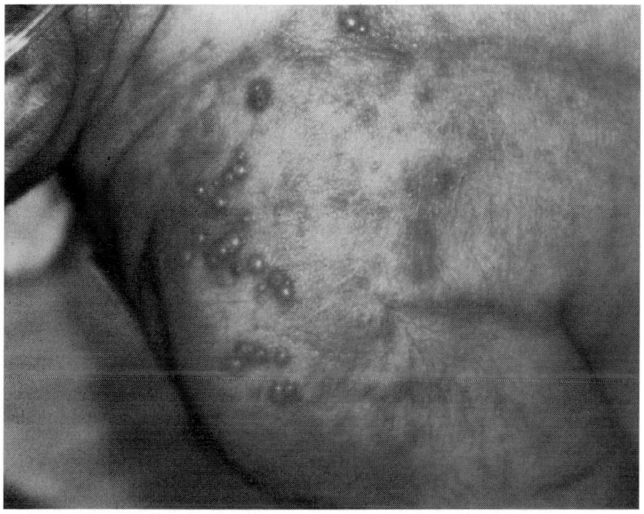

FIGURE 70–6. *Grouped tensed vesicles over the right upper chest and shoulder of a neonate with herpes simplex virus infection.*

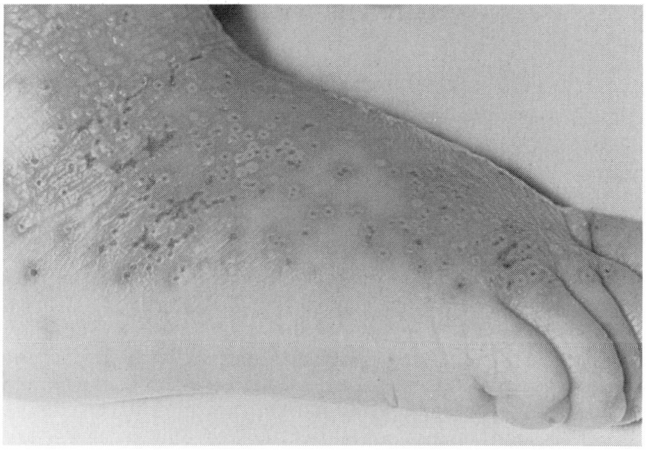

FIGURE 70–8. *Multiple intact vesicles, pustules, and well-circumscribed superficial erosions involving the skin of the foot and ankle of a child with eczema herpeticum.*

colleagues,[210] HSV DNA was found in the skin biopsy specimens of 8 of 10 children with known herpes-associated EM minor and in 8 of 10 children who were described as having idiopathic EM minor (all control biopsy specimens were negative).[210] EM minor usually occurs 1 to 3 weeks after the onset of a recurrent HSV infection and tends to recur with subsequent infections.[125] EM minor presents as characteristic red papules that often involve a concentric zone of color change and characteristically are known as iris or target lesions. Mucous membrane ulceration is seen in addition to the characteristic skin findings in Stevens-Johnson syndrome. Both forms of disease can be recurrent. The pathogenesis of EM is unknown but is believed to be mediated immunologically. Although HSV rarely has been recovered from the lesions of EM, both HSV DNA and HSV glycoprotein B have been recovered, suggesting that an immune mechanism is responsible.[207] One possible mechanism of disease suggests deposition of herpes in the skin by a transient viremia associated with a previous HSV infection.[210] The HSV antigens then would be expressed on the surface of the keratinocytes and in association with a host inflammatory immune response and would result in the EM lesions.[210] Alternatively, the inflammatory response may be to a viral protein produced by HSV that is latent in the skin.[210]

HSV can cause serious infection in the immunocompromised host. Complicated HSV infections have been seen in patients with cancer, HIV infection, organ transplant, and other primary, especially cellular, and secondary immunodeficiency states. The immunodeficient patient is at risk of disseminated HSV infection but also can experience severe forms of the cutaneous and mucocutaneous infections described earlier. Localized cutaneous lesions often may form large, deep necrotizing ulcers and often are chronic or recur frequently.[49, 139, 207] When lesions do heal, patients may be left with severe scars.[49, 139, 207] Flexion contracture and pseudosyndactyly have been reported after a progressive HSV infection of the hand of a child with AIDS.[49] Prompt recognition and treatment of HSV are essential to decrease the risks of dissemination and scarring.

Differential Diagnosis

Because of the multiple ways in which HSV can present, it can be difficult to differentiate from most any vesiculobullous eruption. Herpetic gingivostomatitis can be confused with herpangina due to enteroviral infection. Enteroviral gingivostomatitis usually affects the posterior portion of the oropharynx, and concurrent hand and/or foot lesions may be seen in the hand, foot, and mouth syndrome. Gingivostomatitis also can be confused with Stevens-Johnson syndrome, but absence of the skin lesions of EM helps differentiate these disorders. Occasionally, aphthous ulcers and oral herpes can be confused. Herpetic pharyngitis can be very difficult to differentiate from bacterial and other viral causes of pharyngitis, and the causative organism may have to be identified by culture or other methods. Herpes facialis can mimic impetigo.

Other sexually transmitted diseases must be considered in the differential diagnosis of genital herpes. Herpetic eye infections must be differentiated from infection by *Chlamydia*, herpes zoster virus, and vaccinia virus.[79] Herpetic whitlow can be mistaken for bacterial felon or paronychia. Herpetic skin infections can be confused with other viral infections, such as varicella, and with impetigo and other bacterial skin infections. Noninfectious diseases that sometimes can be confused with cutaneous herpes include epidermolysis bullosa and chronic bullous disease of childhood (linear IgA dermatosis).

Diagnosis

The diagnosis of herpetic infection often is clinical. The Tzanck smear is a commonly used, rapid test that can identify cytopathic changes seen in herpesvirus infection.[54, 79, 140, 144] This test is performed best by scraping the base of a fresh blister, spreading the cells and debris onto a slide, and staining with methylene blue, toluidine blue, or Giemsa or Wright stain.[54, 79, 144, 207] Positive smears should show characteristic cytopathic changes of multinucleated giant cells, atypical keratinocytes with large nuclei, peripheral margination of nuclear chromatin, and ground-glass cytoplasm (Fig. 70–9).[144] Tzanck smears are unable to differentiate between HSV and VZV infections and can be hard to interpret. Tzanck smears are positive in approximately 50 to 80 per cent of HSV and VZV infections.[54, 144] Smears from crusted lesions are the least useful for Tzanck preparations. Electron microscopy also can be used to identify HSV but cannot differentiate HSV and VZV and may not be readily available.[54, 116, 207]

There are multiple specific antigen detection methods that can be used to diagnose HSV infection. Immunofluorescence, immunoperoxidase staining, and enzyme-linked immunosorbent assay can be used to identify antigen in smears or tissue specimens. These tests are rapid and specific. The sensitivity of these methods is reported to be 50 to 90 per cent when compared with tissue culture, but some of the current commercially available tests are reported to have sensitivities and specificities of 90 to 95 per cent.[54, 116]

Serologic tests are not used often in diagnosing HSV. A fourfold or greater rise in titer is diagnostic of primary infection. Most individuals have no increase in titer with recurrent infection.[54] If a diagnosis of recurrent HSV is being questioned, negative antibody titers virtually rule it out as a diagnostic possibility.[54]

Tissue culture of HSV remains the gold standard for diagnosis.[54, 116] Imperfect results can be due to improper transport, specimen contamination, or sampling of lesions with insufficient virus (e.g., crusted lesions).[54, 140] Positive culture results can be obtained in 24 hours to 7 days.[54, 140]

Polymerase chain reaction detection of viral DNA is a rapid diagnostic method. This method is extremely sensitive and is able to differentiate HSV-1, HSV-2, and VZV. Care must be taken in preparing and processing specimens to avoid cross-contamination and false-positive results.[54, 207]

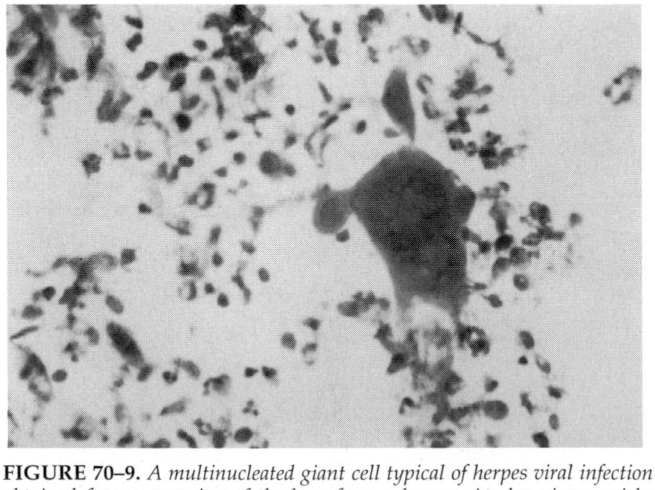

FIGURE 70–9. *A multinucleated giant cell typical of herpes viral infection obtained from a scraping of the base from a herpes simplex virus vesicle. (Wright-Giemsa stain ×400.)*

Treatment

In most cases of primary and recurrent HSV, treatment is supportive. Some children with gingivostomatitis refuse to drink, necessitating hospitalization for intravenous fluids and, in severe cases, pain control. Acyclovir now is the drug of choice for HSV infection. Unfortunately, most studies using acyclovir have been conducted in adults, and few data are available on its use in children with HSV infection. For acyclovir to be maximally beneficial, it must be begun early in infection due to its activity during active HSV replication, which is within 48 hours of new vesicle formation.[207]

The efficacy of topical acyclovir in mucocutaneous HSV has been questionable, and the main modes of therapy have become either oral or intravenous acyclovir.[116, 140, 207] Topical therapy with acyclovir, idoxuridine, trifluridine, or vidarabine in conjunction with ophthalmologic consultation is recommended for HSV keratitis.[116, 140] If topical acyclovir is to be used for recurrent herpes labialis, it must be begun at the first prodromal symptoms of burning or tingling, which usually is not feasible in young children.[145, 207] Topical acyclovir has been shown to decrease viral shedding and speed healing in one study of immunocompromised patients and may be useful in uncomplicated infections in which there is a desire to avoid use of systemic medications.[118] Use of oral acyclovir has been studied most extensively in primary genital HSV. It has been shown to speed healing and decrease the duration of viral shedding.[116, 207] The same effects would be expected in other sites of primary mucocutaneous disease.[23, 116, 207] Oral acyclovir is useful in recurrent genital HSV[116] and probably for recurrent infections in other sites also.[207] Intravenous acyclovir is indicated for severe and disseminated infections, including severe cases of eczema herpeticum.[141] Intravenous acyclovir also frequently is indicated in the immunocompromised patient, in whom persistence or spread of infection can cause major morbidity.

Acyclovir may be used prophylactically to decrease the incidence of recurrences.[79, 118, 207] In adults, this therapy has been used for up to 1 year without significant side effects.[79, 118, 207] Prophylactic acyclovir also is indicated in recurrent EM secondary to HSV infection.[104, 125] EM is not prevented when oral acyclovir is used after a herpes recurrence is evident or after EM has occurred.[104] One study used acyclovir prophylactically to prevent primary HSV infection of children in an outbreak of HSV in a day care facility; 70 per cent of treated children did not show seroconversion.[119] Because prophylaxis must be given with each exposure and because in most instances HSV infection is uncomplicated, this type of prophylaxis should be reserved for cases that could have serious sequelae.[119]

With the increased use of acyclovir, the emergence of resistant strains of HSV has become a problem, most notably in immunocompromised patients. Ganciclovir, foscarnet, vidarabine, and numerous experimental therapies have been tried, but no treatment has been effective universally in the treatment of resistant strains.

Prevention

Avoiding contact with infected lesions is the primary means of prevention, which often is difficult due to frequently asymptomatic shedding of HSV. Gloves should be worn by health care workers and others in contact with active infection. Athletes involved in contact sports should be examined and excluded from competition if lesions are noted.[4] Cleaning wrestling mats with dilute household bleach is recommended.[4] Only children with gingivostomatitis who do not have control of oral secretions and those with severe cutaneous infection that cannot be covered by bandages or clothing should be excluded from school or day care.[4] The prevention of neonatal herpes is discussed in Chapter 76.

The possibility of a HSV vaccine currently is being studied. A 17-year Bulgarian study showed whole viral vaccines to be useful in reducing recurrences and speeding recovery in patients with HSV infection.[64] To date, no vaccine has been completely effective in preventing human disease.[213]

Human Papilloma Virus Infection

Human papilloma virus (HPV), a DNA virus that cannot be grown in tissue culture, is the cause of warts. Warts have been documented as a human disease at least since ancient Greek and Roman times, and the terminology currently used today has ancient origins.[28] Condyloma comes from the Greek word for knuckle or knob, and verrucae means steep place.[28] There are close to 70 subtypes of the virus.[62, 76, 106] There are four main types of warts caused by HPV: common wart (verruca vulgaris), plantar wart (verruca plantaris), flat wart (verruca plana), and venereal wart (condyloma acuminatum).[77, 209] In addition to these common morphologic forms, HPV is the causative agent of laryngeal papillomas and epidermodysplasia verruciformis and has oncogenic potential, as demonstrated by recovery of HPV from squamous cell carcinomas in epidermodysplasia verruciformis patients, Buschke-Löwenstein tumors, bowenoid papulosis, and cervical dysplasias and neoplasias.[106, 121]

Epidemiology

Available information on the prevalence of HPV includes studies that use methods as varied as physical examination and DNA detection in asymptomatic individuals, therefore making an estimate of the true rate of infection with HPV exceedingly difficult. Nongenital warts are estimated to occur in 7 to 10 per cent of the population,[108, 111, 132] with the highest incidence in those 12 to 16 years of age.[108] A study of nongenital warts in 9263 British schoolchildren found warts to be present in 3.9 per cent at 11 years of age and 4.9 per cent at 16 years of age.[214] An earlier 2-year study of 1000 institutionalized, mentally handicapped children reported an incidence of warts in 18 to 25 per cent of the population.[132] Both studies point out that incidence is highly variable in different populations. There is no definite sex difference in nongenital warts, and warts do seem to be more prevalent in situations of increased contact, such as large families,[214] schools, barracks,[121] and locker rooms, with a higher incidence of plantar warts in individuals using communal showers.[111]

A multitude of studies have been conducted on the incidence of anogenital warts, with reported infection rates ranging from 1 per cent based on physical examination of unselected 15- to 49-year-old individuals,[117, 142] to cytologic evidence of HPV infection in 3 to 11 per cent of women, to HPV DNA detection in 11 to 80 per cent of sexually active young women.[142] The problem of varied populations and varied methods of detection again makes it very difficult to determine the incidence of anogenital HPV infection. It is, however, definitively known that in recent years the incidence of anogenital HPV in adults and children has increased precipitously.[76, 106, 117, 147] Because evidence of HPV in females can be detected on routine gynecologic examination and Papanicolaou smear and because of the higher oncogenic risks associated with female genital HPV infection, there is much more information available on genital HPV infection in females. The incidence in men likely is similar, and it has been shown that men whose partners have HPV have the same subtype HPV infection of the penis.[147] No studies have been conducted on the incidence of anogenital HPV in children, although adolescent females have among the highest rates of anogenital HPV infection,[117] ranging from 15 to 54 per cent, with infection being more common in women with multiple sexual partners.[67]

Anogenital warts in children can be caused by sexual abuse, by transmission in utero or at the time of birth, and through autoinoculation and heteroinoculation. The incidence of sexual abuse in children with anogenital warts has been the subject of many studies, with varying conclusions. In a study of 73 children with anogenital warts, it was concluded that 66 had no evidence of sexual abuse.[52] This study has been criticized for using subjective criteria for sexual abuse and for not examining all of the patients' caretakers.[115] Other, smaller studies have reported rates of sexual abuse among children with anogenital warts ranging from 2 of 14 children[92] to 6 of 7 children.[61] Because of differing populations and differing methods used in determining sexual abuse, the true incidence of sexual abuse is difficult to determine. In an attempt to lessen the confusion and present a unified opinion on the subject, the American Academy of Dermatology Task Force on Pediatrics issued a 1984 statement on the incidence of sexual abuse in children with anogenital warts, saying, "... based on the articles written and the experience of those involved in such cases, that the association is significant; at least 50 per cent of the cases can be documented by knowledgeable investigators, meaning the true incidence is probably higher."[3] Perioral and oral condylomata also can be caused by sexual abuse; however, these lesions are rare, and literature on the subject is scarce. One case report of oral condylomata acuminata in a 4-year-old excluded sexual abuse and determined that heteroinoculation from the parents who had a known history of genital warts was the most likely mode of transmission.[154]

Age of the child is one factor in determining if lesions were caused by abuse or transmitted from an infected mother either in utero or at the time of delivery. A nonsexual mode of transmission should be considered strongly in children whose mothers have a history of genital HPV and who are younger than 1 year of age,[61, 142] and it is a possible consideration up to 3 years of age.[52, 76, 106] The subtype of anogenital warts may be beneficial in determining the mode of transmission. If a child has anogenital warts caused by a subtype of HPV that is associated with causation of nongenital warts, the child may have developed the anogenital lesions through autoinoculation or through a caregiver with hand warts.[76, 109] However, fondling, a frequent type of childhood sexual abuse, still is possible.[76] HPV-2, a common cause of hand warts, rarely is found in the adult genital tract,[76, 147] and HPV subtypes 6 and 11, associated with genital warts, are seen very rarely in cutaneous lesions in adults.[33, 92] Location of the warts also can be helpful when evaluating the possibility of sexual abuse. Warts that are somewhat distant from the anus or introitus are less likely to be caused by sexual abuse than are penile, testicular, vulval, vaginal, cervical, and anal lesions.[61, 106] Although these associations are helpful, the most important information in determining whether anogenital warts are due to sexual abuse relies on the physician's thorough history and physical examination, with careful attention to medical and behavioral indicators of abuse, appropriate testing for other sexually transmitted diseases, and interview and assessment of the child and caretakers by skilled personnel.[89] Whether or not anogenital warts are caused by sexual transmission, the increased incidence in children is alarming because of possible long-term infection with potentially oncogenic strains.

Warts are seen more commonly in the immunosuppressed individual.[79] Extensive number and size of warts have been reported in patients with HIV infection and in organ transplant recipients.[114] The incidence of neoplastic transformation in warts in HIV-infected individuals and renal transplant recipients is known to be higher than that of the immunocompetent population.[160] Patients with atopic dermatitis often have more severe cutaneous viral infections possibly secondary to abnormalities in cell-mediated immunity.[214] However, the incidence or severity of warts in patients with atopic dermatitis is not believed to be increased and in some studies has been found to be lower than in individuals without eczema.[214]

Clinical Manifestations

As mentioned previously, there are approximately 70 subtypes of HPV, many of which have been associated with causing specific clinical wart types. The most common associations are listed in Table 70–2. A large variety of common and rare subtypes have been isolated from immunocompromised patients[176] and those with epidermodysplasia verruciformis.[121] The incubation period of HPV may be from 1 to 6 months[106, 121] or longer,[109] and an individual wart may resolve spontaneously in a few months to several years.[106, 132] In Massing and Epstein's study,[132] 40 per cent of single and 42 per cent of multiple warts had resolved without treatment in 1 year and 46 per cent of single and 45 per cent of multiple warts had resolved without treatment in 2 years. In the study by Williams and colleagues,[214] 93 per cent of the children at 11 years of age with warts were free of warts at 16 years of age.

Common warts are solid, papular, scaly, or horny projections that most often are seen on the fingers and hands but can be seen on any area of the skin and occasionally on the oral mucosa. They may be solitary or multiple and vary in size from a few millimeters to more than a centimeter (Fig. 70–10).[106] Filiform warts are a variant of the common wart that have a slender stalk and multiple projections from the surface. They most commonly appear on the eyelids, nose, and lips.

Flat warts are skin-colored, smooth, slightly raised papules that are common on the face and extremities (Fig. 70–11). Flat

TABLE 70–2. Most Common Subtypes of Human Papilloma Virus Associated with Specific Clinical Wart Types

Clinical Manifestation	Human Papilloma Virus	Comments
Common wart	2, 4, 7	4 is seen more commonly in palmar and plantar warts 2 is seen more commonly in hand warts
Plantar wart	1, 4	
Flat wart	3, 10	
Anogenital wart	6, 11, 16, 18, 31, 33, 35 2 in children	6, 11 are seen more commonly in vulvar, penile, and perianal condyloma and are the most common cause of venereal warts in children 16, 18 are associated with neoplasia
Laryngeal papilloma	6, 11	

Data from references 106, 108, 109, 121, 147, 148, 209.

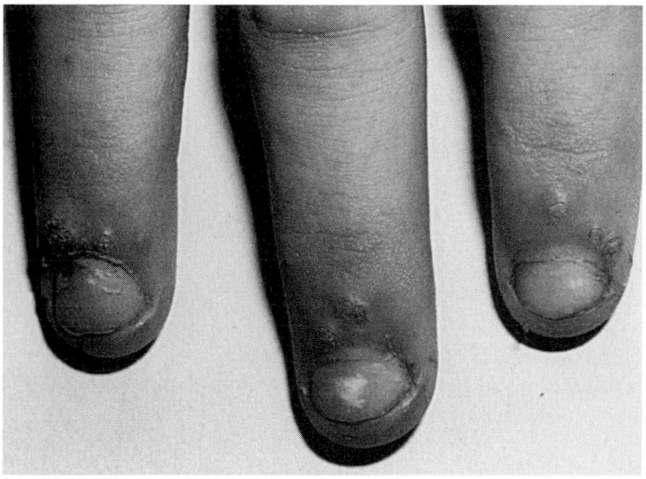

FIGURE 70–10. *Scattered hyperkeratotic papules typical of verruca vulgaris over the dorsum of the distal second, third, and fourth fingers of a child.*

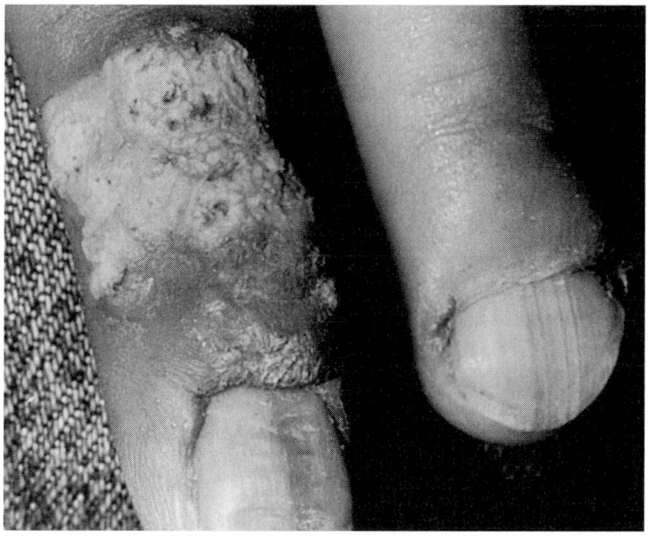

FIGURE 70–12. *Clinical photograph of myrmecia-type human papilloma virus infection over the skin of the middle finger.*

warts often are seen on the beard area in men and on the legs of women and may be spread by shaving.[106] Widespread flat warts, often caused by HPV-5, are seen in patients with epidermodysplasia verruciformis and also have been seen in renal transplant patients and in other patients with defective cellular immune function, including a 10-year-old boy with HIV infection.[168]

Plantar warts occur on the soles of the feet, especially in the weight-bearing areas, and can be very painful. These warts have inverted apices, pressed inward by walking. The warts may be flat with the skin surface or bulge slightly and are covered by thick, hyperkeratotic skin that when removed reveals the characteristic black dot representing thrombosed capillaries. Plantar warts often occur in groups and are termed mosaic warts because of the appearance of the closely approximated hyperkeratotic plaques over the warts' surfaces.

Myrmecia is the term used to describe deep palmoplantar warts, which are very painful and appear on the tips of the fingers and toes periungually and on the palms and soles (Fig. 70–12).[101] They are single or multiple nodules that may

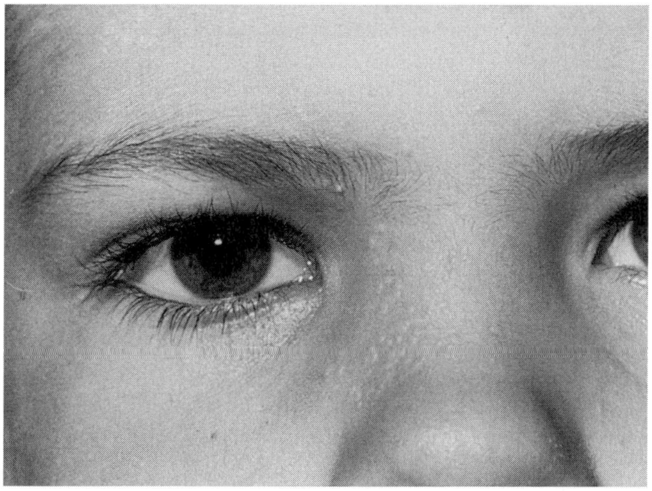

FIGURE 70–11. *Grouped flat-topped, skin-colored papules on the nose skin of a child with flat warts.*

be covered by a callus and surrounded by a hyperkeratotic collar and associated with erythema and edema, making them easy to mistake for paronychia.[101]

The characteristic type of condylomata are pink or skin-colored polypoid masses, which are described as cauliflower-like and typically are multiple lesions that grow in clusters (Fig. 70–13). These lesions can be seen anywhere in the anogenital region but typically occur in the moist areas of the labia, glans penis, prepuce, and urethral meatus. Condyloma planum (atypical condyloma) is more common but less often recognized than the typical form of venereal warts.[87, 142] These lesions can be seen with the aid of the colposcope and acetic acid and appear as white patches. Associated cellular atypia is common, and HPV-16 to -18 often are the causative viral subtypes.[87] Bowenoid papulosis is a term used to describe multiple, small, flat, skin-colored or tan papules that occur in the genital area and show features consistent with carcinoma in situ (see Fig. 67–20, Color Plate IV). The papules spontaneously may regress or progress to squamous cell carcinoma.[87] Although rare, this disorder has been reported in children.[109] Giant condyloma of Buschke and Löwenstein is a locally invasive verrucous carcinoma associated with HPV-6 and -11.[87, 121]

Epidermodysplasia verruciformis is a rare disorder that usually begins in childhood and may be familial.[106] The disease is characterized by disseminated, flat, wart-like lesions and reddish, hyperpigmented or hypopigmented macules,[106] also described as tinea versicolor–like lesions.[168] Malignant degeneration of the lesions to carcinoma in situ with progression to squamous cell carcinoma often occurs in the third decade of life.[106, 168]

HPV infection also may occur on the oral and nasal mucosa. Laryngeal papillomas occur in infants whose mothers are infected with HPV. They occur both in infants who are delivered vaginally and in those delivered by cesarean section, suggesting that transmission in utero is possible.[106]

Diagnosis

Like most other primary viral infections of the skin, the diagnosis of warts usually is clinical. If a nongenital wart is biopsied, epidermal hyperplasia with hyperkeratosis, papillomatosis, acanthosis, koilocytosis, and focal areas of para-

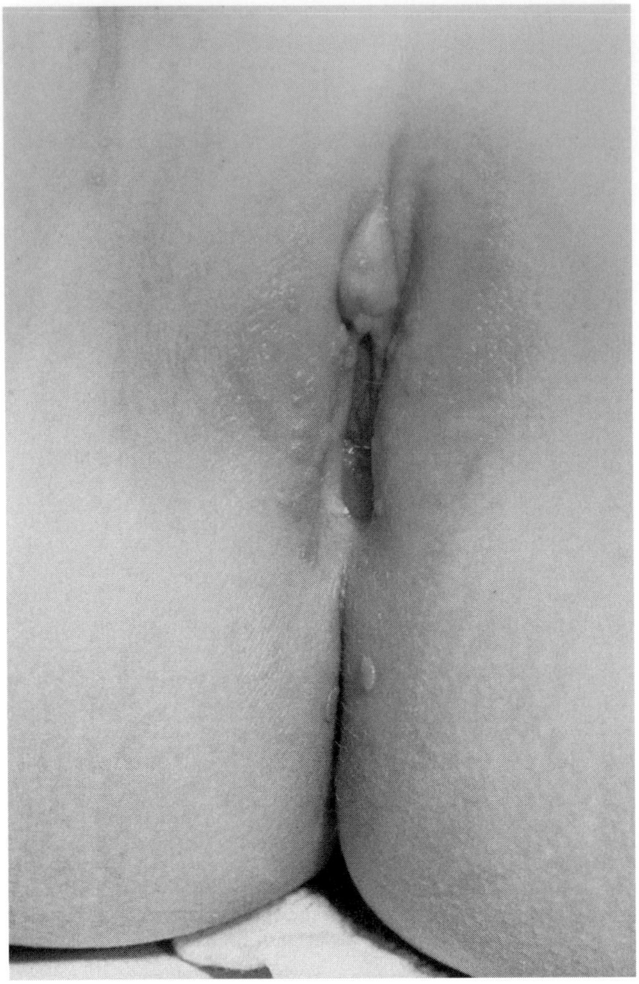

FIGURE 70–13. *Clinical photograph of multiple flat-topped verrucous papules typical of condyloma acuminata over the skin of the perineum of a young girl.*

keratosis will be seen.[79, 106] The characteristic histologic feature of warts that distinguishes them from other types of papillomas is the presence of large vacuolated cells in the upper stratum malpighi and granular layer.[106, 121] Application of 3 to 5 per cent acetic acid produces acetowhitening and will aid in the identification of clinically inapparent anogenital HPV lesions. Colposcopy with acetic acid is helpful in identifying HPV infection. Koilocytosis, which is the presence of mature squamous cells with dense marginal cytoplasm, wrinkled pyknotic nuclei, and perinuclear cavitation,[142] commonly is identified on cytologic specimens that can be obtained by Papanicolaou smear.[87] Histologically, HPV-infected cells show koilocytosis, nuclear atypia, and hyperkeratosis.[142] Direct methods of detecting HPV include electron microscopy[87] and DNA analysis by nucleic acid hybridization and polymerase chain reaction.[142] DNA analysis also can identify the subtype of HPV.[142] Neither of these methods currently is in widespread clinical use.

Differential Diagnosis

Common and filiform warts usually are characteristic in their appearance and usually do not present a diagnostic dilemma. Occasionally, these lesions can be confused with actinic keratosis, seborrheic keratosis, and squamous cell carcinoma.[121] Flat warts can be difficult to differentiate from folliculitis, juvenile xanthogranuloma, granuloma annulare, lichen nitidus, syringomas, milia, and molluscum contagiosum.[79, 121] Plantar warts must be differentiated from corns, calluses, plantar porokeratosis, and black heel (rupture of papillary capillaries by shearing forces in athletes).[79, 121] The differential diagnosis of anogenital warts includes condyloma latum of secondary syphilis, molluscum contagiosum, chronic benign pemphigus (Hailey-Hailey disease), neurofibromas, and certain benign and malignant neoplasms.[76]

Treatment

There have been a multitude of modalities used to treat warts. Because latent HPV infects the normal-appearing epithelium adjacent to the clinically apparent wart and because certain warts may be difficult to perceive clinically (especially flat or anogenital warts), it is impossible to eradicate the virus completely and thus, regardless of therapy, the recurrence rate is high.[76, 106] As mentioned previously, most warts will resolve spontaneously, but because of cosmetic issues, autoinoculation, transmission to others, and in some cases the possibility of neoplastic transformation, warts generally should be treated. It is important to keep in mind that because the virus is not destroyed completely, multiple treatments may be needed and the possibility of neoplastic transformation from areas of subclinical infection still exists. Treatment can be classified as destructive or immunologic. Local keratolytics, such as salicylic acid, lactic acid, bichloroacetic acid, and trichloroacetic acid, can be painted onto the wart or applied by a film or plaster. Trichloroacetic acid is the only one of these preparations indicated for use in genital warts. These preparations are easy to use, and some are available over the counter for home use. Cantharidin is a vesicant, extracted from the blister beetle, that can be useful for treatment of periungual and other common warts. Podophyllin, an alcoholic extract of the resin from the plant *Podophyllum rhizomes*, is a metaphase inhibitor and can be efficacious in treating genital warts. When applied, it must be placed only onto the wart and washed off after 2 to 6 hours to avoid severe local inflammation and systemic absorption and effects (leukopenia, thrombocytopenia, possible carcinogenesis). This drug should not be used during pregnancy.[87] Less toxic formulations containing a purified compound of podophyllotoxin (podofilox) now are available for use and can be self-administered.[87, 106, 160] Cryotherapy, usually with liquid nitrogen, is a common and relatively safe method of local therapy for genital and nongenital warts. Pain, blistering, and need for repeated applications are limitations of this therapy. When treating plantar warts with either keratolytics or cryotherapy, the overlying hyperkeratotic skin should be pared down prior to treatment. Tretinoin 0.01 to 0.05 per cent can be efficacious in treating flat warts.[2, 108, 209] Carbon dioxide and pulsed dye lasers have been used in the treatment of recalcitrant warts and provide an alternative, therapeutic modality when other treatments have failed.[129, 197] Surgical excision may be useful in the treatment of filiform warts but has a high recurrence rate when used in the treatment of other types of warts.[106, 209]

Cimetidine, which is known to have immunomodulatory effects, has been used to treat children with nongenital warts. A study of cimetidine therapy in 32 children with multiple warts showed disappearance and no recurrence of the lesions in 81 per cent of the children after 2 months of treatment at a dosage of 25 to 40 mg/kg/day divided three to four times a day.[151] Various interferon preparations, used topically, intralesionally, and systemically, have been used in the treatment of both nongenital and genital warts. Resolution of 53 to 62 per cent of genital warts[87] and in one study 73 per cent of palmar and plantar warts[22] was seen using intralesional interferon-α. Headache, fever, chills, and malaise are side effects of interferon treatment. Inosine pranobex, an immunomodulating agent not currently available in the United States, has been used in combination with conventional treatments in treating both refractory warts of the hands and feet[13] and genital warts.[87]

Other therapies that have been used include intralesional bleomycin, topical 5-fluorouracil, electrocautery, and radiation, none of which are recommended in children.[79, 209] More aggressive and longer duration of treatment often is necessary in the immunosupressed patient. Finally, the power of suggestion may play a significant role in the treatment of childhood nongenital warts.[106, 108] This may explain how many of the folk remedies that have been used successfully to treat warts have worked. Because no one therapy universally is efficacious in treating warts, the primary principle that should be followed is to select the treatment that has the least toxicity and will cause the patient the least distress.

Prevention

Because of the universal prevalence of HPV, there are no methods other than treatment and good personal hygiene that can help decrease the spread of nongenital warts. Health care workers with, just as those without, genital HPV infection should use good hand washing techniques before contact with patients. Parents and other child caretakers with genital warts also should use good hand washing techniques before changing diapers, feeding, and performing other activities that could spread the virus to the child. Use of condoms can decrease sexual transmission.[5] The development of a vaccine against HPV has been considered, but the oncogenic potential of the virus and other limiting factors must be worked out before this can become a reality.

Orf

Orf, also known as sheep pox and ecthyma contagiosum, is a member of the poxvirus group and causes disease of sheep and goats that can be acquired by humans. Infection occurs in an individual who has contact with the animal or contaminated objects.[122] The incubation period is 4 to 7 days.[36] The lesions usually are located on the hands and fingers and begin as one or occasionally more macules or papules that develop into nodules with erythematous, weeping surfaces (Fig. 70–14).[122] The lesions eventually crust over and evolve into a papillomatous stage and ultimately regress.[122] The average total duration of the lesions is 5 weeks.[122] There may be associated regional lymphadenopathy or lymphadenitis and mild fever, with other complications rarely seen.[79, 122] Treatment is symptomatic, but superficial epidermal excision will reduce healing time and complications.[183]

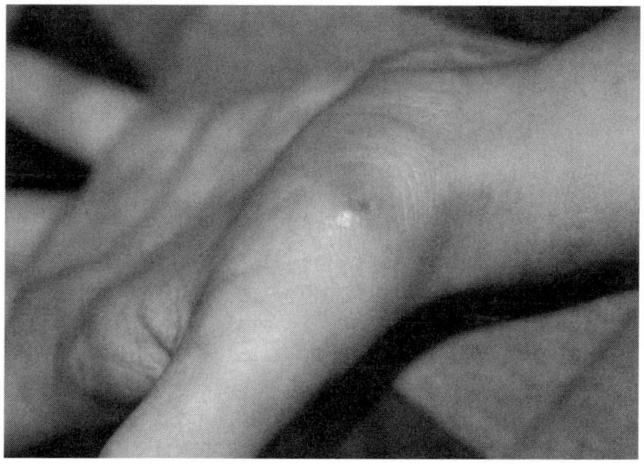

FIGURE 70–14. *Erythematous papules with a small central ulceration involving the base of the left thumb and left hand of a patient with orf.*

Milker's Nodules

Milker's nodules are caused by a paravaccinia virus endemic in cattle that is acquired by humans through contact with the udders of cows. Fomite transmission in patients with first- and second-degree burns[179] and experimental human-to-human infection are rare modes of transmission that have been reported.[123] The clinical and histopathologic manifestations nearly are identical to those of orf.[106] The incubation period is 4 to 7 days.[36] A single or occasionally a few red macules or papules appear most often on the fingers, hand, or forearm. Similar to orf, the lesion then progresses through target, acute weeping, nodular, papillomatous, and regressive stages.[123] Spontaneous healing usually occurs in 6 to 8 weeks.[123] Superficial surgical removal, as in orf, can be used to hasten healing.[183]

Human Herpesvirus 6 and 7 Infections

(Table 70–3)

Human herpesvirus 6 (HHV-6) is the most common cause of roseola (exanthem subitum, sixth disease). HHV-7, a virus first isolated in 1990, also can cause roseola. One study demonstrated HHV-7 to be the etiologic agent in 10 per cent of the cases of 49 patients diagnosed with exanthem subitum.[100] Other viruses, including strains of echovirus, coxsackievirus, adenovirus, parainfluenza virus, and measles vaccine virus, also have been shown to cause roseola.[35, 41]

The most common presentation of roseola is described in Table 70–3 (Fig. 70–15). Not all children with HHV-6 infection develop rash after the febrile phase.[67, 88, 169] In a United States study of 34 children younger than 2 years of age infected with HHV-6, 9 had a macular or maculopapular rash and 6 had other variable rashes, with only 3 of the typical roseola rashes occurring after the fever subsided.[169] However, in a Japanese study of 176 children younger than 2 years of age with HHV-6 infection, 98 per cent had a macular or papular rash and 75 per cent of the eruptions appeared at or after defervescence.[8] The reason for this difference is unknown. The years of the study and the populations used were similar, but one could speculate that there may be slight differences in the viral strains, differences in expression of the rash in Japanese and American children, or, less likely, that unrecognized concomitant infection with another virus was responsible for some of the rashes. There also have been reported cases of rash without fever.[88, 150] Despite the degree of fever (mean, 39.7° C) in roseola, affected children often are happy and playful. Mild systemic symptoms, including pharyngeal injection, cough, coryza, cervical and occipital lymphadenopathy, injection of the tympanic membranes, edematous eyelids, nausea, vomiting, and diarrhea, may accompany roseola infection.[9, 41] Bulging anterior fontanelle, seizures (usually febrile), and encephalitis also can occur.[41, 88, 169] Liver failure secondary to fulminant hepatitis[165] and thrombocytopenic purpura are other complications that have been reported in children with roseola.[41, 88] An enanthem of erythematous

TABLE 70–3. Major Epidemiologic and Clinical Characteristics of Several of the Systemic Viral Diseases that Have Associated Exanthems

Virus	Disease	Age	Season	Incubation Period	Clinical Characteristics	Lesions	Distribution	Timing/Duration	Comments
Parvovirus B19	Erythema infectiosum, fifth disease	School age	Epidemics in winter and spring, peaks of 3 years' duration every 6 years	4–14 days	May have prodrome of fever, malaise, and headache followed by 3–7 days of no symptoms before onset of rash	3 stages: a. Erythematous macular rash	a. Malar rash ("slapped cheek") with circumoral pallor and sparing of nasal bridge		No longer contagious at onset of rash
						b. Macular or papular erythematous rash ± pruritus; evolves into pathognomonic lacy or reticular pattern	b. Any body surface; most frequently limbs and trunk	b. 1–4 days after stage a	
						c. Recurrence	c. 1–3-week period of rash recurrence, especially brought on by heat, cold, and friction		
Human herpesvirus-6 Human herpesvirus-7	Roseola infantum, exanthem subitum, sixth disease	6 months–3 years	Nonseasonal	5–15 days	3–5 days of fever (mean, 39.7); possible mild systemic symptoms (see text)	2–5-mm rose-pink–colored macules or maculopapules	Favors face, neck, and trunk	Rash appears with defervescence and lasts several hours–2 days	
Varicella-zoster	Chickenpox	90% younger then 10 years of age	Late winter/ early spring	11–21 days	Low-grade fever, malaise, and rash occur together (prodromal period of fever, malaise, and myalgias more common in older children and adults)	Erythematous macules with progression to vesicles and then crusted lesions; all stages seen at once; mucous membranes show ulcers (secondary to rapid vesicle breakdown)	Initially scalp and trunk with spread to extremities (distal areas rarely involved)	Occasionally 1–3 lesions appear on trunk 1–2 days before generalized rash; vesicle to crust progression in 6–12 hours; crusts fall off in 5–25 days	Contagious minimum of 2 days prior to and 5 days after onset of rash or until all lesions crusted
	Herpes zoster (shingles)	More common with advancing age			Intense dermatomal paresthesias or pruritus precedes rash by 1–3 days; may have prodrome of malaise, headache, and fever and may be preceded by postherpetic neuralgia	Erythematous macules and papules with progression to vesicles, pustules, and then crusts	Dermatomal; trigeminal (ophthalmic branch), T3-L4 most common	Loss of crusts at 3–4 weeks	
Enterovirus	Many	Young children	Late summer-early fall (year-round in tropical climates)	4–6 days	See text and specific viruses below	Most often vesicular, maculopapular, macular, or morbilliform; may be urticarial, scarlatiniform, zosteriform, petechial, purpuric, or hemangioma-like; usually nonpruritic	Often generalized		
Coxsackievirus A16 and others	Hand, foot, and mouth syndrome				Brief prodrome of low-grade fever, sore mouth, anorexia, malaise, and cervical and submandibular lymphadenopathy	Enanthem: 2–8 mm (up to 20 mm); erythematous macules rapidly progressing to vesicles and ulcers	Enanthem: buccal mucosa, tongue most commonly; also seen on the palate, uvula, and anterior tonsillar pillars	Enanthem: precedes exanthem by 1–4 days and lasts 1–6 days	

						Exanthem: erythematous maculopapules proceeding to 3–7-mm gray vesicles	Exanthem: hands and feet (may be on palms and soles); buttocks of infants	Exanthem: duration, 2–7 days	
Coxsackievirus A9					Fever; frequently aseptic meningitis	Erythematous maculopapular and others (see text)	Starts on face and neck, with spread to trunk and extremities	1–7 days	
Coxsackievirus A4					Fever, anorexia, drooling, herpangina, pharyngitis, coryza, headache, vomiting, and diarrhea	Small macules and papules that disappear or progress to 5–10-mm yellowish, opaque vesicles; regression occurs with brownish discoloration	Face and trunk, with spread of vesicles to the extremities	Rash appears at or after defervescence; maculopapular phase lasts 1–4 days; vesicular phase lasts 1–2 weeks	
Coxsackievirus B5					Fever; aseptic meningitis	Usually maculopapular; may be urticarial or petechial	Begins on face and neck with spread to trunk and extremities	Rash appears at or after defervescence; spreads over 4–24 hours; lasts 36 hours	
Echovirus 9					Fever, headache, nausea, and vomiting; possible pharyngitis, cough, abdominal pain, and cervical lymphadenopathy	Erythematous, maculopapular rash, often associated with petechiae or may be only petechial	Begins on face with spread to neck, trunk, and extremities	3–5 days	
Echovirus 16	Boston exanthem			3–8 days	Fever, anorexia, vomiting, aseptic meningitis, encephalitis, and sepsis-like illness in neonates	Erythematous, discrete, maculopapular lesions	Face, trunk, and extremities	1–5 days	
Adenoviruses		6 months–5 years	Winter and spring	6–9 days	Fever, rhinitis, conjunctivitis, pharyngitis, cough, and adenopathy	Erythematous, maculopapular rash	Rash usually appears 1–2 days after onset of fever; begins on face with spread to trunk and extremities	3–5 days	
Reoviruses					Fever, malaise, anorexia, and pharyngitis; less common: adenopathy, diarrhea, and conjunctivitis	Maculopapular vesicular in 1 case; mildly pruritic	Begins on face and trunk with spread to extremities	3–9 days	Information based on study of 7 children[128]
Multiple (see text)	Gianotti-Crosti syndrome	2–6 years; rare after 10 years of age	Variable	Variable	Adenopathy (mainly inguinal and axillary); may have hepatitis	Multiple skin-colored or erythematous 2–4-mm flat-topped papules (size may be larger in younger children, smaller in older children) ± pruritus; may see Koebner phenomenon	Face, extremities, and buttocks	Develops in 2–3 days; lasts 15–20 days	
Measles	Classic measles, rubeola, first disease	5–9 years of age	Winter and spring	10 days	Malaise, fever, cough, coryza, conjunctivitis, and cervical and preauricular adenopathy	Enanthem: Koplik spots: 1–2-mm papules on an erythematous, granular base	Enanthem: begins on buccal mucosa opposite lower molars; may spread to involve any part of the mucous membranes	Enanthem: appears during prodrome and fades during first 3 days of exanthem	
						Exanthem: erythematous and maculopapular; rapidly becomes confluent; turns coppery or brown with areas of fine desquamation during fading	Exanthem: begins behind ears and at hairline with centrifugal spread from head to foot; also clears centrifugally	Exanthem: spreads over 3 days and lasts 6–7 days	

Table continued on following page

TABLE 70–3. Major Epidemiologic and Clinical Characteristics of Several of the Systemic Viral Diseases that Have Associated Exanthems *Continued*

Virus	Disease	Age	Season	Incubation Period	Clinical Characteristics	Lesions	Distribution	Timing/Duration	Comments
Measles *Continued*	Modified measles				Shortened prodrome; milder illness than classic measles	Variable Koplik spots; exanthem may not be confluent			Occurs in partially immune host (see text)
	Atypical measles			Similar to classic measles	Abrupt onset of high fever, headache, abdominal pain, myalgias, cough, and pneumonia	Koplik spots are rare; erythematous, maculopapular rash	Begins on distal extremities, with concentration on ankles and wrists with spread cephalad	Rash occurs 2–3 days after onset of illness; total illness lasts 1–2 weeks	Occurs in previously immunized individuals (usually with killed vaccine) exposed to the natural virus
Rubella	Rubella, German measles, third disease	Prevaccine: 5–9 years of age; now: older unvaccinated population	Winter and spring	18 ± 3 days	Prodrome (most common in adolescents and adults): eye pain (especially on lateral and upward movement), sore throat, headache, lymphadenopathy, fever, chills, malaise, anorexia, and nausea; exanthem: may occur without other symptoms or with lymphadenopathy (especially postauricular and suboccipital) or fever	Exanthem: erythematous, maculopapular, discrete rash; may become morbilliform; often pruritic in adults Enanthem: seen occasionally; pinhead-size, rose-red macules on uvula and soft palate (Forscheimer spots)	Exanthem: begins on face and spreads centrifugally to trunk and extremities	Prodrome: 1–5 days before rash Exanthem: spreads over 24 hours and usually lasts 3 days (range, 1–5 or more days)	
Mumps		14–21 days	Childhood	Late winter/ early spring	Fever, parotid and submandibular swelling, anorexia, and headache	Exanthem (rare): erythematous, maculopapular, macular, urticarial, and vesicular lesions	Trunk	2–5 days	Based on report of 6 patients[143] (see text)
Epstein-Barr	Infectious mononucleosis	See text		28–49 days	Fever, lymphadenopathy, tonsillopharyngitis, splenomegaly, and hepatomegaly	a. Nonantimicrobial associated: erythematous maculopapular b. Ampicillin associated: erythematous or copper-colored macules and papules; usually pruritic	a. Trunk and proximal upper extremities; occasionally face, forearms, and legs b. Begins on trunk and spreads to face and extremities	a. 1–5 days b. Appears 7–10 days after starting ampicillin and lasts about 1 week	

Data from references 8–10, 16, 20, 24, 25, 30, 35, 36, 38–47, 67, 79, 91, 99, 100, 106, 134, 136, 150, 156, 163, 167, 169, 171, 174, 185, 192–194, 198, 201–203, 206.

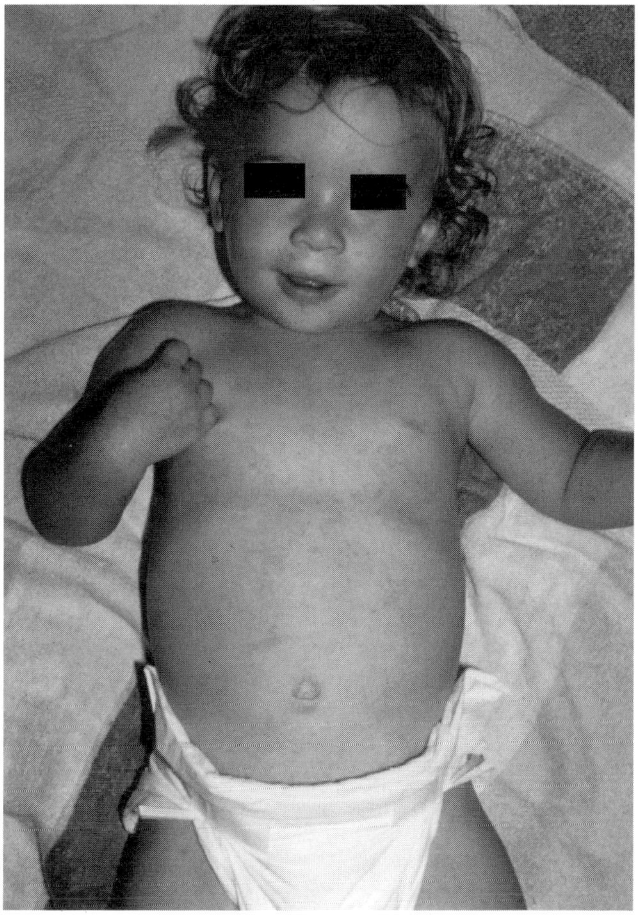

FIGURE 70–15. *Diffusely distributed erythematous macules on the skin of a well-appearing infant with roseola.*

papules on the soft palate and base of the uvula has been reported in children with primary HHV-6 infection.[8] Residual mild skin pigmentation after disappearance of skin rash was seen in 11 of 176 children with primary HHV-6 infection.[8] In the vast majority of patients, roseola is a benign illness without sequelae.

In addition to roseola, antibodies to HHV-6 have been found in a variety of clinical diseases, including Kawasaki syndrome, chronic fatigue syndrome, and mononucleosis, as well as in asymptomatic individuals.[165] There also has been one case report of fatal disseminated HHV-6 infection in an immunocompetent 13-month-old child.[165]

Parvovirus B19 Infection (Table 70–3)

Parvovirus B19 is a single-stranded DNA virus of the family *Parvoviridae*. Infection is spread via contact with respiratory secretions. It is the etiologic agent of erythema infectiosum (fifth disease) and of other diseases, including aplastic crisis in patients with chronic hemolytic anemias and immunodeficiencies. Parvovirus B19 also can cause nonimmune fetal hydrops and fetal demise. The epidemiology and characteristics of erythema infectiosum are described in Table 70–3.

The diagnosis of erythema infectiosum is clinical (Figs. 70–16; 67–6, Color Plate I; and 67–7 and 67–8, Color Plate II). Patients initially may be seen for evaluation of an asymptomatic confluent macular erythema involving the malar areas of the face. More typically, however, information such as history must be sought when physicians are asked to evaluate children for the more commonly encountered reticular macular erythema involving the extremities. This eruption can, in fact, wax and wane over weeks and, sometimes, months after the initial episode. Skin biopsies reveal mild perivascular inflammation or normal skin.[79] Schwarz and colleagues[181] demonstrated B19 capsid proteins and B19 DNA in the nuclei of epidermal cells of a 3-year-old with erythema infectiosum.

Although erythema infectiosum is the disease most commonly associated with parvovirus B19 infection, this viral infection often is asymptomatic[162, 167] or may present with unusual cutaneous manifestations. Parvovirus B19 has been linked to cases of Gianotti-Crosti syndrome, purpuric and petechial rashes, Henoch-Schönlein purpura, and various vasculitides.[170] There is a case report of parvovirus B19 causing Koplik-like spots and a purpuric eruption in a 26-year-old female.[71] An association between active or recent parvovirus B19 infection and Kawasaki disease has been suggested,[146] but other investigators believe that there is no such association,[53, 218] and at this point no definitive study has been conducted to answer the question.

Case reports also have linked parvovirus B19 to the papular-purpuric gloves and socks syndrome (PPGS; also termed petechial gloves and socks syndrome).[90, 170] PPGS first was described in a series of five patients by Harms and colleagues[94] in 1990. A viral etiology was suggested but not shown at that time, but subsequently several cases have been associated with parvovirus B19 infection.[90, 170] There also have been reports of association with measles virus and coxsackievirus B6,[170] but in other cases no etiology was found.[204] Most case reports of PPGS have been in adults, but there is one report of a case of PPGS of unknown etiology in a 9-year-old child.[191] The eruptions in the original patients described by Harms and colleagues all occurred in the spring and summer and consisted of erythematous papules and petechial purpura located on the hands and feet with demarcation at the wrists and ankles, accompanied by edema and pruritus of the region.[94] Lesions also were seen variably on the cheeks, elbows, knees, inner thighs, hips, inguinal area, buttocks, and penis.[94] All of the cases were associated with oral mucosal

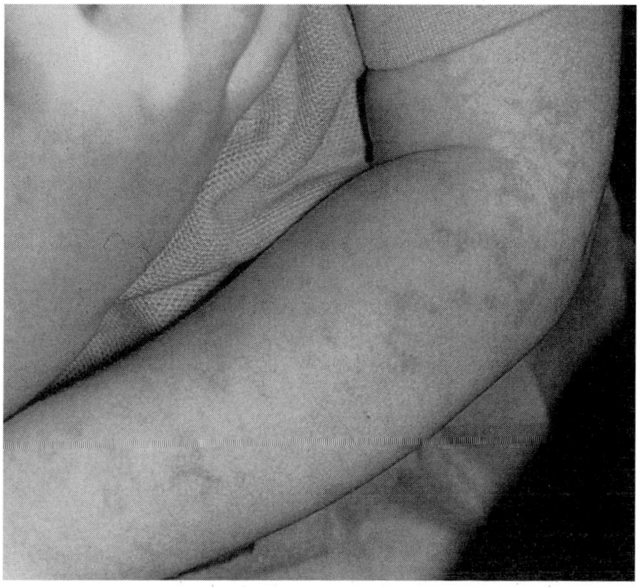

FIGURE 70–16. *Reticulated macular erythema on the skin of the left arm and forearm of a child with erythema infectiosum.*

findings, ranging from pharyngeal erythema to ulcerative lesions, and in many cases there were low-grade fever and lymphadenopathy. Subsequent case reports have described a similar syndrome.[90, 170, 191, 204] Leukopenia often has been reported.[90, 94, 191, 204] The lesions all cleared in 6 to 14 days,[94] and in some cases clearing has been associated with desquamation.[90, 204] Differential diagnoses considered in the original patients included Rocky Mountain spotted fever and other rickettsial diseases, Kawasaki syndrome, acral erythema due to chemotherapy, acral eruption associated with serum sickness, Gianotti-Crosti syndrome, measles, and hand, foot, and mouth disease.[94] Biopsy specimens have shown a lymphocytic and/or monocytic perivascular infiltrate in the upper dermis.[94, 170] Because PPGS is a self-limited disorder, no specific treatment is needed, but emollients and antipruritics may provide symptomatic relief.

Varicella-Zoster Virus Infection (Table 70–3)

VZV (herpesvirus 3) is the etiologic agent of chickenpox and herpes zoster (shingles). Chickenpox is a disease entity with which all pediatricians are exceedingly familiar. The common presentations of chickenpox and herpes zoster are presented in Table 70–3 (Figs. 70–17, 70–18, and 67–4, Color Plate I). Atypical or severe VZV infection may be seen in immunocompromised patients; in neonates of women who developed rash between 5 days before and 2 days after delivery and thus did not benefit from transplacental antibody transfer; as a result of secondary bacterial infection; and in areas of skin trauma, sun exposure, or inflammation. Congenital varicella is another severe form of disease that most often occurs in infants of mothers experiencing primary varicella, especially during the first trimester of pregnancy. Anomalies seen with the syndrome include cutaneous scarring, ocular abnormalities, limb hypoplasia, cortical atrophy, mental retardation and prematurity, and low birth weight.[152, 206] In addition, herpes zoster is being seen more commonly because of the increasing frequency and improved survival of immunocompromised children. With the licensing of the varicella vaccine for general use, herpes zoster may become a more common manifestation of VZV infection than chickenpox. Some of the less common cutaneous manifestations of VZV infection will be reviewed briefly.

Varicella lesions may become infected secondarily with streptococci or staphylococci, leading to impetigo.[167, 206, 212] Bullous varicella may result when secondary staphylococcal

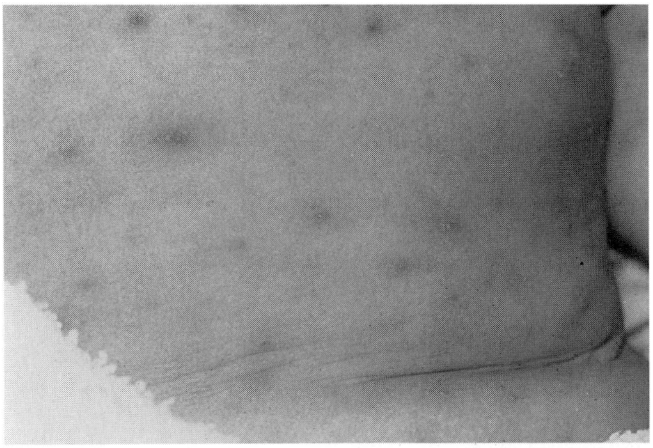

FIGURE 70–17. *Multiple isolated vesicles overlying a mildly inflamed base on the chest of a child with chickenpox.*

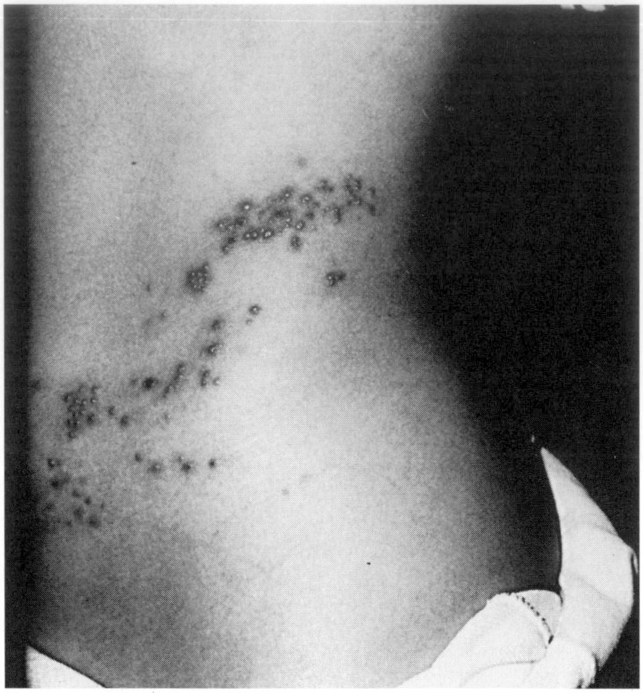

FIGURE 70–18. *A zosteriform distribution of isolated and grouped tense vesicles typical of herpes zoster.*

infection causes bullous impetigo or occasionally secondary to the varicella itself.[167, 212]

Both varicella and herpes zoster may be more severe and lead to disseminated infection in the immunocompromised host. Patients with defects of cellular immunity are at high risk of severe infection.[174] In a study by Srugo and colleagues,[106] HIV-infected children with low CD4 counts and those with advanced stages of HIV infection had a higher incidence of severe, chronic, recurrent, and disseminated varicella infection than did other HIV-infected children,[189] again emphasizing the role of cellular immunity. Chronic and recurrent infections, frequent herpes zoster, hemorrhagic and purpuric lesions, hyperkeratotic nodules and plaques, and chronic verrucous lesions resembling molluscum contagiosum infection[112] are some of the unusual manifestations of varicella seen in HIV-infected patients.[112, 166, 174, 189]

Another well-described but atypical form of varicella occurs in areas of previous skin injury. Photolocalized varicella occurs in skin that recently has been suntanned or sunburned.[10, 20, 163] The lesions initially may begin on the sun-exposed skin, may be more fulminant, and, unlike typical chickenpox lesions, may be of the same stage and size and not show characteristic centripetal spread.[20, 163] A large concentration of atypical lesions also may occur in skin previously affected by insect bites, pressure, inflammation, and other forms of skin trauma.[10] Severe or localized varicella in the diaper area may be seen as a result of previous diaper dermatitis and sometimes may be difficult to differentiate from genital HSV infection or impetigo.[106]

As the varicella vaccine becomes more widely used, it is likely that the manifestations of VZV infection will change. Previous studies have shown that breakthrough varicella in the first few years after immunization occurs in 5 to 12 per cent of healthy children.[81] Breakthrough infections generally are mild, with up to a 90 per cent reduction in the number of skin lesions, many of which may not be vesicular.[81] Rash occurs after immunization in about 5 per cent of healthy children, although VZV rarely has been cultured from the lesions.[81] Approximately 50 per cent of leukemic children develop a vaccine-associated rash 1 month after the first dose of varicella vaccine.[81] The reaction sometimes resembles a case of chickenpox, and acyclovir treatment may be needed.[81]

In healthy children, herpes zoster is a rare infection and occurs no more frequently in vaccinated than unvaccinated children.[55, 81] Herpes zoster is common in children with leukemia, and studies of this population have shown a lower incidence of zoster after vaccine than after natural varicella infection.[55, 81] Leukemic children who experienced a rash after varicella vaccine have a higher incidence of zoster than did those who had no rash, which may be secondary to increased viral access to sensory nerves after skin infection.[81]

Treatment of varicella generally is symptomatic, with use of antipyretics and antipruritics when needed. Application of cool compresses and topical agents, such as calamine lotion, is useful in relieving pruritus. Topical agents containing diphenhydramine should be avoided because of the potential for increased systemic absorption due to disrupted skin and subsequent toxicity. The use of oral acyclovir in normal children with varicella was approved by the Food and Drug Administration in 1992 and has been studied extensively. Early initiation of acyclovir therapy reduces the duration and severity of chickenpox in normal children.[65] Although it is not recommended for routine use in uncomplicated VZV infections, formal recommendations for use in specific circumstances have been made by the Committee on Infectious Disease.[56] Intravenous acyclovir is used for the treatment of severe cases of VZV infection and for VZV infection in immunocompromised patients.

Enterovirus Infections (Table 70–3)

The enteroviruses, a subgroup of picornaviruses, include poliovirus, coxsackieviruses, echoviruses, and enteroviruses. The nonpolio enteroviruses are a very common cause of viral exanthems. Because there are a large number of enteroviruses, many of which cause a variety of exanthems, the nonpolio enteroviruses will be considered as a group, and then the common subtypes and those that are responsible for specific syndromes will be discussed briefly. Chapter 170 presents a detailed discussion on the enteroviruses and their clinical manifestations.

Enteroviral infection is spread from person to person by the fecal-oral and possibly respiratory route.[37, 209] Because of the mode of transmission and because prevalence of antibody to the various enteroviruses rises with age, children are most susceptible to infection.[37, 79] Exanthems caused by enteroviruses also are more common in children and generally are related inversely to age.[37, 43] The subtype of enterovirus prevalent in a specific community will vary year to year, and thus the prevalence and type of associated exanthem also will vary.[43] Asymptomatic infection, as well as a variety of clinical symptoms, are caused by the enteroviruses. Nonspecific febrile illness, herpangina, pharyngitis, mild conjunctivitis, neurologic manifestations (most commonly aseptic meningitis), vomiting, diarrhea, and abdominal pain are some of the more frequent noncutaneous manifestations of enteroviral infection.[37] Epidemic acute hemorrhagic conjunctivitis, pneumonia, pleurodynia, pericarditis, myocarditis, hepatitis, and a host of other manifestations are associated with various types of enterovirus infection.[37] Although illness caused by the nonpolio enteroviruses usually is benign, fatal outcomes, including cases of sudden infant death, can occur.[37, 217]

Hand, foot, and mouth syndrome most frequently is associated with coxsackievirus A16 but can be caused by other enteroviruses, including coxsackieviruses A5, A7, A9, A10, B1, B3, and B5 and enterovirus 71 (Figs. 70–19, 67–9, 67–10, and 67–11, Color Plate II).[79] Enanthem occurs in about 90 per cent of patients[79] and exanthem in about two-thirds of those infected.[39, 79] Diagnosis usually is clinical, but virus can be cultured from the cutaneous or oral lesion.[201] Skin biopsy shows an initial intraepidermal vesicle that rapidly becomes subepidermal, as well as epidermal necrosis, intracellular and intercellular edema, and a lymphohistiocytic perivascular infiltrate of the superficial dermal plexus.[79] Aphthous stomatitis, bacterial infections, and herpetic infections sometimes are hard to differentiate from hand, foot, and mouth syndrome, but the presence of lesions in the three locations virtually is diagnostic. Herpangina, a febrile illness accompanied by papules, vesicles, and ulcerations of the anterior tonsillar pillars, tonsils, pharynx, soft palate, and anterior buccal mucosa, is caused by a variety of coxsackieviruses (including A16), echoviruses, and HSV.[36] There is no associated exanthem that differentiates it from hand, foot, and mouth syndrome. The treatment of this disease is supportive and includes attention to hydration and antipyretics, and, if needed, topical analgesia (such as diphenhydramine/Maalox combinations) can be used. In addition to hand, foot, and mouth syndrome, coxsackievirus A16 has been reported to cause morbilliform eruptions,[79] a papulovesicular acrodermatitis resembling Gianotti-Crosti syndrome,[37, 79] and has been associated with various subacute, chronic, and recurring skin lesions.[37]

Coxsackievirus A5 is a common cause of exanthem and enanthem.[37] The most frequent manifestation of infection is hand, foot, and mouth syndrome, which is indistinguishable from that caused by coxsackievirus A16.[37, 43]

Coxsackievirus A10 also causes hand, foot, and mouth syndrome and also has been reported in one case of Stevens-Johnson syndrome and in one case of ulcerative labial lesions and oral enanthem.[37]

Exanthem occurs in 4 per cent of coxsackievirus A9 infections, but because of the high prevalence of A9 infection, it is a common etiologic agent of viral exanthems.[37, 79] The maculopapular rash described in Table 70–3 is the most commonly associated exanthem, but urticarial, vesicular, petechial, and purpuric lesions mimicking meningococcemia have been reported (see Figs. 67–12, Color Plate II, and 67–14, Color Plate III).[37, 39, 43, 46, 79, 106] As previously mentioned, it also can cause hand, foot, and mouth syndrome.

Coxsackievirus A4 causes herpangina and occasional exan-

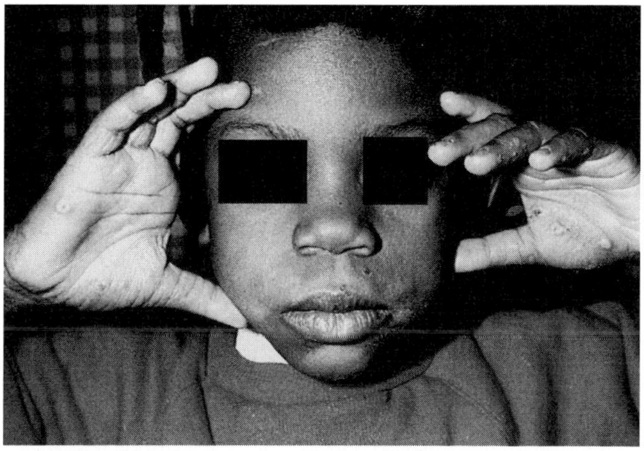

FIGURE 70–19. *Multiple erosions and vesicles present on the skin around the mouth and on the hands of a young girl with hand, foot, and mouth syndrome.*

thems and has been associated with small epidemics of disease.[39] The description of disease in Table 70–3 comes from a study of 11 patients with coxsackievirus A4 infection, 6 of whom had exanthem.[75]

Exanthems have been associated with coxsackieviruses B1 to 5, with exanthem most frequently occurring with coxsackievirus B5 infection.[37] In a study of seven patients with coxsackievirus B5–associated exanthems, symptoms included fever, pharyngitis, conjunctivitis, lymphadenopathy, and pharyngeal irritation.[47] Coxsackievirus B5 has been noted to cause roseola-like illness and, when associated with petechiae and meningitis, mimics meningococcemia.[79] Other manifestations of coxsackievirus B5 infection include hand, foot, and mouth syndrome, encephalitis, pleurodynia, myocarditis, pericarditis, abdominal pain, hepatitis, pancreatitis, and orchitis.[37, 106]

Echovirus 9 is the most frequent echoviral disease, with a common manifestation of infection being exanthem (see Fig. 67–13, Color Plate III).[37, 79] Overall, echovirus 9 causes rash in 35 per cent of infections[39] but, as in other enteroviral infections, exanthem is related inversely to age, with 57 per cent of children younger than 5 years of age exhibiting exanthem and only 6 per cent of those older than 10 years of age manifesting exanthem due to echovirus 9 infection.[37, 79] Photoexaggeration of viral exanthems is known to occur commonly, and this phenomenon is seen frequently with the exanthem of echovirus 9.[106] Like many other enteroviruses, echovirus 9 can cause aseptic meningitis, and because of its association with a petechial eruption, it mimics meningococcal disease.[37, 79, 106]

Boston exanthem is the name given to echovirus 16 infection originally studied by Neva and his colleagues in a 1951 Boston outbreak and was the first echoviral exanthem to be described.[91] Since that time, three other outbreaks have been described, the last in 1974.[37, 91] The illness is described in Table 70–3 and frequently is roseola-like, with rash occurring at or after defervescence.[37, 79, 91] However, the fever usually is of shorter duration.[79] Herpangina also occurs in some cases of echovirus 16 infection.[37, 79]

Echovirus 11 can cause aseptic meningitis, gastroenteritis, upper respiratory infections, croup,[48, 79] and paralytic poliomyelitis.[48] Variable exanthems have been associated with some cases of echovirus 11 infection.[48] Echovirus 11–associated exanthem and maculopapular, urticarial, and vesicular lesions may be limited or widespread,[48] as was determined in a study of seven patients. Associated symptoms of fever, pharyngitis, coryza, rhonchi, cough, and lymphadenopathy were reported, but illness was mild in the seven cases described.[48]

Echovirus 25 is associated with many different exanthems.[37, 79] Most commonly, rashes are maculopapular or morbilliform, but hemangioma-like lesions have been described.[37, 79] These interesting lesions were described as erythematous papules, with a central bright red papule or macule suggestive of a terminal arteriole or capillary surrounded by a 1 to 4 mm wide area of blanched-appearing skin (Fig. 70–20). The entire lesion would blanch with central pressure.[37, 39] Echovirus 32 also has been associated with hemangioma-like lesions.[37]

Adenovirus Infections (Table 70–3)

The adenoviruses cause a wide array of illnesses. Adenoviral types 1 to 4, 7, 7a, and other unknown types have been associated with exanthems.[34, 79] Exanthem is seen most frequently in association with adenoviral-associated respiratory illness, including the common cold, pharyngitis, laryngotracheitis, bronchiolitis, pneumonia, and pharyngoconjunctival fever.[39] Adenoviral rashes may mimic those of rubella, measles, or roseola.[34, 79] Adenoviral type 7 infection has been associated with a petechial exanthem mimicking meningococcemia and with the Stevens-Johnson syndrome.[43, 79]

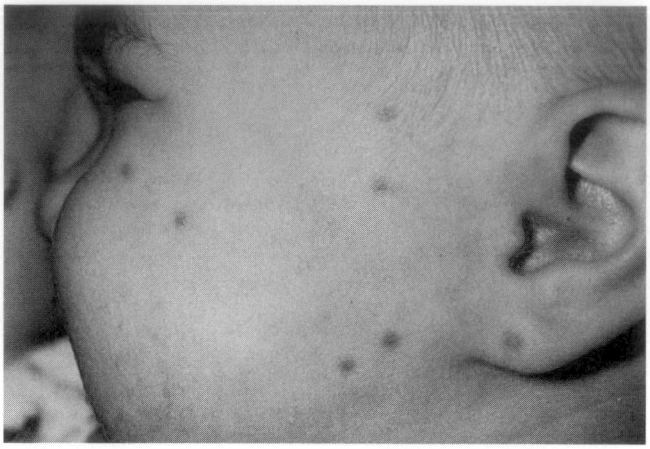

FIGURE 70–20. *Bright red papules on the skin of a child with culture-proven echovirus infection.*

Reovirus Infections (Table 70–3)

Reoviruses are common infectious agents of both animals and humans, but human clinical disease has not been well defined. Exanthem has been noted to be a common manifestation of clinically apparent reoviral disease.[43, 79] In one study, six of seven children with reovirus type 2 infection had associated exanthem.[126]

Gianotti-Crosti Syndrome (Table 70–3)

In 1955, Gianotti first described the distinctive cutaneous eruption that is known today as the Gianotti-Crosti syndrome. All of the initial cases of this syndrome were associated with anicteric hepatitis B (mostly subtype ayw) infection.[167] It was discovered later that a similar eruption could be produced by other viral infections. Initially, all cases caused by agents other than hepatitis B virus were classified by Gianotti as papulovesicular acrolocated syndrome, and all cases due to hepatitis B virus infection were called papular acrodermatitis of childhood.[29] In a retrospective study of 308 patients diagnosed with one of the aforementioned syndromes, Caputo and colleagues[29] showed that the differences between papulovesicular acrolocated syndrome and papular acrodermatitis of childhood probably were due to individual patient characteristics and not to a difference in the causative virus. They proposed that the term Gianotti-Crosti syndrome be used for all cases,[29] and this now generally is accepted as the correct terminology. The viruses that have been reported in association with the Gianotti-Crosti syndrome include various subtypes of hepatitis B virus,[124] EBV,[9] hepatitis A virus,[177] CMV,[11] respiratory syncytial virus,[63] coxsackievirus A16, coxsackieviruses B4 and B5, echoviruses 7 and 9, parainfluenza virus,[188] hepatitis C virus, poliovaccine virus,[63] VZV, rubella virus,[157] and, as previously mentioned, parvovirus B19.[16, 130, 167, 170] There also is a report of two cases of Gianotti-Crosti syndrome in HIV-infected children, but whether it was caused by HIV, another virus the patients had been infected with, or a nonviral agent, such as *Mycobacterium avium-intra-*

cellulare, could not be determined definitively.[16] In addition, two patients have been reported to have Gianotti-Crosti syndrome associated with group A beta-hemolytic streptococcal pharyngitis and negative viral cultures.[63]

The major epidemiologic and clinical features of the Gianotti-Crosti syndrome are described in Table 70–3 (Fig. 70–21). This syndrome mainly affects children younger than 10 years of age[136] but also can affect infants[79] and rarely has been reported in young adults.[136] The clinical features can be highly variable due to the multitude of different agents that are capable of causing disease. There is a hemorrhagic variant of the Gianotti-Crosti syndrome, in which purpuric lesions are seen and are believed to be due to capillary fragility rather than vasculitis.[130] Although Gianotti-Crosti syndrome has been defined as being a nonrecurrent illness, there is one case report of its being associated with a hepatitis B virus infection and recurrence 5 months later in association with rubella virus infection.[157] The diagnosis of Gianotti-Crosti syndrome is made based on the clinical characteristics and evidence of an underlying viral infection. Biopsy of the lesions generally shows spongiosis and epidermal and upper dermal perivascular lymphocytic and histiocytic infiltrates.[11, 16, 130] The differential diagnosis includes contact dermatitis, atopic dermatitis, lichen planus, Henoch-Schönlein purpura, EM, and papular urticaria.[79, 136, 209] Gianotti-Crosti syndrome is a benign, self-limited cutaneous eruption that requires no specific treatment. The underlying viral illness may require therapy, and patients with hepatitis B or C with or without associated Gianotti-Crosti syndrome should be monitored for the development of chronic hepatitis.

Measles (Table 70–3)

The measles virus is discussed in detail in Chapter 183. A few brief comments on the infection, with emphasis on the dermatologic manifestations, will be given in this section.

The exanthem and enanthem of measles are believed to be due to direct infection of the epithelial cells with virus.[196] Histologic examination of the skin reveals focal parakeratosis, dyskeratosis, and spongiosis.[79, 196] Two types of multinucleated giant cells are characteristic: the epidermal syncytial giant cells in the skin, mucous membranes, and respiratory epithelium and the Warthin-Finkeldey cell found in the reticuloendothelial system.[38, 79] The pathogenesis of the lesions of atypical measles is not certain, but an Arthus-type reaction or a delayed-type hypersensitivity reaction may be involved.[44]

Classic or typical measles occurs in an individual who has no prior immunity to the measles virus. The typical exanthem of classic measles is described in Table 70–3 (Figs. 70–22, 70–23, and Fig. 67–2, Color Plate I). Occasionally, the lesions appear purpuric or, in the extremely rare case of "black" or hemorrhagic measles, are confluent and hemorrhagic.[79] In the immunocompromised host, the rash of measles may be diminished or absent, and the disease is very severe and often fatal.[79] Modified measles may occur in a variety of situations in which the host partially is immune. It classically was seen when measles immune serum globulin was administered to a nonimmune individual exposed to measles.[38] It also may be seen in infants younger than 9

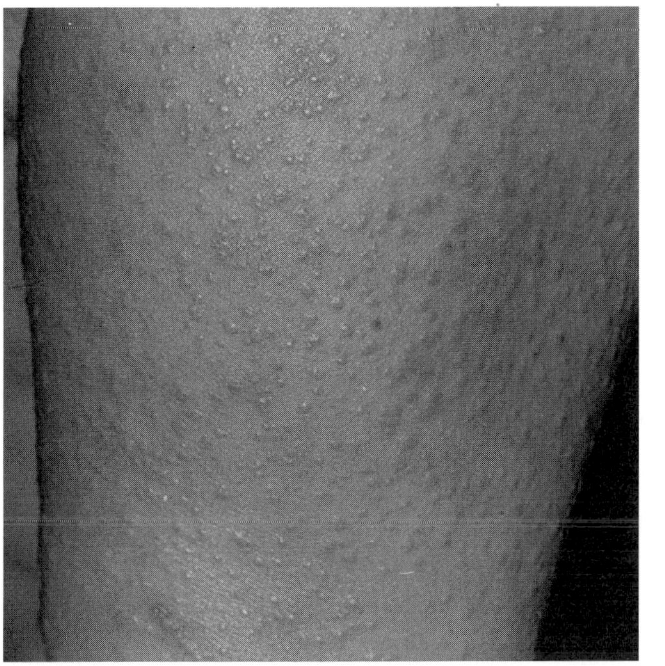

FIGURE 70–21. *Diffusely distributed isolated, monomorphous skin-colored papules on the thigh of a child typical of Gianotti-Crosti syndrome.*

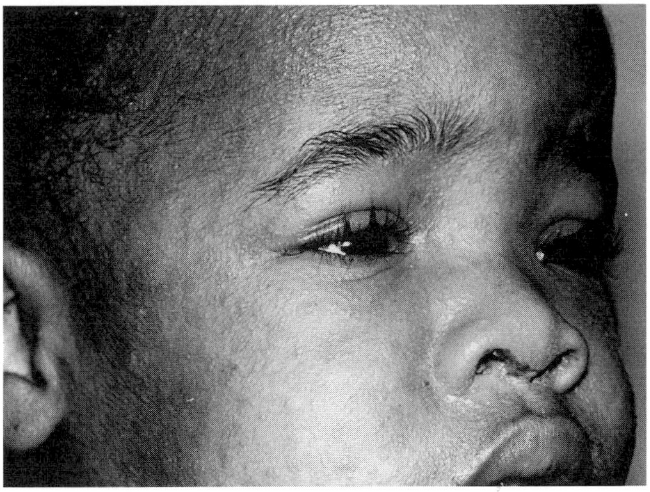

FIGURE 70–22. *Erythematous maculopapular eruption on the skin of a child with measles.*

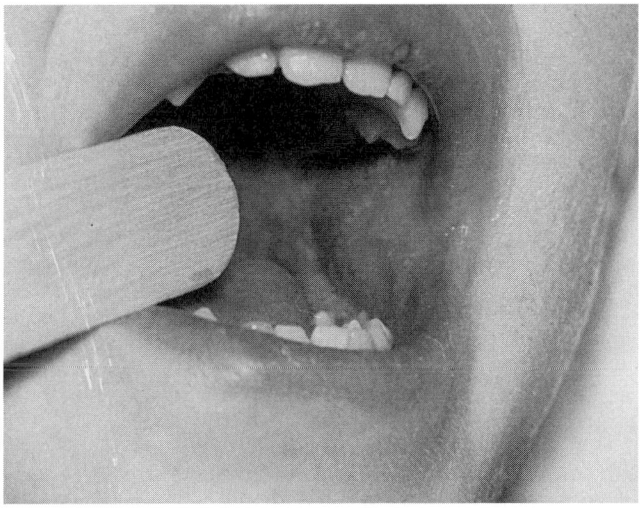

FIGURE 70–23. *Numerous white papules characteristic of Koplik spots present over the posterior buccal mucosa of a child diagnosed with measles.*

months of age with presence of maternal antibodies, cases of partial vaccine failure, and recurrent measles.[38, 79] Features generally are those of classic measles but are milder. Atypical measles occurs when an individual previously vaccinated, usually with inactivated vaccine but occasionally also with live viral vaccine, is exposed to the natural virus.[44] The exanthem is quite variable and may not occur at all.[79] The lesions most often are maculopapular but may be vesicular, petechial, purpuric, or urticarial.[38, 79] A biphasic rash, with an initial transitory rash suggestive of atypical measles and the appearance 2 weeks later of the exanthem commonly seen in atypical measles, has been described.[38, 79] Accompanying edema of the extremities is not an uncommon finding.[38, 79] Atypical measles especially may be difficult to differentiate from Rocky Mountain spotted fever, drug reactions, and Henoch-Schönlein purpura.[44] The final atypical manifestation associated with measles is a faint maculopapular rash that occasionally occurs 7 to 10 days after immunization with the live attenuated vaccine.[79]

Mumps (Table 70–3)

Mumps virus is a paramyxovirus that produces a generalized infection but rarely has been associated with exanthem. The major characteristics of mumps virus infection and the characteristics of the rashes of six patients whose exanthems were thought to be associated with mumps are reported in Table 70–3. In the report of six patients with presumed mumps-associated exanthems, mumps virus was isolated from one of the patients and four had serologic evidence of infection.[45] No other viruses were isolated from any of the patients.[45] EM also has been associated with mumps on rare occasions.[43] Two of the six patients with exanthems also had accompanying enanthems, one with sores under the tongue and the other with anterior buccal ulcerations.[45] Because mumps is not seen often in the postvaccine era, no recent information on the incidence of exanthem is available.

Rubella (Table 70–3)

Rubella generally is a mild disease when acquired postnatally. The incidence has dropped precipitously, and the usual age of onset has increased since the licensing of the vaccine in 1969. The disease may be asymptomatic or present with the clinical manifestations and exanthem described in Table 70–3 (see Fig. 67–3, Color Plate I). The prodromal symptoms and lymphadenopathy associated with rubella may be present without rash.[42] Other reported manifestations of rubella are erythema infectiosum and roseola-like illnesses.[42, 79] The complications of rubella include arthritis and arthralgias (both of which are more common in adults and in females), thrombocytopenic purpura, and encephalitis.[42]

The pathogenesis of the rubella exanthem is not known precisely, but virus has been cultured from the skin in both congenital and postnatal rubella.[79, 96] An inflammatory response to viral infection and/or an antigen-antibody response may be involved in producing the characteristic cutaneous manifestations of the disease.[79, 96]

Congenital rubella is a much more severe form of disease that most commonly occurs when a susceptible woman is infected during the first trimester of pregnancy.[152] Rubella may result in fetal death or clinically may be inapparent at birth but may lead to long-term sequelae within 5 years.[152] The common symptoms of congenital rubella that present in the neonatal period are growth retardation, hepatosplenomegaly, jaundice, thrombocytopenic purpura and petechiae, congenital heart disease, and cataracts.[152] Congenital rubella also may involve the central nervous system, the most common manifestation of which is nerve deafness, which often is not recognized until later in life.[42, 152] Two cutaneous manifestations associated with congenital rubella are blueberry muffin spots, which are purple–dark blue macules, nodules, or papules representing extramedullary hematopoiesis, and thrombocytopenic purpura.[42, 152, 167] Both of these manifestations often are poor prognostic signs because they often are seen in severely affected infants.[42, 152] Children with congenital rubella later may develop a morbilliform rash, similar to that seen in postnatal rubella.[167]

Epstein-Barr Virus Infection (Table 70–3)

EBV is a double-stranded DNA virus that is a member of the herpesvirus family and is the cause of infectious mononucleosis. EBV also is implicated as the cause of Burkitt lymphoma, nasopharyngeal carcinoma, and various lymphoproliferative disorders.[193] Although almost all adults show seroreactivity to EBV antigens, the age of primary infection with EBV varies, with a younger age of primary infection in developing countries and lower socioeconomic groups.[193] Primary EBV infection more often manifests as an asymptomatic or mild viral infection in young children, whereas infectious mononucleosis is more common in adolescents and young adults.[193] However, in a prospective study of 113 patients with infectious mononucleosis, 64 of the patients were between 6 months and 5 years of age, suggesting that infectious mononucleosis may be more common than suspected in young children.[194]

The principal features of infectious mononucleosis are fever, lymphadenopathy (especially cervical), tonsillopharyngitis with or without exudate, splenomegaly, and hepatomegaly.[194] Rhinitis, cough, rash, abdominal pain, and eyelid or periorbital edema also are seen frequently.[194] In the previously mentioned study of 113 children with infectious mononucleosis, rash, upper respiratory infection symptoms, and possibly hepatosplenomegaly were seen more commonly in the younger than 4-year-old age group.[194] The rate of cutaneous manifestations in infectious mononucleosis varies in different studies. In Sumaya and Ench's study, 34 per cent of the children younger than 4 years of age and 16.7 per cent of those 4 to 16 years of age developed a rash as part of the infectious mononucleosis syndrome.[194] Other studies that have included adults report rash in 3[148] to 16 per cent[171] of patients. There is a definite increase in the frequency of rash when ampicillin is administered to an individual with infectious mononucleosis.[156, 171] Incidences of 95[171] to 100 per cent[156] were reported in older studies, but the incidence may be lower[66] and may be recognized less frequently in children because of the higher incidence of rash accompanying infection alone.[193] The association between drug administration and rash is not believed to be related to ampicillin hypersensitivity.[156, 171] The incidence of this association with other antimicrobials is somewhat questionable, but it seems that administration of penicillin during mononucleosis leads to an increased incidence of rash.[79, 171, 209] The clinical manifestations of ampicillin-associated and -nonassociated rashes in infectious mononucleosis are described in Table 70–3. In addition to the typical exanthems described in the table, urticarial, EM-like, petechial, and papulovesicular rashes have been reported (Fig. 70–24).[194] Palatal petechiae appearing between the fifth and seventeenth day of illness are a nonspecific enanthem seen in about one-quarter of the cases of infectious mononucleosis.[134] Because the cutaneous manifestations of EBV infection are nonspecific, the diagnosis must be made

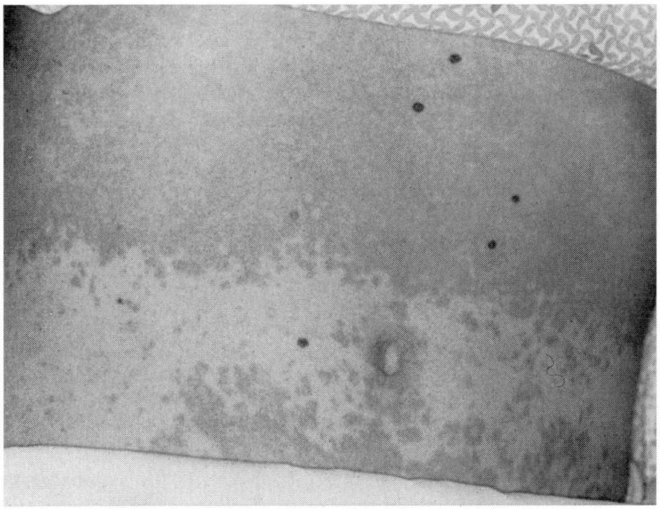

FIGURE 70–24. *Confluent maculopapular erythema on the abdomen of a child with mononucleosis after receiving ampicillin. (Courtesy of Morven Edwards, M.D.)*

in conjunction with the other clinical characteristics and the appropriate laboratory evaluation, including complete blood count and heterophil antibody test. The heterophil antibody response is decreased in children younger than 4 years of age, and EBV serologies may need to be measured in order to make a definitive diagnosis.[195]

EBV also has been associated variably with other cutaneous manifestations. EBV has been found to replicate in the lesions of oral hairy leukoplakia, an AIDS-associated disease (see HIV section).[99] As mentioned previously, EBV is associated with the Gianotti-Crosti syndrome, and there also have been scattered reports associating EBV with other skin diseases, including pityriasis lichenoides[19] and granuloma annulare–like lesions.[99]

Cytomegalovirus Infection (Table 70–3)

CMV is a member of the family *Herpesviridae*. Infection is very common, and, like EBV infection, primary infection occurring during childhood is seen more frequently in children from developing countries and lower socioeconomic groups.[60] Excluding congenital and perinatal infections, CMV in the immunocompetent host usually is an asymptomatic infection. Because of this, cutaneous manifestations of infection are seen almost exclusively in infants and immunosuppressed patients.

CMV may cause a mononucleosis-like syndrome that is seen most frequently in the 20- to 40-year-old age group but may be seen in any age group.[60] A rubelliform or maculopapular rash sometimes is seen with this syndrome.[60, 79, 127] As in EBV-associated mononucleosis, rash is more frequent in CMV mononucleosis in patients given ampicillin.[60, 127] The Gianotti-Crosti syndrome also can be associated with CMV infection with or without hepatitis.[127]

Congenital CMV infection often is not apparent, with 90 per cent of infants being asymptomatic at birth or in the neonatal period.[127, 152] The most common features of congenital infection are microcephaly, intracerebral calcifications, chorioretinitis, low birth weight, hepatosplenomegaly, jaundice, thrombocytopenic purpura or petechiae, and pneumonia.[152, 153] In addition to the petechial or purpuric lesions due to thrombocytopenia, congenitally infected infants may present with so-called blueberry muffin spots, which are dark blue to red papules or nodules of persistent dermal erythropoiesis (see Fig. 67–21, Color Plate IV).[127] There also is a report of cutaneous vesicles in an infant with congenital CMV infection.[15] Perinatally acquired CMV infection often is asymptomatic or may present with hepatosplenomegaly, lymphadenopathy, or pneumonitis[60] but is not associated with specific cutaneous manifestations.

CMV has been associated with a variety of cutaneous manifestations in the immunocompromised host. Most of the cutaneous manifestations of CMV infection seen in the immunocompromised host can be divided into two broad categories: localized, ulcerative lesions and widespread exanthematous eruptions.[155] The ulcerative lesions are demarcated sharply and most often occur in the genital and perineal regions but may occur elsewhere.[155] Biopsy of the lesions shows a cytomegalic vasculitis of the small dermal vessels.[155] The widespread eruptions may be morbilliform, urticarial, petechial, or purpuric.[79, 128, 155] Biopsy shows intranuclear inclusions of CMV in the vascular endothelial cells.[155] In one immunocompromised patient with acute disseminated CMV infection, a morbilliform rash first occurred while the patient was receiving ampicillin and later recurred.[128] At the time of death, there was no rash, but histologic examination of normal-appearing skin showed CMV inclusion bodies in the endothelium of capillaries and small vessels with luminal obliteration, stasis, vasculitis, and thrombus formation, suggesting that CMV disease involving the skin may not be clinically apparent always.[128] There also is a report of an immunocompromised patient with a vesiculobullous eruption due to CMV.[14] There has been some question of a possible role of CMV infection in the neoplastic process of Kaposi sarcoma.[60, 127] Although there is no specific skin lesion associated with CMV, it may play a role in many of the skin lesions seen in immunocompromised patients, and as more studies are conducted, an even wider variety of manifestations may become apparent.

HIV Infection

Infectious, inflammatory, and neoplastic cutaneous diseases are a common problem in HIV-infected patients. Severe, recurrent, or unusual skin diseases may be a presenting sign or later complication of HIV infection. Throughout this chapter, references are made to the presentation and treatment of common viral diseases occurring in HIV-infected and other immunosuppressed patients. There also are rarer, possibly viral-related cutaneous manifestations that are seen in HIV-infected patients. Acute HIV infection in adults may be accompanied by an exanthem.[135, 167] The exanthem appears after several days of flu-like symptoms and most often presents as round to oval maculopapular lesions that occur on the face, neck, and trunk and may involve the extremities.[135] The lesions may desquamate, have necrotic or hemorrhagic centers, or appear urticarial.[135] An ulcerative enanthem also has been reported,[135] although not in children.

Oral hairy leukoplakia is a manifestation of HIV infection believed to be caused by EBV infection of the tongue.[26, 166] It presents as whitish, corrugated plaques on the lateral surfaces of the tongue (Fig. 70–25). Although usually seen in adults, it also has been reported in children.[166] The disease usually is asymptomatic but occasionally is accompanied by a burning sensation within the lesions.[26] Treatments that have been used include superficial shave excision, topical tretinoin, podophyllin, and oral acyclovir.[26] Lesions tend to recur after most treatments.[26]

Kaposi sarcoma is an AIDS-defining neoplastic disease that most often is seen in adults but has been reported in chil-

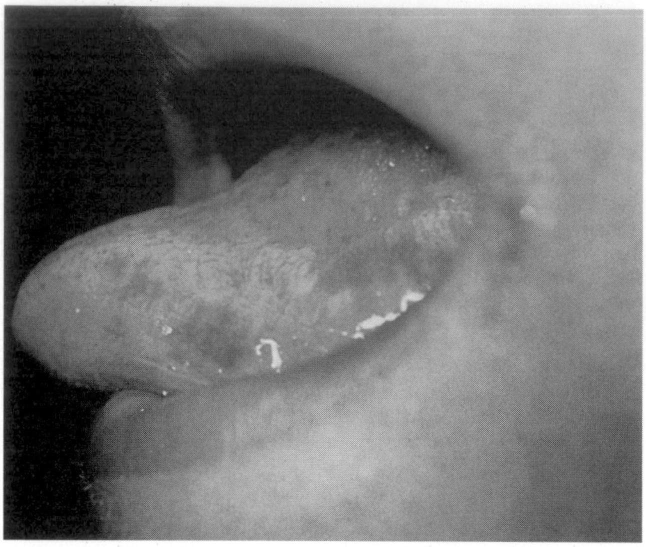

FIGURE 70–25. *Confluent white plaque on the lateral surface of the tongue of a child with HIV infection.*

dren.[93, 167] The cutaneous lesions initially are macular but go on to the plaque stage of thickened, indurated, pink to red or purple papules that may progress to nodules and later develop postinflammatory hyperpigmentation (Fig. 70–26).[135] The pathogenesis of Kaposi sarcoma is not known, but CMV infection may be involved.[60, 93]

Finally, mixed viral, bacterial, and fungal infections may occur in cutaneous lesions of HIV-infected patients.[166] Failure to respond to a therapeutic intervention should prompt a search for both co-infectious and resistant organisms.

FUNGAL INFECTIONS

Most infections caused by fungi involving the skin are superficial in nature. Such infections generally are due to dermatophytes, yeasts, or (rarely) the dematiaceous fungi. Additionally, however, involvement of deeper cutaneous structures and multisystem involvement may occur with fungal infections. An appreciation of a more common clinical presentation of each of these infections, their diagnosis, and therapy is important. This review will focus on the clinical aspects of fungal infections and particularly their appearance when involving the skin. Therapeutic issues of the superficial fungal infections will be summarized briefly.

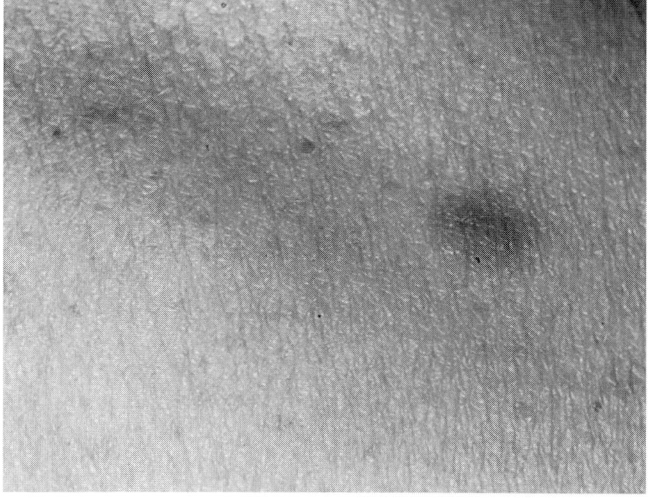

FIGURE 70–26. *An isolated indurated red papule typical of Kaposi sarcoma on the skin of a patient with AIDS.*

Superficial Fungal Infections

Dermatophyte Infections

Dermatophytosis describes infection with organisms belonging to the *Trichophyton*, *Microsporum*, or *Epidermophyton* genus.[131, 208] Infections with these agents generally present with skin involvement. The most common dermatophytes are anthropophilic and can be passed from human to human. The zoophilic agents, although seen in humans, generally infect animals. Lastly, the geophilic dermatophytes come from the soil and can infect both humans and animals.[131] Dermatophyte infections are described using the designation tinea with the body site involved (tinea capitis = scalp, tinea pedis = foot, tinea manum = hand, etc.).

In the general population, tinea corporis is seen with greater frequency than is either tinea pedis or tinea unguium.[50] Because tinea capitis is seen with greater frequency in children than in adults, it will be discussed first.

In North and South America, infection of the scalp with fungi generally is due to *Trichophyton tonsurans*.[50] Tinea capitis is seen primarily in prepubertal children. Its clinical presentation may be that of a diffusely distributed seborrheic-like scaling of the scalp, focal areas of scaling with or without alopecia, alopecia with only black dots representative of broken hairs in affected individuals, or with a kerion representing a hypersensitivity response by the host to the dermatophyte (Fig. 70–27). Kerions more often are seen with either zoophilic or geophilic fungi due to the inflammatory nature of these organisms. "Id" reactions may be seen in some individuals with particularly inflammatory lesions. These represent inflammatory lesions on the skin seen adjacent to or distant from the primary infection (Fig. 70–28). Id reactions are felt to be another immune response to the dermatophyte infections.[131] Tinea corporis refers to fungal infection of the trunk or extremities with a dermatophyte. Clinically, annular scaling patches or plaques (with the scale being present at the periphery or advancing margin of a lesion) are seen (Fig. 70–29). The more central area generally is free of scale. Erythema is distributed throughout such a lesion. Addition-

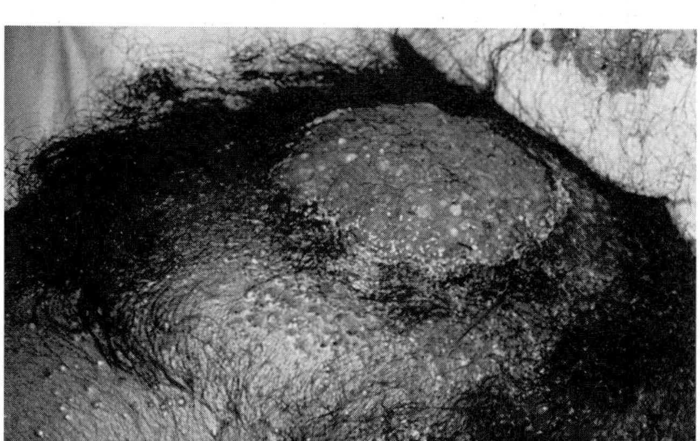

FIGURE 70–27. *Well-circumscribed tender tumor with overlying pustules characteristic of a kerion on the scalp of a child.*

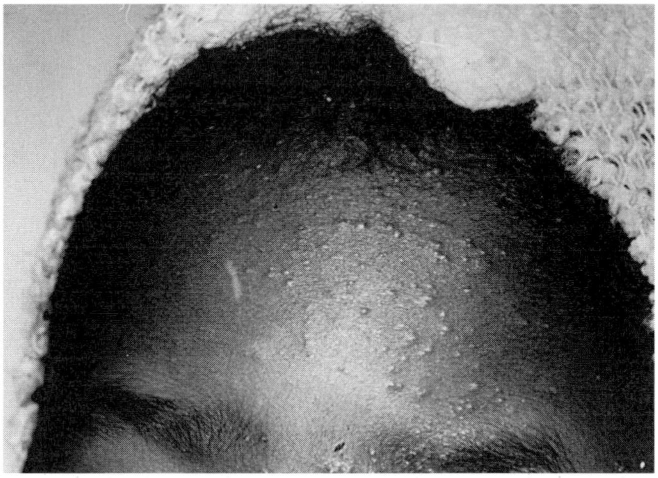

FIGURE 70–28. *Multiple skin-colored papules and pustules on the forehead typical of an "id" reaction to tinea capitis.*

ally, one may see pustules, papules, or nodules in cases of tinea corporis. Infection with *Microsporum canis, Trichophyton rubrum, Epidermophyton floccosum,* and other organisms may prove to be the cause of cases of tinea corporis. Tinea pedis describes infection of the feet with any of a variety of dermatophytes. Most isolates, however, are *T. rubrum* or *Trichophyton mentagrophytes*. Scaling, fissuring, and maceration between toes with erythema surrounding the area of involvement commonly are seen (see Fig. 67–22, Color Plate IV). Additionally, some patients may present with a moccasin-like distribution of tinea pedis involving the soles of the feet. Children and adults also may present with tense, deeply situated vesicles over the instep of the feet. Tinea cruris describes infection of the groin area with any of a variety of dermatophytes. Clinically, affected patients will complain of some discomfort in the involved area and, upon examination, will reveal erythema and maceration in the skin folds with a scaling advancing margin to the area of inflammation. Lastly, infection of the nails with a dermatophyte is described as tinea unguium, and onychomycosis is a generic term used

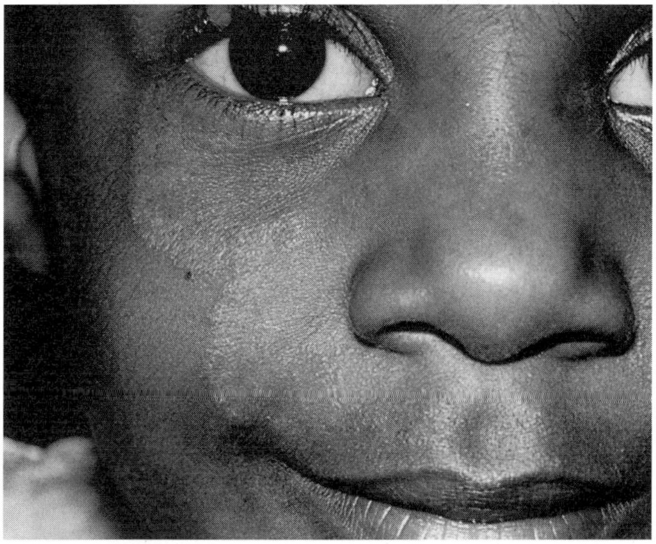

FIGURE 70–29. *An annular plaque with peripheral scale on the face of a child with tinea faciei.*

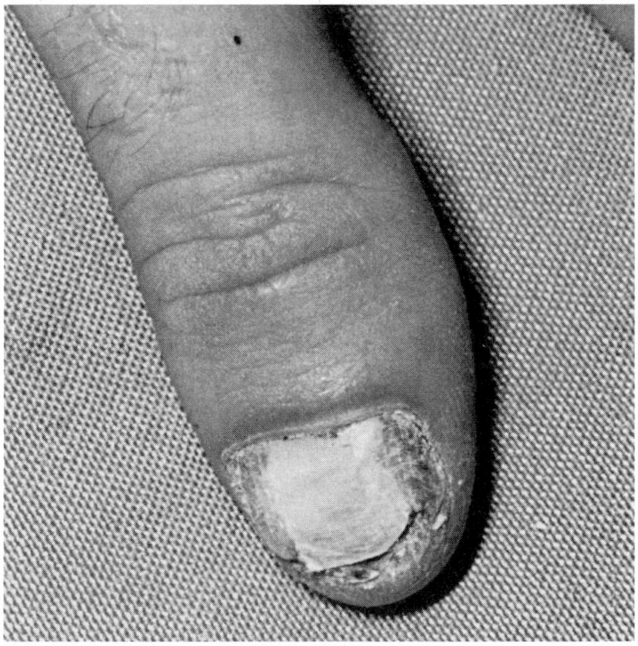

FIGURE 70–30. *Clinical photograph illustrating onychodystrophy and subungual hyperkeratosis involving the left thumb of a child with onychomycosis.*

to describe fungal infection of the nails.[131] Most commonly, patients will present with involvement of the distal finger or toenail with subungual debris and either mild or no inflammation (Fig. 70–30). Involvement of the proximal nail fold is uncommon but can be seen as well. A clinically distinct form of involvement of the fingernails or toenails presenting with superficial white scaling can be seen in some individuals (Fig. 70–31). *T. mentagrophytes* is the most common dermatophyte causing such an infection.

DIAGNOSIS. Although one may suspect the diagnosis of dermatophytosis clinically, it is imperative to confirm the diagnosis, as with any infection. Examination of suitable

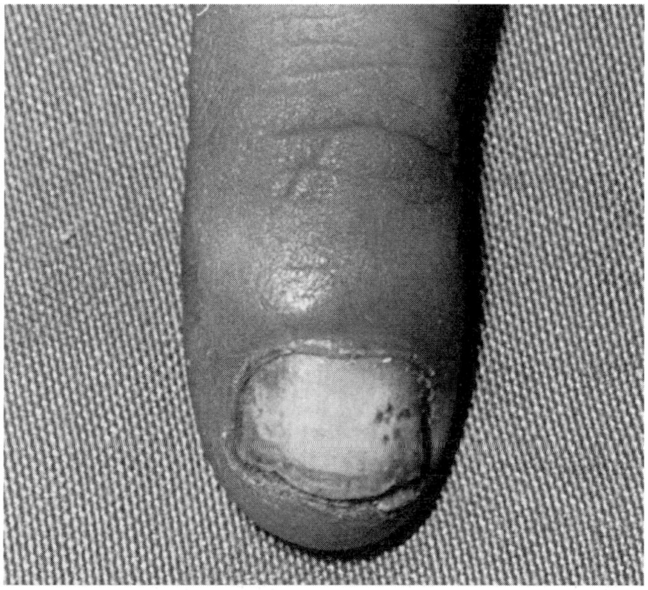

FIGURE 70–31. *Clinical photograph of the fingernail illustrating the superficial white scaling typical of superficial white onychomycosis.*

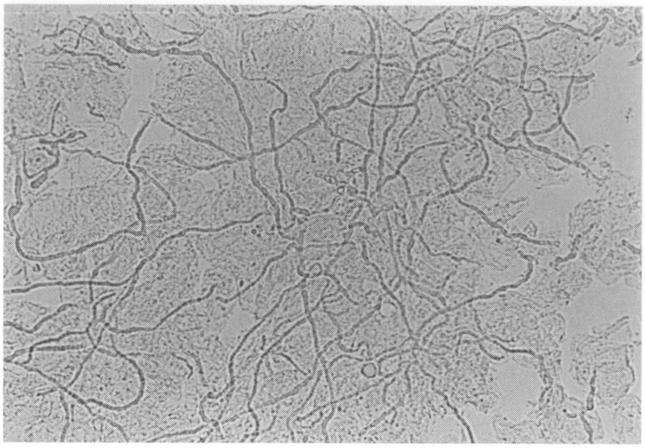

FIGURE 70–32. *Photomicrograph revealing branching hyphae from a case of tinea corporis. (×400.) (Courtesy of J. Tschen, M.D.)*

clinical material (e.g., affected scalp hairs, skin scrapings from the advancing margin of lesions on the body, nails) with potassium hydroxide by standard light microscopy should reveal branching hyphae in cases of tinea corporis or tinea unguium (Fig. 70–32). With suspected cases of tinea capitis, however, branching hyphae generally are not seen. Rather, multiple spores in or around infected hairs should be demonstrated (Fig. 70–33). Endothrix infections of the scalp hair are due to *Trichophyton* organisms, and ectothrix infections generally are due to *Microsporum*.[74] To perform a potassium hydroxide examination, the clinical material is placed on a glass slide, onto which either 10 or 20 per cent potassium hydroxide is applied. After a coverslip is placed over the sample, the epithelial cells will "clear" after a period of 10 to 15 minutes. This period can be shortened by general heating of the slide or by the addition of dimethylsulfoxide. Spores and hyphae are resistant to this "clearing" effect. The specimen then is examined under the 20× or 40× objective to reveal hyphae or spores.

When the clinical appearance of a lesion is uncharacteristic, if the potassium hydroxide examination is negative for evidence of fungal disease, or in unusual clinical situations, cultures for fungi should be performed. Suitable clinical material is inoculated easily onto Sabouraud dextrose agar medium. Chloramphenicol and cycloheximide sometimes are added to Sabouraud to inhibit bacterial or saprophytic growth.

Lastly, biopsy of representative skin lesions occasionally may be required. Such specimens are obtained from suspected lesions and are examined by routine light microscopy utilizing a variety of stains to enhance the recognition of fungal elements. Certainly, biopsy specimens also should be submitted for appropriate cultures.

Although the clinical diagnosis of tinea infections generally is clear, other disorders present some confusion with tinea on occasion. In cases of tinea capitis presenting with diffuse scaling of the scalp, primary inflammatory diseases of the skin, such as seborrheic dermatitis, psoriasis, or eczema, should be considered (Fig. 70–34). These disorders, however, generally will present with clinical features elsewhere on the body. Rarely, scabies can involve the scalp in a manner that might demonstrate diffuse papules and scaling.

On occasion, areas of alopecia on the scalp can be seen due to trauma, bacterial folliculitis, subcutaneous masses, and alopecia areata. Due to the extreme inflammation present with a kerion, some patients may be felt to have a localized (bacterial) scalp abscess. In fact, bacteria frequently are cultured from kerions but generally are felt to be secondary to the primary fungal infection.[102, 103]

Well-defined annular scaling patches of tinea corporis may be confused with a "reactive" scaling annular inflammatory condition known as erythema annulare centrifugum (Fig. 70–35). It is a noninfectious process that has been reported to occur in response to a dermatophyte, as well as other infections. Most commonly, however, it occurs in an idiopathic form. A nonscaling annular condition, common in children, is granuloma annulare (Fig. 70–36). This noninfectious granulomatous process is characterized by its indurated border and depressed center. Lesions typically occur on the dorsa of the hands or feet but may occur anywhere.

Scaling of the feet may be seen in a variety of conditions, including psoriasis, pityriasis rubra pilaris, a variety of bacterial or viral disorders, reactions to medications, endocrinologic diseases, eczema, and ichthyosis. When scaling and maceration are present between toes, *Candida* must be considered in addition to dermatophyte infections. Noninfectious intertrigo also should be considered.

Lastly, onychodystrophy can occur frequently due to fun-

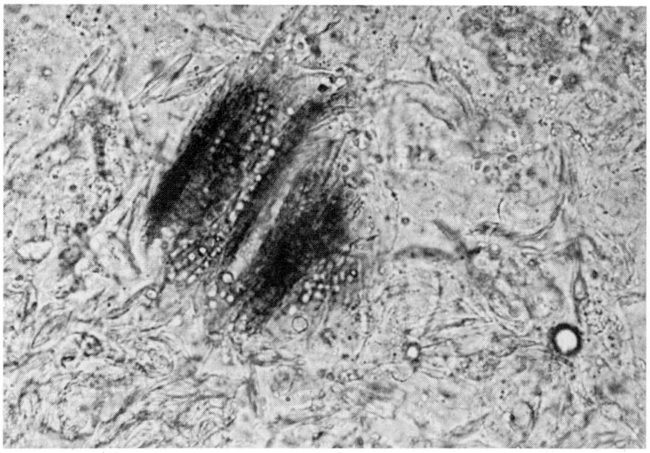

FIGURE 70–33. *Multiple spores present within a hair shaft from a patient diagnosed with tinea capitis. (×400.)*

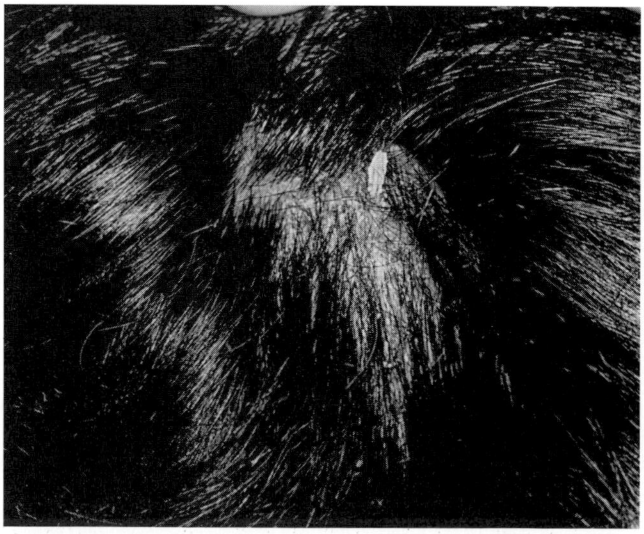

FIGURE 70–34. *A focal area of dense scaling of the scalp typical of psoriasis.*

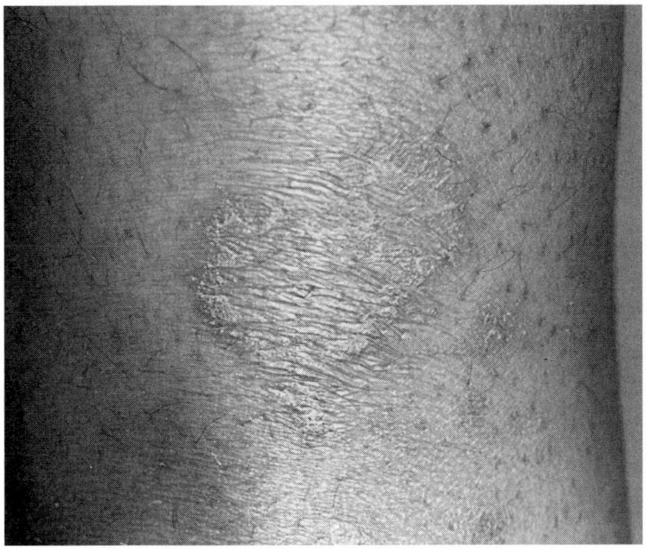

FIGURE 70–35. *A mildly inflammatory scaling patch on the arm of a patient diagnosed with erythema annulare centrifugum.*

gal infections. However, it is important to keep in mind other infectious causes, such as *Candida* and bacterial infections. Many inflammatory diseases of the skin, such as psoriasis, chronic eczema, and lichen planus, also can involve the nails. Patients with alopecia areata may have nail dystrophy as a feature of their disease at various times during their therapy.

TREATMENT. Therapies for dermatophyte infections have changed somewhat in recent years. A variety of over-the-counter preparations currently are available that have variable success in treating uncomplicated dermatophyte infections of the skin. These include Whitfield ointment, which is a mixture of salicylic acid and benzoic acid. This preparation is somewhat useful on dry lesions, such as these found in uncomplicated cases of tinea pedis.[85] Tolnaftate has moderate utility in treating cases of tinea pedis and, perhaps, mild cases of tinea corporis or tinea cruris. Undecylenic acid is available in a variety of preparations and offers only mild to moderate success in the treatment of tinea pedis.

The imidazole class of antifungals offers significantly more effective treatment of dermatophyte infections than do any of the previously mentioned products. Some relatively newer imidazole compounds, such as econazole, sulconazole, ketoconazole, and oxiconazole, have been shown to offer similar efficacy with shorter treatment schedules than the over-the-counter imidazole compounds.[187] These compounds are useful against dermatophytes, yeasts, and dermatiaceous fungi.

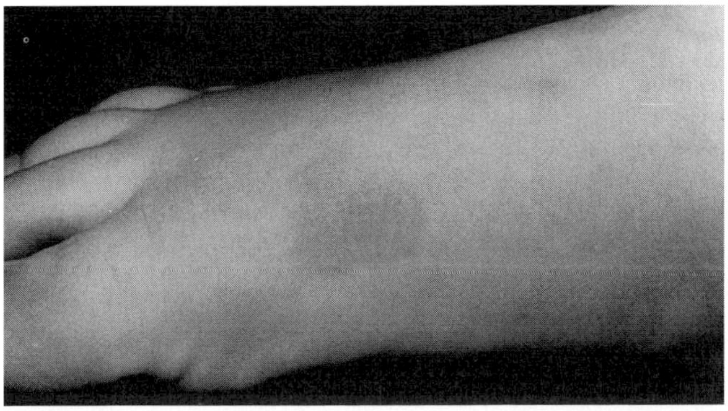

FIGURE 70–36. *Photograph of the right foot illustrating a nonscaling annular erythematous plaque with raised borders and a depressed center typical of granuloma annulare.*

A new class of antifungal medications called allylamines offers fungicidal activity against dermatophytes. The two compounds currently available are naftifine and terbinafine. This group of agents offers fungicidal activity against dermatophytes with only limited utility for infections due to yeast.[12, 138] A double-blind, placebo-controlled study showed a 96 per cent mycologic cure rate in patients treated with a single daily application of terbinafine for 12 weeks.

Systemic therapy is indicated for widespread cases of tinea corporis, tinea unguium, and tinea capitis. Griseofulvin used at a dose of 15 to 20 mg/kg/day in the liquid microsized form or 10 mg/kg/day in the ultramicrosized tablet form continues to be the treatment of choice for most cases of tinea capitis. The drug (in either form) is effective for the treatment of tinea capitis and should be continued for 6 to 8 weeks.[74, 103, 199] Routine testing of blood counts and liver functions is not needed in patients not receiving hepatotoxic drugs and without a history of liver disease.[78] Like griseofulvin, ketoconazole has been shown to have utility in treating widespread or resistant cases of tinea corporis. It is less useful than griseofulvin for treating tinea capitis, although some studies have shown its utility for treating resistant cases of tinea unguium. In the adult population, reports of hepatotoxicity have limited its use in this group of diseases. In children, long-term use should include monitoring of liver functions. Additionally, there may be some concern in children due to its affect on sterol biosynthesis.[182] Fluconazole is a biosynthesis product, i.e., it is an azole product with a similar spectrum of activity as the other compounds in that class.[182] It is unique in that its oral absorption is good and is not affected by gastric acidity.[78] Another azole compound, itraconazole, has proved to be very useful against dermatophyte infections. Because of its lipophilic nature, very high concentrations of the drug are deposited in keratin.[31, 161] For this reason, some studies have suggested its superiority to griseofulvin in the treatment of dermatophyte infections at a variety of sites on the body. It has shown to be of particular utility in the treatment of tinea unguium, in which it can be utilized for shorter courses of therapy than griseofulvin.[58] Lastly, terbinafine demonstrates excellent activity against the wide variety of dermatophyte infections.[95, 161] Like itraconazole, this drug should prove to be particularly useful in view of its ability to clear tinea unguium with shorter courses of therapy than those currently required with griseofulvin.

Yeast Infections

Candidiasis

Clinically, infections with *Candida* can involve the skin or mucous membranes. Mucous membrane involvement can present as oral thrush, vulvovaginitis, or esophagitis. Candidal intertrigo, paronychia, onychomycosis, or folliculitis also may be seen.[83]

Oral thrush generally presents with a white plaque involving the oral mucosa (Fig. 70–37). Infants may be totally asymptomatic or may refuse to eat due to discomfort from the infection. Although more common in infants, oral thrush also can be seen in older patients, particularly those infected with HIV.

Candida also is a frequent cause of intertrigo or diaper dermatitis in healthy children (see Fig. 67–23, Color Plate IV). Affected infants often will demonstrate obvious discomfort when urinating onto skin infected with *Candida*. *Candida* paronychia or nail infection is seen most often in healthy children due to thumb sucking or other trauma to the nail or its

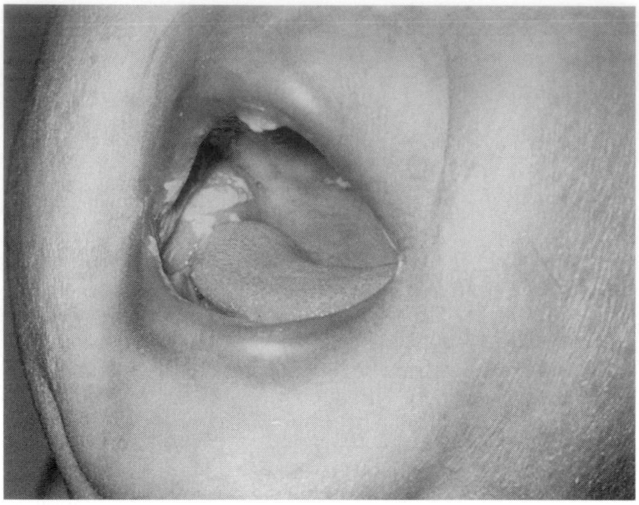

FIGURE 70–37. *A white plaque involving the oral mucosa of a patient diagnosed with oral thrush.*

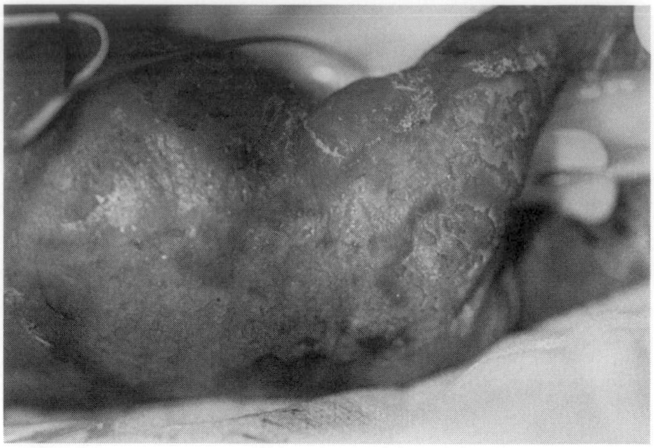

FIGURE 70–39. *Dense crusting overlying the flank and buttocks of a neonate with* Candida *dermatitis. (From Rowen, J. L., Atkins, J. T., Levy, M. L., et al.: Invasive fungal dermatitis in the 1000-gram neonate. Reproduced with permission of Pediatrics 95:682–687, 1995.)*

surrounding tissues. Clinically, profound erythema of the involved tissues is seen (Fig. 70–38). Occasionally, scant purulent discharge may be seen.

Candidal infections of the skin are seen with great frequency in immunocompromised patients.[149] Individuals infected with HIV, patients diagnosed with lymphoproliferative disease, and patients on immunosuppressive medications represent a few examples. As a distinct group demonstrating immunodeficiency, neonates have been seen to present with a distinct clinical type of candidal infection. Very premature infants have been noted to have erythema and crusting over dependent or intertriginous areas of skin (Fig. 70–39). This infection has been assumed to be due to a high rate of maternal colonization with *Candida albicans*. Although other fungi also have been implicated, *C. albicans* proved to be the cause of most cases reported from our institution. Of great importance was the fact that 69 per cent of those children found to have such disease ultimately prove to have disseminated infection.[175] Cheilitis, balanitis, and an interdigital form of cutaneous candidiasis also can be seen.

Tinea Versicolor

A distinctive yeast infection of the skin caused by *Malassezia furfur* can occur. In spite of its name, tinea versicolor is not due to dermatophyte infection. Such infections also occasionally are described as pityriasis versicolor.[200] Hyper- or hypopigmented scaling patches or plaques are seen characteristically over the upper chest, back, face, or neck (Fig. 70–40). Such lesions generally are asymptomatic, although some patients may complain of mild pruritus. Infections due to *M. furfur* may present with follicular papules or pustules involving the same areas.[27, 97]

Diagnosis

As with other fungal infections, potassium hydroxide examination of appropriate clinical material (involved skin or nails) generally will demonstrate yeast-like structures. *Candida* is seen as budding yeast with hyphae or pseudohypha, whereas *M. furfur* will be seen as typical "spaghetti and

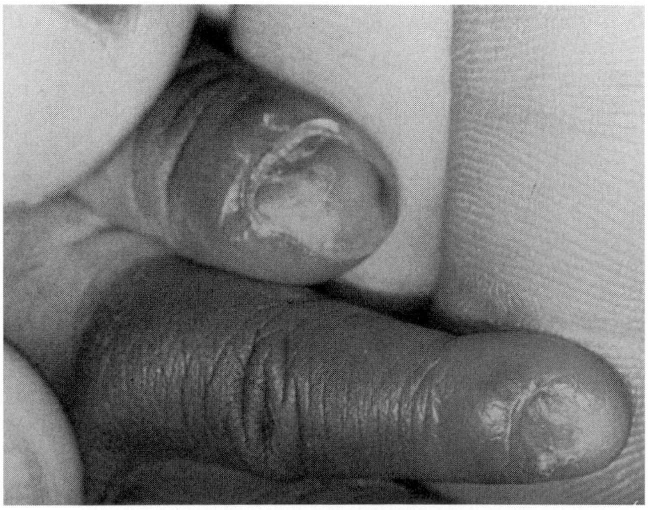

FIGURE 70–38. *Onychodystrophy involving the thumb and index finger, with erythema and edema of the paronychium. These features are typical of* Candida *paronychia.*

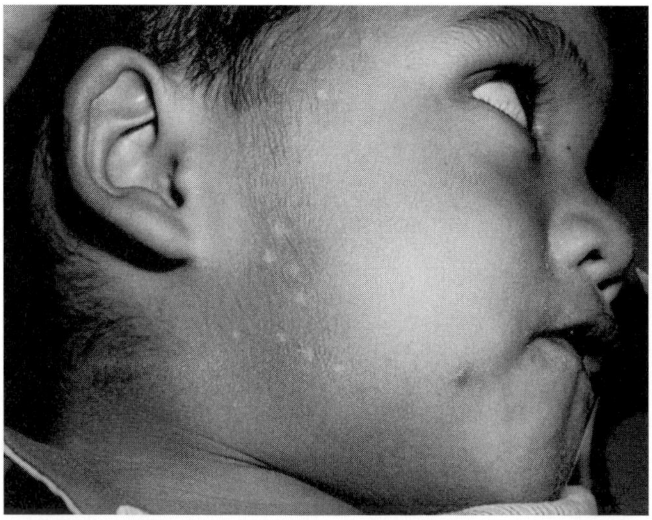

FIGURE 70–40. *Annular hypopigmented scaling macules involving the face of a child with tinea versicolor.*

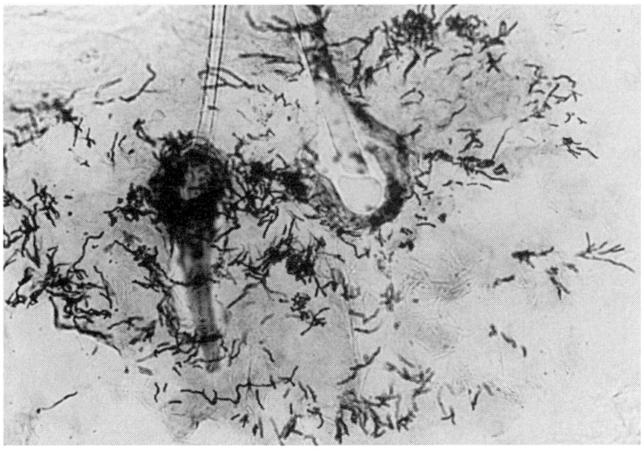

FIGURE 70–41. *Photomicrograph of multiple hyphae and spores ("spaghetti and meatballs") typical of tinea versicolor. (×200, Paragon.) (Courtesy of J. Tschen, M.D.)*

meatballs" (Fig. 70–41). *Candida* grows readily on routine culture media, whereas culture of *M. furfur* requires special media.

DIFFERENTIAL DIAGNOSIS

The adherent white plaques or patches of oral thrush generally are quite classic. However, other conditions, such as lichen planus, trauma, and the rare genetic condition of pachyonychia congenita, also can present with similar oral involvement. With involvement in the intertriginous areas, specifically in the diaper region, an irritant or noninfectious intertrigo should be considered. Similarly, in the diaper area, seborrheic dermatitis or psoriasis can be a potential source of confusion. Nail infection with *Candida*, paronychia, or onychomycosis can be confused with any of the conditions mentioned previously under the dermatophyte section.

The lesions of tinea versicolor, when hypopigmented, can be confused with early lesions of vitiligo or with a postinflammatory hypopigmentation of the skin due to any preexisting infectious or inflammatory condition.

TREATMENT

For the treatment of candidiasis, local hygiene is of importance. Measures attempting to ensure a drier skin environment should be sought. Each of the imidazole compounds is useful in treating candidal infections.

The allylamines, terbinafine, and to a lesser extent naftifine have some utility topically in the management of candidiasis. For the management of systemic infections due to *Candida*, the polyene compound amphotericin B continues to show its utility as a first-line agent for most infections. Nystatin is a topical agent with a long history of utility in the management of candidal infections. Of the azole compounds, ketoconazole, fluconazole, and itraconazole are effective in the management of candidiasis.

In the treatment of tinea versicolor, selenium sulfide shampoo applied as a lotion for limited periods is of proven utility in the management of this chronic disorder. Any of the azole compounds are useful as well.[178] Although the newer oral azole compounds (itraconazole, fluconazole) are useful against this infection, they should not be considered to be of primary indication.[59] Ketoconazole, however, has been utilized in a very short-term (bolus) form for the treatment of very widespread disease resistant to topical therapy.[18, 72]

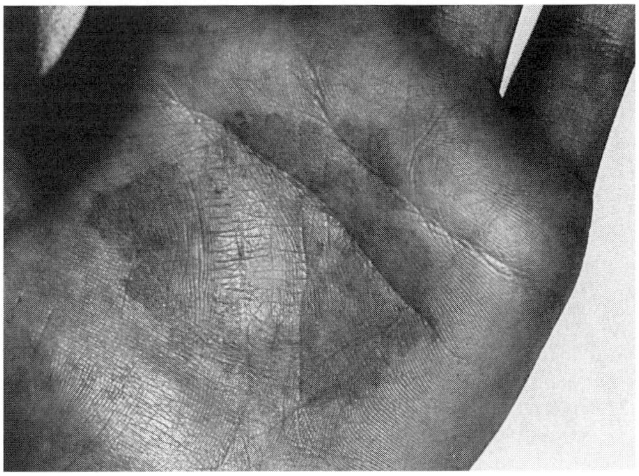

FIGURE 70–42. *A large hyperpigmented patch on the palm of the left hand of a patient with tinea nigra palmaris.*

Dematiaceous Fungal Infections

Dematiaceous fungi are noted for inhabiting the soil and demonstrating a brown to black pigmentation. Infections due to dematiaceous fungi can present in a variety of fashions. Tinea nigra represents a superficial fungal infection most commonly involving the hands, but any areas of the body may be involved.[190] Dark brown to black macules or patches may be seen (Fig. 70–42). This infection is due to *Exophiala werneckii*, which can be cultured easily on Sabouraud agar.

Chromoblastomycosis may present as primarily cutaneous disease, with the organism being visualized within lesions as darkly pigmented flecks. Infiltrated inflammatory plaques, nodules, or tumors may be seen (Fig. 70–43). More deeply situated skin infection may be due to chromoblastomycosis. Most cases of chromoblastomycosis are due to *Fonsecaea pedrosoi*.[32, 172] Diagnosis of suspected lesions can be made by potassium hydroxide examination revealing the characteristic bodies. Culture is indicated to diagnose the causative agent specifically.

When confronted with lesions of chromoblastomycosis, infections due to mycobacteria and the deep fungi should be considered. Additionally, cutaneous malignancies can be a source of confusion.

Treatment of chromoblastomycosis is difficult. Surgical ex-

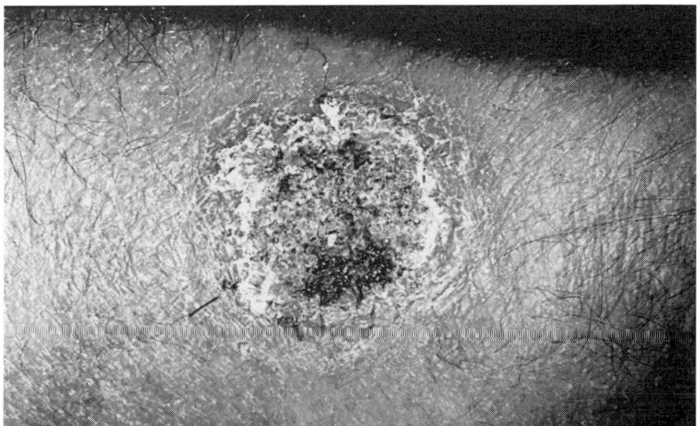

FIGURE 70–43. *Heavily crusted plaque on the arm characteristic of chromoblastomycosis.*

cision, when feasible, probably represents the primary line of therapy.[82] Systemic therapy with ketoconazole or itraconazole shows some utility.[32, 172, 186, 205] Amphotericin B also has shown limited success in the management of chromoblastomycosis.

Deep Fungal Infections

Cryptococcosis

Skin involvement is seen rarely in patients infected with *Cryptococcus neoformans* and usually is consistent with systemic disease. *C. neoformans* is ubiquitous and found in all countries. The organism may be demonstrated in soil, fruits, or avian stool, and human infection is acquired by inhalation. Although disseminated infection generally involves the lungs and central nervous system, the skin may, as mentioned previously, be involved. Skin involvement may be seen in approximately 10 to 20 per cent of infected individuals with the presence of papules, pustules, nodules, crusted erosions, or large vegetating plaques (see Fig. 67–24, Color Plate IV).[158] Cellulitis and purpura-like involvement have been reported. In HIV-infected patients, papules resembling molluscum contagiosum have been seen, as have Kaposi sarcoma–like lesions and acneiform-like lesions.[133, 158]

Smears of infected material examined after application of potassium hydroxide may demonstrate the characteristic organisms. Certainly, material obtained by biopsy for histopathologic examination and culture is preferable. The organism can be cultured easily on Sabouraud agar at both 20° C and 37° C.

Sporotrichosis

Infection with *Sporothrix schenckii* generally presents with cutaneous and subcutaneous disease. There are four recognized clinical forms of this disease.[137] The lymphocutaneous and fixed cutaneous forms are the most common forms of disease; cutaneous dissemination and extra cutaneous disease may occur rarely. Eighty per cent of the cases of sporotrichosis in the United States occurs as the lymphocutaneous variant. At the site of inoculation, one will see firm, nontender, subcutaneous nodules, which ultimately ulcerate and extend proximally (Fig. 70–44). Fixed cutaneous disease may be seen as a single nodule or verrucous plaque in individuals demonstrating high immunity to the organism. Diagnosis of

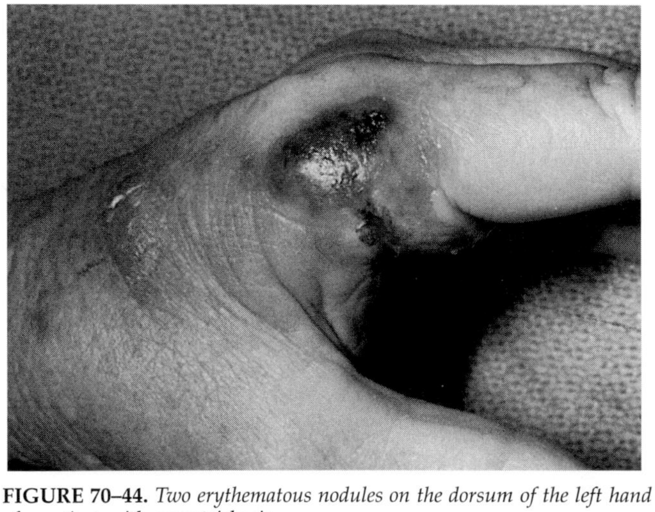

FIGURE 70–44. *Two erythematous nodules on the dorsum of the left hand of a patient with sporotrichosis.*

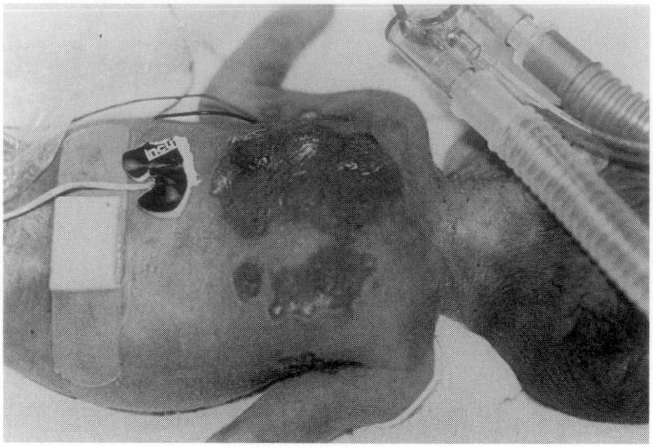

FIGURE 70–45. *An extensive eschar overlying the back of a neonate with aspergillosis. (From Rowen, J. L., Correa, A. G., Sokol, D. M., et al.: Invasive aspergillosis in neonates: Report of five cases and literature review. Pediatr. Infect. Dis. J. 11:576–582, 1992.)*

sporotrichosis should be made by culture of wound material obtained by swab, aspiration, or biopsy. Organisms may be seen free within tissue or within giant cells and appear as cigar-shaped budding yeast. Their recognition may be enhanced by staining of tissue with periodic acid–Schiff or Gomori methenamine silver. When the organisms are surrounded by periodic acid–Schiff positive staining of material, they may be recognized more easily as asteroid bodies. Cultures should be obtained for definitive diagnosis on Sabouraud agar. Mycelial forms will grow at 25° C to 35° C, and the budding yeast will be seen when grown at 37° C.

Aspergillosis

Primary or secondary skin disease may be seen in aspergillosis. Infections due to *Aspergillus fumigatus* or *Aspergillus niger* may occur. Primary skin disease generally is seen in immunocompromised patients, such as children receiving chemotherapy for leukemia, neonates, and any patient demonstrating an immunocompromised state. Many cases have been related to the use of occlusive dressings, casting materials, or taping to arm boards.[32, 143] Inflammatory papules, nodules, or plaques initially are seen. The lesions rapidly enlarge and ulcerate, ultimately becoming covered with a dark eschar (Fig. 70–45).

Skin involvement also may occur secondary to hematogenous spread from internal disease. Lesions in this instance may resemble those of ecthyma gangrenosum in patients infected with *Pseudomonas*. Potassium hydroxide examination of wound material may reveal fungi, but tissue obtained by biopsy for histopathology and culture is preferable for diagnosis.

Histoplasmosis

Infection with *Histoplasma capsulatum* is seen very commonly in the United States, particularly in the Mississippi River Valley. Although most cases of infection due to *H. capsulatum* result in pulmonary disease, primary cutaneous manifestations of histoplasmosis may be seen rarely.[32, 51, 77, 190] Skin manifestations seen more commonly include "reactive" disorders, such as erythema nodosum and EM. Multiple papules, nodules, vesicles, or ulcerated dermal plaques may be seen (Fig. 70–46). Mucosal involvement manifesting as ulcers or plaques is seen with greater frequency than is infection at other cutaneous sites. Diagnosis of histoplasmosis should be obtained by biopsies of involved tissues. Organisms can be demonstrated by appropriate stains, but culture is required for definitive diagnosis.

Blastomycosis

Like histoplasmosis, blastomycosis is seen more commonly as a primary pulmonary infection than as a skin infection. It is due to infection with *Blastomyces dermatitidis*. North American blastomycosis is seen commonly in the United States in the upper Midwest, Kentucky, and North Carolina. Cases have been reported from Mexico and Central and South America. Most cases of cutaneous infection result from hematogenous spread from a pulmonary site. Cutaneous infection due to blastomycosis is seen most commonly as verrucous or ulcerating lesions.[21, 32, 190] The initial lesion may begin as an isolated papule or pustule that ultimately enlarges, ulcerates, and crusts. Small pustules may be seen peripherally on such lesions. Occasionally, abscesses may be seen. As with histoplasmosis, erythema nodosum and EM may be seen with acute blastomycosis.

Diagnosis of suspected cases of blastomycosis occasionally can be made by a potassium hydroxide examination of material obtained from representative lesions. Organisms will demonstrate yeast forms with broad single budding. Cultures of purulent material obtained from lesions or biopsies of representative skin lesions can be grown on Sabouraud agar at 25° C.

Coccidioidomycosis

Infection due to inhalation of *Coccidioides immitis* is seen commonly in the southwestern United States and northern Mexico. Cases have been reported in Texas, Mexico, and Central and South America. A flu-like illness may be seen in primary infection, and in 10 to 40 per cent of these patients, a diffuse erythematous maculopapular eruption may be seen. With progression of this stage of the disease, erythema nodosum or EM may be seen.

Primary inoculation of the skin is rare, but it has been reported that 40 per cent of the patients with disseminated disease can have skin involvement, with the skin being the most frequent extrapulmonary site.[6, 32, 149] Asymptomatic nodules or plaques that may ulcerate are seen with regional adenopathy. Lymphangiectatic spread, such as in sporotrichosis, also may be seen. More commonly, abscesses or verrucous papules or nodules occur in the setting of primary pulmonary disease. Sinus tracts may occur. A verrucous granuloma describes a hyperkeratotic, verrucous nodule that may be seen in coccidioidomycosis.

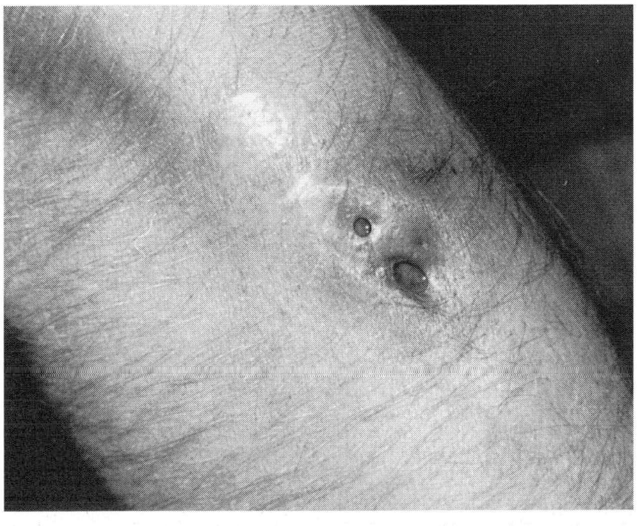

FIGURE 70–46. *An infiltrated dermal plaque with overlying ulceration on the forearm due to histoplasmosis.*

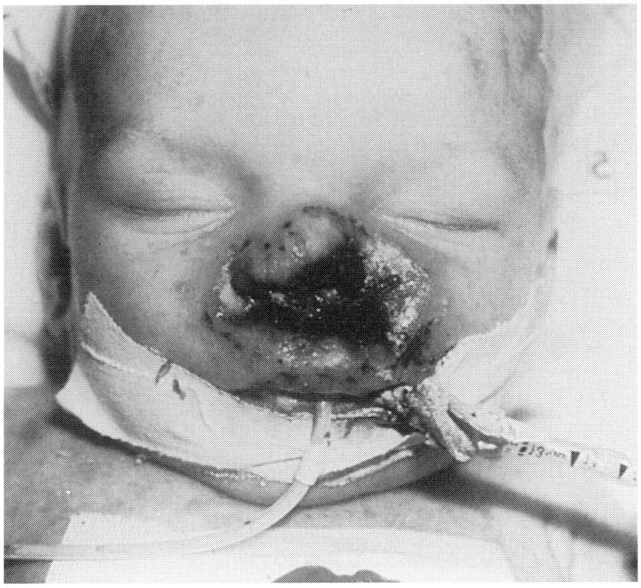

FIGURE 70–47. *An extensive area of ulceration with overlying black eschar over the central face of a child with mucormycosis. (From Lewis, L. L., Hawkins, H. K., and Edwards, M. S.: Disseminated mucormycosis in an infant with methylmalonicaciduria. Pediatr. Infect. Dis. J. 9:851–853, 1991.)*

Mucormycosis

Mucormycosis, or zygomycosis, describes a group of opportunistic infections due to fungi from the order Mucorales. Most infections are due to species from the genus *Mucor* or *Rhizopus*. These fungi are ubiquitous. Patients with extreme immunosuppression due to lymphoproliferative disease, diabetes, burns, or malnutrition particularly are susceptible to mucormycosis.

Cutaneous disease can be primary or secondary. Local skin injury predisposes patients to primary skin disease. As with aspergillosis, patients have developed mucormycosis (due to *Rhizopus*) due to the use of occlusive dressings.[1, 32] Skin necrosis and eschar formation characteristically are seen due to vascular invasion and infarction of affected tissues, which characteristically are seen in this group of fungi (Fig. 70–47). Secondary skin involvement can be seen, as with the other deep fungi, due to hematogenous spread from an internal source. Lesions, in this instance, characteristically appear as a cellulitis that progresses quickly to develop necrosis and eschar formation.

Diagnosis is established by potassium hydroxide examination of infected tissues or by biopsy of involved tissues followed by histopathologic examination and culture on Sabouraud agar.

References

1. Adam, R. D., Hunger, G., DiTomasso, J., et al.: Mucormycosis: Emerging prominence of cutaneous infections. Clin. Infect. Dis. *19*:67–76, 1994.

2. Al-Aboosi, M.: Treatment of plane warts by tretinoin-induced irritant reaction. Int. J. Dermatol. *33*:826–827, 1994.
3. American Academy of Dermatology Task Force: Genital warts and sexual abuse. J. Am. Acad. Dermatol. *11*:529–530, 1984.
4. American Academy of Pediatrics: Herpes simplex. *In* Peter, G. (ed.): 1994 Redbook: Report of the Committee on Infectious Diseases. 23rd ed. Elk Grove Village, IL, American Academy of Pediatrics, 1994, pp. 242–252.
5. American Academy of Pediatrics: Papillomaviruses. *In* Peter, G. (ed): 1994 Redbook: Report of the Committee on Infectious Diseases. 23rd ed. Elk Grove Village, IL, American Academy of Pediatrics, 1994, pp. 337–339.
6. Ampel, N. W., Wieden, M. A., and Galgiani, J. N.: Coccidioidomycosis: Clinical update. Rev. Infect. Dis. *11*:897–911, 1989.
7. Asano, Y., Suga, S., Yoshikawa, T., et al.: Clinical features and viral excretion in an infant with primary human herpesvirus 7 infection. Pediatrics *95*:187–190, 1995.
8. Asano, Y., Yoshikawa, T., Suga, S., et al.: Clinical features of infants with primary human herpesvirus 6 infection (exanthem subitum, roseola infantum). Pediatrics *93*:104–108, 1994.
9. Baldari, U., Monti, A., and Righini, M. G.: An epidemic of infantile papular acrodermatitis (Gianotti-Crosti Syndrome) due to Epstein-Barr virus. Dermatology *188*:203–204, 1994.
10. Belhorn, T. H., and Lucky, A. W.: Atypical varicella exanthems associated with skin injury. Pediatr. Dermatol. *11*:129–132, 1994.
11. Berant, M., Naveh, Y., and Weissman, I.: Papular acrodermatitis with cytomegalovirus hepatitis. Arch. Dis. Child. *58*:1024–1025, 1983.
12. Bergstresser, P., Elewski, B., Hanifin, J., et al.: Topical terbinafine and clotrimazole in interdigital tinea pedis: A multicenter comparison of cure and relapse rates with 1- and 4-week treatment regimens. J. Am. Acad. Dermatol. *28*:648–657, 1993.
13. Berth-Jones, J., and Hutchinson, P. E.: Moderate treatment of warts: Cure rates at 3 and 6 months. Br. J. Dermatol. *127*:262–265, 1992.
14. Bhawan, J., Gellis, S., Ucci, A., et al.: Vesiculobullous lesions caused by cytomegalovirus virus infection in an immunocompromised adult. J. Am. Acad. Dermatol. *11*:743–747, 1984.
15. Blatt, J., Kastner, O., and Hodes, D. S.: Cutaneous vesicles in congenital cytomegalovirus virus infection. J. Pediatr. *92*:509, 1978.
16. Blauvelt, A., and Turner, M. L.: Gianotti-Crosti syndrome and human immunodeficiency virus infection. Arch. Dermatol. *130*:481–483, 1994.
17. Bolton, R. A.: Non-genital warts: Classification and treatment options. Am. J. Fam. Pract. *43*:2049–2056, 1991.
18. Borelli, Jacobs, P. H., and Nall, L.: Tinea versicolor epidemiologic, clinical, and therapeutic aspects. J. Am. Acad. Dermatol. *25*:300–305, 1991.
19. Boss, J. M., Boxley, J. D., Summerly, R., et al.: The detection of Epstein-Barr virus antibody in "exanthematic" dermatoses with special reference to pityriasis lichenoides: A preliminary survey. Clin. Exp. Dermatol. *3*:51–56, 1978.
20. Boyd, A. S., Neldner, K. H., Zemtsov, A., et al.: Photolocalized varicella. J. Am. Acad. Dermatol. *26*:772–774, 1992.
21. Bradsher, R. W.: Blastomycosis. Clin. Infect. Dis. *14*:582–590, 1992.
22. Brodell, R. T., and Bredle, D. L.: The treatment of palmar and plantar warts using natural alpha interferon and a needleless injector. Dermatol. Surg. *21*:213–219, 1995.
23. Brunell, P. A.: Indications for oral acyclovir in children. Pediatr. Infect. Dis. J. *12*:970, 1993.
24. Brunell, P. A.: Mumps. *In* Feigin, R. D., and Cherry, J. D. (eds.): Textbook of Pediatric Infectious Diseases. 3rd ed. Philadelphia, W. B. Saunders, 1992, pp. 1610–1613.
25. Brunell, P. A.: Varicella-zoster infections. *In* Feigin, R. D., and Cherry, J. D. (eds.): Textbook of Pediatric Infectious Diseases. 3rd ed. Philadelphia, W. B. Saunders, 1992, pp. 1587–1591.
26. Buchness, M. R.: Treatment of skin diseases in HIV-infected patients. Dermatol. Clin. *13*:231–238, 1995.
27. Bufill, J. A., Lum, L. G., Caya, J. G., et al.: Pityrosporum folliculitis after bone marrow transplantation: Clinical observations in five patients. Ann. Intern. Med. *108*:560–563, 1988.
28. Burns, D. A.: "Warts and all": The history and folklore of warts: A review. J. R. Soc. Med. *85*:37–40, 1992.
29. Caputo, R., Gelmetti, C., Ermacora, E., et al.: Gianotti-Crosti syndrome: A retrospective analysis of 308 cases. J. Am. Acad. Dermatol. *26*:207, 1992.
30. Caserta, M. T., and Hall, C. B.: Human herpesvirus-6. Annu. Rev. Med. *44*:377–383, 1993.
31. Cavwenberg, G., DeDoncker, P., Stoops, K., et al.: Itraconazole in the treatment of human mycoses: Review of three years of clinical experience. Rev. Infect. Dis. *9*:5146–5152, 1987.
32. Chapman, S. W., and Daniel, C. R.: Cutaneous manifestations of fungal infection. Infect. Dis. Clin. North Am. *8*:879–910, 1994.
33. Chen, S. L., Tsao, Y. P., Lee, J. W., et al.: Characterization and skin analysis of human papillomaviruses of skin warts. Arch. Dermatol. Res. *285*:460–465, 1993.
34. Cherry, J. D.: Adenoviral infection. *In* Feigin, R. D., and Cherry, J. D. (eds.): Textbook of Pediatric Infectious Diseases. 3rd ed. Philadelphia, W. B. Saunders, 1992, pp. 1670–1687.
35. Cherry, J. D.: Contemporary infectious exanthems. Clin. Infect. Dis. *16*:199–205, 1993.
36. Cherry, J. D.: Cutaneous manifestations of systemic disease. *In* Feigin, R. D., and Cherry, J. D. (eds.): Textbook of Pediatric Infectious Diseases. 3rd ed. Philadelphia, W. B. Saunders, 1992, pp. 755–782.
37. Cherry, J. D.: Enteroviruses: Polioviruses (poliomyelitis), coxsackieviruses, echoviruses and enteroviruses. *In* Feigin, R. D., and Cherry, J. D. (eds.): Textbook of Pediatric Infectious Diseases. 3rd ed. Philadelphia, W. B. Saunders, 1992, pp. 1705–1753.
38. Cherry, J. D.: Measles. *In* Feigin, R. D., and Cherry, J. D. (eds.): Textbook of Pediatric Infectious Diseases. 3rd ed. Philadelphia, W. B. Saunders, 1992, pp. 1591–1609.
39. Cherry, J. D.: Newer viral exanthems. *In* Schulman, I. (ed.): Advances in Pediatrics. Vol. 16. Chicago, Year Book Medical Publishers, 1969, pp. 233–286.
40. Cherry, J. D.: Parvoviruses. *In* Feigin, R. D., and Cherry, J. D. (eds.): Textbook of Pediatric Infectious Diseases. 3rd ed. Philadelphia, W. B. Saunders, 1992, pp. 1626–1633.
41. Cherry, J. D.: Roseola in infantum (exanthem subitum). *In* Feigin, R. D., and Cherry, J. D. (eds.): Textbook of Pediatric Infectious Diseases. 3rd ed. Philadelphia, W. B. Saunders, 1992, pp. 1789–1792.
42. Cherry, J. D.: Rubella. *In* Feigin, R. D., and Cherry, J. D. (eds.): Textbook of Pediatric Infectious Diseases. 3rd ed. Philadelphia, W. B. Saunders, 1992, pp. 1792–1817.
43. Cherry, J. D.: Viral exanthems. Curr. Probl. Pediatr. *13*:5–44, 1983.
44. Cherry, J. D., Feigin, R. D., Lobes, L. A., et al.: Atypical measles in children previously immunized with attenuated measle virus vaccine. Pediatrics *50*:712–717, 1972.
45. Cherry, J. D., and Jahn, C. L.: Exanthem and enanthem associated with mumps virus infection. Arch. Environ. Health. *12*:518–521, 1966.
46. Cherry, J. D., Lerner, M., Klein, J. O., et al.: Coxsackie A9 infections with exanthems: With particular reference to urticaria. Pediatrics *31*:819–823, 1963.
47. Cherry, J. D., Lerner, M. L., Klein, J. O., et al.: Coxsackie B5 infections with exanthems. Pediatrics *31*:455–462, 1963.
48. Cherry, J. D., Lerner, M. L., Klein, J. O., et al.: Echo II infections associated with exanthems. Pediatrics *32*:509–516, 1963.
49. Choudhury, S. A., Hodes, D. S., Peters, B., et al.: Cutaneous herpes simplex virus infection in a child with acquired immunodeficiency syndrome. Clin. Pediatr. *33*:698–699, 1994.
50. Chu, T. C.: Fungi. Curr. Opin. Infect. Dis. *8*:310–314, 1995.
51. Cockerell, C. J.: Human immunodeficiency virus infection and the skin. Arch. Intern. Med. *151*:1295–1303, 1991.
52. Cohen, B. A., Honig, P., and Androphy, E.: Anogenital warts in children: Clinical and virologic evaluation for sexual abuse. Arch. Dermatol. *126*:1575–1580, 1990.
53. Cohen, B. J.: Human parvovirus B19 infection in Kawasaki disease. Lancet *344*:59, 1994.
54. Cohen, P. R.: Tests for detecting herpes simplex virus and varicella-zoster virus infections. Dermatol. Clin. *12*:51–68, 1994.
55. Committee on Infectious Diseases: Recommendations for the use of live attenuated varicella vaccine. Pediatrics *95*:791–796, 1995.
56. Committee on Infectious Diseases: The use of oral acyclovir in otherwise healthy children with varicella. Pediatrics *91*:674–676, 1993.
57. David, T. J., and Longson, M.: Herpes simplex infections in atopic eczema. Arch. Dis. Child. *60*:338–343, 1985.
58. DeDoncker, P., Decroix, J., Pierard, G. E., et al.: Antifungal pulse therapy for onychomycosis: A pharmacokinetic and pharmacodynamic investigation of monthly cycles of 1-week pulse therapy with itraconazole. Arch. Dermatol. *132*:34–41, 1996.
59. Delescluse, J.: Itraconazole in tinea versicolor: A review. J. Am. Acad. Dermatol. *23*:551–554, 1990.
60. Demmler, G. J.: Acquired cytomegalovirus infection. *In* Feigin, R. D., and Cherry, J. D. (eds.): Textbook of Pediatric Infectious Diseases. 3rd ed. Philadelphia, W. B. Saunders, 1992, pp. 1532–1547.
61. Derksen, D. J.: Children with condylomata acuminata. J. Fam. Pract. *34*:419–423, 1992.
62. DeVilliers, E. M.: Importance of human papillomavirus DNA typing in the diagnosis of anogenital warts in children. Arch. Dermatol. *131*:366–367, 1995.
63. Draelos, Z. K., Hansen, R. C., and James, W. D.: Gianotti-Crosti syndrome associated with infections other than hepatitis B. J. A. M. A. *256*:2386–2388, 1986.
64. Dundarov, S., and Andonov, P.: Seventeen years of application of herpes vaccines in Bulgaria. Acta. Virol. *38*:205–208, 1994.
65. Dunkle, L. M., Arvin, A. M., Whitley, R. J., et al.: A controlled trial of acyclovir for chickenpox in normal children. N. Engl. J. Med. *325*:1539–1544, 1991.
66. Durbin, W. A., and Sullivan, J. L.: Epstein-Barr virus infection. Pediatr. Rev. *15*:63–68, 1994.
67. Eichenfield, L. F., and Honig, P. J.: New developments in pediatric dermatology. Curr. Probl. Pediatr. *21*:420–427, 1991.
68. Epstein, W. L.: Molluscum contagiosum. Semin. Dermatol. *11*:184–189, 1992.
69. Esterly, N. B.: Viral exanthems: Diagnoses and management. Semin. Dermatol. *3*:140–145, 1984.
70. Evans, E. G. V., Seaman, R. A. J., and James, I. G. V.: Short-duration

therapy with terbinafine 1% cream in dermatophyte skin infections. Br. J. Dermatol. *130*:83–87, 1994.
71. Evans, L. M., Grossman, M. E., and Gregory, N.: Koplik spots and a purpuric eruption associated with parvovirus B19 infection. J. Am. Acad. Dermatol. *21*:466–467, 1992.
72. Faergemann, J.: Pityriasis versicolor. Sci. Dermatol. *12*:276–279, 1993.
73. Feder, H. M., and Geller, R. W.: Herpetic whitlow of the great toe. N. Engl. J. Med. *326*:1295, 1992.
74. Fitzpatrick, R. E., and Newcomer, V. D.: Dermatophytosis and candidiasis. *In* Feigin, R. D., and Cherry, J. D. (eds.): Textbook of Pediatric Infectious Diseases. 3rd ed. Philadelphia, W. B. Saunders, 1992, pp. 782–813.
75. Forman, M. J., and Cherry, J. D.: Exanthems associated with uncommon viral syndromes. Pediatrics *41*:873–882, 1968.
76. Frasier, L. D.: Human papillomavirus infection in children. Pediatr. Ann. *23*:354–360, 1994.
77. Freeman, W. E., O'Quinn, J. L., and Lesher, J. L.: Fever and hypopigmented papules in an intravenous drug abuser: Disseminated histoplasmosis in acquired immunodeficiency syndrome (AIDS). Arch. Dermatol. *125*:692–693, 1989.
78. Frieden, I., and Howard, R.: Tinea capitis: Epidemiology, diagnosis, treatment and control. J. Am. Acad. Dermatol. *31*:542–546, 1994.
79. Frieden, I. J., and Penneys, N. S.: Viral infections. *In* Schachner, L. A., and Hansen, R. C. (eds.): Pediatric Dermatology. New York, Churchill Livingstone, 1988, pp. 1371–1413.
80. Gan, V. N., Petruska, M., and Ginsburg, C. M.: Epidemiology and treatment of tinea capitis: Ketoconazole vs. griseofulvin. Pediatr. Infect. Dis. J. *6*:46–49, 1987.
81. Gershon, A. A., LaRussa, P., Hardy, I., et al.: Varicella vaccine: The American experience. J. Infect. Dis. *166*:S63–S68, 1992.
82. Glorioso, L., and Webster, G. F.: The role of surgery in the management of uncommon skin infections. Dermatol. Surg. *21*:136–144, 1995.
83. Goldgeier, M. H.: Fungal infections of the skin, hair, and nails. Pediatr. Ann. *22*:253–259, 1993.
84. Goodyear, H. M., Laidler, P. W., Price, E. H., et al.: Acute infectious erythemas in children: A clinico-microbiological study. Br. J. Dermatol. *124*:433–438, 1991.
85. Gooskens, V., Ponnighaus, J. M., Clayton, Y., et al.: Treatment of superficial mycoses in the tropics: Whitfield's ointment versus clotrimazole. Int. J. Dermatol. *33*:738–742, 1994.
86. Gottlieb, S. L., and Myskowski, P. L.: Molluscum contagiosum. Int. J. Dermatol. *33*:453–461, 1994.
87. Greene, I.: Therapy for genital warts. Dermatol. Clin. *10*:253–267, 1992.
88. Grossman, K. L., and Rasmussen, J. E.: Recent advances in pediatric infectious disease and their impact on dermatology. J. Am. Acad. Dermatol. *24*:379–389, 1991.
89. Gutman, L. T., Herman-Giddens, M., Prose, N. S., et al.: Diagnosis of child sexual abuse in children with genital warts. Am. J. Dis. Child. *145*:126–127, 1991.
90. Halasz, C. L. G., Cormier, D., and Den, M.: Petechial glove and sock syndrome caused by parvovirus B19. J. Am. Acad. Dermatol. *27*:835–838, 1992.
91. Hall, C. B., Cherry, J. D., Hatch, M. H., et al.: The return of Boston exanthem: Echovirus 16 infections. Am. J. Dis. Child. *131*:323–326, 1977.
92. Handley, J. M., Maw, R. D., Bingham, E. A., et al.: Anogenital warts in children. Clin. Exp. Dermatol. *18*:241–247, 1993.
93. Hanson, C. G., and Shearer, W. T.: Pediatric HIV infection and AIDS. *In* Feigin, R. D., and Cherry, J. D. (eds.): Textbook of Pediatric Infectious Diseases. 3rd ed. Philadelphia, W. B. Saunders, 1992, pp. 990–1011.
94. Harms, M., Feldmann, R., and Saurat, J. H.: Papular-purpuric "gloves and socks" syndrome. J. Am. Acad. Dermatol. *23*:850–854, 1990.
95. Hay, R. J., Logan, R. A., Moore, M. K., et al.: A comparative study for terbinafine versus griseofulvin in "dry-type" dermatophyte infections. J. Am. Acad. Dermatol. *24*:243–246, 1991.
96. Heggie, A. D.: Pathogenesis of the rubella exanthem. N. Engl. J. Med. *12*:664–667, 1971.
97. Helm, K. F., and Lookingbill, D. P.: Pityrosporum folliculitis and severe pruritus in two patients with Hodgkin's disease. Arch. Dermatol. *129*:380–381, 1993.
98. Highet, A. S.: Molluscum contagiosum. Arch. Dis. Child. *67*:1248–1249, 1992.
99. Highet, A. S., and Kurtz, J.: Viral infections. *In* Champion, R. H., Burton, J. L., and Ebling, F. J. G. (eds.): Textbook of Dermatology. 5th ed. Oxford, Blackwell Scientific Publications, 1992, pp. 867–894.
100. Hikada, Y., Okada, K., Kushara, K., et al.: Exanthem subitum and human herpesvirus 7 infection. Pediatr. Infect. Dis. J. *13*:1010–1011, 1994.
101. Holland, T. T., Weber, B. B., and James, W. D.: Tender periungual nodules. Arch. Dermatol. *128*:105–106, 1992.
102. Honig, P. J., Caputo, G. L., Leyden, J. J., et al.: Microbiology of kerions. J. Pediatr. *123*:422–424, 1993.
103. Honig, P. J., Caputo, G. L., Leyden, J. J., et al.: Treatment of kerions. Pediatr. Dermatol. *11*:69–71, 1994.
104. Huff, J. C.: Acyclovir for recurrent erythema multiforme caused by herpes simplex. J. Am. Acad. Dermatol. *18*:197–199, 1988.
105. Hughes, W. P., and Parham, D. M.: Molluscum contagiosum in children with cancer or acquired immunodeficiency syndrome. Pediatr. Infect. Dis. J. *10*:152–156, 1991.
106. Hurwitz, S.: Clinical Pediatric Dermatology. 2nd ed. Philadelphia, W. B. Saunders, 1993, pp. 318–371.
107. Izu, R., Manzano, D., Gardezabal, J., et al.: Giant molluscum contagiosum presenting as a tumor in an HIV-infected patient. Int. J. Dermatol. *33*:266–267, 1994.
108. Janniger, C. K.: Childhood warts. Cutis *50*:15–16, 1992.
109. Janniger, C. K.: Genital warts in children. Cutis *50*:101–102, 1992.
110. Janniger, C. K., and Schwartz, R. A.: Molluscum contagiosum in children. Cutis *52*:194–196, 1993.
111. Johnson, L. W.: Communal showers and the risk of plantar warts. J. Fam. Pract. *40*:136–138, 1995.
112. Jones, Vaughan, S. A., McGibbon, D. H., and Bradbeer, C. S.: Chronic verrucous varicella-zoster infection in a patient with AIDS. Clin. Exp. Dermatol. *19*:327–329, 1994.
113. Jordan, M. B., and Abramo, T. J.: Occurrence of herpetic whitlow in a twelve-day-old infant. Pediatr. Infect. Dis. J. *13*:832–833, 1994.
114. Kang, S., and Fitzpatrick, Y. T. B.: Debilitating verruca vulgaris in a patient infected with human immunodeficiency virus. Arch. Dermatol. *130*:294–296, 1994.
115. Kanzler, M. H., and Gorsulowsky, D. C.: Anogenital warts in children. Arch. Dermatol. *127*:1063–1064, 1991.
116. Kohl, S.: Postnatal herpes simplex virus infection. *In* Feigin, R. D., and Cherry, J. D. (eds.): Textbook of Pediatric Infectious Diseases. 3rd ed. Philadelphia, W. B. Saunders, 1992, pp. 1558–1583.
117. Krowchuk, D. P., and Anglin, T. M.: Genital human papillomavirus infection in adolescents: Implications for evaluation and management. Semin. Dermatol. *11*:24–30, 1992.
118. Krusinski, P. A.: Treatment of mucocutaneous herpes simplex infections with acyclovir. J. Am. Acad. Dermatol. *1*:179–181, 1988.
119. Kuzushima, K., Kudo, T., Kimura, H., et al.: Prophylactic oral acyclovir in outbreaks of primary herpes simplex virus type I infection in a closed community. Pediatrics *89*:379–383, 1992.
120. Landau, J. W., and Gurevitch, A. W.: Molluscum contagiosum. *In* Feigin, R. D., and Cherry, J. D. (eds.): Textbook of Pediatric Infectious Diseases. 3rd ed. Philadelphia, W. B. Saunders, 1992, pp. 818–820.
121. Landau, J. W., and Gurevitch, A. W.: Warts (human papillomavirus). *In* Feigin, R. D., and Cherry, J. D. (eds): Textbook of Pediatric Infectious Diseases. 3rd ed. Philadelphia, W. B. Saunders, 1992, pp. 814–817.
122. Leavell, U. W.: Orf. J. A. M. A. *204*:109–116, 1968.
123. Leavell, U. W., and Phillips, I. A.: Milker's nodules. Arch. Dermatol. *111*:1307–1311, 1975.
124. Lee, S., Kim, K., Hahn, C. S., et al.: Gianotti-Crosti syndrome associated with hepatitis B surface antigen (subtype ADR). J. Am. Acad. Dermatol. *12*:629–633, 1985.
125. Lemak, M. A., Duvic, M., and Bean, S. F.: Oral acyclovir for the prevention of herpes-associated erythema multiforme. J. Am. Acad. Dermatol. *15*:50–54, 1986.
126. Lerner, A. M., Cherry, J. D., Klein, J. O., et al.: Infections with reoviruses. N. Engl. J. Med. *267*:947–952, 1962.
127. Lesher, J. L.: Cytomegalovirus virus infections and the skin. J. Am. Acad. Dermatol. *18*:1333–1338, 1988.
128. Lin, C. S., Penha, P. D., Krishnan, M. N., et al.: Cytomegalic inclusion disease of the skin. Arch. Dermatol. *117*:282–284, 1981.
129. Logan, R. A., and Zachary, C. B.: Outcome of carbon dioxide laser therapy for persistent cutaneous viral warts. Br. J. Dermatol. *129*:99–105, 1989.
130. Lucky, A. W., and Prendiville, J. S.: Acral hemorrhagic eruption in a 3-year-old boy. Pediatr. Dermatol. *8*:169–171, 1991.
131. Martin, A. G., and Kobayashi, G. S.: Superficial fungal infection: Dermatophytosis, tinea, nigra, ridra. *In* Fitzpatrick, T. B., Eisen, A. S., Wolff, K., et al. (eds.): Dermatology in General Medicine. 4th ed. New York, McGraw-Hill, 1993, pp. 2421–2452.
132. Massing, A. M., and Epstein, W. L.: Natural history of warts. Arch. Dermatol. *87*:306–310, 1963.
133. Maurique, P., Mayo, J., Alvarez, J. A., et al.: Polymorphous cutaneous cryptococcosis: Nodular, herpes-like, and molluscum-like lesions in a patient with the acquired immunodeficiency syndrome. J. Am. Acad. Dermatol. *26*:122–124, 1992.
134. McCarthy, J. T., and Hoagland, R. J.: Cutaneous manifestations of infectious mononucleosis. J. A. M. A. *187*:153–154, 1964.
135. McCrossin, I., and Wong, D.: HIV-related skin disease. Med. J. Aust. *158*:179–185, 1993.
136. McElgunn, P. S. J.: Dermatologic manifestation of hepatitis B virus infection. J. Am. Acad. Dermatol. *8*:539–548, 1983.
137. Mercurio, M. G., and Elewski, B. E.: Therapy of sporotrichosis. Semin. Dermatol. *12*:285–289, 1993.
138. Milliken, L., Galen, W., Guwirtzman, J. G., et al.: Naftifine cream 1% versus econazole cream 1% in the treatment of tinea cruris and tinea corporis. J. Am. Acad. Dermatol. *18*:52–56, 1988.
139. Mindel, A.: Cutaneous herpes simplex infection. Scand. J. Infect. Dis. *80*(Suppl.):47–52, 1991.
140. Mofid, M., Dover, J. S., Skerlev, M., et al.: Herpes simplex. Semin. Neurol. *12*:312–321, 1992.

141. Mooney, M. A., Janniger, C. K., and Schwartz, R. A.: Kaposi's varicelliform eruption. Cutis *53*:243–245, 1994.
142. Moscicki, A. B.: Human papillomavirus infection. Adv. Pediatr. *39*:257–281, 1992.
143. Mowad, C. M., Nguyen, T. V., Jaworsky, C., et al.: Primary cutaneous aspergillosis in an immunocompetent child. J. Am. Acad. Dermatol. *33*:136–137, 1995.
144. Nahass, G. T., Goldstein, B. A., Zhu, W. Y., et al.: Comparison of Tzanck smear, viral culture, and DNA diagnostic methods in detection of herpes simplex and varicella-zoster infection. J. A. M. A. *268*:2541–2544, 1992.
145. Nathwani, D., and Wood, M. J.: Herpesvirus infection in childhood. Br. J. Hosp. Med. *50*:234–241, 1993.
146. Nigro, G., Zerbini, M., Kryztofiak, A., et al.: Active or recent parvovirus B19 infection in children with Kawasaki disease. Lancet *343*:1260–1261, 1994.
147. Nuovo, G. J., Lastarria, D. A., Smith, S., et al.: Human papillomavirus segregation patterns in genital and non-genital warts in pre-pubertal children and adults. Am. J. Clin. Pathol. *95*:467–474, 1991.
148. Obalek, S., Misiewicz, J., Jablonska, S., et al.: Childhood condyloma acuminatum: Association with genital and cutaneous human papillomaviruses. Pediatr. Dermatol. *10*:101–106, 1993.
149. Odom, R. B.: Common superficial fungal infections in immunosupressed patients. J. Am. Acad. Dermatol. *31*:556–559, 1994.
150. Okada, K., Ueda, K., Kusuhara, K., et al.: Exanthema subitum and human herpesvirus 6 infection: Clinical observation in fifty-seven cases. Pediatr. Infect. Dis. J. *12*:204–208, 1993.
151. Orlow, S. J., and Paller, A.: Cimetidine therapy for multiple viral warts in children. J. Am. Acad. Dermatol. *28*:794–796, 1993.
152. Overall, J. C.: Viral infection of the fetus and neonate. *In* Feigin, R. D., and Cherry, J. D. (eds.): Textbook of Pediatric Infectious Diseases. 3rd ed. Philadelphia, W. B. Saunders, 1992, pp. 924–959.
153. Panjvani, Z. F. K., and Hanshaw, J. B.: Cytomegalovirus virus in the perinatal period. Am. J. Dis. Child. *135*:56–60, 1981.
154. Paradisi, M., Mostaccioli, F., Celano, G., et al.: Infantile condylomata of the oral cavity. Pediatr. Dermatol. *9*:107–111, 1992.
155. Pariser, R. J.: Histologically specific skin lesions in disseminated cytomegalovirus infection. J. Am. Acad. Dermatol. *9*:937–946, 1983.
156. Patel, B. M.: Skin rash with infectious mononucleosis and ampicillin. Pediatrics *40*:910–911, 1967.
157. Patrizi, A., Di Lernia, V., Neri, I., et al.: An unusual case of recurrent Gianotti-Crosti syndrome. Pediatr. Dermatol. *11*:283–284, 1994.
158. Pema, K., Diaz, J., Guerra, L. G., et al.: Disseminated cutaneous cryptococcosis: Comparison of clinical manifestations in the pre-AIDS and AIDS eras. Arch. Intern. Med. *154*:1032–1034, 1994.
159. Person, J. R.: Generalized granuloma annulare, mononucleosis and positive rheumatoid factor. Int. J. Dermatol. *34*:40–41, 1995.
160. Phillips, T. J., and Dover, J. S.: Recent advances in dermatology. N. Engl. J. Med. *326*:167, 1992.
161. Pierard, G., Arrese, J., and DeDoncker, P.: Antifungal activity of itraconazole and terbinafine in human stratum corneum: A comparative study. J. Am. Acad. Dermatol. *32*:429–435, 1995.
162. Pillay, D., Patou, G., Hurt, S., et al.: Parvovirus B19 outbreak in a children's ward. Lancet *339*:107–109, 1992.
163. Pond, K. E., Feder, H. M., and Tunnessen, W. W.: Atypical presentations of varicella with underlying skin disorders. Arch. Pediatr. Adolesc. Med. *149*:313–314, 1995.
164. Porter, C. D., Blake, N. W., Archard, L. C., et al.: Molluscum contagiosum virus types in genital and non-genital lesions. Br. J. Dermatol. *120*:37–41, 1989.
165. Prezioso, P. J., Cangiarella, J., Lee, M., et al.: Fatal disseminated infection with human herpesvirus-6. J. Pediatr. *120*:921–923, 1992.
166. Prose, N. S.: Cutaneous manifestations of HIV infection in children. Dermatol. Clin. *9*:543–550, 1991.
167. Prose, N. S., and Resnick, S. D.: Cutaneous manifestations of systemic infection in children. Curr. Probl. Pediatr. *21*:92–113, 1991.
168. Prose, N. S., von Knebel-Doeberitz, C., Miller, S., et al.: Widespread flat warts associated with human papillomavirus type 5: A cutaneous manifestation of human immunodeficiency virus infection. J. Am. Acad. Dermatol. *23*:978–981, 1990.
169. Pruksananonda, P., Hall, C. B., Insel, R. A., et al.: Primary human herpesvirus 6 infection in young children. N. Engl. J. Med. *326*:1445–1450, 1992.
170. Puig, L., Diaz, M., Alexandre, R. C., et al.: Petechial glove and sock syndrome caused by parvovirus B19. Cutis *54*:335–340, 1994.
171. Pullen, H., Wright, N., and Murdock, J. McC.: Hypersensitivity reactions to antibacterial drugs in infectious mononucleosis. Lancet *2*:1176–1178, 1967.
172. Restrepo, A.: Treatment of tropical mycoses. J. Am. Acad. Dermatol. *31*:S91–S102, 1994.
173. Robinson, M. R., Udell, I. J., Garber, P. F., et al.: Molluscum contagiosum of the eyelid in patients with acquired immune deficiency syndrome. Ophthalmology *99*:1745–1747, 1992.
174. Rockley, P. S., and Tyring, S. K.: Pathophysiology and clinical manifestations of varicella-zoster infections. Int. J. Dermatol. *33*:227–232, 1994.
175. Rowen, J. L., Atkins, J. T., Levy, M. L., et al.: Invasive fungal dermatitis in the ≤1000-gram neonate. Pediatrics *95*:682–687, 1995.
176. Rübben, A., Krones, R., and Schwetschenau, B., et al.: Common warts from immunocompetent patients show the same distribution of human papillomavirus types as common warts from immunocompromised patients. Br. J. Dermatol. *128*:264–270, 1993.
177. Sagi, E. F., Linder, N., and Shouval, D.: Papular acrodermatitis of childhood associated with hepatitis A virus infection. Pediatr. Dermatol. *3*:31–33, 1985.
178. Savin, R., and Horowitz, S.: Double-blind comparison of 2% ketoconazole cream and placebo in the treatment of tinea versicolor. J. Am. Acad. Dermatol. *15*:500–503, 1986.
179. Schuler, G., Hönigsmann, H., and Wolff, K.: The syndrome of milker's nodules in burn injury. Am. Acad. Dermatol. *6*:334–339, 1982.
180. Schwartz, J. J., and Myskowski, P. L.: Molluscum contagiosum in patients with human immunodeficiency virus infection. J. Am. Acad. Dermatol. *27*:583–588, 1992.
181. Schwarz, T. F., Wiersbitzky, S., and Pambor, M.: Detection of parvovirus B19 in a skin biopsy of a patient with erythema infectiosum. J. Med. Virol. *43*:171–174, 1994.
182. Segal, R., Trattner, A., Alteras, I., et al.: Once weekly treatment with oral ketoconazole for superficial fungal infections. J. Am. Acad. Dermatol. *28*:126–127, 1993.
183. Shelley, W. B., and Shelley, E. D.: Surgical treatment of farmyard pox. Cutis *31*:191–192, 1983.
184. Siegel, D., Golden, E., Washington, A. E., et al.: Prevalence and correlates of herpes simplex infections. J. A. M. A. *268*:1702–1708, 1992.
185. Simon, H. K., and Steele, D. W.: Varicella: Pediatric genital/rectal vesicular lesions of unclear etiology. Ann. Emerg. Med. *25*:111–114, 1995.
186. Smith, C. H., Barker, J. N., and Hay, R. J.: A case of chromoblastomycosis responding to treatment with itraconazole. Br. J. Dermatol. *128*:436–439, 1993.
187. Smith, E.: History of antifungals. J. Am. Acad. Dermatol. *23*:776–778, 1990.
188. Spear, K. L., and Winkelmann, R. K.: Gianotti-Crosti syndrome: A review of 10 cases not associated with hepatitis B. Arch. Dermatol. *120*:891–896, 1984.
189. Srugo, I., Israele, V., Wittek, A. E., et al.: Clinical manifestations of varicella-zoster virus infections in human immunodeficiency virus–infected children. Am. J. Dis. Child. *147*:742–745, 1993.
190. Stein, D. H.: Fungal, protozoan, and helminth infections. *In* Schachner, L. A., and Hansen, R. C. (eds.): Pediatric Dermatology. 2nd ed. New York, Churchill Livingstone, 1995, pp. 1295–1345.
191. Stone, M. S., and Murph, J. R.: Papular-purpuric gloves and socks syndrome: A characteristic viral exanthem. Pediatrics *92*:864–865, 1993.
192. Stratte, E. G., and Esterly, N. B.: Human immunodeficiency virus in the Gianotti-Crosti syndrome. Arch. Dermatol. *131*:108–109, 1995.
193. Sumaya, C. V.: Epstein-Barr virus. *In* Feigin, R. D., and Cherry, J. D. (eds.): Textbook of Pediatric Infectious Diseases. 3rd ed. Philadelphia, W. B. Saunders, 1992, pp. 1547–1557.
194. Sumaya, C. V., and Ench, Y.: Epstein-Barr virus infectious mononucleosis in children. I. Clinical and general laboratory findings. Pediatrics *75*:1003–1018, 1985.
195. Sumaya, C. V., and Ench, Y.: Epstein-Barr virus infectious mononucleosis in children. II. Heterophil antibody and viral-specific responses. Pediatrics *75*:1011–1019, 1985.
196. Suringa, D. W. R., Bank, L. J., and Ackerman, A. B.: Role of measle virus in skin lesions and Koplik's spots. N. Engl. J. Med. *283*:1139–1142, 1970.
197. Tan, O. T., Hurwitz, R. M., and Stafford, T. J.: Pulsed dye laser treatment of recalcitrant verrucae: A preliminary report. Lasers Surg. Med. *13*:127–137, 1993.
198. Tanaka, K., Kondo, T., Torigoe, S., et al.: Human herpesvirus 7: Another causal agent for roseola (exanthem subitum). J. Pediatr. *125*:1–5, 1994.
199. Tanz, R. R., Hebert, A. A., and Esterly, N. B.: Treating tinea capitis: Should ketoconazole replace griseofulvin? J. Pediatr. *112*:987–991, 1988.
200. Terragni, L., Lasagui, A., Oriani, A., et al.: Pityriasis versicolor in the pediatric age. Pediatr. Dermatol. *8*:9–12, 1991.
201. Thomas, I., and Janniger, C. K.: Hand, foot, and mouth disease. Pediatr. Dermatol. *52*:265–266, 1993.
202. Tindall, J. P., and Miller, G. D.: Hand, foot and mouth disease. Cutis *9*:459–463, 1972.
203. Török, T. J.: Parvovirus B19 and human disease. Intern. Med. *37*:431–455, 1992.
204. Trattner, A., and David, M.: Purpuric "gloves-and-socks" syndrome: Histologic, immunofluorescence, and polymerase chain reaction study. J. Am. Acad. Dermatol. *30*:267–268, 1994.
205. Tuffanelli, L., and Milburn, P. B.: Treatment of chromoblastomycosis. J. Am. Acad. Dermatol. *23*:728–732, 1990.
206. Tyring, S. K.: Natural history of varicella-zoster virus. Semin. Dermatol. *11*:211–217, 1992.
207. Vestey, J. P., and Norval, M.: Mucocutaneous infections with herpes simplex virus and their management. Clin. Exp. Dermatol. *17*:221–237, 1992.
208. Weitzman, I., and Summerbell, R. C.: The dermatophytes. Clin. Micro. Rev. *8*:240–259, 1995.
209. Weston, W. L.: Practical Pediatric Dermatology. 2nd ed. Boston, Little, Brown, 1985, pp. 107–143.
210. Weston, W. L., Brice, S. L., Jester, J. D., et al.: Herpes simplex virus in childhood erythema multiforme. Pediatrics *89*:32–35, 1992.

211. Weston, W. L., and Lane, A. T.: Color Textbook of Pediatric Dermatology. St. Louis, Mosby–Year Book, 1991, pp. 74–97.
212. White, G. M., and Broska, P.: Vesicles and bulla in an infant. Arch. Dermatol. *130*:107–108, 1994.
213. Whitley, R. J.: Prospects for vaccination against herpes simplex virus. Pediatr. Ann. *22*:726–732, 1993.
214. Williams, H. C., Pottier, A., and Strachan, D.: Are viral warts seen more commonly in children with eczema? Arch. Dermatol. *129*:717–720,1993.
215. Williams, H. C., Pottier, A., and Strachan, D.: The descriptive epidemiology of warts in British school children. Br. J. Dermatol. *128*:504–511, 1993.
216. Williams, L. R., and Webster, G.: Warts and molluscum contagiosum. Clin. Dermatol. *9*:87–93, 1991.
217. Wright, H. T., Landing, B. H., Lennette, E. H., et al.: Fatal infection in an infant associated with coxsackie virus group A, type 16. N. Engl. J. Med. *268*:1041–1044, 1963.
218. Yoto, Y., Kudoh, T., Haseyama, K., et al: Human parvovirus B19 infection in Kawasaki disease. Lancet *344*:58–59, 1994.

SECTION ELEVEN

OCULAR INFECTIONS

❑ ❑ ❑

71

OCULAR INFECTIONS

Paul G. Steinkuller, Jane C. Edmond, and Ronni M. Chen

The eye may be involved in a wide variety of infections and infestations, some with or because of systemic disease. Many are vision-threatening, and some have implications for generalized disease. It often is helpful for the nonophthalmologist to sort through this group of disorders in an organized way based on the anatomic location of the evident inflammatory response, and this discussion is based on that format. The chapter proceeds systematically from infections involving the eyelids and conjunctiva, through those affecting the orbit, to those involving the cornea, the uvea, and the retina. There is considerable overlap in many of these infections because many organisms affect several components of the eye; some duplication will be noted, despite an attempt to keep this to a minimum.

The clinician will find that with an accurate history and visual acuity testing, the list of appropriate differential diagnoses often can be reduced to a very workable minimum. Thereafter, further distinction commonly can be made by the observation of simple signs evident with a penlight or with a direct ophthalmoscope. Some, however, do require special tests or ophthalmic consultation; these situations are pointed out in the text.

INFECTIONS OF THE EYELIDS

Infection of the skin of the eyelids commonly is called dermatoblepharitis. *Staphylococcus aureus* and *Staphylococcus epidermidis* are the most common bacteria. Angular blepharitis, in which the lids at the lateral canthus are inflamed, frequently is caused by *Moraxella* species. Impetigo or erysipelas of the eyelids may be due to *Streptococcus pyogenes.* Parasites infecting the lids include the mite *Demodex folliculorum, Sarcoptes scabei* (scabies), *Pediculus capitis,* and the pubic louse *Phthirus pubis.*

The eyelids contain dense connective tissue, hair follicles, sweat and sebaceous glands, smooth and striated muscle, sensory and motor nerves, and blood vessels. They are covered by the thinnest skin of the body anteriorly and by palpebral conjunctiva posteriorly. The glands of Zeis are sebaceous glands attached to hair follicles. The meibomian glands also are sebaceous but are located within the tarsal plates. They empty onto the lid margin posterior to the cilia.

Eyelid infections involving the lid margins can be considered as being predominantly anterior or posterior. The anterior infections include staphylococcal blepharitis, skin lesions and conjunctivitis due to *Molluscum contagiosum*, and parasitic disease. Posterior lid infections include those due to chronic meibomian gland dysfunction. Lid infections associated with herpes simplex virus (HSV) and herpes zoster virus are discussed in other sections.

Anterior Lid Disease

Staphylococcal Blepharitis

Staphylococcal disease of the eyelids is quite common. The chronic form usually presents as crusting of the lid margins, especially on awakening. The lid margins may be thickened, and a mild conjunctival injection may be present. A child with this condition may be asymptomatic or may complain of a burning or foreign body sensation. Treatment requires daily cleaning of the lid margins with plain warm water on a clean wash cloth or with dilute baby shampoo on a moistened cotton swab. A short course of erythromycin or Bacitracin ointment applied twice a day may be beneficial.[69]

The acute ulcerative form of staphylococcal blepharitis, rare in children, also may require a 5- to 10-day course of systemic antibiotics, such as cloxacillin.

Molluscum contagiosum *Infection*

M. contagiosum infections of the eyelid usually are unilateral. Signs include mild conjunctival injection and small lid nodules of variable size, usually 1 to 3 mm in diameter. Older lesions are umbilicated with a white or waxy core. Chronic cases may involve corneal epithelial disease and subepithelial infiltrates. There may be a history of exposure to other affected individuals, especially within the family.

The condition is self-limited. Most lesions will disappear spontaneously in 2 to 9 months. Treatment can provide relief from any associated ocular discomfort and will reduce the possibility of corneal involvement. Treatment consists of simple expression, curettage, or excision and cautery. These treatments all appear to be equally effective.[85]

Parasitic Lid Disease

Phthirus pubis *Infestation*

The pubic louse *P. pubis* can live in the cilia of the eyelids as well as in pubic hair. The organism reaches the lids by direct person-to-person contact or by contact with contaminated clothing or bed linen. Patients may be asymptomatic or may complain of redness and swelling of the lid margins or itching. Examination reveals the adult lice firmly attached by the head to the eyelid margin, egg cases (nits) stuck to the proximal ends of the hair shafts, and reddish-brown flecks of louse excreta at the bases of the lashes. Treatment consists of mechanically removing the lice and the nits under slit-lamp or other magnification and smothering the remaining organisms and nits by applying a bland ointment, such as yellow mercuric oxide or petrolatum jelly, four times a day to the lid margins. These applications should be maintained for up to 2 weeks to accommodate the life cycle of the nits. Anticholinesterase ophthalmic ointment (topical physostigmine ointment) applied to the lid margins twice a day for 3 days may facilitate removal of the lice or may kill them directly. The patient also should undergo lindane shampoo scrubs of the scalp, pubic hair, and body. The clothing and bed linen should be laundered carefully, and family members should be examined. A follow-up visit in 4 weeks is recommended to look for reinfestation. In the pediatric population, the possibility of sexual abuse should be considered.[24, 69]

Demodex folliculorum *Infection*

D. folliculorum is a mite that frequently infests the eyelids of humans, most of whom are totally asymptomatic. Although it is postulated that these organisms may cause obstruction of the orifices of the sebaceous glands of the eyelids and therefore increase the frequency of hordeola, their real role in disease production is unknown. Treatment is unnecessary.[32]

Other Parasitic Eyelid Disease

P. humanus capitis rarely infests the eyelids, but some of these lice may appear in the cilia of patients with scalp involvement. The scalp infestation should be treated with permethrin rinse or with pyrethrum or lindane shampoos according to the usual guidelines. The lid organisms then usually will disappear, or they can be treated according to the regimen previously described for *P. pubis*. The chemical agents intended for use on the scalp should not be applied to the eyelids or lid margins; they can be quite toxic to the corneal epithelium. The mite *S. scabei* may infest the scalp in infants and young children. In older individuals, the head usually is spared. In either case, the eyelids rarely are involved. The treatment of the scalp infestation alone probably is adequate to eradicate the organisms from the eyelids.[85]

Posterior Eyelid Disease

Hordeolum (Stye)

A hordeolum is an abscess secondary to an obstructed eyelid sebaceous gland. When the glands of Zeis are obstructed and infected, the patient develops an *external* hordeolum, which tends to point to the skin surface. When the meibomian glands similarly are infected, an *internal* hordeolum forms, pointing either to the skin or to the palpebral conjunctival surface. In either case, the usual organism responsible is *S. aureus*. Patients with chronic staphylococcal blepharitis, seborrhea, and rosacea are more prone than others to develop repeated styes, especially during the first decade of life. A hordeolum presents as a red, elevated, tender nodule in the eyelid. The lesions typically are 5 to 10 mm in diameter. They usually are solitary but may be multiple or bilateral. A patient with recurrent styes may have several in various stages of evolution or resolution.

The treatment of hordeola is the application of warm compresses. Although compliance may be a problem in young children, a useful regimen would call for the application of a clean wash cloth wetted with warm water for 15 minutes at a time several times a day. A stye so treated usually will resolve or drain within a few days. Topical antibiotics do not appear to alter the course. Children with very difficult recurrences can be considered rarely for a course of systemic medications to reduce the indigenous flora. Erythromycin is appropriate for children younger than 12 years of age and tetracycline for those 12 years of age or older. After an initial loading dose course (two or four times a day) for 4 to 6 weeks, a maintenance dose level (every day) may be continued for another 4 to 8 weeks. If such a regimen is warranted, lid margin hygiene efforts should be initiated and continued, as recommended earlier.

Hordeola usually do not need to be drained surgically, especially in the pediatric age group. The hazards of approaching a young and frightened child with a sharp instrument pointed at the eye cannot be overemphasized. Such drainage, when deemed necessary, may require general anesthesia.

Chalazion

A chalazion is a lipogranuloma in an obstructed meibomian gland; it may represent the residual of a resolved internal hordeolum. Chalazia are round, nontender nodules within the substance of lids. They often are solitary but may be multiple and are located in the upper lid more often than in the lower. They range in size from 2 to 10 mm or more.

Small chalazia tend to resolve and disappear completely with no treatment over the course of several months; lesions larger than 10 mm in diameter may not resolve without treatment. If some chronic inflammation is present, warm compresses may help. If a chalazion is large and cosmetically objectionable, causes significant astigmatism by pressing on the cornea, or causes a problematic ptosis, more aggressive intervention may be considered. Intralesional injections of 0.05 to 0.1 mL of triamcinolone acetonide suspension (Kenalog), 5 mg/mL, often accelerate resolution. A side effect of steroid injection may be permanent skin depigmentation, which is worse in darkly pigmented individuals. Such injections are done best with a chalazion clamp, which protects the underlying globe from accidental trauma. Sedation or general anesthesia may be required. If general anesthesia is to be undertaken, it may be better to incise, drain, and curette or to excise the lesion completely rather than to inject it. In older children, it may be possible to do this under local anesthesia but with a chalazion clamp in place.[34, 69]

INFECTIONS OF THE LACRIMAL SYSTEM

Dacryoadenitis

The clinical features include localized tenderness and swelling of the outer half of the upper eyelid, producing an S-shaped deformity of the lid margin. There may be an associated conjunctivitis and preseptal lid edema or cellulitis.[138]

The etiology may be bacterial, viral, solely idiopathic, or idiopathic but associated with a systemic illness. The usual causative bacteria are *S. aureus*, *S. pyogenes*, and *Streptococcus pneumoniae*. The nonsuppurative (viral) form may be due to the Epstein-Barr virus (EBV) or to the mumps virus.

Management depends on the clinical situation and the suspected organism. If a bacterial agent is suspected, a swab of an area of suppuration for Gram stain and culture (blood agar, chocolate agar, thioglycolate broth, or anaerobic plate) should be done. Localized abscesses may require drainage; a computed tomographic (CT) or magnetic resonance imaging scan can be useful in identifying an abscess cavity.

The initial antibiotic choice depends on the results of the Gram stain, on the suspected organism, and eventually on the culture results. If the child is septic, a blood culture should be considered. If the stain shows gram-positive cocci, intravenous nafcillin or vancomycin or oral cloxacillin can be considered. If the stain shows gram-negative bacilli, intravenous ceftazidime or oral ciprofloxacin (not approved for use in patients younger than 18 years of age) would be appropriate. If no organisms are seen on Gram stain, intravenous nafcillin, intravenous vancomycin, or oral cloxacillin would be appropriate.

If the infection appears to be viral (nonsuppurative), appropriate serology should be done for the suspected agent. If infection is due to EBV, the level of viral capsid antibodies (IgM and IgG) is high during the acute infection; nuclear antigen is nondetectable. If mumps is suspected, paired sera should be examined for titer rise by enzyme-linked immunosorbent assay, complement fixation, or hemagglutination inhibition.

For a nonsuppurative dacryoadenitis, antibiotics are not effective, but warm compresses and oral analgesics will make the patient comfortable.

Chronic dacryoadenitis can result from syphilis, tuberculosis, and cysticercosis. Causes of chronic noninfectious dacryoadenitis include sarcoidosis, Sjögren syndrome, leukemia, lymphoma, amyloidosis, eosinophilic granuloma, and pseudotumor. Appropriate laboratory evaluations for chronic dacryoadenitis include a CT scan, complete blood cell count, purified protein derivative skin test, chest film, and a serologic test for syphilis. A lacrimal gland biopsy can be considered in difficult cases.[11, 127]

Dacryocystitis

Obstruction of the lacrimal drainage apparatus (dacryostenosis) may result in infection of the lacrimal sac (dacryocystitis).

Acute dacryocystitis presents as a tender swelling of the lacrimal sac with redness and tense skin just below the medial canthal tendon. Epiphora (increased tearing) and/or purulent discharge from the lacrimal puncta may be present. If the obstruction persists and both ends of the sac become obstructed, there may be a spontaneous perforation of the overlying skin with fistula formation. Most such fistulas close spontaneously; if one persists, surgical excision of the fistulous tract may be necessary after the lacrimal obstruction has been cleared.[109, 116]

Common etiologic agents of dacryocystitis include *S. aureus*, *S. pyogenes*, and the viridans group of streptococci. Uncommon agents include *Escherichia coli*, *Pseudomonas*, *Enterobacter*, *Haemophilus influenzae*, *Pasteurella multocida*, various anaerobes, and fungi. Evaluation includes obtaining smears and cultures of any purulent material that presents. A nasal culture from below the inferior turbinate may be useful. Both aerobic and anaerobic culture media should be plated. The lacrimal sac can be massaged to express material, but heavy pressure should not be employed because the sac may rupture and cause cellulitis. Ophthalmic consultation should be requested to consider drainage of the lacrimal sac and/or probing of the system; general anesthesia commonly is required. The ophthalmologist may elect to decompress the distended lacrimal sac before probing by aspirating the contents with a large bore needle on a 3-cc syringe. Any material so obtained should be stained and cultured.[87, 106, 111]

Initial antibiotic coverage should be selected on the basis of the Gram stain. If gram-positive cocci are found, intravenous nafcillin and/or vancomycin may be considered; in mild cases, oral cloxacillin can be used. If gram-negative bacilli are recovered, intravenous ceftazidime or oral ciprofloxacin (not approved for use in patients younger than 18 years of age) may be appropriate. If no organisms are seen on stain preparations, intravenous nafcillin or intravenous vancomycin may be considered.[69, 145]

PRESEPTAL (PERIORBITAL) CELLULITIS

The orbital septum is a layer of fascia extending vertically from the periosteum of the orbital rim to the tarsal plates within the lids. This septum is penetrated by nerves and by blood and lymphatic vessels, but it does serve to prevent many infections from passing from the preseptal (periorbital) space to the deeper orbital and retroorbital structures.[71]

Preseptal cellulitis refers to infectious inflammation and distention of the eyelids without inflammatory proptosis (Table 71–1). The presenting signs indicate infection anterior to the orbital septum, but the clinician must be aware that sinusitis, especially ethmoiditis, may appear initially as preseptal inflammation without orbital signs.[7, 146, 147]

There are three types of preseptal cellulitis: (1) posttraumatic; (2) that secondary to dermatitis and/or blepharitis; and (3) the nonsuppurative form, which occurs in young children without any preceding break in the skin and without a preceding infectious dermatitis.[66, 69]

Posttraumatic Preseptal Cellulitis

Posttraumatic preseptal cellulitis occurs after puncture wounds and lacerations of the lids, face, or scalp but may occur after blunt trauma without an apparent entry wound. The principal agents are *S. aureus* and *S. pyogenes*. Other bacterial causes include the non–spore-forming anaerobic bacteria, such as *Peptococcus*, *Peptostreptococcus*, and *Bacteroides*. Polymicrobial infections are common, but infections by aerobic gram-negative bacilli are uncommon.[64]

The clinical signs are determined by the severity of the injury, the interval after injury, and the responsible organism(s). There is edema of the upper and/or lower lids and hyperemia of the skin. Fluctuation of subcutaneous tissue may be noted if abscess formation is present. Swelling of the contralateral upper and lower lids may occur due to lymphedema. As with other forms of preseptal cellulitis, the vision is normal, there is no proptosis, and the ocular motility is normal. Chemosis is unlikely but may be present.

Evaluation may require a CT scan if the eyeball cannot be examined adequately, if there is a possibility of perforation of the orbital septum and involvement of orbital tissues, or if an orbital fracture or a retained foreign body may be present. If fluctuation is present, incision and drainage of the abscess are indicated, and appropriate stains and cultures should be obtained. A Gram stain is necessary, and cultures should include a blood agar plate, a chocolate agar plate, and an anaerobic medium, such as thioglycolate broth and/or a solid agar plate. Tetanus prophylaxis should be considered according to standard guidelines. The initial antibiotic

TABLE 71–1. Cardinal Differentiating Signs: Preseptal (Periorbital) versus Orbital Cellulitis

Clinical Finding	Preseptal Cellulitis	Orbital Cellulitis
Ocular motility	Normal	Limited
Proptosis	Absent	Present
Pain on eye movement	None	Present
Chemosis	Usually none	Common

can be selected according to the organism identified on Gram stain, if suitable material for staining is present; otherwise, coverage should be appropriate for gram-positive cocci. The agent(s) chosen can be modified later, depending on the clinical course and on the culture results.[69, 114]

Preseptal Cellulitis Secondary to Skin Infection

Preseptal cellulitis may occur secondarily after local dermatitis due to HSV and varicella-zoster virus (VZV), for example. These entities are addressed in the sections on dermatoblepharitis.

Nonsuppurative Preseptal Cellulitis

Nonsuppurative preseptal cellulitis in children commonly was due to *H. influenzae* type b before the widespread availability of appropriate vaccines. Since 1990, the use of these vaccines has resulted in a marked decrease in preseptal cellulitis caused by this particular organism. It still is quite possible, however, to encounter *H. influenzae* type b infections in developing countries and in situations in which vaccines are not widely available. Currently, in the United States, *S. pneumoniae* is the most common bacterial cause of nontraumatic preseptal cellulitis in the pediatric age group.

Viral causes of preseptal cellulitis are fairly common and usually are preceded by adenoviral conjunctivitis or by keratoconjunctivitis with characteristic clinical signs and symptoms.

The clinical features of nonsuppurative preseptal cellulitis depend on the causative agent. As with posttraumatic preseptal cellulitis, the vision is normal (except when adenoviral keratoconjunctivitis is the cause), there is no proptosis, the ocular motility is normal, and chemosis is possible but unlikely.

If *H. influenzae* type b is the cause, the organism apparently gains access to the subcutaneous tissue from infected nasal passages in the context of a preceding or concurrent upper respiratory tract infection. Two kinds of local soft tissue infection may result: preseptal cellulitis or buccal cellulitis. *H. influenzae* type b infection represents the most ominous form of pediatric preseptal cellulitis because of the association with a devastating meningitis; meningitis can occur in up to 2 per cent of such cases, and subdural or brain abscesses occur in 1 per cent.

Adenoviral conjunctivitis is quite common and may present with inflammation and edema of the eyelids mimicking preseptal cellulitis. It usually can be recognized by its copious serous discharge, preauricular lymphadenopathy, and marked conjunctival hyperemia, occasionally with chemosis and a punctate keratitis. Other family members may be infected.

S. pneumoniae nonsuppurative preseptal cellulitis also is associated with upper respiratory tract infections, but the patient is less ill systemically than with *H. influenzae* infection, and the risks of serious ocular and intracranial complications are reduced markedly. Appropriate clinical measures include ruling out orbital and intraocular inflammation and ensuring that the vision is normal.

Hospital admission for preseptal cellulitis should be considered if the child is younger than 1 year of age, if the child is septic, if there has been no obvious trauma, or if the child has not been immunized adequately. Sepsis work-up would be appropriate if the child appears seriously ill and/or if any meningeal signs are present. Sinus films or orbital CT scan can be useful if orbital cellulitis cannot be ruled out clearly. If a radiographic study is warranted, a CT scan will provide much more adequate information than plain sinus films. Ophthalmic consultation is recommended if there is any doubt whatsoever about the status of the ocular inflammation or vision. Blood and conjunctival cultures may be useful. If adenoviral infection is suspected, hospitalization generally is not indicated, and precautions should be taken to avoid spreading the infection to medical personnel.[147]

Intravenous antibiotics, if necessary, could include cephalosporins effective against *H. influenzae, S. pneumoniae* and other streptococci, and *S. aureus*. If the possibility of meningitis is excluded, cefuroxime can be appropriate; if meningitis is a possibility, consideration should be given to ceftriaxone or cefotaxime. Systemic antibiotics should be continued until clinical improvement is obvious and the patient has been afebrile for at least 24 hours or for 48 hours if the blood culture is positive. If the child has been admitted, the discharge regimen should include oral antibiotics for an additional 7 to 10 days. Augmentin or Bactrim often is appropriate.

Penicillin resistance of the pneumococcus has become a serious and growing problem. All isolates should be tested for resistance to penicillin, cefotaxime, and ceftriaxone.

Since October 1990, an *H. influenzae* type b early vaccination regimen has been available and now is in widespread use in the United States. With any vaccine failure, immune deficiency conditions should be ruled out, including those due to HIV.[69]

The clinician should be acutely aware that an apparent case of preseptal cellulitis in fact may represent the initial manifestations of a developing orbital cellulitis due to sinusitis, a much more ominous situation.[128]

ORBITAL CELLULITIS

Orbital cellulitis means inflammation of the tissues of the orbit behind the orbital septum. The cardinal signs and symptoms of orbital cellulitis include pain on eye movement, proptosis, and ophthalmoplegia (decreased ocular motility). Decreased vision, elevated intraocular pressure, and chemosis are common ancillary signs. (Patients with periorbital cellulitis have normal vision, normal motility, and no proptosis.) Occasionally, the first outward sign of sinusitis is preseptal inflammation, which subsequently progresses to clearly recognizable orbital cellulitis.[20] Almost all cases of orbital cellulitis are due to a preceding/concurrent ethmoid sinus infection; some cases are due to penetrating orbital trauma or skin infections of the middle third of the face or more rarely occur after orbital, ocular, or periocular surgery, such as strabismus procedures. Orbital cellulitis and cavernous sinus thrombosis have been reported after dental infections and dental surgery.[18, 19, 28, 57, 150]

The median age of children admitted for orbital cellulitis due to sinusitis is 7 years. The condition is more common in cold weather, when the frequency of sinusitis increases.

The presumed pathogenesis, when due to sinusitis, includes local irritation and/or infection within the nasal passages; edema of the sinus mucosa; closing of the sinus ostia; proliferation of indigenous facultative aerobic and anaerobic microflora in a reduced oxygen environment; and entrance of the organisms into the orbit through the naturally occurring foramina, dehiscences in bone, and blood vessels. The most common etiologic bacteria are *S. aureus, Streptococcus* species, and nontypable *H. influenzae*. *S. pneumoniae* commonly is implicated. Other organisms involved are *Peptostreptococcus, Veillonella, Bacteroides, Fusobacteria, Eubacteria, Pseudomonas, Klebsiella, Mycobacterium tuberculosis*, and other *Mycobac-*

terium species. In the pediatric age group, the etiologic agents usually are *S. pneumoniae* and nontypeable *H. influenzae*. Polymicrobial infection is common.[75]

The differential diagnosis of inflammatory proptosis in childhood includes (1) infection: orbital cellulitis and/or cavernous sinus thrombosis; (2) idiopathic inflammation: orbital pseudotumor, orbital myositis, hidradenitis, and Wegner granulomatosis; (3) inflammatory neoplasm: sarcoidosis, leukemia, Burkitt lymphoma, rhabdomyosarcoma, retinoblastoma, metastatic carcinoma, and histiocytosis-X (Letterer-Siwe variety); and (4) endocrine dysfunction: dysthyroid exophthalmos.[7, 23, 55, 95]

The clinical features of orbital cellulitis include the expected ancillary signs, symptoms, and associated findings of sinusitis. An antecedent upper respiratory infection is present in almost all cases. The child typically is quite ill, with an oral temperature of 39° to 40° C (102° to 104° F).

Adequate clinical evaluation calls for a complete blood count, a CT scan of the orbits including low narrow cuts of the frontal lobes, and an adequate ocular examination with evaluation of the ocular media and intraocular structures. A necrotic retinoblastoma may present as orbital inflammation.

Stain and culture results may help guide the choice of antibiotics. The most useful culture material will be from the infected ethmoid sinuses or from an associated abscess if surgical drainage is undertaken. Nasal, nasopharyngeal, and blood cultures are indicated but commonly are either negative or noncontributory. A lumbar puncture should be considered if any meningeal and/or cerebral signs develop.

Treatment calls for immediate high-dose intravenous antibiotics after blood, nasal, and/or nasopharyngeal cultures. Prompt evaluation by an otorhinolaryngologist, an ophthalmologist, and a pediatrician is indicated, and a neurosurgeon should be consulted if intracranial suppuration is suspected. The patient should be admitted and watched carefully; progression may be rapid. The initial systemic antibiotics are selected on the basis of the most likely pathogens: *S. pneumoniae* and other streptococci, *S. aureus*, *H. influenzae*, and non–spore-forming anaerobes. Appropriate antibiotics could include nafcillin (*Staphylococcus* and *Streptococcus* species), metronidazole (anaerobes), and cefotaxime (gram-negative organisms, nontypeable *H. influenzae*, *Moraxella*, and pneumococci with intermediate resistance). Nafcillin and chloramphenicol can be considered; in place of chloramphenicol, ceftazidime or ticarcillin-clavulanate can be used. If a penicillin allergy exists, one may substitute cefazolin or vancomycin for nafcillin. Antibiotic coverage should be adjusted as indicated by the clinical course and by the culture results. The mean hospital stay is 10 to 14 days. Ancillary in-hospital management includes frequent and meticulous reevaluation, including vision testing, which can be done easily and quickly at the bedside. These vision checks should be performed by the same examiner to avoid interobserver discrepancies and confusion. Rapid progression and deterioration should be considered possible in all cases. Repeat CT scans may be called for, possibly daily or more often as the clinical picture dictates. If corneal exposure occurs from severe proptosis, an ophthalmologist should be consulted promptly because this amount of proptosis also may cause a secondary glaucoma and compromised ocular circulation. Ocular antihypertensive agents should be used if a secondary glaucoma develops. Nasal decongestants, such as phenylephrine 0.125 per cent drops, may be useful in clearing the sinus ostia and promoting drainage.[153]

The patient and/or family should be made aware that progression, complications, and permanent vision loss may occur, despite the best and most timely treatment.

Surgical intervention should be considered in certain situations. Sinus drainage may be appropriate if the clinical response to conventional treatment is poor or if the sinuses are opacified completely on CT scan. A craniotomy may be indicated if brain abscesses develop and do not respond quickly to systemic antibiotics. A subperiosteal abscess need not be drained always, but such drainage definitely is indicated if an afferent pupillary defect is present or develops, if vision is decreased or decreasing, if the proptosis is severe and/or progressing despite adequate antibiotic treatment, and if the CT scan shows no improvement in the abscess after 48 to 72 hours of appropriate intravenous antibiotics. True orbital abscesses (outside the confines of the subperiosteal space) are unusual; the surgical drainage rules are the same as for subperiosteal abscesses.[21, 54, 120]

When discharged from the hospital, the patient should be kept on oral antibiotics for an extra 7 to 14 days and should be re-evaluated in the interim.

There are two types of significant complications of orbital cellulitis: intracranial and ocular. When the cellulitis is caused by ethmoid sinusitis, intracranial complications include meningitis (2 per cent), cavernous sinus thrombosis (1 per cent), and abscess of the brain parenchyma or of the subdural or epidural space (1 per cent). Orbital complications include subperiosteal and other orbital abscesses (7 per cent) and vision loss (1 per cent). The patient may lose vision by a variety of mechanisms: corneal opacification secondary to exposure, destruction of intraocular tissues by secondary glaucoma, endophthalmitis, or septic uveitis or retinitis. An exudative retinal detachment may occur, and a secondary glaucoma may develop due to elevated orbital pressure or due to inflammation or obstruction of the trabecular meshwork. The optic nerve may be infected directly, or an aseptic optic neuritis may occur. Central retinal vein and central retinal artery occlusions have been reported.[63]

Orbital cellulitis also may be due to fungal infections, particularly mucormycosis or aspergillosis. *Mucor* infections are most common in patients who are diabetic or acidotic from diarrhea and dehydration and in immunocompromised individuals. In this infection, the signs and symptoms of orbital cellulitis may take a subacute or even a chronic course. The orbital apex syndrome (loss of function of all of the cranial nerves traversing the apex of the orbit, i.e., II, III, IV, V, and VI) may be present, and there may be black eschar-like lesions in the oro- or nasopharynx.[49]

Aspergillus orbital infections, most commonly due to *A. flavus*, *A. fumigatus*, or *A. oryvae*, are very rare in children and take a slow, chronic course over months or years. There are no clear predisposing factors, most cases occurring in otherwise healthy individuals. There is some predilection for humid climates. Signs and symptoms of orbital aspergillosis include loss of vision, constant dull pain, decreased or absent ocular motility, and proptosis with a very firm resistance to retropulsion. Palate and nasopharyngeal lesions are rare but may appear; biopsy is required for diagnosis.[43]

The treatment of orbital fungal infections requires correction of any underlying systemic or metabolic disturbance, intravenous amphotericin B, and surgical débridement. The treatment frequently is unrewarding; fatalities are common with mucormycosis and rare with aspergillosis, although vision will not return once lost.[96, 105]

The larva of *Echinococcus granulosus* can produce a hydatid cyst of the orbit. The dog is the definitive host, but the organism also may live in the intestines of sheep, goats, cattle, pigs, and other animals. The disease is endemic in the Middle East, Africa, and Asia. Humans become infested by eating contaminated food, usually meat. Involvement may occur in any age group. Patients present with a noninflammatory proptosis, decreased ocular motility, and dull orbital pain. Surgical excision is the only useful treatment: the cyst is injected with alcohol or hypertonic saline to kill the parasite, then excised.[97]

CONJUNCTIVAL INFECTIONS

The conjunctiva is a mucous membrane covering the front part of the eye except for the cornea, lining the inner surface of the eyelids, and dividing into *bulbar* and *palpebral* portions. It contains numerous small glands that produce most of the aqueous component of tears as well as the mucin responsible for effecting a smooth uniform tear film over the cornea. The conjunctiva may be infected by a wide variety of bacterial and viral agents. It may become inflamed due to noninfectious allergic and toxic events. Primary fungal conjunctival infections probably do not occur.

Patients with conjunctivitis may complain of burning or itching and occasionally of a foreign body sensation. Significant itching usually points to an allergic cause. The affected eye(s) will be reddened, with most of the redness located away from the cornea. Redness accentuated next to the cornea (limbal or ciliary flush) suggests inflammation of the cornea (keratitis) or of the inside of the anterior segment of the eye, as seen with an iritis or iridocyclitis form of uveitis. When the eye is very red, such a differentiating pattern may not be distinguishable. Conjunctivitis usually is accompanied by a discharge that has some diagnostic properties. Purulence suggests a bacterial etiology; mucopurulence or a mucoid discharge most often is seen with viral infections, and a serous discharge with either viral or allergic causes. Patients with conjunctivitis alone will not have any significant decrease in vision. A red eye with poor vision calls for an explanation other than simple conjunctivitis.[39, 40, 94]

Bacterial Conjunctivitis

Bacterial conjunctivitis is the most common form of infectious conjunctivitis in children. It is characterized by a purulent discharge, and it commonly is unilateral. It is useful to divide bacterial conjunctivitis into nonsevere and severe forms.[69]

Nonsevere Bacterial Conjunctivitis

The most common causes of mild, nonsevere bacterial conjunctivitis in children 5 years of age or older are nontypable *H. influenzae, S. pneumoniae*, and *Moraxella* species. *S. aureus* conjunctivitis is seen most frequently after accidental or surgical ocular trauma. Conjunctival stains and cultures often are not necessary because the disease is self-limited and responds so rapidly to topical antibiotics that the eye may be back to normal by the time the culture results are finalized. If cultures are done, swabs from *both* eyes should be plated out on chocolate agar. Culturing both eyes may afford an automatic control. One should be aware that regardless of how well they are done, cultures may not be helpful in determining the causative agent. Appropriate topical treatment may be erythromycin ointment, although many other antibiotics are effective, including tobramycin, gentamicin, gramicidin-neomycin–polymixin B, trimethoprim–polymixin B, ciprofloxacin, norfloxacin, and sulfacetamide drops or ointment. Aminoglycoside containing compounds such as neomycin may cause a dramatic allergic blepharoconjunctivitis that may be much worse than the original problem. The choice of drops or ointment often best is left to whoever will be instilling the medication at home. There is no proven therapeutic advantage of one over the other. An appropriate regimen would call for instillation of a drop or a quarter-inch bead of ointment into the inferior conjunctival fornix four to six times a day for 3 to 5 days, by which time the infection will be gone; persistence calls for a return to the physician and reconsideration of the diagnosis. Untreated bacterial conjunctivitis will resolve spontaneously in 7 to 14 days.[39, 40]

Severe Bacterial Conjunctivitis

Severe bacterial conjunctivitis with a very red eye and a copious discharge may be caused by *Neisseria gonorrhoeae, Neisseria meningitidis, S. aureus, S. pneumoniae*, and, in children younger than 5 years of age, *H. influenzae*. A hyperpurulent state with a very copious discharge suggests infection with *N. gonorrheae*.

Severe conjunctivitis does call for stains and cultures because the causative organisms may cause permanent vision loss and/or systemic morbidity. Both eyes should be tested. Gram stains of conjunctival scrapings are necessary; appropriate culture technique could include the use of a calcium alginate swab (Calgiswab: Spectrum, Houston, TX) rubbed against the palpebral conjunctiva of the lower lid and inoculated onto blood and chocolate agar.

Treatment of severe conjunctivitis is based on the results of the stains and cultures, but if *Neisseria* strongly is suspected, the patient should be treated so, even if the laboratory results are not revealing. Gram-positive cocci call for erythromycin ointment or ciprofloxacin drops topically and nafcillin or cefuroxime parenterally as needed; cloxacillin may be considered for oral use. Gram-negative cocci can be treated with erythromycin ointment topically or cefuroxime or ceftriaxone parenterally. Ocular *N. gonorrhoeae* infections are vision- and life-threatening. They occur in three situations: (1) in the neonate due to passage through an infected birth canal; (2) in sexually active individuals; and (3) in sexually abused individuals. Pediatric infections with *N. gonorrhoeae* usually call for admission and always call for systemic treatment. Due to the prevalence of penicillin-resistant strains, an extended-spectrum (third-generation) cephalosporin, such as ceftriaxone, is the appropriate antibiotic at the time of this writing. The adjunctive topical treatment of *N. gonorrhoeae* conjunctivitis is erythromycin ointment, penicillin G (100,000 units/mL) drops, or simple saline irrigation for the first 1 to 2 days of systemic treatment.[48, 53]

Viral Conjunctivitis

Adenoviral Conjunctivitis

Most cases of viral conjunctivitis in children are caused by various serotypes of the adenovirus. Serotypes 1, 2, 3, 4, 7, and 10 cause an acute form with prominent conjunctival follicles; serotypes 3 and 7 may cause pharyngoconjunctival fever, with fever and pharyngitis in addition to the conjunctivitis; serotypes 8, 19, and 37 can cause epidemic keratoconjunctivitis, with pharyngitis, rhinitis, and corneal inflammation. Pharyngoconjunctival fever is more common in adults than in children.[12]

Adenoviral conjunctivitis occurs after exposure to an infected individual, commonly at home or at school. The incubation period usually is 5 to 10 days but may be up to 21 days; the virus is shed from the conjunctiva for 7 to 12 days after the onset of infection. There often is a prodromal upper respiratory infection with fever, pharyngitis, otitis media, or nausea, vomiting, and diarrhea. Ocular signs and symptoms include photophobia, a foreign body sensation, increased tearing with a watery discharge, redness of the bulbar and palpebral conjunctiva, subconjunctival hemorrhages, the formation of a grayish-pink friable membrane on the palpebral conjunctiva, and an enlarged nontender preauricular lymph node. Slit-lamp examination occasionally reveals a mild diffuse punctate keratitis with subepithelial infiltrates. The corneal involvement may be prolonged, lasting much longer than the conjunctivitis component.

The diagnosis is a clinical one, and only in extraordinary circumstances are laboratory tests indicated; viral cultures probably are the most specific. Treatment of adenoviral conjunctivitis is symptomatic. Cold compresses and acetaminophen are useful, and removal of the conjunctival membranes with a cotton swab may afford very significant relief from the foreign body sensation. A small amount of bleeding may occur after removal of the membranes. The membranes may re-form daily for several days. If the corneal infiltrates cause significant discomfort or unacceptable decrease in vision, the ophthalmologist may elect to treat the patient with a short course of topical steroids. The use of such steroid preparations requires careful and repeated slit-lamp examinations.[148]

Adenoviral conjunctivitis is extremely contagious. The clinician must wear gloves when dealing with such patients, and careful hand washing is essential. Any instruments or equipment used in examining these children should be cleaned with 10 per cent sodium hypochlorite solution, and the patients should be kept as separate as possible from other patients. At home, the families should exercise caution, keeping the towels and bedclothes of the patient separate. Children of school age should be kept home for 5 to 7 days.[68]

Herpes Simplex Virus External Ocular Infections

HSV conjunctivitis may occur primarily or secondarily; it may occur with or without lid vesicles and with or without corneal involvement (keratitis). Ocular infections usually are caused by HSV-1, except in newborns, in whom HSV-2 predominates.

Typical presenting signs of HSV conjunctivitis include a serous discharge, scant follicle formation on the inferior palpebral conjunctiva, and preauricular lymphadenopathy. Eighty per cent of cases are unilateral. Eyelid vesicles may be present. Bulbar conjunctival ulceration is unusual but when present virtually is pathognomonic. Corneal involvement (keratitis) occurs in up to 50 per cent of cases and often is of such characteristic dendritic appearance as to be diagnostic.

The diagnosis usually is made on the basis of the clinical appearance alone. Antigen detection procedures or viral cultures are used only when the diagnosis is in doubt and the case problematic. A MicroTrak (Syva) test is available.

Viral cultures, when necessary, require a specific technique. After swabbing the surface with an alcohol sponge, a tuberculin syringe with a 30-gauge needle is used to aspirate fluid from an intact vesicle. If no vesicles are present, a Dacron swab is wiped on the palpebral conjunctiva of the lower lid. In either case, viral transport medium then is inoculated and taken to the laboratory chilled on ice but not frozen.

Treatment of HSV conjunctivitis alone in the absence of corneal epithelial disease is somewhat controversial. Topical and oral medications have not been proved to prevent corneal involvement, but both are relatively safe and may be beneficial. Oral acyclovir can be considered for severe cases; topical trifluridine 1 per cent (Viroptic) drops every 2 to 4 hours during the day or vidarabine 3 per cent (Vira-A) ointment applied five times daily is appropriate for mild cases.[126]

HSV dermatoblepharitis most commonly is seen in children younger than 6 years of age but may occur at any age. The initial episode may be associated with an upper respiratory infection. Recurrences are common. Clinical signs may include a mild follicular conjunctivitis, preauricular lymphadenopathy, and occasionally an atypical epithelial keratitis. Secondary bacterial infection may occur. Systemic acyclovir is a safe and moderately effective treatment, although the disease is self-limited if left untreated.

When HSV keratitis occurs, a typical dendritic (branched) epithelial lesion usually is present and the cornea is somewhat hypesthetic. A secondary iritis is common, with miosis, photophobia, ocular pain with a foreign body sensation, and decreased vision, especially if the visual axis (center of the cornea) is involved. The disease may be atypical, more severe, and more complicated if the patient has been receiving topical steroids or is immunocompromised or if the infection is recurrent. In such situations, the corneal stroma may be involved, and a hypopyon, iritis, or perforation of the cornea may develop. Topical treatment definitely is indicated in all cases of HSV keratitis, as noted earlier. Ancillary treatment may include cycloplegic agents and pain medications. As with all cases of corneal inflammation or infection, ophthalmic consultation is strongly recommended.

Varicella-Zoster Virus External Ocular Infections

Childhood varicella commonly is accompanied by conjunctivitis, occasionally with vesicles or ulcers on the bulbar or palpebral conjunctiva. Corneal involvement is quite rare.

After primary varicella, the virus may persist in a latent form in the trigeminal ganglia. Herpes zoster ophthalmicus occurs when the ophthalmic division of the fifth cranial nerve is affected; there is trigeminal involvement in 15 per cent of all cases of herpes zoster. Involvement of the nasociliary branch of V-1 does not predict reliably direct involvement of the eyeball. Although it is more common in adults, herpes zoster ophthalmicus does occur in children. The frequency increases if the patient is immunocompromised for any reason, as in leukemia or in patients receiving chemotherapy. HIV testing should be considered. Recurrences are infrequent and may involve another dermatome.

The diagnosis almost always is made on the basis of the typical clinical features: a painful tender vesicular eruption, which occurs in the distribution of a single dermatome. Immunofluorescence testing of vesicular base scrapings or viral cultures can be considered if the presentation is atypical and the diagnosis is in doubt. With recurrences, there is an accompanying rise in antibody titers.

Treatment involves oral or intravenous acyclovir, the latter route especially being indicated in immunocompromised individuals. The treatment is most effective when initiated within 72 hours of the appearance of vesicles. Involvement of the eyeball may include keratitis or uveitis; corneal epithelial lesions may be dendritic with subepithelial infiltrates. The dendritic corneal ulcers of herpes zoster ophthalmicus do not respond to topical antiviral agents. Herpes zoster ophthalmicus uveitis may occur with or without an overlying keratitis. It usually is a mild to moderate iritis, but it may be severe, with the formation of a hypopyon or hyphema. In such cases, topical, periocular, or systemic steroids may be required to prevent permanent vision loss from a secondary glaucoma.[94]

Chlamydial Conjunctivitis and Trachoma

Chlamydia psittaci rarely causes conjunctivitis. *Chlamydia trachomatis* has numerous serotypes that affect the eyes and may cause inclusion conjunctivitis. Serotypes A, B, Ba, and C can cause trachoma, and serotypes B, C, D, Da, D-, E, F, G, H, I, Ia, J, and K can cause conjunctivitis, including the neonatal form. Neonatal chlamydial conjunctivitis is discussed in a subsequent section. Inclusion conjunctivitis in older children and adults presents as a subacute or chronic inflammation with a mucopurulent discharge, the formation of follicles on the bulbar and perilimbal conjunctiva, and preauricular lymphadenopathy. It may be unilateral or bilateral. The cornea may become involved, with a punctate epithelial keratitis, subepithelial infiltrates, and formation of a superior micropannus. Iritis rarely occurs.

The differential diagnosis of inclusion conjunctivitis is sizable, including viral and bacterial conjunctivitis, molluscum contagiosum, and toxic keratoconjunctivitis. Laboratory testing may be necessary for confirmation. Giemsa staining of conjunctival scrapings may show intracytoplasmic inclusions, but false negatives are very common. Antigen detection by fluorescent antibody detection (MicroTrak: Syva) or by enzyme immunoassay is more likely to be appropriately positive. Chlamydial cultures may be considered in difficult or confusing cases.

Treatment calls for systemic erythromycin or doxycycline (not recommended for patients younger than 9 years of age) if systemic disease is suspected or for topical erythromycin or tetracycline ointment four times a day for 7 days if the infection is limited to the conjunctiva.[68, 69]

Trachoma remains one of the leading causes of blindness worldwide, ranking either second or third, depending on the region studied. It is a disease of poverty, exacerbated by inadequate supplies of water and by poor hygiene. It seldom is seen in developed countries; in the United States, it can be encountered on Native American reservations in the Southwest and in individuals arriving from the Middle East and other endemic areas. Trachoma causes blindness by producing a chronic inflammation of the palpebral conjunctiva of the upper eyelid with secondary scar formation, contracture of the scars with entropion, and trichiasis leading to corneal opacification. The cornea also may be infected directly. Children are the reservoir of the disease, and their caregivers—older sisters, mothers, and grandmothers—continuously are reinfected; trachoma-induced blindness therefore usually is much more common in the female population. The complete course of the disease from initial infection to serious vision loss usually takes decades.

The diagnosis of trachoma almost always is clinical, laboratory testing being reserved for study populations. The disease passes through characteristic stages, from inflammation to follicle formation to scarring to entropion and trichiasis. More than one stage may be present. The World Health Organization classification characterizes the stages: TF = trachomatous follicular response (typically on the superior palpebral conjunctiva), TI = diffuse trachomatous conjunctival inflammation, TS = trachomatous scarring of the palpebral conjunctiva (of the upper lid), TT = trachomatous trichiasis, and TO = trachomatous corneal opacification. In the pediatric population, one usually encounters stages TI and TF only and occasionally TS. The scars of the upper lid palpebral conjunctiva are linear and multidirectional and are called Arlt's lines. Slit-lamp examination may show a superior limbal micropannus and Herbert's pits, hollowed out areas in the superior limbus representing the sites of resolved follicles.[142]

Treatment of trachoma calls for topical tetracycline 1 per cent or erythromycin ointment instilled twice a day for 2 months and improved facial hygiene to prevent recurrences. In children older than 8 years of age and in adults who do not respond promptly to topical treatment, systemic treatment also is effective: tetracycline 1.5 to 2.0 g in divided doses daily for 3 weeks. Oral erythromycin can be used in younger children or in patients intolerant of tetracycline. Most patients can be treated adequately by topical means only. The disease often is self-limited if improved hygiene alone is effected.[135]

Neonatal Conjunctivitis

Neonatal conjunctivitis, also called ophthalmia neonatorum, is a common problem for pediatricians throughout the world, representing a persistent threat to vision. Although it has been relegated to a position of secondary importance in the industrialized world, where prophylactic measures are in widespread use, it remains a significant cause of ocular morbidity in childhood in developing countries. Corneal damage accounts for 70 per cent of all pediatric blindness in nonindustrialized nations. Although most of this blindness is due to the ocular complications of vitamin A deficiency, neonatal conjunctivitis, especially that caused by *N. gonorrhoeae*, is a significant threat as well. In 1881, Crede introduced the use of dilute topical silver nitrate solution instilled into the eyes of newborns for prophylaxis, thereby reducing the prevalence of gonococcal ophthalmia neonatorum from 10 to 0.3 per cent of all live births in Europe. With the rise of regional conflicts, increased political instability, and burgeoning refugee populations with concomitant breakdown of entire local health infrastructures, such simple prophylactic measures often are abandoned.[38, 50, 51]

The frequency of neonatal conjunctivitis is highly variable in any population. In hospitals using silver nitrate drops for prophylaxis, chemical conjunctivitis is the most common cause of neonatal conjunctivitis. Infectious conjunctivitis occurs in 0.5 to 6.0 per cent of live births in the United States. The leading infectious cause is *C. trachomatis*. Infection is caused by exposure to contaminated maternal vaginal discharge, although it may occur in infants born by cesarean section if premature rupture of membranes has occurred. The other common infectious causes are *N. gonorrhoeae* and *S. aureus*. Other microorganisms implicated in occasional cases include *Streptococcus* species, *Haemophilus* species, *Pseudomonas aeruginosa*, *Moraxella* species, *Branhamella catarrhalis*, *N. meningitidis*, *E. coli*, and *Enterobacter cloacae*. Viruses also can cause neonatal conjunctivitis. HSV may cause keratoconjunctivitis, but such infections usually are associated with distinctive skin changes and/or systemic signs, and the diagnosis seldom is in doubt. Other viruses that can cause ocular disease in neonates include adenovirus, coxsackievirus A9, cytomegalovirus (CMV), and echovirus.[1, 10, 37, 131, 134]

Certain clinical features may help establish the diagnosis (Table 71–2), but there is considerable overlap in presentation, and the physician must use the entire triad of history, physical examination, and laboratory studies to identify the correct organism. Even when all appropriate investigative modalities are assessed adequately, some doubt may remain. In such cases, it may be prudent to treat for *N. gonorrhoeae*, the worst of the neonatal ocular infections.

Variations in the time of onset after birth, severity of inflammation, and character of the ocular discharge are common, and none of the signs can be considered pathognomonic of a specific etiology. Silver nitrate conjunctivitis begins during the first 48 hours of life and produces a watery discharge with mild inflammation. It is self-limited and resolves within 48 to 72 hours of appearance; no treatment is

TABLE 71–2. Clinical Characteristics of Neonatal Conjunctivitis Caused by Various Agents

Agent	Onset, Day of Life	Discharge
Silver nitrate	1 (0–2)	Serous
Chlamydia trachomatis	7 (1–21)	Mucopurulent
Staphylococcus aureus	5 (1–21)	Mucopurulent
Other bacteria	7 (1–21)	Mucopurulent
Neisseria gonorrhoeae	3 (0–21)	Purulent
Herpes simplex virus	5 (0–21)	Serosanguinous
Other viruses	Not established	Probably serous

required. *C. trachomatis* conjunctivitis begins from day 1 to day 21 after birth and usually is present by day 7; it can produce a moderately copious but highly variable mucopurulent discharge. *S. aureus* conjunctivitis also begins during the first 3 weeks of life and can produce a moderately profuse mucopurulent discharge. Other nongonococcal bacteria have similar characteristics. Conjunctivitis due to *N. gonorrhoeae* ordinarily begins somewhat earlier, usually by day 3, but may appear up to 3 weeks after birth. It usually produces a copious purulent discharge, often so profuse as to warrant the term "hyperpurulent"; pus literally may squirt from the eyes when the lids are separated manually.[102]

Viral neonatal conjunctivitis is rare. HSV infection may begin during the first 3 weeks of life and usually will cause a serous or serosanguinous discharge. Other viruses have highly variable characteristics, but a serous discharge is likely.

The differential diagnosis of neonatal conjunctivitis includes congenital dacryostenosis with or without dacryocystitis and congenital glaucoma. The former two conditions may present with increased tearing, a watery or purulent discharge, and swelling and redness of the periocular tissues. Epiphora due to congenital dacryostenosis ordinarily is not seen until the second or third week of life. Newborns with congenital glaucoma often are photophobic and irritable and may exhibit increased tearing and periocular inflammation. Any condition producing intraocular inflammation may present in a similar fashion, and if any doubt whatsoever exists about the diagnosis, consultation with an ophthalmologist should be considered.

The diagnosis of neonatal conjunctivitis is made by the clinical picture, including the birth history; the maternal history and/or examination and paternal history and/or examination also may be useful. Laboratory testing commonly is used to establish a specific diagnosis. Such testing includes stains and cultures. An appropriate stain protocol for neonatal conjunctivitis includes using a sterile spatula for conjunctival scraping and obtaining a Gram stain and a *Chlamydia* immunoassay. A Giemsa stain can be useful, but it must be read by a skilled technician who is familiar with the technique. Gonococcal immunoassay and HSV immunochemical tests are available but are not yet in widespread use. Cultures should include thioglycolate broth for aerobic and nonaerobic bacteria and a Thayer-Martin preparation (chocolate agar with antibiotics) for *N. gonorrhoeae*. Cotton-tipped swabs should be used to obtain material for cultures, and the nasopharynx should be cultured as well as the conjunctiva. Chocolate agar is useful for detecting aerobic bacteria, *Neisseria* species, and *Haemophilus* species. Viral transport media and a *Chlamydia* culture can be considered but often are not necessary.[137]

A simple practical laboratory work-up would include a Gram stain, a *Chlamydia* immunoassay stain, and a Thayer-Martin culture for *N. gonorrhoeae*. A *Chlamydia* culture and a thioglycolate broth culture for nongonococcal bacteria can be added for completeness as desired, but the physician must be mindful that the main point is to rule in or rule out gonococcal infection, which is the condition representing the most serious and immediate threat to vision, to systemic morbidity, and to life. Only two bacteria can penetrate an initially intact cornea and cause a perforation, with loss of intraocular contents and spread of infection to the inside of the eye: *N. gonorrhoeae* and *P. aeruginosa*.[122, 123]

The treatment of neonatal conjunctivitis depends on the suspected etiologic agent. Silver nitrate–induced conjunctivitis does not require topical or systemic treatment and is self-limited, with no danger of significant sequelae. *C. trachomatis* conjunctivitis calls for tetracycline 1 per cent or erythromycin 0.5 per cent ointment four times a day for 3 weeks, as well as erythromycin systemically for 2 to 3 weeks to prevent or to treat *Chlamydia* pneumonia; sulfonamides can be used if erythromycin is not tolerated. Staphylococcal conjunctivitis calls for erythromycin 0.5 per cent ointment every 4 to 6 hours for 3 to 7 days, and appropriate systemic antibiotic treatment should be considered if the infection is severe. Conjunctivitis caused by other bacteria calls for treatment specific to the organism identified; systemic medications may be necessary.[42, 57]

N. gonorrhoeae infection calls for systemic treatment in all cases. Aqueous penicillin G can be considered if resistant strains are unlikely, but if resistant strains are possible, ceftriaxone, cefotaxime, or another appropriate antibiotic should be considered. Topical treatment of *N. gonorrhoeae* calls for saline irrigation every hour until the discharge clears and then in decreased frequency as necessary; usually, saline irrigation is necessary for 24 to 48 hours after the initiation of systemic treatment. Penicillin G drops, 100,000 units per milliliter every hour, are recommended by some but do not appear to improve the overall prognosis or the rapidity of recovery.[115]

HSV infection calls for acyclovir systemically in appropriate doses for up to 3 weeks, as well as vidarabine ophthalmic ointment four times a day for 2 to 3 weeks. Infection with other viruses is unlikely to need systemic or topical treatment.

If the cornea is seen to be infected, ophthalmic consultation is required, and treatment depends on the specific organism identified.

Prevention of ophthalmia neonatorum requires instillation of an antibiotic or antiseptic agent within the first hour after birth. Silver nitrate 1 per cent drops, erythromycin 0.5 per cent ointment, and tetracycline 1 per cent ointment have proved to be effective against *N. gonorrhoeae* and *C. trachomatis*. Povidone-iodine in a dilute solution has proved to be effective and economical in the prophylaxis against gonococcal neonatal conjunctivitis in a developing country setting.[52, 65, 125]

As with other clinical manifestations of sexually transmitted disease, neonatal conjunctivitis caused by *N. gonorrhoeae*, *C. trachomatis*, and/or HSV should be considered from preventive and public health standpoints and handled according to standard reporting, investigative, and case identification guidelines.

Complications of neonatal conjunctivitis depend on the etiologic agent. Most significant are the complications of *N. gonorrhoeae* infection. Ocular complications include corneal ulceration and perforation with the expected disastrous sequelae: flat anterior chamber, secondary glaucoma, anterior staphyloma, and/or endophthalmitis with blindness. Systemic complications include septicemia, meningitis, and arthritis. Death has been reported.

Ocular complications of neonatal *C. trachomatis* include corneal scarring of various degrees but usually not severe enough to decrease vision significantly. Systemic complications include pharyngitis, otitis media, and pneumonia, which usually is mild in an otherwise healthy infant. Ocular complications of *S. aureus* neonatal conjunctivitis as well as conjunctivitis with other bacteria include corneal scarring and perforation with endophthalmitis and blindness. Systemic complications can include septicemia, meningitis, otitis media, and pneumonia.[98]

If HSV infection is present at birth, numerous organ systems may be involved, and the central nervous system sequelae can be devastating. Up to 50 per cent of infants with disseminated neonatal HSV infection die. Local ocular complications of HSV infection include corneal scarring, infectious retinitis, and optic atrophy.[101]

KERATITIS (CORNEAL INFECTIONS)

The cornea, with its overlying tear film, is the major refracting component of the human eye. Keratitis means "inflammation of the cornea." Any irregularity of its surface or opacity involving the central visual axis will impair vision, which is why keratitis is taken so seriously by ophthalmologists. An incorrect diagnosis, a delay in appropriate treatment, or an improper treatment regimen for corneal inflammation of any cause may have a permanent and devastating effect on vision.

The five layers of the cornea are the epithelium, Bowman's layer, stroma, Descemet membrane, and endothelium. The epithelium is several layers thick and when healthy can regenerate quickly and without scarring. Bowman's layer lies beneath the epithelium and actually is the uppermost part of the stroma, although it is made up of collagen fibers arranged more randomly. Bowman's layer does not regenerate and when injured will heal with a scar. The stroma is the largest part of the cornea, measuring approximately 0.5 mm in thickness. It is composed of regularly arranged collagen fibrils embedded in a matrix of muco- and glycoproteins. The arrangement of the fibrils is more regular in the posterior part of the stroma than in the anterior part. Like Bowman's layer, the stroma heals with scarring. Descemet's membrane is the basement layer of the endothelium. It can be replaced at least partially after an injury and does not opacify. The innermost layer, endothelium, actually is derived from neuroectoderm. It consists of a single layer of cells, which does not have significant regenerative capacity. When endothelial cells are damaged, they are not replaced; the number of endothelial cells continually decreases throughout life. The cornea is an avascular structure that is kept clear by virtue of the regular arrangement of collagen fibers in the stroma and by the pumping action of the endothelium, which keeps the stroma relatively dry. If the endothelium significantly is damaged or diseased, the cornea will opacify.

The external corneal surface is protected from foreign bodies by the cilia and by the reflex of tearing in response to mechanical irritation. The blink response to threat and the antimicrobial properties of various enzymes in the normal tear film further protect the cornea from injury and from infection.

The cornea can become inflamed and infected. Keratitis can be sterile, as when there is an inflammatory response to a retained foreign body, such as suture material, or it can be caused by infection. Most serious cases of keratitis are caused by infection.

The diagnosis of keratitis is based on the presence of a corneal epithelial and/or stromal infiltrate. There also usually is redness of the bulbar conjunctiva in the limbal area surrounding the edge of the cornea, with ocular pain and decreased vision. A corneal infiltrate ordinarily is a grayish-white lesion with indistinct borders. It may be extremely difficult to see in infants and young children due to the accompanying discomfort and photophobia, and sedation or general anesthesia may be needed for an adequate examination. Ideally, the patient will be examined at the slit lamp. Infants or very young or uncooperative children can be examined with a portable slit lamp, although the optical properties of such instruments are not optimal.

Because keratitis is a potentially blinding condition, immediate consultation with an ophthalmologist is recommended. Expertise with the slit-lamp examination and with maneuvers to obtain appropriate material for stains and cultures and extensive experience dealing with these unusual infections are required, and most ophthalmologists will refer patients to subspecialists when possible. A biopsy of the cornea may be needed to obtain culture material, and corneal transplantation occasionally is needed to halt the progression of a fungal lesion. Specific diagnosis is based on clinical presentation and examination of stains and cultures.[70] Treatment includes topical antibiotics and, occasionally, subconjunctival injections (Table 71–3). Systemic medication is required for gonococcal, chlamydial, and onchocercal disease and for bacterial infections in which the cornea is involved extensively or perforated or if the sclera has become infected. Systemic antibiotics are considered if there is actual or threatened perforation of the globe, a large area of involvement, extension of the infection to the sclera, or worsening on topical and/or periocular regimens alone. Adenoviral keratitis usually requires no treatment, but a short course of topical steroids may be beneficial if the patient is extremely uncomfortable or if vision is impaired significantly. HSV keratitis calls for topical medication, as do acanthamoebal and fungal infections. Topical steroids may be called for if the resulting inflammation threatens to destroy the mechanical integrity or the visual function of the cornea. Soft contact lenses, conjunctival covering grafts, or full-thickness corneal transplantation may be needed to enhance healing or to eliminate recalcitrant infections.

Epithelial Keratitis

Keratitis can be classified according to the layer of the cornea involved. Most infections involve either the epithelium or the stroma. The epithelial infections usually are caused by viruses: HSV, herpes zoster virus, adenovirus, or measles virus. The first three organisms have been discussed in a previous section. EBV can cause herpes-like corneal epithelial lesions, including dendrites, and also can cause stromal disease. These lesions do not respond to antiviral agents and are self-limited.[22]

When measles involves the cornea, it usually is in the context of transient epithelial infiltrates, which resolve without permanent sequelae. In malnourished children who also are vitamin A–deficient, however, measles represents not only a serious threat to life but a potentially blinding condition as well. Such children, usually younger than 6 years of age and living in impoverished circumstances in a developing country, may develop deep corneal ulcers during the first few days of measles; these ulcers may progress and deepen rapidly, culminating in corneal perforation and ultimately in loss of the eye. Whether these ulcers are due to the measles virus directly affecting the cornea, to the keratomalacia of the vitamin A deficiency, to secondary bacterial infection of a measles-induced lesion, or to some combination of these factors long has been debated. It is accepted, however, that malnourished children with measles often become blind and that both measles immunization schemes and vitamin A promotion programs can reduce significantly childhood blindness in developing countries. The complications of malnutrition represent the leading cause of blindness in children worldwide.

Stromal Keratitis

Viruses, syphilis, and some parasites will cause a nonsuppurative response, whereas bacteria and fungi typically cause a more rapid, dramatic, and suppurative inflammation. Congenital syphilis may cause an interstitial keratitis (stromal but no epithelial involvement) in childhood but usually not until late in the first decade of life at the earliest. This keratitis manifests as an indolent peripheral corneal haze that progresses centrally and can reduce vision significantly. The condition is bilateral in 80 per cent of the cases and is accompanied by iritis, iridocyclitis, or scleritis that may require topical steroids and cycloplegics. The systemic disease should be treated according to accepted guidelines.[11]

Bacterial Keratitis

Bacterial keratitis usually occurs after trauma that disrupts the normal integrity of the epithelium, with penetration of the stroma or even perforation of the full thickness of the cornea. *S. aureus, S. pneumoniae*, and *P. aeruginosa* are the most common bacterial causes of severe necrotizing keratitis. Other organisms have been implicated in less severe, more slowly progressive keratitis. This group includes *S. epidermidis, Actinomycetales*, the viridans group of streptococci, *Moraxella*, and *Bacteroides*.

Proper treatment requires accurate identification of the responsible agent. Obtaining a specimen from a corneal ulcer is done by scraping the edge of the lesion with a sterile platinum spatula. The best material is obtained from the part of the ulcer farthest from the limbus, under slit-lamp magnification, but it can be done at the bedside when necessary; sedation or general anesthesia may be required for infants or young children. Smears should be fixed in 70 per cent methanol, not by heat. A Gram stain for bacteria and an acridine orange stain (for fungi and *Acanthamoeba*) are recommended in all cases. An acid-fast stain is appropriate when mycobacteria are suspected. Material for cultures should be inoculated to fresh media. Useful media include blood and chocolate agar plates for aerobes and facultative anaerobes, Saboraud's agar (for fungi), and thioglycolate broth for anaerobic bacteria. A Thayer-Martin agar plate for *Neisseria* should be considered when that organism is a possibility. Initial treatment is based on the stain results (Table 71–3) and modified according to the cultures (Table 71–4).[70]

Fungal Keratitis

Fungal keratitis may occur after trauma from plant matter and usually involves *Candida, Aspergillus*, or *Fusarium*. Almost any fungus can infect a traumatized cornea, especially in an immunologically compromised patient or a patient who has been on topical or systemic steroids. Soft contact lens wearers are at increased risk. Fungal ulcers tend to be relatively indolent compared with bacterial ulcers. They typically are white with irregular and indistinct borders; satellite lesions may be evident. There commonly is a mild secondary iritis; severe iritis with hypopyon is possible but unusual in fungal corneal disease. An acridine orange stain is recommended, and a Saboraud agar plate for fungal culture is indicated. Treatment is based on the stain and culture results.

Protozoan Keratitis

Protozoan keratitis most commonly is caused by *Acanthamoeba*. This has been reported with increasing frequency

TABLE 71–3. Treatment of Keratitis Based on Smear Morphology

Organism	Antibiotic: Ocular	Antibiotic: Systemic[5]
Gram-positive cocci, gram-positive bacilli	Cefazolin[1]	Nafcillin IV
Gram-positive filaments	Amikacin[2]	Trimethoprim-sulfamethoxazole IV
Gram-negative cocci	Ceftriaxone[1] or ciprofloxacin[2, 4]	Ceftriaxone IV or IM
Gram-negative bacilli	Tobramycin[1]	Tobramycin IV
Acid-fast bacilli	Amikacin[2]	
Hyphal fragments	Natamycin,[2] fluconazole[3]	Fluconazole orally
Yeasts	Amphotericin B,[2] fluconazole[3]	Fluconazole orally
Cysts, trophozoites	Polyhexamethylene biguanide,[2] paromomycin,[2] propamidine isethionate[2]	Itraconazole orally

[1]Topical and periocular use only.
[2]Topical use only.
[3]Periocular use only.
[4]Use in children 12 years of age or older.
[5]Standard age-appropriate mg/kg dosages.
IM, intramuscularly; IV, intravenously.
From Jones, D. B., Matoba, A. Y., and Wilhelmus, K. R.: Problem solving in corneal and external diseases 1995, part II: Cornea and sclera. American Academy of Ophthalmology Annual Meeting, Course 626, 1995.

TABLE 71–4. Treatment Based on Identification of Organisms

Organism	Antibiotic: Ocular	Antibiotic: Systemic
Micrococcus, *Staphylococcus* (penicillin-resistant)	Cefazolin[1]	Nafcillin IV
Micrococcus, *Staphylococcus* (methicillin-resistant)	Vancomycin[1]	Vancomycin IV
Streptococcus	Penicillin G[1]	Penicillin G IV
Enterococcus	Vancomycin[1] and gentamicin[1]	Vancomycin IV and gentamicin IV
Anaerobic gram-positive coccus	Penicillin G[1]	Penicillin G IV
Corynebacterium species	Penicillin G[1]	Penicillin G IV
Mycobacterium fortuitum-chelonae	Amikacin[2]	Amikacin IV[1] or clarithromycin orally
Nocardia	Amikacin[2]	Trimethoprim-sulfamethoxazole IV
Neisseria gonorrhoeae	Ceftriaxone[1]	Ceftriaxone IV or IM
Pseudomonas species	Ceftazidime[1] ± tobramycin[1]	Ceftazidime IV or IM
Other aerobic, gram-negative bacilli	Ceftazidime[1] ± tobramycin[1]	Ceftazidime IV or IM
Filamentous fungi	Natamycin,[2] fluconazole[3]	Fluconazole orally
Candida species	Amphotericin B,[2] fluconazole[3]	Fluconazole orally
Acanthamoeba	Polyhexamethylene biguanide,[2] paromomycin,[2] and propamidine isethionate[2]	Itraconazole orally

[1]Topical and/or periocular use only.
[2]Topical use only.
[3]Periocular use only.
IM, intramuscularly; IV, intravenously.
From Jones, D. B., Matoba, A. Y., and Wilhelmus, K. R.: Problem solving in corneal and external diseases 1995, part II: Cornea and sclera. American Academy of Ophthalmology Annual Meeting, Course 626, 1995.

among soft contact lens wearers, especially those using homemade saline solutions. *Amoebida* are ubiquitous organisms present in soil, water, and air and have been identified in hot tubs and in the feces of domestic animals. People living in rural areas may be at special risk.

Acanthamoeba corneal ulcers are pleomorphic. Older lesions may exhibit a ring-like infiltrate around the central ulcer. Iritis or iridocyclitis may be intense, and severe pain is common. Corneal perforation may occur. Appropriate stains are acridine orange and calcafluor white. The organism may grow on blood or chocolate agar. Tandem scanning confocal microscopy of specimens may increase the accuracy of diagnosis. The optimal treatment has not been determined, but topical application of polyhexamethylene biguanide 0.02 per cent, chlorhexidine 0.02 per cent, paromomycin (10 mg/mL), or propamidine isethionate (Brolene) 0.1 per cent drops may be effective. Oral itraconazole (Sporanox) has been used in adults. Cycloplegic agents are recommended, and pain medications often are required. Corneal transplantation may be needed if the lesion progresses despite treatment or if the cornea perforates.[73, 79, 88, 92, 93, 113]

Onchocera volvulus is a filarial parasite that causes river blindness, or onchocerciasis. The disease is endemic in Sub-Saharan West Africa and in several areas in Central and South America. The organism is transmitted by the bite of a blackfly of the family *Simuliidae*. The fly bites an infected human and carries the larvae to another human host. There the larvae migrate to the subcutaneous tissue and pass through several molts to become adult worms. The worms encapsulate in nodules and produce the microfilariae that pass to the blood, skin, and other organs, including the eyes. The conjunctiva, cornea, aqueous, vitreous, retina, uveal tract, sclera, and optic nerve all may be infested. At least some of the blindness attributed to this organism is due to corneal opacification, although much of the severe vision loss is due to choroidal and retinal damage and to optic atrophy. At least some of this damage is due to the inflammatory response to the death of the microfilariae within the eye. Although children often are affected, blindness usually does not occur until the third or fourth decade of life.[141, 144]

The current treatment involves the distribution of ivermectin every 6 to 12 months to all individuals living within endemic areas. Ivermectin kills the microfilariae but not the adult worms, which may live 10 years or more. The drug does kill the microfilariae within the uterus of the adult female worm, however, and they will not reform in significant numbers for 6 months.[139]

INFECTIONS PRIMARILY INVOLVING THE UVEA (UVEITIS)

The uveal tract is the vascular middle coat of the eye. It is situated between the sclera and the retina, and its major function is to provide nourishment for the intraocular tissues, including the retina, the lens, and the cornea. The uveal tract is composed of the iris, the ciliary body, and the choroid.

Uveitis is a nonspecific term for inflammation of the uvea. If the inflammatory process primarily affects the iris, it is termed iritis. If the ciliary body primarily is involved, the process is termed cyclitis. If these two structures together are involved, it is termed iridocyclitis or anterior uveitis. The term intermediate uveitis (or pars planitis) applies to inflammation in the region of the ciliary body and peripheral retina with minimal anterior segment and moderate posterior vitreous inflammation. The term posterior uveitis usually applies to combined inflammation of the retina and choroid together and sometimes is called chorioretinitis. If the choroid alone is involved, it is termed choroiditis; inflammation of the retina alone is called retinitis. Vitreous inflammation is termed vitritis.

Inflammation can be defined as a series of local tissue reactions that take place at the site of injury. Although the causes of uveitis are diverse, they can be divided into two general classes: infectious and noninfectious. In this chapter, the infectious causes are discussed. The basic effect of inflammation is to induce vascular dilation, leakage of fluid into extravascular spaces, and migration of leukocytes and other cells into these spaces.

Inflammation primarily involving the anterior segment of the eye may result in pain, conjunctival hyperemia, photophobia, increased lacrimation, and decreased vision. These symptoms often bring the patient to the physician early in the course of the illness. Occasionally, however, the pain may be minimal, the external appearance of the eye is normal, and compromised vision is not discernible to the patient. However, anterior uveitis typically causes hyperemia of the globe. With biomicroscopy (the slit-lamp examination), the hallmark of anterior segment uveitis is the finding of hazy, proteinaceous aqueous humor, termed flare, and the presence of cells in the aqueous humor, which typically are clumps of leukocytes. Both cells and flare generally are graded on a 1 to 4+ scale. The cells can aggregate on the back of the cornea to create fine, medium, and large precipitates known as keratic precipitates. With chronic inflammation, the pupil border often adheres to the anterior surface of the lens. Such adhesions are called posterior synechiae and may cause the pupil to have an irregular shape and size and poor reactivity to light. Chronic or recurrent anterior segment inflammation may lead to cataract formation. Rarely, iris nodules also develop in long-standing inflammation. Cells may spill over into the anterior vitreous, with severe anterior uveitis. The inflammatory effect on the ciliary body generally hinders aqueous humor production and thereby reduces intraocular pressure. However, cellular debris can occlude the aqueous humor outflow channels (trabecular meshwork) and lead to elevated intraocular pressure.

Inflammation primarily involving the posterior segment of the eye often leads to decreased vision, which may be the presenting symptom. Pain may be minimal or absent. Inflammatory lesions of the retina and choroid also may lead to cellular debris in the vitreous, causing the patient to perceive "floaters." The borders of the retinal or choroidal inflammatory focus often are indistinct and cream-colored. In their healing phase, the borders of these lesions increasingly become distinct, and a defined, partially pigmented scar will remain. Inflammatory perivascular sheathing of the retinal vessels may occur. The optic nerve may exhibit an inflammatory response; if the optic disc is so involved, this response is termed papillitis. Inflammatory debris in the vitreous also may be noted.[3, 89, 107, 154]

Viral Uveitis

Herpes Simplex Virus

Most of the uveal inflammation associated with HSV (typically iridocyclitis) is secondary to the corneal disease. On occasion, iritis may occur without noticeable corneal involvement. The iritis may require treatment with topical steroids and a "cover" of topical antivirals to prevent corneal epithelial disease.[22]

Varicella-Zoster Virus

Rarely, varicella (chickenpox) may be associated with a transient iritis that requires no treatment.

Herpes zoster may cause an iridocyclitis during the acute stage of the disease and may recur long after the cutaneous component of the condition has passed. Herpes zoster always should be considered in the differential diagnosis of chronic unilateral iridocyclitis. Topical steroids are indicated for iritis, with the addition of oral or intravenous acyclovir for severe cases. Segmental iris atrophy is a characteristic sequela of herpes zoster uveitis. Glaucoma, hyphema, retinitis, vasculitis, and extraocular muscle palsies occasionally may occur in herpes zoster ophthalmicus.[110]

VZV and HSV-2 both have been implicated as primary causes of the acute retinal necrosis syndrome. Patients diagnosed with this syndrome range from 13 to 71 years of age, with an average age of 43 years. This syndrome typically occurs in healthy patients. The virus causes a triad of an acute vitritis, retinal vasculitis, and a peripheral necrotizing retinitis and is bilateral in 33 per cent of the patients. The treatment is intravenous acyclovir. Prophylactic laser photocoagulation may prevent retinal detachment. The visual prognosis is guarded.[13, 82]

Epstein-Barr Virus

Ocular involvement with EBV has been reported primarily in patients with infectious mononucleosis. A follicular conjunctivitis may be noted in 2 to 40 per cent of patients. Corneal stromal inflammation, iritis, episcleritis, optic neuritis, and chorioretinitis occur less commonly. Systemic corticosteroids and acyclovir may be useful in cases of sight-threatening complications of chronic intraocular inflammation secondary to EBV.[94]

Enteroviruses

Coxsackievirus A24 and enterovirus 70 may cause a painful follicular conjunctivitis termed acute hemorrhagic conjunctivitis. Rarely, chorioretinitis may be noted. The treatment for these infections primarily is supportive.

Rubella Virus

Rubella virus can cause both acquired and congenital infections. Ocular manifestations of acquired rubella include conjunctivitis in 70 per cent of patients, superficial keratitis, and iritis. Rarely, retinitis has been noted.

Congenital rubella syndrome may present with cataracts, glaucoma, iritis, microphthalmia, and retinitis. Cataracts occur in 15 per cent of the patients and glaucoma in 10 per cent. Retinal examination reveals a "salt and pepper fundus" because of the alternating hypopigmented and hyperpigmented changes of the retinal pigment epithelium. The visual prognosis for patients with retinitis alone usually is good, with vision between 20/20 and 20/40. Glaucoma secondary to rubella commonly requires surgery, as do the cataracts.[14]

Mumps Virus

The ocular involvement with mumps includes dacryoadenitis, conjunctivitis, iritis, optic neuritis, and keratitis. Retinitis also has been noted. Prognosis for visual recovery from the retinitis is good.[36]

Measles Virus

The measles virus can cause congenital and acquired infections. In congenital infections, a "salt and pepper" retinopathy and cataract formation may occur, similar to that found in rubella. Ocular manifestations in acquired measles are conjunctivitis and, rarely, retinitis, retinal vasculitis, and optic nerve edema.[9]

Subacute Sclerosing Panencephalitis

Thirty to 75 per cent of patients with subacute sclerosing panencephalitis (Dawson encephalitis) have ocular findings. Optic nerve edema, inflammation, and subsequent optic atrophy have been noted. Retinitis in the macula with overlying vitreous cells is a common finding. The visual prognosis of survivors is poor.[103]

Creutzfeldt-Jakob Disease

The most common ocular manifestation of Creutzfeldt-Jakob disease is cortical blindness. Optic atrophy may occur secondary to degeneration of the neurons of the optic nerve.

HIV and AIDS

Ocular findings are present in 75 per cent of patients with AIDS. Cotton wool spots occur in more than 50 per cent of the patients and are bilateral in more than 80 per cent. Cotton wool patches represent focal infarctions of the neural layer of the retina and are the most common ocular finding in AIDS patients. They generally produce no symptoms and do not decrease vision. These spots are white and fluffy and present most commonly in the macular portion of the retina. They resolve in 4 to 6 weeks with no residual scars. Occasionally, flame-shaped hemorrhages are present as well. The retina in these patients also may become infected with CMV, VZV, syphilis, tuberculosis, ocular histoplasmosis, *Candida*, toxoplasmosis, and pneumocystis.[67]

Cytomegalovirus

CMV infections may occur in preterm neonates and immunosuppressed patients, especially patients with AIDS. Approximately 30 per cent of patients with AIDS develop CMV retinitis. Patients with CMV retinitis have no external ocular signs but may complain of vision loss. Retinal lesions of CMV are white and granular (resembling the classic description of cottage cheese) and often are associated with hemorrhage. These lesions almost always occur in the macular area and lead to vision loss. The retina becomes necrotic and eventually will atrophy, leaving a permanent scar. CMV optic neuritis also may develop. Development of CMV retinitis in an AIDS patient is a poor prognostic sign, and many patients die within months of the onset of the retinal disease. Treatment consists of intravenous or intravitreal ganciclovir or intravenous foscarnet.[29]

Bacterial Uveitis

Syphilis (Treponema Pallidum)

Syphilis is one of the great masqueraders in medicine and always must be considered as a possible etiology in all cases of uveitis. Syphilitic infections may occur congenitally or be acquired.[4] Any patient with syphilitic uveitis should have a lumbar puncture to rule out asymptomatic neurosyphilis.

Acute interstitial keratitis (stromal corneal inflammation) may occur in late congenital syphilis, between 5 and 25 years of age. It is believed to be an allergic response to the treponemal antigen in the cornea. Acutely, patients present with pain and photophobia and manifest a diffusely opaque cornea and an anterior uveitis. Gradually, the inflammation subsides and the cornea partially will clear, but deep ghost (nonperfused) corneal stromal vessels and opacities will remain. Glaucoma may occur. Congenital syphilis also may cause a retinitis that leads to "salt and pepper" fundus appearance.

Patients with secondary syphilis may develop an episcleritis, scleritis, acute chronic or recurrent iridocyclitis, iris capillary dilatation (iris roseata), vascular papules of the iris (iris papulosa), and inflammatory nodules (iris nodosa). Choroiditis, chorioretinitis, and retinal vasculitis have been noted, as well as optic neuritis and subsequent atrophy.

Tertiary syphilis may have associated gumma of the iris and an Argyll Robertson pupil (very miotic pupils with light near dissociation). Intraocular inflammation is uncommon at this stage.

Ocular inflammation secondary to syphilis should be considered and treated as neurosyphilis because the eye and the optic nerve are extensions of the brain. With the appropriate doses of penicillin G, the inflammation typically resolves rapidly. Topical regional steroids sometimes are required to control inflammation.[90]

Lyme Disease (Borrelia Burgdorferi)

A mild follicular conjunctivitis may occur in patients with stage 1 disease. During the second and third stages, neuro-ophthalmic manifestations may be noted, including cranial neuropathy, optic neuritis, bilateral keratitis, bilateral iridocyclitis, diffuse choroiditis, vasculitis, intermediate uveitis, and Parinaud oculoglandular syndrome. Oral tetracycline or doxycycline is the treatment of choice in adults and penicillin V or amoxicillin in children. Antibiotic treatment early in the course of the disease carries a better prognosis than therapy initiated at later stages.[11]

Leptospirosis

Leptospirosis may cause an anterior uveitis that occurs months after the acute infection.

Tuberculosis

Any structure of the eye may be affected by tuberculosis. Both allergic and infectious processes have been implicated as important causes of tuberculous uveitis. An anterior uveitis with or without keratitis has been ascribed to tuberculosis. Choroiditis, optic neuritis, and orbital infections have been noted in miliary tuberculosis. Treatment should be undertaken with the appropriate antituberculous medications; corticosteroids often are necessary in conjunction with the antimicrobial therapy.

Leprosy (Mycobacterium Leprae)

Because *Mycobacterium leprae* grows best at lower temperatures, corneal infections predominate. Corneal infection is associated with the prominence of corneal nerves, interstitial keratitis, and corneal anesthesia. Secondary spread to the iris and ciliary body may lead to an anterior uveitis.

Brucella *Infection*

Ocular manifestations are rare but include an iritis, choroiditis, and panophthalmitis.[107]

Fungal Uveitis

Histoplasmosis

The diagnosis of the presumed ocular histoplasmosis syndrome is based on the clinical picture of disseminated retinal "histo spots," atrophic retinal changes around the optic nerve, and a clear vitreous. Later in the course of the disease, subretinal hemorrhages and retinal detachment are possible. Ocular histoplasmosis often is bilateral and can result in legal blindness from the loss of macular vision. Presumed ocular histoplasmosis syndrome may occur after benign systemic histoplasmosis during childhood. Active inflammation and vitreous cells are not seen in this syndrome. The hallmark "histo spots" appear as white, punched-out, well-demarcated chorioretinal scars representing healed fungal lesions. They usually first appear during adolescence, typically do not reduce vision, and do not require treatment. Macular disease, which severely may reduce vision, does not develop until after the second decade of life. Subretinal neovascularization may develop at the site of a macular histoplasmosis spot, with fluid, blood, and lipid accumulating in the subretinal space. This process, plus local scarring, can result in a marked reduction in central vision. Macular neovascularization may be treated suitably with laser photocoagulation. Antifungal drugs do not play a role in the treatment of the presumed ocular histoplasmosis syndrome.[121]

Candidiasis

Candida species, including *C. albicans*, are fungi with both yeast and filamentous forms. Candidiasis is encountered in immunocompromised patients and in situations involving indwelling catheters, intravenous therapy, chronic antibiotic use, poorly controlled diabetes, and intravenous drug abuse.

In the eye, *Candida* infection usually begins in the choroid and eventually causes multifocal white chorioretinal lesions. As the fungus proliferates, it may break through the retina into the vitreous, producing the classic white snowball-like "fungus ball."

Intravenous amphotericin B is the drug of choice. Other antifungal agents, such as fluconazole, flucytosine, and miconazole, also may be effective, but none dramatically so. The surgical treatment of intraocular *Candida* disease is discussed in the section on endophthalmitis.

Coccidioidomycosis

Coccidioides species have yeast and filamentous forms. Ocular disease consists of a multifocal chorioretinitis that develops during the course of systemic coccidioidomycosis. The lesions initially appear similar to those seen in histoplasmosis; in severe cases, endophthalmitis results, and vitrectomy may be necessary. In less severe cases, the lesions may respond to intravenous amphotericin B.

Cryptococcosis

Cryptococcus neoformans is a yeast-like fungus that can cause a multifocal chorioretinitis and endophthalmitis. Most patients with cryptococcosis are severely immunocompromised; many have AIDS. The central nervous system and eye commonly are involved, and elevated intracranial pressure may cause papilledema and sixth nerve palsies. Intravenous amphotericin B is the treatment of choice.[74]

Helminthic Uveitis

Toxocariasis

Toxocara canis causes visceral larval migrans, which is not associated with ocular disease. Ocular toxocariasis has three classical clinical presentations, almost always involving one eye only. One form occurs in children 2 to 9 years of age and causes an indolent endophthalmitis and leukocoria (white pupil). A tractional retinal detachment may occur. The eye typically shows little or no external evidence of inflammation, and there is no pain.

A second form appears in children between 4 and 14 years of age. These patients present with reduced vision but little or no external inflammation and no pain. The reduced vision may cause strabismus, which may be the first sign. There is an inflammatory granuloma in the macula.

The third form of ocular toxocariasis occurs in patients between 4 and 6 years of age but may not be recognized until much later. The patients have good vision, but a peripheral retinal granuloma is seen on routine eye examination. Vision may be affected if a traction band from the granuloma distorts the macula.

Inactive *Toxocara* granulomas do not respond to medication. When active intraocular inflammation is present and is sufficient to represent a further threat to vision, periocular or systemic steroids may be necessary. Anthelminthic agents do not play a role in the treatment of ocular toxocariasis because it is the death of the larva that incites the inflammation and granuloma formation. Vitrectomy may be helpful if there is significant traction on the retina. The visual prognosis is poor if the macula is involved.[124, 129, 149]

Onchocerciasis

Onchocerciasis often causes a severe choroiditis with an overlying retinitis. The various ocular manifestations of infestation with *O. volvulus* are discussed in the section on keratitis.

Loiasis

The loa loa worm can migrate through the tissues of the eye and cause conjunctivitis, iridocyclitis, vitritis, and chorioretinitis. Vascular obstruction also may occur, with intraretinal hemorrhage and retinal exudation. Medical treatment with diethylcarbamazine can kill both the adult worms and the microfilariae. The adult also can be removed from the eye surgically.

Cysticercosis

Cysticercosis is caused by the tapeworm *Taenia solium*. When the larva gains access to the eye, cysts form in the vitreous or subretinal space in 13 to 46 per cent of patients. The living worm may be seen undulating in these spaces. With death of the organism, severe panuveitis can occur. Orbital and subconjunctival involvement is less common.

Surgical removal of the intraocular cysts may prevent the severe inflammation that occurs with the death of the worm. Praziquantel can kill the organism, but the ensuing increase in inflammation may be dramatic.

Uveitis Caused by Insect-Induced Disease

Ophthalmomyiasis is the ocular disorder caused by infestation with fly larvae, most commonly the larval form of the sheep botfly, *Oestrus ovis*. Maggots may be seen in the conjunctival fornix (cul-de-sac) or in the inside of the eye. Internal ophthalmomyiasis can present with a motile larva in the anterior chamber, vitreous, or subretinal space. The maggot may leave behind trails ("railroad tracks") throughout the retina. There may be a mild inflammatory response in the anterior chamber (iritis, iridocyclitis) or vitreous.

The treatment is surgical removal of the larva; corticosteroids may be used to treat the accompanying intraocular inflammation.[30]

INFECTIONS PRIMARILY INVOLVING THE RETINA

TORCHS

The TORCHS complex is a group of congenital and perinatal infections that can cause severe systemic and ophthalmic abnormalities. The effect of TORCHS—*Toxoplasma*, rubella, CMV, HSV, varicella virus, and syphilis—may be evident at birth or manifest later in childhood or adulthood. Diagnosis can not be made always on clinical grounds alone, and neonatal and maternal serologic testing may be needed to confirm the clinical suspicion.[154]

Toxoplasmosis

Toxoplasma gondii is an obligate intracellular parasite that has an affinity for the central nervous system and the retina. Humans become infected by ingestion of undercooked meat with oocysts or tissue cysts of the toxoplasma or by exposure to feces of infected cats, the definitive host. In adults, primary infection with *T. gondii* usually is asymptomatic. However, pregnant women with primary toxoplasma infection can transmit the parasite transplacentally. In the United States, the incidence of congenital toxoplasmosis infection has been reported to be between 1 in 1000 to 1 in 10,000 births.[6, 25]

Ocular involvement occurs in disseminated, asymptomatic, or subclinical disease. Chorioretinitis is the most common sequela of congenital toxoplasmosis, but most infected newborns are asymptomatic. *T. gondii* causes a focal necrotizing retinitis infiltrated with T-cell lymphocytes, with a secondary choroiditis and vitritis. After the inflammation has resolved, a flat, pigmented chorioretinal scar is seen. In a prospective study, 15 per cent of infected newborns had chorioretinal scars, indicating infection in utero, 4 per cent had active chorioretinitis, and 10 per cent developed retinal lesions by 1 to 2 years of age. Long-term follow-up studies have found that between 82 and 85 per cent of children with subclinical *Toxoplasma* infection developed chorioretinal lesions, some with severe visual loss. Visual loss depends on the location of the retinal lesion: peripheral lesions result in little or no visual disturbance, and macular lesions can produce profound visual loss. In one series, 46 per cent of patients with congenital toxoplasmosis had macular involvement. Ocular toxoplasmosis in adults often is reactivation of a congenital infection and can be seen as a satellite lesion next to the border of a chorioretinal scar.[35, 46, 60, 118]

Microphthalmia has been reported as a rare association with congenital *Toxoplasma* infection. Individuals with macular involvement may have strabismus and nystagmus as results of poor visual acuity. Systemic associations with congenital toxoplasmosis include hydrocephalus, intracranial calcifications, mental retardation, and deafness.[151] Symptomatic neonates with disseminated disease have hepatosplenomegaly, lymphadenopathy, jaundice, fever, anemia, pneumonitis, and a poor prognosis. In the neonate, the differential diagnosis for the inactive scar includes CMV and herpes-virus infections. Active chorioretinitis can suggest Coat disease, retinoblastoma, tuberculosis, and syphilis. Diagnosis is confirmed by identification of IgM antibody specific for toxoplasmosis in the newborn's serum because IgM cannot transfer transplacentally. Treatment for active ocular toxoplasmosis includes pyrimethamine, sulfadiazine, and leucovorin. Infants with asymptomatic toxoplasmosis should have regular ophthalmologic examinations because retinal involvement can occur later in childhood or adulthood.[17, 33, 76]

Rubella

The rubella virion is an RNA virus of the family *Togaviridae* that causes a febrile exanthem. Prior to the advent of the rubella vaccine in 1969, rubella or "German measles" epidemics occurred every 6 to 9 years. With immunization programs of preschool children, most cases reported now occur in individuals between 15 and 24 years of age. Transmission is by instillation of the virus in the nasopharynx. Susceptibility of nonimmunized women of child-bearing age ranges from 10 to 25 per cent. Fetal infection occurs via transplacental transmission of the virus from the mother. The likelihood of transmission from mother to fetus is highest in the first trimester. In a series of 125 congenital rubella patients, the median gestational age at the time of maternal infection was 8 weeks. Rates of infection decreased with gestational age: at 8 weeks, the infection rate was 50 per cent, and at 16 weeks, the rate was 10 per cent.[119]

Pigmentary retinopathy, or "salt and pepper" retinopathy, is the most common ophthalmic complication in the congenital rubella syndrome. Mottling with black irregular clumps of pigment most frequently is observed in the posterior pole; the optic nerve and vessels usually are normal unless there is associated glaucoma. Subretinal neovascularization and macular scarring have been reported. Retinal involvement usually is bilateral.[108]

Nuclear cataracts, affecting between 15 to 27 per cent of patients, are the second most frequent ocular complication. Glaucoma is seen in about 10 per cent of eyes; the combination of cataracts and glaucoma is uncommon. Microphthalmia, which occurs in 10 to 63 per cent of affected individuals, is associated with cataracts and glaucoma. Iris atrophy and iritis have been reported as rare complications.[14]

The classic congenital rubella syndrome is characterized by cardiac defects, ocular abnormalities, and hearing deficits. The incidence of ocular and cardiac defects is higher with exposure early in the first trimester; hearing deficits appear associated with exposure late in the first trimester. Givens and associates[41] reported that 88 per cent had multiorgan involvement.

Although "salt and pepper" retinopathy does not necessitate treatment, its complications of subretinal neovascularization may require laser or subfoveal surgery. Visual rehabilitation is dependent upon early cataract extraction to prevent deprivation amblyopia, correction of the aphakia with spectacles or contact lenses, and careful follow-up. Glaucoma in infants and children can be temporized with topical medications, but definitive treatment to control the intraocular pressure is surgery.

Congenital rubella has long-term consequences for all organs involved. Nearly two-thirds of infants with no manifestations at birth develop subsequent hearing loss or psychomotor deficits. From the ocular standpoint, individuals with congenital rubella need regular ophthalmologic follow-up care.[41]

Cytomegalovirus

CMV is an enveloped DNA virus of the family *Herpesviridae*. It is estimated that 80 per cent of adults have been infected by 40 years of age. In immunocompetent adults, infection is asymptomatic or can cause a mononucleosis syndrome. Individuals can shed virus in saliva, urine, and other body fluids for months to years after acute infection. Transmission is via exposure to body fluids, via transplanted organs, or in utero.

Congenital CMV can result from exposure to the virus in utero or in the birth canal. Infection occurs in 0.5 to 25 per cent of all live births. Maternal infection may be primary or recurrent, but primary infection is a greater risk factor for symptomatic CMV in the newborn. Only 5 per cent of infants with congenital CMV infection are symptomatic and have cytomegalic inclusion disease. Blood transfusions from CMV antibody–positive donors also can result in severe CMV infections in the newborn.

CMV preferentially affects the reticuloendothelial system and the central nervous system. Infected tissues have giant cells with intranuclear and intracytoplasmic viral inclusions. Newborns with cytomegalic inclusion disease have hepatomegaly, splenomegaly, jaundice, petechiae, respiratory difficulties, and intracranial calcifications. Deafness, motor and behavior disabilities, mental retardation, microcephaly, and seizures also can occur. Some manifestations develop later in childhood.

In symptomatic, congenital CMV infection, the retina is the primary site of ocular involvement. Cytomegalic inclusion bodies are seen in all layers of the retina. Patchy white areas of necrotic retina with hemorrhage and vascular sheathing are seen in the peripheral retina, although the posterior pole can be affected as well. Resolution of the retinitis results in an atrophic scar with occasional areas of hyperpigmentation. If the area of involvement is in the periphery, vision may be normal. However, vision may be poor if the posterior pole is affected or if optic atrophy or retinal detachment occurs. CMV retinopathy develops in 5 to 30 per cent of infants with clinically apparent disease. Microphthalmia, optic nerve hypoplasia, optic nerve colobomas, anophthalmia, and anterior segment dysgenesis have been reported in association with congenital CMV infection.[61]

The diagnosis of CMV retinitis is based on the clinical appearance and the constellation of systemic signs and symptoms. Serologic testing and urine cultures may be necessary because many of the multiorgan manifestations of CMV are similar to those of other congenital infections. Complement fixation can identify IgM antibodies to CMV and does not cross-react with other herpesviruses. Immunofluorescence techniques are more sensitive but less specific than complement fixation.[84]

Treatment of neonatal or pediatric CMV retinitis is based on the results of treatment of adults with CMV retinitis. Ganciclovir has been shown to stabilize and prevent the spread of the disease in infants. However, the drug is virustatic and not virucidal, and maintenance therapy is required. Granulocytopenia and thrombocytopenia can result. Retinal detachment requires vitrectomy, membrane peel, and silicone oil to tamponade the detached retina.[62]

Herpes Simplex Virus

HSV is an enveloped DNA virus. Both subtypes, HSV-1 and HSV-2, cause a vesicular skin eruption. HSV-1 typically is isolated from oral-facial infections; HSV-2 usually is isolated from genital infections. After primary infection, HSV can maintain latency in neuronal ganglion cells and reactivate. Transmission is by exposure to infected body fluids, such as saliva, and the risk of transmission is higher when the individual is symptomatic.[101]

Maternal-fetal transmission is via infected genital secretions in the birth canal (HSV-2) or exposure to infected individuals with oral-facial herpetic disease (HSV-1) in the postnatal period. In active genital disease, the risk of transmission to the neonate with vaginal delivery is 50 per cent. Most series report that between 70 and 80 per cent of neonatal HSV infection is caused by HSV-2. Although less than 1 per cent of immunocompetent adults with HSV infection develop ocular sequelae, 17 to 40 per cent of affected neonates have ocular disease.[94, 133]

In acute HSV neonatal infection, conjunctivitis is the most frequent manifestation. Unlike adult HSV conjunctivitis, follicles are absent until 4 to 6 weeks of age. Diffuse epithelial keratitis, geographic ulceration, or alinear dendritic lesions are the next most frequent manifestations. Ocular involvement can be unilateral or bilateral. Conjunctivitis, keratitis, and occasionally retinitis will manifest 2 to 14 days after birth. Keratitis may resolve and leave corneal scarring or can reactivate as recurrent herpetic keratitis. HSV retinitis causes punctate, white-yellow lesions in the periphery and the posterior pole accompanied by choroiditis, vascular sheathing, hemorrhage, and vitritis. Chorioretinal atrophic scars with variable amounts of pigmentation around the border result after resolution of acute infection.

Azazi and colleagues[5] examined individuals with serologically proven HSV infection 1 to 15 years after neonatal exposure and found a higher prevalence of chorioretinal scars than in previous reports: 28 per cent compared with 4 per cent. This may suggest that HSV remains dormant in the retina and reactivates later in childhood or adulthood. Chorioretinitis, cataracts, optic atrophy, and microphthalmia have been reported.[47] Acute retinal necrosis from reactivation of HSV-2 also has occurred.[140]

Ocular HSV infection can be seen in conjunction with a vesicular skin rash or with disseminated disease. Disseminated disease causes encephalitis, seizures, esophagitis, pharyngitis, rhinitis, pneumonitis, hepatitis, thrombocytopenia, lymphadenopathy, necrotizing enteritis, adrenal necrosis, glomerulonephritis, and microcephaly. The differential diagnosis for the ophthalmic complications of HSV consists of TORCHS. Identification of neonatal IgM antibody to HSV confirms the diagnosis of in utero infection.[5]

Acyclovir is the drug of choice to treat neonatal HSV infection. Conjunctival and corneal disease also can be treated with débridement and topical antivirals, such as vidarabine. Topical steroids should be used only if the corneal epithelium is intact. In neonatal HSV infection, systemic acyclovir should be given, regardless of topical treatment. Early diagnosis and treatment can reduce ocular morbidity. Cesarean delivery of mothers with active genital herpes also is indicated to prevent the systemic and ocular complications of neonatal HSV infection.

Varicella-Zoster Virus

VZV is a DNA virus of the family *Herpesviridae*; enveloped virions are the infectious agents. Primary infection results in chickenpox, a highly communicable, febrile illness with a vesicular rash that appears after 48 to 72 hours of incubation. VZV can remain dormant in sensory ganglion neurons and reactivate as herpes zoster, a painful rash in the dermatomal distribution of the sensory ganglion.

Congenital varicella syndrome is considered a rare entity. One prospective series reported a 24 per cent incidence of congenital varicella with serologic or clinical confirmation of maternal infection during pregnancy. Mortality rates can be high if maternal infection develops from 5 days before delivery to 2 days after delivery. Systemic complications of VZV infection include cranial nerve palsies, hemiparesis, cicatricial skin lesions, developmental delay, seizures, neurogenic bladder, and learning difficulties.[110]

Ocular abnormalities in congenital VZV infection include chorioretinitis, cataract, Horner syndrome, optic nerve hypoplasia, retinal coloboma, and microphthalmia. The chorioretinal scars of VZV infection have either a deeply pigmented center with depigmented borders or a gliotic white center with hyperpigmented edges. Lambert and colleagues[78] reported optic nerve atrophy attributed to nerve fiber loss. The neurotropic nature of VZV infection may explain the association of Horner syndrome. Ocular involvement can be unilateral or bilateral. VZV chorioretinitis affects the macula, periphery, or both. Although VZV is a causative agent of acute retinal necrosis, active retinitis in congenital varicella has not been reported.

As with other disease entities with chorioretinal scars, cataract, and microphthalmia, the differential diagnosis encompasses TORCHS. Serologic testing for IgG and IgM antibodies to VZV, history of maternal infection during pregnancy, and the constellation of systemic findings help make the diagnosis. Because active infection may be early in the pregnancy, the neonate may have IgG but no detectable IgM antibodies to VZV by the time of delivery. The persistence of elevated IgG antibodies beyond 6 months of age, when passive immunity via maternal antibodies has waned without evidence of primary VZV infection postnatally, is a helpful indication of infection in utero.

Syphilis

Syphilis is caused by the spirochete *T. pallidum*. The incidence of congenital and acquired syphilis has increased in the United States since 1986. In acquired syphilis, there are three stages of infection. Primary infection is characterized by painless, indurated chancres of the skin or mucous membranes at the site of inoculation. The secondary stage appears as a maculopapular rash, classically involving the palms and soles. Generalized lymphadenopathy, fever, malaise, sore throat, headache, and arthralgias can accompany the rash. Hypertrophic lesions (condyloma lata) occur in moist mucous membranes. The tertiary stage occurs after a variable latent period that may have occasional recurrences of secondary syphilis. Neurologic deficits, aortitis, and gumma of the skin, bone, or viscera typify tertiary syphilis.[3]

Transmission to the fetus can occur with maternal syphilis in any stage of the disease. Forty per cent of pregnancies with early untreated syphilis in the mother result in spontaneous abortion, stillbirth, or perinatal death. Rates of maternal-fetal transmission can be nearly 100 per cent in the secondary stage, although the frequency drops if maternal infection is of more than 2 years' duration. Congenital infection may occur, despite treatment of the mother. Treatment failures result from treatment late in the pregnancy, use of an antibiotic other than penicillin, or inadequate treatment with penicillin.[136]

Pigmentary retinopathy is the most common ocular manifestation of congenital syphilis. The diffuse mottling in the periphery, "salt and pepper retinopathy," is indicative of chorioretinitis in utero. Pigment clumping in the periphery usually has no effect on vision; macular involvement can cause decreased vision. Retinal changes can appear later in adulthood, suggesting that inflammatory changes can happen after birth in congenital infection. Salt and pepper retinopathy is evidence of previous inflammation, and no treatment is required.

Interstitial keratitis is the hallmark of congenital syphilis and is discussed in the section on corneal infections.

Congenital syphilis may be asymptomatic in the first weeks of life. Few infants have the classic stigmata of congenital syphilis: saddle-nose deformities, "snuffles," and shiny-red palms and soles. Neonates may have failure to thrive, prematurity, hepatosplenomegaly, thrombocytopenia, and nonspecific rash. Characteristic x-ray findings of osteochondritis and periostitis can help make the diagnosis. Deafness and dental anomalies are late manifestations. The ocular abnormalities can be seen with or without systemic findings.

Diagnosis of congenital infection is made by testing the serum by nontreponemal and treponemal methods. Nontreponemal tests (Veneral Disease Research Laboratory [VDRL] and rapid plasma reagin [RPR] tests) measure antibody against the lipoidal antigen of *T. pallidum*. Quantitative VDRL tests or RPR tests can be followed to determine response to treatment. Treponemal tests (microhemagglutination for *T. pallidum* and fluorescent treponemal antibody absorption test) are indicative of infection but remain positive, despite adequate treatment. All pregnant women should have syphilis serologies checked during pregnancy and at delivery. Neonates with mothers who are positive by nontreponemal and treponemal testing need to be evaluated for syphilis. The American Academy of Pediatrics recommends physical examination, quantitative nontreponemal serologic testing, cerebrospinal fluid VDRL test, long-bone roentgenograms, and antitreponemal IgM testing, as specified by the Centers for Disease Control and Prevention. Treatment is with penicillin G, intravenously, for 10 to 14 days.[4, 90]

ENDOPHTHALMITIS

Endophthalmitis means "inflammation inside the eyeball" and in ordinary usage means that the entirety of the internal structure is involved. Infectious endophthalmitis may be endogenous, as may occur with septicemia due to various organisms, or it may be exogenous (posttraumatic), including both accidental and surgical traumatic causes.[119, 130]

Endogenous (metastatic) endophthalmitis should be suspected whenever ocular inflammation occurs in a septicemic patient. Clinical signs may include orbital and/or periocular inflammation, decreased vision, proptosis, decreased ocular motility, hazy ocular media, and purulent material in the anterior chamber or in the vitreous compartment. It may be difficult to distinguish such a situation from the much more common periorbital cellulitis or even orbital cellulitis. The patient may or may not complain of ocular discomfort. Any ocular signs and/or symptoms in a septicemic patient should be taken seriously, and appropriate ophthalmic consultation should be requested promptly. Any significant delay in recognition and treatment of endophthalmitis can result in permanent vision loss. Possible etiologic agents in endogenous cases include *H. influenzae, C. albicans, Coccidia* species, *Listeria monocytogenes, Klebsiella, E. coli, S. aureus*, and *S. pneumoniae*.[44, 91, 86]

The physician especially should be alert to the possibility of endogenous endophthalmitis if the immune system is compromised and/or if the patient has an underlying systemic illness, such as diabetes or leukemia.[15, 100, 104]

In posttraumatic or postsurgical exogenous endophthalmitis, the condition ordinarily is diagnosed in a much more timely manner because the ophthalmologist automatically will be looking for this complication. Nonophthalmologists should be aware that apparently minor accidental ocular trauma actually may involve an easily overlooked perforation with or without a retained foreign body. This especially is true in the pediatric setting, in which children are unable or unwilling to provide an accurate history of the event. The likelihood of posttraumatic endophthalmitis increases directly with the extent of the injury and the degree of intraocular contamination. The most common infectious agents involved are *S. epidermidis, Bacillus* species, *Streptococcus* species, *S. aureus,* and various fungi. *Bacillus cereus* is isolated in 30 to 40 per cent of cases and can cause severe ocular morbidity.[2, 26, 27, 56]

Postoperative endophthalmitis is a potentially disastrous but rare complication of ocular surgery, including cataract and glaucoma procedures. Extraocular surgery, such as strabismus surgery and scleral buckling procedures, also rarely can be complicated by endophthalmitis. After every ocular surgical procedure, the condition specifically is sought during the first 48 to 72 postoperative hours.

Clinical evidence of postoperative intraocular infection includes redness and swelling of the eyelids, ocular pain, decreased vision, and hazy ocular media. Intraocular infection after penetrating/perforating ocular trauma will present with similar signs and symptoms. With intraocular foreign bodies, the site of perforation may be quite small and easily can be overlooked. Also, a child may be unwilling to admit that he or she has been engaging in behavior that might lead to a significant ocular injury, and the history may be unreliable. When evidence of any ocular injury is present, the vision is decreased inexplicably, and/or the ocular media are hazy, the patient must be considered as having endophthalmitis until proven otherwise.[112]

An adequate work-up includes a meticulous ocular examination by a qualified ophthalmologist. Radiographic studies may be necessary to rule out a retained intraocular foreign body. An anterior chamber and/or vitreous tap in the operating room under anesthesia usually is required to obtain appropriate material for stains and cultures. Based on the Gram stain results, appropriate antibiotic coverage can be selected and modified later when the culture results are obtained.

When endophthalmitis is suspected, some ophthalmologists advocate starting intravenous antibiotics at once, but this may not be necessary when endophthalmitis occurs postoperatively.[31] Intravitreous antibiotic injections often are called for, and surgical removal of the entire vitreous body may be necessary. Treatment of endophthalmitis also may require periocular and topical antibiotics. Cycloplegic drops, such as atropine 1 per cent or scopolamine 0.25 per cent, may make the patient much more comfortable. Appropriate initial intravenous antibiotics may include gentamicin, cefazolin, vancomycin, or other broad-spectrum preparations. Some authorities recommend systemic or local steroids concurrently with antibiotics for endophthalmitis, but this treatment remains controversial and must be considered on an individual case basis.

Fungal endophthalmitis has become a relatively common form of endophthalmitis in childhood due to the prolonged hospital care of severely ill immunocompromised children. The most common organism is *C. albicans*. Children with a central line or with prolonged intravenous therapy of any type may grow the organism from catheters and occasionally from blood cultures. When such is the case, ophthalmology consultation should be requested. When *Candida* endophthalmitis is present, the vitreous will be hazy, and small, white "snowball" localizations of infected material may appear in the vitreous or on the surface of the retina. Daily careful observation may be required during intravenous amphotericin B therapy. If the endophthalmitis clears, no ocular surgical intervention will be indicated. If the vitreous becomes progressively hazy and the white lesions enlarge, a total vitrectomy under general anesthesia may be required to clear the intraocular infection. Intravitreous amphotericin B is quite toxic to the retina and should be used only when other treatment methods fail.[45]

References

1. Alexander, E. R., and Harrison, H. R.: Role of *Chlamydia trachomatis* in perinatal infection. Rev. Infect. Dis. *5*:713–719, 1983.
2. Alfaro, D. V., Roth, D., and Liggett, P. E.: Posttraumatic endophthalmitis: Causative organisms, treatment, and prevention. Retina *14*:206–211, 1994.
3. American Academy of Ophthalmology: Basic and Clinical Science Course, Section 9: Intraocular Inflammation and Uveitis. San Francisco, pp. 57–61, 1995.
4. American Academy of Pediatrics: 1994 Red Book: Report of the Committee on Infectious Diseases. 23rd ed. Elk Grove Village, 1994, pp. 445–455,.
5. Azazi, M. E., Malm, G., and Forsgren, M.: Late ophthalmologic manifestations of neonatal herpes simplex virus infection. Am. J. Ophthalmol. *109*:1–7, 1990.
6. Bale, J. F., Jr., and Murphy, J. R.: Congenital infections and the nervous system. Pediatr. Clin. North Am. *39*:669–690, 1982.
7. Bardenstein, D. S., Haluschak, J., Gerson, S., et al.: Neutrophilic eccrine hidradenitis simulating orbital cellulitis. Arch. Ophthalmol. *112*:1460–1463, 1994.
8. Barkin, R. M., Todd, J. K., and Amer, J.: Periorbital cellulitis in children. Pediatrics *62*:390–392, 1978.
9. Bedrossian, R. H.: Neuroretinitis following measles. J. Pediatr. *46*:329–331, 1955.
10. Bell, T. A., Kuo, C., Stamm, W. E., et al.: Direct fluorescent monoclonal antibody stain for rapid detection of infant *Chlamydia trachomatis* infections. Pediatrics *74*:224–228, 1984.
11. Bertuch, A. W., Rocco, E., and Schwartz, E.G.: Lyme disease: Ocular manifestations. Ann. Ophthalmol. *20*:376–378, 1988.
12. Birebaum E, Linder N, Varsano N, et al.: Adenovirus type 8 conjunctivitis outbreak in a neonatal intensive care unit. Arch. Dis. Child. *68*:610–611, 1993.
13. Blumenkranz, M., Clarkson, J., Cubertson, W. W., et al.: Visual results and complications after retinal reattachment in the acute retinal necrosis syndrome: The influence of operative technique. Retina *9*:170–174, 1989.
14. Boniuk, M., and Zimmerman, L. E.: Ocular pathology in the rubella syndrome. Arch. Ophthalmol. *77*:455–473, 1967.
15. Borne, M. J., Shields, J. A., Shields, C. L., et al.: Bilateral viral endophthalmitis as the presenting sign of severe combined immunodeficiency. Arch. Ophthalmol. *112*:1280–1281, 1994.
16. Bray, W. H., Giangiacomo, J., and Ide, C. H.: Orbital apex syndrome. Surv. Ophthalmol. *32*:136–140, 1987.
17. Brezin, A. P., Kasner, L., Thulliez, P., et al.: Ocular toxoplasmosis in the fetus: Immunohistochemistry analysis and DNA amplification. Retina *14*:19–26, 1994.
18. Bullock, J. D., and Fleishman, J. A.: Orbital cellulitis following dental extraction. Trans. Am. Ophthalmol. Soc. *82*:111–133, 1984.
19. Cano-Parra, J., Espana, E., Esteban, M., et al.: *Pseudomonas* conjunctival ulcer and secondary orbital cellulitis in a patient with AIDS. Br. J. Ophthalmol. *78*:72–73, 1994.
20. Chandler, J. R., Langebrunner, D. J., and Stevens, E. R.: The pathogenesis of orbital complications in acute sinusitis. Laryngoscope *80*:1414–1423, 1970.
21. Clary, R., Weber, A. L., and Eavey, R.: Orbital cellulitis with abscess formation caused by sinusitis. Ann. Otol. Rhinol. Laryngol. *97*:211–212, 1988.
22. Corey, L.: Herpes simplex viruses. *In* Braunwald, E., Isselbacher, K. J., Petersdorf, R. G., et al. (eds.): Harrison's Principles of Internal Medicine. 13th ed. New York, McGraw-Hill, 1994, pp. 782–787.
23. Cornblath, W. T., Elner, V., and Rolfe, M.: Extraocular muscle involvement in sarcoidosis. Ophthalmology *100*:501–505, 1993.
24. Couch, J. M., Green, W. R., Hirst, L. W., et al.: Diagnosing and treating *Phthirus pubis* palpebrum. Surv. Ophthalmol. 26:219-225, 1982.
25. Daffos, F., Forestier, F., Capella-Pavlovsky, M., et al.: Prenatal management of 746 pregnancies at risk for congenital toxoplasmosis. N. Engl. J. Med. *318*:271–275, 1988.
26. Davey, R. T., and Tauber, W. B.: Post traumatic endophthalmitis: The emerging role of *Bacillus cereus* infection. Rev. Infect. Dis. *9*:110–124, 1987.
27. David, D. B., Kirkby, G. R., and Noble, B. A.: *Bacillus cereus* endophthalmitis. Br. J. Ophthalmol. *78*:577–580, 1994.
28. Deans, R. M., Harris, G. J., and Gonnering, R. S.: Infections of the orbit. *In* Tabbara, K. F., Hyndiuk, R. A. (eds.): Infections of the Eye. 2nd ed. Boston, Little, Brown, and Co., 1996, pp. 546–548.
29. Drew, W. L.: Cytomegalovirus infection in patients with AIDS. J. Infect. Dis. *158*:449–456, 1988.
30. Edwards, K., Meredith, T. A., Hager, W. S., et al.: Ophthalmomyiasis interna causing visual loss. Am. J. Ophthalmol. *97*:605–610, 1984.
31. Endophthalmitis Vitrectomy Study Group: Results of the endophthalmitis vitrectomy study: A randomized trial of immediate vitrectomy and of intravenous antibiotics for the treatment of postoperative bacterial endophthalmitis. Arch. Ophthalmol. *113*:1479–1557, 1995.
32. English, F. P., and Nutting, W. B.: Demodicosis of ophthalmic concern. Am. J. Ophthalmol. *91*:362–372, 1981.
33. Engstrom, R. E., Holland, G. N., Nussenblatt, R. B., et al.: Current practices in the management of ocular toxoplasmosis. Am. J. Ophthalmol. *111*:601–610, 1991.
34. Epstein, G. A., and Putterman, A. M.: Combined excision and drainage with intralesional corticosteroid injection in the treatment of chronic chalazia. Arch. Ophthalmol. *106*:514–516, 1988.

35. Fair, J. R.: Clinical eye findings in congenital toxoplasmosis. Surv. Ophthalmol. *6*:923–935, 1961.
36. Foster, R. E., Lowder, C. Y., Meisler, D. M., et al.: Mumps neuroretinitis in an adolescent. Am. J. Ophthalmol. *110*:91–93, 1990.
37. Fox, K. R., and Golomb, H. S.: Staphylococcal ophthalmia neonatorum and the staphylococcal scalded skin syndrome. Am. J. Ophthalmol. *88*:1052–1055, 1979.
38. Friendly, D. S.: Ophthalmia neonatorum. Pediatr. Clin. North Am. *30*:1033–1042, 1983.
39. Gigliotti, F., Hendley, J. O., Morgan, J., et al.: Efficacy of topical antibiotic therapy in acute conjunctivitis in children. J. Pediatr. *104*:623–626, 1984.
40. Gigliotti, F., Williams, W. T., Hayden, F. G., et al.: Etiology of acute conjunctivitis in children. J. Pediatr. *98*:531–536, 1981.
41. Givens, K. T., Lee, D. A, and Ilstrup, D. M.: Congenital rubella syndrome: Ophthalmic manifestations and associated systemic disorders. Br. J. Ophthalmol. *77*:358–363, 1993.
42. Goscienski, P. J.: Inclusion conjunctivitis in the newborn infant. J. Pediatr. *77*:19–26, 1970.
43. Green, W. R., Font, R. L., and Zimmerman, L. E.: Aspergillosis of the orbit. Arch. Ophthalmol. *82*:302–313, 1969.
44. Greenwald, M. J., Wohl, L. G., and Sell, C. H.: Metastatic bacterial endophthalmitis: A contemporary reappraisal. Surv. Ophthalmol. *31*:81–101, 1986.
45. Griffin, J. R., Pettit, T. H., Fishman, L. S., et al.: Bloodborne *Candida endophthalmitis*: A clinical and pathologic study of 21 cases. Arch. Ophthalmol. *89*:450–456, 1973.
46. Guerina, N. H., Hsu, H. W., Meissner, C., et al.: Neonatal serologic screening and early treatment for congenital *Toxoplasma gondii* infection. N. Engl. J. Med. *330*:1858–1863, 1994.
47. Hagler, W. S., Walters, P. V., and Nahmias, A. J.: Ocular involvement in neonatal herpes simplex virus infection. Arch. Ophthalmol. *82*:109–176, 1969.
48. Haimovicki, R., and Roussel, T. J.: Treatment of gonococcal conjunctivitis with a single injection of intramuscular ceftriaxone. Am. J. Ophthalmol. *107*:511–514, 1989.
49. Hale, L. M.: Orbital-cerebral phycomycosis: Report of a case and a review of the disease in infants. Arch. Ophthalmol. *86*:39–43, 1971
50. Hammerschlag, M. R.: Neonatal conjunctivitis. Pediatr. Ann. *22*:346–351, 1993.
51. Hammerschlag, M. R., Chandler, J. W., Alexander, E. R., et al.: Erythromycin ointment for ocular prophylaxis of neonatal chlamydial infection. J. A. M. A. *244*:2291–2293, 1980.
52. Hammerschlag, M. R., Cummings, C., Robin, P. M., et al.: Efficacy of neonatal ocular prophylaxis for the prevention of chlamydial and gonococcal conjunctivitis. N. Engl. J. Med. *320*:769–772, 1989.
53. Hansen, T., Burns, R. P., and Allen, A.: Gonorrheal conjunctivitis: An old disease returned. J. A. M. A. *195*:1156, 1966.
54. Harris, G. J.: Subperiosteal inflammation of the orbit: A bacteriological analysis of 17 cases. Arch. Ophthalmol. *106*:947–952, 1988.
55. Heier, J. S., Gardner, T. A., Hawes, M. J., et al.: Proptosis as the initial presentation of fungal sinusitis in immunocompetent patients. Ophthalmology *102*:713–717, 1995.
56. Hemady, R., Zaltas, M., Paton, B., et al.: *Bacillus*-induced endophthalmitis: New series of 10 cases and review of the literature. Br. J. Ophthalmol. *74*:26–29, 1990.
57. Hess, D. L.: *Chlamydia* in the neonate. Neonatal Netw. *12*:9–12, 1993.
58. Hierholzer, J. C., and Hatch, M. H.: Acute hemorrhagic conjunctivitis. *In* Darnell, R. W. (ed.): Viral Diseases of the Eye. Philadelphia, Lea & Febiger, 1985, pp. 165–196.
59. Hofbauer, J. D., Gordon, L. K., and Palmer, J.: Acute orbital cellulitis after peribulbar injection. Am. J. Ophthalmol. *118*:391–392, 1994.
60. Hogan, M. J., Kimura, S. J., and O'Connor, G. R.: Ocular toxoplasmosis. Arch. Ophthalmol. *72*:592–600, 1964.
61. Holland, G. N.: Infectious diseases. *In* Isenberg, S. (ed.): The Eye in Infancy. Chicago, Yearbook Medical Publishers, 1989, pp. 387–416.
62. Holland, G. N.: An update on AIDS-related cytomegalovirus retinitis. *In* Focal Points: Clinical Modules for Ophthalmologists. Vol. 9, Module 5. San Francisco, American Academy of Ophthalmology, 1991.
63. Hornblass, A., Herschorn, B. J., Stern, K., et al.: Orbital abscess. Surv. Ophthalmol. *29*:169–178, 1984.
64. Hunter, L. R., Krinsky, A. H., and Fleener, C. H.: Preseptal cellulitis caused by *Nocardia brasiliensis*. Am. J. Ophthalmol. *114*:373–374, 1992.
65. Isenberg, S. J., Apt, L., and Wood, M.: A controlled trial of povidone-iodine as prophylaxis against ophthalmia neonatorum. N. Engl. J. Med. *332*:562–566, 1995.
66. Israele, V., and Nelson, J. D.: Periorbital and orbital cellulitis. Pediatr. Infect. Dis. *6*:404–410, 1987.
67. Jobs, D. A., Green, W. R., Fox, R., et al.: Ocular manifestations of AIDS. Ophthalmology *96*:1092–1099, 1989.
68. Jones, D. B: Viral and chlamydial conjunctivitis. *In* Symposium on Medical and Surgical Diseases of the Cornea: Transactions of the New Orleans Academy of Ophthalmology. St. Louis, CV Mosby, 1980, pp. 497–523.
69. Jones, D. B., Matoba, A. Y., Steinkuller, P. G., et al.: Problem solving in corneal and external diseases 1995, part I: Adnexa and conjunctiva. American Academy of Ophthalmology Annual Meeting, Course 524, pp. 5–23, 26–30, 31–38, 65–74, 79–94, 1995.
70. Jones, D. B., Matoba, A. Y., and Wilhelmus, K. R.: Problem solving in corneal and external diseases 1995, part II: Cornea and sclera. American Academy of Ophthalmology Annual Meeting, Course 626, pp. 69–72, tables, 1995.
71. Jones, D. B., Steinkuller, P. G.: Microbial preseptal and orbital cellulitis. *In* Duane, T. D. (ed.): Clinical Ophthalmology. Vol. 4. Hagerstown, Harper & Row, 1989, pp. 1–24.
72. Jones, D. B., and Steinkuller, P. G.: Strategies for the initial management of acute preseptal and orbital cellulitis. Trans. Am. Ophthal. Soc. *86*:94–112, 1988.
73. Jones, D. B., Visvesvara, G. S., and Robinson, N. M.: *Acanthamoeba polyphagia* keratitis and *Acanthamoeba* uveitis associated with fatal meningoencephalitis. Trans. Ophthal. Soc. U. K. *95*:221–232, 1975.
74. Kestelyn, P., Taelman, H., Bogarts, J., et al.: Ophthalmic manifestations of infections with *Cryptococcus neoformans* in patients with the acquired immunodeficiency syndrome. Am. J. Ophthalmol. *116*:721–727, 1993.
75. Khali, M., Lindley, S., and Matouk, E.: Tuberculosis of the orbit. Ophthalmology *92*:1624–1627, 1985.
76. Koppe, J. G., Kloosterman, G. J., de Roever-Bonnet, H., et al.: Toxoplasmosis and pregnancy, with a long-term follow-up of the children. Eur. J. Obstet. Gynecol. Reprod. Biol. *4*:101–110, 1974.
77. Kruger-Leite, E., Jalkh, A. E., Quiroz, H., et al.: Intraocular cysticercosis. Am. J. Ophthalmol. *99*:252–257, 1985.
78. Lambert, S. R., Taylor, D., Kriss, A., et al.: Ocular manifestations of the congenital varicella syndrome. Arch. Ophthalmol. *107*:52–56, 1989.
79. Larkin, D. F. P., Kilvington, S., and Dart, J. K. T.: Treatment of *Acanthamoeba* keratitis with polyhexamethylene biguanide. Ophthalmology *99*:185–191, 1992.
80. Lessner, A., and Stern, G. A.: Preseptal and orbital cellulitis. Infect. Dis. Clin. North Am. *6*:933–952, 1992.
81. Lieberman, H., and Brem, J.: Syndrome of acute osteomyelitis of the superior maxilla in early infancy. N. Engl. J. Med. *260*:318–322, 1959.
82. Liesgang, T. J.: Diagnosis and therapy of herpes zoster ophthalmicus. Ophthalmology *98*:763–770, 1991.
83. Londer, L., and Nelson, D. L.: Orbital cellulitis due to *Haemophilus influenzae*. Arch. Ophthalmol. *91*:89–91, 1974.
84. Lonn, L. I.: Neonatal cytomegalic inclusion disease: Chorioretinitis. Arch. Ophthalmol. *88*:434–438, 1972.
85. McCulley, J. P., Dougherty, J. M., and Deneau, D. G.: Classification of chronic blepharitis. Ophthalmology *89*:1173–1180, 1982.
86. McDonnell, P. J., McDonnell, J. M., and Brown, R. H.: Ocular involvement in patients with fungal infections. Ophthalmology *92*:706–709, 1985.
87. MacEwen, C. J., Phillips, M. G., and Young, J. D.: Value of bacterial culturing in the course of congenital nasolacrimal duct (NLD) obstruction. J. Pediatr. Ophthalmol. Strabismus *31*:246–250, 1994.
88. Mannis, M. J., Tamaru, R., Roth, A. M., et al.: *Acanthamoeba* sclerokeratitis: Determining diagnostic criteria. Arch. Ophthalmol. *104*:1313–1317, 1986.
89. Marcus, D. M., Frederick, A. R., Jr., Raizman, M. B., et al.: Choroidal and retinal detachment in antineutrophil cytoplasmic antibody-positive scleritis. Am. J. Ophthalmol. *119*:517–519, 1995.
90. Margo, C. E., and Hamed, L. M.: Ocular syphilis. Surv. Ophthalmol. *37*:203–220, 1992.
91. Margo, C. E., Mames, R. N., and Guy, J. R.: Endogenous *Klebsiella* endophthalmitis: Report of two cases and review of the literature. Ophthalmology *101*:1298–1301, 1994.
92. Marines, H. M., Osato, M. S., and Font, R. L.: The value of calcofluor white in the diagnosis of mycotic and acanthamoeba infections of the eye and ocular adnexa. Ophthalmology *94*:23–26, 1987.
93. Mathers, W. D., Sutphin, J. E., Folberg, R., et al.: Outbreak of keratitis presumed to be caused by *Acanthamoeba*. Am. J. Ophthalmol. *121*:129–142, 1996.
94. Matoba, A. Y.: Ocular viral infections. Pediatr. Infect. Dis. *3*:358–368, 1984.
95. Mauriello, J. A., Jr., Hargrave, S., Yee, S., et al.: Infection after insertion of alloplastic orbital floor implants. Am. J. Ophthalmol. *117*:246–252, 1994.
96. Miller, R. D., Steinkuller, P. G., and Nagele, D.: Nonfatal maxillocerebral mucormycosis. Ann. Ophthalmol. *12*:1065–1068, 1980.
97. Morales, A. G., Croxatto, J. O., Crovetto, L., et al.: Hydatid cysts of the orbit: A review of 35 cases. Ophthalmology *95*:1027–1032, 1988.
98. Mordhorst, C. H., and Dawson, C.: Sequelae of neonatal inclusion conjunctivitis and associated disease in parents. Am. J. Ophthalmol. *71*:861–867, 1971.
99. Myles, W., Antoszyk, J. H., and Brownstein, S.: Cysticercosis of the orbit. Can. J. Ophthalmol. *29*:291–294, 1994.
100. Nagelberg, H. P., Petashnick, D. E., and To, K. W.: Group B streptococcal metastatic endophthalmitis. Am. J. Ophthalmol. *117*:498–500, 1994.
101. Nahmias, A. J., and Visintine, A. M.: Eye infections with herpes simplex viruses in neonates. Surv. Ophthalmol. *21*:100–105, 1976.
102. Nishida, H., and Risemberg, H. M.: Silver nitrate ophthalmic solution and chemical conjunctivitis. Pediatrics *56*:368–373, 1975.
103. Obenour, L. C.: Subacute sclerosing panencephalitis. Int. Ophthal. Clin. *12*:215–223, 1972.
104. Okada, A. A., Johnson, R. P., and Liles, W. C.: Endogenous bacterial endophthalmitis: Report of a ten-year retrospective study. Ophthalmology *101*:832–838, 1994.

105. O'Keefe, M., Haining, W. M., Young, J. D. H., et al.: Orbital mucormycosis with survival. Br. J. Ophthalmol. *70*:634–636, 1986.
106. O'Keefe, M., Shaikh, A., and Bowell, R.: Management of congenital dacryocele. Acta Ophthalmol. *72*:122–123, 1994.
107. Opremcak, E. M.: Uveitis: A Clinical Manual for Ocular Inflammation. New York, Springer-Verlag Publishers, 1994, pp. 1–50.
108. Orth, D. H., Fishman, G. A., Segall, M., et al.: Rubella maculopathy. Br. J. Ophthalmol. *64*:201–205, 1980.
109. Paoli, C., Francois, M., Triglia, J. M., et al.: Nasal obstruction in the neonate secondary to nasolacrimal ducts cysts. Laryngoscope *105*:86–89, 1995.
110. Paryani, S. G., and Arvin, A. M.: Intrauterine infection with varicella-zoster virus after maternal varicella. N. Engl. J. Med. *314*:1542–1545, 1986.
111. Peloquin, L., Arcand, P., and Abela, A.: Endonasal dacryocystocele of the newborn. J. Otolaryngol. *24*:84–86, 1995.
112. Peyman, G. A., and Daun, M.: Prophylaxis of endophthalmitis. Ophthalmic Surg. *25*:671–674, 1994.
113. Pfister, D. R., Cameron, J. D., Krachmer, J. H., et al.: Confocal microscopy findings of *Acanthamoeba* keratitis. Am. J. Ophthalmol. *121*:119–128, 1996.
114. Powell, K. R.: Orbital and periorbital cellulitis. Pediatr. Rev. *16*:163–167, 1995.
115. Raucher, H. S., Newton, M. J., and Stearn, R. H.: Ophthalmia neonatorum caused by penicillinase-producing *Neisseria gonorrhoeae*. J. Pediatr. *100*:925–926, 1982.
116. Ravin, J. G.: Pissarro, dacryocystitis, and the development of modern lacrimal surgery. Doc. Ophthalmol. *86*:191–202, 1994.
117. Ray, C. G.: Rubella ("German measles"). *In* Braunwald, E., Isselbacher, K. J., Petersdoft, R. G., et al. (eds.): Harrison's Principles of Internal Medicine. 13th ed. New York, McGraw-Hill, 1994, pp. 827–829.
118. Remington, J. S., and Desmonts, G.: Toxoplasmosis. *In* Remington, J. S., and Klein, J. O. (eds.): Infectious Diseases of the Fetus and Newborn. 3rd ed. Philadelphia, W. B. Saunders, 1990, pp. 89–105.
119. Rowsey, J. J., Jensen, H., and Sexton, D. J.: Clinical diagnosis of endophthalmitis. Int. Ophthalmol. Clin. *27*:82–88, 1987.
120. Rubin, S. E., Rubin, L. G., Zito, J., et al.: Medical management of orbital subperiosteal abscess in children. J. Pediatr. Ophthalmol. Strabismus *26*:21–26, 1989.
121. Ryan, S. J., Jr.: De novo subretinal neovascularization in the histoplasmosis syndrome. Arch. Ophthalmol. *94*:321–327, 1976.
122. Sandstrom, K. I., Bell, T. A., Chandler, J. W., et al.: Diagnosis of neonatal purulent conjunctivitis caused by *Chlamydia trachomatis* and other organisms. *In* Marah, P. A., Holmes, K. K., Oriel, J. D., et al. (eds.): Chlamydial Infections. Amsterdam, Elsevier Biomedical Press, 1982, pp. 217–220.
123. Sandstrom, K. I., Bell, T. A., Chandler, J. W., et al.: Microbial causes of neonatal conjunctivitis. J. Pediatr. *105*:706–711, 1984.
124. Schantz, P. M., and Glickman, L. T.: *Toxocara* visceral larva migrans. N. Engl. J. Med. *298*:436–439, 1978.
125. Schneider, G.: Silver nitrate prophylaxis. Can. Med. Assoc. J. *131*:193–197, 1984.
126. Schwab, I. R.: Oral acyclovir and the management of herpes simplex ocular infections. Ophthalmology *95*:423–430, 1988.
127. Sen, D. K.: Tuberculosis of the orbit and lacrimal gland: A clinical study of 14 cases. J. Pediatr. Ophthalmol. Strabismus *17*:232–238, 1980.
128. Shapiro, E. D., Wald, E. R., and Brozanski, B. A.: Periorbital cellulitis and paranasal sinusitis: A reappraisal. Pediatr. Infect. Dis. *1*:91–94, 1982.
129. Shields, J. A.: Ocular toxocariasis: A review. Surv. Ophthalmol. *28*:361–381, 1984.
130. Shrader, S. K., Band, J. D., and Lauter, C. B.: The clinical spectrum of endophthalmitis: Incidence, predisposing factors, and features influencing outcome. J. Infect. Dis. *162*:115-120, 1990.
131. Snowe, R. J., and Wilfert, C. M.: Epidemic reappearance of gonococcal ophthalmia neonatorum. Pediatrics *51*:110–114, 1973.
132. Spaide, R., Natlis, R., Lipka, A., et al.: Ocular findings in leprosy in the United States. Am. J. Ophthalmol. *100*:411–416, 1985.
133. Stagno, S., and Whitley, R. J.: Herpesvirus infections of pregnancy. Part I. Cytomegalovirus and Epstein-Barr virus infections. N. Engl. J. Med. *313*:1270–1274, 1985.
134. Stenson, S., Newman, R., and Fedukowicz, H.: Conjunctivitis in the newborn: Observations on the incidence, cause, and prophylaxis. Ann. Ophthalmol. *13*:329–334, 1981.
135. Tabbara, K. F.: Trachoma: Have we advanced in the last 20 years? Int. Ophthalmol. Clin. *30*:23–27, 1990.
136. Taber, L. H.: Syphilis. *In* Kaplan, S. L. (ed.): Current Therapy in Pediatric Infectious Disease. 3rd ed. St. Louis, Mosby, 1993, pp. 243–245.
137. Talley, A. R., Garcia-Ferrer, F., and Laycock, K. A.: Comparative diagnosis of neonatal chlamydial conjunctivitis by polymerase chain reaction and McCoy cell culture. Am. J. Ophthalmol. *177*:50–57, 1994.
138. Tanner, O. R.: Ocular manifestations of infectious mono-nucleosis. Arch. Ophthalmol. *51*:229–241, 1954.
139. Taylor, H. R., and Dax, E. M.: Ocular onchocerciasis. *In* Tabbara, K. F., and Hyndiuk, R. A. (eds.): Infections of the Eye. 2nd ed. Boston, Little, Brown and Co., 1996, pp. 673–683.
140. Thompson, W. S., Culbertson, W. W., Smiddy, W. E., et al.: Acute retinal necrosis caused by reactivation of herpes simplex virus type 2. Am. J. Ophthalmol. *118*:205–211, 1994.
141. Thylefors, B.: Onchocerciasis: An overview. Int. Ophthalmol. Clin. *30*:21–22, 1990.
142. Thylefors, B., Dawson, C. R., Jones, B. R., et al.: A simple system for the assessment of trachoma and its complications. Bull. W. H. O. *65*:477–483, 1987.
143. Ullman, S., Pflugfelder, S. C., and Hughes R. S.: *Bacillus cereus* panophthalmitis manifesting as an orbital cellulitis. Am. J. Ophthalmol. *103*:105–106, 1987.
144. von Noorden, G. K., and Buck, A. A.: Ocular onchocerciasis: An ophthalmological and epidemiological study in an African village. Arch. Ophthalmol. *80*:26–34, 1968.
145. Walland, M. J., and Rose, G. E.: Soft tissue infections after open lacrimal surgery. Ophthalmology *101*:608–611, 1994.
146. Weber, A. L., and Mikulis, D. K.: Inflammatory disorders of the periorbital sinuses and their complications. Radiol. Clin. North Am. *25*:615–630, 1987.
147. Weiss, A., Friendly, D., Eglin, K., et al.: Bacterial periorbital and orbital cellulitis in childhood. Ophthalmology *90*:195–203, 1983.
148. Wiley, L., Springer, D., Kowalski, R. P., et al.: Rapid diagnostic test for ocular adenovirus. Ophthalmology *95*:431–433, 1988.
149. Wilkinson, C. P., and Walch, R. B.: Intraocular *Toxocara*. Am. J. Ophthalmol. *71*:921–930, 1971.
150. Wilson, C. B., Remington, J. S., Stagno, S., et al.: Development of adverse sequelae in children born with subclinical congenital *Toxoplasma* infection. Pediatrics *66*:767–774, 1980.
151. Wilson, M. E., and Paul, T. O.: Orbital cellulitis following strabismus surgery. Ophthalmic Surg. *18*:92–94, 1987.
152. Wolf, S. M.: Ocular manifestations of congenital rubella: A prospective study of 328 cases of congenital rubella. J. Pediatr. Ophthalmol. *10*:101–104, 1973.
153. Wong, V. Y., Duncan, N., III, and Edwards, M. S.: Medical management of orbital infection. Pediatr. Infect. Dis. J. *13*:1012–1013, 1994.
154. Yoser, S. L., Forster, D. J., and Rao, N. A.: Systemic viral infections and their retinal and choroidal manifestations. Surv. Ophthalmol. *37*:313–352, 1993.

S E C T I O N   T W E L V E

SYSTEMIC INFECTIOUS DISEASES

❑ ❑ ❑

72

BACTEREMIA AND SEPTIC SHOCK

Sheldon L. Kaplan

One of the most serious and potentially life-threatening infectious diseases in childhood is a bacteremic illness. Bacteremia may be caused by a wide variety of gram-positive or gram-negative microorganisms, and it may or may not be associated with a specific focus of infection, such as pneumonia or meningitis. Some bacteremias are transient and self-limited, and they are not discussed in this chapter. The incidence of bacteremia in children has been studied in both hospital and ambulatory settings. In otherwise normal children, beyond the newborn age group, *Streptococcus pneumoniae, Haemophilus influenzae* type b (unimmunized child), *Staphylococcus aureus,* group A *Streptococcus, Salmonella* species, and *Neisseria meningitidis* are the most common microorganisms causing bacteremia.[170, 194] *S. pneumoniae* and *Salmonella* species are particularly common blood isolates in children with fever, elevated white blood cell counts, and no obvious source of infection on physical examination, i.e., outpatient or unsuspected bacteremia. Children with underlying illnesses that depress the host response to infection may develop illnesses due to these same microorganisms; however, in this population of children, especially when hospitalized, Enterobacteriaceae, *S. aureus, Staphylococcus epidermidis,* and fungi are the most important organisms commonly isolated from the blood cultures.[3, 129, 163] Indwelling vascular lines, urinary catheters, and endotracheal tubes, as well as other foreign material, further predispose to nosocomial infections in already compromised children. In fact, the diagnosis of septicemia has increased over the past 15 years, in part related to improved medical technology and the greater numbers of individuals with immunocompromising conditions who previously would not have survived.[121]

One potential consequence of bacteremia is septic shock, a state characterized by inadequate tissue perfusion that is associated frequently with endotoxemia. Although the majority of children with septic shock have infections due to gram-negative enteric bacteria, *Pseudomonas aeruginosa, H. influenzae* type b, or *N. meningitidis*—organisms with endotoxin or lipopolysaccharide within cell walls—it also has been associated with disease due to gram-positive bacteria (especially *S. aureus* and *Streptococcus pyogenes*), viruses, rickettsiae, and fungi.

The incidence of septic shock in children is unknown. In adults, the frequency of septic shock is thought to be approximately 20-fold that of two decades ago. Dupont and Spink[45] reviewed the cases of 172 children, 30 days to 16 years of age, who were hospitalized at the University of Minnesota Medical Center with gram-negative bacteremia. Infection or manipulation of the urinary tract preceded bacteremia in 20 per cent of these cases, of which 73 per cent had a potentially lethal chronic disease. Shock occurred in 25 per cent of the children, and 98 per cent of those with shock died. In contrast, 42 per cent of children with bacteremia but without shock survived. Corrigan and associates[34] reported that 11 of 36 (31 per cent) children with septicemia developed shock. Eight of these patients were younger than 1 year of age. In meningococcal infections, 11 to 40 per cent of children develop hypotension.[46, 195] Over a 10-month study period, Naqvi and colleagues[118] reported that 5 of 29 (17 per cent) children with meningitis and 1 of 19 (5 per cent) children with extrameningeal infection due to *H. influenzae* type b developed shock. In addition, shock occurred in 5 of 39 (13 per cent) episodes of gram-negative bacillary sepsis with three deaths. Jacobs and associates[78] reviewed the admissions of previously normal children to a pediatric intensive care unit in a large children's hospital over a 30-month period. Hypotension or evidence of peripheral hypoperfusion occurred in 143 children with confirmed bacterial sepsis or apparent meningococcemia (Table 72–1). The overall mortality rate in children with proven sepsis and septic shock was 9.8 per cent (14 of 143). However, in this series, the most common organism was *H. influenzae* type b, which rarely causes systemic infections in the infant or child who has received at least two doses of a conjugate *H. influenzae* type b vaccine.[148] Early-onset group B streptococcal infections in neonates and overwhelming *S. pneumoniae* infections in the child with splenic dysfunction or asplenia are associated with

TABLE 72–1. Confirmed Etiology and Mortality of Septic Shock in Children*

Organism	Number	Mortality
Haemophilus influenzae type b	59	1 (1.7%)
Neisseria meningitidis	26	3 (11.5%)
Apparent meningococcemia	3	3 (100%)
Streptococcus pneumoniae	16	1 (6.3%)
Group B *Streptococcus*	8	1 (12.5%)
Staphylococcus aureus	7	2 (29%)
Gram-negative enteric	8	2 (25%)
Other	16	1 (6.3%)

*Arkansas Children's Hospital (9/84 to 4/87); oncology, burn, and primary immunodeficiency patients excluded from analysis.

Modified from Jacobs, R. F., Sowell, M. K., Moss, M. M., et al.: Septic shock in children: Bacterial etiologies and temporal relationships. Pediatr. Infect. Dis. J. *9*:196–200, 1990.

shock in a high percentage of cases. *S. aureus* or group A *Streptococcus* may cause hypotension in a child with or without other manifestations of toxic shock syndrome.[162, 170]

Over the past decade, many advances in our understanding of the pathogenesis and pathophysiology of septic shock with respect to the host response to infection have required that more precise clinical definitions of "sepsis" and expanded syndromes be developed. Much of the impetus for this effort is related to an ability to identify more readily patients with infections who might benefit from newer (expensive) adjunctive measures. An American College of Chest Physicians/Society of Critical Care Medicine Consensus Conference in 1991 developed new terminology to define sepsis and its sequelae.[15] The terminology may not apply directly to the pediatric population, and modifications for use in children have been proposed[67, 153] (Table 72–2).

PATHOPHYSIOLOGY

The pathophysiology of bacteremia is highly variable and dependent upon the specific microorganism isolated; the nature of the immune status of the host; and other factors, such as the locations of indwelling lines. Highly encapsulated organisms, such as *H. influenzae* type b, *S. pneumoniae,* and *N. meningitidis,* normally may reside in the nasopharynx and for reasons that are poorly understood are capable of invading beyond mucosal barriers into the blood stream. A preceding viral upper respiratory tract infection may play some role in alterations in local host defense mechanisms that result in bacteremia.[83, 106]

Using human columnar nasopharyngeal tissue in organ cultures, Stephens and colleagues[166] demonstrated that *N. meningitidis* organisms were ingested by the columnar cells, then found within phagocytic vacuoles, and later observed within subepithelial tissues, which suggests that the meningococci had penetrated the epithelial layer. In this same model, *H. influenzae* type b organisms attach to nonciliated columnar epithelial cells and subsequently are found in the intercellular spaces in association with a preceding disruption of the tight junctions of epithelial cells.[47] Once past the mucosal barriers, *H. influenzae* type b may enter the blood stream directly through pharyngeal blood vessels.[151] Gram-negative enteric organisms have surface structures called pili or adhesins, which appear to be important in attachment and adherence of these microorganisms to specific receptor sites on epithelial surfaces. The placement of an endotracheal tube unmasks a greater number of these receptor sites, presumably through increased protease activity of secretions and decreased cell-bound fibronectin, and thus leads to colonization of the upper respiratory tract with gram-negative organisms, which are ubiquitous in the environment of an intensive care unit.[197] Again, by mechanisms that are unclear but that certainly are related in part to altered host defenses, these organisms are able to move beyond epithelial surfaces and cause bacteremia.

TABLE 72–2. Terminology of Sepsis and Its Sequelae

Bacteremia—positive blood culture indicating viable bacteria in the blood

Systemic inflammatory response syndrome (SIRS)—severe clinical insult leading to a systemic inflammatory response manifested by ≥2 of the following conditions: (1) temperature >38° C or <36° C; (2) heart rate >2 standard deviations above normal for age; (3) respiratory rate >2 standard deviations above normal for age; (4) peripheral white blood cell count <4000/mm³, >12,000/mm³, or >10 per cent immature forms

Sepsis—SIRS due to an infection

Severe sepsis—sepsis plus organ dysfunction, hypoperfusion, or hypotension. Evidence of hypoperfusion may include oliguria, lactic acidosis, and acute alteration in mental status

Septic shock—sepsis associated with hypotension despite adequate fluid resuscitation in addition to evidence of hypoperfusion as defined under Severe Sepsis. Patients may not be hypotensive at the time perfusion abnormalities are noted if they are receiving inotropic or vasopressor agents. Sepsis-induced hypotension—systolic blood pressure measurement >2 standard deviations below the mean for age in the absence of other causes for hypotension

Multiple organ dysfunction syndrome (MODS)—presence of altered organ function in an acutely ill patient such that homeostasis cannot be maintained without intervention

The gastrointestinal and genitourinary tracts are a major source of gram-negative organisms responsible for bacteremia. These organisms first may cause localized abscesses or peritonitis if intestinal perforation occurs, or they may invade directly through intestinal mucosa, particularly when the mucosa is affected by antineoplastic agents. Microorganisms within the bladder may ascend the genitourinary tract and presumably enter the blood stream via the kidneys. *S. aureus* and *S. pyogenes* are common inhabitants of the skin and skin structures. Any skin wound or foreign matter within the skin tissue makes the skin more susceptible to bacterial invasion. Staphylococci have a unique capability of adhering to solid surfaces, such as catheters, which may be an important prerequisite to colonization and subsequent line-related bacteremia. In fact, in vitro, *S. epidermidis* is capable of proliferating on the surface of polyethylene catheters in the absence of any other nutrients and is covered by a slime-like material.[133]

The pathophysiology of septic shock is very complex. Septic shock associated with gram-negative organisms has been studied most extensively, especially with respect to endotoxin, which has multiple biologic effects. Bacterial lipopolysaccharide or endotoxin has three basic components: (1) terminal side chains, which consist of repeating oligosaccharides that differ from strain to strain and are responsible for the antigenic specificity of the O antigens; (2) a core lipopolysaccharide, which also consists of oligosaccharides but has less diversity in structure among strains than the terminal side chains; and (3) lipid A, which is very similar among the different strains and is responsible for most of the biologic activity of endotoxin.

Endotoxin shock has been the subject of intensive animal research, and much of what is known about the pathogenesis of endotoxin shock has been derived from animal models.[92] Although septic shock in humans is not simulated precisely in these animal models because the animals do not have underlying host defense defects, much of what has been learned about endotoxin shock in animals has been corroborated in the human host.

Endotoxin Shock in Animals

Most animal models of endotoxin shock employ infusions of either live gram-negative bacteria, usually *Escherichia coli*, or purified endotoxin, after which observations are made. The effects of purified endotoxin in part are dependent upon the species of animal being studied. A summary of the effect of endotoxin in animal models is shown in Table 72–3.

It now is clear that several circulating mediators induced by endotoxin play a pivotal role in the pathogenesis of endotoxin shock. Tumor necrosis factor (TNF)/cachectin, a poly-

TABLE 72–3. Endotoxin Shock in Animal Models

	Mediators
Cardiovascular Effects	
Decreased peripheral vascular resistance[141]	Histamine, bradykinin,[107, 108] serotonin, complement activation, prostaglandins, anaphylatoxins
Lowered cardiac output[5]	
Depressed myocardial function[119]	
Decreased systemic blood pressure	
Metabolic Effects	
Hyperglycemia[35]	Hypoinsulinemia
Hypoglycemia[50]	
Increased adrenocorticotropic hormone, growth hormone, and antidiuretic hormone[193]	
Decreased calcium[201]	
Increased triglycerides[84, 176]	
Decreased iron, transferrin, and zinc	
Pulmonary Effects	
Congestive atelectasis[29]	Polymorphonuclear leukocytes
Increased capillary permeability[71]	Polymorphonuclear leukocytes
Vasoconstriction	Thromboxane A_2, prostacyclin
Bronchoconstriction[18]	Leukotrienes
Central Nervous System Effects	
Decreased regional and total cerebral blood flow[140]	
Increased cerebral oxygen consumption[140]	

peptide hormone, appears to be the key cytokine mediating septic shock. The tissue injury induced by TNF largely is a result of other mediators that are stimulated by TNF and include interleukin-1, interleukin-6, eicosanoids, and platelet-activating factor.[42, 73, 173, 175, 177, 178] TNF is synthesized by a wide variety of cells (including monocytes/macrophages, natural killer cells, microglial cells, hepatic Kupffer cells) after stimulation by lipopolysaccharides, C5a, viruses, and enterotoxins, among others. It initiates a cascade of events eventually leading to endothelial cell injury, an enhanced inflammatory response, and ultimately the characteristic findings of endotoxic shock. Furthermore, transgenic mice deficient for the p55-kD TNF receptor are resistant to lipopolysaccharide-induced shock, which supports the critical role of TNF in the pathogenesis of septic shock.[135]

Nitric oxide (endothelium-derived relaxing factor) is the final pathway by which endogenous vasodilators stimulated by endotoxin result in hypotension secondary to altered control of microcirculation. Endotoxin via the release of cytokines induces a form of the enzyme nitric oxide synthase, which leads to increased nitric oxide production.[113] Inhibitors of nitric oxide synthase, such as N^G-monomethyl-L-arginine, can reverse or prevent hypotension in animals after endotoxin administration.[105]

Endotoxin Shock in Humans

The pathophysiology of septic shock is highly complex and is related predominantly to actions of endogenous mediators released as part of the systemic inflammatory response to an infection. The cascade of events is intertwining, with production of one cytokine stimulating the synthesis of others; synergistic in that the activities of certain cytokines act in concert; and sometimes antagonistic, with the production of other molecules to inhibit or compete with various cytokines. This complicated response to an infectious stimulus has been studied best for lipopolysaccharide, but a similar series of events occurs in response to gram-positive infections.

TNF largely is responsible for the biologic effects of lipopolysaccharide in humans, including fever, shock, myocardial suppression, capillary leak (endothelial damage), coagulation alterations, and metabolic changes.[10, 20, 21, 69, 107, 137, 174] In children, including neonates, the role of cytokines in sepsis due to a variety of organisms, but especially *N. meningitidis*, is well documented.[19, 37, 58, 169, 183] Lipopolysaccharide and TNF each can induce the synthesis of other "proinflammatory" cytokines, such as interleukin-1β and interleukin-6.[43] Interleukin-6 levels in plasma correlate with mortality. Interleukin-8 plasma concentrations also are increased after lipopolysaccharide or interleukin-1β infusion.[64]

The "anti-inflammatory" cytokine interleukin-10 is produced after lipopolysaccharide injection and inhibits the production of TNF-α, interleukin-1β, and interleukin-6.[100] Furthermore, naturally occurring inhibitors of TNF or interleukin-1β are measurable in patients with the sepsis syndrome.[39, 40, 60] Interleukin-1 receptor antagonist (interleukin-1ra) binds competitively to the interleukin-1 receptor to block the action of interleukin-1. Soluble TNF receptors bind to circulating TNF, which prevents its proinflammatory actions (Fig. 72–1).

Lipopolysaccharide stimulates a number of different cells to increase production of cytokines, especially mononuclear phagocytes. Mononuclear cells have a surface receptor (CD14) that recognizes and binds a complex of lipopolysaccharide and lipopolysaccharide-binding protein, a glycoprotein that opsonizes lipopolysaccharide and is an acute-phase reactant increased during sepsis.[189, 198] The lipopolysaccharide–lipopolysaccharide-binding protein complex interaction with CD14 promotes mononuclear phagocytes to produce reactive oxygen molecules, cytokines, and arachidonic acid metabolites, including prostaglandin and leukotrienes. A counterregulatory protein is bactericidal/permeability-increasing protein, which is stored in the granules of polymorphonuclear leukocytes and inhibits the effects of lipopolysaccharide.[55]

In humans, gram-negative bacteremia is followed by a decrease in systemic vascular resistance and mean blood pressure and an increase in cardiac output.[11, 190] The decrease

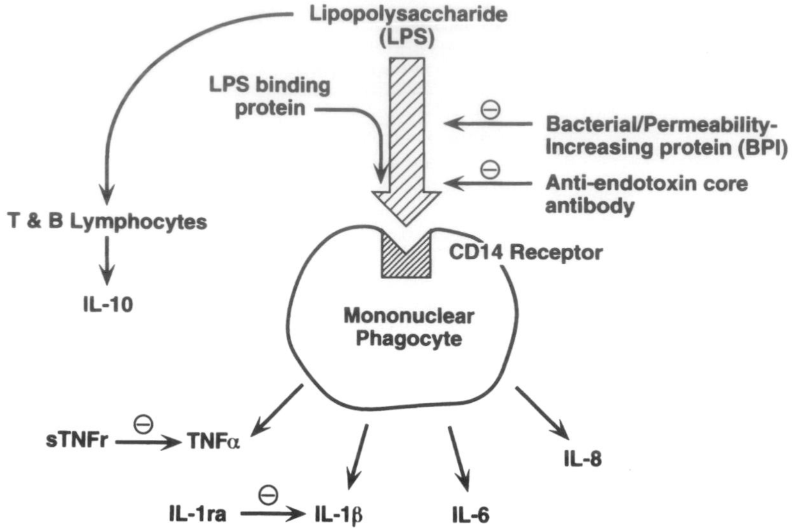

FIGURE 72–1. *Activation of the cytokine network by lipopolysaccharide interaction with mononuclear phagocytes. sTNFr, soluble tumor necrosis factor receptor; IL-1ra, interleukin-1 receptor antagonist; ⊖, antagonistic effect.*

in systemic vascular resistance may be accompanied by activation of the complement and kinin systems.[108] After this early phase, the blood pressure decreases further without change in the central venous pressure. Certain patients are able to maintain their cardiac output and index; this may be associated with increased rates of survival. When peripheral resistance is measured within 12 to 24 hours of the onset of shock, its decrease is significant in patients who survive when compared with those who die.[123] In contrast, cardiac output is reduced significantly in other patients; this is associated with increased concentration of blood lactate, decreased arterial blood pH, and decreased rates of survival.

Depression of myocardial function has been demonstrated in adult patients in septic shock. These patients have a reduced ejection fraction and left ventricular dilatation and significantly altered ventricular performance in response to infusion of volume.[125] However, this depression of myocardial function is transient in survivors, reverting to normal within 1 to 4 days.[126] Parker and colleagues[127] found that patients who did not survive septic shock did not have left ventricular dilatation or reduction in the ejection fraction. Furthermore, when the systemic vascular resistance index was averaged over time, nonsurvivors had a significantly ($p < .05$) lower index than did survivors of septic shock. This study included three children who were 9 to 17 years of age. Abraham and associates[1] sequentially monitored hemodynamic and oxygen transport measurement in 33 patients with septic shock. In the 24-hour period prior to the onset of hypotension, the survivors demonstrated significantly greater cardiac index, left cardiac work index, oxygen delivery, and oxygen consumption than did the nonsurvivors.

The pathogenesis of the myocardial depression in septic shock may be related to some humoral factor. By infusing plasma from patients with septic shock into the coronary arteries of healthy dogs, McConn and colleagues[98] noted a marked fall in the left ventricular work index and two different patterns of myocardial depression—an early and a late phase. Parrillo and colleagues[128] demonstrated a circulation of myocardial depressant substance in humans with septic shock by employing an in vitro preparation of newborn rat heart cell cultures that beat spontaneously. Serum from 20 patients with septic shock (including three patients 9 to 15 years of age) decreased the extent and velocity of myocardial cell shortening during contraction. In a subsequent study in patients with septic shock, patients with myocardial depressant substance–positive assays had lower mean lowest ejection fractions and greater pulmonary artery wedge pressures and peak lactic acid concentrations than patients with negative assays.[142] The myocardial depressant substance has a molecular weight of more than 10,000 daltons. This same group has shown that the infusion of purified *E. coli* endotoxin into normal volunteers results in a depression of left ventricular function and a cardiovascular state similar to that observed in clinical septic shock, which suggests that endotoxin is the major mediator of the cardiovascular dysfunction in septic shock.[168]

Hematologic changes, such as leukocytosis, leukopenia, and thrombocytopenia, have been observed in human volunteers after infusion of endotoxin. Thrombocytopenia commonly occurs in association with septicemia of any etiology. Corrigan[30] noted thrombocytopenia ($<150{,}000$ cells/mm^3) in 57 per cent of children with gram-negative and 77 per cent of children with gram-positive infections. Septic shock is one of the most common causes of disseminated intravascular coagulation in children. Hageman factor, which initiates the coagulation cascade, can be activated directly by endotoxin or through endothelial damage induced by bacteria. In bacterial shock, concentrations of Hageman factor (factor XII), prekallikrein, high-molecular-weight kininogen, and factor VII are decreased, in part, through consumption.[33, 81] Similarly, levels of inactivators of clotting factors, such as C1 esterase inhibitor, α_2-macroglobulin, and antithrombin III, also are diminished. Corrigan and Jordan[33] diagnosed disseminated intravascular coagulation in 24 of 26 children with septic shock and found that improvement in coagulation parameters appeared to be related most to restoration of blood pressure. In addition, gram-negative bacteremia may be associated with a coagulopathy that is not disseminated intravascular coagulation but is characterized by prolongation of the prothrombin and partial thromboplastin times due to a reduction in the vitamin K–dependent coagulation factors.[32]

More recent studies have shown that lipopolysaccharide through cytokine stimulation activates blood coagulation predominantly via the extrinsic pathway. The procoagulant state is enhanced further by decreased protein C activity, which is an important inhibitor of coagulation factors V and VIII. The fibrinolytic system also is altered by endotoxemia mediated by plasminogen activator inhibitor 1–induced suppression. Thus, the coagulopathy associated with septic shock is characterized by both a procoagulant state and inhibition of fibrinolysis.[88, 93]

Endotoxin can activate the complement cascade by either the classic or the alternate pathways. Several investigators have documented that significantly depressed concentrations of C3 occur in human patients with bacteremia and hypotension, when compared with normal individuals or with patients with uncomplicated bacteremia, and that C3 was activated primarily by the alternate pathway.[48, 81, 94] In patients with bacteremia and hypotension, C1, C4, and C2 were not depressed significantly from values found in normal controls or in normotensive patients with bacteremia. In contrast, C3, C5, C6, C9, properdin, and factor B levels were decreased significantly ($p < .05$) in bacteremic patients with shock. In children with meningococcal disease, Tubbs[180] noted a mean C3 concentration (as a percentage of normal values) of 132 ± 21 per cent for survivors versus 91 ± 21 per cent for nonsurvivors. The C3 levels did not correlate with endotoxin levels in sera. Fenton and Strunk[49] have provided evidence that complement activation also occurs during group B streptococcal sepsis in newborns.

Many metabolic alterations have been documented in the human host during endotoxin shock. Hyperglycemia followed by hypoglycemia can complicate the shock state induced by sepsis.[109] Children with underlying liver disease or with reduced glycogen stores are most likely to develop hypoglycemia during septic shock. Lactic acidosis develops as a result of poor tissue perfusion, and lactic acid concentrations are increased in nonsurvivors and those patients with poor or low-flow cardiac output during sepsis. In clinical studies, Clowes and associates[28] identified a subgroup of patients with low-flow septic shock in whom serum insulin concentrations were lower than a control population. They postulated that low insulin concentrations affect the myocardium adversely; in these patients, a beneficial response to glucose-potassium-insulin administration has been observed.

Hypocalcemia and decreased serum ionized calcium concentrations occur frequently during bacterial sepsis. In one study, 12 of 60 (20 per cent) critically ill adults with bacterial sepsis had hypocalcemia.[201] The mortality rate in the hypocalcemic patients was 50 per cent, compared with 30 per cent in the patients who were normocalcemic. Cardenas-Rivero and associates[23] studied calcium homeostasis in 145 children admitted to an intensive care unit. Of eight children with confirmed sepsis and/or meningitis not caused by *H. influenzae* type b, seven had hypocalcemia and six of seven had ionized hypocalcemia. Five of the six children with ionized hypocalcemia had inappropriately normal concentrations of parathyroid hormone, which suggests that transient hypoparathyroidism occurs in some children with sepsis. Hypocalcemia also is noted commonly in patients with toxic shock syndrome.[192] In women with toxic shock syndrome and hypocalcemia, serum concentrations of calcitonin are elevated by mechanisms that are unknown.[25] Hypocalcemia and elevated calcitonin concentrations also have been documented in children with fulminant meningococcemia.[99] These changes in calcium levels especially are critical because the level of ionized calcium and cardiac output in septic shock can be correlated.[196] Other metabolic changes that may occur during septic shock in humans include the following:

1. Increased concentrations of cortisol and growth hormone[184] (including neonates[171])
2. Depression of T_3 and T_4 levels related to poor nutrition[145]
3. Elevations in total amino acid concentrations in plasma and the preferential use of branched-chain amino acids as an energy source for skeletal muscle[54, 110]
4. Elevations of plasma cathepsin D, a lysosomal enzyme[59]
5. Muscle proteolysis, possibly induced by one or more circulating agents in the plasma of patients with serious infections[26]
6. Elevations in plasma thromboxane concentrations, which are noted in nonsurvivors of septic shock[144]
7. Elevation in triglycerides and free fatty acid concentrations during gram-negative bacteremia[56]

Liver dysfunction is an important aspect of endotoxin shock in adults. Banks and colleagues[6] found that clinical jaundice was apparent in 63 per cent of their patients with septic shock, that it was more common in nonsurvivors than survivors, and that the degree of biochemical liver abnormalities was related to the duration of shock. Postmortem findings included focal liver necrosis, Kupffer cell hyperplasia, portal tract inflammation, venous congestion, and intrahepatic cholestasis.

Adult respiratory distress syndrome (ARDS), or shock lung, is a major complication of septic shock in children.[75, 136] The lungs of children with ARDS have characteristic changes consisting of increased lung weight reflecting congestion and atelectasis, alveoli lined with hyaline membranes, microthrombi, hemorrhage, and interstitial edema.[75] Increased capillary permeability and intrapulmonary shunts have been documented in patients with shock lung.[4, 36] C5a, a potent chemotactic factor, causes aggregation of polymorphonuclear neutrophils, is elevated in the sera of patients who ultimately develop ARDS, and is found in increased concentrations in bronchoalveolar lavage fluid obtained from patients with ARDS.[65, 146] It is thought that leukocyte aggregates are trapped in lung tissue and may cause damage to the endothelium of the pulmonary microvasculature through the release of oxygen radicals, lysosomal enzymes, and products of arachidonic acid metabolism. Although neutrophils clearly play a critical role in the pathogenesis of ARDS, other factors also are important, considering that ARDS can develop in patients who are neutropenic.[124, 191] Thromboxane, platelet-activating factor, fibrin, and other substances contribute to the lung injury in ARDS.[149]

The effects of endotoxin shock on the central nervous system have not been studied carefully in humans; however, a study by Graham and associates[61] particularly is intriguing. The brains of six adult patients with both septic shock due to gram-negative bacteremia and neurologic dysfunction, predominantly coma, demonstrated an acute hemorrhagic leukoencephalitis on histologic examination. Microscopic findings included necrosis of vessel walls, perivascular tissue destruction, perivascular edema—especially of white matter—polymorphonuclear leukocyte infiltration into abnormal areas of the brain, and ball or ring hemorrhages. These authors postulated that these histologic findings could be caused by a Shwartzman reaction mediated by endotoxin. The encephalopathy associated with sepsis in general appears, in part, to be due to altered phenylalanine metabolism; concentrations of phenylalanine and its metabolite, phenylacetic acid, are increased in the sera and cerebrospinal fluid of septic adults either stuporous or comatose.[111]

Endotoxin has been implicated in the pathogenesis of acute renal failure associated with septicemia. Wardle[186, 187] showed that 12 of 16 patients with acute tubular necrosis had endotoxemia. Renal arterial blood flow and renal vascular resistance are decreased significantly in baboons 2 to 4 hours after infusion of endotoxin. Inadequate perfusion pressure was associated with renal ischemia and negligible urine output in these animals shortly after administration of endotoxin.[154] Pathologic examination of the kidneys revealed focal necrosis of the proximal tubular epithelium, eosinophilic casts within proximal and distal tubules, and microthrombi in the glomerular capillaries. Endothelin, a potent vasoconstrictor peptide produced by endothelial cells, is elevated in concentration in the plasma of patients with septic shock. Because endothelin contributes to the regulation of regional blood flow, elevated levels suggest that it may relate to renal vasoconstriction and dysfunction.[182]

Endotoxin can be measured in the plasma of patients with gram-negative bacteremia; the presence of circulating endotoxin, however, does not necessarily mean that bacteremia is present or ever has occurred, because endotoxin presumably may be "absorbed or leak" into the circulation from the gastrointestinal tract.[89, 90, 167, 179] However, endotoxemia may be a valid indicator of impending gram-negative septicemia in febrile patients.[41] Preformed antibody to lipopolysaccharide or lipid A is associated with protection against shock and death due to gram-negative bacteremia in adults. McCartney and colleagues[96] detected endotoxin in the blood (after chloroform extraction) of patients with gram-negative septic shock; all 18 patients with persistently positive endotoxin assays died. In contrast, nine patients who initially had endotoxemia, but subsequently had negative assays, survived. There is evidence that human endotoxin is cleared from the circulation by the liver and can be detoxified by neutrophil enzymes (acyloxacyl hydrolases).[104, 115]

The sequence of events in the evolution of endotoxin shock has been outlined by several investigators.[120, 206] Bacteria, endotoxin, or other bacterial products stimulate the production of TNF and other cytokines, which in concert with endotoxin set off a whole series of events. Potent mediators, including C3a, C5a, eicosanoids, platelet-activating factor, histamine, and myocardial depressant substance, are released. Potent vasodilators cause peripheral vasodilatation, and decreased systemic peripheral resistance leads to pooling of blood and a decreased venous return to the heart. Mean blood pressure may be low, or it may be normal if cardiac output increases sufficiently to compensate for these alterations despite depression of ventricular function. The central venous pressure, which partially depends on myocardial competence, may be low or in the normal range.

If intravascular volume is increased by the administration of sufficient fluids, shock may be prevented or corrected. However, continued hypotension and diminished perfusion pressure may lead to cellular hypoxia and increased production of lactic acid from pyruvate. The microcirculation is altered by local tissue acidosis. Capillary beds become congested, and intravascular fluid may leak into the interstitial spaces. Increased catecholamine secretion leads to arteriolar and venular constriction and increased peripheral resistance. Pooling of blood is enhanced, which leads to a further diminution in venous return and a reduction of cardiac output. Oliguria, coagulation abnormalities, and additional metabolic alterations indicate multiple organ system failure and presage the death of the patient.

CLINICAL PRESENTATION AND DIAGNOSIS

The symptoms and signs of bacteremia are highly variable, being greatly dependent upon the age and underlying disease of the patient, the duration of illness, and the specific microorganisms. Young, otherwise healthy children between 6 months and 3 years of age may present with fever and evidence of an upper or lower respiratory tract infection or no focus of infection and yet have unsuspected bacteremia. Most studies have indicated that the risk of bacteremia increases as the body temperature rises and that once the temperature exceeds 41° C, almost 25 per cent of these children may be bacteremic.[8] In the previously healthy child, the persistence of irritability and the inability to console the infant, despite optimal environmental conditions, have been proposed as key points in the physical examination that should alert the clinician to the possibility of a serious infection, such as bacteremia or meningitis.[95, 164] Underlying illnesses with splenic dysfunction place the child at increased risk for infections due to encapsulated organisms, whereas children with leukemia or other immunosuppressive diseases or children in the intensive care unit are more likely to get infections with gram-negative bacilli or *S. aureus.* A history of diarrhea may suggest *Salmonella* species as a possible etiology of illness. Preceding skin infections or wounds are important clues to infection due to *S. aureus* or group A streptococcal organisms. An indwelling vascular catheter may precipitate overlying erythema in the patient with evidence of phlebitis proximally. Both gram-positive cocci and gram-negative bacilli can be associated with catheter-related sepsis.[157] Toxic shock syndrome should be considered in a hypotensive female with a recent menstrual period and history of tampon use, although toxic shock also is associated with *S. aureus* sepsis in males and nonmenstruating females. Intra-abdominal sources of infection increase the likelihood of anaerobic bacteremia. Petechiae may be associated with many microorganisms, especially invasive disease due to *N. meningitidis.*[122] Purpura is an ominous finding and frequently is associated with overwhelming infection due to *N. meningitidis, S. pneumoniae,* and *H. influenzae* type b. *P. aeruginosa* is associated specifically with erythema gangrenosum. Other skin and soft tissue manifestations of gram-negative sepsis include bullous lesions, cellulitis, fasciitis, thrombophlebitis, and symmetric peripheral gangrene with disseminated intravascular coagulation.[116] Signs of meningeal irritation or increased intracranial pressure are important to note because these may modify the approach to fluid management of the child in shock.

The onset of gram-negative bacteremia may be heralded by chills, fever, nausea, vomiting, diarrhea, rashes, and petechiae. Initially, the skin feels warm and appears flushed. A change or impairment in mental status may be the first clue to the presence of shock. Hyperventilation also may occur prior to the onset of clinical shock, which can alert the physician to impending circulatory insufficiency.[12] In time, cold, clammy extremities, a weak pulse, tachycardia, tachypnea, hypotension, and oliguria may be noted. The skin over the extremities, the tip of the nose, and the earlobes especially is prone to cyanosis. Auscultation of the lungs may reveal rales, indicating pneumonia or pulmonary edema. Abnormal distention or tenderness to palpation and guarding may be evidence of peritonitis.

The physician must distinguish between the three main types of shock in children[130]: (1) *hypovolemic* shock, such as occurs with blood loss, fluid and electrolyte loss, adrenal insufficiency, or other causes; (2) *cardiogenic* shock, which is associated with drug intoxication, cardiac surgery, arrhythmias, and pericardial tamponade, among others; and (3) *distributive* shock, which indicates abnormal distribution of blood flow leading to inadequate tissue perfusion (septic shock and anaphylaxis are classic examples).

The laboratory evaluation of the child with bacteremia, septic shock, or both should provide information concerning the etiology as well as data required for optimal supportive management. Several studies have demonstrated that a total white blood cell count exceeding 15,000 cells/mm^3 in a 3- to 36-month-old child with a fever exceeding 39° to 40° C and without a focus of infection is an indication that the child has an increased risk for bacteremia.[7] An erythrocyte sedimentation rate greater than 30 mm/hour also has been suggested as a screening test for such patients. A low peripheral white blood cell count also may suggest septicemia and commonly is observed during overwhelming bacteremic illnesses. The hemoglobin and hematocrit results should help differentiate between septic and hemorrhagic shock. Examination of the peripheral smear may disclose evidence of splenic dysfunction (i.e., Howell-Jolly bodies) or fragmented red blood cells, as seen in disseminated intravascular coagulation. Thrombocytopenia, prolongation of prothrombin time and partial prothrombin time, and the presence of fibrin split products are consistent with disseminated intravascular coagulation.[31] Hyponatremia is common. Serum bicarbonate concentrations may be depressed, which may signify a state of metabolic acidosis. Elevated lactic acid concentrations result from inadequate tissue perfusion and in some reports have been significantly greater in nonsurvivors or those with low-flow states than in survivors or patients with high-flow shock.[28] Hyperglycemia or hypoglycemia may be encountered. Elevated transaminases also can be noted and presumably reflect cellular injury. Serum calcium concentrations, and preferably ionized calcium levels, should be checked periodically because hypocalcemia may interfere with optimal myocardial function.

Arterial blood gases obtained early in the course of endotoxin shock usually reveal hypocapnia and normal to elevated pH.[12, 13] At this point, the patient has a mixed metabolic acidosis and respiratory alkalosis. If the shock state progresses, the metabolic acidosis becomes so severe that respiratory compensation is ineffective, and the patient becomes acidotic. In some patients, respiratory acidosis accompanies metabolic acidosis. In either case, decompensated metabolic acidosis in the patient with septic shock is associated with a grave prognosis. A major consequence of ARDS is hypoxemia. With ARDS, the chest radiograph characteristically shows bilateral and diffuse hazy infiltrates; opacification of all lung fields usually is noted during the late phases of ARDS.

Blood urea nitrogen and serum creatinine concentrations may be elevated. Jones and Weil[80] noted that the ratio of urine to plasma osmolality was the most valuable indicator of renal impairment in adult patients with shock. When this ratio was greater than 1.5, the likelihood of progressive renal failure was remote. A urine osmolality greater than 400 mOsm/kg also indicated adequate renal function. Many white blood cells or white blood cell casts in the urine may suggest the genitourinary tract as the source of bacteremia. If one or more gram-negative rods are seen on the Gram stain of unspun urine, greater than 10^5 colony-forming units per milliliter of bacteria are likely to be present.

Obviously, isolating the organism responsible for bacteremia or septic shock is important for documenting the infection and for providing optimal antimicrobial therapy. Many authorities recommend that a blood culture be obtained in the 3- to 36-month-old child with fever higher than 39° to 40° C and a total white blood cell count greater than or equal to 15,000 cells/mm^3 and without a specific focus of infection. In this way, instances of "unsuspected or outpatient" bacteremia will be identified. When appropriate, cerebrospinal fluid, urine, and other pertinent sites should be cultured prior to initiating antibiotic therapy, if possible. When an intra-abdominal source of infection is likely, blood as well as other cultures should be processed anaerobically. Gram stain or acridine orange stain of a buffy coat smear of peripheral blood may reveal evidence of the causative microorganism, especially in an overwhelming infection.[85] Bacterial polysaccharide antigens can be detected rapidly in many body fluids by latex agglutination tests. Unfortunately, rapid diagnostic procedures for evaluating outpatients with suspected bacteremia are not reliable. Pneumococcal antigenuria is not detected readily when bacteremia occurs without a specific focus of infection. The value of assays for detecting circulating endotoxin is unclear.

TREATMENT

The initial selection of antibiotics for administration to a child with suspected bacteremia is based upon the clinical situation. If untreated initially, children with occult bacteremia are at risk to develop serious complications, such as meningitis or pneumonia.[102, 117] Therefore, empiric antibiotic therapy in children who carefully are selected and followed would seem reasonable.[7] However, two prospective studies of empiric administration of antibiotics in this situation reached different conclusions. Carroll and associates[24] randomly treated children with suspected occult bacteremia with either no antibiotic or 25,000 U/kg of penicillin G benzathine and 25,000 U/kg of penicillin G procaine administered intramuscularly followed by oral penicillin V, 100 mg/kg/day in three or four doses. Four of five children with bacteremia in the expectant treatment group compared with none of five untreated bacteremic children were improved at follow-up ($p < .05$). Four of the five untreated children subsequently developed a local infection, including two with meningitis. In the second study, Jaffe and colleagues[79] randomly treated children with possible occult bacteremia with either a placebo or oral amoxicillin. There were no differences in the incidence of major infectious morbidity associated with bacteremia between the two groups. Differences in the type of expectant antibiotic therapy administered may, in part, explain the opposite conclusions of these studies. Ceftriaxone has been compared with amoxicillin or amoxicillin-clavulanate in two large studies involving children 3 to 36 months of age. Ceftriaxone was marginally superior at best to the oral agents with regard to efficacy.[8, 52]

I favor obtaining a blood culture from children 3 to 36 months of age with a temperature 39° C or higher who have no focal findings and whose peripheral white blood cell count is greater than or equal to 15,000/mm^3. In such patients, the decision to administer antibiotics expectantly may be based on several factors, especially the ability of the parents to observe the child and communicate this information back to the physician in a timely manner. Ceftriaxone parenterally; an oral agent, such as amoxicillin and amoxicillin-clavulanate (if the child has not received two or more conjugate *H. influenzae* type b vaccines); or other oral antibiotics can be administered. If treatment is initiated, a properly collected urine specimen for urinalysis and/or urine culture also should be obtained so that a urinary tract infection will not be treated inadvertently. Occult bacteremia due to *S. pneumoniae* intermediate or resistant to penicillin in an otherwise normal child should resolve with any of the options noted earlier.

Children who subsequently are determined to have *S. pneumoniae* bacteremia and who have been treated with antibiotics expectantly need to be re-evaluated as soon as the results of the blood cultures are known. If the child appears well and has been afebrile for at least 24 hours and the parents can observe the child carefully and are able to communicate frequently with the physician, outpatient management can be continued. Close contact with the parents and patient is mandatory no matter how these children are managed initially. Hospitalization for intravenous antibiotics is indicated if the child appears "toxic" or has other signs suggesting a serious infection.

For children with suspected bacteremia who are ill and thus require admission to the hospital, antibiotics are selected to cover the most serious organisms causing that infection.

In normal children 3 months of age or older, a combination of nafcillin (150 to 200 mg/kg/day) or another semisynthetic antistaphylococcal penicillin plus cefotaxime (150 to 200 mg/kg/day) or ceftriaxone (75 to 100 mg/kg/day) will cover most of the likely pathogens (such as *S. pneumoniae*, *S. aureus*, *S. pyogenes*, *N. meningitidis*, and *H. influenzae* type b). Vancomycin (40 to 60 mg/kg/day) is necessary for infections due to methicillin-resistant *S. aureus*. Bacteremia associated with a genitourinary or gastrointestinal source requires antibiotics to which gram-negative enterics are susceptible. In such cases, initial therapy could consist of an aminoglycoside with an additional antibiotic active against anaerobes for a gastrointestinal focus of infection. Extended-spectrum cephalosporins, such as cefotaxime, are possible alternative drugs for serious gram-negative enteric infections.[82] The optimal management of intra-abdominal or other abscesses usually requires surgical drainage, which should be undertaken as soon as the child's condition allows.

Immunosuppressed children or children with serious illnesses in intensive care settings require a different initial approach to suspected bacteremia. Gram-negative enterics, *P. aeruginosa* and *S. aureus*, are very likely to be isolated from these patients.[3] Empiric therapy of nosocomial infection is based upon the current antibiotic susceptibility pattern within the hospital.[172] In general, a combination of an antistaphylococcal semisynthetic penicillin or vancomycin if a central line is present, an aminoglycoside, and an extended-spectrum penicillin (ticarcillin, piperacillin, mezlocillin) is administered initially until a specific pathogen(s) is isolated.[76] Broad-spectrum penicillins and aminoglycosides frequently exhibit synergy in vitro against gram-negative organisms, especially against *P. aeruginosa*.[87, 156] In the critically ill patient, a synergistic combination of antibiotics is beneficial for treating bacteremia due to *P. aeruginosa* or *Klebsiella* species.[70, 86]

In these patients, it also is important to achieve therapeutic aminoglycoside levels rapidly in the plasma.[114] Therefore, serum concentrations of the aminoglycoside should be measured within 24 hours of initiation of therapy to ensure that therapeutic concentrations have been reached.

The management of endotoxin shock is directed toward three main objectives: (1) control of the infectious process, (2) restoration of adequate tissue perfusion, and (3) maintenance of efficient respiratory function. Details of management have been the subject of numerous reports.[131, 160, 161, 206]

Antibiotics should be administered as soon as the diagnosis of septic shock is suspected. The selection of antibiotics is as for bacteremia.

Restoration of adequate tissue perfusion requires infusions of fluids intravenously. Initially, an isotonic solution, such as 5 per cent dextrose and normal saline or 5 per cent dextrose and lactated Ringer solution, should be infused rapidly at 20 to 40 mL/kg over 15 to 30 minutes. In one study of children presenting in septic shock, the administration of fluid in excess of 40 mL/kg in the first hour in the emergency department was associated with improved survival, decreased occurrence of persistent hypovolemia, and no increased risk of ARDS.[22] Unless the initial fluid administration returns perfusion to normal, all children should have central venous pressure measured to help guide fluid therapy. Urine output should be monitored carefully by bladder catheterization. If hypoproteinemia is documented, albumin or fresh-frozen plasma should be administered with careful monitoring of the central venous pressure. Some individuals may require more than one dose of albumin. If no improvement in blood pressure, urine output, or mental status is noted after the infusion and the central venous pressure has risen less than 5 cm H_2O, additional fluid should be administered. Infusion of isotonic fluids (blood if the hematocrit is < 30 per cent) should be continued at rates sufficient to maintain systolic blood pressure at greater than 80 mm Hg and a urine output greater than 300 mL/m^2/24 hours.

Generally, improvement in mental status accompanies fluid administration. Sodium bicarbonate provided in a dose of 2 to 3 mEq/kg may be helpful if improvement in tissue perfusion with replacement of fluid alone does not correct the metabolic acidosis. A nasogastric tube is inserted so that gastric bleeding can be recognized easily.

When expansion of the extracellular space with fluid administration is not followed by improvement, when central venous pressure increases to more than 5 cm above its initial value or to an absolute value greater than 10 to 15 cm H_2O, or when pulmonary edema develops, the use of vasoactive agents, such as dopamine and dobutamine, may be considered. When such agents are used, optimal management requires careful monitoring of the central venous pressure as well as the pulmonary capillary wedge pressure and cardiac output via pulmonary artery catheterization. The reader is referred to general reviews of the use of vasoactive agents in children for detailed information.[74, 132, 155, 203]

Dopamine is a valuable agent for use in endotoxin shock. Dopamine has beta-adrenergic activity on the myocardium but causes vasodilatation of the renal, coronary, and mesenteric vessels.[44] Blood flow to skeletal muscles is decreased concomitantly. However, dopamine has different effects, depending upon the dose administered. At doses exceeding 10 to 15 μg/kg/minute, dopamine causes peripheral vasoconstriction due to its alpha-adrenergic effects, which may result in both increased systemic vascular resistance and afterload for the heart and decreased urine output. Therefore, dopamine doses between 10 and 15 μg/kg/minute generally are considered optimal for septic shock after smaller doses have been infused initially (2 to 5 μg/kg/minute). Frequently, dobutamine, a cardiac beta-adrenergic agent, is added to the dopamine.[132] Dobutamine increases cardiac contractility without affecting heart rate or vascular tone. The dose of dobutamine is between 2 and 10 μg/kg/minute, depending upon the individual patient's response. Norepinephrine may be useful in treating refractory hypotension in septic shock.[101, 139]

The benefits of therapy with high doses of corticosteroids in the treatment of endotoxin shock remain unproven. Extensive experimental data document the salutary hemodynamic, metabolic, microcirculatory, and cellular effect of steroids in laboratory models of endotoxin shock. Pretreated animals or tissue preparations have been utilized for most of these studies; thus, extrapolation of these data to clinical situations is difficult. Hinshaw and associates[72] have shown that the combination of methylprednisolone, 15 to 30 mg/kg, and gentamicin leads to greater survival ($p < .025$) than gentamicin alone or no therapy in baboons injected with 2 to 3 $\times$ 10^{10} live *E. coli* organisms. In this experiment, therapy was not administered until after the *E. coli* had been infused.

Sprung and colleagues[165] evaluated high-dose corticosteroids in patients with septic shock in a prospective, controlled study. Patients in septic shock were assigned randomly to one of three treatment groups: (1) methylprednisolone sodium succinate, 30 mg/kg; (2) dexamethasone sodium phosphate, 6 mg/kg; and (3) no steroid preparation. If shock persisted, the same dose of steroid was administered in 4 hours. Steroid therapy did result in a greater likelihood of reversal of shock in the first 24 hours after drug administration (26 per cent for steroid-treated patients versus 0 in controls, $p < .05$). In addition, by 133 hours after the drugs were administered, 40 per cent (17 of 43 patients) of steroid-treated patients versus 69 per cent (11 of 16 patients) of the control group had died ($p < .05$). However, the overall survival rate was not changed by the steroid therapy. Although superinfections did occur significantly ($p < .05$) more frequently in corticosteroid-treated patients than in controls, the number of patients at risk for superinfection was diminished in the control group, especially after 2 days following administration of the study drugs.

Two other randomized, controlled multicenter clinical trials of high-dose methylprednisolone in adults with severe sepsis and/or septic shock have been conducted. In both studies, the placebo or corticosteroids were to be administered within 2 hours of the time the patient was considered to have met the entry criteria. In one study, methylprednisolone was administered as a 30 mg/kg dose given every 6 hours for four doses.[17] In the other study, methylprednisolone was administered as an initial 30 mg/kg bolus over 15 minutes followed by a 5 mg/kg/hour constant infusion for 9 hours.[181] In both studies, methylprednisolone did not alter the mortality rates of severe sepsis or septic shock. Reversal or prevention of shock also was not affected. Children were not included in any of these studies.

On the basis of these studies, the routine use of high-dose corticosteroids in children with severe sepsis or septic shock is not recommended.

Every effort should be expended to ensure an adequate airway. This may require periodic suctioning if the patient is unable to clear pooled secretions. A chest radiograph may reveal underlying pneumonia or other pulmonary pathology. Humidified oxygen in concentrations required to maintain an adequate partial pressure of oxygen should be provided early. The method of oxygen administration (mask, ventilator, and so on) will depend upon the clinical state of the patient. Intubation and assisted ventilation are indicated if the child shows evidence of impending respiratory failure.

"Shock lung," usually appearing within 2 days after the onset of shock, may complicate the respiratory and fluid management.[75] Pulmonary edema, atelectasis, decreased pulmonary compliance, and ventilation-perfusion abnormalities are some of the factors that can lead to inadequate oxygenation. Excessive fluid administration may contribute to shock lung. The central venous pressure may remain normal, despite the presence of pulmonary edema. Positive end-expiratory pressure, oxygen, and careful attention to cardiovascular parameters are the mainstays of therapy for ARDS.[75, 136, 150] Steroids are not beneficial once ARDS has been diagnosed.

The general supportive care of the child with septic shock includes attention to nutritional and metabolic requirements.[27, 143] Fluids containing 10 per cent glucose may be necessary to prevent hypoglycemia. Parenteral alimentation may be the only means by which to provide nutrition, although the optimal amount and composition of elemental nutrients for children with septic shock are unknown. Hypocalcemia should be corrected. Platelet transfusions or fresh-frozen plasma may be necessary to correct coagulopathies. Dialysis may be instituted for complications of renal failure, such as fluid overload with pulmonary edema and hyperkalemia.

Investigative Therapies

Antibody to Lipopolysaccharide

Endotoxemia frequently can be documented in patients with gram-negative sepsis. Furthermore, endotoxin is released when bacteria are killed by bactericidal antibiotics.[158] Shenep and associates[159] documented that circulating levels of endotoxin increased shortly after antibiotics were administered to selected children with gram-negative infections. This may help explain why some patients develop shock after parenteral antibiotics are administered.[78] Because endotoxin is responsible directly or through mediators for many of the adverse effects of gram-negative bacteremia, attempts to neutralize endotoxin have been undertaken.

The *E. coli* J5 is a mutant strain that lacks side chains to the core polysaccharide. Thus, the J5 lipopolysaccharide consists of lipid A and other core determinants that are surface exposed. Antibody to the J5 *E. coli* is thought to be broadly reactive with the lipopolysaccharide of a wide variety of gram-negative bacteria, although some studies have questioned the broad-spectrum cross-reactivity by J5 antisera.[63]

Human antisera to *E. coli* J5 mutant harvested from volunteers immunized with *E. coli* J5 in phenol proved to be efficacious in preventing mortality in adults with bacteremia and hypotension or profound shock.[205] However, the antibody titer to *E. coli* J5 was not related conclusively to prevention of mortality. Moreover, human antisera to *E. coli* J5 did not affect the course or mortality of severe infectious purpura (predominantly due to *N. meningitidis*) in children.[77]

Murine and human immunoglobulin monoclonal antibodies to the core-lipid A region of lipopolysaccharide have been developed using the *E. coli* J5 and appear to be broadly reactive with lipid A from other gram-negative organisms.[14, 138] One such murine monoclonal antibody, E-5 (XMMEN-OEJ, XOMA Corp.), is an immunoglobulin antibody that has a serum half-life in humans of 10 to 18 hours, depending upon the dose.[66] In a randomized multicenter trial, patients with gram-negative sepsis received either monoclonal antibody to *E. coli* J5 or placebo, in addition to antibiotics.[62] Mortality was reduced significantly only for patients with gram-negative sepsis without shock. However, a follow-up study focusing on patients with gram-negative sepsis with nonrefractory shock did not demonstrate efficacy.[16] Another multicenter study compared a different human monoclonal immunoglobulin antibody against lipid A HA-1A (Centoxin, Centocor) with human serum albumin in patients with a presumptive diagnosis of gram negative sepsis with hypotension and/or systemic manifestations of infection.[188, 204] Mortality was reduced significantly for patients with gram-negative bacteremia with or without shock who received the human monoclonal antibody. Again, a larger second study of patients with gram-negative bacteremia and septic shock found no efficacy for HA-1A and suggested a greater mortality for patients without gram-negative bacteremia in association with HA-1A.[97] Children were not included in either study, although the pharmacokinetics and safety of HA-1A have been established in children.[147] HA-1A is being evaluated in children with meningococcal disease.

Antibody to TNF-α and recombinant IL-1ra are anticytokine therapies that have undergone evaluation in large clinical trials for adjunctive therapy of adults with sepsis syndrome. Unfortunately, neither measure proved beneficial.[2, 51] It may be that some combination of the antiendotoxin or anticytokine therapies may provide significant benefit in humans with septic shock, as has been demonstrated in animals.[152] Other adjunctive measures that require clinical trials for evaluation include recombinant bactericidal/permeability-increasing protein ($rBPI_{23}$), a human-derived recombinant protein that expresses the amino-terminal half of the whole bactericidal permeability-increasing protein molecule.[112] Using recombinant soluble CD14 is another approach for blocking the action of endotoxin.[68] Inhibition of nitric oxide synthase also has been proposed for patients with septic shock.[134] Carefully designed and conducted clinical trials are necessary to show that any of these adjunctive agents are safe and beneficial in the management of septic shock. A summary of the antiendo-

TABLE 72–4. Antiendotoxin or Anticytokine Therapy for Septic Shock

Therapy	Patient Group		Mortality Rate			p
			Placebo		Agent	
HA-1A[203]	Gram-negative bacteremia	at 14 days	32/95		25/105	.12
		at 28 days	45/92		32/105	.014
	+ shock		27/47		18/54	.017
HA-1A[97]	Gram-negative bacteremia and septic shock	at 14 days	95/293		109/328	.86
	Septic shock without gram-negative bacteremia	at 14 days	292/793		318/785	.07
E-5 monoclonal IgM antibody[62]	Gram-negative sepsis	at 30 days	62/152		62/164	NS
E-5[16]	Gram-negative sepsis, nonrefractory shock		69/266		79/264	NS
Monoclonal antibody to tumor necrosis factor-α[2]	Sepsis syndrome	at 28 days	108/326	95/322[a]	101/323[a]	NS
Recombinant human interleukin-1 receptor antagonist[51]	Sepsis syndrome	at 28 days	102/302	91/298[a]	86/293[a]	NS

[a]Two doses of agents evaluated.

toxin or anticytokine randomized trials in adults is shown in Table 72–4.

Other Potential Adjunctive Therapies

Polymyxin B is an antibiotic that can neutralize endotoxin possibly through a detergent-like action. In experimental models, polymyxin B moderates some of the cardiovascular, metabolic, and lethal consequences of *E. coli* sepsis in rabbits and overwhelming *H. influenzae* type b disease in infant rats, respectively.[53, 185] Clinical studies of polymyxin B have not been conducted in humans with sepsis or septic shock.

Pentoxifylline is a phosphodiesterase inhibitor that now is known to have anti-inflammatory properties, including the ability to suppress endotoxin-induced mononuclear cell production of TNF. Pentoxifylline decreases endotoxin or TNF-induced lung injury as well as increases survival in animals infected with *E. coli* or infused with endotoxin.[91] In a study of human volunteers, a 500-mg dose of pentoxifylline infused 30 minutes before a 100-ng injection of endotoxin from *Salmonella abortus equa* blunted the TNF response but did not affect interleukin-6 serum levels after endotoxin administration.[199] Clinical effects, such as fever, myalgia, and headache, were not affected by pentoxifylline. Clinical studies of pentoxifylline or similar agents are warranted for the adjunctive treatment of sepsis and septic shock.

Plasmapheresis, exchange transfusions, and extracorporeal membrane oxygenation are heroic measures that appear to be beneficial in selected patients not responding to standard management.[9, 38, 57, 200] These procedures may be considered for such patients when in the opinion of experienced clinicians their use is justified and they are the last hope for a successful outcome.

PROGNOSIS

The morbidity and mortality of septic shock in children vary with age, the presence or absence of underlying diseases, and the specific microorganisms responsible for the septicemic state. Dupont and Spink[45] noted a 98 per cent mortality in their series of children with septic shock and gram-negative bacteremia. Jacobs and colleagues[78] reported a 9.8 per cent case fatality rate for otherwise normal children with septic shock. In the pediatric HA-1A study, the overall mortality for severe sepsis or septic shock was 31 per cent.[147] As with many infections, prevention obviously is more desirable than treatment. Careful attention to sterile techniques for insertion and maintenance of intravascular or other lines, as well as other procedures, is critically important and may prevent some episodes of bacteremia and septic shock.

References

1. Abraham, E., Bland, R. D., Cobo, J. C., et al.: Sequential cardiorespiratory patterns associated with outcome in septic shock. Chest *85*:75–80, 1984.
2. Abraham, E., Wunderink, R., Silverman, H., et al.: Efficacy and safety of monoclonal antibody to human tumor necrosis factor α in patients with sepsis syndrome: A randomized, controlled, double-blind, multicenter clinical trial. J. A. M. A. *273*:934–941, 1995.
3. Albano, E. A., and Pizzo, P. A.: Infectious complications in childhood acute leukemias. Pediatr. Clin. North Am. *35*:873–901, 1988.
4. Anderson, R. R., Holliday, R. L., Driedger, A. A., et al.: Documentation of pulmonary capillary permeability in the adult respiratory distress syndrome accompanying human sepsis. Am. Rev. Respir. Dis. *119*:869–877, 1979.
5. Archer, L. T., Benjamin, B. A., Beller-Todd, B. K., et al.: Does LD_{100} *E. coli* shock cause myocardial failure? Cir. Shock *9*:7–16, 1982.
6. Banks, J. G., Foulis, A. K., Ledingham, I. M., et al.: Liver function in septic shock. J. Clin. Pathol. *35*:1249–1252, 1982.
7. Baraff, L. J., Bass, J. W., Fleisher, G. R., et al.: Practice guideline for the management of infants and children 0 to 36 months of age with fever without source. Pediatrics *92*:1–12, 1993.
8. Bass, J. W., Steele, R. W., Wittler, R. R., et al.: Antimicrobial treatment of occult bacteremia: A multicenter cooperative study. Pediatr. Infect. Dis. J. *12*:466–473, 1993.
9. Beca, J., and Butt, W.: Extracorporeal membrane oxygenation for refractory septic shock in children. Pediatrics *93*:726–729, 1994.
10. Beutler, B. A., Milsark, I. W., and Cerami, A.: Cachectin/tumor necrosis factor: Production, distribution, and metabolic fate in vivo. J. Immunol. *135*:3972–3977, 1985.
11. Blain, C. M., Anderson, T. O., Pietras, R. J., et al.: Immediate hemodynamic effects of gram-negative vs. gram-positive bacteremia in man. Arch. Intern. Med. *126*:260–265, 1970.
12. Blair, E.: Hypocapnea and gram-negative bacteremic shock. Am. Surg. J. *119*:433–438, 1970.
13. Blair, E.: Acid-base balance in bacteremic shock. Arch. Intern. Med. *127*:731–739, 1971.
14. Bogard, W. C., Jr., Dunn, D. L., Abernathy, K., et al.: Isolation and characterization of murine monoclonal antibodies specific for gram-negative bacterial lipopolysaccharide: Association of cross-genus reactivity with lipid A specificity. Infect. Immun. *55*:899–908, 1987.
15. Bone, R. C., Balk, R. A., Cerra, F. B., et al.: Definitions for sepsis and

organ failure and guidelines for the use of innovative therapies in sepsis. Chest *101*:1644–1655, 1992.
16. Bone, R. C., Balk, R. A., Fein, A. M., et al.: A second large controlled clinical study of E5, a monoclonal antibody to endotoxin: Results of a prospective, multicenter, randomized, controlled trial: The E5 sepsis study group. Crit. Care Med. *23*:994–1006, 1995.
17. Bone, R. C., Fisher, C. J., Jr., Clemmer, T. P., et al.: A controlled clinical trial of high-dose methylprednisolone in the treatment of severe sepsis and septic shock. N. Engl. J. Med. *317*:653–658, 1987.
18. Brigham, K. L., and Meyrick, B.: Endotoxin and lung injury. Am. Rev. Respir. Dis. *133*:913–927, 1986.
19. Buck, C., Bundschu, J., Gallati, H., et al.: Interleukin-6: A sensitive parameter for early diagnosis of neonatal bacterial infection. Pediatrics *93*:54–58, 1994.
20. Calandra, T., Baumgartner, J. D., Grau, G. E., et al.: Prognostic values of tumor necrosis factor/cachectin, interleukin-1, interferon-alpha, and interferon-gamma in the serum of patients with septic shock. J. Infect. Dis. *161*:982–987, 1990.
21. Cannon, J. G., Tompkins, R. G., Gelfand, J. A., et al.: Circulating interleukin-1 and tumor necrosis factor in septic shock and experimental endotoxin fever. J. Infect. Dis. *161*:79–84, 1990.
22. Carcillo, J. A., Davis, A. L., and Zaritsky, A.: Role of early fluid resuscitation in pediatric septic shock. J. A. M. A. *266*:1242–1245, 1991.
23. Cardenas-Rivero, N., Chernow, B., Stoiko, M. A., et al.: Hypocalcemia in critically ill children. J. Pediatr. *114*:946–951, 1989.
24. Carroll, W. L., Farrell, M. K., Singer, J. L., et al.: Treatment of occult bacteremia: A prospective randomized clinical trial. Pediatrics *72*:608–612, 1983.
25. Chesney, R. W., McCarron, D. M., Haddad, J. G., et al.: Pathogenic mechanisms of the hypocalcemia of the staphylococcal toxic-shock syndrome. J. Lab. Clin. Med. *101*:576–585, 1983.
26. Clowes, G. H. A., George, B. C., Villee, C. A., et al.: Muscle proteolysis induced by a circulating peptide in patients with sepsis or trauma. N. Engl. J. Med. *308*:545–552, 1983.
27. Clowes, G. H. A., Heidman, M., Lindberg, B., et al.: Effects of parenteral alimentation on amino acid metabolism in septic patients. Surgery *88*:531–543, 1980.
28. Clowes, G. H. A., O'Donnell, T. F., Ryan, V. T., et al.: Energy metabolism in sepsis: Treatment based on different patterns in shock and high output stage. Ann. Surg. *179*:684–696, 1974.
29. Coalson, J. J., Archer, L. T., Hall, N. K., et al.: Prolonged shock in the monkey following live *E. coli* organism infusion. Circ. Shock *6*:343–355, 1979.
30. Corrigan, J. J.: Thrombocytopenia: A laboratory sign of septicemia in infants and children. J. Pediatr. *85*:219–221, 1974.
31. Corrigan, J. J.: Disseminated intravascular coagulopathy. Pediatrics *64*:37–45, 1979.
32. Corrigan, J. J.: Vitamin K–dependent coagulation factors in gram-negative septicemia. Am. J. Dis. Child. *138*:240–242, 1984.
33. Corrigan, J. J., and Jordan, C. M.: Heparin therapy in septicemia with disseminated intravascular coagulation. N. Engl. J. Med. *283*:778–782, 1970.
34. Corrigan, J. J., Ray, W. L., and May, N.: Changes in the blood coagulation system associated with septicemia. N. Engl. J. Med. *279*:851–856, 1968.
35. Cryer, P. E., Coran, A. G., Soda, J., et al.: Lethal *Escherichia coli* septicemia in the baboon: Alpha-adrenergic inhibition in insulin secretion and its relationship to the duration of survival. J. Lab. Clin. Med. *79*:622–638, 1972.
36. Dantzsker, D. R., Brook, C. J., Hebart, P., et al.: Ventilation-perfusion distributions in the adult respiratory distress syndrome. Am. Rev. Respir. Dis. *120*:1039–1052, 1979.
37. DeBont, E. S. J. M., Raan, M. J., Samson, G., et al.: Tumor necrosis factor–α, interleukin-1β, and interleukin-6 plasma levels in neonatal sepsis. Pediatr. Res. *33*:330–383, 1993.
38. Deuren, M., Santman, F. W., Dalen, R., et al.: Plasma and whole blood exchange in meningococcal sepsis. Clin. Infect. Dis. *15*:424–430, 1992.
39. Deuren, M., Ven-Jongekrijg, J., Bartelink, A. K. M., et al.: Correlation between proinflammatory cytokines and antiinflammatory mediators and severity of disease in meningococcal infections. J. Infect. Dis. *172*:433–439, 1995.
40. Deuren, M., Ven-Jongekrijg, J., Demacker, P. N. M., et al.: Differential expression of proinflammatory cytokines and their inhibitors during the course of meningococcal infections. J. Infect. Dis. *169*:157–161, 1994.
41. Deventer, S. J. H. V., Bulter, H. R., Cate, J. W. T., et al.: Endotoxaemia: An early predictor of septicaemia in febrile patients. Lancet *1*:605–609, 1988.
42. Dinarello, C. A.: Interleukin-1 and its biologically related cytokines. Adv. Immunol. *44*:153–203, 1989.
43. Dinarello, C. A., and Wolff, S. M.: The role of interleukin-1 in disease. N. Engl. J. Med. *328*:106–113, 1993.
44. Driscoll, D. J., Gillette, P. C., and McNamara, D. G.: The use of dopamine in children. J. Pediatr. *92*:309–314, 1978.
45. Dupont, H. L., and Spink, W. W.: Infections due to gram-negative organisms: An analysis of 860 patients with bacteremia at the University of Minnesota Medical Center, 1958–1966. Medicine *48*:307–332, 1969.
46. Edwards, M. S., and Baker, C. J.: Complications and sequelae of meningococcal infections in children. J. Pediatr. *99*:540–545, 1981.
47. Farley, M. M., Stephens, D. S., Mulks, M. H., et al.: Pathogenesis of IgA1 protease producing and non producing *Haemophilus influenzae* in human nasopharyngeal organ cultures. J. Infect. Dis. *154*:752–759, 1986.
48. Fearson, D. T., Ruddy, S., Schur, P. H., et al.: Activation of the properdin pathway of complement in patients with gram-negative bacteremia. N. Engl. J. Med. *292*:937–940, 1975.
49. Fenton, L. J., and Strunk, R. C.: Complement activation and group B streptococcal infection in the newborn: Similarities to endotoxin shock. Pediatrics *60*:901–907, 1977.
50. Filkins, J. P., and Cornell, R. P.: Depression of hepatic gluconeogenesis and the hypoglycemia of endotoxin shock. Am. J. Physiol. *227*:778–781, 1974.
51. Fisher, C. J., Dhainaut, J.-F. A., Opal, S. M., et al.: Recombinant human interleukin 1 receptor antagonist in the treatment of patients with sepsis syndrome: Results from a randomized, double-blind, placebo-controlled trial. J. A. M. A. *271*:1836–1843, 1995.
52. Fleisher, G. R., Rosenberg, N., Vinci, R., et al.: Intramuscular versus oral antibiotic therapy for the prevention of meningitis and other bacterial sequelae in young, febrile children at risk for occult bacteremia. J. Pediatr. *124*:504–512, 1994.
53. Flynn, P. M., Shenep, J. L., Stokes, D. C., et al.: Polymyxin B moderates acidosis and hypotension in established experimental gram-negative septicemia. J. Infect. Dis. *156*:706–712, 1987.
54. Freund, H. R., Ryan, J. A., and Fischer, J. E.: Amino acid derangements in patients with sepsis. Ann. Surg. *188*:423–430, 1978.
55. Froon, A. H. M., Dentener, M. A., Greve, J. W. M., et al.: Lipopolysaccharide toxicity-regulating proteins in bacteremia. J. Infect. Dis. *171*:1250–1257, 1995.
56. Gallin, J. I., Kaye, D., and O'Leary, W. M.: Serum lipids in infections. N. Engl. J. Med. *281*:1081–1086, 1969.
57. Garlund, B., Sjölin, J., Nilsson, A., et al.: Plasmapheresis in the treatment of primary septic shock in humans. Scand. J. Infect. Dis. *25*:757–761, 1993.
58. Girardin, E., Grau, G. E., Dayer, J. M., et al.: Tumor necrosis factor and interleukin-1 in the serum of children with severe infectious purpura. N. Engl. J. Med. *319*:397–400, 1988.
59. Godin, D. V., Wright, J. M., Tuchek, J. M., et al.: Plasma lysosomal enzymes in experimental and clinical endotoxemia. Clin. Invest. Med. *6*:319–325, 1983.
60. Goldie, A. S., Fearon, K. C. H., Ross, J. A., et al.: Natural cytokine antagonists and endogenous antiendotoxin core antibodies in sepsis syndrome. J. A. M. A. *274*:172–177, 1995.
61. Graham, D. L., Behan, P. O., and More, I. A. R.: Brain damage complicating septic shock: Acute hemorrhagic leukoencephalitis as a complication of the generalized Schwartzman reaction. J. Neurol. Neurosurg. Psychiatr. *42*:19–28, 1979.
62. Greenman, R. L., Schein, R. M., Martin, M. A., et al.: A controlled clinical trial of E5 murine monoclonal IgM antibody to endotoxin in the treatment of gram-negative sepsis. J. A. M. A. *266*:1097–1102, 1991.
63. Greisman, S. E., and Johnston, C. A.: Failure of antisera to J5 and R595 rough mutants to reduce endotoxemic lethality. J. Infect. Dis. *157*:54–64, 1988.
64. Hack, C. E., Hart, M., Strack, R. J. M., et al.: Interleukin-8 in sepsis: Relation to shock and inflammatory mediators. Infect. Immun. *60*:2835–2842, 1992.
65. Hammerschmidt, D. E., Weaver, L. J., Hudson, L. D., et al.: Association of complement activation and elevated plasma-C5a with adult respiratory distress syndrome: Pathophysiologic relevance and possible prognostic value. Lancet *1*:947–949, 1980.
66. Harkonen, S., Scannon, P., Mischak, R. P., et al.: Phase I study of a murine monoclonal antilipid A antibody in bacteremic and nonbacteremic patients. Antimicrob. Agents Chemother. *32*:710–716, 1988.
67. Hayden, W. R.: Sepsis terminology in pediatrics. J. Pediatr. *124*:657–658, 1993.
68. Haziot, A., Rong, G. W., Lin, X.-Y., et al.: Recombinant soluble CD14 prevents mortality in mice treated with endotoxin (lipopolysaccharide). J. Immunol. *154*:6529–6532, 1995.
69. Hesse, D. G., Tracey, K. J., Fong, Y., et al.: Cytokine appearance in human endotoxemia and primate bacteremia. Surg. Gynecol. Obstet. *166*:147–153, 1988.
70. Hilf, M., Yu, V. L., Sharp, J., et al.: Antibiotic therapy for *Pseudomonas aeruginosa* bacteremia: Outcome correlations in a prospective study of 200 patients. Am. J. Med. *87*:540–546, 1989.
71. Hill, S. L., Eblings, V. B., and Lewis, F. R.: Changes in lung water and capillary permeability following sepsis and fluid overload. J. Surg. Res. *28*:140–150, 1980.
72. Hinshaw, L. B., Beller-Todd, B. K., Archer, L. T., et al.: Effectiveness of steroid/antibiotic treatment in primates administered LD_{100} *Escherichia coli*. Ann. Surg. *194*:51–56, 1981.
73. Hinshaw, L. B., Tekamp-Olson, P., Chang, A. C. K., et al.: Survival of primates in LD_{100} septic shock following therapy with antibody to tumor necrosis factor (TNF). Circ. Shock *30*:279–292, 1990.
74. Holbrook, P. R., Mickell, J., Pollack, M. M., et al.: Cardiovascular resuscitation drugs for children. Crit. Care Med. *8*:77–78, 1980.

75. Holbrook, P. R., Taylor, G., Pollack, M. M., et al.: Adult respiratory distress syndrome in children. Pediatr. Clin. North Am. *27*:677–685, 1980.
76. Hughes, W. T., Armstrong, D., Bodey, G. P., et al.: Guidelines for the use of antimicrobial agents in neutropenic patients with unexplained fever. J. Infect. Dis. *161*:381–396, 1990.
77. J5 Study Group: Treatment of severe infectious purpura in children with human plasma from donors immunized with *Escherichia coli* J5: A prospective double-blind study. J. Infect. Dis. *165*:695–701, 1992.
78. Jacobs, R. F., Sowell, M. K., Moss, M. M., et al.: Septic shock in children: Bacterial etiologies and temporal relationships. Pediatr. Infect. Dis. J. *9*:196–200, 1990.
79. Jaffe, D. M., Tanz, R. R., Davis, A. T., et al.: Antibiotic administration to treat possible occult bacteremia in febrile children. N. Engl. J. Med. *317*:1175–1180, 1987.
80. Jones, L. W., and Weil, M. H.: Water, creatinine and sodium excretion following circulatory shock with renal failure. Am. J. Med. *51*:314–318, 1971.
81. Kalter, E. S., Daha, M. R., Cate, J. W. T., et al.: Activation and inhibition of Hageman factor–dependent pathways and the complement system in uncomplicated bacteremia or bacterial shock. J. Infect. Dis. *151*:1019–1027, 1985.
82. Kaplan, S. L.: Serious pediatric infections. Am. J. Med. *88*(Suppl. 4A):18S–24S, 1990.
83. Kaplan, S. L., Taber, L. H., Frank, A. L., et al.: Nasopharyngeal viral isolates in children with *Haemophilus influenzae* type b meningitis. J. Pediatr. *99*:591–593, 1981.
84. Kaufmann, R. L., Matson, C. F., and Beisel, W. R.: Hypertriglyceridemia produced by endotoxin: Role of impaired triglyceride disposal mechanisms. J. Infect. Dis. *133*:548–555, 1976.
85. Kleiman, M. B., Reynolds, J. K., Schreiner, R. L., et al.: Rapid diagnosis of neonatal bacteremia with acridine orange–stained buffy coat smears. J. Pediatr. *105*:419–421, 1984.
86. Korvick, J. A., Bryan, C. S., Farber, B., et al.: Prospective observational study of *Klebsiella* bacteremia in 230 patients: Outcome for antibiotic combinations versus monotherapy. Antimicrob. Agents Chemother. *36*:2639–2644, 1992.
87. Lau, W. K., Young, L. S., Black, R. E., et al.: Comparative efficacy and toxicity of amikacin/carbenicillin versus gentamicin/carbenicillin in leukopenic patients: A randomized prospective trial. Am. J. Med. *62*:959–966, 1977.
88. Levi, M., ten Cate, H., Poll, T., et al.: Pathogenesis of disseminated intravascular coagulation in sepsis. J. A. M. A. *270*:975–979, 1993.
89. Levin, J., Poore, T. E., Young, N. S., et al.: Gram-negative sepsis: Detection of endotoxemia with the Limulus test. Ann. Intern. Med. *76*:1–7, 1972.
90. Levin, J., Poore, T. E., Zauber, N. P., et al.: Detection of endotoxin in the blood of patients with sepsis due to gram-negative bacteria. N. Engl. J. Med. *283*:1313–1316, 1970.
91. Lilly, C. M., Sandhu, J. S., Ishizaka, A., et al.: Pentoxifylline prevents tumor necrosis factor–induced lung injury. Am. Rev. Respir. Dis. *139*:1361–1368, 1989.
92. Loegering, D. J.: RES uptake of red blood cell stroma: Time course of effects on phagocytic function and susceptibility to endotoxin shock. Circ. Shock *11*:319–327, 1983.
93. Lorente, J. A., Garcia-Frade, L. J., Landin, L., et al.: Time course of hemostatic abnormalities in sepsis and its relation to outcome. Chest *103*:1536–1542, 1993.
94. McCabe, M. R.: Serum complement levels in bacteremia due to gram-negative organisms. N. Engl. J. Med. *288*:21–23, 1973.
95. McCarthy, P. L.: Controversies in pediatrics: What tests are indicated for the child under 2 with fever? Pediatr. Rev. *1*:51–56, 1979.
96. McCartney, A. C., Banks, J. G., Clements, G. B., et al.: Endotoxemia in septic shock: Clinical and post-mortem correlations. Intensive Care Med. *9*:117–122, 1983.
97. McCloskey, R. V., Straube, R. C., Sanders, C., et al.: Treatment of septic shock with human monoclonal antibody HA-1A: A randomized, double-blind, placebo-controlled trial. Ann. Intern. Med. *121*:1–5, 1994.
98. McConn, R., Greineder, J. K., Wasserman, F., et al.: Is there a humoral factor that depresses ventricular function in sepsis? Circ. Shock *1*(Suppl.):9–27, 1979.
99. Mallet, E., Lanse, X., Devaux, A. M., et al.: Hypercalcitoninaemia in fulminant meningococcaemia in children. Lancet *1*:294, 1983.
100. Marchant, A., Devière, J., Byl, B., et al.: Interleukin-10 production during septicemia. Lancet *343*:707–708, 1994.
101. Marik, P. E., and Mohedin, M.: The contrasting effects of dopamine and norepinephrine on systemic and splanchnic oxygen utilization in hyperdynamic sepsis. J. A. M. A. *272*:1354–1357, 1994.
102. Marshall, R., Teele, D. W., and Klein, J. O.: Unsuspected bacteremia due to *Haemophilus influenzae*: Outcome in children not initially admitted to hospital. J. Pediatr. *95*:690–695, 1979.
103. Mason, J. W., Kleeberg, V., Dolan, P., et al.: Plasma kallikrein and Hageman factor in gram-negative bacteremia. Ann. Intern. Med. *73*:545–551, 1970.
104. Matuschak, G. M., and Rinaldo, J. E.: Organ interactions in the adult respiratory distress syndrome during sepsis: Role of the liver in host defense. Chest *94*:400–406, 1988.
105. Meyer, J., Traber, L. D., Nelson, S., et al.: Reversal of hyperdynamic response to continuous endotoxin administration by inhibition of NO synthesis. J. Appl. Physiol. *73*:324–328, 1992.
106. Michaels, R. H., Myerowitz, R. L., and Klaw, R.: Potentiation of experimental meningitis due to *Haemophilus influenzae* by influenza A virus. J. Infect. Dis. *135*:641–645, 1977.
107. Michie, H. R., Manoque, K. R., Spriggs, D. R., et al.: Detection of circulating tumor necrosis factor after endotoxin administration. N. Engl. J. Med. *318*:1481–1486, 1988.
108. Miller, R. L., Reichgott, M. J., and Melmon, K. L.: Biochemical mechanisms of generation of bradykinin by endotoxin. J. Infect. Dis. *128*(Suppl.):144–156, 1973.
109. Miller, S. I., Wallace, R. J., Musher, D. M., et al.: Hypoglycemia as a manifestation of sepsis. Am. J. Med. *68*:649–654, 1980.
110. Mizock, B.: Septic shock: A metabolic perspective. Arch. Intern. Med. *144*:579–585, 1984.
111. Mizock, B. A., Sabelli, H. C., Dubin, A., et al.: Septic encephalopathy. Evidence for altered phenylalanine metabolism and comparison with hepatic encephalopathy. Arch. Intern. Med. *150*:443–449, 1990.
112. Möhlen, M. A. M., Kimmings, A. N., Wedel, N. I., et al.: Inhibition of endotoxin-induced cytokine release and neutrophil activation in humans by use of recombinant bactericidal/permeability-increasing protein. J. Infect. Dis. *172*:144–151, 1995.
113. Moncada, S., and Higgs, A.: The L-arginine–nitric oxide pathway. N. Engl. J. Med. *329*:2002–2012, 1993.
114. Moore, R. D., Smith, C. R., and Lietman, P. S.: The association of aminoglycoside plasma levels with mortality in patients with gram-negative bacteremia. J. Infect. Dis. *199*:443–448, 1984.
115. Munford, R. S., and Hall, C. L.: Detoxification of bacterial lipopolysaccharides (endotoxins) by a human neutrophil enzyme. Science *234*:203–205, 1986.
116. Musher, D. M.: Cutaneous and soft-tissue manifestations of sepsis due to gram-negative enteric bacilli. Rev. Infect. Dis. *2*:854–866, 1980.
117. Myers, M. G., Wright, P. F., Smith, A. L., et al.: Complications of occult pneumococcal bacteremia in children. J. Pediatr. *84*:656–660, 1974.
118. Naqvi, S. H., Chundu, K. R., and Friedman, A. D.: Shock in children with gram-negative bacillary sepsis and *Haemophilus influenzae* type b sepsis. Pediatr. Infect. Dis. *5*:512–515, 1986.
119. Natanson, C., Fink, M. P., Ballantyne, H. K., et al.: Gram-negative bacteremia produces both severe systolic and diastolic cardiac dysfunction in a canine model that simulates human septic shock. J. Clin. Invest. *78*:259–270, 1986.
120. Natanson, C., Hoffman, W. D., Suffredini, A. F., et al.: Selected treatment strategies for septic shock based on proposed mechanisms of pathogenesis. Ann. Intern. Med. *120*:771–783, 1994.
121. National Center for Health Statistics: Increase in national hospital discharge survey rates for septicemia: United States, 1979–1987. M. M. W. R. 39:31–34, 1990.
122. Nguyen, Q. V., Nguyen, E. A., and Weiner, L. B.: Incidence of invasive bacterial disease in children with fever and petechiae. Pediatrics *74*:77–80, 1984.
123. Nishijima, J., Weil, M. H., Subin, H., et al.: Hemodynamic and metabolic studies on shock associated with gram-negative bacteremia. Medicine *52*:287–294, 1973.
124. Ognibene, F. P., Martin, S. E., Parker, M. M., et al.: Adult respiratory distress syndrome in patients with severe neutropenia. N. Engl. J. Med. *315*:547–551, 1986.
125. Ognibene, F. P., Parker, M. M., Natanson, C., et al.: Depressed left ventricular performance: Response to volume infusion in patients with sepsis and septic shock. Chest *93*:903–910, 1988.
126. Parker, M. M., and Parillo, J. E.: Septic shock: Hemodynamics and pathogenesis. J. A. M. A. *250*:3324–3327, 1983.
127. Parker, M. M., Shelhamer, J. H., Bacharach, S. L., et al.: Profound but reversible myocardial depression in patients with septic shock. Ann. Intern. Med. *100*:483–490, 1984.
128. Parrillo, J. E., Burch, C., Shelhamer, J. H., et al.: A circulating myocardial depressant substance in humans with septic shock: Septic shock patients with a reduced ejection fraction have a circulating factor that depresses *in vitro* myocardial cell performance. J. Clin. Invest. *76*:1539–1553, 1985.
129. Patrick, C. C.: Coagulase-negative staphylococci: Pathogens with increasing clinical significance. J. Pediatr. *116*:497–507, 1990.
130. Perkin, R. M., and Levin, D. L.: Shock in the pediatric patient. Pt. I. J. Pediatr. *101*:163–169, 1982.
131. Perkin, R. M., and Levin, D. L.: Shock in the pediatric patient. Pt. II. Therapy. J. Pediatr. *101*:319–332, 1982.
132. Perkin, R. M., Levin, D. L., Webb, R., et al.: Dobutamine: A hemodynamic evaluation in children with shock. J. Pediatr. *101*:977–983, 1982.
133. Peters, G., Locci, R., and Pulverer, G.: Adherence and growth of coagulase-negative staphylococci on surfaces of intravenous catheters. J. Infect. Dis. *146*:479–482, 1982.
134. Petros, A., Bennett, D., and Vallance, P.: Effect of nitric oxide synthase inhibitors on hypotension in patients with septic shock. Lancet *338*:1557–1558, 1991.
135. Pfeffer, K., Matsuyama, T., Kundig, T. M., et al.: Mice deficient for the 55-

kD tumor necrosis factor receptor are resistant to endotoxic shock, yet succumb to *L. monocytogenes* infection. Cell *73*:457–467, 1993.

136. Pfenniger, J., Gerber, A., Tschappeler, H., et al.: Adult respiratory distress syndrome in children. J. Pediatr. *101*:352–357, 1982.
137. Poll, T. V. D., Büller, H. R., Cate, H. T., et al.: Activation of coagulation after administration of tumor necrosis factor to normal subjects. N. Engl. J. Med. *322*:1622–1627, 1990.
138. Pollack, M., Raubitschek, A. A., and Larrick, J. W.: Human monoclonal antibodies that recognize conserved epitopes in the core–lipid A region of lipopolysaccharides. J. Clin. Invest. *79*:1421–1430, 1987.
139. Quezado, Z. M. N., and Natanson, C.: Systemic hemodynamic abnormalities and vasopressor therapy in sepsis and septic shock. Am J. Kid. Dis. *20*:214–222, 1992.
140. Raymond, R. M., and Emerson, T. E.: Cerebral metabolism during endotoxin shock in the dog. Circ. Shock *5*:407–414, 1978.
141. Reichgott, M. L., Melmon, K. L., Forsyth, R. P., et al.: Cardiovascular and metabolic effects of whole or fractionated gram-negative bacterial endotoxin in the unanesthetized rhesus monkey. Circ. Res. *33*:346–352, 1973.
142. Reilly, J. M., Cunnion, R. E., Burch-Whitman, C., et al.: A circulating myocardial depressant substance is associated with cardiac dysfunction and peripheral hypoperfusion (lactic acidemia) in patients with septic shock. Chest *95*:1072–1080, 1989.
143. Reimer, S. L., Michener, W. M., and Steiger, E.: Nutritional support of the critically ill child. Pediatr. Clin. North Am. *27*:647–660, 1980.
144. Reines, H. D., Cook, J. A., Halushka, P. V., et al.: Plasma thromboxane concentrations are raised in patients dying with septic shock. Lancet *11*:174–175, 1982.
145. Richmond, D. A., Molitch, M. E., and O'Donnell, T. F.: Altered thyroid hormone levels in bacterial sepsis: The role of nutritional adequacy. Metabolism *29*:936–942, 1980.
146. Robbins, R. A., Russ, W. D., Rasmussen, J. K., et al.: Activation of the complement system in the adult respiratory distress syndrome. Am. Rev. Respir. Dis. *135*:651–658, 1987.
147. Romano, M. J., Kearns, G. L., Kaplan, S. L., et al.: Single-dose pharmacokinetics and safety of HA-1A, a human IgM anti–lipid-A monoclonal antibody, in pediatric patients with sepsis syndrome. J. Pediatr. *122*:974–981, 1993.
148. Rothbrock, G., Smithee, L., Rado, M., et al.: Progress toward elimination of *Haemophilus influenzae* type b disease among infants and children: United States, 1993–1994. M. M. W. R. *44*:545–550, 1995.
149. Royall, J. P., and Levin, D. L.: Adult respiratory distress syndrome in pediatric patients. 1. Clinical aspects, pathophysiology, pathology, and mechanisms of lung injury. J. Pediatr. *112*:169–180, 1988.
150. Royall, J. A., and Levin, D. L.: Adult respiratory distress syndrome in pediatric patients. II. Management. J. Pediatr. *112*:335–347, 1988.
151. Rubin, L. G., and Moxon, E. R.: Pathogenesis of bloodstream invasion with *Haemophilus influenzae* type b. Infect. Immun. *41*:280–284, 1983.
152. Russell, D. A., Tucker, K. K., Chinookoswong, N., et al.: Combined inhibition of interleukin-1 and tumor necrosis factor in rodent endotoxemia: Improved survival and organ function. J. Infect. Dis. *171*:1528–1538, 1995.
153. Sáez-Llorens, X., and McCracken, G. H., Jr.: Sepsis syndrome and septic shock in pediatrics: Current concepts of terminology, pathophysiology, and management. J. Pediatr. *123*:497–508, 1993.
154. Schmyer, J. P., Reynolds, D. G., and Swan, K. G.: Renal blood flow during endotoxin shock in the subhuman primate. Surg. Gynecol. Obstet. *137*:3–6, 1973.
155. Seri, I.: Cardiovascular, renal, and endocrine actions of dopamine in neonates and children. J. Pediatr. *126*:333–344, 1995.
156. Shales, D. M., and Bass, S. N.: Combination antimicrobial therapy. Pediatr. Clin. North Am. *30*:121–134, 1983.
157. Shapiro, E. D., Wald, E. R., Nelson, K. A., et al.: Broviac catheter–related bacteremia in oncology patients. Am. J. Dis. Child. *136*:679–681, 1982.
158. Shenep, J. L., Barton, R. P., and Mogan, K. A.: Role of antibiotic class in the rate of liberation of endotoxin during therapy for experimental gram-negative bacterial sepsis. J. Infect. Dis. *151*:1012–1018, 1985.
159. Shenep, J. L., Flynn, P. M., Barrett, F. F., et al.: Serial quantitation of endotoxemia and bacteremia during therapy for gram-negative bacterial sepsis. J. Infect. Dis. *157*:565–568, 1988.
160. Shine, K. I., Kuhn, M., Young, L. S., et al.: Aspects of the management of shock. Ann. Intern. Med. *93*:723–734, 1980.
161. Shubin, H., and Weil, M. H.: Bacterial shock. J. A. M. A. *235*:421–424, 1976.
162. Shulman, S. T., and Ayoub, E. M.: Severe staphylococcal sepsis in adolescents. Pediatrics *58*:59–66, 1976.
163. Siber, G. R.: Bacteremias due to *Haemophilus influenzae* and *Streptococcus pneumoniae*. Their occurrence and course in children with cancer. Am. J. Dis. Child. *134*:668–672, 1980.
164. Smith, A. L.: Commentary: The febrile infant. Pediatr. Rev. *1*:35–36, 1979.
165. Sprung, C. L., Caralis, P. V., Marcial, E. H., et al.: The effects of high-dose corticosteroids in patients with septic shock: A prospective, controlled study. N. Engl. J. Med. *311*:1137–1143, 1984.
166. Stephens, D. S., Hoffman, L. H., and McGee, Z. A.: Interaction of *Neisseria meningitidis* with human nasopharyngeal mucosa: Attachment and entry into columnar epithelial cells. J. Infect. Dis. *148*:369–376, 1983.
167. Stumacher, R. J., Kovnat, M. J., and McCabe, W. R.: Limitations of the usefulness of the Limulus assay for endotoxin. N. Engl. J. Med. *288*:1261–1264, 1973.
168. Suffredini, A. F., Fromm, R. E., Parker, M. M., et al.: The cardiovascular response of normal humans to the administration of endotoxin. N. Engl. J. Med. *321*:280–287, 1989.
169. Sullivan, J. S., Kilpatrick, L., Costarino, A. T., et al.: Correlation of plasma cytokine elevations with mortality rate in children with sepsis. J. Pediatr. *120*:510–515, 1992.
170. Todd, J., Fishant, M., Kapral, F., et al.: Toxic-shock syndrome associated with phage-group I staphylococci. Lancet *2*:1116–1118, 1978.
171. Togari, H., Sugiyama, S., Ogino, T., et al.: Interactions of endotoxin with cortisol and acute phase proteins in septic shock neonates. Acta Paediatr. Scand. *75*:69–74, 1986.
172. Toltzis, P., and Blumer, J. L.: Antibiotic-resistant gram-negative bacteria in the critical care setting. Pediatr. Clin. North Am. *42*:687–702, 1995.
173. Tracey, K. J., Beutler, B., Lowry, S. F., et al.: Shock and tissue injury induced by recombinant human cachectin. Science *234*:470–474, 1986.
174. Tracey, K. J., and Cerami, A.: Tumor necrosis factor: An updated review of its biology. Crit. Care Med. *21*:5415–5422, 1993.
175. Tracey, K. J., Fong, Y., Hesse, D. G., et al.: Anti-cachectin/TNF monoclonal antibodies prevent septic shock during lethal bacteraemia. Nature *330*:662–664, 1987.
176. Tracey, K. J., Lowry, S. F., and Cerami, A.: Cachectin: A hormone that triggers acute shock and chronic cachexia. J. Infect. Dis. *157*:413–420, 1988.
177. Tracey, K. J., Lowry, S. F., Fahey, T. J., III, et al.: Cachectin/tumor necrosis factor induces lethal shock and stress hormone responses in the dog. Surg. Gynecol. Obstet. *164*:415–422, 1987.
178. Tracey, K. J., Vlassara, H., and Cerami, A.: Cachectin/tumor necrosis factor. Lancet *1*:1122–1126, 1989.
179. Triger, D. R., Boyer, T. D., and Levin, J.: Portal and systemic bacteremia and endotoxaemia in liver disease. Gut *19*:935–939, 1978.
180. Tubbs, H. R.: Endotoxin in meningococcal infections. Arch. Dis. Child. *55*:808 819, 1980.
181. Veterans Administration Systemic Sepsis Cooperative Study Group: Effect of high-dose glucocorticoid therapy on mortality in patients with clinical signs of systemic sepsis. N. Engl. J. Med. *317*:659–665, 1987.
182. Voerman, H. J., Stehouwer, C. D. A., Kamp, G. J., et al.: Plasma endothelin levels are increased during septic shock. Crit. Care Med. *20*:1097–1101, 1992.
183. Waage, A., Brandtzaeg, P., Halstensen, A., et al.: The complex pattern of cytokines in serum from patients with meningococcal septic shock. Association between interleukin 6, interleukin 1, and fatal outcome. J. Exp. Med. *169*:333–338, 1989.
184. Wajchenberg, B., Leme, C. E., Tambascia, M., et al.: The adrenal response to exogenous adrenocorticotrophin in patients with infections due to *Neisseria meningitidis*. J. Infect. Dis. *138*:387–391, 1978.
185. Walterspiel, J. W., Kaplan, S. L., and Mason, E. O., Jr.: Protective effect of subinhibitory polymyxin B alone and in combination with ampicillin for overwhelming *Haemophilus influenzae* type b infection in the infant rat: Evidence for in vivo and in vitro release of free endotoxin after ampicillin treatment. Pediatr. Res. *20*:237–241, 1986.
186. Wardle, E. N.: Endotoxin and acute renal failure. Nephron *14*:321–332, 1975.
187. Wardle, E. N.: Acute renal failure in the 1980's: The importance of septic shock and of endotoxaemia. Nephron *30*:193–200, 1982.
188. Warren, H. S., Danner, R. L., and Munford, R. S.: Anti-endotoxin monoclonal antibodies: A second look. N. Engl. J. Med. *326*:1151–1157, 1992.
189. Watson, R. W. G., Redmond, H. P., and Bouchier-Hayes, D.: Role of endotoxin in mononuclear phagocyte–mediated inflammatory responses. J. Leuk. Biol. *56*:95–103, 1994.
190. Weil, M. H., and Nishijima, H.: Cardiac output in bacterial shock. Am. J. Med. *64*:920–922, 1978.
191. Weiland, J. E., Davis, W. B., Holter, J. F., et al.: Lung neutrophils in the adult respiratory distress syndrome: Clinical and pathophysiologic significance. Am. Rev. Respir. Dis. *133*:218–225, 1986.
192. Wiesenthal, A. M., and Todd, J. K.: Toxic shock syndrome in children aged 10 years or less. Pediatrics *74*:112–117, 1984.
193. Wilson, M. D., Brackett, D. J., Hinshaw, L. B., et al.: Vasopressin release during sepsis and septic shock in baboons and dogs. Surg. Gynecol. Obstet. *153*:869–872, 1981.
194. Winchester, P. D., Todd, J. K., and Roe, M. H.: Bacteremia in hospitalized children. Am. J. Dis. Child. *131*:753–758, 1977.
195. Wong, V. K., Hitchcock, W., and Mason, W. H.: Meningococcal infections in children: A review of 100 cases. Pediatr. Infect. Dis. J. *8*:224–227, 1989.
196. Woo, P., Carpenter, M. A., and Trunkey, D.: Ionized calcium: The effect of septic shock in the human. J. Surg. Res. *26*:605–610, 1979.
197. Woods, D. E., Strauss, D. C., Johanson, W. G., Jr., et al.: Role of salivary protease activity in adherence of gram-negative bacilli to mammalian buccal epithelial cells in vivo. J. Clin. Invest. *68*:1435–1440, 1981.
198. Wright, S. D., Ramos, R. A., Tobias, P. S., et al.: CD14, a receptor for complexes of lipopolysaccharide (LPS) and LPS binding protein. Science *249*:1431–1433, 1990.
199. Zabel, P., Schönharting, M. M., Wolter, D. T., et al.: Oxpentifylline in endotoxaemia. Lancet *2*:1474–1477, 1989.

200. Zaeg, P. B., Sirnes, K., Folsland, B., et al.: Plasmapheresis in the treatment of severe meningococcal or pneumococcal septicemia with DIC and fibrinolysis: Preliminary data on eight patients. Scand. J. Clin. Lab. Invest. *45*(Suppl. 178):53–55, 1985.
201. Zaloga, G. P., and Chernow, B.: The multifactorial basis for hypocalcemia during sepsis: Studies of the parathyroid hormone–vitamin D axis. Ann. Intern. Med. *107*:36–41, 1987.
202. Zaloga, G. P., Malcolm, D., Chernow, B., et al.: Endotoxin-induced hypocalcemia results in defective calcium mobilization in rats. Circ. Shock *24*:143–148, 1988.
203. Zaritsky, A., and Chernow, B.: Use of catecholamines in pediatrics. J. Pediatr. *105*:341–350, 1984.
204. Ziegler, E., Fisher, C., Sprung, C., et al.: Treatment of gram-negative bacteremia and septic shock with HA-1A human monoclonal antibody against endotoxin. N. Engl. J. Med. *324*:429–436, 1991.
205. Ziegler, E. J., McCutchan, J. A., Fierer, J., et al.: Treatment of gram-negative bacteremia and shock with human antiserum to a mutant *Escherichia coli.* N. Engl. J. Med. *307*:1225–1230, 1982.
206. Zimmerman, J. J., and Dietrich, K. A.: Current perspectives on septic shock. Pediatr. Clin. North Am. *34*:131–163, 1987.

73

Fever Without Localizing Signs and Fever of Unknown Origin

Martin I. Lorin and Ralph D. Feigin

Petersdorf and Beeson[64] proposed in 1961 that the term *fever of unknown origin* (FUO) be reserved for persons with an illness persisting for 3 or more weeks and accompanied by temperatures higher than 38.4° C (101.2° F) on at least several occasions. They further specified that the cause of the fever should remain undetermined after at least 1 week of investigation in the hospital. Although this was an arbitrary definition, it was useful at that time, when many of the diagnostic tests now in routine use were unknown. The purpose of their precise definition was to explore the etiology of fever in this select group of *adult* patients and to permit comparison of data from different investigations. It is doubtful that this exacting definition was ever applied rigorously in pediatric practice.

Currently, many authors prefer the term *fever without localizing signs* (FWLS) for those patients with fever of recent onset who have no adequate explanation for the fever, either by history or on physical examination. The term *FUO* is best reserved for children with fever of at least 8 days in duration, in whom no diagnosis is apparent after initial work-up either in the hospital or as an outpatient.

The distinction between FUO and FWLS is of more than academic interest for several reasons: (1) Although there is overlap, the differential diagnoses of these two clinical conditions are distinct, and the most frequent causes of one are different from the most frequent causes of the other. (2) The child with fever of recent onset generally warrants more immediate evaluation than a child with FUO. The latter usually does not present as an emergency and requires timely, but not urgent, diagnostic or therapeutic intervention. (3) Although expectant antibiotic treatment of children with FUO usually is not indicated, expectant treatment of a select group of infants with FWLS generally is recommended. (4) Most patients with FWLS are managed as outpatients, whereas children with documented FUO often require in-hospital investigation.

FEVER WITHOUT LOCALIZING SIGNS

A convenient definition for FWLS is the occurrence of fever for 1 week or less in a child in whom careful history and physical examination fail to reveal a probable cause of the fever. Thus, a child with fever and bloody diarrhea should not be designated as having FWLS, despite a normal physical examination. It has been estimated that between 5 and 10 per cent of children presenting with fever have no localizing signs,[45] although in some series this figure has been as high as 22 per cent.[84] Stein[74] found the peak incidence to occur during the second year of life. On the basis of a review of private pediatric practices in upstate New York, Hoekelman and colleagues[34] predicted that the practicing pediatrician would see one child, between 1 and 24 months of age, with FWLS every 4 to 5 days.

The great majority of children with fever of recent onset have acute infectious diseases, most of which are self-limited.[84] A few of these patients have serious acute infectious diseases, including bacteremia, and a very few turn out to have acute noninfectious diseases or chronic disorders. For example, an occasional patient presenting with FWLS is discovered to have a disorder such as heat illness, drug poisoning, malignancy, or connective tissue disease. However, these occurrences are so infrequent that most series of patients with FWLS include no such patients.[6, 25, 52, 53, 57, 77] The physician faced with a child with FWLS should consider the possibility of a noninfectious cause or the onset of a chronic disease, but unless there is a clinical clue to suggest one of these entities, investigation in this direction is not warranted.

Many children with FWLS are in the prodromal stages of an acute infectious illness and will develop evidence of specific infection, such as pharyngitis, otitis media, or pneumonia, within hours to days of first being seen by a physician. Fever may precede the appearance of specific signs and symptoms by as long as 3 days, as in measles, Rocky Mountain spotted fever, and leptospirosis. In some infections, such as roseola, viral hepatitis, infectious mononucleosis, typhus, typhoid fever, and Kawasaki disease (presumably an infectious disease), the interval between the onset of fever and the appearance of specific findings is even more than 3 days.

Occult Bacteremia

One major concern regarding the young child with FWLS is the possibility of occult bacteremia. The patient does not look particularly ill and is judged clinically well enough to be managed as an outpatient. The child is presumed not to be bacteremic, and yet the blood culture yields a pathogenic bacteria, most commonly *Streptococcus pneumoniae,* less commonly *Neisseria meningitidis, Haemophilus influenzae, Salmo-*

nella, or *Staphylococcus aureus*. Although a few authors define occult bacteremia as bacteremia in the absence of evidence of focal infection, the most useful and the generally accepted definition is a positive blood culture in a child who looks well enough to be treated as an outpatient and does not have an infection commonly associated with bacteremia, such as pneumonia or pyelonephritis. Thus, many series of occult bacteremia include children with upper respiratory tract infection and otitis media.[22, 38, 69, 70] The incidence of occult bacteremia in children with FWLS is about 5 per cent.[6, 17, 47, 60, 77, 84] In most series, occult bacteremia has been found to be more common in children with FWLS than in febrile children of the same age with infections commonly treated on an outpatient basis, such as pharyngitis, otitis media, upper respiratory tract infection, and bronchitis. For example, McCarthy and associates[47] found the incidence of bacteremia among febrile children without an obvious source of infection to be 9.9 per cent, compared with 3.3 per cent in children with otitis media, upper respiratory tract infection, or flu-like syndrome. Teele and colleagues[77] found an incidence of bacteremia of 3.9 per cent among children with FWLS and 1.5 per cent in comparably febrile children with otitis media or pharyngitis.

The entity of occult bacteremia, first recognized and described in indigent children attending inner-city clinics, once was believed to be a problem restricted to that segment of the population. A study by Baron and Fink,[6] however, showed that occult bacteremia occurred with approximately the same frequency in patients seen in a private office, and a study in Chicago found an incidence of occult bacteremia of 3.5 per cent among febrile children seen at an inner-city hospital outpatient department, 1.9 per cent in children at a suburban hospital emergency room, and 5.9 per cent in predominantly white middle-class children in the offices of pediatricians in private practice.[25] These differences were not statistically significant.

The risk of occult bacteremia in a child with FWLS is age-related, with most cases occurring in children between the ages of 6 and 24 months. Other age groups, however, are by no means spared, with numerous studies demonstrating a high risk for bacteremia or other serious bacterial infections in the febrile infant younger than 3 months of age.[47, 52, 68, 76] In one series of pneumococcal bacteremia in children with FWLS, 14 of 15 patients were between 6 and 24 months of age.[14] In another series of 98 children with FWLS and pneumococcal bacteremia, 4 children were younger than 3 months of age, 73 were between 3 and 24 months of age, and 20 were older than 24 months of age.[36] In a group of children with clinically unsuspected meningococcemia reported by Dashefsky and associates,[24] all 12 patients who initially looked well enough to be treated as outpatients were younger than 24 months of age, 9 (75%) of them between 6 and 24 months of age. The incidence of occult *H. influenzae* bacteremia, however, is distributed fairly evenly over the first 4 or 5 years of life. In a series of children with unsuspected bacteremia due to *H. influenzae* described by Marshall and associates in the era prior to *H. influenzae* immunization,[58] 52 per cent of patients who looked well enough to be sent home were between 6 and 24 months of age, 7 per cent were 6 months of age or younger, and 40 per cent were older than 2 years of age. Although it is important to be aware that the highest risk for occult bacteremia is between 6 and 24 months of age, it is equally important not to be unduly complacent outside this age group. The child in the first few months of life is especially at risk for bacteremia due to group B *Streptococcus*.

In a rough sense, the risk of occult bacteremia increases with the severity of fever. In a prospective study of bacteremia in children seen in the outpatient department, McCarthy and colleagues[47] noted a statistically significant, albeit not clinically impressive, difference in the incidence of bacteremia between children with temperatures of 40° C (104° F) or higher and those with temperatures of 40.5° C (104.9° F) or higher (i.e., 8.2 per cent vs. 10.5 per cent). The authors noted that the tendency of positive blood cultures to increase in frequency as the initial temperature increased was most pronounced for pneumococcal and meningococcal bacteremia and less so for *H. influenzae* type b, *Salmonella* species, and other organisms. However, in the series of unsuspected meningococcemia reported by Dashefsky and colleagues,[24] the distribution of cases within the temperature range of 38.7° to 40.9° C was fairly even (101.8° to 105.6° F). In a prospective study in which blood cultures were obtained from all febrile children younger than 2 years of age seen in a walk-in clinic, Teele and colleagues[77] found no positive blood cultures among 44 children with FWLS and rectal temperatures of less than 38.9° C (102° F) and five (3.9%) positive blood cultures among 129 FWLS children with rectal temperatures equal to or greater than 38.9° C (102° F). Other series have reported similar findings.[6, 52]

Of all laboratory tests potentially useful in the diagnosis of occult bacteremia, the white blood cell (WBC) count has been the most studied and probably the most controversial. In 1974, on the basis of a study of hospitalized children, Todd[78] reported that the absolute number of polymorphonuclear leukocytes and the absolute number of nonsegmented polymorphonuclear leukocytes were more sensitive than the total WBC count, the percentage of polymorphonuclear leukocytes, or the percentage of nonsegmented polymorphonuclear leukocytes. It is questionable, however, whether information based on hospitalized children—presumably all of whom had serious localized infections or looked ill enough to warrant hospitalization—can be applied to the child with FWLS who looks well enough to be treated on an ambulatory basis.

Several studies have examined the usefulness of the WBC count in febrile children seen in the outpatient setting. McCarthy and associates[53] concluded that a WBC count equal to or greater than 15,000/mm³ was useful in identifying those patients at greatest risk for bacteremia. Dershewitz[25] noted a direct relationship between total leukocyte count and prevalence of bacteremia and stated that "knowledge of the count was a helpful but limited predictor of patients with positive blood cultures." McGowan and associates[55] found that the incidence of bacteremia increased with increased WBC counts and that bacteremia was most common in patients with counts of 20,000/mm³ or higher.

Several studies have examined the utility of the WBC count specifically in children with FWLS who look well enough to be treated on an outpatient basis. One such study, by Teele and colleagues,[77] found a sensitivity of 1.0 and a positive predictive value of 0.11 for a total WBC of 15,000/mm³. Utilizing a WBC of 20,000/mm³ would have decreased the sensitivity to 0.4 while increasing positive predictive value only to 0.13. In the Baron and Fink series,[6] the sensitivity for a WBC of 15,000/mm³ was 0.87 with a specificity of 0.73. McGowan and colleagues[55] provided data only for a total WBC of 20,000/mm³, which had a sensitivity of 0.35 and positive predictive value of 0.12. Kline and coworkers[40] found that a WBC count of 15,000/mm³ was more sensitive for *S. pneumoniae* bacteremia than for *H. influenzae* bacteremia. Although a total WBC of 15,000/mm³ does not predict accurately which child is or is not bacteremic, it is helpful in dividing the population of children with FWLS into high- and low-risk groups.

The erythrocyte sedimentation rate appears to be no more

useful than the WBC count in predicting bacteremia in ambulatory febrile patients.[53] Determination of serum concentration of C-reactive protein may be more accurate than either the complete blood count or erythrocyte sedimentation rate in distinguishing bacterial from viral infections,[48, 63] but its role in detecting occult bacteremia in FWLS has not been reported.

Other hematologic findings that suggest bacteremia include thrombocytopenia,[21] Döhle inclusion bodies, toxic granulations, and vacuolization of neutrophils. In one study, peripheral blood smears of children younger than 24 months of age with acute febrile illnesses were reviewed the following day by a single investigator to determine whether vacuolization and toxic granulations were present; when both abnormalities were present, the positive predictive value for bacteremia was 0.76.[42] The presence of these findings in febrile children should be considered when estimating the risk of bacteremia.[1, 21, 59]

Several studies have examined the response to acetaminophen and found no difference between bacteremic and nonbacteremic children regarding either the rate of temperature reduction or the improvement in clinical appearance.[3, 79, 86] Mazur and associates,[46] however, found that febrile children 2 months to 6 years of age who did not respond to a dose of acetaminophen by at least 0.8° C in 2 hours had a statistically significant increased risk of occult bacteremia compared with those who did respond.

The most important aspect of assessment of the febrile child is a careful history and physical examination. Laboratory data are secondary and should be ordered on the basis of the clinical assessment. By definition, the child with FWLS has no localizing signs to explain the fever or indicate a site of infection. Many physicians believe that a general impression, or gestalt, can indicate whether or not the child has occult bacteremia. It has been suggested that careful clinical judgment, based on extensive experience, can identify most, if not all, children with serious illnesses.[10] McCarthy and colleagues,[49–51] in a series of carefully designed studies, elucidated those variables of history and observation most useful in assessing febrile children. They found that the observation variable *playfulness* had the strongest correlation with overall assessment.[50] However, they noted that even the experienced attending pediatrician could identify only 57 per cent of seriously ill children by initial impression prior to a full physical examination. Dershewitz[25] found that private pediatricians were no more accurate than pediatric residents in identifying children with occult bacteremia and that, in the private office, pediatricians were no better at predicting bacteremia in familiar patients than they were in first-time patients.

In a study of 292 consecutive febrile children seen in an emergency room, Waskerwitz and Berkelhammer[81] identified a subgroup of patients who had no localizing signs and who looked so well that they were predicted not to have bacteremia. The physicians were assisted in their assessment by a functional scale that gave 0 to 2 points for the child's eating, drinking, sleeping, and play activities, with a best possible score of 8. The group of patients with functional scores equal to or greater than 5, with no localized infection and predicted clinically not to have bacteremia, were indeed free of bacteremia, whereas 14 of 202 patients with functional scores of 4 or less were bacteremic. It must be understood that, in this study, the physicians were not able to identify which patients had bacteremia and which did not; rather, they were able to identify one subgroup at high risk for bacteremia and another at very low risk. Thus, it appears that the clinician's overall assessment of the degree of illness of the child is a valuable, but not infallible, tool in estimating the risk of occult bacteremia in children with FWLS.

Clinical Management of Fever Without Localizing Signs

Approximately 3 to 5 per cent of children with FWLS are bacteremic. A number of studies (all carried out prior to the routine use of *H. influenzae* vaccine) showed that if these children were not treated with antibiotics at the time of the initial clinical encounter, 5 to 10 per cent would return with bacterial meningitis, 10 per cent with localized bacterial infection, and another 30 per cent with continued fever and persistent bacteremia.[6, 12, 33, 47, 53, 55, 58, 77] In all of these retrospective studies, patients initially treated with antibiotics fared better than those not treated initially, although the decision of whether or not to treat was always at the discretion of the treating physician and not randomized.

In a prospective, randomized investigation, Carroll and associates[17] studied 96 children, ages 6 to 24 months, with FWLS and temperature greater than 40° C (104° F). Ten of these patients were bacteremic, five were treated initially with antibiotics on an outpatient basis, and five were not treated. The difference in outcome between the two groups was statistically significant in favor of the treatment group; four of the five treated patients were improved clinically, whereas none of the five untreated patients was improved clinically. None of the treated patients developed bacterial meningitis, whereas two of the five untreated patients developed bacterial meningitis. In a prospective, randomized, placebo-controlled study of empiric treatment with amoxicillin in children at risk for occult bacteremia, Jaffee and colleagues[37] showed no difference between treatment and nontreatment groups. It has been pointed out that the power of this study was low and that a true difference in outcome easily could have been missed.[2] It also should be noted that the dosage of amoxicillin used was 125 mg three times a day for children who weighed 10 kg or less and 250 mg three times a day for those weighing more than 10 kg. This means that some children may have received as little as 37.5 mg/kg/day. Although this is close to the usual recommended dosage of 40 mg/kg/day, Baron and coworkers[8] have suggested that considerably higher doses may be required to treat occult bacteremia. In a retrospective study of a private pediatric practice, these investigators found that none of 11 infants with FWLS and bacteremia who initially received 150 mg/kg/day or more of amoxicillin developed complications. In contrast, 5 of 12 such infants not treated or treated with less than 100 mg/kg/day of amoxicillin (p = .03) developed complications.

It is difficult to be dogmatic about the management of children with FWLS. One reasonable approach, based on a careful history and physical examination and overall clinical impression, is to classify these children as being at either low or high risk for occult bacteremia and other serious bacterial illnesses. For the low-risk group, no laboratory investigation would be required routinely. For the high-risk group, a complete blood count and blood culture should be obtained. Lumbar puncture, chest radiograph, urinalysis, and urine culture are considered on an individual basis. If the patient appears ill, admission to the hospital may be justified, even if all test results are negative. When high-risk children look well enough to be sent home, they are reasonable candidates for expectant antibiotic therapy, pending the outcome of the blood culture. For those patients clinically considered at moderate risk (not clearly high or low risk), the physician has the option of obtaining a WBC count and using the results to decide whether to draw a blood culture and prescribe antibiotics expectantly.

Table 73–1 lists risk factors for occult bacteremia. Current information is not sufficient to warrant the use of scoring systems except as part of investigational series. In the final analysis, the clinician's judgment, taking into account all available clinical and laboratory data about each patient individually, is the guide to selecting which children require diagnostic work-up and expectant therapy with antibiotics.

If the physician elects to prescribe antibiotics while awaiting the results of the blood culture, such antibiotic therapy should provide adequate coverage for *S. pneumoniae, N. meningitidis,* and *H. influenzae,* although the frequency of *H. influenzae* has decreased dramatically with current immunization practice. In geographic areas where ampicillin-resistant *H. influenzae* is common, the physician may wish to use an antibiotic that covers this organism as well. Amoxicillin-clavulanate (20 to 40 mg/kg/day every 8 hours based on amoxicillin content) is a reasonable choice. A single injection of 75 mg/kg of ceftriaxone while awaiting the results of blood culture has been successful in resolving fever, clearing bacteremia, and preventing meningitis and was found to be superior to oral regimens in several series.[5, 7, 30] However, the decreasing frequency of *H. influenzae* type b disease may lessen the need for this drug.[44] For the patient with a significant history of penicillin allergy for whom a cephalosporin is not considered appropriate, trimethoprim-sulfamethoxazole, in a dosage of 8 mg of trimethoprim per kilogram per day, may be an acceptable alternative. Those children in whom the blood culture turns out to be positive should be recalled for re-evaluation, even if they are afebrile.

Infants younger than 90 days of age pose a special problem because of increased risk of serious bacterial infection, more difficult clinical evaluation, and a broader spectrum of invading organisms (e.g., group B *Streptococcus, Escherichia coli,* and *Listeria monocytogenes*). One reasonable practice guideline for infants with FWLS is to hospitalize and treat all who appear "toxic" and all younger than 28 days of age. Those between 28 and 90 days of age may be managed as outpatients if they look well and the blood count, urinalysis, and cerebrospinal fluid are within normal limits.[4]

Although low socioeconomic status does not appear to increase the risk of occult bacteremia, it is believed to impair appropriate follow-up. Many such patients fail to keep return appointments, and it often is difficult to locate them should a blood culture be positive. The potential for adequate follow-up should be assessed for each individual patient and considered when one makes a decision regarding both diagnostic work-up and the use of antibiotics, pending cultures.

FEVER OF UNKNOWN ORIGIN

Currently, pediatricians disagree on the exact definition of the term *FUO,* and series in the pediatric literature differ considerably in their criteria for inclusion. Brewis[13] defined FUO in children as the presence of temperature equal to or greater than 38.3° C (101° F) for 5 to 7 consecutive days without localizing signs or symptoms. In sharp contrast, both McClung[54] and Lohr and Hendley[43] considered children whose fever had been noted for at least 3 weeks on an outpatient basis or 1 week in the hospital to have FUO. Pizzo and associates,[66] however, required only that the fever be present for 2 weeks, with no distinction between outpatient or in-hospital status. We believe that a reasonable working definition of FUO, for clinical purposes, is the presence of fever for 8 or more days in a child in whom a careful and thorough history and physical examination and preliminary laboratory data fail to reveal a probable cause for the fever.

Most cases of FUO in children are caused by relatively common diseases. In four series of FUO, totaling 418 children, only five patients would be considered to have rare disorders (Behçet syndrome, ichthyosis, variant of "blue diaper" syndrome, diencephalic seizure disorder, and "possible chronic lead and/or arsenic intoxication").[13, 43, 54, 66] The adage that an FUO is more likely to be caused by an unusual presentation of a common disorder than a common presentation of a rare disorder certainly is true in pediatrics. The three most common discernible causes of FUO in children, in order of decreasing frequency, are infectious diseases, connective tissue diseases, and neoplasms. In about 10 to 20 per cent of cases, a definitive diagnosis is never established.

In the United States, the systemic infectious diseases most frequently diagnosed in children with FUO include tuberculosis; brucellosis; tularemia; salmonellosis; and infections due to rickettsia, spirochetes (such as leptospirosis), Epstein-Barr virus, cytomegalic inclusion virus, human immunodeficiency virus, hepatitis viruses, and other viruses. The most common causes of localized infection are upper respiratory tract infections (sinusitis, otitis, tonsillitis), urinary tract infection, osteomyelitis, and occult abscesses, including hepatic and pelvic abscesses.

The connective tissue disease most commonly presenting as FUO in children is juvenile rheumatoid arthritis (accounting for more than 90 per cent of connective tissue diseases in most series), followed by systemic lupus erythematosus and, finally, undefined vasculitis.[43, 54, 66] The definitive diagnosis of juvenile rheumatoid arthritis frequently is possible only after an extended period of observation because there may be no findings on physical examination and because the results of specific serologic studies generally are normal or negative.

TABLE 73–1. Risk Factors for Occult Bacteremia

Factor	High Risk	Low Risk
Age	≥ 24 mo	> 36 mo
Magnitude of fever	≥ 40° C (104° F)	≤ 39.4° C (103° F)
White blood cell count	≥ 15,000/mm³	< 15,000/mm³
Peripheral blood smear	Toxic granulation or vacuolization of polymorphonuclear leukocytes; thrombocytopenia	
Underlying chronic disorder	Sickle-cell disease, immunodeficiency, malnutrition	None
History of contact with bacterial disease	Contact with *Neisseria meningitidis* or *Haemophilus influenzae*	No known contact
Clinical appearance	Appears ill, "toxic," or unhappy; inconsolable; irritable or lethargic; not eating or drinking enough	Looks well; playful; eating normally; not irritable

Malignancy is a less frequent cause of FUO in children than in adults but is not rare and usually is the third-largest group, after infectious diseases and connective tissue diseases. Malignancy accounted for 7 per cent of the cases in the series of Pizzo and associates[66] and for 13 per cent in the Lohr and Hendley[43] series. Leukemia and lymphoma are responsible for most cases of cancer presenting as FUO in children. Other tumors less commonly reported as causing FUO include neuroblastoma, hepatoma, sarcoma, and atrial myxoma.

Although the outlook for children with FUO is better than for adults and although most children with FUO have either treatable or self-limited diseases, the overall prognosis is far from benign. Mortality was 9 per cent in the series of Pizzo and associates[66] and 6 per cent in Lohr and Hendley's series.[43] The prognosis for children in whom a definitive diagnosis is not established during the initial hospitalization is mixed. In most cases, fever eventually resolves.[28] In some, a specific diagnosis is made finally, whereas other patients continue to have fever without definitive diagnosis. McClung[54] described 11 such patients, most of whom appeared to do well despite recurrent episodes of fever.

Diagnostic Approach to the Child with Fever of Unknown Origin

When a child with FUO is admitted to the hospital, it is not only for laboratory investigation. Hospitalization also provides an opportunity to observe the child, repeat the history and physical examination, analyze all available data, and follow up on every potential diagnostic lead. In the Lohr and Hendley[43] series of 54 children with FUO, an incomplete history delayed the diagnosis in nine cases, and physical findings that were ignored delayed the diagnosis in four cases. In McClung's[54] report of 99 cases of FUO in children, errors in the history or physical examination obscured the correct diagnosis in at least 10 patients. Failure to utilize existing laboratory data correctly is another common factor preventing early diagnosis in children with FUO.[43, 66]

Clinical Evaluation

The first and most important step in the diagnostic workup of the child with FUO is a complete and detailed history and physical examination. The clinical evaluation not only must be thorough and careful, it must be repeated again and again. Often, a patient or parent eventually recalls information that was omitted or forgotten when the initial history was obtained. Physical findings change, and abnormalities not originally present may appear subsequently. In the series by Lohr and Hendley,[43] more than 25 per cent of children admitted to the hospital with FUO developed significant physical findings not present at the time of admission.

A detailed history should be obtained regarding contact with infected or otherwise ill persons and any exposure to animals, both pets and wild animals. The number of children with zoonotic infections is increasing each year. Immunization against leptospirosis of domestic animals, such as the dog, may prevent canine disease, but it does not prevent the carriage, excretion, and transmission of this infection. A history of travel extending back to birth must be elicited. Reemergence of histoplasmosis, coccidioidomycosis, blastomycosis, or malaria, years after visiting or living in an endemic area, is well known. It is important to inquire about prophylactic immunizations, precautions taken against the ingestion of contaminated food or water, and malarial prophylaxis. Questioning should include the possibility that rocks, soil, or artifacts from geographically distant regions may have been brought into the home, as well as the possibility of contact with persons who have visited distant countries. Even contact with insects can be important. Tick bites can be a clue to Rocky Mountain spotted fever or tick-borne relapsing fever. North American mosquitoes and some ticks carry a variety of arboviruses.

The physician should determine if the patient has eaten game meat, raw meat, or raw shellfish. A history of pica should be sought routinely. Ingestion of dirt may suggest a diagnosis of visceral larva migrans, toxoplasmosis, or other infectious diseases. A detailed history regarding all medications, including topical agents and nonprescription items, must be elicited carefully. Any history of surgical procedures should be explored carefully.

Questions designed to determine the genetic or ethnic background of the patient may reveal information that specifically suggests or largely excludes diagnoses such as nephrogenic diabetes insipidus (found in Ulster Scots), familial Mediterranean fever (found in Armenians, Arabs, and Sephardic Jews), and familial dysautonomia (found in Jews).

The history should be exacting regarding not only the duration, height, and pattern of the fever but also the circumstances under which temperature elevation occurs, whether the child appears ill or develops any signs or symptoms, and how well the fever responds to antipyretic drugs. A history of "fever" occurring only after exercise or late in the afternoon may indicate parental concern about normal variations in body temperature. A history of high fevers in the absence of malaise or other generalized signs may be a clue to factitious fever. The physician also should take a careful history regarding how well the fever has been documented. Has a thermometer been used, by whom, and in whose presence? A history of sweating and heat intolerance may indicate hyperthyroidism, whereas a history of heat intolerance with the absence of sweating may be a clue to ectodermal dysplasia.

Although certain patterns of fever classically have been associated with specific conditions, both Lohr and Hendley[43] and Pizzo and associates[66] found that neither the pattern of fever nor its duration was useful in pointing to or establishing a diagnosis in children with FUO in their series. The authors' experience suggests that the pattern and duration of fever can be helpful, but only rarely. *Intermittent* fever is characterized by the return of temperature to normal at least once daily. If the peak of fever is high and the rate of defervescence quick, this pattern often is referred to as hectic or spiking. Intermittent fevers suggest pyogenic infections but also are seen with tuberculosis, lymphoma, and juvenile rheumatoid arthritis. In *remittent* fever, the temperature fluctuates but does not return to normal. A *sustained* fever pattern is characterized by persistent fever with little or no fluctuation and may occur in typhoid fever or typhus. Antipyretic agents can make a remittent or sustained fever appear intermittent. *Relapsing* fever refers to a pattern in which the patient is afebrile for 1 or more days between episodes of fever and may be seen in malaria, rat-bite fever, infection with the *Borrelia* organism, and lymphomas. Recurrent episodes of fever of more than a year's duration should suggest metabolic defects, central nervous system abnormalities of temperature control, and immunodeficient states.

The general activity and appearance of the patient should be observed, vital signs checked, and growth parameters measured. Weight loss is an important, although nonspecific, finding. Impairment of linear growth or short stature may be a clue to inflammatory bowel disease, an intracranial lesion involving the pituitary gland, or a long-standing chronic disease. It helps to examine the patient during an episode of fever, noting the presence or absence of sweating, the effect of the fever on the heart and respiratory rate, the presence or absence of malaise or other symptoms, and the appearance of "toxicity." The rash of juvenile rheumatoid arthritis is characteristically evanescent and may be present only during periods of temperature elevation.

Some special aspects of the physical examination merit mention. Hypohidrosis, anomalous dentition, and sparse hair, particularly of the eyebrows and eyelashes, suggest anhidrotic ectodermal dysplasia. Red, weeping eyes may be a sign of polyarteritis nodosa. Palpebral conjunctivitis may be a clue to the presence of infectious mononucleosis, Newcastle disease, or lupus erythematosus. Predominantly bulbar conjunctivitis may suggest leptospirosis. Phlyctenular conjunctivitis may signal tuberculosis.

Absence of the pupillary constrictor response may be caused by a deficiency of the constrictor sphincter muscle of the eye. This muscle, derived from ectoderm rather than mesoderm, develops embryologically at the same time that hypothalamic structures and function are undergoing differentiation. The absence of this muscle may suggest that temperature elevation is the result of hypothalamic or autonomic dysfunction. Careful funduscopic examination may disclose evidence of miliary tuberculosis, vasculitis, or toxoplasmosis. Lack of tears, absent corneal reflexes, and a smooth tongue with absence of the fungiform papillae would indicate familial dysautonomia.

Purulent or persistent nasal discharge may be a sign of sinusitis. The physician should palpate for tenderness over the sinuses.

Hyperemia of the pharynx, even in the absence of exudate or specific symptoms, may be a clue to the diagnosis of infectious mononucleosis, cytomegalic inclusion disease, toxoplasmosis, tularemia, or leptospirosis. Gingival hypertrophy, inflammation, or both or loosening or loss of teeth may indicate histiocytosis.

The bones and muscles should be palpated carefully. Tenderness over a bone may be found in osteomyelitis or marrow invasion due to neoplastic disease. Muscle tenderness may be associated with trichinosis, dermatomyositis, polyarteritis, or various arboviral infections.

The search for skin lesions and rashes must be careful, extensive, and repeated. Petechiae may indicate endocarditis or other sources of bacteremia but also may occur with viral and rickettsial infections. A seborrheic rash may be a sign of histiocytosis.

A careful rectal examination is imperative in patients of all ages and may reveal pararectal tenderness or a mass, indicating a pelvic abscess or tumor. A test for occult blood should be performed on any stool found on the examining finger. Examination of the external genitalia should be completed on patients of all ages, and sexually active adolescent females should undergo pelvic examination.

Laboratory Evaluation

The extent of laboratory investigation depends on the age of the patient, duration of fever, and history and physical examination. Laboratory studies should be directed, as much as possible, toward the most likely diagnostic possibilities. The tempo of the diagnostic evaluation should be adjusted to the severity of the illness. In a critically ill child, speed is important. If the patient is less severely ill, however, the evaluation can proceed more slowly; the clinician sometimes may be rewarded by the disappearance of fever without apparent explanation before a definitive diagnosis can be established and before any invasive diagnostic procedures have been undertaken.

A complete blood count and careful examination of the peripheral smear is indicated for all patients. Anemia should be noted and attention paid to thrombocytosis as well as thrombocytopenia. Although mild or moderate changes in the total WBC count or differential count usually are of no help, in some series, children with more than 10,000 polymorphonuclear leukocytes or 500 nonsegmented neutrophils/mm^3 were found to have a high chance of having a severe bacterial infection.[74, 78] Atypical lymphocytes generally indicate viral infections, whereas bizarre or immature forms may suggest leukemia. Although the erythrocyte sedimentation rate is of no specific diagnostic value, it is a general indicator of inflammation and can help in determining the need for further evaluation and in following the progress of the disease process.

Blood cultures should be obtained aerobically and anaerobically from all patients. In select cases, media appropriate to the isolation of *Francisella* organisms, *Leptospira,* and *Spirillum* also should be employed.

All patients should undergo analysis and culture of urine. In one series of FUO in children, failure to perform urinalysis and failure to investigate pyuria adequately were the most common laboratory errors.[54] Radiographic study of the urinary tract, however, should be performed only when indicated.

All patients should undergo radiographic examination of the chest; examinations of the nasal sinuses, mastoids, and gastrointestinal tract are ordered initially only for specific indications but should be done eventually in all children whose fever persists without explanation for a long period. Persistent fever and elevation of the erythrocyte sedimentation rate, with or without anemia, abdominal complaints, anorexia, and weight loss, are sufficient indications for radiographic study to rule out inflammatory bowel disease.

All patients should undergo an intermediate-strength (5 units of purified protein derivative) tuberculin skin test. Control skin tests with antigens such as *Candida* are of limited value because anergy may be specific for tuberculosis rather than universal for all skin-testing materials.[47, 56, 57, 61] Thus, a positive control test result and negative tuberculin test result still do not rule out tuberculosis.

Bone marrow examination is most useful in diagnosing cancer (especially leukemia), histiocytic disorders, and hemophagocytic disease. It is less useful in determining infection. Hayani and associates[32] reviewed the results of 414 bone marrow examinations for FUO in children. In only one case (*Salmonella* group D) was an organism recovered from the marrow not also recovered from blood or another source. Noninfectious causes of FUO were found in 8 per cent of specimens: malignancy (6.7%), hemophagocytic syndromes (0.7%), histiocytosis (0.5%), and hypoplastic anemia (0.2%). In most of these cases, the diagnosis had been suspected clinically prior to the bone marrow examination.

All patients should undergo a serum test for human immunodeficiency virus infection. Other appropriate serologic tests can help to establish a diagnosis of salmonellosis, brucellosis, tularemia, Epstein-Barr virus infections, cytomegalic inclusion virus infection, and other viral infections, toxoplasmosis, and certain fungal infections.

Hepatic enzymes and serum chemistries, including electrolytes, urea nitrogen, and creatinine, should be determined in all patients. Serum antinuclear antibody should be measured in those older than 5 years of age. Serum hepatitis antigens, electrocardiography, electroencephalography, echocardiography, and stool culture and examination for ova and parasites generally should be performed in selected cases. Other tests to be considered for individual patients include ophthalmologic examination by slit lamp, radiographic bone survey, technetium bone scan, liver-spleen scan, and abdominal imaging by ultrasonography or computed tomography.[16, 65] Computed tomographic scanning, gallium scanning, and indium-111 scanning[29] can detect masses as well as organ involvement by tumor, in addition to infection and perhaps other inflammatory processes. Such scanning procedures offer a relatively noninvasive technique for screening patients with FUO for a variety of disorders. Although Steele and associates[73] found that radionucleotide scans seldom led to unsuspected diagnoses in children and suggested that they not be used indiscriminately, gallium scanning has been helpful in adult patients with FUO,[31] and the authors' experience suggests that it also may be a reasonable test in selected children. Lymph node biopsy, liver biopsy, and exploratory laparotomy are reserved for patients with evidence of involvement of these organs.

In general, antibiotics or other medications should not be administered empirically as a diagnostic measure in children with FUO. One exception to this rule is the use of nonsteroidal agents in children with presumed juvenile rheumatoid arthritis. Another exception is the use of antituberculous drugs in critically ill children thought to have disseminated tuberculosis. Empiric trials of broad-spectrum antibiotics generally do more to obscure than illuminate and may mask or delay diagnosis of infections such as meningitis, parameningeal infection, endocarditis, or osteomyelitis.

Examples of disorders that can present as FUO in children are listed in Table 73–2. A number of these are discussed briefly in the following sections.

TABLE 73–2. Causes of Fever of Unknown Origin in Children

Infectious Diseases	Collagen Vascular Diseases
Bacterial	Juvenile rheumatoid arthritis
Brucellosis	Polyarteritis nodosa
Bacterial endocarditis	Systemic lupus erythematosus
Leptospirosis	**Malignancies**
Liver abscess	Hodgkin disease
Mastoiditis (chronic)	Leukemia/lymphoma
Osteomyelitis	Neuroblastoma
Pelvic abscess	**Miscellaneous**
Perinephric abscess	Central diabetes insipidus
Pyelonephritis	Drug fever
Salmonellosis	Ectodermal dysplasia
Sinusitis	Factitious fever
Subdiaphragmatic abscess	Familial dysautonomia
Tuberculosis	Granulomatous colitis
Tularemia	Infantile cortical hyperostosis
Viral	Nephrogenic diabetes insipidus
Cytomegalovirus	Pancreatitis
Hepatitis viruses	Periodic fever
Epstein-Barr virus (infectious mononucleosis)	Serum sickness
Chlamydial	Thyrotoxicosis
Lymphogranuloma venereum	Ulcerative colitis
Psittacosis	
Rickettsial	
Q fever	
Rocky Mountain spotted fever	
Fungal	
Blastomycosis (nonpulmonary)	
Histoplasmosis (disseminated)	
Parasitic	
Malaria	
Toxoplasmosis	
Visceral larva migrans	
Unclassified	
Sarcoidosis	

Examples of Infectious Causes of Fever of Unknown Origin

Infectious causes of FUO can be divided into systemic infections due to a specific organism and localized infection due to one or more of a variety of organisms. In addition, immunodeficient states may be considered under the general classification of infections.

Generalized Infections

BRUCELLOSIS. The presentation of this disease as FUO is explained by the nonspecific symptoms it engenders and by the chronicity of untreated infection. Many physicians, particularly in urban areas, tend to ignore the possibility of this disease and neglect to ask for a history of exposure to animals or animal products. (See Chapter 133.)

LEPTOSPIROSIS. Leptospirosis is caused by a single family of organisms composed of multiple serogroups and serotypes; it is one of the most widespread zoonoses in the world. Transmission of infection from animal to human may follow direct contact with the blood, tissue, organs, or urine of infected animals or indirectly by exposure to an environment that has been contaminated by leptospires. Additionally, the organism may be acquired from soil or from fresh water after ingestion. Reports indicate that leptospirosis is not rare, that most infections no longer are associated with occupational exposure, and that urban and suburban cases now are more prevalent than cases reported from rural areas.[18] Clinical manifestations of leptospirosis usually are not specific. A variety of laboratory aids are available, but proper collection and handling of specimens are imperative. In some cases, it may be impossible to establish a definitive diagnosis; negative cultures or failure to demonstrate a rise in antibody titer does not exclude the possibility of active infection because the organism may not be in the specimens that have been cultured, the antibody titer may have peaked prior to the collection of an acute phase specimen, and antibiotic therapy may suppress the development of positive titers or delay their appearance. (See Chapter 148.)

PARASITIC INFECTIONS. Toxoplasmosis should be considered in any child with persistent fever. Cervical or supraclavicular adenopathy is present in most cases, but occasionally fever is the only manifestation. Diagnosis is established by demonstration of a rising serologic titer; antibody to *Toxoplasma gondii* is so prevalent that demonstration of a high titer alone is not diagnostic of acute infection. Demonstration of toxoplasma in tissue sections or body fluid is highly suggestive, although the organism may persist in tissue for years. Thus, isolation of the parasite is not absolutely diagnostic of recent infection. (See Chapter 221.)

Malaria also should be considered in children with FUO. In addition to fever, splenomegaly usually is present. A history of travel to endemic areas should be sought, although cases have occurred in patients who never left the United States. The disease can become apparent even in persons who have taken antimalarial drugs when they visited the endemic region. There may be a hiatus of several months between infection and onset of symptoms. Additionally, the infection may be transmitted from a person who has visited an endemic area to one who has not when an appropriate mosquito vector is present. Malaria also may be acquired by blood transfusion or by the use of needles and syringes contaminated by the parasite. Demonstration of malarial organisms on appropriately stained thin or thick smears of blood is diagnostic. (See Chapter 217.)

SALMONELLOSIS. *Salmonella* organisms occur as contaminants in many food products. In view of the nonspecific signs and symptoms with which salmonellosis may occur, its association with FUO in children is not surprising. Repetitive blood and stool cultures are most helpful in establishing a diagnosis. Serologic evidence of infection also should be sought. (See Chapter 115.)

TUBERCULOSIS. Tuberculosis is an important cause of FUO in children as well as in adults. Nonpulmonary tuberculosis presents as FUO more frequently than pulmonary tuberculosis, which usually is evident on routine chest radiographs. FUO is most common with disseminated tuberculosis or infection of the liver, peritoneum, pericardium, or genitourinary tract. Active disseminated tuberculosis has been well documented in children with negative results on chest radiography and tuberculin tests.[62, 75] A high index of suspicion and a careful history for possible contacts can be the best tools for diagnosis. Fundoscopic examination may reveal choroid tubercles. Liver and bone marrow frequently are involved in children with miliary tuberculosis; liver biopsy specimens and bone marrow aspirates should be obtained and processed for morphologic evaluation and culture. If the chest radiograph yields abnormal results, cultures of gastric aspirates, sputum, or both should be obtained. Because nontuberculous mycobacteria ("atypical organisms") are present in the gastric contents of normal individuals, demonstration of acid-fast organisms on smears of gastric secretion does not indicate disease necessarily. Rarely, tuberculous pericarditis presents with fever, weight loss, and weakness but without precordial pain or other specific cardiac complaints. Disseminated infection with atypical mycobacteria generally is seen in patients with HIV infections. (See Chapter 101.)

TULAREMIA. Failure to consider tularemia in children with FUO generally may be attributed to a lack of appreciation of the many sources of infection and the varied routes of inoculation. The organism may be acquired from contact with a variety of animal species, as well as from ticks, mosquitoes, lice, fleas, flies, and contaminated water. The organism can penetrate mucous membranes and broken or unbroken skin, or it may be inhaled or swallowed. It is important to question the patients and parents not only about animal contact but also about ingestion of rabbit or squirrel meat. (See Chapter 138.)

VIRAL INFECTIONS. Infection by most viruses produces an illness that is relatively brief. Exceptions to this rule include cytomegalovirus, Epstein-Barr virus, hepatitis viruses, and certain arboviruses. In all of these diseases, symptoms are extremely variable, and signs and symptoms frequently are nonspecific. Diagnosis can be established by appropriate cultures and serologic studies. (See Section 17 and Chapters 244 and 245.)

IMMUNODEFICIENCY. A variety of immunodeficient states, both congenital and acquired, can present as FUO. Patients with immunoglobulin deficiencies (e.g., Bruton agammaglobulinemia) may have a long history of recurrent fevers, with or without evident infections, whereas patients with abnormalities of lymphocyte function are more likely to have prolonged fever due to persistent viral or parasitic infection.

Localized Infections

BACTERIAL ENDOCARDITIS. Infective endocarditis is an infrequent cause of FUO in children. Acute bacterial endocarditis tends to be explosive in onset, but the subacute form begins insidiously, generally at the site of a preexisting cardiac lesion. Subacute bacterial endocarditis is rare in infants and increases in frequency with advancing age. The most commonly encountered organisms are viridans streptococci, enterococci, *S. aureus,* and *S. epidermidis.* The absence of a cardiac murmur does not exclude the possibility of endocarditis and especially is frequent when infection involves the right side of the heart. Endocarditis also may occur in the absence of positive blood cultures, especially in association with the following factors: use of antibiotics for an undefined febrile illness; right-sided cardiac lesions; prolonged duration of disease; infection by unusual organisms, such as *Brucella* or *Coxiella burnetii;* and inadequate culture methods for the detection of infection with anaerobic organisms. Frequently associated laboratory findings include anemia, leukocytosis, and an elevated erythrocyte sedimentation rate. Five or six blood cultures (aerobic and anaerobic) should be obtained over a period of several days. Echocardiography and gallium scan may reveal vegetations, but negative results do not rule out endocarditis. (See Chapter 32.)

BONE AND JOINT INFECTIONS. Infections of the bones and joints usually can be diagnosed clinically, but occasionally they present as FUO. This is more common with osteomyelitis than with septic arthritis. Infection of the pelvic bones most often is implicated in this regard. Radioisotopic bone scan and whole-body gallium scan are more sensitive than plain radiographs of the bones. (See Chapter 64.)

INTRA-ABDOMINAL ABSCESSES. Subphrenic, perinephric, and pelvic abscesses may present as FUO. A history of prior intra-abdominal disease or abdominal surgery or a history of vague abdominal complaints should heighten suspicion of an intra-abdominal collection of pus. The most common organisms involved are *S. aureus,* streptococci, *E. coli,* and anaerobic flora. Perinephric abscesses generally develop during the course of bacteremia, and fever may be the only sign. *S. aureus* is the organism most commonly recovered. Urinalysis generally yields normal results. The mass usually can be demonstrated by ultrasound examination, gallium scan, or computed tomography.

Deep pelvic abscesses are important causes of FUO in children. The source of the abscess cannot be determined always, but possibilities include chronic osteomyelitis of the pelvic bones, infected skin lesions with associated lymphadenitis, appendiceal infection, mesenteric salmonellosis, and pelvic thrombophlebitis. Careful rectal and pelvic examinations are important. Radiographic studies of the genitourinary and gastrointestinal tract, gallium scan, ultrasound examination, and computed tomography may be used to confirm the diagnosis.

LIVER ABSCESS AND OTHER HEPATIC INFECTIONS. Pyogenic liver abscesses are encountered most frequently in the immunocompromised pediatric patient but may be seen in the otherwise normal child.[39] In some patients, persistent fever is the only finding. Blood cultures usually are sterile, and liver function test results generally are within normal limits. Many patients have hepatomegaly and right upper quadrant abdominal tenderness. Diagnosis can be established by examination of the liver by ultrasonography, radioisotope scan, or computed tomography; a body gallium scan also may yield positive results. Bacterial hepatitis as well as bacterial cholangitis can occur in the absence of jaundice and other specific signs of liver dysfunction.[82, 85] Granulomatous hepatitis is not a specific disease but rather a syndrome characterized by granuloma formation within the liver. A specific etiology often cannot be determined. Although most reported cases have been in adults,[71] we have seen examples in children, particularly in children with Epstein-Barr virus infection and with cat-scratch disease. The diagnosis can be established only by liver biopsy. See Chapter 58.

UPPER RESPIRATORY TRACT INFECTIONS. In both published series and our experience, it is surprising how frequently infections of the upper respiratory tract and related organs present as FUO.[43, 54, 66] Although obvious signs or symptoms would be expected, the complaints often appear trivial and thus may be ignored. Occasionally, physical findings may be absent in cases of mastoiditis or sinusitis. Reported cases of FUO in children have included other diagnoses, such as chronic or recurrent otitis media, chronic or recurrent pharyngitis, tonsillitis, peritonsillar abscess, and nonspecific upper respiratory tract infection. Generally, it is not possible to determine from the published material the validity of either the diagnosis or the appellation FUO in these cases.

A syndrome of periodic fever has been associated with aphthous stomatitis, pharyngitis, and cervical adenitis. Symptoms recur at 4- to 6-week intervals, generally beginning abruptly and resolving spontaneously in 4 to 5 days. The cause of this syndrome remains unknown.[27]

A parapharyngeal inflammatory pseudotumor presenting as FUO has been reported in a 3-year-old female who also developed anemia and weight loss. The etiology was never discerned, but the symptoms resolved after surgical removal of the inflammatory mass.[19]

Examples of Noninfectious Causes of Fever of Unknown Origin

Central Nervous System Dysfunction

It is well known that children with severe brain damage may have dysfunction of thermoregulation and that some of these patients may run elevated body temperatures for months. There also are reports of otherwise neurologically normal children who have had fever as a result of central dysfunction. Berger[9] reported a 16-year-old child with recurrent episodes of fever that were believed to represent a form of epilepsy and that disappeared when treatment with phenytoin was begun. Wolff and associates[83] reported a 14-year-old child with cyclic episodes of fever, nausea, vomiting, and emotional disturbance due to a central nervous system lesion.

Diabetes Insipidus

Both central and nephrogenic diabetes insipidus can cause FUO in infants and young children. Polyuria and polydipsia may not be appreciated during infancy. Hyperthermia, weight loss, and peripheral vascular collapse may ensue. Signs of dehydration or an increased serum concentration of sodium suggests the diagnosis. Diagnosis is established by simultaneous measurements of urine and serum electrolytes and osmolality during periods of normal hydration and after carefully controlled periods of water deprivation. Serum levels of antidiuretic hormone also may be measured by radioimmunoassay.

Drug Fever

Nearly any medication can be associated with an allergic reaction, including fever. The offending agent may be a prescribed drug, an over-the-counter preparation, or a street drug, such as amphetamine or PCP. Atropine, whether taken systemically or used topically as eye drops, can cause temperature elevation. Phenothiazines and anticholinergic drugs can inhibit sweating and impair temperature regulation. Epinephrine and related compounds may affect thermoregulatory control mechanisms and produce fever. Generally, drug fever is low-grade but may be high and spiking. Fever may be continuous or intermittent. Discontinuation of the drug generally is followed by disappearance of fever within 48 hours, but the fever sometimes persists for as long as a month as a result of slow excretion of the offending agent.

Factitious Fever

A parent or patient may report falsely the presence of fever that does not exist, or the reading of the thermometer may be increased by immersing the bulb in hot liquids, placing it beside a cigarette, rubbing the bulb vigorously on the bedsheet, or rinsing the mouth with hot liquid immediately before inserting the thermometer. Clues to a factitious fever include (1) absence of tachycardia, malaise, or discomfort, despite a markedly elevated temperature, (2) apparent rapid defervescence unaccompanied by diaphoresis, (3) failure of the temperature curve to follow the normal diurnal variation of body temperature, (4) hyperpyrexia, and (5) normal temperature reading when the temperature is obtained rectally by someone who remains in attendance during the procedure. The presence of fever also may be confirmed or excluded by measuring the temperature of a freshly voided urine specimen. The current use of electronic thermometers in most hospitals decreases the possibility of factitious fever in that setting because the nurse or aide usually brings in the thermometer and stays in attendance during the relatively brief period of insertion. In more unusual cases, the patient or parent actually may induce fever by the injection of infective or foreign materials.

Familial Dysautonomia (Riley-Day Syndrome)

Familial dysautonomia, transmitted as an autosomal recessive trait, is a disorder in autonomic and peripheral sensory nerve function. Eighty per cent of cases have occurred in children of Jewish parentage, particularly Ashkenazi Jews. Defective temperature regulation may result in either hypothermia or hyperthermia.[23]

A careful history and physical examination may reveal the following: poorly coordinated swallowing movements, which lead to recurrent aspiration and pneumonia; recurrent episodes of vomiting; excessive salivation; excessive or diminished sweating; diminished formation of tears; periods of hypotension, hypertension, or both; and erythema or blanching of the skin. The fungiform papillae of the tongue are diminished in number or absent, and the sensation of taste is deficient.[72] Self-mutilation or multiple sites of skin trauma may reflect diminished or absent pain sensation peripherally. Deep-tendon reflexes are diminished; corneal reflexes are impaired; and mental deficiency, dysarthria, and emotional lability are common.

Vanillylmandelic acid excretion in urine may be diminished, and homovanillic acid excretion may be increased. Administration of histamine intradermally may produce a wheal but no flare or pain at the site of injection. Placement of methacholine (2.5 per cent) into the conjunctival sac produces pupillary constriction in children with familial dysautonomia but no response in the normal child. Intravenous infusion of norepinephrine is followed by an exaggerated pressor response, and the hypotensive response to infusion of methacholine is increased.

Inflammatory Bowel Disease

Fever has been associated repeatedly with regional enteritis or granulomatous colitis, and fever has been stressed as a prominent sign in most children with inflammatory bowel disease.[20, 41, 80] A greater percentage of children than adults with regional enteritis have fever. Appropriate radiographic contrast studies of the intestines should be undertaken in children with prolonged FUO, even in the absence of findings specifically referable to the gastrointestinal tract. This especially is true if the erythrocyte sedimentation rate is elevated and if there is anemia, weight loss, failure of linear growth, or a positive result on stool guaiac test.

Ulcerative colitis also may present as FUO, although less commonly than regional enteritis. In patients with ulcerative colitis, symptoms referable to the gastrointestinal tract generally are present at the time the patient is febrile.

Infantile Cortical Hyperostosis (Caffey Disease)

The etiology of this condition is unknown. A decrease in frequency in recent years has suggested an infectious, possibly viral, etiology. Spontaneous hyperplasia of the subperiosteal bone begins during infancy and is associated with swelling of the overlying tissues. The skull, mandible, clavicles, scapula, and ribs are affected most frequently, but in some children the long bones and even the metatarsal bones may be involved. Most patients have persistent fever, usually low-grade but sometimes as high as 40° C (104° F). Tenderness over the affected regions, irritability, elevated erythrocyte sedimentation rate, and leukocytosis are common. The diagnosis is established by the clinical picture in conjunction with radiographically demonstrated periosteal involvement.

Juvenile Rheumatoid Arthritis

This chronic inflammatory disorder generally presents as one of three distinct syndromes: (1) the systemic form, characterized by high, spiking temperatures (generally once or twice a day), evanescent rash, and lymphadenopathy; (2) a polyarticular form; and (3) a monarticular or pauciarticular form. Fever is associated with all three presentations but is most common in the systemic form, in which case it is present in nearly 100 per cent of patients. This also is the form most likely to present as FUO.[15] Arthritis may not develop for months to years after the onset of fever. Diagnosis often needs to be made by exclusion because serologic tests generally are negative.

Periodic Fevers

Reimann[67] called attention to a group of patients with recurrent episodes of fever at intervals of 7 to 21 days. Some of the patients had leukopenia and abdominal or thoracic pain. The reasons for the fever and its periodicity remain unknown. Patients with cyclic neutropenia frequently have fever during acute episodes, but not all the patients reported by Reimann had neutropenia. Familial Mediterranean fever also may be characterized by episodic fever and abdominal pain.[26] This disease, found in persons of Mediterranean ancestry, is inherited as an autosomal recessive trait. The pattern of recurrent fever in familial Mediterranean fever, however, is irregular, with varying periods of normality between episodes of fever. Although recurrent fever has been associated with elevated serum concentrations of etiocholanolone,[11, 35] the concentration of etiocholanolone in the serum of patients with familial Mediterranean fever is normal. Most patients with this set of findings have been of northern or eastern European origin. The relationship, if any, of etiocholanolone to the fever is unknown.

References

1. Adams, K. C., Dixon, J. H., and Eichner, E. R.: Clinical usefulness of polymorphonuclear leukocyte vacuolization in predicting septicemia in febrile children. Pediatrics *62*:67–70, 1978.
2. Ayus, C. J., Krothapalli, R. K., and Arieff, A. I.: Occult bacteremia in febrile children. N. Engl. J. Med. *318*:1338–1339, 1988.
3. Baker, R. C., Tiller, T., Bausher, J. C., et al.: Severity of disease correlated with fever reduction in febrile infants. Pediatrics *83*:1016–1019, 1989.
4. Baraff, L. J., Bass, J. W., Fleisher, G. R., et al.: Practice guidelines for the management of infants and children 0 to 36 months of age with fever without source. Pediatrics *92*:1–12, 1993.
5. Baraff, L. J., Oslund, S., and Prather, M.: Effect of antibiotic therapy and etiologic microorganism on the risk of bacterial meningitis in children with occult bacteremia. Pediatrics *92*:140–143, 1993.
6. Baron, M. A., and Fink, H. D.: Bacteremia in private pediatric practice. Pediatrics *66*:171–175, 1980.
7. Bass, J. W., Steel, R. W., Wittler, R. R., et al.: Antimicrobial treatment of occult bacteremia: A multicenter cooperative study. Pediatr. Infect. Dis. J. *12*:466–473, 1993.
8. Baron, M. A., Fink, H. D., and Cicchetti, D. V.: Blood cultures in private pediatric practice: An eleven-year experience. Pediatr. Infect. Dis. *8*:2–7, 1989.
9. Berger, H.: Fever: An unusual manifestation of epilepsy. Postgrad. Med. *40*:479–481, 1966.
10. Bloom, H. R.: Must we treat clinical judgment? Pediatrics *67*:745–746, 1981.
11. Bondy, P. K., Cohn, G. L., Herrmann, W., et al.: The possible relationship of etiocholanolone to periodic fever. Yale J. Biol. Med. *30*:395–405, 1958.
12. Bratton, L., Teele, D. W., and Klein, J. O.: Outcome of unsuspected pneumococcemia in children not initially admitted to the hospital. J. Pediatr. *90*:703–706, 1977.
13. Brewis, E. C.: Undiagnosed fever. Br. Med. J. *1*:107–110, 1965.
14. Burke, J. P., Klein, J. O., Gezon, H. M., et al.: Pneumococcal bacteremia: Review of 111 cases, 1957–1969, with special reference to cases with undetermined focus. Am. J. Dis. Child. *121*:353–359, 1971.
15. Calabro, J. J., and Marchesano, J. M.: Juvenile rheumatoid arthritis. N. Engl. J. Med. *277*:746–749, 1967.
16. Carey, B. M., Williams, C. E., and Arthur, R. J.: Ultrasound demonstration of pericardial empyema in an infant with pyrexia of undetermined origin. Pediatr. Radiol. *18*:349–350, 1988.
17. Carroll, W. L., Farrell, M. K., Singer, J. I., et al.: Treatment of occult bacteremia: A prospective randomized clinical trial. Pediatrics *72*:608–611, 1983.
18. Centers for Disease Control: Annual Survey of Leptospirosis for 1972. Issued 1974.
19. Chan, Y. F., Ma, L. T., Yeung, L. T., et al.: Parapharyngeal inflammatory pseudotumor presenting as fever of unknown origin in a 3-year-old girl. Pediatr. Pathol. *8*:195–203, 1988.
20. Chron, B. B., and Yarnis, H.: Continuous fever of intestinal origin. Ann. Intern. Med. *26*:858–862, 1947.
21. Corrigan, J. J.: Thrombocytopenia: Laboratory sign of septicemia in infants and children. J. Pediatr. *85*:219–223, 1974.
22. Crocker, P. J., Quick, G., and McCombs, W.: Occult bacteremia in the emergency department: Diagnostic criteria for the young febrile child. Ann. Intern. Med. *14*:71–76, 1995.
23. Dancis, J., and Smith, A. A.: Familial dysautonomia. N. Engl. J. Med. *274*:207–209, 1966.
24. Dashefsky, B., Teele, D. W., and Klein, J. O.: Unsuspected meningococcemia. J. Pediatr. *102*:69–72, 1983.
25. Dershewitz, R. A.: A comparative study of the prevalence, outcome and prediction of bacteremia in children. J. Pediatr. *103*:352–358, 1983.
26. Ehrenfeld, E. N., Eliakin, M., and Rachmilewitz, M.: Recurrent polyserositis (familial Mediterranean fever, periodic disease): A report of 55 cases. Am. J. Med. *31*:107–123, 1961.
27. Feder, H. M. J., and Bialecki, C. A.: Periodic fever associated with aphthous stomatitis, pharyngitis and cervical adenitis. Pediatr. Infect. Dis. *8*:186–189, 1989.
28. Feigin, R. D., and Shearer, W. T.: Fever of unknown origin in children. Curr. Probl. Pediatr. *6*:2–57, 1976.
29. Fineman, D. S., Palestno, C. J., Kim, C. K., et al.: Detection of abnormalities in febrile AIDS patients with In-111-labelled leukocyte and ga-67 scintigraphy. Radiology *170*:677–680, 1989.
30. Fleishner, G. R., Rosenberg, N., Vinci, R., et al.: Intramuscular versus oral antibiotic therapy for the prevention of meningitis and other bacterial sequela in young febrile children at risk for occult bacteremia. J. Pediatr. *124*:504–512, 1994.
31. Habibian, M. R., Staab, E. V., and Matthews, H. A.: Gallium citrate Ga 67 scans in febrile patients. J. A. M. A. *233*:1073–1076, 1975.
32. Hayani, A., Mahoney, D. H., and Fernback, D. J.: Role of bone marrow examination in the child with prolonged fever. J. Pediatr. *116*:919–920, 1990.
33. Heldrich, F. J.: *Diplococcus pneumoniae* bacteremia. Am. J. Dis. Child. *119*:12–17, 1970.
34. Hoekelman, R., Lewin, E. B., and Shapira, M. D., et al.: Potential bacteremia in pediatric practice. Am. J. Dis. Child. *133*:1017–1019, 1979.
35. Jacobs, J. C.: Etiocholanolone fever: Report of a case in childhood with

periodic peritonitis associated with elevated serum etiocholanolone. Pediatrics *33*:284–287, 1964.
36. Jacobs, N. M., Lerdkachornsuk, S., and Metzger, W. I.: Pneumococcal bacteremia in infants and children: A ten-year experience at the Cook County Hospital with special reference to the pneumococcal serotypes isolated. Pediatrics *64*:296–300, 1979.
37. Jaffee, D. M., Tanz, R. R., Davis, T., et al.: Antibiotic administration to treat possible occult bacteremia in febrile children. N. Engl. J. Med. *317*:1175–1180, 1987.
38. Joffe, M., and Avner, J. R.: Follow up of patients with occult bacteremia in pediatric emergency departments. Pediatr. Emerg. Care *8*:258–261, 1992.
39. Kaplan, S. L., and Feigin, R. D.: Pyogenic liver abscess in normal children with fever of unknown origin. Pediatrics *58*:614–616, 1976.
40. Kline, M. W., Smith, E. O., Kaplan, S. L., et al.: Effects of causative organism and presence or absence of meningitis on white blood cell counts in children with bacteremia. J. Emerg. Med. *6*:33–35, 1988.
41. Lee, F. I., and Davies, D. M.: Crohn's disease presenting as pyrexia of unknown origin. Lancet *1*:1205–1206, 1961.
42. Liu, C., Lehan, C., Speer, M. E., et al.: Early detection of bacteremia in an outpatient clinic. Pediatrics *75*:827–831, 1985.
43. Lohr, J. A., and Hendley, J. O.: Prolonged fever of unknown origin: Record of experience with 54 childhood patients. Clin. Pediatr. *16*:768–773, 1977.
44. Long, S. S.: Antibiotic therapy in febrile children: "Best laid schemes...." J. Pediatr. *124*:585–588, 1994.
45. Lorin, M. I.: The Febrile Child: Clinical Management of Fever and Other Types of Pyrexia. New York, John Wiley & Sons, 1982, p. 70.
46. Mazur, L. J., Jones, T., and Kozinetz, C. A.: Temperature response to acetaminophen and risk of occult bacteremia: A case control study. J. Pediatr. *115*:888–891, 1989.
47. McCarthy, P. L., Grundy, G. W., Spiesel, S. Z., et al.: Bacteremia in children: An outpatient review. Pediatrics *57*:861–868, 1976.
48. McCarthy, P. L., Frank, A. L., Ablow, R. C., et al.: Creative protein test in the differentiation of bacterial and viral pneumonia. J. Pediatr. *92*:454–459, 1978.
49. McCarthy, P. L., Jekel, J. F., Stashwick, C. A., et al.: History and observation variables in assessing febrile children. Pediatrics *65*:1090–1095, 1980.
50. McCarthy, P. L., Jekel, J. F., Stashwick, C. A., et al.: Further definition of history and observation variables in assessing febrile children. Pediatrics *67*:687–693, 1981.
51. McCarthy, P. L., Sharpe, M. R., Spiesel, S. Z., et al.: Observation scales to identify serious illness in febrile children. Pediatrics *70*:802–809, 1982.
52. McCarthy, P. L., and Dolan, T. F.: Hyperpyrexia in children: Eight-year emergency room experience. Am. J. Dis. Child. *130*:849–851, 1976.
53. McCarthy, P. L., Jekel, J. F., and Dolan, T. F.: Temperature greater than or equal to 40° C in children less than 24 months of age: A prospective study. Pediatrics *59*:663–668, 1977.
54. McClung, H. J.: Prolonged fever of unknown origin in childhood. Am. J. Dis. Child. *124*:544–550, 1972.
55. McGowan, J. E., Bratton, L., Klein, J. O., et al.: Bacteremia in febrile children seen in a walk-in pediatric clinic. N. Engl. J. Med. *288*:1309–1312, 1973.
56. McMurray, D. N., and Echeverri, A.: Cell-mediated immunity in anergic patients with pulmonary tuberculosis. Am. Rev. Respir. Dis. *118*:827–834, 1978.
57. Margolis, M. T.: Specific anergy in tuberculosis. N. Engl. J. Med. *309*:1388, 1983.
58. Marshall, R., Teele, D. W., and Klein, J. O.: Unsuspected bacteremia due to *Haemophilus influenzae:* Outcome in children not initially admitted to hospital. J. Pediatr. *95*:690–695, 1979.
59. Morens, D. W.: WBC and differential: Value in predicting bacterial disease in children. Am. J. Dis. Child. *133*:25–27, 1979.
60. Murray, D. L., et al.: Relative importance of bacteremia and viremia in the course of acute fevers of unknown origin in outpatient children. Pediatrics *68*:157–160, 1981.
61. Nash, D. R., and Douglas, J. E.: Anergy in active pulmonary tuberculosis: A comparison between positive and negative reactors and an evaluation of 5 TU and 250 TU skin test doses. Chest *77*:32–37, 1980.
62. Ostrow, J. H.: Tuberculin negative tuberculosis. Am. Rev. Respir. Dis. *107*:882–883, 1973.
63. Peltola, H.: C-reactive protein in rapid differentiation of acute epiglottitis from spasmodic croup and acute laryngotracheitis: Preliminary report. J. Pediatr. *102*:713–715, 1983.
64. Petersdorf, R. G., and Beeson, P. B.: Fever of unexplained origin: Report on 100 cases. Medicine *40*:1–30, 1961.
65. Picus, D., Siegel, M. J., and Balfe, D. M.: Abdominal computed tomography in children with unexplained prolonged fever. J. Comput. Assist. Tomogr. *8*:851–856, 1984.
66. Pizzo, P. A., Lovejoy, F. H., and Smith, D. H.: Prolonged fever in children: Review of 100 cases. Pediatrics *55*:468–473, 1975.
67. Reimann, H. A.: Periodic disease, periodic fever, periodic abdominalgia, cyclic neutropenia, intermittent arthralgia, angioneurotic edema, anaphylactoid purpura and periodic paralysis. J. A. M. A. *141*:175–183, 1949.
68. Roberts, K. B., and Borzy, M. S.: Fever in the first eight weeks of life. Johns Hopkins Med. J. *141*:9–13, 1977.
69. Rosenberg N.: Pediatric occult bacteremia. Am. J. Emerg. Med. *2*:231–237, 1983.
70. Shapiro E. D., Aaron, N. H., Wald, E. R., et al.: Risk factors for development of bacterial meningitis among children with occult bacteremia. J. Pediatr. *109*:15–19, 1986.
71. Simon, H. B., and Wolff, S. M.: Granulomatous hepatitis and prolonged fever of unknown origin: A study of 13 patients. Medicine *52*:1–21, 1973.
72. Smith, A. A., Farbman, A., and Dancis, J.: Tongue in familial dysautonomia. Am. J. Dis. Child. *110*:152–153, 1965.
73. Steele, R. W., Jones S. M., Lowe, B. A., et al.: Usefulness of scanning procedures for diagnosis of fever of unknown origin in children. J. Pediatr. *119*:526–530, 1991.
74. Stein, R. C.: The white blood cell count in fevers of unknown origin. Am. J. Dis. Child. *124*:60–63, 1972.
75. Steiner, P., and Portuguleza, C.: Tuberculous meningitis in children. Am. Rev. Respir. Dis. *107*:22–29, 1973.
76. Strickland, A. D.: Serious implications of fever in the young infant. Presentation at Grand Rounds, Ben Taub Hospital, Houston, September 1978.
77. Teele, D. W., Pelton, S. I., Grant, M. J., et al.: Bacteremia in febrile children under 2 years of age: Results of cultures of blood of 600 consecutive febrile children in a "walk-in" clinic. J. Pediatr. *87*:227–230, 1975.
78. Todd, J. K.: Childhood infections: Diagnostic value of peripheral white blood cell and differential cell counts. Am. J. Dis. Child. *127*:810–816, 1974.
79. Torrey, S. B., Henretig, F., Fleisher, G., et al.: Temperature response to antipyretic therapy in children. Am. J. Emerg. Med. *3*:190–192, 1985.
80. Walker, S. H.: Periodic fever in juvenile regional enteritis. J. Pediatr. *60*:561–565, 1962.
81. Waskerwitz, S., and Berkelhammer, J. E.: Outpatient bacteremia: Clinical findings in children under two years with initial temperatures of 39.5° C or higher. J. Pediatr. *99*:231–233, 1981.
82. Weinstein, L.: Bacterial hepatitis: A case report on an unrecognized cause of fever of unknown origin. N. Engl. J. Med. *299*:1052–1054, 1978.
83. Wolff, S. M., Ward, S. B., and Landy, M.: A syndrome of periodic hypothalamic discharge. Am. J. Med. *36*:956–966, 1964.
84. Wright, P. F., Thompson, J., McKee, K. T., Jr., et al.: Patterns of illness in the highly febrile young child: Epidemiologic, clinical and laboratory correlates. Pediatrics *67*:694–700, 1981.
85. Wyllie, R., and Fitzgerald, J. F.: Bacterial cholangitis in a 10-week-old infant with fever of undetermined origin. Pediatrics *65*:164–167, 1980.
86. Yamamoto, L. T., Wigder, H. N., Fligner, D. J., et al.: Relationship of bacteremia to antipyretic therapy in febrile children. Pediatr. Emerg. Care *3*:223–226, 1987.

74

TOXIC SHOCK SYNDROME

P. Joan Chesney and Jeffrey P. Davis

Much has been learned about the pathogenesis and pathophysiology of toxic shock syndrome (TSS) since the initial description in 1978 by Dr. James K. Todd. The clinical illness is defined by the criteria listed in the case definition formulated for epidemiologic studies (Table 74–1). Although often confused with septic shock, TSS has unique clinical manifestations not generally noted in septic shock, including diffuse erythroderma, delayed desquamation of palms and soles, conjunctival and pharyngeal hyperemia, muscle injury, rapidly accelerated renal failure, and gastrointestinal symptoms.

TABLE 74–1. Toxic Shock Syndrome Clinical Case Definition

Fever:	Temperature ≥38.9°C
Rash:	Diffuse macular erythroderma
Desquamation:	1–2 weeks after onset of illness, particularly of palms, soles, fingers, and toes
Hypotension:	Systolic blood pressure ≤90 mm Hg for adults; <5th percentile by age for children <16 years of age; orthostatic drop in diastolic blood pressure ≥15 mm Hg from lying to sitting; orthostatic syncope or orthostatic dizziness

Involvement of three or more of the following organ systems:

A. Gastrointestinal: vomiting or diarrhea at onset of illness
B. Muscular: severe myalgia or creatinine phosphokinase level greater than twice the upper limit of normal for laboratory
C. Mucous membrane: vaginal, oropharyngeal, or conjunctival hyperemia
D. Renal: BUN or serum creatinine greater than twice the upper limit of normal or ≥5 white blood cells per high-power field in the absence of a urinary tract infection
E. Hepatic: total bilirubin, SGOT, or SGPT greater than twice the upper limit of normal for laboratory
F. Hematologic: platelets <100,000/mm^3
G. Central nervous system: disorientation or alterations in consciousness without focal neurologic signs when fever and hypotension are absent

Negative results on the following tests, if obtained:

A. Blood, throat, or cerebrospinal fluid cultures; blood culture may be positive for *Staphylococcus aureus*
B. Serologic tests for Rocky Mountain spotted fever, leptospirosis, or measles

Case Classification

Probable: a case with five of the six clinical findings described above

Confirmed: a case with all six of the clinical findings described above, including desquamation, unless the patient dies before desquamation could occur

From Centers for Disease Control: Case definitions for public health surveillance. M. M. W. R. *39*(No. RR-13):38–39, 1990.

The capillary leak syndrome, or the rapid and massive loss of fluid from capillaries into the interstitial space, loss of peripheral vascular resistance, and subsequent multisystem end-organ failure further characterize this entity. Histopathologic findings are minimal and nonspecific, with extensive interstitial edema of all tissues and a minimal perivascular mononuclear cellular infiltrate. TSS can recur after both menstrual and nonmenstrual cases. The highest recurrence rate of 65 per cent was described in a subset of untreated women with menstrual TSS who continued to use tampons during menses.

When first described, TSS had unique geographic, age, sex, and racial characteristics. It was associated with menses, particularly with tampon use, as well as with a phenotypically distinctive type of *Staphylococcus aureus*. In 1994, at least 42 per cent of reported cases of TSS were nonmenstrual. *S. aureus* exotoxins now recognized to be "superantigens" and the endogenous mediators produced by these exotoxins appear to mediate the disease manifestations.

TSS toxin I (TSST-I) and the staphylococcal enterotoxins are extremely potent stimuli for the in vitro macrophage production of interleukin-1 (IL-1) and tumor necrosis factor–alpha (TNF-α) and the T-lymphocyte production of IL-2, lymphotoxin (TNF-β), and interferon gamma (IFN-γ). These staphylococcal exotoxins are functionally bivalent mitogens that bind highly selectively to the major histocompatibility complex class II receptors on antigen-processing cells and to selected beta elements of the T-cell receptor (TCR) specific for each toxin. They now are known as superantigens.

HISTORY

Illnesses resembling TSS and associated with *S. aureus* have been reported since 1927.[6, 97, 107, 266, 287] The initial description of the illness as a disease of children was published in 1978.[273] A Kawasaki-like syndrome described in adults subsequently was recognized to be TSS.[184] The first 12 cases of TSS identified in Wisconsin and Minnesota between July 1979 and January 1980 were reported by the state epidemiologists to the Centers for Disease Control and Prevention (CDC) in January 1980.[48, 80, 253] All 12 cases had occurred in women, and a possible association with menses was noted. The probable recurrent nature of the illness also was reported.[48, 80] In May 1980, the CDC reported findings of the first 55 nationally reported cases.[48] Ninety-five per cent of the cases were in women. Of 40 patients for whom a menstrual history was obtained, 38 (95 per cent) had onset during menstruation. Thirteen patients had experienced recurrent episodes of TSS.

By June 1980, case-control studies statistically linking the occurrence of menstrual TSS with tampons had been completed by the Wisconsin Division of Health[80] and the CDC,[253] and similar trends had been noted by the Utah Department of Health.[151] In September 1980, the CDC reported that although TSS had been associated with many tampon brands, women using one particular brand of tampon, Rely (Procter & Gamble), were at a greater risk. This brand immediately and voluntarily was withdrawn from the market by the manufacturer.[21, 41, 243] Subsequent frequent updates by the CDC documented a decrease in reported cases.[46, 47, 49]

Microbiologic studies have established that the majority of patients with menses-associated TSS (menstrual TSS) had vaginal or cervical colonization with *S. aureus*.[19] These strains of *S. aureus* made a characteristic marker protein or toxin initially named staphylococcal enterotoxin F (SEF)[20] and pyrogenic exotoxin C[245] and now known as TSST-I.

EPIDEMIOLOGY

Surveillance and Incidence

Statewide surveillance for cases of TSS began in Wisconsin[84] and Minnesota[209] in January 1980, in Utah in February 1980,[162] and in other states after the national communications about TSS in the spring of 1980. In 1982, TSS became a nationally notifiable disease. During the years 1983 through 1994, the CDC had received reports of 4192 cases of TSS through the National Electronic Telecommunications System for Surveillance (NETSS).[43] The National Center for Infectious Diseases at the CDC maintains a database of cases meeting the TSS case definition. This database includes cases reported prior to 1983. Since 1983, a continued downward trend in passively reported cases has been noted (Fig. 74–1).

Of 2509 confirmed cases reported to the CDC through April 1984, 95 per cent were in females.[40] Among the 2295 women with known menstrual histories, 89 per cent had TSS onset associated with menstruation. Of 1716 menses-associated cases for which information related to catamenial product use was available, 99 per cent occurred in tampon users, 1 per cent occurred with the exclusive use of napkins

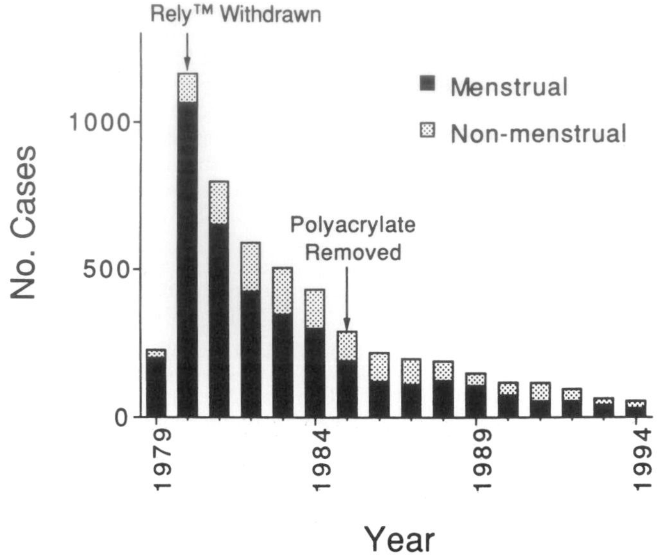

FIGURE 74–1. *Menstrual and nonmenstrual cases of toxic shock syndrome reported to the Centers for Disease Control and Prevention, by year, 1979 to 1994. Indicated are the dates of withdrawal of Rely brand tampons and superabsorbent tampons containing polyacrylate rayon. (From Deresiewicz, R. L.: Staphylococcal toxic shock syndrome. In Leung, D. Y. M., Huber, B. T., and Schlievert, P. M. [eds.]: Superantigens: Molecular Biology, Immunology and Relevance to Human Disease. New York, Marcel Dekker [in press]. By courtesy of Marcel Dekker, Inc.)*

or minipads, and one case occurred after the use of a sea sponge.

Results of an active surveillance study conducted by the CDC in 1986 and 1987 in five states and Los Angeles County confirmed the trends previously noted using the CDC passive surveillance system.[124] The incidence of menstrual TSS was found to be 1 case per 100,000 women 15 to 44 years of age. This is a substantial reduction from the reported rates of 2.4 to 12.3 cases per 100,000 women of menstruating age in 1980.[80, 162, 209, 222] Only 55 per cent of the cases detected in the 1986 and 1987 study were in women, and 45 per cent of all cases were menstrually associated.[35, 124] In 1986 and 1987, the incidence of nonmenstrual, nonvaginal TSS in women (0.25 cases per 100,000 women) and TSS in males (0.16 cases per 100,000 men) had changed little since 1980. In 1994, only 192 cases of TSS were reported to the CDC through the NETSS. The overall passive reported incidence of TSS was 0.1 cases per 100,000 population. Among confirmed cases, 42 per cent were nonmenstrual.[43]

Principal reasons for the striking reduction in the incidence of menstrual TSS include the decrease in tampon absorbency, changes in tampon composition and usage patterns during the 1980s, and the impact of publicity on the early reporting during 1980.[42, 79, 84, 210, 250] There may be other factors that have contributed to the significant decrease in incidence.[42, 250] With enhanced recognition of symptoms of TSS, women may seek medical help sooner, thus obviating development of the severe syndrome. Also, proportionately fewer women now may use tampons continuously or at all.[110]

The nationally reported TSS-related mortality rate generally decreased with time from 10 per cent for the years prior to 1980 to 2.6 per cent in 1983.[35] Among women with menstrual TSS, the reported national case-fatality rate was 5 per cent in 1980 and 0 per cent in 1988 and 1989.[42] During the years 1980 to 1986, an increased mortality rate was observed among nonmenstrual case patients. The increase in mortality rate particularly was noticeable in men (17.1 per cent) and women (13.2 per cent) older than 45 years of age, compared with men (9.5 per cent) or women with nonmenstrual TSS (4.3 per cent) who were between 15 and 44 years of age.[35]

Although cases in the United States have been reported in all 50 states and the District of Columbia, significant differences in incidence were noted among the states through 1983.[40] Through mid-1983, the five states of Wisconsin, Minnesota, Colorado, Utah, and California accounted for 44 per cent of the total reported cases but represented only 16 per cent of the United States population. Although intensified surveillance may have been a factor, regional differences in the degree of immunity to TSS-associated *S. aureus* toxins and in the distribution of toxin-producing organisms may have been important factors.[284] Geographic differences in TSS occurrence continue to exist even with the increase in the relative proportion of nonmenstrual cases.[35]

Risk Factors for Menstrual Toxic Shock Syndrome (Table 74–2)

From early 1980 through 1990, most reported cases of TSS occurred in previously healthy, young, white, menstruating women who were using tampons at the time of onset of illness. The explanation for this combination of risk factors is complex.

Age

The mean age of patients with confirmed menstrual TSS (22.6 years in 1980, 23 years in 1986) has varied little since 1980.[40, 124] Roughly one-third of the cases occur in adolescents 15 to 19 years of age (Fig. 74–2).[40] The mean age of patients with nonmenstrual TSS (27 years through 1982, 30 years in 1986) is significantly higher than that for menses-associated cases.[124, 229] The precise reason for the increased incidence of TSS in adolescent females is not known; however, a lower prevalence of antibody to TSST-I may increase susceptibility in this age group.[286]

Race

A striking race/ethnicity distribution is present for menstrual TSS; 97 per cent of such cases have occurred in whites, who make up 83 per cent of the United States population. This distribution is not as striking for nonmenstrual TSS because 87 per cent of nonmenstrual cases have occurred in whites. The reasons for racial differences are not clear and only partially explained by differences in menses-related practices.[40, 110, 229] Racial differences in antibody to TSST-I partially may explain the differences in the distribution of cases.[284]

Menstruation and Tampon Use

The initial observations in 1980 that a high proportion of patients with TSS had onset during menses now has been well documented. The use of tampons as a significant risk factor for the development of TSS was well established in six case-control studies conducted in 1980[80, 131, 151, 211, 243, 253] and one conducted in 1987.[124] Although these studies varied in design and methodologic technique, all demonstrated that at least 97 per cent of case individuals wore tampons during menstrual periods associated with disease onset. Although 76 to 89 per cent of matched control individuals wore tampons during temporally comparable menstrual periods, the use of tampons was associated with menstrual TSS in each of these studies, with odds ratios ranging from 11 to 18.[35]

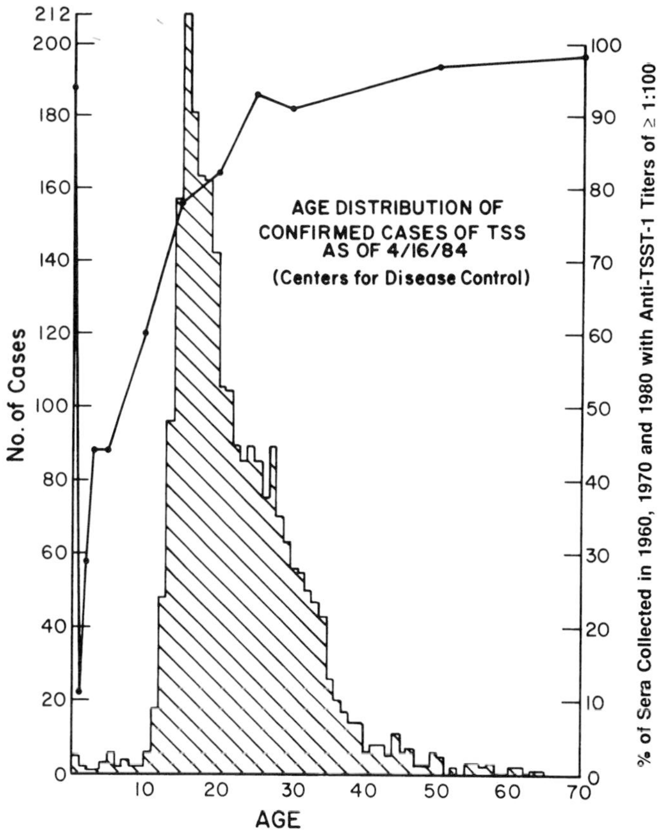

FIGURE 74–2. *Age distribution of patients with confirmed toxic shock syndrome reported to the Centers for Disease Control and Prevention prior to April 16, 1984. The age-specific prevalence of antibodies to toxic shock syndrome toxin I in a normal population in Wisconsin in the years 1960, 1970, and 1980 is indicated by the solid connected line (Data from Vergeront, J. M., Stolz, S. J., Crass, B. A., et al.: Prevalence of serum antibody to staphylococcal enterotoxin F among Wisconsin residents: Implications for toxic shock syndrome. J. Infect. Dis.* 148:692–698, 1983.)

Although TSS has occurred and continues to occur with the use of all brands of tampons, the second CDC case-control study demonstrated a greater relative risk of developing menstrual TSS with use of one tampon brand, Rely, compared with other brands.[41, 243] The Tri-State (Minnesota, Wisconsin, and Iowa) TSS Study established that tampons of increasing absorbency were associated with an increasing relative risk of the development of menstrual TSS and that the risk of menstrual TSS associated with Rely tampons was greater than that predicted by absorbency alone.[211]

Reasons listed earlier for the striking reduction in the incidence of menstrual TSS may be the decrease in tampon absorbency and changes in tampon composition.[42] In 1980, very high absorbency products were used by 42 per cent of tampon users.[209] By 1983, this proportion had decreased to 18 per cent and by 1986 to 1 per cent.[42] Overall, the absorbency of available tampon brand styles, as measured by the syngina test,[200] ranged from 10.3 to 20.5 g in 1980 and from less than 6 to 15 g in 1990, which indicates an industry-wide decrease in tampon absorbency. Tampon composition also has changed since 1980. Currently available tampons are composed of cotton and/or cotton and rayon combinations. In 1980, tampon additives included polyacrylate, polyester foam, cross-linked carboxymethylcellulose, and several surfactants, including pluronic L-92.[248] It is unclear whether these additives enhanced the risk of TSS independently or in combination with or independent of their increasing absorbency.[21, 211, 243]

Two subsequent case-control studies conducted by the CDC involving patients with onset of TSS in 1983 and 1984 (CDC III) and 1986 and 1987 (CDC IV) confirmed the Tri-State TSS Study results of a linear increasing TSS risk related to increasing tampon absorbency; for each 1 g increase in absorbency, the TSS risk increased by 34 to 37 per cent.[21, 114] In addition, the Tri-State TSS Study and the CDC III study both suggested that the effects of tampon absorbency and chemical composition on TSS risk were independent.[21, 35, 211]

Continuous use of tampons was associated with a greater risk of TSS than was noncontinuous use in one case-control study[253]; however, this was not found in a subsequent study.[211] No association between TSS and the frequency of changing tampons has been demonstrated.

As a result of these studies demonstrating the importance of tampons in menses-associated TSS and in addition to the voluntary withdrawal of Rely, several other changes in tampon manufacturing, labeling, and distribution have occurred. After a request by the Food and Drug Administration (FDA) in November 1980 that tampon manufacturers place warnings on tampon packages, on June 22, 1982, an FDA regulation required that information on TSS and tampon-associated risks appear on tampon packages.[92] In April 1985, two additional tampon manufacturers withdrew their superabsorbent tampons containing polyacrylate from the market on the basis of an in vitro study[191] and a judicial decision.[203] In 1990, the FDA published the in vitro rating system to be used by manufacturers to inform the public about tampon absorbency.[117, 167, 200]

Risk Factors for Nonmenstrual Toxic Shock Syndrome (Table 74–2)

Prior to 1986, less than 20 per cent of confirmed cases of TSS reported to the CDC were nonmenstrual. In the 1986 and 1987 multistate active surveillance study (CDC IV), 54 per cent of cases were found to be nonmenstrual.[121] Although the mean age of nonmenstrual cases is higher than that of the general population and the ratio of males to females closer to that in the general population, the clinical findings and complications of nonmenstrual TSS are the same as those occurring in menstrual TSS. The number of confirmed cases of TSS reported in children younger than 10 years of age is surprisingly low, particularly in light of their demonstrated low antibody titers to TSST-I and the increased prevalence of nasal colonization (10 per cent) with TSST-I–positive strains.[35, 142, 286, 295]

Data on risk factors were obtained for 559 nonmenstrual TSS cases reported to the CDC through 1986.[35] Associated infections or procedures included nonsurgical cutaneous and subcutaneous infections, 22 per cent; childbirth or abortion, 15 per cent; infections after a wide variety of surgical procedures, 15 per cent; vaginal infections occurring at times other than during menses, 6 per cent; vaginal contraceptive sponge use, 5 per cent[77]; diaphragm use, 6 per cent; and other or unknown sources of infection, 31 per cent.

In 1994, nonmenstrual cases accounted for at least 42 per cent of all cases of TSS reported to the CDC through the passive surveillance system.[43] The three necessary risk factors for nonmenstrual disease include colonization (or acquisition) of a toxin-producing strain of *S. aureus*, absence of protective antitoxin antibody, and an infected site. TSS has been reported in association with *S. aureus* infections of almost every type, including primary staphylococcal infections and those occurring after surgery, those associated with disruption of skin or a mucous membrane, and those occurring after placement of a foreign body (Table 74–2).[19] A number of patients with TSS have been reported for whom there was no obvious focus of infection.[35, 229] Trauma or surgery at areas of the body frequently colonized with *S. aureus* (nose, skin, vagina) places individuals at enhanced risk for infection and TSS.

CLINICAL SPECTRUM

Acute Phase: Moderate to Severe Disease[54, 62, 81, 112–114, 132, 175, 253, 273, 279]

Multisystem end-organ damage secondary to loss of peripheral vascular resistance, loss of intravascular volume as a result of endothelial damage and the capillary leak syndrome, and interstitial edema constitute the most important mediator-induced changes of TSS. Prolonged hypotension, interstitial edema, and vascular congestion further may result in ischemic organ damage.

The onset of illness for moderate to severe disease is abrupt, with symptoms and signs including fever, chills, malaise, headache, sore throat, myalgias, muscle tenderness, fatigue, vomiting, diarrhea, abdominal pain, and orthostatic dizziness or syncope (Fig. 74–3).

During the first 24 to 48 hours, diffuse erythroderma, severe watery diarrhea, often with incontinence, decreased urine output, cyanosis, and edema of the extremities may be noted. Cerebral ischemia and edema rapidly result in somnolence, confusion, irritability, agitation, and occasionally hallucinations, even in individuals without hypotension. Patients with TSS have presented with signs and symptoms of encephalopathy, cerebral infarct, meningismus,[14, 24, 129, 165, 258] and the cauda equina syndrome.[7]

During initial physical examination of a moderately to severely ill patient, fever, tachycardia, tachypnea, a low or unobtainable blood pressure, erythroderma (generally not seen in patients with severe hypotension) (Fig. 74–4*A* and *B*), and muscle tenderness are noted in conjunction with peripheral cyanosis and edema, conjunctival hyperemia, subconjunctival hemorrhages (see Fig. 74–4*B*), beefy red edematous mucous membranes, somnolence, disorientation, and agitation. In menstrual TSS, edema and erythema of the inner thighs and perineum may be noted in conjunction with a normal uterine and adnexal examination. In nonmenstrual cases, vaginitis or another focus of infection will be present. In most postoperative cases, the surgical wound is not inflamed. If erythroderma is present, it will be most intense surrounding the infected focus.

Surgical wounds colonized or infected with *S. aureus* and responsible for postoperative TSS typically have minimal or no signs of inflammation.[16, 95, 229] The production of TNF-α by macrophages in response to TSST-I inhibits neutrophil mobilization in vitro.[106] This may provide an explanation for the absence of signs of inflammation. The incubation period for postoperative or postpartum TSS may be as short as 12 to 48 hours. Relatively few cases have been associated with deep-tissue infections.[19]

TABLE 74–2. Risk Factors for Nonmenstrual Toxic Shock Syndrome

I. Colonization with toxin-producing *Staphylococcus aureus*
II. Absence of protective antitoxin antibody
III. Infected site
  A. Primary *S. aureus* infection

Carbuncle	Peritonitis
Cellulitis	Peritonsillar abscess
Dental abscess	Pneumonia
Empyema	Pyarthrosis
Endocarditis	Pyomyositis
Folliculitis	Sinusitis
Mastitis	Tracheitis
Osteomyelitis	

  B. After surgery: wound infection

Abdominal	Ear, nose, and throat
Breast	Genitourinary
C-section	Neurosurgery
Dermatologic	Orthopedic

  C. Skin or mucous membrane disruption
    Burns (chemical, scald, etc.)
    Dermatitis
    Postpartum (vaginal delivery)
    Superficial/penetrating trauma (insect bite, needle stick)
    Viral infection
      Influenza
      Pharyngitis
      Varicella
  D. After surgical or nonsurgical foreign body placement
    Augmentation mammoplasty
    Catheters
    Diaphragm
    Sponge (contraceptive)
    Surgical prostheses/stents/packing material/sutures
  E. No obvious focus of infection (vaginal or pharyngeal colonization)

Laboratory Changes

Abnormalities in clinical laboratory tests will reflect the endogenous cytokine release, shock, and organ failure. Leukocytosis may not be present, but the total number of mature and immature neutrophils usually exceeds 90 per cent. The number of immature neutrophils usually is 25 to 50 per cent of the total number of neutrophils and is associated with a profound and absolute lymphopenia. Thrombocytopenia and anemia are present during the first few days, frequently accompanied by prolonged prothrombin and partial thromboplastin times. Disseminated intravascular coagulation may be present. Sterile pyuria and a cerebrospinal fluid pleocytosis reflect the generalized involvement of mucous membranes and serosal surfaces. Elevated blood urea nitrogen and creatinine levels reflect kidney damage,[56] abnormalities in tests of liver function reflect liver damage and acute cholestasis,[126, 140] and profound hypocalcemia may reflect both hypoproteinemia and high serum levels of a calcitonin-like material.[57, 261] Muscle involvement is reflected by an elevated creatine phosphokinase level, and the hypophosphatemia that occurs despite impaired renal function is unexplained.[13, 57, 282] The majority of these tests will return to normal within 7 to 10 days of disease onset. *S. aureus* will be cultured from the cervix or vagina in more than 85 per cent of patients with menstrual TSS and from the focus of infection in patients with nonmenstrual TSS. Antibody to TSST-I or the staphylococcal enterotoxins will be absent at the onset of disease in more than 85 per cent of patients.[20, 28, 71, 238, 267, 293]

Treatment

There are three general principles of treatment of TSS (Table 74–3): (1) identification and drainage of the focus of toxin production; (2) antimicrobial therapy to block synthesis of toxin and to kill *S. aureus;* and (3) management of the systemic multiorgan actions of the toxin(s) or mediators.[54, 62, 80, 81, 113, 114, 132, 175, 243, 278, 279]

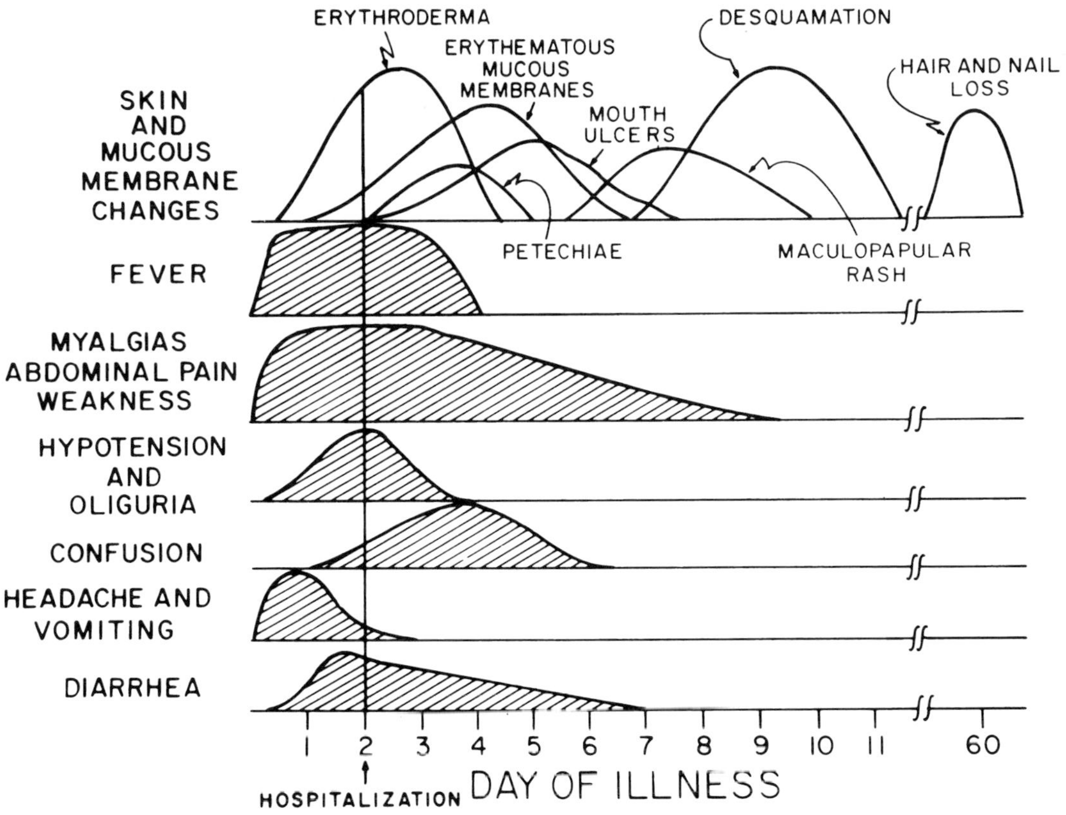

FIGURE 74–3. *Composite drawing of major systemic skin and mucous membrane manifestations of toxic shock syndrome. (From Chesney, P. J., Davis, J. P., Purdy, W. K., et al.: The clinical manifestations of toxic shock syndrome. J. A. M. A. 246:741–748, 1981. Copyright 1981, American Medical Association.)*

Location and Drainage of Infected Site

The focus of infection should be identified rapidly, any foreign bodies should be removed, and the site should be drained or irrigated completely, even if it appears uninflamed. This is of utmost importance because perpetuation of even a small, undrained focus of infection may result in serious clinical consequences. If TSS occurs in the immediate postoperative period, the wound should be assumed to be the source of infection, regardless of its benign appearance.

Antimicrobial Agents

Beta-lactamase–resistant antistaphylococcal antibiotics are indicated to eradicate organisms and to prevent recurrences.[80, 81] The infection may be a superficial or deep-tissue infection and may be associated with *S. aureus* bacteremia or bacteriuria. The antistaphylococcal antimicrobial agents should be used intravenously at maximal doses for age and should be initiated as soon as possible. A first- or second-generation cephalosporin could be used as an alternative in patients allergic to penicillin, with recognition of the 10 per cent cross-reactivity between penicillins and the cephalosporins. Once the patient is stable, no longer having vomiting or diarrhea, and able to take food by mouth, high doses of an oral beta-lactamase–resistant penicillin can be given. Toxin-producing methicillin-resistant *S. aureus* associated with TSS rarely are identified and uncommonly are isolated from the vagina of well women.[150] The predominant clone causing menstrual TSS is methicillin-sensitive.[158] Vancomycin should be used only in patients for whom there is a high suspicion of a methicillin-resistant *S. aureus*.

Subinhibitory concentrations of the protein synthesis inhibitors clindamycin, lincomycin, erythromycin, clarithromycin, kanamycin, gentamicin, and tetracycline have been shown to suppress TSST-I production in vitro.[91, 216, 244] In one study, clindamycin concentrations of 1/64 times the minimal inhibitory concentration were effective at totally blocking TSST I production.[216] Data suggest that subinhibitory concentrations of beta-lactam antibiotics actually may *increase* TSST-I pro-

TABLE 74–3. Therapeutic Principles for Management of Toxic Shock Syndrome

Identify focus of infection: débride and irrigate extensively and remove any foreign material
Parenteral antimicrobial therapy
Stop enzyme/toxin production with protein synthesis inhibitor (e.g., clindamycin, erythromycin, gentamicin)
and
Eradicate organism with bactericidal cell-wall inhibitor (e.g., β-lactamase–resistant antistaphylococcal antimicrobial agent)
Consider intravenous immunoglobulin to provide antitoxin antibodies for a subset of patients, including those with
Disease refractory to initial fluid replacement and several hours of vasopressor support
Presence of a focus of infection that cannot be drained
Persistent oliguria in spite of massive fluid replacement and in the presence of pulmonary edema
Consider methylprednisolone to suppress cytokine production and the inflammatory response
Fluid therapy to maintain adequate venous return and cardiac filling pressures and to prevent end-organ damage
Anticipatory management of multisystem organ failure

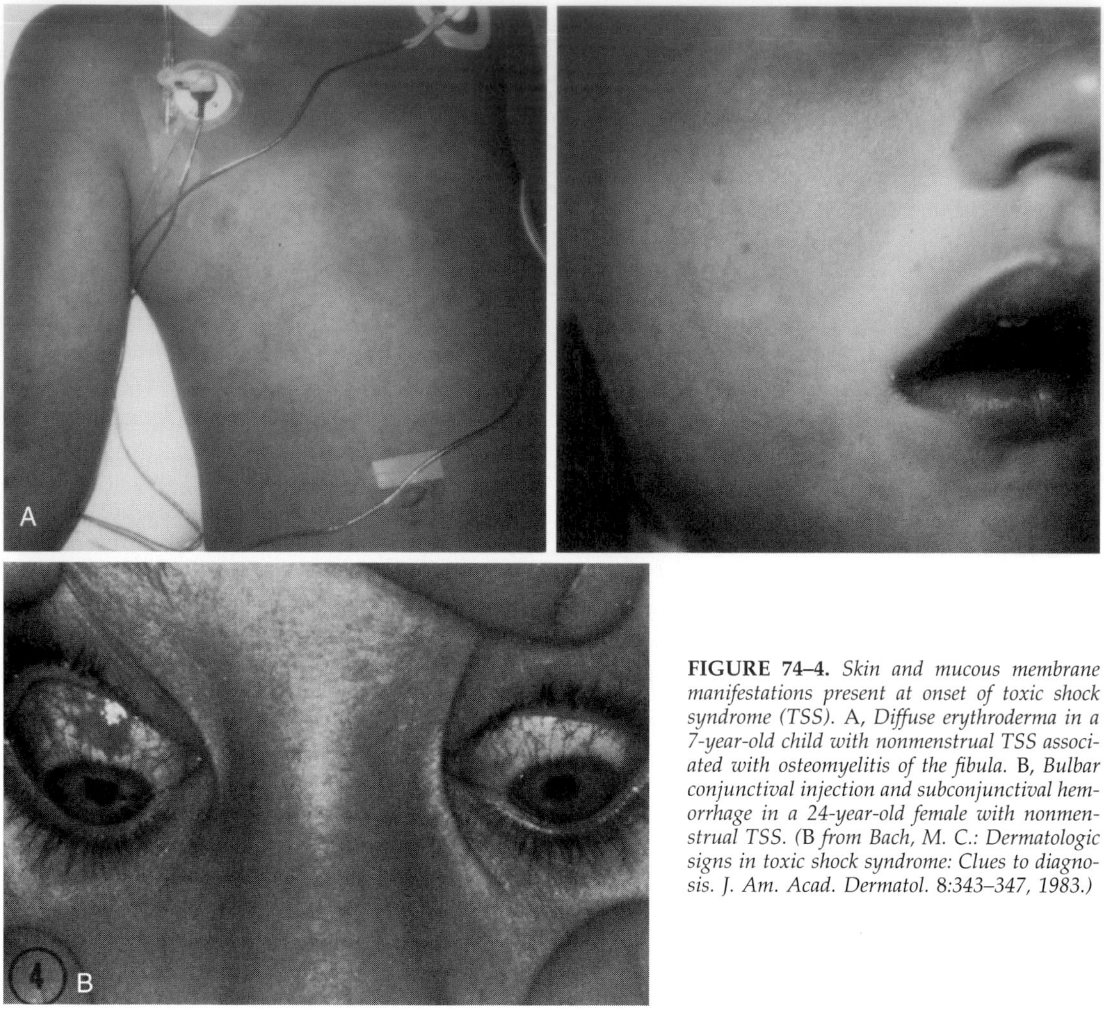

FIGURE 74–4. *Skin and mucous membrane manifestations present at onset of toxic shock syndrome (TSS).* A, *Diffuse erythroderma in a 7-year-old child with nonmenstrual TSS associated with osteomyelitis of the fibula.* B, *Bulbar conjunctival injection and subconjunctival hemorrhage in a 24-year-old female with nonmenstrual TSS. (*B *from Bach, M. C.: Dermatologic signs in toxic shock syndrome: Clues to diagnosis. J. Am. Acad. Dermatol. 8:343–347, 1983.)*

duction by *S. aureus*. At a concentration one half the minimal inhibitory concentration, nafcillin can *increase* toxin production 10-fold more than control conditions.[5] A similar effect has been described for nafcillin and the staphylococcal alpha toxin.[152] The effect is not seen with vancomycin, another cell wall–active drug, suggesting a specificity beyond merely a cell wall effect. The coadministration of a protein synthesis inhibitor with a beta-lactam antibiotic blocks the effect.[5] These preliminary results suggest a potential beneficial effect of adding clindamycin to a beta-lactam drug for therapy of TSS. In a mouse model of myositis caused by *Streptococcus pyogenes*, another superantigen-producing organism, clindamycin and erythromycin were more efficacious than was penicillin.[98, 264, 265]

Fluid Replacement

The most important aspect of the nonspecific treatment of symptomatic patients is fluid replacement.[278] The intravascular volume and cardiac filling pressures must be restored rapidly to achieve adequate tissue perfusion. Because of the ongoing capillary leakage, this fluid replacement far may exceed the calculated fluid requirements, based on calculated maintenance and fluid deficit volumes. Some adults have required vasopressors and up to 12 liters of fluid during the first 24 hours to stabilize the circulating blood pressure. Pleural, pericardial, and peritoneal effusions and interstitial edema inevitably occur as a result of the continued vascular capillary fluid leak. Close monitoring in an intensive care unit will facilitate determining when the correct intravascular volume has been achieved and will facilitate detection and appropriate monitoring and treatment of myocardial dysfunction, hemodynamic derangements, pulmonary edema, adult respiratory distress syndrome, acute renal failure, encephalopathy, and disseminated intravascular coagulation.

Corticosteroids

Short courses of methylprednisolone or dexamethasone have been associated with reduction in duration of fever and severity of illness but no reduction in mortality, if given early in the course of the disease.[275] In vitro, dexamethasone has been shown to down-regulate TSST-I–induced cytokine production.[156] Because no controlled prospective study has demonstrated efficacy, steroid use probably should be restricted to the hypotensive patient unresponsive to fluid resuscitation, antimicrobial agents, and intravenous immunoglobulin (IVIG).

Intravenous Immunoglobulin

Not surprisingly, given the high prevalence of antibodies to TSST-I in adults,[286] high levels of antibody to TSST-I are present in IVIG preparations.[53, 58, 177, 220, 270] Through use of the rabbit subcutaneous Wiffle ball or tampon model of TSS, human IVIG given at the time of inoculation of TSST-I–

positive *S. aureus* prevented TSS. When IVIG was given 8 hours later, it decreased the mortality from 90 per cent in the control rabbits to 16 per cent. When IVIG was given 29 hours after TSST-I administration, the increase in survival among the IVIG-treated animals still was significant. No adverse reactions were noted in the treated animals, and there was no evidence of disease mediated by formation of antigen-antibody complexes.[177, 178, 182, 183] Monoclonal antibodies to TSST-I can prevent manifestations of TSS in the rabbit model completely.[29, 215, 252]

High concentrations of antibodies to TSST-I and the eight staphylococcal enterotoxins (SEA, SEB, $SEC_{1, 2, 3}$, SED, and SEE) have been demonstrated in pooled IVIG.[53, 58, 220, 270] These antibodies may inhibit the binding of toxins to the major histocompatibility complex class II antigen-processing cells or interfere with toxin presentation by these cells to the TCR. As a result, production of TNF-α and TNF-γ is inhibited by these antibodies in vitro in an apparent toxin-specific manner.[270] In vitro down-regulation of lymphokine production induced by streptococcal pyrogenic exotoxin A by IVIG also has been demonstrated.[198, 256]

The results of these in vitro studies have led to the suggestion that IVIG may be valuable in patients with both streptococcal and staphylococcal TSS.[232] Anecdotal case reports have indicated a beneficial effect for both streptococcal[15, 198, 298] and staphylococcal[2, 58, 67, 204, 220] TSS in humans. Until more information is available and because IVIG is expensive and most patients respond rapidly once standard therapeutic measures are initiated, most authors would reserve IVIG use for patients with an inaccessible focus of infection and/or those who continue to deteriorate after several hours of fluid and vasopressor support (see Table 74–3). The dose most often used has been 400 mg/kg given as a single dose over several hours. This dose results in a serum antibody titer of greater than 1:100, much higher than that appearing to provide immunity to TSST-I.[220] Because it is possible that early administration of IVIG could blunt the immune response to TSST-I or other toxins and increase the possibility of a recurrent episode, the potential risks and benefits of this form of therapy must be considered for each patient.

The role of endotoxin in the pathogenesis of TSS is unclear. The failure of polymyxin B and anti-J5 antiserum to alter the course of TSST-I–positive TSS in a rabbit model suggests that endotoxin may not be an important mediator in TSS in humans.[179]

Early and sporadic case reports of TSS have suggested therapeutic benefits of naloxone,[64] calcium,[220] and exchange transfusion in severely ill patients unresponsive to the usual forms of therapy.

Subacute Phase: After Treatment Initiated

Once treatment is initiated, the response usually is rapid. The temperature returns to normal within 48 hours. The hemodynamic changes are observed initially as tachycardia, decreased systemic vascular resistance, decreased central venous pressure, hypovolemia, a normal pulmonary artery wedge pressure, and an increased cardiac index.[12, 37, 72, 113, 115] Once aggressive fluid therapy has been initiated, myocardial edema and potential failure along with pulmonary and cerebral edema in the face of renal failure become the most critical management issues. The reasons for the myocardial failure are unclear but probably are related to perivascular inflammation of the coronary vessels, edema, and postulated myocardial depressant factors.[161, 212] TSST-I has been shown to inhibit systolic function in isolated rabbit atria, although at higher than usual circulating concentrations.[206] Arrhythmias may result from myocardial damage or electrolyte abnormalities.[176, 234] An endomyocardial biopsy from one patient with severe global hypokinesis of the left ventricle revealed no substantial inflammatory infiltrate but a mild to moderate number of T cells scattered diffusely throughout the biopsy specimen.[72]

During the decompensated stage of myocardial dysfunction, the cardiac index falls and pulmonary wedge pressure increases, with both left atrial and ventricular and diastolic diameters at the upper limits of normal.[113] Reversible electrocardiographic findings include sinus tachycardia, diffuse loss of voltage, flattened T waves, and diffuse nonspecific ST-T wave changes. If a fatal arrhythmia does not occur during the decompensated stage, the toxic cardiomyopathy is reversible and rarely results in permanent changes. This process is similar to the "stunned myocardium," a transient, postischemic myocardial dysfunctional state.[72]

Pulmonary edema and the adult respiratory distress syndrome are common in severe disease when massive fluid replacement is necessary and the capillary leak syndrome continues in the lungs. Pulmonary edema appears rapidly once fluid replacement is initiated, often necessitating intubation and respirator management for several days.[278]

The forms of TSS-associated acute renal failure include prerenal azotemia and both nonoliguric and oliguric renal failure.[56] The form of renal failure manifested may be dependent upon the degree of intravascular volume depletion. Unless severe acute tubular necrosis necessitates temporary hemodialysis, repletion of the intravascular volume usually results in rapid restoration of renal function and ultimately diuresis. Permanent renal damage is extremely rare.[53]

The gastrointestinal, musculoskeletal, and hepatic changes resolve rapidly. Sequelae associated with these changes are rare, except for prolonged muscle weakness.[53, 83] Joint manifestations generally are self-limited.[19, 116]

Management of fluids, electrolytes, and metabolic acidosis in a patient with TSS is complex. Although tetany is rare, this common severe hypocalcemia may be life-threatening and should be corrected.[57, 220, 261] Most patients require potassium replacement and management of the metabolic acidosis. Use of colloid for fluid replacement and removal of the toxin stimulus for the capillary leak syndrome ultimately correct the hypoproteinemia.

The typical dermatologic manifestations follow a predictable sequence (see Fig. 74–3). A dandruff-like flaky desquamation begins on the trunk and extremities 5 to 7 days after the onset of symptoms. From days 10 to 12 and for as long as a month, the characteristic full-thickness desquamation of the fingers, toes, palms, and soles occurs (Fig. 74–5). A variety of atypical dermatologic manifestations have been described, including petechiae and subepidermal bullae.[9, 101, 137]

Early in the acute phase, many patients have desquamation of the mucous membranes, which particularly is painful when the oral mucous membranes are involved.[54] In addition, a small number of patients will have reactivated herpes simplex virus 1 or 2 lesions with the acute illness.[54] A late-onset pruritic maculopapular rash with edema and low-grade fever probably unrelated to antimicrobial therapy occurs in more than 50 per cent of menses-associated cases within 7 to 14 days of disease onset.[54, 88] The cause of this late-onset rash is unknown.

Telogen effluvium, a common sequela, is a nonspecific response to severe trauma, sepsis, or stress that results in disturbed metabolism and keratinization of the hair follicles and nails. The hair follicles appear to transform prematurely from the growth, or anlagen, phase to the telogen, or resting, phase. Hair and nail loss occurs 4 to 16 weeks after the onset of illness, with restoration in 5 to 6 months.[19, 23, 54]

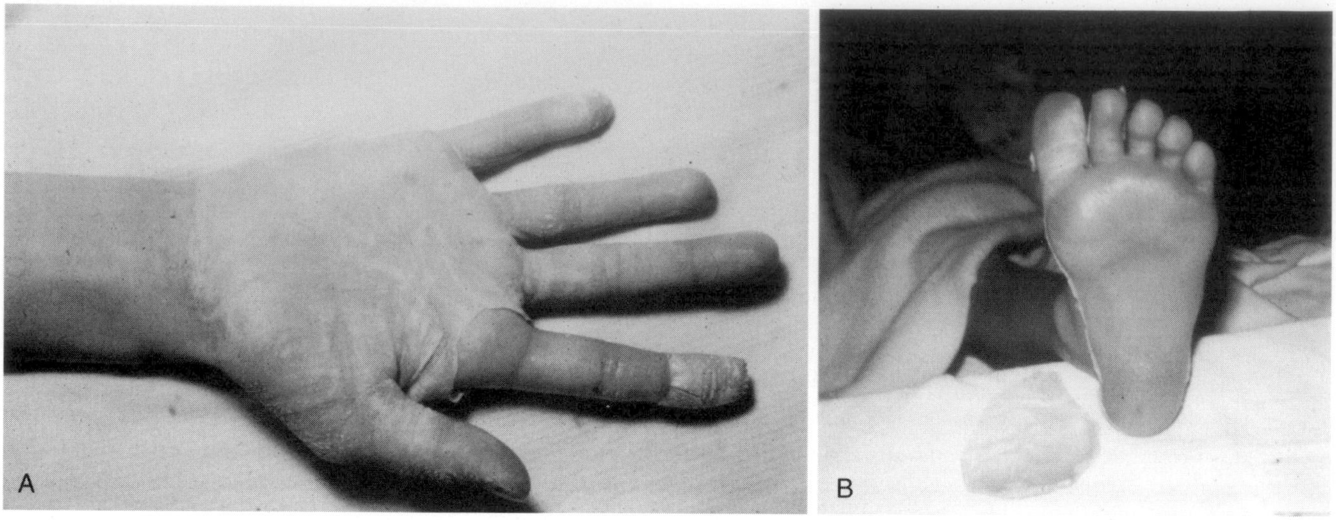

FIGURE 74–5. *Universal full-thickness desquamation of hands (A) and feet (B) first noted 7 to 14 days after disease onset and with persistence for up to 30 days.*

The hematologic system seldom is involved with major complications in TSS. Although disseminated intravascular coagulation may be present, gastrointestinal, uterine, or cerebral bleeding rarely occurs. Thrombocytopenia may be present initially in those patients with disseminated intravascular coagulation; thrombocytosis is characteristic of the recovery phase. Mild to moderate normocytic, normochromic anemia, which probably is dilutional and a result of suppressed red blood cell synthesis, develops in virtually all moderately to severely ill patients with TSS and resolves during convalescence.[52, 54] Hypoferrinemia is common.[52]

The relatively common toxic or ischemic encephalopathy, rarely complicated by seizures, resolves slowly during the first 4 to 5 days of hospitalization.

Outcome and Sequelae

Death associated with TSS usually occurs within the first few days of hospitalization but may occur as late as 15 days after admission. Fatalities have been attributed to refractory cardiac arrhythmias, cardiomyopathy, irreversible respiratory failure, and rarely bleeding due to coagulation defects.[161, 212] Duration of circulation of toxins and mediators and the associated hypotension may predict best the severity of the end-organ damage.

After discharge, prolonged fatigue, muscle weakness, and pain are noted by most patients.[53] Sequelae attributed to TSS that appear to be related to a prolonged period of hypotension have included chronic renal failure, gangrene, and telogen effluvium.[83, 148, 185, 237, 241] Other sequelae, such as neuropsychologic abnormalities, prolonged myalgias and weakness, carpal tunnel syndrome, chronic dermatitis, Raynaud syndrome, new allergies, and recurrences, are explained less easily. Abnormalities such as impaired memory and poorly sustained concentration have been found in patients who did not require any therapy other than intravenous fluids to restore their blood pressure.[237] In one center, patients with nonmenstrual TSS had more serious short- and long-term neuropsychologic complications than did patients with menstrual TSS.[148] Sequelae relating primarily to the neuromuscular system have resulted in speculation that the TSS-associated toxin may have a direct effect on nerve or muscle tissue. One patient with TSS developed a cauda equina syndrome with partial paralysis after a lumbar laminectomy and staphylococcal meningitis, suggesting a neurotoxic effect of the intrathecally produced SEC.[7]

One study compared the sequelae and other long-term effects among 183 (174 menstrual cases) women with TSS and 366 control women hospitalized with appendicitis and appendectomy and matched for age, race, and duration of follow-up.[83] Each subject completed two comprehensive phone interviews. When compared with controls, women with TSS were significantly more likely to report sequelae involving fatigue, the integument (hair loss and nail changes), mental and cognitive skills (problems with concentration, reading difficulty, and memory loss), emotions (menses attitude and emotional change), and multiple organ systems (conditions involving the joint cardiac, muscle, and genitourinary systems). In addition, women with TSS were significantly more likely than were controls to report persistence of symptoms. Fertility patterns and pregnancy outcomes were similar in controls and women with TSS, both before and after the index illness.[83]

Atypical Manifestations

Mild Disease

Recognition of mild episodes of TSS particularly is important in patients with menstrual TSS because repeated tampon use and the risk for recurrences are episodic.[55, 89, 280] Patients with mild or severe menstrual TSS typically do not develop antibody to TSST-I during convalescence[19, 28, 238, 267, 293] and, without appropriate therapy, may have one or more recurrences. Such recurrences may be mild or severe.[80, 81, 175] Patients with nonmenstrual TSS also do not develop antibodies in convalesence. A mild episode may be recognized only in retrospect, after desquamation and/or a recurrent episode develops.[220]

The presence of any combination of fever, headache, sore throat, diarrhea, vomiting, orthostatic dizziness, syncope, and myalgia in a menstruating woman or an individual with a potential *S. aureus* infection, no matter how trivial, should raise the suspicion of TSS. A specific laboratory test to confirm the clinical diagnosis is not available. A bacterial culture positive for *S. aureus* may be helpful but is not diagnostic for menstrual cases because *S. aureus* may be cultured from the cervix or vagina of up to 33 per cent of menstruating women.[171, 218]

Other laboratory data usually do not reflect multisystem involvement in mild disease, and assays for TSST-I in body fluids are investigational.[181, 285] Diagnostic support for the theory that signs and symptoms represent mild TSS often depends on the constellation of findings, including subsequent typical desquamation of the palms, soles, toes, or fingers; the demonstration that *S. aureus* isolates from the site of infection produce TSST-I or an enterotoxin; the absence of antibody to TSST-I or enterotoxins in an acute-phase serum; and recurrent disease, if it develops.

Recurrences

One of the most puzzling aspects of the pathophysiology of TSS is the high rate of recurrence in patients with inadequately treated menstrual or nonmenstrual disease.[54, 80, 81, 174, 175] A small number of patients with menstrual disease and repeated tampon exposure have experienced as many as 6 to 12 recurrences. There is no predictable pattern to recurrences associated with menstrual disease. In most patients, the first episode is the most severe. However, asymptomatic menses may occur between symptomatic episodes, and the most severe episode may occur after one or more milder episodes.[81] The use of appropriate antistaphylococcal antimicrobial therapy for 10 to 14 days and discontinuation of tampon use can be expected to reduce the rate of recurrence significantly.[81] Recurrences after nonmenstrual TSS are well described and usually also associated with inadequate initial therapy.[148, 220] Cisplatin administration resulting in significant hypomagnesemia precipitated several recurrent episodes of TSS in an immunocompromised adult.[22]

The absent or delayed antibody response to TSST-I found in both menstrual and nonmenstrual TSS patients probably accounts for the continued susceptibility to TSS and for the high recurrence rate.[19, 28, 238, 267, 293] The fact that superantigenic toxins are not processed by antigen-processing cells and T lymphocytes as conventional antigens (see later section) may provide an explanation for the poor convalescent antibody response to these antigens.[155]

Culture-negative, menses-associated, recurrent episodes of TSS continue to occur in a small number of patients, despite discontinuation of tampon use and the use of appropriate antimicrobial therapy during the acute episode.[81] Administration of an oral beta-lactamase–resistant antistaphylococcal antimicrobial agent during menses has been tried in an attempt to prevent these recurrences but is not always successful. In recurrent cases resistant to this form of prophylaxis, consideration could be given to the untested and empiric use of rifampin, clindamycin, erythromycin, or IVIG (if the patient has no antibody to TSST-I) or to the use of an oral contraceptive.[174]

Recalcitrant, Erythematous Desquamating Disorder

An atypical, subacute variant of TSS has been described in patients with AIDS and labeled the recalcitrant, erythematous, desquamating disorder. *S. aureus* strains producing TSST-I, SEA, or SEB have been isolated from patients with AIDS and prolonged erythema, extensive cutaneous desquamation, hypotension, tachycardia, and multiple and variable organ involvement.[67, 93, 153] The illness is recalcitrant, prolonged, and characterized by multiple recurrences. In one patient, elevated levels of TNF and IL-6 were found with severe episodes. When antitoxin antibodies have been measured during recurrences, they have been undetectable. Two patients responded well to IVIG.[67, 153] Patients with the combined cellular and humoral immunodeficiencies of AIDS may be at particular risk for severe, frequent, and prolonged recurrent episodes of TSS.[67, 93, 111, 153, 259] TSST-I and the enterotoxins may activate HIV-1 gene expression in vivo, as has been observed in vitro.[120]

Nonmenstrual Disease

The incidence of postoperative cases of TSS after all types of surgery has been estimated to be 3 per 100,000 population.[127] For ear, nose, and throat surgery, the incidence is higher (16.5/100,000 population).[143] A striking feature of most postoperative cases of rapid onset is the absence of any signs of a wound infection.[16, 127, 227, 239] The mean time from surgery to onset of symptoms is 2 to 4 days.[16] Nosocomial acquisition of the TSST-I–positive organisms rarely has been documented for postoperative cases.[8, 157, 195] A wide variety of types of surgery have been associated with TSS.[19, 39, 194, 205, 231, 254, 257]

Burn wounds provide a particularly rich environment for *S. aureus* growth and toxin production.[10, 58, 65, 119, 121, 125, 134, 168, 172, 290] In one large pediatric burn center, *S. aureus* normally was not cultured from any site on admission.[58] However, it was acquired within a few days of admission to become the most common wound pathogen. Of all wound isolates of *S. aureus*, only 16 per cent produced TSST-I. Only half of the children had antibodies to TSST-I on admission, which reflects the low prevalence of antibodies in children.[286] Of administered blood products, 76 per cent had antibodies to TSST-I, and seroconversion occurred in children receiving these products. A TSS-like syndrome developed in 13 per cent (7/53) of children, only one of whom had TSST-I–producing *S. aureus* isolated from the wound. SEA and SEB were produced by isolates from three patients. In burn patients, issues regarding the use of prophylactic antibiotics, occlusive dressings, and enhancement of production of TSST-I by topical antimicrobial agents are unsettled.[99] The mortality of TSS in children with burns may be as high as 57 per cent.[119] Skin disrupted in any way, including by varicella or a tattoo, also may be a focus for TSS.[19, 31, 70]

Patients who have colonization of the anterior nares by *S. aureus* are at particular risk for TSS when the respiratory mucosa is disrupted by surgery, trauma, or a respiratory infection, such as influenza.[19, 44, 68, 166, 281] TSS has been reported in association with sinusitis,[19, 108] pharyngitis,[19, 242] parapharyngeal abscesses,[242] tracheitis,[19, 76, 94, 122, 201] pneumonia,[19, 78] rubeola,[269] and submandibular space abscesses. TSS occurring after ear, nose, and throat surgery has been associated with the use of nasal splints and packing materials and in part may be the result of interruption of the ciliary blanket.[3, 19, 118, 190, 299]

After orthopedic procedures or in association with bone and joint infections, the clinical presentation of TSS may be confusing as a result of the intense and generalized myalgias associated with TSS, which may be misinterpreted as postoperative musculoskeletal symptoms. The wounds usually appear to be benign.[19, 189, 221, 271, 283] Infected abrasions under casts may be focal sites of TSST-I production.[260]

In one center, when cases of nonmenstrual TSS were compared with menstrual cases, patients with nonmenstrual disease were found to have a delayed onset of symptoms after the precipitating event, more frequent central nervous system manifestations, less frequent musculoskeletal involvement (myalgia and arthralgia), and a higher degree of anemia.[148] Recurrences occurred in both groups in untreated patients; mortality was not different. It is suggested that clinical differences between the two categories may be related to differences in the types of toxins produced. TSST-I was produced with comparable frequency in both groups. SEA was produced less often by nonmenstrual isolates, and menstrual isolates more often produced both TSST-I and SEA. SEB was produced more often by nonmenstrual isolates.

Several patients with TSS have been reported to have simultaneous infections with *S. aureus* and *Streptococcus pyogenes*.[100] It was not possible to determine which infection primarily was responsible for the manifestations or if an amplified effect of exotoxins from both organisms was present.

Streptococcal Toxic Shock–Like Syndrome

There has been an increase in the incidence and severity of invasive *S. pyogenes* infections during the last decade. Manifestations of severe disease have included septicemia with or without a focus of infection; severe, painful cellulitis; necrotizing fasciitis; and in some cases a streptococcal toxic shock–like syndrome with or without a focus of infection. Streptococcal toxic shock–like syndrome is similar to staphylococcal TSS in that it appears to be mediated by superantigenic toxins and results in endothelial damage, hypotension, and multisystem organ involvement. Streptococcal toxic shock–like syndrome differs from staphylococcal TSS in a number of respects, including a slower onset over several days; the usual absence of vomiting, profuse diarrhea, and conjunctival infection; the frequent absence of erythroderma or presence only of a sandpaper-like rash; severe generalized hyperesthesia; extreme pain at the site of skin involvement; and a mortality of 40 to 50 per cent.[66, 263]

Diagnosis

Application of the case definition for a single episode or recurrent episodes[81] to the patient's illness currently is the only way to confirm the diagnosis (see Table 74–1). Aggressive attempts always should be made to find the focus of *S. aureus* replication, including cultures of the cervix and vagina in patients with menses-associated illness and other potentially infected sites that may not appear obviously to be infected in patients with nonmenstrual illness. *S. aureus* isolates could be examined, when possible, for their ability to produce TSST-I, although this seldom is indicated. This test is of limited usefulness for nonmenstrual cases because TSST-I is produced by only 40 to 60 per cent of *S. aureus* isolates from such patients.[123] Isolates from these patients could be examined for the presence of the other enterotoxins. Acute and convalescent sera can be tested for the presence of antibodies to TSST-I and the other enterotoxins. Elevated levels of anti–TSST-I in acute-phase serum of a patient with menstrual-associated TSS would be highly unusual.

In most instances, toxin detection tests are of value only for research or for the rare patient with chronic recurrent or otherwise puzzling disease. Genes for TSST-I and the enterotoxins have been detected in *S. aureus* strains using the polymerase chain reaction[147] and hybridization techniques.[146, 199, 208] A noncompetitive enzyme-linked immunosorbent assay allows quantitation of TSST-I in clinical samples.[181, 192] Reversed passive latex agglutination has been used in hospital laboratories to detect TSST-I and in research laboratories to detect enterotoxins.[85, 103]

Differential Diagnosis

The differential diagnosis of TSS includes those clinical entities in which the rapid onset of fever, erythroderma-like rash, hypotension, and multisystem involvement are observed (Table 74–4).[38, 109, 193, 220, 222]

Prevention and Prophylaxis

To decrease the risk of menstrual TSS, in 1982 the Institute of Medicine Committee on TSS recommended that women, and particularly adolescents, minimize their use of high-absorbency tampons.[225] The committee also recommended that women who have had TSS not use tampons because of the increased risk of recurrences and that postpartum women be informed that tampon use might increase their risk of TSS.

Although the frequency of changing tampons during a menstrual period has not been associated with TSS risk, the use of an individual tampon unit for no more than 12 hours at a time might decrease the risk of menstrual TSS. Women using intravaginal contraceptive devices also should be informed of the potential increase in risk for TSS.[251]

Although postoperative TSS is rare, it generally occurs in healthy people. As a result of its unexpected and potentially severe consequences, issues regarding surgical antimicrobial prophylaxis for prevention have been raised. Perioperative systemic antistaphylococcal antibiotics did not prevent TSS in four patients[32, 239] and do not eradicate nasal carriage of *S. aureus*.[144] TSS with onset after 48 hours of amoxicillin was reported in two patients after endonasal sinus surgery.[2] Topical bacitracin ointment on nasal packing does not prevent TSS.[32, 90, 143, 144]

Most authors feel that the rare risk of postoperative TSS is comparable to the risk of a severe antimicrobial reaction and that perioperative antimicrobial prophylaxis is not indicated for clean procedures of short duration.[127, 227] Efforts should be intensified to recognize postoperative cases early; to open,

TABLE 74–4. Differential Diagnosis of Toxic Shock Syndrome Based on Clinical Manifestations

Diagnosis	Fever	Exanthem	Shock
Severe invasive *Streptococcus pyogenes* infections	+	+	+
Meningococcemia	+	+	+
Rocky Mountain spotted fever	+	+	±
Ehrlichiosis	+	+	±
Kawasaki disease	+	+	−
Staphylococcal scalded skin syndrome	+	+	−
Toxic epidermal necrolysis	+	+	−
Viral syndromes	+	+	−
Leptospirosis	+	+	−
Systemic lupus erythematosus	+	+	−
Erythema multiforme	+	+	−
Septic shock	+	−	+
Hantavirus pulmonary syndrome	+	−	+
Salmonella infections	+	−	±
Gastroenteritis	+	−	−
Urinary tract infection	+	−	−
Drug reactions			
Dilantin	+	+	±
Cocaine	+	+	±
Pseudophedrine	+	+	±
Inhalational mercury	+	+	±
Quinidine	+	+	−
Sulfonamides	+	+	−
β-lactam antibiotics	+	+	−
Quinolones	+	+	−

explore extensively, and irrigate wounds; and to provide immediate antimicrobial and supportive therapy for suspected TSS.

HISTOPATHOLOGY[1, 25, 33, 161, 212, 294]

The histopathologic findings found on postmortem examination support the concept that TSS is a toxin-mediated disease. Striking histopathologic similarities exist between patients with TSS and those with "scarlet fever" reported in 1936.[33] Typically, there is a total absence of tissue invasion by bacteria and minimal evidence of an inflammatory reaction in most organs. Findings thought to be due to a direct effect of the toxin and/or mediators and unrelated to hypoperfusion have included subepidermal ulcerations in the cervix, vagina, esophagus, and bladder; lymphocyte depletion in the lymph nodes; a subepidermal cleavage plane in the skin; and the mild inflammatory changes present in the kidney, liver, heart, and muscle.

Cervicovaginal ulcerations are the only characteristic lesions noted in the genital tract of patients with fatal menstrual TSS and also were found in a patient with menstrual TSS who had never used tampons.[161, 220] The ulcerations are superficial. Capillary vasodilation and thrombosis with inflammation of the mucosa are present, but no deep-tissue bacterial invasion is seen. The layer of vacuolization and separation in the ulcers occurs beneath the basal layer. The same type of ulcer also has been found in the bladder and the esophagus, which suggests that these ulcerations may be due to the toxin(s) or mediators and not to tampon use.

Although the myocardium was described as normal in one postmortem series of TSS, in another series of eight fatal cases, all patients had evidence of focal round cell infiltration with variable degrees of congestion, edema, and hemorrhage.[161, 212] Myxoid degeneration was found in all heart valves from four patients in one series. Sections of skeletal muscle have demonstrated only congestion, edema, focal hemorrhage or fiber necrosis, and a mild acute inflammatory infiltrate.

Varying degrees of triaditis or periportal lymphocytic inflammation have been the most consistent findings in the liver; centrilobular congestion with necrosis and mild cellular degeneration also has been described.[140] In the kidney, toxin-mediated mononuclear interstitial nephritis may result from perivasculitis of the adventitia of the renal venules, lesions that probably precede the hypotension-induced acute tubular necrosis. The most characteristic findings in the spleen and lymph nodes have been lymphocyte depletion; inactive hypocellular, hypoplastic lymphoid follicles with edema; marked histiocytosis in the interfollicular areas; and hemophagocytosis.

Perivascular lymphocytic infiltrates and bullae that separate at the basement membrane are characteristic of the early skin changes in TSS.[7, 9, 132] There has been no evidence of vasculitis.

CHARACTERISTICS OF TOXIC SHOCK SYNDROME–ASSOCIATED *STAPHYLOCOCCUS AUREUS* ISOLATES

The ability to produce TSST-I, a previously uncharacterized protein, is the single most distinguishing characteristic of TSS-associated *S. aureus* strains. More than 90 per cent of *S. aureus* isolates from patients with menstrual TSS[20, 245] and 40 to 60 per cent of isolates from patients with nonmenstrual disease[123] produce TSST-I, compared with less than 20 per cent of non-TSS strains.

S. aureus strains isolated from patients with TSS are different phenotypically from other strains of *S. aureus*.[19, 274] They produce less beta-hemolysis on sheep blood agar and less frequently harbor plasmids than do control strains. There is an increase in protease production and proteolytic activity by TSS-associated strains.[274] Next to TSST-I production, protease production is the most characteristic marker for these strains.

Unlike non-TSS *S. aureus* strains, tryptophan is required for growth of most TSST-I–positive strains of *S. aureus* and for TSST-I production.[63] In one study, 91 per cent of 27 TSST-I–positive vaginal *S. aureus* isolates were tryptophan auxotrophs, compared with 6 per cent of 32 TSST-I–negative vaginal *S. aureus* isolates. Eight of 22 TSST-I–producing tryptophan auxotrophs were blocked at the tryptophan synthetase B locus, which suggests that the TSST-I gene cluster may have been inserted into this locus, thus disrupting its function.

Additional differences between TSS and non-TSS strains of *S. aureus* include the resistance of TSS strains to cadmium, arsenate, and penicillin, characteristics that usually are plasmid-mediated but that in the TSS strains are chromosomally mediated. As such, these traits must be the result of heterologous insertions. These characteristics are not cotransferred with and therefore presumably not closely linked to the gene segment responsible for TSST-I production.[19, 274]

ROLE OF THE STAPHYLOCOCCAL EXOTOXINS TOXIC SHOCK SYNDROME TOXIN I AND THE ENTEROTOXINS IN TOXIC SHOCK SYNDROME

Role of Toxic Shock Syndrome Toxin I

TSST-I appears to be an important toxin in TSS. Factors supporting this statement include (1) the observations that greater than 90 per cent of isolates from patients with TSS produce TSST-I; (2) the absence of acute-phase antibody to TSST-I in more than 90 per cent of patients with menstrual TSS; (3) the increase in anti–TSST-I antibody during recovery in nonmenstrual cases; (4) absent or low levels of antibody in patients with recurrent menstrual TSS; (5) comparable illness inducible with TSST-I in in vivo animal models; and (6) the neutralization of IL-1 stimulation and response to TSST-I by antibody to TSST-I.

Most convincing are the experiments in which the ability to cause TSS followed the bacteriophage-mediated transfer of the TSST-I–positive chromosomal segment into a recipient *S. aureus* strain without the segment.[86, 220] Experiments demonstrating the effectiveness of monoclonal antibodies to TSST-I in reversing the effects of TSST-I provide additional strong support.[159]

Role of the Enterotoxins

Because 40 to 60 per cent of nonmenstrual TSS *S. aureus* isolates and 5 to 10 per cent of menstrual TSS isolates do not produce TSST-I, a role for other staphylococcal exotoxins including the enterotoxins has been proposed.[19, 71, 164, 214, 247, 297] Patients with nonmenstrual disease infected with TSST-I–negative strains may have a higher mortality rate.[123] Significant increases in titer of antibody to the staphylococcal enterotoxins during convalescence strongly suggest a role for these proteins in the pathogenesis of TSS.[11]

In rabbit models, the morbidity and mortality after injection of TSST-I–negative TSS isolates were comparable to those after infection with TSST-I–positive strains and significantly greater than those after inoculation with TSST-1–negative non-TSS isolates.[123] The administration of staphylococcal enterotoxins to animals results in many of the manifestations characteristic of TSS.[18, 102]

When large numbers of isolates from patients with TSS have been examined, production of TSST-I alone is the most common toxin pattern identified.[19, 71, 169] Other identified patterns include production of TSST-I in combination with one or more of the identified enterotoxins, production of enterotoxins *only* (one or more), and nonproduction of TSST-I and enterotoxins. Of the TSS strains producing TSST-I, 60.6 per cent also produce an enterotoxin.[71, 169] SEA frequently is coexpressed with TSST-I, particularly in menstrual isolates. A clone producing both TSST-I and SEA is associated with 88 per cent of menstrual TSS cases and may account for up to 54 per cent of isolates from nonmenstrual TSS cases.[50] Seroconversion to SEA is more common in TSS than in non-TSS *S. aureus* infections, further suggesting a role for SEA.

The third most common pattern of toxin production by TSS isolates is that of TSST-I plus SEC. These isolates have been associated with both menstrual and nonmenstrual cases and particularly with severe respiratory tract TSS-associated infections.[71]

The fourth most common pattern of toxin production is that of SEB alone. In one study, strains producing SEB alone accounted for 38 per cent of all nonmenstrual TSS isolates.[164, 247] This is significantly higher than for isolates from non-TSS *S. aureus* infections (15 per cent) or asymptomatic carriers (13 per cent). SEB is never coexpressed with TSST-I. Even though all TSST-I–positive isolates contain the SEB genetic determinant, none produce SEB. SEB is produced only by isolates that have the SEB gene and no TSST-I gene. Because production of both toxins is mutually exclusive and both genes are located close together on the chromosome, it has been suggested that the TSST-I genetic determinant may have a preferred site of insertion within the SEB genetic element. Because the TSST-I gene is associated with a variable genetic element and such mobile genetic elements are known to be capable of gene disruption, it is possible that the gene was inserted within the SEB gene or in a position to interfere with its transcription.[85]

TSS isolates producing TSST-I plus two other enterotoxins in combination are the fifth most common combination, and isolates producing no known toxins are the sixth. The identification of new enterotoxins[230, 268] capable of producing a TSS-like disease in rabbits may account for isolates previously identified as producing no toxins. Isolates producing a non-SEB enterotoxin alone are the least common.

PREVALENCE OF EXOTOXIN-PRODUCING *STAPHYLOCOCCUS AUREUS* STRAINS AND OF ANTIBODY TO THE EXOTOXINS

Prevalence of Exotoxin-Producing Organisms

TSST-I–positive strains of *S. aureus* have been present since at least 1957, and antibody to TSST-I was as prevalent in a general population in 1960 as it was in 1983.[286] Thus, the increase in incidence of TSS from 1980 to 1985 is assumed to have been the result of newly introduced cofactors, rather than the result of an increase in the prevalence of TSST-I–positive organisms.

At any given time, *S. aureus* is present in 20 to 40 per cent of cultures from the anterior nasal vestibule of adults and as many as 33 per cent of nasal cultures of children.[141] In women, the prevalence of *S. aureus* in vaginal cultures is higher during menses than at midcycle.[171, 207] Vaginal carriage rates vary from 7 per cent in premenarcheal and nonmenstruating women to 33 per cent in menstruating women.[218] TSST-I–positive *S. aureus* is present in 1 to 5 per cent of vaginal cultures of women, 7 per cent of nasal cultures of hospitalized patients, and 18 per cent of nasal cultures in children. In prospective studies of *S. aureus* isolates from healthy individuals and from specimens received for other purposes, 14 to 39 per cent of all isolates produced TSST-I and 7 to 14 per cent produced SEB.[89, 220] Overall, between 1 and 4 per cent of healthy individuals at any given time are colonized at a mucosal site with TSST-I–positive *S. aureus.*

Of 60 *S. aureus* isolates from blood cultures of patients who did not have TSS, 28 per cent produced TSST-I.[53] Presumably, these patients had circulating antibody to TSST-I, which prevented them from developing TSS despite an *S. aureus* infection. Adults and children who have persistent nasal carriage with a TSST-I–positive strain have high levels of antibody to TSST-I.[233]

Evidence suggests that a single clone of *S. aureus* causes the majority of cases of TSS.[50, 197] Multilocus enzyme electrophoresis has demonstrated that the TSST-I gene, *tst*H, is distributed widely over the whole spectrum of *S. aureus* genotypes. Of 315 *S. aureus* strains collected from around the world, 88 per cent of menstrual TSS strains and 53 per cent of nonmenstrual strains were indistinguishable by multilocus enzyme electrophoresis. The same clone also was found in 28 per cent of vaginal isolates from asymptomatic women. This remarkable phenomenon may reflect the unique ability of this clone to colonize the urogenital epithelium or the unique capability of this clone to cause disease.

Although TSST-I–positive strains may cluster within families, living units, and hospital settings, the occurrence of TSS clusters is rare.[157, 195] Probable TSS has occurred within 24 hours in a husband and wife[112] and in two mother-daughter pairs. Nosocomial acquisition and transmission of TSST-I–positive organisms have been described.[8, 157, 195]

Prevalence of Antibody to the Exotoxins

The prevalence of antibody to TSST-I in 689 Wisconsin residents was found to be 47 per cent at age 1 year, 58 per cent at age 5 years, 70 per cent at age 10 years, 88 per cent at age 20 years, and 96 per cent for ages 30 to 50 during the years 1960 to 1983 (see Fig. 74–2).[286] The presence of transplacentally acquired antibody in more than 90 per cent of infants also was demonstrated. There were no significant gender differences in antibody prevalence. It is assumed that mucosal colonization with TSST-I–positive *S. aureus* strains results in antibody formation[233] because more than 90 per cent of adults have antibody to TSST-I and have never had TSS. This is supported by data from a burn unit, staffed by a nurse who developed recurrent TSS. Personnel in the unit were demonstrated to be colonized by TSST-I–positive strains and to develop antibody to TSST-I but not TSS during a period of several months.[8] Subclinical and mild, unrecognized disease[55] also may result in antibody formation.

Acquisition of antibodies to the enterotoxins also is age-related. By age 10 years, the per cent of children with antibody titers of 1:100 or higher is 15 per cent for SEA, 65 per cent for SEB, 30 per cent for SEC, 5 per cent for SED, and 20 per cent for SEE. By age 22 years, the numbers increase to 55 per cent for SEA, 77 per cent for SEB, and 98 per cent for SEC.[19]

The prevalence of antibody varies from one area of the country to another. During 1982, of 1017 sera obtained from

U.S. Air Force recruits between the ages of 17 and 26 years, 35 per cent from the Mountain and Pacific states were serosusceptible to TSST-I, compared with 3 per cent from the South Atlantic states and 5 per cent from the East South Central states. Because low titers appear to indicate susceptibility, the findings in this study suggest that differences in TSS incidence between states and regions were explained in part by differences in host susceptibility.[284]

Sera randomly selected from 87 control women were seronegative more frequently for antibody to TSST-I (24 per cent) than were those from 66 control men (9 per cent), leading to the suggestion that women may be more susceptible to TSS than are men.[238] Patients in whom TSS develops have significantly lower levels of antibody to SEB and SEC, as well as to TSST-I when compared with the general population.[19, 71]

As noted in the discussion of recurrences, acute-phase sera of patients with TSS uniformly demonstrate absent or low levels of antibody to TSST-I. The antibody response to TSST-I is absent or delayed in both menstrual and nonmenstrual TSS.[220, 267]

PHYSICOCHEMICAL AND BIOLOGIC CHARACTERISTICS OF TOXIC SHOCK SYNDROME TOXIN I

Physicochemical Properties

The mature secreted TSST-I protein is a single polypeptide chain with a molecular weight of 22,000 daltons and an isoelectric point of 7.2. It is resistant to proteolytic digestion by trypsin but is hydrolyzed by pepsin at pH 4.5. In sterile solution at a neutral pH, it is stable for months. When lyophilized, it is a white powder easily dissolved in distilled water. There is no loss of serologic activity of the lyophilized powder for at least a year. TSST-I can be heated to 100° C for more than an hour without loss of biologic activity.[26]

Purification of TSST-I has yielded diffraction quality crystals that have led to an understanding of the three-dimensional structure.[26] The molecule is folded into two closely associated domains that create two major grooves, the front and backside grooves. The backside groove is larger and more exposed to the external environment.

Regulation of Production

S. aureus is highly adaptable and able to live and grow in extremes of temperature, pH, and oxygen concentrations. TSST-I production, however, is controlled tightly. TSST-I is not produced in unfavorable conditions, including an anaerobic environment, pH values of less than 6.0 and greater than 8.0, concentrations of clindamycin below the minimal inhibitory concentration of the organism, glucose concentrations greater than 3 per cent, and temperatures of less than 37° C or greater than 40° C.[19, 26, 296] Conditions and factors that enhance TSST-I production include uniform aeration of medium through shaking or a roller apparatus, complex medium containing animal protein and low glucose concentrations, a neutral pH, incubation in 5 per cent carbon dioxide (under some in vitro conditions), and temperatures of 37° to 40° C. The role of magnesium is unclear.[91] Twice as much toxin is produced at 40° C as at 37° C. The addition of blood to media does not increase TSST-I production reliably. Depending on in vitro growth conditions, most strains of TSST-I–negative *S. aureus* produce 3 μg/mL of TSST-I, but some may produce up to 30 μg/mL.

Under optimal in vitro growth conditions, TSST-I production lags behind but parallels bacterial growth. Like other *S. aureus* exotoxins, TSST-I is made primarily during the postexponential phase of growth, when nutrients are scarce and cell density is great.[89] Levels of TSST-I remain stable throughout the stationary phase, even after the organisms begin to die. Under less-than-optimal conditions, this synchronous production of TSST-I and growth of *S. aureus* do not occur. For example, bacterial growth may be reduced only twofold in an anaerobic environment, whereas TSST-I production is inhibited. Likewise, clindamycin at concentrations below the minimal inhibitory concentration for the organism will inhibit toxin production without altering growth.[244]

Most strains of *S. aureus* do not have the genes for TSST-I or the enterotoxins. TSST-I thus is not necessary for bacterial homeostasis, and its production is a variable genetic trait.

*tst*H is encoded by a transposon-like mobile genetic element.[63, 85, 138, 158] The chromosomal fragment with the structural gene for TSST-I production is a 10.6-kb unit that has been cloned in *Escherichia coli*. *tst*H has been sequenced and encodes a 234-amino-acid protein that is converted by the removal of a signal peptide of 40 amino acids to the mature exotoxin of 194 amino acids.[26, 89, 158] *tst*H has been inserted in the chromosome to disrupt both the tryptophan synthetase B and SEB genes, preventing production of both proteins.[63, 85]

The production of TSST-I and other postexponential phase virulence factors is regulated by three separate genetic loci: the accessory gene regulator (*agr*), the staphylococcal accessory regulator (*sar*), and the extracellular protein regulator (*xpr*).[11, 26, 89] All three regulators affect gene expression primarily at the level of transcription. During the late log phase of bacterial growth, they activate the expression of TSST-I, the alpha and gamma hemolysins, serine protease, and nuclease and down-regulate the expression of the cell wall–associated proteins, fibronectin-binding protein, protein A, and coagulase. Beta hemolysin, SEB, SEC, and exfoliative toxin A are regulated less tightly by *agr* than is TSST-I. SEA appears to be independent of *agr* in some strains. This complex regulation of exoprotein synthesis probably is the result of a complex interaction between environmental factors and gene products.[26, 89] These regulatory functions explain why TSST-I production is stimulated under some conditions without SEA or SEC stimulation.[296]

Glyceryl monolaurate is a mild surfactant and emulsifier commonly used in the food and cosmetic industries. It is capable of inhibiting production of staphylococcal and streptococcal exotoxins at concentrations subinhibitory to growth.[36, 180, 226, 248] As a lipophilic compound, the mechanism of action appears to be that of insertion into the cell membrane with resulting interruption of signal transduction. Other surfactants used in the tampon industry have been found to both inhibit and enhance[249] TSST-I production in vitro.

Kinetics of Distribution

It is difficult to detect TSST-I in body fluids. In humans, using a radioimmunoassay, nanogram quantities have been detected in the breast milk of a woman with TSS,[285] in serum early during illness in two of four patients,[181] in urine, and in vaginal washings in a small number of patients.[181] By means of the rabbit subcutaneous Wiffle ball abscess model, TSST-I first can be detected in the abscess fluid 4 hours after *S. aureus* has been inoculated into the Wiffle ball and can be detected in urine until 48 hours after inoculation.[181]

For further examination of in vivo target tissues for TSST-I activity, purified TSST-I radiolabeled with iodine-139 has been injected intravenously into rabbits. Measurement of plasma clearance demonstrated a half-life of 1.5 hours. Within 15 minutes of injection, TSST-I was concentrated fourfold in blood cells, compared with plasma. Toxin persisted in the cellular compartment, and plasma concentrations fell. After 3 hours, most of the radiolabel was found in the spleen.

Cellular Interactions

TSST-I has been shown to inhibit systolic function in isolated rabbit atria.[206] It also can bind directly to human and porcine endothelial cells and is cytotoxic for porcine endothelial cells, permitting leakage across endothelial-cell monolayers.[160, 163] However, the concentrations of TSST-I needed to induce these and other diverse cytotoxic changes in vitro are higher than usual tissue and serum levels. The interactions of TSST-I and the enterotoxins with T lymphocytes and antigen-processing cells are described in the next section.

Biologic Functions

Animal Models

Much information regarding pathogenesis has been obtained from both the subcutaneous Wiffle ball and vaginal tampon rabbit models and a primate model.[87] Rabbits, primates, and other species have been examined for sensitivity to TSST-I or TSS-associated strains of *S. aureus*.[219] Rabbits and baboons exhibit clinical and laboratory changes most consistent with the human syndrome, including pyrogenicity and lethality.[30, 31, 86, 87, 177–180, 214, 228, 245, 252] Signs and symptoms observed in these animals after the intravenous injection of purified TSST-I include skin erythema, conjunctivitis, diarrhea, lethargy, tachypnea, respiratory distress, central nervous system changes, and increased capillary permeability, as demonstrated by the skin bluing technique. A variety of laboratory abnormalities consistent with those described in human TSS have been described for these models.

Immunoregulatory Activities

The absence of in vitro cytotoxicity of TSST-I[19, 219] despite potent in vivo biologic effects has suggested an important role for endogenous mediators in TSS. The ability of SEB to induce dramatic T-cell proliferation was recognized a decade ago.[149, 155, 170] Subsequent work has shown this to be a feature of other bacterial exotoxins, including TSST-I, the staphylococcal enterotoxins, the streptococcal pyrogenic exotoxins A and C, a new streptococcal superantigen, and a streptococcal M surface protein.[155] Since the late 1980s, activation of T cells by these bacterial components or products has become an area of intense interest. The term *superantigen* was coined in 1989 to describe antigens that at concentrations lower than those of conventional antigens (picomolar concentrations) can stimulate proliferation of a large percentage of T cells bearing a TCR beta chain variable (Vβ) sequence(s) specific for each superantigen. This activation and proliferation of T cells result in profound alterations in immune system homeostasis by inducing the release of large quantities of both monokines (IL-1, TNF-α) and lymphokines (IL-2, TNF-βγ).[155, 255, 301]

T cells are activated to produce lymphokines as a result of TCR antigen binding and activation of signal transduction.[51] Antigens can bind to the TCR in one of two forms, as conventional antigens or superantigens. Conventional antigens enter antigen-processing cells by endocytosis. They are broken into small peptides in the lysosomal compartments of the antigen-processing cell and targeted to small vesicles, where they form complexes with one of the allele-restricted major histocompatibility complex class II molecules (HLA-DQ, -DP, and -DR).[255] The complex then is transported to the cell surface, where it is bound in the groove on the heavy chain, formed by the alpha and beta chains of the class II molecule. Certain amino acids in residues at critical points in the peptide's sequence anchor the peptides in the groove, and this interaction moderately is specific for each different allelic form of the major histocompatibility complex molecule.[255] This complex of peptide and major histocompatibility complex molecule of the same allelic type as the T cell is recognized by the TCR.

The TCR is composed of both alpha and beta glycoprotein chains, each of which is composed of variable (V) and joining (J) segments. The beta chain has an additional diversity (D) segment. There are up to 50 Vβ and 32 Vα segments present on human T cells. The VαβαββVαβαββ segments each are encoded by different genes that undergo gene rearrangement to give more than 10,000 possible combinations to recognize conventional antigenic peptides presented by the antigen-processing cells.[15, 255] Conventional antigens presented as peptides must be recognized by a specific combination of these elements. Thus, one peptide will activate only 1 in 10^4 to 10^6 T cells, and only CD_4-positive T cells respond to conventional antigens.

In contrast, superantigens are presented to T lymphocytes in a very different fashion. They bind first as intact proteins (small fragments are inactive) to most allelic forms of major histocompatibility complex class II molecules in an unrestricted fashion at a site outside of the peptide-binding groove. They then react with the TCR only through the Vβ element(s) specific for that molecule and will react with all T cells carrying that Vβ element.[136] Because there are only 25 to 50 major families of Vβ genes in humans, each superantigen can interact with 5 to 20 per cent of resting T cells, depending on the frequency of T cells expressing that Vβ family in each individual's repertoire. Both CD_4-positive and CD_8-positive T cells are activated. Features unique to the presentation of superantigens to the TCR Vβ receptor thus include the requirement for initial superantigen binding to the major histocompatibility complex class II molecule (even if unrestricted and not self) outside of the antigen-presenting groove and for an intact superantigen protein.

Once the T cell has recognized the superantigen, both antigen-processing cell and T-cell activation by signal transduction[51] result in cytokine release by the antigen-processing cell (IL-1, TNF-α) and the lymphocyte (IL-2, TNF-βγ). In mice and possibly also in humans, the initial T-cell activation occurs in lymph nodes.[188] Within hours of T-cell activation by superantigens, cytokines are detected in vitro and in serum in vivo.

TSST-I binds only to the $V\beta_2$ element.[235] In humans with TSS caused by TSST-I secreting *S. aureus,* within 10 to 14 days, 30 to 70 per cent of the circulating T-cell population will be T cells bearing the $V\beta_2$ element.[59, 60] The number of circulating $V\beta_2$ T cells does not return to normal for several months. In contrast, for patients with TSS caused by *S. pyogenes,* there is a consistent pattern of depletion of certain Vβ T-cell types after T-cell activation.[155, 202, 289] In mice, such depletion is thought to be the result of programmed cell death (apoptosis).[186, 187]

Thus, activation of T cells by superantigens may result in massive cytokine release with subsequent selected Vβ T-cell expansion, T-cell deletion, or apoptosis, depending on the superantigen and species. The fact that superantigens bind only to selected and specific Vβ elements distinguishes them from the nondiscriminating mitogens.

The activation of monocytes and lymphocytes by superantigens involves signal transduction. Activation of both src protein tyrosine kinases and protein kinase C occurs in a manner common to other immunoglobulin supragene family members. Major histocompatibility complex class II cells also are expressed on beta, endothelial, and dendritic cells. In some instances, superantigens may activate these cells uniquely.

Convincing evidence from the mouse model supports a central role for T-lymphocyte activation in superantigen-mediated disease. Mice that have received cyclosporin A to block T-cell activation and lymphokine production or mice with severe combined immunodeficiency disease are protected against SEB-induced lethal shock. Repopulation with T cells results in susceptibility to SEB. The same mice are not protected against endotoxin-induced shock because lipopolysaccharide activates only the monocyte.[186–188]

Mononuclear production of IL-1 and TNF-α is central to shock induced by endotoxin. Production of these two cytokines in addition to the production of the lymphokines IL-2, IFN-α, and TNF-β may explain the enhanced severity of superantigen-associated TSS.[27, 155] These powerful effects on the immune system may account for the tenacity of shock in otherwise healthy individuals. If more than one superantigen is produced by an organism (e.g., TSST-I plus one or more enterotoxins), then different Vβ specificities would result in an even greater number of T cells being activated with the potential for enhanced disease severity and mortality.

Once the superantigens have resulted in monokine and lymphokine release, subsequent pathophysiologic events appear to be related to the many and complex interactions of these cytokines,[27, 130, 300] ultimately resulting in profound endothelial damage. TNF-αβ and the complex interaction of cytokines, leukotrienes, prostaglandins, adhesion molecules, nitric oxide, platelet-activating factor, complement components, neutrophils, platelets, and endothelium-derived factors appear to be responsible for the extensive endothelial damage with resulting capillary fluid leakage and decrease in peripheral vascular resistance.[27, 130, 300] In a different setting of antineoplastic therapy, high doses of IL-2 and lymphokine-activated killer cells induce the capillary leak syndrome characterized by rapid weight gain, anasarca, pulmonary edema, hypoalbuminemia, and multiple organ dysfunctions in humans.[69, 154]

Endotoxin Enhancement

A striking property of TSST-I is its ability markedly to enhance the susceptibility of some animals to lethal endotoxin shock.[26, 245, 246] Intravenous administration of TSST-I to rabbits at less than one-twentieth of the median lethal dose (LD_{50}) followed 2 hours later by endotoxin at less than one-five hundredth of the LD_{50} results in 50 to 100 per cent mortality, a 10,000-fold enhancement. In vitro, endotoxin enhances IL-1 production by TSST-I–stimulated monocytes.[17] It is not clear if enhanced endotoxin susceptibility plays any role in human disease.[61]

Structure-Function Relationships

Efforts to understand the molecular actions of TSST-I have focused on separating those regions that interact with the TCR from those regions required for lethality.[26, 30, 31, 196] Through use of the TSST-I variants (TSST-ovine and TSST-bovine) and TSST-I molecules with single amino acid mutations, the areas responsible for the binding of TSST-I to both the TCR and to the macrophage class II major histocompatibility complex molecule have been defined.[26] In animal models, lethality, fever induction, and endotoxin susceptibility do not depend on T-cell proliferation as measured by superantigenic activity but must involve toxin interaction with other host-cell receptors in the body.[26]

The majority of secreted bacterial superantigens are small, compact globular proteins of 20 to 30 kDa.[26] They are protease-, heat-, and acid-resistant and share immunologic, biologic, and functional properties. However, they do not share sequence homology. Although they do not share obvious structural features that would predict their superantigen properties, they may share a common conformational structure.[155] The secreted exotoxins can be divided into two groups based on their amino acid sequence homology. In group 1, SEA, SED, and SEE share 54 to 90 per cent homology. In group 2, streptococcal pyrogenic exotoxin A, SEB, and $SEC_{1, 2, 3}$ share 46 to 68 per cent homology. In group 3, TSST-I, the exfoliative toxins, and the streptococcal pyrogenic exotoxin show no significant homology to each other or any of the members of group 1 or 2. However, all of the secreted superantigens may share a three-dimensional conformation that allows them to interact simultaneously with two different receptors on two different cell types.[26, 155]

The structure and binding sites of SEB to the major histocompatibility complex class II molecule have been determined using crystallographic conformation. There are two different major histocompatibility complex class II binding sites for SEB. The amino terminal domain forms most of the contact, but residues at the carboxy terminal domain also contact the major histocompatibility complex class II molecule as well as the TCR. Although TSST-I is very similar to SEB on the basis of crystallographic structure, the two proteins do not compete with each other for the same major histocompatibility complex class II HLA-DR sites. Likewise, SEA and SEE have greater than 90 per cent amino acid sequence homology but have quite distinct patterns of Vβ specificity. TSST-I and the exfoliative toxins A and B are unrelated structurally but have the same $V\beta_2$ specificity.[155, 170]

HOST RISK FACTORS

Colonization with Exotoxin *Staphylococcus aureus*

To develop TSS, an individual must be colonized with or acquire a strain of *S. aureus* that produces TSST-I or one of the staphylococcal enterotoxins. There now is compelling evidence that SEB alone and uncommonly SEA or SEC alone as well as TSST-I may be responsible for the manifestations of TSS. Although many genotypically different strains of *S. aureus* possess the *tst*H gene, one clone has been isolated from 88 per cent of menstrual cases and 54 per cent of nonmenstrual cases.[197] Colonization with this clone, particularly for menstruating women, clearly provides a significant risk factor. Future work may identify other clones with unique adherence properties for other mucosal or skin sites.

Absence of Protective Antibody Levels

A necessary factor for developing TSS is the absence of protective antibody levels for the toxin (TSST-I or enterotoxin) produced by the isolate associated with TSS. Thus, more than 90 per cent of women with menstrual TSS associated with TSST-1–positive strains have antibody titers of 1:10 or lower, whereas a titer of 1:100 or higher is considered protective.[19] Because most adults acquire these antibodies without developing disease, absent antibody levels may be the result of lack of exposure to a toxin-producing organism or a lacunar inability to respond to the toxin. The failure of most patients, menstrual and nonmenstrual, to make antibody during convalescence may reflect this lacunar nonrecognition of staphylococcal protein antigen, or it may be a reflection of the superantigenic nature of these proteins and failure of the toxin proteins to be presented to the TCR as conventional antigens.

Interruption of a Mucosal or Skin Surface

Primary deep-tissue staphylococcal infections (e.g., osteomyelitis, pyarthrosis, pyomyositis,[4] endocarditis,[223, 292] renal carbuncles, bacteremia) rarely are associated with TSS. The majority of nonmenstrual cases occur in patients with alteration of a skin or a mucosal surface. Examples of skin disruption associated with TSS include burns, insect bites, needle sticks, surgical incisions, and varicella. Examples of mucous membrane disruption can be divided into those associated with respiratory and those with genital mucosae. Damaged respiratory mucosa may appear after nasal or other surgery, particularly with placement of stents or packing, in association with a viral respiratory infection, such as influenza, or as a primary sinusitis, tracheitis, or parapharyngeal abscess. Heavy colonization of the pharynx also has been associated with TSS. The vaginal mucosa may be damaged in a number of ways, including placement of tampons or barrier contraceptives,[45, 104, 251] postpartum,[19, 220] or after genital surgery or genital mucosal damage.[105, 213, 236] Heavy colonization of the vagina without any other apparent risk factor also has been associated with TSS.[229] These mucosal infections may provide the right conditions for TSST-I production, including an aerobic environment, a high carbon dioxide concentration, a neutral pH, high protein and low glucose concentrations, and low to normal magnesium concentrations.[276]

Presence of a Foreign Body

Tampons create an aerobic environment in the vagina, which normally is anaerobic. Tampons of three different types have been shown in humans to change the partial pressure of oxygen of the vaginal wall from an anaerobic environment to that of atmospheric air throughout the 90-minute interval after insertion.[288] Because oxygen is required for TSST-I production, it has been suggested that tampons of enhanced absorbency allowed the introduction of increasing concentrations of oxygen to enhance toxin production.

Several alternative explanations for the role of tampons have been proposed. Tampons may remove vaginal substrates that normally inhibit the growth of *S. aureus*.[19] Another suggested role for tampons is that of inducing cervicovaginal ulcerations. It is suggested that these ulcers may enhance bacterial growth or toxin absorption and expose submucosal fibronectin for *S. aureus* binding.[73, 75, 291] Tampons can induce chronic cervicovaginal ulcers after long-term continuous use or superficial microulcerations after a brief insertion in otherwise healthy women. However, vaginal ulcerations of the type typically seen in TSS have been found during postmortem examination in women who had never used tampons. This suggests that vaginal ulcerations, such as those seen in the esophagus and bladder in TSS, may be induced by TSST-I.[161]

Investigations to determine whether individual tampon components can induce or amplify TSST-I production in vitro have provided conflicting data, in part because there is no consensus regarding how best to test tampons and their components to determine their potential to increase the risk of TSS. In one setting, although bacterial growth was unaffected, TSST-I production varied from undetectable levels to levels of 300 μg/mL, depending on the particular brand and style of tampon studied.[19] Other investigators have found that the majority of tampons tested were inhibitory to both bacterial growth and TSST-I production and that none consistently increased the production of TSST-I.[19]

Two studies clearly have demonstrated the enhanced production of TSST-I in vitro by the Rely tampon composed of cross-linked carboxymethylcellulose and polyester foam.[217, 249] Polyacrylate rayon included in two tampons now removed from the market increased TSST-I production under certain conditions,[191] as did the surfactant pluronic L-92 used in at least one tampon.[249] Neither cotton nor rayon amplifies TSST-I production in vitro, nor do cotton tampons adsorb TSST-I or prevent its production.[217, 249] Thus, cotton tampons cannot be claimed to be safer than cotton/rayon combinations, although this has been disputed.[272] The role of magnesium in controlling TSST-I production in the presence of tampons is unclear.[191]

Implanted foreign material, such as sutures, central venous lines, and metallic or polymeric implants, repeatedly have been documented to enhance the risk of bacterial infection.[19, 145] These infections are characterized by limited spread beyond the tissues in immediate contact with the implants, poor response to antibiotics, and poor healing without removal of the foreign material. Two important differences between TSS and other *S. aureus* infections related to foreign material are the added ability of the organism to produce a toxin that readily disseminates and the limited ability of these strains to produce inflammation.[106]

The enhanced risk of infection by *S. aureus* in the presence of foreign material has been defined experimentally in animals. Rats remained asymptomatic after the subcutaneous injection of more than 1×10^6 colony-forming units of *S. aureus*, whereas 3×10^2 colony-forming units invariably led to infection in the presence of a suture. In addition, the ability of the sutured tissue to resist infection varies with the kind of material implanted, particularly its physical or chemical configuration. For example, bacterial adherence is eightfold higher for braided sutures of silk, silicone-heated blue polyester, and absorbable polyglycolic acid than for monofilament nylon.[145]

In addition to sutures, other foreign materials associated with TSS-related wound infections are Teflon splints, gauze packing, and mammary implants.[19]

Other Potential Host Risk Factors

Other factors have been examined in an attempt to identify individuals who may be at increased risk for TSS.[82] Some of these factors have included HLA typing,[19] neutrophil function,[133] adherence of *S. aureus* to vaginal epithelial cells,[19] alteration of the cervicovaginal flora,[19] hormonal factors, and personal hygiene practices.[82] Of all these factors, those of potential importance included the cervicovaginal flora and hormonal factors.

It has been postulated that vaginal cocolonization with *S. aureus* and one of the enterobacteriaceae might enhance the risk of TSS.[61] Prospective examination of 495 healthy women revealed a 7 per cent vaginal colonization rate for *S. aureus* TSST-I–positive strains. Women who were colonized with toxin-producing *S. aureus* also were colonized with *E. coli* or other enterobacteriaceae statistically significantly more often than were women colonized with non–toxin-producing or no *S. aureus*. The *E. coli* isolation rates were 54 per cent in women with TSST-I–positive isolates, 15 per cent in women with TSST-I–negative isolates, and 11 per cent in women with no *S. aureus*. Coisolation of *E. coli* was the only identified factor associated with vaginal carriage of TSST-I–positive *S. aureus*. Additionally, among the 14 TSS patients followed in this study, 9 had *E. coli* as well as TSST-I–positive *S. aureus* coisolated during the acute TSS episode. The significance of these observations and their relationship to postulated roles for endotoxin in TSS is not clear.

Results of early case-control studies suggested that oral contraceptive steroids may have an effect on vaginal *S. aureus* organisms that may produce or release TSS-associated toxin(s)[80, 211] and that this effect was protective. However, one case-control study found no protective effect or enhanced risk associated with oral contraceptive use.[124] Hormonal control is known to be responsible for a number of cycle changes in the vaginal pH and flora; however, the role of hormonal factors in the pathogenesis of TSS has not been well examined.

UNIQUE MANIFESTATIONS OF TOXIC SHOCK SYNDROME

Work with superantigens suggests that the pathophysiologic events observed in TSS are the result of endogenous mediator release after monocyte and T-cell activation by TSST-I or the staphylococcal enterotoxins.

The physiologic changes induced by this dysregulation of the immune system are striking in their rapidity of onset and progression and the involvement of almost all body tissues and organs. The consequent functional disorders of many organs appear to be the result of extensive endothelial damage and loss of peripheral vascular resistance. The generalized decrease in vasomotor tone results in pooling of blood in the peripheral vasculature, vascular congestion, and probable relaxation of the microcirculation. There is rapid, nonhydrostatic leakage of fluid from the intravascular to the interstitial space, or "second-spacing," which is manifested in the patient as extensive generalized anasarca-like, nonpitting edema. The universal hypoproteinemia and hypoalbuminemia in patients with TSS suggest that the fluid that leaks from the vasculature is high in protein.

Unique clinical manifestations include the profuse vomiting and diarrhea often associated with incontinence; generalized erythroderma; intense erythema of mucous membranes, including conjunctival injection and subconjunctival hemorrhages; the absence of inflammation in surgical wounds and other focal sites of infection; the absence of bacteremia; severe hypocalcemia and hypophosphatemia; rapidly accelerated renal dysfunction; universal desquamation of palms, soles, fingers, and toes; and long-term cognitive sequelae.

References

1. Abdul-Karim, F. W., Lederman, M. M., Carter, J. R., et al.: Toxic shock syndrome: Clinicopathologic findings in a fatal case. Hum. Pathol. *12*:16–22, 1981.
2. Abram, A. C., Bellian, K. T., Giles, W. J., et al.: Toxic shock syndrome after functional endonasal sinus surgery: An all or none phenomenon? Laryngoscope *104*:927–931, 1994.
3. Allen, S. T., Liland, J. B., Nichols, C. G., et al.: Toxic shock syndrome associated with use of latex nasal packing. Arch. Intern. Med. *150*:2587–2588, 1990.
4. Alsoub, H.: Toxic shock syndrome associated with pyomyositis. Postgrad. Med. J. Engl. *70*:309–312, 1994.
5. Andrews, M. M., Giacobbe, K. D., and Parsonnet, J.: Induction of toxic shock syndrome toxin-1 (TSST-1) and beta-lactamase by subinhibitory concentrations of beta-lactam antibiotics. Biomedicine '96, Washington, D.C., May 3–6, 1996. Abstract N-IN-0011.
6. Aranow, H., Jr., and Wood, W. B., Jr.: Staphylococcic infection simulating scarlet fever. J. A. M. A. *119*:1491–1495, 1942.
7. Arend, S. M., Steenmeyer, A. V., Mosmans, P. C. M., et al.: Postoperative cauda syndrome caused by *Staphylococcus aureus*. Infection *21*:248–250, 1993.
8. Arnow, P. M., Chou, T., Weil, D., et al.: Spread of a toxic-shock syndrome-associated strain of *Staphylococcus aureus* and measurement of antibodies to staphylooccal enterotoxin F. J. Infect. Dis. *149*:103–107, 1984.
9. Bach, M. C.: Dermatologic signs in toxic shock syndrome: Clues to diagnosis. J. Am. Acad. Dermatol. *8*:343–347, 1983.
10. Bacha, E. A., Sheridan, R. L., Donohue, G. A., et al.: Staphylococcal toxic shock syndrome in a paediatric burn unit. Burns *20*:499–502, 1994.
11. Balaban, N., and Novick, R. P.: Autocrine regulation of toxin synthesis by *Staphylococcus aureus*. Proc. Natl. Acad. Sci. U. S. A. *92*:1619–1623, 1995.
12. Bannister, B., and Platts, A. J.: Some cardiological findings in toxic shock syndrome. J. Infect. *3*:293–294, 1981.
13. Baracos, V., Rodemann, P., Dinarello, C. A., et al.: Stimulation of muscle protein degradation and prostaglandin E2 release by leucocytic pyrogen (interleukin-1). N. Engl. J. Med. *308*:553–558, 1983.
14. Barrett, J. A., and Graham, D. R.: TSS presenting as encephalopathy. J. Infect. *12*:276, 1986.
15. Barry, W., Hudgins, L., Donta, S.T., et al.: Intravenous immunoglobulin therapy for toxic-shock syndrome. J. A. M. A. *267*:3315–3317, 1992.
16. Bartlett, P., Reingold, A. L., Graham, D. R., et al.: Toxic shock syndrome associated with surgical wound infections. J. A. M. A. *247*:1448–1450, 1982.
17. Beezhold, D. H., Best, G. K., Bonventre, P. F., et al.: Endotoxin enhancement of TSST-1-induced secretion of interleukin-1 by murine macrophages. Rev. Infect. Dis. *11*:S289–S293, 1989.
18. Beisel, W. R.: Pathophysiology of staphylococcal enterotoxin, type B, (SEB) toxemia after the intravenous administration to monkeys. Toxicon *10*:433, 1972.
19. Bergdoll, M. S., and Chesney, P. J.: Toxic-Shock Syndrome. Boca Raton, CRC Press, 1991.
20. Bergdoll, M. S., Crass, B. A., Reiser, R. F., et al.: A new staphylococcal enterotoxin, enterotoxin F, associated with toxic-shock syndrome *Staphylococcus aureus* isolates. Lancet *1*:1017–1021, 1981.
21. Berkley, S. F., Hightower, A. W., Broome, C. W., et al.: The relationship of tampon characteristics to menstrual toxic-shock syndrome. J. A. M. A. *258*:917–920, 1987.
22. Berman, A. C., and Boly, L. R.: Cisplatin therapy-associated recurrent toxic shock syndrome. West. J. Med. *155*:415–416, 1991.
23. Bernstein, G. M., Crollick, J. S., and Hassett, J. M., Jr.: Post febrile telogen effluvium in critically ill patients. Crit. Care Med. *16*:98–99, 1988.
24. Black, D. A., and Maw, D. S.: Toxic shock syndrome presenting as cerebral infarct. Corres. J. Neurol. Neurosurg. Psychiatry *47*:568, 1984.
25. Blair, J. D., Livingston, D. G., and Vongsnichakul, R.: Tampon-related toxic-shock syndrome: Histopathologic and clinical findings in a fatal case. Am. J. Clin. Pathol. *78*:372–376, 1982.
26. Bohach, G. A., Dinges, M. M., Mitchell, D. T., et al.: Staphylococcal exotoxins. *In* Leung, D. Y. M., Huber, B. T., and Schlievert, P. M. (eds.): Superantigens: Molecular Biology, Immunology and Relevance to Human Disease. New York, Marcel Dekker (in press).
27. Bone, R. C.: The pathogenesis of sepsis. Ann. Intern. Med. *115*:457–469, 1991.
28. Bonventre, P. F., Linnemann, C., Weckback, L. S., et al.: Antibody responses to toxic-shock-syndrome (TSS) toxin by patients with TSS and by healthy staphylococcal carriers. J. Infect. Dis. *150*:662–666, 1984.
29. Bonventre, P. F., Thompson, M. R., Adinolfi, L. E., et al.: Neutralization of TSST-1 by monoclonal antibodies in vitro and in vivo. Infect. Immun. *50*:135, 1987.
30. Bonventre, P. F., Heeg, H., Cullen, C., et al.: Toxicity of recombinant toxic shock syndrome toxin 1 and mutant toxins produced by *Staphylococcus aureus* in a rabbit infection model of toxic shock syndrome. Infect. Immun. *61*:793–799, 1993.
31. Bonventre, P. F., Heeg, H., Edwards, C. K., III, et al.: A mutation at histidine residue 135 of toxic shock syndrome toxin yields an immunogenic protein with minimal toxicity. Infect. Immun. *63*:509–515, 1995.
32. Breda, S. D., Jacobs, J. B., Lebowitz, A. S., et al.: Toxic shock syndrome in nasal surgery: A physiochemical and microbiologic evaluation of Merocel and NuGauze nasal packing. Laryngoscope *97*:1388, 1987.
33. Brody, H., and Smith, L. W.: The visceral pathology in scarlet fever and related *Streptococcus* infections. Am. J. Pathol. *12*:373, 1936.
34. Brook, M. G., and Bannister, B. A.: Staphylococcal enterotoxins in scarlet fever complicating chicken pox. Postgrad. Med. J. *67*:1013–1014, 1991.
35. Broome, C. V.: Epidemiology of TSS in the United States: Overview. Rev Infect. Dis. *11*:S14–S21, 1989.
36. Brown-Skrobot, S. K., Irving, M. M., and Wojnarowicz, L.: Tampon additives and toxic shock syndrome toxin-1 (TSST-1) production. Abstract B18, p. 28. Abstracts of the Ninety-first General Meeting of the American Society of Microbiology, 1991.
37. Burns, J. R., and Menpace, F. J.: Acute reversible cardiomyopathy complicating toxic shock syndrome. Arch. Intern. Med. *142*:1032–1034, 1982.
38. Cavanah, D. K., and Ballas, Z. K.: Pseudoephedrine reaction presenting as recurrent toxic shock syndrome. Ann. Intern. Med. *119*:302–303, 1993.

39. Cederna, J. P.: Toxic shock syndrome after transverse rectus abdominis musculocutaneous flap breast reconstruction. Ann. Plast. Surg. *34*:73–75, 1995.
40. Centers for Disease Control: Epidemiology of toxic shock syndrome, United States, 1960–1984. M. M. W. R. *33*:19SS–22SS, 1984.
41. Centers for Disease Control: Follow-up on toxic-shock syndrome, United States. M. M. W. R. *29*:441–445, 1980.
42. Centers for Disease Control: Reduced incidence of menstrual toxic-shock syndrome—United States, 1980–1990. M. M. W. R. *39*:421–423, 1990.
42a. Centers for Disease Control: Case definitions for public health surveillance. M. M. W. R. *39*(RR-13):38–39, 1990.
43. Centers for Disease Control and Prevention: Summary of notifiable diseases, United States, 1994. M. M. W. R. *43*:60, 69–73, 1994.
44. Centers for Disease Control: Toxic shock syndrome following influenza—Oregon, United States. M. M. W. R. *36*:64–65, 1987.
45. Centers for Disease Control: Toxic-shock syndrome and the vaginal contraceptive sponge. M. M. W. R. *33*:43–44, 49, 1984.
46. Centers for Disease Control: Toxic-shock syndrome, United States, 1970–1980. M. M. W. R. *30*:25–28, 33, 1981.
47. Centers for Disease Control: Toxic-shock syndrome, United States, 1970–1982. M. M. W. R. *31*:201–204, 1982.
48. Centers for Disease Control: Toxic-shock syndrome, United States. M. M. W. R. *29*:229–230, 1980.
49. Centers for Disease Control: Update: Toxic shock syndrome, United States. M. M. W. R. *32*:397–400, 1983.
50. Chang, A. H., Musser, J. M., and Chow, A. W.: A single clone which produces both TSST-1 and SEA causes the majority of menstrual toxic shock syndrome. Clin. Res. *39*:36A, 1991.
51. Chatila, T., and Geha, R. S.: Signal transduction by microbial superantigens via MHC class II molecules. Immunol. Rev. *131*:43–59, 1993.
52. Chesney, P. J., and Zimmerman, J. J.: Hypoferrinemia in toxic-shock syndrome (TSS). Pediatr. Res. *20*:306A, 1986.
53. Chesney, P. J., Crass, B. A., and Polyak, M. B., et al.: Toxic-shock syndrome: Management and long-term sequelae. Ann. Intern. Med. *96*(Part 2):847–851, 1982.
54. Chesney, P. J., Davis, J. P., Purdy, W. K., et al.: The clinical manifestations of toxic shock syndrome. J. A. M. A. *246*:741–748, 1981.
55. Chesney, P. J., Slama, S. L., Hawkins, R. L., et al.: Outpatient diagnosis and management of toxic-shock syndrome. N. Engl. J. Med. *304*:1426, 1981.
56. Chesney, R. W., Chesney, P. J., Davis, J. P., et al.: Renal manifestations of the staphylococcal toxic-shock syndrome. Am. J. Med. *71*:583–588, 1981.
57. Chesney, R. W., McCarren, D. M., Haddad, J. G., et al.: Pathogenic mechanisms of the hypocalcemia of the staphylococcal toxic-shock syndrome. J. Lab. Clin. Med. *101*:576–585, 1983.
58. Childs, C., Edwards-Jones, V., Healthcote, D. M., et al.: Patterns of *Staphylococcal aureus* colonization, toxin production, immunity and illness in burned children. Burns *20*:514–521, 1994.
59. Choi, Y., Kotzin, B., Herron, L., et al.: Interaction of *Staphylococcus aureus* toxin "superantigens" with human T cells. Proc. Natl. Acad. Sci. U. S. A. *86*:8941–8945, 1989.
60. Choi, Y., Lafferty, J. A., Clements, J. R., et al.: Selective expansion of T cells expressing V beta 2 in toxic-shock syndrome. J. Exp. Med. *172*:981–984, 1990.
61. Chow, A. Microbiology of toxic shock syndrome: Overview. Rev. Infect. Dis. *1*:55–60, 1989.
62. Chow, A. W., Wong, C. K., MacFarlane, A. M., et al.: Toxic shock syndrome: Clinical and laboratory findings in 30 patients. Can. Med. Assoc. J. *130*:425–430, 1984.
63. Chu, M. C., Kreiswirth, B. N., Pattee, P. A., et al.: Association of toxic shock toxin-1 determinant with a heterologous insertion at multiple loci in the *Staphylococcus aureus* chromosome. Infect. Immun. *56*:2702–2708, 1988.
64. Cohen, K. R., Emmons, K. M., and Goldstein, M. F.: Naloxone treatment of toxic shock syndrome. Arch. Intern. Med. *143*:1072, 1983.
65. Cole, R. P., and Shakespeare, P. G.: Toxic-shock syndrome in scalded children. Burns *16*:221–224, 1990.
66. Cone, L. A., Woodard, D. R., Schlievert, P. M., et al.: Clinical and bacteriologic observations of a toxic-shock-like syndrome due to *Streptococcus pyogenes*. N. Engl. J. Med. *317*:146–149, 1987.
67. Cone, L. A., Woodward, D. R., Byrd, R. G., et al.: A recalcitrant, erythematous, desquamating disorder associated with toxin-producing staphylococci in patients with AIDS. J. Infect. Dis. 165:638-643, 1992.
68. Conway, E. E., Jr., Haber, R. S., Gumprecht, J., et al.: Toxic shock syndrome following influenza A in a child. Crit. Care Med. *19*:123–125, 1991.
69. Cotran, R. S., Proba, J. S., Gimbrone, M. A., et al.: Endothelial activation during IL-2 immunotherapy: A possible mechanism for the vascular leak syndrome. J. Immunol. *139*:1883, 1987.
70. Cowan, R. K. and Martens, M. G.: Toxic shock syndrome mimicking pelvic inflammatory disease presumably resulting from tattoo. South. Med. J. *86*:1427–1431, 1993.
71. Crass, B. A., and Bergdoll, M. S.: Toxin involvement in toxic shock syndrome. J. Infect. Dis. *153*:918–926, 1986.
72. Crews, J. R., Harrison, J. K, Corey, G. R., et al.: Stunned myocardium in the toxic shock syndrome. Ann. Intern. Med. *117*:912–913, 1992.
73. Crowder, W. E., and Shannon, F. C.: Colposcopic diagnosis of vaginal ulcerations in toxic-shock syndrome. Obstet. Gynecol. *61*:505–535, 1983.
74. Crowther, M. A., and Ralph, E. D.: Menstrual toxic shock syndrome complicated by persistent bacteremia: Case report and review. Clin. Infect. Dis. *16*:288–289, 1993.
75. Danielson, R. W.: Vaginal ulcers caused by tampons. Am. J. Obstet. Gynecol. *146*:547–549, 1983.
76. Dann, E. J., Weinberger, M., Gillis, S., et al.: Bacterial laryngotracheitis associated with toxic-shock syndrome in an adult. Clin. Infect. Dis. *18*:437–439, 1994.
77. Dart, R. C., and Levitt, M. A.: Toxic-shock syndrome associated with the use of the vaginal contraceptive sponge. J. A. M. A. *253*:1877, 1985.
78. Davidson, A. C., Creach, M., and Cameron, I. R.: Staphylococcal pneumonia, pneumatoceles, and the toxic shock syndrome. Thorax *45*:639–640, 1990.
79. Davis, J. P., and Vergeront, J. M.: A review of toxic shock syndrome surveillance in Wisconsin: The effect of media publicity and laboratory services on reporting of illness. Ann. Intern. Med. *96*:883–886, 1982.
80. Davis, J. P., Chesney, P. J., Wand, P. J., et al.: Toxic shock syndrome: Epidemiologic features, recurrences, risk factors and prevention. N. Engl. J. Med. *303*:1429–1435, 1980.
81. Davis, J. P., Osterholm, M. T., Helms, C. M., et al.: Tri-state toxic-shock syndrome study. II. Clinical and laboratory findings. J. Infect. Dis. *145*:441–448, 1982.
82. Davis, J. P., Vergeront, J. M., and Chesney, P. J.: Possible host-defense mechanisms in toxic shock syndrome. Ann. Intern. Med. *96*:986–991, 1982.
83. Davis, J. P., Vergeront, J. V., Amsterdam, L. E., et al.: Long-term effects of TSS in women: Sequelae, subsequent pregnancy, menstrual history, and long-term trends in catamenial product use. Rev. Infect. Dis. *11*:S50, 1989.
84. Davis, J. P., and Vergeront, J. M.: The effect of publicity on the reporting of toxic-shock syndrome in Wisconsin. J. Infect. Dis. *145*:449–457, 1982.
85. De Boer, M. L., and Chow, A. W.: Toxic shock syndrome toxin 1-producing *Staphylococcus aureus* isolates contain the staphylococcal enterotoxin B genetic element but do not express staphylococcal enterotoxin B. J. Infect. Dis. *170*:818–827, 1994.
86. de Azavedo, J. C. S., Foster, T. J., Hartigan, J., et al.: Expression of the cloned toxic shock syndrome toxin 1 gene (*tst*) in vivo with a rabbit uterine model. Infect. Immun. *50*:304–309, 1985.
87. de Azavedo, J. C. S.: Animal models for toxic-shock syndrome: Overview. Rev. Infect. Dis. *11*:S205–S209, 1989.
88. Deetz, T. R., Reves, R., and Septimus, E.: Secondary rash in toxic shock syndrome. N. Engl. J. Med. *304*:174, 1981.
89. Deresiewicz, R. L.: Staphylococcal toxic shock syndrome. *In* Leung, D. Y. M., Huber, B. T., and Schlievert P. M. (eds.): Superantigens: Molecular Biology, Immunology and Relevance to Human Disease. New York, Marcel Dekker (in press).
90. deVries, N., and Vander Baan, S.: Toxic shock syndrome after nasal surgery: Is prevention possible? A case report and review of literature. Rhinology *27*:125–128, 1989.
91. Dickgiesser, N. and Wallach, U.: Toxic shock syndrome toxin-1 (TSST-1): Influence of its production by subinhibitory antibiotic concentrations. Infection *15*:351–353, 1987.
92. Donawa, M. E., Schmid, G. R., and Osterholm, M. T.: Toxic shock syndrome: Chronology of state and federal epidemiologic studies and regulatory decision-making. Public Health Rep. *99*:342–350, 1984.
93. Dondorp, A. M., Veenstra, J., vanderPoll, T., et al.: Activation of the cytokine network in a patient with AIDS and the recalcitrant erythematous desquamating disorder. Clin. Infect. Dis. *18*:942–945, 1994.
94. Donnelly, B. W., McMillan, J. A., and Weiner, L. B.: Bacterial tracheitis: Report of eight new cases and a review. Rev. Infect. Dis. *12*:729–735, 1990.
95. Dornan, K. J., Thompson, D. M., Conn, A. R., et al.: Toxic shock syndrome in the postoperative patient. Surg. Gynecol. Obstet. *154*:65–68, 1982.
96. Driessen, C., Hirv, K., Kirchner, H., et al.: Zinc regulates cytokine induction by superantigens and lipopolysaccharide. Immunology *84*:272–277, 1995.
97. Dunnet, U. B., and Schallibaum, E. M.: Scarlet fever like illness due to staphylococcal infection. Lancet *2*:1227–1229, 1960.
98. Eagle, H.: Experimental approach to the problem of treatment failure with penicillin. I. Group A streptococcal infection in mice. Am. J. Med. *13*:389–399, 1952.
99. Edwards-Jones, V., and Foster, H. A.: The effect of topical antimicrobial agents on the production of toxic shock syndrome toxin-1. J. Med. Microbiol. *41*:408–413, 1994.
100. Ejlertsen, T., and Porsborg, P. A.: Toxic-shock syndrome related to simultaneous *Staphylococcus aureus* epiglottic abscess and group A streptococcal pharyngitis with bacteremia. A. P. M. I. S. *102*:956–959, 1994.
101. Elbaum, D. J., Wood, C., Abuabara, F., et al.: Bullae in a patient with toxic shock syndrome. J. Am. Acad. Dermatol. *10*:267–272, 1984.
102. Elsberry, D. D., Rhoda, D. A., and Beisel, W. R.: Hemodynamics of staphylococcal B enterotoxemia and other types of shock in monkeys. J. Appl. Physiol. *27*:164, 1969.
103. Espersen F., Baek, L., Kjaeldgaard, P., et al.: Detection of staphylococcal toxic shock syndrome toxin 1 by a latex agglutination kit. Scand. J. Infect. Dis. *20*:449–450, 1988.

104. Faich, G., Pearson, K., and Fleming, D., et al.: Toxic-shock syndrome and the vaginal contraceptive sponge. J. A. M. A. *255*:216–218, 1986.
105. Farley, D. E., Katz, V. L., and Dotters, D. J.: Toxic shock syndrome associated with vulvar necrotizing fasciitis. Obstet. Gynecol. *82*:660–662, 1993.
106. Fast, D. J., Schlievert, P. M., and Nelson, R. D.: Nonpurulent response to toxic shock syndrome toxin-1-producing *Staphylococcus aureus*. J. Immunol. *140*:949–953, 1988.
107. Feldman, C. A.: Staphylococcal scarlet fever. N. Engl. J. Med. *267*:877–888, 1962.
108. Ferguson, M. A., and Todd, J. K.: Toxic-shock syndrome associated with *Staphylococcus aureus* sinusitis in children. J. Infect. Dis. *161*:953–955, 1990.
109. Fichtenbaum, C. J., Peterson, L. R. and Weil, G. J.: Ehrlichiosis presenting as a life-threatening illness with features of the toxic shock syndrome. Am. J. Med. *95*:351–357, 1993.
110. Finkelstein, J. W., and von Eye, A.: Sanitary product use by white, black and Mexican American women. Public Health Rep. *105*:491, 1990.
111. Finkelstein, S., and Hyland, R. H.: Toxic shock syndrome as the AIDS defining diagnosis. Chest *104*:950–951, 1993.
112. Fisher, C. J., Jr., Horowitz, B. Z., and Nolan, S. M.: The clinical spectrum of toxic shock syndrome. West. J. Med. *15*:175–182, 1981.
113. Fisher, C. J., Jr., Horowitz, Z., and Albertson, T. E.: Cardiorespiratory failure in toxic shock syndrome: Effect of dobutamine. Crit. Care Med. *13*:160–165, 1985.
114. Fisher, R. F., Goodpasture, H. C., Peterie, J. D., et al.: Toxic shock syndrome in menstruating women. Ann. Intern. Med. *94*:156–163, 1981.
115. Fitz, J. D., Weeks, K. D., and Duff, P.: Left ventricular dysfunction in a patient with toxic shock syndrome. Am. J. Obstet. Gynecol. *146*:467–468, 1983.
116. Foley-Nolan, D., Coughlan, R. J., and Sugrue, D.: Toxic shock syndrome associated arthropathy. *Staphylococcus aureus*: A further triggering event in reactive arthritis? Ann. Rheum. Dis. *48*:331, 1989.
117. Food and Drug Administration: Tampon packages carry TSS information. FDA Drug Bull. *3*:19–20, 1982.
118. Fornadley, J. A., Gomez, P. J., Crane, R. T., et al.: Toxic shock syndrome following submandibular gland excision. Head Neck *12*:66–68, 1990.
119. Frame, J. D., Eve, M. D., and Hackett, M. E., et al.: The toxic shock syndrome in burned children. Burns, Including Thermal Injury *11*:234–241, 1985.
120. Fuleihan, R., Trede, N., Chatila, T., et al.: Superantigens activate HIV-1 gene expression in monocytic cells. Clin. Immunol. Immunopathol. *72*:357–361, 1994.
121. Galea, P., and Goel, K. M.: Toxic shock syndrome (TSS) in children. Scott. Med. J. *32*:28–29, 1987.
122. Gallagher, P. G., and Myer, C. M.: An approach to the diagnosis and treatment of membranous laryngotracheobronchitis in infants and children. Pediatr. Emerg. Care *7*:337–342, 1991.
123. Garbe, P. L., Arko, R. J., and Reingold, A. L., et al.: *Staphylococcus aureus* isolates from patients with non-menstrual toxic shock syndrome: Evidence for additional toxins. J. A. M. A. *253*:2538–2542, 1985.
124. Gaventa, S., Reingold, A. L., Hightower, A. W., et al.: Active surveillance for TSS in the United States. Rev. Infect. Dis. *11*:S28–S34, 1989.
125. Glazowski, M. J., Ostergaard, G. Z., Arpi, M., et al.: Toxic shock sydrome: A case of a child with burns. Ugeskrift for Laeger *154*:868–869, 1992.
126. Gourley, G. R., Chesney, P. J., Davis, J. P., et al.: Acute cholestasis in patients with toxic-shock syndrome. Gastroenterology *81*:928–931, 1981.
127. Graham, D. R., O'Brien, M., Hayes, J. M., et al.: Postoperative toxic shock syndrome. Clin. Infect. Dis. *20*:895–899, 1995.
128. Hackett, S. P., and Stevens, D. L.: Superantigens associated with staphylococcal and streptococcal toxic shock syndrome are potent inducers of tumore necrosis factor β synthesis. J. Infect. Dis. *168*:232–235, 1993.
129. Hanafiah, S. R., and Chong, S. K. F.: Toxic shock syndrome presenting as an acute encephalopathy and diarrhoea. J. R. Soc. Med. *84*:48–49, 1991.
130. Hauschildt, S., Bessler, W. G., and Scheipers, P.: Engagement of major histocompatibility complex class II molecules leads to nitrite production in bone marrow-derived macrophages. Eur. J. Immunol. *23*:2988–2992, 1993.
131. Helgerson, S. D., and Foster, L. R.: Toxic shock syndrome in Oregon: Epidemiologic findings. Ann. Intern. Med. *96*:909–911, 1982.
132. Helms, C. M., Lengeling, R. W., Pinsky, R. L., et al.: Toxic shock syndrome: A retrospective study of 25 cases from Iowa. Am. J. Med. Sci. *282*:50–60, 1981.
133. Hensler, T., Koller, M., Geoffroy, C., et al.: *Staphylococcus aureus* toxic shock syndrome toxin 1 and *Streptococcus pyogenes* erythrogenic toxin A modulate inflammatory mediator release from human neutrophils. Infect. Immun. *61*:1055–1061, 1993.
134. Heywood, A. J., and al-Essa, S.: Toxic shock syndrome in child with only 2% burn. Lancet *335*:867, 1990.
135. Hirose-Kumagai, A., Whipple, F. H., Ikejima, T., et al.: A comparison of neutralizing and antigen-binding assays for human antibodies against toxic-shock-syndrome 1. J. Infect. Dis. *150*:788, 1984.
136. Hurley, J. M., Shimonkevitz, R., Hanagan, A., et al.: Identification of class II major histocompatibility complex and T cell receptor binding sites in the superantigen toxic shock syndrome toxin 1. J. Exp. Med. *181*:2229, 1995.
137. Hurwitz, R. M., and Ackerman, A. B.: Cutaneous pathology of the toxic shock syndrome. Am. J. Dermatopathol. *7*:563, 1985.
138. Iandolo, J. J.: Genetic analysis of extracellular toxins of *Staphylococcus aureus*. Annu. Rev. Microbiol. *43*:375–402, 1989.
139. Ikejima, T., and Dinarello, C. A.: Distribution of radiolabeled toxic shock syndrome toxin: Implications for the pathogenesis of interleukin-1 mediated-toxic shock syndrome. J. Leukocyte Biol. *37*:714, 1985.
140. Ishak, K. G., and Rogers, W. A.: Cryptogenic acute cholangitis: Association with toxic shock syndrome. Am. J. Clin. Pathol. *76*:619–626, 1981.
141. Jacobson, J. A., Kasworm, E. M., and Bolte, R. G., et al.: Prevalence of nasal carriage of toxigenic *Staphylococcus aureus* and antibody to TSST-1 in Utah children. Rev. Infect. Dis. *11*:S324–S325, 1989.
142. Jacobson, J. A., Kasworm, E. M., Reiser, R. F., et al.: Low incidence of toxic shock syndrome in children with staphylococcal infection. Am. J. Med. Sci. *294*:403–407, 1987.
143. Jacobson, J. A., Kasworm, E., and Daly, J. A.: Risk of developing TSS associated with TSST-1 following nongenital staphylococcal infection. Rev. Infect. Dis. *11*:S8–S13, 1989.
144. Jacobson, J. A., Stevens, M. H., and Kasworm, E. M.: Evaluation of single-dose cefazol in prophylaxis for toxic-shock syndrome. Arch. Otolaryngol. Head Neck Surg. *114*:326–327, 1988.
145. James, R. C., and MacLeod, C. J.: Induction of staphylococcal infections in mice with small inocula introduced on sutures. Br. J. Exp. Pathol. *42*:266, 1961.
146. Jaulhac, B., Bes, M., Bornstein, N., et al.: Synthetic DNA probes for detection of genes for enterotoxins A, B, C, D, E and for TSST-1 in staphylococcal strains. J. Appl. Bacteriol. *72*:386–392, 1992.
147. Johnson, W. M., Tyler, S. D., Ewan, E. P., et al.: Detection of genes for enterotoxins, exfoliative toxins, and toxic shock syndrome toxin 1 in *Staphylococcus aureus* by the polymerase chain reaction. J. Clin. Microbiol. *29*:426–430, 1991.
148. Kain, K. C., Schulzer, M., and Chow, A. W.: Clinical spectrum of nonmenstrual toxic shock syndrome (TSS): Comparison with menstrual TSS by multivariate discriminant analyses. Clin. Infect. Dis. *16*:100–106, 1993.
149. Kappler, J., Kotzin, B., Herron, L., et al.: Vβ-specific stimulation of human T-cells by staphylococcal toxins. Science *244*:811–813, 1989.
150. Kato, K., and Tanaka, T.: MRSA infection and toxic shock syndrome in burn patients. Jpn. J. Clin. Med. *50*:1104–1111, 1992.
151. Kehrberg, M. W., Latham, R. H., Haslam, B. T., et al.: Risk factors for staphylococcal toxic-shock syndrome. Am. J. Epidemiol. *114*:873–879, 1981.
152. Kernodle, D. S., McGraw, P. A., Barg, N. L., et al.: Growth of *Staphylococcus aureus* with nafcillin in vitro induces α-toxin production and increases the lethal activity of sterile broth filtrates in a murine model. J. Infect. Dis. *172*:410–419, 1995.
153. Kline, M. W., and Dunkle, L. M.: Toxic shock syndrome and the acquired immunodefiency syndrome. Pediatr. Infect. Dis. J. *7*:736–738, 1988.
154. Kotasek, D., Vercelloti, G. M., Ochoa, A. C., et al.: Mechanism of cultured endothelial injury induced by lymphokine activated killer cells. Cancer Res. *48*:5528, 1988.
155. Kotb, M.: Bacterial pyrogenic exotoxins as superantigens. Clin. Microbiol. Rev. *8*:411–426, 1995.
156. Krakauer, T.: Inhibition of toxic shock syndrome toxin-1-induced cytokine production and T cell activation by interleukin-10, interleukin-4 and dexamethasone. J. Infect. Dis. *172*:988–992, 1995.
157. Kreiswirth, B. N., Kravitz, G. R., Schlievert, P. M., et al.: Nosocomial transmission of a strain of *Staphylococcus aureus*, causing toxic shock syndrome. Ann. Intern. Med. *105*:704, 1986.
158. Kreiswirth, B. N., Projan, S. J., Schlievert, P. M., et al.: Toxic shock syndrome toxin 1 is encoded by a variable genetic element. Rev. Infect. Dis. *11*:S83–S88, 1989.
159. Ku, W. W. S., and Chow, A. W.: Monoclonal antibodies (MAb5 and MAb4) protect against the lethal effect of toxic shock syndrome toxin-1 in the D-galactosamine sensitized mouse mode. J. Invest. Med. 110A, 1996.
160. Kushnaryov, V. M., MacDonald, H. S., Reiser, R. F., et al.: Reaction of TSST-1 with endothelium of human umbilical cord vein. Rev. Infect. Dis. *11*:S282–S287, 1989.
161. Larkin, S. M., Williams, D. N., Osterholm, M. T., et al.: Toxic shock syndrome: Clinical, laboratory, and pathologic findings in nine fatal cases. Ann. Intern. Med. *96*:858–864, 1982.
162. Latham, R. H., Kehrberg, M. W., Jacobson, J. A., et al.: Toxic shock syndrome in Utah: A case-control and surveillance study. Ann. Intern. Med. *96*:906–908, 1982.
163. Lee, P. K., Vercellotti, G. M., Deringer, J. R., et al.: Effects of staphylococcal toxic shock syndrome toxin 1 on aortic endothelial cells. J. Infect. Dis. *164*:711–719, 1991.
164. Lee, V. T. P., Chang, A. H., and Chow, A. W.: Detection of staphylococcal enterotoxin B among toxic-shock syndrome (TSS) and non-TSS associated *Staphylococcus aureus* isolates. J. Infect. Dis. *166*:911–915, 1992.
165. Lund, L., Nielsen, D., and Anderson, E. S.: Meningismus as the main symptom in toxic shock syndrome. Acta Obstet. Gynecol. Scand. *67*:395, 1988.
166. MacDonald, K. L., Osterholm, M. T., Hedberg, C. W., et al.: Toxic shock syndrome: A newly recognized complication of influenza and influenza like illness. J. A. M. A. *257*:1053–1058, 1987.

167. Marlowe, D. E., Weigle, R. M., and Stauffenberg, R. S.: Measurement of tampon absorbency: Evaluation of tampon brands. Rockville, FDA Bureau of Biologics, 1981.
168. Marodi, L., Kaposzta, R., Rozgonyi, F., et al.: Staphylococcal enterotoxin A involvement in the illness of a 20-month-old burn patient. Pediatr. Infect. Dis. J. *14*:632–634, 1995.
169. Marples, R. R., and Wienecke, A. A.: Enterotoxins and toxic-shock syndrome-1 in non-enteric staphylococcal disease. Epidemiol. Infect. *110*:477–488, 1993.
170. Marrack, P., and Kappler, J.: The staphylococcal enterotoxins and their relatives. Science *248*:705–711, 1990.
171. Martin, R. R., Buttram, V., Besch, P., et al.: Nasal and vaginal *Staphylococcus aureus* in young women: Quantitative studies. Ann. Intern. Med. *96*:951–953, 1982.
172. McAllister, R. M., Mercer, N. S., Morgan, B. D., et al.: Early diagnosis of staphylococcal toxemia in burned children. Burns *19*:22–25, 1993.
173. McGann, V. G., Rollins, J. B. and Mason, D. W.: Evaluation of resistance to staphylococcal enterotoxin B: Naturally acquired antibodies of man and monkey. J. Infect. Dis. *124*:206–213, 1971.
174. McIvor, M. E., and Levin, M. L.: Treatment of recurrent toxic shock syndrome with oral contraceptive agents. Md. Med. J. *31*:56–57, 1982.
175. McKenna, U. G., Meadows, J. A., III, Brewer, N. S., et al.: Toxic shock syndrome, a newly recognized disease entity: Report of 11 cases. Mayo Clin. Proc. *55*:663–672, 1980.
176. McMahon, W. S., Patrenos, M. E., McConnell, M. E., et al.: Complete heart block in toxic shock syndrome. Am. J. Dis. Child. *144*:748, 1990.
177. Melish, M. E., Frogner, K. S., Hirata, S. A., et al.: Use of IVGG for therapy in the rabbit model of TSS. Clin. Res. *35*:220A, 1987.
178. Melish, M. E., Murata, S., Fukunaga, C., et al.: Corticosteroid and immunoglobulin therapy in TSS. Rev. Infect. Dis. *11*::S332–S333, 1989.
179. Melish, M. E., Murata, S., Fukunaga, C., et al.: Endotoxin is not an essential mediator in TSS. Rev. Infect. Dis. *11*:S219–S228, 1989.
180. Melish, M., Murata, S., Frogner, K., et al.: Glyceryl monolaurate (GML) in model toxic shock syndrome (TSS). Abstracts of the Ninety-first General Meeting of the American Society of Microbiology, 1991. Abstract B19, p. 28.
181. Melish, M. E., Chen, F. S., and Murata, M. S.: Quantitative detection of toxic shock marker protein in human and experimental toxic shock ssyndrome. Clin. Res. *31*:122A, 1983.
182. Melish, M. E., Murata, S., Fukunaga, C., et al.: Vaginal tampon model for toxic shock syndrome. Rev. Infect. Dis. *11*:S219–S228, 1989.
183. Melish, M. E., Murata, S., Fukunaga, C., et al.: Corticosteroid and immunoglobulin therapy in toxic shock syndrome (TSS). Clin. Res. *36*:781A, 1988.
184. Michels, T. C.: Mucocutaneous lymph node syndrome in adults: Differentiation from toxic shock syndrome. Am. J. Med. *80*:724, 1986.
185. Michie, C. A., Davis, T., and MacAllister, M.: The sequelae of toxic shock syndrome. Pediatr. Res. *39*:179A, 1996.
186. Miethke, T., Duschek, K., Wahl, C., et al.: Pathogenesis of the toxic shock syndrome: T-cell-mediated lethal shock caused by the superantigen TSST-1. Eur. J. Immunol. *23*:1494–1500, 1993.
187. Miethke, T., Wah, I. C., Heeg, K., et al.: T-cell-mediated lethal shock triggered in mice by the superantigen staphylococcal enterotoxin B: Critical role of tumor necrosis factor. J. Exp. Med. *175*:91–98, 1992.
188. Miethke, T., Wahl, C., Regele, D., et al.: *Staphylococcus aureus* mediated shock: A cytokine release syndrome. Immunobiology *189*:270–284, 1993.
189. Miller, S. D.: Postoperative toxic shock syndrome after lumbar laminectomy in a male patient. Spine *19*:1182–1185, 1994.
190. Miller, W., and Stankiewicz, J. A.: Delayed toxic shock syndrome in sinus surgery. Otolaryngol. Head. Neck Surg. *111*:121–123, 1994.
191. Mills, J. T., Parsonnet, J., Hickman, R. K., et al.: Control of production of toxic-shock syndrome toxin-1 (TSST-1) by magnesium ion. J. Infect. Dis. *151*:1158–1161, 1985.
192. Miwa, K., Fukuyama, M., Kunitomo, T., et al.: Rapid assay for detection of toxic shock syndrome toxin 1 from human sera. J. Clin. Microbiol. *32*:539–542, 1994.
193. Mohan, S. B., Tamilarasan, A., and Buhl, M.: Inhalational mercury poisoning masquerading as toxic shock syndrome. Anaesth. Intensive Care *22*:305–306, 1994.
194. Mohsenipour, M., Deusch, E., Twerdy, K., et al.: Toxic shock syndrome in transsphenoidal neurosurgery. Acta Neurochir. *128*:169–170, 1994.
195. Moyer, M. A., Edwards, L. D., and Bergdoll, M. S.: Nosocomial toxic shock syndrome in two patients after knee surgery. Am. J. Infect. Control *11*:83–87, 1983.
196. Murray, D. L., Earhart, C. A., Mitchell, D. T., et al.: Localization of biologically important regions on toxic shock syndrome toxin-1. Infect. Immun. *64*:371–374, 1996.
197. Musser, J. M., Schlievert, P. M., Chow, A. W., et al.: A single clone of *Staphylococcus aureus* causes the majority of cases of toxic-shock syndrome. Proc. Natl. Acad. Sci. U. S. A. *87*:225–229, 1990.
198. Nadal, D., Lauener, R. P., Braegger, C. P., et al.: T-cell activation and cytokine release in streptococcal toxic shock-like syndrome. J. Pediatr. *122*:727–729, 1993.
199. Neill R. J., Fanning G. R., Delahoz F., et al.: Oligonucleotide probes for detection and differentiation of *Staplylococcus aureus* strains containing genes for enterotoxins A, B, and C and toxic shock syndrome toxin 1. J. Clin. Microbiol. *28*:1514–1518, 1990.
200. Nightingale, S. L.: New requirements for tampon labeling. Am. Fam. Physician *41*:999, 1990.
201. Nijssen-Jordan, C., Donaldson, J. D., and Halperin, S. A.: Bacterial tracheitis associated with respiratory syncytial virus infection and toxic-shock syndrome. Can. Med. Assoc. J. *142*:233–234, 1990.
202. Norrby-Teglund, A., Pauksens, K., Holm, S. E., et al.: Relation between low capacity of human sera to inhibit streptococcal mitogens and serious manifestation of disease. J. Infect. Dis. *170*:585–591, 1994.
203. O'Gilvie vs. International Playtex, No. 83-1845, Vol. 37 (DC Kansas March 21, 1985, posttrial motions and court findings).
204. Ogawa, M., Ueda, S., Anzai, N., et al.: Toxic shock syndrome after staphylococcal pneumonia treated with intravenous immunoglobulin. Vox Sang. *68*:59–60, 1995.
205. Olesen, L. L., Ejlertsen, T., and Nielsen, J.: Toxic shock syndrome following insertion of breast prostheses. Br. J. Surg. *78*:585–586, 1991.
206. Olson, R. D., Stevens, D. L., and Melish, M. E.: Direct effects of purified staphylococcal TSST-1 on myocardial function of isolated rabbit atria. Rev. Infect. Dis. *11*:S313–S315, 1989.
207. Onderdonk, A. B., Delaney, M. L., Zamarchi, G. R., et al.: Normal vaginal microflora during use of various forms of catamenial protection. Rev. Infect. Dis. *11*:S61–S67, 1989.
208. Orden, J. A., Goyache, J., Hernandez, F. J., et al.: Detection of staphylococcal enterotoxin and toxic shock syndrome toxin-1 (TSST-1) by immunoblot combined with a semiautomated electrophoresis system. J. Immunol. Methods *144*:197–202, 1991.
209. Osterholm, M. T., and Forfang, J. C.: Toxic-shock syndrome in Minnesota: Results of an active-passive surveillance system. J. Infect. Dis. *145*:458–464, 1982.
210. Osterholm, M. T., Davis, J. P., Gibson, R. W., et al.: Toxic shock syndrome: Relation to catamenial products, personal health and hygiene, and sexual practices. Ann. Intern. Med. *96*:954–958, 1982.
211. Osterholm, M. T., Davis, J. P., Gibson, R. W., et al.: Tri-state toxic-shock syndrome study. I. Epidemiologic findings. J. Infect. Dis. *145*:431–440, 1982.
212. Paris, A. L., Herwaldt, L. A., Blum, D., et al.: Pathologic findings in twelve fatal cases of toxic-shock syndrome. Ann. Intern. Med. *96*:852–857, 1982.
213. Parkin, D. E.: Fatal toxic shock syndrome following endometrial resection. Br. J. Obstet. Gynaecol. *102*:163–164, 1995.
214. Parsonnet, J., Gillis, Z. A., and Pier, G. B.: Induction of interleukin-1 by strains of *Staphylococcus aureus* from patients with non-menstrual toxic shock syndrome. J. Infect. Dis. *154*:55–63, 1986.
215. Parsonnet, J., Gillis, Z. A., Thompson, M. R., et al.: Effects of monoclonal antibody on biologic function of TSST-1 in vitro and in vivo. Rev. Infect. Dis. *11*:S318–S319, 1989.
216. Parsonnet, J., Modern, P. A., and Giacobbe, K.: Effect of subinhibitory concentrations of antibiotics on production of toxic shock syndrome toxin-1 (TSST-1). Program and Abstracts of the 32nd Annual Meeting of the Infectious Disease Society of America. Washington, Infectious Disease Society of America, 1994. Abstract 29.
217. Parsonnet, J., Modern, P. A., and Giacobbe, K. D.: Effect of tampon composition on production of toxic shock syndrome toxin-1 by *Staphylococcus aureus* in vitro. J. Infect. Dis. *173*:98–103, 1996.
218. Parsonnet, J., Tosteson, A., Modern, P., et al.: Antibody to toxic shock syndrome toxin-1 (TSST-1) and vaginal colonization by TSST-1 producing *S. aureus* among adolescent women. Program and Abstracts of the 33rd Interscience Conference on Antimicrobial Agents and Chemotherapy. Washington, American Society for Microbiology, 1993. Abstract 1327.
219. Parsonnet, J.: Mediators in the pathogenesis of TSS: Overview. Rev. Infect. Dis. *11*:S263–S269, 1989.
220. Parsonnet, J.: Nonmenstrual toxic shock syndrome: New insights into diagnosis, pathogenesis and treatment. Curr. Clin. Top. Infect. Dis. *16*:1–20, 1996.
221. Paterson, M. P., Hoffman, E. B., and Roux, P.: Severe disseminated staphylococcal disease associated with osteitis and septic arthritis. J. Bone Joint Surg. (Br.) *72*:94–97, 1990.
222. Petitti, D. B., Reingold, A., and Chin, J.: The incidence of toxic shock syndrome in northern California: 1972 through 1983. J. A. M. A. *255*:368–372, 1986.
223. Pokriefka, R., Rabah, M., Saravolatz, L., et al.: Toxic shock syndrome in an injection drug user with *Staphylococcus aureus* endocarditis. Infect. Med. *11*:34–36, 48–49, 1994.
224. Potter, T., DiGregorio, F., Stiff, M., et al.: Dilantin hypersensitivity syndrome imitating staphylococcal toxic shock. Arch. Dermatol. *130*:856–858, 1994.
225. Prevention and Recognition of TSS: Institute of Medicine: Toxic shock syndrome: Assessment of current information and future research needs. National Academy Press, 1982, pp. 85–86.
226. Projan, S. J., Brown-Skrobot, S., and Schlievert, P. M.: Glycerol monolaurate inhibits the production of beta-lactamase, toxic shock toxin-1, and other staphylococococcal exoproteins by interfering with signal transduction. J. Bacteriol. *176*:4204–4209, 1994.
227. Raab, M. G., O'Brien, M., Hayes, J. M., et al.: Postoperative toxic shock syndrome. Am. J. Orthop. *24*:130–136, 1995.

228. Rasheed, J. K., Arko, R. J., Feeley, J. C., et al.: Acquired ability of *Staphylococcus aureus* to produce toxic shock-associated protein and resulting illness in a rabbit model. Infect. Immun. *47*:598–604, 1985.
229. Reingold, A. L., Hargrett, N. T., Dan, B. B., et al.: Nonmenstrual toxic shock syndrome: A review of 130 cases. Ann. Intern. Med. *96*:871–874, 1982.
230. Ren, K., Bannan, J. D., Pancholi, V., et al.: Characterization and biological properties of a new staphylococcal exotoxin. J. Exp. Med. *180*:1675–1683, 1994.
231. Rhee, C. A., Smith, R. J., and Jackson, I. T.: Toxic shock syndrome associated with suction-assisted lipectomy. Aesthetic Plast. Surg. *18*:161–163, 1994.
232. Rich, R. R.: Intravenous IgG: Supertherapy for superantigens. J. Clin. Invest. *91*:378, 1993.
233. Ritz, H. L., Kirkland, J. J., Bond, G. G., et al.: Association of high levels of serum antibody to staphyloccal toxic shock antigen with nasal carriage of toxic shock antigen-producing strains of *Staphylococcus aureus*. Infect. Immun. *43*:954–958, 1984.
234. Rolston, R. D., Yabek, S. M., Florman, A. L., et al.: Severe cardiac conduction abnormalities associated with atypical toxic-shock syndrome. J. Pediatr. *117*:89, 1990.
235. Romagne, F., Besnardeau, L., and Malissen, B.: A versatile method to produce antibodies to human T cell receptor V beta segments: Frequency determination of human V beta 2+ T cells that react with toxic-shock syndrome toxin-1. Eur. J. Immunol. *22*:2749–2752, 1992.
236. Rose, P. G., and Wilson, G.: Advanced cervical carcinoma presenting with toxic shock syndrome. Gynecol. Oncol. (U. S.) *52*:264–266, 1994.
237. Rosene, K. A., Copass, M. K., Kastner, L. S., et al.: Persistent neuropsychological sequelae of toxic shock syndrome. Ann. Intern. Med. *96*:865–870, 1982.
238. Rosten, P. M., Bartlett, K. H., and Chow, A. W.: Serologic responses to toxic shock syndrome (TSS) toxin-1 in menstrual and nonmenstrual TSS. Clin. Invest. Med. *11*:187–192, 1988.
239. Rovner, R. A., Baird, R. A., and Malerich, M. M.: Fatal toxic-shock syndrome as a complication of orthopedic surgery. J. Bone Jt. Surg. *66A*:952–954, 1984.
240. Royall, J. A., Berkow, R. L., Beckman, J. S., et al.: Tumor necrosis factor and interleukin 1-α increase vascular endothelial cell permeability. Crit. Care Med. *16*:396, 1988.
241. Sahs, A. L., Helms, C. M., and DuBois, C.: Carpal tunnel syndrome: Complication of toxic shock syndrome. Arch. Neurol. *40*:414–415, 1983.
242. Sales, J. H., Kennedy, K. S., Galantich, P. T., et al.: Toxic shock syndrome associated with pharyngitis and submandibular space abscess. Ann. Otol. Rhinol. Laryngol. *100*:540–543, 1991.
243. Schlech, W. F., III, Shands, K. N., Reingold, A. L., et al.: Risk factors for development of toxic shock syndrome: Association with a tampon brand. J. A. M. A. 7:835–839, 1982.
244. Schlievert, P. M., and Kelly, J. A.: Clindamycin-induced suppression of toxic-shock syndrome-associated exotoxin production. J. Infect. Dis. *149*:471, 1984
245. Schlievert, P. M., Shands, K. N., Dan, B. B., et al.: Identification and characterization of exotoxin from *Staphylococcus aureus* associated with toxic shock syndrome. J. Infect. Dis. *143*:509–516, 1981.
246. Schlievert, P. M.: Enhancement of host susceptibility to lethal endotoxin shock by staphylococcal pyrogenic exotoxin type C. Infect. Immun. *36*:123–128, 1982.
247. Schlievert, P. M.: Staphylococcal enterotoxin B and toxic-shock syndrome toxin-1 are significantly associated with non-menstrual TSS. Lancet *1*:1149, 1986.
248. Schlievert, P. M., Deringer, J. R., Kim, M. H., et al.: Effect of glycerol monolaurate on bacterial growth and toxin production. Antimicrob. Agents Chemother. *36*:626–632, 1992.
249. Schlievert, P. M.: Comparison of cotton and cotton/rayon tampons for effect on production of toxic shock syndrome toxin. J. Infect. Dis. *172*:1112–1114, 1995.
250. Schuchat, A., and Broome, C. V.: Toxic shock syndrome and tampons. Epidemiol. Rev. *13*:99–112, 1991.
251. Schwartz, B., Gaventa, S., Broome, C. V., et al.: Nonmenstrual TSS associated with barrier contraceptives: Report of a case-control study. Rev. Infect. Dis. *11*:S43–S48, 1989.
252. Scott, D. F., Best, G. K., Kling, J. M., et al.: Passive protection of rabbits infected with TSS associated strains of *Staphylococcus aureus* by monoclonal antibody to TSST-1. Rev. Infect. Dis. *11*:S214–S217, 1989.
253. Shands, K. N., Schmid, G. P., Dan, B. B., et al.: Toxic-shock syndrome in menstruating women: Association with tampon use and *Staphylococcus aureus* and clinical features in 52 cases. N. Engl. J. Med. *303*:1436–1442, 1980.
254. Shlasko, E., Harris, M. T., Benjamin, E., et al.: Toxic shock syndrome after pilonidal cystectomy: Report of a case. Dis. Colon Rectum *34*:502–505, 1991.
255. Sissons, J. G.: Superantigens and infectious disease. Lancet *341*:1627–1629, 1993.
256. Skansen-Saphir, U., Andersson, J., Bjork, L., et al.: Lymphokine production induced by streptococcal pyrogenic exotoxin A is selectively down regulated by pooled human IgG. Eur. J. Immunol. *24*:916–922, 1994.
257. Slingluff, C. L., Jr., Burns, W. W., and Cooperberg, C.: Toxic shock syndrome after inguinal hernia repair: Report of a case with patient survival. Am. Surg. *56*:610–612, 1990.
258. Smith, D. B., and Gulinson, J.: Fatal cerebral edema complicating toxic shock syndrome. Neurosurgery *22*:598–599, 1988.
259. Sparano, J., and Ferranti, E.: The acquired immunodeficiency syndrome and non-menstrual toxic shock syndrome. Ann. Intern. Med. *105*:300–301, 1986.
260. Spearman, P. W., and Barson, W. J.: Toxic shock syndrome occurring in children with abrasve injuries beneath casts. J. Pediatr. Orthop. *12*:169–172, 1992.
261. Sperber, S. J., Blevins, D. D., and Francis, J. B.: Hypercalcitonemia, hypocalcemia, and toxic-shock syndrome. Rev. Infect. Dis. *12*:736–739, 1990.
262. Spertini, F., Spits, H., and Geha, R. S.: Staphylococcal exotoxins deliver activation signals to human T-cell clones via major histocompatibility complex class II molecules. Proc. Natl. Acad. Sci. U. S. A. *88*:7533–7537, 1991.
263. Stevens, D. L., Tanner, M. H., Winship, J., et al.: Severe group A streptococcal infections associated with a toxic shock like syndrome and scarlet fever toxin A. N. Engl. J. Med. *321*:1–7, 1989.
264. Stevens, D. L., Gibbons, A. E., Bergstrom, R., et al.: The eagle effect revisited: Efficacy of clindamycin, erythromycin, and penicillin in the treatment of streptococcal myositis. J. Infect. Dis. *158*:23–28, 1988.
265. Stevens, D. L., Yan, S., and Bryant, A. E.: Penicillin-binding protein expression at different growth stages determines penicillin efficacy in vitro and in vivo: An explanation for the inoculum effect. J. Infect. Dis. *167*:1401–1405, 1993.
266. Stevens, F. A.: The occurrence of *Staphylococcus aureus* infection with a scarlatiniform rash. J. A. M. A. *18*:1957–1958, 1927.
267. Stolz, S. J., Davis, J. P., Vergeront, J. M., et al.: Development of serum antibody to toxic shock toxin among individuals with toxic shock syndrome in Wisconsin. J. Infect. Dis. *151*:883–889, 1985.
268. Su, Y. C., and Wong, A. C.: Identification and purification of a new staphylococcal enterotoxin, H. Appl. Environ. Microbiol. *61*:1438–1443, 1995.
269. Swift, J. D., Barruga, M. C., Perkin, R. M., et al: Respiratory failure complicating rubeola. Chest *104*:1786–1787, 1993.
270. Takei, S., Arora, Y. K., and Walker, S. M.: Intravenous immunoglobulin contains specific antibodies inhibitory to activation of T cells by staphylococcal toxin superantigens. J. Clin. Invest. *91*:602–607, 1993.
271. Thompson, T. D., and Friedman, A. L.: Simultaneous occurrence of *Staphylococcus aureus*-associated septic arthritis and toxic shock syndrome. Clin. Pediatr. (Phila.) *33*:243–245, 1994.
272. Tierno, P. M., Jr., and Hanna, B. A.: Propensity of tampons and barrier contraceptives to amplify *Staphylococcus aureus* toxic shock syndrome toxin-1. Infect. Dis. Obstet. Gynecol. 2:140–145, 1994.
273. Todd, J. K., Fishaut, M., and Kapral, F., et al.: Toxic-shock syndrome associated with phage-group 1 staphylococci. Lancet 2:1116–1118, 1978.
274. Todd, J. K., Franco-Buff, A., Lawellin, D. W., et al.: Phenotypic distinctiveness of *Staphylococcus aureus* strains associated with toxic shock syndrome. Infect. Immun. *45*:339–344, 1984.
275. Todd, J. K., Ressman, M., Caston, S. A., et al.: Corticosteroid therapy for patients with toxic shock syndrome. J. A. M. A. *252*:3399–3402, 1984.
276. Todd, J. K., Todd, B. H., Franco-Buff, A., et al.: Influence of focal growth conditions on the pathogenesis of toxic shock syndrome. J. Infect. Dis. *155*:673–681, 1987.
277. Todd, J. K., Weisenthal, A. M., Ressman, M., et al.: Toxic shock syndrome. II. Estimated occurrence in Colorado as influenced by case ascertainment methods. Am. J. Epidemiol. *22*:857–867, 1985.
278. Todd, J. K.: Therapy of toxic shock syndrome. Drugs *39*:856–861, 1990.
279. Tofte, R. W., and Williams, D. N.: Clinical and laboratory manifestations of toxic shock syndrome. Ann. Intern. Med. *96*:843–847, 1982.
280. Tofte, R. W., and Williams, D. N.: Toxic shock syndrome: Evidence of a broad clinical spectrum. J. A. M. A. *246*:2163–2167, 1981.
281. Tolan, R. W., Jr.: Toxic shock syndrome complicating influenza A in a child: Case report and review. Clin. Infect. Dis. *17*:43–45, 1993.
282. Tracey, K. J., Lowry, S. F., Beutler, B., et al.: Cachectin/tumor necrosis factor mediates changes of skeletal muscle plasma membrane potential. J. Exp. Med. *164*:1368–1373, 1986.
283. Turker, R., Lubicky, J. P., and Vogel, L. C.: Toxic shock syndrome in patients with external fixators. J. Pediatr. Orthop. *12*:658–662, 1992.
284. Vergeront, J. M., Blouse, L. E., Crass, B. A., et al.: Regional differences in the prevalence of serum antibody to toxic-shock toxin (anti-TST). Abstracts of the Twenty-Fourth Interscience Conference on Antimicrobial Agents and Chemotherapy, 1984, p. 193. Abstract #610.
285. Vergeront, J. M., Evenson, M. L., Crass, B. A., et al.: Recovery of staphylococcal enterotoxin F from the breast milk of a woman with toxic-shock syndrome. J. Infect. Dis. *146*:456–459, 1982.
286. Vergeront, J. M., Stolz, S. J., Crass, B. A., et al.: Prevalence of serum antibody to staphylococcal enterotoxin F among Wisconsin residents: Implications for toxic shock syndrome. J. Infect. Dis. *148*:692–698, 1983.
287. Vic-Dupont, M. P., Duval, P., and Kamaliv, S. R.: Scarlatiniform staphylococcal diseases. Soc. Med. Hop. Paris *116*:51, 1965.
288. Wagner, G., Bohr, L., Wagner, P., et al.: Tampon-induced changes in

vaginal oxygen and carbon dioxide tensions. Am. J. Obstet. Gynecol. *148*:147–150, 1984.

289. Watanabe-Ohnishi, R., Low, D. E., McGeer, et al.: Selective depletion of Vβ-bearing T cells in patients with severe invasive group A streptococcal infections and streptococcal toxic shock syndrome. J. Infect. Dis. *171*:74–84, 1995.
290. Weinzweig, J., Gottlich, L. J., and Krizek, T. J.: Toxic shock syndrome associated with the use of Biobrane in a scald burn victim. Burns *20*:180–181, 1994.
291. Weissberg, S. M., and Dodson, M. G.: Recurrent vaginal and cervical ulcers associated with tampon use. J. A. M. A. *250*:1430–1431, 1983.
292. Whitby, M., Fraser, S., Gemmell, C. G., et al.: Toxic shock syndrome and endocarditis. Br. Med. J. Clin. Res. Ed. *286*:1613, 1983.
293. Whiting, J. L., Rosten, P. M., and Chow, A. W.: Determination by western blot (immunoblot) of serconversions to toxic shock syndrome (TSS) toxin 1 and enterotoxin A, B, or C during infection with TSS- and non-TSS-associated *Staphylococcus aureus*. Infect. Immun. *57*:231–234, 1989.
294. Wick, M. R., Bahn, R. C., and McKenna, U. G.: Toxic shock syndrome: A fatal case with autopsy findings. Mayo Clin. Proc. *57*:583–589, 1982.
295. Wiesenthal, A. M., and Todd, J. K.: Toxic shock syndrome in children aged 10 years or less. Pediatrics *74*:112–117, 1984.
296. Wong, A. C. L., and Bergdoll, M. S.: Effect of envirnonmental conditions on production of toxic shock syndrome toxin 1 by *Staphylococcus aureus*. Infect. Immun. *58*:1026–1029, 1990.
297. Yagoob, M., McClelland, P., Murray, A. E., et al.: Staphylococcal enterotoxins A and C causing toxic shock syndrome. J. Infect. *20*:176–178, 1990.
298. Yong, J. M.: Necrotising fasciitis. Lancet *343*:1427, 1994.
299. Younis, R. T., Gross, C. W., and Lazar, R. H.: Toxic shock syndrome following functional endonasal sinus surgery: A case report. Head Neck *13*:247–248, 1991.
300. Zembowicz, A., and Vane, J. R.: Induction of nitric oxide synthase activity by toxic shock syndrome toxin 1 in a macrophage-monocyte cell line. Proc. Soc. Natl. Acad. Sci. U. S. A. *89*:2051–2055, 1992.
301. Zumla, A.: Superantigens, T cells and microbes. Clin. Infect. Dis. *15*:313–320, 1992.

75

Adult Respiratory Distress Syndrome in Children

Peter W. Hiatt

Adult respiratory distress syndrome (ARDS) first was described in 1967 by Ashbaugh and associates.[3] It is a clinical syndrome of acute respiratory failure. Both local and systemic diseases can lead to injury of the alveolar-capillary membrane, endothelial cells, and alveolar epithelial cells of the lung. Increased capillary permeability and pulmonary edema develop after cellular damage. Despite the variety of diseases that can cause ARDS, the symptoms remain the same, manifesting with severe hypoxemia, tachypnea, retractions, and tachycardia. Although first described in adults, ARDS is a well-recognized entity in children. The true incidence of pediatric ARDS is unknown. Previous studies have estimated the incidence from 8.5 to 10.4 cases per 100 pediatric intensive care unit admissions.[18] Although treatment has changed during the past 20 years, mortality has remained greater than 50 per cent. Reported ages in children have ranged from 2 months to 17 years.

DEFINITION

There is no universally accepted definition for ARDS. It generally is agreed that ARDS represents a rapidly progressive bilateral process of severe diffuse parenchymal lung injury resulting in pulmonary edema. The most agreed-upon criteria for ARDS are (1) acute respiratory distress after a pulmonary or nonpulmonary insult in a patient with previously normal lungs; (2) severe hypoxemia, decreased lung compliance, and an increased shunt fraction; (3) the presence of diffuse patchy infiltrates on radiographic examination of the chest; and (4) the exclusion of heart disease and left ventricular dysfunction (pulmonary artery occlusion pressure < 18 mm Hg).[16]

PATHOPHYSIOLOGY

The mechanism by which lung injury occurs in ARDS remains unknown, despite intense research efforts. The body's defense mechanisms and response to injury and infection appear to determine the degree of tissue damage.[20] Complement activation, neutrophils, macrophages, and platelets all have been implicated in the host inflammatory response. Complement activation occurs after trauma, pancreatic injury, endothelial damage, and endotoxin exposure. By-products of complement then activate neutrophils, which in turn damage the pulmonary parenchyma. A strong association has been demonstrated between complement activation and the development of ARDS.[9] Other investigators have reported that complement activation is nonspecific in predicting the development of ARDS. Once activated, neutrophils can damage the pulmonary parenchyma by the release of proteolytic enzymes, generation of toxic oxygen radicals, and initiation of arachidonic acid metabolites. Patients with ARDS have elevated levels of elastase and collagenase in bronchoalveolar lavage fluid, increased levels of leukotriene B4, and hydrogen peroxide, all consistent with neutrophil degranulation.[22] Although neutrophils are capable of widespread damage and characteristically are found in ARDS, they are not essential for its development.

Alveolar macrophages may play a role in the pathogenesis of ARDS.[20] Alveolar macrophages are found in abundance in normal airways and synthesize tumor necrosis factor and interleukin-1. Both products promote neutrophil chemotaxis, degranulation, and release of oxygen metabolites. Infusion of tumor necrosis factor in animals produces pulmonary edema, decreased pulmonary compliance, increased cellularity, and increased lung water.[21,25] Anti–tumor necrosis factor antibody offers protection from ARDS in a baboon septicemia model. Increased levels of tumor necrosis factor are found in bronchoalveolar secretions and plasma of patients with ARDS. As with complement and neutrophils, a cause-and-effect relationship has not been established for alveolar macrophages and ARDS.

Increased capillary permeability with accumulation of protein-rich material in the interstitium and alveoli is the initial manifestation of ARDS.[19] Accumulation of edema fluid re-

TABLE 75–1. Noninfectious Conditions Associated with Adult Respiratory Distress Syndrome

Direct Injury to the Lung	Secondary Injury to the Lung
Pulmonary infections	Shock (any cause)
Inhalation	Sepsis
Nitrogen dioxide	Trauma
Chlorine	Multiple trauma
Sulfur dioxide	Fractures
Ammonia	Burns
Phosgene	Head trauma
Smoke	Blood disorders
Oxygen toxicity	Diffuse intravascular coagulation
Aspiration	Massive blood transfusion
Gastric fluid (especially if pH < 2.5)	Drug overdose
Near-drowning (fresh or salt water)	Heroin
Hydrocarbons	Methadone
Emboli	Barbiturates
Air	Ethchlorvynol
Fat	Salicylates
Amniotic fluid	Propoxyphene
Pulmonary contusion	Metabolic disorders
Radiation pneumonitis	Diabetic ketoacidosis
	Uremia
	Pancreatitis
	Increased intracranial pressure
	Postcardiopulmonary bypass
	Posthemodialysis
	Postcardioversion
	Paraquat ingestion

From Royall, J. A., and Levin, D. L.: Adult respiratory distress syndrome in pediatric patients. 1. Clinical aspects, pathophysiology, pathology, and mechanisms of lung injury. J. Pediatr. *112*:169–180, 1988.

sults in decreased lung compliance, a reduction in functional residual capacity, and ventilation-perfusion mismatch. The pathologic changes in the lung can be divided into three stages. The early exudative phase occurs within 12 to 48 hours of ARDS and is characterized by increased fluid in the alveoli and interstitium. The alveolar fluid is protein-rich, often hemorrhagic, and associated with hyaline membranes. Neutrophilic infiltrate is observed in pulmonary capillaries, interstitium, and alveoli. Capillaries have fibrin plugs and microthrombi; however, endothelial cells show only subtle abnormalities. The cellular proliferative phase occurs 3 to 10 days after the onset of ARDS. It is characterized by the proliferation of type II cuboidal epithelial cells. These cells are responsible for the production of surfactant and have the ability to transform into type I epithelial cells. Type I cells normally line the alveolar space. This phase is considered reparative in nature. Phase III, the fibrotic proliferative stage, develops 7 or 10 days after the onset of ARDS. Cellularity is reduced, alveolar fluid organizes, and fibrosis develops in and around the terminal respiratory units. Extensive fibrosis appears and is related to irreversible respiratory failure.[4]

CLINICAL MANIFESTATIONS

The clinical features of ARDS are based on the pathophysiologic changes affecting the lung. The physical examination is remarkable for tachypnea, tachycardia, retractions, and hypoxemia. The chest generally is quiet with few crackles. Hypoxemia refractory to supplemental oxygen is common. The onset of symptoms can be acute (aspiration pneumonitis) or gradual (sepsis). Infectious and noninfectious conditions associated with ARDS are listed in Tables 75–1 and 75–2. The diagnosis is based on a collection of clinical, radiographic, and physiologic measures as just outlined. In children, diseases most commonly associated with ARDS include sepsis, pneumonia, aspiration, trauma, and near-drowning.[24] Radiographic abnormalities initially start with increased interstitial markings and progress over hours to patchy infiltrates with diffuse alveolar disease. Increased lung water leads to a loss of lung compliance, a reduction in functional residual capacity, and increased intrapulmonary shunting. Intubation of patients for profound hypoxemia results in voluminous pink, frothy secretions. Hypoxemia worsens rapidly, despite assisted ventilation. The clinical course thereafter depends on severity and character of the initial illness, development of complications (e.g., sepsis), disseminated intravascular coagulation, and pulmonary air leak syndromes.

TABLE 75–2. Infectious Conditions Associated with Adult Respiratory Distress Syndrome in Children

Authors	Year	No. of Patients	Mortality	Viral Isolates	Bacterial Isolates	Fungal	Other
Lyrene and Troug[13]	1981	15	9/15 (60%)	0	*Enterococcus*	0	0
Pfenninger et al.[17]	1982	20	8/20 (40%)	0	Intra-abdominal process (7/20 NS)	0	0
Nussbaum[15]	1983	7	2/7 (29%)	0	*Haemophilus influenzae* type b	0	0
Katz et al.[11]	1984	23	8/23 (35%)	2/23 NS†	Pneumococcus	0	0
DeBruin et al.*[6]	1989	100	72/100 (72%)	HIV, cytomegalovirus, respiratory syncytial virus	Septic shock syndrome (64/100 NS), *Bordetella pertussis*	5/100 NS	*Pneumocystis carinii* 14/100
Tamburro et al.[23]	1991	37	19/37 (51%)	Adenovirus, cytomegalovirus, varicella virus	*Staphylococcus aureus*	0	0
Davis et al.[5]	1993	60	37/60 (62%)	Respiratory syncytial virus, influenza virus, cytomegalovirus, varicella virus	Sepsis syndrome (22/60 NS)	4/60 NS	0

*Children with malignancy and/or compromised immunity.
†NS, organism not specified.

TREATMENT

Although tremendous energy has been put into defining the mechanism of lung injury in ARDS, treatment remains supportive. The goals of therapy are to treat the underlying predisposing condition, minimize oxygen toxicity and barotrauma to the lung, and treat secondary complicating conditions.[8]

Hypoxemia is profound in patients with ARDS and refractory to supplemental oxygen given by facemask for long periods. The majority of patients with ARDS should be intubated and supported with mechanical ventilation if their inspired oxygen fraction is greater than 0.6. Once the patient is intubated, positive end-expiratory pressure should be applied. Positive end-expiratory pressure acts by increasing functional residual capacity, thereby preventing early airway closure. It also reduces the repetitive expansion and collapse of terminal airways and redistributes alveolar fluid. These changes in lung mechanics improve compliance and decrease ventilation-perfusion mismatch. Supplemental oxygen can be decreased, reducing the potential for oxygen toxicity to the lung.

Although positive end-expiratory pressure significantly improves ventilation-perfusion mismatch, it can affect cardiac output. Decreased venous return to the heart and a shift in the intraventricular cardiac septum can occur with high pressures. This is treated by left ventricular afterload reduction. Positive end-expiratory pressure should be used to maximize oxygen delivery at the lowest pressure that achieves this goal. Peak inspiratory pressure should be limited to 50 cm of water, if possible, to reduce barotrauma. Treatment of bronchospasm with $beta_2$ agonists and pulmonary toilet for airway secretions often can lower peak inspiratory pressure.

Many of the predisposing conditions associated with ARDS result in cardiovascular instability. Colloid or crystalloid is used for volume resuscitation. Once the patient is hemodynamically stable, fluids are restricted in order to decrease lung water via altered alveolar capillary permeability. Patients frequently are given diuretics to reduce fluid in the interstitium and alveolus. Maintaining fluid balance can be very difficult and can lead to destabilization of the patient. Positive inotropic support with dopamine or dobutamine may be required. The overall goal of management is to maintain good cardiac output, limit fluid administration, and optimize oxygen delivery.

Patients unresponsive to conventional mechanical ventilation may benefit from pressure-limited ventilation.[10] The inspiratory:expiratory ratio is changed to 2:1 or longer with this method of ventilation. Improved oxygenation, lower positive end-expiratory pressure, and decreased peak inspiratory pressure have been reported. High-frequency oscillation,[2] liquid ventilation,[16] and extracorporeal membrane oxygenation[14] are newer forms of ventilation that show promise. Integration of these newer forms of ventilation for children with ARDS will require more research and clinical experience. Use of surfactant[12] and inhaled nitric oxide,[1] a potent pulmonary vasodilator, for the treatment of ARDS is being investigated.

Secondary infections in patients with ARDS are frequent. Organisms frequently isolated are *Klebsiella* and *Pseudomonas;* however, *Escherichia coli, Candida albicans,* and *Staphylococcus epidermidis* are not uncommon.[20] The gastrointestinal tract is thought to be the source of many of these organisms. New radiographic infiltrates or change in color of tracheal secretions from yellow to green should increase the suspicion of a secondary bacterial pneumonia. Once suspected, cultures should be obtained and treatment started with broad-spectrum antibiotics.

Although the lung is the primary organ affected with ARDS, other organs can be injured by activation of inflammatory cells. Renal impairment is noted in up to 50 per cent of patients with ARDS.[20] Hepatic failure is uncommon, yet mild elevations in transaminases, increased clotting times, and an elevated bilirubin are observed. Central nervous system abnormalities occur in up to 30 per cent of patients with ARDS, the majority associated with sepsis. Prevention, detection, and treatment of these associated complications are critical in the overall management of children with ARDS.

PROGNOSIS

Mortality has not changed in the last 15 to 20 years since this disease first was described. It remains high, ranging from 40 per cent to 70 per cent (Table 75–2). New forms of mechanical ventilation, use of surfactant, and alteration of the inflammatory cascade should improve outcome. The chest x-rays of most children who survive ARDS eventually normalize. Pulmonary function improves gradually, with mild reduction in forced vital capacity.[7] Long-term physiologic abnormalities show a strong correlation with the level of support required in the acute phase of ARDS.

References

1. Abman, S. H., Griebel, J. L., Parker, D. K., et al.: Acute effects of inhaled nitric oxide in children with severe hypoxemic respiratory failure. J. Pediatr. *124*:881–888, 1994.
2. Arnold, J. H., Harrison, J. H., Toro-Figuero, L. O., et al.: Prospective, randomized comparison of high frequency oscillatory ventilation and conventional mechanical ventilation in pediatric respiratory failure. Crit. Care Med. *20*:1530–1539, 1994.
3. Ashbaugh, D. G., Bigelow, D. B., Petty, T. L., et al.: Acute respiratory distress in adults. Lancet *2*:319–323, 1967.
4. Bachofen, M., and Weibel, E. R.: Structural alterations of lung parenchyma in the adult respiratory distress syndrome. Clin. Chest *3*:35–56, 1982.
5. Davis, S. L., Furman, D. P., and Costarino, A. T.: ARDS in children: Associated disease, clinical course, and predictors of death. J. Pediatr. *123*:35–45, 1993.
6. DeBruin, W., Notterman, D., and Greenwald, B.: Mortality of ARDS in infants and children. Crit. Care Med. *17*:S111, 1989.
7. Fanconi, S., Kraemer, R., Weber, J., et al.: Long-term sequelae in children surviving adult respiratory distress syndrome. J. Pediatr. *106*:218–222, 1985.
8. Fiser, D. H.: Adult respiratory distress syndrome. Pediatr. Rev. *14*:163–167, 1993.
9. Hammerschmidt, D. E., Weaver, L. J., Hudson, L. D., et al.: Association of complement activation and elevated plasma-C5a with adult respiratory distress syndrome. Lancet *1*:947, 1987.
10. Hickling, K. G., Walsh, J., Henderson, S., et al.: Low mortality rate in adult respiratory distress syndrome using low-volume, pressure limited ventilation with permissive hypercapnia: A prospective study. Crit. Care Med. *22*:1568–1578, 1994.
11. Katz, R., Pollack, M., and Spady, D.: Cardiopulmonary abnormalities in severe acute respiratory failure. J. Pediatr. *104*:357–364, 1984.
12. Lewis, J. F., and Jobe, A. H.: Surfactant and the adult respiratory distress syndrome. Am. Rev. Respir. Dis. *147*:218–233, 1993.
13. Lyrene, R. K., and Troug, W. E.: Adult respiratory distress syndrome in a pediatric intensive care unit: Predisposing conditions, clinical course, and outcome. Pediatrics *67*:790–795, 1981.
14. Moler, F. W., Custer, J. R., Bartlett, R. H., et al.: Extracorporeal life support for severe pediatric respiratory failure: An updated experience 1991–1993. J. Pediatr. *124*:875–880, 1994.
15. Nussbaum, E.: Adult type respiratory distress syndrome in children. Clin. Pediatr. *22*:401–406, 1983.
16. Paulson, T. E., Spear, R. M., and Peterson, B. M.: New concepts in the treatment of children with acute respiratory distress syndrome. J. Pediatr. *127*:163–175, 1995.
17. Pfenninger, J., Gerber, A., Tschäppeler, H., et al.: Adult respiratory distress syndrome in children. J. Pediatr. *101*:352–357, 1982.
18. Royall, J. A., and Levin, D. L.: Adult respiratory distress syndrome in pediatric patients. 1. Clinical aspects, pathophysiology, pathology, and mechanisms of lung injury. J. Pediatr. *112*:169–180, 1988.
19. Royall, J. A.: Adult respiratory distress syndrome in children. Semin. Respir. Med. *11*:223–234, 1990.

20. Sarnaik, A. P., and Lieh-Lai, M.: Adult respiratory distress syndrome in children. Pediatr. Clin. North Am. *41*:337–363, 1994.
21. Stephens, K. E., Ishizaka, A., Larrick, J. W., et al.: Tumor necrosis factor causes increased pulmonary permeability and edema: Comparison to septic acute lung injury. Am. Rev. Respir. Dis. *137*:1364–1370, 1988.
22. Swank, D. W., and Moore, S. B.: Roles of the neutrophil and other mediators in adult respiratory distress syndrome. Mayo Clin. Proc. *64*:118–132, 1989.
23. Tamburro, R. F., Bugnitz, M. C., and Stidham, G. L.: Alveolar-arterial oxygen gradient as a predictor of outcome in patients with non-neonatal pediatric respiratory failure. J. Pediatr. *119*:935–938, 1991.
24. Tilden, S. J., and Logan, J. J.: Lung parenchyma. *In* Holbrook, P. R. (ed.): Textbook of Pediatric Critical Care. Philadelphia, W. B. Saunders, 1993, pp. 523–535.
25. Tracey, K. J., Lowry, S. F., Fahey, T. J., III, et al.: Cachectin/tumor necrosis factor induces lethal shock and stress hormone responses in the dog. Surg. Gynecol. Obstet. *164*:415–422, 1987.

SECTION THIRTEEN

INFECTIONS OF THE FETUS AND NEWBORN

❑ ❑ ❑

76

VIRAL INFECTIONS OF THE FETUS AND NEONATE

James C. Overall, Jr.

GENERAL ASPECTS

The fetus and newborn infant highly are susceptible to a number of different viruses, which in most instances cause little or no disease in older age groups. However, relatively few of the hundreds of viruses to which humans constantly are exposed are ever transmitted to the fetus or cause infection in the newborn infant. Nevertheless, viral infections are an important cause of neonatal morbidity and mortality. The cumulative frequency of viral infections that occur in the fetus or the newborn infant may be as much as 6 to 8 per cent of all live births, whereas systemic bacterial disease occurs in only 1 to 2 per cent of neonates.[357]

Contributing to the frequency of viral infections in this age group is the fact that the infection can be acquired at several different periods during intrauterine and neonatal life: in utero (congenital infection), at time of birth (natal infection), or after birth but during the neonatal period (postnatal infection). In addition, a number of different outcomes from infection are possible. Congenital infections can result in resorption of the embryo, abortion, stillbirth, congenital malformation, prematurity, intrauterine growth retardation, acute disease apparent at birth or shortly thereafter, asymptomatic infection in the neonatal period but a persistent postnatal infection with neurologic sequelae later in life, or a normal infant without apparent sequelae. Natal or postnatal infections can cause acute systemic illness leading to death, persistent infection with late sequelae, self-limited disease with no discernible damage, or asymptomatic infection.

Recent developments in the fields of diagnostic virology, epidemiology, and viral immunology have expanded our knowledge tremendously and modified our understanding of fetal and neonatal viral infections and their contribution to disease, not only in the neonatal period but also later in life. In addition, the development of rubella vaccine and antiviral drugs effective against a few of the agents offers hope for prevention or control of these infections. This chapter provides the physician with an approach to the diagnosis and management of and prognostic information about the viral infections that occur in the fetus and newborn infant. The important perinatal viral pathogen, HIV, is covered in Chapters 80 and 192. For more detailed information and more extensive bibliographies, the reader can consult several excellent recent reviews, monographs or chapters, and textbooks.[24, 120, 148, 163, 177]

Pathogenesis

Congenital Viral Infections

Congenital viral infections occur secondary to the exposure of the fetus during maternal viral infection. Evidence from both humans and experimental animals indicates that fetal infection is preceded by a systemic viral infection in the mother with hematogenous spread of the virus to the placenta and subsequently to the fetus (Fig. 76–1). Most viral infections that occur in the mother during pregnancy appear to be limited to the respiratory or gastrointestinal tract and therefore do not pose a risk to the fetus. Even if viremia does

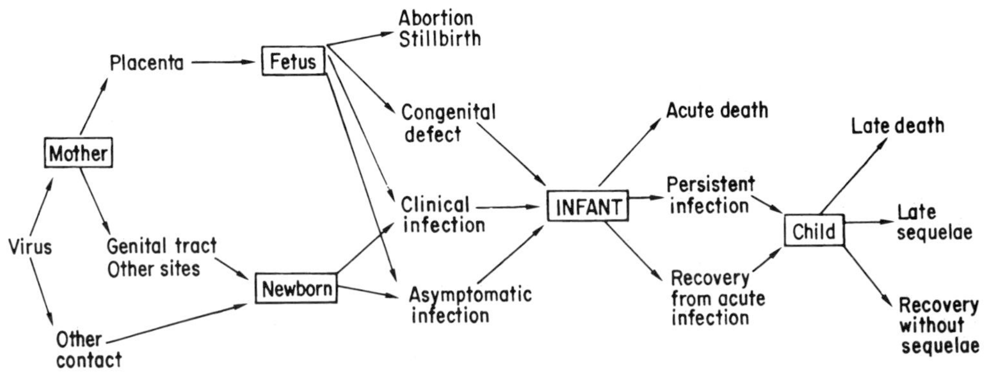

FIGURE 76–1. *Pathogenesis of viral infections in the fetus and newborn.*

TABLE 76–1. Period of Transmission of Viruses to the Fetus or Newborn Infant

Viruses	Congenital	Natal	Postnatal
Cytomegalovirus	+ +	+ +	+
Rubella	+ +	−	−
Hepatitis B	+	+ +	+
Herpes simplex	+	+ +	+
Varicella-zoster	+ +	−	−
Echoviruses	+	+	+
Type B coxsackieviruses	+	+	+
Polioviruses	+	−	−
Mumps	+	−	−
Measles	+	−	−
Vaccinia	+	−	−
Smallpox	+	−	−
Influenza	(+)	−	−
Western equine encephalitis	+	−	−
Epstein-Barr	+	−	−
Parvovirus B19	+	−	−

+ +, major demonstrated route; +, minor demonstrated route; (+), suggested route, few supporting data; −, route not demonstrated.

occur in the mother, maternal host defense mechanisms and the placenta appear to provide a protective barrier for the fetus. With most viruses known to cause fetal infection, placental involvement by the virus also has been documented: cytomegalovirus (CMV), rubella virus, herpes simplex virus (HSV), varicella-zoster virus (VZV), and vaccinia virus.[48] Viruses may reach the fetal circulation by (1) replication through the layers of the placenta, (2) production of virus-induced vascular lesions in the placenta, resulting in abnormal communications between maternal and fetal circulations, or (3) diapedesis of virus-infected maternal leukocytes through the layers of the placenta to the fetal circulation.[48, 326, 431] Damage to the fetus also may occur in the absence of actual fetal viral infection because of severe systemic illness in the mother or alteration of placental function (e.g., abortion or stillbirth in maternal measles, influenza). Those viruses demonstrated to have caused congenital infection are listed in Table 76–1. Proof of congenital infection usually consists of the presence of disease due to the virus or demonstration of the pathogen in the neonate at birth or shortly thereafter.[177, 357]

The effect that congenital infection with various viruses can have on the fetus is shown in Table 76–2.[357, 390–392] Abortion or stillbirth usually occurs when the mother is infected very early in gestation (e.g., rubella) or when the systemic illness in the mother is severe (e.g., measles, influenza). The reasons premature birth occurs in congenital viral infection are not well understood. Infants with congenital viral infection and that are small for gestational age have intrauterine growth retardation, usually the result of decreased numbers of cells in organs.[301, 302]

Developmental malformations result from infection of the fetus with the virus (Table 76–2). Rubella virus is the classic known teratogen; that is, it causes disturbances in organogenesis. VZV has been shown to cause limb hypoplasia and developmental malformations of the eye.[157] The other viruses that result in congenital defects, CMV and HSV, cause inflammatory, destructive lesions of already developed organs.[177] The B coxsackieviruses have been associated with a variety of congenital malformations of the heart[58–60] and mumps with endocardial fibroelastosis,[399] but these associations require further substantiation before a causative role can be assigned.

In Table 76–2, congenital disease refers to any manifestation of illness present at birth or shortly thereafter that is secondary to transplacental infection with the virus. Some of the viruses that result in congenital disease cause a chronic persistent infection (CMV infection, rubella, and hepatitis B), whereas others cause acute, self-limited, or fatal infection (echovirus infections, coxsackievirus B infections, poliovirus infections, measles, vaccinia, smallpox, western equine encephalitis, and parvovirus B19 infection). HSV and VZV can cause a chronic persistent intrauterine infection as well as an acute transplacental infection at the time of delivery. With one virus, HSV, congenital infection has occurred by other than the transplacental route. Ascending amniotic infection with HSV, in association with premature rupture of the membranes and a maternal genital herpes infection, has resulted

TABLE 76–2. Effect of Specific Viruses on the Fetus and Newborn Infant

Viruses	Abortion; Stillbirth	Prematurity	Small for Gestational Age	Developmental Malformations	Congenital Disease	Acute Postnatal Disease	Persistent Postnatal Infection
Cytomegalovirus	+	+	+	+	+ (C)	+	+
Rubella	+	+	+	+	+ (C)	−	+
Hepatitis B	−	+	−	−	+ (C)	+	+
Herpes simplex	+	+	+	+	+ (C, A)	+	+
Varicella-zoster	−	+	+	+	+ (C, A)	+	+
Echoviruses	−	−	−	−	+ (A)	+	−
Type B coxsackieviruses	+	−	−	(+)	+ (A)	+	−
Polioviruses	+	+	−	−	+ (A)	−	−
Mumps	+	−	−	(+)	−	−	−
Measles	+	+	−	−	+ (A)	−	−
Vaccinia	+	+	−	−	+ (A)	−	−
Smallpox	+	+	−	−	+ (A)	−	−
Influenza	+		−	−	−	(+)	−
Western equine encephalitis	−	−	−	−	+ (A)	−	−
Epstein-Barr	−	−	+	+	+ (C)	−	+
Parvovirus B19	+	−	−	−	+ (C, A)	+	+

+, effect established; −, effect not established; (+), effect suggested, but not proved; (C), chronic persistent infection; (A), acute fatal or self-limited infection.

in acute disease at birth because of the short incubation period in the neonate.

Viruses and Congenital Malformation

The role of viruses as etiologic agents in congenital malformations merits special mention. After the recognition by Gregg[164] in 1941 that congenital cataracts and other defects occurred in the offspring of mothers with German measles, the concept of an infectious origin for congenital malformations firmly was established. Major malformations occur in 2 to 3 per cent of all live births.[177] Although great strides have been made in the diagnosis and management of these defects, their etiologic basis remains largely undefined. Approximately 10 per cent are due to environmental causes such as infections, drugs, or radiation. Another 10 per cent are of genetic origin, resulting from familial inheritance or demonstrable chromosomal abnormalities.[326] The remaining 80 per cent are of unknown etiology. The majority of congenital defects may not be caused by environmental or genetic factors acting individually but rather in concert with one another. The genetically predisposed fetus is exposed to the appropriate environmental factor at a particular stage during organogenesis, which then leads to the development of malformations.[177] Because control of the genetic factors contributing to fetal malformation is unlikely to be developed to the point of practical application in the near future, efforts to identify environmental factors that are amenable to control appear warranted.

There are several reasons viruses have been considered to be likely contributors to the 80 per cent of malformations that are of unknown etiology. First, the precedent is established that rubella virus and CMV infections during pregnancy do cause congenital defects. Second, it is expected that most women would have one or more viral infections at some time during pregnancy,[382] so the potential exposure rate is high. Third, a viral infection could be unrecognized in the mother yet produce significant disease in the fetus, which could lead to the occurrence of a "congenital defect of unknown etiology." Fourth, viruses are known to multiply readily in rapidly dividing immature cells, with resultant cell destruction or altered cell function.[290] With more destructive viruses (e.g., measles, vaccinia), fetal death with abortion or stillbirth may occur, whereas with less cytolytic agents (e.g., rubella, CMV), the fetus may survive but defects are produced. Finally, experimental animals provide numerous examples of infection with a virus resulting in little or no disease in the pregnant mother; yet the fetuses are aborted or the newborn offspring are deformed.[134] The physician caring for newborn infants, therefore, should not only be familiar with the patterns of congenital defects currently known to be caused by viruses (CMV, rubella, HSV, and VZV) but also be aware that additional viruses may be added to the list of causative agents in the future.

Natal Viral Infections

Natal viral infections are the result of exposure of the newborn to virus replicating in the genital tract (CMV, HSV, hepatitis B virus [HBV]) or to fecal virus contaminating genital secretions (enteroviruses) (see Fig. 76–1 and Table 76–1). Because the incubation period of HSV and enteroviruses is short, acute postnatal disease may appear in the neonate within 5 to 7 days after natal infection with these agents (see Table 76–2). In contrast, the incubation periods of CMV and HBV are long, and clinically manifest disease, if it occurs, may not be observed for several weeks or even months after birth (see Table 76–2). Persistent postnatal infection can occur after natal infection with CMV, HSV, and HBV.

Postnatal Viral Infections

The source of exposure for postnatal infections of the newborn infant often is the mother, but other sources have been observed, such as personnel or other infants in the nursery or newborn intensive care unit and family members (see Fig. 76–1). Outbreaks of enterovirus[293] and respiratory syncytial virus[171] infections have occurred in nurseries, and nosocomial HSV infections[172, 215, 330, 369, 443] have been reported (see Table 76–1). Although the maternal respiratory and gastrointestinal tracts are the most common sites from which virus can be transmitted to the neonate postnatally, both CMV[185] and HBV[256] have been recovered from breast milk. Finally, both CMV[478] and HBV[128] have been transmitted to newborn infants by blood transfusion.[127, 475] Although most postnatal infections are acute, self-limited processes, fatalities have been reported, and persistent postnatal infection may occur with CMV and HBV (see Table 76–2).

Epidemiology

Factors Influencing Infection Frequency

A number of factors can influence the frequency of infections in the fetus and newborn infant (Table 76–3). Because the mother is the source of virus causing fetal and neonatal infection in most instances, the factors influencing frequency of maternal infection are of major importance. Except for CMV infection, the majority of congenital infections of the fetus occur after primary viral infection in the mother. Congenital CMV infection may occur as frequently with mothers known to be seropositive prior to conception as in seronegative mothers.[405] Congenital rubella, on the other hand, occurs only rarely in immune mothers.[177, 362] Transplacental HBV infection occurs much more frequently in mothers with acute, primary, symptomatic infection, whereas natal infection is the primary route of transmission in chronic carrier mothers.[318, 374] Perinatal enteroviral infections acquired from the mother almost always are the result of primary maternal infection. In contrast, natal infections with CMV, HBV, and HSV may result from persistent or recurrent genital infections in the mother. The frequency of primary viral infection in mothers is influenced by maternal age because susceptibility is related inversely to the age of the mother.

The evidence is clear that the time during pregnancy at which the mother is infected (the gestational age of the fetus) is a major factor influencing both the frequency and the severity of congenital rubella. One hundred per cent of infants with congenital infection during the first 11 weeks of pregnancy have malformations of the congenital rubella syndrome, 30 per cent with congenital infection from 12 to 20 weeks have malformations, and no malformations occur with infections occurring after 20 weeks.[286] The same phenomenon occurs with congenital CMV and VZV infections.[190, 331, 401] In contrast, transplacental HBV infection appears to be more frequent when the acute, symptomatic maternal infection occurs in the third trimester rather than the first or second.[483] With viruses such as polio, measles, vaccinia, and smallpox, early gestation maternal disease results in abortion or stillbirth, whereas late gestation infection results in congenital disease with acute symptoms in the early neonatal period (see Table 76–2).

Several social and environmental factors may influence the likelihood of maternal infection and thereby affect fetal and

TABLE 76–3. Factors Influencing Frequency and Severity of Viral Infections in the Fetus and Newborn Infant

	Time of Fetal or Neonatal Infection		
Factors	***Congenital***	***Natal***	***Postnatal***
Primary infection in mother	++	++	++
Maternal age	++	+	++
Gestational age of fetus	++	+	+
Absence of vaccine	++	−	−
Presence of epidemic in community	++	+	++
Season of year	++	+	++
Geographic location	++	++	++
Socioeconomic status	++	++	++
Sexual promiscuity	+	++	−
Method of case identification	++	++	++

++, major influence; +, minor influence; −, little or no influence.

neonatal infection frequency. The development of rubella vaccine and its licensure in 1969 has reduced significantly the incidence of the congenital rubella syndrome.[33, 320] The successful eradication of smallpox worldwide and the discontinuation of the need for smallpox vaccine (vaccinia virus) have eliminated fetal infection with these viruses. Although measles and mumps vaccines significantly have reduced the occurrence of these diseases in childhood, it is unclear whether waning immunity in women of child-bearing age who were vaccinated as infants will predispose to reinfection in the pregnant woman and consequent fetal or neonatal disease. The presence of epidemics in the community, such as those due to rubella or enteroviruses, certainly can influence maternal and thereby congenital, natal, and postnatal infection frequency. The incidence of infection with some viruses (e.g., rubella, primary VZV, enteroviruses, measles, mumps, influenza) clearly is higher during certain months of the year, so the season can influence maternal and neonatal infection rates. In contrast, other viruses causing congenital or natal infection (CMV, HBV, HSV) do not occur in an epidemic or seasonal fashion. Geographic location also can be influential, probably because of differences in the ethnic (and therefore genetic) origin of populations in different locations. Rates of chronic carriage of hepatitis B surface antigen (HBsAg) in mothers and the frequency of congenital and natal HBV infection in neonates are much higher in Taiwanese than in United States residents.[483] The incidence of a number of maternal viral infections is known to be higher in populations with a lower socioeconomic status, thereby influencing the frequency of congenital, natal, and postnatal infections. Other social factors such as drug abuse, which is associated with higher rates of HBV infection, can influence congenital and natal infection frequency. CMV, HBV, and HSV all have been shown to be transmitted venereally, so sexual promiscuity in the mother can influence frequency of the infection in the neonate.

Although listed last in Table 76–3, the method of case identification is a major factor that can influence the frequency of recognized infection in the neonate. Because most neonates with congenital CMV, rubella virus, and HBV infection are asymptomatic, use of clinical case-finding methods alone underestimates significantly the true frequency of the infections. Epidemiologic observations (e.g., rubella or enterovirus epidemic in the community), clinical or laboratory information about the mother (e.g., viral illness with a rash or presence of HBsAg in the serum), or screening tests in the newborn (e.g., elevated quantitative IgM in cord blood serum) often have been used to select a group of neonates at high risk of congenital infection. The performance of additional laboratory tests in these high-risk neonates to identify potential specific causative agents often has led to the demonstration of infection rates much higher than previously suspected.

Frequency of Infection in the Mother and Neonate

Table 76–4 shows the approximate frequency of the most common viral infections in the mother during pregnancy and in the newborn infant.[24, 177, 357] Although the figures have been obtained by a variety of laboratory methods and some are based on a relatively small or nonrepresentative population sample, they do provide an estimate of the relative frequency of the infections. In many studies, prospective screening of mothers for viral infection during pregnancy or of infants for elevated cord blood serum IgM levels was done to select a population of neonates at high risk of congenital infection for more detailed virologic investigation.

CMV clearly is the most common cause of viral infection, both in the mother and in the neonate. Surveys in the United States indicate that 30 to 110 per 1000 women excrete virus in the urine during pregnancy and that 60 per 1000 are excreters at the time of delivery.[145, 191, 223, 297, 309, 359] Isolation from cervical swabs is even more common: 80 to 120 per 1000 women during pregnancy and 110 to 130 per 1000 at delivery.[79, 223, 297, 359] Most maternal CMV infections during pregnancy are recurrent rather than primary.[403] Extrapolation from data obtained at the same institution[359, 403, 407] suggests that two-thirds to three-quarters of CMV shedding in the cervix or urine during pregnancy is the result of recurrent, rather than primary, CMV infection in the mother. The frequency of primary CMV infection during pregnancy averages 20 to 25 per 1000 (range, 10 to 40), with higher rates occurring in populations with a larger percentage of susceptible persons (seronegative at the beginning of pregnancy).[401] Several factors are known to be associated with increased rates of recurrent urine or cervical shedding: (1) sampling on several occasions rather than a single time, (2) specimen collection during the third rather than the first trimester because shedding rates are known to increase as gestation progresses, (3) Asian, black, or Native American versus white population, (4) younger maternal age, (5) lower socioeconomic status, (6) a greater number of lifetime sexual partners, and (7) a history of sexually transmitted diseases.[79, 223, 309, 409] An even more important source for transmission of CMV to the neonate may be breast milk. Postpartum shedding from colostrum or breast milk, cervix, urine, or saliva was demonstrated in 130 to 280 per 1000 unselected women, and breast

TABLE 76–4. Approximate Frequency of Infections in the Mother During Pregnancy and in the Newborn Infant

Viruses	Mother (No./1000 Pregnancies)	Neonate (No./1000 Live Births)
Cytomegalovirus		
During pregnancy, congenital	30–120	6–24
At delivery, natal	80–130	20–60
After delivery, postnatal	130–280	140–210
Rubella		
1964 epidemic	20–40	3–7
Interepidemic prevaccine	0.1–2.0	0.1–0.7
Postvaccine	0.15–0.3	0.03
Hepatitis B	1–160	0–61
Enteroviruses	90–600	2–38
Herpes simplex	1–7	0.1–0.6

milk was the most common site by far.[130, 401, 407, 408] Because maternal CMV infection usually is asymptomatic, it is not possible to estimate the frequency of clinical disease.

Congenital CMV infection has been documented in 6 to 24 per 1000 live births, as evidenced by the isolation of virus from the urine of the neonate within the first few days of life.[47, 361, 405] In contrast with rubella, congenital infection with CMV occurs in mothers with either primary or recurrent infections during pregnancy.[405] Congenital CMV infection rates are significantly higher in lower socioeconomic groups (1.6 per cent) than in middle to upper ones (0.6 per cent).[403] However, among low-income mothers, the status of immunity to CMV is high (82 per cent), and most congenital infections (81 per cent) are associated with recurrent CMV infection during pregnancy. In contrast, seroimmunity to CMV among middle- to upper-income women is lower (55 per cent), and the frequency of congenital infection associated with recurrent maternal CMV also is lower (47 per cent). Although the rate of total congenital CMV infection is lower among mid- to high-income mothers, the proportion of infants born after primary CMV infection during pregnancy is higher (53 vs. 19 per cent). Pooled data from several studies indicate that 30 to 40 per cent of mothers with primary CMV infection during pregnancy (range, 20 to 52 per cent among the various studies) deliver congenitally infected infants.[6, 7, 165, 242, 401, 403] Congenitally infected babies born to mothers with primary, rather than recurrent, CMV infection during pregnancy have a greater frequency of symptoms of CMV disease at birth, higher levels of IgM in cord serum, higher titers of virus in urine, and a greater likelihood of neurologic sequelae on follow-up.[5, 6, 401, 403] The time during gestation that maternal primary CMV infection occurs does not appear to influence the rate of fetal infection, but fetal damage appears to be more frequent and more severe after maternal infection during the first half than during the second half of pregnancy.[5, 165, 345, 401]

The frequency of natal and postnatal acquisition of CMV by the newborn infant is far greater than that of congenital infection. Natally acquired CMV infection occurs at an incidence of 20 per 1000 live births.[359, 407] Because about one-half of the infants born to mothers known to be cervical excreters at the time of delivery acquire natal infection[359] and because as many as 130 per 1000 mothers from a low socioeconomic group are excreting CMV at this time,[359] the actual rate of natally acquired CMV infection may be as high as 60 per 1000 live births. A more frequent source for infection of the neonate with CMV is postnatal consumption of virus-infected colostrum or breast milk. In two studies, 58 to 69 per cent of infants of nursing mothers excreting CMV in milk acquired infection.[130, 407] Maternal shedding occurred most frequently between 2 and 12 weeks post partum, and onset of infant viruria usually occurred between 1 and 6 months of age. The aforementioned rates of postnatal infection would project to between 140 and 210 infections per 1000 live births in the United States. These rates, of course, would be influenced by all of those factors mentioned earlier that influence maternal CMV infection rates, as well as the frequency and duration of breast feeding.

Yet another source for transmission of CMV to neonates is blood transfusion in infants in neonatal intensive care units. Risk factors include birth weight less than 1250 g, a CMV-seronegative mother, hospitalization for more than 4 weeks, receipt of multiple blood transfusions or a total volume of more than 50 mL, and receipt of blood from a CMV-seropositive donor.[4, 31, 147, 478] The infection rate in high-risk infants may be high: 24 to 31 per cent. Morbidity and mortality rates with these infections also are high: 88 per cent of 34 reported cases developed clinical disease, and 24 per cent died (CMV believed to be causal or contributory).

In summary, several factors contribute to the high rates of fetal and neonatal infection with CMV: (1) virus can be transmitted from both immune mothers (recurrent infection) and nonimmune mothers (primary infection), (2) virus may be shed or carried in many different sites in the mother—blood (for transplacental infection), urine, cervix, breast milk, and saliva, (3) infection may occur at different times—congenital, natal, and postnatal, and (4) infection may come from sources other than the mother (e.g., hospital-acquired infection from blood transfusion).

The use of rubella vaccine has modified the epidemiologic patterns of this disease in the United States,[33, 320] and incidence data from periods prior to licensure of the vaccine in 1969 are not applicable currently. In addition, rates of maternal and congenital rubella during the 1964 epidemic were many times higher than in interepidemic periods. Nevertheless, a comparison of the incidence during the 1964 epidemic, the rates during prevaccine interepidemic periods, and what may be happening currently provides useful information. The frequency of serologically proven clinical rubella among 30,000 pregnant women in the Collaborative Perinatal Research Study was approximately 1 per 1000 during interepidemic years prior to vaccine licensure but rose to 22 per 1000 during the epidemic.[382] The total figure for rubella during pregnancy is likely to be at least two times higher because as many as one-half to two-thirds of maternal rubella infections are subclinical or are not diagnosed as rubella.[380] An incidence of congenital rubella of 0.7 per 1000 live births was demonstrated during the interepidemic period in a study screening cord blood sera from the presence of rubella-specific IgM antibody.[9] During the 1964 epidemic, an estimated

20,000 babies were born with congenital rubella syndrome in the United States among approximately 4 million live births, an incidence of 5 per 1000 live births.[311] During 1980 to 1982, an average of 11 cases of confirmed congenital rubella syndrome were reported to the Centers for Disease Control and Prevention (CDC) each year.[320] Correcting for underreporting and missed cases yielded an annual estimate of 110 cases.[320] With an annual national birth rate of 3.5 million per year, this projects to 0.03 cases of congenital rubella syndrome per 1000 live births currently in the United States. Assuming a 10 to 20 per cent rate of congenital infection with rubella during pregnancy,[177] this translates into a current estimate of 0.15 to 0.3 cases of maternal rubella per 1000 pregnancies. Importantly, however, a resurgence of acquired and congenital rubella, particularly among unvaccinated women in correctional institutions or unimmunized communities,[71, 280] emphasizes the need for continued surveillance for rubella disease and emphasis on proper use of the vaccine.

HBV infection during pregnancy may result in acute clinical disease in the mother or, more commonly, be present as an asymptomatic chronic carrier state.[375] The frequency of HBsAg in the serum of pregnant women varies highly and is influenced by geographic location; ethnic origin; socioeconomic status; and other social factors, such as drug abuse and sexual promiscuity. An incidence of 1 to 160 per 1000 pregnancies has been reported from several series.[19, 42, 117, 129, 227, 256, 317, 329, 375, 415, 471] The frequency of HBV infection in the neonate is even more variable, for several reasons. First, transmission of the virus to the fetus or neonate may occur by several routes: (1) transplacental, (2) natal, from the genital tract, (3) postnatal, by fecal-oral spread or breast feeding, and (4) postnatal, by blood transfusion. Second, infants born to mothers with hepatitis B may follow one of the following courses: (1) Serum from the infant remains negative for HBsAg, and hepatitis B never develops. (2) Cord blood serum is positive for HBsAg, but the antigenemia clears and no disease is evident, presumably representing transplacental transmission of antigen only or insufficient virus to cause true infection of the neonate. (3) Cord blood is HBsAg-positive, and clinical or subclinical infection develops with or without persistent hepatitis B antigenemia. (4) Cord blood is antigen-negative, but infection occurs, sometimes not until several months after birth, and persistent antigenemia may or may not develop. Third, because exposed infants may follow one of several courses and because HBV infection may be demonstrable at various times after birth, serial blood specimens must be obtained for evaluation of the true frequency of neonatal infection. Serial blood specimens are difficult to obtain in this age group, and published reports may have based their estimates of infection on one or two blood specimens per infant. Fourth, transplacental infection is much more common in mothers with acute, symptomatic hepatitis, particularly during the second or third trimester of pregnancy, than in chronic carrier mothers.[375] Finally, even in chronic carrier mothers, there are true differences in the rate of transplacental transmission: Asians have a much higher incidence than whites,[483] and mothers who are HBeAg-positive are much more likely to transmit infection than mothers with anti-HBe antibody or who lack e-antigen markers.[317] Therefore, the incidence of HBV infection in the neonate varies from 0 to 61 per 1000 live births among different reports.[19, 42, 117, 129, 227, 256, 317, 329, 375, 386, 415, 471]

Data from several studies indicate that perinatal enteroviral infections are much more frequent than previously realized.[109, 208, 212, 293, 295, 298, 365] Serologic surveys indicate a surprisingly high rate of seroconversion to at least one enterovirus during pregnancy (first serum at time of enrollment for obstetric care, second serum at delivery): 90 to 600 per 1000 pregnancies.[58–60, 232, 379] Several factors complicate the interpretation of the data concerning frequency of maternal enteroviral infections. First, only 2 to 13 of the almost 70 nonpolio enterovirus serotypes were used for antibody testing, thereby resulting in an underestimate of the true frequency for all enteroviruses. Second, the data are reported as the total number of enteroviral infections for a group of pregnant women rather than the percentage of pregnancies complicated by at least one enteroviral infection. Use of these data for calculating the number of pregnancies per 1000 complicated by enteroviral infection would result in an overestimation because more than 25 per cent of women may have more than one enteroviral infection during the 9 months of pregnancy.[58] Nevertheless, these data represent the best estimates of the frequency of enteroviral infections during pregnancy. Data concerning the actual frequency of neonatal enteroviral infections also are difficult to summarize because of the differences in study design used in the various published results. Modlin and associates[295] reported four echovirus 11 infections among 158 consecutive neonates with stool samples at 3 days and 2 weeks of age during the 3-week period of an outbreak of echovirus 11 infection in Boston. Assuming that live births are distributed evenly throughout the year and that no additional cases of enteroviral infection occurred during the remainder of the year, this translates into two enteroviral infections per 1000 live births. These calculations are likely to underestimate markedly the true frequency because only echovirus 11 was sought in the diagnostic virology laboratory evaluation of these 158 infants, and obviously enteroviral infections occur for more than a 3-week period of the year. A prospective study of all enteroviral infections during the first month of life in Rochester, New York, during the peak enterovirus season (June to October) demonstrated 75 (12.8 per cent) nonpolio enteroviral infections among 586 infants.[208] Fourteen (18.7 per cent) of these 75 infected infants were hospitalized for "suspected sepsis." Using the estimated number of live births per year in the Rochester area and assuming that no additional cases of neonatal enteroviral infection occurred during the remaining 7 months of the year, the authors projected a rate of 7 per 1000 live births for neonatal enteroviral infections serious enough to require hospitalization. If one considered the total 75 enteroviral infections (14 hospitalized and 61 not hospitalized), the rate would be 38 per 1000 live births. A survey by Kaplan and associates[212] of 77 cases of coxsackievirus B infections during the first 3 months of life in infants hospitalized at the Nassau County Medical Center between 1970 and 1979 yielded an estimated rate of 0.5 per 1000 live births. Because coxsackieviruses B account for only 45 per cent of all enteroviral infections during early infancy[298] and because only 18 to 19 per cent of all enterovirus-infected infants may require hospitalization,[208] the actual rate for all enteroviral infections may be 6 per 1000 live births. Despite the variation in the estimates, it is clear that enteroviral infections are a frequent cause of maternal and neonatal infections.

As mentioned earlier, the infected genital tract of the mother is the source of virus for most neonatal HSV infections. Other sources, however, such as nongenital sites in the mother, family members, and even other infants in the nursery through hands of personnel, have been implicated. Both genital and neonatal herpes have increased in frequency in recent years.[43, 423] Current estimates are that culture-positive genital herpes may occur during pregnancy at a rate of 1 to 7 per 1000[49, 50, 61–63, 307] and at the time of delivery at a rate of 1 to 4 per 1000.[61, 63, 306, 349, 428] However, culture is not the most sensitive method to detect genital HSV-2 infection. Seroprevalence studies demonstrated HSV-2–specific antibody among 32 per cent of women in private obstetric practices,[240] and polymerase chain reaction detected HSV DNA among 9 per cent of asymptomatic women in labor.[95] Higher rates are associated with lower socioeconomic status, increased numbers of sexual partners, and occurrence of other sexually transmitted diseases. Rates of neonatal herpes have been estimated at 0.1 to 0.6 per 1000 live births.[61, 307, 423, 456] The greatest risk of neonatal infection appears to be when the mother has an initial genital infection at the time of vaginal delivery.

The frequency of infection with the other viruses listed in Tables 76–1 and 76–2 is so low that numeric estimates per 1000 pregnancies or live births are not possible.

Approach to Diagnosis

The usual set of circumstances leading one to consider the diagnosis of viral infection in the newborn infant is the presence of clinical or laboratory features in the neonate that suggest this possibility (Table 76–5). The observation of congenital defects, icterus, petechiae, or hepatosplenomegaly at the time of birth or shortly thereafter in a small-for-gestational-age infant points toward a chronic viral infection. On the other hand, acute viral infection in this age group usually comes to mind in the infant with suspected sepsis when cultures of blood, spinal fluid, and urine fail to yield a bacterial or fungal agent.

TABLE 76–5. Common Manifestations of Viral Infections in the Newborn Infant

1. Asymptomatic infection
2. Chronic infection (early gestation to midgestation congenital)
   - *General characteristics*
     - Manifestations present at birth or shortly thereafter
     - Presence of congenital defects
   - *Specific features*
     - Small for gestational age
     - Central nervous system: Microcephaly, seizures, cerebral calcification, hyper- or hypotonia, cerebrospinal fluid pleocytosis, encephalitis
     - Skin: Icterus, petechiae, purpura, vesicles, hypopigmentation
     - Eye: Chorioretinitis, cataracts, glaucoma, microphthalmia, optic atrophy
     - Heart: Patent ductus arteriosus, pulmonary artery stenosis
     - Abdomen: Hepatosplenomegaly, hepatitis
     - Lung: Pneumonitis
     - Musculoskeletal: Bone lesions, limb hypoplasia
3. Acute infection (late-gestation congenital, natal, or postnatal)
   - *General characteristics*
     - Manifestations usually appear several days to weeks after birth
     - Absence of congenital defects
   - *Specific features*
     - Hyper- or hypothermia
     - General: Irritability, lethargy, jitters, poor feeding, vomiting
     - Central nervous system: Seizures, hyper- or hypotonia, full fontanelle, meningitis, encephalitis
     - Skin: Icterus, petechiae, purpura, vesicle, maculopapular rash
     - Eye: Conjunctivitis, keratitis
     - Heart: Myocarditis
     - Abdomen: Hepatosplenomegaly, hepatitis
     - Lung: Pneumonitis, respiratory distress, cyanosis

Evaluation of the Mother

Once the suspicion of a viral infection in the newborn infant has been raised, one should proceed with an evaluation of the mother for features that might add further evidence to this possibility. For example, the occurrence of maternal viral illness with an associated maculopapular rash suggests rubella or enterovirus infection in the neonate, whereas ulcerative genital lesions point toward HSV and heterophile-negative infectious mononucleosis toward CMV. It should be noted, however, that most maternal viral infections that lead to fetal or neonatal infection (almost all cases of CMV and HBV infection[412, 471] and one-half to two-thirds of rubella virus and HSV infections[306, 380, 456, 460]) are asymptomatic in the mother. Therefore, the absence of a history of viral infection in the mother certainly does not rule out the possibility of such infection in her neonate.

Specimens from the mother for isolation or detection of the viral agent usually are not available. However, the presence of HBsAg in maternal serum or the isolation of CMV or HSV from the genital tract or an enterovirus from the stool at the time of birth certainly should make one consider these agents in her newborn infant. Serologic documentation of a specific viral illness in the mother during pregnancy requires serum specimens that bracket the illness. Unfortunately, these rarely are available when the pediatrician is considering the possibility of a congenital viral illness in the neonate. Routine antibody determinations on a single specimen obtained from the mother after the birth of an abnormal child with suspected congenital viral infection are not likely to yield useful information. However, the presence of specific IgM antibody against CMV,[166, 179, 410] rubella virus,[159] or HSV[303] in a single maternal serum specimen is highly suggestive of recent infection. On the other hand, if the maternal viral infection occurs near the time of delivery (e.g., enterovirus meningitis, coxsackievirus B pleurodynia, initial genital herpes), acute and convalescent serum specimens may be obtained from the mother that do demonstrate the diagnostic fourfold or greater rise in antibody titer against a specific agent. Documentation of a particular causative agent in the mother does not constitute proof that the same agent is causing disease in the neonate, but it certainly does provide strong suggestive evidence. Definitive proof, therefore, must come from studies in the newborn infant.

Clinical Features in the Neonate

Certain clinical manifestations of viral disease in the neonate may provide helpful clues to the specific etiologic agent. However, most viral infections in the neonate are asymptomatic: more than 95 per cent of CMV, two-thirds of rubella virus, and most HBV. In contrast, less than 1 per cent of HSV infections in the neonate are subclinical.[307] To complicate the effort to pinpoint the diagnosis further, the clinical and laboratory manifestations of symptomatic disease due to a number of agents often have a similar pattern (see Table 76–5; Figs. 76–2 and 76–3). However, infants whose congenital viral infection is incurred in early gestation to midgestation present manifestations of disease at birth or shortly thereafter, whereas infants with late-gestation congenital or natal or postnatal infection usually do not exhibit signs and symptoms for several days to several weeks after birth (see Table 76–5). In addition, newborn infants with congenital infection in early gestation to midgestation exhibit congenital defects and intrauterine growth retardation, whereas neonates who

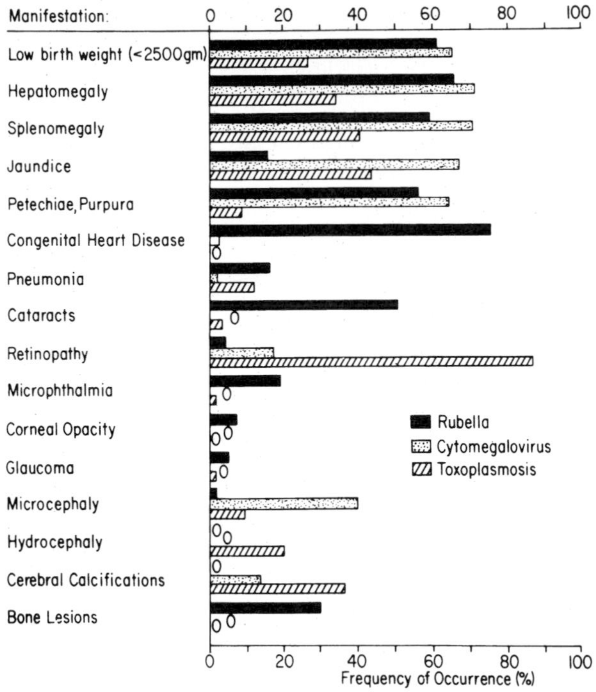

FIGURE 76–2. *Manifestations of symptomatic congenital rubella virus and cytomegalovirus infections and toxoplasmosis.*

acquire viral infection near the time of birth have acute disease resembling bacterial sepsis or the viral syndrome typically seen in older children (e.g., enterovirus exanthem, chickenpox) (see Table 76–5). Because the viral agents that commonly cause chronic intrauterine infection are different from those that result in acute neonatal disease (see Tables 76–1 to 76–3), the recognition of these two different patterns of presentation helps define a specific etiologic agent.

The most common manifestations of congenital CMV and rubella infections in symptomatic newborn infants are shown in Figure 76–2. Also shown in this figure are the features observed in infants with congenital toxoplasmosis because this infection is important to consider in the differential diagnosis. (Infection with *Toxoplasma gondii* is covered in Chapter 221.) Note that many nonspecific manifestations, such as low birth weight due to intrauterine growth retardation, hepatomegaly, splenomegaly, jaundice, and petechiae/purpura, occur with a similar frequency among the three infections. However, certain specific findings may be helpful in the differential diagnosis. The presence of cataracts, congenital heart disease, bone lesions, or microphthalmia is highly suggestive of rubella, whereas chorioretinitis, cerebral calcifications, and hydrocephaly or microcephaly are against this diagnosis. In congenital CMV infection, microcephaly and cerebral calcifications are relatively common, but congenital heart disease, eye abnormalities, and bone lesions are rare. Chorioretinitis, cerebral calcifications, or hydrocephaly should suggest toxoplasmosis. The cerebral calcifications in CMV infection tend to be periventricular, whereas the distribution in toxoplasmosis is scattered through the parietal lobes of the cerebrum. It is important to note that some manifestations may not be evident for several months after birth: congenital heart disease, chorioretinitis, microcephaly, hydrocephaly, and cerebral calcifications.

The most frequent findings in the common acute viral infections of the neonate, HSV and enterovirus infections, are shown in Figure 76–3. Because the features in infants with these two kinds of viral infections resemble bacterial sepsis, the manifestations in neonates with septicemia also are presented. Again, the more common nonspecific features, such as fever or hypothermia, respiratory distress, cyanosis, an-

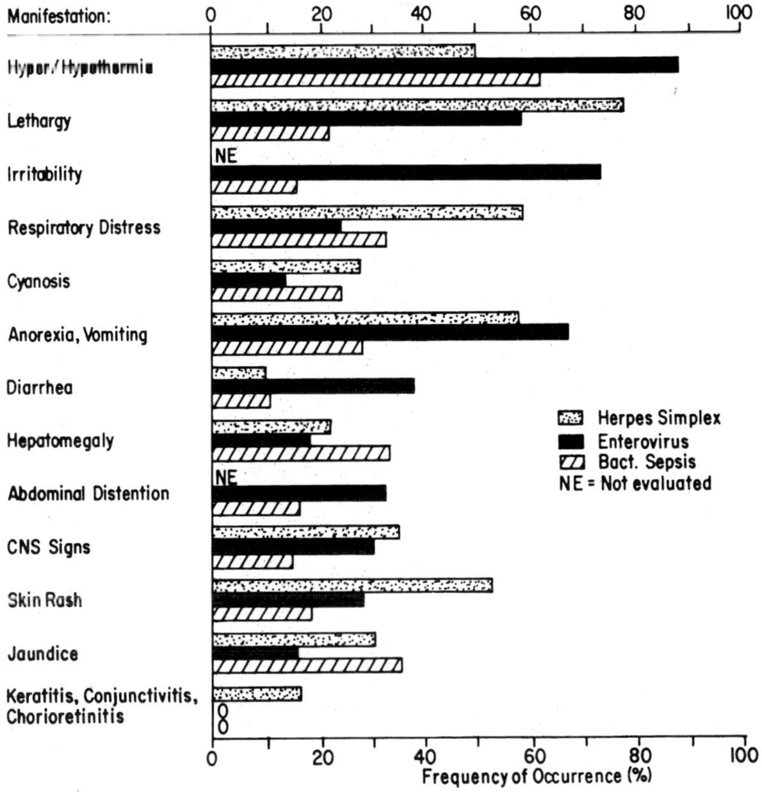

FIGURE 76–3. *Manifestations of herpes simplex virus and enterovirus infections and bacterial sepsis in the neonate.*

orexia or vomiting, and hepatomegaly, occur with a relatively similar frequency among the three infections. Lethargy, irritability, and central nervous system signs are more common in HSV and enterovirus infections, probably because encephalitis and meningitis, respectively, occur more frequently in these two infections. The features that suggest the diagnosis of HSV infection are a vesicular skin rash and keratitis, conjunctivitis, or chorioretinitis, whereas those that bring to mind enterovirus infection include diarrhea and abdominal distention. The rash in enterovirus infection usually is erythematous and maculopapular, but petechiae can occur with overwhelming infection. The skin lesions in bacterial sepsis usually are pustules, abscesses, cellulitis, or purpura.

Differential Diagnosis in the Neonate

The differential diagnosis in the newborn infant with a suspected viral infection is extensive.[177] Many of the manifestations shown in Figures 76–2 and 76–3, such as lethargy, irritability, respiratory distress, cyanosis, and anorexia, can be caused by the most common diseases occurring in the sick newborn infant—hyaline membrane disease, prematurity, intraventricular hemorrhage, metabolic disturbances, and bacterial sepsis. In infants with low birth weight due to intrauterine growth retardation (small for gestational age), one should consider congenital malformations, chromosomal abnormalities, placental insufficiency, and inborn errors of metabolism. Hepatosplenomegaly usually is caused by one of the infectious diseases of the neonate. In infants with jaundice, ABO and Rh hemolytic disease and physiologic jaundice should be considered. Noninfectious causes of petechiae/purpura include idiopathic or drug-induced (including transplacental passage) thrombocytopenia, erythroblastosis fetalis, and disseminated intravascular coagulation.

There is little firm evidence that infectious agents other than rubella can cause congenital heart disease. Diffuse pulmonary infiltrates early in the neonatal period most commonly are hyaline membrane disease, but in older neonates one should consider bronchopulmonary dysplasia and chlamydial infection. Causes of cataracts other than congenital rubella, HSV, and VZV infections include congenital galactosemia and the oculocerebrorenal (Lowe) syndrome. Chorioretinitis or retinopathy usually is caused by infection. Microcephaly also can be caused by infection with HSV or VZV; noninfectious causes include Down syndrome, perinatal anoxia, phenylketonuria, and maternal irradiation. Hydrocephalus usually is due to a congenital malformation of the ventricular aqueductal or subarachnoid space system. In the infant with manifestations of an acute infection, the major diagnostic consideration is a serious bacterial infection, such as sepsis, meningitis, urinary tract infection, or pneumonia. After appropriate cultures have been obtained in the infant, antibiotics should be administered until a bacterial infection has been ruled out.

Laboratory Diagnosis

Because the clinical manifestations in the various neonatal viral infections frequently overlap, specific etiologic diagnosis usually depends on the laboratory. Unfortunately, general laboratory tests, such as the peripheral white blood cell count, urinalysis, and blood chemistries, are not helpful in this regard. The approach to the specific laboratory diagnosis of viral infection in the newborn infant is outlined in Table 76–6. Details of the various methods for each virus are covered in the respective chapters for these agents; only general comments relevant to the diagnosis of infection in the neonate are presented here.

Routine histopathologic methods include the examination of stained cells from urine for CMV inclusions or of cells scraped from the base of a vesicle or from conjunctivae for multinucleated giant cells with intranuclear inclusions characteristic of HSV or VZV. In addition, tissue obtained by biopsy or at postmortem examination may reveal intranuclear inclusions and multinucleated giant cells characteristic of the herpesviruses. Except for the propensity to involve certain organs (e.g., rubella virus, the heart; HBV, the liver), the pathologic changes induced by viruses other than the herpes group rarely are specific enough to enable an etiologic diagnosis. Even for the herpesviruses, the routine histopathologic methods are only one-half to two-thirds as sensitive as isolation of the virus.

The most direct method of establishing the diagnosis is the isolation of the agent from an appropriate site in the infant.

TABLE 76–6. Laboratory Diagnosis of Viral Infection in the Newborn Infant

Procedure	Details, Comments
Routine histopathologic methods	Urine cells stained for inclusions Scraping of vesicle base or conjunctiva for multinucleated giant cells Examination of biopsy or autopsy tissue
Isolation or detection of infectious agents	Isolation of infectious agent in cell culture or animals Detection of viral particles by electron microscopy Detection of viral antigen by immunologic methods Detection of viral nucleic acid by DNA probes, often after amplification by PCR
IgG antiviral antibody	Persistence of antibody in serum of infant beyond age of normal decline of maternal transplacental antibody—usually 4–6 months Variety of methods available (CF, neut, HI, IHA, IFA, ELISA, etc.)—sensitivity of method varies according to the specific virus
IgM-specific antiviral antibody	IgM not normally passed transplacentally, presence in cord blood or neonatal serum diagnostic IgM-specific antibodies not always present in neonate False-positive and false-negative results
Quantitative IgM level	Not a specific diagnostic test, suggests intrauterine infection

Modified from Hanshaw, J. B., Dudgeon, J. A., and Marshall, W. C.: Viral Diseases of the Fetus and Newborn. 2nd ed. Philadelphia, W. B. Saunders, 1985.

CF, complement fixation; ELISA, enzyme-linked immunosorbent assay; HI, hemagglutination inhibition; IFA, immunofluorescent assay; IHA, indirect hemagglutination; neut, neutralization; PCR, polymerase chain reaction.

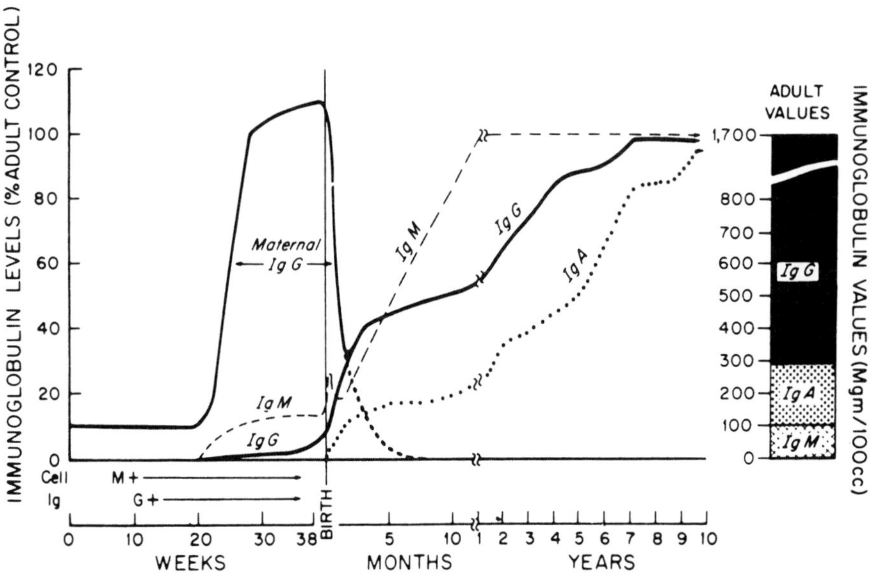

FIGURE 76–4. *Kinetics of fetal and neonatal immunoglobulins. (From Alford, C. A.: Immunoglobulin determinations in the diagnosis of fetal infection. Pediatr. Clin. North Am. 18:99–113, 1971.)*

The following sites usually are used: urine for CMV; throat and occasionally spinal fluid or urine for rubella; skin vesicles, buffy coat, cerebrospinal fluid, or urine for HSV; throat, stool, cerebrospinal fluid, or serum/buffy coat for enteroviruses; and skin vesicles for VZV. In addition, isolation of virus can be attempted from biopsy material or sterile specimens obtained at autopsy. Recovery of a virus from internal body fluids (buffy coat, cerebrospinal fluid, urine), vesicle fluid, or tissue from organs is strong evidence for an etiologic association. One should interpret cautiously, however, the isolation of agents, particularly enteroviruses, from throat swabs or stool specimens. In the latter instance, viral isolation data must be considered in conjunction with the clinical picture and serologic studies. Electron microscopic examination of vesicle fluid can demonstrate typical herpesvirus particles in both HSV and VZV infections but cannot distinguish between the two. Immunofluorescence and immunoperoxidase methods are available for many of the viruses to demonstrate viral antigen in cells scraped from lesions or in biopsy material. HBsAg is demonstrable in serum by radioimmunoassay or enzyme-linked immunosorbent assay.

Methods to amplify a particular segment of a viral genome, such as polymerase chain reaction, followed by probe or gel electrophoresis detection of the particular amplified gene are available for CMV, HBV, HSV, VZV, and enteroviruses.[322] In general, polymerase chain reaction and other amplification methods are more sensitive than is virus isolation and are quite specific but may not be widely available.

Although not as sensitive, immediate, or direct as isolation or detection of the viral agent, serologic studies often are the most readily available means for laboratory diagnosis of viral infection in the newborn infant. The TORCH screen for antibodies (*T*oxoplasma, *O*ther, *R*ubella, *C*ytomegalovirus, and *H*erpes simplex) was developed for this purpose and is available through university medical center and state health laboratories and the CDC in Atlanta. However, proper interpretation of serologic tests in newborn infants requires an understanding of the kinetics of the humoral immune response in the fetus and newborn infant as well as of the transplacental passage of antibodies from mother to fetus. Figure 76–4 illustrates the pattern of immunoglobulin concentrations in the serum of the fetus and newborn infant and in the older infant and child. Maternal IgG, containing antibody against viruses to which the mother has been exposed, passes transplacentally, beginning at midgestation. Peak levels are reached in the fetal serum at the time of birth (cord blood serum); these decline to undetectable levels in the infant by 5 to 6 months of age.

In contrast, maternal IgM antibody normally is not passed transplacentally. Because the fetus is in a "protected" environment and usually does not receive an antigenic challenge in utero, fetal immunoglobulin levels remain low and do not begin to rise until after birth, when exposure to a variety of antigens occurs. However, the fetus is capable of mounting a humoral immune response when exposed to an antigen (a virus) in utero. Elevated levels of fetal immunoglobulins, therefore, can be detected at birth in cord blood serum. Because maternal IgG is present in such high concentration in cord blood serum, assays for IgM are performed. A fetus challenged in utero with a virus can have specific IgM antibodies against the viral agent, as well as elevated levels of the total IgM fraction. There are three usual approaches to the serologic diagnosis of viral infection in the newborn infant: (1) assay of maternal serum and serum specimens from the infant at birth and at 5 to 6 months of age for antiviral antibody (predominantly IgG activity), (2) assay of neonatal serum for IgM antibody against a specific viral agent, and (3) assay of neonatal serum for quantitative IgM levels, a nonspecific indication of antigenic challenge in utero.

For purposes of illustration, the rubella hemagglutination inhibition titers of two mother/infant pairs are shown in Table 76–7. Both mothers were exposed to someone with a rubella-like rash during pregnancy. The first mother was susceptible, developed subclinical rubella, and delivered an infant with congenital rubella, whereas the second mother was immune and delivered an uninfected normal infant. The serum specimen obtained from the first mother at the time of exposure showed no detectable hemagglutination-inhibition titer, whereas the serum at delivery and 6 months postpartum showed high titers, indicating acute rubella virus infection during pregnancy. Both serum specimens from her infant, at birth and at 6 months of age, demonstrated rubella virus hemagglutination-inhibition antibodies at approximately the same level, indicating persistence of antibody formed by the infant and substantiating congenital infection. In the second mother, the rubella hemagglutination-inhibition titers remained unchanged in all three specimens. Her

TABLE 76–7. Mother and Infant Serologic Response in Congenital Rubella

Serum Specimens	Rubella Hemagglutination-Inhibition Antibody Titers			
	Mother	*Infant*	*Mother*	*Infant*
At exposure	<8	—	128	—
At birth	1024	1024	128	256
6 months post partum	1024	2048	250	<8
Comment	Congenital rubella		Passive transfer of antibody; no congenital rubella	

infant had evidence of transplacental maternal antibody in the serum obtained at birth but no detectable antibody at 6 months of age. Similar results could be expected from serologic studies with the other viral agents listed in Tables 76–1 and 76–2, not only in congenital infections but also in natal and postnatal infections in which there was primary viral infection in the mother. Even with natal infections in immune mothers and postnatal infections from nonmaternal sources, the serologic responses in the neonate would be similar to those shown in Table 76–7.

Although the presence of IgM antibodies in neonatal serum against a specific virus usually is considered to be diagnostic of infection with that agent, there can be both false-positive and false-negative results. False-positive results can occur with cross-reaction between viruses, especially the herpesviruses,[313] and the presence of rheumatoid factor (IgM antibody that binds to the Fc portion of IgG) in the serum.[78] False-negative results can occur because of a poor or delayed humoral immune response in the fetus/neonate. For example, CMV IgM antibody was present in the serum of only 70 per cent of congenitally infected infants, which was proved by isolation of virus from urine in the first few days of life.[410]

The performance of a quantitative IgM level on cord blood serum often has been recommended as a screening test for congenital viral infection. Values above 20 mg/dL are considered to be abnormal,[12] but the normal values in local laboratories should be used as a guide. Unfortunately, contamination of cord blood serum samples by maternal blood may occur in one-half to two-thirds of specimens.[9, 289] Contamination is determined by demonstrating that the cord blood serum IgA level, which also is not passed transplacentally, is higher than the IgM level. If one excludes contaminated specimens, the incidence of congenital infection in infants with an elevated IgM level is many times higher than in infants with normal levels. However, as many as 50 per cent of infants with a proven congenital infection have a normal IgM level, particularly those neonates with asymptomatic infection.[177] In two-thirds of infants with elevated IgM, infection with a specific etiologic agent could not be diagnosed.[9, 12] Therefore, there is a high rate of both false-positive and false-negative results. Finally, elevated IgM does not enable a specific etiologic diagnosis; it merely provides strong evidence for an intrauterine infection of some type. A more fruitful approach to the serologic diagnosis of neonatal viral infection, therefore, is the submission of maternal and neonatal serum specimens for the TORCH screen or, in selected instances, a single neonatal specimen for specific IgM antibodies. However, if an elevated quantitative IgM level is found in a neonate, further evaluation for the possibility of a congenital infection should be undertaken. Screening of cord blood serum for elevated IgM levels has been used successfully in research investigations evaluating the frequency of a variety of congenital infections.[12]

CYTOMEGALOVIRUS INFECTION

CMV is a ubiquitous agent that usually causes asymptomatic infection in the normal infant, child, or adult. However, patients with immature or impaired host defenses, such as the fetus, newborn infant, or immunosuppressed patient, may exhibit a variety of clinical manifestations during the acute infection and have a greater potential for long-term neurologic sequelae (see also Chapter 164, Acquired Cytomegalovirus Infection).[11, 116, 147, 174]

Microbiology and Epidemiology

CMV is a member of the herpesvirus group, which includes HSV, VZV, and Epstein-Barr virus. There are several strains of CMV that differ antigenically, and so an individual could have more than one CMV infection.[11, 116, 147] Human CMV is limited to the human host and grows only in human cells in tissue culture.[177] Distribution is worldwide, and there is no predilection for either sex or a particular season of the year.[11, 116, 147] Studies of antibody prevalence and virus isolation have indicated that there are two peak ages for acquisition of infection: (1) infancy and early childhood and (2) early adulthood (in the sexually active).[147, 480] Infection rates are higher, and exposure to the virus occurs earlier in life in developing countries, lower socioeconomic groups in industrial nations, and Asian populations.[147] The major source of infection of young infants is the mother, whereas transmission in the day care setting is an important source for older infants and toddlers.[333] In the young adult, intimate interpersonal contact appears to be necessary for transmission.

Usual sites for isolation of virus are the urine, cervix, and saliva,[147] but CMV also has been recovered from amniotic fluid,[113] semen,[252, 253] breast milk,[130, 185] feces,[103] and autopsy and biopsy tissues.[177] Excretion of virus in urine, saliva, or the cervix may be prolonged after primary infection, particularly with the congenital disease.[11, 116, 177, 405, 409] There also may be intermittent, recurring shedding in a significant proportion of seropositive young adults.[359, 405, 409] Despite this prevalence of virus excretion, CMV appears to be of low communicability.[147] Beyond the neonatal period, infection appears to require prolonged or intimate contact and presumably is transmitted through oropharyngeal or genital secretions.[177] It has been assumed that CMV may be transmitted venereally because of the frequency of isolation of virus from genital secretions and because the prevalence of antibody is higher in sexually active population groups.[11, 116] Finally, transmission of CMV by blood transfusion has been documented, particularly when there are multiple blood donors.[4, 147]

Prenatal transmission of CMV to the fetus presumably is associated with maternal viremia and transplacental passage of the virus, perhaps within virus-infected leukocytes.[11, 116, 177] An important observation is that congenital CMV infection occurs in infants of mothers known to be immune to CMV, indicating that transplacental transmission is possible despite circulating antibody in maternal serum.[403, 405] In addition, mothers have delivered more than one congenitally infected infant in successive pregnancies.[405, 406] Analysis of CMV isolates obtained from the same mothers on repeated occasions antigenically and genetically are identical, whereas the strains from different mothers are not.[203] In addition, the strains obtained from mother/congenitally infected infant pairs, as well as congenitally infected siblings, are identical. These results suggest that most, if not all, CMV transmission from immune mothers to their fetuses or newborns is the result of reactivated latent infection rather than acquisition of a new strain of CMV.

Natal transmission of CMV results from the exposure of the neonate to infected genital secretions at the time of delivery.[11, 359, 360] If the mother is excreting virus at the time of delivery, 40 per cent of exposed infants become infected.[359] The level of maternal antibody did not influence the frequency or time of onset of infection in the neonate. The usual incubation period for natal infection is 5 to 6 weeks.[360]

The importance of breast milk and blood transfusion as sources for postnatal acquisition of CMV was mentioned earlier in the section Frequency of Infection in the Mother and Neonate. Although nosocomial transmission of CMV from baby to baby in the neonatal intensive care unit has been documented,[397] this is rare.

Pathogenesis and Pathology

Congenital infection results from transplacental transmission during maternal viremia.[11, 177] However, CMV placentitis may occur without transplacental transmission of virus.[186] After transplacental transmission, the virus spreads through the fetus by the hematogenous route. It is likely that severity of congenital disease in the neonate correlates with intrauterine infection at an earlier gestational age.[401] With the exception of blood transfusion–associated infection, natal and postnatal infection with CMV usually is acquired secondary to challenge of the nasopharynx or oropharynx of the infant with virus from infected maternal genital secretions or breast milk.[11, 116, 177] Replication of virus in the neonate occurs in the mucosa of the respiratory or gastrointestinal tracts, with subsequent viremic spread to target organs. With blood transfusion–associated infection, virus is inoculated directly into the blood stream. The major target organs are the central nervous system, eyes, lungs, liver, and kidneys.[11, 177] It is of interest that overt disease in the neonate appears to be associated more commonly with the hematogenous route of inoculation: transplacental infection or infection secondary to blood transfusion.

CMV appears to have a particular affinity for epithelial cells, ependymal cells lining the ventricles of the brain, and the organ of Corti and the neurons of the eighth nerve.[177, 404] The characteristic pathologic features of CMV infection are cytolysis, focal necrosis and inflammatory response, the formation of enlarged cells with intranuclear inclusions (cytomegalic cells), and the production of multinucleated giant cells.[177] Healing results in fibrosis and often calcification, which cause structural damage to developing organs in the fetus. Damage may continue after birth because of persistent postnatal viral replication.[11] Replication of CMV in epithelial cells of blood vessels may result in vascular damage and secondary structural defects. Intrauterine growth retardation present in the symptomatic congenital infection appears to be the result of reduction in numbers of cells in various organs, rather than diminution of cell size.[301] Abnormalities resulting from faulty organogenesis secondary to CMV infection are limited primarily to the brain and include microcephaly, optic atrophy, aplasia of various parts of the brain, and microphthalmia.[175, 177] Although a variety of congenital malformations outside the central nervous system have been observed in infants with congenital CMV infection, it is likely that these are coincidental rather than true teratogenic effects of the virus.[175] The extraneural defects in infants with congenital CMV infection have been infrequent, sporadic, and diverse. These include a variety of heart lesions, club foot deformities, indirect inguinal hernias, high arched palate, and hypospadias.[11, 175]

The fetus is capable of a humoral immune response to CMV, as evidenced by the presence of elevated IgM levels and specific CMV IgM antibody in cord serum.[11, 177, 361, 410] Excessive production of IgM and IgG in the presence of virus replication during the early postnatal course of congenital CMV has resulted in the formation of circulating immune complexes and rheumatoid factor, providing the potential risk for immune complex tissue damage.[411] The factors contributing to prolonged replication and excretion of CMV in involved infants are not understood fully, but it does not appear to be a matter of immunologic tolerance, because infants do produce specific antibody against CMV.[11] However, abnormalities of other aspects of the immune response of congenitally infected infants have been observed, including a decreased lymphocyte blastogenesis and immune interferon production in response to CMV antigen,[358, 413] a decreased percentage of T cells in the peripheral blood,[371] and a diminished interferon response in leukocytes challenged with Newcastle disease virus in vitro.[136] The degree of suppression of these responses appears to correlate with the presence and amount of virus excretion and the severity of the disease.[358, 413] Further investigations are required to determine the contribution of these immunologic aberrations to the pathogenesis of congenital CMV infection.

Clinical Manifestations

From 90 to 95 per cent of neonates with congenital CMV infection are asymptomatic in the neonatal period. Babies born to mothers with primary CMV infection during pregnancy are much more likely to be symptomatic as neonates than are newborns of mothers with recurrent infection.[5, 11, 116, 149, 346, 403] The clinical manifestations present in those with overt disease in the neonatal period are shown in Figure 76–2. Typical clinical features include hepatomegaly, splenomegaly, jaundice, petechiae or purpura, pneumonia, microcephaly, chorioretinitis, and cerebral calcifications. The enlargement of the liver and spleen is due to mild hepatitis, a reticuloendothelial response to chronic infection, and extramedullary hematopoiesis.[177] Hepatitis is associated with direct- and indirect-reacting hyperbilirubinemia and mild elevation of the liver enzymes.[177] Liver biopsy specimens have revealed local infiltration and necrosis, multinucleated giant cells, large inclusion-bearing cells, cholangitis, fatty metamorphosis, interstitial fibrosis, and bile stasis.[11, 116, 177] Although hepatomegaly and mild alteration of liver function tests may persist for several months after birth, there is no evidence of severe chronic liver disease.[177] Petechiae and purpura are the result of thrombocytopenia, which usually resolves within a few weeks or months.[177]

Involvement of the central nervous system by CMV results in the most severe sequelae of the disease. The most common ocular abnormalities are chorioretinitis, strabismus, and optic atrophy.[177] Although microphthalmia, cataracts, and other eye abnormalities have been observed, they are rare.[175] The associated chorioretinitis cannot be differentiated from that due to congenital toxoplasmosis, either in appearance or location in the retina.[177] Microcephaly may not be present at birth but may become apparent at 1 year of age or later, when differences in growth rates between the brain and somatic tissues are observed. When associated with cerebral calcification, microcephaly carries a high probability of psychomotor retardation. The cerebral calcifications typically are periventricular, a pattern that may be distinguished from the more diffuse pattern observed in congenital toxoplasmosis.

Most naturally acquired natal and postnatal CMV infections in newborn infants are asymptomatic. However, hepatosplenomegaly, pneumonitis, and lymphadenopathy have been noted in some infants.[243, 457, 479] An important clinical syndrome associated with multiple blood transfusions in lowbirth weight infants in newborn intensive care units has been recognized in recent years.[4, 31, 475, 478] Eighty-eight per cent of babies had hepatosplenomegaly, a "septic" appearance, deterioration of respiratory status, a peculiar gray pallor, and atypical lymphocytosis.[4, 31, 478] Twenty-four per cent died, and CMV was thought to be causal or contributory.

Diagnosis and Differential Diagnosis

The definitive means of diagnosing CMV infection in the mother is isolation of virus from the cervix or urine. However, primary infection cannot be differentiated from recurrent infection unless serologic studies are performed. Because most maternal CMV infections are asymptomatic, acute and convalescent sera bracketing an "illness" rarely are available. Primary CMV infection during pregnancy has been documented by demonstration of IgG seroconversion with sera obtained before or during early pregnancy and at delivery or by detection of anti-CMV IgM in a single specimen.[6, 7, 166, 242, 309, 345, 410]

Because the signs and symptoms of symptomatic CMV infection in newborns so often overlap with those in other diseases during this period of life, definitive diagnosis requires the use of laboratory tests. Isolation of virus from infants within the first 3 weeks of life is considered proof of congenital infection and is the most sensitive means for diagnosis.[11, 116] The usual site for isolation of CMV is urine, but virus has been recovered from cerebrospinal fluid, saliva, buffy coat, and biopsy and postmortem tissue.[177] Congenitally infected infants are known to excrete virus for several years after birth.[177] Isolation of virus in an infant a few months of age does not, by itself, differentiate between natal or postnatal infection and congenital infection, unless negative cultures have been obtained previously. CMV DNA in the cerebrospinal fluid of congenitally infected infants as detected by polymerase chain reaction methods correlates with abnormal neurologic outcome.[438]

If serologic tests that measure predominantly IgG are used, serial serum specimens from birth are required to differentiate congenital from natal or postnatal infection. One observes maintenance of a stable antibody titer over the first 6 months of life in infants with a congenital infection. In contrast, with natal and postnatal infection, there is a drop in antibody titer during the first 2 to 3 months of life as maternal passive antibody declines, followed by a rise by 5 to 6 months of age.[360, 408] If the infant is not evaluated until several months of age and serum specimens from earlier life are not available, it may not be possible to determine whether the infection is congenital, natal, or postnatal in origin.

Examination for inclusion-bearing cells in the urine may be performed, but this test yields positive results in only 20 to 50 per cent of known virus-positive cases.[11, 116] Typical intranuclear inclusions may be seen in biopsy tissue or in megakaryocytes of bone marrow aspirates,[11, 116, 177] but virus may be isolated from tissue when these pathologic findings are absent.

The major diseases to consider in the differential diagnosis include congenital rubella, congenital toxoplasmosis, erythroblastosis fetalis, disseminated HSV infection, neonatal sepsis, congenital syphilis, and enterovirus infections.[177] The presence of congenital heart disease and cataracts suggests rubella, and chorioretinitis suggests toxoplasmosis, but definitive diagnosis depends on the laboratory. In uncomplicated erythroblastosis, the direct bilirubin and liver function study results remain normal. Vesicular skin lesions suggest HSV or VZV infection. Positive blood cultures confirm the diagnosis of neonatal sepsis. It is unusual for congenital CMV infection to be complicated by bacterial sepsis in the newborn.[177] Congenital syphilis is suggested by the presence of osteochondritis and epiphysitis on radiographs of the long bones. Darkfield examination of spirochete-laden nasal secretions in infants with rhinitis or serologic tests confirms the diagnosis. Neonatal enterovirus infections are seasonal, associated with maternal symptoms of enteroviral disease, and characterized by aseptic meningitis, gastroenteritis, or both.

Treatment

Although treatment with idoxuridine,[94] 5-fluorodeoxyuridine,[342] cytosine arabinoside,[235, 274, 342] adenine arabinoside,[34, 86] interferon inducers,[342] human interferon,[26, 137] and acyclovir[341] has been tried in infants with congenital CMV infection, the only effect was transient alteration of viral excretion. There was little or no effect on the clinical course of the disease. Because these agents have appreciable side effects, they should not be used in the treatment of CMV disease in neonates.

Ganciclovir has been licensed for the treatment of life- or sight-threatening CMV disease in immunosuppressed adults.[65] The combination of ganciclovir plus CMV hyperimmune intravenous immunoglobulin has reduced mortality in CMV pneumonitis.[135, 354] Use of ganciclovir to treat infants with congenital CMV disease has been reported,[193, 441] but clinical trials in larger numbers of infants are required to determine safety and efficacy.[116] It is hoped that the use of ganciclovir, perhaps in combination with other forms of antiviral therapy, will retard the progression of central nervous system damage known to occur in congenitally infected infants.[11, 116]

Prognosis

The major long-term sequelae of neonatal CMV infection are mental retardation, hearing loss, and microcephaly.[149, 178, 361, 404] The worst prognosis occurs in neonates born to mothers with primary CMV infection during pregnancy; in infants with symptoms at birth, particularly those of the central nervous system; in infants with microcephaly, intracranial calcification, or both; and in neonates who have elevated quantitative IgM or in whom CMV-specific IgM is present.[11, 116, 149, 167, 177, 244] Of symptomatic, congenitally infected neonates, approximately 30 per cent die during infancy, and up to 90 per cent of survivors have some evidence of central nervous system abnormality, such as microcephaly, impaired intellect or development, neuromuscular disorders (seizures, spasticity, hemiparesis), sensorineural hearing loss, and ocular abnormalities (usually chorioretinitis).[93, 149, 334, 400, 463] Other studies have found less frequent and less severe sequelae in infants born to mothers with primary CMV infections,[165, 244, 368] perhaps because infants were identified by screening of urine for virus rather than serum for IgM antibody. Elevated serum IgM is known to be associated with a poor prognosis.[167] Neurologic sequelae of congenital CMV disease may progress after the first year of life.[52]

Ninety to 95 per cent of infants with congenital CMV infection are asymptomatic in the neonatal period. Several long-term follow-up studies have indicated that these infants may suffer neurologic damage as a result of their infection. The following abnormalities were noted in infected infants when compared with matched control children: IQ less than 90 (32 vs. 16 per cent), significant hearing loss (23 vs. 9 per cent), predicted school failure (36 vs. 14 per cent), and microcephaly (15 vs. 5 per cent).[178, 361] In addition, approximately 6 per cent of infants with asymptomatic congenital infection will have some visual defect.[404] It initially was thought that babies born to mothers with recurrent CMV infection during pregnancy would be asymptomatic at birth and would be free of neurologic sequelae on follow-up.[403] However, a few infants may have neonatal disease, and subsequent neurologic abnormalities occur in up to 8 per cent of infants.[5, 149]

Up to one-third of neonates who acquire CMV natally from maternal cervical secretions may have acute disease associated with the onset of viruria regardless of birth weight.[243, 479] However, birth weight and age of onset of viral excretion appear to influence neurologic sequelae significantly. Full-term neonates with natally acquired CMV do not have significantly altered behavioral, neurologic, audiologic, speech, and language examinations on long-term follow-up compared with uninfected controls.[244] In contrast, infants with birth weight less than 2000 g and onset of CMV excretion before 8 weeks of age have associated severe cardiopulmonary disease during the neonatal intensive care unit stay (perhaps because of CMV worsening the pulmonary disease) and a significantly greater percentage of severe handicaps on long-term follow-up than do matched controls.[332] The relationships between low birth weight, early onset of CMV excretion, lower levels of transplacental antibody, and more severe cardiopulmonary disease and their contribution to neurologic sequelae require further evaluation, but it does appear that natal acquisition of CMV may contribute to sequelae in selected situations. CMV disease acquired from blood transfusion in very low birth weight infants also may contribute to neurologic sequelae.[4, 11, 478]

Prevention

Although limited clinical trials have begun with two live attenuated CMV vaccines (AD-169 and Towne strains), many questions remain to be answered before these vaccines can be considered for use in preventing congenital or natal CMV infection.[11, 116, 177] First, the attenuated live virus vaccine strains could be oncogenic. Second, the duration of protection by vaccine-induced immunity against infection with the wild virus is not known. Third, whether the vaccine virus itself could be passed transplacentally and cause congenital infection in humans is not known. Fourth, because congenital infection is known to occur in mothers with natural immunity, how can one expect vaccine-induced immunity to provide protection? Despite these questions, one can anticipate that evaluation of the CMV vaccines will continue and that answers will come.

Because of the frequency of congenital, natal, and postnatal CMV infection in infants and because of the prolonged excretion of the virus in urine and saliva, there has been concern about potential nosocomial spread of this agent among hospital personnel and hospitalized infants. However, the rate of transmission of CMV in the hospital setting appears to be low,[147] and prolonged or intimate contact appears to be necessary for spread.[11, 116, 147] Nevertheless, neonates with known CMV infection should be isolated.

The frequency of new blood transfusion–associated CMV infection in low birth weight infants in neonatal intensive care units may be reduced by using CMV-seronegative blood donors,[2] but this excludes 40 to 75 per cent of the population.[55] Other preventive measures include use of frozen, deglycerolized red cells[55, 427] and use of donors who are CMV IgG antibody–positive but lack IgM, anti–early antigen antibody, or both.[251, 260]

RUBELLA

Rubella usually is a mild, often subclinical disease involving school age children and young adults. However, rubella virus also can cross the placenta, infect the fetus, and cause fetal death or congenital malformations. Since the original observations by Gregg[164] associating maternal rubella with the birth of offspring with defects of the eye and heart, rubella has been the prototype for congenital viral infection (see also Chapter 177, Rubella).

Microbiology and Epidemiology

Rubella virus is an enveloped RNA virus in the family *Togaviridae* and has only a single antigenic type.[98] Rubella virus grows in tissue culture from a variety of animal species, but commonly, African green monkey kidney cells are used for isolation in the diagnostic virology laboratory.[83] Several serologic tests are available, including complement fixation, hemagglutination inhibition, immunofluorescence, radioimmunoassay, and enzyme immunoassay.[83, 177, 189] Although hemagglutination inhibition[419] is the gold standard, many diagnostic virology laboratories now are using commercially available enzyme-linked immunosorbent assay or fluorescent assay kits.[83]

Rubella is worldwide in distribution. Human beings are the only host, and transmission is from person to person.[98, 465] In the era before rubella vaccine, epidemics occurred at 6- to 9-year intervals, and pandemics occurred every 10 to 20 years.[465] Since licensure of the vaccine in 1969, this epidemic pattern has been interrupted; the last major outbreak in the United States was in 1964.[33, 320] The peak seasonal incidence is in the spring.[465] In the prevaccine era, the peak age incidence was between 5 and 14 years of age,[465] but in the mid-1970s, the peak age was 15 to 19 years.[320] Currently, there is no peak age. Approximately 5 to 25 per cent of women of child-bearing age lack rubella antibody and are susceptible to primary infection.[33, 71, 177] The attack rate for rubella in susceptible populations with prolonged intimate exposure is high—95 to 100 percent.[98, 465] The frequency of transmission after brief exposure, however, is low.[98, 465] The frequency of subclinical infections is much higher in adults than in children, although some serologically diagnosed infections in adults actually may be reinfections rather than primary disease.[199, 200, 378]

The incubation period for acquired rubella is 16 to 21 days.[378] Virus may be isolated from the throat from 1 week before to 2 weeks after the onset of rash. Rubella virus infection may be subclinical in from one-third to one-half of children and in from one-half to two-thirds of adults.[199, 378] Rubella hemagglutination-inhibition antibody is detectable in the serum within 2 to 3 days after the onset of the rash, with peak titers being reached in 3 to 4 weeks.[83, 177] Complement-fixation antibody rises more slowly, reaching a peak titer 4 to 6 weeks after the rash.[177] Primary rubella virus infection is associated with an initial response in IgM-specific antibody, followed by an increase in IgG antibody.[177] Reinfection with rubella virus is known to occur, and rates are higher in vaccine-immune than in naturally immune subjects.[199] The vast majority of congenital rubella virus infections occur with primary infections, but a few cases have been reported after reinfection.[80, 132, 177, 362] If there is no evidence of rubella-specific IgM in cases of subclinical reinfection during pregnancy, the fetus is unlikely to be at risk.[177]

Pathogenesis and Pathology

Transplacental infection of the fetus with rubella virus occurs secondary to maternal viremia during the course of primary infection.[10] Fetal infection appears to result from embolization of pieces of necrotic placental vascular endothelium.[284] However, involvement of the placenta with rubella virus does not result always in fetal infection, particularly after the first trimester.[10, 177] After maternal immunity, the next most critical factor determining the frequency of fetal infection and severity of disease in the neonate is the time during gestation that rubella virus infection occurs.[177] Studies of the frequency of fetal infection and congenital defects according to the gestational age at the time of maternal infection have utilized more sensitive methods to detect maternal and neonatal infection and long-term follow-up to detect abnormalities that were not apparent during infancy.[286] These studies indicated higher fetal infection rates than previously realized: 90 per cent during the first 11 weeks, 50 per cent during 11 to 20 weeks, 37 per cent from 20 to 35 weeks, and 100 per cent during the last month. The congenital defect rate was 100 per cent for the first 11 weeks, 30 per cent during 11 to 20 weeks, and none thereafter. Neonatal purpura and cataracts or glaucoma are observed when maternal rubella occurs during the first 2 months of gestation; congenital heart disease, during the first 3 months; deafness and neurologic deficit, during the first 4 months; and retinopathy, during the first 5 months.[177, 286, 439]

Excretion of rubella virus from the throat of congenitally infected infants may continue for several months after birth, and the virus has been recovered from tissues up to several years later.[10, 99, 177] Persistence of viral replication after birth may result in continuing damage of involved tissues. In fact, hearing loss and neurologic deficits may appear long after birth in children previously considered well, or the clinical severity of these sequelae actually may worsen as the child is followed.[85, 99, 118, 177]

Rubella virus is a proven teratogenic viral agent—that is, one that results in congenital malformations.[326] Hence, knowledge of the mechanisms by which rubella virus causes deformities may lead to basic understanding of the pathogenesis of these malformations. Rubella virus is noncytolytic in certain tissues, in that it does not destroy the cells in which it replicates. This characteristic, if manifested in the fetus, would tend to allow survival but result in disordered function of cells, tissues, and organs. On the other hand, selective cell destruction also may occur in fetal tissues.

In pathologic studies of therapeutically aborted, rubella-infected fetuses, scattered foci of necrotic cellular damage without inflammatory infiltrate were noted in endothelial cells of blood vessels and in myocardial cells.[431] These rubella-induced defects could result in defective formation or function of developing tissues by direct cellular destruction or by hypoxic damage secondary to blood vessel obliteration. For example, alteration of the elastic or muscle fibers in the ductus arteriosus could result in failure of postnatal ductus closure. Studies of tissue obtained from infants with rubella syndrome and maintained in culture show that the cells persistently were infected with rubella virus and had a decreased growth rate and shortened survival time.[353] Naeye and Blanc[302] noted that the growth retardation in infants with the rubella syndrome was the result of decreased numbers of cells in the organs. This impaired cellular growth, if it occurred during a crucial phase in cardiac development, for example, could result in such cardiac anomalies as septal defects.

Increased numbers of chromosome breaks have been noted in leukocyte cultures of children with congenital rubella.[315] It is possible that this chromosomal injury results in cell loss during rapid organ development and is, in part, responsible for the congenital anomalies. It also is possible that persistence of virus may result in continuing cell destruction or immunopathologic damage to tissues.[177] In addition, two studies have demonstrated circulating rubella antigen-antibody complexes in 10 infants with congenital rubella with late-onset manifestations: interstitial pneumonia, hepatosplenomegaly, skin rash, lymphocytic meningitis, and rapid neurologic deterioration.[51, 426] IgG levels were low and IgM levels elevated, with a diminished number of T cells and an increased proportion of B cells. It was postulated that a delayed maturation of the immune response in congenital rubella might predispose to persistent antigenemia complexed with IgM and deposition of circulating immune complexes in tissues. Finally, antibodies against thyroid microsomes or thyroglobulin were found in a much larger percentage of children with the congenital rubella syndrome than in control subjects.[89] A significant number of the congenital rubella patients with thyroid antibodies also had thyroid dysfunction. These observations suggest that autoimmunity, induced in some way by persistent infection with rubella virus, plays a role in the late-onset endocrine dysfunctions that occur in children and young adults with the congenital rubella syndrome.

Specific pathologic lesions in infants with congenital rubella depend on the gestational age at the time of infection and the particular organs that are involved. One common finding is necrosis of vascular endothelium, which may be accompanied by damage to organs secondary to vascular obstruction.[284, 431] Diffuse intimal changes have been observed in the pulmonary and systemic arteries, as well as the ductus arteriosus.[284] Focal inflammation and necrosis have been seen in the myocardium[231] and the structures of the inner ear.[177]

The fetus is capable of an immune response to rubella virus: specific IgM and occasionally IgA have been observed in fetal and cord blood specimens.[177] In fact, hypergammaglobulinemia may be observed during early life in some infants with congenital rubella.[173] On the other hand, hypogammaglobulinemia has been noted in a few infants.[173, 340] In 10 to 20 per cent of infants with congenital rubella, hemagglutination-inhibition antibody declines to undetectable levels between 1 and 4 years of age.[99, 180] Several of these infants failed to respond to immunization with rubella vaccine.[96, 177] In fact, infants with congenital rubella have been reinfected with rubella virus later in life.[282] Several defects in cell-mediated immunity have been observed in infants with congenital rubella. These include diminished responsiveness of peripheral blood leukocytes to phytohemagglutinin and diminished lymphocyte transformation, interferon production, and synthesis of leukocyte migration inhibitory factor in response to challenge with rubella virus antigen.[66, 319] Normal responses were observed in healthy, seropositive children and adults. It is presumed, but has not been proved, that these abnormalities in cell-mediated immunity play a role in persistent viral excretion in congenitally infected infants.

Clinical Manifestations

Although typical clinical features of rubella may occur in the pregnant woman, as many as one-half to two-thirds of these infections are subclinical.[177, 380] Typical features that might occur in the symptomatic postpubertal woman include fever, rash, posterior auricular and postoccipital adenopathy, and arthralgia or arthritis.[177]

As many as two-thirds of infants with proven congenital rubella may be asymptomatic in the neonatal period.[372] However, almost three-quarters of these infants with silent infection in early life developed evidence of long-term sequelae within the first 5 years of life.[372] The clinical manifestations of the congenital rubella syndrome vary highly, not only with regard to the specific features but also in relation to the age during which the specific feature presents. The collected features may be divided into three broad categories: (1) transient—those that are present in the neonatal period and clear after a few months, such as thrombocytopenia and hepatitis, (2) permanent—those major malformations that persist and may even worsen as the child grows older, such as congenital heart lesions, cataracts, or hearing loss, and (3) developmental—those aspects that do not emerge until childhood or young adulthood, such as behavioral disorders or endocrine dysfunctions.[96, 177, 381] This categorization of abnormal features may be useful in the prognosis and management of these children.

The manifestations of congenital rubella that are symptomatic in the neonatal period, combined from several series,[97, 198, 230, 265, 367] are illustrated in Figure 76–2. The low birth weight of infants with rubella syndrome is thought to result from intrauterine growth retardation; even when born prematurely, the infant often is small for estimated gestational age. The frequency of purpura in most series ranges from 15 to 50 per cent. Thrombocytopenia almost always was present in association with the purpura and usually resolved spontaneously in the first month of life. Neonatal thrombocytopenic purpura is a poor prognostic sign because it usually occurs in severely affected infants with multiple manifestations. Thirty-five per cent of 58 patients with purpura in one series[97] died during the first year, in contrast with a mortality rate during the first 18 months of only 13 per cent for patients from the entire series. Although the thrombocytopenia frequently was profound, death due to hemorrhage was rare.

Direct involvement of the liver by rubella virus results in neonatal hepatitis, as evidenced by hepatomegaly, predominantly direct-reacting hyperbilirubinemia, and elevation of liver enzymes.[140] Pathologic studies usually demonstrate hepatocellular disease with necrosis, giant cell formation, bile stasis, and fibrosis, but extrahepatic biliary obstruction also has been demonstrated.[420]

Congenital heart disease occurs frequently and usually is detectable in the neonatal period, although specific lesions may not be defined until later in life. The most commonly occurring lesions are patent ductus arteriosus, pulmonary artery stenosis, valvular pulmonic stenosis, aortic stenosis, aberrant subclavian vessels, and ventricular septal defect.[99] Evidence of active myocardial disease has been noted in some infants.[231]

Interstitial pneumonia with cough, tachypnea, and breathlessness as the major manifestation of congenital rubella has been reported.[337] Six of seven patients with this syndrome died in the first year of life as a result of their pulmonary disease. Cardiac abnormalities also were present but were believed not to be significant either clinically or from autopsy findings. Microscopic studies revealed acute to subacute chronic interstitial pneumonitis. Rubella virus was isolated from four of four lung specimens cultured.

Although cataracts are the most characteristic ocular lesion in rubella syndrome, they may not be visualized until after the neonatal period. The retinopathy is described as widespread, mottled or blotchy, black pigmentary deposits of variable size and location: the "salt and pepper" retinitis.[236] Retinal function usually is not affected adversely. The frequency of occurrence of retinopathy in the combined data from six series of children followed for several years was 36 per cent.

Bone lesions are another finding in congenital rubella in the neonatal period. Radiographic studies reveal small linear areas of radiolucency and increased bone density in a longitudinal axis of the metaphyseal area in the long bones of the lower and upper extremities.[367] The abnormality results from disturbances in laying down and calcification of osteoid and usually resolves by 2 to 3 months of age.

Central nervous system involvement frequently is evident in symptomatic infants. Lethargy, irritability, disturbances of tone, and a bulging fontanelle are common. One or more seizures occurred in 27 of 100 infants in one series.[118, 119] However, these usually occurred after the neonatal period. In the majority of infants with central nervous system involvement, cerebrospinal fluid protein is elevated; increase in cell counts is less frequent. Rubella virus may be isolated from the cerebrospinal fluid; in one series, 25 per cent of 99 cerebrospinal fluid specimens from patients with central nervous system symptoms obtained during the first 3 months of life were positive.[118, 119] The extent of impairment at 18 months of age was not predictable readily on the basis of clinical symptoms or virus isolation in the first few weeks of life. However, severe involvement was more frequent in infants with seizures and with high levels of cerebrospinal fluid protein in the first few months of life.[118, 119] It is important to emphasize the chronic nature of congenital rubella infection and to note that although the majority of infants may be asymptomatic in the neonatal period, as many as 70 per cent developed evidence of disease on follow-up examinations.[177]

Diagnosis and Differential Diagnosis

Because a significant proportion of maternal rubella cases is subclinical and other diseases may mimic symptomatic rubella, definitive diagnosis in the mother depends on the laboratory. Although rubella virus may be isolated from the throat during the acute phase of the illness, such a culture frequently is not a practical means of establishing the diagnosis. Widely used serologic tests include hemagglutination inhibition, enzyme-linked immunosorbent assay, and fluorescent assay.[83] Susceptible persons lack IgG antibody. Detectable antibody is present in the blood within a few days after the onset of the rash, and peak titers are reached within 2 to 3 weeks. If serum specimens are not available until some time after the illness, complement fixation antibody titers may be useful because peak titers are not reached for 4 to 6 weeks after the rash.[177] If only a single specimen is available, rubella-specific IgM antibody may be demonstrable using immunofluorescence methods.[83, 189] These antibodies peak 3 to 6 weeks after infection and persist for several months.[177] Although culturing of amniotic fluid for virus and sampling of fetal blood for antibody have been used in the attempt to make antenatal diagnosis of congenital rubella, both false-positive (viral infection but no fetal damage) and false-negative results may be obtained.

The most characteristic clinical features of congenital rubella are congenital heart disease, cataracts, microphthalmia, corneal opacity, glaucoma, and radiolucent bone lesions. In infants with these classic features, the clinical diagnosis correlates with laboratory confirmation of congenital rubella 80 per cent of the time.[177] However, many of the features, such as low birth weight, hepatosplenomegaly, icterus, and petechiae/purpura, overlap with those found in other infectious diseases of the newborn, and definitive diagnosis requires laboratory confirmation. Rubella virus usually is isolated from the throat or urine, but it also has been recovered from conjunctival swabs, cerebrospinal fluid, feces, bone marrow, and circulating leukocytes.[177] The diagnosis of congenital rubella is made more commonly by serologic means. Because rubella hemagglutination-inhibition antibody is passed transplacentally, levels in serum obtained early in the neonatal period mimic those of the mother. Persistence of hemagglutination-inhibition antibody in the serum of infants 4 to 6 months of age can be considered diagnostic of congenital rubella when the clinical picture is compatible.[177] The presence of specific IgM antibody in a single serum specimen obtained from an infant early in life also can be diagnostic.

The principal diseases to consider in the differential diagnosis include congenital CMV infection, congenital toxoplasmosis, erythroblastosis fetalis, disseminated herpes simplex, neonatal sepsis, and congenital syphilis. Infants with congenital CMV infection more commonly have chorioretinitis and microcephaly, whereas congenital heart disease and eye malformations are unusual. Infants with symptomatic congenital toxoplasmosis have chorioretinitis, hydrocephaly, and cerebral calcifications but not congenital heart disease, cataracts, or glaucoma. In uncomplicated erythroblastosis, the direct bilirubin and liver function studies remain normal. Disseminated herpes simplex should be differentiated on the basis of the characteristic vesicular skin lesions or the presence of keratoconjunctivitis. Positive blood cultures identify neonatal sepsis. The bone lesions in congenital syphilis are associated with periosteal new bone formation; rhinitis and lesions of the skin and mucous membranes also are seen. Because of overlapping clinical features, however, definitive diagnosis requires laboratory confirmation.

Treatment

There is no specific antiviral therapy for congenital rubella. Although amantadine hydrochloride inhibits rubella virus in vitro, treatment with this drug was shown not to alter the clinical or virologic course of the disease.[340]

Prognosis

The most common long-term sequelae of congenital rubella are listed in Table 76–8. Deafness is the most common finding and may not be apparent for several months to several years after birth. In 15 to 20 per cent of children, it may be the only abnormality detectable.[99, 177] Approximately half of the children may have absent or hyporeactive responses to tests of vestibular function.[288] The hearing loss may be profound and thus a major contributor to speech impairment and learning disability. The most common cardiac lesions in 87 catheterized patients with congenital rubella were patent ductus arteriosus in 78 per cent, right pulmonary artery stenosis in 70 per cent, left pulmonary artery stenosis in 56 per cent, valvular pulmonic stenosis in 40 per cent, mild aortic valvular stenosis in 14 per cent, aberrant subclavian artery in 11 per cent, and ventricular septal defect in 10 per cent.[99] In approximately 50 per cent of children with mental retardation, the deficiency is moderate to severe. Although retinopathy is present in a significant proportion of infants, it does not appear to interfere with vision. Cataracts, of course, certainly can interfere with the development of vision, and these should be removed surgically at an early age. Most fatalities from congenital rubella occur in the first year of life and are associated with severe congenital heart disease and general debility from multiple defects.[99]

TABLE 76–8. Frequency of Defects in Children with Congenital Rubella

Defect	Percentage of Cases
No defect	19
Deafness	67
Congenital heart disease	48
Psychomotor retardation	45
Retinopathy	39
Cataracts	29
Neonatal purpura	23
Glaucoma	3
Deaths	16

Data from 376 children studied in the New York Rubella Birth Defect Project. (Modified from Cooper, L. Z., Ziring, P. R., Ockerse, A. B., et al.: Rubella: Clinical manifestations and management. Am. J. Dis. Child. *118*:18–29, 1969.)

Long-term follow-up evaluation of children with congenital rubella syndrome is available.[85, 118, 119, 282, 381] Among 205 children examined at 8 to 9 years of age, 26 per cent had severe mental retardation, 18 per cent had reactive behavior disorder, 12 per cent showed behavior disorder with neurologic damage, and 6 per cent displayed autism. Of 29 children with neurologic manifestations of congenital rubella between birth and 18 months but with normal intelligence, 93 per cent had hearing loss when examined at 9 to 12 years of age; 61 per cent, poor balance; 54 per cent, muscular weakness; 52 per cent, learning deficits; 48 per cent, behavioral disturbance; and 41 per cent, deficits in tactile perception. Head circumference appears to correlate poorly with intellectual function in patients with congenital rubella.[270] Diabetes mellitus has been observed in 15 to 20 per cent of adults with congenital rubella.[283] Onset usually is in the second or third decade of life. Other late manifestations[381] of the congenital rubella syndrome include chronic lymphocytic thyroiditis,[484] thymic hypoplasia,[152] abnormal dermatoglyphics,[99] chromosomal abnormalities,[21] pancreatic insufficiency,[121] and progressive panencephalitis.[437, 449] As one might expect, severity of the long-term sequelae appears to correlate with the number of defects observed in early life.[85, 99]

Prevention

The development and use of rubella vaccine in the United States clearly has reduced the frequency of congenital rubella.[33, 192, 320] The target population in the United States has been preschool and school age children, whereas in Great Britain, selective vaccination of 11- to 14-year-olds and women immediately after delivery has been used. More recently, immunization programs in the United States have emphasized the need to vaccinate susceptible women of child-bearing age.[33, 192, 320] Chapter 177 provides more detailed information about rubella vaccine. However, continuing possible concerns include reinfection with wild rubella virus in vaccine-immune subjects,[199] failure of rubella herd immunity during an epidemic,[222] arthralgia and arthritis as side effects of the vaccine in children and particularly postpubertal women,[219, 448] risk to the fetus in women receiving the vaccine who unknowingly were pregnant,[76, 294] waning immunity that is more profound after immunization than that of natural infection,[33, 192, 320] and, more recently, outbreaks of rubella among unvaccinated pregnant women in custodial institutions or selected communities.[71, 76, 280]

Although gamma-globulin administration to women during pregnancy may reduce the frequency of symptomatic disease in the mother, there appears to be little effect on the frequency or severity of fetal and neonatal disease.[57, 275] Neonates with congenital rubella syndrome are contagious, and isolation precautions should be used for the first several months of life.[177]

HEPATITIS

Since the late 1970s, there has been a veritable explosion of information concerning infection with HAV, HBV, HCV, HDV, and HEV.[69, 70, 74, 107, 161, 197, 202, 226, 234, 239, 343, 384, 416, 442] HAV has been grown in cell cultures, and two purified viral glycoprotein vaccines have been licensed.[90, 195, 258] HBV and HCV are discussed later. HDV is a defective virus that only infects persons with acute or chronic HBV infection.[343] The major cause of enterically transmitted NANB hepatitis, a problem largely confined to developing countries,[444] has been shown to be HEV, an RNA virus not yet classified.[233, 430]

HAV and HDV rarely cause infection of the fetus and newborn.[483] Although a recent preliminary report from India indicated a relatively high rate of vertical transmission among eight women with third-trimester HEV infection,[217] more investigations are needed to determine the true significance of maternal HEV infections for the fetus and newborn infant in the United States. The following section focuses on HBV and HCV.

See also Chapters 55, 162, 172, and 180 on hepatitis viruses.

Microbiology and Epidemiology

HBV, a double-stranded DNA virus with a DNA polymerase, is the prototype member of the family *Hepadnaviridae*.[202, 226] The seroepidemiologic investigation of HBV infections has been enhanced by the identification and development of three major antigen systems, antibody systems, or both: surface antigen (HBsAg and anti-HBs), core antigen (total anti-HBc and IgM anti-HBc), and e antigen (HBeAg and anti-HBe).[202, 226] Tests for HBsAg are used widely for the diagnosis of acute or chronic infection with HBV, anti-HBc is a marker of continuing viral replication in the liver, IgM anti-HBc is present during acute but not chronic HBV infection, and HBeAg is a more specific indicator of infectivity than is HbsAg.[69, 202, 226, 384]

HBV accounts for 40 to 50 per cent of all the cases of hepatitis in the United States and 10 per cent of those associated with blood transfusion.[69, 384] Between 5 and 10 per cent of patients infected with HBV become chronic carriers, and many of these have benign chronic persistent hepatitis or the more serious chronic active hepatitis.[202, 226, 384] There also is a strong association, particularly in Asian males, between chronic carriage of HBsAg and death from cirrhosis or primary hepatocellular carcinoma.[17, 37, 278] The age at which HBV infection occurs has a significant effect on the occurrence of clinically overt hepatitis and the development of a chronic carrier state. The vast majority of neonates who acquire HBV from their mothers have subclinical infection, but 60 to 95 per cent of infected infants become chronic carriers, particularly when the mother is HbeAg-positive.[36, 39, 42, 117, 156, 317, 418, 470]

In the United States, the frequency of surface antigenemia (HBsAg in serum) in the general population is 0.2 to 0.9 per cent.[73] The highest prevalence of HBV antigenemia in the United States is in Asian immigrants/refugees (13 per cent), Alaskan natives/Pacific Islanders (5 to 15 per cent), clients in institutions for the developmentally disabled (10 to 20 per cent), users of illicit parenteral drugs (7 per cent), sexually active homosexual men (6 per cent), household contacts of HBV chronic carriers (3 to 6 per cent), and patients of hemodialysis units (3 to 10 per cent).[73] Only 10 to 15 per cent of the persons reactive for HBsAg have a history of hepatitis. In chronic carriers of HBsAg, antigen has been detected in saliva, feces, urine, vaginal secretions, breast milk, amniotic fluid, and semen.[202, 226, 384] The prevalence of anti-HBs in the general population is approximately 11 per cent; this frequency increases with increasing age and is related inversely to socioeconomic status.[73]

Among children and adults, HBV most commonly is transmitted by the parenteral route (blood transfusion, needle sticks), but infection by nonparenteral routes also occurs.[35, 38, 384, 433] The incubation period for the onset of HBV antigenemia after parenteral inoculation is 2 weeks to 2 months, depending on the dose of virus received. In nonparenteral exposure, the incubation period for antigenemia is 2 to 3 months. Onset of liver enzyme elevation and clinical symptoms follows antigenemia by 2 weeks to 2 months.[226] Clustering of HBV infections in families is known to occur; family members of a known antigen-positive index case have a 10-fold higher prevalence of HBsAg or anti-HBs than do control families of the same ethnic background.[425] Although this clustering within families initially was considered to have a genetic basis,[425] more recent data seem to support "vertical" transmission of HBV infection from the mother to the infant as the major source.[117, 156, 317] Some studies, however, have suggested transmission from fathers or siblings,[35, 433, 483] but the mechanism of transmission is not known.

In the fetus and neonate, transmission by the following routes has been suggested: (1) transplacental, either during pregnancy or at the time of delivery secondary to placental leaks; (2) natal, by exposure to HBsAg in amniotic fluid, vaginal secretions, or maternal blood; and (3) postnatal, by fecal-oral spread, blood transfusion, breast feeding, or other mechanisms. The fetus or newborn infant, therefore, can be infected by hematogenous (transplacental, blood transfusion) or nonparenteral (contamination of oropharynx or breaks in the skin) routes. Differences in the time of exposure (congenital, natal, postnatal) and in the route of viral inoculation (parenteral, nonparenteral) may account for the wide variation in time of onset of antigenemia in the neonate after birth. The usual age at onset of antigenemia in neonates born to chronic carrier mothers is 2 to 5 months,[19, 117, 129, 256, 318, 386, 415] which is consistent with an exposure at the time of birth. Infections secondary to blood transfusion in the neonatal period also are associated with onset of antigenemia at 2 to 4 months of age.[128] Infants with onset of antigenemia at younger than 2 months of age presumably were exposed to HBV in utero.[129, 156, 256, 318, 374, 386] In general, infants of mothers with acute hepatitis near the time of birth have antigenemia at an earlier age (1 to 2 months), suggesting transplacental transmission of HBV.[156, 374] Infants with onset of antigenemia after 6 months of age can be assumed to have a postnatal exposure,[374] but the exact source of virus in these infants is unclear.

In summary, there is good evidence that infection with HBV can occur transplacentally, at the time of birth, and postnatally by blood transfusion and perhaps by contamination of the oropharynx with infected secretions. Several studies indicate that transmission by breast milk is rare.[41, 117, 471] Further substantiation for the mother as the primary source of virus for the neonate comes from observations that the HBV serotype almost always is the same in infants and their carrier mother.[156, 318, 415]

From 0.1 to 15.6 per cent of pregnant women are asymptomatic chronic carriers of HBsAg. The lowest rates occur in

United States and North European populations,[117, 129, 394, 471] and the highest rates occur in Chinese, regardless of the geographic location.[19, 42, 117, 256, 415] Intermediate rates are observed in Japanese,[317, 386] African,[117, 471] South Asian,[117, 471] and Mediterranean populations.[329] The rates of transmission of HBsAg from infected mothers to the neonate vary highly and are influenced by (1) the sensitivity of the assay system for HBsAg used in the study, (2) whether neonatal serum is examined for anti-HBs as well as for HBsAg, (3) the frequency of bleeding and length of follow-up of infants, and (4) the e antigen/antibody status of the mother. In general, HBsAg in a cord blood specimen is thought not to be a reliable indicator of neonatal infection because of the possibility of contamination with antigen-positive maternal blood or vaginal secretions and because of the possibility of transient noninfectious antigenemia from the mother.[117, 256, 328, 471] Demonstration of HBsAg in the serum of the infant during the first several months of life can be considered diagnostic of infection with HBV. Most infants demonstrate antigenemia by 6 months of age, with a peak acquisition at 3 to 4 months of age.[19, 156, 256, 386]

Factors known to be associated with higher rates of HBV transmission to neonates include (1) the presence of HBeAg and the absence of anti-HBe in maternal serum—attack rates of 80 to 95 per cent[42, 117, 156, 256, 317, 328, 471]; (2) an Asian racial origin, particularly Chinese—attack rates of 40 to 70 per cent[19, 117, 256, 386, 415]; (3) maternal acute hepatitis in the third trimester of pregnancy or the immediate postpartum period—attack rates of 60 to 70 per cent[156, 374, 375]; (4) a higher titer of HBsAg in maternal serum—attack rates parallel the titer[42, 256, 415]; and (5) the presence of antigenemia in older siblings.[19, 317, 415] Factors *not* related to transmission include (1) the presence or absence of breast feeding,[41, 117, 471] (2) the particular HBV subtype in the mother,[156, 318, 415] (3) the presence or absence of HBsAg in amniotic fluid,[256] and (4) the presence or a titer of anti-HBc in cord blood.[117, 129, 156] Data conflict regarding the significance of HBsAg in cord blood. Some studies have found no relationship between its presence or absence and subsequent infection of the neonate, and others have found a correlation. The reasons for this difference are not understood.[117, 256, 328, 415, 471]

From 75 to 100 per cent of infants who develop HBsAg in their serum within the first several months of life have persistent or chronic antigenemia.[19, 117, 156, 317, 318, 386, 415] A few may develop anti-HBs after transient carriage of HBsAg, and a few (usually those born to asymptomatic carrier mothers) develop anti-HBs without ever having detectable antigen.[328, 386]

Transmission of HBV to infants in successive pregnancies of the same mother has been documented,[122, 127] and this has, on occasion, been associated with fatal hepatitis.

Pathogenesis and Pathology

It is likely that HBV transmitted to the neonate by the hematogenous route seeds the liver directly, whereas nonparenteral exposure requires replication at the portal of entry before spread to the liver through the blood stream. Electron microscopic studies of liver biopsy specimens from chronic carrier infants indicate that replication of HBV appears to occur in the nuclei of hepatocytes and that 50 to 100 per cent of cells are involved.[126, 374] Histopathologic examination demonstrates a diffuse hydropic appearance to liver cells with an effacement of the normal cord pattern and the creation of a "cobblestone appearance" in the liver lobule.[374] There are only small foci of hepatocytolysis, surrounded by macrophages and lymphocytes. In infants with symptomatic acute hepatitis, there is more widespread hepatic necrosis with surrounding inflammatory infiltrate, including giant cells.[127, 213] In fulminant disease, there is massive necrosis with little or no inflammatory response.[127, 213] In some infants with symptomatic hepatitis, the disease may progress to chronic persistent hepatitis, chronic active hepatitis, cirrhosis, or hepatocellular carcinoma.[53, 128, 213, 271, 432, 440, 472]

Clinical Manifestations

Although clinically typical acute hepatitis may occur in mothers of infants in whom infection with HBV develops, most are asymptomatic chronic carriers of HBsAg. Therefore, screening of serum for antigen in populations likely to be chronic carriers is necessary for the identification of infants at risk for acquiring HBV infection. Maternal HBV infection has not been associated with abortion, stillbirth, congenital malformations, or intrauterine growth retardation.[117, 128, 386] However, prematurity has been observed, particularly when the mother has acute hepatitis during pregnancy.[374]

The fetus or newborn infant exposed to HBV may follow one of several courses: (1) asymptomatic transient hepatitis B antigenemia followed by the production of anti-HBs[129, 328]; (2) asymptomatic persistent antigenemia, variably associated with mild and fluctuating elevations of liver enzymes[19, 129, 156, 374, 386]; (3) symptomatic hepatitis with recovery and clearance of the antigen[128, 129]; (4) symptomatic hepatitis that becomes chronic persistent or chronic active with continued presence of hepatitis B antigenemia[127, 128, 213, 472]; (5) acute fulminant hepatitis with death[128, 143]; and (6) asymptomatic neonatal/infant infection with progression to cirrhosis or liver cancer.[53, 432, 440] The majority of infants with HBsAg in their serum become asymptomatic chronic carriers. However, liver function studies may be abnormal in some of these infants, and liver biopsies usually have shown evidence of mild, unresolved hepatitis.[117, 128, 156, 374, 386] The long-term significance of these persistent abnormalities in asymptomatic chronic carrier infants is unknown. The factors that determine which pattern of HBV infection occurs in a given newborn infant and the mechanisms responsible for chronic carriage of HBsAg in many infants are not understood.

The source of virus for 29 infants with symptomatic HBV infection in the first few months of life was blood transfusion in 15 (52 per cent), a chronic carrier mother in 9 (31 per cent), and unknown in 5 (17 per cent).[128] The type of clinical disease in these infants was acute, self-limited hepatitis in 16 (55 per cent), severe or fulminant hepatitis in 9 (31 per cent), chronic persistent hepatitis in 2 (7 per cent), chronic active hepatitis in 1, and asymptomatic chronic carrier in 1. The majority of the patients with fulminant hepatitis died.

Diagnosis and Differential Diagnosis

HBV infection in an infant usually is diagnosed by the demonstration of HBsAg in the serum. The major diseases to be considered in the differential diagnosis include biliary atresia and acute hepatitis due to other viruses—HAV, CMV, rubella virus, and HSV.

Treatment

Treatment with human interferon has resulted in the termination or transient cessation of hepatitis B antigenemia in chronic hepatitis of adults,[162, 197, 336] but experience in children has been limited.[214, 247, 310] Treatment of established disease in infants with hepatitis B immunoglobulin has not altered the course of illness.[127, 143] Therefore, treatment for neonatal HBV infection primarily is supportive.

Prognosis

The long-term outcome of asymptomatic infants with persistent antigenemia is guarded because chronic active and progressive hepatitis occur and death from cirrhosis, liver failure, and hepatocellular carcinoma occurs. Death from fulminant HBV infection in the neonate or young infant is rare but has occurred, particularly in successive children born to the same chronic carrier mother.[122, 143]

Prevention

There have been remarkable advances in the prophylaxis of neonates born to mothers with HBV infection. Initial studies in infants born to HBeAg-positive chronic carrier mothers demonstrated that administration of hepatitis B immunoglobulin significantly reduced the development of a chronic carrier state.[39, 40, 122, 209, 227, 355] The most successful regimens were those that began as soon as possible after birth and used multiple doses of hepatitis B immunoglobulin. The majority of infants who were protected against becoming chronic carriers developed anti-HBs, indicating that passive/active immunization had occurred. However, protection against persistent antigenemia was only 50 to 75 per cent. Twenty to 30 per cent of infants became infected during their second and third years after the protective effects of the passive immunoglobulin subsided.[39, 40] This suggested that there was a continuing risk of infection beyond the time of birth and that active immunization would be necessary to provide long-term protection.

Hepatitis B vaccine then was demonstrated to be both safe and effective in inducing protective levels of anti-HBs in 95 per cent or more of infants receiving three doses of the vaccine.[32, 257] Because passive/active immunization (hepatitis B immunoglobulin plus three doses of HBV vaccine) in adults was shown to be safe and as effective in inducing long-term protective titers of anti-HBs as three doses of vaccine alone,[481] this regimen was tried in infants. Several investigations have demonstrated 85 to 96 per cent efficacy in preventing chronic antigenemia with the combined hepatitis B immunoglobulin/vaccine regimen.[36, 269, 418, 469] Virtually all protected infants developed persistent antibody against HBsAg. Vaccine failures were believed to occur in babies who already were infected with HBV in utero and hence could not be protected by the hepatitis B immunoglobulin/vaccine regimen initiated at birth. Other studies indicate that neonates also are protected with the recombinant HBV vaccines.[344, 417]

Because of these successful trials, the Immunization Protection Advisory Committee of the U.S. Public Health Service recommended the following regimen for all infants born to chronic carrier mothers: (1) 0.5 mL of hepatitis B immunoglobulin intramuscularly within a few hours of birth and (2) 0.5 mL of HBV vaccine intramuscularly at a different site at birth, with two repeat doses of vaccine according to the manufacturer's recommendations.[73] It would be useful to screen the infant at 12 to 15 months of age for anti-HBs and HBsAg to determine whether there was prophylactic success or failure.[73]

Because most chronic carrier mothers are asymptomatic, serologic screening during pregnancy would be required to identify those neonates needing prophylaxis beginning at birth. Initial recommendations suggested screening high-risk populations during pregnancy: (1) Asian, Alaskan, or Pacific Island descent, (2) birth in Haiti, sub-Saharan Africa, Eastern Europe, the Middle East, the Caribbean, or Central or South America, (3) acute or chronic liver disease, (4) work or treatment in a dialysis unit, (5) work or residence in an institution for the mentally retarded, (6) rejection as a blood donor, (7) blood transfusion on repeated occasions, (8) frequent occupational exposure to blood in medical or dental settings, (9) household contact with an HBV carrier or hemodialysis patient, (10) multiple episodes of sexually transmitted disease, and (11) percutaneous use of illicit drugs.[73, 74, 395] Because routine prenatal history to screen for these risk factors will miss half to two-thirds of asymptomatic chronic carrier mothers,[106, 241] recent recommendations have urged the screening of *all* pregnant women for HbsAg.[22, 23, 68, 72, 416]

Because the rate of perinatal transmission is greatest in mothers who are HBeAg-positive or those who are negative for both HBeAg and anti-HBe, some have suggested prophylaxis in neonates born only to this group of mothers.[364] However, the occurrence of several cases of hepatitis in babies born to mothers with anti-HBe[115, 393] and the demonstration that measurements such as HBV DNA polymerase or HBV DNA by polymerase chain reaction may be more accurate indicators of infectivity than measurements of HBe antigen or antibody[188, 433] indicate that prophylaxis should be given to neonates of all chronic carrier mothers, regardless of e antigen/antibody status. Because the combined hepatitis B immunoglobulin/vaccine regimen appears to result in solid and long-term protection, there is no need to advise against breast feeding in chronic carrier mothers. These significant developments in the prophylaxis against perinatal transmission of hepatitis B should reduce strikingly the frequency of chronic carriers and thereby decrease the number of cases of chronic active or progressive hepatitis and death from cirrhosis, liver failure, and hepatocellular carcinoma.

In 1991, the Advisory Committee on Immunization Practices of the CDC[68] and in 1992 the Committee on Infectious Diseases of the American Academy of Pediatrics[92] recommended the universal use of hepatitis B vaccine in all infants.[416]

Hepatitis C Virus Infection

The remarkable molecular biology effort to isolate and clone the gene of HCV[88] and to express a major nonstructural protein[245] led to the demonstration that HCV is the predominant cause of non-A, non-B hepatitis and a major contributor to chronic hepatitis in developed countries[14–16, 107, 442] (see also Chapter 55). The rates of HCV seroprevalence are highest (60 to 90 per cent) among those with repeated exposure to blood or blood products (e.g., injection drug users, hemophilia patients); intermediate (20 per cent) among those with repeated or inapparent percutaneous exposures (e.g., hemodialysis patients); lower (1 to 10 per cent) among those with high-risk sexual behaviors or household contacts of infected persons; and lowest (less than 0.5 per cent) among blood donors.[15, 107, 442] Among studies of infants born to anti-HCV–positive women, an average of 6 per cent (range, 0 to 13 per cent) of infants were positive persistently for second-generation assay anti-HCV antibody or HCV RNA during a follow-up period of a least 10 months.[250, 263, 272, 314, 316, 356, 366, 429, 450, 451, 482] Risk of vertical transmission correlated with the titer of HCV RNA[263, 316] but not with maternal HIV status.[250, 272] Although HCV RNA has been detected in breast milk, transmission by this route has not been documented.[264]

HCV infection can be diagnosed by (1) antibody titers and (2) molecular methods to detect and quantitate viral RNA.

Antigen detection tests are not available. Antibody titers in the infant are confounded by maternal transplacental antibody; this effect presumably is gone by 10 months of age. Antibody testing involves a screening enzyme immunoassay with repeat positive results confirmed by a recombinant immunoblot assay analogous to what is done for serologic diagnosis of HIV infection. The second-generation enzyme immunoassay and recombinant immunoblot assay are 95 per cent sensitive and 97 per cent specific.[167a] Polymerase chain reaction and other molecular methods to detect HCV RNA in infant serum are available through major medical center and national reference laboratories.[167a] However, these molecular tests are costly, and information on sensitivity and specificity in neonates is not available.

Controlled trials of interferon therapy in children with chronic hepatitis C are limited,[91] and this drug is not approved by the Food and Drug Administration for use in persons younger than 18 years of age. The long-term prognosis for HCV infection in infants and children is not clear, but 85 per cent of adults become chronically infected, and HCV is known to be associated with cirrhosis and hepatocellular carcinoma.[15, 107, 442]

Development of a successful vaccine for hepatitis C must overcome several obstacles, including multiple genotypes of the virus, lack of cross-protective immunity among the genotypes, lack of long-term protection with the same genotype, and lack of successful cultivation of the virus in cell cultures.[15, 107] In February 1994, the Advisory Committee on Immunization Practices reviewed available data and concluded that there was no support for the use of immunoglobulin for postexposure prophylaxis. Routine screening of all pregnant women for HCV infection cannot be recommended now, but screening should be considered in those with known risk factors. Until more is known about the natural history, practical laboratory diagnosis, and therapeutic management of HCV infection in infants, routine testing of infants born to HCV-infected mothers cannot be recommended. Data are not available to permit clear recommendations about breast feeding in women with chronic HCV infection.

HERPES SIMPLEX

HSV, the etiologic agent of cold sores, keratitis, encephalitis, and genital ulcers in older children and adults, causes serious disease in the neonate, with high mortality and severe neurologic sequelae (see also Chapter 163).

Microbiology and Epidemiology

There are two types of HSV, type 1 and type 2, which may be distinguished by antigenic, biochemical, and biologic differences.[101, 453] HSV-1 (the oral strain) causes mouth lesions, eye infections, and encephalitis and is transmitted nonvenereally, whereas HSV-2 (the genital strain) is associated with genital infection and venereal transmission.[101, 453] However, from 8 to 50 per cent of genital disease is caused by HSV-1,[321] perhaps reflecting an increase in orogenital sex.

Antiviral collaborative studies indicate that 4 per cent of neonatal herpes cases are acquired congenitally, 86 per cent natally, and 10 per cent postnatally.[454] Three-quarters of the natal/postnatal cases of neonatal herpes are caused by HSV-2, and the remainder are due to HSV-1 strains.[307, 325] Virtually all neonatal HSV-2 infections are acquired from the mother with an active genital herpes infection at the time of delivery.[307, 324, 423, 454, 460, 476] Importantly, however, 60 to 80 per cent of these mothers have no signs or symptoms of genital herpes at the time of labor and delivery and have a negative past history of genital herpes or sexual contact with a partner with a genital vesicular rash.[454, 455, 459] In a study of 140 pregnant women with cytologically diagnosed genital herpes, only 36 per cent had clinically recognized herpetic lesions.[306] Twenty-one per cent had nonspecific abnormal findings, and 43 per cent were asymptomatic. In addition, 20 to 40 per cent of nonpregnant women from whose genital secretions HSV is isolated are asymptomatic.[207, 464] The use of more sensitive techniques, such as polymerase chain reaction, detects genital HSV shedding in asymptomatic women even more frequently.[95]

Neonates with HSV-1 infection can acquire the virus from several sources: maternal genital, oral, or breast lesions[125, 262, 422, 476]; paternal or other family member oral herpes[123, 423, 476]; or nosocomial transmission from other infected babies.[172, 266] Although HSV-1 cold sores and asymptomatic oral shedding may be common among nursery personnel,[183, 184] transmission to a neonate from this source is rare.[307, 369, 443] If one needs to identify the source clearly, HSV from the infected neonate and from the suspected contact should be typed and examined by molecular techniques.[363, 454]

Because most fetal and neonatal HSV infections are transmitted from the mother, a summary of several aspects of herpes infection during pregnancy is appropriate. Fulminant or disseminated primary HSV disease may occur in pregnancy, but it is not clear whether this occurs more often than with nonpregnant women. A review[335] of seven such cases revealed (1) infection during the third trimester in all, (2) four beginning as a genital HSV infection and three as oral disease, (3) hepatitis in six, encephalitis in two, and pancreatitis in two, (4) maternal death in three (43 per cent)—two from hepatitis and one from encephalitis, and (5) three instances of fetal death—each secondary to severe maternal systemic illness rather than direct infection with HSV. Evidence of visceral disease in a pregnant woman with either genital or oral HSV infection warrants strong consideration of systemic antiviral therapy.[246]

There is an increased rate of spontaneous abortion in women with primary genital herpes during early pregnancy, regardless of socioeconomic status.[181, 182, 306, 325] Premature delivery is not more common in prospectively followed women with recurrent genital herpes,[182, 325, 446, 466] but most reports of neonatal herpes cases find a greater preponderance of premature infants than in the general population.[307, 455, 460, 476] Recurrent genital herpes in middle-class pregnant women is no more severe or frequent than in nonpregnant ones,[181, 446, 466] but older studies demonstrated more frequent and longer episodes in women of lower socioeconomic groups.[306, 312] Between 74 and 88 per cent of middle-class pregnant women with a history of genital herpes had at least one clinical recurrence during an observed pregnancy.[181, 446, 466] There was a mean of 2.7 to 3.0 episodes during gestation, and HSV was isolated from lesions in 56 to 75 per cent of the recurrences and from 0.6 to 12 per cent of concomitant cervical cultures obtained during the recurrence. Asymptomatic shedding of HSV from the cervix, either between clinical recurrences or in the history-positive women with no episodes during the observed pregnancy, was detected in 0.5 to 2.3 per cent of cultures obtained. Importantly, the presence of HSV shedding during the latter weeks of pregnancy did not appear to be predictive of shedding at the time of delivery.[25, 466]

It often has been stated that the number of cases of neonatal herpes occurring in the United States each year is far less than one would expect from the likely number of pregnancies complicated by genital herpes. There are 3.5 million annual pregnancies; from 7000 to 200,000 of these women have genital herpes at some time during the pregnancy, and from 3500 to 14,000 have positive HSV cultures at the time of delivery.[49, 168, 182, 307, 428, 446, 466] The actual number of cases of neonatal herpes per year in Seattle and Atlanta (0.1 and 0.3 per 1000 live births, respectively) would project to a national estimate of 350 to 1050 per year in the United States.[307, 423] Because asymptomatic HSV infection of the neonate is rare,[307] it is unlikely that subclinical cases or missed diagnoses account for the differences between the estimated number of maternal infections and neonatal infections. It is more likely that neonatal infection rates in the babies of mothers with genital herpes are far less than currently assumed. The estimated infection rates most often quoted currently are (1) a 33 to 50 per cent rate for infants vaginally delivered to mothers with primary genital herpes, (2) a 3 to 5 per cent rate in mothers with recurrent lesions, and (3) less than 3 per cent with recurrent asymptomatic shedding at the time of delivery.[49, 61, 100, 325, 466] In the early 1970s, Nahmias and associates[306] reported the following neonatal infection rates in babies born to mothers with genital herpes during pregnancy: (1) 33 per cent in mothers with primary disease after the 32nd week of gestation, (2) 3 per cent in mothers with recurrent episodes after 32 weeks, and (3) 42 per cent in mothers with virus-positive lesions at the time of delivery (primary vs. recurrent episodes not specified). More recent studies have examined the risk of neonatal herpes in babies born to mothers with *asymptomatic* shedding at the time of vaginal delivery: 33 per cent with *subclinical first episodes*[61] and 0 to 3 per cent in recurrent shedding.[61, 327, 347] Accurate knowledge of the actual neonatal infection risks is important for making decisions about management (e.g., cesarean section, prophylactic antiviral therapy).

Several factors influence the risk of neonatal herpes and the severity of neonatal disease once the infection develops. The greater risk of neonatal infection in mothers with primary, as opposed to recurrent, lesions at the time of delivery has been mentioned already. In turn, a woman with virus-positive recurrent lesions at the time of delivery is likely to be a greater risk than the asymptomatic shedder identified only by HSV surveillance cultures. It follows that other aspects of the anatomic site and severity of maternal genital herpes would be associated with greater risk of neonatal disease: (1) cervical as opposed to vulvar or buttock skin involvement—resulting in more virus being shed into vaginal secretions, (2) multiple as opposed to single lesions—again, more virus from multiple lesions, (3) higher titer of virus in vaginal secretions—cultures positive sooner or more intensely positive in the diagnostic virology laboratory, and (4) longer duration of fetal exposure to infected vaginal secretions because of prolonged rupture of membranes.[100, 307, 323, 325] Investigations by Yeager and associates[476, 477] indicate that no anti-HSV antibody or a low titer of such antibody in maternal and neonatal serum is associated with a greater risk of neonatal infection and more serious disease and that high-titered antibody is associated with a lower risk. Studies of HSV antibody titers in neonates enrolled in the collaborative antiviral study group trial do not show an association between antibody titer and disease outcome.[461] More investigations are required, therefore, to determine the potential protective role of maternal transplacental anti-HSV antibody. Premature infants have accounted for 40 to 50 per cent of the cases of neonatal herpes,[307, 454, 455, 461] in contrast with the usual prematurity rates of 6 to 7 per cent for whites and 17 to 18 per cent for nonwhites. It is not known whether the increased frequency of premature babies among neonates with herpes indicates a greater propensity of mothers with genital herpes to deliver prematurely or a greater susceptibility of the premature infant to HSV infection. Premature infants are more likely to have a fatal outcome.[455, 456] Instrumentation of the neonate, particularly with scalp electrodes for fetal monitoring, is known to increase the risk of neonatal HSV infection.[131, 215, 307, 330] Mortality appears to be higher in neonates with HSV-1 than with HSV-2 infection, likely because of the greater proportion of HSV-1–infected babies with dissemination.[456] In neonatal herpes survivors, neurologic damage occurs much more frequently with HSV-2 than with HSV-1 infection.[102, 456] Finally, the body sites of involvement in the neonate clearly influence outcome. Babies with disseminated infection (liver, lungs, adrenals) with or without central nervous system involvement have the highest mortality rates (70 to 80 per cent), those with encephalitis have only intermediate rates (30 to 40 per cent), and those with infection limited to the skin, eye, or mouth have the lowest rates (0 to 10 per cent).[307, 454, 461] The factors that are discussed in this paragraph and that are associated with higher risk of neonatal infection (e.g., type and severity of maternal genital infection, fetal instrumentation) should be kept in mind in the management approach of the infant determined postnatally to have been delivered through a virus- or lesion-positive birth canal. Babies delivered in a high-risk situation might be given anticipatory antiviral chemotherapy after appropriate cultures have been obtained, whereas those in a low-risk situation might be cultured and observed closely for evidence of neonatal herpes.[325, 327]

Pathogenesis and Pathology

As mentioned previously, HSV may be transmitted to the neonate in utero (congenital infection), at the time of birth (natal infection), or after birth (postnatal infection). It is likely that the congenital infection results from transplacental transmission of virus secondary to leukocyte-associated viremia in a mother with genital herpes, but there is no direct evidence to support this hypothesis. HSV-2 viremia has been documented in two women with primary genital herpes.[104] A report of 13 neonates with intrauterine HSV infection indicated that there was primary genital herpes during pregnancy in four mothers, recurrent disease in one, and no history of genital herpes in the remaining eight.[205] In the fetus, HSV appears to be transmitted directly from the placenta through the blood stream to target organs. Because of the known tropism of HSV for the central nervous system, it is not surprising that most infants with congenital infection have evidence of brain involvement at birth.[205]

The natal infection presumably is acquired secondary to aspiration of infected vaginal secretions into the upper respiratory tract of the infant. Other portals of entry for the natal infection include the eyes, scalp, skin, and umbilical cord.[307, 325, 454, 455] In postnatal HSV infection, there is no evidence that the genital tract is a source of virus. Most postnatally acquired infections appear to result from contact with saliva from persons with oral herpes or with virus carried on the hands of personnel.[262, 454, 455, 476] After natal or postnatal acquisition of HSV, initial replication of the virus occurs at the portal of entry with subsequent viremic dissemination to viscera and spread to the central nervous system by both blood and neural routes.[216, 307, 454, 455]

Characteristic pathologic features of neonatal herpes include involvement primarily of the brain, liver, adrenals, and lungs, as manifested by necrosis, eosinophilic intranuclear inclusions, and multinucleated giant cells. It is important to note that virus may be isolated from tissue that does not show evidence of inclusions or giant cells.[307]

Clinical Manifestations

The clinical features of genital herpes in women have been discussed in detail elsewhere.[62, 100, 321] Women with initial or primary infections may have extensive vesicular and ulcerative lesions involving the cervix, vagina, vulva, and skin of the perineal region. With the appearance of lesions, severe pain and tenderness develop. In addition, patients may complain of inguinal or pelvic pain that is due to associated lymphadenopathy. Systemic symptoms consisting of fever, malaise, and myalgia usually are present. The total duration of pain is 10 days to 2 weeks, whereas the total duration of lesions may be from 2 to 3 weeks. Peak lesion virus titers, from 10^4 to 10^5 plaque-forming units/mL, occur during the first week of illness.[62] The total duration of viral shedding lasts from 10 to 14 days.[62, 100] Lesions on dry skin progress through the well-defined vesicle, ulcer, crust, and healed stages described for herpes simplex labialis.[398] On moist mucous membranes, vesicles quickly rupture to form shallow ulcers that persist for days and gradually heal from the periphery.[62]

Recurrent genital herpes in women is milder and of shorter duration, the lesions are more circumscribed and fewer in number, and the disease appears to be limited largely to the external genitals.[62] Peak lesion virus titers occur during the first few days and are lower, 10^3 to 10^4 plaque-forming units/mL. The total duration of pain is 5 to 9 days, of lesions is 8 to 11 days, and of viral shedding is 5 to 8 days.[62, 100] Importantly, women with both primary or initial and recurrent genital herpes may be asymptomatic.[61]

The clinical spectrum in infants with congenital HSV infection is different from that observed in babies with natal or postnatal disease. The most prominent features summarized from 30 cases with congenital infection reported in the literature are shown in Table 76–9.[124, 146, 196, 205, 228, 254, 291, 296, 383, 389, 396, 421] A vesicular rash or bullae present at birth or within a few days of birth were noted in almost all infants. Two-thirds of the infants demonstrated some evidence of extensive involvement of the central nervous system at birth, either clinically or from autopsy findings: diffuse brain damage, microcephaly, or intracranial calcifications. In a number of infants, eye findings more commonly observed in congenital CMV and rubella infections were seen: chorioretinitis, microphthalmia, retinal dysplasia, and cataracts.

As indicated in Figure 76–3, infants with natal or postnatal herpes commonly present a clinical picture resembling that of bacterial sepsis: alterations in temperature, lethargy, respiratory distress, anorexia or vomiting, and cyanosis.[176, 454, 459, 460] There are three general patterns of infection: (1) disseminated infection with or without central nervous system involvement present in 32 per cent of the cases, (2) infection localized to the central nervous system in 33 per cent of cases, and (3) infection localized to the skin, eye, or mouth in 35 per cent of cases.[454] The disseminated form of the infection usually involves the liver, adrenal glands, and lung and most closely resembles the picture of bacterial sepsis.[187, 436, 454] Approximately 60 per cent of all infants with symptomatic infection have prominent signs and symptoms of central nervous system involvement: irritability, bulging fontanelle, localized or generalized seizures, flaccid or spastic paralysis, opisthotonus, decerebrate rigidity, or coma.[307, 454] Approximately 75 per cent of neonates present with skin lesions: usually single vesicles, occasionally vesicle clusters, and rarely a zoster-like rash.[300, 454] Several neonates have had recurrences of skin vesicles during infancy.[201, 456] Approximately 13 per cent of infants have eye involvement; disease is limited to the eye in one-third of these.[307] Common manifestations include conjunctivitis, keratitis, and chorioretinitis.[169, 304] Although one-third of all infants have evidence of herpetic mouth lesions, involvement of this site alone is rare.

TABLE 76–9. Congenital Herpes Simplex Virus (HSV) Infection: Features in 30 Cases*

Feature	Number	Percentage
Low birth weight	22/26	85
Small for gestational age	9/25	36
Microcephaly, seizures, diffuse brain damage, intracranial calcification	20/30	67
Chorioretinitis, microphthalmia	17/30	57
Culture-positive vesicles or bullae	28/30	93
HSV-2	24/27	89
Other features: Retinal dysplasia, scars on skin or digits, cataracts, pneumonitis, hepatomegaly		

*Features present at birth or shortly thereafter.

From Hutto, C., Arvin, A., Jacob, R., et al.: Intrauterine herpes simplex virus infections. J. Pediatr. *110*:97–101, 1987.

Diagnosis and Differential Diagnosis

Importantly, more than 80 per cent of infants have classic features that would suggest herpes simplex, such as skin vesicles, mouth ulcers, or keratoconjunctivitis. Half of the remaining 15 to 20 per cent have either (1) focal or diffuse encephalitis or (2) a sepsis syndrome with pneumonitis, hepatitis, encephalitis, and often disseminated intravascular coagulopathy.[325, 454] A clinical picture of encephalitis certainly should suggest HSV infection; it is unusual to see the combination of pneumonitis, hepatitis, and encephalitis in bacterial sepsis/meningitis.

The major diseases to be considered in the differential diagnosis include bacterial sepsis, enterovirus infection, and, to a lesser extent, congenital infection with CMV, rubella virus, and VZV. Inquiry about illness in the mother and other epidemiologic features may be helpful. For example, mothers of neonates with HSV infection may have a history of genital lesions or sexual contact with someone with genital herpes. Infants with sepsis usually have associated factors known to predispose to bacterial infections, such as maternal peripartum infection, premature rupture of membranes, and procedures carried out in the intensive care unit or nursery. Enterovirus infection of infants tends to occur in the summer and fall and is associated with signs and symptoms of enterovirus disease in the mother.

The most definitive means of establishing the diagnosis of HSV infection in the neonate is isolation or identification of the virus in clinical or autopsy specimens. Samples for virus isolation in cell culture may be obtained from vesicular fluid, swabs of the mouth or eyes, peripheral blood buffy coat, and cerebrospinal fluid. In selected instances, when the infection appears to be localized to the central nervous system and cultures for HSV from the usual sites are negative, polymerase chain reaction for HSV DNA on cerebrospinal fluid specimens may be useful.[249] Ideally, specimens should be processed immediately or frozen at $-70°$ C if testing can not be done until later. However, HSV is stable for 2 to 3 days at 4° C in trypticase soy broth or brain-heart infusion broth.[474] In cell culture, typical HSV cytopathic effect often is evident within 1 to 2 days after inoculation. Studies using centrifugation of the specimen onto a cell monolayer at the bottom of a shell vial, followed by staining for HSV antigen the next day, yielded 99 per cent sensitivity and 100 per cent specificity.[322] In addition, immunofluorescent or immunoperoxidase techniques are available to demonstrate HSV-1 or -2 antigens in cells scraped from the base of vesicles or conjunctivae or in biopsy or autopsy material.[299, 373] However, results of procedures that stain cells scraped from lesions may be falsely negative in 10 to 30 per cent of instances.

In most circumstances, serologic assays are not useful for the diagnosis of maternal or neonatal herpes during the acute phase of the disease. Although antibody assays may be used for documenting initial or primary genital herpes infection in the mother, recurrent disease cannot be identified by this method. Immunofluorescent techniques to quantify HSV-specific IgM antibodies have been developed, but these antibodies usually are not detected in the serum for 2 or more weeks after the onset of the infection in neonates.[303]

Treatment

Placebo-controlled trials demonstrated that adenine arabinoside (vidarabine, ara-A) at doses of 15 or 30 mg/kg/day given as a 12-hour infusion significantly reduced the mortality rate from 62 per cent in historic cases and placebo controls to 35 per cent in treated cases and increased the percentage of normal survivors from 19 to 43 per cent.[461] Results were best in infants with disseminated infection and disease localized to the central nervous system, with the mortality rate reduced from 70 to 40 per cent and the percentage of normal survivors increased from 10 to 30 per cent. There was no difference between the 15-mg and the 30-mg dose in side effects, but the higher dose appeared more effectively to inhibit progression of disease from skin-eye-mouth involvement to disseminated or central nervous system disease.[459] None of the 49 treated patients had significant adverse clinical reactions or laboratory abnormalities attributable to the drug. On the negative side, 21 per cent of infants progressed to more serious disease while on therapy, and 27 per cent of the total developed serious neurologic sequelae. Fifteen per cent of babies with disseminated or central nervous system disease continued to excrete HSV in the throat after 10 days of therapy.

The results of a vidarabine-acyclovir comparison trial in the treatment of neonatal herpes indicated that there was no difference in efficacy and safety between the two drugs.[455] When the results with vidarabine and vidarabine-acyclovir are combined, it can be seen that the mortality rate was reduced from 49 per cent in untreated historical controls[307] to 17 per cent in treated patients (Table 76–10). Normal survivors increased from 26 to 67 per cent. Although the results from the total group of patients are encouraging, the outcome in the group of patients with disseminated disease is not: a mortality rate of 54 per cent in treated patients compared with 76 per cent in untreated historical controls, 59 per cent of treated survivors developing normally compared with 54 per cent in controls (see Table 76–10). Factors that predicted mortality outcome and their relative risks are as follows: disseminated disease, 33; central nervous system disease, 5.8; semicoma or coma, 5.2; disseminated intravascular coagulation, 3.8; prematurity, 3.7; and pneumonitis, 3.6.[456] Factors significantly associated with neurologic sequelae in survivors and their relative risks are as follows: skin-eye-mouth disease with three or more recurrent skin lesions after acute therapy was completed, 21; skin-eye-mouth disease due to HSV-2, 14; HSV-2 infection, regardless of disease category, 4.9; central nervous system disease, 4.4; and seizures, 3.0. Because of greater ease of administration, most centers use acyclovir at the clinical trial dose of 30 mg/kg/day intravenously, divided every 8 hours. Future trials will address (1) whether a higher dose or longer treatment course of acyclovir is more beneficial, (2) whether oral acyclovir suspension should be used after the initial intravenous therapy in an attempt to suppress skin recurrences and potential continuing replication of HSV in the central nervous system, and (3) whether combination antiviral therapy might be synergistic and more beneficial.

Questions have been raised concerning prophylactic or anticipatory antiviral chemotherapy in the neonate delivered through a birth canal discovered postnatally to have active herpes lesions or a positive culture for HSV.[323–325, 327, 347, 376] In the high-risk infant, in whom infection rates may be 30 to 50 per cent, intravenous antiviral chemotherapy might be considered after appropriate viral cultures have been obtained from the neonate. Antiviral therapy could be discontinued after 2 to 3 days in infants when further observation indicates that the diagnosis of HSV infection is unlikely, particularly if another cause for the neonate's illness is found. In the low-risk infant, infection rates probably are less than 3 per cent. Thus, systemic antiviral therapy might be withheld pending results of cultures or development in the neonate of clinical illness that could be due to HSV. In the infant for whom the decision is made to initiate systemic antiviral therapy, the following specimens should be collected: (1) eye swab, nasopharyngeal swab, buffy coat, and cerebrospinal fluid for culture of HSV and (2) acute serum for HSV antibody. In the low-risk infant in whom systemic antivirals will be withheld, a culture of the conjunctivae and then the nasopharynx with the same swab 24 to 48 hours after delivery is recommended. Cultures obtained at birth may indicate only contaminating virus, whereas those obtained 1 to 2 days after birth probably represent HSV newly replicating in the mucous membranes. It should be noted that the sensitivity of this culture in detecting infected infants is not known. Some have recommended continuing weekly surveillance cultures of the eye and nasopharynx for several weeks after

TABLE 76–10. Neonatal Herpes: Antiviral Therapy

Outcome	Total	Skin, Eyes, Mouth	Encephalitis	Disseminated
Mortality				
ACV, Ara-A*	17%	0	14%	54%
Historical controls†	49%	7%	37%	76%
Development normal				
ACV, Ara-A*	67%	94%	36%	59%
Historical controls†	26%	73%	19%	54%

*Data from Whitley, R., Arvin, A., Prober, C., et al.: A controlled trial comparing vidarabine with acyclovir in neonatal herpes simplex virus infection. N. Engl. J. Med. *324*:444–449, 1991.

†Data from Nahmias, A. J., Keyserling, H. L., and Kerrick, G. M.: Herpes simplex. *In* Remington, J. S., and Klein, J. O. (eds.): Infectious Diseases of the Fetus and Newborn Infant. 2nd ed. Philadelphia, W. B. Saunders Co., 1983, pp. 636–678.

ACV, acyclovir; Ara-A, vidarabine (adenine arabinoside).

birth.[347] Low-risk babies should be followed closely for (1) results of cultures and (2) any clinical evidence of HSV disease. Development of positive cultures or the occurrence of signs or symptoms suggesting HSV infection in the neonate should initiate full virologic evaluation and antiviral therapy. Because the presence of a positive HSV culture of vaginal secretions at the time of delivery is important information to have for optimal management of infants, it is critical to obtain this culture for all women at risk for genital herpes: (1) those with a prior history of genital herpes, either prior to or during the current pregnancy, (2) women with a sexual partner with a history of genital herpes, and possibly (3) women with a history of other sexually transmitted diseases or multiple sexual partners.

General supportive measures, such as the maintenance of fluid and electrolyte balance, correction of hypoglycemia, management of disseminated intravascular coagulation and shock, control of seizures with anticonvulsants, mechanical support of the respiratory system, and antimicrobial therapy for complicating bacterial infections, also are critical in improving the outcome for neonates with HSV infection.

Prognosis

As indicated in Table 76–10, the overall mortality rate from untreated neonatal HSV infection is 49 per cent, and only 26 per cent of survivors develop normally. The worst prognosis is in infants with a natal infection that is disseminated or localized to the central nervous system. Occurrence of pneumonia is a particularly poor prognostic sign. Between 50 and 60 per cent of infants who present with HSV infection limited to the skin, eye, and mouth progress to central nervous system or disseminated disease. As shown in Table 76–10, neurologic sequelae develop in an appreciable proportion of survivors. All infants with neonatal herpes, therefore, deserve antiviral chemotherapy, regardless of the mildness of disease at the time of presentation.

The major sequelae in infants surviving neonatal herpes involve the central nervous system. Diffuse brain damage, seizures, microcephaly, spasticity, paralysis, growth retardation, and chorioretinitis with visual loss all have been observed.[454, 461] Serial computed tomography or magnetic resonance imaging of the head may be useful in these infants and provide prognostic information.[454, 459] Infants with skin involvement may have recurrent lesions in subsequent months.[307]

Prevention

The major approaches to the prevention of neonatal herpes involve interruption of transmission from sites of HSV infection (1) at the time of delivery and (2) postnatally from a variety of potential sources. Because congenital infection is so infrequent[455] and because it is not possible to predict the occurrence of congenital infection during pregnancy,[205] consideration of abortion for this purpose is not indicated.

Cesarean section in the mother with active genital herpes at the time of delivery is the major means used to prevent natal infection. Because serial vaginal cultures during the latter stages of pregnancy have failed to predict shedding at the time of delivery,[25, 466] this monitoring has been abandoned and cesarean section is recommended only for those women with active lesions at the time of delivery.[29, 158, 182, 325, 347, 376] It should be recognized that cesarean section is not 100 per cent protective, even if membranes are intact.[182, 307, 325, 347, 376] In addition, a recent analysis questioned the cost-effectiveness of performing a cesarean section in women with recurrent lesions at delivery.[352]

Because 60 to 80 per cent of mothers of babies with neonatal herpes are asymptomatic or have unrecognized infection,[454] it would be optimal to have a screening test to identify women shedding or likely to shed HSV at the time of delivery. Although HSV rapid antigen detection tests continue to be developed commercially,[322] sensitivity in *asymptomatic* women still is only 60 to 75 per cent. Screening of pregnant women for non–type-specific HSV antibody would be confounded by the presence of HSV-1 antibody, which is present in 60 to 80 per cent of the population.[321] The presence of HSV-1 antibody probably represents oral herpes, which poses little risk to the neonate. Although type-specific antibody assays are available to identify pregnant women infected with HSV-2,[210] such an approach would miss those women with genital HSV-1 infection[100, 347] or those with asymptomatic primary HSV-2 infection near the time of delivery before antibody was detectable.[61, 347] Culturing the genital tract of women at the time of vaginal delivery would identify infants exposed to HSV and allow anticipatory management.[323, 325, 347] However, because infection rates are only 0.1 to 0.4 per cent,[61, 306, 349] this would not likely be a cost-effective approach for *all* women. Culturing of *selected* women at delivery could focus on (1) those identified by HSV-2 serologic tests, (2) those with a history of genital herpes in themselves or their sexual partners, and (3) those with a history of another sexually transmitted disease or multiple sexual partners. Further investigation is required to determine whether screening of pregnant women to prevent neonatal herpes is practical and cost-effective.

The prevention of postnatally acquired neonatal infection needs to take into account the potential sources of HSV: (1) maternal oral herpes or breast lesions, (2) paternal or other close contact with oral herpes, and (3) nosocomial transmission from other infected babies.[123, 172, 266, 422, 423, 476] Transmission to the neonate from oral herpes lesions can be interrupted by education and common sense personal hygiene, and nosocomial spread can be interrupted by conventional isolation and infection control measures.[218, 221]

ENTEROVIRUS INFECTIONS

The enteroviruses are members of the family *Picornaviridae* and include the polioviruses, coxsackieviruses A and B, and echoviruses. Enteroviruses are limited to the human host, infections are common, and there is a wide spectrum of clinical manifestations in children and adults as well as in neonates (see Chapter 170). Coxsackievirus and echovirus infections are fairly common in young infants and, as with other viral agents, often result in more severe disease in the neonate. Neonatal poliomyelitis, however, is a rarity in the United States and is not covered in this section.

Microbiology and Epidemiology

There are 23 types of type A coxsackieviruses, 6 types of type B coxsackieviruses, 30 types of echoviruses, and 5 types of enteroviruses (68 to 72).[281] Most strains grow in tissue culture, but some, particularly the type A coxsackieviruses, require inoculation in suckling mice. Because there are no common or group antigens for the enteroviruses, separate antibody titration must be performed for each virus. It is not practical, therefore, to make a laboratory diagnosis of enteroviral infection by serologic means alone. However, antibody titers can be performed after a specific enterovirus has been isolated from the patient or when there is a concurrent epidemic in the community with a known virus.

The attack rate for enteroviral infections is highest during infancy and early childhood.[1, 108–110, 237, 273, 293, 298, 468] In addition, severe disease is much more common in neonates than in older children or adults.[293, 468] Sixty to 70 per cent of infected neonates are males.[212, 248, 293, 298, 351] The enteroviruses are worldwide in distribution, and in temperate climates infections occur predominantly during the summer and fall months with peaks in July, August, and September.[67, 208, 281] The incubation period for enteroviral infections in children and adults usually is 5 to 8 days, with a range of 2 to 12 days.[370, 452] Of the cases reported to the CDC from 1970 to 1979, echoviruses accounted for 57 per cent; type B coxsackieviruses, 25 per cent; polioviruses, 9 per cent; type A coxsackieviruses, 8 per cent; and enterovirus types 68 to 71, 0.1 per cent.[67] In infants younger than 2 months of age, echoviruses accounted for 51 per cent of the infections; type B coxsackieviruses, 45 per cent; and type A coxsackieviruses, 4 per cent.[298] In any given year in the United States, there usually is an epidemic caused by a few enterovirus types: echovirus 11 and coxsackieviruses B2 and B4 in 1979, echoviruses 9 and 4 in 1978, echovirus 6 in 1977, coxsackievirus B4 in 1976, and echovirus 9 in 1975.[67] Outbreaks of enteroviral disease have occurred in normal nurseries and in neonatal intensive care units.[27, 56, 81, 105, 142, 255, 273, 293, 320, 365, 424]

Acute enteroviral infection in the newborn infant may be acquired congenitally, natally, or postnatally.[84, 365] However, there often has been confusion concerning the incubation period and source of virus for neonatal infection. Late-gestation congenital infection is presumed to occur in infants with onset of illness at birth or within the first few days of life, when their mothers had symptoms of enteroviral disease just before or immediately after delivery.[1, 82, 114, 248, 293, 338] Further evidence for congenital infection is the observation that viremia with echoviruses and coxsackieviruses is known to occur in pregnant women,[84] and virus has been isolated from the placenta of infants with onset of disease early in life.[56, 293] Infants with onset of enteroviral disease between 3 and 8 to 10 days of age probably acquired the infection from their mothers at the time of birth (natal infection), whereas those with illness appearing after this time probably acquired it postnatally. The source of virus for most cases in nurseries appears to be the mother because the age of the infants at the time of first symptoms usually is less than 10 days.[1, 248, 255, 293, 351, 424] However, in some cases and outbreaks, the infection clearly appears to be nosocomial in origin, presumably through spread of virus from other infected neonates by the hands of personnel or from infected personnel themselves.[105, 276, 293]

Some investigations indicate that enteroviral infections acquired in the community are a common cause of hospitalization for a febrile illness in young infants.[108–110, 208, 237] Enteroviral infections were estimated to account for 20,000 to 40,000 hospitalizations per year in young infants in the United States. In one study of 182 infants younger than 3 months of age hospitalized for fever over a year, viral pathogens were isolated in 41 per cent and bacteria in only 15 per cent.[237] Enteroviruses accounted for 85 per cent of the viral isolates. Among a cohort of 586 newborns prospectively followed during the enteroviral season in Rochester, New York, 24 (4 per cent) were hospitalized during the first month of life.[208] Two-thirds of these 24 were infected with enteroviruses. Risk factors associated with infection and severity of enteroviral disease included a particular serotype of virus (e.g., echovirus 22, presumably a more virulent strain), lower socioeconomic status probably with associated crowding and increased rate of transmission, bottle feeding (absence of passive antibody in breast milk), and absence of antibody in cord serum.[109, 208, 293, 295]

There is evidence to suggest that coxsackieviral infections in early pregnancy may cause congenital malformations in the fetus. Brown and colleagues[59, 60] demonstrated a significant association between serologic evidence of coxsackievirus A9, B2, B3, and B4 infections in mothers during pregnancy and the birth of infants with anomalies of the cardiovascular, urogenital, and digestive systems. However, specific viral isolation and antibody studies were not performed on the involved infants, and there was no seasonal distribution in their births. In addition, the observations of Brown and colleagues[59, 60] have not been confirmed by others.[133, 232, 339] The association between maternal infections with coxsackieviruses and congenital malformations, therefore, remains suggestive but not proven.

Pathogenesis and Pathology

Our knowledge of the pathogenesis of congenital enteroviral infection is incomplete because the occurrence is relatively infrequent in humans and because there is no satisfactory animal model of transplacental infection. By inference from our understanding of congenital CMV and rubella virus infections, transplacental transmission secondary to maternal viremia is likely. Virus then is transmitted through fetal blood to target organs, principally the central nervous system, liver, heart, lung, kidneys, and adrenal glands. In congenital infections that are fatal in the early neonatal period, type B coxsackieviruses involve primarily the heart, central nervous system, liver, and lungs,[153, 212, 248, 468] and echoviruses involve the liver, adrenals, kidneys, central nervous system, and lungs.[82, 170, 204, 238, 292, 293, 338] Histopathologic findings have consisted of focal myocardial necrosis with type B coxsackieviruses[153, 468]; massive hepatic necrosis with echoviruses[204, 238, 293, 338]; and evidence of disseminated intravascular coagulation with adrenal, pulmonary, and renal hemorrhage with both virus groups.[82, 153, 204, 238, 248, 293, 338, 468] It is of interest that the onset of illness in most of the neonates with fatal coxsackievirus B and echovirus infections occurred at birth or within the first few days of life, suggesting that transplacental infections carry a worse prognosis.[1, 82, 204, 238, 248, 293, 338] In addition, lack of transplacental transfer of maternal antibody prior to delivery could play a role.[292, 293] There have been only a few isolated case reports of congenital coxsackievirus A infections.[84]

Natal infection presumably occurs secondary to aspiration and swallowing of enterovirus-contaminated vaginal secretions at the time of birth. Postnatal acquisition is the result of fecal-oropharyngeal spread of the virus on the hands of the mother, other family members, or hospital personnel.[84, 293] The pathogenesis of natal and postnatal infection is similar to that observed in older infants and children (see Chapter 170). Because most infants with postnatal infection survive, the pathologic features are not well characterized.

Clinical Manifestations

The clinical features in 134 neonates and very young infants with echoviral and coxsackieviral infections are shown in Figure 76–3. The most common findings, hyperthermia or hypothermia, anorexia or vomiting, and lethargy, are relatively nonspecific and are encountered with a similar frequency in neonates with other viral infections or bacterial sepsis. The features that appear to be characteristic of enteroviral infections include signs and symptoms of aseptic meningitis (irritability, central nervous system signs), gastroenteritis (anorexia, vomiting, diarrhea, abdominal distention), and an erythematous, maculopapular skin rash.

Infants with more serious disease may have a biphasic course that begins as a mild illness with slight temperature elevation, coryza, anorexia, and diarrhea. After an apparent recovery period lasting 1 to 5 days, more severe symptoms of aseptic meningitis, myocarditis (tachycardia, tachypnea, respiratory distress, cyanosis), or disseminated infection (abdominal distention, hepatomegaly, petechial rash, disseminated intravascular coagulation) occur.

Milder forms of disease, such as pneumonitis, undifferentiated febrile illness, exanthematous illness, or gastroenteritis lasting only a few days, also occur.[206, 248] In a survey of 338 infants younger than 2 months of age with enteroviral infections reported to the CDC, 74 per cent had severe disease and 26 per cent had mild disease.[298] Five (1 per cent) of these infants died, all in the severe disease group. Asymptomatic infections in neonates have been detected during outbreaks in nurseries or when routine virologic surveillance was being carried out in a nursery.[56] An outbreak of neonatal herpangina due to coxsackievirus A5 was observed in Thailand.[81]

Diagnosis and Differential Diagnosis

The major epidemiologic and clinical features that suggest a diagnosis of enteroviral infection in the neonate are listed in Table 76–11. Because the signs and symptoms in neonates with enteroviral disease often mimic bacterial sepsis and meningitis, antibiotic therapy should be initiated until a bacterial etiology is ruled out. In addition to sepsis and meningitis, the major diseases to be considered in the differential diagnosis include HSV infection and, to a lesser extent, congenital infection with CMV and rubella virus. HSV infection is nonseasonal, endemic, and associated with genital ulcerative lesions in the mother. Symptomatic congenital CMV and rubella infections are associated with intrauterine growth retardation and a chronic rather than an acute infectious clinical picture in the infant.

The most direct means of establishing a diagnosis of enteroviral infection in the neonate is isolation of the virus in tissue culture or suckling mice.[322] Virus may be recovered from throat swab, stool, cerebrospinal fluid, serum or buffy coat, and biopsy and autopsy tissue. Ideally, specimens should be processed immediately, but enteroviruses may remain stable at 4° C for several days if testing cannot be performed until later. Isolation of virus from the cerebrospinal fluid, blood, or tissue can be considered diagnostic. A throat or stool isolate also can be considered etiologic in most neonatal illnesses. Polymerase chain reaction for enterovirus in cerebrospinal fluid or serum is more sensitive than virus isolation[365] and likely will become commercially available in the near future.

TABLE 76–11. Characteristics Associated with Enteroviral Infection of the Neonate

Seasonal occurrence—summer and fall
Presence of known enteroviral epidemic in the community
History of maternal viral illness near time of delivery
Absence of factors predisposing to bacterial sepsis
Nursery outbreak of infectious illness with negative bacterial cultures
Development of culture-negative sepsis or aseptic meningitis in the neonate
Development of myocarditis, hepatitis, or erythematous maculopapular exanthem in the neonate

Treatment

There is no effective antiviral chemotherapy for enteroviruses. Anecdotal reports suggest that infusion of large doses of intravenous immunoglobulin, which contains high titers of antibody to enteroviruses,[111] may improve survival.[211]

Prognosis

The outcome is influenced by several factors: the enterovirus serotype causing the infection, the route of transmission of virus to the neonate, the age at acquisition of the infection, prematurity, and severity of the disease in the neonate. The mortality rates are highest for coxsackievirus B infections, intermediate for echovirus infections, and lowest for coxsackievirus A infections.[84, 153, 212, 248, 293] Most of the neonatal deaths due to enteroviruses reported in recent years have occurred in infants whose onset of disease was at or within a few days of birth and, therefore, was congenital.[82, 204, 238, 248, 293, 338] Infection rates and mortality rates both appear to be higher in premature infants.[56, 293] Death is most likely in infants with myocarditis, encephalitis, or hepatitis.[84, 293] Neurologic sequelae have been observed to follow meningoencephalitis in the neonatal period,[141, 377, 462] but long-term cardiac sequelae do not appear to follow myocarditis.[153]

Prevention

Polio vaccine has reduced maternal and neonatal poliomyelitis to an extremely rare occurrence. There are no prospects for vaccines for the echoviruses or coxsackieviruses. With the appearance of a case of enteroviral disease in a newborn nursery or intensive care unit, vigorous infection control measures are indicated, including enteric isolation for known or suspected cases, renewed emphasis on hand washing, and exclusion of personnel with symptoms of enteroviral disease. It should be emphasized that infection control measures applied in the nursery do not prevent congenital or natal transmission of virus from the mother to the infant. The continued appearance of cases in neonates younger than 8 to 10 days of age may reflect a persistent epidemic among pregnant women rather than a failure of nursery infection control measures and spread within the nursery.[424]

VARICELLA-ZOSTER VIRUS INFECTION

VZV causes both chickenpox, the result of primary exposure to the virus, and zoster, due to reactivation of latent virus.[154, 157, 321] VZV infection of a pregnant woman results in three separate and distinct syndromes that become apparent in the neonate and in infancy: (1) congenital defects secondary to intrauterine VZV infection, (2) neonatal chickenpox, and (3) zoster in infants.[138, 139, 154, 157, 177, 334a] For a discussion of VZV infections beyond infancy, see Chapter 167.

Maternal Varicella

Knowledge of several features of chickenpox in the mother is necessary to understand the pathogenesis of VZV infections in the fetus and neonate. Because antibody to VZV is present in approximately 90 per cent of women of child-bearing age,[157] one would expect chickenpox in pregnancy to be rare. In fact, maternal chickenpox has been reported to occur in only 0.7 per 1000 pregnancies.[382] The incubation period for chickenpox (from exposure to onset of rash) usually is between 13 and 17 days, with a range of 10 to 21 days.[154, 157] Viremia is presumed to occur before the onset of the rash, and antibody production begins shortly thereafter. Fetal infection, therefore, likely occurs during the period of maternal viremia—before the onset of rash.[154, 157]

Congenital Defects Syndrome

In several large prospective studies, no increase in anomalies is apparent in the offspring of women who had VZV infection during pregnancy.[54, 390–392] However, a prospective study[331] of 43 pregnancies complicated by varicella indicated that (1) 21 per cent of the women experienced appreciable morbidity, (2) 24 per cent of 33 infants tested had clinical or immunologic evidence of intrauterine VZV infection, and (3) the congenital varicella syndrome occurred in 9 per cent of 11 women with first-trimester varicella. Maternal zoster was not associated with fetal infection or neonatal morbidity. Pooling of results from several prospective studies indicated a risk of embryopathy due to maternal varicella during the first 20 weeks of pregnancy of approximately 2 per cent.[139, 334a]

The abnormalities present in 37 infants with the congenital varicella syndrome are summarized in Table 76–12. The defects apparently are the result of VZV replication in and destruction of developing fetal ectodermal tissues: skin, peripheral nerves, cervical and lumbosacral spinal cord, brain, and eye. Diagnosis of the syndrome essentially is clinical: history of chickenpox in the mother and recognition of the characteristic defects in the neonate. Virus has not been isolated from these infants, and serologic studies often have not been diagnostic.[157] Damage to the infants has been severe; many died in infancy.[157] Fortunately, the syndrome appears to be relatively rare, although additional cases may be recognized as the syndrome becomes appreciated more widely.

Neonatal Chickenpox

The neonatal varicella syndrome occurs when a pregnant woman suffers from chickenpox during the last 1 to 2 weeks of pregnancy or within the first few days post partum. Disease begins in the neonate within the first 10 days of life. As indicated in Table 76–13, the timing of the onset of disease in the mother and in the neonate is a critical factor influencing outcome in the infant. If the disease onset in the mother is 5 or more days before delivery or in the neonate during the first 4 days of life, the infection is mild. In contrast, if disease onset in the mother is within the 4 days prior to delivery or in the neonate between 5 and 10 days of age, the infection usually is disseminated and fulminant, and approximately one-third of the infants die.[157, 287] Other investigations have found the maternal rash onset risk period to extend from 7 days before to 7 days after delivery.[348] The generally accepted explanation for this observation is that when illness in the mother occurs prior to 5 days before delivery or when illness in the baby occurs during the first 4 days of life, maternal antibody has time to pass transplacentally and to provide passive protection for the infant. However, passive protection does not have time to occur when illness in the mother occurs within 4 days of delivery. Presumably, the immune responses of the neonate are insufficient to retard the growth and dissemination of VZV after intravenous inoculation via the placenta, and disseminated disease results.

TABLE 76–12. Abnormalities in 37 Infants with Congenital Varicella

Features	Percentage
Cutaneous scars	70
Ocular abnormalities*	62
Prematurity, low birth weight	60
Hypoplasia of limb	46
Cortical atrophy, mental retardation	30

*Microphthalmia, chorioretinitis, lenticular cataracts, optic atrophy, anisocoria, nystagmus.

Data from Gershon, A. A.: Chickenpox, measles and mumps. *In* Remington, J. S., and Klein, J. O. (eds.): Infectious Diseases of the Fetus and Newborn Infant. Philadelphia, W. B. Saunders, 1990, pp. 395–445.

TABLE 76–13. Neonatal Varicella Syndrome: Outcome in Relation to Rash Onset in Mother and Neonate

Day of Rash Onset	Neonatal Cases	Neonatal Deaths	
		Number	*Percentage*
Mother, ante partum			
5 or more	23	0	0
0 to 4	13	4	31
Neonate, post delivery			
0 to 4	22	0	0
5 to 10	19	4	21

Modified from Gershon, A. A.: Chickenpox, measles and mumps. *In* Remington, J. S., and Klein, J. O. (eds.): Infectious Diseases of the Fetus and Newborn Infant. Philadelphia, W. B. Saunders, 1990, pp. 395–445, as modified from Meyers, J. D.: Congenital varicella in term infants: Risk reconsidered. J. Infect. Dis. *129*:215, 1974, with permission from the University of Chicago.

The milder form of neonatal chickenpox resembles the disease in normal, older children, whereas the disseminated variety is similar to that seen in immunosuppressed, leukemic children. In the latter, diffuse pneumonia, severe hepatitis, and meningoencephalitis are the most common clinical manifestations. The diagnosis usually can be made clinically from the characteristic appearance of skin vesicles, but VZV may be isolated in tissue culture from vesicular fluid.[177, 322] The major disease to consider in the differential diagnosis is disseminated neonatal HSV infection. With HSV infection, there usually is a history of maternal genital herpes; characteristic keratoconjunctivitis, mouth lesions, or both may be present in the infant, and growth of the virus in cell culture is markedly different.[321, 322]

Varicella-zoster immunoglobulin, 1.25 mL total dose intramuscularly, should be given to the neonate born to the mother with chickenpox rash onset between 5 days before delivery and 2 days after delivery.[348] Varicella-zoster immunoglobulin should be administered as soon as possible after birth. Breakthrough severe varicella has occurred in neonates properly treated with varicella-zoster immunoglobulin.[30] If, despite varicella-zoster immunoglobulin therapy, breakthrough occurs and the neonatal varicella appears to be becoming severe (extensive skin lesions, high fever and toxicity, hepatitis, pneumonitis), treatment with intravenous acyclovir at 1500 mg/m²/day, divided every 8 hours, should be instituted.[385]

Zoster in Infancy and Childhood

Epidemiologic and serologic evidence indicates that zoster is a reactivated latent, rather than an exogenously acquired, infection with VZV.[154, 321] Persons with zoster, therefore, have had a previous episode of chickenpox. The vast majority of zoster occurs in older adult patients. The occurrence of zoster in infants and children is somewhat of a paradox because many of these patients have a negative history of chickenpox.[64, 157, 277] However, with several of these cases of childhood zoster, particularly those occurring in infants and young children, there was a history of chickenpox in the mother during pregnancy.[64, 139, 154, 261] The presumption is that there was fetal VZV infection with recovery and no evidence of disease in the neonate at birth. In a few other instances, the infant born to a VZV-immune mother may be exposed to chickenpox or zoster during early life at a time when maternal transplacental antibody still would be present. This passive antibody could provide protection against chickenpox and modify the disease to a subclinical or mild form that was not recognized.[144] Both situations could result in a patient with (1) an unrecognized episode of varicella and (2) the occurrence of zoster as the first overt manifestation of VZV infection.

Again, the major disease in the differential diagnosis is HSV infection. Patients with neonatal herpes may present a clinical picture resembling zoster,[300] and laboratory evaluation is required to differentiate the two diseases. Both neonatal chickenpox and childhood zoster are contagious, and appropriate isolation procedures should be used when the patient is hospitalized.

PARVOVIRUS B19 INFECTION

Parvovirus B19 has been shown to be the cause of erythema infectiosum, or fifth disease, a mild exanthematous illness in school age children.[20] (See Chapter 158.) There has been great concern about parvovirus infection in pregnant women because of the known associated occurrence of abortion, stillbirth, and hydrops fetalis.[18, 220, 224, 388, 434, 467] A summary of 22 published case reports of parvovirus fetal infection revealed that (1) only half the mothers had parvovirus-like clinical illness 4 to 13 weeks before fetal death, (2) all fetuses had hydrops fetalis and probable myocarditis, and (3) 19 died in utero at 16 to 26 weeks, and the remaining 3 died within 24 hours of delivery.[20] Hydrops fetalis occurs from replication of parvovirus in the bone marrow and resultant profound fetal anemia, with myocarditis playing a potential secondary role.[20]

Laboratory evidence of parvovirus infection included (1) maternal parvovirus IgM antibody, (2) elevated maternal alpha-fetoprotein, and (3) presence of parvovirus DNA in amniotic fluid.[20, 434, 435] Importantly, not all pregnancies complicated by parvovirus infection result in fetal infection, and not all infected fetuses develop hydrops. A British study of 186 pregnant women with parvovirus IgM antibody followed to term demonstrated that (1) fetal loss occurred in 16 per cent (no data on fetal loss rates in a control population) and (2) 43 per cent of 14 fetal tissues tested showed parvovirus DNA.[75, 350] Extrapolation from these figures yielded a maximum parvovirus-associated adverse fetal outcome of 7 per cent in pregnancies with *laboratory-proven* parvovirus infection. Extrapolation to the community level yielded the following estimates of fetal death in a pregnant woman exposed to active parvovirus infection: 1.8 per cent in home exposure and 1.1 per cent or less in school exposure.[75, 350] The figures used in this estimate include the 7 per cent fetal death rate with documented maternal infection cited earlier. Furthermore, only approximately 50 per cent of women of childbearing age are seronegative and therefore susceptible, and infection rates after parvovirus infection exposure are 50 per cent in the home and 30 per cent with a *widespread* school outbreak. More recent studies have indicated a total fetal infection rate of 25 to 30 per cent but an adverse fetal outcome rate of only 1 to 2 per cent.[160, 225] These latter results indicate that most intrauterine parvovirus infections are benign and self-limited.

Although intravenous immunoglobulin therapy has suppressed or controlled parvovirus-associated chronic anemia in immunosuppressed patients,[151] there is no evidence that this would be beneficial in pregnant women with parvovirus infection.

Prevention consists largely of rational use of infection control measures. It makes no sense to isolate or quarantine otherwise normal children who have the rash of erythema infectiosum because viral shedding has ceased by the time the rash appears.[20] On the other hand, hemoglobinopathy patients with parvovirus-induced aplastic crisis or immunosuppressed patients with parvovirus-associated chronic anemia may be highly infectious,[45] so respiratory isolation should be observed.

References

1. Abzug, M. J., Levin, M. J., and Rotbart, H. A.: Profile of enterovirus disease in the first two weeks of life. Pediatr. Infect. Dis. J. *12*:820–824, 1993.
2. Adler, S. P.: Transfusion-associated cytomegalovirus infections. Rev. Infect. Dis. *5*:977–993, 1983.
3. Adler, S. P., Baggett, J., Wilson, M., et al.: Molecular epidemiology of cytomegalovirus in a nursery: Lack of evidence for nosocomial transmission. J. Pediatr. *108*:117–123, 1986.
4. Adler, S. P., Tattamangalam, C., Lawrence, L., et al.: Cytomegalovirus infections in neonates acquired by blood transfusions. Pediatr. Infect. Dis. *2*:114–118, 1983.
5. Ahlfors, K., Forsgren, M., Ivarsson, S. A., et al.: Congenital cytomegalovirus infection: On the relation between type and time of maternal infection and infant's symptoms. Scand. J. Infect. Dis. *15*:129–138, 1983.
6. Ahlfors, K., Ivarsson, S. A., Harris, S., et al.: Congenital cytomegalovirus infection and disease in Sweden and the relative importance of primary and secondary maternal infections. Scand. J. Infect. Dis. *16*:129–137, 1984.
7. Ahlfors, K., Ivarsson, S. A., Johnsson, T., et al.: Primary and secondary maternal cytomegalovirus infections and their relation to congenital infection. Acta Paediatr. Scand. *71*:109–113, 1982.
8. Alestig, K., Bartsch, F. K., Nilsson, L.-A., et al.: Studies of amniotic fluid in women infected with rubella. J. Infect. Dis. *129*:79–81, 1974.
9. Alford, C. A., Jr., Foft, J. W., Blankenship, W. J., et al.: Subclinical central nervous system disease of neonates: A prospective study of infants born with increased levels of IgM. J. Pediatr. *75*:1167–1178, 1969.
10. Alford, C. A., Jr., Neva, F. A., and Weller, T. H.: Virologic and serologic studies on human products of conception after maternal rubella. N. Engl. J. Med. *271*:1275–1281, 1964.
11. Alford, C. A., Stagno, S., Pass, R. F., et al.: Congenital and perinatal cytomegalovirus infections. Rev. Infect. Dis. *12*(Suppl. 7):S745–S753, 1990.
12. Alford, C. A., Jr., Stagno, S., and Reynolds, D. W.: Diagnosis of chronic perinatal infections. Am. J. Dis. Child. *129*:455–463, 1975.
13. Alkalay, A. L., Pomerance, J. J., and Rimoin, D. L.: Fetal varicella syndrome. J. Pediatr. *111*:320–323, 1987.
14. Alter, H. J., Purcell, R. H., Shih, J. W., et al.: Detection of antibody to hepatitis C virus in prospectively followed transfusion recipients with acute and chronic non-A, non-B hepatitis. N. Engl. J. Med. *321*:1492–1500, 1989.
15. Alter, M. J.: The detection, transmission, and outcome of hepatitis C virus infection. Infect. Agents Dis. *2*:155–166, 1993.
16. Alter, M. J., Hadler, S. C., Judson, F. N., et al.: Risk factors for acute non-A, non-B hepatitis in the United States and association with hepatitis C virus infection. J. A. M. A. *264*:2231–2235, 1990.
17. Alward, W. L. M., McMahon, B. J., Hall, D. B., et al.: The long-term serological course of asymptomatic hepatitis B virus carriers and the

development of primary hepatocellular carcinoma. J. Infect. Dis. *151*:604–609, 1985.
18. Anand, A., Gray, E. S., Brown, T., et al.: Human parvovirus infection in pregnancy and hydrops fetalis. N. Engl. J. Med. *316*:183–186, 1987.
19. Anderson, K. E., Stevens, C. E., Tsuei, J. J., et al.: Hepatitis B antigen in infants born to mothers with chronic hepatitis B antigenemia in Taiwan. Am. J. Dis. Child. *129*:1389–1392, 1975.
20. Anderson, L. J.: Human parvoviruses. J. Infect. Dis. *161*:603–608, 1990.
21. Ansari, B. M., and Mason, M. K.: Chromosomal abnormality in congenital rubella. Pediatrics *59*:13–15, 1977.
22. Arevalo, J. A.: Hepatitis B in pregnancy. West. J. Med. *150*:668–674, 1989.
23. Arevalo, J. A., and Washington, A. E.: Cost-effectiveness of prenatal screening and immunization for hepatitis B virus. J. A. M. A. *259*:365–369, 1988.
24. Arvin, A. M., and Alford, C. A., Jr.: Chronic intrauterine and perinatal infections. *In* Galasso, G. J., Whitley, R. J., and Merigan, T. C. (eds.): Antiviral Agents and Viral Diseases of Man. 3rd ed. New York, Raven Press, 1990, pp. 497–580.
25. Arvin, A. M., Hensleigh, P. A., Prober, C. G., et al.: Failure of antepartum maternal cultures to predict the infant's risk of exposure to herpes simplex virus at delivery. N. Engl. J. Med. *315*:796–800, 1986.
26. Arvin, A. M., Yeager, A. S., and Merigan, T. C.: Effect of leukocyte interferon on urinary excretion of cytomegalovirus by infants. J. Infect. Dis. *133*(Suppl.):A205–A210, 1976.
27. Bacon, C. J., and Sims, D. G.: Echovirus 19 infection in infants under six months. Arch. Dis. Child. *51*:631–633, 1976.
28. Bai, P. V. A., and John, T. J.: Congenital skin ulcers following varicella in late pregnancy. J. Pediatr. *94*:65–67, 1979.
29. Baker, D. A.: Herpes and pregnancy: New management. Clin. Obstet. Gynecol. *33*:253–257, 1990.
30. Bakshi, S. S., Miller, T. C., Kaplan, M., et al.: Failure of varicella-zoster immunoglobulin in modification of severe congenital varicella. Pediatr. Infect. Dis. *5*:699–702, 1986.
31. Ballard, R. A., Drew, W. L., Hufnagle, K. G., et al.: Acquired cytomegalovirus infection in preterm infants. Am. J. Dis. Child. *133*:482–485, 1979.
32. Barin, F., Goudeau, A., Denis, F., et al.: Immune response in neonates to hepatitis B vaccine. Lancet *1*:251–253, 1982.
33. Bart, K. J., Orenstein, W. A., Preblud, S. R., et al.: Elimination of rubella and congenital rubella from the United States. Pediatr. Infect. Dis. *4*:14–21, 1985.
34. Baublis, J. V., Whitley, R. J., Ch'ien, L. T., et al.: Treatment of cytomegalovirus infection in infants and adults. *In* Pavan-Langston, D., and Buchanan, R. A. (eds.): Adenine Arabinoside: An Antiviral Agent. New York, Raven Press, 1975, pp. 247–260.
35. Beasley, R. P., and Hwang, L.-Y.: Postnatal infectivity of hepatitis B surface antigen-carrier mothers. J. Infect. Dis. *147*:185–190, 1983.
36. Beasley, R. P., Hwang, L.-Y., Lee, G. C.-Y., et al.: Prevention of perinatally transmitted hepatitis B virus infections with hepatitis B immune globulin and hepatitis B vaccine. Lancet 2:1099–1102, 1983.
37. Beasley, R. P., Hwang, L.-Y., Lin, C.-C., et al.: Hepatocellular carcinoma and hepatitis B virus: A prospective study of 22,707 men in Taiwan. Lancet *2*:1129–1133, 1981.
38. Beasley, R. P., Hwang, L.-Y., Lin, C.-C., et al.: Incidence of hepatitis B virus infections in preschool children in Taiwan. J. Infect. Dis. *146*:198–204, 1982.
39. Beasley, R. P., Hwang, L.-Y., Lin, C.-C., et al.: Hepatitis B immune globulin (HBIG) efficacy in the interruption of perinatal transmission of hepatitis B virus carrier state. Lancet 2:388–393, 1981.
40. Beasley, R. P., Hwang, L.-Y., Stevens, C. E., et al.: Efficacy of hepatitis B immune globulin for prevention of perinatal transmission of the hepatitis B virus carrier state: Final report of a randomized double-blind, placebo-controlled trial. Hepatology *3*:135–141, 1983.
41. Beasley, R. P., Shiao, I.-S., Stevens, C. E., et al.: Evidence against breast-feeding as a mechanism for vertical transmission of hepatitis B. Lancet 2:740–741, 1975.
42. Beasley, R. P., Trepo, C., Stevens, C. E., et al.: The e antigen and vertical transmission of hepatitis B surface antigen. Am. J. Epidemiol. *105*:94–98, 1977.
43. Becker, T. M., Blount, J. H., and Guinan, M. E.: Genital herpes infections in private practice in the United States, 1966 to 1981. J. A. M. A. *253*:1601–1603, 1985.
44. Behrman, R. E.: The high-risk infant. *In* Vaughan, V. C., III, McKay, R. J., Jr., and Behrman, R. E. (eds.): Nelson Textbook of Pediatrics. Philadelphia, W. B. Saunders, 1979, pp. 398–414.
45. Bell, L. M., Naides, S. J., Stoffman, P., et al.: Human parvovirus B19 infection among hospital staff members after contact with infected patients. N. Engl. J. Med. *321*:485–491, 1989.
46. Binkin, N. J., Koplan, J. P., and Cates, W., Jr.: Preventing neonatal herpes: The value of weekly viral cultures in pregnant women with recurrent genital herpes. J. A. M. A. *251*:2816–2821, 1984.
47. Birnbaum, G., Lynch, J. I., Margileth, A. M., et al.: Cytomegalovirus infections in newborn infants. J. Pediatr. *75*:789–795, 1969.
48. Blanc, W. A.: Pathology of the placenta and cord in some viral infections. *In* Hanshaw, J. B., and Dudgeon, J. A. (eds.): Viral Diseases of the Fetus and Newborn. Philadelphia, W. B. Saunders, 1978, pp. 237–258.
49. Boehm, F. H., Estes, W., Wright, P. F., et al.: Management of genital herpes simplex virus infection occurring during pregnancy. Am. J. Obstet. Gynecol. *141*:735–740, 1981.
50. Bolognese, R. J., Corson, S. L., Fuccillo, D. A., et al.: Herpesvirus hominis type II infections in asymptomatic pregnant women. Obstet. Gynecol. *48*:507–510, 1976.
51. Boner, A., Wilmott, R. W., Dinwiddie, R., et al.: Desquamative interstitial pneumonia and antigen-antibody complexes in two infants with congenital rubella. Pediatrics *72*:835–839, 1983.
52. Boppana, S., Amos, C., Britt, W., et al.: Late onset and reactivation of chorioretinitis in children with congenital cytomegalovirus infection. Pediatr. Infect. Dis. J. *13*:1139–1142, 1994.
53. Bortolotti, F., Caizia, R., Cadrobbi, P., et al.: Liver cirrhosis associated with chronic hepatitis B virus infection in childhood. J. Pediatr. *108*:224–227, 1986.
54. Bradford-Hill, A., Doll, R., Galloway, T. M., et al.: Virus diseases in pregnancy and congenital defects. Br. J. Prev. Soc. Med. *12*:1–7, 1958.
55. Brady, M. T., Milam, J. D., Anderson, D. C., et al.: Use of deglycerolized red blood cells to prevent posttransfusion infection with cytomegalovirus in neonates. J. Infect. Dis. *150*:334–339, 1984.
56. Brightman, V. J., Scott, T. F. M., Westphal, M., et al.: An outbreak of coxsackie B-5 virus infection in a newborn nursery. J. Pediatr. *69*:179–192, 1966.
57. Brody, J. A., Sever, J. L., and Schiff, G. M.: Prevention of rubella by gamma globulin during an epidemic in Barrow, Alaska, in 1964. N. Engl. J. Med. *272*:127–129, 1965.
58. Brown, G. C.: Maternal virus infection and congenital anomalies. Arch. Environ. Health *21*:362–365, 1970.
59. Brown, G. C., and Evans, T. N.: Serologic evidence of coxsackievirus etiology of congenital heart disease. J. A. M. A. *199*:183–187, 1967.
60. Brown, G. C., and Karunas, R. S.: Relationship of congenital anomalies and maternal infection with selected enteroviruses. Am. J. Epidemiol. *95*:207–217, 1972.
61. Brown, Z. A., Benedetti, J., Ashley, R., et al.: Neonatal herpes simplex virus infection in relation to asymptomatic maternal infection at the time of labor. N. Engl. J. Med. *324*:1247–1252, 1991.
62. Brown, Z. A., Kern, E. R., Spruance, S. L., et al.: Clinical and virologic course of herpes simplex genitalis. West. J. Med. *130*:414–421, 1979.
63. Brown, Z. A., Vontver, L. A., Benedetti, J., et al.: Effects on infants of a first episode of genital herpes during pregnancy. N. Engl. J. Med. *317*:1246–1251, 1987.
64. Brunell, P. A., Miller, L. H., and Lovejoy, F.: Zoster in children. Am. J. Dis. Child. *115*:432–437, 1968.
65. Buhles, W. C., Jr., Mastre, B. J., Tinker, A. J., et al.: Ganciclovir treatment of life- or sight-threatening cytomegalovirus infection: Experience in 314 immunocompromised patients. Rev. Infect. Dis. *10*(Suppl. 3):S495–S506, 1988.
66. Buimovici-Klein, E., Lang, P. B., Ziring, P. R., et al.: Impaired cell-mediated immune response in patients with congenital rubella: Correlation with gestational age at time of infection. Pediatrics *64*:620–626, 1979.
67. Centers for Disease Control: Enterovirus Surveillance Report, 1970–1979. Issued November 1981.
68. Centers for Disease Control: Hepatitis B virus: A comprehensive strategy for eliminating transmission in the United States through universal childhood vaccination. M. M. W. R. *40*(RR-13):1–25, 1991.
69. Centers for Disease Control: Hepatitis Surveillance Report No. 55, 1994, pp. 1–34.
70. Centers for Disease Control: Immune globulins for protection against viral hepatitis. M. M. W. R. *30*:423–435, 1981.
71. Centers for Disease Control: Increase in rubella and congenital rubella. J. A. M. A. *265*:1076–1077, 1991.
72. Centers for Disease Control: Prevention of perinatal transmission of hepatitis B virus: Prenatal screening of all pregnant women for hepatitis B surface antigen. M. M. W. R. *37*:341–346, 1988.
73. Centers for Disease Control: Protection against viral hepatitis. M. M. W. R. *39*(RR-2):1–26, 1990.
74. Centers for Disease Control: Recommendations for protection against viral hepatitis. M. M. W. R. *34*:313–335, 1985.
75. Centers for Disease Control: Risks associated with human parvovirus B19 infection. M. M. W. R. *38*:81–97, 1989.
76. Centers for Disease Control: Rubella vaccination during pregnancy: United States, 1971–1988. M. M. W. R. *38*:289–293, 1989.
77. Chairez, R., Cesario, A. J., Barrett, J. E., et al.: Evaluation of CMV antibody EIA: An enzyme immunoassay for detection of antibodies to cytomegalovirus. Diagn. Microbiol. Infect. Dis. *3*:403–410, 1985.
78. Champsaur, H., Fattal-German, M., and Arranhado, R.: Sensitivity and specificity of viral immunoglobulin M determination by indirect enzyme linked immunosorbent assay. J. Clin. Microbiol. *26*:328–332, 1988.
79. Chandler, S. H., Alexander, E. R., and Holmes, K. K.: Epidemiology of cytomegaloviral infection in a heterogeneous population of pregnant women. J. Infect. Dis. *2*:249–256, 1985.
80. Chang, T. W.: Rubella reinfection and intrauterine involvement. J. Pediatr. *84*:617–618, 1974.
81. Chawareewong, S., Kiangsiri, S., Lokaphadhana, K., et al.: Neonatal herpangina caused by Coxsackie A-5 virus. J. Pediatr. *93*:492–494, 1978.

82. Cheeseman, S. H., Hirsch, M. S., Keller, E. W., et al.: Fatal neonatal pneumonia caused by echovirus type 9. Am. J. Dis. Child. *131*:1169, 1977.
83. Chernesky, M. A., and Mahony, J. B.: Rubella virus. *In* Murray, P. R., Barron, E. J., Pfaller, M. A., et al.: (eds.): Manual of Clinical Microbiology. Washington, D. C., American Society of Microbiology, 1995, pp. 968–973.
84. Cherry, J. D.: Enteroviruses. *In* Remington, J. S., and Klein, J. O. (eds.): Infectious Diseases of the Fetus and Newborn Infant. 4th ed. Philadelphia, W. B. Saunders, 1995, pp. 404–446.
85. Chess, S., Fernandez, P., and Korn, S.: Behavioral consequences of congenital rubella. J. Pediatr. *93*:699–703, 1978.
86. Ch'ien, L. T., Cannon, N. J., Whitley, R. J., et al.: Effect of adenine arabinoside on cytomegalovirus infections. J. Infect. Dis. *130*:32–39, 1974.
87. Ch'ien, L. T., Whitley, R. J., Nahmias, A. J., et al.: Antiviral chemotherapy and neonatal herpes simplex virus infection: A pilot study—Experience with adenine arabinoside (ARA-A). Pediatrics *55*:678–685, 1975.
88. Choo, Q.-L., Kuo, G., Weiner, A. J., et al.: Isolation of a cDNA clone derived from a blood-borne non-A, non-B viral hepatitis genome. Science *244*:359–362, 1989.
89. Clarke, W. L., Shaver, K. A., Bright, G. M., et al.: Autoimmunity in congenital rubella syndrome. J. Pediatr. *104*:370–373, 1984.
90. Clemens, R., Safary, A., Hepburn A., et al.: Clinical experience with an inactivated hepatitis A vaccine. J. Infect. Dis. *171*(Suppl. 1):S44–S49, 1995.
91. Clemente, M. G., Congia, M., Lai, M. E., et al.: Effect of iron overload on the response to recombinant interferon-alfa treatment in transfusion dependent patients with thalassemia major and chronic hepatitis C. J. Pediatr. *125*:123–128, 1994.
92. Committee on Infectious Diseases: Universal hepatitis B immunization. Pediatrics *89*:795–800, 1992.
93. Conboy, T. J., Pass, R. F., Stagno, S., et al.: Early clinical manifestations and intellectual outcome in children with symptomatic congenital cytomegalovirus infection. J. Pediatr. *111*:343–348, 1987.
94. Conchie, A. F., Barton, B. W., and Tobin, J. O.: Congenital cytomegalovirus infection treated with idoxuridine. B. M. J. *4*:162–163, 1968.
95. Cone, R. W., Hobson, A. C., Brown. Z., et al.: Frequent detection of genital herpes simplex virus DNA by polymerase chain reaction among pregnant women. J. A. M. A. *272*:792–796, 1994.
96. Cooper, L. Z.: The history and medical consequences of rubella. Rev. Infect. Dis. *7*(Suppl. 1):S2–S10, 1985.
97. Cooper, L. Z., Green, R. H., Krugman, S., et al.: Neonatal thrombocytopenic purpura and other manifestations of rubella contracted in utero. Am. J. Dis. Child. *110*:416–427, 1965.
98. Cooper, L. Z., Preblud, S. R., and Alford, C. A., Jr.: Rubella. *In* Remington, J. S., and Klein, J. O. (eds.): Infections of the Fetus and Newborn Infant. Philadelphia, W. B. Saunders, 1995, pp. 268–311.
99. Cooper, L. Z., Ziring, P. R., Ockerse, A. B., et al.: Rubella: Clinical manifestations and management. Am. J. Dis. Child. *118*:18–29, 1969.
100. Corey, L., Adams, H. G., Brown, Z. A., et al.: Genital herpes simplex virus infections: Clinical manifestations, course, and complications. Ann. Intern. Med. *98*:958–972, 1983.
101. Corey, L., and Spear, P. G.: Infections of herpes simplex viruses. N. Engl. J. Med. *314*:686–691; 749–757, 1986.
102. Corey, L., Whitley, R. J., Stone, E. F., et al.: Difference between herpes simplex virus type 1 and type 2 neonatal encephalitis in neurological outcome. Lancet *1*:1–4, 1988.
103. Cox, F., and Hughes, W. T.: Fecal excretion of cytomegalovirus in disseminated cytomegalic inclusion disease. J. Infect. Dis. *129*:732–736, 1974.
104. Craig, C. P., and Nahmias, A. J.: Different patterns of neurologic involvement with herpes simplex virus types 1 and 2: Isolation of herpes simplex virus type 2 from the buffy coat of two adults with meningitis. J. Infect. Dis. *127*:365–372, 1973.
105. Cramblett, H. G., Haynes, R. E., Azimi, P. H., et al.: Nosocomial infection with echovirus type 11 in handicapped and premature infants. Pediatrics *51*:603–607, 1973.
106. Cruz, A. C., Frentzen, B. H., and Behnke, M.: Hepatitis B: A case for prenatal screening of all patients. Am. J. Obstet. Gynecol. *156*:1180–1183, 1987.
107. Cuthbert, J. A.: Hepatitis C: Progress and problems. Clin. Microbiol. Rev. *7*:505–552, 1994.
108. Dagan, R., Hall, C. B., Powell, K. R., et al.: Epidemiology and laboratory diagnosis of infection with viral and bacterial pathogens in infants hospitalized for suspected sepsis. J. Pediatr. *115*:351–356, 1989.
109. Dagan, R., Jenista, J. A., and Menegus, M. A.: Clinical, epidemiological, and laboratory aspects of enterovirus infection in young infants. *In* de la Maza, L. M., and Peterson, E. M. (eds.): Medical Virology IV. Hillsdale, N. J., L. Erlbaum Assoc., 1985, pp. 123–151.
110. Dagan, R., Jenista, J. A., Prather, S. L., et al.: Viremia in hospitalized children with enterovirus infections. J. Pediatr. *106*:397–401, 1985.
111. Dagan, R., Prather, S. L., Powell, K. R., et al.: Neutralizing antibodies to non-polio enteroviruses in human immune serum globulin. Pediatr. Infect. Dis. *2*:454–456, 1983.
112. Daling, J. A., and Wolf, M. E.: The role of decision and cost analyses in the treatment of pregnant women with recurrent genital herpes. J. A. M. A. *251*:2828–2829, 1984.
113. Davis, L. E., Tweed, G. V., Chin, T. D. Y., et al.: Intrauterine diagnosis of cytomegalovirus infection: Viral recovery from amniocentesis fluid. Am. J. Obstet. Gynecol. *109*:1217–1219, 1971.
114. De Backer, S., Samule, K., Carton, D., et al.: Neonatal Coxsackie B3 sepsis. Acta Paediatr. Belg. *29*:55–57, 1976.
115. Delaplane, D., Yogev, R., Crussi, F., et al.: Fatal hepatitis B in early infancy: The importance of identifying HBsAg-positive pregnant women and providing immunoprophylaxis to their newborns. Pediatrics *72*:176–180, 1983.
116. Demmler, G. J.: Summary of a workshop on surveillance for congenital cytomegalovirus disease. Rev. Infect. Dis. *13*:315–329, 1991.
117. Derso, A., Boxall, E. H., Tarlow, M. J., et al.: Transmission of HBsAg from mother to infant in four ethnic groups. B. M. J. *1*:949–952, 1978.
118. Desmond, M. M., Fisher, E. S., Vorderman, A. L., et al.: The longitudinal course of congenital rubella encephalitis in nonretarded children. J. Pediatr. *93*:584–591, 1978.
119. Desmond, M. M., Wilson, G. S., and Melnick, J. L.: Congenital rubella encephalitis. J. Pediatr. *71*:311–331, 1967.
120. Dickinson, J., and Gonik, B.: Teratogenic viral infections. Clin. Obstet. Gynecol. *33*:242–252, 1990.
121. Donowitz, M., and Gryboski, J. D.: Pancreatic insufficiency and the congenital rubella syndrome. J. Pediatr. *87*:241–243, 1975.
122. Dosik, H., and Jhaveri, R.: Prevention of neonatal hepatitis B infection by high-dose hepatitis B immune globulin. N. Engl. J. Med. *298*:602–603, 1978.
123. Douglas, J. M., Schmidt, O., and Corey, L.: Acquisition of neonatal HSV-1 infection from a paternal source contact. J. Pediatr. *103*:908–910, 1983.
124. Dublin, A. B., and Merten, D. F.: Computed tomography in the evaluation of herpes simplex encephalitis. Radiology *125*:133–134, 1977.
125. Dunkle, L. M., Schmidt, R. R., and O'Connor, D. M.: Neonatal herpes simplex infection possibly acquired via maternal breast milk. Pediatrics *63*:250–251, 1979.
126. Dunn, A. E. G., Peters, R. L., Schweitzer, I. L., et al.: Virus-like particles in livers of infants with vertically transmitted hepatitis. Arch. Pathol. *94*:258–264, 1972.
127. Dupuy, J. M., Frommel, D., and Alagille, D.: Severe viral hepatitis type B in infancy. Lancet *1*:191–194, 1975.
128. Dupuy, J. M., Kostewicz, E., and Alagille, D.: Hepatitis B in children. I. Analysis of 80 cases of acute and chronic hepatitis B. J. Pediatr. *92*:17–20, 1978.
129. Dupuy, J. M., Giraud, P., Dupuy, C., et al.: Hepatitis B in children. II. Study of children born to chronic HBsAg carrier mothers. J. Pediatr. *92*:200–204, 1978.
130. Dworsky, M., Yow, M., Stagno, S., et al.: Cytomegalovirus infection of breast milk and transmission in infancy. Pediatrics *72*:295–299, 1983.
131. Echeverria, P., Miller, G., Campbell, A. G. M., et al.: Scalp vesicles within the first week of life: A clue to early diagnosis of herpes neonatorum. J. Pediatr. *83*:1062–1064, 1973.
132. Eilard, T., and Strannegard, Ö.: Rubella reinfection in pregnancy followed by transmission to the fetus. J. Infect. Dis. *129*:594–596, 1974.
133. Elizan, T. S., Ajero-Froehlich, L., Fabiyi, A., et al.: Viral infection in pregnancy and congenital CNS malformations in man. Arch. Neurol. *20*:115–119, 1969.
134. Elizan, T. S., and Fabiyi, A.: Congenital and neonatal anomalies linked with viral infections in experimental animals. Am. J. Obstet. Gynecol. *106*:147–165, 1970.
135. Emanuel, D., Cunningham, I., Jules-Elysee, K., et al.: Cytomegalovirus pneumonia after bone marrow transplantation successfully treated with the combination of ganciclovir and high-dose intravenous immune globulin. Ann. Intern. Med. *109*:777–782, 1988.
136. Em'di, G., and Just, M.: Impaired interferon response of children with congenital cytomegalovirus disease. Acta Paediatr. Scand. *63*:183–187, 1974.
137. Em'di, G., O'Reilly, R., Müller, A., et al.: Effect of human exogenous leukocyte interferon in cytomegalovirus infections. J. Infect. Dis. *133*(Suppl.):A199–A203, 1976.
138. Enders, G.: Varicella-zoster virus infection in pregnancy. Prog. Med. Virol. *29*:166–196, 1984.
139. Enders, G., Miller, E., and Cradock-Watson, J.: Consequences of varicella and herpes zoster in pregnancy: Prospective study of 1379 cases. Lancet *343*:1547–1560, 1994.
140. Esterly, J. R., Slusser, R. J., and Ruebner, B. H.: Hepatic lesions in the congenital rubella syndrome. J. Pediatr. *71*:676–685, 1967.
141. Farmer, K., MacArthur, B. A., and Clay, M. M.: A follow-up study of 15 cases of neonatal meningoencephalitis due to coxsackievirus B5. J. Pediatr. *87*:568–571, 1975.
142. Faulkner, R. S., and van Rooyen, C. E.: Echovirus type 17 in the neonate. Can. Med. Assoc. J. *108*:878–882, 1973.
143. Fawaz, K. A., Grady, G. F., Kaplan, M. M., et al.: Repetitive maternal-fetal transmission of fatal hepatitis B. N. Engl. J. Med. *293*:1357–1359, 1975.
144. Feldman, G. V.: Herpes zoster neonatorum. Arch. Dis. Child. *27*:126–127, 1952.
145. Feldman, R. A.: Cytomegalovirus infection during pregnancy. Am. J. Dis. Child. *117*:517–521, 1969.
146. Florman, A. L., Gershon, A. A., Blackett, P. R., et al.: Intrauterine infection with herpes simplex virus. J. A. M. A. *225*:129–132, 1973.

147. Forbes, B. A.: Acquisition of cytomegalovirus infection: An update. Clin. Microbiol. Rev. *2*:204–216, 1989.
148. Forbes, B. A.: Perinatal viral infections. Clin. Microbiol. Newsl. *14*:169–173, 1992.
149. Fowler, K. B., Stagno, S., and Pass, R. F., et al.: The outcome of congenital cytomegalovirus infection in relation to maternal antibody status. N. Engl. J. Med. *326*:663–667, 1992.
150. Frey, H. M., Bailkin, G., and Gershon, A. A.: Congenital varicella: Case report of a serologically proved long-term survivor. Pediatrics *59*:110–112, 1977.
151. Frickhofen, N., Abkowitz, J. L., Safford, M., et al.: Persistent B19 parvovirus infection in patients infected with human immunodeficiency virus type-1 (HIV-1): A treatable cause of anemia in AIDS. Ann. Intern. Med. *113*:926–933, 1990.
152. Garcia, A. G. P., Olinto, F., and Fortes, T. G. O.: Thymic hypoplasia due to congenital rubella. Arch. Dis. Child. *49*:181–185, 1974.
153. Gear, J. H. S., and Measroch, V.: Coxsackievirus infections of the newborn. Prog. Med. Virol. *15*:42–62, 1973.
154. Gelb, L. D.: Varicella-zoster virus. *In* Fields, B. N., and Knipe, D. M. (eds.): Virology. New York, Raven Press, 1990, pp. 2011–2054.
155. Gerety, R. J., Hoofnagle, J. H., Markenson, J. A., et al.: Exposure to hepatitis B virus and development of the chronic HBAg carrier state in children. J. Pediatr. *84*:661–665, 1974.
156. Gerety, R. J., and Schweitzer, I. L.: Viral hepatitis type B during pregnancy, the neonatal period, and infancy. J. Pediatr. *90*:368–374, 1977.
157. Gershon, A. A.: Chickenpox, measles and mumps. *In* Remington, J. S., and Klein, J. O. (eds.): Infectious Diseases of the Fetus and Newborn Infant. 4th ed. Philadelphia, W. B. Saunders, 1995, pp. 555–618.
158. Gibbs, R. S., Amstey, M. S., Sweet, R. L., et al.: Editorial: Management of genital herpes infection in pregnancy. Obstet. Gynecol. *71*:779–780, 1988.
159. Grangeot-Keros, L., Pillot, J., Daffos, F., et al.: Prenatal and postnatal production of IgM and IgA antibodies to rubella virus studied by antibody capture immunoassay. J. Infect. Dis. *158*:138–143, 1988.
160. Gratacos, E., Torres, P.-J., Vidal, J., et al.: The incidence of human parvovirus B19 infection during pregnancy and its impact on perinatal outcome. J. Infect. Dis. *171*:1360–1363, 1995.
161. Greenberg, D. P.: Pediatric experience with recombinant hepatitis B vaccines and relevant safety and immunogenicity studies. Pediatr. Infect. Dis. J. *12*:438–445, 1993.
162. Greenberg, H. B., Pollard, R. B., Lutwick, L. L., et al.: Effect of human leukocyte interferon on hepatitis B virus infection in patients with chronic active hepatitis. N. Engl. J. Med. *295*:517–522, 1976.
163. Greenough, A., Osborne, J., and Sutherland, S.: Congenital, Perinatal and Neonatal Infections. Edinburgh, Churchill Livingstone, 1992.
164. Gregg, N. M.: Congenital cataract following German measles in the mother. Trans. Ophthalmol. Soc. Aust. *3*:35–46, 1941.
165. Griffiths, P. D., and Baboonian, C.: A prospective study of primary cytomegalovirus infection during pregnancy: Final report. Br. J. Obstet. Gynecol. *91*:307–315, 1984.
166. Griffiths, P. D., Stagno, S., Pass, R. F., et al.: Infection with cytomegalovirus during pregnancy. Specific IgM antibodies as a marker of recent primary infection. J. Infect. Dis. *145*:647–653, 1982.
167. Griffiths, P. D., Stagno, S., Pass, R. F., et al.: Congenital cytomegalovirus infection: Diagnostic and prognostic significance of the detection of specific immunoglobulin M antibodies in cord serum. Pediatrics *69*:544–549, 1982.
167a. Gross, J. B., Jr., and Persing, D. H.: Hepatitis C: Advances in diagnosis. Mayo Clin. Proc. *70*:296–297, 1995.
168. Grossman, J. H., III: Herpes simplex virus (HSV) infections. Clin. Obstet. Gynecol. *25*:555–561, 1982.
169. Hagler, W. S., Walters, P. V., and Nahmias, A. J.: Ocular involvement in neonatal herpes simplex virus infection. Arch. Ophthalmol. *82*:169–176, 1969.
170. Halfon, N., and Spector, S. A.: Fatal echovirus type 11 infections. Am. J. Dis. Child. *135*:1017–1020, 1981.
171. Hall, C. B., Douglas, R. G., Jr., Gelman, J. M., et al.: Nosocomial respiratory syncytial virus infections. N. Engl. J. Med. *293*:1343–1346, 1975.
172. Hammerberg, O., Watts, J., Chernesky, M., et al.: An outbreak of herpes simplex virus type I in an intensive care nursery. Pediatr. Infect. Dis. *2*:290–294, 1983.
173. Hancock, M. P., Huntley, C. C., and Sever, J. L.: Congenital rubella syndrome with immunoglobulin disorder. J. Pediatr. *72*:636–645, 1968.
174. Hanshaw, J. B.: Congenital cytomegalovirus infection. Pediatr. Ann. *23*:124–128, 1994.
175. Hanshaw, J. B.: Developmental abnormalities associated with congenital cytomegalovirus infection. Adv. Teratol. *4*:64–93, 1970.
176. Hanshaw, J. B.: Herpesvirus hominis infections in the fetus and the newborn. Am J. Dis. Child. *126*:546–555, 1973.
177. Hanshaw, J. B., Dudgeon, J. A., and Marshall, W. C.: Viral Diseases of the Fetus and Newborn. 2nd ed. Philadelphia, W. B. Saunders, 1985.
178. Hanshaw, J. B., Scheiner, A. P., Moxley, A. W., et al.: School failure and deafness after "silent" congenital cytomegalovirus infection. N. Engl. J. Med. *295*:468–470, 1976.
179. Hanshaw, J. B., Steinfeld, H. J., and White, C. J.: Fluorescent-antibody test for cytomegalovirus macroglobulin. N. Engl. J. Med. *279*:566–570, 1968.
180. Hardy, J. B., Sever, J. L., and Gilkeson, M. R.: Declining antibody titers in children with congenital rubella. J. Pediatr. *75*:213–220, 1969.
181. Harger, J. H.: Indications for antepartum HSV screening cultures. Infect. Surg. *8*:24–33, 1989.
182. Harger, J. H., Pazin, G. J., Armstrong, J. A., et al.: Characteristics and management of pregnancy in women with genital herpes simplex virus infection. Am. J. Obstet. Gynecol. *145*:784–791, 1983.
183. Hatherley, L. I., Hay, K., Hennessy, E. M., et al.: Herpesvirus in an obstetric hospital. I. Herpetic eruptions. Med. J. Aust. *2*:205–208, 1980.
184. Hatherley, L. I., Hayes, K., and Jack, I.: Herpesvirus in an obstetric hospital. II. Asymptomatic virus excretion in staff members. Med. J. Aust. *2*:273–275, 1980.
185. Hayes, K., Danks, D. M., Gibas, H., et al.: Cytomegalovirus in human milk. N. Engl. J. Med. *287*:177–178, 1972.
186. Hayes, K., and Gibas, H.: Placental cytomegalovirus infection without fetal involvement following primary infection in pregnancy. J. Pediatr. *79*:401–405, 1971.
187. Haynes, R. E., Azimi, P. H., and Cramblett, H. G.: Fatal herpesvirus hominis (herpes simplex virus) infections in children: Clinical, pathologic, and virologic characteristics. J. A. M. A. *206*:312–319, 1968.
188. Heijtink, R. A., Boender, P. J., Schalm, S. W., et al.: Hepatitis B virus DNA in serum of pregnant women with HBsAg and HBeAg or antibodies to HBe. J. Infect. Dis. *150*:462, 1984.
189. Herrmann, K. L.: Available rubella serologic tests. Rev. Infect. Dis. *7*(Suppl. 1):S108–S112, 1985.
190. Higa, K., Dan, K., and Manabe, H.: Varicella-zoster virus infections during pregnancy: Hypothesis concerning the mechanisms of congenital malformations. Obstet. Gynecol. *69*:214–222, 1987.
191. Hildebrandt, R. J., Sever, J. L., Margileth, A. M., et al.: Cytomegalovirus in the normal pregnant woman. Am. J. Obstet. Gynecol. *98*:1125–1128, 1967.
192. Hinman, A. R.: Prevention of congenital rubella infection: Symposium summary. Pediatrics *75*:1162–1165, 1985.
193. Hocker, J. R., Cook, L. N., Adams, G., et al.: Ganciclovir therapy of congenital cytomegalovirus pneumonia. Pediatr. Infect. Dis. J. *9*:743–745,1990.
194. Hollinger, F. B.: Serologic evaluation of viral hepatitis. Hosp. Pract. *22*:101–114, 1987.
195. Holzer, B R., and Egger, M.: Hepatitis A vaccine. Curr. Opin. Infect. Dis. *8*:186–190, 1995.
196. Honig, P. J., and Brown, D.: Congenital herpes simplex virus infection initially resembling epidermolysis bullosa. J. Pediatr. *101*:958–959, 1982.
197. Hoofnagle, J. H.: Therapy of acute and chronic viral hepatitis. Adv. Intern. Med. *39*:241–275, 1994.
198. Horstmann, D. M., Banatvala, J. E., Riordan, J. T., et al.: Maternal rubella and the rubella syndrome in infants: Epidemiologic, clinical, and virologic observations. Am. J. Dis. Child. *110*:408–415, 1965.
199. Horstmann, D. M., Liebhaber, H., Le Bouvier, G. L., et al.: Rubella: Reinfection of vaccinated and naturally immune persons exposed in an epidemic. N. Engl. J. Med. *283*:771–778, 1970.
200. Horstmann, D. M., Pajot, T. G., and Liebhaber, H.: Epidemiology of rubella: Subclinical infection and occurrence of reinfection. Am. J. Dis. Child. *118*:133–136, 1969.
201. Hovig, D. E., Hodgman, J. E., Mathies, A. W., Jr., et al.: Herpesvirus hominis (simplex) infection: With recurrences during infancy. Am. J. Dis. Child. *115*:438–444, 1968.
202. Hsu, H. H., Feinstone, S. M., and Hoofnagle, J. H.: Acute viral hepatitis. *In* Mandell, G. L., Bennett, J. E., and Dolin, R. (eds.): Principles and Practice of Infectious Diseases. 4th ed. New York, Churchill Livingstone, 1995, pp. 1136–1153.
203. Huang, E.-S., Alford, C. A., Reynolds, D. W., et al.: Molecular epidemiology of cytomegalovirus infections in women and their infants. N. Engl. J. Med. *303*:958–962, 1980.
204. Hughes, J. R., Wilfert, C. M., Moore, M., et al.: Echovirus 14 infection associated with fatal neonatal hepatic necrosis. Am. J. Dis. Child. *123*:61–67, 1972.
205. Hutto, C., Arvin, A., Jacob, R., et al.: Intrauterine herpes simplex virus infections. J. Pediatr. *110*:97–101, 1987.
206. Jahn, C. L., and Cherry, J. D.: Mild neonatal illness associated with heavy enterovirus infection. N. Engl. J. Med. *274*:394–395, 1966.
207. Jeansson, S., and Molin, L.: On the occurrence of genital herpes simplex virus infection: Clinical and virological findings and relation to gonorrhoea. Acta Derm. Venereol. (Stockh.) *54*:479–485, 1974.
208. Jenista, J. A., Powell, K. R., and Menegus, M. A.,: Epidemiology of neonatal enterovirus infection. J. Pediatr. *104*:685–690, 1984.
209. Jhaveri, R., Rosenfeld, W., Salazar, J. D., et al.: High titer multiple dose therapy with HBIG in newborn infants of HBsAg positive mothers. J. Pediatr. *97*:305–308, 1980.
210. Johnson, R. E., Nahmias, A. J., Magder, L. S., et al.: A seroepidemiologic survey of the prevalence of herpes simplex virus type 2 infection in the United States. N. Engl. J. Med. *321*:7–12, 1989.
211. Johnston, J. M., and Overall, J. C., Jr.: Intravaneous immunoglobulin in disseminated neonatal echovirus 11 infection. Pediatr. Infect. Dis. J. *8*:254–256, 1989.
212. Kaplan, M. H., Klein, S. W., McPhee, J., and Harper, R. G.: Group B

coxsackie infections in infants younger than three months of age: A serious childhood illness. Rev. Infect. Dis. *5*:1019–1032, 1983.
213. Kattamis, C. A., Demetrios, D., and Matsaniotis, N. S.: Australia antigen and neonatal hepatitis syndrome. Pediatrics *54*:157–164, 1974.
214. Kay, M. H., Wyllie, R., Deimler, C., et al.: Alpha interferon therapy in children with chronic active hepatitis B and delta virus infection. J. Pediatr. *123*:1001–1004, 1993.
215. Kaye, E. M., and Dooling, E. C.: Neonatal herpes simplex meningoencephalitis associated with fetal monitor scalp electrodes. Neurology *31*:1045–1047, 1981.
216. Kern, E. R., Overall, J. C., Jr., and Glasgow, L. A.: Herpesvirus hominis infection in newborn mice. I. An experimental model and therapy with iododeoxyuridine. J. Infect. Dis. *128*:290–299, 1973.
217. Khuroo, M. S., Kamili, S., and Jameel, S.: Vertical transmission of hepatitis E virus. Lancet *345*:1025–1026, 1995.
218. Kibrick, S.: Herpes simplex infection at term: What to do with mother, newborn, and nursery personnel. J. A. M. A. *243*:157–160, 1980.
219. Kilroy, A. W., Schaffner, W., Fleet, W. F., Jr., et al.: Two syndromes following rubella immunization: Clinical observations and epidemiological studies. J. A. M. A. *214*:2287–2292, 1980.
220. Kinney, J. S., Anderson, L. J., Farrar, J., et al.: Risk of adverse outcomes of pregnancy after human parvovirus B19 infection. J. Infect. Dis. *157*:663–667, 1988.
221. Kleiman, M. B., Schreiner, R. L., Eitzen, H., et al.: Oral herpesvirus infection in nursery personnel: Infection control policy. Pediatrics *70*:609–612, 1982.
222. Klock, L. E., and Rachelefsky, G. S.: Failure of rubella herd immunity during an epidemic. N. Engl. J. Med. *288*:69–72, 1973.
223. Knox, G. E., Pass, R. F., Reynolds, D. W., et al.: Comparative prevalence of subclinical cytomegalovirus and herpes simplex virus infections in the genital and urinary tracts of low-income, urban women. J. Infect. Dis. *140*:419–422, 1979.
224. Koch, W. C., and Adler, S. P.: Human parvovirus B19 infections in women of childbearing age and within families. Pediatr. Infect. Dis. J. *8*:83–87, 1989.
225. Koch, W. C., Adler, S., P., and Harger, J.: Intrauterine parvovirus B19 infection may cause an asymptomatic or recurrent postnatal infection. Pediatr. Infect. Dis. J. *12*:747–750, 1993.
226. Koff, R. S.: Hepatitis B today: Clinical and diagnostic overview. Pediatr. Infect. Dis J. *12*:428–432, 1993.
227. Kohler, P. F., Dubois, R. S., Merrill, D. A., et al.: Prevention of chronic neonatal hepatitis B virus infection with antibody to the hepatitis B surface antigen. N. Engl. J. Med. *291*:1378–1380, 1974.
228. Komorous, J. M., Wheeler, C. E., Briggaman, R. A., et al.: Intrauterine herpes simplex infections. Arch. Dermatol. *113*:918–922, 1977.
229. Kono, R., Hayakawa, Y., Hibi, M., et al.: Experimental vertical transmission of rubella virus in rabbits. Lancet *1*:343–347, 1969.
230. Korones, S. B., Ainger, L. E., Monif, G. R. G., et al.: Congenital rubella syndrome: New clinical aspects with recovery of virus from affected infants. J. Pediatr. *67*:166–181, 1965.
231. Korones, S. B., Ainger, L. E., Monif, G. R. G., et al.: Congenital rubella syndrome: Study of 22 infants. Myocardial damage and other new clinical aspects. Am. J. Dis. Child. *110*:434–440, 1965.
232. Koskimies, O., Lapinleimu, K., and Saxén, L.: Infections and other maternal factors as risk indicators for congenital malformations: A case-control study with paired serum samples. Pediatrics *61*:832–837, 1978.
233. Krawczynski, K., and Bradley, D. W.: Enterically transmitted non-A, non-B hepatitis: Identification of virus-associated antigen in experimentally infected cynomolgus macaques. J. Infect. Dis. *159*:1042–1049, 1989.
234. Krawitt, E. L.: Chronic hepatitis. *In* Mandell, G. L., Bennett, J. E., and Dolin, R. (eds.): Principals and Practice of Infectious Diseases. 4th ed. New York, Churchill Livingstone, 1995, pp. 1153–1159.
235. Kraybill, E. N., Sever, J. L., Avery, G. B., et al.: Experimental use of cytosine arabinoside in congenital cytomegalovirus infection. J. Pediatr. *80*:485–487, 1972.
236. Krill, A. E.: The retinal disease of rubella. Arch. Ophthalmol. *77*:445–449, 1967.
237. Krober, M. S., Bass, J. W., Powell, J. M., et al.: Bacterial and viral pathogens causing fever in infants less than 3 months old. Am. J. Dis. Child. *139*:889–892, 1985.
238. Krous, H. F., Dietzman, D., and Ray, C. G.: Fatal infections with echovirus types 6 and 11 in early infancy. Am. J. Dis. Child. *126*:842–846, 1973.
239. Krugman, S.: Viral hepatitis: A, B, C, D and E infection. Pediatr. Rev. *13*:203–212, 1992.
240. Kulhanjian, J. A., Soroush, V., Au, D. S., et al.: Identification of women at unsuspected risk of primary infection with herpes simplex virus during pregnancy. N. Engl. J. Med. *326*:916–920, 1992.
241. Kumar, M. L., Dawson, N. V., McCullough, A. J., et al.: Should all pregnant women be screened for hepatitis B? Ann. Intern. Med. *107*:273–277, 1987.
242. Kumar, M. L., Gold, E., Jacobs, I. B., et al.: Primary cytomegalovirus infection in adolescent pregnancy. Pediatrics *74*:493–500, 1984.
243. Kumar, M. L., Nankervis, G. A., Cooper, A. R., et al.: Postnatally acquired cytomegalovirus infections in infants of CMV-excreting mothers. J. Pediatr. *104*:669–673, 1984.
244. Kumar, M. L., Nankervis, G. A., Jacobs, I. B., et al.: Congenital and postnatally acquired cytomegalovirus infections: Long-term follow-up. J. Pediatr. *104*:674–679, 1984.
245. Kuo, G., Choo, Q.-L., Alter, H. J., et al.: An assay for circulating antibodies to a major etiologic virus of human non-A, non-B hepatitis. Science *244*:362–364, 1989.
246. Lagrew, D. C., Jr., Furlow, T. G., Harger, W. D., et al.: Disseminated herpes simplex virus infection in pregnancy: Successful treatment with acyclovir. J. A. M. A. *252*:2058–2059, 1984.
247. Lai, C.-L., Lin, H.-J., Yeoh, E.-K., et al.: Placebo-controlled trial of recombinant α_2 interferon in Chinese HBsAg-carrier children. Lancet *2*:877–880, 1987.
248. Lake, A. M., Lauer, B. A., Clark, J. C., et al.: Enterovirus infections in neonates. J. Pediatr. *89*:787–791, 1976.
249. Lakeman, F. D., Whitley, R., J., and NIAID Collaborative Antiviral Study Group: Diagnosis of herpes simplex encephalitis: Application of polymerase chain reaction to cerebrospinal fluid from brain-biopsied patients and correlation with disease. J. Infect. Dis. *171*:857–863, 1995.
250. Lam, J. P. H., McOmish, F., Burns, S. M., et al.: Infrequent vertical transmission of hepatitis C virus. J. Infect. Dis. *167*:572–576, 1993.
251. Lamberson, H. V., Jr., McMillan, J. A., Weiner, L. B., et al.: Prevention of transfusion-associated cytomegalovirus (CMV) infection in neonates by screening blood donors for IgM to CMV. J. Infect. Dis. *157*:820–823, 1988.
252. Lang, D. J., and Kummer, J. F.: Cytomegalovirus in semen: Observations in selected populations. J. Infect. Dis. *132*:472–473, 1975.
253. Lang, D. J., Kummer, J. F., and Hartley, D. P.: Cytomegalovirus in semen: Persistence and demonstration in extracellular fluids. N. Engl. J. Med. *291*:121–124, 1974.
254. Lapinleimu, K., Cantell, K., Koskimies, O., et al.: Association between maternal herpesvirus infections and congenital malformations. Lancet *1*:1127–1129, 1974.
255. Lapinleimu, K., and Hakulinen, A.: A hospital outbreak caused by echovirus type 11 among newborn infants. Ann. Clin. Res. *4*:183–187, 1972.
256. Lee, A. K. Y., Ip, H. M. H., and Wong, V. C. W.: Mechanisms of maternal-fetal transmission of hepatitis B virus. J. Infect. Dis. *138*:668–671, 1978.
257. Lee, G. C.-Y., Hwang, L.-Y., Beasley, R. P., et al.: Immunogenicity of hepatitis B virus vaccine in healthy Chinese neonates. J. Infect. Dis. *148*:526–529, 1983.
258. Lemon, S. M.: Inactivated hepatitis A vaccines. J. A. M. A. *271*:1363–1364, 1994.
259. Lemon, S. M.: Type A viral hepatitis: New developments in an old disease. N. Engl. J. Med. *313*:1059–1067, 1985.
260. Lentz, E. B., Dock, N. L., McMahon, C. A., et al.: Detection of antibody to cytomegalovirus-induced early antigens and comparison with four serologic assays and presence of viruria in blood donors. J. Clin. Microbiol. *26*:133–135, 1988.
261. Lewkonia, I. K., and Jackson, A. A.: Infantile herpes zoster after intrauterine exposure to varicella. B. M. J. *3*:149, 1973.
262. Light, I. J.: Postnatal acquisition of herpes simplex by the newborn infant: A review of the literature. Pediatrics *63*:480–482, 1979.
263. Lin, H.-H., Kao, J.-H., Hsu, H.-Y., et al.: Possible role of high titered maternal viremia in perinatal transmission of hepatitis C virus. J. Infect. Dis. *169*:638–641, 1994.
264. Lin, H.-H., Kao, J.-H., Hsu, H.-Y., et al.: Absence of infection in breast-fed infants born to hepatitis C virus–infected mothers. J. Pediatr. *126*:589–591, 1995.
265. Lindquist, J. M., Plotkin, S. A., Shaw, L., et al.: Congenital rubella syndrome as a systemic infection: Studies of affected infants born in Philadelphia, U. S. A. B. M. J. *2*:1401–1406, 1965.
266. Linnemann, C. C., Jr., Light, I. J., Buchman, T. G., et al.: Transmission of herpes simplex virus type 1 in a nursery for the newborn identification of viral isolates by D.N.A. "fingerprinting." Lancet *1*:964–966, 1978.
267. Linnemann, C. C., Jr., Steichen, J., Sherman, W. G., et al.: Febrile illness in early infancy associated with ECHO virus infection. J. Pediatr. *84*:49–54, 1974.
268. Lo, K.-J., Tong, M. J., Chien, M.-C., et al.: The natural course of hepatitis B surface antigen–positive chronic active hepatitis in Taiwan. J. Infect. Dis. *146*:205–210, 1982.
269. Lo, K.-J., Tsai, Y.-T., Lee, S.-D., et al.: Immunoprophylaxis of infection with hepatitis B virus in infants born to hepatitis B surface antigen–positive carrier mothers. J. Infect. Dis. *152*:817–822, 1985.
270. Macfarlane, D. W., Boyd, R. D., Dodrill, C. B., et al.: Intrauterine rubella, head size, and intellect. Pediatrics *55*:797–801, 1975.
271. Maggiore, G., De Giacomo, C., Marzani, D., et al.: Chronic viral hepatitis B in infancy. J. Pediatr. *103*:749–752, 1983.
272. Manzini, P., Saracco, G., Cerchier, A., et al.: Human immunodeficiency virus infection as risk factor for mother-to-child hepatitis C virus transmission: Persistence of anti-hepatitis C virus in children is associated with mother's anti-hepatitis C virus immunoblotting pattern. Hepatology *21*:328–332, 1995.
273. Marier, R., Rodriguez, W., Chloupek, R. J., et al.: Coxsackievirus B5 infection and aseptic meningitis in neonates and children. Am. J. Dis. Child. *129*:321–325, 1975.
274. McCracken, G. H., Jr., and Luby, J. P.: Cytosine arabinoside in the treat-

ment of congenital cytomegalic inclusion disease. J. Pediatr. *80*:488–495, 1972.

275. McDonald, J. C., and Peckham, C. S.: Gammaglobulin in prevention of rubella and congenital defect: A study of 30,000 pregnancies. B. M. J. *3*:633–637, 1967.
276. McDonald, L. L., St. Geme, J. W., Jr., and Arnold, B. H.: Nosocomial infection with echovirus type 31 in a neonatal intensive care unit. Pediatrics *47*:995–999, 1971.
277. McKendrick, G. D. W., and Raychoudhury, S. C.: Herpes zoster in childhood. Scand. J. Infect. Dis. *4*:23–25, 1972.
278. McMahon, B. J., Alberts, S. R., Wainwright, R. B., et al.: Hepatitis B-related sequelae: Prospective study in 1400 hepatitis B surface antigen-positive Alaska native carriers. Arch. Intern. Med. *150*:1051–1054, 1990.
279. McMahon, B. J., Alward, W. L. M., Hall, D. B., et al.: Acute hepatitis B virus infection: Relation of age to the clinical expression of disease and subsequent development of the carrier state. J. Infect. Dis. *151*:599–603, 1985.
280. Mellinger, A. K., Cragan, J. D., Atkinson, W. L., et al.: High incidence of congenital rubella syndrome after a rubella outbreak. Pediatr. Infect. Dis. J. *14*:573–578, 1995.
281. Melnick, J. L.: Enteroviruses: Polioviruses, coxsackieviruses, echoviruses, and newer enteroviruses. *In*: Fields, B. N., and Knipe, D. M. (eds.): Virology. 2nd ed. New York, Raven Press, 1990, pp. 549–605.
282. Menser, M. A., Dods, L., and Harley, J. D.: A twenty-five year follow-up of congenital rubella. Lancet *2*:1347–1350, 1967.
283. Menser, M. A., Forrest, J. M., and Bransby, R. D.: Rubella infection and diabetes mellitus. Lancet *1*:57–60, 1978.
284. Menser, M. A., and Reye, R. D. K.: The pathology of congenital rubella: A review written by request. Pathology *6*:215–222, 1974.
285. Meyers, J. D.: Congenital varicella in term infants: Risk reconsidered. J. Infect. Dis. *129*:215–217, 1974.
286. Miller, E., Cradock-Watson, J. E., and Pollock, T. M.: Consequences of confirmed maternal rubella at successive stages of pregnancy. Lancet *2*:781–784, 1982.
287. Miller, E., Cradock-Watson, J. E., and Ridehalgh, M. K. S.: Outcome in newborn babies given anti–varicella-zoster immunoglobulin after perinatal maternal infection with varicella-zoster virus. Lancet *2*:371–373, 1989.
288. Miller, M. H., Rabinowitz, M. A., Frost, J. O., and Seager, G. M.: Audiological problems associated with maternal rubella. Laryngoscope *79*:417–426, 1969.
289. Miller, M. J., Sunshine, P. J., and Remington, J. S.: Quantitation of cord serum IgM and IgA as a screening procedure to detect congenital infection: Results of 5006 infants. J. Pediatr. *75*:1287–1291, 1969.
290. Mims, C. A.: Pathogenesis of viral infections of the fetus. Prog. Med. Virol. *10*:194–237, 1968.
291. Mitchell, J. E., and McCall, F. C.: Transplacental infection by herpes simplex virus. Am. J. Dis. Child. *106*:207–209, 1963.
292. Modlin, J. F.: Fatal echovirus 11 disease in premature neonates. Pediatrics *66*:775–780, 1980.
293. Modlin, J. F.: Perinatal echovirus infection: Insights from a literature review of 61 cases of serious infection and 16 outbreaks in nurseries. Rev. Infect. Dis. *8*:918–926, 1986.
294. Modlin, J. F., Herrmann, K., Brandling-Bennett, A. D., et al.: Risk of congenital abnormality after inadvertent rubella vaccination of pregnant women. N. Engl. J. Med. *294*:972–974, 1976.
295. Modlin, J. F., Polk, B. F., Horton, P., et al.: Perinatal echovirus infection: Risk of transmission during a community outbreak. N. Engl. J. Med. *305*:368–371, 1981.
296. Montgomery, J. R., Flanders, R. W., and Yow, M. D.: Congenital anomalies and herpesvirus infection. Am. J. Dis Child. *126*:364–366, 1973.
297. Montgomery, R., Youngblood, L., and Medearis, D. N., Jr.: Recovery of cytomegalovirus from the cervix in pregnancy. Pediatrics *49*:524–530, 1972.
298. Morens, D. M.: Enteroviral disease in early infancy. J. Pediatr. *92*:374–377, 1978.
299. Moseley, R. C., Corey, L., Benjamin, D., et al.: Comparison of viral isolation, direct immunofluorescence, and indirect immunoperoxidase techniques for detection of genital herpes simplex virus infection. J. Clin. Microbiol. *13*:913–918, 1981.
300. Music, S. T., Fine, E. M., and Togo, Y.: Zoster-like disease in the newborn due to herpes-simplex virus. N. Engl. J. Med. *284*:24–26, 1971.
301. Naeye, R. L.: Cytomegalic inclusion disease: The fetal disorder. Am. J. Clin. Pathol. *47*:738–744, 1967.
302. Naeye, R. L., and Blanc, W.: Pathogenesis of congenital rubella. J. A. M. A. *194*:1277–1283, 1965.
303. Nahmias, A. J., Dowdle, W. R., Josey, W. E., et al.: Newborn infection with herpesvirus hominis types 1 and 2. J. Pediatr. *75*:1194–1203, 1969.
304. Nahmias, A. J., and Hagler, W. S.: Ocular manifestations of herpes simplex in the newborn (neonatal ocular herpes). Int. Ophthalmol. Clin. *12*:191–213, 1972.
305. Nahmias, A. J., Josey, W. E., and Naib, Z. M.: Significance of herpes simplex virus infection during pregnancy. Clin. Obstet. Gynecol. *15*:929–938, 1972.
306. Nahmias, A. J., Josey, W. E., Naib, Z. M., et al.: Perinatal risk associated with maternal genital herpes simplex virus infection. Am. J. Obstet. Gynecol. *110*:825–836, 1971.
307. Nahmias, A. J., Keyserling, H. L., and Kerrick, G. M.: Herpes simplex. *In* Remington, J. S., and Klein, J. O. (eds.): Infectious Diseases of the Fetus and Newborn Infant. 2nd ed. Philadelphia, W. B. Saunders, 1983, pp. 636–678.
308. Nankervis, G. A.: Cytomegaloviral infections: Epidemiology, therapy, and prevention. Pediatr. Rev. *7*:169–175, 1985.
309. Nankervis, G. A., Kumar, M. L., Cox, F. E., et al.: A prospective study of maternal cytomegalovirus infection and its effect on the fetus. Am. J. Obstet. Gynecol. *149*:435–440, 1984.
310. Narkiewicz, M. R., Smith, D., Silverman, A., et al.: Clearance of chronic hepatitis B virus infection in young children after alpha interferon treatment. J. Pediatr. *127*:815–818, 1995.
311. National Communicable Disease Center: Rubella Surveillance, June, 1969.
312. Ng, A. B. P., Reagan, J. W., and Yen, S. S. C.: Herpes genitalis. Obstet. Gynecol. *36*:645–651, 1970.
313. Nielsen, C. M., Hansen, K., Andersen, H. M. K., et al.: An enzyme labeled nuclear antigen immunoassay for detection of cytomegalovirus IgM antibodies in human serum: Specific and nonspecific reaction. J. Med. Virol. *7*:111–113, 1987.
314. Novati, R., Thiers, V., Monforte, A. D., et al.: Mother-to-child transmission of hepatitis C virus detected by nested polymerase chain reaction. J. Infect. Dis. *165*:720–723, 1992.
315. Nusbacher, J., Hirschhorn, K., and Cooper, L. Z.: Chromosomal abnormalities in congenital rubella. N. Engl. J. Med. *276*:1409–1413, 1967.
316. Ohto, H., Terazawa, S., Sasaki, N., et al.: Transmission of hepatitis C virus from mothers to infants. N. Engl. J. Med. *330*:744–750, 1994.
317. Okada, K., Kamiyama, I., Inomata, M., et al.: e Antigen and anti-e in the serum of asymptomatic carrier mothers as indicators of positive and negative transmission of hepatitis B virus to their infants. N. Engl. J. Med. *294*:746–749, 1976.
318. Okada, K., Yamada, T., Miyakawa, Y., et al.: Hepatitis B surface antigen in the serum of infants after delivery from asymptomatic carrier mothers. J. Pediatr. *87*:360–363, 1975.
319. Olson, G. B., Dent, P. B., Rawls, W. E., et al.: Abnormalities of in vitro lymphocyte responses during rubella virus infections. J. Exp. Med. *128*:47–68, 1968.
320. Orenstein, W. A., Bart, K. J., Hinman, A. R., et al.: The opportunity and obligation to eliminate rubella from the United States. J. A. M. A. *251*:1988–1994, 1984.
321. Overall, J. C., Jr.: Dermatologic viral diseases. *In* Galasso, G. J., Merigan, T. C., and Buchanan, R. A. (eds.): Antiviral Agents and Viral Diseases of Man. 2nd ed. New York, Raven Press, 1984, pp. 247–312.
322. Overall, J. C., Jr.: Diagnostic virology. *In* McClatchy, K. D. (ed.): Clinical Laboratory Medicine. Baltimore, Williams & Wilkins, 1994, pp. 1359–1385.
323. Overall, J. C., Jr.: Empiric therapy with acyclovir for suspected neonatal herpes simplex infections. Pediatr. Infect. Dis. J. *8*:808–809, 1989.
324. Overall, J. C., Jr.: Genital and perinatal herpes simplex virus infections. *In* de la Maza, L. M., and Peterson, E. M. (eds.): Medical Virology. IV. Hillsdale, NJ, L. Erlbaum Assoc., 1985, pp. 253–304.
325. Overall, J. C., Jr.: Herpes simplex virus infection of the fetus and newborn. Pediatr. Ann. *23*:131–136, 1994.
326. Overall, J. C., Jr.: Intrauterine virus infections and congenital heart disease. Am. Heart J. *84*:823–833, 1972.
327. Overall, J. C., Jr., Whitley, R. J., Yeager, A. S., et al.: Prophylactic or anticipatory antiviral therapy for newborns exposed to herpes simplex infection. Pediatr. Infect. Dis. *3*:193–195, 1984.
328. Papaevangelou, G., and Hoofnagle, J. H.: Transmission of hepatitis B virus infection by asymptomatic chronic HBsAg carrier mothers. Pediatrics *63*:602–605, 1979.
329. Papaevangelou, G., Hoofnagle, J., and Kremastinou, J.: Transplacental transmission of hepatitis-B virus by symptom-free chronic carrier mothers. Lancet *2*:746–748, 1974.
330. Parvey, L. S., and Ch'ien, L. T.: Neonatal herpes simplex virus infection introduced by fetal-monitor scalp electrodes. Pediatrics *65*:1150–1153, 1980.
331. Paryani, S. G., and Arvin, A. M.: Intrauterine infection with varicella-zoster virus after maternal varicella. N. Engl. J. Med. *314*:1542–1546, 1986.
332. Paryani, S. G., Yeager, A. S., Hosford-Dunn, H., et al.: Sequelae of acquired cytomegalovirus infection in premature and sick term infants. J. Pediatr. *107*:451–456, 1985.
333. Pass, R. F., August, A. M., Dworsky, M., et al.: Cytomegalovirus infection in a day-care center. N. Engl. J. Med. *307*:477–479, 1982.
334. Pass, R. F., Stagno, S., Myers, G. J., et al.: Outcome of symptomatic congenital cytomegalovirus infection: Results of long term longitudinal follow-up. Pediatrics *66*:758–762, 1980.

334a. Pastuszak, A. L., Levy, M., Schick, B., et al.: Outcome after maternal varicella infection in the first 20 weeks of pregnancy. N. Engl. J. Med. *330*:901–905, 1994.

335. Peacock, J. E., Jr., and Sarubbi, F. A.: Disseminated herpes simplex virus infection during pregnancy. Obstet. Gynecol. *61*(Suppl.):13S–18S, 1983.
336. Perrillo, R. P., Schiff, E. R., Davis, G. L., et al.: A randomized, controlled trial of interferon alpha-2b alone and after prednisone withdrawal for the treatment of chronic hepatitis B. N. Engl. J. Med. *323*:295–301, 1990.

337. Phelan, P., and Campbell, P.: Pulmonary complications of rubella embryopathy. J. Pediatr. *75*:202–212, 1969.
338. Philip, A. G. S., and Larson, E. J.: Overwhelming neonatal infection with ECHO 19 virus. J. Pediatr. *82*:391–397, 1973.
339. Plager, H., Beebe, R., and Miller, J. K.: Coxsackie B-5 pericarditis in pregnancy. Arch. Intern. Med. *110*:735–738, 1962.
340. Plotkin, S. A., Klaus, R. M., and Whitely, J. P.: Hypogammaglobulinemia in an infant with congenital rubella syndrome: Failure of 1-adamantanamine to stop virus excretion. J. Pediatr. *69*:1085–1091, 1966.
341. Plotkin, S. A., Starr, S. E., and Bryan, C. K.: In vitro and in vivo responses of cytomegalovirus to acyclovir. Am. J. Med. *73*(Suppl. 1A):257–261, 1982.
342. Plotkin, S. A., and Stetler, H.: Treatment of congenital cytomegalic inclusion disease with antiviral agents. Antimicrob. Agents Chemother. *9*:372–379, 1969.
343. Polish, L. B., Gallagher, M., Fields, H. A., et al.: Delta hepatitis: Molecular biology and clinical and epidemiologic features. Clin. Microbiol. Rev. *6*:211–229, 1993.
344. Poovorawan, Y., Sanpavat, S., Pongpunlert, W., et al.: Protective efficacy of a recombinant DNA hepatitis B vaccine in neonates of HBe antigen–positive mothers. J. A. M. A. *261*:3278–3281, 1989.
345. Preece, P. M., Blount, J. M., Glover, J., et al.: The consequences of primary cytomegalovirus infection in pregnancy. Arch. Dis. Child. *58*:970–975, 1983.
346. Preece, P. M., Pearl, K. N., and Peckham, C. S.: Congenital cytomegalovirus infection. Arch. Dis. Child. *59*:1120–1126, 1984.
347. Prober, C. G., Corey, L., Brown, Z. A., et al.: The management of pregnancies complicated by genital infection with herpes simplex virus. Clin. Infect. Dis. *15*:1031–1038, 1992.
348. Prober, C. G., Gershon, A. A., Grose, C., et al.: Consensus: Varicella-zoster infections in pregnancy and the perinatal period. Pediatr. Infect. Dis. J. *9*:865–869, 1990.
349. Prober, C. G., Hensleigh, P. A., Boucher, F. D., et al.: Use of routine viral cultures at delivery to identify neonates exposed to herpes simplex virus. N. Engl. J. Med. *318*:887–891, 1988.
350. Public Health Laboratory Service Working Party on Fifth Disease: Prospective study of human parvovirus B19 infection in pregnancy. B. M. J. *300*:1166–1170, 1990.
351. Purdham, D. R., Purdham, P. A., Wood, B. S. B., et al.: Severe echo 19 virus infection in a neonatal unit. Arch. Dis. Child. *51*:634–636, 1976.
352. Randolph, A. G., Washington, A. E., and Prober, C. G.: Cesarean delivery for women presenting with genital herpes lesions: Efficacy, risks, and costs. J. A. M. A. *270*:77–82, 1993.
353. Rawls, W. E., and Melnick, J. L.: Rubella virus carrier cultures derived from congenitally infected infants. J. Exp. Med. *123*:795–816, 1966.
354. Reed, E. C., Bowden, R. A., Dandliker, P. S., et al.: Treatment of cytomegalovirus pneumonia with ganciclovir and intravenous cytomegalovirus immunoglobulin in patients with bone marrow transplants. Ann. Intern. Med. *109*:783–788, 1988.
355. Reesink, H. W., Reerink-Brongers, E. E., Lafeber-Schut, B. J. T., et al.: Prevention of chronic HBsAg carrier state in infants of HBsAg-positive mothers by hepatitis B immunoglobulin. Lancet *2*:436–438, 1979.
356. Reinus, J. F., Leikin, E. L., Alter, H. J., et al.: Failure to detect vertical transmission of hepatitis C virus. Ann. Intern. Med. *117*:881–886, 1992.
357. Remington, J. S., and Klein, J. O. (eds.): Infectious Diseases of the Fetus and Newborn Infant. 4th ed. Philadelphia, W. B. Saunders, 1995.
358. Reynolds, D. W., Dean, P. H., Pass, R. F., et al.: Specific cell-mediated immunity in children with congenital and neonatal cytomegalovirus infection and their mothers. J. Infect. Dis. *140*:493–499, 1979.
359. Reynolds, D. W., Stagno, S., Hosty, T. S., et al.: Maternal cytomegalovirus excretion and perinatal infection. N. Engl. J. Med. *289*:1–5, 1973.
360. Reynolds, D. W., Stagno, S., Reynolds, R., et al.: Perinatal cytomegalovirus infection: Influence of placentally transferred maternal antibody. J. Infect. Dis. *137*:564–567, 1978.
361. Reynolds, D. W., Stagno, S., Stubbs, G., et al.: Inapparent congenital cytomegalovirus infection with elevated cord IgM levels. N. Engl. J. Med. *290*:291–296, 1974.
362. Robinson, J., Lemay, M., and Vaudry, W. L.: Congenital rubella after anticipated maternal immunity: Two cases and a review of the literature. Pediatr. Infect. Dis. J. *13*:812–815, 1994.
363. Roizman, B., and Buchman, T.: The molecular epidemiology of herpes simplex viruses. Hosp. Pract. *14*:95–104, 1979.
364. Rosendahl, C., Kochen, M. M., Kretschmer, R., et al.: Avoidance of perinatal transmission of hepatitis B virus: Is passive immunisation always necessary? Lancet *1*:1127–1129, 1983.
365. Rotbart, H. A.: Human Enterovirus Infections. Washington, ASM Press, 1995.
366. Roudot-Thoraval, F., Pawlotsky, J.-M., Thiers, V., et al.: Lack of mother-to-infant transmission of hepatitis C virus in human immunodeficiency virus–seronegative women: A prospective study with hepatitis C virus RNA testing. Hepatology *17*:772–777, 1993.
367. Rudolph, A. J., Singleton, E. B., Rosenberg, H. S., et al.: Osseous manifestations of the congenital rubella syndrome. Am. J. Dis. Child. *110*:428–433, 1965.
368. Saigal, S., Lunyk, O., Larke, R. P. B., et al.: The outcome in children with congenital cytomegalovirus infection: A longitudinal follow-up study. Am. J. Dis. Child. *136*:896–901, 1982.
369. Sakaoka, H., Saheki, Y., Uzuki, K., et al.: Two outbreaks of herpes simplex virus type 1 nosocomial infection among newborns. J. Clin. Microbiol. *24*:36–40, 1986.
370. Sanford, J. P.: Coxsackievirus and echovirus infections. *In* Hoeprich, P. D. (ed.): Infectious Diseases. New York, Harper & Row, 1977, pp. 1107–1117.
371. Schauf, V., Strelkauskas, A. J., and Deveikis, A.: Alteration of lymphocyte subpopulations with cytomegalovirus infection in infancy. Clin. Exp. Immunol. *26*:478–483, 1976.
372. Schiff, G. M., Sutherland, J., and Light, I.: Congenital rubella. *In* Thalhammer, O. (ed.): Prenatal Infections. Stuttgart, Georg Thieme Verlag, 1971, pp. 31–36.
373. Schmidt, N. J., Dennis, J., Devlin, V., et al.: Comparison of direct immunofluorescence and direct immunoperoxidase procedures for detection of herpes simplex virus antigen in lesion specimens. J. Clin. Microbiol. *18*:445–448, 1983.
374. Schweitzer, I. L., Dunn, A. E. G., Peters, R. L., et al.: Viral hepatitis B in neonates and infants. Am. J. Med. *55*:762–771, 1973.
375. Schweitzer, I. L., Mosley, J. W., Ashcaval, M., et al.: Factors influencing neonatal infection by hepatitis B virus. Gastroenterology *65*:277–283, 1973.
376. Scott, L. L.: Perinatal herpes: Current status and obstetric management strategies. Pediatr. Infect. Dis. J. *14*:827–832, 1995.
377. Sells, C. J., Carpenter, R. L., and Ray, C. G.: Sequelae of central-nervous-system enterovirus infections. N. Engl. J. Med. *293*:1–4, 1975.
378. Sever, J. L., Brody, J. A., Schiff, G. M., et al.: Rubella epidemic on St. Paul Island in the Pribilofs, 1963. II. Clinical and laboratory findings for the intensive study population. J. A. M. A. *191*:624–626, 1965.
379. Sever, J. L., Huebner, R. J., Castellano, G. A., et al.: Serologic diagnosis "en masse" with multiple antigens. II. Am. Rev. Respir. Dis. *88*:342–359, 1963.
380. Sever, J. L., Nelson, K. B., and Gilkeson, M. R.: Rubella epidemic, 1964: Effect on 6000 pregnancies. I. Preliminary clinical and laboratory findings through the neonatal period: A report from the Collaborative Study on Cerebral Palsy. Am. J. Dis. Child. *110*:395–407, 1965.
381. Sever, J. L., South, M. A., and Shaver, K. A.: Delayed manifestations of congenital rubella. Rev. Infect. Dis. *7*(Suppl. 1):S164–S169, 1985.
382. Sever, J., and White, L. R.: Intrauterine viral infections. Annu. Rev. Med. *19*:471–486, 1968.
383. Shackelford, G. D., and Kirks, D. R.: Neonatal hepatic calcification secondary to transplacental infection. Radiology *122*:753–757, 1977.
384. Shapiro, C. N.: Epidemiology of hepatitis B. Pediatr. Infect. Dis. J. *12*:433–437, 1993.
385. Shepp, D. H., Dandliker, P. S., and Meyers, J. D.: Treatment of varicella-zoster virus infection in severely immunocompromised patients: A randomized comparison of acyclovir and vidarabine. N. Engl. J. Med. *314*:208–212, 1986.
386. Shiraki, K., Yoshihara, N., Kawana, T., et al.: Hepatitis B surface antigen and chronic hepatitis in infants born to asymptomatic carrier mothers. Am. J. Dis. Child. *131*:644–647, 1977.
387. Shiraki, K., Yoshihara, N., Sakurai, M., et al.: Acute hepatitis B in infants born to carrier mothers with the antibody to hepatitis B e antigen. J. Pediatr. *97*:768–770, 1980.
388. Shmoys, S., and Kaplan, C.: Parvovirus and pregnancy. Clin. Obstet. Gynecol. *33*:268–275, 1990.
389. Sieber, O. F., Fulginiti, V. A., Brazie, J., et al.: In utero infection of the fetus by herpes simplex virus. J. Pediatr. *69*:30–34, 1966.
390. Siegel, M.: Congenital malformations following chickenpox, measles, mumps, and hepatitis: Results of a cohort study. J. A. M. A. *226*:1521–1524, 1973.
391. Siegel, M., and Fuerst, H. T.: Low birth weight and maternal virus diseases: A prospective study of rubella, measles, mumps, chickenpox, and hepatitis. J. A. M. A. *197*:680–681, 1966.
392. Siegel, M., Fuerst, H. T., and Peress, N. S.: Comparative fetal mortality in maternal virus diseases: A prospective study on rubella, measles, mumps, chickenpox, and hepatitis. N. Engl. J. Med. *274*:768–771, 1966.
393. Sinatra, F. R., Shah, P., Weissman, J. Y., et al.: Perinatal transmitted acute icteric hepatitis B in infants born to hepatitis B surface antigen-positive and anti-hepatitis Be-positive carrier mothers. Pediatrics *70*:557–559, 1982.
394. Skinhoj, P., Sardemann, H., Cohn, J., et al.: Hepatitis-associated antigen (HAA) in pregnant women and their newborn infants. Am. J. Dis. Child. *123*:380–381, 1972.
395. Snydman, D. R.: Hepatitis in pregnancy. N. Engl. J. Med. *313*:1398–1401, 1985.
396. South, M. A., Tompkins, W. A. F., Morris, C. R., et al.: Congenital malformation of the central nervous system associated with genital type (type 2) herpesvirus. J. Pediatr. *75*:13–18, 1969.
397. Spector, S. A.: Transmission of cytomegalovirus among infants in hospital documented by restriction-endonuclease-digestion analyses. Lancet *1*:378–381, 1983.
398. Spruance, S. L., Overall, J. C., Jr., Kern, E. R., et al.: The natural history of recurrent herpes simplex labialis: Implications for antiviral therapy. N. Engl. J. Med. *297*:69–75, 1977.
399. St. Geme, J. W., Jr., Noren, G. R., and Adams, P., Jr.: Proposed embryopathic relation between mumps virus and primary endocardial fibroelastosis. N. Engl. J. Med. *275*:339–346, 1966.

400. Stagno, S.: Cytomegalovirus. *In* Remington, J. S., and Klein, J. O. (eds.): Infectious Diseases of the Fetus and Newborn Infant. 3rd ed. Philadelphia, W. B. Saunders, 1990, pp. 241–281.
401. Stagno, S., Pass, R. F., Cloud, G., et al.: Primary cytomegalovirus infection in pregnancy: Incidence, transmission to fetus, and clinical outcome. J. A. M. A. *256*:1904–1908, 1986.
402. Stagno, S., Pass, R. F., Dworsky, M. E., et al.: Congenital and perinatal cytomegalovirus infections. Semin. Perinatol. *7*:31–42, 1983.
403. Stagno, S., Pass, R. F., Dworsky, M. E., et al.: Congenital cytomegalovirus infection: The relative importance of primary and recurrent maternal infection. N. Engl. J. Med. *306*:945–949, 1982.
404. Stagno, S., Reynolds, D. W., Amos, C. S., et al.: Auditory and visual defects resulting from symptomatic and subclinical congenital cytomegalovirus and *Toxoplasma* infections. Pediatrics *59*:669–678, 1977.
405. Stagno, S., Reynolds, D. W., Huang, E.-S., et al.: Congenital cytomegalovirus infection: Occurrence in an immune population. N. Engl. J. Med. *296*:1254–1258, 1977.
406. Stagno, S., Reynolds, D. W., Lakeman, A., et al.: Congenital cytomegalovirus infection: Consecutive occurrence due to viruses with similar antigenic compositions. Pediatrics *52*:788–794, 1973.
407. Stagno, S., Reynolds, D. W., Pass, R. F., et al.: Breast milk and the risk of cytomegalovirus infection. N. Engl. J. Med. *302*:1073–1076, 1980.
408. Stagno, S., Reynolds, D. W., Tsiantos, A., et al.: Comparative serial virologic and serologic studies of symptomatic and subclinical congenitally and natally acquired cytomegalovirus infections. J. Infect. Dis. *132*:568–577, 1975.
409. Stagno, S., Reynolds, D., Tsiantos, A., et al.: Cervical cytomegalovirus excretion in pregnant and nonpregnant women: Suppression in early gestation. J. Infect. Dis. *131*:522–527, 1975.
410. Stagno, S., Tinker, M. K., Elrod, C., et al.: Immunoglobulin M antibodies detected by enzyme-linked immunosorbent assay and radioimmunoassay in the diagnosis of cytomegalovirus infections in pregnant women and newborn infants. J. Clin. Microbiol. *21*:930–935, 1985.
411. Stagno, S., Volanakis, J. E., Reynolds, D. W., et al.: Immune complexes in congenital and natal cytomegalovirus infections of man. J. Clin. Invest. *60*:838–845, 1977.
412. Starr, J. G.: Cytomegalovirus infection in pregnancy. N. Engl. J. Med. *282*:50–51, 1970.
413. Starr, S. E., Tolpin, M. D., Friedman, H. M., et al.: Impaired cellular immunity to cytomegalovirus in congenitally infected children and their mothers. J. Infect. Dis. *140*:500–505, 1979.
414. Stevens, C. E.: In utero and perinatal transmission of hepatitis viruses. Pediatr. Ann. *23*:152–158, 1994.
415. Stevens, C. E., Beasley, R. P., Tsui, J., et al.: Vertical transmission of hepatitis B antigen in Taiwan. N. Engl. J. Med. *292*:771–774, 1975.
416. Stevens, C. E., Toy, P. T., Taylor, P. E., et al.: Prospects for control of hepatitis B virus infection: Implications of childhood vaccination and long-term protection. Pediatrics *90*:170–173, 1992.
417. Stevens, C. E., Taylor, P. E., Tong, M. J., et al.: Yeast-recombinant hepatitis B vaccine: Efficacy with hepatitis B immune globulin in prevention of perinatal hepatitis B transmission. J. A. M. A. *257*:2612–2616, 1989.
418. Stevens, C. E., Toy, P. T., Tong, M. J., et al.: Perinatal hepatitis B virus transmission in the United States: Prevention by passive-active immunization. J. A. M. A. *253*:1740–1745, 1985.
419. Stewart, G. L., Parkman, P. D., Hopps, H. E., et al.: Rubella-virus hemagglutination-inhibition test. N. Engl. J. Med. *276*:554–557, 1967.
420. Strauss, L., and Bernstein, J.: Neonatal hepatitis in congenital rubella. Arch. Pathol. *86*:317–327, 1968.
421. Strawn, E. Y., and Scrimenti, R. J.: Intrauterine herpes simplex infection. Am. J. Obstet. Gynecol. *115*:581–582, 1973.
422. Sullivan-Bolyai, J. Z., Fife, K. H., Jacobs, R. F., et al.: Disseminated neonatal herpes simplex virus type 1 from a maternal breast lesion. Pediatrics *71*:455–457, 1983.
423. Sullivan-Bolyai, J. Z., Hull, H. F., Wilson, C., et al.: Neonatal herpes simplex virus infection in King County, Washington: Increasing incidence and epidemiologic correlates. J. A. M. A. *250*:3059–3062, 1983.
424. Swender, P. T., Shott, R. J., and Williams, M. L.: A community and intensive care nursery outbreak of coxsackievirus B5 meningitis. Am. J. Dis. Child. *127*:42–45, 1974.
425. Szmuness, W., Harley, E. J., and Prince, A. M.: Intrafamilial spread of asymptomatic hepatitis B. Am. J. Med. Sci. *270*:292–304, 1975.
426. Tardieu, M., Grospierre, B., Durandy, A., et al.: Circulating immune complexes containing rubella antigens in late-onset rubella syndrome. J. Pediatr. *97*:370–373, 1980.
427. Taylor, B. J., Jacobs, R. F., Baker, R. L., et al.: Frozen deglycerolyzed blood prevents transfusion-acquired cytomegalovirus infections in neonates. Pediatr. Infect. Dis. *5*:188–191, 1986.
428. Tejani, N., Klein, S. W., and Kaplan, M.: Subclinical herpes simplex genitalis infections in the perinatal period. Am. J. Obstet. Gynecol. *135*:547, 1979.
429. Thaler, M. M., Park, C.-K., Landers, D. V., et al.: Vertical transmission of hepatitis C virus. Lancet *338*:17–18, 1991.
430. Ticehurst, J.: Hepatitis E virus. *In* Murray, P. R., Baron, E. J., Pfaller, M. A., et al. (eds.): Manual of Clinical Microbiology. 6th ed. Washington, ASM Press, 1995, pp. 1056–1067.
431. Töndury, G., and Smith, D. W.: Fetal rubella pathology. J. Pediatr. *68*:867–879, 1966.
432. Tong, M. J., and Govindarajan, S.: Primary hepatocellular carcinoma following perinatal transmission of hepatitis B. West. J. Med. *148*:205–208, 1988.
433. Tong, M. J., Thursby, M. W., Lin, J.-H., et al.: Studies on the maternal-infant transmission of the hepatitis B virus and HBV infection within families. Prog. Med. Virol. *27*:137–147, 1981.
434. Torok, T. J.: Human parvovirus B19 infections in pregnancy. Pediatr. Infect. Dis. J. *9*:772–776, 1990.
435. Torok, T. J., Wang, Q.-Y., Gary, G. W., Jr., et al.: Prenatal diagnosis of intrauterine infection with parvovirus B19 by the polymerase chain reaction technique. J. Infect. Dis. *14*:149–155, 1992.
436. Torphy, D. E., Ray, C. G., McAlister, R., et al.: Herpes simplex virus infection in infants: A spectrum of disease. J. Pediatr. *76*:405–408, 1970.
437. Townsend, J. J., Baringer, J. R., Wolinsky, J. S., et al.: Progressive rubella panencephalitis: Late onset after congenital rubella. N. Engl. J. Med. *292*:990–993, 1975.
438. Troendle-Atkins, J., Demmler, G. J., Williamson, W. D., et al.: Polymerase chain reaction to detect cytomegalovirus DNA in the cerebrospinal fluid of neonates with congenital infection. J. Infect. Dis. *169*:1334–1377, 1994.
439. Ueda, K., Nishida, Y., Oshima, K., et al.: Congenital rubella syndrome: Correlation of gestational age at time of maternal rubella with type of defect. J. Pediatr. *94*:763–765, 1979.
440. Vajro, P., Hadchouel, P., Hadchouel, M., et al.: Incidence of cirrhosis in children with chronic hepatitis. J. Pediatr. *117*:392–396, 1990.
441. Vallejo, J. G., Englund, J. A., Garcia-Prats, J. A., et al.: Ganciclovir treatment of steroid-associated cytomegalovirus disease in a congenitally-infected neonate. Pediatr. Infect. Dis. J. *13*:239–241, 1994.
442. Van der Poel, C. L., Cuypers, H. T., and Reesink, H. W.: Hepatitis C virus 6 years on. Lancet *344*:1475–1479, 1994.
443. Van Dyke, R. B., and Spector, S.: Transmission of herpes simplex virus type 1 to a newborn infant during endotracheal suctioning for meconium aspiration. Pediatr. Infect. Dis. *3*:153–156, 1984.
444. Velazquez, O., Stetler, H. C., Avila, C., et al.: Epidemic transmission of enterically transmitted non-A, non-B hepatitis in Mexico, 1986 1987. J. A. M. A. *263*:3281–3285, 1990.
445. Verano, L., and Michalski, F. J.: Herpes simplex virus antigen direct detection in standard virus transport medium by DuPont Herpchek enzyme-linked immunosorbent assay. J. Clin. Microbiol. *28*:2555–2558, 1990.
446. Vontver, L. A., Hickok, D. E., Brown, Z., et al.: Recurrent genital herpes simplex virus infection in pregnancy: Infant outcome and frequency of asymptomatic recurrences. Am. J. Obstet. Gynecol. *143*:75–84, 1982.
447. Waner, J. L., Weller, T. H., and Kevy, S. V.: Patterns of cytomegaloviral complement-fixing antibody activity: A longitudinal study of blood donors. J. Infect. Dis. *127*:538–543, 1973.
448. Weibel, R. E., Stokes, J., Jr., Buynak, E. B., et al.: Rubella vaccination in adult females. N. Engl. J. Med. *280*:682–685, 1969.
449. Weil, M. L., Itabashi, H. H., Cremer, N. E., et al.: Chronic progressive panencephalitis due to rubella virus simulating subacute sclerosing panencephalitis. N. Engl. J. Med. *292*:994–998, 1975.
450. Weinstock, H. S., Bolan, G., Reingold, A. L., et al.: Hepatitis C virus infection among patients attending a clinic for sexually transmitted diseases. J. A. M. A. *269*:392–394, 1993.
451. Wejstal, R., Widell, A., Mansson, A.-S., et al.: Mother-to-infant transmission of hepatitis C virus. Ann. Intern. Med. *117*:887–890, 1992.
452. Wenner, H. A.: Viral meningitis. *In* Hoeprich, P. D. (ed.): Infectious Diseases. New York, Harper & Row, 1977, pp. 881–888.
453. Whitley, R. J.: Herpes simplex viruses. *In* Fields, B. N., and Knipe, D. M. (eds.): Virology. 2nd ed. New York, Raven Press, 1990, pp. 1843–1887.
454. Whitley, R. J., and Arvin, A. M.: Herpes simplex virus infections. *In* Remington, J. S., and Klein, J. O. (eds.): Infectious Diseases of the Fetus and Newborn Infant. 4th ed. Philadelphia, W. B. Saunders, 1995, pp. 354–376.
455. Whitley, R., Arvin, A., Prober, C., et al.: A controlled trial comparing vidarabine with acyclovir in neonatal herpes simplex virus infection. N. Engl. J. Med. *324*:444–449, 1991.
456. Whitley, R., Arvin, A., Prober, C., et al.: Predictors of morbidity and mortality in neonates with herpes simplex virus infections. N. Engl. J. Med. *324*:450–454, 1991.
457. Whitley, R. J., Brasfield, D., Reynolds, D. W., et al.: Protracted pneumonitis in young infants associated with perinatally acquired cytomegaloviral infection. J. Pediatr. *89*:16–22, 1976.
458. Whitley, R. J., Corey, L., Arvin, A., et al.: Changing presentation of herpes simplex virus infection in neonates. J. Infect. Dis. *158*:109–116, 1988.
459. Whitley, R. J., and Hutto, C.: Neonatal herpes simplex virus infections. Pediatr. Rev. *7*:119–126, 1985.
460. Whitley, R. J., Nahmias, A. J., Visintine, A. M., et al.: The natural history of herpes simplex virus infection of mother and newborn. Pediatrics *66*:489–494, 1980.
461. Whitley, R. J., Yeager, A., Kartus, P., et al.: Neonatal herpes simplex virus infection: Follow-up evaluation of vidarabine therapy. Pediatrics *72*:778–785, 1983.
462. Wilfert, C. M., Thompson, R. J., Sunder, T. R., et al.: Longitudinal assess-

ment of children with enteroviral meningitis during the first three months of life. Pediatrics *67*:811–815, 1981.
463. Williamson, W. D., Desmond, M. M., LaFevers, N., et al.: Symptomatic congenital cytomegalovirus: Disorders of language, learning, and hearing. Am. J. Dis. Child. *136*:896–901, 1982.
464. Willmott, F. E., and Mair, H. J.: Genital herpesvirus infection in women attending a venereal diseases clinic. Br. J. Vener. Dis. *54*:341–343, 1978.
465. Witte, J. J., Karchmer, A. W., Herrmann, K. L., et al.: Epidemiology of rubella. Am. J. Dis. Child. *118*:107–111, 1969.
466. Wittek, A. E., Yeager, A. S., Au, D. S., et al.: Asymptomatic shedding of herpes simplex virus from the cervix and lesion site during pregnancy: Correlation of antepartum shedding with shedding at delivery. Am. J. Dis. Child. *138*:439–442, 1984.
467. Woernle, C. H., Anderson, L. J., Tattersall, P., et al.: Human parvovirus B19 infection during pregnancy. J. Infect. Dis. *156*:17–20, 1987.
468. Wong, S. N., Tam, A. Y. C., Ng, T. H. K., et al.: Fatal coxsackie B1 virus infection in neonates. Pediatr. Infect. Dis. J. *8*:638–641, 1989.
469. Wong, V. C. W., Ip, H. M. H., Reesink, H. W., et al.: Prevention of the HBsAg carrier state in newborn infants of mothers who are chronic carriers of HBsAg and HBeAg by administration of hepatitis-B vaccine and hepatitis-B immunoglobulin. Lancet *1*:921–926, 1984.
470. Wong, V. C. W., Lee, A. K. Y., and Ip, H. M. H.: Transmission of hepatitis B antigens from symptom free carrier mothers to the fetus and the infant. Br. J. Obstet. Gynaecol. *87*:958–965, 1980.
471. Woo, D., Cummins, M., Davies, P. A., et al.: Vertical transmission of hepatitis B surface antigen in carrier mothers in two west London hospitals. Arch. Dis. Child. *54*:670–675, 1979.
472. Wright, R., Perkins, J. R., Bower, B. D., et al.: Cirrhosis associated with the Australia antigen in an infant who acquired hepatitis from her mother. B. M. J. *4*:719–721, 1970.
473. Yeager, A. S.: Longitudinal, serological study of cytomegalovirus infections in nurses and in personnel without patient contact. J. Clin. Microbiol. *2*:448–452, 1975.
474. Yeager, A. S.: Storage and transport of cultures for herpes simplex virus type 2. Am. J. Clin. Pathol. *72*:977–979, 1979.
475. Yeager, A. S.: Transfusion-acquired cytomegalovirus infection in newborn infants. Am. J. Dis. Child. *128*:478–483, 1974.
476. Yeager, A. S., and Arvin, A. M.: Reasons for the absence of a history of recurrent genital infections in mothers of neonates infected with herpes simplex virus. Pediatrics *73*:188–193, 1984.
477. Yeager, A. S., Arvin, A. M., Urbani, L. J., et al.: Relationship of antibody to outcome in neonatal herpes simplex virus infections. Infect. Immun. *29*:532–538, 1980.
478. Yeager, A. S., Grumet, F. C., Hafleigh, E. B., et al.: Prevention of transfusion-acquired cytomegalovirus infections in newborn infants. J. Pediatr. *98*:281–287, 1981.
479. Yeager, A. S., Palumbo, P. E., Malachowski, N., et al.: Sequelae of maternally derived cytomegalovirus infections in premature infants. J. Pediatr. *102*:918–922, 1983.
480. Yow, M. D., White, N. H., Taber, L. H., et al.: Acquisition of cytomegalovirus infection from birth to 10 years: A longitudinal serologic study. J. Pediatr. *110*:37–42, 1987.
481. Zachoval, R., Jilg, W., Lorbeer, B., et al.: Passive/active immunization against hepatitis B. J. Infect. Dis. *150*:112–117, 1984.
482. Zanetti, A. R., Tanzi, E., Paccagnini, S., et al.: Mother-to-infant transmission of hepatitis C virus. Lancet *345*:289–291, 1995.
483. Zeldis, J. B., and Crumpacker, C. S.: Hepatitis. *In* Remington, J. S., and Klein, J. O. (eds.): Infectious Diseases of the Fetus and Newborn Infant. 4th ed. Philadelphia, W. B. Saunders, 1995, pp. 805–834.
484. Ziring, P. R., Gallo, G., Finegold, M., et al.: Chronic lymphocytic thyroiditis: Identification of rubella virus antigen in the thyroid of a child with congenital rubella. J. Pediatr. *90*:419–420, 1977.

77

Perinatal Bacterial Diseases

Xavier Sáez-Llorens and George H. McCracken, Jr.

In this chapter, we update relevant information on neonatal bacterial infections, with emphasis on epidemiology, pathogenesis, diagnosis, treatment, and prevention strategies. Those aspects of the clinical manifestations, laboratory features, and management that are peculiar to the newborn infant are stressed. A more complete description of the bacterial pathogens, host-parasite inter-relationships, and spectrum of diseases in older infants and children is presented elsewhere in the text.

ANTIBIOTIC DOSAGE SCHEDULES IN NEONATES

Much has been written about the irrational use of antimicrobial agents in newborn infants. The "therapeutic misadventures" (the gray syndrome of chloramphenicol, kernicterus associated with sulfisoxazole, enamel hypoplasia following tetracycline therapy, and deafness secondary to streptomycin and kanamycin) of past decades resulted primarily from the lack of knowledge about pharmacologic concepts in neonates. Dosage recommendations in babies were calculated from simplified formulas that pared down the usual dosage in adults or from armchair reasoning based on information obtained from healthy men and women. In either case, the amount of antibiotic administered to neonates was as often subtherapeutic as it was toxic.

Physicians have come to realize that many of the physiologic and metabolic processes of the newborn constantly change during the first few days of life and that these alterations profoundly affect pharmacokinetics of antibiotics. During the past 20 years, systematic investigations of these drugs have produced a clearer understanding of the factors influencing absorption, distribution, metabolism, and excretion of antimicrobials in newborn infants. As a result, the dosage and intervals of administration for the most commonly used drugs have been defined (Table 77–1).[195, 278] These dosage schedules are offered as a guide to safe and effective use of antibiotics in newborn infants. It must be realized that these suggested regimens have to be modified in premature babies weighing less than 1200 g at birth, in patients with reduced renal or hepatic function, and in infants with altered metabolic or physiologic states (congestive heart failure, shock, hypothyroidism, during exchange-transfusions and extracorporeal membrane oxygenation treatment) in whom the volume of drug distribution in the body may be affected profoundly. Under such circumstances, the most effective means of prescribing antibiotics is to monitor serum concentrations and to adjust the dosage accordingly.

EPIDEMIOLOGY AND PATHOGENESIS

Throughout pregnancy and until the membranes rupture, the infant's environment usually is sterile. Not until delivery and in the immediate neonatal period is the infant exposed to many microorganisms. The human birth canal is host to large numbers of aerobic and anaerobic bacteria, *Mycoplasma*, *Ureaplasma*, *Chlamydia*, fungi, yeast, and viruses. *Staphylococcus epidermidis*, lactobacilli, diphtheroids, and alpha-hemo-

TABLE 77–1. Antibiotic Dosage Schedules in Neonates

		Individual Dose (mg/kg) and Frequency of Administration				
		Weight <1200 g	Weight 1200–2000 g		Weight >2000 g	
Antibiotics	Route	*Ages: 0–4 Weeks*	*0–7 Days*	*>7 Days*	*0–7 Days*	*>7 Days*
Amikacin	IV, IM	7.5 q12h	7.5 q12h	7.5 q8h	10 q12h	10 q8h
Ampicillin*	IV, IM	25 q12h	25 q12h	25 q8h	25 q8h	25 q6h
Cefazolin	IV, IM	20 q12h	20 q12h	20 q12h	20 q12h	20 q8h
Cefotaxime	IV, IM	50 q12h	50 q12h	50 q8h	50 q12h	50 q8h
Ceftazidime	IV, IM	50 q12h	50 q12h	50 q8h	50 q12h	50 q8h
Ceftriaxone	IV, IM	50 q24h	50 q24h	50 q24h	50 q24h	75 q24h
Cephalothin	IV	20 q12h	20 q12h	20 q8h	20 q8h	20 q6h
Clindamycin	IV, IM, PO	5 q12h	5 q12h	5 q8h	5 q8h	5 q6h
Erythromycin	PO	10 q12h	10 q12h	10 q8h	10 q12h	10 q8h
Gentamicin	IV, IM	2.5 q18h	2.5 q12h	2.5 q8h	2.5 q12h	2.5 q8h
Methicillin*	IV, IM	25 q12h	25 q12h	25 q8h	25 q8h	25 q6h
Metronidazole	IV, PO	7.5 q48h	7.5 q24h	7.5 q12h	7.5 q12h	7.5 q8h
Mezlocillin	IV, IM	7.5 q12h	7.5 q12h	7.5 q8h	7.5 q12h	7.5 q8h
Nafcillin*	IV	25 q12h	25 q12h	25 q8h	25 q8h	25 q6h
Netilmicin	IV, IM	2.5 q18h	2.5 q12h	2.5 q8h	2.5 q12h	2.5 q8h
Oxacillin*	IV, IM	25 q12h	25 q12h	25 q8h	25 q8h	25 q6h
Penicillin G (units/kg)*	IV	25,000 q12h	25,000 q12h	25,000 q8h	25,000 q8h	25,000 q6h
Piperacillin	IV, IM	75 q12h	75 q12h	75 q8h	75 q8h	75 q6h
Ticarcillin	IV, IM	75 q12h	75 q12h	75 q8h	75 q8h	75 q6h
Tobramycin	IV, IM	2.5 q18h	2 q12h	2 q8h	2 q12h	2 q8h
Vancomycin	IV	15 q24h	10 q12h	10 q12h	10 q8h	10 q8h

*For meningitis, double the recommended dosage.

lytic streptococci are found in 50 to 100 per cent of the vaginal cultures of pregnant women and constitute the predominant aerobic flora.[33, 170, 320] Significant but less common isolates include *Gardnerella vaginalis*, *Proteus* and *Klebsiella* species, and group B and D streptococci; miscellaneous organisms, such as *Citrobacter*, *Acinetobacter*, and the *Campylobacter* group, are less common.

Obligate anaerobes are present in most vaginal cultures of normal, healthy women.[125] Commonly, multiple anaerobic and aerobic species are present in the same host. Approximately 85 per cent of women with genital colonization by anaerobes harbor *Bacteroides* species, including *Bacteroides fragilis* in one-third of cases. Anaerobic streptococci, *Peptostreptococcus* and *Peptococcus*, are found in about 40 per cent of women, and *Clostridium* is found in 20 per cent. Uncommon anaerobic isolates include *Veillonella*, *Bifidobacterium*, and *Eubacterium*. Vaginal cultures of pregnant women also yield mixed aerobic and anaerobic species, but the number of anaerobes decreases from early pregnancy to delivery.[170]

During the process of delivery, encounters with some of these bacteria initiate colonization of the infant's respiratory and gastrointestinal tracts. In most infants, the microbial flora is established without incident; however, disease caused by one of these organisms develops occasionally in an infant. The factors influencing conversion from colonization to disease are not understood well.

The incidence of neonatal sepsis ranges from 1 to 10 per 1000 live births. This rate varies from country to country, nursery to nursery, and within the same nursery at different times. The incidence also varies according to conditions that predispose to infection, prominent among which are prematurity and low birth weight. Between 1962 and 1987, the overall incidence of neonatal sepsis in Panorama City, California, was 2.2 per 1000 live births, whereas it was 18.6 in infants with birth weights less than 2500 g, compared with 1.2 with birth weights equal to or greater than 2500 g.[166] In the same study, the incidence of meningitis was 0.3 per 1000 live births and 2.8 and 0.07 in those with birth weights less than and greater than 2500 g, respectively. The highest age-specific incidence of bacterial meningitis of 99.5 per 100,000 population occurs during the first month of life.[165]

Socioeconomic factors appear to be important in determining whether infants are at risk of infection. Premature infants and infants with low birth weight are born more frequently to mothers of low socioeconomic class than to those of average or high socioeconomic class.

Although there is no noticeable sex predilection in infants with intrauterine infections, a male predominance is noted in almost all reported studies. The greater susceptibility of male infants is more evident in cases of sepsis caused by gram-negative enteric bacilli. The reasons behind this male predominance are not known but may be related to sex-linked factors in host susceptibility.

The bacterial cause of neonatal sepsis and meningitis varies from one geographic area to another. Although the bacterial causes of neonatal sepsis in countries of western Europe are similar to those in the United States, a different pattern has been noted in other countries, such as Saudi Arabia,[229] Nigeria,[29] Mexico,[77] and Panama.[209] In these countries, gram-negative enteric bacilli are the predominant organisms causing neonatal sepsis and meningitis. The worldwide prevalence of group B streptococcal genital colonization among pregnant women varies from 5 to 30 per cent, but group B streptococci are reported more frequently as a cause of neonatal sepsis in developed countries than in developing areas. In a recent report from Panama,[209] only 5 per cent of poor pregnant women seen in a public hospital were colonized by group B streptococci, and approximately 2 per cent of documented neonatal sepsis cases were caused by these organisms; in contrast, almost 20 per cent of "septic" neonates born to mothers with better socioeconomic status and higher vaginal colonization (seen in a hospital that is only 5 miles away) had group B streptococcal disease (Rosinda de Espino, M.D., personal communication). It is possible, but unproved, that better hygienic practices contribute to eradication of many microorganisms from vaginal sites, thus allowing group B streptococci to colonize the vagina without interference by other microbes.

The bacterial pathogens that cause infections that occur in the nursery are different from those encountered when the infant arrives home. In the nursery, besides organisms acquired vertically from mothers, staphylococci (coagulase-positive and -negative) and gram-negative bacilli constitute the predominate etiologic agents causing nosocomial disease. At home, the infant is exposed to a different environment and to members and pets of the household, which provides opportunity for infection in the newborn and probably in the household from the newborn.

The three most common bacterial pathogens of the neonatal period are group B beta-hemolytic streptococci, *Escherichia coli*, and *Listeria monocytogenes*. These three organisms account for approximately 65 to 70 per cent of all systemic neonatal bacterial diseases. The bacteria usually are acquired from the mother during the intrapartum period. The acute septicemic form of group B streptococcal disease can be caused by any of the group B types (B_I to B_V), and the specific B-type causing disease in the infant usually is found in the maternal vaginal tract.[17, 18] Epidemiologic studies have shown that about 35 per cent of pregnant women in the United States are colonized vaginally, rectally, or in both ways with group B streptococci.[89] Vertical transmission from mother to infant occurs in 40 to 70 per cent of women colonized with this organism.[1, 28, 106, 355] Infants born to heavily colonized women are more likely to harbor the organism, frequently at multiple sites, than are those born to lightly colonized women.[9, 157, 238] Some mothers of group B *Streptococcus*–infected infants are at high risk of having future babies similarly infected. A low titer of serum antibodies to the type of infecting group B *Streptococcus* and persistence of the organism in the mother have been demonstrated.[64]

Although intrapartum mother-to-infant transfer is the initial mode of acquisition of group B streptococci for the newborn, it is not the sole way in which the baby becomes colonized.[1, 11, 28, 237] In a Houston nursery, infant colonization rates increased from 20 to 25 per cent at 1 day of age to 60 to 65 per cent at 3 to 5 days of age without a concomitant increase in parturient colonization rates.[237] It seems likely that nosocomial spread of organisms from the hands of nursery personnel to the infant explains the remarkable increase in colonization rates in this nursery. Analysis of serotype distribution of group B streptococci discloses no significant differences among parturients, 1-day-old infants, nursery personnel, and infants at hospital discharge.

The major sites of colonization in infants are the skin, nasopharynx, and rectum. The group B *Streptococcus* persists in the nasopharynx for weeks to months, whereas its cutaneous location usually is lost by several weeks of age. It has been estimated that for every 100 infants colonized with group B streptococci, one or two infants will develop disease caused by this organism.

Group B streptococcal meningitis is caused almost exclusively by the B_{III} organism.[18] These organisms may be acquired from nonmaternal sites. Clusters of three or four cases of group B streptococcal meningitis have occurred in nurseries during short intervals, suggesting nosocomial acquisition.[1, 22, 313]

E. coli is the second most common agent implicated in neonatal bacterial disease, with an annual incidence of approximately one case per 1000 live births. The *Escherichia* genus is antigenically complex, comprising at least 160 somatic (O), 100 capsular (K), and 50 flagellar (H) antigens. The epidemiology of this agent in relation to newborn infection was defined more clearly with the discovery of the association between the K1 capsular polysaccharide antigen and invasive disease.[262] At present, strains with K1 antigen cause approximately 75 per cent of neonatal meningitis cases caused by *E. coli* and 40 per cent of sepsis cases.[210, 282] Furthermore, K1 strains are associated with more severe disease than are non-K1 strains.[196]

The explanation for the association between *E. coli* K1 strains and neonatal meningitis is unknown. Animal studies have demonstrated that *E. coli* strains with K1 are highly virulent for mice and that this lethal effect can be prevented completely by pretreatment of mice with minute amounts of specific K1 antibody.[262] The proclivity of K1 strains for the meninges also has been demonstrated in infant rats, in which oral feedings of *E. coli* K1 strains resulted in septicemia and meningitis in approximately 20 per cent of experimental animals.[121] Similar feeding experiments with *E. coli* K92 and K100 strains did not cause disease in this animal model.

The highest prevalence rates for rectal colonization with *E. coli* K1 strains are found in pregnant and nonpregnant women who are 16 to 31 years of age. Approximately 45 to 50 per cent of this population have K1 organisms on rectal culture.[282] Studies of pediatric populations have disclosed colonization rates of 20 to 30 per cent for newborns on the second day of life, 40 per cent for infants 4 weeks to 1 year of age, and 35 per cent for children 1 year to 16 years of age. As expected, the organism is dispersed widely among hospital personnel, who have rectal carriage rates of approximately 40 per cent.

Both vertical (mother-to-infant) and horizontal (nursery staff–to-infant, infant-to-infant) modes of transmission have been proved for *E. coli* K1 infections.[46, 282] Approximately 70 per cent of infants born to culture-positive women acquire *E. coli* K1 strains during the first 48 hours of life; in these instances of vertical transmission, there is serologic concordance for O and H types of the *E. coli* cultured from mother and baby. Approximately 10 to 15 per cent of infants colonized with K1 strains are born to K1-negative mothers. For this group of babies, *E. coli* is acquired at a later age (3 to 4 days), presumably from horizontal transmission. Additionally, vertical acquisition of K1 organisms has been documented in approximately three-fourths of neonates with *E. coli* K1 meningitis. Based on a colonization rate of approximately 200 to 300 infants per 1000 live births and an attack rate of 1 per 1000 live births, the colonization-to-disease ratio for *E. coli* is approximately 200:1 to 300:1.

Our knowledge of the epidemiology of *Listeria* remains relatively incomplete. It is a ubiquitous soil organism, and although the animal reservoir for this organism is large, transfer from animal to human is rare and occurs in high-risk persons, such as farmers and veterinarians.[236] Epidemiologic information implicating food as a vehicle for transmission of listeriosis from animals to humans now appears to be established firmly. Food-borne outbreaks have been traced to cabbage, dairy products, and vegetables. In an outbreak in Canada,[290] *Listeria*-contaminated sheep manure was used to fertilize locally grown cabbage that was stored for the winter in the cold, where the organism is known to survive for long periods. Clinical disease occurred among pregnant women who consumed the processed cabbage months after its original contamination. In 1985, the first well-documented outbreak of listeriosis in humans via contaminated milk products was reported.[111] The milk, which came from a group of farms where listeriosis among dairy cattle was known to have occurred, was pasteurized well, which indicated that pasteurization might not be enough to eradicate a large inoculum of *L. monocytogenes*. Linnan and associates[182] reported a large outbreak of perinatal listeriosis in Southern California that appeared to be due to Mexican-style cheese contaminated with raw milk. In a recent report from Costa Rica, a nosocomial outbreak of listeriosis was associated with the use of contaminated mineral oil for bathing neonates.[293]

Several large prospective epidemiologic studies have demonstrated that few women during pregnancy are colonized with *Listeria* strains and that the organism is cultured infrequently from healthy premature and term infants or from stillborn fetuses.[149, 347] From these studies, it would appear that human carriage of this bacterium is not of the same magnitude as for group B *Streptococcus* and *E. coli* K1. This is not to deny that asymptomatic colonization with *Listeria* does occur. *Listeria* has been found occasionally in the genitourinary tracts of pregnant women, in the throats of children, and in the noses of adult males.[131] *L. monocytogenes* rectal carriage rates of from 1 to 30 per cent of all pregnant or nonpregnant women have been reported.[175] The possible venereal nature of listerial colonization has been suggested.[130]

Since the 1980s, epidemic and endemic colonization and disease of the newborn infant with methicillin-resistant *S. aureus* (MRSA) have been reported with increasing frequency in the United States and Europe. Table 77–2 demonstrates the relative frequency of infections caused by MRSA, compared with those caused by other common neonatal pathogens in nurseries at Parkland Memorial Hospital in Dallas. In addition, epidemics of disease caused by MRSA have been reported in the United States and in several other countries. Risk factors associated with development of MRSA infections include lengthy hospitalization; previous antibiotic administration; overcrowding and understaffing; and the presence of predisposing factors, such as indwelling central venous catheters, cerebrospinal shunts, mechanical ventilation, and prematurity.[167]

Potential reservoirs of MRSA in the hospital environment include colonized or infected neonates, hospital personnel, and the hospital inanimate environment. Although chronic nasal carriage of MRSA by hospital personnel has been implicated in several hospital outbreaks, it generally is uncommon and is not necessary for initiation or propagation of hospital outbreaks.[323] Limited data suggest that the hospital inanimate environment may become contaminated with MRSA, possibly sustaining outbreaks of infection.[323] Colonized patients without clinical disease, on the other hand, contribute substantially to the inpatient reservoir of MRSA.

TABLE 77–2. Etiology and Outcome of Neonatal Bacterial Systemic Infections at Parkland Memorial Hospital from 1969 to 1989

Organisms	No.	(%)	Death	(%)
Group B *Streptococcus*	277	(37)	47	(17)
Escherichia coli	127	(17)	43	(34)
Other coliforms	76	(10)	28	(37)
*Staphylococcus aureus**	94	(13)	20	(21)
Enterococci	79	(10)	6	(8)
Coagulase-negative *Staphylococcus*	56	(7)	3	(5)
Pseudomonas aeruginosa	17	(2)	13	(76)
Listeria monocytogenes	5	(1)	1	(20)
Streptococcus pneumoniae	4	(1)	0	
Haemophilus influenzae type b	3	(1)	1	(33)
Nontypable *H. influenzae*	5	(1)	1	(20)
Neisseria meningitidis	1	(0)	0	
Miscellaneous	5	(1)	2	(40)
Polymicrobial†	50	(6)	15	(30)
Totals	799	(100)	180	(23)

*51 (54%) of *S. aureus* strains exhibited methicillin resistance.
†Mostly caused by gram-negative rods and anaerobes.

Coagulase-negative staphylococci also have been increasingly important neonatal pathogens. They are the most common species of the normal flora on the skin, nasal mucosa, and umbilicus of the newborn. With sensitive culture techniques, colonization rates with coagulase-negative staphylococci of the nose, umbilicus, gastrointestinal tract, and cutaneous areas of the neonate can be as high as 83 per cent at 4 days of age.[305] The ubiquitous presence of the organisms and their tolerance to both drying and temperature changes contribute to the increased presence of coagulase-negative staphylococci in neonates. In some neonatal intensive care units, disease caused by coagulase-negative staphylococci exceeds that of group B streptococci and *E. coli*.[251]

Prematurity, high rates of colonization, and aggressive treatment of the newborn infant in intensive care units (such as placement of umbilical catheters, central venous catheters, intravenous parenteral nutrition, and mechanical ventilation) account for coagulase-negative staphylococci becoming important invasive nosocomial pathogens. Despite plausible evidence of their increasing prevalence as neonatal pathogens, it often is difficult to distinguish between infection and contamination of blood cultures by these organisms.[138]

Group D streptococci are normal inhabitants of the gastrointestinal tract and can cause invasive disease. From 1969 to 1989,[273] approximately 10 per cent of neonatal infections in nurseries at Parkland Memorial Hospital in Dallas were caused by group D streptococci (see Table 76–2). Dobson and Baker[91] reported an increase in the number of blood culture isolates of enterococci from neonates in Jefferson Davis Hospital in Houston and described differences in incidence rates for early-onset and late-onset diseases. The increased incidence between 1973 and 1986 was attributed to infections in infants older than 1 week of age. In support of this is our experience at Parkland Memorial Hospital in Dallas, where 80 per cent of enterococcal infections occurred in infants older than 1 week of age. Outbreaks of bacteremia and meningitis related to *Streptococcus faecium* were reported from the neonatal intensive care units at the Medical College of Virginia and Children's Hospital of Denver.[79] These organisms have become resistant to ampicillin and vancomycin in many hospitals. Disease caused by these multiple, resistant enterococci often is difficult to treat.

Maternal, environmental, and host factors determine which infants exposed to a potentially pathogenic organism will develop invasive bacterial infections. The presence of any of the following factors can be associated with a 10-fold or greater increased risk of developing systemic infection: premature onset of labor, prolonged rupture of fetal membranes, chorioamnionitis, and maternal fever. Twin pregnancy remains an independent risk factor for group B *Streptococcus* infection and other organisms after correction for low birth weight. The first-born of twins is at a higher risk of contracting ascending intrauterine infection than is the second-born. Infection developed in 3 of 56 twin births or 54 per 1000 live births, compared with 7 infections in 603 single births, or 12 per 1000 live births.[239] The basis for increased risk of infection in twins includes the common features of virulent organisms, absence of protective antibody, and similar genetic heritage. Substance abuse by the mother (e.g., heroin) has been shown to alter significantly T-cell activity in the neonate that persists through the first year of life.[80] Although numerous microorganisms have been documented to cause maternal bacteremia before delivery, infants born to mothers with bacteremia usually remain well. This most likely is explained by a balance between the presence of maternal antibody, the virulence of the organism, and the effectiveness of the placenta in preventing transmission of the organism to the fetus.

All arms of the defense system are relatively immature (i.e., lack of prior experience with microorganisms) in the healthy neonate and are impaired further by such conditions as prematurity, hypoxia, acidosis, jaundice, and metabolic derangements. Infants with galactosemia particularly are susceptible to sepsis by gram-negative enteric bacilli.[177] *E. coli* is by far the most commonly encountered organism causing sepsis and meningitis in these infants. The umbilical stump may serve as the portal of entry of microorganisms to the blood stream. Closure of the umbilical vessels and the subsequent aseptic necrosis of the cord, which begins soon after birth, result in an ideal environment for microorganisms to multiply and invade deeper tissues, with resultant omphalitis. Complications of omphalitis include septic umbilical arteritis, suppurative thrombophlebitis of the umbilical or portal vein, peritonitis, liver abscess, and endocarditis.

Of the various microbial virulence factors, the polysaccharide capsule has been studied most thoroughly. Blood stream infections in infant rats and mice caused by *E. coli* K1 or any of the group B streptococcal serotypes can be prevented by pretreatment with type-specific capsular polysaccharide antibody. In infants, mortality and long-term sequelae have been increased in cases of meningitis caused by *E. coli* K1 strains, compared with those caused by non-K1 strains.[144] Furthermore, K1 capsular polysaccharide has been detected in cerebrospinal fluid (CSF) by counterimmunoelectrophoresis in higher concentrations and for longer durations in those patients who died or were impaired neurologically, compared with those who were normal survivors.[144] Concentrations and persistence of K1 capsular polysaccharide in the CSF of neonates with *E. coli* meningitis have been correlated with concentrations and persistence of endotoxin and interleukin-1β in CSF.[194] *E. coli* strains also have been found to resist phagocytosis by normal adult polymorphonuclear leukocytes, resulting in delayed clearance of bacteria from the blood stream. This allows the organism to multiply and achieve the concentration of 1000 colony-forming units per milliliter of blood or more, an inoculum that generally is considered essential for invasion of the meninges. The presence of K1 antigen by itself, however, does not appear to account fully for an organism's virulence because nonpathogenic *E. coli* K12 strains that are transformed by plasmid containing the cloned K1 antigen gene do not become virulent upon expression of the K1 antigen.[304] In addition, because clones of pyelonephritis strains have been identified in which specific K types occur in association with O antigens, pili, and an alpha-hemolysin, it appears that the virulence of an organism is multifactorial and that for certain infections, specific K types, in conjunction with other bacterial properties, determine pathogenicity.

Detailed studies of the type III group B *Streptococcus* demonstrated that both the quantity of sialic acid residues in the capsular polysaccharide and the spatial conformation of the antigenic molecule determine the antiphagocytic properties of this organism. A gene sequence that is specific for type III group B *Streptococcus* has been identified and cloned. Those strains with multiple copies of the gene sequence repeated within the chromosome have a lower LD_{50} (lethal dose required to kill 50 per cent of the infected animals) in the infant rat model of disease and are more resistant to opsonophagocytosis than strains that do not contain the gene structure or have only one or two copies of that sequence.[269]

Studies in children and adults have demonstrated clearly that protection from disease caused by bacteria (*Haemophilus influenzae* type b, *Neisseria meningitidis*, and *Streptococcus pneumoniae*) possessing polysaccharide capsules is afforded by specific antibody directed against these structures.[206, 291] Resistance to blood stream clearance probably relates, in part, to relative complement resistance of the encapsulated organisms. The capsule may protect the deep somatic antigen structures capable of activating the alternative complement pathway. Opsonization is essential for phagocytosis and intracellular killing of these organisms and depends primarily on anticapsular antibody. Studies indicate that levels of B_{III} antibody correlate with in vitro opsonic activity[10] and with in vivo protection in animals experimentally infected with group B streptococci.[332] The lack of type-specific maternal opsonizing antibody is a significant risk factor for the development of systemic disease caused by group B streptococcal organisms in the mother and infant.[22, 146]

Most pregnant women colonized with group B_{III} organisms have increased concentrations of antibody in the circulation, which pass transplacentally to the fetus. Both mother and baby in this instance are protected against disease by that specific B type. Conversely, infants born to mothers with undetectable concentrations of antibody are susceptible to invasion by the group B organisms. In one study, protective B_{III} antibody titers were detected in 73 per cent of women whose newborns were well, compared with 17 per cent of mothers whose newborn infants developed group B streptococcal sepsis or meningitis.[20] The same study documented lower concentrations of B_{III} antibody in sick neonates compared with those in healthy infants born to mothers with vaginal colonization. Other studies have shown that premature infants have lower B_{Ia}, B_{II}, and B_{III} antibody concentrations, compared with full-term neonates.[54, 70] This partly may explain the higher incidence and larger case-fatality rates of group B streptococcal disease observed in premature infants. It is likely, but by no means proved to date, that a lack of K1 antibody in the sera of neonates predisposes to *E. coli* K1 disease as well.[197] Mouse protection studies lend credence to this contention.[262]

Thus, there are strong parallels between the host-parasite relationships found with the group B *Streptococcus* and with *E. coli*. Both organisms possess immunochemical structures as components of the surface polysaccharide capsule that appear to confer virulence. In both, neonatal immunity is mediated, at least in part, by maternally derived serum antibody. For both organisms, asymptomatic infection (colonization) occurs commonly and clinical disease rarely (colonization-to-disease ratios of 100:1 to 200:1). Questions concerning the precise role of the complement system in opsonization of these and other bacterial pathogens, the exact concentration of antibody that confers protection, and the feasibility of screening large populations for absence of antibody need further investigation. The role of local immunity in determining invasion of these bacteria from their sites of colonization (respiratory and gastrointestinal tracts) needs clarification.

The meninges can be invaded directly from an infected adjacent site, such as skin lesions, meningomyelocele, and a skull fracture. Most cases of meningitis, however, result from bacteremia. After gaining access to the blood, bacteria probably enter the CSF space via the choroid plexus of the lateral ventricle and then spread to the subarachnoid space along normal paths of CSF flow. Because of the absence of antibody and complement in the subarachnoid space, bacteria multiply logarithmically, and as many as 10^8 colony-forming units/mL can be cultured from lumbar CSF. The larger the number of bacteria in CSF, the poorer the prognosis.

As a response to the interaction of bacteria or their cell-wall components with central nervous system tissues, the local production of inflammatory mediators, such as tumor necrosis factor and interleukin-1β, is an initial step in the cascade of events leading to inflammation and tissue destruction.[214, 257, 277] Experiments in animals demonstrated that interleukin-1β, tumor necrosis factor, and other mediators can act synergistically in altering the function of the cerebral capillary endothelium (i.e., the blood-brain barrier) and in promoting attachment of leukocytes through the expression of adhesion receptors.[277, 288] The net result is injury and increased permeability of the usually highly efficient blood-brain barrier that allows transendothelial passage of phagocytic cells and low-molecular-weight serum proteins, including complement. Despite this influx, the opsonic activity of the CSF remains low; as a result, phagocytosis is inefficient, allowing continued bacterial growth and meningeal inflammation.

Accumulation of inflammatory exudate and inflammation of the arachnoid villi can alter CSF flow, which, coupled with loss of autoregulation of cerebral blood flow, can result in increased intracranial pressure. Hydrocephalus results either from aqueductal obstruction by fibrinous debris or from reduced CSF outflow caused by inflammation of the arachnoid villi. The raised intracranial pressure, occlusion of blood vessels traversing the subarachnoid space, and edema of vascular endothelial cells can result in cerebral ischemia and possibly in cerebral infarction. Anaerobic glycolysis by poorly perfused cerebral tissues results in increased CSF lactate concentrations and hypoglycorrhachia, which further potentiate swelling of glial and neuronal cells through failure of the adenosine triphosphate–dependent sodium pump, which results in accumulation of intracellular sodium. Inappropriate secretion of antidiuretic hormone also can contribute to cerebral edema.

SEPSIS NEONATORUM

Sepsis neonatorum is a bacterial disease of infants 30 days of age or younger. It involves primarily the blood stream, although spread to the meninges or other organs occurs in a substantial portion of affected infants. No obvious focus of infection of the blood stream can be found in most cases. The presence of clinical and laboratory findings distinguishes this condition from the transient bacteremia observed in some healthy neonates. Recently, new terminology guidelines have been proposed[275, 276] to classify infants and children with a systemic inflammatory response syndrome secondary to an infectious process; the terms *sepsis, severe sepsis, septic shock,* and *multiple organ dysfunction syndrome* have been validated in large retrospective reviews.[275] Their application to septic newborns, however, needs careful assessment.

The incidence of sepsis neonatorum ranges from 1 to 10 cases per 1000 live births.[300] This rate varies from nursery to nursery and depends on conditions predisposing to infection.

Predisposing Factors

Many prepartum and intrapartum obstetric complications are associated with an increased risk of infection in newborn infants. Among these are premature onset of labor, prolonged rupture of the fetal membranes, uterine inertia with high forceps extraction, and maternal pyrexia.[41, 198, 234]

Sophisticated equipment for respiratory and nutritional support combined with invasive techniques provides life support to the ill infant. Arterial and venous umbilical catheters, central venous catheters, peripheral arterial and venous cannulas, urinary indwelling catheters, and tracheal intubation provide enormous opportunity for relatively nonvirulent pathogens to establish infection and to invade the host.[3, 26, 56, 76, 144, 155, 168, 317] The frequency of these infections varies and usually is sporadic. It may be difficult to recognize these opportunistic infections because of the severe underlying illnesses requiring intensive therapy and the frequent use of antimicrobial agents in these infants.

Clinical Manifestations

The newborn infant responds to many varieties of noxious stimuli (infectious, metabolic, respiratory, traumatic) with a limited repertoire of stereotyped reactions. As a result, many of the manifestations of sepsis have their counterparts in hypoglycemia, hypocalcemia, hypoxemia, hemolytic blood disorders, drug reactions, and surgical events. Most infectious problems in infants can not be differentiated from other neonatal disorders on the basis of the presenting clinical manifestations. The major signs and symptoms of sepsis relate to disturbances of thermoregulation, respiration, and gastrointestinal function.[93, 198, 226, 306]

Abnormalities of temperature regulation frequently are observed as initial complaints. These may take the form of hyperthermia (approximately 40 per cent of cases) or, less commonly, hypothermia.[81, 99, 333] With the introduction of Isolette care of the premature infant to maintain an optimal thermic environment, thermoregulatory disturbances commonly become obvious when the nurse reports the need to make frequent changes in the Isolette's thermostat to accommodate the infant's loss of regulatory control. Fever, on the other hand, can result from a variety of noninfectious reasons, such as dehydration, elevation in ambient temperature, and hematomas, or fever can be of central origins from such neonatal conditions as anoxia, central nervous system hemorrhage, and kernicterus.

Another frequent mode of presentation is respiratory distress manifested as tachypnea, grunting respirations, cyanosis, intercostal and substernal retractions, and apnea. A heart rate persistently in excess of 160 beats per minute can be a sensitive indicator of early-onset neonatal sepsis.[129] Although these findings particularly are indicative of early-onset group B streptococcal disease, they have been associated with infection caused by all of the pathogens commonly encountered in the neonatal period.

Approximately one-third of infants have gastrointestinal findings, including poor feeding, regurgitation, vomiting, weak suck, abdominal distention, diarrhea, and, rarely, gallbladder distention.[242] Although in most cases conditions other than sepsis explain these findings, bacterial disease always must be considered. In most patients, it is impossible to rule out sepsis on clinical grounds alone. Therefore, appropriate laboratory studies and therapeutic intervention frequently are necessary in the assessment of these nonspecific clinical manifestations.

Only a small percentage of infants show cutaneous findings (except for jaundice). These include cellulitis, impetiginous lesions, furunculosis, papular lesions (listeriosis), vascular lesions *(Pseudomonas)*, and exfoliative dermatitis (phage group II staphylococcal disease). Jaundice is present in approximately one-third of infants with sepsis and can occur in infants with urinary tract infection. Occasionally, jaundice is the only sign of infection and occurs in septic infants, regardless of the type of bacterial pathogen.

In utero infection is identified by the presence of bacteria in blood obtained at delivery. Signs of fetal distress may be the first indication of infection in the newborn. Schiano and associates[289] have suggested fetal tachycardia in the second stage of labor as a sign of intrauterine infection. Pneumonia or sepsis occurred in 3 of 8 infants with fetal heart beats of more than 180 per minute, in 7 of 32 infants with 160 to

179 beats per minute, and in 1 of 167 infants with lower heart rates.

Etiology

Since the middle of the century, there has been a shift in the microorganisms responsible for neonatal septicemia and meningitis.[93, 114, 122, 198, 226] In the 1930s and 1940s, the predominant organism was the group A beta-hemolytic *Streptococcus*. This was replaced in the 1950s by the phage group I *S. aureus* and by coliform organisms. By the late 1950s to the present, *E. coli* and group B beta-hemolytic streptococci accounted for approximately 60 to 70 per cent of all infections. *S. epidermidis* recently has emerged as an important pathogen for neonates and is responsible for at least 10 per cent of cases of sepsis in newborn intensive care facilities.[32, 65, 211] The apparent increased incidence of *S. epidermidis* sepsis has been associated with increased survival of very small premature infants and the introduction of invasive procedures.[138] MRSA also has emerged as a nosocomial pathogen of major importance in some nurseries. The prevalence rates for a specific bacterial pathogen vary from nursery to nursery and may change abruptly in any one unit.[31, 114, 122, 146] Knowledge of the most commonly isolated bacteria in a nursery or intensive care unit, as well as the antimicrobial susceptibility of these organisms, is invaluable in treating infants with suspected sepsis neonatorum.

Table 77–3 presents the bacterial agents responsible for neonatal sepsis in three nurseries from different areas of the world.[147, 209, 273] Group B *Streptococcus* has remained the most common single etiologic agent of neonatal sepsis and meningitis in Dallas, it was the second most frequent in Mallorca, Spain, and it was isolated uncommonly in Panama City, Panama.

Coliform bacteria, including *E. coli* and *Klebsiella* and *Enterobacter* species, were recovered more frequently in Panama and Mallorca than in Dallas. *S. aureus* was recovered relatively commonly in the three nurseries; a large percentage of the strains isolated in the United States were methicillin-resistant, which underscores the importance of these organisms in some neonatal units. Coagulase-negative staphylococci also were recovered frequently in infants with neonatal sepsis. Anaerobes were responsible for a small percentage of cases of septicemia. Because special techniques for isolation of these relatively fastidious organisms were not used, it is possible that we underestimated considerably the actual contribution of these bacteria in causing sepsis.

H. influenzae, S. pneumoniae, and *N. meningitidis* are occasional causes of neonatal sepsis. Viridans streptococci are being isolated with increased frequency and in one series were the major pathogens in neonates with streptococcal septicemia. From 1987 to 1989, viridans streptococci were recovered from the blood of 20 of 273 infants with neonatal sepsis in nurseries at Parkland Memorial Hospital in Dallas.

The changing distribution of etiologic agents over time has been demonstrated in developed and in developing countries. In United States nurseries, gram-negative enteric organisms were the most frequent isolates two decades ago; presently, gram-positive bacteria (mostly group B streptococci and staphylococci) constitute the predominant pathogens. In the largest public hospital of Panama, during an 18-year period (1975 to 1992), the proportional incidence of gram-negative infections also declined with time, whereas that of gram-positive infections increased.[209]

Specific Clinical Syndromes

Group B Beta-Hemolytic Streptococcus

Group B streptococcal infection may become evident in a variety of ways, ranging from asymptomatic bacteremia to septicemia, pneumonia, and meningitis. Skin infections, such as impetigo, cellulitis, erythema nodosum–like lesions, adenitis, breast abscess, and scalp abscesses, also may occur.[15, 151, 219] Group B streptococci may present first as conjunctivitis, orbital cellulitis, otitis media, or ethmoiditis. These organisms are responsible for an increasing proportion of suppurative arthritis and osteomyelitis cases during the newborn period and have been incriminated in such unusual infections as retropharyngeal cellulitis, pleural empyema, endocarditis, peritonitis, and adrenal abscess.[13, 66, 151, 335, 342]

Two clinically and epidemiologically distinct forms of illness have been described.[19, 30, 113, 151] The early- or acute-onset form is seen in the first 5 days of life (usually within the first 6 to 12 hours) and is characterized by a high incidence of

TABLE 77–3. Etiology of Bacterial Sepsis in Newborns from Three Different Areas of the World

	Number and Percentage of Isolates		
Organisms	*Dallas (U.S.) (1969–1989) n = 744*	*Mallorca (Spain) (1977–1991) n = 332*	*Panama (Panama) (1975–1992) n = 577*
Gram-negative	229 (30%)	151 (45%)	361 (63%)
Escherichia coli	17%	10%	14%
Klebsiella species	7%	15%	20%
Other enteric rods	3%	10%	20%
Pseudomonas species	2%	6%	6%
Haemophilus influenzae	1%	1%	<1%
Others	<1%	3%	2%
Gram-positive	515 (70%)	181 (55%)	216 (37%)
Group B *Streptococcus*	37%	22%	2%
Coagulase-negative *Staphylococcus*	9%	15%	20%
S. aureus	12%	8%	12%
Enterococci	10%	7%	1%
Listeria monocytogenes	1%	2%	<1%
S. pneumoniae	<1%	<1%	<1%
Others	<1%	<1%	<1%

maternal complications. These infants usually are very ill within hours of delivery and exhibit unexplained apnea or tachypnea, respiratory distress, hypoxemia, and shock. Chest radiographs reveal either a diffuse pulmonary infiltrate similar to that seen after aspiration or findings indistinguishable from hyaline membrane disease. One of the major diagnostic problems with the acute-onset syndrome is its clinical differentiation from respiratory distress syndrome. Several features of early-onset group B streptococcal disease may be helpful in differentiating it from the respiratory distress syndrome. Obstetric complications are encountered commonly in mothers of those with group B streptococcal disease, whereas this is uncommon in mothers of those with respiratory distress syndrome.[30, 113] In fact, there is evidence that prenatal complications may protect the infant from respiratory distress syndrome because of increased corticosteroid secretion by the mother.

Compared with infants with respiratory distress syndrome, infants with streptococcal disease usually are sicker early in the course of illness, and apnea, shock, or both occur within 12 to 24 hours of onset of infection. Infants with respiratory distress syndrome experience a more gradual evolution of events. In some infants with group B streptococcal disease, rapid progression to respiratory failure and death occurs within 12 hours. This is unusual in the infants with uncomplicated respiratory distress syndrome. The peak inspiratory pressures required to ventilate babies with streptococcal disease are said to be lower than those necessary for infants with respiratory distress syndrome.[2] In preterm infants, leukopenia with increased numbers of band forms is common in the infected cases.[2, 185]

The chest radiograph may be helpful in differentiating these two illnesses. Neonatal pneumonia is found in approximately 40 per cent of infants with group B streptococcal disease. In the others, a diffuse reticulogranular pattern with air bronchograms is seen and cannot be distinguished from that observed in infants with the respiratory distress syndrome. Hyaline membranes are seen pathologically in both illnesses.

The second major form of neonatal group B streptococcal disease is the late-onset syndrome. In contrast with the acute fulminant disease of the first day of life, the late-onset syndrome has an insidious onset after 5 to 7 days of age, although it occasionally may be fulminant.[19, 153] The disease almost invariably involves the meninges. Most infants present in the second through fourth weeks of life, but documented cases have occurred at up to 12 weeks of age. A history of maternal obstetric complications usually is lacking, and the infants almost always have an unremarkable early neonatal history, although late-onset disease does occur occasionally among premature infants,[90] and the case-fatality rate is low, on the order of 5 to 15 per cent.

In contrast with the uniform distribution of all five major serotypes causing early-onset disease, the group B_{III} organism is responsible for approximately 90 per cent of all late-onset cases[18] (irrespective of clinical manifestation) and of cases of infants with meningitis (irrespective of age of onset). This apparently virulent effect of type III strains, which account for two-thirds of group B streptococcal infections in infants, appears to be restricted to young infants. In contrast, type II strains are predominant among isolates from adults with meningitis, a serotype rarely ever isolated from CSF of infants with meningitis. The mode of acquisition is uncertain because the B_{III} organism usually can not be recovered from maternal sites at onset of the infant's illness. Horizontal transmission of the pathogen from nursery personnel, caregivers at home, and others to the newborn has been proposed as the most reasonable mode of acquisition.[1, 18, 240]

The clinical features of illness are indistinguishable from the other forms of purulent meningitis of this age group. An exception to the normal pattern for late-onset infection is the intensive care unit setting, where nosocomially acquired clusters of disease among low birth weight infants have been reported.[225, 341] In such circumstances, the spectrum of clinical expression is similar to that of early-onset disease, although serotype III still predominates.[225]

Other Streptococci

Group A beta-hemolytic streptococcal disease is not as common now as in previous decades. Disease caused by this organism varies from a low-grade chronic omphalitis to fulminant septicemia and meningitis. Because of the explosive nature of this organism in nursery settings, constant surveillance for colonized infants and prompt recognition of illness are mandatory to avert a nursery outbreak of group A streptococcal disease.[118]

Group D and G streptococci have been reported to cause an illness indistinguishable from early-onset group B streptococcal sepsis.[94, 299] On the other hand, viridans streptococci usually cause a less severe illness with a lower incidence of respiratory distress, shock, and white blood cell count abnormalities.[309] Dobson and Baker,[91] in a review of 56 neonates with enterococcal septicemia from a single hospital in Houston from 1977 through 1986, described two distinct clinical syndromes. Infants older than 7 days were more premature, had lower birth weights, and in most cases had infections characterized by a nosocomial origin. Compared with early-onset disease (5 days of age or younger), which was characterized by mild illness with respiratory distress or diarrhea without focal infection, the late-onset enterococcal sepsis was heralded by severe apnea, bradycardia, circulatory collapse, and increased ventilation requirements. Focal infections, such as meningitis, pneumonia, scalp abscess, and catheter-related illnesses, were common.

Staphylococcus

In the mid-1950s, phage group I *S. aureus* was the most common bacterial agent causing serious bacterial diseases in newborn infants. Its unique invasive properties caused disseminated disease with widespread manifestations, including mastitis, furunculosis, suppurative arthritis, osteomyelitis, septicemia, and meningitis. Because blood stream infection usually is secondary to local invasion, the primary focus must be searched for carefully in all septic babies. Changes in the epidemiologic characteristics of the organism, coupled with intensified microbial surveillance and infection control measures, have reduced colonization and disease rates caused by the phage group I *Staphylococcus*.

Coagulase-positive staphylococcal disease in nurseries also has been caused by phage group II organisms.[200] These organisms produce an exotoxin (exfoliatin) that results in intraepidermal cleavage through the granular cell layer because of the disruption of desmosomes.[201] Clinical disease may take one of several forms, including bullous impetigo, toxic epidermal necrolysis (Ritter disease), and nonstreptococcal scarlatina. The initial finding in Ritter disease is intense, painful erythema followed by bulla formation, which, when ruptured, leaves a tender, weeping erythematous area. A characteristic desquamation of large epidermal sheets occurs approximately 3 to 5 days after the onset of disease. A fine desquamation is observed commonly in the perioral region. Bullous impetigo has been the most common disease associated with nursery outbreaks of group II staphylococcal infections.[5]

In the 1980s, MRSA emerged as a nosocomial pathogen of considerable importance. MRSA describes resistance to the penicillinase-resistant penicillin class of antibiotics, which includes methicillin, nafcillin, oxacillin, cloxacillin, and dicloxacillin. The mechanism of resistance, in part, involves alteration of penicillin-binding proteins in the periplasm of the bacterium, resulting in a decrease in affinity for those antibiotics. The spectrum of clinical disease that is caused by MRSA is similar to that caused by methicillin-susceptible *S. aureus*, except that patients with MRSA bacteremia were reported to be less likely to have bone or joint infection.[316] Of 44 cases of MRSA infections in the nurseries of Parkland Memorial Hospital in Dallas from 1987 to 1990, the organism was recovered from the blood in 35, from CSF in 4, from peritoneal fluid in 4, and from joint fluid in 1. Of the 35 patients with bacteremia, 7 had pneumonia, 2 had meningitis, 2 had arthritis/osteomyelitis, 1 had urinary tract infection, and 1 had a soft tissue abscess (J. D. Siegel, personal communication).

Coagulase-negative staphylococci are being identified more often in blood cultures of neonates with signs and symptoms of sepsis[31, 110] but frequently are dismissed as contaminants. The isolation of these organisms should be considered significant when they grow in both aerobic and anaerobic blood culture bottles, when growth occurs within 72 hours, or when they are isolated from two or more sites or from the same site at different times.[32, 211, 224] *S. epidermidis* disease tends to occur as a late-onset infection (i.e., nosocomial acquisition) and is associated with the usual signs and symptoms of sepsis. White blood cell count abnormalities are found in about half of all infected infants. Major risk factors include prematurity, low birth weight, invasive procedures, central venous catheters, and total parenteral nutrition. These infections frequently are associated with colonization of the central venous catheters and involvement of other sites, such as the central nervous system. The patients usually are not very ill and respond well to antimicrobial therapy, but the central venous catheters frequently have to be removed to prevent further seeding of the blood stream. The mortality rate is low and ranges between 0 and 15 per cent in different series.[32, 110, 211, 224]

Escherichia coli

E. coli strains are the most common gram-negative bacteria causing septicemia during the neonatal period. Annual incidence rates for the past 15 years in Dallas have remained reasonably constant at 0.5 to 1.5 cases per 1000 live births.[151] This etiologic agent still remains the single most frequent cause of neonatal sepsis and meningitis in many developing countries (*Klebsiella* species is more common in some countries).[209] Unlike illnesses caused by group B streptococci and *L. monocytogenes*, *E. coli* infections do not fit into distinct clinical syndromes of early- and late-onset disease. Approximately 40 per cent of *E. coli* strains causing septicemia possess K1 capsular antigen.[282] The clinical features of *E. coli* sepsis generally are similar to those observed in infants with disease caused by other pathogens. Localized *E. coli* infections have included breast abscess, cellulitis, meningitis, pneumonia, lung abscess, empyema, osteomyelitis, septic arthritis, urinary tract infection, ascending cholangitis, and otitis media.

Listeria monocytogenes

The pathogenesis and clinical spectrum of diseases caused by *L. monocytogenes* are similar to those caused by group B streptococci. Because the most common foci for neonatal infection are lung and gut, the fetus probably is infected by the mother's swallowing contaminated liquor as well as through the transplacental route. Chorioamnionitis diagnosed by transabdominal amniocentesis in pregnant women with intact fetal membranes has been reported,[244] thus favoring the blood-borne route of infection. Nevertheless, an ascending pathway from the lower genital tract is possible. Early gestational *Listeria* can be associated with abortion or stillbirth. Premature labor in mothers with *Listeria* infection is common; in approximately 70 per cent, delivery occurs before 35 weeks' gestation.

Evidence of preceding maternal illness often is described in infants with early-onset disease. Symptoms in mothers can be vague (malaise and myalgia) or distinctive (fever and chills) and may alert the physician to a risk of *Listeria* infection. Blood cultures often (35 per cent) are positive for *Listeria* in such mothers. A fulminant, disseminated disease may occur during the first several days of life (granulomatosis infantiseptica). The pathogen is acquired transplacentally[330] or by aspiration at the time of vaginal delivery; multiple organ systems are involved.[35] The infant frequently has hypothermia, is lethargic, and feeds poorly.[294] A characteristic rash consisting of small, salmon-colored papules scattered primarily on the trunk may be observed in some infants.

Listeria infection should be suspected in premature infants with early passage of meconium. Because meconium is extremely unusual in premature infants younger than 32 weeks of gestational age, if it is present, the physician should suspect *Listeria* infection. Chest radiographs show parenchymal infiltrates suggestive of aspiration pneumonitis in most infants. A miliary type of bronchopneumonia also can be seen in some cases. There are no reports of acute-onset listeriosis mimicking the radiographic picture of hyaline membrane disease. *Listeria* serotypes Ia, Ib, and IVb produce the early-onset disease, whereas serotype IVb is the predominant type in late-onset meningitic disease.[6]

A delayed form of neonatal listeriosis occurs during the second through eighth week of life and involves the meninges in almost all cases. The infected infant usually is the full-term product of an uncomplicated labor and delivery. Onset of symptoms and signs is relatively insidious, and it is indistinguishable from those observed with meningitis caused by other pathogens. Acute *Listeria* encephalitis, which usually is fatal within a few days, is a rare disease in humans. Other clinical forms of disease at this age include *Listeria*-induced colitis with associated diarrhea and sepsis without meningitis. The bacteriology laboratory should be forewarned of the clinical suspicion of listerial meningitis because these microorganisms frequently are discarded as contaminants because of their tinctorial and morphologic similarities with diphtheroids. Overnight refrigeration of spinal fluid specimens frequently enhances growth of this organism.

The peripheral white blood cell count usually shows a brisk leukocytosis with a predominance of polymorphonuclear leukocytes in the differential count. A significant elevation in the number of monocytes to 7 to 21 per cent of the total white blood cell count has been documented on admission laboratory evaluation of infected infants.[331] Likewise, a monocytosis of this magnitude can be demonstrated in most remaining infants on repetitive testing of the peripheral white blood cell count. In contrast, monocytes are not found typically in the spinal fluid of infants infected with *L. monocytogenes*. Polymorphonuclear leukocytes predominate in about 75 per cent of cases, with a relative lymphocytosis noted in the remaining 25 per cent. As with other pyogenic meningitides, hypoglycorrhachia and elevated protein concentrations are frequent findings. Examination of the stained smear of spinal fluid has not been rewarding in more than 50 per cent of cases. This is a reflection of the relatively low concentrations of organisms in the fluid,[105] the atypical morphology, and the variable decoloration resulting from the Gram staining procedure, which may result in organisms appearing as gram-negative rods or gram-positive cocci.

Pseudomonas aeruginosa

Pseudomonas septicemia may show a characteristic violaceous papular lesion or lesions, in which central necrosis develops after several days (ichthyma gangrenous). Noma (gangrenous lesions of the nose, lips, and mouth) has been associated with bacteremia caused by *P. aeruginosa*. This is caused by a suppurative vasculitis, and deep-seated abscess formation is common.[260] The neonate who is treated with broad-spectrum antimicrobial agents while in an environment potentially contaminated by "water bugs" (respirators, moist oxygen) particularly is prone to disease caused by *Pseudomonas* species or other fastidious commensals. Thus, the organism usually is a cause of late-onset disease.[174] Stevens and associates,[315] however, reported nine cases of *Pseudomonas* sepsis, four of which presented in the first 72 hours of life. The clinical and radiologic findings in these four infants were similar to those of hyaline membrane disease.

Diagnosis

The diagnosis of sepsis neonatorum relies heavily on the clinical judgment and diagnostic acumen of the physician. Signs and symptoms may be vague and frequently misleading. Bacterial infection may masquerade as metabolic disease, respiratory distress, environmental stress, and other noninfectious conditions. The physician confronted by an infant with possible sepsis must be guided by a complete perinatal history eliciting those factors that place the infant at high risk, by a thorough physical examination attentive to signs suggestive of infection, and by clinical experience. When infection is likely, a laboratory work-up is indicated. When infection is unlikely and not substantiated by history, physical examination, and clinical judgment, investigation for an infectious process usually is unnecessary. If doubt exists, as frequently is the case, it is good practice to proceed with a laboratory work-up.

Recovery of an organism from a meaningful site, such as blood, CSF, urine, abscesses, pleural and peritoneal spaces, joints, bones, and middle ear cavities, substantiates the clinical impression of systemic bacterial disease. Isolation of an organism from mucocutaneous sites, such as skin, ear canal, nasopharynx, gastric aspirate, and rectum, usually does not reflect the microbiological status of normally sterile body fluids or tissues.[107] It must be emphasized that the colonization-to-disease ratio for the major pathogens of the neonate is approximately 100:1 to 200:1. That is, for every infant with proved systemic bacterial disease, there are 100 or more infants who are colonized superficially with this organism but who are free of systemic bacterial disease.

Several sites for sampling blood for culture give reliable results: peripheral vein, umbilical artery, and capillary blood. The preferred site is the peripheral vein. Venipuncture should be performed after the skin has been prepared properly by cleansing with an iodine-containing solution.[98] A two-phase antisepsis procedure using 70 per cent isopropyl alcohol followed by chlorhexidine or povidone-iodine has been shown to be superior to one using chlorhexidine or povidone-iodine alone in reducing skin colonization by *S. epidermidis*.[67] The theoretic minimal amount of blood needed for detecting bacteremia is a function of the number of organisms circulating at any given time. Infants with *E. coli* sepsis have 5 to more than 1000 colony-forming units per milliliter of blood.[87] Thus, culturing as little as 0.2 mL of blood should be sufficient for detecting *E. coli* bacteremia in these patients. On the basis of experimental *E. coli* sepsis in rabbits, a cultured volume of blood of 0.2 mL is as sensitive as 1 mL in detecting bacteremia at a threshold level of 5 organisms per milliliter of circulating blood.[108] Similar data for the other pathogens of neonatal sepsis are not available. Until additional studies have been reported, it is prudent to obtain 0.5 to 1 mL of blood for culture. Optimal results are obtained when the cultured volume of blood is 5 to 10 per cent of the total amount of liquid growth medium to be inoculated.

Bacterial growth is evidenced in the vast majority of blood cultures within 48 hours. With the use of conventional culture techniques and subcultures at 4 and 14 hours, only 4 per cent of cultures that had positive results required more than 48 hours of incubation.[248] With the use of radiometric technique, 98 per cent of cultures growing group B *Streptococcus* and *E. coli* were identified within 24 hours.[268] The number of blood cultures required to document sepsis in newborn infants is unknown. We generally recommend one or two blood cultures before initiating antibiotic therapy. Additionally, urine and CSF should be obtained for examination and culture before starting therapy.

Many laboratory tests have been recommended for the evaluation of suspected bacterial diseases in neonates. The white blood cell count is a simple, readily available test that can help in the early detection of sepsis.[38, 185, 186] Elevated total white blood cell counts, absolute neutrophil counts, and absolute band counts usually are not helpful singly as indicators of sepsis. Although neutropenia in neonates most often is due to infection, it frequently is associated with other conditions, such as birth asphyxia and pregnancy-induced hypertension.[100]

The usefulness of abnormal white blood cell counts in the detection of sepsis is enhanced by measurement of the immature-to-total (I:T) neutrophil ratio; a ratio of 0.2 or greater is a relatively sensitive indicator of neonatal sepsis.[245, 246] A large number of studies that evaluated the I:T neutrophil ratio have shown that the ratio is too unreliable to achieve more than limited clinical usefulness. Sensitivities ranging from 90 to 60 per cent or less have been reported.[44, 45] Furthermore, elevated ratios caused by a variety of perinatal conditions have been seen in 25 to 50 per cent of noninfected, ill infants.[117, 163] The ratio's greatest value is believed to be in its good negative predictive value; if the ratio is normal, the likelihood that infection is absent is very high.[117, 163] An I:T ratio of 0.8 or greater indicates depletion of bone marrow neutrophil reserves and is a poor prognostic indicator. A combination of all these laboratory findings (hematologic scoring system), rather than those of any test alone, increases the diagnostic specificity of a bacterial infection.[263] This scoring system is of limited value in late-onset, coagulase-negative staphylococcal infections.[83]

It is important to repeat a white blood cell count and I:T ratio determination 6 to 8 hours after the initial evaluation because studies in both animals and human infants have demonstrated that the white blood cell count can be normal at the onset of group B streptococcal sepsis and abnormal 4 to 8 hours later. Morphologic changes in neutrophils, such as vacuolization and toxic granulation, suggest the presence of infection. The degree of these degenerative changes in neutrophils of infected neonates has no implication as to the severity or potential outcome of the illness.[183] Identical morphologic findings can occur as artifacts in citrated blood samples stored for longer than 1 hour before smears are made. The platelet count is unreliable for establishing the diagnosis of bacterial infection during the neonatal period.

The erythrocyte sedimentation rate in infected patients usually is elevated above the normal range of 1 to 2 mm/hour at 12 hours of age to 17 to 20 mm/hour at 14 days of age.[4] Elevated rates usually are not observed until 24 to 48 hours after clinical signs of disease first occur. Other acute-phase reactants, such as C-reactive protein, haptoglobin, prealbumin, orosomucoid, and transferrin, may be useful in the diagnosis of neonatal sepsis and in following the course of the infection.[247] The most extensively studied of these acute-phase reactants is the C-reactive protein. Concentrations of this protein increase significantly within a few hours of the onset of infection. In general, other perinatal events have little impact on C-reactive protein neonatal values.[292] C-reactive protein concentrations decrease rapidly in infected neonates who respond to therapy and, conversely, persistently are elevated in neonates whose infections fail to respond to therapy.[281] Reliance on a single C-reactive protein determination as an early indicator of neonatal bacterial infections is not recommended. Serial determinations are helpful, especially in combination with other hematologic tests, when making a decision to stop antimicrobial therapy safely.

Fibronectin is a glycoprotein that has been identified on cell surfaces and in extracellular fluids. The concentration of it in fetal plasma increases with gestational age to values at term of approximately one-half of those found in healthy adults. Plasma concentrations fall significantly during sepsis[117] but may decrease in noninfectious neonatal conditions, such as perinatal asphyxia and respiratory distress syndrome.[354] More data are needed for determining the value of fibronectin concentrations as indicators of bacterial sepsis.

Recently, detection of interleukin-6 in plasma samples of newborns has been suggested as a reliable early indicator of sepsis.[58, 134, 145] Interleukin-6 is a pleiotropic cytokine involved in many aspects of the immune system. It is synthesized and released in response to inflammatory stimuli by monocytes, endothelial cells, and fibroblasts after production of tumor necrosis factor and interleukin-1. Interleukin-6 is the major inducer of hepatic protein synthesis including C-reactive protein, fibrinogen, and other acute-phase reactants. Its sensitivity in the diagnosis of sepsis and necrotizing enterocolitis appears to be high.[145] More studies are needed, however, to evaluate the precise role of interleukin-6 measurement in guiding physicians to a better diagnostic approach of systemic neonatal infections.

The detection of bacterial antigens in blood, urine, or CSF confirms the presence of systemic bacterial disease. Diagnostic techniques include countercurrent immunoelectrophoresis, latex particle agglutination, and coagglutination procedures. Countercurrent immunoelectrophoresis is specific but has low sensitivity and can be used to detect infections caused by *E. coli* K1 and group B streptococci.[24, 143] Latex particle agglutination and coagglutination tests are more sensitive than countercurrent immunoelectrophoresis but have been associated with a small percentage of both false-positive and false-negative reactions.[115, 143] They can be used for the detection of disease caused by group B streptococci, *N. meningitidis*, *S. pneumoniae*, and *H. influenzae* type b. The highest yield is achieved by testing concentrated heat-treated urine specimens and CSF. The sensitivity of this test is 90 to 98 per cent, with an average false-positive rate of 2 to 6 per cent. Perineal contamination may cause false-positive results in healthy colonized infants in the absence of invasive disease when the urine tested is obtained by bag collection.[279] The absence of antigen does not rule out infection. A positive result in the urine antigen test with negative results in the blood culture can imply occult infection (e.g., osteomyelitis), partial treatment by intrapartum antibiotic therapy, or a false-positive result. The *E. coli* K1 antigen is identical immunologically to the *N. meningitidis* group B antigen and therefore can be detected by *N. meningitidis* group B kits. The usefulness of this test is much decreased, however, by its low sensitivity and the high contamination rates of urine collected by bag with *E. coli* from the gastrointestinal tract.

Direct examination of Gram-stained or methylene blue buffy-coat smears can help in the early detection of neonatal bacteremia if bacteria engulfed by neutrophils are visualized.[102] Some authors consider only those smears with intragranulocytic bacteria to be positive. Bacteria are seen more readily when acridine orange stain is used.[164] This technique requires a smaller volume of blood but can not distinguish between gram-positive and gram-negative bacteria. Identification of bacteria on Gram-stained smears of tracheal secretions obtained in the first 12 hours of life from infants who require intubation is associated with bacteremia in about half of these cases.[295]

Endotoxin elaborated from gram-negative bacteria circulates in blood and is present in urine for considerable periods after sterilization of these fluids. Detection of endotoxin by the *Limulus* amebocyte lysate assay may be helpful in the early identification of infected infants.[161, 287] Endotoxin may be present in blood of septic-appearing infants who have sterile blood cultures. It is possible that transient endotoxemia is responsible for "clinical sepsis" in these infants. The source of endotoxin may be the gram-negative bacterial flora of the bowel. It is possible that endotoxin entered the circulation through an injured and permeable gastrointestinal mucosa.

Several serologic tests for the diagnosis of listeriosis have been described, but none has become an established means of routine diagnosis. Agglutination reactions, complement fixation, enzyme-linked immunosorbent assay, precipitin, indirect hemagglutination, and antigen fixation tests are available and may help occasionally. Caution is warranted, however, in attempts to use these tests for diagnostic purposes. Genetic studies showed that an extracellular hemolysin, listeriolysin O, is essential for intracellular multiplication of *Listeria*.

In a French study,[39] investigators examined whether detection of specific anti–listeriolysin O could be used for serodiagnosis of human listeriosis. Sera from 28 patients (13 were newborn) infected with *L. monocytogenes* and 101 controls were tested by dot-blot titration with purified listeriolysin O. Twenty-seven patients (96 per cent) with *Listeria* infection produced specific anti–listeriolysin O, which was detected in low titers in 16 per cent of healthy controls and in 12 per cent of persons who had various bacterial, fungal, and viral infections. Anti–listeriolysin O could be detected soon after infection and persisted for at least several months. Although this test might be useful for epidemiologic surveys and for serodiagnosis of listeriosis, more data are needed before it can be used routinely for serodiagnosis of human listeriosis.

Treatment

Once the diagnosis of sepsis is suspected or proved and the appropriate cultures have been obtained, antibiotic therapy should be instituted. When the infant's condition prompts an evaluation for sepsis, it usually is prudent to initiate empiric parenteral antibiotic treatment, despite the fact that only 5 to 10 per cent of blood cultures are positive.

Infants with suspected sepsis should be treated with a combination that includes a penicillin and an aminoglycoside. The choice of antibiotics must be based on the historic experience of the nursery, the antimicrobial susceptibilities of bacteria recently isolated from both sick and healthy neonates, the likely etiologic agent, CSF penetration of antibiotics, and the infant's hepatic and renal functions. Factors that determine the likely infecting organism include patient age and birth weight; environment (home versus hospital); prior antibiotic therapy; perinatal or nosocomial exposure to pathogens (e.g., MRSA); presence of central lines, drains, or endotracheal tube; and identification of specific infections, such as meningitis, necrotizing enterocolitis, peritonitis, thrombophlebitis, pneumonia, and soft-tissue infections.

For early-onset sepsis neonatorum, we recommend ampicillin and gentamicin for the reasons that follow. Ampicillin is effective in vitro and clinically against group B streptococci, *Listeria, Proteus,* and most enterococci and is active against approximately 50 per cent of *E. coli* strains. The aminoglycosides have broader antimicrobial activity against many Enterobacteriaceae, including most *E. coli, Klebsiella-Enterobacter,* and *Proteus* strains, and, with the exception of kanamycin, against *Pseudomonas aeruginosa.* Although gentamicin frequently is used, the choice of the aminoglycoside (e.g., amikacin, tobramycin, netilmicin) should be based on antimicrobial susceptibilities of nosocomial bacteria within individual nurseries. For infections caused by gentamicin-resistant coliforms, amikacin or third-generation cephalosporins, such as cefotaxime and ceftazidime, should be used.[152, 159, 285]

Cephalosporins are not active against *Listeria* or enterococci and should not be used without concomitant administration of ampicillin. Moreover, when used with ampicillin, cephalosporins do not offer the advantage of synergism that aminoglycosides do against strains of enterococci. Staphylococci, nosocomial gram-negative organisms, and fungi rarely are encountered in early-onset sepsis neonatorum, and empiric coverage for them usually is not required. When the epidemiologic experience of the nursery or cutaneous lesions suggest *Pseudomonas,* an extended-spectrum penicillin (i.e., ticarcillin or piperacillin) or ceftazidime combined with an aminoglycoside should be used (see Table 77–1 for dosages). Therapeutic drug monitoring is recommended when aminoglycosides are used, especially in low birth weight neonates, and dosage adjustment is essential in infants with impaired renal function.

Because late-onset sepsis neonatorum is more heterogeneous in its epidemiology than is early-onset disease and may reflect maternal, family, community, or nosocomial sources for the infecting pathogen, the organisms involved cover a broad taxonomic spectrum. As a result, empiric antimicrobial regimens vary. In the previously healthy infant who already has been discharged from the hospital, ampicillin and an aminoglycoside or cefotaxime are recommended unless staphylococcal infection is highly suspected, in which case an antistaphylococcal agent (e.g., methicillin, nafcillin) should replace ampicillin. In contrast, selection of empiric antibiotic regimens can be more difficult for a septic premature infant who has had a prolonged hospitalization, previous antibiotic administration, possible prolonged tracheal intubation, and placement of a central or peripheral intravascular catheter.

In these patients, major pathogens include coagulase-negative and -positive staphylococci (including MRSA), aminoglycoside-resistant coliforms, highly resistant opportunistic organisms (such as *Pseudomonas* and *Serratia),* fungi, and possibly enterococci. As a result, empiric regimens in this situation should be individualized. Examples include ampicillin, amikacin, and clindamycin for suspected necrotizing enterocolitis, vancomycin and an aminoglycoside or cefotaxime for patients with indwelling central vascular lines, and nafcillin and an aminoglycoside for babies with skin infection. Of paramount importance, we always must keep in mind the potential empiric use of amphotericin in these infants. Ceftazidime and cefotaxime should not be used routinely in neonatal units because of the potential for emergence of resistant *Enterobacter* and *Serratia* species. Empiric treatment with aztreonam, a monobactam antibiotic, in combination with ampicillin has been shown to be as effective as the standard ampicillin and aminoglycoside regimen.[328] Aztreonam has not been approved yet by the Food and Drug Administration for use in newborn infants.

Once the culture and susceptibility studies are available, changes in therapy may be necessary. Ampicillin alone is preferred for enterococcal and *Listeria* infections, whereas either ampicillin or penicillin can be used for group B streptococcal disease. Infants infected with these organisms usually receive the combination of ampicillin and an aminoglycoside for the first 3 to 5 days followed by ampicillin for the balance of 7 to 10 days. The minimal inhibitory concentration and minimal bactericidal concentration of ampicillin or penicillin against streptococci and of nafcillin or methicillin against *S. aureus* should be determined for the purpose of detecting tolerant strains of these organisms.[162, 265, 272, 303] Tolerant strains are inhibited but not killed by concentrations of these antibiotics that usually can be achieved in body fluids and are treated best by the addition of an aminoglycoside to ampicillin or methicillin. For *S. epidermidis* infections, vancomycin is the drug of choice unless the isolate demonstrates in vitro susceptibility to nafcillin or methicillin; most are resistant to these latter drugs.

Central venous catheters or other foreign bodies frequently must be removed to eliminate the source of these organisms. If a gram-negative enteric isolate is susceptible to both ampicillin and aminoglycosides, treatment with either antibiotic alone can be adequate, but we prefer treatment with both drugs for at least a portion of the treatment period. For *Pseudomonas* infections, combined therapy with ticarcillin, piperacillin, or ceftazidime and an aminoglycoside should be used for the total duration of therapy.

Although the third-generation cephalosporins have attractive features for therapy of sepsis neonatorum, such as excellent in vitro activity against group B streptococci and gram-negative enteric bacilli, provision of high serum and CSF concentrations, and no dose-related toxicity, we do not recommend their routine use in the nursery. Clinical studies suggest that they are comparable with but not superior to ampicillin and gentamicin and that gram-negative enteric bacilli rapidly can become resistant when the third-generation cephalosporins are used for presumptive therapy of neonatal sepsis.

In a 1991 survey of directors of programs in pediatric infectious disease in the United States and Canada, most physicians favored the traditional regimen of ampicillin and gentamicin for initial empiric treatment of sepsis and meningitis.[353] Use of a cephalosporin (cefotaxime in most cases) in combination with ampicillin was considered to be appropriate alternative therapy when meningitis was diagnosed. Antibiotics, such as ceftriaxone and sulfonamides, that have the potential of displacing bilirubin from albumin-binding sites should be avoided in the newborn period.[212] Currently, there is no rationale for routine use of chloramphenicol in newborn infants because of the individual variations in pharmacokinetics in neonates that are associated with increased risk of toxicity and that necessitate monitoring of serum drug concentrations, its bacteriostatic action against most gram-negative enteric pathogens in vitro, antagonism with ampicillin against enteric gram-negative rods and group B streptococci, and the availability of equally potent and safer beta-lactam antibiotics.

The duration of antimicrobial therapy for neonatal sepsis usually is 7 to 10 days or for approximately 5 to 7 days after clinical signs and symptoms of infection have disappeared. Delayed clinical improvement or persistently positive blood cultures during therapy may indicate either that inappropriate antibiotics have been selected or that occult sites of infection exist (e.g., endocarditis, abscesses, infected foreign bodies).

Blood cultures in bacteremic neonates become positive in 96 per cent of infants by 48 hours and in 98 per cent by 72 hours.[248] Thus, in infants whose initial bacterial cultures are sterile after 48 to 72 hours of incubation, antimicrobial therapy can be stopped. If no pathogen has been isolated but bacterial sepsis cannot be excluded, a negative C-reactive protein test at 72 hours can help support the decision to discontinue antibiotics.[311] Because postmortem blood cultures can be negative (in 18 per cent of patients in one study[310]) in infants with unequivocal evidence of sepsis, it is likely that blood cultures from septic infants are sterile in some at the time of initial evaluation.

Careful attention to fluid and electrolyte balance; correction of hypoxia, acidosis, hypoglycemia, and other metabolic abnormalities; and nutritional support all are critical for a good outcome. The use of fresh-frozen plasma and exchange transfusions as adjunctive therapy in severe neonatal sepsis has not been studied adequately, and no recommendations for their use can be made.[340] The infusion of intravenous immunoglobulin with functional activity against group B streptococci to neonates produces a significant increase in group B *Streptococcus*–specific immunoglobulin G that is sustained for several days.[109] The potential therapeutic benefits of intravenous immunoglobulin include enhanced chemotaxis and opsonophagocytosis and improved bactericidal activity of neonatal sera for these organisms. In animal models, a therapeutic effect is achieved only when immunoglobulins are given early in the course of disease.[259]

To date, experience with human immunoglobulin for intravenous use in septic neonates is limited, but such use appears safe. In a recent double-blind, placebo-controlled study, Weisman and associates[346] evaluated the effect of intravenous immunoglobulin (500 mg/kg) in the outcome of 31 premature infants with early-onset sepsis. During the first 7 days after therapy, 5 (30 per cent) of 17 albumin-treated patients and none of 14 patients treated with intravenous immunoglobulin died ($p < .05$). The survival rate at 56 days of age, however, was not improved significantly. It is important to note that very large doses of intravenous immunoglobulin may cause a blockade of neutrophil receptors that are necessary for opsonophagocytosis of group B streptococci. Additional studies are required to demonstrate efficacy, safety, and optimal dosage before immunoglobulin therapy can be recommended confidently.

The efficacy of granulocyte transfusions in reducing mortality from severe neonatal sepsis has been reported by several researchers.[62, 72, 171] Christensen and associates[72] conducted a randomized, prospective, controlled trial of granulocyte transfusions in 16 septic neonates with depleted bone marrow reserves. None of seven infants receiving the transfusions died, whereas only one of nine neonates survived among those not receiving granulocyte transfusions. Cairo and associates[62] evaluated the early administration of granulocyte transfusions to neonates with clinical sepsis. Of 23 infants in their study, only 3 had depleted neutrophil storage pools. These workers also found that survival was improved in neonates with sepsis who received these transfusions compared with control neonates. Only infants with granulocyte-depleted storage pools are likely to benefit from transfusion. Neither clinical severity nor the degree of neutropenia predicted neutrophil storage pool depletion in septic infants; thus, bone marrow aspiration is required for determining the granulocyte storage pool.[27]

Although these studies are encouraging, they involve a small number of patients, and larger, carefully designed studies are needed. Currently, this strategy is used sporadically in a few nurseries around the world. The granulocytes normally are obtained from healthy adult volunteers by leukapheresis and then irradiated for prevention of graft-versus-host disease. Approximately 0.5 to 1 $\times$ 10^9 granulocytes per kilogram of recipient body weight is transfused in 20 to 30 minutes.[340] These transfusions usually are tolerated well by neonates, but potential risks include blood group sensitization, graft-versus-host disease, transmission of cytomegalovirus and hepatitis viruses, and volume overload from hydroxyethyl starch.

Other nonconventional therapeutic approaches that are being evaluated include extracorporeal membrane oxygenation of neonates with early-onset group B streptococcal disease,[148] administration of colony-stimulating factors to neutropenic infants,[62a] and immunomodulating strategies (e.g., anticytokine agents, steroids, pentoxifylline, nitric oxide inhibitors).[276] The precise role, if any, of these approaches for management of newborns with systemic infections will need to be demonstrated in rigorous, carefully designed, double-blinded clinical studies.

Prevention

Studies on prevention of neonatal infections have focused on those caused by group B *Streptococcus* because of its greater prevalence and immunogenicity, compared with other common neonatal pathogens. Methods proposed for the prevention of neonatal group B streptococcal disease are aimed either at decreasing the likelihood of exposure of the infant to group B *Streptococcus* by use of antibiotic chemoprophylaxis or at decreasing the susceptibility of the exposed infant through improved host defenses by passive or active immunoprophylaxis.

The efficacy of antepartum, intrapartum, or postpartum administration of ampicillin or penicillin has been evaluated in numerous studies. It now is established that selective intrapartum chemoprophylaxis can prevent colonization and disease caused by group B streptococci in the first days of life and prevent postpartum maternal infection caused by this organism.

A number of investigators have attempted to eradicate group B streptococcal colonization from pregnant women during the last trimester. In a prospective randomized study of women known to be colonized with group B *Streptococcus*, Hall and associates[139] demonstrated that treatment with ampicillin (500 mg four times daily for 1 week) briefly reduced maternal colonization, but there was no difference in maternal or infant colonization at the time of delivery. Reinfection from the untreated sexual partner or reemergence of group B *Streptococcus* from an undetectably low population of organisms remaining after antibiotic treatment probably explains failure of antepartum chemoprophylaxis. Gardner and associates[116] treated colonized women in the last trimester of pregnancy and their husbands simultaneously with oral penicillin for 12 to 14 days. Before therapy, 63 per cent of husbands also were colonized with group B *Streptococcus* in the genital tract with concordance of isolated serotypes in 88 per cent of colonized couples. Such treatment was found to have no effect on the colonization rate of the maternal genital tract at delivery. Other studies also demonstrated that antibiotic therapy had little effect on carriage of group B *Streptococcus*.

In contrast, Merenstein and associates[202] demonstrated that treatment of colonized pregnant women with 500 mg of penicillin four times daily at 38 weeks' gestation until delivery resulted in a significant reduction in maternal and infant colonization. Such an approach may eliminate colonization in infants delivered after 38 weeks' gestation; however, because 30 per cent of infants with early-onset disease are preterm, the timing of such treatment is inappropriate. Thus, the bulk of evidence indicates that antepartum oral antibiotic prophylaxis generally is unacceptable for prevention of early-onset group B streptococcal disease.

The parenteral administration of antibiotics during labor has been examined in an attempt to overcome the potential shortcomings of antibiotic administration during pregnancy. In the first published study of intrapartum therapy, 34 women with group B streptococcal genital colonization early in the third trimester were treated at term with intravenously administered ampicillin (500 mg every 6 hours until delivery) at hospital admission.[356] This approach interrupted uniformly vertical transmission of the organism to the infants of treated mothers, which would be expected in approximately 50 per cent of infants born to genitally colonized women. Easmon and associates[95] conducted a prospective, controlled trial of 87 colonized parturient patients based on vaginal and anorectal cultures obtained at 36 weeks' gestation. Intrapartum prophylaxis with benzyl penicillin during labor significantly reduced the rate of transmission of group B *Streptococcus* from mothers to their babies from 45 per cent (untreated controls) to 3 per cent ($p < .001$). Additionally, Allerdice and associates[7] identified prospectively 57 women with prenatal colonization with group B *Streptococcus* and treated them intrapartum with ampicillin. Seven per cent of infants born to treated women acquired group B streptococcal colonization, and none had invasive disease; 46 per cent of infants born to untreated women acquired colonization, and 7 per cent had invasive disease.

Intrapartum chemoprophylaxis given to women with proven group B *Streptococcus* colonization reliably prevents colonization of the newborn in the postpartum period. Universal prophylaxis given to all pregnant women with group B *Streptococcus* colonization, however, would result in a large number of pregnant women being treated unnecessarily and clearly is unacceptable. Realizing this limitation, researchers started to investigate the feasibility of selective, rather than universal, intrapartum chemoprophylaxis.

Boyer and Gotoff[53] were the first to document the efficacy of maternal chemoprophylaxis in high-risk parturients for the prevention of neonatal sepsis. Infants born to women with prenatal cultures positive for group B *Streptococcus* and gestation of less than 37 weeks, rupture of amniotic membranes more than 12 hours before delivery, or both were studied. Eighty women were randomized to receive either ampicillin (2 g intravenously and then 1 g every 4 hours until delivery) or no therapy. Infants whose mothers had received ampicillin also were given ampicillin, 50 mg/kg body weight every 12 hours intramuscularly for 4 days. Only 1 (2 per cent) of 43 infants born to treated mothers was colonized, compared with 13 (35 per cent) of 37 born to untreated mothers. Boyer and associates,[52, 53] in a randomized controlled trial of selective intrapartum chemoprophylaxis using the same selection criteria, demonstrated the efficacy of this approach in prevention of neonatal sepsis and postpartum maternal febrile morbidity.[51] None of the 85 infants born to mothers in the treatment group versus 5 (6 per cent) of 79 infants born to mothers in the untreated control group developed group B streptococcal bacteremia ($p = .024$). Additionally, none of the parturient women developed an intrapartum temperature of more than 37.5° C in the ampicillin-treated group versus four in the control group ($p < .01$). The authors estimated that their approach had the potential to eliminate more than 50 per cent of early-onset group B streptococcal disease and 75 per cent of associated deaths in the United States.

A prospective epidemiologic study of early-onset group B *Streptococcus* disease for a 9-year period has provided additional data regarding risk factors for early-onset disease.[52] In this study, the relative risk of early-onset disease was 7.3 for infants whose birth weight was 2500 g or less (compared with those weighing more than 2500 g), 7.2 for infants delivered more than 18 hours after rupture of membranes, and 4.0 for those born to women with intrapartum fever. Overall, 74 per cent of the 61 infants had one of those perinatal risk factors at the time the pregnant women were admitted to the hospital in labor. In Finland, Tupperainen and associates[327] selected patients solely on the basis of healthy intrapartum colonization, using a rapid latex agglutination test. Seven (12 per cent) of 58 babies born to mothers who did not receive penicillin developed early-onset group B streptococcal sepsis, whereas only 1 (3 per cent) of 36 infants whose mothers received penicillin developed infection. That one infant had intrauterine pneumonia thought probably to be caused by group B *Streptococcus*.

Morales and associates[208] selected patients in labor who had positive results on serial coagglutination tests on vaginal secretions performed prenatally. Patients were stratified according to whether their test results were positive after 5 hours' preincubation, which indicated heavy colonization, or after 20 hours' preincubation, which indicated light colonization. None of the infants born to treated, highly colonized mothers were colonized at birth, compared with 35 per cent of the control babies ($p < .001$). No infant in either group developed group B streptococcal invasive disease. Additionally, none of the infants born to treated, heavily colonized mothers were colonized at birth or developed early-onset disease, compared with 80 per cent colonization of the control babies whose mothers were untreated ($p < .001$), and three control infants developed early-onset group B streptococcal disease ($p = .08$). In another study by the same group,[207] only preterm patients who had premature rupture of membranes were studied again with the use of the results of rapid coagglutination test on vaginal secretions obtained at the time of hospital admission. Ampicillin treatment of 36 women resulted in no cases of chorioamnionitis or neonatal sepsis, whereas 23 per cent of untreated mothers developed chorioamnionitis, and 27 per cent of babies developed early-onset group B streptococcal sepsis.

Altogether, these studies establish the efficacy of selective treatment to chemoprophylaxis to prevent early-onset group B streptococcal disease in neonates and of postpartum infections in their mothers. Despite endorsement of this approach by the American Academy of Pediatrics and the American College of Obstetricians and Gynecologists, many physicians involved in the management of mothers and their infants are not aware of or do not follow widely published guidelines to prevent group B streptococcal disease.[154]

Chemoprophylaxis also has been targeted for neonates at birth. The observation in 1978 that infants born at Mount Sinai Hospital in New York who received intramuscular penicillin at birth for the prevention of gonococcal ophthalmia did not develop early-onset group B streptococcal disease prompted two prospective randomized studies using this regimen. Siegel and associates[301, 302] studied both preterm and term infants and demonstrated the efficacy of a single dose of penicillin administered at birth. The population in this study was characterized by group B streptococcal infections mostly in term infants who acquired infection at the time of delivery, as evidenced by the delayed onset of symptoms. Because blood cultures were not obtained before administration of penicillin, it was not known whether some infections were suppressed inadvertently. The other study of chemoprophylaxis at birth was reported by Pyati and associates.[252] They studied only infants weighing 2000 g or less at birth and found no beneficial effect of penicillin administered at birth. These infants were infected in utero, as evidenced by the presence of positive blood cultures at the time of delivery in 21 of 24 infants with group B streptococcal disease. Therefore, infection had been established before the administration of penicillin at delivery. The population in each of these studies had unique characteristics, and therefore the results may not be broadly applicable to all nurseries.

Three special circumstances merit chemoprophylaxis. The first is the asymptomatic twin of an infant with group B streptococcal disease. This twin has an approximately 25-fold increased risk for the development of invasive group B streptococcal disease.[96] Cultures of blood and CSF should be obtained from the twin, and close observation in the hospital with or without treatment is indicated until cultures have been sterile for 72 hours. The second situation is chemoprophylaxis for the pregnant woman who previously has delivered an infant with invasive group B streptococcal disease. Starting at the end of the second trimester, rectal and vaginal cultures are recommended on three occasions at regular intervals for isolation of group B streptococci. If cultures are negative and delivery occurs at term in the absence of maternal risk factors for neonatal infection, prophylaxis can be withheld. If one or more cultures are positive or delivery occurs before 37 weeks of gestation, intrapartum ampicillin should be administered intravenously. The condition of the newborn infant should be assessed; clinical findings and maternal obstetric factors may warrant further laboratory evaluation and antimicrobial therapy. Finally, it seems prudent to initiate chemoprophylaxis in all women colonized with group B *Streptococcus* who have two or more risk factors for invasive infection of the neonate.[21, 119, 253]

Recently, we demonstrated that a single 1-g parenteral injection of ceftriaxone given to high-risk Panamanian pregnant women (i.e., gestations of less than 37 weeks, prolonged rupture of membranes of more than 12 hours, or both) during labor is associated with decreased bacterial colonization and early-onset infection caused by gram-negative enteric bacilli and, possibly, by group B streptococci.[274] Although this prophylactic strategy seems safe and attractive, cost-effective analysis and careful evaluation of potential emergence of ceftriaxone-resistant organisms must be done before recommending it for routine use in selected mothers.

Immunoprophylaxis

Effective immunoprophylaxis would be preferable to chemoprophylaxis, not only because of the limitations of antibiotic prophylaxis but also because an immunologic approach is more likely to prevent late-onset as well as early-onset group B streptococcal disease in neonates and postpartum febrile morbidity in the pregnant woman. The underlying principle is that IgG antibody directed against the type-specific polysaccharide antigen critical to protection against invasive group B streptococcal disease would be provided by passive or active immunization. Group B *Streptococcus* type-specific polysaccharide vaccines have been developed and were found to be associated with low rates of side effects.[23] However, the immune response was unsatisfactory in up to 40 per cent of nonimmune pregnant women who received type III polysaccharide vaccine. These nonresponders did not develop specific antibody, even after repeated vaccine challenges.[23] It is possible that response to vaccine is determined genetically and that some of the women in whom antibodies do not respond to vaginal colonization by group B streptococci may be the same women in whom the vaccine will fail. Thus, pregnant women with the highest risk may not benefit from vaccination. It is likely that a second-generation vaccine consisting of polysaccharide antigen conjugated to a protein carrier will be immunogenic, as observed with *H. influenzae* vaccines in young infants. Maternal immunization, however, no matter how successful, does not prevent disease in neonates who are born so prematurely (<32 weeks) that sufficient amounts of antibody would not have passed transplacentally. Administration of hyperimmunoglobulin to newborns, provided they are not already seriously ill at birth, might help these particular infants.

Prevention of late-onset infection, compared with early-onset disease, in neonates by the administration of intravenous immunoglobulin to preterm babies recently has undergone intense clinical scrutiny.[16, 25, 103, 344] Premature babies, particularly those born before 32 weeks' gestation, are relatively hypogammaglobulinemic at birth and become more so during the first several weeks of life. Because these same infants are at high risk of infection beyond the first week of life (late-onset), intravenous immunoglobulin infusions might provide opsonizing antibody to prevent late-onset infections. Three of the five early clinical trials that examined the efficacy of intravenous immunoglobulin administration in preventing infection in neonates demonstrated significant favorable responses.[69, 75, 137, 312] Problems with these studies included a small sample size, definition of infection, and the lack of a blind design.

A recent well-controlled multicenter study demonstrated efficacy of intravenous immunoglobulin infusions in reducing late-onset infection rates.[16] Study infants received either intravenous immunoglobulin, 500 mg/kg, or placebo at 3 to 7 days of age, 1 week later, and every 2 weeks for a total of five infusions or until hospital discharge. Infusions were tolerated well. Although there were no significant differences in mortality or reduction of infections in infants weighing more than 1500 g, bacterial infections were reduced significantly in infants weighing less than 1500 g at birth, and the duration of hospitalization was significantly shorter among intravenous immunoglobulin recipients. Most infections were bacterial in origin, and approximately 70 per cent of these were caused by gram-positive organisms, primarily staphylococci. In contrast with the beneficial effect found in this study, two recent, larger, multicenter, well-designed trials showed no significant differences in the rate of nosocomial infection or in the mortality rate between control and treated groups.[103, 344] Thus, at this time intravenous immunoglobulin cannot be recommended as routine prophylaxis for low birth weight infants. Investigations now are directed at evaluating the usefulness of pathogen-specific hyperimmunoglobulin for the prevention and treatment of sepsis caused by the most common etiologic agents.[345]

PURULENT MENINGITIS

Up to one-fourth of neonates with bacterial sepsis have a simultaneous meningeal infection. The incidence of neonatal meningitis varies greatly among institutions in North America. Rates are approximately 0.2 to 0.4 cases per 1000 live births but may be as high as 1 case per 1000 live births in some nurseries. In general, group B beta-hemolytic streptococci and *E. coli* strains account for two-thirds of all cases of neonatal meningitis in North America. Gram-negative enteric bacilli predominate in many developing areas of the world.

Information about the bacteria isolated from CSF cultures of 257 neonates with meningitis treated at Children's Medical Center or Parkland Memorial Hospital in Dallas from 1969 to 1989 is presented in Table 77–4. One hundred twenty-one (49 per cent) of these 249 infants had disease caused by group B streptococci. An additional 46 infants (18 per cent) had meningitis caused by *E. coli* strains. *L. monocytogenes* added an additional 7 per cent of cases. These three agents accounted for 74 per cent of cases seen during the 20-year period. *E. coli* and *Klebsiella-Enterobacter* strains accounted for 68 per cent of gram-negative organisms causing meningitis. For an etiologic comparison, the distribution of meningeal pathogens in a developing setting[209] also is displayed in the same table.

Pathology

The pathologic findings are similar, regardless of bacterial etiology. Studies of the fulminant, early-onset form of group B streptococcal disease have shown primarily a bronchopneumonia with or without hyaline membranes and usually no histologic evidence of meningeal involvement. The most consistent finding at necropsy of meningitis cases is a purulent exudate of the meninges and ependymal surfaces of the ventricles.[44] The inflammatory response of neonates is similar to that observed in adults with meningitis, with the exception that babies have a scarcity of plasma cells and lymphocytes during the subacute stage of meningeal reactions. Perivascular inflammation also is noted. Hydrocephalus and a noninfectious encephalopathy can be demonstrated in approximately 50 per cent of infants dying of meningitis.

Subdural effusions occur rarely in neonates. In contrast, effusions are observed commonly (i.e., by computed tomography or magnetic resonance imaging) in infants with meningitis who are 3 to 12 months of age. Varying degrees of phlebitis and arteritis of intracranial vessels can be found in all infants. Thrombophlebitis with occlusions of veins may occur in the subependymal zone. K1 antigen has been demonstrated in brain tissue of infants succumbing to *E. coli* K1 infection.[282] High concentrations of interleukin-1β have been detected in brain and meningeal tissues of infants succumbing to meningitis.[27]

TABLE 77–4. Etiologic Agents of Neonatal Meningitis in a Developed and in a Developing Nursery

Organisms	Isolation Rate (%) in Dallas (U.S.) (1969–1989) n = 257	Isolation Rate (%) in Panama (Panama) (1975–1992) n = 105
Gram-negative bacteria	88 (35%)	68 (64%)
Escherichia coli	19%	16%
Klebsiella species	8%	25%
Other gram-negative rods	4%	16%
Pseudomonas aeruginosa	2%	5%
Haemophilus influenzae	1%	1%
Neisseria meningitidis	1%	1%
Gram-positive bacteria	169 (65%)	37 (36%)
Group B *Streptococcus*	53%	5%
Coagulase-negative *Staphylococcus*	<1%	18%
S. aureus	2%	10%
Listeria monocytogenes	7%	1%
Enterococci	2%	1%
S. pneumoniae	1%	<1%

Clinical Manifestations

The early signs and symptoms of neonatal meningitis frequently are indistinguishable from those of septicemia and other disorders occurring in the neonatal period. The most frequent signs are temperature instability, respiratory distress, irritability, lethargy, and poor feeding or vomiting. Group B *Streptococcus* occasionally has been reported to present as hydrocephalus without other signs of infection. Signs suggestive of meningeal involvement, such as stiff neck, bulging fontanelle, convulsions, and opisthotonus, are the exception in neonates with meningitis. The frequency of these findings as culled from the literature is 17 per cent for bulging fontanelle, 33 per cent for opisthotonos, 23 per cent for stiff neck, and 12 per cent for convulsions.[44, 198, 234] The sensitivity of these findings to distinguish infection of the pia-arachnoid is poor. Therefore, all newborns being evaluated for sepsis should undergo examination of the CSF, especially if antimicrobial therapy is to be instituted.

Diagnosis

Interpretation of CSF values in newborn infants may be difficult. During the first several days of life, the mean white blood cell count is 15 ± 30 (95 per cent limit, 12 to 18 cells/mm^3) in the spinal fluid of healthy or high-risk uninfected babies.[233, 283] Approximately 60 per cent of these cells are polymorphonuclear leukocytes. During the first week of life, the cell count slowly diminishes in term infants and increases in premature infants. Cell counts in the range of 0 to 10 cells/mm^3 (median, 4 cells/mm^3) are observed at approximately 2 to 4 weeks of age. The white blood cell count is uncertain when bleeding occurs after the lumbar puncture. The fixed relationship between the number of white blood cells in CSF and peripheral blood has been disputed. A repeat lumbar puncture in 12 to 24 hours may be necessary to resolve the ambiguity of the traumatic lumbar puncture.

The mean cerebrospinal protein concentration in the first month of life is 64 ± 24, although individual values can be as great as 170 mg/dL, especially in low birth weight, premature infants. The percentage ratio of cerebrospinal glucose to blood glucose is 60 to 70 per cent and can be greater than 100 per cent in term and preterm infants.[283] The upper normal limits of cellular and chemistry values are higher in very low birth weight, uninfected infants.[49]

It is apparent from these data that CSF values must be interpreted in relation to these normal findings if an early diagnosis of neonatal meningitis is to be made. When the results of initial CSF evaluations obtained from newborns with proven bacterial meningitis were compared with those from normal or high-risk infants, there was considerable overlap in the findings.[283] For example, approximately 30 per cent of infants with group B streptococcal meningitis had normal spinal fluid leukocyte counts (<32 cells/mm^3), whereas only 4 per cent of neonates with meningitis caused by gram-negative organisms had normal counts. The ratio of CSF to blood glucose was normal in 45 per cent and 15 per cent of patients with streptococcal and coliform meningitis, respectively. However, when the total CSF evaluation (including Gram-stained smears) was considered, less than 1 per cent of babies with bacteriologically proven meningitis had a totally normal CSF on initial lumbar tap. Thus, the likelihood of suppurative meningitis is diminished greatly but not impossible if the evaluation of CSF discloses no abnormalities. In some patients in whom the diagnosis is obscured, a repeat CSF examination 4 to 6 hours after the initial tap (whether or not therapy has been instituted in the interim) may help to establish the diagnosis. In premature infants with meningitis caused by *S. epidermidis*, the CSF analysis can be only mildly abnormal, despite compatible clinical findings.[135]

It is important to examine carefully the stained smears of CSF from every infant with suspected meningitis. Grossly clear fluid may contain few white blood cells and many bacteria. The stained smears from approximately 20 per cent of neonates with proven meningitis are interpreted as showing no bacteria. Because of the low concentrations of organisms, most Gram-stained smears of CSF from infants with *L. monocytogenes* meningitis do not reveal bacteria. The CSF findings in the infant with a brain abscess may have a pleocytosis of up to a few hundred cells with a predominance of mononuclear cells and with an elevated protein concentration. Bacteria may not be seen in a Gram-stained smear of CSF if meningitis is not present. Ventriculitis is diagnosed on the basis of elevated white blood cell count (>100 cells/mm^3), identification of organism by culture, Gram-stained smear antigen detection, increased intraventricular pressure, and dilated ventricles. A cranial computed tomogram with contrast material may show enhancement of the lining tissue of the ventricles.

Several new techniques to diagnose rapidly bacterial meningitis have been described. The first, counterimmunoelectrophoresis, is used to detect bacterial capsular antigens in CSF and other body fluids. Depending on the source of antisera used in this method, meningitis can be diagnosed with counterimmunoelectrophoresis in almost all patients with *H. influenzae* type b and meningococcal groups B and C meningitis if spinal fluid, serum, and urine are tested.[104] Approximately 70 per cent of infants with *E. coli* K1 meningitis have detectable K1 antigen in CSF, serum, or both.[186] Group B_{III} streptococcal antigen has been detected in CSF, serum, and urine of about 90 per cent of infected infants.[24] Quantitation of antigen is helpful in the prognosis of infants with *E. coli* K1 and type III group B streptococcal meningitis.[24, 196]

Latex particle agglutination and staphylococcal coagglutination tests have been developed for detection of bacterial antigens in body fluid. The latex particle agglutination method has been found useful in detecting antigen in the CSF of older infants and children with meningitis caused by *H. influenzae* type b; *N. meningitidis* groups A, B, and C; and *S. pneumoniae*.[223, 348] This method is more sensitive than counterimmunoelectrophoresis for measuring capsular antigen of *H. influenzae*.[338] The staphylococcal coagglutination test has not been used extensively in pediatric patients. The polyribose phosphate antigen of *H. influenzae* has been detected in body fluids by this method.[318] Both of these methods can be used for the detection of group B streptococcal infection, as mentioned previously.

The *Limulus* lysate test detects the presence of endotoxin, a soluble lipopolysaccharide constituent of the cell wall of gram-negative bacteria.[176] Endotoxin can be measured in the CSF of patients with meningitis caused by coliform bacteria, *H. influenzae*, and *N. meningitidis*.[192] Endotoxin has been detected in initial CSF specimens obtained from infants with meningitis caused by *E. coli* and other coliforms. Both counterimmunoelectrophoresis and the *Limulus* lysate techniques require approximately 1 hour to run and can be established in most hospital laboratories. If both methods are used, approximately 80 per cent of neonates with coliform meningitis can be identified as having disease within an hour of the initial lumbar tap. However, these results are no better than those from a carefully prepared and examined stained smear of CSF, in which bacteria can be identified in approximately 80 per cent of patients with documented bacterial meningitis.[283]

Treatment

Selection of appropriate antibiotic therapy for meningitis is based in part on achievable CSF concentrations of these drugs in relation to the susceptibility of the pathogens causing disease. The highest concentrations of penicillin or ampicillin in CSF are at least 10 to 100 times greater than the susceptibilities (minimal inhibitory concentrations) of group B streptococci and *L. monocytogenes*. As a result, sufficient activity remains in CSF for at least 40 to 60 per cent of the dosing interval, and most infants with meningitis caused by these two organisms respond promptly to ampicillin or penicillin therapy. CSF cultures usually are sterile within 24 to 36 hours of initiation of therapy. In contrast, the concentrations of the aminoglycosides (kanamycin, gentamicin, tobramycin, and amikacin) in CSF usually are equal to or several times greater than the minimal inhibitory concentrations for coliform organisms and *P. aeruginosa*. Because killing of bacteria by the aminoglycosides is concentration-dependent, requiring drug concentrations in the CSF at least four- to eightfold the minimal bactericidal concentration, cultures of CSF from infants with meningitis caused by these organisms often remain positive for 2 or 3 days or longer. It is important to document bacteriologic cure in patients with meningitis because outcome is correlated with the time necessary to eradicate the bacterial pathogen.

Ampicillin and gentamicin or cefotaxime are recommended for initial empiric therapy of neonatal meningitis (for dosages, see Table 77–1). All infants should undergo repeat CSF examination and culture at 24 to 36 hours after initiation of therapy. If organisms are observed on methylene blue or Gram-stained smears of fluid, modification of the therapeutic regimen should be considered. For many years, physicians have attempted to increase antibiotic concentrations in CSF by instilling drugs directly into the lumbar intrathecal space. The first Neonatal Meningitis Cooperative Study evaluated 117 prospectively enrolled, randomly treated infants to determine the role of intrathecal gentamicin therapy in the management of neonatal meningitis caused by coliform bacilli.[192] There were no statistically significant differences in mortality, long-term morbidity, or days that CSF cultures remained positive among infants who received lumbar intrathecal gentamicin plus systemic therapy and those who were treated with systemic drugs only.

Data from the Neonatal Meningitis Cooperative Study and from adult neurosurgical patients with meningitis demonstrated that lumbar CSF concentrations of aminoglycosidic drugs administered locally usually exceed the minimal inhibitory concentration values for coliform organisms by 10 to 50 times.[192, 255] However, lumbar instillation does not result consistently in diffusion of these drugs to the level of the cisterna or into ventricular fluid. In contrast, instillation of aminoglycosides into unobstructed ventricles results in rapid and uniform distribution of drug throughout the CSF space.

Data obtained from the second Neonatal Meningitis Cooperative Study demonstrated ventricular fluid gentamicin concentrations of 10 to 130 μg/mL at 1 to 6 hours after a 2.5-mg intraventricular dose and from 1 to 24 μg/mL 16 to 24 hours later.[191, 193] The concentrations in lumbar CSF at comparable intervals after intraventricular administration were 8 to 85 μg/mL and 1.8 to 4.2 μg/mL, respectively. However, results of the intraventricular regimen were inferior to those obtained with systemic therapy alone. The mortality rate was significantly higher in infants who had meningitis and ventriculitis and who received intraventricular gentamicin and systemic antibiotics (43 per cent) than in those who were given systemic therapy only (12.5 per cent). The duration of positive CSF cultures was 1 day shorter in those receiving intraventricular therapy. Using serial CSF samples from patients enrolled in this study, we demonstrated some years later that intraventricular gentamicin therapy, which resulted in higher gentamicin CSF concentrations, was associated with higher ventricular CSF endotoxin and interleukin 1-β concentrations and greater central nervous system inflammation (higher CSF leukocyte count, higher protein concentration, and lower glucose concentration), most likely as a result of lysis of organisms.[213] This possibly could explain the poor outcome in those patients compared with that in infants who received parenteral antibiotic therapy only.[213]

On the basis of the findings from the second Neonatal Meningitis Cooperative Study, intraventricular therapy cannot be recommended for the routine management of neonatal meningitis caused by gram-negative enteric bacilli. A controlled study[199] found that ampicillin and moxalactam therapy (a broad-spectrum cephalosporin no longer available) in neonatal coliform meningitis was as effective as a conventional regimen of ampicillin and amikacin. In that study, moxalactam achieved greater CSF and ventricular fluid concentrations, and the bactericidal titers were considerably greater than those achieved with conventional therapy, but this did not translate into more rapid sterilization of the CSF, lower case-fatality rates, or improved neurologic outcome for survivors. Although no large controlled trials have evaluated the use of cefotaxime, clinical experience indicates that it can be used safely and effectively for the treatment of gram-negative meningitis in neonates. CSF examination and culture should be repeated 48 to 72 hours after initiation of therapy. If the results still are positive, computed axial tomography should be performed to rule out the possibility of subdural empyema, brain abscess, or ventriculitis. In all cases caused by *Citrobacter diversus*, cranial computed tomograms should be obtained early because of the frequent association with brain abscess. The duration of antibiotic therapy should be extended, depending on clinical evolution and resolution of the lesion based on repeated tomography. A neurosurgeon should be consulted early for needle aspiration or excision of the abscess. Aminoglycosides probably should not be used because of decreased activity in abscess cavities that have a low pH and anaerobic conditions.

Third-generation cephalosporins possess attractive features for therapy of bacterial meningitis in newborn infants, which include lower minimal inhibitory concentrations for gram-negative enteric bacilli than for aminoglycosides, good penetration into CSF in the presence of inflamed meninges, and a wide therapeutic index. These agents are active against most streptococci but inactive against *L. monocytogenes* and enterococci. Only ceftazidime provides adequate activity against *P. aeruginosa*. Among these agents, cefotaxime is preferred for therapy of neonatal meningitis because of the extensive experience with this drug in the neonatal period and because it does not alter substantially the bowel flora. Cefotaxime can be used singly or in combination with an aminoglycoside. Ceftazidime has been shown to be effective in treating patients with *P. aeruginosa* meningitis. Because of high biliary excretion and marked alteration of the normal intestinal flora and because of potential concern for displacement of bilirubin, we do not recommend routine use of ceftriaxone during the neonatal period.

For premature infants hospitalized in the nursery for prolonged periods, staphylococci, enterococci, and gentamicin-resistant gram-negative organisms are potential pathogens; an alternative antimicrobial regimen should be considered for initial empiric treatment. A combination of methicillin or oxacillin and amikacin or ceftazidime or cefotaxime could be used as initial empiric therapy. When MRSA or *S. epidermidis* is a potential cause of infection, vancomycin and amikacin or cefotaxime can be used initially.

Once the pathogen has been identified and susceptibility studies are available, the single drug or combination of drugs that is most effective should be used. In general, penicillin G or ampicillin is preferred for group B streptococcal meningitis, ampicillin for *L. monocytogenes* and enterococci, ampicillin plus an aminoglycoside or cefotaxime for coliforms, and ceftazidime or ticarcillin and an aminoglycoside for *Pseudomonas* infections. The duration of systemic therapy in neonatal meningitis depends on the causative agent and the time necessary to sterilize CSF cultures. As a rule, therapy is given for approximately 2 weeks after bacteriologic cure. For meningitis caused by group B streptococci or *Listeria*, approximately 2 weeks of therapy usually is satisfactory. Because delayed sterilization is common in infants with gram-negative enteric disease, systemic therapy is given for a minimum of 3 weeks and in some babies for many additional weeks. Final judgment as to when to stop therapy must be based on the clinical course of illness and on CSF findings at the time this decision is to be made.

Despite the beneficial effects of dexamethasone found in several recent studies for the treatment of infants and children with bacterial meningitis,[277, 286] no data are available for its use in newborns; thus, utilization of steroids in neonatal meningitis cannot be recommended at present.

Prognosis

The acute complications of bacterial meningitis include communicating and noncommunicating hydrocephalus, subdural effusions (approximately 1 per cent of patients), deafness, and blindness. Ventriculitis occurs in approximately 70 per cent of neonates with coliform meningitis and usually is present at the time of initial diagnosis. Brain abscess is an infrequent complication except in infants with *C. diversus* meningitis, in whom it develops about 70 per cent of the time.[128, 192, 193, 199] Although gross retardation and neurologic deficits may be obvious in some infants at discharge, most babies appear "well" at this time. It is only after prolonged and careful follow-up that perceptual difficulties, behavioral problems, and other subtle neurologic signs become apparent. Within 4 to 6 weeks of recovering from meningitis, hearing should be evaluated by evoked response audiometry.

The case-fatality rates in neonates with meningitis range from 15 to more than 30 per cent.[198, 234] A mortality rate of 30 per cent was observed in 117 neonates with coliform meningitis enrolled in the first Neonatal Meningitis Cooperative Study.[192] In this project, term infants had a significantly lower rate (18 per cent) than that observed in low birth weight (<2500 g) babies (45 per cent) and in infants older than 30 days of age (48 per cent). Poor outcome after gram-negative enteric meningitis is correlated directly with the presence of ventriculitis, the persistence of positive CSF cultures, the presence and persistence of elevated endotoxin and interleukin-1β concentrations in CSF, CSF cell count of more than 10,000/mm^3, and a CSF protein concentration of more than 500 mg/dL. When meningitis is caused by *E. coli* K1, poor outcome is associated with persistence of large quantities of K1 capsular polysaccharide antigen in CSF.[194, 196]

In a 20-year period, the mortality rate of neonatal meningitis at Parkland Memorial Hospital and Children's Medical Center in Dallas did not changed appreciably. Approximately 15 per cent of infants died during the 4-year periods of 1956 to 1959, 1969 to 1972, and 1973 to 1976. During the 8 years from 1969 to 1976, 17 (14 per cent) of 123 neonates with bacterial meningitis died, and this did not change appreciably through 1984.[191] The first 24 hours of management are critical; the case-fatality rate for infants who survive the first 24 hours of therapy is approximately 5 per cent.

Long-term follow-up studies of babies with coliform meningitis enrolled in the Neonatal Meningitis Cooperative Study have revealed that approximately 65 per cent of survivors were normal at 3 to 7 years after illness. An additional 30 per cent were classified as having mild to moderate neurologic sequelae. Many of these latter patients had only slightly abnormal neurologic or psychologic evaluations and were considered normal on routine physical examination. Approximately 5 to 10 per cent of survivors had severe neurologic or mental impairment requiring custodial care. Approximately 15 to 20 per cent of survivors of group B streptococcal meningitis have major sequelae, including spastic quadriplegia, profound mental retardation, hemiparesis, deafness, and blindness.[72] Hydrocephalus develops in 11 per cent, and 13 per cent have a seizure disorder. The survivors without major sequelae on physical examination, however, appear to function within normal limits and comparably with their siblings.

Edwards and associates[97] reported a 21 per cent morbidity rate after group B streptococcal meningitis. Of the survivors, 29 per cent had severe neurologic sequelae, 21 per cent had minor deficits, and 50 per cent were functioning normally. Factors associated with death or severe disability at presentation included coma, decreased perfusion, CSF protein greater than 300 mg/dL, an absolute neutrophil count less than 1000, and a total leukocyte count less than 5000/mm^3. Recently, our experience with gram-negative enteric bacillary meningitis in newborns managed from 1969 through 1989 in Dallas was published.[329] In 98 identified neonates, the case-fatality rate was 17 per cent, and 61 per cent of survivors had long-term sequelae that included seizure disorders, hydrocephalus, physical disability, developmental delay, and hearing loss.

OTITIS MEDIA

Otitis media (see also Chapter 19) is diagnosed infrequently in neonates because of the paucity of clinical findings and the difficulty in examining the infant's tympanic membrane. The external canal is narrow and tortuous and often is filled with debris. Because the healthy baby's membrane may appear thickened and dull, mobility of the drum determined by pneumatoscopy should be used as the single most reliable indicator of middle ear abnormalities. The examiner must beware of mistaking the movement of the distal interior canal wall for movement of the tympanic membrane. Movement of the normal membrane is seen best in the posterior portion. A reddish or reddish-orange color of the tympanic membrane usually indicates infection, provided that the infant is not crying.

The exact incidence of disease is unknown, but a recent prospective study found that 34 per cent of 70 infants followed from birth developed their first episode of otitis media before 2 months of age.[187] Otitis media is more common in premature than in term infants and occurs almost exclusively in bottle-fed babies. It is a frequent finding in neonates receiving intensive care, especially those with prolonged nasotracheal intubation.[45] Warren and Stool[339] examined the ears of 127 infants with birth weights of less than 2300 g thrice weekly until discharge from the nursery and found that only 3 (2 per cent) developed otitis media. In contrast, in a study of 125 premature infants in a neonatal intensive care unit, Berman and associates[45] found that 38 infants (30 per cent) had middle ear fluid compatible with the diagnosis of otitis media; this was confirmed by tympanocentesis in 13 patients in whom the procedure was done. Development of otitis media was correlated significantly with nasotracheal intubation for longer than 7 days.

Meconium staining of amniotic fluid and prolonged rupture of membranes are two other risk factors for subsequent development of middle ear disease.[243] Neonates with cleft palate, Down syndrome, or maxillofacial anomalies are at high risk for chronic middle ear disease. Onset of illness is insidious, and the most common manifestations are rhinorrhea, irritability, and failure to thrive. Fever greater than 38° C is rare. The presence of lethargy, hypotonia, hypothermia, high fever, or jaundice suggests septic complications, such as bacteremia or meningitis.

The cause of neonatal otitis media is similar to that observed in older infants and children. *S. pneumoniae, H. influenzae,* and *Moraxella catarrhalis* account for more than 50 per cent of cases.[47, 298, 321] The important difference from disease in older patients is that 10 to 15 per cent of neonates have disease caused by coliforms, group B streptococci, or *S. aureus.* Pathogens isolated from middle ear fluid of 169 infants 6 weeks of age or younger were *S. pneumoniae* in 18 per cent of cases, *H. influenzae* in 12 per cent, *S. aureus* in 8 per cent, *E. coli* in 6 per cent, *Klebsiella-Enterobacter* species in 5 per cent, *M. catarrhalis* in 5 per cent, group A or B streptococci in 3 per cent, and *P. aeruginosa* in 2 per cent; no pathogen was isolated in 32 per cent.[48] We occasionally have encountered neonates with otitis media associated with septicemia and either pneumonia or meningitis. Group B streptococci or coliform organisms were the causative agents in these cases.

The importance of establishing the diagnosis and cause of otitis media in neonates and of employing appropriate therapy cannot be overemphasized. When the otologic examination demonstrates middle ear disease, the infant should be examined carefully for other sites of infection. If none is found, which is the usual case, the infant can be treated on an outpatient basis. Because a small percentage of these cases are caused by coliform bacilli or *S. aureus,* drugs that include those organisms in their spectrum (a second-generation cephalosporin or amoxicillin-clavulanate) are preferable to the aminopenicillins. The patient's condition should be reevaluated 8 to 72 hours after initiation of therapy to determine whether clinical improvement has occurred and that middle ear infection is resolving. In patients demonstrating no improvement, tympanocentesis should be performed for examination of stained smears of middle ear fluid and for culture of the contents. Alteration of therapy should be based on the findings of these examinations. If gram-negative organisms or staphylococci are observed, the infant probably is managed best in the hospital by means of parenteral therapy, with an aminoglycoside if coliforms are suspected or with an antistaphylococcal penicillin for *S. aureus.* If organisms are not observed in infants with unresolving disease, methicillin and gentamicin or cefuroxime can be used until results of cultures and susceptibility studies are available. A CSF examination should be performed before initiation of parenteral therapy.

All infants with otitis media should be followed carefully for many months after illness. Misdiagnosis or improper therapy may result in chronic middle ear disease and, occasionally, extension of infection to adjacent structures, such as the mastoid or central nervous system. Infants who develop their first episode of otitis media before 2 months of age may require 3 to 4 months to clear the effusions, and a third of them are said to develop recurrent or chronic otitis media.[187]

DIARRHEAL DISEASE

Although diarrheal disease during the neonatal period usually is brief and self-limited, it may cause significant morbidity in some infants and represents a potential danger to other infants in the nursery. The advent of modern sterilization practices and increased emphasis on hospital infection control measures have reduced significantly the incidence of nosocomial diarrheal disease.

A number of factors contribute to an increased susceptibility of neonate enteric infections, including underdevelopment of local and systemic immune responses; lack of a fully developed aerobic and anaerobic enteric flora, which protects the gastrointestinal tract of older infants and children; a less effective gastric bactericidal barrier; less intestinal mucus; and less motility.[229] The infant may have been fed powdered formula that could have been mixed with contaminated water, or the critically ill newborn may have received a broad-spectrum antibiotic in intensive care, in which case highly resistant nosocomial flora pose a special risk.

The importance of breast feeding in prevention of diarrheal diseases in infants cannot be overemphasized. The protective effects of breast feeding have been confirmed in surveys of sporadic gastroenteritis, in community epidemics, and in outbreaks in newborn nurseries. Antibacterial and antiviral factors in breast milk have been documented well, including lactoferrin, lysozyme, phagocytes, specific secretory immunoglobulins, and lymphocytes sensitive to such organisms as *E. coli, Salmonella, Shigella, Clostridium difficile* toxin A and B, and rotavirus.[131, 229] Breast-fed infants are less susceptible to diarrheal diseases than are bottle-fed infants.[136, 229]

Etiology and Pathogenesis

The most common cause of diarrhea in young infants is alteration of diet and feeding practices rather than specific bacterial or viral pathogens. Diarrhea can be a nonspecific symptom of sepsis or urinary tract infection in the newborn infant. Of the infectious causes, rotaviruses are important causative agents in infantile diarrheal disease.[204, 271] They have been associated with nursery outbreaks of gastroenteritis and necrotizing enterocolitis.[74, 266] Studies from France have shown that about one-third of all neonates shed rotavirus in their stools; of these infants, only 29 per cent have associated diarrhea.[68]

The transplacental transfer of rotaviral group-specific or type-specific maternal antibodies to neonates appears to have little effect on the incidence of infection or illness by the rotaviruses.[89, 90] The essential pathogenic feature of rotavirus infection is destruction of the absorptive cells lining the duodenum, the jejunum, and possibly the ileum.[203] It has been suggested that lactase, which is present only in the brush borders of the differentiated epithelial cells at these sites, acts as a combined receptor and uncoating enzyme for the virus. This may explain why rotavirus infection is less common in infants of less than 32 weeks' gestation than in more mature infants.[63] Between 26 and 34 weeks of gestational age, lactase activity is approximately 30 per cent of that found in full-term infants.[173]

Enteropathogenic *E. coli* serotypes once were considered the most common bacterial agents responsible for diarrhea in young infants. Failure to demonstrate on rectal cultures specific serotypes of *E. coli* designated as enteropathogenic does not rule out coliform disease. Enterotoxigenic strains of *E. coli* possessing nonenteropathogenic serotypes have been identified in nursery outbreaks of diarrheal disease.[55, 231] These organisms inhabit the small bowel, where they attach to but do not invade the intestinal mucosa. The enterotoxin produced by these organisms stimulates cyclic adenosine monophosphate, which, in turn, inhibits sodium and chloride transport across the intestinal wall. As a result, these salts are lost into the lumen of the upper bowel, followed passively by water, which causes a net loss of stools containing high concentrations of electrolytes. *Vibrio cholerae,* some *E. coli* serotypes (almost exclusively nonenteropathogenic strains), *Vibrio parahaemolyticus, Aeromonas,* and possibly some *Campylobacter* and *Yersinia* strains are examples of bacteria that cause diarrhea by this mechanism.

The importance of recognizing this form of diarrheal disease was emphasized in a nursery outbreak in the southwestern United States. Severe, watery diarrhea was observed in 59 infants during a 9-month period; in the 7 per cent of infants who died, death was secondary to altered hepatic function and a hemorrhagic diathesis.[55] An O142/K86/H6 *E. coli* strain was responsible for the outbreak. Because this organism is not a classic enteropathogenic serotype, it was not identified as a pathogen, which thereby delayed definitive diagnosis and institution of proper infection control techniques. It was only by special laboratory techniques that this *E. coli* strain was shown to produce labile enterotoxin.

A second mechanism for bacterial diarrhea involves invasion of the intestinal mucosa. *Shigella* dysentery is the classic example of this disease. Colonic invasion with subsequent destruction of the mucosa causes an outpouring of polymorphonuclear cells and mucus. The resultant diarrhea usually is bloody and contains mucus and pus. *Salmonella* species also invade the intestinal mucosa, but destruction is not extensive. The epithelial lining is left intact, and the organisms reach the lamina propria, where an inflammatory response is elicited.[319] *Campylobacter, Yersinia,* and *Aeromonas* species and *C. difficile* also can cause bloody diarrhea.

Although serotyping of *E. coli* to identify the traditional enteropathogenic strains no longer is available routinely, the epidemiologic evidence is strong enough to support a pathogenic role for these strains, even though the mechanism of pathogenicity is unknown. When an index case of diarrhea caused by enteropathogenic *E. coli* or other pathogens is recognized in a nursery, secondary cases are likely. In any nursery infant with diarrhea, a potentially communicable disease should be suspected. With all infants in proximity to the index case, rectal swabs should be tested by culture or by fluorescent antibody technique, which is more sensitive for identifying asymptomatic carriers of enteropathogenic *E. coli.* Ill and healthy colonized infants should be segregated and treated with orally administered neomycin (100 mg/kg/day in three or four divided doses) or with colistin sulfate (15 mg/kg/day in three or four divided doses) for 5 days. Neomycin causes rapid disappearance of the organism and abbreviates the period of diarrhea, but approximately 20 per cent of infants revert to an asymptomatic carrier state.[217] Repeated surveillance of infants is necessary until it has been shown that the pathogenic strain has been eliminated from the nursery.

Campylobacter, a curved gram-negative bacterium, has been recognized increasingly as a common cause of enteritis. Of the 14 known species, *Campylobacter fetus* and *Campylobacter jejuni* cause human disease most frequently. *C. fetus* causes prenatal and neonatal infections that result in abortion, premature delivery, bacteremia, and meningitis. Infections caused by *C. fetus* appear to be the most common type of *Campylobacter* infection in the first 3 weeks of life and are associated with a high incidence of fetal and neonatal morbidity.[136] In contrast, the most common syndrome produced by a *Campylobacter* species is enteritis caused by *C. jejuni*. Unlike the serious neonatal disease caused by *C. fetus*, infections with *C. jejuni* usually result in mild gastroenteritis, although meningitis occurs rarely. Nursery outbreaks of gastroenteritis caused by *C. jejuni* have been documented well.[136]

Although it is likely that some diarrheal episodes in neonates can be caused by *C. difficile*, the diagnostic criteria used in older children and adults are inadequate to establish a definitive diagnosis in this age group. *C. difficile* is a gram-positive anaerobic bacillus that produces an enterotoxin (toxin A) that causes fluid secretion and a cytotoxin that damages cells (toxin B).[60, 178] *C. difficile* colonic overgrowth and toxin production can result from the selective pressure of antibiotic therapy. A wide variety of antibiotic, antifungal, and antituberculous agents have been associated with *C. difficile* colitis.[136] Although healthy children older than 1 year of age and healthy adults rarely carry the organisms, as many as two-thirds of neonates can be demonstrated to have both *C. difficile* and its cytotoxins in their stools.[136] This high frequency of colonization and the presence of cytotoxin have led to skepticism about the pathogenic potential of this organism in the neonate.

Clinical Manifestations

Although the etiology of diarrhea in infants and children may be suspected on clinical grounds, this usually is not possible in newborn infants. As a general rule, diarrhea caused by enteropathogenic strains of *E. coli* is insidious in onset, is associated with 7 to 10 green, watery stools daily, and usually is without blood or mucus. The infants do not appear to be acutely ill. Complications are rare and primarily are related to dehydration and electrolyte disturbances. *Shigella* infection is uncommon, usually is episodic in neonates, and usually does not spread within nurseries.[141] Shigellosis in the newborn may occur as a diarrheic or dysenteric syndrome or may be evidenced only by a septic or toxic infant. Suppurative complications are rare, but dehydration and electrolyte disturbances are common and need immediate and constant attention. *C. jejuni* infection typically involves the gastrointestinal tract, producing watery diarrhea or a dysentery-like illness with fever and bloody mucoid stools. Extraintestinal infections related to *C. jejuni* other than bacteremia are rare but include cholecystitis, urinary tract infection, and meningitis.[136] The clinical manifestations in neonates with *C. fetus* infection are similar to those caused by the common neonatal pathogens.[136] *C. jejuni* has been reported to cause bloody diarrhea in otherwise asymptomatic neonates.[59]

A useful procedure for differentiating enteroinvasive from enterotoxigenic diarrhea is examination of fecal material for polymorphonuclear cells. Feces from many patients with dysentery show significant numbers of polymorphonuclear leukocytes, whereas those from patients with enterotoxigenic disease usually show few neutrophils.

Treatment

The most important aspect of therapy for diarrheal disease of newborn infants is maintenance of hydration and electrolyte balance. As a rule, parenteral solutions containing appropriate electrolytes should be administered during the time of active diarrhea, and the infant should be examined and weighed frequently to ensure proper rehydration and prevention of complications. Estimation of fluid loss from diarrhea and vomiting should be recorded carefully and used as a basis for replacement therapy.

Selection of appropriate antimicrobial therapy depends in part on the mechanism of diarrhea. In general, an orally administered, absorbable antibiotic, such as ampicillin and trimethoprim-sulfamethoxazole, is indicated for disease caused by invasive bacteria (shigellosis), whereas orally administered, nonabsorbable drugs, such as neomycin and colistin sulfate, are used for noninvasive organisms that produce enterotoxin (some *E. coli*).

Antimicrobial therapy for *Salmonella* gastroenteritis is controversial. We do not recommend antibiotics for most infants and children with uncomplicated *Salmonella* disease because such therapy does not shorten the course of illness and can be associated with an increased likelihood of prolonged asymptomatic excretion of the organism. On the other hand, neonates and infants younger than 3 or 4 months of age should be treated with a 7-day course of amoxicillin because of their propensity to develop a protracted illness or blood stream invasion with distant foci of infection.[85] Trimethoprim-sulfamethoxazole is a suitable alternative for ampicillin-resistant strains. The asymptomatic carrier state requires no therapy.

Ampicillin formerly was the antibiotic of choice for shigellosis, but in recent years, significant resistance to this agent has been observed in many areas of the country. Most strains are susceptible to trimethoprim-sulfamethoxazole in a daily dosage of 10 mg trimethoprim, 50 mg sulfamethoxazole/kg/day in two divided doses. Sulfa drugs are contraindicated in jaundiced newborns. For multiresistant *Shigella* strains, some authorities recommend third-generation cephalosporins given parenterally (e.g., ceftriaxone) or orally (e.g., cefixime).

Erythromycin is the preferred drug for treating symptomatic *C. jejuni* enteritis. Often, if erythromycin therapy is initiated within the first 4 days of illness, excretion of the organism is reduced and symptoms resolve rapidly. An aminoglycoside is the drug of choice for *C. fetus* infections; chloramphenicol is an alternative.

Any infant with diarrhea must be isolated from the other babies in the nursery. Surveillance of all infants in contact with the index case and institution of infection control measures are mandatory (as discussed earlier).

URINARY TRACT INFECTIONS

The incidence of bacteriuria in newborn infants ranges from 0.5 to 1 per cent for term infants and is approximately 3 per cent for premature infants.[222] Urinary tract infections are more common in babies born to bacteriuric mothers and in males during the neonatal period. The latter observation is contrasted with the predominance in females beyond the first months of life. The frequencies of urinary tract infection and bacteremia are significantly higher in uncircumcised male neonates and young infants.[351] Circumcision reduces the frequency of urinary tract infection by approximately 90 per cent. Bacterial colonization of both the prepuce and female perineum may occur because of the presence of maternal urinary tract infection. This was shown in a study in which 24 per cent of infants were bacteriuric when delivered to mothers who had bacteriuria, whereas control infants whose mothers had not been bacteriuric had no bacteriuria. Clinical pyelonephritis occurred in 3 per cent of these bacteriuric infants, whereas only 0.2 per cent of 500 control infants of nonbacteriuric mothers had pyelonephritis.[241]

Etiology

E. coli is the most common etiologic agent of urinary tract infections, accounting for approximately 90 per cent of acute infections and 70 to 80 per cent of recurrent disease. About 70 per cent of *E. coli* strains belong to one of eight common somatic (O) antigen groups similar to those found in older persons. Several capsular polysaccharide antigens (K1, K2, K12, and K13) are found more often in children with upper tract disease than in those with cystitis.[160, 349] The association between K1 antigen and upper tract disease is found significantly more often in newborn and young infants than in older infants and children with *E. coli* urinary tract infections.[349] Fimbriated *E. coli* can attach to specific receptors or uroepithelial cells. Glycolipids of the P blood group constitute a specific receptor that is believed to be associated with pyelonephritis in patients who do not have reflux. Compared with asymptomatic bacteriuric infants, those with febrile urinary tract infections were found to have significantly increased inflammatory signs (e.g., C-reactive protein value, microsedimentation rate) and attaching *E. coli*.[189] This suggests that bacterial properties determine not only the location of urinary tract infection but also the severity of inflammation in individual patients.

Proteus, Klebsiella, and *Pseudomonas* species are encountered in patients with recurrent disease, particularly those receiving prolonged antimicrobial prophylaxis. Gram-positive bacteria, with the exception of enterococci, rarely are encountered as pathogens for the urinary tract. Only a few neonatal cases of renal abscess have been reported in the literature. *S. aureus* and coliforms were the predominant etiologic agents.[307]

Clinical Manifestations

Most infants with significant bacteriuria either are asymptomatic or have nonspecific signs and symptoms. The neonate may appear septic or may have decreased activity, feeding problems, and the other constitutional signs that are seen with infections of other organ systems as well. Jaundice, hepatomegaly, and thrombocytopenia may be observed in a few infants with urinary tract infection; these findings are associated with septicemia or cholestatic hepatitis in some babies.[42] Localizing signs suggesting urinary tract involvement are unusual. When present, they usually consist of a weak urinary stream on voiding or an abdominal tumor from bladder distention, hydronephrosis, or both.

Diagnosis

The diagnosis of urinary tract infection is confirmed by examination and culture of urine. The results of these tests depend largely on the method of urine collection. Most pediatricians obtain urine with a sterile, plastic receptacle applied to the cleansed perineum. However, urine obtained by this method may have an elevated cell count because of recent circumcision, vaginal reflux of urine, or contamination from the perineum. Neonatal asphyxia also may increase the urine cell count. Furthermore, white blood cells must be differentiated from round epithelial cells, which appear in the urine in significant numbers during the early days of life. Although pyuria commonly accompanies significant bacteriuria, cells can be few or absent. Direct microscopic examination of uncentrifuged, fresh urine is useful. If bacteria are seen readily in each high-power field, they generally number greater than 10^5/mL. Glitter cells are thought by many to be diagnostic of urinary tract infections.

Quantitative urine cultures from infants with documented disease usually contain more than 100,000 colonies/mL of a single bacterial species. Any number of bacteria in a urine specimen obtained by percutaneous needle puncture of the bladder should be considered significant. This latter procedure is the single best source of urine for culture and is safe in most newborn infants.[222] The procedure should not be performed in infants who are dehydrated or have bleeding problems. Minor, transient hematuria is uncommon, and serious problems from hemorrhage or perforation of the bowel have been exceedingly rare. If a "bagged urine specimen" contains fewer than 100,000 colonies/mL of a single species of bacteria or if the culture yields a mixed bacterial population, a repeat urine specimen should be obtained for culture by suprapubic bladder aspiration or catheterization.

Examination of the urinary sediment for antibody-coated bacteria has been found useful in differentiating upper tract disease from cystitis in adult patients.[158] Some reports have suggested, however, that this technique is not applicable to infants and children.[349] These studies have demonstrated false-positive and false-negative rates of approximately 30 per cent. Because acute pyelonephritis is associated with enlargement of the kidneys resulting from edema and acute inflammatory infiltrate of the medulla and the pelvis, volume measurements of the kidneys, by means of ultrasonography, provide a noninvasive method for identifying the probable site of urinary tract infection.[156] Fifteen of 18 children with upper urinary tract infection had volume increases of 30 per cent or more in at least one kidney, whereas only 4 of 21 children with lower urinary tract infection had increases of greater than 30 per cent ($p < .005$).

Treatment

Blood and urine cultures should be obtained from all newborn infants with suspected or proven urinary tract infection before antimicrobial therapy is initiated. Antibiotics initially are administered parenterally because sepsis occurs in association with urinary tract infection in 20 to 30 per cent of infants,[120] and antibiotic absorption after oral administration is erratic in some babies. Therapy is initiated with an aminoglycoside and ampicillin to provide antibacterial coverage for the anticipated coliforms, enterococci, and group B streptococci. If renal impairment is present, ampicillin and cefotaxime is an alternative empiric regimen. Because urine concentrations of these drugs exceed many times the minimal inhibitory concentration values of the urinary pathogens, the usual dosages may be reduced after septicemia has been ruled out.[195] Infants with renal or perineal abscesses require percutaneous drainage under sonographic guidance or open surgical drainage if the former fails.

A repeat urine culture taken 48 to 72 hours after initiation of appropriate therapy should be sterile or show a substantial reduction in the bacterial count. Infants with persistent bacteriuria should be evaluated for the possibility of inappropriate therapy, obstruction, or perinephric abscess. In uncomplicated disease, therapy usually is continued for a period of 7 to 10 days. Approximately 1 week after discontinuing therapy, a repeat urine culture is obtained.

All infants with documented infection should undergo radiologic evaluation of the urinary tract. An intravenous pyelogram or renal sonograph is obtained during the course of therapy to rule out the possibility of gross congenital abnormalities of the urinary system. Renal sonography is preferred over intravenous pyelography in the acute phase of disease. Congenital malformations are unusual in the first week of life but may be found in a significant portion of infants with urinary tract infections after this age. If obstruction is demonstrated, urologic procedures to ensure proper drainage are mandatory if therapy is to be successful. A voiding cystourethrogram or a radionuclide cystourethrogram should be obtained several weeks after therapy is stopped. Radiologic abnormalities are found in about 45 per cent of infants, especially in girls.[50, 120]

It is the physician's responsibility to be certain that neonates with urinary tract infections do not have congenital abnormalities of the urinary system. In such patients, recurrent urinary tract infections are common, and physical growth may be retarded until definitive surgery has been performed. Every infant with urinary tract infection should undergo long-term follow-up studies for detection of recurrent infections, many of which are asymptomatic.

Infants identified to have anatomic abnormalities (e.g., vesicoureteral reflux) must be protected from reinfection by prophylactic administration of trimethoprim-sulfamethoxazole or nitrofurantoin, and urine cultures or urinary nitrite tests in children should be performed soon thereafter. Although there is no absolute medical indication for routine circumcision of the newborn, cumulative data suggest that circumcision protects against urinary tract infections during early infancy.[352] Compared with complications of urinary tract infections, short-term complications of circumcision are rare and mostly minor.[351]

SUPPURATIVE ARTHRITIS AND OSTEOMYELITIS

Osteomyelitis and suppurative arthritis rarely occur in the first 4 weeks of life. The incidence has not changed for many years and is estimated to be 1 to 3 cases of bone or joint infections per 1000 nursery admissions. According to the Dallas experience, there were 18 cases (3 per cent) of neonatal arthritis and 18 cases (5 per cent) of osteomyelitis among 632 arthritis and 365 osteomyelitis cases in infants and children managed from 1959 to 1986.[216] Male infants are affected more often than female (1.6:1), and the incidence is higher in premature than in term infants.

Bone and joint infections can be difficult to detect in neonates and young infants. Early diagnosis and appropriate management are vital to prevent orthopedic abnormalities later in life.

Etiology and Pathogenesis

The infecting organisms in osteomyelitis and septic arthritis are varied, but the predominant ones are *S. aureus*, group B *Streptococcus*, and gram-negative enteric organisms, such as *Klebsiella, Proteus,* and *E. coli. S. aureus* was the etiologic agent in 50 and 44 per cent of cases of osteomyelitis and arthritis in neonates in Dallas, respectively, whereas streptococci were responsible for 6 and 22 per cent of cases, respectively. Group B *Streptococcus*, on the other hand, had become the single most common agent associated with arthritis in many areas of the United States.[112] Osteomyelitis and arthritis caused by gram-negative enteric bacilli have remained uncommon, despite the frequency of neonatal bacteremia caused by these organisms. Coliforms caused 11 per cent of cases in Dallas and 5 per cent in a children's hospital in Stockholm.[37] In Africa and Asia, rates as high as 45 per cent have been reported.[169] In Panama, we reported recently that coliforms and *S. aureus* accounted for two-thirds of isolates in neonates with osteoarticular infections.[278a] Gonococcal arthritis and tenosynovitis were common in previous decades, but they are seen only occasionally today.[78] Other causative agents associated infrequently with newborn infection are *Salmonella, Pseudomonas,* and *Candida albicans*.[82, 250]

Osteomyelitis and arthritis have been reported consequent to several invasive procedures in newborns. These include heel puncture, femoral venipuncture, exchange transfusions, fetal monitoring using electrodes, serial lumbar punctures, and umbilical artery catheterization.[14, 40, 180, 215, 235, 250, 254] Osteomyelitis of cranial bones has complicated infected cephalohematomas. The use of peripheral as well as central intravascular catheters in neonates has been associated with bacterial and fungal osteomyelitis.[112] Septic embolization from catheter tip thrombi together with local hypoxia from partial occlusion of the vessel by the catheter may explain this association.[112, 181] There is very strong correlation between the site of the catheter and localization of infection in the limb; for example, the knees and hips are involved in most cases associated with aortic catheters.[181] Usually, the origin is unknown and presumed to be hematogenous.

During the first month of life, the epiphyseal plate is traversed by multiple small transepiphyseal vessels that provide a direct communication between the articular space and the metaphysis of the long bones.[228] As a result, infection of the metaphysis (osteomyelitis) can spread across the growth plate to penetrate the epiphysis or enter the joint space. Because the perforating vessels disappear at approximately 1 year of age, septic arthritis usually is not associated with osteomyelitis in older infants and children. There are two exceptions to this rule: osteomyelitis of the proximal femur and of the proximal humerus. The capsule of the hip and shoulder attaches below the proximal metaphysis of the femur and humerus, respectively. Infection of the epiphyseal cartilage may rupture through the periosteum and enter the joint space, producing purulent arthritis. Because the capsular articulation of the hip and shoulder is permanent, osteomyelitis and septic arthritis may coexist, making the origin of infection difficult to establish.

The large vascular spaces and thin spongy structure of the metaphyseal cortex in infants permit early decompression of the primary abscess into the subperiosteal space. The abscess then dissects rapidly between the loosely attached periosteum. As pressure increases from the accumulating pus, a subcutaneous abscess can form that may point and drain spontaneously through the skin, forming a sinus tract. Free communication between the original site of osteomyelitis and subperiosteal space prevents the necrosis and extensive spread of infection within bone that occurs frequently in older children and adults.

Clinical Manifestations

Two distinct clinical syndromes that may be associated with osteomyelitis in the newborn period have been described.[86, 133, 324] The first is a benign form in which the earliest sign of bone and joint infections of newborns is failure to move an extremity spontaneously or apparent pain on movement without systemic evidence of infection. Swelling, erythema, and heat localized to the affected part are late findings. Multiple bones or joints can be involved, especially when disease is caused by *S. aureus*. Thus, the striking feature of this form is the satisfactory general condition of the infant despite the intensity of the local process. The fatality rate is exceedingly low, and healing is prompt. The second syndrome, a severe form, is characterized by systemic manifestations of sepsis; only later are multiple sites of bone and visceral involvement noted.

Two other clinical entities unique to the newborn are maxillary bone involvement and osteomyelitis caused by group

B *Streptococcus*. Maxillitis or osteomyelitis of the superior maxilla is an unusual form of bone infection in newborn infants.[180] More than 85 per cent of all maxillary infections in infants occur in the first 3 months of life, the peak incidence occurring in the second to fourth weeks of life.[188] Swelling of the cheek, associated with unilateral nasal discharge of pus, and swelling of the alveolar ridge of the maxilla should alert the physician to this entity. Initially, dacryocystitis or orbital cellulitis may be suspected. The etiologic agent usually is *S. aureus*. Septicemia and death are common in untreated cases.

Group B streptococcal osteomyelitis presents during the third and fourth weeks of life (late-onset) and is caused predominantly by type III strains. It affects females more often than males, and the humerus is the most common site of involvement. In contrast with the fulminant onset and poor outcome that occur in some infants with late-onset meningitis, group B streptococcal bone and joint infection has an indolent nature and an almost uniformly good outcome. Occasionally, a diagnosis of Erb palsy may be entertained when inflammatory signs are minimal and diminished use of an arm is marked. Manipulations known to predispose neonates to bone and joint infections caused by other organisms have not been reported among infants with group B streptococcal arthritis or osteomyelitis.[188]

Diagnosis

Conventional radiography remains the most useful way of establishing the diagnosis in patients with suspected suppurative arthritis; radiographs may be normal or show enlargement of the joint space. Later in the course of disease, subluxation and destruction of the joint are common. In early osteomyelitis, the normal radiographic water markings of tissues adjacent to the affected bone may be obliterated, indicating deep tissue inflammation and swelling. Lifting of the periosteum also may be observed, but cortical bone destruction is unusual before the second week of illness. A complete skeletal survey should be performed because of the frequent involvement of multiple sites.[112, 205] In approximately 10 per cent of patients, radiographic abnormalities are not seen during the course of disease. Although radionuclide bone scans are useful in early diagnosis of osteomyelitis in infants and children, they can be normal in newborn and young infants with proven infection. Magnetic resonance imaging has been used successfully for diagnosis of osteomyelitis in the newborn period.

Blood cultures should be obtained from all infants with osteomyelitis or septic arthritis. Considering the varied etiologic bacteria, it is imperative to get specimens of bone or a joint aspirate for culture. Therefore, a percutaneous needle aspiration of intra-articular pus in patients with suspected suppurative arthritis or of sequestrum in those with suspected osteomyelitis is imperative. If pus is obtained, the material should be Gram stained and cultured.

Treatment

Selection of initial antimicrobial therapy is guided by preliminary identification of the pathogen from stained smears of material obtained from needle aspirations. If no microorganisms are seen, it is advisable to begin treatment with two drugs, a penicillinase-resistant penicillin (e.g., methicillin, oxacillin) and cefotaxime. Use of an aminoglycoside with the antistaphylococcal penicillin does not provide adequate coverage for group B *Streptococcus*. Definitive treatment is based on culture and susceptibility results. Direct instillation of an antibiotic into the joint space is unnecessary because most drugs penetrate the inflamed synovium and adequate concentrations are achieved in purulent material.[218] This also applies to treatment of osteomyelitis; direct instillation of antibiotics into acutely inflamed bone is unnecessary.[322]

Surgical removal of infected material is an integral part of treatment. Open drainage is essential for management of septic hip disease. As emphasized previously, inflammation in osteomyelitis or in septic arthritis can occupy the epiphyseal and metaphyseal sides of the growth plate, resulting in ischemia and necrosis of the plate and in permanent orthopedic damage. For other joints, repeated daily evacuation of fluid with needle and syringe usually is adequate. In patients with osteomyelitis, the subperiosteal space and the metaphysis should be drained if pus is obtained during diagnostic aspiration. If only a small amount of bloody material is obtained at aspiration, immediate surgery is not necessary, and the patient usually can be managed with antibiotic therapy alone as long as local and systemic signs resolve. If improvement is not satisfactory, repeat aspirations or open surgical drainage may be necessary.

Antimicrobial therapy of neonatal musculoskeletal infections caused by staphylococci or coliform organisms is continued for a minimum of 3 weeks. Group B streptococcal infection is treated with penicillin G or ampicillin for at least 2 weeks. Ten days of therapy usually is adequate for gonococcal infection. Use of oral antibiotics as a substitute for parenteral therapy during the second and third weeks of treatment is unwise unless compliance can be ensured, and serum bactericidal activity or antibiotic concentration is satisfactory, indicating adequate absorption of the orally administered drug. Parenteral antibiotic therapy can be administered at home if the infant can be assessed routinely by a physician.

As a general rule, systemic symptoms disappear within several days of initiating therapy and of adequate surgical drainage, although such local signs as heat, erythema, and swelling may persist for 4 to 7 days. Full range of motion may not return to the involved limb for several months. The erythrocyte sedimentation rate is a useful guide for determining duration of therapy. The rate usually returns to within the normal range within 2 to 4 weeks compared with the C-reactive protein value that becomes normal earlier. As recently reported in older infants and children, it is possible that serial determinations of C-reactive protein can be valuable in assessing the clinical course, but experience is inadequate to use this test in guiding duration of antimicrobial therapy in neonatal osteoarticular infections.[264] Complete resolution of the radiographic changes may take several months.

Physical therapy to ensure full range of motion should be started as soon as pain has abated. It frequently is difficult to assess residual joint abnormalities and abnormal bone growth patterns in infants until many months or years have passed. It is important to have good long-term follow-up after treatment has been concluded.

CONJUNCTIVITIS AND ORBITAL CELLULITIS

Infections of the eye of the newborn can be caused by a variety of microorganisms, including *Neisseria gonorrhoeae*, *Chlamydia trachomatis*, *S. aureus*, and *P. aeruginosa*. From a review of more than 300 cases of eye infections in newborns at Grady Memorial Hospital in Atlanta,[12] it was determined that 29 per cent were caused by *Chlamydia*, 14 per cent by gonococci, 10 per cent by staphylococci, 2 per cent by chemical reactions, and 1 per cent by mixed gonococcal and chlamydial infections. The remaining 44 per cent were of uncertain cause. A prospective, controlled study found that the major microbial causes of neonatal conjunctivitis were *Haemophilus* species in 17 per cent, *S. aureus* in 17 per cent, *C. trachomatis* in 14 per cent, *S. pneumoniae* in 11 per cent, and enterococci in 8 per cent.[280] Other less frequently encountered organisms included *M. catarrhalis, Pasteurella multocida, N. meningitidis,* and herpes simplex virus.

The incidence of ophthalmia neonatorum has not paralleled the large increase in gonococcal disease rates among adolescent and young adults. This almost certainly is a result of universal neonatal prophylaxis with 1 per cent silver nitrate solution, antibiotic ointment, or systemic penicillin G. Today, we rarely see the invasive, destructive ophthalmitis described so vividly in the old literature.[191]

A number of agents have been shown to be effective prophylactically against gonococci. The largest series was published by Greenberg and Vandow[132] and involved 250,000 infants treated with 1 per cent silver nitrate. A failure rate of 6.6/100,000 infants treated with silver nitrate compared favorably with the 22.5/100,000 rate in 86,000 infants who received no prophylaxis. Of the topical antimicrobial agents, tetracycline or erythromycin appears to be comparable in efficacy to silver nitrate and has the advantage of causing fewer cases of chemical conjunctivitis.[232] Penicillin applied topically or given intramuscularly also is effective, although the ointment no longer is available commercially. Bacitracin ointment is ineffective.[73, 190] Ceftriaxone as a single dose of 50 mg/kg (for low birth weight infants, 25 to 50 mg/kg) can be useful for prophylaxis when the risk is high. Infants born to mothers with active gonorrhea should receive a single dose of ceftriaxone, 125 mg intravenously or intramuscularly. Ceftriaxone should be given cautiously to hyperbilirubinemic infants, especially premature infants.

A study by Hammerschlag and associates[141] showed that neonatal ocular prophylaxis with either erythromycin or tetracycline ophthalmic ointment does not reduce significantly the incidence of chlamydial conjunctivitis in the offspring of mothers with *Chlamydia* infection, compared with silver nitrate. The authors concluded that better management of maternal *Chlamydia* infection is required if the incidence of conjunctivitis caused by this organism is to be reduced. Additionally, they suggested that a small but appreciable incidence of neonatal gonococcal ophthalmia could be prevented by better prenatal screening and treatment of maternal gonococcal infections.

Diagnosis

Any infant with a conjunctival discharge should be evaluated carefully to determine the etiology. Three tests should be performed: (1) Gram and methylene blue stain of the exudate, (2) culture of the exudate, and (3) Giemsa stain and culture for *Chlamydia,* if available, of scrapings made from the lower palpebral conjunctiva after exudate has been wiped away. The results of the stained smears determine the appropriate therapy. Direct detection of chlamydial antigens in eye scrapings now is possible by means of a commercially available enzyme-linked immunoassay (Chlamydiazime). Limited experience in neonates suggests that it is a sensitive and specific test that can provide rapid and reliable results.[142]

Differential Diagnosis

Conjunctivitis occurring in the first days of life can be either chemical or bacterial. Chemical irritants, such as silver nitrate, cause transient conjunctival hyperemia and a watery discharge that rarely turns purulent.

Gonococcal ophthalmia usually becomes apparent within the first 5 days of life and is characterized initially by a clear watery discharge. Conjunctival hyperemia and chemosis are associated with a copious discharge of thick, white, purulent material. Both eyes usually are involved but not necessarily to the same degree. Untreated gonococcal ophthalmia may extend to involve the cornea (keratitis) and the anterior chamber of the eye. Corneal perforation and blindness can result. Before the introduction of adequate prophylactic measures, ophthalmia neonatorum was the most frequent cause of acquired blindness in the United States.

If gram-negative rods are seen in the stained exudate, the greatest concern is *P. aeruginosa* because of the virulent necrotizing endophthalmitis that can result. In this condition, a relatively mild conjunctivitis can progress to infection of the entire globe within 12 to 24 hours. Invasion of the cornea by small blood vessels (pannus) is characteristic of *Pseudomonas* conjunctivitis. Perforation of the cornea may occur, and blindness from corneal opacity is common. The ophthalmic disease occasionally can be followed by bacteremia and septic foci in other organs.[61] Prompt diagnosis and immediate institution of appropriate antimicrobial therapy are mandatory.[61]

Conjunctivitis during the second or third week of life can be caused by viral, bacterial, or chlamydial agents. Viral conjunctivitis frequently is associated with other symptoms of respiratory tract disease, such as rhinorrhea, cough, and rash, and several individuals in the family or nursery may have simultaneous disease. The discharge in viral conjunctivitis usually is watery or mucopurulent but rarely purulent. A hemorrhagic discharge can be seen with adenoviral infection. Preauricular adenopathy is common. Staphylococci, streptococci, *Haemophilus,* and, occasionally, gonococci cause conjunctivitis in this age group. A smear of purulent material helps to differentiate these bacterial agents. However, the presence of bacteria on a Gram-stained smear of exudate is not necessarily related etiologically to the conjunctivitis. The exudate may contain normal inhabitants of the skin and mucous membranes, such as staphylococci, diphtheroids, and *Neisseria* species.

Chlamydial eye infection may begin in the first days of life but usually does not come to the attention of the physician until the second or third week. Clinical manifestations of chlamydial infection (inclusion blennorrhea) vary from mild conjunctivitis to intense inflammation and swelling of the lids, associated with copious purulent discharge.[126, 267] Pseudomembrane formation and a diffuse "matte" injection of the tarsal conjunctiva are common. The cornea rarely is affected, and preauricular adenopathy is unusual. In the early stages of disease, one eye may appear more swollen and infected than the other, but both eyes almost invariably are involved.

Diagnosis is made by scraping the tarsal conjunctiva and looking for typical cytoplasmic inclusions within epithelial cells (not in the exudate). Specially prepared tissue culture cells for *Chlamydia* are available in some centers, and immunoassays are available commercially for a rapid and specific diagnosis. An opened paper clip usually is satisfactory to scrape the conjunctiva, and the material is layered carefully onto a microscope slide and stained by the Giemsa method. Without treatment, the acute inflammation continues for several weeks, merging into a subacute phase of slight conjunctival infection with scant purulent material. Occasionally, chronicity develops; some cases persist for longer than a year.

Treatment

Initial therapy is based on the results of stained smears of exudate and epithelial cells. If gonococci are seen, parenteral penicillin or ceftriaxone therapy is employed. If staphylococci are seen, methicillin or another penicillinase-resistant penicillin analogue is used. The necessity for topical antibiotics in these two bacterial infections is dubious. In the presence of acute inflammation, ample antibiotic is present in eye secretions to inhibit bacteria.

Since the beginning of the 1980s, gonococci resistant to penicillin have appeared in the United States and other parts of the world.[92, 258] These strains are susceptible to spectinomycin, erythromycin, and to the new-generation cephalosporins (e.g., ceftriaxone, cefotaxime). Experience in treating gonococcal ophthalmia with these drugs is limited, as are pharmacologic data for spectinomycin in the newborn. Infants with documented gonococcal infections at any site, including the eye, should be examined for disseminated gonococcal infection. This should include a careful physical examination, especially of the joints, as well as blood and CSF cultures. Infants with gonococcal ophthalmia should be treated for 4 to 7 days with ceftriaxone, 50 mg/kg intravenously or intramuscularly every 24 hours. Limited data suggest that uncomplicated gonococcal ophthalmia in infants can be cured with a single injection of ceftriaxone (50 mg/kg up to 125 mg). If the gonococcal isolate is susceptible to penicillin, crystalline penicillin G can be given. The dose is 100,000 units/kg/day given in two doses (or four doses in infants older than 1 week of age). The eye should be irrigated with buffered saline solution until eye discharge has cleared. In patients who do not respond satisfactorily, co-infection with *Chlamydia* should be considered. The mother and infant should be tested routinely for *Chlamydia* infection.

Pseudomonas eye infection always should be treated with parenteral therapy consisting of ticarcillin or ceftriaxone and gentamicin. Additionally, gentamicin ophthalmic drops are used for simple *Pseudomonas* conjunctivitis, and subtenon injections of gentamicin may be indicated when endophthalmitis is present.[124]

Orally administered erythromycin is superior to topically applied tetracycline or sodium sulfacetamide in the therapy of chlamydial conjunctivitis. Topical therapy suppresses chlamydial growth only, whereas erythromycin eradicates the organism in most patients. Topical and oral erythromycin regimens have comparable efficacies, but oral therapy has the advantage of eradicating nasopharyngeal carriage of *Chlamydia*.[240] Most cases heal without residua.[127] Approximately one-quarter of infants with gonococcal ophthalmia have concomitant infection with *Chlamydia* that requires therapy.

Patients with gonococcal ophthalmia should be segregated, and strict hand washing techniques should be employed because the exudate is highly contagious.

CUTANEOUS AND GLANDULAR INFECTIONS

Pustular and Vesicular Lesions

Superficial pustular staphylococcal disease (impetigo neonatorum) is the most common skin infection of neonates. The lesions tend to concentrate in the periumbilical and diaper areas and rarely become invasive, except when extensive areas are involved or when monitoring devices, catheters, or other invasive devices are used in the gravely ill infant. The lesions respond to simple topical measures; systemic antibiotic treatment usually is not indicated unless there is extensive involvement of the skin. The organisms should be phage typed (they usually belong to group I), so that if additional cases are encountered in the same nursery, the infected infants and their cohorts can be evaluated for the possibility of nosocomial staphylococcal disease. If these infections are caused by the same staphylococcal phage type, prompt measures should be instituted for determining the source and extent of infection for prevention of further colonization and disease.

A second form of staphylococcal disease has been recognized with increased frequency in recent years. The disease takes one of several clinical forms, including bullous impetigo, the most common manifestation, and Ritter disease, the eponymic equivalent in newborns of toxic epidermal necrolysis of older infants.[200] These illnesses usually are caused by phage group II staphylococci, which produce an exotoxin (exfoliatin) that causes intraepidermal cleavage through the granular cell layer resulting from disruption of desmosomes.[201] The initial finding in Ritter disease is intense, painful erythema, not unlike a severe sunburn. Over the next hours, bullous formations occur, and when these rupture, they leave a tender, weeping, erythematous area. A characteristic desquamation of large epidermal sheets occurs approximately 3 to 5 days after onset of illness. A finer desquamation commonly is seen periorally.

Bacteremic complications are more common in neonates than in older infants with the scalded skin syndrome. Treatment is with systemically administered, penicillinase-resistant penicillin because most phage group II staphylococci are resistant to penicillin. Because the cleavage plane in this syndrome is very superficial in the epidermis, there is little risk of superinfection. Steroids are contraindicated. Maceration may occur in intertriginous areas that should be treated by local soaks with Burow solution.

Cellulitis and Fasciitis

Group A streptococci are the usual cause of diffuse, well-demarcated cellulitis (or erysipelas), although we have seen the same diseases caused by group B organisms as well. The involved skin usually is intensely red, hot, and moderately indurated. Occasionally, streptococci can be recovered from material aspirated from the lesion, but the blood culture rarely is positive. Parenteral therapy is with penicillin G, and although the borders continue to advance for the first 12 to 24 hours, stabilization of body temperature and improvement in general appearance of the infant give reassurance that the diagnosis and therapy are correct.

Necrotizing fasciitis is a virulent form of cellulitis that is rare in newborns. Initially, it resembles uncomplicated cellulitis, but the baby rapidly becomes "toxic," the lesion advances progressively, and the central portion becomes discolored and anesthetic. The lesion has borders that usually are indistinct, compared with erysipelas, in which the borders are raised and palpated easily. The disease may be associated with surgical procedures, birth trauma, or cutaneous infection and has been reported after circumcision. The trunk and the extremities are the areas involved most commonly. Causative agents include streptococci, *S. aureus*, *P. aeruginosa*, *E. coli*, and anaerobic bacteria.[256, 343, 350] In this condition, subcutaneous tissues, including muscle layers, are invaded, and the organism spreads along the fascial planes. Extensive surgery involving resection of destroyed tissue is imperative in treating necrotizing fasciitis.[350] Blood and tissue cultures should be obtained, and initial antibiotic therapy should be with a penicillinase-resistant penicillin or clindamycin and an aminoglycosidic drug, pending results of these cultures. Hypocalcemia and hypoproteinemia may complicate the illness. If the infant survives the first days, extensive skin grafting generally is necessary.

Funisitis and Omphalitis

The umbilical cord may be colonized with a number of different potential bacterial pathogens, some of which may have significant epidemiologic importance. Hexachlorophene was used in many institutions in an attempt to reduce or eliminate staphylococci that were responsible for nursery epidemics in the late 1950s and early 1960s. Although this antiseptic is effective in reducing staphylococcal colony counts, the agent is not effective in controlling nosocomial staphylococcal disease in nursery units. Furthermore, its widespread use occasionally has been associated with central nervous system spongiform degeneration, particularly in premature infants.[297] A single application of triple dye to the cord results in significant reduction of all bacteria, particularly staphylococci, streptococci, and coliforms.[221, 249] Mupirocin ointment also is effective in eradicating staphylococcal carriage.

Group A streptococci may colonize the umbilical cord and be important as a focal point for epidemic streptococcal disease in a nursery. Unlike staphylococci, they tend to cause an inflammatory reaction.[88, 221] Streptococcal funisitis (inflammation of the cord) is mild and is characterized by a wet, malodorous umbilical stump with minimal inflammation. Disseminated disease is uncommon, but, when present, it occurs secondary to blood stream invasion or by direct extension to the peritoneal cavity by way of the umbilical vessels. Treatment is with systemic penicillin G and topical therapy with antibiotic ointment or with triple dye. Local therapy is provided for epidemiologic reasons to eliminate surface colonization. Identification of a single infant with group A streptococcal disease in a nursery necessitates immediate infection control measures for identification and segregation of all colonized persons. When a nursery outbreak is suspected, specific M and T typing of the organism is useful in defining the source and spread of infection. A single injection of benzathine penicillin G is satisfactory for mild superficial infection or for elimination of the organism from colonized persons.[118, 221]

Omphalitis, or infection of the umbilicus, has many causes and occurs more frequently in low birth weight infants and in those with complicated deliveries. The incidence is estimated to be approximately 2 per cent, and symptoms start at an average age of 3 days. Culture and susceptibility test results are necessary for the selection of an appropriate antibiotic.

Breast Abscess

Breast abscesses are encountered most frequently during the second or third week of life and are more common in females, particularly those older than 2 weeks of age.[270] The disease does not occur in premature infants, presumably because of underdevelopment of the mammary glands in these infants. Bilateral disease is rare, but a case caused by group B streptococci has been reported.[219]

The major clinical finding is swelling of the affected breast with or without accompanying erythema and warmth. Systemic manifestations are uncommon, and only a fourth of patients have low-grade fever. The disease sometimes can progress rapidly and involve not only the breast tissue but the entire subcutaneous tissue beyond the breast's anatomic area.[296] This is associated with considerable toxicity and systemic signs and symptoms. *S. aureus* is the major pathogen, but coliform bacteria and group B streptococci have become more common in the past decade.[270, 314] Mixed infection is rare. In 36 infants with mastitis seen in Dallas during a 16-year period, 32 cases were caused by *S. aureus*, 1 case by *E. coli*, 2 cases by *Salmonella* species, and 1 case by both *S. aureus* and *E. coli*.

Breast abscess is diagnosed by examination of stained purulent material obtained from gentle manipulation of the nipple or by needle aspiration of the abscess. If gram-positive cocci are seen, methicillin or another penicillinase-resistant penicillin is given. For gram-negative bacilli, an aminoglycoside or cefotaxime is appropriate. When no organisms are seen, methicillin and an aminoglycoside or cefotaxime should be used initially until results of the culture are available. Bacteremia is rare in this condition.

If there is only mild cellulitis and no discernible fluctuance, antibiotic treatment alone may suffice. We have managed successfully several patients with group B streptococcal mastitis in this fashion. In most instances, however, surgical incision and drainage by a skilled surgeon are required. Duration of treatment depends on the rate of response. It generally is rapid, and we have found that healing is complete within 5 to 7 days in most instances. Long-term follow-up studies suggest that some girls will have diminished breast tissue on the affected side.[270]

Suppurative Parotitis

Suppurative parotitis of the newborn usually is easy to recognize, although occasionally it is confused with infection of a preauricular or superior anterior cervical lymph node. We have encountered one instance in which delay in initiating therapy was caused by attributing the swelling to trauma from obstetric forceps. Infection is more common in low birth weight infants than in term infants and in males. Dehydration predisposes to stasis of parotid secretions and subsequent infection. Bilateral infection is rare.

Although *S. aureus* accounts for most cases, disease may be caused by coliform bacteria, *Pseudomonas*, pneumococci, and group A streptococci.[84, 172] The clinical manifestations include fever, anorexia, irritability, and failure to gain weight. There may be erythema, swelling, and tenderness over the involved gland. Diagnosis can be confirmed by expressing pus through the parotid duct or by needle aspiration of a fluctuant area. Gram staining of this material helps identify the causative agent; however, it should be recognized that material expressed from the duct may be contaminated by mouth microflora.

Selection of antimicrobial therapy should be based on interpretation of the Gram-stained smear of expressed pus. If gram-positive cocci are seen, methicillin or another penicillinase-resistant penicillin should be used. Gram-negative organisms are treated best with an aminoglycoside, cefotaxime, or ceftazidime to cover both coliform bacteria and *Pseudomonas*. If no organisms are seen in the purulent material, a combination of methicillin and gentamicin or cefotaxime should be used until results of the culture are available. In most cases, antibiotic therapy alone suffices, and surgical incision and drainage are not necessary. The gland should not be extirpated. Response to therapy generally is rapid. Most patients require only 7 to 10 days of therapy until healing is complete.

Scalp Abscess

Scalp abscesses usually are a complication of fetal monitoring using scalp electrodes.[57, 334] The number of vaginal examinations, use of more than one electrode, and fetal scalp blood sampling are risk factors for its development. Pathogens incriminated include staphylococci, gonococci, and gram-negative enteric bacteria. A polymicrobial flora, including anaerobic organisms, frequently is isolated in scalp abscesses secondary to electronic fetal monitoring electrodes. Incision and drainage of the infected site usually are sufficient. If there is an associated cellulitis, antibiotics are used and are continued for 5 to 7 days.

LOWER RESPIRATORY TRACT INFECTIONS

Neonatal lower respiratory tract infections may be acquired congenitally or postnatally. Perinatal infection results either from transplacental transfer of the agent (congenital infection) or from inhalation of infected amniotic fluid (usually associated with prolonged rupture of membranes) or of infected vaginal secretions during delivery. Viruses, bacteria, *Chlamydia,* and spirochetes are the most common causative agents that produce perinatal pneumonias. The common viral agents include cytomegalovirus, rubella, and herpes simplex virus. The common bacterial agents are group B streptococci, *L. monocytogenes*, and coliform bacilli. *Chlamydia* have been implicated as the cause of a chronic interstitial pneumonitis of early infancy (eosinophilic pertussis-like pneumonia).[36] *Treponema pallidum* produces a severe, sometimes fatal pneumonitis, and mycoplasmas have caused a rare form of fatal congenital pneumonia. Of note, we also have seen in Panama a few cases of congenital pneumonia caused by *Candida* species in the last 4 years (unpublished observation).

Perinatal lower respiratory tract disease usually becomes apparent clinically from birth to 7 days, occasionally up to 2 weeks of age. It should be emphasized that inhalation of amniotic fluid or of maternal vaginal secretions usually is not associated with infection. This also is true of meconium inhalation, in which the pneumonitis has a chemical cause. Only a small percentage of inhalation pneumonias are bacterial in origin; the pathogens most commonly encountered in such cases are group B streptococci and coliform organisms. The clinical signs of inhalation pneumonia are caused by obstruction, chemical inflammation, or both.

The second category of pneumonias is acquired postnatally and usually beyond the first week of life. These diseases may be caused by viral or bacterial agents and most frequently are bronchopneumonic in type. Viral disease may be sporadic or occur as part of a nosocomial nursery outbreak. The respiratory syncytial virus is the most important pathogen of lower respiratory tract disease in young infants.[43] This agent causes particularly severe disease in infants with congenital heart disease. The parainfluenza viruses and adenoviruses also cause bronchiolitis and pneumonia during early infancy. An obliterating, necrotizing bronchiolitis may be caused by adenoviruses and result in radiographic hyperlucency of a segment or a lobe in later infancy and childhood.[123]

Documented nursery outbreaks of lower respiratory tract disease have been associated with respiratory syncytial virus, adenoviruses, echoviruses, influenza A and B viruses, and parainfluenza virus infections. During these outbreaks, many infants are colonized with the epidemic strains, but only a few have clinical disease.

The common bacterial pathogens causing postnatally acquired pneumonia are *S. aureus*, coliform bacilli, and *Pseudomonas.* These infections occur sporadically or epidemically and often are of nosocomial origin. They may be rapidly progressive, necrotic pneumonias that result in pyogenic complications (e.g., empyema, pulmonary abscesses), and metastatic disease in the bones or meninges.

Clinical Manifestations

The early signs of respiratory disease in the neonate and young infant frequently are nonspecific and include change in feeding status, listlessness or irritability, and poor color. More specific findings that may not be present at the onset of illness are tachypnea, dyspnea, cyanosis, alteration of temperature (hypothermia or fever), cough, and grunting. Accentuation of the normal irregularity of breathing is a common finding in neonates.

The physical findings of pneumonia are variable. Flaring of the alae nasi, rapid respirations, and sternal and subcostal retractions are common. Coughing indicates lower respiratory tract involvement; brassy coughing is found frequently in viral disease. Percussion dullness is difficult to demonstrate but, when present, indicates consolidation or effusion. Breath sounds also may be diminished over the affected area. Crackles or wheezes usually can be heard on deep inspiration (or when the baby is crying) but may be absent early in disease. The clinician frequently is surprised by the meager clinical signs in the face of clearly demonstrable and sometimes extensive radiographic findings of pneumonitis.

Diagnosis

The white blood cell count usually does not help to differentiate viral from bacterial pneumonia. An exception is seen in premature infants with acute respiratory distress syndrome caused by group B streptococci. In these patients, the white blood cell count often reveals a leukopenia with an increased proportion of band forms.[191]

Cultures of blood and material from the trachea frequently help in defining the etiologic agent of neonatal pneumonia. Results of cultures from the ear canal, throat, and other external sites usually are unreliable in defining the etiology of pneumonia; more often, they are misleading. Lung puncture should be considered in severely ill infants with consolidated pneumonia when the etiology is unknown or in an infant who fails to respond to conventional antimicrobial therapy. Material obtained by needle aspiration is Gram stained for direct visualization and cultured.

A chest radiograph should be obtained for all babies with suspected lower respiratory tract disease. Radiographic evidence of pneumonia may not be present in the absence of specific physical findings. Although it usually is possible to determine the etiology of neonatal pneumonia from a radiograph, certain radiologic patterns are associated with specific diseases. With acute-onset group B streptococcal disease, the radiograph may mimic one showing hyaline membrane disease. A consolidating bronchopneumonia with pneumatoceles with or without empyema suggests staphylococcal disease. When a lobar infiltrate is associated with expansion of the lobe, *Klebsiella pneumoniae* infection should be considered. A miliary type of bronchopneumonia in a septic neonate is characteristic of listeriosis.

Specific Clinical Syndromes

Staphylococcal Pneumonia

Primary staphylococcal pneumonia is most common in young infants. Epidemics of staphylococcal disease caused by phage group I organisms are rare today. In the epidemic setting, many infants are colonized with a virulent strain, but only a few have disease. It is possible, but unproved, that concomitant viral respiratory tract infections play a role in promoting dissemination of staphylococci among infants and in converting colonization to disease.

Staphylococci cause a confluent bronchopneumonia consisting of extensive areas of hemorrhagic necrosis and irregular areas of cavitation. The pleural surface usually is covered by a thick layer of fibrinopurulent exudate. Multiple small abscesses are scattered throughout the affected lung. Rupture of a small subpleural abscess may result in a pyopneumothorax. If there is erosion into a large bronchus, a bronchopleural fistula results.

Most patients with staphylococcal pneumonia have radiographic evidence of bronchopneumonia early in the illness. The infiltrate may be patchy and limited in extent or dense and homogeneous, involving an entire lobe or hemithorax. Bilateral disease occurs in half the patients. Pleural effusion or empyema is noted in most infants. Pneumatoceles of varying size are common. Although no radiographic picture can be considered absolutely diagnostic, progression over a few hours from bronchopneumonia to empyema or pyopneumothorax, with or without pneumatoceles, is highly suggestive of staphylococcal disease.

Klebsiella pneumoniae *Pneumonia*

Primary *K. pneumoniae* infection is unusual in infants and young children. However, nursery epidemics of *Klebsiella* infection have been reported. During these epidemics, colonization rates are high, but most infants remain asymptomatic. Contaminated fomites are the primary source of nosocomial infection with this organism.

K. pneumoniae pneumonia may be difficult to distinguish clinically from pneumonia due to other causes. The disease may have a fulminant course characterized by copious, thick, purulent secretions and the formation of pulmonary abscesses and cavitation. The case-fatality rate in sporadic cases is about 50 per cent but is considerably lower during epidemics.

Pertussis

Based on approximately 400 confirmed cases in Dallas from 1959 to 1977, the annual incidence of disease has decreased more than 50 per cent, but the proportion of cases in infants younger than 3 months of age has doubled from 15 to 30 per cent.[220] More recently, approximately 35 per cent of cases have occurred in infants younger than 6 months and 50 per cent in those younger than 12 months of age. Although infants formerly acquired disease from siblings, in the past 10 to 15 years, infection usually has been acquired from one or both parents whose illnesses have not been diagnosed correctly as pertussis. The reason for these epidemiologic changes most likely is better vaccination in schoolchildren. Because immunity starts to wane in adolescence, parents of young infants are susceptible to infection. The infants of these women also are susceptible to infection because of the lack of transplacental immunity.

The onset of disease usually is in the second to sixth weeks of life; the earliest onset reported was at 10 days of age. Most young infants do not have a characteristic whoop. Pertussis should be suspected when an infant has a paroxysmal cough with excessive mucus. Because apneic spells are common in these infants, as they are also in those with respiratory syncytial virus, *Chlamydia*, or influenza virus infection, all infants with pertussis are admitted to the hospital for management. Fluorescent antibody testing provides a means of rapid diagnosis, but false-negative and false-positive results are common. Cultures for *Bordetella* should be performed in all infants. Mucus for examination is obtained from patients with a nasopharyngeal flexible wire swab or by nasopharyngeal washing or aspiration.

The greatest hazards to an infant with pertussis are asphyxia and secondary bacterial pneumonias. Supportive care is essential. Excessive mucus must be suctioned, and equipment for emergency airway intubation should be at hand. Fluid therapy is necessary, and maintaining adequate nutritional intake may present the greatest challenge. Infants with pertussis should not be placed in mist tents. Mist therapy provides no substantial amelioration of paroxysmal coughing episodes, and it increases the risk of secondary infection with *P. aeruginosa* (or with other commensals).

Atelectasis secondary to mucus plugs is a common complication of pertussis in small babies. Once the infant has passed the stage of severe paroxysms, chest physiotherapy can be employed; in almost all cases atelectasis will resolve within 2 to 3 weeks.

Chlamydial Pneumonia

Chlamydial pneumonia presents between the fourth and eleventh weeks of life in most infants.[325] Infants typically are afebrile and tachypneic and have a characteristic staccato cough. Only half the patients have a history of conjunctivitis. On chest auscultation, rales may be heard, but wheezes are uncommon. The chest radiograph reveals hyperexpanded lungs with bilateral interstitial infiltrates. Peripheral eosinophilia is noted in about half of these infants. A definitive diagnosis made by isolating the organism from the respiratory tract is not possible in many institutions. The role of immunologic techniques to identify *Chlamydia* in throat swabs is yet to be determined. Serologic testing more readily is available. These infants usually respond to therapy with erythromycin. Both the clinical course and duration of nasopharyngeal shedding of *Chlamydia* are shortened by treatment with this antibiotic. If left untreated, these infants remain sick for several weeks but do not become acutely ill. Death from this infection is rare.

Treatment

Initial antibiotic therapy of suspected bacterial pneumonia should be with ampicillin or methicillin and an aminoglycoside or cefotaxime. The most suitable combination of these drugs depends on the clinical features of illness and the recent historical experience with bacterial diseases in the local nursery or community. For patients in whom the cause is never defined and staphylococcal disease cannot be ruled out, therapy with methicillin or vancomycin and an aminoglycoside or cefotaxime is indicated. If the organism is identified, the single most effective drug should be used. Penicillin G or ampicillin is effective against group B streptococci and penicillin-susceptible staphylococci, ampicillin against *Listeria*, and methicillin or another suitable antistaphylococcal penicillin against penicillinase-producing *S. aureus*. Vancomycin should be used for disease caused by MRSA or coagulase-negative staphylococci. For pneumonia caused by gram-negative bacilli (*K. pneumoniae* and others), an aminoglycoside or a third-generation cephalosporin should be used. *Pseudomonas* pneumonia is treated best with ticarcillin or ceftazidime in combination with an aminoglycoside. Therapy is continued for 10 to 14 days for disease caused by group B streptococci and *Listeria* and for a minimum of 3 weeks for pneumonia caused by staphylococci or gram-negative bacilli.

Empyema is managed best with closed drainage, using chest tubes of the largest possible caliber. It generally is necessary to place one tube high and anteriorly and the second tube low and posterolaterally for optimal drainage. Pyopneumothorax is another indication for immediate insertion of a catheter into the pleural space. Once the infant has improved clinically and the amount of drainage is minimal, the tubes should be removed. In general, they should not remain in the chest for more than 5 to 7 days. The instillation of antimicrobial agents or enzymes into the pleural space does not help control infection or promote drainage.

Pneumonia may be one manifestation of generalized congenital viral infection. It is important to distinguish these infections from congenital syphilis and bacterial pneumonias resulting from inhalation.

Most infants with inhalation pneumonia do not require antimicrobial therapy. It frequently is difficult to differentiate infants inhaling sterile fluid from those inhaling infected materials. If doubt exists, therapy with ampicillin and an aminoglycoside should be initiated and continued until results of cultures are available.

Therapy for pertussis is with erythromycin administered orally. Antibiotic therapy may lessen the symptoms of pertussis if administered early in the paroxysmal stage and is valuable for rendering the patient noncontagious. Hyperimmune serum probably is not beneficial.

Finally, an association between bronchopulmonary dysplasia and respiratory colonization by species of *Ureaplasma* or *Mycoplasma* has received considerable attention. A few case reports have suggested that eradication of *Ureaplasma* with erythromycin contributes to faster resolution of symptoms and to better outcome for neonates with this chronic disease.[7, 150, 337] Controlled studies are needed to verify these preliminary observations. There is no experience with the use of new macrolides in neonates.

References

1. Aber, R. C., Allen, N., Howell, J. T., et al.: Nosocomial transmission of group B streptococci. Pediatrics *58*:346, 1976.
2. Ablow, R. C., Driscoll, S. G., Effmann, E. L., et al.: A comparison of early-onset group B streptococcal neonatal infection and the respiratory-distress syndrome of the newborn. N. Engl. J. Med. *294*:65, 1976.
3. Adams, J. M., Speer, M. E., and Rudolph, A. J.: Bacterial colonization of radial artery catheters. Pediatrics *65*:94, 1980.
4. Adler, S. M., and Denton, R. L.: The erythrocyte sedimentation rate in the newborn period. J. Pediatr. *86*:942, 1975.
5. Albert, S., Baldwin, R., Czekajewski, S., et al.: Bullous impetigo due to group II *Staphylococcus aureus*: An epidemic in a normal newborn nursery. Am. J. Dis. Child. *120*:10, 1970.
6. Albritton, W. L., Wiggins, G. L., and Feeley, J. C.: Neonatal listeriosis: Distribution of serotypes in relation to age at onset of disease. J. Pediatr. *88*:481, 1976.
7. Alfa, M. J., Embree J. E., Degagne P., et al.: Transmission of *Ureaplasma urealyticum* from mothers to full and preterm infants. Pediatr. Infect. Dis. J. *14*:341, 1995.
8. Allerdice, J. G., Baskett, T. F., Seshia M. M. K., et al.: Perinatal group B streptococcal colonization and infection. Am. J. Obstet. Gynecol. *142*:617, 1982.
9. Ancona, R. J., Ferrieri, P., and Williams, P. P.: Maternal factors that enhance the acquisition of group B streptococci by newborn infants. J. Med. Microbiol. *13*:273, 1980.
10. Anderson, D. C., Edwards, M. S., and Baker, C. J.: Luminol-enhanced chemiluminescence for evaluation of type III group B streptococcal opsonins in human sera. J. Infect. Dis. *141*:370, 1980.
11. Anthony, B. F., Okada, D. M., and Hobel, C. J.: Epidemiology of the group B *Streptococcus*: Maternal and nosocomial sources for infant acquisitions. J. Pediatr. *95*:431, 1979.
12. Armstrong, J. H., Zacarias, F., and Rein, M. F.: Ophthalmia neonatorum: A chart review. Pediatrics *57*:884, 1976.
13. Asmar, B. I.: Neonatal retropharyngeal cellulitis due to group B *Streptococcus*. Clin. Pediatr. *26*:183, 1987.
14. Asnes, R. S., and Arendar, G. M.: Septic arthritis of the hip: A complication of femoral venipuncture. Pediatrics *38*:837, 1966.
15. Baker, C. J.: Group B streptococcal cellulitis-adenitis in infants. Am. J. Dis. Child. *136*:631, 1982.
16. Baker, C. J., and the Neonatal IVIG Collaborative Study Group: Multicenter trial of intravenous immunoglobulin (IVIG) to present late-onset infection in preterm infants: Preliminary results. Pediatr. Res. *25*:275A, 1989.
17. Baker, C. J., and Barrett, F. F.: Transmission of group B streptococci among parturient women and their neonates. J. Pediatr. *83*:919, 1973.
18. Baker, C. J., and Barrett, F. F.: Group B streptococcal infections in infants: The importance of the various serotypes. J. A. M. A. *230*:1158, 1974.
19. Baker, C. J., Barrett, F. F., Gordon, R. C., et al.: Suppurative meningitis due to streptococci of Lancefield group B: A study of 33 infants. J. Pediatr. *82*:724, 1973.
20. Baker, C. J., Edwards, M. S., and Kasper, D. L.: Role of antibody to native type III polysaccharide of group B *Streptococcus* in infant infection. Pediatrics *68*:544, 1981.
21. Baker, C. J., and Edwards, M. S.: Group B streptococcal infections. *In* Remington, J. S., and Klein, J. O. (eds.): Infectious Diseases of the Fetus and Newborn Infants. 3rd ed. Philadelphia, W. B. Saunders, 1990, pp. 742–811.
22. Baker, C. J., and Kasper, D. L.: Correlation of maternal antibody deficiency with susceptibility to neonatal group B streptococcal infection. N. Engl. J. Med. *294*:753, 1976.
23. Baker, C. J., and Kasper, D. L.: Group B streptococcal vaccines. Rev. Infect. Dis. *7*:458, 1985.
24. Baker, C. J., Webb, B. J., Jackson, C. V., et al.: Counter-current immunoelectrophoresis in the evaluation of infants with group B streptococcal disease. Pediatrics *65*:1110, 1980.
25. Baker C. J., Melish M. E., Hall R. T., et al.: Intravenous immune globulin for the prevention of nosocomial infection in low–birth-weight neonates. N. Engl. J. Med. *327*:213, 1992.
26. Balagtas, R. C., Bell, C. E., Edwards, L. D., et al.: Risk of local and systemic infections associated with umbilical vein catheterization: A prospective study in 86 newborn patients. Pediatrics *48*:359, 1971.
27. Baley, J. E., Stork, E. K., Warkentin, P. I., et al.: Buffy coat transfusions in neutropenic neonates with presumed sepsis: A prospective, randomized trial. Pediatrics *80*:712, 1987.
28. Band, J. D., Clegg, H. W., II, Hayes, P. S., et al.: Transmission of group B streptococci: Traced by use of multiple epidemiologic markers. Am. J. Dis. Child. *135*:355, 1981.
29. Barclay, N.: High frequency of *Salmonella* species as a cause of neonatal meningitis in Ibadan, Nigeria: A review of thirty-eight cases. Acta Paediatr. Scand. *60*:540, 1971.
30. Barton, L. L., Feigin, R. D., and Lins, R.: Group B beta hemolytic streptococcal meningitis in infants. J. Pediatr. *82*:719, 1973.
31. Battisti, O., Mitchison, R., and Davies, P. A.: Changing blood culture isolates in a referral neonatal intensive care unit. Arch. Dis. Child. *56*:775, 1981.
32. Baumgart, S., Hall, S. E., Campos, J. M., et al.: Sepsis with coagulase-negative staphylococci in critically ill newborns. Am. J. Dis. Child. *137*:461, 1983.
33. Beargie, R., Lynd, P., Tucker, E., et al.: Perinatal infection and vaginal flora. Am. J. Obstet. Gynecol. *122*:31, 1975.
34. Beck-Sague, C. M., Azimi P., Fonseca, S. N., et al.: Bloodstream infections in neonatal intensive care unit patients: Results of a multicenter study. Pediatr. Infect. Dis. J. *13*:1110, 1994.
35. Becroft, D. M. O., Farmer, K., Seddon, R. J., et al.: Epidemic listeriosis in the newborn. Br. Med. J. *3*:747, 1971.
36. Beem, M. O., and Saxon, E. M.: Respiratory-tract colonization and a distinctive pneumonia syndrome in infants with *Chlamydia trachomatis*. N. Engl. J. Med. *296*:306, 1977.
37. Bennet, R., Eriksson, M., and Zetterström, R.: Increasing incidence of neonatal septicemia: Causative organisms and predisposing risk factors. Acta Paediatr. Scand. *70*:207, 1981.
38. Benuck, I., and David, R. J.: Sensitivity of published neutrophil indexes in identifying newborn infants with sepsis. J. Pediatr. *103*:961, 1983.
39. Berche, P., Reich, K. A., Bonnichon, M., et al.: Detection of anti-listeriolysin O for serodiagnosis of human listeriosis. Lancet *335*:624, 1990.
40. Bergman, I., Wald, E. R., Meyer, J. D., et al.: Epidural abscess and vertebral osteomyelitis following serial lumbar punctures. Pediatrics *72*:476, 1983.
41. Bergqvist, G., Eriksson, M., and Zetterström, R.: Neonatal septicemia and perinatal risk factors. Acta Paediatr. Scand. *68*:337, 1979.
42. Bergstrom, T., Larson, H., Lincoln, K., et al.: Studies of urinary tract infections in infancy and childhood. XII. Eighty consecutive patients with neonatal infection. J. Pediatr. *80*:858, 1972.
43. Berkovich, S., and Taranko, L.: Acute respiratory illness in the premature nursery associated with respiratory syncytial virus infections. Pediatrics *34*:753, 1964.
44. Berman, P. H., and Banker, B. Q.: Neonatal meningitis: A clinical and pathological study of 29 cases. Pediatrics *38*:6, 1966.
45. Berman, S. A., Balkany, T. J., and Simmons, M. A.: Otitis media in the neonatal intensive care unit. Pediatrics *62*:198, 1978.
46. Bettelheim, K. A., and Lennox-King, S. M. J.: The acquisition of *Escherichia coli* by new-born babies. Infection *4*:174, 1976.
47. Bland, R. D.: Otitis media in the first six weeks of life: Diagnosis, bacteriology, and management. Pediatrics *49*:187, 1972.
48. Bluestone, C. D., and Klein, J. O.: Otitis Media in Infants and Children. Philadelphia, W. B. Saunders, 1988.
49. Bonadio, W. A., Stanco, L., Bruce, R., et al.: Reference values of normal cerebrospinal fluid composition in infants ages 0 to 8 weeks. Pediatr. Infect. Dis. J. *11*:589, 1992.
50. Bourchier, D., Abbott, G. D., and Maling, T. M. J.: Radiological abnormalities in infants with urinary tract infections. Arch. Dis. Child. *59*:620, 1984.

51. Boyer, K. M., Gadzala, C. A., Kelly, P. D., et al.: Selective intrapartum chemoprophylaxis of neonatal group B streptococcal early-onset disease. III. Interruption of mother-to-infant transmission. J. Infect. Dis. *148*:810, 1983.
52. Boyer, K. M., Gadzala, C. A., Burd, L. I., et al.: Selective intrapartum chemoprophylaxis of neonatal group B streptococcal early-onset disease. I. Epidemiologic rationale. J. Infect. Dis. *148*:795, 1983.
53. Boyer, K. M., and Gotoff, S. P.: Prevention of early-onset neonatal group B streptococcal disease with selective intrapartum chemoprophylaxis. N. Engl. J. Med. *314*:1665, 1986.
54. Boyer, K. M., Papierniak, C. K., Gadzala, C. A., et al.: Transplacental passage of IgG antibody to group B *Streptococcus* serotype Ia. J. Pediatr. *104*:618, 1984.
55. Boyer, K. M., Petersen, N. J., Farzaneh, I., et al.: An outbreak of gastroenteritis due to *E. coli* 0142 in a neonatal nursery. J. Pediatr. *86*:919, 1975.
56. Brans, Y. W., Ceballos, R., and Cassady, G.: Umbilical catheters and hepatic abscesses. Pediatrics *53*:264, 1974.
57. Brook I., and Frazier, E. H.: Microbiology of scalp abscess in newborns. Pediatr. Infect. Dis. J. *11*:766, 1992.
58. Buck, C., Bundschu, J., Gallati, H., et al.: Interleukin-6: A sensitive parameter for the early diagnosis of neonatal bacterial infection. Pediatrics *93*:54, 1994.
59. Buck, G. E., Kelly, M. T., Pichanick, A. M., et al.: *Campylobacter jejuni* in newborns: A cause of asymptomatic bloody diarrhea. Am. J. Dis. Child. *136*:744, 1982.
60. Burdon, D. W., Thompson, H., Candy, D. C. A., et al.: Enterotoxin(s) of *Clostridium difficile*. Lancet 2:258, 1981.
61. Burns, R. P., and Rhodes, D. H., Jr.: *Pseudomonas* eye infection as a cause of death in premature infants. Arch. Ophthalmol. *65*:517, 1961.
62. Cairo, M. S., Rucker, R., Bennetts, G. A., et al.: Improved survival of newborns receiving leukocyte transfusions for sepsis. Pediatrics *74*:887, 1984.
62a. Cairo, M. S.: Review of G-CSF and GM-CSF effects on neonatal neutrophil kinetics. Am. J. Pediatr. Hematol. Oncol. *11*:238, 1989.
63. Cameron, D. J. S., Bishop, R. F., Veenstra, A., et al.: Nonculturable viruses and neonatal diarrhea: Fifteen-month survey in a newborn special care nursery. J. Clin. Microbiol. *8*:93, 1978.
64. Carstensen, H., Christensen, K. K., Grennert, I., et al.: Early-onset neonatal group B streptococcal septicemia in siblings. J. Infect. *17*:201, 1988.
65. Centers for Disease Control: Nosocomial infection surveillance, 1980–1982. CDC Surveillance Summaries *32*(No. 4SS):1SS, 1983.
66. Chadwick, E. G., Shulman, S. T., and Yogev, R.: Peritonitis as a late manifestation of group B streptococcal disease in newborns. Pediatr. Infect. Dis. *2*:142, 1983.
67. Champagne, S., Fussell, S., and Scheifele, D.: Evaluation of skin antisepsis prior to blood culture in neonates. Infect. Control *5*:489, 1984.
68. Champsaur, H., Questiaux, E., Prevot, J., et al.: Rotavirus carriage, asymptomatic infection, and disease in the first two years of life. I. Virus shedding. J. Infect. Dis. *149*:667, 1984.
69. Chirico, G., Rondini, G., Plebani, A., et al.: Intravenous gammaglobulin therapy for prophylaxis of infection in high-risk neonates. J. Pediatr. *110*:437, 1987.
70. Christensen, K. K., Christensen, P., Duc, G., et al.: Correlation between serum antibody-levels against group B streptococci and gestational age in newborns. Eur. J. Pediatr. *142*:86, 1984.
71. Christensen, R. D., Bradley, P. P., and Rothstein, G.: The leukocyte left shift in clinical and experimental neonatal sepsis. J. Pediatr. *98*:101, 1981.
72. Christensen, R. D., Rothstein, G., Anstall, H. B., et al.: Granulocyte transfusions in neonates with bacterial infection, neutropenia, and depletion of mature marrow neutrophils. Pediatrics *70*:1, 1982.
73. Christian, J. R.: Comparison of ocular reactions with the use of silver nitrate and erythromycin ointment in ophthalmia neonatorum prophylaxis. J. Pediatr. *57*:55, 1960.
74. Chrystie, I. L., Totterdell, B., Baker, M. J., et al.: Rotavirus infections in a maternity unit. Lancet *2*:79, 1975.
75. Clapp, D. W., Kliegman, R. M., Baley, J. E., et al.: The use of intravenously administered immune globulin to prevent nosocomial sepsis in low birth weight infants: Report of a pilot study. J. Pediatr. *115*:973, 1989.
76. Cochran, W. D., Davis, H. T., and Smith, C. A.: Advantages and complications of umbilical artery catheterization in the newborn. Pediatrics *42*:769, 1968.
77. Collado, M., Kretschmer, R. R., Becker, I., et al.: Colonization of Mexican pregnant women with group B *Streptococcus*. J. Infect. Dis. *143*:134, 1981.
78. Cooperman, M. B.: *Gonococcus* arthritis in infancy: A clinical study of forty-four cases. Am. J. Dis. Child. *33*:932, 1927.
79. Coudron, P. E., Mayhall, C. G., Facklam, R. R., et al.: *Streptococcus faecium* outbreak in a neonatal intensive care unit. J. Clin. Microbiol. *20*:1044, 1984.
80. Culver, K. W., Ammann, A. J., Partridge, J. C., et al.: Lymphocyte abnormalities in infants born to drug-abusing mothers. J. Pediatr. *111*:230, 1987.
81. Dagan, R., and Gorodischer, R.: Infections in hypothermic infants younger than 3 months old. Am. J. Dis. Child. *138*:483, 1984.
82. Dan, M.: Septic arthritis in young infants: Clinical and microbiologic correlations and therapeutic implications. Rev. Infect. Dis. *6*:147, 1984.
83. DaSilva, O., and Hammerberg, O.: Diagnostic value of leukocyte indices in late neonatal sepsis. Pediatr. Infect. Dis. J. *13*:409, 1994.
84. David, R. B., and O'Connell, E. J.: Suppurative parotitis in children. Am. J. Dis. Child. *119*:332, 1970.
85. Davis, R. C.: *Salmonella* sepsis in infancy. Am. J. Dis. Child. *135*:1096, 1981.
86. Dennison, W. M.: Haematogenous osteomyelitis of the newborn. Lancet *2*:474, 1955.
87. Dietzman, D. E., Fischer, G. W., and Schoenknecht, F. D.: Neonatal *Escherichia coli* septicemia: Bacterial counts in blood. J. Pediatr. *85*:128, 1974.
88. Dillon, H. C., Jr.: Group A type 12 streptococcal infection in a newborn nursery: Successfully treated neonatal meningitis. Am. J. Dis. Child. *112*:177, 1966.
89. Dillon, H. C., Jr., Gray, E., Pass, M. A., et al.: Anorectal and vaginal carriage of group B streptococci during pregnancy. J. Infect. Dis. *145*:794, 1982.
90. Dillon, H. C., Jr., Khane, S., and Gary, B. M.: Group B streptococcal carriage and disease: A 6-year prospective study. J. Pediatr. *110*:31, 1987.
91. Dobson, S. R. M., and Baker, C. J.: Enterococcal sepsis in neonates: Features by age at onset and occurrence of focal infection. Pediatrics *85*:165, 1990.
92. Doraiswamy, B., Hammerschlag, M. R., Pringle, G. F., et al.: Ophthalmia neonatorum caused by β-lactamase–producing *Neisseria gonorrhoeae*. JAMA *250*:790, 1983.
93. Dunham, E. C.: Septicemia in the new-born. Am. J. Dis. Child. *45*:229, 1933.
94. Dyson, A. E., and Read, S. E.: Group G streptococcal colonization and sepsis in neonates. J. Pediatr. *99*:944, 1981.
95. Easmon, C. S. F., Hastings, M. J. G., Deeley, J., et al.: The effect of intrapartum chemoprophylaxis on the vertical transmission of group B streptococci. Br. J. Obstet. Gynaecol. *90*:633, 1983.
96. Edwards, M. S., Jackson, C. V., and Baker, C. J.: Increased risk of group B streptococcal disease in twins. J. A. M. A. *245*:2044, 1981.
97. Edwards, M. S., Rench, M. A., Haffar, A. A. M., et al.: Long-term sequelae of group B streptococcal meningitis in infants. J. Pediatr. *106*:717, 1985.
98. Eitzman, D. V., and Smith, R. T.: The significance of blood cultures in the newborn period. Am. J. Dis. Child. *94*:601, 1957.
99. El-Radhi, A. S., Jawad, M. H., Mansor, N., et al.: Infection in neonatal hypothermia. Arch. Dis. Child. *58*:143, 1983.
100. Engle, W. D., and Rosenfeld, C. R.: Neutropenia in high-risk neonates. J. Pediatr. *105*:982, 1984.
101. Evanston, R. T., and Maunsell, H.: A Practical Treatise on the Management and Diseases of Children (first American edition from the first Irish edition in 1836). Philadelphia, Haswell, Barrington, and Haswell, 1838, p. 115.
102. Faden, H. S.: Early diagnosis of neonatal bacteremia by buffy-coat examination. J. Pediatr. *88*:1032, 1976.
103. Fanaroff, A. A., Korones, S. B., Wright, L. L., et al.: Controlled trial of intravenous immune-globulin to reduce nosocomial infections in very low–birth-weight infants. N. Engl. J. Med. *330*:1107–1113, 1994.
104. Feigin, R. D., Wong, M., Shackelford, P. G., et al.: Countercurrent immunoelectrophoresis of urine as well as of CSF and blood for diagnosis of bacterial meningitis. J. Pediatr. *89*:773, 1976.
105. Feldman, W. E.: Relation of concentrations of bacteria and bacterial antigen in cerebrospinal fluid to prognosis in patients with bacterial meningitis. N. Engl. J. Med. *296*:433, 1977.
106. Ferrieri, P., Cleary, P. P., and Seeds, A. E.: Epidemiology of group-B streptococcal carriage in pregnant women and newborn infants. J. Med. Microbiol. *10*:103, 1977.
107. Finelli, L., Livengood, J. R., and Saiman, L.: Surveillance of pharyngeal colonization: Detection and control of serious bacterial illness in low birth weight infants. Pediatr. Infect. Dis. J. *13*:854, 1994.
108. Fischer, G. W., Crumrine, M. H., and Jennings, P. B.: Experimental *Escherichia coli* sepsis in rabbits. J. Pediatr. *85*:117, 1974.
109. Fischer, G. W., Weisman, L. B., Hemming, V. G., et al.: Intravenous immunoglobulin in neonatal group B streptococcal disease: Pharmacokinetic and safety studies in monkeys and humans. Am. J. Med. *76*(Suppl. 3A):117, 1984.
110. Fleer, A., Senders, R. C., Visser, M. R., et al.: Septicemia due to coagulase-negative staphylococci in a neonatal intensive care unit: Clinical and bacteriological features and contaminated parenteral fluids as a source of sepsis. Pediatr. Infect. Dis. *2*:426, 1983.
111. Fleming, D. W., Cochi, S. L., MacDonald, K. L., et al.: Pasteurized milk as a vehicle of infection in an outbreak of listeriosis. N. Engl. J. Med. *312*:404, 1985.
112. Fox, L., and Sprunt, K.: Neonatal osteomyelitis. Pediatrics *62*:535, 1978.
113. Franciosi, R. A., Knostman, J. D., and Zimmerman, R. A.: Group B streptococcal neonatal and infant infections. J. Pediatr. *82*:707, 1973.
114. Freedman, R. M., Ingram, D. L., Gross, I., et al.: A half century of neonatal sepsis at Yale: 1928 to 1978. Am. J. Dis. Child. *135*:140, 1981.
115. Friedman, C. A., Wender, D. F., and Rawson, J. E.: Rapid diagnosis of group B streptococcal infection utilizing a commercially available latex agglutination assay. Pediatrics *73*:27, 1984.
116. Gardner, S. E., Yow, M. D., Leeds, L. J., et al.: Failure of penicillin to eradicate group B streptococcal colonization in the pregnant woman: A couple study. Am. J. Obstet. Gynecol. *135*:1062, 1979.
117. Gerdes, J. S., and Polin, R. A.: Sepsis screen in neonates with evaluation of plasma fibronectin. Pediatr. Infect. Dis. J. *6*:443, 1987.

118. Gezon, H. M., Schaberg, M. J., and Klein, J. O.: Concurrent epidemics of *Staphylococcus aureus* and group A *Streptococcus* disease in a newborn nursery: Control with penicillin G and hexachlorophene bathing. Pediatrics *51*:383, 1973.
119. Gibbs, R. S., Hall, R. T., Yow, M. D., et al.: Consensus: Perinatal prophylaxis for group B streptococcal infection. Pediatr. Infect. Dis. J. *11*:179, 1992.
120. Ginsburg, C. M., and McCracken, G. H., Jr.: Urinary tract infections in young infants. Pediatrics *69*:409, 1982.
121. Glode, M. P., Sutton, A., Moxon, E. R., et al.: Pathogenesis of neonatal *Escherichia coli* meningitis: Induction of bacteremia and meningitis in infant rats fed *E. coli* K1. Infect. Immun. *16*:75, 1977.
122. Gluck, L., Wood, H. F., and Fousek, M. D.: Septicemia of the newborn. Pediatr. Clin. North Am. *13*:1131, 1966.
123. Gold, R., Wilt, J. C., Adhikari, P. K., et al.: Adenoviral pneumonia and its complications in infancy and childhood. J. Can. Assoc. Radiol. *20*:218, 1969.
124. Golden, B.: Subtenon injection of gentamicin for bacterial infections of the eye. J. Infect. Dis. *124*:S271, 1971.
125. Gorbach, S. L., Menda, K. B., Thadepalli, H., et al.: Anaerobic microflora of the cervix in healthy women. Am. J. Obstet. Gynecol. *117*:1053, 1973.
126. Goscienski, P. J.: Inclusion conjunctivitis in the newborn infant. J. Pediatr. *77*:19, 1970.
127. Goscienski, P. J., and Sexton, R. R.: Follow-up studies in neonatal inclusion conjunctivitis. Am. J. Dis. Child. *124*:180, 1972.
128. Graham, D. R., Anderson, R. L., Ariel, F. E., et al.: Epidemic nosocomial meningitis due to *Citrobacter diversus* in neonates. J. Infect. Dis. *144*:203, 1981.
129. Graves, G. R., and Rhodes, P. G.: Tachycardia as a sign of early onset neonatal sepsis. Pediatr. Infect. Dis. *3*:404, 1984.
130. Gray, M. L.: Genital listeriosis as a cause of repeated abortion. Lancet *2*:315, 1960.
131. Gray, M. L.: Epidemiological aspects of listeriosis. Am. J. Public Health *53*:554, 1963.
132. Greenberg, M., and Vandow, J. E.: Ophthalmia neonatorum: Evaluation of different methods of prophylaxis in New York City. Am. J. Public Health *51*:836, 1961.
133. Greengard, J.: Acute hematogenous osteomyelitis in infancy. Med. Clin. North Am. *30*:135, 1946.
134. Groll, A. H., Meiser, A., Weise, M., et al.: Interleukin-6 as early mediator in neonatal sepsis. Pediatr. Infect. Dis. J. *11*:496, 1992.
135. Gruskay, J., Harris, M. C., Costarino, A. T., et al.: Neonatal *Staphylococcus epidermidis* meningitis with unremarkable CSF examination results. Am. J. Dis. Child. *143*:580, 1989.
136. Guerrant, R. L., Cleary, T. G., and Pickering, L. K.: Microorganisms responsible for neonatal diarrhea. *In* Remington, J. S., and Klein, J. O. (eds.): Infectious Diseases of the Fetus and Newborn Infant. 3rd ed. Philadelphia, W. B. Saunders, 1990, pp. 901–989.
137. Hague, K. N., Zaidi, M. H., Hazne, S. K., et al.: Intravenous immunoglobulin for prevention of sepsis in preterm and low birth weight infants. Pediatr. Infect. Dis. J. *5*:622, 1986.
138. Hall, S. L.: Coagulase-negative staphylococcal infections in neonates. Pediatr. Infect. Dis. J. *10*:57, 1991.
139. Hall, R. T., Barnes, W., Krishnan, et al.: Antibiotic treatment of parturient women colonized with group B streptococci. Am. J. Obstet. Gynecol. *124*:630, 1976.
140. Haltalin, K. C.: Neonatal shigellosis: Report of 16 cases and review of the literature. Am. J. Dis. Child. *114*:603, 1967.
141. Hammerschlag, M. R., Cummings, C., Roblin, P. M., et al.: Efficacy of neonatal ocular prophylaxis for the prevention of *Chlamydia* and gonococcal conjunctivitis. N. Engl. J. Med. *320*:769, 1989.
142. Hammerschlag, M. R., Herrmann, J. E., Cox, P., et al.: Prospective comparison of Chlamydiazyme to chlamydial cultures for the diagnosis of neonatal conjunctivitis. Presented at the Twenty-Fourth Interscience Conference on Antimicrobial Agents and Chemotherapy, Washington, D. C., October, 1984.
143. Hamoudi, A. C., Marcon, M. J., Cannon, H. J., et al.: Comparison of three major antigen detection methods for the diagnosis of group B streptococcal sepsis in neonates. Pediatr. Infect. Dis. *2*:432, 1983.
144. Harris, H., Wirtschafter, D., and Cassady, G.: Endotracheal intubation and its relationship to bacterial colonization and systemic infection of newborn infants. Pediatrics *58*:816, 1976.
145. Harris, M. C., Costarino, A. T., Sullivan, J. S., et al.: Cytokine elevations in critically ill infants with sepsis and necrotizing enterocolitis. J. Pediatr. *124*:105, 1994.
146. Hemming, V. G., Hall, R. T., Rhodes, P. G., et al.: Assessment of group B streptococcal opsonins in human and rabbit serum by neutrophil chemiluminescence. J. Clin. Invest. *58*:1379, 1976.
147. Hervás, J. A., Alomar, A., Salvá, F., et al.: Neonatal sepsis and meningitis in Mallorca, Spain, 1977–1991. Clin. Infect. Dis. *16*:719, 1993.
148. Hocker, J. R., Simpson, P. M., Rabalais, G. P., et al.: Extracorporeal membrane oxygenation and early-onset group B streptococcal sepsis. Pediatrics *89*:1, 1992.
149. Hood, M.: Listeriosis as an infection of pregnancy manifested in the newborn. Pediatrics *27*:390, 1961.
150. Horowitz, S., Landau, D., Shinwell, E. S., et al.: Respiratory tract colonization with *Ureaplasma urealyticum* and bronchopulmonary dysplasia in neonates in southern Israel. Pediatr. Infect. Dis. J. *11*:847, 1992.
151. Howard, J. B., and McCracken, G. H., Jr.: The spectrum of group B streptococcal infections in infancy. Am. J. Dis. Child. *128*:815, 1974.
152. Howard, J. B., and McCracken, G. H., Jr.: Reappraisal of kanamycin usage in neonates. J. Pediatr. *86*:949, 1975.
153. Isaacman, S. H., Heroman, W. M., and Lightsey, A. L.: Purpura fulminans following late-onset group B β-hemolytic streptococcal sepsis. Am. J. Dis. Child. *138*:915, 1984.
154. Jafari, H. S., Schuchat, A., Hildson, R., et al.: Barriers to prevention of perinatal group B streptococcal disease. Pediatr. Infect. Dis. J. *14*:662, 1995.
155. Johns, A. W., Kitchen, W. H., and Leslie, D. W.: Complications of umbilical vessel catheters. Med. J. Aust. *2*:810, 1972.
156. Johnson, C. E., DeBaz, B. P., Shurin, P. A., et al.: Renal ultrasound evaluation of urinary tract infection in children. Pediatrics *78*:871, 1986.
157. Jones, D. E., Kanarek, K. S., and Lim, D. V.: Group B streptococcal colonization patterns in mothers and their infants. J. Clin. Microbiol. *20*:438, 1984.
158. Jones, S. R., Smith, J. W., and Sanford, J. P.: Localization of urinary-tract infections by detection of antibody-coated bacteria in urine sediment. N. Engl. J. Med. *290*:591, 1974.
159. Kafetzis, D. A., Brater, D. C., Kapiki, A. N., et al.: Treatment of severe neonatal infections with cefotaxime: Efficacy and pharmacokinetics. J. Pediatr. *100*:483, 1982.
160. Kaijser, B., Hanson, L. A., Jodal, U., et al.: Frequency of *E. coli* K antigens in urinary-tract infections in children. Lancet *1*:663, 1977.
161. Kelsey, M. C., Lipscomb, A. P., and Mowles, J. M.: *Limulus* amoebocyte lysate endotoxin test: An aid to the diagnosis in the septic neonate? J. Infect. *4*:69, 1982.
162. Kim, K. S., and Anthony, B. F.: Penicillin tolerance in group B streptococci isolated from infected neonates. J. Infect. Dis. *144*:411, 1981.
163. King, J. C., Berman, E. D., and Wright, P. F.: Evaluation of fever in infants less than 8 weeks old. South. Med. J. *80*:948, 1987.
164. Kleiman, M. B., Reynolds, J. K., Schreiner, R. L., et al.: Rapid diagnosis of neonatal bacteremia with acridine orange-stained buffy coat smears. J. Pediatr. *105*:419, 1984.
165. Klein, J. O., Feigin, R. D., and McCracken, G. H., Jr.: Report of the task force on diagnosis and management of meningitis. Pediatrics *78*(S):959, 1986.
166. Klein, J. O., and Marcy, S. M.: Bacterial sepsis and meningitis. *In* Remington, J. S., and Klein, J. O. (eds.): Infectious Diseases of the Fetus and Newborn Infant. 3rd ed. Philadelphia, W. B. Saunders, 1990, p. 60.
167. Kline, M. W., and Mason, E. O., Jr.: Methicillin-resistant *Staphylococcus aureus*: Pediatric perspective. Pediatr. Clin. North Am. *35*:613, 1988.
168. Krauss, A. N., Albert, R. F., and Kannan, M. M.: Contamination of umbilical catheters in the newborn infant. J. Pediatr. *77*:965, 1970.
169. Kumari, S., Bhargava, S. K., Baijal, V. N., et al.: Neonatal osteomyelitis: A clinical and follow-up study. Indian Pediatr. *15*:393, 1978.
170. Larsen, B., and Galask, R. P.: Vaginal microbial flora: Practical and theoretic relevance. Obstet. Gynecol. *55*:100S, 1980.
171. Laurenti, F., Ferro, R., Isacchi, G., et al.: Polymorphonuclear leukocyte transfusion for the treatment of sepsis in the newborn infant. J. Pediatr. *98*:118, 1981.
172. Leake, D., and Leake, R.: Neonatal suppurative parotitis. Pediatrics *46*:203, 1970.
173. Lebenthal, E.: Lactose malabsorption and milk consumption in infants and children. Am. J. Dis. Child. *133*:21, 1979.
174. Leigh, L., Stoll, B. J., Rahman M., et al.: *Pseudomonas aeruginosa* infection in very low birth weight infants: A case-control study. Pediatr. Infect. Dis. J. *14*:367, 1995.
175. Lennon, D., Lewis, B., Mantell, C., et al.: Epidemic perinatal listeriosis. Pediatr. Infect. Dis. *3*:30, 1984.
176. Levin, J., and Bang, F. B.: Clottable protein in *Limulus*: Its localization and kinetics of its coagulation by endotoxin. Thromb. Diath. Haemorrh. *19*:186, 1968.
177. Levy, H. L., Sepe, S. J., Shih, V. E., et al.: Sepsis due to *Escherichia coli* in neonates with galactosemia. N. Engl. J. Med. *297*:1403, 1977.
178. Libby, J. M., Donta, S. T., and Wilkins, T. D.: *Clostridium difficile* toxin A in infants. J. Infect. Dis. *148*:606, 1983.
179. Lieberman, H., and Brem, J.: Syndrome of acute osteomyelitis of the superior maxilla in early infancy. N. Engl. J. Med. *260*:318, 1959.
180. Lilien, L. D., Harris, V. J., Ramamurthy, R. S., et al.: Neonatal osteomyelitis of the calcaneus: Complication of heel puncture. J. Pediatr. *88*:478, 1976.
181. Lim, M. O., Gresham, E. L., Franken, E. A., Jr., et al.: Osteomyelitis as a complication of umbilical artery catheterization. Am. J. Dis. Child. *131*:142, 1977.
182. Linnan, M. J., Mascola, L., Lou, X. D., et al.: Epidemic listeriosis associated with Mexican-style cheese. N. Engl. J. Med. *319*:823, 1988.
183. Liu, C.-H., Lehan, C., Speer, M. E., et al.: Degenerative changes in neutrophils: An indicator of bacterial infection. Pediatrics *74*:823, 1984.
184. MacFarlane, D. E.: Neonatal group B streptococcal septicemia in a developing country. Acta Pediatr. Scand. *76*:470, 1987.
185. Manroe, B. L., Rosenfeld, C. R., Weinberg, A. G., et al.: The differential

leukocyte count in the assessment and outcome of early-onset neonatal group B streptococcal disease. J. Pediatr. *91*:632, 1977.
186. Manroe, B. L., Weinberg, A. G., Rosenfeld, C. R., et al.: The neonatal blood count in health and disease. I. Reference values for neutrophilic cells. J. Pediatr. *95*:89, 1979.
187. Marchant, C. D., Shurin, P. A., Turczyk, V. A., et al.: Course and outcome of otitis media in early infancy: A prospective study. J. Pediatr. *104*:826, 1984.
188. Marcy, S. M.: Bacterial infections of the bones and joints. *In* Remington, J. S., and Klein, J. O. (eds.): Infectious Diseases of the Fetus and Newborn Infant. 3rd ed. Philadelphia, W. B. Saunders, 1990, p. 674.
189. Marild, S., Wettergren, B., Hellstrom, M., et al.: Bacterial virulence and inflammatory response in infants with febrile urinary tract infection or screening bacteriuria. J. Pediatr. *112*:348, 1988.
190. Mathieu, P. L.: Comparison study: Silver nitrate and oxytetracycline in newborn eyes: A comparison of the incidence of conjunctivitis following the instillation of silver nitrate or oxytetracycline into the eyes of newborn infants. Am. J. Dis. Child. *95*:609, 1958.
191. McCracken, G. H., Jr.: Intraventricular treatment of neonatal meningitis due to gram-negative bacilli. J. Pediatr. *91*:1037, 1977.
192. McCracken, G. H., Jr., and Mize, S. G.: A controlled study of intrathecal antibiotic therapy in gram-negative enteric meningitis of infancy: Report of the Neonatal Cooperative Study Group. J. Pediatr. *89*:66, 1976.
193. McCracken, G. H., Jr., Mize, S. G., and Threlkeld, N.: Intraventricular gentamicin therapy in gram-negative bacillary meningitis of infancy: Report of the Second Neonatal Meningitis Cooperative Study Group. Lancet *1*:787, 1980.
194. McCracken, G. H., Jr., Mustafa, M. M., Ramilo, O., et al.: Cerebrospinal fluid interleukin-1β and tumor necrosis factor concentrations and outcome from neonatal gram-negative enteric bacillary meningitis. Pediatr. Infect. Dis. J. *8*:155, 1989.
195. McCracken, G. H., Jr., and Nelson, J. D.: Antimicrobial Therapy for Newborns. 2nd ed. New York, Grune & Stratton, 1983.
196. McCracken, G. H., Jr., Sarff, L. D., Glode, M. P., et al.: Relation between *Escherichia coli* K1 capsular polysaccharide antigen and clinical outcome in neonatal meningitis. Lancet *2*:246, 1974.
197. McCracken, G. H., Jr., Sarff, L. D., Robbins, J. B., et al.: Ontogeny of serum and secretory K1 antibodies. Presented to the American Pediatric Society, St. Louis, April, 1976.
198. McCracken, G. H., Jr., and Shinefield, H. R.: Changes in the pattern of neonatal septicemia and meningitis. Am. J. Dis. Child. *112*:33, 1966.
199. McCracken, G. H., Jr., Threlkeld, N., Mize, S., et al.: Moxalactam therapy for neonatal meningitis due to gram-negative enteric bacilli: A prospective controlled evaluation. J. A. M. A. *252*:1427, 1984.
200. Melish, M. E., and Glasgow, L. A.: Staphylococcal scalded skin syndrome: The expanded clinical syndrome. J. Pediatr. *78*:958, 1971.
201. Melish, M. E., Glasgow, L. A., and Turner, M. D.: The staphylococcal scalded-skin syndrome: Isolation and partial characterization of the exfoliative toxin. J. Infect. Dis. *125*:129, 1972.
202. Merenstein, G. B., Todd, W. A., Brown, G., et al.: Group B β-hemolytic *Streptococcus:* Randomized controlled treatment study at term. Obstet. Gynecol. *55*:315, 1980.
203. Middelton, P. J.: Pathogenesis of rotaviral infection. J. Am. Vet. Med. Assoc. *173*:544, 1978.
204. Middelton, P. J., Szymanski, M. T., and Petric, M.: Viruses associated with acute gastroenteritis in young children. Am. J. Dis. Child. *131*:733, 1977.
205. Mok, P. M., Reilly, B. J., and Ash, J. M.: Osteomyelitis in the neonate. Radiology *145*:677, 1982.
206. Monto, A. S., Brandt, B. L., and Artenstein, M. S.: Response of children to *Neisseria meningitidis* polysaccharide vaccines. J. Infect. Dis. *127*:394, 1973.
207. Morales, W. J., and Lim, D. V.: Reduction of group B streptococcal maternal and neonatal infections in preterm pregnancies with premature rupture of membranes through a rapid identification test. Am. J. Obstet. Gynecol. *157*:13, 1987.
208. Morales, W. J., Lim, D. V., and Walsh, A. F.: Prevention of neonatal group B streptococcal sepsis by the use of rapid screening test and selective intrapartum chemoprophylaxis. Am. J. Obstet. Gynecol. *155*:979, 1986.
209. Moreno, M. T., Vargas, S., Poveda, R., et al.: Neonatal sepsis and meningitis in a developing Latin American country. Pediatr. Infect. Dis. J. *13*:516, 1994.
210. Mulder, C. J. J., van Alphen, L., and Zanen, H. C.: Neonatal meningitis caused by *Escherichia coli* in the Netherlands. J. Infect. Dis. *150*:935, 1984.
211. Munson, D. P., Thompson, T. R., Johnson, D. E., et al.: Coagulase-negative staphylococcal septicemia: Experience in a newborn intensive care unit. J. Pediatr. *101*:602, 1982.
212. Mustafa, M. M., and McCracken, G. H., Jr.: Antimicrobial agents in pediatrics. Infect. Dis. Clin. North Am. *3*:491, 1989.
213. Mustafa, M. M., Mertsola, J., Ramilo, O., et al.: Increased endotoxin and interleukin-1β concentrations in cerebrospinal fluid of infants with coliform meningitis and ventriculitis associated with intraventricular gentamicin therapy. J. Infect. Dis. *160*:891, 1989.
214. Mustafa, M. M., Ramilo, O., Olsen, K. D., et al.: Tumor necrosis factor in mediating experimental *Haemophilus influenzae* type b meningitis. J. Clin. Invest. *84*:1253, 1989.
215. Nelson, D. L., Hable, K. A., and Matsen, J. M.: *Proteus mirabilis* osteomyelitis in two neonates following needle puncture: Successful treatment with ampicillin. Am. J. Dis. Child. *125*:109, 1973.
216. Nelson, J. D.: Personal communication, 1990.
217. Nelson, J. D.: Duration of neomycin therapy for enteropathogenic *Escherichia coli* diarrheal disease: A comparative study of 113 cases. Pediatrics *48*:248, 1971.
218. Nelson, J. D.: Antibiotic concentrations in septic joint effusions. N. Engl. J. Med. *284*:349, 1971.
219. Nelson, J. D.: Bilateral breast abscess due to group B *Streptococcus*. Am. J. Dis. Child. *130*:567, 1976.
220. Nelson, J. D.: The changing epidemiology of pertussis in young infants: The role of adults as reservoirs of infection. Am. J. Dis. Child. *132*:371, 1978.
221. Nelson, J. D., Dillon, Jr., H. C., and Howard, J. B.: A prolonged nursery epidemic associated with a newly recognized type of group A *Streptococcus*. J. Pediatr. *89*:792, 1976.
222. Nelson, J. D., and Peters, P. C.: Suprapubic aspiration of urine in premature and term infants. Pediatrics *36*:132, 1965.
223. Newman, R. B., Stevens, R. W., and Gaafar, H. A.: Latex agglutination test for the diagnosis of *Haemophilus influenzae* meningitis. J. Lab. Clin. Med. *76*:107, 1970.
224. Noel, G. J., and Edelson, P. J.: *Staphylococcus epidermidis* bacteremia in neonates: Further observations and the occurrence of focal infection. Pediatrics *74*:832, 1984.
225. Noya, F. J. D., Rench, M. N., Metzger, T. A., et al.: Unusual occurrence of an epidemic of type Ib/c group B streptococcal sepsis in a neonatal intensive care unit. J. Infect. Dis. *115*:1135, 1987.
226. Nyhan, W. L., and Fousek, M. D.: Septicemia of the newborn. Pediatrics *22*:268, 1958.
227. Offit, P. A., and Clarke, H. F.: Protection against rotavirus-induced gastroenteritis in a marine model by passively acquired gastrointestinal but not circulatory antibodies. J. Virol. *54*:58, 1985.
228. Ogden, J. A., and Lister, G.: The pathology of neonatal osteomyelitis. Pediatrics *55*:474, 1975.
229. Ogra, P. L., and Fishaut, M.: Human breast milk. *In* Remington, J. S., and Klein, J. O. (eds.): Infectious Diseases of the Fetus and Newborn Infant. 3rd ed. Philadelphia, W. B. Saunders, 1990, pp 68–88.
230. Ohlsson, A., Baily, T., and Takiedine, F.: Changing etiology and outcome of neonatal septicemia in Riyadh, Saudi Arabia. Acta Paediatr. Scand. *75*:540, 1986.
231. Olarte, J., and Ramos-Alvares, M.: Epidemic diarrhea in premature infants: Etiologic significance of a newly recognized type of *Escherichia coli* (0142:K86[B]:H6). Am. J. Dis. Child. *109*:436, 1965.
232. Oriel, J. D.: Ophthalmia neonatorum: Relative efficacy of current prophylactic practices and treatment. J. Antimicrob. Chemother. *14*:209, 1984.
233. Otila, E.: Studies on the cerebrospinal fluid in premature infants. Acta Paediatr. *35*(Suppl. 8):9, 1948.
234. Overall, J. C., Jr.: Neonatal bacterial meningitis: Analysis of predisposing factors and outcome compared with matched control subjects. J. Pediatr. *76*:499, 1970.
235. Overturf, G. D., and Balfour, G.: Osteomyelitis and sepsis: Severe complications of fetal monitoring. Pediatrics *55*:244, 1975.
236. Owen, C. R., Meis, A., Jackson, J. W., et al.: A case of primary cutaneous listeriosis. N. Engl. J. Med. *262*:1026, 1960.
237. Paredes, A., Wong, P., Mason, E. O., Jr., et al.: Nosocomial transmission of group B streptococci in a newborn nursery. Pediatrics *59*:679, 1977.
238. Pass, M. A., Gray, B. M., Khare, S., et al.: Prospective studies of group B streptococcal infections in infants. J. Pediatr. *95*:437, 1979.
239. Pass, M. A., Khare, S., and Dillon, H. C., Jr.: Twin pregnancies: Incidence of group B streptococcal colonization and disease. J. Pediatr. *97*:635, 1980.
240. Patamasucon, P., Rettig, P. J., Faust, K. L., et al.: Oral *v* topical erythromycin therapies for chlamydial conjunctivitis. Am. J. Dis. Child. *136*:817, 1982.
241. Patrick, M. J.: Influence of maternal renal infection on the fetus and infant. Arch. Dis. Child. *42*:208, 1967.
242. Peevy, K. J., and Wiseman, H. J.: Gallbladder distension in septic neonates. Arch. Dis. Child. *57*:75, 1982.
243. Pestalozza, G.: Otitis media in newborn infants. Int. J. Pediatr. Otorhinolaryngol. *8*:109, 1984.
244. Petrilli, E. S., d'Ablaig, G., and Ledger, W. J.: *Listeria monocytogenes* chorioamnionitis: Diagnosis by transabdominal amniocentesis. Obstet. Gynecol. *55*:5S, 1980.
245. Philip, A. G. S.: Decreased use of antibiotics using a neonatal sepsis screening technique. J. Pediatr. *98*:795, 1981.
246. Philip, A. G. S.: Detection of neonatal sepsis of late onset. J. A. M. A. *247*:489, 1982.
247. Philip, A. G. S.: Acute-phase proteins in neonatal infection. J. Pediatr. *105*:940, 1984.
248. Pichichero, M. E., and Todd, J. K.: Detection of neonatal bacteremia. J. Pediatr. *94*:958, 1979.
249. Pildes, R. S., Ramamurthy, R. S., and Vidyasagar, D.: Effect of triple dye on staphylococcal colonization in the newborn infant. J. Pediatr. *82*:987, 1973.
250. Pittard, W. B., III, Thullen, J. D., and Fanaroff, A. A.: Neonatal septic arthritis. J. Pediatr. *88*:621, 1976.

251. Placezek, M. M., and Whitelaw, A.: Early and late septicemia. Arch. Dis. Child. *58*:728, 1983.
252. Pyati, S. P., Pildes, R. S., Jacobs, N. M., et al.: Penicillin in infants weighing two kilograms or less with early-onset group B streptococcal disease. N. Engl. J. Med. *308*:1383, 1983.
253. Pylipow, M., Gaddis, M., and Kinney, J. S.: Selective intrapartum prophylaxis for group B *Streptococcus* colonization: Management and outcome of newborns. Pediatrics *93*:631, 1994.
254. Qureshi, M. E., and Puri, S. P.: Osteomyelitis after exchange transfusion. Br. Med. J. *2*:28, 1971.
255. Rahal, J. J., Jr., Hyams, P. J., Simberkoff, M. S., et al.: Combined intrathecal and intramuscular gentamicin for gram-negative meningitis: Pharmacologic study of 21 patients. N. Engl. J. Med. *290*:1394, 1974.
256. Ramamurthy, R. S., Srinivasan, G., and Jacobs, N. M.: Necrotizing fasciitis and necrotizing cellulitis due to group B *Streptococcus*. Am. J. Dis. Child. *131*:1169, 1977.
257. Ramilo, O., Mertsola, J., Mustafa, M. M., et al.: Interleukin-1β appears to mediate CSF inflammation in rabbits [Abstract No. 708]. Presented to the 29th Interscience Conference on Antimicrobial Agents and Chemotherapy, Houston, September, 1989.
258. Raucher, H. S., Newton, M. J., and Stern, R. H.: Ophthalmia neonatorum caused by penicillinase-producing *Neisseria gonorrhoeae*. J. Pediatr. *100*:925, 1982.
259. Redd, H., Christensen, R. D., and Fisher, C. W.: Circulating and storage neutrophils in septic neonatal rats treated with immunoglobulin. J. Infect. Dis. *157*:705, 1988.
260. Reed, R. K., Larter, W. E., Sieber, O. F., et al.: Peripheral nodular lesions in *Pseudomonas* sepsis: The importance of incision and drainage. J. Pediatr. *88*:977, 1976.
261. Reid, B. S., Binder, T. M.: Radiographic evaluation of children with urinary tract infections. Radiol. Clin. North Am. *26*:933, 1988.
262. Robbins, J. B., McCracken, G. H., Jr., Gotschlich, E. C., et al.: *Escherichia coli* K1 capsular polysaccharide associated with neonatal meningitis. N. Engl. J. Med. *290*:1216, 1974.
263. Rodwell, R. L., Faims, K., Taylor, K., et al.: Hematologic scoring system in early diagnosis of sepsis in neutropenic newborns. Pediatr. Infect. Dis. J. *12*:372, 1993.
264. Roine, I., Faingezicht, I., Arguedas, A., et al.: Serial serum C-reactive protein to monitor recovery from acute hematogenous osteomyelitis in children. Pediatr. Infect. Dis. J. *14*:40, 1995.
265. Rolston, K. V. I., Chandrasekar, P. H., and LeFrock, J. L.: Antimicrobial tolerance in group C and group G streptococci. J. Antimicrob. Chemother. *13*:389, 1984.
266. Rotbart, H. A., Levin, M. J., Yolken, R. H., et al.: An outbreak of rotavirus-associated neonatal necrotizing enterocolitis. J. Pediatr. *103*:454, 1983.
267. Rowe, D. S., Aicardi, E. Z., Dawson, C. R., et al.: Purulent ocular discharge in neonates: Significance of *Chlamydia trachomatis*. Pediatrics *63*:628, 1979.
268. Rowley, A. H., and Wald, E. R.: Incubation period necessary to detect bacteremia in neonates. Pediatr. Infect. Dis. J. *5*:590, 1986.
269. Rubens, C. E., Heggan, L., and Wessels, M.: A genetic marker for virulence of the type III group B streptococci [Abstract No. 1076]. Pediatr. Res. *23*:380A, 1988.
270. Rudoy, R. C., and Nelson, J. D.: Breast abscess during the neonatal period: A review. Am. J. Dis. Child. *129*:1031, 1975.
271. Ryder, R. W., McGowan, J. E., Hatch, M. H., et al.: Reovirus-like agent as a cause of nosocomial diarrhea in infants. J. Pediatr. *90*:698, 1977.
272. Sabath, L. D., Wheeler, N., Laverdiere, M., et al.: A new type of penicillin resistance of *Staphylococcus aureus*. Lancet *1*:443, 1977.
273. Sáez-Llorens, X., and Siegel, J. D.: Neonatal septicemia, meningitis, and pneumonia. *In* Gellis & Kagan's Current Pediatric Therapy. 14th ed. Philadelphia, W. B. Saunders, 1993, pp. 544–549.
274. Sáez-Llorens, X., Ah Chu, M. S., CastaZo, E., et al.: Intrapartum prophylaxis with ceftriaxone decreases rates of bacterial colonization and early-onset infection in newborns. Clin. Infect. Dis. *21*:876, 1995.
275. Sáez-Llorens, X., Vargas, S., Guerra, F., et al.: Application of new sepsis definitions to evaluate outcome of pediatric patients with severe systemic infections. Pediatr. Infect. Dis. J. *14*:557, 1995.
276. Sáez-Llorens, X., and McCracken, G. H.: Sepsis syndrome and septic shock in pediatrics: Current concepts on terminology, pathophysiology, and management. J. Pediatr. *123*:497, 1993.
277. Sáez-Llorens, X., Ramilo, O., Mustafa, M., et al.: The molecular pathophysiology of bacterial meningitis: Current concepts and therapeutic implications. J. Pediatr. *116*:671, 1990.
278. Sáez-Llorens, X., and McCracken, G. H.: Clinical pharmacology of antibacterial agents. *In* Remington, J. S., and Klein, J. O. (eds.): Infectious Diseases of the Fetus and Newborn Infant. 4th ed. Philadephia, W. B. Saunders, 1995, pp. 1287–1336.
278a. Sáez-Llorens, X., Velarde, J., and Cantón, C.: Pediatric osteomyelitis in a developing country. Clin. Infect. Dis. *19*:323, 1994.
279. Sánchez, P. J., Siegel, J. D., Cushion, N. B., et al.: Significance of a positive urine group B streptococcal latex agglutination test in neonates. J. Pediatr. *116*:601, 1990.
280. Sandström, K. I., Bell, T. A., Chandler, J. W., et al.: Microbial causes of neonatal conjunctivitis. J. Pediatr. *105*:706, 1984.
281. Sann, L., Bienvenu, F., Bienvenu, J., et al.: Evolution of serum prealbumin, C-reactive protein, and orosomucoid in neonates with bacterial infection. J. Pediatr. *105*:977, 1984.
282. Sarff, L. D., McCracken, G. H., Jr., Schiffer, M. S., et al.: Epidemiology of *Escherichia coli* K1 in healthy and diseased newborns. Lancet *1*:1099, 1975.
283. Sarff, L. D., Platt, L. H., and McCracken, G. H., Jr.: Cerebrospinal fluid evaluation in neonates: Comparison of high-risk infants with and without meningitis. J. Pediatr. *88*:473, 1976.
284. Sarman, G., Moise, A. A., and Edwards, M. S.: Meningeal inflammation in neonatal gram-negative bacteremia. Pediatr. Infect. Dis. J. *14*:701, 1995.
285. Schaad, U. B., McCracken, G. H., Jr., Threlkeld, N., et al.: Clinical evaluation of a new broad-spectrum oxa-beta-lactam antibiotic, moxalactam, in neonates and infants. J. Pediatr. *98*:129, 1981.
286. Schaad, U. B., Kaplan, S. L., and McCracken, G. H.: Steroid therapy for bacterial meningitis. Clin. Infect. Dis. *20*:685, 1995.
287. Scheifele, D. W., Melton, P., and Whitchelo, V.: Evaluation of the *Limulus* test for endotoxemia in neonates with suspected sepsis. J. Pediatr. *98*:899, 1981.
288. Scheld, W. M., Quagliarello, V. J., and Wispelwey, B.: The potential role of host cytokines in *Haemophilus influenzae* lipopolysaccharide-induced blood-brain barrier permeability. Pediatr. Infect. Dis. J. *8*:910, 1989.
289. Schiano, M. A., Hauth, J. C., and Gilstrap, L. C.: Second-stage fetal tachycardia and neonatal infection. Am. J. Obstet. Gynecol. *148*:779, 1984.
290. Schlech, W. F., III, Lavigne, P. M., Bortolussi, R., et al.: Epidemic listeriosis: Evidence of transmission by food. N. Engl. J. Med. *308*:203, 1983.
291. Schneerson, R., Rodrigues, L. P., Parke, J. C., Jr., et al.: Immunity to disease caused by *Hemophilus influenzae* type b. II. Specificity and some biologic characteristics of "natural," infection-acquired, and immunization-induced antibodies to the capsular polysaccharide of *Hemophilus influenzae* type b. J. Immunol. *107*:1081, 1971.
292. Schouten-Van Meeteren, N. Y., Rietveld, A., Moolenaar, A. J., et al.: Influence of perinatal conditions on C-reactive protein production. J. Pediatr. *120*:621, 1992.
293. Schuchat, A., Lizano, C., Broome, C. V., et al.: Outbreak of neonatal listeriosis associated with mineral oil. Pediatr. Infect. Dis. J. *10*:183, 1991.
294. Seeliger, H. P. R.: Listeriosis. New York, Hafner, 1961.
295. Sherman, M. P., Chance, K. H., and Goetzman, B. W.: Gram's stains of tracheal secretions predict neonatal bacteremia. Am. J. Dis. Child. *138*:848, 1984.
296. Shinefield, H. R.: Staphylococcal infections. *In* Remington, J. S., and Klein, J. O. (eds.): Infectious Diseases of the Fetus and Newborn Infant. 3rd ed. Philadelphia, W. B. Saunders, 1990, pp. 866–900.
297. Shuman, R. M., Leech, R. W., and Alvord, E. C., Jr.: Neurotoxicity of hexachlorophene in the human. I. A clinicopathologic study of 248 children. Pediatrics *54*:689, 1974.
298. Shurin, P. A., Howie, V. M., Pelton, S. I., et al.: Bacterial etiology of otitis media during the first six weeks of life. J. Pediatr. *92*:893, 1978.
299. Siegel, J. D., and McCracken, G. H., Jr.: Group D streptococcal infections. J. Pediatr. *93*:542, 1978.
300. Siegel, J. D., and McCracken, G. H., Jr.: Sepsis neonatorum. N. Engl. J. Med. *304*:642, 1981.
301. Siegel, J. D., McCracken, G. H., Jr., Threlkeld, N., et al.: Single-dose penicillin prophylaxis against neonatal group B streptococcal infection. N. Engl. J. Med. *303*:769, 1980.
302. Siegel, J. D., McCracken, G. H., Jr., Threlkeld, N., et al.: Single-dose penicillin prophylaxis of neonatal group-B streptococcal disease: Conclusion of a 41 month controlled trial. Lancet *1*:1426, 1982.
303. Siegel, J. D., Shannon, K. M., and DePasse, B. M.: Recurrent infection associated with penicillin-tolerant group B streptococci: A report of two cases. J. Pediatr. *99*:920, 1981.
304. Silver, R. P., Finn, C. W., Vann, W. F., et al.: Molecular cloning of the K1 capsular polysaccharide genes of *E. coli*. Nature *289*:696, 1981.
305. Simpson, R. A., Spencer, A. F., Speller, D. C. E., et al.: Colonization by gentamicin-resistant *Staphylococcus epidermidis* in a special care baby unit. J. Hosp. Infect. *7*:108, 1986.
306. Smith, R. T., Platou, E. S., and Good, R. A.: Septicemia of the newborn: Current status of the problem. Pediatrics *17*:549, 1956.
307. Sood, K., Mulvihill, D., and Daum, R. S.: Intrarenal abscess caused by *Klebsiella pneumoniae* in a neonate: Modern management and diagnosis. Am. J. Perinatol. *6*:367, 1989.
308. Speer, C. P., Hauptmann, D., Stubbe, P., et al.: Neonatal septicemia and meningitis in Göttingen, West Germany. Pediatr. Infect. Dis. *4*:36, 1985.
309. Spigelblatt, L., Saintonge, J., Chicoine, R., et al.: Changing pattern of neonatal streptococcal septicemia. Pediatr. Infect. Dis. *4*:56, 1985.
310. Squire, E., Favara, B., and Todd, J.: Diagnosis of neonatal bacterial infection: Hematologic and pathologic findings in fatal and nonfatal cases. Pediatrics *64*:60, 1979.
311. Squire, E. N., Jr., Reich, H. M., Merenstein, G. B., et al.: Criteria for the discontinuation of antibiotic therapy during presumptive treatment of suspected neonatal infection. Pediatr. Infect. Dis. *1*:85, 1982.
312. Stabile, A., Miceli Sopo, S., Romanelli, V., et al.: Intravenous immunoglobulin for prophylaxis of neonatal sepsis in premature infants. Arch. Dis. Child. *63*:441, 1988.
313. Steere, A. C., Aber, R. C., Warford, L. R., et al.: Possible nosocomial transmission of group B streptococci in a newborn nursery. J. Pediatr. *87*:784, 1975.

314. Stetler, H., Martin, E., Plotkin, S., et al.: Neonatal mastitis due to *Escherichia coli*. J. Pediatr. *76*:611, 1970.
315. Stevens, D. C., Kleiman, M. B., and Schreiner, R. L.: Early onset *Pseudomonas* sepsis of the neonate. Perinatol. Neonatol. *6*:75, 1982.
316. Storch, G. A., and Rajagopalan, L.: Methicillin-resistant *Staphylococcus aureus* bacteremia in children. Pediatr. Infect. Dis. J. *5*:59, 1986.
317. Storm, W.: Transient bacteremia following endotracheal suctioning in ventilated newborns. Pediatrics *65*:487, 1980.
318. Suksanong, M., and Dajani, A. S.: Detection of *Haemophilus influenzae* type b antigens in body fluids, using specific antibody-coated staphylococci. J. Clin. Microbiol. *5*:81, 1977.
319. Szanton, V. L.: Epidemic salmonellosis: A 30-month study of 80 cases of *Salmonella oranienburg* infection. Pediatrics *20*:794, 1957.
320. Tashjian, J. H., Coulam, C. B., and Washington, J. A: II. Vaginal flora in asymptomatic women. Mayo Clin. Proc. *51*:557, 1976.
321. Tetzlaff, T. R., Ashworth, C., and Nelson, J. D.: Otitis media in children less than 12 weeks of age. Pediatrics *59*:827, 1977.
322. Tetzlaff, T. R., Howard, J. B., McCracken, G. H., Jr., et al.: Antibiotic concentrations in pus and bone of children with osteomyelitis. J. Pediatr. *92*:135, 1978.
323. Thompson, R. L., Cabezudo, I., and Wenzel, R. P.: Epidemiology of nosocomial infections caused by methicillin-resistant *Staphylococcus aureus*. Ann. Intern. Med. *97*:309, 1982.
324. Thomson, J., and Lewis, I. C.: Osteomyelitis in the newborn. Arch. Dis. Child. *25*:273, 1950.
325. Tipple, M. A., Beem, M. O., and Saxon, E. M.: Clinical characteristics of the afebrile pneumonia associated with *Chlamydia trachomatis* infection in infants less than 6 months of age. Pediatrics *63*:192, 1979.
326. Totterdell, B. M., Chrystie, I. L., and Banatvala, J. E.: Cord blood and breast milk antibodies in neonatal rotavirus infection. Br. Med. J. *1*:828, 1980.
327. Tupperainen, N., Osterlund, K., and Hallman, M.: Selective intrapartum penicillin prophylaxis of early onset group B streptococcal disease. Pediatr. Res. *20*:403A, 1986.
328. UmaZa, M. A., Odio, C. M., Salas, J. L., et al.: Comparative evaluation of aztreonam/ampicillin versus amikacin/ampicillin in neonates with bacterial infections. Presented at the 27th Interscience Conference on Antimicrobial Agents and Chemotherapy, New York, October, 1987.
329. Unhanand, M., Mustafa, M. M., McCracken, G. H., et al.: Gram-negative enteric bacillary meningitis: A twenty-one–year experience. J. Pediatr. *122*:15, 1993.
330. Vawter, G. F.: Perinatal listeriosis. *In* Rosenberg, H. S., and Bernstein, J. (eds.): Perspectives in Pediatric Pathology. Vol. 6. New York, Masson Publishing, 1981, p. 153.
331. Visintine, A. M., Oleske, J. M., and Nahmias, A. J.: *Listeria monocytogenes* infection in infants and children. Am. J. Dis. Child. *131*:393, 1977.
332. Vogel, L. C., Kretschmer, R. R., Boyer, K. M., et al.: Human immunity to group B steptococci measured by indirect immunofluorescence: Correlation with protection in chick embyros. J. Infect. Dis. *140*:682, 1979.
333. Voora, S., Srinivasan, G., Lilien, L. D., et al.: Fever in full-term newborns in the first four days of life. Pediatrics *69*:40, 1982.
334. Wagener, M. M., Rycheck, R. R., Yee, R. B., et al.: Septic dermatitis of the neonatal scalp and maternal endomyometritis with intrapartum internal fetal monitoring. Pediatrics *74*:81, 1984.
335. Walker, K. M., and Coyer, W. F.: Suprarenal abscess due to group B *Streptococcus*. J. Pediatr. *94*:970, 1979.
336. Walsh, W. F., Stanley, S., Lally, K. P., et al.: *Ureaplasma urealyticum* demonstrated by open lung biopsy in newborns with chronic lung disease. Pediatr. Infect. Dis. J. *10*:823, 1991.
337. Wang, E. L., Cassell, G. H., Sánchez, P. J., et al.: *Ureaplasma urealyticum* and chronic lung disease of prematurity: Critical appraisal of the literature on causation. Clin. Infect. Dis. *17*:S112, 1993.
338. Ward, J. I., Siber, G. R., Scheifele, D. W., et al.: Rapid diagnosis of *Hemophilus influenzae* type b infections by latex particle agglutination and counterimmunoelectrophoresis. J. Pediatr. *93*:37, 1978.
339. Warren, W. S., and Stool, S. E.: Otitis media in low-birth weight infants. J. Pediatr. *79*:740, 1971.
340. Wasserman, R. L.: Unconventional therapies for neonatal sepsis. Pediatr. Infect. Dis. *2*:421, 1983.
341. Weems, J. J., Jr., Jarvis, W. R., and Colman, G.: A cluster of late onset group B streptococcal infections in low birth weight premature infants: No evidence of horizontal transmission. Pediatr. Infect. Dis. J. *5*:715, 1986.
342. Weinberg, A. G., and Laird, W. P.: Group B streptococcal endocarditis detected by echocardiography. J. Pediatr. *92*:335, 1978.
343. Weinberger, M., Haynes, R. E., and Morse, T. S.: Necrotizing fasciitis in a neonate. Am. J. Dis. Child. *123*:591, 1972.
344. Weissman, C. L. E., Stoll, B. J., Kueser, T. J., et al.: Intravenous immune globulin prophylaxis of late-onset sepsis in premature neonates. J. Pediatr. *125*:922, 1994.
345. Weissman C. L. E., Anthony B. F., Hemming, V. G., et al.: Comparison of group B streptococcal hyperimmune globulin and standard intravenously administered immune globulin in neonates. J. Pediatr. *122*:929, 1993.
346. Weissman, C. L. E., Stoll, B. J., Kueser, T. J., et al.: Intravenous immune globulin therapy for early-onset sepsis in premature neonates. J. Pediatr. *121*:434, 1992.
347. Welshimer, H. J., and Winglewish, N. G.: Listeriosis: Summary of seven cases of *Listeria* meningitis. J. A. M. A. *171*:1319, 1959.
348. Whittle, H. C., Tugwell, P., Egler, L. J., et al.: Rapid bacteriological diagnosis of pyogenic meningitis by latex agglutination. Lancet *2*:619, 1974.
349. Wientzen, R. L., McCracken, G. H., Jr., Petruska, M. L., et al.: Localization and therapy of urinary tract infections of childhood. Pediatrics *63*:467, 1979.
350. Wilson, H. D., and Haltalin, K. C.: Acute necrotizing fasciitis in childhood: Report of 11 cases. Am. J. Dis. Child. *125*:591, 1973.
351. Wiswell, T. E., and Geschke, D. W.: Risk from circumcision during the first month of life compared with those for uncircumcized boys. Pediatrics *83*:1011, 1989.
352. Wiswell, T. E., and Roscelli, J. D.: Corroborative evidence for the decreased incidence of urinary tract infections in circumcized male infants. Pediatrics *78*:96, 1986.
353. Word, B. M., and Klein, J. O.: Therapy of bacterial sepsis and meningitis in infants and children: 1989 poll of directors of programs in pediatric infectious diseases. Pediatr. Infect. Dis. J. *8*:635, 1989.
354. Yoder, M. C., Douglas, S. D., Gerdes, J., et al.: Plasma fibronectin in healthy newborn infants: Respiratory diseases syndrome and perinatal asphyxia. J. Pediatr. *102*:777, 1983.
355. Yow, M. D., Leeds, L. J., Thompson, P. K., et al.: The natural history of group B streptococcal colonization in the pregnant woman and her offspring. I. Colonization studies. Am. J. Obstet. Gynecol. *137*:34, 1980.
356. Yow, M. D., Mason, E. O., Leeds, L. J., et al.: Ampicillin prevents intrapartum transmission of group B *Streptococcus*. J. A. M. A. *241*:1245, 1979.

78

MISCELLANEOUS INFECTIONS OF THE NEWBORN

Pablo J. Sánchez

Chlamydia trachomatis Infection

Chlamydiae are obligate intracellular bacterial parasites dependent on the host cell for high-energy compounds such as adenosine triphosphate. Of the three species—*Chlamydia psittaci*, *Chlamydia pneumoniae*, and *Chlamydia trachomatis*—only the latter is a genital pathogen associated with neonatal infection.[1] *C. trachomatis* has 14 serotypes that are divided into two groups: oculogenital serovars A to K and lymphogranuloma serovars L-1 to L-3. The oculogenital serovars are divided further into trachoma serovars A to C, which cause hyperendemic blinding trachoma in the Far East, and genital serovars D to K, which result in genital and neonatal infections.

C. trachomatis is the most common sexually transmitted pathogen in the United States.[2–6] The rate of cervical colonization with *C. trachomatis* during pregnancy varies from 1 to 37 per cent, with the highest rates found in young, unmarried, nonwhite women of lower socioeconomic status.[5] Characteristically, genital chlamydial infection in women results in mucopurulent cervicitis,[6] although infection often is asymptomatic. Chlamydial infection also has been associated with ectopic pregnancy and tubal infertility.[7] Pregnant women with cervical chlamydial infection who have IgM antibody against *C. trachomatis* may be at increased risk for premature rupture of amniotic membranes and delivery of low birth weight infants.[8, 9]

TRANSMISSION

Transmission of *C. trachomatis* from an infected mother to the newborn can result in neonatal inclusion conjunctivitis as well as respiratory tract disease, including pneumonia.[1, 5] Chlamydial infection of the newborn occurs most often intrapartum during vaginal delivery by passage through an infected cervix. After delivery to a colonized mother, 53 per cent of infants born vaginally and 19 per cent of infants delivered by cesarean section will be colonized.[10] Neonatal infection after delivery by cesarean section reflects an ascending route of infection. This usually occurs after prolonged rupture of fetal membranes, but neonatal infection has been described in infants delivered by cesarean section with intact membranes at delivery.[11–13] Transplacental transmission is doubtful because *C. trachomatis* is not associated with abnormalities present at birth that are characteristic of other congenital infections and because IgM antibody directed against *C. trachomatis* has not been detected in umbilical cord blood.

Schachter and associates[14] reported that approximately two-thirds of infants delivered vaginally by mothers colonized with *C. trachomatis* will develop IgM antibody or exhibit a persistence or rise in IgG antibodies to *C. trachomatis* beyond 9 to 12 months of age. Approximately 25 to 50 per cent of exposed infants will be colonized in the conjunctivae, 25 to 50 per cent in the nasopharynx or throat, 10 to 20 per cent in the vagina, and 20 per cent in the rectum.[1, 15, 16] Initial colonization with *C. trachomatis* occurs in the conjunctiva and pharynx, and the rectum and vagina usually become colonized in the second through sixth months of life. Colonization at these sites may persist for as long as 28 months.[17] Of exposed infants, 25 to 50 per cent will develop conjunctivitis and 5 to 20 per cent will develop pneumonia.[18]

Nosocomial transmission has not been reported.

CLINICAL MANIFESTATIONS

Many infected infants have no clinical signs or symptoms suggestive of chlamydial infection.[15] The most common clinical manifestations are conjunctivitis and pneumonia.

Conjunctivitis

C. trachomatis is the most common cause of ophthalmia neonatorum in developed countries, where it causes 6 to 74 per cent (mean, 29 per cent) of neonatal conjunctivitis.[19–22] Its onset usually is 5 to 14 days after birth. It is rare in the first day of life but can occur after prolonged rupture of fetal membranes.

Clinical illness varies from a mild mucoid or watery eye discharge without significant conjunctival erythema to profuse, purulent bilateral discharge with severe chemosis and red, friable conjunctivae. In the most severe cases, the clinical findings are indistinguishable from those associated with *Neisseria gonorrhoeae* infection. Pseudomembranes may occur as inflammatory exudate adheres to the inflamed surface of the conjunctiva. Subconjunctival lymphoid hypertrophy and follicular conjunctivitis rarely occur in the neonatal period because most newborns lack lymphoid follicles. Some 19 to 83 per cent of infants with conjunctivitis have nasopharyngeal carriage of *C. trachomatis* when first examined.

Untreated chlamydial conjunctivitis usually will resolve spontaneously after several weeks to months, although ocular carriage of the organism may persist for up to 2.5 years.[17] Persistent conjunctivitis can occur and may result in mild conjunctival scars with punctate keratitis and micropannus.[23] Normal visual acuity is preserved in most cases.

Pneumonia

In 1977, *C. trachomatis* was recovered from lung biopsy, proving its ability to infect and cause pneumonia.[24] It is thought that the organism may gain access to the lower respiratory tract by either drainage of infected conjunctival secretions or direct inoculation of the nasopharynx or airway during birth. There is no evidence to support blood stream invasion.

C. trachomatis accounts for 15 to 73 per cent of afebrile pneumonia in infants between 2 and 19 weeks of age, usually occurring at 3 to 11 weeks of age.[25–29] There often is a history of conjunctivitis (80 per cent) or mucoid rhinorrhea or nasal congestion (80 per cent), followed by gradually worsening tachypnea and a characteristic staccato cough.[25, 28, 29] Most infants are afebrile or have only mild temperature elevation. On occasion, infants may present with apnea in the absence of other signs of respiratory involvement, or they may develop apnea during the course of the pneumonia.[30, 31] Auscultation of the chest reveals diffuse rales; only 16 per cent of infants have expiratory wheezes. On chest roentgenogram, hyperexpansion and diffuse bilateral interstitial infiltrates are present; lobar consolidation and pleural effusion are unusual but have been reported.[32] Blood gas values may show mild hypoxia, but carbon dioxide retention is uncommon. About half of infected infants will have middle ear abnormalities, with *C. trachomatis* isolated from some middle ear aspirates.[33] Total leukocyte count usually is normal, but 50 to 70 per cent of infants have eosinophil counts greater than $300/mm^3$. Serum levels of IgM, IgG, and IgA usually are elevated. Untreated infants gradually improve after 24 to 61 days with an average of 43 days.

Chlamydial pneumonia in premature infants may be severe and require mechanical ventilatory support resulting in chronic lung disease.[34–36] There is an increased risk of development of long-term pulmonary sequelae such as reactive airway disease, chronic cough, and abnormal pulmonary function tests in children who require hospitalization for chlamydial pneumonia in early infancy.[37]

Other

Chlamydia is an uncommon cause of myocarditis[38] and otitis media.[33] Nasopharyngeal colonization has been associated with rhinitis and nasopharyngitis with nasal congestion without rhinorrhea lasting for weeks or months.[1, 39] The clinical significance of vaginal and rectal colonization with *C. trachomatis* in infancy remains unknown.

DIAGNOSIS

The diagnosis of chlamydial infection is confirmed by inoculation of McCoy cells in tissue culture with conjunctival scrapings, nasopharyngeal secretions, pleural fluid, or lung tissue with subsequent demonstration of the characteristic intracytoplasmic inclusions by immunofluorescence microscopy. Although tissue culture is the gold standard for chlamydial diagnosis and particularly is useful for the diagnosis of pneumonia, rapid detection tests for chlamydial antigen are available for accurate diagnosis of conjunctivitis.

Conjunctivitis

Chlamydial conjunctivitis is diagnosed by sampling the inflamed lower conjunctiva and not the purulent drainage because the organism resides within the epithelial cells of the conjunctiva. Gram stain examination of the ocular discharge reveals both polymorphonuclear leukocytes and mononuclear cells. A Giemsa stain examination of a conjunctival scraping that contains a large number of epithelial cells detects chlamydial inclusions in the cytoplasm of the epithelial cells in approximately 40 per cent of cases. A monoclonal antibody directed against chlamydial elementary bodies in a direct immunofluorescent stain of conjunctival scraping has shown a sensitivity and specificity of 100 per cent.[1, 40] A second method is an enzyme-linked immunoassay that offers the advantage of semiautomation and has demonstrated sensitivity and specificity of 93 and 97 per cent, respectively, in examination of conjunctival smears.[41] Due to their ease of performance and their general availability in most clinical laboratories, these rapid tests have become the preferred methods for diagnosis of chlamydial conjunctivitis.

A microimmunofluorescence test for detection of both IgG and IgM antibodies is available.[42–45] However, serologic evaluation is not useful in the diagnosis of chlamydial conjunctivitis because most infants do not develop specific IgM antibodies and their antichlamydial IgG is of maternal origin.

Pneumonia

The diagnosis of pneumonia often is made on the basis of a typical clinical syndrome, although all attempts should be made to establish the infection either by tissue culture or rapid tests or by serology. This will allow for the identification of an infected mother and sexual partner and result in their treatment before complications occur.[4]

Rapid antigen testing of nasopharyngeal specimens for the diagnosis of pneumonia is not often helpful; the direct antigen assays have a sensitivity of 85 per cent and specificity of 75 per cent.[1, 45] It is best to perform tissue culture on available clinical specimens (e.g., nasopharyngeal and endotracheal secretions, lung tissue, pleural fluid) for optimal recovery of the organism. Schachter and Grossman[1] reported that infants with chlamydial pneumonia have a specific IgM antibody response as detected by microimmunofluorescence technique, with a titer greater than 1:64 being diagnostic of chlamydial pneumonia. They report a sensitivity and specificity of 100 per cent with the use of this test.[44] Its general lack of availability has limited the usefulness of this test in clinical practice.

Polymerase chain reaction and ligase chain reaction have been developed for the diagnosis of chlamydial infection in infants[46] and adults.[47–50] These tests amplify a region of a plasmid that is present in all strains of *C. trachomatis* and a region of the genome coding for a chlamydial outer-membrane protein. They have yielded excellent sensitivity and specificity on infant conjunctival samples and adult urine and cervical specimens. It is hoped that these tests will provide a convenient method for screening high-risk populations and help identify women with chlamydial infection so that they receive treatment before delivery. Their use in neonates has yet to be evaluated fully, although they may be helpful for diagnosis of chlamydial pneumonia.

TREATMENT

The recommended treatment for both chlamydial conjunctivitis and pneumonia is a 10- to 14-day course of either erythromycin estolate (10 mg/kg body weight every 8 hours or 15 to 20 mg/kg body weight every 12 hours) or erythromycin ethylsuccinate (13 mg/kg body weight every 8 hours) administered orally.[51, 52] The advantage of orally administered erythromycin for treatment of chlamydial conjunctivitis is the eradication of *C. trachomatis* from the nasopharynx in infants. Moreover, a shorter clinical course with lower relapse rates after oral therapy for conjunctivitis has been observed. Topical therapy alone has been associated with a failure rate of greater than 50 per cent. Topical therapy in addition to oral erythromycin is not necessary because therapeutic levels of the drug are achieved in tears after oral administration. The efficacy of oral erythromycin therapy for conjunctivitis and pneumonia has been estimated at 80 per cent. Alternative regimens include sulfisoxazole (150 mg/kg/day) and clarithromycin, which at a dosage of 7.5 mg/kg every 12 hours for 21 days showed an efficacy of 95 per cent for conjunctival and nasopharyngeal chlamydial infection.

Treatment of the mother and her sexual partner with doxycycline (100 mg twice a day for 7 days) or azithromycin (1 g orally in a single dose) is recommended at the time of diagnosis of the infant's infection.[51, 54]

PREVENTION

Current ophthalmic prophylaxis at birth does not prevent chlamydial conjunctivitis reliably, and it does not eliminate nasopharyngeal carriage and prevent pneumonia.[55–58] Hammerschlag and associates[55] reported that ophthalmic prophylaxis at birth with 1 per cent silver nitrate, 0.5 per cent erythromycin ointment, or 1 per cent tetracycline ointment resulted in 20, 14, and 11 per cent incidence, respectively, of chlamydial eye infection among 230 infants born to *Chlamydia*-infected mothers. Infants born to mothers known to have untreated chlamydial infection should be followed closely for the development of signs and symptoms suggestive of chlamydial infection or, alternatively, have screening conjunctival and nasopharyngeal chlamydial cultures performed at 7 to 14 days of age.[51]

Identification and treatment of pregnant women colonized with *C. trachomatis* and their sexual partners is believed to be the most efficacious method of preventing infection and disease in neonates.[59–61] Screening of high-risk women (younger than 25 years of age with new or multiple sexual partners) during pregnancy has been advocated, although the optimal time of such screening has not been identified. Among women infected with *N. gonorrhoeae*, presumptive therapy for chlamydial infection also should be provided because as many as 50 per cent of such individuals will have concomitant infection with *C. trachomatis*.[51]

References

1. Schachter, J., and Grossman, M.: *Chlamydia*. *In* Remington, J. S., and Klein, J. O. (eds.): Infectious Diseases of the Fetus and Newborn Infant. 4th ed. Philadelphia, W. B. Saunders, 1995, pp. 657–667.

2. Schachter, J.: Chlamydial infections. N. Engl. J. Med. *298*:428, 1978.
3. Weinstock, H., Dean, D., and Bolan, G.: *Chlamydia trachomatis* infection. Infect. Dis. Clin. North Am. *8*:797, 1994.
4. Scholes, D., Stergachis, A., Heidrich, F. R., et al.: Prevention of pelvic inflammatory disease by screening for cervical chlamydial infection. N. Engl. J. Med. *334*:1362, 1996.
5. Hammerschlag, M. R.: Chlamydial infections. J. Pediatr. *114*:727, 1989.
6. Brunham, R. C., Paavonen, J., Stevens, C. E., et al.: Mucopurulent cervicitis: The ignored counterpart in women of urethritis in men. N. Engl. J. Med. *311*:1, 1984.
7. Cates, W., Jr., Rolfs, R. T., Jr., and Aral, S. O.: Sexually transmitted disease, pelvic inflammatory disease, and infertility: An epidemiologic update. Epidemiol. Rev. *12*:199, 1990.
8. Gencay, M., Koskiniemi, M., Saikku, P., et al.: *Chlamydia trachomatis* seropositivity during pregnancy is associated with perinatal complications. Clin. Infect. Dis. *21*:424, 1995.
9. Harrison, H. R., Alexander, E. R., Weinstein, L., et al.: Cervical *Chlamydia trachomatis* and mycoplasmal infections in pregnancy. J. A. M. A. *250*:1721, 1983.
10. Bell, T. A., Stamm, W. E., Kuo, C. C., et al.: Risk of perinatal transmission of *Chlamydia trachomatis* by mode of delivery. J. Infect. *29*:165, 1994.
11. Givner, L. B., Rennels, M. B., Woodward, C. L., et al.: *Chlamydia trachomatis* infection in an infant delivered by cesarean section. Pediatrics *68*:420, 1981.
12. La Scolea, L. J., Jr., Paroski, J. S., Burzynski, L., et al.: *Chlamydia trachomatis* infection in infants delivered by cesarean section. Clin. Pediatr. *23*:118, 1984.
13. Shariot, H., Young, M., and Abedin, M.: An interesting case presentation: A possible new route for perinatal acquisition of *Chlamydia*. J. Perinatol. *12*:300, 1992.
14. Schachter, J., Grossman, M., Holt, J., et al.: Prospective study of chlamydial infection in neonates. Lancet *2*:377, 1979.
15. Schachter, J., Grossman, M., Sweet, R. L., et al.: Prospective study of perinatal transmission of *Chlamydia trachomatis*. J. A. M. A. *255*:3374, 1986.
16. Schachter, J., Grossman, M., Holt, J., et al.: Infection with *Chlamydia trachomatis*: Involvement of multiple anatomic sites in neonates. J. Infect. Dis. *139*:232, 1979.
17. Bell, T. A., Stamm, W. E., Wang, S. P., et al.: Chronic *Chlamydia trachomatis* infections in infants. J. A. M. A. *267*:400, 1992.
18. Hammerschlag, M. R., Anderka, M., Semine, D. Z., et al.: Prospective study of maternal and infantile infection with *Chlamydia trachomatis*. Pediatrics *64*:142, 1979.
19. Chandler, W. J., Alexander, E. R., Pheiffer, T. A., et al.: Ophthalmia neonatorum associated with maternal chlamydial infections. Trans. Am. Acad. Ophthalmol. Otolaryngol. *83*:302, 1977.
20. Frommell, G. T, Rothenberg, R., Wang, S.-P., et al.: Chlamydial infection of mothers and their infants. J. Pediatr. *95*:28, 1979.
21. Rowe, S., Aicardi, E., Dawson, C. R., et al.: Purulent ocular discharge in neonates: Significance of *Chlamydia trachomatis*. Pediatr. Pediatr. *63*:628, 1979.
22. Dannevig, L., Straume, B., and Melby, K.: Ophthalmia neonatorum in northern Norway. II. Microbiology with emphasis on *Chlamydia trachomatis*. Acta Ophthalmol. 19, 1992.
23. Mordhorst, C. H., and Dawson, C.: Sequelae of neonatal inclusion conjunctivitis and associated disease in parents. Am. J. Ophthalmol. *71*:861, 1971.
24. Frommell, G. T., Bruhn, F. W., and Schwartzman, J. D.: Isolation of *Chlamydia trachomatis* from infant lung tissue. N. Engl. J. Med. *296*:1150, 1977.
25. Beem, M. O., and Saxon, E. M.: Respiratory tract colonization and a distinctive pneumonia syndrome in infants infected with *Chlamydia trachomatis*. N. Engl. J. Med. *296*:306, 1977.
26. Arth, C., Von Schmidt, B., Grossman, M., et al.: Chlamydial pneumonitis. J. Pediatr. *93*:447, 1978.
27. Schachter, J., Lum, L., Gooding, C. A., et al.: Pneumonitis following inclusion blennorrhea. J. Pediatr. *87*:779, 1975.
28. Tipple, M., Beem, M. O., and Saxon, E.: Clinical characteristics of the afebrile pneumonia associated with *Chlamydia trachomatis* infection in infants less than 6 months of age. Pediatrics *63*:192, 1979.
29. Harrison, H. R., English, M. G., Lee, C. K., et al.: *Chlamydia trachomatis* infant pneumonitis: Comparison with matched controls and other infant pneumonitis. N. Engl. J. Med. *298*:702, 1978.
30. Cohen, S. D., Azimi, P. H., and Schachter, J.: *Chlamydia trachomatis* associated with severe rhinitis and apneic episodes in a one-month-old infant. Clin. Pediatr. *21*:498, 1982.
31. Brayden, R. M., Paisley, J. W., Lauer, B. A., et al.: Apnea in infants with *Chlamydia trachomatis* pneumonia. Pediatr. Infect. Dis. J. *6*:423, 1987.
32. Stutman, H. R., Rettig, P. H., and Reyes, S.: *Chlamydia trachomatis* as a cause of pneumonitis and pleural effusion. J. Pediatr. *104*:588, 1984.
33. Hammerschlag, M. R., Hammerschlag, P. E., and Alexander, E. R.: The role of *Chlamydia trachomatis* in middle ear effusions in children. Pediatrics *66*:615, 1980.
34. Mardh, P. A., Johansson, P. J. H., and Svenningsen, N.: Intrauterine lung infection with *Chlamydia trachomatis* in a premature infant. Acta Paediatr. Scand. *73*:569, 1984.
35. Attenburrow, A. A., and Barker, C. M.: Chlamydial pneumonia in the low-birthweight neonate. Arch. Dis. Child. *60*:1169, 1985.
36. Sollecito, D., Midulla, M., Bavastrelli, M., et al.: *Chlamydia trachomatis* in neonatal respiratory distress of very preterm babies: Biphasic clinical picture. Acta Paediatr. *81*:788, 1992.
37. Weiss, S. G., Newcomb, R. W., and Beem, M. O.: Pulmonary assessment of children after chlamydial pneumonia in infancy. J. Pediatr. *108*:659, 1986.
38. Ringel, R. E., Givner, L. B., Brenner, J. I., et al.: Myocarditis as a complication of infantile *Chlamydia trachomatis* pneumonitis. Clin. Pediatr. *22*:631, 1983.
39. Shinkwin, C. A., and Gibbin, K. P.: Neonatal upper airway obstruction caused by chlamydial rhinitis. J. Laryngol. Otol. *109*:58, 1995.
40. Bell, T. A., Kuo, C. C., Stamm, W. E., et al.: Direct fluorescent monoclonal antibody stain for rapid detection of infant *Chlamydia trachomatis* infections. Pediatrics *74*:224, 1984.
41. Hammerschlag, M. R., Herrmann, J. E., Cox, P., et al.: Enzyme immunoassay for diagnosis of neonatal chlamydial conjunctivitis. J. Pediatr. *107*:741, 1985.
42. Wang, S.-P., Grayston, J. T., Alexander, E. R., et al.: Simplified microimmunofluorescence test with trachoma–lymphogranuloma venereum *(Chlamydia trachomatis)* antigens for use as a screening test for antibody. J. Clin. Microbiol. *1*:250, 1975.
43. Yong, E. C., Chinn, J. S., Caldwell, H. D., et al.: Reticulate body as a single antigen in *Chlamydia trachomatis* serology with microimmunofluorescence. J. Clin. Microbiol. *10*:351, 1979.
44. Schachter, J., Grossman, M, and Azimi, P. H.: Serology of *Chlamydia trachomatis* in infants. J. Infect. Dis. *146*:530, 1982.
45. Paisley, J. W., Lauer, B. A., Melinkovich, P., et al.: Rapid diagnosis of *Chlamydia trachomatis* pneumonia in infants by direct immunofluorescence microscopy of nasopharyngeal secretions. J. Pediatr. *109*:653, 1986.
46. Talley, A. R., Garcia-Ferrer, F., Laycock, K. A., et al.: Comparative diagnosis of neonatal chlamydial conjunctivitis by polymerase chain reaction and McCoy cell culture. Am. J. Ophthalmol. *117*:50, 1994.
47. Skulnick, M., Chua, R., Simor, A. E., et al.: Use of the polymerase chain reaction for the detection of *Chlamydia trachomatis* from endocervical and urine specimens in an asymptomatic low-prevalence population of women. Diagn. Microbiol. Infect. Dis. *20*:195, 1994.
48. Martin, J. L., Alexander, S. Y., Selwood, T. S., et al.: Use of the polymerase chain reaction for the detection of *Chlamydia trachomatis* in clinical specimens and its comparison to commercially available tests. Genitourin. Med. *71*:169, 1995.
49. Schachter, J., Stamm, W. E., Quinn, T. C., et al.: Ligase chain reaction to detect *Chlamydia trachomatis* infection of the cervix. J. Clin. Microbiol. *32*:2540, 1994.
50. Lee, H. H., Chernesky, M. A., Schachter, J., et al.: Diagnosis of *Chlamydia trachomatis* genitourinary infection in women by ligase chain reaction assay of urine. Lancet *345*:213, 1995.
51. Centers for Disease Control and Prevention: 1993 sexually transmitted diseases treatment guidelines. M. M. W. R. *42*:50, 1993.
52. Beem, M. O., Saxon, E. M., and Tipple, M.: Treatment of chlamydial pneumonia in infancy. Pediatrics *63*:198, 1979.
53. Hess, D. L.: *Chlamydia* in the neonate. Neonat. Network *12*:9, 1993.
54. Martin, D. H., Mroczkowski, T. F., Dalu, Z. A., et al.: A controlled trial of a single dose of azithromycin for the treatment of chlamydial urethritis and cervicitis: The Azithromycin for Chlamydial Infections Study Group. N. Engl. J. Med. *327*:921, 1992.
55. Hammerschlag, M. R., Cummings, C., Roblin, P. M., et al.: Efficacy of neonatal ocular prophylaxis for the prevention of chlamydial and gonococcal conjunctivitis. N. Engl. J. Med. *320*:769, 1989.
56. Chen, J.-Y.: Prophylaxis of ophthalmia neonatorum: Comparison of silver nitrate, tetracycline, erythromycin and no prophylaxis. Pediatr. Infect. Dis. J. *11*:1026, 1992.
57. Bell, T. A., Sandstrom, K. I., Gravett, M. G., et al.: Comparison of ophthalmic silver nitrate solution and erythromycin ointment for prevention of natally acquired *Chlamydia trachomatis*. Sex. Transm. Dis. *14*:195, 1987.
58. Zanoni, D., Isenberg, S. J., and Apt, L.: A comparison of silver nitrate with erythromycin for prophylaxis against ophthalmia neonatorum. Clin. Pediatr. *31*:295, 1992.
59. Schachter, J., Sweet, R. L., Grossman, M., et al.: Experience with the routine use of erythromycin for chlamydial infections in pregnancy. N. Engl. J. Med. *314*:276, 1986.
60. Weber, J. T., and Johnson, R. E.: New treatments for *Chlamydia trachomatis* genital infection. Clin. Infect. Dis. *20*(Suppl. 1):S66, 1995.
61. Turrentine, M. A., and Newton, E. R.: Amoxicillin or erythromycin for the treatment of antenatal chlamydial infection: A meta-analysis. Obstet. Gynecol. *86*:1021, 1995.

Genital *Mycoplasma* Infections

The genital mycoplasmas consist of *Mycoplasma hominis*, *Mycoplasma fermentans*, *Mycoplasma genitalium*, and *Urea-*

plasma urealyticum (T-strain *Mycoplasma*), with only *M. hominis* and *U. urealyticum* being of clinical significance in neonatal disease.[1] Mycoplasmas are the smallest free-living microorganisms and are characterized by the lack of a cell wall. Serologic studies have demonstrated seven serotypes of *M. hominis* and at least 14 serotypes of *U. urealyticum*. *M. hominis* and *U. urealyticum* are sexually transmitted organisms accounting for female urogenital colonization rates of 20 to 50 per cent and 40 to 80 per cent, respectively.[2–4] Colonization rates are similar among pregnant and nonpregnant women. Colonization has been associated with younger age, lower socioeconomic status, sexual activity with multiple sexual partners, black ethnicity, and oral contraceptive use.

Cervicovaginal colonization with *U. urealyticum* and *M. hominis* is not predictive of such adverse pregnancy outcomes as prematurity, low birth weight, and spontaneous abortion.[5, 6] However, each organism appears capable of invading the upper genital tract, as evidenced by their isolation from endometrium,[7] placenta,[8, 9] amniotic fluid,[10–15] and even blood[16] in a subpopulation of women. *U. urealyticum* has been associated strongly with histologic chorioamnionitis, postpartum fever, and endometritis.[5, 11, 17–20] *M. hominis* is a recognized cause of pelvic inflammatory disease, postpartum septicemia, and endometritis.[1, 21–24] It also has been associated with surgical wound infection after cesarean delivery.[25, 26] The role of these organisms in causing spontaneous abortion and premature birth, however, remains controversial and currently unproved.[27]

TRANSMISSION

Vertical transmission of *U. urealyticum* and *M. hominis* from a colonized mother to the newborn occurs in utero or during delivery.[28–30] The relative frequency of occurrence at each time-point is not known. In utero transmission occurs either transplacentally or by an ascending route from a colonized maternal genital tract, and it is supported by the isolation of mycoplasmas from maternal blood at the time of delivery, umbilical cord blood, amniotic fluid, endometrium, chorioamnion, placenta, and aborted fetal tissue and by the detection of specific IgM antibody response in neonatal serum. Mycoplasmas also have been isolated from mucosal surfaces of newborn infants delivered by cesarean section performed before the onset of labor and rupture of amniotic membranes.[31, 32] Acquisition of mycoplasmas by newborn infants also can occur at the time of delivery through contact with a colonized birth canal. Postpartum or nosocomial transmission probably occurs, but definitive proof is lacking. It has been suggested by the finding of initial ureaplasmal colonization at 3 to 4 weeks of age in some infants who previously had been shown not to be colonized with *U. urealyticum* while in a neonatal intensive care unit (NICU).[32]

The rate of vertical transmission of *U. urealyticum* is 45 to 55 per cent in full-term and 58 per cent in preterm infants.[28, 31, 32] Similar data are lacking for *M. hominis*. The rate of vertical transmission is not affected by method of delivery or duration of rupture of membranes; colonization of infants occurs despite cesarean delivery with intact fetal membranes. Vertical transmission is increased significantly in the presence of chorioamnionitis and intraamniotic infection.[34, 35] Colonization of newborn infants increases with decreasing gestational age and birth weight, and it is highest among infants weighing less than 1000 g at birth.[32] Female newborns also are more likely than males to be colonized with *U. urealyticum* due to the vagina being a common site of colonization.[33, 36]

Colonization with *U. urealyticum* persists through early infancy; 68, 33, and 37 per cent of full-term newborns colonized in the throat, eye, and vagina, respectively, still are colonized at 3 months of age.[31] However, most lose colonization by 2 years of age.[36] Among preterm infants, 65 per cent remain colonized at discharge from the NICU or at 28 days of life.[32] Overall, the prevalence of ureaplasmal colonization varies from 2 to 86 per cent among infants admitted to NICUs, and as many as 14 to 41 per cent of infants have endotracheal aspirate cultures positive for *U. urealyticum*.[28, 37, 38] Ultimately, however, mycoplasmal colonization of newborns will depend on the prevalence of maternal colonization in that population.

CLINICAL MANIFESTATIONS

The role of *U. urealyticum* and *M. hominis* in neonatal disease continues to be investigated and defined. *M. hominis* and *U. urealyticum* have been recovered from the lungs, brain, heart, and viscera of aborted fetuses and stillborn infants, with histologic findings of bronchopneumonia present in the lungs of these fetuses.[39, 40] The genital mycoplasmas also have been isolated from blood, urine, cerebrospinal fluid, and lung tissue of newborn infants with clinical signs of infection. Because these organisms frequently colonize mucosal surfaces of newborns,[41] it often is difficult to ascribe disease. However, their isolation from normally sterile body fluids has led to their recognition as neonatal pathogens.

The following clinical associations with *U. urealyticum* have been made: (1) isolation of *U. urealyticum* from blood in as many as 34 per cent of infants younger than 34 weeks of gestational age[42] and 26 per cent of preterm infants with positive endotracheal aspirate cultures for *U. urealyticum*[43]; (2) fatal neonatal pneumonia in a term infant documented by isolation of the organism from lung at autopsy and demonstration of elevated serum IgG and IgM titers to *U. urealyticum* in the infant[44]; (3) pneumonia and persistent pulmonary hypertension in five infants from whom *U. urealyticum* was isolated from blood, endotracheal aspirate, pleural fluid, and/or lung at autopsy[45]; (4) afebrile pneumonitis in infants younger than 3 months of age[46]; (5) development of chronic lung disease in low birth weight infants whose respiratory tracts are colonized with *U. urealyticum* in the first week of life[43, 47–53]; (6) isolation of *U. urealyticum* from lung biopsy tissue of four infants with chronic lung disease[54]; (7) isolation of *U. urealyticum* from the cerebrosphinal fluid of both preterm and full-term infants[55–61]; (8) osteomyelitis of the femur in association with isolation of *U. urealyticum* from blood in a preterm infant[62]; (9) nonimmune hydrops fetalis in a newborn at 32 weeks' gestation in which *U. urealyticum* was isolated from bronchial secretions, lung, and brain at autopsy[63]; and (10) scalp abscess at the site of an internal fetal electrode monitor.[64]

The potential role of *U. urealyticum* in neonatal pneumonia[65–67] has been strengthened by the production of histologic evidence of pneumonia in lungs of newborn mice and premature baboons using ureaplasmal isolates obtained from pleural fluid, lung biopsy samples, and lung tissue of infants with pneumonia.[1, 68, 69] Crouse and colleagues[70] demonstrated that pneumonia is produced in newborn mice but significantly less in those older than 14 days of age and is potentiated by oxygen therapy. Moreover, *U. urealyticum* has been shown to induce ciliostasis and mucosal lesions in human fetal tracheal organ cultures.[1]

Isolation of *U. urealyticum* from endotracheal secretions, nasopharynx, throat, and/or gastric aspirate also has been associated with chronic lung disease of prematurity. A meta-analysis performed by Wang and associates[71] involving 17 publications supported a significant association between ureaplasmal colonization and subsequent development of chronic lung disease, even with the use of surfactant therapy for respiratory distress syndrome. Crouse and colleagues[72, 73] have shown that among infants who weigh 1250 g at birth or less and who have respiratory disease, those colonized with *U. urealyticum* in their tracheal secretions have radiographic evidence of more severe pulmonary disease than those who are not colonized. The isolation of *U. urealyticum* from lungs of infants with chronic lung disease by Walsh and associates[54] also implies an invasive bacterial process as part of the pathogenesis of lung injury. However, the possibility of ureaplasmal colonization of the respiratory tract inducing an inflammatory response without direct pulmonary invasion cannot be excluded. It has been supported by the finding of elevated levels of interleukins-6 and -8 in tracheal secretions of colonized infants[1, 74] as well as by elevated white blood cell counts and eosinophilia among infants colonized with *U. urealyticum* in their respiratory tracts.[75, 76] Anecdotally, it is believed by some investigators that it is the *Ureaplasma*-colonized infants who respond best to steroid therapy for bronchopulmonary dysplasia (Crouse, D. T., personal communication).

M. hominis has been associated with neonatal septicemia,[1, 77] meningitis,[45, 55, 78–84] pneumonia,[77] pericarditis,[85] and conjunctivitis.[86] Other manifestations of infection with *M. hominis* are brain and scalp abscess, ventriculitis, submandibular adenitis, and abscesses of the subcutaneous tissue.[87–89]

Both *U. urealyticum* and *M. hominis* have been isolated from the cerebrospinal fluid of both full-term and preterm infants. Their repeated isolation from cerebrospinal fluid and their ability to result in cerebrospinal fluid pleocytosis consisting of a polymorphonuclear or mononuclear cellular response, hypoglycorrhachia, and elevated protein content in predominantly preterm infants with suspected meningitis support their role in causing neonatal meningitis. Waites and coworkers[55] have noted hemiplegia, hydrocephalus, and developmental delay among survivors. The isolation of *U. urealyticum* from the cerebrospinal fluid of preterm infants also has been associated with severe intraventricular hemorrhage.[55, 90] However, primarily among full-term infants, isolation of *U. urealyticum* and *M. hominis* often has been associated with minimal if any cerebrospinal fluid abnormalities, and the infants do well without specific antimicrobial therapy.[58–60, 91, 92] In these instances, their isolation remains of unclear clinical significance, and their role in producing disease is questionable.

The clinical significance of the isolation of genital mycoplasmas from urine obtained by suprapubic bladder aspiration in infants remains to be determined.[93] In these instances, analysis of the urinary sediment has been normal.

DIAGNOSIS

The diagnosis of mycoplasmal infection is made by the isolation of the organism from a normally sterile body fluid or suppurative focus. Because colonization of newborn infants with mycoplasmas occurs frequently, an etiologic role for these agents cannot be supported by isolation from mucosal surfaces only. Genital mycoplasmas may be isolated on special broth and solid media that are commercially available. Shepard 10 broth and A8 agar have been employed successfully for cultivation of both *U. urealyticum* and *M. hominis*.[1] Cultures generally become positive within 2 to 5 days. *M. hominis* but not *U. urealyticum* may be identified presumptively on blood agar as tiny pinpoint colonies.

Cassell and associates[1, 94] have recommended that mucosal specimens be obtained with a Dacron or calcium alginate swab and placed in a specific mycoplasmal transport medium such as Shepard 10B broth. Specimens should be refrigerated at 4° C until transported to the laboratory and protected from drying. Alternatively, specimens in appropriate transport media can be frozen at −70° C because both *U. urealyticum* and *M. hominis* are stable for long periods under these conditions. Specimens should be diluted serially in 10B broth to at least 10^{-3} (preferably to 10^{-5}) in order to overcome any potential inhibitory substances or metabolites, and an aliquot of the original sample and dilution should be plated directly onto A8 agar. Body fluids (e.g., blood, cerebrospinal fluids, pleural fluid) should be inoculated into 10B broth in an approximately 1:10 ratio (usually 0.1 mL of fluid per 0.9 mL of 10B broth). Blood should be collected free of anticoagulants. Broth cultures and agar plates are incubated under 95 per cent nitrogen and 5 per cent carbon dioxide. The presence of mycoplasmal growth in 10B medium is indicated by a color change from yellow to pink, which is due to an alkaline shift in the media due to either the urease activity of ureaplasmas or arginine hydrolysis by *M. hominis*. Growth of mycoplasmas in broth cultures as indicated by color change should be confirmed by inoculation of a broth specimen onto A8 agar. Characteristic colonies of *U. urealyticum* and *M. hominis* can be identified readily on A8 agar after 24 to 72 hours of incubation.

Serologic tests have been used to measure antibody to genital mycoplasmas. These include metabolic-inhibition assay, enzyme-linked immunoassay, mycoplasmacidal test, indirect hemagglutination, indirect immunofluorescence, and IgG and IgM immunoblotting.[1, 95–97] The use of these tests for the diagnosis of mycoplasmal infection in infants remains problematic and is not well established. None are commercially available, and in newborns, diagnosis rests on culture results.

Polymerase chain reaction utilizing the urease structural gene or the MB (multiple-banded) ureaplasmal surface antigen has been used to detect *U. urealyticum* in neonatal clinical specimens.[98–99a] On endotracheal secretions, Blanchard and associates[98] have reported a sensitivity of 100 per cent and specificity of 99 per cent, compared with ureaplasmal culture.

TREATMENT

The decision to treat an infant for possible mycoplasmal infection should be based on the clinical symptomatology and culture results. In general, isolation of mycoplasmas from a normally sterile site in an ill neonate is an indication for consideration of treatment. The problem lies in that there are no clinical trials to determine the efficacy of treatment in neonates and there is very little experience on which to base treatment decisions, choice of drug, and duration of therapy.

In preterm infants with clinical evidence of sepsis in whom routine bacterial and viral cultures are sterile and the infant is not responding to antibacterial or antiviral therapy, the diagnosis should be suspected and appropriate cultures for mycoplasmas obtained. Also, cerebrospinal fluid from neonates who have abnormal indices but whose cultures are sterile should be cultured for mycoplasmas. Recovery of mycoplasmas from endotracheal secretions is not diagnostic of pneumonia, and the majority of these infants do not require any antimycoplasmal therapy. However, if pneumonia is suspected and the infant's clinical condition is deteriorating, a trial of therapy may be indicated, although the efficacy of treatment remains unknown. Likewise, treatment of very low birth weight infants who have respiratory tract colonization with *U. urealyticum* in order to prevent chronic lung disease cannot be recommended at present. Steroid therapy for chronic lung disease has been administered to colonized infants without resulting in disseminated ureaplasmal infection.

Mycoplasmas are not susceptible to antimicrobial agents routinely used to treat neonatal infections.[100–103] Because mycoplasmas lack a cell wall, they are insensitive to penicillins, cephalosporins, polymyxins, sulfonamides, and vancomycin. Although they may have moderate sensitivity to the aminoglycosides, the minimum inhibitory concentrations (MICs) of these agents for the genital mycoplasmas usually are too high for therapeutic use. The drugs of choice for treatment of infection due to *M. hominis* are chloramphenicol, clindamycin, doxycycline, and tetracycline; for treatment of ureaplasmal infections, erythromycin, doxycycline, tetracycline, and chloramphenicol are recommended.[103, 104] Whenever possible, antibiotic susceptibility testing should be performed on all clinically significant isolates because multidrug resistance occurs.

M. hominis is resistant to erythromycin. High-level resistance of *U. urealyticum* to erythromycin (MIC $\geq$ 32 μg/mL) is very infrequent. Cardiac toxicity consisting of acute cardiorespiratory deterioration possibly secondary to cardiac arrhythmias has been reported among neonates treated with intravenous erythromycin lactobionate for presumed ureaplasmal pneumonia.[105] Ototoxicity also has been seen in adults but not in neonates.[106] Although the exact duration of therapy is not known, a 10- to 14-day course seems reasonable when there is associated clinical improvement and microbiologic eradication during that period.

Azithromycin and clarithromycin are active against both *U. urealyticum* and *M. hominis,* but their use in neonates has not been evaluated.[104] When given orally to very low birth weight infants colonized with *U. urealyticum*, serum levels of clarithromycin at a dose of 7.5 mg/kg every 12 hours were subtherapeutic (personal observation, unpublished data).

PREVENTION

Erythromycin administered between 26 and 35 weeks' gestation to pregnant women colonized with *U. urealyticum* has not been effective in reducing adverse outcomes such as preterm delivery, low birth weight, or premature rupture of membranes.[6] Because erythromycin therapy is not effective in eliminating *U. urealyticum* from the lower genital tract, it most likely also will not prevent neonatal ureaplasmal colonization. Its effect on prevention of neonatal disease has not been studied. It also is not known whether administration of an antiureaplasmal agent such as erythromycin to very low birth weight infants colonized with *U. urealyticum* will prevent or ameliorate chronic lung disease of prematurity.

References

1. Cassell, G. H., Waites, K. B., and Crouse, D. T.: Mycoplasmal infections. *In* Remington, J. S., and Klein, J. O. (eds.): Infectious Diseases of the Fetus and Newborn Infant. 4th ed. Philadelphia, W. B. Saunders, 1995, pp. 619–655.
2. Braun, P., Klein, J. O., Lee, Y. H., et al.: Methodologic investigations and prevalence of genital mycoplasmas in pregnancy. J. Infect. Dis. *121*:391, 1970.
3. Taylor-Robinson, D., and McCormack, W. M.: The genital mycoplasmas. N. Engl. J. Med. *302*:1003, 1980.
4. McCormack, W. M., Rosner, B., Alpert, S, et al.: Vaginal colonization with *Mycoplasma hominis* and *Ureaplasma urealyticum*. Sex. Transm. Dis. *134*:67, 1986.
5. Cassell, G. H., Waites, K. B., Watson, H. L., et al.: *Ureaplasma urealyticum* intrauterine infection: Role in prematurity and disease in newborns. Clin. Microbiol. Rev. *6*:69, 1993.
6. Eschenbach, D. A., Nugent, R. P., Rao, A. V., et al.: A randomized placebo-controlled trial of erythromycin for the treatment of *Ureaplasma urealyticum* to prevent premature delivery. Am. J. Obstet. Gynecol. *164*:734, 1991.
7. Lamey, J. R., Foy, H. M., and Kenny, G. E.: Infection with *Mycoplasma hominis* and T-strains in the female genital tract. Obstet. Gynecol. *44*:703, 1974.
8. Embree, J. E., Krause, V. W., Embil, J. A., et al.: Placental infection with *Mycoplasma hominis* and *Ureaplasma urealyticum:* Clinical correlation. Obstet. Gynecol. *56*:475, 1980.
9. Kundsin, R. B., Driscoll, S. G., Monson, R. R., et al.: Association of *Ureaplasma urealyticum* in the placenta with perinatal morbidity and mortality. N. Engl. J. Med. *310*:941, 1984.
10. Cassell, G. H., Davis, R. O., Waites, K. B., et al.: Isolation of *Mycoplasma hominis* and *Ureaplasma urealyticum* from amniotic fluid at 16–20 weeks gestation. Potential effect on pregnancy outcome. Sex. Transm. Dis. *10*:294, 1983.
11. Cassell, G. H., Waites, K. B., Gibbs, R. S., et al.: The role of *Ureaplasma urealyticum* in amnionitis. Pediatr. Infect. Dis. J. *5*(Suppl.):247, 1986.
12. Thomsen, A. C., Taylor-Robinson, D., Hanson, K. B., et al.: The infrequent occurrence of mycoplasmas in amniotic fluid from women with intact fetal membranes. Acta Obstet. Gynecol. Scand. *3*:425, 1983.
13. Gray, D. J., Robinson, H. B., Malone, J., et al.: Adverse outcome in pregnancy following amniotic fluid isolation of *Ureaplasma urealyticum.* Prenat. Diagn. *12*:111, 1992.
14. Foulon, W., Naessens, A., Dewaele, M., et al.: Chronic *Ureaplasma urealyticum* amnionitis associated with abruptio placentae. Obstet. Gynecol. *68*:280, 1986.
15. Horowitz, S., Mazor, M., Romero, R., et al.: Infection of the amniotic cavity with *Ureaplasma urealyticum* in the midtrimester of pregnancy. J. Reprod. Med. *40*:375, 1995.
16. Caspi, E., Herczeg, E., Solomon, F., et al.: Amnionitis and T strain mycoplasmemia. Am. J. Obstet. Gynecol. *111*:1102, 1971.
17. Cassell, G. H., Clyde, W. A., Kenny, G. E., et al.: Ureaplasmas of humans with emphasis on maternal and neonatal infections. Pediatr. Infect. Dis. J. *6*(Suppl.):S221, 1986.
18. Sompolinsky, D., Solomon, F., Leiba, H., et al.: Puerperal sepsis due to T-strain *Mycoplasma*. Isr. J. Med. Sci. *7*:745, 1971.
19. Andrews, W., Shah, S., Goldenberg, R., et al.: Post-cesarean endometritis: Role of asymptomatic antenatal colonization of the chorioamnion with *Ureaplasma urealyticum*. Am. J. Obstet. Gynecol. *170*:416, 1994.
20. Andrews, W. W., Shah, S. R., Goldenberg, R.. L., et al.: Association of post–cesarean delivery endometritis with colonization of the chorioamnion by *Ureaplasma urealyticum*. Obstet. Gynecol. *85*:509, 1995.
21. Edelin, K. C., and McCormack, W. M.: Infection with *Mycoplasma hominis* in postpartum fever. Lancet *2*:1217, 1980.
22. McCormack, W. M., Rosner, B., Lee, Y. H., et al.: Isolation of genital mycoplasmas from blood obtained shortly after vaginal delivery. Lancet *1*:596, 1975.
23. Kelly, V. N., Garland, S. M., and Gilbert, G. L.: Isolation of genital mycoplasmas from the blood of neonates and women with pelvic infection using conventional SPS-free blood culture media. Pathology *19*:277, 1987.
24. Neman-Simha, V., Renaudin, H., de Barbeyrac, B., et al.: Isolation of genital mycoplasmas from blood of febrile obstetrical-gynecologic patients and neonates. Scand. J. Infect. Dis. *24*:317, 1992.
25. Roberts, S., Maccato, M., Faro, S., et al.: The microbiology of post–cesarean wound morbidity. Obstet. Gynecol. *81*:383, 1993.
26. Maccato, M., Faro, S., and Summers, K. L.: Wound infections after cesarean section with *Mycoplasma hominis* and *Ureaplasma urealyticum*: A report of three cases. Diagn. Microbiol. Infect. Dis. *13*:363, 1990.
27. Eschenbach, D. A.: *Ureaplasma urealyticum* and premature birth. Clin. Infect. Dis. *17*(Suppl. 1):S100, 1993.
28. Sanchez, P. J.: Perinatal transmission of *Ureaplasma urealyticum*: Current concepts based on review of the literature. Clin. Infect. Dis. *17*(Suppl. 1):S107, 1993.
29. Alfa, M. J., Embree, J. E., Degagne, P., et al.: Transmission of *Ureaplasma urealyticum* from mothers to full and preterm infants. Pediatr. Infect. Dis. J. *14*:341, 1995.
30. Grattard, F., Soleihac, B., de Barbeyrac, B., et al.: Epidemiologic and molecular investigations of genital mycoplasmas from women and neonates at delivery. Pediatr. Infect. Dis. J. *14*:853, 1995.
31. Syrogiannopoulos, G. A., Kapatais-Zoumbox, K., Decavalas, G. O., et al.: *Ureaplasma urealyticum* colonization of full term infants: Perinatal acquisition and persistence during early infancy. Pediatr. Infect. Dis. J. *9*:236, 1990.
32. Sanchez, P. J., and Regan, J. A.: Vertical transmission of *Ureaplasma urealyticum* in preterm infants. Pediatr. Infect. Dis. J. *9*:398, 1990.
33. Sanchez, P., and Regan, J. A.: Vertical transmission of *Ureaplasma urealyticum* in full term infants. Pediatr. Infect. Dis. J. *6*:825, 1988.
34. Shurin, P. A., Alpert, S., Rosner, B., et al.: Chorioamnionitis and colonization of the newborn infant with genital mycoplasmas. N. Engl. J. Med. *293*:5, 1975.
35. Dinsmoor, M. J., Ramamurty, R. S., and Gibbs, R. S.: Transmission of genital mycoplasmas from mother to neonate in women with prolonged membrane rupture. Pediatr. Infect. Dis. J. *8*:483, 1989.

36. Foy, H. M., Kenny, G. E., Levinsohn, E. M., et al.: Acquisition of mycoplasmata and T-strains during infancy. J. Infect. Dis. *121*:579, 1970.
37. Dyke, M. P., Grauaug, A., Kohan, R., et al.: *Ureaplasma urealyticum* in a neonatal intensive care population. J. Paediatr. Child Health *29*:295, 1993.
38. Izraeli, S., Samra, Z., Sirota, L., et al.: Genital mycoplasmas in preterm infants: Prevalence and clinical significance. Eur. J. Pediatr. *150*:804, 1991.
39. Tafari, N., Ross, S., Naeye, R. L., et al.: *Mycoplasma* "T" strains and perinatal death. Lancet *1*:108, 1976.
40. Madan, E., Meyer, M. P., and Amortegui, A. J.: Isolation of genital mycoplasmas and *Chlamydia trachomatis* in stillborn and neonatal autopsy material. Arch. Pathol. Lab. Med. *112*:749, 1988.
41. Klein, J. O., Buckland, D. O., and Finland, M.: Colonization of newborn infants by mycoplasmas. N. Engl. J. Med. *20*:1025, 1969.
42. Ollikainen, J., Heikkaniemi, H., Korppi, M., et al.: *Ureaplasma urealyticum* infection associated with acute respiratory insufficiency and death in premature infants. J. Pediatr. *122*:756, 1993.
43. Cassell, G. H., Waites, K. B., Crouse, D. T., et al.: Association of *Ureaplasma urealyticum* infection of the lower respiratory tract with chronic lung disease and death in very low birthweight infants. Lancet *2*:240, 1988.
44. Quinn, P. A., Gillian, J. E., Markestad, T., et al.: Intrauterine infection with *Ureaplasma urealyticum* as a cause of fatal neonatal pneumonia. Pediatr. Infect. Dis. J. *4*:538, 1985.
45. Waites, K. B., Crouse, D. T., Phillips, J. G., et al.: *Ureaplasma* pneumonia and sepsis associated with persistent pulmonary hypertension of the newborn. Pediatrics *83*:84, 1991.
46. Stagno, S., Brasfield, D. M., Brown, M. B., et al.: Infant pneumonitis associated with cytomegalovirus, *Chlamydia, Pneumocystis*, and *Ureaplasma*: A prospective study. Pediatrics *68*:322, 1981.
47. Sanchez, P. J., and Regan, J. A.: *Ureaplasma urealyticum* colonization and chronic lung disease in low birth weight infants. Pediatr. Infect. Dis. J. *78*:542, 1988.
48. Wang, E. E., Frayha, H., Watts, J., et al.: The role of *Ureaplasma urealyticum* and other pathogens in the development of chronic lung disease of prematurity. Pediatr. Infect. Dis. J. *7*:547, 1988.
49. Horowitz, S., Landau, D., Shinwell, E. S., et al.: Respiratory tract colonization with *Ureaplasma urealyticum* and bronchopulmonary dysplasia in neonates in southern Israel. Pediatr. Infect. Dis. J. *11*:847, 1992.
50. Payne, N. R., Steinberg, S., Stefan, H., et al.: New prospective studies of the association of *Ureaplasma urealyticum* colonization and chronic lung disease. Clin. Infect. Dis. *17*(Suppl. 1):S117, 1993.
51. Wang, E. L., Cassell, G. H., Sanchez, P., et al.: *Ureaplasma urealyticum* and chronic lung disease of prematurity: Critical appraisal of the literature on causation. Clin. Infect. Dis. *17*(Suppl. 1):S112, 1993.
52. Jonsson, B., Karell, A. C., Ringertz, S., et al.: Neonatal *Ureaplasma urealyticum* colonization and chronic lung disease. Acta Paediatr. *83*:927, 1994.
53. Smyth, A. R., Shaw, N. J., Pratt, B. C., et al.: *Ureaplasma urealyticum* and chronic lung disease. Eur. J. Pediat. *152*:931, 1993.
54. Walsh, W. F., Stanley, S., Lally, K. P., et al.: *Ureaplasma urealyticum* demonstrated by open lung biopsy in newborns with chronic lung disease. Pediatr. Infect. Dis. J. *10*:823, 1991.
55. Waites, K. B., Rudd, P. T., Crouse, D. T., et al.: Chronic *Ureaplasma urealyticum* and *Mycoplasma hominis* infections of central nervous systems in preterm infants. Lancet *2*:17, 1988.
56. Garland, S., and Murton, L. J.: Neonatal meningitis caused by *Ureaplasma urealyticum*. Pediatr. Infect. Dis. J. *6*:868, 1987.
57. Hentschel, J., Abele-Horn, M., and Peters, J.: *Ureaplasma urealyticum* in the cerebrospinal fluid of a premature infant. Acta Paediatr. Scand. *82*:690, 1993.
58. Waites, K. B., Duffy, L. B., Crouse, D. T., et al.: Mycoplasmal infection of cerebrospinal fluid in newborn infants from a community hospital population. Pediatr. Infect. Dis. J. *9*:241, 1990.
59. Valencia, G. B., Banzon, F., Cummings, M., et al.: *Mycoplasma hominis* and *Ureaplasma urealyticum* in neonates with suspected infection. Pediatr. Infect. Dis. J. *12*:571, 1993.
60. Neal, T. J., Roe, M. F., and Shaw, N. J.: Spontaneously resolving *Ureaplasma urealyticum* meningitis. Eur. J. Pediatr. *153*:342, 1994.
61. Stahelin-Massik, J., Levy, F., Friderich, P., et al.: Meningitis caused by *Ureaplasma urealyticum* in a full term neonate. Pediatr. Infect. Dis. J. *13*:419, 1994.
62. Gjuric, G., Prislin-Muskic, M., Nikolic, E., et al.: *Ureaplasma urealyticum* osteomyelitis in a very low birth weight infant. J. Perinat. Med. *22*:79, 1994.
63. Ollikainen, J., Hiekkaniemi, H., Korppi, M., et al.: Hydrops fetalis associated with *Ureaplasma urealyticum*. Acta Paediatr. Scand. *81*:851, 1992.
64. Hamrick, H. J., and Mangum, M. E.: *Ureaplasma urealyticum* abscess at site of an internal fetal heart rate monitor. Pediatr. Infect. Dis. J. *12*:410, 1993.
65. Gannon, H.: *Ureaplasma urealyticum* and its role in neonatal lung disease. Neonat. Network *12*:13, 1993.
66. Brus, F., van Waarde, W. M., Schoots, C., et al.: Fatal ureaplasmal pneumonia and sepsis in a newborn infant. Eur. J. Pediatr. *150*:782, 1991.
67. Gjuric, G., Prislin-Muskic, M., Zurga, B., et al.: *Ureaplasma urealyticum* infection in newborns: Three case reports. Eur. J. Pediatr. *152*:599, 1993.
68. Walsh, W. F., Butler, J., Coalson, J., et al.: A primate model of *Ureaplasma urealyticum* infection in the premature infant with hyaline membrane disease. Clin. Infect. Dis. *17*(Suppl. 1):S158, 1993.
69. Rudd, P. T., Cassell, G. H., Waites, K. B., et al.: Experimental production of *Ureaplasma urealyticum* pneumonia and demonstration of age-related susceptibility. Infect. Immun. *57*:918, 1989.
70. Crouse, D. T., Cassell, G. H., Waites, K. B., et al.: Hyperoxia potentiates *Ureaplasma urealyticum* pneumonia in newborn mice. Infect. Immun. *58*:3487, 1990.
71. Wang, E. E. L., Ohlsson, A., and Kellner, J. D.: Association of *Ureaplasma urealyticum* colonization with chronic lung disease of prematurity: Results of a metaanalysis. J. Pediatr. *127*:640, 1995.
72. Crouse, D. T., Odrezin, G. T., Cutter, G. R., et al.: Radiographic changes associated with tracheal isolation of *Ureaplasma urealyticum* in a neonatal intensive care population. J. Paediatr. Child Health *29*:295, 1993.
73. Crouse, D. T., Odrezin, G. T., Cutter, G. R., et al.: Radiographic changes associated with tracheal isolation of *Ureaplasma urealyticum* from neonates. Clin. Infect. Dis. *17*(Suppl. 1):S122–S130, 1993.
74. Stancombe, B. B., Walsh, W. F., Derdak, S., et al.: Induction of human neonatal pulmonary fibroblast cytokines by hyperoxia and *Ureaplasma urealyticum*. Clin. Infect. Dis. *17*(Suppl. 1):S154, 1993.
75. Ohlsson, A., Wang, E., and Vearncombe, M.: Leukocyte counts and colonization with *Ureaplasma urealyticum* in preterm neonates. Clin. Infect. Dis. *17*(Suppl. 1):S144, 1993.
76. Panero, A., Pacifico, L., Rossi, N., et al.: *Ureaplasma urealyticum* as a cause of pneumonia in preterm infants: Analysis of the white cell response. Arch. Dis. Child. Fetal Neonat. Educ. *73*:F37–F40, 1995.
77. Unsworth, P. F., Taylor-Robinson, D., Sho, E. E., et al.: Neonatal mycoplasmemia: *Mycoplasma hominis* as a significant cause of disease? J. Infect. *10*:163, 1985.
78. Mardh, P. A.: *Mycoplasma hominis* infection of the central nervous system in newborn infants. Sex. Transm. Dis. *10*:332, 1983.
79. McDonald, J. C.: *Mycoplasma hominis* meningitis in a premature infant. Pediatr. Infect. Dis. J. *7*:795, 1988.
80. Siber, G. R., Alpert, S., Smith, D. L., et al.: Neonatal central nervous system infection due to *Mycoplasma hominis*. J. Pediatr. *90*:625, 1977.
81. Kirk, N., and Kovar, I.: *Mycoplasma hominis* meningitis in a preterm infant. J. Infect. *15*:109, 1987.
82. Hjelm, E., Jousell, E., Linglof, T., et al.: Meningitis in a newborn infant caused by *Mycoplasma hominis*. Acta Paediatr. Scand. *68*:415, 1980.
83. Gewitz, M., Dinwiddle, R., Rees, L., et al.: *Mycoplasma hominis*: A cause of neonatal meningitis. Arch. Dis. Child. *54*:231, 1979.
84. Gilbert, G. L., Law, F., and Macinnes, S. J.: Chronic *Mycoplasma hominis* infection complicating severe intraventricular hemorrhage in a premature neonate. Pediatr. Infect. Dis. *5*:285, 1973.
85. Miller, T. C., Baman, S. I., and Albers, W. H.: Massive pericardial effusion due to *Mycoplasma hominis* in a newborn. Am. J. Dis. Child. *136*:271, 1982.
86. Jones, D. M., and Tobin, B.: Neonatal eye infections due to *Mycoplasma hominis*. Br. Med. J. *2*:467, 1968.
87. Glaser, J. B., Engelbert, M., and Hammerschlag, M.: Scalp abscess associated with *Mycoplasma hominis* infection complicating intrapartum monitoring. Pediatr. Infect. Dis. J. *2*:468, 1983.
88. Sacker, I., and Brunnell, P. A.: Abscess in newborn infants caused by *Mycoplasma*. Pediatrics *46*:303, 1970.
89. Powell, D. A., Miller, K., and Clyde, W. A., Jr.: Submandibular adenitis in a newborn caused by *Mycoplasma hominis*. Pediatrics *63*:789, 1979.
90. Ollikainen, J., Hiekkaniemi, H., Korppi, M., et al.: *Ureaplasma urealyticum* cultured from brain tissue of preterm twins who die of intraventricular hemorrhage. Scand J. Infect. Dis. *25*:528, 1993.
91. Shaw, N. J., Pratt, B. C., and Weindling, A. M.: *Ureaplasma* and *Mycoplasma* infections of the central nervous system in preterm infants. Lancet *23*:1530, 1989.
92. Heggie, A. D., Jacobs, M. R., Butler, V. T., et al.: Frequency and significance of isolation of *Ureaplasma urealyticum* and *Mycoplasma hominis* from cerebrospinal fluid and tracheal aspirate specimens from low birth weight infants. J. Pediatr. *124*:956, 1994.
93. Likitnukul, S., Kusmiesz, H., Nelson, J. D., et al.: Role of genital mycoplasmas in young infants with suspected sepsis. J. Pediatr. *109*:971, 1986.
94. Cassell, G. H., Blanchard, A., Duffy, L., et al.: Mycoplasmas. *In* Howard B. J., Klaas, J., III, Rubin S. J., et al. (eds.): Clinical and Pathogenic Microbiology. St. Louis, Mosby–Year Book, 1994, pp. 491–502.
95. Quinn, P. A., Li, H. C., Th'ng, C., et al.: Serological response to *Ureaplasma urealyticum* in the neonate. Clin. Infect. Dis. *17*(Suppl. 1):S136, 1993.
96. Dinsmoore, M. J., Ramamurthy, R. S., Cassell, G. H., et al.: Neonatal serologic response at term to the genital mycoplasmas. Pediatr. Infect. Dis. J. *8*:487, 1989.
97. Gallo, D., Dupuis, K. W., Schmidt, N. J., et al.: Broadly reactive immunofluorescence test for measurement of immunoglobulin M and G antibodies to *Ureaplasma urealyticum* in infant and adult sera. J. Clin. Microbiol. *17*:614, 1983.
98. Blanchard, A., Hentschel J., Duffy, L., et al.: Detection of *Ureaplasma urealyticum* by polymerase chain reaction in the urogenital tract of adults, in amniotic fluid, and in the respiratory tract of newborns. Clin. Infect. Dis. *17*(Suppl. 1):S148, 1993.
99. Scheurlen, W., Frauendienst, G., Schrod, L., et al.: Polymerase chain reaction–amplification of urease genes: Rapid screening for *Ureaplasma urealyticum* infection in endotracheal aspirates of ventilated newborns. Eur. J. Pediatr. *151*:740, 1992.

99a. Cunliffe, N. A., Fergusson, S., Davidson, F., et al.: Comparison of culture with the polymerase chain reaction for detection of *Ureaplasma urealyticum* in endotracheal aspirates of preterm infants. J. Med. Microbiol. *45*:27, 1996.
100. Braun, P., Klein, J. O., and Kass, E. H.: Susceptibility of *Mycoplasma hominis* and T-strains to 14 antimicrobial agents. Appl. Microbiol. *19*:62, 1970.
101. Waites, K. B., Crouse, D. T., and Cassell, G. H.: Therapeutic consideration for *Ureaplasma urealyticum* infections in neonates. Clin. Infect. Dis. *17*(Suppl. 1):S208, 1993.
102. Waites, K. B., Figarola, T. A., Schmid, T., et al.: Comparison of agar versus broth dilution techniques for determining antibiotic susceptibilities of *Ureaplasma urealyticum*. Diagn. Microbiol. Infect. Dis. *14*:265, 1991.
103. Waites, K. B., Crouse, D. T., and Cassell, G. H.: Antibiotic susceptibilities and therapeutic options for *Ureaplasma urealyticum* infections in neonates. Pediatr. Infect. Dis. J. *11*:23, 1992.
104. Waites, K. B., Sims, P. J., Crouse, D. T., et al.: Serum concentrations of erythromycin after intravenous infusion in preterm neonates treated for *Ureaplasma urealyticum* infection. Pediatr. Infect. Dis. J. *13*:287, 1994.
105. Farrar, H. C., Walsh-Sukys, M. C., Pharmd, K. K., et al.: Cardiac toxicity associated with intravenous erythromycin lactobionate: Two case reports and a review of the literature. Pediatr. Infect. Dis. J. *12*:688, 1993.
106. Crouse, D. T., Waites, K. B., Geerts, M. H., et al.: Parenteral erythromycin is not associated with hearing loss in preterm infants. Clin. Res. *39*:832A, 1991.
107. Waites, K. B., Cassell, G. H., Canupp, K. C., et al.: In vitro susceptibilities of mycoplasmas and ureaplasmas to new macrolides and aryl-fluoroquinolones. Antimicrob. Agents Chemother. *32*:1500, 1988.

Candida Infections

The improved survival of preterm infants since the early 1980s has resulted in the emergence of *Candida* as a significant pathogen in the NICU.[1–7] *Candida* species account for approximately 9 per cent of nosocomial infections in the NICU, affecting about 1 to 3 per cent of infants with birth weight less than 1500 g.[6, 8] The most frequently isolated species is *C. albicans*,[1, 6] although *C. tropicalis*,[1] *C. parapsilosis*,[9] and *C. lusitaniae*[10] also have been shown to cause neonatal infection. The disease manifestations range from the commonly encountered and relatively benign oral and cutaneous candidiasis to the more severe and even fatal congenital and systemic candidiasis. The latter, representing a disseminated form of candidal infection, remains one of the most vexing infectious problems in the NICU. Delays in recognition of infection and in institution of antifungal therapy often lead to significant morbidity and mortality among high-risk infants.[1]

TRANSMISSION

Candida may be transmitted to the fetus in utero by an ascending route from the colonized vagina of the mother. Transplacental infection has not been described. In utero transmission results in either pulmonary or mucocutaneous infection termed congenital candidiasis.[11–18] More commonly, transmission to the newborn occurs during birth from contact with an infected birth canal,[19] which results in the infant developing oral candidiasis, or thrush.[20] Subsequent colonization of the gastrointestinal tract and its presence in stool lead to superficial cutaneous infection primarily involving the perineal area.[19] Among high-risk neonates, gastrointestinal colonization also may lead to blood stream dissemination, particularly if the integrity of the intestinal mucosal lining is disrupted by surgery, ischemia, or enterocolitis.[6, 21] Candidal dissemination in neonates is aided further by the impaired ability of neonatal polymorphonuclear leukocytes to adhere to, ingest, and kill *Candida*.[7]

Candida also may be acquired by the infant during breast feeding if the mother's skin is colonized as well as from inadequate sterilization of feeding bottles and nipples.[22] Nosocomial transmission occurs, but it is believed to be uncommon except in instances of catheter-related candidemia.[7, 23–25]

Candidal colonization of the neonatal oropharynx is common, occurring in approximately 4 to 19 per cent of infants in the first few days of life. Baley and colleagues[19] in 1986 studied 146 infants with birth weight less than 1500 g during an 11-month period. She performed fungal cultures of pharynx, rectum, and endotracheal aspirate within 24 hours of birth and then weekly while in the NICU. The overall colonization rate was 27 per cent, although by 2 weeks of age, 85 per cent of infants were colonized with the majority of isolates being *Candida* species. Mucocutaneous disease developed in 28 per cent of colonized infants, while systemic candidiasis was seen in 8 per cent.

CLINICAL MANIFESTATIONS

Oral Candidiasis

Oral candidiasis is the most common form of infection.[22] Lesions on the mucous membranes of the mouth and oropharynx usually appear on the seventh to tenth day of life as whitish-gray plaques that easily are scraped from the mucosa, exposing an erythematous base but no blood. Persistent infection may be due to continued use of bottle nipples and pacifiers that have been used before initiation of antifungal therapy, as *Candida* may be recovered readily from these sources. However, the need to consider immunodeficiency states, including infection with HIV, when oral thrush fails to clear cannot be overemphasized.

Cutaneous Candidiasis

This typically is manifested by erythematous, vesiculopustular lesions found primarily on the skin of the perineum, axilla, and intertriginous areas but also can involve the axilla and periumbilical area.[22] So-called satellite lesions are common, and the peak incidence occurs at 3 to 4 months of age.

Congenital Candidiasis

This form of candidal infection presents at birth or within 24 hours of life with a widespread, erythematous maculopapular or vesiculopustular rash with or without pneumonia.[11–18] A presumptive diagnosis can be made by potassium hydroxide preparations or Gram stain of pustular or vesicular contents. *Candida* can be isolated from these skin lesions. Pneumonia as a sole manifestation of congenital candidiasis has been reported. Histologic chorioamnionitis and funisitis also may be present. Risk factors include a maternal history of vaginitis, antibiotic use, cervical cerclage, and prolonged rupture of fetal membranes, although usually none are present. Poor prognostic factors include the presence of pneumonia and prematurity. At autopsy, *Candida* has been isolated only from lung, gastrointestinal tract, and skin, and therefore hematogenous dissemination is considered to be uncommon except in preterm, low birth weight infants.

Systemic Candidiasis

Systemic candidiasis refers to the isolation of *Candida* from or its histopathologic demonstration in a normally sterile body site. Butler and Baker[6] have proposed two forms of this clinical syndrome: (1) catheter-associated sepsis in which *Candida* is isolated from the blood of infants who have central venous catheters but no evidence of focal infection or disseminated disease and (2) disseminated candidiasis in which there is fungemia in association with other foci of infection irrespective of whether the infant has a central venous catheter. Several risk factors have been associated with systemic candidiasis.[1, 6, 7, 26, 27] The most common are prematurity and very low birth weight, with its attendant impairment of host defense mechanisms, and prolonged use of broad-spectrum antimicrobial therapy. Antibiotics have a suppressive effect on normal gastrointestinal flora, with the concomitant overgrowth of *Candida*.[28] Gastrointestinal surgery and/or illness further can facilitate the passage of the fungus across the bowel mucosa and into the blood stream. Prolonged use of intravascular catheters and the use of hyperalimentation solutions also play a role in development of systemic candidiasis. Other risk factors associated with the development of candidal infections include malnutrition, prolonged endotracheal intubation, and use of corticosteroids. The early use of steroids for treatment of hypotension has been associated with development of fungal infections in extremely low birth weight infants.[29, 30] Although aminophylline is able to inhibit the candicidal activity of human granulocytes, its use has not been associated with development of neonatal fungal infection.

The clinical and laboratory signs of systemic candidiasis usually are nonspecific and resemble those seen with bacterial sepsis.[6, 7] Respiratory deterioration (74 per cent), apnea and bradycardia (60 per cent), carbohydrate intolerance (56 per cent), skin manifestations (53 per cent),[30, 31] abdominal distention (49 per cent), temperature instability (35 per cent), guaiac-positive stools (26 per cent), and hypotension (21 per cent) are the most commonly seen signs and symptoms.[6] The sites most commonly involved include blood (60 to 80 per cent), central nervous system with meningitis (40 to 60 per cent),[26, 32, 33] pneumonia (70 per cent),[1, 34, 35] renal candidiasis (60 per cent),[1, 26, 36–39] and endophthalmitis (30 per cent).[40] Other less common but significant manifestations include brain abscess, intracranial calcifications, endocarditis,[41–45] osteoarthritis,[33, 46–48] peritonitis,[49, 50] and liver abscess.

DIAGNOSIS

The diagnosis of systemic candidiasis is established by the isolation of *Candida* species in culture from a normally sterile body fluid or site. There is no reliable, sensitive, or specific rapid antigen or serologic test available to aid in its diagnosis. Therefore, it is not surprising that as many as 20 to 50 per cent of infants are diagnosed at autopsy.[1] Similarly, a mean delay of 11 days has been reported between onset of symptomatic disease and initiation of antifungal therapy.

The diagnosis often is made when a routine blood culture from an infant evaluated for possible bacterial sepsis yields a *Candida* species. *Candida* will demonstrate growth in the Bactec blood culture system that is used by the majority of clinical laboratories. However, for optimal recovery of more fastidious fungi, specific fungal blood cultures should be obtained and held in the laboratory for up to 4 weeks. On occasion, yeast may be detected in smears of blood even before incubation in culture media.[51] Reddy and colleagues[51a] have reported the usefulness of buffy coat smear and culture for detection of fungal infection in high-risk neonates. These tests showed a sensitivity of 62 and 85 per cent, respectively, and excellent specificity when compared with the recovery of fungi from routine blood culture.

In the evaluation of an infant for possible candidemia, blood cultures should be obtained from a peripheral vein or artery as well as through all intravascular catheters in place at the time. The isolation of *Candida* from blood obtained through any vascular catheter requires the prompt removal of that device.[52] *Candida* is difficult to eradicate from such catheters. Moreover, the longer these infected devices remain in place, the greater likelihood of fungal dissemination with involvement of other body sites and resulting in significant morbidity and mortality. Examination and culture of the cerebrospinal fluid (CSF) also should be performed. Abnormal CSF analysis may be the only indicator of fungal invasion of the central nervous system (CNS).[26]

Urine obtained by suprapubic bladder aspiration is an excellent source for recovery of *Candida*.[52a] Bag specimens of urine should not be used due to the high rate of perineal candidal colonization in infants. Catheterized urine specimens, although preferable to those obtained by bag, nonetheless may be contaminated due to improper cleansing of the perineum and penis. The need for obtaining an adequate urine sample from the bladder, even if by ultrasound guidance, cannot be overemphasized, because results of urine cultures will help determine the duration of antifungal therapy. Fungal culture of urine may yield candidal growth when other body fluids such as blood and CSF are sterile. A potassium hydroxide preparation of freshly obtained urine may show evidence of fungi, thereby leading to a presumptive diagnosis and early initiation of antifungal therapy.

In addition to cultures of blood, CSF, and urine, cultures of all involved sites such as joint, bone, catheter exit site, catheter tip, and abscess should be performed. In addition, peritoneal fluid from infants with necrotizing enterocolitis who require surgical intervention should be examined. If these cultures are positive, antifungal therapy should be instituted. Endotracheal fungal cultures are of questionable value due to the frequent candidal colonization of the neonatal respiratory tract. Thrombocytopenia is a frequent early finding in infants with systemic candidiasis. Additional laboratory tests such as a complete blood cell count, liver function tests, and determination of serum glucose, blood urea nitrogen, and creatinine may be helpful in assessing the degree of systemic involvement.

Infants whose cultures yield *Candida* should have further evaluation performed to detect any evidence of dissemination that will influence prognosis and duration of antifungal therapy. Ultrasonographic evaluation of the abdomen for evaluation of possible liver or splenic abscess as well as of the kidneys and bladder for evidence of fungal balls should be performed. Cranial ultrasonography may be a useful screen for CNS pathology such as hydrocephalus.[53–55] However, in infants with a positive CSF candidal culture, computed tomography of the head probably is best for detection of possible abscess or infarction. Careful ophthalmologic examination will detect endophthalmitis. Infants with a central venous catheter or persistent candidemia should have an echocardiogram performed for possible endocarditis.[42]

TREATMENT

Thrush is treated with oral nystatin suspension or gentian violet. Superficial cutaneous candidiasis is treated with topical nystatin cream. When the diaper area is involved, oral nystatin therapy may be administered as well in an attempt to eliminate the yeast from the gastrointestinal tract. Congenital candidiasis generally does not require treatment, or possibly it requires only topical antifungal therapy, except in preterm infants and those with pulmonary involvement who are at greater risk for dissemination and a poor outcome.[6, 22] In these instances, amphotericin B should be used for about 5 to 10 days until clinical signs and symptoms have resolved.

Amphotericin B remains the drug of choice for systemic candidiasis.[6, 7, 56–59] It is tolerated better in neonates than in older children and adults. The initial dose is 0.25 to 0.5 mg/kg, and it is increased by a similar amount on a daily basis until a dosage of 1 mg/kg/day is reached. No initial test dose or premedication is necessary, and it is infused over 2 to 4 hours. For severe infections, more rapid increases in daily dosages can be administered. The duration of therapy varies by the severity and type of candidal infection. For catheter-associated candidiasis in which prompt removal of the intravascular device results in rapid clinical and laboratory improvement, a cumulative dose of 7 to 10 mg/kg is sufficient.[6] However, for disseminated infection, cumulative doses of 15 to 20 mg/kg is necessary. Specifically for meningitis, 25 to 30 mg/kg cumulative dose is preferred, while for endocarditis, cumulative doses as high as 40 to 50 mg/kg have been administered.[42] Adverse effects of amphotericin B include nephrotoxicity manifested by oliguria, azotemia, and elevated serum creatinine concentration.[58, 60] Hypokalemia is common and reflects tubular injury resulting in increased urinary excretion of potassium.[6, 58] Hepatic enzyme abnormalities, anemia, and thrombocytopenia[61] have been reported but occur rarely in neonates. Similarly, neonates do not experience the fever, chills, and vomiting that are common in older individuals.

The addition of oral 5-fluorocytosine (5-FC, 100 to 150 mg/kg/day divided every 6 hours) to amphotericin B therapy has been advocated when persistent candidemia, meningitis,[62] or endocarditis occurs. Synergy of 5-FC with amphotericin B has been documented.[63] Moreover, 5-FC is well absorbed from the gastrointestinal tract and diffuses well into the CSF.[64] Side effects of 5-FC include hepatotoxicity, bone marrow suppression, and gastrointestinal intolerance as well as a hemorrhagic enterocolitis.[42, 65] These usually are the result of elevated serum levels in excess of 100 μg/mL. Because of the potential for significant toxicity, need for oral administration, and drug level monitoring, as well as excellent clinical experience with amphotericin B monotherapy,[56] the routine use of 5-FC has been discouraged and generally is used only for the most difficult to treat cases. Other antifungal agents such as liposomal amphotericin B, fluconazole, and itraconazole have been used successfully in neonates, but because of limited experience, these cannot be recommended for routine use at present.[64–74] Liposomal amphotericin B is distributed mainly to organs such as liver, spleen, and lung, which contain large numbers of reticuloendothelial cells; this preparation may be beneficial when candidal infection involves these sites.

References

1. Baley, J. E., Kliegman, R. M., and Fanaroff, A. A.: Disseminated fungal infections in very low birth weight infants: Clinical manifestations and epidemiology. Pediatrics 73:144, 1984.
2. Ho, N. K.: Systemic candidiasis in premature infants. Aust. Pediatr. J. *20*:127, 1984.
3. Johnson, D. E., Thompson, T. R., Green, T. P., et al.: Systemic candidiasis in very low-birth-weight infants (<1500 grams). Pediatrics *73*:138,1984.
4. Keller, M..A., Sellers, B..B., Melish, M..E., et al.: Systemic candidiasis in infants. Am. J. Dis. Child. *131*:1260, 1977.
5. Smith, H., and Congdon, P.: Neonatal systemic candidiasis. Arch. Dis. Child. 60:365, 1985
6. Butler, K. N., and Baker, C. J.: *Candida*: An increasingly important pathogen in the nursery. Pediatr. Clin. North Am. *35*:543, 1988.
7. Bendel, C. M., and Hostetter, M. K.: Systemic candidiasis and other fungal infections in the newborn. Semin. Pediatr. Infect. Dis. *5*:35, 1994.
8. Stoll, B. J., Gordon, T., Korones, S. B., et al.: Late-onset sepsis in very low birth weight neonates: A report from the National Institute of Child Health and Human Development Neonatal Research Network. J. Pediatr. *129*:63, 1996.
9. Faix, R. G.: Invasive neonatal candidiasis: Comparison of albicans and parapsilosis infection. Pediatr. Infect. Dis. J. *11*:88, 1992.
10. Sanchez, P. J., and Cooper, B. H.: *Candida lusitaniae:* Sepsis and meningitis in a neonate. Pediatr Infect. Dis. *6*:758, 1987.
11. Sonnenschein, H., Clark, H. L., and Taschdjian, C. L.: Congenital cutaneous candidiasis in a premature infant. Am. J. Dis. Child. *99*:81, 1960.
12. Sonnenschein, H., Taschdjian, C. L., and Clark, D. H.: Congenital cutaneous candidiasis in a premature infant. Am. J. Dis. Child. *107*:260, 1964.
13. Dvorak, A. M., and Gavaller, B.: Congenital systemic candidiasis. N. Engl. J. Med. *10*:540, 1966.
14. Jahn, C. L., and Cherry, J. D.: Congenital cutaneous candidiasis. Pediatrics *33*:440, 1966.
15. Johnson, D. E., Thompson, T. R., and Ferrieri, P.: Congenital candidiasis. Am. J. Dis. Child. *135*:273, 1981.
16. Kam, L. A., and Giaoia, G. P.: Congenital cutaneous candidiasis. Am. J. Dis. Child. *129*:1215, 1975.
17. Lopez, E. R., and Aterman, K.: Intra-uterine infection by *Candida*. Am. J. Dis. Child. *115*:663, 1968.
18. Mamlok, R. J., Richardson, C. J., Mamlok, V., et al.: A case of intrauterine pulmonary candidiasis. Pediatr. Infect. Dis. *4*:692, 1985.
19. Baley, J. E., Kliegman, R. M., Boxerbaum, B., et al.: Fungal colonization in the very low birth weight infant. Pediatrics *78*:225, 1986.
20. Anderson, N. A., Sage, D. N., and Spaulding, E. H.: Oral moniliasis in newborn infants. Am. J. Dis. Child. *67*:450, 1944.
21. Ekenna, O., and Sherertz, R. J: Factors affecting colonization and dissemination of *Candida albicans* from the gastrointestinal tract of mice. Infect. Immun. *55*:1558, 1987.
22. Miller, M. J: Fungal infections. *In* Remington, J. S., and Klein, J. O. (eds.): Infectious Diseases of the Fetus and Newborn Infant. 4th ed. Philadelphia, W. B. Saunders, 1995, pp. 703–744.
23. Vaudry, W. L., Tierney, A. J., and Wenman, W. M.: Investigation of a cluster of systemic *Candida albicans* infections in a neonatal intensive care unit. J. Infect. Dis. *158*:1375, 1988.
24. Leibovitz, E., Iuster-Reicher, A., Amitai, M., et al.: Systemic candidal infections associated with the use of peripheral venous catheters in neonates: A 9-year experience. Clin. Infect. Dis. *14*:485, 1992.
25. Sherertz, R. J., Gledhill, K. S., Hampton, K. D., et al.: Outbreak of *Candida* bloodstream infections associated with retrograde medication administration in a neonatal intensive care unit. J. Pediatr. *120*:455, 1992.
26. Faix, R. G.: Systemic *Candida* infections in infants in intensive care nurseries. High incidence of central nervous system involvement. J. Pediatr. *105*:616–6522, 1984.
27. Weese-Mayer, D. E., Fondriest, D. W., Brouillette R. T., et al.: Risk factors associated with candidemia in the neonatal intensive care unit: A case-control study. Pediatr. Infect. Dis. *6*:190, 1987.
28. Seelig, M. S.: The role of antibiotics in the pathogenesis of *Candida* infections. Am J. Med. *40*:887, 1966.
29. Botas, C. M., Kurlat, I., Young, S. M., et al.: Disseminated candidal infections and intravenous hydrocortisone in preterm infants. Pediatrics *95*:883, 1995.
30. Rowen, J. L., Atkins, J. T., Levy, M. L., et al.: Invasive fungal dermatitis in the ≤1000-gram neonate. Pediatrics *95*:682, 1995.
31. Baley, J. E., and Silverman, R. A.: Systemic candidiasis: Cutaneous manifestations in low birth weight infants. Pediatrics *82*:211, 1988.
32. Faix, R. G.: *Candida* parapsilosis meningitis in premature infant. Pediatr. Infect. Dis. 2:462, 1983.
33. Klein, J. D., Yamauchi, T., and Horlick, S. P.: Neonatal candidiasis, meningitis and arthritis: Observations and a review of the literature. J. Pediatr. *81*:31, 1972.
34. Kassner, E. G., Kauffman, S. L., Yoon, J. J., et al.: Pulmonary candidiasis in infants: Clinical, radiologic and pathologic features. A. J. R. Am. J. Roentgenol. *137*:707, 1981.
35. Patriquin, H., Lebowitz, R., Perreault, G., et al.: Neonatal candidiasis: Renal and pulmonary manifestations. A. J. R. Am. J. Roentgenol. *135*:1205, 1980.
36. Eckstein, C. J., and Kass, E. J.: Anuria in a newborn secondary to bilateral uteropelvic fungus balls. J. Urol. *127*:109, 1982.
37. Fisher, J. F., Chew, W. H., Shadomy, S., et al.: Urinary tract infections due to *Candida albicans*. Rev. Infect. Dis. *4*:1107, 1982.
38. Khan, M. Y.: Anuria from *Candida* pyelonephritis and obstructing fungal balls. Urology *21*:421, 1983.
39. Pappu, L. D., Purohit, D. M., Bradford, B. F., et al.: Primary renal candidiasis in two preterm neonates. Am. J. Dis. Child. *138*:923, 1984.
40. Baley, J. E., Annable, W. L., and Kliegman, R. M.: *Candida* endophthalmitis in the premature infant. J. Pediatr. *98*:458, 1981.
41. Faix, R. G., Feick, H. J., Frommelt, P., et al.: Successful medical treatment of *Candida parapsilosis* endocarditis in a premature infant. Am J. Perinatol. *7*:272, 1990.
42. Sanchez, P. J., Siegel, J. D., and Fishbein, J.: *Candida* endocarditis: Successful medical management in three preterm infants and review of the literature. Pediatr. Infect. Dis. J. *10*:239, 1991.
43. Zenker, P. N., Rosenberg, E. M., Van Dyke, R. B., et al.: Successful medical treatment of presumed *Candida* endocarditis in critically ill infants. J. Pediatr. *119*:472, 1991.
44. Foker, J. E., Bass, J. L., Thompson, T., et al.: Management of intracardiac fungal masses in premature infants. J. Thorac. Cardiovasc. Surg. *87*:244, 1984.
45. Johnson, D. E., Bass, J. L., Thompson, T. R., et al.: *Candida* septicemia and right atrial mass secondary to umbilical vein catheterization. Am. J. Dis. Child. *135*:275, 1981.
46. Adler, S., Randall, J., and Plotkin, S. A.: Candidal osteomyelitis and arthritis in a neonate. Am. J. Dis. Child. *123*:595, 1972.

47. Svirsky-Fein, S., Langer, L., Milbauer, B., et al.: Neonatal osteomyelitis caused by *Candida tropicalis*. J. Bone Joint Surg [Am.] *61*:455, 1979.
48. Ward, R. M., Sattler, R. F., and Dalton, A. S.: Assessment of antifungal therapy in an 800 gram infant with candidal arthritis and osteomyelitis. Pediatrics *72*:234, 1983.
49. Bayer, A. S., Blumenkrantz, M. J., Montgamerie, J. Z., et al.: *Candida* peritonitis: Report of 22 cases and review of the English literature. Am J. Med. *61*:832, 1976.
50. Johnson, D. E., Conroy, M. M., Foker, J. E., et al.: *Candida* peritonitis in the newborn infant. J. Pediatr. *97*:298, 1980.
51. Portnoy, J., Wolf, P. L., Webb, M., et al.: *Candida* blastospores and pseudohyphae in blood smears. N. Engl. J. Med. *285*:1010, 1971.
51a. Reddy, T. C. S., Chakrabarti, A., Singh, M., et al: Role of buffy coat examination in the diagnosis of neonatal candidemia. Pediatr. Infect. Dis. J. *15*:718, 1996.
52. Eppes, S. C., Troutman, J. L., and Gutman, L. T.: Outcome of treatment of candidemia in children whose central catheters were removed or retained. Pediatr. Infect. Dis. J. *8*:99, 1989.
52a. Phillips, J. R., and Karlowicz, M. G.: Prevalence of *Candida* species in hospital-acquired urinary tract infections in a neonatal intensive care unit. Pediatr. Infect. Dis. J. *16*:190, 1997.
53. Kirpekar, M., Abiri, M. M., Hilfer, C., et al.: Ultrasound in the diagnosis of systemic candidiasis (renal and cranial) in very low birth weight premature infants. Pediatr. Radiol. *16*:17, 1986.
54. Boxynski, M. E., Naglie, R. A., and Russell, E. J.: Real-time ultrasonographic surveillance in the detection of CNS involvement in systemic candidiasis. Pediatr. Radiol. *16*:235, 1986.
55. Kintanar, C., Cramer, B. C., Reid, W. D., et al.: Neonatal candidiasis: Sonographic diagnosis. A. J. R. Am. J. Roentgenol. *147*:801, 1986.
56. Butler, K. M., Rench, M. A., and Baker, C. J.: Amphotericin B as a single agent in the treatment of systemic candidiasis in neonates. Pediatr. Infect. Dis. J. *9*:51, 1990.
57. Baley, J. E., Meyers, C., Kliegman, R. M., et al.: The pharmacokinetics, outcome and toxicity of amphotericin B and 5-fluorocytosine in neonates. J. Pediatr. *116*:791, 1990.
58. Baley, J. E., Kliegman, R. M., and Fanaroff, A. A.: Disseminated fungal infections in very low birth weight infants: Therapeutic toxicity. Pediatrics *73*:152, 1984.
59. Starke, J. R., Mason, E. O., Kramer, W. G., et al.: Pharmacokinetics of amphotericin B in infants and children. J. Infect. Dis. *155*:766, 1987.
60. Cherry, J. D., Lloyd, C. A., Quilty, J. F., et al.: Amphotericin B therapy in children. J. Pediatr. *75*:1063, 1969.
61. Chan, C. S., Tuazon, C. U., and Lessin, L. S.: Amphotericin-B–induced thrombocytopenia. Ann. Intern. Med. *96*:332, 1982.
62. Chesney, P. J., Teets, K. C., Mulvihill, J. J., et al.: Successful treatment of *Candida* meningitis with amphotericin B and 5-fluorocytosine in combination. J. Pediatr. *89*:1017, 1976.
63. Montgomery, J. A., Edwards, J. E., and Guze, L. B.: Synergism of amphotericin B and 5-fluorocytosine for *Candida* species. J. Infect. Dis. *132*:82, 1975.
64. Bhandari, V., Narang, A., Kumar, B., et al.: Itraconazole therapy for disseminated candidiasis in very low birth weight neonate. J. Pediatr. Child Health *28*:323, 1992.
65. van den Anker, J. N.: Treatment of neonatal *Candida albicans* septicemia with itraconazole. Pediatr. Infect. Dis. J. *11*:684, 1992.
66. Bode, S., Pederson-Bjergaard, L., and Hjelt, K.: *Candida albicans* septicemia in a premature infant successfully treated with oral fluconazole. Scand. J. Infect. Dis. *24*:673, 1992.
67. Block, E. R., and Bennett, J. E.: Pharmacological studies with 5-fluorocytosine. Antimicrob. Agents Chemother. *1*:476, 1972.
68. Kauffman, C. A., and Frame, P. T.: Bone marrow toxicity associated with 5-fluorocytosine therapy. Antimicrob. Agents Chemother. *11*:244, 1977.
69. Clarke, M., and Davies, D. P.: Neonatal systemic candidiasis treated with miconazole. Br. Med. J. [Clin. Res.] *281*:354, 1980.
70. Sung, J. P., Rajani, K., Chopra, D. R., et al.: Miconazole therapy for systemic candidiasis in conjoined (siamese) twin and a premature newborn. Am. J. Surg. *138*:688, 1979.
71. Tuck, S.: Neonatal systemic candidiasis treated with miconazole. Arch. Dis. Child. *55*:903, 1980.
72. Lackner, H., Schwinger, W., Urban, C., et al.: Liposomal amphotericin-B (AmBisome) for treatment of disseminated fungal infections in two infants of very low birth weight. Pediatrics *89*:1259, 1992.
73. Saxen, H., Hoppu, K., and Pohjavuori, M.: Pharmacokinetics of fluconazole in very low birth weight infants during the first two weeks of life. Clin. Pharmacol. Ther. *54*:269, 1993.
74. Driessen, M., Ellis, J. B., Cooper, P. A., et al.: Fluconazole vs. amphotericin B for the treatment of neonatal fungal septicemia: A prospective randomized trial. Pediatr. Infect. Dis. J. *15*:1107, 1996.

Congenital Toxoplasmosis

Congenital toxoplasmosis results from placental infection and subsequent hematogenous infection of the fetus by the obligate intracellular protozoan parasite *Toxoplasma gondii*.[1] *Toxoplasma* is a coccidian that is ubiquitious in nature with the cat family being the definitive host.[2] The organism exists in three forms: (1) an oocyst that produces sporozoites, (2) a proliferative form that formerly was referred to as a trophozoite but more recently as an endozoite or tachyzoite, and (3) a tissue cyst that has an intracystic form termed cystozoite or bradyzoite. Nonfeline mammals or birds ingest infective oocysts from contaminated soil. Tissue cysts then accumulate in the organs and skeletal muscle of these animals. The possible routes of transmission from animal to human are direct contact with cat feces, ingestion of undercooked meat containing infective cysts, and ingestion of fruits or vegetables that have been in contaminated soil.

The prevalence of antibody to *T. gondii* among women of child-bearing age in the United States varies from approximately 3 to 30 per cent, depending on the region of the country.[1, 3] The lowest seroprevalence rates have been found in the Mountain and Pacific states, and the highest rates have been seen in the Northeastern and Southeastern states. In contrast, the seropositivity rate for women in Paris is as high as 70 per cent. These widely disparate seroprevalence rates among different adult populations throughout the world have been explained by differences in eating and sanitation practices that contribute to acquisition of infection.

The prevalence of congenital infection in the United States has been documented to be 0.08 per 1000 births by IgM screening of blood specimens collected on filter paper among newborns in Massachusetts and New Hampshire.[4] This compares with a rate of 3 to 10 per 1000 live births in Paris and Vienna.

TRANSMISSION

Infection of the fetus occurs during maternal parasitemia with subsequent infection of the placenta by the tachyzoites.[1, 3] Placental infection represents an important intermediary step between maternal and fetal infection. A delay of as long as 16 weeks between placental infection and subsequent infection of the fetus has been noted; it has been termed the prenatal incubation period.[1] Fetal infection occurs as a consequence of maternal primary infection during pregnancy or, rarely, just before conception. Reactivation of latent *Toxoplasma* infection during pregnancy does not lead to fetal infection except among immunocompromised women such as those infected with HIV.[1, 5–9] In these instances, congenital infection has been documented. Maternal reinfection leading to congenital toxoplasmosis also has been reported.[9a, 9b] Congenital toxoplasmosis has occurred in twins[10, 11] and triplets.[12] Among monozygotic twins, the clinical manifestations usually are similar, whereas among dizygotic twins, discrepancies in clinical findings are frequent.

The overall fetal infection rate from untreated maternal infection during pregnancy is approximately 40 per cent, although it depends when in pregnancy the mother became infected (Table 78–1).[1, 7] Although the actual rate of fetal infection increases as pregnancy advances, the severity of clinical manifestations is greatest when maternal infection is acquired during the first trimester.

Transmission during breast feeding in humans has not been demonstrated, although the organism has been detected in human milk.

CLINICAL MANIFESTATIONS

Acute maternal infection usually acquired early in pregnancy may lead to fulminant fetal infection resulting in still-

TABLE 78–1. Vertical Transmission of Congenital Toxoplasmosis by the Timing of Maternal Infection during Pregnancy

	Fetal Infection Rate		
Trimester of pregnancy	1st	2nd	3rd
Overall transmission rate	15%	30%	60%
Rate by disease severity			
Subclinical	18%	67%	90%
Mild	6%	18%	10%
Severe	41%	8%	0
Stillborn/perinatal death	35%	7%	0

birth, nonimmune fetal hydrops, preterm birth, and perinatal death.[7,13] On the other hand, chronic *Toxoplasma* infection only rarely has been associated with sporadic abortion.[14]

The majority of infants born with congenital *Toxoplasma* infection are asymptomatic in the neonatal period with clinical signs and symptoms being present in only approximately 25 per cent of infants.[4,15,16] However, long-term follow-up of these asymptomatically infected infants reveals eye and/or neurologic disease in as many as 80 to 90 per cent by adulthood.[17–20] The clinical manifestations of congenital toxoplasmosis in the newborn generally are indistinguishable from those associated with other agents of congenital infection such as cytomegalovirus (CMV) and *Treponema pallidum*. The most characteristic clinical findings, frequently referred to as the classic triad of congenital toxoplasmosis, are chorioretinitis, intracranial calcifications, and hydrocephalus.[1,3,21] These are seen in approximately 86, 37, and 20 per cent of symptomatic infants, respectively. Moreover, they often are accompanied by a combination of such signs and symptoms as anemia (59 per cent), jaundice (43 per cent), splenomegaly (41 per cent), seizures (41 per cent), fever (40 per cent), hepatomegaly (34 per cent), lymphadenopathy (32 per cent), microcephaly (9 per cent), and eosinophilia (9 per cent).[3,21]

Central nervous system involvement is a hallmark of congenital *Toxoplasma* infection.[1,22,23] Hydrocephalus usually is obstructive, often requiring ventriculoperitoneal shunting.[23,24] It may be the only manifestation of disease. Abnormalities of the cerebrospinal fluid (CSF) occur in about 63 per cent of infected infants; characteristically, they consist of lymphocytic pleocytosis and an elevated protein content. The markedly high protein concentrations in ventricular fluid, often exceeding 1 g per 100 mL, and hydrocephalus are explained by periaqueductal and periventricular vasculitis with necrosis that specifically are associated with toxoplasmosis.[1] Inflammation and necrosis involving the hypothalamus surrounding the third ventricle have resulted in both hypothermia and hyperthermia. When microcephaly is present, it is indicative of severe brain damage. Intracranial calcifications may be single or multiple but typically are generalized and located in the caudate nucleus, choroid plexus, meninges, and subependyma.[25] Periventricular calcifications similar to those of CMV also have been described. They are visualized best by computed tomography,[23] although ultrasonography also has been helpful. They may resolve with appropriate antimicrobial therapy.[23] Neurologic sequelae from untreated congenital toxoplasmosis include mental retardation (87 per cent), seizures (82 per cent), spasticity and palsies (71 per cent), and deafness (15 per cent).[21,23,26,27] *Toxoplasma* has been detected in the inner ear and mastoid with the associated inflammation resulting in deafness.

Chorioretinitis due to *Toxoplasma* at any age is considered to be a result of congenital infection.[1] In infants, the most common presentation is strabismus, whereas in older children and adults, defects in visual acuity predominates. The characteristic lesion consists of a focal necrotizing retinitis that often is bilateral. Organisms are present in the retina, and there is a predilection for the macula, with resultant loss of vision. There also may be involvement of the optic nerve. Other complications include iridocyclitis and cataracts.[23]

Other manifestations of congenital toxoplasmosis include nonspecific maculopapular or petechial rash, myocarditis, pneumonitis, thrombocytopenia, nephrotic syndrome, and abnormalities in immunoglobulin production.[1,21] Bony abnormalities consisting of metaphyseal lucencies similar to those seen in congenital syphilis also have been reported.[28] A variety of endocrine abnormalities may occur, including hypothyroidism, diabetes insipidus, precocious puberty, and growth hormone deficiency. These all are related to the fact that the organism is capable of widespread dissemination throughout the body with involvement of virtually all organ systems.

DIAGNOSIS

The diagnosis of congenital toxoplasmosis can be established by the isolation of the organism from infected body fluids and tissues such as placenta, amniotic fluid, fetal blood obtained by cordocentesis, umbilical cord blood, infant blood, and CSF.[1,7] This involves inoculation of the specimen intraperitoneally into laboratory mice and requires approximately 4 to 6 weeks for confirmation. Although not a practical method, it is available at the *Toxoplasma* Serology Laboratory, Palo Alto Medical Foundation (860 Bryant St., Palo Alto, CA 94301; 415-326-8120). Alternatively, a diagnosis can be made by histopathologic examination of the placenta that reveals the tachyzoites. Polymerase chain reaction (PCR) has been used successfully to detect *Toxoplasma* DNA in amniotic fluid, placenta, CSF, and fetal and infant blood.[29,30] PCR performed on amniotic fluid obtained by amniocentesis currently is the preferred method of confirming in utero infection.

The most practical and usual method of making the diagnosis is by serologic techniques.[4,7,30–38] The major problems associated with serologic diagnosis are determining the acuity of the maternal infection and differentiating endogenous from transplacentally acquired antibodies in neonatal/fetal infection. Because of this, a battery of serologic tests need to be utilized. These are commercially available at the *Toxoplasma* Serology Laboratory. Those tests that detect *T. gondii*–specific IgG include the Sabin-Feldman dye test, which is considered to be the gold standard but requires live organisms/tachyzoites, indirect immunofluorescent antibody test, IgG enzyme-linked immunosorbent assay (ELISA), and direct agglutination. An AC/HS differential agglutination test has been developed as a confirmatory test to differentiate acute versus chronic maternal infection.[37,38] This test compares the IgG serologic titer obtained with the use of formalin-fixed tachyzoites (HS antigen) to those obtained with acetone- or methanol-fixed tachyzoites (AC antigen). The latter preparation contains stage-specific *Toxoplasma* antigens that are recognized by IgG antibodies only during early infection.

Tests that detect *T. gondii*–specific IgM include (1) the double-sandwich IgM ELISA, which has a sensitivity of 75 per cent and specificity of 100 per cent[4]; (2) the IgM immunosorbent agglutination assay, which is the most sensitive test but should not be performed on umbilical cord blood because even small quantities of maternal IgM antibodies contaminating the specimen will result in a falsely positive test result[3]; and (3) the IgM immunofluorescent antibody test, which is not recommended due to lower sensitivity than either the IgM ELISA or IgM immunosorbent agglutination assay and poor specificity secondary to rheumatoid factors and antinuclear antibodies contributing to false-positive test results. Other tests that remain under research investigation include a *T. gondii*–specific IgA ELISA and IgA immunofiltration assay; a *T. gondii*–specific IgE immunofiltration assay; and IgG, IgM, and IgA immunoblotting tests.

Evaluation of the pregnant woman and fetus first is prompted by either seroconversion or the finding of an elevated *Toxoplasma* IgG titer.[38a, 38b] Because the latter may reflect only chronic infection, the acuity of the maternal infection is determined best serologically by means of the AC/HS differential agglutination test. If recent maternal infection is documented, the fetus should be evaluated by ultrasound and amniotic fluid should be tested for specific *Toxoplasma* DNA by PCR. The latter has supplanted the need for cordocentesis, and a positive result confirms fetal infection.[29] Postnatally, serologic testing of paired maternal and infant sera should be performed at a reliable laboratory that will include assays for IgG and IgM antibodies. Subinoculation of placental tissue, amniotic fluid, and umbilical cord blood into mice should be considered. The newborn should be evaluated fully by complete blood cell count and platelet determination, liver function tests, CSF evaluation (including tests for IgG and IgM antibodies and PCR), ophthalmologic examination, and computed tomography of the head. The presence of neonatal IgM antibody in serum or CSF, increasing serum IgG titers during the first year of life, or a positive PCR in serum or CSF is indicative of congenital infection.

Low IgG titers and an AC/HS differential agglutination test that indicates remote maternal infection do not require further evaluation of the mother or infant unless the mother is infected with HIV. Because fetal infection has occurred during chronic *Toxoplasma* infection in HIV-infected pregnant women, their infants should be evaluated serologically at birth for evidence of congenital infection. It has been suggested that HIV-infected pregnant women who have low CD4 counts and who are seropositive for *Toxoplasma* antibody receive empiric therapy in order to prevent fetal infection.[7, 39] However, at present, insufficient data are available to recommend routinely such therapy.

TREATMENT

Pregnant women with acute toxoplasmosis and infants with congenital toxoplasmosis, even if they have no clinical signs or symptoms, should receive treatment.[7, 23–27, 38a, 38b, 40, 41] Based on comparison with historical controls, outcome is improved substantially by maternal and fetal treatment. Neonatal treatment also has resulted in reductions in sensorineural hearing loss[41] and neurodevelopmental and visual handicaps.[23] Current therapies, however, are not effective against encysted bradyzoites and therefore do not prevent reactivation of chorioretinitis and neurologic disease.[1]

Table 78–2 shows the recommended guidelines for the treatment of congenital toxoplasmosis. In infants with congenital toxoplasmosis, the treatment consists of pyrimethamine, sulfadiazine, and folinic acid.[1, 3, 42] Complete blood

TABLE 78–2. Treatment Guidelines for Congenital Toxoplasmosis

Manifestation of Disease	Therapy	Dosage (Oral Unless Specified)	Duration
In pregnant women with acute toxoplasmosis in first 21 weeks of gestation or until term if fetus not infected	Spiramycin*	1.5 g q 12 hr without food	Until fetal infection documented or excluded at 21 wk; if documented, replaced with pyrimethamine, leucovorin, and sulfadiazine
If fetal infection confirmed after 17th week of gestation or if infection acquired in last few weeks of gestation	Pyrimethamine	Loading dose: 100 mg/d in divided doses for 2 d followed by 50 mg/d	Until delivery
	and Sulfadiazine	Loading dose: 75 mg/kg/d in 2 divided doses (maximum, 4 g/d) for 2 d, then 100 mg/kg/d in 2 divided doses (maximum, 4 g/d)	Until delivery
	and Leucovorin†	5–20 mg q d	Until delivery
Congenital toxoplasmosis‡	Pyrimethamine*	Loading dose: 2 mg/kg/d for 2 d, then 1 mg/kg/d for 2 or 6 mo, then this on each Mon, Wed, and Fri	1 yr
	and Sulfadiazine*	100 mg/kg/d in 2 daily divided doses	1 yr
	and Leucovorin (folinic acid)‡	5–10 mg 3 times weekly	1 yr
	Corticosteroids (prednisone)§	1 mg/kd/d in 2 daily divided doses	Until resolution of elevated (≥1 g/dL) cerebrospinal fluid protein or active chorioretinitis that threatens vision

*Available only on request from the Food and Drug Administration (301-443-9550).
†Monitor blood cell counts and platelets weekly and adjust for megaloblastic anemia, granulocytopenia, or thrombocytopenia.
‡Optimal dosage and feasibility currently being evaluated in ongoing National Collaborative Treatment Trial (312-791-4152).
§Corticosteroids should be continued until signs of inflammation (cerebrospinal fluid protein ≥1 g/dL) or active chorioretinitis that threatens vision have subsided; dosage then can be tapered and discontinued; use only in conjunction with pyrimethamine, sulfadiazine, and leucovorin.
Modified from Boyer, K. M., and McAuley, J. B.: Congenital toxoplasmosis. Semin. Pediatr. Infect. Dis. *5*:42, 1994.

cell counts and platelet determination need to be monitored closely while the patient is receiving therapy because granulocytopenia, thrombocytopenia, and megaloblastic anemia may occur. These usually improve quickly once an increased dosage of folinic acid is administered or pyrimethamine and sulfadiazine are discontinued temporarily. Spiramycin has been used in alternate months in place of the aforementioned regimen in France.

The indications for corticosteroid therapy with prednisone (0.5 mg/kg twice a day) are CSF protein concentration ≥1 g/dL and chorioretinitis that threatens vision, and it is continued until these resolve.

PREVENTION

The focus of prevention should be on the education of women of child-bearing age to avoid ingesting oocysts in cat feces, fruits, or vegetables and encysted bradyzoites in raw meat.[1, 43] Routine serologic screening of women during pregnancy has been an effective means of prevention in France and Austria, and it has been advocated in other areas where the incidence of congenital toxoplasmosis remains high. Neonatal screening for IgM antibody also has been advocated so that asymptomatic infants can be detected and treated before neurologic symptoms develop. This strategy, however, has been hampered by the lack of readily available and reliable IgM test kits. Moreover, it will not detect approximately 25 per cent of infected infants who lack anti-*Toxoplasma* IgM antibody.

References

1. Remington, J. S., McLeod, R., and Desmonts, G.: Toxoplasmosis. *In* Remington, J. S., and Klein, J. O. (eds.): Infectious Diseases of the Fetus and Newborn Infant. 4th ed. Philadelphia, W. B. Saunders, 1995, pp. 140–267.
2. Frenkel, J. K.: Toxoplasmosis: Parasite life cycle, pathology and immunology. *In* Hammond, D. M. (ed.): The Coccidia. Baltimore, University Park Press, 1973, pp. 343–410.
3. Boyer, K. M., and McAuley, J. B.: Congenital toxoplasmosis. Semin. Pediatr. Infect. Dis. *5*:42, 1994.
4. Guerina, N. G., Hsu, H.-W., Meissner, H. C., et al.: Neonatal serologic screening and early treatment for congenital *Toxoplasma gondii* infection. N. Engl. J. Med. *330*:1858, 1994.
5. Mitchell, C. D., Erlich, S. S., Mastrucci, M. T., et al.: Congenital toxoplasmosis occurring in infants perinatally infected with human immunodeficiency virus 1. Pediatr. Infect. Dis. *9*:512, 1990.
6. O'Donohoe, J. M., Brueton, M. J., and Holliman, R. E.: Concurrent congenital human immunodeficiency virus infection and toxoplasmosis. Pediatr. Infect. Dis. J. *10*:627, 1991.
7. Wong, S.-Y., and Remington, J. S.: Toxoplasmosis in pregnancy. Clin. Infect. Dis. *18*:853, 1994.
8. Langer, H.: Repeated congenital infection with *Toxoplasma gondii*. Obstet. Gynecol. *21*:318, 1983.
9. Cohen-Addad, N. E., Joshi, V. V., Sharer, L. R., et al.: Congenital acquired immunodeficiency syndrome and congenital toxoplasmosis: Pathologic support for a chronology of events. J. Perinatol. *8*:328, 1988.

9a. Fortier, B., Aissi, E., Ajana, F., et al.: Spontaneous abortion and reinfection by *Toxoplasma gondii*. Lancet *338*:444, 1991.

9b. Hennequin, C., Dureau, P., N'Guyen, L., et al.: Congenital toxoplasmosis acquired from an immune woman. Pediatr. Infect. Dis. J. *16*:75, 1997.

10. Sibalic, D., Djurkovic-Djakovic, O., and Nikolic, R.: Congenital toxoplasmosis in premature twins. Folia Parasitol. (Praha) *33*:1, 1986.
11. Couvreur J., Thulliez P., Daffos F., et al.: Six cases of toxoplasmosis in twins. Ann. Pediatr. (Paris) *38*:63, 1991.
12. Wiswell, T. E., Fajardo, J. E., Bass, J. W., et al.: Congenital toxoplasmosis in triplets. J. Pediatr. *105*:59, 1984.
13. Kimball, A. C., Dean, B. H., and Fuchs, F.: The role of toxoplasmosis in abortion. Am. J. Obstet. Gynecol. *111*:219, 1971.
14. Remington, J. S., Newell, J. W., and Cavanaugh, E.: Spontaneous abortion and chronic toxoplasmosis. Report of a case, with isolation of the parasite. Obstet. Gynecol. *24*:25, 1964.
15. Alford, C. A., Jr., Stagno, S., and Reynolds, D. W.: Congenital toxoplasmosis: Clinical, laboratory and therapeutic considerations, with special reference to subclinical disease. Bull. N. Y. Acad. Med. *50*:160, 1974.
16. Alford, C. A., Jr., Foft, J. W., Blanckenship, W. J., et al.: Subclinical central nervous system disease of neonates: A prospective study of infants born with increased levels of IgM. J. Pediatr. *75*:1167, 1969.
17. Saxon, S. A., Knight, N., Reynolds, D. W., et al.: Intellectual deficits in children born with subclinical congenital toxoplasmosis: A preliminary report. J. Pediatr. *82*:792, 1973.
18. Wilson, C. B., Remington, J. S., Stagno, S., et al.: Development of adverse sequelae in children born with subclinical congenital *Toxoplasma* infection. Pediatrics *66*:767, 1980.
19. Couvreur, J., and Desmonts, G.: Congenital and maternal toxoplasmosis: A review of 300 congenital cases. Dev. Med. Child Neurol. *4*:519, 1962.
20. Couvreur, J., Desmonts, G., Tournier, G., et al.: Study of a homogeneous series of 210 cases of congenital toxoplasmosis in infants aged 0 to 11 months detected prospectively. Ann. Pediatr. *31*:815, 1984.
21. Eichenwald, H. G.: A study of congenital toxoplasmosis, with particular emphasis on clinical manifestations, sequelae, and therapy. *In* Siim, J. C. (ed.): Human Toxoplasmosis. Copenhagen, Munksgaard, 1960, pp. 41–49.
22. Diebler, C., Dusser, A., and Dulac, O.: Congenital toxoplasmosis: Clinical and neuroradiologic evaluation of the cerebral lesions. Neuroradiology *27*:125, 1985.
23. McAuley, J., Boyer, K. M., Patel, D., et al.: Early and longitudinal evaluations of treated infants and children and untreated historical patients with congenital toxoplasmosis: The Chicago collaborative treatment trial. Clin. Infect. Dis. *18*:38, 1994.
24. Martinovic, J., Sibalic, D., Djordjevic, M., et al.: Frequency of toxoplasmosis in the appearance of congenital hydrocephalus. J. Neurosurg. *56*:830, 1982.
25. Müssbichler, H.: Radiologic study of intracranial calcifications in congenital toxoplasmosis. Acta Radiol. *7*:369–379, 1968.
26. Koppe, J. G., Loewer-Sieger, D. H., and DeRoever-Bonnet, H.: Result of 20-year follow-up of congenital toxoplasmosis. Lancet *1*:254, 1986.
27. Hohlfeld, P., Daffos, F., Thurlliez, P., et al.: Fetal toxoplasmosis: Outcome of pregnancy and infant follow-up after in utero treatment. J. Pediatr. *115*:765, 1989.
28. Milgram, J. W.: Osseous changes in congenital toxoplasmosis. Arch. Pathol. *97*:150, 1974.
29. Hohlfeld, P., Daffos, F., Costa, J.-M., et al.: Prenatal diagnosis of congenital toxoplasmosis with a polymerase-chain-reaction test on amniotic fluid. N. Engl. J. Med. *331*:695, 1994.
30. Grover, C. M., Thulliez, P., Remington, J. S., et al.: Rapid prenatal diagnosis of congenital *Toxoplasma* infection by using polymerase chain reaction and amniotic fluid. J. Clin. Microbiol. *28*:2297, 1990.
31. Wilson, M., and McAuley, J. B.: Laboratory diagnosis of congenital toxoplasmosis. Clin. Lab. Med. *11*:923, 1991.
32. Naot, Y., Desmonts, G., and Remington, J. S.: IgM enzyme-linked immunosorbent assay test for the diagnosis of congenital Toxoplasma infection. J. Pediatr. *98*:32,1991.
33. Desmonts, G., Naot, Y., and Remington, J. S.: Immunoglobulin M–immunosorbent agglutination assay for diagnosis of infectious diseases: Diagnosis of acute congenital and acquired Toxoplasma infections. J. Clin. Microbiol. *11*:186, 1981.
34. Stepick-Bick, P., Thulliez, P., Araujo, F. G., and Remington, J. S: IgA antibodies for diagnosis of acute congenital and acquired toxoplasmosis. J. Infect. Dis. *162*:270, 1990.
35. Decoster, A., Darcy, F., Caron, A., et al.: IgA antibodies against P30 as markers of congenital and acute toxoplasmosis. Lancet *2*:1104, 1988.
36. Remington, J., Araujo, F. G., and Desmonts, G.: Recognition of different toxoplasma antigen by IgM and IgG antibodies in mothers and their congenitally infected newborns. J. Infect. Dis. *152*:1020, 1985.
37. Dannemann, B. R., Vaughan, W. C., Thurlliez, P., et al.: Differential agglutination test for diagnosis of recently acquired infection with *Toxoplasma gondii*. J. Clin. Microbiol. *28*:1928, 1990.
38. Lappalainen, M., Koskela, P., Koskiniemi, M., et al.: Toxoplasmosis acquired during pregnancy: Improved serodiagnosis based on avidity of IgG. J. Infect. Dis. *167*:691, 1993.

38a. Couvreur, J., Desmonts, G., and Thulliez, P.: Prophylaxis of congenital toxoplasmosis. Effect of spiramycin on placental infection. J. Antimicrob. Chemother. *22*:193, 1988.

38b. Daffos, F., Forestier, F., Capella-Pavlovsky, M., et al.: Prenatal management of 746 pregnancies at risk for congenital toxoplasmosis. N. Engl. J. Med. *318*:271, 1988.

39. Beaman, M. H., Luft, B. J., and Remington, J. S.: Prophylaxis for toxoplasmosis in AIDS. Ann. Intern. Med. *117*:163, 1992.
40. Roizen, N., Swisher, C. N., Stein, M. A., et al.: Neurologic and developmental outcome in treated congenital toxoplasmosis. Pediatrics *95*:11, 1995.
41. McGee, T., Wolters, C., Stein, L., et al.: Absence of sensorineural hearing abnormalities in treated infants with congenital toxoplasmosis. Otolaryngol. Head Neck Surg. *106*:75, 1992.
42. McLeod, R., Mack, D., Foss, R., et al.: The Toxoplasmosis Study Group: Levels of pyrimethamine in sera and cerebrospinal and ventricular fluids from infants treated for congenital toxoplasmosis. Antimicrob. Agents Chemother. *36*:1040, 1992.
43. Wilson, C. B., and Remington, J. S.: What can be done to prevent congenital toxoplasmosis? Am. J. Obstet. Gynecol. *138*:357, 1980.

SECTION FOURTEEN

INFECTIONS OF THE COMPROMISED HOST

❑ ❑ ❑

79

CONGENITAL IMMUNE DEFICIENCY

Mark W. Kline and William T. Shearer

The term *congenital (primary) immune deficiency* encompasses a broad range of hereditary disorders having in common a principal effect on immune system development or function and a predisposition to recurrent or unusual infections. As the term implies, these disorders are present from birth, although clinical manifestations may not be evident until much later in life. In contrast, the secondary immune deficiencies are acquired disorders, with immune dysfunction occurring as a result of exogenous factors or along with some other primary disease process. Causes of secondary immune deficiency include infection (e.g., HIV), medications (e.g., chronic corticosteroid administration), malnutrition, and infiltrative or metabolic diseases (e.g., Hodgkin disease or diabetes mellitus). Many secondary immune deficiency disorders are far more common than any of the congenital immune deficiencies.

Children generally are referred for immunologic evaluation because of unusually frequent or severe infections or infections caused by unusual organisms. Only a small percentage of children who undergo evaluation have demonstrable immune deficiency. This chapter focuses on medical history and physical examination findings that serve to differentiate those few children with congenital immune deficiency from the many other children with normal immune function. Screening laboratory tests that are useful in excluding clinically significant immune dysfunction are discussed, and some of the more common or distinctive primary antibody, cellular, complement, and phagocyte deficiencies are described.

INITIAL EVALUATION FOR SUSPECTED CONGENITAL IMMUNE DEFICIENCY

Medical History

Minor infections occur commonly throughout childhood. For example, otherwise healthy children younger than 5 years of age average between three and eight episodes of upper respiratory infection annually.[9, 12, 30] By 1 year of age, 62 per cent of children have had at least one episode of acute otitis media, and 17 per cent have had three or more episodes.[80] By 3 years of age, more than 80 per cent of children have had at least one episode of acute otitis media, and 46 per cent have had three or more episodes. About 2 per cent of children 1 to 5 years of age develop symptomatic urinary tract infection.[71] The incidence of gastroenteritis among U.S. children is about two to three episodes per child-year, with rates as high as five episodes per child-year among children attending day care centers.[10, 34] Occurrence of these infections during infancy or early childhood is the result of several factors, including immunologic immaturity or naivete (lack of prior exposure to infectious agents); poor hygiene; mouthing behavior; and frequent exposure to ill contacts in the home, school, or day care settings.

Medical history is the key element in distinguishing children with congenital immune deficiency from those with frequent infections but normal immune function. Children with congenital immune deficiency often have a history of infections that are not only frequent but also severe (e.g., pneumonia, meningitis, septicemia, osteomyelitis, or abscess of soft tissue or an internal organ). The course of individual episodes of infection may be unusually prolonged or associated with unexpected complications (e.g., lung abscess in a child with pneumonia or skull bone osteomyelitis as a complication of sinusitis). In general, infections over time at multiple body sites are more suggestive of immune deficiency than are infections occurring at only one site (e.g., recurrent otitis media). In the latter circumstance, a mechanical or anatomic explanation for the infections should be considered (e.g., foreign body or occult tracheoesophageal fistula in the child with recurrent pneumonia or a congenital fistulous tract to the middle ear in the child with recurrent bacterial meningitis).

A history of recurrent infections of defined etiology may be more meaningful than one of frequent, self-limited infections of presumed viral etiology (Table 79–1). Children with primary antibody deficiencies typically experience infections caused by extracellular bacteria with polysaccharide capsules (e.g., *Streptococcus pneumoniae* or *Haemophilus influenzae* type b). In contrast, children with primary cellular immune deficiencies often have infections with unusual or opportunistic viruses, fungi, protozoa, and mycobacteria. Because of impairment of T-cell–dependent antibody responses, infections with common bacteria also may be observed. Children with congenital deficiencies of late-acting complement components typically have recurrent neisserial infections, and those with phagocyte deficiencies have infections with a variety of bacterial (e.g., *Staphylococcus aureus, Pseudomonas aeruginosa, Serratia marcescens*) and fungal (e.g., *Candida, Aspergillus*) organisms.

In addition to the microbial etiology of infections, several other items of historical information may help to define the risk for and possible nature of a congenital immune deficiency. Because young infants are afforded some protection by the presence of maternal IgG, children with primary anti-

TABLE 79–1. Common Pathogens in Children with Congenital Immune Deficiency

Immune Deficiency	Common Pathogens
Antibody Deficiencies	
X-linked agammaglobulinemia	*Streptococcus pneumoniae, Haemophilus influenzae, Staphylococcus aureus, Pseudomonas aeruginosa, Mycoplasma, Salmonella, Shigella, Campylobacter, Giardia,* rotavirus, enteroviruses
Immunoglobulin deficiency with increased IgM	Same as X-linked agammaglobulinemia, *Pneumocystis carinii*
Common variable immunodeficiency	Same as X-linked agammaglobulinemia
IgA deficiency	Common viral and bacterial respiratory pathogens, *Giardia*
IgG subclass deficiency	*S. pneumoniae, H. influenzae,* other common bacterial respiratory pathogens
Transient hypogammaglobulinemia of infancy	Common bacterial respiratory pathogens
Cellular and Combined Immune Deficiencies	
DiGeorge anomaly	*Candida,* herpesviruses, *P. carinii,* mycobacteria, *S. pneumoniae, P. aeruginosa*
Wiskott-Aldrich syndrome	*S. pneumoniae, H. influenzae, Candida,* herpesviruses, *P. carinii* less commonly
Ataxia telangiectasia	*S. pneumoniae, H. influenzae,* other common bacterial respiratory pathogens
Severe combined immune deficiency	Same as DiGeorge anomaly
Complement Deficiencies	
C3, C1, C4, or C2 deficiency	*S. pneumoniae, H. influenzae*
C5 through C9 deficiency	*Neisseria meningitidis*
Phagocyte Deficiencies	
Quantitative abnormalities	*S. aureus, P. aeruginosa,* enteric gram-negative bacilli, *Candida, Aspergillus*
Chronic granulomatous disease	Catalase-positive bacteria and fungi
Leukocyte adhesion deficiency	Same as for quantitative abnormalities

body deficiencies generally have an initial period of relative well-being, with onset of infections between 3 and 18 months of age. On the other hand, children with severe congenital cellular, complement, or phagocyte deficiencies may have onset of infections in the first days or weeks of life. Delayed cord separation and poor wound healing suggest congenital phagocyte deficiency. Hypocalcemic seizures in the neonatal period and congenital heart disease may be clues to the presence of DiGeorge anomaly. Severe disease associated with live virus vaccines (e.g., measles, poliomyelitis, varicella) may be observed in children with severe congenital antibody or cellular immune deficiencies.

Family history can offer important clues to the presence of congenital immune deficiency. A history of consanguinity or deaths from infection or unexplained causes during infancy

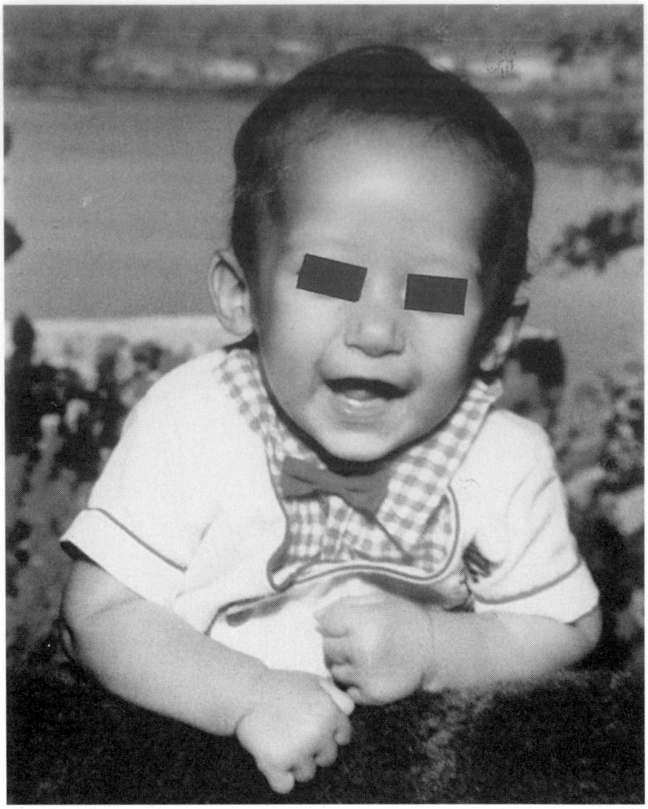

FIGURE 79–1. *Typical facial appearance of a child with DiGeorge anomaly. Note the presence of microstomia, hypertelorism, upturned nose, and posteriorly rotated and small, low-set ears.*

or early childhood should be sought. Many of the better-defined immune deficiency syndromes have X-linked inheritance patterns (Table 79–2), resulting in an overall male-to-female ratio of 5:1 among children with congenital immune deficiency.

Physical Examination

The physical examination often is unrevealing in children with congenital immune deficiency. Short stature is a feature of some of these congenital disorders (e.g., chronic granulomatous disease), and wasting or failure to thrive is observed in some children with severe primary antibody or cellular immune deficiencies, because of either recurrent infections or chronic intestinal malabsorption. A paucity of lymphoid tissues (e.g., tonsils, superficial lymph nodes) suggests X-linked agammaglobulinemia.

Several congenital immune deficiency syndromes are associated with highly characteristic physical stigmata. For exam-

TABLE 79–2. X-linked Congenital Immune Deficiency Disorders

- X-linked agammaglobulinemia (Bruton disease)
- Immunodeficiency with hyper-IgM (some forms)
- Severe combined immune deficiency (some forms)
- Wiskott-Aldrich syndrome
- Chronic granulomatous disease (most)

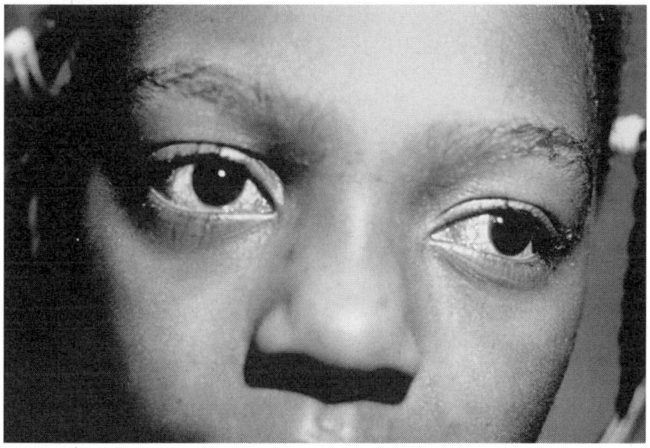

FIGURE 79–2. *Telangiectases of the bulbar conjunctivae in a child with ataxia telangiectasia. (Courtesy of Dr. Martin Lorin, Texas Children's Hospital.)*

TABLE 79–3. Screening Tests for Suspected Congenital Immune Deficiency

Type of Immune Deficiency	Recommended Screening Tests
All types	Complete blood count Peripheral blood smear
Primary antibody deficiency	Quantitative serum immunoglobulins Postimmunization antibody titers Isohemagglutinins
Primary cellular immune deficiency	Chest roentgenography Delayed hypersensitivity skin tests
Primary complement deficiency	Total hemolytic complement (CH_{50}) assay
Primary phagocyte deficiency	Nitroblue tetrazolium (NBT) dye test Neutrophil $CD11_{a,b,c}$/CD18 expression

ple, children with DiGeorge anomaly often have characteristic facial features (Fig. 79–1). Telangiectases of the bulbar conjunctivae (Fig. 79–2), nasal bridge, ears, and flexor surfaces of the extremities, with or without ataxia, suggest ataxia telangiectasia. Chronic eczema is observed in the hyperimmunoglobulinemia E and Wiskott-Aldrich syndromes, and severe gingivitis and periodontitis with loss of alveolar bone and dentition can occur in children with leukocyte adhesion deficiency (Fig. 79–3).

Laboratory Tests

Screening laboratory evaluations for immune deficiency should be undertaken selectively. Possible indications for screening include unusually frequent, severe, or complicated infections; infection caused by an opportunistic organism; or recognition of a specific syndrome that has been associated with immune deficiency.

A screening evaluation for congenital immune deficiency employs generally available, relatively inexpensive laboratory tests to exclude common and serious disorders (Table 79–3). If possible, the evaluation should be targeted to the type of immune deficiency (e.g., primary antibody deficiency) suggested by the child's medical history and physical examination findings. Laboratory test results must be interpreted in the context of the child's age.

The initial evaluation for immune deficiency should include a complete blood count and examination of the peripheral blood smear. Because 50 to 70 per cent of circulating lymphocytes are T cells, children with severe cellular (e.g., DiGeorge anomaly) or combined (e.g., severe combined immunodeficiency [SCID]) immune deficiencies may have lymphopenia. Children with Wiskott-Aldrich syndrome have reduced numbers of platelets, which are small in size (decreased mean platelet volume), and large neutrophil cytoplasmic granules are observed in children with Chédiak-Higashi syndrome.

A complete blood count also is useful in excluding congenital neutropenia. Children with leukocyte adhesion deficiency often have markedly increased neutrophil and total white blood cell counts. Finally, the presence of Howell-Jolly bodies, with or without thrombocytosis, suggests anatomic or functional asplenia.

EVALUATION OF HUMORAL (ANTIBODY) IMMUNITY. Screening evaluation of the child with suspected primary antibody deficiency should include both quantitative

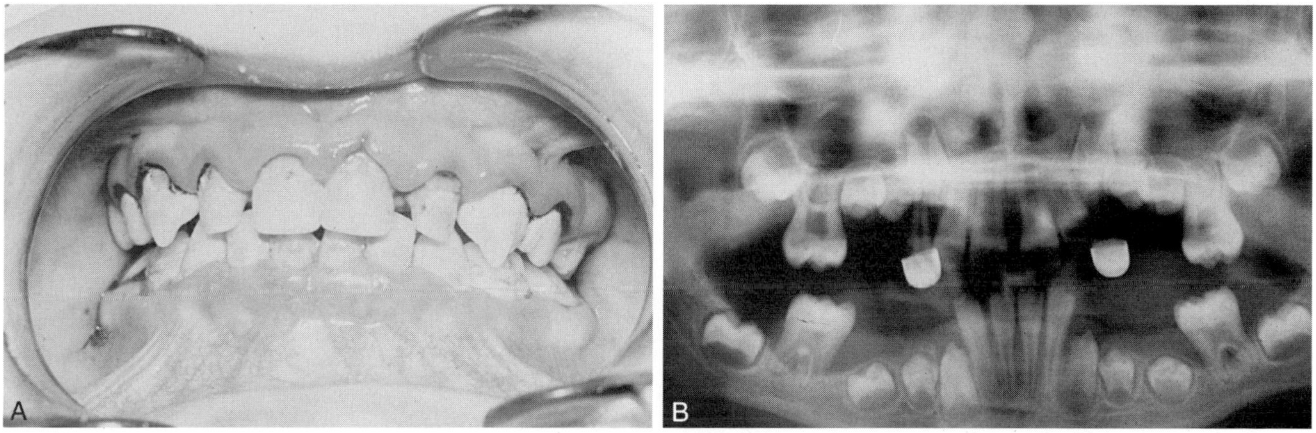

FIGURE 79–3. A, *Chronic periodontitis in a boy with leukocyte adhesion deficiency.* B, *Roentgenogram from the same patient shows extensive alveolar bone loss. (Courtesy of Dr. Bruce Carter, Texas Children's Hospital.)*

measurement of serum immunoglobulins and functional assessment of specific antibody production. Most children with primary antibody deficiencies have abnormalities of serum immunoglobulin concentrations. Measurement of serum IgG, IgA, and IgM concentrations will identify children with panhypogammaglobulinemia as well as those with deficiency of a particular immunoglobulin isotype, such as selective IgA deficiency. Because there are marked age-related changes in serum immunoglobulin concentrations, it is important to use age-appropriate normal values for purposes of comparison.

In infants, functional antibody production usually is assessed by measuring antibody titers generated in response to immunization with diphtheria and tetanus toxoids. Assessment of antibody responses to polysaccharide antigens is problematic in infants because of functional immaturity in the ability to respond to this class of antigens. After 18 to 24 months of age, antibody responses to pneumococcal polysaccharide (Pneumovax) immunization can be employed. Alternatively, because ABO blood group antigens are polysaccharides, antipolysaccharide antibody production can be assessed by measuring serum isohemagglutinin titers. Children with blood type AB will not form isohemagglutinins. Because they are not pure polysaccharides, the conjugate *Haemophilus* vaccines are not suitable for use in assessment of antipolysaccharide antibody responses.

Measurement of serum IgG subclasses may be indicated in children with apparent abnormalities in functional antibody production. Evaluation of children whose screening tests indicate significant quantitative and functional antibody abnormalities should include enumeration of B cells in the peripheral blood and in vitro studies of mitogen- or antigen-induced B-cell proliferation.

EVALUATION OF CELLULAR IMMUNITY. The screening evaluation for primary cellular immune deficiency generally consists of delayed hypersensitivity skin tests and, in the young infant, posteroanterior and lateral chest roentgenograms for assessment of a thymic shadow (Fig. 79–4).

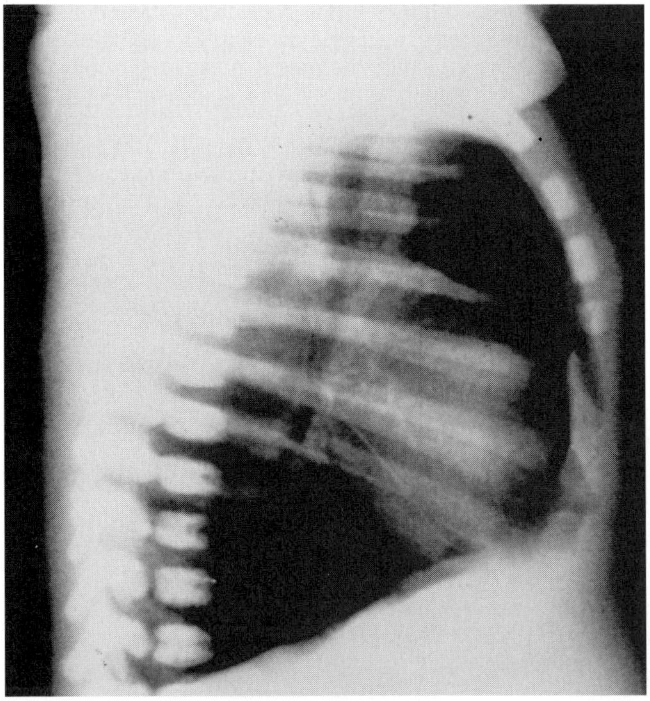

FIGURE 79–4. *Lateral chest roentgenogram of an infant with severe combined immune deficiency. Note absence of the normal thymic shadow.*

Delayed hypersensitivity skin tests are performed using vaccine or microbial antigens to which the child has had prior exposure. Commonly used antigens include tetanus toxoid and *Candida albicans*. Standard initial dilutions are 1:100 for both antigens, but a *C. albicans* dilution of 1:10 may be more appropriate for children 5 years of age or younger. The diluted antigen is administered intradermally in a volume of 0.1 mL.

Unfortunately, delayed hypersensitivity skin test responses often are absent in children younger than 1 year of age, and the thymus gland involutes with age or stress, sometimes giving the radiographic appearance of thymic aplasia. As a consequence, enumeration of peripheral blood T cells, T-cell subset analysis (e.g., CD4+ or CD8+ lymphocyte counts), and mitogen- and antigen-induced lymphocyte proliferation studies may be needed for definitive determination of cellular immune function.

EVALUATION OF THE COMPLEMENT SYSTEM. Primary deficiencies of components of the classic complement pathway can be detected with the total serum hemolytic complement (CH_{50}) assay. This test measures the ability of fresh patient serum to lyse antibody-coated sheep erythrocytes and reflects the activity of all numbered components of the classic complement pathway from C1 through C9. Complete deficiency of any of these components results in a CH_{50} approaching 0. Specific immunochemical and functional testing is necessary for identification of the deficient component.

EVALUATION OF PHAGOCYTE FUNCTION. Evaluation of children with suspected primary phagocyte deficiencies should begin with examination of the total and differential white blood cell counts and the peripheral smear. A variety of assays are available for assessment of phagocyte function. The nitroblue tetrazolium (NBT) dye test uses reduction of NBT to formazan by activated phagocytes to measure the oxidative metabolic responses that accompany phagocytosis. Children with chronic granulomatous disease (CGD) show very little dye reduction (<10 per cent of cells formazan-positive); carriers of X-linked CGD typically have between 10 and 90 per cent formazan-positive cells.

More sophisticated tests, including chemiluminescence and assays of chemotaxis, phagocytosis, and bactericidal activity, may be indicated for children in whom a disorder of phagocyte function is strongly suspected. Enumeration of $CD11_{a,b,c}+/CD18+$ white blood cells is useful in diagnosis of leukocyte adhesion deficiency.

PRIMARY ANTIBODY DEFICIENCIES

X-Linked Agammaglobulinemia

CLINICAL FEATURES. Boys with X-linked agammaglobulinemia (Bruton disease) often are healthy during the first several months of life because of the protective presence of transplacentally acquired maternal IgG. As maternal immunoglobulin disappears, chronic or recurrent infections develop.[14, 38, 45] Otitis media, sinusitis, pneumonia, and diarrhea are most common, but infections are not limited to mucosal surfaces, and bacteremia, meningitis, and osteomyelitis also may occur. The mean age at diagnosis in a retrospective study of 96 patients with X-linked agammaglobulinemia was 2.5 years in cases where there was a family history of the disease and 3.5 years where there was not.[45]

S. pneumoniae, *H. influenzae* type b, *S. aureus*, and *P. aeruginosa* are bacterial pathogens observed commonly in the setting of X-linked agammaglobulinemia. *Mycoplasma* species infections also occur with increased frequency. These organisms have been implicated as a cause of a subacute, destructive arthritis.[38, 46] Gastrointestinal infections may be caused by *Salmonella*, *Shigella*, *Campylobacter*, or rotavirus.[38, 64] Chronic giardiasis with intestinal malabsorption has been described.[58]

Children with X-linked agammaglobulinemia are susceptible to chronic enteroviral meningoencephalitis.[38, 50] Diverse signs and symptoms are observed, including fever, headache, altered mental status, seizures, ataxia, myoclonus, paresthesias, peripheral neuropathy, aphasia or dysarthria, and visual disturbances. Intrathecal and intravenous immunoglobulin (IVIG) therapy has been attempted, but most reported cases have had a fatal outcome. Vaccine-associated paralytic poliomyelitis also has been reported.

An unusual disorder resembling juvenile dermatomyositis, with myositis and extremity edema and erythema, has been reported in children with X-linked agammaglobulinemia and enteroviral infection of skeletal muscle.[21]

PATHOGENESIS. X-linked agammaglobulinemia results from developmental arrest of B-cell maturation. As a consequence, blood, lymph nodes, and bone marrow contain markedly diminished numbers of B cells and plasma cells, resulting in hypogammaglobulinemia. Other components of the immune system are normal.

The defective gene maps to the midportion of the long arm of the X chromosome. The gene encodes a cytoplasmic protein-tyrosine kinase, the normal function of which is necessary for expansion of B-cell populations during their maturation.[82, 85] Inactivating mutations of the gene have been found in all affected individuals studied.

DIAGNOSIS. Because of the confounding presence of transplacentally acquired maternal IgG, use of quantitative serum immunoglobulin determinations for diagnosis of X-linked agammaglobulinemia in the first 6 months of life is problematic. Infants with X-linked agammaglobulinemia also have low concentrations of other immunoglobulin isotypes (e.g., IgA, IgM), but it is difficult to define values that clearly differentiate between infants with the disease and normal infants. As a consequence, definitive diagnosis during early infancy generally relies on immunophenotyping and flow cytometry to demonstrate absence of B cells in the patient's peripheral blood. After 6 months of age, serum IgG concentrations usually are less than 100 mg/dL, and concentrations of other immunoglobulin isotypes are low or undetectable. Isohemagglutinins are absent, and specific antibodies are not produced in response to immunization or natural infection.

TREATMENT AND PROGNOSIS. Lifetime replacement therapy with IVIG is indicated for all patients with X-linked agammaglobulinemia.[15, 61] This form of therapy decreases the frequency of serious infections, reduces the need for hospitalization, and may help to prevent chronic bronchiectasis.[47] The dose and frequency of administration of IVIG are adjusted to produce serum IgG trough concentrations of at least 400 to 500 mg/dL. For most patients, IVIG doses of 300 to 600 mg/kg, given every 3 or 4 weeks, are required.

Because patients with X-linked agammaglobulinemia do not make antibody in response to immunization and because of the risk of adverse effects, vaccination is not recommended.

Acute infections should be treated aggressively in patients with X-linked agammaglobulinemia. Minor middle ear, sinus, and skin infections usually can be treated with oral antibiotics. Pneumonia, other serious focal or systemic infections, and chronic otitis media and sinusitis should be treated initially with intravenous antibiotics. Empiric antibiotic therapy is directed against common bacterial pathogens, including *S. pneumoniae*, *H. influenzae*, and *S. aureus*. If possible, etiologic diagnosis should be obtained, particularly in cases of severe or chronic infection. Because serum IgG concentrations often decrease during acute infection, the serum IgG concentration should be measured; additional doses of IVIG may be indicated.

Chronic pulmonary disease with bronchiectasis is an important cause of death in patients with X-linked agammaglobulinemia. Long-term antibiotic therapy, similar to that employed in patients with cystic fibrosis, may be helpful in individual cases. Long-term survivors of X-linked agammaglobulinemia are at increased risk for lymphoreticular malignancies.[74]

Immunoglobulin Deficiency with Increased IgM

CLINICAL FEATURES. Most cases of immunoglobulin deficiency with increased IgM are associated with X-linked transmission, but autosomal recessive and dominant inheritance also has been reported. Patients with this disorder develop recurrent pyogenic infections during infancy as transplacentally acquired IgG wanes. Respiratory tract infections and chronic diarrhea with failure to thrive are common; septicemia, meningitis, and other serious systemic infections also occur.[57] *Pneumocystis carinii* pneumonia, an unusual infection in children with other primary antibody deficiencies, also has been reported.

Neutropenia is present in half of patients with immunoglobulin deficiency with increased IgM. It can be intermittent but lacks the precise periodicity of cyclic neutropenia. Aphthous ulcers occur commonly. Perirectal ulcers and abscess also have been reported.

Hyperplasia of superficial and deep lymph nodes is common. Intestinal nodular lymphoid hyperplasia may lead to malabsorption and protein-losing enteropathy. Diffuse lymphoid infiltration of other organs also may occur. Autoimmune conditions, including arthritis and nephritis, have been described, and there is an increased incidence of lymphoreticular malignancies.

PATHOGENESIS. Most males with immunoglobulin deficiency with increased IgM have mutations of a gene on the X chromosome that encodes the T-cell ligand for B-cell CD40.[3, 7] Several patients with normal expression of the CD40 ligand and defects in the B-cell CD40 signaling pathway also have been described.[19] Interaction of B-cell CD40 with the CD40 ligand is essential to B-cell proliferation, isotype switching, and terminal differentiation of B cells to antibody-secreting plasma cells. The described mutations therefore provide an explanation for the observed B-cell dysfunction.

DIAGNOSIS. Patients with this disorder have a characteristic increase in serum IgM concentrations in association with low to absent concentrations of serum IgA and IgG. Serum IgM concentrations may exceed 1000 mg/dL. Circulating B cells expressing surface IgM are found in normal numbers, but there is a paucity of circulating cells bearing IgA or IgG. Antibody responses to immunization often are present but consist predominantly or exclusively of IgM; isotype switching does not occur.

Evaluation of males with suspected immunoglobulin deficiency with increased IgM should include a determination of whether activated T cells bind CD40. This is done by flow cytometry using recombinant CD40 fusion protein.[3, 7]

TREATMENT AND PROGNOSIS. Patients with this disorder usually have a more favorable clinical course than do patients with X-linked agammaglobulinemia, but long-term studies have not been performed. Replacement therapy with IVIG is indicated. This often results in a decrease in serum IgM concentrations.

Common Variable Immunodeficiency

CLINICAL FEATURES. The term *common variable immunodeficiency* (CVID) encompasses a heterogeneous group of disorders having in common hypogammaglobulinemia, abnormal antibody production, recurrent infections, and a propensity for autoimmune conditions. Onset can occur at any time from infancy to old age, but symptoms frequently begin during the second or third decades of life.

The clinical manifestations of CVID are similar to those of X-linked agammaglobulinemia, with recurrent infections of the respiratory tract, bacteremia, meningitis, osteomyelitis, and septic arthritis. The most common infecting organisms are *S. pneumoniae, H. influenzae,* and *S. aureus. Mycoplasma* and *Ureaplasma* are important considerations in the patient with CVID and arthritis.[29]

Many individuals with CVID suffer from chronic diarrhea and intestinal malabsorption, either on an infectious or autoimmune basis.[20, 22, 37] This may exacerbate underlying hypogammaglobulinemia. Organisms implicated in these chronic gastrointestinal infections include *Giardia, Campylobacter, Salmonella,* and *Cryptosporidium*. Bacterial overgrowth syndrome occurs commonly. Ulcerative colitis and Crohn disease occur with increased frequency in CVID, as do atrophic gastritis with achlorhydria, viral or autoimmune chronic active hepatitis, and cholelithiasis.

A variety of nongastrointestinal autoimmune conditions also have been reported in individuals with CVID, including a chronic arthritis resembling juvenile rheumatoid arthritis; scleroderma, a lupus-like syndrome; and neutropenia, anemia, and thrombocytopenia.[20, 22, 37]

A pseudolymphoma syndrome, with lymphoid hyperplasia of the lung (lymphoid interstitial pneumonia) and intestine (nodular lymphoid hyperplasia), massive splenomegaly, and mediastinal adenopathy, occurs in CVID. Malignancies, including lymphomas and gastric carcinoma, are common among adults with CVID.[22, 23, 73] Cancer is observed infrequently in children with CVID.

PATHOGENESIS. The pathogenesis of CVID is poorly defined. Unlike X-linked agammaglobulinemia, B-cell maturation is intact and normal numbers of B cells are present in peripheral blood and lymph nodes. However, antibody production clearly is impaired.[76] Many patients with CVID appear to have an intrinsic B-cell defect that impairs the ability of these cells to differentiate into immunoglobulin-secreting plasma cells, but a variety of T-cell functional abnormalities also have been described.[22, 76] A separate T-cell defect could explain the increased risk of malignancy and autoimmunity in CVID.

Possession of rare alleles of complement genes within major histocompatibility complex III on chromosome 6 is associated strongly with development of CVID and selective IgA deficiency, suggesting that these two disorders may be related mechanistically.[86] In fact, some individuals with selective IgA deficiency subsequently develop CVID.

DIAGNOSIS. Quantitative immunoglobulin determination generally reveals a serum IgG concentration less than 250 mg/dL, with comparable decreases in other immunoglobulin isotypes. Immunophenotyping of peripheral blood lymphocytes demonstrates normal numbers of mature B cells expressing surface immunoglobulin. Antibody responses to immunization are subnormal or absent.

TREATMENT AND PROGNOSIS. Treatment of patients with CVID is similar to that of patients with X-linked agammaglobulinemia. Replacement therapy with IVIG is indicated. Patients with enteropathy may require unusually large IVIG doses to maintain trough serum IgG concentrations of 400 to 500 mg/dL or higher. Acute infections should be treated aggressively. Some patients will require therapy for associated autoimmune conditions.

IgA Deficiency

CLINICAL FEATURES. Most individuals with selective IgA deficiency are clinically normal. Some patients have frequent, noninvasive viral and bacterial infections of the respiratory tract. Chronic diarrhea may occur, with *Giardia* being a commonly implicated pathogen. Infections in patients with IgA deficiency usually are less severe than those observed in patients with X-linked agammaglobulinemia or CVID. Individuals with more severe or chronic infections often have another associated immune deficiency, such as IgG subclass deficiency[59] or, rarely, ataxia telangiectasia.

It has been reported that there is a higher incidence of atopy in patients with IgA deficiency than in the general population. Autoimmune disorders, including systemic lupus erythematosus, rheumatoid arthritis, and pernicious anemia, and lymphoreticular and gastrointestinal malignancies also may be more prevalent.[66]

PATHOGENESIS. The pathogenesis of IgA deficiency has clear parallels with that of CVID. The fundamental defect in both disorders is a failure of B cells to differentiate into immunoglobulin-secreting plasma cells. In addition, as mentioned previously, both disorders are associated with inheritance of a restricted set of extended major histocompatibility complex haplotypes.[86]

DIAGNOSIS. Selective IgA deficiency is diagnosed by a simple quantitative serum immunoglobulin determination showing a subnormal concentration or absence of circulating IgA. In interpreting test results, it is important to remember that serum IgA concentrations are undetectable (<5 to 7 mg/dL) in some normal infants younger than 6 to 9 months of age. Determination of IgG subclass concentrations should be included in the evaluation of all IgA-deficient individuals.

TREATMENT AND PROGNOSIS. IVIG generally is not recommended in the management of patients with selective IgA deficiency. Most blood products, including IVIG, contain trace amounts of IgA. Patients who are totally IgA-deficient are at risk for IgE-mediated anaphylactic reactions if blood products containing these exogenous IgA neoantigens are administered.[16]

Sinopulmonary infections in individuals with IgA deficiency often require unusually long courses of therapy for cure. Parenteral antibiotic therapy sometimes is necessary for refractory cases of sinusitis or pneumonia.

IgG Subclass Deficiency

CLINICAL FEATURES. Commonly reported IgG subclass deficiencies include IgG2, sometimes in association with deficiency of IgG4 or IgA, and IgG3, which may occur in association with IgG1 deficiency.[68, 83] Many individuals with IgG subclass deficiencies are asymptomatic; others have recurrent or chronic bacterial infections, usually of the respiratory tract. Commonly implicated pathogens include *S. pneumoniae, H. influenzae* type b, and other encapsulated bacteria. Children with selective IgG subclass deficiency usually do not have problems with intestinal malabsorption or autoimmunity.

PATHOGENESIS. The pathogenesis of IgG subclass deficiency is unknown. Genetic factors have been implicated by studies showing linkage to certain immunoglobulin allotypes.[36] Slow, age-related increases in serum IgG2 and IgG4 concentrations suggest some sort of developmental control mechanism. T-cell immunity generally is intact in patients with IgG subclass deficiency.

DIAGNOSIS. A diagnosis of clinically relevant IgG subclass deficiency is supported by finding a marked decrease from age-adjusted normal values in the serum concentrations of one or more IgG subclasses, together with evidence for a functional impairment in antibody production. The total serum IgG concentration may be normal, decreased, or even elevated as a result of a compensatory increase in production of unaffected IgG subclasses.

Some children with IgG2 subclass deficiency respond poorly to pure polysaccharide vaccines (e.g., pneumococcal vaccine).[68, 69, 83] Responses to protein antigens (e.g., tetanus toxoid) and protein-conjugated polysaccharide vaccines (e.g., *H. influenzae* type b conjugate vaccines) also may be abnormal.[68, 69] In contrast, patients with IgG3 subclass deficiency may respond poorly to protein antigens, but responses to polysaccharides generally are normal.[83] Assessment of the patient's antibody responses to vaccination with polysaccharide and protein antigens can help to establish the functional significance of an IgG subclass deficiency. Because of the age-dependent nature of antipolysaccharide antibody responses, such testing is not feasible in children younger than 2 years of age.

TREATMENT AND PROGNOSIS. Antibiotic prophylaxis of recurrent sinopulmonary infections and aggressive treatment of intercurrent illnesses form the cornerstone of management for patients with symptomatic IgG subclass deficiency. Because most individuals with IgG subclass deficiency are not at increased risk for infection, IVIG replacement therapy is reserved for patients with abnormal vaccination-induced antibody responses and a demonstrated propensity for frequent or chronic infections. The perceived effectiveness and continued need for IVIG should be reassessed at regular intervals (e.g., annually). IVIG must be administered with caution to patients who have concomitant IgG subclass and IgA deficiency.

Transient Hypogammaglobulinemia of Infancy

CLINICAL FEATURES. Transient hypogammaglobulinemia of infancy is a developmental disorder wherein there is delay in normal physiologic maturation of immunoglobulin synthesis during infancy, resulting in an exaggeration and prolongation of the relative hypogammaglobulinemia observed in most normal infants at 4 or 5 months of age. Many of these infants come to medical attention because of recurrent respiratory tract infections (e.g., otitis media, sinusitis). Septicemia, meningitis, and other serious systemic infections are rare. In other cases, hypogammaglobulinemia is an incidental finding in an otherwise normal and healthy infant.

PATHOGENESIS. Patients with transient hypogammaglobulinemia of infancy do not appear to have any inherent defects of B-cell maturation or function. One report suggests that patients have decreased numbers and function of circulating CD4+ T cells,[70] but a subsequent report did not confirm this finding.[25]

DIAGNOSIS. Transient hypogammaglobulinemia of infancy is a diagnosis that can be made with certainty only in retrospect. Serum immunoglobulin concentrations may remain low (>2 standard deviations below the age-adjusted mean) to several years of age in some cases.[49] In contrast to children with X-linked agammaglobulinemia, infants with transient hypogammaglobulinemia have normal numbers of circulating mature B cells and generate normal antibody responses to diphtheria, tetanus, and pertussis vaccines.

Infants with suspected transient hypogammaglobulinemia should be followed clinically, and serial serum immunoglobulin concentration measurements should be performed. Some children who initially appear to have transient hypogammaglobulinemia continue to have persistent abnormalities of humoral function and eventually are diagnosed as having CVID, selective IgA deficiency, or some other disorder.

TREATMENT AND PROGNOSIS. Because transient hypogammaglobulinemia of infancy is self-limited and specific antibody production usually is normal, ordinarily there is no indication for replacement therapy with IVIG. Antibiotic prophylaxis for recurrent respiratory infections occasionally is indicated.

PRIMARY CELLULAR AND COMBINED IMMUNE DEFICIENCIES

DiGeorge Anomaly

CLINICAL FEATURES. The DiGeorge anomaly includes facial, cardiac, parathyroid, and thymic defects.[44] Patients with DiGeorge anomaly usually present early in infancy with findings unrelated to immune deficiency. Hypoparathyroidism occurs in almost all infants with DiGeorge anomaly, and hypocalcemic tetany is the most common presenting feature. Congenital heart disease, particularly truncus arteriosus and interrupted aortic arch, also may bring the infant to medical attention in the first few weeks of life.[84] Characteristic facial features include microstomia; hypertelorism; upturned nose; posteriorly rotated and small, low-set ears with notched pinnae; and antimongoloid slant of the eyes (see Fig. 79–1). Hypothyroidism, esophageal atresia, tracheoesophageal fistula, and bifid uvula also have been described.

Only a minority of individuals with DiGeorge anomaly have clinically significant immune deficiency. Clinical manifestations of the immune deficiency may include predisposition to a wide variety of common and opportunistic infectious diseases. Recurrent or chronic pneumonias; chronic diarrhea; and candidiasis of the skin, mouth, or esophagus particularly are common. Recurrent or severe herpesvirus infections (e.g., herpes simplex virus, cytomegalovirus); *P. carinii* pneumonia; and other opportunistic viral, fungal, protozoal, and mycobacterial infections sometimes are observed. Fatal graft-versus-host disease may occur if infants receive blood products containing viable lymphocytes during surgical correction of heart defects.

PATHOGENESIS. The syndrome is classified as a developmental field defect resulting from faulty embryologic development of the third and fourth branchial arches and their derivatives, including parathyroid glands, aortic arch structures, and thymus gland.[44] Both males and females are affected. Most cases occur sporadically, but several families have been reported in which more than one child was affected. A variety of teratogens (e.g., retinoids, alcohol) and chromosomal abnormalities (e.g., partial monosomy of chromosome 22 or 10) have been implicated etiologically.

DIAGNOSIS. Hypocalcemia, congenital heart disease, and characteristic facies may lead to suspicion of DiGeorge anomaly in the newborn period. The immune defect is variable. Lymphopenia may be present. A decrease in the number of circulating CD4+ cells (<400/μL) and a decrease in phytohemagglutinin responsiveness may be useful in discriminating patients with immunodeficiency from those without. Quantitative serum immunoglobulin determinations often are normal, but antibody responses after immunization usually are diminished.

TREATMENT AND PROGNOSIS. Initial management should focus on treatment of hypocalcemia and surgical correction of congenital heart disease. Only irradiated blood products should be administered. Children with CD4+ lymphopenia or evidence of cellular immune dysfunction should receive trimethoprim-sulfamethoxazole or a suitable alternative for *P. carinii* pneumonia prophylaxis. Severe immune deficiency may require bone marrow or thymus transplantation.

Wiskott-Aldrich Syndrome

CLINICAL FEATURES. Wiskott-Aldrich syndrome is an X-linked disorder classically characterized by recurrent infection, bleeding, and eczema. However, only a minority of patients has this classic triad of features, and some patients have infectious manifestations alone.[78] Patients may come to medical attention because of recurrent otitis media or pneumonia caused by encapsulated bacteria (e.g., *S. pneumoniae, H. influenzae*). Septicemia, meningitis, and other serious systemic bacterial infections also may occur. Common opportunistic pathogens include *Candida*, cytomegalovirus and other herpesviruses, and *P. carinii.*

Gastrointestinal bleeding in the first few months of life is a common presenting feature of Wiskott-Aldrich syndrome. Life-threatening gastrointestinal or intracranial hemorrhage may occur. Individuals with Wiskott-Aldrich syndrome often have severely depressed platelet counts of 10,000/μL or less. A unique feature of the syndrome is the presence of small platelets in about 50 per cent of cases. Eczema, when present, initially resembles the typical allergic form of the condition. Over time, it may become more generalized and prone to superinfection.

There is a high incidence of autoimmune disorders in patients with Wiskott-Aldrich syndrome. Hemolytic anemia, a juvenile rheumatoid arthritis–like condition, and large or small vessel vasculitis all have been reported. In addition to the intrinsic thrombocytopenia, some patients develop autoimmune thrombocytopenia as their disease progresses. Lymphoreticular malignancies, especially non-Hodgkin lymphomas involving the brain, are common.

PATHOGENESIS. The genetic defect of Wiskott-Aldrich syndrome maps to the proximal part of the short arm of the X chromosome. The molecular basis for the syndrome is not understood completely. T-cell morphologic and membrane abnormalities and signal transduction defects have been described.[52, 60] One group of investigators isolated a novel gene *(WASP)* that is mutated in individuals with Wiskott-Aldrich syndrome.[24] This gene encodes a 501-amino-acid product that appears to be a key regulator of lymphocyte and platelet function.

DIAGNOSIS. Wiskott-Aldrich syndrome should be strongly suspected in a boy with thrombocytopenia and small platelets. Serum immunoglobulin concentrations are variable, with the most typical pattern showing normal IgG, increased IgA, and decreased IgM. Antibody responses to protein antigens (e.g., tetanus) usually are normal, but responses to polysaccharides (e.g., *S. pneumoniae, H. influenzae* type b, isohemagglutinins) are absent.

Patients with Wiskott-Aldrich syndrome typically show delayed hypersensitivity skin test anergy. There are near-normal numbers of circulating T cells, and in vitro proliferative responses to mitogens (e.g., phytohemagglutinin) are normal. However, responses to specific antigens are decreased. Monocytes exhibit abnormal chemotaxis and antibody-dependent cellular cytotoxicity.

TREATMENT AND PROGNOSIS. Human leukocyte antigen–matched bone marrow transplantation results in normalization of cellular immunity, specific antibody responses, and platelet count. Therefore, if an appropriate donor (usually a sibling) can be identified, bone marrow transplantation is the definitive treatment of choice. T-cell–depleted, haploidentical bone marrow transplantation also may be curative, but more formidable difficulties are entailed, including a high incidence of graft failure, graft-versus-host disease, and B-cell proliferative disease.

Splenectomy is curative of thrombocytopenia and can simplify medical management and improve quality of life. As with all primary cellular immune deficiencies, only irradiated blood products should be administered.

Replacement therapy with IVIG is indicated for prophylaxis of infections. Most patients also should receive *P. carinii* pneumonia prophylaxis. Daily antibiotic prophylaxis directed against *S. pneumoniae* and *H. influenzae* may be indicated for patients who have undergone splenectomy. Acute infections should be treated aggressively.

The prognosis of Wiskott-Aldrich syndrome has improved in recent years, with some patients surviving to adulthood.[78] Infection, malignancy, and hemorrhage are the leading causes of death.

Ataxia Telangiectasia

CLINICAL FEATURES. Ataxia telangiectasia is characterized by the presence of cerebellar ataxia, oculocutaneous telangiectases, variable immunodeficiency with frequent infections, and a high incidence of malignancy.[87] Neurologic signs and symptoms often dominate the clinical picture. Ataxia usually becomes evident about the time the child begins to walk. Progressive choreoathetosis, myoclonic jerking movements, and oculomotor abnormalities subsequently develop, resulting ultimately in severe disability.

Telangiectases appear first on the bulbar conjunctivae, usually between 2 and 5 years of age (see Fig. 79–2). They subsequently appear on the nasal bridge, ears, and other areas of sun exposure or trauma. Other cutaneous manifestations of ataxia telangiectasia include café-au-lait spots, vitiligo, and prematurely gray hair.

Recurrent infections are a major feature of ataxia telangiectasia in many patients; other individuals with the disease have relatively few infections. Sinopulmonary infections predominate. Commonly implicated organisms include *S. pneumoniae* and *H. influenzae*. Opportunistic infections are rare.

Up to 15 per cent of patients with ataxia telangiectasia develop malignancy. Non-Hodgkin lymphomas occur most commonly. Carcinomas (especially of the stomach) occur commonly among adults with ataxia telangiectasia.

PATHOGENESIS. Ataxia telangiectasia is inherited in an autosomal recessive manner. The gene defect maps to chromosome 11.[42, 79] The defective gene responsible for the disorder *(ATM)* has been identified.[65] One domain of the ATM protein resembles the phosphatidylinositol-3 kinases, which appear to be important in a number of cellular responses, including cytokine signaling. Another region of the protein is similar to yeast proteins (Rad3 and Mec1) involved in DNA repair. Disease manifestations may result from a major defect in one or more DNA repair mechanisms. Chromosomal instability, with breakage and rearrangements at the sites of the T-cell receptor genes and immunoglobulin heavy-chain genes on chromosomes 7 and 14, may explain the observed immunodeficiency.

DIAGNOSIS. A clinical diagnosis of ataxia telangiectasia is possible when the disease is fully manifest. However, because several years may elapse between onset of signs and symptoms and full disease expression, laboratory studies are necessary for early diagnosis. Increased serum alpha-fetoprotein concentrations are observed in essentially all patients older than 6 months of age. Most patients have deficiencies in serum IgA and IgE; immunoglobulin subclass (especially IgG2) deficiency also may be present. Specific antibody responses usually decline as the patient ages. Most patients have serum IgM in a monomeric 7S form rather than the pentameric 19S molecule usually observed. Common manifestations of cellular immune deficiency include delayed hypersensitivity skin test anergy and decreased in vitro lymphocyte proliferative responses to mitogens and antigens.

TREATMENT AND PROGNOSIS. There is no specific treatment for ataxia telangiectasia. Sinopulmonary infections should be treated aggressively with oral or parenteral antibiotics. Continuous prophylactic antibiotic therapy may be of benefit to individual patients. Replacement therapy with IVIG is reserved for those patients with recurrent infections and abnormal specific antibody responses.

The clinical course and prognosis of ataxia telangiectasia are variable. Some patients survive to adulthood. Death from chronic pulmonary disease or malignancy is common.

Severe Combined Immune Deficiency

CLINICAL FEATURES. Infants with SCID generally present during the first few months of life with infections.[77] Recurrent pneumonias, other respiratory tract infections, and persistent oral and cutaneous candidiasis are common, as are chronic diarrhea and failure to thrive. Septicemia and other serious systemic bacterial infections also occur. Causative organisms include routine pathogens (e.g., *S. pneumoniae, H. influenzae* type b), as well as more unusual organisms, such as *P. aeruginosa*. Life-threatening opportunistic infections, including *P. carinii* pneumonia, sometimes occur early in infancy. Fatal Epstein-Barr virus–associated lymphocyte proliferative disease has been observed in both bone marrow transplant recipients and untreated SCID patients.[28]

PATHOGENESIS. The term *SCID* encompasses a heterogeneous group of disorders having in common defects that lead to profound immunodeficiency with failure of both cellular and humoral immune function. No single pathogenetic mechanism is common to all patients with SCID. Various types of SCID have been defined on the basis of enzymatic, genetic, and immunologic criteria, including (1) reticular dysgenesis, with impaired lymphoid, myeloid, and erythroid differentiation; (2) absence of both T-cell and B-cell differentiation; (3) selective absence of T-cell differentiation; and (4) adenosine deaminase deficiency. Both autosomal and X-linked recessive inheritance patterns have been recognized. Individuals with X-linked SCID have a defect in the gamma chain of the interleukin-2 receptor.[56] This same chain also is a functional component of the interleukin-4 and interleukin-7 receptors.[56, 63] These findings help to explain why a defect in the gamma chain has such a profound effect on lymphoid development and function.

DIAGNOSIS. Infants with SCID typically lack palpable lymph nodes, visible tonsils, and roentgenographic evidence of a thymus gland. Lymphocytopenia often is noted.[77] Serum immunoglobulin concentrations are variable; some patients have panhypogammaglobulinemia, whereas others have depressed concentrations of only one or two immunoglobulin isotypes. Antibody responses almost always are profoundly impaired or absent. Lymphocyte monoclonal phenotyping may or may not reveal the presence of circulating mature B cells. Particularly in boys with X-linked SCID, B cells may account for all circulating lymphocytes.

Circulating T-cell counts are profoundly diminished (<10 per cent of normal) in most patients with SCID. Delayed hypersensitivity skin test anergy is present, and in vitro proliferative responses to mitogens and antigens are depressed severely.

TREATMENT AND PROGNOSIS. Bone marrow transplantation is the treatment of choice for most patients with SCID. Both enzyme replacement[39] and gene therapy[11] have been used for treatment of SCID secondary to adenosine deaminase deficiency.

As with all children who have primary cellular immune deficiencies, live virus vaccines should be avoided. All blood products should be irradiated before transfusion.

Miscellaneous Cellular Immune Deficiencies

Many other disorders of cellular immunity have been described. Two lacunar cellular immune deficiencies are particularly noteworthy. The X-linked lymphoproliferative syndrome represents a defect in control of Epstein-Barr virus infection.[33] Patients may present with severe and often fatal infectious mononucleosis or with B-cell lymphoma.

Chronic mucocutaneous candidiasis, as the name implies, is a condition characterized by chronic, severe candidal infection of mucous membranes, skin, and nails, often in association with autoimmune polyendocrinopathy.[1] T-cell numbers and function usually are normal, but most patients do not manifest delayed hypersensitivity skin test responses to *Candida*, and their lymphocytes fail to proliferate to *Candida* antigen in vitro.

PRIMARY COMPLEMENT DEFICIENCIES

CLINICAL FEATURES. Individuals with primary complement deficiencies may present with frequent infections, rheumatologic disorders, or angioedema, depending on the particular complement component that is deficient.

Complement-deficient individuals are most susceptible to bacterial infections. Serious systemic infections, including septicemia, meningitis, septic arthritis, and osteomyelitis, occur frequently. Recurrent episodes of septicemia and meningitis especially are common.[27, 43, 62] Patients with deficiencies of early-acting complement components (e.g., C3, C1, C4, C2) particularly are susceptible to infection with encapsulated bacteria, including *S. pneumoniae* and *H. influenzae. Neisseria meningitidis* is the most important bacterial pathogen observed in patients with deficiencies of terminal complement components (C5 through C9). Although patients with deficiencies of late-acting complement components are at increased risk for meningococcal septicemia and meningitis, they appear to suffer paradoxically lower rates of morbidity and mortality than do immunologically normal individuals with systemic meningococcal infection. The frequency of primary complement deficiencies among patients with invasive meningococcal disease is about 5 to 10 per cent,[27] although the likelihood of complement deficiency increases dramatically (31 per cent) among individuals who have had more than one episode of invasive disease.[51]

PATHOGENESIS. Various heterozygous and homozygous gene defects are responsible for the many distinct primary complement deficiencies. The particular bacteria that cause infection in these patients reflect the specific role of the missing component in host defense. For example, C3b, the major cleavage product of C3, is an important opsonic ligand that promotes ingestion and killing of bacteria. As a consequence, patients with C3 deficiency have increased susceptibility to infection with bacteria (e.g., *S. pneumoniae, H. influenzae*), for which opsonization is the primary mechanism of host defense.[27, 62] Individuals with deficiencies of C1, C4, or C2 also have increased susceptibility to these same encapsulated bacteria because these components are necessary for activation of C3 via the classic pathway. Activation of terminal complement components C5, C6, C7, C8, and C9 results in assembly of the membrane attack complex C5b-9, a multicomponent macromolecule capable of bactericidal activity. Only gram-negative bacteria are susceptible to this bactericidal effect. Thus, infections in patients with deficiencies of terminal complement components are limited to gram-negative bacteria, such as *N. meningitidis*.[27, 62]

DIAGNOSIS. The screening test used most commonly for primary complement deficiencies is the CH_{50} assay, which reflects the activity of all numbered components of the classic complement pathway from C1 through C9. Primary deficiency of one of the classic complement pathway components results in a CH_{50} approaching 0. Specific immunochemical and functional testing can be performed for identification of the deficient component.

TREATMENT AND PROGNOSIS. There is no specific therapy for primary complement deficiencies. Meningococcal vaccine is recommended for children with terminal complement component deficiencies.[5] Antibiotic prophylaxis is of doubtful benefit. Febrile illnesses should be approached with caution and early institution of expectant antibiotic therapy.

PRIMARY PHAGOCYTE DEFICIENCIES

The primary phagocyte deficiencies are a heterogeneous group of disorders having in common a propensity for frequent infections, resulting either from a decreased number of phagocytic cells (e.g., neutropenia) or because of impaired adhesion, chemotaxis, opsonization and phagocytosis, or intracellular killing (Table 79–4). Infections resulting from quantitative or qualitative phagocyte deficiencies tend to be prolonged and recurrent, with a slower than expected response to antibiotic therapy. Common pathogens include *S. aureus, P. aeruginosa*, enteric gram-negative bacteria, and certain fungi (e.g., *Candida, Aspergillus*).

TABLE 79–4. Primary Phagocyte Deficiencies

Quantitative Defects
Infantile agranulocytosis
Familial granulocytopenia
Cyclic neutropenia
Qualitative Defects
Adhesion defects
Leukocyte adhesion deficiency
Type I, integrin deficiency
Type II, E- and P-selectin ligand deficiency
Chemotactic defects
Humoral
Complement deficiency
Hyperimmunoglobulinemia E
Cellular
Chédiak-Higashi syndrome
Defects of opsonization and phagocytosis
Complement deficiency
Antibody deficiency
Intracellular killing defects
Chronic granulomatous disease
Glucose-6-phosphate dehydrogenase deficiency
Myeloperoxidase deficiency
Chédiak-Higashi syndrome
Specific granule deficiency

Quantitative Phagocyte Abnormalities

As a class, the most common phagocyte deficiencies encountered in clinical practice are quantitative in origin. However, most of these disorders are acquired (e.g., drug-induced or autoimmune neutropenia) rather than primary. In general, risk of infection increases progressively with both duration and magnitude of granulocytopenia below 1500/μL, with a dramatic increase in risk for those patients with granulocyte counts less than 500/μL.

Primary quantitative phagocyte deficiencies can be observed either as solitary defects or in association with other disorders (e.g., Schwachman syndrome). Infantile agranulocytosis (Kostmann syndrome) is an autosomal recessive disorder characterized by granulocyte maturation arrest, markedly decreased numbers of circulating granulocytes (typically <100/μL), and severe infection and death, often in early infancy. More benign familial granulocytopenia (or neutropenia) syndromes also are recognized. Affected individuals present at various ages from infancy to adulthood, usually with indolent skin and soft tissue infections.

Cyclic neutropenia is an autosomal dominant defect of myelopoiesis in which there is periodic disappearance of granulocytes from the circulation.[73] Early granulocyte precursors are present in the bone marrow during periods of granulocytopenia, suggesting transient maturation arrest. Periods of granulocytopenia usually last 5 to 7 days and occur at 14- to 35-day intervals. The cycle length generally is constant for any given individual. Fever, malaise, aphthous stomatitis, and skin and soft tissue infections often are observed during periods of granulocytopenia.

Some of the primary quantitative phagocyte deficiencies, particularly familial granulocytopenia and cyclic neutropenia, respond to therapy with recombinant granulocyte colony-stimulating factor.[31, 35, 41] Alternate-day corticosteroid therapy also has been used with some success in cyclic neutropenia.[88]

Chronic Granulomatous Disease

CLINICAL FEATURES. The physical findings of patients with CGD are nonspecific. Lymphadenopathy and hepatomegaly are common. Aphthous stomatitis may be present. Infectious complications dominate the clinical picture. Infections often begin during infancy and recur throughout the patient's life. Occasional patients have a relatively mild disease course and come to medical attention only during adolescence or adulthood.[67]

Patients with CGD may have infections of virtually any organ or body site. Suppurative lymphadenitis, soft tissue abscesses, pneumonia, lung abscess, hepatic abscess, and osteomyelitis especially are common. Perirectal abscess may occur during early infancy. Most infections in patients with CGD have an indolent course. Granuloma formation may occur, possibly because of persistence of viable intracellular bacteria or fungi.

Patients with CGD generally have infections caused by catalase-positive bacteria and fungi.[18, 53] *S. aureus* accounts for almost one-third of all infections of determined etiology. *Salmonella*, *S. marcescens*, *Pseudomonas* (especially *Pseudomonas cepacia*[75]), and certain enteric gram-negative bacilli also are common. *S. marcescens* osteomyelitis particularly is suggestive of the diagnosis of CGD. Fungi, especially *Aspergillus*, account for nearly one-fifth of all defined infections in patients with CGD (Fig. 79–5).

Patients with CGD often have poor wound healing. Granulomatous obstructive lesions of the urinary[2] and gastrointestinal[4] tracts have been reported. Corticosteroid therapy may be effective in relieving these sometimes life-threatening obstructions.[17] Granulomatous bowel involvement may resemble Crohn disease. Boys with X-linked CGD sometimes have the McLeod blood phenotype, which results in difficulty in transfusion crossmatching and the potential for hemolytic transfusion reactions.[13]

PATHOGENESIS. Both X-linked and autosomal recessive forms of CGD have been described. The various gene defects result in abnormalities of membrane or cytosolic components of the cellular nicotinamide adenine dinucleotide phosphate (reduced form) oxidase system. Despite the genetic heterogeneity, all individuals with CGD have in common failure of the cellular respiratory burst, which ordinarily accompanies phagocytosis and various soluble stimuli. All phagocytic cells are affected. As a consequence, oxygen-derived microbicidal factors (e.g., superoxide, hydrogen peroxide) are not formed, and intracellular killing of phagocytized microorganisms is severely impaired. Catalase-negative microorganisms (e.g., streptococci, *H. influenzae*), because they produce hydrogen peroxide that can accumulate within the phagocytic vacuole, are killed normally, despite failure of the phagocyte itself to produce hydrogen peroxide.

DIAGNOSIS. The diagnosis of CGD usually is made with the NBT dye test.[8] Neutrophils are stimulated in the presence of NBT, a soluble yellow dye that is reduced by cellular superoxide to formazan, an insoluble blue precipitate. Neutrophils from normal individuals show virtually 100 per cent reduction of NBT to formazan, whereas patients with CGD show essentially no dye reduction.

TREATMENT AND PROGNOSIS. Complicating infections should be treated aggressively in the patient with CGD. Specific microbiologic diagnosis should be established whenever possible. Empiric therapy is directed against the bacterial organisms known to be common causes of infection, namely, *S. aureus*, *Pseudomonas*, and enteric gram-negative bacilli. Surgical drainage or débridement of sites of infection often is required. The ultimate duration of antimicrobial therapy is individualized, but, compared with non-immunocompromised individuals with similar infections, substantially longer treatment courses usually are required in the CGD patient. Anecdotal reports suggest beneficial effects of granulocyte transfusions in some CGD patients with serious bacterial or fungal infections. However, in a retrospective analysis, there was not a significant reduction in the rate of persistent infection or death for CGD patients treated with granulocyte transfusions as an adjunct to antifungal therapy for pulmonary or disseminated fungal infection.[18]

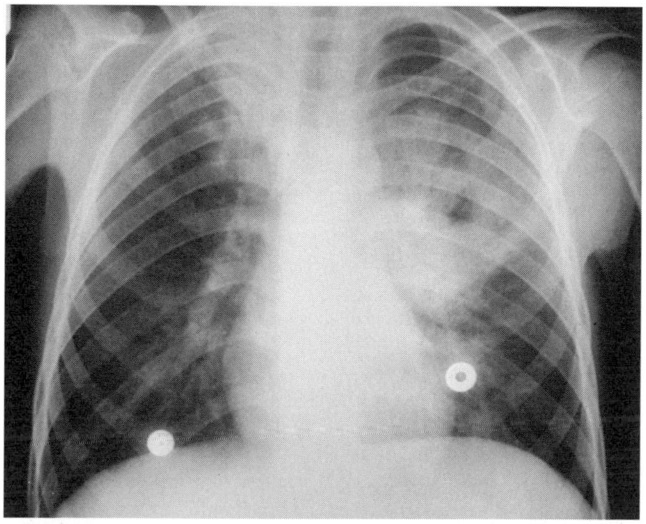

FIGURE 79–5. *Chest roentgenogram of a 10-year-old boy with chronic granulomatous disease showing a left-sided pulmonary infiltrate and cavitary lung lesion. Biopsy revealed* Aspergillus fumigatus *infection.*

Antibiotic prophylaxis is of benefit in reducing the frequency of bacterial infections in patients with CGD.[48] Daily trimethoprim-sulfamethoxazole usually is used for this purpose. It has been suggested that daily itraconazole also may be effective when used in a similar fashion for prevention of *Aspergillus* infections.[54] Interferon-γ, given by subcutaneous injection three times weekly, may reduce the incidence of serious infections in CGD by up to two-thirds without causing major deleterious side effects.[40] This agent should be offered routinely to all individuals with any of the recognized forms of CGD.

The prognosis of CGD has improved remarkably over the past several decades. Most patients now survive to adulthood.

Leukocyte Adhesion Deficiency

CLINICAL FEATURES. Patients with leukocyte adhesion deficiency (LAD) suffer severe and recurrent bacterial infections of the skin and soft tissues, mucosal surfaces, and gastrointestinal tract, often beginning during early infancy.[81] Common causative microorganisms include staphylococci and *Pseudomonas*. Moderate and severe phenotypes are recognized.[6] Infants with the severe phenotype may have delayed separation of the umbilical cord or omphalitis. Poor wound healing also is observed. Cutaneous infections may become necrotic, initially resembling the lesions of ecthyma gangrenosum. Later, lesions may develop a pyoderma gangrenosum–like appearance. Individuals surviving infancy typically develop severe gingivitis and periodontitis with progressive alveolar bone loss (see Fig. 79–3).

Marked granulocytosis is a hallmark of LAD. Circulating granulocyte counts may range between 15,000/μL and 75,000/μL, even in the absence of infection, and counts of 100,000/μL or greater are common during intercurrent episodes of infection. Despite this granulocytosis, pus formation is poor, and abscesses are "cold."

PATHOGENESIS. LAD is an autosomal recessive disorder that maps to chromosome 21. Neutrophils from individuals with LAD are defective in their expression of several surface glycoproteins known as the leukocyte integrin (CD11/CD18) complex. These molecules are critical for adhesion-dependent functions, and their absence is responsible for defects in adherence, chemotaxis, and phagocytosis that are observed in the disorder.

The severity of infectious complications of LAD is related directly to the degree of CD18 expression.[6, 14] Patients with the severe clinical phenotype have undetectable expression of CD11/CD18 complexes on their phagocytes, whereas individuals with the moderate phenotype generally have 2 to 8 per cent expression.

A second form of LAD has been described in two patients with craniofacial dysmorphism, neurologic deficits, recurrent respiratory infections, and marked granulocytosis.[26, 32] Both individuals manifested the Bombay (hh) blood phenotype. In vitro studies revealed defects of random and directed neutrophil migration and aggregation. Unlike patients with

LAD type I, neutrophils from patients with this second type of LAD had normal surface expression of CD18. The molecular basis for the phagocyte dysfunction appears to be a glycosylation defect influencing expression of sialyl-Lewis X, a carbohydrate ligand for the endothelial adhesion molecules E-selectin and P-selectin.

DIAGNOSIS. The diagnosis of LAD type I is made using fluorescence-labeled monoclonal anti-CD11/CD18 antibody and flow cytometry. In vitro studies reveal abnormalities of phagocyte adherence, chemotaxis, and phagocytosis. Individuals with the second recognized type of LAD have similar phagocyte function abnormalities, but expression of phagocyte surface integrins is normal.

TREATMENT AND PROGNOSIS. Intercurrent bacterial infections in patients with LAD must be treated aggressively with prolonged courses of parenteral antibiotics. Although survival to adulthood is described, almost half of affected individuals die before 2 years of age. Bone marrow transplantation offers the best hope for long-term survival.

Other Primary Phagocyte Deficiencies

A variety of other defects of phagocyte chemotaxis, phagocytosis, and intracellular killing have been described. The Chédiak-Higashi syndrome is a rare autosomal recessive disorder characterized by partial oculocutaneous albinism, rotatory nystagmus, and peripheral neuropathy. Affected individuals develop recurrent serious or life-threatening infections caused by a wide variety of catalase-positive and catalase-negative bacteria. In the accelerated phase of the illness, hepatosplenomegaly, lymphadenopathy, lymphocytic infiltration of multiple body organs, and unexplained febrile illnesses are common. Giant granules are found in a number of different cell types in the body, including leukocytes. Neutrophils exhibit defective chemotaxis and abnormal bactericidal activity.

Hyperimmunoglobulinemia E with impaired chemotaxis (Job syndrome) is characterized by eczema, recurrent "cold" staphylococcal abscesses, sinusitis, and otitis media. Coarse facial features are common. In addition to staphylococcal abscesses, recurrent pneumonia and mucocutaneous candidiasis are common. All patients have markedly increased serum IgE concentrations. A variable neutrophil chemotactic defect also is present.

Myeloperoxidase deficiency generally is a mild disorder of phagocyte intracellular killing. Systemic candidiasis has been reported in a few patients with myeloperoxidase deficiency, usually in conjunction with diabetes mellitus.[55] Because affected phagocytes are devoid of meloperoxidase-dependent but not other oxidative killing mechanisms, there is delay in, but not absence of, intracellular killing.

References

1. Ahonen, P., Myllarniemi, S., Sipila I., et al.: Clinical variations of autoimmune polyendocrinopathy-candidiasis-ectoderm dystrophy (APECED) in a series of 68 patients. N. Engl. J. Med. *322*:1829–1836, 1990.
2. Aliabadi, H., Gonzalez, R., and Quie, P. G.: Urinary tract disorders in patients with chronic granulomatous disease. N. Engl. J. Med. *321*:706–708, 1989.
3. Allen, R. C., Armitage, R. J., Conley, M. E., et al.: CD40 ligand gene defects responsible for X-linked hyper-IgM syndrome. Science *259*:990–993, 1993.
4. Ament, M. E., and Ochs, H. D.: Gastrointestinal manifestations of chronic granulomatous disease. N. Engl. J. Med. *288*:382–387, 1973.
5. American Academy of Pediatrics: Meningococcal infections. *In* Peter, G. (ed.): 1994 Red Book: Report of the Committee on Infectious Diseases. 23rd ed. Elk Grove Village, IL, American Academy of Pediatrics, 1994, p. 323.
6. Anderson, D. C., Schmalstieg, F. C., Finegold, M. J., et al.: The severe and moderate phenotypes of heritable MAC-1, LFA-1, P150,95 deficiency: Their quantitative definition and relation to leukocyte dysfunction and clinical features. J. Infect. Dis. *152*:668–689, 1985.
7. Aruffo, A., Farrington, M., Hollenbaugh, D., et al.: The CD40 ligand, gp39, is defective in activated T cells from patients with X-linked hyper-IgM syndrome. Cell *72*:291–300, 1993.
8. Axtell, R. A.: Evaluation of the patient with a possible phagocytic disorder. Hematol. Oncol. Clin. North Am. *2*:1–12, 1988.
9. Badger, G. F., Dingle, J. H., Feller, A. E., et al.: A study of illness in a group of Cleveland families. II. Incidence of the common respiratory diseases. Am. J. Hyg. *58*:31, 1953.
10. Bartlett, A. V., Moore, M., Gary, G. W., et al.: Diarrheal illness among infants and toddlers in day care centers. II. Comparison with day care homes and households. J. Pediatr. *107*:503–509, 1985.
11. Blaese, R. M.: Development of gene therapy for immunodeficiency: Adenosine deaminase deficiency. Pediatr. Res. *33*(Suppl. 1):S49–S53, 1993.
12. Brimblecombe, F. S. W., Cruickshank, R., Masters, P. L., et al.: Family studies of respiratory infections. Br. Med. J. *1*:119, 1958.
13. Brzica, S. M., Jr., Pineda, A. A., Taswell, H. F., et al.: Chronic granulomatous disease and the McLeod phenotype: Successful treatment of infection with granulocyte transfusions resulting in subsequent hemolytic transfusion reaction. Mayo Clin. Proc. *52*:153–156, 1977.
14. Buckley, R. H.: Immunodeficiency diseases. J. A. M. A. *268*:2797–2806, 1992.
15. Buckley, R. H., and Schiff, R. I.: The use of intravenous immune globulin in immunodeficiency diseases. N. Engl. J. Med. *325*:110–117, 1991.
16. Burks, A. W., Sampson, H. A., and Buckley, R. H.: Anaphylactic reactions after gamma globulin administration in patients with hypogammaglobulinemia: Detection of IgE antibodies to IgA. N. Engl. J. Med. *314*:560–564, 1986.
17. Chin, T. W., Stiehm, E. R., Falloon, J., et al.: Corticosteroids in treatment of obstructive lesions of chronic granulomatous disease. J. Pediatr. *111*:349–352, 1987.
18. Cohen, M. S., Isturiz, R. E., Malech, H. L., et al.: Fungal infection in chronic granulomatous disease: The importance of the phagocyte in defense against fungi. Am. J. Med. *71*:59–66, 1981.
19. Conley, M. E., Larche, M., Bonagura, V. R., et al.: Hyper IgM syndrome associated with defective CD40-mediated B cell activation. J. Clin. Invest. *94*:1404–1409, 1994.
20. Conley, M. E., Park, C. L., and Douglas, S. D.: Childhood common variable immunodeficiency with autoimmune disease. J. Pediatr. *108*:915–922, 1986.
21. Crennan, J. M., Van Scoy, R. E., McKenna, C. H., et al.: Echovirus polymyositis in patients with hypogammaglobulinemia: Failure of high-dose intravenous gammaglobulin therapy and review of the literature. Am. J. Med. *81*:35–42, 1986.
22. Cunningham-Rundles, C.: Clinical and immunologic analyses of 103 patients with common variable immunodeficiency. J. Clin. Immunol. *9*:22–33, 1989.
23. Cunningham-Rundles, C., Siegal, F. P., Cunningham-Rundles, S., et al.: Incidence of cancer in 98 patients with common varied immunodeficiency. J. Clin. Immunol. *7*:294–299, 1987.
24. Derry, J. M. J., Ochs, H. D., and Francke, U.: Isolation of a novel gene mutated in Wiskott-Aldrich syndrome. Cell *78*:635–644, 1994.
25. Dressler, F., Peter, H. H., Muller, W., et al.: Transient hypogammaglobulinemia of infancy. Acta Paediatr. Scand. *78*:767–774, 1989.
26. Etzioni, A., Frydman, M., Pollack, S., et al.: Brief report: Recurrent severe infections caused by a novel leukocyte adhesion deficiency. N. Engl. J. Med. *327*:1789–1792, 1992.
27. Figueroa, J. E., and Densen, P.: Infectious diseases associated with complement deficiencies. Clin. Microbiol. Rev. *4*:359–395, 1991.
28. Filipovich, A. H., Mathur, A., Kamat, D., et al.: Lymphoproliferative disorders and other tumors complicating immunodeficiencies. Immunodeficiency *5*:91–112, 1994.
29. Forgacs, P., Kundsin, R. B., Margles, S. W., et al.: A case of *Ureaplasma urealyticum* septic arthritis in a patient with hypogammaglobulinemia. Clin. Infect. Dis. *16*:293–294, 1993.
30. Fox, J. P., Hall, C. E., Cooney, M. K., et al.: The Seattle virus watch. II. Objectives, study population and its observation, data processing and summary of illnesses. Am. J. Epidemiol. *96*:270–285, 1972.
31. Frampton, J. E., Lee, C. R., and Faulds, D.: Filgrastim: A review of its pharmacological properties and therapeutic efficacy in neutropenia. Drugs *48*:731–760, 1994.
32. Frydman, M., Etzioni, A., Eidlitz-Markus, T., et al.: Rambam-Hasharon syndrome of psychomotor retardation, short stature, defective neutrophil motility, and Bombay phenotype. Am. J. Med. Genet. *44*:297–302, 1992.
33. Grierson, H., and Purtilo, D. T.: Epstein-Barr virus infections in males with the X-linked proliferative syndrome. Ann. Intern. Med. *106*:538–545, 1987.
34. Guerrant, R. L., Lohr, J. A., and Williams, E. K.: Acute infectious diarrhea. I. Epidemiology, etiology, and pathogenesis. Pediatr. Infect. Dis. *5*:353–359, 1986.
35. Hammond, W. P., IV, Price, T. H., Souza, L. M., et al.: Treatment of cyclic neutropenia with granulocyte colony-stimulating factor. N. Engl. J. Med. *320*:1306–1311, 1989.
36. Hanson, L. A., Soderstrom, R., Nilssen, D. E., et al.: IgG subclass deficiency with or without IgA deficiency. Clin. Immunol. Immunopathol. *61*:S70–S77, 1991.
37. Hausser, C., Virelizier, J. L., Buriot, D., et al.: Common variable hypogam-

maglobulinemia in children: Clinical and immunologic observations in 30 patients. Am. J. Dis. Child. *137*:833–837, 1983.
38. Hermaszewski, R. A., and Webster, A. D.: Primary hypogammaglobuliaemia: A survey of clinical manifestations and complications. Q. J. Med. *86*:31–42, 1993.
39. Hershfield, M. S., Chaffee, S., and Sorensen, R. V.: Enzyme replacement therapy with polyethylene glycol–adenosine deaminase in adenosine deaminase deficiency: Overview and case reports of three patients, including two now receiving gene therapy. Pediatr. Res. *33*:S42–S47, 1993.
40. International Chronic Granulomatous Disease Cooperative Study Group: A controlled trial of interferon gamma to prevent infection in chronic granulomatous disease. N. Engl. J. Med. *324*:509–516, 1991.
41. Jayabose, S., Tugal, O., Sandoval, C., et al.: Recombinant human granulocyte colony stimulating factor in cyclic neutropenia: Use of a new 3-day-a-week regimen. Am. J. Pediatr. Hematol. Oncol. *16*:338–340, 1994.
42. Kapp, L. N., Painter, R. B., Yu, L. C., et al.: Cloning of a candidate gene for ataxia-telangiectasia group D. Am. J. Hum. Genet. *51*:45–54, 1992.
43. Kline, M. W.: Recurrent bacterial meningitis. Antibiot. Chemother. *45*:254–261, 1992.
44. Lammer, E. J., and Opitz, J. M.: The DiGeorge anomaly as a developmental field defect. Am. J. Med. Genet. 2(Suppl.):113–127, 1986.
45. Lederman, H. M., and Winkelstein, J. A.: X-linked agammaglobulinemia: An analysis of 96 patients. Medicine *64*:145–156, 1985.
46. Lee, A. H., Levinson, A. I., and Schumacher, H. R.: Hypogammaglobulinemia and rheumatic disease. Semin. Arthritis Rheum. *22*:252–264, 1993.
47. Liese, J. G., Wintergerst, J., Tympner, K. D., et al.: High- vs low-dose immunoglobulin therapy in the long-term treatment of X-linked agammaglobulinemia. Am. J. Dis. Child. *146*:335–339, 1992.
48. Margolis, D. M., Melnick, D. A., Alling, D. W., et al.: Trimethoprim-sulfamethoxazole prophylaxis in the management of chronic granulomatous disease. J. Infect. Dis. *162*:723–726, 1990.
49. McGeady, S. J.: Transient hypogammaglobulinemia of infancy: Need to reconsider name and definition. J. Pediatr. *110*:47–50, 1987.
50. McKinney, R. E., Jr., Katz, S. L., and Wilfert, C. M.: Chronic enteroviral meningoencephalitis in agammaglobulinemic patients. Rev. Infect. Dis. *9*:334–356, 1987.
51. Merino, J., Rodriguez-Valverde, V., Lamelas, J. A., et al.: Prevalence of deficits of complement components in patients with recurrent meningococcal infections. J. Infect. Dis. *148*:331, 1983.
52. Molina, I. J., Kenney, D. M., Rosen, F. S., et al.: T cell lines characterize events in the pathogenesis of the Wiskott-Aldrich syndrome. J. Exp. Med. *176*:867–874, 1992.
53. Mouy, R., Fischer, A., Vilmer, E., et al.: Incidence, severity, and prevention of infections in chronic granulomatous disease. J. Pediatr. *114*:555–560, 1989.
54. Mouy, R., Veber, F., Blanche, S., et al.: Long-term itraconazole prophylaxis against *Aspergillus* infections in thirty-two patients with chronic granulomatous disease. J. Pediatr. *125*:998–1003, 1994.
55. Nauseef, W. M.: Myeloperoxidase deficiency. Hematol. Oncol. Clin. North Am. *2*:135–158, 1988.
56. Noguchi, M., Nakamura, Y., Russell, S. M., et al.: Interleukin-2 receptor gamma chain: A functional component of the interleukin-7 receptor. Science *262*:1877–1880, 1993.
57. Notarangelo, L. D., Duse, M., and Ugazio, A. G.: Immunodeficiency with hyper-IgM (HIM). Immunodefic. Rev. *3*:101–121, 1992.
58. Ochs, H. D., Ament, M. E., and Davis, S. D.: Giardiasis with malabsorption in X-linked agammaglobulinemia. N. Engl. J. Med. *287*:341–342, 1972.
59. Oxelius, V. A., Laurell, A. B., Lindquist, B., et al.: IgG subclasses in selective IgA deficiency: Importance of IgG2-IgA deficiency. N. Engl. J. Med. *302*:1476–1477, 1981.
60. Remold-O'Donnell, E., Van Brocklyn, J., and Kenney, D. M.: Effect of platelet calpain on normal T lymphocyte CD43: Hypothesis of events in the Wiskott-Aldrich syndrome. Blood *79*:1754–1762, 1992.
61. Rosenblatt, H. M.: Primary immunodeficiency disorders and the rational use of intravenous immunoglobulin. Semin. Pediatr. Infect. Dis. *3*:150–156, 1992.
62. Ross, S. C., and Densen, P.: Complement deficiency states and infection: Epidemiology, pathogenesis and consequences of neisserial and other infections in an immune deficiency. Medicine *63*:243–273, 1984.
63. Russell, S. M., Keegan, A. D., Harada, N., et al.: Interleukin-2 receptor gamma chain: A functional component of the interleukin-4 receptor. Science *262*:1880–1883, 1993.
64. Saulsbury, F. T., Winkelstein, J. A., and Yolken, R. H.: Chronic rotavirus infection in immunodeficiency. J. Pediatr. *97*:61–65, 1980.
65. Savitsky, K., Bar-Shira, A., Gilad, S., et al.: A single ataxia-telangiectasia gene with a product similar to PI-3 kinase. Science *268*:1749–1753, 1995.
66. Schaffer, F. M., Monteiro, R. C., Volanakis, J. E., et al.: IgA deficiency. Immunodeficiency Rev. *3*:15–44, 1991.
67. Schapiro, B. L., Newburger, P. E., Klempner, M. S., et al.: Chronic granulomatous disease presenting in a 69-year-old man. N. Engl. J. Med. *325*:1786–1790, 1991.
68. Shackelford, P. G., Granoff, D. M., Polmar, S. H., et al.: Subnormal serum concentrations of IgG2 in children with frequent infections associated with varied patterns of immunologic dysfunction. J. Pediatr. *116*:529–538, 1990.
69. Shackelford, P. G., Polmar, S. H., Mayus, J. L., et al.: Spectrum of IgG2 subclass deficiency in children with recurrent infections: Prospective study. J. Pediatr. *108*:647–653, 1986.
70. Siegel, R. L., Issekutz, T., Schwaber, J., et al.: Deficiency of helper T cells in transient hypogammaglobulinemia of infancy. N. Engl. J. Med. *305*:1307–1313, 1981.
71. Siegel, S. R., Siegel, B., Sokoloff, B. Z., et al.: Urinary tract infection in infants and preschool children. Am. J. Dis. Child. *134*:369–372, 1980.
72. Sneller, M. C., Strober, W., Eisenstein, E., et al.: New insights into common variable immunodeficiency. Ann. Intern. Med. *118*:720–730, 1993.
73. Souid, A. K.: Congenital cyclic neutropenia. Clin. Pediatr. *34*:151–155, 1995.
74. Spector, B. D., Perry, G. S., III, and Kersey, J. H.: Genetically determined immunodeficiency disease (GDID) and malignancy: Report from the Immunodeficiency-Cancer Registry. Clin. Immunol. Immunopathol. *11*:12–29, 1978.
75. Speert, D. P., Bond, M., Woodman, R. C., et al.: Infection with *Pseudomonas cepacia* in chronic granulomatous disease: Role of nonoxidative killing by neutrophils in host defense. J. Infect. Dis. *170*:1524–1531, 1994.
76. Spickett, G. P., Webster, A. D., and Farrant, J.: Cellular abnormalities in common variable immunodeficiency. Immunodeficiency Rev. *2*:199–219, 1990.
77. Stephan, J. L., Vlekova, V., Le Deist, F., et al.: Severe combined immunodeficiency: A retrospective single-center study of clinical presentation and outcome in 117 cases. J. Pediatr. *123*:564–572, 1993.
78. Sullivan, K. E., Mullen, C. A., Blaese, R. M., et al.: A multiinstitutional survey of the Wiskott-Aldrich syndrome. J. Pediatr. *125*:876–885, 1994.
79. Taylor, A. M., Jaspers, N. G., and Gatti, R. A.: Fifth International Workshop on Ataxia-Telangiectasia. Cancer Res. *53*:438–441, 1993.
80. Teele, D. W., Klein, J. O., Rosner, B., et al.: Epidemiology of otitis media during the first seven years of life in children in greater Boston: A prospective cohort study. J. Infect. Dis. *160*:83–94, 1989.
81. Todd, R. F., III, and Freyer, D. R.: The CD11/18 leukocyte glycoprotein deficiency. Hematol. Oncol. Clin. North Am. *2*:13–31, 1988.
82. Tsukada, S., Saffran, D. C., Rawlings, D. J., et al.: Deficient expression of a B cell cytoplasmic tyrosine kinase in human X-linked agammaglobulinemia. Cell *72*:279–290, 1993.
83. Umetsu, D. T., Ambrosino, D. M., Quinti, I., et al.: Recurrent sinopulmonary infection and impaired antibody response to bacterial capsular polysaccharide antigen in children with selective IgG-subclass deficiency. N. Engl. J. Med. *313*:1247–1251, 1985.
84. Van Mierop, L. H., and Kutsche, L. M.: Cardiovascular anomalies in DiGeorge syndrome and importance of neural crest as a possible pathogenetic factor. Am. J. Cardiol. *58*:133–137, 1986.
85. Vetrie, D., Vorechovsky, I., Sideras, P., et al.: The gene involved in X-linked agammaglobulinemia is a member of the src family of protein-tyrosine kinases. Nature *316*:226–233, 1993.
86. Volanakis, J. E., Zhu, Z. B., Schaffer, F. M., et al.: Major histocompatibility complex class III genes and susceptibility to immunoglobulin A deficiency and common variable immunodeficiency. J. Clin. Invest. *89*:1914–1922, 1992.
87. Woods, C. G., and Taylor, A. M.: Ataxia-telangiectasia in the British Isles: The clinical and laboratory features of 70 affected individuals. Q. J. Med. *82*:169–179, 1992.
88. Wright, D. G., Fauci, A. S., Dale, D. C., et al.: Correction of human cyclic neutropenia and prednisolone. N. Engl. J. Med. *298*:295–300, 1978.

80

AIDS AND OTHER ACQUIRED IMMUNODEFICIENCY DISEASES

I. Celine Hanson and William T. Shearer

In contrast with the primary or congenital immunodeficiencies, pediatric secondary or acquired immunodeficiencies make up the majority of immunodeficiency disorders in childhood and affect the greatest number of children. Table 80–1 outlines the most common of the childhood acquired immunodeficiency disorders.[192] This chapter provides an overview of the newest pediatric acquired immunodeficiency, HIV infection, and the resultant AIDS; it also broadly describes infectious diseases that commonly have been associated with other acquired immunodeficiencies, namely the newborn and premature infant, malnutrition, and oncologic diseases.

AIDS

HIV infection and AIDS have had a significant clinical impact on children worldwide. The World Health Organization has estimated that by the year 2000, in sub-Saharan Africa alone, 3 to 4 million children may be HIV-infected.[209] The ever-increasing incidence of HIV infection and AIDS in children closely follows that in young women of child-bearing years (15 to 49 years of age).[53] The global specter of HIV infection in women, and consequently in their children, is presented in Figure 80–1; the numbers of motherless infants and adolescents in the United States is estimated to exceed 150,000 through the year 2000.[155]

The few early cases of pediatric HIV infection/AIDS in the United States have been replaced with increasing numbers (6611 AIDS cases in children younger than 13 years of age through June 1995). AIDS currently is the sixth leading cause of death among women of child-bearing age and the seventh for children 1 to 4 years of age.[195] HIV infection/AIDS looms, then, as a significant health care threat to infants and children of all nations, including the United States. Because HIV infection/AIDS has such a wide spectrum of clinical manifestations and expression, every clinician and health care specialist (including primary caregivers, pediatric subspecialists, nursing personnel, and social service professionals) who provide care to children should familiarize themselves with HIV infection, develop expertise, and anticipate service provision to this population.

Epidemiology and Transmission

Pediatric AIDS first was described to the Centers for Disease Control and Prevention (CDC) in 1982 and appeared at the same time as an epidemic of adult AIDS.[51] The first definitions of pediatric AIDS in 1985 proved cumbersome, and in 1987, the CDC developed a classification system that more accurately and adequately represented infants; by then, it was recognized that HIV was the etiology of adult and pediatric AIDS.[40] In 1994, the classification system again was revised to include more advanced viral diagnostic technology and a system for staging pediatric HIV disease using both clinical and immunologic axes.[46] This new staging system accommodates the criticisms of many clinicians who believed that the 1987 strict pediatric AIDS definition did not allow for reporting of infants and children with significant morbidity from HIV infection without an AIDS diagnosis.[39] Table 80–2 outlines the clinical axis of the staging system, which is composed of four clinical categories (N, A, B, C).[46] The clinical axis is intended for unidirectional use for any individual child—that is, disease severity proceeds from N (asymptomatic) ⇒ A (mildly asymptomatic) ⇒ B (moderately symptom-

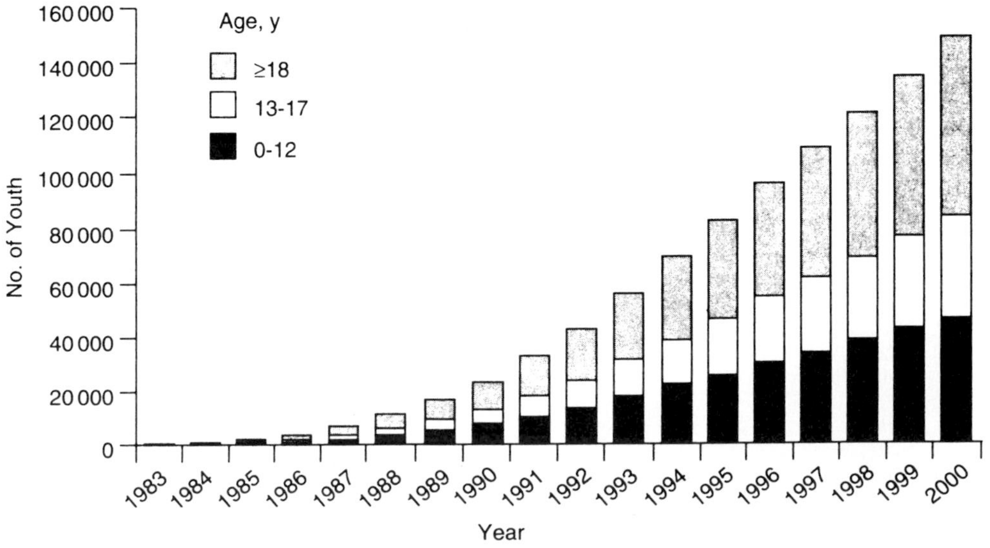

FIGURE 80–1. *Estimation of the cumulative number of motherless children, adolescents, and young adults orphaned by the HIV/AIDS epidemic in the United States, 1983 through 2000. (From Michaels, D., and Levine, C.: Estimates of the number of motherless youth orphaned by AIDS in the United States. J. A. M. A. 268:3456–3461, 1992. Copyright 1992, American Medical Association.)*

TABLE 80–1. Secondary Immunodeficiencies

I. Premature and newborn infant
II. AIDS
III. Infiltrative and hematologic diseases
  A. Histiocytosis
  B. Lymphoid malignancy
  C. Sarcoidosis
  D. Leukemia
  E. Hodgkin disease
  F. Lymphoproliferative disease
  G. Agranulocytosis and aplastic anemia
IV. Hereditary diseases
  A. Chromosomal abnormalities
  B. Chromosome instability syndromes
  C. Enzyme deficiencies
  D. Sickle-cell disease
  E. Myotonic dystrophy
  F. Congenital asplenia
  G. Skeletal dysplasias
V. Specific organ system dysfunction
  A. Diabetes mellitus
  B. Protein-losing enteropathy
  C. Nephrotic syndrome
  D. Uremia
VI. Nutritional deficiency
  A. Protein-calorie malnutrition
  B. Iron deficiency
  C. Vitamin A deficiency
VII. Immunosuppressive agents
  A. Radiation
  B. Antibodies
  C. Glucocorticosteroids
  D. Cyclosporine
  E. Cytotoxic drugs
  F. Anticonvulsant drugs
VIII. Infectious diseases
  A. Bacterial infection
  B. Fungal infection
  C. Viral infection
  D. Parasitic infection
IX. Surgery and trauma
  A. Burns
  B. Splenectomy
  C. Head injury

From Sandburg, E. T., Kline, M. W., and Shearer, W. T.: The secondary immunodeficiencies. *In* Steihm, E. R. (ed.): Immunologic Disorders of Infants and Children. 4th ed. Philadelphia, W. B. Saunders, 1996, pp. 553–602.

atic) ⇒ C (severely symptomatic) ⇒ HIV-associated death. Clinical category C describes children with AIDS-defining characteristics, namely wasting, encephalopathy, opportunistic infections, and malignancies, but excludes lymphoid interstitial pneumonitis/pulmonary lymphoid hyperplasia (LIP/PLH). Clinical category B describes children with other specific HIV-associated illnesses (e.g., single episodes of bacteremia, leiomyosarcomas, LIP/PLH, anemia, thrombocytopenia) and excludes children with a clinical category C event. Clinical category A describes children with two or more specific HIV-associated illnesses, namely lymphadenopathy, hepatomegaly, splenomegaly, upper respiratory tract infections/sinusitis/otitis media, parotitis, and dermatitis, and excludes children with a clinical category C or B event. Clinical category N describes children without clinical category C, B, or A events; these children may or may not be completely asymptomatic (single category A events may exist, i.e., lymphadenopathy).

Table 80–3 provides an expanded description of the immunologic axis of the staging system, which includes categories 1 (no evidence of immune suppression), 2 (moderate immunosuppression), and 3 (severe immunosuppression).[46] The immune axis is limited to quantitative assessment (absolute count, percentage, or both) of the peripheral blood T-helper cell (CD4) population. Each category is linked to age-matched CD4 counts and percentages; age groups include 0 to 11 months, 12 to 71 months, and 72 months or more. Age-matched CD4 percentages and count standards for moderate to severe immunosuppression are identical to those provided in the 1995 revised guidelines for pediatric *Pneumocystis carinii* prophylaxis interventions.[48]

Pediatric HIV transmission has been documented by blood and blood products predominantly prior to the spring of 1985 (transfusion-associated AIDS and hemophilia-associated AIDS), perinatal transmission by mothers with identified risk behavior, sexual transmission to children and adolescents, and breast milk transmission.[68, 89] The first case report of transfusion-associated AIDS was linked to a transfusion in 1977. Demographic characteristics of 72 children with neonatal transfusion-associated HIV infection have documented a 54 per cent incidence in children of color (Hispanic and black children) and equal gender representation.[82] In the hemophiliac population, the incidence of HIV seropositivity approaches 80 per cent for persons born prior to 1985 (before adaptation of HIV screening techniques to pooled blood products, namely factor concentrate therapy). The demographic data of hemophiliac patients with AIDS closely resemble the characteristics of the hemophiliac population as a whole (predominance of affected white males).[118] In transfusion-associated pediatric AIDS cases and hemophiliac-associated AIDS cases, the symptom-free period has been reported to range from a median of 18 months to 5 years and more nearly approximates the adult HIV experience of greater than 10 years.[60, 82]

Perinatal transmission of HIV infection accounts for more than 90 per cent of newly reported pediatric AIDS cases.[188] Through June 1995, the United States reported 5925 cases of perinatally transmitted AIDS to the CDC. This perinatal predominance is mimicked worldwide, especially in countries where adult heterosexual transmission uniquely is prevalent (e.g., Africa).[34, 68, 191, 209] The transmission rate for perinatally acquired HIV infection without perinatal antiretroviral intervention has been reported to be between 12 and 25 per

TABLE 80–2. Pediatric HIV Classification—Clinical Categories

Immunologic Categories	N: No Signs/Symptoms	A: Mild Signs/Symptoms	B: Moderate Signs/Symptoms	C: Severe Signs/Symptoms
1. No evidence of suppression	N1	A1	B1	C1
2. Evidence of moderate suppression	N2	A2	B2	C2
3. Severe suppression	N3	A3	B3	C3

Adapted from Centers for Disease Control and Prevention: 1994 revised classification system for human immunodeficiency virus infection in children less than 13 years of age. M. M. W. R. *43*:2, 1994.

TABLE 80–3. Immunologic Categories Based on Age-Specific CD4+ T-Lymphocyte Counts and Percentage of Total Lymphocytes

	Age of Child					
	<12 mos		1–5 yrs		6–12 yrs	
Immunologic Category	μL	(%)	μL	(%)	μL	(%)
1. No evidence of suppression	≥1500	(≥25)	≥1000	(≥25)	≥500	(≥25)
2. Evidence of moderate suppression	750–1499	(15–24)	500–999	(15–24)	200–499	(15–24)
3. Severe suppression	<750	(<15)	<500	(<15)	<200	(<15)

Adapted from Centers for Disease Control and Prevention: 1994 revised classification system for human immunodeficiency virus infection in children less than 13 years of age. M. M. W. R. *43*:4, 1994.

cent in the United States and Europe and probably is higher in Africa.[51, 57, 185, 216, 218] Recent advances in perinatal primary antiretroviral therapy (antepartum, peripartum, and postpartum delivery of zidovudine in HIV-infected women without severe immunosuppression) have documented a decrease in perinatal transmission rates to approximately 8 per cent.[57] Implementation of published guidelines promoting the use of zidovudine in pregnant HIV-infected women promises a marked reduction in future perinatal HIV transmission rates for developing countries.[47] Targeting such interventions can be nationwide or geographic. The incidence of perinatal pediatric AIDS cases in the United States can be predicted in communities with the highest maternal seroprevalence rates.[188] Maternal HIV seroprevalence rates vary by site and can be matched to trends documenting increasing rates of sexually transmitted diseases (e.g., syphilis).[188] This especially is true in urban centers and in the southeastern United States. Described perinatal transmission rates define transmission only in the context of live infant outcomes. The incidence of spontaneous fetal loss in HIV-infected pregnant women has been suggested to be increased and may represent increased HIV perinatal morbidity.[133]

Maternal risk factors as identified through national surveillance in reported AIDS cases include drug abuse, heterosexual infection by sexual partners with risk factors for HIV disease, and maternal transfusion prior to 1985.[188, 197]

Prospective and retrospective evaluations of maternal predictors for perinatal HIV transmission have been the focus of multiple studies. Proposed maternal predictors to date include maternal viremia (measured as serum p24 antigen levels and quantitative RNA or DNA polymerase chain reaction for HIV),[73, 86, 208] maternal immunosuppression or inadequate immune response (CD4 count, neutralizing antibody production),[63, 64, 73, 86, 208] viral characteristics (maternal virus at delivery/infant virus at birth [syncytium formation, zidovudine resistance]),[25, 228] and pregnancy and placental variables (delivery mode, duration of rupture of membranes, vitamin A deficiency, chorioamnionitis).[74, 131, 196, 208] Infant variables under evaluation as predictors of HIV transmission include human leukocyte antigen frequency and the infant cellular immune response (cytokine production, cytotoxic T-cell function).[63, 72, 75, 121, 144, 172]

The timing of perinatal HIV transmission has been proposed to take place in the antepartum, peripartum, and postpartum periods.[6, 68, 90, 205, 217] However, the distribution of transmission across these timing periods has not been defined precisely. The timing of the first positive culture for perinatally infected infants—that is, early (the first 7 days of life) versus late (second week of life or later)—has been used to identify epidemiologically those children potentially infected in utero from those with intrapartum infection.[31] Such distinctions and a need for more precise definition of the timing distribution of perinatal transmission are of paramount importance in defining interventions for transmission interruption.

The demographics of the perinatally infected pediatric cohort include enhanced prevalence in black and Hispanic children and no significant distinction between male and female cases.[188] In contrast with transfusion-associated pediatric AIDS, perinatally infected infants exhibit symptoms shortly after birth (6.4 versus 17.8 months).[82] Scott and associates[194] reported the onset of symptoms at a mean of 8 months in one perinatally HIV-infected cohort of 177 patients. Attempts to assess disease progression have led to descriptions of subpopulations of HIV-infected children: rapid, usual, and slow progressors.[18, 65, 96, 117, 125, 221] Standardized definitions for rapid or usual progressors are lacking. A stringent definition of slow progressors has been proposed (≤8 years of age without evidence of clinical or immunologic decline).[96, 117] Multicenter studies to assess the demographic, virologic, and immunologic characteristics of these rapid, usual, and slow progressors are ongoing. In addition, isolated reports of children with documented HIV infection with evidence of clearance have prompted careful study of perinatally exposed but uninfected infants with evidence of HIV-indeterminant status as documented by a single positive HIV culture.[32, 101]

In the adult population, acquisition of HIV infection through sexual relations is the predominant transmission pattern. The intersection of pediatric sexual abuse and HIV transmission increasingly has been reported in the 1990s.[89, 97] Sexual abuse in young children and infants may be associated with traditional sexual disease transmission (syphilis, gonorrhea), and HIV infection should be considered in the list of sexually transmitted diseases under assessment. In contrast with the infrequent reports of sexual transmission in infants and children younger than 13 years of age, adolescents, who account for 1 per cent of U.S. AIDS cases, are infected frequently by sexual transmission.[140] Because the symptom-free period for clinical expression of HIV infection in adolescents may approach adult standards (i.e., more than 10 years), many young adults (20 to 29 years of age) with AIDS may have become HIV-infected during adolescence.[140] Adolescents with AIDS, like affected infants and children, are more likely to be poor and black or Hispanic. Reported transmission risks in adolescents vary by age, sex, and race or ethnicity. The youngest teenage AIDS cases more often are linked to receipt of blood products for hemophilia or coagulopathies and the oldest to sexual transmission (men who have sex with men and heterosexual contact). However, female adolescents with AIDS (all ages) have reported heterosexual contact as their most frequent transmission risk (52 per cent of cumulative cases through 1992). In 1991 and 1992, the category of heterosexual contact accounted for the largest proportional increase of reported transmission risk for both female and male adolescent AIDS cases. The nature of youth (experimentation, search for self and sexual identity, and inability to access health care easily) has prompted many clinicians to suggest that adolescents and heterosexual transmission of HIV infection may constitute the "second wave" of the HIV epidemic.[28]

Less frequently reported transmission routes of HIV infection are important for pediatric health care providers to acknowledge and target. The risk of HIV transmission through breast feeding has been reported infrequently. In a study of HIV-infected breast-feeding mothers and their exposed infants, Dunn and associates[66] documented a 14 per cent risk of HIV transmission through breast feeding above and beyond the established perinatal transmission risk. These studies have prompted the adoption of guidelines for preventing transmission via this route by avoiding breast feeding in HIV-seropositive postpartum mothers in the United States.[37] Guidelines adapted by the American Academy of Pediatrics for children in the United States should not be extrapolated necessarily to children of developing countries, where malnutrition continues to affect significantly infant mortality and where restriction of breast feeding might exacerbate the problem.

The pediatric population has undergone careful epidemiologic assessment for casual (household contact) transmission of HIV. Isolated cases of transmission of HIV among children have been reported, but blood exposure has been implicated in these cases, and casual transmission has *not* been documented.[80, 200] To date, *no* data suggest that HIV infection is transmitted casually from HIV-infected children to siblings, playmates, or caregivers.[83, 187, 200] In addition, no evidence suggests that exposed noninfected children would be at greater risk of HIV acquisition than the noninfected immunologically mature adult. Documentation of transmission routes and lack of casual transmission have prompted guidelines from the American Academy of Pediatrics and CDC for appropriate "mainstreaming" of HIV-infected children and families.[36, 177] These guidelines include school, day care, and foster care placement for HIV-infected children and promote social incorporation of these children.

Etiology

Identification of the etiology of AIDS followed closely behind the clinical description of this complex immunodeficiency. In 1983, investigators worldwide identified a viral etiology for AIDS and described human lymphotropic virus III, lymphadenopathy-associated virus, and a virus associated with persistent generalized lymphadenopathy.[55, 88] These viruses subsequently have been identified as similar and now are called HIV-1 or simply HIV (Fig. 80–2).[61] Two species of HIV have been identified: HIV-1 and HIV-2. HIV-1 has been the more prevalent pathogenic species and, especially in the United States, almost uniformly has been associated with reported AIDS cases.[41, 43]

HIV belongs to the family of retroviruses first described almost 50 years ago. This RNA virus acts as an infectious agent by penetrating cell membranes and utilizing a pivotal and integral enzyme, reverse transcriptase, which is carried in its core to become integrated into the host-cell genome.[76] Genetic mapping of HIV has identified genes common to human retroviruses (*gag, pol,* and *env)* and necessary for replication. Considerable heterogeneity of the *env* gene, which codes for viral envelope proteins, has been noted in multiple HIV isolates. The *env* gene produces a glycosylated protein (gp160) that can be divided between an external component (gp120) and a transmembrane component (gp41).

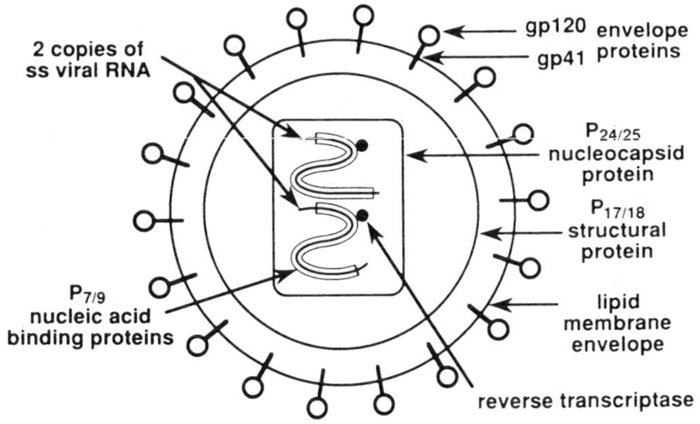

FIGURE 80–2. *Diagram of the virion of HIV-1. (From Demmler, G. J., and Taber, L. H.: Virology of HIV-1. Semin. Pediatr. Infect. Dis. 1:17–20, 1990.)*

The *env* gene heterogeneity and resulting gp120 structural variability make effective vaccine preparation difficult. The group-specific antigen or *gag* gene codes for a precursor protein (p55) that is converted enzymatically to the three principal core or nucleocapsid proteins (p15, p18, p24).[61] The *pol* gene codes for the production of a number of enzymes important for the life cycle of HIV, namely a reverse transcriptase (p51/66), endonuclease (p31/32), integrase, and protease. At least five other HIV genes—*tat, rev, vif, nef,* and *vpr*—play a regulatory role in HIV activation and replication. For example, the *tat* (transactivator of transcription) gene binds to a specific protein sequence within the viral RNA, TAR, and the result is an increase in provirus transcription by cellular RNA polymerase II.[92] *nef* appears to modify host cells to enable better HIV virion manufacturing; *rev* appears to activate viral structural and enzymatic protein production. Newer HIV intervention therapy has targeted these HIV genes; for example, *tat* inhibitors are the subject of active clinical trials.

Many investigators have compared HIV with the lentivirus, visna, which infects sheep, because both share a tropism for lymphocytes and central nervous tissue. Comparisons with simian immunodeficiency virus infection in primates has provided important information about early infection and potentials for interruption of infection.[222] In animal models, introduction of HIV has led to rapid seroconversion; however, clinical disease with immune defects and opportunistic infection has not been reproduced. Despite these problems, continued exploration of the effects of HIV infection in animal models, such as the immunodeficient mouse model, may yield new insights into the pathogenesis of HIV disease in humans.

Pathogenesis

Vulnerability of the Fetal/Neonatal Immune System to HIV Infection

The human fetus and neonate particularly are susceptible to the devastating effects of HIV infection because the normal networking of components of the immune system has not developed.[156] Although it is known that B- and T-lymphocyte differentiation can begin as early as 10 weeks of gestational life, HIV transmission from mother to fetus can occur even earlier.[207] It is possible that this early HIV infection in a host characterized by immunologic naiveté leads to rapid and full expression of the fatal illness by the early age of 2 to 3 years.[96, 117] Undoubtedly, the longer survival of HIV-infected adults can be accounted for, at least in part, by the fully developed T- and B-cell repertoire, immune memory of humoral and cellular responses, mature complement components, and intact phagocytic system of monocytes, macrophages, and polymorphonuclear leukocytes.[74] All of these defense mechanisms have been shown to be impaired in normal newborns, and it is reasonable that this secondary state of immunodeficiency of the newborn lends itself to the early establishment and rapid development of full-blown HIV infection.[4, 156] It is to be expected that at every level of the immune response—inflammation, antigen presentation, primary immune response, secondary immune response—the newborn is unable to protect itself against HIV infection and against the secondary infections that inexorably follow.

The Developing Immune System and HIV Infection

Perhaps the easiest way to envision the disruption that HIV creates in the newborn immune system is to consider the intricate normal differentiation pathways of the bone marrow stem cell as it creates the many cellular components of the immune system (Fig. 80–3).[223] The T- and B-lymphocyte differentiation pathways present multiple opportunities for genetic defects, such as occurs in states of congenital immunodeficiency (see Fig. 80–3). Most certainly the precise differentiation of lymphocyte subsets and secretion and interaction of interleukins are disrupted severely by HIV infection. Most important among these lymphocyte subsets is the helper T or CD4 lymphocyte, whose central role in the production of normal immune responses has been compared with that of a symphony conductor in the production of beautiful music.[76] For some inexplicable reason, this all-important CD4 lymphocyte bears a receptor (the CD4 molecule itself) for the gp120 of the HIV virion coat, rendering it particularly susceptible to attack, paralysis, and destruction by HIV.[76] One can understand the pathogenesis of HIV infection best by considering all of the important roles the CD4 lymphocyte plays in the immune symphony (Fig. 80–4).[76] In many regards, the immunodeficiency of neonatal HIV infection parallels that of genetically inherited immune disorders.

In addition to its central role in the pathogenesis of pediatric HIV infection, the immune system also seems to contribute directly to perhaps the most devastating aspect of pediatric HIV infection, that of HIV-induced encephalopathy (Fig. 80–5).[30, 104] HIV-induced encephalopathy also is important in adults, but it particularly is devastating in young infants who fail to reach early motor milestones or, worse, regress from acquired early development. Possibly the incomplete state of myelination of central nervous tissue accounts for this extraordinary susceptibility to neurologic effects of HIV infection. HIV-infected CD4 lymphocytes and HIV-containing macrophages, which may serve as HIV reservoirs, are thought to transport HIV into the central nervous system, where it is thought that the virus can infect nerve cells directly.[104] It also is plausible that release of cytokines by HIV-infected lymphocytes and macrophages may damage nerve cells indirectly, the "innocent bystander" effect.

Immune Dysfunction in HIV Infection—Adults Versus Children

Immune abnormalities of the HIV-infected adult host are characterized better than those of the HIV-infected pediatric patient. Classically, abnormalities in adult HIV infection include leukopenia, lymphopenia, and decreased CD4 helper-inducer cells with an expanded CD8 cell population, which results in an inverted CD4/CD8 ratio, usually with a number much less than 1.0. Early in infection, T-lymphocyte function has been noted to be diminished (<50 per cent) with decreased in vitro responses to soluble antigens preceding CD4 cell depletion.[102] Although in vitro responses to common mitogens, such as phytohemagglutinin, concanavalin A, and pokeweed, appear normal early in HIV infection, these responses begin to decrease with clinical decline; characteristically, pokeweed mitogen responses disappear first. Also, in vivo T-lymphocyte function typically reveals cutaneous anergy to *Candida*, tetanus, and mumps antigens.[76] Because of HIV-related paralysis of CD4 cells, interleukin-2 (IL-2)

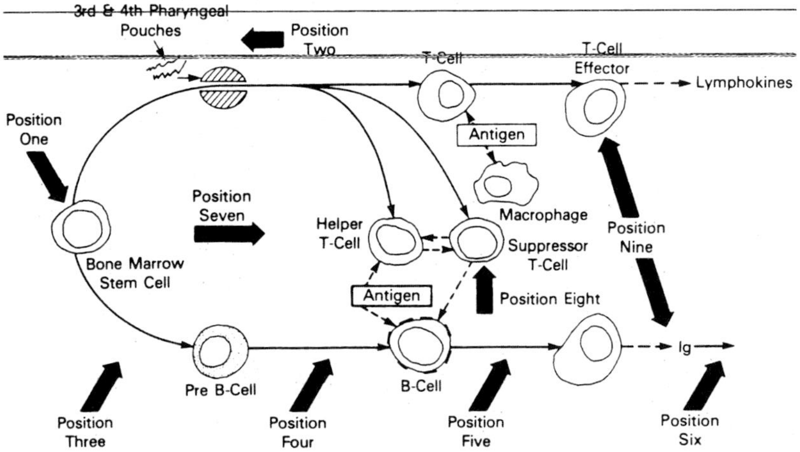

FIGURE 80–3. *Model of events of cellular maturation, cellular interaction, and cellular biosynthesis required for normal immune response. The arrows indicate presumed defects in various immunodeficiency states. Position 1: Failure of B- and T-cell development (e.g., severe combined immunodeficiency disease). Position 2: Failure of development of thymus (e.g., DiGeorge syndrome). Position 3: Failure of maturation of stem cells into pre-B cells (e.g., thymoma, hypogammaglobulinemia). Position 4: Failure of maturation of pre-B cells into B cells (e.g., X-linked hypogammaglobulinemia). Position 5: Failure of maturation of B cells into plasma cells (e.g., common variable hypogammaglobulinemia). Position 6: Hypercatabolism of immunoglobulin (e.g., myotonic dystrophy). Position 7: Reduced helper T cells (e.g., subset of common variable hypogammaglobulinemia). Position 8: Increase in suppressor T-cell activity (e.g., subset of common variable hypogammaglobulinemia). Position 9: Excessive loss of immunoglobulins and lymphocytes (e.g., intestinal lymphangiectasia). (From Waldmann, T. A.: Immunodeficiency diseases: Primary and acquired.* In *Samter, M., Talmage, D. W., Frank, M. M., et al. [eds.]: Immunological Diseases. 4th ed. Boston, Little, Brown, 1988, pp. 411–465.)*

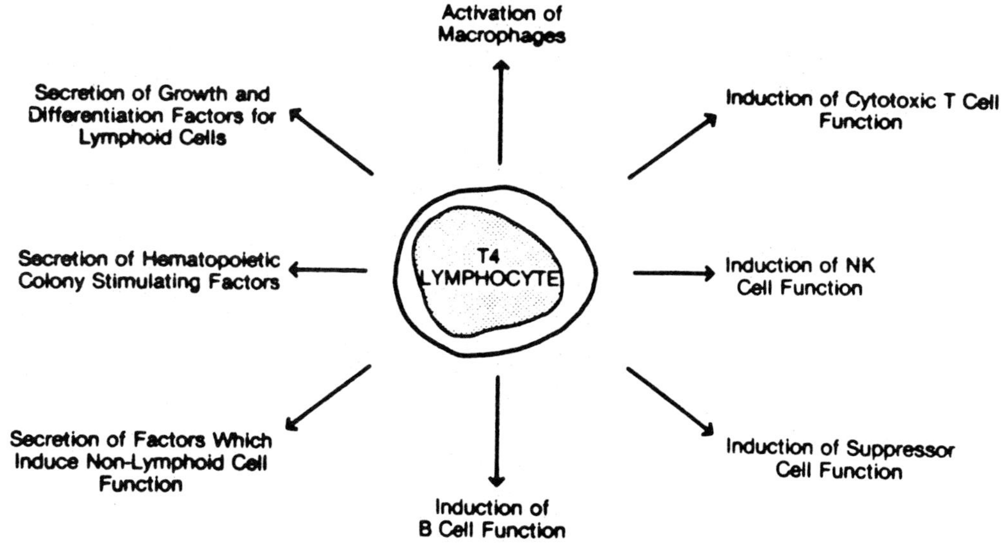

FIGURE 80–4. *Critical role of the T4 (CD4) lymphocyte in the human response. The T4 cell is responsible directly or indirectly for the induction of a wide array of functions of multiple limbs of the immune response as well as for certain nonlymphoid cell functions. This is effected for the most part by the secretion of a variety of soluble factors that have trophic or inductive effects (or both) on the cells in question. (Reprinted from Fauci, A. S.: The human immunodeficiency virus: Infectivity and mechanisms of pathogenesis. Science 239:617–622, 1988. Copyright 1988, American Association for the Advancement of Science.)*

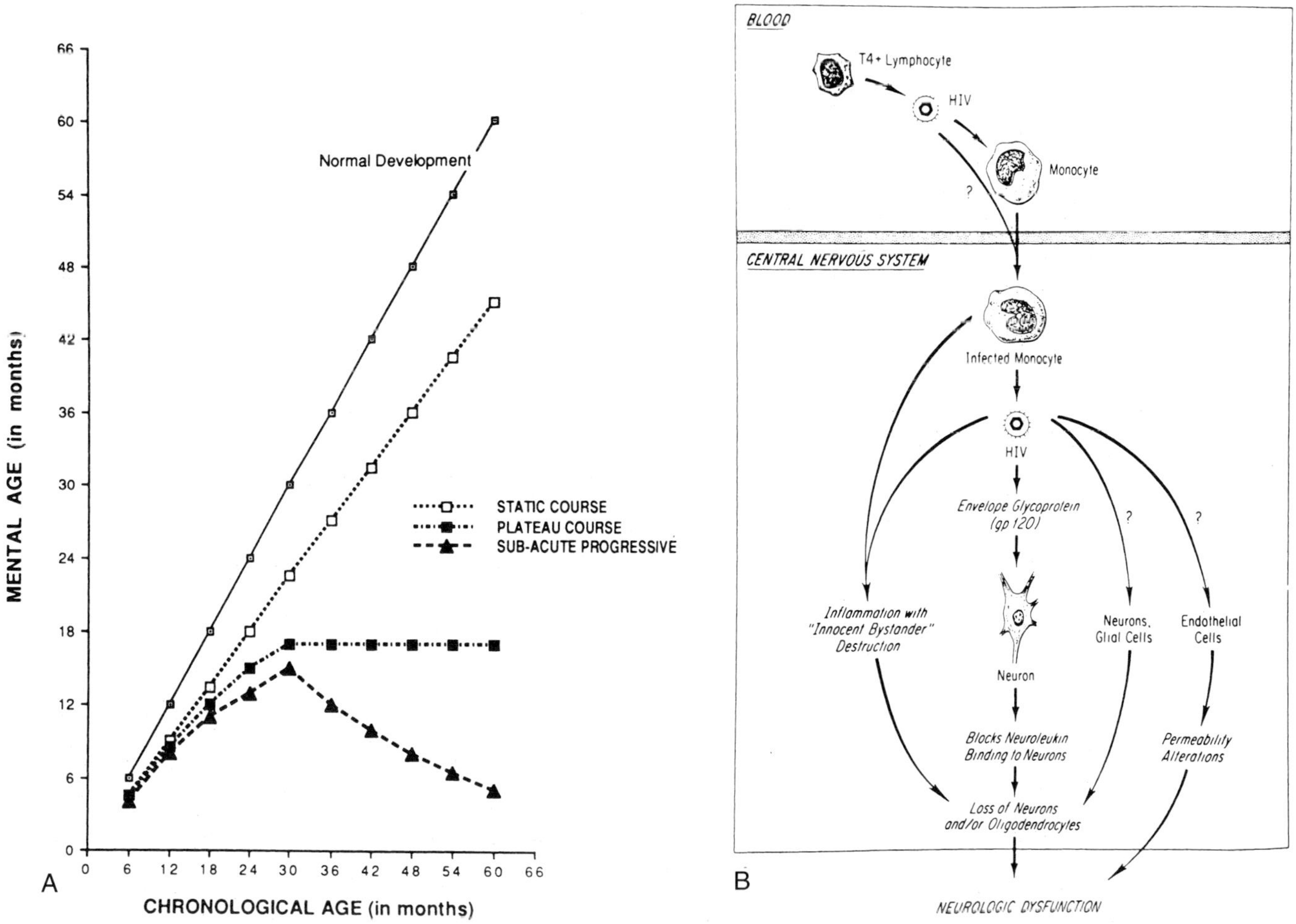

FIGURE 80–5. *Role of the immune system in pediatric HIV-induced encephalopathy.* A, *Schematic representation of different encephalopathic courses. (From Brouwers, P., Belman, A., and Epstein, L. G.: Central nervous system involvement: Manifestations, evaluation and immunopathogenesis.* In *Pizzo, P. A., and Wilfert, C. M. [eds.]: Pediatric AIDS: The Challenge of HIV Infection in Infants, Children, and Adolescents. Baltimore, Williams & Wilkins, 1994, pp. 435–455.)* B, *Entry of HIV-infected CD4 lymphocytes and macrophages into the central nervous system. HIV may escape from these transport cells and infect nerve cells directly or cause indirect damage to neurons by the release of cytokines, such as tumor necrosis factor and interleukin-2. (From Ho, D., Pomerantz, R. J., and Kaplan, J. C.: Pathogenesis of infection with human immunodeficiency virus. N. Engl. J. Med. 317:278–286, 1987.)*

TABLE 80–4. Comparison of Immune Dysfunction in Symptomatic HIV Infection in Adults and Children

		Infants	Children
	Adults	*0–2 yrs*	*>2 yrs*
Lymphopenia	+ + + +[a]	+	+
CD4+ cellular depletion			
<400 cells/mm³	+ + +	+	+
<1000 cells/mm³		+[b]	
Inverted CD4/CD8 ratio	+ +	+ +	+ +
Hypergammaglobulinemia	+ +	+ + + +	+ + + +
CD8+ cellular dysfuncton	+ + +	c	c
Reduced interleukin-2 production	+ +	+ +	+ +
Cutaneous anergy	+ + +	d	+ + + +
Reduced natural killer cell function	+ + +	+ + +	+ + +
Elevated soluble interleukin-2 receptors	+ + +	+ +	+ +
Defective monocyte function	+ +	c	c

a, + + + + indicates common, + indicates occasional.
b, Because of relative normal lymphocytosis in infants, a CD4 count of 1000 is a better discriminator of depletion in perinatally infected patients.
c, Not fully evaluated.
d, Normal infants younger than 2 years of age (and particularly younger than 1 year of age) can have cutaneous anergy.

production is reduced, thereby weakening the immune amplification system.[76] HIV-infected CD4 cells release soluble IL-2 receptors. These elevated serum IL-2 receptor levels produce a blockade of cell-bound IL-2 receptors by competition for IL-2.

In addition to T-lymphocyte dysfunction in HIV-infected adults, B-cell dysfunction similarly is marked (e.g., hypergammaglobulinemia occurs in adults and can be used to monitor disease progression). HIV-infected adults also demonstrate circulating immune complexes and autoantibody production secondary to polyclonal activation of B cells by HIV itself or concomitant viral infections with cytomegalovirus or Epstein-Barr virus.[132] Other host defense cells are affected by HIV infection[21, 203] (e.g., natural killer cells in HIV infection have been shown to be unable to kill target cells normally, despite adequate binding, and cytotoxic T-cell function has been demonstrated to be diminished, although patients have sufficient numbers of precursor cytoxic T lymphocytes).[120, 145] Monocytes and macrophages most likely play a major role in the pathogenesis of HIV infection, serving as HIV reservoirs that are spared the cytopathic effects of HIV. Defective chemotaxis and bacterial killing have been observed in HIV-infected monocytes and macrophages, as well as defective induction of IL-1, possibly accounting for the decreased IL-2 response in CD4 cells.[203]

Similar changes in immunologic function in the presence of HIV infection have been observed in infants and children (Table 80–4). Children with HIV infection infrequently are lymphopenic in terms of values observed in adults.[51] If lymphopenia is observed in children with HIV infection, it usually is seen in older children with transfusion-associated infection or in children with end-stage HIV-disease progression. CD4 cell depletion may be less dramatic in children as a consequence of their relative lymphocytosis. In fact, CD4 cell counts in HIV-infected children commonly exceed 400 cells/mm³. Moreover, Denny and associates[62] have shown that in infants 12 to 24 months of age, a CD4 value of less than 1000 cells/mm³ is significant for HIV-related CD4 depletion; in infants younger than 12 months of age, a value of less than 1500 cells/mm³ similarly applies. Because of altered relative proportions of CD4 and CD8 cells, an inverted CD4/CD8 ratio observed in children is similar to that in adults. As in the adult, lymphoproliferative responses to recall antigens have been documented as relatively normal early in infection; decline is correlated with the onset of clinical symptoms.[23] HIV-1–specific CD8 cytotoxic-suppressor cell function has been documented as nondetectable in infants with primary infection (early perinatal infection).[144] The impact of cytotoxic cell function on disease progression currently is under analysis.[85]

Cutaneous anergy is a usual finding for children with HIV infection; however, interpretation in children younger than 2 years of age may be difficult because of the relative degree of anergy in very young normal children. Hypergammaglobulinemia particularly is prominent in infants and children with HIV infection, frequently serving as the herald sign of HIV infection at a time when the HIV enzyme-linked immunosorbent assay and Western blot tests are nondiagnostic because of the presence of maternal antibody. This evidence of B-cell activation or dysregulation often precedes other evidence for immune dysfunction, namely CD4 depletion, inverted CD4/CD8 ratio, or in vitro evidence of T-cell dysfunction. In particular, IgG levels may rise to 2 to 3 standard deviations above the mean of normal values, and serum IgA, IgM, and IgE levels may be elevated as well. This extreme hypergammaglobulinemia in children may be caused by polyclonal stimulation of B cells by HIV or coinfection with cytomegalovirus or Epstein-Barr virus, or it may be caused by the absence of normal CD4 immunoregulatory cells.[173] Our experience with more than 350 HIV-infected infants and children demonstrates that only a small percentage (<2 per cent) of children with HIV infection present with hypogammaglobulinemia. In terms of functional activity, it has been documented in some children with HIV infection that specific antibody production is inadequate for host protection, despite elevation of serum immunoglobulin levels.[3, 17, 22, 23]

Origin of Immunodeficiency in HIV Infection

Hypotheses have been proposed to explain the immune aberrations, specifically CD4 depletion and dysfunction, noted in HIV infection; Table 80–5 lists several of these hypotheses.[172] None of these proposals is satisfactory entirely in explaining the secondary immunodeficiency of HIV infection in adults or children. Probably the first and second of these (CD4 cell depletion and CD4 cell syncytial formation) are the easiest to comprehend because removal of CD4 cells

TABLE 80–5. Potential Mechanisms of the Functional and Quantitative Depletion of CD4 T Lymphocytes

Direct HIV-mediated cytopathic effects (single-cell killing)
HIV-mediated formation of syncytia
Virus-specific immune responses
  HIV-specific cytolytic T lymphocytes
  Antibody-dependent cellular cytotoxicity
  Natural-killer cells
Autoimmune mechanisms
Anergy caused by inappropriate cell signaling through gp120-CD4 interaction
Superantigen-mediated perturbation of T-cell subgroups
Programmed cell death (apoptosis)

From Pantaleo, G., Grazosi, C., and Fauci, A. S.: The immunopathogenesis of human immunodeficiency virus infection. N. Engl. J. Med. *328*:330, 1993.

or CD4 function from the immune system would render it progressively weaker and unable to thwart secondary infections. However, more recent data elucidating the immunopathogenesis of HIV infection document that HIV-1 replication in vivo is continuous and drives rapid and constant turnover of CD4 lymphocytes, in contrast with the notion that inconstant HIV replication affects circulating CD4 lymphocytes by stepwise decline.[106, 224] Rabin and associates[181] and Roederer and colleagues[184] described concomitant depletion of CD8-naive T cells with CD4 depletion in children and adults, respectively. CD8 expansion, characteristic of early asymptomatic infection, was noted especially with CD8-memory T cells. CD4 depletion preferentially involved naive T cells. These findings suggest a relationship between depletion of naive CD4 T cells and poor new T-cell–mediated responses. The idea that immunopathogenesis may be related to syncytial formation is provocative because of already existing immunopathologic viral models of infection, such as respiratory syncytial virus infection.[199]

In most children, there is the additional complexity of maternal-fetal transmission of HIV to consider, and few data define the immunopathogenesis of HIV infection in this transplacental or perinatal event. The maternal immunologic status and the role of the placenta in affording protection or permitting infection should be defined, and potential perinatal cofactors (such as intravenous drug abuse, sexually transmitted diseases, maternal malnutrition) should be understood better. Langston and associates[133] suggest that HIV may be fetotoxic, with impact most notably reported in the thymus, where precocious involution, epithelial injury, and, occasionally, severe thymitis are described. Loss of lymphocytes at the corticomedullary junction of the thymus implies a defect induced by HIV in the immunologic selection process. Pediatric virus-specific immune responses (i.e., the roles of CD8+ cytotoxic cells and monocytes and neutralizing antibody production) are being studied. Normal mechanisms of cell death, programmed cell death or apoptosis, may be enhanced by cross-linking of the CD4 molecule by HIV gp120 complexes or circulating immune complexes.[95, 172] Vigano and associates[221] documented the predominant production of type 2 cytokines (IL-4, IL-10) in children with symptomatic infection and proposed that this might increase clinical progression and CD4 depletion by enhancing apoptosis or enhancing HIV replication.

Abundant epidemiologic information clearly documents that children with perinatally acquired HIV infection and immune dysfunction more rapidly develop serious and life-threatening clinical manifestations than do adults, who typically are symptom-free for approximately 10 years after HIV infection prior to emergence of clinical manifestations.[188, 226] In the case of perinatal HIV infection, symptoms typically occur by 2 years and ultimately lead to death.[185, 194] These epidemiologic data indicate that the immunologically naive, pediatric host defense system is affected more quickly by HIV infection, most likely on the basis of several defects in host defense.[226]

Clinical Manifestations

HIV infection in children and adults is manifested by a spectrum of postnatal clinical presentations that affect multiorgan systems and include the symptom constellation of AIDS. Table 80–6 includes many of the presumed or documented opportunistic infections that satisfy the current criteria for a pediatric AIDS diagnosis.[40] Wasting, encephalopathy, lymphoproliferative lung disorders, and oncologic processes also are diagnostic of AIDS. Infection with HIV, independent of an AIDS diagnosis, may be attended by nonspecific clinical findings. These include mild failure to thrive (not sufficient enough to meet the AIDS wasting definition), hepatosplenomegaly, acquired microcephaly, parotitis, generalized lymphadenopathy, nonspecific intermittent diarrhea, intermittent fever, and chronic skin disease.[169] These clinical symptoms that are shared by other pediatric disease processes can, when manifested singly in the HIV-infected host, delay diagnosis. However, a careful and detailed history should provide helpful insight into potential HIV risk factors, prompting inclusion of HIV infection in the differential diagnosis. The major clinical features of AIDS are discussed here by broad categories: opportunistic infections, pulmonary complications, central nervous system complications, and so forth.

TABLE 80–6. Opportunistic Infections That Establish the Diagnosis of AIDS

Documented HIV Infection
Presumptive diagnosis
Esophageal candidiasis
Cytomegalovirus retinitis
Pneumocystis carinii pneumonia
Toxoplasmosis of the brain (after 1 month of age)
Disseminated atypical mycobacterial infection
Definitive histologically confirmed diagnosis
Disseminated coccidioidomycosis
Disseminated histoplasmosis
Isosporiasis
Extrapulmonary cryptococcosis
Extrapulmonary *Mycobacterium tuberculosis*
Recurrent *Salmonella* septicemia
Disseminated/persistent herpes simplex
Indeterminate HIV Infection
All opportunists listed above are applicable but definitively must be diagnosed, i.e., histologic confirmation

Opportunistic Infections

Opportunistic infections plague the HIV-infected child and are the most prominent cause of both morbidity and mortality in this cohort. In children with AIDS, *Pneumocystis carinii* pneumonia (PCP) ranks second only to lymphoid interstitial pneumonitis as the most common pulmonary disease.[99, 201] PCP has a fulminant course in the pediatric population, with highest mortality rates in affected children younger than 1 year of age.[201] In a study of 172 children with perinatal HIV infection, 9 per cent had PCP when younger than 1 year of age, with a median survival of 1 month.[194] The clinical expression of pediatric PCP often can be distinguished from other pulmonary diseases by severity of hypoxemia (higher alveolar-arterial oxygen gradients), elevated serum lactate dehydrogenase levels, rapidity of disease progression with tachypnea and fever, characteristic diffuse interstitial infiltrates on radiography, and the usual lack of digital clubbing.[98] The more insidious presentation of PCP characteristic of HIV-infected adults, namely prolonged fever (>7 weeks) and cough and dyspnea (averaging 3 weeks), is appreciated less commonly in infants and children. Radiographically, pediatric PCP presents with diffuse interstitial markings progressing to the "white-out" picture of adult respiratory distress syndrome (Fig. 80–6). However, PCP initially can present as a unilateral streaky pneumonic infiltrate, as lobar consolidation, or with accompanying pleural effusions.

As in primary immunodeficiency disorders, aggressive diagnostic measures may be indicated to establish a diagnosis

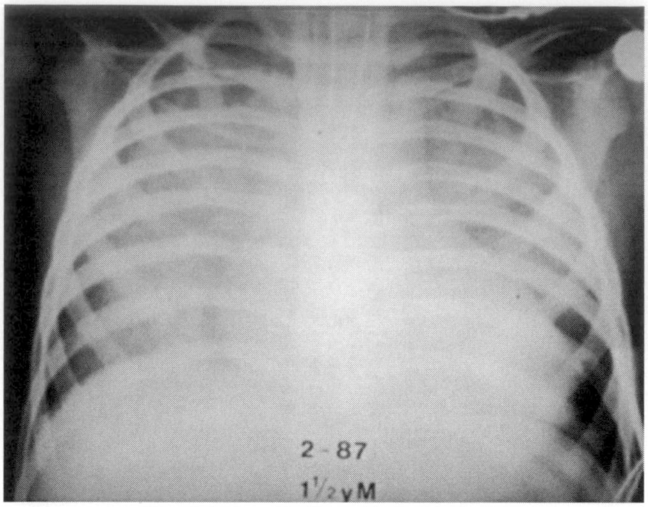

FIGURE 80–6. *Classic diffuse interstitial infiltrates of acute and fatal* Pneumocystis carinii *pneumonia in a 15-month-old child with perinatal AIDS. (From Hanson, I. C.: Respiratory infections in HIV-infected children. Immunol. Allerg. Clin. North Am. 13:205–217, 1993.)*

of PCP. Lung biopsy remains the gold standard of distinguishing PCP from other lung diseases in AIDS. However, bronchoscopic alveolar lavage has been proved a useful diagnostic tool in adults and children and should be considered a first diagnostic choice for presumed PCP.[98] In older children and adults, evaluation of sputum for PCP with appropriate stains or monoclonal antibodies may pre-empt the need for invasive diagnostic measures.

Acute PCP traditionally is treated with parenteral trimethoprim-sulfamethoxazole (TMP-SMZ) or pentamidine. Adjunctive corticosteroid therapy early in moderate to severe PCP may provide significant benefit with only limited evidence for concomitant immune suppression and attendant infectious complications.[87, 202, 214]

Secondary PCP prophylaxis (therapy initiated after resolution and complete treatment of acute PCP) for adults and children is accepted as standard care.[42, 48, 110] Proposed pediatric regimens include: TMP-SMZ at 150 mg/m^2/day and 750 mg/m^2/day, respectively, three times a week (single dose on 3 consecutive days a week; two divided doses on 3 alternate days a week; two divided doses daily), dapsone at 2 mg/kg (single dosing not to exceed 100 mg/day), and pentamidine (aerosolized [300 mg via Respirgard II inhaler monthly] or intravenously [4 mg/kg administered every 2 to 4 weeks]).[48, 111] Primary PCP prophylaxis for adults and children is well defined by the CDC.[45, 48] Newer medications for use in PCP prophylaxis, atovaquone and azithromycin, are the subject of ongoing clinical trials in HIV-infected children nationally (AIDS Clinical Trials Group, protocol 254).[113] In 1993, the CDC published the first PCP prophylaxis guidelines for HIV-infected children, which linked the institution of therapy to the level of immunosuppression as measured by CD4 count or percentage.[42, 136] After implementation of these guidelines, Simonds and associates[201] reviewed the incidence of reported PCP cases to the CDC and noted no decline in case numbers. Of 300 children with PCP reported to the CDC between January 1991 and June 1993, 66 per cent had never received prophylaxis. In addition, 18 per cent of infants younger than 1 year of age experienced PCP with CD4 counts that were above guideline thresholds for immunosuppression. Based on these data, the guidelines for PCP prophylaxis for children were modified in 1995, and Table 80–7 outlines the institution of therapy by age and CD4 monitoring.[48] The most significant changes in the revised guidelines include (1) emphasis on early HIV infection detection in infants for optimal guideline implementation, (2) provision of PCP prophylaxis to all HIV-exposed infants in the first months of life, and (3) emphasis on quarterly CD4 monitoring, with immunosuppression thresholds for HIV-infected children. The low potential for associated morbidity from PCP prophylaxis therapy allows for implementation of therapy to all infants, independent of HIV status in the first months of life, when their risk has been documented to be highest and is least likely to correlate with CD4 monitoring.[201]

Mycobacterium avium-intracellulare complex (MAC) causes disseminated infections in both adults and children with HIV infection. In one review reported to the CDC of opportunistic infections in pediatric AIDS patients, 43 of 552 (7.8 per cent) children 0 to 9 years of age were found to have disseminated MAC.[98] Epidemiologically, MAC has been linked to evidence for significant immunosuppression (CD4 counts well below 100 cells/mm^3) in adults.[45, 109] It has been noted that the development of MAC in children may be associated with CD4 counts greater than 100 cells/mm^3, especially for those younger than 2 years of age.[122, 190] The clinical presentation of MAC includes fever, malaise, weight loss, anorexia, and night sweats. Gastrointestinal manifestations are not uncommon and have included abdominal pain, diarrhea, malabsorption, and intestinal perforation. Rarely, MAC has been reported with extrabiliary obstructive jaundice (presumed to be sec-

TABLE 80–7. Recommendations for *Pneumocystis carinii* Pneumonia Prophylaxis and CD4+ Monitoring for HIV-Exposed Infants and HIV-Infected Children, by Age and HIV Infection Status

Age/HIV Infection Status	PCP Prophylaxis	CD4+ Monitoring
Birth to 4–6 wk, HIV-exposed	No prophylaxis	1 mo
4–6 wk to 4 mo, HIV-exposed	Prophylaxis	3 mo
4–12 mo		
HIV-infected or indeterminate	Prophylaxis	6, 9, and 12 mo
HIV infection reasonably excluded	No prophylaxis	None
1–5 yr, HIV-infected	Prophylaxis *if:* CD4+ count is <500 cells/μL or CD4+ percentage is <15%	Every 3–4 mo
6–12 yr, HIV-infected	Prophylaxis *if:* CD4+ count is <200 cells/μL or CD4+ percentage is <15%	Every 3–4 mo

From Centers for Disease Control and Prevention: 1995 revised guidelines for prophylaxis against *Pneumocystis carinii* pneumonia for children infected with or perinatally exposed to human immunodeficiency virus. M. M. W. R. *44*:6, 1995.

ondary to lymphadenopathy) and endobronchial masses. The diagnosis of disseminated MAC relies on identification of these microorganisms from blood, lymph tissue, bone marrow, liver, lung, and gastrointestinal tract. Therapy of disseminated MAC in the pediatric population remains suboptimal, but most clinicians use some combination of rifabutin, clofazimine, ethambutol, amikacin, ciprofloxacin, azithromycin, and clarithromycin.[99, 108] The epidemiologic link with severe immunosuppression and the advent of therapeutic prophylactic interventions (rifabutin, clarithromycin) has prompted implementation of MAC prophylaxis guidelines for adults, adolescents, and older children with CD4 counts less than 100 cells/mm^3.[45]

In reports to the CDC, disseminated cytomegalovirus infection has occurred in 19 per cent of pediatric AIDS patients.[185] The adult spectrum of cytomegalovirus disease, including retinitis, pneumonitis, esophagitis, gastritis, colitis, hepatitis, cholangitis, and encephalitis, is not defined as precisely in the pediatric AIDS literature. Cytomegalovirus clearly can cause primary pneumonitis in children or be found in association with other pulmonary pathogens, especially *P. carinii.* Unusual gastrointestinal manifestations have included pyloric obstruction, enterocolitis, and oral and esophageal ulcers. Cytomegalovirus retinitis in children, in contrast with that of adults, infrequently is described. This discrepancy may reflect the lack of good subjective complaints in the pediatric population or early demise from other infections, such as PCP. Ganciclovir, an antiviral analogue of acyclovir with anti-cytomegalovirus activity, has been administered intravenously to adult AIDS patients with disseminated cytomegalovirus infection and has been documented to have some benefit in cytomegalovirus colitis at doses of 5 mg/kg every 12 hours (14 days).[66] Although many adults describe subjective and objective improvement on therapy, drug discontinuation is associated with high relapse rates, independent of the affected site. Common adverse reactions to ganciclovir therapy include neutropenia, thrombocytopenia, and nausea, which often limit its utility. Careful monitoring of children receiving ganciclovir and antiretroviral therapy (zidovudine) is mandatory because both agents may depress bone marrow function. Guidelines to prevent opportunistic infections in HIV-infected persons have been published and include cytomegalovirus infection. No chemotherapeutic agent has been described for use in prophylaxis, so outlined measures include careful monitoring for onset of clinical disease, specifically eye disease.[49]

Chronic *Candida* infection plagues HIV-infected children.[51, 169] Affected mucous membranes or skin often does not respond well to treatment with topical antifungal agents, although some patients may respond to treatment with miconazole. Ketoconazole is an effective antifungal agent that may be used orally but is associated with an increased incidence of hepatitis. Because many patients with AIDS have preexisting hepatitis, this drug should be used with caution. Fluconazole has been documented in an open multicenter study to be as effective and safe as ketoconazole in the treatment of oropharyngeal candidiasis.[103] In severe fungal infections, amphotericin B should be administered intravenously. Suggestions for candidal prophylaxis span the use of nystatin after first opportunistic infection to fluconazole or ketoconazole for recurrences of opportunistic infection with *Candida*.[49]

Disseminated histoplasmosis less commonly affects pediatric AIDS patients but may be prevalent in the midwestern United States, where *Histoplasma capsulatum* is endemic.[225] Symptoms include fever, rash, cough, lymphadenopathy, splenomegaly, thrombocytopenia, low-grade disseminated intravascular coagulopathy, adult respiratory distress syndrome, meningoencephalitis, and neurologic abnormalities consistent with intracranial mass lesions. Treatment consists of a full course of systemic antifungal therapy (amphotericin B 40 mg/kg total dose) followed by maintenance therapy. No outlined course of maintenance has emerged as completely successful in the prevention of relapses; however, weekly doses of amphotericin B or daily itraconazole or fluconazole have been attempted.[49] Figure 80–7 documents in a 12-year-old hemophiliac patient the progression of disseminated histoplasmosis to development of central nervous system disease with intracranial mass lesions histologically positive for *H. capsulatum* despite induction and maintenance amphotericin B therapy.

Cryptococcosis has been reported infrequently in pediatric AIDS patients (1 per cent in a CDC cohort).[185] At Baylor College of Medicine, cryptococcosis has been documented in three pediatric patients with AIDS since 1986 and has prompted more rigorous evaluation of HIV-infected children with vague complaints of fever and headache or a clinical picture of bacterial sepsis. After treatment of acute disease, daily fluconazole or itraconazole has been suggested as prophylaxis for recurrences.[49]

Unlike adult patients with AIDS, pediatric patients have an increased incidence of severe bacterial infections, including *Streptococcus pneumoniae, Staphylococcus aureus,* and various gram-negative organisms. The risk of community-acquired invasive bacterial infections has been estimated as three times higher than the rate in non–HIV-infected children.[5] In a study of 372 HIV-infected children followed for a median of 17 months, 14 per cent experienced one or more laboratory-proven serious bacterial infections.[215] Clinical infections included bacteremia, pneumonia, osteomyelitis, meningitis, and sinusitis. In this study, the use of intravenous immunoglobulin (400 mg/kg every 28 days) reduced the time free from serious bacterial infections for those children with CD4 counts exceeding 199 cells/mm^3. A crossover study of the

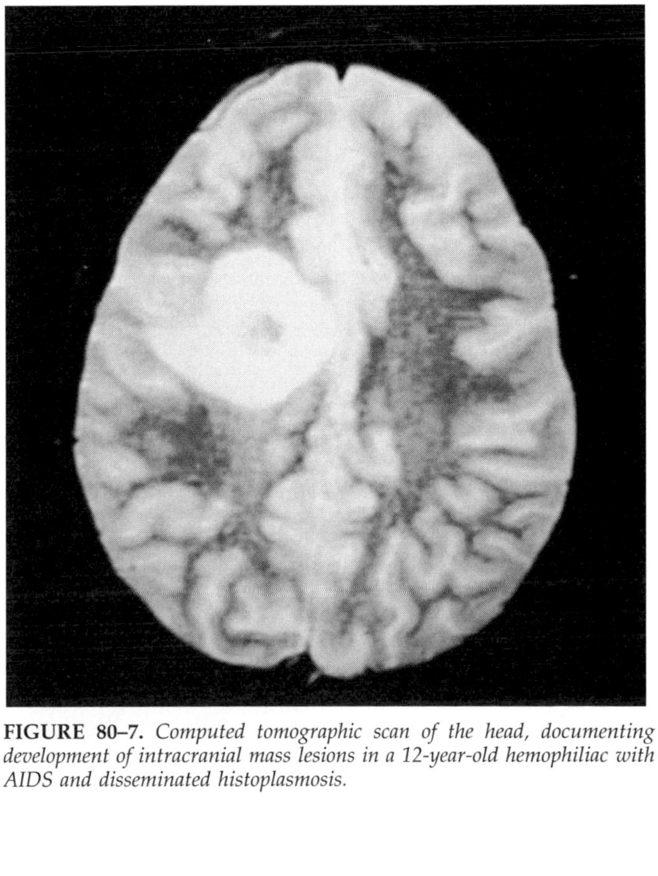

FIGURE 80–7. *Computed tomographic scan of the head, documenting development of intracranial mass lesions in a 12-year-old hemophiliac with AIDS and disseminated histoplasmosis.*

same population again documented the efficacy of exogenous immunoglobulin administration for prophylaxis of bacterial infections and a decrease in morbidity as measured by hospitalizations.[160]

An increasing incidence of tuberculosis nationwide since the mid-1980s has affected the HIV-infected population because factors that increase the transmission of tuberculosis also are responsible for risk factors that affect HIV transmission.[159] In a cohort of pregnant and nonpregnant HIV-infected women followed in a multicenter longitudinal study, the prevalence of tuberculosis by medical history or positive skin test was 14 per cent.[161] Factors associated with pediatric tuberculosis acquisition primarily have included family and caregiver risks. In a study of 60 HIV-infected families, the incidence of tuberculosis was approximately 6 per cent, with both HIV-infected and uninfected children affected.[13] The vector for transmission was identified as an infected family member or caregiver. Tuberculosis should be considered in the differential diagnosis of pulmonary disease in HIV-exposed children, and routine testing for tuberculosis should be standard care for this population.

Infections of the herpesvirus family are prevalent in HIV-infected children, with 5 per cent of children with AIDS reporting chronic herpes simplex virus infection.[185] In general, herpes simplex virus infection in pediatric AIDS has been limited to mild-to-severe localized infections without reports of dissemination. Varicella-zoster and herpes-zoster virus infections have contributed significant morbidity to HIV-infected persons. Disseminated herpes-zoster virus and chronic herpes-zoster virus infection are reported in pediatric AIDS patients. The judicious use of acyclovir in chronic infection is warranted to lessen the probability of emergence of resistant strains. Prevention of herpes infections in school age children especially is important because varicella exposure may be considerable. Varicella-zoster immunoglobulin is indicated for HIV-infected children with varicella-zoster virus exposure.

Pulmonary Complications

In addition to PCP and chronic sinopulmonary infection, the noninfectious pulmonary complications of pediatric AIDS are associated with significant morbidity. In a series of more than 150 children with perinatal HIV infection, the lymphoproliferative lung disorders LIP/PLH most frequently were reported, affecting 17 per cent of these children.[194] Histopathologically, LIP and PLH appear to be distinct entities, although whether these disorders represent a continuum of reactive hyperplasia of lymphoid tissue is somewhat controversial.[99] In LIP, small lymphoid infiltrates are dispersed throughout parenchymal lung tissue and often are accompanied by alveolar epithelial hyperplasia and interstitial widening. PLH describes larger, dense, nodular aggregates of lymphoid tissue both in distal parenchymal tissue and in the walls of bronchi and bronchioles (Fig. 80–8*A*). Compression of blood and lymphatic vessels by these nodules may contribute to the accompanying clinical interstitial widening. The etiology of LIP/PLH is not defined. Associations with in situ Epstein-Barr virus and HIV genome have been noted, and an increase in local nonspecific and HIV-specific IgG and IgA production is described.[99]

Clinically, LIP/PLH is characterized by a nonproductive cough and the insidious onset of progressive hypoxia. Hypoxemia may be subtle and best appreciated during febrile, upper respiratory tract illnesses. Digital clubbing, generalized lymphadenopathy, chronic parotitis, or failure to thrive may accompany LIP/PLH. Radiographically, LIP/PLH often presents characteristic interstitial infiltrates with a nodular pattern (Fig. 80–8*B*). This radiographic picture often mimics that of miliary tuberculosis and warrants exclusion of this pulmonary infection. In the immunocompromised, anergic, HIV-positive child, simple delayed hypersensitivity skin testing for tuberculosis exclusion may not suffice, and bronchoalveolar lavage or gastric aspirates for acid-fast microorganisms may be necessary. Lung biopsy is the definitive diagnostic procedure for LIP/PLH. However, in HIV-infected children, a presumed diagnosis of LIP/PLH by less invasive exclusion of infectious pathogens is preferred.

The therapy of LIP/PLH is not defined clearly because the clinical outcome is variable. HIV-infected children with LIP/PLH have been noted to have spontaneous remissions without therapeutic intervention, whereas other affected children progress to respiratory insufficiency and failure. Therapeutic intervention has included intravenous immunoglobulin supplementation; antiretroviral therapy, specifically zidovudine and corticosteroids (daily or alternate-day dosing ranging from 0.5 to 2.0 mg/kg/day); and observation.[99] No significant associated infectious sequelae (bacteremia, fungemia) of corticosteroid use were reported in treated children. Supportive therapy with oxygen supplementation, chest physiotherapy, and attention to adequate nutritional intake is helpful adjunctive treatment.

In general, children with LIP/PLH have prolonged survival, compared with those with PCP or other AIDS-defining events. Of note, LIP/PLH is included as a category B event in the 1994 revised pediatric classification and staging system.[46] Scott and associates[194] described a median survival time of 72 months for children with LIP/PLH. This contrasts with median survival times of 12 and 11 months for children with *Candida* esophagitis and HIV encephalopathy, respectively.

Other noninfectious pulmonary complications have been reported less frequently in the pediatric HIV-infected population and include bronchiectasis, vasculitis, and diffuse interstitial pneumonitis. Pulmonary B-cell lymphoproliferative disorders (non-Hodgkin lymphoma) have been described in pediatric AIDS cases, often associated with described lymphoproliferative lung disorders (LIP/PLH) with Epstein-Barr virus detection by polymerase chain reaction, immunochemistry, and Southern blot analysis.[149, 167]

Central Nervous System Complications

Neurologic abnormalities have been documented in persons with HIV and can be attributed to opportunistic infections, adverse events of primary treatment, or primary infection with HIV, especially in light of HIV's described tropism for monocytes. Ten per cent of adults with AIDS present with neurologic symptoms, and 40 per cent are affected during their clinical course.[148] An appreciation of pediatric AIDS neurologic abnormalities lagged behind documentation of immunodeficiency and concomitant opportunistic infections and lung disease in the literature. Belman and associates (1985)[13] and Epstein and associates (1986)[71] described significant neurologic complications in association with HIV disease, including seizure disorders, attention deficit disorders, developmental delay, and acquired microcephaly and encephalopathy. In 1987, expansion of the CDC surveillance criteria for AIDS diagnosis incorporated and acknowledged neurologic deficits by defining AIDS dementia or encephalopathy.[40] In adults, *dementia* described "clinical findings of disabling cognitive and/or motor dysfunction interfering with occupation or activities of daily living." In children, this definition incorporated progressive loss of behavioral developmental milestones. A diagnosis of AIDS dementia in adults and HIV encephalopathy in children requires exclu-

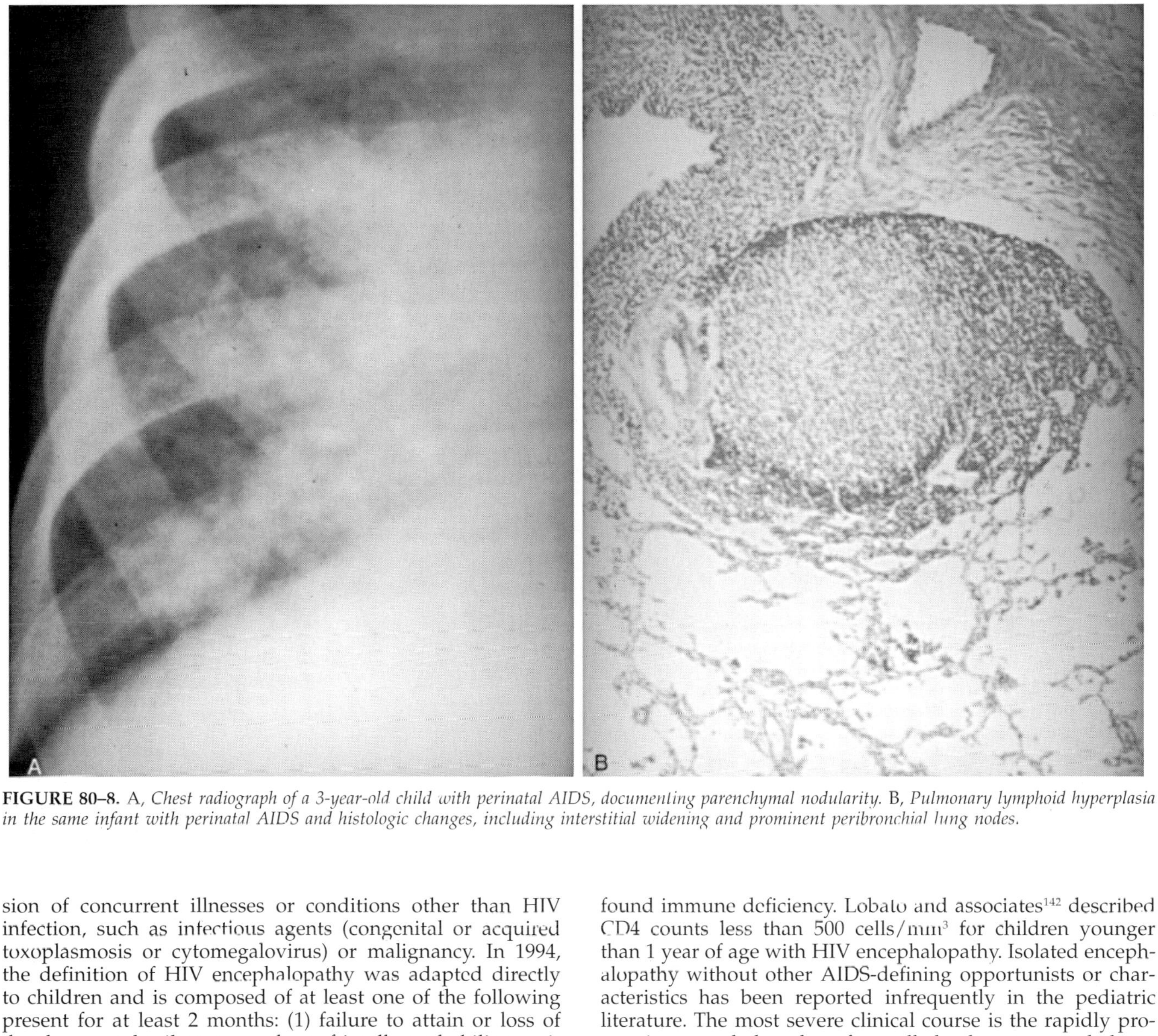

FIGURE 80–8. A, *Chest radiograph of a 3-year-old child with perinatal AIDS, documenting parenchymal nodularity.* B, *Pulmonary lymphoid hyperplasia in the same infant with perinatal AIDS and histologic changes, including interstitial widening and prominent peribronchial lung nodes.*

sion of concurrent illnesses or conditions other than HIV infection, such as infectious agents (congenital or acquired toxoplasmosis or cytomegalovirus) or malignancy. In 1994, the definition of HIV encephalopathy was adapted directly to children and is composed of at least one of the following present for at least 2 months: (1) failure to attain or loss of developmental milestones or loss of intellectual ability, verified by standard developmental scale or neuropsychological tests, (2) impaired brain growth or acquired microcephaly demonstrated by head circumference measurements or brain atrophy demonstrated by computerized tomography or magnetic resonance imaging (serial imaging is required for children younger than 2 years of age), (3) acquired symmetric motor deficit manifested by two or more of the following: paresis, pathologic reflexes, ataxia, or gait disturbance.[46] The incidence of HIV encephalopathy in the pediatric AIDS population is high. In a large multicenter surveillance cohort of perinatal HIV-infected children, 23 per cent exhibited clinical symptoms consistent with the diagnosis of HIV encephalopathy.[142] Other neurologic abnormalities described in adult AIDS patients, including neuropathy, myopathy, radiculopathy, and vacuolar myelopathy, have been reported infrequently in the pediatric AIDS cohort.

The encephalopathy of AIDS has been described as static, slowly progressive, or rapidly progressive with accompanying deterioration of motor and developmental skills and the onset of abnormal neurologic signs (pseudobulbar palsy, ataxia, myoclonic jerks, and seizures).[15, 71] The onset of encephalopathy has been described in association with profound immune deficiency. Lobato and associates[142] described CD4 counts less than 500 cells/mm^3 for children younger than 1 year of age with HIV encephalopathy. Isolated encephalopathy without other AIDS-defining opportunists or characteristics has been reported infrequently in the pediatric literature. The most severe clinical course is the rapidly progressive encephalopathy, often called subacute encephalopathy, with death usually weeks to months after the onset of symptoms. Figure 80–9 documents by nuclear imaging rapid progression of cerebral cortical atrophy in a 5-year-old with transfusion-associated AIDS and subacute encephalopathy. For this child, who presented with a seizure disorder and progression over 3 months to significant motor dysfunction, death was from aspiration secondary to swallowing incoordination and not from opportunistic infection.

The precise pathogenesis of the encephalopathic changes of HIV infection remains elusive, although HIV with cellular tropism clearly is implicated.[10] At histopathology, most children with central nervous system involvement (not related to malignancy or opportunistic infection) show significant brain atrophy. Of note, inflammatory lesions usually are sparse and alone cannot account for the significant amount of observed atrophy. Other purported factors potentially contributing to diminished brain size have included the following: (1) direct or indirect interference of HIV with brain growth (HIV toxic effect versus competition with brain growth factors such as neuroleukin), (2) severe malnutrition, (3) severe hypoxia from cardiac and pulmonary compromise, and (4) therapeutic regimens for infectious or noninfectious

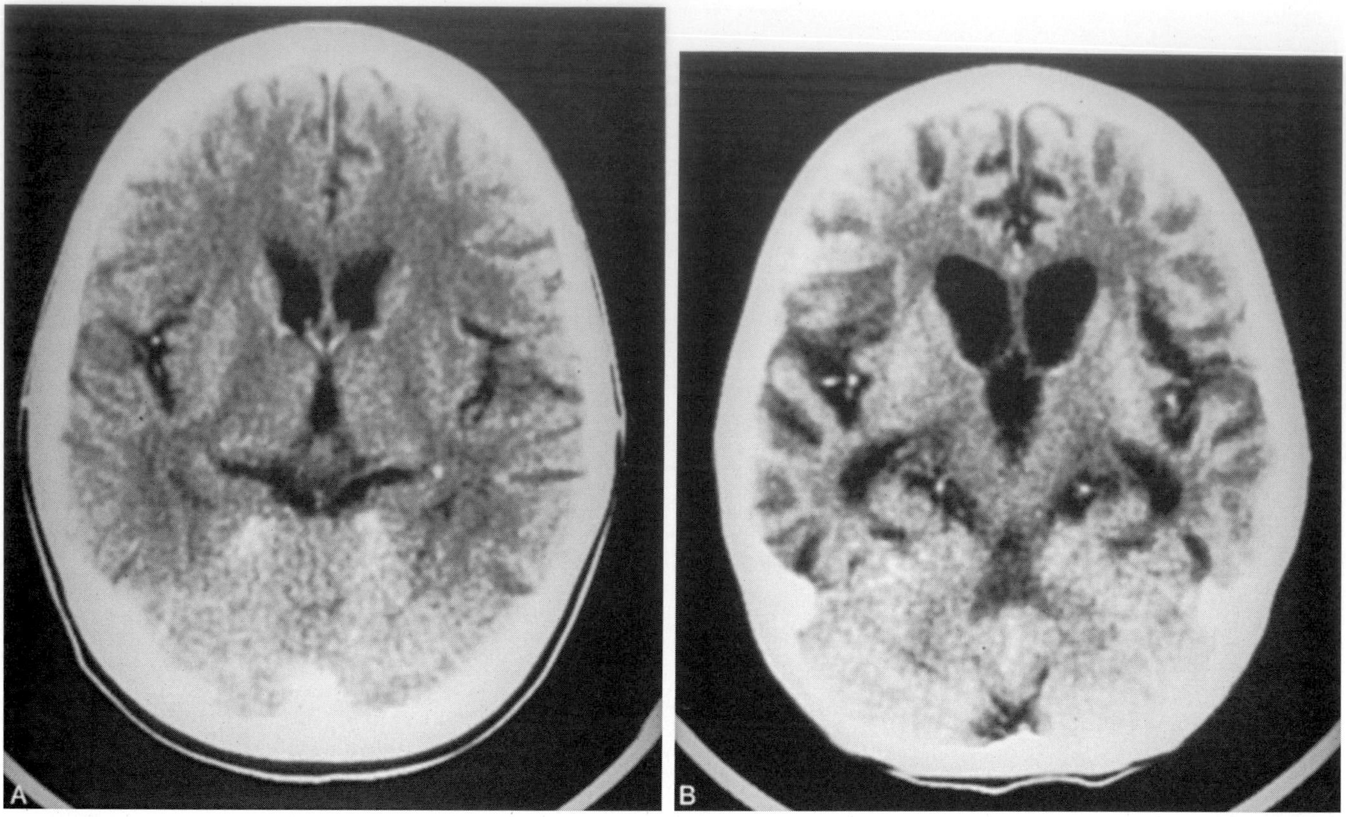

FIGURE 80–9. *Successive computed tomographic scans in a 5-year-old child with transfusion-associated AIDS and dementia.* A, *Significant cortical atrophy and myelin pallor are noted at diagnosis.* B, *Over 3 months, significant neurologic decline correlates with radiographic documentation of progressive cortical atrophy.*

processes that mandate the prolonged use of medications that may inhibit brain growth.[10] In addition to cortical atrophy, myelin pallor and basal ganglia calcifications are not reported infrequently at histology or by use of nuclear imaging techniques (computed tomography or magnetic resonance imaging). These latter findings often have no correlation with clinical neurologic abnormality and suggest that further study of central nervous system involvement in pediatric patients is warranted.

Behavioral abnormalities, so common in early HIV disease in adults, are not described as well in the literature in the pediatric cohort. Attention deficit hyperactivity disorder has been described in small numbers of affected children, and systematic behavioral assessment along with neurodevelopmental evaluation clearly is warranted.[158]

Therapy for central nervous system involvement of noninfectious and nonmalignant encephalopathy has included antiretroviral therapy.[152, 175] Behavioral, neurodevelopmental, and, occasionally, imaging improvement has been documented with nucleoside analogue intervention. Clearly, antiviral therapy not only must achieve effective serum and plasma concentrations but also must be able to cross the blood-brain barrier and affect HIV-infected central nervous system monocytes. Currently, no surrogate markers predictive of central nervous system involvement exist. Mintz[157] has evaluated tumor necrosis factor as a possible marker of progressive encephalopathy in pediatric AIDS, but only serum and not cerebrospinal fluid tumor necrosis factor levels have shown clinical correlation.

A clinical syndrome of aseptic meningitis, often recurring and presumed to be solely related to HIV infection, has been described in adults.[148] Clinical trials assessing the efficacy of zidovudine in HIV-associated aseptic meningitis currently are under way. In pediatric AIDS, bacterial pathogens predominate as the most common cause of meningitis, and the aforementioned recurrent aseptic meningitis syndrome appears to be rare.[11] Assessments of cerebrospinal fluid in HIV-infected children without overt clinical central nervous system involvement usually are normal but occasionally reveal pleocytosis, elevated protein content, and elevated intrathecal antibody synthesis directed toward HIV or HIV antigen itself.[91] Isolation of HIV from cerebrospinal fluid is rare. Other pathogens reported in the pediatric HIV-infected population include *Candida* species, cytomegalovirus, tuberculosis, toxoplasma, and *Cryptococcus*.[158]

Gastrointestinal Complications

Gastrointestinal complications of HIV disease frequently are encountered in both children and adults. Among children with AIDS reported to the CDC in 1988 and 1989, wasting syndrome was reported in 16 per cent.[188] Wasting has been revised from the 1987 definition to its present definition (1994): (1) persistent weight loss greater than 10 per cent of baseline *or* (2) downward crossing of at least two of the following percentile lines on the weight-for-age chart in a child 1 year of age or older *or* (3) less than the 5th percentile on weight-for-height chart on two consecutive measurements, greater than or equal to 30 days apart *plus* (a) chronic diarrhea (at least two loose stools per day for $\geq$30 days) *or* (b) documented fever (for $\geq$30 days, intermittent or constant).[40, 46] Associated protein and micronutrient (zinc, selenium) deficiencies have been documented in HIV-infected adults and children.[164] Nutritional defects may be related to inadequate caloric intake (anorexia from concomitant infection such as MAC or tuberculosis, neuropsychiatric abnormalities, or dysphagia from infectious etiologies, such as chronic oral herpes or *Candida* esophagitis), malabsorption with or without diarrhea, or increased energy expenditure (persistent fever with resultant increased metabolic rates). Macallan and associates[146] documented, in a recent study of 27 adults with HIV wasting, that reduced energy intake and not elevated energy expenditure was the prime determinant in weight loss. Data comparing energy expenditure with intake are scant in the pediatric literature.

In two separate analyses of HIV-infected children, somatic growth (weight-for-age and length-for-age) has been shown to decline by 4 to 6 months of age and to be significantly different from that of HIV-uninfected but exposed controls.[153, 164] These studies have prompted careful attention to the nutritional needs of HIV-infected children. In addition to provision of optimal caloric and nutritional supplementation, therapies that serve as appetite stimulants increasingly have been used and include cyproheptadine, megestrol acetate (Megace), and dronabinol (Marinol). The documented efficacy of these agents usually is not permanent, especially when concomitant opportunistic infections are evident.[7, 214]

Opportunistic infections commonly affect the gastrointestinal tract. Diarrhea, malabsorption, intestinal perforation, and colitis have been associated with isosporiasis, cryptosporidiosis, *Mycobacterium avium-intracellulare* infection, cytomegalovirus infection, *Giardia* infection, and bacterial infections (*Salmonella, Shigella, Campylobacter*). Specific therapeutic intervention should be designed to treat the pathogens that have been isolated. Long-term maintenance therapy often is required to keep the patient as free of infection as possible.

Malignancy

Adults with HIV infection are afflicted not uncommonly by oncologic processes. B-cell non-Hodgkin lymphomas occur in 3 to 4 per cent of patients, and Kaposi sarcoma occurs in as many as 40 per cent of HIV-infected male homosexuals.[149] Malignancy, originally reported infrequently in pediatric AIDS, increasingly is reported as children live longer (improved antiretroviral and supportive therapy) and as the numbers of children with HIV infection increase. In a study of 1300 Italian children with HIV infection, approximately 0.2 per cent had documented malignancies: non-Hodgkin lymphoma (n = 4) and Kaposi sarcoma (n = 1), hepatoblastoma (n = 1), and acute B-cell lymphoblastic leukemia (n = 1).[9] McClain and Rosenblatt[149] reviewed the literature and documented 26 pediatric AIDS cases (younger than 13 years of age) with lymphomas. The most prevalent symptom complex included fever, weight loss, hepatomegaly, and abdominal distention. Of note, seven patients had presenting neurologic complaints. Respiratory complaints were noted in a handful of children with pulmonary lymphoma in association with the lymphoproliferative lung disorders, LIP/PLH. Associated in situ infection with HIV, Epstein-Barr virus, or both has been documented, although its precise role in pathogenesis is not defined. Early chemotherapeutic intervention has enhanced the quality of life and longevity and has been provided often in conjunction with antiretroviral therapy.

Kaposi sarcoma was described in 11 pediatric AIDS patients through 1989.[149] This disease clearly is much less common in HIV-infected children than in their adult counterparts. The pathogenesis of Kaposi sarcoma more recently has been elucidated, and herpes-like DNA sequences have been documented in lesions that most likely represent a new human herpesvirus.[162] This virus has been identified in both HIV-infected and non–HIV-infected persons with Kaposi sarcoma, suggesting that the immunopathogenesis of Kaposi sarcoma may not be linked uniquely to the HIV-1 virus itself. The clinical manifestations of Kaposi sarcoma associated with AIDS affect multiple organs. Skin, gastrointestinal tract, lung, and heart have been affected with Kaposi sarcoma proliferations. The prognosis for Kaposi sarcoma in adults has been linked to clinical progression of the underlying HIV disease with poorer responses in patients with more profound immunodeficiency (lowered CD4 counts) or opportunistic infections. The treatment of Kaposi sarcoma in adults has included antiretroviral therapy (zidovudine), chemotherapy (vinca alkaloids), radiation therapy, and most recently interferon-α therapy.[94, 128]

Since 1987, more than 13 children with AIDS have been reported with smooth muscle malignancies, leiomyosarcomas of the gastrointestinal tract.[50, 150] Previously described in small numbers of children in the world's literature, this upsurge of such an uncommon malignancy in pediatric AIDS patients suggests a distinct relationship to HIV infection or other concomitant infections. McClain and associates[150] documented the association of Epstein-Barr virus (by polymerase chain reaction and in situ hybridization techniques) with leiomyosarcoma in children with AIDS.

Such unusual clinical manifestations have prompted pediatric oncologists nationwide to establish a pediatric AIDS cancer registry to define and understand better oncologic processes in HIV-infected children. Such efforts should be helpful in the development of concerted oncologic intervention as the number of pediatric AIDS cases continues to grow.

Other Complications

Cardiac Abnormalities

The importance of cardiac manifestations of HIV infection in children only recently has been recognized.[141] The National Institutes of Health have funded a national multicenter study to evaluate the onset and clinical implications of cardiac and pulmonary complications in pediatric HIV disease. In this study of almost 600 HIV-infected infants, progressive left ventricular dysfunction as measured by diminished shortening fraction was associated with decreased CD4 lymphocyte counts.[26] Clearly, opportunistic infections (cryptococcosis, aspergillosis) and malignancy (Kaposi sarcoma) have affected cardiac disease and AIDS in children and adults. Clinically, HIV-infected children have been described with congestive heart failure and cardiomegaly, cardiac tamponade, nonbacterial thrombotic endocarditis, conduction disturbances, and sudden death, presumably secondary to primary ventricular arrhythmia associated with severe cardiomyopathy. In one study, four of six HIV-infected infants with cardiac abnormalities showed focal myocarditis when myocardial histologic studies were performed.[139] No precise etiology for this associated myocarditis was defined.

In a study of 81 HIV-infected children, unexpected cardiorespiratory arrests occurred in 9 per cent, chronic congestive heart failure in 10 per cent, and dysrhythmias in 35 per cent of children.[143] Asymptomatic children with HIV infection additionally have been documented to exhibit cardiac abnormalities, including ventricular dysfunction and dilation and pericardial effusions. There is no evidence to suggest that HIV directly is cardiotoxic, although HIV has been documented within myocardial cells by in situ hybridization. Decreased left ventricular function associated with antiretroviral therapy has been reported. In one study of HIV-infected children on antiretroviral nucleoside analogue therapy, zidovudine or didanosine, the odds for cardiomyopathy development were 8.4 times greater for children receiving zidovudine but *not* didanosine.[67] As clinical drug trials to combat opportunistic infections, malignancy, and underlying HIV disease progress and as potentially cardiotoxic therapeutic intervention is defined, understanding the pathogenesis of HIV-associated cardiac complications becomes integral.

RENAL DYSFUNCTION

Renal disease is yet another clinical manifestation of HIV infection. In a retrospective evaluation of 155 pediatric AIDS patients, 12 were noted to have significant proteinuria.[210] Described renal abnormalities in this cohort included nephritis (focal glomerulosclerosis and mesangial hyperplasia) and nephrosis. In fact, focal sclerosis and segmental sclerosis have been described in more than one-half of reported children.[211] Immunopathologic characteristics of HIV-associated nephropathy include inflammatory infiltrations predominantly composed of activated T cells (CD4 cells usually exceeding CD8 cells).[183] Renal disease in HIV-infected children appears often in concert with profound immunodeficiency and end-stage HIV disease. Toxic therapy, concomitant infection, HIV alone, and circulating immune complexes have been implicated in the pathogenesis of this entity. Because most pediatric AIDS patients with renal disease have vertically acquired HIV infection, the importance of congenital or early concomitant infections (e.g., cytomegalovirus) has been postulated to affect pathogenesis. Lending further credence to this postulate is documentation of concurrent viral illnesses in both primarily immunodeficient and HIV-infected children with renal disease.[81] Of note, renal disease manifested histologically as focal glomerulosclerosis in both populations. The uniqueness of HIV nephropathy then becomes questionable. The nephrosis of HIV disease particularly can be difficult to treat in the already malnourished, hypoproteinemic, HIV-infected child. Corticosteroid therapy may be attempted but often ameliorates symptoms with variable efficacy. Nutritional supplementation and dietary restriction may be supportive adjunctive therapy.

BONE MARROW SUPPRESSION

The hematologic abnormalities of HIV infection in children include leukopenia, anemia, and thrombocytopenia. Of note, leukopenia and in particular lymphopenia, so characteristic of the HIV-infected adult, is an uncharacteristic clinical finding early in pediatric HIV infection, especially in perinatally infected infants.[50] Neutropenia has been described often in association with circulating antineutrophil antibodies and may respond to blockade therapy with intravenous immunoglobulin. Granulocyte colony-stimulating factor has been used successfully in neutropenia, both drug-induced and HIV-associated.[93, 165] The anemia of HIV infection may be microcytic, hypochromic as seen in chronic infection, autoimmune with positive Coombs testing, or typical of nutritional deprivation (iron deficiency or B_{12} deficiency). The etiology of anemia in AIDS cases is difficult to sort out and is confounded by multiple cofactors that affect red blood cell counts—that is, poor nutritional status and concomitant use of toxic therapeutic agents (zidovudine). In adults and children, recombinant erythropoietin has been beneficial for anemia associated with zidovudine therapy.[27, 79, 139]

Immune thrombocytopenia has been reported in 13 per cent of children with symptomatic HIV infection with onset as early as the first year of life.[69] This phenomenon appears to be mediated immunologically, although pathogenesis is not defined clearly. Two proposed explanations are (1) nonspecific binding of platelets to circulating antibody complexes, which are documented so commonly in HIV-infected adults and children, and (2) production of antibodies specifically targeted toward platelets and triggered by the same stimulus that produces almost universal hypergammaglobulinemia in HIV-infected children. The presence of platelet-associated IgG in HIV-infected children has been reported to have a sensitivity of 93 per cent; however, specificity is only 13 per cent, suggesting that platelet-associated IgG is unlikely to be a cause of thrombocytopenia.[70] Therapy of thrombocytopenia in children and adults has included no intervention, platelet transfusions, systemic corticosteroids, intravenous immunoglobulin, antiretroviral therapy (zidovudine), and most recently in adults, interferon-α. Results have been variable. Immune thrombocytopenia has resolved spontaneously in some children with simple supportive measures. Listed therapeutic interventions have documented individual variability in responses. Current placebo-controlled trials of intravenous immunoglobulin and trials of zidovudine alone or in combination with immunoglobulin supplementation may provide helpful information and insight into the definition of the most efficacious treatment route of HIV-immune thrombocytopenia.

Diagnosis of HIV Infection in Infants and Children

Early Transmission of HIV to Fetus

There is a serious lack of information on the role of the human placenta in transmitting HIV infection from mother to fetus, although a few studies have suggested that fetal infection can take place as early as 9 to 11 weeks of gestational age.[29, 52, 147, 207, 219] In one study, 16- to 24-week-old fetal tissue obtained from HIV-infected mothers was examined for the presence of HIV DNA using polymerase chain reaction amplification.[207] HIV DNA was found in 19 of 31 thymic samples and 22 of 33 spleen samples studied, which indicated that HIV can be transmitted early in gestation. Preliminary examination of birth placental tissue from HIV-infected mothers in another study indicates that HIV core antigens can be detected in about 50 per cent of the cases studied (23 of 51); furthermore, HIV antigens were localized in the Hofbauer cells.[219] Another group suggests that HIV infection does not cause significant pathology in the placenta and that HIV antigens and RNA synthesis only rarely were detected in the placental tissue.[52] Finally, it has been documented that placental tissue expresses the CD4 molecule for HIV and therefore can be infected experimentally.[114] Thus, there is little doubt that HIV can be transmitted in utero to the fetus and result in an infected infant,[134, 193] although other modes of HIV transmission from mother to infant have been observed, such as exposure to infected amniotic fluid, mixing of maternal blood with fetal blood at the time of delivery, exposure to infected cervical secretions in the birth canal, and infection by breast milk.[68, 230] Because the rate of transmission of HIV from infected mother to fetus or infant is estimated to range from 12 to 25 per cent,[51, 59, 218] it seems reasonable to suspect that some pathologic HIV-related effect on the placenta permits such an extraordinary transmission rate of virus.

An increase in intrauterine fetal demise has been demonstrated in the literature in HIV-infected pregnant women.[133] For HIV-negative fetuses, placental or fetal lesions known to be associated with fetal demise were identified: abruption, infarction, and other infections (cytomegalovirus). For HIV-positive fetuses, no such placental lesions could be identified and death was attributed to HIV detection in fetal tissue as measured by in situ hybridization. Two hypotheses for transmission are proposed: (1) direct cell-to-cell spread of

TABLE 80–8. Guidelines for the Diagnosis of HIV Infection in Infants Born to HIV-Infected Mothers

Definitive HIV diagnosis for infants 18 months of age or older
- Two positive enzyme-linked immunosorbent assays and a positive confirmatory serological test, e.g., Western blot or immunofluorescence assay

OR

- Any two positive viral detection assays on separate specimens:
  - HIV culture
  - HIV polymerase chain reaction
  - p24 antigen test

OR

- Documentation of a pediatric AIDS-defining illness

Presumptive diagnosis for infants younger than 18 months of age
- A single positive viral detection assay (excluding cord blood):
  - HIV culture
  - HIV polymerase chain reaction
  - p24 antigen assay

Definitive diagnosis for infants younger than 18 months of age
- Any two positive viral detection assays on separate specimens:
  - HIV culture
  - HIV polymerase chain reaction
  - p24 antigen test

OR

- Documentation of a pediatric AIDS-defining illness

From Hanson, I. C., and Shearer, W. T.: Diagnosis of HIV infection. Semin. Pediatr. Infect. Dis. *5*:269, 1994.

HIV from infected maternal mononuclear cells through placental cells eventually to fetal tissue itself or (2) infected maternal cells that gain access to the fetal circulation.

Methods Used to Diagnose HIV Infection in Children Older than 18 Months of Age

In children older than 18 months of age in whom the presence of maternal anti-HIV antibody no longer is a confounding variable, the conventional tests used to diagnose HIV infection in adults are applicable (Table 80–8).[100] Thus, enzyme-linked immunosorbent assay, Western blot analysis, indirect fluorescent antibody assay, p24 HIV antigen analysis (p24Ag), HIV culture, and HIV polymerase chain reaction may be used. Of these, enzyme-linked immunosorbent assay and Western blot analysis are the most practical, and two positive enzyme-linked immunosorbent assays plus a positive Western blot test confirm a diagnosis of HIV infection.

The enzyme-linked immunosorbent assay for serum antibodies to HIV is a standardized screening test for detecting present or past infection with HIV. It is a test that is overly sensitive because it tends to overpredict the number of positive subjects and must be confirmed by the more specific Western blot test. A number of commercial testing kits have been approved by the Food and Drug Administration and CDC for the screening of individuals, and, more recently, combination kits that test for both HIV-1 and HIV-2 have been made available.[213] The method consists of adding patient serum to microwells in a plastic plate that have been coated with native or recombinant HIV antigens. After reaction and washing, reagents containing a colored dye are added to the microwells, and the resulting solutions are read at a certain wavelength in a special spectrophotometer.

The Western blot assay is a method in which individual proteins of an HIV lysate are separated according to size by polyacrylamide gel electrophoresis. The viral proteins then are transferred onto nitrocellulose paper and reacted with the patient's serum. Any antibody from the patient's serum is detected by an antihuman IgG antibody conjugated with an enzyme that in the presence of substrate will produce a colored band. Positive and negative control specimens are run simultaneously to allow identification of viral proteins. Western blot results are interpreted as positive, negative, or indeterminate (Table 80–9).[100]

Methods Used to Make an Early Diagnosis of HIV Infection in Infants and Children Younger than 18 Months of Age

The clinical manifestations of HIV infection in children are varied and nonspecific, including chronic pneumonitis, failure to thrive, hepatosplenomegaly, thrombocytopenia, and chronic diarrhea. In children younger than 18 months of age, positive serologic determination for HIV is not accepted as indicative of HIV infection because passive maternal antibody confuses the serologic picture. In children younger than 18 months of age, symptomatic or not, documentation of HIV infection requires more thorough investigation of the immune system with CD4 (helper T lymphocyte) determination, exclusion of congenital immunodeficiency, and identification of viral components from serum or cerebrospinal fluid—that is, p24 HIV antigen determination (including the immune complex dissociated p24 antigen), HIV culture (blood or cerebrospinal fluid) utilizing reverse transcriptase assay or p24 HIV antigen determination, or HIV polymerase chain reaction.[46]

Table 80–8 outlines the current guidelines for determining positive HIV infection status for infants younger than 18 months of age who are born to HIV-infected mothers.[46, 100] Diagnostic distinctions are made by infant age and the number and type of positive virologic assays. Note that a single positive diagnostic test does *not* confirm HIV infection, except in the presence of clinical AIDS-defining events. To date, the methods that have been utilized to make early diagnosis in high-risk infants include culture of peripheral blood mononuclear cells for HIV[149, 180]; DNA polymerase chain reaction of peripheral blood mononuclear cells for HIV[56, 170, 186]; detection of HIV antigen (p24Ag or immune complex–dissociated p24Ag) in blood or spinal fluid[78, 173, 184]; assays for neonatal IgA, IgM, and IgG and for neonatal IgG_3 specific for HIV[35, 180]; and in vitro assays to determine the ability of neonatal peripheral blood mononuclear cells to secrete HIV-specific IgG antibody.[2, 174, 182] Table 80–10 summarizes the sensitivity of each assay by infant age, and it is notable that the sensitivities of HIV culture and HIV polymerase chain reaction approach adult standards by 3 to 6 months of age.[100, 182]

Despite advances in diagnostic technology, there still is a

TABLE 80–9. The Association of State and Territorial Public Health Laboratory Directors (ASTPHLD)/Centers for Disease Control and Prevention Criteria for Positive Interpretation of Western Blot Assays

Any two of:
- p24
- gp41
- gp120/160*

*Distinction of the 120/160 bands is not required, and these bands may be considered as a single reactant for interpretation of Western blot.

From Hanson, I. C., and Shearer, W. T.: Diagnosis of HIV infection. Semin. Pediatr. Infect. Dis. *5*:267, 1994.

TABLE 80–10. Sensitivity (Expressed as a Percentage) of Early Diagnostic Tests by Infant Age

	Birth–1 wk	1–2 mo	3–6 mo	>6 mo
HIV culture	30–50	70–90	>90	>90
HIV polymerase chain reaction	30–50	50–90	>90	>90
p24 antigen tests				
p24 Ag	10–25	20–60	30–50	20–40
ICD p24 Ag	63	100		

Modified from Hanson, I. C., and Shearer, W. T.: Diagnosis of HIV infection. Semin. Infect. Pediatr. Dis. *5*:268, 1994.

problem with sensitivity in all assays in the first few days and weeks of life (see Table 80–10).[100, 182] Cord blood determinations for HIV are problematic because of maternal cell contamination. Experience with use of the polymerase chain reaction or culture technology in neonates born to HIV-infected women has shown that there is a high false-negative rate in polymerase chain reaction tests and HIV culture on early blood specimens in infants who later "test positive" (confirmed by HIV culture, clinical disease, or both). It is possible that poor detection is associated with a low virus load, possibly as the result of infection near the time of delivery rather than earlier in gestation.

In the past, the exclusion of HIV infection for infants born to HIV-infected mothers (~80 per cent of children born to HIV-infected mothers) temporally was delayed to 15 to 18 months when HIV serology was determined to be negative. Based on evaluation of the specificity and sensitivity of viral diagnostic tests, the current pediatric PCP prophylaxis guidelines suggest that infants with two negative virologic assays (HIV culture or HIV polymerase chain reaction), both at 1 month of age or older and one at 4 months of age or older, most likely are not HIV-infected and warrant interruption of therapeutic intervention.[48] Hence, early diagnosis for HIV-exposed infants has been improved both for identification of HIV-infected children (as early as the first month of life) and for uninfected children labeled as seroreverters (as early as the fourth month of life). Schedules for testing of HIV-exposed infants vary nationally. However, advancements in diagnostic technology allow for early testing of HIV-exposed infants, including shortly after birth, every 3 months in the first year of life, and every 6 months until HIV infection status can be determined.

As demonstrated, the viral diagnostic assays listed appear to be most sensitive in those older than 1 month of age. Clearly, there is a need to develop and perfect rapid, reliable, and reproducible tests for the presence of HIV in newborns and infants born to HIV-infected mothers. Not only is it important to make an early diagnosis for purposes of symptomatic treatment intervention, but it is equally compelling to make an early registry of affected infants for accurate population studies and enrollment in national clinical trials of antiretroviral agents and immunomodulators and implementation of appropriate prophylactic regimens.

Treatment

Secondary and Supportive Treatments

Therapeutic intervention for HIV-infected children includes prompt and aggressive treatment of acute infections, particularly opportunistic infections. Because immunodeficiency often precludes complete microorganism eradication, long-term, chronic maintenance therapy often is required. Relapses with and without preventive therapy are not uncommon. With its high morbidity and mortality in children, PCP has focused clinicians on preventive or prophylactic regimens. Of note, other opportunists frequently may recur and may require prophylactic therapeutic regimens (herpes zoster, pneumococcosis). Other preventive measures applicable to all immunodeficient children particularly are important in the HIV-infected host. Examples include measles, influenza, and varicella prophylaxis after exposures. Additionally, routine childhood health care preventive measures, including adequate nutritional support, age and developmentally appropriate stimulation, dental and skin hygiene, and immunizations, should be offered to the child with HIV infection/AIDS.[38, 49] Table 80–11 outlines suggested immunizations for HIV-infected children.

The efficacy of intravenous immunoglobulin in reducing the development of serious laboratory-proven bacterial and clinically diagnosed infections recently has been documented in symptomatic HIV-infected children with CD4 counts of more than 200/mm^3.[160, 215] Although morbidity was reduced, mortality was not affected. The efficacy of intravenous immunoglobulin therapy in conjunction with zidovudine therapy has been reviewed in a multicenter, placebo-controlled trial sponsored by the National Institute of Allergy and Infectious Diseases.[206] In this study of 255 HIV-infected children, intravenous immunoglobulin again demonstrated a reduction in morbidity from serious bacterial infections but only in those children not concomitantly receiving TMP-SMZ as PCP prophylaxis. For children receiving TMP-SMZ, no differences in morbidity from bacterial infections were noted between the immunoglobulin-treated group and placebo (albumin) controls. Current indications for immunoglobulin intervention as suggested by the CDC guidelines for prophylaxis of HIV-infected children include (1) all children with documentation of hypogammaglobulinemia and (2) children with more than two invasive bacterial infections in a 1-year period.[49] Many investigators limit immunoglobulin administration to children with previously outlined clinical indications whose CD4 counts exceed 199 cells/mm^3.

Primary (Anti–HIV) Treatment

Much effort has been expended to evaluate rapidly and safely chemotherapeutic agents with purported antiretroviral activity. Large multicenter efforts to assess antiretroviral agents in adults and children have been the focus of the National Institutes of Health, AIDS Clinical Trial Group (ACTG). Many important collaborative studies documenting efficacy of antiretroviral and opportunistic therapy are the results of these efforts.[57, 152, 206, 215]

Current antiretroviral intervention has targeted different steps in HIV's replication cycle (Fig. 80–10).[14, 126] Because of

TABLE 80–11. Suggested Immunizations for HIV-Infected or HIV-Suspect Children*

TOPV	No
IPV	Yes
DTP	Yes
MMR	Yes
HBV	Yes
Hib	Yes
Pneumovax	Yes
Influenza	Yes

*Authors' recommendations compiled from guidelines suggested by the Centers for Disease Control and Prevention.[38]

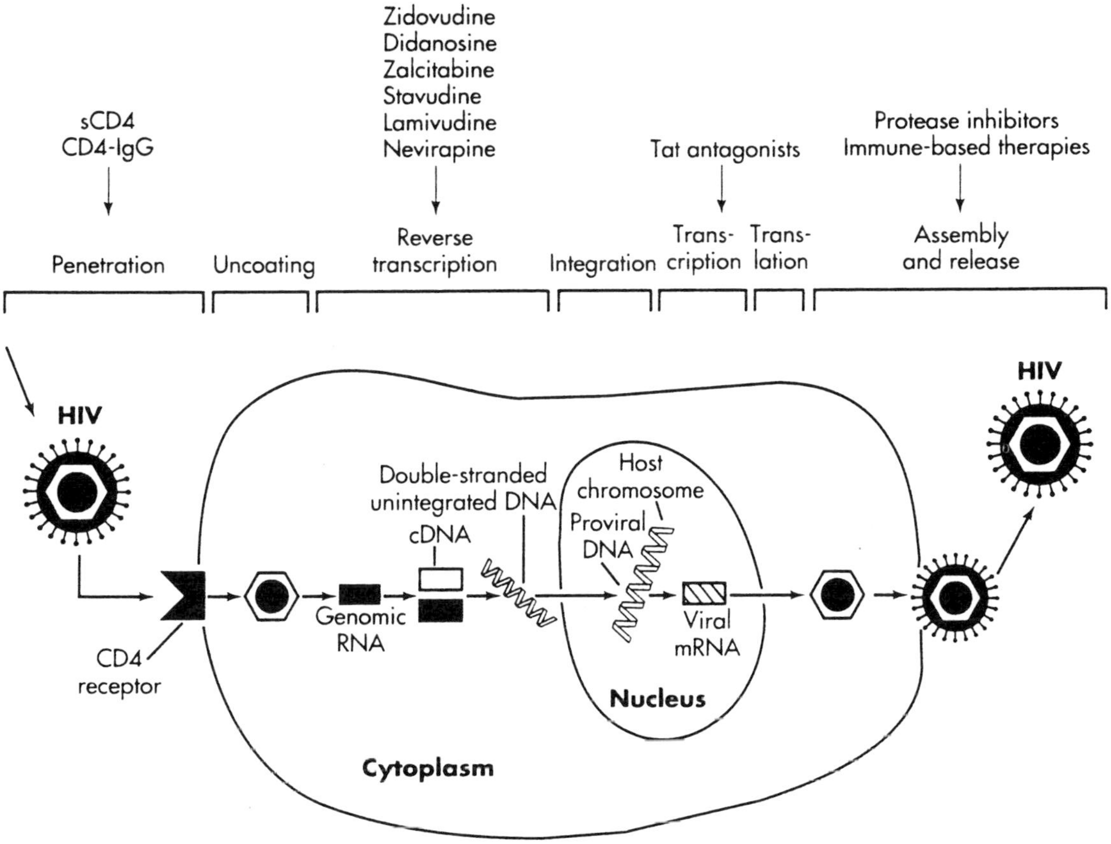

FIGURE 80–10. *Life cycle of HIV, illustrating targets for pharmacologic intervention. (From Kline, M. W., and Shearer, W. T.: HIV infection and AIDS in children.* In *Rich, R. R., Fleischer, T. A., Schwartz, W. T., et al. [eds.]: Clinical Immunology. St. Louis, Mosby, 1996, pp. 739–750.)*

the special nature and challenge of pediatric HIV infection, few of the steps in the HIV life cycle have been approached therapeutically in contrast with the situation in adults with HIV infection, in whom many experimental regimens have been attempted. Nevertheless, with the ever-increasing number of children being afflicted by HIV infection, more public and private resources are accelerating the pace of experimental antiretroviral and immunomodulatory treatment in children. The discussion of therapy should be considered not only in the context of the HIV replication cycle but also by designed impact on the targeted population (i.e., interruption of perinatal transmission or impact on already established pediatric HIV infection).

Blockade of HIV by CD4

Because HIV first attaches by binding its gp120 envelope protein to cellular CD4, antiretroviral therapy has been proposed to block the target binding site, CD4.[114] Recombinant human CD4 (rCD4) molecules have been evaluated in animal models and humans for safety and pharmacokinetics as target binders[119] but have been hampered by their short half-life. In an effort to prolong half-life and perhaps enhance efficacy, rCD4 has been constructed to include the Fc region of human IgG_1, which produces a chimeric molecule rCD4-IgG.[107] For use in children, rCD4-IgG may cross the placenta in similar fashion to native IgG and offer potential protection to the HIV-exposed fetus. Shearer and associates[198] studied the pharmacokinetics and safety of rCD4-IgG in six mother-infant pairs and documented safety and clear evidence for placental transfer of rCD4-IgG and appropriate elimination. Studies of rCD4-IgG in adults have demonstrated a potential for immune modulation but no evidence to date for short-term activity in halting disease progression.[54]

Blockade of HIV by Passive HIV Antibody

In immunodeficient children and adults, intervention with specific immunoglobulin therapy has proved useful adjunctive or prophylactic therapy in combating or preventing infections. A classic example is the use of high-titer cytomegalovirus-specific immunoglobulin in solid organ and bone marrow transplants and resultant reduction in morbidity from cytomegalovirus pneumonitis.[77, 154] Preliminary attempts to use such a "blocking" concept in animal models have been promising.[179] Such a blocking therapeutic concept currently is under evaluation in HIV-infected pregnant women and their offspring in a multicenter, double-blinded, placebo-controlled trial (ACTG protocol 185) utilizing anti-HIV immunoglobulin versus pooled immunoglobulin in combination with zidovudine delivery. Antepartum, peripartum, and postpartum zidovudine delivery has become the standard of care and has been incorporated into all perinatal transmission interruption research trials in the United States because of its recent success in reducing perinatal transmission. Combination therapeutic approaches, in this case passive immunization and reverse-transcriptase inhibition, appear to be the future for pediatric HIV intervention. Establishing the efficacy of anti-HIV immunoglobulin in children with documented HIV infection is ongoing as a clinical trial (ACTG protocol 273). Monoclonal anti-HIV antibodies are being prepared for clinical trials in pediatric as well as adult patients.

Humanizing these previously murine antibodies reduces the chance of immune response by patients to foreign protein.

Nucleosides (Proviral DNA Reverse-Transcriptase Inhibitors)

Several investigational efforts have been directed toward inhibition of the formation of proviral DNA by HIV reverse transcriptase. Although nucleosides have no effect on reverse transcriptase itself but affect the elongation of its proviral DNA product, these drugs are considered reverse-transcriptase inhibitors. Because this antiviral approach best inhibits only actively replicating cells, latently infected, resting cells may derive little benefit from reverse-transcriptase inhibition alone.

ZIDOVUDINE. Zidovudine (azidothymidine, AZT, Retrovir) was the first nucleoside analogue to be evaluated in adults and children. Early placebo-controlled trials in homosexual adults with AIDS documented a significant reduction in mortality and prompted licensure of zidovudine for adults in 1987.[78] Initial recommended doses (1200 mg/day) were reassessed in dose-controlled trials in adults with AIDS and placebo-controlled trials in asymptomatic HIV-infected adults. Current standard of care for adults in the United States includes lowered dose intervention (500 mg/day) at the onset of symptoms or significant immunodeficiency (CD4 $<500/mm^3$).[8] Controversy continues to exist regarding the efficacy of zidovudine in adults with asymptomatic disease.[105, 138, 222] In pediatric studies utilizing the perspective of historical controls and clinical status of patients before and after drug treatment, zidovudine has been documented to be efficacious both by continuous infusion and by oral intermittent dosing.[152, 175] Parameters defining efficacy in children included enhanced sense of well-being, improvement in dementia (especially in cognitive abilities), reduced hepatosplenomegaly and lymphadenopathy, and increased appetite and weight gain. Immunologically, zidovudine has been associated in children with a decline in serum immunoglobulin levels and a transient increase in CD4 helper T-lymphocyte numbers. This latter phenomenon is observed best in children initiating therapy with CD4 cell counts more than $100/mm^3$. However, the immunologic changes noted with zidovudine, particularly changes in CD4 counts, have not been sustained consistently. Most children's CD4 counts drift back to baseline within several months of therapy.

Zidovudine pharmacokinetics by oral, intermittent dosing document good oral bioavailability (65 per cent) and central nervous system penetration with a mean half-life of 1 to 1.5 hours. Because zidovudine requires phosphorylation to be active against HIV infection, the active metabolite (zidovudine triphosphate) accumulates intracellularly and has a longer half-life. Zidovudine is metabolized hepatically, and 25 per cent of its clearance is via renal secretion and glomerular filtration. Hence, primary renal or hepatic compromise or drugs that affect flow or hepatic glucuronidation (acetaminophen) may alter the metabolism of zidovudine and result in accumulation and toxicity.

Zidovudine has documented toxic effects with prominent macrocytic anemia, leukopenia/neutropenia, and chemical hepatitis. Leukopenia and particularly neutropenia is the most common dose-limiting toxicity. Most clinicians rely on bimonthly blood counts to monitor bone marrow suppression. Human granulocyte colony-stimulating factor has been used in adults and children with AIDS to enhance myelopoiesis and correct both HIV and zidovudine-induced neutropenia.[93, 165] Transfusion-dependent anemia is not uncommon and often responds to dose reduction. Recombinant erythropoietin has proved efficacious in adults and children with zidovudine-induced anemia.[27, 139]

Zidovudine was licensed in the United States for pediatric use in 1990. Indications for use include asymptomatic HIV-infected children with evidence of immune dysregulation and symptomatic HIV-infected children, including those with AIDS. Licensing closely followed the documentation of efficacy of intermittent oral zidovudine therapy in pediatric clinical trials. Not surprisingly, recommended dosing for children was the same as that used in these trials, 180 mg/m^2/dose every 6 hours, not to exceed 500 mg/day.[152] The efficacy of lowered doses of intermittent oral zidovudine dosing (90 to 120 mg/m^2/dose every 6 hours) is the subject of a current clinical trial comparing the toxicity and efficacy of 90 versus 180 mg/m^2/dose every 6 hours in mildly symptomatic HIV-infected children. Most clinicians have lumped children older than 13 years of age into adult standards—that is, zidovudine intervention at 500 mg/day (100 mg five times/day). Because specific guidelines are lacking, intrainstitutional variability in dosing for children younger than 13 years of age is not surprising.

Yet another population considered for antiretroviral therapeutic intervention is the fetal population. Early pharmacokinetic and safety trials of zidovudine documented safety with only mild reversible anemia in infants. Pharmacokinetic data suggested that doses of 1.5 mg/kg (intravenous) or 2.0 mg/kg (oral) were safe and associated with minimal toxicity. Connor and associates,[57] in ACTG protocol 076, dramatically demonstrated the efficacy of zidovudine delivered during gestation (500 mg/day, orally), during labor and delivery (intravenous loading dose of 2 mg/kg followed by a continuous infusion of 1 mg/kg), and to the newborn infant (2.0 mg/kg/dose every 6 hours, orally, or for infants not able to tolerate oral dosing, 1.5 mg/kg/dose every 6 hours, intravenously) in reducing perinatal transmission (Fig. 80–11). This reduction from 25 to 8 per cent documented a 66 per cent reduction in vertical transmission and has altered the standard of care for HIV-infected pregnant women and for their exposed fetuses.[47] The short-term toxicity of therapy was linked to reversible anemia not requiring transfusion. Clinical trials to provide long-term follow-up of the infants and

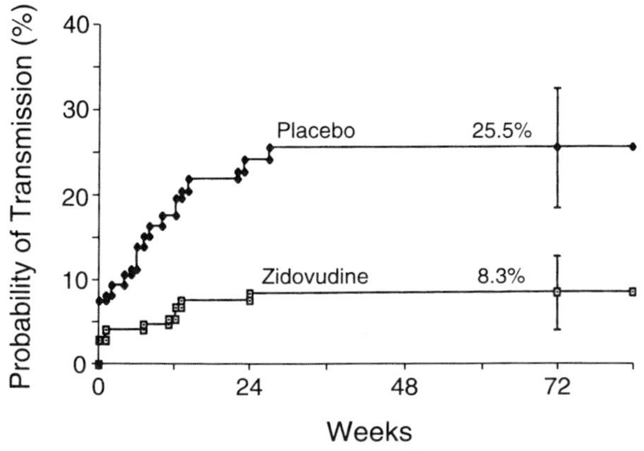

Placebo	183	84	42	37
Zidovudine	180	105	51	43

FIGURE 80–11. *Analysis demonstrating a 66 per cent reduction in perinatal transmission rates from 25 to 8 per cent with antepartum, peripartum, and postpartum zidovudine therapy in HIV-infected pregnant women and their infants. (From Connor, E. M., Sperling, R. S., Gelber, R., et al.: Reduction of maternal-infant transmission of human immunodeficiency virus type 1 with zidovudine treatment: Pediatric AIDS Clinical Trials Group Protocol 076 Study Group. N. Engl. J. Med. 331:1173–1180, 1994.)*

women previously enrolled in ACTG protocol 076 are ongoing and seek to examine evidence for delay in HIV infection status determination in treated infants, the potential for zidovudine resistance in treated women, and the potential for longer-term adverse events associated with infant zidovudine use.

Zidovudine resistance has been described in HIV-1 isolates of patients receiving long-term therapy. Mutations at codon 215 of the HIV-1 reverse transcriptase have been described as characteristic of zidovudine resistance in both adults and children.[115] Resistance to didanosine or zalcitabine is reported less frequently, and clinical significance is not understood fully. Nielsen and associates[168] examined 34 children for evidence of zidovudine-resistant isolates and documented increased disease progression (failure to thrive; onset of opportunistic infections), compared with children with nonresistant isolates. Evidence of such resistance has fueled the development of combination therapies to reduce not only toxicity but also the potential for resistance development.

In a recent clinical trial (ACTG protocol 152) comparing monotherapy zidovudine, monotherapy didanosine, and combination zidovudine and didanosine (reduced-dose zidovudine), the monotherapy zidovudine arm was halted secondary to an increase in clinical disease progression at a mean of 1 year after therapy initiation. Well-documented toxicities attributable to zidovudine were documented in the monotherapy zidovudine-treated group but were not seen in the other two arms. These data have affected other developed clinical trials that have been modified to halt continued monotherapy zidovudine in children with symptomatic disease. Studies currently are under way to elucidate these differences.

DIDEOXYINOSINE. Dideoxyinosine (ddI) has been evaluated in phase I/II trials both at the National Cancer Institute (NCI) by Butler and associates[33] and at the National Institute for Allergy and Infectious Diseases by Lambert and colleagues.[130] Both adults and children have been reported with ddI-associated, dose-limiting neuropathy. In the NCI's clinical studies, cases of clinical pancreatitis were documented, none with demise; in contrast with those in adults, risk factors for pancreatitis in children receiving ddI are unknown. ddI is an attractive alternative or adjunct to zidovudine therapy for several reasons: (1) infrequent description of leukopenia/anemia/thrombocytopenia and (2) alternating or concomitant combination chemotherapy (zidovudine and ddI) offer a unique and hopeful approach to abating HIV disease. A nucleoside analogue, ddI has a prolonged intracellular half-life (approximately 12 hours), which allows for twice-daily and thrice-daily dosing. Blanche and associates[17] described the efficacy of ddI in an open-label trial in children. In July 1991, the Food and Drug Administration approved the use of ddI in adults and children based on available clinical data and the urgent need for alternative drugs for HIV infection. The current recommended dose is 200 $mg/m^2/24$ hours in two divided doses. For optimal absorption, ddI should be administered on an empty stomach. Periodic assessment of liver function tests, amylase, neurologic examination, and ophthalmologic examination (retinal depigmentation has been described) is warranted.

DIDEOXYCYTIDINE. Dideoxycytidine (ddC), a nucleoside analogue akin to ddI, is a potent in vitro inhibitor of HIV replication. Initially limited by administration route (intravenous, subcutaneous) and high-dose toxicity (peripheral neuropathy), ddC has produced palliation of clinical symptoms, decreased virologic parameters (serum p24 Ag levels), and improved immunologic status at lower, oral doses in adults.[1] The most frequent reported adverse effects of ddC include aphthous ulcers, painful peripheral neuropathy, and rash. Studies of ddC in children have been limited. Pizzo and associates[176] have concluded that ddC alone or in combination with zidovudine appears to have antiretroviral activity and is safe in HIV-infected children. Because of poor central nervous system penetration, it seems likely that ddC may be limited in use for children with zidovudine or ddI failure or in combination regimens.

STAVUDINE. Stavudine (d4T) has been evaluated recently in phase I/II trials in children with HIV infection. Like zidovudine, ddI, and ddC, d4T is a potent inhibitor of in vitro HIV replication and functions as a nucleoside analogue.[124] Pharmacokinetic studies document that the oral bioavailability of the drug ranges from 61 to 78 per cent. d4T crosses the blood-brain barrier, and cerebrospinal fluid concentrations ranged from 16 to 97 per cent 2 to 3 hours after an oral dose. In this cohort of 37 children (7 months to 15 years of age), d4T was well tolerated and no drug-associated adverse events were noted. Limited efficacy data suggested that patients showed improvement by increase in CD4 count, decrease in serum p24Ag levels, and no evidence for clinical disease progression. The efficacy of monotherapy d4T currently is being assessed in a national clinical trial (ACTG protocol 240).

COMBINATION NUCLEOSIDE THERAPY. Combination antiviral therapy has been proposed, and multiple clinical trials are ongoing in the pediatric HIV-infected population. To date, these trials include comparisons of monotherapy zidovudine and monotherapy ddI with combination zidovudine and ddI, comparisons of combination therapy (zidovudine and ddI, ddI and nevaripine) with triple therapy with zidovudine, ddI, and nevaripine, and combination *tat* inhibitor and nucleoside inhibitor therapy. Alternating antivirals such as zidovudine and ddI may be preferred over single-agent therapy because it (1) minimizes toxicity from any single agent by allowing single-agent dose reduction in combination regimens, (2) enhances antiviral activity through the use of distinct agents, which may have preferential clinical impact, and (3) diminishes the risk of in vitro/in vivo viral resistance to a constant single agent by offering an alternating regimen schedule.[159] Husson and associates[116] described potent in vivo antiviral activity with combination zidovudine and ddI in 68 HIV-infected children. This therapeutic combination was well tolerated, and no new or enhanced toxicity was documented.

IMMUNOMODULATORS. Because antiretroviral therapy has not been shown to eradicate HIV infection, many investigators have turned their attention to the restoration of the secondary immunodeficiency that attends HIV infection in an attempt to augment natural antiretroviral defenses. Immune modulators have been assessed as single therapeutic agents or in combination regimens in adult clinical trials. Kovacs and associates[127] documented increases in CD4 T lymphocytes after intermittent infusions of IL-2 in adults with HIV infection with CD4 counts greater than or equal to 200 cells/mm^3. Of note, in patients with lower CD4 counts, infusions of IL-2 were attended with evidence for viral activation and no improvement of CD4 counts. Combination zidovudine and immunomodulator therapy is promising and is the subject of ongoing trials (IL-2 and nucleoside analogues, interferon-γ and nucleoside analogues).

Interferons, especially interferon-α, have been documented to produce in vitro antiretroviral activity.[189] It is presumed that interferons inhibit HIV replication by diminishing assembly and release of mature virus particles (virion budding) from an infected cell surface. Trials to assess the efficacy of interferons in vivo have documented increases in CD4 counts with combination therapy compared with monotherapy zidovudine.[84] Alternating zidovudine and interferon-α regimens for children have been proposed and approved in principle by the Pediatric Core Committee of the ACTG. The toxicity of interferon-α is not insignificant and includes fever, malaise, myalgia, and bone marrow suppression. Of note, interferon-α is licensed for use in adults with Kaposi sarcoma,[94] and clinical trials are ongoing to assess its role in ameliorating HIV-induced immune thrombocytopenia.

VACCINES. Significant problems attend the development of vaccines against HIV.[20, 159] Effective viral vaccines afford protection by production of functional neutralizing antibodies in the immunized host. Neutralizing antibodies to HIV have been detected in 10 to 80 per cent of HIV-infected patients. Currently, there is no clear method to decipher whether these circulating antibodies with in vitro activity afford in vivo protection from HIV and diminish progression of disease. The current paucity of animals that seroconvert to HIV and develop immunodeficiency and clinical manifestations makes the process of evaluating antibody function more difficult to approach. Complicating this issue is the heterogeneity of the HIV envelope glycoprotein, which additionally makes vaccine development problematic.

Despite obstacles and in the face of a growing HIV epidemic, vaccine development is progressing. Killed or synthetic virus vaccine trials utilizing gp120 candidate vaccines in animal models[16, 166, 178] and more recently in HIV-infected pregnant women and their offspring are under way.[58] Considering that the vast majority of children infected with HIV acquire their infection at birth, the construct of a vaccine for perinatal interruption is a high priority.

Because perinatal transmission occurs at a period of intimate mucosal contact of infants and their mothers, interest in the research area of mucosal immunity in HIV infection has grown. Twin studies suggest that mode of delivery (cesarean section versus vaginal delivery), at least for twins, may affect transmission outcome. Active interest on the impact of cleansing the vaginal vault has led to the implementation of international studies of chlorhexidine in interrupting perinatal transmission.[58]

Prognosis

Once established, T-cell immunodeficiency persists in patients with AIDS. Mortality rates for adult patients with AIDS have been described, with one report documenting median survival for all patients as 12.5 months.[135] These rates have been modified by the advent of effective antiretroviral therapy for adults and are reflected in a decrease in recent AIDS patient mortality numbers from projected CDC statistics.

Mortality rates in children with AIDS reported to the CDC approach 60 per cent.[185] A number of primary and secondary therapies have become available, but no alteration in mortality or disease progression rates in large numbers of pediatric patients has been described yet. Pediatric HIV infection clearly is expressed in differing patterns; rapid, usual, or slow progressors and factors that influence any individual child's clinical course are not defined precisely yet.

With accelerating research efforts directed toward early diagnostic methods for documenting HIV infection, it is hoped that earlier diagnosis will lead to early primary viral therapy and prompt treatment and prevention of opportunistic infection. This should have a positive impact, with diminished morbidity and mortality rates in HIV-infected children, particularly those with more rapid onset of symptoms and abrupt clinical and immunologic decline. In addition, pediatric research emphasizes continuing evaluation of new therapeutic interventions that might reduce even further perinatal transmission rates. For example, effective vaccine development would clearly have a significant impact on adults and children worldwide exposed to HIV.

Significant research efforts and expenditures are warranted in the face of an HIV epidemic that has affected so many over such a short time and that is a sexually transmitted disease. For children and women, the shift in transmission patterns to prominent heterosexual transmission makes this infectious process a clear and persistent future threat. When viewed from this perspective, it is imperative to place the highest priority on the global confrontation of this epidemic that threatens the future of our children.

OTHER ACQUIRED IMMUNODEFICIENCIES

The Neonate and Premature Infant

More than 4 million infants are born each year in the United States, and it is estimated that almost 7 per cent of these infants weigh less than 2500 g at birth.[23] The evolving immune system of the newborn and children was discussed earlier. It is these inherent deficits that make the newborn and premature infant susceptible to infectious processes that their older counterparts handle with ease. Neonatal bacteremia is suggested to affect approximately 5 of every 1000 infants.[122] Causative agents include gram-positive organisms, group B streptococci, *S. aureus, S. epidermidis,* gram-negative organisms, *Escherichia coli, Klebsiella* species, *Pseudomonas* species, *Enterobacter* species, fungi, and *Candida albicans*. Particularly bothersome for the premature infant are infections related to invasive devices that are required for optimal care, such as scalp electrode skin infections, catheter infections, endotracheal tube infections, chest tube infections, and ventriculoperitoneal shunt infections. Portals of entry for the outlined infectious agents include the maternal genital tract, the infant's respiratory tract, the gastrointestinal and urinary tracts, and the skin. The central nervous system is a common site for hematogenous spread of sepsis, and, for this reason, evaluation of cerebrospinal fluid commonly is included in the evaluation of neonatal sepsis. Antimicrobial agents should be delivered in age-appropriate doses in the neonatal period to ensure that the pharmacokinetics for each agent have been assessed.

Malnutrition

Malnutrition is accompanied by a host of immunologic defects, including normal to elevated serum immunoglobulins, compromise of cellular immunity (anergy; diminished numbers of circulating T cells; diminished lymphoproliferative responses to mitogens, specific antigens, or both; impaired cytokine production), impaired leukocyte function, and reduced complement levels.[129] The clinical impact of such complex and diverse immunologic functions has been documented worldwide by epidemic outbreaks of common infectious diseases in malnourished children.[204, 212] In addition, malnourished children require frequent hospital admissions; bacterial infection is common.[202] Malnutrition can be separated into two clinical entities: marasmus, poor caloric intake in general, and kwashiorkor, protein-deficient diet independent of caloric intake. Table 80–12 documents organisms that commonly cause serious infections in infants with kwashiorkor.[112]

Oncologic Disorders

Childhood cancers are common causes of death in children younger than 13 years of age. According to one estimate of

TABLE 80–12. Organisms Causing Serious Infections in Kwashiorkor and Other Causes of Impaired Cell-Mediated Immunity

Herpesviruses	*Plasmodium* species
Hepatitis viruses	*Mycobacterium tuberculosis*
Measles virus	*Pneumocystis carinii*
Gram-negative bacilli	*Candida albicans*

From Hughes, W. T.: Malnutrition. *In* Patrick, C. C. (ed.): Infection in Immunocompromised Infants and Children. New York, Churchill Livingstone, 1992, pp. 329–333.

oncologic diseases in childhood, more than 6500 occur each year, with more than 50 per cent attributed to leukemias and lymphomas.[135] As with the other acquired immunodeficiencies of childhood, the immunologic defects of oncologic diseases are diverse and affect multiple arms of the immune system concomitantly. Granulocytopenia particularly is problematic for children with childhood cancers, and the nonspecific finding of fever often heralds serious infectious processes. Lee and Pizzo[135] describe bacteremia in 10 to 20 per cent of febrile and granulocytopenic pediatric cancer patients.

TABLE 80–13. Differential Diagnosis of Pneumonia in Cancer Patients

Localized Infiltrate	Diffuse Infiltrate
Nonneutropenic Patients	
Bacteria: *Streptococcus pneumoniae, Haemophilus,* mycobacteria	Parasites: *Pneumocystis carinii, Toxoplasma gondii, Strongyloides*
Mycoplasma	Bacteria: *Mycobacterium, Nocardia, Legionella, Chlamydia* (including TWAR)
Fungi: *Cryptococcus, Histoplasma, Coccidioides*	*Mycoplasma*
Viruses: respiratory syncytial, adenovirus	Viruses: herpes simplex, varicella-zoster, cytomegalovirus, measles, influenza, adenovirus
Underlying tumor	Fungi: *Aspergillus, Candida, Zygomycetes, Cryptococcus*
Drugs: busulfan, bleomycin, cyclophosphamide, methotrexate, cytosine arabinoside	Radiation pneumonitis
Radiation	Drugs
Neutropenic Patients	
Bacteria: any gram-positive or gram-negative *Mycobacterium, Nocardia*	Bacteria: any gram-positive or gram-negative *Mycobacterium, Nocardia, Legionella, Chlamydia*
Fungi: *Aspergillus, Zygomycetes, Candida, Cryptococcus, Histoplasma*	*Mycoplasma*
Viruses: herpes simplex, varicella-zoster	Fungi: *Candida, Aspergillus, Zygomycetes, Cryptococcus, Histoplasma*
Drugs: (see above)	Parasites: *P. carinii, T. gondii, Strongyloides*
Radiation	Viruses: herpes simplex, varicella-zoster, cytomegalovirus, measles, influenza, adenovirus, respiratory syncytial
	Radiation pneumonitis
	Drugs

From Lee, J. W., and Pizzo, P. A.: Management of specific problems in children with leukemias and lymphomas. *In* Patrick, C. C. (ed.): Infection in Immunocompromised Infants and Children. New York, Churchill Livingstone, 1992, p. 201.

Common sources for bacteremia include the respiratory tract, skin, gastrointestinal tract, and invasive devices placed for optimal care (e.g., indwelling catheters). Pulmonary infections are estimated to make up more than 25 per cent of all bacteremic events. Table 80–13 outlines those microorganisms that should be included in the differential diagnosis of pneumonia for cancer patients with neutropenia.[133] Many of the same secondary infections described in the pediatric patient with HIV infection also are common in cancer patients (i.e., *Candida* esophagitis, PCP, cytomegalovirus pneumonitis, herpes simplex virus esophagitis, primary varicella, and cryptococcal meningitis).[105, 163] Fulminant fungal infection is a common cause of morbidity and mortality, and *C. albicans* and *Aspergillus fumigatus* are not uncommon isolated pathogens. Hematogenous spread of fungal infections is not uncommon, and careful investigation for dissemination is warranted. Specific therapy should be tailored to isolated organism sensitivities, suggesting that active search for a pathogen is warranted in the child with cancer, granulocytopenia, and fever. Therapy usually is extended for cancer patients (i.e., 14 to 28 days, depending on the isolated organism).

The large number of children affected by the few acquired immunodeficiencies elucidated in this chapter mandates that health care providers be familiar with acquired immunodeficiencies and their predilection for extraordinary clinical presentation. Knowledge of the clinical diseases that attend these disorders allows for life-saving acute care and opportunities to offer preventive interventions to affected children.

Acknowledgments

The following grants supported in part the clinical research contained in this chapter: grant numbers U01-AI-27551, U01-AI-27551-03S, and UO1-AI-34840-03 from the National Institute of Allergy and Infectious Diseases; contract number N01-HD-72925 and grant number R01-HD-26603 from the National Institute of Child Health and Human Development; contract number N01-HR-96040 from the National Heart, Lung, and Blood Institute; and grant number RR-00188 from the General Clinical Research Center.

References

1. Abrams, D. I., Goldman, A. I., Launer, C., et al.: A comparative trial of didanosine or zalcitabine after treatment with zidovudine in patients with human immunodeficiency virus infection: The Terry Beirn Community Programs for Clinical Research on AIDS. N. Engl. J. Med. *330*:657–662, 1994.
2. Amadori, A., de Rossi, A., Giaquinto, C., et al.: In vitro production of HIV-specific antibody in children at risk of AIDS. Lancet *1*:852–854, 1988.
3. Ammann, A. J., Schiffman, G., Abrams, D., et al.: B cell immunodeficiency in acquired immunodeficiency syndrome. J. A. M. A. *251*:1447–1449, 1984.
4. Anderson, D. C., Hughes, B. J., and Smith, C. W.: Abnormal mobility of neonatal polymorphonuclear leukocytes: Relationship to impaired redistribution of surface adhesion sites by chemotactic factor or colchicine. J. Clin. Invest. *63*:863–874, 1981.
5. Andiman, W. A., Mezger, J., and Shapiro, E.: Invasive bacterial infections in children born to women infected with human immunodeficiency virus type 1. J. Pediatr. *124*:846–852, 1994.
6. Anonymous: Report of a consensus workshop, Siena, Italy, January 17 to 18, 1992: Early diagnosis of HIV infection in infants. J. Acquir. Immune Defic. Syndr. *5*:1169–1178, 1992.
7. Anonymous: Drug approval for weight loss in AIDS news. Am. Fam. Physician *47*:997, 1993.
8. Anonymous: State of the art conference on azidothymidine therapy for early HIV infection. Am. J. Med. *89*:335–344, 1990.
9. Arico, M., Caselli, D., D'Argenio, P., et al.: Malignancies in children with human immunodeficiency virus type 1 infection: The Italian multicenter study on human immunodeficiency virus infection in children. Cancer *68*:2473–2477, 1991.
10. Armstrong, D. D., and Kirkpatrick, J. B.: Neuropathology of pediatric AIDS. Semin. Pediatr. Infect. Dis. *1*:112–123, 1990.
11. Ashkenazi, S., and Kohl, S.: Central nervous system abnormalities in

pediatric HIV infection and AIDS. Semin. Pediatr. Infect. Dis. *1*:94–106, 1990.
12. The Association of State and Territorial Public Health Laboratory Directors: Seventh Annual Conference on Human Retrovirus Testing, Chicago, March 1992, Report. *1*:1–26, 1992.
13. Bakshi, S. S., Alvarez, D., Hilfer, C. L., et al.: Tuberculosis in human immunodeficiency virus–infected children: A family infection. Am. J. Dis. Child. *147*:320–324, 1993.
14. Balis, F. M., and Poplack, D. G.: Drug development and clinical pharmacology. *In* Pizzo, P. A., and Wilfert, C. M. (eds.): Pediatric AIDS: The Challenge of HIV Infection in Infants, Children, and Adolescents. Baltimore, Williams and Wilkins, 1990, pp. 457–477.
15. Belman, A. L., Diamond, G., Dickson, D., et al.: Pediatric acquired immunodeficiency syndrome: Neurologic syndromes. Am. J. Dis. Child. *142*:29–35, 1988.
16. Berman, P. W., Gregory, T. J., Riddle, L., et al.: Protection of chimpanzees from infection by HIV-1 after vaccination with recombinant glycoprotein gp120 but not gp160. Nature *345*:622–625, 1990.
17. Bernstein, L. J., Ochs, H. D., Wedgwood, R. J., et al.: Defective humoral immunity in pediatric acquired immune deficiency syndrome. J. Pediatr. *107*:352–356, 1985.
18. Blanche, S., Tardieu, M., Duliege, A. M., et al.: Longitudinal study of 94 symptomatic infants with perinatally acquired human immunodeficiency virus infection: Evidence for a bimodal expression of clinical and biological symptoms. Am. J. Dis. Child. *144*:1210–1215, 1990.
19. Blanche, S., Calvez, T., Rouzioux, C., et al.: Randomized study of two doses of didanosine in children infected with human immunodeficiency virus. J. Pediatr. *122*:966–973, 1993.
20. Bolognesi, D. P.: AIDS vaccines: Progress and unmet challenges. Ann. Intern. Med. *114*:161–162, 1991.
21. Bonavida, B., Katy, J., and Gottlieb, M.: Mechanism of defective NK cell activity in patients with acquired immunodeficiency syndrome (AIDS) and AIDS-related complex. I. Defective trigger of NK cells for NKLF production by target cells, and partial restoration by IL-2. J. Immunol. *137*:1157–1163, 1986.
22. Borkowsky, W., Steele, C. J., Grubman, S., et al.: Antibody responses to bacterial toxoids in children infected with human immunodeficiency virus. J. Pediatr. *110*:563–566, 1987.
23. Borkowsky, W., Rigaud, M., Krasinski, K., et al.: Cell-mediated and humoral immune responses in children infected with human immunodeficiency virus during the first four years of life. J. Pediatr. *120*:371–375, 1992.
24. Boyer, K. M.: Premature infants. *In* Patrick, C. C. (ed.): Infections in Immunocompromised Infants and Children. New York, Churchill Livingstone, 1992, pp. 137–159.
25. Brenner, T. J., Dahl, K. E., Olson, B., et al.: Relation between HIV-1 synctium inhibition antibodies and clinical outcome in children. Lancet *337*:1001–1005, 1991.
26. Bricker, J. T., for the P^2C^2 HIV Study Group: Transmission, immunodeficiency, and infectious complications [Abstract]. Seattle, American Thoracic Society, May 1995.
27. Brigitta, U. M., Jacobsen, F., Butler, K. M., et al.: Combination treatment with azidothymidine and granulocyte colony-stimulating factor in children with human immunodeficiency virus infection. J. Pediatr. *121*:797–802, 1992.
28. Brookmeyer, R.: Reconstruction and future trends of the AIDS epidemic in the United States. Science *253*:37–42, 1991.
29. Brossard, Y., Aubin, J. T., Madnelbrot, L., et al.: Frequency of early in utero HIV-1 infection: A blind DNA polymerase chain reaction study on 100 fetal thymuses. AIDS *9*:359–366, 1995.
30. Brouwers, P., Belman, A., and Epstein, L. G.: Central nervous system involvement: Manifestations, evaluation and pathogenesis. *In* Pizzo, P. A., and Wilfert, C. M., (eds.): Pediatric AIDS: The Challenge of HIV Infection in Infants, Children, and Adolescents. Baltimore, Williams & Wilkins, 1994, pp. 433–455.
31. Bryson, Y. J., Luzuriaga, K., Sullivan, J. L., et al.: Proposed definitions for in utero versus intrapartum transmission of HIV-1. N. Engl. J. Med. *327*:1246–1247, 1992.
32. Bryson, Y. J., Pang, S., Wei, L. S., et al.: Clearance of HIV infection in a perinatally infected infant. N. Engl. J. Med. *332*:833–838, 1995.
33. Butler, K., Husson, R. N., Balis, F. M. et al.: Dideoxyinosine (ddI) in children with symptomatic HIV infection. N. Engl. J. Med. *324*:137–144, 1991.
34. Canosa, C. A.: Epidemiology of HIV infection in children in Europe. Acta Paediatr. *400*:8–14, 1994.
35. Caselli, D., Marconi, M., Maccabruni, A., et al.: HIV-specific IgG3 in cord blood: Predictive value for seroreversion. Ann. N. Y. Acad. Sci. *693*:262–263, 1993.
36. Centers for Disease Control and Prevention: Education and foster care of children infected with human T-lymphotropic virus type III/lymphadenopathy-associated virus. M. M. W. R. *34*:517–521, 1985.
37. Centers for Disease Control and Prevention: Recommendations for assisting in the prevention of perinatal transmission of human T-lymphotropic virus type III/lymphadenopathy-associated virus and acquired immunodeficiency syndrome. M. M. W. R. *34*:721–732, 1985.
38. Centers for Disease Control and Prevention: Immunization of children infected with human T-lymphotropic virus type III/lymphadenopathy-associated virus. M. M. W. R. *35*:595–606, 1986.
39. Centers for Disease Control and Prevention: Revision of the CDC surveillance case definition for acquired immunodeficiency syndrome. Council of State and Territorial Epidemiologists; AIDS Program, Center for Infectious Diseases. M. M. W. R. *36*:1S–15S, 1987.
40. Centers for Disease Control and Prevention: Classification system for human immunodeficiency virus (HIV) infection in children under 13 years of age. M. M. W. R. *36*:225–230, 1987.
41. Centers for Disease Control and Prevention: First 100,000 cases of acquired immunodeficiency syndrome—United States. M. M. W. R. *38*:561–563, 1989.
42. Centers for Disease Control and Prevention: Guidelines for prophylaxis against *Pneumocystis carinii* pneumonia for children infected with human immunodeficiency virus. M. M. W. R. *40*:1–13, 1991.
43. Centers for Disease Control and Prevention: Summary of notifiable diseases, United States, 1991. M. M. W. R. *40*:45, 1992.
44. Centers for Disease Control and Prevention: Recommendations for prophylaxis against *Pneumocystis carinii* pneumonia for adults and adolescents infected with human immunodeficiency virus. M. M. W. R. *41*:1–10, 1992.
45. Centers for Disease Control and Prevention: Recommendations on prophylaxis and therapy for disseminated *Mycobacterium avium* complex for adults and adolescents infected with human immunodeficiency virus. M. M. W. R. *42*:14–20, 1993.
46. Centers for Disease Control and Prevention: 1994 revised classification system for human immunodeficiency virus infection in children less than 13 years of age. M. M. W. R. *43*:1–17, 1994.
47. Centers for Disease Control and Prevention: Recommendations of the U.S. Public Health Service Task Force on the use of zidovudine to reduce perinatal transmission of human immunodeficiency virus. M. M. W. R. *43*:1–20, 1995.
48. Centers for Disease Control and Prevention: 1995 revised guidelines for prophylaxis against *Pneumocystis carinii* pneumonia for children infected with or perinatally exposed to human immunodeficiency virus. M. M. W. R. *44*:1–10, 1995.
49. Centers for Disease Control and Prevention: USPHA/IDSA guidelines for the prevention of opportunistic infections in persons infected with human immunodeficiency virus: A summary. M. M. W. R. *44*:1–34, 1995.
50. Chadwick, E. G., Connor, E. J., Hanson, I. C., et al.: Tumors of smooth muscle origin in pediatric HIV-infected patients: A new association of AIDS and cancer. J. A. M. A. *263*:3182–3184, 1990.
51. Chadwick, E. G., and Yogev, R.: Pediatric AIDS. Pediatr. Clin. North Am. *42*:969–992, 1995.
52. Chandwani, E., Greco, M. A., Mittal, K., et al.: Pathology and HIV expression in term placentas from seropositive women. Abstract MBP 20 of the Fifth International Conference on AIDS, Montreal, June 1989, p. 225.
53. Chin, J.: Current and future dimensions of the HIV/AIDS pandemic in women and children. Lancet *336*:221–224, 1990.
54. Chowdhury, I. H., Koyanagi, Y., Takamatsu, K., et al.: Evaluation of anti-human immunodeficiency virus effect of recombinant CD4-immunoglobulin in vitro: A good candidate for AIDS treatment. Med. Micro. Immunol. *180*:183–192, 1991.
55. Clavel, F., Guetard, D., Brun-Vezinet, F., et al.: Isolation of a new human retrovirus from West African patients with AIDS. Science *233*:343–346, 1986.
56. Comeau, A. M., Hsu, H.-W., Schwerzier, M., et al.: Identifying human immunodeficiency virus infection at birth: Application of polymerase chain reaction to guthrie cards. J. Pediatr. *123*:252–258, 1993.
57. Connor, E. M., Sperling, R. S., Gelber, R., et al.: Reduction of maternal-infant transmission of human immunodeficiency virus type 1 with zidovudine treatment: Pediatric AIDS Clinical Trials Group Protocol 076 Study Group. N. Engl. J. Med. *331*:1173–1180, 1994.
58. Connor, E. M., and McSherry G.: Immune-based interventions in perinatal human immunodeficiency virus infection. Pediatr. Infect. Dis. J. *13*:440–448, 1994.
59. Cowan, M. J., Hellman, D., Chudwin, D., et al.: Maternal transmission of acquired immune deficiency syndrome. Pediatrics *73*:382–386, 1984.
60. Curran, J. W., Lawrence, D. N., Jaffe, H., et al.: Acquired immunodeficiency syndrome (AIDS) associated with transfusions. N. Engl. J. Med. *310*:492–497, 1984.
61. Demmler, G. J., and Taber, L. H.: Virology of HIV-1. Semin. Pediatr. Infect. Dis. *1*:17–20, 1990.
62. Denny, T. N., Yogev, R., Gelman, R., et al.: Lymphocyte subsets in healthy children during the first 5 years of life. J. A. M. A. *267*:1484–1488, 1992.
63. DeRossi, A., Zanotto, C., Mammano, F., et al.: Pattern of antibody response against the v3 loop in children with vertically acquired immunodeficiency type-1 (HIV-1) infection. AIDS Res. Hum. Retroviruses *9*:221–228, 1993.
64. Devash, Y., Calvelli, T. A., Wood, D. G., et al.: Vertical transmission of human immunodeficiency virus is correlated with the absence of high-affinity/avidity maternal antibodies to the gp120 principal neutralizing domain. Proc. Natl. Acad. Sci. U. S. A. *87*:3445–3449, 1990.
65. Dickover, R. E., Dillon, M., Gillete, S. G., et al.: Rapid increases in load of human immunodeficiency virus correlate with early disease progression

and loss of CD4 cells in vertically infected infants. J. Infect. Dis. *170*:1279–1284, 1994.
66. Dieterich, D. T., Kotler, D. P., Busch, D. F., et al: Ganciclovir treatment of cytomegalovirus colitis in AIDS: A randomized, double-blind, placebo-controlled multicenter study. J. Infect. Dis. *167*:278–282, 1993.
67. Domanski, M. J., Sloas, M. M., Follmann, D. A., et al.: Effect of zidovudine and didanosine treatment on heart function in children infected with human immunodeficiency virus. J. Pediatr. *127*:137–146, 1995.
68. Dunn, D. T., Newell, M. L., Ades, A. E., et al.: Risk of human immunodeficiency virus type 1 transmission through breastfeeding. Lancet *340*:585–588, 1992.
69. Ellaurie, M., Burns, E. R., Bernstein, L. J., et al.: Thrombocytopenia and human immunodeficiency virus in children. Pediatrics *82*:905–908, 1988.
70. Ellaurie, M., Burns, E. R., and Rubinstein, A.: Platelet-associated IgG in pediatric HIV infection. Pediatr. Hematol. Oncol. *8*:179–185, 1991.
71. Epstein, L. G., Sharer, L. R., Oleske, J. M., et al.: Neurologic manifestations of HIV infection in children. Pediatrics *78*:678–687, 1986.
72. European Collaborative Study: Children born to women with HIV-1 infection: Natural history and transmission. Lancet *337*:253–260, 1991.
73. European Collaborative Study: Risk factors for mother-to-child transmission of HIV-1. Lancet *339*:1007–1012, 1992.
74. European Collaborative Study: Caesarean section and risk of vertical transmission of HIV-1 infection. Lancet *343*:1464–1467, 1994.
75. Fabio, G., Scorza, R., Lazzarin, A., et al.: HLA-associated susceptibility to HIV-1 infection. Clin. Exp. Immunol. *87*:20–23, 1992.
76. Fauci, A. S.: The human immunodeficiency virus: Infectivity and mechanisms of pathogenesis. Science *239*:617–622, 1988.
77. Fehir, K. M., Decker, W. A., Samo, T., et al.: Immune globulin (GAMMAGARD) prophylaxis of CMV infections in patients undergoing organ transplantation and allogeneic bone marrow transplantation. Transplant. Proc. *21*:3107–3109, 1989.
78. Fischl, M. A., Richman, D. D., Grieco, M. H., et al.: The efficacy of azidothymidine (AZT) in the treatment of patients with AIDS and AIDS-related complex. N. Engl. J. Med. *313*:192–197, 1987.
79. Fischl, M. A., Galpin, J. E., Levine, J. D., et al.: Recombinant human erythropoietin for patient with AIDS treated with zidovudine. N. Engl. J. Med. *322*:488–493, 1990.
80. Fitzgibbon, J. E., Gaur, S., Frenkel, L. D., et al.: Transmission from one child to another of human immunodeficiency virus type 1 with a zidovudine-resistance mutation. N. Engl. J. Med. *329*:1835–1841, 1993.
81. Foster, S., Hawkins, E., Hanson, C. G., et al.: Pathology of the kidney in childhood immunodeficiency: Is AIDS-related nephropathy unique? Pediatr. Pathol. *11*:63–74, 1991.
82. Frederick, T., Mascola, L., Eller, A., et al.: Progression of human immunodeficiency virus disease among infants and children infected perinatally with human immunodeficiency virus or through neonatal blood transfusion. Pediatr. Infect. Dis. J. *13*:1091–1097, 1994.
83. Friedland, G., Kahl, P., Slatzman, B., et al.: Additional evidence for lack of transmission of HIV infection by close interpersonal (casual) contact. AIDS *4*:639–644, 1990.
84. Frissen, P. H., Van der Ende, M. E., ten Napel, C. H., et al.: Zidovudine and interferon-alpha combination therapy versus zidovudine monotherapy in subjects with symptomatic human immunodeficiency virus type 1 infection. J. Infect. Dis. *169*:1351–1355, 1994.
85. Froebel, K. S., Aldhous, M. C., Mok, J. Y., et al.: Cytotoxic T lymphocyte activity in children infected with HIV. AIDS Res. Hum. Retroviruses *10*:83–88, 1994.
86. Gabiano, C., Tovo, P., de Martino, M., et al.: Mother-to-child transmission of human immunodeficiency virus type-1: Risk of infection and correlates of transmission. Pediatrics *90*:369–374, 1992.
87. Gagnon, S., Boota, A. M., Fischl, M. A., et al.: Corticosteroids as adjunctive therapy for severe *Pneumocystis carinii* pneumonia in the acquired immunodeficiency syndrome: A double-blind, placebo-controlled trial. N. Engl. J. Med. *323*:1444–1450, 1990.
88. Gallo, R. C., Salahuddin, S. Z., Shearer, G. M., et al.: Frequent detection and isolation of cytopathic retroviruses (HTLV-III) from patients with AIDS and at risk for AIDS. Science *224*:500–503, 1984.
89. Gellert, G. A., Durfee, M. J., Berkowith, C. D., et al.: Situational and sociodemographic characteristics of children infected with human immunodeficiency virus from pediatric sexual abuse. Pediatrics *91*:39–44, 1993.
90. Goedert, J. J., Duliege, A., Amos, C. I., et al.: High risk of HIV-1 infection for first-born twins. Lancet *338*:1471–1475, 1991.
91. Goudsmit, J., de Wolf, F., Paul, D. A., et al.: Expression of human immunodeficiency virus antigen (HIV-Ag) in serum and cerebrospinal fluid during acute and chronic infection. Lancet *2*:177–180, 1986.
92. Greene, W. C.: AIDS and the immune system. Sci. Am. *269*:105–117, 1993.
93. Groopman, J. E., Mitsuyasu, R. T., Delco, M. J., et al.: Effect of recombinant human granulocyte-macrophage colony-stimulating factor on myelopoiesis in the acquired immunodeficiency syndrome. N. Engl. J. Med. *317*:593–598, 1987.
94. Groopman, J. E., and Scadden, D. T.: Interferon therapy for Kaposi sarcoma associated with the acquired immunodeficiency syndrome (AIDS). Ann. Intern. Med. *110*:335–337, 1989.
95. Groux, H., Torpier, G., Monte, D., et al.: Activation-induced death by apoptosis in CD4+ T cells from human immunodeficiency virus–infected asymptomatic individuals. J. Exp. Med. *175*:331–340, 1992.
96. Grubman, S., Gross, E., Lerner-Weiss, N., et al.: Older children and adolescents living with perinatally acquired human immunodeficiency virus infection. Pediatrics *95*:657–663, 1995.
97. Gutman, L. T., St. Claire, K. K., Weedy, C., et al.: Human immunodeficiency virus transmission by child sexual abuse. Am. J. Dis. Child. *145*:137–141, 1991.
98. Hanson, I. C., and Kaplan, S. L.: Opportunistic infections. Semin. Pediatr. Infect. Dis. *1*:31–39, 1990.
99. Hanson, I. C.: Respiratory infections in HIV-infected children. Immunol. Allerg. Clin. North Am. *13*:205–217, 1993.
100. Hanson, I. C., and Shearer, W. T.: Diagnosis of HIV infection. Semin. Pediatr. Infect. Dis. *5*:266–271, 1994.
101. Hanson, I. C., Pitt, J., Sherrieb, K., et al.: Followup of single positive or indeterminate HIV cultures among infants in a multisite perinatal HIV study [Abstract]. San Francisco, Infectious Disease Society of America, September 16, 1995.
102. Hay, J. F., Lewis, D. E., and Miller, G. G.: Functional versus phenotypic analysis of T cells in subjects seropositive for the human immunodeficiency virus: A prospective study of in vitro responses to *Cryptococcus neoformans*. J. Infect. Dis. *158*:1071–1078, 1988.
103. Hernandez-Sampelayo, T.: Fluconazole versus ketoconazole in the treatment of oropharyngeal candidiasis in HIV-infected children: Multicentre study group. Eur. J. Clin. Microbiol. Infect. Dis. *13*:340–344, 1994.
104. Ho, D., Pomerantz, R. J., and Kaplan, J. C.: Pathogenesis of infection with human immunodeficiency virus. N. Engl. J. Med. *317*:278–286, 1987.
105. Ho, D. D.: Time to hit HIV, early and hard. N. Engl. J. Med. *333*:450–451, 1995.
106. Ho, D. D., Neumann, A. U., Perelson, A. S., et al.: Rapid turnover of plasma virions and CD4 lymphocytes in HIV-1 infection. Nature *373*:123–126, 1995.
107. Hodges, T. L., Kahn, J. O., Kaplan, L. D., et al.: Phase 1 study of recombinant CD4-immunoglobulin G therapy of patients with AIDS and AIDS-related complex. Antimicrob. Agents Chemother. *35*:2580–2586, 1991.
108. Horsburgh, C. R., Havlik, J. A., Metchock, B. G., et al.: Oral therapy of disseminated *Mycobacterium avium* complex infection in AIDS relieves symptoms and is well tolerated. Am. Rev. Respir. Dis. *143*:115, 1991.
109. Horsburgh, C. R.: *Mycobacterium avium* complex infection in the acquired immunodeficiency syndrome. N. Engl. J. Med. *324*:1332–1338, 1991.
110. Hughes, W. T.: *Pneumocystis carinii* pneumonia. N. Engl. J. Med. *297*:1381, 1971.
111. Hughes, W. T., Rivera, G. K., Schell, M. J., et al.: Successful intermittent chemoprophylaxis for *Pneumocystis carinii* pneumonitis. N. Engl. J. Med *316*:1627–1632, 1987.
112. Hughes, W. T.: Malnutrition. *In* Patrick, C. C. (ed.): Infections in Immunocompromised Infants and Children. New York, Churchill Livingstone, 1992, pp. 329–333.
113. Hughes, W. T., Leoung, G., Dramer, F., et al.: Comparison of atovaquone (566C80) with trimethoprim-sulfamethoxazole to PCP in patients with AIDS. N. Engl. J. Med. *328*:1521–1527, 1993.
114. Hussey, R. E., Richardson, N. E., Kowalski, M., et al.: A soluble CD4 protein selectively inhibits HIV replication and syncytium formation. Nature *331*:78–81, 1988.
115. Husson, R. N., Shirasaka, T., Butler, K. M., et al.: High-level resistance to zidovudine but not to zalcitabine or didanosine in human immunodeficiency virus from children receiving antiretroviral therapy. J. Pediatr. *123*:9–16, 1993.
116. Husson, R. N., Mueller, B. U., Farley, M., et al.: Zidovudine and didanosine combination therapy in children with human immunodeficiency virus infection. Pediatrics *93*:316–322, 1994.
117. Italian Register for HIV Infection in Children.: Features of children perinatally infected with HIV-1 surviving longer than 5 years. Lancet *343*:191–195, 1994.
118. Jason, J. M., Stehr-Green, J., Holman, R. C., et al.: Human immunodeficiency virus infection in hemophilic children. Pediatrics *82*:565–570, 1988.
119. Kahn, J. O., Allan, J. D., Hodges, T. L., et al.: The safety and pharmokinetics of recombinant soluble CD4 (rCD4) in subjects with the acquired immunodeficiency syndrome (AIDS) and AIDS-related complex: A phase 1 study. Ann. Intern. Med. *112*:254–261, 1990.
120. Katzman, M., and Lederman, M. M.: Defective postbinding lysis underlies the impaired natural killer activity in factor VIII-treated human T-lymphotropic virus type III seropositive hemophiliacs. J. Clin. Invest. *77*:1067–1062, 1986.
121. Kilpatrick, D. C., Hague, R. A., Yap, P. L., et al.: HLA antigen frequencies in children born to HIV-infected mothers. Dis. Mark. *9*:21–26, 1991.
122. Kirkpatrick, S., Hanson, I. C., Bohannon, B., et al.: *Mycobacterium avium* complex (MAC) in HIV-infected children less than 13 years of age [Abstract]. San Francisco, Infectious Disease Society of America, September 16, 1995.
123. Klein, J. O., and March, S. M.: Bacterial sepsis and meningitis. *In* Remington, J. S., and Klein, J. O. (eds.): Infectious Diseases of the Fetus and Newborn Infant. Philadelphia, W. B. Saunders, 1990, p. 601.
124. Kline, M. W., Dunkle, L. M., Church, J. A., et al.: A phase I/II evaluation

of stavudine (d4T) in children with human immunodeficiency virus infection. Pediatrics *96*:247–252, 1995.
125. Kline, M. W., Paul, M. E., Bohannon, B., et al.: Characteristics of children surviving to five years of age or older with vertically acquired human immunodeficiency. Pediatr. AIDS *6*:350–353, 1995.
126. Kline, M. W., and Shearer, W. T.: HIV infection and AIDS in children. *In* Rich, R. R., Fleischer, T. A., Schwartz, W. T., et al. (eds.): Clinical Immunology. St. Louis, Mosby, 1996, pp. 739–750.
127. Kovacs, J. A., Baseler, M., Dewar, R. J., et al.: Increases in CD4 T lymphocytes with intermittent courses of interleukin-2 in patients with human immunodeficiency virus infection. N. Engl. J. Med. *332*:567–575, 1995.
128. Krown, S. E.: AIDS-associated Kaposi sarcoma: Pathogenesis, clinical course and treatment. AIDS *2*:71–80, 1980.
129. Kuvibidila, S., Yu, L., Ode, D., et al.: The immune response in protein-energy malnutrition and single-nutrient deficiencies. *In* Klurfeld, D. M. (ed.): Nutrition and Immunology. New York, Plenum Press, 1993, pp. 121–155.
130. Lambert, J. S., Seidlin, M., Reichman, R. C., et al.: 2'3'-dideoxyinosine (ddI) in patients with the acquired immunodeficiency syndrome or AIDS-related complex. N. Engl. J. Med. *322*:1333–1340, 1990.
131. Landesman, S. A., Kalish, L. A., Burns, D., et al.: Obstetrical factors in vertical transmission of HIV: Role of duration of ruptured membranes. N. Engl. J. Med. *334*:1617–1623, 1996.
132. Lane, H. C., Depper, J. M., Green, W. C., et al.: Qualitative analysis of immune function in patients with the acquired immunodeficiency syndrome: Evidence for a selective defect in soluble antigen recognition. N. Engl. J. Med. *313*:79–84, 1985.
133. Langston, C., Lewis, D. E., Hammill, H. A., et al.: Excess intrauterine fetal demise associated with maternal HIV infection. J. Infect. Dis. *172*:1451–1460, 1995.
134. Lapointe, N., Michaud, J., Pekovic, D., et al.: Transplacental transmission of HTLV-III virus. N. Engl. J. Med. *312*:1325–1326, 1985.
135. Lee, J. W., and Pizzo, P. A.: Management of specific problems in children with leukemias and lymphomas. *In* Patrick, C. C. (ed.): Infections in Immunocompromised Infants and Children. New York, Churchill Livingstone, 1992, pp. 195–214.
136. Leibovitz, E., Rigaud, M., Pollack, H., et al.: *Pneumocystis carinii* pneumonia in infants infected with the human immunodeficiency virus with more than 450 CD4 T-lymphocytes per cubic millimeter. N. Engl. J. Med. *323*:631–633, 1990.
137. Lemp, G. F., Payne, S. F., Neal, D., et al.: Survival trends for patients with AIDS. J. A. M. A. *263*:402–406, 1990.
138. Lenderking, W. R., Gelber, R. D., Cotton, D. J., et al.: Evaluation of the quality of life associated with zidovudine treatment in asymptomatic human immunodeficiency virus infection: The AIDS Clinical Trials Group. N. Engl. J. Med. *330*:738–743, 1994.
139. Levine, R. L., Englard, A., McKinley, G. F., et al.: The efficacy and lack of toxicity of escalating doses of recombinant erythropoietin (rHuEPO) in anemic AIDS patients on zidovudine (AZT). Blood *74*:1–7, 1989.
140. Lindegren, M. L., Hanson, C., Miller, K., et al.: Epidemiology of human immunodeficiency virus infection in adolescents, United States. Pediatr. Infect. Dis. J. *13*:525–535, 1994.
141. Lipshultz, S. E., Chanock, S., Sanders, S. P., et al.: Cardiovascular manifestations of human immunodeficiency virus infection in infants and children. Am. J. Cardiol. *63*:1489–1497, 1989.
142. Lobato, M. N., Caldwell, M. B., and Oxtoby, M. J.: Encephalopathy in children with perinatally acquired human immunodeficiency virus infection: Pediatric spectrum of disease clinical consortium. J. Pediatr. *126*:710–715, 1995.
143. Luginbuhl, L. M., Orav, E., McIntosh, K., et al.: Cardiac morbidity and related mortality in children with HIV infection. J. A. M. A. *269*:2869–2875, 1993.
144. Luzuriaga, K., Koup, R. A., Pikora, C. A., et al.: Deficiency human immunodeficiency virus type-1 specific cytotoxic T-cell responses in vertically infected children. Pediatrics *119*:230–236, 1991.
145. Luzuriaga, K., McQuilken, P., Alimenti, A., et al.: Early viremia and immune responses in vertical human immunodeficiency virus type 1 infection. J. Infect. Dis. *167*:1008–1013, 1993.
146. Macallan, D. C., Noble, C., Baldwin, C., et al.: Energy expenditure and wasting in human immunodeficiency virus infection. N. Engl. J. Med. *333*:83–88, 1995.
147. Maury, W., Potts, B. J., and Rabson, A. B.: HIV-1 infection of first trimester and term human placental tissue: A possible mode of maternal-fetal transmission. J. Infect. Dis. *160*:583–588, 1989.
148. McArthur, J. C.: Neurologic manifestations of AIDS. Medicine *66*:407–437, 1987.
149. McClain, K. L., and Rosenblatt, H.: Pediatric HIV Infection and AIDS: Clinical expression of malignancy. Semin. Pediatr. Infect. Dis. *1*:124–129, 1990.
150. McClain, K. L., Leach, C. T., Jenson, H. B., et al.: Association of Epstein-Barr virus with leiomyosarcomas in children with AIDS. N. Engl. J. Med. *332*:12–18, 1995.
151. McIntosh, K., Pitt, J., Brambilla, D., et al.: Blood culture in the first 6 months of life for the diagnosis of vertically transmitted human immunodeficiency virus infection: The Women and Infants Transmission Study Group. J. Infect. Dis. *170*:996–1000, 1994.
152. McKinney, R. E., Pizzo, P. A., Scott, G. B., et al.: Safety and tolerance of intermittent intravenous and oral zidovudine therapy in human immunodeficiency virus–infected pediatric patients. J. Pediatr. *116*:640–647, 1990.
153. McKinney, R. E., and Robertson, J. W.: Effect of human immunodeficiency virus infection on the growth of young children: Duke Pediatric AIDS Clinical Trials Unit. J. Pediatr. *123*:579–582, 1993.
154. Metselaar, H. J., Velzing, J., Rothbarth, P. H., et al.: Prophylactic use of anti-CMV immunoglobulins in heart transplant recipients: A study on its safety. Transplant. Proc. *21*:2504–2505, 1989.
155. Michaels, D., and Levine, C.: Estimates of the number of motherless youth orphaned by AIDS in the United States. J. A. M. A. *268*:3456–3461, 1992.
156. Miller, M. E.: Immunodeficiencies of immaturity. *In* Stiehm E. R. (ed.): Immunologic Disorders of Infants and Children. 3rd ed. Philadelphia, W. B. Saunders, 1989, pp. 196–225.
157. Mintz, M.: Elevated serum levels of tumor necrosis factor are associated with progressive encephalopathy in children with acquired immunodeficiency syndrome. Am. J. Dis. Child. *143*:771–774, 1989.
158. Mintz, M., and Epstein, L. G.: Neurologic manifestation of pediatric acquired immunodeficiency syndrome: Clinical features and therapeutic approaches. Semin. Neurol. *12*:51–56, 1992.
159. Mitsuya, H., and Broder, S.: Strategies for antiviral therapy in AIDS. Nature *325*:773–778, 1987.
160. Mofenson, L. M., Moye, J., Korelitz, J., et al.: Crossover of placebo patients to intravenous immunoglobulin confirms efficacy for prophylaxis of bacterial infections and reduction of hospitalizations in human immunodeficiency virus–infected children. Pediatr. Infect. Dis. J. *13*:477–484, 1994.
161. Mofenson, L. M., Rodriguez, E. M., Hershow, R., et al.: *Mycobacterium tuberculosis* infection in pregnant and nonpregnant women infected with HIV in the women and infants transmission study. Arch. Intern. Med. *155*:1066–1072, 1995.
162. Moore, P. S., and Chang, Y.: Detection of herpesvirus-like DNA sequences in Kaposi sarcoma in patients with and those without HIV infection. N. Engl. J. Med. *332*:1181–1185, 1995.
163. Morgan, E. T., and Smalley, L. A.: Varicella in immunocompromised children: Incidence of abdominal pain and organ involvement. Am. J. Dis. Child. *137*:883, 1983.
164. Moye, J. M., Rich, K. C., Kalish, L. A., et al.: Natural history of somatic growth in pediatric HIV infection. J. Pediatr. *128*:58–69, 1996.
165. Mueller, B. U., Jacobsen, F., Butler, K. M., et al.: Combination treatment with azidothymidine and granulocyte colony–stimulating factor in children with human immunodeficiency virus infection. J. Pediatr. *121*:797–802, 1992.
166. Murphey-Corb, M., Martin, L., Davison-Fairburn, B., et al.: A formalin-inactivated whole SIV vaccine confers protection in macaques. Science *246*:1293–1297, 1989.
167. Nadal, D., Caduff, R., Frey, E., et al.: Non-Hodgkin lymphoma in four children infected with the human immunodeficiency virus: Association with Epstein-Barr virus and treatment. Cancer *73*:224–230, 1994.
168. Nielsen, K., Wei, L. S., Sim, M. S., et al.: Correlation of clinical progression in human immunodeficiency virus–infected children with in vitro zidovudine resistance measured by a direct quantitative peripheral blood lymphocyte assay. J. Infect. Dis. *172*:359–364, 1995.
169. Oleske, J. M., Minnefor, A. B., Cooper, R., et al.: Immune deficiency syndrome in children. J. A. M. A. *249*:2345–2349, 1983.
170. Ou, C. Y., Kwok, S., Mitchell, S. W., et al.: DNA amplification for direct detection of HIV-1 in DNA of peripheral blood mononuclear cells. Science *239*:295–297, 1988.
171. Palomba, E., Gay, V., DeMartino, M., et al.: Early diagnosis of human immunodeficiency virus infection in infants by detection of free and complexed p24 antigen. J. Infect. Dis. *165*:394–395, 1992.
172. Pantaleo, G., Grazosi, C., and Fauci, A. S.: The immunopathogenesis of human immunodeficiency virus infection. N. Engl. J. Med. *328*:327–335, 1993.
173. Pawha, S., Fikrig, S., Mesey, R., et al.: Pediatric acquired immunodeficiency syndrome: Demonstration of B lymphocyte defects in vivo. Diagn. Immunol. *4*:24–30, 1986.
174. Pawha, S., Chirmule, N., Leombruno, C., et al.: In vitro synthesis of human immunodeficiency virus–specific antibodies in peripheral blood lymphoctyes of infants. Proc. Natl. Acad. Sci. U. S. A. *86*:7532–7536, 1989.
175. Pizzo, P. A., Eddy, J., Falloon, J., et al.: Effect of continuous intravenous infusion of zidovudine (AZT) in children with symptomatic HIV infection. N. Engl. J. Med. *319*:889–896, 1988.
176. Pizzo, P. A., Butler, K., Balis, F., et al.: Dideoxycytidine alone and in an alternating schedule with zodivudine in children with symptomatic human immunodeficiency virus infection. J. Pediatr. *117*:799–808, 1990.
177. Plotkin, S. A., and the Task Force on Pediatric AIDS: Pediatric guidelines for infection control of human immunodeficiency virus infection (acquired immunodeficiency virus) in hospitals, medical offices, schools and other settings. Pediatrics *82*:801–807, 1988.
178. Purcell, R. H.: Animal models for the development of a vaccine for the acquired immunodeficiency syndrome. Ann. Intern. Med. *110*:381–385, 1989.
179. Putkonen, P., Thorstensson, R., Ghavamzadeh, L., et al.: Prevention of

HIV-2 and SIVsm infection by passive immunization in cynomolgus monkeys. Nature *352*:436–438, 1991.
180. Quinn, T. C., Kline, R. L., Halsey, N., et al.: Early diagnosis of perinatal HIV infection by detection of viral-specific IgA antibodies. J. A. M. A. *24*:3439–3442, 1991.
181. Rabin, R. L., Roederer, M., Maldonado, Y., et al.: Altered presentation of naive and memory CD8 T cell subsets in HIV-infected children. J. Clin. Invest. *95*:2054–2060, 1995.
182. Report of a consensus workshop (Rossi, P., Albert, J., Biberfeld, G., et al.) Siena, Italy, January 17–18, 1992: Early diagnosis of HIV infection in infants. J. Acquir. Immune Defic. Syndr. *5*:1169–1178, 1992.
183. Rey, L., Viciana, A., and Ruiz, P.: Immunopathological characteristics of in situ T-cell subpopulations in human immunodeficiency virus-associated nephropathy. Hum. Pathol. *26*:408–415, 1995.
184. Roederer, M., Dubs, J. G., Anderson, M. T., et al.: CD8 naive T cell counts decrease progressively in HIV-infected adults. J. Clin. Invest. *95*:2061–2066, 1995.
185. Rogers, M. F., Thomas, P. A., Starcher, E. T., et al.: Acquired immunodeficiency syndrome in children: Report of the Centers for Disease Control National Surveillance, 1982 to 1985. Pediatrics *79*:1008–1014, 1987.
186. Rogers, M. F., Ou, C. Y., Rayfield, M., et al.: Use of the polymerase chain reaction for early detection of the proviral sequences of human immunodeficiency virus in infants born to seropositive mothers. N. Engl. J. Med. *320*:1649–1654, 1989.
187. Rogers, M. F., White, C. R., Sanders, R., et al.: Lack of transmission of human immunodeficiency virus from infected children to their household contacts. Pediatrics *85*:210–215, 1990.
188. Rogers, M. F., Caldwell, M. B., Gwinn, M. L., et al.: Epidemiology of pediatric human immunodeficiency virus infection in the United States. Acta Paediatr. *400*:5–7, 1994.
189. Rusconi, S., Merrill, D. P., Hirsch, M. S., et al.: Inhibition of human immunodeficiency virus type 1 replication in cytokine-stimulated monocytes/macrophages by combination therapy. J. Infect. Dis. *170*:1361–1366, 1994.
190. Rutstein, R., Cobb, P., McGowan, K., et al.: *Mycobacterium avium-intracellulare* complex in HIV-infected children. AIDS *7*:507–512, 1993.
191. Ryder, R. W., Nsa, W., Hassig, S. E., et al.: Perinatal transmission of the human immunodeficiency virus type 1 to infant of seropositive women in Zaire. N. Engl. J. Med. *320*:1637–1642, 1989.
192. Sandberg, E. T., Kline M. W., and Shearer, W. T.: The secondary immunodeficiencies. *In* Stiehm, E. R. (ed.): Immunologic Disorders of Infants and Children. Philadelphia, W. B. Saunders, 1996, pp. 553–602.
193. Scott, G. B., Fischl, M. A., Klimas, N., et al.: Mothers of infants with the acquired immunodeficiency syndrome: Evidence for both symptomatic and asymptomatic carriers. J. A. M. A. *253*:363–365, 1985.
194. Scott, G. B., Hutto, C., McKuch, R. W., et al.: Survival in children with perinatally acquired human immunodeficiency virus type 1 infection. N. Engl. J. Med. *321*:1791–1796, 1989.
195. Selik, R. M., Chu, S., and Buehler, J. S.: HIV infection as leading cause of death among young adults in US cities and states. J. A. M. A. *269*:2991–2994, 1993.
196. Semba, R. D., Miotti, P. G., Chiphangwi, J. D., et al.: Maternal vitamin A deficiency and mother-to-child transmission of HIV-1. Lancet *343*:1593–1597, 1994.
197. Semprini, A. E., Vucetich, A., Pardi, G., et al.: HIV infection and AIDS in newborn babies of mothers positive for HIV antibody. Br. Med. J. *294*:610, 1987.
198. Shearer, W. T., Duliege, A. M., Kline, M. W., et al.: Transport of recombinant human CD4-immunoglobulin G across the human placenta: Pharmacokinetics and safety in six mother-infant pairs in AIDS clinical trial group protocol 146. Clin. Diag. Lab. Immunol. 2:281–285, 1995.
199. Shigita, S., Henuima, Y., Suto, T., et al.: The cell to cell infection of respiratory syncytial virus in HEp-2 monolayer cultures. J. Gen. Virol. *3*:129–131, 1968.
200. Simonds, R. J., and Chanock, S.: Medical issues related to caring for human immunodeficiency virus-infected children in and out of the home. Pediatr. Infect. Dis. J. *12*:845–852, 1993.
201. Simonds, R. J., Lindegren, M. L., Thomas, P., et al.: Prophylaxis against *Pneumocystis carinii* pneumonia among children with perinatally acquired human immunodeficiency virus infection in the United States. N. Engl. J. Med. *332*:786–790, 1995.
202. Sleasman, J. W., Hemenway, C., Klein, A. S., et al.: Corticosteroids improve survival of children with AIDS and *Pneumocystis carinii* pneumonia. Am. J. Dis. Child. *147*:30–34, 1993.
203. Smith, P. D., Ohura, K., Masur, H., et al.: Monocyte function in the acquired immunodeficiency syndrome: Defective chemotaxis. J. Clin. Invest. *74*:2121–2128, 1984.
204. Smythe, P. M., Brereton Stiles, G. G., Grace, H. J., et al: Thymolymphatic deficiency and depression of cell-mediated immunity in protein-calorie malnutrition. Lancet *2*:939–943, 1971.
205. Soeiro, R., Rubinstein, A., Rashburn, W. K., et al.: Maternofetal transmission of AIDS: Frequency of human immunodeficiency virus type 1 nucleic acid sequences in human fetal DNA. J. Infect. Dis. *166*:699–703, 1992.
206. Spector, S. A., Gelber, R. D., McGrath, N., et al.: A controlled trial of intravenous immune globulin for the prevention of serious bacterial infections in children receiving zidovudine for advanced human immunodeficiency virus infection. N. Eng. J. Med. *331*:1181–1187, 1994.
207. Sprecher, S., Soumenkoff, G., Pussant, F., et al.: Vertical transmission of HIV in 15-week fetus. Lancet *2*:288–289, 1986.
208. St. Louis, M. E., Kamenga, M., Brown, C., et al.: Risk of perinatal transmission according to maternal immunologic, virologic, and placental factors. J. A. M. A. *269*:2853–2859, 1993.
209. Stoneburner, R., Sato, P., Burton, A., et al.: The global HIV pandemic. Acta. Paediatr. *400*(Suppl):1–4, 1994.
210. Strauss, J., Abitbol, C., Zilleruelo, G., et al.: Renal disease in children with the acquired immunodeficiency syndrome. N. Engl. J. Med. *321*:625–630, 1989.
211. Strauss, J., Zilleruelo, G., Abitbol, C., et al.: Human immunodeficiency virus nephropathy. Pediatr. Nephrol. *7*:220–225, 1993.
212. Suskind, R. M., Olson, L. C., and Olson, R. E.: Protein calorie malnutrition and infection with hepatitis-associated antigen. Pediatrics *51*:525–530, 1973.
213. Tchekmedyian, N. S., Hickman, M., and Heber, D.: Treatment of anorexia and weight loss with megestrol acetate in patients with cancer or acquired imunodeficiency syndrome. Semin. Oncol. *18*:35–42, 1991.
214. The National Institutes of Health—University of California Expert Panel for Corticosteroids as Adjunctive Therapy for Pneumocystis Pneumonia: SPECIAL REPORT consensus statement on the use of corticosteroids as adjunctive therapy for pneumocystis pneumonia in the acquired immunodeficiency syndrome. N. Engl. J. Med. *323*:1500–1504, 1990.
215. The National Institute of Child Health and Human Development Intravenous Immunoglobulin Study Group: Intravenous immune globulin for the prevention of bacterial infections in children with symptomatic human immunodeficiency virus infection. N. Engl. J. Med. *325*:73–80, 1991.
216. The Working Group on Mother to Child Transmission of HIV: Rates of mother-to-child transmission of HIV-1 in Africa, America, and Europe: Results from 13 perinatal studies. J. Acquir. Immune Defic. Syndr. Hum. Retrovirol. *8*:506–510, 1995.
217. Thiry, L., Sprecher-Goldberger, S., Jonckheer, T., et al.: Isolation of AIDS virus from cell free breast milk of three healthy virus carriers. Lancet *2*:891–892, 1985.
218. Thomas, P. A., Weedon, J., Krasinski, K., et al.: Maternal predictors of perinatal human immunodeficiency virus transmission: The New York City Perinatal HIV Transmission Collaborative Study Group. Pediatr. Infect. Dis. J. *13*:489–495, 1994.
219. Unger, M., Jimenez, E., Backe, E., et al.: Allantoic vasculopathy of the placenta in HIV-exposed pregnancies: Correlation to clinical findings. Abstract FB452 of the Sixth International Conference on AIDS, San Francisco, June 1990, p. 191.
220. VanRompay, K. K., Otsyula, M. G., Marthas, M. L., et al.: Immediate zidovudine treatment protects simian immunodeficiency virus-infected newborn macaques against rapid onset of AIDS. Antimicrob. Agents Chemother. *39*:125–131, 1995.
221. Vigano, A., Principi, N., Villa, M. L., et al.: Immunologic characterization of children vertically infected with human immunodeficiency virus, with slow or rapid disease progression. J. Pediatr. *126*:368–374, 1995.
222. Volberding, P. A., Lagakos, S. W., Grimes, J. M., et al.: A comparison of immediate with deferred zidovudine therapy for asymptomatic HIV-infected adults with CD4 cell counts of 500 or more per cubic millimeter: AIDS Clinical Trials Group. N. Engl. J. Med. *333*:401–407, 1995.
223. Waldmann, T. A.: Immunodeficiency diseases: Primary and acquired. *In* Samter, M., Talmage, D. W., Frank, M. M., et al. (eds.): Immunological Diseases. 4th ed. Boston, Little Brown, 1988, pp. 411–465.
224. Wei, X., Sajal, K. G., Taylor, M. E., et al.: Viral dynamics in human immunodeficiency virus type 1 infection. Nature *373*:117–122, 1995.
225. Wheat, L. J., Salma, T. G., and Zechkel, M. L.: Histoplasmosis in the acquired immune deficiency syndrome. Am. J. Med. *78*:203–210, 1985.
226. Wilfert, C. M., Wilson, C., Luzuriaga, K., et al.: Pathogenesis of pediatric human immunodeficiency virus type 1 infection. J. Infect. Dis. *170*:286–292, 1994.
227. Wofsy, C. B., Cohen, J. B., Hauer, L. B., et al.: Isolation of AIDS-associated retrovirus from genital secretions of women with antibodies to the virus. Lancet *1*:527–529, 1986.
228. Wolinsky, S. M., Wike, C. M., Korber, B. T., et al.: Selective transmission of human immunodeficiency virus type 1 variants from mothers to infants. Science *5048*:1134–1137, 1992.

81

Opportunistic Infections in the Compromised Host

Christian C. Patrick and Karen S. Slobod

The immunocompromised host has one or more deficits in host defenses, increasing the patient's risk of infection.[84] There is a growing pool of immunocompromised patients due to the increasing use of immunosuppressive drugs for a variety of illnesses (e.g., malignancies, connective tissue diseases, transplants); infections causing an immunocompromised state (e.g., disseminated viral infections); and congenital immunodeficiency disease (e.g., severe combined immunodeficiency disease) (Table 81–1). This chapter does not discuss patients infected with HIV because this is discussed in Chapter 80.

Microorganisms infecting immunocompromised patients include not only the well-recognized pathogens but also organisms that once were considered nonpathogenic (Table 81–2). These latter organisms also can cause life-threatening disease in the immunocompromised host. Thus, therapy and diagnosis can become problematic because commensal organisms can assume a pathogenic role.

These opportunistic infections are predictable somewhat based on the type of immune deficiency. This chapter is divided into sections discussing infections that occur in patients with immune dysfunctions of phagocytosis, cellular-mediated immunity, humoral immunity, and complement dysfunction. We briefly describe specific disorders of immune function and the organisms to which patients are susceptible. We also include sections on infections associated with prosthetic devices (central venous catheters [CVCs]) because of their increased use in immunocompromised patients. Infections associated with blood product transfusions are important and also are discussed in this chapter. Finally, antimicrobial therapy and preventive mechanisms are discussed.

IMMUNE DYSFUNCTIONS

Neutrophil Dysfunction

Other than physical barriers to infection, the phagocytic system and predominantly the polymorphonuclear cell or neutrophil constitute the first-line defense against infecting organisms. The neutrophil is the cell with the greatest capacity to contain and eliminate bacterial infections. Cytokine stimulation causes the differentiation of myeloid progenitors and the release of neutrophils into the circulation.[45] This evolution involves both proliferation and differentiation. Mature neutrophils, once in the blood stream, reside either in the circulation or in a marginated pool of cells.[4] These two pools are in dynamic exchange. The evolution of progenitor cells into neutrophils also is a dynamic process, given that the half-life of normal neutrophils in the circulation is approximately 6 to 10 hours.

Neutrophils are evaluated initially through an assessment of neutrophil morphology.[80] The examination should include cell morphology and the presence of primary and secondary granules. Expression of surface receptors, detected by either specific antibodies or ligands, chemotaxis by Rebuck Skin Window or Boyden Chamber, assays for neutrophil adhesion and orientation, neutrophil aggregation, phagocytosis, and microbicidal activity also can be assessed.

Neutrophil function can be diminished by either quantitative or qualitative defects. Quantitative defects (hereditary or acquired) are more common than qualitative disorders. Qualitative deficiencies can be classified as defects in microbicidal activity or those involving cell migration.

Significant neutropenia is a state of decreased neutrophil number and is defined as an absolute neutrophil count of 1000/μL or less.[60] This neutrophil count includes mature neutrophils, band forms, and metamyelocytes.

The causes of neutropenia can be classified by a variety of methods but have been described here by function and cause (Tables 81–3 and 81–4). Functional classifications of neutropenia (see Table 81–3) refer to defects that affect a particular progenitor cell or metabolic disturbances or disorders associated with decreased neutrophil survival. The acquired neutropenias most commonly are associated with disorders of committed myeloid stem cells.

Causes of acquired neutropenias (see Table 81–2) can include infections, drugs, chemical or environmental toxins, anticancer chemotherapy, or bone marrow infiltration. Infectious etiologies include viral, bacterial, rickettsial, and protozoan. More commonly used drugs such as trimethoprim-sulfamethoxazole (TMP-SMX) and other sulfa drugs, anticonvulsants such as phenytoin, or miscellaneous drugs such as the thiazides have been known to cause neutropenia. Chemical or environmental toxins include benzene, carbon tetrachloride, or DDT and anticancer chemotherapy, including such drugs as doxorubicin (Adriamycin), cytoarabinoside, daunomycin, and methotrexate.

The spectrum of bacterial isolates from neutropenic cancer patients with bacteremia has changed over the last 40 years. In the 1950s and early 1960s, gram-positive bacteria, specifically *Staphylococcus aureus,* were the predominant organisms. This changed markedly in the mid-1960s and 1970s to a gram-negative flora consisting mainly of *Pseudomonas aeruginosa, Escherichia coli,* and *Klebsiella pneumoniae.*[12] Since 1980, the frequency of infections caused by gram-positive bacteria has increased markedly, with coagulase-negative staphylococci, viridans streptococci, and *S. aureus* being the predominant isolates.[11] The common microbial causes of infection in febrile, neutropenic patients are shown in Table 81–2. *Corynebacterium jeikeium,* previously known as *Corynebacterium* JK, also is recognized with catheter-related infections. Of the gram-negative organisms, the Enterobacteriaceae *(E. coli, K. pneumoniae,* and *Enterobacter* species) are becoming isolated more frequently. *Enterobacter* species is of great concern because of the ease of inducibility of β-lactamase and the rapidity at which it becomes resistant to cephalosporins and penicillin.[14] *P. aeruginosa* has decreased in some centers but is devastating when it occurs.[15, 39] Fungal infections that occur after a period of neutropenia in patients on broad-spectrum antibiotics mainly are caused by *Candida* species, with *Aspergillus* species being second and *Histoplasma capsulatum* seen occasionally.[3, 63] Microorganisms causing infections

TABLE 81–1. Compromised Patients at Risk for Opportunistic Infections

Underlying Defect (Selected Examples)	Deficit(s)	Examples of Organisms Most Frequently Isolated
Anatomic defects		
Dermal sinus tract	No skin barrier	*Staphylococcus epidermidis*, diphtheroids
Central venous catheters	Deficient skin barrier; catheter as nidus	*S. epidermidis, Staphylococcus aureus,* Enterobacteriaceae
Urinary catheters	Serves as nidus of infection	Enterobacteriaceae, *Pseudomonas* species, *Serratia, Candida* species
Respirators	Serves as portal of entry	*Pseudomonas* species, *Serratia*
General surgery	Bypasses skin barrier	*S. aureus, S. epidermidis,* Enterobacteriaceae, *Pseudomonas* species, *Candida* species
Inherited immunodeficiencies		
Phagocytic defects (chronic granulomatous disease, Job syndrome, Chédiak-Higashi syndrome)	Defect in bactericidal killing, chemotaxis	*S. aureus, Nocardia, Serratia, Candida*
Cellular immunity defects (DiGeorge syndrome, chronic mucocutaneous candidiasis)	Reduced T-cell numbers; diminished lymphoproliferative responses	*Pneumocystis carinii, Candida* species
Humoral immunity defects (X-linked agammaglobulinemia and common variable immunodeficiency, selective IgA deficiency, hyper-IgM syndrome, IgG subclass deficiency)	Low to absent levels of antibody	*Streptococcus pneumoniae, Haemophilus influenzae, Neisseria meningitidis*
Combined cellular and humoral defects (severe combined immunodeficiency, Wiskott-Aldrich syndrome, ataxia telangiectasia)	Reduced lymphocyte counts, aberrant T-cell function	Herpesviruses, *P. carinii,* enteroviruses
Complement defects (C3 deficiency in terminal complement components, C4B defects)	Deficient opsonization, reduced chemotaxis	*S. pneumoniae, N. meningitidis, H. influenzae*
Acquired immunodeficiencies		
Viral infections (HIV, cytomegalovirus, Epstein-Barr virus)	Cytopenia, T-cell deficits	Herpesviruses, bacterial infection
Immunosuppressive therapy (steroids, chemotherapy)	Depends on type of agent used	*P. carinii,* bacterial and fungal infections
Malignancies (leukemia, lymphoma)	T-cell deficits	*P. carinii,* viral infections (herpesviruses), bacterial infection
Transplantation	Temporally correlated with transplant	Bacterial and fungal infections during neutropenic phase; *P. carinii* and viral infections (cytomegalovirus, Epstein-Barr virus) after engraftment
Splenic deficiencies (sickle-cell anemia, congenital asplenia)	Loss of opsonic activity, decrease in phagocytosis	*S. pneumoniae, H. influenzae*
Collagen vascular diseases (systemic lupus erythematosus, rheumatoid arthritis)	Deficits in reticuloendothelial system	Fungal infection *(Candida, Aspergillus, Mucor), Staphylococcus* species, *Pseudomonas* species
Trauma (burns, splenectomy, surgery)	Loss of skin protection (burns), neutrophil dysfunction	*Pseudomonas* species, *Staphylococcus* species, *Serratia* (burns)
Other (malnutrition, renal disease, cystic fibrosis, premature neonates, diabetes mellitus, uremia, endocrine abnormalities)	Impaired T-cell function (malnutrition, uremia), impaired ciliary function (cystic fibrosis)	Measles virus, herpes simplex virus, varicella-zoster virus, *Mycobacterium* species (malnutrition), *S. aureus, Pseudomonas* species (cystic fibrosis)

TABLE 81–2. Etiologic Organisms Most Commonly Associated with Defects in Host Defense

Neutrophil Dysfunction

Bacteria
- Gram-positive
  - Coagulase-negative staphylococci
  - Viridans streptococci
  - *Staphylococcus aureus*
  - *Corynebacterium jeikeium*
- Gram-negative
  - Enterobacteriaceae
  - *Pseudomonas aeruginosa*

Fungi
- *Candida* species
- *Aspergillus* species
- *Histoplasma capsulatum*

Cellular Immune Dysfunction

Bacteria
- *Legionella pneumophila*
- *Listeria monocytogenes*
- *Mycobacterium tuberculosis*
- *Mycobacterium avium* complex
- *Nocardia* species
- *Salmonella* species
- *Serratia marcescens*

Fungi
- *Candida* species
- *Cryptococcus neoformans*
- *Coccidioides immitis*
- *H. capsulatum*

Viruses
- Cytomegalovirus
- Epstein-Barr virus
- Herpes simplex virus
- Rotavirus
- Varicella-zoster virus

Protozoa
- *Cryptosporidium*
- *Pneumocystis carinii*
- *Toxoplasma gondii*

Helminth
- *Strongyloides stercoralis*

Humoral Immune Dysfunction

Bacteria
- *Haemophilus influenzae*
- *Neisseria meningitidis*
- *Streptococcus pneumoniae*

Viruses
- Echoviruses
- Coxsackieviruses
- Adenoviruses
- Other respiratory viruses

in the immunocompromised host most often are acquired from the endogenous flora.[103] Thus, one of the more common sites for dissemination is the alimentary tract, including the oral cavity, esophagus, colon, and rectum. Additionally, damage to these areas can lead to translocation of organisms from the mucosae to the blood stream. Drug-induced vomiting with stomach-acid reflux may help to explain the increased risk in the distal third of the esophagus, although direct viral reactivation can occur as well. Damage to ciliary function and tracheobronchial mucosa in the respiratory tract may help to explain the high frequency of pneumonia and sinusitis in patients with granulocytopenia.

A hallmark study by Bodey and colleagues[13] in 1966 was the first to demonstrate a relationship between the incidence of infection and the magnitude of neutropenia. The frequency of infection increased when the absolute neutrophil count was 500/μL or less. At an absolute neutrophil count of 100/μL or less, patients were at an extremely high risk of severe infection, including gram-negative bacteremia. Also, the risk of infection is higher with a rapidly declining absolute neutrophil count than with a slow decline, such as that observed with aplastic anemia.

The duration of neutropenia is an additional risk factor for infection.[13, 25, 38] The number of infectious episodes is correlated directly to the length of neutropenia. Thus, patients with neutropenia lasting more than 1 week are at a substantially higher risk than patients with neutropenia lasting only a few days.

Qualitative defects in neutrophils also can place the patient at risk for infection. Patients with leukemia or lymphoma have qualitative defects in neutrophil function consisting of deficits in chemotaxis, phagocytosis, and bactericidal activity. Certain chemotherapeutic agents, such as methotrexate and

TABLE 81–3. Functional Classification of Neutropenias

Disorders of proliferation of committed stem cells
- Reticular dysgenesis
- Cyclic neutropenia

Disorders of committed myeloid stem cells
- Infantile genetic agranulocytosis of Kostmann
- Familial benign chronic neutropenia
- Chronic neutropenia of childhood
- Acquired neutropenias

Disorders associated with immune dysfunctions or metabolic disturbances
- Cartilage hair hypoplasia
- Disorders of immunoglobulin production
- Metabolic disorders

Disorders associated with decreased neutrophil survival
- Viral infections
- Immune neutropenias

TABLE 81–4. Etiologic Causes of Acquired Neutropenias

Infection
- *Viral*: hepatitis A and B viruses, measles virus, rubella virus, influenza A virus, varicella virus, cytomegalovirus, Epstein-Barr virus, herpes simplex virus, respiratory syncytial virus, HIV
- *Bacterial*: overwhelming sepsis, typhoid, tularemia, brucellosis
- *Rickettsial*: Rocky Mountain spotted fever, scrub typhus, epidemic typhus, rickettsialpox
- *Protozoan*: malaria, toxoplasmosis

Drugs
- *Antibiotics*: sulfa, trimethoprim-sulfamethoxazole, penicillin, cephalosporins, amphotericin B, etc.
- *Anticonvulsants*: phenytoin, valproic acid, barbiturates, etc.
- *Miscellaneous*: thiazides, propranolol, imipramine, etc.

Chemical/environmental toxins

Anticancer chemotherapy

Bone marrow infiltration—leukemia, lymphoma, neuroblastoma, etc.

anthracyclines, can decrease phagocytic and bactericidal activity.[87] Corticosteroids can decrease phagocytosis.[33] Impaired bactericidal activity has been observed after craniospinal radiation therapy.[6]

A definition of fever must be accurate so that care of the neutropenic patient can be standardized. At St. Jude Children's Research Hospital (Memphis, Tennessee), fever is defined as a single, oral temperature of at least 38.3° C or two oral temperatures at least 38.0° C taken 1 hour apart.[83] Fever is the most important indicator of infection. It must be kept in mind, however, that fever can occur as a result of noninfectious causes such as tumors, can be associated with tissue necrosis such as Ewing sarcoma, can result from tumor-producing pyrogens such as lymphoma, or can be the result of drug side effects, drug reaction (drug allergy), blood transfusion reactions, metastatic diseases to the central nervous system, or radiation therapy.[24] Clinical findings may not be prominent in infected neutropenic patients because the inflammatory response is muted. Pain is a reliable symptom and should be pursued aggressively. Serial physical examinations are important.

The management of febrile patients who are neutropenic can include both antibiotics and supportive care. The selection of antibiotic therapy should include broad-spectrum antibiotics that have bactericidal activity; the antibiotic susceptibility data of the hospital, the geographic area, and the patient's colonizing isolates; the pharmacokinetic properties of the antibiotics to be used; the potential for emergence of resistance (especially important with the use of monotherapy); the possibilities for drug interaction with toxicities associated with the antibiotics; and the presence of a focal site of infection, such as intra-abdominal or possible central venous catheter infection.

With these caveats in mind, it is imperative that a standardized system be used. The advantages of such a system allow areas of therapeutic deficiencies to be identified. Such a system also circumvents inappropriate therapy.

Although a myriad of drug combinations is possible, an Infectious Disease Society of America working committee categorized these combinations into four broad areas:[60] (1) aminoglycoside plus an antipseudomonal β-lactam antibiotic (e.g., ticarcillin), (2) two β-lactam antibiotics, a third-generation cephalosporin (e.g., ceftazidime) plus an antipseudomonal β-lactam antibiotic (e.g., ticarcillin) or ureidopenicillin (e.g., piperacillin), (3) monotherapy (e.g., ceftazidime, imipenem), or (4) vancomycin plus an aminoglycoside plus an antipseudomonal β-lactam antibiotic (e.g., ticarcillin) or vancomycin plus a third-generation cephalosporin (e.g., ceftazidime). The decision on an antibiotic regimen should be predicated on the patient's status, including renal function, focal findings, and the epidemiology of infecting organisms in the environment.

The microbicidal mechanisms can be divided into oxygen-dependent and oxygen-independent mechanisms of the phagolysosome. No deficiency of the oxygen-independent mechanism has been described. Chronic granulomatous disease is the prototype of microbicidal deficiency. This disease represents a heterogeneous group of biochemical and genetic disorders of the phagocytic NADPH oxidase complex originally described by Berendes and colleagues and Landing and Shirkey.[5, 9, 44, 70] The defect results in an inability of phagocytes to generate superoxide anion and other oxygen species.[58] Infections are prolonged and recurrent and are caused by bacteria and fungi that produce catalase because these organisms degrade their own hydrogen peroxide and thus survive within phagocytic cells.[72] Thus, organisms infecting these patients include staphylococci, gram-negative enteric bacteria (e.g., *Salmonella* species and *Serratia marcescens*), *Pseudomonas* species, *Nocardia*, yeasts, and filamentous fungi (*Aspergillus fumigatus*).[82] *Pneumocystis carinii* has been reported as an infecting agent but appears to be rare.[85]

Patients usually present with infections early in life. Suppurative lymphadenitis, pneumonia, lung abscesses, liver abscesses, osteomyelitis, and skin and soft-tissue infection are common.[67] Sinopulmonary disease accounts for approximately 80 per cent of serious localized infections. Hepatic abscesses always should alert the physician to consider chronic granulomatous disease. Obstructive lesions of the genitourinary and gastrointestinal tracts can occur.

Diagnosis usually is based on clinical findings and can be confirmed by nitroblue tetrazolium test.[7] Windhorst and colleagues[121] showed that 50 per cent of neutrophils from female carriers of the disease reduce nitroblue tetrazolium, in contrast with 5 per cent from males with chronic granulomatous disease.

Treatment of any infection must be managed aggressively with early and sometimes prolonged antibiotic therapy. Prophylactic antibiotics routinely are used, although prospective controlled clinical trials are lacking. Dicloxacillin or TMP-SMX commonly is used prophylactically, with TMP-SMX used more frequently because of its broader spectrum of activity.[46] Granulocyte transfusions have been utilized with variable success.[21, 28] Interferon has shown a clinical benefit and partially can reverse the defect.[65, 106]

Glutathione synthetase deficiency, myeloperoxidase deficiency, deficiencies of glucose-6-phosphate dehydrogenase, and glutathione peroxidase deficiency are other microbicidal mechanism disorders.[31, 75, 113]

Defects in neutrophil migration can be due to intrinsic or extrinsic factors. Leukocyte adhesion deficiency first was proposed in patients with recurrent bacterial infections and marked diminished neutrophil mobility.[53] The biologic defect was described as deficits in leukocyte integrins, including the three glycoproteins Mac-1, LFA-1, and P150,95.[107]

Patients have recurrent necrotic skin and soft-tissue infections, severe gingivitis and periodontal disease, and poor wound healing.[2] Laboratory features show leukocytosis. Diagnosis is by demonstration of absent expression of CD11/CD18 glycoproteins on circulating leukocytes.[2]

Infections should be treated aggressively with antibiotics. Recurrent infections with staphylococci and gram-negative rods are common. Some advocate antimicrobial prophylaxis with TMP-SMX.[2]

Chédiak-Higashi syndrome is a rare autosomal recessive disorder, characterized by recurrent pyogenic infections, neutropenia, peripheral neuropathy, and partial oculocutaneous albinism.[10] Infections occur early in life and include pneumonia, bronchitis, skin infections (cellulitis, pyoderma, impetigo), sinusitis, and otitis media. More than 70 per cent of infections are due to *S. aureus*. Other organisms include group A *Streptococcus*, *Haemophilus influenzae*, *Haemophilus parainfluenzae*, *Shigella flexneri*, *Klebsiella* species, *Pseudomonas* species, *Proteus* species, *Neisseria* species, and fungal organisms, including *Aspergillus* species and *Candida* species. Phagocytosis is normal, but leukocyte dysfunctions include impaired chemotaxis, delayed intracellular killing, and defective natural killer cell activity.[57] Definitive laboratory diagnosis consists of demonstrating defective cell migration. Therapy with ascorbic acid has been suggested but is controversial.[18, 120]

Intrinsic defects of neutrophil migration include specific granule deficiency syndrome, actin dysfunction, Job syndrome, lazy leukocyte syndrome, and glycogen storage disease (type 1B). Extrinsic factors relating to defects in neutrophil migration include hyperimmunoglobulin E syndrome and impaired generation of serum-derived chemotaxis.

Cellular Immune Dysfunction

The specific immune system is made up of two arms: antibody-mediated or humoral immunity (B cell), and cell-mediated or cellular immunity (T cell). Aspects of humoral immunity, so named because of the secretion of antibodies in body fluids, are discussed in the following section. Cell-mediated immunity involves thymus-derived, or T, lymphocytes. Although we separate these two components of the immune system for the purpose of discussion, such separation is artificial. T cells, derived from pluripotent bone marrow progenitors after "education" and maturation in the thymus, function directly in the elimination of certain pathogens, and they provide essential assistance to B cells. Thus, defects in cell-mediated immunity often result in secondary defects in humoral immunity. Indeed, isolated defects in cellular immunity are rare.

Relevant to our understanding of defects in cell-mediated immunity is knowledge of the complicated process of T-cell development and function. Bone marrow–derived pre–T cells colonize the thymus (derived from the third branchial cleft and the third branchial pouch), which is detectable near the fourth week of gestation. Thymocyte maturation involves progressive steps resulting in the selection of a widely diverse repertoire of T cells capable of differentiating self from nonself. In the thymus, T cells are selected to express either the CD4 or the CD8 molecule on their cell surface, glycoproteins important in the normal functioning of the different T-cell subsets. T cells recognize and can destroy host cells that express foreign antigens. The thymus is the site where T-cell receptor genes are rearranged. T-cell receptor gene rearrangement is the means by which a broad diversity of T cells, each with a unique specificity, is generated. The complete T-cell receptor complex includes the CD3 molecule, which serves as an identifier of T-cell numbers in clinical laboratories.

The cellular immune system thus is a highly evolved and specific immune system. T cells "learn" to discriminate self (healthy tissues) from nonself (infected, cancerous, or damaged tissues) through positive and negative selection in the thymus. This discriminatory ability lies in the T-cell receptor, which recognizes antigens only when associated with glycoproteins encoded by the major histocompatibility complex. Multiple genetic loci within the major histocompatibility complex encode the human leukocyte antigen proteins, which are found on the surface of nearly all cells. T cells recognize foreign antigens only by their association with human leukocyte antigen molecules (also known as histocompatibility antigens because of their role in transplantation rejection). After recognition of an altered host target cell, the T cell is activated. T-cell activation results in various functions generally dependent on the T-cell subset that is activated. CD4+ T-cell activation leads to the production of cytokines that modulate immunologic processes, including antibody production by B cells. CD8+ T cells are capable of target-cell cytolysis, as well as the secretion of cytokines.

Deficiencies in cellular immunity are both congenital and acquired. The manifestations of T-cell deficiency have become appreciated more widely in this era of infection with HIV.

Understanding the nature of T-cell immunity largely assists in the prediction of the infectious complications expected in disorders of cellular immunity. Intracellular pathogens are particular targets of T-cell–mediated immunity (see Table 81–1). Thus, defects in cellular immunity result in particular susceptibility to viral infections, which often are difficult to clear in the compromised host. Such susceptible persons also are plagued by fungal and protozoal infections. Associated humoral immunodeficiency results in recurrent bacterial infections, often otitis media and pneumonia.

Initial evaluation of the immune system should include a simple measure of the total lymphocyte number. At any age, this value should be greater than 1200 cells/μL of blood. Lymphopenia may be present in a number of congenital and acquired disorders.

Flow cytometry is a powerful technique in which the flow cytometer (instrument consisting of a laser source and fluorescence detectors) is used to analyze a population of cells for the expression of various surface markers. Such markers are detected by their binding to various monoclonal antibodies conjugated to particular colored fluorochromes. A wide array of monoclonal antibodies directed toward numerous human T-cell markers are available for such studies. Antibodies used in the analysis of T-cell number include (1) anti-CD3, a pan–T-cell marker; (2) anti-CD4, a marker for CD4-positive cells, which include human T cells and monocytes; and (3) anti-CD8, a marker identifying cytotoxic T cells. CD4 and CD8 molecules may be expressed by cells other than T cells; however, all T cells are identified by the expression of the CD3 molecule because it is an essential component of the T-cell receptor. In combination with the results of the Coulter counter, the absolute number of T cells and subsets in the blood can be determined.

Lymphocyte activation is an in vitro technique used to assess cellular immunity. It estimates the functional ability of T cells to proliferate in response to antigenic stimulation. Thus, it is superior to T-cell enumeration in indicating immunocompetence. Evaluation of lymphocyte activation or stimulation usually involves a measure of the degree of proliferation of lymphocytes after incubation with mitogens or specific antigens.

Mitogens are substances, generally plant lectins or bacterial proteins, able to activate T or B cells nonspecifically. Phytohemagglutinin and concanavalin A (Con A) are two plant lectins that act predominantly as T-cell mitogens, whereas the plant derivative pokeweed mitogen stimulates B cells. In this procedure, lymphocytes are purified from peripheral blood and established in culture with a titrated concentration of mitogens. After 72 hours, the degree of lymphocyte proliferation generally is determined by measuring the amount of tritiated thymidine incorporated into replicating cells.

Unlike mitogens, which stimulate large numbers of lymphocytes nonspecifically, antigens stimulate only those cells specific to the particular antigen. Moreover, in most cases, only T cells proliferate under these conditions. The antigens used in tests of lymphocyte activation are similar to those used for tests of delayed hypersensitivity skin testing (purified protein derivative, *Candida,* tetanus toxoid). Indeed, the two tests measure similar responses. However, in vitro analysis often is a more sensitive measure of specific T-cell function than is skin testing. The technique is similar to mitogen stimulation, except that the cultures must be maintained for 5 to 7 days and lower maximal responses are obtained because fewer lymphocytes are stimulated. It is important to understand that these responses develop only after an encounter with the specific antigen and thus poorly are developed in young, naive infants.

Because of the associated abnormalities, congenital thymic aplasia, or DiGeorge syndrome, is one of the few immunodeficiency disorders that can be detected immediately after birth. This syndrome represents interference in the normal embryonic development at approximately 12 weeks of gestation, when the thymus and parathyroid glands are developing from the third and fourth pharyngeal pouches. The syndrome consists of hypoparathyroidism and cellular immunodeficiency, as well as a characteristic abnormal facies and congenital heart disease.[30] The latter two components of the syndrome reflect the contemporaneous development of facial features and aortic arch structures. Thus, initial symptoms may consist of hypocalcemia and congestive heart failure, warranting examination of T-cell function in such infants.

These infants usually have low total lymphocyte counts (< 1200/μL), often have an absent thymic shadow radiologically, and fail to show normal lymphocyte activation in response to mitogen stimulation. They often have an associated impairment in specific antibody production explained by a failure in the normal collaboration of T and B cells, although concentrations of serum immunoglobulins may be normal.

Accordingly, this population is susceptible to infections with facultative intracellular organisms (e.g., *Mycobacterium tuberculosis, Listeria monocytogenes),* viruses (e.g., cytomegalovirus, varicella-zoster virus, measles, adenovirus, enterovirus, rotavirus, vaccinia virus), fungi (e.g., *Cryptococcus neoformans, Histoplasma capsulatum),* and pathogenic bacteria *(Streptococcus pneumoniae, H. influenzae).*[114, 124] *P. carinii* pulmonary infections are not uncommon.

Chronic mucocutaneous candidiasis is considered to be an isolated defect in T-cell immunity specific for *Candida* species, usually *C. albicans.* This disorder probably represents a spectrum of diseases that affects both males and females, has a familial occurrence, and often is associated with an endocrinopathy (e.g., hypoparathyroidism, hypothyroidism, diabetes mellitus, pernicious anemia).[55] The candidal susceptibility usually is manifested as a chronic infection of the skin, nails, and mucous membranes, rather than as a systemic infection. Patients rarely are infected with other fungal pathogens.

Patients usually have a normal total lymphocyte count and normal mitogen response but abnormal T-cell responses to *Candida* antigens. B-cell immunity generally is intact, with normal production of antibody to *Candida.* For patients presenting with chronic candidal infection and hypoparathyroidism, studies of T-cell immunity differentiate chronic mucocutaneous candidiasis from DiGeorge syndrome.

The X-linked recessive immunodeficiency known as Wiskott-Aldrich syndrome can present with recurrent infections and an eczematoid rash in childhood.[86] Patients may present with petechiae in infancy. Immunologic abnormalities include T-cell and antibody defects. Infection is the primary cause of mortality, followed by bleeding.[86] Approximately one-third of these infections involve the respiratory tract. Other infections include skin infections and sinopulmonary disease. Pathogens include cytomegalovirus, varicella, herpes simplex virus, enteroviruses, Epstein-Barr viruses, and *P. carinii.* Therapy includes pathogen-specific antibiotics. Some advocate gamma-globulin to prevent infections.

Ataxia telangiectasia is an autosomal-recessive primary immunodeficiency that includes defects in cell-mediated and humoral immunity plus cerebellar ataxia and telangiectasias.[118, 127] Infections present late, with neurologic abnormalities often noted at the end of the second year of life and oculocutaneous abnormalities manifesting as telangiectases of the bulbar conjunctivae presenting in the fifth year. Sinopulmonary disease leading to bronchiectasis is most common.

Severe combined immunodeficiency disease is characterized by an absence of both T- and B-cell immunity. It can occur in X-linked, autosomal, or sporadic forms.[29, 96] A deficiency of adenosine deaminase, an enzyme used to catabolize purines, is found in approximately 50 per cent of patients. Serum immunoglobulin is low to nondetectable.

Patients with severe combined immunodeficiency disease usually present with failure to thrive, diaper dermatitis, thrush, or a combination thereof. Additionally, chronic respiratory tract infections or diarrhea is common.

These patients particularly are prone to infection with fungi *(Candida* species), viruses (cytomegalovirus, Epstein-Barr virus, enterovirus), bacteria (both gram-negative and gram-positive), and protozoa *(P. carinii).*[71] Specific therapy and supportive care are needed. A human leukocyte antigen–compatible bone marrow transplant is the treatment of choice for a patient with severe combined immunodeficiency disease.[93]

Secondary T-cell defects are far more common than the primary defects. These include malnutrition, immunosuppressive therapy (e.g., corticosteroids, irradiation, cyclosporine, cytotoxic drugs), and infection (measles, HIV, tuberculosis).[8, 26, 64, 66, 94, 102, 109]

The management of infecting organisms involves the use of specific antimicrobial agents. The length of therapy depends on the severity of the underlying defect and the extent of the infection. Prophylactic therapy often is utilized, with the paradigm being TMP-SMX for *P. carinii* prophylaxis.

Humoral Immune Dysfunction

The elaboration of antibodies specific to soluble antigens is known as humoral immunity. Antigens generally can be divided into two groups: those that depend on T-cell help (T-dependent) and those that do not (T-independent). T-independent antigens usually are polysaccharides with repeating units of structure and elicit predominantly IgM isotype antibodies, whereas T-dependent antigens are proteins with little structural repetition and induce IgG isotype antibodies.

B-cell or humoral immunodeficiencies often are heralded by repeated pyogenic infections, including tonsillitis, otitis media, sinusitis, and pneumonia. Encapsulated bacteria, such as *S. pneumoniae, H. influenzae* type b, and *N. meningitidis,* are the most frequent infecting agents (see Table 81–2). Infection with respiratory viruses is common in these patients. Interestingly, children with humoral immunodeficiency often fail to eradicate infections with echovirus, adenovirus, and coxsackievirus, which therefore can result in chronic meningoencephalitis.

The evaluation of humoral immunity should begin with assays of immunoglobulin quantitation, isohemagglutinin titers, T- and B-cell enumeration, and CH_{50} determination if complement deficiencies are considered. The humoral immune response can be studied further by quantitation of antibodies after antigenic challenge using antigens such as ØX174.

X-linked agammaglobulinemia is a pure B-cell deficiency, originally described by Bruton,[20] characterized by low serum immunoglobulin concentrations of all antibody subclasses. A peripheral blood lymphocyte count usually is normal, with absent or reduced B cells. Infections begin in the first 6 months of life concurrent with depletion of maternal antibody. The most common infections, such as otitis media and pneumonia in infancy and sinusitis and mastoiditis as the sinuses develop, are of the upper and lower respiratory tract.[108] Response to antibiotics usually is prompt. Gastrointestinal infections are second to respiratory infections, and together they make up approximately 90 per cent of infections in these patients.[73] Diarrhea is common, often resulting in the presentation as a failure to thrive. As mentioned earlier, viral infections of the central nervous system are significant and can persist in children.[79] Chronic sinopulmonary disease is common because of IgA deficiency.

Repeated infections can cause chronic lung disease, prompting the use of prophylactic antibiotics, such as amoxicillin or TMP-SMX, in conjunction with gamma-globulin replacement in the management of these children.

Common variable immunodeficiency actually refers to a

heterogeneous collection of disorders that by definition have a muted or absent response to B-cell mitogens with normal B-cell numbers. The onset of symptoms can vary from early childhood to early adulthood. Specific pathogens are similar to those implicated in X-linked agammaglobulinemia.

Complement Dysfunction

The complement system consists of several proteins that interact to solubilize and clear immune complexes and to promote bacterial lysis and immunologic hemostasis. Deficiencies of complement components are associated with autoimmune disease, recurrent infections, and glomerulonephritis.

C3 deficiency is a rare disease transmitted as an autosomal recessive trait. Patients present with recurrent pyogenic infections with *N. meningitidis, Neisseria gonorrhoeae,* and *S. pneumoniae.*[16] This defect often is associated with collagen vascular disease and membranoproliferative glomerulonephritis.

C5 to C9 deficiencies of the terminal components of complement are associated with recurrent and disseminated infection, mainly with *N. meningitidis* and *N. gonorrhoeae.*[36, 40] An association with collagen vascular disease has been noted.

CENTRAL VENOUS CATHETERS

CVCs increasingly are used in clinical medicine. These foreign bodies can become infected predominantly by the surrounding microbial flora. Occasionally, a persistent infection necessitates removal of the CVC.

CVCs have been utilized since 1973 for a variety of long-term intravenous needs of hospitalized patients.[19, 56] Infection rates vary among studies primarily because of a lack of a standard definition of a catheter-related infection, the underlying illness, and the age of the patient. The overall infection rate of oncology patients with Hickman/Broviac catheters is 2.7 infectious episodes per 1000 catheter-days.[52, 116, 125]

Catheter-related infections can be stratified into three types according to their anatomic location relative to the catheter. Hickman/Broviac CVCs have a skin entrance site, a subcutaneous tunnel tract usually containing a Dacron cuff (the cuff fibroses to stabilize the catheter and to prevent migration of infection), and a vessel insertion site. Septic infections occur at the vessel insertion site, whereas superficial infections are divided in either exit-site or tunnel-tract infections. Exit-site infections are defined as the presence of erythema, tenderness, induration, or purulence within 2 cm of the exit site of the catheter.[89]

Patients with totally implanted vascular access devices have a subcutaneous pocket in which a portal is placed instead of an exit site. Thus, these patients can have portal infections, tunnel-tract infections, and septic infections.[81]

Organisms causing infections in patients with CVCs primarily are gram-positive bacteria, which cause approximately two-thirds of all infections (Table 81–5).[34, 92] Of the gram-positive bacteria, *Staphylococcus* predominates, with *Staphylococcus epidermidis* being the most common. Enterobacteriaceae are the most predominant gram-negative bacteria, although *Pseudomonas* species is prevalent.

TABLE 81–5. Microbial Agents Isolated from Patients with Catheter-Related Septic Episodes

Agent	Prevalence
Bacteria	
Coagulase-negative staphylococci	36%
Staphylococcus	16%
Streptococcus species (e.g., *S. pneumoniae, S. bovis, S. pyogenes*)	6%
Enterococcus faecalis	5%
Bacillus species	1%
Enterobacteriaceae (e.g., *Escherichia coli, Klebsiella pneumoniae, Enterobacter* species)	14%
Pseudomonas species	3%
Other bacteria	13%
Fungi	
Candida species	5%
Malassezia furfur	1%

Evaluation

An infection of the catheter always should be considered in a patient who has a CVC and presents with a fever.[68] Exit-site infections commonly present with erythema, tenderness, induration, purulence, or a combination thereof. However, these symptoms may not be as apparent in the neutropenic host. Pain may be the only manifestation. Tunnel-tract infections have similar symptoms as exit-site infections, except that the signs extend along the subcutaneous tract.

Septic infections present as bacteremia, with fever being the most common symptom. Patients may present with septic syndrome, which might be induced iatrogenically by flushing the catheter, causing the release of large amounts of endotoxin if gram-negative bacteria are the etiologic agents.

Superficial catheter-related infections usually are diagnosed by a physical examination. Aspirated purulent materials should be submitted for Gram and acid-fast stains along with culture.

The diagnosis of a septic infection requires differentiation of a CVC-related septic episode from a bacteremia not associated with a catheter. Blood cultures should be obtained from all lumens. Maki and colleagues[77] were the first to distinguish a CVC-related infection by culturing the distal 5 to 7 cm of the catheter on a 5 per cent sheep red blood cell agar plate; more than 15 colonies denoted a CVC-related infection. However, this technique requires the removal of the catheter. Several investigators have shown since that quantitative blood cultures drawn from a peripheral site and from each lumen of the CVC can diagnose a CVC-related infection without removal of the catheter.[42, 99] If the number of colony-forming units from the catheter is 5 to 10 times that of the peripheral blood, a catheter-related infection is indicated.

Management

Exit-site infections usually can be managed with local care and an oral antibiotic.[23] If the patient is neutropenic, parenteral antibiotics should be administered. *P. aeruginosa* often is difficult to eradicate and usually requires line removal.[81]

Tunnel-tract infections and portal infections are difficult to eradicate.[41, 97, 116] Cure rates are approximately one-third for tunnel-tract infections and one-half for portal infections.[81, 89] Broad-spectrum antibiotics should be administered parenterally. Often the catheter must be removed.

Septic infections in neutropenic patients require broad-spectrum parenteral antibiotics. Vancomycin should be considered for the treatment of coagulase-negative *Staphylococcus* infections. The typical antibiotic regimen includes vancomycin plus an aminoglycoside or vancomycin plus a third-generation cephalosporin.[34] This therapy needs to be administered for at least 10 to 14 days; if multiple lumens are present, the antibiotics should be rotated through each lumen.[34, 41]

The catheter should be removed if the catheter is no longer needed, the patient's clinical status deteriorates, or the blood cultures remain positive consistently for more than 72 hours on appropriate therapy.[90] If the infection is due to *Candida* species or *Malassezia* species, early catheter removal should be considered because these organisms are extremely difficult to eradicate.[37, 76] Additionally, methicillin-resistant *S. aureus*, *Bacillus* species, and atypical *Mycobacterium* have been reported to be difficult infections to clear.

Prevention

The best method to prevent infections is meticulous care of the catheter. This requires education of the patient and parents. The use of dry gauze dressings is preferred over transparent occlusive dressings for lowering bacterial colonization of the site and thus lowering site infections. Antibiotic ointment can reduce bacterial colonization but can cause increased rates in fungal colonization.

Antibiotic-impregnated catheters have been shown to reduce infection rates, but their effect is short-lived. The use of vancomycin as part of the heparin dwell fluid has shown a decrease in catheter-related bacteremias, but this is not condoned by the Hospitals' Infection Controls Practice Advisory Committees and Centers for Disease Control and Prevention because of the risk of increasing the prevalence of vancomycin-resistant enterococci.[105]

INFECTIONS INVOLVING BLOOD OR BLOOD PRODUCT TRANSFUSIONS

Transfusion medicine involving all aspects of the administration of blood and blood products is in increasing demand, partially because of the need of immunocompromised patients. This increased use of blood or blood product transfusions has increased the risk of infecting microbial pathogens (Table 81–6). Currently, donor screening consists of searching for antibodies to HIV, hepatitis B surface antigen, core antibody to hepatitis B, antibody to hepatitis C, rapid plasma reagin for syphilis, and antibodies to human T-cell leukemia virus types 1 and 2 as mandated by the American Association of Blood Banks and the Center for Blood Evaluation and Research of the Food and Drug Administration. Historically, viral hepatitis has been a major cause of blood transfusion reactions and has served as a model for the management of transfusion-acquired infections. Although a variety of hepatitis viruses can cause infections, hepatitis C has been shown to be responsible for approximately 85 per cent of non-A, non-B hepatitis.[69] With testing for hepatitis C, current estimates place the incidence of posttransfusion hepatitis of any etiology at less than 5 per cent.

Antibody to cytomegalovirus is not tested for routinely in blood banks but is important in selected immunocompromised patient populations, such as persons undergoing transplantation and neonates. Serologic testing of blood and blood products is necessary for these select patient populations.

The possible transmission of HIV-1 brought tremendous attention to blood banking.[22] Since April 1985, blood and blood products have been screened routinely for antibodies to HIV by solid-phase enzyme immunoassay methodology and confirmed by Western blot analysis. Currently, specificity exceeds 99.5 per cent. Samples that are reactive are retested in duplicate. If there is a positive, the unit is destroyed. Western blot analysis is performed to verify HIV antibodies for purposes of donor notification. Persons at high risk for HIV are encouraged not to donate blood; however, this latter point is becoming problematic because the proportion of acquired immunodeficiency syndrome cases due to heterosexual transmission is increasing.

TABLE 81–6. Etiology of Infectious Agents Contaminating Blood or Blood Products

Agent	Etiology
Viruses	Hepatitis virus (A, B, C, D, and E)
	HIV-1 and HIV-2
	Human T-cell leukemia virus 1 and 2
	Cytomegalovirus
	Epstein-Barr virus
	Parvovirus B19
	Colorado tick fever virus
Bacteria	*Escherichia coli*
	Brucella species
	Bacillus species
	Staphylococcus epidermidis
	Pseudomonas fluorescens
	Serratia liquefaciens
	Serratia marcescens
	Syphilis
	Yersinia enterocolitica
Parasites	Babesiosis
	Leishmaniasis
	Malaria
	Toxoplasmosis
	Trypanosomiasis
Rickettsia	Q fever
	Rocky Mountain spotted fever

HIV-2 can be acquired by transfusion but is rare in the United States. However, the Food and Drug Administration has mandated a combined HIV-1 and HIV-2 antibody test since June 1992.[27] The use of enzyme-linked immunosorbent assay technology or polymerase chain reaction techniques to reduce the seronegative "window" between infection and seropositive currently is being studied.

Acute hepatitis C virus produces infection that may go unnoticed.[88] However, 70 per cent of patients may develop chronic liver dysfunction, with 6 to 8 per cent being fatal. Primary hepatocellular carcinoma may occur from a protracted course of hepatitis C.[88] Enzyme immunoassay for hepatitis C antibodies has evolved with "second- and third-generation" enzyme immunoassay tests that currently are in use.[126] A confirmatory strip immunoblot assay (RIBA-2) is licensed. The risk per unit of a second-generation test is 0.06 per cent.

Infection with hepatitis B is less likely to result in chronic disease.[74] Hepatitis B infection historically has been a serious consequence of blood transfusions.[43] Testing for hepatitis B surface antigen began in 1972 and has reduced the risk of hepatitis B infection after transfusion to 0.002 per cent per person infused.[43] Additionally, the elimination of paid donors and the institution of donor questionnaires and examinations greatly have diminished the risk of hepatitis B. Currently, hepatitis B surface antigen antibody tests to the hepatitis B core antigen are performed.

Hepatitis A is transmitted infrequently by blood transfusion because of its short duration of viremia.[35] Hepatitis D and E can cause posttransfusion hepatitis but rarely. The possibility of non-A, non-B, and non-C hepatitis causing transfusion-related infection is debated.[1]

TABLE 81–7. Selected Agents Useful in Treating Severe Bacterial Infections in Immunologically Compromised Children*

Agent	Dose	Usual Susceptible Organisms	Comments
Amikacin	15–22.5 mg/kg/d q8h IM or IV	*Enterobacter* species, *Escherichia coli, Klebsiella pneumoniae, Proteus* species, *Providencia, Serratia, Acinetobacter, Pseudomonas aeruginosa,* nontuberculous mycobacteria	Blood levels 1 and 8 hr (peak and trough) after administration necessary to ensure adequate concentration without toxicity†
Ampicillin	100–400 mg/kg/d q4–6h IM or IV	Enterococci, *Listeria monocytogenes, E. coli, Proteus mirabilis, Salmonella* species, *Shigella* species, *Haemophilus influenzae*	When administered in conjunction with an aminoglycoside, synergism frequently occurs
Chlorampenicol	50–100 mg/kg/d q6h PO or IV	*Salmonella* species, *Shigella* species, *H. influenzae,* anaerobes, gram-negative bacilli	
Clindamycin	10–40 mg/kg/d q6h IM or IV (30-min infusion)	Anaerobes	
Erythromycin	30–50 mg/kg/d q6h PO or IV	*Staphylococcus aureus, Streptococcus* species, *Chlamydia* species, *Legionella* species, *Mycoplasma pneumoniae*	
Ethambutol	25 mg/kg/d for 2 mo, then 15 mg/kg/d PO	*Mycobacterium* species	
Ethionamide	15 mg/kg/d (max, 500 mg/d) bid PO	*Mycobacterium* species	
Gentamicin	5–7.5 mg/kg/d q8h IM or IV	*Enterobacter* species, *E. coli, K. pneumoniae, Proteus* species, *Providencia, Serratia, Acinetobacter, P. aeruginosa*	Blood levels 1 and 8 hr (peak and trough) after administration necessary to ensure adequate concentration without toxicity†
Isoniazid	10–20 mg/kg/d (max, 300 mg/d) PO or IM	*Mycobacterium* species	Use in conjunction with ethionamide or rifampin; three-drug therapy with ethambutol, streptomycin, or pyrazinamide
Metronidazole	15–35 mg/kg/d q8h IV or PO	Anaerobes	
Nafcillin	100–150 mg/kg/d q4–6h IM, IV, or PO	*S. aureus*	
Oxacillin	50–200 mg/kg/d q4–6h IM or IV	*S. aureus*	
Penicillin	50,000–300,000 U/kg/d q4h IM or IV	*Streptococcus* species, *Neisseria* species, *Clostridium* species, *Pasteurella multocida,* oropharyngeal anaerobes, *Streptobacillus moniliformis*	
Piperacillin	200–300 mg/kg/d q4–6h IV or IM	Streptococci, including enterococci, *K. pneumoniae, Enterobacter* species, *Pseudomonas* species, some *Providencia* and *Serratia,* anaerobes	Frequently used in combination with an aminoglycoside
Pyrazinamide	20–30 mg/kg/d or 20 mg/kg twice/wk PO	*Mycobacterium* species	Fourth drug in tuberculous meningitis. Useful in selected patients with isoniazid-resistant *Mycobacterium tuberculosis*
Rifampin	10–20 mg/kg/d PO (max, 600 mg/d)	*Mycobacterium* species; other susceptible organisms	For tuberculosis, usse in conjunction with isoniazid or ethionamide; three-drug therapy with streptomycin or ethambutol
Streptomycin	15–30 mg/kg/d q8–12h IM	*Mycobacterium* species	Use in three-drug therapy with isoniazid and rifampin; has synergistic role in therapy of bacterial endocarditis
Tetracycline	25–50 mg/kg/d q6h PO	*M. pneumoniae;* other susceptible organisms	
Tobramycin	3–7.5 mg/kg/d q8h IM or IV	*Enterobacter* species, *E. coli, K. pneumoniae, Proteus* species, *Providencia, Serratia, Acinetobacter, P. aeruginosa*	Blood levels 1 and 8 hr (peak and trough) after administration necessary to ensure adequate concentration without toxicity†
Trimethoprim-sulfamethoxazole	Trimethoprim, 8–20 mg/kg/d; sulfamethoxazole, 50–100 mg/kg/d q12h PO or IV	*Providencia, Salmonella* species, *Serratia, Shigella* species	Useful when organism is resistant to aminoglycosides
Vancomycin	20–40 mg/kg/d q6h IV	*S. aureus, Streptococcus* species	Oral route restricted to intraintestinal infections

*Consult drug product information sheets (package inserts) and other sources for more complete administration and toxicity data.
†Patients with cystic fibrosis frequently require higher doses of aminoglycosides to achieve therapeutic blood levels.

TABLE 81–8. Agents Used in Treating Viral Infections in Immunologically Compromised Children*

Agent	Dose	Usual Susceptible Viruses	Comments
Acyclovir	25–50 mg/kg/d (420–1350 mg/m²/d) q8h IV (1-hr infusion); 5% ointment six times/d for 7 d	Herpes simplex, varicella-zoster	Oral therapy may be beneficial in certain situations
Amantadine	1–9 yr: 4.4–8.8 mg/kg/d (125–250 mg/m²/d) q12h PO (max, 200 mg/d); 9–12 yr: 100 mg PO q12h	Influenza A	Most effective when given within hours of first symptoms
Foscarnet	60 mg/kg/d q8h IV	Acyclovir-resistant herpes simplex, varicella-zoster; ganciclovir-resistant cytomegalovirus	
Ganciclovir	7.5 mg/kg/d (210 mg/m²/d) q8h IV for 14 d	Cytomegalovirus	Symptoms likely to recur when therapy is stopped
Methisazone	200 mg/kg/d (560 mg/m²/d) q6h PO (initial dose, 200 mg/kg)	Vaccinia	
Ribavirin	Ribavirin (Virazole) supplied as 6 g of the lyophilized drug per vial; to reconstitute the therapeutic concentration (20 mg of ribavirin/mL of sterile water), add by sterile technique 300 mL of sterile United States Pharmacopeia water for injection or inhalation *Important:* This water should not have had any antimicrobial agent or other substance added. Pour solution into clean, sterilized 500-mL widemouth Erlenmeyer flask (reservoir) Ribavirin not to be administered with any other device or in conjunction with any other drugs using SPAG-2 aerosol generator See product insert for additional information	Respiratory syncytial	Has proved useful in therapy of respiratory syncytial viral infections in children and adults In vitro, has shown efficacy against influenza, parainfluenza, and measles viruses; clinical studies of this agent for treatment of influenza and parainfluenza viruses are in progress
Rimantadine	6.6 mg/kg/d (185 mg/m²/d) q12h PO for 5 d (max, 150 mg/d)	Influenza A	Experimental for this indication
Vidarabine (adenine arabinoside)	15–30 mg/kg/d (20–740 mg/m²/d) IV (12-hr infusion) for 10–14 d; 3% ointment, 1/2″, 5 times/d for 7 d after complete reepithelialization for herpes simplex keratitis	Herpes simplex, varicella-zoster	Experimental for this indication

*Consult drug product information sheets (package insert) and other sources for more complete administration and toxicity data.

Bacterial contamination of red blood cell components primarily is due to contamination of blood collection devices or transient bacteremia in an asymptomatic donor.[91] Contamination of red blood cell products is related to the storage time. The predominant contaminating organism is *Yersinia enterocolitica,* although *S. marcescens, Serratia liquefaciens, Pseudomonas* species, and *Enterobacter* species also have been implicated.[54, 112] Contamination of platelets is a more frequent problem than is red blood cell contamination. Platelets can be contaminated by commensal skin flora; thus, common organisms include *S. epidermidis* and *Bacillus cereus*.[47, 101] Fresh frozen plasma and cryoprecipitates are at low risk of bacterial contamination because the freezing process reduces bacterial growth.

ANTIMICROBIAL THERAPY

Treatment of opportunistic infections in compromised patients is governed by the type of defect and the infectious agent(s). The use of antimicrobial therapy is based on the patient's colonizing isolates, the hospital environment, and the microbial resistance pattern within the hospital and community. Standard agents and dosages are given in Tables 81–7 through 81–10.

PREVENTION

Prevention in the immunocompromised host varies with the type of immune defect. Prophylaxis usually involves the use of an antibiotic to prevent bacterial infections but also can include prophylaxis with antiviral, antifungal, or antiprotozoal agents. Additionally, the use of immunoglobulin and most recently adoptive therapy using cytotoxic T cells is being evaluated.

The use of selected antimicrobial antibiotics already has been alluded to with immune deficiencies. In patients with neutropenias, the principle of colonization resistance, in which the autochthonous anaerobic bacterial flora in the gastrointestinal tract limit the colonization by potentially pathogenic microorganisms, is being explored.[117] Antibiotics with minimal or no activity against anaerobic bacteria are administered, allowing colonization resistance to occur.[115] The antibiotics predominantly used are the quinolones, although TMP-SMX can be used.[17, 32, 51, 62, 111] The quinolones have been shown

TABLE 81–9. Selected Agents Useful in Treating Fungal Infections in Immunologically Compromised Children*

Agent	Dose	Usual Susceptible Organisms	Comments
Amphotericin B	0.5–1.5 mg/kg/d qd or qod (2–6-hr infusion)	*Aspergillus* species, *Blastomyces*, *Candida* species, *Coccidioides immitis*, *Cryptococcus neoformans*, *Histoplasma capsulatum*, *Mucor*	
Clotrimazole	1% ointment or solution bid to qid	*Candida* species	
Fluconazole	3–6 mg/kg/d q12h PO or IV	*Candida*, *Cryptococcus*	Primary use is in suppressive therapy
Flucytosine	50–150 mg/kg/d q6h PO	*Candida* species, *C. neoformans*	Use in conjunction with amphotericin B
Ketoconazole	5–10 mg/kg/d q12h or qd PO	*Blastomyces*, *Candida* species, *C. immitis*, *C. neoformans*, *H. capsulatum*	Cerebrospinal fluid penetration inadequate for treatment of fungal meningitis
Itraconazole	200–400 mg/d (adult dosage) qd PO	*Aspergillus* species, *Blastomyces*, *C. immitis*, *Paracoccidia*	
Nystatin	Cream, ointment, powder, oral suspension, oral tablets, and vaginal tablets, 100,000 to 1 million U/d qid	*Candida* species	

*Consult drug product information sheets (package insert) and other sources for more complete administration and toxicity data.

TABLE 81–10. Selected Agents Useful in Treating Parasitic Infections in Immunologically Compromised Children*

Agent	Dose	Usual Susceptible Organisms	Comments
Amphotericin B	1 mg/kg/d (28 mg/m²/d) IV	*Acanthamoeba* species, *Naegleria* species	Investigational for this indication
Chloroquine phosphate	10 mg base/kg/d (280 mg/m²/d) PO for 2–3 wk	*Entamoeba histolytica*	Maximum dose, 300 mg/d in combination therapy
Dehydroemetine	1.0–1.5 mg/kg/d (28–42 mg/m²/d) bid IM, for up to 5 d	*E. histolytica*	Maximum dose, 90 mg/d; followed by chloroquine or iodoquinol
Emetine	1 mg/kg/d (28 mg/m²/d) bid IM for up to 5 d	*E. histolytica*	Maximum dose, 60 mg/d; followed by chloroquine or iodoquinol
Iodoquinol	30–40 mg/kg/d (0.8–1.1 g/m²/d) tid PO for 20 d	*E. histolytica* and others	Maximum dose, 2 g/d; dosage and duration should not be exceeded because of possibility of causing optic neuritis
Mebendazole	100 mg bid PO for 3 d	*Ascaris* and others	
Metronidazole	15–50 mg/kg/d (420–1400 mg/m²/d) q8h PO	*E. histolytica, Giardia lamblia*	For *E. histolytica* use 50 mg/kg/d; for *G. lamblia* use 15 mg/kg/d
Pentamidine	4 mg/kg/d IV (112 mg/m²/d) for 14 d	*Pneumocystis carinii*	
Praziquantel	40 mg/kg/d (112 mg/m²/d) bid PO for 14 d	Cysticercosis, schistosomiasis	Single day for schistosomiasis
Pyrantel pamoate	11 mg/kg/d (310 mg/m²/d) PO for 3 d	*Ascaria,* hookworm	Single dose for *Ascaris*
Pyrimethamine	2 mg/kg/d (56 mg/m²/d) for 3 d, then 1 mg/kg/d (28 mg/m²/d) PO	*Toxoplasma gondii, Isospora belli*	Use with trisulfapyrimidines or sulfadiazine. To prevent hematologic toxicity, administer leucovorin 10 mg/d PO or IV; administer with triple sulfonamides (150 mg/kg/d q6h). For ocular toxoplasmosis, administer corticosteroids to reduce ocular inflammation
Quinacrine hydrochloride	6 mg/kg/d (56 mg/m²/d) tid PO	*G. lamblia*	Maximum dose, 300 mg/d
Spiramycin	50–100 mg/kg/d (1.4–2.8 g/m³/d) PO for 3–4 wk	*T. gondii*	Use with pyrimethamine
Thiabendazole	50 mg/kg/d (1400 mg/m²/d) bid PO for 2–5 d	Creeping eruption, *Strongyloides*	
Trimethoprim-sulfamethoxazole	Trimethoprim, 20 mg/kg/d (560 mg/m²/d); sulfamethoxazole, 100 mg/kg/d (2.8 g/m²/d) q6h PO or IV	*I. belli, P. carinii*	For *Isospora:* quadruple dose for 10 d, then double dose for 3 wk
Trisulfapyrimidines	100–200 mg/kg/d (2.8 to 5.6 g/m²/d) q6h PO for 4 wk	*T. gondii*	Use with pyrimethamine

*Consult drug product information sheets (package insert) and other sources for more complete administration and toxicity data.

in several controlled trials to prevent gram-negative bacterial infections; however, gram-positive bacteria, against which the quinolones have varying activity, can cause infections.[17]

Intravenous immunoglobulin has been used to prevent infections in immunocompromised patients. This especially is common in bone marrow transplant patients. Studies have yielded mixed results, with a randomized study in bone marrow transplant patients showing no prevention of infection.[123]

Preventive antiviral therapy has been focused primarily in bone marrow transplant patients. Reactivation of herpes simplex virus can be prevented with acyclovir, although it is not used by all physicians because of the low mortality of herpes simplex virus infection and patients' rapid response to acyclovir if such infection is diagnosed.[100] Ganciclovir has made a significant difference in cytomegalovirus disease in bone marrow transplant patients. This drug is administered after engraftment and continues until day +100 to +120.[50, 104] Caution must be taken because ganciclovir has been shown to cause neutropenia, which in one study resulted in an increased risk of bacterial infections.

Fluconazole has been evaluated for prophylaxis against fungal infections in bone marrow transplant patients and in one study showed a marked reduction in both disseminated and superficial fungal infection.[48] However, this imidazole has no activity against *Aspergillus* species or *Candida krusei,* resulting in reports of *C. krusei* breakthrough infections in patients receiving fluconazole prophylaxis.[122] Other preventive measures are low-dose amphotericin B or aerosolized amphotericin B to reduce *Aspergillus* in the respiratory tract.[98]

Antiprotozoal prophylaxis has been focused on the prevention of *P. carinii* infections. The drug most commonly used for this purpose is TMP-SMX, although other drugs are available for this purpose.[59, 61, 78]

Adoptive therapy is showing promise in the prevention of viral infections. Epstein-Barr virus–specific cytotoxic lymphocytes have been shown to prevent Epstein-Barr virus–associated lymphoproliferative disorder in bone marrow transplant patients.[95] Also, cytotoxic T cells against cytomegalovirus can prevent cytomegalovirus disease in the bone marrow transplant recipient.[119]

Acknowledgments

Support was provided in part by the National Cancer Institute (CA21765) and the American-Lebanese-Syrian Associated Charities (ALSAC).

References

1. Alter, H. J., Purcell, R. H., Holland, P. V., et al.: Donor transaminase and recipient hepatitis. Impact on blood transfusion services. J. A. M. A. *236*:630–634, 1981.
2. Anderson, D. C., Schmalstieg, F., Finegold, M. J., et al.: The severe and moderate phenotypes of inheritable MAC-1, LFA-1, P150,195 deficiency: Their quantitative definition and relation to leukocyte dysfunction and clinical features. J. Infect. Dis. *152*:668–689, 1985.
3. Annaissee, E., Bodey, G. P., Kantarjian, H., et al.: New spectrum of fungal infections in patients with cancer. Rev. Infect. Dis. *11*:369–378, 1989.
4. Athens, J. W., Haab, O. P., Raab, S. O., et al.: Leukokinetic studies. IV. The total blood, circulating and marginal granulocyte pools and the granulocyte turnover rate in normal subsets. J. Clin. Invest. *40*:989–996, 1961.
5. Babior, B. M., and Woodman, R. C.: Chronic granulomatous disease. Semin. Hematol. *27*:247–259, 1990.
6. Baehner, R. L., Neiburger, R. G., Johnson, D. G., et al.: Transient bactericidal defect of peripheral blood phagocytes from children with acute lymphoblastic leukemia receiving craniospinal irradiation. N. Engl. J. Med. *289*:1209–1213, 1973.
7. Baehner, R. L, and Nathan, D. G.: Quantitative nitroblue tetrazolium test in chronic granulomatous disease. N. Engl. J. Med. *278*:971–976, 1968.
8. Becker, W., Naude, D. T., Kipps, A., et al.: Virus studies in disseminated herpes simplex infections: Associated with malnutrition in children. S. Afr. Med. J. *37*:74–76, 1963.
9. Berendes, H., Bridges, R. A., and Good, R. A.: A fatal granulomatosis of childhood: The clinical study of a new syndrome. Minn. Med. *40*:309–312, 1957.
10. Blume, R. S., and Wolff, S. M.: The Chediak-Higashi syndrome studies in four patients and a review of the literature. Medicine *51*:247–280, 1972.
11. Bodey, G. P.: Infection in cancer patients: A continuing association. Am. J. Med. *81*(Suppl. 1A):11–26, 1986.
12. Bodey, G. P., Bolivar, R., and Fainstein, V.: Infectious complications in leukemic patients. Semin. Hematol. *19*:193–226, 1982.
13. Bodey, G. P., Buckley, M., Sathe, Y. S., et al.: Qualitative relationships between circulating leukocytes and infections in patients with acute leukemia. Ann. Intern. Med. *64*:328–340, 1966.
14. Bodey, G. P., Elting, L. S., and Rodriguez, S.: Bacteremia caused by *Enterobacter*: 15 years of experience in a cancer hospital. Rev. Infect. Dis. *13*:550–558, 1991.
15. Bodey, G. P., Jadeja, L., and Elting, L.: Pseudomonas bacteremia: Retrospective analysis of 410 episodes. Arch. Intern. Med. *145*:1621–1629, 1985.
16. Borzy, M. S., Gewurz, A., Wolff, L., et al.: Inherited C3 deficiency with recurrent infections and glomerulonephritis. Am. J. Dis. Child. *142*:79–83, 1988.
17. Bow, E. J., Rayner, E., and Louie, T. J.: Comparison of norfloxacin with cotrimoxazole for infection prophylaxis in acute leukemia: The trade-off for reduced gram-negative sepsis. Am. J. Med. *84*:847–854, 1988.
18. Boxer, L. A., Watanabe, A. M., Rister, M., et al.: Correction of leukocyte function in Chediak-Higashi syndrome by ascorbate. N. Engl. J. Med. *295*:1041–1045, 1976.
19. Broviac, J. W., Cole, J. J., and Scribner, B. H.: A silicone rubber atrial catheter for prolonged parenteral alimentation. Surg. Gynecol. Obstet. *136*:602–606, 1973.
20. Bruton, O. C.: Agammaglobulinemia. Pediatrics *9*:722–727, 1952.
21. Buescher, E. S., and Gallin, J. I.: Leukocyte transfusions chronic granulomatous disease: Persistence of transfused leukocytes in sputum. N. Engl. J. Med. *307*:800–803, 1982.
22. Busch, M. P.: HIV and blood transfusion: Focus on seroconversion. Vox Sang. *67*:13–18, 1994.
23. Cameron, G. S.: Central venous catheters for children with malignant disease: Surgical issues. J. Pediatr. Surg. *22*:702–704, 1987.
24. Chang, J. C.: Neoplastic fever: A proposal for diagnosis. Arch. Intern. Med. *149*:1728–1730, 1989.
25. Chang, H.-Y., Rodriguez, V., Narboni, G., et al.: Causes of death in adults with acute leukemia. Medicine *55*:259–268, 1976.
26. Claman, H. N.: Corticosteroids and lymphoid cells. N. Engl. J. Med. *287*:388–397, 1972.
27. Clavel, F., Guetard, D., Brun-Vezinet, F. B., et al.: Isolation of a new human retrovirus from west African patients with AIDS. Science *233*:343–347, 1986.
28. Cohen, M. S., Isturiz, R. E., Malech, H. L., et al.: Fungal infection in chronic granulomatous disease. Am. J. Med. *71*:59–66, 1981.
29. Conley, M. E., Brown, P., Picard, et al.: Expression of the gene defective in X-linked agammaglobulinemia. N. Engl. J. Med. *315*:564–567, 1986.
30. Conley, M. E., Beckwith, J. B., Mancer, J. F. K., et al.: The spectrum of DiGeorge syndrome. J. Pediatr. *94*:883–890, 1979.
31. Cooper, M. R., DeChatelet, L. R., LaVia, M. T., et al.: Complete deficiency of leukocyte glucose-6-phosphate dehydrogenase with defective bactericidal activity. J. Clin. Invest. *51*:769–778, 1972.
32. Cruciani, M., Concia, E., Navarra, A., et al.: Prophylactic co-trimoxazole versus norfloxacin in neutropenic children: Perspective randomized study. Infection *17*:65–69, 1989.
33. Dale, D. C., and Petersdorf, R. G.: Corticosteroids and infectious disease. Med. Clin. North Am. *57*:1277–1287, 1973.
34. Decker, M. D., and Edwards, K. M.: Central venous catheter infections. Pediatr. Clin. North Am. *35*:579–612, 1988.
35. Dodd, R. Y.: The risk of transfusion-transmitted infection. N. Engl. J. Med. *327*:419–421, 1992.
36. Ellison, R. T., III, Kohler, P. F., Curd, J. G., et al.: Prevalence of congenital or acquired complement deficiency in patients with sporadic meningococcal disease. N. Engl. J. Med. *308*:913–916, 1983.
37. Eppes, S. C., Troutman, J. L., and Gutman, L. T.: Outcome of treatment of candidemia in children whose central catheters were removed or retained. Pediatr. Infect. Dis. J. *8*:99–104, 1989.
38. Feld, R., Bodey, G. P., Rodriguez, V., et al.: Causes of death in patients with malignant lymphoma. Am. J. Med. Sci. *268*:97–106, 1974.
39. Fergie, J. E., Shema, S. J., Lott, L., et al.: *Pseudomonas aeruginosa* bacteremia in immunocompromised children: Analysis of factors associated with a poor outcome. Clin. Infect. Dis. *18*:390–394, 1994.
40. Fijen, C. A., Kuijper, E. J., Hannema, A. J., et al.: Complement deficiencies in patients over ten years old with meningococcal disease due to uncommon serogroups. Lancet 2:585–588, 1989.
41. Flynn, P. M., Shenep, J. L., Stokes, D. C., et al.: *In situ* management of confirmed central venous catheter-related bacteremia. Pediatr. Infect. Dis. *6*:729–734, 1987.
42. Flynn, P. M., Shenep, J. L., and Barrett, F. F.: Differential quantitation with a commercial blood culture tube for diagnosis of catheter-related infection. J. Clin. Microbiol. *26*:1045–1046, 1988.
43. Fritelson, M.: Hepatitis B virus infection and primary hepatocellular carcinoma. Clin. Microbiol. Rev. *5*:275–301, 1992.
44. Gallin, J. I., Buesher, E. S., Seligmann, B. E., et al.: NIH Conference: Recent advances in chronic granulomatous disease. Ann. Intern. Med. *99*:657–674, 1983.
45. Glasser, L., and Friederlein, R. L.: Functional differentiation of normal human neutrophils. Blood *69*:937–944, 1987.
46. Gmunder, F. K., and Seger, R. A.: Chronic granulomatous disease: Mode of action of sulfamethoxazole/trimethoprim. Pediatr. Res. *15*:1533–1537, 1981.
47. Goldman, M., and Blajchman, M. A.: Blood product-associated bacterial sepsis. Transfusion Med. Rev. *5*:73–83, 1991.
48. Goodman, J. L., Winston, D. J., Greenfield, R. A., et al.: A controlled trial of fluconazole to prevent fungal infections in patients undergoing bone marrow transplantation. N. Engl. J. Med. *326*:845–851, 1992.
49. Goodrich, J. M., Bowden, R. A., Fisher, L, et al.: Ganciclovor prophylaxis to prevent cytomegalovirus disease after allogeneic bone marrow transplantation. Ann. Intern. Med. *118*:173–178, 1993.
50. Goodrich, J. M., Mori, M., Gleaves, C. A., et al.: Early treatment with ganciclovir to prevent cytomegalovirus disease after allogeneic bone marrow transplantation. N. Engl. J. Med. *325*:1601–1607, 1991.
51. Gurwith, M. J., Brunton, J. L., Lank, B. A., et al.: A prospective controlled investigation of prophylactic trimethoprim-sulfamethoxazole in hospitalized granulocytopenic patients. Am. J. Med. *66*:248–256, 1979.
52. Hartman, G. E., and Schochat, S. J.: Management of septic complications associated with Silastic® catheters in childhood malignancy. Pediatr. Infect. Dis. *6*:1042–1047, 1987.
53. Hayward, A. R., Harvey, B. A., Leonard, J., et al.: Delayed separation of the umbilical cord, widespread infections, and defective neutrophil mobility. Lancet *1*:1099–1101, 1979.
54. Heltberg, O., Skov, F., Gerner-Smidt, P., et al.: Nosocomial epidemic of *Serratia marcescens* septicemia ascribed to contaminated blood transfusion bags. Transfusion *33*:221–227, 1993.
55. Herrod, H. G.: Chronic mucocutaneous candidiasis (CMC) in childhood:

Complications of non-*Candida* infection: A report of the Pediatric Immunodeficiency Collaborative Study Group. J. Pediatr. *116*:377–382, 1990.
56. Hickman, R. O., Bucker, C. D., Clift, R. A., et al.: A modified right atrial catheter for access to the venous system in marrow transplant recipients. Surg. Gynecol. Obstet. *148*:871–875, 1979.
57. Holcombe, R. F., van de Griend, R., Ang, S. L., et al.: Gamma-delta T cells in Chédiak-Higashi syndrome. Acta Haematol. *83*:193–197, 1990.
58. Holmes, B., Page, A. R., and Good, R. A.: Studies of the metabolic activity of leukocytes from patients with a genetic abnormality of phagocytic function. J. Clin. Invest. *46*:1422–1432, 1967.
59. Hughes, W. T.: *Pneumocystis carinii* pneumonia: New approaches to diagnosis, treatment and prevention. Pediatr. Infect. Dis. J. *10*:391–399, 1991.
60. Hughes, W. T., Armstrong, D., Bodey, G. P., et al.: Guidelines for the use of antimicrobial agents in neutropenic patients with unexplained fever. J. Infect. Dis. *161*:381–396, 1990.
61. Hughes, W. T., Rivera, G. K. Schell, M. J., et al.: Successful intermittent chemoprophylaxis for *Pneumocystis carinii* pneumonitis. N. Engl. J. Med. *316*:1627–1632, 1987.
62. Hughes, W. T., Kuhn, S., Chaudhary, S. C., et al.: Successful chemoprophylaxis for *Pneumocystis carinii* pneumonitis. N. Engl. J. Med. *297*:1419–1426, 1977.
63. Hughes, W. T.: Hematogenous histoplasmosis in the immunocompromised child. J. Pediatr. *105*:569–575, 1984.
64. Hughes, W. T., Price, R. A., Sisko, F., et al.: Protein-calorie malnutrition: A host determinant for *Pneumocystis carinii* infection. Am. J. Dis. Child. *128*:44–52, 1974.
65. International Chronic Granulomatous Disease Cooperative Study Group: A controlled trial of interferon gamma to prevent infection in chronic granulomatous disease. N. Engl. J. Med. *324*:509–516, 1991.
66. James, J. W.: Longitudinal study of the morbidity of diarrheal and respiratory infections in malnourished children. Am. J. Clin. Nutr. *25*:690–694, 1972.
67. Johnston, Jr., R. B., and McMurray, J. S.: Chronic familial granulomatosis: Report of five cases and review of the literature. Am. J. Dis. Child. *114*:370–378, 1967.
68. King, D. R., Komer, M., Hoffman, J., et al.: Broviac catheter sepsis: The natural history of an iatrogenic infection. J. Pediatr. Surg. *20*:728–733, 1985.
69. Kuo, G., Choo, Q.-L., Alter, H. J., et al.: An assay for circulating antibodies to a major etiologic virus or human non-A, non-B hepatitis. Science *244*:362–364, 1989.
70. Landing, B. H., and Shirkey, H. S.: A syndrome of recurrent infection and infiltration of viscera by pigmented lipid histiocytes. Pediatrics *20*:431–438, 1957.
71. Lauzon, D., DeLage, G., Brochu, P., et al.: Pathogens in children with severe combined immune deficiency disease on AIDS. Can. Med. Assoc. J. *135*:33–38, 1986.
72. Lazarus, G. M., and Neu, H. C.: Agents responsible for infection in chronic granulomatous disease of childhood. J. Pediatr. *86*:415–417, 1975.
73. Lederman, H. M., and Winkelstein, J. A.: X-linked agammaglobulinemia: An analysis of 96 patients. Medicine *64*:145 156, 1985.
74. Lok, A. S., Chien, D., Choo, D. L., et al.: Antibody response to core, envelope and nonstructural hepatitis C virus antigens: Comparison of immunocompetent and immunosuppressed. Hepatology *18*:497–502, 1993.
75. Lomax, K. J., Malech, H. L., and Gallin, J. I.: The molecular biology of selected phagocyte defects. Blood Rev. *3*:94–104, 1989.
76. Long, J. G., and Keyserling, H. L.: Catheter-related infection in infants due to an unusual lipophilic yeast: *Malassezia furfur*. Pediatrics *76*:896–900, 1985.
77. Maki, D. G., Weise, C. E., and Sarafin, H. W.: A semiquantitative culture method for identifying intravenous-catheter-related infection. N. Engl. J. Med. *296*:1305–1309, 1977.
78. Masur, H.: Prevention and treatment of penumocystic pneumonia. N. Engl. J. Med. *327*:1853–1860, 1992.
79. McKinney, R. E., Katz, S. L., and Wilfert, C. M.: Chronic enteroviral meningoencephalitis in agammaglobulinemic patients. Rev. Infect. Dis. *9*:334–356, 1987.
80. Metcalf, J. A., Gallin, J. I., Nauseef, W. M., et al.: Laboratory Manual of Neutrophil Function. New York, Raven Press, 1986.
81. Mirro, J., Jr., Rao, B. N., Stokes, D. C., et al.: A prospective study of Hickman/Broviac catheters and implantable port in oncology patients. J. Clin. Oncol. *7*:214–222, 1989.
82. Mouy, R., Fischer, A., Vilmer, E., et al.: Incidence, severity, and prevention of infections in chronic granulomatous disease. J. Pediatr. *114*:555–560, 1989.
83. Patrick, C. C., and Shenep, J. L.: Fever and infection in the child with cancer. *In* Kaplan, S. L. (ed.): Current Therapy in Pediatric Infectious Diseases. St. Louis, Mosby–Year Book, 1993, pp. 287–291.
84. Patrick, C. C. (ed.): Infections in Immunocompromised Infants and Children. New York, Churchill Livingstone, 1992.
85. Pedersen, F. K., Johansen, K. S., Rosenkvist, J., et al.: Refractory *Pneumocystis carinii* infection in chronic granulomatous disease: Successful treatment with granulocytes. Pediatrics *64*:935–938, 1979.
86. Perry, G. S., III, Spector, B. D., Schuman, L. M., et al.: The Wiskott-Aldrich syndrome in the United States and Canada (1892–1979). J. Pediatr. *97*:72–73, 1980.
87. Pickering, L. K., Ericsson, C. D., and Kohl, S.: Effect of chemotherapeutic agents on metabolic and bactericidal activity of polymorphonuclear leukocytes. Cancer *42*:1741–1746, 1978.
88. Plagemann, P. G. W.: Hepatitis C virus. Arch. Virol. *120*:165–180, 1991.
89. Press, O. W., Ramsey, P. G., Larson, E. B., et al.: Hickman catheter infections in patients with malignancies. Medicine *63*:189–200, 1984.
90. Prince, A., Heller, B., Levy, J., et al.: Management of fever in patients with central vein catheters. Pediatr. Infect. Dis. *5*:20–24, 1986.
91. Purcell, R. H.: Hepatitis viruses: Changing patterns of human disease. Proc. Natl. Acad. Sci. U. S. A. *91*:2401–2406, 1994.
92. Raad, I. I., and Bodey, G. P.: Infectious complications of indwelling vascular catheters. Clin. Infect. Dis. *15*:197–210, 1992.
93. Reinherz, E. L., Geha, R., Rappeport, J. M., et al.: Reconstitution after transplantation with T-lymphocyte–depleted HLA haplotype-mismatched bone marrow for severe combined immunodeficiency. Proc. Natl. Acad. Sci. U. S. A. *79*:6047–6051, 1982.
94. Rinehart, J. J., Sagone, A. L., Balcerzak, S. P., et al.: Effects of corticosteroid therapy on human monocyte function. N. Engl. J. Med. *292*:236–241, 1975.
95. Rooney, C. M., Smith, C. A., Ng, C. Y. C., et al.: Use of gene-modified virus-specific T lymphocytes to control Epstein-Barr virus–related lymphoproliferation. Lancet *345*:9–13, 1995.
96. Rosen, F. S., Wedgwood, R. J., Eibl, M. C., et al.: Primary immunodeficiency diseases: Report of a WHO scientific group. Immunodeficiency Rev. *3*:195–236, 1992.
97. Ross, M. N., Haase, G. M., Poole, M. A., et al.: Comparison of totally implanted reservoirs with external catheters as venous access devices in pediatric oncologic patients. Surg. Gynecol. Obstet. *167*:141–144, 1988.
98. Rousey, S. R., Russler, S., Gottlieb, M., et al.: Low-dose amphotericin B prophylaxis against invasive *Aspergillus* infections in allogeneic marrow transplantation. Am. J. Med. *91*:484–492, 1991.
99. Ruderman, J. W., Morgan, M. A., and Klein, A. H.: Quantitative blood cultures in the diagnosis of sepsis in infants with umbilical and Broviac catheters. J. Pediatr. *112*:748–751, 1988.
100. Saral, R., Burns, W. H., Larkin, O. L., et al.: Acyclovir prophylaxis of herpes-simplex infections: A randomized, double-blinded controlled trial in bone marrow transplant recipients. N. Engl. J. Med. *305*:63–67, 1981.
101. Sazama, K.: Bacteria in blood for transfusions: A review. Arch. Pathol. Lab. Med. *118*:350–365, 1994.
102. Schaffner, A., Douglas, H., and Braude, A.: Selective protection against conidia by mononuclear and against mycelia by polymorphonuclear phagocytes in resistance to *Aspergillus*: Observations on these two lines of defense *in vivo* and *in vitro* with human and mouse phagocytes. J. Clin. Invest. *69*:617–631, 1982.
103. Schimpff, S. C., Young, V. M., Greene, W. H., et al.: Origin of infection in acute non-lymphocytic leukemia: Significance of hospital acquisition of potential pathogens. Ann. Intern. Med. *77*:707–714, 1972.
104. Schmidt, G. M., Horak, D. A., Niland, J. C., et al.: A randomized, controlled trial of prophylactic ganciclovir for cytomegalovirus pulmonary infection in recipients of allogeneic bone marrow transplant. N. Engl. J. Med. *324*:1005–1011, 1991.
105. Schwartz, C., Hendrickson, K. J., Roghmann, K., et al.: Prevention of bacteremia attributed to luminal colonization of tunneled central venous catheters with vancomycin-susceptible organisms. J. Clin. Oncol. *8*:1591–1597, 1990.
106. Sechler, J. M., Malech, H. L., White, C. J., et al.: Recombinant human interferon-gamma reconstitutes defective phagocyte function in patients with chronic granulomatous disease of childhood. Proc. Natl. Acad. Sci. U. S. A. *85*:4874–4878, 1988.
107. Springer, T. A., Thompson, W. S., Miller, L. J., et al.: Inherited deficiency of the Mac-1, LFA-1, P150,95 glycoprotein family and its molecular basis. J. Exp. Med. *160*:1901–1918, 1984.
108. Stiehm, E. R., Chin, T. W., Haas, A., et al.: Infectious complications of the primary immunodeficiencies. Clin. Immunol. Immunopathol. *40*:69–86, 1986.
109. Sugarman, B.: Zinc and infection. Rev. Infect. Dis. *5*:137–147, 1983.
110. Surgenor, D. M., Wallace, E. L., Hao, S. H. S., et al.: Collection and transfusion of blood in the United States, 1982–1988. N. Engl. J. Med. *322*:1646–1651, 1990.
111. The Giemema Infection Program: Prevention of bacterial infection in neutropenic patients with hematologic malignancies: A randomized, multicenter trial comparing norfloxacin with ciprofloxacin. Ann. Intern. Med. *115*:7–12, 1991.
112. Tipple, M. A., Bland, L. A., Murphy, J. J., et al.: Sepsis associated with transfusion of red blood cells contaminated with *Yersinia enterocolitica*. Transfusion *30*:207–213, 1990.
113. Tobler, A., Selsted, M. E., Miller, C. W., et al.: Evidence for a pretranslational defect in hereditary and acquired myeloperoxidase deficiency. Blood *73*:1981–1986, 1989.
114. Tuvia, J., Weisselberg, B., Shif, I., et al.: Aplastic anemia complicating adenovirus infection with DiGeorge syndrome. Eur. J. Pediatr. *147*:643–644, 1988.

115. Van der Waaij, D.: Selective decontamination of the digestive tract: General principles. Eur. J. Cancer Clin. Oncol. *24*(Suppl. 1):51–54, 1988.
116. Viscoli, C., Garaventa, A., Boni, L., et al.: Role of Broviac catheters in infections in children with cancer. Pediatr. Infect. Dis. J. *7*:556–560, 1988.
117. Vollaard, E. J., and Clasener, H. A. L.: Colonization resistance. Antimicrob. Agents Chemother. *38*:409–414, 1994.
118. Waldmann, T. A., Misiti, J., Nelson, D. L., et al.: Ataxia-telangiectasia: A multisystem hereditary disease with immunodeficiency, impaired organ maturation, x-ray hypersensitivity, and a high incidence of neoplasia. Ann. Intern. Med. *99*:367–379, 1983.
119. Walter, E. A., Greenberg, P. D., and Gilbert, M. J.: Reconstitution of cellular immunity against cytomegalovirus in recipients of allogeneic bone marrow by transfer of T-cell clones from the donor. N. Engl. J. Med. *333*:1038–1044, 1995.
120. Weening, R. S., Schoorel, E. P., Roos, D., et al.: Effects of ascorbate on abnormal neutrophil, platelet and lymphocytic function in a patient with the Chediak-Higashi syndrome. Blood *57*:856–865, 1981.
121. Windhorst, D. B., Holmes, B., and Good, R. A.: A newly defined X-linked trait in man with demonstration of the Lyon effect in carrier females. Lancet *1*:737–739, 1967.
122. Wingard, J. R., Merz, W. G., Rinaldi, M. G., et al.: Increase in *Candida krusei* infection among patients with bone marrow transplantation and neutropenia treated prophylactically with fluconazole. N. Engl. J. Med. *325*:1274–1277, 1991.
123. Wolff, S. N., Fay, J. W., Herzig, R. H., et al.: High-dose weekly intravenous immunoglobulin to prevent infections in patients undergoing autologous bone marrow transplantation or severe myelosuppressive therapy. Ann. Intern. Med. *118*:937–942, 1993.
124. Wood, D. J., David, T. J., Chrystie, I. L., et al.: Chronic enteric virus infection in two T-cell immunodeficient children. J. Med. Virol. *24*:435–444, 1988.
125. Wurzel, C. L., Halom, K., Feldman, J. G., et al.: Infection rates of Broviac-Hickman catheters and implantable venous devices. Am. J. Dis. Child. *142*:536–540, 1988.
126. Yano, M., Yatsuhashi, H., Inoue, O., et al.: Epidemiology and long-term prognosis of hepatitis C virus infection in Japan. Gut *34*:513–516, 1993.
127. Yount, W. J.: IgG2 deficiency and ataxia-telangiectasia. N. Engl. J. Med. *306*:541–543, 1982.

S E C T I O N   F I F T E E N

UNCLASSIFIED INFECTIOUS DISEASES

❑ ❑ ❑

82

KAWASAKI DISEASE

David M. Morens and Marian E. Melish

Kawasaki disease is an acute febrile multisystem vasculitic syndrome of unknown etiology occurring predominantly in infants and young children. Although based entirely on clinical features, the diagnosis is straightforward when characteristic cutaneous and mucosal changes are expressed fully. Serious complications include coronary arteritis, coronary artery aneurysms, and aneurysmal thrombosis or rupture.

Synonyms for Kawasaki disease include Kawasaki syndrome and mucocutaneous lymph node syndrome (MCLS, MLNS, or MCLNS). It also has been referred to as lymphomucocutaneous syndrome and a variety of other similar terms. As discussed later, infantile periarteritis nodosa is indistinguishable from fatal Kawasaki disease. The ninth revision of the International Classification of Diseases (ICD-9) designates the condition as both Kawasaki disease and mucocutaneous lymph node syndrome (acute) (febrile) (infantile) under rubric 446.1. Until 1983, the National Library of Medicine listed Kawasaki disease publications under various subject headings, notably "Lymphatic Diseases." Since 1984, publications are listed under "Mucocutaneous Lymph Node Syndrome."

HISTORY

The disease bearing his name first was recognized as a clinical entity in 1961 by Dr. Tomisaku Kawasaki, Chairman of the Department of Pediatrics at Tokyo's Japan Red Cross Medical Center. In that year, Kawasaki began to identify infants and young children with a distinctive constellation of signs that included prolonged high fever, cervical adenopathy, bilateral conjunctival suffusion, erythematous rash, desquamation, changes of the mucosa of the upper respiratory tract, and edema and erythema of the extremities. Although the syndrome was impressive, its signs were nonspecific and occurred in other diseases seen commonly or occasionally by pediatricians. Tests to rule out these other disease possibilities invariably were negative. Believing he had observed a unique and distinct clinical syndrome, in 1967 Kawasaki published a report of his experience with 50 cases of "febrile oculo-oro-cutaneo-acrodesquamatous syndrome with or without acute nonsuppurative cervical lymphadenitis."[152, 155, 156] So quick were other Japanese physicians to recognize the syndrome that it soon was observed and diagnosed throughout the country. A Japan MCLS Research Committee was formed, undertaking its first biennial national epidemiologic survey in 1970. Kawasaki's clear description of the syndrome, which was based on the six clinical criteria noted earlier, remains the foundation of diagnosis 30 years later (1997) and the basis of all clinical and epidemiologic case definitions in use today.

In 1971, without knowledge of the body of information gathered by Japanese investigators, a group of American physicians working independently at the University of Hawaii began gathering clinical and laboratory information about an unusual Reiter-like syndrome. After publication of information about Kawasaki disease in the English language literature, it became apparent that the Japanese and American diseases were identical.[107, 156, 237, 238] An exchange of information between Japanese and American investigators led to the publication of English-language articles by both groups,[156, 237, 238] triggering worldwide recognition of cases. It also was recognized in the early 1970s that death from myocardial infarction occurred in approximately 2 per cent of cases and later that approximately 30 per cent develop clinical evidence of cardiac disease, with 20 per cent developing coronary artery abnormalities of sufficient magnitude to be detected by echocardiogram, and that 30 per cent develop inflammatory arthritis.

Although Kawasaki disease had been publicized as a new entity, it readily was apparent that there were strong clinical and pathologic similarities between the fatal form and infantile periarteritis nodosa, a condition recognized in North America since the 1940s, if not before. Coronary and peripheral arterial aneurysms in adults and children had been well documented in the European medical literature for centuries, and in the late nineteenth century occasionally were linked to clinical presentations compatible with Kawasaki disease or other conditions, such as streptococcal infection. It has been suggested that in previous decades, cases of Kawasaki disease may have occurred and been misdiagnosed as measles.[296] It seems equally likely that cases could have been attributed to scarlet fever, rubella, or other conditions once more prevalent than they are today. The novelty of Kawasaki disease thus is an open question.

In North America, Kawasaki disease now is a more common cause of both acquired heart disease and inflammatory arthritis than is acute poststreptococcal rheumatic fever.[345, 346] It has been recognized on all continents in children of all racial groups. Although the etiology of the disorder remains unknown, administration of intravenous gamma globulin during the first week of illness has a dramatic effect on the clinical illness and reduces the likelihood of coronary abnormalities from more than 20 per cent to less than 5 per cent.[91, 252, 257, 258, 265, 318]

EPIDEMIOLOGY

Sources of Epidemiologic Data on Kawasaki Disease

Available epidemiologic data on Kawasaki disease come from national surveillance, local passive surveillance, hospital-based case series, and case reports in the medical literature. Because Kawasaki disease is notifiable in most states, all observed cases should be reported. As with most notifiable diseases, however, reporting is incomplete. Such surveillance data may be helpful in monitoring secular trends in disease occurrence and in identifying epidemics but are of little value in estimating disease incidence. Outbreak investigations are more sensitive in determining local disease incidence and in characterizing the disease clinically and epidemiologically. They also offer the chance to study potential risk factors.

Although both clinical and epidemiologic case definitions of Kawasaki disease are based on Kawasaki's original (1967) criteria, they should not be regarded as comparable, because they are designed for different purposes. In the past, physicians have refrained from making a diagnosis of Kawasaki disease when epidemiologic case criteria were not met. It should be emphasized strongly, however, that the epidemiologic case definitions were not intended for clinical application. This is a critical point now that effective treatment is available. A contemporary clinical case definition of Kawasaki disease, slightly modified from Kawasaki's original criteria, is shown in Table 82–1. However, the diagnosis of Kawasaki disease should be made in consideration of all available clinical information. Because formes frustes and atypical cases probably are common in Kawasaki disease,[27, 75, 132, 210, 294] the diagnosis should be suspected in cases with similar features that do not meet case criteria. This especially may be true in infancy because, as is true for many infectious and noninfectious diseases, the signs in infantile Kawasaki disease may be less specific and more variable.[132, 294] A more liberal application of clinical case criteria[132] may be beneficial in light of new appreciation of disease severity and recent advances in treatment (see later). Epidemiologic criteria may need to be stricter in order to exclude from health department surveillance data the many undiagnosed exanthematous conditions that otherwise would dilute the "true" cases of Kawasaki disease, thus obscuring secular trends in its occurrence. In the United States, the Centers for Disease Control and Prevention (CDC) case definition usually is used for epidemiologic purposes.[246] The Japanese epidemiologic case definition, an earlier version of which served as a model for the CDC case definition, is more complex.[365] Both epidemiologic case definitions have been revised, so that earlier data may not be strictly comparable to data collected currently. The present Japanese epidemiologic case definition has been in use since 1984.[367] The CDC epidemiologic case definition was modified slightly in 1978[246] to specify reasonable attempts to exclude other causes of the documented signs and symptoms.

TABLE 82–1. Principal Diagnostic Criteria for Kawasaki Disease*

Fever
Conjunctival injection
Changes in the mouth
Erythema, fissuring, and crusting of the lips
Diffuse oropharyngeal erythema
Strawberry tongue
Changes in the peripheral extremities
Induration of hands and feet
Erythema of palms and soles
Desquamation of fingertips and toetips, approximately 2 weeks after onset
Transverse grooves across fingernails, 2 to 3 months after onset
Erythematous rash
Enlarged lymph node mass measuring more than 1.5 cm in diameter

*Five of six criteria needed for secure diagnosis.

Gender

In virtually all countries where it has been studied, the ratio of males to females with uncomplicated Kawasaki disease is around 1.5:1. Male-to-female ratios reported from several countries include Japan (1.4), the United States (1.4), Canada (1.7), England (1.3), Korea (1.8), Germany (1.5), and Finland (1.2). The preponderance of males is notable.[44, 368] It is not accounted for entirely by excess male births. Proponents of a genetic predisposition to Kawasaki disease frequently cite the different incidences by gender. However, differences in exposures by gender are difficult to rule out for older infants and children. As is true for many disease complications, serious and fatal Kawasaki disease is much more common in males than females[44, 368]; examination of death certificates in the third Japanese national survey found an overall male-to-female ratio of Kawasaki disease–related deaths of 4.5:1, with an 8:1 or 9:1 ratio in infancy. The preponderance of males and the apparent differences in incidence by racial background (see later), both characteristic of Kawasaki disease, raise questions about its etiology. Infectious diseases such as poliomyelitis, for example, affect male and female infants with about the same incidence, although serious complications are more common in males.

Race/Ethnic Background

Because the first cases were seen in Japanese children and American children of predominantly Japanese background, Kawasaki disease initially was presumed to occur most commonly in Japanese persons. That assumption has not been disproved.[103, 285] The annual incidence rates in Japan and Korea are about 50 to 100 cases per 100,000 children 4 years of age or younger.[369] In epidemic years in Japan, however, the annual age-specific incidence rates, calculated by peak risk-years of age, have reached or exceeded 200 per 100,000 children younger than 5 years of age.[365] Incidence rates in white children determined by active surveillance in many communities are lower, clustering around 5 to 10 per 100,000 children 4 years of age or younger.[28, 36, 50, 95, 279, 324] In the United States, where national surveillance is based on passive reporting that underestimates the actual incidence to a considerable degree, the annual incidence of Kawasaki disease in children 4 years of age or younger has been estimated to be approximately 5 per 100,000 for children of Asian ancestry, 1.5 for black children, and less than 1.0 for white and Hispanic children combined.[284] In Washington State, ethnic group-specific incidence rates per 100,000 children 4 years of age or younger were estimated to be 33.3 for Asian Americans, 23.4 for blacks, and 12.7 for whites.[50] In Hawaii, with a "cosmopolitan" racial-ethnic makeup and excellent case recognition, Kawasaki disease is seen significantly more often in children of Japanese background. The overall annual incidence in Hawaii is 45 per 100,000 children younger than 5 years of age. The yearly incidence in Japanese and Korean children in Hawaii is 140 cases per 100,000 children and 9 per 100,000 whites, with intermediate rates for Hawaii children of black, Hispanic, Chinese, Filipino, and Polynesian ancestry.[51] In New Zealand, incidence differences between white and Polynesian children were not apparent,[95] but in Singapore, an increased occurrence of Kawasaki disease in Chinese versus Malay children was suggested.[259] Projecting the Hawaii figures to the United States as a whole would suggest 3000 to

5000 annual cases of Kawasaki disease. One thousand to 1500 annual U.S. cases were reported in a national survey of hospitals with large children's services.[345, 346]

No single HLA antigen is common to all or most cases of Kawasaki disease. Preliminary suggestions[149, 171, 231] that Kawasaki disease is associated with HLA-Bw 22 (or subtype Bw 54) have not been confirmed by subsequent studies in Japan, Hong Kong, or in the Boston area, where HLA-Bw 51 and HLA-B 44 were found to be more common.[38, 102, 172] The incidence of HLA-Bw 51 antigen also was increased in one series of Israeli patients.[159] A smaller Maryland study suggested that despite an association between Kawasaki disease and B 44, the A2 B 44 Cw 5 triplet, carried as a haplotype, was a more likely and more specific risk factor.[141] Studies of HLA class II genes have detected no association.[19, 63] To date, no specific HLA type conclusively has been proved to be a risk factor for Kawasaki disease. Evidence that immunoglobulin allotypic markers may be correlated with Kawasaki disease are unconfirmed.[320]

Age

Kawasaki disease is seen almost exclusively in children. In the United States and Japan, reports of adult cases are viewed with skepticism, although some adult cases have been diagnosed using accepted diagnostic criteria.[10, 15, 32, 34, 60, 99, 193, 241, 281, 312] In several adult cases, the reported diseases appeared to be related more closely to toxic shock syndrome than to Kawasaki disease.[351] Adult cases probably are extremely rare. Because the signs and symptoms are nonspecific, suspected adult cases of Kawasaki disease should be evaluated carefully for infectious, toxic, and other possible causes of the disease episodes. Occurrence by age in childhood is illustrated in Figure 82–1. The disease virtually is restricted to young children: 50 per cent are younger than 2 years of age, 80 per cent are younger than 4 years of age, and cases are rare in individuals older than 12 years of age. Although national surveillance data from Japan and the United States have shown a peak age of about 18 months, more recent figures from both Japan and Hawaii, where disease recognition and reporting currently are better than elsewhere, identify the ages of peak incidence as before 1 year of age (e.g., 9 to 11 months of age for males and 3 to 8 months of age for females in Japan).[368] Presumably, the better-defined age-incidence patterns reported from Japan and Hawaii reflect improved recognition in infants, in whom Kawasaki disease, like many other infectious diseases, may present a more nonspecific clinical picture.[132] The pattern of the age-incidence curve also may be helpful in elucidating risk factors for Kawasaki disease. Such a pattern nearly is pathognomonic for highly transmissible infectious agents, particularly respiratory agents. However, the Kawasaki disease age-incidence pattern also is consistent with an environmental exposure linked to a restricted age range in infancy and early childhood. Among the many age-restricted behaviors that come to mind (pica, teething, cow's milk ingestion, solid food exposures, vaccinations, physician's office visits), none has been linked yet to Kawasaki disease. The question has been raised as to whether the Kawasaki disease age-incidence pattern may not be consistent with a syndrome associated with multiple etiologies (as is seen, for example, with aseptic meningitis). This suggestion merits further consideration.

The age-incidence patterns of uncomplicated and fatal Kawasaki disease are dissimilar to those most common in infancy. Japanese data, based on information from death certificates, suggest that 23 per cent of all reported Kawasaki disease deaths occur in infants, 45 per cent in children younger than 2 years of age, and 75 per cent in children 3 years of age or younger. Extrapolations of Japanese data suggest that the combined case-fatality ratio for all children 1 year of age or older may be less than 1 per cent, whereas for infants it may be as high as 4 per cent or more. Males account for a disproportionate number of deaths in infants and older children. In Japan, Kawasaki disease causes an overall doubling of the mortality rate in boys.[255] However, based on vital statistics data, within the first 2 months of illness onset, boys are about 13 times and girls 4 times more likely to die than expected.[255] This difference almost entirely is due to development of coronary artery aneurysms.

Recurrent Cases

Recurrence is defined as a new episode meeting Kawasaki disease case criteria that begins more than 3 months after the

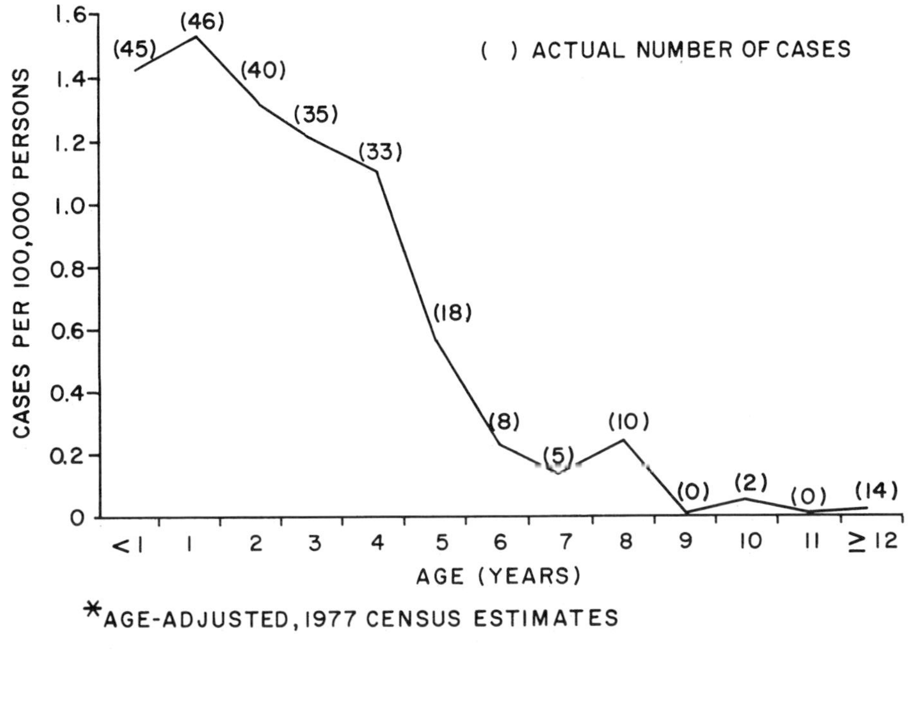

FIGURE 82–1. *Occurrence of Kawasaki disease, by age, in the United States.*

initial episode and after the erythrocyte sedimentation rate and platelet count have returned to normal. Recurrent cases of Kawasaki disease have been documented with increasing frequency.[364, 365] The frequency of recurrences in reported first cases of Kawasaki disease in Japan has been estimated to be about 1.9 per cent in 3-year follow-up, with about 0.07 per cent experiencing a third episode.[256] This corresponds to an incidence rate for one or more recurrences of 5.21 per 1000 person-years.[256] With longer follow-up, eventual recurrence rates reach 3 per cent or more.[368] Recurrences appear to be most frequent within the first 2 years after the initial episode, especially in males and in children who had the initial episode before their second birthday.[256] The frequency distributions of intervals between initial and recurrent episodes are unimodal for both genders; curiously, however, the mode is seen at 3 to 5 months for males but at 9 to 11 months for females.[368] The incidence of recurrences in the United States has been estimated to be less than 1 per cent, although recurrences have been documented in 2.3 per cent of Hawaii cases followed during a 15-year period (1973–1987). Without any means to prove a diagnosis of Kawasaki disease, it is impossible to establish that the second episode represents the same disease as the first.

Family Cases

Simultaneous or sequential cases of Kawasaki disease in siblings, twin siblings, or other family contacts also have been reported with increasing frequency.[68, 124, 228] Japanese investigators have documented secondary sibling cases in about 1 per cent of all cases,[368] but such figures are difficult to interpret because the denominator of siblings at risk has not been available in most studies. Such data also may be suspected of suffering from various recognition and reporting biases. Sibling cases are reported to be more common in twins than nontwins. An apparently higher frequency of family cases during outbreaks also has been noted.[369]

Epidemics and Outbreaks

Japanese investigators have noted nationwide epidemics of Kawasaki disease in 1979, 1982, and 1985 to 1986.[367] Localized outbreaks also have been observed. In the United States and other countries where community-wide outbreaks are the rule, outbreaks have been documented with increasing frequency, including sudden peaks of case detection in 1977 to 1978 (Hawaii, New York), 1979 (Japan), 1979 to 1980 (Hawaii; Los Angeles, California; northern Louisiana; Rochester, New York; eastern Massachusetts and New England; Quebec Province, Canada; East Germany; Korea), 1981 (Australia, Hawaii), 1981 to 1982 (Finland, West Germany, northeast Italy), 1982 (Denver, Colorado; Japan), 1982 to 1983 (Wisconsin; Illinois; Michigan; New York; Ontario, Canada; London, England), 1984 (Washington; Oakland/San Francisco, California; Harris County, Texas; Indiana; Tennessee; eastern North Carolina; Virginia; Washington, D.C.; Massachusetts), 1984 to 1985 (Colorado, Wyoming), 1985 (Ohio), 1985 to 1986 (Japan), and 1986 (Los Angeles, possibly Australia). Although investigation of such outbreaks provides an opportunity to study potential risk factors, to date no proven risk factor has been identified.[22] Clustering of cases within families, schools, or neighborhoods is unusual, even in the midst of large-scale epidemics. Japanese investigators have associated epidemics with a statistically increased likelihood of second family cases, fatalities, and relapsed cases, but the implications of these findings are uncertain. It is curious that in recent years (1987–1995), outbreaks have not been identified, suggesting either that earlier outbreaks were outbreaks of recognition, rather than occurrence, or that the epidemiology of Kawasaki disease has changed.[372]

Geography

Kawasaki disease has been diagnosed in all of the United States and in all 47 prefectures of Japan. Thousands of cases also have been reported from most developed and many developing countries on all continents, including temperate and tropical zones.[28, 36, 38, 304] No striking rural-urban differences have been noted. Elevation, longitude, and latitude have not been implicated, although most reports have come from countries with temperate climates. Travel histories of cases have not been remarkable, although one anecdotal report of a 7-month-old infant in Australia documents Kawasaki disease onset 17 days after leaving Japan during that country's 1982 epidemic.[324]

In some epidemics, geographic spread has been noted, for example, in Finland in 1981 to 1982[279] and in Japan in 1979, 1982, and 1985 to 1986.[254, 366] The 1982 Japanese epidemic[366] broke out simultaneously in four different places, spreading outward from each of them, in much the same way that epidemic influenza has been noted to spread in Europe and America. In the 1985 to 1986 Japanese epidemic, investigators identified epidemic "waves" that spread outward from an initial focus in the Tokyo metropolitan area, heading simultaneously northward and southward to involve most of the country within about 4 months.[364] In each of the nine districts studied in this epidemic, the epidemic curves were similar except for their temporal patterns. A similar but less distinctive pattern of interprefectural progression in waves had been noted in the 1982 Japanese epidemic, which began as a multifocal outbreak. Within the northern Tohoku District, for example, Kawasaki disease spread from prefecture to prefecture over a period of about 7 months.[364] After the Japanese epidemics of 1979 and 1985 to 1986, Korean epidemics were detected 7 and 15 months later, respectively.[190, 364]

Seasonality

In Japan, Kawasaki disease occurs year-round but tends to predominate in the winter-spring, with incidence peaks usually falling within the December to May period,[367] especially in December and January.[368] Even so, Japan and Korea have documented annual increases in cases in June or July.[191, 368] A similarly imprecise pattern appears to prevail in the United States as a whole, in various locales within the United States,[23, 284] and in other countries.[306] Seasonal incidence data from the Southern Hemisphere have not established clear seasonal patterns.[95, 324] That sporadic cases commonly are recognized year-round is unlike the pattern seen with highly transmissible respiratory viral diseases that peak in the winter-spring (e.g., measles, rubella, influenza). Nevertheless, outbreaks in many locales have tended to begin in the winter and continue into the spring.[369]

Communicability

There is no evidence that the syndrome recognized as Kawasaki disease is transmissible from person to person. Nosocomial and secondary or coprimary cases in families are documented uncommonly. Often, concomitant nonspecific illnesses are seen in siblings,[300] but there is no evidence that this is due to anything other than chance. Previous exposure of children with Kawasaki disease to clothes, food, or toys from Japan or elsewhere in Asia and Southeast Asia is common, but the ubiquity of such product exposures makes interpretation difficult. Japanese family data suggest that sibling cases cluster either on the same day as onset in the index case or 7 days later.[68] Because these results are based on questionnaire data, however, the possibility of bias is great; thus, it is difficult to estimate whether the majority of the Japanese family cases are coprimary or actual secondary cases.

Other Risk Factors

In addition to the demographic risk factors for Kawasaki disease, epidemiologic investigations have linked some cases to specific exposures that could be markers or indicators for an etiologic agent of Kawasaki disease. The first of these to be identified was a history of more frequent antecedent respiratory illnesses in cases compared with control patients. As noted later, many viral agents are prevalent during the seasons when Kawasaki disease is most prevalent, and isolations of many different viruses from patients (and from matched control children) are to be expected. The most widely discussed of the Kawasaki disease associations are prior carpet cleaning/shampooing, exposure to house dust mites, and residence near bodies of water, particularly septic water. Of these, the most intriguing may be the association of some Kawasaki disease outbreaks with rug or carpet cleaning/shampooing in the houses of patients. The association has been documented in some American outbreaks[61, 101, 122, 266, 278, 281, 288] but not in others[166, 215, 284, 292, 293, 347] and also has been associated with non-outbreak cases.[25] In Japan, where carpets are uncommon, Kawasaki disease has been associated with ownership of rugs or tatamis (traditional straw mats). In three of the carpet shampoo–associated outbreaks investigated by the CDC, the shampooing events had clustered in 2- to 4-week intervals prior to disease onset, with few cases in the 2-week interval immediately preceding disease onset. Of 35 cases with rug shampooing exposure in the preceding month investigated by the CDC, 33 reported the exposure to have occurred 13 to 30 days before onset, with only 2 reporting such exposure 0 to 12 days before onset, a finding of high statistical significance. A fourth study, although not discussing specific intervals between shampooing and disease onset, noted clustering of the shampooing event around 3 weeks before disease onset.[61] The meaning of the shampooing association is unclear.[49, 248] In some well-studied outbreaks, it has been absent entirely. Furthermore, because rug shampoos contain mostly water, anionic detergents, and inert ingredients, they seem unlikely agents of Kawasaki disease. Conceivably, shampooing is a confounded risk factor, perhaps serving as a marker for aerosolization of an actual microbial or sensitizing agent already in the carpet. Carpets normally are virtual culture media for a variety of microbial agents, for mites, and for many other substances. Vacuuming of carpets, whether or not associated with shampooing, may be a highly efficient mechanism for aerosolizing particles or infectious agents in the carpet.[135] Alternatively, carpet hydration could activate some agent or enhance its growth, allowing it eventually to find its way into the mouth of an infant or toddler who later plays on the floor. Future outbreak investigations should take particular care to document the child's specific exposures during and in the first week or so after carpet cleaning.

A possible link between Kawasaki disease and house dust mites (chiefly *Dermatophagoides farinae* and *Dermatophagoides pteronyssimus*), proposed as an allergic hypothesis before the carpet shampoo association was suggested,[92] gained further impetus when it was realized that mites and mite antigens are significant components of carpets, rugs, and tatamis. A Japanese group claimed to have identified *Rickettsia*-like bodies in the digestive systems of mites taken from the house dust of Kawasaki disease patients.[109] Other investigators supported the notion that Kawasaki disease might result from an infectious organism found in house dust mites.[67] However, house dust mite counts were found not to be significantly different in the houses of case and control patients,[101, 127] and investigators found no evidence of specific anti-mite IgE, IgG, or antibodies to *D. pteronyssimus* in Kawasaki disease patients.[101, 136] Interestingly, *Propionibacterium acnes,* a common organism found in the human skin scales that mites feed on and in the mites themselves, has been proposed as a cause of Kawasaki disease. However, convincing data have not been provided.

CDC investigators also have studied several outbreaks in which they claim Kawasaki disease case patients lived closer to bodies of water than did control patients.[284, 287, 288] If confirmed, this association could indicate an actual risk factor, such as an insect vector or a water-associated organism. Cautious interpretation is advisable, however, until more sophisticated epidemiologic studies rule out effects of bias or confounding.

In a Washington State incidence study of endemic cases, proximity to water was not associated with Kawasaki disease.[50]

ETIOLOGY

The etiology of Kawasaki disease remains unknown. Many investigators believe that the disease has an infectious cause or is the result of an immune response to an infectious agent or agents. In support of this hypothesis are such aspects as sudden onset with the early appearance of oropharyngeal inflammation and cervical adenitis, consistent with airborne acquisition of a replicating agent; the toxic appearance of the child with fever and evidence of inflammation of the respiratory tract mucosa, central nervous system, cardiovascular system, and joints; and the laboratory picture of an elevated white blood cell count with a "left shift," elevated acute-phase reactants, meatitis, pyuria, and the generally self-limited nature of most cases. Furthermore, systemic vasculitis with inflammatory cell infiltration could be infectious or the result of an immune reaction to infection. On epidemiologic grounds, the age-incidence pattern (see Fig. 82–1) is consistent with a transmissible disease of childhood, as are seasonality (winter-spring), the occurrence of definite community-wide outbreaks with geographic spreading, and apparent epidemic cycles. In fact, if a large percentage of mild or subclinical cases is postulated, the epidemiology of Kawasaki disease would not be remarkably different from other highly transmissible childhood diseases in which only rare or occasional complications, perhaps in genetically susceptible children, are detected. This is analogous to poliomyelitis, which is an uncommon complication of poliovirus infection occurring in only about 1 of 200 infected children. Attempts to incriminate an infectious agent, however, have failed so far, including attempts to culture bacteria on artificial media and to detect viruses in cell culture, primates, mice, and guinea pigs, as well as by electron microscopy. No infectious agent has been isolated consistently or frequently from a normally sterile site.

A wide variety of microorganisms have been suspected of causing Kawasaki disease, including bacteria, leptospires, spirochetes, rickettsia, and viruses. All of the following agents have been proposed as causative agents and have been investigated moderately or thoroughly with little or no evidence of an etiologic relationship: group A streptococci,[4, 173] *P. acnes*,[148, 353] leptospires,[24, 62, 221] *Borrelia*,[37, 221] *Pseudomonas*,[158] *Klebsiella pneumoniae*,[134] *Mycoplasma*,[26, 52, 66, 115, 133, 140, 236, 237, 299, 322] parvovirus,[76, 261, 269] cytomegalovirus,[58, 219] Epstein-Barr virus,[13, 15, 128, 161, 162, 219, 271, 313] varicella-zoster virus,[219] human herpesviruses 6 and 7,[58, 219, 272] and multiple other fungi, bacteria, viruses, or vaccines.[57, 113, 157, 195, 196, 232, 251, 313, 336, 358]

A hypothesis that Kawasaki disease may be caused by *Rickettsia*-like agents has been neither proved nor disproved conclusively.[23, 35, 56, 71, 107, 108, 111, 178, 218, 244, 247, 333, 342, 343, 360] This hypothesis originally was based upon observation of structures thought to resemble rickettsiae on electron micrographs of skin, arterial walls, lymph nodes, and blood from Kawasaki disease patients. These structures have not been identified definitively, and no convincing serologic link to any known *Rickettsia* has been demonstrated.

The possibility that Kawasaki disease might be caused by a novel retrovirus was raised when two groups reported finding reverse transcriptase activity in cultured peripheral blood mononuclear cells from patients with active Kawasaki disease.[30, 317] Other studies have failed to support this claim.[240, 270] Serologic studies for the retroviruses HIV-1, human T-cell lymphotropic virus types I and II, simian immunodeficiency virus, and feline T-cell lymphotrophic virus have been negative,[260, 270, 286, 297] although occasionally Kawasaki disease has occurred in HIV-positive persons.[358]

Yersinia organisms, particularly *Yersinia pseudotuberculosis*, are capable of causing a systemic illness resembling Kawasaki disease. This organism has been recovered from some patients with Kawasaki disease–like illness in Japan.[40, 185, 308] However, convincing evidence of an etiologic association is lacking at present. Newer molecular tools have been developed that ultimately may lead to an understanding of whether this organism is related etiologically and what proportion of patients have a link to this organism.[335]

A number of investigators have been evaluating a hypothesis that Kawasaki disease might be the result of a bacterial superantigen toxin. Superantigens have the ability to bind to MHC class II molecules on monocytes and B cells and to the T-cell receptor. This superantigen binding has the potential to activate large numbers of immunoreactive cells and to cause the release of large amounts of inflammatory cytokines. Superantigens potentially cause expansion of autoreactive T cells.[112, 160] These features of T-cell activation and elevated serum levels of the cytokines, tumor necrosis factor–alpha, and interleukin-6 characterize the acute phase of Kawasaki disease. Staphylococcal toxic shock syndrome caused by the superantigen toxic shock syndrome toxin-1 is a prime example of a superantigen-mediated disease. Toxic shock syndrome and Kawasaki disease share the features of fever, rash, conjunctival injection, hand and foot erythema and edema, and convalescent desquamation.[110, 280] One group of investigators has reported selective expansion of $V\beta_2$ and $V\beta_8$ families on the T cells of patients with acute Kawasaki disease.[1, 2] This group also found that 11 of 16 Kawasaki disease patients were colonized with toxic shock syndrome toxin-1–producing staphylococci, usually in the throat or rectum.[209] This hypothesis has been investigated quite thoroughly by several groups. The finding of selective expansion of $V\beta_2$ and $V\beta_8$ families on T cells has not been confirmed.[3, 262, 282, 355] Colonization with *Staphylococcus aureus*, including toxic shock syndrome toxin-1–producing staphylococci, has been found to be equal among Kawasaki disease cases and well controls in two other studies.[222, 350] Most studies fail to show *any* disturbance of Vβ T-cell utilization in Kawasaki disease,[355] calling into question the entire hypothesis of a superantigen etiology.

An additional possibility raised by several investigators[220, 245, 361] is that Kawasaki disease may be an immunologic response triggered by any of a number of viral or other microbial agents. Consistent with this hypothesis is documentation of infection of different individual cases with a variety of different microorganisms, documentation of specific immunologic abnormalities in Kawasaki disease (vide infra), failure to detect any single microbiologic or environmental agent after more than two decades of searching, and analogies to other multifactorial syndromes, for example, that of aseptic meningitis. However, this hypothesis may be difficult to reconcile with the relatively distinctive clinical-laboratory picture of Kawasaki disease and by such epidemiologic features as documented epidemics and geographic spread.

Kawasaki disease has not been associated consistently with exposure to drugs[121] or to such environmental pollutants as toxins, pesticides, chemicals, and heavy metals, although the similarities between Kawasaki disease and acrodynia (mercury poisoning) have been noted.[5, 14, 39, 45, 153, 275] Kawasaki disease does not appear to be related to known adult vasculitides.[131, 192, 289, 310]

As of mid-1996, the etiology of Kawasaki disease remained undiscovered. The identification of the so-far elusive etiologic agent by either serendipity or the focused application of newer molecular techniques will be a major step forward in understanding the pathogenesis and will bring improved methods of treatment and prevention.

PATHOLOGY AND PATHOGENESIS

Relationship to Infantile Periarteritis Nodosa and Coronary Artery Aneurysms of Unknown Cause

Japanese and American investigators were quick to recognize the pathologic similarities between infantile periarteritis nodosa and fatal infantile Kawasaki disease,[339] neither of which was seen in Japan prior to 1960.[6, 20, 21, 98, 179, 186, 338, 341] Because, however, the etiologies of both entirely are unknown, the spectra of both diseases are vague and experience with gross and histologic investigation still is incomplete. It currently is impossible to distinguish pathologically between infantile periarteritis nodosa with coronary artery involvement and fatal infantile Kawasaki disease.[186] Although most patients with infantile periarteritis nodosa and coronary artery involvement previously reported in the medical literature have not met Kawasaki disease case criteria applied retrospectively, this failure is likely to be caused by a combination of documentation bias and the young age of the victims—infants with Kawasaki disease are less likely to have a classic presentation than are older children. Even when pathologic and clinical criteria are combined, the two diseases appear to be indistinguishable, which raises interesting questions about the novelty of Kawasaki disease, especially in the United States, where infantile periarteritis nodosa has been documented reasonably well since the 1940s and where Kawasaki disease was not recognized as a distinct entity until the 1970s. It is of uncertain significance that cases of both adult- and classic-type periarteritis nodosa and of childhood coronary artery aneurysms were reported long before recognition of Kawasaki disease as a clinical entity. Childhood periarteritis nodosa began to be reported after 1866, when adult-type periarteritis nodosa first was described, but it is difficult to ascertain retrospectively whether these children suffered from the adult or infantile type of disease.

Adult-type periarteritis nodosa appears, however, to be a different disease, one that commonly leads to hypertension, renal disease, and pulmonary disease and that most often involves small and medium muscular arteries, especially in the lung, kidney, and intestines.[64, 69, 74, 179, 340, 341] The earliest recorded case of possible infantile periarteritis nodosa was reported in 1899.[175] It was not until 1959, however, that Munro-Faure[250] delineated a syndrome of infantile necrotizing arteritis with coronary artery involvement, fever, rash, conjunctival and pharyngeal injection, and cervical adenitis. Roberts and Fetterman[291] expanded on these observations to define a distinct clinical-pathologic syndrome of infantile periarteritis nodosa.

Coronary artery aneurysms had been detected in persons of all ages since the early nineteenth century,[46, 277, 314] with a male-to-female ratio of roughly 3:1, including a male preponderance in childhood cases. Childhood death from multiple coronary artery aneurysms was known at least as early as 1871.[94] The heart from this case, formalin-fixed for more than 120 years in the Pathology Museum at St. Bartholomew's Hospital, London, recently has been sectioned. The coronary arteries showed the characteristic findings of fatal Kawasaki disease and infantile periarteritis nodosa.[321] In 1899, however, Capps[33] reviewed all 19 published cases with which he was familiar (cases having occurred between 1812 and 1897) and found that only two were in children. A more exhaustive 1948 literature review documented the rarity of coronary artery aneurysms; the author noted that in his series of 19,403 autopsies, only one case was identified.[314] Whether any of these early cases of periarteritis nodosa or childhood coronary artery aneurysms represented early examples of Kawasaki disease is highly speculative; histories usually were scanty, and deaths often were attributed, perhaps erroneously, to better understood diseases, such as scarlet fever.[94, 283] However, some of these cases, although not meeting Kawasaki disease diagnostic criteria applied retrospectively, greatly resembled Kawasaki disease.[46 [case 2], 250, 283] When various findings from many such early case reports are combined, it is possible to assemble a reasonably accurate picture of Kawasaki disease as recognized today. Most clinicians and pediatric infectious disease specialists deny having seen children with illnesses compatible with Kawasaki disease before 1970. If infantile periarteritis nodosa is indeed a tip-of-the-iceberg phenomenon, Kawasaki disease has been prevalent longer than previously suspected. As noted earlier, it is likely that in prior decades cases of Kawasaki disease were misdiagnosed as measles, scarlet fever, or other more common conditions.

General Pathologic Features in Kawasaki Disease

Kawasaki disease originally was described as benign mucocutaneous lymph node syndrome[152] and initially was not linked to periarteritis nodosa or coronary aneurysms. However, it became evident by the mid-1970s that approximately 2 per cent of children with Kawasaki disease died suddenly, generally in the subacute or convalescent stages of illness,[155] and that 80 per cent of these deaths occurred within 40 days of fever onset.

At autopsy, the major finding in Kawasaki disease is multisystem vasculitis with a predilection for the coronary arteries.[8, 9, 69, 179, 340, 341] In more than 80 per cent of fatal cases, the immediate cause of death is acute thrombosis of inflamed coronary arteries. In some early deaths (within the first 2 weeks after onset), pancarditis with inflammation in the atrioventricular conduction system apparently causes fatal arrhythmia or intractable congestive heart failure. Some late deaths (months to years after the acute episode) appear to be secondary to coronary stenosis with chronic myocardial ischemia or, rarely, to rupture of a coronary aneurysm. Variable and scattered involvement of other arteries during the initial episode particularly includes large and medium muscular arteries. The evolution of vascular lesions is related directly to the stage of illness at the time of death, indicating that the insult in Kawasaki disease is a part of the otherwise self-limited acute illness rather than being chronic or progressive.

The general pathologic findings in autopsied cases of Kawasaki disease have been described by Landing and Larson,[179, 186] who stress not only the similarities to infantile periarteritis nodosa with coronary artery involvement but also the marked differences from adult or classic periarteritis nodosa, which occurs rarely in children. Excellent descriptions also have been provided by Tanaka and associates[338, 341] and Fujiwara and Hamashima.[70] Gross anatomic findings usually include cardiac hypertrophy and multiple or single bead-like or fusiform aneurysms of the coronary arteries and their branches, with or without thrombotic occlusion. Aneurysms of other arteries, such as the brachial, renal, and iliac, may be present as well. Although phlebitis is found commonly, vascular inflammation more typically, and more severely, affects larger musculoelastic arteries in their extraparenchymal portions. Sites of arteritis include the kidney, testes, mesentery, lung, pancreas, spleen, adrenal gland, and gastrointestinal tract. Panarteritis with mononuclear cell infiltration is typical.

Tanaka and associates[338, 339, 341] describe proliferative granulation and thickening of both the intima and media, associated with edema, collagen fiber proliferation, and destruction of muscle cells of the coronary arteries. They also describe fibrinoid necrosis, especially of the intima but sometimes intensive and involving all layers.[338, 339, 341] Landing and Larson,[179, 186] who note that fibrinoid necrosis is more consistent with adult periarteritis nodosa, did not detect significant fibrinoid necrosis in their series. Most investigators have described vascular lesions in roughly the same stage of development. Inflammation and necrosis of the media result in true aneurysms, which at autopsy may show histologic evidence of thrombus organization and granulation. Tanaka and associates[338, 339, 341] have stressed the frequency of severe involvement of the arcuate and interlobular branches of the renal arteries associated with focal fibrinoid necrosis and intimal thickening.

Other documented findings include renal infarcts and glomerular histologic changes, possible evidence of immune complex deposition,[302] including mesangial deposition of IgM and C3, and multifocal periglomerular infiltration of lymphocytes and plasma cells. Changes found in other arteries, the thymus, and lymph nodes have been noted. Tanaka[338] has described thymic atrophy (although most patients probably had been treated with steroids) and nondiagnostic lymph node biopsies. Other reports have described early lymph node biopsies showing multiple foci of necrosis and fibrin thrombi within the microvasculature,[97] as well as T-zone hyperplasia, B-zone macrophage infiltration, and immunoblast proliferation.[97, 179, 265]

From biopsy study of 27 patients, Hirose and Hamashima[120] concluded that the acute histologic findings of papillary edema, dilation of superficial vascular plexuses and intrapapillary capillary loops, endothelial necrosis that spread outward, modest perivascular mononuclear cell infiltration, and appearance of mast cells and mast cell degranulation are suggestive of a delayed-type hypersensitivity reaction. These investigators theorized that the vascular changes in Kawasaki disease are initiated by circulating noxious agents (presumably infectious or toxic) that directly damage the capillary endothelium. They concluded that direct damage began in all vessels in the endothelium and progressed outward and on to larger vessels as well. In this view, the inflammatory response, subendothelial edema, and muscle cell changes occurred secondarily. Although small vessel changes had disappeared after several days in biopsy specimens taken at autopsy of fatal cases, large vessel involvement still was detectable many days after onset. However, patients whose deaths occur more than 2 months after Kawasaki disease onset generally show little or no evidence of inflammation in the vessel walls or the heart. Autopsy findings more typically include arterial stenosis and myocardial infarction, both recent and remote. The cause of death in these late cases usually is acute infarction or chronic myocardial ischemia.[70]

Cardiac Pathology

Fujiwara and Hamashima[70] reported pathologic findings in the hearts of patients dying of Kawasaki disease and attempted to identify sequential stages of involvement. They observed early vasculitis (days 0 to 9) involving the coronary artery intima, characterized by intense adventitial perivasculitis of small vessels supplying the arterial wall associated with perivasculitis and endarteritis of the coronary arteries, but with medial sparing, pericarditis, myocarditis, endocarditis, valvulitis, and conduction system inflammation. These changes were followed by coronary artery panvasculitis and aneurysm formation (days 12 to 25), coronary artery granulation and resolution of inflammation in the smaller cardiac vessels (days 28 to 30), and coronary artery scarring and stenosis with endocardial fibroelastosis (day 40 and beyond).

Clinical correlation by serial echocardiography shows that initial evidence of coronary dilation appears at around 10 days in children ultimately developing coronary aneurysms. At this early stage, there is carditis associated with histologic evidence of an acute polymorphonuclear infiltrate in the pericardium, in the perivascular spaces of the myocardium, and in the endothelium, especially the mitral, tricuspid, and aortic valves. Polymorphonuclear leukocyte infiltration also is notable in the atrioventricular conduction system.[70] From the second week of illness through the sixth week, there is a progressive change in the intensity and nature of the inflammatory infiltrate, which matures from a dominance of polymorphonuclear cells to a less intense infiltrate composed predominantly of plasma cells and lymphocytes. The inflammation of the pericardium, myocardium, and endocardium gradually subsides. Destruction of the media appears, along with multiple fractures of the internal elastic lamina and development of aneurysmal dilation. Death at this stage of disease usually results from coronary thrombosis close to the origin of the vessel, which leads to myocardial infarction. Such deaths exhibit the typical cardiac pathology of Kawasaki disease, indistinguishable from infantile periarteritis nodosa.[70, 179, 341]

In a separate study of the hearts of 10 childhood deaths from Kawasaki disease, 8 because of coronary aneurysms, Fujiwara and associates[72] found luminal stenosis or scarring of the sinoatrial or atrioventricular nodal artery in 4 of the 10; inflammation of the main, left, or right bundle branch or the bundle of His in 7; mitral valvulitis in 4; and tricuspid valvulitis in 3. Overall, significant atrioventricular conduction system lesions were present in five of the children. The authors also noted a strong correlation between the electrocardiographic findings and lesions in the conduction system, especially between PQ prolongation and acute inflammation of the atrioventricular conduction system. Severe acute changes were most pronounced at 21 to 31 days after onset. Changes similar to those seen in acute rheumatic fever (without Aschoff bodies) also were reported. Tomisawa and colleagues[352] reported right ventricular endomyocardial biopsy of 10 children with Kawasaki disease, most of whom were beyond the acute stages and had some evidence of coronary artery or cardiac abnormalities. Light and electron microscopic examination of biopsied tissue revealed microinfarction and focal inflammatory and nonspecific degenerative changes that persisted for months after onset of the disease. In another study of right ventricular endomyocardial biopsies, Yutani and associates[375] noted myocarditis and cellular infiltration in every one of 201 specimens taken from patients up to 11 years after the onset of Kawasaki disease. However, 1 year earlier, the same authors had reported myocarditis in only 13 of 50 biopsies.[376] These findings need to be evaluated further because of the possibility that chronic myocarditis leads to chronic cardiomyopathy. Residual myocardial fibrosis apparently may be a common finding after the stages of active myocarditis (the first 3 weeks). Fibrosis may be due to infarcts by platelet emboli from the dilated and inflamed coronary arteries or from resolving myocarditis. Patchy fibrosis was found in 36 per cent of patients in the study of Yutani and associates.[376] Extensive fibrosis may affect myocardial function permanently; persistently decreased left ventricular function has been demonstrated by echocardiography in one study[11] but not in another.[102]

In general, after the acute phase of the illness and in the absence of ischemic events or infarction, there has been imperfect correlation between the degree of coronary artery involvement and left ventricular performance as indicated by the echocardiogram.[11, 102] Neither has there been a good correlation between the development of coronary artery aneurysms and the clinical signs of cardiovascular involvement.[118] A recent pathologic study of the coronary arteries of fatal cases without autopsy evidence of aneurysms showed coronary artery vasculitis without dilation similar in appearance to vasculitis in cases with aneurysms,[73] which suggests that Kawasaki disease with coronary artery aneurysm is the same entity as Kawasaki disease without aneurysm. Pancarditis and ventricular wall rupture also have been noted with increasing frequency in Kawasaki disease. Immunofluorescent staining has demonstrated deposition of IgG in the walls of the coronary arteries and in the myocardium.

One histologic/immunochemical study examined the intercostal arteries, which arise directly from the aorta but have no connections to the heart, in order to compare the nature and developmental processes of lesions with those of the coronary arteries.[225] Although the lesions were similar, they appeared somewhat later in the intercostal arteries. The investigators suggested that a general feature of arterial lesions in Kawasaki disease may be degeneration of medial smooth muscle cells followed by proliferation, in some cases leading to destruction of the medial structure associated with mononuclear cell infiltration, and eventually to aneurysm formation, consistent with many earlier observations.

Immunologic Findings

Studies of children with Kawasaki disease reveal widespread alterations in the humoral and cell-mediated immune systems.[16] The cause or causes of these changes are unknown but presumably reflect responses to antigens involved in the pathogenesis of the disease, secondary responses to vasculitic changes, or both. The early phase of Kawasaki disease is characterized by marked activation of polymorphonuclear neutrophils, T cells, B cells, and monocytes, with nonspecifically increased TH_1 and TH_2 cytokine production and with polyclonal elevations in serum immunoglobulins. Despite such markers of general immune activation as activated cells and presence of cell receptor markers and secretion of cytokines and monokines, CD8+ T-suppressor cells may be deficient in the circulation and in the tissues,[89, 119, 253, 349] including the coronary endothelium, with evidence for suppression of both cell-mediated cytotoxic[82] and natural killer cell activity.[82] Some data suggest that activated T cells leave the circulation to become sequestered in tissues, presumably including vascular tissue.[86, 87] Increased levels of cytokines also have been detected at sites of prior bacillus Calmette-Guérin vaccination.[309] There has been considerable interest in the possibility that cytokines such as gamma interferon expose endothelial cell antigens to the lytic effects of antiendothelial cell antibodies and also may induce endothelial cells to act as antigen-presenting cells and to produce interleukins-1 and -6. Cytokines such as interleukin-1, tumor necrosis factor–alpha, and gamma interferon also can lead to endothelial inflammatory and prothrombotic changes and induce leukocyte adhesion molecules and leukocyte chemoattractants. Histologic studies of coronary arteries, veins, and capillaries in Kawasaki disease have revealed expression of HLA-DR antigens (possible antigen-presenting cells) at the inflammatory site.[348] Immunologic abnormalities in Kawasaki disease, many of which have been associated with development of coronary artery aneurysms,[17, 41, 84, 88, 123, 213, 216, 217, 226, 253, 357] reverse as the disease progresses or after treatment with immunoglobulin.[199, 205, 223] Early treatment with aspirin and gamma globulin may be beneficial because it moderates the immune activation responses.

Evidence for activation of polymorphonuclear neutrophils is of interest because these cells, along with monocytes/macrophages, have been postulated to mediate endothelial cell damage in Kawasaki disease via production of such oxyradical intermediates as oxygen and hydrogen peroxide.[188, 189, 263, 342, 356] Kawasaki disease also is associated with widespread activation of monocytes/macrophages,[79, 80, 84, 123] T lymphocytes,[89, 309, 371] and B lymphocytes.[54, 81] Cytokine production in Kawasaki disease includes increased production of interleukins-1 and -2, tumor necrosis factors–alpha and –beta, and gamma interferon.[78, 163, 180–183, 202, 214, 216, 217, 226, 229, 233, 234] Enhanced interleukin-6 production apparently stimulates B cells,[55, 81, 85, 163, 217] leading to polyclonal antibody production. Jejunal mucosal changes similar to delayed type hypersensitivity in the epithelium and lamina propria have been detected,[253] including decreases in CD8+ cells coupled with increases in CD4+ and HLA-DR+ cells. Delayed hypersensitivity skin test responsiveness to *Candida*, streptokinase/streptodornose, phytohemagglutinin, and purified protein derivative is suppressed during the acute stage of Kawasaki disease but normalizes within 1 to 2 months.[370] As noted, Kawasaki disease is associated with inflammatory reactivation of bacillus Calmette-Guérin sites, apparently reflecting both cellular and humoral responses.[374] Plasma fibronectin levels have been reported to be decreased early in illness but to rebound to high levels in the fourth week of illness.[315, 316]

An acute rise and convalescent fall of all classes of serum immunoglobulins occurs in Kawasaki disease. Serum IgE levels are elevated frequently,[140, 171, 174, 176, 239] with 50 per cent of IgE values and 80 per cent of IgM values exceeding two standard deviations above mean values for age-matched children. The increase in serum immunoglobulin is polyclonal and associated with a very high proportion of activated B cells. These abnormalities, linked to T cell–derived B-cell factors, such as interleukin-6,[165] have been reversed by aspirin/gamma globulin treatment.[198] Autoantibodies to type III collagen have been detected in some Kawasaki disease patients,[167] but their association with coronary complications is questionable. Complement 3 universally is elevated in the first through the third weeks of illness and then becomes normal.[65, 90, 114, 208, 224, 268, 303, 373] Complement appears to be activated through the classical pathway.[168]

Deposition of IgM and complement in skin biopsy specimens has been reported.[47] The quantity of circulating immune complexes (IgG, IgM, and IgA) in Kawasaki disease is lower than in systemic lupus erythematosus but higher than in normal, afebrile children.[207, 223, 243, 269, 276, 359] Opinions differ over whether immune complexes in Kawasaki disease are associated with coronary artery aneurysm formation or with arthritis or carditis.[224] Most IgG circulating immune complexes in Kawasaki disease contain antibodies of the IgG1 and IgG3 subclasses,[54, 212, 274, 337] whose Fc portions can bind to monocytes and platelets. These IgG subclasses are common in various viral and bacterial infections, as well as in systemic lupus erythematosus, juvenile rheumatoid arthritis, and drug-induced autoimmunity. Immune complexes in Kawasaki disease may aggregate platelets, causing release of vasoactive factors[207]; thus, it is conceivable that they bind directly to the vascular endothelium to induce inflammatory reactions.

A number of studies have shown IgM or IgG antiendothelial cell antibodies in Kawasaki disease, a nonspecific finding also seen in systemic lupus erythematosus, scleroderma, juvenile rheumatoid arthritis, hemolytic-uremic syndrome, allograft rejection, and other acute and chronic conditions involving the immune system. Anti–endothelial cell antibodies might injure cells directly or participate in complement-mediated injury or in antibody-mediated cellular cytotoxic reactions.[12, 139, 200, 203, 206] Among the endothelial cell antigens of interest are adhesion molecules, E-selectin, and endothelin, all of which may be elevated in Kawasaki disease.[83, 125, 164, 249, 264] It is not known whether immunologic reactions to endothelial cells play a part in the pathogenesis of Kawasaki disease. However, the correlation of immune activation, endothelial cell "activation,"[203] and development of coronary artery lesions, all of which are suppressed by administration of immunoglobulin, is consistent with a powerful immune stimulator triggering an immunologic cascade leading to vascular damage via cytokine-induced exposure of endothelial proteins that are recognized as antigens in destructive autoimmune responses. In at least one study, antiendothelial cell antibodies were cytotoxic to endothelial cells even without cytokine prestimulation.[139]

Controversial evidence for the involvement in Kawasaki disease of superantigens, bacterial or viral proteins capable of activating large numbers of T cells via stimulation of the T-cell receptor Vβ region, has been discussed in the Etiology section. Both IgM and IgG antineutrophil cytoplasm antibodies[290, 310, 325] and antimyeloperoxidase antibodies[290] are elevated in Kawasaki disease. Although detection of these antibodies conceivably may be of diagnostic value, they do not appear to be correlated with coronary involvement.

Production of leukotriene B_4 by polymorphonuclear cells reportedly is increased from 13 to 29 days after Kawasaki disease onset.[106] Although apparently not associated with aneurysm formation, this powerful endogenous chemoattractant, released by cells at an inflammatory site, may play a role in attracting more inflammatory cells to the site, thus prolonging the period of intense inflammation.[105] Leukotriene E_4 and prostaglandin E_2 also have been shown to be elevated in Kawasaki disease,[77, 194, 230] as have increased platelet synthesis of thromboxane A_2[117] and plasma thromboxane B_2.

In almost all of these studies of immune activation, the period of most intense immune activation and cytokine elaboration is detected during the acute and early subacute phase, the period of most intense vascular inflammation and of aneurysm formation. Yet despite the many studies that seem to support broad and complex immune activation in Kawasaki disease, some investigators have raised legitimate questions about the nature and spectrum of the immune response,[282, 301] suggesting that Kawasaki disease may be merely a "typical" disease associated with conventional antigens.[282]

The strongest evidence of the importance of immunologic factors in the pathogenesis of vasculitis in Kawasaki disease is provided by the remarkable beneficial effect, discussed later, of intravenous gamma globulin on both the acute febrile illness and the development of coronary aneurysms.[252, 257, 258, 265, 318] Investigators also have associated immunoglobulin treatment with reduction in B-cell activation, more rapid normalization of T-cell activity, reduction in cytokine secretion, and disappearance of endothelial cell activation antigens.[197, 203] Theories attempting to explain the beneficial action of gamma globulin in this disease include the shutting off of endothelial cell "activation," "down-regulation" of immunoglobulin production by a negative feedback mechanism, specific immunoglobulin neutralization of an unknown etiologic agent or toxin, and nonspecific blockage of an attachment site for immune complexes or of harmful autoantibodies on the vascular endothelium affecting attachment of platelets or white blood cells.[319] Although the expanding body of descriptive immunologic data are of interest, they do not point to any specific mechanism of immunopathogenesis.

CLINICAL MANIFESTATIONS

In its fully expressed state, Kawasaki disease is a distinctive clinical entity with a predictable course. As with any condition, there undoubtedly is a spectrum of clinical effects. Children who do not fulfill all criteria for Kawasaki disease in fact may have the illness and may develop complications of arthritis and coronary artery disease. The principal clinical diagnostic criteria are presented in Table 82–1. Kawasaki disease should be considered in the differential diagnosis of infants and children with fever and any of the following: generalized polymorphous erythematous rash, conjunctival injection, characteristic changes in the mouth, characteristic changes in the hands and feet, or unilateral cervical lymph node swelling measuring greater than 1.5 cm. A secure diagnosis, according to accepted clinical criteria (see Table 82–1), is made in patients who fulfill five of the six clinical criteria and have exclusion of other illnesses that mimic Kawasaki disease. The most commonly encountered diseases to be excluded are (1) nonspecific exanthems, actually or presumably viral; (2) measles; (3) streptococcal and staphylococcal scarlatiniform eruptions; (4) infectious mononucleosis; and (5) hypersensitivity reactions. There apparently are many incomplete cases of Kawasaki disease that do not fulfill diagnostic criteria but are associated with risk of coronary artery aneurysms.[27, 75, 210, 211] Children younger than 6 months of age have been reported to be particularly likely to develop coronary abnormalities although not completely fulfilling diagnostic criteria,[31, 294] so a more liberal application of clinical diagnostic criteria in infancy is warranted. In Hawaii, most young infants diagnosed as having Kawasaki disease have fulfilled diagnostic criteria but with milder and more subtle manifestations than usually seen in older children. Therefore, we believe that the diagnosis should be considered even if clinical diagnostic criteria are not fulfilled.

Of the diagnostic symptoms, fever typically is hectic and remittent, with peak temperatures frequently exceeding 39.9° C (104° F) and in many cases exceeding 40.5° C (105° F). Unless treated with aspirin or intravenous gamma globulin, fever persists for a mean of 11 days.[116]

Vascular injection of the bulbar conjunctivae, more severe than injection of the palpebral conjunctivae, also is seen in the first week of illness. Patients sometimes have follicular palpebral conjunctivitis. There is no associated exudate, nor does edema of the conjunctivae or corneal ulceration occur, which distinguishes the conjunctivitis of Kawasaki disease from the purulent conjunctivitis of Stevens-Johnson syndrome. Mild acute iridocyclitis or anterior uveitis, which occurs early in the acute phase, rapidly resolves and rarely is associated with photophobia or eye pain.[29, 96, 184, 267, 323] Less common ocular findings include superficial punctate keratitis, vitreous opacities, vitreous and chorioretinal inflammation, and papilledema.[129]

Changes in the mouth consist of (1) erythema progressing to fissuring, cracking, and bleeding of the lips; (2) a "strawberry tongue" indistinguishable from that associated with streptococcal scarlet fever; and (3) diffuse erythema of the oropharynx. Concomitant tympanitis, especially common with high fever and marked oropharyngeal erythema, is not an exclusionary finding.

Changes in the extremities are among the most distinctive features of Kawasaki disease. In the acute phase, the hands and feet become indurated and swollen slightly with stretched, shiny skin. The palms and soles diffusely and deeply are erythematous. In the subacute phase, these changes are followed by a distinctive pattern of desquamation in thick sheets that are different from the fine, branny, flaking characteristic of digital peeling following scarlet fever.

The erythematous rash associated with Kawasaki disease may take any of several forms, most commonly raised, red, pruritic plaques or morbilliform erythematous papules. Occasionally, the skin shows diffuse scarlatiniform erythroderma or has an exanthem reminiscent of erythema marginatum. A variety of other exanthems have been reported, including rashes resembling erythema multiforme and urticaria. Perineal rashes have been emphasized by many observers. Rashes in Kawasaki disease tend to be most prominent on the trunk but frequently also involve the face and extremities.

Lymph node swelling is the least common of the principal diagnostic criteria, occurring in about 50 to 75 per cent of patients. It usually is unilateral and confined to the anterior cervical triangle. The enlarged node or mass of nodes usually is larger than 1.5 cm, is nonfluctuant, may or may not be associated with erythema of the overlying skin, and only moderately is tender. Lymphadenopathy generally is benign and transient.

The associated features of Kawasaki disease attest to its multisystem nature (Table 82–2). Sterile pyuria reflecting urethritis is found in three-quarters of patients. Meatitis and vulvitis are common. Arthritis developing in the first week of illness tends to involve multiple joints, including the small interphalangeal joints as well as large weight-bearing joints. Arthrocentesis during this phase reveals thick purulent-

TABLE 82–2. Associated Features of Kawasaki Disease (in Order of Frequency)

Pyuria and urethritis	Pericardial effusion
Arthralgia and arthritis	Obstructive jaundice
Aseptic meningitis	Hydrops of the gallbladder
Diarrhea	Acute mitral insufficiency
Abdominal pain	Myocardial infarction
Myocardiopathy	

appearing fluid, often in large volume, with a mean white blood cell count of 125,000 to 300,000 per cubic millimeter. Glucose determinations of the joint fluid are within normal limits; Gram stain and bacterial cultures invariably are negative. Approximately one-third of patients with arthritis have onset in the first 10 days of illness. Arthritis developing after 10 days has a predilection for large weight-bearing joints, especially the knees and ankles, and is associated with a slightly lower white blood cell count in the joint fluid. Gastrointestinal complaints, seen in approximately one-third of cases during the early stages, include nausea, abdominal pain, and severe diarrhea. Central nervous system involvement with severe lethargy, semicoma, and aseptic meningitis occurs in one-quarter of patients. Obstructive jaundice and acute gallbladder hydrops are seen in approximately 5 per cent.

The most important associated feature of Kawasaki disease is cardiac involvement. Clinical cardiac disease is detected in approximately 20 per cent of affected children and most often is manifest as pericardial effusion, transient myocardiopathy with congestive heart failure, and arrhythmia.[142] Angiographic and two-dimensional echocardiographic studies performed on a routine basis 4 to 8 weeks after onset demonstrate coronary artery aneurysms in 20 per cent or more of patients.[144, 146] There is an imperfect correlation between clinically apparent cardiac involvement and echocardiographic evidence of cardiac involvement.

The clinical course of Kawasaki disease, divided into acute, subacute, and late or convalescent phases, begins with fever, rash, conjunctival injection, strawberry tongue, edema and erythema of the hands and feet, lymphadenitis, and sometimes aseptic meningitis and mild hepatic dysfunction. Arrhythmias and congestive heart failure due to myocardiopathy may develop during the acute febrile phase or the subacute phase. Without aspirin or intravenous gamma globulin treatment, this acute phase generally lasts for 8 to 30 days (mean, 11 days). After defervescence, the physical findings rapidly disappear, but the child may remain irritable and anorectic. Arthritis is most likely to develop in this subacute phase, which is marked also by desquamation and thrombocytosis. The subacute phase persists until the child returns to normal at approximately 3 to 4 weeks. The subacute and early convalescent periods (2 to 6 weeks after onset) constitute the time of greatest risk of sudden death from acute coronary artery thrombosis.

CLINICAL LABORATORY PICTURE

Kawasaki disease is characterized by leukocytosis, especially granulocytosis with high band form counts, by elevated platelets in the second and third weeks of illness, and in the acute and subacute phases by general elevation of such "acute-phase reactants" as the erythrocyte sedimentation rate, C-reactive protein, alpha$_2$-globulin, alpha$_1$-antitrypsin, and percentage of nitro blue tetrazolium-positive cells. These return to normal by 8 to 12 weeks after illness onset. The white blood cell count nearly always is elevated, with a predominance of immature and mature granulocytes. Counts in excess of 30,000 per cubic millimeter occur in about 15 per cent of patients and in excess of 15,000 per cubic millimeter in about 50 per cent. Toxic granulation and Döhle bodies have been seen on peripheral blood smear.[66] Mild anemia may develop with normal or microcytic/hypochromic red blood cell indices. Severe hemolytic anemia, requiring multiple transfusions, is unusual[43, 100] and probably results from extensive systemic vasculitis. The serum complement generally is normal or slightly elevated. Modest elevation in transaminase values is seen in 40 per cent. Elevated bilirubin values are present in 10 per cent. Hypoalbuminemia appears to mark more severe disease.[188, 295] Urinalysis often reveals mild to moderate pyuria and proteinuria, although suprapubic bladder puncture reveals few or no white blood cells in the urine,[53, 237] which indicates urethritis. Another constant feature of the later phases of illness is thrombocytosis with platelet counts ranging from 300,000 to 3,000,000 per cubic millimeter.[244] Thrombocytosis rarely is seen in the first week of illness, usually appears in the second week, and peaks in the third with a gradual return to normal by a month after onset in uncomplicated cases. The average peak platelet count, reached in the second or third week of illness, is around 700,000 per cubic millimeter. There are no differences in ^{65}Cr-labeled autologous platelet survival between cases and controls and no correlation between thrombocytosis and accelerated platelet aggregation, which has been detected in patients with Kawasaki disease from a few days until a year after onset.[150, 363] During the course of Kawasaki disease, increases in fibrinogen and prolongation of the partial thromboplastin time have been reported. Examination of bone marrow reveals the normal number and morphology of megakaryocytes. Bone marrow changes rarely are remarkable.[43, 187, 326] Serum high-density lipoprotein and total cholesterol sometimes may be depressed, with elevated triglycerides.[305]

Laboratory tests can provide diagnostic support in otherwise nondiagnostic cases. An elevated C-reactive protein or erythrocyte sedimentation rate, almost universal in Kawasaki disease, is uncommon in viral exanthems, hypersensitivity reactions, and measles. Platelet counts higher than 450,000 per cubic millimeter usually are seen in patients presenting after the seventh day of illness. An analysis of reported cases of atypical Kawasaki disease with coronary abnormalities demonstrated that platelet elevation and elevated sedimentation rate were universal in these cases.[210] Our experience in Hawaii and with 900 patients evaluated in a United States multicenter treatment study further suggests that Kawasaki disease is extremely unlikely if platelet counts and a full panel of acute-phase inflammatory reactants (e.g., erythrocyte sedimentation rate, C-reactive protein, alpha$_1$-antitrypsin) are normal after the seventh day of illness.

TREATMENT

Intravenous Gamma Globulin

As soon as the condition can be diagnosed, patients with Kawasaki disease should undergo a baseline echocardiogram and begin receiving intravenous gamma globulin, 2 g/kg, given in a 10- to 12-hour infusion. This dosage schedule has been demonstrated to be of equal efficacy in reducing the risk of coronary disease to a schedule of 400 mg/kg/day given over 4 consecutive days. The single-dose schedule is superior to the four-dose schedule in rapidity of defervescence and return of acute-phase reactants to normal.[257, 265] Single-dose infusion is safe, having been given to 273 children in a controlled trial without significant adverse effects; pulse, heart rate, and blood pressure should be monitored at the beginning of infusion and at 30 minutes, 1 hour, and every 2 hours thereafter during infusion. Despite the substantial fluid and protein load associated with this dosage, it has not been found to increase the risk of congestive heart failure, even in patients with decreased myocardial function.

No substantial clinical experience has demonstrated efficacy of single-infusion therapy at dosages less than 2 g/kg. Although a 1-g/kg dose was reported in two pilot trials, the numbers of patients studied were too small to prove efficacy.[18, 59] Multiple studies in Japan also have demonstrated efficacy for multiple-dose regimens of greater than 1 g/kg,[59] but total doses at or less than 1 g/kg have not been shown to be effective in reducing the incidence of coronary abnormalities.[273]

No data are available to guide therapy of patients encountered more than 10 days after onset of Kawasaki disease. If patients still are febrile or have such other signs of active disease as progressive coronary dilation, gamma globulin therapy probably should be instituted because it may result in prompt clinical improvement. Patients who have become afebrile and have normal coronary arteries by 3 weeks after illness onset, however, are unlikely to benefit from gamma globulin. Such children instead should be given aspirin, 3 to 5 mg/kg once daily. In patients who already have developed coronary aneurysms and already have passed beyond 4 weeks from onset, there is no evidence to suggest any beneficial effect of gamma globulin.

Aspirin

On the same day that gamma globulin is administered, aspirin therapy also should be started. The aspirin dosage most thoroughly studied in the United States is 100 mg/kg/day until defervescence or until the fourteenth day of illness, followed by a daily dose of 5 to 10 mg/kg until the erythrocyte sedimentation rate and platelet counts return to normal, usually by about 3 months after illness onset. The optimal dose of aspirin in Kawasaki disease is controversial. High-dose aspirin (greater than 80 mg/kg/day), adjusted to produce a serum salicylate level of 18 to 28 mg/dL, theoretically might decrease the intensity of vasculitis, whereas much lower doses (e.g., 3 to 10 mg/kg/day) might be expected to provide optimal inhibition of platelet aggregation. Both dosage regimens have been endorsed by different American investigators. Japanese clinicians generally have used an intermediate antipyretic dose of 30 to 50 mg/kg/day.[177] Two retrospective studies suggested that children who received early treatment with high-dose aspirin had a lower rate of aneurysm development than did those who did not receive aspirin at all or those whose therapy was started late.[48, 169] Difficulty in obtaining therapeutic anti-inflammatory serum salicylate levels during the acute phase of illness may complicate aspirin treatment.[130] Koren and associates[170] linked this phenomenon to impaired bioavailability and enhanced salicylate clearance. Salicylate levels should be obtained if symptoms of vomiting, hyperpnea, lethargy, or liver function abnormalities develop in children receiving aspirin. To decrease the risk of Reye syndrome, aspirin can be interrupted if patients develop varicella, influenza B, or influenza A during the follow-up phase.

Initial Management

All patients with Kawasaki disease should be admitted to a hospital to receive gamma globulin infusion and to be observed until fever is controlled. Cardiovascular function should be monitored carefully. Once a child's fever has subsided, it is unlikely that significant congestive heart failure or myocardial dysfunction will occur. All patients should be evaluated within 1 week after discharge and should have an echocardiogram between 21 and 28 days after onset of fever. If baseline and 3- to 4-week echocardiograms fail to detect evidence of coronary abnormality, further echocardiograms are unnecessary. In a study of more than 800 patients, abnormalities at 8 weeks were not detected in patients who had normal 3- to 4-week echocardiograms. Patients with no evidence of coronary abnormalities should receive 3 to 5 mg/kg (maximum, 80 mg) of aspirin per day for approximately 3 months, the period required for both platelet count and sedimentation rate to return to normal.

Cardiovascular Evaluations

The development of coronary artery stenosis that may result in myocardial ischemia and infarction remains the most important clinical problem in following patients with Kawasaki disease. Patients with medium (6 to 8 mm) and large (>8 mm) aneurysms are at greater risk for development of stenosis.[138] Noninvasive methods, such as echocardiography and electrocardiography, are not sufficiently sensitive to detect stenotic lesions directly. It has been found that exercise and dypyridamole stress thallium 201 myocardial nuclear scanning and electron beam tomography are the most sensitive noninvasive measures to detect myocardial ischemia.[137] Coronary arteriography remains the most definitive method to determine the degree of stenosis and the adequacy of collateral circulation. Intravascular ultrasound is an effective method to evaluate vascular wall morphology during angiography.[327, 331] The indications for and timing of angiography remain unclear, although all patients with evidence of myocardial ischemia and infarction should be studied by angiography to determine the need for and type of intervention.

LONG-TERM MANAGEMENT

Patients with No Evidence of Coronary Artery Abnormalities

For patients without coronary artery involvement there is no need for aspirin or other antiplatelet medication beyond 3 months after illness onset or for restriction of physical activities in the convalescent stage. Cardiac evaluation and electrocardiography every 2 to 3 years may be prudent.

Patients with Transient or Small Coronary Aneurysms

Patients with coronary artery involvement that does not include giant aneurysms should be started on long-term therapy with aspirin, 3 to 5 mg/kg/day, at least until resolution of abnormalities, and preferably indefinitely. Such patients should be followed with yearly cardiac evaluations and undergo periodic stress testing after they reach the age of 5 years. There is no need for restriction of physical activities in patients without stress test abnormalities. Angiography is indicated if electrocardiographic or stress test abnormalities develop.

Patients with Giant Coronary Aneurysms (Greater than 8 mm in Diameter)

Therapy with aspirin, 3 to 5 mg/kg once daily, with or without dipyridamole, 3 to 4 mg/kg/day in three doses, is indicated for children with giant coronary aneurysms and should be continued indefinitely. All such patients should be under the care of a cardiologist, preferably a pediatric cardiologist with extensive experience in managing Kawasaki disease patients. Anticoagulant therapy with warfarin sodium should be added for most of these patients, especially during the first 2 years after disease onset. Cardiac evaluation should be performed every 6 months with periodic stress testing. Angiography should be performed initially to define the extent of disease and whenever symptoms or stress tests indicate myocardial ischemia. Physical activity should be regulated on the basis of stress test results and level of anticoagulation.

Patients with obstructive lesions or signs of ischemia may need to be evaluated for possible surgical intervention. Balloon angioplasty, rotablator angioplasty, coronary artery bypass grafting, and cardiac transplantation all have been employed for patients with serious coronary artery pathology.

COMPLICATIONS

Myocardial Infarction

Myocardial infarction is the most common cause of death in Kawasaki disease. A cooperative study in Japan involving 195 cases found that the first myocardial infarction was fatal in 22 per cent and asymptomatic in 37 per cent. It was most common in the first year after onset of disease. Major symptoms were shock, vomiting, and abdominal pain with chest pain found primarily in children older than 4 years of age. Of those surviving the first attack, 16 per cent had a second myocardial infarction.[145, 151] Fatal infarctions tended to involve the left main coronary artery or a combination of the right main and left anterior descending arteries; survivors were most likely to have isolated right coronary involvement. Approximately half of the survivors of acute myocardial infarction had one or more complications, such as ventricular dysfunction, mitral regurgitation, and arrhythmias. Patients with large coronary aneurysms are at greatest risk. Parents of all children with coronary abnormalities should be instructed to contact a physician and alert the emergency medical system if chest pain, dyspnea, extreme lethargy, or syncope develops. Prompt fibrinolytic therapy with streptokinase, urokinase, or tissue plasminogen activator should be attempted at a tertiary care center if acute coronary thrombosis is diagnosed.[143]

Other Cardiac Complications

As noted earlier, other cardiac complications include myocardial fibrosis, myocardial failure, and valvulitis. A recent study has suggested valvular disease in more than 1 per cent of cases, most of which resulted in mitral regurgitation.[7]

Peripheral Vascular Compromise

A rare complication seen in the acute febrile stage is peripheral vasoconstriction and gangrene of distal extremities.[354] This usually occurs only in severe systemic illness with widespread vascular involvement and has been managed with either prostaglandin E_1 infusion, 0.007 to 0.03 mg/kg/minute, maintained over several days in an intensive care unit with constant hemodynamic monitoring,[362] or with systemic heparinization and corticosteroid pulse therapy (methylprednisolone, 25 mg/kg administered by rapid intravenous infusion). Success with both approaches has been reported anecdotally.

Noncardiac Complications

Although Kawasaki disease is a multisystem disease, severe systemic involvement generally is self-limited. Although intense and painful, acute-stage arthritis has self-limited involvement, usually less than 2 weeks. Despite treatment of arthritic Kawasaki disease patients with both high-dose aspirin (100 mg/kg/day) and with other nonsteroidal anti-inflammatory drugs, such as tolmetin sodium (20 mg/kg/day in three divided doses), we have not seen impressive clinical responses. Many patients with large effusions appear to benefit most from arthrocentesis, which usually has to be done only once. Abdominal pain and diarrhea in the early acute stage usually respond to intravenous hydration and supportive care. Gallbladder hydrops, presenting clinically as a right upper quadrant mass with or without obstructive jaundice, can be confirmed and monitored by ultrasonography until its resolution. Surgical removal of the dilated gallbladder is not necessary. Hepatic involvement appears to be entirely self-limited (lasting less than 3 months) and is not associated with chronic or progressive disability.

Rare events reported to have occurred in association with Kawasaki disease include hearing loss and various transient or secondary complications. Some of these may be unassociated with the disease process. These include facial nerve palsy[93] and, more rarely, cerebral embolus, subarachnoid hemorrhage, ataxia, encephalopathy, hemiparesis, renal infarct, nephritis, and nephrosis. Telephone consultation with a center treating large numbers of Kawasaki disease patients should be sought by the physician faced with rare or serious complications.

PROGNOSIS

Kawasaki disease normally is acute and self-limited; however, cardiac damage sustained when the disease is active may be progressive. From multiple studies, it is clear that approximately 20 per cent of all patients not treated with intravenous gamma globulin develop coronary artery aneurysms that are detectable by angiography or two-dimensional echocardiography. These abnormalities may appear as early as 7 days and as late as 4 weeks after onset. The risk of coronary aneurysms now has been lowered to about 3 per cent when gamma globulin is given in the first 10 days of illness.[257, 258] However, for infants, even with gamma globulin treatment, the risk of coronary abnormalities at 8 weeks still is 15 per cent. Patients with coronary artery abnormalities are at risk of myocardial infarction, sudden death, and myocardial ischemia for a period of at least 5 years after onset of illness.[145] Regression of small and medium aneurysms appears to be common. Although one-third of children continue to have coronary artery dilation, approximately one-half with coronary aneurysms at 8 weeks post onset have regression by 1 year, as shown by apparently normal vessels on angiography or echocardiography.[151] Regression of the internal lumen of the aneurysm to normal diameter may occur by intimal proliferation or by thrombus organization and recanalization. Regression usually occurs within 2 years of onset. Previously aneurysmal segments are known to have an abnormal functional response with decreased ability to dilate in response to exercise or pharmacologic agents.[307, 329] Most patients with regressed aneurysms do not progress to stenosis, but tortuosity and coronary thrombosis still may occur.[147, 330, 332]

Patients with giant aneurysms are known to be at risk for the development of significant stenosis with resultant myocardial ischemia.[344] The risk of developing significant stenosis in the area of a large or medium coronary aneurysm shows a steady rise over 15 to 20 years of observation.[138, 328] These markedly abnormal vessels are subject to calcification and thrombosis and may cause myocardial ischemia or infarction. The giant aneurysm risk, 3 to 7 per cent of untreated patients, also has been lowered dramatically by gamma globulin therapy.[298] The U.S. Multicenter Kawasaki Disease Study Group has administered gamma globulin to more than 800 patients. Six of these patients developed giant aneurysms, but only three developed coronary artery dilation after gamma globulin was begun.[42]

To date, there is no evidence for significant cardiovascular sequelae in patients with no evidence of coronary artery abnormalities in the first month after onset. One study, however, has demonstrated functional abnormalities of coronary vessel endothelium relaxation compared with a mean of 6 years since onset of Kawasaki disease.[242] Newer imaging methods (ultrafast computed tomography and intravenous ultrasound) have demonstrated internal changes in patients with no history of abnormalities in the acute phase. The meaning of these persistent, pervasive vascular abnormalities in those thought to have escaped coronary abnormalities with acute Kawasaki disease and their long-term significance completely are unclear at this time.

Although a Kawasaki disease mortality rate of approximately 2 per cent was reported in the mid-1970s, in Japan the mortality rate has dropped to approximately 0.1 per cent.[154, 368] This improvement coincided with widespread use of aspirin and greater awareness of cardiac complications, which led to more intensive follow-up, better supportive care, and increased recognition of Kawasaki disease, possibly leading to the inclusion of milder cases in the total. The true long-term prognosis of Kawasaki disease is not known because follow-up studies into the second and third decades after disease are not completed.

Ten- to 20-year follow-up studies of Kawasaki disease are beginning to be performed.[138, 328] These studies demonstrate that large and medium aneurysms may progress to stenosis usually at the inlet or outlet throughout the follow-up period. The arteries most likely to develop stenosis are the right main and left anterior descending arteries. A very limited number of postmortem studies of adults who had a history of diagnosed Kawasaki disease or a compatible clinical illness have been performed. Fatty deposits from cells and advanced changes similar to atherosclerotic disease have been found,[334] raising the important issue of whether Kawasaki disease patients may be at an increased risk for earlier or more severe atherosclerosis. Intravascular ultrasound studies show that thickened arteries and coronary calcification are present in areas of regressed aneurysms. These changes resemble those of atherosclerosis.[104, 330]

A survey of adult cardiologists throughout Japan found 130 adult patients with coronary aneurysms.[126] These aneurysms were detected by angiography performed to evaluate myocardial infarction or ischemia. Twenty-one of these patients, with a mean age of 34 years (range, 20 to 63 years), had a history compatible with Kawasaki syndrome in childhood. These patients had severe clinical coronary artery disease with myocardial infarction, angina pectoris, mitral regurgitation, arrhythmias, a need for coronary bypass grafting, and congestive heart failure. This study indicates that the coronary artery sequelae of Kawasaki disease may be an important cause of ischemic heart disease in young adults.

The arteritis of Kawasaki syndrome may cause long-lasting changes in blood vessel function, even in those with no evidence of coronary artery abnormalities in the acute and subacute phases. For those with acute coronary artery abnormalities, the highest risk is for children with large and medium aneurysms, who are at risk for myocardial ischemia, infarction, and sudden death, particularly in the first year after onset. In the first 2 years after onset, regression of aneurysms with restoration of a normal lumen size occurs in one-third to one-half of those with aneurysms. These patients have persistent functional and structural abnormalities but appear to have a good short-term prognosis without evidence of ischemia. Those with persistent coronary aneurysms are at risk for the ultimate development of hemodynamically significant stenosis and the need for medical and surgical intervention.

The important question about whether childhood Kawasaki disease increases the risk for coronary atherosclerosis for all or most patients can be answered only by long-term prospective cohort studies.

References

1. Abe, J., Kotzin, B. L., Jujo, K., et al.: Selective expansion of T cells expressing T-cell receptor variable regions V beta 2 and V beta 8 in Kawasaki disease. Proc. Natl. Acad. Sci. U. S. A. *89*:4066–4070, 1992.
2. Abe, J., Kotzin, B. L., Meissner, C., et al.: Characterization of T cell repertoire changes in acute Kawasaki disease. J. Exp. Med. *177*:791–796, 1993.
3. Abe, J., Takeda, T., Ito, Y., et al.: TCR-V specificity of *Staphylococcus aureus* isolated from acute patients with Kawasaki syndrome. *In* Kato, H. (ed.): Kawasaki Disease. Amsterdam, Elsevier Science, 1995, pp. 127–132.
4. Abe, Y., Nakano, S., Nakahara, T., et al.: Detection of serum antibody by the antimitogen assay against streptococcal erythrogenic toxins: Age distribution in children and the relation to Kawasaki disease. Pediatr. Res. *27*:11–15, 1990.
5. Adler, R., Boxstein, D., Schaff, P., et al.: Metallic mercury vapor poisoning stimulating mucocutaneous lymph node syndrome. J. Pediatr. *107*:967–968, 1982.
6. Ahlström, H., Lundström, N. R., Mortensson, W., et al.: Infantile periarteritis nodosa or mucocutaneous lymph node syndrome: A report of four cases and diagnostic considerations. Acta Paediatr. Scand. *66*:193–198, 1977.
7. Akagi, T., Kato, H., Inoue, O., et al.: Valvular heart disease in Kawasaki syndrome: Incidence and natural history. Am. Heart J. *120*:366–372, 1990.
8. Amano, S., Hazama, F., and Hamashima, Y.: Pathology of Kawasaki disease. I. Pathology and morphogenesis of the vascular changes. Jpn. Circ. J. *43*:633–643, 1979.
9. Amano, S., Hazama, F., and Hamashima, Y.: Pathology of Kawasaki disease. II. Distribution and incidence of the vascular lesions. Jpn. Circ. J. *43*:741–748, 1979.
10. Anderson, L. J., Morens, D. M., and Hurwitz, E. S.: Kawasaki disease in a young adult. Arch. Intern. Med. *140*:280–281, 1980.
11. Anderson, T., Meyer, R. A., and Kaplan, S.: Long-term evaluation of cardiac size and function in patients with Kawasaki disease. J. Am. Coll. Cardiol. *1*:714, 1983.
12. Anonymous: Antibodies to endothelial cells. Lancet *337*:649–650, 1991.
13. Arita, K., Ikuta, K., Nishi, Y., et al.: Heterophile Hanganutziu-Deicher antibodies in sera of patients with Kawasaki diseases. Biken J. *25*:157–162, 1982.
14. Aschner, M., and Aschner, J. L.: Mucocutaneous lymph node syndrome: Is there a relationship to mercury exposure? Am. J. Dis. Child. *143*:1133–1134, 1989.
15. Barbour, A. G., Krueger, G. G., Feorino, P. M., et al.: Kawasaki-like disease in a young adult: Association with primary Epstein-Barr virus infection. J. A. M. A. *241*:397–398, 1979.
16. Barron, K., DeCunton, C., Montalvo, J., et al.: Abnormalities of immunoregulation in Kawasaki syndrome. J. Rheumatol. *15*:1243–1249, 1988.
17. Barron, K. S., Montalvo, J. F., Joseph, A. K., et al.: Soluble interleukin-2 receptors in children with Kawasaki syndrome. Arthritis Rheum. *33*:1371–1377, 1990.
18. Barron, K. S., Murphy, D. J., Silverman, E. D., et al.: Treatment of Kawasaki syndrome: A comparison of two dosage regimens of intravenously administered globulins. J. Pediatr. *117*:638–644, 1990.
19. Barron, K. S., Silverman, E. D., Gonzales, J. C., et al.: Major histocompatibility complex class II alleles in Kawasaki syndrome: Lack of consistent correlation with disease or cardiac involvement. J. Rheumatol. *19*:1790–1793, 1992.
20. Becker, A. E.: Kawasaki disease. Lancet *1*:864, 1976.
21. Becker, A. E., Beekman, R. P., and van der Hal, A. L.: De infantiele polyarteritis nodosa en de ziekte van Kawasaki ("muco-cutaneous lymph node syndrome"): Twee verschillende ziekten of uitingen van een zelfde ziekteproces? Ned. Tijdschr. Geneeskd. *120*:2147–2151, 1976.
22. Bell, D. M., Brink, E. W., Nitzkin, J., et al.: Kawasaki syndrome: Description of two outbreaks in the United States. N. Engl. J. Med. *304*:1568–1575, 1981.
23. Bell, D. M., Morens, D. M., Holman, R. C., et al.: Kawasaki syndrome in the United States. Am. J. Dis. Child. *137*:211–224, 1983.
24. Bergeson, P. S., Serlin, S. P., and Corman, L. I.: Mucocutaneous lymph-node syndrome with a positive Weil-Felix reaction but negative *Leptospira* studies. Lancet *1*:720–721, 1978.

25. Blum-Hoffmann, E., Hoffman, G. F., Wessel, A., et al.: Kawasaki syndrome: Association mit der exposition von teppichshampoo und erfolgreiche therapie mit immunoglobulinen in der zweiten krankheitswoche. Monatsschr. Kinderheilk. *140*:273–276, 1992.
26. Bos, S. E., and Kooi-Voskuyl, M. J. P.: Het mucocutane lymfkliersyndroom, de ziekte van Kawasaki. Ned. Tijdschr. Geneeskd. *122*:1184–1187, 1978.
27. Boven, K., De Fraeff-Meeder, E. R., Spliet, W., et al.: Atypical Kawasaki disease: An often missed diagnosis. Eur. J. Pediatr. *151*:577–580, 1992.
28. Bülow, S. L., Hansen, U. S., Hansen, D., et al.: Kawasaki's sygdom: Forekomst i Danmark i perioden 1981–1990. Ugeskr. Laeger. *156*:4813–4816, 1994.
29. Burke, M. J., and Rennebohm, R. M.: Eye involvement in Kawasaki disease. J. Pediatr. Ophthalmol. Strabismus *18*:7–11, 1981.
30. Burns, J. C., Geha, R. S., Schneeberger, E. E., et al.: Polymerase activity in lymphocyte culture supernatants from patients with Kawasaki disease. Nature *323*:814–816, 1987.
31. Burns, J. C., Wiggins, J. W., Toews, W. H., et al.: Clinical spectrum of Kawasaki syndrome in infants younger than 6 months of age. J. Pediatr. *109*:759–763, 1986.
32. Butler, D. F., Hough, D. R., Friedman, S. J., et al.: Adult Kawasaki syndrome. Arch. Dermatol. *123*:1356–1361, 1987.
33. Capps, J. A.: Aneurysm of the coronary artery: A report of two cases. Am. J. Med. Sci. *118*:312–318, 1989.
34. Caron, G. A.: Kawasaki disease in an adult. J. A. M. A. *243*:430, 1980.
35. Carter, R. F., Haynes, M. E., and Morton, J.: *Rickettsia*-like bodies and splenitis in Kawasaki disease. Lancet *2*:1254–1255, 1976.
36. Casey, F., Craig, B., Shanks, D., et al.: Kawasaki disease: The Northern Ireland experience. Ir. J. Med. Sci. *162*:397–400, 1993.
37. Centers for Disease Control: Lyme disease. M. M. W. R. *30*:668–672, 1989.
38. Chang, C. C., Hawkins, B. R., Kao, H. K., et al.: Human leucocyte antigens in Southern Chinese with Kawasaki disease. Eur. J. Pediatr. *151*:866, 1992.
39. Cheek, D. B.: Comment on mucocutaneous lymph node syndrome: Could it be a heavy metal poisoning? Pediatrics *56*:335–336, 1973.
40. Chiba, S., Kaneko, K., Hashimoto, N., et al.: *Yersinia pseudotuberculosis* and Kawasaki disease. Pediatr. Infect. Dis. *2*:494, 1983.
41. Chow, Y. M., Lin, C. Y., and Hwang, B.: Serum and urinary interleukin-6 (IL-6) levels as predicting factors of Kawasaki disease activity. Acta Paediatr. Sin. *34*:77–83, 1993.
42. Chung, K. J., and U.S. Multicenter Kawasaki Study Group: Incidence and prognosis of giant coronary artery aneurysms in Kawasaki disease. Circulation *80*(Suppl.):II–282, 1989.
43. Chusid, M. J., and Tang, T. T.: Fever, diarrhea, anemia, rash, and acrocyanosis in a 2-month-old girl. J. Pediatr. *93*:1052–1057, 1978.
44. Cook, D. H., Antia, A., Attie, F., et al.: Results from an international survey of Kawasaki disease in 1979–1982. Can. J. Cardiol. *5*:389–394, 1989.
45. Corbeel, L., Delmotte, E., Standaert, L., et al.: Kawasaki disease in Europe. Lancet *1*:797, 1977.
46. Crocker, D. W., Sobin, S., and Thomas, W. C.: Aneurysms of the coronary arteries: Report of three cases in infants and review of the literature. Am. J. Pathol. *33*:819–843, 1957.
47. Damiano, A., Zulaica, D., Cuadrado, E., et al.: Immunologic findings in Kawasaki disease. Ann. Intern. Med. *94*:138–139, 1981.
48. Daniels, S. R., Specker, B., Capannari, T. E., et al.: Predictors of coronary artery aneurysms in patients with Kawasaki disease. Pediatr. Res. *20*:169A, 1986.
49. Daniels, S. R., and Specker, B.: Association of rug shampooing and Kawasaki disease. J. Pediatr. *118*:485–488, 1991.
50. Davis, R. L., Waller, P. L., Mueller, B. A., et al.: Kawasaki syndrome in Washington State: Race-specific incidence rates and residential proximity to water. Arch. Pediatr. Adolesc. Med. *149*:66–69, 1995.
51. Dean, A. G., Melish, M. E., Hicks, R. V., et al.: An epidemic of Kawasaki syndrome in Hawaii. J. Pediatr. *100*:552–557, 1982.
52. Della Porta, G. G., and Alberta, A.: Kawasaki disease in Europe. Lancet *1*:797–798, 1977.
53. Dennis, M. K., Ayoub, E. M., Graham, T., et al.: Mucocutaneous lymph node syndrome in Florida. J. Fla. Med. Assoc. *64*:21–26, 1977.
54. Ding, X. T., Yang, X. Q., Li, C. R., et al.: Immunologic abnormalities in children with acute Kawasaki disease. Chin. Med. J. (Engl.) *106*:688–692, 1993.
55. Eberhard, B. A., Anderson, U., Laxer, R. M., et al.: Evaluation of the cytokine response in Kawasaki disease. Pediatr. Infect. Dis. J. *14*:199–203, 1995.
56. Edlinger, E. A., Benichou, J. J., and Labrune, B.: Positive *Erlichia canis* serology in Kawasaki disease. Lancet *1*:1146–1147, 1980.
57. Embil, J. A., McFarlane, E. S., Murphy, D. M., et al.: Adenovirus type 2 isolated from a patient with fatal Kawasaki disease. Can. Med. Assoc. J. *132*:1400, 1985.
58. Enders, G., Biber, M., Meyer, G., et al.: Prevalence of antibodies to human herpesvirus 6 in different age groups, in children with exanthem subitum, other acute exanthematous childhood diseases, Kawasaki syndrome, and acute infections with other herpesviruses and HIV. Infection *18*:12–15, 1990.
59. Engle, M. A., Fatica, N. S., Bussel, J. B., et al.: Clinical trial of single dose intravenous gamma globulin in Kawasaki disease: Preliminary report. Am. J. Dis. Child. *143*:1300–1304, 1989.
60. Everett, E. D.: Mucocutaneous lymph node syndrome (Kawasaki's disease) in adults. J. A. M. A. *242*:542–543, 1979.
61. Fatica, N. S., Ichida, F., Engle, M. A., et al.: Rug shampoo and Kawasaki disease. Pediatrics *84*:231–234, 1989.
62. Feigin, R. D., and Schleien, C. L.: Kawasaki disease. *In* Remington, J. S., and Swartz, M. N. (eds.): Current Topics in Infectious Diseases. New York, McGraw-Hill, 1983, pp. 30–63.
63. Fildes, N., Burns, J. C., Newburger, J. W., et al.: The HLA class II region and susceptibility to Kawasaki disease. Tissue Antigens *39*:99–101, 1992.
64. Fink, C. W.: Childhood polyarteritis. *In* Hicks, R. V. (ed.): Vasculopathies of Childhood. Littleton, MA, PSG Publishing, 1988, pp. 272–283.
65. Fossard, C., and Thompson, R. A.: Mucocutaneous lymph-node syndrome (Kawasaki disease): Probable soluble-complex disorder. Br. Med. J. *1*:883, 1977.
66. Fowler, R. N., Stevenson, R. E., Burton, O. M., et al.: Mucocutaneous lymph node syndrome in South Carolina. J. South Carolina Med. Assoc. *75*:11–14, 1979.
67. Fujimoto, T., Kato, H., Ichiose, E., et al.: Immune complex and mite antigen in Kawasaki disease. Lancet *2*:980–981, 1982.
68. Fujita, Y., Nakamura, Y., Sakata, K., et al.: Kawasaki disease in families. Pediatrics *84*:666–669, 1989.
69. Fujiwara, H., Fujiwara, T., Kao, T. C., et al.: Pathology of Kawasaki disease in the healed stage: Relationships between typical and atypical cases of Kawasaki disease. Acta Pathol. Jpn. *36*:857–867, 1986.
70. Fujiwara, H., and Hamashima, Y.: Pathology of the heart in Kawasaki disease. Pediatrics *61*:100–107, 1978.
71. Fujiwara, H., Kao, T. C., Shimizu, J., et al.: Microorganism in the heart in Kawasaki disease. Lancet *2*:620–621, 1983.
72. Fujiwara, H., Kawai, C., and Hamashima, Y.: Clinico-pathologic study of the conduction systems in 10 patients with Kawasaki's disease (mucocutaneous lymph node syndrome). Am. Heart J. *96*:744–750, 1978.
73. Fujiwara, T., Fujiwara, H., and Nakano, H.: Pathological features of coronary arteries in children with Kawasaki disease in which coronary arterial aneurysm was absent at autopsy: Quantitative analysis. Circulation *78*:345–350, 1988.
74. Fukushige, J., Nihill, M. R., and McNamara, D. G.: Spectrum of cardiovascular lesions in mucocutaneous lymph node syndrome: Analysis of eight cases. Am. J. Cardiol. *45*:98–107, 1980.
75. Fukushige, J., Takahashi, N., and Ueda, Y.: Incidence and clinical features of incomplete Kawasaki disease. Acta Paediatr. *83*:1057–1060, 1994.
76. Fukushige, J., Takahashi, N., Ueda K., et al.: Kawasaki disease and parvovirus B19 antibody: Role of immunoglobulin therapy in Kawasaki disease. *In* Kato, H. (ed.): Kawasaki Disease. Amsterdam, Elsevier Science, 1995, pp. 170–173.
77. Fulton, D. R.: Effects of current therapy of Kawasaki disease on eicosanoid metabolism. Am. J. Cardiol. *61*:1323–1327, 1988.
78. Furukawa, S., Matsubara, T., Jujoh, K., et al.: Peripheral blood monocyte/macrophages and serum tumor necrosis factor in Kawasaki disease. Clin. Immunol. Immunopathol. *48*:247–251, 1988.
79. Furukawa, S., Matsubara, T., Motohashi, T., et al.: Expression of FcεR2/CD23 on peripheral blood macrophages/monocytes in Kawasaki disease. Clin. Immunol. Immunopathol. *56*:280–286, 1990.
80. Furukawa, S., Matsubara, T., Jujoh, K., et al.: Reduction of peripheral blood macrophages/monocytes in Kawasaki disease by intravenous gamma globulin. Eur. J. Pediatr. *150*:43–47, 1990.
81. Furukawa, S., Matsubara, T., Motohashi, T., et al.: Increased expression of FcεR2/CD23 on peripheral blood B lymphocytes and serum IgE levels in Kawasaki disease. Int. Arch. Allergy Appl. Immunol. *95*:7–12, 1991.
82. Furukawa, S., Matsubara, T., Tsuji, K., et al.: Comparison of Kawasaki disease and infectious mononucleosis in terms of natural killer cell and CD8+ T cell subsets. J. Infect. Dis. *163*:416–417, 1991.
83. Furukawa, S., Imai, K., Matsubara, T., et al.: Increased levels of intercellular adhesion molecule 1 in Kawasaki disease. Arthritis Rheum. *35*:672–677, 1992.
84. Furukawa, S., Matsubara, T., and Yabuta, K.: Mononuclear cell subsets and coronary artery lesions in Kawasaki disease. Arch. Dis. Child. *67*:706–708, 1992.
85. Furukawa, S., Matsubara, T., Yone, K., et al.: Kawasaki disease differs from anaphylactoid purpura and measles with regard to tumour necrosis factor-α and interleukin 6 in serum. Eur. J. Pediatr. *151*:44–47, 1992.
86. Furukawa, S., Matsubara, T., Okumura, K., et al.: Decreased expression of CD23 on peripheral blood macrophages/monocytes during acute Kawasaki disease with coronary artery lesions. Int. Arch. Allergy Immunol. *102*:335–339, 1993.
87. Furukawa, S., Matsubara, T., Tsuji, K., et al.: Transient depletion of T cells with Bright CD11a/CD18 expression from peripheral circulation during acute Kawasaki disease. Scand. J. Immunol. *37*:377–380, 1993.
88. Furukawa, S., Matsubara, T., Umezawa, Y., et al.: Serum levels of p60 soluble tumor necrosis factor receptor during acute Kawasaki disease. J. Pediatr. *124*:721–725, 1994.
89. Furumoto, H., Sakano, T., Tanabe, A., et al.: Serum soluble CD8 antigen level is not elevated in mucocutaneous lymph node syndrome (Kawasaki

disease) in spite of an increase in serum soluble interleukin 2 receptors. Eur. J. Pediatr. *149*:448–449, 1990.
90. Furuse, A., and Matsuda, I.: Circulating immune complex in the mucocutaneous lymph node syndrome. Eur. J. Pediatr. *141*:50–51, 1983.
91. Furusho, K., Kamiya, T., Nakano, H., et al.: High-dose intravenous gamma globulin for Kawasaki disease. Lancet *2*:1055–1058, 1984.
92. Furusho, K., Ohba, T., Soeda, T., et al.: Possible role for mite antigen in Kawasaki disease. Lancet *2*:194–195, 1981.
93. Gallagher, P. G.: Facial nerve paralysis and Kawasaki disease. Rev. Infect. Dis. *12*:403–405, 1990.
94. Gee, S. J.: Aneurysms of the coronary arteries in a boy. St. Barth. Hosp. Rep. Lond. *7*:148, 1871.
95. Gentles, T. L., Clarkson, P. M., Trenholme, A. A., et al.: Kawasaki disease in Auckland, 1979–1988. N. Z. Med. J. *103*:389–391, 1990.
96. Germain, B. F., Moroney, J. D., Guggino, G. S., et al.: Anterior uveitis in Kawasaki disease. J. Pediatr. *97*:780–781, 1980.
97. Giesker, D. W., Krause, P. J., Pastuszak, W. T., et al.: Lymph node biopsy for early diagnosis in Kawasaki disease. Am. J. Surg. Pathol. *6*:493–501, 1982.
98. Glanz, S., Bittner, S. J., Berman, M. A., et al.: Regression of coronary artery aneurysms in infantile polyartertis nodosa. N. Engl. J. Med. *294*:939–941, 1976.
99. Glanzer, J. M., Galbraith, W. B., and Jacobs, J. P.: Kawasaki disease in a 28-year-old man. J. A. M. A. *244*:1604–1606, 1980.
100. Gleason, S. C., and Overton, R. W.: A possible case of mucocutaneous lymph node syndrome in Iowa. J. Iowa Med. Soc. *67*:396–397, 1977.
101. Glode, M. P., Brogden, R., Joffe, L. S., et al.: Kawasaki syndrome and house dust mite exposure. Pediatr. Infect. Dis. J. *5*:644–648, 1986.
102. Grenadier, E., Allen, H., Goldberg, S. J., et al.: Left ventricular wall motion abnormalities in Kawasaki disease. J. Am. Coll. Cardiol. *1*:714, 1982.
103. Hall, S. M.: Surveillance of Kawasaki disease in the British Isles. Arch. Dis. Child. *64*:1218, 1989.
104. Hamada, R., Uehara, R., and Fuyama, Y.: CT detection of coronary calcification in Kawasaki disease. *In* Kato, H. (ed.): Kawasaki Disease. Amsterdam, Elsevier Science, 1995, pp. 598–602.
105. Hamasaki, Y., Ichimaru, T., Koga, H., et al.: Increased in vitro leukotriene B4 production by stimulated polymorphonuclear cells in Kawasaki disease. Acta Paediatr. Jpn. *31*:346–348, 1989.
106. Hamasaki, Y., and Miyazaki, S.: Leukotriene B4 and Kawasaki disease. Acta Paediatr. Jpn. *33*:771–777, 1991.
107. Hamashima, Y., Kishi, K., and Tasaka, K.: *Rickettsia*-like bodies in infantile acute febrile mucocutaneous lymph-node syndrome. Lancet *2*:42, 1973.
108. Hamashima, Y., Kishi, K., Tasaka, K., et al.: Isolation of rickettsia-like particles in infantile acute febrile mucocutaneous lymph node syndrome (MCLS, so-called Kawasaki fever). Jpn. J. Clin. Med. *31*:3491–3505, 1973.
109. Hamashima, Y., Tasaka, K., Hoshino, T., et al.: Mite-associated particles in Kawasaki disease. Lancet *2*:266, 1982.
110. Hansen, R. C.: Staphylococcal scaled skin syndrome, toxic shock syndrome, and Kawasaki disease. Pediatr. Clin. North Am. *30*:533–544, 1983.
111. Headings, D. L., and Santosham, M.: Kawasaki disease associated with serologic evidence of Rocky Mountain spotted fever. Johns Hopkins Med. J. *149*:220–221, 1981.
112. Herman, A., Keppler, J. W., Marrack, P., et al.: Superantigens: Mechanism of T cell stimulation and role in immunologic responses. Ann. Rev. Immunol. *9*:745–772, 1991.
113. Herman, J.: Mucocutaneous lymph node syndrome in general practice. Practitioner *22*:261–262, 1979.
114. Herold, B. C., Davis, A. T., Arroyave, C. M., et al.: Cryoprecipitates in Kawasaki syndrome: Association with coronary artery aneurysms. Pediatr. Infect. Dis. J. *7*:255–257, 1988.
115. Hewitt, C. J.: Case of Kawasaki disease. Br. Med. J. *1*:883–884, 1977.
116. Hicks, R. V., and Melish, M. E.: Kawasaki syndrome: Rheumatic complaints and analysis of salicylate therapy. Arthritis Rheum. *22*:621–622, 1979.
117. Hidaka, T., Nakano, M., Ueta, T., et al.: Increased synthesis of thromboxane A2 by platelets from patients with Kawasaki disease. J. Pediatr. *102*:94–96, 1983.
118. Hiraishi, S., Yashiro, K., Oguchi, K., et al.: Clinical course of cardiovascular involvement in the mucocutaneous lymph node syndrome: Relation between clinical signs of carditis and development of coronary arterial aneurysm. Am. J. Cardiol. *47*:323–330, 1981.
119. Hirao, J., Yoshimura, N., Homma, N., et al.: Immunological studies on Kawasaki disease. II. Isolation and characterization of an immunosuppressive factor in acute phase sera. Clin. Exp. Immunol. *67*:433–440, 1987.
120. Hirose, S., and Hamashima, Y.: Morphological observations on the vasculitis in the mucocutaneous lymph node syndrome: A skin biopsy study of 27 patients. Eur. J. Pediatr. *129*:17–27, 1978.
121. Hurvitz, H., Branski, D., Gross-Kieselstein, E., et al.: Acetamenophen hypersensitivity resembling Kawasaki disease. Israel J. Med. Sci. *20*:145–147, 1984.
122. Ichida, F., Fatica, N. S., O'Loughlin, J. E., et al.: Epidemiologic aspects of Kawasaki disease in a Manhattan hospital. Pediatrics *84*:235–241, 1989.
123. Iizuka, T., Minatogawa, Y., Suzuki, H., et al.: Urinary neopterin as a predictive marker of coronary artery abnormalities in Kawasaki syndrome. Clin. Chem. *39*:600–604, 1993.
124. Imada, Y., Kawasaki, T., and Nakamura, Y.: Cousin cases of Kawasaki disease suggesting person-to-person transmission. Pediatrics *85*:1127, 1990.
125. Ino, T., Ohkubo, M., Shimazaki, S., et al.: Plasma endothelin concentration: Relation with vascular resistance and comparison before and after balloon dilatation procedures. Eur. J. Pediatr. *151*:416–419, 1992.
126. Inoue, O., Akagi, T., and Kato, H.: Fate of giant coronary artery aneurysms in Kawasaki disease. Circulation *80*(Suppl.):II–262, 1989.
127. Ishii, A., Yatani, T., Kato, H., et al.: Mite fauna, housedust, and Kawasaki disease. Lancet *2*:102–103, 1983.
128. Iwanaga, M., Takada, K., Osato, T., et al.: Kawasaki disease and Epstein-Barr virus. Lancet *1*:938–939, 1981.
129. Jacob, J. L., Polomeno, R. C., Chad, Z., et al.: Ocular manifestations of Kawasaki disease (mucocutaneous lymph node syndrome). Can. J. Ophthalmol. *17*:199–202, 1982.
130. Jacobs, J. C.: Salicylate treatment of epidemic Kawasaki disease in New York City. Ther. Drug Monit. *1*:123–130, 1979.
131. Jayne, D. R. W., and Lockwood, C. M.: Pathogenesis of acute Kawasaki disease. Lancet *335*:410–411, 1990.
132. Joffe, A., Kabani, A., and Jadavji, T.: Atypical and complicated Kawasaki disease in infants: Do we need criteria? West. J. Med. *162*:322–327, 1995.
133. John, T. J., DeBenedetti, C. D., and Zee, M. L.: Mucocutaneous lymph node syndrome in Arizona. Am. J. Dis. Child. *130*:613–614, 1976.
134. Johnson, D., and Azimi, P.: Kawasaki disease associated with *Klebsiella pneumoniae* bacteremia and parainfluenza type 3 virus infection. Pediatr. Infect. Dis. J. *4*:100, 1985.
135. Kalra, S., Owen, S. J., Hepworth, J., et al.: Airborne house dust mite antigen after vacuum cleaning. Lancet *336*:449, 1990.
136. Jordan, S. C., Platts-Mills, T. A., Mason, W., et al.: Lack of evidence for mite-antigen–mediated pathogenesis in Kawasaki disease. Lancet *1*:931, 1983.
137. Kamiya, T.: How to evaluate myocardial ischemia in Kawasaki disease. *In* Kato, H. (ed.): Kawasaki Disease. Amsterdam, Elsevier Science, 1995, pp. 447–450.
138. Kamiya, T., Suzuki, A., Ono, Y., et al.: Angiographic follow-up study of coronary artery lesion in the cases with a history of Kawasaki disease: With a focus on the follow-up more than 10 years after the onset of the disease. *In* Kato, H. (ed.): Kawasaki Disease. Amsterdam, Elsevier Science, 1995, pp. 569–573.
139. Kaneko, K., Savage, C. O., Pottinger, B. E., et al.: Antiendothelial cell antibodies can be cytotoxic to endothelial cells without cytokine prestimulation and correlate with ELISA antibody measurement in Kawasaki disease. Clin. Exp. Immunol. *98*:264–269, 1994.
140. Kantor, N. M.: Mucocutaneous lymph node syndrome (Kawasaki disease): Report of four cases. J. Am. Osteopath. Assoc. *77*:901–906, 1978.
141. Kaslow, R. A., Bailowitz, A., Lin, F. Y. C., et al.: Association of epidemic Kawasaki syndrome with the HLA-A2, B44, Cw5 antigen combination. Arthritis Rheum. *28*:938–940, 1985.
142. Kato, H.: Natural history of Kawasaki disease. *In* Shiokawa Y. (ed.): Vascular Lesions of Collagen Diseases and Related Conditions. Baltimore, University Park Press, 1977, pp. 281–286.
143. Kato, H.: Intracoronary thrombolytic therapy in Kawasaki disease: Treatment and prevention of acute myocardial infarction. Prog. Clin. Biol. Res. *250*:445–454, 1987.
144. Kato, H., and Ichinose, E.: Cardiovascular involvement in Kawasaki disease. Acta Paediatr. Jpn. *26*:132–145, 1984.
145. Kato, H., Ichinose, E., and Kawasaki, T.: Myocardial infarction in Kawasaki disease. J. Pediatr. *108*:923–928, 1986.
146. Kato, H., Ichinose, E., Yoshioka, F., et al.: Fate of coronary aneurysms in Kawasaki disease: Serial coronary angiography and long-term follow-up study. Am. J. Cardiol. *49*:1758–1766, 1982.
147. Kato, H., Inoue, O., and Akagi, T.: Kawasaki disease: Cardiac problems and management. Pediatr. Rev. *9*:209–217, 1988.
148. Kato, H., Inoue, O., Koga, Y., et al.: Variant strain of *Propionibacterium acnes*: A clue to the aetiology of Kawasaki disease. Lancet *2*:1383–1387, 1983.
149. Kato, S., Kimura, M., Tsuji, K., et al.: HLA antigens in Kawasaki disease. Pediatrics *61*:252–255, 1978.
150. Kato, H., Koike, S., and Yokoyama, T.: Kawasaki disease: Effect of treatment of coronary artery involvement. Pediatrics *63*:175–179, 1979.
151. Kato, A.: Long-term consequences of Kawasaki disease: Pediatrics to adults. *In* Kato, H. (ed.): Kawasaki Disease. Amsterdam, Elsevier Science, 1995, pp. 557–566.
152. Kawasaki, T.: Acute febrile mucocutaneous syndrome with lymphoid involvement with specific desquamation of the fingers and toes in children. Jpn. J. Allerg. *16*:178–222, 1967.
153. Kawasaki, T.: Dr. Kawasaki replies. Pediatrics *56*:336–337, 1975.
154. Kawasaki, T.: Kawasaki disease. Asian Med. J. *32*:497–506, 1989.
155. Kawasaki, T., and Kosaki, F.: Febrile oculo-oro-cutaneo-acrodesquamatous syndrome with or without acute nonsuppurative cervical lymphadenitis in infancy and children: Clinical observations of 30 cases. Jpn. J. Allerg. *16*:225, 1967.
156. Kawasaki, T., Kosaki, F., Okawa, S., et al.: A new infantile acute febrile mucocutaneous lymph node syndrome (MLNS) prevailing in Japan. Pediatrics *54*:271–276, 1974.

157. Keim, D. E., Keller, E. W., and Hirsch, M. S.: Mucocutaneous lymph-node syndrome and parainfluenza 2 virus infection. Lancet 2:303, 1977.
158. Keren, G., Barzilay, G., Alpert, G., et al.: Mucocutaneous lymph node syndrome (Kawasaki disease) in Israel. Acta Paediatr. Scand. *72*:455–458, 1983.
159. Keren, G., Danon, Y. L., Orgad, S., et al.: HLA Bw 51 is increased in mucocutaneous lymph node syndrome in Israeli patients. Tissue Antigens *20*:144–146, 1982.
160. Kotb, M.: Superantigens: A possible link between infection and autoimmunity. *In* Kato, H. (ed.): Kawasaki Disease. Amsterdam, Elsevier Science, 1995, pp. 111–119.
161. Kikuta, H., Mizuno, F., and Osato, T.: Kawasaki disease and an unusual primary infection with Epstein-Barr virus. Pediatrics *73*:413–414, 1984.
162. Kikuta, H., Taguchi, Y., Tomizawa, K., et al.: Epstein-Barr virus genome-positive T lymphocytes in a boy with chronic active EBV infection associated with Kawasaki-like disease. Nature *333*:455–457, 1988.
163. Kim, D. S.: Serum interleukin-6 in Kawasaki disease. Yonsei Med. J. *33*:183–188, 1992.
164. Kim, D. S., and Lee, K. Y.: Serum soluble E-selectin levels in Kawasaki disease. Scand. J. Rheumatol. *23*:283–286, 1995.
165. Kisimoto, T.: B-cell stimulatory factors (BSFs): Molecular structure, biological function, and regulation of expression. J. Clin. Immunol. *7*:343–355, 1987.
166. Klein, B. S., Rogers, M. F., Patrican, L. A., et al.: Kawasaki syndrome: A controlled study of an outbreak in Wisconsin. Am. J. Epidemiol. *124*:306–316, 1986.
167. Kobayashi, S., Wada, N., and Kubo, M.: Antibodies to native type III collagen in the serum of patients with Kawasaki disease. Eur. J. Pediatr. *151*:183–187, 1992.
168. Kohsaka, T., Abe, J., Asahina, T., et al.: Classical pathway complement activation in Kawasaki syndrome. J. Allergy Clin. Immunol. *93*:520–525, 1994.
169. Koren, G., Rose, V., and Levi, S.: Probable efficacy of high dose salicylates in reducing coronary involvement in Kawasaki disease. J. A. M. A. *254*:767, 1985.
170. Koren, G., Schaffer, F., Silverman, E. D., et al.: Determinants of low serum salicylates in patients with Kawasaki disease. J. Pediatr. *112*:663–667, 1988.
171. Krensky, A. M., Berenberg, W., Shanley, K., et al.: HLA antigens in mucocutaneous lymph node syndrome in New England. Pediatrics *67*:741–744, 1981.
172. Krensky, A. M., Grady, S., Shanley, K. M., et al.: Epidemic and endemic HLA-B and DR associations in mucocutaneous lymph node syndrome. Hum. Immunol. *6*:75–77, 1983.
173. Krensky, A. M., Teele, R., Watkins, J., et al.: Streptococcal antigenicity in mucocutaneous lymph node syndrome and hydropic gallbladders. Pediatrics *64*:979–980, 1979.
174. Krous, H. F., Clausen, C. R., and Ray, C. G.: Elevated immunoglobulin E in infantile polyarteritis nodosa. Pediatrics *84*:841–845, 1974.
175. Krzyszkowski, J.: Periarteritis nodosa. Przegl. Post. Nauk. Lek. (Warsaw) *38*:30, 45, 58, 1899.
176. Kusakawa, S., and Heiner, D. C.: Elevated levels of immunoglobulin E in the acute febrile mucocutaneous lymph node syndrome. Pediatr. Res. *10*:108–111, 1976.
177. Kusakawa, S., and Tatara, K.: Efficacies and risks of aspirin in the treatment of Kawasaki disease. Prog. Clin. Biol. Res. *20*:401–413, 1987.
178. Lambert, H. P., Fisher-Hoch, S. P., and Grover, S. A.: Kawasaki disease and *Coxiella burnetii*. Lancet 2:844, 1985.
179. Landing, B. H., and Larson, E. J.: Are infantile periarteritis nodosa with coronary artery involvement and fatal mucocutaneous lymph node syndrome the same?: Comparison of 20 patients from North America with patients from Hawaii and Japan. Pediatrics *59*:651–662, 1977.
180. Lang, B. A., Silverman, E. D., Laxer, R. M., et al.: Spontaneous tumor necrosis factor production in Kawasaki disease. J. Pediatr. *115*:939–943, 1989.
181. Lang, B. A., Silverman, E. D., Laxer, R. M., et al.: Spontaneous tumor necrosis factor production in Kawasaki disease. J. Pediatr. *115*:939–943, 1989.
182. Lang, B. A., Silverman, E. D., Laxer, R. M., et al.: Serum-soluble interleukin-2 receptor levels in Kawasaki disease. J. Pediatr. *116*:592–596, 1990.
183. Lang, B. A., Silverman, E. D., Laxer, R. M., et al.: Serum-soluble interleukin-2 receptor levels in Kawasaki disease. J. Pediatr. *116*:592–596, 1990.
184. Lapointe, N., Chad, Z., Lacroix, J., et al.: Kawasaki disease: Association with uveitis in seven patients. Pediatrics *69*:376–379, 1982.
185. Larsen, J. H.: Kawasaki disease: A yersiniosis? J. Infect. Dis. *160*:900, 1989.
186. Larson, E. J.: Comparison of pathology of infantile periarteritis nodosa (IPN) with coronary artery disease in North America with Kawasaki disease (MCLS) in Hawaii and Japan. *In* Japan Medical Research Foundation (ed.): Vascular Lesions of Collagen Diseases and Related Conditions. Tokyo, University of Tokyo Press, 1977, pp. 322–334.
187. Lauer, B. A., Bruhn, F. W., Todd, J. K., et al.: Mucocutaneous lymph node syndrome in Denver. Am. J. Dis. Child. *130*:610–612, 1976.
188. Laxer, R. M., and Petty, R. E.: Hyponatremia in Kawasaki disease. Pediatrics *70*:655, 1982.
189. Lebranchu, Y., Malvy, D., Richard, M. J., et al.: Kawasaki disease and oxidative metabolism. Clin. Chim. Acta *187*:193–198, 1990.
190. Lee, D. B.: Epidemiological survey of Kawasaki syndrome in Korea (1976–1984). J. Cath. Med. Coll. *38*:13–19, 1985.
191. Lee, D. B.: Epidemiologic study of Kawasaki disease in Korea. Prog. Clin. Biol. Res. *250*:55–60, 1987.
192. Lee, L. A., Burns, J., Glode, M., et al.: No autoantibodies to nuclear antigens in the Kawasaki syndrome. N. Engl. J. Med. *308*:1034, 1983.
193. Lee, T. J., and Vaughan, D.: Mucocutaneous lymph node syndrome in a young adult. Arch. Intern. Med. *139*:104–105, 1979.
194. Lee, T., Furukawa, S., Fukuda, Y., et al.: Plasma prostaglandin E2 level in Kawasaki disease. Prostaglandins Leukotrienes Essential Fatty Acids *31*:53–57, 1988.
195. Lehman, T. J. A., and Mahnovski, V.: Animal models of vasculitis: Lessons we can learn to improve our understanding of Kawasaki disease. Rheum. Dis. Clin. North Am. *14*:479–487, 1988.
196. Lehman, T. J. A., Warren, R., Gietl, D., et al.: Variable expression of *Lactobacillus casei* wall-induced coronary arteritis: An animal model of Kawasaki's disease in selected inbred mouse strains. Clin. Immunol. Immunopathol. *48*:108–118, 1988.
197. Leung, D. Y. M.: Immunomodulation by intravenous immune globulin in Kawasaki disease. J. Allergy Clin. Immunol. *84*:588–594, 1989.
198. Leung, D. Y. M., Burns, J. C., Newburger, J. W., et al.: Reversal of lymphocyte activation in vivo in the Kawasaki syndrome by intravenous gammaglobulin. J. Clin. Invest. *79*:468–472, 1987.
199. Leung, D. Y. M., Chu, E. T., Wood, N., et al.: Immunoregulatory T cell abnormalities in mucocutaneous lymph node syndrome. J. Immunol. *130*:2002–2004, 1983.
200. Leung, D. Y. M., Collins, T., LaPierre, L. A., et al.: Immunoglobulin M antibodies present in the acute phase of Kawasaki syndrome lyse cultured vascular endothelial cells stimulated by gamma interferon. J. Clin. Invest. *77*:1428–1435, 1986.
201. Leung, D. Y. M., Collins, T., LaPierre, L. A., et al.: Immunoglobulin M antibodies present in the acute phase of Kawasaki syndrome lyse cultured vascular endothelial cells stimulated by gamma interferon. J. Clin. Invest. *77*:1428–1435, 1986.
202. Leung, D. Y. M., Geha, R., and Newberger, J.: Two monokines, interleukin-1 and tumor necrosis factor, render cultured vascular endothelial cells susceptible to lysis by antibodies circulating during Kawasaki syndrome. J. Exp. Med. *164*:1958–1972, 1986.
203. Leung, D. Y. M., Kurt-Jones, E., Newberger, J. W., et al.: Endothelial cell activation and high interleukin-1 secretion in the pathogenesis of acute Kawasaki disease. Lancet 2:1298–1302, 1989.
204. Leung, D. Y. M., Cotran, R. S., Kurt-Jones, E., et al.: Endothelial cell activation and high interleukin-1 secretion in the pathogenesis of acute Kawasaki disease. Lancet 2:1298–1302, 1989.
205. Leung, D. Y. M., Seigel, R. L., Grady, S., et al.: Immunoregulatory abnormalities in mucocutaneous lymph node syndrome. Clin. Immunol. Immunopathol. *23*:100–112, 1982.
206. Leung, D. Y. M.: The potential role of cytokine-mediated vascular endothelial activation in the pathogenesis of Kawasaki disease. Acta Paediatr. Jpn. *33*:739–744, 1991.
207. Levin, M., Holland, P. C., Nokes, T. J. C., et al.: Platelet immune complex interaction in pathogenesis of Kawasaki disease and childhood polyarteritis. Br. Med. J. *290*:1456–1460, 1985.
208. Levinsky, R., and Marshall, W. C.: Circulating immune complexes in mucocutaneous lymph node syndrome (Kawasaki disease). Arch. Dis. Child. *54*:240–245, 1979.
209. Leung, D. Y., Meissner, H. C., Fulton, D. R., et al.: Toxic shock syndrome toxin-secreting *Staphylococcus aureus* in Kawasaki syndrome. Lancet *342*:1385–1388, 1993.
210. Levy, M., and Koren, G.: Atypical Kawasaki disease: Analysis of clinical presentation and diagnostic clues. Pediatr. Infect. Dis. J. *9*:122–126, 1990.
211. Levy, M., and Koren, G.: Atypical Kawasaki disease: Analysis of clinical presentation and diagnostic clues. Pediatr. Infect. Dis. J. *9*:122–126, 1990.
212. Li, C. R., Yang, X. Q., Shen, J., et al.: Immunoglobulin G subclasses in serum and circulating immune complexes in patients with Kawasaki syndrome. Pediatr. Infect. Dis. J. *9*:544–547, 1990.
213. Lin, C. Y., Lin, C. C., Hwang, B., et al.: The changes of interleukin-2, tumor necrotic factor and gamma-interferon production among patients with Kawasaki disease. Eur. J. Pediatr. *150*:179–182, 1991.
214. Lin, C. Y., and Hwang, B.: Serial immunologic studies in patients with mucocutaneous lymph node syndrome (Kawasaki disease). Ann. Allergy *59*:291–297, 1987.
215. Lin, F. Y. C., Bailowitz, A., Koslowe, P., et al.: Kawasaki syndrome: A case-control study during an outbreak in Maryland. Am. J. Dis. Child. *139*:277–279, 1985.
216. Lin, C. Y., Lin, C. C., Hwang, B., et al.: Serial changes of serum interleukin-6, interleukin-8, and tumor necrosis factor alpha among patients with Kawasaki disease. J. Pediatr. *121*:924–926, 1992.
217. Lin, C Y., Lin, C. C., Hwang, B., et al.: Cytokines predict coronary aneurysm formation in Kawasaki disease patients. Eur. J. Pediatr. *152*:309–312, 1993.
218. Maeda, T., Yoshida, H., and Funabashi, T.: Subcostal 2-dimensional echocardiographic imaging of peripheral left coronary aneurysms in Kawasaki disease. Am. J. Cardiol. *52*:48–52, 1983.
219. Marchette, N. J., Melish, M. E., Hicks, R., et al.: Epstein-Barr virus and

other herpesvirus infections in Kawasaki syndrome. J. Infect. Dis. *161*:680–684, 1990.
220. Marchette, N. J., Melish, M. E., and Kihara, S.: Viral etiology of Kawasaki syndrome. Proc. Fourth Int. Kawasaki Dis. Symp. (in press).
221. Marchette, N. J., Melish, M. E., James, J. F., et al.: Spirochaetal studies in Kawasaki syndrome. Prog. Clin. Biol. Res. *250*:87–99, 1987.
222. Marchette, N. J., Cao, Y., Kihara, S., et al.: Staphylococcal toxic shock syndrome toxin-1, one possible cause of Kawasaki syndrome. *In* Kato, H. (ed.): Kawasaki Disease. Amsterdam, Elsevier Science, 1995, pp. 149–155.
223. Mason, W. H., Jordan, S. C., Sakai, R., et al.: Circulating immune complexes in Kawasaki syndrome. Pediatr. Infect. Dis. *4*:48–51, 1985.
224. Mason, W., Jordan, S., Sakai, R., et al.: Lack of effect of gamma-globulin infusion on circulating immune complexes in patients with Kawasaki syndrome. Pediatr. Infect. Dis. J. *7*:94–99, 1988.
225. Masuda, H., Shozawa, T., Naoe, S., et al.: The intercostal artery in Kawasaki disease: A pathologic study of 17 autopsy cases. Arch. Pathol. Lab. Med. *110*:1136–1142, 1986.
226. Matsubara, T., Furukawa, S., and Yabuta, K.: Serum levels of tumor necrosis factor, interleukin-2 receptor, and interferon-gamma in Kawasaki disease involved coronary artery lesions. Clin. Immunol. Immunopathol. *56*:29–36, 1990.
227. Matsubara, T., Furukawa, S., and Yabuta, K.: Serum levels of tumor necrosis factor, interleukin 2 receptor, and interferon-γ in Kawasaki disease involved coronary-artery lesions. Clin. Immunol. Immunopathol. *56*:29–36, 1990.
228. Matsubara, T., Furukawa, S., Ino, T., et al.: A sibship with recurrent Kawasaki disease and coronary artery lesion. Acta Paediatr. *83*:1002–1004, 1994.
229. Maury, C. P. J., Salo, E., and Pelkonen, P.: Elevated circulating tumor necrosis factor-α in patients with Kawasaki disease. J. Lab. Clin. Med. *113*:651–654, 1989.
230. Mayatepek, E., and Lehmann, W. D: Increased generation of cysteinyl leukotrienes in Kawasaki disease. Arch. Dis. Child. *72*:526–527, 1995.
231. Matsuda, I., Hattori, S., Nagata, N., et al.: HLA antigens in mucocutaneous lymph node syndrome. Am. J. Dis. Child. *131*:1417–1418, 1977.
232. Matsuno, S., Utagawa, E., and Sugiura, A.: Association of rotavirus infection with Kawasaki syndrome. J. Infect. Dis. *148*:177, 1983.
233. Maury, C. P. J., Salo, E., and Pelkonen, P.: Circulating interleukin-1 beta in patients with Kawasaki disease. N. Engl. J. Med. *312*:1670–1671, 1988.
234. Maury, C. P. J., Salo, E., and Pelkonen, P.: Elevated circulating tumor necrosis factor-alpha in patients with Kawasaki disease. J. Lab. Clin. Med. *113*:651–654, 1989.
235. Melekian, B.: Kawasaki-like infectious mononucleosis. Acta Paediatr. Scand. *71*:843–844, 1982.
236. Melish, M. E.: Kawasaki syndrome (the mucocutaneous lymph node syndrome). Pediatr. Ann. *11*:255–268, 1982.
237. Melish, M. E., Hicks, R. M., and Larson, E. J.: Mucocutaneous lymph node syndrome (MCLS) in the U.S. Pediatr. Res. *8*:427, 1974.
238. Melish, M. E., Hicks, R. M., and Larson, E. J.: Mucocutaneous lymph node syndrome in the United States. Am. J. Dis. Child. *130*:599–607, 1976.
239. Melish, M. E., Hicks, R. M., and Reddy, V.: Kawasaki syndrome: An update. Hosp. Pract. *17*:99–106, 1982.
240. Melish, M. E., Marchette, N. J., Kaplan, J. C., et al.: Absence of significant RNA-dependent DNA polymerase activity in lymphocytes from patients with Kawasaki syndrome. Nature *337*:288–290, 1989.
241. Milgrom, H., Palmer, E. L., Slovin, S. F., et al.: Kawasaki disease in a healthy young adult. Ann. Intern. Med. *92*:467–470, 1980.
242. Mitani, Y., Okada, Y., Inoue, M., et al.: Impaired endothelium dependent relaxation of angiographically normal coronary arteries in patients after Kawasaki disease in the long-term follow-up period. *In* Kato, H. (ed.): Kawasaki Disease. Amsterdam, Elsevier Science, 1995, pp. 587–591.
243. Miyata, K., Kawakami, K., Onimaru, T., et al.: Circulating immune complexes and granulocytes chemotaxis in Kawasaki disease. Jpn. Circ. J. *48*:1350–1353, 1984.
244. Morens, D. M.: National surveillance of Kawasaki disease. Pediatrics *65*:21–25, 1980.
245. Morens, D. M.: Thoughts on Kawasaki disease etiology. J. A. M. A. *241*:399, 1979.
246. Morens, D. M., and Nahmias, A. J.: Kawasaki disease: A "new" pediatric enigma. Hosp. Pract. *13*:109–120, 1978.
247. Morens, D. M., and O'Brien, R. J.: Kawasaki disease in the United States. J. Infect. Dis. *137*:91–93, 1978.
248. Morens, D. M.: Kawasaki disease and rug shampooing. J. Pediatr. *120*:333–334, 1992.
249. Morise, T., Takeuchi, Y., Takeda, R., et al.: Increased plasma endothelin levels in Kawasaki disease: A possible marker for Kawasaki disease. Angiology *44*:719–723, 1993.
250. Munro-Faure, H.: Necrotizing arteritis of the coronary vessels in infancy: Case report and review of the literature. Pediatrics *23*:914–926, 1959.
251. Murata, H.: Experimental arteritis on murine with *Candida*: In relation to arteritis in MCLS (author's translation). Kansenshogaku Zasshi *52*:331–337, 1978.
252. Nagashima, M., Matsushima, M., Matsuoka, H., et al.: High-dose gamma globulin therapy for Kawasaki disease. J. Pediatr. *110*:710–712, 1987.
253. Nagata, S., Yamashiro, Y., Maeda, M., et al.: Immunohistochemical studies on small intestinal mucosa in Kawasaki disease. Pediatr. Res. *33*:557–563, 1993.
254. Nakamura, Y., Yanagawa, H., and Kawasaki, T.: Temporal and geographical clustering of Kawasaki disease in Japan. Prog. Clin. Biol. Res. *250*:19–32, 1987.
255. Nakamura, Y., Yanagawa, H., and Kawasaki, T.: Mortality among children with Kawasaki disease in Japan. N. Engl. J. Med. *326*:1246–1249, 1992.
256. Nakamura, Y., Hirose, K., Yanagawa, H., et al.: Incidence rate of recurrent Kawasaki disease in Japan. Acta Paediatr. *83*:1061–1064, 1994.
257. Newburger, J. W., and the United States Multicenter Kawasaki Study Group: A single infusion of intravenous gamma globulin compared to four daily doses in the treatment of acute Kawasaki syndrome. N. Engl. J. Med. *324*:1633–1639, 1991.
258. Newburger, J. W., Takahashi, M., Burns, J. C., et al.: The treatment of Kawasaki syndrome with intravenous gamma globulin. N. Engl. J. Med. *315*:341–347, 1986.
259. Ng, M. P., Wong, K. Y., Tan, C. L., et al.: Kawasaki disease: The Singapore experience. Ann. Acad. Med. *18*:15–18, 1989.
260. Nigro, G., and Midulla, M.: Retrovirus and Kawasaki disease. Lancet *2*:1045, 1986.
261. Nigro, G., Zerbine, M., Krzystofia, K., et al.: Active or recent parvovirus B_{19} infection in children with Kawasaki disease. Lancet *343*:1260–1261, 1994.
262. Nishiyori, A., Sakaguchi, M., Kato, H., et al.: Toxic shock syndrome toxin 1 and Vβ2 expression on T cells in Kawasaki disease. *In* Kato, H. (ed.): Kawasaki Disease. Amsterdam, Elsevier Science, 1995, pp. 139–143.
263. Niwa, Y., and Sohmiya, K.: Enhanced neutrophilic functions in mucocutaneous lymph node syndrome, with special reference to the possible role of increased oxygen intermediate generation in the pathogenesis of coronary thromboarteritis. J. Pediatr. *104*:56–60, 1984.
264. Ogawa, S., Zhang, J., Yuge, K., et al.: Increased plasma endothelin-1 concentration in Kawasaki disease. J. Cardiovasc. Pharmacol. *22*(Suppl. 8):S364–S366, 1993.
265. Ogino, H., Ogawa, M., Harima, Y., et al.: Clinical evaluation of gamma-globulin preparations for the treatment of Kawasaki disease. Prog. Clin. Biol. Res. *250*:555–556, 1987.
266. Ohga, K., Yamanaha, R., Kinumaki, H., et al.: Kawasaki disease and rug shampoo. Lancet *1*:930, 1983.
267. Ohno, S., Miyajima, T., Higuchi, M., et al.: Ocular manifestations of Kawasaki disease (mucocutaneous lymph node syndrome). Am. J. Ophthalmol. *93*:713–717, 1982.
268. Ohshio, G., Furukawa, F., Khine, M., et al.: High levels of IgA-containing circulating immune complex and secretory IgA in Kawasaki disease. Microbiol. Immunol. *31*:891–898, 1987.
269. Okabe, N., Koboyashi, S., Tatsuzawa, O., et al.: Detection of antibodies to human parvovirus in erythema infectiosum (fifth disease). Arch. Dis. Child. *59*:1016–1019, 1984.
270. Okamoto, T., Kuwabara, H., Shimotohno, K., et al.: Lack of evidence of retroviral involvement in Kawasaki disease. Pediatrics *81*:599, 1988.
271. Okano, M., Hase, N., Sakiyama, Y., et al.: Long-term observation in patients with Kawasaki syndrome and their relation to Epstein-Barr virus infection. Pediatr. Infect. Dis. J. *9*:139–141, 1990.
272. Okano, M., Luka, J., Thiele, G. M., et al.: Human herpesvirus 6 infection and Kawasaki disease. J. Clin. Microbiol. *27*:2379–2380, 1989.
273. Okuni, M., Harada, K., Yamaguchi, H., et al.: Intravenous gamma globulin therapy in Kawasaki disease: Trial of low-dose gamma globulin. Prog. Clin. Biol. Res. *250*:433–439, 1987.
274. Ono, S., Onimaru, T., Kawakami, K., et al.: Impaired granulocyte chemotaxis and increased circulating immune complexes in Kawasaki disease. J. Pediatr. *106*:567–570, 1985.
275. Orlowski, J. P., and Mercer, R. D.: Urine mercury levels in Kawasaki disease. Pediatrics *66*:633–636, 1980.
276. Pachman, L. M., Herold, B. C., and Davis, A. T.: Immune complexes in Kawasaki syndrome: A review. Prog. Clin. Biol. Res. *250*:193–207, 1987.
277. Packard, M., and Wechsler, H. F.: Aneurysm of the coronary arteries. Arch. Intern. Med. *43*:1–14, 1929.
278. Patriarca, P. A., Rogers, M. F., Morens, D. M., et al.: Kawasaki syndrome: Association with the application of rug shampoo. Lancet *2*:578–580, 1982.
279. Pelkonen, P., and Salo, E.: Epidemiology of Kawasaki disease. Clin. Exp. Rheumatol. *12*(Suppl. 10):S83–S85, 1994.
280. Person, J. R.: Kawasaki disease and staphylococcal exotoxins. Arch. Dermatol. *116*:986, 1980.
281. Phillips, W. G., and Marsden, J. R.: Adult Kawasaki syndrome. Br. J. Dermatol. *129*:330–333, 1993.
282. Pietra, B. A., De Inocencio J., Giannini, E. H., et al.: TCR Vβ family repertoire and T cell activation markers in Kawasaki disease. J. Immunol. *153*:1881–1888, 1994.
283. Rae, M. V.: Coronary aneurysms with thrombosis in rheumatic carditis: Unusual occurrence accompanied by hyperleukocytosis in a child. Arch. Pathol. *24*:369–376, 1937.
284. Rauch, A. M.: Kawasaki syndrome: Critical review of U.S. epidemiology. Prog. Clin. Biol. Res. *250*:33–44, 1987.
285. Rauch, A. M.: Kawasaki syndrome: Issues in etiology and treatment advances. Pediatr. Infect. Dis. J. *4*:163–182, 1989.

286. Rauch, A. M., Fultz, P. N., and Kalyanaraman, V. S.: Retrovirus serology and Kawasaki syndrome. Lancet *1*:1431, 1987.
287. Rauch, A. M.. Kaplan, S. L., Nihill, M. R., et al.: Kawasaki syndrome clusters in Harris County, Texas, and eastern North Carolina. Am. J. Dis. Child. 142:441–444, 1988.
288. Rauch, A. M., Glode, M. P., Wiggins, J. W., et al.: Outbreak of Kawasaki syndrome in Denver, Colorado: Association with rug and carpet cleaning. Pediatrics *87*:663–669, 1991.
289. Reddy, A. B.: Mucocutaneous lymph node syndrome. Illinois Med. J. 153:326–328, 1978.
290. Rider, L. G., Wener, M. H., French, J., et al.: Autoantibody production in Kawasaki syndrome. Clin. Exp. Rheumatol. *11*:445–449, 1993.
291. Roberts, F. B., and Fetterman, G. H.: Polyarteritis nodosa in infancy. J. Pediatr. *63*:519–529, 1963.
292. Rogers, M. F.: Kawasaki syndrome. Am. J. Dis. Child. *140*:191, 1986.
293. Rogers, M. F., Kochel, R. L., Hurwitz, E. S., et al.: Kawasaki syndrome: Is exposure to rug shampoo important? Am. J. Dis. Child. *139*:777–779, 1985.
294. Rosenfeld, E. A., Corydon, K. E., and Shulman, S. T.: Kawasaki disease in infants less than one year of age. J. Pediatr. *126*:524–529, 1995.
295. Ross, L., Mason, W., and Wright, T. J.: Mucocutaneous lymph node syndrome: Recent new laboratory observations. Pediatr. Res. *13*:467, 1979.
296. Rowe, R. D., Rose, V., Wilson, G. J., et al.: Kawasaki disease: A measles cover-up? Can. Med. Assoc. J. *136*:1146, 1987.
297. Rowley, A. H., Preble, O. T., Poiesz, B. J., et al.: Serum interferon concentrations and retroviral serology in Kawasaki syndrome. Pediatr. Infect. Dis. J. *7*:663–665. 1988.
298. Rowley, A. H., Duffy, E., and Shulman, S. T.: Prevention of giant aneurysms in Kawasaki disease by intravenous gamma globulin therapy. J. Pediatr. *113*:290–294, 1988.
299. Ruiz, D., and Krober, M. S.: Mucocutaneous lymph node syndrome. J. Oklahoma State Med. Assoc. *70*:351–353, 1977.
300. Russell, A. S., Zaragosa, A. J., and Shea, R.: Mucocutaneous lymph node syndrome in Canada. Can. Med. Assoc. J. *112*:1210–1211, 1975.
301. Sakaguchi, M., Kato, H., Nishiyori, A., et al.: Characterization of CD4+ T helper cells in patients with Kawasaki disease (KD): Preferential production of tumor necrosis factor-alpha (TNF α) by Vβ2− or Vβ8− CD4+ T helper cells. Clin. Exp. Immunol. *99*:276–282, 1995.
302. Salcedo, J. R., Greenberg, L., and Kapur, S.: Renal histology of mucocutaneous lymph node syndrome. Clin. Nephrol. *29*:47–51, 1988.
303. Salo, E., Kekomaki, R., Pelkonen, P., et al.: Kawasaki disease: Monitoring of circulating immune complexes. Eur. J. Pediatr. *147*:377–380, 1988.
304. Salo, E., Pelkonen, P., and Pettay, O.: Outbreak of Kawasaki syndrome in Finland. Acta Paediatr. Scand. *75*:75–80, 1986.
305. Salo, E., Pesonen, E., and Viikari, J.: Serum cholesterol levels during and after Kawasaki disease. J. Pediatr. *119*:557–561, 1991.
306. Salo, E.: Kawasaki disease in Finland in 1982–1992. Scand. J. Infect. Dis. *25*:497–502, 1993.
307. Sasaguri, Y., and Kato, H.: Regression of aneurysms in Kawasaki disease: A pathologic study. Pediatrics *100*:225–231, 1982.
308. Sato, K., Ouchi, K., and Taki, M.: *Yersinia pseudotuberculosis* infection in children, resembling Izumi fever and Kawasaki syndrome. Pediatr. Infect. Dis. 2:123–126, 1983.
309. Sato, N., Sagawa, K., Sasaguri, Y., et al.: Immunopathology and cytokine detection in the skin lesions of patients with Kawasaki disease. J. Pediatr. *122*:198–203, 1993.
310. Savage, C. O. S., Tizard, J., Jayne, D., et al.: Antineutrophil cytoplasm antibodies in Kawasaki disease. Arch. Dis. Child. *64*:360–363, 1989.
311. See references 310, 312.
312. Saxe, N., Horak, K., and Goldblatt, J.: Mucocutaneous lymph node syndrome in a young adult. S. Afr. Med. J. *68*:1011–1013, 1980.
313. Schnaar, D. A., and Bell, D. M.: Kawasaki syndrome in two cousins with parainfluenza virus infection. Am. J. Dis. Child. *136*:554–555, 1982.
314. Scott, D. H.: Aneurysm of the coronary arteries. Am. Heart J. *36*:403–421, 1948.
315. Shimizu, S.: Plasma fibronectin concentrations in mucocutaneous lymph node syndrome. Arch. Dis. Child. *61*:312, 1986.
316. Shimizu, S., Kuratsuji, T., and Ojima, T.: Plasma fibronectin concentrations in mucocutaneous lymph node syndrome. Arch. Dis. Child. *61*:72–74, 1986.
317. Shulman, S. T., and Rowley, A. H.: Does Kawasaki disease have a retroviral aetiology? Lancet *2*:545–546, 1986.
318. Anonymous: Management of Kawasaki syndrome: A consensus statement prepared by North American participants of the Third International Kawasaki Disease Symposium: Tokyo, Japan, December, 1988. Pediatr. Infect. Dis. J. *8*:663–667, 1989.
319. Shulman, S. T.: IVGG therapy in Kawasaki disease: Mechanism(s) of action. Clin. Immunol. Immunopathol. *53*:5141–5146, 1989.
320. Shulman, S. T., Melish, M., Inoue, O., et al.: Immunoglobulin allotypic markers in Kawasaki disease. J. Pediatr. *122*:84–86, 1993.
321. Shulman, S. T.: A commentary on disease mechanism. *In* Takahashi, M., and Taubert, K. (eds.): Proceedings of the Fourth International Symposium on Kawasaki Disease. Am. Heart Assoc., Dallas, Texas, 1993.
322. Siegel, C. J., and Wenner, H. A.: The mucocutaneous lymph node syndrome: Description of an affected 21-month-old child in Kansas City. Clin. Pediatr. *15*:1105–1106, 1976.
323. Smith, L. B., and Burns, J. C.: Kawasaki syndrome and the eye. Pediatr. Infect. Dis. J. *8*:116–118, 1989.
324. Smith, P. K., and Goldwater, P. N.: Kawasaki disease in Adelaide: A review. J. Paediatr. Child Health *29*:126–131, 1993.
325. Soppi, E., Salo, E., and Pelkonen, P.: Antibodies against neutrophil cytoplasmic components in Kawasaki disease. APMIS *100*:269–272, 1992.
326. Strauss, M.: Acute febrile mucocutaneous lymph node syndrome. Trans. Pennsylvania Acad. Ophthalmol. Otolaryngol. *30*:156–160, 1977.
327. Sugimura, T., Kato, H., Yokoi, H., et al.: Intravascular ultrasound study in Kawasaki disease: Assessment of coronary and systemic arterial pathology and application for coronary intervention. *In* Kato, H. (ed.): Kawasaki Disease. Amsterdam, Elsevier Science, 1995, p. 460.
328. Sugimura, T., Kato, H., Inoue, O., et al.: Long-term consequences of Kawasaki disease: Serial coronary angiography and 10-20 years follow-up study. *In* Kato, H. (ed.): Kawasaki Disease. Amsterdam, Elsevier Science, 1995, pp. 574–579.
329. Sugimura, T., Kato, H., Inoue, O., et al.: Vasodilatory response of the coronary arteries after Kawasaki disease: Evaluation by intracoronary injection of isosorbide dinitrate. Pediatrics *121*:684–688, 1992.
330. Sugimura, T., Kato, H., Inoue, O., et al.: Intravascular ultrasound of coronary arteries in children: Assessment of the wall morphology and the lumen after Kawasaki disease. Circulation *89*:258–265, 1994.
331. Suzuki, A., Arakaki, Y., Sugiyama, H., et al.: Observation of coronary arterial lesion due to Kawasaki disease by intravascular ultrasound. *In* Kato, H. (ed.): Kawasaki Disease. Amsterdam, Elsevier Science, 1995, pp. 451–459.
332. Suzuki, A., Kamiya, T., Arakaki, Y., et al.: Fate of coronary aneurysms in Kawasaki disease. Am. J. Cardiol. *74*:822–824, 1994.
333. Swaby, E. D., Fisher-Hoch, S. P., Lambert, H. P., et al.: Is Kawasaki disease a variant of Q fever? Lancet *2*:146, 1980.
334. Takahashi, K., Naoe, S., Wakayama, M., et al.: Pathologic study of coronary aneurysms in adults who had Kawasaki disease in childhood. *In* Kato, H. (ed.): Kawasaki Disease. Amsterdam, Elsevier Science, 1995, pp. 592–597.
335. Takeda, T., Abe, J., Yoshino, K., et al.: Establishment of a novel superantigen produced by *Yersinia pseudotuberculosis* and its association with systemic Kawasaki disease–like symptoms. *In* Kato, H. (ed.): Kawasaki Disease. Amsterdam, Elsevier Science, Amsterdam, 1995, pp. 193–199.
336. Takeuchi, Y., Suma, K., Shiroma, K., et al.: Coronary artery changes in Kawasaki disease and its surgical treatment by aorto-coronary bypass grafting. Kyobu Geka *31*:356–361, 1978.
337. Takiguchi, M., Tamura, T., Goto, M., et al.: Immunological studies on Kawasaki disease. I. Appearance of Hanganutziu-Deicher antibodies. Clin. Exp. Immunol. *56*:345–352, 1984.
338. Tanaka, N.: Kawasaki disease (acute febrile mucocutaneous lymph node syndrome) in Japan: Relationship with infantile periarteritis nodosa. Pathol. Microbiol. *43*:204–218, 1975.
339. Tanaka, N., Naoe, S., and Kawasaki, T.: Pathological study of autopsy cases of MCLS: Relationship with infantile periarteritis nodosa. J. Jpn. Red Cross Center Hosp. 2:85–94, 1971.
340. Tanaka, N., Sekimoto, K., Fukushima, T., et al.: Pathological study of fatal MCLS cases of Kawasaki disease: Relationship with infantile polyarteritis nodosa. *In* Shiokawa, Y. (ed.): Vascular Lesions of Collagen Diseases and Related Conditions. Baltimore, University Park Press, 1977, p. 44.
341. Tanaka, N., Sekimoto, K., and Naoe, S.: Kawasaki disease: Relationship with infantile periarteritis nodosa. Arch. Pathol. Lab. Med. *100*:81–86, 1976.
342. Tasaka, K., and Hamashima, Y.: Function of phagocytosis and intracellular killing of peripheral neutrophils in Kawasaki disease. Acta Pathol. Jpn. *28*:247–252, 1978.
343. Tasaka, K., Kishi, K., Hirose, S., et al.: *Rickettsia*-like bodies in Kawasaki disease. *In* Shiokawa, Y. (ed.): Vascular Lesions of Collagen Diseases and Related Conditions. Baltimore, University Park Press, 1977, pp. 311–321.
344. Tatara, K., and Kusukawa, S.: Long-term prognosis of Kawasaki disease patients with coronary artery obstruction. J. Pediatr. *111*:705–710, 1987.
345. Taubert, K. A., Rowley, A. H., and Shulman, S. T.: Seven-year national survey of Kawasaki disease and acute rheumatic fever. Pediatr. Infect. Dis. J. *13*:704–708, 1994.
346. Taubert, K. A., Rowley, A. H., and Shulman, S. T.: A 10-year (1984–1993) United States hospital survey of Kawasaki disease. *In* Kato, H. (ed.): Kawasaki Disease. Amsterdam, Elsevier Science, 1995, pp. 34–38.
347. Teixeira, O. H. P., and Quinn, A.: Kawasaki syndrome. Am. J. Dis. Child. *140*:190–191, 1986.
348. Terai, M., Kohno, Y., Namba, M., et al.: Class II major histocompatibility antigen expression on coronary arterial endothelium in a patient with Kawasaki disease. Hum. Pathol. *21*:231–234, 1990.
349. Terai, M., Kohno, Y., Niwa, K., et al.: Imbalance among T cell subsets in patients with coronary arterial aneurysms in Kawasaki disease. Am. J. Cardiol. *60*:555–559, 1987.
350. Terai, M., Miwa, K., Williams, T., et al.: Failure to confirm involvement of staphylococcal toxin in the pathogenesis of Kawasaki disease. *In* Kato, H. (ed.): Kawasaki Disease. Amsterdam, Elsevier Science, Amsterdam, 1995, pp. 144–148.
351. Todd, J. K.: Mucocutaneous lymph node syndrome (Kawasaki disease) in adults. J. A. M. A. *243*:1631, 1980.

352. Tomisawa, M., Onouchi, Z., Goto, M., et al.: Ultrastructure of the myocardium in acute febrile mucocutaneous lymph node syndrome. Jpn. Circ. J. *41*:151–157, 1977.
353. Tomita, S., Kato, H., Fujimoto, T., et al.: Cytopathogenic protein in filtrates from cultures of *Propionibacterium acnes* isolated from patients with Kawasaki disease. Br. Med. J. *295*:1229–1232, 1987.
354. Tomita, S., Chung, K., Mas, M., et al.: Peripheral gangrene associated with Kawasaki disease. Clin. Infect. Dis. *14*:121–126, 1992.
355. Tristani-Fironzi, M., Kamango-Sollo, E. D., Sun, S., et al.: TCR Vβ gene family repertoire and humoral immunity in Kawasaki syndrome. *In* Kato, H. (ed.): Kawasaki Disease. Amsterdam, Elsevier Science, 1995, pp. 200–205.
356. Uchida, N., Asayama, K., Dobashi, K., et al.: Antioxidant enzymes and lipoperoxide in blood in patients with Kawasaki disease: Comparison with the changes in acute infections. Acta Paediatr. Jpn. *32*:242–248, 1990.
357. Vaarala, O., Salo, E., Pelkonen, P., et al.: Anticardiolipin response in Kawasaki disease. Acta Paediatr. Scand. *79*:804–809, 1990.
358. Viraben, R., and Dupre, A.: Kawasaki disease associated with HIV infection. Lancet *1*:1430–1431, 1987.
359. Weindling, A. M., Levinsky, R. J., and Marshall, W. C.: Circulating immune complexes in mucocutaneous lymph node syndrome (Kawasaki disease). Arch. Dis. Child. *54*:241–242, 1979.
360. Weir, W. R., Bouchet, V. A., Mitford, E., et al.: Kawasaki disease in European adult associated with serological response to *Coxiella burnetii*. Lancet *2*:504, 1985.
361. Weston, W. L., and Huff, J. C.: The mucocutaneous lymph node syndrome: A critical re-examination. Clin. Exp. Dermatol. *6*:167–178, 1981.
362. Westphalen, M. A., McGrath, M. A., Kelly, W., et al.: Kawasaki disease with severe peripheral ischemia: Treatment with prostaglandin E1 infusion. J. Pediatr. *112*:431–433, 1988.
363. Yamada, K., Fukumoto, T., Shinkai, A., et al.: The platelet functions in acute febrile mucocutaneous lymph node syndrome and a trial of prevention for thrombosis by antiplatelet agent. Acta Hematol. Jpn. *41*:791–802, 1978.
364. Yanagawa, H.: Epidemiology of Kawasaki disease in Japan. Prog. Clin. Biol. Res. *250*:5–17, 1987.
365. Yanagawa, H., Kawasaki, T., and Shigematsu, I.: Nationwide survey on Kawasaki disease in Japan. Pediatrics *80*:58–62, 1987.
366. Yanagawa, H., Nakamura, Y., Kawasaki, T., et al.: Nationwide epidemic of Kawasaki disease in Japan during winter of 1985–86. Lancet *2*:1138–1139, 1986.
367. Yanagawa, H., Nakamura, Y., Yashiro, M., et al.: A nationwide incidence survey of Kawasaki disease in 1985–1986 in Japan. J. Infect. Dis. *158*:1296–1301, 1988.
368. Yanagawa, H., Yashiro, M., Nakamura, Y., et al.: Epidemiologic pictures of Kawasaki disease in Japan: From the nationwide incidence survey in 1991 and 1992. Pediatrics *95*:475–479, 1995.
369. Yanagawa, H., Yashiro, M., Nakamura, Y., et al.: Results of 12 nationwide epidemiological incidence surveys of Kawasaki disease in Japan. Arch. Pediatr. Adolesc. Med. *149*:779–783, 1995.
370. Yanase, Y., Takayama, J., Aso, S., et al.: Studies on serum immunoglobulins and delayed skin tests in patients with MCLS. Acta Paediatr. Jpn. *24*:408–409, 1982.
371. Yanase, Y., Tango, T., Okumura, K., et al.: A comparative study of alteration in lymphocyte subsets among varicella, hand-foot-and-mouth disease, scarlet fever, measles, and Kawasaki disease. Microbiol. Immunol. *31*:701–710, 1987.
372. Yashiro, M., Nakamura, Y., Hirose, K., Yanagawa, H.: Surveillance of Kawasaki disease in Japan, 1984–1994. *In* Kato, H. (ed.): Kawasaki Disease. Amsterdam, Elsevier Science, 1995, pp. 15–21.
373. Yata, J., Nakagawa, T., and Sawa, F.: Some immunological studies on Kawasaki disease. *In* Shiokawa, Y. (ed.): Vascular Lesions of Collagen Diseases and Related Conditions. Baltimore, University Park Press, 1977, pp. 335–336.
374. Yokota, S.: Heat shock protein as a predisposing and immunopotentiating factor in Kawasaki disease. Acta Paediatr. Jpn. *33*:756–764, 1991.
375. Yutani, C., Go, S., Kamiya, F., et al.: Cardiac biopsy of Kawasaki disease. Arch. Pathol. Lab. Med. *105*:470–473, 1981.
376. Yutani, C., Okano, K., Kamiya, T., et al.: Histopatholgical study on right endomyocardial biopsy of Kawasaki disease. Br. Heart J. *43*:589–592, 1980.

83

CHRONIC FATIGUE SYNDROME

Ciro V. Sumaya

Several reports appeared in the mid-1980s that described a chronic fatiguing condition associated with a constellation of manifestations, such as neuropsychiatric problems, pharyngitis, low-grade fever, myalgias, mild lymphadenopathy, and other nonspecific problems.[22, 44, 79, 85] This condition seemingly was linked with Epstein-Barr virus (EBV) and infectious mononucleosis: (1) the disorder often was noticed after a bout of infectious mononucleosis, (2) many of the manifestations were those seen in infectious mononucleosis, and (3) the affected persons commonly had abnormal EBV antibody patterns. This heralded a flurry of other reports in the scientific and public press on this disorder and its putative association with EBV.

Similarities were noted between this chronic disorder and prior reports of patients with suspected persistent or recurrent episodes of infectious mononucleosis.[6, 28, 41] However, in these latter cases, EBV laboratory testing was not available yet to determine whether unusual immune responses to the virus correlated with the "chronic or recurrent mononucleosis." Previously described accounts of sporadic and epidemic episodes of various chronic debilitating conditions, often associated with precipitating infectious processes (i.e., neurasthenia,[4] epidemic neuromyasthenia,[71] Iceland disease,[88] benign myalgic encephalitis,[24] and chronic brucellosis[15]), also were resurrected and considered to resemble this modern-day chronic fatiguing disorder. Although this disorder has been described predominantly in young adults, several reports have identified adolescents and young children with similar debilitating manifestations.

More recent findings dispute the earlier-held notion that EBV played a major role in this chronic debilitating disorder, by consensus now labeled chronic fatigue syndrome (CFS). Considerable attention still is being placed on ascertaining the clinical validity of CFS and its possible association with any infectious agent, psychologic aberrations, and interplay between these or other as yet unknown factors and the immunologic system. This chapter focuses principally on the status of relationships studied or proposed between CFS and infectious processes; pediatric issues receive specific attention.

EPIDEMIOLOGY

As a group, the patients with CFS, particularly those reported from the United States, share some common features. They typically are from middle-class, well-educated white families, and females outnumber males 3 to 1.[22, 44, 79, 85] In pediatric patients, an overrepresentation of whites from middle and upper socioeconomic settings, females, and those from early teenage years also has been noted.[12, 58, 87] As further cases have been described across the country and world, some variations have emerged.

From surveillance studies in selected cities in the United

States, it has been estimated that the prevalence rate for CFS (or that approximated CFS) ranged from 2 to nearly 8 per 100,000 of the general population.[29, 63] One study[29] calculated that more than 80 per cent of the CFS cases were female, most were white, and the average age at onset was approximately 30 years.

Epidemiologic data related to childhood cases of CFS are less well defined in part because the case definitions used in surveillance studies did not take into account any differences that may exist in chronic fatigue in children. Moreover, children with severe chronic fatigue and dysfunction may not be manifesting the same disease process as are adults with CFS.[13]

It also is unclear how limited access or sociocultural factors related to the health care of economically disadvantaged or minority persons affect the epidemiologic statistics. Furthermore, comparisons among studies often are hampered by the lack of uniform definition for the syndrome. It is, therefore, difficult to interpret the findings in other countries, indicating that, in contrast with the experience in the United States, there may be no difference in distribution among social classes[54] or even a relatively lower rate in professional workers.[21]

ETIOLOGY

Infections

EBV has the general property of producing a lifelong latent infection after the primary nonsymptomatic or symptomatic infection of the human host.[60, 73] Reactivation of the quiescent, latent state is presumed to occur periodically and without accompanying symptoms.[14, 80] In some persons (i.e., those associated with immunocompromised states or selected genetic or environmental influences), the reactivation is suspected of occasionally leading to such serious, chronic manifestations as lymphoproliferative lesions, cancer, or multiorgan dysfunction.[2, 19, 20, 33, 34, 59, 65, 70, 73] (For additional details on chronic EBV infections, see Chapter 165.)

Aside from the feature of latency that links EBV with a variety of chronic human disorders, there do exist a number of EBV-related clinical, serologic, virologic, and immunologic findings that denote an as yet obscure and perplexing association of this virus and CFS. CFS often has been reported after an infectious mononucleosis–like illness in the recent past, and some of the clinical manifestations, although usually symptoms as opposed to signs, are those noted in acute infectious mononucleosis.[22, 44, 79, 85] Patients with CFS as a group may have elevated antibody titers to EBV capsid antigen and early antigen,[38, 81] abnormal antibody responses to components of EBV nuclear antigen,[31] high ratios of antibodies to early antigen/EBV nuclear antigen,[46] enhanced spontaneous (EBV-induced) proliferation of peripheral blood lymphocytes,[81] and some mildly aberrant cell-mediated immune responses to EBV.[7, 48, 84]

However, all of these associations of EBV and CFS are tempered by other evidence revealing that similar unusual clinical or laboratory findings may be noted in healthy persons, many of the CFS patients may not exhibit unusual EBV findings or associations, confirmation of results in various laboratories is insufficient, and comparability of patient groups studied may be unclear.[10, 25, 30, 36, 38, 44, 79–81]

With additional patient groups reported, it was noted that there were other viruses besides EBV that had some type of association with CFS. Elevated antibody titers to multiple viruses have been found in patients, albeit a selected subgroup, in a CFS-like epidemic in Nevada.[36] A high seroprevalence of antibodies to the recently discovered herpesvirus human herpesvirus 6 (HHV-6) has been found in some[75, 86] but not other[25] patient groups with CFS. Evidence of an active HHV-6 infection and increased detection of HHV-6 DNA in peripheral blood mononuclear cells also have been reported in adult patients.[9, 91] At least two outbreaks of a chronic fatigue condition have been associated with coxsackievirus B infections,[11, 23] a virus with well-known muscle tropism. British investigators also have reported evidence of a persisting enteroviral or EBV infection of muscle in patients with "postviral" CFS.[8, 53] Recent interest in human retrovirus causality was stimulated when DeFreitas and colleagues[17] found human T-lymphotropic virus type 2 *gag* gene sequences in adults and children with CFS. However, several other laboratories subsequently have been unable to detect retroviral markers that distinguish CFS patients from control subjects.[27, 37, 47] A lack of association of hepatitis C virus infection with CFS has been reported.[16] Currently, the enthusiasm initially generated that CFS was caused by EBV or another virus appears to be subsiding, while the possibility that any viral association merely is an epiphenomenon is being considered increasingly.

Immunologic Dysfunctions

Abnormalities in both the humoral and the cellular immune systems have been detected to a variable degree in patients with CFS, including levels of circulating immune complexes, IgG, and antinuclear antibodies[3]; T-cell function and T-cell phenotypic populations[49, 52, 56, 78, 83]; and aberrant antibody or other immune responses to a number of latent viruses, as described earlier. On the whole, these immunologic abnormalities suggest a chronic, low-level dysfunction or unusual activation of the immune system in patients with CFS. The direct or indirect effects of these findings on the pathogenesis and course of CFS are not defined well. Furthermore, it is important to recognize that these immune abnormalities are not present consistently in CFS patients and may not correlate with severity of symptoms.

Psychiatric Disorders

The possibility that CFS is a psychiatric disorder has been considered by several investigators. A significant prevalence of neuropsychologic complaints and psychiatric diagnoses, mostly depression, abound in CFS patients,[51, 57] including children and adolescents.[74, 87] Many of the manifestations of depression resemble those of CFS, making a separation of these two conditions difficult in individual patients. The contribution in terms of interaction or influence of each condition on the other has not been elucidated well.

Other

Central nervous system anomalies have been uncovered by magnetic resonance imaging and advanced computed tomography[9, 39]; abnormalities in the metabolites of neurotransmitters have been reported by one group of investigators.[18] Additional abnormalities have been detected in pituitary and hypothalamic function, basal plasma levels of certain neurotransmitter metabolites, and cerebral perfusion of patients with CFS.[5] It is unknown whether these findings play any role in CFS; the reason for these abnormalities is unclear (i.e., it could be a primary dysfunction or perhaps one induced by a persistent viral infection).

PATHOGENESIS

The circumstances that produce and perpetuate CFS are obscure. There is a growing opinion that the relationship of CFS with infectious agents as cited in the previous section is a nonspecific and noncontributory consequence of an idiopathic generalized immune dysfunction in patients with CFS. In this context, the findings showing aberrant host immune responses to EBV and other latent viruses evidently would not be specific for the virus but would reflect the enhanced latent infection of these infectious agents. Alternatively, but probably of lesser validity, a viral infection (acute or reactivated) or infection from some other organism or organisms could initiate the development of the syndrome and contribute to its evolution and clinical course. It also has been speculated that there may be subsets of patients with varying causes for their condition, such as acute infection from various agents, persistent active viral infections or lymphokine disturbances secondary to a significant underlying immunologic dysfunction, a predominantly psychologic basis, or other etiologic or contributing factors as yet unknown.

Some investigators,[51, 82] but not others,[32] have noted an apparent association between preceding psychiatric impairment and subsequent CFS. Patients with depression also have been noted to have significantly higher rates of somatic symptoms and medical utilization, compared with nondepressed patients.[45] The consequences of the association of CFS with psychiatric disturbances are not clear but raise the issue of the potential role of psychologic factors in influencing immunologic mechanisms and human susceptibility to infectious diseases.[42] Depression has been shown in some studies, although not consistently, to be associated with modifications in cellular immune responses.[1, 68] Preexisting depressive symptoms may lead to delayed convalescence from viral infections.[40]

TABLE 83–1. Approximate Percentage of Patients with Chronic Fatigue Syndrome Reporting Symptoms

Symptom	Percentage
Easy fatigability	100
Difficulty concentrating	90
Headache	90
Sore throat	85
Tender lymph nodes	80
Muscle aches	80
Joint aches	75
Feverishness	75
Difficulty sleeping	70
Psychiatric problems	65
Allergies	55
Abdominal cramps	40
Weight loss	20
Rash	10
Rapid pulse	10
Weight gain	5
Chest pain	5
Night sweats	5

From Straus, S. E.: The chronic mononucleosis syndrome. J. Infect. Dis. *157*:405–412, 1988.

DIAGNOSIS

Historical Clinical Picture

A chronic, debilitating illness linked initially with a persistent EBV infection was reported by several groups in the mid-1980s.[22, 44, 79, 85] A rather characteristic pattern of manifestations, most notably significant fatigue, was described in the patient groups in the United States (Table 83–1). Other symptoms included neuropsychiatric problems (depression, moodiness, sleep disturbances, paresthesias), pharyngitis, low-grade fever, myalgias, mild lymphadenopathy, and other nonspecific problems. The chronic fatigue condition often started within 1 year of an episode of infectious mononucleosis. Occasionally, there was no antecedent episode of infectious mononucleosis or, possibly, a prior nonspecific illness with no known relation to EBV. Some patients experienced a persistent debilitating condition with only its intensity varying throughout the course. Others had more intermittent symptoms, with periods of well-being interspersed between the recurrent episodes of illness. With the exception of the group described by Tobi and colleagues,[85] the patients in most of these early reports had a predominance of symptoms unassociated with discrete physical or documentable signs. Laboratory findings characteristic of acute infectious mononucleosis, such as lymphocytosis, atypical lymphocyte formation, elevated levels of liver transaminases, and heterophil antibodies, were not found commonly. General immunologic abnormalities found in some patients included low levels of immunoglobulins (in particular, mild IgA deficiencies), increased rates of circulating immune complexes, and a deficiency of circulating interferon. As a group, these patients had elevated antibody responses to some EBV antigens, suggesting an enhanced EBV carrier state or possibly a reactivation of a previously latent EBV infection.[80]

Subsequently, an outbreak of a chronic fatiguing condition after an acute infectious-type illness was described in more than 200 persons living in neighboring communities near Lake Tahoe, Nevada. After further investigation, a report by Holmes and colleagues[36] noted that most of these persons did not have a chronic illness and had other possible explanations for their symptoms. In a much smaller number (n = 15) of the initially described outbreak group, the illness was determined to have lasted more than 1 month and to have been associated with an increased frequency of splenomegaly. Elevated antibody titers to a number of viruses (EBV, cytomegalovirus, measles virus, and herpes simplex virus) were found in this selected subgroup of patients. A number of circumstances surrounding this outbreak remain unclear.

With the evaluation of a larger pool of patients after the initial reports, additional manifestations were found and considered part of this chronic, debilitating disorder. These manifestations included various cognitive disorders, neurologic problems, and arthritis episodes.[25, 36, 43] In another study group, it was reported that 70 per cent of the patients had persistent, diffuse musculoskeletal pain, a finding similar to that in patients with fibromyalgia.[26] An increased frequency of allergic complaints also was noted in patients diagnosed as having the chronic fatiguing condition[61]; atopy was reported to exist concurrently in greater than 50 per cent of patients.[77]

Case Definition

A group of experts developed a working case definition of CFS and published it in 1988[35] (Table 83–2). This improved the management and research efforts through better identification and comparability of patients. The nomenclature adopted, CFS, justifiably lacks the reference to an EBV relationship—earlier names for this condition included chronic EBV infection and chronic mononucleosis—or to any other specific etiologic agent. The name also incorporates the primary clinical manifestation: fatigue.

TABLE 83–2. Case Definition for Chronic Fatigue Syndrome*

Major Criteria	New onset of persistent or relapsing, debilitating fatigue (≥6 months) not resolved by bed rest and severe enough to impair daily activity below 50%
	Exclusion of other conditions that may produce similar symptoms
Minor Criteria	
Symptom (onset on or after fatigability; duration ≥6 months)	Mild fever (37.6°–38.6° C oral) or chills
	Sore throat
	Painful lymph nodes (anterior or posterior cervical, axillary)
	Unexplained generalized muscle weakness
	Muscle discomfort or myalgia
	Prolonged fatigue (≥24 hours) after exercise previously tolerated
	Generalized headaches (new or different from premorbid state)
	Migratory arthralgia
	Neuropsychologic complaints (photophobia, transient visual scotomata, forgetfulness, excessive irritability, confusion, difficulty thinking, inability to concentrate, or depression)
	Sleep disturbance
	Main sympton complex developed over a few hours to days
Physical (to be documented by physician on at least 2 occasions, at least 1 month apart)	Low-grade fever (37.6°–38.6° C oral)
	Nonexudative pharyngitis
	Palpable or tender anterior or posterior cervical or axillary lymph nodes (usually <2 cm diameter)

*A case of chronic fatigue syndrome must fulfill the major criteria and the following minor criteria: 6 or more of the 11 symptom criteria and 2 or more of the 3 physical criteria or 8 or more of the 11 symptoms.

From Holmes, G. P., Kaplan, J. E., Gantz, N. M., et al.: Chronic fatigue syndrome: A working case definition. Ann. Intern. Med. *108*:387–389, 1988.

However, the working case definition was criticized by some investigators because of the problems with insufficient exclusion of other causes of chronic fatigue (particularly psychiatric disorders), the lack of objective findings, and the variable interpretations of the major and minor criteria. Subsequently, another workshop of experts developed a modification that did not dismantle the earlier case definition criteria but complemented it by providing additional exclusions or inclusions of various illness categories for those persons meeting the initial case definition[69] (Table 83–3). Laboratory tests conforming to the exclusion of various diseases and adapted to the individual patient's symptoms were included in the modified scheme. It also was recognized that the earlier case definition was developed principally for research and comparative study purposes and not intended for rigid adherence by clinicians.

Despite these improved diagnostic measures, it still may be difficult to distinguish patients with CFS from patients with depression and other severe psychiatric disorders.[53] Depressive episodes and anxiety disorders predominate in women in the same age group as those with CFS.[67] Furthermore, the often intimate association between CFS and affective illness as described in some studies[50, 82] suggests to some clinicians that depression may be the primary disorder in some patients.

The case definition with its modification may have diagnostic and epidemiologic limitations in children and adolescents with a chronic fatiguing condition because of differences as yet unclear associated with fatigue in varying age groups (see the subsequent section, Pediatric Cases, for more information).

The status and eventual outcome of what may be a broader cohort of patients that do not fulfill completely the formal criteria for inclusion as a case of CFS remain an additional enigma that warrants further scrutiny.

The early phases of oncogenic processes, chronic infectious illnesses, diseases resulting from endocrine or neurologic abnormalities, and autoimmune disorders may mimic some of the manifestations of CFS,[35] although a search in patients for other specific diseases that fit the CFS criteria usually is not revealing. Certain signs, however, such as fever documented above 38.6° C (oral), weight change of greater than 10 per cent, and lymph nodes enlarged more than 2 cm, should be considered atypical for CFS and prompt studies for other diseases.

The extent of the evaluation of patients with possible CFS should be based on the history, physical examination, and selected laboratory findings. A recommended evaluation can include some of the following measures: serial weights; serial morning and afternoon body temperatures; complete blood count and differential; serum electrolytes; glucose; creatinine and blood urea nitrogen; calcium, phosphorus, total bilirubin, alkaline phosphatase, serum aspartate aminotransferase, and serum alanine aminotransferase; creatine phosphokinase or aldolase; urinalysis; posteroanterior and lateral chest radiographs; erythrocyte sedimentation rate; antinuclear antibody; thyroid-stimulating hormone; HIV antibody test; and intermediate-strength purified protein derivative skin test.[35] A detailed personal and family psychiatric history should be obtained; self-report instruments also can be used to screen for psychiatric disorders. If after the evaluation no other conditions are detected, the criteria for CFS may be satisfied. Serologic tests for EBV antibody are not indicated in patients with possible CFS because these titers are not of diagnostic value.

In the modification of the initial case definition (see Table 83–3),[69] similar laboratory and psychologic tests are recommended, corresponding to illness categories being excluded (or included) according to patient history and physical findings.

Pediatric Cases

Most of the reports on CFS involve young adult patients. The data available on pediatric patients diagnosed as having CFS or a CFS-like condition[44, 53, 58, 74, 87] indicate that, in general, children may have manifestations relatively similar to those of the adult patient. One study[53] detected a lower frequency of emotional symptoms along with a greater frequency of somatic symptoms in pediatric compared with adult patients. School performance may be affected severely, with about one-third of the affected children missing at least 6 months of school.

It should be kept in mind, however, that the manifestation of chronic, debilitating fatigue in children (and making the diagnosis of CFS in children) may need to be considered in a different context from that in adults. Although relatively

TABLE 83–3. Recommended Modification of Case Definition for Chronic Fatigue Syndrome

Illness Category	Exclusions	Inclusions*	Recommended Tests†
Chronic medical conditions	Major conditions to be considered in differential diagnoses are listed in the study by Holmes et al.[35] and include malignancy, autoimmune disease, inflammatory disease, endocrine disease, neurologic disease, and chronic disease		*Standard:* Urinalysis, complete blood count with differential, serum electrolytes, blood urea nitrogen, glucose, creatinine, calcium, thyroid function tests, erythrocyte sedimentation rate, and antinuclear antibodies
		Fibromyalgia‡	Tender-point examination‡ *Optional or as clinically indicated:* Serum cortisol, rheumatoid factor, and immunoglobulin levels
Postinfectious disease	Chronic active hepatitis B or C; Lyme borreliosis, inadequately treated; HIV infection; tuberculosis	Infectious mononucleosis, adequately treated infection that is not associated typically with chronicity; toxoplasmosis; brucellosis; Lyme borreliosis§	Tuberculin skin test; Lyme serology in endemic area; HIV serology when indicated
Psychiatric and behavioral disorders	Psychoses: psychotic depression, bipolar disorder, schizophrenia Substance abuse	Nonpsychotic depression: concurrent, 1 month after onset, or 6 months or more before onset: recurrent or nonrecurrent; somatoform disorders; anxiety disorders; generalized or panic disorder	*Screen:* General Health Questionnaire combination of self-report instruments¶ For patients with positive screening results: *Structured interview:* Diagnostic Interview Schedule version III A or Structured Clinical Interview for the *Diagnostic and Statistical Manual of Mental Disorders,* Third Edition Revised (DSM-III-R)

Adapted from Schluederberg, A., Straus, S. E., Peterson, P., et al.: Chronic fatigue syndrome research: Definition and medical outcome assessment. Ann. Intern. Med. *117*:325–331, 1992.

*Stratified by individual category in analysis.

†Tests are to be used in conjunction with complete detailed medical history and comprehensive physician examination.[22]

‡See report by Wolfe, F., Smythe, H. A., Yunus, M. B., et al.: Criteria for fibromyalgia. Arthritis Rheum. *32*(Suppl.):S47, 1989.

§Recognized recrudescence and chronicity of active *Borrelia* infection were considered an exception.

¶Zung Self-Rating Anxiety Scale, Symptom Checklist-90, Beck Depression Inventory.

few studies have been published on pediatric CFS, fatigue is a common complaint in the pediatric age group, particularly among adolescents.[72] It has been reported that chronic fatigue sufferers may account for 15 per cent of new referral outpatients to a pediatric infectious disease subspecialty group.[12] Because there are differences in physical, psychosocial, and developmental stressors between children/adolescents and adults, dysfunctional fatigue in these two age groups may be from different factors and respond to different management. The relative lack of information on chronic fatigue in children results in a significant disadvantage for practitioners caring for children with this condition. As an additional hurdle, none of the attempts at case definitions of CFS by expert groups as cited earlier specifically accounted for issues pertaining to chronic fatigue in children.

MANAGEMENT AND TREATMENT

Although some investigators and practitioners question whether CFS is a valid diagnosis, it is evident in adults as well as in children[13, 58, 74] that chronic fatigue can have a major adverse effect on a person's state of being. In pediatric patients, effective intervention strategies are needed to contain the disruptive effects on the child's or adolescent's opportunity to complete crucial psychosocial developmental tasks.

Patients should be reassured and advised to remain as active as possible within their individual tolerance limits. Appropriate psychiatric evaluation and counseling may be needed (1) to identify psychologic features that adversely may affect development and (2) when the neuropsychiatric complaints are significant. In selected patients, antidepressants may provide some benefit, although not abating all symptoms (personal communication, Stephen Straus, *Infectious Disease News,* July 1990). Acyclovir does not alter the clinical course.[76] Despite advocacy by some clinicians, data are insufficient to indicate that immune serum globulin or intravenous gamma-globulin benefits patients with CFS. Two controlled clinic trials have shown contrasting results.[55, 62] It is prudent to avoid the use of parenteral gamma-globulin until adequately controlled trials determine clearly that this drug is of benefit. Patients should be counseled against using nontraditional or inadequately evaluated medications, particularly because progression to a life-threatening illness is not likely and recovery does occur. Individual, family, or group therapy, as well as constructive support group services, may be helpful.

PROGNOSIS

An accurate evaluation of the long-term outcomes in CFS is handicapped by a lack of sufficient surveillance of a well-defined homogeneous patient population. However, evidence indicates that in general the natural history of CFS (or of CSF-like conditions) is favorable in children and adolescents[12, 58, 74] (as in adults[25, 50, 89]), with many or the majority of study patients showing improvement even to the point of resolution after 6 to 12 months. In a minority of patients, though, the symptoms have persisted for many months or years. It also is apparent that pediatric patients with chronic fatigue are at considerable risk for significant psychologic morbidity and social dysfunction.[12, 58, 74, 87] A study focused on adolescent patients noted that the lost schooling, diminished peer contact, family disruption, and lowered self-esteem resulting from CFS may pose a major problem during a vulnerable life phase and possibly continue to affect future development.[66] There is no definite evidence that CFS can progress to a life-threatening form or to a malignant process.

References

1. Albrecht, J., Helderman, J. H., Schlesser, M. A., et al.: A controlled study of cellular immune function in affective disorders before and during somatic therapy. Psychiatr. Res. *15*:185–193, 1985.
2. Andiman, W. A., Eastman, R., Martin, K., et al.: Opportunistic lymphoproliferations associated with Epstein-Barr viral DNA in infants and children with AIDS. Lancet *2*:1390, 1985.
3. Bates, D. W., Buchwald, D., Lee, J., et al.: Clinical laboratory test findings in patients with chronic fatigue syndrome. Arch. Intern. Med. *155*:97–103, 1995.
4. Beard, G.: Neurasthenia, or nervous exhaustion. Boston Med. Surg. J. *3*(new series):217–220, 1869.
5. Bell, D. S.: Chronic fatigue syndrome update. Postgrad. Med. *96*:73–81, 1994.
6. Bender, C. E.: Recurrent mononucleosis. J. A. M. A. *182*:954, 1962.
7. Borysiewicz, L. K., Haworth, S. J., Cohen, J., et al.: Epstein-Barr virus–specific immune defects in patients with persistent symptoms following infectious mononucleosis. Q. J. Med. *58*:111–121, 1986.
8. Bowles, N. E., Bayston, T. A., Zhang, H.-Y., et al.: Persistence of enterovirus RNA in muscle biopsy samples suggests that some cases of chronic fatigue syndrome result from a previous, inflammatory viral myopathy. J. Med. *24*:145–160, 1993.
9. Buchwald, D., Cheney, P. R., Peterson, D. L., et al.: A chronic illness characterized by fatigue, neurologic and immunologic disorders, and active herpes virus type 6 infection. Ann. Intern. Med. *116*:103–113, 1992.
10. Buchwald, D., Sullivan, J. L., and Komaroff, A. L.: Frequency of "chronic active Epstein-Barr virus infection" in a general medical practice. J. A. M. A. *257*:2303–2307, 1987.
11. Calder, B. D., and Warnock, P. J.: Coxsackie B infection in a Scottish general practice. J. R. Coll. Gen. Pract. *34*:15–19, 1984.
12. Carter B. D., Edwards, J. F., Kronenberger, W. G., et al.: Case control study of chronic fatigue in pediatric patients. Pediatrics *95*:179–186, 1995.
13. Carter, B. D., Edwards, J. F., and Marshall, G. S.: Chronic fatigue in children: Illness or disease? Pediatrics *91*:163–164, 1993.
14. Chang, R. S., Lewis, J. P., Reynolds, R. D., et al.: Oropharyngeal excretion of Epstein-Barr virus by patients with lymphoproliferative disorders and by recipients of renal homografts. Ann. Intern. Med. *88*:34–40, 1978.
15. Cluff, L. E., Trever, R. W., Imboden, J. B., et al.: Brucellosis. II. Medical aspects of delayed convalescence. Arch. Intern. Med. *103*:398–405, 1959.
16. Dale, J. K., Di Bisceglie, A. M., Hoofnagle, J. H., et al.: Chronic fatigue syndrome: Lack of association with hepatitis C virus infection. J. Med. Virol. *34*:119–121, 1991.
17. Defreitas, E., Hilliard, B., Cheney, P. R., et al.: Retroviral sequences related to human T-lymphotropic virus type II in patients with chronic fatigue immune dysfunction syndrome. Proc. Natl. Acad. Sci. U. S. A. *88*:2922–2926, 1991.
18. Demitrack, M. A., Gold, P. W., Dale, J. K., et al.: Plasma and cerebrospinal fluid monoamine metabolism in patients with chronic fatigue syndrome: Preliminary findings. Biol. Psychiatry *32*:1065–1077, 1992.
19. de-The, G.: Is Burkitt's lymphoma related to perinatal infection by Epstein-Barr virus? Lancet *1*:335, 1977.
20. de-The, G., Geser, A., Day, N. E., et al.: Epidemiological evidence for causal relationship between Epstein-Barr virus and Burkitt's lymphoma from Ugandan prospective study. Nature *274*:756–761, 1978.
21. Dowsett, E. G., Ramsay, A. M., McCartney, R. A., et al.: Myalgic encephalomyelitis: A persistent enteroviral infection. Postgrad. Med. J. *66*:526–530, 1990.
22. Dubois, R. E., Seeley, J. K., Brus, I., et al.: Chronic mononucleosis syndrome. South Med. J. *77*:1376–1382, 1984.
23. Fegan, K. G., Behan, P. O., and Bell, E. J.: Myalgic encephalomyelitis: Report of an epidemic. J. R. Coll. Gen. Pract. *33*:335–337, 1983.
24. Galpine, J. F., and Brady, C.: Benign myalgic encephalomyelitis. Lancet *1*:757, 1957.
25. Gold, D., Bowden, R., Sixbey, J., et al.: Chronic fatigue: A prospective clinical and virologic study. J. A. M. A. *264*:48–53, 1990.
26. Goldenberg, D. L., Simms, R. W., Geiger, A., et al.: High frequency of fibromyalgia in patients with chronic fatigue seen in a primary care practice. Arth. Rheum. *33*:381–387, 1990.
27. Gow, J. W., Simpson, K., Schliephake, A., et al.: Search for retrovirus in the chronic fatigue syndrome. J. Clin. Pathol. *45*:1058–1061, 1992.
28. Graves, S., Jr.: Recurrent infectious mononucleosis. J. Ky. Med. Assoc. *1*:790, 1970.
29. Gunn, W. J., Connell, D. B., and Randall, B.: Epidemiology of chronic fatigue syndrome: The Centers for Disease Control study. Ciba Found. Symp. *172*:83–93, 1993.
30. Henle, W., and Henle, G.: Epstein-Barr virus–specific serology in immunologically compromised individuals. Cancer Res. *41*:4222–4225, 1981.
31. Henle, W., Henle, G., Andersson, J., et al.: Antibody responses to Epstein-Barr virus–determined nuclear antigen (EBNA)-1 and EBNA-2 in acute and chronic Epstein-Barr virus infection. Proc. Natl. Acad. Sci. U. S. A. *84*:570–574, 1987.
32. Hickie, I., Lloyd, A., Wakefield, D., et al.: The psychiatric status of patients with the chronic fatigue syndrome [see comments]. Br. J. Psychiatry 534–540, 1990.
33. Ho, H. C., Ng, M. H., Kwan, H. C., et al.: Epstein-Barr virus–specific IgA and IgG serum antibodies in nasopharyngeal carcinoma. Br. J. Cancer *34*:655–660, 1976.
34. Ho, M., Miller, G., Athison, R. W., et al.: Epstein-Barr virus infections and DNA hybridization studies in post-transplantation lymphoma and lymphoproliferative lesions: The role of primary infection. J. Infect. Dis. *152*:876–886, 1985.
35. Holmes, G. P., Kaplan, J. E., Gantz, N. M., et al.: Chronic fatigue syndrome: A working case definition. Ann. Intern. Med. *108*:387–389, 1988.
36. Holmes, G. P., Kaplan, J. E., Stewart, J. A., et al.: A cluster of patients with a mononucleosis-like syndrome: Is Epstein-Barr virus the cause? J. A. M. A. *25*:2297–2302, 1987.
37. Honda, M., Kitamura, K., Nakasone, T., et al.: Japanese patients with chronic fatigue syndrome are negative for known retrovirus infections. Microbiol. Immunol. *37*:779–784, 1993.
38. Horwitz, C. A., Henle, W., Henle, G., et al.: Long-term serologic follow-up of patients for Epstein-Barr virus after recovery from infectious mononucleosis. J. Infect. Dis. *151*:1150–1153, 1985.
39. Ichise, M., Salit, I. E., Abbey, S. E., et al.: Assessment of regional cerebral perfusion by $^{99}Tc^{m}$-HMPAO SPECT in chronic fatigue syndrome. Nucl. Med. Commun. *13*:767–772, 1992.
40. Imboden, J. B., and Canter, A.: Convalescence from influenza: A study of the psychological and clinical determinants. Arch. Intern. Med. *108*:393–399, 1961.
41. Isaacs, R.: Chronic infectious mononucleosis. Blood *3*:858–861, 1948.
42. Jemmott, J. B., and Locke, S. E.: Psychol. Bull. *95*:78–108, 1984.
43. Jones, J. F., Friedman, A. D., and Larson, M. D.: Chronic/recurrent Epstein-Barr virus infections. Clin. Res. *31*:122A, 1983.
44. Jones, J. F., Ray, C. G., Minnich, L. L., et al.: Evidence for active Epstein-Barr virus infection in patients with persistent, unexplained illnesses: Elevated anti-early antigen antibodies. Ann. Intern. Med. *102*:1–7, 1985.
45. Katon, W., Berg, A. O., Robins, A. J., et al.: Depression: Medical utilization and somatization. West. J. Med. *144*:564–568, 1986.
46. Kawai, K., and Kawai, A.: Studies on the relationship between chronic fatigue syndrome and Epstein-Barr virus in Japan. Intern. Med. *31*:313–318, 1992.
47. Khan, A. S., Heneine, W. M., Chapman, L. E., et al.: Assessment of a retrovirus sequence and other possible risk factors for the chronic fatigue syndrome in adults. Ann. Intern. Med. *118*:241–245, 1993.
48. Kibler, R., Lucas, D. O., Hicks, M. J., et al.: Immune function in chronic active Epstein-Barr virus infection. J. Clin. Immunol. *5*:46–54, 1985.
49. Klimas, N. G., Salvato, F. R., Morgan, R., et al.: Immunological abnormalities in chronic fatigue syndrome. J. Clin. Microbiol. *28*:1403–1410, 1990.
50. Kroenke, K., Wood, D. R., Mangelsdorff, A. D., et al.: Chronic fatigue in primary care: Prevalence, patient characteristics and outcome. J. A. M. A. *260*:929–934, 1988.
51. Kruesi, M. J. P., Dale, J., and Straus, S. E.: Psychiatric diagnoses in patients who have chronic fatigue syndrome. J. Clin. Psychiatry *50*:53–56, 1989.
52. Landay, A. L., Jessop, C., Lennette, E. T., et al.: Chronic fatigue syndrome: Clinical condition associated with immune activation. Lancet *338*:707–712, 1991.
53. Levine, P. H., Krueger, G. R. F., and Straus, S. E.: The postviral chronic fatigue syndrome: A roundtable. J. Infect. Dis. *160*:722–724, 1989.
54. Lloyd, A. R., Hickie, I., Boughton, C. R., et al.: Prevalence of chronic fatigue syndrome in an Australian population. Med. J. Aust. *153*:522–528, 1990.
55. Lloyd, A., Hickie, I., Wakefield, D., et al.: A double-blind, placebo-controlled trial of intravenous immunoglobulin therapy in patients with chronic fatigue syndrome. Am. J. Med. *89*:561–568, 1990.

56. Lloyd, A. R., Wakefield, D., Boughton, C. R., et al.: Immunological abnormalities in the chronic fatigue syndrome. Med. J. Aust. *151*:122–124, 1989.
57. Manu, P., Matthews, D. A., and Lane, T. J.: The mental health of patients with a chief complaint of chronic fatigue: A prospective evaluation and follow-up. Arch. Intern. Med. *148*:2213–2217, 1988.
58. Marshall, G. S., Gesser, R. M., Yamanishi, K., et al.: Chronic fatigue in children: Clinical features, Epstein-Barr virus and human herpesvirus 6 serology and long-term follow-up. Pediatr. Infect. Dis. J. *10*:287–290, 1991.
59. Miller, G., Grogin E., Rowe, D., et al.: Selective lack of antibody to a component of EB nuclear antigen in patients with chronic active EBV infection. J. Infect. Dis. *156*:26, 1987.
60. Nilsson, K., Klein, G., Henle, W., et al.: The establishment of lymphoblastoid lines from adult and fetal human tissue and its dependence in EBV. Int. J. Cancer *8*:443, 1971.
61. Olson, G. B., Kanaan, M. N., Gersuk, G. M., et al.: Correlation between allergy and persistent Epstein-Barr virus infections in chronic-active Epstein-Barr virus–infected patients. J. Allergy Clin. Immunol. *78*:308–314, 1986.
62. Peterson, P. K., Shepard, J., Macres, M., et al.: A controlled trial of intravenous immunoglobulin G in chronic fatigue syndrome. Am. J. Med. *89*:554–560, 1990.
63. Price, R. K., North, C. S., Wessley, S., et al.: Estimating the prevalence of chronic fatigue syndrome and associated symptoms in the community. Public Health Rep. *107*:514–522, 1992.
64. Purtilo, D. T.: X-linked lymphoproliferative syndrome. J. A. M. A. *105*:119, 1981.
65. Purtilo, D. T., and Linder, J.: Oncological consequences of impaired immune surveillance against ubiquitous viruses. J. Clin. Immunol. *3*:197, 1983.
66. Rickard-Bell, C. J., and Waters, B. G.: Psychosocial management of chronic fatigue syndrome in adolescence. Aust. N. Z. J. Psychiatry *26*:64–72, 1992.
67. Robins, L. N., Helzer, J. E., Weissman, M. M., et al.: Lifetime prevalence of specific psychiatric disorders in three sites. Arch. Gen. Psychiatry *41*:949–967, 1984.
68. Schleifer, S. J., Keller, S. E., Sirism, S. G., et al.: Depression and immunity: Lymphocyte function in ambulatory depressed patients, hospitalized schizophrenic patients, and patients hospitalized for herniorrhaphy. Arch. Gen. Psychiatry *42*:129–133, 1985.
69. Schluederberg, A., Straus, S. E., Peterson, P., et al.: Chronic fatigue syndrome research: Definition and medical outcome assessment. Ann. Intern. Med. *117*:325–331, 1992.
70. Schooley, R. T., Carey, R. W., Miller, G., et al.: Chronic Epstein-Barr virus infection associated with fever and interstitial pneumonitis. Ann. Intern. Med. *104*:636, 1986.
71. Shelokov, A., Habel, K., Verder, E., et al.: Epidemic neuromyasthenia: An outbreak of poliomyelitis-like illness in student nurses. N. Engl. J. Med. *257*:345, 1957.
72. Sigler, A. T.: Fatigue and weakness. *In* Hoekelman, R. A., Friedman, S. B., Nelson, N. M., et al. (eds.): Primary Pediatric Care. St. Louis, C. V. Mosby, 1987, pp. 952–955.
73. Sixbey, J. W., Nedruff, J. G., Raab-Traub, N., et al.: Epstein-Barr virus replication in oropharyngeal epithelial cells. N. Engl. J. Med. *310*:1225, 1984.
74. Smith, M. S., Mitchell, J., Corey, L., et al.: Chronic fatigue in adolescents. Pediatrics *88*:195–202, 1991.
75. Straus, S. E.: The chronic mononucleosis syndrome. J. Infect. Dis. *157*:405–412, 1988.
76. Straus, S. E., Dale, J. K., Tobi, M., et al.: Acyclovir treatment of the chronic fatigue syndrome: Lack of efficacy in a placebo-controlled trial. N. Engl. J. Med. *319*:1692–1698, 1988.
77. Straus, S. E., Dale, J. K., Wright, R., et al.: Allergy and the chronic fatigue syndrome. J. Allergy Clin. Immunol. *81*:791–795, 1988.
78. Straus, S. E., Fritz, S., Dale, J. K., et al.: Lymphocyte phenotype and function in the chronic fatigue syndrome. J. Clin. Immunol. *13*:30–40, 1993.
79. Straus, S. E., Tosato, G., Armstrong G., et al.: Persisting illness and fatigue in adults with evidence of Epstein-Barr virus infection. Ann. Intern. Med. *102*:7–16, 1985.
80. Sumaya, C. V.: Serologic testing for Epstein-Barr virus: Developments in interpretation. J. Infect. Dis. *151*:984–987, 1985.
81. Sumaya, C. V.: Serologic and virologic epidemiology of Epstein-Barr virus: Relevance to chronic fatigue syndrome. Rev. Infect. Dis. *13*:S19–S25, 1991.
82. Taerk, G. S., Toner, B. B., Salit, I. E., et al.: Depression in patients with neuromyasthenia benign myalgic encephalomyelitis. Int. J. Psychiatry Med. *17*:49–56, 1987.
83. Tirelli, U., Marota, G., Improta, S., et al.: Immunological abnormalities in patients with chronic fatigue syndrome. Scand. J. Immunol. *40*:601–608, 1994.
84. Tosato, G., Straus, S., Henle, W., et al.: Characteristic T cell dysfunction in patients with chronic active Epstein-Barr virus infection (chronic infectious mononucleosis). J. Immunol. *134*:3082–3088, 1985.
85. Tobi, M., Morag, A., Ravid, Z., et al.: Prolonged atypical illness associated with serological evidence of persistent Epstein-Barr virus infection. Lancet *1*:61–63, 1982.
86. Wakefield, D., Lloyd, A., Dwyer, J., et al.: Human herpesvirus 6 and myalgic encephalomyelitis. Lancet *1*:1059, 1988.
87. Walford, G. A., Nelson, W. M., and McCluskey, D. R.: Fatigue, depression, and social adjustment in chronic fatigue syndrome. Arch. Dis. Child. *68*:384–388, 1993.
88. White, D. N., and Burtch, R. B.: Iceland disease: New infection simulating acute anterior poliomyelitis. Neurology *4*:506, 1954.
89. Wilson, A., Hickie, I., Lloyd, A., et al: Longitudinal study of outcomes of chronic fatigue syndrome. Br. Med. J. *308*:756–759, 1994.
90. Wolfe, F., Smythe, H. A., Yunus, M. B., et al.: Criteria for fibromyalgia. Arthritis Rheum. *32*(Suppl.):S47, 1989.
91. Yalcin, S., Kuratsune, H., Yamaguchi, K., et al.: Prevalence of human herpesvirus 6 variants A and B in patients with chronic fatigue syndrome. Microbiol. Immunol. *38*:587–590, 1994.

PART 3

INFECTIONS WITH SPECIFIC MICROORGANISMS

SECTION SIXTEEN

BACTERIAL INFECTIONS

84

NOMENCLATURE OF AEROBIC AND ANAEROBIC BACTERIA

David A. Bruckner

The only relevant classification for bacteria is the one that is accepted widely and used by the microbiology community. Bacterial taxonomy is composed of three interrelated areas: classification, nomenclature, and identification. The most comprehensive taxonomic information available for bacteriologic classification can be found in *Bergey's Manual of Determinative Bacteriology*, ninth edition, and in *Bergey's Manual of Systematic Bacteriology*, volumes 1 through 4. Leading journals that contain up-to-date information on nomenclature and new species include the *International Journal of Systematic Bacteriology, Annales de Microbiologie (Institute Pasteur), Current Microbiology, Journal of Clinical Microbiology,* and *Systematic and Applied Microbiology.*

Taxonomic ranks for naming bacterial organisms include kingdom, division, class, order, family, genus, species, and subspecies. All of these ranks have official standing in nomenclature. Ranks below subspecies have no official standing but are used to indicate groups of strains or isolates that can be distinguished by some special characters (Table 84–1).

Nomenclature priorities for bacteriologic names have dated back to May 1753. Because of difficulties in searching literature and limited available information on described species, approved lists of bacterial names were published in the *International Journal of Systematic Bacteriology* in 1980. Names not included on those lists have lost all standing in nomenclature status.

Historically, bacterial classification has been based on phenotypic characteristics. Multivariate analysis has played a large role in classification since the 1950s. This analysis used biochemical, cultural, and morphologic characteristics and susceptibilities to antibiotics and inorganic compounds to define the degrees of similarities between organisms. More recently, molecular techniques (DNA hybridization, gene sequence analysis, et al.) have played a major role in determining phylogenetic relationships.

The DNA molecular weight for most bacteria is 1×10^9 to 8×10^9, enough to specify 1500 to 6000 genes. Using nucleic acids, a number of parameters have been used to determine taxonomic relationships. These parameters include genome size, mole per cent guanine plus cytosine content, DNA relatedness under optimal and supraoptimal conditions for DNA reassociation, and rRNA oglionucleotide sequences. By correlating phenotypic results with DNA homology and rRNA sequence analysis, it has been possible to select phenotypic tests that can be used more accurately to identify organisms belonging to specific groups.

Within the past few years, there have been many taxonomic name changes and new infectious agents described. In some cases, newly recognized species have resulted from better delineation of a species, such as the separation of *Klebsiella oxytoca* from *Klebsiella pneumoniae* by indole reactions. Although some name changes may be confusing at first, their overall impact could improve medical care when pathogenic strains can be differentiated from nonpathogenic strains of the same species through the use of simplified clinical laboratory tests or to establish more predictable antibiograms.

The following bacterial classification is based upon the organism's morphologic and stain characteristics. Organisms included are those that often are associated with pathologic processes or those that are significant medically. The current names are those either officially recognized or proposed for recognition and currently used in the literature.

TABLE 84–1. Bacterial Ranks Below Subspecies

Preferred Name	Synonym	When Applied
Biovar	Biotype	Special biochemical or physiologic features
Serovar	Serotype	Distinct antigenic features
Pathovar	Pathotype	Host-specific pathogenic features
Phagovar	Phagotype	Lysis by distinct bacteriophages
Morphovar	Morphotype	Special morphologic features

I. AEROBIC GRAM-POSITIVE COCCI

Characteristics: occur singly or in pairs, tetrads, chains, or clusters; can be catalase-positive or -negative. Organisms positive for coagulase or clumping factor include Staphylococcus aureus, Staphylococcus hyicus, Staphylococcus intermedius, Staphylococcus lugdunensis, *and* Staphylococcus schleiferi *subspecies* coagulans. Aerococcus *species,* Alloiococcus *species, and* Stomatococcus *species may have a weak positive to negative catalase reaction.*

Current Name	Synonym
Catalase-Positive	
Alloiococcus otitis	
Micrococcus spp.	
Staphylococcus aureus	
Staphylococcus auricularis	
Staphylococcus capitis subsp. *capitis*	
Staphylococcus capitis subsp. *ureolyticus*	
Staphylococcus caprae	
Staphylococcus cohnii subsp. *cohnii*	
Staphylococcus cohnii subsp. *urealyticum*	
Staphylococcus epidermidis	*Staphylococcus albus*
Staphylococcus gallinarum	
Staphylococcus haemolyticus	
Staphylococcus hominis	
Staphylococcus hyicus	
Staphylococcus intermedius	
Staphylococcus lentus	
Staphylococcus lugdunensis	
Staphylococcus pasteuri	
Staphylococcus pulvereri	
Staphylococcus saccharolyticus	*Peptococcus saccharolyticus*
Staphylococcus saprophyticus	*Micrococcus* subgroup 3
Staphylococcus schleiferi subsp. *coagulans*	
Staphylococcus schleiferi subsp. *schleiferi*	
Staphylococcus simulans	
Staphylococcus warneri	
Staphylococcus xylosus	
Staphylococcus mucilaginosus	
Catalase-Negative	
Abiotrophia adiacens	Nutritionally variant streptococci *Staphylococcus adjacens*
Abiotrophia defectiva	Nutritionally variant streptococci *Streptococcus defectivus*
Aerococcus viridans	*Gaffkya homari* *Pediococcus homari*
Aerococcus urinae	ALO
Dolosigranulum pigrum	
Enterococcus avium	*Streptococcus avium* (group D *Enterococcus*)
Enterococcus casseliflavus	
Enterococcus dispar	
Enterococcus durans	*Streptococcus durans* (group D *Enterococcus*)
Enterococcus faecalis	*Streptococcus faecalis* (group D *Enterococcus*)
Enterococcus faecium	*Streptococcus faecium* (group D *Enterococcus*)
Enterococcus flavescens	
Enterococcus gallinarum	
Enterococcus hirae	
Enterococcus malodoratus	
Enterococcus mundtii	
Enterococcus pseudoavium	
Enterococcus raffinosus	
Enterococcus solitaries	
Gemella haemolysans	*Neisseria haemolysans*
Gemella morbillorum	*Streptococcus morbillorum* *Peptostreptococcus morbillorum*
Globicatella sanguis	Salt-tolerant viridans streptococci
Helcococcus kunzii	
Lactococcus garvieae	Lancefield group N

Current Name	Synonym
Catalase-Negative *Continued*	
Lactococcus lactis subsp. *lactis*	
Leuconostoc citreum	
Leuconostoc cremoris	
Leuconostoc dextranicum	
Leuconostoc lactis	
Leuconostoc mesenteroides	
Leuconostoc pseudomesenteroides	
Pediococcus acidilactici	
Pediococcus pentosaceus	
***Streptococcus* Groups**	
Anginosus Group	Viridans streptococci
Streptococcus anginosus	
Streptococcus constellatus	
Streptococcus intermedius	
Bovis Group	
Streptococcus bovis	Group D nonenterococcus
Mitis Group	Viridans streptococci
Streptococcus crista	*Streptococcus sanguis* I
Streptococcus gordonii	
Streptococcus mitis	*Streptococcus mitior*
Streptococcus oralis	
Streptococcus parasanguis	
Streptococcus pneumoniae	*Diplococcus pneumoniae*
Streptococcus sanguis II	
Mutans Group	Viridans streptococci
Streptococcus cricetus	
Streptococcus mutans	
Streptococcus sobrinus	
Streptococcus rattus	
Pyogenic Group	
Streptococcus agalactiae	Group B streptococci
Streptococcus dysgalactiae	Group C streptococci *Streptococcus equi* *Streptococcus equi* subsp. *zooepidemicus* *Streptococcus equisimilis* Group G streptococci *Streptococcus dysgalactiae* *Streptococcus canis*
Streptococcus porcinus	
Streptococcus pyogenes	Group A streptococci
Streptococcus zooepidemicus	Group C streptococci
Salivarius Group	Viridans streptococci
Streptococcus salivarius	
Streptococcus vestibularis	
Vagococcus fluvialis	
Weissella paramesenteroides	*Leuconostoc paramesenteroides*

II. ANAEROBIC GRAM-POSITIVE COCCI

Characteristic: occur singly or in pairs, chains, or clumps.

Current Name	Synonym
Peptococcus niger	*Micrococcus niger*
Peptostreptococcus anaerobius	*Streptococcus anaerobius*
Peptostreptococcus asaccharolyticus	*Peptococcus asaccharolyticus*
Peptostreptococcus hydrogenalis	
Peptostreptococcus indolicus	*Peptococcus indolicus*
Peptostreptococcus lacrimalis	
Peptostreptococcus lactolyticus	

Current Name	Synonym
Peptostreptococcus magnus	*Peptococcus magnus*
	Peptococcus variabilis
Peptostreptococcus micros	*Peptococcus glycinophilus*
Peptostreptococcus prevotii	*Peptococcus prevotii*
Peptostreptococcus tetradius	*Gappkya anaerobia*
Peptostreptococcus vaginalis	
Ruminococcus hansenii	*Streptococcus hansenii*
Ruminococcus productus	*Peptostreptococcus productus*

III. AEROBIC GRAM-NEGATIVE COCCI

Characteristics: occur singly or in pairs or clumps; are catalase- and oxidase-positive.

Current Name	Synonym
Moraxella catarrhalis	*Branhamella catarrhalis*
	Neisseria catarrhalis
Neisseria canis	
Neisseria cinerea	*Micrococcus cinereus*
	Neisseria pharyngis
Neisseria elongata subsp. *elongata*	*Neisseria elongata*
Neisseria elongata subsp. *glycolytica*	*Neisseria elongata*
Neisseria elongata subsp. *nitroreducens*	*Neisseria elongata*
	CDC group M-6
Neisseria flavescens	
Neisseria gonorrhoeae	
Neisseria kochii	
Neisseria lactamica	
Neisseria meningitidis	
Neisseria mucosa	
Neisseria parelongata	
Neisseria polysaccharea	
Neisseria sicca	
Neisseria subflava biovar *flava*	*Neisseria subflava*
Neisseria subflava biovar *perflava*	*Neisseria subflava*
Neisseria subflava biovar *subflava*	*Neisseria subflava*
Neisseria weaveri	*Moraxella* spp. M-5
	CDC group M-5

IV. ANAEROBIC GRAM-NEGATIVE COCCI

Characteristic: occur in pairs or clumps.

Current Name	Synonym
Acidaminococcus fermentans	
Megasphaera elsdenfi	
Veillonella parvula	*Veillonella alkalescens*

V. AEROBIC GRAM-POSITIVE BACILLI

Characteristics: are rod-like and diphtheroid or branching; are catalase-negative or -positive; some are positive for acid-fast stain; only Bacillus *species produce spores.*

Current Name	Synonym
Arcanobacterium haemolyticum	*Corynebacterium haemolyticum*
Aureobacterium spp.	
Bacillus alvei	
Bacillus anthracis	
Bacillus brevis	
Bacillus cereus	
Bacillus circulans	
Bacillus coagulans	
Bacillus licheniformis	

Current Name	Synonym
Bacillus macerans	
Bacillus megaterium	
Bacillus pumilus	
Bacillus sphaericus	
Bacillus subtilis	
Bacillus thuringiensis	
Brevibacterium casei	
Brevibacterium epidermidis	
Brevibacterium mcbrellneri	
Cellumonas hominis	CDC coryneform group A-3
Cellulomonas turbata	*Oerskovia turbata*
Corynebacterium afermentans	*Corynebacterium* ANF-1
Corynebacterium auris	CDC group ANF-1–like
Corynebacterium bovis	
Corynebacterium cystitidis	
Corynebacterium diphtheriae	
Corynebacterium glucuronolyticum	
Corynebacterium glutamicum	
Corynebacterium group G-2	
Corynebacterium jeikeium	*Corynebacterium* group JK CDC group JK
Corynebacterium kutscheri	
Corynebacterium macginleyi	CDC coryneform group G-1
Corynebacterium matruchotii	*Bacterionema matruchotii*
Corynebacterium minutissimum	
Corynebacterium mycetoides	
Corynebacterium pilosum	
Corynebacterium pseudodiphtheriticum	*Corynebacterium hofmannii*
Corynebacterium pseudotuberculosis	
Corynebacterium renale	
Corynebacterium seminale	
Corynebacterium striatum	
Corynebacterium ulcerans	
Corynebacterium urealyticum	*Corynebacterium* group D2 CDC group D2
Corynebacterium xerosis	
Dermabacter hominis	CDC fermentative coryneform groups 3 and 5
Erysipelothrix rhusiopathiae	*Erysipelothrix insidiosa*
Gardnerella vaginalis	*Haemophilus vaginalis* *Corynebacterium vaginalis*
Gordona aichiensis	*Tsukamura aichiensis*
Gordona bronchialis	*Rhodococcus bronchialis*
Gordona rubropertincta	*Rhodococcus rubropertinctus*
Gordona sputi	*Rhodococcus chubuensis*
Kurthia bessonii	
Lactobacillus acidophilus	
Lactobacillus amylovorus	
Lactobacillus brevis	
Lactobacillus casei	
Lactobacillus catenaforme	
Lactobacillus crispatus	
Lactobacillus gasseri	
Lactobacillus jensenii	
Lactobacillus johnsonii	
Lactobacillus oris	
Lactobacillus reuteri	
Lactobacillus uli	
Lactobacillus vaginalis	
Listeria grayi	*Listeria murrayi*
Listeria ivanovii	
Listeria monocytogenes	*Listeria monocytogenes* serovar 5
Microbacterium spp.	CDC coryneform groups A-4 and A-5
Microbacterium arborescens	CDC coryneform group A-4
Microbacterium imperiale	CDC coryneform group A-4
Mycobacterium abscessus	*Mycobacterium chelonae* subsp. *abscessus*

Current Name	Synonym
Mycobacterium africanum	
Mycobacterium alvei	
Mycobacterium asiaticum	
Mycobacterium aurum	
Mycobacterium avium	
Mycobacterium bovis	
Mycobacterium brumae	
Mycobacterium celatum	
Mycobacterium chelonae	*Mycobacterium chelonae* subsp. *chelonae* *Mycobacterium chelonei*
Mycobacterium confluentis	
Mycobacterium flavescens	
Mycobacterium fortuitum	*Mycobacterium fortuitum* subsp. *fortuitum* Third biovariant complex sorbitol-positive Third biovariant complex sorbitol-negative
Mycobacterium gastri	
Mycobacterium genavense	
Mycobacterium gordonae	*Mycobacterium aquae*
Mycobacterium haemophilum	
Mycobacterium intracellulare	
Mycobacterium interjectum	
Mycobacterium kansasii	
Mycobacterium leprae	
Mycobacterium malmoense	
Mycobacterium marinum	*Mycobacterium balnei*
Mycobacterium mucogenicum	*Mycobacterium chelonae*–like organism (MCLO)
Mycobacterium neoaurum	
Mycobacterium nonchromogenicum	
Mycobacterium peregrinum	*Mycobacterium fortuitum* complex
Mycobacterium phlei	
Mycobacterium scrofulaceum	
Mycobacterium shimoidei	
Mycobacterium simiae	*Mycobacterium habana*
Mycobacterium smegmatis	
Mycobacterium szulgai	
Mycobacterium terrae	
Mycobacterium triviale	
Mycobacterium tuberculosis	
Mycobacterium ulcerans	*Mycobacterium buruli*
Mycobacterium vaccae	
Mycobacterium xenopi	
Nocardia asteroides	
Nocardia brasiliensis	
Nocardia carnea	
Nocardia farcinica	
Nocardia nova	
Nocardia otitidiscaviarum	*Nocardia caviae*
Nocardia transvalensis	
Oerskovia xanthineolytica	
Rhodococcus equi	*Corynebacterium equi*
Rothia dentocariosa	*Nocardia dentocariosus*
Tsukamurella inchonensis	
Tsukamurella paurometabola	*Gordona aurantiaca*
Turicella otitidis	*Rhodococcus aurantiazus*

VI. ANAEROBIC GRAM-POSITIVE NON–SPORE-FORMING BACILLI

Characteristic: may be long-branching bacilli or pleomorphic coccobacilli.

Current Name	Synonym
Actinomyces bernardiae	
Actinomyces georgiae	*Actinomyces* DO8

Current Name	Synonym
Actinomyces gerencseriae	*Actinomyces israelii* serotype II
Actinomyces israelii	
Actinomyces meyeri	
Actinomyces naeslundii	
Actinomyces neuii subsp. *anitratus*	CDC coryneform group 1
Actinomyces neuii subsp. *neuii*	CDC coryneform group 1
Actinomyces odontolyticus	
Actinomyces pyogenes	*Corynebacterium pyogenes*
Actinomyces radingae	CDC coryneform group E
Actinomyces turicensis	CDC coryneform group E
Actinomyces viscosus	
Atopobium minutum	*Lactobacillus minutus*
Atopobium parvulum	*Streptococcus parvulus* *Peptostreptococcus parvulus*
Atopobium rimae	*Lactobacillus rimae*
Bifidobacterium breve	
Bifidobacterium dentium	*Bifdobacterium eriksonii* *Bifdobacterium appendicitis*
Bifdobacterium longum	
Eubacterium aerofaciens	
Eubacterium alactolyticum	
Eubacterium barkeri	*Clostridium barkeri*
Eubacterium brachy	
Eubacterium combesii	
Eubacterium contortum	
Eubacterium lentum	
Eubacterium limosum	
Eubacterium moniliforme	
Eubacterium nitrogenes	
Eubacterium nodatum	
Eubacterium saburreum	
Eubacterium saphenum	
Eubacterium tenue	
Eubacterium timidum	
Eubacterium yurii subsp. *yurii*	
Eubacterium yurii subsp. *margaretiae*	
Eubacterium yurii subsp. *schtitka*	
Mobiluncus curtsii subsp. *curtsii*	
Mobiluncus curtsii subsp. *holmesii*	
Mobiluncus mulieris	
Propionibacterium acnes	
Propionibacterium avidum	
Propionibacterium granulosum	
Propionibacterium lymphophilum	
Propionibacterium propionicum	*Arachnia propionica* *Actinomyces propionicus*

VII. ANAEROBIC GRAM-POSITIVE SPORE-FORMING BACILLI

Characteristics: are broad, short bacilli with blunt ends; most organisms readily produce spores, except Clostridium perfringens.

Current Name	Synonym
Clostridium absonum	
Clostridium argentinense	*Clostridium botulinum* type G *Clostridium subterminale* *Clostridium hastiforme*
Clostridium baratti	*Clostridium barati* *Clostridium paraperfringens* *Clostridium perenne*
Clostridium bifermentans	
Clostridium botulinum	Toxigenic strains *Clostridium putrificum* *Clostridium lentoputrescens*
Clostridium butyricum	*Clostridium pseudotetanicum*

Current Name	Synonym
Clostridium cadaveris	
Clostridium carnis	
Clostridium clostridioforme	*Clostridium clostridiiforme*
Clostridium cochlearium	*Clostridium lentoputrescens*
Clostridium difficile	*Clostridium difficilis*
Clostridium fallax	*Clostridium pseudofallax*
Clostridium ghonii	*Clostridium ghoni*
Clostridium glycolicum	
Clostridium haemolyticum	*Clostridium novyi* type D
Clostridium hastiforme	
Clostridium histolyticum	
Clostridium indolis	
Clostridium innocuum	
Clostridium irregulare	*Clostridium irregularis*
Clostridium limosum	
Clostridium malenominatum	
Clostridium novyi	
Clostridium oroticum	*Zymobacterium oroticum*
Clostridium paraputrificum	
Clostridium perfringens	*Clostridium welchii* *Welchia perfringens*
Clostridium piliforme	*Bacillus piliformis*
Clostridium putrefaciens	
Clostridium ramosum	*Eubacterium filamentosum* *Ramibacterium ramosum* *Actinomyces ramosus* *Eubacterium ramosum*
Clostridium septicum	
Clostridium sordellii	
Clostridium sphenoides	
Clostridium sporogenes	Nontoxigenic strains
Clostridium subterminale	
Clostridium symbiosum	*Fusobacterium symbiosum* *Fusobacterium biacutus* *Bacteroides symbiosus*
Clostridium tertium	
Clostridium tetani	
Filifactor villosus	*Clostridium villosum*

VIII. AEROBIC GRAM-NEGATIVE BACILLI: ENTEROBACTERIACEAE

Characteristics: ferment sugars; are oxidase-negative; most reduce nitrate to nitrite.

Current Name	Synonym
Budvicia aquatica	
Cedecea davisae	CDC enteric group 15
Cedecea lapagei	
Cedecea neteri	*Cedecea* spp. 4
Cedecea spp. 3	
Cedecea spp. 5	
Citrobacter amalonaticus	*Levinea amalonatica*
Citrobacter braakii	*Citrobacter freundii*
Citrobacter farmeri	*Citrobacter amalonaticus* biogroup 1
Citrobacter freundii	*Colobactrum freundii*
Citrobacter genomospecies 9	*Citrobacter freundii*
Citrobacter genomospecies 10	*Citrobacter freundii*
Citrobacter genomospecies 11	*Citrobacter freundii*
Citrobacter koseri	*Citrobacter diversus*
Citrobacter sedlakii	*Citrobacter freundii*
Citrobacter werkmanii	*Citrobacter freundii*
Citrobacter youngae	*Citrobacter amalonaticus*
Edwardsiella hoshinae	
Edwardsiella ictaluri	
Edwardsiella tarda	

Current Name	Synonym
Enterobacter aerogenes	*Aerobacter aerogenes*
Enterobacter amnigenus	
Enterobacter asburiae	CDC enteric group 17
Enterobacter cancerogenus	*Enterobacter taylorae*
Enterobacter cloacae	
Enterobacter gergoviae	
Enterobacter hormaechei	CDC enteric group 75
Enterobacter sakazakii	
Escherichia blattae	
Escherichia coli	
Escherichia fergusonii	CDC enteric group 10
Escherichia hermannii	CDC enteric group 11
Escherichia vulneris	CDC enteric group 1
Ewingella americana	
Hafnia alvei	
Klebsiella ornithinolytica	*Klebsiella oxytoca* ornithine-positive
Klebsiella oxytoca	
Klebsiella ozaenae	
Klebsiella planticola	
Klebsiella pneumoniae	
Klebsiella rhinoscleromatis	
Klebsiella terrigena	
Kluyvera ascorbata	
Kluyvera cryocrescens	
Leclercia adecarboxylata	*Escherichia adecarboxylata*
Leminorella grimontii	CDC enteric group 57
Leminorella richardii	
Moellerella wisconsensis	CDC enteric group 46
Morganella morganii subsp. *morganii*	*Proteus morganii*
Morganella morganii subsp. *sibonii*	*Proteus morganii*
Pantoea agglomerans	*Enterobacter agglomerans*
Proteus mirabilis	
Proteus penneri	*Proteus vulgaris* indole-negative
Proteus vulgaris	
Providencia alcalifaciens	*Proteus inconstans*
Providencia rettgeri	*Proteus rettgeri*
Providencia rustigianii	*Providencia alcalifaciens* biogroup 3
Providencia stuartii	*Proteus inconstans*
Rahnella aquatilis	
Salmonella subgroup I serotypes	*Salmonella choleraesuis* *Salmonella enteritidis* *Salmonella gallinarum* *Salmonella paratyphi* A *Salmonella pullorum* *Salmonella typhi*
Salmonella subgroup 2	
Salmonella subgroup 3a	
Salmonella subgroup 3b	
Salmonella subgroup 4	
Salmonella subgroup 5	
Serratia ficaria	
Serratia fonticola	
Serratia grimesii	*Serratia liquefaciens*
Serratia liquefaciens	*Enterobacter liquefaciens*
Serratia marcescens	
Serratia odorifera	
Serratia plymuthica	
Serratia proteamaculans subsp. *proteamaculans*	*Serratia liquefaciens*
Serratia proteamaculans subsp. *quinovora*	*Serratia liquefaciens*
Serratia rubidaea	
Shigella boydii	*Shigella* biogroup C
Shigella dysenteriae	*Shigella* biogroup A
Shigella flexneri	*Shigella* biogroup B
Shigella sonnei	*Shigella* biogroup D
Tatumella ptyseos	CDC group EF-9

Current Name	Synonym
Trabulsiella guamensis	CDC enteric group 90
Yersinia aldovae	
Yersinia bercovieri	*Yersinia enterocolitica* biogroup 3b
Yersinia enterocolitica	*Pasteurella enterocolitica*
Yersinia frederiksenii	
Yersinia intermedia	
Yersinia kristensenii	
Yersinia mollaretii	*Yersinia enterocolitica* biogroup 3a
Yersinia pestis	*Pasteurella pestis*
Yersinia pseudotuberculosis	*Pasteurella pseudotuberculosis*
Yersinia rohdei	
Yokenella regensburgei	*Koserella trabulsii* CDC enteric group 45

IX. AEROBIC GRAM-NEGATIVE BACILLI: NONENTERO-BACTERIACEAE—FERMENTATIVE

Characteristics: ferment sugars; are oxidase-positive.

Current Name	Synonym
Aeromonas caviae	
Aeromonas hydrophila	*Pseudomonas hydrophila*
Aeromonas jandaei	
Aeromonas media	
Aeromonas salmonicida	
Aeromonas schubertii	
Aeromonas trota	
Aeromonas veronii biovar *sobria*	
Aeromonas veronii biovar *veronii*	
Chromobacterium violaceum	*Bacillus violaceus*
Pasteurella aerogenes	
Pasteurella bettyae	CDC group HB-5
Pasteurella canis	*Pasteurella multocida* biotype 6
Pasteurella dagmatis	*Pasteurella* new species 1 *Pasteurella* "gas"
Pasteurella gallinarum	
Pasteurella haemolytica	
Pasteurella-like	CDC group EF-4
Pasteurella multocida	*Pasteurella septica*
Pasteurella pneumotropica	
Pasteurella stomatis	
Plesiomonas shigelloides	*Aeromonas shigelloides*
Vibrio alginolyticus	*Vibrio parahaemolyticus* biotype 2
Vibrio carchariae	
Vibrio cholerae	*Vibrio comma*
Vibrio cincinnatiensis	
Vibrio damsela	CDC group EF-5
Vibrio fluvialis	CDC group EF-6
Vibrio furnissii	*Vibrio fluvialis* biogroup 2
Vibrio hollisae	CDC group EF-13 CDC enteric group 42
Vibrio metschnikovii	CDC enteric group 16 *Vibrio cholerae* biovar proteus
Vibrio mimicus	*Vibrio cholerae* sucrose-negative
Vibrio parahaemolyticus	
Vibrio vulnificus	CDC group EF-3 *Beneckea vulnifica*

X. AEROBIC GRAM-NEGATIVE BACILLI: NONENTERO-BACTERIACEAE—NONFERMENTATIVE

Characteristics: may or may not oxidize sugars; are catalase-positive; are oxidase-variable.

Current Name	Synonym
Acinetobacter baumannii	*Acinetobacter anitratus*
Acinetobacter calcoaceticus	*Acinetobacter anitratus*

Current Name	Synonym
Acinetobacter calcoaceticus Continued	*Acinetobacter calcoaceticus* subsp. *calcoaceticus*
Acinetobacter haemolyticus	*Acinetobacter anitratus*
Acinetobacter johnsonii	
Acinetobacter junii	
Acinetobacter lwoffii	*Acinetobacter anitratus*
	Acinetobacter calcoaceticus subsp. *lwoffii*
Agrobacterium tumefaciens	*Agrobacterium radiobacter*
	CDC group Vd-3
Alcaligenes denitrificans	*Alcaligenes xylosoxidans denitrificans*
	CDC group Vc
Alcaligenes faecalis	*Alcaligenes odorans*
	Pseudomonas odorans
Alcaligenes piechaudii	
Alcaligenes xylosoxidans	*Alcaligenes denitrificans* subsp. *xylosoxidans*
	Achromobacter xylosoxidans
	CDC group IIIa, IIIb
Bergeyella zoohelcum	*Weeksella zoohelcum*
	CDC group IIj
Brevundimonas diminuta	*Pseudomonas diminuta*
	CDC group Ia
Brevundimonas vesicularis	*Pseudomonas vesicularis*
	Corynebacterium vesiculare
Burkholderia cepacia	*Pseudomonas cepacia*
	Pseudomonas multivorans
	Pseudomonas kingae
	CDC group EO-1
Burkholderia gladioli	*Pseudomonas gladioli*
	Pseudomonas marginata
Burkholderia mallei	*Pseudomonas mallei*
	Actinobacillus mallei
	Burkholderia pickettii
	Pseudomonas pickettii
	CDC groups Va-1, Va-2
	Pseudomonas thomasii
Burkholderia pseudomallei	*Pseudomonas pseudomallei*
Chryseobacterium gleum	*Flavobacterium gleum*
	CDC group IIb
Chryseobacterium indologenes	*Flavobacterium indologenes*
	CDC group IIb
Chryseobacterium meningosepticum	*Flavobacterium meningosepticum*
	CDC group IIa
Chryseobacterium odoratum	*Flavobacterium odoratum*
	CDC group M-4f
Chryseomonas luteola	*Pseudomonas luteola*
	CDC group Ve-1
Comamonas acidovorans	*Pseudomonas acidovorans*
Comamonas testosteroni	*Pseudomonas testosteroni*
Comamonas terrigena	CDC group EF-19
Empedobacter brevis	*Flavobacterium breve*
Flavimonas oryzihabitans	*Pseudomonas oryzihabitans*
	CDC group Ve-2
Flavobacterium spp. group IIe	CDC group IIe
Flavobacterium spp. group IIh	CDC group IIh
Flavobacterium spp. group IIi	CDC group IIi
Methylobacterium spp.	
Moraxella atlantae	CDC group M-3
Moraxella catarrhalis	*Branhamella catarrhalis*
Moraxella lacunata	*Moraxella liquefaciens*
Moraxella nonliquefaciens	
Moraxella osloensis	
Moraxella phenylpyruvica	CDC group M-2
Ochrobactrum anthropi	*Achromobacter* spp. biotypes 1 and 2
	CDC groups Vd-1, Vd-2

Current Name	Synonym
Oligella ureolytica	CDC group IVe
Oligella urethralis	*Moraxella urethralis*
	CDC group M-4
Pseudomonas aeruginosa	
Pseudomonas alcaligenes	
Pseudomonas chlororaphis	*Pseudomonas aureofaciens*
Pseudomonas delafieldii	
Pseudomonas fluorescens	
Pseudomonas mendocina	CDC group Vb-2
Pseudomonas pertucinogena	*Bordetella pertussis* rough phase IV
Pseudomonas pseudoalcaligenes	*Pseudomonas alcaligenes* biotype B
Pseudomonas putida	CDC group Vb-1
Pseudomonas stutzeri	CDC group Vb-3
Pseudomonas stutzeri-like	*Pseudomonas dentrificans*
Pseudomonas spp. group 1	CDC group Ivd
Pseudomonas-like group 2	CDC group EF-1
Ralstonia pickettii	
Roseomonas cervicalis	CDC "pink coccoid" group
Roseomonas fauriae	CDC "pink coccoid" group
Roseomonas genomospecies 4	CDC "pink coccoid" group
Roseomonas genomospecies 5	CDC "pink coccoid" group
Roseomonas genomospecies 6	CDC "pink coccoid" group
Roseomonas gilardii	
Shewanella alga	
Shewanella putrefaciens	*Alteromonas putrefaciens*
	Pseudomonas putrefaciens
	CDC groups Ib-1, Ib-2
Sphingobacterium mizutaii	*Flavobacterium mizutae*
Sphingobacterium multivorum	*Flavobacterium multivorum*
	CDC group IIk-2
Sphingobacterium spiritivorum	*Flavobacterium spiritivorum*
	Sphingobacterium versatilis
	CDC group IIk-3
Sphingobacterium thalpophilum	*Flavobacterium thalpophilum*
Sphingobacterium yabuuchiae	
Sphingomonas paucimobilis	*Pseudomonas paucimobilis*
	CDC group IIk-I
Stenotrophomonas maltophilia	*Xanthomonas maltophilia*
	Pseudomonas maltophilia
Weeksella virosa	*Flavobacterium genitale*
	CDC group IIf

XI. ANAEROBIC GRAM-NEGATIVE BACILLI

Characteristic: may appear as rods with rounded ends, curved rods, coccobacilli, or slender, spindle-shaped rods with tapered ends. Dialister *and* Johnsonella *belong to the* Clostridium *subphylum.*

Current Name	Synonym
Anerobiospirinum succiniciproducens	
Anaerorhabdus furcosus	*Bacteroides furcosus*
Bacteroides fragilis group	
Bacteroides caccae	*Bacteroides fragilis* group 3452A
Bacteroides distasonis	
Bacteroides eggerthii	
Bacteroides fragilis	
Bacteroides merdae	*Bacteroides fragilis* T4-1
Bacteroides ovatus	
Bacteroides stercoris	*Bacteroides fragilis* subsp. A
Bacteroides thetaiotaomicron	
Bacteroides uniformis	
Bacteroides vulgatus	

Current Name	Synonym
Bacteroides species, other	
Bacteroides capillosus	
Bacteroides coagulans	
Bacteroides forsythus	
Bacteroides putredinis	
Bacteroides splanchnicus	
Bacteroides tectum	
Bacteroides ureolyticus	
Bilophila wadsworthia	
Catonella morbi	*Bacteroides* D42
Centipeda periodontii	
Desulfomonas pigra	
Desulfovibrio desulfuricans	
Dialister pneumosintes	*Bacteroides pneumosintes*
Dichelobacter nodosus	*Bacteroides nodosus*
	Bacteroides corrodens
Fusobacterium alocis	
Fusobacterium gonidiaformans	*Bacteroides varius*
Fusobacterium mortiferum	*Fusobacterium ridiculosum*
	Sphaerophorus mortiferus
Fusobacterium naviforme	*Fusobacterium fusiforme*
	Bacillus fusiforme
	Sphaerophorus funduliformis
Fusobacterium necrogenes	
Fusobacterium necrophorum subsp. *funduliforme*	
Fusobacterium necrophorum subsp. *necrophorum*	
Fusobacterium nucleatum subsp. *fusiforme*	
Fusobacterium nucleatum subsp. *nucleatum*	
Fusobacterium nucleatum subsp. *polymorphum*	
Fusobacterium nucleatum subsp. *vincentii*	
Fusobacterium periodonticum	
Fusobacterium russii	
Fusobacterium sulci	
Fusobacterium ulcerans	
Fusobacterium varium	
Johnsonella ignava	*Bacteroides* D19
Leptotrichia buccalis	
Mitsuokella multiacidus	*Bacteroides mutiacidus*
Porphyromonas asaccharolytica	*Bacteroides asaccharolyticus*
	Bacteroides melaninogenicus subsp. *asaccharolyticus*
Porphyromonas cangingivalis	
Porphyromonas canoris	
Porphyromonas cansulci	
Porphyromona catoniae	*Oribaculum catoniae*
	Bacteroides D26
Porphyromonas circumdentaria	
Porphyromonas crevioricanis	
Porphyromonas endodontalis	*Bacteroides endodontalis*
Porphyromonas gingivalis	*Bacteroides gingivalis*
Porphyromonas gingivicanis	
Porphyromona levii	*Bacteroides levii*
	Bacteroides melaninogenicus subsp. *levi*
Porphyromonas macacae	*Bacteroides macacae*
Porphyromonas salivosa	*Bacteroides salivosus*
Prevotella bivia	*Bacteroides bivius*
Prevotella buccae	*Bacteroides buccae*
	Bacteroides rumincola subsp. *brevis*
	Bacteroides capillus
	Bacteroides pentosaceus
Prevotella buccalis	*Bacteroides buccalis*
Prevotella corporis	*Bacteroides corporis*

Current Name	Synonym
Prevotella dentalis	*Hallella seregens*
	Mitsuokella dentalis
Prevotella denticola	*Bacteroides denticola*
Prevotella disiens	*Bacteroides disiens*
Prevotella enoeca	
Prevotella heparinolytica	*Bacteroides heparinolyheus*
Prevotella intermedia	*Bacteroides intermedius*
	Bacteroides melaninogenicus subsp. *intermedius*
Prevotella loescheii	*Bacteroides loescheii*
Prevotella melaninogenica	*Bacteroides melaninogenicus*
	Bacteroides melaninogenicus subsp. *melaninogenicus*
Prevotella nigrescens	
Prevotella oralis	*Bacteroides oralis*
Prevotella oris	*Bacteroides oris*
	Bacteroides ruminicola subsp. *brevis*
Prevotella oulorum	*Bacteroides oulorum*
	Prevotella oulora
Prevotella tannerae	
Prevotella veroralis	*Bacteroides veroralis*
Prevotella zoogleoformans	*Bacteroides zoogleoformans*
Selenomonas artemidis	
Selenomonas dianae	
Selenomonas flueggei	
Selenomonas infelix	
Selenomonas noxia	
Selenomonas suptigena	
Tissierella creatinini	*Tissierella praeacuta*
	Bacteroides praeacutus

XII. AEROBIC GRAM-NEGATIVE COCCOBACILLI

Characteristics: small, gram-negative bacilli or coccobacilli; may require carbon dioxide and enriched media or special conditions for adequate growth.

Current Name	Synonym
Actinobacillus actinomycetemcomitans	CDC groups HB-3, HB-4
Actinobacillus lignieresii	
Actinobacillus suis	
Actinobacillus ureae	*Pasteurella ureae*
Afipia felis	
Afipia clevelandensis	
Afipia broomeae	
Arcobacter butzleri	*Campylobacter butzleri*
Arcobacter cryaerophilus	*Campylobacter cryaerophilus*
Arcobacter nitrofigilis	
Bartonella bacilliformis	
Bartonella elizabethae	*Rochalimaea elizabethae*
Bartonella henselae	*Rochalimaea henselae*
Bartonella quintana	*Rochalimaea quintana*
Bartonella vinsonii	*Rochalimea vinsonii*
Brucella abortus	
Brucella canis	
Brucella melitensis	
Brucella suis	
Bordetella avium	
Bordetella bronchiseptica	CDC group IVa
Bordetella hinzii	
Bordetella holmesii	CDC group NO-2
Bordetella-like *species*	CDC group EF-26
Bordetella parapertussis	
Bordetella pertussis	
Calymmatobacterium granulomatis	
Campylobacter coli	

Current Name	Synonym
Campylobacter concisus	CDC group EF-22
Campylobacter curvus	*Wolinella curva*
Campylobacter fetus subsp. *fetus*	*Vibrio fetus*
Campylobacter gracilis	*Bacteroides gracilis*
Campylobacter hyointestinalis	
Campylobacter lari	*Campylobacter laridis*
Campylobacter jejuni subsp. *doylei*	
Campylobacter jejuni subsp. *jejuni*	
Campylobacter jejuni subsp. *venerealis*	
Campylobacter mucosalis	
Campylobacter rectus	*Wolinella recta*
Campylobacter showae	
Campylobacter sputorum subsp. *sputorum*	
Campylobacter upsaliensis	
Capnocytophaga canimorsus	CDC group DF-2
Capnocytophaga cynodegmi	CDC group DF-2–like
Capnocytophaga gingivalis	CDC group DF-1
Capnocytophaga granulosa	
Capnocytophaga haemolytica	
Capnocytophaga ochracea	CDC group DF-1
Capnocytophaga sputigena	CDC group DF-1
Cardiobacterium hominis	CDC group IId
Chlamydia pneumoniae	TWAR
Chlamydia psittaci	
Chlamydia trachomatis	
Coxiella burnetii	
Eikenella corrodens	CDC group HB-1
Ehrlichia canis	
Ehrlichia chaffeensis	
Ehrlichia sennetsu	
Francisella philomiragia	*Yersinia philomiragia*
Francisella tularenesis biovar *novicida*	*Francisella novicida* *Pasteurella tularensis* *Bacterium tularense*
Francisella tularensis biovar *palearctica*	*Francisella tularensis* type B *Bacterium tularense*
Francisella tularensis biovar *tularensis*	*Francisella tularensis* type A *Pasteurella tularensis* *Bacterium tularense*
Haemophilus aegyptius	
Haemophilus aphrophilus	CDC group HB-2
Haemophilus ducreyi	
Haemophilus haemolyticus	
Haemophilus influenzae	
Haemophilus parahaemolyticus	
Haemophilus parainfluenzae	
Haemophilus paraphrophilus	
Haemophilus segnis	
Helicobacter cinaedi	*Campylobacter cinaedi*
Helicobacter fennelliae	*Campylobacter fennelliae*
Helicobacter pullorum	
Helicobacter pylori	*Campylobacter pylori*
Kingella denitrificans	CDC group TM-1
Kingella kingae	*Moraxella kingae* *Moraxella kingii*
Kingella oralis	
Legionella anisa	
Legionella birminghamensis	
Legionella bozemanii	*Fluoribacter bozemanae*
Legionella brunensis	
Legionella cherii	
Legionella cincinnatiensis	
Legionella dumoffii	*Fluoribacter dumoffii*
Legionella erythra	
Legionella feeleii	
Legionella geestiana	
Legionella gormanii	

Current Name	Synonym
Legionella hackeliae	
Legionella israelensis	
Legionella jamestowniensis	
Legionella jordanis	
Legionella lansingensis	
Legionella londoniensis	
Legionella longbeachae	
Legionella maceachernii	
Legionella micdadei	*Tatlockia micdadei*
Legionella moravica	
Legionella nautarum	
Legionella oakridgensis	
Legionella parisiensis	
Legionella pneumophila	
Legionella quateriensis	
Legionella quinlivanii	
Legionella rubrilucens	
Legionella sainthelensi	
Legionella santicrucis	
Legionella shakespearei	
Legionella spiritensis	
Legionella steigerwaltii	
Legionella tucsonensis	
Legionella wadsworthii	
Legionella worsliensis	
Orientia tsutsugamushi	*Rickettsia tsutsugamushi*
Psychrobacter immobilis	*Micrococcus cryophilus*
Rickettsia akari	
Rickettsia conorii	
Rickettsia japonica	
Rickettsia mooseri	
Rickettsia prowazekii	
Rickettsia rickettsii	
Rickettsia typhi	
Streptobacillus moniliformis	*Haverhillia multiformis*
Suttonella indologenes	*Kingella indologenes*

XIII. *MYCOPLASMA* (PLEUROPNEUMONIA-LIKE ORGANISMS [PPLOs])

Characteristics: small, highly pleomorphic organisms that are difficult to observe with routine stains; require complex medium for growth.

Current Name	Synonym
Mycoplasma arginini	
Mycoplasma buccale	
Mycoplasma faucium	
Mycoplasma fermentans	
Mycoplasma genitalium	
Mycoplasma hominis	
Mycoplasma incognitus	
Mycoplasma lipophilum	
Mycoplasma orale	
Mycoplasma penetrans	
Mycoplasma pneumoniae	
Mycoplasma primatum	
Mycoplasma salivarium	
Mycoplasma spermatophilum	
Ureaplasma urealyticum	T-*Mycoplasma*

XIV. *TREPONEMATACEAE* (SPIRAL ORGANISMS)

Characteristics: filamentous, spiral organisms that may or may not stain with usual laboratory stains; require complex media or animal host for growth.

Current Name	Synonym
Anguillina coli	*Serpulina jonesii* *Treponema jonesii*

Current Name	Synonym
Borrelia afzelii	Lyme disease agent, Africa, Europe
Borrelia burgdorferi	Lyme disease agent, North America
Borrelia duttoni	
Borrelia garinii	Lyme disease agent, Europe
Borrelia hermsii	
Borrelia parkeri	
Borrelia recurrentis	
Borrelia turicatae	
Brachyspira aalborgii	
Leptospira borgpetersenii	
Leptospira inadai	
Leptospira interrogans	
Leptospira interrogans serogroup *autumnalis*	
Leptospira interrogans serogroup *ballum*	
Leptospira interrogans serogroup *bataviae*	
Leptospira interrogans serogroup *canicola*	
Leptospira interrogans serogroup *grippotyphosa*	
Leptospira interrogans serogroup *icterohaemorrhagiae*	
Leptospira interrogans serogroup *pomona*	
Leptospira kirschneri	
Leptospira noguchii	
Leptospira santarosai	
Leptospira weilii	
Spirillum minus	*Spirillum minor*
Treponema carateum	
Treponema denticola	
Treponema pallidum subsp. *endemicum*	
Treponema pallidum subsp. *pallidum*	*Treponema pallidum*
Treponema pallidum subsp. *pertenue*	
Treponema phagedenis	
Treponema refringens	
Treponema vincentii	

Bibliography

1. Brenner, D. J., O'Connor, S. P., Winkler, H. H., et al.: Proposals to unify the genera *Bartonella* and *Rochalimaea,* with descriptions of *Bartonella quintana* comb. nov., *Bartonella vinsonii* comb. nov., *Bartonella henselae* comb. nov., and *Bartonella elizabethae* comb. nov., and to remove the family Bartonellaceae from the order Rickettsiales. Int. J. Syst. Bacteriol. *43:*777–786, 1993.
2. Coykendall, A. L.: Classification and identification of the viridans streptococci. Clin. Microbiol. Rev. *2:*315–328, 1989.
3. Facklam, R., and Elliott, J. A.: Idenitification, classification, and clinical relevance of catalase-negative, gram-positive cocci, excluding the streptococci and enterococci. Clin. Microbiol Rev. *8:*479–495, 1995.
4. Farmer, J. J., III, Davis, B. R., Hickman-Brenner, F. W., et al.: Biochemical identification of new species and biogroups of Enterobacteriaceae isolated from clinical specimens. J. Clin. Microbiol. *21:*46–76, 1985.
5. Holt, J. G. (ed.): Bergey's Manual of Systematic Bacteriology. Vol. 1, 1984. Vol. 2, 1986, Vol. 3, 1989. Vol. 4, 1989, Baltimore, Williams & Wilkins.
6. Holt, J. G., Krieg, N. R., Sneath, P. H. A., et al.: Bergey's Manual of Determinative Bacteriology. 9th ed. Baltimore, Williams & Wilkins, 1994.
7. Kawamura, Y., Hou, X., Sultana, F., et al.: Transfer of *Streptococcus adjacens* and *Streptococcus defectivus* to *Abiotrophia* gen. nov. as *Abiotrophia adjacens* comb. nov. and *Abiotrophia defectiva* comb. nov., respectively. Int. J. Syst. Bacteriol. *45:*798–803, 1995.
8. Kawamura, Y., Hou, X., Sultana, F., et al.: Determination of 16S rRNA sequences of *Streptococcus mitis* and *Streptococcus gordonii* and phylogenetic relationships among members of the genus *Streptococcus.* Int. J. Syst. Bacteriol. *45:*406–408, 1995.
9. McNeil, M. M., and Brown, J. M.: The medically important aerobic actinomycetes: Epidemiology and microbiology. Clin. Microbiol. Rev. *7:*357–417, 1994.
10. Palleroni, N. J., and Bradbury, J. F.: *Stenotrophomonas,* a new bacterial genus for *Xanthomonas maltophilia* (Hugh 1980) Swings et al. 1983. Int. J. Syst. Bacteriol. *43:*606–609, 1993.
11. Ruimy, R., Boiron, P., Boivin, V., Christen, R.: A phylogeny of the genus *Nocardia* deduced from the analysis of small-subunit ribosomal DNA sequences, including transfer of *Nocardia amarae* to the genus *Gordona* as *Gordona amarae* comb. FEMS Microbiol. Letters *123:*261–268, 1994.
12. Ruoff, K. L.: Recent taxonomic changes in the genus *Enterococcus.* Eur. J. Clin. Microbiol. Infect. Dis. *9:*75–79, 1990.
13. Shah, H. N., and Collins, M. D.: Proposal for reclassification of *Bacteroides asaccharolyticus, Bacteroides gingivalis,* and *Bacteroides endotalis* in a new genus, *Porphyromonas.* Int. J. Syst. Bacteriol. *38:*128–131, 1988.
14. Shah, H. N., and Collins, M. D.: *Prevotella,* a new genus, to include *Bacteroides melaninogenicus* and related species formerly classified in the genus, *Bacteroides.* Int. J. Syst. Bacteriol. *40:*205–208, 1990.
15. Shinnick, T. M., and Good, R. C.: Mycobacterial taxonomy. Eur. J. Clin. Microbiol. *13:*884–901, 1994.
16. Stackebrandt, E., and Goebel, B. M.: Taxonomic note: A place for DNA-DNA reassociation and 16S rRNA sequence analysis in the present species definition in bacteriology. Int. J. Syst. Bacteriol. *44:*846–849, 1994.

❑ ❑ ❑

SUBSECTION ONE

GRAM-POSITIVE COCCI

85

COAGULASE-POSITIVE STAPHYLOCOCCAL INFECTIONS

Marian E. Melish and Kathleen A. Campbell

Staphylococci are ubiquitous microorganisms, pathogenic for humans and animals, and distributed widely in the environment. They are part of the normal human flora. Coagulase-negative staphylococci *(Staphylococcus epidermidis)* are found universally on the skin and frequently in the nasopharynx, whereas coagulase-positive staphylococci occasionally are carried on the skin, particularly of the face; they rapidly colonize small abrasions and are found in the nose and fingernails of approximately 30 per cent of normal adults. Staphylococcal organisms are responsible for an impressive variety of diseases, ranging from minor nuisances to major life-threatening and fatal infections. Coagulase-positive staphylococci are responsible for superficial skin infections, cellulitis, furuncles, wound infections, deep-tissue abscesses, phlebitis, endocarditis, pericarditis, pneumonia, empyema, osteomyelitis, and septic arthritis. Coagulase-negative staphylococci may be responsible for urinary tract infections, bacteremia in the newborn and the compromised host, and infections associated with foreign bodies (particularly cerebrospinal fluid shunt devices and cardiac and vascular prostheses) (see Chapter 86).

THE ORGANISMS

Staphylococci are nonmotile aerobic or facultatively anaerobic cocci that are cultivated readily in simple microbiologic media. They are spherical organisms ranging from 0.7 to 1.2 μm in diameter and stain gram-positive. In smears of infected tissue, they can be recognized as occurring in pairs and grape-like clusters (Fig. 85–1). Indeed, their appearance prompted their name, from the Greek words *staphylo* (bunch of grapes) and *kokkus* (grain or berry). Staphylococci do not have fastidious growth requirements and multiply well in foodstuffs. They are more resistant to high salt concentrations than are most other pathogenic bacteria, surviving well in ham and salt pork, for example. Staphylococci resist drying and can survive in dust and soil for years. They are tolerant of temperatures to 50° C; this and resistance to drying allow prolonged survival on fomites and clothing.

On blood agar, these organisms form round, convex, shiny, opaque colonies 1 to 2 mm in diameter. On this medium, a zone of clear hemolysis surrounding the colony can be recognized for most coagulase-positive strains and some coagulase-negative strains. Pigment production varies; strains exhibiting a deep yellow or golden pigment generally are coagulase-positive and are known as *Staphylococcus aureus;* those of lesser pathogenicity generally are chalk-white and are known as *S. epidermidis* or *Staphylococcus albus.* Classification by pigment production is unreliable and has been superseded completely by coagulase determination, which provides a much better basis for general determination of virulence and species differentiation.

Virulent human staphylococci secrete free coagulase into the broth medium. This free coagulase reacts with coagulase-reacting factor in plasma, resulting in the conversion of fibrinogen to fibrin and the formation of a fibrin clot. Coagulase also can be evaluated by the use of a test for bound coagulase or clumping factor (Fig. 85–2). This substance is bound to the organism; acts directly on fibrinogen, converting it to fibrin; and is detected by the easily visible clumping or agglutination reaction when a suspension of organisms is incubated with plasma. The bound coagulase test is employed most commonly in clinical laboratories. The bound and free coagulases are distinct immunologically but nearly always are present together in virulent organisms. Because fully virulent staphylococci may be nonpigmented, "coagulase-positive staphylococcus" is preferred to "*S. aureus*" and now is considered synonymous.

IDENTIFICATION OF STAPHYLOCOCCI

Three species of staphylococci of major clinical importance can be identified by certain characteristics, which are listed in Table 85–1.[211] For routine clinical purposes, carefully performed slide and tube coagulase tests are sufficient to distinguish coagulase-positive staphylococci from coagulase-negative species.

Structure

Ultrastructural analysis of staphylococci reveals the relatively simple structure typical of prokaryotic cells. The cell wall is composed of inner and outer dense layers apposed to

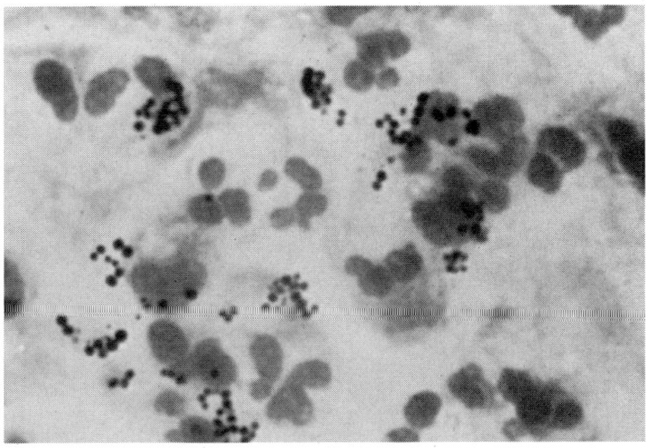

FIGURE 85–1. *Staphylococci in pus. The organisms tend to form clusters, are round, and stain purple with Gram stain (positive), looking like bunches of grapes.*

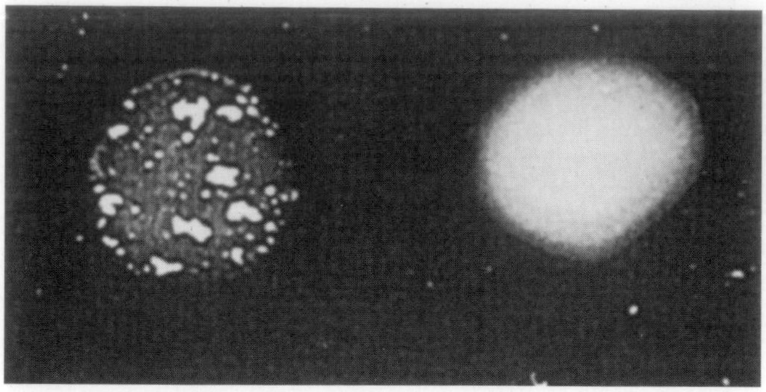

FIGURE 85–2. *Bound (slide) coagulase test. A suspension of organisms is mixed with plasma. Immediate clumping (reaction on the left) indicates both the presence of bound coagulase and the fact that the organism is coagulase-positive.*

the plasma membrane. Cells divide by binary fission, a cross-wall composed of three dense layers forming through the center of the cell. The internal structure is relatively simple. Nuclear material is identified as an area of reduced density containing delicate filaments lacking a well-defined nuclear membrane. Membranous structures or mesosomes arise from the plasma membrane and are found variously in contact with plasma membrane, free in cytoplasm, and in association with the nuclear material. The cytoplasm is populated thickly with ribosomes.[241]

Organisms usually are not encapsulated. Naturally occurring polysaccharide capsules have been demonstrated in human strains and mouse strains. Four different antigenic types have been identified. In experimental animals, encapsulated organisms appear to be of increased virulence. However, the majority of fully virulent staphylococci isolated from severe human infections are not encapsulated. Coagulase-positive staphylococci possess a cell wall with three main components: peptidoglycan, ribitol teichoic acids, and protein A. *S. epidermidis* has a similar cell wall structure, except that the teichoic acids contain glycerol instead of ribitol and protein A is absent. Antibodies to teichoic acids and peptidoglycan are formed in the course of infection. The presence of these antibodies may be useful in the diagnosis of occult infection, particularly osteomyelitis and endocarditis.

Protein A

Staphylococcal protein A, a major component of the cell wall of coagulase-positive staphylococci, has been found to bind to the Fc portion of IgG. This binding is nonimmune. It differs from specific antigen-antibody reactions because the reaction is nonspecific, although both precipitation and agglutination are observed. Protein A binds the IgG of many mammalian species. This property has made protein A a major reagent in many immune assays.

TABLE 85–1. Identification of Staphylococci

Characteristics	*S. aureus*	*S. epidermidis*	*S. saprophyticus*
Coagulase	+	−	−
Acid aerobically from			
Sucrose	+	+	+
Trehalose	+	−	+
Mannitol	+	−	+
Phosphatase	+	+	−
Novobiocin	Sensitive	Sensitive	Resistant

Extracellular Products

Coagulase-positive staphylococci elaborate a wide variety of extracellular toxins, many of which have potent biologic effects in the isolated state on intact animals, tissues, cells, and membranes. These toxins generally are believed to be responsible for the virulence of coagulase-positive staphylococci, and their role in staphylococcal infection in humans has been proved definitively. The important staphylococcal extracellular products include alpha-, beta-, and delta-hemolysins; coagulases; leukocidin; hyaluronidase; staphylokinase; bacteriocins; the epidermolytic toxins; toxic shock syndrome toxin I (TSST-I); and the enterotoxins.

Hemolysins

Alpha-hemolysin is produced by most coagulase-positive organisms. Because of impressive hemolytic, dermonecrotic, and lethal properties of the purified toxin, it has received the lion's share of attention given to all the staphylococcal extracellular products. Most, but not all, coagulase-positive staphylococci produce alpha-hemolysin. Advances in protein purification have allowed the production of pure toxin; this, in turn, has led to better understanding of its properties.

The protein interacts with and damages a variety of cell membranes, releases hemoglobin from erythrocytes of various mammalian and avian species, and is cytotoxic to various cell lines in tissue culture. It lyses rabbit and human platelets and disrupts lysosomes. It causes contraction in skeletal and vascular smooth muscle—the latter action perhaps explains its property of causing localized dermal necrosis. Injection of alpha-toxin is lethal to mammals and reptiles, causing death within 2 to 5 minutes. Human death has been attributed to preformed alpha-toxin on at least one occasion. In a disaster occurring in Bundaberg, Australia, 12 of 21 children died after receiving diphtheria vaccine that had been contaminated with a heavy growth of staphylococci and in which high levels of hemolysin were found.

Anti–alpha-toxin can be demonstrated in normal persons; the level of anti–alpha-hemolysin is high in approximately 70 per cent of patients with staphylococcal osteomyelitis.[243] In humans and in experimental animals, the presence of anti–alpha-hemolysin neither modifies nor prevents staphylococcal infection.

Other hemolytic toxins, the beta- and delta-hemolysins, also possess hemolytic and cytotoxic activities, beta-toxin showing lethal and dermonecrotic effects in addition. Eighty to 100 per cent of adults possess antibody to beta-hemolysin.

Despite evidence that these toxins are produced during infection, their role in the production of the typical staphylococcal tissue lesion remains unclear.[191] Although these toxins, interacting with each other and with other biologically active staphylococcal products, may play an important role in the establishment of infection, this has not been proved; infection is not prevented by antitoxic antibody, and virulent staphylococci that lack one or more of these toxins are encountered.[279]

Leukocidin

Although certain hemolysins are toxic to various leukocytes, the Panton-Valentine leukocidin is the only known extracellular toxin that attacks the leukocyte exclusively.[193] It consists of two protein components, which synergistically kill human polymorphonuclear leukocytes and macrophages.[81] Leukocidin injected into rabbits causes a marked fall in levels of circulating and bone marrow leukocytes, followed by marked granulocytosis; these changes occur without death to the rabbits. Leukocidin interacts with the membrane phospholipid, causing depolarization, increased permeability, and cell death. Local secretion of leukocidin might appear to confer an advantage to the staphylococcus by killing leukocytes, thereby preventing phagocytosis and intracellular killing. This proposition remains unproven. Levels of antileukocidin rise rapidly in the course of infection,[89, 116] and there is some evidence that infants and mothers with high antileukocidin antibodies are less likely to develop staphylococcal disease in high-risk epidemiologic situations.[18] However, leukocidin is likely to confer only a slight advantage because at least 25 per cent of pathogenic staphylococci are leukocidin-negative.

Enzymes

Staphylococci elaborate a variety of enzymes that might play a role in local tissue aggression or the establishment of a nidus of infection. These include hyaluronidase, nuclease, proteases, lipase, catalase, lysozyme, and lactic dehydrogenase.

Other biologically active extracellular products, as yet unidentified, undoubtedly are produced by the staphylococcus. At the time of this writing, no single one of the extracellular products has emerged as the long-sought "virulence factor." The potency and number of these weapons in the armamentarium of the coagulase-positive staphylococcus, compared with the small number of extracellular products associated with the much less virulent coagulase-negative staphylococcus, suggest that the synergistic action of these toxins and enzymes may explain the superior ability of coagulase-positive staphylococci to establish infection and cause tissue necrosis.

Several extracellular toxins have been proved to have specific roles in staphylococcal infection or disease: the epidermolytic toxins, TSST-I, and the enterotoxins.

Epidermolytic Toxins

Two biochemically and immunologically distinct exotoxins, epidermolytic toxins A and B (epidermolysins, exfoliatins), can separate adjacent cell layers within the epidermis, causing the various skin manifestations of the staphylococcal scalded skin syndrome. The toxin acts extracellularly and does not cause cell death directly or lysis of the cell membrane or elicit an inflammatory response. It does not damage any organ or cell, except those of the upper epidermis.[69, 146, 149, 168] These low-molecular-weight (approximately 24,000 daltons) protein exotoxins are elaborated primarily by strains belonging to phage group II (types 3A, 3B, 3C, 55, and 71) but also by nontypable strains and those belonging to other phage groups.

Toxic Shock Syndrome Toxin I

TSST-I was discovered independently in 1981 by two research groups. One group called it low-molecular-weight (approximately 24,000 daltons) neutral protein staphylococcal enterotoxin F, and the other called it pyrogenic exotoxin C. It was proved to be an excellent marker for staphylococci associated with vaginal TSS, correctly identifying more than 90 per cent of strains in blinded testing. In experimental animal models, purified TSST-I can reproduce the major physiologic changes of TSS: fever, mucous membrane suffusion, renal impairment, hepatic damage, hypocalcemia, lymphocytopenia, and hypotension.[165] TSST-I can be detected in blood, pus, urine, and tissues during human and experimental model TSS.

Enterotoxins

Five antigenically different staphylococcal exotoxins (enterotoxins A to E) with the property of causing emesis in primates have been identified. The majority of coagulase-positive staphylococci can elaborate at least one enterotoxin under the appropriate circumstances. The toxins are heat-stable and resist boiling. Therefore, once sufficient toxin has formed within food, even heating or boiling will not inactivate the toxin. Food involved in outbreaks of food poisoning has been inoculated frequently by a lesion on the hand of a food worker and then held at temperatures that allow bacterial growth between 25° and 60° C for some time before serving. Foods that particularly are implicated are ham, salads with starch and mayonnaise, salami, poultry, cream sauces, pastry, and dairy products. The mode of action of enterotoxins is not understood completely, but vomiting appears to be induced through action on the central nervous system. Intravenous injection of purified enterotoxins in laboratory animals causes hypotension, cardiovascular collapse, and death. The significance of these properties of enterotoxins in naturally occurring human infections is unknown, although they may be linked to clinical syndromes, including TSS. Enterotoxin A often is elaborated with TSST-I in menstrual-associated TSS. It also is elaborated without TSST-I in patients with septicemia who do not develop TSS. Staphylococcal enterotoxin B, most often isolated in phage group V organisms, is associated with local infections and pneumonia.[160] Staphylococcal enterotoxin C has been demonstrated by immunohistologic methods in the proximal convoluted tubular cells of the kidney of 36 per cent of patients with sudden infant death syndrome versus 18 per cent of control patients.[157]

Staphylococcal L-Forms

L-forms are staphylococcal variants with impaired or absent cell walls. L-forms can be induced in vitro by growing staphylococci in hypertonic media, in the presence of the muralytic enzyme lysostaphin, or in the presence of cell wall inhibiting antibiotics, such as the penicillin-methicillin group, cycloserine, or vancomycin. These L-forms or protoplasts require hypertonic environments for survival, do not accept Gram stain, and are resistant to cell wall–inhibiting antibiotics. Under favorable conditions, L-forms revert to complete cell wall–containing bacteria. These bacteria, however, differ significantly from the parent strain, many of them losing such markers as coagulase production, mannitol fermentation, penicillinase elaboration, and phage-typing pattern. Reverted organisms appear to be much less able to colonize and infect experimental animals. Therefore, L-form revertants appear to be considerably deficient in pathogenic potential.

Clinical interest in L-forms has arisen because of concern that antibiotics might induce these forms in vivo. L-forms then might persist in the host in a latent or less virulent phase, reverting to a fully virulent state at some time when antibiotics no longer are present. Overt experimental infections have been produced with difficulty with L-forms, reversion to intact staphylococci being demonstrated in these situations. Identification of L forms in specimens from human infection or in infected animals treated with antibiotics has been reported exceedingly rarely, despite considerable searching.[268] The presence of latent L-forms remains an attractive hypothesis to explain the well-known tendency of staphylococcal infections to persist and recur. Despite extensive laboratory and clinical investigation, there is no evidence that L-forms are important causes of bacterial persistence in clinical infections. Extensive searches and special therapy for L-forms rarely are productive.

Phage Typing

Coagulase-positive staphylococci are susceptible to lysis when exposed to bacteriophages. The particular pattern of bacteriophage lysis can be used to identify strains of staphylococci. Bacteriophage typing has been used primarily as an epidemiologic tool for identifying related strains in epidemics. An international system for strain identification by bacteriophage typing has been established, and this method is in widespread use. Another method, serologic typing based on type-specific agglutinogens, is used less frequently. Bacteriophage typing has few clinical correlations and generally is made available through state health departments only for the identification of strains involved in staphylococcal outbreaks. In exceptional cases, it can be used in determining whether a particular infection is a recurrence or a reinfection if organisms from the present and prior infections are available. Staphylococci of phage group 80/81 were widespread during the pandemic of staphylococcal disease in the late 1950s. At present, a wide variety of phage types are involved in staphylococcal disease.

The major clinical correlate of staphylococcal phage typing at present is the association of the phage group II strains with the various forms of the staphylococcal scalded skin syndrome. Phage group I 29/52 complex is associated with TSS strains, phage group V with enterotoxin B, and phage type 95 with enterotoxin C.[160] In no case is the association absolute; many strains of these phage types are nontoxigenic, and toxigenic strains are prevalent among nontypable staphylococci and those belonging to other phage groups.

EPIDEMIOLOGY

Coagulase-positive staphylococci are responsible both for sporadic infections and for epidemics of varying size, ranging from the commonly encountered intrafamily outbreaks of staphylococcal disease to large and often prolonged hospital-associated outbreaks, such as those emanating from a newborn nursery or a surgical service. Epidemic spread of staphylococci of phage type 80/81 was so widespread in hospitals across North America and the world in the period encompassing the mid-1950s through the early 1960s that it constituted a pandemic. It has been suggested that a few "epidemiologically virulent" strains, such as 80/81, particularly are capable of spreading widely and causing disease.

However, just as the factors responsible for the appearance of this staphylococcal pandemic and for other cyclical variations in the prevalence of staphylococcal disease remain unexplained, so do the reasons for its decline. The introduction of the penicillinase-resistant penicillins, the establishment of hospital nosocomial infection surveillance, and the introduction of control measures within hospitals have been cited as responsible for the decline, as has genetic change within the epidemic strain, but there are problems in accepting any or all of these hypotheses. Because we remain largely ignorant of the factors responsible for pandemic spread, we currently cannot prevent or predict recurrence. However, much has been learned about modes of spread of staphylococci and of various effective control measures that can be applied to the control of more limited outbreaks.

Staphylococci may be transmitted by multiple routes, including contact with infected persons, contact with asymptomatic carriers, airborne spread, and contact with contaminated objects. Of these, contact with a person with a staphylococcal lesion appears to be particularly important in the spread of staphylococci. Persons with open draining lesions disseminate organisms into their environment and to others via direct contact. In a hospital, staphylococcal spread may occur from an infected patient to another on the hands of caretakers, such as physicians or nurses. Hospital personnel with mild or inapparent lesions, such as styes, furuncles, or paronychia, themselves may spread organisms. In family and small community outbreaks, multiple secondary cases frequently can be traced to an individual with a draining lesion. Secondary cases tend to appear for months after the initiating case within these small epidemiologic units.[236]

Staphylococci also may be spread by asymptomatic carriers who have staphylococci in one or more body sites, including the nose, skin, hair, nails, axillae, and perineum. Detailed studies have been performed to delineate factors regulating the carrier state and its establishment and perpetuation, as well as factors responsible for organism dispersion from carriers. The asymptomatic carrier may be a source of disease for himself and others. For example, a hospitalized patient who becomes a carrier appears to be more likely to develop a wound infection than does a noncarrier. In the past, much attention has been devoted to detecting and attempting to treat nasal carriers of staphylococci. Studies of nursery outbreaks have indicated that nasal carriage is not as important as is hand transmission in the dispersal of staphylococci.[275] Transmission by hand contact can be minimized by effective hand washing.[90] The problem of hair carriage of staphylococci for operating room personnel has been minimized by improved head coverings.

Staphylococci are widespread in the environment and can be cultured from clothing, carpets, toiletries (e.g., hairbrushes, razors), and virtually all environmental surfaces. Airborne dissemination of organisms is possible, particularly in operating rooms with poor ventilation and heavy traffic; improved methods of ventilating operating rooms may have reduced the sepsis or colonization rate. Environmental staphylococci may serve as an important reservoir, but direct human-to-human transfer probably is a much more important means of transmission in epidemic situations than is airborne spread or contact with contaminated objects. Various methods are used to identify epidemiologic markers in nosocomial outbreaks of staphylococcal infections. These include phage typing, serotyping, esterase activity, antimicrobial susceptibility patterns, immunoblotting of exported proteins, sodium dodecyl sulfate gel electrophoresis, and toxin production. Molecular typing techniques include plasmid DNA analysis, restriction endonuclease fingerprinting of chromosome DNA, and rapid field inversion gel electrophoresis. Molecular methods of typing, although often more time-consuming, can offer adjunctive or novel information useful in characterizing strains involved in outbreaks.[172]

The neonatal nursery has been an area of particular concern in transmission of staphylococci. Until the 1980s, coagulase-positive staphylococci were the major concern. During the pandemic of strain 80/81 disease, outbreaks of serious neonatal disease were commonplace, high colonization rates were found in infants upon discharge from the nursery, and in some outbreaks the subsequent incidence of disease was as high as 50 to 70 per cent. Skin disease and infant and maternal mastitis usually appear within 1 to 4 weeks after discharge. Staphylococcal pneumonia, far more common during that period than at present, may not be seen for months after delivery, even though the infecting strain was acquired in a hospital. During the experience with 80/81 disease, a particularly high attack rate for staphylococcal disease was seen in the families of colonized infants. The epidemiology of neonatal staphylococcal infections has been reviewed by Baker[15] and Shinefeld.[228]

Various control measures were used successfully to terminate individual outbreaks during this period. Measures to protect the infant from colonization and subsequent diseases by establishing a barrier at the site of initial colonization included hexachlorophene bathing, application of antibiotic ointment to the umbilicus and circumcision site, and application of an antiseptic dye to the umbilicus. Another approach, deliberate colonization of the umbilicus with an interfering "avirulent" strain, was successful in controlling several epidemics but itself has caused skin disease and, in one case, fatal septicemia.[25, 229] Hexachlorophene bathing became a widespread practice during the period in which nosocomial staphylococcal infections were declining.[90, 202] After approximately a decade of hexachlorophene use, it was recognized that cutaneous absorption of hexachlorophene resulting in potentially toxic hexachlorophene blood levels may occur in infants, particularly premature infants, subjected to repeated daily baths over a period. Brain-stem abnormalities associated with hexachlorophene have been demonstrated in premature infants. For these reasons, controls were placed on hexachlorophene sale, and its routine use was discouraged in 1973. In one neonatal nursery outbreak of methicillin-resistant *S. aureus* (MRSA), the use of 0.3 per cent triclosan (Bactistat) was associated with cessation of an outbreak.[285]

Coincident with widespread discontinuation of hexachlorophene bathing but not necessarily causally related to it, an increased incidence of nursery outbreaks of coagulase-positive staphylococcal disease was reported. Many of these have been caused by epidermolytic toxin–producing strains of staphylococci belonging to phage group II. In these outbreaks, the majority of children have developed limited areas of bullous impetigo within 1 to 4 weeks after discharge, a small number showing the more dramatic manifestations of generalized exfoliative disease. Contemporary epidemics appear to have a much lower incidence of septicemia, pneumonia, and osteomyelitis and less potential for spread to other family members. Personal experience with four such outbreaks in different hospital nurseries demonstrates that they may arise under various conditions and can be controlled by diverse means.[164]

Patterns of crowding of infants and understaffing contribute to outbreaks. Active clinical and bacteriologic surveillance and cohorting of infants may be effective in reducing outbreaks.[15, 95]

Although nosocomial coagulase-positive staphylococcal infection was not as prevalent in the 1970s and 1980s as in the 1950s, new challenges have become apparent. The frequency of bacteremia related to intravenous catheters and prosthetic devices has increased considerably.[155, 156] Methicillin-resistant staphylococci have become more prevalent in the community and now are responsible for widespread nosocomial outbreaks of disease in hospitals.[34, 40, 50, 58, 73, 134, 219, 240, 272] Coagulase-negative staphylococci have become the most commonly encountered cause of nosocomial bacteremia among neonates in neonatal intensive care services.[73, 79, 82, 83, 97, 112, 123, 180, 222]

HOST DEFENSES

Coagulase-positive staphylococci are ubiquitous in the environment, and approximately 30 per cent of the population are carriers. A major defense against staphylococcal infection is intact skin. Minor wounds frequently become colonized and infected and serve as portals to deeper, more significant staphylococcal infections. In some cases, the integumentary infection may be of major significance; in others, minor skin punctures may serve to introduce infection to distant internal sites. Burns, varicella virus and cutaneous herpesvirus infections, primary skin diseases (e.g., atopic eczema), epidermolysis bullosa, and surgical wounds are important portals of entry for staphylococci. In hospitalized patients, intravenous needles and catheters may be sources of staphylococcal infection.[155, 156]

Foreign bodies reduce local resistance to staphylococcal engraftment and are important in the pathogenesis and perpetuation of infection. Important foreign bodies are cerebrospinal fluid shunts, prosthetic cardiac valves, nonabsorbable sutures, vascular prostheses (including arteriovenous shunts for hemodialysis), orthopedic prostheses, nails, and wires.

Among neonates, the umbilicus and circumcision sites, which may be colonized within the first few hours of life and from which both local and distant infections may be established, are important portals of entry.

Among adults, diabetes mellitus appears to predispose to staphylococcal infections, probably for multiple reasons, of which vascular insufficiency is prominent.

Viral respiratory diseases, such as measles and influenza, predispose to pulmonary infection, again predominantly by damaging the integrity of the barrier at the portal of entry. Disruption of the respiratory epithelium and impairment of ciliary motion and other local defenses may allow secondary staphylococcal invasion.

Once the integumental barrier has been breached, the polymorphonuclear leukocyte appears to be the most important line of defense. Successful phagocytosis involves chemotaxis, opsonization, and intracellular killing. The incidence of difficulty with staphylococcal infection is highest in patients with defects in this area of host defense. Granulocytopenia of any origin predisposes to infection, particularly with the host's endogenous bacteria, including staphylococci, *Escherichia coli*, *Pseudomonas*, and *Klebsiella*.[13]

Disorders in neutrophil chemotaxis have been recognized only recently, but patients with these disorders particularly are subject to recurrent and severe staphylococcal infections. A heterogeneous group of patients has been described with abnormalities in chemotactic factor generation and with serum inhibitors of white blood cell movement.[230] A disorder of neutrophil movement was reported by Miller and associates[175] in 1971; it is called the lazy leukocyte syndrome. The patients have recurrent respiratory infections, gingivitis, and stomatitis. Their leukocytes exhibit normal phagocytosis and intracellular killing but are deficient both in motility toward a chemotactic stimulant and in random motility. Despite normal marrow reserves, peripheral neutropenia and depression of neutrophil migration, as measured by the Rebuck skin window, may be noted.

Leukocyte adhesion deficiency is a rare autosomal recessive disorder of leukocytes. Leukocyte adhesion deficiency I presents with recurrent necrotic and indolent infections of soft tissue, delayed wound healing, and severely impaired pus formation, despite marked peripheral blood neutrophilia. Staphylococcal or gram-negative enteric bacterial organisms may be cultured from lesions for up to several weeks, despite antimicrobial therapy. Persons with leukocyte adhesion deficiency have a decreased or absent expression of a family of structurally and functionally related leukocyte surface glycoproteins designated the CD11/CD18 complex. Diminished or absent expression of the CD11/CD18 complex accounts for the failure of the patient's neutrophils to adhere to endothelium and subsequently migrate to specific sites of inflammation.

Diagnosis is made by flow cytometry and measurement of surface CD11/CD18 in stimulated and unstimulated neutrophils using monoclonal antibodies directed against the

CD11/CD18 complex. Treatment of the disorder largely is supportive. Prophylactic antibiotics given in an attempt to prevent recurrent infections and human leukocyte antigen-compatible bone marrow transplantation have been used in patients with the severe phenotype.

Patients with the Chédiak-Higashi syndrome have recurrent infection in association with neutrophils that are abnormal morphologically, with giant lysosomes present in decreased number. Neutrophils from these patients show depressed chemotaxis, probably on the basis of decreased neutrophil deformability.[260] The lysosomes alter cell motility by compromising the ability of the neutrophils to traverse between endothelial cells.

Abnormal neutrophil behavior, with decreased phagocytosis and decreased random and directed migration, in a patient with recurrent infection has been ascribed to abnormalities of the actin filaments.[33] Treatment consists of prophylactic antibiotics, as well as appropriate antibiotics for specific infections. Ascorbic acid (10 to 20 mg/kg/day) has been shown to rectify the microbicidal effect in some patients.

The disease in another group of patients with profound susceptibility to staphylococcal infection colorfully has been called Job syndrome, or, more prosaically, hyper-IgE syndrome. The severe, recurrent staphylococcal infections of the subcutaneous-skin and deep-skin tissues are similar to the boils that plagued Job of the Old Testament. These patients characteristically have severe staphylococcal infections with little overt inflammation, suggestive of tuberculous "cold abscesses." Concomitant features of their disease are chronic eczematoid skin disorders, elevated levels of immunoglobulins, extremely elevated IgE levels, eosinophilia, and a generally normal infection history for other bacteria and viruses. Neutrophils from these patients are adequate in number and show normal phagocytosis and intracellular killing but are deficient in migration toward a chemotactic stimulant, as measured in the Boyden chamber assay.[104, 223] The defect in chemotaxis is associated with production of a chemotactic inhibitor released by mononuclear cells that inhibits normal neutrophil and monocyte chemotaxis. Judicious use of antistaphylococcal antibiotics is the mainstay of management. A small uncontrolled study of interferon-γ and interferon-α demonstrated attenuation of the frequency of infections and reduction in severity scores of patients with atopic dermatitis.[205]

Other patients with recurrent severe staphylococcal abscesses and extremely elevated IgE levels have been reported. It appears likely that these patients, whose histories nearly are indistinguishable from those of patients with Job syndrome, share the same chemotactic defect.[48] Two of these patients also had partial abnormalities of cell-mediated immunity. These patients have been shown to have extremely high antistaphylococcus-specific IgE, an excess of antistaphylococcus IgM, and deficient *S. aureus* IgA, compared with normal subjects.[66, 223] It has been postulated that the high level of antistaphylococcal IgE in serum may create an abnormal local environment surrounding an invading staphylococcus, such that mast-cell degranulation may be stimulated and polymorphonuclear responses affected adversely.

Once the staphylococcus and the leukocyte are close to one another, opsonization of the bacterium must proceed in order for phagocytosis to take place. Two systems for opsonization of staphylococci have been described. Serum from normal adults has good opsonic activity unheated but generally is inactive after heating at 56° C for 1 hour. The heat lability of the normal opsonin and observation of normal or only slightly decreased opsonic activity in unheated sera from patients with agammaglobulinemia[277] indicate that the major opsonin is complement. A few sera, generally from patients convalescing from serious staphylococcal disease, contain heat-stable opsonins, presumably antibody directed at the staphylococcal cell-wall components.[141] Therefore, either complement or antibody can provide opsonins for staphylococci; specific antibody is helpful but not required. The clinical correlate to these observations may be found in patients with defective defenses; patients with agammaglobulinemia and defective antibody generally have more severe problems with organisms other than staphylococci, whereas patients with deficiencies in complement components have been reported to have repeated and severe staphylococcal infection.[3, 6, 7, 174, 200]

Once the bacterium has been ingested, intracellular killing normally proceeds. Coagulase-positive staphylococci can survive within the polymorphonuclear leukocyte for a considerably longer period than can coagulase-negative organisms. In in vitro studies, after 90 minutes of intracellular residence, 5 per cent of coagulase-positive staphylococci remain viable, whereas coagulase-negative strains are killed within 20 minutes.[171] Prolonged intracellular survival may be an important virulence factor separating coagulase-negative from coagulase-positive strains and may provide a mechanism whereby surviving organisms may be carried to distant body sites to set up metastatic foci of infection.

Patients with chronic granulomatous disease of childhood have an inborn error in intraleukocytic killing of catalase-positive bacteria and fungi. These patients have early onset of recurrent purulent infections of skin, subcutaneous tissues, lungs, and reticuloendothelial organs, particularly the liver. Persistent purulent lesions with extensive tissue necrosis and granuloma formation are pathologic characteristics.[206] A wide range of catalase-positive organisms, including staphylococci, gram-negative enterics and anaerobes, mycobacteria, and fungi, are etiologic agents of their multiple infections. Catalase-negative organisms, notably pneumococci and streptococci, are not a problem to these patients because these organisms cannot break down the hydrogen peroxide produced by their own metabolism within the phagocytic vacuole. The buildup of hydrogen peroxide is toxic to the organisms, whose death is caused by this buildup.[38, 127]

The leukocytes of patients with this disorder have normal chemotactic and increased phagocytic capacity but cannot generate a normal burst of oxidative metabolic activity.[171] In normal polymorphonuclear leukocytes, this metabolic burst converts oxygen into metabolites that are toxic to bacteria and fungi. Leukocytes from patients with chronic granulomatous disease are deficient in their ability to kill bacteria and to reduce oxidative chemicals, such as nitroblue tetrazolium dye. The qualitative nitroblue tetrazolium dye reduction test has become a standard diagnostic test for detection of these patients and is as sensitive as tests that employ live bacteria or measure biochemical activity are. Although the fundamental enzyme defect has not been elucidated clearly yet, studies have demonstrated a failure in the activation of nicotinamide adenine dinucleotide phosphate (NADPH) oxidase.[57, 163, 225] Chronic granulomatous disease is caused by mutations involving several genes that encode the components of NADPH oxidase. Approximately 55 per cent of the patients have the X-linked variety and have an abnormality in gp91phox, the membrane-associated heavy chain of the cytochrome b558. Those who inherit the disease in an autosomal recessive pattern have defects in one of the three recently identified cytosolic factors (p47phox, p22phox, and p47 phox). Staphylococci are prominent pathogens in chronic granulomatous disease, producing skin, subcutaneous, and lymph node abscesses; metastatic lung and liver abscesses; and osteomyelitis. The response of these patients to therapy is slow and poor, demonstrating the absolute necessity of an intact polymorphonuclear bactericidal system in host defense against staphylococci.

In contrast with the primacy of the polymorphonuclear defense against staphylococci, evidence for an important role for specific humoral and cellular immunity in host defense against staphylococci is either lacking or contradictory.

Specific antibody is not required for opsonization of unencapsulated strains of staphylococci. The opsonic activity of serum from patients recovering from staphylococcal endocarditis or other serious disease is greater than that of normal persons.[141, 276] Despite the presence of humoral antibodies to cell-wall teichoic acids and to various toxins and enzymes, which are found regularly in convalescents from serious staphylococcal infection, the patient remains liable to recurrence of infection with the same strain of staphylococci. Staphylococcal infections generally occur and proceed in the face of some degree of humoral immunity. Specific antibody to one or more staphylococcal components or products does not protect against infection.

Studies of the importance of cell-mediated immunity to the pathogenesis of staphylococcal infection are in their infancy. Evidence from animal studies is fragmentary and not directly applicable to human disease. After induction of delayed hypersensitivity, both increased resistance and increased susceptibility to staphylococcal tissue invasion have been found. Once infection is established, there may be increased tissue destruction in the presence of delayed hypersensitivity.

Clinical evidence from patients with deficient cell-mediated immunity (combined immunodeficiency, thymic aplasia, Nezelof syndrome) suggests that staphylococcal infections are not among the most important pathogens for these patients.

Present evidence suggests, therefore, that intact local skin and mucous membrane barriers are the most important defense against the establishment of staphylococcal infection. Once infection is established, an intact polymorphonuclear response is essential for containment of infection and for clearance of the organisms.

PATHOGENESIS

Staphylococci cause disease by two mechanisms: direct invasion of tissues and liberation of toxins, which may have effects at sites distant from the focus of infection or colonization. The hallmark of the staphylococcal lesion is the abscess. Local tissue destruction at the site of inoculation is followed rapidly by hyperemia and a vigorous inflammatory response marked by accumulation of large numbers of polymorphonuclear leukocytes. Tissue necrosis in the center of the lesion follows. At the site of intensive hyperemia surrounding the lesions, a fibrin wall is formed. Liquefaction necrosis occurs centrally; the mature lesion consists of a fibrin wall surrounded by inflamed tissues enclosing a central core of pus consisting of organisms and leukocytes. Live bacteria may persist within these lesions for a considerable period. As pus accumulates, it may drain toward the skin surface or into adjacent tissues, where it forms sinus tracts and secondary abscesses. In the presence of an intact host inflammatory response, this type of reaction may be seen in diverse areas, including the skin and subcutaneous tissues, lymph nodes, joints, renal tissues, liver, parotid glands, muscles, lung, and long bones.

In addition to local extension, coagulase-positive staphylococci may be disseminated hematogenously from this focus of infection, even from abscesses that are trivial in size. Through hematogenous dissemination, infection of bones, joints, and heart valves may result. Given the ubiquitous nature of staphylococci, skin and wounds that are the usual ports of entry appear remarkably resistant to infection. This natural resistance is affected dramatically by the presence of foreign bodies within the wound, such as sutures and bits of soil or gravel. Natural resistance also is affected by the presence of compromised tissue after ecchymosis or hemorrhage or in the presence of vascular insufficiency. Poor personal hygiene also predisposes to staphylococcal skin infection. Moist, macerated skin is invaded more easily, contributing to the increased frequency of staphylococcal skin infection in intertriginous areas and in tropical climates.

Toxigenic staphylococcal disease includes staphylococcal scalded skin syndrome, TSS, and staphylococcal food poisoning. The major manifestations of these diseases are caused by the effects of specific toxins.

CLINICAL MANIFESTATIONS

Skin Infections

The simplest and most superficial staphylococcal infection is impetigo. Impetigo can be recognized clinically: it generally begins with a slightly tender, erythematous patch or papule, frequently at the site of a minor abrasion, insect bite, or excoriated or macerated area, such as that around the nares or mouth. The erythematous papule may have a transient vesicular stage but rapidly becomes covered with a characteristic dirty-looking, honey-colored crust consisting of dried serous material. Local spread generally is observed, with satellite erythematous papules crusting over and becoming confluent with the parent lesion. Suppuration generally is not seen or occurs late in the evolution of the lesion. The lesions of impetigo are moderately painful but frequently are neglected or ignored; several studies show that patients wait 2 weeks or longer before seeking medical care. In the United States, staphylococci appear to participate with streptococci in common impetiginous lesions. Previous studies in the United States have indicated that streptococci are found alone in approximately 30 per cent of typical impetigo lesions, streptococci and staphylococci are found together in approximately 60 per cent; and a pure culture of staphylococci is found in approximately 10 per cent.

The epidemiology of impetigo appears to be changing. Impetigo classically was described as a streptococcal or combined staphylococcal and streptococcal disease. Multiple studies now reveal *S. aureus* to be the sole organism in between 46 and 64 per cent of cases.[21, 22, 59] *S. aureus* may be resistant to erythromycin in up to 28 per cent of cases of impetigo; however, the clinical failure rates usually are less than 28 per cent. Erythromycin continues to be a useful therapeutic agent, but mupirocin is a reasonable alternative in clinical failures or with known erythromycin-resistant strains of *Staphylococcus*.[59, 176] The prevalence of staphylococci has been found to increase with the increasing age of the lesion, suggesting that the streptococcal infection may be primary, with staphylococci a secondary colonizer or, less frequently, an invader. Moreover, many studies of therapy suggest that penicillin directed against the streptococcus generally is effective, even when penicillin-resistant staphylococci also are present. In some long-neglected lesions, staphylococci may have become the dominant pathogen; for these cases, a course of specific antistaphylococcal therapy may be needed if penicillin has failed.

An etiologic role for *S. aureus* in patients with atopic dermatitis has never been established; however, up to 93 per cent of patients with atopic dermatitis are colonized with this organism.[106] Bacterial colonization has been attributed to hyperkeratosis and dyskeratosis, increased transepidermal loss of water, local immunologic defects inherent to atopic dermatitis, and depressed polymorphonuclear leukocyte chemotaxis. Despite this high rate of colonization, particularly with toxigenic strains,[106] the incidence of severe or systemic infections is relatively low, perhaps because of the enhanced polymorphonuclear leukocyte oxidative metabolism.[107] The degree of colonization increases with the severity of eczema, and lesions that appear to be infected may contain *S. aureus* at rates of 10^7 colony-forming units/cm^2 or greater. Antibacterial treatment without topical steroids reduces the colony count of staphylococci but has little effect on eczema, suggesting that staphylococci play a secondary rather than primary role. Oral antibiotic therapy is indicated in the presence of pyoderma, superficial pustules, impetiginized lesions, bullous impetigo, or folliculitis. Topical treatment of eczematous areas with class III steroids is associated with decreased bacterial colonization and improved clinical response.[184, 235]

Furuncles or boils are acute circumscribed abscesses of the skin and the immediately underlying subcutaneous tissues. When only a hair follicle is involved, it is called folliculitis; involvement of sweat glands is called hidradenitis. These infections are found commonly in the breasts, axillae, buttocks, thighs, and perineum, with a predilection for moist intertriginous areas. As inflammation progresses, the overlying skin becomes thinned, stretched, and shiny, and exquisite tenderness appears. There usually are no systemic signs in small circumscribed abscesses, although even the most minor folliculitis may be followed by bacteremia and dissemination. Larger lesions, called carbuncles, made of interconnecting abscesses, may be associated with fever and signs of systemic illness.

In the newborn infant, the clinical picture may be altered. Multiple abscesses are common. These may be associated with little inflammation for some time, but the infant then rapidly may develop signs of severe systemic illness, septicemia, and shock.

Cellulitis is a poorly localized, soft tissue infection occurring with or without a focus of overlying skin infection. Contrary to popular belief, there are no clues on physical examination that lead to a microbiologic diagnosis. Although it is true that staphylococcal infections *tend* to be localized, streptococcal infections *tend* to be spreading and diffuse, and *Haemophilus influenzae* type b infections *tend* to have a blue or violaceous hue, none of these observations is of help in evaluating a single patient. Coagulase-positive staphylococcal cellulitis may be extensive and rapidly progressive. Suppuration may occur late or be prevented by early treatment. Careful aspiration of the lesion, together with blood cultures, offers the best approach to an etiologic diagnosis. It should be remembered that cellulitis may be the external manifestation of underlying osteomyelitis, and this diagnosis should be pursued by serial radiographs or bone scans during the course of therapy.

Breast Abscesses

Coagulase-positive staphylococci are the leading cause of the breast abscesses that are relatively common among newborn infants and nursing mothers.[131, 216]

Infantile breast abscess usually is unilateral, occurs primarily in term infants, particularly girls with physiologic breast enlargement, and is seen primarily within the first 2 weeks of life. Occasionally, patients up to 8 weeks of age are found. The most prominent feature is marked erythema and induration of the affected breast. Fever and constitutional signs are absent in the majority of cases, although progressive cellulitis and bacteremia may occur. Surgical drainage nearly always is required except when spontaneous rupture ensues. Gram stain and culture of pus are important for diagnosis and therapy because gram-negative organisms (particularly *Salmonella* and *E. coli)* also may cause breast abscesses.[42, 216, 238] Because blood culture may be positive (2 of 20 cases in which these were obtained in the series reported by Rudoy and Nelson[216]), parenteral antibiotics should be started after blood cultures are obtained. Adequate surgical drainage appears to be of greatest importance for cure. In some cases, tissue destruction is extensive enough to cause permanent damage with reduction in size and function in adult life.

Maternal mastitis and breast abscess also are of concern to the physician caring for children. Although breast abscesses may occur at any time in girls or women at any age, more than two-thirds of cases are seen in nursing mothers from 2 to 8 weeks post partum. Maternal breast abscesses were seen especially frequently during nursery epidemics of staphylococcal infection.[281] Important factors appear to be engorgement of the mammary gland from incomplete emptying of the breast and, in epidemics, colonization of the mother's breast from the infant. In its early stages, mastitis can be recognized as a limited area of tenderness and erythema of the breast, frequently associated with fever. At this stage, culture of breast milk may be misleading because staphylococci can be recovered from the milk of women without infection.[81] Early mastitis is treated best with oral antistaphylococcal antibiotics and frequent and complete emptying of the affected breast. Continued nursing of the affected side has been advocated.[137] When milk secretion is mixed with frank pus, continued lactation may not be wise, and manual expression of milk should be used until the infection is under control. Whenever suppuration occurs, incision and drainage are required.

Wound Infections

The infection of surgical wounds with coagulase-positive staphylococci has been less of a problem since the mid-1980s, partly because of improved prophylactic measures employed in the hospitals. In large measure, however, the decline appears to be part of a general decline in the prevalence of nosocomial staphylococcal infections. Surgical wound infections continue to occur, with reduced frequency, because conditions in wounds especially are favorable to staphylococcal proliferation. Sutures, serum exudation, and tissues with impaired perfusion all promote the growth of staphylococci. Daily careful inspection of wounds, frequent dressing changes, and early removal of sutures are indicated in the general care of the postoperative patient. In the work-up for postoperative fever, nonsurgical clinicians often have a peculiar reluctance to examine the wound. Inspection of the wound and culture and Gram stain of the exudate may be of invaluable help in inpatient management. In our experience, superficial but troublesome wound infection occurs frequently at the site of venous cutdowns days to weeks after removal of the catheter; superficial silk sutures are shown to have been left in place by oversight.

Eye Infections

Purulent conjunctivitis may result from coagulase-positive staphylococcal infection. In these cases, Gram stain of the exudate shows polymorphonuclear leukocytes and gram-positive cocci, and staphylococci can be grown in pure culture. The coexistence of coagulase-negative staphylococci and conjunctivitis does not imply causality, except in unusual circumstances. Another common infection, the hordeolum, or stye, involves the sebaceous glands or eyelash follicles. When well localized in patients without fever or systemic symptoms, styes may be treated successfully by hot soaks to produce drainage and with antibiotic ophthalmic ointments to prevent secondary conjunctivitis. *S. aureus* colonization of the lids is common in atopic patients; however, this does not appear to play a role in chronic allergic conjunctivitis.[256] Whenever there is associated eyelid cellulitis, systemic antibiotics should be prescribed after culture of pus. In cases of minor inflammation, oral therapy may suffice, provided the patient has rapid access to the physician or hospital in the event of extension of cellulitis.

Staphylococcal cellulitis or skin infection near the eye always should be considered a serious infection because there may be extension of infection into the periorbital tissues, causing orbital cellulitis, and from there through venous drainage into the cavernous sinus. A diagnosis of cavernous sinus thrombosis cannot be established always in the presence of orbital cellulitis, but this complication, as well as ethmoid sinusitis and meningeal extension of infection, is a possible complication of orbital infection. Cavernous sinus thrombophlebitis is a rapidly progressive disease that continues to yield high morbidity rates (up to 34 per cent[245]) and mortality despite the availability of effective antibiotics. Approximately two-thirds of the cases are caused by *S. aureus,* predominantly from infections occurring on the medial one-third of the face.[245] It can be recognized by paralysis of cranial nerves III, IV, and VI; proptosis; retinal venous obstruction; and acute visual deterioration, in addition to periorbital swelling and inflammation. Extension to the meninges is common, as are manifestations of systemic septicemia.

In addition to extension from facial infection, orbital cellulitis may arise from dental abscesses, maxillary sinusitis, and particularly ethmoid sinusitis. Pneumococci are frequent etiologic agents, particularly if the orbital cellulitis arises from sinusitis. In children younger than 5 years of age, *H. influenzae* type b and *Streptococcus pneumoniae* may be more frequent etiologic agents than are staphylococci, so that initial antibiotic therapy must be directed toward treatment of these organisms in addition to coverage for staphylococci. Nasopharyngeal, eye, and skin or pus cultures of facial infection may be valuable, and blood cultures always should be obtained.[203, 262, 271, 281]

Ear, Nose, and Throat Infections

Staphylococci do not appear to be important pathogens in acute suppurative otitis media,[23, 219] except perhaps in neonates, a group that has been studied inadequately. In the report by Bland,[27] middle ear pathogens of neonates differed markedly from those of older children. Coagulase-positive staphylococci were prominent offenders, being found in 5 of 18 aspirates but not in the external canal. In the presence of a perforated eardrum, coagulase-positive staphylococci may be secondary invaders but can become serious pathogens, especially for mastoiditis. There is little evidence that staphylococci are responsible for pharyngitis. Recovery of staphylococci from throat cultures, of course, is common in asymptomatic persons. Staphylococci cause other frank suppurative processes of the nasopharynx, including the paranasal sinuses, peritonsillar abscesses, and retropharyngeal abscess.

With the publication of several well-documented series of cases,[68, 121, 148] bacterial tracheitis appears to be "an old disease which is becoming prevalent again."[232] Possibly representing a superinfection of larynx and trachea damaged by viral tracheitis, this syndrome is life-threatening, may be rapidly progressive, and holds an intermediate position between epiglottitis and viral tracheobronchitis in most of its clinical manifestations and severity. Severe respiratory difficulty is related to the accumulation of thick purulent secretion in the trachea as well as marked subglottic edema. It most often is caused by *S. aureus* or *H. influenzae.* The illness begins with hoarseness and inspiratory stridor. High fever and severe respiratory distress develop subsequently. Diagnosis is made by direct laryngoscopy or bronchoscopy showing purulent secretions and subglottic edema. Pneumonia is a frequent association. Antibiotic therapy and an artificial airway by intubation or tracheostomy are required. The illness is severe and may be fatal because of difficulties in controlling the airway, septic complications, or both.

Acute suppurative parotitis is infrequent in children. When present, it occurs in newborns, premature infants, and those with underlying systemic disease. The most common organism isolated is *S. aureus,* with *Bacteroides* the predominant anaerobic organism.[188]

Thrombophlebitis

Thrombophlebitis and thromboembolism have constituted a neglected area in pediatrics, although deep vein thrombosis does occur in children, particularly in association with septicemia and trauma.[120] In adults, bacteremic consequences of infected intravenous catheters and needles are so well recognized that specific prophylactic regimens are in common practice. A comprehensive review of infection associated with intravenous therapy demonstrates that coagulase-negative and coagulase-positive staphylococci and the gram-negative organisms *Klebsiella, Enterobacter,* and *Serratia* were isolated from intravenous needles and catheters, whereas *S. aureus* was the leading organism associated with bacteremia. Colonization rates ranged from 4 to 50 per cent, with associated sepsis in 0 to 8 per cent.[155, 156]

In both adults and children, the pediatric scalp vein needle has been associated with a markedly decreased risk of infection.[55, 56, 198] Major factors in the relative safety of scalp vein needles appear to be lesser trauma to the vein because of small bore and shorter length, lesser incidence of local thrombi, and shorter duration of cannulation because of frequent infiltration. This last aspect may be of major importance, for the rate of positive scalp vein needles equals that of catheters when both are left in place for more than 102 hours. Only 50 per cent of patients with bacteremia associated with intravenous infusions have clinically evident phlebitis in the cannulated vein; it therefore is obvious that serious bacteremia occurs in the absence of local signs. Based on the considerable experience in adults, reasonable guidelines for prevention of infusion-related sepsis can be formulated:

1. Scalp vein needles or short over-the-needle catheters should be used whenever possible. Longer catheters should be reserved for the critically ill, when a secure line is essential, and should be removed when the danger has passed.
2. The skin should be prepared carefully prior to insertion of the intravenous needle or catheter. Iodine or iodophor is preferred to alcohol or benzalkonium.
3. Dressings should be changed daily, and the puncture site and cannulated vein should be inspected carefully for signs of inflammation.
4. Whenever possible, intravenous solutions should be mixed in the hospital pharmacy rather than on the ward.
5. The catheter should be removed at the earliest sign of phlebitis or local inflammation, and the catheter tip or intravenous needle should be cultured.
6. The date and time of insertion of the intravenous needle

should be recorded on the dressing to ensure mandatory removal after 72 hours.[91]

Physicians caring for children have an understandable reluctance to remove a functional intravenous infusion, but iatrogenic phlebitis frequently is a major setback or life-threatening complication in the already seriously ill child.

When phlebitis, recurrent fever, or persistent fever is encountered in a patient receiving intravenous therapy, the following procedures should be carried out:

1. The entire infusion system—bottle, tubing, and needle or cannula—should be removed.
2. The infusion fluid and the needle or cannula tip should be cultured in blood culture media.
3. Pus, if present, should be Gram stained and cultured.
4. Blood cultures should be obtained from two independent venipunctures.[91]

Infusion-associated bacteremia frequently responds to removal of the infected needle or cannula. In serious illness, or if phlebitis is present or pus is seen at cannula removal, systemic antibiotic therapy should be initiated empirically. Antibiotic coverage should include drugs effective in the treatment of infection due to staphylococci and gram-negative enteric organisms, particularly *Klebsiella. Candida* frequently has been the cause of infection associated with total parenteral nutrition.

Particularly severe and frequently lethal suppurative thrombophlebitis has been reported in burned patients who had infected cannulas or intravenous cutdowns. Fewer than half of diagnoses were made while patients were alive. In the absence of other foci of infection, the venotomy site should be examined, and, if no pus is encountered, exploratory proximal venotomy should be performed for evidence of suppuration. When suppurative thrombophlebitis is encountered, surgical removal of the infected vein offers the best chance for survival. In this series, the majority of responsible organisms were gram-negative, but *S. aureus* was encountered frequently.[237] Suppurative thrombophlebitis should be considered in seriously ill immunocompromised or burned patients, especially when catheter-associated bacteremia fails to respond to catheter removal and antibiotic therapy.

Semipermanent indwelling catheters (Hickman, Broviac, Port-A-Cath) now are used widely in children undergoing chemotherapy and long-term hyperalimentation. Over the weeks to months that these devices are in place, 20 to 30 per cent of sites become infected and may develop local phlebitis or serious bacteremia. Because these catheters are tunneled subcutaneously for several centimeters from the skin site to the entry into vein, are implanted under strict asepsis, and are designed to form a barrier preventing in-migration of bacteria, they are less prone to infection than are conventional intravascular devices. Because replacement of these devices requires general anesthesia and the sites available for catheter placement are limited, a trial of antibiotic treatment with the catheter in place sometimes may be desirable.[226] Patients who are severely ill with infection or who are neutropenic should undergo immediate catheter removal with antibiotic therapy. For mild to moderately ill patients, blood cultures through the catheter as well as at a peripheral site should be drawn. A trial of antibiotic therapy through the catheter then may be attempted. This form of therapy may be successful with coagulase-negative staphylococci but has failed to yield satisfactory results when infection is caused by *S. aureus* and *Pseudomonas aeruginosa* or *Candida albicans.*[92] Organisms most commonly recovered are *S. aureus, S. epidermidis,* and gram-negative enterics.[94, 226] Because these are the predominant organisms encountered, vancomycin plus an aminoglycoside is the choice for initial empiric therapy.[267]

Lymphadenitis

Acute cervical adenitis in both infants[12, 83, 103, 224] and children frequently is of staphylococcal origin. Despite both the widespread clinical assumption that the etiology overwhelmingly is streptococcal and the common clinical practice of prescribing penicillin without diagnostic cultures, series of infections have shown a prominent[61] or preeminent role for the staphylococci.[20, 224] Several investigators have demonstrated the value of needle aspiration of enlarged, inflamed lymph nodes even in the absence of fluctuation on clinical examination.[20, 61] Culture of lymph node aspirates and provision of antistaphylococcal antibiotics appear to be the best initial treatment plan for most cases of acute cervical adenitis. Infants with staphylococcal adenitis have been reported, particularly in association with nursery epidemics, with attack rates of 2 and 6 per cent in the first few months of life.[12, 63] Although the disease generally has remained limited to the lymph glands, rapid development of staphylococcal pneumonia and bacteremia may occur if patients are untreated or are receiving ineffective therapy with penicillin or ampicillin.[103]

Pneumonia

Staphylococcal pneumonia generally is a rapidly progressive process in all age groups. Two main forms are recognized: primary pneumonia due to direct inoculation through the respiratory tract and secondary or metastatic hematogenous lung infection due to bacteremic seeding of the lung during the course of endocarditis or septicemia associated with infection at other sites.

Primary staphylococcal pneumonia chiefly is a disease of infancy and early childhood: infants younger than 1 year of age consistently account for three-quarters of cases.[29, 45, 65, 78, 80, 100, 113, 126, 136, 204, 210, 212, 257] Predisposing factors include cystic fibrosis; chronic lung disease; leukemia; prior antibiotic treatment; preexisting skin infection; and viral respiratory diseases, particularly measles, influenza, and adenovirus infection. In addition, *S. aureus* may be the etiologic organism in nearly one-third of malnourished patients with pneumonia. This finding most likely is related to the relative acquired immunodeficiency of this population.[75]

The majority of patients come to their physician with acute, severe symptoms of fever, lethargy, and significant respiratory distress. The respiratory difficulties consist of tachypnea, grunting, retractions, and cyanosis. Many also have gastrointestinal disturbances, chiefly anorexia, vomiting, and abdominal distention from air swallowing. Occasionally, the distention and gastrointestinal symptoms are so impressive that a primary gastrointestinal etiology is sought. Physical signs on initial examination frequently suggest empyema or pneumothorax. The chest radiograph gives valuable clues to the diagnosis. A characteristic group of radiographic changes has been defined, together with a pattern of progression.[43]

At very early stages, the chest radiograph may look normal or show only minimal focal segmental or lobar infiltration (Fig. 85–3). In children seen at this stage, rapid progression of radiographic findings within hours is common. A high proportion of patients either have pleural effusion when first seen or develop it early in the course of illness. Rebhan and Edwards[210] reported that 59 per cent of 329 patients demonstrated effusion on their initial chest radiograph and that an additional 19 per cent developed subsequent effusion.

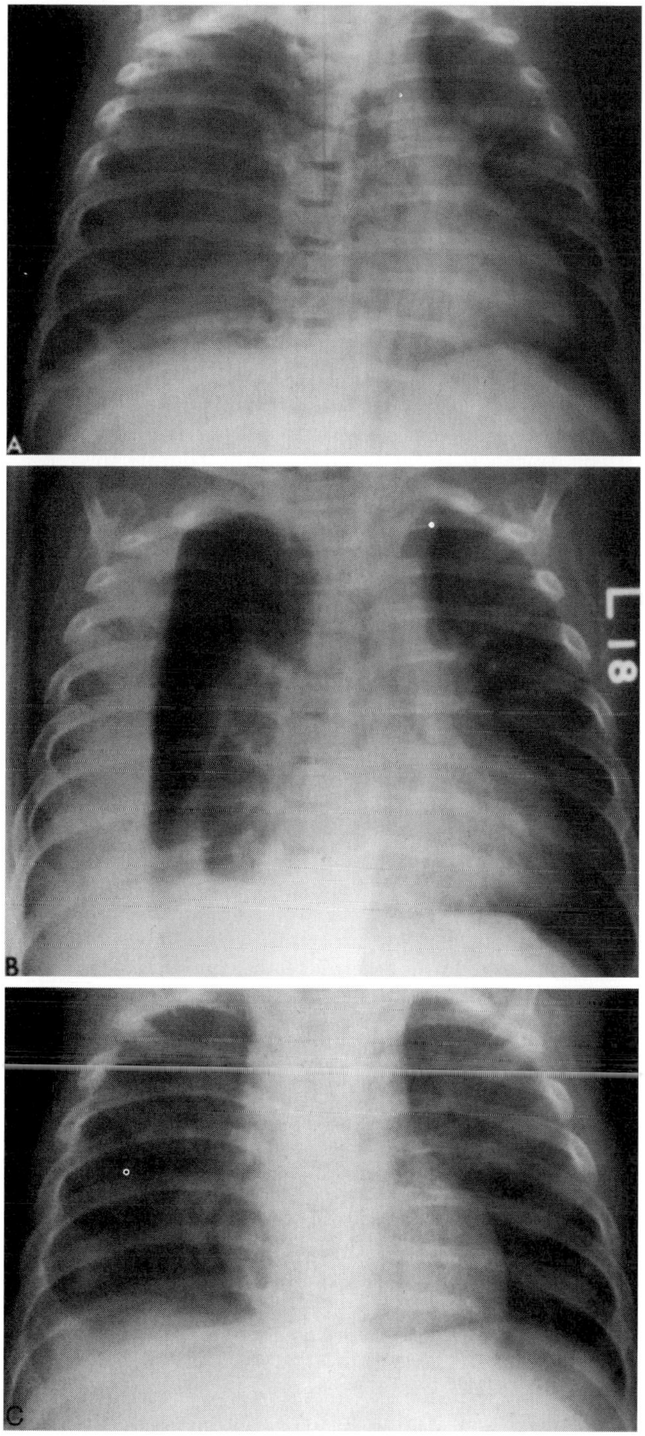

FIGURE 85–3. *Staphylococcal pneumonia.* A, *Radiograph of an 8-month-old boy acutely ill with fever and respiratory disease of several hours' duration. AP supine view.* B, *Decubitus view of same patient reveals the presence of a right tension pyopneumothorax with collapsed right lung and shift of the mediastinum to the left.* C, *Follow-up film 5 weeks after intravenous oxacillin therapy for 4 weeks showed marked resolution with minimal residual pleural thickening.*

Hendren and Haggerty[100] noted that 71 per cent of patients had effusion at some time in the course of the disease. The finding of effusion in a majority of cases has been a common experience. Pneumothorax is another relatively common manifestation of staphylococcal pneumonia; 42 per cent of the patients described by Hendren and Haggerty[100] experienced this complication. The sudden development of tension pneumothorax is a particularly severe but relatively frequent clinical event responsible for sudden, severe decompensation. The combination of pneumothorax and empyema—pyopneumonothorax—is highly suggestive of staphylococcal pneumonia.

Pulmonary pneumatoceles generally are seen after the initial stages. They can be recognized as single, although more often multiple, thin-walled, cyst-like, air-filled cavities in the pulmonary parenchyma. Pneumatoceles are believed to result from localized areas of bronchiolar and alveolar necrosis, which allow one-way passage of air into the interstitial space. Pneumatocele rupture is one of two mechanisms producing pneumothorax; the other is the formation of a bronchopleural fistula caused by localized bronchial wall necrosis. The frequency of pneumatoceles may exceed 85 per cent.[100] In most cases, pneumatoceles occur during the course of infection; a few patients have a pneumatocele at the time of admission.

Diagnosis is established best by isolation of an organism from blood, pleural fluid, or lung tap. The finding of staphylococci in upper respiratory secretions or "sputum" is not sufficient because of their frequent presence in the normal pharynx. A more reliable culture can be obtained by performing deep tracheal suction through an endotracheal tube. For a secure etiologic diagnosis, empyema fluid or lung tap aspirate from an area of infiltration is preferable. Blood cultures frequently are negative in staphylococcal pneumonia. An adequate specimen for culture of the respiratory tract, as well as at least two blood specimens, should be obtained before initiating therapy. In recent years, it has been recognized that empyema and even pneumatoceles may be seen with gram-negative infection, particularly those due to *Klebsiella.* In order to guide the prolonged antibiotic therapy needed for these serious and slowly resolving pneumonias, one should make every attempt to obtain adequate culture specimens from the pleural space or blood at the time of starting antibiotic therapy.

Management of patients with staphylococcal pneumonia requires more than antibiotics. Early consultation with a thoracic surgeon or pediatric surgeon should be obtained and a joint management plan discussed. It is important to have surgical opinion and expertise available for the immediate management of complications such as pneumothorax or bronchopleural fistula. Close observation, preferably in an intensive care unit, is indicated during the acute phase of the disease. Empyema generally is managed best with the implantation of a chest tube for constant drainage. The response to combined drainage and antibiotic therapy generally is slow; fever usually persists beyond 1 week and frequently for at least 2 weeks. High-dose antibiotic therapy should be continued for a minimum of 3 to 4 weeks. The clinical course of the patients is such that hospital care usually is required for most of this period.

Despite the severe illness and mortality rate of approximately 10 per cent,[100, 210] the long-term prognosis of the survivors is excellent. Two large series showed no pulmonary function abnormalities on long-term follow-up.[45, 113] Resolution of pulmonary changes may seem slow, however, because pleural thickening, parenchymal fibrous stranding, and pneumatoceles may persist on chest radiographs for many months. In view of the natural history of slow resolution of these changes and the excellent long-term prognosis, the general consensus now is that decortication operations should be avoided. There is no evidence that they influence the course favorably, and pleural thickening resolves without surgery. In children with staphylococcal pneumonia, "fibrous entrapment" of lung has not been a problem in practice.[29]

Large series of patients with staphylococcal pneumonia were compiled from several locations in the United States and Europe from the early 1950s to the mid-1960s, a period when hospital outbreaks of staphylococcal neonatal and wound infections were common. In some localities, staphylococcal pneumonia again has become a rather rare and sporadic event.[257] In other areas, particularly where staphylococcal infections remain common, primary staphylococcal pneumonia continues to be relatively common. In any case, because this is a particularly severe and rapidly progressive disease, the possibility of a staphylococcal etiology should be considered when one is evaluating the condition of any child with fever and respiratory distress.

Secondary metastatic staphylococcal lung infection is encountered with increasing frequency. In this condition, the lungs are infected hematogenously in a patient with widespread focal infections, persistent bacteremia, endocarditis, or some combination thereof.[179] This form of lung infection always is bilateral and multifocal, starting with round, large or small consolidated infiltrates, which represent septic emboli. Pleural effusion and bronchopleural complications frequently develop. This form of disease has been reported in children and adolescents with severe focal staphylococcal infections, as well as in intravenous drug abusers with right-sided endocarditis. Most reported patients have not been immunocompromised.

Bacteremia

Unlike pneumococcal and *H. influenzae* type b bacteremia in childhood, staphylococcal bacteremia is recognized rarely in the absence of a focus of infection. The focus may be inapparent or exceedingly minor, such as an infected blister or a small furuncle. Bacteremia may occur in the course of a primary infection of the skin or respiratory tract or as a result of intravenous therapy. Frequently, it is not recognized until it has set up a secondary, hematogenously disseminated focus of infection, such as osteomyelitis, septic arthritis, or a deep-tissue infection. Staphylococcal bacteremia should be respected under all circumstances: on one hand, it can be an extremely fulminant disease with shock and disseminated intravascular coagulation, and on the other hand, it may persist and recur over a considerable period, establishing metastatic foci of infection.[71] In every case of staphylococcal bacteremia, careful consideration should be given to the possibility that endocarditis may have developed so that prolonged parenteral therapy may be given if necessary.

Endocarditis

During the period in which hospital-associated staphylococcal infections and staphylococcal pneumonia have declined, staphylococcal endocarditis in infants, children, and adolescents has increased.[117, 195, 259, 286] For infants and children, this increase has occurred primarily in children with congenital heart disease and is related to the performance of cardiac surgery and cardiac catheterization. Adolescent drug abusers have developed staphylococcal endocarditis on normal valves, associated with intravenous drug injection and cutaneous abscesses from "skin popping." The mortality rate from infective endocarditis ranges from 20 to 30 per cent.

S. aureus may cause endocarditis in patients with no preexisting heart disease, in those with congenital or rheumatic lesions, and in patients convalescing from cardiac surgery. In four series of pediatric patients with endocarditis, *S. aureus* was responsible for 16 to 45 per cent of the cases of endocarditis.[30, 117, 186, 246, 259, 286] When cases from the period between 1963 and the early 1990s are analyzed, *S. aureus* was the cause of 35 to 40 per cent of all cases.[117, 259] In neonates, the incidence may be more than 50 per cent, a finding related to the increased incidence of *S. aureus* bacteremia in this population.[60] A prospective study in France found the risk of endocarditis with staphyloccocal bacteremia to be 11 per cent (4 of 36). Clinical signs were absent in all of the children with endocarditis. In this study, the diagnosis was made on the basis of bacteremia and vegetations seen on the echocardiogram.[84] Cardiac surgery and cardiac catheterization have been associated with staphylococcal endocarditis more frequently in recent years. Repair of congenital lesions without implantation of prosthetic valves, conduits, or patches is associated with a lower incidence of subsequent endocarditis. Coagulase-positive staphylococcal endocarditis generally occurs within 60 days of surgery. *S. epidermidis* also is an important causative agent in endocarditis complicating heart surgery.

Diagnosis depends on having a high index of suspicion of endocarditis, finding a positive blood culture or serologic evidence of staphylococcal infection, and demonstrating intracardiac location of disease whenever possible. Patients are likely to be ill. They are febrile and lethargic, and disease progresses rapidly. Fever and cardiac decompensation are common, but classic changes of endocarditis—anemia, splenomegaly, petechiae, splinter and conjunctival hemorrhages, and Janeway spots—may not be noted initially, in part because the serious symptoms and rapid progression of staphylococcal endocarditis are recognized early, before embolic phenomena or more chronic changes occur. It is important to note that one-fourth of all patients with endocarditis may have no murmur and one-third may have no leukocytosis.[270]

The most important diagnostic signs distinguishing *S. aureus* endocarditis from bacteremia associated with other foci are new or changing murmur, evidence of vegetations on two-dimensional echocardiograms, and the presence of embolic phenomena.[248] Two-dimensional echocardiography had a sensitivity of 25 to 82 per cent in detecting vegetations in three series of pediatric patients with endocarditis.[37, 130, 259] Transesophageal echocardiography yields a greater sensitivity than does the transthoracic approach. Two studies demonstrated sensitivities of 90 to 100 per cent using transesophageal echocardiography, compared with 50 to 58 per cent with the transthoracic approach.[178, 196] The presence of elevated titers of antibodies to teichoic acid[122, 128, 143, 247, 254] and to peptidoglycan[47, 261, 274] has been used to distinguish endocarditis from simple bacteremia with varying degrees of specificity and sensitivity.

Infective endocarditis has become a frequently recognized infectious complication of illicit drug use. The majority of patients are male, and their age reflects that of the general population of addicts. The frequency of endocarditis in addicts younger than 20 years of age has been increasing.[268] The majority of the patients develop endocarditis on previously normal heart valves. Right-sided endocarditis particularly is prevalent, and patients may have multiple pulmonary abscesses or shifting infiltrates and bacteremia.

Endocardial infection may occur at any time during a period of staphylococcal bacteremia. This fact should be kept in mind and the need for a prolonged course of antibiotic therapy considered for every patient with severe or persistent signs of illness during septicemia. If staphylococcal bacteremia associated with any other focus of infection occurs in a patient with a history of recent cardiac surgery or cardiac catheterization or with any intracardiac foreign body, that patient should be treated as for endocarditis.

Treatment of staphylococcal endocarditis requires a minimum of 4 to 6 weeks of high-dose intravenous antibiotic therapy, preferably with a semisynthetic penicillin (penicillin G, if the organism is sensitive). Antibiotic levels should be obtained to guide therapy and ensure that the peak serum level is at least 8 to 16 times the minimum inhibitory level for that organism. The aim of this therapy is to eradicate a focus of infection from a relatively avascular area. Response to therapy characteristically is slow, with fever and leukocytosis generally persisting for more than 1 week. After therapy is discontinued, repeat blood cultures should be obtained. If endocarditis occurs in the presence of an intracardiac foreign body, surgical removal may be necessary for bacteriologic cure.

Surgical therapy, such as valve replacement, may be required in patients with severe or progressive cardiac failure.

Purulent Pericarditis

Acute bacterial pericarditis is a rare and extremely serious complication of primary bacterial infection. Associated illness is seen in nearly all patients, respiratory tract infections most frequently, followed by meningitis, osteomyelitis, and skin infections. Coagulase-positive staphylococci are the most common etiologic agents, followed by *H. influenzae* type b meningococci, gram-negative enterics, pneumococci, and beta-hemolytic streptococci.

Common presenting signs are fever and respiratory distress, including cough, tachypnea, and dyspnea. A considerable proportion of the patients have signs of congestive heart failure when seen. Signs of pericardial tamponade are common. Pericardial friction rub may or may not be present initially. An electrocardiogram, chest radiograph, and echocardiogram help to establish a diagnosis. ST-segment abnormalities are seen most often, but a few patients show decreased voltage. Cardiomegaly, with a globular heart shape, is seen on chest radiograph in nearly all patients.

Mortality rates have been high (66 per cent in the children reported up to 1967).[87] Mortality rates were lower (25 per cent) in a more recent series.[280] There is general agreement that pericardial drainage by pericardiocentesis, pericardiectomy, or both should be done for both diagnosis and therapy. High-dose antibiotic therapy also must be provided intravenously. Medical treatment without surgical drainage clearly is inferior to combined therapy.[77, 87, 191, 260] Constrictive pericarditis develops in a small minority of patients and requires surgery.[189]

Meningitis

S. aureus is an unusual cause of meningitis, occurring predominantly in patients with abnormalities of the central nervous system or those who have undergone neurosurgical procedures or who have sustained trauma to the central nervous system. A review of 40 pediatric patients with *S. aureus* meningitis found that 32 (80 per cent) had an abnormality of the central nervous system (i.e., recent neurosurgery), 4 (10 per cent) were immunocompromised, and the remaining 4 (10 per cent) had an occult central nervous system abnormality demonstrated in a subsequent workup.[88] This study emphasizes the importance of undertaking the search for an abnormality of the central nervous system or an immunologic defect when staphylococcal meningitis is diagnosed.

Osteomyelitis

Osteomyelitis continues to be caused primarily by coagulase-positive staphylococci, although the proportion of infections caused by other organisms, particularly gram-negative enterics, may be increasing.[52, 73, 265] In children, osteomyelitis occurs by two major routes: acute hematogenous spread and spread from a contiguous focus of infection.

Acute hematogenous osteomyelitis has different manifestations, depending on the age of the affected patient. These differences are due to the differing nature of the vascular bone pattern in (1) infants, up to 1 year of age, (2) children, between 1 year of age and puberty, and (3) adults, after the cessation of bone growth.[253] In the infant, membranous bones are affected as well as long bones. Although acute illness with fever has been noted, the infant with osteomyelitis generally has little evidence of systemic toxicity. Local signs generally are absent except for pseudoparalysis or failure to move the affected limb, and multiple bones may be involved. *S. aureus* is the dominant organism, with only a few reports of gram-negative infection, despite the hazard these organisms generally present in neonates.[135, 147, 273] Antecedent or concomitant infections are common, particularly of the skin.

In addition to the benign, poorly localized clinical presentation, the distinctive feature of infantile osteomyelitis is the tendency to develop adjacent septic arthritis, permanent arrest of bone growth, or both. This is because the infantile bone has vessels that perforate the growth plate, thereby delivering infection to the epiphysis and possibly causing both joint disease and permanent epiphyseal damage.[105, 135, 147]

Hematogenous osteomyelitis in children beyond the neonatal period may occur either as an abrupt illness with fever and systemic signs of toxicity dominating the clinical picture or subacutely, with local complaints at the involved bone dominating the clinical picture and normal temperature or low-grade fever. Careful examination of bone, with particular attention to signs of local tenderness, is mandatory in evaluating children with either type. In children, osteomyelitis most often localizes in the long bones (Fig. 85–4), but osteomyelitis of the pelvis, patella, and small bones of the hands and feet certainly occurs and must be kept in mind because it may be particularly difficult to diagnose.[28, 64]

In childhood, the last ramifications of the nutrient artery to the long bones are the capillary loops located in the metaphysis of the bone just below the growth plate. Bacteria localize in the venous lakes just below these capillaries, causing thrombosis and retrograde spread of infection. In children older than 1 year of age, vessels no longer cross the cartilaginous growth plate, and the blood supply to the epiphysis largely is separate from that to the metaphysis. For this reason, infection from metaphyseal infection rarely reaches the joint or the epiphysis, thus explaining why children older than 1 year of age rarely have joint involvement or growth arrest.[253]

Children do develop osteomyelitis secondary to open trauma and contiguous infection. Although these cases still are caused predominantly by staphylococci, the range of other possibilities is even wider than in hematogenous osteomyelitis and includes soil and water organisms of generally low pathogenicity, such as *Pseudomonas.* In following patients with contaminated wounds and tissue infections adjacent to bone, the possibility of an associated osteomyelitis should be entertained and diligently investigated.

Hematogenous osteomyelitis of long bones primarily is a disease of infants and children. Adults are more likely to have osteomyelitis secondary to infection from a contiguous focus of infection.[265]

A particular type of hematogenous osteomyelitis involving the vertebrae occurs in adolescents and adults. Clinically, vertebral osteomyelitis is notable for its insidious onset, vague symptoms, and lack of fever or systemic toxicity. Patients usually report vague back pain present for several

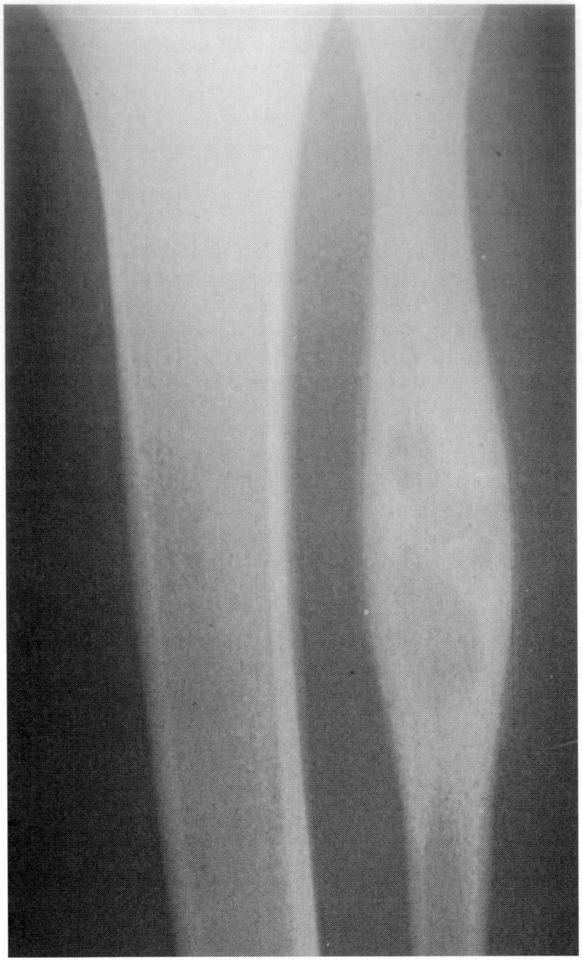

FIGURE 85–4. *Chronic staphylococcal osteomyelitis. A well-defined Brodie abscess in the fibula of a 7-year-old boy who had a history of several months of pain in the limb without fever. Lytic changes can be seen in the center of the lesion with remodeling of bone and periosteal elevation.*

weeks. The staphylococcus is the usual cause, but streptococci are prominent, and gram-negative enteric organisms may cause disease, particularly when there is an associated urinary tract infection.[239, 265] An increased frequency of vertebral osteomyelitis caused by *Pseudomonas* has been reported in heroin addicts.[239, 279] Cervical osteomyelitis, either as a consequence of hematogenous spread or direct extension from a contiguous site, may result in a prevertebral space infection. Symptoms of such infections include fever, localized pain, and neck stiffness. The symptoms of prevertebral space infections, such as dysphagia, drooling, and shortness of breath, may not be present. Complications can be life-threatening and include cervical spine subluxation or dislocation, mechanical compression of the spinal cord, and vascular compromise from mechanical compression or thrombosis.[24]

Children younger than 5 years of age may present with diskitis, now recognized as an early finding in the spectrum of osteomyelitis.[54]

The diagnosis of osteomyelitis must be pursued with vigor. Careful examination should reveal marked tenderness over the involved bone; the tender areas may be small and sharply limited. The total white blood cell count frequently is normal and generally of no help in diagnosis. The erythrocyte sedimentation rate, although nonspecific, nearly always is elevated. It is of help in monitoring the progress of the patient, as well as in diagnosis, with the caveat that the erythrocyte sedimentation rate may remain elevated in the first week of treatment. Serum C-reactive protein may be a better monitoring test because it almost always is elevated at presentation and its normalization may follow the clinical course closely.[258] The radionuclide bone scan has been shown to be of value in the early diagnosis of osteomyelitis prior to the appearance of bone changes on radiographs.[85, 252] Radiographic changes generally are not seen until 10 to 16 days after onset of infection. Magnetic resonance imaging is becoming a more widely used modality for the diagnosis of musculoskeletal disorders. Magnetic resonance imaging has the advantage of defining the extent and location of the inflammatory process. The sensitivity is 97 per cent, and the specificity ranges from 75 to 92 per cent.[161] Blood cultures frequently yield the etiologic agent and should be performed in all cases. Blood culture was positive in 50 and 57 per cent, respectively, of cases of osteomyelitis in children in two series.[28, 64] The sensitivity for retrieval of an organism with combined blood culture and bone aspiration approaches 80 per cent.[214]

Bone aspiration or bone biopsy is important in the confirmation of osteomyelitis and the determination of the etiologic agent. Aspiration is simple, performed by direct needle puncture into the bone at the point of maximum tenderness or site of radiographic change. If pus is returned, it is Gram stained and cultured. The results of Gram staining guide the choice of parenteral antibiotic therapy. If the aspiration does not yield pus, surgical bone biopsy should be performed for culture and drainage. Needle aspiration does not cause significant changes on bone scans and therefore should not be postponed for this reason.[44] Because the diagnosis of osteomyelitis mandates a prolonged course of therapy, considerable effort should be extended in the original evaluation to obtain an etiologic diagnosis. Adequate specimens for culture from more than one site give the highest yield. Throughout the process of diagnosis, management, and follow-up of the child with osteomyelitis, close cooperation and joint decision making with an orthopedic surgeon are required for optimal care of the patient.

After the diagnostic efforts, parenteral antibiotic therapy should be started, based on results of the Gram stain of bone aspirate or biopsy, clinical considerations, or both. Initial coverage should be provided against penicillinase-producing staphylococci. Coverage should be provided for gram-negative enterics in patients with soil-contaminated contiguous wounds or for *Salmonella* in cases of osteomyelitis in children who have hemoglobin S diseases. Fever and local tenderness generally show prompt resolution within 48 hours. Continued hectic fever after therapy is begun requires careful consideration of complete surgical drainage of the involved bone and careful search for other undrained foci of infection.

Therapy for osteomyelitis appears to require a prolonged period and a considerable amount of antibiotic in serum to provide adequate levels in the bone. Neither optimum has been defined adequately, and few series reporting "successful" treatment with one or another regimen have had adequate follow-up data. High-dose intravenous antibiotic therapy has been preferred because serum antibiotic levels several times above the minimum inhibitory concentration of most organisms responsible for osteomyelitis can be achieved reliably. Two retrospective studies provide evidence to support this view. Waldvogel and associates[265] defined intensive therapy as consisting of 4 weeks of high-dose intravenous therapy and found a treatment failure rate of 4 per cent for 26 patients on this regimen. Five of six patients receiving less intensive therapy developed chronic infection. In children, Dich and colleagues[64] found that 19 per cent of 37 children treated with parenteral therapy for less than 3 weeks developed chronic or recurrent disease, compared with only 1 of 48 treated for more than 3 weeks. At present, therefore, the optimal standard of therapy appears to be parenteral high-dose therapy directed against the organism isolated or empirically against penicillinase-producing staphylococci for a minimum of 4 weeks. After this period, the decision to discontinue therapy should be based on review of the patient's course, radiographic evidence of healing, and a sedimentation rate that has returned to normal. Oral therapy may be provided after 4 weeks of intravenous therapy for certain patients who are doing well but have persistent sedimentation rate elevation. Dicloxacillin at a dose of 100 mg/kg/24 hours gives good serum levels, which should provide adequate bone levels.

It theoretically is possible to obtain antistaphylococcal serum antibiotic levels from 10 to 20 times the minimum inhibitory concentration of the organism with extremely high oral doses of certain antibiotics. Providing equivalent oral antibiotic therapy should shorten hospitalization, but patient tolerance of high doses, patient compliance, and adequate follow-up once a patient has been discharged must be ensured.[41] At present, for patients not involved in carefully conducted treatment trials, at least *4 weeks of intravenous therapy provides the best chance for cure and is the standard by which other treatment programs must be measured.* Treatment for chronic osteomyelitis continues to be surgical primarily, although antibiotics are a useful adjunct and may be required for prolonged periods.

Septic Arthritis

Staphylococci are frequent etiologic agents of septic arthritis in patients in all age groups, although many other agents also are involved. In the neonate, the staphylococcus is the most common etiologic agent, but gram-negative enteric organisms also are found.[103, 182, 183] In the child from 2 months to 4 years of age, *H. influenzae* type b now is the most frequent causative agent, followed by staphylococci, streptococci, pneumococci, and meningococci. Beyond 41 years of age, *Staphylococcus* is predominant among a great variety of other organisms. Sexually active adolescents may have gonococcal arthritis or sterile inflammatory arthritis associated with gonococcal disease. Septic arthritis most often occurs in only one joint, but more than one may be involved, particularly in the neonate or in association with neglected and prolonged multifocal bacteremic illness. The large joints—knee, hip, ankle, and elbow—account for 90 per cent of infected joints.[32]

Differential diagnoses include acute rheumatic fever, the inflammatory noninfectious arthropathies associated with rheumatoid arthritis, lupus erythematosus, serum sickness, and vasculitis syndromes. The work-up should include blood cultures, culture of associated septic foci, and joint aspiration. In septic arthritis, the blood culture is positive in approximately 50 per cent of cases. Joint fluid should be examined for total and differential cell counts, glucose and protein content, and mucin clot formation, in addition to Gram stain and culture. Counterimmunoelectrophoresis of joint fluid may be of help in the diagnosis of type b *H. influenzae* and pneumococcal, meningococcal, and group B streptococcal arthritides. In some cases, culture may be sterile, even when organisms are seen clearly on Gram stain.

The hip joint presents special problems in diagnosis. In the neonate or young infant, clinical signs of hip involvement may be minimal. Warmth, erythema, and swelling may not be appreciated because of the considerable amount of soft tissue surrounding the joint. Pain on movement and refusal to move the limb may be the only signs. On physical examination, the range of movement may appear normal because the strength of the examiner may overcome the resistance of the infant. By the time signs of joint dislocation appear, the damage may be irreparable.[46, 105, 158]

When a diagnosis of septic arthritis has been made by aspiration (joint fluid generally shows >30,000 white blood cells/mm^3, >75 per cent polymorphonuclear leukocytes, glucose two-thirds of the serum value, and poor mucin clot), systemic antibiotics should be administered. The choice of antibiotic should be based on Gram stain and a consideration of the likely agents in a child of that age. Antibiotic irrigation of the joint space is unnecessary, except in the case of fungal arthritis, because adequate antibiotic levels can be achieved by systemic therapy.[181] Surgical drainage should be performed immediately in the case of hip joint involvement. The special characteristics of this joint mandate drainage for the following reasons:

1. The joint capsule limits the amount of expansion possible, which may compromise blood flow to the head of the femur.
2. Osteomyelitis from the spread of infection to adjacent bone is a possibility in the hip joint because the articular cartilage covers only the articular surface of the head of the femur. The periosteum of the neck of the femur therefore is exposed and in contact with the infected fluid. Surgical drainage of other joints may be required when rapid reaccumulation of fluid occurs after needle drainage.

The minimum effective duration of therapy of septic arthritis has not been determined yet. At present, it appears prudent to continue high-dose, preferably intravenous, therapy for 14 to 21 days in most cases. Hip disease should be treated as osteomyelitis with at least 4 weeks of therapy.

Deep-Tissue Abscesses

During the course of bacteremia, staphylococci may establish multiple metastatic foci in a wide variety of tissues. Abscesses of liver, spleen, and pancreas have been reported in association with staphylococcal bacteremia and have been detected at autopsy more often than while patients were alive. Liver abscess has been a rare complication of bacteremia or ascending septic cholangitis. In children, hematogenous spread appears to be most important because patients generally have abscesses in other organs. In the preantibiotic era, liver abscess was seen most often in normal children with an uncontrolled focal infection, such as osteomyelitis or infected wounds. However, liver abscess has been seen primarily in children with leukopenia as in treated leukemia and with white cell dysfunction syndromes (e.g., chronic granulomatous disease).[62, 119] Liver abscess also has been a problem in neonates with bacteremia and after umbilical vein catheterization.[36] Staphylococci and the enteric organisms are encountered most frequently.

Although uncommon, hepatic abscess should be considered, even in normal patients with persistent liver enlargement associated with bacteremia; liver function tests may be normal or abnormal. Large abscesses are apparent on liver scan, ultrasonography, or computed tomography. Surgical drainage, along with antibiotic therapy, is needed for resolution.[142]

Bacterial muscle abscesses are so common in tropical countries that they form an appreciable proportion of hospital admissions; they are rare in other areas.[109, 227] From sporadic reports from the United States, it appears that the clinical behavior is similar in various locales, although muscle abscess is more likely to be misdiagnosed where it is encountered infrequently.[8, 67, 145] Pyomyositis occurs in all groups.[154] The onset generally is subacute, with patients complaining of muscle pain of days' to weeks' duration, followed by fever. Abscesses are found in large striated muscles, particularly the quadriceps. Muscle masses involved, in decreasing order of frequency, are thigh, buttocks, arm, lower legs, groin, chest wall, flank, and shoulder. Two cases of abdominal wall muscle abscesses in children presented as acute abdominal pain suggesting peritonitis.[25] These abscesses first manifest themselves as firm indurated swellings without significant erythema or heat. Staphylococci practically are the only etiologic agents identified and can be discovered from single or multiple abscesses. Surgical drainage of the mass is diagnostic and therapeutic; large volumes of pus often are recovered. Antistaphylococcal antibiotic therapy should be employed as an adjunct. The pathogenesis of the lesion is unexplained, but localization of bacteria within a traumatized or parasitized area has been suggested.

Staphylococcal Enterocolitis

Enterocolitis due to staphylococci is an uncommon disease that generally has been described in adult patients given broad-spectrum antibiotics, particularly tetracycline.[99] Patients with debilitating diseases, such as cirrhosis, or recuperating from gastrointestinal surgery develop diarrhea while receiving broad-spectrum antibiotics. Stool examination shows polymorphonuclear leukocytes in large numbers, with

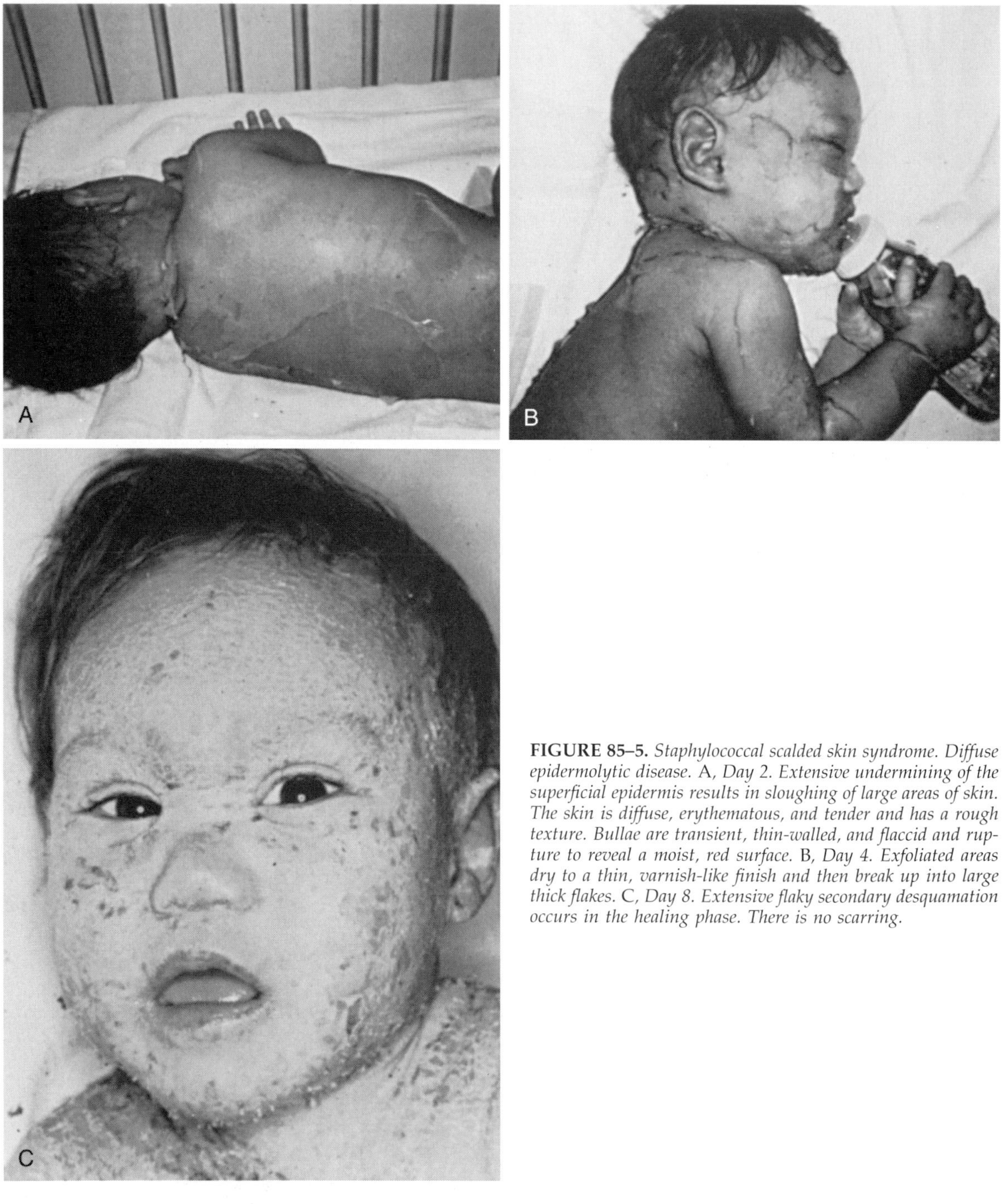

FIGURE 85–5. *Staphylococcal scalded skin syndrome. Diffuse epidermolytic disease.* A, *Day 2. Extensive undermining of the superficial epidermis results in sloughing of large areas of skin. The skin is diffuse, erythematous, and tender and has a rough texture. Bullae are transient, thin-walled, and flaccid and rupture to reveal a moist, red surface.* B, *Day 4. Exfoliated areas dry to a thin, varnish-like finish and then break up into large thick flakes.* C, *Day 8. Extensive flaky secondary desquamation occurs in the healing phase. There is no scarring.*

gram-positive cocci as the only, or heavily predominant, stool organisms. Stool cultures confirm that staphylococci are the predominant organisms.[124]

Staphylococci should be the predominant organisms on both smear and culture in persons with staphylococcal enterocolitis. Staphylococci can be cultured from the stool in smaller numbers from many normal persons. Persons who merely are colonized never have a predominantly staphylococcal fecal flora.

Staphylococcal enterocolitis has been reported to be severe and occasionally fatal, with deaths due to overwhelming septicemia or gastrointestinal ulceration. Staphylococci have been recovered from multiple ulcers at all levels of the intestinal tract in fatal cases.[99] In two series of carefully selected patients with staphylococcal enterocolitis, all isolates were found to produce enterotoxin.[98, 124] For this reason, in vivo elaboration of enterotoxin was presumed to be important in the pathogenesis of the diarrhea.

Reports of well-documented staphylococcal enterocolitis are extremely rare in infants and children.[93, 99] Oral and systemic antistaphylococcal antibiotic therapy is indicated whenever a firm diagnosis can be made.

Staphylococcal Toxin-Mediated Diseases

Staphylococcal Food Poisoning

Within 2 to 6 hours after ingestion of preformed enterotoxin contaminating various foodstuffs, patients develop the sudden onset of recurrent vomiting, which usually ceases by 12 hours after ingestion. Diarrhea also may occur during this period. Fever is not a part of this syndrome.

Staphylococcal Scalded Skin Syndrome

The staphylococcal scalded skin syndrome comprises a spectrum of dermatologic disease associated with staphylococcal infection. The dermatologic manifestations of the illness differ in degree and extent, but all bear a superficial resemblance to skin lesions caused by scalding.[159, 168] The skin changes are caused by the action of a soluble exotoxin, the epidermolytic toxin produced by certain strains of staphylococci.[146, 169] Epidermolytic toxin is the preferred name for this relatively recently discovered toxin; this provides a more precise description of the skin pathology than do the other terms, exfoliative toxin and exfoliatin.

The most severe and generalized form of the scalded skin syndrome is an acute, dramatic, bullous desquamation of large areas of skin (Fig. 85–5). It has been known as Ritter disease and pemphigus neonatorum when it occurs in neonates and as toxic epidermal necrolysis or Lyell disease when it occurs in older children and adults. The onset usually is abrupt, with the sudden appearance of diffuse, tender erythroderma. Within 1 to 3 days, a positive Nikolsky sign develops and flaccid, thin-walled bullae appear. Within hours, the bullae spontaneously rupture and the superficial epidermis separates in large sheets, revealing widespread areas of moist red surface. Within 1 to 3 days, these denuded areas dry and the entire body surface undergoes a secondary flaky desquamation. Unless infection or other skin irritation supervenes, the entire skin heals without scarring within 14 days of the onset of the process.[151, 152, 168]

The second generalized form of the scalded skin syndrome is that of diffuse scarlatiniform erythroderma. Patients with this manifestation also show the abrupt development of diffuse, tender erythroderma, which is indistinguishable from the initial stages of the diffuse, epidermolytic form of the disease. The skin appearance also is similar to that of streptococcal scarlet fever, with diffuse erythroderma, sandpaper texture, and increased erythema in skin creases (similar to Pastia lines). Even at the beginning there are important clinical differences from streptococcal scarlet fever: the skin is tender to the touch, and there is no strawberry tongue or palatal exanthem. Within 2 to 5 days after the onset of erythroderma, cracks appear about the eyes and mouth; over the next 5 days, the entire skin surface undergoes a thick flaky desquamation, which also is identical with the final and healing phase of the most severe form. Therefore, it appears that the initial and concluding phases are identical to those of the epidermolytic form but that the intermediate stages of Nikolsky sign formation, flaccid bullae, and extensive epidermal loss do not occur. We have noted that many children with both generalized forms of the disease have been misdiagnosed by experienced physicians as having streptococcal scarlet fever in the early stages. Recognition of the tender or painful skin problem and the early appearance of flaky desquamation lead to a diagnosis of staphylococcal scarlatiniform eruption. Children with either of these two forms of disease generally are febrile and irritable and appear moderately ill. Their skin is tender, and they are uncomfortable when handled or held.

Staphylococci can be isolated from some focus of infection in children presenting with this problem. The focus of infection frequently is distant from the skin, and fluid aspirated from intact bullae repeatedly is found to be sterile. The denuded skin, however, is colonized rapidly. The infected focus most often is minor; conjunctivitis or infected superficial abrasions are encountered most frequently. In neonates, an infected circumcision site is common. On the other hand, the infection itself may be severe and life-threatening; patients with associated endocarditis, septicemia, omphalitis, and severe surgical wound infection have been described.

There are two localized forms of the scalded skin syndrome, bullous impetigo and bullous varicella, which truly are skin infections. Unlike the two generalized forms, staphylococci are present at the site of the skin manifestations.

Bullous impetigo (Fig. 85–6) is a condition in which single or multiple flaccid bullae arise from normal-appearing skin. Fluid within the bulla may be turbid, cloudy, or frankly purulent. When bullae rupture, their base is moist and erythematous but soon dries to a varnish-like finish. In neonates,

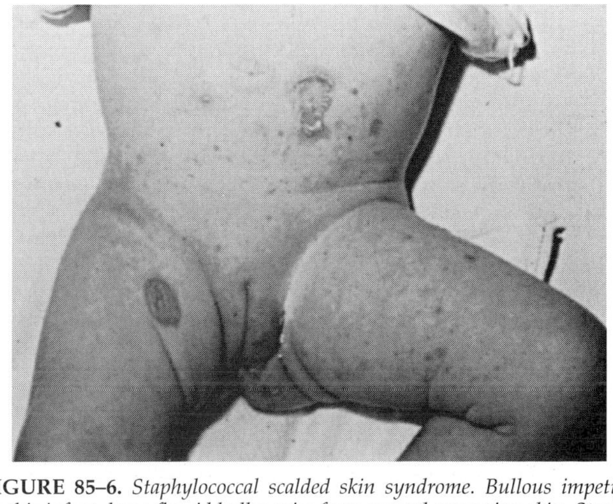

FIGURE 85–6. *Staphylococcal scalded skin syndrome. Bullous impetigo. In this infant, large flaccid bullae arise from normal-appearing skin. Staphylococci are present within the lesions in bullous impetigo, unlike in the generalized forms.*

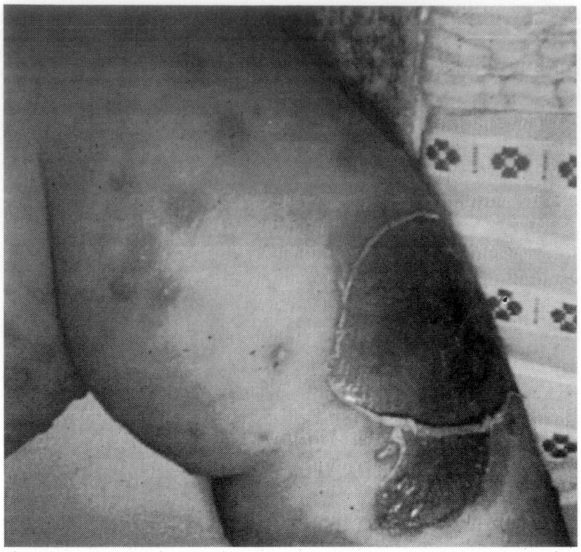

FIGURE 85–7. *Staphylococcal scalded skin syndrome. Bullous varicella. A large, ruptured bullous lesion is seen among typical smaller varicella vesicles. Bullous lesions appeared 3 days after the onset of the varicella rash and represent a distinctive superinfection.*

lesions of bullous impetigo generally are found around the umbilicus and perineum. If unrecognized and untreated, involvement may be extensive.

Bullous varicella (Fig. 85–7) is an example of viral-bacterial synergism. One to 5 days after the onset of typical lesions of varicella, a sudden change occurs, with the appearance of large flaccid bullae interspersed among the more typical varicella lesions. The bullous lesions usually are multiple and seen in diverse areas of the body, creating an unusual appearance that generally calls the original diagnosis of varicella into question. Proof of varicella virus infection can be obtained by scraping the base of a vesicle; the Tzanck preparation reveals herpetic giant cells, and varicella virus can be isolated from the typical varicella lesions. Staphylococci can be isolated from the bullous lesions, which have a histologic appearance identical to that of bullous impetigo.[166, 263]

Staphylococci isolated from patients with any of the forms of the scalded skin syndrome have the unique property of inducing epidermolysis in newborn mice. This experimental model is indistinguishable clinically, histologically, and ultrastructurally from the most severe form of the disease seen in humans.[146, 173] The mouse model provided a bioassay system that led to the discovery of the epidermolytic toxin. The toxin is a low-molecular-weight (26,000 daltons) protein, which causes lysis of the intracellular attachment between cells of the granular layer of the epidermis.[69, 146, 169] The toxin does not cause cell death primarily and does not elicit an inflammatory response. Although the precise site of action is known, the mechanism of action remains elusive. In the generalized forms of staphylococcal scalded skin syndrome, the toxin is released from the site of infection, is disseminated hematogenously, and acts on the granular layers of cells of the superficial epidermis. There is no evidence of epidermolytic toxin action on other cells of epidermal origin. In bullous impetigo and bullous varicella, conditions in which staphylococci are present in the skin, the toxin is produced locally and acts locally.

In the United States, the majority of toxin-producing strains associated with staphylococcal scalded skin syndrome belong to phage group II (phage types 3A, 3B, 3C, 55, and 71), but in Japan, strains of other phage groups appear to be more prevalent. Prior to the discovery of the epidermolytic toxin, some investigators had noted a relationship between a phage group II strain type 71, bullous impetigo, and toxic epidermal necrolysis, but until the discovery of epidermolytic toxin, the relationship was not proved nor the mechanism that induces the skin changes elucidated.

Staphylococcal scalded skin syndrome, in all its forms, primarily is a disease of childhood, although in recent years it has occurred increasingly in adults, generally those with immunosuppression, renal impairment, or both. Adult skin is sensitive to the effects of toxin, so it appears that the adult protection from staphylococcal scalded skin syndrome may be related to some combination of increased prevalence of preformed antitoxin, metabolic differences, or greater ability to contain infection.[69, 70] Adults are more likely to develop another form of toxic epidermal necrolysis, which is idiopathic or associated with hypersensitivity to drugs. This form is similar clinically but different histologically and is associated with a higher mortality rate.

Diagnosis may be made on clinical grounds in some patients. However, because the other form of toxic epidermal necrolysis responds to steroids and not to antibiotics, skin biopsy may be necessary in some cases (Fig. 85–8). In staphylococcal toxic epidermal necrolysis, a cleavage plane is seen high in the epidermis, and there is no significant inflammatory reaction. In drug-induced or idiopathic toxic epidermal necrolysis, a cleavage plane is seen either at the level of the dermal-epidermal junction or within the dermis, and there is intense polymorphonuclear infiltration with extensive epidermal necrosis. An effective diagnostic procedure, simpler even than skin biopsy, is to excise some exfoliated skin for frozen and permanent histologic section (Fig. 85–9).[9, 108] In staphylococcal toxic epidermal necrolysis, only the cornified layer is seen, whereas the entire necrotic epidermis can be recognized in the idiopathic or drug-induced form of toxic epidermal necrolysis. Diagnosis is confirmed either by isolation of staphylococci and demonstration of toxin production or by histologic study.

Therapy for all of the forms of staphylococcal scalded skin syndrome should be directed at eradicating staphylococci from the focus of infection, thereby ending toxin production. Parenteral antibiotics in large doses should be given to those with extensive skin disease and those with serious infection, whereas oral therapy generally is sufficient for the limited bullous impetigo. Neither topical nor systemic steroids should be employed because they have no effect on toxin-

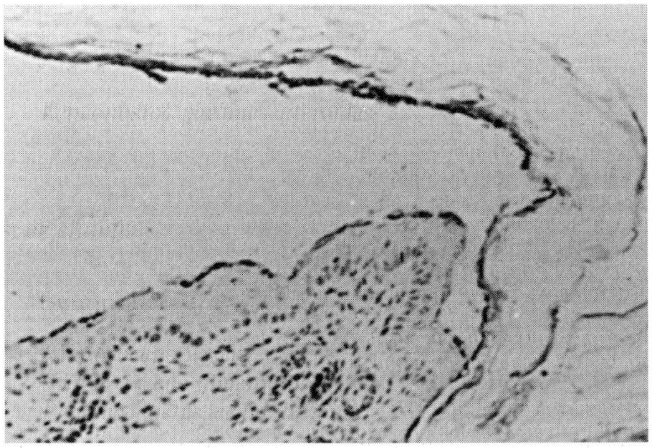

FIGURE 85–8. *Staphylococcal scalded skin syndrome. Photomicrograph of skin biopsy at the margin of a bulla showing the cleavage plane high in the epidermis with no inflammatory reaction or other changes in the epidermis or dermis.*

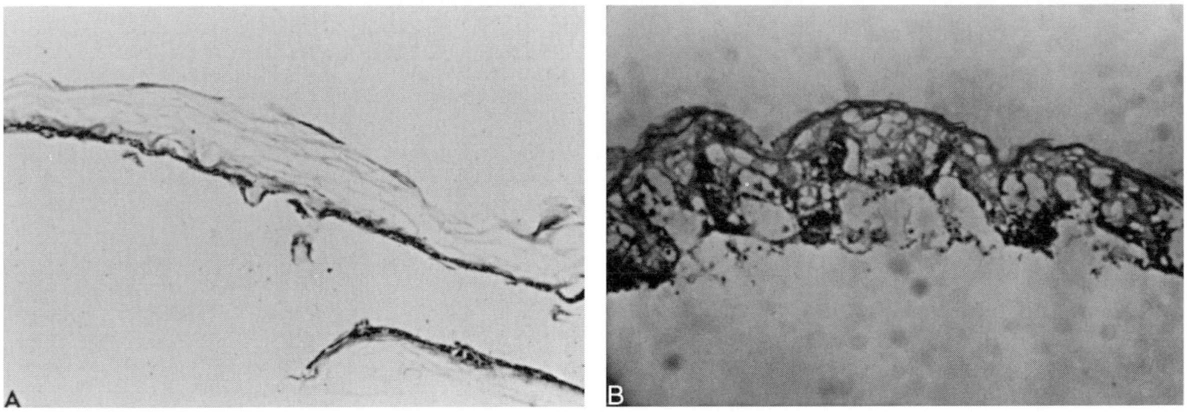

FIGURE 85–9. *Differentiation of staphylococcal from idiopathic toxic epidermal necrolysis by section of spontaneously exfoliated skin.* A, *Exfoliated skin from a patient with staphylococcal scalded skin syndrome shows only the stratum corneum and one-cell layer of the stratum granulosum demonstrating the subcorneal level of the cleavage plane.* B, *Shed skin from a patient with idiopathic nonstaphylococcal toxic epidermal necrolysis shows the entire epidermis involved in a necrotic inflammatory reaction. This process obviously involves deeper layers of skin. (From Honig, P. J., Gaisin, A., and Buck, B. E.: Frozen section differentiation of drug-induced and staphylococcal-induced toxic epidermal necrolysis. J. Pediatr. 92:504, 1978.)*

mediated skin changes but do enhance infection in the experimental model.[167] A clinical study confirms the detrimental effect of steroids.[215] Children with extensively denuded skin should be allowed to rest on sterile linen unclothed and should be handled as little as possible. Topical preparations are without benefit and should not be employed because the epidermal damage is self-limited once adequate antibiotics are given.

Toxic Shock Syndrome

TSS is discussed separately in Chapter 74.

Kawasaki Disease

Kawasaki disease is an acute multisystemic vasculitis of infancy and childhood and is the most common cause of acquired heart disease in Japan and the United States. The diagnosis is made when certain clinical criteria are fulfilled, including high fever, rash, nonexudative conjunctivitis, inflammation of the mucous membranes, erythematous induration of the hands and feet, and cervical lymphadenopathy. An infectious etiology for Kawasaki disease has never been proved. Recent investigations demonstrate an association of Kawasaki disease with selective expansion of VB2+ T cells in the peripheral blood, a known consequence of superantigens.[1, 2] This finding has been challenged subsequently. It has been suggested that Kawasaki disease may be caused by a staphylococcal antigen acting as a superantigen. Lueng and associates[144] recovered *S. aureus* that produced TSST-I in a significantly greater proportion of Kawasaki disease patients compared with controls and suggested a causal link between TSST-I and Kawasaki disease. Melish and associates[170] and Terai and colleagues[244] have found no association between *S. aureus* that produces TSST-I and Kawasaki disease. Additional studies are required to evaluate a potential role for toxin-producing bacteria and Kawasaki disease.

DIAGNOSIS

The diagnosis of significant staphylococcal infections should be pursued with vigor. Collections of pus, whether superficial or deep, should be aspirated or drained surgically for diagnostic and therapeutic purposes. Gram stain and culture should be obtained. An aggressive approach to the diagnosis of osteomyelitis by bone aspiration and bone biopsy provides an etiologic security that is helpful during the prolonged treatment phase that necessarily follows. When infection is associated with a foreign body, such as an intravenous catheter or suture, removal and culture of the foreign body help.

At least two blood cultures should be obtained before starting therapy in all serious infections. One need not wait for fever spikes or delay therapy to obtain cultures. Blood cultures frequently are negative in serious staphylococcal infection, a fact that demonstrates the need for other cultures. Blood cultures are positive in most cases of staphylococcal endocarditis, approximately half of cases of osteomyelitis and septic arthritis, and less than half of cases of pneumonia and deep-tissue abscesses. Measurement of nonspecific indicators of inflammation (e.g., erythrocyte sedimentation rate and C-reactive protein), although of limited value in diagnosis, can be helpful in following the clinical course of infection and response to intervention. A pilot study of patients with *S. aureus* septicemia revealed that changes in cytokine interleukin-6 levels correlated with the clinical course. The advantage of this test over other nonspecific markers is that interleukin-6 may be detected in the early phase of infection, before the indicators of inflammation have begun to rise.[231]

Accurate, sensitive serologic methods for the diagnosis of serious staphylococcal infections would be of great clinical usefulness. An ideal test or battery of tests would detect both bacteremia and invasive nonbacteremic staphylococcal disease but would not be positive in patients with simple superficial infections. This would allow certain etiologic diagnosis of patients with multiple, severe staphylococcal diseases that may not be bacteremic and in which direct culture is difficult, such as osteomyelitis, septic arthritis, pneumonia, and liver abscess. Multiple antigens have been used in the search for this ideal test, but at present none has been useful enough to be made widely available in the clinical laboratory.

Enzyme-linked immunosorbent assay, gel diffusion, and counterimmunoelectrophoresis methods for the detection of antibodies to teichoic acid (a cell-wall constituent) have been demonstrated to be highly specific for detection soon after the onset of infection and to disappear in late convalescence. More than 90 per cent of patients with staphylococcal endocarditis, approximately 70 per cent of patients with staphylococcal osteomyelitis, and up to 50 per cent of patients with

TABLE 85–2. Therapy for Staphylococcal Infection in Infants and Children (Excluding Neonates)

	Oral (Mild–Moderate Infection)		Parenteral (Moderate–Severe Infection)	
	<40 kg	*Children >40 kg and Adults*	*<40 kg*	*Children >40 kg and Adults*
Penicillins				
Methicillin	—	—	200 mg/kg/24 hr in 6 doses q 4 hr IV	6–12 g/24 hr in 6 doses q 4 hr IV
Oxacillin			100–200 mg/kg/24 hr in 6 doses q 4 hr IV	4–8 g/24 hr in 6 doses q 4 hr IV
Nafcillin			100–200 mg/kg/24 hr in 6 doses q 4 hr IV	4–8 g/24 hr in 6 doses q 4 hr IV
Cloxacillin	50–100 mg/kg/24 hr in 4 doses	1–2 g/24 hr in 4 doses	—	—
Dicloxacillin	12.5–25 mg/kg/24 hr in 4 doses	1 g/24 hr in 4 doses	—	—
Cephalosporins				
Cephalothin (Keflin)	—	—	100 mg/kg/24 hr in 6 doses q 4 hr IV	3–12 g/24 hr in 6 doses q 4 hr IV
Cefazolin (Ancef; Kefzol)	—	—	50–100 mg/kg/24 hr in 3 doses q 8 hr	2–4 g/24 hr in 3 doses
Cephalexin (Keflex)	25–50 mg/kg/24 hr in 4 doses	1.4 g/24 hr in 4 doses	—	—
Cefadroxil (Duricef; Ultracef)	30 mg/kg/24 hr in 2 doses	1–2 g/24 hr in 2 doses	—	—
Other Agents				
Erythromycin	35–50 mg/kg/24 hr in 4 doses	1–2 g/24 hr in 4 doses	20–30 mg/kg/24 hr q 6 hr (lactobionate)	10–20 mg/kg/24 hr q 6 hr
Clindamycin	12–16 mg/kg/24 hr in 4 doses	600–1200 mg/24 hr in 4 doses	15–40 mg/kg/24 hr q 6 hr IV	600–2400 mg/24 hr q 6 hr IV
Vancomycin	—	—	40–60 mg/kg/24 hr by continuous IV drip or q 6 hr by drip over 1 hr	1–2 g/24 hr by continuous drip or q 6 hr by drip over 1 hr

simple uncomplicated bacteremia have detectable antibodies, whereas these cannot be detected in persons without staphylococcal disease or superficial infections. Antibodies may be detected in nonbacteremic patients with serious invasive disease, such as staphylococcal osteomyelitis, septic arthritis, and pneumonia.[122, 128, 129, 254, 255] An IgG response to *S. aureus* collagen-binding protein is present in 60 per cent of patients with septic arthritis. Serologic studies therefore may be helpful in detecting staphylococcal infections, but the hope that these tests reliably would differentiate between patients with serious infections and those with uncomplicated bacteremia has not been fulfilled. Tests for antibody to alpha-hemolysin have similar limitations.[243] More recently, the antibody response to staphylococcal peptidoglycan has been studied. Virtually all adults have detectable antibodies to this substance. However, with quantitative studies, a threshold level for antibody can be established so that elevated levels can be correlated with recent severe disease.[47, 261, 274] To date, none of these tests is widely available, and we still need serologic tests similar to those used for the diagnosis of streptococcal infection. Evaluation and development of more sensitive and easily performed serologic tests may make diagnosis of staphylococcal infection easier and more secure in the future.

Enterotoxins can be identified by a variety of methods. Immunoassay is used routinely but may lack the sensitivity required to detect levels seen in staphylococcal food poisoning. DNA oligonucleotide probes are highly sensitive, but their clinical utility is limited by the identification of nonexpressed genes.[190]

TREATMENT

General Principles

Successful treatment of staphylococcal infections depends on adequate drainage of collections of pus and on the rational use of antibiotic therapy. Staphylococcal infections have a particular tendency to persist and recur; for these reasons, prolonged antibiotic therapy usually is required for all but minor infections. Surgical drainage is extremely important and in some cases of minor superficial abscesses may be all that is required. For most infections, a period of antibiotic therapy after surgical drainage better ensures that the infection has been contained. Failure to provide surgical drainage is an important reason for organism persistence or recurrence. Antibiotics cannot be expected to penetrate into the avascular center of abscess cavities. When abscess cavities are undrained or when antibiotic therapy is discontinued before an area is sterilized, live bacteria may persist and be disseminated, causing later recurrence at that site or metastatically.

For moderate to severe staphylococcal infections, the patient should be hospitalized for intravenous therapy, which generally should be given by intermittent infusion. This strategy ensures peak antibiotic levels, which may allow greater penetration into relatively avascular areas and eliminates potential problems with antibiotic inactivation in intravenous solutions. Intramuscular injections rarely are indicated in children because intermittent injections are far more painful than is intravenous administration of drugs. A heparin lock may be inserted to provide an intravenous route in the active patient not requiring parenteral fluids.

Coagulase-Positive Staphylococci

(Table 85–2)

Since the mid-1960s, it has been apparent that the majority of coagulase-positive staphylococci from most sections of North America and Europe are penicillinase producers and therefore penicillin-resistant. In addition, the distinction formerly drawn between hospital-acquired and community-acquired staphylococci has disappeared. The proportion of penicillin-resistant staphylococci from both sources approaches 90 per cent. When coagulase-positive staphylococci are likely to be the cause of infection, treatment with a penicillinase-resistant penicillin or cephalosporin should be initiated prior to bacterial isolation and sensitivity testing. In some locations, methicillin resistance is widespread. Methicillin-resistant organisms cannot be treated adequately with cephalosporins; vancomycin therefore is indicated for MRSA. Vancomycin also is the drug of choice for *S. epidermidis* prior to the return of sensitivity test reports. When staphylococci are presumed to be the cause of infection, it is mandatory to treat the patient with a penicillinase-resistant antibiotic prior to isolation and adequate sensitivity testing. Coagulase-negative staphylococci also show a high percentage of resistance to penicillin. Remarks about the treatment of coagulase-positive staphylococci apply to treatment of coagulase-negative strains as well.

Penicillin G is the treatment of choice for penicillin-sensitive, nonpenicillinase-producing organisms. When properly performed sensitivity tests indicate penicillin sensitivity, therapy should be changed to this antibiotic, which has far greater specific activity than do the alternatives. Conversion from penicillin sensitivity to resistance during the course of infection has not been a clinical problem.

In the far more common situation in which a penicillin-resistant organism is isolated, the semisynthetic penicillinase-resistant penicillins are the drugs of choice. Methicillin, oxacillin, and nafcillin are available for parenteral use. Of drugs available for oral use, cloxacillin and dicloxacillin are preferred; they are absorbed well and cause less gastrointestinal discomfort. Much discussion is heard about which of these drugs is superior. Protein binding in vivo affects the amount of antibiotic available for therapy. Methicillin has the least degree of protein binding, followed by penicillin G, nafcillin, oxacillin, cloxacillin, and dicloxacillin. On the other hand, nafcillin, oxacillin, cloxacillin, and dicloxacillin show greater specific activity against penicillinase-producing staphylococci than does methicillin. No clinical evidence for the therapeutic superiority of one of these antibiotics over another exists.

For neonates with coagulase-positive staphylococcal infections (Table 85–3), methicillin continues to be the drug of choice; it is the antistaphylococcal drug that has been studied most completely.[11, 31, 220] For most infections, 25 mg/kg/dose is indicated, the frequency of administration being varied according to postnatal age and birth weight. This dose can be doubled safely for severe, disseminated infections. Low-birth-weight infants (<2000 g) receive a dose every 12 hours for the first week, then every 8 hours from 1 to 4 weeks of age. Infants who weigh more than 2000 g receive 25 to 50 mg/kg/dose every 8 hours for the first week and every 6 hours for from 1 to 4 weeks.

In all serious staphylococcal infections, it is desirable to assess serum bactericidal activity against the patient's organism and adjust dosage and schedule to maintain a peak serum level at least eight times the minimum inhibitory concentration. The clinician should become familiar with the use of one parenteral and one oral antistaphylococcal penicillin. If clinical response appears slow, nothing is to be gained by switching to another antibiotic within this category; instead, microbiologic data should be reviewed and serum antibiotic levels obtained.

"Methicillin" Nephropathy

A syndrome consisting of fever, eosinophilia, erythematous rash, proteinuria, and hematuria has been reported in patients receiving methicillin therapy.[14, 218, 284] In a small number of patients with this complication, renal biopsy specimens have provided evidence of interstitial nephritis. In one patient, immune complexes consisting of IgG and the major methicillin hapten were demonstrated in the tubular and glomerular basement membrane. Although a hypersensitivity reaction has been postulated to be the cause, the appearance of this complication definitely also was related to the dose of drug and duration of therapy and was more common in patients receiving more than 200 mg/kg/24 hours for longer than 2 weeks.[76]

This syndrome appears to be rare in children in the United States, even when large doses of methicillin are used for a prolonged period, and has been found to be reversible when antibiotics are discontinued.[162, 284] Yow and associates[284] estimate that all adverse reactions to methicillin occur in less than 1.5 per cent of treated children. Although the syndrome of fever, eosinophilia, and interstitial nephritis has been reported most frequently with methicillin therapy, it also is

TABLE 85–3. Antistaphylococcal Therapy in Neonates with Moderate to Severe Infection

	Premature Infants (<2000 g)		Term Infants	
	<1 Week	*1–4 Weeks*	*<1 Week*	*1–4 Weeks*
Penicillin IM or IV	50,000–100,000 units/kg/24 hr in 2 doses q 12 hr	75,000–225,000 units/kg/24 hr in 3 doses q 8 hr	75,000–150,000 units/kg/24 hr in 3 doses q 8 hr	100,000–200,000 units/kg/24 hr in 4 doses q 6 hr
Methicillin IM or IV	50–100 mg/kg/24 hr in 2 doses q 12 hr	75–150 mg/kg/24 hr in 3 doses q 8 hr	75–150 mg/kg/24 hr in 3 doses q 8 hr	100–200 mg/kg/24 hr in 4 doses q 6 hr
Gentamicin IM	2.5 mg per dose q 12–24 hr*	2.5 mg per dose q 8–18 hr	5 mg/kg/24 hr in 2 doses q 12 hr*	7.5 mg/kg/24 hr in 3 doses q 8 hr*
Vancomycin IM	15 mg/kg/dose q 12–24 hr*	15 mg/kg/dose q 8–24 hr*	30 mg/kg/24 hr in 2 doses q 12 hr*	45 mg/kg/24 hr in 3 doses q 8 hr*

*Administer over 1 hour.

associated with penicillin,[14] ampicillin,[217] nafcillin, and the cephalosporins.[218]

Lesser degrees of toxicity consisting only of proteinuria and microscopic hematuria may be encountered more frequently than may the complete syndrome; hemorrhagic cystitis also has been reported.[35, 220] At this time, it appears prudent to monitor urinalyses two times a week in patients receiving high-dose penicillin, methicillin, or other homologues and to discontinue therapy with drugs of this group if definite evidence of nephritis occurs, particularly when associated with fever, rash, and eosinophilia.

Nafcillin has been shown to have less renal toxicity than has methicillin. This is related to its pharmacology because it is excreted primarily by the liver rather than the kidneys. Its pharmacokinetics are erratic in newborns, who should not receive this drug, but it appears to be the antistaphylococcal drug of choice beyond the newborn period.

Alternative Drugs

Ampicillin has no place in the therapy of staphylococcal infections. Less active than penicillin, it also is susceptible to attack by penicillinase. The cephalosporin antibiotics are active against penicillinase-producing staphylococci but offer no particular advantages over the penicillinase-resistant penicillins. A potential disadvantage lies in their broader spectrum of activity, which may promote superinfection with cephalosporin-resistant, gram-negative organisms in the debilitated patient with serious staphylococcal disease. Cephalosporins have been advocated widely for use in patients allergic to penicillin, but because of considerable cross-reactivity, they should be used extremely cautiously, if at all, in patients with a clear history of serious penicillin allergy or anaphylaxis. Among this group of antibiotics, cefazolin appears to have significant advantages over cephalothin for parenteral use. Serum concentrations of cefazolin are higher, and effective tissue levels appear easier to attain. Cephaloridine has been associated with nephrotoxicity. The efficacy of the second- and third-generation cephalosporins against *S. aureus* is reduced. Therefore, these drugs, especially moxalactam, cefotaxime, and cefuroxime, should be given in addition to penicillinase-resistant penicillins or a first general cephalosporin if *S. aureus* strongly is suspected.

Methicillin-Resistant Staphylococci

MRSA first was detected in England in 1961 and was encountered with increasing frequency in the United Kingdom and Europe over the next decade and a half.[138, 174] During that period, MRSA remained rare in the United States, despite a few sporadic cases and epidemic outbreaks.[14, 134, 138] However, the period from 1975 to the present has witnessed a considerable increase in both nosocomial outbreaks and community-acquired infections due to MRSA in North America.[34, 40, 49–51, 58, 73, 96, 177, 185, 213, 219, 240, 249, 269, 272]

MRSA appears to be fully virulent, with in vitro characteristics similar to those of methicillin-sensitive staphylococci. It has equivalent virulence in studies of experimental infection with mice, and clinical studies confirm comparable mortality rates.[102, 249] These strains characteristically are multiresistant, usually showing little or no sensitivity to cephalosporins, aminoglycosides, erythromycin, lincomycin, and tetracyclines.[4, 269] Strains that appear sensitive to cephalosporins by standard disk sensitivity tests are proved resistant in quantitative dilution tests. The clinical efficacy of cephalosporins against methicillin-resistant strains has been poor.[269] Vancomycin is the drug of choice for MRSA, alone or together with an aminoglycoside or rifampin. Coagulase-negative staphylococci have a high frequency of methicillin resistance.

MRSA infections in children are more likely to be nosocomial than community-acquired and particularly are likely to be associated with neonatal or pediatric intensive care units. MRSA bacteremias therefore are likely to be superimposed on critical or severe underlying diseases. Prolonged hospital stay, invasive procedures, indwelling catheters, endotracheal tubes, and prolonged or recurrent exposure to antibiotics appear to be predisposing factors. Characteristics most commonly associated with community-acquired MRSA infections include prior hospitalization, previous antibiotic use, and intravenous drug abuse.[142]

Epidemic outbreaks have occurred. In these outbreaks, it has been noted that patients developed nasopharyngeal colonization with MRSA before becoming infected. A high rate of nasal and hand carriage has been noted in health care workers associated with units having MRSA outbreaks.[177] The usual approach to outbreaks has been to emphasize hand washing between seeing patients. Strict isolation in a private room usually is advocated, although there is no scientific information to justify this approach. Single-room isolation usually is impractical in neonatal and pediatric intensive care units, where isolation facilities are in short supply and a single MRSA-colonized patient may occupy a room for months. Strict adherence to universal precautions (body substance isolation) with all moist body fluids and strict hand washing between seeing patients appear to be rational alternatives to "strict isolation."[153] A new approach, that of intranasal application of mupirocin ointment, has been found to be capable of eliminating nasal and hand carriage of both colonized patients and of hospital staff.[209] Because of its simplicity and reported effectiveness, this measure should be tried in preference to prolonged strict isolation of MRSA-colonized patients. If mupirocin treatment of MRSA-colonized patients is insufficient to curb an outbreak, culturing of health care workers and extension of mupirocin to colonized health care personnel may be tried. Alternatively, systemic antibiotics may be used. Rifampin has a high degree of activity against MRSA, but the development of resistance remains a problem when this antibiotic is used alone. The combination of novobiocin and rifampin is associated with the development of less resistance than that noted with rifampin alone or when used in combination with trimethoprim-sulfamethoxazole.[266] These combinations are not more efficacious in the clearance of MRSA carriage than is application of mupirocin ointment.

PREVENTION

Staphylococcal infections are so common that virtually everyone has had at least some minor encounters. Skin infections occur more commonly in tropical climates or during warm, humid weather in temperate areas and are likely to arise in moist areas of the body, such as the axillae, and in skin creases. High standards of personal hygiene, careful cleaning, and adequate protection of abrasions and minor lacerations reduce the likelihood of skin infection.[242] Early attention to minor infection in these small wounds with careful cleaning and antibiotic ointment may help to prevent more serious or invasive infection. We have been impressed repeatedly with the minor nature of the cutaneous source of infection in serious staphylococcal osteomyelitis, pneumonia, and endocarditis.

Person-to-person spread from an overt lesion is a major route for dissemination of infection within families, in hospitals, and in schools. The person with an infected, purulent wound should receive prompt treatment and should be excused from school and from such occupations as hospital worker or food handler while the infection is open or draining. At home, special precautions should be taken in the care and dressing of the wound. Disposable gauze pads should be used to wash and dry it, and towels and washcloths should not be shared with other members of the family.

Nosocomial Infection

Prevention of transmission of staphylococci within hospitals remains a challenge. Routine environmental cultures and routine personnel cultures for the identification of asymptomatic carriers have not been found effective in identifying problems or pointing the way to solutions. Recognition of an outbreak or cluster of infections on a surgical or medical service is the essential first step in control. Hospital-based infection surveillance systems may detect hospital-acquired infections under some circumstances; but frequently, as among newborns or after simple surgical procedures, the stay in the hospital is short and infection is not apparent until after discharge. Unless an easy mechanism for reporting such infections back to the hospital infection control committee is set up and utilized, a cross-infection problem of considerable size may be present before being recognized. For epidemic outbreaks involving medical or surgical patients, an individualized approach to control must be taken after analyzing the characteristics of the outbreak.[140]

Prevention of MRSA outbreaks is likely to be optimized by strict adherence to hand washing between seeing patients and the faithful performance of universal precautions or body substance isolation. Studies have shown that MRSA nasal colonization precedes MRSA infection in chronically ill patients.[177] Other studies have demonstrated that nasal application of mupirocin ointment eradicates nasal and hand MRSA carriage. Therefore, in an MRSA outbreak, patients at risk should be surveyed for nasal MRSA colonization. Mupirocin should be tried in an attempt to eradicate carriage in addition to appropriate treatment of patients with established infections.[209] If new infections continue to appear, survey and mupirocin treatment of colonized hospital staff may be effective.

Certain procedures expose individual patients to a higher risk of staphylococcal infection. These include intravenous therapy; cardiac surgical procedures, particularly those involving valve replacement; and cerebrospinal fluid shunt placement. Prevention of these infections has been discussed in preceding sections. Simple adherence to accepted surgical principles in the care of wounds and burns is important in the prevention of infection at these sites.

Neonatal Care Units

The neonatal nursery once again has become a source of nosocomial infection. Since 1972, an increasing number of nursery outbreaks of staphylococcal disease have been reported. In many of these outbreaks, the predominant manifestation has been bullous impetigo. To date, there appears to be less severe invasive disease than was reported in the outbreaks of the 1950s and a lower risk of spread to other family members. An intelligent approach to preventing neonatal infection consists of the following elements:

1. Strict hand washing techniques for all persons handling infants in the nursery, including nursing personnel, physicians, and parents. An effective antistaphylococcal preparation, such as chlorhexidine, povidone-iodine, or 0.3 per cent triclosan, should be used upon entering the nursery and hands rewashed between handling babies. Hand washing has been demonstrated to be effective in decreasing the organisms transferred from baby to baby.[232]

2. Absolute prohibition from the nursery of personnel or parents with draining skin lesions.

3. Careful daily examination of infants for pustules, periumbilical or perineal erythema, and bullous lesions, with prompt culture and strict isolation of infected infants. The circumcision site in boys particularly is likely to become infected.

4. A mechanism for prompt reporting of infection, both major and minor, to the hospital by parents and local pediatricians.

5. Determination of the staphylococcal colonization rate by discharge culture surveillance. This may be done conveniently by culturing every fifth or tenth infant or by culturing all infants discharged on a certain day of the week. The umbilicus and circumcision site are more likely to be colonized than is the nose; therefore, these are preferred sites for surveillance. A level or percentage of colonization above which epidemic skin infections are likely has not been established; in fact, epidemic outbreaks have arisen at relatively low colonization rates and in some instances have not been noted in nurseries with high colonization rates. However, if a nursery maintains a profile or relatively stable colonization rate and then experiences a sudden increase in colonization, it can modify its procedures to reduce colonization. Sudden increases in colonization have been noted repeatedly prior to epidemic outbreaks. Limited culture surveillance for coagulase-positive staphylococci only, as described earlier, is simple, feasible, and relatively inexpensive and provides continually useful information.

When an outbreak of staphylococcal infections is recognized or when colonization rates are higher than 20 to 30 per cent, review of procedures and institution of control measures are indicated. Among the more effective control measures available that can reduce the carrier rate to less than 10 per cent are the following:

1. Routine application of a triple-dye mixture to the umbilicus. This method has been shown to be useful in reducing colonization and terminating an epidemic and has been used widely.[224] Despite the sanctification of this method by time and wide use, the possibility of systemic absorption and toxicity of the dyes have not been evaluated.

2. Routine daily application of antibiotic ointment to the cord and circumcision site.[118, 133] Potential disadvantages with this approach include the possibility of sensitization of some infants to the antibiotic and the potential for altering the microbiologic ecology of the nursery and enhancing the development of antibiotic resistance. Use of bacitracin ointment minimizes both problems. Bacitracin is unlikely to be used systemically in the future. Concerns about serious drug allergy and clinically important microbial resistance, therefore, will be eliminated.

All of the foregoing approaches reduce colonization of the infants by creating a barrier to the establishment of staphylococci at favored sites for colonization.[115] Another approach, which has been effective in controlling epidemics, has been to colonize infants deliberately with a less pathogenic staphylococcus, strain 502A, and thereby prevent the establishment of more pathogenic strains.[229] This technique of bacterial interference is a potential source of iatrogenic disease because 502A has caused episodes of skin infection, serious disease, and death in one case of fatal septicemia.[26, 110]

Procedures of lesser value in dealing with outbreaks of disease are those that reduce the degree of contacts of infants within a central nursery by use of earlier discharge, rooming-in programs, and establishment of a strict cohort system so that infants remain with a small group of other babies during their hospital stay. Searching for and treating nasal carriers among nursery personnel are a waste of time and money. Nasal carriers appear to be insignificant factors in the propagation of epidemics and colonization of newborns.

The optimal approach to prevention of nosocomial "late-onset" coagulase-negative staphylococcal sepsis remains unclear. Although there is a strong association of coagulase-negative bacteremia with prolonged venous catheterization and the use of lipid emulsions for hyperalimentation, the benefits of hyperalimentation appear to outweigh the risks. Further investigation is needed to determine safer methods of intravenous lipid administration. A preliminary report of a carefully controlled multicenter trial has demonstrated that prophylactic intravenous gamma-globulin therapy administered to infants weighing less than 1500 g in the first week of life, 1 week later, and then every 2 weeks while in intensive care units reduced the incidence of nosocomial bacteremia by approximately one-third.[16] Staphylococci, both coagulase-negative and coagulase-positive, were the dominant pathogens in the control group. Another study has demonstrated opsonic activity against coagulase-negative staphylococci in gamma-globulin preparations.[72] Prophylactic intravenous gamma-globulin therapy may confer significant benefit and may become standard in neonatal intensive care.

In summary, the staphylococcus is a ubiquitous agent and a frequent cause of disease. Prevention of sporadic infections belongs with the individual patient. Prevention of nosocomial disease depends on the vigilance of hospital personnel in services as diverse as the operating room, intravenous therapy, and the neonatal nursery in recognizing the potential for infection and developing and maintaining effective control measures.

References

1. Abe, J. K., Kotzin, B. L., and Jujo, K.: Selective expansion of T cells expressing T-cell receptor variable regions VB2 and VB8 in Kawasaki disease. Proc. Natl. Acad. Sci. U. S. A. *89*:4066–4070, 1992.
2. Abe, J. K., Kotzin, B. L., Meissener, C., et al.: Characterization of T-cell repertoire changes in acute Kawasaki disease. J. Exp. Med. *177*:791–796, 1993.
3. Abramson, N., Alper, C. A., Lachman, P. J., et al.: Deficiency of C3 inactivation in man. J. Immunol. *107*:19–27, 1971.
4. Acar, J. F., and Chabbert, Y. A.: Methicillin-resistant staphylococcemia: Bacteriological failure of treatment with cephalosporins. Antimicrob. Agents Chemother. *10*:280–285, 1972.
5. Almquist, E. E.: The changing epidemiology of septic arthritis in children. Clin. Orthop. *68*:96–99, 1970.
6. Alper, C. A., Abramson, N., Johnston, R. B., et al.: Increased susceptibility to infection associated with abnormalities of complement-mediated functions and of the third component of complement (C3). N. Engl. J. Med. *282*:350–354, 1970.
7. Alper, C. A., Colten, R. H., and Rosen, F. S.: Homozygous deficiency of C3 in a patient with repeated infections. Lancet 2:1179–1181, 1972.
8. Altrocchi, P. H.: Spontaneous bacterial myositis. J. A. M. A. *217*:819–820, 1971.
9. Amon, R. B., and Dimond, R.: Toxic epidermal necrolysis: Rapid differentiation between staphylococcal and drug-induced diseases. Arch. Dermatol. *111*:1433–1437, 1975.
10. Arbuthnott, J. P., Kent, K., Lyell, A., et al.: Studies on staphylococcal toxins in relation to toxic epidermal necrolysis (the scalded skin syndrome). Br. J. Dermatol. *86*(Suppl. 8):35–39, 1972.
11. Axline, S. G., Yaffe, S. J., and Simon, H. J.: Clinical pharmacology of antimicrobials in premature infants. II. Ampicillin, methicillin, oxacillin, neomycin and colistin. Pediatrics *39*:97–107, 1967.
12. Ayliffe, G. A. J., Brightwell, K. M., Ball, P. M., et al.: Staphylococcal infection in cervical glands of infants. Lancet 2:479–484, 1972.
13. Baehner, R. L.: Neutrophil dysfunction associated with states of chronic and recurrent infection. Pediatr. Clin. North Am. *27*:377–401, 1980.
14. Baehner, R. L., Boxer, L. A., and Davis, J.: The biochemical basis of nitroblue tetrazolium reduction in normal human and chronic granulomatous disease and polymorphonuclear leukocytes. Blood *48*:309–313, 1977.
15. Baker, C. J.: Nosocomial septicemia and meningitis in neonates. Am. J. Med. *70*:698–701, 1981.
16. Baker, C. J., and the Neonatal IVIG Collaborative Study Group: Multicenter trial of intravenous immunoglobulin (IVIG) to prevent preterm infants. Pediatr. Res. *25*:1633, 1989.
17. Baldwin, D. S., Levin, B. B., McCluskey, R. T., et al.: Renal failure and interstitial nephritis due to penicillin and methicillin. N. Engl. J. Med. *279*:1245–1249, 1968.
18. Banffer, J. R.: Anti-leucocidin and mastitis puerperalis. B. M. J. *2*:1224, 1962.
19. Barrett, F. F., McGehee, R. F., and Finland, M.: Methicillin-resistant *Staphylococcus aureus* at Boston City Hospital: Bacteriologic and epidemiologic observations. N. Engl. J. Med. *279*:441–448, 1968.
20. Barton, L. L., and Feigin, R. D.: Childhood cervical lymphadenitis: A reappraisal. J. Pediatr. *84*:846–852, 1974.
21. Barton, L. L., Freidman, A. D., Sharkey, A. M., et al.: Impetigo contagiosa. III. Comparative efficacy of oral erythromycin and topical mupiricin. Pediatr. Dermatol. *6*:134–138, 1989.
22. Barton, L. L., Freidman, A. D., and Portilla, M. G.: Impetigo contagiosa: A comparison of erythromycin and dicloxacillin therapy. Pediatr. Dermatol. *5*:88–91, 1988.
23. Bass, J. W., Cohen, S. H., Corless, J. D., et al.: Ampicillin compared to other antimicrobials in acute otitis media. J. A. M. A. *202*:697–702, 1967.
24. Batista, R. A., Baredes, S., and Krieger, A.: Prevertebral space infections associated with cervical osteomyelitis. Otolaryngol. Head Neck Surg. *108*:160–166, 1993.
25. Beck, W., and Grose, C.: Pyomyositis presenting as acute abdominal pain. Pediatr. Infect. Dis. *3*:445–448, 1984.
26. Blair, E. B., and Tull, A. H.: Multiple infections among newborns resulting from colonization with *Staphylococcus aureus* 502A. Am. J. Clin. Pathol. *52*:42–49, 1969.
27. Bland, R. D.: Otitis media in the first six weeks of life: Diagnosis, bacteriology and management. Pediatrics *49*:187–197, 1972.
28. Blockley, N. J., and Watson, J. T.: Acute osteomyelitis in children. J. Bone Joint Surg. [Br.] *52*:77–87, 1970.
29. Bloomer, W. E., Giammona, S., Lindskog, C. F., et al.: Staphylococcal pneumonia and empyema in infancy. J. Thorac. Surg. *30*:265–274, 1955.
30. Blumenthal, S., Griffiths, S. P., and Morgan, B. C.: Bacterial endocarditis in children with heart disease. Pediatrics *26*:993–998, 1960.
31. Boe, R. W., Williams, C. P. S., Bennett, J. V., et al.: Serum levels of methicillin and ampicillin in newborn and premature infants in relation to post-natal age. Pediatrics *39*:194–198, 1967.
32. Borella, L., Goobar, J. E., Summitt, R. L., et al.: Septic arthritis in childhood. J. Pediatr. *62*:742–747, 1963.
33. Boxer, L. A., Hedley-Whyte, E. T., and Stossel, T. P.: Neutrophil action dysfunction and abnormal neutrophil behavior. N. Engl. J. Med. *291*:1093–1099, 1974.
34. Boyce, J. M.: Methicillin-resistant *Staphylococcus aureus*: Detection, epidemiology, and control measures. Infect. Dis. Clin. North Am. *3*:901-B, 1989.
35. Bracis, R., Sandus, C., Kimbrough, R., et al.: Methicillin hemorrhagic cystitis. Presented to the 16th Interscience Conference on Antimicrobial Agents and Chemotherapy. Chicago, October 1976.
36. Brans, Y. W., Aballos, R., and Cassady, G.: Umbilical catheters and hepatic abscesses. Pediatrics *53*:264–268, 1974.
37. Bricker, T., Gutgesell, H. P., Latson, L. A., et al.: Echocardiographic evaluation of endocarditis in children. Pediatr. Cardiol. *3*:350, 1982.
38. Bridges, R. A., Berendes, H., and Good, R. A.: A fatal granulomatous disease of childhood. Am. J. Dis. Child. *97*:387–391, 1959.
39. Brown, J. D., and Wheeler, B.: Pyomyositis: Report of 18 cases in Hawaii. Arch. Intern. Med. *144*:1749–1751, 1984.
40. Brumfitt, W., and Hamilton-Miller, J.: Methicillin-resistant *Staphylococcus aureus*. N. Engl. J. Med. *320*:1188–1196, 1989.
41. Bryson, Y. J., Connor, J. D., Leclerc, M., et al.: Oral dicloxacillin as a mode of therapy of treatment of acute staphylococcal osteomyelitis. Pediatr. Res. *9*:339–345, 1975.
42. Burry, V. F., and Beezley, M.: Infant mastitis due to gram-negative organisms. Am. J. Dis. Child. *124*:736–737, 1972.
43. Campbell, J. A., Gastineau, D. C., and Velias, F.: Roentgen studies in suppurative pneumonia in infants and children. J. A. M. A. *154*:468–472, 1954.
44. Cannale, S. T., Harkness, R. M., Thomas, P. A., et al.: Does aspiration of bones and joints affect results of later bone scanning? J. Pediatr. Orthop. *5*:23–26, 1985.
45. Ceruti, E., Contreras, J., and Neira, M.: Staphylococcal pneumonia in childhood. Am. J. Dis. Child. *122*:386–392, 1971.
46. Chacha, P. B.: Suppurative arthritis of the hip joint in infancy. J. Bone Joint Surg. [Am.] *53*:538–544, 1971.
47. Christensson, B., Esperson, F., Hedstrom, S. A., et al.: Solid-phase radioimmunoassay of immunoglobulin G antibodies to *Staphylococcus aureus* peptidoglycan in patients with staphylococcal infections. Acta Pathol. Microbiol. Immunol. Scand. *91*:401–406, 1983.
48. Clark, R. A., Root, R. K., Kimball, H. R., et al.: Defective neutrophil

chemotaxis and cellular immunity in a child with recurrent infection. Ann. Intern. Med. *78*:515–519, 1972.
49. Coello, R., Jimenez, J., Garcia, M., et al.: Prospective study of infection, colonization, and carriage of methicillin-resistant *Staphylococcus aureus* in an outbreak affecting 990 patients. Eur. J. Clin. Microbiol. Infect. Dis. *13*:74–81, 1994.
50. Coovadia, Y. M., Bhana, R. H., Johnson, A. P., et al.: Laboratory-confirmed outbreak of rifampicin methicillin-resistant *Staphylococcus aureus* in a newborn nursery. J. Hosp. Infect. *14*:303–312, 1989.
51. Cox, R. A., Conquest, C., Mallaghan, C., et al.: A major outbreak of methicillin-resistant *Staphylococcus aureus* caused by a new phage-type (EMRSA-16). J. Hosp. Infect. *29*:87–106, 1995.
52. Craigen, M. A., Watters, J., and Hackett, J. S.: The changing epidemiology of osteomyelitis in children. J. Bone Joint Surg. [Br.] *74*:541–545, 1992.
53. Craven, D. E., Reed, C., Kollisch, N., et al.: A large outbreak of infections caused by a strain of *Staphylococcus aureus* resistant to oxacillin and aminoglycosides. Am. J. Med. *71*:53–58, 1981.
54. Crawford, A. H., Kucharzyk, D. W., Ruda, R., et al.: Diskitis in children. Clin. Orthop. *266*:70–79, 1991.
55. Crenshaw, C. A., Kelly, L., and Turner, R. I.: Prevention of infections at scalp vein sites of needle insertion during intravenous therapy. Am. J. Surg. *124*:43–45, 1972.
56. Crossley, K., and Matson, J. M.: The scalp vein needle: A prospective study of associated complications. J. A. M. A. *220*:985–987, 1972.
57. Curnett, J. P., Kipnes, R. S., and Bevior, B. M.: Defect in pyridine nucleotide-dependent superoxide production by a particulate fraction from the granulocytes of patients with chronic granulomatous disease. N. Engl. J. Med. *293*:628–632, 1975.
58. Dacre, J., Emmerson, A. M., and Jenner, E. A.: Gentamicin methicillin-resistant *Staphylococcus aureus*: Epidemiology and containment of an outbreak. J. Hosp. Infect. *7*:130–136, 1986.
59. Dagan, R., and Bar-David, Y.: Double-blind study comparing erythromycin and mupirocin for treatment of impetigo in children: Implications of a high prevalence of erythromycin-resistant *Staphylococcus aureus* strains. Antimicrob. Agents Chemother. *36*:287–290, 1992.
60. Daher, A. H., and Berkowitz, F. E.: Infective endocarditis in neonates. Clin. Pediatr. *34*:198–206, 1995.
61. Dajani, A. S., Garcia, R. E., and Wolinsky, E.: Etiology of cervical lymphadenitis in children. N. Engl. J. Med. *268*:1329–1333, 1963.
62. Dehner, L. P., and Kissane, J. M.: Pyogenic hepatic abscesses in infancy and childhood. J. Pediatr. *74*:763–773, 1969.
63. Dewar, J., Porter, I. A., and Smylie, H. G.: Staphylococcal infection in cervical glands of infants. Lancet *2*:712–717, 1972.
64. Dich, V. Q., Nelson, J. D., and Haltalin, G.: Osteomyelitis in infants and children: A review of 163 cases. Am. J. Dis. Child. *129*:1273–1278, 1975.
65. Disney, M. E., Wolff, J., and Wood, B. S. B.: Staphylococcal pneumonia in infants. Lancet *1*:767–771, 1956.
66. Dreskin, S. C., Goldsmith, P. K., and Gullin, J. I.: Immunoglobulin E and recurrent infection (Job's) syndrome. J. Clin. Invest. *75*:26–31, 1985.
67. Echeverria, P., and Vaughn, M. C.: Tropical pyomyositis: A diagnostic problem in temperate climates. Am. J. Dis. Child. *129*:856–857, 1975.
68. Edwards, K. M., Dundon, C., and Altemeier, W. A.: Bacterial tracheitis as a complication of viral croup. Pediatr. Infect. Dis. *2*:390–391, 1983.
69. Elias, P. M., Fritsch, P., Dahl, M. V., et al.: Staphylococcal exfoliative toxin: Pathogenesis and subcellular site of action. J. Invest. Dermatol. *65*:501–512, 1975.
70. Elias, P. M., Mittermayer, H., Tappeiner, G., et al.: Staphylococcal toxic epidermal necrolysis (TEN): The expanded mouse model. J. Invest. Dermatol. *63*:467–472, 1974.
71. Esperson, F., Fremodt-Miller, N., Thamdrup Rosendal, V., et al.: *Staphylococcus aureus* bacteremia in children below the age of one year: A review of 407 cases. Acta Pediatr. Scand. *78*:56–61, 1989.
72. Etzioni, A., Obedeanui, S., Blazer, S., et al.: Effect of an intravenous gamma globulin preparation on the opsonophagocytic activity of preterm serum against coagulase-negative staphylococci. Acta Pediatr. Scand. *79*:156–161, 1990.
73. Eykyn, S. J.: Staphylococcal sepsis: The changing pattern of disease and therapy. Lancet *1*:100–103, 1988.
74. Faden, H., and Grossi, M.: Acute osteomyelitis in children: Reassessment of etiologic agents and their clinical characteristics. Am. J. Dis. Child. *145*:65–69, 1991.
75. Fagbule, D. O.: Bacterial pathogens in malnourished children with pneumonia. Trop. Geogr. Med. *45*:294–296, 1993.
76. Feigin, R. D., VanReken, D. E., and Pickering, L. L.: Dosage in methicillin-associated nephropathy. J. Pediatr. *85*:734, 1974.
77. Feldman, W. E.: Bacterial etiologies and mortality of purulent pericarditis in pediatric patients. Am. J. Dis. Child. *133*:641–644, 1979.
78. Fisher, J. H., and Swenson, O.: Surgical complications of staphylococcal pneumonia. Pediatrics *20*:835–847, 1957.
79. Fleer, A., Senders, R. C., Visser, M. R., et al.: Septicemia due to coagulase-negative staphylococci in a neonatal intensive care unit: Clinical and bacteriologic features and contaminated parenteral fluids as a source of sepsis. Pediatr. Infect. Dis. *2*:426–431, 1983.
80. Forbes, G. B., and Emerson, G. L.: Staphylococcal pneumonia and empyema. Pediatr. Clin. North Am. *4*:215–230, 1957.
81. Foster, D., and Harris, R. E.: The incidence of *Staphylococcus pyogenes* in normal human breast milk. J. Obstet. Gynecol. *67*:463–466, 1960.
82. Freeman, J., Epstein, M. F., Smith, N. E., et al.: Extra hospital stay and antibiotic usage with nosocomial coagulase negative staphylococcal bacteremia in two neonatal intensive care unit populations. Am. J. Dis. Child. *144*:324–329, 1990.
83. Freeman, J., Goldmann, D. A., Smith, N. E., et al.: Association of intravenous lipid emulsion and coagulase-negative staphylococcal bacteremia in neonatal intensive care units. N. Engl. J. Med. *323*:301–308, 1990.
84. Freidland, I. R., du Pless, J., and Cilliers, A.: Cardiac complications in children with *Staphylococcus aureus* bacteremia. J. Pediatr. *127*:746–748,1995.
85. Gelfand, M. J., and Silberstein, E. G.: Radionuclide imaging use in diagnosis of osteomyelitis in children. J. A. M. A. *237*:245–247, 1977.
86. George, R., Leibrock, L., and Epstein, M.: Long-term analysis of cerebrospinal fluid shunt infections: A 25-year experience. J. Neurosurg. *51*:804–811, 1979.
87. Gersony, W. M., and McCracken, G. H.: Purulent pericarditis in infancy. Pediatrics *40*:224–232, 1967.
88. Givner, L. B., and Kaplan, S. L.: Meningitis due to *Staphylococcus aureus* in children. Clin. Infect. Dis. *16*:766–771, 1993.
89. Gladstone, G. P., and Mudd, S.: The assay of antistaphylococcal leukocidal components in human sera. Br. J. Exp. Pathol. *43*:295–298, 1962.
90. Gluck, L., and Wood, H. F.: Effect of an antiseptic skin care regimen in reducing staphylococcal colonization in newborn infants. N. Engl. J. Med. *265*:1177–1181, 1961.
91. Goldmann, D. A., Maki, D. G., Phame, F. S., et al.: Guidelines for infection control in intravenous therapy. Am. J. Med. *79*:848–850, 1973.
92. Guggenbichler, J. P., Berchtold, D., Allerberger, F., et al.: In vitro and in vivo effect of antibiotics on catheters colonized by staphylococci. Eur. J. Clin. Microbiol. Infect. Dis. *11*:408–415, 1992.
93. Gutman, L. T., Idriss, Z. H., Gehlbach, S., et al.: Neonatal staphylococcal enterocolitis: Association with indwelling feeding catheters and *S. aureus* colonization. J. Pediatr. *88*:836–839, 1976.
94. Haffar, A. A., Rench, M. A., Ferry, G. D., et al.: Failure of urokinase to resolve Broviac catheter-related bacteremia in children. J. Pediatr. *104*:256–258, 1984.
95. Haley, R. W., and Bregman, D. A.: The role of understaffing and overcrowding in recurrent outbreaks of staphylococcal infection in a neonatal special care unit. J. Infect. Dis. *145*:875–885, 1982.
96. Haley, R. W., Hightower, A. W., Khabbaz, R. F., et al.: The emergence of methicillin-resistant *Staphylococcus aureus* infections in United States hospitals. Ann. Intern. Med. *97*:297–308, 1982.
97. Hall, S. L.: Coagulase-negative staphylococcal infections in neonates. Pediatr. Infect. Dis. *10*:51–67, 1991.
98. Hallander, H. O., and Korloff, B.: Enterotoxin-producing staphylococci. Acta Pathol. Microbiol. Scand. *71*:359–362, 1967.
99. Hay, P., and McKenzie, P.: Side effects of oxytetracycline therapy. Lancet *1*:945–949, 1954.
100. Hendren, W. H., and Haggerty, R. J.: Staphylococcal pneumonia in infancy and childhood: Analysis of 75 cases. J. A. M. A. *168*:6–16, 1958.
101. Hermansson, G., Bollgren, I., Bugstrom, T., et al.: Coagulase-negative staphylococci as a cause of symptomatic urinary infections in children. J. Pediatr. *84*:807–810, 1974.
102. Hershow, R. C., Khayr, W. F., and Smith, N. L.: A comparison of clinical virulence of nosocomially acquired methicillin-resistant and methicillin-sensitive *Staphylococcus aureus* infections in a university hospital. Infect. Control Hosp. Epidemiol. *13*:587–593, 1992.
103. Hieber, J. P., and Davis, A. T.: Staphylococcal cervical adenitis in young infants. Pediatrics *57*:424–426, 1976.
104. Hill, H. R., and Quie, P. G.: Raised IgE levels and defective neutrophil chemotaxis with eczema and recurrent bacterial infections. Lancet *1*:183–186, 1974.
105. Ho, N. K., Low, Y. P., and See, H. F.: Septic arthritis in the newborn: A 17-year clinical experience. Singapore Med. J. *30*:356–358, 1989.
106. Hoeger, P. H., Lens, A. B., and Fournier, J. M.: Staphylococcal skin colonization in children with atopic dermatitis: Prevalence, persistence, and transmission of toxigenic and non-toxigenic strains. J. Infect. Dis. *165*:1064–1068, 1992.
107. Hoeger, P. H., Niggermann, B., and Schoeder, C.: Enhanced basal and stimulated PMN chemiluminescence activity in children with atopic dermatitis: Stimulatory role of colonizing staphylococci? Acta Paediatr. *81*:562–546, 1992.
108. Honig, P. J., Gaisin, A., and Buck, B. E.: Frozen section differentiation of drug-induced and staphylococcal-induced toxic epidermal necrolysis. J. Pediatr. *92*:504, 1978.
109. Horn, C. V., and Master, S.: Pyomyositis tropicans in Uganda. East Afr. Med. J. *45*:563–571, 1968.
110. Houck, P. W., Nelson, J. D., and Kay, J. L.: Fatal septicemia due to *Staphylococcus aureus* 502A. Am. J. Dis. Child. *123*:45–48, 1972.
111. Howie, V. M., Ploussand, J. H., and Lester, R. L.: Otitis media: A clinical and bacteriologic correlation. Pediatrics *45*:29–35, 1970.
112. Huebner, J., Pier, G. B., Maslow, J. N., et al.: Endemic nosocomial transmission of *Staphylococcus epidermidis* bacteremia isolates in a neonatal intensive care unit over 10 years. J. Infect. Dis. *169*:526–531, 1994.

113. Huxtable, K. A., Tucker, A. S., and Wedgwood, R. J.: Staphylococcal pneumonia in childhood. Am. J. Dis. Child. *108*:262–269, 1964.
114. Issekutz, A. C., Lee, K. Y., and Biggar, W. D.: Neutrophil chemotaxis in two patients with recurrent staphylococcal skin infections and hyperimmunoglobulin E. J. Lab. Clin. Med. *92*:640–647, 1978.
115. Jellard, J.: Umbilical cord as a reservoir of infection in a maternity hospital. B. M. J. *1*:925–929, 1957.
116. Johanovsky, J.: Importance of anti-leucocidin and anti-toxin in immunity against staphylococcal infections. Immunotactsforschung *116*:318–320, 1959.
117. Johnson, D. H., Rosenthal, A., and Nadas, A. S.: A forty-year review of bacterial endocarditis in infancy and childhood. Circulation *51*:581–588, 1975.
118. Johnson, J. D., Malachowski, N. C., Vosti, K. L., et al.: A sequential study of various modes of skin and umbilical care and the incidence of staphylococcal colonization and infection in the neonate. Pediatrics *58*:354–361, 1976.
119. Johnston, R. B., and Baehner, R. L.: Chronic granulomatous disease: Correlation between pathogenesis and clinical findings. Pediatrics *48*:730–733, 1971.
120. Jones, D. R. B., and MacIntyre, K.: Venous thromboembolism in infancy and childhood. Arch. Dis. Child. *50*:153–155, 1975.
121. Jones, R., Santos, J. I., and Overall, J. C., Jr.: Bacterial tracheitis. J. A. M. A. *242*:721–726, 1979.
122. Julander, I. G., Grandstrom, M., Hedstrom, S. A., et al.: The role of antibodies against alpha-toxin and teichoic acid in the diagnosis of staphylococcal infections. Infection *11*:77–83, 1983.
123. Kacica, M. A., Horgan, M. J., and Preston, K. E.: Relatedness of coagulase-negative staphylococci causing bacteremia in low-birthweight infants. Infect. Control Hosp. Epidemiol. *15*:658–662, 1994.
124. Kahn, M. Y., and Hall, W. H.: Staphylococcal enterocolitis treatment with oral vancomycin. Ann. Intern. Med. *65*:1–8, 1966.
125. Kallen, P., Nies, K. M., Louie, J. S., et al.: Tropical pyomyositis. Arthritis Rheum. *25*:107–110, 1982.
126. Kanoff, A., Epstein, B., and Kromes, B.: Staphylococcal pneumonia and empyema. Pediatrics *11*:385–391, 1953.
127. Kaplan, E. K., Laxdal, T., and Quie, P. G.: Studies of polymorphonuclear leukocytes from patients with chronic granulomatous disease of childhood: Bactericidal capacity for streptococci. Pediatrics *41*:591–597, 1968.
128. Kaplan, J. E., Palmer, D. L., Tung, K. S. K.: Teichoic acid antibody and circulating immune complexes in the management of *Staphylococcus aureus* bacteremia. Am. J. Med. *70*:769–774, 1981.
129. Kaplan, S. L., and Feigin, R. D.: Pyogenic liver abscesses in normal children with fever of unknown origin. Pediatrics *58*:614–616, 1976.
130. Kavey, R. E., Frank, D. M., Byrum, C. J., et al.: Two-dimensional echocardiographic assessment of infective endocarditis in children. Pediatr. Cardiol. *3*:349, 1982.
131. Keelen, W. C., and Stoltz, C. R.: An unusual epidemic of neonatal mastitis. Am. J. Obstet. Gynecol. *59*:642–647, 1950.
132. Khan, A. J., Evans, H. E., Bombeck, E., et al.: Coagulase-negative staphylococcal bacteriuria: A rarity in infants and children. J. Pediatr. *86*:309–313, 1975.
133. Klainer, L. M., Agrawal, H. S., Mortimer, E. A., et al.: Bacitracin ointment and neonatal staphylococci. Am. J. Dis. Child. *103*:72–76, 1962.
134. Klimek, J. J., Marsik, F. J., Bartlett, R. C., et al.: Clinical, epidemiologic and bacteriologic observations of an outbreak of methicillin-resistant *Staphylococcus aureus* at a large community hospital. Am. J. Med. *61*:340–345, 1976.
135. Knudsen, C. J. M., and Hoffman, E. B.: Neonatal osteomyelitis. J. Bone Joint Surg. [Br.] *72*:846–851, 1990.
136. Koch, R., Carson, M. J., and Donnell, G.: Staphylococcal pneumonia in children: A review of 83 cases. J. Pediatrics *55*:473–480, 1959.
137. La Leche League International: The Womanly Art of Breastfeeding. 2nd ed. Franklin Park, 1963.
138. Lacey, R. W.: Genetic basis: Epidemiology and future significance of antibiotic resistance in *Staphylococcus aureus:* A review. J. Clin. Pathol. *26*:899–913, 1973.
139. Latham, R. H., Running, K., and Stamm, W. E.: Urinary tract infections in young adult women caused by *Staphylococcus saprophyticus*. J. A. M. A. *250*:3063–3066, 1983.
140. Lavine, D., Hurst, V., Grossman, M., et al.: Staphylococcus of a newly recognized bacteriophage type: Report of a hospital outbreak. J. A. M. A. *192*:935–938, 1965.
141. Laxdal, T., Melsner, R. P., Williams, R. G., et al.: Opsonic agglutinating and complement-fixing antibodies in patients with subacute bacterial endocarditis. J. Lab. Clin. Med. *71*:638–653, 1968.
142. Layton, M. C., Hierholzer, W. J., and Patterson, J.: The evolving epidemiology of methicillin-resistant *Staphylococcus aureus* at a university hospital. Infect. Control Hosp. Epidemiol. *16*:12–17, 1995.
143. Lee, C. T., and Lewin, E. B.: Teichoic acid serology in various staphylococcal coagulase-positive infections in infants and children. Pediatr. Res. *11*:502–507, 1977.
144. Leung, D. Y., Meissner, H. C., Fulton, D. R., et al.: Toxic shock syndrome toxin-secreting *Staphylococcus aureus* in Kawasaki syndrome. Lancet *342*:1385–1388, 1993.
145. Levin, M. J., Gardner, P., and Waldvogel, F. A.: Tropical pyomyositis: An unusual infection due to *Staphylococcus aureus*. N. Engl. J. Med. *284*:196–198, 1971.
146. Lillibridge, C. B., Melish, M. E., and Glasgow, L. A.: Site of action of exfoliative toxin in the staphylococcal scalded-skin syndrome. Pediatrics *50*:728–738, 1972.
147. Lindblade, B., Ekingren, K., and Aurelius, G.: The prognosis of acute hematogenous osteomyelitis and its complications during early infancy after the advent of antibiotics. Acta Paediatr. Scand. *54*:24–32, 1965.
148. Liston, S. L., Gehrz, R. C., Siegel, L. G., et al.: Bacterial tracheitis. Am. J. Dis. Child. *137*:764–767, 1983.
149. Lowder, J. N., Lazarus, H. M., and Herzig, R. H.: Bacteremias and fungemias in oncologic patients with central venous catheters: Changing spectrum of infection. Arch. Intern. Med. *142*:1456–1459, 1982.
150. Lowenbraun, S., Young, V., and Kenton, D.: Infection from venous scalp vein needles in a susceptible population. J. A. M. A. *212*:451–453, 1970.
151. Lowney, E. D., Baublis, J. V., Kreye, G. M., et al.: The scalded skin syndrome in small children. Arch. Dermatol. *75*:359–369, 1967.
152. Lyell, A.: A review of toxic epidermal necrolysis in Britain. Br. J. Dermatol. *9*:661–669, 1967.
153. Lynch, P., Cummings, M. J., Herriott, M. J., et al.: Implementing and evaluating a system of generic infection control precautions: Body substance isolation. Am. J. Infect. Control *18*:1–12, 1990.
154. Maddox, J. L., Riordan, T. P., and Odom, R. B.: Pyomyositis in a neonate. J. Am. Acad. Dermatol. *10*:391–394, 1984.
155. Maki, D. G.: Nosocomial bacteremia: An epidemiologic overview. Am. J. Med. *70*:719–732, 1981.
156. Maki, D. G., Goldman, D. A., and Rhame, F. S.: Infection control of intravenous therapy. Ann. Intern. Med. *79*:867–889, 1973.
157. Malam, J. E., Carrick, G. F., Telford, D. R., et al.: Staphylococcal toxins and sudden infant death syndrome. J. Clin. Pathol. *45*:716–721, 1992.
158. March, A. W., Riley, L. H., and Robinson, R. A.: Retroperitoneal abscess and septic arthritis of the hip in children. J. Bone Joint Surg. [Am.] *54*:67–74, 1972.
159. Margileth, A. M.: Scalded skin syndrome: Diagnosis, differential diagnosis and management of 42 children. South. Med. J. *68*:447–452, 1975.
160. Marples, R. R., and Wieneke, A. A.: Enterotoxins and toxic-shock syndrome toxin-1 in non-enteric staphylococcal disease. Epidemiol. Infect. *110*:477–488, 1993.
161. Mazur, J. M., Ross, G., Cummings, R. J., et al.: Usefulness of magnetic resonance imaging for the diagnosis of acute musculoskeletal infections in children. J. Pediatr. Orthop. *15*:144–147, 1995.
162. McCracken, G.: Commentary. J. Pediatr. *84*:882–883, 1974.
163. McPhail, L. C., DeChatelet, L. R., Shirley, P. S., et al.: Deficiency of NADPH oxidase activity in chronic granulomatous disease. J. Pediatr. *90*:213–217, 1977.
164. Melish, M. E.: Bullous varicella: Its association with the staphylococcal scalded skin syndrome. J. Pediatr. *82*:1010–1021, 1973.
165. Melish, M. E., Bertrando, R., and Gluck, L.: Unpublished observations. 1975.
166. Melish, M. E., Frogner, K. S., Hirata, S. A., et al.: Pathogenesis of toxic shock syndrome. Pediatr. Res. *19*:301A, 1985.
167. Melish, M. E., and Glasgow, L. A.: The staphylococcal scalded skin syndrome: Development of an experimental model. N. Engl. J. Med. *282*:1114–1119, 1970.
168. Melish, M. E., and Glasgow, L. A.: The staphylococcal scalded skin syndrome: The expanded clinical syndrome. J. Pediatr. *78*:959–965, 1971.
169. Melish, M. E., Glasgow, L. A., and Turner, M. E.: The staphylococcal scalded skin syndrome: Isolation and partial characterization of the exfoliative toxin. J. Infect. Dis. *125*:129–140, 1972.
170. Melish, M. E., Parsonett, J., and Marchette, N.: Kawasaki syndrome is not caused by toxic shock syndrome-1 staphylococci. Pediatr. Res. *35*:187A, 1994.
171. Melley, M. A., Throison, J. B., and Rogus, D. E.: Fate of staphylococci with human leukocytes. J. Exp. Med. *112*:1121–1130, 1974.
172. Meugnier, H., Fernandez, M. P., Bes, M., et al.: rRNA gene restriction patterns as an epidemiological marker in nosocomial outbreaks of *Staphylococcus aureus* infections. Res. Microbiol. *144*:25–33, 1993.
173. Mickenberg, I. D., Root, R. K., and Wolf, S. M.: Leukocyte function in hypergammaglobulinemia. J. Clin. Invest. *49*:1529–1538, 1970.
174. Miller, M. E., and Nilsson, U. R.: A familial deficiency in the phagocytosis enhancing activity of serum related to a dysfunction of the 5th component of complement (C5). N. Engl. J. Med. *282*:354–358, 1970.
175. Miller, M. E., Oski, F. A., and Harris, M. B.: Lazy leukocyte syndrome. Lancet *1*:665–669, 1971.
176. Misko, M. L., Terracina, J. R., and Divin, D. G.: The frequency of erythromycin-resistant *Staphylococcus aureus* in impetiginized dermatoses. Pediatr. Dermatol. *12*:12–15, 1995.
177. Muder, R., Brennen, C., Wagener, M. M., et al.: Methicillin-resistant staphylococcal colonization and infection in a long-term care facility. Ann. Intern. Med. *114*:107–112, 1991.
178. Muggae, A., Daniel, W. G., Frank, G., et al.: Echocardiography in infective endocarditis: Reassessment of prognostic implications of vegetation size determined by the transthoracic and transesophageal approach. J. Am. Coll. Cardiol. *14*:631–638, 1989.

179. Naraqi, S., and McDonnell, G.: Hematogenous staphylococcal pneumonia secondary to soft tissue infection. Chest *79*:173–175, 1981.
180. Nataro, J. P., Corcoran, L., Zirin, S., et al.: Prospective analysis of coagulase-negative staphylococcal infection in hospitalized infants. J. Pediatr. *125*:798–804, 1994.
181. Nelson, J. D.: Antibiotic concentrations in septic joint effusion. N. Engl. J. Med. *285*:178–181, 1971.
182. Nelson, J. D.: The bacterial etiology and antibiotic management of septic arthritis in infants and children. Pediatrics *50*:437–441, 1972.
183. Nelson, J. D., and Koontz, W. B.: Septic arthritis in infants and children: A review of 117 cases. Pediatrics *38*:967–971, 1966.
184. Nilsson, E. J., Henning, C. G., and Magnusson, J.: Topical corticosteriods and *Staphylococcus aureus* in atopic dermatitis. J. Am. Acad. Dermatol. *27*:29–34, 1992.
185. Noel, G. J., Kreiswirth, B. N., Edelson, P. J., et al.: Multiple methicillin-resistant *Staphylococcus aureus* strains as a cause for a single outbreak of severe disease in hospitalized neonates. Pediatr. Infect. Dis. J. *11*:184–188, 1992.
186. Normand, J., Bozio, A., Etienne, J., et al.: Changing patterns and prognosis of infective endocarditis in childhood. Eur. Heart J. *16*(Suppl. B):28–31, 1995.
187. Nowel, G. J., and Edelson, P. J.: *Staphylococcus epidermidis* bacteremia in neonates: Further observations and the occurrence of focal infection. Pediatrics *74*:832–837, 1984.
188. Nusem-Horowitz, S., Wolf, M., Coret, A. et al.: Acute suppurative parotitis and parotid abscess in children. Int. J. Pediatr. Otorhinolaryngol. *32*:123–127, 1995.
189. O'Toole, R. D., Drew, W. L., and Dahygren, B. J.: An outbreak of methicillin-resistant *Staphylococcus aureus* infection. J. A. M. A. *213*:257–263, 1970.
190. Okoji, C. N., Inglis, B., and Stewart, P. R.: Potential problems in the use of oligonucleotide probes for staphylococcal enterotoxin genes. J. Appl. Bacteriol. *74*:637–644, 1993.
191. Okoroma, E. O., Perry, L. W., and Scott, L. P.: Acute bacterial pericarditis in children: Report of 25 cases. Am. Heart J. *90*:709–713, 1975.
192. Overturf, G. D., Sherman, M. P., Scheifele, D. W., et al.: Neonatal necrotizing enterocolitis associated with delta toxin-producing methicillin-resistant *Staphylococcus aureus*. Pediatr. Infect. Dis. J. *9*:88–91, 1990.
193. Panton, P. N., and Valentine, F. C. O.: Staphylococcal toxins. Lancet *1*:506–510, 1932.
194. Parker, M. T., and Hewitt, J. H.: Methicillin resistance in *Staphylococcus aureus*. Lancet *1*:800–804, 1970.
195. Parres, F., Bouza, E., Romero, J., et al.: Infectious endocarditis in children. Pediatr. Cardiol. *11*:77–81, 1990.
196. Pederson, W. R., Walker, M., Olson, J. D., et al.: Value of transesophageal echocardiography as an adjunct to transthoracic echocardiography in the evaluation of native and prosthetic valve endocarditis. Chest *100*:351–356, 1991.
197. Perlman, B. B., and Freedman, L. R.: Experimental endocarditis. III. Natural history of catheter-induced staphylococcal endocarditis following catheter removal. Yale J. Biol. Med. *44*:214–224, 1971.
198. Peter, G., Lloyd-Still, J. D., and Lovejoy, F. H.: Local infection and bacteremia from scalp vein needles and polyethylene catheters in children. J. Pediatr. *80*:78–83, 1972.
199. Peters, G., Locci, R., and Pulverer, G.: Adherence and growth of coagulase-negative staphylococci on the surface of intravenous catheters. J. Infect. Dis. *146*:479–482, 1982.
200. Peterson, P. K., Quie, P. G., Kim, Y., et al.: Recognition of *Staphylococcus aureus* by human phagocytes: Signals and disguises of the bacterial surface. Scand. J. Infect. Dis. *41*(Suppl.):67–78, 1983.
201. Pildes, R. S., Ramamurthy, R. S., and Vidyasagar, D.: Effect of triple dye on staphylococcal colonization of newborn infants. J. Pediatr. *82*:987–990, 1973.
202. Pleuckhahn, V. D.: Hexachlorophene and the control of staphylococcal sepsis in a maternity unit in Geelong, Australia. Pediatrics *51*(Suppl.):368–372, 1973.
203. Price, C. D., Hameroff, S. B., and Richards, R. D.: Cavernous sinus thrombosis and orbital cellulitis. South. Med. J. *64*:1243–1247, 1971.
204. Pryles, C. V.: Staphylococcal pneumonia in infancy and childhood. Pediatrics *21*:609–623, 1958.
205. Pung, Y. H., Vetro, S. W., and Bellanti, J. A.: Use of interferons in atopic (IgE-mediated) diseases. Ann. Allergy *71*:234–238, 1993.
206. Quie, P. G.: Chronic granulomatous disease in childhood. Adv. Pediatr. *16*:287–300, 1969.
207. Raimondi, A. J., Robinson, J. S., and Kuwamura, K.: Complications of ventriculoperitoneal shunting and a critical comparison of the three-piece system and one-piece systems. Child's Brain *3*:321–342, 1977.
208. Raucher, H. S., Hyatt, A. C., Barzilai, A., et al.: Quantitative blood cultures in the evaluation of septicemia in children with Broviac catheters. J. Pediatr. *104*:29–33, 1984.
209. Reagan, D. R., Doebbling, B. N., Pfaller, M. A., et al.: Elimination of coincident *Staphylococcus aureus* nasal and hand carriage with contranasal application of mupirocin calcium ointment. Ann. Intern. Med. *114*:101–106, 1991.
210. Rebhan, A. W., and Edwards, H. E.: Staphylococcal pneumonia: A review of 329 cases. Can. Med. Assoc. J. *82*:513–517, 1960.
211. Recommendation: ICSB Subcommittee on Taxonomy of Staphylococcal Micrococci. Zentralbl. Bakteriol. (Naturwissenschaft) *5*(Suppl.):129–133, 1976.
212. Riley, P. M.: Staphylococcal empyema in infants and children. J. Pediatr. *24*:577–581, 1944.
213. Rosenfeld, C. R., Laptook, A. R., and Jeffrey, J.: Limited effectiveness of triple dye in preventing colonization with methicillin: Resistant *Staphylococcus aureus* in a special care nursery. Pediatr. Infect. Dis. J. *9*:290–291, 1990.
214. Roy, D. R.: Osteomyelitis. Pediatr. Rev. *16*:380–384, 1995.
215. Rudolph, R. I., Schwartz, W., and Leyden, J. J.: Treatment of staphylococcal toxic epidermal necrolysis. Arch. Dermatol. *110*:559–562, 1974.
216. Rudoy, R. C., and Nelson, T. D.: Breast abscess in the neonatal period. Am. J. Dis. Child. *129*:1031–1034, 1975.
217. Ruley, E. J., and Lisi, L. M.: Interstitial nephritis and renal failure due to ampicillin. J. Pediatr. *84*:878–881, 1974.
218. Sanjad, S. A., Hadded, G. G., and Nassar, V. H.: Nephropathy, an underestimated complication of methicillin therapy. J. Pediatr. *84*:873–875, 1974.
219. Saravoltz, L. D., Pohlod, D. J., and Arking, L. M.: Community-acquired methicillin-resistant *Staphylococcus aureus* infections: A new source for nosocomial outbreaks. Ann. Intern. Med. *97*:325–329, 1982.
220. Sarff, L. D., and McCracken, G. H.: Methicillin-associated nephropathy or cystitis. J. Pediatr. *90*:1031–1032, 1977.
221. Sarff, L. D., McCracken, G. H., Thomas, M. L., et al.: Clinical pharmacology of methicillin in neonates. J. Pediatr. *90*:1005–1008, 1977.
222. Schmidt, B. K., Kirpalani, H. M., Corey, M., et al.: Coagulase-negative staphylococci as true pathogens in newborn infants: A cohort study. Pediatr. Infect. Dis. *6*:1026–1031, 1987.
223. Schopfer, K., Baerlocker, K., Price, P., et al.: Staphylococcal IgE antibodies, hyperimmunoglobulinemia E and *Staphylococcus aureus* infections. N. Engl. J. Med. *300*:835–838, 1979.
224. Scobie, W.: Acute cervical adenitis in children. Scott. Med. J. *14*:352–355, 1969.
225. Segal, A. W., and Peters, T. J.: Characterization of the enzyme defect in chronic granulomatous disease. Lancet *1*:1363–1365, 1976.
226. Shapiro, E. D., Wald, E. R., Nelson, J. A., et al.: Broviac catheter-related bacteremia in oncology patients. Am. J. Dis. Child. *136*:679–681, 1982.
227. Shepherd, J. J.: Tropical myositis: Is it an entity and what is its cause? Lancet *2*:1240–1242, 1983.
228. Shinefeld, H. R.: Staphylococcal infections. *In* Remington, J., and Klein, J. O. (eds.): Infectious Diseases of the Fetus and Newborn Infant. New York, Harper & Row, 1977.
229. Shinefeld, H. R., Ribble, J. C., Boris, M., et al.: Bacterial interference: Its effect on nursery-acquired infection with *Staphylococcus aureus*. IV. Am. J. Dis. Child. *105*:683–688, 1963.
230. Snyderman, R., and Pike, M. C.: Disorders of leukocyte chemotaxis. Pediatr. Clin. North Am. *24*:377–393, 1977.
231. Soderquist, B., Sundquist, K., and Vikerfors, T.: Kinetics of serum levels of interleukin-6 in *Staphylococcus aureus* septicemia. Scand. J. Infect. Dis. *24*:607–612, 1992.
232. Sofer, S., Duncan, P., and Cuernick, V.: Bacterial tracheitis: An old disease rediscovered. Clin. Pediatr. *22*:407–411, 1983.
233. Sprunt, K., Redman, W., and Leidy, G.: Antibacterial effectiveness of routine hand washing. Pediatrics *52*:264–271, 1973.
234. St. Geme, J. W., III, Bell, L. M., Baumgart, S., et al.: Distinguishing sepsis from blood culture contamination in young infants with blood cultures growing coagulase-negative staphylococci. Pediatrics *86*:157–162, 1990.
235. Stalder, J. F., Fleury, M., Sourisse, M., et al.: Local steroid therapy and bacterial skin flora in atopic dermatitis. Br. J. Dermatol. *131*:536–540, 1994.
236. Steel, R. W., Ashcraft, E. W., Payton, T. S., et al.: Recurrent staphylococcal infection in a pediatric residential care facility. Am. J. Infect. Control *11*:217–220, 1983.
237. Stein, J. M., and Pruitt, B. A.: Suppurative thrombophlebitis: A lethal iatrogenic disease. N. Engl. J. Med. *282*:1452–1455, 1970.
238. Stether, H., Martin, E., and Plotkin, H.: Neonatal mastitis due to *Escherichia coli*. J. Pediatr. *76*:611–613, 1970.
239. Stone, D. B., and Bonfigli, M. L.: Pyogenic vertebral osteomyelitis: A diagnostic pitfall for the internist. Arch. Intern. Med. *112*:491–500, 1963.
240. Storch, G., and Rajogopalan, L.: Methicillin-resistant *Staphylococcus aureus* bacteremia in children. Pediatr. Infect. Dis. *5*:59–67, 1986.
241. Suganuma, A.: Fine structure of staphylococci: Electron microscopy in the staphylococci. *In* Cohen, J. O. (ed.): The Staphylococci. New York, Wiley-Interscience, 1972, pp. 21–40.
242. Taplin, D., Lansdell, L., and Allen, A. M.: Prevalence of streptococcal pyoderma in relation to climate and hygiene. Lancet *1*:501–503, 1973.
243. Taylor, A. G., Cook, J., Finclan, W. J., et al.: Serologic tests in the differentiation of staphylococcal and tuberculous bone disease. J. Clin. Pathol. *28*:284–288, 1975.
244. Terai, M., Miwa, K., Williams, T., et al.: The absence of evidence of staphylococcal toxin involvement in the pathogenesis of Kawasaki disease. J. Infect. Dis. *172*:558–561, 1995.
245. Thatai, D., Chandy, L., and Dhar, K. L.: Septic cavernous sinus thrombophlebitis: A review of 35 cases. J. Indian Med. Assoc. *90*:290–292, 1992.
246. Thekekara, A. G., Denham, B., and Duff, D. F.: Eleven-year review of infective endocarditis. Irish Med. J. *87*:80–82, 1994.

247. Thisyakorn, U. S. A., Shelton, S., Tzou-Yien, L., et al.: Detection of teichoic acid antibodies in children with staphylococcal infections. Pediatr. Infect. Dis. *3*:222–225, 1984.
248. Thompson, R. L.: Staphylococcal infective endocarditis. Mayo Clin. Proc. *57*:106–114, 1982.
249. Thompson, R. L., Cabezudo, I., and Wenzel, R. P.: Epidemiology of nosocomial infections caused by methicillin-resistant *Staphylococcus aureus*. Ann. Intern. Med. *97*:309–317, 1982.
250. Todd, J., and Fishaut, M.: Toxic-shock syndrome associated with phage-group-I staphylococci. Lancet *2*:1116–1118, 1978.
251. Tojo, M., Yamashita, N., Goldmann, D. A., et al.: Isolation and characterization of a capsular polysaccharide adhesion from *Staphylococcus epidermidis*. J. Infect. Dis. *157*:713–722, 1988.
252. Treves, S., Khethy, J., Broker, R. H., et al.: Osteomyelitis: Early scintigraphic detection in children. Pediatrics *57*:173–186, 1976.
253. Trueta, J.: The three types of acute hematogenous osteomyelitis: A clinical and vascular study. J. Bone Joint Surg. [Br.] *41*:671–680, 1959.
254. Tuazon, C. U.: Teichoic acid antibodies in osteomyelitis and septic arthritis caused by *Staphylococcus aureus*. J. Bone Joint Surg. *64*:762–765, 1982.
255. Tuazon, C. U., and Sheagren, J. M.: Teichoic acid antibodies in the diagnosis of serious infections with *Staphylococcus aureus*. Ann. Intern. Med. *84*:543–546, 1976.
256. Tuft, S. J., Ramakrishnan, M., Seal, D. V., et al.: Role of *Staphylococcus aureus* in chronic allergic conjunctivitis. Ophthomology *99*:180–184, 1992.
257. Turner, J. A. P.: Staphylococcal pneumonia: A contemporary rarity. Clin. Pediatr. *11*:69–71, 1972.
258. Ukhila-Kallio, L., Kallio, M. J., Eskola, J., et al.: Serum C-reactive protein, erythrocyte sedimentation rate, and white blood cell count in acute hematogenous osteomyelitis of children. Pediatrics *93*:59–62, 1994.
259. Van Hare, G. F., Ben-Shachar, G., Liebman, J., et al.: Infective endocarditis in infants and children during the past 10 years: A decade of change. Am. Heart J. *107*:1235–1240, 1984.
260. Van Reken, D., Strauss, A., Hernandez, A., et al.: Infectious pericarditis in children. J. Pediatr. *85*:165–169, 1974.
261. Verbrugh, H. A., Peters, R., Rozenberg-Arska, M., et al.: Antibodies to cell wall peptidoglycan of *Staphylococcus aureus* in patients with serious staphylococcal infections. J. Infect. Dis. *144*:1–9, 1981.
262. Vinnick, L., Cooper, E. B., and Overholt, L. L.: Cavernous sinus thrombosis. Arch. Otolaryngol. *82*:303–306, 1975.
263. Wald, E. R., Levine, M. M., and Togo, Y.: Concomitant varicella and staphylococcal scalded skin syndrome. J. Pediatr. *83*:1011–1019, 1973.
264. Waldman, I. S.: Medical Mycology. Philadelphia, W. B. Saunders, 1974.
265. Waldvogel, F. A., Medoff, G., and Swartz, M. V.: Osteomyelitis: A review of clinical features, therapeutic considerations and unusual aspects. N. Engl. J. Med. *282*:206, 260–266, 316–322, 1970.
266. Walsh, T. J., Standiford, H. C., Reboli, A. C., et al.: Randomized double-blinded trial of rifampin with either novobiocin or trimethoprim-sulfamethoxazole against methicillin-resistant *Staphylococcus aureus* colonization: Prevention of antimicrobial resistance and effect of host factors on outcome. Antimicrob. Agents Chemother. *37*:1334–1342, 1993.
267. Wang, E. E., Prober, C. G., Ford-Jones, L., et al.: The management of central intravenous catheter infections. Pediatr. Infect. Dis. *3*:110–113, 1984.
268. Watanakunakorn, C.: Changing epidemiology of infective endocarditis. Adv. Intern. Med. *22*:21–29, 1977.
269. Watanakunakorn, C.: Treatment of infections due to methicillin-resistant *Staphylococcus aureus*. Ann. Intern. Med. *97*:376–378, 1982.
270. Watanakunakorn, C.: *Staphylococcus aureus* endocarditis at a community teaching hospital, 1980–1991. Arch. Intern. Med. *154*:2330–2335, 1994.
271. Watters, E. C., Wallar, P. H., Hiles, D. A., et al.: Acute orbital cellulitis. Arch. Ophthalmol. *94*:785–788, 1976.
272. Webster, J., and Faogali, S. L.: Endemic methicillin-resistant *Staphylococcus aureus* in a special care baby unit: A 2-year review. J. Pediatr. Child Health *26*:160–163, 1990.
273. Weissberg, E. D., Smith, A. L., and Smith, D. H.: Clinical features of neonatal osteomyelitis. Pediatrics *53*:505–510, 1974.
274. Wheat, L. J., Wilkinson, B. J., Kohler, R. B., et al.: Antibody response to peptidoglycan during staphylococcal infections. J. Infect. Dis. *147*:16–22, 1983.
275. Williams, C. P. S., and Oliver, T. K. P.: Nursery routines and staphylococcal colonization of the newborn. Pediatrics *44*:640–645, 1969.
276. Williams, R. C., Dossett, J. H., and Quie, P. G.: Comparative studies of immunoglobulin opsonins in osteomyelitis and other established infections. Immunology *17*:249–265, 1969.
277. Williams, R. C., and Quie, P. G.: Opsonic activity of agammaglobulinemic human sera. J. Immunol. *106*:51–55, 1971.
278. Wiseman, G. M.: The hemolysins of *Staphylococcus aureus*. Bacteriol. Rev. *39*:317–344, 1975.
279. Wisseman, G. J., Wood, V. E., and Kroll, L. L.: Pseudomonas vertebral osteomyelitis in heroin addicts. J. Bone Joint Surg. [Am.] *55*:1416–1424, 1973.
280. Wolff, S. M., Dale, D. C., and Clark, R. A.: The Chèdiak-Higashi syndrome: Studies of host defense. Ann. Intern. Med. *76*:293–306, 1972.
281. Wysham, D. N., Mulhern, M. E., Navarre, G. C., et al.: Staphylococcal infections in an obstetric unit. II. Epidemic studies of puerperal mastitis. N. Engl. J. Med. *257*:304–308, 1957.
282 Yarrington, C. T.: The prognosis and treatment of cavernous sinus thrombosis: A review of 878 cases in the literature. Ann. Otol. Rhinol. Laryngol. *70*:263–267, 1961.
283. Yogev, R., and Davis, A. T.: Neurosurgical shunt infections: A review. Child's Brain *6*:74–81, 1980.
284. Yow, M. D., Taber, L. H., Barrett, F. F., et al.: A ten-year assessment of methicillin-associated side effects. Pediatrics *58*:329–334, 1976.
285. Zafar, A. B., Butler, R. C., Reese, D. J., et al.: Use of 0.3% triclosan (Bacto-stat) to eradicate an outbreak of methicillin-resistant *Staphylococcus aureus* in a neonatal nursery. Am. J. Infect. Control *23*:201–208, 1995.
286. Zakrzewski, T., and Keith, J. D.: Bacterial endocarditis in infants and children. J. Pediatr. *67*:1179–1181, 1965.

86

Coagulase-Negative Staphylococcal Infections

Christian C. Patrick

Coagulase-negative staphylococci increasingly are implicated as causative agents of nosocomial infections. These organisms are part of the normal flora of the skin and mucous membranes. This ecologic niche hampers studies on this group of bacteria because they also are frequent contaminants in the clinical microbiology laboratory. Coagulase-negative staphylococci infections occur mainly in immunocompromised patients, particularly those with indwelling medical devices.[133, 150, 171] Epidemiologic investigations are problematic because of unreliable strain markers. The pathogenesis of these organisms is advanced, with several possible virulence factors identified. Effective therapy can be difficult because of the high proportion of isolates resistant to antibiotics. This chapter reviews the classification, pathogenesis, diagnosis, clinical manifestations, and therapy of infections caused by these ubiquitous organisms.

HISTORICAL BACKGROUND

Staphylococcus albus was the descriptive term used to define all coagulase-negative staphylococci prior to 1960. This generic designation was used because there were so few techniques for species definition. Rosenbach in 1884 used the term *S. albus* for coagulase-negative staphylococci to denote the white color imparted by the colony on an agar plate in contrast with the pathogenic *Staphylococcus aureus*, which had a yellow colony color. Interestingly, although *S. albus* was considered nonpathogenic at that time, one article published in 1958 described 90 retrospective cases of coagulase-negative staphylococcal infections.[193]

In the 1960s, coagulase-negative staphylococci clearly were identified in association with infections in certain patient populations. Coagulase-negative staphylococci were implicated as the etiologic agent of infections in patients with atrioventricular shunts and peritoneal catheters and in neonatal sepsis.[22, 24, 108, 124, 180]

During the 1960s, *Staphylococcus saprophyticus* was recognized as a singular species and found to be a pathogen in urinary tract infections. Additionally, *Staphylococcus epidermidis* supplanted *S. albus* as a generic term for all coagulase-negative staphylococci other than *S. saprophyticus*. The association of disease with coagulase-negative staphylococci highlighted the need for further specification. Work in the 1970s focused on coagulase-negative staphylococci biotyping (differentiation based on biochemical reactions), and this work continues. Currently, 29 species of coagulase-negative staphylococci are recognized. Now that individual species can be identified, *S. epidermidis* is used as a specific species term and not as a generic term. This has prompted the use of *S. epidermidis sensu stricto* to provide a distinction for a specific species. In this chapter, *S. epidermidis* is synonymous with *S. epidermidis sensu stricto*.

MICROBIOLOGY

Staphylococci are nonmotile, non spore-forming, gram-positive bacteria belonging to the Micrococcaceae family.[102] Staphylococci usually are catalase-positive. Staphylococci can be divided by the ability to produce or not produce coagulase, an extracellular enzyme that promotes the congealing of rabbit plasma. *S. aureus* also can be differentiated from the majority of coagulase-negative staphylococci by the fermentation of mannitol and the production of thermonucleases. Currently, 32 species of staphylococci are recognized, 29 being coagulase-negative staphylococci, which are identified by the following criteria: (1) colony morphology, (2) oxygen requirements, (3) novobiocin resistance, (4) aerobic acid production from carbohydrates, and (5) selected liability to enzymatic activities.[101, 102] Susceptibility to novobiocin is a convenient assay to differentiate *S. saprophyticus* from the majority of coagulase-negative staphylococci from human specimens, including *S. epidermidis*. *S. saprophyticus*, the uncommon pathogen *Staphylococcus cohnii*, and the rare pathogen *Staphylococcus xylosus* are novobiocin-resistant.[157] One should be warned that commercial kits used to identify species of coagulase-negative staphylococci have various degrees of confidence: an identification is made 60 to 95 per cent of the time, depending on the species. Most systems are developed to identify especially *S. epidermidis* and *S. saprophyticus* because these are the species clearly associated with clinical diseases.[160] Additionally, DNA-pairing studies have identified intraspecies differences with strains considered to be *S. epidermidis* by biotyping.[221]

Coagulase-negative staphylococci are prototypic, gram-positive bacteria. The outermost structure is a cell wall primarily composed of peptidoglycan with teichoic acid molecules and an assortment of interspersed proteins. The teichoic acid has a glycerol backbone, compared with the ribitol of *S. aureus*.[139] Approximately 20 to 30 proteins are located within the cell wall, 15 to 20 of these surface-exposed and thus able to interact with the host.[152]

S. epidermidis and other coagulase-negative staphylococci produce a capsule that appears to be a virulence factor in animal models.[85, 140, 217] However, its presence has been demonstrated in only 9 per cent of fresh clinical isolates.[84]

A glycocalyx or slime-layer substance is produced by most strains of *S. epidermidis*. This substance is considered a virulence factor that inhibits phagocytosis.[30, 40]

EPIDEMIOLOGY

Epidemiologic studies involving strain delineation of coagulase-negative staphylococci have proven difficult because of the organism's commensal nature on the human body. *S. epidermidis* is the prominent species, accounting for 60 to 90 per cent of all staphylococci recovered from humans. The ecologic niches of coagulase-negative staphylococci have allowed a classification, as shown in Table 86–1.

Coagulase-negative staphylococci, except for *S. saprophyticus*, primarily cause nosocomial infections. Antibiotic resistance of coagulase-negative staphylococci is common because of selective antibiotic use in the hospital setting. Coagulase-negative staphylococci primarily gain access to the blood

TABLE 86–1. Staphylococci That Are Part of the Normal Flora, Including Common Sites of Habitation and Pathogenic Potential

Species	Common Anatomic Site of Habitation	Pathogenic Potential
S. aureus	Nares	Common
S. epidermidis	Nares; axillae; skin of head, arms, and legs	Common
S. saprophyticus	Occasionally from skin	Common
S. haemolyticus	Skin of head, arms, and legs	Uncommon
S. hominis	Axillae; skin of head, arms, and legs	Uncommon
S. lugdunensis	Widely distributed on body	Uncommon
S. simulans	Occasionally from skin	Uncommon
S. cohnii	Occasionally from skin	Uncommon
S. warneri	Occasionally from skin	Uncommon
S. saccharolyticus	Rarely from skin	Uncommon
S. caprae	Occasionally from skin	Rare
S. capitis	Skin of head, face, ear, and arms	Rare
S. auricularis	Ear	Rare
S. schleiferi	? Skin	Rare
S. xylosus	Occasionally from skin	Rare

Modified from Pfaller, M. A., and Herwaldt, L. A.: Laboratory, clinical, and epidemiological aspects of coagulase-negative staphylococci. Clin. Microbiol. Rev. *1*:281–299, 1988.

stream by a breakdown of skin or mucocutaneous barriers, by following a prosthetic catheter tract, or via the hub of a central venous catheter.

Two studies have addressed the acquisition of *S. epidermidis* as a colonizing organism in low birth weight neonates.[36, 76] Both reports described rapid colonization, 75 per cent of neonates being colonized by 2 weeks of age, but differed in their findings of increased slime-layer production or antibiotic-resistant organisms with increased colonization time.[36, 76]

Epidemiologic techniques are of paramount importance in coagulase-negative staphylococci infections to identify a strain causing (1) a common-source outbreak or (2) repeated infections within an individual.[160] Techniques currently available are divided into conventional or molecular and are listed in Table 86–2. Conventional methods are fraught with poor standardization, sensitivity, and specificity. However, a combination of these techniques has been used for strain delineation. With the molecular techniques, plasmid analysis has been used most frequently because of its ease of performance and availability.[78] This latter technique is hampered by the loss of gain of plasmids. The use of analysis of chromosomal DNA analysis by restriction enzymes, using specific probes or polymerase chain amplification, is promising.

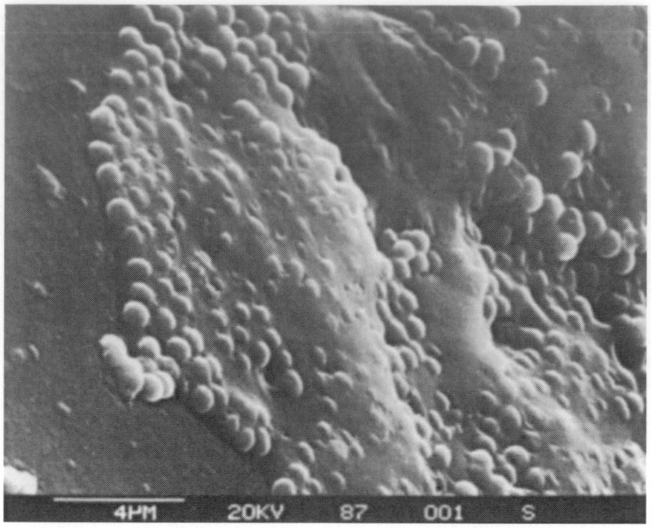

FIGURE 86–1. *Scanning electron microscopy of slime-producing coagulase-negative staphylococci. (From Peters, G., Locci, R., and Pulverer, G.: Adherence and growth of coagulase-negative staphylococci on surfaces of intravenous catheters. J. Infect. Dis. 4:479–482, 1982. University of Chicago, publishers.)*

PATHOGENESIS

Several virulence factors of *S. epidermidis* have been postulated. Most studies have investigated coagulase-negative staphylococci infections involving prosthetic devices.[63] Adherence of organisms to the catheter is the initial step in pathogenesis.[31, 32, 220] Coagulase-negative staphylococci can gain access to the device by either contiguous or bacteremic spread after traversing cutaneous or mucocutaneous barriers. Adherence then is followed by colonization and, subsequently, an infection.[68] It is thought that nonspecific electrostatic and hydrophobic interaction promotes initial attachment.[82] Specific binding by adhesions, including a polysaccharide surface antigen, other surface polysaccharides, or proteins,[115, 184, 203, 204] can occur with the catheter material or host fibronectin and other proteins.[109, 170, 211]

Once coagulase-negative staphylococci are bound, a slime-like substance is extruded, forming a biofilm that covers the organism (Fig. 86–1).[31, 220] The slime-like layer is not a capsule, and the chemical structure is unclear.[46] Reports conflict as to the antiphagocytic properties of the slime-like layer,[104, 158, 206] but it does not appear to inhibit *S. epidermidis* from nutrient sources. The slime-like layer also protects the organism from certain antibiotics.[50, 183, 207] The reported effect of the slime on coagulation[26] and the immune system[66, 90] has been challenged.[46] Shiro and associates[185] reported that *S. epidermidis* mutated to delete the production of polysaccharide surface antigen and slime is avirulent in a rabbit model of endocarditis.

TABLE 86–2. Current Methods of Epidemiologic Analysis of Coagulase-Negative Staphylococci

Method	Reference
Conventional	
Biotyping	80, 146, 160
Colony morphology	102
Antibiograms	4, 29, 30, 77, 78, 119, 129, 144, 145
Serologic	1, 154, 219
Polypeptide analysis	23, 25, 33, 47, 151, 202
Slime-layer production	30, 37, 220
Phage typing	29, 147, 191, 197
Pyrolysis mass spectrometry	58
Molecular	
Multilocus enzyme electrophoresis	222
Plasmid analysis	5, 6, 144, 145, 176, 177, 199, 209
Chromosomal analysis	17, 62, 86

A number of exotoxins are produced by coagulase-negative staphylococci, including hemolysins, cytotoxins, and proteinases.[60] Delta toxin, an enteropathogenic toxin, has been linked to necrotizing enterocolitis in infants.[178]

Surface-exposed proteins have received little attention as to their role in pathogenesis, which is unknown.[152]

Several risk factors for coagulase-negative staphylococci infection are caused by changes in host defense. Initial risk factors include a breakdown of the mucocutaneous barrier,[210, 216] immunosuppression,[54, 95, 210, 216] and prior antibiotic therapy.[96, 181] Also, the presence of a prosthetic device, such as an indwelling central venous catheter, cerebrospinal fluid shunt, or peritoneal dialysis catheter, can increase the susceptibility to infection.[10, 16, 49, 210, 216]

Opsonophagocytosis is the most important immune defense against coagulase-negative staphylococci.[54, 96, 216] An increased rate of infection has been noted in patients with a dysfunctional opsonophagocytosis system, including neonates[54] and patients receiving continuous ambulatory at peritoneal dialysis.[64, 96] Initially, this inhibition of opsonophagocytosis was believed to be due to the slime-like layer,[96] but this contention has been questioned.[104]

CLINICAL MANIFESTATIONS

Coagulase-negative staphylococci have been implicated in a variety of clinical infections in immunocompetent and immunocompromised persons (Table 86–3).[101, 150, 171] There is a basic difficulty in interpreting clinical studies of coagulase-negative staphylococci because of the different criteria used

TABLE 86–3. Clinically Important Coagulase-Negative *Staphylococcus* Infections

Infection	Reference
Bacteremia	122, 196
Neonates	13, 44, 55, 72, 75, 131, 134, 137, 138, 151, 169, 178, 195
Leukemia/lymphoma patients	59, 105, 113, 114, 157–159, 174, 182, 210, 216
Bone marrow transplant patients	15, 23, 128
Infections in patients with indwelling medical devices	
Central venous catheters	16, 79, 83, 112, 117, 130, 184, 186, 188, 190, 205, 210
Cerebrospinal fluid shunts	97, 127, 132, 135, 141, 187, 218, 220
Peritoneal dialysis catheter	52, 70, 158
Prosthetic valves	2, 42, 43, 61, 94, 123, 212, 214
Other	
Prosthetic joints	53, 93
Vascular grafts and prosthesis	11, 45
Hemodialysis shunt	149, 179
Pacemaker	28, 87, 118, 156
Scalp electrode	142
Native valve endocarditis	3, 14, 89
Urinary tract infections	73, 74, 91, 106, 110, 120, 124, 136
Miscellaneous	
Infections after ocular surgery	12, 20, 159
Postoperative wound infections	19, 48, 69
Osteomyelitis	143
Toxic shock syndrome	34

Modified from Patrick, C. C.: Coagulase-negative staphylococci: Pathogens with increasing clinical significance. J. Pediatr. *116*:497–507, 1990.

to define a clinically significant culture.[44] This must be kept in mind when analyzing the data that follow.

Bacteremia

Coagulase-negative staphylococci, particularly *S. epidermidis*, have become the major nosocomial pathogens in most studies.[44, 122, 196] The National Nosocomial Infections Study reported an increase, from 1980 to 1989, of 70 per cent in large teaching hospitals and 279 per cent in small nonteaching hospitals in nosocomial bacteremia as primarily due to *S. epidermidis*.[175] This trend has been reported from other centers.[29, 57, 122, 196, 210, 216] These infections occur primarily with the use of indwelling vascular catheters. In febrile immunocompromised pediatric cancer patients, coagulase-negative staphylococci can account for 35 per cent of all positive blood culture isolates.[105, 153]

Neonatal Bacteremias

Coagulase-negative staphylococci have become the prominent pathogen causing bacteremia in low birth weight infants.[13, 55, 75, 151] Table 86–4 lists the salient features from six large studies.[13, 55, 75, 131, 138, 151] These infections are found predominantly in premature infants with a gestational age of less than 35 weeks. Nosocomial infection risk for low birth weight infants can be correlated with an assessment of illness severity score.[65, 67] Premature infants have an immature immune system, particularly in both quantitative and qualitative neutrophil function.[27, 214] Central venous catheters have been implicated in approximately half of neonatal coagulase-negative staphylococci bacteremias.[13, 75, 138, 146]

Signs and symptoms of coagulase-negative staphylococci bacteremia are subtle, as are other systemic insults in this patient population. The most common are bradycardia and temperature instability, but these are not uniform (see Table 86–4). We have noted skin abscesses in more than 40 per cent of neonates with coagulase-negative staphylococci bacteremia.[151]

Laboratory studies usually are not helpful in identifying patients with coagulase-negative staphylococci bacteremia.[134] Leukocytosis is an inconsistent finding. Reports have conflicted about slime production, a possible virulence factor, as a marker for infection.[75, 151] One study successfully correlated quantitative blood cultures with specific clinical information to distinguish a true pathogen.[195]

Two unusual clinical entities merit comment. We have described persistent coagulase-negative staphylococci bacteremia (mean duration of 13 days) in spite of adequate antibiotic therapy.[151] This occurred in neonates without central venous catheters. No clinical or laboratory evidence was found consistently. Additionally, coagulase-negative staphylococci meningitis has been reported in low birth weight neonates with normal cerebrospinal fluid profiles.[71] This latter finding has prompted a recommendation that neonates with coagulase-negative staphylococci bacteremia undergo one or more cerebrospinal fluid examinations to determine the duration of therapy.

Coagulase-negative staphylococci also have been implicated as etiologic agents of necrotizing enterocolitis.[72, 178] At least two studies have shown an association between coagulase-negative staphylococci and necrotizing enterocolitis; one report showed no association.[169] Scheifele and associates[178] have shown that delta toxin, an exoprotein with enteropathic effects, is present in *S. epidermidis*.

Noel and associates[137] have described five cases of right-sided endocarditis in catheterized infants. This can lead to prolonged bacteremia with an associated thrombocytopenia.

Leukemia and Lymphoma

Immunocompromised patients with leukemia, lymphoma, or both are a group at risk for the development of coagulase-negative staphylococci bacteremia.[59, 105, 161, 162, 182, 210, 216] The occurrence of coagulase-negative staphylococci bacteremia in this patient population is increasing (Table 86–5). The most common portal of entry is the gastrointestinal tract, where chemotherapy causes defects.[210] Coagulase-negative staphylococci were the most common isolates causing bacteremia in pediatric cancer patients, accounting for 35 per cent of all initial isolates.[105, 153] One-third of these patients did not have central venous catheters at the time of their bacteremia.[59]

Morbidity from coagulase-negative staphylococci bacteremia was appreciable because of the organism's acquisition of multiple antibiotic resistance, requiring the use of vancomycin or combination antibiotic therapy with potentially toxic effects.[59, 95, 105, 113, 114, 163, 174, 210, 216] We reported no mortality in our study, but two other children's series had 10.5 and 11 per cent mortality rates.[59, 105, 153]

Bone Marrow Transplantation

Coagulase-negative staphylococci have become the primary pathogen causing bacteremia in bone marrow trans-

TABLE 86–4. Salient Aspects of Six Studies of Coagulase-Negative Staphylococci Bacteremia in Neonates

	Munson et al. (1982)[31] (n = 27)	Baumgart et al. (1983)[13] (n = 14)	Fleer et al. (1983)[55] (n = 30)	Noel et al. (1984)[138] (n = 23)	Hall et al. (1985)[75] (n = 29)	Patrick et al. (1989)[151] (n = 32)
Patient characteristics						
Mean birth weight (g)	1130	1910	1564	NR	1607	1172
Gestational age (wk)	28.9	34.0	32.1	32.2	31.0	28.6
Central lines (% patients)	85	54 (7/13)	NR	26	34	19
TPN (% patients)	78	92 (12/13)	77 (20/26)	NR	NR	91
Clinical characteristics						
Apnea/bradycardia (%)	>50	38 (5/13)	100	17	62	78
Temperature instability (%)	<50	NR	70	35	7	22
Tachycardia (%)	>50	NR	100	NR	NR	6
Mortality (%)	0	15 (2/13)	0 (0/13)	0	0	0
Laboratory characteristics						
Slime production (% patients isolates)	NR	NR	NR	NR	79	54 (6/13)
Antibiotic susceptibility	100% S to cephalothin	57% R to semisynthetic PCN 100% S to vancomycin and cephalothin	100% S to cephalothin	74% S to methicillin 100% S to vancomycin	83% S to methicillin 100% S to vancomycin	100% S to vancomycin

NR, not reported; S, susceptible; R, resistant; PCN, pregnenolone carbonitrile; TPN, total parenteral nutrition.

plantation patients.[23, 128] These episodes occur most often during periods of agranulocytosis prior to marrow engraftment[23] and can be fatal.[15] Most of these episodes are due to the universal use of central venous catheters and the use of broad-spectrum antibiotics.

Indwelling Medical Devices

Central Venous Catheters

Infections associated with central venous catheters are caused primarily by coagulase-negative staphylococci. Coagulase-negative staphylococci also can cause infections in peripheral catheters composed of steel or polyethylene.[205] Central venous catheters are of increasing importance in pediatrics for long-term hyperalimentation or medication administration.[83] Two types of devices are in common use: Broviac and Hickman catheters, which have an external port, and totally implanted vascular access devices.[21, 81, 168] Broviac and Hickman catheters have an exit site where the catheter enters the skin, whereas the totally implanted vascular devices have a subcutaneous tract; all three types have a Dacron cuff that promotes fibrosis, limiting the trafficking of potential pathogens, and an insert site into the major vessel. Thus, infection can occur at the exit site, along the catheter tunnel, or at the catheter vessel insertion site. Infection at the vessel insertion site can lead to bacteremia or a septic thrombophlebitis, with further complications caused by metastatic spread.[164]

Infectious complications involving central venous catheters have a variable reported frequency of 2.7 to 47 per cent[16, 79, 112, 130, 190, 208]; coagulase-negative staphylococci are the pathogen in approximately half. This variability depends on the definition of a catheter-related infection, the type of catheter used, and the presence of hyperalimentation fluid and lipid in the infusion.[117, 184, 186] The use of a guide wire for catheter placement or a multilumen catheter leads to higher infection rates.[188]

S. epidermidis is the species associated most often with central venous catheter infections, identified in approximately 70 per cent of coagulase-negative staphylococci central venous catheter infections.[16, 79] This is not unexpected, because it is the major species colonizing the skin.[103] Other implicated coagulase-negative staphylococci species include *S. haemolyticus*, *S. warneri*, and *S. hominis*.[79]

The diagnosis of a true infection caused by *S. epidermidis* versus a contaminated specimen is difficult. Making the diagnosis depends on the patient's clinical status and the isolation of identical isolate strains in repeated cultures. Proper ther-

TABLE 86–5. Clinical Characteristics of Coagulase-Negative Staphylococci Bacteremia in Childhood Cancer Patients*

	Friedman et al. (1984)[59] (n = 150 +)	Langley and Gold (1988)[105] (n = 100)	Patrick et al. (1989)[153] (n = 207)
Coagulase-negative staphylococci among total bacteremias (%)	12.7	35	35
Patients with central venous catheters (%)	32.0	53	61
Mortality (%)	10.5	38	30
Patients susceptible to:			
Methicillin (%)	17.0	38	30
Vancomycin (%)	100.0	100	100

*Percentages are based on the number of episodes of coagulase-negative staphylococcal sepsis.

apy, possibly including removal of a catheter, requires an accurate diagnosis.[165] Additionally, distinction of a central venous catheter–related bacteremia from a bacteremia not associated with a central venous catheter is important. The use of quantitative blood cultures using the DuPont isolator system has shown that catheter-related bacteremias have a 5- to 10-fold difference in bacterial concentration compared with peripheral cultures.[56, 166] Maki and associates[116] have determined that catheter-related bacteremia can be confirmed after catheter removal by rolling the distal 5 to 7 cm of the catheter on a culture plate and finding greater than 15 colony-forming units.

Therapy for coagulase-negative staphylococci infections involving central venous catheters should include catheter removal if the catheter is no longer necessary. Exit site infections usually can be managed without removal of the catheter.[165] Approximately one-third of tunnel tract infections can be managed without catheter removal, but the remaining patients have continued bacteremia or relapse of their bacteremia requiring catheter removal. Catheters should be removed immediately if the patient's clinical status deteriorates.[216] The duration of therapy depends on whether or not the catheter was removed and on the patient's underlying immune status.

Central Nervous System Shunts

Central nervous system shunts are used commonly to divert or shunt central nervous system fluid to relieve hydrocephalus.[97] Other prosthetic devices within the central nervous system have been used to monitor ventricular pressure or to administer chemotherapy.[41] Two types of central nervous system shunts have been used commonly. The earlier shunts diverted ventricular fluid into the right atrium; this technique is used infrequently because of its high complication rate.[127, 141] Ventriculoperitoneal shunts that divert ventricular fluid into the peritoneal cavity have been used since the 1960s because of their lower rate of mechanical complications.[97, 132, 141] However, the incidences of infection involving both the ventriculoperitoneal and the ventriculoatrial shunts are comparable.[97, 111, 187] Infection rates are higher in neonates. In both central nervous system shunts, *S. epidermidis* is the principal microorganism implicated, with a 5 to 12 per cent infection rate. Coagulase-negative staphylococci account for 60 to 75 per cent of all bacterial causes of shunt infection.[97, 135, 187]

The pathogenesis of central nervous system infections primarily occurs at the insertion site by contamination of the catheter from the patient's skin flora.[187] Seventy per cent of ventriculoperitoneal shunt infections occur within 2 months of shunt placement.[135] The pathogenesis of this infection appears to be similar to the catheter-related infection, described in the pathogenesis section. Two other modes of infection involve hematogenous seeding or retrograde migration from the distal end of the shunt.

The diagnosis of central nervous system shunt infections is difficult owing to the differentiation between a true infection and a contaminating organism. The Gram stain of ventricular fluid often is negative, but culture is sensitive. Subtle changes are noted in cerebrospinal and ventricular fluid cell counts or cytochemical findings.[218] Patients with ventriculoatrial shunts often have signs and symptoms compatible with septicemia and the additional complications of glomerulonephritis secondary to immune complexes. In patients with ventriculoperitoneal shunts, because of the distal placement of the catheter into the peritoneum, an intra-abdominal cyst may develop at the distal end of the catheter. Shunt dysfunctions secondary to infections often are noted because of signs and symptoms consistent with increased intracranial pressure.

Standard therapy for ventriculoperitoneal shunt infections has been removal of the shunt system and administration of systemic antibiotics.[187, 218] However, this mode of therapy has been challenged, after successful treatment by externalization of the peritoneal end of the ventriculoperitoneal shunt and administration of both intraventricular and systemic antibiotics.[127]

Peritoneal Dialysis Catheters

In 1968, Tenckhoff and Schechter[201] devised a catheter that allowed for peritoneal dialysis with a low infection rate. Infection remains the most common complication of peritoneal dialysis, and *S. epidermidis* is the most common bacterial pathogen isolated.[70, 158] It represents up to 50 per cent of infecting organisms.[158] The pathogenesis of infections involving the peritoneal dialysis catheter is similar to that of catheter-related infections with infections involving the exit site, along the subcutaneous catheter tunnel and peritonitis.[158] The prevalence of peritonitis in patients undergoing continuous ambulatory peritoneal dialysis is approximately 60 per cent. Signs of peritonitis include fever, abdominal pain, and cloudy peritoneal dialysis, fever being variable. The removal of the catheter is not usually necessary as part of the therapy but may be necessary in refractory cases or when the catheter malfunctions. Antibiotics are administered in the dialysis fluid, and systemic antibiotics also can be used.[52]

Prosthetic Devices

S. epidermidis is the most common cause of prosthetic valve endocarditis, accounting for 25 to 40 per cent of all cases.[42, 61, 123, 212] The mortality rate from *S. epidermidis* prosthetic valve endocarditis approaches 70 per cent.[2, 43, 94, 123, 124] Commonly, *S. epidermidis* prosthetic valve endocarditis occurs within 60 days after implanting the device and is defined as early prosthetic valve endocarditis. Pathogenesis is believed to involve contamination at the time of surgery leading to an abscess of the mechanical valve ring. No sign or symptom is consistently diagnostic of prosthetic valve endocarditis, but fever is the most common finding. Anemia is the most common abnormality identified by laboratory tests. Blood cultures are imperative in diagnosing prosthetic valve endocarditis. Therapy should include vancomycin and rifampin or an aminoglycoside, with surgical intervention as indicated.[94]

Other Indwelling Medical Devices

Coagulase-negative staphylococci are involved in an expanded spectrum of infections involving indwelling medical devices.[41] These include infections of prosthetic joints,[53, 93] vascular grafts,[11, 45] hemodialysis shunts,[148, 179] and pacemaker pockets.[28, 87, 118, 156] Additionally, osteomyelitis secondary to *S. epidermidis* has been reported to occur after hemodialysis and in neonates after the use of a monitoring scalp electrode.[142]

Native Valve Endocarditis

Native valve endocarditis is the only non-nosocomial infection other than *S. saprophyticus* urinary tract infection that is caused by coagulase-negative staphylococci. Coagulase-negative staphylococci are the etiologic agents involved in 22 per cent of native valve endocarditis in pediatric patients with previously normal heart valves.[89] These infections usually are subacute and arise from transient bacteremia. Pathogenesis is believed to involve seeding of a previously damaged valve or endocarditis that previously had not been identified.[3, 14]

Urinary Tract Infections

S. saprophyticus is the most common coagulase-negative *Staphylococcus* causing urinary tract infections in both the upper and the lower urinary tracts.[106] These infections predominantly occur in young, healthy, sexually active women.[91, 106, 120] *S. epidermidis* and other coagulase-negative staphylococci rarely cause urinary tract infections but have been noted to produce disease in older adults with urinary tract complications.[73, 110, 136] McDonald and Lohr[125] and Hall and Snitzer[74] have described healthy children with pyelonephritis caused by *S. epidermidis*.

Miscellaneous

Numerous case reports have described *S. epidermidis* as an etiologic agent in a variety of infections. Endophthalmitis secondary to *S. epidermidis* has been reported in patients undergoing ocular surgery or trauma.[12, 20, 159] Postoperative mediastinitis after median sternotomy for open heart surgery can be caused by *S. epidermidis*.[19, 48, 69] Primary osteomyelitis secondary to coagulase-negative staphylococci is rare in healthy children.[143] Of note, coagulase-negative staphylococci have been implicated as a possible cause of toxic shock syndrome.[34]

TREATMENT

The treatment of coagulase-negative staphylococci infections depends on the patient's immunologic status, the presence of an indwelling medical device, and the results of antimicrobial testing. Many coagulase-negative staphylococci, particularly *S. epidermidis* and *S. haemolyticus*, are resistant to antimicrobial therapy.[7, 9, 29, 38, 51, 65, 181, 194, 213] Methicillin resistance especially is prevalent in nosocomial infections and occurs in approximately 60 per cent of cases.[18, 172, 189] Methicillin resistance is most prevalent in patients with prosthetic valve endocarditis.[94] There is a high degree of resistance among methicillin-resistant *S. epidermidis* to other antibiotics, such as clindamycin, erythromycin, and gentamicin.[7]

Penicillin is an active drug in susceptible strains of *S. epidermidis*. For organisms that are resistant to penicillin but susceptible to semisynthetic penicillins, nafcillin is the most active antibiotic.[160, 173]

There is a degree of cross-resistance between the semisynthetic penicillin-resistant penicillins and cephalosporins.[172] Thus, routine susceptibility testing can indicate that a strain is susceptible to a cephalosporin when in fact it is resistant.[70, 107] As a rule, methicillin resistance can be interpreted as resistance to all β-lactam antibiotics.[88]

Vancomycin is the drug of choice for methicillin-resistant organisms and is recommended for treating severe infections.[99] Coagulase-negative staphylococci can exhibit heteroresistance, defined as a culture population comprising two subpopulations, one susceptible to methicillin and the other resistant.[172] Enhanced detection of this admixture of organisms can be obtained by change in the culture conditions.[126] The clinical significance of this heteroresistance in coagulase-negative staphylococci is unknown, but in a study of *S. aureus* it was shown not to affect outcome.[100]

Several newer antibiotics, including the quinolones and teicoplanin, have shown activity against coagulase-negative staphylococci and could be useful in therapy of multiresistant organisms.[111, 184] However, resistance to these agents also has been observed.[9, 181, 194, 213]

Gentamicin and rifampin are active against coagulase-negative staphylococci, but rapid emergence of resistance has limited their use as single drugs.[29, 121, 173] These two antibiotics have been shown to be synergistic with vancomycin against methicillin-resistant, coagulase-negative staphylococci.[113] Additionally, rifampin has been used in neonates with persistent bacteremia to eradicate the organisms.[198] Arditi and Yogev[8] reported a novel antibiotic combination using clindamycin and rifampin. This combination in vitro has allowed rifampin to exert its activity without the development of rifampin resistance.

PREVENTION

Prevention of coagulase-negative staphylococci infection is difficult because of these organisms' ubiquitous nature as predominant skin commensals. Hand washing can limit the spread of infection from staff to patient or patient to patient.[167] Additionally, proper surgical techniques help minimize these infections associated with installation of indwelling medical devices.

There has been an increased effort toward developing catheters that are both inert and resistant to bacterial colonization adherence; however, these attempts have been only marginally successful.[98, 149, 155] Catheters with antibiotics or disinfectants impregnated in their surfaces appear promising, but their effect is short-lived.[200]

The use of prophylactic antibiotics during the implantation of an indwelling medical device has not been studied in a controlled manner and appears to promote antibiotic resistance.[4, 5, 35] This idea was challenged in two studies involving cardiovascular surgery patients in whom prophylactic cephalosporins were shown to reduce postoperative wound infections due to *S. epidermidis*.[92, 192]

CONCLUSION

Coagulase-negative staphylococci, particularly *S. epidermidis*, are a major source of nosocomial infection in a variety of clinical situations. Most infections occur in patients who are immunosuppressed or have an indwelling medical device. Epidemiologic studies are difficult because of the organisms' commensal existence and the limitations of available epidemiologic techniques. The pathogenesis of coagulase-negative staphylococci infection is being defined in the context of a catheter-related infection. Therapy is difficult because of the usual presence of an indwelling medical device and the multiple antimicrobial resistance of the organisms.

Acknowledgment

Supported in part by the National Cancer Institute (CA 21765) and the American Lebanese Syrian Associated Charities (ALSAC).

References

1. Aasen, J., and Oeding, P.: Antigenic studies on *Staphylococcus epidermidis*. Acta Pathol. Microbiol. Scand. [B] *79*:827–834, 1972.
2. Anderson, D. J., Bulkley, B. H., and Hutchins, G. M.: A clinicopathologic study of prosthetic valve endocarditis in 22 patients: Morphologic basis for diagnosis and therapy. Am. Heart J. *94*:325–332, 1977.

3. Archer, G. L.: *Staphylococcus epidermidis* and other coagulase-negative staphylococci. *In* Mandell, G. L., Bennett, J. E., and Dolin, R. (eds.): Principles and Practice of Infectious Diseases. 4th ed. New York, Churchill Livingstone, 1995, pp. 1777–1784.
4. Archer, G.: Antimicrobial susceptibility and selection of resistance among *Staphylococcus epidermidis* isolates recovered from patients with infections of indwelling foreign devices. Antimicrob. Agents Chemother. *14*:353–359, 1987.
5. Archer, G. L., Dietrick, D. R., and Johnston, J. L.: Molecular epidemiology of transmissible gentamicin resistance among coagulase-negative staphylococci in a cardiac surgery unit. J. Infect. Dis. *151*:243–251, 1985.
6. Archer, G. L., Karchmer, A. W., Vishniavsky, N., et al.: Plasmid-pattern analysis for the differentiation of infecting from noninfecting *Staphylococcus epidermidis*. J. Infect. Dis. *149*:913–920, 1984.
7. Archer, G. L., and Climo, M. W.: Antimicrobial susceptibility of coagulase-negative staphylococci. Antimicrob. Agents Chemother. *38*:2231–2237, 1994.
8. Arditi, M., and Yogev, R.: In vitro interaction between rifampin and clindamycin against pathogenic coagulase-negative staphylococci. Antimicrob. Agents Chemother. *33*:245–247, 1989.
9. Arioli, V., and Pallanza, R.: Teicoplanin-resistant coagulase-negative staphylococci. Lancet *1*:39, 1987.
10. Baddour, L. M., Smalley, D. L., Kraus, A. P., Jr., et al.: Comparison of microbiologic characteristics of pathogenic and saprophytic coagulase-negative staphylococci from patients on continuous ambulatory peritoneal dialysis. Diagn. Microbiol. Infect. Dis. *5*:197–205, 1986.
11. Bandyk D. F., Berni, G. A., Thiele, B. L., et al.: Aortofemoral graft infection due to *Staphylococcus epidermidis*. Arch. Surg. *119*:102–108, 1984.
12. Baum, J. L.: Current concepts in ophthalmology: Ocular infections. N. Engl. J. Med. *299*:28–31, 1978.
13. Baumgart, S., Hall, S. E., Campos, J. M., et al.: Sepsis with coagulase-negative staphylococci in critically ill newborns. Am. J. Dis. Child *137*:461–463, 1983.
14. Belik, J., Finn, G., Rivera, G., et al.: Successful management of bacterial endocarditis of the mitral valve due to *Staphylococcus epidermidis* in an immunocompromised host. Acta Paediatr. Scand. *69*:731–734, 1980.
15. Bender, J. W., and Hughes, W. T.: Fatal *Staphylococcus epidermidis* sepsis following bone marrow transplantation. Johns Hopkins Med. J. *146*:13–15, 1980.
16. Benezra, D., Kiehn, T. E., Gold, J. W. M., et al.: Prospective study of infections in indwelling central venous catheters using quantitative blood cultures. Am. J. Med. *85*:495–498, 1988.
17. Bialkowska-Hobrzanska, H., Jaskor, D., and Hammerberg, O.: Evaluation of restriction endonuclease fingerprinting of chromosomal DNA and plasmid profile analysis for characterization of multiresistant coagulase-negative staphylococci in bacteremic neonates. J. Clin. Microbiol. *28*:269–275, 1990.
18. Blum, R. A., and Rodvold, K. A.: Recognition and importance of *Staphylococcus epidermidis* infections. Clin. Pharm. *6*:464–475, 1987.
19. Bor, D. H., Rose, R. M., and Modlin, J. F.: Mediastinitis after cardiovascular surgery. Rev. Infect. Dis. *5*:885–896, 1983.
20. Brinton, G. S., Topping, T. M., and Hyndiuk, R. A.: Posttraumatic endophthalmitis. Arch. Ophthalmol. *102*:547–550, 1984.
21. Broviac, J. W., Cole, J. J., and Scribner, B. H.: A silicone rubber atrial catheter for prolonged parenteral alimentation. Surg. Gynecol. Obstet. *136*:602–606, 1973.
22. Bruce, A. M., Lorber, J., Shedden, W. I. H., et al.: Persistent bacteremia following ventriculo-caval shunt operations for hydrocephalus in infants. Dev. Med. Child. Neurol. *5*:461–470, 1963.
23. Buckner, C. D., Clift, R. A., Sanders, J. E., et al.: Protective environment for bone marrow transplant recipients: A prospective study. Ann. Intern. Med. *89*:893–901, 1978.
24. Buetow, K. C., Klein, S. W., and Lane, R. B.: Septicemia in premature infants. Am. J. Dis. Child. *110*:29–41, 1965.
25. Burnie, J. P., Lee, W., Matthews, R. C., et al.: Immunoblot fingerprinting of coagulase-negative staphylococci. J. Clin. Pathol. *41*:103–110, 1988.
26. Bykowska, K., Ludwicka, A., and Wegrzynowicz, Z.: Anticoagulant properties of extracellular slime substance produced by *Staphylococcus epidermidis*. Thromb. Haemost. *54*:853–856, 1985.
27. Cairo, M. S.: Neonatal neutrophic host defense: Prospects for immunologic enhancement during neonatal sepsis. Am. J. Dis. Child. *143*:40–46, 1989.
28. Choo, M. H., Holmes, D. R., Jr., Gersh, B. J., et al.: Permanent pacemaker infections: Characterization and management. Am. J. Cardiol. *48*:559–564, 1981.
29. Christensen, G. D., Bisno, A. L., and Parisi, J. T., et al.: Nosocomial septicemia due to multiply antibiotic-resistant *Staphylococcus epidermidis*. Ann. Intern. Med. *96*:1–10, 1982.
30. Christensen, G. D., Parisi, J. T., Bisno, A. L., et al.: Characterization of clinically significant strains of coagulase-negative staphylococci. J. Clin. Microbiol. *18*:258–269, 1983.
31. Christensen, G. D., Simpson, W. A., Bisno, A. L., et al.: Adherence of slime-producing strains of *Staphylococcus epidermidis* to smooth surfaces. Infect. Immun. *37*:318–326, 1982.
32. Christensen, G. D., Simpson, W. A., Bisno, A. L., et al.: Experimental foreign body infections in mice challenged with slime-producing *Staphylococcus epidermidis*. Infect. Immun. *40*:407–410, 1983.
33. Clink, J., and Pennington, T. H.: Staphylococcal whole-cell polypeptide analysis: Evaluation as a taxonomic and typing tool. J. Med. Microbiol. *23*:41–44, 1987.
34. Crass, B. A., and Bergdoll, M. S.: Involvement of coagulase-negative staphylococci in toxic shock syndrome. J. Clin. Microbiol. *23*:43–45, 1986.
35. Dandalides, P. C., Rutala, W. A., Thomann, C. A., et al.: Serious postoperative infections caused by coagulase-negative staphylococci: An epidemiological and clinical study. J. Hosp. Infect. *8*:233–241, 1986.
36. D'Angio, C. T., McGowan, K. L., and Baumgart, S.: Surface colonization with coagulase-negative staphylococci in premature neonates. J. Pediatr. *114*:1029–1034, 1989.
37. Davenport, D. S., Massanari, R. M., Pfaller, M. A., et al.: Usefulness of a test for slime production as a marker for clinically significant infections with coagulase-negative staphylococci. J. Infect. Dis. *153*:332–339, 1986.
38. Del Bene, V. E., John, J. F., Jr., Twitty, J. A., et al.: Antistaphylococcal activity of teicoplanin, vancomycin, and other antimicrobial agents: The significance of methicillin resistance. J. Infect. Dis. *154*:349–352, 1986.
39. de Saxe, M. J., Crees-Morris, J. A., Marples, R. R., et al.: Evaluation of current phage-typing systems for coagulase-negative staphylococci. *In* Jeljaszewicz, J. (ed.): Staphylococci and Staphylococcal Infections. Stuttgart, Gustave Fischer Verlag, 1981, pp. 197–204.
40. Dickinson, G. M., and Bisno, A. L.: Infections associated with indwelling devices: Concepts of pathogenesis: Infections associated with intravascular devices. Antimicrob. Agents Chemother. *33*:597–601, 1989.
41. Dickinson, G. M., and Bisno, A. L.: Infections associated with indwelling devices: Infections related to extravascular devices. Antimicrob. Agents Chemother. *33*:602–607, 1989.
42. Dismukes, W. E.: Prosthetic valve endocarditis factors influencing outcome and recommendations for therapy. *In* Bisno, A. L. (ed.): Treatment of Infective Endocarditis. New York, Grune & Stratton, 1981, pp. 167–191.
43. Dismukes, W. E., Karchmer, A. W., Buckley, M. J., et al.: Prosthetic valve endocarditis: Analysis of 38 cases. Circulation *48*:365–377, 1973.
44. Donowitz, L. C., Haley, C. E., Gregory, W. W., et al.: Neonatal intensive care unit bacteremia: Emergence of gram-positive bacteria as major pathogens. Am. J. Infect. Control *15*:141–147, 1987.
45. Dougherty, S. H., and Simmons, R. L.: Infections in bionic man: The pathobiology of infections in prosthetic devices: Parts I and II. Curr. Problems Surg. *19*:217–319, 1982.
46. Drewry, D. T., Galbraith, L., Wilkinson, B. J., et al.: Staphylococcal slime: A cautionary tale. J. Clin. Microbiol. *28*:1292–1296, 1990.
47. Dryden, M. S., Talsania, H. G., Martin, S., et al.: Evaluation of methods for typing coagulase-negative staphylococci. J. Med. Microbiol. *37*:109–117, 1992.
48. Edwards, M. S., and Baker, C. J.: Median sternotomy wound infections in children. Pediatr. Infect. Dis. *2*:105–109, 1987.
49. Etienne, J., Brun, Y., and El Solh, N., et al.: Characterization of clinically significant isolates of *Staphylococcus epidermidis* from patients with endocarditis. J. Clin. Microbiol. *26*:613–617, 1988.
50. Farber, B. F., Kaplan, M. H., and Clogston, A. G.: *Staphylococcus epidermidis* extracted slime inhibits the antimicrobial action of glycopeptide antibiotics. J. Infect. Dis. *161*:27–40, 1990.
51. Fass, R. J., Helsel, V. L., Barnishan, J., et al.: In vitro susceptibilities of four species of coagulase-negative staphylococci. Antimicrob. Agents Chemother. *30*:545–552, 1986.
52. Fine, R. N., Salusky, I. B., Hall, T., et al.: Peritonitis in children undergoing continuous ambulatory peritoneal dialysis. Pediatrics *71*:806–809, 1983.
53. Fitzgerald, R. H., Jr., Nolan, D. R., Ilstrup, D. M., et al.: Deep wound sepsis following total hip arthroplasty. J. Bone Joint Surg. *59*:847–855, 1977.
54. Fleer, A., Gerards, L. J., Aerts, P., et al.: Opsonic defense to *Staphylococcus epidermidis* in the premature neonate. J. Infect. Dis. *152*:930–937, 1985.
55. Fleer, A., Senders, R. C., Visser, M. R., et al.: Septicemia due to coagulase-negative staphylococci in a neonatal intensive care unit: Clinical and bacteriological features and contaminated parenteral fluids as a source of sepsis. Pediatr. Infect. Dis. *2*:426–431, 1983.
56. Flynn, P. M., Shenep, J. L., Stokes, D. C., et al.: *In situ* management of confirmed central venous catheter–related bacteremia. Pediatr. Infect. Dis. J. *6*:729–734, 1987.
57. Freeman, J., Platt, R., Sidebottom, D. G., et al.: Coagulase-negative staphylococcal bacteremia in the changing neonatal intensive care unit population. JAMA *258*:2548–2552, 1987.
58. Freeman, R., Goodfellow, M., Ward, A. C., et al.: Epidemiological typing of coagulase-negative staphylococci by pyrolysis mass spectrometry. J. Med. Microbiol. *34*:245–248, 1991.
59. Friedman, L. E., Brown, A. E., Miller, D. R., et al.: *Staphylococcus epidermidis* septicemia in children with leukemia and lymphoma. Am. J. Dis. Child. *138*:715–719, 1984.
60. Gemmell, C. G.: Virulence characteristics of *Staphylococcus epidermidis*. J. Med. Microbiol. *22*:287–289, 1986.
61. Gnann, J. W., Jr., and Cobbs, C. G.: Infections of prosthetic valves and intravascular devices. *In* Mandell, G. L., Douglas, R. G., Jr., and Bennett, J. E. (eds.): Principles and Practice of Infectious Diseases. 2nd ed. New York, John Wiley and Sons, 1985, pp. 530–539.
62. Goering, R. V., and Winters, M. A.: Rapid method for epidemiologic

evaluation of gram-positive cocci by field inversion gel electrophoresis. J. Clin. Microbiol. *30*:577–580, 1992.
63. Goldman, D. A., and Pier, G. B.: Pathogenesis of infections relapsed to intravascular catheterization. Clin. Microbiol. Rev. *6*:176–192, 1993.
64. Gordon, D. L., Rice, J. L., and Avery, V. M.: Surface phagocytosis and host defence in the peritoneal cavity during continuous ambulatory peritoneal dialysis. Eur. J. Clin. Microbiol. Infect. Dis. *9*:191–197, 1990.
65. Graninger, W., Wenish, C., and Hasenhündl, M.: Treatment of staphylococcal infections. Curr. Opin. Infect. Dis. *8*(Suppl. 1):520–528, 1995.
66. Gray, E. D., Peters, G., Verstegen, M., et al.: Effect of extracellular slime substance from *Staphylococcus epidermidis* on the human cellular immune response. Lancet *1*:365–367, 1984.
67. Gray, J. E., Richardson, D. K., McCormick, M. C., et al.: Coagulase-negative staphylococcal bacteremia among very low birth weight infants: Relation to admission illness severity, resource use, and outcome. Pediatrics *95*:225–230, 1995.
68. Gristina, A. G.: Biomaterial-centered infection: Microbial adhesion versus tissue integration. Science *237*:1588–1595, 1987.
69. Grossi, E. A., Culliford, A. T., and Krieger, K. H., et al.: A survey of 77 major infectious complications of median sternotomy: A review of 7,949 consecutive operative procedures. Ann. Thorac. Surg. *40*:214–223, 1985.
70. Gruer, L. D., Bartlett, R., and Ayliffe, G. A. J.: Species identification and antibiotic sensitivity of coagulase-negative staphylococci from CAPD peritonitis. J. Antimicrob. Chemother. *13*:577–583, 1984.
71. Gruskay, J., Harris, M. C., Costarino, A. T., et al.: Neonatal *Staphylococcus epidermidis* meningitis with unremarkable CSF examination results. Am. J. Dis. Child. *143*:580–582, 1989.
72. Gruskay, J. A., Abbasi, S., Anday, E., et al.: *Staphylococcus epidermidis*-associated enterocolitis. J. Pediatr. *109*:520–524, 1986.
73. Gunn, B. A., and Davis, C. E., Jr.: *Staphylococcus haemolyticus* urinary tract infection in a male patient. J. Clin. Microbiol. *26*:1055–1057, 1988.
74. Hall, D. E., and Snitzer, J. A., III: *Staphylococcus epidermidis* as a cause of urinary tract infections in children. J. Pediatr. *124*:437–438, 1994.
75. Hall, R. T., Hall, S. L., Barnes, W. G., et al.: Characteristics of coagulase-negative staphylococci from infants with bacteremia. Pediatr. Infect. Dis. J. *6*:377–383, 1987.
76. Hall, S. L., Riddell, S. W., Barnes, W. G., et al.: Evaluation of coagulase-negative staphylococcal isolates from serial nasopharyngeal cultures of premature infants. Diagn. Microbiol. Infect. Dis. *13*:17–23, 1990.
77. Hamilton-Miller, J. M. T., and Iliffe, A.: Antimicrobial resistance in coagulase negative staphylococci. J. Med. Microbiol. *19*:217–226, 1985.
78. Hamory, B. H., Parisi, J. T., and Hutton, J. P.: *Staphylococcus epidermidis:* A significant nosocomial pathogen. Am. J. Infect. Control. *15*:59–74, 1987.
79. Haslett, T. M., Isenberg, H. D., Hilton, E., et al.: Microbiology of indwelling central intravascular catheters. J. Clin. Microbiol. *26*:696–701, 1988.
80. Hebert, G. A., Cooksey, R. C., Clark, N. C., et al.: Biotyping coagulase-negative staphylococci. J. Clin. Microbiol. *26*:1950–1956, 1988.
81. Hickman, R. O., Buckner, C. D., Clift, R. A., et al.: A modified right atrial catheter for access to the venous system in marrow transplant recipients. Surg. Gynecol. Obstet. *148*:871–875, 1979.
82. Hogt, A. H., Dankert, J., Hulstaert, C. E., et al.: Cell surface characteristics of coagulase-negative staphylococci and their adherence to fluorinated poly (ethyleneprophylene). Infect. Immun. *51*:294–301, 1986.
83. Iannacci, L., and Piomelli, S.: Supportive care for children with cancer: Guidelines of the Children's Cancer Study Group: Use of venous access lines. Am. J. Pediatr. Hematol. Oncol. *6*:277–281, 1984.
84. Ichiman, Y.: Applications of fluorescent antibody for detecting capsular substance in *Staphylococcus epidermidis*. J. Appl. Bacteriol. *56*:311–316, 1984.
85. Ichiman, Y., and Yoshida, K.: The relationship of capsular-type of *Staphylococcus epidermidis* to virulence and induction of resistance in the mouse. J. Appl. Bacteriol. *51*:229–241, 1981.
86. Izard, N. C., Hachler, H., Grehn, M., et al.: Ribotyping of coagulase-negative staphylococci with special emphasis on intraspecific typing of *Staphylococcus epidermidis*. J. Clin. Microbiol. *30*:817–823, 1992.
87. Jara, F. M., Toledo-Pereyra, L., Lewis, J. W., Jr., et al.: The infected pacemaker pocket. J. Thorac. Cardiovasc. Surg. *78*:298–300, 1979.
88. John, J. F., and McNeill, W. F.: Activity of cephalosporins against methicillin-susceptible and methicillin-resistant, coagulase-negative staphylococci: Minimal effect of beta-lactamases. Antimicrob. Agents Chemother. *17*:179–183, 1980.
89. Johnson, C. M., and Rhodes, K. H.: Pediatric endocarditis. Mayo Clin. Proc. *57*:86–94, 1982.
90. Johnson, G. M., Lee, D. A., Regelmann, W. E., et al.: Interference with granulocyte function by *Staphylococcus epidermidis* slime. Infect. Immun. *54*:13–20, 1986.
91. Jordan, P. A., Iravani, A., Richard, G. A., et al.: Urinary tract infection caused by *Staphylococcus saprophyticus*. J. Infect. Dis. *142*:510–515, 1980.
92. Kaiser, A. B., Petracek, M. R., Lea, J. W., IV, et al.: Efficacy of cefazolin, cefamandole, and gentamicin as prophylactic agents in cardiac surgery: Results of a prospective, randomized, double-blind trial in 1030 patients. Ann. Surg. *206*:791–797, 1987.
93. Kamme, C., and Lindberg, L.: Aerobic and anaerobic bacteria in deep infections after total hip arthroplasty: Differential diagnosis between infectious and non-infectious loosening. Clin. Orthop. *154*:201–207, 1981.
94. Karchmer, A. W., Archer, G. L., and Dismukes, W. E.: *Staphylococcus epidermidis* causing prosthetic valve endocarditis: Microbiologic and clinical observations as guides to therapy. Ann. Intern. Med. *98*:447–455, 1983.
95. Karp, J. E., Dick, J. D., Angelopulos, C., et al.: Empiric use of vancomycin during prolonged treatment-induced granulocytopenia: Randomized, double-blind, placebo-controlled clinical trial in patients with acute leukemia. Am. J. Med. *81*:237–242, 1986.
96. Keane, W. F., Comty, C. M., Verbrugh, H. A., et al.: Opsonic deficiency of peritoneal dialysis effluent in continuous ambulatory peritoneal dialysis. Kidney Int. *25*:539–543, 1984.
97. Keucher, T. R., and Mealey, J., Jr.: Long-term results after ventriculoatrial and ventriculoperitoneal shunting for infantile hydrocephalus. J. Neurosurg. *50*:79–186, 1979.
98. Kingston, D., Seal, D., and Hill, I. D.: Self-disinfecting plastics for intravenous catheters and prosthetic inserts. J. Hyg. *96*:185–198, 1986.
99. Kirby, W. M. M.: Vancomycin therapy in severe staphylococcal infections. Rev. Infect. Dis. *3*(Suppl.):236–239, 1981.
100. Kline, M. W., Mason, E. O., Jr., and Kaplan, S. L.: Outcome of heteroresistant *Staphylococcus aureus* infections in children. J. Infect. Dis. *156*:205–208, 1987.
101. Kloos, W. E., and Bannerman, T. L.: Update of clinical significance of coagulase-negative staphylococci. Clin. Microbiol. Rev. *7*:117–140, 1994.
102. Kloos, W. E., and Bannerman, T. L.: *Staphylococcus* and *Micrococcus*. *In* Murray, P. R, Baron, E. J., Pfaller, M. A., et al. (eds.): Manual of Clinical Microbiology. 4th ed. Washington, D. C., American Society for Microbiology, 1995, pp. 282–298.
103. Kloos, W. E., and Musselwhite, M. S.: Distribution and persistence of *Staphylococcus* and *Micrococcus* species and other aerobic bacteria on human skin. Appl. Microbiol. *30*:381–385, 1975.
104. Kristinsson, K. G., Hastings, J. G. M., and Spencer, R. C.: The role of extracellular slime in opsonophagocytosis of *Staphylococcus epidermidis*. J. Med. Microbiol. *27*:207–213, 1988.
105. Langley, J., and Gold, R.: Sepsis in febrile neutropenic children with cancer. Pediatr. Infect. Dis. J. *7*:34–37, 1988.
106. Latham, R. H., Running, K., and Stamm, W. E.: Urinary tract infections in young adult women caused by *Staphylococcus saprophyticus*. J. A. M. A. *250*:3063–3066, 1983.
107. Laverdiere, M., Peterson, P. K., and Verhoef, J.: In vitro activity of cephalosporins against methicillin-resistant coagulase-negative staphylococci. J. Infect. Dis. *137*:245–250, 1978.
108. Levison, M. E., and Bush, L.M.: Peritonitis and other intra-abdominal infections. *In* Mandell, G. L., Bennett, J. E., and Dolin, R. (eds.): Principles and Practice of Infectious Diseases. New York, Churchill Livingstone, 1995, pp. 705–740.
109. Lew, D. P.: Physiopathology of foreign body infections. Eur. J. Cancer Clin. Oncol. *25*:1379–1382, 1989.
110. Lewis, J. F., Brake, S. R., Anderson, D. J., et al.: Urinary tract infection due to coagulase-negative *Staphylococcus*. Am. J. Clin. Pathol. *77*:736–739, 1982.
111. Low, D. E., McGeer, A., and Poon, R.: Activities of daptomycin and teicoplanin against *Staphylococcus haemolyticus* and *Staphylococcus epidermidis,* including evaluation of susceptibility testing recommendation. Antimicrob. Agents Chemother. *33*:585–588, 1989.
112. Lowder, J. N., Lazarus, H. M., and Herzig, R. H.: Bacteremias and fungemias in oncologic patients with central venous catheters: Changing spectrum of infection. Arch. Intern. Med. *142*:1456–1459, 1982.
113. Lowy, F. D., Chang, D. S., and Lash, P. R.: Synergy of combinations of vancomycin, gentamicin, and rifampin against methicillin-resistant, coagulase-negative staphylococci. Antimicrob. Agents Chemother. *23*:932–934, 1983.
114. Lowy, F. D., Walsh, J. A., and Mayers, M. M.: Antibiotic activity in-vitro against methicillin-resistant *Staphylococcus epidermidis* and therapy of an experimental infection. Antimicrob. Agents Chemother. *16*:314–321, 1979.
115. Mack, D., Siemssen, N., and Laufs, R.: Parallel induction by glucose of adherence and a polysaccharide antigen specific for plastic-adherent *Staphylococcus epidermidis:* Evidence for functional relation to intracellular adhesion. Infect. Immun. *60*:2048–2057, 1992.
116. Maki, D., Weise, C. E., and Safarin, H. W.: A semi-quantitative culture method for identifying intravenous-catheter-related infection. N. Engl. J. Med. *296*:1305–1309, 1977.
117. Maki, D., Goldman, D., and Rhame, F. S.: Infection control in intravenous therapy. Ann. Intern. Med. *79*:867–887, 1973.
118. Mansour, K. A., Kauten, J. R., and Hatcher, C. R., Jr.: Management of the infected pacemaker: Explanation, sterilization, and reimplantation. Ann. Thorac. Surg. *40*:617–619, 1985.
119. Marples, R. R.: Laboratory assessment in the epidemiology of infections caused by coagulase-negative staphylococci. J. Med. Microbiol. *22*:285–287, 1986.
120. Marrie, T. J., Kwan, C., and Noble, A.: *Staphylococcus saprophyticus* as a cause of urinary tract infections. J. Clin. Microbiol. *16*:427–431, 1982.
121. Marsik, F. J., and Brake, S.: Species identification and susceptibility to 17 antibiotics of coagulase-negative staphylococci isolated from clinical specimens. J. Clin. Microbiol. *15*:640–645, 1982.
122. Martin, M. A., Pfaller, M. A., and Wenzel, R. P.: Coagulase-negative staphylococcal bacteremia: Mortality and hospital stay. Ann. Intern. Med. *110*:9–16, 1989.

123. Masur, H., and Johnson, W. D., Jr.: Prosthetic valve endocarditis. J. Thorac. Cardiovasc. Surg. *80*:31–37, 1980.
124. McCracken, G. H., Jr., and Shinefield, H. R.: Changes in the pattern of neonatal septicemia and meningitis. Am. J. Dis. Child. *112*:33–39, 1966.
125. McDonald, J. A., and Lohr, J. A.: *Staphylococcus epidermidis* pyelonephritis in a previously healthy child. Pediatr. Infect. Dis. J. *13*:1155–1156, 1994.
126. McDougal, L. K., and Thornsberry, C.: New recommendations for disk diffusion antimicrobial susceptibility tests for methicillin-resistant (heteroresistant) staphylococci. J. Clin. Microbiol. *19*:482–488, 1984.
127. McLaurin, R. L., and Frame, P. T.: Treatment of infections of cerebrospinal fluid shunts. Rev. Infect. Dis. *9*:595–603, 1987.
128. Meyers, J. D.: Infection in bone marrow transplant recipients. Am. J. Med. *81*(Suppl. 1A):27–38, 1986.
129. Mickelsen, P. A., Plorde, J. J., Gordon, K. P., et al.: Instability of antibiotic resistance in a strain of *Staphylococcus epidermidis* isolated from an outbreak of prosthetic valve endocarditis. J. Infect. Dis. *152*:50–58, 1985.
130. Mirro, J., Jr., Rao, B. N., Stokes, D. C., et al.: A prospective study of Hickman/Broviac catheters and implantable ports in pediatric oncology patients. J. Clin. Oncol. *7*:214–222, 1989.
131. Munson, D. P., Thompson, T. R., Johnson, D. E., et al.: Coagulase-negative staphylococci septicemia: Experience in a newborn intensive care unit. J. Pediatr. *101*:602–605, 1982.
132. Murtagh, F., and Lehman, R.: Peritoneal shunts in the management of hydrocephalus. J. A. M. A. *202*:1010–1014, 1967.
133. Nafziger, D. A., and Wenzel, R. P.: Coagulase-negative staphylococci: Epidemiology, evaluation, and therapy. Infect. Dis. Clin. North Am. *3*:915–928, 1989.
134. Nataro, J. P., Corcoran, L., Zirin, S., et al.: Prospective analysis of coagulase-negative staphylococcal infections in hospitalized infants. J. Pediatr. *125*:798–804, 1994.
135. Nelson, J. D.: Cerebrospinal fluid shunt infections. Pediatr. Infect. Dis. *3*(Suppl.):S30–S32, 1984.
136. Nicolle, L. E., Hoban, S. A., and Harding, G. K. M.: Characterization of coagulase-negative staphylococci from urinary tract infections. J. Clin. Microbiol. *17*:267–271, 1983.
137. Noel, G. J., O'Loughlin, J. E., and Edelson, P. J.: Neonatal *Staphylococcus epidermidis* right-sided endocarditis: Description of five catheterized infants. Pediatrics *82*:234–239, 1988.
138. Noel, G. J., and Edelson, P. J.: *Staphylococcus epidermidis* bacteremia in neonates: Further observations and the occurrence of focal infection. Pediatrics *74*:832–837, 1984.
139. Oeding, P.: Genus staphylococci. *In* Gergan, T., and Norris, J. R. (eds.): Methods in Microbiology. Vol. 12. New York, Academic Press, 1978, pp. 130–133.
140. Ohshima, Y., Schumacher-Perdreau, F., and Peters, G.: Antiphagocytic effect of the capsule of *Staphylococcus simulans*. Infect. Immun. *58*:1350–1354, 1990.
141. Olsen, L., and Frykberg, T.: Complications in the treatment of hydrocephalus in children: A comparison of ventriculoatrial and ventriculoperitoneal shunts in a 20-year material. Acta Paediatr. Scand. *72*:385–390, 1983.
142. Overturf, G. D., and Balfour, G.: Osteomyelitis and sepsis: Severe complications of fetal monitoring. Pediatrics *55*:244–247, 1975.
143. Paley, D., Moseley, C. F., Armstrong, P., et al.: Primary osteomyelitis caused by coagulase-negative staphylococci. J. Pediatr. Orthop. *6*:622–626, 1986.
144. Parisi, J. T.: Coagulase-negative staphylococci and the epidemiological typing of *Staphylococcus epidermidis*. Microbiol. Rev. *49*:126–139, 1985.
145. Parisi, J. T., and Hecht, D. W.: Plasmid profiles in epidemiologic studies of infections by *Staphylococcus epidermidis*. J. Infect. Dis. *141*:637–643, 1980.
146. Parisi, J. T., Lampson, B. C., Hoover, D. L., et al.: Comparison of epidemiologic markers for *Staphylococcus epidermidis*. J. Clin. Microbiol. *24*:56–60, 1986.
147. Parisi, J. T., Talbot, H. W., Jr., and Skahan, J. M.: Development of a phage typing set for *Staphylococcus epidermidis* in the United States. Zentralbl. Bakteriol. [A] *241*:60–67, 1978.
148. Parker, M. A., and Tuazon, C. U.: Cervical osteomyelitis: Infection due to *Staphylococcus epidermidis* in hemodialysis patients. J. A. M. A. *240*:50–51, 1978.
149. Pascual, A., Fleer, A., Westerdaal, N. A. C., et al.: Modulation of adherence of coagulase-negative staphylococci to teflon catheters in vitro. Eur. J. Clin. Microbiol. *5*:518–522, 1986.
150. Patrick C. C.: Coagulase-negative staphylococci: Pathogens with increasing clinical significance. J. Pediatr. *116*:497–507, 1990.
151. Patrick, C. C., Kaplan, S. L., Baker, C. J., et al.: Persistent bacteremia due to coagulase-negative staphylococci in low birth weight neonates. Pediatrics *84*:977–985, 1989.
152. Patrick, C. C., Plaunt, M. R., Sweet, S. M., et al.: Defining *Staphylococcus epidermidis* cell wall proteins. J. Clin. Microbiol. *28*:2757–2760, 1990.
153. Patrick, C. C., Shenep, J. L., and Crawford, R.: Coagulase-negative *Staphylococcus* (ConS) bacteremia in a children's cancer hospital [Abstract]. Houston, Texas, Interscience Conference on Antimicrobial Agents and Chemotherapy, Abstract 644, 1989, p. 209.
154. Pereira, A. T.: Coagulase-negative strains of *Staphylococcus* possessing antigen 51 as agents of urinary tract infection. J. Clin. Pathol. *15*:252–253, 1962.
155. Peters, G., and Pulverer, G.: Pathogenesis and management of *Staphylococcus epidermidis* "plastic" foreign body infections. J. Antimicrob. Chemother. *14*(Suppl. D):67–71, 1984.
156. Peters, G., Saborowski, F., Locci, R., et al.: Investigations on staphylococcal infection of transvenous endocardial pacemaker electrodes. Am. Heart J. *108*:359–365, 1984.
157. Peters, G., von Eiff, C., and Herrmann, M.: The changing pattern of coagulase-negative staphylococci as infectious pathogens. Curr. Opin. Infect. Dis. *8*(Suppl. 1):512–519, 1995.
158. Peterson, P. K., Matzke, G., and Keane, W. F.: Current concepts in the management of peritonitis in patients undergoing continuous ambulatory peritoneal dialysis. Rev. Infect. Dis. *9*:604–612, 1987.
159. Peyman, G. A., Carroll, C. P., and Raichand, M.: Prevention and management of traumatic endophthalmitis. Ophthalmology *87*:320–324, 1980.
160. Pfaller, M. A, and Herwaldt, L. A.: Laboratory, clinical, and epidemiological aspects of coagulase-negative staphylococci. Clin. Microbiol. Rev. *1*:281–299, 1988.
161. Pizzo, P. A., Hathorn, J. W., Hiemenz, J., et al.: A randomized trial comparing ceftazidime alone with combination antibiotic therapy in cancer patients with fever and neutropenia. N. Engl. J. Med. *315*:552–558, 1986.
162. Pizzo, P. A, Ladisch, S., Simon, R. M., et al.: Increasing incidence of gram-positive sepsis in cancer patients. Med. Pediatr. Oncol. *5*:241–244, 1978.
163. Ponce De Leon, S., and Wenzel, R. P.: Hospital-acquired bloodstream infections with *Staphylococcus epidermidis:* Review of 100 cases. Am. J. Med. *77*:639–644, 1984.
164. Power, J., Wing, E. J., Talamo, T. S., et al.: Fatal bacterial endocarditis as a complication of permanent indwelling catheters: Report of two cases. Am. J. Med. *81*:166–168, 1986.
165. Press, O. W., Ramsey, P. G., Larson, E. B., et al.: Hickman catheter infections in patients with malignancies. Medicine (Baltimore) *63*:189–200, 1984.
166. Raucher, H. S., Hyatt, A. C., and Barzilai, A.: Quantitative blood cultures in the evaluation of septicemia in children with Broviac catheters. J. Pediatr. *104*:29–33, 1984.
167. Reybrouck, G.: Handwashing and hand disinfection. J. Hosp. Infect. *8*:5–23, 1986.
168. Ross, M. N., Haase, G. M., and Poole, M. A.: Comparison of totally implanted reservoirs with external catheters as venous access devices in pediatric oncologic patients. Surg. Gynecol. Obstet. *167*:141, 1988.
169. Rotbart, H. A., Johnson, Z. T., and Reller, L. B.: Analysis of enteric coagulase-negative staphylococci from neonates with necrotizing enterocolitis. Pediatr. Infect. Dis. J. *8*:140–142, 1989.
170. Rupp, M. E., and Archer, G.: Hemagglutination and adherence to plastic by *Staphylococcus epidermidis*. Infect. Immun. *60*:1055–1060, 1992.
171. Rupp, M. E., and Archer, G. L.: Coagulase-negative staphylococci: Pathogens associated with medical progress. Clin. Infect. Dis. *19*:231–245, 1994.
172. Sabath, L. D.: Reappraisal of the antistaphylococcal activities of first-generation (narrow-spectrum) and second-generation (expanded-spectrum) cephalosporins. Antimicrob. Agents Chemother. *33*:407–411, 1989.
173. Sabath, L. D., Garner, C., Wilcox, C., et al.: Susceptibility of *Staphylococcus aureus* and *Staphylococcus epidermidis* to 65 antibiotics. Antimicrob. Agents Chemother. *9*:962–969, 1976.
174. Sattler, F. R., Foderaro, J. B., and Aber, R. C.: *Staphylococcus epidermidis* bacteremia associated with vascular catheters: An important cause of febrile morbidity in hospitalized patients. Infect. Control *5*:279–283, 1984.
175. Schaberg, D. R., Culver, D. H., and Gaynes, R. P.: Major trends in the microbial etiology of nosocomial infections. Am. J. Med. *91*(Suppl. 3B):72–75, 1991.
176. Schaberg, D. R., and Zervos, M. J.: Intergeneric and interspecies gene exchange in gram-positive cocci. Antimicrob. Agents Chemother. *30*:817–822, 1986.
177. Schaberg, D. R., and Zervos, M.: Plasmid analysis in the study of the epidemiology of nosocomial gram-positive cocci. Rev. Infect. Dis. *8*:705–712, 1986.
178. Scheifele, D. W., Bjornson, G. L., Dyer, R. A., et al.: Delta-like toxin produced by coagulase-negative staphylococci is associated with neonatal necrotizing enterocolitis. Infect. Immun. *55*:2268–2273, 1987.
179. Scheretz, R. J., Falk, R. J., Huffman, K. A., et al.: Infections associated with subclavian Udall catheters. Arch. Intern. Med. *143*:52–56, 1983.
180. Schimke, R. T., Black, P. H., Mark, V. H., et al.: Indolent *Staphylococcus albus* or *aureus* bacteremia after ventriculoatriostomy: Role of foreign body in its initiation and perpetuation. N. Engl. J. Med. *264*:264–270, 1961.
181. Schwalbe, R. S., Stapleton, J. T., and Gilligan, P. H.: Emergence of vancomycin resistance in coagulase-negative staphylococci. N. Engl. J. Med. *316*:927–931, 1987.
182. Shenep, J. L., Hughes, W. T., Robertson, P. K., et al.: Vancomycin, ticarcillin and amikacin compared with ticarcillin-clavulanate and amikacin in the empirical treatment of febrile, neutropenic children with cancer. N. Engl. J. Med. *319*:1053–1058, 1988.
183. Sheth, N. K., Franson, T. R., Rose, H. D., et al.: Colonization of bacteria on polyvinyl chloride and Teflon intravascular catheters in hospitalized patients. J. Clin. Microbiol. *18*:1061–1063, 1983.
184. Sheth, N. K., Franson, T. R., and Sohnle, P. G.: Influence of bacterial

adherence to intravascular catheters on *in vitro* antibiotic susceptibility. Lancet 2:1266–1268, 1985.
185. Shiro, H., Muller, E., Guttierrez, N., et al.: Transposon mutants or *Staphylococcus epidermidis* deficient in elaboration of capsular polysaccharide/adhesion and slime are avirulent in a rabbit model or endocarditis. J. Infect. Dis. *169*:1042–1049, 1994.
186. Shiro, H., Muller, E., Takeda, S., et al.: Potentiation of *Staphylococcus epidermidis* catheter-related bacteremia by lipid infusions. J. Infect. Dis. *171*:220–224, 1995.
187. Shoenbaum, S. C., Gardner, P., and Shillito, J.: Infections of cerebrospinal fluid shunts: Epidemiology, clinical manifestations, and therapy. J. Infect. Dis. *131*:543–552, 1975.
188. Shulman, R. J., Smith, E. O., Rahman, S., et al.: Single- vs double-lumen central venous catheters in pediatric oncology patients. Am. J. Dis. Child. *142*:893–895, 1988.
189. Siebert, W. T., Moreland, N., and Williams, T. W., Jr.: Methicillin-resistant *Staphylococcus epidermidis*. South. Med. J. *71*:1353–1355, 1978.
190. Sitges-Serra, A., Puig, P., and Jaurrieta, E.: Catheter sepsis due to *Staphylococcus epidermidis* during parenteral nutrition. Surg. Gynecol. Obstet. *151*:481–483, 1980.
191. Skahan, J. M., and Parisi, J. T.: Development of a bacteriophage-typing set for *Staphylococcus epidermidis*. J. Clin. Microbiol. *6*:16–18, 1977.
192. Slama, T. G., Sklar, S. J., Misinski, J., et al.: Randomized comparison of cefamandole, cefazolin, and cefuroxime prophylaxis in open-heart surgery. Antimicrob. Agents Chemother. *29*:744–747, 1986.
193. Smith, I. M., Beals, P. D., Kinsbury, K. R., et al.: Observations on *Staphylococcus albus* septicemia in mice and men. Arch. Intern. Med. *102*:375–388, 1958.
194. Smith, J. A., Henry, D. A., Bourgault, A., et al: Comparison of agar disk diffusion, microdilution broth, and agar dilution for testing antimicrobial susceptibility of coagulase-negative staphylococci. J. Clin. Microbiol. *25*:1741–1746, 1987.
195. St. Geme, J. W., III, Bell, L. M., Baumgart, S., et al.: Distinguishing sepsis from blood culture contamination in young infants with blood cultures growing coagulase-negative staphylococci. Pediatrics *86*:157–162, 1990.
196. Stillman, R. I., Wenzel, R. P., and Donowitz, L. C.: Emergence of coagulase-negative staphylococci as major nosocomial bloodstream pathogens. Infect. Control *8*:108–112, 1987.
197. Talbot, H. W., Jr., and Parisi, J. T.: Phage typing of *Staphylococcus epidermidis*. J. Clin. Microbiol. *3*:519–523, 1976.
198. Tan, T. Q., Mason, E. O., Jr., Ou, C. N., et al.: Use of intravenous rifampin in neonates with persistent staphylococcal bacteremia. Antimicrob. Agents Chemother. *37*:2401–2406, 1993.
199. Tan, T. Q., Musser, J. M., Shulman, R. J., et al.: Molecular epidemiology of coagulase-negative staphylococcus blood isolated from neonates with persistent bacteremia and children with central venous catheter infections. J. Infect. Dis. *169*:1393–1397, 1994.
200. Tebbs, S. E., and Elliott, T. S. J.: Modification of central venous catheter polymers to prevent in vitro microbial colonization. Eur. J. Clin. Microbiol. Inf. Dis. *13*:111–117, 1994.
201. Tenckhoff, H., and Schechter, H.: A bacteriologically safe peritoneal access device. Trans. Am. Soc. Artif. Intern. Organs *14*:181–187, 1968.
202. Thomson-Carter, F. M., and Pennington, T. H.: Characterization of coagulase-negative staphylococci by sodium dodecyl sulfate-polyacrylamide gel electrophoresis and immunoblot analysis. J. Clin. Microbiol. *27*:2199–2203, 1989.
203. Timmermann, C. P., Fleer, A., Besnier, J. M., et al.: Characterization of a proteinaceous adhesion of *Staphylococcus epidermidis* which mediates attachment to polystyrene. Infect. Immun. *59*:4187–4192, 1991.
204. Tojo, M., Yamashita, N., Goldmann, D. A., et al.: Isolation and characterization of a capsular polysaccharide adhesion from *Staphylococcus epidermidis*. J. Infect. Dis. *157*:713–722, 1988.
205. Tully, J. L., Friedland, G. H., Baldini, L. M., et al.: Complications of intravenous therapy with steel needles and small-bore Teflon catheters: A comparative study. Am. J. Med. *70*:702–706, 1981.
206. Van Bronswijk, H., Verbrugh, H. A., Heezius, C. J. M., et al.: Heterogeneity in opsonic requirements of *Staphylococcus epidermidis:* Relative importance of surface hydrophobicity, capsules and slime. Immunology *67*:81–86, 1989.
207. Venditti, M., Santini, C., Serra, P., et al.: Comparative *in vitro* activities of new fluorinated quinolones and other antibiotics against coagulase-negative *Staphylococcus* blood isolates from neutropenic patients, and relationship between susceptibility and slime production. Antimicrob. Agents Chemother. *33*:209–211, 1989.
208. Viscoli, C., Garaventa, A., Boni, L., et al.: Role of Broviac catheters in infections in children with cancer. Pediatr. Infect. Dis. J. *7*:556–560, 1988.
209. Wachsmuth, K.: Molecular epidemiology of bacterial infections: Examples of methodology and investigations of outbreaks. Rev. Infect. Dis. *8*:682–692, 1986.
210. Wade, J. C., Schimpft, S. C., Newman, K. A., et al.: *Staphylococcus epidermidis:* An increasing cause of infection in patients with granulocytopenia. Ann. Intern. Med. *97*:503–508, 1982.
211. Wadstrom, T., and Rozgonyi, F.: Virulence determinants of coagulase-negative staphylococci. *In* Mardh, P. A., and Schleifer, K. H. (eds.): Coagulase-Negative Staphylococci. Stockholm, Almquist and Wiksel International, 1986, pp. 123–130.
212. Watanakunakorn, C.: Prosthetic valve infection endocarditis. Prog. Cardiovasc. Dis. *22*:181–192, 1979.
213. Wilson, A. P. R., O'Hare, M. D., Felmingham, D., et al.: Teicoplanin-resistant coagulase-negative *Staphylococcus*. Lancet *2*:973, 1986.
214. Wilson, C. B.: Immunologic basis for increased susceptibility of the neonate to infection. J. Pediatr. *108*:1–12, 1986.
215. Wilson, W. R., Jaumin, P. M., Danielson, G. K., et al.: Prosthetic valve endocarditis. Ann. Intern. Med. *82*:751–756, 1975.
216. Winston, D. J., Dudnick, D. V., Chapin, M., et al.: Coagulase-negative staphylococcal bacteremia in patients receiving immunosuppressive therapy. Arch. Intern. Med. *143*:32–36, 1983.
217. Yamada, T., Ichiman, Y., and Yoshida, K.: Possible common biological and immunological properties for detecting encapsulated strains of *Staphylococcus epidermidis*. J. Clin. Microbiol. *26*:2167–2172, 1988.
218. Yogev, R.: Cerebrospinal fluid shunt infections: A personal view. Pediatr. Infect. Dis. *4*:113–118, 1985.
219. Yoshida, K., Umeda, A., Ichiman, T., et al.: Cross protection between a strain of *Staphylococcus epidermidis* and eight other species of coagulase-negative staphylococci. Can. J. Microbiol. *34*:913–915, 1988.
220. Younger, J. J., Christensen, G. D., Bartley, D. L., et al.: Coagulase-negative staphylococci isolated from cerebrospinal fluid shunts: Importance of slime production, species identification and shunt removal to clinical outcome. J. Infect. Dis. *156*:548–554, 1987.
221. Zakrzewska-Czerwinska, J., Mordarski, M., Goodfellow, M., et al.: Deoxyribonucleic acid relatedness amongst *Staphylococcus epidermidis* and *Staphylococcus saprophyticus* strains. Zentralbl. Bakteriol. Mikrobiol. Hyg. *269*:179–187, 1988.
222. Zimmerman, R. J., and Kloos, W. E.: Comparative zone electrophoresis of esterases of *Staphylococcus* species isolated from mammalian skin. Can. J. Microbiol. *22*:771–779, 1976.

87

GROUP A, GROUP C, AND GROUP G BETA-HEMOLYTIC STREPTOCOCCAL INFECTIONS

Edward L. Kaplan and Michael A. Gerber

GROUP A STREPTOCOCCAL INFECTIONS

Group A beta-hemolytic streptococci are among the most common pathogenic bacteria isolated from children. They are associated with a wide variety of infections and disease states. Although uniformly sensitive to penicillin and exquisitely sensitive to many other antibiotics, group A streptococcal infections continue to present formidable clinical and public health problems for pediatricians and other primary care physicians. Although the vast majority of group A streptococcal infections are of short duration and relatively benign, they may be fulminating and life-threatening. The importance of group A streptococcal infections has been reinforced at the close of the twentieth century by the resurgence of acute rheumatic fever in the United States[90] as well as the appearance of a group A streptococcal toxic shock syndrome with very high morbidity and mortality.[120] Additionally, the bacterium is different from other pyogenic bacteria because of the potential for delayed, nonsuppurative sequelae (e.g., acute glomerulonephritis, acute rheumatic fever).

The Organism

Streptococcus pyogenes (group A *Streptococcus*) is a gram-positive coccus, forming either short or long chains. Group A streptococci produce clear (beta) hemolysis on blood agar, a bacteriologic feature important in their recognition and in their differentiation from nonhemolytic (gamma) streptococci and from viridans (alpha) streptococci, which cause partial or green hemolysis on blood agar. Although hemolysis is produced on culture plates containing blood from a variety of mammalian species, sheep or horse blood gives the clearest differentiation. Some strains of group A streptococci hemolyze red blood cells slowly or even result in almost greenish hemolysis on the surface of blood agar plates incubated aerobically. These strains can be recognized by their ability to produce clear hemolysis under anaerobic conditions. This is achieved readily by routinely making a short cut or stab into the blood agar at the time of inoculation. Incubation with carbon dioxide or in a candle jar also can be helpful in enhancing beta hemolysis. Rare strains of group A streptococci are not hemolytic.[64, 69]

More than 80 different serotypes of group A streptococci have been recognized on the basis of a series of serologically distinct surface proteins, the M proteins.[88] The M serotypes of streptococci associated with impetigo and pyoderma are different from those associated with clinical pharyngitis, although a few M types have the capacity to produce both kinds of infection.[6] The M protein renders the group A *Streptococcus* resistant to phagocytosis and therefore is a major virulence factor for these organisms. There is new evidence that many more serotypes exist that have not been characterized yet.[78]

The group A streptococcal cell is a complex structure. In rapidly dividing strains (e.g., young cultures, epidemic strains), the cell is covered with a hyaluronic acid capsule, which gives the colonies a mucoid appearance. Protruding from the cell surface and into the hyaluronic capsular layer are hairlike fimbriae, which are responsible for adherence of group A streptococci to epithelial cells. A basic chemical component of these fimbriae is lipoteichoic acid.[11] The M protein also is associated with these fimbriae.[47] Other surface proteins of interest are the T and R proteins, the SOR (serum opacity reaction) proteins, and proteins that bind nonspecifically to the Fc fragment of gamma globulins. The function and the exact location of these other proteins on the surface of the organism have not been identified precisely. However, they may be useful epidemiologic markers, particularly in strains difficult to M type. Strains of a particular M type generally are associated with a particular T pattern,[68] and in strains producing serum opacity, the serologically specific SOR protein correlates closely with the M type of the strain. At present, there are almost 30 recognized opacity factor–positive types of group A streptococci; undoubtedly, there are others that have not been characterized yet. All of these characteristics are very useful in epidemiologic studies of streptococcal infections, either in an individual or in a community.

In addition to these surface proteins, the carbohydrate moiety responsible for group specificity (e.g., group A carbohydrate) also is found in the cell wall in a position sufficiently superficial to permit reaction with antibody specifically directed toward it. The group A carbohydrate is a polymer of rhamnose units with side chains of N-acetyl-glucosamine, which is responsible for its group specificity.[94] The structure providing rigidity for the cell wall is another large polymer, a peptidoglycan, consisting of glycan strands cross-linked by peptide bridges. Its role in the pathogenesis of infection is poorly defined.

Within the cell wall of the group A *Streptococcus* lies the cell membrane, composed mainly of lipoprotein or lipid-protein complexes. This membrane is the outer surface of the osmotically fragile protoplasts or L forms of streptococci. These wall-less forms of group A streptococci are resistant to penicillin and other cell wall–inhibiting antibiotics.[49]

Intracellular constituents of the group A streptococci include, in addition to DNA and RNA, a number of enzymes and hemolysins.[23] Plasmids have been identified that control resistance to certain antibiotics, for example, erythromycin.[89] Bacteriophages play an important role in the genetics of group A streptococci, including the transfer of the determinants of antibiotic resistance and the control of erythrogenic toxin production.[131, 136]

Group A streptococci produce and release into the surrounding medium a large number of biologically active extracellular products. Some of these are toxic for human and other mammalian cells. Both streptolysin O (the oxygen-labile hemolysin) and streptolysin S (the oxygen-stable hemolysin) injure cell membranes, lysing not only red blood cells but also damaging other eukaryotic cells and membranous subcellular organelles, including myocardial cells.[14] Streptolysin O is antigenic; streptolysin S is not. The latter hemolysin is bound loosely to the streptococcal cell and is released in a complexed, stable form with a variety of carrier molecules. The erythrogenic or pyrogenic exotoxins resemble endotoxin in exhibiting both a primary or intrinsic toxicity and a secondary toxicity resulting from the acquisition of host hypersensitivity.[83] The late 1980s outbreak of the streptococcal toxic shock syndrome has been reported to be associated with the reappearance of strains making pyrogenic exotoxin A, but a number of unanswered questions remain about the precise pathogenesis.[117] Group A streptococci also produce bacteriocins,[121] low-molecular-weight proteins that can kill a variety of other gram-positive bacterial species and thus may play a role in promoting infection or even persistence of colonization.

Many of the other extracellular products of group A streptococci are specific enzymes that do not appear to be directly toxic for mammalian or bacterial cells but digest or initiate the breakdown of important biologic substrates. These include the deoxyribonucleases (nucleases A, B, C, and D), the streptokinases (which activate the fibrinolytic or plasmin-plasminogen system), a hyaluronidase, an amylase, a proteinase, an esterase, and an NADase (nicotinamide adenine dinucleotidase). Several of these are antigenic; measuring their antibodies can be useful clinically (e.g., DNase B, streptokinase, hyaluronidase, NADase).

Transmission

The mechanism of spread of streptococci from one person to another and from one body site to another varies according to the clinical manifestations of the infection.

Epidemiologic studies of patients with streptococcal sore throat indicate that airborne routes of spread (by small droplet nuclei, dust) and environmental contamination (e.g., contaminated clothing or bedding) play little, if any, role in spread of this kind of group A streptococcal infection.[103] Close contact is required for transmission of streptococcal pharyngitis to occur, apparently by direct projection of large droplets or by physical transfer of respiratory secretions containing the infectious bacteria. Spread within family units, school rooms, or other crowded facilities, such as military barracks, is common.

The period of greatest contagiousness of streptococcal pharyngitis and scarlet fever is during the acute stage of the illness. Most antibiotic therapy (especially penicillin) rapidly suppresses the growth of group A streptococci and, if continued, usually eradicates them from the upper respiratory tract; the patient can be considered much less contagious after 36 to 48 hours of antimicrobial therapy. Most physicians believe that children can return to school by that time, especially if they are afebrile, with little risk of spread of the organism to close contacts.[117]

Although humans with active but subclinical infection also may contribute to the spread of group A streptococci, the role of throat "carriers" is less certain. Most secondary spread occurs during the first 2 weeks after acquisition.[130] It is rare for streptococcal upper respiratory tract carriers to spread the organism.[72] In contrast to throat carriage, which may persist for weeks or months, the prolonged presence of group A streptococci in the anterior nares is unusual and, when present, suggests chronic sinusitis.

Contaminated food or milk also may result in group A streptococcal infection of the throat, producing a common source outbreak.[61] Salads containing hard-boiled eggs (e.g., egg salad) appear to be a special problem.

Anal carriers have been identified as the source of contagion in several hospital outbreaks of streptococcal wound infections. Some studies have suggested that rectal or anal carriers may be more common than suspected.[84]

In contrast to the upper respiratory tract, where group A *Streptococcus* readily can establish infection on an intact epithelial surface, the production of streptococcal impetigo or pyoderma appears to require prior disruption of the skin by trauma, insects, or some preexisting skin disorder. Group A streptococci may be found on the normal skin for several days to 2 weeks before infection develops,[46] requiring some other means of access. It does not seem likely that the source of infection for streptococcal skin infections is the upper respiratory tract. Group A streptococci causing impetigo may be found in the nose or throat, but they usually do not reach this site until several weeks after the establishment of cutaneous infection. One possible source is a skin lesion in another child, with spread occurring by direct contact. There even are data to suggest spread by small flies that feed on such lesions.[10] However, the exact role of environmental contamination in the spread of streptococcal impetigo and pyoderma and in secondary infection of wounds, burns, and eczema and other dermatoses is not known. The mechanism of transmission of erysipelas also is poorly understood but may involve spread via the respiratory tract.

Measures to prevent spread of group A streptococcal infections are variable in their effectiveness. Spread of throat or skin infection within a family unit often occurs before the index case is identified and isolated or treated. In epidemic situations, especially when there are cases of rheumatic fever or acute nephritis, a culture survey with treatment of all individuals with positive cultures (mass prophylaxis) may be indicated. Reduction of crowding, especially in sleeping quarters, seems to be an effective long-term method of minimizing spread of streptococcal sore throat among some population groups. In families in which persistence or recurrence of streptococcal infection is a problem, simultaneous throat culture and/or culture of skin lesions of all members and treatment of all positives has been successful. Some have advocated a role for family pets (dogs) in transmission of streptococcal infections. However, available data do not support such transmission as a common occurrence.[15, 32, 134] Control of environmental contamination would be expected to have little or no influence on the spread of group A streptococcal respiratory infections, although it possibly may have an effect in controlling skin or wound infections.

Epidemiology

Group A streptococci appear to have a narrow host range. They are one of the pathogenic bacteria identified most frequently in man but rarely are found in other species.[88] In considering the epidemiology of group A streptococcal infections, it is necessary to recognize the differences between throat and skin infections.[126]

Streptococcal impetigo occurs with greatest frequency in preschool children, whereas streptococcal pharyngitis predominantly is a disease of school-age children. Outbreaks of streptococcal respiratory tract infections also have been observed in day care centers.[116] On the average, streptococcal respiratory infections occur at the rate of one every 3 to 5 years during childhood. Among preschool and early school-age children of certain population groups, streptococcal impetigo also tends to be a recurrent disease.

The seasonal occurrence and geographic distribution are different for throat and skin infections. Tonsillitis and pharyngitis caused by streptococci are common in temperate and cold climates; streptococcal pyoderma and impetigo appear to occur with greater frequency in hot or tropical climates. Streptococcal sore throat is more frequent in late autumn, winter, and spring months. In tropical climates, pharyngeal colonization appears to be more common during the rainy season. Streptococcal impetigo usually is a disease of the summer months in temperate climates but may occur with equal frequency year-round in tropical countries. In some tropical countries, groups C and G hemolytic streptococci are isolated more frequently from the upper respiratory tract than group A.

Pathogenesis

No complete explanation is available for the predilection of certain body sites for infection by group A streptococci or for the ability of strains of certain M types to produce pharyngitis or tonsillitis and of others to produce impetigo or pyoderma.

In the establishment of throat infection, a primary requisite is a method of attachment to the epithelial cells of the pharynx. The group A streptococci accomplish this by means of their fimbriae (see earlier). In order to initiate an infection, group A streptococci also must compete with the resident pharyngeal flora, notably the alpha-hemolytic or viridans streptococci, which may interfere with the colonization of group A streptococci in the throat,[33] perhaps as a result of the production of a bacteriocin-like substance.[38] However, the importance of bacterial interference in preventing colonization of the upper respiratory tract with group A streptococci is not entirely clear. In fact, the influence of bacteriocin-like substance producers may be minimal in certain situations.[63]

In the production of impetigo, group A streptococci also

must vie with other local bacterial flora. Removal of the normal flora increases the time of survival of group A streptococci applied to the skin.[3] Skin lipids, which are lethal for group A streptococci in vitro, also may provide a natural barrier against the establishment of streptococcal infection.

Invasion of the tissues by group A streptococci may be facilitated by a combination of bacteriologic properties. Damage to leukocytes and to fixed tissue cells may result from any of the several toxins produced, and the spread of infection may be aided by specific enzymes that attack hyaluronic acid and fibrin (see earlier). The M protein, a surface component of virulent strains, is antiphagocytic and also contains a moiety that is cytotoxic in the presence of non–type-specific antibody.[13] The hyaluronic acid capsule of group A *Streptococcus* may serve as a camouflage because it resembles mammalian hyaluronic acid. In addition, several streptococcal substances (the streptococcal pyrogenic exotoxins and the peptidoglycan) have been shown to have endotoxin-like properties. A role for the pyrogenic exotoxins has been postulated for streptococcal toxic shock syndrome and for necrotizing fasciitis.[119]

The factors responsible for the early host defense against group A streptococci (before the development of antibody) are poorly understood. Type-specific antibody against M protein, which greatly promotes phagocytosis, usually is not detectable until 6 to 8 weeks after the initiation of infection[39]; therefore, its primary role may not be in the limitation or termination of active infection but rather in the prevention of reinfection by the same serologic type. Surface phagocytosis, first by monocytes and later by polymorphonuclear leukocytes, may be the primary mechanism of defense in the early stages of infection.[109] In streptococcal skin infections, an increase in the leukotactic activity of polymorphonuclear leukocytes has been reported.[52]

About 30 minutes after ingestion by a polymorphonuclear leukocyte, the streptococcus may be killed. Occasionally, the reverse occurs due to a phenomenon known as leukotoxicity, which apparently is related to the production of streptolysin S.[97] Degradation of the streptococcus within phagocytes or in tissues is a much slower process, suggesting that the human host may not be able to break down the streptococcal cell wall in an efficient manner.[52]

Spread of streptococci to the regional lymph nodes is common, especially in infections of the pharynx and tonsils.[38] Bacteremia occurs in the absence of underlying systemic disease, such as leukemia or other malignancies,[43, 56] but it is uncommon in older children and adults. The reason(s) for the apparent increase of severe systemic group A streptococcal infections in the 1980s and 1990s remains incompletely explained.

The rash and other toxic manifestations of scarlet fever have been attributed to the development of hypersensitivity to the erythrogenic (pyrogenic) toxins.[93] Toxic manifestations that have been noted in the group A streptococcal toxic shock syndrome also may result from a direct influence of the pyrogenic exotoxins on lymphokines, such as tumor necrosis factor.[119] Hypersensitivity to other streptococcal products also may contribute to the manifestations of streptococcal disease.

There are many theories about the pathogenetic mechanism(s) leading to the development of the nonsuppurative complications of streptococcal infections, acute rheumatic fever, and acute glomerulonephritis. Most of these hypotheses invoke immunologic processes in one way or another.[93]

Clinical Manifestations

Streptococcal pharyngitis or tonsillitis usually is a short-term illness with a short incubation period (12 hours to 4 days). It varies greatly in its severity, from a subclinical or almost subclinical form, occurring in 30 to 50 per cent of infections, to a very toxic form with high fever, nausea, vomiting, and collapse. Extreme toxicity may be more frequent in epidemic situations, especially food-borne outbreaks, suggesting the importance of the rapid passage of the infecting organism in determining the severity of infection. The onset is acute and may be marked by fever, sore throat, headache, or abdominal pain (more common in children). The tonsils and pharynx may appear inflamed or infected but in the presence of marked edema may look pale. Exudate is common (50 to 90 per cent). It usually appears by the second day and typically is discrete and whitish yellow and may become confluent by the following day. Swollen, tender anterior cervical lymph nodes (adenitis) also can be observed in 30 to 60 per cent of the patients.

The clinical manifestations subside spontaneously in 3 to 5 days unless suppurative complications (otitis media, sinusitis, peritonsillar abscess) develop. In the relatively few patients who develop nonsuppurative sequelae, there usually is a latent period of several days to several weeks during which the child or adult seems completely well. After streptococcal infection of the upper respiratory tract, the average latent period for acute glomerulonephritis is 10 days; for acute rheumatic fever, the average latent period is 18 days.[126]

An infantile form of streptococcal infection, referred to as streptococcal fever, may take a more prolonged course, with chronic low-grade fever, generalized effect on the lymph nodes, and a persistent serous nasal discharge; there is little or no evidence of localized inflammation in the pharyngeal area. The term streptococcosis, which sometimes has been used to refer specifically to this infantile form, should be employed more correctly to indicate the broad spectrum of clinical pictures that change with age in a manner somewhat analogous to tuberculosis.[102]

Scarlet fever is rare in infancy. Initially, this may be because of the possibility of placental transfer of maternal antibody to the erythrogenic (pyrogenic) toxins. A more basic reason appears to be the necessity for hypersensitization to these exotoxins to develop before this manifestation of streptococcal disease can be expressed.[83] The severe toxic form of scarlet fever was rare in most countries; milder forms of the disease were prevalent. However, in the late 1980s, an increase in scarlet fever also was seen in Western Europe. In the late 1980s, numerous reports of an illness characterized by scarlet fever–like rash but with severe systemic manifestations, including fasciitis, myositis, adult respiratory distress syndrome, and very high mortality (up to 30 per cent), became more evident in the United States.[19]

The characteristic rash is red and finely punctate, appearing initially on the trunk and spreading peripherally to cover almost the entire body in full-blown cases within several hours to several days. A typical feature of the rash is that it fades on pressure and almost always leads to desquamation. Petechiae may develop in the folds of the joints (Pastia lines) or in other areas of the extremities. The strawberry tongue of scarlet fever has a swollen, red, and mottled appearance and eventually peels. A scarlatiniform rash also may occur with streptococcal impetigo and streptococcal wound infections. An enanthema of stippled, bright red or hemorrhagic spots may appear on the soft palate or the anterior pillars of the tonsillar fossae. Exudate and tender cervical nodes may be present as in streptococcal pharyngitis without a rash, but the pharyngeal signs sometimes are minimal.

Streptococcal impetigo may develop a few days up to several weeks after deposition of the infecting strain on the normal skin; the average latent period is 10 days.[46] In contrast to pharyngitis, this form of group A streptococcal infection frequently is painless, and the patient usually is afebrile. The initial lesion is a superficial vesicle with little surrounding erythema. This rapidly progresses to a pustule and then to a thick, honey-colored crust; this stage may last for a few days to several weeks. Secondary infection with staphylococci is common in the pustular and crust stages.[37, 40] Removal of the crusts by trauma or as part of local therapy reveals a moist or purulent undersurface in the earlier stages. The infection does not involve the dermis. On healing, depigmentation may be seen, but rarely is there permanent scarring. The lesions are most common on the lower extremities but may occur on other exposed portions of the body, such as the upper extremities and the face.

Acute poststreptococcal glomerulonephritis may follow impetigo or other forms of cutaneous streptococcal infection produced by a nephritogenic strain; curiously, however, rheumatic fever has not been associated with streptococcal skin infections.[129] The latent period for acute nephritis is much longer after skin infection (3 weeks on average) than after throat infection (10 days on average).[75] The serologic types associated with nephritis after skin infection usually are different from those causing nephritis after throat infection.[126] For example, M-12 has been the classic nephritogenic serotype associated with pharyngitis, whereas serotypes such as M-49, M-55, and M-57 have been associated more frequently with nephritis occurring after skin infection.[126]

Impetigo and more nondescript forms of streptococcal pyoderma may be superimposed upon scabies, eczema, other dermatoses, burns, and wounds, which afford a means of access through the cutaneous barrier. Ecthyma is a more deep-seated and chronic form of streptococcal pyoderma found predominantly in tropical climates.[1]

Erysipelas is a peculiar type of streptococcal infection involving the skin and sometimes the adjacent mucous membranes. It is an elevated erythematous lesion, sometimes exhibiting blebs filled with yellowish fluid, which may crust over after rupture. The lesion is characterized by a well-demarcated advancing border, more reddened and edematous than the central area, which may fade and become more normal in appearance as the lesion progresses. Erysipelas most often involves the face (especially in children), the extremities, or the body. The lesion may surround a surgical or traumatic wound, an area of dermatosis, or the umbilical stump in a newborn infant. Erysipelas tends not to spread from one body region to another. In erysipelas, the onset is acute and often is accompanied by the manifestations of systemic toxicity characteristic of other febrile forms of streptococcal infection. The lesion may last for a few days to several weeks. Relapses are rather common, with recurrences frequently at the same body site.

In addition to the infections described earlier, group A streptococci may produce a variety of other clinical pictures. Other infections associated with upper respiratory tract infections by these organisms include otitis media, sinusitis, mastoiditis, pneumonia, and empyema. Beta-hemolytic streptococci are recoverable from about 50 per cent of patients with peritonsillar abscess and may act in concert with anaerobic bacteria in the production of this clinical picture.[48] Acute puerperal sepsis, now fortunately rare, classically has been associated with group A streptococci. Nursery outbreaks of omphalitis, bacteremia, and meningitis still are reported on occasion.[122] Fatal gangrene,[53] disseminated intravascular coagulopathy,[66] and purpura fulminans[31] may be associated with infection by group A streptococci. These bacteria also are a common cause of perianal cellulitis and vaginitis in children.[4, 84] Subpectoral abscesses and pleural effusion may develop as complications of streptococcal infections of the thumb because of lymphocytic drainage.[4] Septic complications of varicella, including varicella gangrenosa,[22, 115] osteomyelitis (especially in infants),[57] the hand-foot syndrome,[58] blistering distal dactylitis,[59] and the toxic shock syndrome, are associated with beta-hemolytic streptococci. Some evidence also has accumulated suggesting that streptococcal infections may be responsible for episodes of acute guttate psoriasis, perhaps on the basis of a genetic predisposition.[8]

Streptococcal Upper Respiratory Tract Carrier State

One of the most puzzling aspects of the relationship of group A streptococci and the human host is the streptococcal "carrier" state. Not only does it represent both a diagnostic and a therapeutic enigma for both the clinician and public health authorities, but the theoretical implications relating to pathogenesis of nonsuppurative sequelae are intriguing.[72] Data in the literature suggest that group A upper respiratory tract carriers are less dangerous to others because carriers only rarely spread the organism to close contacts. In addition, the risk of developing nonsuppurative sequelae, such as rheumatic fever, appears to be significantly reduced in carriers.[71]

Much of this confusion has resulted from the definition of the carrier state. In contrast to true infection, in which there are both presence of an organism and evidence of a host immune response, group A streptococcal upper respiratory tract carriers may harbor the organism in the upper respiratory tract for prolonged periods without evidence of an immunologic response as measured by a rise in antibody to streptococcal antigens.

The explanation for this prolonged persistence of group A streptococci in the upper respiratory tract is unknown. Whether this is due to bacterial or host factors remains unexplained. For clinicians, the diagnosis and management of streptococcal upper respiratory tract carriers remain a controversial, but practical, problem.[71, 125]

Immunologic Response

The large number of somatic constituents and extracellular products of group A streptococci, most of which are antigenic, accounts for the complex nature of the host immune response after group A streptococcal infection. Both humoral and cellular immune responses have been studied, the former more thoroughly than the latter.[127]

Skin and in vitro tests suggest that most adults are hypersensitive to a variety of streptococcal preparations, whereas infants more often are nonreactive. Lymphocyte transformation responses to most streptococcal substances probably are specific in nature, resulting from prior sensitization. However, some studies indicate that a nonspecific (mitogenic) response may occur with certain extracellular and cellular fractions. Migration inhibition of leukocytes has been demonstrated with fractions of streptococcal culture supernates and with cell membrane and cell wall fractions.[105, 112] There is some evidence in humans suggesting that the cellular immune response to a streptococcal extracellular antigen is controlled genetically.[112]

Humoral immune responses have been demonstrated in humans to a number of somatic components of the group A streptococcal cell. Of particular interest are antibodies to the group A carbohydrate that serologically are cross-reactive with the glycoprotein of human and bovine heart valves and antibodies to protein components of the group A cell wall or cell membrane that have been reported to be cross-reactive with the sarcolemma of heart muscle.[9]

Antibody to the M protein (type-specific antibody) is of special importance because it is the basis of immunity/protection against reinfection with the same serologic type.[87, 130] Type-specific antibody may be transferred across the placenta from mother to fetus.[137] The development of type-specific antibody can be inhibited partially by prompt penicillin treatment of the streptococcal infection.[35]

Humoral antibodies to specific streptococcal extracellular products can be demonstrated readily by neutralization assays.[18] They have been especially useful in allowing a more precise method of defining streptococcal infection in clinical and epidemiologic studies and in documenting the occurrence of a preceding streptococcal infection in patients with a suspected nonsuppurative complication.

The antistreptolysin O assay is the streptococcal antibody test most commonly used. Because streptolysin O also is produced by group C and G streptococci, the test is not specific for group A infection. The antistreptolysin O response can be feeble in patients with streptococcal impetigo or pyoderma[76]; its usefulness for this latter condition is limited. In contrast, the anti-deoxyribonuclease B (anti-DNase B) and the anti-hyaluronidase responses are reliable after both skin and throat infections.

Another antibody test, the Streptozyme agglutination test, is based on antibody agglutination of erythrocytes coated with a mixture of streptococcal extracellular antigens. It has the theoretical appeal of simplicity, speed, and reaction with a number of streptococcal antigens.[65] Peak titers for an immune response as measured by the Streptozyme test have been demonstrated within the first week or 10 days after onset of infection,[98] whereas neutralizing antibody titers to streptolysin O (3 to 6 weeks) or anti-DNase B (6 to 8 weeks) do not peak until later. However, because of documented problems of standardization of this reagent (variable results may be obtained with different lots) and because of problems with group specificity, this test should be interpreted with caution.[77, 127] In fact, some studies have indicated problems in interpretation of this test; the World Health Organization has recommended that it not be used.[5]

Diagnosis and Differential Diagnosis

In patients presenting with acute pharyngitis or tonsillitis, the practicing physician must rely on a combination of the clinical appearance, identification of the organism, and the epidemiologic findings to confirm the probability of group A streptococcal infection. The problem especially is difficult because most of the clinical manifestations of streptococcal pharyngitis also can be associated with a variety of other etiologic agents.[16] Moreover, group A streptococci can be found in the throats of normal children and in children whose clinical findings are due to one of these other agents.[128] (See also Chapter 10, Pharyngitis.) Exudative sore throat may be caused by a number of viruses, *Corynebacterium diphtheriae*, gonococci, and groups C and G as well as group A streptococci.[16]

Viral pharyngitis closely may mimic streptococcal pharyngitis, which only can be ruled out by the absence of a positive culture for group A streptococci. In children, the white blood cell count may be elevated in viral infections, but a low count makes it unlikely that the infection is streptococcal. The C-reactive protein test is marginally useful in the acute phase of the illness.[80]

Because most streptococcal infections are short-term illnesses and antibody responses can be slow in appearing, streptococcal antibody titers are useful only retrospectively in diagnosing acute group A streptococcal infection. However, in addition to their primary role in supporting the diagnosis of nonsuppurative complications (acute nephritis and acute rheumatic fever), occasionally they may be useful clinically in diagnosing infections in which it is difficult to culture the primary site (e.g., streptococcal pneumonia or osteomyelitis) or in infections that have been treated or partially treated with antibiotics.

A number of schemes have been proposed for differentiating streptococcal from nonstreptococcal pharyngitis, but none of them are entirely satisfactory in making this distinction or in differentiating streptococcal carriers with an intervening nonstreptococcal pharyngitis from those with active streptococcal disease.[74] Clinical manifestations that are most suggestive of a group A streptococcal cause include the scarlatiniform rash (which, however, occasionally is associated with staphylococcal, rather than streptococcal, infection), excoriated nares (especially in infants), tender (not merely enlarged) anterior cervical lymph nodes, and a history of close contact with a well-documented case of group A streptococcal infection. The presence of cough, hoarseness, or conjunctivitis makes the diagnosis of streptococcal pharyngitis unlikely. It is important to note that exudative pharyngitis in infants usually is nonstreptococcal in etiology.[2] In addition, a number of clinical scoring systems have been found to be helpful to the clinician in some circumstances, but even these are not entirely reliable.[125]

Cultures may yield invalid results unless they are obtained and processed carefully. For cultures of the throat, the affected areas (tonsils and posterior pharynx) should be rubbed firmly with the cotton culture swab. Impetiginous lesions should be cleansed with alcohol and the vesicle punctured or the crust lifted by a sterile needle so that purulent material or the moist base can be touched by the swab. Group A streptococci sometimes can be recovered even from dry crusted lesions if the swab is moistened with culture broth before touching the exposed base of the lesion. Because streptococcal impetigo lesions commonly contain secondarily invading staphylococci, which may overgrow and obscure the colonies of streptococci, cultures should be examined carefully with a hand lens; alternatively, gentian violet may be incorporated in the blood agar plates as an inhibitor of staphylococci. If the culture swab cannot be plated onto agar within a few hours, the swab can be inoculated onto sterile filter paper and sent through the mail. Although this and several other transport methods generally are satisfactory, quantitation of the number of colonies is less accurate than when there is direct plating.

Presumptive differentiation of group A from other hemolytic streptococci can be achieved by the sensitivity of the former (but relatively few of the latter) to bacitracin but only when tested by a disc designed specifically for this purpose. Definite identification of group A streptococci can be accomplished by several serologic techniques employing group-specific antisera, for example, by (1) extraction of the organism by boiling in hydrochloric acid or by several other extraction methods with examination of the resulting extract in a precipitin test, (2) fluorescent antibody test on isolated colonies or broth cultures, and (3) agglutination of the organisms by group-specific antisera bound to protein A–containing staphylococci. Direct and rapid identification of group A streptococcal antigens from throat swabs has become quite popular. The specificity of these tests usually is very good, but published reports indicate that the sensitivity has varied widely.[73, 113]

On the basis of cost-effectiveness, analyses by some authors have suggested that throat cultures should not be performed, except when the percentage of positive cultures is between 15 and 20 per cent. There are many theoretic and practical objections attached to this recommendation,[17, 100] not the least of which is that it is necessary to do throat cultures anyway in order to determine whether one is within this range.

A number of rapid techniques for direct identification of group A streptococci from the upper respiratory tract are commercially available. These techniques employ extraction of the group-specific carbohydrate from the cell wall of the organism. Available data suggest that the specificity for these tests generally is greater than 90 per cent, but the sensitivity has ranged from less than 60 per cent to greater than 90 per cent.[73]

The advantages of these tests include the ability to identify group A streptococci rapidly and treat the patient at the time the patient is in the physician's office or emergency room. This advantage has appeal, especially in view of the data suggesting that in children, the more quickly the patient is treated, the more rapid is the clinical response.[104] Studies also have suggested that rapid antigen detection tests can be useful in the detection of group A streptococci in streptococcal pyoderma-like lesions.[79]

Data suggest that the sensitivity of the new tests may be improved. This has led many to suggest that a positive rapid antigen detection test is sufficient proof of group A infection but that a negative rapid antigen detection test should be confirmed with a conventional throat culture on sheep blood agar. Most believe that the throat culture still is the "gold standard" for identifying group A streptococci in the upper respiratory tract. It also must be recognized that, just as with any other laboratory test, there is a "learning curve effect" with streptococcal rapid antigen detection tests.[79]

The pharyngeal exudate of infectious mononucleosis tends to be more extensive, thicker, whiter, and more membranous and shaggy than that of streptococcal pharyngitis. The clinical impression usually can be confirmed quickly by the heterophil "spot test" (see Chapter 10).

In diphtheritic pharyngitis, the membrane is adherent and may tend to extend onto the uvula. It has a sweet-fetid odor recognized by experienced clinicians. Simultaneous infection with both *C. diphtheriae* and streptococci occurs in some patients and may result in the clinical picture of "bull neck" diphtheria.

It generally is safer to make a diagnosis of streptococcal impetigo than it is to make a diagnosis of streptococcal pharyngitis on clinical findings alone. Impetigo in which *Staphylococcus* is the primary invader generally is bullous rather than vesicular in type, and on rupture of the bulla a crust appears that is paper-thin and white rather than thick and honey-colored. Some confusion may result from reports of cultures performed on patients with primary streptococcal impetigo. Staphylococci, often present as secondary invaders, may overgrow the streptococci, which consequently may be missed unless the colonies are well isolated and the bacteriologist has an unusually sharp eye or unless a culture medium inhibitory for staphylococci is used.

The vesicles of chickenpox may resemble those of streptococcal impetigo superficially, but they are less transient, are surrounded by a red areola, are more centripetal in distribution (tending to involve the trunk and the proximal portions of the extremities), frequently itch, occur in crops, and often are accompanied by constitutional symptoms. The crusts are not so thick as those of streptococcal impetigo. It is worth noting that the lesions of chickenpox can be infected with streptococci secondarily and that varicella has been identified as an important risk factor in the development of severe and invasive group A streptococcal infections.

Prognosis

Patients with streptococcal sore throat or streptococcal impetigo recover spontaneously. A few may develop suppurative complications, and an occasional patient may have a nonsuppurative sequel.

In the general population, the risk of developing rheumatic fever after an untreated streptococcal infection of the upper respiratory tract is about 3 per cent under epidemic conditions but appears to be considerably less (about 0.3 per cent) in endemic situations,[114] owing, at least in part, to differences in definition of infection.[81] Patients who have had one attack of rheumatic fever are at high risk of a rheumatic fever recurrence when reinfected with group A streptococci (15 to 50 per cent). There appears to be no risk of rheumatic fever after a streptococcal infection of the skin.

The risk of acute glomerulonephritis is dependent upon whether the infection is caused by a nephritogenic or a non-nephritogenic strain. With a nephritogenic strain, the attack rate appears to be about 10 to 15 per cent and can occur after either throat or skin infection.[126]

In contrast to the usual short and often benign course of throat and superficial skin infections, streptococcal cellulitis spreads rapidly both locally and to the regional lymph nodes and blood stream. In immunosuppressed patients and patients with streptococcal infection superimposed on leukemia, lymphoma, or other malignancies, bacteremia may develop, and the patients may have serious life-threatening problems. Patients with puerperal sepsis, neonatal infection, streptococcal toxic shock–like syndrome, or gangrene due to group A streptococci also have a high mortality rate despite timely and high doses of penicillin therapy.

The prognosis for complete recovery in patients with the group A streptococcal toxic shock syndrome and in patients with necrotizing fasciitis varies. Early series reported a mortality of at least 30 per cent in patients with toxic shock syndrome.[120] The mortality with necrotizing fasciitis is even greater.[119]

Treatment

Although group A streptococci generally are susceptible to a number of antibiotics,[30, 44, 92] penicillin remains the drug of choice for treatment except in those patients allergic to it. No group A streptococcal strains have been identified yet that are resistant to penicillin. Although penicillin tolerance has been described in group A streptococci, its clinical significance has not been defined.[82]

It sometimes is difficult, however, to eradicate group A streptococci from the upper respiratory tract (especially from carriers) with penicillin or other antibiotics.[70] This observation has not been explained adequately, but possible explanations include the presence of β-lactamase–producing organisms in the upper respiratory tract, the presence of group A streptococci tolerant to penicillin, and the production of inhibitory substances by certain of the normal upper respiratory tract flora, which influence persistence of the organism. In addition, there even is evidence to suggest microbial differences in organisms isolated from carriers.[85]

Erythromycin remains the drug of choice in patients allergic to penicillin. Resistance to erythromycin still is rare in most countries (less than 5 per cent). The incidence was high in Japan in the 1960s,[41] and this also has been noted in Finland.[111] There are no advantages and potential disadvantages in the use of broad-spectrum antibiotics for group A streptococcal infections. Group A streptococci most frequently are resistant to tetracyclines and the sulfonamides. β-lactamase–resistant antibiotics have been advocated in some studies[20]; a role for β-lactamase production by normal flora in penicillin treatment failures has not been clarified yet.

In the treatment of true streptococcal sore throat, it is

necessary to eradicate the group A streptococcus in order to prevent the development of acute rheumatic fever.[26] High doses usually are not required, but the penicillin must be present for a rather long period in order to kill all of the infecting organisms. Administration of a single intramuscular injection of benzathine penicillin G (1,200,000 units in adults and in children more than 60 lb; 600,000 units in children less than 60 lb) is one method of accomplishing this objective. If a combination of benzathine penicillin and procaine penicillin is used, its dosage should be based upon the amount of benzathine used. If oral medication (penicillin or erythromycin) is used, the patient and parent must be impressed with the importance of continuing the medication for a full 10 days, which usually is many days beyond the period when the patient feels entirely well. Oral penicillin V (two to three times a day) is the treatment of choice. In patients with a suspected allergy to penicillin, erythromycin (250 mg four times a day in adults; in children, 40 mg/kg per day in four doses, not to exceed the adult dose) should be used.[36] Other antibiotics that have been used successfully in the therapy of group A beta-hemolytic streptococcal pharyngitis or tonsillitis include clindamycin, amoxicillin or a mixture of amoxicillin with clavulanate acid, and other cephalosporins. Erythromycin resistance has not been a clinically significant problem in the United States, but occasionally reports of increases in erythromycin resistance have appeared in the literature.[60, 135]

In patients with strong clinical or epidemiologic evidence of streptococcal infection, the physician may decide to begin therapy before the result of the throat culture is available. If oral therapy is used for initiating treatment, it may be continued or discontinued, depending on the culture report. Alternatively, an injection of benzathine penicillin G may be administered at that time if the report is positive. For patients who may not return for a culture report or who may be difficult to contact, it may be necessary to make an immediate clinical judgment whether to prescribe penicillin therapy. In these situations, the use of the rapid direct techniques for detection of group A streptococci is advantageous. Because such patients also may be less reliable with respect to completing a course of oral therapy, the use of intramuscular benzathine penicillin G may be preferable in these patients. Intramuscular benzathine penicillin G also is advantageous in epidemic situations. Even if the decision to treat or not to treat must be made on clinical grounds, throat cultures can be very useful in indicating to the physician the current prevalence and clinical features of streptococcal and nonstreptococcal respiratory illnesses.

In the past, it was believed that it was good clinical practice to repeat throat cultures after completion of oral therapy to ensure that the group A streptococci had been eradicated. Because studies have shown that many penicillin treatment failures appear to be group A streptococcal upper respiratory tract carriers,[72] in areas where rheumatic fever has not reappeared, most physicians now believe it is unnecessary to reculture asymptomatic individuals routinely after antibiotic therapy unless there are unusual epidemiologic circumstances, such as a rheumatic individual in the household or epidemic streptococcal disease in the community. Other regimens that have been used for treatment of those patients with persistently positive cultures include dicloxacillin, clindamycin, a mixture of amoxicillin and clavulanate acid, and rifampin along with an injection of benzathine penicillin G.

In those symptomatic patients for whom cultures are performed and who have persistently positive cultures, benzathine penicillin G frequently is used for re-treatment; other clinicians use clindamycin, dicloxacillin, or a semisynthetic penicillin. In patients who show a repeated clinical pattern of treatment failure, it may be helpful to determine the serologic group and type of the strains recovered in order to ascertain whether the isolates are the same or are different serologic types.

If the throat culture remains positive after a second course of therapy and the patient is not symptomatic, the routine need for additional cultures or antibiotic therapy is doubtful, except in high-risk situations. At this time, the patient probably is beyond the period of greatest risk of rheumatic fever or of spreading the infection. However, it is important in "problem" families, in which intrafamilial spread is a possibility, to culture the throats of all members of the family simultaneously and to treat all of those with positive results. Routine culturing in asymptomatic siblings is controversial; most physicians do not culture in these circumstances. The main problem of the persisting carrier is that this may complicate interpretation of throat cultures obtained at the time of future nonstreptococcal respiratory tract infections.

It has been suggested in the literature that the rapid treatment of group A streptococcal upper respiratory tract infection tends to promote recurrent streptococcal infections in the future because of the suppression of the type-specific antibody response. Some studies, however, have demonstrated no difference in the frequency of recurrences of streptococcal infections whether therapy is started upon diagnosis or delayed up to 48 hours.[50]

In contrast to group A streptococcal pharyngitis or tonsillitis, no authoritative guidelines have been developed for the treatment of streptococcal impetigo.[132] The effectiveness of hygienic measures and local skin care (removal of crusts and use of antibacterial soaps) probably is dependent on the thoroughness and perseverance with which they are carried out. These measures and the use of local antimicrobial ointments can be sufficient for the management of patients with only a few lesions. However, systemic antibiotics have been associated with rapid clearing of the lesions. Oral or parenteral penicillin or oral erythromycin (in the amounts prescribed for the treatment of streptococcal pharyngitis) should be administered to patients with more severe or persistent infections. First-generation cephalosporins and semisynthetic penicillins also are effective. Antibiotic therapy probably does help prevent the spread of streptococcal impetigo in the family.

Whether penicillin or other antibiotic treatment reduces the risk of development of acute nephritis is unclear.[133] One study suggests that penicillin therapy may lower the risk of this complication in patients with streptococcal sore throat due to a nephritogenic strain.[118] However, there is no proof that penicillin treatment reduces the frequency of acute nephritis after treatment of skin infections. Furthermore, clinical experience indicates that patients with cutaneous infection due to a nephritogenic strain of group A streptococci may develop this complication despite adequate penicillin therapy.[75]

Otitis media or cervical adenitis due to group A streptococci usually responds to the regimens prescribed for treatment of streptococcal sore throat. Patients with peritonsillar abscess require surgical drainage in addition to vigorous parenteral antibiotic therapy. Patients with more serious infections (e.g., mastoiditis, pneumonia, empyema) also should be given intensive systemic therapy. Those with meningitis, arthritis, or osteomyelitis require high-dose intravenous penicillin administered for a relatively long period (see Chapters 38 and 64). Patients with streptococcal toxic shock syndrome and patients with necrotizing fasciitis may be treated with parenteral penicillin, but recent evidence suggests that clindamycin, either alone or in combination with penicillin, has advantages.[119] In patients sensitive to penicillin, clindamycin is an excellent alternative. Because of cross-reactions with penicillin, the cephalosporins should be used only cautiously in penicillin-allergic patients.

Prevention

Antimicrobial agents have been helpful in controlling group A streptococcal infections and their sequelae, but they do not provide an encompassing solution for this group of diseases, either in industrialized countries or in the developing world. This has been evident from the "resurgence" of rheumatic fever and the appearance of the streptococcal toxic shock syndrome in the United States during the 1980s and 1990s. Penicillin's greatest impact has been on the prevention of recurrences of rheumatic fever (see Chapter 35). Prevention of first attacks of rheumatic fever is a problem of greater dimensions because it involves detection, diagnosis, and appropriate treatment in the general population. One cost-effective program can be obtained from well-conceived secondary prevention programs in defined rheumatics and perhaps from primary prevention programs in school-age children of lower socioeconomic status.

The prevention of spread by isolation, limiting population density, and antibiotic treatment of known cases is discussed in the section on transmission (see earlier). Mass penicillin prophylaxis has been used in epidemics with a well-defined streptococcal etiology,[21] but in actual practice, the epidemic often is subsiding by the time a large-scale prophylactic effort can be mounted. Intramuscular benzathine penicillin G is very effective for this purpose.[21] The dose is the same as recommended for treating streptococcal pharyngitis. In populations in which streptococcal infections occur at epidemic or near-epidemic levels over a long period (e.g., certain military populations), it may be necessary to repeat the injections of benzathine penicillin at monthly intervals and to administer them to all new arrivals.

The role of antibiotic prophylaxis for contacts and families of individuals with streptococcal toxic shock syndrome has not been examined carefully in controlled studies. However, even though clusters of severe infections have been described in such situations, the risk of recurring infections must be very low. Nevertheless, many choose to culture the upper respiratory tract of all individuals in close contact with severely ill patients, especially if they have been exposed to their secretions. All culture-positive individuals should be treated with antibiotics. In fact, some would treat all such contacts whether or not the cultures reveal group A streptococci. Many follow the same approach for family contacts of such patients. The approach to school contacts is even less clear at this time. A single case in a school or other similar population probably does not necessitate culturing of the entire population. Again, recommendations for more than a single case in such a population are not available, but as the number of cases increases in a school or other defined population, culture and antibiotic therapy of those with positive cultures appear to be more justified.

The question of the possible advantages of tonsillectomy for the prevention of streptococcal infections and their sequelae also has not been settled by well-controlled studies. From the information available, it would appear that tonsillectomy may reduce the frequency of clinically apparent streptococcal infections, perhaps making it less likely that they receive appropriate treatment.[27] However, one study indicates that recurrences are more frequent in individuals who have had rheumatic fever and who have large tonsils.[45]

No satisfactory method of manipulating host defenses to prevent streptococcal infections has been devised. Because immunity to streptococcal infections is type-specific, considerable efforts have been spent on purifying M proteins for vaccine studies.[12, 62] The problem is difficult because of the complexity, the potential toxicity, and the large number of M proteins. With the differentiation of "cross-reactive" from "protective" epitopes on the M protein, the concept of a vaccine becomes more feasible. Furthermore, the finding of conserved regions on the M protein molecule raises the possibility that vaccines using this portion of the M protein can induce protection against multiple serotypes.[47] Early studies in experimental animals are promising in demonstrating the efficacy of vaccines, but extensive human clinical trials obviously are necessary. Studies also are being directed toward the prevention of adherence of group A streptococci to epithelial cells.[11, 34]

The inability of antibiotics to influence the epidemiology of group A streptococcal infections and their sequelae consistently and favorably is reflected by the concentration of sequelae recently occurring in middle class populations with ready access to medical care.[124] Control measures would be much more effective were a group A streptococcal vaccine available. Issues relating to the more than 80 known serotypes of group A streptococci and the recognized similarities between group A streptococci and mammalian tissues remain to be resolved before clinical trials can be undertaken. In fact, recent data indicating that there are numerous group A streptococci of as yet undefined serotypes in many parts of the world make this even more complicated in terms of preparing a suitable multivalent vaccine.

GROUP C AND GROUP G STREPTOCOCCAL INFECTIONS

The Organisms

The characterization of beta-hemolytic streptococci on the basis of group-specific carbohydrate antigens is complicated by the presence of similar antigens among streptococci that, on the basis of biochemical and genetic testing, have been demonstrated to be different species. Organisms that possess either the group C or group G Lancefield antigens can be divided into groups based on colony size. The strains that produce small or minute colonies ($<$0.5 mm in diameter) have been placed in the *Streptococcus anginosus* group (classified as *Streptococcus milleri* by British taxonomists), whereas the strains that produce large-sized colonies ($\geq$0 to 5 mm in diameter) have been referred to as "true" or "large colony" group C or group G, depending on the nature of their carbohydrate antigen. However, the taxonomic classification of these streptococci still is unsettled, and undoubtedly more changes will occur before a universally agreed-upon scheme is established.[7, 28, 55]

Most group C streptococci are beta-hemolytic on blood agar plates, but all types of hemolysis have been observed. Group C streptococci are aerobic, facultatively anaerobic, coprophilic, and catalase-negative organisms. Rhamnose-N-acetylgalactosamine is the group C antigenic determinant in the cell wall, and four species possessing this determinant have been described. Although most group C streptococci are resistant to bacitracin, at least one-third (and in one study up to 62 per cent) of group C streptococci are bacitracin-sensitive.[7]

Streptococcus equisimilis is the species of group C streptococci that most often colonizes and causes infections in humans. It has been isolated from the nose, throat, and genital tract of asymptomatic carriers and from the umbilicus of asymptomatic newborns. *S. equisimilis* produces streptokinase and streptolysin O, and infection may elicit an antibody response to these extracellular antigens similar to that seen with a group A streptococcal infection. This organism also can cause infections in a variety of domestic animals (e.g., horses, cattle, pigs, chickens).

Streptococcus zooepidemicus can cause significant, often epidemic infections in domestic animals (e.g., horses, cattle, pigs, sheep) but is an uncommon pathogen in humans. Most human infections have been associated with consumption of homemade cheese or unpasteurized cow's milk.

Streptococcus equi rarely is isolated from humans but does cause a serious and highly contagious respiratory disease in horses known as strangles.

Streptococcus dysgalactiae rarely is found in humans but does cause a serious mastitis in cows and a suppurative polyarthritis in lambs.

The vast majority of group G streptococci are beta-hemolytic on blood agar plates. L-rhamnose is the group G antigenic determinant in the cell wall. Many group G streptococci isolated from infected humans (but not from animals) express an M protein in their cell wall with biologic, immunochemical, and genetic features similar to those of the M protein of group A streptococci.[24, 29] As with group A streptococci, the M protein of group G streptococci is a virulence factor that helps the organism resist phagocytosis. There are a number of antigenic variants of the group G M protein, and type-specific opsonic antibodies are produced in response to the M protein of the infecting strain.

Several schemes for typing group G streptococci have been described based on biochemical properties or bacteriocin typing. Although no association between particular types and infections in humans has been identified, these schemes have been useful in distinguishing human from animal strains and in epidemiologic investigations. T-typing and M-typing schemes similar to those used for group A streptococci also have been devised for group G streptococci. Although most group G streptococci are resistant to bacitracin, various reports have determined anywhere from 8 to 67 per cent of group G streptococci to be bacitracin-sensitive.[55]

In addition to M protein, human isolates of group G streptococci share other virulence factors with group A streptococci, such as a streptokinase, a hyaluronidase, and a C5a peptidase. Group G streptococci also produce a streptolysin that is similar antigenically to the streptolysin O produced by group A streptococci. Patients with group G streptococcal infections may demonstrate a significant increase in antistreptolysin O titers.

Epidemiology

Group C streptococci are an uncommon cause of human infections but more commonly are pathogenic in animals. Humans infected with this organism often will have had some animal contact. Both group C and group G streptococci often can be part of the normal human flora of the nasopharynx, skin, and/or genital tract. Group C streptococci also can be cultured from the umbilicus of asymptomatic newborns as well as from routine puerperal vaginal cultures. Group G streptococci also can be cultured from the gastrointestinal tract. The relatively low virulence of group C and group G streptococci is indicated by the fact that most humans infected with either of these organisms will have some underlying medical disorder (e.g., diabetes mellitus, malignancy, alcohol abuse, immunosuppression).[25, 86]

Clinical Manifestations

The clinical features of both group C and group G streptococcal pharyngitis are similar to those of group A streptococcal pharyngitis with fever, mild to moderate sore throat, pharyngeal exudate, and cervical adenitis.

It has been reported that between 1 and 18 per cent of asymptomatic people in temperate climates harbor group C streptococci in their upper respiratory tract. The proportion of carriers among people living in the tropics is even greater.[99] Such carrier rates make it difficult to establish the etiologic role of group C streptococci in acute pharyngitis. Several studies have been performed comparing the isolation rates of group C streptococci from patients with acute pharyngitis with rates in asymptomatic controls; the results have been contradictory.[7, 28] However, two investigations established a strong epidemiologic association between group C streptococci and endemic acute pharyngitis. In the first investigation, group C streptococci were isolated significantly more often from college students with acute pharyngitis (26 per cent) than from asymptomatic controls (11 per cent).[123] In the other investigation, group C streptococci were isolated significantly more often from adults who came to an emergency room with acute pharyngitis (6 per cent) than from asymptomatic controls (1.4 per cent).[96]

In contrast to endemic pharyngitis, group C streptococci can cause epidemic food-borne pharyngitis after ingestion of contaminated products, such as unpasteurized cow's milk. Epidemics have been reported from Great Britain, Romania, the United States, and Israel.[7, 28] In one report of a milk-borne epidemic of pharyngitis caused by *S. zooepidemicus*, approximately one-third of the patients developed signs of acute glomerulonephritis.[42] This outbreak was related to the consumption of unpasteurized milk from cattle with mastitis. There were no cases of acute rheumatic fever. Family outbreaks of group C streptococcal pharyngitis as well as an outbreak in a residential school for boys have been described.

Group C streptococci also have been reported as the cause of a number of other uncommon infections, including skin and soft tissue infections, septic arthritis, osteomyelitis, pneumonitis, infective endocarditis, bacteremia and septicemia, meningitis, epiglottitis, pericarditis, urinary tract infections, and sinusitis. These organisms also have been associated with epidemic and nonepidemic cases of puerperal sepsis and endometritis.[67]

It has been reported that 1 to 23 per cent of asymptomatic people may carry group G streptococci in their upper respiratory tract. As with group C streptococci, the carrier rates of group G streptococci appear to be even higher in the tropics.[99] Such carrier rates also make it difficult to establish the etiologic role of group G streptococci in acute pharyngitis. Several studies have been performed comparing the isolation rates of group G streptococci from patients with acute pharyngitis with rates from asymptomatic controls. The results of these studies showed little difference in the isolation rates, suggesting that group G streptococci may not play an important role in endemic acute pharyngitis. Few of these studies were adequately controlled, prospective investigations, however, and in many, the incidence of group G streptococci in the symptomatic group was so low as to preclude any possibility of demonstrating a statistically significant difference. Support for an etiologic role of group G streptococci in acute pharyngitis comes primarily from anecdotes, small case clusters, and a few large outbreaks, most of which were food-borne. To date, there have been several reported food-borne outbreaks of group G streptococcal pharyngitis, all of which occurred in semiclosed populations, including one outbreak at a college cafeteria.[91] In the first reported respiratory outbreak of group G streptococcal pharyngitis in the United States, McCue[95] described 68 cases of acute pharyngitis on a college campus seen during a 9-day period in 1981. The possibility of food-borne spread could not be eliminated completely but seemed unlikely, and airborne droplet transmission appeared to be the most likely mechanism of spread.

Despite the evidence supporting the etiologic role of group G streptococci in epidemic pharyngitis, the role of group G streptococci in acute, endemic pharyngitis remains unclear. Previous outbreaks of group G streptococcal pharyngitis had been reported in university-aged or older patients, and all had occurred in semiclosed communities. However, a community-wide, respiratory outbreak of group G streptococcal pharyngitis in a pediatric population was described.[51] During a 6-month period, group G streptococci were isolated from 56 of 222 (25 per cent) consecutive children with acute pharyngitis seen at a private pediatric office. Results of DNA fingerprinting of the group G streptococcal isolates suggested that 75 per cent of them were the same strain. The patients with group G streptococcal pharyngitis were comparable to those with group A streptococcal pharyngitis with respect to clinical findings, antistreptolysin O titer response, and clinical response to antibiotic therapy. However, patients with group G streptococci were significantly older. The findings suggested that antibiotic therapy has a dramatic impact on the clinical course of group G streptococcal pharyngitis. These findings lend support to the belief that group G streptococci may be a more important cause of acute, endemic pharyngitis than had been recognized previously.

The actual role of group C and group G streptococci in acute pharyngitis may be underestimated for several reasons. Anaerobic incubation increases the yield of these organisms, but most clinicians do not use anaerobic incubation for throat cultures routinely.[110] Because clinicians generally disregard beta-hemolytic streptococci that are bacitracin-resistant (and most strains of group C and group G streptococci are bacitracin-resistant), many group C and group G streptococci would be missed.

Acute rheumatic fever has not been described as a complication of either group C or group G streptococcal pharyngitis, and, although there have been reports attempting to link acute glomerulonephritis with group G streptococcal pharyngitis, the evidence is anecdotal and a causal relationship has not been established.[101, 106] Although acute glomerulonephritis has been reported as a complication of group C streptococcal pharyngitis, it is extremely unusual.[42] Therefore, the primary reason to identify either group C or group G streptococci as the etiologic agent of acute pharyngitis is to initiate antibiotic therapy that may reduce the clinical impact of the illness. However, there is no convincing evidence as yet from controlled studies of a clinical response to antibiotic therapy in patients with acute pharyngitis and either group C or group G streptococci isolated from their upper respiratory tract.

Group G streptococci also have been reported to be an uncommon cause of puerperal sepsis and occasionally may cause a neonatal infection that is clinically very similar to early-onset group B streptococcal infections. Other infections occasionally caused by group G streptococci include bacteremia, endocarditis, septic arthritis, osteomyelitis, pneumonia, skin and soft tissue infections, and meningitis.[67]

Treatment

Penicillin is the antibiotic of choice for treating infections due to either group C or group G streptococci.[108] Some strains of group C and group G streptococci have been shown to be tolerant to penicillin in laboratory studies, but the clinical significance of this finding is not known.[107] Synergism in producing in vitro killing of group C and group G streptococci has been demonstrated with gentamicin and various β-lactam antibiotics, but no controlled trials have been performed to establish the clinical significance of this finding. Group C and group G streptococci also are susceptible to most β-lactam antibiotics, as well as to macrolides, vancomycin, clindamycin, and chloramphenicol. Pharyngitis usually is treated in a similar manner to group A streptococcal upper respiratory infections. More severe infection requires parenteral therapy.

References

1. Allan, A. M., Taplin, D., and Twigg, L.: Cutaneous streptococcal infections in Vietnam. Arch. Dermatol. *104*:271–280, 1971.
2. Alpert, J. J., Pickering, M. R., and Warren, R. J.: Failure to isolate streptococci from children under the age of 3 years with exudative tonsillitis. Pediatrics *38*:663–666, 1966.
3. Aly, R., Maibach, H. I., Shinefield, H. R., et al.: Survival of pathogenic microorganisms on human skin. J. Invest. Dermatol. *58*:205–210, 1972.
4. Amren, D. P.: Unusual forms of streptococcal disease. *In* Wannamaker, L. W., and Matsen, J. M. (eds.): Streptococci and Streptococcal Diseases. Recognition, Understanding, and Management. New York, Academic Press, 1972, pp. 545–556.
5. Anonymous: Evaluation of the Streptozyme test for streptococcal antibodies. Bull. W. H. O. *64*:504, 1986.
6. Anthony, B. F., Kaplan, E. L., Wannamaker, L. W., et al.: The dynamics of streptococcal infections in a defined population of children: Serotypes associated with skin and respiratory infections. Am. J. Epidemiol. *104*:652–666, 1976.
7. Arditi, M., Shulman, S. T., Davis, A. T., et al.: Group C beta-hemolytic streptococcal infections in children: Nine pediatric cases and review. Rev. Infect. Dis. *11*:34–45, 1989.
8. Asboe-Hansen, G.: Psoriasis in childhood. *In* Farber, E. M., and Cox, A. J. (eds.): Psoriasis. Proceedings of the International Symposium, Stanford University. Stanford, Stanford University Press, 1971, pp. 53–59.
9. Ayoub, E. M.: Cross-reacting antibodies in the pathogenesis of rheumatic myocardial and valvular disease. *In* Wannamaker, L. W., and Matsen, J. M. (eds.): Streptococci and Streptococcal Diseases: Recognition, Understanding, and Management. New York, Academic Press, 1972, pp. 451–464.
10. Bassett, D. C. J.: Hippelates flies and acute nephritis. Lancet *i*:503, 1967.
11. Beachey, E. H., and Ofek, I.: Epithelial cell binding of group A streptococci by lipoteichoic acid on fimbriae denuded of M protein. J. Exp. Med. *143*:759–771, 1976.
12. Beachey, E. H., Seyer, J. M., Dale, J. B., et al.: Type-specific protective immunity evoked by synthetic peptide of Streptococcus pyogenes M protein. Nature *292*:457–459, 1981.
13. Beachey, E. H., and Stollerman, G. H.: Mediation of cytotoxic effects of streptococcal M protein by nontype-specific antibody in human sera. J. Clin. Invest. *52*:2563–2570, 1973.
14. Bernheimer, A. W.: Hemolysins of streptococci: Characterization and effects on biological membranes. *In* Wannamaker, L. W., and Matsen, J. M. (eds.): Streptococci and Streptococcal Diseases: Recognition, Understanding, and Management. New York, Academic Press, 1972, pp. 19–31.
15. Biberstein, E. L., Brown, C., and Smith, T.: Serogroups and biotypes among beta-hemolytic streptococci of canine origin. J. Clin. Microbiol. *11*:558–561, 1980.
16. Bisno, A. L.: Acute pharyngitis: Etiology and diagnosis. Pediatrics *97*:949–954, 1996.
17. Bisno, A. L.: Therapeutic strategies for the prevention of rheumatic fever. Ann. Intern. Med. 86:494–496, 1977.
18. Bisno, A. L., and Stollerman, G. H.: Streptococcal antibodies in the diagnosis of rheumatic fever. *In* Cohen, A. S. (ed.): Laboratory Diagnostic Procedures in the Rheumatic Diseases. Boston, Little, Brown and Co., 1975, pp. 207–263.
19. Breiman, R. F., David, J. P., Facklam, R. R., et al.: Defining the group A streptococcal toxic shock syndrome: Rationale and consensus definition. J. A. M. A. *269*:390–391, 1993.
20. Brook, I.: The role of beta-lactamase-producing bacteria in the persistence of streptococcal tonsillar infection. Rev. Infect. Dis. *6*:601–607, 1984.
21. Brundage, J. F., Gunzenhauser, J. D., Longfield, J. N., et al.: Epidemiology and control of acute respiratory diseases with emphasis on group A beta-hemolytic streptococcus: A decade of U.S. Army experience. Pediatrics *97*:964–970, 1996.
22. Bullowa, J. G. M., and Wishik, S. M.: Complications of varicella: Their occurrence among 2,534 patients. Am. J. Dis. Child. *49*:923–926, 1935.
23. Calandra, G. B., Whitt, R. S., and Cole, R. M.: Relationship of cellular potential hemolysin in group A Streptococci to extracellular streptolysin S. Infect. Immun. *13*:813–817, 1976.
24. Campo, R. E., Schultz, D. R., and Bisno, A. L.: M proteins of group G streptococci: Mechanisms of resistance to phagocytosis. J. Infect. Dis. *171*:601–606, 1995.
25. Carmeli, Y., Schapiro, J. M., Neeman, D., et al.: Streptococcal group C

bacteremia: Survey in Israel and analytic review. Arch. Intern. Med. *155*:1170–1176, 1996.

26. Catanzaro, F. J., Rammelkamp, C. H., Jr., and Chamovitz, R.: Prevention of rheumatic fever by treatment of streptococcal infections. II. Factors responsible for failures. N. Engl. J. Med. *259*:51–57, 1958.
27. Chamovitz, R., Rammelkamp, C. H., Jr., Wannamaker, L. W., et al.: The effect of tonsillectomy on the incidence of streptococcal respiratory disease and its complications. Pediatrics *26*:355–367, 1960.
28. Cimolai, N., Elford, R. W., Bryan, L., et al.: Do the beta-hemolytic non-group A streptococci cause pharyngitis? Rev. Infect. Dis. *10*:587–601, 1988.
29. Collins, C. M., Kimura, A., and Bisno, A. L.: Group G streptococcal M protein exhibits structural features analogous to those of class I M protein of group A streptococci. Infect. Immun. *60*:3689–3696, 1992.
30. Coonan, K. M., and Kaplan, E. L.: In vitro susceptibility of recent North American group A streptococcal isolates to eleven oral antibiotics. Pediatr. Infect. Dis. J. *13*:630–635, 1994.
31. Crawford, S. E., and Riddler, J. G.: Purpura fulminans. Am. J. Dis. Child. *97*:197–201, 1959.
32. Crowder, H. R., Dorn, C. R., and Smith, R. E.: Group A *Streptococcus* in pets and group A streptococcal disease in man. Int. J. Zoonoses *5*:45–54, 1978.
33. Crowe, C. C., Sanders, W. E., Jr., and Longley, S.: Bacterial interference. II. Role of the normal throat flora in prevention of colonization by group A *Streptococcus*. J. Infect. Dis. *128*:527–532, 1973.
34. Cunningham, M. W., and Beachey, E. H.: Peptic digestion of streptococcal M protein. I. Effect of digestion at suboptimal pH upon the biological and immunochemical properties of purified M protein extracts. Infect. Immun. *9*:244–248, 1974.
35. Daikos, G., and Weinstein, L.: Streptococci bacteriostatic antibody in patients treated with penicillin. Proc. Soc. Exp. Biol. Med. *78*:160–163, 1951.
36. Dajani, A. S., Bisno, A. L., Chung, K. J., et al.: Prevention of rheumatic fever: A statement for health professionals by the Committee on Rheumatic Fever, Endocarditis and Kawasaki Disease of the Council on Cardiovascular Disease in the Young, the American Heart Association. Pediatr. Infect. Dis. J. *8*:263–266, 1989.
37. Dajani, A. S., Ferrieri, P., and Wannamaker, L. W.: Endemic superficial pyoderma in children. Arch. Dermatol. *108*:517–522, 1973.
38. Dajani, A. S., Garcia, R. E., and Wolinsky, E.: Etiology of cervical lymphadenitis in children. N. Engl. J. Med. *268*:1329–1333, 1963.
39. Denny, F. W., Jr., Perry, W. D., and Wannamaker, L. W.: Type-specific streptococcal antibody. J. Clin. Invest. *36*:1092–1100, 1957.
40. Dillon, H. C., Jr.: Impetigo contagiosa: Suppurative and non-suppurative complications. I. Clinical, bacteriologic, and epidemiologic characteristics of impetigo. Am. J. Dis. Child. *115*:530–541, 1968.
41. Dixon, J. M., and Lipinski, A. E.: Infections with beta-hemolytic streptococcus resistant to lincomycin and erythromycin and observations on zonal-pattern resistance to lincomycin. J. Infect. Dis. *130*:351–356, 1974.
42. Duca, E., Teodorovici, G., Radu, C., et al.: A new nephritogenic streptococcus. J. Hyg. *67*:691–698, 1969.
43. Dudding, B., Humphrey, G. B., and Nesbit, M. E.: Beta-hemolytic streptococcal septicemias in childhood leukemia. Pediatrics *43*:359–364, 1969.
44. Eickhoff, T. C., and Finland, M.: In vitro susceptibility of group A beta hemolytic streptococci to 18 antibiotics. Am. J. Med. Sci., *249*:261–268, 1965.
45. Feinstein, A. R., and Levitt, M.: The role of tonsils in predisposing to streptococcal infections and recurrences of rheumatic fever. N. Engl. J. Med. *282*:285–291, 1970.
46. Ferrieri, P., Dajani, A. S., Wannamaker, L. W., et al.: Natural history of impetigo. I. Site sequence of acquisition and familial patterns of spread of cutaneous streptococci. J. Clin. Invest. *51*:2851–2862, 1972.
47. Fischetti, V. A.: Streptococcal M protein: Molecular design and biological behavior. Clin. Microbiol. Rev. *2*:285, 1989.
48. Flodstrom, A., and Hallander, H. O.: Microbiological aspects on peritonsillar abscesses. Scand. J. Infect. Dis., *8*:157–160, 1976.
49. Freimer, E. H.: Studies of L forms and protoplasts of group A streptococci. II. Chemical and immunological properties of the cell membrane. J. Exp. Med. *117*: 377–399, 1963.
50. Gerber, M. A., Deleo, K., Randolph, M. A., et al.: Lack of impact of early antibiotic therapy for streptococcal pharyngitis on recurrence rates. J. Pediatr. (in press).
51. Gerber, M. A., Randolph, M. F., Martin, N. J., et al.: Community-wide outbreak of group G streptococcal pharyngitis. Pediatrics 87:598–603, 1991.
52. Ginsburg, I., and Sela, M. N.: The role of leukocytes and their hydrolases in the persistence, degradation, and transport of bacterial constituents in tissues: Relation to chronic inflammatory processes in staphylococcal, streptococcal, and mycobacterial infections and in chronic periodontal disease. CRC Crit. Rev. Microbiol. *4*:249–322, 1976.
53. Graybill, J. R., Pierson, D. N., and Charache, P.: Tissue antibiotic penetration in streptococcal gangrene. Johns Hopkins Med. J. *133*:45–50, 1973.
54. Greenberg, L. J., Gray, E. D., and Yunis, E. J.: Association of HL-A 5 and immune responsiveness in vitro to streptococcal antigens. J. Exp. Med. *141*:935–943, 1975.
55. See reference 54.
56. Hable, K. A., Horstmeier, C., Wold, A. D., et al.: Group A β-hemolytic streptococcemia: Bacteriologic and clinical study of 44 cases. Mayo Clin. Proc. *48*:336–339, 1973.
57. Hall, J. E., and Silverstein, E. A.: Acute hematogenous osteomyelitis. Pediatrics *31*:1033–1038, 1963.
58. Haltalin, K. C., and Nelson, J. D.: Hand-foot syndrome due to streptococcal infection. Am. J. Dis. Child. *109*:156–159, 1965.
59. Hays, G. C., and Mullard, J. E.: Blistering distal dactylitis: A clinically recognizable streptococcal infection. Pediatrics *56*:129–131, 1975.
60. Henderson, R. J., Bares, G. J., Rambin, E. D., et al.: Typing and plasmid analysis of clinical isolates of group A beta hemolytic streptococcus with increased resistance to erythromycin. Clin. Res. *38*:55A, 1990.
61. Hill, H. R., Zimmerman, R. A., Reid, G. V., et al.: Food-borne epidemic of streptoccal pharyngitis at the United States Air Force Academy. N. Engl. J. Med., *280*:917–921, 1969.
62. Hosein, B., McCarty, M., and Fischetti, V. A.: Amino acid sequence and physicochemical similarities between streptococcal M protein and mammalian tropomyosin. Proc. Natl. Acad. Sci. U. S. A. *76*:3765–3768, 1976.
63. Huskins, W. C., and Kaplan, E. L.: Inhibitory substances produced by *Streptococcus salivarius* and colonization of the upper respiratory tract with group A streptococci. Epidemiol. Infect. *102*:401–412, 1989.
64. James, L., and McFarland, R. B.: An epidemic of pharyngitis due to a nonhemolytic group A *Streptococcus* at Lowry Air Force Base. N. Engl. J. Med. *284*:750–752, 1971.
65. Janeff, J., Janeff, D., Taranta, A., et al.: A screening test for streptococcal antibodies. Lab. Med. *2*:38–40, 1971.
66. Jewett, J. F.: Coagulopathy syndrome due to streptococci. N. Engl. J. Med. *289*: 43–44, 1973.
67. Johnson, C. C., and Tunkel, A. R.: Viridans streptococci and groups C and G streptococci. *In* Mandell, G. L., Bennett, J. E., and Dolin, R. (eds.): Principles and Practice of Infectious Diseases. New York, Churchill Livingstone, 1995.
68. Johnson, D. R., and Kaplan, E. L.: A review of the correlation of T-agglutination patterns and M-protein typing and opacity factor production in the identification of group A streptococci. J. Med. Microbiol. *38*:311 315, 1993.
69. Johnson, D. R., Kaplan, E. L., and Ferrieri, P.: Pharyngitis-associated M-12 group A *Streptococcus* satellite strain: Association with *Neisseria subflava*. Pediatr. Infect. Dis. J. *8*:800–802, 1989.
70. Kaplan, E. L.: Benzathine penicillin G for treatment of group A streptococcal pharyngitis: A reappraisal in 1985. Pediatr. Infect. Dis. *4*:592–596, 1985.
71. Kaplan, E. L.: Group A streptococcal carriers and contacts: (When) is retreatment necessary? *In* Shulman, S. (ed.): Management of Pharyngitis in an Era of Declining Rheumatic Fever. Columbus, Ross Conference of Pediatric Research, 1984, p. 92.
72. Kaplan, E. L.: The group A streptococcal upper respiratory tract carrier state: An enigma. J. Pediatr. *97*:337–345, 1980.
73. Kaplan, E. L.: The rapid identification of group A beta-hemolytic streptococci in the upper respiratory tract: Current status. Pediatr. Clin. North Am. *35*:535–542, 1988.
74. Kaplan, E. L.: Unresolved problems in diagnosis and epidemiology of streptococcal infection. *In* Wannamaker, L. W., and Matsen, J. M. (eds.): Streptococci and Streptococcal Diseases. Recognition, Understanding, and Management. New York, Academic Press, 1972, pp. 557–570.
75. Kaplan, E. L., Anthony, B. F., Chapman, S. S., et al.: Epidemic acute glomerulonephritis associated with type 49 streptococcal pyoderma. I. Clinical and laboratory findings. Am. J. Med. *48*:9–27, 1970.
76. Kaplan, E. L., Anthony, B. F., Chapman, S. S., et al.: The influence of the site of infection on the immune response to group A streptococci. J. Clin. Invest. *49*:1405–1414, 1970.
77. Kaplan, E. L., and Kunde, C.: Quantitative evaluation of variation in composition of the streptozyme agglutination reagent for detection of antibodies to group A streptococcal extracellular antigens. J. Clin. Microbiol. *14*:678–680, 1981.
78. Kaplan, E. L., Johnson, D. R., Nanthapisud, P., et al.: A comparison of group A streptococcal serotypes isolated from the upper respiratory tract in the USA and Thailand: Implications. Bull. W. H. O. *70*:433–437, 1992.
79. Kaplan, E. L., Reid, H. F., Johnson, D. R., et al.: Rapid antigen detection in the diagnosis of group A streptococcal pyoderma: Influence of a "learning curve effect" on sensitivity and specificity. Pediatr. Infect. Dis. J. *8*:591–593, 1989.
80. Kaplan, E. L., and Wannamaker, L. W.: C-reactive protein in streptococcal pharyngitis. Pediatrics *60*:28–32, 1977.
81. Kaplan, E. L., Top, F. H., Jr., Dudding, B. A., et al.: Diagnosis of streptococcal pharyngitis: Differentiation of active infection from the carrier state in the symptomatic child. J. Infect. Dis. *123*:490–501, 1971.
82. Kim, K. S.: Clinical perspectives on penicillin tolerance. J. Pediatr. *112*:509–514, 1988.
83. Kim, Y. B., and Watson, D. W., Streptococcal exotoxins: Biological and pathological properties. *In* Wannamaker, L. W., and Matsen, J. M. (eds.): Streptococci and Streptococcal Diseases: Recognition, Understanding, and Management. New York, Academic Press, 1972, pp. 33–50.
84. Kokx, N. P., Comstock, J. A., and Facklam, R. R.: Streptococcal perianal disease in children. Pediatrics *80*:659–663, 1987.
85. Krause, R. M., and Rammelkamp, C. H., Jr.: Studies of the carrier state following infection with group A streptococci. J. Clin. Invest. *41*:575, 1962.

86. Kristensen, B., and Schonheyder, H. C.: A 13-year survey of bacteraemia due to beta-haemolytic streptococci in a Danish county. J. Med. Microbiol. *43*:63–67, 1995.
87. Lancefield, R. C.: Current knowledge of type-specific M antigens of group A streptococci. J. Immunol. *89*:307–313, 1962.
88. Lancefield, R. C.: Group A streptococcal infections in animals: Natural and experimental. *In* Wannamaker, L. W., and Matsen, J. M. (eds.): Streptococci and Streptococcal Diseases: Recognition, Understanding, and Management, 1972, New York, Academic Press, 1972, pp. 313–326.
89. Malke, H., Jacob, H. E., and Störl, K.: Characterization of the antibiotic resistance plasmid ERL1 from *Streptococcus pyogenes*. Mol. Gen. Genet. *144*:333–338, 1976.
90. Markowitz, M., and Kaplan, E. L.: Reappearance of rheumatic fever. *In* Barness, L. A. (ed.): Advances in Pediatrics. Chicago, Year Book Medical Publishers, 1989, pp. 39–66.
91. Martin, N. J., Kaplan, E. L., Gerber, M. A., et al.: Comparison of epidemic and endemic group G streptococci by restriction enzyme analysis. J. Clin. Microbiol. *28*:1881–1886, 1990.
92. Matsen, J. M., and Coghlan, C. R.: Antibiotic testing and susceptibility patterns of streptococci. *In* Wannamaker, L. W., and Matsen, J. M. (eds.): Streptococci and Streptococcal Diseases: Recognition, Understanding, and Management. New York, Academic Press, 1972, pp. 189–204.
93. McCarty, M.: Theories of pathogenesis of streptococcal complications. *In* Wannamaker, L. W., and Matsen, J. M. (eds.): Streptococci and Streptococcal Diseases: Recognition, Understanding, and Management. New York, Academic Press, 1972, pp. 517–526.
94. McCarty, M.: The Streptococcal Cell Wall. Harvey Lectures, 1971, *65*:73–96.
95. McCue, J. D.: Group G streptococcal pharyngitis: Analysis of an outbreak at a college. J. A. M. A. *248*:1333–1336, 1982.
96. Meier, F. A., Centor, R. M., Graham, L., Jr., et al.: Clinical and microbiological evidence for endemic pharyngitis among adults due to group C streptococci. Arch. Intern. Med. *150*:825–829, 1990.
97. Ofek, I., Bergner-Rabinowitz, S., and Ginsburg, I.: Oxygen-stable hemolysins of group A streptococci. VII. The relation of the leukotoxic factor to streptolysin S. J. Infect. Dis. *122*:517–522, 1970.
98. Ofek, I., Kaplan, O., Bergner-Rabinowitz, S., et al.: Antibody tests in streptococcal pharyngitis: Streptozyme versus conventional methods. Clin. Pediatr. *12*:341–344, 1973.
99. Ogunbi, O., Lasi, Q., and Lawal, S. F.: An epidemiological study of beta-hemolytic streptococcal infections in a Nigerian (Lagos) urban population. *In* Haverkorn, M. J. (ed.): Streptococcal Disease and the Community. Amsterdam, Excerpta Medica, 1974, pp. 282–284.
100. Pantell, R. H.: Cost-effectiveness of pharyngitis management and prevention of rheumatic fever. Ann. Intern. Med. *86*:497–499, 1977.
101. Poon-King, T., Mohammed, I., Cox, R., et al.: Recurrent epidemic nephritis in South Trinidad. N. Engl. J. Med. *277*:728–733, 1967.
102. Powers, G. F., and Boisvert, P. L.: Tuberculosis and streptococcosis. Yale J. Biol. Med. *15*:517–530, 1943.
103. Rammelkamp, C. H., Jr.: Epidemiology of Streptococcal Infections. Harvey Lectures *51*:113–142, 1957.
104. Randolph, M. F., Gerber, M. A., DeMeo, K. K., et al.: Effect of antibiotic therapy on the clinical course of streptococcal pharyngitis. J. Pediatr. *106*:870–875, 1985.
105. Read, S. E., Fischetti, V. A., Utermohlen, V., et al.: Cellular reactivity studies to streptococcal antigens: Migration inhibition studies in patients with streptococcal infections and rheumatic fever. J. Clin. Invest. *54*:439–450, 1974.
106. Reid, H. F., Bassett, D. C., Poon-King, T., et al.: Group G streptococci in healthy school-children and in patients with glomerulonephritis in Trinidad. J. Hyg. *94*:61–68, 1985.
107. Rolston, K. V., Chandrasekar, P. H., and LeFrock, J. L.: Antimicrobial tolerance in group C and group G streptococci. J. Antimicrob. Chemother. *13*:389–392, 1984.
108. Rolston, K. V., LeFrock, J. L., and Schell, R. F.: Activity of nine antimicrobial agents against Lancefield group C and group G streptococci. Antimicrob. Agents Chemother. *22*:930–932, 1982.
109. Sawyer, W. D., Smith, M. R., and Wood, W. B., Jr.: The mechanisms by which macrophages phagocyte encapsulated bacteria in the absence of antibody. J. Exp. Med. *100*:417–424, 1954.
110. Schwartz, R. H., Gerber, M. A., and McCoy, P.: Effect of atmosphere of incubation on the isolation of group A streptococci from throat cultures. J. Lab. Clin. Med. *106*:88–92, 1985.
111. Seppala, H., Nissinen, A., Jarvinen, H., et al.: Resistance to erythromycin in group A streptococci. N. Engl. J. Med. *326*:292–297, 1992.
112. Seravalli, E., and Taranta, A.: Lymphocyte transformation and macrophage migration inhibition by electrofocused and gel-filtered fractions of group A streptococcal filtrate. Cell. Immunol. *14*:366–375, 1974.
113. Shulman, S. T.: Streptococcal pharyngitis: Diagnostic considerations. Pediatr. Infect. Dis. J. *13*:567–571, 1994.
114. Siegel, A. C., Johnson, E. E., and Stollerman, G. H.: Conrolled studies of streptococcal pharyngitis in a pediatric population. I. Factors related to the attack rate of rheumatic fever. N. Engl. J. Med. *265*:559–566, 1961.
115. Smith, E. W., Garson, A., Jr., Boyleston, J. A., et al.: Varicella gangrenosa due to group A beta-hemolytic *Streptococcus*. Pediatrics *57*:306–310, 1976.
116. Smith, T. D., Wilkinson, V., and Kaplan, E. L.: Group A *Streptococcus*–associated upper respiratory tract infections in a day-care center. Pediatrics *83*:380–384, 1989.
117. Snellman, L. W., Stang, H. J., Stang, J. M., et al.: Duration of positive throat cultures for group A streptococci after initiation of antibiotic therapy. Pediatrics *91*:1166–1170, 1993.
118. Stetson, C. A., Rammelkamp, C. H., Jr., Krause, R. M., et al.: Epidemic acute nephritis: Studies on etiology, natural history and prevention. Medicine *34*:431–450, 1955.
119. Stevens, D. L.: Streptococcal toxic-shock syndrome: Spectrum of disease, pathogenesis, and new concepts in treatment. Emerg. Infect. Dis. *1*:69–78, 1995.
120. Stevens, D. L., Tanner, M. H., Winship, J., et al.: Severe group A streptococcal infections associated with a toxic shock–like syndrome and scarlet fever toxin A. N. Engl. J. Med. *321*:1–7, 1989.
121. Tagg, J. R., Dajani, A. S., Wannamaker, L. W., et al.: Group A streptococcal bacteriocin: Production, purification, and mode of action. J. Exp. Med. *138*:1168–1183, 1973.
122. Tancer, M. L., McManus, J. E., and Bellotti, G.: Group A, type 33, beta-hemolytic streptococcal outbreak on a maternity and newborn service. Am. J. Obstet. Gynecol. *103*:1028–1033, 1969.
123. Turner, J. C., Hayden, G. F., Kiselica, D., et al.: Association of group C beta-hemolytic streptococci with endemic pharyngitis among college students. J. A. M. A. *264*:2644–2647, 1990.
124. Veasy, L. G., Tani, L. Y., and Hill, H. R.: Persistence of acute rheumatic fever in the intermountain area of the United States. J. Pediatr. *124*:9–16, 1994.
125. Wannamaker, L. W.: Diagnosis of pharyngitis: Clinical and epidemiologic features. *In* Shulman, S. (ed.): Management of Pharyngitis in an Era of Declining Rheumatic Fever. Columbus, Ross Conference on Pediatric Research, 1984, p. 25.
126. Wannamaker, L. W.: Differences between streptococcal infections of the throat and of the skin. I. N. Engl. J. Med. *282*:23–31, 1970.
127. Wannamaker, L. W.: Immunology of streptococci. *In* Good, R. A., Nahmias, A. J., and O'Reilly, R. J. (eds.): Comprehensive Immunology: Immunology of Human Infection. New York, Plenum, 1981, pp. 47–72.
128. Wannamaker, L. W.: Perplexity and precision in the diagnosis of streptococcal pharyngitis. Am. J. Dis. Child. *124*:352–358, 1972.
129. Wannamaker, L. W.: The chain that links the heart to the throat. Circulation *48*:9–18, 1973.
130. Wannamaker, L. W.: The epidemiology of streptococcal infections. *In* McCarty, M. (ed.): Streptococcal Infections. New York, Columbia University Press, 1954, 157–175.
131. Wannamaker, L. W., Almquist, S., and Skjold, S.: Intergroup phage reactions and transduction between group C and group A streptococci. J. Exp. Med. *137*:1338–1353, 1973.
132. Wannamaker, L. W., and Ferrieri, P.: Streptococcal infections: Updated. Disease-A-Month, pp. 1–40, 1975.
133. Weinstein, L., and Le Frock, J.: Does antimicrobial therapy of streptococcal pharyngitis or pyoderma alter the risk of glomerulonephritis? J. Infect. Dis. *124*:229–231, 1971.
134. Wesley, T. B., Johnson, D. R., Diesch, S. L., et al.: Do beta hemolytic streptococci in the upper respiratory tract (URT) of household dogs constitute a significant zoonotic threat? Abstracts of the Interscience Conference on Antibiotics and Chemotherapy, 1995.
135. Wittler, R. R., Yamada, S. M., Bass, J. W., et al.: Penicillin tolerance and erythromycin resistance of group A beta-hemolytic streptococci in Hawaii and the Philippines. Am. J. Dis. Child. *144*:587–589, 1990.
136. Zabriski, J. B.: The role of temperate bacteriophage in the production of erythrogenic toxin by group A streptococci. J. Exp. Med. *119*:761–779, 1964.
137. Zimmerman, R. A., and Hill, H. R.: Placental transfer of group A type-specific streptococcal antibody. Pediatrics *43*:809–814, 1969.

88

GROUP B STREPTOCOCCAL INFECTIONS

Judith L. Rowen and Carol J. Baker

HISTORY

The organism we know as group B *Streptococcus,* or *Streptococcus agalactiae,* first was isolated by Nocard in 1887[214] and for decades was recognized as a cause of bovine mastitis[205] but not of human infection. Serologic techniques for differentiating beta-hemolytic streptococci were developed by Lancefield,[169] who also described isolation of group B streptococci from parturient women in 1935. In that same year, Congdon[79] included one fatal puerperal case of group B streptococcal sepsis and pneumonia in a report of streptococcal infections associated with childbirth. The significance of this organism as a human pathogen first was reported in 1938, when Fry[112] described three cases of fatal puerperal sepsis. Group B streptococcal infections continued to be reported sporadically until the 1960s, when maternal and neonatal infections increasingly were ascribed to this pathogen.[70, 95, 138] In the 1970s, group B *Streptococcus* emerged as the predominant organism causing bacteremia and meningitis in neonates.[19, 33, 110, 142, 223] Since then, the incidence of neonatal infection has remained stable, with reported attack rates ranging from 0.2 to 5.4 per 1000 live births.[35, 223, 269, 327] Systemic infection does occur beyond the neonatal period in pregnant women, and group B streptococci have been recognized as significant pathogens in nonpregnant adults.[99, 143, 217]

MICROBIOLOGY

Isolation and Identification

Group B streptococci are facultative gram-positive diplococci that grow on a variety of bacteriologic media. Colonies are 3 to 4 mm in diameter, grayish-white, flat, and somewhat mucoid. Colonies are surrounded by a narrow zone of beta-hemolysis that for some strains is detectable only when the colony is lifted from the agar. Nonhemolytic strains account for 1 to 2 per cent of isolates and may cause human disease.[19, 253] Differentiation of hemolytic streptococci relies on detection of group-specific antigens within the cell wall. The standard method, as described by Lancefield,[168] requires acid treatment of the bacteria to solubilize the carbohydrate group B antigen, followed by capillary precipitation with hyperimmune rabbit serum. Several newer methods utilizing hyperimmune antisera have been developed, but latex agglutination is used widely because of the commercial availability of test kits, the ease of performing the assay, and the specificity of the results when organisms in pure culture are tested.[277] Other laboratory methods for presumptive identification include testing for resistance to bacitracin or trimethoprim-sulfamethoxazole, hydrolysis of sodium hippurate broth, failure to hydrolyze bile esculin, production of orange pigment when cultured under certain conditions, and CAMP testing. CAMP is an acronym of the names of the authors who first described synergistic hemolysis on sheep blood agar when group B streptococci are grown in the presence of the beta-toxin of *Staphylococcus aureus.*[78]

Serologic Classification and Antigenic Structure

Just as beta-hemolytic streptococci are divided into groups based on cell wall antigens, group B streptococci are divided further into serotypes based on type-specific capsular polysaccharides. The type-specific polysaccharides of group B streptococci are repeating units of five to seven monosaccharides (glucose, galactose, glucosamine, and *N*-acetylneuraminic acid). All of the characterized polysaccharides include an *N*-acetylneuraminic acid (sialic acid) residue, which may be important in the pathogenesis of human infection.[40, 272, 311] Seven such polysaccharides are characterized: Ia, Ib, and II to VI. This number may increase because a new serotype from Japan, previously known as JM9, is being characterized[300] and provisional types VII and IX are being considered. A small proportion of strains do not react with hyperimmune sera to the characterized capsular polysaccharides and are called nontypable. Further differentiation of type Ia strains was based on the presence or absence of a protein antigen known as c, leading to the nomenclature of Ia and Ia/c serotypes. This c protein is present on many other serotypes as well, but it is rare in type III strains.[108] Table 88–1 reviews the major surface antigens of group B streptococci, including R and X, which may not be related to the virulence of these organisms.

Extracellular Products

Several bacterial products are elaborated by group B streptococci. Type-specific capsular polysaccharide is released from cells, and the amount elaborated has been correlated with virulence.[166, 322] These soluble polysaccharides inhibit opsonophagocytic killing in vitro, providing a mechanism for the documented increase in virulence.[175] Most strains possess C5a-ase, an enzyme of the serine esterase class that inactivates complement component C5a.[136] Because C5a is a potent chemoattractant for neutrophils, this enzyme helps the bacteria to evade the host immune system by hindering the accumulation of neutrophils at the site of infection. Other bacterial products of group B streptococci have been described, including hemolysin, CAMP factor, lipoteichoic acid, pigment, hippuricase, neuraminidase, hyaluronidase, and nucleases, but the contribution of these substances to pathogenesis is not clear.[106, 107, 118, 155, 188, 196, 211, 212, 289, 305]

Antimicrobial Susceptibility

To date, human isolates of group B streptococci have remained uniformly susceptible to penicillin G. However, approximately 10-fold greater concentrations are required for inhibition and killing of group B streptococci than of group A streptococci. Group B streptococci also are susceptible to other β-lactams, cephalosporins, vancomycin, and imipenem. Resistance to the macrolides (erythromycin, clindamycin, clarithromycin) occurs in 1 to 3 per cent of isolates.[54, 254] Nearly 90 per cent of strains are resistant to tetracycline, and

TABLE 88–1. Antigenic Determinants of Group B *Streptococcus*

	Serotypes	Structure/Composition	Comments	Reference
Polysaccharides				
Group B	All	Highly branched; 4 oligosaccharides; probably linked to cell wall peptidoglycan	Antibody not protective	170, 202
Ia	Ia, Ia/c	5-monosaccharide repeating unit		150
Ib	Ib	5-monosaccharide repeating unit; identical to Ia except 1-3 instead of 1-4 linkage at galactose side chain	Homology with oligosaccharides from human milk	150, 236
II	II	7-monosaccharide repeating unit	2 side chains; sialic acid linked directly to repeating unit	152
III	III	5-monosaccharide repeating unit	Removal of terminal sialic acid results in a polysaccharide identical to type 14 *S. pneumoniae*	109, 151
IV	IV	6-monosaccharide repeating unit		308
V	V	7-monosaccharide repeating unit		309
VI	VI	5-monosaccharide repeating unit; lacks *N*-acetylglucosamine		299
Proteins*				
c	Ia/c, Ib, up to 60% of II, many IV, occasional V	Alpha (trypsin-resistant) and beta (trypsin-sensitive) antigens may be present singly or in combination	Beta binds Fc portion of human IgA	64, 108, 153, 228
R	37% of II, 80% of III, occasional IV, many V	5 species known	Found also on groups A and C streptococci; immunologically cross-reactive with X antigen	108, 312
X	Occasional III and IV, many nontypable strains		Found on 47% of bovine strains	108, 312

*Protein constituents of type VI strains not yet evaluated.

resistance to bacitracin, nalidixic acid, trimethoprim-sulfamethoxazole, and metronidazole is uniform.[231] Low-level gentamicin resistance is typical, but when gentamicin is combined with either penicillin G or ampicillin, there is synergistic killing of group B streptococci in vitro and in vivo.[263, 264, 286]

Up to 5 per cent of group B streptococcal isolates have been reported to be tolerant to penicillin.[163] Expression of tolerance requires laboratory conditions that promote a greater than 16-fold discrepancy between minimal inhibitory concentrations and minimal bactericidal concentrations. Tolerant strains are characterized in vitro by delayed penicillin killing, similar rates of killing by penicillin whether growth is exponential or stationary, an additive rather than a synergistic response to the combination of penicillin and gentamicin, and deficient autolysis. The clinical significance, if any, of these laboratory-induced properties remains unknown.[26, 162]

EPIDEMIOLOGY

Incidence

Reported attack rates for group B streptococcal disease in infants range from 0.2 to 5.4 per 1000 live births.[32, 223, 306, 327] Early-onset disease accounts for approximately 80 per cent of cases.[267] Late-onset disease attack rates range from 0.3 to 1.8 per 1000 live births.[84, 223] A multistate active surveillance program encompassing a population of 10.1 million persons in five U.S. states indicated attack rates of 1.4 and 0.3 per 1000 live births, respectively, for early- and late-onset disease.[327] When these rates are applied to the U.S. population as a whole, a minimum of 6200 early- and 1400 late-onset cases can be expected each year.[327] As the use of maternal intrapartum chemoprophylaxis to prevent early-onset disease increases, these rates may diminish.[35, 235]

Information relating to infants with onset of group B streptococcal disease beyond 3 months of age is sparse. Several reported infants have had concomitant infection with HIV or have been born before 34 weeks' gestation.[82, 143] Group B streptococcal disease also is common in pregnant women, with clinical presentations that include urinary tract infection (usually asymptomatic bacteriuria), intra-amniotic infection, endometritis (often with bacteremia), puerperal sepsis, and occasionally meningitis, septic thrombophlebitis, or other serious complications.[25, 102, 222, 269] Attack rates of 2 per 1000 deliveries have been reported.[222] However, nonpregnant adults actually made up the majority of cases (68 per cent) of group B streptococcal infection from the greater Atlanta metropolitan region.[99] In these patients, underlying medical conditions are the rule, and these include diabetes mellitus, malignancy (especially solid tumors), HIV infection, liver disease, stroke and other neurologic disorders, decubitus ulcer, neurogenic bladder, and advanced age.[99, 146, 217]

Maternal Colonization

Infection in the neonate with group B streptococci results from the presence of the organism in the maternal genital tract at delivery.[32] In most cases, the mother asymptomatically is infected or colonized. Maternal colonization rates vary widely and relate to body sites sampled, microbiologic techniques employed, and the period of gestation in which cultures are performed.

The site chosen for culture is critical, and sampling of multiple sites improves detection.[25, 30, 83] The distal vagina more frequently yields group B streptococci than does the cervix.[186, 246] Concomitant sampling of the rectal site results in detection of virtually all carriers. Several investigators have suggested the gastrointestinal tract as the principal reservoir for this organism,[17, 25, 139] and not uncommonly the rectal site is the only one that yields group B streptococci.[32, 83, 139, 232, 326] The urinary tract is an important site of infection (asymptomatic bacteriuria) because it is a surrogate for high ($>10^5$ colony-forming units/mL) genital inoculum.[209, 319]

The manner in which swab specimens from the vagina and rectum are processed also is important in accurately assessing colonization. Swabs may be placed in transport media at environmental temperatures for up to 96 hours. Once they reach the laboratory, however, they should be placed in antibiotic-containing broth rather than on solid media because the latter "misses" detection of up to 50 per cent of group B streptococcal positive cultures.[30, 37] The addition of antibiotics to the broth (selective broth medium) limits growth of competing flora and enhances detection.[7, 37, 193] Todd Hewitt broth with gentamicin (selective broth medium)[34] or colistin and nalidixic acid (Lim broth)[179] are recommended for detection of group B streptococcal colonization.[8, 235] After overnight incubation, the broth is subcultured onto a 5 per cent sheep blood agar plate and processed conventionally.

The proximity to delivery also affects the accuracy of predicting colonization at delivery. Ninety-two per cent of culture-positive women are identified if lower vaginal and rectal cultures are obtained at a single visit.[87] Furthermore, although rates are similar by trimester, cultures obtained at 35 and 37 weeks' gestation predict colonization at delivery with nearly 100 per cent accuracy.[60, 235] Reported colonization rates vary widely, but if the aforementioned methods are used, the overall rate is about 25 per cent.[30, 87]

Risk Factors for Colonization During Pregnancy

Much effort has been spent trying to define groups of women at enhanced risk for colonization with group B streptococci. Nonpregnant women have similar colonization rates, suggesting that pregnancy does not affect colonization.[38, 97] Women younger than 20 years of age have higher and multiparous (≥ 3 pregnancies) women have lower colonization rates.[18, 38, 246, 324, 326] Although group B streptococci are sexually transmissible, the number of sexual partners or frequency of sexual activity does not influence colonization status.[38, 246] Ethnicity does affect the likelihood of colonization. In a survey of 2929 women, 36.7 per cent of black women were colonized, a rate significantly greater than the 23.3 per cent in women belonging to other ethnic groups.[326] In the same study, Asian women had a significantly lower rate of group B streptococcal colonization (14 per cent) than any other ethnic group. The multicenter study conducted by the Vaginal Infections and Prematurity Study Group evaluated 7742 women at 23 to 26 weeks' gestation and reported that black race, age younger than 20 years, and lower educational level were correlated independently with high group B streptococcal colonization rates.[246]

Infant Colonization

Acquisition of the organism by infants born to colonized mothers (vertical transmission) occurs in 29 to 72 per cent of cases.[5, 18, 32, 81, 87, 223, 274] As with maternal colonization, detection depends on sites sampled, culture method, and timing. Acquisition is presumed to occur either by the ascending route through ruptured membranes or from contact with the organism in the genital tract during parturition. Nosocomial transmission and community acquisition may occur, although uncommonly.[1, 18, 115, 215] If cultures are obtained immediately after birth, positive results reflect contamination with infected maternal secretions and high inoculum. Twenty-four to 48 hours is an appropriate age to determine whether the infant has become colonized in the gastrointestinal or respiratory tract after exposure to maternal group B *Streptococcus*. Many sites have been utilized for neonatal cultures, including the ear canal, throat, umbilicus, and rectum. Historically, the umbilicus was a reliable site, but its routine treatment with triple dye and other antiseptics diminishes recovery of group B streptococci.[48, 281] Isolation of the organism from the throat or rectum implies replication of organisms at respiratory or gastrointestinal tract sites after ingestion of infected amniotic fluid or genital secretions. One study determined that sampling of the throat and rectum at 24 to 48 hours of age identified all colonized infants.[135]

Factors Influencing Infant Colonization Rates

The single factor most clearly associated with the likelihood of vertical transmission and subsequent neonatal colonization is the number of organisms (inoculum) in the maternal genital tract. Mothers with high group B streptococcal inocula ($>10^5$ colony-forming units/mL) are more likely to transmit the organism to their baby.[12, 18, 139, 154] However, maternal intrapartum antibiotic therapy substantially diminishes the vertical transmission of group B streptococci.[61, 62, 274, 325] In one study, infant colonization was significantly lower (8 per cent vs. 20 per cent) in an obstetric population in which 35 per cent of colonized mothers received intrapartum antibiotics than in another group in which only 15 per cent were treated.[135]

Risk Factors for Infant Disease

Vertical transmission is a prerequisite for the development of invasive, early-onset infection.[32, 195, 223] There is evidence that the majority of late-onset infections also occur after vertical transmission.[84] The degree of colonization or inoculum also increases the likelihood of infant disease; heavily colonized mothers are more likely to have symptomatically infected infants, and heavily colonized infants are more likely to develop either early- or late-onset disease.[60, 84, 154, 178] Other maternal factors associated with the development of early-onset disease include labor prior to 37 weeks' gestation, premature rupture of membranes or rupture of membranes more than 18 hours before delivery at any gestation, and intrapartum fever.[19, 60, 84, 110, 223] The association with premature rupture of membranes or premature labor may be a "chicken and egg" phenomenon because colonization with group B streptococci, especially in high inoculum, has been associated with premature rupture of membranes and preterm labor.[4, 137, 194, 198, 245] Other maternal factors associated with an increased attack rate of early-onset infection are black race, age younger than 20 years, history of previous fetal loss, history of urinary tract infection with group B streptococci, and primiparity.[268] Late-onset disease also is associated with young maternal age and black race.[269] Infants who are the product of a multiple pregnancy (e.g., twins) have been shown to be at some enhanced risk of early- and late-onset group B streptococcal disease,[91, 224] but this association has not been demonstrated consistently.[269]

Serotypes Causing Disease

Reports from the 1970s indicated that the group B streptococcal serotypes colonizing pregnant women and neonates were fairly evenly divided among types I, II, and III.[25, 31, 313, 314] However, a new serotype, type V, has emerged.[56, 135, 250] The representation of serotypes in invasive disease is less balanced, however. When meningitis is present, either as a focus of early-onset disease or as the manifestation of late-onset infection, type III is implicated in the majority of cases (80 to 93 per cent).[31, 314] In contrast, type II was the predominant isolate in adult cases of meningitis.[174, 314] The serotype distribution is relatively balanced when other manifestations of early-onset disease (e.g., bacteremia without a focus or pneumonia) are considered, but type III strains still dominate late-onset infections.[31] Type V causes both early- and late-onset infant disease and serious infections in adults but appears to lag behind types Ia and III.[56, 250] The least common serotypes causing human disease are types Ib/c, IV, and VI.

PATHOGENESIS

For pediatricians, group B streptococcal disease predominantly afflicts neonates, a predilection that results from a unique combination of maternal, bacterial, and host factors. A proposed scheme for the pathogenesis of early-onset infection is outlined in Figure 88–1. First, an organism carried by an asymptomatically colonized mother is transmitted to her neonate. Evidence suggests that this may occur in utero or during parturition. This continuum in the time of acquisition is reflected in the time of onset of symptoms; infected neonates often are symptomatic within 6 hours of birth (up to 70 per cent), whereas others may not evidence disease for a few days.[33, 269] The organism successfully colonizes about 50 per cent of all infants born to group B streptococcal carriers, yet only 1 to 2 per cent of these infants develop disease.[19, 32, 267] A breach in the delicate interplay of maternal, infant, and bacterial factors allows the organism to invade. Once invasion occurs, a combination of host defenses and therapeutic interventions may halt progression of disease, or the infant's defenses may fail and the disease may progress and result in tissue damage or death.

Maternal Factors

The bacterial inoculum in the maternal genital tract determines the likelihood that the organism will be transmitted vertically. Infants born to heavily colonized women are more likely to be colonized themselves and are more likely to develop early-onset disease.[12, 18, 60, 84, 139, 154] Infants delivered prematurely have an increased risk for developing early-onset disease. Heavy maternal colonization may instigate preterm delivery,[194, 208, 245] with the infant more likely to develop disease in this setting of exposure to high bacterial inoculum combined with immunologic immaturity. Invasive disease also has been reported in neonates delivered by elective cesarean (intact membranes).[19, 95, 222]

In addition to bacterial load, the other critical maternal factor is the concentration of antibody to the serotype-specific polysaccharide capsule of the colonizing strain of group B *Streptococcus* in serum at delivery. Antibody to the type-specific antigen is protective against the homologous serotype in the mouse model; antibody to the group B polysaccharide is not.[170] Baker and associates[36, 41] determined that invasive disease with type III group B streptococci occurred primarily in infants born to women with low concentrations

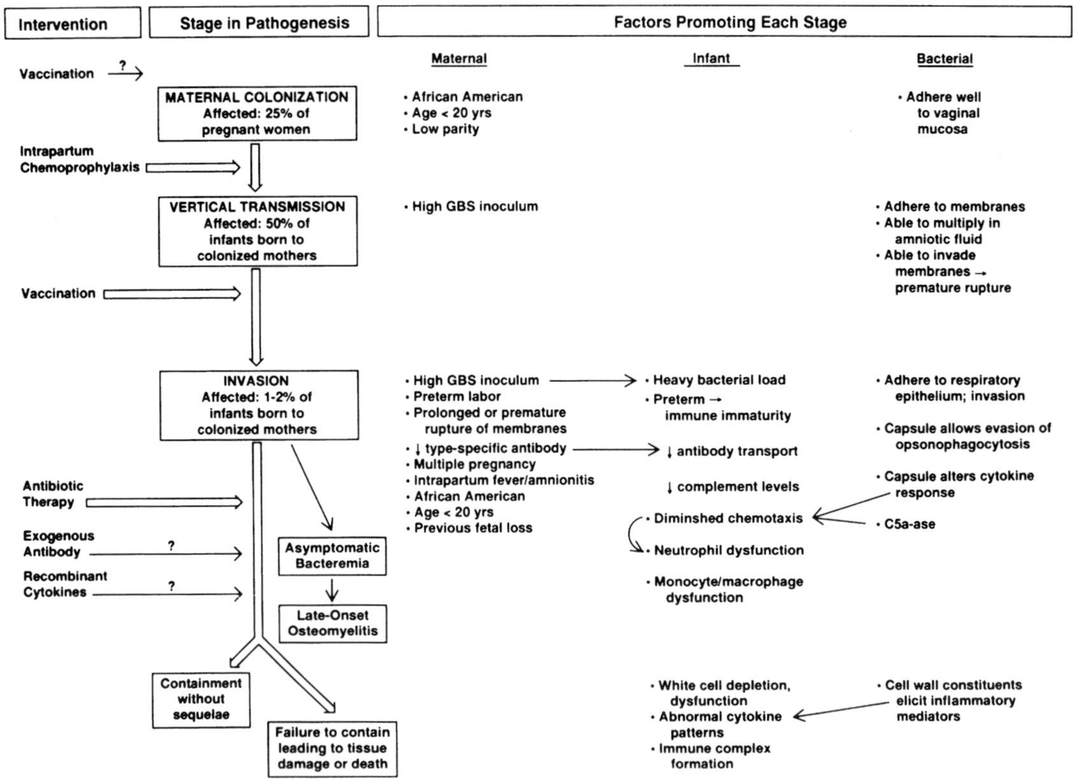

FIGURE 88–1. *Proposed scheme for the pathophysiology of group B streptococcal infections in infants.*

of anti–type III capsular antibody in their sera. Several other investigators also have reported a correlation between low concentrations of antibody to types Ia, Ib, II, and III polysaccharides in maternal delivery sera and occurrence of early- and late-onset group B streptococcal infant disease.[122, 123] A correlation between antibody concentration and maternal age may explain the epidemiologic association of young maternal age and increased likelihood of neonatal disease.[16] Animal models have demonstrated that antibody directed against the alpha or beta determinants of c protein is protective,[170, 201] but definitive human studies are lacking. Antibody to other protein determinants in some serotypes has been postulated to be partially protective. Titers of antibody to R protein were found to be higher in maternal serum from mothers colonized with R protein–bearing strains whose infants were healthy than from mothers whose infants were ill; such antibodies were protective in a mouse model against some strains.[180, 181]

Bacterial Factors

In order to colonize the genital tract or cause disease effectively, the organisms must be able to adhere to host tissues. Group B streptococci adhere well to many types of epithelium, including vaginal epithelium and chorioamnionic membranes.[113, 189, 278, 288] Type III strains adhere more avidly to vaginal cells than do other serotypes in vitro.[59] Furthermore, invasive strains adhere better to epithelial tissues than do colonizing strains.[132] This capacity to adhere to, and possibly invade, chorioamnionic cells may explain the association of group B streptococcal colonization with preterm labor and premature rupture of membranes.[137] If a breach occurs in the membranes, the bacteria can multiply in amniotic fluid.[133] After transmission and colonization, the capacity of the bacteria to adhere to neonatal epithelial cells may allow them to invade and disseminate. The lung, after aspiration of infected maternal fluids, is a frequent initial site of infection in the newborn. Group B streptococci can adhere to and invade respiratory epithelial cell lines.[258] Also, they can invade endothelial cells, which may be a mechanism for some of the pathologic features of disseminated disease.[118] Some have postulated that the bacterial cell wall component, lipoteichoic acid, confers adherence properties to group B streptococci,[212] but others have suggested other surface proteins.[69, 288]

A well-defined virulence structure of group B streptococci is the capsular polysaccharide. Mouse virulent strains are able to synthesize greater amounts of surface-bound type-specific polysaccharide than are avirulent strains.[322] An unencapsulated mutant, created by inserting a transposon into the gene regulating capsule expression, has significantly less virulence in neonatal rats than does the parent type III strain.[259] As with other encapsulated organisms, the capsule is thought to confer virulence primarily by interfering with opsonophagocytosis. In vitro, the capsule of type III group B streptococci has been shown to prevent deposition of C3,[191] and the presence of the terminal sialic acid residue on the repeating unit of the polysaccharide is crucial to this interference.[93] Removal of sialic acid residues from the polysaccharide leads to diminished virulence, and a desialylated mutant loses virulence when compared with the parent strain.[311] Furthermore, the presence of this sialic acid moiety prevents activation of the alternative complement pathway, the predominant pathway utilized by the human host when minimal type-specific antibody is present.[93] Also, when bacteria grow in the presence of human serum, the quantity of sialic acid increases, thereby potentiating its contribution to virulence.[234] Opsonization may be affected by cell surface components other than capsular sialic acid. C protein also lends relative resistance to opsonization to strains bearing the antigen.[228]

Sialic acid residues on the capsule may interfere with another component of the immune system. In a serum-free system, the desialylated mutant of type III group B streptococci elicited much larger quantities of leukotriene B_4 from macrophages than the parent strain did.[256] Leukotriene B_4 is a potent neutrophil chemoattractant, so this effect may result in diminished influx of effector cells. Similarly, C5a-ase may disable C5a, another host product capable of eliciting neutrophil influx. C5a also has direct stimulatory effects on the neutrophil, enhancing phagocytosis and killing of group B streptococci, so bacterial elaboration of C5a-ase may affect both the accumulation of neutrophils and the efficiency of neutrophil function.[287]

Once invasive infection is established, ongoing replication and digestion of the bacteria can instigate host inflammatory responses that may be deleterious. Neonates recovering from group B streptococcal disease have circulating immune complexes for a prolonged period; immune complexes can contribute to end-organ damage.[293] Additionally, immune complexes containing group B streptococcal components elicit inflammatory mediators, such as leukotriene B_4 and interleukin (IL)-6. The cytokine response to gram-positive pathogens is not as clearly delineated as is that to gram-negative bacteria, partly because of the greater heterogeneity in structure of the latter.[57] Both the group B and the type III capsular polysaccharides induce IL-6 release from monocytes[294]; the group B antigen also causes tumor necrosis factor (TNF)-α release.[295] As with other gram-positive pathogens, the cell walls of group B streptococci contain peptidoglycan and lipoteichoic acid. Peptidoglycans from other gram-positive organisms elicit a variety of proinflammatory cytokines, such as TNF-α, IL-1, IL-6, and granulocyte colony-stimulating factor.[85, 134, 247] Lipoteichoic acid also induces release of IL-1β, IL-6, and TNF-α.[55, 159] Group B streptococcal cell wall components also exert similar effects. Elaboration of these cytokines has been implicated in the clinical, hemodynamic effects of sepsis.[57] Specifically, blockade of IL-1 activity by administration of IL-1 receptor antagonist in a piglet model of group B streptococcal sepsis ameliorated systemic hypotension and prolonged survival.[296]

Infant Host Factors

Neonates have several domains of immune dysfunction that affect their ability to mount a sufficient defense against group B streptococci. Neutrophils are the primary effector cell in host defense against extracellular bacterial pathogens. Neutrophils from neonates have functional abnormalities,[176] including impaired migration to a chemotactic stimulus.[15] The generation of chemotactic activity in neonatal serum in response to group B streptococci is diminished, as is the release of chemotactic factors by neonatal monocytes.[14, 257] Thus, the diminished ability of neutrophils to migrate is amplified by a diminished level of chemotactic stimulation. Phagocytosis and bacterial killing also are impaired when opsonic activity is poor, which is the usual pattern in neonates with sepsis.[176] The neutrophil storage pools of neonates rapidly become depleted during invasive infection, leading to profound neutropenia,[77] an ominous prognostic indicator.[227] These defects in neonatal neutrophils are even more pronounced in infants born prematurely.[176]

Cells of the monocyte/macrophage lineage also may have a role in host defense against group B streptococci, especially in the lung, where the alveolar macrophage is the first effector cell to encounter pathogens. Defects in the function of these cells have been described in neonates. Cord blood monocytes have impaired phagocytosis and killing of group B streptococci.[190] In animal models, oxidative metabolism, bacterial uptake, and migration to the site of infection by neonatal macrophages are diminished in response to group B streptococci.[192, 270, 271]

Humoral immunity is compromised in neonates. Both the alternative and classic complement pathways are affected, and premature neonates are impaired more severely.[80, 90] Both pathways are important in opsonization of group B streptococci.[35] The concentration of type-specific antibody passively acquired from the mother is an important protective factor. Because passive transfer of IgG increases dramatically in the final 8 weeks of pregnancy, premature neonates again are at a disadvantage because they may not receive sufficient amounts of antibodies if born before protective levels are transferred.[76]

The pattern of cytokine production by neonatal immune cells frequently is altered compared with that of adults. For example, in response to group B streptococci, the level of TNF-α released by neonatal monocytes is increased relative to adults,[295, 315] but levels of IL-8 and leukotriene B_4 are decreased.[257, 265] Cytokine networks are important both in the manifestations of sepsis and in the stimulation of an appropriate immune response, so alterations in cytokine expression may affect the neonate's response to this pathogen both clinically and immunologically.

CLINICAL MANIFESTATIONS

Age Onset

The paradigm of early- versus late-onset disease in neonates and young infants first was described in 1973 by Baker and associates,[33] when they and investigators from Colorado[110] noted the bimodal distribution of group B streptococcal infections. The syndromes of early- and late-onset disease differ in epidemiologic characteristics, pathogenesis, clinical presentation, and prognosis. Their major clinical features are detailed in Table 88–2. Early-onset disease occurs in the first week of life, but the majority of neonates present at or within 12 hours of birth.[27, 267] Infants with late-onset infection present between 8 and 90 days of age (median, 27 days; mean, 36 days).[269] Originally, 3 months of age was considered the end of the risk period, but late, late–onset disease, although rare, has been reported.[143, 320]

Early-onset disease often, but not universally, occurs in the setting of maternal complications known to increase the risk for neonatal sepsis. These include labor before 37 weeks' gestation, prolonged rupture of membranes for more than 18 hours, chorioamnionitis, and early postpartum febrile morbidity.[33, 35, 50, 60, 84, 239, 306] The three most frequent clinical presentations are bacteremia or septicemia without a focus, pneumonia, and meningitis.[19, 35, 306, 320] The signs are similar for each, and these range from shock and respiratory failure at delivery to asymptomatic infection detected during evaluation of the term neonate because of maternal risk factors known to increase sepsis risk.[229, 306] Respiratory signs predominate and include apnea, grunting respirations, tachypnea, and cyanosis.[27, 33] Other signs include lethargy, poor feeding, abdominal distention, pallor, tachycardia, and jaundice. Fever usually is present in term neonates, but premature infants often are normothermic or hypothermic.[306] The case-fatality rate is 6 to 15 per cent.[269, 306, 320, 327]

Late-onset disease primarily affects term infants with an unremarkable maternal history and early neonatal course.[33, 84] However, more recent case series suggest that a larger number of infants born quite prematurely (<32 weeks' gestation) develop late, late–onset infection beyond 3 months of age. "Epidemics" of late-onset disease also have occurred in neonatal intensive care units, usually in preterm neonates infected through nosocomial transmission.[47, 215] Meningitis and bacteremia without focus are the two most common manifestations of late-onset disease.[110, 320, 327] Osteoarticular infections and cellulitis are additional clinical presentations.[28, 89, 320] Whereas early-onset disease most frequently presents acutely with apnea and hypotension, late-onset disease often presents with fever, irritability, and other nonspecific signs.[35] More fulminant, rapidly progressive cases do occur, however.[33] The case-fatality rate ranges from 0 to 6 per cent.[269, 320, 327]

Bacteremia

Bacteremia without a focus is present in 27 to 87 per cent of neonates with early-onset disease.[269, 306, 320] Signs of septicemia, such as respiratory distress and poor perfusion, often are present, especially in prematurely born neonates.[306] Asymptomatic bacteremia also may occur in term infants, and, in one series, this made up 22 per cent of cases.[142, 306, 320] It is likely that these infants remained asymptomatic because of early evaluation and institution of empiric therapy.[306] Bacteremia without a focus was the presentation in 46 per cent of late-onset infections reported by Yagupsky and associates.[320]

TABLE 88–2. Features of Group B Streptococcal Disease in Infants

Feature (Reference)	Early-Onset	Late-Onset	Late, Late–Onset
Age at onset (35, 269)	≤7 days; mean, 8 hours; median, 1 hour	≥7–90 days; mean, 36 days; median, 27 days	>90 days
Infants affected (33, 91, 269, 306)	Premature neonates, births after maternal obstetric complications	Term infants predominate	Premature neonates <1500 g, immune deficiency
Presentation (35)	Acute respiratory distress, apnea and hypotension common	Fever, irritability, nonspecific signs; occasionally fulminant	Fever, irritability, nonspecific signs
Manifestations (19, 28, 89, 110, 306, 320)	Septicemia or bacteremia (40–55%), pneumonia (30–45%), meningitis (6–15%)	Bacteremia without a focus (55%), meningitis (35%), osteoarthritis (~5%), cellulitis/adenitis (~2%)	Bacteremia without a focus, focal infections as in late-onset
Serotypes isolated (31, 313)	All (Ia, II, III, and V most frequent)	Type III predominates	All
Case-fatality ratio (269, 306, 320, 327)	6–15%	0–6%	<5%

Generally, these infants are mildly ill and present with fever and nonspecific signs that should prompt a bacteriologic evaluation.

Meningitis

Meningitis is documented in 6 to 15 per cent of neonates with early-onset disease.[35, 269, 306, 320] As a rule, there are no signs that specifically indicate its presence, underscoring the need to evaluate all neonates with presumed early-onset disease for the possibility of meningeal involvement.[306, 317] Early in the course, the cerebrospinal fluid white blood cell count may be normal despite isolation of group B streptococci.[75] Respiratory distress is the most frequent clinical finding.[27, 33, 306] Seizures rarely are the presenting feature but do occur in up to 50 per cent of affected neonates early in the course of therapy.[33, 75] Postmortem evaluation of infants who died of early-onset group B streptococcal meningitis revealed hemorrhage, prominent basilar involvement, and abundant bacteria with relatively sparse inflammation.[110, 239]

Late-onset meningitis most typically presents with fever and lethargy, although respiratory distress, coma, and shock also may occur.[33] Classic signs of meningitis, such as a bulging fontanelle or nuchal rigidity, are more common in neonates with late-onset meningitis. Subdural effusions occur in up to 20 per cent of cases, but subdural empyema is rare.[19, 33, 104, 199, 262] Infants who die of late-onset meningitis have purulent leptomeningitis at postmortem examination.[110]

Sequelae occur in 25 to 50 per cent of survivors of early- and late-onset meningitis. These sequelae include mental retardation, spastic quadriplegia, cortical blindness, deafness, uncontrolled seizures, hydrocephalus, and speech and language delay.[75, 94, 130, 141, 301] Signs at admission that are correlated with a high likelihood of poor outcome include hypotension, coma or semicoma, status epilepticus, neutropenia, cerebrospinal fluid protein levels greater that 300 mg/dL, and high levels of bacterial antigen in cerebrospinal fluid.[45, 94, 227]

Pneumonia

Respiratory distress is a common manifestation at presentation in all forms of early-onset group B streptococcal disease.[27, 33, 110, 298, 320] Radiographic findings may include infiltrates suggestive of congenital pneumonia, small pleural effusions, a pattern similar to that of hyaline membrane disease or respiratory distress syndrome, or increased vascular markings as seen in transient tachypnea of the newborn; the radiographs also may appear normal despite pulmonary symptoms.[177, 183, 298, 307] In preterm neonates, the presentation frequently is identical to that of respiratory distress syndrome, and at autopsy, hyaline membranes containing bacteria and minimal inflammatory infiltrates have been described.[2, 158]

Septic Arthritis and Osteomyelitis

Osteoarthritis occurs in about 5 per cent of late-onset infections.[35, 320] Among neonates and young infants with osteomyelitis, group B streptococci have been identified as the causal agent in 5 to 38 per cent of cases.[89, 208, 318] The presentation of osteoarticular disease usually is more indolent than that caused by other etiologic agents causing osteomyelitis in young infants. Decreased motion of the involved extremity and pain with manipulation are common signs. Warmth and redness are uncommon but have been described.[89, 241] Systemic signs and symptoms, including fever, are unusual.[13, 22, 89, 197, 200]

The mean age at diagnosis for infants who have septic arthritis without osteomyelitis is 20 days. The presentation typically is acute, with a mean of 2 days of abnormal findings before diagnosis.[35] The lower extremities most often are involved, with the hip joint predominating. Concomitant bacteremia occurs in more than 50 per cent of cases.[89]

As stated earlier, osteomyelitis is more indolent, with a mean of 9 days of findings before the diagnosis is made at a mean age of 31 days.[35] The humerus, usually the proximal humerus, is the bone most frequently involved. The femur is the second most commonly involved bone. Unlike other forms of neonatal osteomyelitis, infection of a single bone is the rule.[89] Blood cultures infrequently are positive, which contrasts again with neonatal osteomyelitis caused by other etiologic agents. However, involvement of the adjacent joint is typical. A lytic lesion often is found on radiographs at admission (Fig. 88–2), implying that the process began weeks before. This suggests that this manifestation may be a late presentation developing after seeding of the metaphysis during an episode of asymptomatic, early-onset bacteremia.[35]

Cellulitis/Adenitis

In one case series, 2 per cent of late-onset group B streptococcal infections presented with cellulitis/adenitis syndrome.[320] The most frequent sites involved are the face and neck.[28, 131, 225] The mean age at presentation is 5 weeks, and there is a male predominance.[28] The typical presentation is one of fever, irritability, poor feeding, and swelling of the affected soft-tissue area. Enlarged adjacent lymph nodes become palpable within a few days. When this happens, the most common site of involvement is the submandibular area.

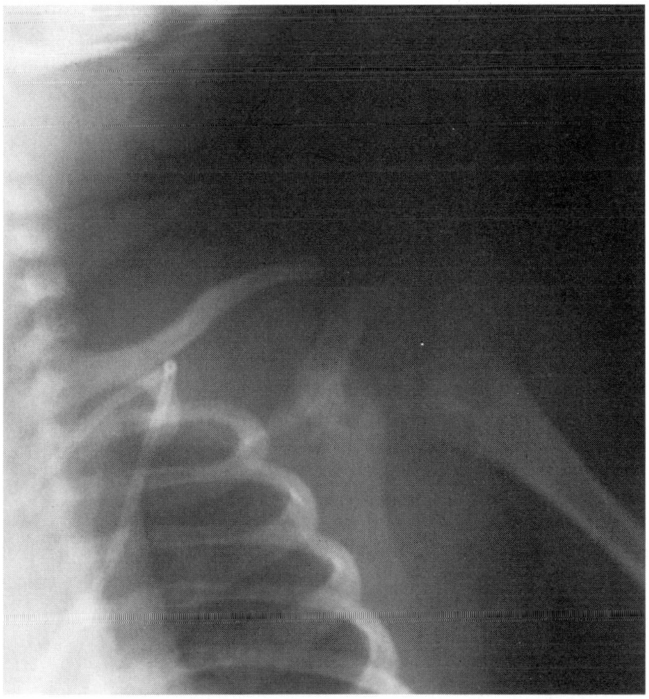

FIGURE 88–2. *Radiograph of the left arm of a 26-day-old infant with a 2-day history of diminished movement of that extremity, demonstrating a well-defined, lytic lesion in the proximal humerus. Necrotic material from this area surgically was débrided and grew group B streptococci.*

Ipsilateral otitis media was noted in four of five infants with facial or submandibular cellulitis in one case series.[28] Less commonly affected areas reported include the genital or inguinal region (Fig. 88–3), hand, and prepatellar bursa.[28, 35, 65, 216, 244] Aspiration of the affected area of cellulitis often yields group B streptococci, and concomitant bacteremia almost always is present.

Nearly every organ has been reported to be a site of group B streptococcal infection in young infants. Table 88–3 lists these reported unusual manifestations of early- and late-onset disease.

Late, Late–Onset Infections

Late, late–onset infection was reported in 19 per cent of cases of late-onset group B streptococcal disease in one case series.[320] Another report of group B streptococcal disease in three HIV-infected children presenting beyond 3 months of age supports the recommendation that immunodeficiency be considered in any child presenting beyond the usual period of risk.[82] Two of the 18 children reported by Hussain and associates[143] were infected with HIV, and 1 patient had transient hypogammaglobulinemia. The clinical manifestations in these older infants are similar to those in patients with typical late-onset infection; bacteremia without a focus and meningitis are the most common presentations.[82, 143] Endocarditis, cellulitis, and central venous catheter infection also have been noted.[102, 143]

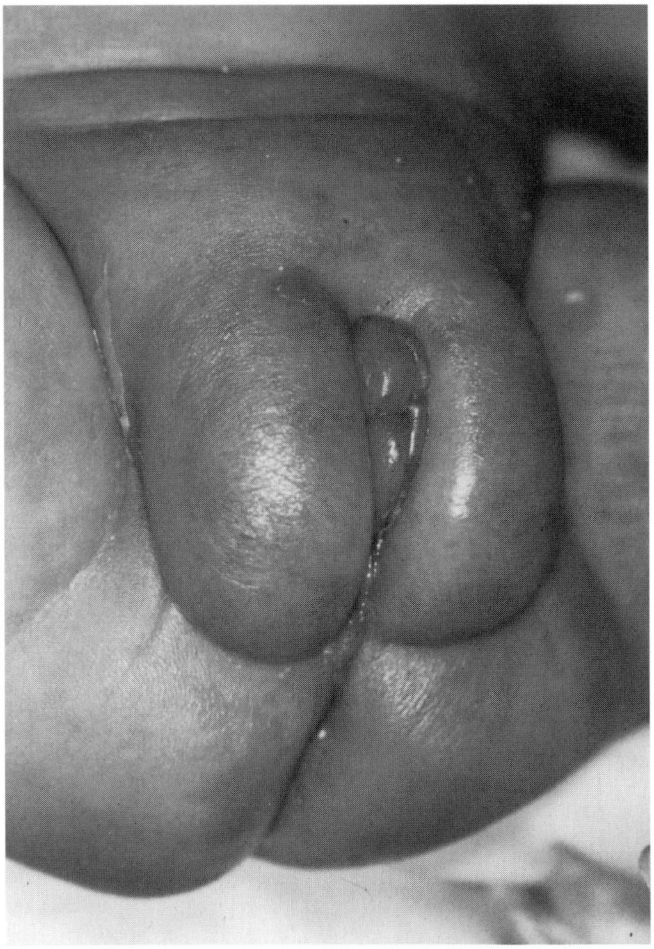

FIGURE 88–3. *This 3-month-old female infant who was born after 28 weeks of gestation presented with fever, lethargy, swelling of the external genitalia, and erythema that extended to the lower abdomen and to the thigh. The blood culture grew type Ib/c group B streptococci. (Courtesy of Morven S. Edwards, M.D.)*

TABLE 88–3. Unusual Clinical Manifestations of Group B Streptococcal Disease in Infants

Site and Manifestation	Reference
Brain	
Abscess	276
Cerebritis	164
Chronic meningitis	280
Eosinophilic meningitis	206
Subdural empyema	104, 199, 262
Ventriculitis complicating myelomeningocele	96
Eye	
Conjunctivitis	20, 110
Endophthalmitis	52, 125
Ear and Sinus	
Ethmoiditis	142
Otitis media/mastoiditis	28, 98, 262, 273, 290
Cardiovascular/Hematologic	
Asymptomatic bacteremia	142, 243, 251, 283
Acquired protein c deficiency	23
Endocarditis	49, 74, 140, 215, 304
Myocarditis	13
Mycotic aneurysm	3
Pericarditis	129
Respiratory Tract	
Epiglottitis	323
Supraglottitis	182
Tracheitis	221
Pleural empyema	142, 172, 279
Skin and Soft Tissue	
Abscess of cystic hygroma	316
Breast abscess	213, 248
Bursitis	67
Cellulitis/adenitis	11, 28, 102, 131, 142, 225, 226, 260
Dactylitis	111
Fasciitis	120, 242
Impetigo neonatorum	51, 167, 184
Purpura fulminans	145, 185
Omphalitis	53, 147, 297
Rhabdomyolysis	292
Scalp abscess	101, 128
Abdomen	
Adrenal abscess	24, 72, 173, 302
Delayed diaphragmatic hernia	21, 46, 160, 233, 285
Gallbladder distention	230
Infected meconium pseudocyst	121
Peritonitis	71, 73
Urinary Tract	
Renal abscess	302
Urinary tract infection	282, 320

Adapted and reprinted with permission from Baker, C. J., and Edwards, M. S.: Group B streptococcal infections. *In* Remington, J. S., and Klein, J. O. (eds.): Infectious Diseases of the Fetus and Newborn Infant. 4th ed. Philadelphia, W. B. Saunders, 1995, pp. 980–1054.

Recurrent Infections

Second (and sometimes third) episodes of group B streptococcal infection occur in up to 8.8 per cent of cases,[124, 327] but most estimates are about 1 per cent. In a case series from Houston, the mean age at recurrence was 44 days, with the mean duration of the interval between the first course of therapy and recurrence being 19 days.[124] Molecular epidemiologic techniques indicated that most, but not all, of these recurrent infections are due to the strain implicated in the first episode. This suggests that persistent mucosal colonization after treatment of the first episode is followed by invasion of the blood stream. No specific risk factors are evident in these infants, but the majority are born prematurely.[124]

DIAGNOSIS AND DIFFERENTIAL DIAGNOSIS

Laboratory Studies

The diagnosis of group B streptococcal infection is confirmed by isolation of this pathogen from a normally sterile body site, such as blood, cerebrospinal fluid, aspirate of bone, joint fluid, or soft tissue. Meningitis in early-onset disease is indistinguishable clinically from bacteremia without a focus, and 10 to 38 per cent of neonates with meningitis have negative blood culture results,[317] so lumbar puncture is necessary to determine the presence or absence of meningeal involvement.[35] Tracheal aspirate cultures that grow group B streptococci indicate neonatal colonization but do not prove pulmonary invasion (pneumonia). Rather, isolation of the organism from the blood (or, in rare circumstances, the lung tissue or pleural space) is required.

Several methods for detecting group B polysaccharide antigen in body fluid specimens have been developed. Those most commonly employed are countercurrent immunoelectrophoresis, latex particle agglutination, and enzyme immunoassay.[45, 58, 127, 210, 275] The advantage of these methods is their simplicity, rapidity, and ability to detect antigen, even after cultures are rendered sterile by antimicrobial therapy. Their disadvantage is the frequency (up to 10 per cent) of false-positive results, especially when they are used to "screen" asymptomatic infants for sepsis. Their proper use should be limited to the setting of the symptomatic infant in whom rapid diagnosis may alter therapy or allow proper tailoring of antibiotic choice—for example, the sick neonate with cerebrospinal fluid pleocytosis and prior antibiotic administration. These tests are never useful in asymptomatic infants.

Concentrated urine is the best specimen for antigen detection tests, with a sensitivity of 84 to 97 per cent, in identifying neonates with positive blood or cerebrospinal fluid cultures.[45, 249, 275] The cerebrospinal fluid has had detectable group B antigen in 72 to 89 per cent of neonates with meningitis, and serum is the least likely specimen to be positive. Latex agglutination assays are somewhat more sensitive than is countercurrent immunoelectrophoresis, but they also are less specific.[42, 92, 240, 275] Positive urine latex agglutination tests often are found in specimens from asymptomatic neonates who have perineal contamination from group B streptococcal colonized rectal or genital sites.[261]

The finding of gram-positive cocci on Gram stain of a gastric aspirate has been reported in neonates with group B streptococcal sepsis and respiratory distress.[88, 144] However, positive Gram stains also are found in neonates with noninfectious causes of respiratory distress. Furthermore, some aspirates with gram-positive cocci by Gram stain grow gram-positive organisms other than group B *Streptococcus,* and some are gram-negative from infants with group B streptococcal bacteremia. Thus, this test has a low specificity and is not recommended for routine use.

The white blood cell count of the neonate with proven group B streptococcal sepsis may reflect leukopenia, neutropenia, or leukocytosis.[158, 187, 227, 298] Manroe and associates[187] found the ratio of absolute immature neutrophils to absolute total neutrophils (I:T index) to be the most reliable index for distinguishing respiratory distress caused by group B streptococcal infection from that with noninfectious etiologies. Most infected neonates had an elevation greater than 0.20 (91 per cent vs. 4 per cent of uninfected infants).

Differential Diagnosis

The presentation of early-onset group B streptococcal disease is indistinguishable clinically from neonatal sepsis caused by other bacterial pathogens. The timing may be somewhat different, with group B streptococcal disease presenting earlier and leading to death earlier in fatal cases.[149] The prominence of respiratory signs in early-onset disease has led to confusion with noninfectious causes of respiratory distress, such as respiratory distress syndrome, transient tachypnea of the newborn, and persistent fetal circulation.[2, 27, 158, 227, 298] Clinical features that suggest group B streptococcal infection rather than noninfectious etiologies are a history of prolonged rupture of membranes, apnea, and shock in the first 24 hours of life; a 1-minute Apgar score of 5 or less; and rapid progression of pulmonary disease.[2, 27, 298]

The differential diagnosis of late-onset disease depends on the focus of infection. Meningitis in infants of this age also is caused by *Listeria, Haemophilus influenzae* type b, *Streptococcus pneumoniae, Neisseria meningitidis,* or viruses. If the results of cerebrospinal fluid Gram stain analysis are inconclusive, other potential pathogens should be considered when therapy is selected. The presentation of osteomyelitis may be subtle, with refusal to move the arm ascribed to neuromuscular disease or Erb palsy.[22, 89] Careful physical examination usually reveals tenderness over the involved area, and radiographs usually reveal a lytic defect in the metaphyses.[89] If the organism is isolated from a bone aspirate, the diagnosis is definitive. Finally, as seen in Table 88–3, many unusual manifestations of group B streptococcal infection have been described, so this organism should be included in the differential diagnosis of any focal infection occurring in the age group at risk.

TREATMENT

Empiric Treatment

The antimicrobial regimens recommended for treatment of group B streptococcal infections in infants are summarized in Table 88–4. Penicillin G remains the drug of choice because susceptibility is uniform. In the usual circumstance, however, antimicrobial therapy for group B streptococcal infection is initiated before culture results are known. Initial empiric therapy for early-onset disease would include ampicillin and gentamicin for treatment of neonatal pathogens in addition to group B streptococci. Irrespective of gestational age, neonates with suspected meningitis and those in whom the clinical condition will not permit a lumbar puncture should receive high doses of ampicillin (300 mg/kg/day).[9] This combination is more effective than is either ampicillin or penicillin G alone in the killing of most group B streptococcal strains in vitro[263] and in vivo.[286] For suspected late-onset disease, the usual initial therapy would include intravenous ampicillin in combination with cefotaxime or ceftriaxone.[9] If an infant is receiving empiric vancomycin therapy and group B streptococcal meningitis has not been excluded, penicillin G or ampicillin should be added to the regimen because vancomy-

TABLE 88–4. Treatment of Group B Streptococcal Infections in Infants

Focus of Infection	Antibiotic Dose	Duration
Suspected meningitis (initial empiric therapy)	Ampicillin (300 mg/kg/day) *plus* Gentamicin	Until cerebrospinal fluid sterility or penicillin G susceptibility documented (MIC ≤0.6 μg/mL)
Suspected sepsis* (initial empiric therapy)	Ampicillin (100–150 mg/kg/day) *plus* Gentamicin	Until blood stream sterility documented
Bacteremia	Penicillin G (200,000 units/kg/day)	10 days
Meningitis	Penicillin G (450,000–500,000 units/kg/day)	14 days minimum†
Arthritis	Penicillin G (200,000–300,000 units/kg/day)	2 to 3 weeks
Osteomyelitis	Penicillin G (200,000–300,000 units/kg/day)	3 to 4 weeks
Endocarditis	Penicillin G (200,000–300,000 units/kg/day)	4 weeks

*Assumes that lumbar puncture has been performed and that cerebrospinal fluid has no abnormalities.
†This should be extended to 21 days or longer if ventriculitis, cerebritis, subdural empyema, or other suppurative complications occur.

cin is inhibitory in vitro rather than bactericidal, and cerebrospinal fluid concentrations may not exceed the minimum inhibitory concentration if a high inoculum of group B streptococci is present.[35]

Specific Treatment

Once group B streptococci have been identified from blood, cerebrospinal fluid, or other normally sterile body site cultures and penicillin susceptibility has been verified, penicillin G alone should be used to complete therapy. Recommendations concerning optimal dose and duration have varied, but these should be dictated by the focus and severity of the infection (see Table 88–4). Facts to consider when selecting the appropriate dose are (1) the usual minimal bactericidal concentration of penicillin for group B streptococci ranges from 0.04 to 0.8 μg/mL,[35, 161] (2) only 10 to 20 per cent of penicillin serum levels reach the cerebrospinal fluid, (3) the inoculum of group B streptococci in the cerebrospinal fluid of infants with meningitis may reach 10^7 to 10^8 colony-forming units/mL,[103] and (4) high doses of penicillin G and ampicillin are safe in the neonate.[35] To ensure rapid bacterial killing, especially in infants with meningitis, relatively high doses of penicillin are recommended both for early- and for late-onset infections.

The infant with meningitis should undergo a second lumbar puncture 24 to 48 hours into therapy to document cerebrospinal fluid sterility.[35] Infants with positive cerebrospinal fluid cultures should be considered to have ventriculitis with obstruction, severe infection with cerebritis and vasculitis, a very high inoculum, or a penicillin-resistant strain; in this circumstance, appropriate studies should be initiated to determine which of these conditions is present. When cerebrospinal fluid sterility and penicillin G susceptibility are verified, penicillin G alone is given for a minimum of 14 days,[9] longer if the course is severe, the infant has ventriculitis, or if there is delayed cerebrospinal fluid sterilization. At the anticipated completion of therapy, contrast-enhanced computed tomography of the head should be performed in complicated cases. These include infants who have prolonged fever (>5 days), cerebritis, abscess, subdural empyema, or venous thrombosis. Such complications often correlate with neurologic abnormalities that lead to a poor prognosis for complete central nervous system recovery.[35, 75, 94]

Infants with bacteremia without a focus should receive intravenous therapy for a total of 10 days.[9] A shorter duration has not been documented to be efficacious, and relapses, although rare, have been reported under these circumstances.[68, 86, 303] Patients with septic arthritis, osteomyelitis, or endocarditis should be treated for the durations summarized in Table 88–4. Oral therapy has no place in the management of infants with group B streptococcal disease.[9, 35] Alternative agents, such as the cephalosporins and vancomycin, are active against group B streptococci in vitro,[54, 161] but their efficacy is unknown and they are not recommended.

Supportive Treatment

The importance of prompt, vigorous, and careful supportive therapy in the successful treatment of infant group B streptococcal infections cannot be overemphasized. Neonates with early-onset disease accompanied by pneumonia should be suspected of having early respiratory failure, and ventilatory support should precede onset of apnea, septic shock, or frank respiratory failure. Persistent metabolic acidosis and delayed capillary refill should prompt treatment of shock. All patients with signs of impending respiratory or circulatory failure or meningitis should be treated in an intensive care unit. When present, hypoxemia, severe anemia, and acidosis should be corrected, and seizures should be controlled with anticonvulsants. In addition, fluid and electrolyte status should be monitored meticulously. Finally, if the infant has persistent pulmonary hypertension or the conventional ventilatory therapy has failed, extracorporeal membrane oxygenation may be considered, if available.

Adjunctive Treatments

Adjunctive treatments of life-threatening group B streptococcal disease are aimed at correcting poor host defenses and are under investigation. These include intravenous human immunoglobulin; monoclonal antibodies to group B streptococcal polysaccharide antigen; leukocyte transfusion; and growth factors, such as granulocyte colony–stimulating factor and granulocyte monocyte–stimulating factor, for neutropenia. The efficacy of these agents is unknown, and although they may be employed occasionally, their use should be considered experimental.

Recurrent Infections

In those few infants who experience a recurrence, suppurative foci should be excluded or treated, if present, as should humoral immune deficiency. Quantitative immunoglobulins should be determined to exclude the latter. Although it may be too early to document humoral immune deficiency unequivocally, the total IgG usually is significantly lower than would be expected for age in weeks.[124] Tube dilution susceptibility of isolates from the first and recurrent episodes should be determined to ensure in vitro susceptibility to penicillin. If the reason for the recurrence remains unknown, it is likely that persistent mucous membrane infection with group B streptococci is the source.[35] β-Lactam antibiotics, even when administered by the parenteral route, do not eradicate group B streptococcal colonization reliably.[220] Because rifampin has eradicated mucosal group B streptococcal colonization in a few human cases,[203] this treatment (20 mg/kg/day) may be useful and may be given orally during the last 4 days of parenteral therapy.[124]

PROGNOSIS

The outcome of group B streptococcal disease is related closely to the severity and site of infection at presentation. Improved outcome from early-onset infection has resulted from greater awareness among pediatricians, allowing earlier intervention, and from improved obstetric management. The latter includes the use of intrapartum antibiotic prophylaxis in women at risk for delivering an infant with early-onset group B streptococcal infection. However, the mortality rate remains substantial at 2 to 8 per cent, especially among neonates born at less than 37 weeks' gestation, in whom the mortality rate often exceeds 20 per cent.[35, 267] It is hoped that greater implementation of strategies to identify women for chemoprophylaxis will reduce further not only incidence but also mortality.

Little information is available concerning the long-term prognosis for survivors of group B streptococcal sepsis without meningitis. Among infants with septic shock, the development of periventricular leukomalacia has been reported and associated with neurodevelopmental sequelae. However, the frequency of this association is not known.

For infants with early- or late-onset meningitis, 20 to 30 per cent have permanent neurologic sequelae, and 20 per cent of these impaired survivors have global mental retardation, cortical blindness, spasticity, or paresis.[75, 94, 130, 141, 301] Whether these rates that were reported more than a decade ago can be applied to infants currently being treated is unknown. One might hope that improvements in both specific and supportive therapy have diminished the frequency of lasting impairments.

To date, the prognosis for infants with osteoarticular or soft tissue infections with group B streptococci has been excellent.[28, 89] However, it is possible that omission of early surgical intervention for infections that involve either the hip or shoulder joints might result in epiphyseal injury.

PREVENTION

The continuing magnitude and severity of group B streptococcal disease and its attendant mortality and morbidity have led to investigations aimed at their prevention. Certainly, decreasing the number of neonates born before 37 weeks' gestation would itself diminish the number of cases. Two general approaches have been proposed: chemoprophylaxis and immunoprophylaxis.

Chemoprophylaxis

Three approaches to prevent early-onset group B streptococcal disease through chemoprophylaxis have been evaluated. The first, antenatal treatment of group B streptococcal maternal carriers, temporarily suppresses colonization but does not eradicate it at delivery or interrupt vertical transmission of group B streptococci to neonates.[114, 126] The second, single-dose intramuscular penicillin given to newborns shortly after birth, is controversial.

The two controlled trials evaluating neonatal prophylaxis reached contradictory conclusions.[237, 274] In the first, more than 16,000 newborns received either intramuscular penicillin G or topical tetracycline (prophylaxis for gonococcal ophthalmia) within an hour of birth during alternating weeks.[274] In penicillin-treated newborns, the incidence of proven group B streptococcal disease decreased significantly during the first 4 days of life; death rates were similar. In contrast with experiences published elsewhere, few of the neonates with proven group B streptococcal disease who presented within the first few hours of life had septic shock or severe infection. Furthermore, because no bacterial cultures were obtained before penicillin therapy, it is possible that early-onset disease cases occurred but were not documented. In fact, in a second controlled study, blood cultures were obtained before penicillin therapy, and the rates of group B streptococcal bacteremia were similar in treatment and control groups.[237] In this study of nearly 1200 neonates weighing 2000 g or less at birth, intramuscular penicillin (or no treatment) was given in the first hour of life and continued for 3 days. Penicillin prophylaxis probably was ineffective because almost 90 per cent of neonates with early-onset group B streptococcal disease were bacteremic immediately after birth. The results of the second study are supported by numerous observations, indicating that early-onset disease begins in utero.[28, 61, 223, 267, 269]

The third approach, maternal intrapartum chemoprophylaxis, has been demonstrated to be efficacious in the prevention of vertical transmission of group B streptococci from colonized mothers to their neonates, of early-onset disease, and of maternal febrile morbidity. Its impact on late-onset disease, if any, has not been documented. Four controlled trials involving thousands of deliveries have indicated that intrapartum penicillin G or ampicillin given intravenously to group B streptococcal carriers prevents early-onset disease in neonates.[62, 116, 195, 291] The first was designed to identify group B streptococcal carriers using vaginal and rectal cultures obtained at 26 to 28 weeks' gestation.[62] Those women who were culture-positive and had labor at less than 37 weeks' gestation, rupture of membranes more than 12 hours before delivery, or intrapartum fever (>37.5° C) were randomized to receive intravenous ampicillin during labor or conventional care. Ampicillin reduced the rate of vertical transmission from 51 to 9 per cent and that of early-onset disease from 6 to 0 per cent.[62] This approach—intrapartum chemoprophylaxis for group B streptococcal carriers selected because of one or more risk factors for early-onset disease—was recommended in 1992 by the American Academy of Pediatrics.[8] These guidelines provoked controversy,[10, 71] and their implementation has been problematic.[148] New recommendations have been published[235] and are supported both by the American Academy of Pediatrics and the American College of Obstetricians and Gynecologists. Key features of these new guidelines include a choice of prevention strategies, use of penicillin G rather than ampicillin as the prophylactic agent, and an empiric algorithm for management of the infant (Table 88–5). Maternal chemoprophylaxis begins at hospital admission for delivery or rupture of membranes and consists of intravenous penicillin G (initial dose, 5 million units, subsequent doses, 2.5 million units every 4 hours) until delivery.[291] Penicillin-allergic women are given intravenous clindamycin (900 mg) every 8 hours or erythromycin (500 mg) every 6 hours until delivery, although neither drug has been

TABLE 88–5. Strategies to Prevent Early-Onset Group B Streptococcal (GBS) Disease by Intrapartum Maternal Chemoprophylaxis

Strategy	Antenatal Screening	Selection Criteria	Estimated Proportion of Cases Prevented*	Agent/Dose	Optimal Timing
Culture-based	Vaginal and rectal cultures at 35–37 weeks' gestation	All women with (1) previous GBS infant, (2) GBS bacteriuria, or (3) labor at <37 weeks *without* culture screening GBS carriers with membrane rupture >18 hours before delivery or intrapartum fever (≥38° C) Other GBS carriers†	85–90%	Penicillin G 5 million units IV (initial), then 2.5 million units every 4 hours Clindamycin‡ 900 mg every 8 hours	At admission to ensure ≥2 doses before delivery
Risk factor–based	None	All women with (1) previous GBS infant, (2) GBS bacteriuria, (3) labor at <37 weeks, (4) membrane rupture >18 hours before delivery, (5) intrapartum fever (≥38° C)	68%	Same	Same

*Reference 235.
†Carriers without a risk factor should have the opportunity to choose chemoprophylaxis, if desired.
‡If penicillin-allergic.

evaluated for efficacy in this setting. Criteria for selection of women for chemoprophylaxis is based either on group B streptococcal culture screening at 35 to 37 weeks' gestation or on the presence of a factor known to increase significantly the risk of early-onset disease in the neonate. The risk factors include (1) previous delivery of an infant with documented group B streptococcal disease, (2) group B streptococcal bacteriuria during pregnancy, (3) labor onset or membrane rupture before 37 weeks' gestation, (4) rupture of membranes more than 18 hours before delivery, and (5) intrapartum fever (38.0° C). Women who have the first three risk factors need not be screened because they all should receive chemoprophylaxis. Women who are positive for group B streptococci but have no risk factors should have the opportunity to discuss chemoprophylaxis with their obstetric caregiver. Such women, delivering at term with no apparent risk factors, account for 25 to 30 per cent of the cases of early-onset disease.[35, 62, 268] Group B streptococcal carriers who have either intrapartum fever or rupture of membranes more than 18 hours before delivery always should receive penicillin G prophylaxis. Women in whom culture screening is negative and who have no risk factors should be managed routinely (approximately 75 to 80 per cent of obstetrical patients).[235]

Although these two strategies have not been compared in clinical trials for safety, efficacy, and cost-effectiveness, each is thought to be cost-beneficial.[6, 207, 255, 321]

Management of the infant born to the mother given intrapartum penicillin G prophylaxis depends on clinical findings at birth, gestational age, and number of doses administered to the mother. If the infant is asymptomatic, has a gestational age of 35 weeks or more, and has a mother given two or more doses before delivery, neither a diagnostic evaluation nor empiric antimicrobial therapy is required. However, to ensure their asymptomatic status, such infants are observed in the hospital for 48 hours. Neonates with signs of sepsis are evaluated and empirically treated for sepsis. Healthy-appearing neonates who are either born at less than 35 weeks' gestation or have been born to women given fewer than two doses of penicillin G undergo a limited laboratory evaluation (complete blood count and blood culture) and observation in the hospital for 48 hours without therapy, unless either the subsequent clinical course or the laboratory results suggest infection. In the latter circumstance, a full diagnostic evaluation for sepsis should be undertaken and empiric therapy initiated. The reasons for the decision based on two or more doses of maternal penicillin before delivery are that amniotic fluid levels of penicillin that will kill group B streptococci are not achieved until at least 3 hours after the first dose,[66] and infants born after only one maternal dose have been shown to be bacteremic.[238]

Immunoprophylaxis

Although efforts to implement intrapartum chemoprophylaxis are ongoing, the most promising and potentially lasting method for prevention of early- and late-onset infant infections is immunoprophylaxis. This approach remains investigational, and several reviews have summarized the rationale.[35, 39, 99, 268] It is based on the observation that immunity to group B streptococci correlates with antibody directed against the type-specific capsular polysaccharides of these organisms. These IgG class antibodies, in combination with complement and polymorphonuclear leukocytes, promote opsonization, phagocytosis, and bacterial killing of group B streptococci and protect animals against lethal challenge.[218, 219, 311] Thus, provision of protective levels of type-specific immunity to the infant could be achieved through active immunization of the mother. Baker and associates[43] immunized women at a mean gestation of 31 weeks with purified type III polysaccharide vaccine. Although immune response was not optimal (54 per cent), placental transport of maternal antibodies (when stimulated) was about 70 per cent, and among neonates born to women who did respond to vaccination, 75 per cent had protective levels of antibodies in their sera at 2 months of age.[43] Other studies immunizing nonpregnant adults with purified capsular polysaccharide vaccines indicated their safety but also variable immunogenicity.

Because most pregnant women (estimated at 85 to 90 per cent) have nonprotective levels of these antibodies in their sera at delivery, active immunization of women with improved vaccines has been proposed.[35] Initial results using candidate polysaccharide-protein conjugate vaccines in nonpregnant women suggest their safety and excellent immunogenicity.[44, 157] However, this method of prevention requires investigation in pregnant women to ensure safety, immunogenicity, stimulation of class and IgG subclass of antibodies that efficiently are transported to the neonate, and a duration of passively acquired antibodies in protective concentrations that extends up through 3 months of age. Furthermore, because maternal immunization is unlikely to be used in the United States, vaccine strategies that avoid use in pregnancy should be considered. Because immunoprophylaxis should be the most cost-effective and beneficial prevention strategy for group B streptococcal disease,[207, 235] it should be promoted by physicians, public health officials, parents, pharmaceutical manufacturers, and legislators.

References

1. Aber, R. C., Allen, N., Howell, J. T., et al.: Nosocomial transmission of group B streptococci. Pediatrics 58:346–353, 1976.
2. Ablow, R. C., Driscoll, S. G., Effmann, E. L., et al.: A comparison of early-onset group B streptococcal neonatal infection and the respiratory-distress syndrome of the newborn. N. Engl. J. Med. *294*:65–70, 1976.
3. Agarwala, B. N.: Group B streptococcal endocarditis in a neonate. Pediatr. Cardiol. *9*:51–53, 1988.
4. Alger, L. S., Lovchik, J. C., Hebel, J. R., et al.: The association of *Chlamydia trachomatis, Neisseria gonorrhoeae*, and group B streptococci with preterm rupture of the membranes and pregnancy outcome. Am. J. Obstet. Gynecol. *159*:397–404, 1988.
5. Allardice, J. G., Baskett, T. F., Seshia, M. M. K., et al.: Perinatal group B streptococcal colonization and infection. Am. J. Obstet. Gynecol. *142*:617–620, 1982.
6. Allen, U. D., Navas, L., and King, S. M.: Effectiveness of intrapartum penicillin prophylaxis in preventing early-onset group B streptococcal infection: Results of a meta-analysis. Can. Med. Assoc. J. *149*:1659–1665, 1993.
7. Altaie, S. S., and Dryja, D.: Detection of group B *Streptococcus*: Comparison of solid and liquid culture media with and without antibiotics. Diagn. Microbiol. Infect. Dis. *18*:141–144, 1994.
8. American Academy of Pediatrics: Guidelines for prevention of group B streptococcal infection by chemoprophylaxis. Pediatrics *90*:775–778, 1992.
9. American Academy of Pediatrics: Group B streptococcal infections. *In* Peter, G. (ed.): Red Book: Report of the Committee on Infectious Diseases. 23rd ed. Elk Grove Village, 1994, pp. 439–442.
10. American College of Obstetricians and Gynecologists: Group B streptococcal infections in pregnancy: ACOG's recommendations. ACOG Newsletter *37*:1, 1993.
11. Amoury, R. A., Barth, G. W., Hall, R. T., et al.: Scrotal ecchymosis: Sign of intraperitoneal hemorrhage in the newborn. South. Med. J. *75*:1471–1478, 1982.
12. Ancona, R. J., Ferrieri, P., Williams, P. P.: Maternal factors that enhance the acquisition of group B streptococci by newborn infants. J. Med. Microbiol. *13*:273–280, 1980.
13. Ancona, R. J., McAuliffe, J., Thompson, T. R., et al.: Group B streptococcal sepsis with osteomyelitis and arthritis. Am. J. Dis. Child. *133*:919–920, 1979.
14. Anderson, D. C., Hughes, B. J., Edwards, M. S., et al.: Impaired chemotaxigenesis by type III group B streptococci in neonatal sera: Relationship to diminished concentration of specific anticapsular antibody and abnormalities of serum complement. Pediatr. Res. *17*:496–502, 1983.
15. Anderson, D. C., Hughes, B. J., and Smith, C. W.: Abnormal mobility of neonatal polymorphonuclear leukocytes. J. Clin. Invest. *59*:810–818, 1981.
16. Anthony, B. F., Concepcion, I. E., Concepcion, N. F., et al.: Relation between maternal age and serum concentration of IgG antibody to type III group B streptococci. J. Infect. Dis. *170*:717–720, 1994.
17. Anthony, B. F., Okada, D. M., and Hobel, C. J.: Epidemiology of group B *Streptococcus*: Longitudinal observations during pregnancy. J. Infect. Dis. *137*:524–530, 1978.
18. Anthony, B. F., Okada, D. M., and Hobel, C. J.: Epidemiology of the group B *Streptococcus*: Maternal and nosocomial sources for infant acquisitions. J. Pediatr. *95*:431–436, 1979.
19. Anthony, B. F., and Okada, D. M.: The emergence of group B streptococci in infections of the newborn infant. Ann. Rev. Med. *28*:355–369, 1977.
20. Armstrong, J. H., Zacarias, F., and Rein, M. F.: Ophthalmia neonatorum: A chart review. Pediatrics *57*:884–892, 1976.
21. Ashcraft, K. W., Holder, T. M., Amoury, R. A., et al.: Diagnosis and treatment of right Bochdalek hernia associated with group B streptococcal pneumonia and sepsis in the neonate. J. Pediatr. Surg. *18*:480–485, 1983.
22. Ashdown, L. R., Hewson, P. H., and Suleman, S. K.: Neonatal osteomyelitis and meningitis caused by group B streptococci. Med. J. Aust. *2*:500–501, 1977.
23. Atalay, S., Imamoglu, A., Ikizler, C., et al.: Mitral valve and left ventricular thrombi in an infant with acquired protein C deficiency. Angiology *46*:87–90, 1995.
24. Atkinson, G. O., Jr., Kodroff, M. B., Gay, B. B., et al.: Adrenal abscess in the neonate. Radiology *155*:101–104, 1985.
25. Badri, M. S., Zawaneh, S., Cruz, A. C., et al.: Rectal colonization with group B *Streptococcus*: Relation to vaginal colonization of pregnant women. J. Infect. Dis. *135*:308–312, 1977.
26. Baker, C. J.: Antibiotic susceptibility testing in the management of an infant with group B streptococcal meningitis. Pediatr. Infect. Dis. J. *6*:1073–1074, 1987.
27. Baker, C. J.: Early onset group B streptococcal disease. J. Pediatr. *93*:124–125, 1978.
28. Baker, C. J.: Group B streptococcal cellulitis/adenitis in infants. Am. J. Dis. Child. *136*:631–633, 1982.
29. Baker, C. J.: Immunization to prevent group B streptococcal disease: Victories and vexations. J. Infect. Dis. *161*:917–921, 1990.
30. Baker, C. J.: Inadequacy of rapid immunoassays for intrapartum detection of group B streptococcal carriers. Obstet. Gynecol. *88*:51–55, 1996.
31. Baker, C. J., and Barrett, F. F.: Group B streptococcal infections in infants: The importance of the various serotypes. J. A. M. A. *230*:1158–1160, 1974.
32. Baker, C. J., and Barrett, F. F.: Transmission of group B streptococci among parturient women and their neonates. J. Pediatr. *83*:919–925, 1973.
33. Baker, C. J., and Barrett, F. F., Gordon, R. C., et al.: Suppurative meningitis due to streptococci of Lancefield group B: A study of 33 infants. J. Pediatr. *82*:724–729, 1973.
34. Baker, C. J., Clark, D. J., and Barrett, F. F.: Selective broth medium for isolation of group B streptococci. Appl. Microbiol. *26*:884–885, 1973.
35. Baker, C. J., and Edwards, M. S.: Group B streptococcal infections. *In* Remington, J. S., and Klein, J. O. (eds.): Infectious Diseases of the Fetus & Newborn Infant. 4th ed. Philadelphia, W. B. Saunders, 1995, pp. 980–1054.
36. Baker, C. J., Edwards, M. S., and Kasper, D. L.: Role of antibody to native type III polysaccharide of group B *Streptococcus* to infant infection. Pediatrics *68*:544–549, 1981.
37. Baker, C. J., Goroff, D. K., Alpert, S. L., et al.: Comparison of bacteriological methods for the isolation of group B *Streptococcus* from vaginal cultures. J. Clin. Microbiol. *4*:46–48, 1976.
38. Baker, C. J., Goroff, D. K., Alpert, S., et al.: Vaginal colonization with group B *Streptococcus*: A study in college women. J. Infect. Dis. *135*:392–397, 1977.
39. Baker, C. J., and Kasper, D. L.: Group B streptococcal vaccines. Rev. Infect. Dis. *7*:458–467, 1985.
40. Baker, C. J., Kasper, D. L., and Davis, C. E.: Immunochemical characterization of the native type III polysaccharide of group B *Streptococcus*. J. Exp. Med. *143*:258–270, 1976.
41. Baker, C. J., Kasper, D. L., Tager, I. B., et al.: Quantitative determination of antibody to capsular polysaccharide in infection with type III strains of group B *Streptococcus*. J. Clin. Med. *59*:810–811, 1977.
42. Baker, C. J., and Rench, M. A.: Commercial latex agglutination for detection of group B streptococcal antigen in body fluids. J. Pediatr. *102*:393–395, 1983.
43. Baker, C. J., Rench, M. A., Edwards, M. S., et al.: Immunization of pregnant women with a polysaccharide vaccine of group B *Streptococcus*. N. Engl. J. Med. *319*:1180–1185, 1988.
44. Baker, C. J., Rench, M. A., Hickman, M. E., et al.: Safety and immunogenicity of group B streptococcal (GBS) polysaccharide types Ia and Ib-tetanus toxoid conjugate vaccines in women. Pediatr. Res. *39*:980A, 1996.
45. Baker, C. J., Webb, B. J., Jackson, C. V., et al.: Countercurrent immunoelectrophoresis in the evaluation of infants with group B streptococcal disease. Pediatrics *65*:1110–1114, 1980.
46. Banagale, R. C., and Watter, J. H.: Delayed right-sided diaphragmatic hernia following group B streptococcal infection: A discussion of its pathogenesis, with a review of the literature. Hum. Pathol. *14*:67–69, 1983.
47. Band, J. D., Clegg, H. W., Haynes, P. S., et al.: Transmission of group B streptococci. Am. J. Dis. Child. *135*:355–358, 1981.
48. Barrett, F. F., Mason, E. O., Jr., and Fleming, D.: The effect of three cord-care regimens on bacterial colonization of normal newborn infants. J. Pediatr. *94*:796–800, 1979.
49. Barton, C. W., Crowley, D. C., Uzardk, K., et al.: A neonatal survivor of group B beta-hemolytic streptococcal endocarditis. Am. J. Perinatol. *1*:214–215, 1984.
50. Becroft, D. M. O., Farmer, K., Mason, G. H., et al.: Perinatal infections by group B β-haemolytic streptococci. Br. J. Obstet. Gynaecol. *83*:960–966, 1976.
51. Belgaumkar, T. K.: Impetigo neonatorum congenita due to group B beta-hemolytic *Streptococcus* infection. J. Pediatr. *86*:982–983, 1975.
52. Berger, B. B.: Endophthalmitis complicating group B streptococcal septicemia. Am. J. Ophthalmol. *92*:681–684, 1981.
53. Bergqvist, G., Hurvall, B., Thal, E., et al.: Neonatal infections caused by group B streptococci. Scand. J. Infect. Dis. *3*:209–212, 1971.

54. Berkowitz, K., Regan, J. A., and Greenberg, E.: Antibiotic resistance patterns of group B streptococci in pregnant women. J. Clin. Microbiol. *28*:5–7, 1990.
55. Bhakdi, S., Klonisch, T., Nuber, P., et al.: Stimulation of monokine production by lipoteichoic acids. Infect. Immun. *59*:4616–4620, 1991.
56. Blumberg, H. M., Stephens, D. S., Modansky, M., et al.: Invasive group B streptococcal disease: The emergence of serotype V. J. Infect. Dis. *173*:365–373, 1996.
57. Bone, R. C.: Gram-positive organisms and sepsis. Arch. Intern. Med. *154*:26–34, 1994.
58. Bortolussi, R., Wort, A. J., and Casey, S.: The latex agglutination test versus counterimmunoelectrophoresis for rapid diagnosis of bacterial meningitis. Can. Med. Assoc. J. *127*:489–493, 1982.
59. Botta, G. A.: Hormonal and type-dependent adhesion of group B streptococci to human vaginal cells. Infect. Immun. *25*:1084–1086, 1979.
60. Boyer, K. M., Gadzala, C. A., Kelly, P. D., et al.: Selective intrapartum chemoprophylaxis of neonatal group B streptococcal early-onset disease. II. Predictive value of prenatal cultures. J. Infect. Dis. *148*:802–809, 1983.
61. Boyer, K. M., Gadzala, C. A., Kelly, P. D., et al.: Selective intrapartum chemoprophylaxis of neonatal group B streptococcal early-onset disease. III. Interruption of mother-to-infant transmission. J. Infect. Dis. *148*:810–816, 1983.
62. Boyer, K. M., and Gotoff, S. P.: Prevention of early-onset neonatal group B streptococcal disease with selective intrapartum chemoprophylaxis. N. Engl. J. Med. *314*:1665–1669, 1986.
63. Boyer, K. M., Kendall, L. S., Papierniak, C. K., et al.: Protective levels of human immunoglobulin G antibody to group B *Streptococcus* type Ib. Infect. Immun. *45*:618–624, 1984.
64. Brady, L. J., Daphtary, U. D., Ayoub, E. M., et al.: Two novel antigens associated with group B streptococci identified by a rapid two-stage radioimmunoassay. J. Infect. Dis. *158*:965–972, 1988.
65. Brady, M. T.: Cellulitis of the penis and scrotum due to group B *Streptococcus*. J. Urol. *137*:736–737, 1987.
66. Bray, R. E., Boe, R. W., and Johnson, W. L.: Transfer of ampicillin into fetus and amniotic fluid from maternal plasma in late pregnancy. Am. J. Obstet. Gynecol. *96*:965–967, 1966.
67. Brian, M. J., O'Ryan, M., and Waagner, D.: Prepatellar bursitis in an infant caused by group B *Streptococcus*. Pediatr. Infect. Dis. J. *11*:502–503, 1992.
68. Broughton, D. D., Mitchell, W. G., Grossman, M., et al.: Recurrence of group B streptococcal infection. J. Pediatr. *89*:183–185, 1976.
69. Bulgakova, T. N., Grabovskaya, K. B., Roc, M., et al.: The adhesin structures involved in the adherence of group B streptococci to human vaginal cells. Folia. Microbiol. *31*:394–401, 1986.
70. Butter, M. N. W., and DeMoor, C. E.: *Streptococcus agalactiae* as a cause of meningitis in the newborn, and of bacteremia in adults. Antonie van Leeuwenhoek *33*:439–450, 1967.
71. Callanan, D. O., and Harris, G. G.: Group B streptococcal infection in children with liver disease. Clin. Pediatr. *21*:99–100, 1982.
72. Carty, A., and Stanley, P.: Bilateral adrenal abscesses in a neonate. Pediatr. Radiol. *1*:63–64, 1973.
73. Chadwick, E. G., Shulman, S. T., and Yogev, R.: Peritonitis as a late manifestation of group B streptococcal disease in newborns. Pediatr. Infect. Dis. J. *2*:142–143, 1983.
74. Chattopadhyay, B.: Fatal neonatal meningitis due to group B streptococci. Postgrad. Med. J. *51*:240–243, 1975.
75. Chin, K. C., and Fitzhardinge, P. M.: Sequelae of early-onset group B streptococcal neonatal meningitis. J. Pediatr. *106*:819–822, 1985.
76. Christensen, K. K., Christensen, P., Duc, G., et al.: Correlation between serum antibody-levels against group B streptococci and gestational age in newborns. Eur. J. Pediatr. *142*:86–88, 1984.
77. Christensen, R. D., and Rothstein, G.: Exhaustion of mature marrow neutrophils in neonates with sepsis. J. Pediatr. *96*:316–318, 1980.
78. Christie, R., Atkins, N. E., and Munch-Petersen, E.: A note on a lytic phenomenon shown by group B streptococci. Aust. J. Exp. Biol. Med. Sci. *22*:197–200, 1944.
79. Congdon, P. M.: Streptococcal infection in childbirth and septic abortion. Lancet 2:1287–1288, 1935.
80. Davis, C. A., Vallota, E. H., and Forristal, J.: Serum complement levels in infancy: Age-related changes. Pediatr. Res. *13*:1043–1046, 1979.
81. Dawodu, A. H., Damole, I. O., and Onile, B. A.: Epidemiology of group B streptococcal carriage among pregnant women and their neonates: An African experience. Trop. Geogr. Med. *35*:145–150, 1983.
82. DiJohn, D., Krasinski, K., and Lawrence, R.: Very late onset of group B streptococcal disease in infants infected with the human immunodeficiency virus. Pediatr. Infect. Dis. J. *9*:925–928, 1990.
83. Dillon, H. C., Jr., Gray, E., Pass, M. A., et al.: Anorectal and vaginal carriage of group B streptococci during pregnancy. J. Infect. Dis. *145*:794–799, 1982.
84. Dillon, H. C., Jr., Khare, S., and Gray, B. M.: Group B streptococcal carriage and disease: A 6-year prospective study. J. Pediatr. *110*:31–36, 1987.
85. Dokter, W. H. A., Dijkstra, A. J., Koopmans, S. B., et al.: G(Anh)MTetra, a naturally occurring 1,6-anhydro muramyl dipeptide, induces granulocyte colony-stimulating factor expression in human monocytes: A molecular analysis. Infect. Immun. *62*:2953–2957, 1994.
86. Dorand, R. D., and Adams, G.: Relapse during penicillin treatment of group B streptococcal meningitis. J. Pediatr. *89*:188–190, 1976.
87. Easmon, C. S. F., Hastings, M. J. G., Neill. J., et al.: Is group B streptococcal screening during pregnancy justified? Br. J. Obstet. Gynaecol. *92*:197–201, 1985.
88. Echeverria, P.: Observations concerning infections with beta-hemolytic streptococci, not group A or D, in neonates. J. Pediatr. *83*:499–500, 1973.
89. Edwards, M. S., Baker, C. J., Wagner, M. L., et al.: An etiologic shift in infantile osteomyelitis: The emergence of the group B *Streptococcus*. J. Pediatr. *93*:578–583, 1978.
90. Edwards, M. S., Buffone, G. J., Fuselier, P. A., et al.: Deficient classical complement pathway activity in newborn sera. Pediatr. Res. *17*:685–688, 1983.
91. Edwards, M. S., Jackson, C. V., and Baker, C. J.: Increased risk of group B streptococcal disease in twins. J. A. M. A. *245*:2044–2046, 1981.
92. Edwards, M. S., Kasper, D. L., and Baker, C. J.: Rapid diagnosis of type III group B streptococcal meningitis by latex particle agglutination. J. Pediatr. *95*:202–205, 1979.
93. Edwards, M. S., Kasper, D. L., Jennings, H. J., et al.: Capsular sialic acid prevents activation of the alternative complement pathway by type III, group B streptococci. J. Immunol. *128*:1278–1283, 1982.
94. Edwards, M. S., Rench, M. A., Haffar, A. A. M., et al.: Long-term sequelae of group B streptococcal meningitis in infants. J. Pediatr. *106*:717–722, 1985.
95. Eickhoff, T. C., Klein, J. O., Daly, A. L., et al.: Neonatal sepsis and other infections due to group B beta-hemolytic streptococci. N. Engl. J. Med. *271*:1221–1228, 1964.
96. Ellenbogen, R. G., Goldmann, D. A., and Winston, K. R.: Group B streptococcal infections of the central nervous system in infants with myelomeningocele. Surg. Neurol. *29*:237–242, 1988.
97. Embil, J. A., Martin, T. R., Hansen, N. H., et al.: Group B beta haemolytic streptococci in the female genital tract: A study of four clinic populations. Br. J. Obstet. Gynaecol. *85*:783–786, 1978.
98. Ermocilla, R., Cassady, G., and Ceballos, R.: Otitis media in the pathogenesis of neonatal meningitis with group B beta-hemolytic *Streptococcus*. Pediatrics *54*:643–644, 1974.
99. Farley, M. M., Harvey, C., Stull, T., et al.: A population-based assessment of invasive disease due to group B *Streptococcus* in nonpregnant adults. N. Engl. J. Med. *328*:1807–1811, 1993.
100. Faro, S.: Group B beta-hemolytic streptococci and puerperal infections. Am. J. Obstet. Gynecol. *139*:686–689, 1981.
101. Feder, H. M., Jr., MacLean, W. C., and Moxon, R.: Scalp abscess secondary to fetal scalp electrode. J. Pediatr. *89*:808–809, 1976.
102. Feder, H. M., Jr., and Pae, K.: Group B streptococcal cellulitis-adenitis in a previously normal child. Pediatr. Infect. Dis. J. *11*:768–769, 1992.
103. Felman, W. E.: Concentrations of bacteria in cerebrospinal fluid of patients with bacterial meningitis. J. Pediatr. *88*:549–552, 1976.
104. Ferguson, L., and Gotoff, S. P.: Subdural empyema in an infant due to group B beta-hemolytic *Streptococcus*. Am. J. Dis. Child. *131*:97, 1977.
105. Ferrieri, P., Cleary, P. P., and Seeds, A. E.: Epidemiology of group B streptococcal carriage in pregnant women and newborn infants. J. Med. Microbiol. *10*:103–114, 1976.
106. Ferrieri, P., Gray, E. D., and Wannamaker, L. W.: Biochemical and immunological characterization of the extracellular nucleases of group B streptococci. J. Exp. Med. *151*:56–68, 1980.
107. Ferrieri, P., Wannamaker, L. W., and Nelson, J.: Localization and characterization of the hippuricase activity of group B streptococci. Infect. Immun. *7*:747–752, 1973.
108. Ferrieri, P.: Surface-localized protein antigens of group B streptococci. Rev. Infect. Dis. *10*:S363–S366, 1988.
109. Fischer, G. W., Lowell, G. H., Crumrine, M. H., et al.: Demonstration of opsonic activity and in vivo protection against group B streptococci type III by *Streptococcus pneumoniae* type 14 antisera. J. Exp. Med. *148*:776–786, 1978.
110. Franciosi, R. A., Knostman, J. D., and Zimmerman, R. A.: Group B streptococcal neonatal and infant infections. J. Pediatr. *82*:707–718, 1973.
111. Frieden, I. J.: Blistering dactylitis caused by group B streptococci. Pediatr. Dermatol. *6*:300–302, 1989.
112. Fry, R. M.: Fatal infections by haemolytic *Streptococcus* group B. Lancet *1*:199–201, 1938.
113. Galask, R. P., Varner, M. W., Petzold, C. R., et al.: Bacterial attachment to the chorioamniotic membranes. Am. J. Obstet. Gynecol. *148*:915–928, 1984.
114. Gardner, S. E., Yow, M. D., Leeds, L. J., et al.: Failure of penicillin to eradicate group B streptococcal colonization in the pregnant woman. Am. J. Obstet. Gynecol. *135*:1062–1065, 1979.
115. Gardner, S. E., Mason, E. O., Jr., and Yow, M. D.: Community acquisition of group B *Streptococcus* by infants of colonized mothers. Pediatrics *66*:873–875, 1980.
116. Garland, S. M., and Fliegner, J. R.: Group B *Streptococcus* and neonatal infections: The case for intrapartum chemoprophylaxis. Aust. N. Z. J. Obstet. Gynaecol. *31*:119–122, 1991.
117. Gibbs, R. S., McDLuffie, R. S., McNabb, et al.: Neonatal group B streptococcal sepsis during 2 years of a universal screening program. Obstet. Gynecol. *84*:496–500, 1994.
118. Gibson, R. L., Lee, M.K., Soderland, C., et al.: Group B streptococci invade

endothelial cells: Type III capsular polysaccharide attenuates invasion. Infect. Immun. *61*:478–485, 1993.

119. Gilbert, W. L., Isaacs, D., Burgess, M. A., et al.: Prevention of neonatal group B streptococcal sepsis: Is routine antenatal screening appropriate? Aust. N. Z. J. Obstet. Gynaecol. *35*:120–126, 1995.
120. Goldberg, G. N., Hansen, R. C., and Lynch, P. J.: Necrotizing fasciitis in infancy: Report of three cases and review of the literature. Pediatr. Dermatol. *2*:55–63, 1984.
121. Goldstein, M.: Neonatal fellowship: Group B streptococcal disease of a meconium pseudocyst in a neonate presenting with *E. coli* sepsis. J. Perinatol. *14*:234–236, 1994.
122. Gotoff, S. P., Papierniak, C. K., Klegerman, M. E., et al.: Quantitation of IgG antibody to the type-specific polysaccharide of group B *Streptococcus* type Ib in pregnant women and infected infants. J. Pediatr. *105*:628–630, 1984.
123. Gray, B. M., Pritchard, D. G., and Dillon, H. C., Jr.: Seroepidemiological studies of group B *Streptococcus* type II. J. Infect. Dis. *151*:1073–1080, 1985.
124. Green, P. A., Singh, K. V., Murray, B. E., et al.: Recurrent group B streptococcal infections in infants: Clinical and microbiologic aspects. J. Pediatr. *125*:931–938, 1994.
125. Greene, G. R., Carroll, W. L., Morozumi, P. A., et al.: Endophthalmitis associated with group B streptococcal meningitis in an infant. Am. J. Dis. Child. *133*:752, 1979.
126. Hall, R. T., Barnes, W., Krishnan, L., et al.: Antibiotic treatment of parturient women colonized with group B streptococci. Am. J. Obstet. Gynecol. *124*:630–634, 1976.
127. Hamoudi, A. C., Marcon, M. J., Cannon, H. J., et al.: Comparison of three major antigen detection methods for the diagnosis of group B streptococcal sepsis in neonates. Pediatr. Infect. Dis. J. *2*:432–435, 1983.
128. Handrick, V. W., Spencker F.-B., and Künzel, R.: Scalp infection caused by B-streptococci in a newborn infant following internal cardiotocography. Zentrabl. Gynäkol. *106*:1544–1546, 1984.
129. Harper, I. A.: The importance of group B streptococci as human pathogens in the British Isles. J. Clin. Pathol. *24*:438–441, 1971.
130. Haslam, R. H. A., Allen, J. R., Dorsen, M. M., et al.: The sequelae of group B β-hemolytic streptococcal meningitis in early infancy. Am. J. Dis. Child. *131*:845–849, 1977.
131. Hauger, S. B.: Facial cellulitis: An early indicator of group B streptococcal bacteremia. Pediatrics *67*:376–377, 1981.
132. Helmig, R., Halaburt, J. T., Uldbjerg, N., et al.: Increased cell adherence of group B streptococci from preterm infants with neonatal sepsis. Obstet. Gynecol. *76*:825–828, 1990.
133. Hemming, V. G., Nagarajan, K., Hess, L. W., et al.: Rapid in vitro replication of group B *Streptococcus* in term human amniotic fluid. Gynecol. Obstet. Invest. *19*:124–129, 1985.
134. Heumann, D., Barras, C., Severin, A., et al.: Gram-positive cell walls stimulate synthesis of tumor necrosis factor alpha and interleukin-6 by human monocytes. Infect. Immun. *62*:2715–2721, 1994.
135. Hickman, M. F., Rench, M. A., Ferrieri, P., et al.: Obstetrical practices (OP) significantly influence neonatal group B streptococcal (GBS) colonization. Abstracts of the 35th ICAAC. Abstract K190, 322, 1995.
136. Hill, H. R., Bohnsack, J. F., Morris, E. Z., et al.: Group B streptococci inhibit the chemotactic activity of the fifth component of complement. J. Immunol. *141*:3551–3556, 1988.
137. Hillier, S. L., Krohn, M. A., Thwin, S. S., et al.: The association of high-density vaginal colonization by group B *Streptococcus* and preterm birth. Abstracts of the 35th ICAAC. Abstract K189, 322, 1995.
138. Hood, M., Janney, A., and Dameron, G.: Beta hemolytic *Streptococcus* group B associated with problems of the perinatal period. Am. J. Obstet. Gynecol. *82*:809–818, 1961.
139. Hoogkamp-Korstanje, J. A. A., Gerards, L. J., and Cats, B. P.: Maternal carriage and neonatal acquisition of group B streptococci. J. Infect. Dis. *145*:800–803, 1982.
140. Horigome, H., Ikada, Y., Hirano, T., et al.: Group B streptococcal endocarditis in infancy with a giant vegetation on the pulmonary valve. Eur. J. Pediatr. *153*:140–141, 1994.
141. Horn, K. A., Zimmerman, R. A., Knostman, J. S., et al.: Neurological sequelae of group B streptococcal neonatal infection. Pediatrics *53*:501–504, 1974.
142. Howard, J. B., and McCracken, G. H., Jr.: The spectrum of group B streptococcal infections in infancy. Am. J. Dis. Child. *128*:815–818, 1974.
143. Hussain, S. M., Luedtke, G. S., Baker, C. J., et al.: Invasive group B streptococcal disease in children beyond early infancy. Pediatr. Infect. Dis. J. *14*:278–281, 1995.
144. Ingram, D. L., Pendergrass, E. L., Bromberger, P. I., et al.: Group B streptococcal disease: Its diagnosis with use of antigen detection, Gram's stain, and the presence of apnea, hypotension. Am. J. Dis. Child. *134*:754–758, 1980.
145. Isaacman, S. H., Heroman, W. M., and Lightsey, A. L.: Purpura fulminans following late-onset group B beta-hemolytic streptococcal sepsis. Am. J. Dis. Child. *138*:915–916, 1984.
146. Jackson, L. A., Hilsdon, R., Farley, M. M., et al.: Risk factors for group B streptococcal disease in adults. Ann. Intern. Med. *123*:415–420, 1995.
147. Jacobs, M. R., Koornhof, H. J., and Stein, H.: Group B streptococcal infections in neonates and infants. S. Afr. Med. J. *54*:154–158, 1978.
148. Jafari, H. S., Schuchat, A., Hilsdon, R., et al.: Barriers to prevention of perinatal group B streptococcal disease. Pediatr. Infect. Dis. J. *14*:662–665, 1995.
149. Jeffery, H., Mitchison, R., Wigglesworth, J. S., et al.: Early neonatal bacteraemia. Arch. Dis. Child. *52*:683–686, 1977.
150. Jennings, H. J., Katzenellenbogen, E., Lugowski, C., et al.: Structure of native polysaccharide antigens of type Ia and type Ib group B *Streptococcus*. Biochemistry *22*:1258–1264, 1983.
151. Jennings, H. J., Rosell, K.-G., and Kasper, D. L.: Structural determination and serology of the native polysaccharide antigen of the type III group B *Streptococcus*. Can. J. Biochem. *58*:112–120, 1980.
152. Jennings, H. J., Rosell K.-G., Katzenellenbogen, E., et al.: Structural determination of the capsular polysaccharide antigen of type II group B *Streptococcus*. J. Biol. Chem. *258*:1793–1798, 1983.
153. Jerlström, P. G., Chhatwal, G. S., and Timmis, K. N.: The IgA-binding β antigen of the c protein complex of group B streptococci: Sequence determination of its gene and detection of two binding regions. Mol. Microbiol. *5*:843–849, 1991.
154. Jones, D. E., Kanarek, K. S., and Lim, D. V.: Group B streptococcal colonization patterns in mothers and their infants. J. Clin. Microbiol. *20*:438–440, 1984.
155. Jürgens, D., Sterzik, B., and Fehrenbach, F. J.: Unspecific binding of group B streptococcal cocytolysin (CAMP factor) to immunoglobulins and its possible role in pathogenicity. J. Exp. Med. *165*:720–732, 1987.
156. Kasper, D. L., Baker, C. J., Baltimore, R. S., et al.: Immunodeterminant specificity of human immunity to type III group B *Streptococcus*. J. Exp. Med. *149*:327–339, 1979.
157. Kasper, D. L., Paoletti, L. C., Jennings, H. J., et al.: Immunogenicity and safety of a type III group B *Streptococcus* polysaccharide-tetanus toxoid conjugate vaccine in women. Infectious Diseases Society of America 33rd Annual Meeting. 422A, 1995.
158. Katzenstein, A.-L., Davis, C., and Braude, A.: Pulmonary changes in neonatal sepsis due to group B β-hemolytic *Streptococcus*: Relation to hyaline membrane disease. J. Infect. Dis. *133*:430–435, 1976.
159. Keller, R., Fischer, W., Keist, R., et al.: Macrophage response to bacteria. Induction of marked secretory and cellular activities by lipoteichoic acids. Infect. Immun. *60*:3664–3672, 1992.
160. Kenny, J. D.: Right-sided diaphragmatic hernia of delayed onset in the newborn infant. South. Med. J. *70*:373–375, 1977.
161. Kim, K. S.: Antimicrobial susceptibility of group B streptococci. Antimicrob. Agents Chemother. *35*:83–89, 1985.
162. Kim, K. S.: Clinical perspectives on penicillin tolerance. J. Pediatr. *112*:214–216, 1988.
163. Kim, K. S., and Anthony, B. F.: Penicillin tolerance in group B streptococci isolated from infection neonates. J. Infect. Dis. *144*:411–419, 1981.
164. Kim, K. S., Kaye, K. L., Itabashi, H. H., et al.: Cerebritis due to group B *Streptococcus*. Scand. J. Infect. Dis. *14*:305–308, 1982.
165. Klegerman, M. E., Boyer, K. M., Papierniak, C. K., et al.: Estimation of the protective level of human IgG antibody to the type-specific polysaccharide of group B *Streptococcus* type Ia. J. Infect. Dis. *148*:648–655, 1983.
166. Klegerman, M. E., Boyer, K. M., Papierniak, C. K., et al.: Type-specific capsular antigen is associated with virulence in late-onset group B streptococcal type III disease. Infect. Immun. *44*:124–129, 1984.
167. Kline, A., and O'Donnell, E.: Group B *Streptococcus* as a cause of neonatal bullous skin lesions. Pediatr. Infect. Dis. J. *12*:165–166, 1993.
168. Lancefield, R. C.: A serological differentiation of human and other groups of hemolytic streptococci. J. Exp. Med. *57*:571–595, 1933.
169. Lancefield, R. C., and Hare, R.: The serological differentiation of pathogenic and non-pathogenic strains of hemolytic streptococci from parturient women. J. Exp. Med. *61*:335–349, 1935.
170. Lancefield, R. C., McCarty, M., and Everly, W. N.: Multiple mouse-protective antibodies directed against group B streptococci. J. Exp. Med. *142*:165–179, 1975.
171. Larsen, J. W., and Dooley, S. L.: Group B streptococcal infections: An obstetrical viewpoint. Pediatrics *91*:148–149, 1994.
172. LeBovar, Y., Trung, P. H., and Mozziconacci, P.: Neonatal meningitis due to group B streptococci. Ann. Pediatr. *17*:207–213, 1970.
173. Leitner, M., Clarke, T. A., and Feldman, B. H.: Hyperbilirubinemia in association with late onset group B β-hemolytic streptococcal infection. Pediatrics *63*:686, 1979.
174. Lerner, P. I., Gopalakrishna, K. V., Wolinsky, E., et al.: Group B *Streptococcus (S. agalactiae)* bacteremia in adults: Analysis of 32 cases and review of the literature. Medicine *56*:457–473, 1977.
175. Levy, N. J., Nicholson-Weller, A., Baker, C. J., et al.: Potentiation of virulence by group B streptococcal polysaccharides. J. Infect. Dis. *149*:851–860, 1984.
176. Lewis, D. B., and Wilson, C. B.: Developmental immunology and role of host defenses in neonatal susceptibility to infection. *In* Remington, J. S., and Klein, J. O. (eds.): Infectious Diseases of the Fetus & Newborn Infant. 4th ed. Philadelphia, W. B. Saunders, 1995, pp. 20–98.
177. Lilien, L. D., Harris, V. J., and Pildes, R. S.: Significance of radiographic findings in early-onset group B streptococcal infection. Pediatrics *60*:360–365, 1977.
178. Lim, D. V., Kanarek, K. S., and Peterson, M. E.: Magnitude of colonization

and sepsis by group B streptococci in newborn infants. Curr. Microbiol. *7*:99–101, 1982.
179. Lim, D. V., Morales, W. J., and Walsh, A. F.: Lim group B Strep Broth and coagglutination for rapid identification of group B streptococci in preterm pregnant women. J. Clin. Microbiol. *25*:452–453, 1987.
180. Lindén, V., Christensen, K. K., and Christensen, P.: Correlation between low levels of maternal IgG antibodies to R protein and neonatal septicemia with group B streptococci carrying R protein. Int. Archs. Allergy Appl. Immunol. *71*:168–172, 1983.
181. Lindén, V.: Mouse-protective effect of rabbit anti-R-protein antibodies against group B streptococci type II carrying R-protein. Acta Pathol. Microbiol. Immunol. Scand. Sect. B *91*:145–151, 1983.
182. Lipson, A., Kronick, J. B., Tewfik, L., et al.: Group B streptococcal supraglottitis in a 3-month-old infant. Am. J. Dis. Child. *140*:411–412, 1986.
183. Long, W. A., Lawson, E. E., Harned, H. S., Jr., et al.: Pleural effusion in the first days of life: A prospective study. Am. J. Perinatol. *1*:190–194, 1984.
184. Lopez, J. B., Gross, P., and Boggs, T. R.: Skin lesions in association with β-hemolytic *Streptococcus* group B. Pediatrics *58*:859–860, 1976.
185. Lynn, N. J., Pauly, T. H., and Desai, N. S.: Purpura fulminans in three cases of early-onset neonatal group B streptococcal meningitis. J. Perinatol. *11*:144–146, 1991.
186. MacDonald, S. W., Manuel, F. R., and Embil, J. A.: Localization of group B beta-hemolytic streptococci in the female urogenital tract. Am. J. Obstet. Gynecol. *133*:57–59, 1979.
187. Manroe, B. L., Rosenfeld, C. R., Weinberg, A. G., et al.: The differential leukocyte count in the assessment and outcome of early-onset neonatal group B streptococcal disease. J. Pediatr. *91*:632–637, 1977.
188. Marchlewicz, B. A., and Duncan, J. L.: Properties of a hemolysin produced by group B streptococci. Infect. Immun. *30*:805–813, 1980.
189. Måardh, P.-A., and Weström, L.: Adherence of bacteria to vaginal epithelial cells. Infect. Immun. *13*:661–666, 1976.
190. Marodi, L., Leijh, P. C. J., and van Furth, R.: Characteristics and functional capacities of human cord blood granulocytes and monocytes. Pediatr. Res. *18*:1127–1131, 1984.
191. Marques, M. B., Kasper, D. L., Pangburn, M. K., et al.: Prevention of C3 deposition by capsular polysaccharide is a virulence mechanism of type III group B streptococci. Infect. Immun. *60*:3986–3993, 1992.
192. Martin, T. R., Rubens, C. E., and Wilson, C. B.: Lung antibacterial defense mechanisms in infant and adult rats: Implications for the pathogenesis of group B streptococcal infections in the neonatal lung. J. Infect. Dis. *157*:91–100, 1988.
193. Mason, E. O., Wong, P., and Barrett, F. F.: Evaluation of four methods for detection of group B streptococcal colonization. J. Clin. Microbiol. *4*:429–431, 1976.
194. Matorras, R., Garcia-Perea, A., Omẽnaca, F., et al.: Group B *Streptococcus* and premature rupture of membranes and preterm delivery. Gynecol. Obstet. Invest. *27*:14–18, 1989.
195. Matorras, R., Garcia-Perea, A., Omenaca, F., et al.: Intrapartum chemoprophylaxis of early-onset group B streptococcal disease. Eur. J. Obstet. Gynecol. Reprod. Biol. *40*:57–62, 1991.
196. McClean, D.: The capsulation of streptococci and its relation to diffusion factor (hyaluronidase). J. Pathol. Bacteriol. *53*:13–27, 1941.
197. McCook, T. A., Felman, A. H., and Ayoub, E. M.: Streptococcal skeletal infections: observations in four infants. Roentgenology *130*:465–467, 1978.
198. McDonald, H., Vigneswaran, R., and O'Loughlin, J. A.: Group B streptococcal colonization and preterm labour. Aust. N. Z. J. Obstet. Gynaecol. *29*:291–293, 1989.
199. McReynolds, E. W., and Shane, R.: Diabetes insipidus secondary to group B beta streptococcal meningitis. J. Tenn. Med. Assoc. *67*:117–120, 1974.
200. Memon, I. A., Jacobs, N. M., Yeh, T. F., et al.: Group B streptococcal osteomyelitis and septic arthritis. Am. J. Dis. Child. *133*:921–923, 1979.
201. Michel, J. L., Madoff, L. C., Kling, D. E., et al.: Cloned alpha and beta C-protein antigens of group B streptococci elicit protective immunity. Infect. Immun. *59*:2023–2028, 1991.
202. Michon, F., Brisson, J.-R., Dell, A., et al.: Multiantennary group-specific polysaccharide of group B *Streptococcus*. Biochemistry *27*:5341–5351, 1988.
203. Millard, D. D., Bussey, M. E., Shulman, S. T., et al.: Multiple group B streptococcal infections in a premature infant: Eradication of nasal colonization with rifampin. Am. J. Dis. Child. *139*:964–965, 1985.
204. Milligan, T. W., Mattingly, S. J., and Straus, D. C.: Purification and partial characterization of neuraminidase from type III group B streptococci. J. Bacteriol. *144*:164–172, 1980.
205. Minett, F. C., Stableforth, A. W., and Edwards, S. J.: Studies on bovine mastitis. 1. The bacteriology of mastitis. J. Comp. Pathol. *42*:213–231, 1929.
206. Miron, D., Snelling, L. K., Josephson, S. L., et al.: Eosinophilic meningitis in a newborn with group B streptococcal infection. Pediatr. Infect. Dis. J. *12*:966–967, 1993.
207. Mohle-Boetani, J. C., Schuchat, A., Plikaytis, B. D., et al.: Comparison of prevention strategies for neonatal group B streptococcal infection: A population-based economic analysis. J. A. M. A. *270*:1442–1448, 1993.
208. Mok, P. M., Reilly, B. J., and Ash, J. M.: Osteomyelitis in the neonate. Radiology *145*:677–682, 1982.
209. Moller, M., Thomsen, A. C., Borch, K., et al.: Rupture of fetal membranes and premature delivery associated with group B streptococci in urine of pregnant women. Lancet *2*:69–70, 1984.
210. Morrow, D. L., Kline, J. B., Douglas, S. D., et al.: Rapid detection of group B streptococcal antigen by monoclonal antibody sandwich enzyme assay. J. Clin. Microbiol. *19*:457–459, 1984.
211. Nealon, T. J., and Mattingly, S. J.: Association of elevated levels of cellular lipoteichoic acids of group B streptococci with human neonatal disease. Infect. Immun. *39*:1243–1251, 1983.
212. Nealon, T. J., and Mattingly, S. J.: Role of cellular lipoteichoic acids in mediating adherence of serotype III strains of group B streptococci to human embryonic, fetal, and adult epithelial cells. Infect. Immun. *43*:523–530, 1984.
213. Nelson, J. D.: Bilateral breast abscess due to group B *Streptococcus*. Am. J. Dis. Child. *130*:567, 1976.
214. Nocard, M.: Sur une mammite contagieuse des vaches laitières. Ann. Inst. Pasteur *1*:109–127, 1887.
215. Noya, F. J. D., Rench, M. A., Metzger, T. G., et al.: Unusual occurrence of an epidemic of type Ib/c group B streptococcal sepsis in a neonatal intensive care unit. J. Infect. Dis. *155*:1135–1144, 1987.
216. Nudelman, R., Bral, M., Sakhai, Y., et al.: Violaceous cellulitis. Pediatrics *70*:157–158, 1982.
217. Opal, S. M., Cross, A., Palmo, M., et al.: Group B streptococcal sepsis in adults and infants: Contrasts and comparisons. Arch. Intern. Med. *148*:641–645, 1988.
218. Paoletti, L. C., Wessels, M. R., Michon, R., et al.: Group B *Streptococcus* type II polysaccharide-tetanus toxoid conjugate vaccine. Infect. Immun. *60*:4009–4011, 1992.
219. Paoletti, L. C., Wessels, M. R., Rodewald, A. K., et al.: Neonatal mouse protection against infection with multiple group B streptococcal serotypes by maternal immunization with a tetravalent GBS polysaccharide-tetanus toxoid conjugate vaccine. Infect. Immun. *62*:3236–3243, 1994.
220. Paredes, A. B., Wong, P., and Yow, M. D.: Failure of penicillin to eradicate the carrier state of group B *Streptococcus* in infants. J. Pediatr. *89*:191–193, 1976.
221. Park, J. W.: Bacterial tracheitis caused by *Streptococcus agalactiae*. Pediatr. Infect. Dis. J. *9*:450–451, 1990.
222. Pass, M. A., Gray, B. M., and Dillon, H. C., Jr.: Puerperal and perinatal infections with group B streptococci. Am. J. Obstet. Gynecol. *143*:147–152, 1982.
223. Pass, M. A., Gray, B. M., Khare, S., et al.: Prospective studies of group B streptococcal infections in infants. J. Pediatr. *95*:437–443, 1979.
224. Pass, M. A., Khare, S., and Dillon, H. C.: Twin pregnancies: Incidence of group B streptococcal colonization and disease. J. Pediatr. *97*:635–637, 1980.
225. Patamasucon, P., Siegel, J. D., and McCracken, G. H., Jr.: Streptococcal submandibular cellulitis in young infants. Pediatrics *67*:378–380, 1981.
226. Pathak, A., and Hwu, H.-H.: Group B streptococcal cellulitis. South. Med. J. *78*:67–68, 1985.
227. Payne, N. R., Burke, B. A., Day, D. L., et al.: Correlation of clinical and pathologic findings in early onset neonatal group B streptococcal infection with disease severity and prediction of outcome. Pediatr. Infect. Dis. J. *7*:836–847, 1988.
228. Payne, N. R., and Ferrieri, P.: The relation of the Ib/c protein antigen to the opsonization differences between strains of type II group B streptococci. J. Infect. Dis. *151*:672–681, 1985.
229. Peevy, K. J., and Chalhub, E. G.: Occult group B streptococcal infection: An important cause of intrauterine asphyxia. Am. J. Obstet. Gynecol. *146*:989–990, 1983.
230. Peevy, K. J., and Wiseman, H. J.: Gallbladder distention in septic neonates. Arch. Dis. Child. *57*:75–76, 1982.
231. Persson, K. M.-S., and Forsgren, A.: Antimicrobial susceptibility of group B streptococci. Eur. J. Clin. Microbiol. *5*:165–167, 1986.
232. Persson, K., Bjerre, B., Elfström, L., et al.: Longitudinal study of group B streptococcal carriage during late pregnancy. Scand. J. Infect. Dis. *19*:325–329, 1987.
233. Philipps, A. F., Bierney, J.-P., and Crowe, C. P., Jr.: Neonatal radiology: Acquired diaphragmatic hernia with group B streptococcal pneumonia. J. Perinatol. *15*:160–162, 1995.
234. Platt, M. W., Correa, N., Jr., and Mold, C.: Growth of group B streptococci in human serum leads to increased cell surface sialic acid and decreased activation of the alternative complement pathway. Can. J. Microbiol. *40*:99–105, 1994.
235. Prevention of perinatal group B streptococcal disease: A public health perspective. M. M. W. R. *45*:1–24 (No. RR-7), 1996.
236. Pritchard, D. G., Gray, B. M., and Egan, M. L.: Murine monoclonal antibodies to type Ib polysaccharide of group B streptococci bind to human milk oligosaccharides. Infect. Immun. *60*:1598–1602, 1992.
237. Pyati, S. P., Pildes, R. S., Macobs, N. M., et al.: Penicillin in infants weighing two kilograms or less with early-onset group B streptococcal disease. N. Engl. J. Med. *308*:1383–1389, 1983.
238. Pylipow, M., Gaddis, M., and Kinney, J. S.: Selective intrapartum prophylaxis for group B *Streptococcus* colonization: Management and outcome of newborns. Pediatrics *93*:631–635, 1994.
239. Quirante, J., Ceballos, R., and Cassady, G.: Group B β-hemolytic streptococcal infection in the newborn. Am. J. Dis. Child. *128*:659–665, 1974.
240. Rabalais, G. P., Bronfin, D. R., and Daum, R. S.: Evaluation of a commer-

cially available latex agglutination test for rapid diagnosis of group B streptococcal infection. Pediatr. Infect. Dis. J. *6*:177–181, 1987.

241. Ragnhildstreit, E., and Ose, L.: Neonatal osteomyelitis caused by group B streptococci. Scand. J. Infect. Dis. *8*:219–221, 1976.
242. Ramamurthy, R. S., Srinivasan, G., and Jacobs, N. M.: Necrotizing fasciitis and necrotizing cellulitis due to group B *Streptococcus*. Am. J. Dis. Child. *131*:1169–1170, 1977.
243. Ramsey, P. G., and Zwerdling, R.: Asymptomatic neonatal bacteremia. N. Engl. J. Med. *295*:225, 1977.
244. Rand, T. H.: Group B streptococcal cellulitis in infants: A disease modified by prior antibiotic therapy or hospitalization? Pediatrics *81*:63–65, 1988.
245. Regan, J. A., Chao, S., and James, L. S.: Premature rupture of membranes, preterm delivery, and group B streptococcal colonization of mothers. Am. J. Obstet. Gynecol. *141*:184–186, 1981.
246. Regan, J. A., Klebanoff, M. A., and Nugent, R. P.: The epidemiology of group B streptococcal colonization in pregnancy. Obstet. Gynecol. *77*:604–610, 1991.
247. Reisenfeld-Orn, I., Wolpe, S., Garcia-Bustos, J. F., et al.: Production of interleukin-1 but no tumor necrosis factor by human monocytes stimulated with pneumococcal cell surface components. Infect. Immun. *57*:1890–1893, 1989.
248. Rench, M. A., and Baker, C. J.: Group B streptococcal breast abscess in a mother and mastitis in her infant. Obstet. Gynecol. *73*:875–877, 1989.
249. Rench, M. A., Metzger, T. G., and Baker, C. J.: Detection of group B streptococcal antigen in body fluids by a latex-coupled monoclonal antibody assay. J. Clin. Microbiol. *20*:852–854, 1984.
250. Rench, M. A., and Baker, C. J.: Neonatal sepsis caused by a new group B streptococcal serotype. J. Pediatr. *122*:638–640, 1993.
251. Roberts, K. B.: Persistent group B *Streptococcus* bacteremia without clinical "sepsis" in infants. J. Pediatr. *88*:1059–1060, 1976.
252. Rodewald, A. K., Onderdonk, A. B., Warren, H. B., et al.: Neonatal mouse model of group B streptococcal infection. J. Infect. Dis. *166*:635–639, 1992.
253. Roe, M. H., Todd, J. K., and Favara, B. E.: Non-hemolytic group B streptococcal infections. J. Pediatr. *89*:75–77, 1976.
254. Rolston, K. V. I.: Susceptibility of group B and group G streptococci to newer antimicrobial agents. Eur. J. Clin. Microbiol. *5*:534–536, 1986.
255. Rouse, D. J., Goldenberg, R. L., Cliver, S. P., et al.: Strategies for the prevention of early-onset group B streptococcal sepsis: A decision analysis. Obstet. Gynecol. *83*:483–494, 1994.
256. Rowen, J. L., Smith, C. W., and Edwards, M. S.: Capsule delays elaboration of leukotriene B_4 (LTB_4) by monocytes stimulated with type III group B streptococci (GBS). Pediatr. Res. *37*:187A, 1995.
257. Rowen, J. L., Smith, C. W., and Edwards, M. S.: Group B streptococci elicit leukotriene B_4 and interleukin-8 from human monocytes: Neonates exhibit a diminished response. J. Infect. Dis. *172*:420–426, 1995.
258. Rubens, C. E., Smith, S., Hulse, M., et al.: Respiratory epithelial cell invasion by group B streptococci. Infect. Immun. *60*:5157–5163, 1992.
259. Rubens, C. E., Wessels, M. R., Heggen, L. M., et al.: Transposon mutagenesis of type III group B *Streptococcus*: Correlation of capsule expression with virulence. Proc. Natl. Acad. Sci. U. S. A. *84*:7208–7212, 1987.
260. Ruiz-Gomez, D., Tarpay, M., and Riley, H. D.: Recurrent group B streptococcal infections: Report of three cases. Scand. J. Infect. Dis. *11*:35–38, 1979.
261. Sánchez, P. J., Siegel, J. D., Cushion, N. B., et al.: Significance of a positive urine group B streptococcal latex agglutination test in neonates. J. Pediatr. *116*:601–606, 1990.
262. Sapir-Ellis, S., Johnson, A., and Austin, T. L.: Group B streptococcal meningitis associated with otitis media. Am. J. Dis. Child. *130*:1003–1004, 1976.
263. Schauf, V., Deveikis, A., Riff, L., et al.: Antibiotic-killing kinetics of group B streptococci. J. Pediatr. *89*:194–198, 1976.
264. Scheld, W. M., Alliegro, G. M., Field, M. R., et al.: Synergy between penicillins and low concentrations of gentamicin in experimental meningitis due to group B streptococci. J. Infect. Dis. *146*:100, 1982.
265. Schibler, K. R., Trautman, M. S., Liechty, K. W., et al.: Diminished transcription of interleukin-8 by monocytes from preterm neonates. J. Leukoc. Biol. *53*:399–403, 1993.
266. Schlievert, P. M., Gocke, J. E., and Deringer, J. R.: Group B streptococcal toxic shock-like syndrome: Report of a case and purification of an associated pyrogenic toxin. Clin. Infect. Dis. *17*:26–31, 1993.
267. Schuchat, A.: Group B streptococcal disease in newborns: A global perspective on prevention. Biomed. Pharmacother. *49*:19–25, 1995.
268. Schuchat, A., Deaver-Robinson, K., Plikaytis, B. D., et al.: Multistate case-control study of maternal risk factors for neonatal group B streptococcal disease. Pediatr. Infect. Dis. J. *13*:623–629, 1994.
269. Schuchat, A., Oxtoby, M., Cochi, S., et al.: Population-based risk factors for neonatal group B streptococcal disease: Results of a cohort study in metropolitan Atlanta. J. Infect. Dis. *162*:672–677, 1990.
270. Schuit, K. E., and DeBasio, R.: Kinetics of phagocyte response to group B streptococcal infections in newborn rats. Infect. Immun. *28*:319–324, 1980.
271. Sherman, M. P., and Lehrer, R. I.: Oxidative metabolism of neonatal and adult rabbit lung macrophages stimulated with opsonized group B streptococci. Infect. Immun. *47*:26–30, 1985.
272. Shigeoka, A. O., Rote, N. S., Santos, J. I., et al.: Assessment of the virulence factors of group B streptococci: Correlation with sialic acid content. J. Infect. Dis. *147*:857–863, 1983.
273. Shurin, P. A., Howie, V. M., Pelton, S. I., et al.: Bacterial etiology of otitis media during the first six weeks of life. J. Pediatr. *92*:893–896, 1978.
274. Siegel, J. D., McCracken, G. H., Jr., Threlkeld, N., et al.: Single-dose penicillin prophylaxis against neonatal group B streptococcal infections. N. Engl. J. Med. *303*:769–775, 1980.
275. Siegel, J. D., and McCracken, G. H., Jr.: Detection of group B streptococcal antigens in body fluids of neonates. J. Pediatr. *93*:491–492, 1978.
276. Siegel, J. D., Shannon, K. M., and De Passe, B. M.: Recurrent infection associated with penicillin-tolerant group B streptococci: A report of two cases. J. Pediatr. *99*:920–924, 1981.
277. Slifkin, M., and Pouchet-Melvin, G. R.: Evaluation of three commercially available test products for serogrouping beta-hemolytic streptococci. J. Clin. Microbiol. *11*:249–255, 1980.
278. Sobel, J. D., Myers, P., Levison, M. E., et al.: Comparison of bacterial and fungal adherence to vaginal exfoliated epithelial cells and human vaginal epithelial tissue culture cells. Infect. Immun. *35*:697–701, 1982.
279. Sokal, M. M., Nagaraj, A., Fisher, B. J., et al.: Neonatal empyema caused by group B beta-hemolytic *Streptococcus*. Chest *81*:390–391, 1982.
280. Sokol, D. M., Demmler, G. J., and Baker, C. J.: Unusual presentation of group B streptococcal ventriculitis. Pediatr. Infect. Dis. J. *9*:525–527, 1990.
281. Speck, W. T., Driscol, J. M., Polin, R. A., et al.: Staphylococcal and streptococcal colonization of the newborn infant: Effect of antiseptic cord care. Am. J. Dis. Child. *131*:1005–1008, 1977.
282. St. Laurent-Gagnon, T., and Weber, M. L.: Urinary tract *Streptococcus* group B infection in a 6-week-old infant. J. A. M. A. *140*:1269, 1978.
283. Stewardson-Krieger, P. B., and Gotoff, S. P.: Risk factors in early-onset neonatal group B streptococcal infections. Infection *6*:50–53, 1978.
284. Suara, R. O., Adegbola, R. A., Baker, C. J., et al.: Carriage of group B streptococci in pregnant Gambian mothers and their infants. J. Infect. Dis. *170*:1316–1319, 1994.
285. Suresh, B. R., Rios, A., Brion, L. P., et al.: Delayed onset right-sided diaphragmatic hernia secondary to group B streptococcal infection. Pediatr. Infect. Dis. J. *10*:166–168, 1991.
286. Swingle, H. M., Bucciarelli, R. L., and Ayoub, E. M.: Synergy between penicillins and low concentrations of gentamicin in the killing of group B streptococci. J. Infect. Dis. *152*:58–66, 1985.
287. Takahashi, S., Nagano, Y., Nagano, N., et al.: Role of C5a-ase in group B streptococcal resistance to opsonophagocytic killing. Infect. Immun. *63*:4764–4769, 1995.
288. Tamura, G. S., Kuypers, J. M., Smith, S., et al.: Adherence of group B streptococci to cultured epithelial cells: Roles of environmental factors and bacterial surface components. Infect. Immun. *62*:2450–2458, 1994.
289. Tapsall, J. W.: Pigment production by Lancefield-group B streptococci (*Streptococcus agalactiae*). J. Med. Microbiol. *21*:75–81, 1986.
290. Tetzlaff, T. R., Ashworth, C., and Nelson, J. D.: Otitis media in children less than 12 weeks of age. Pediatrics *59*:827–832, 1977.
291. Tuppurainen, N., and Hallman, M.: Prevention of neonatal group B streptococcal disease: Intrapartum detection and chemoprophylaxis of heavily colonized parturients. Obstet. Gynecol. *73*:583–587, 1989.
292. Turner, M. C., and Naumburg, E. G.: Acute renal failure in the neonate: Two fatal cases due to group B streptococci with rhabdomyolysis. Clin. Pediatr. *25*:189–190, 1987.
293. Vallejo, J. G., Baker, C. J., and Edwards, M. S.: Demonstration of circulating group B streptococcal immune complexes in neonates with meningitis. J. Clin. Microbiol. *32*:2041–2045, 1994.
294. Vallejo, J. G., Baker, C. J., and Edwards, M. S.: Interleukin-6 production by human neonatal monocytes stimulated by type III group B streptococci. J. Infect. Dis. *174*:332–337, 1996.
295. Vallejo, J. G., Baker, C. J., and Edwards, M. S.: The role of bacterial cell wall and capsule in the induction of tumor necrosis factor alpha by type III group B streptococci. Infect. Immun. *64*:5042–5046, 1996.
296. Vallette, J. D., Jr., Goldberg, R. N., Suguihara, C., et al.: Effect of an interleukin-1 receptor antagonist on the hemodynamic manifestations of group B streptococcal sepsis. Pediatr. Res. *38*:704–708, 1995.
297. Van Peenen, P. F., Cannon, R. E., and Seibert, D. J.: Group B beta-hemolytic streptococci causing fatal meningitis. Mil. Med. *130*:65–67, 1965.
298. Vollman, J. H., Smith, W. L., Ballard, E. T., et al.: Early onset group B streptococcal disease: Clinical, roentgenographic, and pathologic features. J. Pediatr. *89*:199–203, 1976.
299. von Hunolstein, C., D'Ascenzi, S., Wagner, B., et al.: Immunochemistry of capsular type polysaccharide and virulence properties of type VI *Streptococcus agalactiae* (group B streptococci). Infect. Immun. *61*:1272–1280, 1993.
300. Wagner, M., Murai, T., Wagner, B., et al.: JM9 strains, a new type of group B streptococci from Japan. Int. J. Med. Microbiol. Virol. Parasitol. Infect. Dis. *280*:488–496, 1994.
301. Wald, E. R., Bergman, I., Taylor, H. G., et al.: Long-term outcome of group B streptococcal meningitis. Pediatrics *77*:217–221, 1986.
302. Walker, K. M., and Coyer, W. F.: Suprarenal abscess due to group B *Streptococcus*. J. Pediatr. *94*:970–971, 1979.
303. Walker, S. H., Santos, A. Q., and Quintero, B. A.: Recurrence of group B III streptococcal meningitis. J. Pediatr. *89*:187–188, 1976.
304. Weinberg, A. G., and Laird, W. P.: Group B streptococcal endocarditis detected by echocardiography. J. Pediatr. *92*:334–336, 1978.
305. Weiser, J. N., and Rubens, C. E.: Transposon mutagenesis of group B

Streptococcus beta-hemolysin biosynthesis. Infect. Immun. *55*:2314–2316, 1987.
306. Weisman, L. E., Stoll, B. J., Cruess, D. F., et al.: Early-onset group B streptococcal sepsis: A current assessment. J. Pediatr. *121*:428–433, 1992.
307. Weller, M. H., and Katzenstein, A.: Radiological findings in group B streptococcal sepsis. Radiology *118*:385–387, 1976.
308. Wessels, M. R., Benedí, V.-J., Jennings, H. J., et al.: Isolation and characterization of type IV group B *Streptococcus* capsular polysaccharide. Infect. Immun. *57*:1089–1094, 1989.
309. Wessels, M. R., DiFabio, J. L., Benedí, V-J., et al.: Structural determination and immunochemical characterization of the type V group B *Streptococcus* capsular polysaccharide. J. Biol. Chem. *266*:6714–6719, 1991.
310. Wessels, M. R., Rubens, C. E., Benedí, V.-J., et al.: Definition of a bacterial virulence factor: Sialylation of the group B streptococcal capsule. Proc. Natl. Acad. Sci. U. S. A. *86*:8983–8987, 1989.
311. Wessels, M. R., Paoletti, L. C., Kasper, D. L., et al.: Immunogenicity in animals of a polysaccharide-protein conjugate vaccine against type III group B *Streptococcus*. J. Clin. Invest. *86*:1428–1433, 1990.
312. Wibawan, I. W. T., and Lämmler, C.: Properties of group B streptococci with protein surface antigens X and R. J. Clin. Microbiol. *28*:2834–2836, 1990.
313. Wilkinson, H. W.: Analysis of group B streptococcal types associated with disease in human infants and adults. J. Clin. Microbiol. *7*:176–179, 1978.
314. Wilkinson, H. W., Facklam, R. R., and Wortham, E. C.: Distribution by serological type of group B streptococci isolated from a variety of clinical material over a five-year period (with special reference to neonatal sepsis and meningitis). Infect. Immun. *8*:228–235, 1973.
315. Williams, P. A., Bohnsack, J. F., Augustine, N. H., et al.: Production of tumor necrosis factor by human cells in vitro and in vivo, induced by group B streptococci. J. Pediatr. *123*:292–300, 1993.
316. Wiswell, T. E., and Miller, J. A.: Infections of congenital cervical neck masses associated with bacteremia. J. Pediatr. Surg. *21*:173–174, 1986.
317. Wiswell, T. E., Baumgart, S., Gannon, C. M., et al.: No lumbar puncture in the evaluation for early neonatal sepsis: Will meningitis be missed? Pediatrics *95*:803–806, 1995.
318. Wong, M., Isaacs, D., Howman-Giles, R., et al.: Clinical and diagnostic features of osteomyelitis occurring in the first three months of life. Pediatr. Infect. Dis. J. *14*:1047–1053, 1995.
319. Wood, E. G., and Dillon, H. C., Jr.: A prospective study of group B streptococcal bacteriuria in pregnancy. Am. J. Obstet. Gynecol. *140*:515–520, 1981.
320. Yagupsky, P., Menegus, M. A., and Powell, K. R.: The changing spectrum of group B streptococcal disease in infants: An eleven-year experience in a tertiary care hospital. Pediatr. Infect. Dis. J. *10*:801–808, 1991.
321. Yancy, M. K., and Duff, P.: An analysis of the cost-effectiveness of selected protocols for the prevention of neonatal group B streptococcal infection. Obstet. Gynecol. *83*:367–371, 1994.
322. Yeung, M. K., and Mattingly, S. J.: Biosynthetic capacity for type-specific antigen synthesis determines the virulence of serotype III strains of group B streptococci. Infect. Immun. *44*:217–221, 1984.
323. Young, N., Finn, A., and Powell, C.: Group B streptococcal epiglottitis. Pediatr. Infect. Dis. J. *15*:95–96, 1996.
324. Yow, M. D., Leeds, L. J., Thompson, P. K., et al.: The natural history of group B streptococcal colonization in the pregnant woman and her offspring. I. Colonization studies. Am. J. Obstet. Gynecol. *137*:34–38, 1980.
325. Yow, M. D., Mason, E. O., Leeds, L. J., et al.: Ampicillin prevents intrapartum transmission of group B *Streptococcus*. J. A. M. A. *241*:1245–1247, 1979.
326. Zaleznik, D. F., Krohn, M. A., Hillier, S. L., et al.: Group B streptococcal colonization in parturient women differs among racial groups. Abstracts of the 35th ICAAC. Abstract K188, 322, 1995.
327. Zangwill, K. M., Schuchat, A., and Wenger, J. D.: Group B streptococcal disease in the United States, 1990: Report from a multistate active surveillance system. M. M. W. R. *41*(SS-6):25–32, 1992.

89

Enterococcal and Viridans Streptococcal Infections

B. Keith English and Jerry L. Shenep

Enterococcal Infections

The enterococci are gram-positive ovoid bacteria that are related closely to the streptococci but now are known to be phylogenetically distinct, making up the genus *Enterococcus*. These organisms are found in the normal bowel flora of humans and many animals and are isolated commonly from environmental sources. Enterococci generally are considered to be of low virulence but have been known to cause human infections for almost a century (reviewed by Murray[108]). These ubiquitous bacteria have become recognized increasingly as important causes of both community-acquired and nosocomial infections in adults[18, 102, 103, 108, 110, 125] and children,[6, 12, 17, 25, 37, 125, 130, 133, 135] yet the role of *Enterococcus* species as a copathogen in certain clinical settings—particularly intra-abdominal and pelvic infections—remains uncertain.

Enterococci intrinsically are resistant to many antimicrobial agents (including the cephalosporins, oxacillin, clindamycin, and the aminoglycosides). Since the emergence of high-level aminoglycoside resistance in *Enterococcus* species more than 25 years ago,[99] increasing percentages of these organisms have acquired clinically significant high-level resistance to β-lactam antibiotics and to vancomycin and other glycopeptides, as well as aminoglycosides. Infections due to vancomycin-resistant enterococci (VRE) are of particular concern because VRE isolates frequently are resistant to all available bactericidal antimicrobial agents.[110] The dramatic increase in nosocomial infections due to VRE[18, 110] has resulted in failures of antimicrobial therapy[81, 153] and has inspired comparisons with the pre-antibiotic period[3] and even speculation about a "post-antimicrobial era."[27] Concerns about additional nosocomial spread of VRE and the potential for transfer of vancomycin resistance determinants to other pathogens (pneumococci, staphylococci) have led to the development of stringent hospital infection control guidelines designed to interrupt the spread of vancomycin-resistant organisms.[19] Although the impact of VRE infections in children has been less dramatic, increasing numbers of pediatric centers now are reporting infections due to these organisms.[6, 12, 17, 25, 125, 130, 133, 135]

MICROBIOLOGY

The genus *Enterococcus* consists of gram-positive cocci that are catalase-negative and occur singly, in pairs, and in short chains. Morphologically, enterococci are indistinguishable from streptococci and traditionally have been classified as members of the genus *Streptococcus*. Sherman's early classification scheme[147] divided the streptococci into four groups: pyogenic, viridans, lactic, and enterococcal. By the Lancefield criteria, enterococci were classified as group D streptococci along with the "nonenterococcal" *Streptococcus bovis* group. However, genetic evidence has indicated that the enterococci sufficiently are different from the streptococci to merit the establishment of a separate genus.[44]

Figure 89–1 is a scheme for the differentiation of enterococci from other gram-positive cocci. Catalase-negative gram-positive cocci that have been isolated from human sources include the streptococci, the enterococci, *Lactococcus, Leuconostoc, Pediococcus,* and *Gemella*. Most enterococci produce no (gamma) or partial (alpha) hemolysis on blood agar; the differentiation between enterococci and certain alpha-hemolytic or nonhemolytic streptococci and other nonstreptoccal gram-positive cocci may require a series of biochemical tests.[42, 44] Clinical laboratories presumptively may identify an organism on a primary isolation plate as an enterococcus based on colony morphology, Gram stain, and a pyrrolidonyl arylamidase (PYR) test. Enterococci produce PYR, as do *Streptococcus pyogenes* and nutritionally variant streptococci, but not other streptococci. The PYR test particularly is useful for differentiating enterococci from group D streptococci and from *Leuconostoc* species (see Fig. 89–1). *S. pyogenes* and the nutritionally deficient streptococci are distinguished easily from enterococci based on colony morphology, hemolysis, and special growth requirements.

Enterococci are able to hydrolyze esculin in the presence of 40 per cent bile salts; of the true streptococci, only group D streptococci (*S. bovis* group) and approximately 5 to 10 per cent of viridans streptococci share this characteristic.[44] Enterococci are facultatively anaerobic and grow under harsh conditions that inhibit the growth of streptococci; growth in 6.5 per cent sodium chloride at 45° C is a useful confirmatory test. Enterococci produce leucine aminopeptidase, as do the streptococci, lactococci, pediococci, and some *Gemella* strains. Presence of the group D streptococcal antigen is of limited value because the *S. bovis* group, most pediococci, and half of clinical *Leuconostoc* isolates share this antigen.[44]

Occasional clinical isolates of *Leuconostoc, Pediococcus,* and *Lactococcus* may be difficult to distinguish from the enterococci. Some strains of *Leuconostoc* and *Pediococcus* may grow in 6.5 per cent sodium chloride at 45° C but are PYR-negative. Lactococci are PYR-positive, and some isolates will grow in 6.5 per cent sodium chloride; however, most lactococci fail to grow (or grow very slowly) at 45° C. Definitive confirmation of an organism as an enterococcus may require complete identification to the species level. Fortunately, molecular techniques promise to provide rapid, reliable identification and speciation of enterococci.[35, 38, 39]

The genus *Enterococcus* now includes at least 14 "typical" species and 3 additional "atypical" species (the latter are PYR-negative and grow very slowly in the presence of 6.5 per cent sodium chloride) (Table 89–1). However, most human clinical isolates are either *Enterococcus faecalis* (74 to 90 per cent) or *Enterococcus faecium* (5 to 16 per cent), although clusters of human infections due to *Enterococcus raffinosus*,[23] *Enterococcus casseliflavus*,[117] *Enterococcus avium*,[124] and *Enterococcus durans*[144] have been reported. Occasional human infections due to *Enterococcus gallinarum, Enterococcus mundtii,* and *Enterococcus flavescens* have been described.[43] Although *E. faecalis* and *E. faecium* continue to make up the majority of clinical isolates, the percentage of *E. faecalis* isolates has been

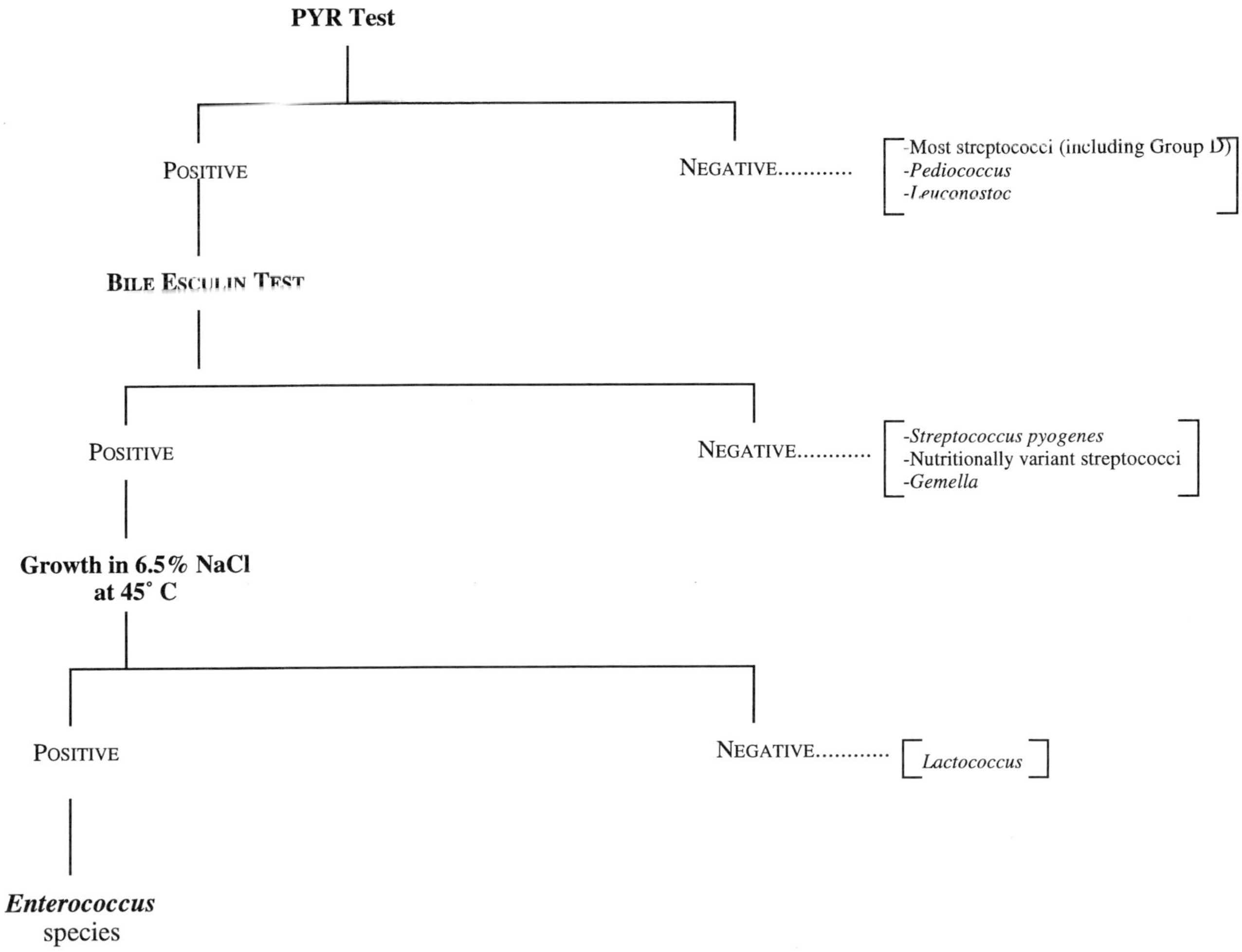

FIGURE 89–1. *Differentiation of enterococci from other catalase-negative gram-positive cocci. PYR, pyrrolidonyl arylamidase.*

TABLE 89–1. *Enterococcus* Species

Typical enterococci (PYR+)	*E. faecalis*
	E. faecium
	E. avium
	E. casseliflavus
	E. durans
	E. raffinosus
	E. gallinarum
	E. malodoratus
	E. hirae
	E. mundtii
	E. pseudoavium
	E. dispar
	E. flavescens
	E. sulfureus
Atypical enterococci (PYR−)	*E. cecorum*
	E. columbae
	E. saccharolyticus

PYR, pyrrolidonyl arylamidase.

decreasing, and relatively more isolates of *E. faecium* and "other" (non-*faecalis*, non-*faecium*) enterococcal species are being identified by clinical laboratories.[71]

Speciation of enterococci is useful primarily for epidemiologic purposes, but the distinction between the more antibiotic-susceptible *E. faecalis* and the more antibiotic-resistant *E. faecium* may be helpful in planning the therapy of endocarditis and other serious enterococcal infections. A panel of biochemical tests readily can differentiate these two common enterococcal species.[44, 75, 108] Most *E. faecalis* isolates (unlike those of *E. faecium*) grow in the presence of 0.04 per cent tellurite, reduce tetrazolium to formazan, and produce acid from sorbitol and glycerol.

A variety of molecular techniques now are available to assist in the identification of enterococci and the determination of the relatedness of enterococcal isolates, including a modification of pulsed-field gel electrophoresis known as the CHEF (contour-clamped homogeneous electric-field electrophoresis) technique[25, 26, 38, 105, 171] and the polymerase chain reaction.[39] These molecular techniques particularly have been valuable in investigations of nosocomial transmission of multidrug-resistant enterococci.[25, 26, 38, 39, 44, 105, 136, 171]

EPIDEMIOLOGY

Enterococci are normal flora of the gastrointestinal tract of most humans and have been found in as many as 97 per cent of fecal samples from adults from Europe, Asia, and North America (reviewed by Murray[108]). Approximately half of newborn infants have acquired colonization with enterococci by 1 week of age.[120] Enterococci are isolated less commonly (<20 per cent of specimens) from other sites, such as the vagina, the oral cavity, and the skin. These organisms also are common inhabitants of the bowel flora of many animals and frequently are present in soil, water, and foods. Enterococci are hardy organisms and may persist for long periods on environmental surfaces, contributing to the potential nosocomial spread of these bacteria.

Human infections due to enterococci were reported before the turn of the 20th century, but the initial patients had infections that uncommonly are associated with the enterococcus today: enteritis, meningitis, and appendicitis (reviewed by Murray[108]). The ubiquitous presence of enterococci in fecal samples led to the mistaken impression that these organisms caused enteritis and food poisoning. Enterococci commonly are isolated as part of mixed flora in intra-abdominal and pelvic infections, but the contribution of these organisms to the pathogenesis of these infections remains uncertain.[52, 118] However, the identification of enterococci as pathogens causing urinary tract infections and endocarditis was made as early as 1906[2] and later confirmed in many studies. Subsequently, enterococci have been documented to cause invasive infections in neonates,[37, 50, 76] patients with malignancies,[12, 55, 104, 146] recipients of bone marrow and solid organ transplants,[139] burn victims,[82] patients with indwelling catheters,[125, 133] and other immunosuppressed or debilitated patients.[94, 103, 108, 125, 133]

In general, enterococcal infections are less frequent in children (outside the neonatal period) than in adults, and enterococci are less important causes of pediatric urinary tract infections[174] and endocarditis.[155] Much of the published experience with enterococcal infections in children focuses on the neonatal period.[31, 37, 90, 130] Some evidence suggests that late-onset (but not early-onset) neonatal infections due to enterococci may be increasing in frequency.[25, 37] Relatively few series of pediatric enterococcal infections have been published.[8, 9, 25, 135]

Enterococci fairly recently have emerged as important nosocomial agents, ranking as either the second or third most common hospital-acquired pathogens in the United States.[18, 66, 102, 140] Evidence for the nosocomial spread of enterococci is relatively recent. Initially, all enterococci isolated from hospitalized patients were thought to have originated from the patients' endogenous bowel flora. However, the emergence of multiply antibiotic-resistant enterococci prompted careful epidemiologic studies that documented the nosocomial spread of these organisms.[10, 11, 18, 40, 74, 86, 104, 130, 133, 135, 144–146] These studies indicated that enterococci may persist for long periods in the environment and may be spread by either direct patient-to-patient contact, via the hands of colonized health care personnel,[130] or through contaminated patient equipment, including thermometers.[10, 74, 86]

It must be emphasized that the growing problem of VRE is multifactorial; the diversity of isolates found in many hospitals indicates that resistant organisms may be introduced via multiple sources.[6, 25, 40, 106, 133, 146] The major risk factors for VRE acquisition and/or infection appear to be severity of underlying illness or immunosuppression, increasing length of hospital stay, recent cardiothoracic or abdominal surgery, the presence of indwelling central venous or urinary catheters, and prior treatment with vancomycin and/or broad-spectrum antibiotics.[10, 19, 60, 86, 104, 106, 135] It is likely that the factors contributing to the nosocomial spread of these organisms differ from those responsible for the gradual overall increase in resistant strains.[133]

Since the first report of VRE in 1988,[83] VRE infection and colonization in the United States have been observed primarily in the intensive care units of large teaching hospitals.[18, 110] Data reported to the Centers for Disease Control and Prevention's (CDC's) National Nosocomial Infections Surveillance System (NNIS) from January 1989 through March 1993 revealed no vancomycin resistance in hospitals with fewer than 200 beds, a resistance rate of 1.8 per cent in hospitals with 200 to 500 beds, and a resistance rate of 3.6 per cent in hospitals with more than 500 beds.[18] A report from a multicenter *Enterococcus* study group analyzed 1936 isolates collected from 97 laboratories in 47 states during the last quarter of 1992 and generally confirmed the findings of the NNIS survey.[71] Experience with VRE in children is less extensive, although a number of pediatric centers have reported VRE infections. In the United States, VRE generally have not been detected in environmental sources or in patients who have not had exposure to hospitals.[110] However, the ecology of VRE in Europe differs: VRE have been detected in the feces of nonhospitalized patients and healthy volunteers in several European studies. The more widespread occurrence of VRE strains in Europe may be related to the use of oral glycopeptides in animal feeds and/or the oral administration of bacterial preparations (possibly contaminated with resistant enterococci) to humans and animals for therapeutic purposes.[110]

Initial reports of VRE in the United States were clustered in the Northeast region, particularly New York, Maryland, and Pennsylvania.[18] Jones and associates[72] and the *Enterococcus* Study Group found that all participating laboratories reporting VRE isolates in late 1992 were east of the Mississippi River; most were focused around New York City. However, a follow-up telephone survey in March 1994 revealed that 37 of 75 medical centers not previously reporting VRE subsequently had identified these organisms from one or more clinical specimens, expanding the geographic distribution of VRE to include the West Coast (California and Washington), the South (Texas, Florida, and Louisiana), and the North (North Dakota, Michigan, and Wisconsin).[72]

Nosocomial enterococcal bacteremia in adults frequently is associated with urinary tract and wound infections, but catheter-related bacteremia is of increasing importance. Enterococcal bacteremia without a source is relatively more common in children,[9, 133] although Bonadio[8] reported that many children with enterococcal bacteremia had an identifiable focus of infection. Enterococcal bacteremia is more common in patients with severe underlying disease and may be life-threatening. The precise contribution of enterococcal bacteremia to morbidity and mortality in this setting remains controversial. Adult intensive care unit patients with enterococcal bacteremia have a very high mortality rate,[54] but the isolation of *Enterococcus* from the blood may serve merely to identify a very high-risk group of patients.[108] Clearance of enterococci from the blood does not reduce the mortality rates in these high-risk patients necessarily, and spontaneous resolution of enterococcal bacteremia has been reported, suggesting that transient bacteremia and/or pseudobacteremia due to enterococci may occur.[165] However, studies indicate that effective therapy of enterococcal bacteremia reduces overall mortality in these high-risk patient groups.[40, 62, 125]

PATHOGENESIS AND VIRULENCE

Enterococci are organisms of low virulence, and their ubiquitous presence in the human gastrointestinal tract likely has contributed to both the spurious association of these organisms with some illnesses (e.g., enteritis) and the failure to recognize other situations in which enterococci are true pathogens (e.g., immunosuppressed and debilitated patients, neonates). Compared with organisms such as *S. pyogenes* and *Staphylococcus aureus*, enterococci are much less virulent in animal models of infection,[67, 102] although they are capable of causing disease at a higher inoculum.

Enterococci rarely cause primary cellulitis or abscesses, although they are isolated frequently as components of polymicrobial wound infections and intra-abdominal and pelvic infections. The contribution of enterococci to the pathogenesis of these polymicrobial infections remains uncertain.[52, 118] In animal models, synergy between enterococci and a variety of other organisms (particularly anaerobes) can be demonstrated, although enterococci injected alone have little propensity to cause either peritonitis or subcutaneous infection.[67, 68, 108, 123] However, several clinical trials have concluded that the provision of antienterococcal therapy generally is not necessary to effect the cure of human intra-abdominal and pelvic infections, even though *Enterococcus* frequently (14 to 33 per cent of cases) is isolated from primary peritoneal cultures.[52]

Enterococci are important causes of urinary tract infections in adults (particularly in elderly men, patients with structural abnormalities of the urinary tract, and patients with indwelling urinary catheters) but are associated less frequently with urinary tract infections in children.[5, 174] Enterococci also are important but less frequent causes of endocarditis in children (compared with adults).[97, 155] Adherence of bacteria to tissue is a necessary first step in the pathogenesis of both urinary tract infections and endocarditis, and there is evidence that pathogenic enterococci produce factors that mediate adherence to urinary epithelial cells and endocardial tissue, respectively (reviewed by Jett and colleagues[67] and Johnson[68]). Enterococcal adhesins include an enterococcal surface protein known as aggregation substance[24, 78] and one or more surface carbohydrates. Lipoteichoic acid, an important adhesin for *S. pyogenes*, does not appear to mediate adhesion of enterococci[152] but may trigger the host inflammatory response to these organisms.[159]

CLINICAL MANIFESTATIONS

Enterococcal infections generally are less common in children than in adults, although the enterococcus is a relatively frequent cause of neonatal infections.[37] The types of infections caused by enterococci in children are similar to those in adults.[8, 9, 133] Enterococci have become increasingly important nosocomial pathogens.[9, 18, 25, 102] As in adults, enterococci are important causes of endocarditis, urinary tract infections, and bacteremia (particularly catheter-related bacteremia), and these organisms commonly are isolated as components of polymicrobial wound, intra-abdominal, and pelvic infections.[8, 9, 103, 108] Meningitis[156] and septic arthritis[129] are rare manifestations of enterococcal infection. Respiratory infections due to enterococci are extremely uncommon, although many neonates with enterococcal infection do have pulmonary symptoms.[37]

Urinary Tract Infection

Urinary tract infections are the most common enterococcal infections in adults,[103] and enterococci are important urinary pathogens in children.[36] Most enterococcal urinary tract infections occur in elderly men after urinary catheterization and/or instrumentation.[46, 107] Enterococci are infrequent (<5 per cent of isolates) causes of cystitis and pyelonephritis in otherwise healthy children, infants, and neonates[5, 174] and are unusual causes of urinary tract infections in young women.[108] However, some centers are reporting an increasing incidence of both community-acquired and nosocomial urinary tract infections caused by enterococci.[46]

Most enterococcal urinary tract infections in children[5, 36, 87] and adults[46, 102] are nosocomial. Risk factors for urinary tract infections caused by *Enterococcus* include indwelling urinary catheters, instrumentation of the urinary tract, structural abnormalities of the urinary tract, and previous broad-spectrum antimicrobial therapy.[107, 108] The increasing problem of nosocomial enterococcal urinary tract infections[46] is compounded by the growing problem of multiply antibiotic-resistant enterococci.[18]

The genitourinary tract reportedly is the most common entry site for enterococcal bacteremia in adults[54, 79] but is implicated much less frequently in the etiology of enterococcal bacteremia in children.[8, 9] However, Christie and colleagues[25] noted urosepsis as the etiology of 12 per cent of episodes of nosocomial enterococcal bacteremia in a children's hospital. Other complications of enterococcal urinary tract infections in adults are prostatitis and perinephric abscess.[103]

Endocarditis

Enterococcal endocarditis was reported first in 1906,[2] and these organisms are important causes of native-valve and prosthetic-valve endocarditis in children and adults.[1, 97, 132] Either normal or previously damaged valves may be involved. Enterococci cause approximately 5 to 20 per cent of cases of native-valve endocarditis in adults (excluding cases in intravenous drug users).[97] Enterococci cause approximately 6 to 7 per cent of prosthetic-valve endocarditis.[97, 163] Approximately 5 to 10 per cent of endocarditis in intravenous drug users is due to enterococci and usually involves the aortic or mitral valves, unlike staphylococcal endocarditis in this setting, which generally involves the tricuspid valve.[108] As with other enterococcal infections, *E. faecalis* causes the majority of cases of endocarditis.

Enterococcal endocarditis primarily is a disease of older males, and the genitourinary tract is the most commonly identified source of the initial bacteremia. Enterococci are relatively less frequent causes of endocarditis in children, causing less than 5 per cent of cases in most series.[69, 70, 154, 155, 160, 177] Typically, enterococcal endocarditis follows a subacute course and is indistinguishable clinically from that caused by the streptococci.[97] Although the enterococcus is a common neonatal pathogen,[37] reports of neonatal endocarditis due to enterococci are extremely rare.[160] The prognosis of enterococcal prosthetic valve endocarditis is somewhat better than that of native-valve endocarditis caused by these organisms.[1, 132] Aortic valve involvement is associated with increased morbidity and mortality.[97]

Bacteremia

Enterococcal bacteremia often represents a conundrum. Bacteremia in severely ill hospitalized patients, particularly that due to VRE, is associated with considerable morbidity and mortality. However, only a portion of that morbidity and mortality can be attributed to enterococcal bacteremia per se. Enterococcal bacteremia frequently occurs as a component of polymicrobial bacteremia in the hospital setting; from 21 to 45 per cent of blood stream isolates of *Enterococcus* are accompanied by one or more other pathogens.[92, 125, 148] As many as half of catheter-related enterococcal bacteremias are polymicrobial.[125] Many[59, 92] but not all[62] series of patients with enterococcal bacteremia have reported increased mortality in patients with polymicrobial bacteremia (including *Enterococcus*) versus isolated enterococcal bacteremia. Mortality in adults with nosocomial enterococcal bacteremia has ranged from 23 to 46 per cent,[92, 93, 125] but patients at risk for nosocomial enterococcal bacteremia are severely ill and have a poor prognosis independent of the bacteremic event. Hospital-acquired enterococcal infections can be life-threatening,[40, 108, 125] and specific therapy does appear to reduce the mortality rate.[40, 62, 125] However, some episodes of enterococcal bacteremia in high-risk patients may resolve in the absence of specific therapy.[62, 165]

In adults, the majority of cases of enterococcal bacteremia are associated with a primary focus, most commonly a urinary tract infection.[54, 79] In contrast, most episodes of enterococcal bacteremia in children have not been associated with an identifiable focus.[9, 133] However, Christie and associates[25] identified a primary focus in 21 of 57 children (37 per cent) with nosocomial enterococcal bacteremia, including 7 patients with urosepsis and 6 patients with peritonitis. In addition, many children with enterococcal bacteremia do have underlying diseases involving the gastrointestinal or respiratory tracts.[8, 9] Central venous catheter–related enterococcal bacteremia is a growing problem in both children[8, 9, 25, 37, 125] and adults.[54, 125] In earlier series, infections of vascular catheters were reported to account for only 2 to 14 per cent of enterococcal bacteremias (reviewed by Graninger and Ragette[54]), but more recent reports have implicated indwelling central venous catheters in up to 28 per cent of these episodes.[125]

Most episodes of enterococcal bacteremia do not lead to endocarditis,[92, 108, 125] and endocarditis particularly is uncommon in the setting of nosocomial enterococcal bacteremia. Maki and Agger[92] identified only one case of endocarditis in 118 episodes of hospital-acquired enterococcal bacteremia, whereas endocarditis was diagnosed in 12 of 35 patients with community-acquired enterococcal bacteremia.

Intra-abdominal Infections

Most of the published information about the role of *Enterococcus* in intra-abdominal and pelvic infections comes from series of adult patients. Enterococci commonly are isolated as components of polymicrobial infections involving the abdomen or pelvis,[52] and animal models suggest that these organisms can play a synergistic role in the pathogenesis of such infections.[67] However, there is no compelling evidence that the addition of specific antienterococcal therapy improves the outcome of human intra-abdominal and pelvic infections, even when enterococci are isolated from peritoneal cultures.[52]

Children with enterococcal bacteremia frequently have underlying conditions related to the gastrointestinal tract.[8, 9, 25] Bonadio[8] reported five cases of enterococcal bacteremia in previously healthy infants with gastroenteritis, six cases associated with bowel obstruction, and one case associated with acute appendicitis without perforation. Boulanger and associates[9] identified underlying conditions affecting the gastrointestinal system in 8 of 32 pediatric patients with enterococcal bacteremia but were unable to implicate specifically any of these conditions as the source of the bacteremia.

Meningitis

Enterococci are rare causes of bacterial meningitis in adults and children. Stevenson and colleagues[156] found only four cases of enterococcal meningitis among 493 episodes (0.8 per cent) of bacterial meningitis in adults and identified an additional 90 cases in a literature search of the interval 1966 to 1992. These authors reviewed 16 published cases of enterococcal meningitis in children: 11 of these 16 pediatric cases were complications of central nervous system trauma or surgery, but four children (three of the four were neonates) had primary meningitis.[156] Enterococci are uncommon but well-recognized causes of infections involving cerebrospinal fluid shunts and related devices.[77, 112, 143] Meningitis rarely complicates nosocomial bacteremia in adults[92, 125] but was noted to occur in 4 of 57 (7 per cent) episodes of nosocomial enterococcal bacteremia in children in Cincinnati[25] and in 4 of 26 (15 per cent) premature neonates with late-onset enterococcal sepsis in Houston.[37]

Stevenson and associates[156] found that most adults with

enterococcal meningitis were immunocompromised (most were receiving steroids) and many had a history of central nervous system trauma or surgery. Enterococcal meningitis has been reported in one adult patient with HIV infection who had completed a course of steroids for presumed *Pneumocystis* pneumonia.[127] Although many children with enterococcal meningitis do have a history of central nervous system trauma or surgery and some are premature neonates, most do not have other identifiable predisposing conditions or a history of immunosuppressive therapy.

As with most enterococcal infections, most cerebrospinal fluid isolates are *E. faecalis*, although meningitis and ventriculoperitoneal shunt infections due to *E. faecium* have been reported in children.[112, 113]

Neonatal Infections

Enterococci are important neonatal pathogens,[8, 9, 31, 37, 50, 76, 90, 130, 151] and the published experience with neonatal enterococcal infections constitutes much of the pediatric literature concerning these organisms. Although several large series of neonatal sepsis included few cases of enterococcal infection (reviewed by Klein and Marcy[76]), many centers have reported that *Enterococcus* is a relatively frequent cause of neonatal bacteremia. Siegel and McCracken[151] found that enterococci were second only to group B streptococci as causes of neonatal sepsis at Parkland Hospital in Dallas from 1974 to 1977, with an incidence rate of approximately 1.0 case per 1000 live births. Gladstone and colleagues[50] reported that *Enterococcus* caused 18 of 270 (6.7 per cent) episodes of neonatal sepsis at Yale–New Haven Hospital during the period from 1979 to 1988, ranking fourth in incidence behind group B *Streptococcus* (64 cases, 23.7 per cent), *Escherichia coli* (46 cases, 17.0 per cent), and coagulase-negative staphylococci (36 cases, 13.3 per cent). Reports from Houston[37] and Cincinnati[25] documented a sharp increase in the rate of late-onset neonatal infections due to enterococci, in both hospitalized high-risk premature neonates and infants[37] and in otherwise healthy term newborns with "community-acquired" infections.[25]

Enterococci cause both early-onset (<7 days of age) and late-onset (>7 days of age) neonatal sepsis. Early onset disease is indistinguishable from that caused by other neonatal pathogens but tends to be less severe.[37] Rates of early-onset disease have remained relatively stable, but several centers are reporting increasing rates of late-onset infection. Dobson and Baker[37] identified 56 neonates with enterococcal sepsis over a 10-year period at Jefferson Davis Hospital in Houston: 18 of 56 (32 per cent) had early-onset sepsis, 26 of 56 (46 per cent) had late-onset sepsis, and 12 of 56 (21 per cent) had sepsis associated with necrotizing enterocolitis (2 early-onset, 10 late-onset).[37] In this study, 25 of the 26 (96 per cent) infants with late-onset enterococcal sepsis were premature infants. Christie and colleagues[25] identified 83 cases of enterococcal bacteremia between 1986 and 1992 at Children's Hospital of Cincinnati: 58 of those 83 episodes occurred in neonates. Most cases (57 of 83, 68.7 per cent) were nosocomial, but many (26 of 83, 31.3 per cent) were community acquired. Young infants (<3 months of age) accounted for almost all (24 of 26, 92.3 per cent) of the community-acquired episodes and for many (34 of 57, 59.6 per cent) of the nosocomial infections. Bonadio[8] and Boulanger and colleagues[9] also have reported community-acquired enterococcal bacteremia in young infants. Nosocomial outbreaks of enterococcal infections, including those due to VRE, have been reported in neonates from several U.S. centers.[25, 31, 90, 130] Indwelling central venous catheters, necrotizing enterocolitis, and intra-abdominal surgery are important predisposing factors for nosocomial enterococcal bacteremia in the neonate, whereas the genitourinary tract is implicated less frequently as a source.[25]

Enterococcal bacteremia in neonates and young infants has been associated with diarrhea[8, 37] and with respiratory disease,[8, 37] but a causative role for *Enterococcus* in the pathogenesis of gastroenteritis or pneumonia remains undefined. Enterococci rarely cause urinary tract infections in neonates,[8, 25, 37] but nosocomial and community-acquired cases have been reported. Enterococci have been reported to cause a variety of other neonatal infections, including focal skin and soft-tissue infections (e.g., scalp abscess),[37] brain abscess,[134] omphalitis,[37] and conjunctivitis.[168]

Most neonatal enterococcal infections are caused by *E. faecalis*, but outbreaks of infection due to *E. faecium* have been reported.[31] In the series from Cincinnati reported by Christie and associates,[25] largely composed of neonates, 82 per cent of enterococcal isolates were *E. faecalis* and 14 per cent were *E. faecium*.

Septic Arthritis

Enterococci rarely have been reported to cause septic arthritis but can infect native or prosthetic joints. Raymond and colleagues[129] reported a case of enterococcal septic arthritis involving a prosthetic hip and reviewed an additional 18 cases from the literature. Eleven of these 19 episodes involved prosthetic joints (2 hips, 9 knees), and 8 involved native joints; only 1 of the 8 individuals with native joint arthritis had an underlying abnormality of the joint. In 7 of the 19 episodes, *Enterococcus* was isolated from a joint isolate along with a second organism (3 with coagulase-negative staphylococci, 1 with group B *Streptococcus*, 1 with *Pseudomonas* species, 1 with *Streptococcus* species, and 1 with *Kingella kingae*). Only one pediatric case was identified: a 21-month-old girl with septic arthritis of the wrist whose joint aspirate grew *Enterococcus* species and *K. kingae*.[150]

DIAGNOSIS

Enterococcal infections usually are diagnosed by the isolation of *Enterococcus* from a culture of blood or another normally sterile site. As discussed earlier, enterococci are ubiquitous inhabitants of the human gastrointestinal tract, and the isolation of these organisms from stool and surface cultures is not evidence of invasive infection. Although enterococci are uncommon blood culture contaminants, transient bacteremia and/or pseudobacteremia due to these organisms may occur.[62, 165]

More problematic is the interpretation of a positive culture for *Enterococcus* as a component of polymicrobial infections, particularly intra-abdominal and pelvic infections. In this setting, the role of the enterococcus in pathogenesis is uncertain, and therapeutic regimens that do not include antienterococcal agents usually suffice to effect a clinical cure.[52] However, cases of breakthrough enterococcal bacteremia have been reported on these regimens, and one study found a decreased rate of abdominal surgical wound infections when antienterococcal coverage was provided in a prophylactic regimen.[169]

ANTIMICROBIAL SUSCEPTIBILITY AND RESISTANCE

The increasing importance of *Enterococcus* as a pathogen, especially in the nosocomial setting,[18, 102] is of particular concern because of the concomitant development of antimicrobial resistance by these organisms. Some enterococci have acquired high-level resistance to all three classes of antimicrobial agents that are used to treat life-threatening enterococcal infections—the β-lactams, the aminoglycosides, and the glycopeptides. This acquired resistance has occurred in the context of intrinsic (usually lower-level) resistance of enterococci to many antibiotics and has confronted physicians with the possibility of infectious diseases that may fail to respond to any currently available antibiotics.

Intrinsic Resistance

β-Lactam Antibiotics

Relative resistance to β-lactam antibiotics is an intrinsic characteristic of enterococci, occurring even in human populations without previous exposure to antibiotics,[101] and is due to the lower affinity of enterococcal (versus streptococcal) penicillin-binding proteins, especially penicillin-binding protein 5.[103, 172] In general, the penicillin minimal inhibitory concentration (MIC) for most *E. faecalis* isolates (2 to 8 μg/mL) is at least 10 to 100 times higher than that of most streptococci, and *E. faecium* is even more resistant (MIC, 8 to 32 μg/mL or higher).[108] Ampicillin is the most active of the β-lactam antibiotics versus enterococci, with average MIC values about twofold lower than those for penicillin.[103, 108] Nafcillin generally is less active than penicillin, and methicillin is much less active (MIC, >50 μg/mL for *E. faecalis*), as are carbenicillin and ticarcillin. Enterococci exposed to β-lactam antibiotics rapidly develop tolerance to the killing effects of these agents.[103, 108] Along with intrinsic resistance to these antibiotics, this limits the utility of β-lactam monotherapy in the treatment of life-threatening enterococcal infections.

Imipenem has some activity against *E. faecalis* but is much less active against *E. faecium*.[103, 108] None of the currently available cephalosporins have clinically useful activity against the enterococci, and the frequent use of broad-spectrum cephalosporins and imipenem has been identified as a risk factor for nosocomial enterococcal infections.

Aminoglycosides

Enterococci intrinsically are resistant to all aminoglycosides because of diminished uptake of these drugs. For most *E. faecalis* isolates, the MIC for gentamicin or tobramycin ranges from 8 to 64 μg/mL, and that to streptomycin ranges from 12 to 250 μg/mL.[96, 126, 164] Moellering and colleagues[100, 179] first demonstrated that the addition of a cell wall–active antibiotic resulted in dramatically increased aminoglycoside uptake by enterococci and led to synergistic killing of these organisms. All *E. faecium* strains exhibit higher MICs (compared with *E. faecalis*) to certain aminoglycosides, including tobramycin, netilmicin, kanamycin, and sissomicin, and these aminoglycosides do not exhibit synergy with β-lactam antibiotics against *E. faecium*.[108]

Other Antibiotics

Under carefully standardized laboratory conditions, enterococci are inhibited but not killed[114] by the combination of trimethoprim and sulfamethoxazole (TMP-SMZ). However, *Enterococcus* isolates should be considered resistant to TMP-SMZ. Enterococci are capable of utilizing exogenous folinic acid to evade the antimicrobial action of TMP-SMZ.[178] TMP-SMZ fails to eradicate enterococci in animal models of infection,[21, 57] and breakthrough enterococcal bacteremias have occurred in patients being treated with TMP-SMZ for enterococcal urinary tract infections.[51] Enterococci also intrinsically are resistant to clindamycin, a drug with excellent activity against many other gram-positive cocci. Most enterococci exhibit a clindamycin MIC of 12.5 to 100 μg/mL.[108] As with low-level β-lactam resistance, clindamycin resistance is found in enterococcal isolates from human populations with no prior antibiotic exposure.[101]

Acquired Resistance

Enterococci have acquired resistance to antibiotics by acquisition of both narrow-host range and broad-host range plasmids and via the exchange of conjugative transposons (reviewed by Murray[108]). Resistance mediated by broad-host range plasmids is of particular concern because glycopeptide resistance encoded by broad-host range plasmids has been transferred to staphylococci in vitro[121] and theoretically could be transmitted to important human pathogens, such as *S. aureus* and *Streptococcus pneumoniae*. Vancomycin-resistant strains of *Staphylococcus haemolyticus* have been identified in clinical specimens.[167]

High-Level Resistance to Aminoglycosides

Intrinsic resistance of enterococci to aminoglycosides is due to poor drug uptake and can be overcome effectively both in vitro and in vivo by the addition of cell wall–active antibiotics. However, high-level resistance to aminoglycosides results when enterococci acquire plasmids coding for aminoglycoside-modifying enzymes (affecting all aminoglycosides via several different enzymes) or develop ribosomal mutations (streptomycin only). High-level aminoglycoside resistance is of great clinical importance because it eliminates synergism between the affected aminoglycoside(s) and β-lactam or glycopeptide antibiotics.[80, 108, 126]

Enterococci with high-level resistance (MIC, ≥2000 μg/mL) to streptomycin, kanamycin, and several other aminoglycosides (excluding gentamicin) were identified more than 25 years ago[99] and were prevalent widely in the United States by the mid-1970s.[14] High-level resistance to streptomycin occurs via two mechanisms: ribosomal mutation or enzymatic modification by a 6′-adenylyltransferase; high-level resistance to kanamycin (but not to gentamicin) is mediated by a 3′-phosphotransferase (reviewed by Murray[108]). All enterococci resistant to kanamycin also should be considered resistant to amikacin, although high-level resistance to amikacin is not found when MICs are performed. Amikacin does not exhibit synergy with β-lactams against kanamycin-resistant enterococci and actually may antagonize the effects of β-lactam antibiotics against these strains.[14, 80]

Horodniceanu and colleagues[64] first reported high-level resistance to gentamicin in *E. faecalis* in 1979. High-level resistance to gentamicin is mediated by a fusion enzyme containing both 6′-acetyltransferase and 2′-phosphotransferase activity and confers resistance to all clinically useful aminoglycosides except streptomycin.[84, 85] Thus, enterococci expressing this fusion enzyme and the 6′-adenylyltransferase mediating streptomycin resistance (or chromosomally mediated streptomycin resistance) are highly resistant to all available aminoglycosides and fail to be killed synergistically by any combinations of β-lactam antibiotics and aminoglycosides. Strains of *E. faecalis* resistant to both streptomycin and gentamicin (thus, to all aminoglycosides) first were detected in Houston, Bangkok, and Santiago in 1983.[96, 108] Subsequently, strains of *E. faecalis*, *E. faecium*, and other enterococci resistant to gentamicin, streptomycin, or both (all) aminoglycosides have become increasingly prevalent (Table 89–2).[22, 29, 53, 72, 126, 131]

All *E. faecium* strains are resistant to synergistic killing when certain aminoglycosides (including tobramycin, kanamycin, netilmicin, and sissomicin) are combined with β-lactam antibiotics. Costa and associates[30] found that all strains of *E. faecium* produce a chromosomally encoded (nontransferable) 6′-adenylyltransferase that is responsible for this resistance. Importantly, the rate of aminoglycoside modification by this enzyme is not sufficient to result in high-level resistance but does abrogate synergy with β-lactams. Consequently, these particular aminoglycosides should not be used to treat infections caused by *E. faecium*. Although high-level resistance to streptomycin and gentamicin first was described in *E. faecalis*, the *Enterococcus* Study Group recently found relatively more high-level resistance to streptomycin in *E. faecium* isolates and comparable amounts of high-level resistance to gentamicin among strains of *E. faecalis* and *E. faecium* (see Table 89–2).[72]

High-Level Resistance to β-Lactams and Production of β-Lactamase

The mechanism of resistance to penicillin, ampicillin, and other β-lactam antibiotics differs among enterococcal species. High-level β-lactam resistance (ampicillin MIC, ≥16 μg/mL) of *E. faecium*[10, 56, 95] and some other non-*faecalis* enterococcal strains[11] has increased dramatically over the past decade (see Table 89–2) and is mediated by additional alterations of penicillin-binding proteins, particularly penicillin-binding protein 5.[47, 56] Thus, high-level resistance to ampicillin and other β-lactams in *E. faecium* (and other non-*faecalis* strains) represents an exaggerated form of intrinsic β-lactam resistance. *E. faecalis* isolates also intrinsically are resistant to β-lactams (although less so than *E. faecium*), but there has been little change in the level of this resistance in recent years. However, some strains of *E. faecalis*[109, 111] and, rarely, *E. faecium*[32] have developed clinically significant resistance to ampicillin and penicillin via the plasmid-mediated, constitutive production of a β-lactamase enzyme identical to that of *S. aureus*.[180] β-Lactamase–producing strains of *E. faecalis* and *E. faecium* will not be detected by routine susceptibility testing because of a pronounced inoculum effect. Therefore, enzymatic methods, such as the nitrocefin test, must be employed to screen for β-lactamase–producing strains.[75, 109]

Glycopeptide Resistance

VRE first were identified in 1988[83, 166] and rapidly have become a major nosocomial problem. Data collected by the NNIS of the CDC revealed a dramatic increase in the rate of vancomycin resistance in nosocomial isolates of *Enterococcus* during the interval from 1989 to 1993.[18] The NNIS survey documented a 26-fold increase in vancomycin resistance among all nosocomial isolates (from 0.3 per cent of enterococcal isolates in 1989 to 7.9 per cent in 1993) and a 34-fold increase in vancomycin resistance among isolates obtained from patients in intensive care units (from 0.4 per cent of isolates in 1989 to 13.6 per cent in 1993). Vancomycin-resistant strains, particularly those of *E. faecium*, also may exhibit high-level resistance to both β-lactam antibiotics and aminoglycosides (see Table 89–2), making the treatment of these infections extremely challenging.[3, 15–17, 20, 31, 40, 45, 60, 74, 82, 84, 103, 104, 110, 119, 133, 135]

Vancomycin resistance among enterococci phenotypically and genotypically is heterogeneous (reviewed by Arthur and Courvalin[4]) and may or may not be associated with resistance to other glycopeptides, including teicoplanin. Three major phenotypes of vancomycin resistance have been described in enterococci. The VanA phenotype is characterized by high-level resistance to vancomycin and teicoplanin, whereas strains with the VanB phenotype exhibit variable levels of resistance to vancomycin but not teicoplanin.[4] The VanC phenotype is limited to *E. gallinarum* and *E. casseliflavus* and is associated with constitutive, low-level, chromosomally mediated (nontransferable) resistance to vancomycin but not teicoplanin.[133]

High-level resistance to both vancomycin and teicoplanin (the VanA phenotype) is found primarily in strains of *E. faecium*, whereas most vancomycin-resistant strains of *E. faecalis* express the VanB phenotype, remaining susceptible to teicoplanin. Jones and associates[72] and the *Enterococcus* Study Group found that 10 of 11 (91 per cent) of vancomycin-resistant strains of *E. faecalis* remained susceptible to teicoplanin (VanB phenotype), whereas 49 of 62 (79 per cent) of vancomycin-resistant strains of *E. faecium* were resistant to teicoplanin (VanA phenotype).[72] Both VanA and VanB pheno-

TABLE 89–2. Antimicrobial Resistance Patterns of Enterococci

	Gordon et al.[53] [July 1988–April 1989]				Jones et al.[72] (The *Enterococcus* Study Group) [October 1992–December 1992]			
	E. faecalis (n = 632)	E. faecium (n = 58)	*Other (n = 15)*	*Total (n = 705)*	E. faecalis (n = 1428)	E. faecium (n = 306)	*Other (n = 202)*	*Total (n = 1936)*
Ampicillin resistance (MIC ≥16 μg/mL)	0%*	41%†	7%	4%	0.6–0.7%‡	58.7–59.3%	19.0%	12%
Streptomycin high-level resistance (MIC >2000 μg/mL)	14%	33%	7%	16%	31.5%	55.7%	35.0%	36%
Gentamicin high-level resistance (MIC >500 μg/mL)	11%	2%	7%	10%	26.0%	30.8%	27.5%	27%
Vancomycin resistance (MIC >4 μg/mL)	0.3%	0%	0%	0.3%	2.0%	21.9%	7%	5.6%
Teicoplanin resistance (MIC >4 μg/mL)	0%	0%	0%	0%	0.1%	16%	6%	3.2%

*However, 11/632 (1.7%) of *E. faecalis* isolates were β-lactamase producers.
†No β-lactamase–producing strains were identified.
‡Only two β-lactamase–producing isolates were identified.

types are mediated by homologous enzymes that catalyze the formation of an altered, vancomycin-resistant depsipeptide that is incorporated into cell wall peptidoglycan.[4, 133] VanA resistance is transferable by either transposition (via the transposon Tn1545) or conjugative plasmids; VanB resistance generally is found on the bacterial chromosome but can be transferred on plasmids; VanC resistance is not transferable (reviewed by Rice and Schlaes[133]).

The peculiar phenomenon of infection due to vancomycin-dependent enterococci has been described. Fraimow and colleagues[48] reported a urinary tract infection due to a strain of *E. faecalis* that would grow only in the presence of vancomycin, and Green and associates[58] have reported breakthrough bacteremia with a vancomycin-dependent strain of *E. faecium* during therapy for bacteremia. The mechanisms responsible for vancomycin dependence remain undefined.

TESTING FOR ANTIMICROBIAL RESISTANCE IN ENTEROCOCCI

All enterococci isolated from cultures of blood, cerebrospinal fluid, or other normally sterile sites (with the possible exception of urine) should be tested for resistance to β-lactam antibiotics (ampicillin and/or penicillin, including a test for β-lactamase production), vancomycin, and high levels of aminoglycosides (streptomycin and gentamicin),[19, 44, 133] employing the methodology and interpretative guidelines published by the National Committee for Clinical Laboratory Standards.[115, 116] For multiply antibiotic-resistant isolates, testing for susceptibility to alternate agents, including chloramphenicol, ciprofloxacin, erythromycin, novobiocin, and quinupristin and dalfopristin, should be considered.[44, 71]

Testing of enterococci for ampicillin (or penicillin) resistance must involve (1) determination of the MIC of these agents and (2) a test for β-lactamase production. Jones and colleagues[72] and the *Enterococcus* Study Group compared three techniques that commonly are used to determine the ampicillin MIC of enterococcal isolates—disk diffusion, broth microdilution, and Etest strips—and found excellent agreement among the three methods. Enterococcal isolates with an MIC of 16 μg/mL to ampicillin or penicillin are considered resistant to these agents.[116] β-Lactamase–producing enterococci cannot be detected by these methods but are identified routinely by performance of the chromogenic nitrocefin assay.[157]

High-level resistance to gentamicin and streptomycin may be detected by agar dilution (high-level resistance to gentamicin $>$ 500 μg/mL, high-level resistance to streptomycin $>$ 2000 μg/mL), broth microdilution (high-level resistance to gentamicin $>$ 500 μg/mL, high-level resistance to streptomycin $>$ 1000 μg/mL), disk diffusion using high-content aminoglycoside disks (120-μg gentamicin disk, 300-μg streptomycin disks, $\geq$10-mm zone = susceptible),[115, 157] or use of high-range Etest strips.[72, 138]

Vancomycin resistance in enterococci, particularly the VanB phenotype of moderate resistance, is not detected reliably by many commercially available antimicrobial susceptibility testing methods, including the Vitek and MicroScan systems.[157, 161, 162, 176] Routine disk diffusion testing is more reliable but requires an extended incubation time and the use of transmitted light to examine zone sizes in order to be highly accurate.[158, 162] Agar dilution screening using brain heart infusion agar supplemented with 16 μg vancomycin/mL does identify VRE strains reliably,[157, 170] as does the standard broth microdilution method.[71, 162] Etest glycopeptide strips are a promising alternative to the more cumbersome broth dilution methodology and were a highly reliable method for detecting vancomycin resistance in the experience of the *Enterococcus* Study Group.[71] However, additional evaluation of the Etest glycopeptide strips is necessary because some variability is observed in Etest estimates of vancomycin MICs in reference strains of *E. faecalis*.[162]

TREATMENT OF ENTEROCOCCAL INFECTIONS

Treatment of Endocarditis

The difficulty of treating enterococcal endocarditis has been apparent since early reports that penicillin alone failed to cure as many as two-thirds of patients with enterococcal endocarditis but was highly effective in the treatment of streptococcal endocarditis (reviewed by Murray[108]). These early failures of penicillin stimulated studies of the in vitro and in vivo effects of β-lactam antibiotics on enterococci, leading to the discovery that enterococci were "tolerant" to the killing effects of cell wall–active agents and providing evidence that bactericidal therapy was required to cure bacterial endocarditis reliably.

For nearly half a century, standard therapy for enterococcal endocarditis has included the addition of an aminoglycoside to a cell wall–active agent. Hunter[65] first reported clinical evidence of synergism between penicillin and streptomycin in the treatment of enterococcal endocarditis in 1947, and this subsequently was confirmed for combinations of penicillin or ampicillin and streptomycin or gentamicin both in vitro and in vivo (reviewed by Murray[108]). Moellering and Weinberg[100] first demonstrated that synergy between β-lactams and aminoglycosides was a consequence of increased aminoglycoside uptake by enterococci exposed to cell wall–active agents. Glycopeptides and aminoglycosides also exhibit in vitro and in vivo synergy against "susceptible" (not expressing high-level resistance) strains of enterococci.[63, 97]

Preferred therapy for endocarditis due to "susceptible" strains of enterococci in both adults[7, 97, 103, 132] and children[34, 155] consists of combination therapy with parenteral ampicillin (or penicillin G) plus parenteral gentamicin (or streptomycin) for a minimum duration of 4 to 6 weeks. Patients with severe penicillin allergy should be treated with vancomycin plus gentamicin or streptomycin. Selected adult patients with a short duration of symptoms and an uncomplicated course may be treated with 4-week regimens[173]; most other patients, including those with mitral valve involvement, longer durations of symptoms (especially those with symptoms for $>$3 months), or prosthetic-valve endocarditis, probably should receive 6-week courses of therapy.[97] Interestingly, several reports indicate that the prognosis of enterococcal prosthetic-valve endocarditis is better than that of native-valve disease, perhaps because of the generally shorter duration of symptoms prior to diagnosis.[97, 132] Many patients with prosthetic-valve endocarditis due to enterococci can be cured without surgery. Rice and colleagues[132] reported a 69 per cent cure rate with medical therapy in those patients who survived enterococcal endocarditis.

Unfortunately, the emergence of enterococci with clinically significant high-level resistance to aminoglycosides, β-lactams, and glycopeptides has complicated the management of endocarditis due to these organisms. Endocarditis caused by enterococci with high-level resistance to either streptomycin or gentamicin may be treated by substituting the other aminoglycoside in a combination regimen, but the isolation of strains with high-level resistance to both aminoglycosides means that no available aminoglycosides will provide synergistic killing in concert with cell wall–active agents.[97, 108] Enterococci resistant to all aminoglycosides have been isolated at an increasing rate from clinical specimens: Jones and associates[72] and the *Enterococcus* Study Group found that fully 20 per cent of 1936 enterococcal isolates (from 97 participating laboratories in 47 states) exhibited high-level resistance to both gentamicin and streptomycin. No reliably bactericidal regimen is available for treatment of endocarditis due to these strains. Based on animal studies, prolonged treatment (8 to 12 weeks, or more) with high-dose intravenous ampicillin given by continuous infusion can be tried in this situation[41, 103]; surgical excision of infected valves may be required.[132] Alternative drugs for treatment of these infections greatly are needed.

Endocarditis and other serious infections due to enterococci resistant to β-lactam antibiotics also are increasing in frequency.[56] Endocarditis due to enterococci highly resistant to β-lactams (usually *E. faecium*) may be treated with vancomycin or teicoplanin plus an aminoglycoside (if the strain is not highly resistant to these agents). Endocarditis due to β-lactamase–producing strains of *E. faecalis* (or, rarely, *E. faecium*) would be expected to respond to ampicillin-sulbactam because this combination is highly effective in animal models.[41] One report suggested that ampicillin-sulbactam was more active than ampicillin alone against some non–β-lactamase–producing, ampicillin-resistant strains of *E. faecium* and found that this combination was effective in clearing one case of persistent bacteremia due to such a strain.[98]

Enterococci resistant to vancomycin may remain susceptible to teicoplanin (VanB phenotype). Teicoplanin with or without the addition of an aminoglycoside has been used successfully in the treatment of serious enterococcal infections due to susceptible isolates,[142] including some cases of endocarditis[128, 142, 175] and meningitis.[88] However, teicoplanin therapy of endocarditis due to susceptible strains of enterococci has been associated with both treatment failure and relapse,[128, 142] and the emergence of high-level teicoplanin resistance in a VanB strain of *E. faecium* has been reported (in a patient who had not received teicoplanin).[61] Endocarditis due to VanB strains of enterococci should be treated with high-dose ampicillin plus gentamicin or streptomycin if resistance to these agents is not present. If the VanB isolate is also highly resistant to ampicillin (primarily a problem in *E. faecium*), teicoplanin plus an aminoglycoside should be used.

Similarly, endocarditis due to enterococci highly resistant to both vancomycin and teicoplanin (VanA phenotype) but susceptible to β-lactams should be treated with ampicillin plus an aminoglycoside (if high-level resistance to aminoglycosides is not present). Unfortunately, the VanA phenotype is associated primarily with strains of *E. faecium*, which increasingly are resistant to β-lactams.[47, 56, 72] Endocarditis due to enterococci highly resistant to both glycopeptides and β-lactams especially is difficult to treat. Combinations of ampicillin and vancomycin are not bactericidal against these isolates but may[149] or may not[20] provide additive or synergistic inhibition in vitro. However, if high-level resistance to aminoglycosides is not present, triple-combination therapy with β-lactams, glycopeptides, and aminoglycosides may achieve bactericidal activity; such combinations are reported to be highly effective in animal models of endocarditis due to ampicillin- and vancomycin-resistant *E. faecium*.[16] For endocarditis due to enterococci exhibiting high-level resistance to both gentamicin and streptomycin along with high-level resistance to β-lactams and glycopeptides, no proven effective therapies are available.

Some multiply antibiotic-resistant enterococci are susceptible to chloramphenicol, tetracycline, or ciprofloxacin, but these agents are not bactericidal and have not been reported to cure enterococcal endocarditis. Chloramphenicol has been effective in the treatment of other serious enterococcal infections.[122] Ciprofloxacin is of limited utility, and increasing numbers of enterococci are resistant to this agent.[72, 141] However, new classes of antimicrobials may prove effective in the treatment of infections due to multiresistant enterococci. In particular, the streptogramin class of protein-synthesis inhibitors is a promising agent for the treatment of infections due to multiply antibiotic-resistant *E. faecium*. Streptogramins are natural combinations of two chemically unrelated molecules and include the recently developed parenteral combination of quinupristin-dalfopristin (RP59500).[89] Quinupristin-dalfopristin is highly active against most clinical isolates of vancomycin-resistant and vancomycin-susceptible *E. faecium* but generally is ineffective against *E. faecalis* isolates at clinically achievable concentrations.[28, 89] Although time-kill curves indicate that quinupristin-dalfopristin is not reliably bactericidal against strains of *E. faecium*,[28] it may provide bactericidal activity against some multiresistant clinical isolates.[91, 112, 137] Quinupristin-dalfopristin has been reported to effect clinical cures of several serious infections due to multiply resistant *E. faecium*, including a ventriculoperitoneal shunt infection in an 8-month-old infant,[112] an aortic graft infection in an adult,[137] and three cases of peritonitis in adults.[91] However, the lack of a consistent bactericidal effect may limit the utility of this agent in the treatment of endocarditis, as predicted by Collins and associates,[28] and the development of a quinupristin-dalfopristin–tolerant strain of *E. faecium* during therapy with this agent already has been reported.[137]

Treatment of Meningitis and Sepsis

There is a general consensus that other life-threatening enterococcal infections, including meningitis and septicemia, should be treated with bactericidal regimens, based on the experience with enterococcal endocarditis.[102, 108, 156] The duration of therapy for uncommon enterococcal infections, such as meningitis, must be individualized, although 2- to 3- week courses of antibiotics have been reported to cure enterococcal meningitis.[156] The optimal treatment of enterococcal bacteremia, particularly that occurring in the nosocomial setting, remains controversial. In adults, single-drug regimens generally are successful in the treatment of enterococcal bacteremia, indicating that bactericidal therapy often is not required.[102, 108]

Treatment of Urinary Tract Infections and Other Less Serious Enterococcal Infections

Considerable clinical experience supports the routine use of single-drug therapy for uncomplicated urinary tract infections and soft tissue infections due to enterococci. Urinary tract infections due to susceptible strains of enterococci generally respond promptly to ampicillin, penicillin, nitrofurantoin, or vancomycin.[102, 107, 108] Single-drug therapy also is effective therapy for most cases of enterococcal bacteremia without endocarditis.[108]

PREVENTION OF ENTEROCOCCAL INFECTIONS

The explosive increase in nosocomial infections due to VRE and multiply antibiotic-resistant enterococci[18] has made the prevention of enterococcal infections, particularly those due to VRE, a public health priority in the United States.[13, 19, 145]

The Hospital Infection Control Practices Advisory Committee (HICPAC) has recommended a series of overlapping strategies designed to prevent serious enterococcal infections.[19] These strategies aim simultaneously to interrupt the dramatic increase in VRE (and multiply antibiotic-resistant enterococci) and to prevent nosocomial infections due to enterococci.

Reversing the Trend Toward Vancomycin and Multiple-Antibiotic Resistance in Enterococci

Vancomycin use[10, 49, 60, 73, 86, 104–106, 135, 145, 146] and the use of broad-spectrum antibiotics[40, 49, 55, 105, 106, 110, 118] are risk factors for the development of colonization and infection with VRE. Consequently, the HICPAC and the CDC have recommended that all hospitals, even those at which VRE have not been isolated, should (1) develop a comprehensive antimicrobial-utilization plan, (2) oversee surgical prophylaxis, and (3) develop institution-specific guidelines for the proper use of vancomycin.[19]

Efforts to eliminate unnecessary vancomycin use are critical.[19, 145] The HICPAC has recommended that the use of vancomycin be considered appropriate or acceptable for (1) treatment of serious infections due to β-lactam–resistant gram-positive microorganisms, (2) treatment of gram-positive infections in patients with serious allergies to β-lactams, (3) treatment of antibiotic-associated colitis only when it fails to respond to metronidazole or is severe and potentially life-threatening, (4) endocarditis prophylaxis after certain procedures in high-risk patients according to American Heart Association guidelines, and (5) prophylaxis for major surgical procedures involving implantation of prosthetic materials or devices (single-dose prophylaxis usually is adequate).[19]

The HICPAC has recommended that vancomycin usage be discouraged in the following situations: (1) routine surgical prophylaxis other than in a patient with life-threatening allergy to β-lactams; (2) empiric therapy for febrile neutropenic patients unless there is presumptive evidence of an infection caused by gram-positive organisms, such as a Hickman catheter exit site infection, and the local prevalence of methicillin-resistant *S. aureus* strains is substantial; (3) treatment of an isolated single blood culture positive for coagulase-negative *Staphylococcus*; (4) continued empiric use for presumed infection in patients whose cultures are negative for β-lactam–resistant gram-positive microorganisms; (5) systemic or local prophylaxis for infection of indwelling intravascular catheters; (6) selective decontamination of the gastrointestinal tract; (7) eradication of methicillin-resistant *S. aureus* colonization; (8) primary treatment of antibiotic-associated diarrhea; (9) routine prophylaxis for very low birth weight infants; (10) routine prophylaxis for dialysis patients (peritoneal dialysis or hemodialysis); (11) treatment (chosen for dosing convenience) of infections due to β-lactam–susceptible gram-positive microorganisms in patients who have renal failure; and (12) use of vancomycin solution for topical application or irrigation.[19]

In addition, efforts should be made to reduce the unnecessary use of broad-spectrum antibiotics, particularly in settings with high rates of nosocomial infections (such as intensive care units).

Preventing and Controlling the Spread of Nosocomial Infections Due to Vancomycin-Resistant Enterococci

The increasing prevalence of *Enterococcus* in nosocomial infections is related to the intrinsic and acquired antimicrobial resistance of these organisms, but the factors leading to increased antibiotic resistance in enterococci are not identical to those that predispose to enterococcal colonization and/or infection. Enterococcal infections increasingly are concentrated in debilitated and immunocompromised patients, including those with malignancies, recipients of bone marrow and solid organ transplants, burn victims, premature neonates, and critically ill patients with indwelling intravascular catheters. Consequently, special attention should be paid to potential outbreaks of VRE infection in those hospital wards caring for these high-risk patients.

Efforts to prevent the spread of VRE colonization and/or infection will be more successful if VRE isolates are confined to a few patients in a single area of the hospital. Unfortunately, widespread colonization with VRE may precede the identification of infections due to these organisms. Consequently, all hospitals should institute active surveillance for VRE and formulate a multidisciplinary plan to prevent nosocomial spread of VRE if such organisms are identified. In hospitals that have not isolated VRE, periodic antimicrobial susceptibility testing should be performed on enterococcal isolates from all sources, particularly from high-risk patient populations, such as those in intensive care or transplant units. If VRE are identified, a comprehensive plan to prevent nosocomial spread of these organisms should be implemented immediately. The HICPAC has summarized the essential elements of such a plan.[19] Hospital infection control staff and clinical staff must be notified promptly when VRE are isolated from a clinical sample, and isolation precautions should be implemented immediately to prevent patient-to-patient transmission of VRE. These precautions include gown and glove isolation, vigorous hand washing, dedicated use of noncritical patient items (e.g., thermometers, stethoscopes), and prompt surveillance of any possibly exposed patients for VRE colonization. Additional measures may be necessary in hospitals with endemic VRE or continued VRE transmission, despite the implementation of the aforementioned measures.[19, 145]

Once VRE become endemic in a hospital unit, complete eradication is very difficult. The measures recommended by the HICPAC aim to prevent the initial establishment of VRE in hospitals. Implementation of these policies will require the involvement of hospital pharmacy and therapeutics committees, quality assurance programs, and medical staff. Ongoing monitoring of these policies will be necessary.

Prevention of Enterococcal Endocarditis

The American Heart Association has provided guidelines for the prevention of bacterial endocarditis in patients with damaged or abnormal heart valves.[33] Bacterial endocarditis that occurs after manipulation (instrumentation or surgery) of the genitourinary or gastrointestinal tracts most frequently is due to enterococci.[33, 97] Consequently, the American Heart Association recommends a standard prophylactic regimen for these procedures that consists of (1) ampicillin (50 mg/kg, not to exceed 2 g, intravenously or intramuscularly) and gentamicin (2 mg/kg, not to exceed 80 mg, intravenously or intramuscularly) 30 minutes before the procedure and (2) ampicillin (50 mg/kg, not to exceed 2 g, intravenously or intramuscularly) or amoxicillin (50 mg/kg, not to exceed 2 g, orally) in a single dose 6 hours after the initial dose.[33, 34] Patients with a history of serious allergic reactions to β-lactam antibiotics may receive vancomycin plus gentamicin as recommended.[33, 34] Fortunately, endocarditis rarely complicates nosocomial bacteremia, the setting in which multiply antibiotic-resistant enterococci usually are found.

References

1. Alminrante, B., Tornos, M., Gurgui, M., et al.: Prognosis of enterococcal endocarditis. Rev. Infect. Dis. *13*:1248–1249, 1991.
2. Andrewes, F. W., and Horder, T. J.: A study of the streptococci pathogenic for man. Lancet *ii*:708–713, 1906.
3. Armstrong, D., Neu, H., Peterson, L. R., et al.: The prospects of treatment failure in the chemotherapy of infectious diseases in the 1990s. Microb. Drug Resistance *1*:1–4, 1995.
4. Arthur, M., and Courvalin, P.: Genetics and mechanisms of glycopeptide resistance in enterococci. Antimicrob. Agents Chemother. *37*:1563–1571, 1993.
5. Ashkenazi, S., Even-Tov, S., Samra, Z., et al.: Uropathogens of various childhood populations and their antibiotic susceptibility. Pediatr. Infect. Dis J. *10*:742–746, 1991.
6. Bingen, E. H., Denamur, E., and Lambert-Zechovsky, N. Y.: Evidence for the genetic unrelatedness of nosocomial vancomycin-resistant *Enterococcus faecium* strains in a pediatric hospital. J. Clin. Microbiol. *29*:1888, 1991.
7. Bisno, A. L., Dismukes, W. E., Durack, D. T., et al.: Antimicrobial treatment of infective endocarditis due to viridans streptococci, enterococci, and staphylococci. J. A. M. A. *261*:1471–1477, 1989.
8. Bonadio, W. A.: Group D streptococcal bacteremia in children: A review of 72 cases in 12 years. Clin. Pediatr. *32*:20–24, 1993.
9. Boulanger, J. M., Ford-Jones, E. L., and Matlow, A. G.: Enterococcal bacteremia in a pediatric insitutution: A four-year review. Rev. Infect. Dis. *13*:847–851, 1991.
10. Boyce, J. M., Opal, S. M., Chow, J. W., et al.: Outbreak of multi-drug resistant *Enterococcus faecium* with transferable vanB class vancomycin resistance. J. Clin. Microbiol. *32*:1148–1153, 1994.
11. Boyce, J. M., Opal, S. M., Potter-Bynoe, G., et al.: Emergence and nosocomial transmission of ampicillin-resistant enterococci. Antimicrob. Agents Chemother. *36*:1032–1039, 1992.
12. Brown, A. E., de Lancastre, H., Henning, K., et al.: Epidemic nosocomial vancomycin-resistant *Enterococcus faecium* (VREF) on a pediatric oncology unit. *In* Proceedings of the 33rd Annual Meeting of the Infectious Diseases Society of America, 1995.
13. Burgert, S. J., and Burke, J. P.: Antibiotic resistance: Will infection control meet the challenge? Am. J. Infect. Control *22*:195–201, 1994.
14. Calderwood, S. A., Wennersten, C., and Moellering, R. C., Jr.: Resistance to six aminoglycosidic aminocyclitol antibiotics among enterococci: Prevalence, evolution, and relationship to synergism with penicillin. Antimicrob. Agents Chemother. *12*:401–405, 1977.
15. Caron, F., Lemeland, J.-F., Humbert, G., et al.: Triple combination penicillin-vancomycin-gentamicin for experimental endocarditis caused by a highly penicillin- and glycopeptide-resistant isolate of *Enterococcus faecium*. J. Infect. Dis. *168*:681–686, 1993.
16. Caron, F., Pestel, M., Kitzis, M. D., et al.: Comparison of different β-lactam–glycopeptide-gentamicin combinations for and experimental endocarditis caused by highly β-lactam–resistant and highly glycopeptide-resistant isolate of *Enterococcus faecium*. J. Infect. Dis. *171*:106—112, 1995.
17. Cavalieri, S. J., Hostetter, J. K., Rupp, M. E., et al.: Synergy studies on and therapy for multiply antibiotic-resistant *Enterococcus faecium* from a recent outbreak. *In* Proceedings of the 32nd Annual Meeting of the Infectious Diseases Society of America, 1994.
18. Centers for Disease Control and Prevention: Nosocomial enterococci resistant to vancomycin. M. M. W. R. *42*:597–599, 1993.
19. Centers for Disease Control and Prevention: Recommendations for preventing the spread of vancomycin resistance: Recommendations of the Hospital Infection Control Practices Advisory Committee (HICPAC). M. M. W. R. *44*(No. RR-12):1–13, 1995.
20. Cercenado, E., Eliopoulos, G. M., Wennersten, C. B., et al.: Absence of synergistic activity between ampicillin and vancomycin against highly vancomycin-resistant enterococci. Antimicrob. Agents Chemother. *36*:2201–2203, 1992.
21. Chenoweth, C. E., Robinson, K. A., and Schaberg, D. R.: Efficacy of ampicillin versus trimethoprim-sulfamethoxazole in a mouse model of lethal enterococcal peritonitis. Antimicrob. Agents Chemother. *34*:1800–1802, 1990.
22. Chenoweth, C. E., Bradley, S. F., Terpenning, M. S., et al.: Colonization and transmission of high-level gentamicin-resistant enterococci in a long-term care facility. Infect. Control Hosp. Epidemiol. *15*:703–709, 1994.
23. Chirurgi, V. A., Oster, S. E., Goldberg, A. A., et al.: Ampicillin-resistant *Enterococcus raffinosus* in an acute-care hospital: Case-control study and antimicrobial susceptibilities. J. Clin. Microbiol. *29*:2663–2665, 1991.
24. Chow, J. W., Thal, L. A., Perri, M. B., et al.: Plasmid-associated hemolysin and aggregation substance production contributes to virulence in experimental enterococcal endocarditis. Antimicrob. Agents Chemother. *37*:2474–2477, 1993.
25. Christie, C., Hammond, J., Reising, S., et al..: Clinical and molecular epidemiology of enterococcal bacteremia in a pediatric teaching hospital. J. Pediatr. *125*:392–399, 1994.
26. Clark, N. C., Cooksey, R. C., Hill, B. C., et al.: Characterization of glycopeptide-resistant enterococci from U.S. hospitals. Antimicrob. Agents Chemother. *37*:2311–2317, 1993.
27. Cohen, M. L.: Epidemiology of drug resistance: Implications for a post-antibiotic era. Science *257*:1050–1055, 1992.
28. Collins, L. A., Malanoski, G. J., Eliopoulos, G. M., et al.: In vitro activity of RP59500, an injectable streptogramin antibiotic, against vancomycin-resistant gram-positive organisms. Antimicrob. Agents Chemother. *37*:598–601, 1993.
29. Coque, T. M., Arduino, R. C., and Murray, B. E.: High-level resistance to aminoglycosides: Comparison of community and nosocomial fecal isolates of enterococci. Clin. Infect. Dis. *20*:1048–1051, 1995.
30. Costa, Y., Galimand, M., LeClercq, R., et al.: Characterization of the chromosomal aac (6')0-Ii gene specific for *Enterococcus faecium*. Antimicrob. Agents Chemother. *37*:1896–1903, 1993.
31. Coudron, P. E., Mayhall, C. G., and Facklam, R. R.: *Streptococcus faecium* outbreak in a neonatal intensive care unit. J. Clin. Microbiol. *20*:1044, 1984.
32. Coudron, P. E., Markowitz, S. M., and Wong, E. S.: Isolation of a beta-lactamase–producing, aminoglycoside-resistant strain of *Enterococcus faecium*. Antimicrob. Agents Chemother. *36*:1125–1126, 1992.
33. Dajani, A. S., Bisno, A. L., Chung, K. J., et al.: Prevention of bacterial endocarditis: Recommendations by the American Heart Association. J. A. M. A. *264*:2919–2922, 1990.
34. Dajani, A. S.: Infective endocarditis. *In* Kaplan, S. L. (ed.): Current Therapy in Pediatric Infectious Diseases. 3rd ed. St. Louis, Mosby–Year Book, 1993, pp. 129–133.
35. Daly, J. A., Clifton, N. L., and Seskin, K. C.: Use of rapid, nonradioactive DNA probes in culture confirmation tests to detect *Streptococcus agalactiae*, *Haemophilus influenzae*, and *Enterococcus* spp. from pediatric patients with significant infections. J. Clin. Microbiol. *29*:80, 1991.
36. Davies, H., Jones, E., Sheng, R. Y., et al.: Nosocomial urinary tract infections at a pediatric hospital. Pediatr. Infect. Dis. J. *11*:349–354, 1992.
37. Dobson, S. R. M., and Baker, C. J.: Enterococcal sepsis in neonates: Features by age of onset and occurrence of focal infection. Pediatrics *85*:165, 1990.
38. Donabedian, S., Chow, J. W., Shales, D. M., et al.: DNA hybridization and contour-clamped homogeneous electric field electrophoresis for identification of enterococci to the species level. J. Clin. Microbiol. *33*:141–145, 1995.
39. Dutka-Malen, S., Evers, S., and Courvalin, P.: Detection of glycopeptide resistance genotypes and identification to the species level of clinically relevant enterococci by PCR. J. Clin. Microbiol. *33*:24–27, 1995.
40. Edmond, M. B., Ober, J. F., Weinbaum, D. L., et al.: Vancomycin-resistant *Enterococcus faecium* bacteremia: Risk factors for infection. Clin. Infect. Dis. *20*:1126–1133, 1995.
41. Eliopoulos, G. M., Thauvin-Eliopoulos, C., and Moellering, R. C., Jr.: Contribution of animal models in the search for effective therapy for endocarditis due to enterococci with high level resistance to gentamicin. Clin. Infect. Dis. *15*:58–62, 1992.
42. Facklam, R., Pigott, N., Franklin, R., et al.: Evaluation of three disk tests for identification of enterococci, leuconostocs, and pediococci. J. Clin. Microbiol. *33*:885–887, 1995.
43. Facklam, R. R., and Collins, M. D.: Identification of *Enterococcus* species isolated from human infections by a conventional test scheme. J. Clin. Microbiol. *27*:731–734, 1989
44. Facklam, R. R., and Sahm, D. R.: *Enterococcus*. *In* Murray, P. R., Baron, E. J., Pfaller, M. A., et al. (eds.): Manual of Clinical Microbiology. 6th ed. Washington, D.C., American Society for Microbiology, 1995, pp. 308–314.
45. Fasola, E. L., Moody, J. A., Shanholtzer, C. J., et al.: Bactericidal action of gentamicin against enterococci that are sensitive, or exhibit low- or high-level resistance to gentamicin. Diagn. Microbiol. Infect. Dis. *19*:57–60, 1994.
46. Felmingham, D., Wilson, A. P. R., Quintana, A. L., et al.: *Enterococcus* species in urinary tract infection. Clin. Infect. Dis. *15*:295–301, 1992.
47. Fontana, R., Amalfitano, G., Rossi, L., et al.: Mechanisms of resistance to growth inhibition and killing by β-lactam antibiotics in enterococci. Clin. Infect. Dis. *15*:486–489, 1992.
48. Fraimow, H. S., Jungkind, D. L., Lander, D. W., et al.: Urinary tract infection with an *Enterococcus faecalis* isolate that requires vancomycin for growth. Ann. Intern. Med. *121*:22–26, 1994.
49. Frieden, T. R., Munsiff, S. S., Low, D. E., et al.: Emergence of vancomycin-resistant enterococci in New York City. Lancet *342*:76–79, 1993.
50. Gladstone, I. J., Ehrenkranz, R. A., Edberg, S. C., et al.: A ten-year review of neonatal sepsis and comparison with the previous fifty-year experience. Pediatr. Infect. Dis. J. *9*:819–825, 1990.
51. Goodhard, G. L.: In vivo vs. in vitro susceptibility of *Enterococcus* to trimethoprim-sulfamethoxazole. J. A. M. A. *252*:2748–2749, 1984.
52. Gorbach, S. L.: Intraabdominal infections. Clin. Infect. Dis. *17*:961–967, 1993.
53. Gordon, S., Swenson, J. M., Hill, B. C., et al.: Antimicrobial susceptibility patterns of common and unusual species of enterococci causing infections in the United States: Enterococcal study group. J. Clin. Microbiol. *30*:2373–2378, 1992.
54. Graninger, W., and Ragette, R.: Nosocomial bacteremia due to *Enterococcus faecalis* without endocarditis. Clin. Infect. Dis. *15*:49–57, 1992.
55. Gray, J. W., Pedler, S., Kernahan, J., et al.: Enterococcal superinfection in paediatric oncology patients treated with imipenem. Lancet *13*:1487–1488, 1992.

56. Grayson, M. L., Eliopoulos, G. M., Wennersten, C. B., et al.: Increasing resistance to beta-lactam antibiotics among clinical isolates of *Enterococcus faecium*: A 22-year review at one institution. Antimicrob. Agents Chemother. *35*:2180–2184, 1991.
57. Grayson, M. L., Thauvin-Eliopoulos, C., Eliopoulos, G. M., et al.: Failure of trimethoprim-sulfamethoxazole therapy in experimental enterococcal endocarditis. Antimicrob. Agents Chemother. *34*:1792–1794, 1990.
58. Green, M., Shlaes, J. H., Barbadora, K., et al.: Bacteremia due to vancomycin-dependent *Enterococcus faecium*. Clin. Infect. Dis. *20*:712–714, 1995.
59. Gullberg, R. M., Homann, S. R., and Phair, J. P.: Enterococcal bacteremia: Analysis of 75 episodes. Rev. Infect. Dis. *11*:74–85, 1989.
60. Handwerger, S., Raucher, B., Altarac, D., et al.: Nosocomial outbreak due to *Enterococcus faecium* highly resistant to vancomycin, penicillin and gentamicin. Clin. Infect. Dis. *16*:750–755, 1993.
61. Hayden, M. K., Trenholme, G. M., Schultz, J. E., et al.: In vivo development of teicoplanin resistance in a VanB *Enterococcus faecium* isolate. J. Infect. Dis. *167*:1224–1227, 1993.
62. Hoge, C. W., Adams, J., Buchanan, B., et al.: Enterococcal bacteremia: To treat or not to treat, a reappraisal. Rev. Infect. Dis. *13*:600–605, 1991.
63. Hook, E. W. I., Roberts, R. B., and Sande, M. A.: Antimicrobial therapy of experimental endocarditis. Antimicrob. Agents Chemother. *8*:564–570, 1975.
64. Horodniceanu, T., Bougueleret, T., El-Solh, N., et al.: High-level, plasmid-borne resistance to gentamicin in *Streptococcus faecalis* subsp. *zymogenes*. Antimicrob. Agents Chemother. *16*:686–689, 1979.
65. Hunter, T. H.: Use of streptomycin in treatment of bacterial endocarditis. Am. J. Med. *2*:436–442, 1947.
66. Jarvis, W. R., and Martone, W. J.: Predominant pathogens in hospital infections. J. Antimicrob. Chemother. *29*(Suppl. A):19–24, 1992.
67. Jett, B. D., Huycke, M. M., and Gilmore, M. S.: Virulence of enterococci. Clin. Microbiol. Rev. *7*:462–478, 1994.
68. Johnson, A. P.: The pathogenicity of enterococci. J. Antimicrob. Chemother. *33*:1083–1089, 1994.
69. Johnson, D. H., Rosenthal, A., and Nadas, A. S.: Bacterial endocarditis in children under 2 years of age. Am. J. Dis. Child. *129*:183–186, 1975.
70. Johnson, D. H., Rosenthal, A., and Nadas, A. S.: A forty-year review of bacterial endocarditis in infants and children. Circulation *51*:581–588, 1975.
71. Jones, R. N., Erwin, M. E., and Anderson, S. C.: Emerging multiply resistant enterococci among clinical isolates. II. Validation of the Etest to recognize glycopeptide-resistant strains. Diagn. Microbiol. Infect. Dis. *21*:95–100, 1995.
72. Jones, R. N., Sader, H. S., Erwin, M. E., et al.: Emerging multiply resistant enterococci among clinical isolates. I. Prevalence data from 97 medical center surveillance study in the United States. *Enterococcus* Study Group. Diagn. Microbiol. Infect. Dis. *21*:85–93, 1995.
73. Kaplan, A. H., Gilligan, P. H., and Facklam, R. R.: Recovery of resistant enterococci during vancomycin prophylaxis. J. Clin. Microbiol. *26*:1216–1218, 1988.
74. Karanfil, L. V., Murphy, M., and Josephson, A.: A cluster of vancomycin-resistant *Enterococcus faecium* in an intensive care unit. Infect. Control Hosp. Epidemiol. *13*:195–200, 1993.
75. Kaufhold, A., and Ferrieri, P.: The microbiologic aspects, including diagnosis, of beta-hemolytic streptococcal and enterococcal infections. Infect. Dis. Clin. North Am. *7*:235–256, 1993.
76. Klein, J. O., and Marcy, S. M.: Bacterial sepsis and meningitis. *In* Remington, J. S., and Klein, J. O. (eds.): Infectious Diseases of the Fetus and Newborn Infant. 4th ed. Philadelphia, W. B. Saunders, 1995, pp. 835–890.
77. Koorevaar, C. T., Scherpenzeel, P. G., Neijens, H. J., et al.: Childhood meningitis caused by enterococci and viridans streptococci. Infection *20*:118–121, 1992.
78. Kreft, B., Marre, R., Schramm, U., et al.: Aggregation substance of *Enterococcus faecalis* mediates adhesion to cultured renal tubular cells. Infect. Immun. *60*:25–30, 1992.
79. Krieger, J. N., Kaiser, D. L., and Wenzel, R. P.: Urinary tract etiology of bloodstream infections in hospitalized patients. J. Infect. Dis. *146*:719–723, 1983.
80. Krogstad, D. J., Korfhagen, T. R., Moellering, R. C., Jr., et al.: Aminoglycoside-inactivating enzymes in clinical isolates of *Streptococcus faecalis*: An explanation for antibiotic synergism. J. Clin. Invest. *62*:480–486, 1978.
81. Kunin, C. M.: Resistance to antimicrobial drugs: A worldwide calamity. Ann. Intern. Med. *118*:557–561, 1993.
82. Law, E. J., Blecher, K., and Still, J. M.: Enterococcal infections as a cause of mortality and morbidity in patients with burns. J. Burn Care Rehab. *15*:236–239, 1994.
83. LeClercq, R., Derlot, E., Duval, J., et al.: Plasmid-mediated resistance to vancomycin and teicoplanin in *Enterococcus faecium*. N. Engl. J. Med. *319*:157–161, 1988.
84. LeClercq, R., Dutka-Malen, S., Brisson-Noel, A., et al.: Resistance of enterococci to aminoglycosides and glycopeptides. Clin. Infect. Dis. *15*:495–501, 1992.
85. LeClercq, R., Dutka-Malen, S., Brisson-Noel, A., et al.: Resistance of enterococci to aminoglycosides and glycopeptides. Clin. Infect. Dis. *16*:331, 1993.
86. Livornese, L. L., Jr., Dias, S., Samel, C., et al.: Hospital-acquired infection with vancomycin-resistant *Enterococcus faecium* transmitted by electronic thermometers. Ann. Intern. Med. *117*:112–116, 1992.
87. Lohr, J. A., Donowitz, L. G., and Sadler, J. E., III: Hospital-acquired urinary tract infection. Pediatrics *83*:193–199, 1989.
88. Losonsky, G., Wolf, A., Schwalbe, R., et al.: Successful treatment of meningitis due to multiply resistant *Enterococcus faecium* with a combination of intrathecal teicoplanin and intravenous antimicrobial agents. Clin. Infect. Dis. *19*:163–165, 1994.
89. Low, D. E.: Quinupristin/dalfopristin: Spectrum of activity, pharmacokinetics, and initial clinical experience. Microb. Drug Resistance *1*:223–234, 1995.
90. Luginbuhl, L. M., Rotbart, H. A., Facklam, R. R., et al.: Neonatal enterococcal sepsis: Case-control study and description of an outbreak. Pediatr. Infect. Dis. J. *6*:1022–1030, 1987.
91. Lynn, W. A., Clutterbuck, E., Want, S., et al.: Treatment of CAPD-peritonitis due to glycopeptide-resistant *Enterococcus faecium* with quinupristin/dalfopristin. Lancet *344*:1025–1026, 1994.
92. Maki, D. G., and Agger, W. A.: Enterococcal bacteremia: Clinical features, the risk of endocarditis, and management. Medicine *67*:248–269, 1988.
93. Malone, D. A., Wagner, R. A., Myers, J. P., et al.: Enterococccal bacteremia in two large community teaching hospitals. Am. J. Med. *81*:601–606, 1986.
94. Mazzulli, T., King, S. M., and Richardson, S. E.: Bacteremia due to beta-lactamase–producing *Enterococcus faecalis* with high-level resistance to gentamicin in a child with Wiskott-Aldrich syndrome. Clin. Infect. Dis. *14*:780–781, 1992.
95. McCarthy, A., Victor, G., Ramotar, K., et al.: Risk factors for acquiring ampicillin-resistant enterococci and clinical outcomes at a Canadian tertiary-care hospital. J. Clin. Microbiol. *32*:2671–2676, 1994.
96. Mederski-Samoraj, B. D., and Murray, B. E.: High-level resistance to gentamicin in clinical isolates of enterococci. J. Infect. Dis. *147*:751–757, 1983.
97. Megran, D. W.: Enterococcal endocarditis. Clin. Infect. Dis. *15*:63–71, 1992.
98. Mekonen, E. T., Noskin, G. A., Hacek, D. M., et al.: Successful treatment of persistent bacteremia due to vancomycin-resistant, ampicillin-resistant *Enterococcus faecium*. Microb. Drug Resistance *1*:249–253, 1995.
99. Moellering, R. C., Jr., Wennersten, C., and Medrek, T.: Prevalence of high-level resistance to aminoglycosides in clinical isolates of enterococci. Antimicrob. Agents Chemother. *1*:335–340, 1970.
100. Moellering, R. C., Jr., and Weinberg, A. N.: Studies on antibiotic synergism against enterococci. II. Effect of various antibiotics on the uptake of C14-labeled streptomycin by enterococci. J. Clin. Invest. *50*:2580–2584, 1971.
101. Moellering, R. C., Jr., and Krogstad, D. J.: Antibiotic resistance in enterococci. *In* Schlessinger, D. (ed.): Microbiology—1979. Washington, D.C., American Society for Microbiology, 1979, pp. 293–298.
102. Moellering, R. C., Jr.: Emergence of *Enterococcus* as a significant pathogen. Clin. Infect. Dis. *14*:1173–1176, 1992.
103. Moellering, R. C., Jr.: *Enterococcus* species, *Streptococcus bovis*, and *Leuconostoc* species. *In* Mandell, G. L., Bennett, J. E., and Dolin, R. (eds.): Principles and Practice of Infectious Diseases. 4th ed. New York, Churchill Livingstone, 1995, pp. 1826–1835.
104. Montecalvo, M. A., Horowitz, H., and Gedris, C.: Outbreak of vancomycin-, ampicillin-, and aminoglycoside-resistant *Enterococcus faecium* bacteremia in an adult oncology unit. Antimicrob. Agents Chemother. *38*:1363–1367, 1994.
105. Moreno, F., Grota, P., Crisp, C., et al.: Clinical and molecular epidemiology of vancomycin-resistant *Enterococcus faecium* during its emergence in a city in southern Texas. Clin. Infect. Dis. *21*:1234–1237, 1995.
106. Morris, J. G., Jr., Shay, D. K., Hebden, J. N., et al.: Enterococci resistant to multiple antimicrobial agents, including vancomycin. Ann. Intern. Med. *123*:250–259, 1995.
107. Morrison, A. J., Jr., and Wenzel, R. P.: Nosocomial urinary tract infections due to *Enterococcus*: Ten years' experience at a university hospital. Arch. Intern. Med. *146*:1549–1551, 1986.
108. Murray, B. E.: The life and times of the *Enterococcus*. Clin. Microbiol. Rev. *3*:46–65, 1990.
109. Murray, B. E.: Beta-lactamase–producing enterococci. Antimicrob. Agents Chemother. *36*:2355–2359, 1992.
110. Murray, B. E.: Editorial response: What can we do about vancomycin-resistant enterococci. Clin. Infect. Dis. *20*:1134–1136, 1995.
111. Murray, B. E., and Mederski-Samoraj, B.: Transferable beta-lactamase: A new mechanism for in vitro penicillin resistance in *Streptococcus faecalis*. J. Clin. Invest. *72*:1168, 1983.
112. Nachman, S. A., Verma, R., and Egnor, M.: Vancomycin-resistant *Enterococcus faecium* shunt infection in an infant: An antibiotic cure. Microb. Drug Resistance *1*:95–96, 1995.
113. Nagai, K., Yuge, K., Ono, E., et al.: *Enterococcus faecium* meningitis in a child. Pediatr. Infect. Dis. J. *13*:1016–1017, 1994.
114. Najjar, A., and Murray, B. E.: Failure to demonstrate a consistent in vitro bactericidal effect of trimethoprim-sulfamethoxazole against enterococci. Antimicrob. Agents Chemother. *31*:808–810, 1987.
115. National Committee for Clinical Laboratory Standards: Methods for Dilution Antimicrobial Susceptibility Tests for Bacteria That Grow Aerobically. 3rd ed. Villanova, PA, NCCLS publication M7-A3, 1993.
116. National Committee for Clinical Laboratory Standards: Minimum Inhibitory Concentration (MIC) Interpretative Standards (μg/ml) for Organisms

Other Than *Haemophilus* spp., *Neisseria gonorrhoeae*, and *Streptococcus pneumoniae*. Fifth Informational Supplement. NCCLS Document M100-S5. Vol. 14, No. 16, Table 89–2–(M7-A3), 1994.

117. Nauschuetz, W. F., Trevino, S. B., Harrison, L. S., et al.: *Enterococcus casseliflavus* as an agent of nosocomial bloodstream infections. Med. Microbiol. Lett. *2*:102–108, 1993.
118. Nichols, R. L., and Muzik, A. C.: Enterococcal infections in surgical patients: The mystery continues. Clin. Infect. Dis. *15*:72–76, 1992.
119. Nicoletti, G., and Stefain, S.: Enterococci: Susceptibility patterns and therapeutic options. Eur. J. Clin. Microbiol. Infect. Dis. *14*:S33–S37, 1995.
120. Noble, C. J.: Carriage of group D streptococci in the human bowel. J. Clin. Pathol. *31*:1182–1186, 1978.
121. Noble, W. C., Virani, Z., and Cree, R.: Cotransfer of vancomycin and other resistance genes from *Enterococcus faecalis* NCTC12201 to *Staphylococcus aureus*. FEMS Microbiol. Lett. *93*:195–198, 1992.
122. Norris, A. H., Reilly, J. P., Edelstein, P. H., et al.: Chloramphenicol for the treatment of vancomycin-resistant enterococcal infections. Clin. Infect. Dis. *20*:1137–1144, 1995.
123. Onderdonk, A. B., Bartlett, J. G., Louie, T. J., et al.: Microbial synergy in experimental intra-abdominal abscess. Infect. Immun. *12*:22–26, 1976.
124. Patel, R., Keating, M. R., Cockerill, F. R., III, et al.: Bacteremia due to *Enterococcus avium*. Clin. Infect. Dis. *17*:1006–1011, 1993.
125. Patterson, J. E., Sweeney, A. H., Simms, M., et al.: An analysis of 110 serious enterococcal infections, epidemiology, antibiotic susceptibility, and outcome. Medicine *74*:191–200, 1995.
126. Patterson, J. E., and Zervos, M. J.: High-level gentamicin resistance in *Enterococcus*: Microbiology, genetic basis, and epidemiology. Rev. Infect. Dis. *12*:644, 1990.
127. Patton, W. N., Bienz, N., Franklin, I. M., et al.: Enterococcal meningitis in an HIV-positive hemophilic patient. J. Clin. Pathol. *44*:608–609, 1991.
128. Presterl, E., Graninger, W., and Georgopoulos, A.: The efficacy of teicoplanin in the treatment of endocarditis caused by gram-positive bacteria. J. Antimicrob. Chemother. *31*:755–766, 1993.
129. Raymond, N. J., Henry, J., and Workowski, K. A.: Enterococcal arthritis: Case report and review. Clin. Infect. Dis. *21*:516–522, 1995.
130. Rhinehart, E., Smith, N. E., Wennersten, C., et al.: Rapid dissemination of beta-lactamase–producing, aminoglycoside-resistant *Enterococcus faecalis* among patients and staff on an infant-toddler surgical ward. N. Engl. J. Med. *323*:1814–1818, 1990.
131. Rice, E. W., Messer, J. W., Johnson, C. H., et al.: Occurrence of high-level aminoglycoside resistance in environmental isolates of enterococci. Appl. Environ. Microbiol. *61*:374–376, 1995.
132. Rice, L. B., Calderwood, S. B., Eliopoulos, G. M., et al.: Enterococcal endocarditis: A comparison of prosthetic and native valve disease. Rev. Infect. Dis. *13*:1–7, 1991.
133. Rice, L. B., and Shlaes, D. M.: Vancomycin resistance in the *Enterococcus*. Pediatr. Clin. North Am. *42*:601–618, 1995.
134. Ries, M., Deeg, K. H., Heininger, U., et al.: Brain abscesses in neonates: Report of three cases. Eur. J. Pediatr. *152*:1993.
135. Rubin, L. G., Tucci, V., Cercenado, E., et al.: Vancomycin-resistant *Enterococcus faecium* in hospitalized children. Infect. Control Hosp. Epidemiol. *13*:700–705, 1992.
136. Sader, H. S., Pfaller, M. A., Tenover, F. C., et al.: Evaluation and characterization of multiresistant *Enterococcus faecium* from 12 U.S. medical centers. J. Clin. Microbiol. *31*:2840–2842, 1994.
137. Sahgal, V. S., Urban, C., Mariano, N., et al.: Quinupristin/dalfopristin (RP 59500) therapy for vancomycin-resistant *Enterococcus faecium* aortic graft infection: Case report. Microb. Drug Resistance *1*:245–247, 1995.
138. Sanchez, M. L., Barrett, M. S., and Jones, R. N.: The Etest applied to susceptibility tests of gonococci, multiply resistant enterococci, and Enterobacteriaceae producing potent beta-lactamases. Diagn. Microbiol. Infect. Dis. *15*:459–462, 1992.
139. Sastry, V., Brennan, P. J., Levy, M. M., et al.: Vancomycin-resistant enterococci: An emerging pathogen in immunosuppressed transplant recipients. Transplant. Proc. *27*:954–955, 1995.
140. Schaberg, D. R., Culver, D. H., and Gaynes, R. P.: Major trends in the microbial etiology of nosocomial infection. Am. J. Med. *91*(Suppl. 3B):72S–75S, 1991.
141. Schaberg, D. R., Dillon, W. I., Terpenning, M. S., et al.: Increasing resistance of enterococci to ciprofloxacin. Antimicrob. Agents Chemother. *36*:2533–2535, 1992.
142. Schmit, J.: Efficacy of teiocoplanin for enterococcal infections: 63 cases and review. Clin. Infect. Dis. *15*:302–306, 1992.
143. Schoenbaum, S. C., Gardner, P., and Shillito, J.: Infections of cerebrospinal fluid shunts: Epidemiology, clinical manifestations, and therapy. J. Infect. Dis. *131*:543–552, 1975.
144. Schwartz, M., Slavoski, L., Dash, G., et al.: Nosocomial outbreak of multiresistant *Enterococcus durans* (VRED): Description of the epidemiology and antimicrobial sensitivity testing. *In* Proceedings of the 33rd Annual Meeting of the Infectious Diseases Society of America, 1995, Abstract 68.
145. Shay, D. K., Goldman, D. A., and Jarvis, W. R.: Reducing the spread of antimicrobial-resistant microorganisms: Control of vancomycin-resistant enterococci. Pediatr. Clin. North Am. *42*:703–716, 1995.
146. Shay, D. K., Maloney, S. A., Montecalvo, M., et al.: Epidemiology and mortality risk of vancomycin-resistant enterococcal bloodstream infections. J. Infect. Dis. *172*:993–1000, 1995.
147. Sherman, J. M.: The streptococci. Bacteriol. Rev. *1*:3–97, 1937.
148. Shlaes, D. M., Levy, J., and Wolinsky, E.: Enterococcal bacteremia without endocarditis. Arch. Intern. Med. *141*:578–581, 1981.
149. Shlaes, D. M., Etter, L., and Gutmann, L.: Synergistic killing of vancomycin-resistant enterococci of classes A, B, and C by combinations of vancomycin, penicillin and gentamicin. Antimicrob. Agents Chemother. *35*:776–779, 1991.
150. Shuler, T. E., Riddle, C. D., Jr., and Potts, D. W.: Polymicrobic septic arthritis caused by *Kingella kingae* and *Enterococcus*. Orthopedics *13*:254–256, 1990.
151. Siegel, J. S., and McCracken, G. H., Jr.: Group D streptococcal Infections. J. Pediatr. *93*:542–543, 1978.
152. Simpson, W. A., Courtney, H. S., and Ofek, I.: Interactions of fibronectin with streptococci: The role of fibronectin as a receptor for *Streptococcus pyogenes*. Rev. Infect. Dis. *9*(Suppl.):351–359, 1987.
153. Spera, R. V., and Faber, B. F.: Multiply-resistant *Enterococcus faecium*: The nosocomial pathogen of the 1990s. J. A. M. A. *268*:2563–2564, 1992.
154. Stanton, B. F., Baltimore, R. S., and Clemens, J. D.: Changing spectrum of infective endocarditis in children. Am. J. Dis. Child. *138*:720–725, 1984.
155. Starke, J. R.: Infective endocarditis. *In* Feigin, R. D., and Cherry, J. D. (eds.): Textbook of Pediatric Infectious Diseases. 3rd ed. Philadelphia, W. B. Saunders, 1993, pp. 326–343.
156. Stevenson, K. B., Murray, E. W., and Sarubbi, F. A.: Enterococcal meningitis: Report of four cases and review. Clin. Infect. Dis. *18*:233–239, 1994.
157. Swenson, J. M., Hindler, J. A., and Peterson, L. R.: Special tests for detecting antibacterial resistance. *In* Murray, P. R., Baron, E. J., Pfaller, M. A., et al. (eds.): Manual of Clinical Microbiology. 6th ed. Washington, D.C., American Society for Microbiology, 1955, pp. 1356–1367.
158. Swenson, J. M., Ferraro, M. J., Sahm, D. F., et al.: New vancomycin disk diffusion breakpoints for enterococci: The National Committee for Clinical Laboratory Standards Working Group on Enterococci. J. Clin. Microbiol. *30*:2525–2528, 1992.
159. Takada, H., Kawabata, Y., Arakaki, R., et al.: Molecular and structural requirements of a lipoteichoic acid from *Enterococcus hirae* ATCC 9790 for cytokine-inducing, anititumor, and antigenic activities. Infect. Immun. *63*:57–65, 1995.
160. Teixeira, O. H., and Francis, C. K.: Enterococcal endocarditis in early infancy. Can. Med. Assoc. J. *127:612–613*, 1982.
161. Tenover, F. C., Tokars, J., Swenson, J., Paul, et al.: Ability of clinical laboratories to detect antimicrobial agent–resistant enterococci. J. Clin. Microbiol. *31*:1695–1699, 1993.
162. Tenover, F. C., Swenson, J. M., O-Hara, C. M., et al.: Ability of commercial and reference antimicrobial susceptibility testing methods to detect vancomcyin resistance in enterococci. J. Clin. Microbiol. *33*:1524–1527, 1995.
163. Threlkeld, M. G., and Cobbs, C. G.: Infectious disorders of prosthetic valves and intravascular devices. *In* Mandell, G. L., Bennett, J. E., and Dolin, R. (eds.): Principles and Practice of Infectious Diseases. 4th ed. New York, Churchill Livingstone, 1995, pp. 783–793.
164. Tofte, R. W., Solliday, J., and Crossley, K. B.: Susceptibilities of enterococci to twelve antibiotics. Antimicrob. Agents Chemother. *25*:532–533, 1984.
165. Urdaneta, M., Hollis, F., and Sperber, S. J.: Vancomycin-resistant enterococci in the blood: Do we need to treat? *In* Proceedings of the 33rd Annual Meeting of the Infectious Diseases Society of America, 1995, Abstract 65.
166. Uttley, A. H., Collins, C. H., Naidoo, J., et al.: Vancomycin-resistant enterococci. Lancet *1*:57–58, 1988.
167. Veach, L. A., Pfaller, M. A., Barrett, M., et al.: Vancomycin resistance in *Staphylococcus haemolyticus* causing colonization and bloodstream infection. J. Clin. Microbiol. *28*:2064–2068, 1990.
168. Verma, M., Chatwal, J., and Varughese, P.: Neonatal conjunctivitis: A profile. Indian Pediatr. *31*:1357–1361, 1994.
169. Weigelt, J. A., Easley, S. M., Thal, E. R., et al.: Abdominal surgical wound infection is lowered with improved perioperative *Enterococcus* and *Bacteroides* therapy. J. Trauma 34:579–584, 1993.
170. Willey, B. M., Kreiswirth, B. N., Simor, A. E., et al.: Detection of vancomycin resistance in *Enterococcus* species. J. Clin. Microbiol. *30*:1621–1624, 1992.
171. Willey, B. M., McGeer, A. J., Ostrowski, M. A., et al.: The use of the molecular typing techniques in the epidemiologic investigation of resistant enterococci. Infect. Control Hosp. Epidemiol. *15*:548–556, 1994.
172. Williamson, R., LeBouguenec, C., Gutmann, L., et al.: One or two low affinity penicillin-binding proteins may be responsible for the range of susceptibility of *Enterococcus faecium* to benzylpenicillin. J. Gen. Microbiol. *131*:1933–1940, 1985.
173. Wilson, W. R., Wilkowske, C. J., Wright, A. J., et al.: Treatment of streptomycin susceptible and streptomycin-resistant enterococcal endocarditis. Ann. Intern. Med. *100*:816–823, 1984.
174. Winberg, J., Anderson, H. J., and Bergstrom, T.: Epidemiology of symptomatic urinary tract infection in childhood. Acta Paediatr. Scand. *252*(Suppl.):1, 1974.
175. Yao, J. D., Thauvin-Eliopoulos, C., Eliopoulos, G. M., et al.: Efficacy of teicoplanin in two dosage regimens for experimental endocarditis caused by a beta-lactamase–producing strain of *Enterococcus faecalis* with high-

level resistance to gentamicin. Antimicrob. Agents Chemother. 34:827–830, 1990.
176. Zabransky, R. J., DiNuzzo, A. R., Huber, M. B., et al.: Detection of vancomycin resistance in enterococci by the Vitek AMS system. Diagn. Microbiol. Infect. Dis. 20:113–116, 1994.
177. Zakrzewski, T., and Keith, J. D.: Bacterial endocarditis in infants and children. J. Pediatr. 67:1179–1193, 1965.
178. Zervos, M. J., and Schaberg, D. S.: Reversal of the in vitro susceptibility of enterococci to trimethoprim-sulfamethoxazole by folinic acid. Antimicrob. Agents Chemother. 28:446–448, 1985.
179. Zimmerman, R. A., Moellering, R. C., Jr., and Weinberg, A. N.: Mechanism of resistance to antibiotic synergism in enterococci. J. Bacteriol. 105:873–879, 1971.
180. Zscheck, K. K., and Murray, B. E.: Genes involved in the regulation of beta-lactamase production in enterococci and staphylococci. Antimicrob. Agents Chemother. 37:1966–1970, 1993.

Viridans Streptococcal Infections

A group of *Streptococcus* species known as viridans, α-hemolytic, or oral streptococci are present ubiquitously on the oral mucosa of virtually all humans. These organisms are important pathogens in children and adults alike, causing infections ranging from caries and subacute endocarditis in immunocompetent hosts to fatal sepsis in neutropenic individuals. Although commonly a cause of infection, viridans streptococci isolated from clinical specimens often are discounted unless endocarditis is suspected. This indifference may reflect the difficulty microbiologists have experienced in defining and classifying the members of this group of streptococci and the ensuing challenges in assimilating clinical and microbiologic data.

Each of the terms applied to this group is problematic. Not all members of the α-hemolytic streptococci are α-hemolytic, some being γ(non)-hemolytic or even β-hemolytic. *Streptococcus pneumoniae*, which is α-hemolytic, is considered to be a separate group of organisms. The term viridans streptococci equally is problematic because this term is derived from the Latin *viridis*, or green, referring to the sheen caused by partial hemolysis around α-hemolytic colonies on sheep blood agar. The term oral streptococci circumvents the problem of outliers in the hemolytic classification schema but also is confusing because viridans streptococci are found in sites other than the oral cavity and nonviridans streptococcal species frequently are present in the oral cavity. In accordance with the American Society of Microbiology's most recent efforts in this field,[138] the term viridans streptococci will be used here in referring to this diverse group of bacteria, recognizing that the member organisms typically, but not invariably, are α-hemolytic. It also should be emphasized that viridans does not refer to a species of streptococci but rather a group of species, erroneous references to *Streptococcus viridans* notwithstanding.[151]

Streptococci have been reclassified based on molecular and genetic studies,[37, 138] which adds to the clinical confusion, at least temporarily. For example, under the new classification system, certain small-colony β-hemolytic streptococci, including some that are Lancefield group A, now are considered to be viridans streptococci. It is hoped that classification based on molecular relatedness eventually will led to a clearer understanding of the infectious diseases associated with these organisms. One should recognize, however, that current knowledge of viridans streptococcal infections is based predominantly on observations of the α-hemolytic members of the viridans group.

MICROBIOLOGY

Streptococci are gram-positive, catalase-negative bacteria that are spherical or ovoid and less than 2 μm in diameter. They are facultatively anaerobic and nonmotile and do not produce spores or gas. Some strains require an atmosphere enriched with carbon dioxide (5 per cent). The enterococci (distinguished by their ability to grow in 6.5 per cent sodium chloride) and lactococci (formerly Lancefield group N streptococci) once were considered to be streptococci but now are classified as separate genera.

Figure 89–2 is a schema for classifying the clinically important streptococcal species. Hemolysis of blood agar remains a key tool for classifying streptococci. Strains that are β-hemolytic are characterized further according to colony size and Lancefield group (a serologic classification system based on cell wall carbohydrate). Group B *Streptococcus agalactiae* strains typically can be identified by β-hemolysis and a positive CAMP test[138]; however, some strains of *S. agalactiae* that are α- or γ-hemolytic also are recognized by a positive CAMP test. Large colony, β-hemolytic, group A streptococci make up the species *Streptococcus pyogenes*. Other large-colony, β-hemolytic streptococci occasionally are pathogenic, and the majority of these are group C or G streptococci. Small-colony, β-hemolytic streptococci, including groups A, C, G, F, and nongroupable strains, partially constitute the *Streptococcus milleri* group of organisms within the viridans streptococci group. Among the α- or γ-hemolytic streptococci, *S. agalactiae* (group B streptococci) and *S. pneumoniae* generally are identified by a positive CAMP test and optochin test, respectively. Bile solubility confirms an optochin-susceptible isolate as *S. pneumoniae*. Nutritionally deficient streptococci are recognized by the requirement of the presence of a second bacterial species (*Staphylococcus aureus* typically is used in testing) to maintain growth on agar. These streptococci generally will grow in blood culture media in the absence of NADH produced by a second bacterial species and may have some growth on agar in the absence of other bacteria. Nutritionally deficient streptococci once were classified as viridans streptococci, but more recent studies have identified these organisms as separate species: *Streptococcus adjacens* and *Streptococcus defectivus*.[138] *Enterococcus* species apart, streptococci that are α- or γ-hemolytic possess Lancefield group D antigen, and are bile esculin–positive may be identified tentatively as *Streptococcus bovis*. Although once included among viridans streptococci, this species now is classified apart from the viridans group. Strains of one species of group C streptococci, *Streptococcus dysgalactiae*, are α- or γ-hemolytic. These strains also must be distinguished from the viridans group streptococci. A former streptococcal species included in the viridans group—*Streptococcus morbillorum*—was reclassified as *Gemella morbillorum*.[84] The remaining streptococcal organisms tentatively may be identified as viridans group streptococci. Thus, in practice, viridans streptococci continue to be characterized by the absence of features that distinguish the other major streptococcal pathogens. There are no characteristics that can be used to confirm definitively the identity of viridans streptococci in the standard microbiology laboratory.

Classification of species within the viridans streptococci group also has been problematic. Several schemata have been developed over the years, including those of Carlsson,[28] Coleman and Williams,[35] Facklam,[53] Ruoff and Kunz,[139, 140] and Coykendall.[37] Each of these classification schemata lack reliable markers of member species, resulting in inconsistent classification of clinical isolates. Consequently, efforts to characterize the clinical features of infections with individual species of viridans streptococci have had marginal results.

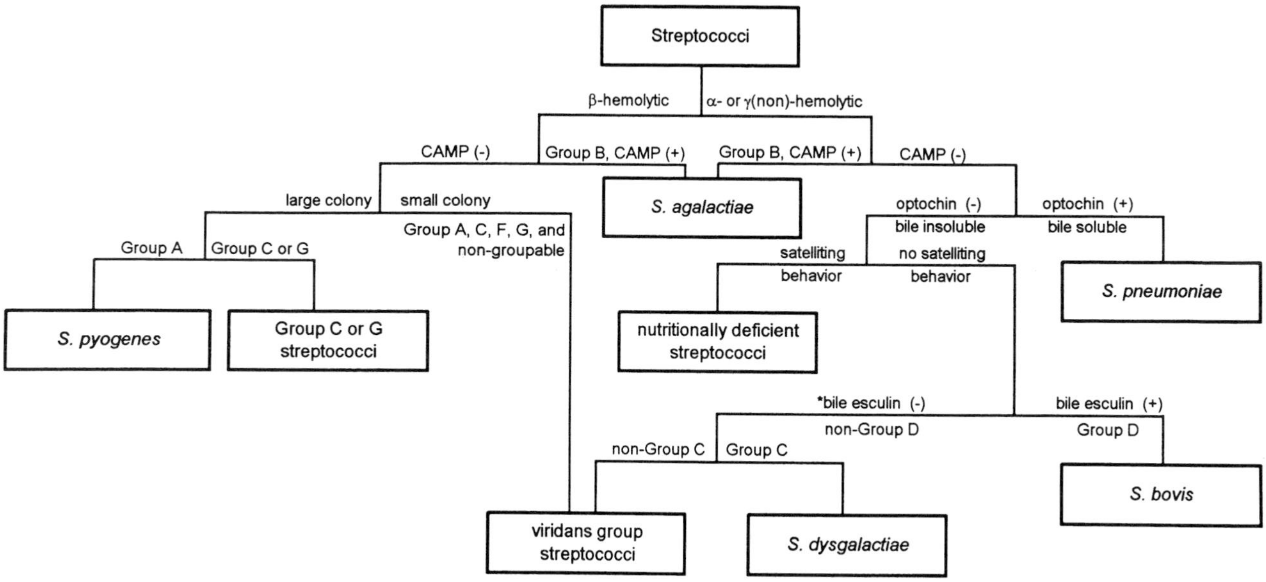

*Occasional viridans streptococcal strains are positive or weakly positive.

FIGURE 89–2. *Schema for the identification of clinically important streptococcal species. Viridans group species are, in general, those remaining after identification of other streptococcal species.*

Molecular taxonomy has been used to classify viridans streptococci,[37] but this technique generally is not available in the clinical laboratory. Given the current flux in the taxonomy of these organisms, a simplified, practical approach to classifying viridans streptococci as outlined in Table 89–3 has been advocated.[138] Biochemical tests available in many clinical microbiology laboratories can be used to assign clinical isolates to one of five groups that encompass the 14 clinically important viridans streptococcal species listed in Table 89–3. Rapid tests are available for tentative identification of individual viridans streptococcal species[56, 118, 140]; however, at this time, precise species identification has little clinical significance except as an epidemiologic tool.

EPIDEMIOLOGY

Viridans streptococci dominate the oral flora of humans. These organisms also are found commonly in other areas of the upper respiratory tract, throughout the gastrointestinal tract, and in the female genital tract. Occasionally, viridans streptococci are found as members of the skin flora. The predominance of viridans streptococci in the oral flora accounts for the origin of most infections caused by these organisms. In a study of 36 children who underwent extraction of normal or abscessed teeth, 11 (30 per cent) had post-extraction positive blood cultures.[155] In all 11, viridans streptococci exclusively were isolated. Bacteremia was more

TABLE 89–3. A Simplified Classification Schema for Viridans Streptococci

Group	Species	Hemolysis	Sorbitol	Arginine	Voges-Proskaner	Mannitol	Esculin
S. milleri	*S. anginosus*	α, β, γ	−	+	+	±	±
	S. constellatus					−	
	S. intermedius					±	
S. mutans	*S. mutans*	β, γ, α	+	−	+	+	+
	S. sobrinus						
	S. rattus						
	S. cricetus						
S. salivarius	*S. salivarius*	γ, α	−	−	+	−	+
	S. vestibularis						
S. sanguis	*S. sanguis*	α	−	+	−	−	+
	S. gordonii						+
	S. parasanguis						±
	S. crista						−
S. mitis	*S. mitis**	α	−	−	−	−	−

*Previously included *S. mitis, S. sanguis* II, and *S. oralis.*
Data from Coykendall, A. L.: Classification and identification of the viridans streptococci. Clin. Microbiol. Rev. *2*:315–328, 1989; Ruoff, K. L.: *Streptococcus. In* Murray, P. R., Baron, E. J., Pfaller, M. A., et al. (eds.): Manual of Clinical Microbiology. 6th ed. Washington, D.C., ASM Press, 1995, pp. 299–307.

common after removal of diseased teeth (37 per cent) but also occurred after removal of normal teeth (23 per cent). A separate study of 58 children undergoing dental extraction included 26 who received penicillin, amoxicillin, or erythromycin prophylaxis because of risk for endocarditis.[36] Only 9 (35 per cent) of the 26 children who received prophylaxis had bacteremia detected, compared with 20 (63 per cent) of 32 children not receiving prophylaxis ($p < .05$). In this study, viridans streptococci accounted for 37 per cent of the blood isolates, strict anaerobes accounted for 26.5 per cent, and a variety of organisms accounted for the remainder. The number of colony-forming units per milliliter of blood ranged from 2 to 12. Even within a single colony-forming unit, more than one bacterial species sometimes was found after subculture. Although these two studies were dissimilar in the diversity of organisms isolated, both indicate that viridans streptococci are the organisms most likely to invade the blood after trauma to the oral cavity.

Viridans streptococci begin colonizing neonates shortly after birth. By 1 month of age, virtually all infants are colonized with at least one species of viridans streptococci.[116] The mix of colonizing viridans streptococcal species varies with ontogeny. For example, *Streptococcus mutans*, a species that plays an important role in the development of caries, rarely is found in predentate children but is common after the eruption of teeth.[29, 48, 164] The ecology of other viridans streptococcal species also appears to be affected by the eruption of teeth.[48, 152, 164] In addition to these temporal factors in colonization of infants and children, viridans streptococci have species-specific predilections for certain anatomic areas of the oral cavity and pharynx. For example, *Streptococcus sanguis* is the predominant isolate of the buccal mucosa but rarely is found on the dorsum of the tongue, where *Streptococcus mitis* is the predominant species.[60] Diet also may affect the viridans streptococcal ecology. The consumption of sugar-containing beverages, for example, favors colonization with caries-producing *S. mutans*.[66]

Little is known about the transmission of viridans streptococci, but studies of the transmission of *S. mutans* within families indicates that intrafamily transmission is common.[2, 69, 141] Toothbrushes may be an important vehicle of transmission of viridans streptococci in children.[92] The hands of hospital personnel, especially those with skin disorders such as eczema, also may be a vehicle of transmission of viridans streptococci.[32]

Viridans streptococci have an important role in the ecology of the oral flora, protecting against potentially more invasive pathogens via colonization resistance.[13] This mechanism is demonstrated by a double-blind study in which patients were treated with either a preparation containing four species of viridans streptococci or a placebo after antibiotic therapy for group A streptococcal pharyngitis. In the treated group, none of 17 patients experienced recurrence of group A streptococcal pharyngitis. In contrast, the pharyngitis recurred in 7 (37 per cent) of 19 patients in the placebo group.[133] Viridans streptococci also may have a role in colonization resistance to pathogens such as *Neisseria gonorrhoeae* in the female genital tract.[99] In addition to competition for mucosal adherence sites, viridans streptococci produce bacteriocins that exert a bactericidal effect on certain competing bacteria and may contribute to colonization resistance.[38, 39]

PATHOGENESIS

Viridans streptococci are organisms of low virulence. They are involved most often in localized infections of the sinuses and oral cavity, including the teeth. Caries is a disease of teeth that develops over a period of years, often in association with *S. mutans* infection. Viridans streptococci also have a role in a variety of gingival diseases, possibly including the development of gingival hyperplasia accompanying chronic administration of phenytoin. In an experimental animal model, phenytoin-induced gingival hyperplasia was enhanced in rats infected with *Streptococcus sobrinus*, compared with uninfected control animals.[111] Typically, viridans streptococci cause life-threatening infection only in settings in which the oral mucosa is disrupted and the host's mechanisms of clearance are compromised, such as in patients with neutropenia or cardiac valve disease. Occasionally, viridans streptococci, usually *S. milleri* group organisms, cause pyogenic infections, including brain, lung, and abdominal abscesses.

The ability of viridans streptococci to bind to oral mucosa, tooth surfaces, and dental plaque via interaction of specific microbial and host "receptors" accounts for the preferential colonization of the oral cavity by these organisms.[172] This interaction also helps to explain the localization of the various viridans streptococcal species to distinct anatomic sites, as well as ontologic factors in colonization. The precise nature of bacterial adherence to the oral mucosa is not defined but appears to involve streptococcal lipoteichoic acid.[74] The host's immunologic status also may be an important determinant of adherence and subsequent invasion. For example, immunocompetent individuals produce secretory IgA to *S. mutans*,[7] and such antibody is capable of preventing caries.[106]

At the University of Texas M. D. Anderson Cancer Center in Houston, the incidence of viridans streptococcal bacteremia increased extraordinarily between 1972 and 1989, from 1 to 47 cases per 10,000 admissions.[50] An analysis of the risk factors associated with viridans streptococcal bacteremia indicated that prophylactic administration of trimethoprim-sulfamethoxazole or a fluoroquinolone, profound neutropenia, and administration of antacids or histamine type 2 antagonists each significantly predisposed to the development of bacteremia.[50] Presumably, administration of the implicated antibiotics and antacids favored overgrowth of viridans streptococci and their proliferation throughout the gastrointestinal tract. This, in turn, would favor viridans streptococcal bacteremia in an immunocompromised host, especially if the mucosal barrier were disrupted by cytotoxic chemotherapy and the host was neutropenic.

The ability to adhere to damaged cardiac valves and vegetations is a principal factor in the predominance of viridans streptococcal endocarditis. Strains of viridans streptococci carried by healthy children adhered less well to both buccal and endocardial cells than did disease-producing strains isolated from children with endocarditis.[143, 144] Lipoteichoic acid is thought to help mediate adhesion of viridans streptococci to endocardium, and penicillin prophylaxis may be effective in part because of its reduction of lipoteichoic acid on the bacterial cell surface.[90] The ability of antibiotics to alter surface properties of bacteria, even when the bacteria are resistant to the bactericidal action of the drug, may be an important determinant in the effectiveness of prophylactic antibiotics.[90, 149] In the host, fibronectin is an important determinate of viridans streptococcal binding to damaged endothelium. Viridans streptococci do not bind to soluble fibronectin, but a reactive domain becomes available for binding when the fibronectin molecule is immobilized, as is the case in endocarditis.[89] Mutant viridans streptococci that cannot bind to fibronectin are significantly less virulent in an animal model of endocarditis.[89] The ability of viridans streptococci to induce platelet aggregation also may be involved in the pathogenesis of endocarditis.[57, 93] Viridans streptococci–challenged, anticoagulated rabbits developed only microscopic vegetations despite fulminant sepsis. In contrast, viridans streptococci–challenged, nonanticoagulated animals tended to develop large vegetations and a subacute course.[77] These finding are concordant with those of a separate study in which viridans streptococci–challenged thrombocytopenic rabbits had a greater density of bacteria within vegetations than did nonthrombocytopenic control animals, suggesting that platelets limit disease progression.[160] Surprisingly, neutropenia appears to have little effect on the susceptibility to endocarditis in animal models but does have a role in containing the infection.[102, 103]

In neutropenic cancer and bone marrow transplant patients, viridans streptococci cause septic shock and adult respiratory distress syndrome. Viridans streptococci also induce nephritis.[3, 167] In either circumstance, little is known about the mechanisms involved. Viridans streptococci produce no endotoxin and are not known to produce exotoxins. Nevertheless, products of these organisms can activate complement[109] and induce production of tumor necrosis factor–α; interleukins-1, -2, and -6; γ-interferon; and nitric oxide.[14, 52, 98, 153, 163] Viridans streptococcal lipoteichoic acid is known to induce cytokine and nitric oxide production in vitro,[52, 109] but the clinical significance of these observations is not known.

CLINICAL MANIFESTATIONS

The viridans streptococcal species are a diverse group of bacteria, and, consequently, a variety of clinical presentations are associated with the infections they cause. Typically, the viridans streptococci cause nonpyogenic infections, such as bacteremia and endocarditis, but the *S. milleri* group, also referred to as the *Streptococcus intermedius* group, tends to cause invasive pyogenic infections, including bone infections, brain abscesses, appendicitis, and pulmonary and abdominal abscesses.[112]

Sepsis in the Immunocompromised Host

For obscure reasons, over the past two or three decades the relative incidence of gram-positive bacterial infections, and especially viridans streptococcal infections, has increased in immunocompromised hosts. Viridans streptococci first were perceived as an important cause of sepsis in the neutropenic cancer patient in 1978, when 29 episodes in adults and children at the National Cancer Institute[120] and 6 episodes in children at M. D. Anderson Cancer Center[73] were reported. Prior to these reports, the significance of blood isolates of viridans streptococci in this setting generally was not appreciated. No deaths occurred in the original National Cancer Institute series or in a subsequent series from that center,[136] suggesting that viridans streptococci produce a benign bacteremia similar to that seen with coagulase-negative staphylococci. In contrast, three of the six children diagnosed at M. D. Anderson died. Several other centers in Europe and North America have reported fulminant, sometimes fatal, viridans streptococcal sepsis in cancer and transplant patients.[6, 9, 19, 20, 27, 34, 50, 67, 70, 86, 104, 128, 130, 148, 154, 158, 176] Overall, the death rate associated with viridans streptococcal sepsis has ranged from 0 to 50 per cent, with most centers reporting mortality of around 10 per cent. In some centers, viridans streptococci are the most common cause of fatal sepsis.[19] The incidence of viridans streptococcal sepsis appears to be higher in children than in adults.[97, 158]

The oral cavity is the most common portal of entry in the immunocompromised host. Catheter-related viridans streptococcal bacteremia is unusual. However, because antacid administration is a risk factor,[50] it seems likely that the lower gastrointestinal tract may be a portal of entry in some patients. Several factors predispose to the development of viridans streptococcal sepsis. Profound neutropenia clearly is a predisposing factor,[19, 50] although cancer patients with absolute neutrophil counts greater than 1000 cells/μL occasionally develop viridans streptococcal bacteremia. Mucositis, especially oral mucositis, is a definitive risk factor.[19, 20, 50, 104] Cytarabine (cytosine arabinoside or Ara-C) appears to be a risk factor beyond its predisposition to produce clinically evident mucositis,[19, 20, 27, 43, 78, 104, 130] although this drug was not found to be an independent risk factor in one large study.[50] The use of prophylactic trimethoprim-sulfamethoxazole or quinolones also is an important risk factor.[19, 20, 33, 50] The observation that acyclovir administration may decrease the incidence of viridans streptococcal bacteremia in transplant patients suggests that herpes simplex virus infection may be a risk factor as well.[131] An association between viridans streptococcal sepsis and menstruation has been noted.[50]

The hallmark clinical feature of viridans streptococcal sepsis in the immunocompromised host is fever, which typically is high, occurs in the presence of neutropenia and mucositis, and frequently lasts for several days after viable organisms are cleared from the blood. The majority of patients recover uneventfully. However, fulminant septic shock may occur. Shock may appear early, although it often is delayed for 2 or 3 days after onset, occurring despite prompt sterilization of the blood by effective antibiotics.[158] Adult respiratory distress syndrome is common in severe cases, usually occurring 2 or 3 days after the initial bacteremia.[6, 50, 78, 165] Focal complications, including pneumonia and meningitis, are uncommon but do occur. Rash and palmar desquamation may be present.[50]

Several studies have implicated *S. mitis* as a more pathogenic species of viridans streptococci with a predilection to cause shock and adult respiratory distress syndrome,[6, 20, 34, 100, 158, 165] but other studies have not found a clear relation between clinical features and species.[50] Given the uncertainty in classifying viridans streptococcal species, reported species associations should be viewed cautiously.

Neonatal Sepsis and Meningitis

Viridans streptococci are normal inhabitants of the female genital tract and are a common cause of chorioamnionitis and resulting abortions.[5] Viridans streptococci are a common cause of neonatal sepsis and meningitis, although this is not recognized universally.[1, 17, 25, 61, 88, 110] Viridans streptococci ordinarily do not colonize newborns' skin and should not be dismissed as contaminants when isolated from normally sterile sites.[1] In some newborn centers, the incidence of viridans streptococcal bacteremia and meningitis has approached or exceeded that seen from group B streptococci, although viridans streptococcal infections tend to be less severe.[25, 110] The portal of entry of the organism generally is unknown in this setting, but a fetal scalp electrode has been implicated in one case.[62] Unusual manifestations in the newborn include pharyngitis and epiglottitis,[22] endocarditis,[101] and conjunctivitis.[85]

Caries

Although caries was recognized as an infectious disease in 1890 by workers trained in Robert Koch's laboratory, its infectious nature still is not accepted universally.[4, 8, 47] There is substantial evidence that *S. mutans* is the major cause of caries in children and adults alike,[4, 8, 23, 147, 166, 169, 173] although other viridans streptococci and *Actinomyces* species also have cariogenic potential.[147, 173] *S. mutans*, which colonizes the oral cavity only after the eruption of teeth, has a predilection for the dental surfaces, metabolizes sucrose, and produces a strong acid that weakens the mineral matrix of teeth, allowing the organisms to penetrate the structure of the teeth.[30, 147] Fluoridation of the water supply has been credited with strengthening tooth enamel, thereby fostering resistance to the harsh acids produced by *S. mutans*.[147] Fluoride has potent antibacterial action against *S. mutans*, particularly at low pH.[30, 174] Thus, our efforts at fluoridation of water supplies may represent, in one form or another, the most widespread and successful use of antibacterial prophylaxis. Topical treatments also provide protection against the cariogenic actions of *S. mutans* and in some circumstances depend on the antibacterial action of fluoride.[72, 168, 171, 180] Short courses of oral antibiotics can reduce colonization with *S. mutans* substantially and may be an important adjunct to treatment of caries.[157] Specially designed culture systems are available to detect the presence and measure the concentration of *S. mutans* in plaque, permitting the effects of therapy to be monitored.[23, 177] Because the development of cavities typically requires a few years of infection, there is ample opportunity to interrupt the pathogenesis of this disease.[4]

Endocarditis

Viridans streptococci are the most common cause of endocarditis at all ages, reflecting the organism's ability to adhere to diseased endocardium and its frequent implication in bacteremia during dental procedures and routine mouth care. Viridans streptococci tend to cause subacute endocarditis; blood cultures may be positive only intermittently. *S. sanguis* and *S. mitis* are the most commonly identified species.[44, 127, 132, 161] Complications of viridans streptococcal endocarditis include septic pulmonary emboli, congestive heart failure, pericarditis, meningitis, osteomyelitis, and glomerulonephritis.[127]

Pneumonia

Pulmonary infiltrates frequently complicate viridans streptococcal sepsis in the neutropenic host. In most cases, these infiltrates represent adult respiratory distress syndrome, not primary pneumonia. However, there have been several reports of previously healthy individuals developing primary viridans streptococcal pneumonia.[65, 94, 124, 142] In some cases, the diagnosis was supported by multiple blood isolates of viridans streptococci in the absence of endocarditis. The incidence of viridans streptococcal pneumonia significantly may be underestimated because tracheal isolates of viridans streptococci usually are discounted as contaminants. Nevertheless, tracheal isolates probably do represent contamination of the specimen with oral flora in many cases.[134] Given the increasing incidence of viridans streptococcal infections and the increasing prevalence of antibiotic resistance among these organisms, clinicians should consider viridans streptococci as potential causes of pneumonia when they are isolated in the absence of other pathogens.

Osteomyelitis and Septic Arthritis

Viridans streptococci are unusual causes of osteomyelitis and septic arthritis. Extension of an oral infection into the mandible or maxilla is the most common circumstance in which viridans streptococci cause osteomyelitis,[115] but vertebral osteomyelitis due to these organisms has been described on several occasions.[26, 41, 137, 170] Infection of the long bones[129] and septic arthritis[10] occur infrequently.

Abscesses

Suppurative infections due to viridans streptococci typically are caused by the *S. milleri* group: *Streptococcus anginosus*, *Streptococcus constellatus*, and *Streptococcus intermedius*. Because *S. milleri* bacteria inhabit the upper respiratory tract and the gastrointestinal tract and are relatively invasive, these organisms cause sinusitis, otitis media, meningitis, and abdominal abscesses and often are present in brain abscesses.[51, 107, 108, 112] *S. milleri* group organisms may infect the brain via a hematogenous route, originating in the oral cavity or intestinal tract or by direct invasion through the upper respiratory tract. Lung abscesses due to viridans streptococci may result from aspiration of saliva.[124] Viridans streptococci also are found occasionally in liver abscess[12, 58] and appendicitis.[121]

DIAGNOSIS

Viridans streptococcal infections typically are diagnosed by culture of blood or other normally sterile tissues. The organisms may be present in low concentration. A volume of 30 mL of blood has been suggested as the optimal volume for culture.[145] The addition of agents that neutralize the antibacterial effects of fresh blood, such as sodium polyanethole sulfonate, significantly improves the yield of blood cultures.[146] Chemotherapy agents may interfere with the detection of viridans streptococci in blood.[117]

Viridans streptococci normally are not part of the skin flora and ordinarily should not be considered contaminants. Viridans streptococci have been reported to cross-react with *S. pneumoniae* omnisera, potentially leading to false-positive omnisera test results.[76]

Clinically, infections due to viridans streptococci can not be distinguished from infections due to other gram-positive and gram-negative bacteria. Collection of adequate culture specimens is essential for diagnosis.

ANTIBIOTIC SUSCEPTIBILITY

In the past, viridans streptococci have been considered penicillin-sensitive. Today, penicillin-resistant and -tolerant viridans streptococci are found worldwide as causes of sepsis, endocarditis, meningitis, and other infections, including conjunctivitis of newborns.[21, 49, 54, 64, 75, 85, 122, 126] Penicillin resistance particularly is common in patients receiving long-term penicillin therapy.[114, 156, 159] Ominously, viridans streptococci resistant to aminoglycosides,[82] vancomycin,[150] and other antibiotics[24, 178] also have been reported. *S. mutans*, however, rarely exhibits antibiotic resistance.[80]

Resistance of viridans streptococci to penicillin appears to involve chromosomally mediated alterations in the organisms' penicillin-binding proteins.[126, 181] Initially, it was suspected that genes conferring penicillin resistance might have been acquired from *S. pneumoniae*.[46] Subsequent studies, however, indicate that penicillin resistance may have evolved first in *S. mitis* and that *S. pneumoniae* acquired genes mediating penicillin resistance from this and other closely related viridans streptococcal species.[31, 45, 123]

The clinical impact of the development of penicillin resistance among viridans streptococci has been far-reaching.

Emergence of penicillin-resistant viridans streptococci incidentally may be encouraging the development of vancomycin-resistant enterococci because of the increased use of vancomycin to prevent and treat viridans streptococcal infection.

TREATMENT

Empiric antibiotic therapy for viridans streptococci should be based on the local pattern of antibiotic susceptibilities among recent clinical isolates. Antimicrobial susceptibility testing of viridans streptococcal isolates is necessary. Although vancomycin-resistant clinical isolates currently are very rare, inclusion of vancomycin in susceptibility testing is advisable. For infections other than endocarditis and meningitis, single-antibiotic therapy usually is preferred. An exception is the neutropenic cancer patient because restricting antibiotic therapy to drugs active against gram-positive bacteria exclusively may predispose to the development of gram-negative bacterial infections.[119] Combination therapy often is advocated for the treatment of viridans streptococcal endocarditis[18, 59, 96, 175] and may be considered for the treatment of meningitis, especially when the infecting organism is tolerant to penicillin. Combinations of penicillins and aminoglycosides or vancomycin and aminoglycosides are used most commonly. Penicillin and vancomycin are thought to increase the uptake of aminoglycosides, leading to synergistic bactericidal activity.[179] Frequent dosing of antibiotics generally has been recommended; however, viridans streptococci exposed to penicillin appear to be susceptible to a postantibiotic effect.[83] Consequently, longer dosing intervals may be satisfactory, but there currently are insufficient data to support a recommendation. Viridans streptococcal endocarditis usually is treated for 4 to 6 weeks; the duration of therapy for infections at other sites has not been studied but generally can be guided by site-specific practice and individual clinical response.

In the treatment of endocarditis, the penetration of antibiotics into the fibrin vegetation may be impeded markedly. Viridans streptococci produce an exopolysaccharide, composed predominantly of dextran, which may limit the penetration. Experimental studies indicate that the degree of exopolysaccharide production by viridans streptococcal strains affects the success rate of antimicrobial therapy.[125] In accord with this observation, administration of dextranase to animals with experimental viridans streptococcal endocarditis enhances antibiotic efficacy.[105] In the future, such adjuvant therapies designed to reduce the size or density of valvular vegetations may offer promise for patients not helped by conventional antibiotic therapy for endocarditis.

Another setting in which adjuvant therapy may be considered is viridans streptococcal sepsis in the neutropenic patient after cytarabine chemotherapy. One uncontrolled trial suggests that early addition of high doses of corticosteroids to the antimicrobial therapeutic regimen may reduce the incidence of associated adult respiratory distress syndrome and death.[42] However, there are insufficient data to recommend this approach routinely.

PREVENTION

Attempts to prevent viridans streptococcal infections have focused on three distinct settings: prevention of caries, prevention of endocarditis, and prevention of sepsis in the neutropenic cancer patient. Efforts have been successful in the former two settings. However, the emergence of penicillin-resistant viridans streptococci and concern about the possible emergence of vancomycin resistance highlight the need for new approaches to preventing infection with these ubiquitous organisms. In developing such methods, investigators should not forget that colonization resistance provided by viridans streptococci can protect the host from more virulent pathogens (see Epidemiology section).

The incidence of caries in the United States has been reduced sharply by fluoridation of water supplies, inclusion of fluoride in toothpaste, and diet modification (e.g., use of sugar substitutes). Fluoride acts as an antibacterial agent while strengthening resistance of the teeth to invasion by bacteria. Use of dental varnishes, gels, and rinses that contain fluoride or other antibacterials, such as chlorhexidine or vancomycin, may be beneficial in selected cases.[55, 81, 95, 113]

The American Heart Association has led a successful effort to prevent endocarditis by systemic antibiotic prophylaxis of patients with known endocardial defects who are undergoing dental procedures. These efforts are aimed especially at preventing viridans streptococcal endocarditis, and penicillin is the antibiotic most commonly utilized. The mechanism(s) by which antibiotic prophylaxis prevents endocarditis is not understood completely. In animals, endocarditis can be prevented by bacteriostatic antibiotics and by serum levels of bactericidal antibiotics that are well below the minimal bactericidal concentration for the colonizing viridans streptococci.[63] Vancomycin has been observed to prevent vancomycin-tolerant *S. sanguis* endocarditis in experimentally challenged animals without reducing the incidence or level of bacteremia, suggesting that antibiotics may prevent endocarditis by reducing bacterial adherence to the endocardium.[15] This hypothesis is supported by a study in which 21 per cent of children receiving antibiotic prophylaxis developed bacteremia, in some cases with antibiotic-resistant organisms, but endocarditis was rare.[71] However, studies in animals indicate that the probability of preventing endocarditis is correlated with the antibiotic susceptibility of the challenging streptococcal strains.[71]

Prophylaxis should be administered immediately prior to dental procedures. Increased numbers of antibiotic-resistant viridans streptococci can be detected within 6 hours of antibiotic treatment, and they persist for 9 days or longer.[87] Experimental studies on the prevention of endocarditis via antibiotic administration after challenge with bacterial inocula have yielded inconsistent results,[16, 79, 91] and the clinical utility of this approach is not known. Topical treatment with vancomycin or chlorhexidine has been advocated as an adjuvant to prevent endocarditis, but the efficacy of this approach is not proven.[162]

Viridans streptococcal infections have become a major problem in neutropenic cancer patients and in bone marrow transplant patients in recent years. Because penicillin-resistant viridans streptococci are widespread, some cancer centers include vancomycin in the initial empiric antibiotic regimen for neutropenic patients with unexplained fever.[148] In addition, despite concerns about the possibility of inducing vancomycin-resistant bacterial strains, physicians managing bone marrow transplant units are administering intravenous vancomycin prophylactically to high-risk patients in an effort to prevent viridans streptococcal sepsis. A noncontrolled trial of oral vancomycin paste in children receiving cytotoxic chemotherapy suggested efficacy in the prevention of viridans streptococcal infections,[11] and a placebo-controlled, double-blind trial of oral prophylaxis is under way. However, increased colonization and infection with vancomycin-resistant enterococci are a predictable consequence of increased vancomycin usage, prompting Centers for Disease Control and Prevention recommendations to avoid the use of empiric vancomycin therapy when feasible and leading investigators to explore alternatives to the use of empiric or prophylactic vancomycin. In a comparative trial, penicillin prophylaxis was superior to trimethoprim-sulfamethoxazole prophylaxis in preventing viridans streptococcal infections in cancer patients, despite extensive colonization with penicillin-resistant streptococci.[68] In other studies, oral administration of a macrolide antibiotic, roxithromycin, also appeared to reduce the incidence of viridans streptococcal infections in cancer patients compared with historical controls.[40, 135] Although these studies are promising, large controlled trials are needed to assess the overall effect of this approach on the cancer patient.

References

1. Adams, J. T., and Faix, R. G.: *Streptococcus mitis* infection in newborns. J. Perinatol. *14*:473–478, 1994.
2. Alaluusua, S.: Transmission of mutans streptococci. Proc. Finn. Dent. Soc. *87*:443–447, 1991.
3. Albini, B., Nisengard, R. J., Glurich, I., et al.: *Streptococcus mutans*–induced nephritis in rabbits. Am. J. Pathol. *118*:408–418, 1985.
4. Anderson, M. H., Molvar, M. P., and Powell, L. V.: Treating dental caries as an infectious disease. Oper. Dent. *16*:21–28, 1991.
5. Ariel, I., and Singer, D. B.: *Streptococcus viridans* infections in midgestation. Pediatr. Pathol. *11*:75–83, 1991.
6. Arning, M., Gehrt, A., Aul, C., et al.: Septicemia due to *Streptococcus mitis* in neutropenic patients with acute leukemia. Blut *61*:364–368, 1990.
7. Arnold, R. R., Mestecky, J., and McGhee, J. R.: Naturally occurring secretory immunoglobulin A antibodies to *Streptococcus mutans* in human colostrum and saliva. Infect. Immun. *14*:355–362, 1976.
8. Asikainen, S., and Alaluusua, S.: Bacteriology of dental infections. Eur. Heart J. *14*(Suppl. K):43–50, 1993.
9. Awada, A., van der Auwera, P., Meunier, F., et al.: Streptococcal and enterococcal bacteremia in patients with cancer. Clin. Infect. Dis. *15*:33–48, 1992.
10. Barbadillo, C., Trujillo, A., Cuende, E., et al.: Septic arthritis due to *Streptococcus viridans*. Clin. Exp. Rheumatol. *8*:520–521, 1990.
11. Barker, G. J., Call, S. K., and Gamis, A. S.: Oral care with vancomycin paste for reduction in incidence of alpha-hemolytic streptococcal (AHS) sepsis (Meeting abstract). Cancer Therapies for the 21st Century 9th Annual Meeting, 1994.
12. Bateman, N. T., Eykyn, S. J., and Phillips, I.: Pyogenic liver abscess caused by *Streptococcus milleri*. Lancet *1*:657–659, 1975.
13. Beck, A.: Interference by an alpha-hemolytic *Streptococcus* of beta-hemolytic pathogenic streptococci. Inflammation *3*:463–465, 1979.
14. Benabdelmoumene, S., Dumont, S., Petit, C., et al.: Activation of human monocytes by *Streptococcus mutans* serotype f polysaccharide: Immunoglobulin G Fc receptor expression and tumor necrosis factor and interleukin-1 production. Infect. Immun. *59*:3261–3266, 1991.
15. Bernard, J. P., Francioli, P., and Glauser, M. P.: Vancomycin prophylaxis of experimental *Streptococcus sanguis*: Inhibition of bacterial adherence rather than bacterial killing. J. Clin. Invest. *68*:1113–1116, 1981.
16. Berney, P., and Francioli, P.: Successful prophylaxis of experimental streptococcal endocarditis with single-dose amoxicillin administered after bacterial challenge. J. Infect. Dis. *161*:281–285, 1990.
17. Bignardi, G. E., and Isaacs, D.: Neonatal meningitis due to *Streptococcus mitis*. Rev. Infect. Dis. *11*:86–88, 1989.
18. Bisno, A. L., Dismukes, W. E., Durack, D. T., et al.: Antimicrobial treatment of infective endocarditis due to viridans streptococci, enterococci, and staphylococci. J. A. M. A. *261*:1471–1477, 1989.
19. Bochud, P. Y., Calandra, T., and Francioli, P.: Bacteremia due to viridans streptococci in neutropenic patients: A review. Am. J. Med. *97*:256–264, 1994.
20. Bochud, P. Y., Eggiman, P., Calandra, T., et al.: Bacteremia due to viridans *Streptococcus* in neutropenic patients with cancer: Clinical spectrum and risk factors. Clin. Infect. Dis. *18*:25–31, 1994.
21. Boenning, D. A., Nelson, L. P., and Campos, J. M.: Relatively penicillin-resistant *Streptococcus sanguis* endocarditis in an adolescent. Pediatr. Infect. Dis. J. *7*:205–207, 1988.
22. Bos, A. P., Fetter, W. P., Baerts, W., et al.: Streptococcal pharyngitis and epiglottitis in a newborn infant. Eur. J. Pediatr. *151*:874–875, 1992.
23. Bratthall, D.: Mutans streptococci: Dental, oral and global aspects. J. Indian Soc. Pedod. Prev. Dent. *9*:4–12, 1991.
24. Bromberg, K., Orson, J. M., Triedman, R., et al.: Erythromycin-resistant *Streptococcus viridans* in oral flora with prolonged erythromycin therapy. Ann. Intern. Med. *93*:931–932, 1980.
25. Broughton, R. A., Krafka, R., and Baker, C. J.: Non–group D alpha-hemolytic streptococci: New neonatal pathogens. J. Pediatr. *99*:450–454, 1981.
26. Buchman, A. L.: *Streptococcus viridans* osteomyelitis with endocarditis presenting as acute onset lower back pain. J. Emerg. Med. *8*:291–294, 1990.
27. Burden, A. D., Oppenheim, B. A., Crowther, D., et al.: Viridans streptococcal bacteraemia in patients with haematological and solid malignancies. Eur. J. Cancer *27*:409–411, 1991.
28. Carlsson, J.: A numerical taxonomic study of human oral streptococci. Odontol. Rev. *19*:137–160, 1968.
29. Caufield, P. W., Cutter, G. R., and Dasanayake, A. P.: Initial acquisition of mutans streptococci by infants: Evidence for a discrete window of infectivity. J. Dent. Res. *72*:37–45, 1993.
30. Caufield, P. W., and Wannemuehler, Y. M.: In vitro susceptibility of *Streptococcus mutans* 6715 to iodine and sodium fluoride, singly and in combination, at various pH values. Antimicrob. Agents Chemother. *22*:115–119, 1982.
31. Chalkley, L., Schuster, C., Potgieter, E., et al.: Relatedness between *Streptococcus pneumoniae* and viridans streptococci: Transfer of penicillin resistance determinants and immunological similarities of penicillin-binding proteins. FEMS Microbiol. Lett. *69*:35–42, 1991.
32. Church, D. L., and Bryant, H. E.: Investigation of a *Streptococcus viridans* pseudobacteremia epidemic at a university teaching hospital. Infect. Control Hosp. Epidemiol. *10*:416–421, 1989.
33. Classen, D. C., Burke, J. P., Ford, C. D., et al.: *Streptococcus mitis* sepsis in bone marrow transplant patients receiving oral antimicrobial prophylaxis. Am. J. Med. *89*:441–446, 1990.
34. Cohen, J., Donnelly, J. P., Worsley, A. M., et al.: Septicaemia caused by viridans streptococci in neutropenic patients with leukaemia. Lancet *2*:1452–1454, 1983.
35. Coleman, G., and Williams, R. E. A.: Taxonomy of some human viridans streptococci. *In* Wannamaker, L. W., and Matsen, J. M. (eds.): Streptococci and Streptococcal Diseases: Recognition, Understanding, and Management. New York, Academic Press, 1972, pp. 282–299.
36. Coulter, W. A., Coffey, A., Saunders, I. D., et al.: Bacteremia in children following dental extraction. J. Dent. Res. *69*:1691–1695, 1990.
37. Coykendall, A. L.: Classification and identification of the viridans streptococci. Clin. Microbiol. Rev. *2*:315–328, 1989.
38. Dajani, A. S., Law, D. J., Bollinger, R. O., et al.: Ultrastructural and biochemical alterations effected by viridin B, a bacterocin of alpha-hemolytic streptococci. Infect. Immun. *14*:776–782, 1976.
39. Dajani, A. S., Tom, M. C., and Law, D. J.: Viridins, bacteriocins of alpha-hemolytic streptococci: Isolation, characterization, and partial purification. Antimicrob. Agents Chemother. *9*:81–88, 1976.
40. Dekker, A. W., Rozenberg-Arska, M., and Verdonck, L. F.: Prevention of bacteremias caused by alpha-hemolytic streptococci by roxithromycin in patients treated with intensive cytotoxic treatment. Hämatol. Bluttransfusion *33*:551–554, 1990.
41. Demers, C., Tremblay, M., and Lacourciere, Y.: Acute vertebral osteomyelitis complicating *Streptococcus sanguis* endocarditis. Ann. Rheum. Dis. *47*:333–336, 1988.
42. Dompeling, E. C., Donnelly, J. P., Raemaekers, J. M., et al.: Pre-emptive administration of corticosteroids prevents the development of ARDS associated with *Streptococcus mitis* bacteremia following chemotherapy with high-dose cytarabine. Ann. Hematol. *69*:69–71, 1994.
43. Donnelly, J. P., Dompeling, E. C., Meis, J. F., et al.: Bacteremia due to oral viridans streptococci in neutropenic patients with cancer: Cytostatics are a more important risk factor than antibacterial prophylaxis. Clin. Infect. Dis. *20*:469–470, 1995.
44. Douglas, C. W., Heath, J., Hampton, K. K., et al.: Identity of viridans streptococci isolated from cases of infective endocarditis. J. Med. Microbiol. *39*:179–182, 1993.
45. Dowson, C. G., Coffey, T. J., Kell, C., et al.: Evolution of penicillin resistance in *Streptococcus pneumoniae*: The role of *Streptococcus mitis* in the formation of a low-affinity PBP2B in *S. pneumoniae*. Mol. Microbiol. *9*:635–643, 1993.
46. Dowson, C. G., Hutchison, A., Woodford, N., et al.: Penicillin-resistant viridans streptococci have obtained altered penicillin-binding protein genes from penicillin-resistant strains of *Streptococcus pneumoniae*. Proc. Natl. Acad. Sci. U. S. A. *87*:5858–5862, 1990.
47. Edelstein, B. L.: The medical management of dental caries. J. Am. Dent. Assoc. *125*(Suppl):31S–39S, 1994.
48. Edwardsson, S., and Mejare, B.: *Streptococcus milleri* (Guthof) and *Streptococcus mutans* in the mouths of infants before and after tooth eruption. Arch. Oral Biol. *23*:811–814, 1978.
49. Elliott, R. H., and Dunbar, J. M.: Antibiotic sensitivity of oral alpha-haemolytic *Streptococcus* from children with congenital or acquired cardiac disease: A prolonged survey. Br. Dent. J. *142*:283–285, 1977.
50. Elting, L. S., Bodey, G. P., and Keefe, B. H.: Septicemia and shock syndrome due to viridans streptococci: A case-control study of predisposing factors. Clin. Infect. Dis. *14*:1201–1207, 1992.
51. Eng, R. H., Mangia, A. J., Smith, S. M., et al.: Meningitis following bacteremia with *Streptococcus sanguis*. N.Y. State. J. Med. *89*:625–626, 1989.
52. English, B. K., Patrick, C. C., Orlicek, S. L., et al.: Lipoteichoic acid from viridans streptococci induces the production of tumor necrosis factor and nitric oxide by the murine macrophage cell line RAW 264.7. J. Invest. Med. *43*(Suppl. 1):68A, 1995.

53. Facklam, R. R.: Physiological differentiation of viridans streptococci. J. Clin. Microbiol. *5*:184–201, 1977.
54. Farber, B. F., Eliopoulos, G. M., Ward, J. I., et al.: Multiply resistant viridans streptococci: Susceptibility to beta-lactam antibiotics and comparison of penicillin-binding protein patterns. Antimicrob. Agents Chemother. *24*:702–705, 1983.
55. Fine, J. B., Harper, D. S., Gordon, J. M., et al.: Short-term microbiological and clinical effects of subgingival irrigation with an antimicrobial mouthrinse. J. Periodontol. *65*:30–36, 1994.
56. Flynn, C. E., and Ruoff, K. L.: Identification of *"Streptococcus milleri"* group isolates to the species level with a commercially available rapid test system. J. Clin. Microbiol. *33*:2704–2706, 1995.
57. Ford, I., Douglas, C. W., Preston, F. E., et al.: Mechanisms of platelet aggregation by *Streptococcus sanguis*, a causative organism in infective endocarditis. Br. J. Haematol. *84*:95–100, 1993.
58. Ford, J. M., and DuBois, R. E.: Multiloculated hepatic abscess caused by alpha-hemolytic *Streptococcus*. South. Med. J. *77*:514–516, 1984.
59. Francioli, P. B., and Glauser, M. P.: Synergistic activity of ceftriaxone combined with netilmicin administered once daily for treatment of experimental streptococcal endocarditis. Antimicrob. Agents Chemother. *37*:207–212, 1993.
60. Frandsen, E. V., Pedrazzoli, V., and Kilian, M.: Ecology of viridans streptococci in the oral cavity and pharynx. Oral Microbiol. Immunol. *6*:129–133, 1991.
61. Fraser, Jr., J. J., Marks, M. I., and Welch, D. F.: Neonatal sepsis and meningitis due to alpha-hemolytic *Streptococcus*. South. Med. J. *76*:401–402, 1983.
62. Freedman, R. M., and Baltimore, R.: Fatal *Streptococcus viridans* septicemia and meningitis: Relationship to fetal scalp electrode monitoring. J. Perinatol. *10*:272–274, 1990.
63. Glauser, M. P., and Francioli, P.: Successful prophylaxis against experimental streptococcal endocarditis with bacteriostatic antibiotics. J. Infect. Dis. *146*:806–810, 1982.
64. Goldfarb, J., Wormser, G. P., and Glaser, J. H.: Meningitis caused by multiply antibiotic-resistant viridans streptococci. J. Pediatr. *105*:891–895, 1984.
65. Goolam Mahomed, A., Feldman, C., Smith, C., et al.: Does primary *Streptococcus viridans* pneumonia exist? S. Afr. Med. J. *82*:432–434, 1992.
66. Grindefjord, M., Dahllof, G., Wikner, S., et al.: Prevalence of mutans streptococci in one-year-old children. Oral Microbiol. Immunol. *6*:280–283, 1991.
67. Groot-Loonen, J. J., van der Noordaa, J., de Kraker, J., et al.: Alpha-hemolytic streptococcal septicemia with severe complications during neutropenia in childhood cancer. Pediatr. Hematol. Oncol. *4*:323–328, 1987.
68. Guiot, H. F., van der Meer, J. W., van den Broek, P. J., et al.: Prevention of viridans-group streptococcal septicemia in oncohematologic patients: A controlled comparative study on the effect of penicillin G and cotrimoxazole. Ann. Hematol. *64*:260–265, 1992.
69. Hamada, S., Masuda, N., and Kotani, S.: Isolation and serotyping of *Streptococcus mutans* from teeth and feces of children. J. Clin. Microbiol. *11*:314–318, 1980.
70. Henslee, J., Bostrom, B., Weisdorf, D., et al.: Streptococcal sepsis in bone marrow transplant patients. Lancet *1*:393, 1984.
71. Hess, J., Dankert, J., and Durack, D.: Significance of penicillin tolerance in vivo: Prevention of experimental *Streptococcus sanguis* endocarditis. J. Antimicrob. Chemother. *11*:555–564, 1983.
72. Hirschfeld, Z., Friedman, M., Golomb, G., et al.: New sustained release dosage form of chlorhexidine for dental use: Use for plaque control in partial denture wearers. J. Oral Rehab. *11*:477–482, 1984.
73. Hoecker, J. L., Pickering, L. K., Groschel, D., et al.: *Streptococcus salivarius* sepsis in children with malignancies. J. Pediatr. *92*:337–338, 1978.
74. Hogg, S. D., and Manning, J. E.: Inhibition of adhesion of viridans streptococci to fibronectin-coated hydroxyapatite beads by lipoteichoic acid. J. Appl. Bacteriol. *65*:483–489, 1988.
75. Holbrook, W. P., Olafsdottir, D., Magnusson, H. B., et al.: Penicillin tolerance among oral streptococci. J. Med. Microbiol. *27*:17–22, 1988.
76. Holmberg, H., Danielsson, D., Hardie, J., et al.: Cross-reactions between alpha-streptococci and Omniserum, a polyvalent pneumococcal serum, demonstrated by direct immunofluorescence, immunoelectroosmophoresis, and latex agglutination. J. Clin. Microbiol. *21*:745–748, 1985.
77. Hook, E. W., III, and Sande, M. A.: Role of the vegetation in experimental *Streptococcus viridans* endocarditis. Infect. Immun. *10*:1433–1438, 1974.
78. Inoue, S., Boyer, D., and Gordon, R.: Interstitial pneumonia and alpha-hemolytic *Streptococcus* sepsis in a child with malignancy who recently received cytosine arabinoside. Pediatr. Infect. Dis. J. *9*:598–600, 1990.
79. James, J., MacFarlane, T. W., McGowan, D. A., et al.: Failure of post-bacteraemia delayed antibiotic prophylaxis of experimental rabbit endocarditis. J. Antimicrob. Chemother. *20*:883–885, 1987.
80. Järvinen, H., Tenovuo, J., and Huovinen, P.: In vitro susceptibility of *Streptococcus mutans* to chlorhexidine and six other antimicrobial agents. Antimicrob. Agents Chemother. *37*:1158–1159, 1993.
81. Jordan, H. V., and De Paola, P. F.: Effect of a topically applied 3 percent vancomycin gel on *Streptococcus mutans* on different tooth surfaces. J. Dent. Res. *53*:115–120, 1974.
82. Kaufhold, A., and Potgieter, E.: Chromosomally mediated high-level gentamicin resistance in *Streptococcus mitis*. Antimicrob. Agents Chemother. *37*:2740–2742, 1993.
83. Kikuchi, K., Enari, T., Minami, S., et al.: Postantibiotic effects and postantibiotic sub-MIC effects of benzylpenicillin on viridans streptococci isolated from patients with infective endocarditis. J. Antimicrob. Chemother. *34*:687–696, 1994.
84. Kilpper-Balz, R., and Schleifer, K.-H.: Transfer of *Streptococcus morbillorum* to the genus *Gemella* as *Gemella haemolysans*. Int. J. Syst. Bacteriol. *38*:442–443, 1988.
85. Kontiainen, S., and Sivonen, A.: Multiply resistant *Streptococcus mitis* isolated from conjunctival exudate of newborns. Eur. J. Clin. Microbiol. *6*:53–55, 1987.
86. Leblanc, T., Leverger, G., Arlet, G., et al.: Frequency and severity of systemic infections caused by *Streptococcus mitis* and *sanguis* II in neutropenic children. Pathol. Biol. (Paris) *37*:459–464, 1989.
87. Leviner, E., Tzukert, A. A., Benoliel, R., et al.: Development of resistant oral viridans streptococci after administration of prophylactic antibiotics: Time management in the dental treatment of patients susceptible to infective endocarditis. Oral Surg. Oral Med. Oral Pathol. *64*:417–420, 1987.
88. Lilien, L. D., Wilks, A. K., and Yeh, T. F.: *Streptococcus sanguis* biotype II meningitis in a premature infant. Clin. Pediatr. *21*:465, 1982.
89. Lowrance, J. H., Baddour, L. M., and Simpson, W. A.: The role of fibronectin binding in the rat model of experimental endocarditis caused by *Streptococcus sanguis*. J. Clin. Invest. *86*:7–13, 1990.
90. Lowy, F. D., Chang, D. S., Neuhaus, E. G., et al.: Effect of penicillin on the adherence of *Streptococcus sanguis* in vitro and in the rabbit model of endocarditis. J. Clin. Invest. *71*:668–675, 1983.
91. Malinverni, R., Bille, J., and Glauser, M. P.: Single-dose rifampin prophylaxis for experimental endocarditis induced by high bacterial inocula of viridans streptococci. J. Infect. Dis. *156*:151–157, 1987.
92. Malmberg, E., Birkhed, D., Norvenius, G., et al.: Microorganisms on toothbrushes at day-care centers. Acta Odontol. Scand. *52*:93–98, 1994.
93. Manning, J. E., Hume, E. B., Hunter, N., et al.: An appraisal of the virulence factors associated with streptococcal endocarditis. J. Med. Microbiol. *40*:110–114, 1994.
94. Marrie, T. J.: Bacteremic community-acquired pneumonia due to viridans group streptococci. Clin. Invest. Med. *16*:38–44, 1993.
95. Marsh, P. D.: Antimicrobial strategies in the prevention of dental caries. Caries Res. *27*(Suppl. 1):72–76, 1993.
96. Martinez, F., Martin-Luengo, F., Garcia, A., et al.: Treatment with imipenem of experimental endocarditis caused by penicillin-resistant *Streptococcus sanguis*. J. Antimicrob. Chemother. *33*:1201–1207, 1994.
97. Martino, R., Subira, M., Manteiga, R., et al.: Viridans streptococcal bacteremia and viridans streptococcal shock syndrome in neutropenic patients: Comparison between children and adults receiving chemotherapy or undergoing bone marrow transplantation. Clin. Infect. Dis. *20*:476–477, 1995.
98. Matsushita, K., Fujimaki, W., Kato, H., et al.: Immunopathological activities of extracellular products of *Streptococcus mitis*, particularly a superantigenic fraction. Infect. Immun. *63*:785–793, 1995.
99. McBride, M. E., Duncan, W. C., and Knox, J. M.: Bacterial interference of *Neisseria gonorrhoeae* by alpha-haemolytic streptococci. Br. J. Vener. Dis. *56*:235–238, 1980.
100. McWhinney, P. H., Gillespie, S. H., Kibbler, C. C., et al.: *Streptococcus mitis* and ARDS in neutropenic patients. Lancet *337*:429, 1991.
101. Mecrow, I. K., and Ladusans, E. J.: Infective endocarditis in newborn infants with structurally normal hearts. Acta Paediatr. *83*:35–39, 1994.
102. Meddens, M. J., Thompson, J., Eulderink, F., et al.: Role of granulocytes in experimental *Streptococcus sanguis* endocarditis. Infect. Immun. *36*:325–332, 1982.
103. Meddens, M. J., Thompson, J., Mattie, H., et al.: Role of granulocytes in the prevention and therapy of experimental *Streptococcus sanguis* endocarditis in rabbits. Antimicrob. Agents Chemother. *25*:263–267, 1984.
104. Menichetti, F., Del Favero, A., Guerciolini, R., et al.: Viridans streptococci septicemia in cancer patients: A clinical study. Eur. J. Epidemiol. *3*:316–318, 1987.
105. Mghir, A. S., Cremieux, A. C., Jambou, R., et al.: Dextranase enhances antibiotic efficacy in experimental viridans streptococcal endocarditis. Antimicrob. Agents Chemother. *38*:953–958, 1994.
106. Michalek, S. M., McGhee, J. R., Mestecky, J., et al.: Ingestion of *Streptococcus mutans* induces secretory immunoglobulin A and caries immunity. Science *192*:1238–1240, 1976.
107. Michel, R. S., DeFlora, E., Jefferies, J., et al.: Recurrent meningitis in a child with inner ear dysplasia. Pediatr. Infect. Dis. J. *11*:336–338, 1992.
108. Molina, J. M., Leport, C., Bure, A., et al.: Clinical and bacterial features of infections caused by *Streptococcus milleri*. Scand. J. Infect. Dis. *23*:659–666, 1991.
109. Monefeldt, K., Helgeland, K., and Tollefsen, T.: In vitro activation of the classical pathway of complement by a streptococcal lipoteichoic acid. Oral Microbiol. Immunol. *9*:70–76, 1994.
110. Moomjian, A. S., Sokal, M. M., and Vijayan, S.: Pathogenicity of alpha-hemolytic streptococci in the neonate. Am. J. Perinatol. *1*:319–321, 1984.
111. Morisaki, I., Mihara, J., Kato, K., et al.: Phenytoin-induced gingival overgrowth in rats infected with *Streptococcus sobrinus* 6715. Arch. Oral Biol. *35*:753–758, 1990.

112. Murray, H. W., Gross, K. C., Masur, H., et al.: Serious infections caused by *Streptococcus milleri*. Am. J. Med. *64*:759–764, 1978.
113. Newbrun, E.: Preventing dental caries: Breaking the chain of transmission. J. Am. Dent. Assoc. *123*:55–59, 1992.
114. Parrillo, J. E., Borst, G. C., Mazur, M. H., et al.: Endocarditis due to resistant viridans streptococci during oral penicillin chemoprophylaxis. N. Engl. J. Med. *300*:296–300, 1979.
115. Parrish, L. C., Kretzschmar, D. P., and Swan, R. H.: Osteomyelitis associated with chronic periodontitis: A report of three cases. J. Periodontol. *60*:716–722, 1989.
116. Pearce, C., Bowden, G. H., Evans, M., et al.: Identification of pioneer viridans streptococci in the oral cavity of human neonates. J. Med. Microbiol. *42*:67–72, 1995.
117. Peiris, V., and Oppenheim, B. A.: Antimicrobial activity of cytotoxic drugs may influence isolation of bacteria and fungi from blood cultures. J. Clin. Pathol. *46*:1124–1125, 1993.
118. Peterson, E. M., Shigei, J. T., Woolard, A., et al.: Identification of viridans streptococci by three commercial systems. Am. J. Clin. Pathol. *90*:87–91, 1988.
119. Pizzo, P. A., Ladisch, S., and Ribichaud, K.: Treatment of gram-positive septicemia in cancer patients. Cancer *45*:206–207, 1980.
120. Pizzo, P. A., Ladisch, S., and Witebsky, F. G.: Alpha-hemolytic streptococci: Clinical significance in the cancer patient. Med. Pediatr. Oncol. *4*:367–370, 1978.
121. Poole, P. M., and Wilson, G.: *Streptococcus milleri* in the appendix. J. Clin. Pathol. *30*:937–942, 1977.
122. Potgieter, E., Carmichael, M., Koornhof, H. J., et al.: In vitro antimicrobial susceptibility of *viridans* streptococci isolated from blood cultures. Eur. J. Clin. Microbiol. Infect. Dis. *11*:543–546, 1992.
123. Potgieter, E., and Chalkley, L. J.: Reciprocal transfer of penicillin resistance genes between *Streptococcus pneumoniae*, *Streptococcus mitior* and *Streptococcus sanguis*. J. Antimicrob. Chemother. *28*:463–465, 1991.
124. Pratter, M. R., and Irwin, R. S.: Viridans streptococcal pulmonary parenchymal infections. J. A. M. A. *243*:2515–2517, 1980.
125. Pulliam, L., Dall, L., Inokuchi, S., et al.: Effects of exopolysaccharide production by viridans streptococci on penicillin therapy of experimental endocarditis. J. Infect. Dis. *151*:153–156, 1985.
126. Quinn, J. P., DiVincenzo, C. A., Lucks, D. A., et al.: Serious infections due to penicillin-resistant strains of viridans streptococci with altered penicillin-binding proteins. J. Infect. Dis. *157*:764–769, 1988.
127. Rapeport, K. B., Giron, J. A., and Rosner, F.: *Streptococcus mitis* endocarditis: Report of 17 cases. Arch. Intern. Med. *146*:2361–2363, 1986.
128. Reed, E., Arneson, M., Vaughan, W., et al.: *Streptococcus viridans* (SV): A significant cause of neutropenic fever (NF) that caused death in some patients not empirically treated for gram-positive (GP) bacteria. Proc. Annu. Meeting Am. Soc. Clin. Oncol. *9*:A1239, 1990.
129. Ribner, B. S., and Freimer, E. H.: Osteomyelitis caused by viridans streptococci. Arch. Intern. Med. *142*:1739, 1982.
130. Richard, P., Amador Del Valle, G., Moreau, P., et al.: Viridans streptococcal bacteraemia in patients with neutropenia. Lancet *345*:1607–1609, 1995.
131. Ringden, O., Heimdahl, A., Lonnqvist, B., et al.: Decreased incidence of viridans streptococcal septicaemia in allogeneic bone marrow transplant recipients after the introduction of acyclovir. Lancet *1*:744, 1984.
132. Roberts, R. B., Krieger, A. G., Schiller, N. L., et al.: Viridans streptococcal endocarditis: The role of various species, including pyridoxal-dependent streptococci. Rev. Infect. Dis. *1*:955–966, 1979.
133. Roos, K., Holm, S. E., Grahn, E., et al.: Alpha-streptococci as supplementary treatment of recurrent streptococcal tonsillitis: A randomized placebo-controlled study. Scand. J. Infect. Dis. *25*:31–35, 1993.
134. Rose, H. D.: Viridans streptococcal pneumonia. J. A. M. A. *245*:32, 1981.
135. Rozenberg-Arska, M., Dekker, A., Verdonck, L., et al.: Prevention of bacteremia caused by alpha-hemolytic streptococci by roxithromycin (RU-28 965) in granulocytopenic patients receiving ciprofloxacin. Infection *17*:240–244, 1989.
136. Rubin, M., Hathorn, J. W., Marshall, D., et al.: Gram-positive infections and the use of vancomycin in 550 episodes of fever and neutropenia. Ann. Intern. Med. *108*:30–35, 1988.
137. Rubin, M. M., Sanfilippo, R. J., and Sadoff, R. S.: Vertebral osteomyelitis secondary to an oral infection. J. Oral Maxillofac. Surg. *49*:897–900, 1991.
138. Ruoff, K. L.: *Streptococcus. In* Murray, P. R., Baron, E. J., Pfaller, M. A., et al. (eds.): Manual of Clinical Microbiology. 6th ed. Washington, D.C., ASM Press, 1995, pp. 299–307.
139. Ruoff, K. L., and Kunz, L. J.: Identification of viridans streptococci isolated from clinical specimens. J. Clin. Microbiol. *15*:920–925, 1982.
140. Ruoff, K. L., and Kunz, L. J.: Use of the Rapid STREP system for identification of viridans streptococcal species. J. Clin. Microbiol. *18*:1138–1140, 1983.
141. Saarela, M., von Troil-Linden, B., Torkko, H., et al.: Transmission of oral bacterial species between spouses. Oral Microbiol. Immunol. *8*:349–354, 1993.
142. Sarkar, T. K., Murarka, R. S., and Gilardi, G. L.: Primary *Streptococcus* viridans pneumonia. Chest *96*:831–834, 1989.
143. Schollin, J.: Adherence of alpha-hemolytic streptococci to human endocardial, endothelial and buccal cells. Acta Paediatr. Scand. *77*:705–710, 1988.
144. Schollin, J., and Danielsson, D.: Bacterial adherence to endothelial cells from rat heart, with special regard to alpha-hemolytic streptococci. APMIS *96*:428–432, 1988.
145. Shanson, D. C., Thomas, F., and Wilson, D.: Effect of volume of blood cultured on detection of *Streptococcus* viridans bacteraemia. J. Clin. Pathol. *37*:568–570, 1984.
146. Shanson, D. C., Thomas, F. D., and Johnstone, D.: Improving detection of "viridans *Streptococcus*" bacteraemia by adding sodium polyanethol sulphonate to blood cultures. J. Clin. Pathol. *38*:1346–1348, 1985.
147. Shaw, J. H.: Causes and control of dental caries. N. Engl. J. Med. *317*:996–1004, 1987.
148. Shenep, J. L., Hughes, W. T., Roberson, P. K., et al.: Vancomycin, ticarcillin, and amikacin compared with ticarcillin-clavulanate and amikacin in the empirical treatment of febrile, neutropenic children with cancer. N. Engl. J. Med. *319*:1053–1058, 1988.
149. Shibl, A. M.: Effect of antibiotics on adherence of microorganisms to epithelial cell surfaces. Rev. Infect. Dis. *7*:51–65, 1985.
150. Shlaes, D. M., Marino, J., and Jacobs, M. R.: Infection caused by vancomycin-resistant *Streptococcus sanguis* II. Antimicrob. Agents Chemother. *25*:527–528, 1984.
151. Shulman, S. T.: *Streptococcus viridans*—not! Am. J. Dis. Child. *147*:611, 1993.
152. Smith, D. J., Anderson, J. M., King, W. F., et al.: Oral streptococcal colonization of infants. Oral. Microbiol. Immunol. *8*:1–4, 1993.
153. Soell, M., Holveck, F., Scholler, M., et al.: Binding of *Streptococcus mutans* SR protein to human monocytes: Production of tumor necrosis factor, interleukin 1, and interleukin 6. Infect. Immun. *62*:1805–1812, 1994.
154. Sotiropoulos, S. V., Jackson, M. A., Woods, G. M., et al.: Alpha-streptococcal septicemia in leukemic children treated with continuous or large dosage intermittent cytosine arabinoside. Pediatr. Infect. Dis. J. *8*:755–758, 1989.
155. Speck, W. T., Spear, S. S., Krongrad, E., et al.: Transient bacteremia in pediatric patients after dental extraction. Am. J. Dis. Child *130*:406–407, 1976.
156. Sprunt, K., Redman, W., and Leidy, G.: Penicillin-resistant alpha streptococci in pharynx of patients given oral penicillin. Pediatrics *42*:957–968, 1968.
157. Staves, E., and Tinanoff, N.: Decline in salivary *S. mutans* levels in children who have received short-term antibiotic therapy. Pediatr. Dent. *13*:176–178, 1991.
158. Steiner, M., Villablanca, J., Kersey, J., et al.: Viridans streptococcal shock in bone marrow transplantation patients. Am. J. Hematol. *42*:354–358, 1993.
159. Stimmel, H. M., Orchen, J. J., Skaff, D. M., et al.: Penicillin-resistant alpha-hemolytic streptococci in children with heart disease who take penicillin daily. ASDC J. Dent. Child *48*:29–32, 1981.
160. Sullam, P. M., Frank, U., Yeaman, M. R., et al.: Effect of thrombocytopenia on the early course of streptococcal endocarditis. J. Infect. Dis. *168*:910–914, 1993.
161. Sussman, J. I., Baron, E. J., Tenenbaum, M. J., et al.: Viridans streptococcal endocarditis: Clinical, microbiological, and echocardiographic correlations. J. Infect. Dis. *154*:597–603, 1986.
162. Svinhufvud, L. B., Heimdahl, A., and Nord, C. E.: Effect of topical administration of vancomycin versus chlorhexidine on alpha-hemolytic streptococci in oral cavity. Oral Med. *66*:304–309, 1988.
163. Takada, H., Kawabata, Y., Tamura, M., et al.: Cytokine induction by extracellular products of oral viridans group streptococci. Infect. Immun. *61*:5252–5260, 1993.
164. Tappuni, A. R., and Challacombe, S. J.: Distribution and isolation frequency of eight streptococcal species in saliva from predentate and dentate children and adults. J. Dent. Res. *72*:31-36, 1993.
165. Tasaka, T., Nagai, M., Sasaki, K., et al.: *Streptococcus mitis* septicemia in leukemia patients: Clinical features and outcome. Intern. Med. *32*:221–224, 1993.
166. Thibodeau, E. A., and O'Sullivan, D. M.: Salivary mutans streptococci and incidence of caries in preschool children. Caries Res. *29*:148–153, 1995.
167. Thorig, L., Daha, M. R., Eulderink, F., et al.: Experimental *Streptococcus sanguis* endocarditis: Immune complexes and renal involvement. Clin. Exp. Immunol. *40*:469–477, 1980.
168. Tinanoff, N.: Review of the antimicrobial action of stannous fluoride. J. Clin. Dent. *2*:22–27, 1990.
169. Twetman, S., Mattiasson, A., Varela, J. R., et al.: Mutans streptococci in saliva and dental caries in children living in a high and a low fluoride area. Oral Microbiol. Immunol. *5*:169–171, 1990.
170. Ullman, R. F., Strampfer, M. J., and Cunha, B. A.: *Streptococcus mutans* vertebral osteomyelitis. Heart Lung *17*:319–321, 1988.
171. Ullsfoss, B. N., Ogaard, B., Arends, J., et al.: Effect of a combined chlorhexidine and NaF mouthrinse: An in vivo human caries model study. Scand. J. Dent. Res. *102*:109–112, 1994.
172. van Houte, J.: Bacterial adherence in the mouth. Rev. Infect. Dis. *5*(Suppl. 4):S659–S669, 1983.
173. van Houte, J.: Role of micro-organisms in caries etiology. J. Dent. Res. *73*:672–681, 1994.

174. Van Loveren, C., Van de Plassche-Simons, Y. M., De Soet, J. J., et al.: Acidogenesis in relation to fluoride resistance of *Streptococcus mutans*. Oral Microbiol. Immunol. *6*:288–291, 1991.
175. Vicente, M. V., Olay, T., and Rodriguez, A.: Experimental endocarditis caused by *Streptococcus sanguis*: Single and combined antibiotic therapy. Antimicrob. Agents Chemother. *20*:10–14, 1981.
176. Watanakunakorn, C., and Pantelakis, J.: Alpha-hemolytic streptococcal bacteremia: A review of 203 episodes during 1980–1991. Scand. J. Infect. Dis. *25*:403–408, 1993.
177. Weinberger, S. J., and Wright, G. Z.: A comparison of *S. mutans* clinical assessment methods. Pediatr. Dent. *12*:375–379, 1990.
178. Wilcox, M. H., Winstanley, T. G., Douglas, C. W., et al.: Susceptibility of alpha-haemolytic streptococci causing endocarditis to benzylpenicillin and ten cephalosporins. J. Antimicrob. Chemother. *32*:63–69, 1993.
179. Yee, Y., Farber, B., and Mates, S.: Mechanism of penicillin-streptomycin synergy for clinical isolates of viridans streptococci. J. Infect. Dis. *154*:531–534, 1986.
180. Zickert, I., Emilson, C. G., Ekblom, K., et al.: Prolonged oral reduction of *Streptococcus mutans* in humans after chlorhexidine disinfection followed by fluoride treatment. Scand. J. Dent. Res. *95*:315–319, 1987.
181. Zito, E. T., and Daneo-Moore, L.: Transformation of *Streptococcus sanguis* to intrinsic penicillin resistance. J. Gen. Microbiol. *134*:1237–1249, 1988.

90

PNEUMOCOCCAL INFECTIONS

David W. Teele

The pneumococcus *Streptococcus pneumoniae* continues to be a leading cause of morbidity and mortality in persons of all ages. Most children experience some form of pneumococcal infection (e.g., otitis media or pneumonia), and some develop sepsis or meningitis. Despite more than a century of research, many aspects of pneumococcal disease remain obscure. The continued frequency and severity of pneumococcal diseases, coupled with the knowledge that antimicrobial therapy invariably does not prevent illness or death, and the emergence of strains of pneumococci resistant to most antimicrobial agents serve to underscore the need for better understanding of pneumococcal infections. Currently, attention is concentrated on efforts to prevent these infections by the development and use of appropriate vaccines.

HISTORY

Interested readers should consult both White's *Biology of the Pneumococcus* and Heffron's *Pneumonia, with Special Reference to* Pneumococcus *Lobar Pneumonia* for a complete account of the long and fascinating history of this organism.[29, 66] Pasteur and Sternberg, working independently in 1880 and 1881, discovered the pneumococcus. Each recovered pneumococci from rabbits injected with human saliva. Friedlander demonstrated pneumococci in tissue from humans with pneumonia in 1882 and in the following year found them in most cases of "acute pneumonia." Friedlander described both the characteristic capsule and colonial morphologic features. In 1884, for the first time, he recovered pneumococci from the blood of patients with pneumonia. During the next few years, pneumococci were found in virtually all types of infection, including meningitis and otitis media. Thus, by 1890, researchers had established the pneumococcus as the most common cause of acute pneumonia as well as a principal cause of meningitis and other serious infections.

During the next decade, researchers immunized animals with cell-free filtrates of pneumococci, demonstrated that serum from immune animals could protect against experimental pneumococcal infection, deduced the role of immunity in promoting phagocytosis, and noted agglutination of pneumococci by serum from immune animals. In 1897, Pane treated humans suffering from pneumonia with serum from such animals. By 1900, researchers had laid the foundation for immunotherapy of pneumococcal pneumonia, the only effective treatment until the advent of chemotherapy.

Over the next few years, investigators noted that agglutination of pneumococci appeared to depend on the strain isolated. In 1910, Neufeld and Haendel classified pneumococci into several discrete serotypes on the basis of the appearance of capsular swelling, the quellung reaction. Only strains exposed to homologous serum showed capsular swelling. Their work made possible all subsequent epidemiologic investigations of pneumococcal infection, immunotherapy with type-specific serum, and development of vaccines capable of preventing infection.

After these discoveries, researchers concentrated on several aspects of pneumococcal disease, including identification of multiple serotypes and their roles in disease, production and clinical use of antisera, and development of pneumococcal vaccines.

Original classification of pneumococci was limited to types I, II, III, and IV (others). Currently, more than 80 serotypes have been identified. Certain serotypes proved to be more virulent than others, and virulence depended, to some extent, on the species of animal infected.

Antisera used to treat pneumococcal pneumonia proved strikingly effective when type-specific sera were used. As early as 1913, Cole and associates showed that treatment with antisera lowered fatality rates from 25 to 30 per cent for untreated pneumonia to 10.5 per cent for treated cases. In addition to all types of allergic reactions, difficulties associated with this treatment included the necessity of identifying the causative serotype and the need for the earliest possible administration of antisera. White compared the efficacy of early antisera therapy with results of delayed treatment; the death rate was 403/1614 (25 per cent) with no therapy, 32/377 (8.5 per cent) with therapy within 3 days of onset, and 24/127 (18.9 per cent) with therapy at 4 or more days after onset. Unfortunately, therapy with antisera had no beneficial effect on localized pneumococcal infections, such as meningitis or endocarditis. Despite these drawbacks, use of antisera soon became widespread. The advent of chemotherapy—first sulfa compounds, then penicillin—was followed by a precipitous decline in the use of antisera. Antimicrobial agents killed or inhibited pneumococci, regardless of serotype, and cured patients with previously incurable localized infections.[66]

Coincident with research resulting in general use of antisera came research into the efficacy of pneumococcal vaccines. Proof of efficacy lagged, so that indisputable evidence of protection induced by vaccination was not available until 1945. The ability of pneumococci to cause epidemic pneumococcal pneumonia in young men crowded into army camps or in gold mines allowed large-scale trials. Highlights of the development of effective vaccines include the trial of Wright and associates[67] in South Africa, beginning in 1911. Using a vaccine made with whole, killed pneumococci, this trial produced inconclusive results. Many trials followed; some showed trends toward protection. In 1930, Francis and Tillett[21] showed capsular polysaccharides to be immunogenic for humans. Ekwurzel and colleagues,[19] during 1933 to 1937, used a vaccine containing such polysaccharides and showed it to be probably effective.

Finally, in 1945, MacLeod and associates[47] published results of a trial carried out in recruits in the U.S. Army Air Force. This trial showed vaccination to be strikingly effective in preventing pneumococcal pneumonia due to serotypes contained in the vaccine. Regrettably, interest in vaccination waned rapidly with the general availability of penicillin. Manufacturers voluntarily withdrew their vaccines from the market. This unfortunate attitude persisted for the next two decades, until there came realization of the inability of chemotherapy to prevent many deaths from pneumococcal disease.[3] Fortunately, a few farsighted individuals continued to maintain surveillance of those serotypes causing human disease. Their work allowed reintroduction of a pneumococcal vaccine. The current status of vaccinations is discussed later in this chapter.

MORPHOLOGY

For a number of years, in the United States, pneumococci carried the designation *Diplococcus pneumoniae*; the change to *S. pneumoniae* reflects a close kinship between pneumococci and other streptococci. Microscopic examination showed pneumococci to be gram-positive, lance-ovate cocci, usually in pairs, with the long axes forming a straight line. Elongated or pointed forms are common. Under certain conditions, pneumococci form chains, the length of which depends on the type of media. As cultures age, autolytic enzymes cause first a change to gram-negative staining and then dissolution of the cocci. Proper use of methylene blue or electron microscopy shows virulent isolates to have a capsule. Capsular size varies considerably, with types 3 and 37 having thick capsules. Pneumococci strikingly resemble other usually nonpathogenic, alpha-hemolytic streptococci when Gram stained and observed by microscopy. This similarly presents a diagnostic pitfall because such streptococci normally are resident in the oropharynx and may contaminate specimens of sputum.

In broth, pneumococci grow diffusely and sediment only as the broth becomes acidic. Nonencapsulated strains sediment rapidly. On solid media, encapsulated pneumococci produce characteristic round, shiny colonies about 1 mm in diameter. Types 3 and 37 produce much larger mucoid colonies. As cultures age (often within 24 hours), the center of the colony subsides, causing a central dimple. Rough strains produce small, dull colonies. When grown on media containing blood, all pneumococci cause partial (alpha) hemolysis of surrounding erythrocytes. Alpha-hemolytic streptococci may show similar morphologic colonial features, although they usually do not develop the central dimples.

Culture Requirements

Pneumococci require multiple nutritional factors. The pH must be adjusted carefully to an ideal of 7.2 to 7.4. Equine or ovine erythrocytes, which contain catalase, are added to the broth to destroy hydrogen peroxide produced by pneumococci. Blood must be added if pneumococci are to be stored for any length of time.

Pneumococci are facultative anaerobes, growing either aerobically or anaerobically. Rare strains are obligate anaerobes.[68] Optimum growth occurs in an atmosphere with reduced oxygen and increased carbon dioxide. Some strains grow poorly, if at all, in the absence of carbon dioxide.[2]

Identification of Pneumococci

Most laboratories employ several tests for the identification of isolates with appropriate colonial morphologic features. As in all of microbiology, many new and apparently simpler tests have appeared (see later). However, a review of more traditional methods is in order. Optochin (optoquine), a derivative of quinine, was used first to treat pneumococcal infections, but toxicity and rapid development of resistance limited such use. Optochin, however, may be used to help identify pneumococci because they generally are sensitive and alpha-hemolytic streptococci generally are resistant. Paper disks impregnated with optochin are laid on a lawn of pneumococci, and the plate is incubated overnight. With currently available 6-mm disks, inhibition, with a zone greater than 14 mm, identifies an isolate as a pneumococcus with greater than 90 per cent accuracy. Limitations include the time required and the inability to identify the serotype.

Neufeld, the discoverer of the quellung reaction, also reported the lytic effect of bile salts on pneumococci. Addition of an equal volume of bile broth to a broth culture of pneumococci results in prompt lysis of the cocci. Alpha-hemolytic streptococci do not lyse.

Injection of most serotypes of pneumococci into mice causes rapid death, and "mouse virulence" has been used to identify pneumococci. Alpha-hemolytic streptococci are avirulent for mice. Unfortunately, so are certain strains of pneumococci; type 14, the most common invasive strain in children, is almost avirulent for mice.

Fermentation of inulin is a characteristic of most pneumococci, but certain other streptococci ferment inulin as well.

Thus, none of these tests identifies pneumococci with certainty, and all are time-consuming. Neufeld's quellung reaction avoids all of these problems and allows immediate, accurate identification. One mixes equal volumes of a suspension of bacteria, methylene blue, and antiserum on a slide, applies a coverslip, and examines the bacteria by light microscopy. Appearance of the quellung reaction (capsular swelling) identifies genus, species, and serotype. Regrettably, most laboratories neglect Neufeld's quellung reaction. Its use allows immediate, accurate identification of pneumococci, either in body fluids or in culture. Currently, researchers have identified more than 80 serotypes, although many share antigens and are closely related. Table 90–1 enumerates the American and Danish systems of serotyping.[46] Only Danish antisera are available at present, but many older publications relied on the American system of enumeration. Identification of infecting serotypes monitors those responsible for disease in humans and is essential for proper use of pneumococcal vaccines.

Recently introduced rapid tests for the identification of pneumococci growing in liquid bacteriologic cultures employ latex particles coated with antibodies to all 84 currently identified serotypes. When these pneumococci are mixed with fluid containing pneumococcal antigen, agglutination occurs.[9]

Identification of Carriers of Pneumococci

Study of the epidemiology of pneumococcal infection requires identification of those carrying pneumococci in the

TABLE 90–1. Correlation between the American and the Danish Nomenclature of the Genus *Pneumococcus*

United States	Denmark	United States	Denmark
1	1	42	33B
2	2	43	11A
3	3	44	18A
4	4	45	40
5	5	46	23A
6	6A	47	35A
7	7A	48	7B
8	8	49	9L
9	9N	50	7C
10	10	51	7
11	11	52	47
12	12	53	11C
13	13	54	15B
14	14	55	18B
15	15	56	18C
16	16	57	19A
17	17	58	19B
18	18	59	19C
19	19	60	24B?
20	20	61	35C
21	21	62	35A
22	22	63	22A
23	23	64	23B
24	24	65	24A
25	25	66	35B
26	6B	67	32A
27	27	68	9V
28	28	69	39
29	29	70	33
30	15A	71	38
31	31	72	45
32	32	73	46
33	9A	74	41A
34	10A	75	43
35	35	76	11B
36	36	77	15C
37	37	78	17A
38	41	79	28A
39	33C	80	42
40	33A	81	44
41	34		

upper respiratory tract. Certain techniques maximize the yield of pneumococci and permit detection of most carriers.

Most investigators interested in identification of carriers obtain cultures from both the nasopharynx and the throat. Whereas some have found one location more likely to yield pneumococci,[31] others found no difference.[7] Usual microbiologic methods, that is, plating a single swab on blood agar and incubating with carbon dioxide, fail to identify many persons colonized by pneumococci. The addition of a gentamicin or neomycin disk to the primary plate may increase the yield. Inoculation of respiratory tract secretions into mice enhances the yield of pneumococci, but certain serotypes commonly found in children are almost avirulent for mice. Addition of 5 μg/mL of gentamicin to agar suppresses many bacteria from the nasopharynx and significantly increases the rate of isolation of pneumococci.[15] Multiple cultures from the same site may increase isolation of pneumococci.[17]

EPIDEMIOLOGY

Pneumococci normally reside in the pharynx of healthy people in all parts of the world. Pneumococci spread from person to person in droplets of respiratory tract secretions, and infection of the upper respiratory tract aids spread.[27] Thus, both colonization and disease due to pneumococci are more common in winter and spring.

Rates of colonization depend on a number of variables, including age, race, exposure to young children, and population studied. Maximum rates usually occur in young children in institutions.[45] Attendance at day care is associated strongly with increased of rates of carriage in general and with increased rates of carriage of penicillin-resistant strains in particular. For other young children, studies have found the prevalence of colonization as high as 97 per cent,[7] but most report rates of 25 to 50 per cent. Most children are colonized at some time during the course of a year. Adults with no contact with young children have the lowest rate of colonization, approximately 5 per cent.

Serotypes isolated from well children mirror, in general, serotypes causing disease in children. Results vary somewhat with the time and the location of studies, but types 6, 14, 18, 19, and 23 account for a large majority of isolates. Of 1205 episodes of pneumococcal otitis media, 63 per cent were due to these five serotypes.[4] These same five caused 76 per cent of episodes of pneumococcal bacteremia occurring in children at Boston City Hospital (Teele, D. W., unpublished data). Over the years, some shifts have occurred in serotypes causing disease. For example, type 1 pneumococci once caused more than 50 per cent of pneumococcal pneumonia in children at Boston City Hospital; in 1978, pneumonia in children due to this serotype was rare.[20] Such data allow preparation of pneumococcal vaccines containing a limited number of antigens and offering protection against most pneumococcal disease. Internationally, some variation occurs in the distribution of serotypes, thus complicating further the task of manufacturers of vaccines.

Several factors determine risk for pneumococcal disease. Age may be the most important because natural immunity strongly depends on age. Such immunity may be acquired either by simple carriage of pneumococci or by pneumococcal disease. In 1932, Sutliff and Finland[57] demonstrated the relationship between age and the bactericidal capacity of blood; Figure 90–1 shows this relationship. Immunity in the first few months of life apparently derives from maternal antibody passively transferred to the fetus. Children younger than 2 years of age respond erratically to pneumococcal antigens administered as vaccines.[14] Presumably, they respond poorly as well to antigens resulting from carriage or disease. These phenomena may explain the frequency of pneumococcal disease in young children. Pneumococcal bacteremia is most common in children 6 months to 24 months of age. The elderly also are at increased risk due to diminished immunologic capacity and to effects of underlying illness.

Race appears important, although data are limited. Blacks have been found to be at higher risk for pneumococcal meningitis, a finding explained only in part by the exquisite susceptibility of children with sickle-cell disease.[22]

Lack of data hinders calculations of rates of pneumococcal disease in children. Approximately 80 per cent of all children experience at least one attack of otitis media by age 3 years,[60] and pneumococci account for about half of all cases of bacterial otitis media. Because bacteria may be isolated from the middle ear of about 75 per cent of children with otitis media, one can calculate that about one-third of children have at least one attack of pneumococcal otitis media by age 3 years. Many experience repeated attacks. Despite the poor response of such children to pneumococcal polysaccharides, repeated episodes of otitis media to the same or closely related serotype are uncommon. The multiplicity of serotypes, however, may account for repeated attacks. In South Carolina, the

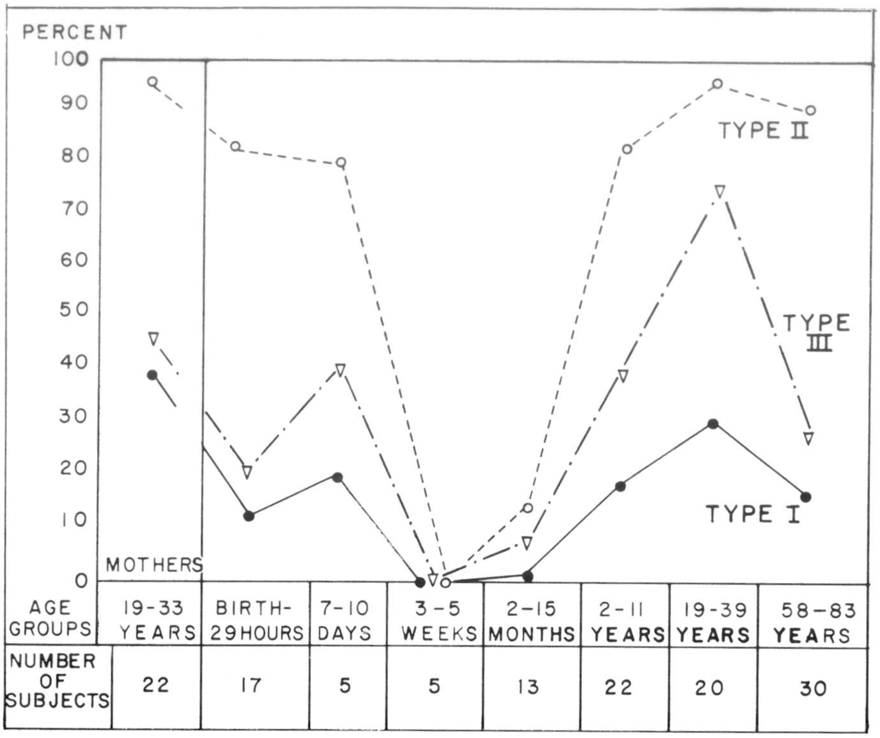

FIGURE 90–1. *Percentage of subjects in different age groups whose blood is pneumococcidal.*

average annual incidence for pneumococcal meningitis in persons of all ages was 0.89 per 100,000 for whites and 4.9 per 100,000 for blacks.[22] Similar data for pneumococcal pneumonia in childhood do not exist. The inability of young children to produce adequate specimens of sputum accounts for part of the scarcity of data; additionally, the rate of colonization by pneumococci in young children is so high as to cast suspicion on the validity of samples from the upper respiratory tract. Nonetheless, on the basis of isolates from the blood of young children with pneumonia, the pneumococcus accounts for most cases of bacterial pneumonia of childhood.

PATHOGENESIS

Pneumococci reach their target within the body either by hematogenous spread or by direct extension from colonized mucosal surfaces. Thus, whereas most cases of pneumococcal meningitis follow pneumococcal bacteremia, some cases result from direct spread to the meninges via a basilar or temporal fracture of the skull. Conversely, most cases of pneumococcal otitis media are not accompanied by bacteremia and result from extension from the nasopharynx to the middle ear via the eustachian tube. Pneumococcal pneumonia results, in most cases, from aspiration of pneumococci resident in the pharynx. Commonly, a preceding viral infection has compromised pulmonary mechanisms of defense by causing shedding of respiratory tract epithelium and increasing production of mucin.[6] Older data suggested that chance, in terms of the colonizing serotype, helped determine who developed pneumonia. Thus, uncommonly, certain virulent serotypes (e.g., type 3) simply colonized adults; more commonly, pneumonia followed acquisition of these serotypes. The high rates of carriage in well children suggest that this chain of events may be less important in children. Having infected the lung, pneumococci gain access to blood via lymphatics. Experimental pneumonia in rabbits indicated that lymph becomes infected before blood.

Although pneumococci most commonly cause bacteremia, otitis media, pneumonia, and meningitis, they can produce disease in virtually any organ. Before immunotherapy and chemotherapy, such "unusual" infections were relatively common. Today, they are less so. Nonetheless, as Table 90–2 shows, pneumococci infect many different organs.[20]

For more than a century, investigators have sought to identify the substances that initiate the inflammatory response. Capsular polysaccharide essentially is nontoxic; vaccines containing large amounts of this material cause minimal reactions. Whereas a serotype characterized by possession of a large capsule, e.g., type 3, is notably virulent, type 37, with a similarly large capsule, has little virulence.

On the other hand, most researchers now incriminate elements of the cell wall (peptidoglycan and techoic acid) in the development of the inflammatory response seen in pneumococcal infections. This topic has been reviewed by Bruyn and colleagues.[10]

Survival of a patient with disease due to pneumococci depends on a number of variables, including site of infection, underlying disease, and age of patient. Before chemotherapy, pneumococcal meningitis was universally fatal, whereas pneumococcal pneumonia killed only about 25 per cent of patients. Austrian and Gold,[3] in 1964, dramatically illustrated the role of age and underlying disease when their survey of mortality associated with bacteremic pneumococcal pneumonia destroyed the complacency of decades induced by chemotherapy. The aged and infirm were likely to die, despite immediate and appropriate therapy with penicillin.

Today, normal children rarely die of pneumococcal disease; thus, prognosis must be related to the likelihood of permanent sequelae. Pneumococci do not cause necrosis in pulmonary tissue, and survivors rapidly regain normal pulmonary function.[36] Many children recovering from pneumococcal meningitis are found to have neurologic sequelae. Some investigators believe that the first attack of pneumococcal otitis media in some way predisposes to subsequent attacks of otitis media.[35]

TABLE 90–2. Occurrence of Specific Types of Pneumococci in 152 "Other" Infected Foci and Body Fluids* at Boston City Hospital during Selected Years between 1935 and 1974

Infected Site	Number of Strains	Specific Types† (Number of Strains)
Brain abscess	2	3, 4
Atrioventricular shunt	1	22
Mastoid	3	3 (2), 19
Ethmoid sinus	2	2, 3
Lacrimal duct	2	4, P
Alveolar abscess	1	3
Tonsillar abscess	1	3
Esophagus	1	3
Peritoneum	32	3 (4), 4, 6 (2), 7 (3), 8, 9 (2), 10 (3), 12, 13, 14 + 18, 18 (2), 19, 22 (2), 25, P (5), U
Gallbladder	2	3 (2)
Perirectal abscess	1	3
Feces	2	3, 19
Urine	17	3 (5), 6, 8 (2), 9 (2), 18, 19, 20 (2), 23, 28, P
Prostatic fluid	1	34
Vagina	5	3, 6, 9, 19, 23
Bartholin gland	1	11
Uterus	1	6
Placenta	1	14
Vernix caseosa	1	6
Bone marrow	1	21
Subcutaneous abscess	18	2,‡ 3 (3), 4, 6, 12, 14, 17 (2), 19, 20, 23, 31, 41, P (2), U
Infected or draining wound	31	3 (7), 6, 9, 11, 13 (2), 14, 14 + 18, 15 (2), 19, 20, 21, 23 (4), 24, 29, 31, 35, P (2)
Breast abscess	1	3
Abscess of hand	2	3, U
Abscess or ulcer of foot	4	3, 19 (2), 31
Synovial fluid	16	1, 3 (2), 4, 7, 9, 10, 12 18, 19 (2), 20, P (4)
"Cyst"	1	3
Source (?)	1	18

*From other than blood, cerebrospinal fluid, otitic fluid, or eye.
†The number of strains (if more than one) per type is given in parentheses. P, strains identified with one of the pooled sera but not further identified with specific serotypes. U, untypable; strain failed to react with any of the available pooled typing zero.
‡Isolated in 1965.

Before the availability of chemotherapy, recovery of a patient with pneumococcal pneumonia depended on the development of type-specific antibody. Although serum and white blood cells from nonimmune children kill pneumococci, probably by use of the alternative pathway for activation of complement, they do so slowly. The importance of this pathway is illustrated best by the inability of children with sickle-cell disease to handle pneumococcal infection.[16, 37, 51] These children and others with asplenia may die rapidly, despite prompt, vigorous therapy.[38, 40, 56]

DIAGNOSIS

Isolation of pneumococci from certain fluids establishes a firm diagnosis; thus, pneumococci should be sought in cerebrospinal fluid, blood, pleural fluid, or effusions of the middle ear. Examination with Gram stain offers prompt, suggestive information, but both alpha-hemolytic streptococci and group B streptococci may mimic closely the appearance of pneumococci. Thus, when Gram stain reveals organisms compatible with pneumococci, one should use the quellung reaction or other methods, such as latex agglutination, in an attempt to confirm the identification. Standard culture techniques require 24 to 48 hours. Neufeld's quellung reaction often allows confirmation in less than an hour.

Whereas most patients with pneumococcal meningitis have cerebrospinal fluid yielding pneumococci, only a minority of those with pneumococcal pneumonia have a demonstrated bacteremia. The exact prevalence of bacteremia associated with pneumococcal pneumonia is unknown. Limitations include the timing of cultures (e.g., taking of blood for culture before or after bacteremia) as well as the volume of blood drawn for culture (the number of pneumococci per cubic centimeter of blood varies from several to many thousand).[63, 65] Data from the era preceding chemotherapy suggest that about one-third of patients with pneumococcal pneumonia have an accompanying bacteremia. Some believe that all patients with pneumococcal pneumonia are bacteremic, however transiently.[29]

While awaiting results of cultures of blood, clinicians turn to microscopic examination and culture of sputum. Even when used for adults, this method is beset with controversy.[5, 62] Difficulties are compounded for pediatricians by the inability of children to produce sputum and the high rates of colonization by pneumococci. Thus, pediatricians generally must use other methods to diagnose pneumococcal pneumonia. Direct aspiration of fluid from the affected lung allows rapid, accurate diagnosis,[41] but most perform this procedure reluctantly, if at all. Therefore, researchers have sought constellations of signs and symptoms significantly associated with bacteremia. Such searches are handicapped by the very problem they are trying to solve: how to diagnose nonbacteremic pneumococcal pneumonia. Features associated with bacteremic pneumococcal pneumonia in children include high temperature (>38.9° C [102° F]), leukocytosis (>15,000/mm^3), and lobar or segmental consolidation.[61] How often these features are associated with nonbacteremic pneumococcal pneumonia remains unknown.

In order to solve this dilemma, efforts have turned to the detection of pneumococcal antigens in blood, sputum, urine, or cerebrospinal fluid. Methods used include counterimmunoelectrophoresis,[12, 13] latex agglutination,[11] and radioimmunoassay. These efforts have met with limited success owing to both the multiplicity of serotypes and the various technical difficulties. Currently, unless a child already has received therapy with antimicrobial agents, these indirect methods are of only adjunctive importance. Nonetheless, these methods have great potential and must be pursued.

More recently, the new tools of the molecular biologist have been turned to the same task of diagnosis. Considerable work has been accomplished, and is being done as this chapter is written, using the technique of polymerase chain reaction. Efforts have concentrated on serum and sputum,[26, 28, 54, 55, 69] but, obviously, urine and cerebrospinal fluid also will be tested.

TREATMENT

For sensitive strains of pneumococci, penicillin remains the drug of choice for pneumococcal infections. The prevalence of resistant strains has increased alarmingly and, in some cases, explosively. This problem is discussed later in this chapter.

Sensitive strains of pneumococci are inhibited and killed by an average concentration of about 0.01 μg/mL. Ordinary doses of penicillin produce levels of drug in blood and most other fluids that exceed this concentration by many hundredfold. Currently recommended dosages of penicillin G for pneumococcal infections of childhood are as follows: for minor infections (e.g., otitis media), 50,000 units/kg/day; for serious infections other than meningitis (e.g., sepsis), 100,000 to 200,000 units/kg/day; for meningitis, 300,000 units/kg/day. Penicillin V, available only in a form suitable for oral dosage, should be used only for less serious infections, such as otitis media or pneumonia. Recommended dosage of penicillin V is 50 to 100 mg/kg/day. Many other penicillins, such as ampicillin and related compounds or methicillin and related compounds, show great activity against pneumococci. In practice, these agents add nothing but additional cost and toxicity and are not drugs of choice for pneumococcal infection. In parts of the world where resistance is relatively uncommon, erythromycin remains an effective, safe alternative to penicillin, as do the cephalosporins for patients who can tolerate these agents. Concern for diffusion into cerebrospinal fluid makes the older cephalosporins undesirable alternatives to penicillin for serious infections. Recently, some third-generation cephalosporins, such as ceftriaxone, have established a record of proven safety and efficacy for all types of disease, including meningitis.

Many other agents are active against pneumococci. Tetracyclines inhibit many pneumococci, but some organisms are resistant. Clindamycin shares the deficiencies of the cephalosporins. Many strains of pneumococci are resistant to sulfa drugs, but trimethoprim-sulfamethoxazole offers promise in areas where resistance remains uncommon. Aminoglycosides and polymyxins do not inhibit or kill pneumococci and must not be used to treat such infections.

In the last decade, two varieties of resistance to penicillin have appeared in pneumococci from various parts of the world. Moderately or relatively resistant strains (minimal inhibitory concentration [MIC] > 0.1 μg/mL to 1.0 μg/mL) (now termed intermediately resistant strains) have appeared rather abruptly in most parts of the world. Recently, 18 per cent of isolates from children in Atlanta had such resistance.[32] In the past, these strains have proved most troublesome when they caused meningitis. Highly resistant strains (MIC ≥2.0) (now termed resistant strains) accounted for 8 per cent of isolates in this same study from Atlanta. In parts of Europe and Africa as well as Iceland, resistant strains have become highly prevalent.

Resistance in penicillin stems from modification of penicillin-binding proteins, probably through the use of DNA obtained from other species. These may then have been shared horizontally with other pneumococci. Finally, resistant strains have spread geographically, probably encouraged by misuse of antimicrobial agents.[64]

In the United States and elsewhere, children appear especially likely to become infected by these resistant pneumococci. Day care centers seem to provide unusually good opportunities for spread to other children.[8, 18, 30, 53]

Unfortunately, these organisms also have learned to become resistant to many other useful agents, including cephalosporins, trimethoprim-sulfamethoxazole, and the macrolides, to name a few. Recently, in Spain, 29 per cent of patients with pneumococcal pneumonia were infected with resistant strains and 6 per cent of strains were resistant to the cephalosporins.[50] In 1989, in Hungary, 49 per cent of pneumococci tested were resistant.[48]

Treatment of infections due to resistant pneumococci must be considered to be in a state of flux. First, the prevalence of resistance is changing rapidly in most parts of the world. Second, data from clinical investigations will continue to become available in the near future. Friedland and McCracken[24] have reviewed this topic.

For meningitis, penicillin has been replaced by ceftriaxone or cefotaxime. In many parts of the world, vancomycin must be added until susceptibility of the infecting strain is known. Dexamethasone has been shown experimentally to decrease penetration of vancomycin into the central nervous system. Thus, doubt has increased about the use of steroids for treatment of pneumococcal meningitis in children.

Chloramphenicol, although generally being active against most pneumococci, seems likely to fail in the treatment of pneumococcal meningitis.[23]

Treatment of infections of soft tissues, pneumonia, otitis media, and sinusitis due to pneumococci of intermediate resistance may be simpler than treatment of infections of the central nervous system.

Anecdotal data suggest that conventional high-dose penicillin may prove adequate. Levels in serum, and in the middle ear, range from very high (serum) to well above the cut-off for characterizing a strain as having intermediate resistance. Pallares and associates[50] reported no difference in terms of mortality for adults with pneumococcal pneumonia who had disease caused by sensitive and resistant pneumococci. Several caveats are in order. First, no children were so treated. Second, high-dose penicillin was used, i.e., 150,000 to 200,000 units/kg/day. Third, resistant strains had MICs that reached a ceiling of 4.0 μg/mL. Finally, it was not a randomized, controlled trial. Nonetheless, the data do suggest that many patients will respond to high-dose conventional treatment. Tan and coworkers[58] reported success in the treatment (usually with amoxicillin or cefuroxime) in 18 of 19 children with pneumococcal infections due to strains of intermediate resistance. Additional studies in children and adults are awaited.

Other antimicrobial agents also may prove useful. Among the parenteral cephalosporins, ceftriaxone, cefotaxime, and cefuroxime are some that are the most active against resistant pneumococci. Cefpodoxime, an oral agent, also belongs to this group of active agents, as does cefuroxime axetil. However, we can expect that no oral β-lactam will be significantly more effective than either penicillin V or amoxicillin.

The prevalence of resistance to erythromycin (and other macrolides) varies with time and place. Unfortunately, resistance to one member of this class often means resistance to all.

Clindamycin is active in vitro against most resistant strains and may prove useful, although it, like many alternatives, may not be useful against some of the other likely pathogens in otitis media or sinusitis.

Resistance to cotrimoxazole also varies around the world but has become highly prevalent in many areas.

Treatment of otitis media or sinusitis due to resistant strains may be more problematic. Data suggest that pneumococcal otitis media has a low spontaneous rate of cure.[34] Thus, it seems likely that as the prevalence of these strains increases, we will see more clinical failures. Where such strains remain susceptible, it is likely that one or more doses of ceftriaxone may prove effective. Myringotomy also may regain some of its former utility.

These rising rates of resistance, coupled with the understanding that many patients still die in spite of effective therapy, mean that recent efforts have been directed toward prevention of pneumococcal infection.

PROSPECTS FOR PREVENTION

Although Austrian and Gold[3] showed that elderly and infirm patients were those most likely to die in spite of appropriate therapy, pediatricians cannot be complacent. Children who survive pneumococcal meningitis may have severe sequelae, particularly significant hearing deficits. Children with recurrent otitis media may suffer a delay in development of speech and language as well as in cognitive function.[33, 39, 44, 59] Children with asplenia, either congenital or acquired, may die suddenly, overwhelmed by pneumococcal sepsis. Children with sickle-cell disease are at an extraordinarily high risk for severe pneumococcal infection. Thus, pediatricians should be as interested in prevention of pneumococcal infections as are their colleagues who care for adults.

Considerable success in prevention of recurrent otitis media has been achieved with the use of chronic administration of either ampicillin[49] or sulfisoxazole.[52] Such studies have not employed microbiologic techniques, and the mechanism by which preventive therapy works remains unknown. Data now exist to support the common practice of prescribing regular doses of penicillin for children with asplenia or sickle-cell disease.[25] The extent to which the efficacy of such practices will be diminished by increasing rates of resistance remains to be seen.

The resurgence of interest in prevention led to many trials using polyvalent pneumococcal vaccines in children. Results suggest that for children older than 2 years of age, these vaccines offer protection against bacteremic and mucosal infections.[1, 43] For these reasons, current recommendations for use of pneumococcal vaccine limit recipients to children older than 2 years of age with asplenia from whatever cause, nephrotic syndrome, and sickle-cell disease and related hemoglobinopathies.[42]

Despite the need for an effective vaccine suitable for use in younger children, efficacy may be hard to achieve. Many pneumococcal polysaccharides are poor immunogens in young children. Type 3 antigen produces a superb response, even in very young children, but type 14 antigen produces a minimal response. Unfortunately, the type 14 pneumococcus is the most commonly invasive serotype, accounting for up to one-third of bacteremias in children. Type 3 is, today, a rather uncommon cause of bacteremia in children. Effective vaccines for young children, if feasible, will have to contain more complex antigens, probably with protein content.

Such vaccines now are entering the stages of clinical investigation, having shown great promise in studies of immunogenicity.

Pneumococcal disease continues to be a leading cause of morbidity and mortality in persons of all ages. Antimicrobial therapy, although strikingly effective, cannot prevent many deaths or much sickness. This knowledge, coupled with the recent appearance of strains of pneumococci resistant to most antimicrobial agents, requires renewed efforts for preventing the development of pneumococcal infections.

References

1. Ammann, A. J., Addiego, J., Wara, D. W., et al.: Polyvalent pneumococcal-polysaccharide immunization of patients with sickle-cell anemia and patients with splenectomy. N. Engl. J. Med. *297*:897–900, 1977.
2. Austrian, R., and Collins, P.: Importance of carbon dioxide in the isolation of pneumococci. J. Bacteriol. *92*:1281–1284, 1966.
3. Austrian, R., and Gold, J.: Pneumococcal bacteremia with a special reference to bacteremic pneumococcal pneumonia. Ann. Intern. Med. *60*:759–776, 1964.
4. Austrian, R., Howie, V. M., and Ploussard, J. H.: The bacteriology of pneumococcal otitis media. Johns Hopkins Med. J. *141*:104–111, 1977.
5. Barrett-Connor, E.: The nonvalue of sputum culture in the diagnosis of pneumococcal pneumonia. Am. Rev. Respir. Dis. *103*:845–848, 1971.
6. Berendt, R. F., Long, G. G., and Walker, J. S.: Influenza alone and in sequence with pneumonia due to *Streptococcus pneumoniae* in the squirrel monkey. J. Infect. Dis. *132*:689–693, 1975.
7. Box, Q. T., Cleveland, R. T., and Willard, C. Y.: Bacterial flora of the upper respiratory tract. 1. Comparative evaluation by anterior nasal, oropharyngeal, and nasopharyngeal swabs. Am. J. Dis. Child *102*:293–301, 1961.
8. Broome, C. V.: Use of bacterial vaccines for prevention of pneumococcal and meningococcal disease in the day care setting. Rev. Infect. Dis. *8*:584–588, 1986.
9. Browne, K., Miegel, J., and Stottmeier, K. D.: Detection of pneumococci in blood cultures by latex agglutination. J. of Clin. Microbiol. *19*:649–650, 1984.
10. Bruyn, G. A., Zegers, B. J., and van Furth, R.: Mechanisms of host defense against infection with *Streptococcus pneumoniae*. Clin. Infect. Dis. *14*:251–262, 1992.
11. Coonrod, J. D., and Rylko-Bauer, B.: Latex agglutination in the diagnosis of pneumococcal infection. J. Clin. Microbiol. *4*:168–174, 1976.
12. Coonrod, J. D., and Rytel, M.: Detection of type-specific pneumococcal antigens by counterimmunoelectrophoresis. I. Methodology and immunologic properties of pneumococcal antigens. J. Lab. Clin. Med. *81*:770–777, 1973.
13. Coonrod, J. D., and Rytel, M.: Detection of type-specific pneumococcal antigens by counterimmunolectrophoresis. II. Etiologic diagnosis of pneumonia. J. Lab. Clin. Med. *81*:778–786, 1973.
14. Davies, J. A. V.: The response of infants to inoculation with type I pneumococcus carbohydrate. J. Immunol. *33*:1–7, 1937.
15. Dilworth, J. A., Stewart, P., and Gwaltney, J. M., Jr.: Methods to improve detection of pneumococci in respiratory secretions. J. Clin. Microbiol. *2*:453–455, 1975.
16. Dimitrov, N. V., Douwes, F. R., and Bartoletta, B.: Metabolic activity of polymorphonuclear leukocytes in sickle cell anemia. Acta Haematol. *47*:283–291, 1972.
17. Dowling, J. N., Sheehe, P. R., and Feldman, H. A.: Pharyngeal pneumococcal acquisitions in "normal" families: A longitudinal study. J. Infect. Dis. *124*:9–16, 1971.
18. Doyle, M. G., Morrow, A. L., Van, R., et al.: Intermediate resistance of *Streptococcus pneumoniae* to penicillin in children in day-care centers [published erratum appears in Pediatr. Infect. Dis. J. *12*:32, 1993]. Pediatr. Infect. Dis. J. 11:831–835, 1992.
19. Ekwurzel, G. M., Simmons, J. S., Dublin, L. I., et al.: Studies on immunizing substances in pneumococci. VIII. Report on field tests to determine prophylactic value of a pneumococcus antigen. Public Health Rep. *53*:1877–1893, 1938.
20. Finland, M., and Barnes, M. W.: Changes in occurrence of capsular serotypes of *Streptococcus pneumoniae* at Boston City Hospital during selected years between 1935 and 1974. J. Clin. Microbiol. *5*:154–166, 1977.
21. Francis, Jr., T., and Tillett, W. S.: Cutaneous reactions in pneumonia. The development of antibodies following the intradermal injection of type-specific polysaccharide. J. Exp. Med. *52*:573–585, 1930.
22. Fraser, D. W., Darby, C. P., and Koehler, R. E.: Risk factors in bacterial meningitis: Charleston County, South Carolina. J. Infect. Dis. *127*:271–277, 1973.
23. Friedland, I. R., and Klugman, K. P.: Failure of chloramphenicol therapy in penicillin-resistant pneumococcal meningitis. Lancet *339*:405–408, 1992.
24. Friedland, I. R., and McCracken, G. H., Jr.: Management of infections caused by antibiotic-resistant *Streptococcus pneumoniae*. N. Engl. J. Med. *333*:377–381, 1995.
25. Gaston, M. H., Verter, J. I., Woods, G., et al.: Prophylaxis with oral penicillin in children with sickle cell anemia: A randomized trial. N. Engl. J. Med. *314*:1593–1599, 1986.
26. Gillespie, S. H., Ullman, C., Smith, M. D., et al.: Detection of *Streptococcus pneumoniae* in sputum samples by PCR. J. Clin. Microbiol. *32*:1308–1311, 1994.
27. Gwaltney, J. M., Jr., Sande, M. A., Austrian, R., et al.: Spread of *Streptococcus pneumoniae* in families. II. Relationship of transfer of *S. pneumoniae* to incidence of colds and serum antibody. J. Infect. Dis. *132*:62–68, 1975.
28. Hassan-King, M., Baldeh, I., Secka, O., et al.: Detection of *Streptococcus pneumoniae* DNA in blood cultures by PCR. J. Clin. Microbiol. *32*:1721–1724, 1994.
29. Heffron, R.: Pneumonia, With Special Reference to Pneumococcus Lobar Pneumonia. New York, Commonwealth Fund, 1939.
30. Henderson, F. W., Gilligan, P. H., Wait, K., et al.: Nasopharyngeal carriage of antibiotic-resistant pneumococci by children in group day care. J. Infect. Dis. *157*:256–263, 1988.
31. Hendley, J. O., Sande, M. A., Stewart, P. M., et al.: Spread of *Streptococcus pneumoniae* in families. I. Carriage rates and distribution of types. J. Infect. Dis. *132*:55–61, 1975.
32. Hofmann, J., Cetron, M. S., Farley, M. M., et al.: The prevalence of drug-resistant *Streptococcus pneumoniae* in Atlanta. N. Engl. J. Med. *333*:481–486, 1995.
33. Holm, V. A., and Kunze, L. H.: Effect of chronic otitis media on language and speech development. Pediatrics *43*:833–839, 1969.
34. Howie, V. M.: Eradication of bacterial pathogens from middle ear infections. Clin. Infect. Dis. *14*(Suppl. 2):209–210, 1992.
35. Howie, V. M., Ploussard, J. H., and Sloyer, Jr., J. L.: The "otitis prone" condition. Am. J. Dis. Child *129*:676–678, 1969.
36. Jay, S. J., Johanson, W. G., Jr., and Pierce, A. K.: The radiographic resolution of *Streptococcus pneumoniae* pneumonia. N. Engl. J. Med. *293*:798–801, 1975.

37. Johnson, R. B., Jr., Newman, S. L., and Struth, A. G.: An abnormality of the alternate pathway of complement activation in sickle-cell disease. N. Engl. J. Med. 288:803–808, 1973.
38. Kabins, S. A., and Lerner, C.: Fulminant pneumococcemia and sickle-cell anemia. J. A. M. A. 211:467–471, 1970.
39. Kaplan, G. J., Fleshman, J. K., Bender, T. R., et al.: Long-term effects of otitis media: A ten-year cohort study of Alaskan Eskimo children. Pediatrics 52:577–585, 1973.
40. King, H., and Schumacker, H. B., Jr.: Splenic studies. I. Susceptibility to infection after splenectomy performed in infancy. Ann. Surg. 136:239–242, 1952.
41. Klein, J. O.: Diagnostic lung puncture in the pneumonia of infants and children. Pediatrics 44:486–492, 1969.
42. Klein, J. O., and Mortimer, E. A., Jr.: Use of pneumococcal vaccine in children. Pediatrics 61:321–322, 1978.
43. Klein, J. O., Teele, D. W., Sloyer, J. L., Jr., et al.: Use of pneumococcal vaccine for prevention of recurrent episodes of otitis media. *In* Robbins, J. B., Hill, J. C., and Sadoff, J. C. (eds.): Seminars in Infectious Diseases. Volume IV: Bacterial Vaccines. New York, Thieme-Stratton, 1982, pp. 305–310.
44. Lewis, N.: Otitis media and linguistic incompetence. Arch. Otolaryngol. 102:387–390, 1976.
45. Loda, F. A., Collier, A. M., Glezen, W. P., et al.: Occurrence of *Diplococcus pneumoniae* in the upper respiratory tract of children. J. Pediatr. 87:1087–1093, 1975.
46. Lund, E.: Laboratory diagnosis of pneumococcus infections. Bull. W. H. O. 23:5–13, 1960.
47. MacLeod, C. M., Hodges, R. G., Heidelberger, M., et al.: Prevention of pneumococcal pneumonia by immunization with specific capsular polysaccharides. J. Exp. Med. 82:445–465, 1945.
48. Marton, A.: Pneumococcal antimicrobial resistance: The problem in Hungary. Clin. Infect. Dis. 15:106–111, 1992.
49. Maynard, J. E., Fleshman, J. K., and Tschopp, C. F.: Otitis media in Alaskan Eskimo children: Prospective evaluation of chemoprophylaxis. J. A. M. A. 219:597–599, 1972.
50. Pallares, R., Linares, J., Vadillo, M., et al.: Resistance to penicillin and cephalosporin and mortality from severe pneumococcal pneumonia in Barcelona, Spain. N. Engl. J. Med. 333:474–480, 1995.
51. Pearson, H. A., Cornelius, E. A., Schwartz, A. D., et al.: Transfusion-reversible functional asplenia in children with sickle-cell anemia. N. Engl. J. Med. 283:334–337, 1970.
52. Perrin, J. M., Charney, E., MacWhinney, J. B., Jr., et al.: Sulfisoxazole as chemoprophylaxis for recurrent otitis media: A double-blind crossover study in pediatric practice. N. Engl. J. Med. 291:664–667, 1974.
53. Rauch, A. M., O'Ryan, M., Van, R., et al.: Invasive disease due to multiply resistant *Streptococcus pneumoniae* in a Houston, Texas, day-care center. Am. J. Dis. Child 144:923–927, 1990.
54. Rudolph, K. M., Parkinson, A. J., Black, C. M., et al.: Evaluation of polymerase chain reaction for diagnosis of pneumococcal pneumonia. J. Clin. Microbiol. 31:2661–2666, 1993.
55. Salo, P., Ortqvist, A., and Leinonen, M.: Diagnosis of bacteremic pneumococcal pneumonia by amplification of pneumolysin gene fragment in serum. J. Infect. Dis. 171:479–482, 1995.
56. Seeler, R. A., Metzger, W., and Mufson, M. A.: *Diplococcus pneumoniae* infections in children with sickle cell anemia. Am. J. Dis. Child 123:8–10, 1972.
57. Sutliff, W. D., and Finland, M.: Antipneumococci immunity reactions in individuals of different ages. J. Exp. Med. 55:837–852, 1932.
58. Tan, T. Q., Mason, E. O., Jr., and Kaplan, S. L.: Systemic infections due to *Streptococcus pneumoniae* relatively resistant to penicillin in a children's hospital: Clinical management and outcome. Pediatrics 90:928–933, 1992.
59. Teele, D. W., Klein, J. O., Chase, C., et al.: Otitis media in infancy and intellectual ability, school achievement, speech, and language at age 7 years. J. Infect. Dis. 162:685–694, 1990.
60. Teele, D. W., Klein, J. O., and Rosner, B.: Epidemiology of otitis media during the first seven years of life in children in greater Boston: A prospective, cohort study. J. Infect. Dis. 160:83–94, 1989.
61. Teele, D. W., Pelton, S. I., Grant, M. J., et al.: Bacteremia in febrile children under 2 years of age: Results of cultures of blood of 600 consecutive febrile children seen in a "walk-in" clinic. J. Pediatr. 87:227–230, 1975.
62. Tempest, B., Morgan, R., Davidson, M., et al.: The value of respiratory tract bacteriology in pneumococcal pneumonia in Navajo Indians. Am. Rev. Respir. Dis. 109:577–578, 1974.
63. Tilghman, R. C., and Finland, M.: Clinical significance of bacteremia in pneumococcal pneumonia. Arch. Intern. Med. 59:602–619, 1937.
64. Tomasz, A.: The pneumococcus at the gates. N. Engl. J. Med. 333:514–515, 1955.
65. Trask, J. D., O'Donovan, C., Jr., Moore, D. M., et al.: Studies on pneumonia in children. I. Mortality, blood cultures, and humoral antibodies in pneumococcus pneumonia. J. Clin. Invest. 8:623–653, 1930.
66. White, B.: Biology of the Pneumococcus. New York, Commonwealth Fund, 1938.
67. Wright, A. E., Morgan, W. P., Colebrook, L., et al.: Observations on prophylactic inoculation against pneumococcus infections, and on the results which have been achieved by it. Lancet 1:87–95, 1914.
68. Yatabe, J. A. H., Baldwin, K. L., and Martin, W. J.: Isolation of an obligately anaerobic *Streptococcus pneumoniae* from blood culture. J. Clin. Microbiol. 6:181–182, 1977.
69. Zhang, Y., Isaacman, D. J., Wadowsky, R. M., et al.: Detection of *Streptococcus pneumoniae* in whole blood by PCR. J. Clin. Microbiol. 33:596–601, 1995.

91

MISCELLANEOUS GRAM-POSITIVE COCCI

Randall G. Fisher and William C. Gruber

This chapter discusses relatively uncommon gram-positive cocci that are of importance because of their unusual antimicrobial sensitivities and because of their increasing recognition as pathogens in hospitalized patients.

LEUCONOSTOC SPECIES

Bacteriology

Leuconostoc species are facultatively anaerobic gram-positive cocci that usually appear in pairs or chains. They are catalase-negative, Vogues-Proskauer–positive, and leucine-aminopeptidase–positive. In addition, colonies often are alpha-hemolytic on blood agar and also may react with group D streptococcal antiserum. These properties are shared by viridans streptococci, with which *Leuconostoc* species often are confused.[11] They also may resemble enterococci, except that they are pyrrolidone carboxylyl peptidase–negative. Differences include the production of gas from glucose and high-level vancomycin resistance.

Epidemiology

Leuconostoc species are found commonly on plants, especially sugar cane and leafy vegetables. They also are found in dairy products and wine.[32] They are employed in the food industry as starter cultures in food production.[22, 40] Although not a part of the normal human flora,[2] they occasionally are recovered from vaginal swabs in healthy individuals.[35] Studies also have shown colonization of mucosal surfaces in some hospitalized individuals.[17] Case reports of pediatric infection began to appear in the 1980s.[9, 19, 21, 44]

Pathophysiology

Leuconostocs rarely are pathogenic. Underlying disease states or immune compromise, gastrointestinal tract disease, prior or current antibiotic therapy (especially vancomycin), venous or gastointestinal tract access devices, recent invasive procedures, and infancy are thought to be risk factors.[17, 32] Of the first 21 cases reported in the English literature, 12 were in children, and 10 of those were in patients younger than 1 year of age. Documented portals of entry include central lines[2, 19] and gastrostomy tubes.[21] Contaminated enteral formula also has been implicated.[5, 21, 28] Occasional sporadic cases without a known risk factor have been reported,[9, 17] which underscores the pathogenic potential of *Leuconostoc* infection.

Clinical Manifestations

Bacteremia is by far the most common clinical manifestation of *Leuconostoc* infection, heralded by fever and usually leukocytosis in patients with risk factors outlined earlier. Gastrointestinal disturbances are common, especially diarrhea.[2] Infants are prone to emesis. *Leuconostoc* bacteremia, in association with cough and chest x-ray findings consistent with pneumonia, was reported in a child with AIDS.[32] *Leuconostoc citreum* has been isolated from lung tissue of a 33-year-old with AIDS who also had *Pneumocystis carinii* pneumonia.[15] Small necrotic cavities scattered through both lungs were associated with gram-positive cocci in tissue. Patients with dental infections,[44] peritonitis, and meningitis[9, 13] also have been described. Meningitis has been reported in an otherwise healthy 16-year old and in a neonate with fatal infection, despite high cerebrospinal fluid bactericidal antibiotic titers.[9, 13]

Diagnosis

Cultures usually are positive within 24 to 48 hours. Leuconostocs are somewhat fastidious. The identification of vancomycin-resistant *Streptococcus* should raise suspicion of *Leuconostoc* infection and prompt additional biochemical studies,[32] including evaluation for the production of gas in MRS broth, failure to hydrolyze arginine, and delayed esculin hydrolysis.

Treatment

Treatment with relatively high doses of penicillin or ampicillin frequently is successful at eradicating infection. When possible, access devices should be removed. Leuconostocs are most sensitive to the primitive beta-lactam antibiotics, especially penicillin and ampicillin, although penicillin tolerance is common.[21, 41] They also frequently are sensitive to erythromycin, cephalothin, and the aminoglycosides. *Leuconostoc* species are variably resistant to clindamycin and trimethoprim-sulfamethoxazole. Resistance increases with later generations of cephalosporins.[17, 41] *Leuconostoc* species are intrinsically vancomycin-resistant because their pentapeptide cell-wall precursors end in D-Ala-lactate rather than the usual D-Ala-alanine.[18] Vancomycin can not bind the lactate. This is the same mode of resistance possessed by vancomycin-resistant enterococci. However, whereas resistance in enterococci is plasmid-derived and transferable, in leuconostocs it is chromosomally mediated, constitutional, and not transferable.

PEDIOCOCCUS SPECIES

Bacteriology

Pediococci also are intrinsically vancomycin-resistant, facultatively anaerobic gram-positive cocci. They appear most characteristically in tetrads on Gram stain, although they may appear in pairs or clusters.[16] The genus name *Pediococcus* is derived from the Greek word *pedium*, which means "plane." The name suggests, therefore, that they are a genus of cocci that grow in a single plane. It is a misnomer, however, because pediococci are the only lactic acid bacteria that divide in two planes.[14] They are catalase- and oxidase-negative. They do not reduce nitrates, and no gas is produced in MRS broth.[38] They are pyrrolidone carboxylyl peptidase–negative.[12] Most isolates react with Lancefield group D streptococcal antibodies.[38] They are leucine-aminopeptidase–positive, which distinguishes them from *Leuconostoc* species.[12] They produce white, opaque, nonhemolytic colonies on sheep's blood agar.

Pediococci produce powerful bacteriocins, which are substances that kill other bacteria. The bacteriocins of pediococci particularly are active against other gram-positive organisms[8] but also are active against *Clostridium botulinum* spores,[29] some gram-negative organisms,[39] and *Listeria monocytogenes*.

Epidemiology

Like leuconostocs and other lactic acid bacteria, pediococci are found on plants, in dairy products, and in alcohol-containing beverages.[42] They also are utilized in the formation of silage[38] and as starter cultures for some meat products. They are not thought to be part of normal flora.

They have been isolated from saliva and stool on rare occasions.[36] Although formerly thought to be nonpathogenic, they now are considered rare opportunistic pathogens of minimal virulence.

Pathophysiology

Pediococci rarely are pathogenic. Many cases of blood isolates are in patients without symptoms of infection or in polymicrobial cultures in which the significance of the isolate could not be assessed adequately.[26] There is one case report of a patient with a clinical picture of septic shock in whom the only organism recovered was *Pediococcus pentosaceus*.[10] Risk factors for bacteremia, with or without symptoms, appear to be extremes of age, recent abdominal surgery or tube feedings, broad-spectrum antimicrobial therapy, and the presence of severe underlying disease states.[26] However, because the overall number of reported cases is small, the relative risks of these factors are uncertain.

Clinical Manifestations and Diagnosis

Most patients are either asymptomatic or have fever as the only symptom. Six of the first 12 reported cases of *Pediococcus* bacteremia had concomitant pneumonia. Fifty-six per cent of adult patients either were receiving tube feedings or had undergone abdominal surgery within 30 days of isolation of the organism.[26] The two reported pediatric cases were infants (16 and 64 days of age), and both had underlying gastrointestinal tract anomalies. The 16-day-old had congenital jejunoileal atresia and had undergone surgical repair just 8 days prior to presentation.[26] Her acute illness was characterized by emesis and a 200-g weight loss. She was afebrile at presentation. The second patient was a 64-day-old with gastroschisis who had undergone two abdominal surgical procedures.[1] His fever reached 101.5° F, and his peripheral white blood cell count was 38,000 with a significant left shift.

Isolation of pediococci in localized infections is common,

especially from abdominal sites, but virtually always is part of a polymicrobial process. The relative importance of pediococci in these sites is difficult to assess.

Diagnosis of infection with pediococci is made by identifying vancomycin-resistant, gram-positive cocci in its characteristic tetrads. Many pediococci are misidentified initially as *Streptococcus equinus*, *S. constellatus*, or group D *Streptococcus*, not *Enterococcus*. Reported cases of pediococcal infection may, therefore, represent only a fraction of the total number of infections.

Treatment

Pediococci generally are susceptible to penicillin, ampicillin, imipenem, and first- and second-generation cephalosporins. Although both imipenem and penicillin are highly active against pediococci, they do not appear to be bactericidal. Pediococci are moderately resistant to the quinolones, tetracycline,[42] and trimethoprim-sulfamethoxazole.[34] Pediococci, like leuconostocs, are instrinsically resistant to vancomycin. Resistance is not plasmid-mediated, nor can it be transferred to other bacteria.[42] Sensitivity to ticarcillin and cefotaxime, when measured by agar dilution, is poor, despite large zones of inhibition on disk susceptibility testing.[42] There is occasional inducible resistance to erythromycin, although most isolates remain sensitive. Aminoglycoside sensitivity is variable.

AEROCOCCUS SPECIES

Bacteriology

The genus *Aerococcus* contains two species, *viridans* and *urinae*. Until recently, *viridans* was considered the only species, and in earlier papers, *A. urinae* was referred to as *Aerococcus*-like organism, or ALO.[6] Aerococci are catalase-negative, nonmotile, gram-positive cocci that appear preferentially in tetrads but sometimes in pairs or clusters. These relatively slow-growing organisms produce small, well-delineated, translucent, and alpha-hemolytic colonies on blood agar.[7] They also are weakly bile-esculin–positive and pyrrolidone carboxylyl peptidase–negative. They ferment mannose and mannitol.[33] Like enterococci, most aerococci will grow in 6.5 per cent salt.[25]

Epidemiology

Aerococci are distributed throughout the world and are contaminants of air and dust.[20] They also have been found on meats, on raw vegetables, and in small numbers on human skin.[4] In hospitals, aerococci have been cultured from all areas, including operating suites and delivery rooms.[23] They also are found in salt water, where they cause a fatal disease in lobsters.[30]

Disease in humans is uncommon, and the organism usually is recovered from the blood stream in patients with infective endocarditis. Most patients are elderly, but infection of infants and neonates also has been reported.[27, 30] A rapidly fatal bacteremia has been described in patients with profound neutropenia.[24]

Pathophysiology

In most circumstances, aerococci are saprophytic. The exact conditions that favor infection have not been elucidated clearly. Some cases of *A. urinae* infection have occurred after genitourinary tract surgery. One case of septic arthritis occurred after a therapeutic abortion.[43] Immunocompromised patients are at higher risk, but infection in otherwise well persons has been described.[33] One report of meningitis in newborns found adherence of aerococci to inflammatory cells and suggested a role of as-yet-undefined adhesion factors.[27] Work in laboratory animals also has shown that a protease isolated from *A. viridans* cleaves the hemagglutinin of influenza virus and potentiates both viral replication and disease in mice.[37] It has been noted that *A. viridans* can be isolated in 0.9 per cent of patients with pneumonia.[45]

Clinical Manifestations

Most cases of *A. viridans* bacteremia have been found in association with signs and symptoms of subacute infective endocarditis, although septic emboli and cardiac failure have not been described. *A. urinae* causes urinary tract infection with dysuria and frequency, usually in the absence of fever.[7] *Aerococcus* infection in childhood is uncommon. One case of bacteremia in a 1-month-old has been reported.[30] The patient presented with a 2-day history of loose stools, irritability, and drowsiness and on physical examination was noted to have mottled skin, circumoral cyanosis, and agitation. Cerebrospinal fluid and urine were normal, but blood cultures grew a pure growth of *A. viridans*. No predisposing factors were identified. Nathavitharana and associates[27] reported three cases of meningitis due to *A. viridans*: a 7-month-old female with jerking movements of the extremities, irritability, and a bulging fontanelle; a 5-month-old female who presented with fever, decreased appetite, and generalized convulsions; and a 24-month-old female whose illness manifested as fever, vomiting, and the neurologic signs of truncal ataxia, flaccidity, and hypoactive deep-tendon reflexes. All three patients had elevated cerebrospinal fluid white blood cell counts with from 55 to 93 per cent segmented forms. Remarkably, all of these patients had a history of prolonged illness (1 week to 2 months) prior to presentation, in contrast to patients with other causes of bacterial meningitis. No risk factors for infection were identified in any of these patients, who were thought to have normal immune function.

Bone and joint infections and wound or other localized infections are exceedingly rare and not distinguishable from similar syndromes caused by more common organisms.

Diagnosis

Careful observation of both appearance on Gram stain and growth in culture is key to the diagnosis of aerococcal infection. On Gram stain, aerococci resemble staphylococci. On blood agar, they resemble viridans group streptococci. One series revealed that 1 per cent of 719 cultures called streptococci actually were aerococci[31]; another study reclassified 3 per cent of 168 cultures.[4] In their propensity toward tetrad formation they mimic pediococci. However, all aerococci are vancomycin-sensitive. In their bile-esculin hydrolysis and growth in 6.5 per cent salt they resemble enterococci; unlike enterococci, however, aerococci are pyrrolidone carboxylyl peptidase–negative and do not form chains.

Treatment

Aerococci generally are sensitive to penicillin, ampicillin, the cephalosporins, chloramphenicol, and the macrolides.

They usually are intermediately susceptible or resistant to sulfonamides and aminoglycosides.[4, 20] One report suggests that *A. viridans* and *A. urinae* have distinct antibiograms,[25] that is, that *A. urinae* is more sensitive to penicillin and resistant to sulfonamides, whereas *A. viridans* is more resistant to penicillin and sensitive to the sulfonamides.[3] Individual case reports do not confirm these in vitro observations, and there are no large clinical trials of antimicrobial susceptibility.

References

1. Atkins, J. T., Tillman, J., Tan, T. Q., et al.: *Pediococcus pentosaceus* catheter-associated infection in an infant with gastroschisis. Pediatr. Infect. Dis. J. *13*:75–76, 1994.
2. Bernaldo de Quiros, J. C., Munoz, P., Cercenado, E., et al.: *Leuconostoc* species as a cause of bacteremia: Two case reports and a literature review. Eur. J. Clin. Microbiol. Infect. Dis. *10*:505–509, 1991.
3. Buu-Hoi, A., Le Bouguenec, C., and Horaud, T.: Genetic basis of antibiotic resistance in *Aerococcus viridans*. Antimicrob. Agents Chemother. *33*:529–534, 1989.
4. Buu-Hoi, A., Branger, C., and Acar, J. F.: Vancomycin-resistant streptococci or *Leuconostoc* sp. Antimicrob. Agents Chemother. *28*:458–460, 1985.
5. Carapetis, J., Bishop, S., Davis, J., et al.: *Leuconostoc* sepsis in association with continuous enteral feeding: Two case reports and a review. Pediatr. Infect. Dis. J. *13*:816–823, 1994.
6. Christensen, J. J., Vibits, H., Ursing, J., et al.: *Aerococcus*-like organism, a newly recognized potential urinary tract pathogen. J. Clin. Microbiol. *29*:1049–1053, 1991.
7. Christensen, J. J., Gutschık, E., Friis-Moller, A., et al.: Urosepticemia and fatal endocarditis caused by *Aerococcus*-like organisms. Scand. J. Infect. Dis. *23*:717–721, 1991.
8. Cintas, L. M., Rodriguez, J. M., Fernandez, M. F., et al.: Isolation and characterization of pediocin L50, a new bacteriocin from *Pediococcus acidilactici* with a broad inhibitory spectrum. Appl. Environ. Microbiol. *61*:2643–2648, 1995.
9. Coovadia, Y. M., Salwa, Z., and van den Ende, J.: Meningitis caused by vancomycin-resistant *Leuconostoc* sp. J. Clin. Microbiol. *25*:1784–1785, 1987.
10. Corcoran, G. D., Gibbons, N., and Mulvihill, T. E.: Septicaemia caused by *Pediococcus pentosaceus*: A new opportunistic pathogen. J. Infect. *23*:179–182, 1991.
11. Facklam, R., Pigott, N., Franklin, R., et al.: Evaluation of three disk tests for identification of enterococci, leuconostocs, and pediococci. J. Clin. Microbiol. *33*:885–887, 1995.
12. Facklam, R., Hollis, D., and Collins, M. D.: Identification of gram positive coccal and coccobacillary vancomycin-resistant bacteria. J. Clin. Microbiol. *27*:724–730, 1984.
13. Friedland, I. R., Snipelisky, M., and Khoosal, M.: Meningitis in a neonate caused by *Leuconostoc* sp. J. Clin. Microbiol. *28*:2125–2126, 1990.
14. Garvie, E. I.: Genus *Pediococcus*. *In* Krieg, N. R., and Holt, J. G. (eds.): Bergey's Manual of Systematic Bacteriology, Vol. 1. Baltimore, Williams & Wilkins, 1984, pp.1075–1079.
15. Giacometti, A., Ranaldi, R., Siquini, F. M., et al.: *Leuconostoc citreum* isolated from lung in AIDS patient. Lancet *342*:622, 1993.
16. Green, M., Barbadora, K., and Michaels, M.: Recovery of vancomycin-resistant gram-positive cocci from pediatric liver transplant recipients. J. Clin. Microbiol. *29*:2503–2506, 1991.
17. Handwerger, S., Pucci, M. J., Volk, K. J., et al.: Vancomycin-resistant *Leuconostoc mesenteroides* and *Lactobacillus casei* synthesize cytoplasmic peptidoglycan precursors that terminate in lactate. J. Bacteriol. *176*:260–264, 1994.
18. Handwerger, S., Horowitz, H., Coburn, K., et al.: Infection due to *Leuconostoc* species: Six cases and review. Rev. Infect. Dis. *12*:602, 1990.
19. Hardy, S., Ruoff, K. L., Catlin, E. A., et al.: Catheter-associated infection with a vancomycin-resistant gram-positive coccus of the *Leuconostoc* sp. Pediatr. Infect. Dis. J. *7*:519–520, 1988.
20. Heilesen, A. M.: Septicaemia due to *Aerococcus urinae*. Scand. J. Infect. Dis. *26*:759–760, 1994.
21. Isenberg, H. D., Vellozzi, E. M., Shapiro, J., et al.: Clinical laboratory challenges in the recognition of *Leuconostoc* spp. J. Clin. Microbiol. *26*:479–483, 1988.
22. Jeppesen, V. F., and Huss, H. H.: Characteristics and antagonistic activity of lactic acid bacteria isolated from chilled fish products. Int. J. Food Microbiol. *18*:305–320, 1993.
23. Kerbaugh, M. A., and Evans, J. B.: *Aerococcus viridans* in the hospital environment. Appl. Microbiol. *16*:519–523, 1968.
24. Kern, W., and Vanek, E.: *Aerococcus* bacteremia associated with granulocytopenia. Eur. J. Clin. Microbiol. *6*:670–673, 1987.
25. Kristensen, B., and Nielsen, G.: Endocarditis caused by *Aerococcus urinae*, a newly recognized pathogen. Eur. J. Clin. Microbiol. Infect. Dis. *14*:49–51, 1995.
26. Mastro, T. D., Spika, J. S., Lozano, P., et al.: Vancomycin-resistant *Pediococcus acidilactici*: Nine cases of bacteremia. J. Infect. Dis. *161*:956–960, 1990.
27. Nathavitharana, K. A., Arseculeratne, S. N., Aponso, H. A., et al.: Acute meningitis in early childhood caused by *Aerococcus viridans*. Br. Med. J. Clin. Res. Ed. *286*:1248, 1983.
28. Noriega, F. R., Kotloff, K. L., Martin, M. A., et al.: Nosocomial bacteremia caused by *Enterobacter sakazaki* and *Leuconostoc mesenteroides* resulting from extrinsic contamination of infant formula. Pediatr. Infect. Dis. J. *9*:447–449, 1990.
29. Okereke, A., and Montville, T. J.: Bacteriocin-mediated inhibition of *Clostridium botulinum* spores by lactic acid bacteria at refrigeration and abuse temperatures. Appl. Environ. Microbiol. *57*:3423–3428, 1991.
30. Park, J. W., and Grossman, O.: *Aerococcus viridans* infection: Case report and review. Clin. Pediatr. *29*:525–526, 1990.
31. Parker, M. T., and Ball, L. C.: Streptococci and aerococci associated with systemic infection in man. J. Med. Microbiol. *9*:275–302, 1976.
32. Peters, V. B., Bottone, E. J., Barzilae, A., et al.: *Leuconostoc* species bacteremia in a child with acquired immunodeficiency syndrome. Clin. Pediatr. *31*:699–701, 1992.
33. Pien, F. D., Wilson, W. R., Kunz, K., et al.: *Aerococcus viridans* endocarditis. Mayo Clin. Proc. *59*:47–48, 1984.
34. Riebel, W. J., and Washington, J. A.: Clinical and microbiologic characteristics of pediococci. J. Clin. Microbiol. *28*:1348–1355, 1990.
35. Rogosa, M., and Sharpe, M. E.: Species differentiation of human vaginal lactobacilli. J. Gen. Microbiol. *23*:197, 1960.
36. Ruoff, K. L., Kuritzkes, D. R., Wolfson, J. S., et al.: Vancomycin-resistant gram positive bacteria isolated from human sources. J. Clin. Microbiol. *26*:2064–2068, 1988.
37. Scheiblauer, H., Reinacher, M., Tashiro, M., et al.: Interactions between bacteria and influenza A virus in the development of influenza pneumonia. J. Infect. Dis. *166*:783–791, 1992.
38. Sire, J. M., Donnio, P. Y., Mesnard, R., et al.: Septicemia and hepatic abscess caused by *Pediococcus acidilactici*. Eur. J. Clin. Microbiol. Infect. Dis. *11*:623–625, 1992.
39. Skytta, E., Haikara, A., and Mattila-Sandholm, T.: Production and characterization of antibacterial compounds produced by *Pediococcus damnosus* and *Pediococcus pentosaceus*. J. Appl. Bacteriol. *74*:134–142, 1993.
40. Stiles, M. E.: Bacteriocins produced by *Leuconostoc* species. J. Dairy Sci. *77*:2718–2724, 1994.
41. Swenson, J. M., Facklam, R. R., and Thornsberry, C. Antimicrobial susceptibility of vancomycin-resistant *Leuconostoc*, *Pediococcus*, and *Lactobacillus* species. Antimicrob. Agents Chemother. *34*:543–549, 1990.
42. Tankovic, J., Leclerq, R., and Duval, J.: Antimicrobial susceptibility of *Pediococcus* spp. and genetic basis of macrolide resistance in *Pediococcus acidilactici* HM3020. Antimicrob. Agents Chemother. *37*:789–792, 1993.
43. Taylor, P. W., and Trueblood, M. C.: Septic arthritis due to *Aerococcus viridans*. J. Rheum. *12*:1004–1005, 1985.
44. Wenocur, H. S., Smith, M. A., Vellozzi, E. M., et al.: Odontogenic infection secondary to *Leuconostoc* species. J. Clin. Microbiol. *26*:1893–1894, 1988.
45. Werk, R.: Medizinische Bakteriologie und Infektiologie. 1st ed. Berlin, Springer-Verlag, 1990, p. 86.

❑ ❑ ❑

SUBSECTION TWO

GRAM-NEGATIVE COCCI

92

MORAXELLA CATARRHALIS

Barbara W. Stechenberg

Once thought to be an unimportant commensal organism in the human respiratory tract, *Moraxella catarrhalis* now is recognized as an important pathogen in respiratory tract disease, particularly otitis, sinusitis, and lower tract disease. The initial paper by Ghon and Pfeiffer[21] in 1902 described gram-negative cocci in sputum referred to as *Micrococcus catarrhalis.* Since then, the organism has undergone several changes in nomenclature, first to *Neisseria catarrhalis* because of the resemblance to other *Neisseria* organisms. In 1970, in recognition of the contributions of Sarah Branham, the name was changed to *Branhamella catarrhalis.*[8] More recently, it has become clear that this organism should be a member of the genus *Moraxella.* Thus, the name was changed to *M. catarrhalis.* With the transition in nomenclature, the last two decades have seen a parallel rebirth of this organism as a mucosal pathogen.

MICROBIOLOGY

M. catarrhalis is a gram-negative diplococcus that morphologically is indistinguishable from *Neisseria.* It has a tendency to resist decolorizing.[1] The organism is kidney shaped, with the flat sides abutting each other. The size varies but may be larger than the meningococcus or gonococcus. However, the resemblance to gonococcus of a sputum Gram stain or conjunctival smear can be striking and confusing clinically.

The organism grows well on blood or chocolate agar, forming small, opaque, grayish colonies that are circular and nonhemolytic. They have poor adhesion to the agar surface, acting like hockey pucks when pushed over the surface of the agar plate.[13] The use of selective media, such as modified Thayer-Martin or TV broth (Mueller-Hinton broth supplemented with trimethoprim and vancomycin), increases the likelihood of recovering the *M. catarrhalis* organism from the complex flora of the mucosal surfaces.

Isolates of *M. catarrhalis* cannot utilize maltose, glucose, lactose, or sucrose as carbohydrate sources. *M. catarrhalis* is oxidase-positive and produces deoxyribonuclease. Hydrolysis of DNA and tributyrin are valuable differentiating tests. Several rapid tests have been described, such as butyrate hydrolysis, Tween 80 hydrolysis, and selective DNase agar.[45, 51] Fatty-acid analysis also has been used to identify atypical strains.

The surface of *M. catarrhalis* is composed of outer-membrane proteins, lipo-oligosaccharide, and pili. The organism does not appear to have a capsule, and the role of the pili is not defined well. Initial attempts to isolate outer-membrane proteins using detergent fractionations of cell envelopes were unsuccessful. Using a technique involving the collection of outer-membrane vesicles, which are released into culture media, and then examination by sodium dodecyl sulfate–polyacrylamide gel electrophoresis (SDS-PAGE), Bartos and Murphy[4] identified eight proteins designated outer-membrane proteins A through H. The outer-membrane protein patterns from strains from diverse geographic and clinical sources were strikingly homogeneous.

Preliminary studies of lipo-oligosaccharide of *M. catarrhalis* show that it is more antigenically conserved than that of other gram-negative bacteria, making it a reasonable candidate for vaccine studies.[35, 48]

Restriction-endonuclease analysis has been used as an epidemiologic tool to distinguish strains of *M. catarrhalis.* Patterson and associates[38] used the technique to evaluate a nosocomial outbreak and to demonstrate the lack of association of other strains. Dickinson and coworkers[12] used a similar technique to study isolates from children with otitis media.

PATHOGENESIS

The ability of *M. catarrhalis* to produce disease, particularly in sequestered areas, such as the ear and lung, indicates that this organism possesses virulence mechanisms that allow it not only to grow in these anatomic sites but also to produce pathologic effects. The presence of endotoxin in the *M. catarrhalis* outer membrane undoubtedly is important to its pathogenic potential, especially in situations in which inflammation plays a major role. Very little is known about the mechanisms involved in colonization and disease production.

There is a rapidly accumulating body of literature concerning the immune response to *M. catarrhalis* and the antigenic composition of this organism.[9, 10, 30] Goldblatt and associates[22] demonstrated that children younger than 4 years of age possessed IgG1 and IgG2, which recognize an 82-kD outer-membrane protein exclusively, but older children developed an IgG3 response to a broad range of outer-membrane proteins. Faden and colleagues[19] developed a technique to measure opsonic antibody using outer-membrane, antigen-coated beads. Convalescent sera opsonized homologous, antigen-coated sera significantly more often than acute sera.

Unhanand and coworkers[47] have used a murine model to study the pulmonary clearance of *M. catarrhalis* from infected lungs. Using 10 strains, they found marked variability in clearance rates and phagocytic cell recruitment. With this model, Maciver and associates[32] actively immunized animals with outer-membrane vesicles of *M. catarrhalis* and passively immunized animals with rabbit antiserum raised against these vesicles. Both experiments resulted in enhanced pulmonary clearance of both homologous and heterologous strains. The same model has been used to evaluate the role of a large, antigenically conserved protein of *M. catarrhalis* in pulmonary clearance as well as the role of outer-membrane protein B in the defense mechanism of the lung.[26] The contribution of these proteins as well as lipo-oligosaccharide in the host defenses continues to unfold.

EPIDEMIOLOGY

M. catarrhalis is a normal inhabitant of the upper respiratory tract. The rate of colonization is highest in the early years and then declines steadily to less than 5 per cent in adult life.[49] Prevalence studies report as many as 50 per cent of children are colonized with *M. catarrhalis*.[28, 33] Faden and associates[18] followed a large cohort of children from birth to 2 years of age. Sixty-six per cent became colonized by 1 year of age and 77.5 per cent by 2 years of age. Nasopharyngeal colonization was increased during visits for otitis media compared with well visits. Otitis-prone children were colonized by 6 months of age. Restriction-endonuclease analysis showed marked heterogeneity, with children acquiring and eliminating over time a number of different strains.[16]

Multiple studies have documented the increased prevalence of *M. catarrhalis* as a pathogen in otitis media.[28, 50] Shurin and colleagues[43] noted that isolation of the *M. catarrhalis* organism from middle ear exudates increased from 6.4 per cent between 1979 and 1980 to 26.5 per cent between 1980 and 1982. A similar increase in *M. catarrhalis* as a pathogen in sinusitis has been reported.[52]

Once colonization of the oropharynx occurs, colonization of the tracheobronchial tree may follow, but usually only if other risk factors are operative. In adults, these risk factors include previous cardiorespiratory disease, smoking, corticosteroids, immunosuppression agents, malignancy, and intercurrent viral illnesses.[24, 51] In children, many of the cases of pneumonia are associated with a preceding viral illness, prematurity, underlying lung disease, IgG deficiency, or other risk factors.

Nosocomial transmission has been well documented by DNA restriction-endonuclease analysis.[11, 38] In pediatric intensive care units, endotracheal intubation and frequent suctioning have been identified as risk factors for pneumonia and bacterial tracheitis.[11, 17]

Other interesting associations need to be investigated further. Seddon and associates[42] noted that colonization with *M. catarrhalis* was more common in asthmatic than in normal children. Whether the organism might be a trigger or pathogenic in these children remains to be seen. Gottfarb and Brauner[23] found a high carriage rate of *M. catarrhalis* in children with severe persistent cough.

There is a seasonality to infection with *M. catarrhalis* in both adults and children.[24, 43, 50] Infection is much more likely in the winter-spring months.

CLINICAL MANIFESTATIONS AND DIAGNOSIS

Otitis media caused by *M. catarrhalis* is indistinguishable clinically from otitis caused by other pathogens, such as *Streptococcus pneumoniae* and *Haemophilus influenzae*. *M. catarrhalis* may be isolated as a single agent or in combination with other organisms. In one study, children with *M. catarrhalis* were less likely to have a serum C-reactive protein greater than 1.0 mg/dL than children with either of the other two major pathogens.[50]

Because tympanocentesis usually is not performed in routine cases, the exact etiology of an episode of acute otitis media usually is not known. One study found that *Moraxella* was an unusual organism as a single agent in children whose acute otitis media had been treated recently.[25] Nevertheless, in a study of persistent otitis, Pichichero and Pichichero[39] demonstrated *Moraxella* in 7 per cent of specimens. The spontaneous resolution rate of *M. catarrhalis* may be high[2]; this fact should be considered when therapy is planned.

The clinical manifestations of acute sinusitis caused by *M. catarrhalis* are similar to those of other organisms; therefore, the choice of antibiotics should be made with consideration of this organism as a potential pathogen.

Lower respiratory tract disease caused by *M. catarrhalis* may have a broad clinical spectrum; however, because sputum samples often are not available in children, many cases documented in the literature have been severe. Berg and Bartley[5] described five premature infants, all younger than 6 months of age, who developed precipitous clinical deterioration after 2 to 4 days of a prodrome consisting of cough, tachypnea, and intercostal retractions. They all required assisted ventilation, which is common in young infants with severe pneumonia.[5, 11, 16] Some cases of *M. catarrhalis* pneumonia have been associated with bacteremia.

Underlying conditions, such as leukemia, AIDS, and trauma, have been reported to predispose a patient to infection with *M. catarrhalis*.[33, 53] An association with immunoglobulin deficiency has been demonstrated in some patients with disease caused by this organism.[9] In adults, cases of *M. catarrhalis* pneumonia are more common in patients with HIV infection, malignancy, or chronic lung problems.[22, 51] The role of this organism in less severe presentations probably is limited.[29]

Bacterial tracheitis caused by *M. catarrhalis* has been reported in both immunocompromised hosts and hosts with normal immune systems.[17]

M. catarrhalis also has caused a wide variety of other infections. Urethritis caused by this organism can be mistaken for infection with *Neisseria gonorrhoeae*.[44] There are several reports of conjunctivitis; when present in the newborn period, *M. catarrhalis* can mimic ophthalmia neonatorum caused by *N. gonorrhoeae*.[46] The relationship of neonatal infections to maternal vaginal carriage of *Moraxella* has not been proved.[37]

More severe infections with *M. catarrhalis* include meningitis and bacteremia and should be considered, especially in immunocompromised children.

Children with *M. catarrhalis* bacteremia may present with many different manifestations. Some patients present with petechial or purpuric rashes, making their clinical picture indistinguishable from that of meningococcemia. Others have been neutropenic and have required mechanical ventilation.[6] Baron and Shapiro[3] reported two cases of unsuspected bacteremia in children with nonspecific symptoms. Their presentation was similar to that of children with occult pneumococcal bacteremia. An immunocompetent child with *M. catarrhalis* bacteremia and preseptal cellulitis has been reported.[41]

Meningitis can occur from hematogenous spread of *M. catarrhalis* from the nasopharynx or as a consequence of ventriculoperitoneal shunt placement or surgery. Rarely, suppurative arthritis has been seen in children and adults.[27, 34] Endocarditis is rare, as is peritonitis.

TREATMENT

In the past, *M. catarrhalis* was susceptible to all β-lactam antibiotics. In the late 1970s, however, β-lactamase–producing strains of *M. catarrhalis* were isolated in Europe. In the United States, there has been a parallel increase in the frequency of isolation of β-lactamase–producing *M. catarrhalis*.

The β-lactamases, BRO-1, BRO-2, and BRO-3, most probably are of chromosomal origin. The laboratory detection of β-lactamase activity depends on the assay used; chromogenic cephalosporin nitrocefin usually is recommended.[15] The β-lactamase inhibitors, clavulanic acid and sulbactam, are active against the enzymes produced by *Moraxella*. Most β-lactamase–positive isolates will respond to achievable concentrations of β-lactam/β-lactamase–inhibitor antimicrobial combinations, cephalosporins, and cephamycins.[14, 20] However, antimicrobial therapy should be guided by in vitro susceptibility tests, particularly for deep infections.

Among the oral cephalosporins active against β-lactamase–positive strains of *Moraxella*, the minimal inhibitory concentration increases two- to fourfold in the presence of β-lactamase BRO-1 but not β-lactamase BRO-2; cefixime is more active than the older cephalosporins.[36] Resistance to tetracycline (by the nontransferable Tet B determinant) and erythromycin have been reported, but such resistance is rare.[7, 40]

In vitro, *M. catarrhalis* usually is susceptible to ampicillin-sulbactam, amoxicillin-clavulanate, erythromycin, azithromycin, clarithromycin, trimethoprim-sulfamethoxazole, aztreonam, tetracyclines, chloramphenicol, fluoroquinolones (e.g., ciprofloxacin), aminoglycosides, and second- or third-generation cephalosporins, such as cefprozil, cefpodoxime, cefixime, and loracarbef. *M. catarrhalis* also is susceptible to cefuroxime and cefaclor, although the latter may be less active. The *Moraxella* organism is resistant to clindamycin, vancomycin, and oxacillin. β-lactamase–producing *M. catarrhalis* may be reported by a clinical laboratory as susceptible to penicillin G or ampicillin because of the relatively low activity of the enzyme, particularly in rapid-testing systems. Clinical treatment failures with such organisms suggest that they should be considered resistant, and alternative antibiotics should be used.

PREVENTION

Prevention of nosocomial *M. catarrhalis* infection is dependent upon sound infection control practices, especially in regard to pulmonary toilet. Prevention of other infections with this organism has not been attempted, except for the use of prophylactic antibiotics for recurrent otitis media.

References

1. Ainsworth, S. M., Nagy, S. B., Morgan, L. A., et al.: Interpretation of gram-stained sputa containing *Moraxella (Branhamella) catarrhalis*. Clin. Microbiol. *28*:2559–2560, 1990.
2. Barnett, E. D., and Klein, J. O.: The problem of resistant bacteria for the management of acute otitis media. Pediatr. Clin. North Am. *42*:509–518, 1995.
3. Baron, J., and Shapiro, E. D.: Unsuspected bacteremia caused by *Branhamella catarrhalis*. Pediatr. Infect. Dis. J. *4*:100–101, 1985.
4. Bartos, L. C., and Murphy, T. F.: Comparison of the outer membrane proteins of 50 strains of *Branhamella catarrhalis*. J. Infect. Dis. *158*:761–765, 1988.
5. Berg, R. A., and Bartley, D. L.: Pneumonia associated with *Branhamella catarrhalis* in infants. Pediatr. Infect. Dis. J. *6*:569–573, 1987.
6. Bonadio, W. A.: *Branhamella catarrhalis* bacteremia in children. Pediatr. Infect. Dis. J. *7*:738–739, 1988.
7. Brown, B. A., Wallace, R. J., Flanagan, C. W., et al.: Tetracycline and erythromycin resistance among clinical isolates of *Branhamella catarrhalis*. Antimicrob. Agents Chemother. *33*:1631–1633, 1989.
8. Catlin, B. W.: Transfer of the organism named *Neisseria catarrhalis* to *Branhamella* gen. nov. Int. J. Syst. Bacteriol. *20*:155–159, 1970.
9. Catlin, B. W.: *Branhamella catarrhalis*: An organism gaining respect as a pathogen. Clin. Microbiol. Rev. *3*:293–320, 1990.
10. Chapman, A. J., Musher, D. M., Jonsson, S., et al.: Development of bactericidal antibody during *Branhamella catarrhalis* infection. J. Infect. Dis. *151*:878–882, 1985.
11. Cook, P. P., Heent, D. W., and Syndman, D. R.: Nosocomial *Branhamella catarrhalis* in a pediatric intensive care unit: Risk factors for disease. J. Hosp. Infect. *13*:299–307, 1989.
12. Dickinson, D. P., Loos, B. G., Dryja, D. M., et al.: Restriction fragment mapping of *Branhamella catarrhalis:* A new tool for studying the epidemiology of this middle ear pathogen. J. Infect. Dis. *158*:208, 1988.
13. Doern, G. V.: *Branhamella catarrhalis*: Phenotypic characteristics. Am. J. Med. *88*:335–355, 1990.
14. Doern, G. V., and Jones, R. N.: Antimicrobial susceptibility testing of *Haemophilus influenzae, Branhamella catarrhalis* and *Neisseria gonorrhoeae*. Antimicrob. Agents Chemother. *32*:1747–1753, 1988.
15. Doern, G. V., and Tubert, A. T.: Detection of β-lactamase activity among clinical isolates of *Branhamella catarrhalis* with six different β-lactamase assays. J. Clin. Microbiol. *25*:1380–1383, 1987.
16. Dyson, C., Poonyth, H. O., Watkinson, et al.: Life threatening *Branhamella catarrhalis* pneumonia in young infants. J. Infect. *21*:305–307, 1990.
17. Ernst, T. N., and Philp, M.: Bacterial tracheitis caused by *Branhamella catarrhalis*. Pediatr. Infect. Dis. J. *6*:574, 1987.
18. Faden, H., Harabuchi, Y., Hong, J. J., et al.: Epidemiology of *Moraxella catarrhalis* in children during the first 2 years of life: Relationship to otitis media. J. Infect. Dis. *169*:1312–1317, 1994.
19. Faden, H., Hong, J. J., and Pahade, N.: Immune response to *Moraxella catarrhalis* in children with otitis media: Opsonophagocytosis with antigen-coated latex beads. Ann. Otol. Rhinol. Laryngol. *103*:522–524, 1994.
20. Fung, C.-P., Yeo, S.-F., and Livermore, D. M.: Susceptibility of *Moraxella catarrhalis* isolates to β-lactam antibiotics in relation to β-lactamase pattern. J. Antimicrob. Chemother. *33*:215–222, 1994.
21. Ghon, A., and Pfeiffer, H.: Der *Mikvococcus catarrhalis* (R. Pfeiffer) als krankheitserreger. Z. Klin. Med. *44*:263–281, 1902.
22. Goldblatt, D., Turner, M. W., and Levinsky, R. J.: *Branhamella catarrhalis*: Antigenic determinants and the development of the IgG subclass response in childhood. J. Infect. Dis. *162*:1128–1135, 1990.
23. Gottfarb, P., and Brauner, A.: Children with persistent cough: Outcome with treatment and role of *Moraxella catarrhalis?* Scand. J. Infect. Dis. *26*:545–551, 1994.
24. Hager, H., Verghese, A., Alvarez, S., et al.: *Branhamella catarrhalis* respiratory infections. Rev. Infect. Dis. *9*:1140–1149, 1987.
25. Harrison, C. J., Marks, J. I., and Welch, D. F.: Microbiology of recently treated acute otitis media compared with previously untreated acute otitis media. Pediatr. Infect. Dis. J. *4*:641–646, 1985.
26. Helminen, M. E., Maciver, I., Paris, M., et al.: A mutation affecting expression of a major outer protein of *Moraxella catarrhalis* alters resistance and survival in vivo. J. Infect. Dis. *168*:1194–1201, 1993.
27. Izraeli, S., Flasterstein, B., Shamir, R., et al.: *Branhamella catarrhalis* as a cause of suppurative arthritis. Pediatr. Infect. Dis. J. *8*:256–257, 1989.
28. Klein, J. O.: Otitis media. Clin. Infect. Dis. *19*:823–833, 1994.
29. Korppi, M., Katila, M. L., Jaaskelainen, J., et al.: Role of *Morraxella (Branhamella) catarrhalis* as a respiratory pathogen in children. Acta Paediatr. *81*:993–996, 1992.
30. Leinonen, M., Luotonen, J., Herva, E., et al.: Preliminary serologic evidence for a pathogenic role of *Branhamella catarrhalis*. J. Infect. Dis. *144*:570–574, 1981.
31. Lemmen, S. W., Anding, K., Engels, I., et al.: Bactericidal activity of clarithromycin and cefaclor against *Streptococcus pneumoniae* and *Moraxella catarrhalis* in healthy volunteers. J. Antimicrob. Chemother. *33*:673–674, 1994.
32. Maciver, I., Unhanand, M., McCracken, G. H., et al.: Effect of immunization on pulmonary clearance of *Moraxella catarrhalis* in animal model. J. Infect. Dis. *168*:469–472, 1993.
33. Marchant, C. D.: Spectrum of disease due to *Branhamella catarrhalis* in children with particular reference to acute otitis media. Am. J. Med. *88*(Suppl. 5A):155–195, 1990.
34. Melendez, P. R., and Johnson, R. H.: Bacteremia and septic arthritis caused by *Moraxella catarrhalis*. Rev. Infect. Dis. *13*:428–429, 1991.
35. Murphy, T. F.: The surface of *Branhamella catarrhalis*: A systematic approach to the surface antigens of an emerging pathogen. Pediatr. Infect. Dis. J. *8*:575–577, 1989.
36. Nash, D. R., Flanagan, C., Steele, L. C., et al.: Comparison of the activity of cefixime and activities of other oral antibiotics against adult clinical isolates of *Moraxella (Branhamella) catarrhalis* containing BRO-1 and BRO-2 and *Haemophilus influenzae*. Antimicrob. Agents Chemother. *35*:192–194, 1991.
37. Ohlsson, A., and Bailey, T.: Neonatal pneumonia caused by *Branhamella catarrhalis*. Scand. J. Infect. Dis. *17*:225–228, 1985.
38. Patterson, J. E., Patterson, T. F., Farrel, P., et al.: Evaluation of restrictions endonuclease analysis as an epidemiologic typing system for *Branhamella catarrhalis*. J. Clin. Microbiol. *27*:994–946, 1989.
39. Pichichero, M. E., and Pichichero, C. L.: Persistent acute otitis media. I. Causative organisms. Pediatr. Infect. Dis. J. *14*:178–183, 1995.
40. Roberts, M. C., Pang, Y., Spencer, R. C., et al.: Tetracycline resistance in *Moraxella (Branhamella) catarrhalis*: Demonstration of two clonal outbreaks by using pulsed-field gel electrophoresis. Antimicrob. Agents Chemother. *35*:2453–2455, 1991.
41. Rotta, A. T., and Asmar, B. I.: *Moraxella catarrhalis* bacteremia and preseptal cellulitis. South. Med. J. *87*:541–542, 1994.
42. Seddon, P. C., Sunderland, D., O'Halloran, S. M., et al.: *Branhamella catarrhalis* colonization in preschool asthmatics. Pediatr. Pulmonol. *13*:133–135, 1992.
43. Shurin, P. A., Marchant, C. D., Kim, C. H., et al.: Emergence of beta-lactamase–producing strains of *Branhamella catarrhalis* as important agents of otitis media. Pediatr. Infect. Dis. J. *2*:34–38, 1983.
44. Smith, G.: *Branhamella catarrhalis* infection imitating gonorrhea in a man. N. Engl. J. Med. *326*:1277, 1987.
45. Speeleveld, E., Fossépré, J. M., Gordts, B., et al.: Comparison of three rapid methods, tributyrine, 4-methylumbelliferyl butyrate, and indoxyl acetate, for rapid identification of *Moraxella catarrhalis*. J. Clin. Microbiol. *32*:1362–1363, 1994.
46. Stull, T. L., and Stanford, E. J.: Pseudogonococcal ophthalmia neonatorum caused by *Branhamella catarrhalis*. Pediatr. Infect. Dis. J. *5*:104–105, 1986.

47. Unhanand, M., Maciver, I., Ramilo, O., et al.: Pulmonary clearance of *Moraxella catarrhalis* in an animal model. J. Infect. Dis. *165*:644–650, 1992.
48. Vaneechoutte, M., Verschraegen, G., Claeys, G., et al.: Serologic typing of *Branhamella catarrhalis* strains on the basis of lipopolysaccharide antigens. J. Clin. Microbiol. *28*:182–187, 1990.
49. Vaneechoutte, M., Verschraegen, G., Claeys, G., et al.: Respiratory tract carrier rates of *Moraxella Branhamella catarrhalis* in adults and children and interpretation of the isolation of *Moraxella catarrhalis* from sputum. J. Clin. Microbiol. *28*:2674–2680, 1990.
50. Van Hare, G. F., Shurin, P. A., Marchant, C. D., et al.: Acute otitis media caused by *Branhamella catarrhalis*: Biology and therapy. Rev. Infect. Dis. *9*:16–27, 1987.
51. Verghese, A., and Berk, S. L.: *Moraxella (Branhamella) catarrhalis*. Infect. Dis. Clin. North Am. *5*:523–538, 1991.
52. Wald, E. R., Reilly, J. S., Casselbrant, M., et al.: Treatment of acute maxillary sinusitis in childhood: A comparative study of amoxicillin and cefaclor. J. Pediatr. *104*:297–302, 1984.
53. Wong, V. K., and Ross, L. A.: *Branhamella catarrhalis* septicemia in an infant with AIDS. Scand. J. Infect. Dis. *20*:559–560, 1988.

93

MENINGOCOCCAL DISEASE

Marsha S. Anderson, Mary P. Glodé, and Arnold L. Smith

Epidemic meningococcal meningitis first was described by Gaspard Vieusseux in Geneva in the spring of 1805. In a monograph entitled "The Disease Which Raged During the Spring of 1805," he wrote:

> It commences suddenly with prostration of strength, often extreme: the face is distorted, the pulse feeble. There appears a violent pain in the head, especially over the forehead; then there comes pain of the heart or vomiting of greenish material, stiffness of the spine, and in infants, convulsions. In cases which were fatal, loss of consciousness occurred. The course of the disease is very rapid, termination by death or by cure. In most of the patients who died in 24 hours or a little after, the body is covered with purple spots at the moment of death or very little time afterward.[137]

Today, meningococcus continues to be a cause of endemic and epidemic disease. In the United States, approximately 3000 sporadic cases occur each year. However, epidemics in Brazil in the early 1970s and in Finland in 1975 serve as a reminder of the potential virulence of this organism. In São Paulo, Brazil, during the epidemic period, almost 1 in every 300 inhabitants developed invasive meningococcal disease during a 1-year period.[48]

MICROBIOLOGY

The family Neisseriaceae contains five genera: *Neisseria, Kingella, Eikenella, Simonsiella,* and *Alysiella*. In addition, it includes three Centers for Disease Control and Prevention (CDC) groups that commonly are found as normal mouth flora in dogs: CDC groups EF-4a, EF-4b, and M-5. Previously, the family contained the genera *Acinetobacter, Moxarella,* and *Psychrobacter*; however, these have not been included in the most recent classification.[76]

The *Neisseria* genus was named for Dr. Albert Neisser, who described the organism of gonorrhea in 1879. The 14 species included in the genus of *Neisseria* are *N. gonorrhoeae, N. meningitidis, N. kochii, N. sicca, N. lactamica, N. subflava, N. flavescens, N. mucosa, N. cinerea, N. polysacchreae, N. elongata, N. macacae, N. canis,* and *N. dentrificans*. *N. kochii* is classified by some as a subspecies. They are distinguished from one another by a series of biochemical tests.[76]

N. meningitidis is a gram-negative coccus, usually less than 1 μm in diameter. It classically occurs in pairs, with adjacent sides flattened, resembling kidney beans. Occasionally, the organism divides in two planes at right angles to one another, which results in the formation of tetrads. The organisms are nonmotile and aerobic (or facultatively anaerobic), produce catalase and oxidase, and may be encapsulated. The organisms may autolyse when exposed to drying or sunlight. *N. meningitidis* ferments glucose and maltose. This distinguishes it from *N. gonorrhoeae*, which ferments glucose only. However, certain rare strains of *N. meningitidis* have been reported that fail to produce acid from either glucose or maltose. Fresh isolates have complex nutritional requirements, growing best on chocolate or blood agar. Incubation in 10 per cent carbon dioxide is not essential but enhances growth. Morphologically, the colonies are bluish-gray in appearance and will produce beta-hemolysis after 48 to 72 hours of incubation on 5 per cent horse blood agar.[16]

In order to survive, pathogenic neisseriae require iron, which they must obtain from the host. Neisseriae possess outer-membrane proteins that bind to host heme, transferrin, and lactoferrin, enabling the organism to acquire the iron it needs for growth. A study in mice showed iron loading increased the likelihood of a fatal infection.[63]

Like other gram-negative bacteria, neisseriae's outer and inner cell membranes are phospholipid bilayers. These membranes sandwich a layer of peptidoglycan. Lipo-oligosaccharide, which is similar to the lipopolysaccharide seen in gram-negative enteric bacteria, is associated with the outer leaflet of the outer cell membrane. Outer-membrane proteins, which function as porins, are an integral part of the outer membrane. Some of these outer-membrane proteins are opacity proteins and may have a role in adherence and invasion.[96] Outside the outer membrane is a polysaccharide capsule, which protects the organism from phagocytosis.

Meningococci also have pili, which seem to be important in some phases of adherence to host cells, colonization, and invasion. The genes that code for pili can be turned on and off, so that the organism at times may not express pili. This may help the meningococci to detach and allow the organism to be transmitted to another site or another host.[56] Antigenic variation of pili occurs, probably in an attempt to escape the host's immune system.[51] In addition, both outer-membrane proteins and lipo-oligopolysaccharide display antigenic variation.

Meningococci can be divided into serogroups, serotypes, subtypes, immunotypes, and multilocus enzyme electrophoresis types. Differences in capsular polysaccharides, outer-membrane proteins, lipo-oligosaccharides, and cytoplasmic isoenzymes constitute the basis for these classifications. Thirteen serogroups currently are recognized: A, B, C, D, H, I, K, L, X, Y, Z, W135, and 29E.[5] Serogroups A, B, and C are the most common causes of invasive disease worldwide. Table 93–1 lists the chemical composition of the capsule from the serogroups most commonly associated with meningococcal disease.[10, 69] The capsular polysaccharides are antigenic and the basis for serogroup designation.

Serotyping of organisms is based on antigenic differences in class 2 and 3 outer-membrane proteins. Subtypes are differentiated based on class 1 outer-membrane protein variation. More than 20 serotypes and 10 subtypes have been identified so far. Antigenic specificity is achieved by the generation of monoclonal antibodies to the major protein (primarily class 2 or 3), lipo-oligosaccharide, and class 1 protein. The designation B:2a:P1.1:L3,7 indicates that the serogroup B strain is an "a" subtype of class 2 proteins, is a "one" of class 1 protein, and possesses two lipo-oligosaccharide antigens: 3 and 7.[42]

Serogroup B isolates can be classified into antigenically distinct serotypes on the basis of outer-membrane protein antigens.[36] Type 2 protein antigen is isolated from more than 50 per cent of cases in the United States and Canada and also is an antigenic determinant in group C strains. These protein antigens not only are important as epidemiologic markers but also may induce protective bactericidal antibodies.[40]

EPIDEMIOLOGY

The incidence of meningococcal disease varies significantly by geographic location. Endemic disease, which occurs in developed countries such as the United States and Europe, has an incidence range of 1 to 3 per 100,000 inhabitants per year.[108] In developing countries, the incidence rate is about 10 times higher (10–25/100,000 inhabitants/year). The highest rate of meningococcal disease appears to be in a multicountry belt across sub-Saharan Africa, which has been termed the *meningitis belt*. Serogroup A meningococcal disease is prevalent here and occurs in epidemics. During epidemics, the incidence of meningococcal disease is as high as 1000 per 100,000 inhibitants (1 per cent). Spread of clonal strains of group A meningococcus may be a factor in Africa's unusually high rate of epidemic disease. Clonal strains can migrate transcontinentally and cause epidemics, as is evidenced by the clonal group A meningococcus, electrophoretic type III-1 (ET III-1), that caused epidemics in China, Nepal, Saudi Arabia, Chad, and Kenya in the 1980s.[93, 107]

A classic case of an epidemic of serogroup A (ET III-1) *N. meningitidis* infection occurred in 1987 in Saudi Arabia and was associated with Muslims making the annual pilgrimage to Mecca. South Asian pilgrims had the highest attack rate, but the disease spread to persons of all nationalities represented, some of whom returned home prior to becoming ill.[93] Nine cases in United States citizens were identified, eight of which were Muslim pilgrims. Two persons became ill prior to leaving Saudi Arabia, and seven persons became symptomatic shortly after their return to the United States. Additionally, a nasopharyngeal carriage rate (of the responsible strain) of 11 per cent was demonstrated in those persons who had visited Mecca and returned to the United States on flights from Saudi Arabia.[91, 4]

Serogroups A, B, and C account for more than 90 per cent of meningococcal disease worldwide. Serogroup A, which causes periodic epidemics in developing countries, is responsible for only 3 per cent of meningococcal disease in the United States.[6] Serogroup B usually causes sporadic disease but occasionally is associated with outbreaks.[6] Serogroup C, although also a cause of sporadic disease, has been associated with numerous outbreaks in the United States, Canada, and Europe.[66]

In the United States, group B and C meningococcal disease each account for 45 per cent of invasive disease. Serotype Y, although rare, has been associated with meningococcal pneumonia in military recruits.[122] Serogroup C disease appears to be on the rise in the United States. Jackson and colleagues[66] reported 21 outbreaks of serogroup C meningococcal disease between 1980 and 1993. However, more than one-third (8 outbreaks) occurred between 1991 and 1993. Multilocus enzyme electrophoresis identified many of the strains in these outbreaks to be clonal and ET-15.[66, 142] ET-15 meningococci also were shown to be the predominant agents causing serogroup C disease in Canada in the early 1990s and were associated with an increase in mortality there.[142] School-related outbreaks of serogroup C meningococcal disease also have been reported.[94]

Meningococcal disease, in the United States, peaks during the months November through March.[117, 126] The highest attack rate is seen in February, and the lowest attack rate occurs in September. In Africa, epidemic disease occurs during the dry season and decreases once the rainy season starts.[107] Males and females are affected equally.

The risk of meningococcal disease is related inversely to age, with 49 per cent of the cases occurring in children 2 years of age or younger. However, in epidemics, there is an age shift, with older children, adolescents, and young adults more often affected.[6, 142] Studies have shown that there is a progressive increase in the development of protective antibodies against meningococci between the ages of 2 and 12 years. Neonates usually are protected, if the mother has antimeningococcal antibody, by passive IgG transfer in utero. In general, the development of bactericidal antibodies to meningococci increases in children at a rate of about 5 per cent per year.[47]

The precise epidemiology of meningococcal disease in recruit populations was defined elegantly in a series of observations in New Jersey. In these studies, an inverse correlation was noted between the age-related incidence of meningococcal disease in the United States and the prevalence of serum bactericidal activity against three pathogenic strains of *N. meningitidis*.[46]

The investigators prospectively studied all incoming recruits to Fort Dix. The sera of 54 of 492 recruits lacked bactericidal activity to the case strains. Twenty-four (45 per cent) of those men acquired a meningococcus group C; 11 of the 24 developed bactericidal antibody to this strain. Of the 13 who were antibody-negative and acquired group C strains in the nasopharynx, 5 became ill with meningococcal meningitis. This corresponds to an attack rate of 38 per cent in the susceptible, exposed population.[46]

In the Fort Dix study, nasopharyngeal carriage was shown

TABLE 93–1. Chemical Structure of Group-Specific Polysaccharide Capsules of Meningococci

Group	Chemical Composition of Capsule
A	2-Acetamido-2-deoxy-D-mannopyranosyl phosphate
B	α-2,8 *N*-acetylneuraminic acid
C	α-2,9 O-acetylneuraminic acid
D	Composition not known
X	2-Acetamido-2-deoxy-D-glucopyranosyl phosphate
Y	4-O-α-D-glucopyranosyl-*N*-acetylneuraminic acid
Z	Composition not known
29E	3-deoxy-D-manno-octulosonic acid
W135	4-O-α-D-galactopyranosyl-*N*-acetylneuraminic acid

to be an immunizing process. Carriage induced the formation of protective antibodies against homologous strains but also produced cross-reacting antibodies to heterologous strains of pathogenic meningococci.[46] Certain strains of cross-reacting bacteria, such as *Escherichia coli* and *Bacillus*, produce capsular polysaccharides that immunologically are identical to the capsules of meningococci serogroups A, B, and C. This is another potential immunizing source against invasive disease in the general population.[47, 73, 136] It seems clear from many studies that the vast majority of persons who are exposed to pathogenic meningococci become carriers, rather than become ill, and that susceptibility to disease correlates with lack of bactericidal antibody.

Nasopharyngeal carriage of *N. meningitidis* is relatively common, with 2.4 per cent of randomly cultured asymptomatic infants and children yielding a positive culture for *N. meningitidis* during a nonepidemic period in a Canadian study.[84] Age seems to affect carriage, with infants and children having lower carriage rates and young to middle-aged adults having the highest incidence. A study of 1500 randomly sampled Norwegians found the overall carriage rate to be 9.6 per cent, but the carriage rate in persons 20 to 24 years of age was 32.7 per cent. Beyond 25 years of age, the carriage rate again was around 10 per cent.[19] The strains were not typed, so it is likely that some strains were not pathogenic, but the trend remains that the young adult appears to be a likely reservoir of infection. Other investigators have shown that approximately 20 per cent of children harbor meningococcal species in their nasopharynx, but the majority of these isolates are atypical, nontypable strains, which ferment lactose in addition to glucose and maltose.[47]

Nasopharyngeal meningococcal carriage in household contacts of persons with documented meningococcal disease has been shown to be about 10 per cent.[84, 100, 113] However, one study showed that the carriage rate is affected by the presence of infants or children in the home.[100] In 1972, an epidemic of serogroup C meningococcal disease occurred in São Paulo.[73] The carriage rate there was 14.2 per cent in households without a case. Carriage rates were 37.8 per cent in households with a case in an infant, 17.5 per cent in households with a case in a child 1 to 14 years of age, and 6.9 per cent in households with disease in an adult. The reason for this is unclear. However, because meningococcal disease is transmitted by the respiratory route and in general children are not as fastidious about controlling their respiratory secretions, young children in a home may facilitate colonization of others.

Marks and colleagues[84] looked at nasopharyngeal carriage after household contact with an index case. Without chemoprophylaxis, 35 per cent of contacts become colonized by the eighth week. The median duration of carriage was 9 months. However, in 38 per cent, it exceeded 16 months.[49] Greenfield and colleagues[44] found that the highest incidence of carriage was in adult males and that 50 per cent of the time, the organism entered the household in this manner. An association between smoking and increased rate of meningococcal carriage has been demonstrated.[125, 127] In addition, passive smoke has been implicated in increasing the risk of meningococcal disease in children younger than 5 years of age by 7.5 times that of the general population.[125]

The factors responsible for converting nasopharyngeal colonization to invasive disease have not been elucidated firmly. There is some evidence that many persons who subsequently develop invasive disease were colonized shortly before their illness began. This ties in with the older Fort Dix studies, in that there are certain susceptible individuals in a population who do not have protective antibody to pathogenic meningococci. Shortly after colonization (if neutralizing antibodies do not develop), they become infected and ill.

Speculation as to the role of other upper respiratory pathogens in meningococcal disease prompted several studies. It was noted that the peak incidence of meningococcal infection mirrors the peaks of such agents as influenza and mycoplasma. Several studies have shown an association between colonization or infection with respiratory viruses or mycoplasma and the increased risk of development of meningococcal disease.[17, 64, 92] Simultaneous outbreaks of meningococcal and influenza or echovirus infections have been documented.[82, 148] In addition, one study suggested that the incidence of meningococcal disease and the resultant morbidity and mortality increased in the 5 weeks following influenza-like syndromes.[92] Although the mechanism of this interaction has not been defined precisely, it has been postulated that viral pathogens temporarily may affect the immune response and facilitate meningococcal disease. It also is possible that disruption of the normal respiratory epithelium occurs with viral infections, and this increases the likelihood that colonizing meningococci might become invasive.[92] Preceding viral respiratory disease is not a prerequisite for the establishment of meningococcal carriage or disease. However, its occurrence may increase the risk of invasive meningococcal disease.

Individuals with late complement component deficiencies (C5, C6, C7, C8, or C9) and properdin pathway deficiencies are at risk for meningococcal disease.[38] This usually is an inherited defect, and there may be a history of other members of the family with meningococcal disease or repeated meningococcal infections. Acquired complement deficiencies associated with diseases such as systemic lupus erythematosus, nephrotic syndrome, and chronic liver disease also are associated with increased risk of meningococcal disease.[80] A Russian study found the incidence of complement deficiency in first episodes of meningococcal disease to be about 1 per cent.[110] In Italy, the prevalence of complement deficiency in patients with meningococcal meningitis was 17 per cent.[23] The decision of who to screen for complement deficiency should be made partly based on the prevalence of meningococcal disease in a given country. In countries where the incidence of meningococcal disease is high, complement deficiency is less likely to be found. In countries such as the United States, where the incidence is relatively low, complement screening may be justified.

The chance of finding a complement or alternate pathway (properdin) deficiency substantially increases in patients who present with recurrent meningococcal disease or with uncommon serogroups. The prevalence of complement or properdin deficiency in a patient with infection by an unusual serogroup was found to range from 31 to 50 per cent.[37, 98] Therefore, screening all individuals who present with unusual serogroups is reasonable. CH_{50} is a generally available test and will screen for combined activity of C1 to C9. If complement deficiency is found, the individual should receive the meningococcal vaccine. In addition, family members who are found to be complement-deficient also should receive vaccine.

Some investigators have shown that although persons with complement deficiency are more at risk for meningococcal disease, the disease they get often is mild. Meningococcal infection activates the complement system, and lipo-oligosaccharides present in the bacteria's outer membrane probably are responsible for the activation. In fatal cases, intense activation has continued until the time of death.[15] The case-fatality rate in complement-deficient individuals is about 3 per cent.[118] It is thought that complement-deficient individuals are unable to maintain the high level complement pathway activation and therefore have less severe disease.

Properdin deficiency, which impairs activation of the alternate complement pathway, is X-linked and has been associated with fulminant meningococcal disease.[26, 123] The case-fatality rate in one kindred was 75 per cent for persons with meningococcal disease.[21] Screening of individuals with exceptionally fulminant disease or individuals who have a family history of meningococcal infections should be considered. AP50 will screen for properdin deficiency in the alternate complement pathway. If a deficiency is documented, those individuals could receive the quadrivalent meningococcal vaccine to prevent at least some serogroups of meningococcus.

PATHOLOGY AND PATHOGENESIS

The mechanisms by which meningococci invade humans are understood only partially at present. We do know that encapsulated, typable meningococci are virulent, whereas nonencapsulated strains are relatively nonpathogenic. Even among encapsulated strains, differences in virulence between case and carrier strains of *N. meningitidis* have been demonstrated in an animal model.[62] It is believed that the presence of a polysaccharide capsule confers some degree of invasiveness to the organism by such mechanisms as resistance to opsonization and phagocytosis, perhaps by inhibiting complement activation via the alternative pathway.

Once pathogenic meningococci have colonized the respiratory tract, they may become invasive or the individual may develop antibody to the organism, conferring immunity against invasive disease. If no antibody develops and invasion occurs, the individual may become bacteremic. A small number of cases have been reported in which unsuspected meningococcal bacteremia has been detected on blood culture and spontaneously cleared on a follow-up culture without antibiotics.[128] However, in most cases, this does not occur and the individual becomes progressively sicker. Bacteria in the blood may seed the meninges and cause meningitis.

Studies have shown that those individuals presenting with meningitis have a better prognosis than do those presenting with only bacteremia. Presumably, this is a function of virulence of the organism, ability of the immune system to contain the infection, or both.

The pathologic lesions seen in fulminant meningococcal disease are similar to those that the generalized Shwartzman reaction induces in rabbits by endotoxin. Pathogenesis of tissue injury in meningococcal disease is mediated through the effects of endotoxin. Davis and Arnold[24] investigated the relative potency of meningococcal endotoxins, compared with *E. coli* and *Salmonella typhimurium* endotoxin. Meningococcal and enteric endotoxins were equally potent in mouse lethality assays and in their ability to induce a generalized Shwartzman reaction. However, the meningococcal endotoxins were 5- to 10-fold more potent in eliciting the dermal Shwartzman reaction. The authors postulate that the greater skin potency of endotoxin preparations from meningococci may explain the prominence of purpuric skin lesions in meningococcemia.

Studies have confirmed the release of mediators, such as tumor necrosis factor and interleukins-1, -6, and -8 in patients with meningococcal disease.[53, 133, 138, 139] Tumor necrosis factor, interleukin-1, and gamma interferon levels are higher in patients who ultimately die than in those patients who survive.[44] It currently is thought that the release of these substances is triggered by endotoxin. These cytokines, in addition to the lipid A portion of the lipo-oligopolysaccharide on the outer cell membrane, likely are responsible for inducing shock that often accompanies meningococcal infections.

Shortly after administration of cidal antibiotics, some patients have marked clinical deterioration, including hypotension and sometimes death. Rapid liberation of endotoxin (and resultant stimulation of cytokine release) from lysing organisms may be the cause of this phenomenon.[89] There may be variation in the amount of endotoxin liberated by a given isolate. In one study, strains from individuals with invasive disease released higher amounts of endotoxin than did isolates from carriers.[88]

The disseminated intravascular coagulation frequently seen in meningococcemia also is believed to be a consequence of activation of the coagulation system by endotoxin.[116] Experimental animal work has suggested a synergistic effect of meningococcal endotoxin and materials egested from leukocytes containing meningococci in the initiation of disseminated intravascular coagulation.[28]

A pathologic study of 200 fatal meningococcal infections, published by Hardman,[54] illustrates the ability of the meningococcus to affect virtually any organ, either directly or indirectly. Approximately 40 per cent of the patients had meningococcemia and meningitis. Except for adults with meningitis, the average survival time for all cases was 72 hours or less. The major organ systems involved at autopsy in these 200 cases were heart, central nervous system, skin, mucous and serous membranes, and adrenals.

Myocarditis occurred in 78 per cent of cases (the histology of this lesion is discussed separately; see Pericarditis and Myocarditis section). In the patients with myocarditis, pulmonary edema also was noted, and pleural effusions were found in 30 per cent. Acute myocarditis was felt to be the primary factor responsible for the fatal outcome.

Cutaneous hemorrhages occurred in 69 per cent of the fatal infections and ranged from isolated petechiae to diffuse purpura. The extent or location of hemorrhage did not correlate with infection due to any particular serotype of *N. meningitidis*. Hemorrhage frequently was associated with acute vasculitis and with fibrin deposition in arterioles, capillaries, and glomeruli.

Acute meningitis was noted at autopsy in 68 per cent of the infections. Acute inflammatory cells were present in the leptomeninges and perivascular spaces; vasculitis of small meningeal veins also was noted. Encephalitis was seen primarily in adult patients who developed meningitis without meningococcemia. Brain abscesses were noted in two patients. In almost half the cases with acute meningococcemia, *N. meningitidis* was isolated from otherwise normal cerebrospinal fluid.

Adrenal hemorrhage and necrosis were found in 48 per cent of autopsy cases. Diffuse adrenal hemorrhage occurred in approximately 50 per cent of adult cases and in more than 80 per cent of pediatric cases. Adrenal vasculitis and acute inflammation were not seen. In this study, some patients had a typical Waterhouse-Friderichsen syndrome (purpura and circulatory collapse) but had normal adrenals on gross and microscopic examination. Hardman[54] postulated that circulatory failure was due to endotoxic shock rather than to adrenal insufficiency.

Focal areas of inflammation and petechial hemorrhage were seen in many other tissues, including synovium, skeletal muscle, and the tracheobronchial tree.

There was an association between the pathologic findings and the infecting serotype of *N. meningitidis*. Group A infections most frequently were associated with encephalitis; groups B and C infections were associated with necrotizing myocarditis.

CLINICAL MANIFESTATIONS

The spectrum of disease caused by *N. meningitidis* ranges from asymptomatic transient bacteremia, which clears spon-

TABLE 93–2. Signs and Symptoms in Serious Meningococcal Disease

Clinical Feature	Per Cent at Presentation
Fever	71–88.8
Rash	68.4–71
Shock	38–42
Vomiting	34–67
Lethargy	30–55
Headache	34
Irritability	21–34
Poor feeding	18
Cough or rhinorrhea	18
Seizures	8–10

Data from references 70, 74, 146.

taneously, to fulminant sepsis resulting in death only a few hours after the first symptoms occur.

Serious/Invasive Disease

Serious or invasive disease usually presents in one of three ways: occult bacteremia, meningococcemia, or meningitis (either with or without meningococcemia).

Occult bacteremia is found when a nontoxic child presents with fever and a blood culture is noted to be positive for *N. meningitidis*. Some of these patients have not received any oral or parenteral antibiotics and have cleared their bacteremia spontaneously.[128] Others go on to develop meningitis or severe meningococcemia.

The signs and symptoms of meningococcemia are variable. Early on, there may be evidence of an upper respiratory infection, including coryza, pharyngitis, tonsillitis, and laryngitis. Patients generally are febrile, with complaints of headache, lethargy, and vomiting. Severe myalgias with muscle tenderness and joint pain also may be the presenting complaint.[11, 29] The typical patient with meningococcemia presents with a short history of upper respiratory symptoms, fever,

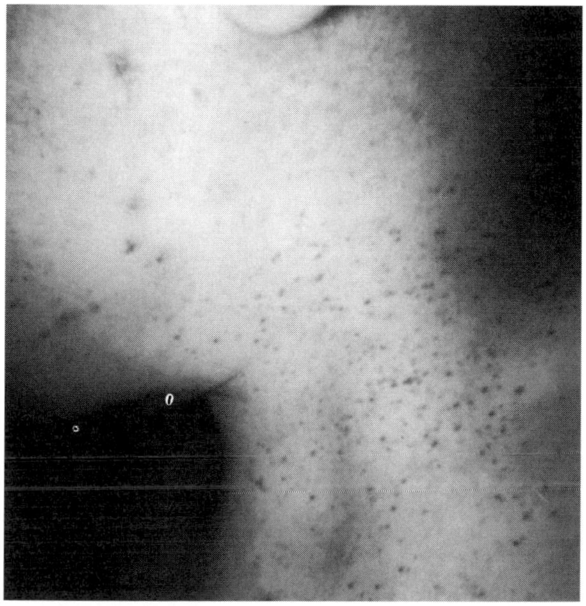

FIGURE 93–1. *Petechial lesions are seen on the face and neck of a young child with meningococcemia.*

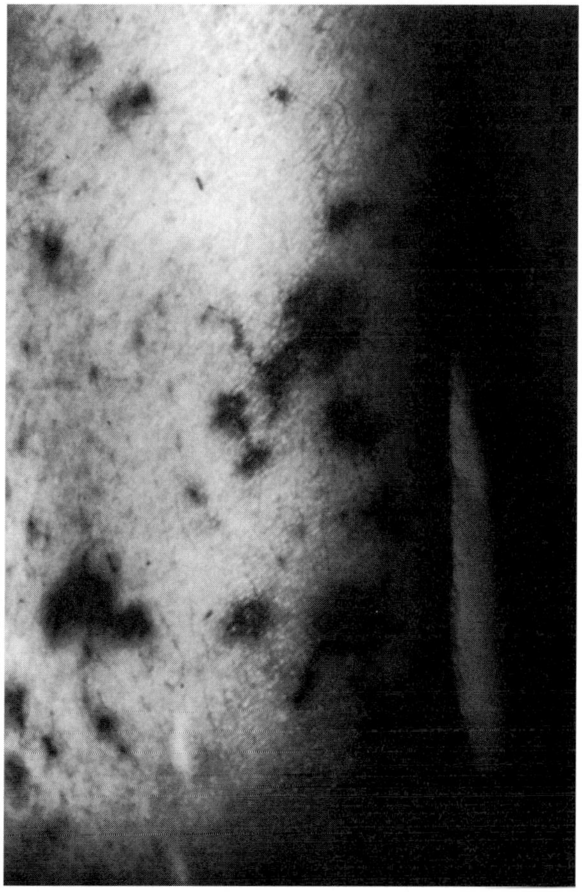

FIGURE 93–2. *Extensive purpuric lesions occurring in a child with overwhelming meningococcemia and disseminated intravascular coagulation.*

and a hemorrhagic rash. The patient often develops signs of severe circulatory collapse. It is not unusual for purpura and shock to develop within hours of the first onset of symptoms.

Patients who present with meningitis often are febrile, with headache, vomiting, irritability, stiff neck, and sometimes seizures. There may be a history of lethargy, or the patient may present obtunded. The same prodromal symptoms that are seen in meningococcemia often are present. Infants may present with fever, irritablility, increased sleeping, and poor feeding. Table 93–2 lists the common signs and symptoms on presentation with serious meningococcal disease.

On physical examination, the findings depend on whether the patient has meningococcemia with or without meningitis. The major physical findings include fever, rash, meningeal signs, and circulatory collapse. In neonates, physical findings of meningismus, such as Kernig's and Brudzinski's signs, often are absent. The anterior fontanelle, if open, may be full and tense.

The skin manifestations of this disease range from a diffuse mottling to extensive purpuric lesions (Figs. 93–1 and 93–2). Unfortunately, there is some variation to the type of rash seen. Petechiae are present in 50 to 60 per cent of patients.[74] However, 7 per cent have fewer than 12 petechiae, and 1 to 2 per cent have no rash at all.[85] One prospective multicenter study found that 13 per cent of children had only a maculopapular rash and did not develop the classic hemorrhagic rash.[85] This makes differentiation from a viral exanthem particularly difficult. A pink macular rash resembling early varicella is another variant sometimes seen in children; these lesions often are tender. They may occur in crops, as do the petechiae, and are seen most frequently on the trunk and extremities.[29, 60] The finding of petechiae or purpura in a febrile child should increase the index of suspicion for meningococcemia or other serious disease (e.g., infectious, neoplastic, immunologic). Acral distribution of a rash particularly is worrisome for meningococcemia or another infectious vasculitic process. A study of 129 febrile patients with petechiae found that 20.2 per cent had invasive bacterial disease.[135] Ten per cent of the total group had infections caused by *N. meningitidis*. Therefore, it seems reasonable to obtain blood cultures on all febrile patients who present with petechiae. Lumbar puncture should be performed if clinically indicated or if the blood culture ultimately is positive. Antibiotic therapy in these patients should include coverage for meningococcus.

Purpura is a feature of fulminant cases and does not arise from the petechiae but is a separate and distinct lesion.[74] Pathologically, it consists of microvascular dermal thrombosis and hemorrhage, sometimes progressing to frank necrosis. Purpura is noted in 16 to 24 per cent of patients.[111, 117, 146] Acquired protein S and C deficiencies have been described in some patients presenting with purpura fulminans.[111, 112] One study showed a mortality rate of 50 per cent in patients who developed purpura. Progressive purpura was accompanied by declining protein C levels, and the level of protein C was related inversely to the clinical severity of the disease.[111]

Neonatal meningococcemia and/or meningitis is uncommon but has been reported. In one report, a 2-week-old infant died after a brief febrile illness with both cerebrospinal fluid and blood cultures positive for meningococcus. Maternal endocervical colonization was documented. In addition, the mother's pharyngeal culture grew *N. meningitidis*.[71] If endocervical colonization by *N. meningitidis* is found prenatally, treatment with antibiotics probably should be initiated in an attempt to eradicate colonization prior to delivery, or intrapartum antibiotics should be given. Ceftriaxone would seem to be a reasonable choice. Rifampin and ciprofloxacin are not advocated for use during pregnancy.

Conjunctivitis

Primary meningococcal conjunctivitis is indistinguishable clinically from acute bacterial conjunctivitis caused by other organisms. Usually, it presents in children as the acute onset of unilateral purulent conjunctivitis.[8] It has been reported in individuals from 2 days of age to adulthood.[4] Gram stain of the purulent material typically shows gram-negative diplococci that may sometimes be confused with gonococcal conjunctivitis. Barquet and colleagues[8] showed that 44 per cent of the isolates were serogroup B meningococci.

The complications of primary meningococcal conjunctivitis reported by Barquet and colleagues[8] included sepsis or meningitis in approximately 18 per cent. The symptoms of systemic meningococcal disease occurred 3 to 96 hours after the onset of the conjunctivitis (mean, 41 hours). Patients treated only with topical therapy at the time they presented with conjunctivitis were 19 times more likely to develop systemic disease than were patients treated with systemic therapy (p = .001). Ocular complications occurred in 15.5 per cent of patients and included corneal ulcers (10.7 per cent), keratitis, hemorrhage, and iritis.

Pharyngitis

The diagnosis of meningococcal pharyngitis is difficult because, like group A beta-hemolytic streptococci, the isolation of meningococcus from the pharynx does not establish that this organism is the etiologic agent. In fact, most individuals who harbor meningococci in their nasopharynges are asymptomatic carriers. However, Banks[7] noted overt nasopharyngitis in one-third of patients with meningococcal sepsis or meningitis. Pizzi,[109] describing a severe epidemic of meningococcal meningitis, noted that individuals with sore throats often had a pure culture of meningococci. Olcén and associates[100] cultured family members of 21 consecutive cases of meningococcal disease and found that 61 per cent of family members with sore throat or other upper respiratory symptoms were meningococcal carriers, compared with 14 per cent of asymptomatic family members.

Meningococcal Pneumonia

Meningococcal pneumonia occurs in conjunction with meningococcemia or meningitis in 8 to 15 per cent of cases.[77] However, the meningococcus also can play a role as a primary respiratory pathogen.

Primary meningococcal pneumonia, once considered a rare disease, now is recognized as the most common form of meningococcal disease in certain military recruit populations and has been reported to cause 4.5 per cent of all bacterial pneumonias in a general hospital population.[77, 83]

Patients with preceding viral pneumonias are at risk for meningococcal pneumonia; more than 100 cases of meningococcal pneumonia occurred during the influenza pandemic of 1918 and 1919. In addition to disease among military recruits, nosocomial acquisition of meningococcal pneumonia in hospitalized patients has been reported.[20]

The diagnosis of meningococcal pneumonia is difficult because isolation of the organism from the sputum does not distinguish a meningococcal carrier from the individual with meningococcal pneumonia. In addition, routine sputum cultures do not include media selective for the meningococcus. Blood cultures are positive in only 15 per cent.[77]

Koppes and associates[77] reported on 68 cases of meningococcal pneumonia; diagnostic criteria included (1) a compatible clinical syndrome, (2) a radiograph demonstrating infiltrates or effusion, (3) culture of transtracheal aspirate yielding the organism and a consistent Gram stain, and (4) isolation of *N. meningitidis* from pleural fluid or blood. All 68 meningococcal pneumonia cases were group Y; during the same period, there were 10 cases of meningococcemia and 6 cases of meningitis due to group Y. The high ratio of pneumonia to meningitis in this study suggested that group Y organisms may be more likely to cause pneumonia than are other serogroups. Pneumonia due to group B or C meningococci has been reported, usually in association with meningococcemia or meningitis.[145]

Primary meningococcal pneumonia usually is associated with a gradual onset of symptoms and a history of an antecedent upper respiratory infection. Rales and fever are found in most patients, and 80 per cent have pharyngitis. The radiograph often shows involvement of lower lobes with patchy alveolar infiltrates. More than one lobe is involved in 40 per cent. Twenty-five per cent have pleural effusions. Petechiae, purpura, or shock was not present in any of the patients with pneumonia reported by Koppes and colleagues.[77]

The pathogenesis of this disease is felt to be pulmonary infection via droplet inhalation. The epidemiologic importance of meningococcal pneumonia was emphasized in a report from the CDC discussing nosocomial transmission of group Y *N. meningitidis* in oncology patients.[20] The index case had meningococcal pneumonia. One other patient in an adjacent room developed meningococcal bacteremia; in three additional patients, group Y *N. meningitidis* was isolated from nasopharyngeal cultures. Airborne dissemination seemed to be the mode of transmission. Respiratory isolation for a patient with suspected meningococcal pneumonia is indicated.

Meningococcal Pericarditis

Pericarditis usually is seen as a complication of meningococcal disease but occasionally has been reported in primary infection. One case report was of an 18-year-old boy who presented with fever, pleuritic chest pain, progressive dyspnea, and orthopnea. Evidence of cardiac tamponade, including cyanosis, jugular venous distention, and distant heart sounds, was noted on physical examination. Meningitis and bacteremia were not found. Pericardial fluid grew *N. meningitidis*, serogroup C.[135]

Mesenteric Adenitis and Peritionitis

Meningococcal mesenteric adenitis and peritonitis are rare but have been reported. The clinical presentation is that of appendicitis, with a normal appendix found at surgery. Enlarged mesenteric nodes may be seen intraoperatively. In the patient reported by Kunkel and colleagues,[78] peritoneal fluid cultures grew *N. meningitidis*.

Infections of the Genitourinary Tract

N. meningitidis is isolated infrequently from the genitourinary tract of asymptomatic or symptomatic individuals. However, the number of isolates from the cervix, urethra, or anus has increased.[36] About 40 per cent of the patients have asymptomatic colonization, with the rest presenting with symptoms of proctitis, urethritis, or cervicitis.[45] Many of the urethral and anal isolates were from homosexual men. Changing sexual habits may be one explanation for the apparent increase in isolation of meningococci from the genitourinary tract and suggest that the changing epidemiology may have important clinical implications, particularly in pregnant women and neonates. One group elected to treat meningococcal anogenital infection as if it were gonococcal infection and was able to eradicate the organism in all patients.[45]

Chronic Meningococcemia

Chronic meningococcemia, first described in 1902, is defined as a meningococcal septicemia without meningeal symptoms in which fever has persisted for at least a week before any antibiotic therapy.[31, 99] Benoit[9] reviewed 148 cases of chronic meningococcemia in the United States in 1963; patients ranged in age from 3 months to 62 years. The major symptoms included fever and chills (present in 100 per cent of patients), skin rash (93.2 per cent), arthralgias (70.3 per cent), and headache (61.5 per cent). The patients generally were not toxic and were in good health before becoming infected. The mean duration of illness prior to diagnosis was 6 to 8 weeks (range, 1 to 40 weeks). Symptoms tended to be intermittent; the rash often appeared in association with fever and then disappeared over the next several days. Bacteremia also may be intermittent. In the Benoit study, in the average patient, five blood cultures were obtained before meningococci were isolated. However, after a blood culture yielded the organism, most subsequent cultures were positive. In children, some investigators report that it is common to isolate the organism in the first blood culture.[81] The arthralgias also tended to be intermittent in nature.

Table 93–3 presents the differential diagnosis of chronic meningococcemia.

In Benoit's series,[9] almost 40 per cent of the patients with chronic meningococcemia developed localizing complications. The meninges were the most common site of localization; meningitis developed in 15.5 per cent of patients. Other localized infection included carditis, nephritis, epididymitis, conjunctivitis, iritis, and retinitis. In only one instance was an organism recovered from the joint. The average duration of meningococcemia in those patients with complications was 10.2 weeks, compared with 4 to 8 weeks in those patients without any localization.

The diagnosis is established by identifying the organism in blood cultures. Antibiotic therapy results in prompt defervescence and dramatic recovery.

The pathophysiologic mechanisms permitting chronic meningococcemia remain unclear. There is no evidence that the organisms are less virulent than are other meningococci; thus, a defect in host immunity has been suggested. A hypersensitivity basis for this disease has been postulated, and it is theorized that the skin changes and arthritis may be secondary to antigen-antibody complexes.[99] In contrast to acute meningococcemia, bacteria almost never are found by biopsy or culture of skin lesions in patients with chronic meningococcemia, and the histologic type is distinct from that seen in skin lesions of patients with acute meningococcemia.[9, 61, 99]

LABORATORY FINDINGS

Wong and colleagues[146] reviewed 100 cases of meningococcal infections in children seen at their institution between 1985 and 1988. Leukopenia (white blood cell count <5000/mm^3) was present in 21 per cent, and thrombocytopenia was noted in 14 per cent. Fifty-five patients had meningitis. Eleven per cent of those with culture-positive meningitis had no cerebrospinal fluid abnormalities on chemistries or examination.

Hyponatremia is seen in some patients with meningitis. Inappropriate secretion of antidiuretic hormone is the mechanism. In one study of 43 children with meningococcal meningitis, 7 per cent developed syndrome of inappropriate secretion of antidiuretic hormone.[35]

Other laboratory abnormalities seen in patients with sepsis

TABLE 93–3. Differential Diagnosis of Chronic Meningococcemia

Acute rheumatic fever
Subacute bacterial endocarditis
Henoch-Schönlein purpura
Malaria
Typhoid
Miliary tuberculosis
Gonococcemia
Erythema multiforme
Erythema nodosum
Secondary syphilis
Haverhill fever
Rocky Mountain spotted fever
Typhus
Collagen vascular disease
Neoplastic processes

or shock include abnormal coagulation panels (disseminated intravascular coagulation), acidosis, and abnormal liver function studies.

DIAGNOSIS

The gold standard for diagnosis is based on recovering the organism from blood, cerebrospinal fluid, or petechiae. Blood culture alone is positive about 50 per cent of the time in patients who have not received antibiotics.[146] Rapid diagnosis often can be made by Gram stain of the cerebrospinal fluid in patients with meningitis. Characteristic gram-negative diplococci are seen. Caution should be exercised in relying solely on the Gram stain and initiating broad therapy until the organism is identified by culture. Overdecolorized gram-positive cocci of *Streptococcus pneumoniae* on occasion have been confused with meningococci on Gram stain.

In patients who have skin lesions, a rapid presumptive diagnosis of meningococcemia often can be made by needle aspiration and Gram stain of a skin lesion. Needle aspiration yields gram-negative diplococci on the Gram-stained specimen in about 50 per cent of patients with acute meningococcal infections.[134] Culturing the obtained aspirate increases the yield further. Correlation of the Gram stain with the clinical presentation is important because disseminated gonococcal infections also may present with skin lesions that yield gram-negative diplococci on Gram stain.

Counterimmunoelectrophoresis and latex agglutination have been used to detect circulating antigen in serum, cerebrospinal fluid, and urine of patients with meningococcal disease.[143] These tests are of particular benefit in cases of partially treated meningococcal meningitis in which culture and Gram stain may be negative. Cross-reactions with certain *E. coli* or *Bacillus* strains may occur. Fecal contamination is more likely to occur with bag collection of the urine specimen. This may have important clinical significance in a neonate with meningitis because *E. coli* strains possessing the K1 capsular antigen are a common cause of neonatal meningitis. These K1 *E. coli* have a capsule that is identical immunochemically to the meningococcus group B capsule, and thus the use of meningococcus group B antisera as a reagent also will detect *E. coli* K1 antigen in body fluids.[87]

Polymerase chain reaction is one of the newer tests for detection of *N. meningitidis*. It may turn out to be very helpful in those patients who have partially treated meningococcemia or meningitis. Once antibiotics have been given, the chances that a blood culture will be positive decrease to less than 5 per cent.[18] One study showed the sensitivity and specificity of polymerase chain reaction for *N. meningitidis* to be 91 per cent in cerebrospinal fluid specimens. Treatment with antibiotics prior to the test did not decrease the test's sensitivity or specificity.[97] Use of this test in confirming meningococcal infections in patients pretreated with antibiotics may be valuable in subsequent patient management, follow-up, and prompt institution of chemoprophylaxis to contacts.

TREATMENT

Therapy for meningococcal disease has evolved over the last century. In the early 1900s, treatment consisted of administration of intravenous and intrathecal horse serum and cerebrospinal fluid drainage. Mortality associated with this therapy was 26 per cent.[60] The use of sulfonamides lowered the death rate to 5 or 10 per cent.[52] With the emergence of sulfa-resistant strains, penicillin was added to the regimen and still is used for susceptible meningococcal infections.[1] Uniformly penicillin-susceptible isolates of meningococci no longer are the rule. Relatively resistant strains have been reported in the United States, Spain, the United Kingdom, Greece, Switzerland, Romania, Belgium, South Africa, and Canada.[67, 104, 129, 147] Isolates that are absolutely resistant to penicillin (minimum inhibitory concentration >1.0 μg/mL) have been documented from Spain and the United Kingdom.[104, 129] In a 1990 article, investigators from Spain noted that 46 per cent of 131 strains examined during the first 4 months of 1990 were moderately resistant to penicillin (minimum inhibitory concentrations between 0.1 and 1.0 μg/mL). In 1991, 3.6 per cent of isolates in the United States were moderately resistant to penicillin. Genotypic and phenotypic studies of resistant isolates from Spain revealed that the strains were genetically diverse and did not arise from a single clone.[150] In addition, Mendelman and colleagues[90] demonstrated that these strains have a penicillin-binding protein (PBP3) with a reduced penicillin-binding capacity, compared with sensitive strains. These strains appear to have arisen by acquisition of segments of genes (by transformation) of naturally resistant commensal *Neisseria*, *N. flavescens*, and *N. lactamica*.[124] The gene encoding PBP2, *penA* in commensal *Neisseria*, encodes for a protein that has less avidity for penicillin G. Transformation of *N. meningitidis* with *penA* from these strains leads to a slight decrease in penicillin G susceptibility; repeated transformation will yield a penicillin-resistant strain.

In 1988, penicillin-resistant meningococci also were reported from South Africa and from the United Kingdom; these strains had acquired a gonococcal plasmid encoding for the production of β-lactamase.[129]

For penicillin-susceptible meningococcemia or meningitis, intravenous penicillin G, 250,000 units/kg/day given in divided doses every 4 hours for 7 days, is effective. Third-generation cephalosporins, ceftriaxone (100 mg/kg/day intravenously in two divided doses) and cefotaxime (200 mg/kg/day intravenously in four divided doses), have been used with success as initial intravenous therapy for meningitis outside the neonatal period. In confirmed cases of meningococcal disease, comparisons of penicillin G with ceftriaxone have shown ceftriaxone to be as efficacious. Necrotic skin lesions were seen more commonly in the penicillin group, but otherwise complication and mortality rates were equivalent.[131] Meningococcal disease has been treated successfully with ceftriaxone intravenously in both the once-a-day (80 to 100 mg/kg/day) and twice-a-day (100 mg/kg/day in two divided doses) dosing regimens.[131] Chloramphenicol is an alternative drug in patients with penicillin and cephalosporin allergies. With all cases of meningococcal disease, eradicating colonization of the index case is important. Rifampin, 10 mg/kg/dose (maximum, 600 mg/dose) every 12 hours for 2 days, is the usual drug used. Typically, these agents are added during the last days of therapy. Rifampin alternatives include ceftriaxone (125 mg intramuscularly for children younger than 12 years of age or 250 mg intramuscularly for those older than 12 years of age) as a single intramuscular injection. If the patient was treated for meningococcal disease with a third-generation cephalosporin (cefotaxime or ceftriaxone), additional prophylactic agents (such as rifampin) are not necessary for the index case.

Steroid administration is somewhat controversial. For patients with Waterhouse-Friderichsen syndrome, treatment with steroids is indicated. However, treatment of meningococcal meningitis with steroids has been debated in the literature for years. Steroid proponents point to the *Haemophilus influenzae* type b meningitis studies, in which treatment with steroids decreases hearing loss. The belief is that steroids, through anti-inflammatory effects, will decrease polymorphonuclear neutrophils, macrophages, and cytokines in the central nervous system and thus decrease central nervous system immune-mediated damage and hearing loss. Steroid opponents say that no conclusive studies show steroids to be of benefit in meningococcal meningitis and that risks include gastrointestinal ulceration, decreased penetration of antibiotics into the central nervous system (because of decreased meningeal inflammation), and steroid psychosis. If steroids are used, it seems prudent to use them early (preferably close to the time the first dose of antibiotic is administered). However, antibiotics should never be withheld due to waiting for steroids to be given.

Additional supportive measures such as prophylactic low-dose heparin, protein C concentrate, plasmapheresis, and topical nitroglycerin also are potential therapies.[144] Hathaway[57] reviewed 63 patients 2 months to 43 years of age with severe meningococcemia and shock who had laboratory evidence of disseminated intravascular coagulation. These patients received heparin in addition to antibiotics and had a mortality rate of 57 per cent. Historical data derived from patients with similar prognostic criteria suggested a mortality rate of 100 per cent.[126] A retrospective chart review of 24 patients with purpura fulminans showed less necrosis of the digits and extremities in patients treated with heparin, but the results were not statistically significant.[79]

The efficacy of heparin therapy in patients with fulminant meningococcemia remains unsettled. Serious side effects directly attributed to heparin therapy have been reported rarely, particularly if the dose of heparin used is that required to maintain normal blood coagulability rather than hypocoagulability.[43] The difficulty in adjusting the dose in small infants may lead to heparin intoxication. Two instances of heparin-induced bleeding diathesis at the Children's Hospital Medical Center, Boston, Massachusetts, led to retinal hemorrhage and blindness; both patients received heparin "prophylactically" during treatment of meningococcal sepsis. A large, prospective, randomized trial needs to be conducted to address the value of heparin in meningococcal disease.

A number of other experimental therapies have been attempted in patients with fulminant meningococcemia. Anecdotal reports have suggested that plasmapheresis may improve survival, and one report showed a dramatic decrease in plasma levels of tumor necrosis factor and interleukin-1 in association with this procedure.[32] Hyperbaric oxygen also has been used to increase oxygen delivery to compromised tissue. Tissue plasminogen activator infused locally has been reported to reverse ischemia.[75] Two patients were reported who received recombinant tissue plasminogen activator systemically for meningococcemia with shock and purpura. Both patients received vigorous cardiovascular and pressor support at the same time, but the authors felt the drug was beneficial in restoring perfusion.[149] Continuous caudal block has been used to restore lower extremity perfusion.[130] A report described two children with purpura fulminans with documented improvement in skin blood flow after the topical application of nitroglycerin.[65] Protein C concentrate use in purpura fulminans has been reported in a small number of patients. Treatment with the protein C concentrate increased plasma protein C levels to normal in these patients. Protein C is a "natural anticoagulant," and it has been shown that protein C levels are low in patients with purpura fulminans. It is speculated that acquired deficiency of protein C may play a role in the pathogenesis of purpura fulminans. However, the number of patients treated with this modality is too small to evaluate therapeutic benefit.[114]

Some patients require surgical procedures for necrosis of skin, digits, or limbs associated with purpura fulminans. In one study of infectious purpura fulminans (of which meningococcemia was a subset), 72 per cent of patients required at least one surgical procedure, including amputations, local débridement, skin grafting, or skin flaps.[59]

Treatment of Miscellaneous Meningococcal Infections

Meningococcal conjunctivitis should be treated with systemic antibiotics. Patients with conjunctivitis are more likely to develop invasive disease if topical therapy is used alone. In addition, we recommend ophthalmologic examination of all patients with meningococcal conjunctivitis because about 15 per cent go on to develop ocular complications. Fortunately, even patients who develop corneal ulcerations rarely are left with corneal opacities.[8]

Encapsulated, pathogenic meningococci isolated from the pharynx of a symptomatic individual also should be treated with systemic therapy. It is problematic because there is a chance that the meningococci isolated are only colonizing and not the infectious agents causing the pharyngitis. If the patient is febrile, a blood culture (and cerebrospinal fluid culture if clinically indicated) should be obtained before beginning systemic therapy. At the end of therapy, it is important to give chemoprophylaxis to eradicate colonization.

Penicillin therapy of penicillin-sensitive meningococcal pneumonia results in a prompt clinical response. Ninety-three per cent of the patients reported by Koppes and colleagues[77] were afebrile after 3 days of therapy. Third-generation cephalosporins, such as ceftriaxone and cefotaxime, may be the current drugs of choice pending sensitivity testing.

Urogenital infections, such as cervicitis, urethritis, and proctitis, have been treated like gonococcal infections by some physicians with good results.

With all meningococcal therapy, it is important to consider whether or not the organism produces β-lactamase and the susceptibility of the organism to penicillin. In addition, colonization must be eradicated with rifampin or an alternative drug to prevent further transmission, unless third-generation cephalosporins are used for therapy.

CHEMOPROPHYLAXIS

The ability of *N. meningitidis* to spread from person to person and cause epidemic disease has been recognized since the 1800s. The secondary attack rate in households with an index case is approximately 3 per 1000, a rate 1000 times the attack rate in the general population.[125] Household crowding and young age are factors that increase the secondary attack rate. The mode of transmission is direct contact with respiratory droplets or secretions. For these reasons, chemoprophylaxis is recommended for household contacts of an index case and for young day care center contacts. Several epidemiologic studies suggested that casual acquaintances (such as school-aged classmates) were not at increased risk, although a number of authors have reported secondary cases in this population.[68, 72] Prophylaxis is indicated for health care workers who have had intimate exposure to nasopharyngeal secretions (e.g., mouth-to-mouth resuscitation). The period of communicability of the index patient is not well established. Most public health authorities recommend that persons in contact with the patient up to 7 days prior to onset of illness be considered for prophylaxis.

There are differing opinions regarding treatment of the index case with a drug designed to eliminate nasopharyngeal carriage. Abramson and Spika[2] reported that 4 of 14 (29 per cent) patients with meningococcal infection treated with intravenous penicillin were culture-positive from the respiratory tract 1 week after completion of therapy. However, Alvez and colleagues[3] found that only 3 of 48 (6.25 per cent) appropriately treated children had positive respiratory cultures at discharge. It is possible that the discharge cultures were done when nasopharyngeal carriage still was suppressed but not eradicated by the penicillin in Alvez's study. We would recommend chemoprophylaxis for index patients if they have been treated with penicillin for their meningococcal infection.

Secondary cases originally were defined as those cases occurring more than 24 but less than 31 days after onset in the index case. Using this definition, approximately 50 per cent of secondary cases will occur in the first 7 days after presentation of the index case. It is essential to initiate prophylaxis as soon as possible, based on clinical presentation of the index case (e.g., fulminant meningococcemia) or on laboratory culture data if the disease presents as bacterial meningitis, septic arthritis, etc.

The original drug used for chemoprophylaxis was sulfadiazine. However, a large percentage of strains now are resistant to sulfa, and rifampin currently is the drug of choice for chemoprophylaxis. Table 93–4 lists three antibiotics that are highly effective in eradicating meningococcus from the nasopharynx. Rifampin generally is well tolerated but has a number of side effects, including orange urine, orange staining of contact lenses, stimulation of liver microsomal enzymes, and reduction in levels of other concurrent medications (e.g., oral contraceptives, anticoagulants, digoxin, phenytoin). Development of resistant strains has been reported rarely.[21] Ciprofloxacin, ceftriaxone, and rifampin have been evaluated in a randomized, comparative study.[22] All three drugs were highly effective in carriage eradication. Ceftriaxone probably is the drug of choice for a pregnant contact and also may be indicated for children because a single intramuscular injection may result in greater compliance than may four doses of rifampin. Ciprofloxacin is contraindicated in children due to evidence of cartilage damage in juvenile beagles.

As mentioned in the section on meningococcal vaccines, secondary disease also can be prevented by immunization of contacts. We recommend both immunization and chemoprophylaxis whenever possible (realizing that no protection against group B meningococci currently is provided by immunization).

The single most important element of chemoprophylaxis is education of contacts regarding the need for immediate medical attention if they develop signs or symptoms of a febrile illness. No prophylactic strategy is 100 per cent effective, and ill contacts should be evaluated with a high suspicion for meningococcal disease.

MORTALITY AND PROGNOSIS

Several scoring systems have been devised in an attempt to predict prognosis in patients with meningococcal disease.

TABLE 93–4. Chemoprophylaxis

Drug	Age Group	Dose	Duration
Rifampin	<1 month	5 mg/kg q 12 hr	2 days
	>1 month	10 mg/kg q 12 hr	2 days
	Adults	600 mg q 12 hr	2 days
Ciprofloxacin	Adults	500 mg	Single dose
Ceftriaxone	<15 years	125 mg IM	Single dose
	Adults	250 mg IM	Single dose

TABLE 93–5. Presenting Features of Meningococcal Infection Associated with Poor Prognosis

Presence of petechiae for less than 12 hours before admission
Presence of hypotension (systolic <70 mm Hg)
Absence of meningitis (<20 white blood cells/mm³)
Peripheral white blood cell count <10,000/mm³
Erythrocyte sedimentation rate <10 mm/hour

Adapted from Stiehm, E. R., and Damrosch, D. S.: Factors in the prognosis of meningococcal infection. J. Pediatr. *68*:457–467, 1966.

Stiehm and Damrosch[126] developed a prognostic scoring system based on five features that indicated a grave prognosis. These features are listed in Table 93–5. The mortality in patients with three or more of these features was 90 per cent, whereas the mortality for patients with two or fewer of these criteria was 9 per cent.

Rosenblatt and colleagues[117] also attempted to define prognostic criteria for meningococcal disease they reviewed. They found ecchymoses or purpura to be a more reliable indicator of poor prognosis than was duration of petechiae.

In a review of 100 cases of meningococcal disease at the Los Angeles Children's Hospital, Los Angeles, California, five features were identified that were correlated with poor prognosis: shock or seizures on presentation, hypothermia, total white blood cell count less than 5000/mm³, platelet count less than 100,000/mm³, and development of purpura fulminans. The overall mortality in this series was 10 per cent.[146]

Most prognostic scoring systems agree that purpura fulminans and shock uniformly are poor prognostic signs. Other signs that also might portend a rocky course are absence of meningitis, relative leukopenia (<5000/mm³), and coma.

COMPLICATIONS OF MENINGOCOCCAL DISEASE

About one-fourth of patients with invasive meningococcal disease experience one or more complications. These can be infectious, neurologic, or immunologic in nature.[33]

Arthritis

Meningococcal arthritis occurs primarily in adults. The overall incidence, as a complication of bacteremia, is about 2 to 14 per cent.[50, 146] There are two forms of meningococcal arthritis. The first is seen within the first few days of treatment and is characterized by severe arthralgias and few objective signs of joint inflammation. It is suggested that the pathogenesis of this arthritis is an inflammatory response to viable organisms, which have seeded the synovium during the initial bacteremia. The second, more common form appears to be a hypersensitivity phenomenon. It usually is noted 3 to 7 days after the recognition of meningococcemia, often at a time when the patient appears to be improving from the meningitis or sepsis. The knee, wrist, elbow, and ankle joints are involved most commonly.[50]

In both forms, the arthritis usually is mono- or oligoarticular with an effusion, with minimal pain, erythema, and limitation of motion. It is very unusual to culture organisms from the effusion; joint fluid culture yields meningococci in less than 10 per cent of cases. The exception to this is a child with suppurative arthritis on initial presentation. In one study, 8 per cent of patients with meningococcal infections presented with arthritis; 75 per cent were culture-positive when cultured prior to receiving antibiotics.[146]

Synovial fluid leukocyte counts vary widely, but counts greater than 100,000/m^3 occur in the early form.[106] The mean leukocyte count in synovial fluid was 43,000 ± 33,000 in a study by Greenwood and Whittle.[51] The appearance of arthritis often is accompanied by a rise in temperature; in 7 of 47 patients with arthritis, a characteristic skin lesion appeared at the same time.[51] These lesions began as skin hyperpigmentation but progressed to vesiculation and ulceration; biopsies showed vasculitis. Additional evidence of concurrent vasculitis is suggested by reports of patients developing episcleritis and mild proteinuria simultaneously with arthritis.[51]

On histologic examination, the synovium is infiltrated with mononuclear cells that contain IgM, C3, and meningococcal antigen.[51] This strongly suggests an immune complex–mediated disease. No specific therapy is indicated, and the arthritis resolves spontaneously. Controversy exists regarding the role of intermittent closed drainage of the joint space.[12] Permanent joint deformity is uncommon in this disease, occurring in approximately 10 per cent of cases.[120] Edwards and Baker[33] reported allergic complications of meningococcal disease in 10 per cent of the 86 children followed prospectively. More than 83 per cent of the 86 cases they studied were serogroup B, although late-onset arthritis and vasculitis also have been reported with serogroup A and C disease.

Permanent joint damage is unusual, occurring in about 1.5 per cent of patients with arthritis. Potential sequelae include ankylosis, decreased range of motion, and bone necrosis.[80]

Pericarditis and Myocarditis

Pericarditis, as a complication of meningococcal disease, occurs in 3 to 5 per cent of cases, although one series reported a 19 per cent incidence in 32 patients with meningococcal meningitis.[30, 95] It generally occurs in patients with meningococcemia but has been reported as an isolated event without septicemia or meningitis.[58]

Pericarditis is presumed to be a late complication of meningococcal disease because clinical symptoms such as fever, dyspnea, or substernal chest pain (or even cardiac tamponade) usually do not appear until the fourth to the seventh day of illness. However, several investigators have noted early evidence of pericarditis based on electrocardiographic or roentgenographic data of patients examined at the time of hospital admission.

Because most symptomatic pericardial effusions develop late in the course of the illness, are serous in nature, and are sterile, the pathophysiologic mechanism is presumed to be a hypersensitivity reaction. Uncontrolled studies report the successful use of steroids in the treatment of this complication.[105] However, other reports document pericarditis and the development of tamponade in a patient receiving steroids.[103]

The clinical course of meningococcal pericarditis usually is benign, but pericardial compression requiring pericardiocentesis occurs.[72, 103] Early relapses also have been reported, but these were self-limited. There are reports of the development of constrictive pericarditis requiring pericardectomy.[103, 121, 141]

Myocarditis was noted at autopsy in 78 per cent of patients with fatal meningococcal disease.[54] Myocarditis was noted most often in adults but was more severe than in children. Rosenblatt and colleagues[117] noted myocarditis at autopsy in 10 of 12 children with fatal meningococcal infection. On pathologic examination, these cases showed collections of inflammatory cells in the myocardial interstitium and focal extravasation of erythrocytes with acute vasculitis. Abscesses and endocarditis were not seen. Inflammation occasionally may involve the atrioventricular node and has been reported as a cause of sudden death in a patient recovering from meningococcal meningitis.[115]

Neurologic Complications

The most common neurologic complications seen are hydrocephalus, cranial nerve palsies (especially hearing loss), subdural effusions or empyemas, cerebral edema, cortical vein thrombosis, and cerebral infarctions. Neurologic sequelae are much more common in patients with meningitis, but complications such as cerebral infarction also can be seen in children with meningococcemia and shock.[101]

Cerebral edema and cranial nerve palsies may be seen at presentation or develop shortly thereafter. Sixth nerve or third nerve palsies are suggestive of increased intracranial pressure and impending herniation, respectively. The development of either of these signs indicates an urgent intracranial process.[101] Hearing loss occurs in 5 to 10 per cent of patients with meningitis. Auditory testing should be performed on all patients with meningitis after recovery.

Subdural effusions or empyemas should be considered in patients with fever persisting after 8 days of therapy (in the absence of a sterile repeat cerebrospinal fluid culture), vomiting, or development of signs of increased intracranial pressure after the initial few days of treatment. Drainage is recommended only if the effusions are infected (empyemas) or are large enough to produce either focal neurologic signs or increased intracranial pressure.[101]

Vascular thrombosis and/or cerebral infarction can be due to arterial or venous thrombosis. Venous thrombosis is more common and generally is not seen before the second week. Hemorrhagic infarction of the brain may occur then. Cerebral infarction also may be seen in those patients without arterial or venous thrombosis who present in shock with prolonged hypotension and cerebral ischemia. Cerebral infarction in these individuals is an early event.

Hydrocephalus occurs most frequently in young children and those with delayed diagnosis or severe disease. It tends to present 3 to 4 weeks after the onset of illness. Inflammation, with collagen deposition and proliferation of fibroblasts in the meninges, produces an obstruction to the flow of cerebrospinal fluid. Progressive increase in head circumference should alert the clinician to the possibility of hydrocephalus.[101] Imaging (computed tomography, magnetic resonance imaging) studies are diagnostic.

Other Complications

Numerous other complications of meningococcal disease have been reported and were summarized best in the paper by Banks[7] in 1948. Radiculitis, hemiplegia, seizure disorders, endophthalmitis, associated herpetic lesions (developing on day 4 or 5 of disease), and arachnoiditis were seen in some patients. Orchitis, epididymitis, and salpingitis are rare complications.

MENINGOCOCCAL VACCINES

Primary prevention of meningococcal disease is essential for several reasons. The presentation may be fulminant, with no opportunity for antibiotics to influence the course of the disease. Antibiotic-resistant strains now are recognized, and chemoprophylaxis of contacts is a cumbersome and often ineffective public health measure. Mass immunization offers the opportunity to prevent both endemic and epidemic disease worldwide.

The primary approach to the development of meningococcal vaccines has been to purify capsular polysaccharides from the cell surface of the organism. These polysaccharides can be well defined chemically and physically, and it has been possible to isolate the capsular polysaccharide from other components of the cell wall, producing a product that is free of contaminating endotoxin and cell-surface proteins.

Early clinical studies of a bivalent vaccine consisting of meningococcal A and C polysaccharides demonstrated that the vaccine was safe and effective in adults and older children. Subsequently, a quadravalent vaccine composed of groups A, C, W135, and Y was licensed and is used routinely by the U.S. military; it is recommended for travelers who are visiting countries with a high incidence of meningococcal disease. The tetravalent vaccine also is used in individuals with functional or anatomic asplenia and in persons with complement or properdin deficiencies.

Meningococcal vaccines have been effective in the control of epidemic disease.[102] In addition, a meningococcal A/C polysaccharide vaccine was effective in preventing secondary cases of meningococcal disease in household contacts.[50] In this study, vaccination was given to household contacts on the day after admission of the index case. There were nine cases of confirmed or probable meningococcal disease in the control group vaccinated with tetanus toxoid, and only one case of possible meningococcal infection in the 520 contacts who received meningococcal vaccine. Approximately 50 per cent of secondary cases may present 5 or more days after presentation of the index case. Immunization of contacts may be useful as a supplement to chemoprophylaxis of contacts.

Two major problems remain with meningococcal vaccines. The pure polysaccharide vaccines are not immunogenic or protective in young children, and an effective and immunogenic group B vaccine is not available yet. In order to overcome the lack of adequate immunogenicity of plain polysaccharide vaccines in infants, protein-polysaccharide conjugate vaccines have been developed. A group A/C conjugate vaccine was safe and immunogenic when administered to 2-month-old African infants in multiple doses.[39] Clinical trials of the safety and immunogenicity of these conjugate vaccines currently are under way in the United States.

Development of an immunogenic group B meningococcal vaccine has been problematic because the polysaccharide capsule of meningococcus group B is not immunogenic in animals or man. Teleologic explanations for this lack of immunogenicity have led to a number of interesting hypotheses. The chemical composition of the group B capsule is a polymer of two to eight neuraminic acids. In 1983, Finnish investigators reported that horse antiserum to meningococcus group B reacted with glycoproteins isolated from human and rat brains.[14] Furthermore, the binding was higher in human fetal brain than in postnatal brain, a finding consistent with the fact that fetal brain contains more polysialosyl glycopeptides than does postnatal brain. Based on this experimental evidence, the authors recommended caution in vaccine development due to concerns for induction of cross-reacting antibodies against neuronal tissue.

Several different strategies have been employed in the development of a meningococcal group B vaccine. A serotype protein vaccine was constructed using membrane vesicles from a serotype 2b strain and noncovalently complexing this protein with the group B capsular polysaccharide. This vaccine induced bactericidal antibody but did not induce antibodies against the polysaccharide capsule as measured by an enzyme-linked immunosorbent assay. A similar vaccine was studied in 171,800 students in Norway, and the calculated rate of protection was 57.2 per cent.[14] The authors concluded that the effect was insufficient to justify a public vaccination program. A similar vaccine was given to 2.4 million children 3 months to 6 years of age in São Paulo. A case-control study showed that the estimated vaccine efficacy for children 48 months of age or older was 74 per cent.[25] The vaccine was much less effective in younger children. Another approach has been to develop a protein-polysaccharide conjugate vaccine utilizing the capsular polysaccharide of *E. coli* K92, an organism with a capsular polysaccharide that cross-reacts with both meningococcus group B and group C. This vaccine induces antibody in animals and will be tested in humans.

A better understanding of the pathophysiologic mechanism of meningococcal disease may lead to a better understanding of the bacterial structures critical for antigenicity and immunogenicity in humans. A safe and effective vaccine that could induce protection against all encapsulated meningococci in all age groups is the ultimate goal.

References

1. Abramowicz, M. (ed.): Medical Letter Handbook of Antimicrobial Therapy, New Rochelle, 1978, p. 16.
2. Abramson, J. S., and Spika, J. S.: Persistence of *Neisseria meningitidis* in the upper respiratory tract after intravenous antibiotic therapy for systemic meningococcal disease. J. Infect. Dis. *151*:370–371, 1985.
3. Alvez, F., Aguilera A., Garcie-Zabarte, A., et al.: Effect of chemoprophylaxis on the meningococcal carrier state after systemic infection. Pediatr. Infect. Dis. J. *10*:700, 1991.
4. Anonymous: Meningococcal disease among travelers returning from Saudi Arabia. M. M. W. R. *36*:559, 1987.
5. Anonymous: Meningococcal Disease Surveillance Group: Analysis of endemic meningococcal disease by serogroup and evaluation of chemoprophylaxis. J. Infect. Dis. *134*:201–204, 1976.
6. Anonymous: Serogroup B meningococcal disease: Oregon, 1994. M. M. W. R. *44*:121–124, 1995.
7. Banks, H. S.: Meningococcosis: A protean disease. Lancet 2:635–640, 1948.
8. Barquet, N., Gasser, I., Domingo, P., et al.: Primary meningococcal conjunctivitis: Report of 21 patients and review. Rev. Infect. Dis. *12*:838–847, 1990.
9. Benoit, F. L.: Chronic meningococcemia. Medicine *35*:103, 1963.
10. Bhattacharjee, A. K., Jennings, H. J., and Kenny, C. P.: Characterization of 3-deoxy-D-manno octulosonic acid as a component of the capsular polysaccharide antigen from *Neisseria meningitidis* serogroup 29-E. Biochem. Biophys. Res. Commun. *61*:489–493, 1974.
11. Boger, W. P.: Fulminating meningococcemia. N. Engl. J. Med. *231*:385–387, 1944.
12. Boger, W. P.: Purulent meningococcal arthritis. Am. J. Med. Sci. *208*:708–717, 1944.
13. Botha P.: Penicillin-resistant *Neisseria meningitidis* in southern Africa. Lancet 2:54, 1988.
14. Bjune, G., Høiby E. A., Grønnesby, J. K., et al.: Effect of outer membrane vesicle vaccine against group B meningococcal disease in Norway. Lancet *338*:1093–1096, 1991.
15. Brandtzaeg, P., Mollnes, T. E., and Kierulk, P.: Complement activation and endotoxin levels in systemic meningococcal disease. J. Infect. Dis. *160*:58–64, 1989.
16. Buchanan, R. E., and Gibbons, N. E. (eds.): Bergey's Manual of Determinative Bacteriology. 8th ed. Baltimore, Williams & Wilkins, 1974, p. 427.
17. Cartwright, K. A., Jones, D. M., Smith, A. J., et al.: Influenza A and meningococcal disease. Lancet *338*:554–557, 1991.
18. Cartwright, K., Reilly, S., White, D., et al.: Early treatment with parenteral penicillin in meningococcal disease. Br. Med. J. *305*:143–147, 1992.
19. Caugant, D. A., Høiby, E. A., Mangus, P., et al.: Asymptomatic carriage of *Neisseria meningitidis* in a randomly sampled population. J. Clin. Microbiol. *32*:323–330, 1994.
20. Cohen, M. S., Steere, A. C., Baltimore, R., et al.: Possible nosocomial transmission of group Y *Neisseria meningitidis* among oncology patients. Ann. Intern. Med. *91*:7–12, 1979.
21. Cooper, E. R., Ellison, R. T., III, Smith, G. S., et al.: Rifampin-resistant meningococcal disease in a contact patient given prophylactic rifampin. J. Pediatr. *108*:93–96, 1986.
22. Cuevas, L. E., Kazembe, P., Mughogho, G. K., et al.: Eradication of nasopharyngeal carriage of *Neisseria meningitidis* in children and adults in rural Africa: A comparison of ciprofloxacin and rifampin. J. Infect. Dis. *171*:728–731, 1995.

23. D'Amelio, R., Agostoni, A., Biselli, R., et al.: Complement deficiency and antibody profile in survivors of meningococcal meningitis due to common serogroups in Italy. Scand. J. Immunol. *35*:589–595, 1992.
24. Davis, C. E., and Arnold, K.: Role of meningococcal endotoxin in meningococcal purpura. J. Exp. Med. *140*:159–171, 1974.
25. de Moraes, J. C., Perkins, B. A., Camargo, M. C., et al.: Protective efficacy of a serogroup B meningococcal vaccine in São Paulo, Brazil. Lancet *340*:1074–1078. 1992.
26. Densen, P., Weiler, J. M., Griffiss, J. M., et al.: Familial properdin deficiency and fatal meningococcemia: Correction of the bactericidal defect by vaccination. N. Engl. J. Med. *316*:922–926, 1987.
27. De wals, P., Hertoghe, L., Borlee-Grimee, L., et al.: Meningococcal disease in Belgium: Secondary attack rate among household, day-care nursery, and pre-elementary school contacts. J. Infect. *3*(Suppl. 1):53–61, 1981.
28. DeVoe, I. W., and Gilka, F.: Disseminated intravascular coagulation in rabbits: Synergistic activity of meningococcal endotoxin and materials egested from leukocytes containing meningococci. J. Med. Microbiol. *9*:451–458, 1976.
29. Dickson, R. C., McKinnon, N. E., Magner, D., et al.: Meningococcal infection. Lancet *2*:631–634, 1941.
30. Dixon, L. M., and Sanford, H. S.: Meningococcal pericarditis in the antibiotic era. Milit. Med. *136*:433–438, 1971.
31. Dock, W.: Intermittent fever of seven months duration due to meningococcemia. J. A. M. A. *83*:31–33, 1924.
32. Drapkin, M. S., Wisch, J. S., Gelfand, J. A., et al.: Plasmapheresis for fulminant meningococcemia. Lancet *8*:399–400, 1989.
33. Edwards, M. S., and Baker, C. J.: Complications and sequelae of meningococcal infections in children. J. Pediatr. *99*:540–545, 1981.
34. Ellis, M., Weindling, A. M., Davidson, D. C., et al.: Neonatal meningococcal conjunctivitis associated with meningococcal meningitis. Arch. Dis. Child. *67*:1219–1222, 1992.
35. Ellsworth, J., Marks, M. I., and Vose, A.: Meningococcal meningitis in children. Can. Med. Assoc. J. *120*:155–158, 1979.
36. Faur, Y. C., Weisburd, M. H., and Wilson, M. E.: Isolation of *Neisseria meningitidis* from the genitourinary tract and anal canal. J. Clin. Microbiol. *2*:178–182, 1975.
37. Fijen, C. A., Kuijper, E. J., Hannema, A. J., et al.: Complement deficiencies in patients over ten years old with meningococcal disease due to uncommon serogroups. Lancet 2:585–588, 1989.
38. Figueroa, J. E., and Densen, P.: Infectious diseases associated with complement deficiencies. Clin. Microbiol. Rev. *4*:359–395, 1991.
39. Finne, J., Leinonen, M., and Makela, P. H.: Antigenic similarities between brain components and bacteria causing meningitis. Lancet *2*:355–357, 1983.
40. Frasch, C. E.: Role of protein serotype antigens in protection against disease due to *Neisseria meningitidis*. J. Infect. Dis. *136*(Suppl.):S84–S90, 1977.
41. Frasch, C. E., and Chapman, S. S.: Classification of *Neisseria meningitidis* group B into distinct serotypes. Infect. Immun. *5*:98–102, 1972.
42. Frasch, C. E., and Gotschlich, E. C.: An outer membrane protein of *Neisseria meningitidis* group B responsible for serotype specificity. J. Exp. Med. *140*:87–104, 1974.
43. Gerard, P., Morian, M., Bachy, A., et al.: Meningococcal purpura: Report of 19 patients treated with heparin. J. Pediatr. *82*:780–786, 1973.
44. Girardin, E., Grau, G. E., Dayer, J. M., et al.: Tumor necrosis factor and interleukin-1 in the serum of children with severe infectious purpura. N. Engl. J. Med. *319*:397–400, 1988.
45. Givan, K. F., Thomas, B. W., and Johnston, A. G.: Isolation of *Neisseria meningitidis* from the urethra, cervix, and anal canal: Further observations. Br. J. Vener. Dis. *53*:109–112, 1977.
46. Goldschneider, I., Gotschlich, E. C., and Artenstein, M. S.: Human immunity to the meningococcus. I. The role of humoral antibodies. J. Exp. Med. *129*:1307–1326, 1969.
47. Goldschneider, I., Gotschlich, E. C., and Artenstein, M. S.: Human immunity to the meningococcus. II. Development of natural immunity. J. Exp. Med. *129*:1327–1348, 1969.
48. Gotschlich, E. C., Goldschneider, I., Lepow, M. L., et al.: The immune response to bacterial polysaccharides in man. *In* Haber, E., and Krause, R. M. (eds.): Antibodies in Human Diagnosis and Therapy. New York, Raven Press, 1977, pp. 391–402.
49. Greenfield, S., Sheehe, P. R., and Feldman, H. A., et al.: Meningococcal carriage in a population of normal families. J. Infect. Dis. *123*:67–73, 1971.
50. Greenwood, B. M., Hassan-King, M., and Whittle, H. C.: Prevention of secondary cases of meningococcal disease in household contacts by vaccination. Br. Med. J. *1*:1317–1319, 1978.
51. Greenwood, B. M., and Whittle, H. C.: The pathogenesis of meningococcal arthritis. *In* Dumonde, D. C., and Path, M. R. (eds.): Infection and Immunology in the Rheumatic Diseases. Philadelphia, Lippincott (Blackwell), 1976, pp. 119–127.
52. Haggerty, R., and Zaia, M.: Acute bacterial meningitis. Adv. Pediatr. *13*:129–173, 1964.
53. Halstensen, A., Ceska, M. Brandtzaeg, P., et al.: Interleukin-8 in serum and cerebrospinal fluid from patients with meningococcal disease. J. Infect. Dis. *167*:471–475, 1993.
54. Hardman, J. M.: Fatal meningococcal infections: The changing pathologic picture in the '60's. Milit. Med. *133*:951–964, 1968.
55. Harrison, L. H., Armstrong, C. W., Jenkins, S. R., et al.: A cluster of meningococcal disease on a school bus following epidemic influenza. Arch. Intern. Med. *141*:1005–1009, 1991.
56. Hart, C. A., and Rogers, T. R.: Meningococcal disease. J. Med. Microbiol. *39*:3–25, 1993.
57. Hathaway, W. E.: Heparin therapy in acute meningococcemia. J. Pediatr. *82*:900–901, 1973.
58. Herman, R. A., and Rubin, H. A.: Meningococcal pericarditis without meningitis presenting as tamponade. N. Engl. J. Med. *290*:143–144, 1974.
59. Herrera, R., Hobar, P. C., and Ginsburg, C. M.: Surgical intervention for the complications of meningococcal-induced purpura fulminans. Pediatr. Infect. Dis. J. *13*:734–737, 1994.
60. Herrick, W. W.: Extrameningeal meningococcus infections. Arch. Intern. Med. *23*:409–418, 1919.
61. Hoagland, R. J., Bartelloni, P., and Cataldo, J. R.: Meningococcemia: Cause of prolonged fever. U. S. Armed Forces Med. J. *11*:1190, 1960.
62. Holbein, B. E.: Differences in virulence for mice between disease and carrier strains of *Neisseria meningitidis*. Can. J. Microbiol. *27*:738–741, 1981.
63. Holbein, B. E.: Enhancement of *Neisseria meningitidis* infection in mice by addition of iron bound to transferrin. Infect. Immun. *34*:120–125, 1981.
64. Hubert, B., Watier, L., Garnerin, P., et al.: Meningococcal disease and influenza-like syndrome: A new approach to an old question. J. Infect. Dis. *166*:542–545, 1992.
65. Irazuzta, J., and McManus, M. L.: Use of topically applied nitroglycerin in the treatment of purpura fulminans. J. Pediatr. *117*:993–995, 1990.
66. Jackson, L. A., Schuchat, A., Reeves, M. W., et al.: Serogroup C meningococcal outbreaks in the United States: An emerging threat. J. A. M. A. *273*:383–388, 1995.
67. Jackson, L. A., Tenover, F. C., Baker, C., et al.: Prevalence of *Neisseria meningitidis* relatively resistant to penicillin in the United States. J. Infect. Dis. *169*:438–441, 1994.
68. Jacobson, J. A., Camargos, P. A., Ferreira, J. T., et al.: The risk of meningitis among classroom contacts during an epidemic of meningococcal disease. Am. J. Epidemiol. *104*:552–555, 1976.
69. Jennings, H. J., Bhattacharjee, A. K., Bundle, D. R., et al.: Structures of the capsular polysaccharides of *Neisseria meningitidis* as determined by ^{13}C-nuclear magnetic resonance spectroscopy. J. Infect. Dis. *136*(Suppl.):S78–S83, 1977.
70. Jones, D. M., and Kaczmarski, E. B., et al.: Meningococcal infections in England and Wales: Report of the Meningococcal Reference Laboratory for 1990. CDR *1*:R76–R78, 1991.
71. Jones, R. N., Slepack, J., and Eades, A.: Fatal neonatal meningococcal meningitis. J. A. M. A. *236*:2652–2653, 1976.
72. Kaiser, A. B., Hennekens, C. H., Saslaw, M. S., et al.: Seroepidemiology and chemoprophylaxis of disease due to sulfonamide-resistant *Neisseria meningitidis* in a civilian population. J. Infect. Dis. *130*:217–224, 1974.
73. Kasper, D. L., Winkelhake, J. L., Zollinger, W. D., et al.: Immunochemical similarity between polysaccharide antigens of *Escherichia coli* 07:K1(L):NM and group B *Neisseria meningitidis*. J. Immunol. *110*:262–268, 1973.
74. Kaufman, B., Levy, H., Zaleznak, B., et al.: Statistical analysis of 242 cases of meningococcus meningitis. Pediatrics *38*:705–716, 1951.
75. Keeley, S. R., Matthews, N. T., and Buist, M.: Tissue plasminogen activator for gangrene in fulminant meningococcemia. Lancet *337*:1359, 1991.
76. Koneman, E. W., and Allen, S. D., et al.: *Neisseria* species and *Moraxella catarrhalis*. *In* Koneman, E. W. (ed.): Color Atlas and Textbook of Diagnostic Microbiology. 4th ed. Philadelphia, J. B. Lippincott, 1992, pp. 369–399.
77. Koppes, G. M., Ellenbogen, E., and Gebhart, R. J.: Group Y meningococcal disease in United States Air Force recruits. Am. J. Med. *62*:661–666, 1977.
78. Kunkel, M. J., Brown, L. G., Banta, H., et al.: Meningococcal mesenteric adenitis and peritonitis in a child. Pediatr. Infect. Dis. *3*:327–328, 1984.
79. Kuppermann, N., Inkelis, S. H., and Saladino, R.: The role of heparin in the prevention of extremity and digit necrosis in meningococcal purpura fulminans. Pediatr. Infect. Dis. J. *13*:867–873, 1994.
80. Lehman, T. J. A., Bernstein, B., Hanson, V., et. al.: Meningococcal infection complicating systemic lupus erythematosus. J. Pediatr. *99*:94–95, 1981.
81. Leibel, R. L., Fangman, J. J., and Ostrovsky, M. C.: Chronic meningococcemia in childhood. Am. J. Dis. Child. *127*:94–98, 1974.
82. Levitt, L. P., Bond, J. O., Hall, I. E., et al.: Meningococcal and ECHO-9 meningitis. Neurology *20*:45–51, 1970.
83. Lewis, J. F., Arnold, C., and Alexander, J.: Meningococcal pneumonia. Am. J. Clin. Pathol. *59*:388–390, 1973.
84. Marks, M. I., Frasch, C. E., and Shapera, R. M.: Meningococcal colonization and infection in children and their household contacts. Am. J. Epidemiol. *109*:563–571, 1979.
85. Marzouk, O., Thomson, A. P., Sills, J. A., et al.: Features and outcome in meningococcal disease presenting with maculopapular rash. Arch. Dis. Child. *66*:485–487, 1991.
86. McCormick, J. B., and Bennett, J. V.: Public health considerations in the management of meningococcal disease. Ann. Intern. Med. *83*:883–886, 1975.
87. McCracken, G. H., Sarff, L. D., Glode, M. P., et al.: Relation between *E. coli* K1 capsular polysaccharide antigen and clinical outcome in neonatal meningitis. Lancet *2*:246–250, 1974.

88. Mellado, M. C., Rodriguez-Contreras, R., Fernandez-Crehuet, M., et al.: Endotoxin liberation by strains of *N. meningitidis* isolated from patients and healthy carriers. Epidemiol. Infect. *106*:289–295, 1991.
89. Mellado, M. C., Rodriguez-Contreras, R., Mariscal, A., et al.: Effect of penicillin and chloramphenicol on the growth and endotoxin release by *N. meningitidis*. Epidemiol. Infect. *106*:283–288, 1991.
90. Mendelman, P. A., Campos, J., Chaffin, D. O., et al.: Relative penicillin G resistance in *Neisseria meningitidis* and reduced affinity of penicillin-binding protein 3. Antimicrob. Agents Chemother. *32*:706–709, 1988.
91. Moore, P. S., Harrison, L. H., Telzak, E. E., et al.: Group A meningococcal carriage in travelers returning from Saudi Arabia. J. A. M. A. *260*:2686–2689, 1988.
92. Moore, P. S., Hierholzer, J., DeWitt, W., et al.: Respiratory viruses and mycoplasma as cofactors for epidemic group A meningococcal meningitis. J. A. M. A. *264*:1271–1275, 1990.
93. Moore, P. S., Reeves, M. W., Schwartz, B., et al.: Intercontinental spread of an epidemic Group A *Neisseria meningitidis* strain. Lancet *21*:260–263, 1989.
94. Morrow, H. W., Slaten, D. D., Reingold, A. L., et al.: Risk factors associated with a school-related outbreak of serogroup C meningococcal disease. Pediatr. Infect. Dis. J. *9*:394–398, 1990.
95. Morse, J. R., Oretsky, M. I., and Hudson, J. S.: Pericarditis as a complication of meningococcal meningitis. Ann. Intern. Med. *74*:212–217, 1971.
96. Nassif, X., and So, M.: Interaction of pathogenic Neisseriae with non-phagocytic cells. Clin. Microbiol. Rev. *8*:376–388, 1995.
97. Ni, H., Knight, A. I., Cartwright K., et al.: Polymerase chain reaction for diagnosis of meningococcal meningitis. Lancet *340*:1432–1434, 1993.
98. Nielsen, H. E., Koch, C., Magnussen, P., et al.: Complement deficiencies in selected groups of patients with meningococcal disease. Scand. J. Infect. Dis. *21*:389–396, 1989.
99. Ognibene, A. J., and Dito, W. R.: Chronic meningococcemia. Arch. Intern. Med. *114*:29–32, 1964.
100. Olcén, P., Kjellander, J., Danielsson, D., et al.: Epidemiology of *Neisseria meningitidis*: Prevalence and symptoms from the upper respiratory tract in family members to patients with meningococcal disease. Scand. J. Infect. Dis. *13*:105–109, 1981.
101. Oppenheimer, E. Y., and Rosman, N. P.: Bacterial meningitis in childhood: Neurologic complications and their management. Pediatr. Neurol. *287*:285–298, 1976.
102. Peltola, H., Mäkelä, H., Kayhty, H., et al.: Clinical efficacy of meningococcus group A capsular polysaccharide vaccine in children three months to five years of age. N. Engl. J. Med. *297*:686–691, 1977.
103. Penny, J. L., Grace, W. J., and Kennedy, R. J.: Meningococcal pericarditis. Am. J. Cardiol. *18*:281–285, 1966.
104. Perez-Trallero, E., Aldamiz-Echeverria, L., and Perez-Yarza, E. G.: Meningococci with increased resistance to penicillin. Lancet *335*:1096, 1990.
105. Pierce, H. I., and Cooper, E. B.: Meningococcal pericarditis: Clinical features and therapy in five patients. Arch. Intern. Med. *129*:918–922, 1972.
106. Pinals, R. S., and Ropes, M. W.: Meningococcal arthritis. Arthritis Rheum. *7*:241–258, 1964.
107. Pinner, R. W., Onyango, F., Perkins, B. A., et al.: Epidemic meningococcal disease in Nairobi, Kenya, 1989: The Kenya/Centers for Disease Control (CDC) Meningitis Study Group. J. Infect. Dis. *166*:359–364, 1992.
108. Pinner, R. W., Gellin, B. G., Bibb, W. F., et al.: Meningococcal disease in the United States: 1986. J. Infect. Dis. *164*:368–374, 1986.
109. Pizzi, M.: A severe epidemic of meningococcus meningitis in Chile, 1941–1942. Am. J. Public Health *34*:231–238, 1944.
110. Platonov, A. E., Beloborodov, V. B., and Vershinina, I. V.: Meningoccocal disease in patients with late complement deficiency: Studies in the U.S.S.R. Medicine *72*:374–392, 1993.
111. Powars, D. Larsen, R., Johnson, J., et al.: Epidemic meningococcemia and purpura fulminans with induced protein C deficiency. Clin. Infect. Dis. *17*:254–261, 1993.
112. Powars, D. R., Rogers, Z. R., Patch, M. J. et al.: Purpura fulminans in meningococcemia: Association with acquired deficiencies of Proteins C and S. N. Engl. J. Med. *317*:571–572, 1987.
113. Riedo, F. X., Plikaytis, M. S., and Broome C. V.: Epidemiology and prevention of meningococcal disease. Pediatr. Infect. Dis. J. *14*:643–657, 1995.
114. Rivard, G. E., David, M., Farrell, C., et al.: Treatment of purpura fulminans in meningococcemia with protein C concentrate. J. Pediatr. *126*:646–652, 1995.
115. Robboy, S. J.: Atrioventricular node inflammation: Mechanism of sudden death in protracted meningococcemia. N. Engl. J. Med. *286*:1091–1093, 1972.
116. Rodriguez-Erdmann, F.: Intravascular activation of the clotting system with phospholipids. Blood *26*:541–553, 1965.
117. Rosenblatt, J. E., Ray, C. G., Enquist, R. W., et al.: Meningococcal infections in children: Observations on prognosis and therapy. Personal communication, 1978.
118. Ross, S. C., and Densen, P.: Complement deficiency states and infection: Epidemiology, pathogenesis and consequences of neisserial and other infections in an immune deficiency. Medicine (Baltimore) *63*:243–273, 1984.
119. Rowe, P. C., McLean, R. H., Wood, R. A., et al.: Association of homozygous C4B deficiency with bacterial meningitis. J. Infect. Dis. *160*:448–451, 1989.
120. Scheim, A. J.: Articular manifestations of meningococcic infections. Arch. Intern. Med. *62*:963–978, 1938.
121. Scott, L. P., Knox, D., Perry, L. W., et al.: Meningococcal pericarditis. Am. J. Cardiol. *29*:104–108, 1972.
122. Similack, J. D.: Group Y meningococcal disease: Twelve cases at an army training center. Ann. Intern. Med. *81*:740–745, 1971.
123. Sjoholm, A. G., Kuijper, E. J., et. al. Dysfunctional properdin in a Dutch family with meningococcal disease. N. Engl. J. Med. *319*:33–37, 1988.
124. Spratt, B. G., Zhang, Q.-Y., Jones, D. M., et al.: Recruitment of a penicillin-binding protein gene from *Neisseria flavescens* during the emergence of penicillin-resistant *Neisseria meningitidis*. Proc. Natl. Acad. Sci. U. S. A. *86*:8988–8992, 1989.
125. Stanwell-Smith, R. E., Stuart, J. M., Hughes, A. O., et al.: Smoking, the environment and meningococcal disease: A case control study. Epidemiol. Infect. *112*:315–328, 1994.
126. Stiehm, E. R., and Damrosch, D. S.: Factors in the prognosis of meningococcal infection. J. Pediatr. *68*:457–467, 1966.
127. Stuart J. M., Cartwright K. A.,. Robinson, P. M., et al.: Effect of smoking on meningococcal carriage. Lancet *2*:723–725, 1989.
128. Sullivan, T. D., and La Scolea, L. J.: *Neisseria meningitidis* bacteremia in children: Quantitation of bacteremia and spontaneous clinical recovery without antibiotic therapy. Pediatrics *80*:63–67, 1987.
129. Sutcliffe, E. M., Jones, D. M., El-Sheikh, S., et al.: Penicillin-insensitive meningococci in the UK. Lancet *1*:657–658, 1988.
130. Tobias, J. D., Haun, S. E., Helfaer, M., et al.: Use of continuous caudal block to relieve lower extremity ischemia caused by vasculitis in a child with meningococcemia. J. Pediatr. *115*:1019–1021, 1989.
131. Tuncer, A. M., Gür, I., Ertem, U., et al.: Once daily ceftriaxone for meningococcemia and meningococcal meningitis. Pediatr. Infect. Dis. J. *7*:711–713, 1988.
132. Twumasi, P. A., Jr., Kumah S., Leach, A., et al: A trial of a group A plus group C meningococcal polysaccharide-protein conjugate vaccine in African infants. J. Infect. Dis. *171*:632–638, 1995.
133. van Deuren, M., van der ven-Jongekrijg, J., Bartelink, A. K., et al.: Correlation between proinflammatory cytokines and antiinflammatory mediators and the severity of disease in meningococcal infections. J. Infect. Dis. *172*:433–439. 1995.
134. van Deuren, M., van Dijke, B. J., et. al.: Rapid diagnosis of acute meningococcal infections by needle aspiration or biopsy of skin lesions. Br. Med. J. *307*:127, 1993.
135. Van Nguyen, Q., Nguyen, E. A., and Weiner, L. B.: Incidence of invasive bacterial disease in children with fever and petechiae. Pediatrics *74*:77–80, 1984.
136. Vann, W. F., Liu, T. Y., and Robbins, J. B.: *Bacillus pumilus* polysaccharide cross-reactive with meningococcal group A polysaccharide. Infect. Immun. *13*:1654–1662, 1976.
137. Vieusseux, G.: Memoire sur la maladie qui a regre a Geneve au printemps de 1805. J. Med. Chir. Pharm. *11*:163, 1806.
138. Waage, A., Brandtzaeg, P., Halstensen, A., et al.: The complex pattern of cytokines in serum from patients with meningococcal septic shock. J. Exp. Med. *169*:333–338, 1989.
139. Waage, A., Halstensen, A. and Esperik, T.: Association between tumour necrosis factor in serum and fatal outcome in patients with meningococcal disease. Lancet *1*:355–357, 1987.
140. Wahdan, M. H., Rizk, F., el-Alkkad, A. M., et al.: A controlled field trial of a serogroup A meningococcal polysaccharide vaccine. Bull. W. H. O. *48*:667–673, 1973.
141. Weis, E. J., and Silber, E. N.: Acute constrictive pericarditis. J. Pediatr. *58*:548–553, 1961.
142. Whalen, C. M., Hockin, J. C., Ryan, A., et al.: The changing epidemiology of invasive meningococcal disease in Canada, 1985 through 1992: Emergence of a virulent clone of *Neisseria meningitidis*. J. A. M. A. *273*:390–394, 1995.
143. Whittle, H., Tugwell, P., Egler, L., et al.: Rapid bacteriologic diagnosis of pyogenic meningitis by latex agglutination. Lancet *2*:619–621, 1974.
144. Wilson, F. E., and Morse, S. R.: Therapy of acute meningococcal infections: Early volume expansion and prophylactic low dose heparin. Am. J. Med. Sci. *264*:445–455, 1972.
145. Wolf, R. E., and Birbara, C. A.: Meningococcal infections at an Army training center. Am. J. Med. *44*:243–255, 1968.
146. Wong, V. K., Hitchcock, W., and Mason, W. H.: Meningococcal infections in children: A review of 100 cases. Pediatr. Infect. Dis. J. *8*:224–227, 1989.
147. Woods, C. R., Smith, A. L., Wasilauskas, B. L., et al.: Invasive disease caused by *Neisseria meningitidis* relatively resistant to penicillin in North Carolina. J. Infect. Dis. *170*:453–456, 1994.
148. Young, L. S., LaForce, M., Head, J. J., et al.: A simultaneous outbreak of meningococcal and influenza infections: Epidemiologic, clinical and laboratory findings. N. Engl. J. Med. *287*:5–9, 1972.
149. Zenz, W., and Muntean, W.: Recombinant tissue plasminogen activator treatment in two infants with fulminant meningococcemia. Pediatrics *96*:144–147, 1995.
150. Zhang, Q. Y., Jones, D. M., Saez-Nieto, J. A., et al.: Genetic diversity of penicillin-binding protein 2 genes of penicillin-resistant strains of *Neisseria meningitidis* revealed by fingerprinting of amplified DNA. Antimicrob. Agents Chemother. *34*:1523–1528, 1990.

94

GONORRHEA

Laura T. Gutman

Gonorrhea in children includes gonococcal ophthalmia neonatorum, sepsis and arthritis, vaginitis, proctitis, perihepatitis, wound infection, and funisitis.

EPIDEMIOLOGIC OBSERVATIONS OF INFECTION IN CHILDREN

Concern over the ongoing epidemic of gonococcal infection has begun to include recognition that higher rates in adults are associated with increased rates of infection in children. However, there remains a paucity of information available from prospective studies in children. The following data pertain largely to information from adult clinics but draw attention to several significant aspects of gonococcal epidemiology that pertain to children.

The reported cases of gonorrhea in the United States declined from 204 per 100,000 in 1950 to a low of 129 per 100,000 in 1958. Subsequently, there was a gradual yearly increase of approximately 8 to 16 per cent, reaching a peak of 472 per 100,000 in 1975. Since then, there have been small yearly decreases, and the rate was 168 per 100,000 in 1994.

Data gathered in a recent 12-year experience report the rates of gonorrhea by age group in children and early adolescent youth based primarily on the detection of symptomatic infection. Data also indicate that asymptomatic infection occurs in children, including in the prepubertal period.[3, 55, 73, 80] These studies document rapid rises in rates of the reported cases of gonococcal infection in children from 10 to 14 years of age to those in adolescence from 15 to 19 years of age. Age- and sex-specific rates of gonorrhea in the early 1980s showed overall declines in rates. However, among white girls 10 to 19 years of age, there was an increase in rates between 1975 and 1984[119] and between 1981 and 1991, an increase from 66 to 99/100,000.[27] Some geographic areas have much higher rates of pediatric disease.[50, 60]

The age-specific rates of gonococcal infection reported in 1991 by sex were as follows:

Age	*Male*	*Female*
10–14 years	32	92
15–19 years	882	1043

These observations show the higher rates of gonococcal infection in female children and adolescents, compared with those in males. In young adulthood, rates in males begin to exceed females in many populations. Rates in black adolescents of both genders greatly exceed those of white adolescents.

SEXUAL ABUSE OF CHILDREN

Sexually transmitted disease (STD) in children other than newborns should be assumed to be sexually transmitted unless proven otherwise. Sexual abuse of children has been defined as the involvement of dependent, developmentally immature children and adolescents in sexual activities that they do not comprehend fully, for which they are unable to give informed consent, or that violate the social taboos of family roles. Sexual abuse includes all forms of adult involvement in sexual relations with children, including rape, incest, child pornography, and child prostitution. Other forms include nonviolent fondling, viewing, and orogenital contact. Exposing a child to adult sexual intercourse or pornography represents sexual abuse or exploitation in many jurisdictions. Each state has specific civil and criminal laws defining which acts and situations are forms of sexual abuse or sexual assault of children. Each clinician must familiarize himself or herself with the laws of the state in which he or she practices.

The incidence of sexual abuse is unknown, but many medical facilities find that increased efforts at recognition lead to identification of very significant numbers of involved children. Sexual abuse has been reported in approximately 10 per cent of all self-reporting populations of females during childhood in numerous studies, and rates in male children appear to be approximately 3 per cent.[10, 122a] It appears that approximately 1 per cent of children experience serious forms of sexual abuse yearly.[35] Reluctance on the part of the perpetrator, family, medical community, and legal system to acknowledge the possibility of sexual abuse of children undoubtedly has hindered the understanding of this problem. Age-appropriate interviewing techniques, including skilled interviewing, the use of anatomically correct dolls, child art, and repeat interviews, are allowing a more complete assessment of suspected cases. Statements from young children are gaining credibility; ". . . molestation may leave no evidence, except the child's story. This must be believed! Children do not fabricate stories of detailed sexual activities unless they have witnessed them, and they have indeed been witness to their abuse."[88] There is a rapidly developing appreciation of the association between sexual abuse, other forms of child abuse, and other forms of behavioral disturbances in children, including truancy, running away, depression, low self-esteem, fears, many other somatic complaints, attention deficit disorder, poor school performance, adolescent pregnancy, interpersonal violence, and sexual violence.

Rates of STDs in sexually abused children have been reported to be approximately 5 to 20 per cent (Table 94–1). Gonorrhea was the most frequently recognized disease when that infection was highly prevalent in the general population. As a result of the improved control of gonorrhea in the 1980s, fewer pediatric cases are being recognized in the United States. Nevertheless, it appears that female children who are exposed to an infected male have a high rate of acquired disease. In an outbreak in an orphanage, 53 of 95 abused girls were found to have contracted infection.[2]

Although only the minority of children who have experienced sexual abuse contract an STD as a consequence, the diagnosis of an STD is a very important indication that the child has been in an abusive setting, and an STD may be the sole finding on physical examination.[78] For this reason, the examination should be thorough, all mucous membranes should be cultured appropriately, and the cultures should be handled in such a way as to ensure legal acceptance if that should be needed. Table 94–1 summarizes the STD diagnoses in 2934 children from six studies who had been evaluated for suspected sexual abuse.

Gonorrhea and acquired syphilis are accepted by the

TABLE 94–1. Sexually Transmitted Diseases in Prepubertal Children Evaluated for Suspected Sexual Abuse

Reference	No. of Children Evaluated	Number (%) Who Had Diagnosis of:				
		Gonorrhea	Chlamydia	*Syphilis*	Trichomonas	*Condylomata Acuminata*
Wald et al., 1980[141]	189	28 (14.8%)	ND	ND	ND	ND
Rimsza and Niggemann, 1982[120]	285	21 (7.4%)	ND	0	ND	ND
White et al., 1983[145]	409	46 (10%)	ND	6 (5.5%)	4 (18%)	3 (5.6%)
Ingram et al., 1984[77]	50	10 (20%)	3 (6%)	ND	2 (4%)	ND
DeJong, 1986[47]	532	25 (4.7%)	ND	1 (0.2%)	ND	3 (0.6%)
Ingram et al., 1992[80]	1469	41 (2.8%)	17 (1.2%)	1 (0.1%)	3 (2%)	28 (2%)

ND, no data.

American Academy of Pediatrics to be infections that, when diagnosed, also provide a confirmed diagnosis of sexual abuse.[35]

The infections of adults that frequently or primarily are transmitted by a sexual route are numerous, and many of the infections are transmitted primarily through male homosexual contact. In contrast, there is a relatively limited number of infections for which a child who is suspected of having been exposed to sexual contact routinely may be examined. These include syphilis,[63] gonorrhea,[59] condyloma acuminatum,[68, 74] herpes simplex of the genitalia,[59] *Chlamydia trachomatis* infection,[45, 116] *Trichomonas vaginalis* infection,[85] and bacterial vaginosis.[69] All children infected with an STD should be evaluated for other STDs, including HIV infection.[67]

The following general issues should be noted:

1. Many institutions have a service that particularly is skilled in the interview and examination of children suspected of having experienced sexual abuse. This may be a child protection team within the pediatric department or a person or group in obstetrics. This group, if available, should be involved in the work-up from the first contact.[109]
2. If the child is symptomatic, all available and appropriate cultures and examinations should be completed before the child receives therapy. For example, if the child has conjunctivitis, cultures of other mucosal areas should be taken before therapy is started.
3. All culture and examination samples must be labeled thoroughly and clearly. Timely delivery to the appropriate laboratory must be ensured by personal delivery if necessary. The clinician should have a policy regarding the identification of specimens and should establish a chain of custody, such that results can be supported in court procedures when issues of the child's safety are being considered.
4. Testing for gonorrhea in infants and children should use only standard culture systems of isolation. Rapid nonculture tests, which have been evaluated in adults, have not been evaluated adequately in children and are not approved for diagnosis of pediatric infection.
5. If sexual abuse is recognized by the presence of spermatozoa, by one of the listed STDs, or by social history, the child should not leave the clinic until his or her safety has been assured. Safety issues usually are assessed by the Department of Social Services or assured by hospitalization of the child pending further investigation.
6. The Child Abuse Reporting Law applies to sexual abuse or assault. Therefore, it is mandatory to report suspected and confirmed cases to the social service of the county in which the child resides.
7. The majority of children who have been the victims of sexual abuse will not have specific physical findings to confirm the diagnosis. Subtle findings such as bruising may be present, but the physical examination is likely to reveal no abnormality. However, the absence of abnormalities on physical examination does not make a diagnosis of sexual abuse unlikely. Oral sexual contact is a common form of abuse, as are fondling and external genital contact, all of which may not result in apparent injuries.
8. If the child has gonorrhea, other members of the family usually are infected as well. In particular, other female children are especially likely to be infected and should be examined.[55, 60]
9. Internal pelvic examinations are indicated very rarely. Exceptions are instances of foreign body presence or major trauma. If an internal examination of a prepubertal girl is requested, it should be performed by an experienced examiner. The manipulation of the hymen of girls of this age causes serious pain and will be viewed by the child as an assault.
10. Children often have compelling reasons to deny abuse and to fail to disclose sexual abuse, even to skillful diagnostic interviewers. The diagnosis of sexual abuse may be based on findings other than the child's disclosure, and denial is not compelling disproof of abuse. For example, in a study of the rate of disclosure among children who presented with physical complaints related to acquired genital gonorrhea, only 43 per cent were able to provide valid verbal disclosure during the first interview.[96]
11. Sexual abuse of children usually is a chronic and recurring condition. Consequently, if the child remains unprotected, reabuse is very likely. If the perpetrator has an STD, the child may present with recurrent episodes of that STD.[95]

Cultures that should be taken from children who are known to have or suspected of having been victims of sexual abuse are as follows:

1. Rectal, throat, and vaginal (females) or urethral (males) cultures for *Neisseria gonorrhoeae* should be plated on Thayer-Martin medium. Vaginal cultures are satisfactory in prepubertal females, and attempts to obtain endocervical specimens should not be made. Only after puberty should endocervical cultures be obtained. Blood cultures should be taken if there is reason to consider disseminated disease. Other sites (conjunctivae, joint fluid) should be cultured if clinically indicated.

In order to achieve satisfactory results from cultures, specimens from children require meticulous handling. Specimens should be plated immediately on prewarmed media. In addition, it appears that it may improve the rate of isolation when two complete plates (one inhibitory, one chocolate agar) are used for each specimen, thus increasing the surface area available to the technician for recognition of sparse organisms. Finally, the plates must be introduced promptly in a carbon dioxide–containing environment.

Among children being evaluated for sexual abuse, some clincians advocate restricting the collection of specimens for gonorrhea to those children who have signs of clinical disease.[131] However, in numerous studies, asymptomatic infection has made up significant proportion of all cases of gonorrhea.[15, 55, 73] Consequently, strong consideration should be given to obtaining cultures, even when the child is asymptomatic.

2. Vulvovaginal, urethral, rectal, and throat cultures for *Chlamydia trachomatis* are indicated.

3. Serum for a VDRL test should be collected at the first examination and repeated in 6 to 12 weeks. HIV serology is recommended by some investigators and should be repeated in 12 to 24 weeks. Perceived risk may determine whether or not the test is performed.

4. A serum sample should be collected and stored frozen.

5. Presence of venereal warts should be sought and noted.

6. Urinalysis and wet preparation of vaginal secretions with attention to the presence of *Trichomonas* should be considered. Cultures for *Trichomonas* species are superior to direct examination.

7. Pregnancy should be determined if indicated.

8. A wet preparation of vaginal secretions of symptomatic girls should be examined for clue cells and amine odor with 10 per cent potassium hydroxide.

The subject of child abuse and sexual abuse of children is one of the most rapidly advancing fields of pediatric interest, and physicians must give attention to emerging changes in concepts concerning diagnosis and management.[11, 55, 77, 79, 99, 106, 120, 123, 137 139]

THE ORGANISM

Neisseria species are aerobic, gram-negative diplococci occurring in pairs with adjacent sides flattened. Catalase and cytochrome oxidase are produced by most species in the genus. Important in vitro growth characteristics include a requirement for free iron, enhanced survival conferred by provision of carbon dioxide in the incubating atmosphere, and relative sensitivity to cold.

The organisms usually are cultured on chocolate blood agar in an atmosphere enriched by carbon dioxide. If the isolate has been made from a highly contaminated site (e.g., rectum, cervix), selective medium or chocolate agar containing nystatin, vancomycin, and colistin to suppress contaminating flora allows growth of most *Neisseria* species, although occasional strains of gonococci are inhibited.[16] Chocolate agar without antimicrobial agents therefore is preferred if the culture is from a usually sterile area, such as blood, cerebrospinal fluid, synovial fluid, or a skin lesion.

It is important to speciate all *Neisseria* organisms cultured from children. This is true because *Neisseria meningitidis, N. gonorrhoeae,* and others of the Neisseriaceae family are morphologically similar and may be isolated from sites such as the vagina, blood, and nasopharynx. Accurate speciation of *Neisseria* organisms is essential in the identification of *N. gonorrhoeae* from any pediatric specimen because misidentification may lead to very serious social consequences for the child by precipitating concerns regarding sexual abuse.[49, 51, 146] The most common method of speciating members of the *Neisseria* genus is by sugar fermentation pattern, and the characteristic reactions are given in Table 94–2. Two other techniques confirm the identification of *N. gonorrhoeae.*[87] One uses enzyme-substrate tests that identify the enzymes 1-hydroxy-prolylaminopeptidase, γ-glutamylaminotransferase, and β-galactosidase. The second method is immunogenic and employs a fluorescent antibody stain. It is recommended that isolates that appear to be *N. gonorrhoeae* and come from a pediatric patient should be confirmed by at least one test using either enzyme-substrate methods or immunofluorescent methods.[146]

At present, there are several methods of distinguishing strains of *N. gonorrhoeae.* Strain differentiation permits study of both the epidemiology of transmission of gonorrhea and the virulence factors.

The following methods have been developed for the characterization of strains:

1. Gonococcal pili have been shown to be antigenically heterologous, and strains may be characterized by their pili.

2. Auxotyping has permitted discrimination of approximately 20 types, which are based upon growth or absence of growth on 11 chemically defined media. Selected compounds that are omitted include L-proline, L-arginine, L-ornithine, L-methionine, hypoxanthine, uracil, thiamine, and thiamine phosphate. Auxotypes are stable in vitro. It has been found that organisms cultured from sexual partners are of a similar auxotype.[23, 25]

3. The serologic specificity of gonococcal strains may be demonstrated by a system that is based upon the antigenic heterogeneity of the protein I molecule contained in the outer membrane of the gonococcus.[7, 83, 124, 125] These serogroups are termed WI, WII, and WIII, as determined by their reactivity with adsorbed polyvalent antibodies. Peptide mapping has demonstrated two protein I molecules designated IA (PrIA) and protein IB (PrIB). The serogroup WI contains PrIA, whereas WII and WIII possess PrIB.

4. Development of a series of 12 monoclonal antibodies to

TABLE 94–2. Biochemical Characteristics Differentiating the Species of Genus *Neisseria*

	N. gonorrhoeae	*N. meningitidis*	*N. sicca*	*N. subflava*	*N. flavescens*	*N. mucosa*	*N. lactamica*
Acid from:							
Glucose	+	+	+	+	−	+	+
Maltose	−	+	+	+	−	+	−
Sucrose	−	−	+	±	−	+	−
Lactose	−	−	−	−	−	−	+
Polysaccharide Produced from 5% sucrose	0	0	+	±	+	+	0
Reduction of:							
Nitrate	−	−	−	−	−	+	−
Nitrite	−	±	+	+	+	+	+
Pigment	−	−	±	+	+	+	−
Extra CO_2 for growth	+	+	−	−	−	−	−

protein I has allowed further classification of gonococcal strains into 18 PrIA and 28 PrIB serovars. Serovars are stable in vitro. Combined use of auxotype and serovar typing has permitted classification of some 107 distinct categories of *N. gonorrhoeae* after testing 1433 isolates.[90] This system permits analysis of geographic distribution and migration of strains. Alternatively, a second panel of monoclonal antibodies also may provide extensive identification of individual strains.[103]

VIRULENCE FACTORS

Extensive studies have described the pathophysiology of *N. gonorrhoeae*.[33] These studies have included data regarding the adaptation of organisms to specific anatomic areas (rectum, blood, endocervix, etc.).[102] No data have been gathered regarding the adaptations of *N. gonorrhoeae* infections of children, and consequently all information pertains only to adults.

Characteristics of *N. gonorrhoeae* strains thought to be of particular interest because of their role in virulence are (1) the presence of pili, (2) opacity proteins, (3) the ability to utilize iron, (4) IgA protease, (5) the lipo-oligosaccharide, and (6) the cell wall peptidoglycan.

1. *The presence of pili.* Bacterial pili are hairlike structures that are protein in content, attach to and extend from the outermost layer of the cell, usually are very profuse in number, and are not involved in motility of the cell. Newly isolated *N. gonorrhoeae* grown on translucent agar medium produces four different colony types.[16, 20] Colony types 1 and 2 predominate and are small, compact, and composed of piliated organisms. Colony types 3 and 4 are larger and granular and contain nonpiliated organisms. Microscopic selection of individual piliated colonies permits propagation of piliated strains. Piliated strains maintained virulence and were responsible for disease, whereas the nonpiliated strains were avirulent.

Pili participate in the adherence of organisms to cells, and close interactions of *N. gonorrhoeae* with mucosal cells, erythrocytes, spermatozoa, and polymorphonuclear cells are well described. Pili thus may initiate contact with the host cell, and species specificity is demonstrated by greater adherence to human cells than nonhuman cells. Of great interest and relevance to virulence is the antigenic diversity of pili, as well as the ability of the organism to switch reversibly from a piliated to a nonpiliated phenotype.[136] In addition, piliated strains are not ingested by phagocytes as well as nonpiliated strains are. Polymorphonuclear cells may discharge specific granule contents but do not kill piliated gonococci in the absence of antibody.

2. *Opacity proteins.* A set of related proteins that are present variably in gonococcal isolates is protein II. Opacity protein (protein II) constituents confer increased opacity on colonies of organisms by promoting adherence of the organisms to one another. Each opacity protein complex shares some antigenic sites inserted in the outer membrane and also has a unique portion on the gonococcal surface. The isolation of particular opacity protein phenotypes from different anatomic sites or from different times during the menstrual cycle has suggested that these proteins contribute to the ability of the organism to succeed in a given niche. Opacity protein influences adherence of the gonococcus. As with pili, there is great variability in opacity protein and consequently in "adherence" properties. Thus, this organism has the capacity to alter both pili and opacity protein rapidly and thereby present different properties and antigenicity to the host.[130]

Protein I is thought to be a porin—that is, a trimer of the protein inserted in the bacterial membrane allows entry of small, water-soluble molecules. Protein I has been shown actually to penetrate the membrane of the host cell, thus anchoring the gonococcus to the cell.

3. *The ability to utilize iron.* Iron is an essential nutrient for *N. gonorrhoeae,* and in host tissues this essential nutrient is sequestered in hemin compounds, as ferritin, or bound to lactoferrin or transferrin. Thus, the efficiency of obtaining iron may contribute to pathogenicity. *N. gonorrhoeae* and *N. meningitidis* can obtain iron from transferrin, whereas the commensal *Neisseria* species can do so with much less consistency—and, in fact, most strains are inhibited by transferrin. The ability to utilize iron from transferrin is a general property of pathogenic *Neisseria* species.

4. *IgA protease.* All *N. gonorrhoeae* make a protease that cleaves IgA1 at the hinge region with Fab_2 and Fc pieces. Nonpathogenic *Neisseria* species lack such an enzyme, and the enzyme and its function—that is, escape from the host protection afforded by local antibody—is associated with strain virulence.

5. *The lipo-oligosaccharide.* Lipo-oligosaccharide is a typical lipid A–containing endotoxin and target antigen for the bactericidal activity mediated by normal human serum. Because strains of *N. gonorrhoeae* isolated from the blood are serum-resistant, this property may be important to invasion of the host. Also, patients with defects in the complement cascade are susceptible to recurrent episodes of gonococcemia, suggesting that the bactericidal qualities of serum are important. Thus, lipo-oligosaccharide should be considered a virulence factor. There is evidence that lipo-oligosaccharide from serum-sensitive strains can activate the classic complement pathway and may do so in the absence of antibody.[130] An adaptation of gonococci during infection includes sialyliation of lipo-oligosaccharide, leading to resistance to binding of complement and thus evasion of the host bactericidal effect of serum.[144] It also is thought that lipo-oligosaccharide contributes to the heat-stable cytotoxicity observed in organ cultures infected with *N. gonorrhoeae.*

6. *The cell wall peptidoglycan.* Gonococci shed soluble peptidoglycan fragments during exponential growth. These peptidoglycan monomers have a number of biologic properties, including activation of complement and modulation of mononuclear cell proliferation. These fragments also damage fallopian tube mucosa in organ culture, suggesting a role for the compounds in invasive disease.[65, 100]

Heightened clinical virulence of some strains is suggested by observations such as those of Handsfield and Holmes,[71] who recorded a microepidemic of gonorrhea involving one asymptomatically infected male and eight female contacts. Seven of the women were infected symptomatically, and four of them experienced disseminated infection. This contrasts with a great deal of information indicating that the majority of infected women have asymptomatic infection and the estimate that only 3 per cent of infected women will manifest disseminated disease.

Strains of *N. gonorrhoeae* obtained from adult patients with disseminated disease have been characterized in the laboratory in an effort to define the basis of the increased virulence:

1. Isolates of *N. gonorrhoeae* from patients with disseminated gonococcal infection are not susceptible to the bactericidal activity of sera[17, 33, 117, 118, 130] (see earlier discussion of lipo-oligosaccharide).

2. These strains have an atypical growth pattern on agar.[102] The presence of opacity protein confers increased opacity on colonies of *N. gonorrhoeae* because organisms adhere to one another. The presence of opacity protein increases attachment to epithelial cells, whereas the absence seems to correlate with invasiveness—for example, salpingitis and bacteremia.

The high frequency of genetic variation provides rapid adaptation to different niches and probably helps organisms to elude the host response.[14]

3. Nutritional requirements usually include arginine, uracil, and hypoxanthine, which are not required for growth of other strains.[89]

4. A high degree of sensitivity to penicillin has characterized strains from patients with disseminated disease.[147]

Morphologic descriptions of invasive disease have used fallopian tube mucosa in organ culture for models.[100] *N. gonorrhoeae* attaches preferentially to microvilli of nonciliated cells. The organisms then are enclosed in a vesicle within the cytoplasm and transported to the base of the cell, where they can multiply and vesicles can fuse. Subsequently, the basilar membrane parts to allow exocytosis of organisms into subepithelial tissues. Adjacent nonepithelial cells are sloughed, probably because of the toxicity of lipo-oligosaccharide and peptidoglycans.[65]

HOST RESPONSE

Extensive investigation has been given to the adult responses to local and systemic infection with *N. gonorrhoeae*.[33] There have been no such studies of infected children, and all information pertains only to adults.

Multiple episodes of gonorrhea may occur in a single individual in a short time. This observation has led to the inference that one episode of *N. gonorrhoeae* infection does not confer protection against subsequent infection. Because this issue is fundamental to understanding the pathophysiology of infection, research is being directed toward understanding the variability of the organism and the elucidation of the host response to infection with *N. gonorrhoeae*. The antigenic diversity and ease of altering the antigenicity of both pili and opacity proteins undoubtedly contribute to the lack of immunity by the host to reinfection.

Circulating humoral antibody to the infecting strain is measured by an assay of bactericidal antibody and is present in the majority of persons who have prolonged mucosal colonization with *N. gonorrhoeae*.[77, 86] In addition, women who develop pelvic inflammatory disease usually develop bactericidal antibody during the infection. IgA- and IgG-blocking antibodies may develop and prevent killing of the bacteria by IgG- and IgM-cidal antibodies.[117]

Secretory IgA antibody occurs in the urethral exudate of men with gonorrhea and in genital secretions of women with gonorrhea.[108] The development of local IgA antibody occurs more rapidly and is more transient than the development of the serum bactericidal response. However, the organism produces an IgA protease capable of destroying IgA. As mentioned previously, an intact complement system is essential for successful eradication of this organism.

PERINATAL GONOCOCCAL INFECTION

Prevention of disease in infants is achieved best through detection and eradication of gonorrhea in the mother. The epidemiology of gonorrhea in women of child-bearing age therefore must be considered.

In teenagers, pregnancy and menstruation are associated with disseminated disease.[75] The highest rates of clinically apparent disease occur at times of low progesterone activity, and progesterone significantly inhibits growth of *N. gonorrhoeae*. The direct effects of hormonal forms of contraception on the inhibition of gonococci have not been studied but must be considered. In addition, intrauterine devices (IUDs) may increase the severity of gonorrhea. Disseminated gonococcal infection may accompany asymptomatic infection of an IUD,[34] and the rate of acute pelvic inflammatory disease in women who use IUDs may be increased.

Since the 1970s, health clinics have encouraged the routine screening of sexually active women for gonorrhea. This especially is important during pregnancy, and rates of gonorrhea in pregnant women range from rare to about 10 per cent. Teenagers may have an even higher prevalence of gonorrhea, as evidenced by studies in Table 94–3. Recognition of gonorrhea early in pregnancy identifies a population at risk that should be followed sequentially throughout pregnancy.[84]

The spectrum of infection with *N. gonorrhoeae* appears to be similar in pregnant and nonpregnant women. Most women are asymptomatic. Pharyngeal infection appears to be more common during pregnancy, perhaps reflecting altered sexual practices. One study had reported that 39 per cent of patients with *N. gonorrhoeae* at any site had pharyngeal infections and 30 per cent had pharyngeal infection as the sole site.[39]

Gonorrheal infections put both the mother and infant at risk for other forms of gonococcal disease:

1. For the mother, there is the risk of gonococcal septic arthritis. Most cases of this disease during pregnancy occur in the third trimester or in the immediate postpartum period.[18, 75] Although the incidence of gonococcal arthritis has been low, many cases have occurred in teenage patients.

2. Gonococcal pelvic inflammatory disease (PID) and acute salpingitis also may complicate the pregnancy of an infected woman.[61] Onset of these diseases usually occurs during the first trimester and has been associated with a high rate of fetal loss. There also is an increased incidence of postpartum fever in women with untreated gonorrhea.

3. Maternal gonococcal infection has been associated with abnormalities of labor and delivery that adversely may affect the infant. Prolonged rupture of the membranes, premature delivery, chorioamnionitis, funisitis, and a clinical diagnosis of sepsis occur frequently in infants with *N. gonorrhoeae* detected in the gastric aspirate during delivery.[5, 52, 70] Intrapartum gonococcal amnionitis was observed at cesarean section

TABLE 94–3. Prevalence of Gonorrhea and Other Sexually Transmitted Diseases in Clinics for Adolescents

Reference	Location	Total Clinic Population Studied	Gonorrhea (%)	*Chlamydia* Infection (%)	Other
Shafer et al., 1984[129]	California	366	15	4	*Trichomonas* infection
Golden et al., 1984[63]	New York	186	10	10	Syphilis *Trichomonas* infection
Demetriou et al., 1984[48]	Oklahoma	839	14	—	
Mulcahy and Lacey, 1987[105]	Leeds	210	14	16	*Trichomonas* infection
Jamison et al., 1995[82]	Colorado	632	7	—	Human papilloma virus infection

TABLE 94–4. Outcome of Pregnancy in Mothers Who Were Infected with *Neisseria gonorrhoeae* at Delivery

Outcome	Charles et al.[30] (N = 14)*	Sarrel and Pruett[126] (N = 37)	Israel et al.[81] (N = 39)	Amstey and Steadman[5] (N = 222)*	Edwards et al.[52] (N = 19)*	Handsfield and Holmes[71] (N = 12)*
Normal or term infant	—	13 (35%)	30 (77%)	142 (64%)	7 (37%)	—
Aborted	—	13 (35%)	1 (2%)	24 (11%)	—	—
Perinatal death	—	3 (8%)	1 (2%)	15 (8%)	2 (11%)	—
Premature	—	6 (17%)	5 (13%)	49 (22%)	8 (42%)	8 (67%)
Perinatal distress	—	—	2 (5%)	—	2 (10%)	—
Premature rupture of membranes	6 (43%)	8 (21%)	—	52 (26%)	12 (63%)	9 (75%)

*Data were provided showing that the outcomes of pregnancies of mothers not infected with *N. gonorrhoeae* were significantly more favorable.

in a woman with premature rupture of the membranes and a preceding, treated episode of gonorrhea.[121]

The hazards to the fetus that are posed by maternal gonorrhea include the neonatal complications of abortion, perinatal death, prematurity, perinatal distress, and premature rupture of the membranes. Table 94–4 tabulates the proportions of infants who were born to infected mothers who experienced these problems in six studies, including the two studies in which a control, noninfected population was presented. A controlled study in an area of high prevalence of gonorrhea found that maternal infection with *N. gonorrhoeae* was associated significantly with preterm birth and that the attributable risk of gonococcal infections was 14 per cent.[53] In addition, maternal complications of peripartum gonorrhea, such as fever and chorioamnionitis, may make it difficult for a new mother to care for her child.[81]

Gonococcal Ophthalmia Neonatorum

Epidemiology—Prevention

It was recognized for several centuries that ophthalmia neonatorum occurred in infants born to women with a vaginal discharge; recommendations for flushing the eyes of a newborn were common prior to the twentieth century.[101] In the last quarter of the nineteenth century, Neisser helped to establish the relationship between the gonococcus and neonatal ophthalmia.

In 1881, Dr. Carl Sigmund Franz Credé[43] published a paper discussing several aspects of gonococcal ophthalmia neonatorum (GON), which still pertain. He recognized that asymptomatic disease in the mother was a potential source of infection. Gonorrhea was highly prevalent in Europe, and Credé described an increased incidence in patients from lower socioeconomic backgrounds. Mechanical cleansing of the birth canal failed to protect the infant from GON, which was occurring in approximately 10 per cent of newborns in major cities. The infection was the cause of a large proportion of admissions to schools for the blind.[12] Finally, he described the method of instillation of 2 per cent silver nitrate ($AgNO_3$) into the infant's conjunctival sac; this still is one basis for recommended preventive procedures.

By 1930, the majority of the states of the United States required that all newborns receive $AgNO_3$ prophylaxis—that is, the Credé procedure. At present, prophylaxis of some form is required by most states. GON decreased as a cause of admissions to schools for the blind in the United States from an average of 24 per cent from 1906 to 1911 to 0.5 per cent from 1951 to 1955.

Worldwide declines of adult gonorrhea in the 1950s probably contributed to the decreased recognition of disease in newborns during that period. The incidence of GON rose in the 1960s and 1970s along with the increased incidence in the general population and was very high in some developing nations.[92] In Los Angeles, California, the rate rose from 9 per 100,000 live births in 1957 to 1958 to 56 per 100,000 live births in 1962 to 1963. In a New York hospital between 1970 and 1973, a rate of 145 per 100,000 births was reported, and in a hospital in North Carolina during 1969 and 1970, a rate of 265.1 per 100,000 live births was proved by culture.[135] In the late 1970s and 1980s, GON again subsided in developed countries but has remained a major problem in underdeveloped nations.

Factors that are associated with higher rates of GON include the following:

1. Lower socioeconomic class of the mother has been an associated condition. In Glasgow, Scotland, from 1963 to 1968, the rate of GON in social class I infants was 0 per 100,000; in social class II infants, 1.8 per 100,000; and in social class V infants 8.6 per 100,000. A related finding was an increased incidence of GON among infants of unwed mothers and among mothers who had not had prenatal care.[134]
2. Prior treatment for gonorrhea during pregnancy is associated with an increased incidence of GON.[84]
3. The incidence of prematurity in infants with GON often is reported to be higher. Whether this is due to an adverse effect of gonorrhea on the pregnancy or because GON may be recognized more readily in the premature infant has not been established.
4. Premature rupture of the membranes appears to increase the risk of GON.

At present, prophylaxis for GON continues to be accomplished mainly through the local instillation of 1 per cent $AgNO_3$ or of several antimicrobial agents. Numerous studies have compared the efficacy of $AgNO_3$ vs. no prophylaxis or vs. another agent. One early study showed that the risk of GON was significantly lower after $AgNO_3$ prophylaxis compared with no prophylaxis and that bacitracin ointment had no value as a prophylactic.[64]

The major advantages to the use of $AgNO_3$ for prophylaxis are the lack of allergic potential and the absence of development of bacterial resistance to the compound. For example, two hospital-based outbreaks in a newborn nursery of erythromycin-resistant staphylococcal conjunctivitis have been associated with the use of erythromycin eye ointment as ocular prophylaxis, and the outbreaks remitted when $AgNO_3$ was substituted.[52] Disadvantages include the problem of conjunctival irritation with the development of exudate in numerous babies and the fact that it is not good treatment if infection already is established when drops are instilled into the eye. A solution of $AgNO_3$ that becomes concentrated may cause ophthalmic injury, but this problem for the most part has been circumvented by dispensing each dose in ampules, which prevent evaporation.

Failures of $AgNO_3$ prophylaxis are not rare. Several factors probably contribute to failures. First, if gonococcal infection of the eye has occurred before birth, $AgNO_3$ is not expected to prevent further progression. Therefore, the increased risk of infection that has been observed in association with premature rupture of the membranes could be predicted because of the exposure to infection prior to actual delivery. In further support of this hypothesis, apparent disease has been reported at the time of birth. Second, administration of $AgNO_3$ is difficult, and the solution may not reach the conjunctival sac. Finally, if prophylaxis is omitted for any reason, protection could not occur.

In spite of these problems, use of 1 per cent $AgNO_3$ remains a widely accepted, carefully evaluated, and safe form of GON prophylaxis. The occasional failure of $AgNO_3$ prophylaxis emphasizes that it is preferable to prevent GON through identification and treatment of the pregnant woman. Alternative ophthalmic prophylactic regimens that have been demonstrated to be efficacious are 0.5 per cent erythromycin ophthalmic ointment and 1 per cent tetracycline ointment given as a single application.

Several investigators since the 1980s have examined the question of whether or not specific regimens that were employed to prevent gonococcal ophthalmia were or were not also efficacious in the prevention of chlamydial ophthalmia. Data from several of these studies are tabulated in Table 94–5, and in all instances the $AgNO_3$ regimen statistically was equivalent to the antimicrobial regimen in preventing chlamydial ophthalmia and conjunctivitis.

Clinical Features

The newborn eye is subject to infections with numerous bacterial organisms that usually cause infections that are clinically mild, nonprogressive, and characterized by conjunctival discharge. A case-control study from Seattle, Washington, identified pathogens in order of prevalence to be *Haemophilus influenzae, Streptococcus pneumoniae, Neisseria cinerea, Klebsiella pneumoniae,* and *C. trachomatis.*[91a] Viral causes include herpes simplex virus and adenoviruses. In contrast to the usually mild disease due to many bacteria, infection of the eye of the newborn with *N. gonorrhoeae* results in disease of a severity that ranges from mild to rapidly destructive. Because of the possibility that GON may lead to scarring and blindness, prevention is a primary concern to pediatricians and obstetricians.

Infection during delivery is followed by an incubation period of usually less than 3 days, but cases occasionally may be recognized for 2 to 3 weeks after delivery.[58] The baby usually develops a discharge that initially is watery but usually becomes thick and mucopurulent within a short time and may contain blood. The disease usually is bilateral. Early findings include prominent edema of the conjunctivae and lids, followed by edema and later ulceration of the cornea or spread to wider areas. Rapid arrest of the disease is essential because the degree of corneal involvement determines whether or not vision will be preserved. Some cases are self-limited and have a benign outcome. Asymptomatic GON even has been discovered during routine screening.[114] Perforation of the globe and panophthalmitis are results of extensive local disease, and the conjunctivae may serve as a portal of entry for gonococcal septicemia, arthritis, and even endocarditis.

A presumptive diagnosis may be made by demonstrating typical gram-negative diplococci by Gram stain of conjunctival exudate. Because other organisms also may cause exudative infection of the conjunctivae, the laboratory confirmation of the diagnosis of GON depends on the culture of *N. gonorrhoeae* from the exudate. In addition, thorough physical examination and a blood culture should be done to evaluate the infant for the presence of other distant foci of gonococcal disease or systemic disease.

Gonococcal Scalp Abscess

Gonococcal infections of scalp wounds that occur after fetal monitoring have been observed quite frequently.[44] The lesions may produce extensive local inflammatory disease and necrosis and can be a focus for disseminated infection. A scalp wound in a neonate should be cultured for gonococci as well as other likely pathogens, which include *Staphylococcus* species, group B streptococci, *H. influenzae,* and gram-negative enteric flora. Herpes simplex also may present in areas of injury to the scalp of newborns. Overall, approximately 1 in 200 births that are monitored with fetal scalp electrodes has been complicated by infections at the monitoring site.[113]

A summary of some studies on the incidence of neonatal gonococcal disease in exposed infants is seen in Table 94–6.

GONOCOCCAL DISEASE BEYOND INFANCY

Vaginitis

Prepubertal vaginitis has been attributed to numerous irritative and infectious agents, such as pinworms, foreign bodies, streptococci, *Trichomonas vaginalis,* diphtheroids, *N. gonorrhoeae,* and other bacteria.[91] Excluding the neonatal period, gonococcal vaginitis is the most common form of gonorrhea in children. In contrast to adults, in prepubertal girls the anestrogenic alkaline vaginal mucosa may be colonized and infected with *N. gonorrhoeae.* Gonococcal vaginitis may be a

TABLE 94–5. Efficacy of Prophylaxis of Gonococcal Neonatal Ophthalmia

Reference	Study Drug	Rate of Maternal Gonorrhea (%)	No. of Infants Studied	Rate of Ophthalmia/ 1000 Neonates	% Reduction
Greenberg and Vandow, 1961, New York (various hospitals not randomized)[64]	1% $AgNO_3$	Unknown	7219	0.28	?
	Bacitracin	Unknown	1935	3.63	?
	No prophylaxis	Unknown	1996	4.0	—
Laga et al., 1988, Kenya (randomized)[94]	1% $AgNO_3$	100	71	70	83
	1% tetracycline	100	66	30	93
	No prophylaxis	100	—	420	—

TABLE 94–6. Incidence of Neonatal Gonococcal Disease in Exposed Infants

Site of Neonatal Infection	Incidence of Infection	Population	Reference
Conjunctiva	5%; 0%; 2%; 9.6%	Exposed infants who had $AgNO_3$ ocular prophylaxis	Edwards et al.[52]; Allen and Barrere[4]; Armstrong et al.[8]; Laga et al.[94]
	2–48%	Exposed infants who had no ocular prophylaxis	Rothenberg[122]; Fransen et al.[57]; Laga et al.[94]
Orogastric fluid	40%; 26%	Infants of infected mothers	Handsfield et al.[70]; Edwards et al.[52]
Oropharynx	35%	Infants with gonococcal ophthalmia	Laga et al.[93]
Disseminated disease as a proportion of all neonatal gonorrhea	0–1% (rare)	Reported series of neonatal gonococcal disease	Folland et al.[56]; Tomeh and Wilfert[140]; Wald et al.[141]; Edwards et al.[52]; Fransen et al.[57]

mild disease or asymptomatic but usually is symptomatic with a profuse vaginal discharge.[15]

The incidences of gonorrhea, genitourinary *Chlamydia* infection, and syphilis in several studies of children who were known to have been sexually abused or adolescents who were sexually active are tabulated in Table 94–1. Gonococcal vaginitis is the most frequently recognized of these. Not all children are symptomatic; Hein and associates[73] demonstrated a 7 per cent prevalence of asymptomatic gonorrhea in sexually active adolescent females and a 1.9 per cent rate in males. The majority of children have vaginal itching, a minor crusting discharge that may discolor the underwear, and minimal to absent signs of systemic infection. Dysuria and polymorphonuclear leukocytes in the urine may accompany this infection. A Gram stain of the vaginal secretions may suggest a diagnosis. Alternatively, the symptoms may include profuse purulent vaginal discharge and significant systemic illness.

A review of reported complications of 1232 cases of gonococcal vaginitis in the preantibiotic era revealed that 35 per cent had urethritis, 19 per cent had proctitis, and 6 per cent had peritonitis.[13] Although ascending infection is uncommon, it may result in salpingitis or peritonitis. A study from Missouri showed that 10 per cent of girls with gonorrhea had signs compatible with peritonitis, including fever, diffuse abdominal pain, leukocytosis, and decreased bowel sounds.[22] Salpingitis and periappendicitis may present findings similar to those of appendicitis, and for these reasons a perineal examination for vaginal irritation, discharge, or both is important prior to abdominal surgery in young girls.[9]

Pelvic Inflammatory Disease and Salpingitis

Vaginal infection of females who are adolescent or younger may progress to involve the fallopian tubes or may disseminate to the pelvis, leading to perihepatitis[98] and PID. Salpingitis appears to be a disease of multiple microbiologic causes, the end result of which is purulent infection of the fallopian tubes causing scarring during healing.[54] It has been estimated that 15 per cent of women may be sterile after a single infection and 50 per cent after three infections. Because of the fibrosis, patency is compromised and fertility jeopardized.[24] PID in adolescents is particularly likely to result in infertility and ectopic pregnancy, and PID is the single most common cause of infertility in young women.[21, 104] Between 1970 and 1980, the rate of ectopic pregnancies per 1000 live births increased from 4.8 to 14.5, and between 1975 and 1981, the rate of hospitalization for salpingitis of women 15 to 19 years of age was 4 per 100,000.[141] Data from some studies of gonococcal disease in adolescent women are found in Table 94–3.

The identification of the cause of PID is complicated by the difficulty of obtaining fallopian tube specimens prior to therapy. Women with acute PID have had recovery of *N. gonorrhoeae* from the endocervix in approximately 35 to 80 per cent of cases and in a smaller proportion of samples of fallopian tube aspirates. It appears that gonococcal infections are one cause of acute PID but not necessarily the only one. Other causes include *C. trachomatis* and *Ureaplasma urealyticum.* After the acute event, chronic polymicrobial disease develops in the scarred areas. Mixed aerobic and anaerobic flora, especially *Peptostreptococcus* and *Peptococcus* species, often is recovered.

Risk factors for PID and acute salpingitis have been shown to include young age at acquisition of gonococcal disease or other STD, a history of previous PID, multiple sexual partners, and use of an IUD for contraception. Approximately 15 per cent of teenagers who develop gonorrhea will develop PID. The immature cervix may be at particular risk of progression to upper tract disease.[133]

Diagnosis of PID may be difficult, and the differential diagnosis includes numerous other conditions of the lower abdomen, such as appendicitis, ectopic pregnancy, cholecystitis, mesenteric adenitis, pyelonephritis, and septic abortion. Laparoscopy may assist in establishing a diagnosis. Recommendations by Shafer and associates[128] suggest that a clinical diagnosis of PID be supported by the presence of lower abdominal pain, tenderness with motion of the cervix, and adnexal tenderness. Fever, leukocytosis, elevated sedimentation rate, and adnexal mass on abdominal ultrasonography support the diagnosis. Culdocentesis may reveal evidence of purulent reaction in the peritoneal cavity. It is probable that the outcome for fertility is improved with prompt and vigorous therapy. Indications for hospitalization for therapy of PID include young age of patients and are listed in Table 94–7.

Therapeutic regimens are not established, and no single antimicrobial agent is effective for all common pathogens for this disease. However, all courses of therapy should include treatment that is appropriate for *C. trachomatis* because a

TABLE 94–7. Indications for Hospitalization of Children with Suspected Salpingitis

All adolescents	Fever, peritoneal signs
Diagnostic uncertainty	Adnexal mass
Failure to respond to prior regimen	IUD use
Pregnancy	Noncompliance

significant proportion of persons who acquire gonococcal disease also acquire a second infection with *C. trachomatis*.

Urethritis

Gonococcal urethritis in prepubertal males is much less common than is vaginitis in girls. When recognized, the disease usually is symptomatic and resembles gonococcal urethritis in the adult male.[42, 61] As with vaginitis, asymptomatic pyuria is a presentation with which the pediatrician should be familiar.[46] In children with gonorrheal infection of the genitourinary tract in the 1970s, concomitant anorectal and tonsillopharyngeal colonization was common. This colonization usually is asymptomatic, as in adults,[107, 148] but may be symptomatic.[1, 137] Whether there are differences in risk of acquiring gonorrhea after sexual contact with infected persons for children compared with adults[76] is not known.

Disseminated Disease

Dissemination of gonorrhea in infants and children is not a rare event. Virulence factors associated with disseminated disease were enumerated earlier. A group of specific deficits in the terminal components of the complement system has been associated with disseminated disease in adults. Disseminated disease has been reported to occur after asymptomatic genitourinary infection more often than symptomatic genitourinary infection, again lending support to the observation that asymptomatic disease is more common than symptomatic disease.

Gonococcal arthritis of the newborn was described extensively between 1900 and 1930 by Cooperman[37, 38] and Wehrbein,[143] and recent case reports suggest that the disease remains similar. It is the form of disseminated disease that is most common in children, although the incidence among children with gonorrhea has been highly variable. In a review of cases of gonorrhea in a teaching hospital in North Carolina between 1961 and 1970, 1 of 19 children (5 per cent) had gonococcal polyarthritis, and this occurred in a neonate.[140] In marked contrast is the report by Cooperman[37] of a hospital-associated outbreak of gonococcal polyarthritis in 1927, in which 53 of 67 infected infants (79 per cent) developed joint complications. During the epidemic, there were 182 infants born in the hospital; hence, the lowest possible rate of joint disease, if all infants were infected, was 67 per 182 (36 per cent). Other studies of outbreaks have indicated that perhaps 15 per cent of children with gonorrhea acquire gonococcal arthritis. These rates are probably considerably greater than the estimated 1 to 3 per cent incidence in adults and suggest an increased risk of dissemination in children. Variations in incidence also may reflect the rate of acquisition of more virulent strains by children. For example, case reports document gonococcal arthritis in both mother and newborn infant.[66] Some studies note a male predominance of cases.

Seventy-nine per cent of Cooperman's cases had involvement of multiple joints, most frequently the ankles, knees, wrists, and hands.[37] Involvement of a joint may include suppurative arthritis, inflammatory disease of the periarticular structures, and tenosynovitis of a joint. Osteomyelitis occasionally is reported in all age groups.[6] Leukocytosis is usual, and most infants have a positive culture and compatible Gram stain from the synovial fluid of the involved joint.[62] Other mucous membranes also may yield a positive culture for gonococci.

Onset of disease in the newborn begins with a prodrome of fever and irritability at approximately 1 or more weeks of age. The mother frequently has symptomatic disease. Although arthritis usually is the first indication of gonococcal disease, infants also may have ophthalmia, vaginitis, and involvement at other sites.

Gonococcal arthritis in older children resembles that of adults and may be accompanied by cutaneous lesions.[4] Multiple septic involvement of joints is not as common as in the newborn period, although a migratory polyarthritis may be part of the prodrome.[40] However, there typically is a single, most severely affected joint, and myositis and tenosynovitis may be prominent.

Treatment of gonococcal arthritis depends on prompt recognition of the disease. Cultures of all mucous membranes (nasopharynx, rectal, vaginal or endocervical, conjunctival), blood culture, and aspiration of the involved joint should be performed. In the newborn period, the gastric aspirate may be cultured to determine contamination from a maternal source.

Each patient must be evaluated for the need for drainage of an involved joint. Because complete response to medical therapy may not occur for several days, most physicians attempt to avoid an open drainage procedure and manage the need for relief from pain with needle aspirations if possible. An exception is purulent arthritis of the hips, in which early drainage is indicated in order to prevent necrosis of the femoral head.

Pharyngeal Gonorrhea

Oropharyngeal gonorrhea was reported in 4 to 6 per cent of one study of abused prepubertal children,[145] and the pharynx was a site of infection in 3 of 11 (27 per cent) of infected children in another study.[47] In the latter study,[47] the pharynx was not colonized in any of the children with symptomatic infection. Another study of children with pharyngeal gonorrhea reported on 16 children 3 to 18 years of age; 75 per cent had asymptomatic colonization, whereas only 25 per cent had clinically apparent disease.[132] The source of the infection is presumed to be orogenital contact because all of 42 adult patients with pharyngeal gonorrhea reported that they had had orogenital contact.[110] The diagnosis of gonococcal pharyngitis is important because the infection has been treated less readily than other forms of gonococcal disease (see treatment section) and because it may be the source of subsequently disseminated gonorrhea.[41] Therefore, high-risk groups should be screened for pharyngeal gonorrhea as well as genital colonization or disease.[19, 29]

Other Forms of Gonococcal Disease

Other complications of gonorrhea very rarely or almost never are reported in the pediatric literature. Gonococcal meningitis, shunt infection, endocarditis, myocarditis, conjunctivitis, and hepatitis occur in adults and may be expected to occur in children. The disease may be fatal.[97, 111] However, the pediatric experience with these conditions is minimal.

ANTIMICROBIAL SENSITIVITY PATTERNS

Until 1976, almost all strains of *N. gonorrhoeae* were sensitive to penicillin. Although there had been a gradual increase in mean minimal inhibitory concentration (MIC) to penicillin during the prior two decades, almost all strains had an MIC to penicillin of less than 0.5 μg/mL. In 1976, strains of *N. gonorrhoeae* that had acquired a plasmid-conferring resistance to penicillin through production of penicillinase were discovered. These strains were found in many parts of the Far East and London, and in the Far East they constituted approximately 30 per cent of the isolates in some cities. The strains caused the expected spectrum of clinical disease, and treatment with penicillin was inefficacious. In 1983, an outbreak of chromosomally mediated, penicillin-resistant gonococci was reported from North Carolina and subsequently occurred in most areas of the country. The organisms do not produce penicillinase.

In 1986, the Centers for Disease Control and Prevention initiated a system to monitor the antimicrobial sensitivities of *N. gonorrhoeae* in 21 clinics for STDs in 21 cities. In 1989, penicillinase-producing *N. gonorrhoeae* accounted for 7.4 per cent of all isolates; tetracycline-resistant *N. gonorrhoeae* accounted for 4.9 per cent of isolates; and combined penicillinase-producing and tetracycline-resistant *N. gonorrhoeae* accounted for 0.9 per cent of isolates.[26] These rates of resistant strains had increased throughout the late 1980s, and because of that, use of single-dose penicillin therapy for gonorrhea was abandoned in 1987.

TREATMENT

Recommendations for therapy of childhood gonorrhea based on 1993 guidelines from the Centers for Disease Control and Prevention[28] are as follows:

Pediatric patients encompass children from birth to adolescence. When a child is postpubertal or weighs more than 45.4 kg (100 lb), he or she should be treated with dosage regimens as defined for adults.

The efficacy of therapeutic regimens for uncomplicated and complicated gonococcal infections of childhood is unproved at present.

Prevention of Neonatal Infection

All pregnant women should have endocervical culture examinations for gonococci as an integral part of prenatal care at the first prenatal visit. A second culture late in pregnancy should be obtained from women who are at high risk of gonococcal infection.

Prevention of Ophthalmia Neonatorum

Instillation of a prophylactic agent into the eyes of all newborn infants is recommended to prevent GON and is required by law in most states. Although all regimens listed below effectively prevent gonococcal eye disease, their efficacy in preventing chlamydial eye disease is not clear. Furthermore, they do not eliminate nasopharyngeal colonization with *C. trachomatis*. Treatment of gonococcal and chlamydial infections in pregnant women is the best method for preventing neonatal gonococcal and chlamydial disease.

RECOMMENDED REGIMEN. Erythromycin (0.5 per cent) ophthalmic ointment, once, tetracycline (1 per cent) ophthalmic ointment, once, or $AgNO_3$ (1 per cent) aqueous solution, once, is effective. One of these should be instilled into the eyes of every neonate as soon as possible after delivery and definitely within 1 hour after birth. Single-use tubes or ampules are preferable to multiple-use tubes.

The efficacy of tetracycline and erythromycin in the prevention of tetracycline-resistant and penicillinase-producing *N. gonorrhoeae* ophthalmia is unknown, although both probably are effective because of the high concentrations of drug in these preparations. Bacitracin is not recommended.

Treatment of Infants Born to Mothers with Gonococcal Infection

Infants born to mothers with untreated gonorrhea are at high risk of infection (e.g., ophthalmia, disseminated gonococcal infection) and should be treated with a single injection of ceftriaxone (25 to 50 mg/kg intravenously or intramuscularly, not to exceed 125 mg). Ceftriaxone should be given cautiously to hyperbilirubinemic infants, especially premature infants. Topical prophylaxis for neonatal ophthalmia is not adequate treatment for documented infections of the eye or other sites.

Treatment of Infants with Gonococcal Infection

Infants with documented gonococcal infections at any site (e.g., eye) should be evaluated for disseminated disease. This evaluation should include a careful physical examination, especially of the joints, as well as blood and cerebrospinal fluid cultures. Infants with gonococcal ophthalmia or disseminated disease should be treated for 7 days (10 to 14 days if meningitis is present) with one of the following regimens:

RECOMMENDED REGIMEN. Ceftriaxone, 25 to 50 mg/kg/day intravenously or intramuscularly in a single daily dose, or cefotaxime, 25 mg/kg intravenously or intramuscularly every 12 hours.

ALTERNATIVE REGIMEN. Data suggest that uncomplicated gonococcal ophthalmia among infants may be cured with a single injection of ceftriaxone (50 mg/kg up to 125 mg). This regimen also may be used for infants with gonococcal disease of rectum, pharynx, vagina, and urethra.[115]

Infants with gonococcal ophthalmia should receive eye irrigation with buffered saline solutions until discharge has cleared. Topical antibiotic therapy alone is inadequate. Simultaneous infection with *C. trachomatis* has been reported and should be considered for patients who do not respond satisfactorily. Therefore, the mother and infant should be tested for chlamydial infection.

Gonococcal Infections of Children Beyond the Neonatal Period

Children who weigh 45 kg or more should be treated with adult regimens. Children who weigh less than 45 kg who have uncomplicated vulvovaginitis, cervicitis, urethritis, pharyngitis, or proctitis may be treated as follows:

RECOMMENDED REGIMEN. Ceftriaxone, 125 mg intramuscularly, once, is effective. However, patients who can not tolerate ceftriaxone may be treated with spectinomycin, 40 mg/kg intramuscularly, once. Patients weighing less than 45 kg with bacteremia or disseminated disease should be treated with ceftriaxone, 50 mg/kg/day (maximum, 1 g) for 7 to 14 days. For meningitis, the duration of treatment is increased to 10 to 14 days, and the dose is 50 to 100 mg/kg/day (maximum, 2 g). Children 8 years of age or older who have gonococcal disease have high rates of concomitant chlamydial disease and therefore also should be given doxycycline, 100 mg, two times a day for 7 days.

All patients should be evaluated for coinfection with syphilis, HIV, and *C. trachomatis*. Recent data indicate that posttherapy test-of-cure cultures are not required in children.[32]

Treatment of Salpingitis

Co-infection with both *Chlamydia* and gonococci is common in children as well as adults. In female adolescents, treatment of gonococcal cervicitis with drug regimens that are effective against gonococci but not *Chlamydia* has led to a high incidence of residual salpingitis in females, and in males of urethritis, both of which are associated with continued disease due to *Chlamydia*.[112, 115, 116, 128] Optimal therapy for known or possible co-infection with both diseases is not certain in adults and also has not been explored in children. The reader is advised to look for recommendations in the report from the Centers for Disease Control and Prevention.

Penicillin, amoxicillin, ceftriaxone, and spectinomycin alone will fail to eradicate *Chlamydia*. Trimethoprim-sulfamethoxazole, tetracycline, and erythromycin are effective in vitro and in many clinical forms of *Chlamydia* disease. The pediatrician may elect to treat the child with a combination of ceftriaxone and to add a 14-day course of erythromycin or doxycycline orally. Unless there are reasons to elect another regimen, erythromycin, 50 mg/kg/day, is the customary choice. Azithromycin, 1 g orally, in older children also has been chosen.

References

1. Abbott, S. L.: Gonococcal tonsillitis–pharyngitis in a 5-year-old girl. Pediatrics *52*:287–289, 1973.
2. Ahmed, H. J., Ilardi, I., Antognoli, A., et al.: An epidemic of *Neisseria gonorrhoeae* in a Somali orphanage. Int. J. STD and AIDS 3:52–53, 1992.
3. Alexander, W. J., Griffith, H., Housch, J. G., et al.: Infections in sexual contacts and associates of children with gonorrhea. Sex. Transm. Dis. *11*:156–158, 1984.
4. Allen, J. H., and Barrere, L. E.: Prophylaxis of gonorrhea ophthalmia of the newborn. J. A. M. A. *141*:522–525, 1949.
5. Amstey, M. S., and Steadman, K. T.: Asymptomatic gonorrhea and pregnancy. J. Am. Vener. Dis. Assoc. *3*:14–16, 1976.
6. Angevine, C. D., Hall, C. B., and Jacox, R. F.: A case of gonococcal osteomyelitis: A complication of gonococcal arthritis. J. Dis. Child. *130*:1013–1014, 1976.
7. Apicella, M. A.: Serogrouping of *Neisseria gonorrhoeae*: Identification of four immunologically distinct acidic polysaccharides. J. Infect. Dis. *134*:377 383, 1976.
8. Armstrong, J. H., Zacarias, F., and Rein, M. F.: Ophthalmia neonatorum: A chart review. Pediatrics *57*:884–892, 1976.
9. Auman, G. L., and Waldenberg, L. M.: Gonococcal periappendicitis and salpingitis in a prepubertal girl. Pediatrics *58*:287–288, 1976.
10. Badgley, R. F., et al.: Sexual Offenses Against Children. Ottawa, Canada, Minister of Supply and Services, 1984.
11. Baker, C. J.: Sexually transmitted diseases and child abuse. J. Am. Vener. Dis. Assoc. *5*:169–171, 1978.
12. Barsam, P. C.: Specific prophylaxis of gonorrheal ophthalmia neonatorum: A review. N. Engl. J. Med. *274*:731–734, 1966.
13. Benson, R. A., and Weinstock, E.: Gonorrheal vaginitis in children: A review of the literature. Am. J. Dis. Child. *59*:1083–1096, 1940.
14. Birji, M., and Everson, J. J.: Comparative virulence of opacity variance of *Neisseria gonorrhoeae* strain P9. Infect. Immun. *31*:965–970, 1981.
15. Bogaerts, J., Lepage, P., DeClercq, A., et al.: Etiology and outcome of acute pelvic inflammatory disease. J. Infect. Dis. *158*:510–517, 1988.
16. Bronson, J. E., Holmberg, I., Nygren, B., et al.: Vancomycin-sensitive strains of *Neisseria gonorrhoeae*: A problem for the diagnostic laboratory. Pont. J. Vener. Dis. *49*:452–453, 1973.
17. Brooks, F., Israel, K. S., and Petersen, B. H.: Bactericidal and opsonic activity against *Neisseria gonorrhoeae* in sera from patients with disseminated gonococcal infection. J. Infect. Dis. *134*:450–462, 1976.
18. Brown, D.: Gonococcal arthritis in pregnancy. South. Med. J. *66*:693–695, 1973.
19. Brown, R. T., Lossick, J. G., Mosure, D. J., et al.: Pharyngeal gonorrhea screening in adolescents: Is it necessary? Pediatrics *84*:623–625, 1989.
20. Brown, W. J., and Kraus, S. J.: Gonococcal colony types. J. A. M. A. *228*:862–863, 1974.
21. Brunham, R. C., Binns, B., Guijon, F., et al.: Etiology and outcome of acute pelvic inflammatory disease. J. Infect. Dis. *158*:510–517, 1988.
22. Burry, V. F.: Gonococcal vulvovaginitis and possible peritonitis in prepubertal girls. Am. J. Dis. Child. *121*:536–537, 1971.
23. Carifo, K., and Catlin, B. W.: *Neisseria gonorrhoeae* autotyping: Differentiation of clinical isolates based on growth responses on chemically defined media. Appl. Microbiol. *26*:223–230, 1973.
24. Cates, W.: Sexually transmitted organisms and infertility: The proof of the pudding. Sex. Transm. Dis. *11*:113–116, 1984.
25. Catlin, B. W.: Nutritional profiles of *Neisseria gonorrhoeae, Neisseria meningitidis*, and *Neisseria lactamica* in chemically defined media and the use of growth requirements for gonococcal typing. J. Infect. Dis. *128*:178–194, 1973.
26. Centers for Disease Control: Plasmid-mediated antimicrobial resistance in *Neisseria gonorrhoeae*—United States, 1988 and 1989. M. M. W. R. *39*:284–293, 1990.
27. Centers for Disease Control: Special focus: Surveillance for sexually transmitted diseases. M. M. W. R. *42*(SS-3):1–39, 1993.
28. Centers for Disease Control: 1993 Sexually Transmitted Diseases Treatment Guidelines. M. M. W. R. *42*(RR-14):1–102, 1993.
29. Chacko, M. R., Phillips, S., and Jacobson, M. S.: Screening for pharyngeal gonorrhea in the urban teenager. Pediatrics *70*:620–623, 1982.
30. Charles, A. G., Cohen, S., Kass, M. B., et al.: Asymptomatic gonorrhea in prenatal patients. Am. J. Obstet. Gynecol. *108*:595–599, 1970.
31. Chen J.-Y.: Prophylaxis of ophthalmia neonatorum: Comparison of silver nitrate, tetracycline, erythromycin, and no prophylaxis. Pediatr. Infect. Dis. *11*:1026–1030, 1992.
32. Christian, C. W., Pinto-Martin, J. A., and McGowan, K. L.: The management of prepubertal children with gonorrhea. Clin. Pediatr. *34*:415–418, 1995.
33. Cohen, M. S., and Sparling, P. F.: Mucosal infection with *Neisseria gonorrhoeae*. J. Clin. Invest. 89:1699–1707, 1992.
34. Colin, M. J., and Weissmann, G.: Disseminated gonococcal infection and tenosynovitis from an asymptomatically infected intrauterine contraceptive device. N. Engl. J. Med. *294*:598–599, 1976.
35. Committee on Child Abuse Neglect: Guidelines for the evaluation of sexual abuse of children. Pediatrics *87*:254–260, 1991.
36. Committee on Infectious Diseases American Academy of Pediatrics: 1994 Red Book. 23rd ed. Evanston, American Academy of Pediatrics, 1994, pp. 533–535.
37. Cooperman, M. B.: *Gonococcus* arthritis in infancy: A clinical study of forty-four cases. Am. J. Dis. Child. *33*:932–948, 1927.
38. Cooperman, M. B.: End results of gonorrheal arthritis: A review of seventy cases. Am. J. Surg. *5*:241–251, 1928.
39. Corman, L. C., Levison, M. E., Knight, R., et al.: The high frequency of pharyngeal gonococcal infection in a prenatal clinic population. J. A. M. A. *230*:568–570, 1974.
40. Coulter, K.: Migratory polyarthritis in a nine-year-old girl. Pediatr. Infect. Dis. J.: *9*:856–857, 1990.
41. Cramolini, G. M., and Litt, I. F.: The pharynx as the only positive culture site in an adolescent with disseminated gonorrhea. J. Pediatr. *100*:644–646, 1982.
42. Crawford, G., Knapp, J. S., Hale, J., et al.: Asymptomatic gonorrhea in men caused by gonococci with unique nutritional requirements. Science 196:1352, 1977.
43. Credé, C. S. F.: Reports from the obstetrical clinic in Leipzig: Prevention of eye inflammation in the newborn. Am. J. Dis. Child. *121*:3–4, 1971.
44. D'Auria, A., Tan, L., Kreitzer, M., et al.: Gonococcal scalp-wound infection. M. M. W. R. *24*:115–116, 1975.
45. Dattel, B. J., Landers, D. V., Coulter, K., et al.: Isolation of *Chlamydia trachomatis* from sexually abused female adolescents. Obstet. Gynecol. *72*:240–242, 1988.
46. Dawar, S., and Hellerstein, S.: Gonorrhea as a cause of asymptomatic pyuria in adolescent boys. J. Pediatr. *81*:357–358, 1972.
47. DeJong, A. R.: Sexually transmitted diseases in sexually abused children. Sex. Transm. Dis. *13*:123–126, 1986.
48. Demetriou, E., Sackett, R., Welch, D. F., et al.: Evaluation of an enzyme immunoassay for detection of *Neisseria gonorrhoea* in an adolescent population. J. A. M. A. *252*:247–250, 1984.
49. Denison, M. R., Perlman, S., and Anderson, R. D.: Misidentification of *Neisseria* species in a neonate with conjunctivitis. Pediatrics *81*:877–888, 1988.
50. Desenclos, J.-C. A., Garrity, D., and Wroten, J.: Pediatric gonococcal infection, Florida, 1984 to 1988. Am J. Public Health *82*:426–428, 1992.
51. Dossett, J. H., Appelbaum, P. C., Knapp, J. S., et al.: Proctitis associated with *Neisseria cinerea* misidentified as *Neisseria gonorrhoeae* in a child. J. Clin. Microbiol. *21*:575–577, 1985.
52. Edwards, L. E., Barrada, M. I., Hamann, A. A., et al.: Gonorrhea in pregnancy. Am. J. Obstet. Gynecol. *132*:637–641, 1978.
53. Elliott, B., Brunham, R. C., Laga, M., et al.: Maternal gonococcal infection as a preventable risk factor for low birth weight. J. Infect. Dis. *161*:531–536, 1990.
54. Eschenbach, D. A., Buchanan, T. M., Pollock, H. M., et al.: Polymicrobial etiology of acute pelvic inflammatory disease. N. Engl. J. Med. *293*:166–171, 1975.
55. Farrell, M. K., Billimire, M. E., Shamroy, J. A., et al.: Prepubertal gonorrhea: A multidisciplinary approach. Pediatrics *67*:151–153, 1981.
56. Folland, D. S., Burke, R. E., Hinman, A. R., et al.: Gonorrhea in preadolescent children: An inquiry into source of infection and mode of transmission. Pediatrics *60*:153–156, 1977.
57. Fransen, L., Nsanze, H., Klaus, V., et al.: Ophthalmia neonatorum in

Nairobi, Kenya: The roles of *Neisseria gonorrhoeae* and *Chlamydia trachomatis*. J. Infect. Dis. *153*:862–869, 1986.
58. Friendly, D. S.: Gonococcal conjunctivitis of the newborn. Clin. Prac. Child. Hosp. *25*:1–9, 1969.
59. Gardner, M., and Jones, J. G.: Genital herpes acquired by sexual abuse of children. J. Pediatr. *104*:243–244, 1984.
60. Geidinghagen, D. H., Hoff, G. L., and Biery, R. M.: Gonorrhea in children: Epidemiologic unit analysis. Pediatr. Infect. Dis. J. *11*:973–974, 1992.
61. Genadry, R. R., Thompson, B. H., and Niebyl, J. R.: Gonococcal salpingitis in pregnancy. Am. J. Obstet. Gynecol. *126*:512–513, 1976.
62. Glaser, S., Boxerbaum, B., and Kennell, J. H.: Gonococcal arthritis in the newborn: Report of a case and review of the literature. Am. J. Dis. Child. *112*:135–138, 1966.
63. Golden, N., Hammerschlag, M., Hewkoff, S., et al.: Prevalence of *Chlamydia trachomatis* cervical infections in female adolescents. Am. J. Dis. Child. *138*:562–564, 1984.
64. Greenberg, M., and Vandow, J. E.: Ophthalmia neonatorum: Evaluation of different methods of prophylaxis in New York City. Am. J. Public Health *51*:836–845, 1961.
65. Gregg, C. R., Melly, M. A., Hellerqvist, C. G., et al.: Toxic activity of purified lipopolysaccharide as *N. gonorrhoeae* for human fallopian tube mucosa. J. Infect. Dis. *143*:432–439, 1983.
66. Gregory, J. E., Chisom, J. L., and Meadows, A. T.: Gonococcal arthritis in an infant. Br. J. Vener. Dis. *48*:306–307, 1972.
67. Gutman, L. G., Herman-Giddens, M. E., and McKinney, Jr., R. E.: Pediatric acquired immunodeficiency syndrome: Barriers to recognizing the role of child sexual abuse. Am. J. Dis. Child. *147*:775–780, 1993.
68. Gutman, L. T., Herman-Giddens, M. E., and Phelps, W. C.: Transmission of human genital papillomavirus disease: Comparison of data from adults and children. Pediatrics *91*:31–38, 1993.
69. Hammerschlag, M. R., Cummings, M., Doraiswamy, B., et al.: Nonspecific vaginitis following sexual abuse in children. Pediatrics *75*:1028–1031, 1985.
70. Handsfield, H. H., Hodson, W. A., and Holmes, K. K.: Neonatal gonococcal infection. 1. Orogastric contamination with *Neisseria gonorrhoeae*. J. A. M. A. *225*:697–701, 1973.
71. Handsfield, H. H., and Holmes, K. K.: Microepidemic of virulent gonococcal infection. J. Am. Vener. Dis. Assoc. *1*:20–22, 1974.
72. Hedberg, K., Ristinen, T. L., Solar, J. T., et al.: Outbreak of erythromycin-resistant staphylococcal conjunctivitis in a newborn nursery. Pediatr. Infect. Dis. *9*:268–273, 1990.
73. Hein, K., Marks, A., and Cohen, M. I.: Asymptomatic gonorrhea: Prevalence in a population of urban adolescents. J. Pediatr. *90*:634–635, 1977.
74. Herman-Giddens, M. E., Gutman, L. T., Benson, H. C., et al.: Association of coexisting vaginal infections and multiple abusers in female children with genital warts. Sex. Transm. Dis. *15*:63–67, 1988.
75. Holmes, K. K., Counts, G. W., and Beaty, H. N.: Disseminated gonococcal infection. Ann. Intern. Med. *74*:979–993, 1971.
76. Holmes, K. K., Johnson, D. W., and Trostle, H. J.: An estimate of the risk of men acquiring gonorrhea by sexual contact with infected females. Am. J. Epidemiol. *91*:170–174, 1970.
77. Ingram, D. L., Runyan, D. K., Collins, A. D., et al.: Vaginal *Chlamydia trachomatis* infection in children with sexual contact. Pediatr. Infect. Dis. *3*:97–99, 1984.
78. Ingram, D. L.: The gonococcus and the toilet seat revisited. Pediatr. Infect. Dis. *8*:191, 1989.
79. Ingram, D. L., White, S. T., Durfee, M. F., et al.: Sexual contact in children with gonorrhea. Am. J. Dis. Child. *136*:994–996, 1982.
80. Ingram, D. L., Everett, V. D., Lyna, P. R., et al.: Epidemiology of adult sexually transmitted disease agents in children being evaluated for sexual abuse. Pediatr. Infect. Dis. J. *11*:945–950, 1992.
81. Israel, K. S., Rissing, K. B., and Brooks, G. F.: Neonatal and childhood gonococcal infections. Clin. Obstet. Gynecol. *18*:143–151, 1975.
82. Jamison, J. H., Kaplan, D. W., Hamman, R., et al.: Spectrum of genital human papillomavirus infection in a female adolescent population. Sex. Transm. Dis. *22*:236, 1995.
83. Johnston, K. H., Holmes, K. K., and Gotschlich, E. C.: The serological classification of *Neisseria gonorrhoeae*. 1. Isolation of the outer membrane complex responsible for serotypic specificity. J. Exp. Med. *143*:741–758, 1976.
84. Jones, D. E. D., Brame, R. G., and Jones, C. P.: Gonorrhea in obstetric patients. J. Am. Vener. Dis. Assoc. *2*:30–32, 1976.
85. Jones, J. G., Yamauchi, T., and Lambert, B.: *Trichomonas vaginalis* infestation in sexually abused girls. Am. J. Dis. Child. *139*:846–847, 1985.
86. Kasper, D. L., Rice, P. A., and McCormack, W. M.: Bactericidal antibody in genital infections due to *Neisseria gonorrhoeae*. J. Infect. Dis. *135*:243–251, 1977.
87. Kellogg, J. A., and Orwig, L. K.: Comparison of Gonogen, Gono Gen II and Micro Trak Direct Fluorescent-Antibody Test with carbohydrate fermentation for confirmation of culture isolates of *Neisseria gonorrhoeae*. J. Clin. Microbiol. *33*:474–476, 1995.
88. Kempe, C. H.: Sexual abuse, another hidden pediatric problem. Pediatrics *62*:382–389, 1978.
89. Knapp, J. S., and Holmes, K. K.: Disseminated gonococcal infections caused by *Neisseria gonorrhoeae* with unique nutritional requirements. J. Infect. Dis. *132*:204–208, 1975.
90. Knapp, J. S., Tam, M. R., Nowinski, R. C., et al.: Serological classification of *Neisseria gonorrhoeae* with use of monoclonal antibodies to gonococcal outer membrane protein I. J. Infect. Dis. *150*:44–48, 1984.
91. Kotcher, E., Keller, K., and Gray, L. A.: A microbiological study of pediatric vaginitis. J. Pediatr. *53*:210–218, 1958.
91a. Krohn, M. A., Hillier, S. L., Bell, J. A., et al.: The bacterial etiology of conjunctivitis in early infancy. Am. J. Epidemiol. *138*:326–332, 1993.
92. Laga, M., Meheus, A., and Piot, P.: Epidemiology and control of gonococcal ophthalmia neonatorum. Bull. W. H. O. *67*:471–477, 1989.
93. Laga, M., Naamara, W., Brunham, R. C., et al.: Single-dose therapy of gonococcal ophthalmia neonatorum with ceftriaxone. N. Engl. J. Med. *315*:1382–1385, 1986.
94. Laga, M., Plummer, F. A., Piot, P., et al.: Prophylaxis of gonococcal and chlamydial ophthalmia neonatorum. N. Engl. J. Med. *318*:653–657, 1988.
95. Laras, L., Craighill, M., Woods, E. R., et al.: Epidemiologic observations of adolescents with *Neisseria gonorrhoeae* genital infections treated at a children's hospital. Adolesc. Pediatr. Gynecol. *7*:9–12, 1994.
96. Lawson, L., and Chaffin, M.: False negatives in sexual abuse disclosure interviews. J. Interpersonal Violence *7*:532–542, 1992.
97. Lewis, L. S., Glauser, T. A., and Joffe, M. D.: Gonococcal conjunctivitis in prepubertal children. Am. J. Dis. Child. *144*:546–548, 1990.
98. Litt, I. F., and Cohen, M. I.: Perihepatitis associated with salpingitis in adolescents. J. A. M. A. *240*:1253, 1978.
99. Litt, I. F., Edberg, S. C., and Finberg, L.: Gonorrhea in children and adolescents: A current review. J. Pediatr. *85*:595–607, 1974.
100. McGee, Z. A., Stephens, D. S., Hoffman, L. H., et al.: Mechanisms of mucosal invasion by pathogenic *Neisseria*. Rev. Infect. Dis. *5*(Suppl. 4, September–October):S708, 1983.
101. Mellin, G. W.: Ophthalmia neonatorum: Yesterday, today, tomorrow. Sight-Saver Rev. *31*:102–113, 1961.
102. Morello, J. A., Lerner, S. A., and Bohnhoff, M.: Characteristics of atypical *Neisseria gonorrhoeae* from disseminated and localized infections. Infect. Immunol. *13*:1510–1516, 1976.
103. Moyes, A., and Young, H.: Epidemiological typing of *Neisseria gonorrhoeae*: A comparative analysis of three monoclonal antibody typing panels. Eur. J. Epidemiol. *7*:311–319, 1991.
104. Mueller, B. A., Luz-Jimenez, M., Daling, J. R., et al.: Risk factors for tubal infertility. Sex. Transm. Dis. *19*:28–34, 1992.
105. Mulcahy, F. M., and Lacey, C. J. N.: Sexually transmitted infections in adolescent girls. Genitourin. Med. *63*:119–121, 1987.
106. Neinstein, L. S., Goldenring, J., and Carpenter, S.: Nonsexual transmission of sexually transmitted diseases: An infrequent occurrence. Pediatrics *74*:67–76, 1984.
107. Nelson, J. D., Mohs, E., Dajani, A. S., et al.: Gonorrhea in preschool and school-age children: Report of the prepubertal gonorrhea cooperative study group. J. A. M. A. *236*:1359–1364, 1976.
108. O'Reilly, R. J., Lee, L., and Welch, B. G.: Secretory IgA antibody responses to *Neisseria gonorrhoeae* in the genital secretions of infected females. J. Infect. Dis. *133*:113–125, 1976.
109. Orr, D. P., and Prietto, S. V.: Emergency management of sexually abused children: The role of the pediatric resident. Am. J. Dis. Child. *133*:628–631, 1979.
110. Osborne, N. G., and Grubin, L.: Colonization of the pharynx with *Neisseria gonorrhoeae*. Sex. Transm. Dis. *6*:253–256, 1979.
111. Pasquariello, C. A., Plotkin, S. A., Rice, R. J., et al.: Fatal gonococcal septicemia. Pediatr. Infect. Dis. *4*:204–206, 1985.
112. Patamasucon, P., Rettig, P. J., and Nelson, J. D.: Cefuroxime therapy of gonorrhea and co-infection with *Chlamydia trachomatis* in children. Pediatrics *68*:534–538, 1981.
113. Plavidal, F. J., and Werch, A.: Fetal scalp abscess secondary to intrauterine monitoring. Am. J. Obstet. Gynecol. *125*:65–68, 1976.
114. Podgore, J. K., and Holmes, K. K.: Ocular gonococcal infection with minimal or no inflammatory response. J. A. M. A. *246*:242–243, 1981.
115. Rawstrom, S. A., Hammerschlag, M. R., Gullans, C., et al.: Ceftriaxone treatment of penicillinase-producing *Neisseria gonorrhoeae* infections in children. Pediatr. Infect. Dis. *8*:445–448, 1989.
116. Rettig, P. J., and Nelson, J. D.: Genital tract infection with *Chlamydia trachomatis* in prepubertal children. J. Pediatr. *99*:206–210, 1981.
117. Rice, P. A., and Kasper, D. L.: Characterization of serum resistance of *Neisseria gonorrhoeae* that disseminate: Roles of blocking antibody in gonococcal outer membrane protein. J. Clin. Invest. *70*:157–167, 1982.
118. Rice, P. A., McCormack, W. M., and Kasper, D. L.: Natural serum bactericidal activity against *N. gonorrhoeae* isolates from disseminated, locally invasive, and uncomplicated disease. J. Immunol. *124*:2105–2109, 1980.
119. Rice, R. J., Aral, S. O., Blount, J. H., et al.: Gonorrhea in the United States 1975–1989: Is the giant only sleeping? Sex. Transm. Dis. *14*:83–87, 1987.
120. Rimsza, M. E., and Niggemann, E. H.: Medical evaluation of sexually abused children: A review of 311 cases. Pediatrics *69*:8–14, 1982.
121. Rothbard, M. J., Gregory, T., and Salerno, L. J.: Intrapartum gonococcal amnionitis. Am. J. Obstet. Gynecol. *121*:565–566, 1975.
122. Rothenberg, R.: Ophthalmia neonatorum due to *Neisseria gonorrhoeae*: Prevention and treatment. Sex. Transm. Dis. *6*(Suppl. 2):187–191, 1979.
122a. Russell, D. E. H.: The incidence and prevalence of intrafamilial and

extrafamilial sexual abuse of female children. Child Abuse Negl. *7*:133–142, 1983.
123. Sanders, J. M., Brookman, R. R., Brown, R. C., et al.: Committee on Adolescence: Role of the pediatrician in management of sexually transmitted diseases in children and adolescents. Pediatrics *79*:454–456, 1987.
124. Sandström, E. G., and Danielsson, D.: Serology of *Neisseria gonorrhoeae*: Classification by coagglutination. Acta Pathol. Microbiol. Scand. *88*:27–38, 1980.
125. Sandström, E. G., Knapp, J. S., and Buchanan, T. M.: Serology of *Neisseria gonorrhoeae*: W-antigen serogrouping by coagglutination and protein I serotyping by enzyme-linked immunosorbent assay both detect protein I antigens. Infect. Immun. *35*:229–239, 1982.
126. Sarrel, P. M., and Pruett, K. A.: Symptomatic gonorrhea during pregnancy. Obstet. Gynecol. *32*:670–673, 1968.
127. Sgroi, S. M.: Pediatric gonorrhea beyond infancy. Pediatr. Ann. *8*:326–336, 1979.
128. Shafer, M.-A. B., Irwin, C. E., and Sweet, R. L.: Acute salpingitis in the adolescent female. J. Pediatr. *100*:339–350, 1982.
129. Shafer, M. A., Beck, A., Blain, B., et al.: *Chlamydia trachomatis*: Important relationships to race, contraception, lower genital tract infection, and Papanicolaou smear. J. Pediatr. *104*:141–146, 1984.
130. Shafer, W. M., Joiner, K., Guymon, L. F., et al.: Serum sensitivity of *Neisseria gonorrhoeae*: The role of lipopolysaccharide. J. Infect. Dis. *149*:175–183, 1984.
131. Sicoli, R. A., Losek, J. D., Hudlett, J. M., et al.: Indications for *Neisseria gonorrhoeae* cultures in children with suspected sexual abuse. Arch. Pediatr. Adolesc. Med. *149*:86–89, 1995.
132. Silber, T. J., and Controni, G.: Clinical spectrum of pharyngeal gonorrhea in children and adolescents: A report of sixteen patients. J. Adolesc. Health Care *4*:51–54, 1983.
133. Singer, A.: The uterine cervix adolescence to the menopause. Br. J. Obstet. Gynaecol. *82*:81–99, 1975.
134. Smith, J. A.: Ophthalmia neonatorum in Glasgow. Scott. Med. J. *14*:272–279, 1969.
135. Snowe, R. J., and Wilfert, C. M.: Epidemic reappearance of gonococcal ophthalmia neonatorum. Pediatrics *57*:110–114, 1973.
136. Sparling, P. F., Cannon, J. G., and So, M.: Phase and antigenic variation of pili and outer membrane protein II of *Neisseria gonorrhoeae*. J. Infect. Dis. *153*:196–201, 1986.
137. Speck, W. T., and Lawsky, A. R.: Symptomatic anorectal gonorrhea in an adolescent female. Am. J. Dis. Child. *122*:438–439, 1971.
138. Summit, R. C.: The child sexual abuse accommodation syndrome. Child Abuse Negl. *7*:177–193, 1983.
139. Tilelli, J. A., Turek, D., and Jaffe, A. C.: Sexual abuse of children: Clinical findings and implications for management. N. Engl. J. Med. *302*:319–323, 1980.
140. Tomeh, M. O., and Wilfert, C. M.: Venereal diseases of infants and children at Duke University Medical Center. N. C. Med. J. *34*:109–113, 1973.
141. Wald, E. R., Woodward, C. L., Marston, G., et al.: Gonorrheal disease among children in a university hospital. Sex. Transm. Dis. *7*:41–43, 1980.
142. Washington, A. E., Cates, W., and Zaidi, A. A.: Hospitalization for pelvic inflammatory disease. J. A. M. A. *251*:2529–2533, 1984.
143. Wehrbein, H. L.: Gonococcus arthritis: A study of six hundred cases. Surg. Gynecol. Obstet. *49*:105–113, 1929.
144. Wetzler, L. M., Barry, K., Blake, M.S., et al.: Gonococcal lipooligosaccharide sialylation prevents complement-dependent killing by immune sera. Infect. Immun. *60*:39–43, 1992.
145. White, S. T., Loda, F. A., Ingram, D. L., et al.: Sexually transmitted diseases in sexually abused children. Pediatrics *72*:16–21, 1983.
146. Whittington, W. L., Rice, R. J., Biddle, J. W., et al.: Incorrect identification of *Neisseria gonorrhoeae* from infants and children. Pediatr. Infect. Dis. *7*:3–10, 1988.
147. Wiesner, P. J., Handsfield, H. H., and Holmes, K. K.: Low antibiotic resistance of gonococci causing systemic infection. N. Engl. J. Med. *288*:1221–1222, 1973.
148. Wiesner, P. J., Tronca, E., Bonin, P., et al.: Clinical spectrum of pharyngeal gonococcal infection. N. Engl. J. Med. *288*:181, 1973.

❑ ❑ ❑

SUBSECTION THREE

GRAM-POSITIVE BACILLI

95

DIPHTHERIA

Ralph D. Feigin, Barbara W. Stechenberg, and Laura K. Aguilar

Diphtheria is an acute infectious disease caused by *Corynebacterium diphtheriae*. Generalized or localized symptoms appear after production and elaboration of a toxin that is an extracellular protein metabolite of toxinogenic strains of *C. diphtheriae*. Nontoxigenic strains also cause disease, which usually is less severe.

Before the discovery of antitoxin at the turn of the century, the "strangling angel of children," as diphtheria once was called, was a significant cause of mortality in children and adults. Apparent reference to diphtheria can be traced to as early as the fourth century B.C. It was recognized as a specific entity in 1821 by Pierre Brettoneau, who suggested that the disease was caused by a germ and could be transmitted from person to person. In 1883, the causative agent was identified by Klebs in stained smears from diphtheritic membranes; a year later, Loeffler grew the organism on artificial media and showed that it caused a fatal infection in guinea pigs closely resembling the human disease.

The toxin was purified in 1889 by Roux and Yersin, who found that toxin alone could cause the disease. Shortly thereafter, Behring and Kitasato discovered antitoxins when they immunized animals with toxins rather than bacteria. The use of antitoxin to treat children with diphtheria at the turn of the century resulted in one of the largest decreases in mortality by a therapeutic intervention. It is estimated that in Germany alone 45,000 lives were saved each year.[19]

ETIOLOGY

C. diphtheriae (Klebs-Loeffler bacilli) are irregularly staining, gram-positive, nonmotile, nonsporulating, pleomorphic bacilli. The club-shaped appearance of the bacillus is not a true morphologic feature but results from attempting to grow the bacillus on media that are nutritionally inadequate (Loeffler media). The organism can be recovered most readily on media containing selective inhibitors that retard the growth of other microorganisms (tellurite).

Colonies of *C. diphtheriae* appear grayish-white on Loeffler medium. On tellurite media, three colony types can be distinguished: mitis, gravis, and intermedius. Mitis colonies are smooth, black, and convex; they do not ferment starch or glycogen and are hemolytic. Gravis colonies are gray and semirough, ferment starch and glycogen, and are not hemolytic. Intermedius colonies are small and smooth and have a black center; they do not ferment starch or glycogen and are not hemolytic. Sodium dodecyl sulfate polyacrylamide gel electrophoresis permits more specific typing within each biotype and aids the epidemiologic study of diphtheria outbreaks.

Both smooth and rough strains may be either nontoxigenic or toxigenic. Intermedius was the biotype isolated most commonly in the United States between 1971 and 1981. Furthermore, of those strains isolated, intermedius was found to be toxigenic more often than either mitis or gravis.[11] No differences have been detected in the exotoxins elaborated by the three strains of *C. diphtheriae.* Only those strains of *C. diphtheriae* that are lysogenic for beta-prophage or a closely related phage carrying the gene for toxin production produce diphtheria toxin. Phage multiplication is not a necessary prerequisite for toxin production. The capacity to synthesize toxin depends on both genetic and nutritional factors. Toxin-producing cells apparently are those in which spontaneous induction of the prophage to the phage occurs.[17] The most important factor controlling the yield of toxin is the concentration of inorganic iron in the culture medium.[13] Growth of *C. diphtheriae* in iron-deficient media prolongs the duration of induction lysis and is associated with a high yield of toxin. High concentrations of iron inhibit toxin production. Toxin production also can be increased by use of ultraviolet irradiation. Conversion to a toxigenic strain occurs in nature, as has been demonstrated by restriction enzyme studies of carriers of both toxigenic and nontoxigenic strains in Manchester, England.

The ability of a strain of *C. diphtheriae* to elaborate toxin can be demonstrated by either of two tests: necrosis of tissue in guinea pigs or gel diffusion in agar. The latter test depends on demonstration of a precipitin band between toxin and antitoxin. Diphtheria toxin is lethal to humans in an amount of about 130 μg/kg body weight. Cytoplasmic internalization of as little as one molecule of toxin has been shown to cause cell death.[3]

Both toxigenic and nontoxigenic strains of *C. diphtheriae* can cause disease. Only strains that produce toxin, however, cause disease with symptoms of myocarditis and neuritis.

EPIDEMIOLOGY

Diphtheria is acquired by contact with either a carrier of or a person with the disease. The bacteria may be transmitted via droplets during coughing, sneezing, or talking. Some reports suggest that skin carriers of *C. diphtheriae* are more infectious than either nose or throat carriers.[4, 7] In areas where skin infections are endemic, levels of natural immunization may be high.[8] Environmental contamination is rare, and although fomites and dust may serve as vehicles of transmission, this is comparatively unimportant.

Diphtheria is distributed worldwide and remains endemic in many developing countries, including those in areas of Africa, Asia, and South America. The incidence of diphtheria declined markedly after the extensive use of diphtheria toxoid after World War II. From 1970 through 1976, the average number of cases of diphtheria reported annually in the United States was 248.[30] From 1980 to 1992, only 40 cases of diphtheria were reported in the United States, 70 per cent of which were in patients older than 15 years of age.[25, 33] Three of these cases were fatal and involved unimmunized children. Maintenance of immunity in adults requires a booster vaccination every 10 years. The Centers for Disease Control and Prevention estimate that less than half of adults in the United States have received their 10-year booster and that 40 to 50 per cent of adults are susceptible to diphtheria.[30, 33] In addition, the toxoid vaccine does not provide any protection against nontoxigenic strains.

The incidence peaks during the cooler autumn and winter months. However, several epidemics, in the southern United States primarily, have occurred in late summer and fall, corresponding to a high prevalence of *C. diphtheriae* skin infections. Between the years 1971 and 1981, the incidence of diphtheria was highest in the western United States. It also is noteworthy that there is a 100-fold greater incidence of diphtheria in Native Americans than in the general population.[12] This difference may not reflect a race difference so much as socioeconomic factors. Between 1972 and 1982, three outbreaks occurred in the indigent alcoholic population living in Seattle's Skid Road.[20] Cutaneous infections accounted for 86 per cent of the 1100 total cases. The first outbreak was caused by a single toxigenic, intermedius biotype clone, whereas the other two involved nontoxigenic mitis and gravis strains. The incidence was highest in winter and spring. During 1974 and 1975, 27 per cent of Native Americans in the Skid Road population were affected, compared with 5 per cent of the white population.

A major epidemic began in 1990 in the New Independent States of the former Soviet Union, where 47,802 cases were reported in 1994, with 1746 fatalities.[18] In the Russian Federation, approximately 70 per cent of reported cases have been in persons 15 years of age or older. As in the United States, many adults probably are susceptible because of waning immunity. Most children in the Russian Federation younger than 6 years of age reportedly have received their primary immunization series; however, up to 50 per cent in some areas may have received tetanus and diphtheria toxoids rather than diphtheria and tetanus toxoids and pertussis vaccine or diphtheria and tetanus toxoids. Efforts are under way to control the epidemic by providing adequate immunization of children and rapidly vaccinating adolescents and adults with tetanus and diphtheria toxoids throughout the New Independent States. Already the epidemic appears to be spreading throughout Europe, with cases reported in Bulgaria, Finland, Germany, Norway, and Poland. As a result, many laboratories in Europe routinely are culturing all throat swabs for *C. diphtheriae.*

PATHOGENESIS AND PATHOLOGY

Diphtheria is initiated by entry of *C. diphtheriae* into the nose or mouth, where the bacilli remain localized on the mucosal surfaces of the upper respiratory tract. Occasionally, the ocular or genital mucous membranes serve as the site of localization. The bacilli are unable to invade intact skin but may infect preexisting skin lesions. After a 2- to 4-day period of incubation, lysogenized strains may elaborate toxin.

Diphtheria toxin is secreted as a single polypeptide with a molecular weight of 60,525. The toxin is absorbed initially to the target cell membrane and then undergoes receptor-mediated endocytosis with subsequent release into the cytoplasm. The toxin is composed of two subunits. The larger B subunit is involved in receptor binding, whereas the A subunit is enzymatically active. The A subunit catalyzes the linkage of the ADP-ribosyl group of NAD to elongation factor 2 (ADP-ribosylation), which inactivates elongation factor 2 and thereby inhibits protein synthesis. ADP-ribosylation also is the mechanism of action of other toxins, including cholera and pertussis toxins. It has been shown that diphtheria toxin also mediates DNA fragmentation and cytolysis by a mechanism independent of the inhibition of protein synthesis and similar to that of tumor necrosis factor.[10]

Toxin-mediated tissue necrosis is most marked in the vicinity of colonization. A local inflammatory response follows, and this, coupled with the necrotic tissue, produces a patchy exudate that initially can be removed. As toxin production increases, the area of infection widens and deepens, and a fibrinous exudate develops. A tough adherent membrane is formed that varies from gray to black, depending on the amount of blood it contains. In addition to fibrin, the membrane contains inflammatory cells, red blood cells, and superficial epithelial cells. Because the latter are an integral part of the membrane, attempts to remove the membrane are followed by bleeding. Edema of the soft tissues beneath the membrane may be marked. The edematous tissue and the diphtheritic membrane may encroach upon the airway. The membrane sloughs spontaneously during the recovery period. Occasionally, secondary bacterial infection (classically due to *Streptococcus pyogenes)* develops. Respiratory embarrassment or suffocation may occur after extension of disease to the larynx or into the tracheobronchial tree.

Toxin produced at the site of infection is distributed via the blood stream and the lymphatics throughout the body. This occurs most readily when the pharynx and tonsils are covered by a diphtheritic membrane. Any organ or tissue can be damaged as a result of diphtheria toxin, but lesions of the heart, nervous system, and kidneys particularly are prominent. Clinical manifestations appear after a variable latent period, ranging, for example, from 10 to 14 days for myocarditis and from 3 to 7 weeks for nervous system manifestations, such as peripheral neuritis. Antitoxin can neutralize circulating toxin or toxin that is absorbed to cells but is ineffective once cells have been penetrated. Thus, early treatment is essential to limiting tissue damage.

The most prominent pathologic findings are necrosis and toxic hyaline degeneration of various organs and tissues. In the heart, edema, congestion, mononuclear cell infiltration, and fatty accumulation in muscle fibers and the conducting system may be observed.[29] Burch and associates[9] demonstrated mitochondrial damage with depletion of glycogen and accumulation of lipid droplets in the damaged myofibrils. If the patient survives, muscle regeneration and interstitial fibrosis can be seen. A toxic neuritis with fatty degeneration of myelin sheaths can be noted. Liver necrosis may occur, possibly associated with hypoglycemia. Adrenal hemorrhage and acute tubular necrosis of the kidney can be noted.

CLINICAL MANIFESTATIONS

The signs and symptoms of diphtheria depend on the site of infection, the immunization status of the host, and whether or not toxin has been distributed to the systemic circulation.

The incubation period ranges from 1 to 6 days. Diphtheria can be classified clinically on the basis of the anatomic location of the initial infection and of the diphtheritic membrane (nasal, tonsillar, pharyngeal, laryngeal or laryngotracheal, conjunctival, skin, and genital). More than one anatomic site may be involved simultaneously.

Nasal diphtheria initially resembles a common cold and is characterized by mild rhinorrhea and a paucity of systemic symptoms. Gradually, the nasal discharge becomes serosanguineous and then mucopurulent, and it excoriates the nares and upper lip. A foul odor may be noticed, and careful inspection reveals a white membrane on the nasal septum. Absorption of toxin usually is slow, and this, coupled with the lack of systemic symptoms, frequently delays an accurate diagnosis. The nasal form of the disease occurs most often in infants.

Tonsillar and pharyngeal diphtherias begin as an insidious but more severe form of the disease. Anorexia, malaise, low-grade fever, and pharyngitis are noted initially. Within 1 or 2 days, a membrane appears that varies in extent, depending on the immune status of the host. In some partially immune persons, a membrane may not develop. The white or gray adherent membrane may cover the tonsils and pharyngeal walls and extend into the uvula and soft palate or down into the larynx and trachea. Attempts to remove the membrane are followed by bleeding. Cervical lymphadenitis is variable. In some cases, it is associated with edema of the soft tissues of the neck and may be so severe that it gives the appearance of a "bull neck." In a 1970 epidemic, "erasure" edema of the neck was noted in patients with pharyngeal diphtheria.[24] Patients with erasure edema did not have a classic bull neck appearance, but the edema was characterized by obliteration of the sternocleidomastoid muscle border, the mandible, and the median border of the clavicle. The edema was brawny, pitting, warm to the touch, and tender to palpation. Erasure edema was noted in 29 per cent of immunized patients and in 30 per cent of nonimmunized or inadequately immunized persons. It was most common in children older than 6 years of age and generally was associated with infection due to the gravis or intermedius strains of *C. diphtheriae.*

The course of pharyngeal diphtheria depends on the degree of toxin elaboration and the extent of the membrane. In severe cases, respiratory and circulatory collapse may occur. The pulse rate is increased disproportionately to the body temperature, which generally remains normal or slightly elevated. The palate may be paralyzed. This paralysis may be unilateral or bilateral and associated with difficulty in swallowing and regurgitation.[14] Stupor, coma, and death may occur within a week to 10 days. In less severe cases, recovery may be slow and may be complicated by the development of myocarditis or neuritis. In mild cases, the membrane sloughs off in 7 to 10 days, and the recovery is uneventful.

Laryngeal diphtheria generally reflects a downward extension of the membrane from the pharynx. Occasionally, only the larynx is involved, and in these patients toxicity is less prominent. The clinical findings are indistinguishable from other types of infectious croup. Noisy breathing, progressive stridor, hoarseness, and a dry cough may be noted. Suprasternal, subcostal, and supraclavicular retractions reflect severe laryngeal obstruction, which may be fatal unless alleviated. Occasionally, in a mild case, an acute and fatal obstruction may occur because of a partially detached piece of membrane that occludes the airway. In severe cases of laryngeal diphtheria, the membrane may extend downward and invade the entire tracheobronchial tree. Rarely, laryngeal diphtheria is primary and does not reflect an extension of disease from the pharynx. In these cases, toxicity and signs of toxemia generally are less prominent.

Cutaneous disease, unlike pharyngeal, is more common in warmer climates and often is due to nontoxigenic strains. In some tropical and subtropical climate countries, such as Uganda, Tanzania, Sri Lanka, and Samoa, *C. diphtheriae* has been isolated from up to 60 per cent of skin lesions in children.[21] This form of the disease may be an important source of person-to-person transmission of diphtheritic organisms and of outbreaks in indigenous populations in which overcrowding and poor hygiene are important risk factors.[4, 8, 21] The skin lesions begin as vesicles or pustules that progress to typical ulcers with sharply defined borders, membranous bases, and surrounding erythema and edema. The lesions are most common on legs, feet, and hands. For the first 1 to 2 weeks, the lesions are painful. Spontaneous healing generally takes 6 to 12 weeks, but lesions have been reported to persist up to a year.[21]

Conjunctival, aural, and vulvovaginal diphtheria may be noted. Conjunctival lesions usually are limited to the palpebral conjunctiva, which appears red, edematous, and membranous. Rarely, conjunctival lesions have been associated with corneal erosion.[35] Aural diphtheria is characterized by the development of otitis externa with a persistent purulent and frequently foul-smelling discharge.

Clinical syndromes other than typical diphtheria have been associated with the isolation of the organism, including meningitis, endocarditis, osteomyelitis, and hepatitis. In most cases, these have occurred in patients with underlying problems.[38] An immunocompetent child with bacterial arthritis caused by *C. diphtheriae* has been reported.[1]

Several cases of septic arthritis caused by nontoxigenic *C. diphtheriae* have been described.[1, 38] A 27-month-old child had septic arthritis of the hip and skin lesions on the lower extremities, which were the presumed portal of entry for the organism.[1] This child had received four doses of diphtheria and tetanus toxoids and pertussis vaccine, but because the *C. diphtheriae* strain was nontoxigenic, immunization with toxoid would not provide protection. In this case, the organism was sensitive to penicillin, cefuroxime, cephalothin, and clindamycin but was resistant to oxacillin, an antistaphylococcal antibiotic often used for treatment of septic arthritis when the causative organism cannot be identified. Four cases of septic arthritis complicating endocarditis caused by nontoxigenic *C. diphtheriae* var gravis were reported in addition to three cases of endocarditis caused by the same strain but without septic arthritis.[38] All seven cases occurred in the state of New South Wales, Australia, in a 12-month period. One case was in a 12-year-old boy who died, five of the patients were in their 20s, and the seventh patient was 49 years old. Three of the patients had underlying cardiac abnormalities, and one used intravenous drugs.

Complications secondary to elaborated diphtheria toxin may affect any system, but myocarditis and nervous system involvement are most characteristic. Myocarditis may occur after both mild and severe cases of diphtheria. Generally, it occurs in patients in whom administration of antitoxin is delayed. Myocarditis most commonly appears in the second week of the disease but can appear as early as the first or as late as the sixth week of illness. Tachycardia, a muffled first heart sound, murmurs, and arrhythmias, such as atrioventricular dissociation, indicate myocardial involvement. Although some cases may result in cardiac failure, most myocardial complications are temporary.

Neurologic complications appear after a variable latent period, are predominantly bilateral, are motor rather than sensory, and usually resolve completely. Paralysis of the soft palate is most common and generally appears in the third week. This is manifested by a nasal quality in the voice, nasal regurgitation, and difficulty in swallowing. Ocular paralysis usually occurs around the fifth week of illness and is characterized by blurring of vision and difficulty with accommodation. Internal strabismus also may be noted. Paralysis of the diaphragm, peripheral neuropathy involving the limbs, and loss of deep tendon reflexes also are reported as complications of diphtheria. When these occur and an elevated cerebrospinal fluid protein also is documented, the syndrome is indistinguishable clinically from Guillain-Barré syndrome.

Rarely, 2 or 3 weeks after the onset of illness, the vasomotor centers are affected, which results in hypotension and cardiac failure. Gastritis, hepatitis, nephritis, and hemolytic uremic syndrome also have been reported as complications of diphtheria.[36]

Information on the effects, if any, of diphtheria during pregnancy on the fetus was not available until fairly recently. El Seed and associates[16] reported a case of pharyngeal diphtheria in a pregnant woman that occurred during the first trimester of pregnancy. Apart from vaginal bleeding, no complications of pregnancy were noted. Severe diphtheritic toxemia in the mother was characterized by quadriparesis, from which she fully recovered. A physically normal female infant was delivered at term. In this single case, severe diphtheritic toxemia during pregnancy was not associated with any teratogenic effect in the fetus and did not impair intrauterine fetal growth.

DIAGNOSIS

The diagnosis of diphtheria should be based on clinical findings, because any delay in therapy poses a serious risk to the patient.

An accurate diagnosis depends on isolation of *C. diphtheriae.* Examination of direct smears of diphtheritic lesions remains an important, although often inaccurate, supplement to the clinical examination. Identification by fluorescent antibody technique may be reliable but only in the hands of highly experienced personnel. Counterimmunoelectrophoresis has been shown to have high validity and predictivity.[31] However, because of the nature of the disease, it is not practical to wait for laboratory confirmation.

Material obtained from beneath the membrane or a portion of the membrane itself should be obtained for culture. *C. diphtheriae* is relatively resistant to drying. Use of non-nutritive, moisture-reducing transport medium helps to prevent the overgrowth of other microorganisms. The laboratory should be notified about the possibility of diphtheria so that appropriate culture media are inoculated. A Loeffler slant, a tellurite plate, and a blood agar plate should be inoculated.

Diphtheria bacilli that are recovered should be tested for toxigenicity. An immunodiffusion assay, the Elek test, is used most commonly.[15] Other methods include the guinea pig or rabbit neutralization test or neutralization in Vero cells. The standard guinea pig or rabbit neutralization test is carried out as follows: Two animals are inoculated intracutaneously with a broth suspension of the microorganism. One of the animals is given diphtheria antitoxin prior to intracutaneous challenge. An inflammatory lesion appears at the site of inoculation in 24 hours, and it becomes necrotic in 72 hours in the control animal if the strain being tested is toxigenic. No skin reaction should occur in the animal given antitoxin. Rapid tests for diphtheria toxin using polymerase chain reaction or coagglutination have been described.[22, 32] The immune status of patients can be determined by toxin neutralization in Vero cells.[28] Levels of diphtheria antitoxin greater than or equal to 0.01 IU/mL generally are accepted as protective. A skin-testing method, the Schick test, also has been used to assess immunity.

The Schick test has been utilized previously to determine the immune status of the patient. It is not helpful in early diagnosis because it cannot be read for several days. In the Schick test, a measured amount of purified diphtheria toxin (0.1 mL) is injected intracutaneously. In the absence of circulating antitoxin, the injected toxin causes a local inflammatory response characterized by erythema, swelling, and tenderness that peaks at about 5 days, as well as central pigmentation, which remains. If sufficient antitoxin is present, no reaction should occur. Many persons become hypersensitive to the toxin itself or to other antigens in the toxin preparation. For this reason, a control injection of toxoid (0.005 Lf) is administered intradermally in the opposite arm. Persons with adequate circulating antitoxin but who are sensitive to the toxin preparation react to both the toxin and the toxoid. Those skin reactions due to hypersensitivity generally are maximal at 48 to 72 hours and then fade. If the person has no antitoxin in his or her serum and is allergic to the toxin preparation, a reaction also will be noted on both arms, but the reaction at the site of toxin injection peaks on day 5 and persists. In contrast, the reaction to toxoid peaks and subsides by 5 days. A positive Schick test consists of more than 10 mm of induration and indicates susceptibility to diphtheria. Although a negative Schick test indicates adequate antitoxin levels, infection with diphtheria still may occur.

The Schick test has been employed since the 1970s to determine whether specific antibody production is developing in immunodeficient patients.

Other laboratory studies are of little diagnostic value. The white blood cell count may be normal or elevated. Rarely, anemia develops as a result of rapid hemolysis of red blood cells. Examination of the cerebrospinal fluid may reveal a minimal elevation of protein and, rarely, a mild pleocytosis in patients with diphtheritic neuritis. Hypoglycemia, glucosuria, or both may occur and reflect hepatic toxicity. An elevation in blood urea nitrogen may develop in patients with acute tubular necrosis. An electrocardiogram should be obtained and may reveal ST-segment and T-wave changes or arrhythmias indicative of myocarditis.

DIFFERENTIAL DIAGNOSIS

Mild forms of nasal diphtheria in the partially immunized host may resemble the common cold. When nasal discharge is more serosanguineous or purulent, nasal diphtheria must be distinguished from a foreign body in the nose, sinusitis, adenoiditis, or the snuffles of congenital syphilis. Careful examination of the nose with a nasal speculum, sinus radiographs, and appropriate serologic tests for syphilis are helpful in excluding these disorders.

Tonsillar or pharyngeal diphtheria must be differentiated from streptococcal pharyngitis. Generally, streptococcal pharyngitis is associated with more severe pain on swallowing, higher temperature, and a relatively nonadherent membrane limited to the tonsils. In some patients, pharyngeal diphtheria and streptococcal pharyngitis coexist.

Tonsillar and pharyngeal diphtheria also must be differentiated from infectious mononucleosis (lymphadenopathy and splenomegaly are common, atypical lymphocytes generally are present, and heterophile antibody may be present); nonbacterial membranous tonsillitis (white blood cell count generally is low, throat cultures reveal normal flora, and the course is unaffected by antibiotics); primary herpetic tonsillitis (the presence of gingivitis, stomatitis, and discrete lesions of the tongue and palate may be helpful); Vincent angina (may be indistinguishable); and thrush (constitutional symptoms are absent, and lesions are present on the buccal mucosa and tongue). Tonsillar and pharyngeal diphtheria also must be differentiated from blood dyscrasias, such as agranulocytosis and leukemia (complete blood count and bone marrow study are helpful); posttonsillectomy faucial membranes (membranes are stationary and do not spread); and oropharyngeal involvement caused by toxoplasmosis, cytomegalovirus, tularemia, and salmonellosis (associated signs and symptoms and appropriate cultures and serologic tests may be diagnostic).

Laryngeal diphtheria must be differentiated from spasmodic or nonspasmodic croup; acute epiglottitis; laryngotracheobronchitis; aspirated foreign bodies; peripharyngeal and retropharyngeal abscesses; and laryngeal papillomas, hemangiomas, or lymphangiomas. A careful history, followed by careful visualization in hospital under controlled conditions, aids correct diagnosis.

PREVENTION

Diphtheria is prevented on a community-wide basis most effectively by active immunization. The preferred immunizing agent for children younger than 6 years of age is diphtheria toxoid given in combination with tetanus toxoid and pertussis antigen. Primary immunization is carried out conveniently and effectively by giving diphtheria and tetanus toxoids and pertussis vaccine at 2, 4, and 6 months of age, with booster doses at 12 to 18 months of age and again between 4 and 6 years of age. Booster doses with adult-type diphtheria and tetanus toxoids adsorbed (Td) should be given at 10-year intervals to all immunized persons. Td contains no more than 2 Lf of diphtheria toxoid per dose, compared with the 7 to 25 Lf in the pediatric diphtheria and tetanus toxoids and pertussis vaccine–adsorbed preparations. Primary immunization of children more than 7 years of age may be carried out with Td. Two doses are given intramuscularly at least 4 weeks apart, with a booster dose provided 1 year later. An oral diphtheria toxoid vaccine is being tested in animals.[27]

The majority of local and systemic reactions to the diphtheria and tetanus toxoids and pertussis vaccine, including fever, have been related to the pertussis component.[2, 12] Administration of tetanus and diphtheria toxoids is not followed by the high incidence of reactions associated with the use of pediatric diphtheria and tetanus toxoids and pertussis vaccine (or diphtheria and tetanus toxoids). For this reason, tetanus and diphtheria toxoids may be administered safely without an earlier skin test. At least one study showed that 7.5 Lf toxoid can be given safely to adults without a higher risk of reactions.[5] Primary immunization against diphtheria for infants with progressive neurologic disorders as well as completion of the primary immunization series in patients who have experienced an untoward reaction to an earlier diphtheria and tetanus toxoids and pertussis vaccine injection may be carried out using diphtheria and tetanus toxoids with adjuvant rather than diphtheria and tetanus toxoids and pertussis vaccine.[34]

Booster doses of tetanus and diphtheria toxoids should be given at 10-year intervals to all immunized persons. Levels of diphtheria antitoxin greater than or equal to 0.01 IU/mL generally are accepted as protective.

Diphtheria immunization is not always followed by complete protection.[23] Immunization is directed against the phage-mediated toxin, not against infection. Therefore, fully immunized persons may be carriers or may have disease secondary to nontoxigenic strains. An investigation during an epidemic in Texas showed no statistical difference in the risk of diphtheria infection among those with full, lapsed, inadequate, or no previous diphtheria immunization; however, there was a 30-fold increased risk of symptomatic diphtheria in those with no immunization and an 11.5-fold increase in those with inadequate immunization.[26] The most important health problem in the United States today is inadequate immunization of the population. Immunization rates in adults are poorer than those in infants and children because of failure to maintain adequate immunity through appropriate booster immunization. A 70 to 80 per cent immunization level is thought to be required to prevent epidemic spread.[11]

Prevention of diphtheria also depends on management of contacts of known cases of diphtheria and carriers of the organism and on isolation of the patient to minimize spread of disease. The patient is infectious until diphtheria bacilli no longer can be cultured from the site of infection. Three consecutive negative cultures are required before the patient is released from isolation.

Cultures should be taken from the nose and throat of all close contacts. Those carriers with prior immunization should be given a booster injection of diphtheria toxoid. They should be treated with aqueous procaine penicillin, 600,000 units daily for 4 days; benzathine penicillin G, 600,000 units intramuscularly as a single dose; or erythromycin, 40 mg/kg/day for 7 to 10 days. The immune status of each contact should be determined; if inadequate, the person should receive an injection of diphtheria toxoid. In addition, patients with diphtheria should be immunized during convalescence because infection may not confer immunity. Asymptomatic carriers who were not immunized previously against diphtheria should have cultures taken, receive diphtheria toxoid and penicillin or erythromycin (as described earlier), and be seen daily by a physician. If daily surveillance is not possible, 10,000 units of diphtheria antitoxin may be administered intramuscularly. The risk of allergic reactions to horse serum restricts prophylactic antitoxin use. When it is used, appropriate skin testing for sensitivity at a site separate from that of the toxoid injection should be carried out. The efficacy of chemoprophylaxis in preventing disease has not been established.[34] If a contact is experiencing symptoms when seen, treatment for diphtheria is indicated. It is important to initiate prophylactic therapy in contacts who have not been immunized before the culture results are received.

TREATMENT

Treatment of diphtheria is predicated on neutralization of free toxin and eradication of *C. diphtheriae* by the use of antibiotics. Antitoxin of equine origin is used in the United States, whereas antitoxin of human origin is available in some countries.[6] Antitoxin should be administered on the basis of the site and size of the membrane, the degree of toxicity, and the duration of illness.

Antitoxin must be administered as early as possible by the intravenous route and in a dosage sufficient to neutralize all free toxin. A single dose is used to avoid the risk of sensitization from repeated doses of horse serum. Tests for sensitivity to horse serum must be performed before administration of antitoxin. For this purpose, 0.1 mL of a 1:1000 dilution of antitoxin in saline can be given intracutaneously or may be placed in the conjunctival sac. A positive reaction of greater than 10 mm of erythema at the site of injection within 20 minutes or the development of conjunctivitis and tearing necessitates desensitization.

If a patient has been shown to be sensitive to horse serum, the serum should be provided in a slowly increasing dosage given at 20-minute intervals. Several regimens have been recommended. One commonly employed regimen is as follows:

0.05 mL of a 1:20 dilution subcutaneously
0.1 mL of a 1:20 dilution subcutaneously
0.1 mL of a 1:10 dilution subcutaneously
0.1 mL undiluted subcutaneously
0.3 mL undiluted intramuscularly
0.5 mL undiluted intramuscularly
0.1 mL undiluted intravenously

If no reaction has occurred, the remaining material is given by slow intravenous infusion. Intravenous administration results in more rapid excretion of antitoxin into saliva, rendering it atoxic and preventing further absorption of toxin in the oropharynx, but does not result in more rapid systemic elimination of antitoxin than intramuscular administration.[37] Reactions should be treated with aqueous epinephrine (1:1000) provided intravenously.

Antitoxin dosage is empiric. Mild nasal or pharyngeal diphtheria can be treated with 40,000 units of antitoxin; 80,000 units should be used for moderately severe pharyngeal diphtheria. Severe pharyngeal or laryngeal diphtheria should be treated with 120,000 units. The latter dose also should be given to patients with mixed clinical symptoms, as well as to those with brawny edema or disease of longer than 48 hours' duration.

Antibiotics are not a substitute for treatment with antitoxin. Still, penicillin and erythromycin are effective against most strains of *C. diphtheriae* and should be provided. Penicillin and erythromycin also are effective in eradicating group A hemolytic streptococci, which may complicate up to 30 per cent of cases of diphtheria. Penicillin may be given as aqueous procaine penicillin G, 600,000 units intramuscularly once daily for 14 days. Patients who are sensitive to penicillin should be given erythromycin in a daily dosage of 40 mg/kg/day in four divided doses for 7 to 10 days. Amoxicillin, rifampin, and clindamycin provided in appropriate dosages also may be effective. Lincomycin and tetracycline have proved to be less effective, and cephalexin, oxacillin, and colistin have been shown to be ineffective against *C. diphtheriae*. The end-point of therapy is three consecutive, negative cultures taken at least 24 hours apart.

The carrier state has been treated effectively with benzathine penicillin G or oral erythromycin.

Supportive Treatment

Bed rest is extremely important and should be required for 2 to 3 weeks. Serial electrocardiograms should be obtained two or three times each week for 4 to 6 weeks to detect myocarditis as early as possible. Absolute bed rest must be enforced if myocarditis is detected because sudden death has been precipitated by excessive activity. The patient with myocarditis may undergo digitalization if congestive heart failure develops. However, digitalization for arrhythmias due to diphtheria may be contraindicated. In severe disease, prednisone, 1.0 to 1.5 mg/kg/day for 2 weeks, has been shown to lessen the incidence of myocarditis.

Hydration should be maintained and a high-calorie liquid or soft diet provided. Secretions should be suctioned as needed to prevent aspiration. Palatal and pharyngeal paralysis increases the risk of aspiration. Gavage via a polyethylene tube is indicated in these patients.

The quality of the voice and the gag reflex should be checked regularly for assessment of progression of the disease. Laryngeal diphtheria may require relief of obstruction with a tracheostomy. This procedure should be carried out before the patient has become exhausted.

At least half of the patients who recover from diphtheria do not develop adequate immunity and remain subject to reinfection. Therefore, immunization is indicated after the recovery of the patient.

PROGNOSIS

Many factors affect the prognosis in cases of diphtheria. The most important of these is the immunization status of the host. Both morbidity and mortality are increased significantly in patients who are unimmunized or inadequately immunized. The rapidity with which medical care is sought and the diagnosis of diphtheria suggested have a great impact on the outcome. If specific treatment is provided on the first day of disease, mortality may be reduced to less than 1 per cent; delay in treatment until day 4 may be associated with a 20-fold increase in the mortality rate.

The virulence of the infecting organism and the location of

infection are important prognostic factors. Infection with a nontoxigenic *C. diphtheriae* strain may cause disease but does not lead to myocarditis, neuritis, and other toxin-related phenomena. All three subtypes of *C. diphtheriae* may produce toxin, and the resulting disease may vary from mild to severe. In cases of mild diphtheria, membrane sloughing and full recovery generally occur within 7 days. Disease caused by toxigenic gravis strains tends to be more severe and carry a poorer prognosis. Although diphtheria may affect the skin, nasopharynx, and other mucous membranes, involvement of the larynx heralds a more complicated course. Laryngeal diphtheria increases the risk of airway obstruction and promotes systemic absorption of the toxin. These patients require close monitoring for respiratory function and for involvement of other organ systems. Laryngeal diphtheria is more likely to be fatal in infants.

Few laboratory parameters indicate the severity of diphtheria. However, the development of amegakaryocytic thrombocytopenia and leukocytosis greater than 25,000/mm^3 have been associated with a poor outcome.

The prognosis in the patient with diphtheria remains guarded until recovery is full. At any time during the course of the illness, complications such as laryngeal obstruction, shock, and ventricular fibrillation may occur suddenly and unexpectedly. In patients with myocardial involvement, permanent damage to the heart, specifically fibrosis, may occur and may lead to later complications. It also must be kept in mind that potentially severe neurologic manifestations, such as phrenic nerve paralysis, may appear late in the course of the disease.

Persistence of *C. diphtheriae* may be noted in the nasopharynx of 5 to 10 per cent of convalescing patients. Recovery from diphtheria is followed by immunity that is demonstrable for at least a year after illness in 50 per cent of patients. Second attacks are rare; nevertheless, immunization should be carried out after recovery.

Before the use of antitoxin and the availability of antibiotics, the mortality rate from diphtheria was 30 to 50 per cent. Death was most common in children younger than 4 years of age and was the result of suffocation. At present, the mortality rate is less than 5 per cent, and there is no clear association with age.

References

1. Afghani, B., and Stutman, H. R.: Bacterial arthritis caused by *Corynebacterium diphtheriae*. Pediatr. Infect. Dis. J. *12*:881–882, 1993.
2. Baraff, L. J., Manclark, C. R., Cherry, J. D., et al.: Analyses of adverse reactions to diphtheria and tetanus toxoids and pertussis vaccine by vaccine lot, endotoxin content, pertussis vaccine potency and percentage of mouse weight gain. Pediatr. Infect. Dis. J. *8*:502–507, 1989.
3. Battistini, A., Curatola, A. M., Gallinare, P., et al.: Inhibition of protein synthesis by diphtheria toxin induces a peculiar pattern of synthesized protein species. Exp. Cell Res. *176*:174–179, 1988.
4. Belsey, M. A., Sinclair, M., Roder, M. R., et al.: *Corynebacterium diphtheriae* skin infections in Alabama and Louisiana: A factor in the epidemiology of diphtheria. N. Engl. J. Med. *280*:135–141, 1969.
5. Bjorkholm, B., Granstrom, M., Wahl, M., et al.: Adverse reactions and immunogenicity in adults to regular and increased dosage of diphtheria vaccine. Eur. J. Clin. Microbiol. *6*:637–640, 1987.
6. Bjorkholm, B., Olling, S., Larsson, P., et al.: An outbreak of diphtheria among Swedish alcoholics. Infection *15*:354–358, 1987.
7. Bowler, C. J., Mandal, B. K., Schlecht, B., et al.: Diphtheria: The continuing hazard. Arch. Dis. Child. *63*:194–195, 1988.
8. Bray, J. P., Burt, E. G., Potter, E. J., et al.: Epidemic diphtheria and skin infections in Trinidad. J. Infect. Dis. *126*:34–40, 1972.
9. Burch, G. E., Sun, S. C., Sohal, R. S., et al.: Diphtheritic myocarditis: A histochemical and electron microscopic study. Am. J. Cardiol. *21*:261–268, 1968.
10. Chang, M. P., Bramhall, J., Graves, S., et al.: Internucleosomal DNA cleavage precedes diphtheria toxin-induced cytolysis: Evidence that cell lysis is not a simple consequence of translation inhibition. J. Biol. Chem. *264*:15261–15267, 1989.
11. Chen, R. T., Broome, C. V., Weinstein, R. A., et al.: Diphtheria in the United States, 1971–1981. Am. J. Public Health *75*:1393–1397, 1985.
12. Cherry, J. D., Baraff, L. J., and Hewlett, E.: The past, present, and future of pertussis: The role of adults in epidemiology and future control. West. J. Med. *150*:319–328, 1989.
13. Collier, R. J., and Kandel, J.: Structure and activity of diphtheria toxin. I. Thiol-dependent dissociation of a fraction of toxin into enzymatically active and inactive fragments. J. Biol. Chem. *246*:1496–1503, 1971.
14. Dietze, W. E., and Sudderth, J. F.: Post-diphtheria polyneuritis: Three case reports. Laryngoscope *82*:765–770, 1972.
15. Elek, S. D.: The plate virulence test for diphtheria. J. Clin. Pathol. *2*:250–258, 1949.
16. El Seed, A. M., Dafalla, A. A., and Abboud, O. I.: Fetal immune response following maternal diphtheria during pregnancy. Ann. Trop. Pediatr. *1*:217–219, 1981.
17. Freeman, V. J.: Studies on virulence of bacteriophage-infected strains of *Corynebacterium diphtheriae*. J. Bacteriol. *61*:675–688, 1951.
18. From the Centers for Disease Control and Prevention: Leads from the Morbidity and Mortality Weekly Report: Diphtheria epidemic—New Independent States of the former Soviet Union, 1990–1994. J. A. M. A. *273*:1250–1251, 1995.
19. Grundbacher, F. J.: Behring's discovery of diphtheria and tetanus antitoxins. Immunol. Today *13*:188–190, 1992.
20. Harnisch, J. P., Tronca, E., Nolan, C. M., et al.: Diphtheria among alcoholic urban adults: A decade of experience in Seattle. Ann. Intern. Med. *111*:71–82, 1989.
21. Hofler, W.: Cutaneous diphtheria. Int. J. Dermatol. *30*:845–847, 1991.
22. Jalgaonkar, S. V., and Saoji, A. M.: Coagglutination for rapid testing of toxin producing *Corynebacterium diphtheriae*. Indian J. Med. Res. *97*:35–36, 1993.
23. McCloskey, R. V.: Diphtheria antitoxin titers in hospital workers after a single dose of adult-type diphtheria tetanus toxoid. Am. J. Med. Sci. *258*:209–213, 1969.
24. McCloskey, R. V., Eller, J. J., Green, M., et al.: The 1970 epidemic of diphtheria in San Antonio. Ann. Intern. Med. *75*:495–503, 1971.
25. Miller, L. W., Older, J. J., Drake, J., et al.: Diphtheria immunization: Effect upon carriers and the control of outbreaks. Am. J. Dis. Child. *123*:197–199, 1972.
26. Mirchamsy, H., Hamedi, M., Fateh, G., et al.: Oral immunization against diphtheria and tetanus infections by fluid diphtheria and tetanus toxoids. Vaccine *12*:1167–1172, 1994.
27. Miyamura, K., Nishio, S., Ito, A., et al.: Micro cell culture method for determination of diphtheria toxin and antitoxin titres using VERO cells. I. Studies on factors affecting the toxin and antitoxin titration. J. Biol. Stand. *2*:189–201, 1974.
28. Morales, A. R., Vichitbandha, P., Chandruang, P., et al.: Pathological features of cardiac conduction disturbances in diphtheric myocarditis. Arch. Pathol. *91*:1–7, 1971.
29. Morbidity and Mortality Weekly Report: Diphtheria, tetanus and pertussis: Guidelines for vaccine prophylaxis and other preventive measures. M. M. W. R. *30*:392–407, 1981.
30. Medical News and Perspectives: Diphtheria in Russia: A reminder of risk. J. A. M. A. *273*:1245, 1995.
31. Natu, M., Borole, D., Shaikh, N., et al.: Comparative assessment of laboratory procedures: Diphtheria. Indian J. Pathol. Microbiol. *29*:31–35, 1986.
32. Pallen, M. J., Hay, A. J., Puckey, L. H., et al.: Polymerase chain reaction for screening clinical isolates of corynebacteria for the production of diphtheria toxin. J. Clin. Pathol. *47*:353–356, 1994.
33. Popovic, T., Wharton, M., Wenger, J. D., et al.: Are we ready for diphtheria? A report from the Diphtheria Diagnostic Workshop, Atlanta, 11 and 12 July 1994. J. Infect. Dis. *171*:765–767, 1995.
34. Report of the Committee on Infectious Diseases, American Academy of Pediatrics. 22nd ed. 1991, pp. 195–199.
35. Rysselaere, M., and Vanneste, L.: Diphtheria of the eye. Bull. Soc. Belge. Ophtalmol. *201*:89–92, 1982.
36. Sheth, K. J., and Sarff, L. D.: Hemolytic uremic syndrome associated with *Corynebacterium diphtheria* infection. Int. J. Pediatr. Nephrol. *7*:17–20, 1986.
37. Tasman, A., Minkenhof, J. E., Vink, H. H., et al.: Importance of intravenous injection of diphtheria antiserum. Lancet *1*:1299–1304, 1958.
38. Tiley, S. M., Kociuba, K. R., Heron, L. G., et al.: Infective endocarditis due to nontoxigenic *Corynebacterium diphtheriae*: Report of seven cases and review. Clin. Infect. Dis. *16*:271–275, 1993.

ADDITIONAL READING

Barksdale, L.: *Corynebacterium diphtheriae* and its relatives. Bacteriol. Rev. *34*:378–422, 1970.

Pappenheimer, A. M., Jr.: Diphtheria toxin. *In* Ajl, S. J., Kadis, S., and Montie, T. C. (eds.): Microbial Toxins. Vol. 11B. New York, Academic Press, 1973.

Wood, W. B., Jr.: From Miasmas to Molecules. New York, Columbia University Press, 1961.

96

ANTHRAX

Morven S. Edwards

Anthrax is a toxigenic disease of herbivores in which humans are an incidental host. The term *anthrax*, derived from the Greek *anthrakos*, or coal, refers to the black eschar characteristic of cutaneous anthrax. There are three human forms of anthrax: cutaneous, which accounts for 95 per cent of infections in the United States, inhalation, and gastrointestinal, which has not been reported in the United States. Each may occur in children.[15, 19, 27, 33] Any form may be complicated by the development of meningitis.

HISTORICAL ASPECTS

Anthrax has been recognized since antiquity. The earliest recorded reference to a disease believed to be anthrax is a description in Exodus of a plague that caused the death of all of the cattle in Egypt.[4] Hippocrates described carbuncles, which are considered to represent the cutaneous form of anthrax. In the early seventeenth century, an anthrax pandemic referred to as the "Black Bane" caused 60,000 human deaths in Europe.[4] By the eighteenth century, there were several excellent descriptions of the clinical disease in humans.

Bacillus anthracis occupies a unique position in the history of infectious diseases. The organism first was seen microscopically by Delafond in 1838. It was isolated and cultivated in 1877 by Robert Koch, who demonstrated its proliferation in vivo, thus establishing a model for causation of infectious disease. In 1881, both Louis Pasteur and W. S. Greenfield[30] demonstrated the protective value of a live vaccine of anthrax bacilli (attenuated by heating) in animal immunization studies. These initial demonstrations of the efficacy of a bacterial vaccine provided the basis for the prevention of infectious diseases by immunization.

BACTERIOLOGY

B. anthracis is an aerobic, nonmotile, spore-forming rod in the family Bacillaceae. Optimal growth occurs at 36° C in nonselective media. Colonies are gray-white, rough, and flat and may have comma-shaped projections resulting from the outgrowth of chains of bacilli from the edges of the colony, which give it a "Medusa head" appearance. Individual colonies are 4 to 5 mm in diameter, with a ground-glass appearance, and exhibit tenacity or a "beaten egg white" appearance when lifted with an inoculating loop.[11] A three-layered capsule, which is associated with virulence and toxin production, may be delineated by electron microscopy.[12] Encapsulation occurs with growth on enriched media. Gram stain of clinical material reveals large, square-ended, gram-positive rods, which occur singly or in short chains without a visible capsule. The equatorial or paracentral spores are not visible in smears fixed promptly after collection. After 24 to 48 hours of aerobic incubation, strands of rods are arranged in "boxcar" or "bamboo" fashion, and sporulation occurs. Small numbers of bacteria are pathogenic for mice, guinea pigs, and rabbits, and death usually occurs 2 to 5 days after inoculation. Currently, there is no method for serologically classifying strains of *B. anthracis*.

TRANSMISSION AND EPIDEMIOLOGY

Domestic herbivores—cattle, sheep, horses, goats, and swine—are the most important agricultural sources of anthrax, but all domestic and many wild animals may serve as hosts. Animals are infected commonly by ingestion of spores from infected pastures. Spores germinate in vivo, and death, associated with massive septicemia, usually occurs in 1 or 2 days. Anthrax is endemic in areas where an animal-soil-animal cycle is established, because the spores can survive indefinitely in a dry environment. Uncultivated soils with a pH greater than 6.0 and ambient temperature greater than 15.5° C provide an environment favorable for the persistence of spores.[32] Direct contact with contaminated animal meat or carcasses or with contaminated animal products, such as hides, hair, wool, bone meal, and animal feeds, can transmit anthrax spores to humans.[9] Commercially processed products, such as shaving brushes and saddle blankets, have been implicated as sources of infection. Cutaneous anthrax may be transmitted through the deposition of spores or bacilli into abrasions or cuts in the skin by nonbiting insects, such as houseflies.[20] Rubbing with contaminated fingers or possibly an insect vector may lead to cutaneous involvement of the eyelids.[36] Although discharges from cutaneous lesions potentially are infectious, there have been no confirmed cases of person-to-person transmission. Bloodsucking insects, including mosquitoes and stable flies, may be vectors of the disease.[31, 32]

Inhalation anthrax, or woolsorters' disease, results from inhalation of spores. The most recently reported case of inhalation anthrax in the United States occurred in a weaver whose imported yarn was contaminated with *B. anthracis*.[5] Gastrointestinal anthrax is caused by ingestion of contaminated meat. Children of industrial workers have acquired infection, presumably from contaminated clothing.[4] A newborn acquiring anthrax meningitis from his mother, who was septicemic at the time of delivery, has been reported.[13]

An estimated 2000 to 20,000 human cases of anthrax occur yearly.[14] Areas of high prevalence include the Near and Middle East, Africa, and parts of South America and Europe.[14] The incidence probably correlates with the enzootic status of the disease in the livestock of these countries. Familial clustering has been associated with exposure to diseased animals.[1, 23] A large outbreak of inhalation anthrax that occurred in 1979 in Sverdlovsk in the former Soviet Union was likely due to release of a biologic agent from a military facility in the district.[2] In endemic areas, children frequently contract cutaneous anthrax from direct contact with animals.[26] More than 50 per cent of 448 patients with cutaneous anthrax reported from Gambia were younger than 15 years of age, and 11 per cent were younger than 2 years of age.[15] Both sexes are affected equally.

In the United States, epizootics of anthrax occur in the lower Mississippi valley and in parts of California, Texas, Missouri, Nebraska, and South Dakota[34]; sporadic cases have been reported from almost every state. The incidence of human anthrax in this country has decreased significantly since the early 1900s, when more than 100 cases were reported annually. Between 1984 and 1993, only three cases of anthrax, all cutaneous, were reported to the Centers for Disease Control and Prevention.[16] Cases often are associated with exposure to contaminated animal products in commercial preparation, but exposure to indigenous animal anthrax does occur in the United States.[28] In children, a history of exposure may be difficult to elicit. For example, the only known source in an 11-year-old child with a cutaneous lesion was proximity to a bone meal factory, which he passed on the way to school.[17]

PATHOGENESIS AND PATHOLOGY

Three virulence factors have been described for *B. anthracis*: edema toxin, lethal toxin, and a poly-D-glutamic acid capsule. One plasmid regulates production of the toxins, and another plasmid regulates capsule production. Toxemia is the critical factor in determining morbidity. The toxins are composed of three proteins—protective antigen (PA), lethal factor (LF), and edema factor (EF)—that individually are not toxic. EF is a calmodulin-dependent adenylate cyclase.[18] PA combines with EF or LF to form the two toxins of *B. anthracis*, edema toxin and lethal toxin, respectively. Edema toxin induces an increase in intracellular cyclic-AMP levels and elicits skin edema, and lethal toxin causes death in experimental animals. PA is the receptor-binding component mediating entry of either LF or EF into target cells.[18] The capsule inhibits phagocytosis, and each of the toxins inhibits priming of neutrophils by lipopolysaccharide, thereby modulating the inflammatory response.[35]

Interstitial edema, lymphatic dilatation, and thrombosis and necrosis of blood vessels are characteristic microscopic features of cutaneous anthrax lesions. Erythrocytes extravasate freely into the interstitial fluid. Few neutrophils or other inflammatory cells are present, unless the lesion is infected secondarily. Hemorrhagic lymphadenitis involving regional lymph nodes occurs in all forms of anthrax. In pulmonary anthrax, spores entering the alveoli are carried through lymphatic channels to the hilar lymph nodes, where germination occurs. The massive hemorrhagic mediastinal lymphadenitis that follows may cause blockage of lymphatic drainage routes and may be related causally to the pulmonary edema and respiratory distress observed clinically.[33] Primary focal hemorrhagic necrotizing pneumonia may be observed at the pulmonary portal of entry.[2] Edema and small necrotic ulcers of the mucosa of the gastrointestinal tract are characteristic autopsy findings in intestinal anthrax. Dissemination to the central nervous system may occur by hematogenous or lymphatic routes. Hemorrhage involving the meninges and intense arteritis are uniform findings in patients who die of anthrax meningitis, but pathologic changes in brain tissue have not been observed.

CLINICAL MANIFESTATIONS

Cutaneous Anthrax

The lesions of cutaneous anthrax occur mainly on exposed areas of the body. In one report, the distribution among young children was head and neck (52 per cent), trunk (28 per cent), and extremities (20 per cent) and among older children was 70 per cent, 16 per cent, and 14 per cent, respectively.[15] Skin lesions develop after the implantation of anthrax spores through epidermal defects. Lesions usually are single and are associated with regional adenitis. After an incubation period of 2 to 5 days, a small, nontender, but frequently pruritic papule develops at the site of inoculation. Progression to a serous or serosanguineous vesicle is rapid. A central black eschar surrounded by a ring of secondary vesicles, sometimes called the "pearly wreath,"[36] and intensive nonpitting edema evolve within 36 hours. The term *malignant edema* is used to describe severe lesions, particularly those involving the head and neck, which may be associated with systemic toxicity and occlusion of the airway. Small children may appear acutely ill, with a temperature of 39° to 40° C and leukocytosis of 20,000 to 30,000 cells/mm^3.[26] Approximately 5 per cent of patients are bacteremic. With appropriate therapy, edema usually resolves within 2 to 3 days, but the central lesion continues its evolution unaffected. The eschar usually is 1 to 3 cm in diameter with sharply defined margins 1 week to 10 days after onset. Separation of the eschar may take several weeks, and healing occurs with variable central scarring.[17]

Inhalation Anthrax

Inhalation anthrax is a biphasic illness. Symptoms in the initial stage—malaise, low-grade fever, myalgia, and nonproductive cough—are nonspecific and resemble a viral upper respiratory illness or bronchitis. After several days, dyspnea and stridor initiate the onset of the second stage, which usually terminates fatally within 24 hours. Widening of the mediastinum with smooth borders and lack of pulmonary infiltrates are radiographic features suggestive of anthrax during the second stage.[33] Pulmonary hemorrhage or edema and pleural effusion may be evident radiographically. Pulmonary infiltrates are usually the result of superimposed bacterial infection. Patchy infiltrates consistent with septic pulmonary emboli may be observed in patients who are septicemic in association with primary cutaneous anthrax.[33]

Gastrointestinal Anthrax

After an incubation period of 2 to 5 days after the ingestion of contaminated meat, symptoms of diffuse abdominal pain with rebound tenderness and fever develop. Vomiting of blood-tinged or coffee ground–like material and melena are common and are secondary to ulceration of the intestinal mucosa.[22] Pain decreases and patients develop massive ascites 24 to 48 hours after the onset of symptoms. Abdominal radiographs at this time show edematous loops of bowel and decreased air. If the abdomen is explored, findings include enlarged, erythematous mesenteric lymph nodes and straw-colored to purulent ascitic fluid in which organisms are readily visible.[3] Death usually occurs in association with significant blood loss, fluid and electrolyte imbalance, and subsequent shock. If the patient survives the acute illness, edema and melena subside in 10 to 14 days.

Involvement of the oral cavity, the oropharynx, or both with anthrax lesions has been reported in association with ingestion of contaminated water buffalo meat.[24] The initial symptoms include neck swelling due to edema and enlargement of cervical lymph nodes, dysphagia, and respiratory difficulty. Lesions on the tonsils or posterior pharynx progress from an area of edema to a pseudomembrane-covered ulcer over a 1- to 2-week period. The oropharyngeal form of anthrax, although uncommon, has a more favorable prognosis than the classic gastrointestinal disease.

Meningitis

The primary focus in anthrax meningitis usually is the skin, although involvement of the lungs or intestines has been reported. In one report of 70 patients ranging in age from newborn to 71 years, no primary focus could be found in 11.5 per cent of patients.[13] Young and middle-aged males are affected most frequently as a result of occupational exposure. The onset of meningitis is sudden. In addition to meningeal signs, clinical features include nausea and vomiting, myalgia, chills, dizziness, and, occasionally, a petechial rash. Progressive neurologic deterioration with delirium, convulsions, and coma usually occurs in 2 to 4 days. Although less than 5 per cent of patients survive the acute illness, there are reports of survival without apparent neurologic sequelae in at least three children, two of whom had cutaneous lesions at the time of diagnosis.[25, 27, 29]

Examination of the cerebrospinal fluid reveals (1) gross or microscopic hemorrhage, (2) leukocytosis consisting predominantly of polymorphonuclear leukocytes, (3) elevated protein, and (4) depressed glucose levels. Gram-positive rods can be seen easily on smears of cerebrospinal fluid. Peripheral leukocytosis is common, and the white blood cell count may be as high as 60,000 to 80,000 cells/mm^3. Blood cultures yield the organism in 70 per cent and cerebrospinal fluid in virtually 100 per cent of patients.[13]

DIAGNOSIS AND DIFFERENTIAL DIAGNOSIS

B. anthracis may be demonstrated by direct smear and cultured from vesicular fluid or exudate from cutaneous lesions and from pleural fluid, blood, and cerebrospinal fluid in systemic infections. The diagnosis may be confirmed by a fourfold rise in titer in paired sera or by a single titer greater than 1:32. More than 90 per cent of patients have a significant antibody titer in serum obtained between 3 weeks and 6 months after onset of illness.[7] Immunoblot and an enzyme-linked immunosorbent assay for detection of capsular antibody are promising newer diagnostic methods.[14]

The lesion of cutaneous anthrax must be differentiated from ecthyma gangrenosum and from ulcerative skin lesions with regional lymphadenopathy, including rat-bite fever, ulceroglandular tularemia, plague, glanders, rickettsialpox, cowpox, and orf. Staphylococcal lymphangitis may be distinguished from anthrax by the discharge of purulent material and by the inflammatory response observed microscopically. The first stage of inhalation anthrax and the clinical presentation of the intestinal form are nonspecific, and a history of exposure is extremely important for establishing the diagnosis. Gastrointestinal anthrax must be differentiated from other causes of abdominal catastrophe and, if bleeding is associated, from duodenal ulcer, typhoid, and intestinal tularemia. Anthrax causes a hemorrhagic meningitis, which must be differentiated from subarachnoid hemorrhage.[13]

TREATMENT

Penicillin, the antibiotic of choice, should be administered intravenously in a dose of 300,000 to 400,000 U/kg/day for systemic anthrax and for cutaneous infection if (1) there are signs of systemic toxicity, (2) lesions are located on the head and neck, and (3) extensive edema is present.[26] Penicillin combined with streptomycin or, possibly, parenteral ciprofloxacin should be used for treating inhalation anthrax or anthrax meningitis. The risk-benefit ratio should be considered in initiating ciprofloxacin, because it is not approved for use in patients younger than 18 years of age.[10] Treatment should be continued for at least 14 days in systemic infections. The lesion of cutaneous anthrax becomes sterile after 24 hours, and edema subsides within 2 to 5 days, but progression to the eschar phase occurs despite appropriate therapy. Treatment should be continued for 3 to 5 days after sterilization. The cutaneous lesion should be cleansed and covered, but local excision is contraindicated. It is not necessary to continue therapy until the eschar has sloughed or until regional adenopathy has resolved. Penicillin by the oral route at a dosage of 50,000 units/kg/day for 7 to 10 days is adequate for therapy of mild cutaneous anthrax. Alternative effective antimicrobial agents for patients with penicillin allergy include erythromycin, tetracycline, chloramphenicol, and ciprofloxacin.[10] Resistance to penicillin has been reported but is rare.[6]

Supportive therapy includes attention to details of fluid and electrolyte balance, endotracheal intubation if indicated to maintain a patent airway, and local care for cutaneous lesions. Systemic steroids may reduce the severity of infections in patients with massive edema[26] or meningitis.[27] A specific anthrax antitoxin is not available.

PROGNOSIS

Prior to the introduction of penicillin, cutaneous anthrax was fatal in approximately 20 per cent of patients. With effective treatment, the mortality rate has been reduced to less than 1 per cent. Cutaneous anthrax of the eyelid may be complicated by ectropion of the upper lid and corneal scarring with blindness.[36] Immunity probably is lifelong in most patients. Although second attacks of cutaneous anthrax have been recorded, these have not been confirmed serologically and usually are mild.[8, 15] Fatality rates are high for all forms of systemic anthrax, ranging from 50 to 100 per cent for gastrointestinal anthrax to virtually 100 per cent for inhalation anthrax, but children who survive these infections have no apparent sequelae.

PREVENTION

A cell-free anthrax vaccine may be obtained from the Division of Biologic Products, Michigan Department of Public Health, Lansing, MI. Its recommended administration is limited to those persons who process potentially contaminated imported animal products (especially goat hair) and to laboratory workers who have contact with *B. anthracis*.[21] Use of penicillin prophylactically for 7 days may prevent infection after known exposure.[7] Hospitalized patients should be kept under strict isolation until lesions are bacteriologically sterile. Contaminated dressings and clothing must be burned or sterilized and the patient's room disinfected to destroy spores.

Procedures to prevent spread of anthrax in animals include disposal of contaminated carcasses by burning and annual vaccination of livestock in known enzootic areas. All suspected or proven cases of anthrax should be reported to public health officials.

References

1. Abdenour, D., Larouze, B., Dalichaouche, M., et al.: Familial occurrence of anthrax in Eastern Algeria. J. Infect. Dis. *155*:1083, 1987.
2. Abramova, F. A., Grinberg, L. M., Yampolskaya, O. V., et al.: Pathology of inhalational anthrax in 42 cases from the Sverdlovsk outbreak of 1979. Proc. Natl. Acad. Sci. U. S. A. *90*:2291, 1993.
3. Alizad, A., Ayoub, E. M., and Makki, N.: Intestinal anthrax in a two-year-old child. Pediatr. Infect. Dis. J. *14*:394, 1995.
4. Brachman, P. S.: Anthrax. Ann. N. Y. Acad. Sci. *174*:577, 1970.
5. Brachman, P. S.: Inhalation anthrax. Ann. N. Y. Acad. Sci. *353*:83, 1980.

6. Bradarić, N., and Punda-Polić, V.: Cutaneous anthrax due to penicillin-resistant *Bacillus anthracis* transmitted by an insect bite. Lancet *340*:306, 1992.
7. Buchanan, T. M., Feeley, J. C., Hayes, P. S., et al.: Anthrax indirect microhemagglutination test. J. Immunol. *107*:1631, 1971.
8. Christie, A. B.: The clinical aspects of anthrax. Postgrad. Med. J. *49*:565, 1973.
9. Christie, A. B.: Anthrax. Practitioner *191*:588, 1963.
10. Committee on Infectious Diseases, American Academy of Pediatrics. *In* Peter, G. (ed.): 1994 Red Book. 23rd ed. Elk Grove Village, IL, 1994, pp. 121–123.
11. Doyle, R. J., Keller, K. F., and Ezzell, J. W.: *Bacillus*. *In* Lennette, E. H., Balows, A., Hauser, W. J., Jr., et al. (eds.): Manual of Clinical Microbiology. 4th ed. Washington, D.C., American Society for Microbiology, 1985, pp. 211–215.
12. Gerhardt, P.: Cytology of *Bacillus anthracis*. Fed. Proc. *26*:1504, 1967.
13. Haight, T. H.: Anthrax meningitis: Review of literature and report of two cases with autopsies. Am. J. Med. Sci. *224*:57, 1952.
14. Harrison, L. H., Ezzell, J. W., Veterinary Laboratory Investigation Center, et al.: Evaluation of serologic tests for diagnosis of anthrax after an outbreak of cutaneous anthrax in Paraguay. J. Infect. Dis. *160*:706, 1989.
15. Heyworth, B., Ropp, M. E., Voos, U. G., et al.: Anthrax in the Gambia: An epidemiological study. Br. Med. J. *4*:79, 1975.
16. LaForce, F. M.: Anthrax. Clin. Infect. Dis. *19*:1009, 1994.
17. Lamb, R.: Anthrax. Br. Med. J. *1*:157, 1973.
18. Leppla, S. H.: *Bacillus anthracis* calmodulin dependent adenylate cyclase: Chemical and enzymatic properties and interactions with eucaryotic cells. Adv. Cyclic Nucleotite Protein Phosphorylation Res. *17*:189, 1984.
19. Manios, S., and Kavaliotis, I.: Anthrax in children: A long forgotten, potentially fatal infection. Scand. J. Infect. Dis. *11*:203, 1979.
20. McKendrick, D. R. A.: Anthrax and its transmission to humans. Cent. Afr. J. Med. *26*:126, 1980.
21. Morbidity and Mortality Weekly Report: Recommendations of the Immunization Practices Advisory Committee, 1984: Anthrax and anthrax vaccine. M. M. W. R. *33*(Suppl. 1):33, 1985.
22. Nalin, D. R., Sultana, B., Sahunja, R., et al.: Survival of a patient with intestinal anthrax. Am. J. Med. *62*:130, 1977.
23. Seboxa, T., and Goldhagen, J.: Anthrax in Ethiopia. Trop. Geogr. Med. *41*:108, 1989.
24. Sirisanthana, T., Navachareon, N., Tharavichitkul, P., et al.: Outbreak of oral-pharyngeal anthrax: An unusual manifestation of human infection with *Bacillus anthracis*. Am. J. Med. Hyg. *33*:144, 1984.
25. Tabatabaie, P., and Syadati, A.: *Bacillus anthracis* as a cause of bacterial meningitis. Pediatr. Infect. Dis. J. *12*:1035, 1993.
26. Tahernia, A. C.: Treatment of anthrax in children. Arch. Dis. Child. *42*:181, 1967.
27. Tahernia, A. C., and Hashemi, G.: Survival in anthrax meningitis. Pediatrics *50*:329, 1972.
28. Taylor, J. P., Dimmitt, D. C., Ezzell, J. W., et al.: Indigenous human cutaneous anthrax in Texas. South. Med. J. *86*:1, 1993.
29. Tengio, F. U.: Anthrax meningitis: Report of two cases. East Afr. Med. J. *50*:337, 1973
30. Tigertt, W. D.: Anthrax. William Smith Greenfield, M.D., F.R.C.P., Professor Superintendent, The Brown Animal Sanatory Institution (1878–1881). Concerning the priority due to him for the production of the first vaccine against anthrax. J. Hyg. Camb. *85*:415, 1980.
31. Turell, M. J., and Knudson, G. B.: Mechanical transmission of *Bacillus anthracis* by stable flies *(Stomoxys calcitrans)* and mosquitoes *(Aedes aegypti* and *Aedes taeniorhynchus)*. Infect. Immun. *55*:1859, 1987.
32. Van Ness, G. B.: Ecology of anthrax. Science *172*:1303, 1971.
33. Vessal, K., Yeganehdoust, J., Dutz, W., et al.: Radiological changes in inhalation anthrax: A report of radiological and pathological correlation in two cases. Clin. Radiol. *26*:471, 1975.
34. Wolff, A. H., and Heimann, H.: Industrial anthrax in the United States. Am. J. Hyg. *53*:80, 1951.
35. Wright, G. G., and Mandell, G. L.: Anthrax toxin blocks priming of neutrophils by lipopolysaccharide and by muramyl dipeptide. J. Exp. Med. *164*:1700, 1986.
36. Yorston, D., and Foster, A.: Cutaneous anthrax leading to corneal scarring from cicatricial ectropion. Br. J. Ophthalmol. *73*:809, 1989.

97

BACILLUS CEREUS

Enrique Caceres and Thomas G. Cleary

The recognition of *Bacillus cereus* pathogenicity was delayed until the clarification in the early 1950s of the taxonomy of the genus *Bacillus*. It is likely that multiple early reports of food poisoning and other infections, including gastroenteritis, bacteremia-septicemia, cellulitis, ear and eye infections, endocarditis, and urinary tract infection, attributed to *B. subtilis* or to other *Bacillus* species were in fact due to *B. cereus*.[77] Now it is recognized widely that *B. cereus* can give rise to two distinct forms of food-borne disease, the emetic and the diarrheal syndromes, related to different toxins, as well as occasional localized and systemic disease.[34]

The diarrheal syndrome first was recognized by Hauge[39] in 1955 after four clinically similar outbreaks in Norway. This common form of disease was related to a great variety of foods, such as meat and vegetable soups, poultry, puddings, sauces, pastas, cakes, and milk. In 1974, Mortimer and McCann[58] described a vomiting syndrome associated with consumption of fried rice in Chinese restaurants. Despite widespread recognition in Europe, *B. cereus* outbreaks have been reported infrequently in the United States. The first documented outbreak in the United States was in 1970.[55]

BACTERIOLOGY

Members of the genus *Bacillus* are aerobic or facultative anaerobic, gram-positive or gram-variable, spore-forming rods. They are distributed widely in the environment because of the high resistance of their endospores to extreme conditions, including heat, cold, desiccation, salinity, and radiation.[26, 66] Based on the high guanine plus cytosine content variability, from 32 per cent to 69 per cent, there is debate regarding classification of *Bacillus* species.[81]

B. cereus, together with other recognized pathogens (*B. anthracis*, *B. megaterium*, *B. thuringiensis*, *B. subtilis*, *B. pumilus*, and *B. licheniformis*), belongs to the subgroup 1 of the genus, that is, gram-positive rods that produce central or terminal ellipsoid or cylindrical spores that do not distend the sporangia.[81] Studies of DNA-DNA hybridization, 16s-rRNA and 23s-rRNA sequencing, as well as enzyme electrophoretic patterns, have shown a close relationship among subgroup 1 species. Differentiation sometimes is difficult in the diagnostic laboratory, particularly between *B. cereus* and the insect pathogen *B. thuringiensis*. Polymerase chain reaction technology has been applied for the identification of species.[15]

B. cereus is a flagellated, motile, gram-positive rod, typically 1.0 to 1.2 μm in diameter by 3.0 to 5.0 μm in length. The organism sporulates freely on many media under well-aerated conditions, but vegetative cells also can grow anaerobically. It is able to metabolize glucose, fructose, and sucrose but not pentoses and other sugar alcohols. It produces acid from glucose but not from arabinose, xylose, or mannitol. Starch hydrolysis and catalase production are similar to those of the other members of the genus. The presence of lipid globules or protoplasts is a characteristic it shares with *B. megaterium*.[49] The colonies on blood agar are large, flat, granular, and slightly green-tinged. *B. cereus* is differentiated from *B. anthracis* by motility, hemolysis, lack of lysis by gamma phage, penicillin resistance, and absence of a capsule in *B. cereus*.[26] However, morphologic differentiation may be difficult with nonmotile *B. cereus* strains and *B. anthracis* strains that occasionally are weakly hemolytic.

Growth and multiplication of vegetative cells occur in a temperature range of 10° C to 50° C, with an optimum of 28° C to 35° C. Some strains responsible for milk spoilage can grow at as low as 5° C.[49, 66] Few strains are able to produce toxin at temperature levels below 7° C.[66] Variations in toxic levels found in certain foods also can be related to pH levels, sugar content, presence of other lactic acid bacteria, and aeration.[71, 72]

Serologic differentiation of *Bacillus* species is hampered by cross-reactive antigens and autoagglutination of spores due to hydrophobic surface properties. Serologic typing based on the flagellar (H) antigen can be used to distinguish between strains and to determine the similarity of isolates obtained from humans during an outbreak with the strains isolated from suspect foods.[26] The serotype scheme is based on 42 H antisera raised against prototype strains. It has been suggested that a common flagellar antigenic epitope exists. Detection of the flagellar antigen by enzyme-linked immunosorbent assay is perhaps more sensitive than that by the agglutination method.[59] In addition to serology and biotyping (based on biochemical typing), plasmid analysis and phage typing have proved useful epidemiologically.[2, 49, 69, 86] New techniques, such as pyrolysis mass spectrometry and gas liquid chromatography of whole cell fatty acids, are showing promise.[26]

Diagnosis of the rare extraintestinal infection is made by isolation from normally sterile sites (blood or tissue) after overnight incubation on nutrient or blood agar; clinical specimens from normally nonsterile sites (feces, vomitus) and food or environmental samples require selective techniques. Polymyxin B is used as a selective agent, and the lecithinase reaction of the organism on egg yolk and its inability to catabolize mannitol permit presumptive identification using a variety of media: mannitol–egg yolk–polymyxin-B, Kim and Goepfert medium, and polymyxin-B–pyruvate–egg yolk–mannitol with bromothimol blue or bromocresol purple.[26]

EPIDEMIOLOGY

B. cereus in the spore and vegetative form is a ubiquitous organism, found in soil, water, vegetation, and food products, especially cereals, dairy products, dried foods, spices, meat products, and vegetables.[49]

The emetic syndrome typically is associated with cooked rice, usually fried, from Chinese restaurants.[58] It used to be the practice to save portions of boiled rice at room temperature over night until required for frying. Refrigerating boiled rice makes the grains stick together and hence less convenient for frying.[73] The spores of *B. cereus* survive cooking and are capable of germination and outgrowth.[35, 37] The optimum temperature for growth in boiled rice is between 30° C and 37° C, although growth occurs during storage at 15° C to 43° C.[35] Most samples of uncooked rice contain multiple serotypes of *B. cereus,* and there is little difference in the growth rate of the various serotypes in boiled rice at 22° C, but spores of serotype 1 strains are more resistant to heating at 95° C. This is the likely reason this serotype usually is implicated in outbreaks.[60]

Starchy dried foods other than rice, including pulse and cereals, frequently are contaminated.[14] Tortillas can be contaminated with the water used in preparation and from the hands of producers.[18] A specific food has been incriminated in 49 of 58 recent U.S. outbreaks. Chinese food accounted for 50 per cent of those, followed by Mexican food, beef, fruits, and vegetables.[7] Other implicated foods included beef stew,[25] turkey loaf,[33] barbecued pork,[52] macaroni and cheese,[42] and potatoes.[46] Among the factors thought to contribute in the outbreaks, the most frequent were improper storage or holding temperature (94 per cent), contaminated equipment (53 per cent), inadequate cooking (32 per cent), and poor personal hygiene (24 per cent).[7, 8]

Studies in three different populations in South Africa and London including school age children found the organism in 18 to 43 per cent of fecal samples.[82] The organism thus can be part of the normal intestinal flora. *B. cereus* does not persist in the intestine after ingestion.[32] *B. cereus* outbreaks have been recognized widely in Europe but rarely in the United States. In the Netherlands, *B. cereus* reportedly was the cause of 22.4 per cent of food-borne disease outbreaks of known bacterial cause. Similarly, in Finland, it accounted for 11.9 per cent of outbreaks. However, in most places, *B. cereus* is incriminated in 0.9 to 7 per cent of outbreaks of food-related disease and 0.7 to 3 per cent of cases.[49] In the United States, 10 outbreaks of *B. cereus* gastroenteritis affecting 133 persons were reported to the Centers for Disease Control and Prevention between 1966 and 1975. Seven of the outbreaks were of the diarrheal syndrome, and three were of the emetic type.[73] For the period 1973 to 1987, 58 of 2841 (2 per cent) food-borne disease outbreaks of known etiology and 1123 of 124,994 (1 per cent) of total cases related to them were attributed to *B. cereus*.[7] The susceptibility of children to this pathogen is evident from the report of an outbreak involving two day care centers,[48] as well as other reports including neonates, children, and adolescents.[29, 41, 45, 61, 65, 78, 89] Only a small fraction of outbreaks are reported to the Centers for Disease Control and Prevention. Small outbreaks of mild, brief illness are less likely to be reported.

For infections not related to food, groups at risk include neonates,[29, 61] immunocompromised hosts,[4, 28, 37, 41, 45, 69, 75] intravenous drug abusers,[21, 75] and patients with intravascular devices or artificial prostheses.[4, 5, 28, 29, 69, 70]

PATHOGENESIS

B. cereus produces an enormous range of extracellular metabolites, including peptides with antibiotic properties (biocerin, cerein, thiocillins), beta-lactamases, hydrolases, nuclease, urease, and proteases.[77] Two different toxins, known as diarrheal toxin (also called diarrheagenic factor, intestinonecrotic toxin, dermonecrotic toxin, and mouse lethal factor #1) and emetic toxin, are responsible for the clinical syndromes of food poisoning.[54, 83] It is likely that the amount of the pertinent toxin secreted by a particular strain determines which clinical syndrome occurs. Some strains may be able to produce both toxins, based on the evidence that occasionally culture filtrates derived from strains isolated from emetic poisoning are able to produce a positive rabbit ileal loop assay.[66]

Biologic activities of the diarrheal toxin can be demonstrated in multiple different assay systems. The purification and isolation of multiple toxic fractions with some but not all of these activities have caused confusion.[26,76] The evaluation of toxic activity of whole-cell suspension, cell-free culture filtrates, and the purified enterotoxin complex classically has included the rabbit ileal loop fluid accumulation assay, vascular permeability in rabbit skin, dermonecrosis and intestinonecrosis, mouse lethality, cytotoxicity, and hemolysis.[10, 17, 51, 74, 79, 84] Toxin assays initially were difficult to interpret because different strains and different growth media and conditions of isolation produce various degrees of activity.[36] In general, there is good correlation between the rabbit ileal loop activity and the vascular permeability assay.

Complete characterization of the diarrheal toxin is not available, but it is a relatively unstable protein, thermolabile, that has a molecular weight of approximately 50,000 daltons and a pI of 4.8, is susceptible to protease digestion, and is synthesized during the late logarithmic growth phase at an optimum temperature of 32° C to 37° C and at a pH of 7.5.[26, 49, 77]

The emetic toxin has been characterized partially. It is a heat-stable protein (126° C for 90 minutes) with a molecular weight of less than 15,000 daltons, stable at a pH between 2 and 11, and protease-resistant. Unlike the diarrheal toxin, it is preformed in foods, so the presence of living organisms at the ingestion time is not necessary to cause symptoms.[34, 77] A new assay in HEp-2 (larynx carcinoma) tissue culture shows that rice culture filtrates derived from emetic syndrome–associated strains cause cytoplasmic vacuolation and swollen mitochondria, suggesting uncoupling of oxidative phosphorylation.[63] A novel dodecadepsipeptide, cereulide, is a fairly recently characterized HEp-2 cell vacuolation factor of *B. cereus*, with emetic activity acting through the 5-HT3 receptor and stimulation of the vagus afferent nerve; it may be the emetic toxin.[1]

Among the multiple other substances with relevant activity, two groups are associated with local infection.[79, 80] Cereolysin, or hemolysin I, is a thiol-activated cytolysin. There are also phospholipase-C– or lecithinase-like substances, including a sphingomyelinase and two hydrolases with preferences for phosphatidylcholine and phosphatidylinositol. These enzymes cause release of lysosomal enzymes from neutrophils that probably are involved in tissue damage, especially in wound and ocular infections.[26, 90]

CLINICAL MANIFESTATIONS

Food Poisoning

DIARRHEAL SYNDROME. The enterotoxin preformed in the food or produced in vivo in the intestine after ingestion of bacilli causes profuse, watery, nonbloody diarrhea accompanied by abdominal pain and cramps, nausea, and, in a few occasions, vomiting or low-grade fever.[3, 25, 33, 46, 49, 53, 68] The typical incubation period is 8 to 16 hours, and the clinical characteristics resemble the food poisoning of *Clostridium perfringes*. The symptoms resolve within approximately 12 to 24 hours but occasionally can last 2 days to 2 weeks.[33] The diarrhea (3 to 10 bowel movements per day) rarely leads to dehydration in healthy individuals. In the elderly, bloody stools can occur.[33] The most prevalent flagellar H serotypes are 1, 2, 6, 8, 10, 12, and 19. Serotyping is available at research laboratories.[14, 25, 52, 82]

EMETIC SYNDROME. The usual illness is characterized by rapid onset (within 1 to 5 hours after ingestion of contaminated food) of nausea, vomiting, and malaise, occasionally followed by diarrhea hours later.[58] Infrequently, the diarrhea is reported to last several days.[87]

Extraintestinal Infections

EYE INFECTION. Keratitis, conjunctivitis, endophthalmitis, and panophthalmitis can be produced by *B. cereus*. Posttraumatic endophthalmitis is caused by this organism in 27 to 46 per cent of cases.[23, 85] A history of soil contamination or presence of a metal foreign body should raise clinical suspicion. Less frequently, corneal ulcers and surgical procedures are the predisposing factors.[40, 85] Exogenous endophthalmitis usually progresses rapidly, with deterioration of vision in less than 48 hours. Severe pain is accompanied by chemosis, periorbital swelling, proptosis, and pus in the anterior chamber. The classic lesion is a corneal ring abscess, similar to that produced by *Pseudomonas* and *Proteus* species. Endogenous cases may present with subretinal exudation, retinal hemorrhages, and perivasculitis. Associated systemic symptoms are not unusual.[21] The outcome is poor, with almost half of the patients left with a visual acuity no better than simple light perception.[85] Many patients require enucleation. Endogenous ophthalmitis is linked with the use of illicit intravenous drugs or transfusion of contaminated blood products resulting in bacteremic seeding of one eye.[21, 69, 75, 85]

The pathogenesis of *B. cereus* on the ocular tissue has been linked to lecithinase activity of the phospholipase C. A new toxin fraction, hemolysin BL, which is formed by three separate components, produces similar destruction of retinal tissue in vitro and in animal experiments.[9] Its relation with the diarrheal enterotoxin is not clear.[10]

WOUND INFECTIONS AND SOFT TISSUE INFECTIONS. Wound infections of variable severity related to trauma, burns, or postsurgical complications occasionally are reported.[78, 79, 80, 89] Because *Bacillus* is a common environmental contaminant, proof of relevance of a *B. cereus* isolate is clearer if the organism is obtained from deep tissue in heavy pure growth. Severe infections in persons involved in motor vehicle accidents can be complicated by necrotizing fasciitis and require extensive débridement.[89] Superficial, benign, infected wounds are common in the tropics.[27] Immunosuppressed patients may present with a severe gas gangrene–like infection requiring amputation[38] or with a less severe primary cutaneous infection manifested by vesicles, pustules, or cellulitis.[41]

MUSCULOSKELETAL INFECTIONS. Cases of chronic osteomyelitis are rare and result from accidental or surgical trauma. Radical débridement and antibiotic treatment are required.[69] *B. cereus* can be found as a copathogen with other more frequent pathogenic bacteria, delaying the resolution of symptoms until its eradication.[65] Acute osteomyelitis may occur in drug abusers.[69, 75]

BACTEREMIA AND SEPTICEMIA. Bacteremia occurs with indwelling catheters and other foreign bodies, contaminated intravenous drugs (e.g., heroin), and blood products, particularly platelets.[16, 28, 92] Immunosuppression and impaired neutrophil killing, such as those caused by neutropenia due to malignancy or chemotherapy and immaturity of the immune system in neonates, are major contributors to morbidity in systemic *B. cereus* infection.[4, 43, 61, 62] Endocarditis is an infrequent complication of bacteremia that usually occurs in intravenous drug abusers or in individuals with a chronic intravascular device.[69, 75] Vegetations can be formed over mechanical prosthetic valves or pacemaker wires, requiring their replacement.[69, 70] Morbidity and mortality rates are high among patients with valvular heart disease. Fatal serosanguineous pericarditis in a patient undergoing hemodialysis has been reported.[30]

PNEUMONIA. Primary pulmonary disease rarely has been recorded. The presentation can be subacute with cough, fever, dyspnea, chest pain, and hemoptysis, with progression to necrotizing pneumonia, cavitation, and empyema. The pleural fluid may appear serosanguineous or sanguinopurulent.[12, 43] Underlying predisposing conditions include leukemia, alcohol abuse, chronic hepatitis, and steroid use.[12, 28, 43, 69]

Multiorgan disease in premature neonates with necrotizing pneumonia usually is fatal.[47] Blood culture is positive in 75 per cent of cases, followed by pleural fluid and sputum culture in 40 to 60 per cent of cases.[12] The pleural space may become contaminated with *B. cereus* by mishandling of the thoracic drainage system in patients with other causes of pleuritis.[44]

CENTRAL NERVOUS SYSTEM INFECTION. Intracranial shunts and penetrating surgical or traumatic cranial wounds expose the central nervous system to environmental *B. cereus*.[29, 67] Spinal anesthesia[28] was associated with *Bacillus* infection in the past. Contamination in the operating room through the linen is a potential source.[5, 6] Premature neonates are susceptible to seeding in the meninges secondary to dissemination of intravascular infection related to catheters.[61] As in patients with other serious infections, those with immunosuppression are at a higher risk.[43] The cerebrospinal fluid in *B. cereus* meningitis is purulent, with white blood cell counts more than 1000/mm^3, polymorphonuclear leukocytes predominating, and moderate increments in protein content. Gram stain is positive in 70 per cent of cases. Multiple brain abscesses may result from hematogenous spread in leukemic patients.[43, 45] Sequelae include hydrocephalus and brain damage. Often, the infection is fatal unless caused by a contaminated spinal anesthetic, in which case the course usually is more benign.

PSEUDOINFECTIONS. Pseudoepidemics with *B. cereus* are a challenge for the clinical microbiologist.[56] Because these spore formers are so hardy, they are common laboratory contaminants. Isolation of *Bacillus* species from clinical specimens usually should be considered a contaminant, although the pathogenic potential is well known.[22, 28, 43, 62, 69, 75, 79, 80] Pseudoinfections have been associated with contaminated blood culture media, syringes, blood culture analyzers, and fiberoptic bronchoscopes.[22] Colonization of umbilical cord stumps and eye surfaces by contaminated diapers may cause pseudo-outbreaks in nurseries.[91]

COMPLICATIONS

Death rarely or never complicates the food poisoning syndromes. Rapidly spreading wound infections may require amputation of extremities,[37] and ocular infections can lead to loss of vision with or without enucleation.[40, 85, 90] The risk of death in septicemia, endocarditis, and meningitis is related to the underlying condition and severity of the disease.[4, 41, 57, 61, 70]

DIAGNOSIS

The laboratory finding of *B. cereus* in a foodstuff without quantitative cultures and without epidemiologic data is insufficient to establish its role in an outbreak.[87] In practice, appropriate specimens often are either unavailable or submitted long after the incident, making their microbiologic significance questionable. Investigation for *B. cereus* should be requested specifically, inasmuch as many state public health laboratories do not make *B. cereus* testing routinely available.[48] During analysis of foods not involved in food-borne illness, the bacteria may be found in counts from 10^1 to 10^6 organisms per gram.[13, 14, 18, 35, 60, 71] The diagnosis of the diarrheal form of *B. cereus* food poisoning is supported by isolation of 10^5 or more organisms per gram from epidemiologically incriminated food.[57, 73] The levels of *B. cereus* found in the implicated foods usually are in the range of 5×10^5 to 9.5×10^8 colony-forming units per gram. With the exception of milk, the products rarely appear to be spoiled, in spite of the bacteria's high density. Isolation of more than 10^5 organisms per gram in the feces during the acute attack provides supportive evidence for the presumed diagnosis and confirms the association if the same serotype is isolated from incriminated food.

The organisms that produce emetic toxin are present in concentrations from 1.0×10^3 to 5.0×10^{10} colony-forming units per gram. Reheating may decrease or eliminate the organisms, leaving toxin intact but making isolation of the organism difficult.[26, 87]

Commercial immunoassay kits (reversed passive latex agglutination test, enzyme-linked immunosorbent assay, and microslide immunodiffusion assay) for detection of *B. cereus* diarrheal toxin are available. The kits may detect a variety of proteins.[11, 24] Experimental techniques based on the detection of genes for phospholipase C and sphingomyelinase by polymerase chain reaction have been developed for the identification of *B. cereus* in food products.[64]

The relevance of clinical isolates in extraintestinal syndromes can be assessed by the degree of growth (heavy vs. scanty), the number of occasions that growth was obtained, the source of the material cultured, and the predisposing or underlying conditions.[80] For suspected endophthalmitis, both aqueous and vitreous samples should be obtained if possible before institution of antibiotics.[23]

TREATMENT (Table 97–1)

During the mild, self-limited attack of food poisoning, patients require only supportive therapy.[73] Usually, oral fluid and electrolyte replacement is adequate.[33]

TABLE 97–1. Management of and Complications Associated with *Bacillus cereus* Infections

Condition	Management	Complications
Food poisoning	Supportive measures; hydration	None
Ocular	Systemic, topical, intravitreal antibiotics: vancomycin or clindamycin ± aminoglycosides; surgical: early vitrectomy	Severe decreased visual acuity, blindness, enucleation
Septicemia	Removal of IV device, foreign body; antibiotics IV (according to sensitivity); vancomycin	Localization of infection: endophthalmitis, endocarditis, meningitis; death
Pneumonia/pleuritis	IV antibiotics; drainage of pleural space; resection of necrotic tissue	Death
Meningitis	IV antibiotics; removal of infected intracranial shunts or cerebrospinal fluid reservoirs	Hydrocephalus, brain damage, death
Wound/subcutaneous infection	IV antibiotics; surgical débridement	Amputation, death

No antibiotic therapy is required, except in cases of non-gastrointestinal infections. The production of beta-lactamases by the majority of organisms renders penicillin derivatives and cephalosporins ineffective against *B. cereus*. Most strains are susceptible to chloramphenicol, vancomycin, clindamycin, aminoglycosides, erythromycin, tetracycline, imipenem, and ciprofloxacin.[4, 19, 79, 80, 88] Definitive antibiotic therapy should be based on the antibiogram susceptibility, but initial empiric therapy with clindamycin or vancomycin with or without an aminoglycoside is appropriate, pending susceptibility data.[4, 12, 22, 45, 65, 89] Ciprofloxacin has been reported to be useful in the treatment of recurrent pneumonia and bacteremia[31] and may have advantages in the penetration of respiratory and eye secretions,[50] but other options for children younger than 18 years of age are preferred.

Immediate empiric coverage for *B. cereus* is indicated for endophthalmitis in groups at risk. The selection of the antibiotic and the appropriate means of administration are subjects of controversy.[23] Clindamycin and an aminoglycoside[90] or vancomycin[85] are the best options. Together with parenterally administered antibiotics, topical and periocular antibiotics are considered adjunctive therapy. In cases of penetrating trauma, early vitrectomy and intravitreal antibiotics (1000 μg vancomycin in combination with 400 μg amikacin) should be considered.[23, 85]

Surgical débridement of necrotic tissue, drainage of closed space infections, and prompt removal of foreign bodies and indwelling catheters are important aspects of successful therapy.[12, 20, 65] Some bacteremic patients may be cured by intravenous catheter removal only.[69]

PREVENTION AND CONTROL

Low-level contamination in food products is difficult to avoid, but proper food handling should diminish the proliferation of bacilli.[66] Practical precautions for handling of cereals and rice include not preparing large quantities at a single time and maintaining the food at a hot temperature (>63° C) or cooling it quickly. The food must not be stored under warm conditions, especially in the range of 15° C to 50° C.[14, 35]

References

1. Agata, N., Ohta, M., Mori, M., et al.: A novel dodecadepsipeptide, cereulide, is an emetic toxin of *Bacillus cereus*. FEMS Microbiol. Letters *129*:17–20, 1995.
2. Ahmed, R., Sankar-Mistry, P., Jackson, S., et al.: *Bacillus cereus* phage typing as an epidemiological tool in outbreaks of food poisoning. J. Clin. Microbiol. *33*:636–640, 1995.
3. Baddour, L. M., Gala, S. M., Griffin, R., et al.: A hospital cafeteria–related food-borne outbreak due to *Bacillus cereus*: Unique features. Infect. Control *7*:462–465, 1986.
4. Banerjee, C., Bustamante, C. I., Wharton, R., et al.: *Bacillus* infections in patients with cancer. Arch. Intern. Med. *148*:1769–1774, 1988.
5. Barrie, D., Wilson, J. A., Hoffman, P. N., et al.: *Bacillus cereus* meningitis in two neurosurgical patients: An investigation into the source of the organism. J. Infect. *25*:291–297, 1992.
6. Barrie, D., Hoffman, P. N., Wilson, J. A., et al.: Contamination of hospital linen by *Bacillus cereus*. Epidemiol. Infect. *113*:297–306, 1994.
7. Bean, N. H., and Griffin, P. M.: Foodborne disease outbreaks in the United States, 1973–1987: Pathogens, vehicles and trends. J. Food Protect. *53*:804–817, 1990.
8. Bean, N. H., Griffin, P. M., Goulding, J. S., et al.: Foodborne Disease Outbreaks, 5 year summary, 1983–1987. M. M. W. R. CDC Surveillance Summaries *39*:15–55, 1990.
9. Beecher, D. J., Pulido, J. S., Barney, N. P., et al.: Extracellular virulence factors in *Bacillus cereus* endophthalmitis: Methods and implication of involvement of hemolysin BL. Infect. Immun. *63*:632–639, 1995.
10. Beecher, D. J., and Wong, A. C.: Improved purification and characterization of hemolysin BL, a hemolytic dermonecrotic vascular permeability factor from *Bacillus cereus*. Infect. Immun. *62*:980–986, 1994.
11. Beecher, D. J., and Wong, A. C.: Identification and analysis of the antigens detected by two commercial *Bacillus cereus* diarrheal enterotoxin immunoassay kits. Appl. Environ. Microbiol. *60*:4614–4616, 1994.
12. Bekemeyer, W. B., and Zimmerman, G. A.: Life threatening complications associated with *Bacillus cereus* pneumonia. Am. Rev. Respir. Dis. *131*:466–469, 1985.
13. Beuchat, L. R., and Ann Ma-Lin, C. F.: Growth of *Bacillus cereus* in media containing plant seed materials and ingredients used in Chinese cookery. J. Appl. Bacteriol. *48*:397–407, 1980.
14. Blakey, L. J., and Priest, F. G.: The occurrence of *Bacillus cereus* in some dried foods including pulses and cereals. J. Appl. Bacteriol. *48*:397–407, 1980.
15. Brousseau, R., Saint-Onge, A., Prefontaine, G., et al.: Arbitrary primer polymerase chain reaction, a powerful method to identify *Bacillus thuringiensis* serovars and strains. Appl. Environ. Microbiol. *59*:114–119, 1993.
16. Bryce, E. A., Smith, J. A., Tweeddale, M., et al.: Dissemination of *Bacillus cereus* in an intensive care unit. Infect. Contr. Hosp. Epidemiol. *14*:459–462, 1993.
17. Burdon, A. L., Davis, J. S., and Wende, R. D.: Experimental infection of mice with *Bacillus cereus*: Studies of pathogenesis and pathologic changes. J. Infect. Dis. *117*:307–316, 1967.
18. Capparelli, E., and Mata, L.: Microflora of maize prepared as tortillas. Appl. Microbiol. *29*:802–806, 1975.
19. Conrod, J. D., Leadley, P. J., and Eickhoff, T. C.: Antibiotic susceptibility of *Bacillus* species. J. Infect. Dis. *123*:102–105, 1971.
20. Cotton, D. J., Gill, V. J., Marshal, D. J., et al.: Clinical features and therapeutic interventions in 17 cases of *Bacillus* bacteremia in an immunosuppressed patient population. J. Clin. Microbiol. *25*:672–674, 1987.
21. Cowan, C. L., Jr., Madden, W. M., Hatem, G. F., et al.: Endogenous *Bacillus cereus* panophthalmitis. Ann. Ophthalmol. *19*:65–68, 1987.
22. Cunha, B. A.: Pseudomeningitis: Another nosocomial headache. Infect. Control. Hosp. Epidemiol. *9*:391–393, 1988.
23. David, D. B., Kirkby, G. R., and Noble, B. A.: *Bacillus cereus* endophthalmitis. Br. J. Ophthalmol. *78*:577–580, 1994.
24. Day, T. L., Tatani, S. R., Notermans, S., et al.: A comparison of ELISA and RPLA for detection of *Bacillus cereus* diarrhoeal enterotoxin. J. Appl. Bacteriol. *77*:9–13, 1994.
25. DeBuono, B. A., Brondum, J., Kramer, J. M., et al.: Plasmid, serotypic and enterotoxin analysis of *Bacillus cereus* in an outbreak setting. J. Clin. Microbiol. *26*:1571–1574, 1988.
26. Drobniewski, F. A.: *Bacillus cereus* and related species. Clin. Microbiol. Rev. *6*:324–338, 1993.
27. Dryden, M. S., and Kramer, J. M.: Toxigenic *Bacillus cereus* as a cause of wound infections in the tropics. J. Infect. *15*:207–212, 1987.
28. Farrar, W. E., Jr.: Serious infections due to "non-pathogenic" organisms of the genus *Bacillus*. Am. J. Med. *34*:134–141, 1963.
29. Feder, H. M., Garibaldi, R. A., Nurse, B. A., et al.: *Bacillus* species isolates from cerebrospinal fluid in patients without shunts. Pediatrics *82*:909–913, 1988.
30. Fricchione, L. F., Sepkowitz, D. V., Gradon, J. D., et al.: Pericarditis due to *Bacillus cereus* in an intravenous drug user. Rev. Infect. Dis. *13*:774, 1991.
31. Gascoigne, A. D., Richards, J., Gould, K., et al.: Successful treatment of *Bacillus cereus* infection with ciprofloxacin. Thorax *46*:220–221, 1991.
32. Ghosh, A. C.: Prevalence of *Bacillus cereus* in the faeces of healthy adults. J. Hyg. *80*:233–236, 1978.
33. Giannella, R. A., and Brasile, L.: A hospital food-borne outbreak of diarrhea caused by *Bacillus cereus*: Clinical, epidemiologic, and microbiologic studies. J. Infect. Dis. *139*:366–370, 1979.
34. Gilbert, R. J., and Kramer, J. M.: *Bacillus cereus* enterotoxins: Present status. Biochem. Soc. Trans. *12*:198–200, 1984.
35. Gilbert, R. J., Stringer, M. F., and Peace, T. C.: The survival and growth of *Bacillus cereus* in boiled and fried rice in relation to outbreaks of food poisoning. J. Hyg. *73*:433–444, 1974.
36. Glatz, B. A., and Goepfert, J. M.: Defined conditions for synthesis of *Bacillus cereus* enterotoxin by fermenter-grown cultures. Appl. Environ. Microbiol. *32*:400–404, 1976.
37. Gonzalez, I., Lopez, M., Mazas, M., et al.: The effect of recovery conditions on the apparent heat resistance of *Bacillus cereus* spores. J. Appl. Bacteriol. *78*:548–554, 1995.
38. Groschell, D., Burgess, M. A., and Bodey, G. P.: Gas gangrene–like infection with *Bacillus cereus* in a lymphoma patient. Cancer *37*:988–992, 1976.
39. Hauge, S.: Food poisoning caused by aerobic spore-forming bacilli. J. Appl. Bacteriol. *18*:591–595, 1955.
40. Hemadi, R., Zaltas, M., Paton, B., et al.: Bacillus-induced endophthalmitis: New series of 10 cases and review of the literature. Br. J. Ophthalmol. *74*:26–29, 1990.
41. Henrickson, K. J., Shenep, J. L., Flynn, P. M., et al.: Primary cutaneous *Bacillus cereus* infection in neutropenic children. Lancet *i*:601–603, 1989.
42. Holmes, J. R., Plunkett, T., Pate, P., et al.: Emetic food poisoning caused by *Bacillus cereus*. Arch. Intern. Med. *141*:766–767, 1981.
43. Ihde, D. C., and Armstrong, D.: Clinical spectrum of infection due to *Bacillus* species. Am. J. Med. *55*:839–846, 1973.
44. Jacobs, J. A., and Stobberingh, E. E.: Infection due to a contaminated thoracic drainage system. J. Hosp. Infect. *24*:23–28, 1993.
45. Jenson, H. B., Levy, S. R., Duncan, C., et al.: Treatment of multiple brain abscesses caused by *Bacillus cereus*. Pediatr. Infect. Dis. J. *8*:795–798, 1989.

46. Jephcott, A. E., Barton, B. W., Gilbert, R. J., et al.: An unusual outbreak of food poisoning associated with meals-on-wheels. Lancet *ii*:129–130, 1977.
47. Jevon, G. P., Dunne, W. M., Hicks, M. J., et al.: *Bacillus cereus* pneumonia in premature neonates: A report of two cases. Pediatr. Infect. Dis. J. *12*:251–253, 1993.
48. Khodr, M., Hill, S., Perkins, L., et al.: *Bacillus cereus* food poisoning associated with fried rice at two child day care centers: Virginia, 1993. M. M. W. R. *43*:177–178, 1994.
49. Kramer, J. M., and Gilbert, R. J.: *Bacillus cereus* and other *Bacillus* species. *In* Doyle, M. P. (ed.): Foodborne Bacterial Pathogens. 1st ed. New York, Marcel Dekker, Inc., 1989, pp. 21–70.
50. Lesk, M. R., Ammann, H., Marcil, G., et al.: The penetration of oral ciprofloxacin into the aqueous humor, vitreous and subretinal fluid of humans. Am. J. Ophthalmol. *115*:623–628, 1993.
51. Lettau, L. A., Benjamin, D., Cantrell, H. F., et al.: *Bacillus* species pseudomeningitis. Infect. Control Hosp. Epidemiol. *9*:394–398, 1988.
52. Luby, S., Jones, J., Dowda, H., et al.: A large outbreak of gastroenteritis caused by diarrheal toxin-producing *Bacillus cereus*. J. Infect. Dis. *167*:1452–1455, 1993.
53. Lund, B. M.: Foodborne disease due to *Bacillus* and *Clostridium* species. Lancet *336*:982–987, 1990.
54. Melling, J., Capel, B. J., Turnbul, P. C., et al.: Identification of a novel enterotoxigenic activity associated with *Bacillus cereus*. J. Clin. Pathol. *29*:938–940, 1976.
55. Midura, T., Gerber, M., Wood, R., et al.: Outbreak of food poisoning caused by *Bacillus cereus*. Public Health Rep. *85*:45–48, 1970.
56. Morrell, R. M., Jr., and Wasilauskas, B. L.: Tracking laboratory contamination by using a *Bacillus cereus* pseudoepidemic as an example. J. Clin. Microbiol. *30*:1469–1473, 1992.
57. Morris, J. G., Jr.: *Bacillus cereus* food poisoning. Arch. Intern. Med. *141*:711, 1981.
58. Mortimer, P. R., and McCann, G.: Food poisoning episodes associated with *Bacillus cereus* in fried rice. Lancet *i*:1043–1045, 1974.
59. Murakami, T., Hiraoka, K., Mikami, T., et al.: Detection of *Bacillus cereus* flagellar antigen by enzyme-linked immunosorbent assay (ELISA). Microbiol. Immunol. *35*:223–234, 1991.
60. Parry, J. M., and Gilbert, R. J.: Studies on the heat resistance of *Bacillus cereus* spores and growth of the organism in boiled rice. J. Hyg. *84*:77–82, 1980.
61. Patrick, C. C., Langston, C., and Baker, C. J.: *Bacillus* species infections in neonates. Rev. Infect. Dis. *111*:612–615, 1989.
62. Richard, V., Van der Auwera, P., Snoeck, R., et al.: Nosocomial bacteremia caused by *Bacillus* species. Eur. J. Clin. Microbiol. Infect. Dis. *7*:783–785, 1988.
63. Sakurai, N., Koike, K. A., Irie, Y., et al.: The rice culture filtrate of *Bacillus cereus* isolated from emetic-type food poisoning causes mitochondrial swelling in a HEp-2 cell. Microbiol. Immunol. *38*:337–340, 1994.
64. Schraft, H., and Griffiths, M. W.: Specific oligonucleotide primers for detection of lecithinase-positive *Bacillus* spp. by PCR. Appl. Environ. Microbiol. *61*:98–102, 1995.
65. Schricker, M. E., Thompson, G. H., and Schreiber, J. R.: Osteomyelitis due to *Bacillus cereus* in an adolescent: Case report and review. Clin. Infect. Dis. *18*:863–867, 1994.
66. Schultz, F. J., and Smith, J. L.: *Bacillus*: Recent advances in *Bacillus cereus* food poisoning research. *In* Hui, Y. H., Gorham, J. R., and Murrel, K. D. (eds.): Foodborne Disease Handbook. New York, Marcel Dekker, Inc., 1994, pp. 29–62.
67. Siegman-Igra, Y., Lavochkin, J., Schwartz, D., et al.: Meningitis and bacteremia due to *Bacillus cereus*: A case report and a review of *Bacillus* infections. Isr. J. Med. Sci. *19*:546–551, 1983.
68. Slaten, D. D., Oropeza, R. I., and Werner, S. B.: An outbreak of *Bacillus cereus* food poisoning: Are caterers supervised sufficiently? Public Health Rep. *107*:477–480, 1992.
69. Sliman, R., Rehm, S., and Shlaes, D. M.: Serious infections caused by *Bacillus* species. Medicine *66*:218–223, 1987.
70. Steen, M. K., Bruno-Murtha, L. A., Chaux, G., et al.: *Bacillus cereus* endocarditis: Report of a case and review. Clin. Infect. Dis. *14*:945–946, 1992.
71. Sutherland, A. D.: Toxin production by *Bacillus cereus* in dairy products. J. Dairy Res. *60*:569–574, 1993.
72. Sutherland, A. D., and Limond, A. M.: Influence of pH and sugars on the growth and production of diarrhoeagenic toxin by *Bacillus cereus*. J. Dairy Res. *60*:575–580, 1993.
73. Terranova, W., and Blake, P. A.: *Bacillus cereus* food poisoning. N. Engl. J. Med. *298*:143–144, 1978.
74. Thompson, N. E., Ketterhagen, M. J., Bergdoll, M. S., et al.: Isolation and some properties of an enterotoxin produced by *Bacillus cereus*. Infect. Immun. *43*:887–894, 1984.
75. Tuazon, C. U., Murray, H. W., Levy, C., et al.: Serious infections from *Bacillus* sp. J. A. M. A. *241*:1137–1140, 1979.
76. Turnbull, P. C.: Studies on the production of enterotoxins by *Bacillus cereus*. J. Clin. Pathol. *29*:941–948, 1976.
77. Turnbull, P. C.: *Bacillus cereus* toxins. Pharmacol. Ther. *13*:453–505, 1981.
78. Turnbull, P. C., French, T. A., and Dowsett, E. G.: Severe systemic and pyogenic infections with *Bacillus cereus*. Br. Med. J. *1*:1628–1629, 1977.
79. Turnbull, P. C., Jorgensen, K., Kramer, J. M., et al.: Severe clinical conditions associated with *Bacillus cereus* and the apparent involvement of exotoxins. J. Clin. Pathol. *32*:289–293, 1979.
80. Turnbull, P. C., and Kramer, J. M.: Non-gastrointestinal *Bacillus cereus* infections: An analysis of exotoxin production by strains isolated over a two year period. J. Clin. Pathol. *36*:1091–1096, 1983.
81. Turnbull, P. C., and Kramer, J. M.: *Bacillus*. *In* Murray, P. R., Baron, E. J., and Pfaller, M. A. (eds.): Manual of Clinical Microbiology. 6th ed. Washington, D.C., American Society for Micobiology, 1995, pp. 349–356.
82. Turnbull, P. C., and Kramer, J. M.: Intestinal carriage of *Bacillus cereus*: Faecal isolation studies in three population groups. J. Hyg. *95*:629–638, 1985.
83. Turnbull, P. C., Kramer, J. M., Jorgensen, K., et al.: Properties and production characteristics of vomiting, diarrheal and necrotizing toxins of *Bacillus cereus*. Am. J. Clin. Nutr. *32*:219–228, 1979.
84. Turnbull, P. C., Nottingham, J. F., and Ghosh, A. C.: A severe necrotic enterotoxin produced by certain food, food poisoning and other clinical isolates of *Bacillus cereus*. Br. J. Exper. Pathol. *58*:273–280, 1977.
85. Vahey, J. B., and Flynn, H. W., Jr.: Results in the management of *Bacillus* endophthalmitis. Ophthalmol. Surg. *22*:681–686, 1991.
86. Vaisanen, O. M., Mwaisumo, N. J., and Salkinoja-Salonen, M. S.: Differentiation of dairy strains of the *Bacillus cereus* group by phage typing, minimum growth temperature, and fatty acid analysis. J. Appl. Bacteriol. *70*:315–324, 1991.
87. Vandeloski, J., and Gensheimer, K. F.: *Bacillus cereus:* Maine. M. M. W. R. *35*:408–410, 1986.
88. Weber, D. J., Saviteer, S. M., Rutala, W. A., et al.: In vitro susceptibility of *Bacillus* spp to selected antimicrobial agents. Antimicrob. Agents Chemother. *32*:642–645, 1988.
89. Wong, M. T., and Dolan, M. J.: Significant infections due to *Bacillus* species following abrasions associated with motor vehicle–related trauma. Clin. Infect. Dis. *15*:855–857, 1992.
90. Young, E. J., Wallace, R. J., Ericsson, C. D., et al.: Panophthalmitis due to *Bacillus cereus*. Arch. Intern. Med. *140*:559–560, 1980.
91. Youngs, E. R., Roberts, C., Kramer, J. M., et al.: Dissemination of *Bacillus cereus* in a maternity unit. J. Infect. *10*:228–232, 1985.
92. Zaza, S., Tokars, J. I., Yomtovian, R., et al.: Bacterial contamination of platelets at a university hospital: Increased identification due to intensified surveillance. Infect. Control Hosp. Epidemiol. *15*:82–87, 1994.

98

ARCANOBACTERIUM HAEMOLYTICUM

James D. Cherry

Arcanobacterium haemolyticum is a pleomorphic gram-positive coryneform rod that causes pharyngitis and exanthem in children and young adults.[10, 26, 28]

HISTORY

This diphtheroid first was noted by MacLean and colleagues[26] in association with exudative pharyngitis in American servicemen in the South Pacific during World War II. The organism originally was named *Corynebacterium haemolyticum* but was reclassified in 1986 as *A. haemolyticum* on the basis of phenetic, peptidoglycan, fatty acid, menaquinone, and DNA data.[8–10] The association between infection with *A. haemolyticum* and pharyngitis was observed repeatedly over the years, but a cause-and-effect relationship between the organism and illness has been established only recently.[26]

THE ORGANISM

Microbiology[10, 11, 39, 42]

A. haemolyticum is a gram-positive to gram-variable pleomorphic rod. Its laboratory characteristics are presented in Table 98–1. The organism grows best at 37° C on a blood- or serum-enriched medium with the addition of 5 per cent carbon dioxide. Alternatively, it also grows well anaerobically. On rabbit or human blood agar, colonies are pinpoint (0.5 mm) at 24 hours; they increase to 1 to 1.5 mm after 48 hours. At this time, a unique black opaque dot is noted in the center of the colony, and this dot remains on the agar when the colony is scraped away.

A 1-mm zone of hemolysis occurs at 24 hours around colonies grown on human or rabbit blood agar. The hemolytic zone increases to 3 to 5 mm by 48 hours. Both growth and red cell hemolysis are minimal on horse and sheep blood agar. Because throat cultures usually are carried out on sheep blood agar plates, the hemolytic activity of *A. haemolyticum* may be missed.

A. haemolyticum resembles *Actinomyces pyogenes* (formerly *Corynebacterium pyogenes*), which is a common cause of bovine mastitis and a rare cause of skin ulcers in children.[20] These organisms can be differentiated by the ability of *A. pyogenes* to hydrolyze gelatin.

TABLE 98–1. Identification Characteristics of *Arcanobacterium haemolyticum*

Test or Characteristic	Finding
Catalase	Negative
Beta-hemolysis	Positive (a narrow zone of slight hemolysis after 48 hours on sheep blood)
Nitrate reduction	Negative
Pigment production	White or gray
Urease	Negative
Gelatin hydrolysis	Negative
Motility	Negative
Esculin hydrolysis	Negative
Carbohydrate utilization	
Glucose	Positive
Maltose	Positive
Sucrose	Positive (requires a rabbit serum for growth in peptone water)
Mannitol	Negative
Xylose	Negative

Data from Collins, M. D., and Cummins, C. S.: Genus *Corynebacterium*. *In* Sneath, P. H. A., Main, N. S., Sharpe, M. E., et al. (eds.): Bergey's Manual of Systemic Bacteriology. Vol. 2. Baltimore, Williams & Wilkins, 1986, pp. 266–276.

Toxin Production

A. haemolyticum liberates three toxins: phospholipase D, a hemolysin, and neuraminidase.[10] Phospholipase D is a dermonecrotic toxin that, after intradermal inoculation in rabbits and guinea pigs, causes local hemorrhagic necrosis; its injection also is lethal in rabbits.[34] It also has been noted that *A. haemolyticum* carries a gene similar to the gene for the erythrogenic toxin of *Streptococcus pyogenes*.[10]

Antimicrobial Susceptibility

All *A. haemolyticum* strains are highly susceptible to erythromycin (minimum inhibitory concentration, <0.06 μg/mL). However, erythromycin is not bactericidal.[6, 26, 39] Waagner[39] noted that of 100 pharyngeal isolates, all were inhibited by concentrations of ≤ 0.25 μg/mL of penicillin G and by 1.0 μg/mL of penicillin V.[39] However, penicillin tolerance has been observed.[26, 32] In one study, the minimum bactericidal concentration:minimum inhibitory concentration ratio varied from 1:1 to 1:8.[26] In addition to being sensitive to penicillin and erythromycin, *A. haemolyticum* also is sensitive to clindamycin, chloramphenicol, azithromycin, vancomycin, ciprofloxacin, and tetracyclines; most strains are resistant to sulfonamides and trimethoprim-sulfamethoxazole.[6, 39]

EPIDEMIOLOGY

Although similar organisms are common causes of infection in animals, humans appear to be the primary host of *A. haemolyticum*.[35, 39] The organism is isolated primarily from throat specimens from patients with pharyngitis,[26, 28, 39] although it also may be a commensal of human skin.[25] It also may be a commensal in the throat but overlooked because laboratories often do not differentiate diphtheroids because they are considered "normal flora."

Although no definitive data are available, it must be assumed that spread from person to person is from throat discharges of an infected person to the throat of a susceptible host. Transmission could occur directly or indirectly by fomites. Secondary cases in families indicate that spread is from person to person rather than from an environmental source.[13, 28]

In an 8-year study, the organism was found to be isolated from throat specimens in each year, with isolation rates varying from 0.2 to 0.7 per cent.[28] The peak age of illness due to *A. haemolyticum* is during the second decade of life; in contrast, the peak age of pharyngitis due to *S. pyogenes* is during the first decade of life.[13, 26, 28] In two studies, illnesses were more common in females than in males.[13, 28] No seasonal prevalence has been reported.

PATHOGENESIS AND PATHOLOGY

Few data are available regarding pathogenesis and pathology. It seems likely that the dermonecrotic toxin plays a role in pharyngitis. Skin biopsies have been done on the exanthem in two patients, and both showed only a mild lymphohistiocytic perivascular infiltrate.[28] Cultures of both biopsies were negative, and no IgG, IgA, or IgM depositions were noted. These findings suggest that the rash may be toxin-mediated, such as the rash in group A streptococcal infection is.

A. haemolyticum has been found to persist intracellularly.[33] This might be a reason for failure of penicillin treatment in some cases.

In one study, 5 of 42 patients were found to have apparent dual infections with Epstein-Barr virus and *A. haemolyticum*.[26] The authors of this study suggested that immune suppression by the virus contributes to more marked effect of the bacterial infection in the throat.

CLINICAL MANIFESTATIONS

Pharyngitis

Pharyngitis[2, 7, 13, 14, 16, 17, 19, 25, 26, 28, 30, 31, 36–39] is the most common finding in *A. haemolyticum* infection. Signs and symptoms associated with pharyngitis are presented in Table 98–2. The illness is indistinguishable from that caused by group A streptococci; frequently, the illness resembles Epstein-Barr virus infectious mononucleosis. Several cases with typical infectious mononucleosis had laboratory evidence of infection with both Epstein-Barr virus and *A. haemolyticum*.[15, 16, 26] Peritonsillar abscess due to *A. haemolyticum* has been reported on several occasions.[3, 22, 23, 27] The most common exanthem is scarlatiniform and has its onset 1 to 4 days after the beginning of pharyngeal symptoms. The rash is most prominent on the extensor surfaces of the arms and legs (see Fig. 67–19). Circumoral pallor, which occurs with group A streptococcal scarlet fever, does not seem to occur with *A. haemolyticum* infection. The rash may progress to involve the chest and back; the rash usually spares the palms, soles, and face, and it rarely involves the abdomen and buttocks.

The rash frequently is pruritic and may be urticarial. Erythema multiforme has been described.[2] Recently, Gaston and Zurowski[14] reported a 20-year-old man who in addition to pharyngitis had a rash involving mainly the hands and feet. His feet were swollen, and on the soles were erythematous macules, petechiae, and vesicles. His palms were tender, and there were 2- to 4-mm erythematous macular lesions that contained small central vesicles.

The duration of the exanthem has not been described adequately in the literature. In one study, exanthem was noted to persist for longer than 2 days in 69 per cent of the patients.[28]

TABLE 98–2. Signs and Symptoms in Children, Adolescents, and Young Adults with *Arcanobacterium haemolyticum* Infections

	Frequency
Symptoms	
Sore throat	100%
Rash	40–70%
Pruritus	50%
Fever	40–75%
Hoarseness	60%
Cough (nonproductive)	40–60%
Vomiting	30%
Signs	
Pharyngitis or tonsillitis	100%
Exudative	50–70%
Palatal petechiae	30%
Glossitis	25%
Cervical lymphadenitis	40–75%
Rash	40–70%
Scarlatiniform	50%
Urticarial	5%
Maculopapular	25%

Data from references 13, 19, 26, 28, and 39.

Skin Infections

In the initial report of infections with *A. haemolyticum* in 1946, MacLean and associates[26] noted both pharyngitis in U.S. servicemen and skin infections in the native populations of the South Pacific Islands. Cutaneous infections have been noted mainly in tropical countries.[39] The most common manifestations are ulcerative lesions that resemble ecthyma. Cellulitis, wound infections, and paronychia all have been noted.[5, 12, 13, 21, 27, 29, 39, 43] In wound infections, mixed infections with *A. haemolyticum* and other organisms are common.

Other Manifestations

Isolated instances of septicemia, brain abscess, meningitis, endocarditis, osteomyelitis, pleural empyema, cavitary pneumonia, and sinusitis have been attributed to *A. haemolyticum* infections.[1, 4, 15, 16, 18, 24, 39–41, 44] The majority of these serious infections have occurred in adults and frequently in association with an underlying problem, such as diabetes or intravenous drug use.

DIFFERENTIAL DIAGNOSIS

Pharyngitis due to *A. haemolyticum* must be differentiated from all other causes of pharyngitis (see Chapter 10). Of particular importance is discerning *A. haemolyticum* pharyngitis from *S. pyogenes* pharyngitis. This only can be done with certainty by specific culture. In *A. haemolyticum* infections, the rapid group A streptococcal antigen tests will be negative, as will the usual group A streptococcal culture. These negative tests in specimens from adolescents strongly should suggest the possibility of pharyngitis due to *A. haemolyticum*.

When exanthem occurs, the confusion with illness due to *S. pyogenes* is more pronounced. In many cases, the rash in infection due to *A. haemolyticum* is scarlatiniform. However, the lack of typical circumoral pallor and a tendency for more discrete lesions in *A. haemolyticum* infections occasionally may help in the clinical diagnosis.

Other common causes of pharyngitis and exanthem in adolescents and young adults are *Mycoplasma pneumoniae* and Epstein-Barr virus infections. As noted by Mackenzie and colleagues,[25] *A. haemolyticum* and Epstein-Barr virus co-infections are not uncommon.

Cutaneous infections, including subacute ulcerations, wound infections, cellulitis, and paronychia due to *A. haemolyticum*, must be differentiated from those caused by other organisms, such as staphylococci and streptococci.

SPECIFIC DIAGNOSIS

Specific diagnosis is made by culturing *A. haemolyticum* from the pharynx, a skin lesion, or a sterile body site in invasive infections. This is done best using rabbit or human blood agar with the addition of 5 per cent carbon dioxide.[10, 11, 39, 42] It is important to note that horse or sheep blood agar, which usually is used for culture of *S. pyogenes*, is not satisfactory for the growth and identification of *A. haemolyticum*.

TREATMENT

A. haemolyticum is highly sensitive to a number of antibiotics.[6, 26, 32, 39] Although no specific treatment studies have been carried out, the experience in several large studies suggests that both penicillin and erythromycin are effective.[6, 19, 26, 28] Clinical failure with penicillin has been noted.[2, 33, 39]

PROGNOSIS

The prognosis in instances of pharyngitis due to *A. haemolyticum* is good, even in the untreated patient. However, invasive disease can be fatal, and peritonsillar abscess needs prompt surgical intervention and appropriate antimicrobial therapy.

References

1. Altmann, G., and Bogokovsky, B.: Brain abscess due to *Corynebacterium haemolyticum*. Lancet *1*:338–339, 1973.
2. Banck, G., and Nyman, M.: Tonsillitis and rash associated with *Corynebacterium haemolyticum*. J. Infect. Dis. *154*:1037–1040, 1986.
3. Barnham, M., and Bradwell, R. A.: Acute peritonsillar abscess caused by *Arcanobacterium haemolyticum*. J. Laryngol. Otol. *106*:1000–1001, 1992.
4. Ben-Yaacob, D., Waron, M., Boldur, I., et al.: Septicemia due to *Corynebacterium haemolyticum*. Israel J. Med. Sci. *20*:431–433, 1984.
5. Bowness, P., Bower, M., Montgomery, J., et al.: The bacteriology of skin sores in Goroka children. Papua New Guinea Med. J. *27*:83–87, 1984.
6. Carlson, P., Kontiainen, S., and Renkonen, O. V.: Antimicrobial susceptibility of *Arcanobacterium haemolyticum*. Antimicrob. Agents Chemother. *38*:142–143, 1994.
7. Carlson, P., Kontianinen, S., Renkonen, O. V., et al.: *Arcanobacterium haemolyticum* and streptococcal pharyngitis in army conscripts. Scand. J. Infect. Dis. *27*:17–18, 1995.
8. Collins, M. D., Jones, D., and Schofield, G. M.: Reclassification of *Corynebacterium haemolyticum* (MacLean, Liebow and Rosenberg) in the genus *Arcanobacterium* gen. nov. as *Arcanobacterium haemolyticum* nom. rev., comb. nov. J. Gen. Microbiol. *128*:1279–1281, 1982.
9. Collins, M. D., and Cummins, C. S.: Genus *Corynebacterium*. *In* Sneath, P. H. A., Mair, N. S., Sharpe, M. E., et al. (eds.): Bergey's Manual of Systemic Bacteriology. Vol. 2. Baltimore, Williams & Wilkins, 1986, pp. 266–276.
10. Coyle, M. B., and Lipsky, B. A.: Coryneform bacteria in infectious diseases: Clinical and laboratory aspects. Clin. Microbiol. Rev. *3*:227–246, 1990.
11. Cummings, L. A., Wu, W. K., Larson, A. M., et al.: Effects of media, atmosphere, and incubation time on colonial morphology of *Arcanobacterium haemolyticum*. J. Clin. Microbiol. *31*:3223–3226, 1993.
12. Esteban, J., Zapardiel, J., and Soriano, F.: Two cases of soft-tissue infection caused by *Arcanobacterium haemolyticum*. Clin. Infect. Dis. *18*:835–836, 1994.
13. Fell, H. W. K., Nagington, J., Naylor, G. R. E., et al.: *Corynebacterium haemolyticum* infections in Cambridgeshire. J. Hyg. Camb. *79*:269–275, 1977.
14. Gaston, D. A., and Zurowski, S. M.: *Arcanobacterium haemolyticum* pharyngitis and exanthem. Arch. Dermatol. *132*:61–64, 1996.
15. Givner, L. B., McGehee, D., Taber, L. H., et al.: Sinusitis, orbital cellulitis and polymicrobial bacteremia in a patient with primary Epstein-Barr virus infection. Pediatr. Infect. Dis. J. *3*:254–256, 1984.
16. Goudswaard, J., van de Merwe, D. W., van der Sluys, P., et al.: *Corynebacterium haemolyticum* septicemia in a girl with mononucleosis infectiosa. Scand. J. Infect. Dis. *20*:339–340, 1988.
17. Green, S. L., and LaPeter, K. S.: Pseudodiphtheritic membranous pharyngitis caused by *Corynebacterium haemolyticum*. J. A. M. A. *245*:2330–2331, 1981.
18. Jobanputra, R. S., and Swain, C. P.: Septicaemia due to *Corynebacterum haemolyticum*. J. Clin. Pathol. *28*:798–800, 1975.
19. Karpathios, T., Drakonaki, S., Zervoudaki, A., et al.: *Arcanobacterium haemolyticum* in children with presumed streptococcal pharyngotonsillitis or scarlet fever. J. Pediatr. *121*:735–737, 1992.
20. Kotrajaras, R. P., Buddhavudhikral, S., Sukroongreung, S., et al.: Endemic leg ulcers caused by *Corynebacterium pyogenes* in Thailand. Int. J. Dermatol. *21*:407–409, 1982.
21. Kotrajaras, R., and Tagami, H.: *Corynebacterium pyogenes:* Its pathogenic mechanism in epidemic leg ulcers in Thailand. Int. J. Dermatol. *26*:45–50, 1987.
22. Kovatch, A. L., Schuit, K. E., and Michaels, R. H.: *Corynebacterium haemolyticum* peritonsillar abscess mimicking diphtheria. J. A. M. A. *249*:1757–1758, 1983.
23. Lipsky, B. A., Goldberger, A. C., Tompkins, L. S., et al.: Infections caused by nondiphtheria corynebacteria. Rev. Infect. Dis. *4*:1220–1235, 1982.
24. Locksley, R. M.: The lowly diphtheroid: Nondiphtheria corynebacterial infections in humans. West J. Med. *137*:45–52, 1982.
25. Mackenzie, A., Fuite, L. A., Chan, F. T. H., et al.: Incidence and pathogenicity of *Arcanobacterium haemolyticum* during a 2-year study in Ottawa. Clin. Infect. Dis. *21*:177–181, 1995.
26. MacLean, P. D., Liebow, A. A., and Rosenberg, A. A.: A hemolytic corynebacterium resembling *Corynebacterium ovis* and *Corynebacterium pyogenes* in man. J. Infect. Dis. *79*:69–90, 1946.
27. Miller, R. A., and Brancato, F.: Peritonsillar abscess associated with *Corynebacterium haemolyticum*. West. J. Med. *140*:449–451, 1984
28. Miller, R. A., Brancato, F., and Holmes, K. K.: *Corynebacterium haemolyticum* as a cause of pharyngitis and scarlatiniform rash in young adults. Ann. Intern. Med. *105*: 867–872, 1986.
29. Montgomery, J.: The aerobic bacteriology of infected skin lesions in children of the Eastern Highlands Province. Papua New Guinea Med. J. *28*:93–103, 1985.
30. Moreno, M. M., Valle, V. A., and Aguillar, A. L.: Pharyngitis caused by *Arcanobacterium hemolyticum*. Anales Espanoles de Pediatria *30*:209–210, 1989.
31. Nyman, M., and Banck, G.: The clinical picture in throat infections caused by *Corynebacterium haemolyticum*. Hygiea Swedish Med. Assoc. 109–110, 1984.
32. Nyman, M., Banck, G., and Thore, M.: Penicillin tolerance in *Arcanobacterium haemolyticum*. J. Infect. Dis. *161*:261–265, 1990.
33. Osterlund, A.: Are penicillin treatment failures in *Arcanobacterium haemolyticum* pharyngotonsillitis caused by intracellularly residing bacteria? Scand. J. Infect. Dis. 27:131–134, 1995.
34. Patocka, F., Mara, M., Soucek, A., et al.: Observations on the biological properties of atypical haemolytic corynbacteria isolated from man as compared with *Corynebacterium haemolyticum*, *Corynebacterium pyogenes bovis* and *Corynebacterium ovis*. J. Hyg. Epidemiol. Microbiol. Imunol. *6*:1–12, 1962.
35. Roberts, R. J.: Isolation of *Corynebacterium haemolyticum* from a case of ovine pneumonia. Vet. Rec. *84*:490, 1969.
36. Robinson, B. E., and Murray, D. L.: *Corynebacterium haemolyticum* and pharyngitis. Ann. Intern. Med. *106*:778–779, 1987.
37. Ryan, W. J.: Throat infection and rash associated with an unusual corynebacterium. Lancet 2:1345–1347, 1972.
38. Selander, B., and Ljungh, A.: *Corynebacterium haemolyticum* as a cause of nonstreptococcal pharyngitis. J. Infect. Dis. *154*:1041, 1986.
39. Waagner, D. C.: *Arcanobacterium haemolyticum*: Biology of the organism and diseases in man. Pediatr. Infect. Dis. J. *10*:933–939, 1991.
40. Waller, K. S., and Wood, B. P.: Cavitary pneumonia due to *Arcanobacterium hemolyticum*. Am. J. Dis. Child. *145*:209–210, 1991.
41. Washington, J. A., Martin, W. J., and Spiekerman, R. E.: Brain abscess with *Corynebacterium haemolyticum*: Report of a case. Am. J. Clin. Pathol. *56*: 212–215, 1971.
42. Wat, L. L., Fleming, C. A., Hodge, D. S., et al.: Selective medium for isolation of *Arcanobacterium haemolyticum* and *Streptococcus pyogenes*. Eur. J. Clin. Microbiol. Infect. Dis. *10*:443–446, 1991.
43. Wickremesinghe, R. S. B.: *Corynebacterium haemolyticum* infections in Sri Lanka. J. Hyg. Camb. *87*:271–277, 1981.
44. Worthington, M. G., Daly, B. D. T., and Smith, F. E.: *Corynebacterium haemolyticum* endocarditis on a native valve. South. Med. J. *78*:1261–1262, 1985.

99

ERYSIPELOTHRIX RHUSIOPATHIAE

William C. Gruber and Randall G. Fisher

Erysipelothrix rhusiopathiae (insidiosa) first was identified definitively by Rosenbach[23] in 1884 as a cause of the cutaneous disease erysipeloid. Although most commonly associated with localized skin infection in humans, this organism has been associated with sepsis,[8, 21, 26] chronic skin eruption,[6, 11] and endocarditis.[1, 8, 16, 17, 22, 26]

BACTERIOLOGY

E. rhusiopathiae is a slender, pleomorphic, gram-positive, unencapsulated rod that produces 0.1-mm bluish colonies on blood agar. Some strains produce alpha-hemolysis in 48 to 72 hours. Gelatin inoculated by stab inconsistently forms a "test-tube brush" appearance diagnostic for this organism.[8] *Erysipelothrix* is differentiated from morphologically similar *Listeria monocytogenes* and diphtheroids by the absence of motility and catalase production and the presence of hydrogen sulfide production in triple sugar iron.[8, 26]

EPIDEMIOLOGY

First isolated from mice in 1880 by Koch, *Erysipelothrix* is a common commensal of wild and domestic mammals, birds, and fish.[8, 26] The *Erysipelothrix* organism may lead a saphrophytic existence in soil. First identified by Löffler in 1882 as the causative agent of swine erysipelas, it remains an important epidemic cause of disease in these animals, with losses in excess of $25 million annually to this industry.[8] Sheep, rabbits, cattle, turkeys, and rats are subject to infection with this organism. *Erysipelothrix* has been recovered from wild moose and domestic emus.[3, 9] *E. rhusiopathiae* survives salting and smoking procedures. Pieces of meat may contain the organism for 170 days after pickling, but exposure to moist heat for 15 minutes at 55° C[25] will kill most strains.[8] Not surprisingly, fish handlers, meat processors, poultry workers, veterinarians, abattoir workers, and food handlers are at risk for exposure to *Erysipelothrix*.[19] Isolates of the same serotype may demonstrate genetic diversity, so serotyping may not be completely reliable as an epidemiologic tool for tracking outbreaks.[4]

PATHOPHYSIOLOGY

Human infection is largely accidental and results from contamination of skin abrasions during handling of infected material. Males are infected more commonly than females, perhaps because of an increased exposure risk. The presence of an antiphagocytic capsule may be a virulence factor for *E. rhusiopathiae*.[24] Disease usually is self-limited, most often involving the hands. Biopsy of skin lesions shows a marked inflammatory response. Difficulty of bacteriologic confirmation has been attributed to the organism's location in the deep part of the pars reticularis of the corium.[5]

CLINICAL MANIFESTATIONS

Human disease typically manifests itself as a mild, localized cutaneous eruption; a more severe, generalized cutaneous form; or a septicemia often associated with endocarditis. Localized cutaneous infection, the erysipeloid of Rosenbach,[23] is the most common manifestation of *Erysipelothrix* disease.[19] After a 1- to 4-day incubation period, an acute localized lesion appears at the site of an abrasion contaminated with *E. rhusiopathiae*–colonized material. Slowly progressive, purplish-red, painful induration is typical. Absence of suppuration and involution without desquamation help to distinguish this lesion from streptococcal or staphylococcal infection. Occasionally, the skin may show sharply circumscribed bluish-red lesions, which are similar to the cutaneous manifestations in swine.[8, 26] Fever and other constitutional symptoms are uncommon, occurring in less than 10 per cent of cases, unless bacteremia supervenes.[6, 19] Untreated infection usually is self-limited, with an average duration of 3 weeks. Lymphangitis and adenitis occur in 10 per cent of cases, and in 20 per cent of cases progression of disease extends from lesions on the hand to the wrist and forearm.[12] A 7-week-old infant with localized *E. rhusiopathiae* infection of the knee without a known source of exposure has been reported,[14] and a 6-year-old girl with *Erysipelothrix* pyopneumothorax has been described.[20]

Cutaneous eruptions rarely may occur in areas distant from the site of inoculation,[13] appearing as violaceous lesions with advancing pink borders. Bullous vesiculation has been described.[6] In 1921, Prausnitz[21] reported the first case of apparent septicemia in childhood, isolating the organism from the blood of a 10-year-old boy.

An uncommon but important complication of *Erysipelothrix* infection is endocarditis. Presumed or proven endocarditis accounts for 90 per cent of serious *E. rhusiopathiae* infection.[7] Patients with congenital heart disease or heart valve damage secondary to acute rheumatic fever are at the greatest risk for endocarditis. However, previously normal heart valves can be infected.[8, 16] Unlike diphtheroid endocarditis, *E. rhusiopathiae* endocarditis usually does not involve prosthetic valves, and, unlike *Bacillus* species endocarditis, it is not associated with intravenous drug abuse.[7] In a review of 1989 cases of endocarditis from 13 series,[1] *Erysipelothrix* was documented in two patients. *Erysipelothrix* endocarditis commonly involved the aortic valve. Overall mortality in reported cases is 38 per cent. Curiously, no history or physical evidence of cutaneous lesions is found in up to 50 per cent of cases of endocarditis, and history of exposure to contaminated material often is lacking. Although immunocompromised individuals[17] may be at increased risk, serious infection also occurs in otherwise normal hosts,[2, 8, 16] particularly in association with occupational exposure.

DIAGNOSIS

For localized disease, diagnosis is dependent largely on clinical appearance of the lesion in association with an appropriate history of exposure. Attempts to culture the organism from material collected by swab or aspirate of a local lesion almost always are unsuccessful, presumably because of the bacteria's location deep within the skin.[5, 26] However, biopsies of affected skin cultured in broth generally will yield the offending bacteria. Amplification and detection of *Erysipelothrix* DNA by polymerase chain reaction show promise in animal models of infection.[15] *Erysipelothrix* is isolated commonly from the blood of patients with septicemia or endocarditis and can be found in affected heart valves at autopsy or at the time of valve replacement.[6] A high index of suspicion is important for the diagnosis of endocarditis. The organism has been misidentified as a viridans group streptococcus because of its pleomorphic coccoid appearance, alpha-hemolysis, and catalase-negative character.

TREATMENT

E. rhusiopathiae is exquisitely sensitive to penicillin. Localized disease usually can be treated with oral medication, but high parenteral doses occasionally are necessary, particularly for disseminated disease.[8] Treatment of endocarditis is similar to treatment of endocarditis caused by viridans streptococci. At least 12 million units of penicillin administered for 4 weeks has been curative in adult patients, but many cases have been treated for 6 weeks or longer. Concomitant administration of an aminoglycoside has been used in some cases. *Erysipelothrix* is resistant to vancomycin.[10] Prompt microbiologic differentiation of *E. rhusiopathiae* from other gram-positive organisms is important in guiding antimicrobial choice, because vancomycin often is employed in empiric therapy for endocarditis. Hyperimmune serum, which at one time was advocated for therapy, is of little value. Risk of disease is minimized by protecting those persons exposed to potentially contaminated materials.

References

1. Ben-Chetrit, E., Muiad, N., and Levo, Y.: Infective endocarditis caused by uncommon bacteria. Scand. J. Infect. Dis. *15*:179–183, 1983.
2. Callon, R. A. J., and Brady, P. G.: Toothpick perforation of the sigmoid colon: An unusual case associated with *Erysipelothrix rhusiopathiae* septicemia. Gastrointest. Endosc. *36*:141–143, 1990.
3. Campbell, G. D., Addison, E. M., Barker, I. K., et al.: *Erysipelothrix rhusiopathiae*, serotype 17, septicemia in moose (*Alces alces*) from Algonquin Park, Ontario. J. Wild. Dis. *30*:436–438, 1994.
4. Chooromoney, K. N., Hampson, D. J., Eamens, G. J., et al.: Analysis of *Erysipelothrix rhusiopathiae* and *Erysipelothrix tonsillarum* by multilocus enzyme electrophoresis. J. Clin. Microbiol. *32*:371–376, 1994.
5. Dhttman, G.: Schweinrotlauf und erysipeloid. Beitr. Klin. Chir. *123*:461–470, 1921.
6. Ehrlich, J. C.: *Erysipelothrix rhusiopathiae* infection in man. Arch. Intern. Med. *78*:565–577, 1944.
7. Gorby, G. L., and Peacock, J. E. J.: *Erysipelothrix rhusiopathiae* endocarditis: Microbiologic, epidemiologic, and clinical features of an occupational disease. Rev. Infect. Dis. *10*:317–325, 1988.
8. Grieco, M. H., and Sheldon, C.: *Erysipelothrix rhusiopathiae*. Ann. N.Y. Acad. Sci. *174*:523–532, 1970.
9. Griffiths, G. L., and Buller, N.: *Erysipelothrix rhusiopathiae* infection in semi-intensively farmed emus. Austr. Vet. J. *68*:121–122, 1991.
10. Johnson, A. P., Uttley, A. H., Woodford, N., et al.: Resistance to vancomycin and teicoplanin: An emerging clinical problem. Clin. Microbiol. Rev. *3*:280–291, 1990.
11. Klauder, J. V.: Erysipeloid as an occupational disease. J. A. M. A. *111*:1345–1348, 1938.
12. Klauder, J. V.: *Erysipelothrix rhusiopathiae* infection in swine and in human beings. Arch. Dermatol. Syph. *50*:151–159, 1944.
13. Kramer, M. R., Gombert, M. E., Corrado, M. L., et al.: *Erysipelothrix rhusiopathiae* endocarditis. South. Med. J. *75*:892, 1982.
14. Lacroix, J., Delage, G., and Mitchell, G.: Erysipeloid in an infant. J. Pediatr. *99*:745–746, 1981.
15. Makino, S., Okada, Y., Maruyama, T., et al.: Direct and rapid detection of *Erysipelothrix rhusiopathiae* DNA in animals by PCR. J. Clin. Microbiol. *32*:1526–1531, 1994.
16. Morris, C. A., Schwabacher, H., Lynch, P. G., et al.: Two fatal cases of septicaemia due to *Erysipelothrix insidiosa*. J. Clin. Pathol. *18*:614–617, 1965.
17. Muirhead, N., and Reid, T. M. S.: *Erysipelothrix rhusiopathiae* endocarditis. J. Infect. *2*:83–85, 1980.
18. Mutalib, A., Keirs, R., and Austin, F.: Erysipelas in quail and suspected erysipeloid in processing plant employees. Avian Dis. *39*:191–193, 1995.
19. Nelson, E.: Five hundred cases of erysipeloid. Rocky Mountain Med. J. *52*:40–42, 1955.
20. Panhotra, B. R., Agarwal, K. C., Kumar, L., et al.: *Erysipelothrix rhusiopathiae* infection in a child: A case report with review of literature. Indian Pediatr. *16*:547–549, 1979.
21. Prausnitz, C.: Bakteriologische untersuchung über schweinrotlauf beim menschen. Zentralbl. Bakteriol. Mikrobiol. Hyg. *85*:362, 1921.
22. Reboli, A. C., and Farrar, W. E.: *Erysipelothrix rhusiopathiae*: An occupational pathogen. Clin. Microbiol. Rev. *2*:354–359, 1989.
23. Rosenbach, F. J.: Experimentelle morphologische und klinische studie über die (krankheitserregenden) mikroorganismen des schweinrotlaufs, des erysipeloids und der mäuse sepsis. Z. Hyg. Infektionskrankheit. *63*:343–371, 1909.
24. Shimoji, Y., Yokomizo, Y., Sekizaki, T., et al.: Presence of a capsule in *Erysipelothrix rhusiopathiae* and its relationship to virulence for mice. Infect. Immun. *62*:2806–2810, 1994.
25. Watarai, M., Sawada, T., Nakagomi, M., et al.: Comparison of etiological and immunological characteristics of two attenuated *Erysipelothrix rhusiopathiae* strains of serotypes 1a and 2. J. Vet. Med. Sci. 55:595–600, 1993.
26. Woodbine, M.: *Erysipelothrix rhusiopathiae*: Bacteriology and chemotherapy. Bacteriol. Rev. *14*:161–178, 1947.

100

LISTERIOSIS

Robert Bortolussi and William A. Kennedy

Listeria monocytogenes first was isolated by Murray and associates[89] more than 65 years ago during their investigation of an epidemic of perinatal infection with monocytosis among laboratory rabbits. The first reported human disease due to *Listeria* was published in 1929.[97] Since then, the organism has been isolated with increasing frequency among the elderly, in immunocompromised individuals, and in perinates. Neonatal *Listeria* infection was not described until 1936 but now represents the largest single identifiable group of listeriosis.[19, 37] A large body of information has been accumulated, with several comprehensive reviews.[13, 37, 107]

THE ORGANISM

Listeria is described as a regular, short, non–spore-forming, gram-positive rod that is motile and forms bluish-gray colonies on solid agar. The genus was named in honor of Lord Lister, the father of antiseptic technique. Of the seven *Listeria* species (*L. monocytogenes, L. murrayi, L. innocua, L. grayi, L. welshimeri, L. seeligeri,* and *L. ivanovii*), only *L. monocytogenes* and *L. ivanovii* have been reported to infect humans.[49, 72] Various characteristics of *L. monocytogenes* have been used to separate the organism from nonpathogenic *Listeria* species or other genera of bacteria with which it may be confused.[111] The four most commonly employed characteristics are the following: (1) *Listeria* is motile (characteristic tumbling motility at 25° C [77° F], with reduced motility at 37° C [98.6° F]); (2) it grows with a narrow zone of beta-hemolysis (certain strains are nonhemolytic but rarely are seen in clinical material) with a rectangular area of increased hemolysis in the adenosine 3′,5′-cyclic phosphate test in association with *Staphylococcus aureus*; (3) it is catalase-positive; and (4) it ferments α-methyl-D-mannoside and L-rhamnose but not D-xylose. Cold enrichment procedures have been used to improve the isolation rate from clinical material but generally are not recommended.[10, 37, 107]

A number of bacterial products and their genes have been defined,[97] but their exact role in the four steps in pathogenesis (internalization, vacuole escape, actin polymerization, ejection into adjacent cells) still largely is unknown. Because all strains of *L. monocytogenes* isolated from natural infections produce hemolysis on blood agar, much attention has focused on this as a potential virulence factor. The hemolysin secreted by *L. monocytogenes*, termed *listerolysin O*, has been purified, and the gene responsible *(hly)* has been sequenced.[23, 97] It is a sulfhydryl-activated, pore-forming protein that most likely causes lysis of host-cell vacuole, allowing it to replicate freely in its cytoplasm. It is antigenically similar to the streptolysin O that is produced by group A streptococci. This organism possesses intrinsic properties of tolerance to low temperature as well as high pH and salt concentrations that allow it to replicate in soil, water, sewage, manure, animal feed, and contaminated, decaying refrigerated foods.

After the early work of Paterson,[95] Seeliger and Finger[112] carried out extensive work on the serologic characterization of *L. monocytogenes*. At least 17 serotypes have been identified on the basis of somatic and flagellar antigens, but three (1a, 1b, 4b) account for the vast majority of clinical isolates and also are the most common serotypes found in food.[83, 96]

TRANSMISSION

An understanding of the factors involved in transmission is far from complete. Early recognition of the disease in animals led to the belief that listeriosis primarily was a zoonosis. Although direct transmission has been reported in such high-risk occupational groups as veterinarians and farm workers, most infections reported in North America occur in urban areas with no epidemiologic explanation.[18, 88] However, a cycle described by Schlech and colleagues[105] involving consumption of cabbage contaminated with *Listeria* from animal manure suggested that food-borne transmission may occur. Since that time, a number of outbreaks have been linked to food-borne listeriosis.[5, 37, 54, 58, 73, 84, 109] Most outbreaks have been associated with consumption of contaminated dairy products.[37, 73] However, paté, pork tongue in jelly, ready-cooked chicken, and even hot dogs also have been implicated.[54, 58, 84, 109] The potential for nosocomial spread is supported by a few reports of small nursery outbreaks.[31, 41, 69, 106]

EPIDEMIOLOGY

Listeriosis is worldwide in distribution and affects a variety of mammals.[111] The age distribution of human cases reported in the United States is not uniform; most cases occur among pregnant women, their newborns, and the elderly (Fig. 100–1). Between these extremes of age, listeriosis also occurs in patients with underlying immune deficiency states, in patients with lymphoreticular malignancies, among renal transplant recipients,[88, 92, 115] and occasionally among healthy subjects.[107, 126] Several major North American and European outbreaks of food-borne listeriosis have been described.[37, 54, 84, 107] Perinatal attack rates during such outbreaks reach as high as 1.3 per cent of all deliveries.[105] In the United States, the overall estimated incidence was 4.2 cases per 10^6 population, based on results from a population-based active surveillance project conducted by the Centers for Disease Control and Prevention in 1993.[118] For perinatal cases, the attack rate was 8.6 per 100,000 deliveries. Surveillance studies in Canada in 1988 estimated an attack rate of 2.3 cases per 10^6 population.[124] The rate in the first month of life was 385 cases per 10^6 population.[124] The mean incubation period for food-borne listeriosis is about 3 weeks. Molecular techniques using multilocus enzyme electrophoresis and gene restriction fragment length polymorphism have been used successfully to track epidemic and sporadic strains found in food from index

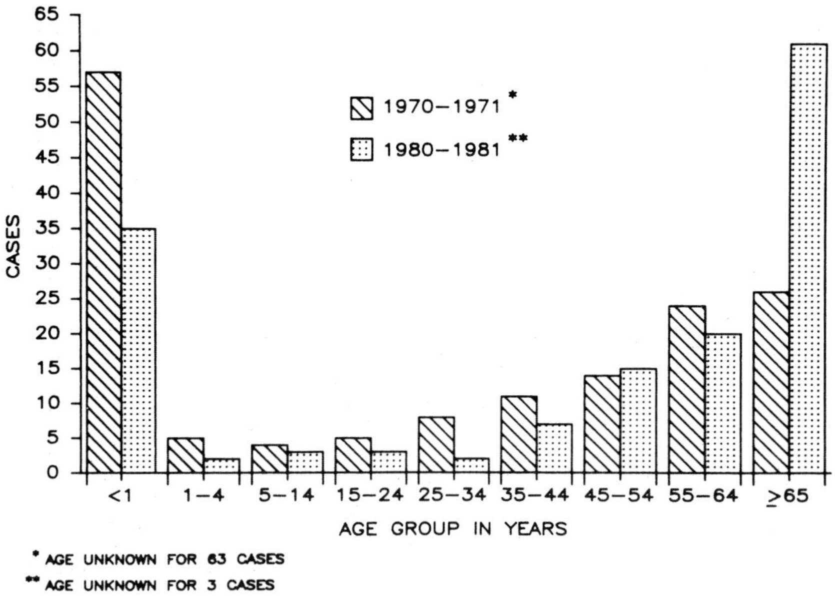

FIGURE 100–1. *Human listeriosis cases by age group for the United States, 1970–1971 and 1980–1981. (From Albritton, W. L., Cochi, S. L., and Feeley, J. C.: Overview of neonatal listeriosis. Clin. Invest. Med. 7:311–314, 1984.)*

TABLE 100–1. Features of Early- and Late-Onset Neonatal Listeriosis*

	Early-Onset[1, 2, 30, 73, 119]	Late-Onset[2, 32, 63, 73, 106, 126]
Age at onset (median in days)	<0.1 (<0.1–1.3)	28 (7–140)
Birth weight (median in grams)	2250 (1800–2540)	3100 (3000–3150)
Per cent of isolates from		
Cerebrospinal fluid	5 (2–7)	63 (30–87)
Blood and cerebrospinal fluid	10 (6–26)	25 (13–4)
Blood alone	74 (45–88)	12 (0–30)
Other only†	5 (0–24)	0
Newborn and maternal	72 (54–93)	4 (0–8)
Per cent mortality	38 (22–63)	3 (0–10)
Per cent with obstetrical complication	63 (38–87)	3 (0–7)

*This table shows the median values and ranges of results from various publications.
†Sources other than blood and cerebrospinal fluid included cutaneous, gastric, throat, urine, and rectal sources.

patients' refrigerators.[54, 96, 102] More rapid techniques using a variation of polymerase chain reaction may be available in the future.[3, 78]

PATHOGENESIS AND PATHOLOGY

The gross and microscopic findings in listeriosis are well documented. Although multiple granulomas are characteristic of disseminated disease, the basic pathologic change of suppurative inflammation is nonspecific.[64] Examination of the placenta of infants with early-onset infection reveals macroabscesses, funisitis, and villitis in most cases.[120]

L. monocytogenes is a facultative intracellular pathogen that has been used extensively to study cell-mediated immunity and the biochemical and pharmacologic abnormalities associated with infection.[6, 79, 82, 117, 128] Resident macrophages in the liver and spleen provide an environment for intracellular growth; however, nonprofessional phagocytic cells (hepatocytes, enterocytes, and fibroblasts) also permit intracellular proliferation.[24, 35, 46, 59, 67] The molecular determinants of intracellular invasion have been reviewed.[97] Two products attached to the bacterial cell wall, "internalin" and a 60-kDa protein (p60), contribute to the invasion of nonphagocytic cells.[47] After internalization, the organism escapes from the host vacuoles and enters the cytoplasm. The ability to escape a phagocytic vacuole is due to listeriolysin O, a 60-kDa cytotoxin with sequence similarity to the hemolysin of other gram-positive pathogens, such as group A *Streptococcus*.[15, 60, 98, 130] The gene encoding listeriolysin has been named *hly*. *L. monocytogenes* mutants lacking *hly* are nonvirulent. After escaping the vacuole, *L. monocytogenes* multiplies rapidly and moves through the cytoplasm to invade adjacent cells by polymerizing host-cell actin filaments. The gene encoding for this factor has been designated *actA*. As bacteria move to the surface of the cell, they are extruded laterally from the cell in pseudopod-like structures that are recognized by neighboring cells and phagocytosed.

Resistance to *L. monocytogenes* and to other facultative intracellular bacteria appears to be mediated through activated macrophages[44, 53, 79] and other mononuclear cells, such as lymphocytes and natural killer cells, that migrate to the site of *Listeria* infection.[66, 99]

Peak immunity to *Listeria* in adults is expressed after 5 to 6 days of infection, a time that coincides with maximal T-cell synthesis of interferon-γ.[14, 17, 113] Other cytokines, such as granulocyte colony-stimulating factor, tumor necrosis factor, and interleukins-6, -10 and -12, are induced and implicated as mediators of *Listeria* clearance.[25, 62, 68, 74, 91, 123, 127]

In newborn animals, susceptibility to *L. monocytogenes* appears to be associated with delayed activation of macrophages.[12] The afferent and efferent arms of the immune system in newborn mice have been studied by Lu and associates,[76, 77] who showed that macrophage–T-lymphocyte interaction was impaired. The relevance of such animal studies to human infection with *L. monocytogenes* remains to be determined[11]; however, Issekutz and colleagues[56] have demonstrated a similar defect among infants surviving natural *Listeria* infection. Synthesis of interferon-γ, interferon-α, and interleukin-2, all of which modulate the immune response and macrophage activation, also is deficient in newborns.[34, 65, 113] Newborn and adult animals are protected against *L. monocytogenes* infection by pretreatment with interferon or inducers of interferon.[14, 21, 68]

The factors associated with the host or the organism necessary to establish mucosal colonization are poorly understood. Extrauterine infections presumably result from initial invasion of colonized mucosal surfaces.[59, 94, 96, 102] In older children and young adults, *Listeria* infection is rare; however, underlying diseases or medications that interfere with cell-mediated immunity may increase susceptibility.[110] Cyclosporine, which blocks cytokine production, is associated with increased susceptibility.[52]

CLINICAL MANIFESTATIONS

Although a variety of clinical manifestations are described in *L. monocytogenes* infections, the vast majority of pediatric infections occur in the first months of life. The clinical presenting features are similar to those of the more prevalent group B streptococcal infection.[7] The serotype distribution of *L. monocytogenes* appears to differ, depending on the age of presentation. Serotypes 1a and 1b are more common in the early-onset form of disease (<7 days of age), and serotype 4b in the late-onset form (>7 days of age).[2]

Infants with the early-onset form of neonatal listeriosis usually are diagnosed within the first 24 hours of life with respiratory distress or pneumonia, septicemia, and occasionally meningitis (Table 100–1).[1, 2, 30, 73, 119, 126] Mothers of these infants frequently have an influenza-like illness with fever, malaise, headache, gastrointestinal symptoms, or pharyngitis in the few days preceding delivery.[50, 73, 100] During labor, maternal fever and green- or brown-stained amniotic fluid may be seen.[1, 70, 71] The more severely affected infants are infected in utero, born prematurely, and often are critically ill at birth. Widespread micro- and macroabscesses, demonstrable externally as discrete roseolar or pustular lesions on the skin and pharynx, may occur. The rash has been termed *granulomatosis infantisepticum* (Fig. 100–2). Depression at

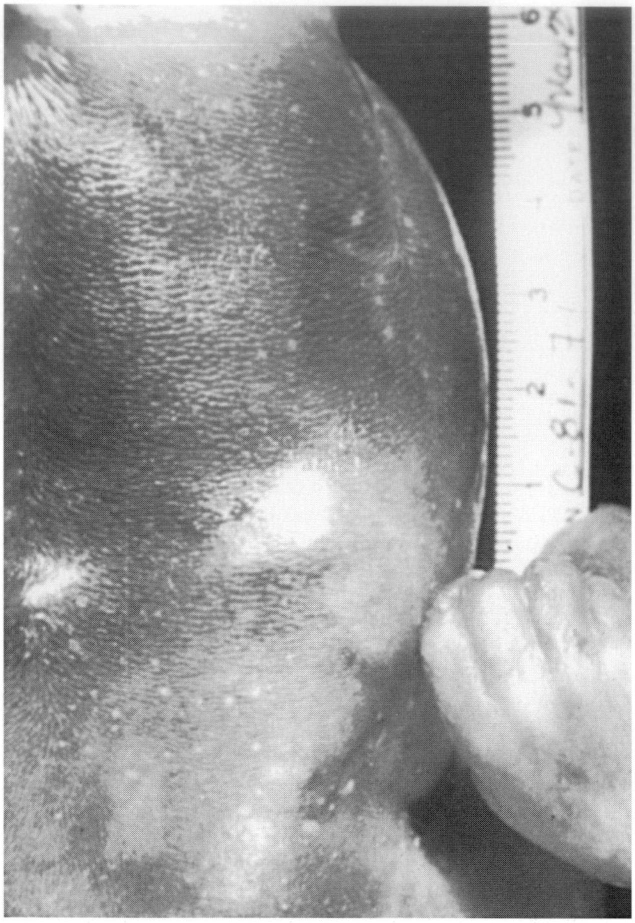

FIGURE 100–2. *Typical pustular rash on abdomen of stillborn infant with listeriosis. Note the small pale granuloma measuring 1 to 3 mm and the dark erythema surrounding these lesions.*

birth, respiratory distress, apnea, lethargy, and fever are common presenting features, but diarrhea, conjunctivitis, and myocarditis all have been described.[71] Respiratory symptoms may mimic those of respiratory distress syndrome. Patchy bronchopneumonic infiltrates, likely due to aspiration of infected amniotic fluid, may be seen on chest roentgenograms. Intrauterine infection also may result in spontaneous abortion or stillbirth.[50] However, colonized asymptomatic neonates[70] have been reported, as well as colonized household contacts.[108]

The late-onset form of neonatal listeriosis is less common than the early-onset form and usually affects term infants who appear healthy until the onset of meningitis or, less commonly, septicemia 1 to 8 weeks after birth.[2, 32, 50, 63, 106] Enterocolitis due to *L. monocytogenes* has been seen.[69] Clinical manifestations in late-onset meningitis may be quite subtle and include fever, irritability, lethargy, and poor feeding.[63, 106] Cerebrospinal fluid findings are variable. Although pleocytosis usually is significant, not all cases will have a polymorphonuclear cell predominance. Maternal history in these cases usually is negative. An outbreak of neonatal listeriosis associated with mineral oil reported by Schuchat and associates[106] provides insight into the pathophysiology of the late-onset form of disease. During the outbreak, babies were bathed after birth with mineral oil, which was applied liberally over the entire body, including the face. A strain identical to one causing the infection was isolated from a mineral oil container in the delivery room. Despite intensive investigation, no other sources of infection were identified. The incubation period before development of symptoms was 5 days, whereas the median age at first positive culture for infants was 7 days. The presenting symptoms and signs in infants were those of the late-onset form of infection: fever and meningitis. Seven of 10 infants had a positive cerebral fluid culture.

Other less common clinical settings in which listeriosis may occur include renal transplantation, malignancy states, and the acquired immune deficiency syndrome.[43, 57, 92, 115] Immunocompromised patients can present with a variety of clinical features, most commonly meningitis or septicemia. Although patients receiving immunosuppressive therapy have a high incidence of infection, their clinical features are similar to those of nonimmunosuppressed patients with *Listeria* infection.[110] Rhombencephalitis, brain abscess, arthritis, osteomyelitis, endocarditis, endophthalmitis, liver abscess, and peritonitis also have been reported in nonpediatric patients.[4, 16, 20, 27, 75, 80, 90, 115] Rarely, listeriosis has been seen in children who are otherwise well.[80, 83, 107, 126]

DIAGNOSIS

Listeriosis should be considered in the differential diagnosis for a variety of clinical problems. Appropriate specimens for staining and culture vary with the clinical syndrome, but investigation from the usual sources, such as blood, cerebrospinal fluid, amniotic fluid, genital tract secretions, and pathologic specimens (e.g., biopsy material, placental or fetal tissue), is most productive. Because prompt recognition is essential, examination of Gram-stained material from newborns (ear, meconium, and placenta) is recommended in suspected early-onset sepsis.[70] Selective culture media for isolation from such contaminated material as stool or vaginal secretions may be helpful.[81, 96] Laboratories undertaking primary isolation must be aware of the similarities between *L. monocytogenes* and frequently discarded "commensals."[83]

Despite extensive attempts to develop serologic techniques for the diagnosis of listeriosis, none has proved satisfactory, and few centers attempt serodiagnosis. A standardized agglutination test may be used[51] but appears to be of no value in neonatal infections. A complement-fixation test has been used and shown to have specificity.[51] High-titered single sera in certain groups, such as mothers of infected neonates, may be suggestive, and a fourfold or greater rise in titer between acute and convalescent specimens may be presumptive; however, at present, a confirmed diagnosis requires isolation of the organism. Berche and colleagues[9] have suggested that measurement of antibody to specific *Listeria* hemolysin may help provide a serodiagnosis.

Histologic diagnosis from pathologic material should be attempted if the organism is not cultured. Specific fluorescent antibody staining,[22] nucleic acid hybridization,[116] and polymerase chain reaction[3, 55] generally are not employed in the routine diagnostic laboratory but do offer potential for development in the future, especially in cases pretreated with antibiotics and for rapid food surveillance.

TREATMENT

Prompt antibiotic therapy is required in most cases of listeriosis for the prevention of death or severe sequelae. Unfortunately, antibiotic susceptibility of clinical isolates of *L. monocytogenes* is variable. Bactericidal activity of the commonly used antibiotics is influenced in vitro by such factors as inoculum size, type of media, and the definition of end points.[28, 75] Similar to a few other bacteria, *L. monocytogenes* demonstrates tolerance to some antibiotics in vitro; the minimum bactericidal concentration is more than fourfold the minimum inhibitory concentration.[28, 86] Thus, the antibiotics commonly recommended for treatment—ampicillin, penicillin, erythromycin, and tetracycline—are only bacteriostatic at concentrations usually achieved in blood.[28, 38, 39, 122, 125]

Newer antibiotics have been considered for possible therapy. Some studies have shown trimethoprim-sulfamethoxazole and rifampin to be effective in eradicating *Listeria* in vivo.[45, 48, 85, 104] These drugs appear to be bactericidal and have been used successfully in a few cases of human listeriosis.[42, 114] Rifampin and trimethoprim-sulfamethoxazole offer theoretic advantage over other drugs because of their better intracellular penetration. New antibiotics, such as quinolones, macrolides, and imipenem, have only moderate activity in vitro against *Listeria*. Quinolone and macrolide antibiotics are bacteriostatic only. The small number of in vivo studies with these agents is not promising.[103] In addition, *L. monocytogenes* is resistant to cephalosporin antibiotics.[28] Vancomycin has been used in a few penicillin- and sulfa-allergic patients with some success, but the experience with this drug is limited.[101]

Combination of antibiotics for therapy or in vitro testing also has shown varying results. Ampicillin plus gentamicin has a synergistic effect on most *Listeria* strains,[26, 85, 87, 121] although at least one in vivo study has found no evidence of synergy.[48] A combination of vancomycin and gentamicin has shown activity similar to that of ampicillin and gentamicin[85] and has been used successfully in one reported case.[36] In addition, penicillin has been reported to be synergistic with sulfonamides, streptomycin, and other aminoglycosides. There appears to be partial synergy with combinations of ampicillin or vancomycin with rifampin, but combinations of penicillin G and rifampin have shown activity ranging from synergy to antagonism.[85] Although controversy exists, there also appears to be antagonism between a number of other antibiotic combinations (trimethoprim-sulfamethoxazole and rifampin, erythromycin and penicillins, erythromycin and aminoglycosides, penicillin and chloramphenicol, and penicillins and tetracycline).[28, 38, 85] On the basis of results of in vitro susceptibility testing and in vivo models, ampicillin plus gentamicin has proved to be the most reliable synergistic combination and remains the recommended initial therapy for patients suspected of having listeriosis. Trimethoprim-sulfamethoxazole may be considered for use in nonperinatal listeriosis, particularly in the presence of penicillin allergy, but it cannot be recommended for use in perinatal infections because of the concern of bilirubin toxicity with sulfonamides. The use of rifampin alone or in combination requires further study. The duration of therapy depends on the clinical syndrome, the presence of underlying disease, and the response to treatment. In the newborn, 2 weeks of antibiotic therapy usually appears to be adequate.

Some animal studies raise new possibilities for the treatment of listeriosis. Nanoparticle-bound ampicillin can be transported into the intracellular space and has been found to be significantly more effective than is free ampicillin in eradicating *Listeria* in an animal model.[129] Liposomal encapsulation also results in a marked enhancement in therapeutic activity of ampicillin.[8]

PROGNOSIS

Precise morbidity and mortality data in *L. monocytogenes* infection are not available. Maternal listeriosis may result in abortion or stillbirth. Fetal mortality probably is high with gestational listeriosis, although the relative risk of intrauterine death is not known. Convincing evidence that *L. monocytogenes* is associated with repeated abortions is lacking.[40]

Among reported cases of early-onset sepsis, the recent mortality rate in North America is about 30 per cent (see Table 100–1).[1, 30] Most survivors appear to be normal.[29, 30, 119] Sequelae are related to associated complications of prematurity, pneumonia, and sepsis; hydrocephalus and cerebral palsy have been reported.[29, 61] Early treatment of maternal disease would appear to affect fetal and neonatal outcome favorably.[30, 61]

Late-onset *Listeria* meningitis has a mortality rate of less than 10 per cent. The outcome after *Listeria* meningitis may be more favorable than with other types of bacterial meningitis.[63, 126] Major sequelae are hydrocephalus and mental retardation. Beyond the newborn period, the outcome of listeriosis depends on the nature of any underlying disease and the availability of intensive medical care.

PREVENTION

The sporadic nature of the disease in North America emphasized the need for collaborative investigation and reporting of infections by physicians and veterinarians to public health authorities.[10, 37] In 1989, epidemiologists in the United States and Canada endorsed making listeriosis a notifiable disease.[96, 118] Since that time, the important role of food in transmission of sporadic cases has been linked firmly.[107] Aggressive investigation of cases and close inspection and testing of food and food-handling facilities in the United States have been under way since the early 1990s.[78, 118] By tracking strains of *L. monocytogenes* from patients' refrigerators to retail sources, specific foods have been identified. Strict adherence to regulations for pasteurization of raw milk is important to inactivate the organism and prevent listeriosis.[33] However, contamination of foods can occur during preparation and processing of pasteurized milk products and ready-to-eat meat or poultry products. Recommendations for persons at high risk, such as pregnant women and immunocompromised patients, include (1) avoiding soft cheeses, (2) reheating leftover foods or ready-to-eat foods (e.g., hot dogs), and (3) avoiding delicatessen meats.[96, 118] Preventive strategies involving food and facility inspection and dissemination of recommendations and educational materials appear to have reduced the incidence of listeriosis in the United States since 1989.[3, 118]

During a *Listeria* outbreak, prompt investigation and treatment of pregnant women with a febrile "influenza-like" illness have been advocated.[10, 61] The attack rate for late-onset disease among colonized infants is not known, and there are no data to demonstrate that treatment of colonized infants can either eradicate asymptomatic carriage or prevent infection.

Careful attention to the handling of infected infants in a neonatal unit in an attempt to prevent transmission is of the utmost importance for preventing nosocomial infection.[31, 106]

References

1. Ahlfors, C. E., Goetzman, B. W., Halsted, C. C., et al.: Neonatal listeriosis. Am. J. Dis. Child. *131*:405–408, 1977.
2. Albritton, W. L., Wiggins, G. L., and Feeley, J. C.: Neonatal listeriosis: Distribution of serotypes in relation to age at onset of disease. J. Pediatr. *88*:481–483, 1976.
3. Allmann, M., Hofelein, C., Koppel, E., et al.: Polymerase chain reaction (PCR) for detection of pathogenic microorganisms in bacteriological monitoring of dairy products. Res. Microbiol. *146*:85–97, 1995.
4. Armstrong, R. W., and Fung, P. C.: Brainstem encephalitis (rhombenceph-

alitis) due to *Listeria monocytogenes*: Case report and review. Clin. Infect. Dis. *16*:689–702, 1993.
5. Ashton, F. E., Ewan, E. P., and Farber, J. M.: Evidence for *Listeria* transmission by food. Can. Dis. Weekly Rep. *15*:216–220, 1988.
6. Azri, S., and Renton, K. W.: Depression of murine hepatic mixed function oxidase during infection with *Listeria monocytogenes*. J. Pharmacol. Exp. Ther. *243*:1089–1094, 1987.
7. Baker, C. J., and Barrett, F. F.: Group B streptococcal infections in infants: The importance of serotypes. J. A. M. A. *230*:1158–1160, 1974.
8. Bakker-Woundenberg, I. A. J. M., Lokerse, A. F., Vink-van den Berg, J. C., et al.: Liposome-encapsulated ampicillin against *Listeria monocytogenes* in vivo and in vitro. Infection *16*(Suppl. 2):S165–S170, 1988.
9. Berche, P., Reich, K. A., Bonnichon, M., et al.: Detection of anti-listerolysin O for serodiagnosis of human listeriosis. Lancet *335*:624–627, 1990.
10. Bortolussi, R.: An ongoing problem: Perinatal infection due to *Listeria monocytogenes*, an old pathogen reborn. J. Clin. Invest. Med. *7*:213–215, 1984.
11. Bortolussi, R.: Neonatal listeriosis: Where do we go from here? Pediatr. Infect. Dis. *4*:228–229, 1985.
12. Bortolussi, R., Campbell, N., and Krause, V.: Dynamics of *Listeria monocytogenes* type 4b infection in pregnant and infant rats. J. Clin. Invest. Med. *7*:273–279, 1984.
13. Bortolussi, R., McGregor, D. D., Kongshavn, P. A. L., et al.: Host defense mechanisms to perinatal and neonatal *Listeria monocytogenes* infection. Surv. Synth. Pathol. Res. *3*:311–332, 1984.
14. Bortolussi, R., Issekutz, T., Burbridge, S., et al.: Neonatal host defense mechanisms against *Listeria monocytogenes* infection: The role of lipopolysaccharides and interferons. Pediatr. Res. *25*:311–315, 1989.
15. Bouwer, H. G. A., Gibbins, B. L., Jones, S., et al.: Antilisterial immunity includes specificity to listeriolysin O (LLO) and non-LLO-derived determinants. Infect. Immun. *62*:1039–1045, 1994.
16. Braun, T. I., Travis, D., Dee, R. R., et al.: Liver abscess due to *Listeria monocytogenes*: Case report and review. Clin. Infect. Dis. *17*:267–269, 1993.
17. Buchmeier, N. A., and Schreiber, R. D.: Immunology: Requirement of endogenous interferon-γ production for resolution of *Listeria monocytogenes* infection. Proc. Natl. Acad. Sci. U. S. A. *82*:7404–7408, 1985.
18. Buchner, L. H., and Schneirson, S. S.: Clinical and laboratory aspects of *Listeria monocytogenes* infections. Am. J. Med. *45*:904–921, 1968.
19. Burn, C. G.: Clinical and pathological features of an infection caused by a new pathogen of the genus *Listerella*. Am. J. Pathol. *12*:341–348, 1936.
20. Carvajal, A., and Frederiksen, W.: Fatal endocarditis due to *Listeria monocytogenes*. Rev. Infect. Dis. *10*:616–623, 1988.
21. Chen, Y., Nakane, A., and Minagawa, T.: Recombinant murine gamma interferon induces enhanced resistance to *Listeria monocytogenes* infection in neonatal mice. Infect. Immun. *57*:2345–2349, 1989.
22. Cherry, W. B., and Moody, M. D.: Fluorescent antibody techniques in diagnostic microbiology. Bacteriol. Rev. *29*:222–250, 1965.
23. Cossart, P.: The listeriolysin O gene: A chromosomal locus crucial for the virulence of *Listeria monocytogenes*. Infection *16*(Suppl. 2):S157–S159, 1988.
24. Cowart, R. E., Lashmet, J., McIntosh, M. E., et al.: Adherence of a virulent strain of *Listeria monocytogenes* to the surface of a hepatocarcinoma cell line via lectin-substrate interaction. Arch. Microbiol. *153*:282–286, 1990.
25. Desiderio, J. V., Kiener, P. A., Lin, P.-F., et al.: Protection of mice against *Listeria monocytogenes* infection by recombinant human tumor necrosis factor alpha. Infect. Immun. *57*:1615–1617, 1989.
26. Edmiston, C. E., and Gordon, R. C.: Evaluation of gentamicin and penicillin as a synergistic combination in experimental murine listeriosis. Antimicrob. Agents Chemother. *16*:862–863, 1979.
27. Ellis, L. C., Gitelis, S., and Huber, J. F.: Joint infections due to *Listeria monocytogenes*: Case report and review. Clin. Infect. Dis. *20*:1548–1550, 1995.
28. Espaze, E. P., and Reynaud, A. E.: Antibiotic susceptibilities of Listeria: In vitro studies. Infection *16*(Suppl. 2):S160–164, 1988.
29. Evans, J. R., Allen, A. C., Bortolussi, R., et al.: Follow-up study of survivors of fetal and early-onset neonatal listeriosis. J. Clin. Invest. Med. *7*:329–334, 1984.
30. Evans, J. R., Allen, A. C., Stinson, D. A., et al.: Perinatal listeriosis: Report of an outbreak. Pediatr. Infect. Dis. *4*:237–241, 1985.
31. Facinelli, B., Varaldo, P. E., Casolari, C., et al.: Cross-infection with *Listeria monocytogenes* confirmed by DNA fingerprinting. Lancet *2*:1247–1248, 1988.
32. Filice, A. G., Cantrell, H. F., Smith, A. B., et al.: *Listeria monocytogenes* infection in neonates: Investigation of an epidemic. J. Infect. Dis. *138*:17–23, 1978.
33. Food and Drug Administration, Milk and Safety Branch. Center for Infectious Diseases, CDC: Update: Listeriosis and pasteurized milk. M. M. W. R. *37*:764–765, 1988.
34. Frenkel, L., and Bryson, Y. J.: Ontogeny of phytohemagglutinin-induced gamma interferon by leukocytes of healthy infants and children: Evidence for decreased production in infants younger than 2 months of age. J. Pediatr. *111*:97–100, 1987.
35. Gaillard, J.-L., Berche, P., Mounier, J., et al.: In vitro model of penetration and intracellular growth of *Listeria monocytogenes* in the human enterocyte-like cell line caco-2. Infect. Immun. *55*:2822–2829, 1987.
36. Gallagher, P. G., Amedia, C. A., and Watankunakom, C.: *L. monocytogenes* endocarditis in a patient on chronic hemodialysis, successfully treated with vancomycin and gentamicin. Infection *14*:125, 1986.
37. Gellin, B. G.: Listeriosis. J. A. M. A. *261*:1313–1319, 1989.
38. Gordon, R. C., Barrett, F. F., and Clark, D. J.: Influence of several antibiotics, singly and in combination, on the growth of *Listeria monocytogenes*. J. Pediatr. *80*:667–670, 1972.
39. Gordon, R. C., Barrett, F. F., and Yow, M. D.: Ampicillin treatment of listeriosis. J. Pediatr. *77*:1067–1070, 1970.
40. Gray, M. L., Seeliger, H. P. R., and Potel, J.: Perinatal infections due to *Listeria monocytogenes*: Do these affect subsequent pregnancies? Clin. Pediatr. *2*:614–623, 1963.
41. Green, H. T., and Macaulay, M. B.: Hospital outbreak of *Listeria monocytogenes* septicemia: A problem of cross infection? Lancet *2*:1039–1040, 1978.
42. Günther, G., and Philipson, A.: Oral trimethoprim as follow-up treatment of meningitis caused by *Listeria monocytogenes*. Rev. Infect. Dis. *10*:53, 1988.
43. Harris, J. O., Marquez, J., Swerdloff, M. A., et al.: *Listeria* brain abscess in the acquired immunodeficiency syndrome. Arch. Neurol. *46*:250, 1989.
44. Hauf, N., Goebel, W., Serfling, E., et al.: *Listeria monocytogenes* infection enhances transcription factor NF-kB in P388D$_1$ macrophage-like cells. Infect. Immun. *62*:2740–2747, 1994.
45. Hawkins, A. E., Bortolussi, R., and Issekutz, A. C.: *In vitro* and *in vivo* activity of various antibiotics against *Listeria monocytogenes* type 4b. Clin. Invest. Med. *7*:335–341, 1984.
46. Hess, C. B., Niesel, D. W., Cho, Y. J., et al.: Bacterial invasion of fibroblasts induces interferon production. J. Immunol. *138*:3949–3953, 1987.
47. Hess, J., Gentschev, I., Szalay, G., et al.: *Listeria monocytogenes* p60 supports host cell invasion by and in vivo survival of attenuated *Salmonella typhimurium*. Infect. Immun. *63*:2047–2053, 1995.
48. Hof, H., and Waldenmeier, G.: Therapy of experimental listeriosis: An evaluation of different antibiotics. Infection *16*(Suppl. 2):S171–S174, 1988.
49. Holt, J. G., Krieg, N. R., Sneath, P. H. A., et al. (eds.): *In* Bergey's Manual of Determinative Bacteriology. Baltimore, Williams & Wilkins, 1994, pp. 566–567.
50. Hood, M.: Listeriosis as an infection of pregnancy manifested in the newborn. Pediatrics *27*:390–396, 1961.
51. Hudak, A. P., Lee, S. H., Issekutz, A. C., et al.: Comparison of three serological methods—enzyme-linked immunosorbent assay, complement fixation, and microagglutination—in diagnosis of human perinatal *Listeria monocytogenes* infection. Clin. Invest. Med. *7*:349–354, 1984.
52. Hügin, A. W., Cerny, A., Wrann, M., et al.: Effect of cyclosporin A on immunity to *Listeria monocytogenes*. Infect. Immun. *52*:12–17, 1986.
53. Inoue, S., Itagaki, S., and Amano, F.: Intracellular killing of *Listeria monocytogenes* in the J774.1 macrophage-like cell line and the lipopolysaccharide (LPS)-resistant mutant LPS1916 cell line defective in the generation of reactive oxygen intermediates after LPS treatment. Infect. Immun. *63*:1876–1886, 1995.
54. Jacquet, C., Catimel, B., Brosch, R., et al.: Investigations related to the epidemic strain involved in the French listeriosis outbreak in 1992. Appl. Environ. Microbiol. *61*:2242–2246, 1995.
55. Jaton, K., Sahli, R. and Bille, J.: Development of polymerase chain reaction assays for detection of *Listeria monocytogenes* in clinical cerebrospinal fluid samples. J. Clin. Microbiol. *30*:1931–1936, 1992.
56. Issekutz, T., Evans, J., and Bortolussi, R.: The immune response of human neonates to *Listeria monocytogenes* infection. Clin. Invest. Med. *7*:281–286, 1984.
57. Jurado, R. L., Farley, M. M., Pereira, E., et al.: Increased risk of meningitis and bacteremia due to *Listeria monocytogenes* in patients with human immunodeficiency virus infection. Clin. Infect. Dis. *17*:224–227, 1993.
58. Kaczmarski, E. B., and Jones, D. M.: Listeriosis and ready-cooked chicken. Lancet *1*:549, 1989.
59. Karunasagar, I., Senghaas, B., Krohne, G., et al.: Ultrastructural study of *Listeria monocytogenes* entry into cultured human colonic epithelial cells. Infect. Immun. *62*:3554–3558, 1994.
60. Kathariou, S., Rocourt, J., Hof, H., et al.: Levels of *Listeria monocytogenes* hemolysin are not directly proportional to virulence in experimental infections of mice. Infect. Immun. *56*:534–536, 1988.
61. Katz, V. L., and Weinstein, L.: Antepartum treatment of *Listeria monocytogenes* septicemia. South. Med. J. *75*:1353–1354, 1982.
62. Kayashima, S., Tsuru, S., Hata, N., et al.: Therapeutic effect of granulocyte colony-stimulating factor (G-CSF) on the protection against *Listeria* infection in SCID mice. Immunology *80*:471–476, 1993.
63. Kessler, S. L., and Dajani, A. S.: *Listeria* meningitis in infants and children. Pediatr. Infect. Dis. J. *9*:61–62, 1990.
64. Klatt, E. C., Pavlova, Z., Teberg, A. J., et al.: Epidemic perinatal listeriosis at autopsy. Hum. Pathol. *17*:1278–1281, 1986.
65. Kohl, S., West, M. S., and Loo, L. S.: Defects in interleukin-2 stimulation of neonatal natural killer cytotoxicity to herpes simplex virus–infected cells. J. Pediatr. *112*:976–981, 1988.
66. Kongshaven, P. A. A., and Skamene, E.: The role of natural resistance in protection of the murine host from listeriosis. Clin. Invest. Med. *7*:253–257, 1984.
67. Kuhn, M., and Goebel, W.: Identification of an extracellular protein of *Listeria monocytogenes* possibly involved in intracellular uptake by mammalian cells. Infect. Immun. *57*:55–61, 1989.
68. Langermans, J. A. M., Mayanski, D. M., Nibbering, P. H., et al.: Effect of

IFN-γ and endogenous TNF on the histopathological changes in the liver of *Listeria monocytogenes*-infected mice. Immunology *81*:192–197, 1994.
69. Larsson, S., Cederberg, A., Ivarsson, S., et al.: *Listeria monocytogenes* causing hospital acquired enterocolitis and meningitis in newborn infants. Br. Med. J. 2:473–474, 1978.
70. Lennon, D., Lewis, B., Mantell, C., et al.: Epidemic perinatal listeriosis. Pediatr. Infect. Dis. 3:30–34, 1984.
71. LeSouef, P. N., and Walters, B. N. J.: Neonatal listeriosis. Med. J. Aust. 2:188–191, 1981.
72. Lessing, M. P., Curtis, G. D., and Bowler, I. C.: *Listeria ivanovii* infection. J. Infect. *29*:230–231, 1994.
73. Linnan, M. J., Mascola, L., Lou, X. D., et al.: Epidemic listeriosis associated with Mexican-style cheese. N. Engl. J. Med. *319*:823–828, 1988.
74. Liu, A., Simpson, R. J., and Cheers, C.: Role of interleukin-6 in T-cell activation during primary and secondary infection with *Listeria monocytogenes*. Infect. Immun. *63*:2790–2792, 1995.
75. Louthrenoo, W., and Schumacher, H. R.: *Listeria monocytogenes* osteomyelitis complicating leukemia: Report and literature review of *Listeria* osteoarticular infections. J. Rheumatol. *17*:107–110, 1990.
76. Lu, C. Y.: The delayed ontogenesis of 1a-positive macrophages: Implications for host defense and self-tolerance in the neonate. Clin. Invest. Med. 7:263–267, 1984.
77. Lu, C. Y., and Unanue, E. R.: Ontogeny of murine macrophages: Functions related to antigen presentation. Infect. Immun. *36*:169–175, 1982.
78. MacGowan, A. P., O'Donaghue, K., Nicholls, S., et al.: Typing of *Listeria* spp. by random amplified polymorphic DNA (RAPD) analysis. J. Med. Microbiol. *38*:322–327, 1993.
79. Mackaness, G. B.: The immunological basis of acquired cellular resistance. J. Exp. Med. *120*:105–119, 1964.
80. Massarotti, E. M., and Dinerman, H.: Septic arthritis due to *Listeria monocytogenes*: Report and review of the literature. J. Rheumatol. *17*:111–113, 1990.
81. McBride, M. E., and Girard, K. F.: Procedure for the selective isolation of *Listeria monocytogenes*. J. Lab. Clin. Med. *55*:153–157, 1960.
82. McCallum, R. E., and Sword, C. P.: Mechanisms of pathogenesis in *Listeria monocytogenes* infection. V. Early imbalance in host energy metabolism during experimental listeriosis. Infect. Immun. 5:863–871, 1972.
83. McLauchlin, J.: Distribution of serovars of *Listeria monocytogenes* isolated from different categories of patients with listeriosis. Eur. J. Clin. Microbiol. Infect. Dis. *9*:210–213, 1990.
84. McLauchlin, J., Hall, S. M., Velani, S. K., et al.: Human listeriosis and paté: A possible association. B. M. J. *303*:773–775, 1991.
85. Meyer, R. D., and Liu, S.: Determination of the effect of antimicrobics in combination against *Listeria monocytogenes*. Diagn. Microbiol. Infect. Dis. 6:199–206, 1986.
86. Moellering, R. C., Medoff, G., Leech, I., et al.: Antibiotic synergism against *Listeria monocytogenes*. Antimicrob. Agents Chemother. *1*:30–34, 1972.
87. Mohan, K., Gordon, R. C., Beaman, T. C., et al.: Synergism of penicillin and gentamicin against *Listeria monocytogenes* in *ex vivo* hemodialysis culture. J. Infect. Dis. *135*:51–54, 1977.
88. Moore, R. M., and Zehmer, R. B.: Listeriosis in the United States, 1971. J. Infect. Dis. *127*:610–611, 1973.
89. Murray, E. G. D., Webb, R. A., and Swann, M. B. R.: A disease of rabbits characterized by large mononuclear leucocytosis, caused by a hitherto undescribed bacillus *Bacterium monocytogenes* (n. sp.). J. Pathol. Bacteriol. *29*:407–439, 1926.
90. Myers, J. P., Peterson, G., and Rashid, A.: Peritonitis due to *Listeria monocytogenes* complicating continuous ambulatory peritoneal dialysis. J. Infect. Dis. *148*:1130, 1983.
91. Nakane, A., Okamoto, M., Asano, M., et al.: An anti-CD3 monoclonal antibody protects mice against a lethal infection with *Listeria monocytogenes* through induction of endogenous cytokines. Infect. Immun. *61*:2786–2793, 1993.
92. Nieman, R. E., and Lorber, B.: Listeriosis in adults: A changing pattern: Report of eight cases and review of the literature, 1968–1978. Rev. Infect. Dis. 2:207–227, 1980.
93. Nyfeldt, A.: Etiologie de la mononucleose infectieuse. Compt. Rend. Soc. Biol. *101*:590–591, 1929.
94. Okamoto, M., Nakane, A., and Minagawa, T.: Host resistance to an intragastric infection with *Listeria monocytogenes* in mice depends on cellular immunity and intestinal bacterial flora. Infect. Immun. *62*:3080–3085, 1994.
95. Paterson, J. S.: The antigenic structure of organisms of the genus *Listerella*. J. Pathol. Bacteriol. *51*:427–436, 1940.
96. Pinner, R. W., Schuchat, A., Swaminathan, B., et al.: Role of foods in sporadic listeriosis. II. Microbiologic and epidemiologic investigation. J. A. M. A. *267*:2046–2050, 1992.
97. Portnoy, D. A., Chakraborty, T., Goebel, W., et al.: Molecular determinants of *Listeria monocytogenes* pathogenesis. Infect. Immun. *60*:1263–1267, 1992.
98. Portnoy, D. A., Jacks, P. S., and Hinrichs, D. J.: Role of hemolysin for the intracellular growth of *Listeria monocytogenes*. J. Exp. Med. *167*:1459–1471, 1988.
99. Rakhmilevich, A. L.: Evidence for a significant role of CD4+ T cells in adoptive immunity to *Listeria monocytogenes* in the liver. Immunology *82*:249–254, 1994.
100. Ray, C. G., and Wedgewood, R. J.: Neonatal listeriosis. Pediatrics *34*:378–392, 1964.
101. Renoult, E., Chabot, F., Aymard, B., et al.: Treatment of *Listeria* bacteremia with vancomycin. Rev. Infect. Dis. *13*:181–182, 1991.
102. Riedo, F. X., Pinner, R. W., de Lourdes Tosca, M., et al.: A point-source foodborne listeriosis outbreak: Documented incubation period and possible mild illness. J. Infect. Dis. *170*:693–696, 1994.
103. Rolston, K. V. I., and Bodey, G. P.: Activity of new antimicrobial agents against *Listeria monocytogenes*. Eur. J. Clin. Microbial. *6*:686–688, 1987.
104. Scheld, W. M.: Evaluation of rifampin and other antibiotics against *Listeria monocytogenes in vitro* and *in vivo*. Rev. Infect. Dis. *5*(Suppl. 3):S593–S599, 1983.
105. Schlech, W. F., Lavigne, P. M., Bortolussi, R. A., et al.: Epidemic listeriosis: Evidence for transmission by food. N. Engl. J. Med. *308*:203–206, 1983.
106. Schuchat, A., Lizano, C., Broome, C. V., et al.: Outbreak of neonatal listeriosis associated with mineral oil. Pediatr. Infect. Dis. J. *10*:183–189, 1991.
107. Schuchat, A., Swaminathan, B., and Broome, C. V.: Epidemiology of human listeriosis. Clin. Microbiol. Rev. *4*:169–183, 1991.
108. Schuchat, A.: Gastrointestinal carriage of *Listeria monocytogenes* in household contacts of patients with listeriosis. J. Infect. Dis. *167*:1261–1262, 1993.
109. Schwartz, B., Broome, C. V., Brown, G. R., et al.: Association of sporadic listeriosis with consumption of uncooked hot dogs and undercooked chicken. Lancet 2:779–782, 1988.
110. Skogberg, K., Syrjanen, J., Jahkota, M., et al.: Clinical presentation and outcome of listeriosis in patients with and without immunosuppressive therapy. Clin. Infect. Dis. *14*:815–821, 1992.
111. Seeliger, H. P. R.: Listeriosis. Basel–New York, S. Karger, 1961.
112. Seeliger, H. P. R., and Finger, H.: Analytical serology of *Listeria*. *In* Kwapinski, J. B. G. (ed.): Analytical Serology of Microorganisms. New York, John Wiley & Sons, 1969, pp. 549–608.
113. Serushago, B., MacDonald, C., Lee, S. H. S., et al.: Interferon-γ detection in cultures of newborn cells exposed to *Listeria monocytogenes*. J. Interferon Cytokine Res. *15*:633–635, 1995.
114. Spitzer, P. G., and Hammer, S. M.: Treatment of *Listeria monocytogenes* infection with trimethoprim-sulfamethoxazole: Case report and review of the literature. Rev. Infect. Dis. *8*:427, 1986.
115. Stamm, A. M., Dismukes, W. E., Simmons, B. P., et al.: Listeriosis in renal transplant recipients: Report of an outbreak and review of 102 cases. Rev. Infect. Dis. *4*:665–682, 1982.
116. Steinman, C. R.: Specific detection and semiquantitation of microorganisms in tissue by nucleic acid hybridization. I. Characterization of the method and application to model systems. J. Lab. Clin. Med. *86*:164–174, 1975.
117. Sword, C. P.: Mechanisms of pathogenesis in *Listeria monocytogenes* infection. I. The influence of iron. J. Bacteriol. *92*:536–542, 1966.
118. Tappero, J. W., Schuchat, A., Deaver, K. A., et al.: Reduction in the incidence of human listeriosis in the United States: Effectiveness of prevention efforts? J. A. M. A. *273*:1118–1122, 1995.
119. Teberg, A. J., Yonekura, M. L., Salminen, C., et al.: Clinical manifestations of epidemic neonatal listeriosis. Pediatr. Infect. Dis. J. *6*:817–820, 1987.
120. Topalovski, M., Yang, S. S., and Boonpasat, Y.: Listeriosis of the placenta: Clinicopathologic study of seven cases. Am. J. Obstet. Gynecol. *169*:616–620, 1993.
121. Traub, W. H.: Perinatal listeriosis. Chemotherapy *27*:423–431, 1981.
122. Tsai, Y. H., Hirth, R. S., and Leitner, F.: A murine model for listerial meningitis and meningoencephalomyelitis: Therapeutic evaluation of drugs in mice. Chemotherapy *26*:196–206, 1980.
123. van Furth, R., van Zwet, T. L., Buisman, A. M., et al.: Anti-tumor necrosis factor antibodies inhibit the influx of granulocytes and monocytes into an inflammatory exudate and enhance the growth of *Listeria monocytogenes* in various organs. J. Infect. Dis. *170*:234–237, 1994.
124. Varughese, P. V., and Carter, A. O.: Human listeriosis in Canada. Can. Dis. Weekly Rep. *15*:213–215, 1988.
125. Vischer, W. A., and Rominger, C.: Rifampicin against experimental listeriosis in the mouse. Chemotherapy *24*:104–111, 1978.
126. Visintine, A. M., Oleske, J. M., and Nahmias, A. J.: *Listeria monocytogenes* infection in infants and children. Am. J. Dis. Child. *131*:393–397, 1977.
127. Wagner, R. D., Maroushek, N. M., Brown, J. F., et al.: Treatment with anti–interleukin-10 monoclonal antibody enhances early resistance to but impairs complete clearance of *Listeria monocytogenes* infection in mice. Infect. Immun. *62*:2345–2353, 1994.
128. Wilder, M. S., and Sword, C. P.: Mechanisms of pathogenesis in *Listeria monocytogenes* infection. II. Characterization of listeriosis in the CD-1 mouse and survey of biochemical lesions. J. Bacteriol. *93*:531–542, 1967.
129. Youssef, M., Fattal, E., Alonso, M.-J., et al.: Effectiveness of nanoparticle-bound ampicillin in the treatment of *Listeria monocytogenes* infection in athymic nude mice. Antimicrob. Agents Chemother. *32*:1204–1207, 1988.
130. Zhan, Y., and Cheers, C.: Differential induction of macrophage-derived cytokines by live and dead intracellular bacteria in vitro. Infect. Immun. *63*:720–723, 1995.

101

TUBERCULOSIS

Jeffrey R. Starke and Margaret H. D. Smith

Tuberculosis still ranks as "Captain of the Men of Death"—the most important infectious disease in the world in terms of morbidity and mortality. Recognizable in skeletons from the Stone Age and in mummified corpses from the Egyptian Old Kingdom, tuberculosis became more widespread in Western Europe after the plague years of the Middle Ages and epidemic during the era of urbanization and industrialization in the eighteenth and nineteenth centuries.[135] At that time, scrofula affected more than half of the young inhabitants of workhouses and orphanages.

As similar social trends developed outside Europe, tuberculosis followed. In the eastern cities of the United States (Boston, New York, and Philadelphia), the mortality from tuberculosis was about 400 per 100,000 population. With improving socioeconomic conditions, the mortality fell to 200 per 100,000 around 1900 and to 26 per 100,000 by 1950. Stress in all its forms—famine, war, rationing, long working hours, child labor, population displacements, crowded living and working conditions—favors the spread of tuberculosis in human beings, whereas years of peace and plenty favor its rapid decline.[134, 402] The decrease in the Western world in the incidence of tuberculosis was accentuated by the discovery, development, and widespread use of antituberculosis drugs, beginning in the late 1940s.

Another important factor leading to the decline of tuberculosis in Western countries was the recognition in the 1920s of the importance of bovine tuberculosis and its successful eradication as a public health problem in the United States by gradual slaughter of infected cattle and almost universal pasteurization of milk.

Tuberculosis was recognized as a clinical entity in the early 19th century by Schönlein, who first used the term *tuberculosis* in 1830, and by Laennec in Paris, among others. Another Frenchman, Parrot, first recognized that "whenever a bronchial node is tuberculous, there is a parenchymal lesion" (Parrot's law, 1876), although credit for extensively detailed descriptions of the primary focus goes to Anton Ghon (1866–1936), professor of pathology in Prague.[62] In 1882, Koch identified *Mycobacterium tuberculosis.* The special diagnostic tools essential to understanding the disease in children were provided by Escherich, who in 1898 set up in Graz the first diagnostic roentgenography for children; by von Pirquet, Mantoux, Mandel, and Moro, who developed tuberculin testing between 1907 and 1910; and by Meunier and DeLille, who in 1898 taught the usefulness of gastric lavage in children.[62] Revealing long-term studies on the natural history of tuberculosis in children and in chemotherapy and prevention came principally from Scandinavia (Wallgren, Ustvedt, Holm, Hyge) and the United States (Brailey, Hardy, Lincoln, Hsu, Ferrebee).

Tuberculosis currently seems to be in a rapidly shifting position worldwide. After years of steady decline in its incidence in the United States, the Centers for Disease Control and Prevention (CDC) in 1989 formed the Advisory Committee for Elimination of Tuberculosis and set the year 2010 as the goal for elimination. Unfortunately, the AIDS epidemic was just getting under way, and no one realized at first the devastatingly stimulating effect that these two diseases have on each other, thereby making the elimination of tuberculosis infinitely more difficult than it first appeared to be. Moreover, the World Health Organization (WHO) has developed a new tuberculosis control strategy and has declared tuberculosis to be a "global health emergency," the first infectious disease to receive this designation.[268] Thus, it behooves every physician and public health worker to keep up to date on all facets of tuberculosis: epidemiology, diagnosis, treatment, and prevention.

TERMINOLOGY—EXPOSURE, INFECTION, DISEASE

The pathophysiology of tuberculosis is complicated, and the delay between infection and disease makes certain pathophysiologic events less distinct. This chapter will consider three major stages of tuberculosis: exposure, infection, and disease (Table 101–1).[119, 481]

Exposure means that the child has had significant contact with an adult or adolescent with infectious pulmonary tuberculosis. The contact investigation—examining those individuals close to a suspected case of tuberculosis with a tuberculin skin test, chest roentgenogram, and physical examination—is the most important activity in a community to prevent cases of tuberculosis in children.[47, 210] The most frequent setting for exposure of a child is the household, but it can occur in a school, day care center, or other closed setting.[202] In this stage, the tuberculin skin test is negative, the chest roentgenogram is normal, and the child lacks signs or symptoms of disease. Some exposed children may have inhaled droplet nuclei infected with *M. tuberculosis* and have early infection, but the clinician cannot know it because it takes up to 3 months for delayed hypersensitivity to tuberculin—a positive skin test—to develop. Children younger than 5 years of age in the exposure stage are treated in the United States to prevent the rapid development of disseminated or meningeal tuberculosis, which can occur before the skin test becomes reactive.[333, 364]

Infection occurs when the individual inhales droplet nuclei containing *M. tuberculosis*, which becomes established intracellularly within the lung and associated lymphoid tissue. The hallmark of tuberculosis infection is a reactive tuberculin skin test. In this stage, the child has no signs or symptoms and the chest roentgenogram is either normal or reveals only granuloma or calcifications in the lung parenchyma and/or regional lymph nodes. In developed countries, virtually all children with tuberculosis infection should receive treatment, usually with isoniazid (INH), to prevent the development of disease in the near or distant future.

Disease occurs when signs or symptoms or roentgenographic manifestations caused by *M. tuberculosis* become apparent. The word *tuberculosis* refers to disease. Not all infected individuals have the same risk of developing disease. An immunocompetent adult with untreated tuberculosis infection has approximately a 5 to 10 per cent *lifetime* risk of developing disease; one-half of the risk occurs in the first 2 to 3 years after infection. Adults with tuberculosis infection who then become infected with HIV have a 5 to 10 per cent

TABLE 101–1. Characteristics of the Stages of Tuberculosis in Children

	Stage		
	Exposure	*Infection*	*Disease*
CDC classification	I	II	III
Skin test results	Negative	Positive	90% positive
Chest radiograph	Normal	Usually normal*	Usually abnormal†
Physical examination	Normal	Normal	Usually abnormal‡
Treatment?	If ≤5 years of age	Always	Always
Number of drugs	Usually 1	Usually 1	Usually 3 or 4

*If the chest radiograph reveals only pulmonary granuloma or calcification in a child with a positive tuberculin skin test, this is considered to be infection, not disease.

†Some children with extrapulmonary tuberculosis have a normal chest radiograph.

‡Some children with pulmonary tuberculosis have a normal physical examination but an abnormal chest radiograph.

CDC, Centers for Disease Control and Prevention.

annual risk of developing tuberculosis disease.[438] Historical studies have shown that up to 40 per cent of immunocompetent infants with untreated tuberculosis infection develop disease, often serious, life-threatening forms, within 1 to 2 years.

EPIDEMIOLOGY

Tuberculosis remains the leading infectious disease in the world. The WHO estimates that during the 1990s there will be 90 million new cases of tuberculosis worldwide and 30 million deaths caused by the disease.[403, 472] About 13 million new cases and 5 million deaths will occur among children younger than 15 years of age.[268] In many developing countries, the annual risk of infection with *M. tuberculosis* is 2 to 5 per cent.[151] More than 40 per cent of the world's population (2 billion people) are infected with tubercle bacilli. Over the past decade, the number of tuberculosis cases has increased in every region of the world except Western Europe. The inability to control tuberculosis despite the availability of effective, relatively inexpensive therapy probably is the greatest medical failure of mankind.

The incidence and mortality of tuberculosis in the United States declined steadily during this century until the year 1985, when the overall case rate was approximately 10 per 100,000, for a total of 22,201 new active cases. At that time, the incidence curve flattened out (Fig. 101–1), and case numbers and rates increased to a recent high of 26,673 cases in 1992. Although total tuberculosis case numbers rose 20 per cent in the United States from 1985 to 1992, the number of pediatric tuberculosis cases rose 40 per cent.[524] Most experts cite four likely causes for these increases: (1) the coepidemic of HIV infection, because immunosuppression from HIV infection is the most potent risk factor for development of tuberculosis disease in a previously infected adult[266, 545]; (2) increasing rates of tuberculosis in foreign-born individuals in the United States, caused by both an increased number of infected individuals entering the country and more persons developing tuberculosis after arrival; (3) increased transmission of *M. tuberculosis* among adults in congregate settings, including jails and prisons, nursing homes, homeless shelters, HIV treatment facilities, hospitals, and, rarely, schools; and (4) a decline in the tuberculosis public health infrastructure in many regions and cities.[59, 93, 482] By 1995, after several years of intense and expensive effort,[158] the number of tuberculosis cases in the United States had declined again to 22,813.[80]

High tuberculosis rates always have occurred among the socioeconomically deprived,[67] as can be seen in Figure 101–2. In upstate New York in 1973, the case rate among the lowest socioeconomic class was 129 per 100,000, compared with only 4.6 per 100,000 in the highest socioeconomic class.[198] In a South Philadelphia ghetto between 1970 and 1972, there was a tuberculosis new-case rate of 177 per 100,000.

That factors other than socioeconomic status also influence susceptibility to tuberculosis was shown many years ago. In the United States, highly urbanized immigrants, such as Jews from European ghettos, fared much better than their rural Irish and African counterparts, presumably because generations of exposure to the disease had selected in favor of the more resistant individuals.[133, 397] Moreover, inherited susceptibility to tuberculosis has been shown, particularly by studies on twins, to exist among humans as well as among laboratory animals.[310, 441]

According to the CDC, the highest tuberculosis rates are found among the nonwhite segments of the population (Fig. 101–3).[67, 412] In 1995, the new active case rate among non-Hispanic whites was only 3.1 per 100,000 but was 45.9 among Asian/Pacific Islanders, 23.9 among blacks, 18.0 among Hispanics, and 16.5 among Native American/Alaskan natives. The greatest number of cases actually occurred in the black population because of its relative size. A study on tuberculosis in the pediatric population of Houston, Texas, showed the majority of cases occurring among Hispanics.[484] Other ways

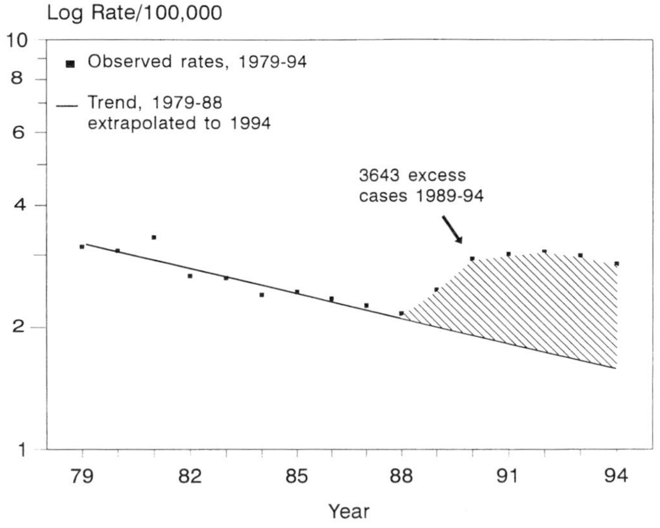

FIGURE 101–1. *Observed and expected tuberculosis cases in children younger than 15 years of age in the United States, 1979–1994.*

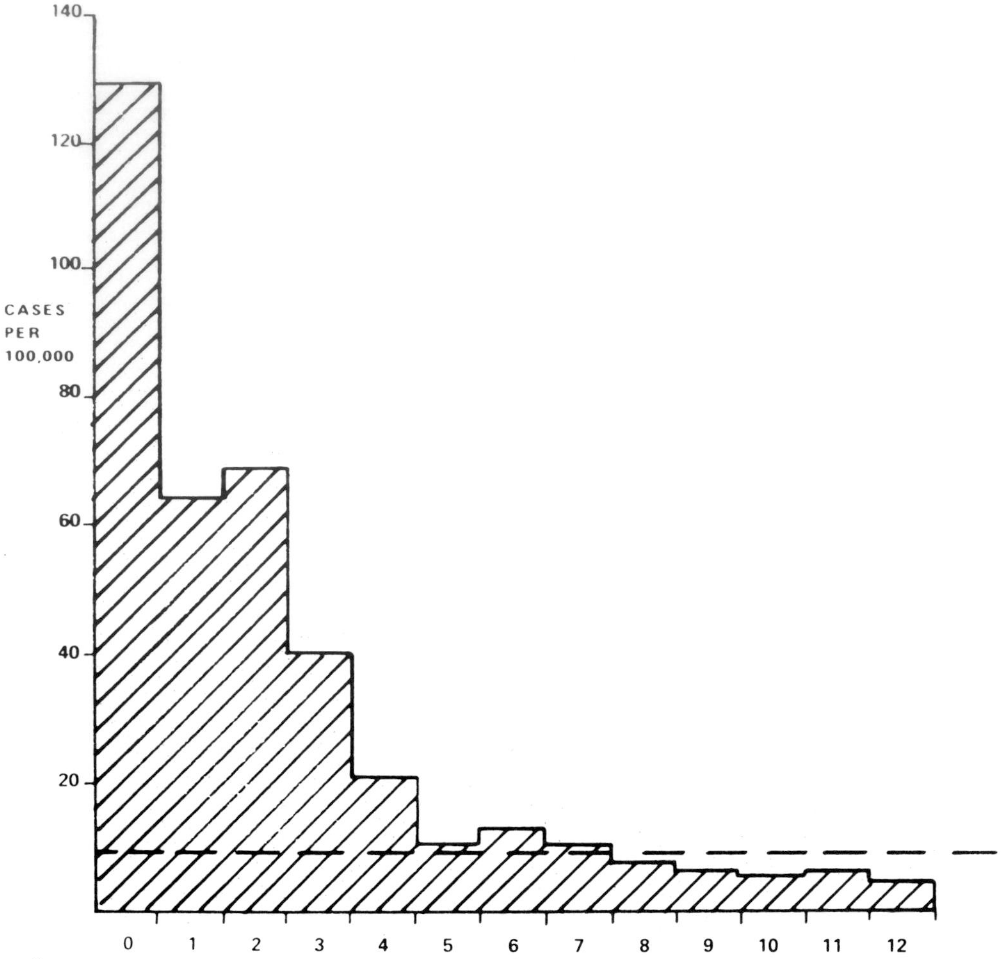

FIGURE 101–2. *Incidence rates of tuberculosis (new active cases per 100,000) according to socioeconomic level. Upstate New York, 1973. (From Hinman, A. R., Judd, J. M., Kolnik, J. P., et al.: Changing risks in tuberculosis. Am. J. Epidemiol. 103:486–497, 1976.)*

of looking at the population show "nests" of active disease, particularly among immigrants during the first year after arrival as well as among the homeless; migrant workers; the elderly, particularly those in nursing homes; current and former inmates of correctional institutions[32]; the HIV-infected; some hospitalized patients (nosocomial)[31, 49, 335, 384]; and individuals with any form of immunodepression (e.g., steroid therapy, lymphoma). Between 30 and 50 per cent of recent immigrants to the United States have tuberculosis infection.[325] It is clear that children from these population groups (particularly foreign-born children) or children who have contact,

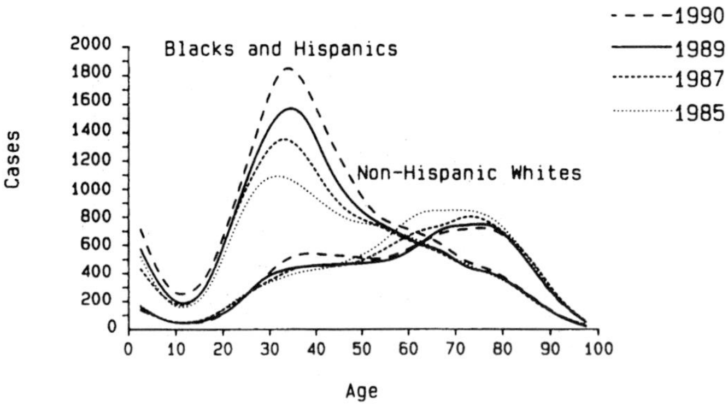

FIGURE 101–3. *Tuberculosis cases among Hispanics and blacks compared with non-Hispanic whites in the United States, 1985–1990.*

direct or indirect, with these groups (e.g., contact with a grandparent in a nursing home, with a father in prison, with an HIV-infected relative) are at higher-than-average risk for tuberculosis infection. In addition, the high-risk pediatric group includes foreign-born adoptees[280] and some foster children.

The relatively high incidence of tuberculosis among minority groups is important from the point of view of children because it occurs largely among people in their twenties, thirties, and forties, at a time when many of these highly infectious individuals are likely to be in contact with children (see Fig. 101–3). That children in the United States population continue to be infected is shown in Table 101–2. The highest rates of pediatric tuberculosis occur in children younger than 5 years of age. Children 5 to 14 years of age (the age termed in the older German literature "the favorable school age period") have a consistently lower case rate than does any other segment of the population. Table 101–2 depicts the striking association of ethnicity with the case rate in children. In early childhood, there is no significant difference in incidence between the sexes, although adolescent girls have a higher rate than adolescent boys. Childhood tuberculosis geographically is focal in the United States (Fig. 101–4) and especially is concentrated in large urban areas.

Throughout the world, tuberculosis case rates tend to be higher among immigrant and migrant populations. In 1995 in the United States, 35 per cent of tuberculosis cases occurred among foreign-born individuals, up from 22 per cent in 1986.[325] The estimated tuberculosis case rates are 13 to 15 times higher in foreign-born compared with U.S.–born persons.

TABLE 101–2. Tuberculosis Cases and Case Rates Among Children Younger Than 15 Years of Age by Race and Ethnicity, United States, 1985 and 1994

	1985			1994		
Race/Ethnicity	*Cases*	*Rate**	*RR†*	*Cases*	*Rate**	*RR†*
White, non-Hispanic	254	0.69	1.0	232	0.61	1.0
Black	450	5.95	8.62	574	6.76	11.08
Hispanic	349	6.33	9.17	650	8.15	13.36
Asian/Pacific Islander	155	11.64	16.87	185	8.92	14.62
Native American/Alaskan native	47	10.00	14.49	31	5.52	9.05

*Rate per 100,000 children per year.
†Rate relative to white, non-Hispanic children.
From Ussery, X. T., Valway, S. E., McKenna, M., et al.: Epidemiology of tuberculosis among children in the United States. Pediatr. Infect. Dis. J. *15*:697–704, 1996.

Individuals from six countries—Mexico, the Philippines, Vietnam, South Korea, Haiti, and China—accounted for about 60 per cent of these cases. The majority of cases occur within 5 years of immigration, indicating that many cases could be prevented if appropriate screening and treatment programs were carried out.[325, 362]

In most U.S. locales that have experienced recent increases in tuberculosis, the demographic groups with the greatest tuberculosis morbidity also have large numbers of HIV-infected persons.[87, 201, 353] The HIV epidemic has had a profound effect on the epidemiology of tuberculosis in children by two mechanisms:[423] (1) most important, HIV-infected adults with tuberculosis may transmit *M. tuberculosis* to children in their environment, some of whom will develop tuberculosis disease, and (2) children with HIV infection are at increased risk of progressing from asymptomatic tuberculosis infection to disease.[309] Several studies have demonstrated increased rates of childhood tuberculosis associated with increased rates of disease among HIV-infected adults in the community.[188, 245] Tuberculosis probably is underdiagnosed in HIV-infected children, especially in the developing world, because of the similarity of its clinical presentation with other opportunistic pulmonary diseases and the difficulty confirming the diagnosis with the skin test or cultures. All children with suspected tuberculosis disease should have HIV serotesting because the two infections are linked epidemiologically and many experts prolong treatment in HIV-infected children with tuberculosis.[183, 546]

The seasonal occurrence of active tuberculosis among children, strikingly higher from January to June in the Northern Hemisphere, long has been noted by clinicians.[204] Closer contact among family members indoors during inclement weather and more frequent coughing produced by winter and spring respiratory infections must be determining factors in this pattern.

Transmission of tuberculosis is from one human to another, usually in infected droplets of mucus that become airborne when an individual coughs, sneezes, or laughs. The droplets dry and become droplet nuclei, which may remain suspended in the air for hours. A single droplet nucleus containing one to three organisms can initiate infection. Only particles less than 10 μm in diameter are small enough to reach the alveoli.[414] Transmission sometimes occurs by direct contact with infected discharges (sputum, saliva, urine, or drainage from an open sinus or abscess); it occasionally occurs by means of heavily contaminated fomites, such as shoes, gastric lavage tubes, bronchoscopes, or syringes prepared by someone with a positive sputum.[114, 196] Rare cases

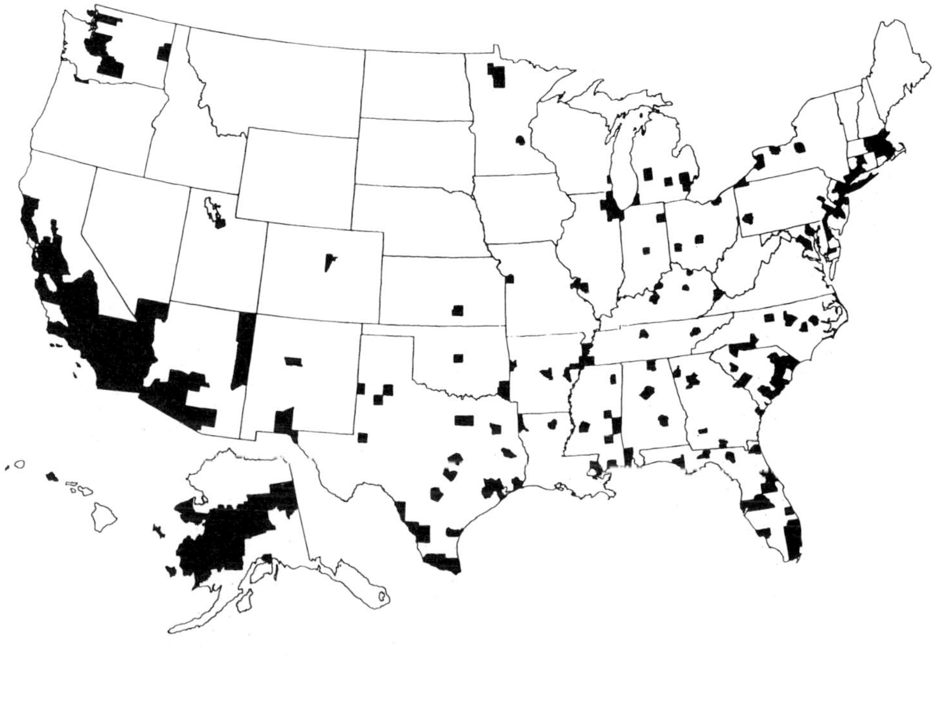

FIGURE 101–4. *U.S. counties reporting tuberculosis in children younger than 15 years of age, 1985–1994.*

of tuberculosis transmitted via a lung transplant have been reported.[340, 411] Dogs may be a source of infection for children because dogs are susceptible to the human type of tubercle bacillus.[409, 475]

The collective experience of many clinicians is that children usually are infected by an adult or adolescent in the immediate household, most often a parent, grandparent, older sibling, boarder, or household employee. Casual extrafamilial contact is the source of infection much less often, but babysitters, schoolteachers, music teachers, school-bus drivers, parishioners, nurses, gardeners, and candy-store keepers have been implicated in individual cases and in hundreds of miniepidemics within limited population groups.[52, 138, 287, 293] Attention has been drawn to the prevalence of active tuberculosis among the residents of nursing homes for the elderly. Children visiting their grandparents have contracted tuberculosis in this setting. Dwellings where tuberculous individuals have resided previously probably are rare sources of infection for children. Within the household of an infectious adult, the infants and toddlers almost always are infected. Also at high risk are the older children and teenagers who wait on the ailing adult, whereas children between 6 and 12 years of age often escape infection. Adults with pulmonary disease who are receiving regular, appropriate chemotherapy probably rarely infect children; much more dangerous are those with chronic tuberculous disease that is unrecognized, inadequately treated, or in relapse because of development of resistance.

Wallgren[539] was the first to point out that children with tuberculosis rarely, if ever, infect other children. Many children with the disease have tuberculin-negative siblings and parents. Children with tuberculosis often have been cared for by their families or in hospitals and institutions without infecting their contacts. When transmission of *M. tuberculosis* has been documented in children's hospitals, it almost invariably has come from an adult with undiagnosed pulmonary tuberculosis.[16, 164, 543] In tuberculous children, tubercle bacilli in endobronchial secretions are relatively sparse, and cough is not at all characteristic of endothoracic tuberculosis or of miliary disease. When young children cough, they lack the tussive force of adults. Children nevertheless play an extremely important role in the transmission of tuberculosis, not so much because they are likely to contaminate their immediate environment, but rather because they may harbor a partially healed infection that lies dormant, only to reactivate as infectious pulmonary tuberculosis many years later under the social, emotional, and physiologic stresses arising during adolescence, pregnancy, or old age. Thus, children infected with *M. tuberculosis* constitute a long-lasting reservoir of tuberculosis in the population.

The risk of infection for child contacts of adults receiving antituberculosis chemotherapy often is a matter of practical concern. Several studies reveal that most contacts are infected by the index case before diagnosis and the start of treatment. Although it is not possible to carry out a definitive clinical study, the evidence indicates that patients on effective chemotherapy rarely transmit *M. tuberculosis*. Nevertheless, it seems prudent to avoid exposing children to adults with positive sputum smears or positive cultures and to assume that adults positive by smear or culture remain infectious for at least several weeks after the start of chemotherapy.

MYCOBACTERIOLOGY

The genus *Mycobacterium*, closely related by its cell wall antigens to the genera *Corynebacterium* and *Nocardia*, presently is classified in the order of Actinomycetales and the family Mycobacteriaceae.[21] Mycobacteria are nonmotile, non–spore-forming, pleomorphic, weakly gram-positive rods, 1 to 5 μm long, typically slender, and slightly "bent." Some appear beaded, and some are clumped. Although *M. tuberculosis* and *M. bovis* show no filaments, others, such as *M. fortuitum*, are characterized by filamentation. In general, species pathogenic for humans are more acid-fast, have more exacting nutritional requirements, grow more slowly, form less pigment, and are more sensitive to chemotherapeutic agents than are the saprophytic species.

The cell wall constituents of mycobacteria determine their most striking biologic properties. The cell walls contain 20 to 60 per cent lipids by dry weight, largely bound to proteins and carbohydrates. These organisms are more resistant than most others to light, alkali, acid, and the bactericidal action of antibodies. Their growth is slow, with a generation time of 14 to 24 hours, perhaps because of the slow metabolic exchange through the waxy "capsule." Their hydrophobic properties make them difficult to study.

Acid-fastness, that is, the capacity to form stable mycolate complexes with certain aryl methane dyes (specifically, carbol-fuchsin, crystal violet, auramine, and rhodamine, which then are not removed readily even by rinsing with 95 per cent ethanol plus hydrochloric acid), is "regarded by many as the hallmark of mycobacteria."[21] The cells appear red when stained with fuchsin (as with the Ziehl-Neelsen or Kinyoun stains), appear purple with crystal violet, or exhibit yellow-green fluorescence under ultraviolet light (when stained with auramine and rhodamine, as in Truant stain). Truant stain, in experienced hands, is considered the best stain for specimens expected to contain small numbers of organisms.

Identification of mycobacteria depends on their staining properties and on their biochemical and metabolic characteristics. Mycobacteria are obligate aerobes. On the whole, their growth requirements are simple (the great exception being *M. leprae*, whose growth requirements have never been defined). *M. tuberculosis* can grow in "classic" media, whose essential ingredients are egg yolk and glycerin (Loewenstein-Jensen, Petragnani, Dorset); often a dye such as malachite green to inhibit contaminants; and sometimes potatoes, charcoal, and so on, which probably neutralize growth inhibitors. They also can grow in simple synthetic media, often with admixture of asparagine, glutamate, or amino acid mixtures (Middlebrook 7H9, Tween-albumin). Once grown, they can be replated on media also containing antituberculosis drugs to determine drug susceptibilities. Isolation on solid media often takes 3 to 6 weeks, followed by another 2 to 4 weeks for drug susceptibility results. Recent improvements in laboratory methods now permit more rapid culture, identification, and drug susceptibility testing of mycobacteria by an automatic radiometric method known as the BACTEC (Becton Dickinson, Towson, MD) method, in which a decontaminated, concentrated specimen is inoculated into a bottle of medium containing carbon-14–labeled palmitic acid as the substrate.[449] As mycobacteria metabolize the carbon-14 palmitic acid, carbon dioxide 14 accumulates in the head space of the bottle, where radioactivity can be measured. Unfortunately, cross-contamination of bottles has been reported, resulting in false-positive cultures.[136] The addition of appropriate dilutions of antituberculosis drugs permits the evaluation of drug susceptibility.[192] The time for identification and drug susceptibility testing can be reduced to 1 to 3 weeks, depending on the size of the inoculum.

Bacteriophage typing to determine relatedness of isolates has advanced slowly. Progress is being made, however, in standardization of techniques, so that phage typing already is of use in strain identification for epidemiologic purposes.[26, 177, 247, 470] However, a newer technique, restriction fragment length polymorphism analysis of mycobacterial DNA, has become a powerful tool for determining strain relatedness in both outbreaks and routine epidemiology of tuberculosis in a community.[7, 455]

RESISTANCE AND IMMUNITY

Natural resistance to tuberculosis infection varies greatly among animal species: humans, guinea pigs, and rabbits are highly susceptible. However, Lurie[310] experimentally bred resistant races of rabbits and showed that although the virulent tubercle bacilli disseminated just as well in the resistant rabbits, their multiplication within the tissues was inhibited. Thus, the differences between resistant and susceptible rabbits appeared to lie in the ability of the former to produce an effective immune response, and this ability appeared to be controlled genetically.

Additional evidence that genetic factors influence susceptibility comes from data in twins. Kallmann and Reisner[250] noted that when one homozygous twin suffered from tuberculosis, the other twin had a higher chance of being affected than was the case with heterozygous twins. Gender affects resistance, and females appear to be especially susceptible during adolescence. The negative nitrogen and calcium balance that can arise during adolescence may account in part for susceptibility at this age.[243]

Likewise, young age appears to predispose to tuberculosis.[427, 526] However, it is impossible to be sure that the apparent susceptibility is not due to a larger dose of bacteria because of more intimate contact between very young children and their infectors. Although diabetes mellitus affects the resistance of adults, it is not clear that it affects that of children. Many viral infections depress tuberculin reactivity, but only measles and perhaps influenza have been incriminated in lowering resistance to tuberculosis.[33, 58, 194, 485, 557] Unfortunately, natural resistance is ill-defined and poorly understood.

Marfan noted in 1886 that acquired resistance to tuberculosis does occur. He commented on the infrequency with which people who have scrofula develop pulmonary tuberculosis in later life, provided the scrofula heals before adolescence (Marfan's law). As in other infections characterized by intracellular parasitism *(Brucella, Listeria, Salmonella)*, macrophages become altered conspicuously through the action of an intermediate product (lymphokine) released when antigen interacts with sensitive lymphoid cells.[314] Synchronously with the appearance of hypersensitivity, the macrophages develop the ability to ingest and kill enormous numbers of organisms. Studies also suggest that delayed hypersensitivity plays a determining role in the mechanism of acquired resistance to *M. tuberculosis* and to other facultative and preferential intracellular parasites, such as *Listeria.* The spread of tuberculosis in experimental animals and in people in whom tuberculin hypersensitivity has been suppressed with steroids accidentally or intentionally suggests that tuberculin hypersensitivity indeed is a desirable accompaniment of tuberculosis infection.

Cell-mediated immunity is regarded as most important in host defense against *M. tuberculosis.*[108] The T-cell–mediated immune response involves a variety of cell subsets that are involved in numerous functions, including protection, delayed hypersensitivity, cytolysis, and establishing memory immunity.[376] The functions also involve an array of cytokines, several of which direct cells of the monocyte/macrophage axis to contain and destroy the invading bacilli. The exact role of individual cytokines is not yet clear, but an emerging concept is that much of the clinical response to the presence of *M. tuberculosis* is determined by the balance of the cellular-cytokine response that, to some degree, is under genetic influence.[376]

PATHOGENESIS

Portal of Entry

The tubercle bacillus usually is inhaled. The observations of Riley[414] suggest that a single tubercle bacillus initiates infection. Ghon, Kuedlich, and their associates[166] (Table 101–3) reported that the primary focus found in 2114 autopsies on children was in the lung in 95.93 per cent of the cases. It especially is significant that their study was done in a time when bovine tuberculosis, which might have produced many primary gastrointestinal foci, was much more common than it is today. Ingestion probably accounts for a small percentage of primary pulmonary foci and for some gastrointestinal foci, particularly in infants who have consumed milk containing bovine tubercle bacilli. Contamination of a superficial skin or mucous membrane lesion, such as an abrasion of the sole of the foot or of the elbow, an insect bite, a ritual circumcision, or infection of the vulva, may lead to infection. Infection by inoculation with a sputum-contaminated syringe has been reported in more recent years.[114, 196] True congenital infection, although rare, may occur either when the mother suffers lymphohematogenous spread during pregnancy or has smoldering endometritis.[528]

Incubation Period

The incubation period from the time the tubercle bacillus enters the body until cutaneous sensitivity develops has been found, in cases in which exposure lasted only 1 day, to be 19 to 56 days. With both bacille Calmette-Guérin (BCG) and experimental infections, the incubation period is shorter when the inoculum is large, and clinical experience suggests that the same is true in humans. Debré, for example, noted long ago that tuberculosis acquired by an infant from its mother was likely to be much more severe than an infection acquired from a visitor to the home. Animal experiments support this concept. The end of the incubation period coincides with the onset of tuberculin hypersensitivity and often is accompanied by what Wallgren called fever of onset or fever of invasion that lasts from 1 to 3 weeks. At this time, the tissue reaction intensifies throughout the primary complex and may permit the complex to be visible on x-ray films.

TABLE 101–3. Portal of Entry of Tubercle Bacilli

Respiratory (%)		Nonrespiratory (%)	
Lung	95.93*	Bowel	1.14
Tonsils	0.09	Skin	0.14
Nose	0.09	Eye	0.05
Middle ear	0.09	Parotid	0.05
Total†	96.20	Total	1.38

*Of 2114 autopsies on children.
†Undetermined, 2.4%.
Data from Ghon, A., and Kuedlich, H.: Die eintrittspforten der infektion. *In* Engel, S., and Pirquet, C. (eds.): Handbuch der Kindertuberkulose. Stuttgart, Georg Thieme Verlag, 1930.

The "Timetable" of Tuberculosis

Wallgren's tremendous experience with tuberculous children in institutions permitted him to recognize and describe the usual early course and timing of the initial infection and of each of its best-known complications.[542] His timetable concept is an extremely useful one for the clinician, permitting a realistic prognosis, an understanding of what complications to look for and when, and a more productive approach to finding the infectious contact (Fig. 101–5).

Symptomatic, massive lymphohematogenous spread, that is, miliary or acute meningeal tuberculosis, is seen in only 0.5 to 3 per cent of infected children. When it does occur, the usual onset is 2 to 6 months after initial infection. Endobronchial tuberculosis, possibly with segmental pulmonary lesions, develops on the average slightly later. The metastatic lesions of bones and joints, which can be expected in 5 per cent of untreated infected children, usually do not appear until about 1 year after infection at the earliest.[183] Renal lesions come later still, 5 to 25 years after initial infection. The relationship between the anatomic site of tuberculosis and the median age of onset in children is shown in Table 101–4. The interval between the initial infection and the appearance of chronic pulmonary tuberculosis is extremely variable but can be months to decades, depending mainly on the age of the child at the time of infection. In adolescents, the interval is likely to be short, but in infants, much longer.

In summary, the first 5 years after initial tuberculosis infection in childhood, but especially the first year, are the time when complications usually occur. Later in life, during times of stress, a previously silent or arrested lesion may reactivate and become dangerous to the patient as well as highly infectious to others.

TABLE 101–4. Median Age of Children* with Tuberculosis by Predominant Site of Involvement, United States, 1988

Site	No. of Cases (%)	Median Age (yr)
Pulmonary	1213 (77.5)	6
Lymphatic	209 (13.3)	5
Pleural	49 (3.1)	16
Meningeal	29 (1.9)	2
Bone/joint	19 (1.2)	8
Other	15 (1.0)	12
Miliary	14 (0.9)	1
Genitourinary	13 (0.8)	16
Peritoneal	4 (0.3)	13
Not stated	1 (0.1)	—
Total	1566 (100.0)	6

*Younger than 20 years of age.

CLINICAL FORMS OF TUBERCULOSIS IN CHILDREN

Endothoracic

Asymptomatic Tuberculosis Infection

Asymptomatic (or latent) infection can be defined as infection associated with tuberculin hypersensitivity and a positive tuberculin test but with no striking clinical or roentgenographic manifestations. Computed tomography may reveal enlarged lymph nodes in the chest, even though the plain roentgenogram is normal.[117] Occasionally, low-grade fever is found at the onset, usually by chance, and a chest roentgeno-

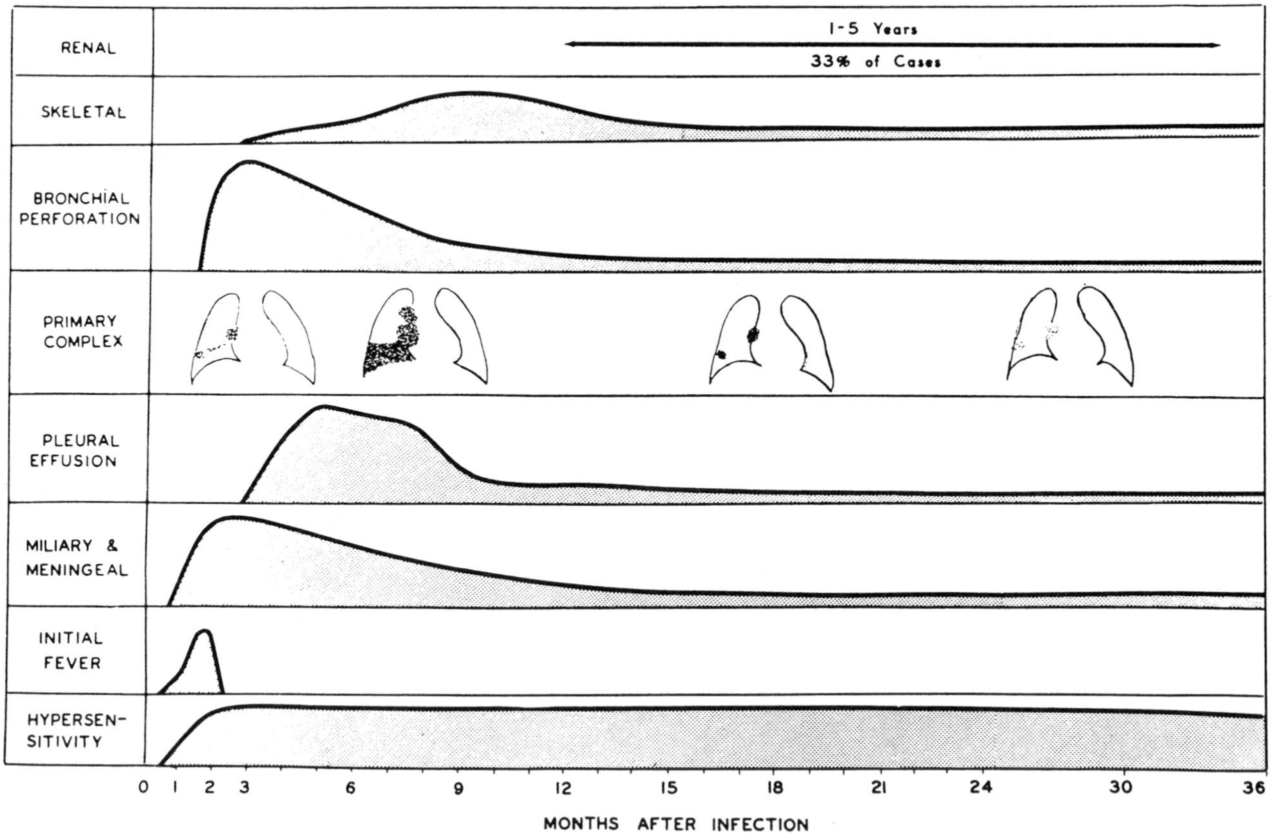

FIGURE 101–5. *The timetable of tuberculosis.*

gram usually will show few if any changes. If the child has been in recent contact with a person who has contagious tuberculosis and the tuberculin test is positive, disease should be ruled out immediately with a chest roentgenogram and a thorough physical examination (because up to 25 per cent of childhood tuberculosis cases are extrapulmonary). Asymptomatic tuberculosis infection occurs more frequently in children of elementary school age than in adolescents or infants. Some 40 to 50 per cent of infections in infants younger than 1 year of age and 80 to 95 per cent in older children can be expected to cause no specific recognizable symptom or roentgenographic findings.[383] Gastric washings in these patients, even when done with great care, yield a very low percentage of positive results.

The clinician making the diagnosis of tuberculosis infection in a child must assume, however, that the patient might be in the earliest stage of infection and at risk for development of symptomatic disease in the near future. Careful history and investigation of contacts must be undertaken immediately for determination, if possible, of the date of exposure. Chemotherapy must be started and the patient closely followed at monthly intervals, not only to detect any toxic effect of chemotherapy and monitor adherence with treatment, but also to be sure disease does not develop.

The Endothoracic Primary Complex and Its Complications

The primary complex, described by Ghon,[165] usually is said to include three elements: the primary focus, lymphangitis, and regional lymphadenitis. This holds true for every primary infection, regardless of the portal of entry. Ghon noted that at least 70 per cent of primary pulmonary foci are subpleural. Thus, pleurisy almost is a regular feature of the primary complex, and Caffey[64] has suggested that it be considered as such.

The evolution of the primary pulmonary focus begins with an acute inflammatory reaction around the tubercle bacilli inhaled into an alveolus, a localized alveolar consolidation varying from the size of a pea to the size of a walnut. Usually, macrophages appear within hours in the inflammatory exudate and change into clusters of epithelioid cells to form tubercles. In turn, these tubercles may resolve and disappear, or central caseation, consisting of incomplete cell autolysis, may develop. The caseous lesion contains large numbers of multiplying tubercle bacilli, which spread rapidly from the primary focus via the regional lymphatic vessels to the regional lymph nodes, setting up along the way areas of inflammation that later may caseate and calcify.[394]

The primary pulmonary focus has been studied carefully by numerous investigators (Table 101–5). Medlar[332] evaluated 100 cases in which there was a single calcified primary complex with a parenchymal lesion of at least 2 mm in diameter. By plotting their locations on a normal chest roentgenogram, he found that "the resulting pattern resembled the scatter of bird-shot on a paper target." Thus, all parts of the lung apparently are at equal risk of being seeded. The belief that the primary focus has a predilection for the lower fields of the lung probably arises from the fact that the lung is pyramid-shaped, with more basilar than apical lung tissue.

TABLE 101–5. Location of the Primary Pulmonary Focus

	No. of Patients	%
Right upper lobe	138	27
Right middle lobe	40	7
Right lower lobe	107	20
Left upper lobe	122	24
Left lower lobe	104	20
Total	511	98

Data from Ghon, A., and Kuedlich, H.: Die eintrittspforten der infektion. *In* Engel, S., and Pirquet, C. (eds.): Handbuch der Kindertuberkulose. Stuttgart, Georg Thieme Verlag, 1930.

TABLE 101–6. Lymphatic Drainage of the Lung

Right upper lobe	→	Right paratracheal chain
Right middle lobe	→	Right and left paratracheal nodes
Right lower lobe	→	Subcarinal nodes
Left upper lobe	→	Left paratracheal nodes
Left lower lobe	→	Left paratracheal nodes
Lingula	→	Subcarinal nodes
Subcarinal nodes	→	Right paratracheal chain

Based on the data of Rouviere, quoted by Courtice, F. C., and Simmonds, W. J.: Physiological significance of lymph drainage of the serous cavities and lungs. Physiol. Rev. *34*:419–442, 1954.

Many investigators, including Ghon,[165] Sweany,[502] and Payne,[383] concurred that 70 to 85 per cent of primary infections are initiated by one focus. In a study of 170 cases, Ghon[165] found two foci in 15 per cent, three in 7 per cent, four in 3 per cent, and five in 2 per cent. Multiple lung foci can result, although rarely, from ingestion and inhalation of tubercle bacilli. This was shown clearly in the results of pathologic studies on the 71 infants who died in the "Lübeck disaster" of the 1930s, an incident in which 251 newborn infants mistakenly had been given live tubercle bacilli by mouth instead of BCG vaccine. Fifteen of the infants were found to have primary lung lesions at autopsy, and all 251 had primary intestinal lesions.

Although the lymphadenitis can not be detected clinically and rarely even on roentgenogram, it is true universally that the hallmark of initial tuberculosis infection is the relatively large size and importance of the adenitis, compared with the relatively insignificant size of the initial focus in the lung, skin, or elsewhere. The development of tuberculin hypersensitivity within 3 to 10 weeks after initial infection enhances the cellular reaction throughout the primary complex, particularly affecting the primary focus and the regional lymph nodes. At this time, the infection may spread along nearby lymphatic chains to involve more distant nodes. The lymphatic drainage of the lungs is outlined in Table 101–6. It occurs predominantly from left to right.[98] It is not surprising, therefore, that the nodes in the right upper paratracheal area appear to be the ones most often affected. Many primary lesions are subpleural, and the lymphatic drainage of the apical pleura is to cervical nodes. Moreover, the paratracheal chains have communications both with the deep cervical nodes and with the abdominal nodes, as shown in Figure 101–6. Among 54 patients with the primary lesion in the right upper lobe, Blacklock[44] found that 14 had involvement of the deep cervical nodes on the same side and 3 had involvement of the abdominal nodes.

Bronchial obstruction due to enlargement of peribronchial lymph nodes was reported by Ghon[165] and others. It was not until the 1920s that Wallgren[540] and others elucidated the role of these large nodes in producing the roentgenographic shadows variously called epituberculosis, collapse-consolidation, and segmental lesions that so often are seen in cases of childhood tuberculosis.[165, 296, 436, 540] At the end of the incubation period, as tuberculin sensitivity develops, the hilar lymph nodes enlarge greatly, and in many cases caseous foci

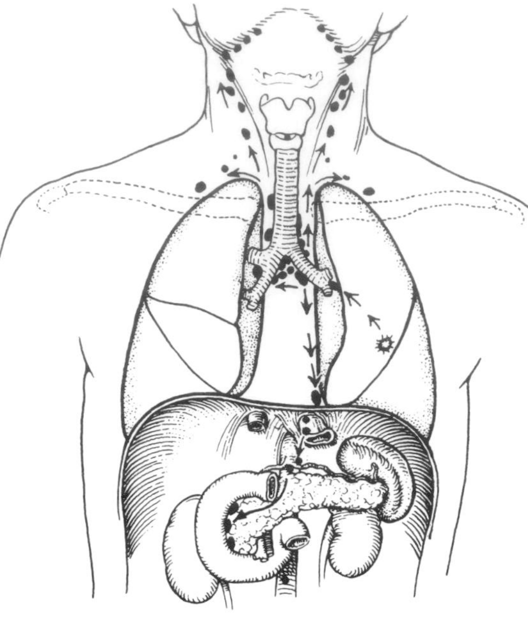

FIGURE 101–6. *Schematic composite drawing illustrating wide lymphogenic spread of the tuberculous infection from a primary pulmonary focus in the base of the left upper lobe. The infection extended cephalad to the submandibular nodes in the head and caudad as far as the pancreatic nodes in the abdomen. Theoretically, there is no reason why lymphogenic spread should be confined even to these wide limits; further spread could carry the infection into the lymphatic tracts in the pelvis (and upper and lower extremities). (Reproduced with permission from Caffey, J.: Pediatric X-Ray Diagnosis. 7th ed. Chicago, Year Book Medical Publishers, 1978.)*

appear within them. Acid-fast studies of smears and sections have confirmed that this caseum has few tubercle bacilli. As the nodes enlarge, they frequently impinge on the neighboring regional bronchus, compressing it and causing diffuse inflammation of its wall, even to the point of obstructing the lumen.[434–436, 478] Daly and colleagues,[105] in their study of endobronchial tuberculosis in children at Bellevue, found this to be the mechanism of obstruction in half of their patients. Other causes of obstruction include damage to the bronchial cartilage that leads to gradual (or rarely, abrupt) perforation of the bronchus and formation of plugs of semiliquid toothpaste-like caseum that partially or completely occlude the bronchus. In some cases, endobronchial granulomatous tissue forms around the stoma of the fistula, obstructing the lumen.

Three immediate results of bronchial obstruction are possible.[296, 511]

The first is sudden death by asphyxia, fortunately an extremely rare event.[282]

The second is obstructive hyperaeration (also called obstructive emphysema) of a lobar segment, a lobe, or even an entire lung.[322, 396] This is unusual (in Walker's series,[536] it occurred in 7 of 538 children with primary tuberculosis of the lungs, whereas half had segmental lesions). When it does occur, it usually is in children younger than 2 years of age, and it may be accompanied by wheezing. Physical examination usually is of little help; roentgenograms, best taken on expiration, show hyperaeration, which usually is not accompanied by mediastinal displacement, probably because of fixation by the tuberculous mediastinal nodes (Fig. 101–7). Aspiration of a foreign body always must be considered in the differential diagnosis. The obstruction ultimately will resolve by itself; however, corticosteroids may be added to the chemotherapeutic regimen to hasten recovery.[356, 357, 514] Surgical removal of the obstructing nodes has been successful but rarely is performed.[113]

The third possible result of bronchial obstruction is the appearance of a segmental lesion, fan-shaped on a roentgenogram, representing mainly atelectasis and almost always involving the very segment occupied by the primary pulmonary focus (Fig. 101–8).[278, 349] Actually, the roentgenographic opacity results from a combination of several elements: the primary pulmonary focus, the caseous material from an eroded bronchus, the inflammatory response elicited by the caseum, and atelectasis. In some instances, acute secondary infection plays a part. Children with a secondary bacterial pneumonia often present with high fever, cough, and rales; the signs and symptoms respond to conventional antibiotics, but the chest roentgenogram findings usually do not clear, due to the underlying tuberculosis. The relative roles of these

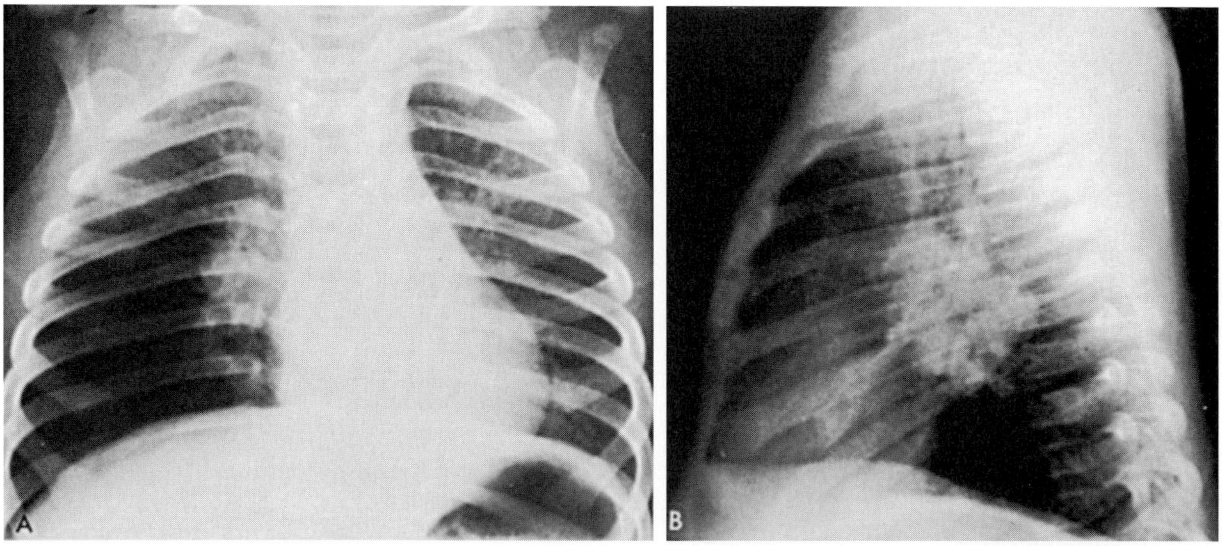

FIGURE 101–7. *X-ray film of an 8-month-old girl with obstructive hyperaeration of the right lower lobe due to tuberculosis.* A, *Note hyperlucent right lower lung and shift of heart and mediastinum away from the ball valve obstruction to the left.* B, *Note large hilar lymph nodes, which are compressing the right lower lobe bronchi. Tuberculosis should be considered in patients with hyperaeration of unknown etiology.*

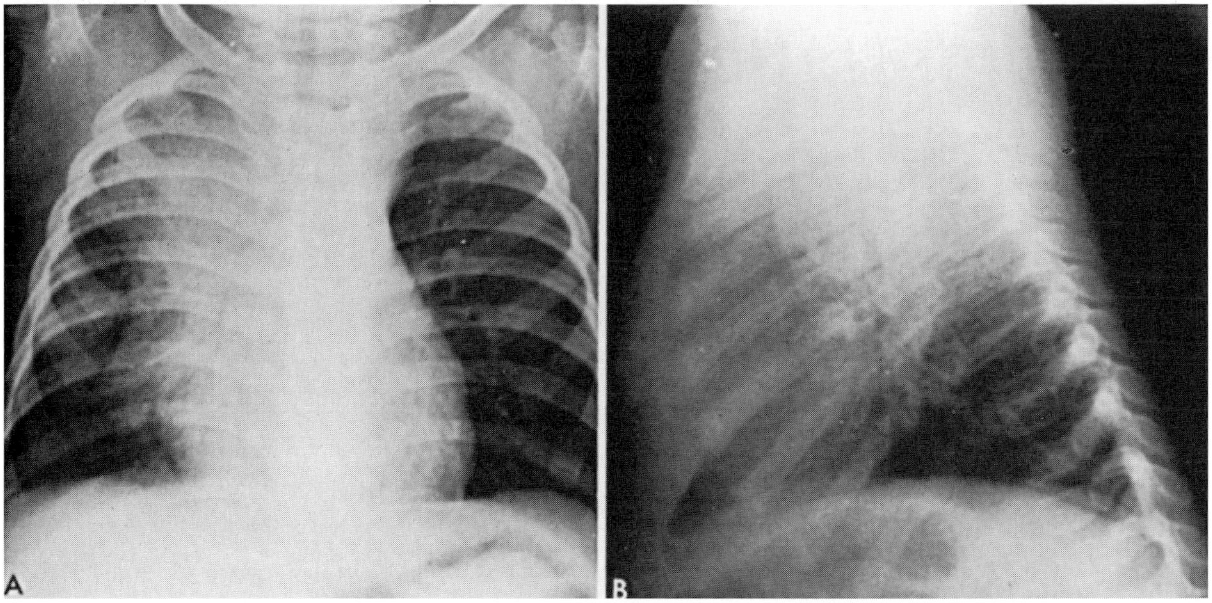

FIGURE 101–8. A *and* B, *Roentgenogram of an 8-month-old boy with primary tuberculosis infection. Posteroanterior film shows collapse-consolidation of the right upper lobe, hilar and paratracheal adenopathy, and pleural reaction. Note narrowed right bronchi.*

various elements often cannot be assessed; sometimes atelectasis is conspicuous, sometimes consolidation is the salient pathologic process, with the volume of the segment undiminished or even increased (hence the descriptive term *collapse-consolidation lesion*, preferred by some clinicians to the less accurate term *atelectasis*).

The percentage of infected children in whom segmental lesions develop has been estimated by several investigators. All agree that the younger the child, the more common are collapse-consolidation lesions (Table 101–7). The segmental lesion is likely to form during the first 3 to 6 months after infection (50 of 65 in Payne's series).[383] Multiple segmental lesions can occur simultaneously (and did in 18 of 160 children in Payne's experience). When this happens, the segmental lesions usually form in one lung, but occasionally lobes or segments of both lungs are affected. Sometimes segmental lesions and obstructive hyperaeration occur simultaneously. Physical signs and symptoms of segmental lesions—cough, rales, localized wheezing, egophony—surprisingly are meager but are more common in infants due to the smaller size of their airways.

Although segmental lesions and hyperaeration are the most common findings produced by enlarging thoracic lymph nodes, others do occur. Enlarged peritracheal nodes may cause stridor and respiratory distress. Subcarinal nodes may impinge on the esophagus and cause difficulty in swallowing, followed occasionally by formation of a diverticulum of the esophagus, or the nodes may rupture directly into the esophagus and produce a bronchoesophageal fistula. Enlarged lymph nodes may compress the subclavian vein, producing edema of the hand and arm, or may erode major blood vessels, including the aorta. They also may rupture into the mediastinum and point in the left, or more often in the right, supraclavicular fossa. Compression of the left recurrent laryngeal nerve has been reported. Compression of the left phrenic nerve leads to paralysis of the left leaf of the diaphragm in an estimated 0.1 to 0.3 per cent of tuberculous children. Rupture into the pericardial sac will be described later.

The late results of bronchial obstruction include the following possibilities: (1) complete re-expansion of the lung and resolution of the roentgenographic findings; (2) disappearance of the segmental lesion, with residual calcification of the primary focus or the regional lymph nodes; or (3) scarring and progressive contraction of the lobe or segment, usually associated with bronchiectasis.[296] Permanent anatomic sequelae result from segmental lesions in about 60 per cent of all cases, even though the abnormality usually is not apparent on roentgenograms. Cylindrical (rarely saccular) bronchiectasis, sometimes stenoses, and elongation or shortenings can be demonstrated on bronchography. Fortunately, most of these abnormalities are asymptomatic in the upper lobes. However, secondary infection may occur in the middle and lower lobes, causing the middle lobe syndrome, an expression that came into use after Brock's report[57] in 1950 on posttuberculous bronchostenosis and bronchiectasis of the middle lobe. Occasionally, the chronic vascularity that accompanies bronchiectasis leads to poor oxygen saturation during exercise and to restricted body growth. Also, bronchogenic carcinoma may arise years later in the old scarred lesions remaining in the bronchus.

Calcification of the primary complex, when it appears, always results from caseation. In calcified caseum, as in bone, the predominant calcium salt is tribasic calcium phosphate.

TABLE 101–7. Percentage of Tuberculin Converters Developing Segmental Lesions (SL) at Different Ages

Age at Infection (yr)	Converters Developing SL No.	Converters Developing SL %	Total Converters (Number)
0–1	77	43	180
1–5	35	24	147
6–10	31	25	121
11–15	16	16	97
Total	159	29	545

After Payne, M., quoted by Miller, F. J. W., Seale, R. M. E., and Taylor, M. D.: Tuberculosis in Children. Boston, Little, Brown, 1963.

Calcification of caseous lesions occurs much more readily in children than in adults, probably because children's calcium and phosphorus plasma levels are higher. In the infants who were victims of the Lübeck disaster, autopsy showed calcification to be present as early as 58 days after the onset of massive infection. Payne,[383] in a study of calcification in 299 children from Newcastle-on-Tyne, reported calcification visible on chest roentgenograms of 1 child within 6 months of infection, 38 within 12 months, 104 within 18 months, 165 within 24 months, 252 within 3 years, and 299 within 4 years.

Calcium usually is deposited as fine particles, creating a stippled effect (Fig. 101–9), but it may be deposited in large, even enormous masses.[450] Calcification may persist without much change, or it may start resorbing within about 5 years and eventually disappear completely. Occasionally, it progresses to ossification with formation of true bone and functional bone marrow. Calcification, if visible at all on roentgenograms, most often involves the regional lymph nodes.[53] Sometimes, however, the primary pulmonary focus or the entire primary complex, including the lymphangitis, calcifies (Fig. 101–10).

Calcification took place in 75 to 80 per cent of the 525 children with pulmonary tuberculosis monitored by Payne.[383] Currently, extensive calcification occurs uncommonly in the Western world, probably because tuberculous lesions treated early with INH rarely caseate, and caseation is a prerequisite for calcification.

Pleural Effusion

Pleural effusion can be localized or generalized, unilateral or bilateral.[294] Localized pleural effusion so frequently accompanies the primary pulmonary focus that it practically is a component of the primary complex. All tuberculous serous effusions probably originate in the discharge of bacilli into the cavity from an adjacent lesion—in the case of the pleura,

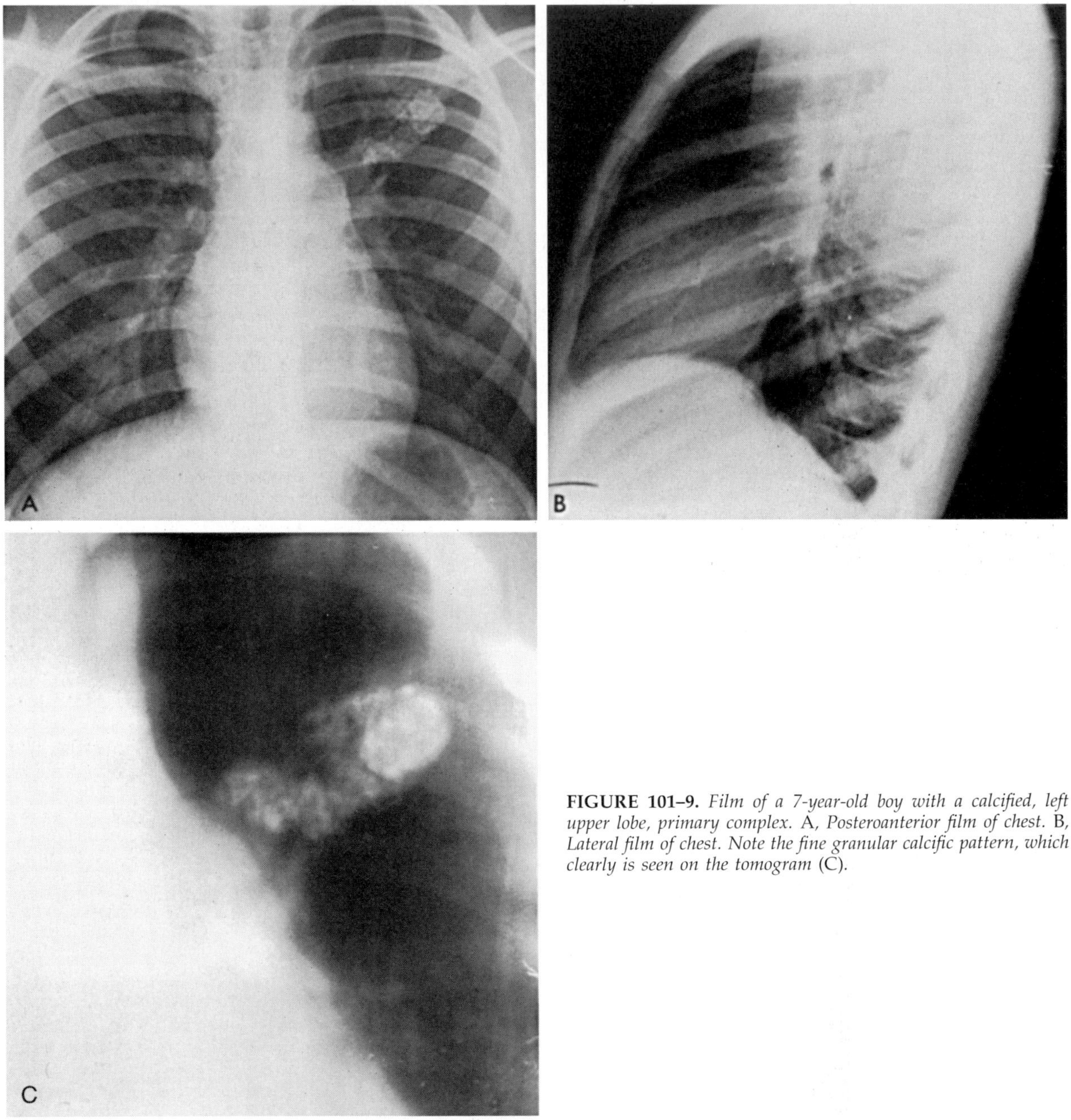

FIGURE 101–9. *Film of a 7-year-old boy with a calcified, left upper lobe, primary complex.* A, *Posteroanterior film of chest.* B, *Lateral film of chest. Note the fine granular calcific pattern, which clearly is seen on the tomogram* (C).

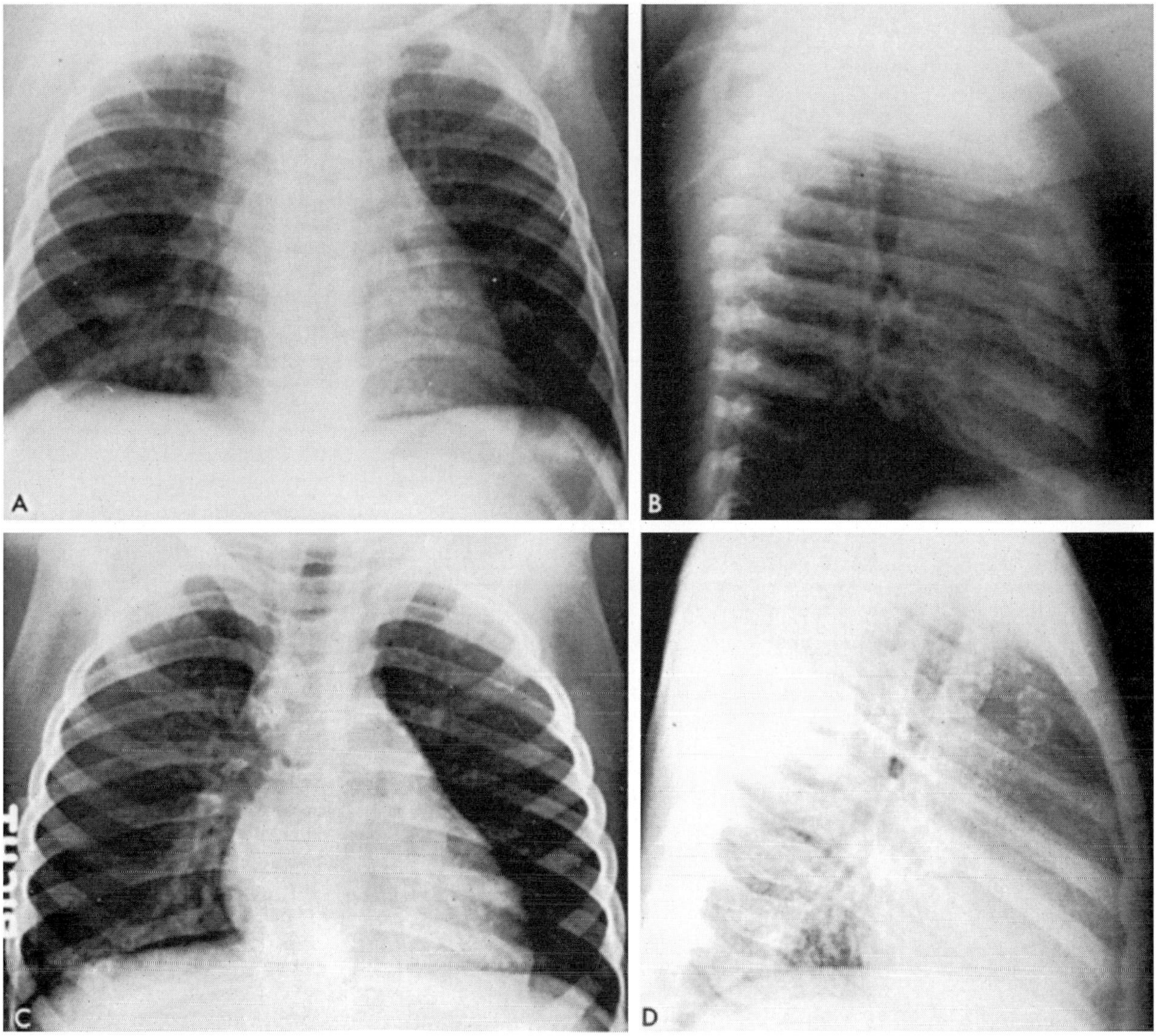

FIGURE 101–10. A *and* B, *Roentgenograms of a 7-month-old girl with mild fullness of the right upper mediastinum and a hazy infiltrate in the right lower lobe. Skin test for tuberculosis was positive. She was treated for tuberculosis and clinically improved.* C, *The same patient 3.5 years later shows a calcified primary complex in the right upper and lower lobes over the diaphragm.* D, *The anterior location of the upper lobe complex clearly is seen on the lateral chest film.*

from a subpleural pulmonary focus or from subpleural caseous lymph nodes. The breakthrough may be small and the pleuritis localized and asymptomatic, or it may occur in the form of a generalized effusion, usually 3 to 6 months after infection (Fig. 101–11). In 75 per cent of Wallgren's cases,[540] later calcification of the pulmonary focus or regional lymph nodes proved the effusion to be on the same side as the original primary focus. Miller and associates[339] postulated that in the 5 per cent or less of cases in which effusions are bilateral, the primary complexes are bilateral. Seemingly without logical explanation are the following clinical observations: tuberculous pleural effusion is rare in children younger than 2 years of age and uncommon in children younger than 5 years of age (perhaps because sensitivity to tuberculin is lower in the very young), is more common in boys than in girls, almost never is associated with a segmental lesion, and rarely is associated with miliary tuberculosis.

The onset of pleurisy usually is abrupt, resembling bacterial pneumonia, with fever, chest pain, shortness of breath, and, on physical examination, dullness to percussion and diminished breath sounds. Fever may be high and, in untreated cases, last for several weeks. Occasionally, it is difficult to differentiate an effusion from an extensive pneumonic lesion; lateral decubitus roentgenographic views are helpful in confirming the presence of pleural fluid.

Thoracentesis is, of course, the essential diagnostic procedure. The puncture should be made in the area shown on the roentgenogram to have the greatest fluid accumulation. No more than 30 mL of pleural fluid should be withdrawn; otherwise, the protein loss from this usually protein-rich fluid may be considerable. The fluid generally is greenish yellow, occasionally blood-tinged, with a specific gravity of 1.012 to 1.022, a high protein content, often a low glucose level (<30 mg/dL), and has several hundred white cells per mm^3 with a predominance of neutrophils or lymphocytes, depending on the age of the effusion. The cells in tuberculous pleural effusion usually predominantly are T lymphocytes, which are present in higher proportion than in the blood simultaneously.[149, 447] Tubercle bacilli usually are present in such small numbers that results from direct smears and cultures are apt to be disappointing; smears almost always are negative, and pleural fluid cultures are positive in less than 30 per cent of

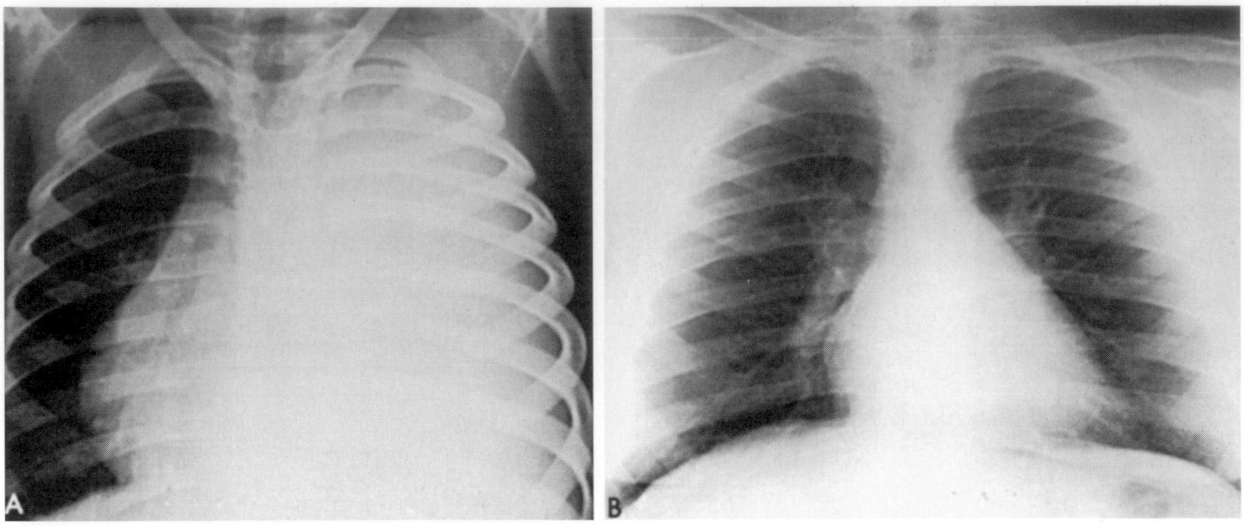

FIGURE 101–11. *Roentgenograms of a 5-year-old boy with massive left pleural effusion due to tuberculosis.* A, *Posteroanterior film of chest.* B, *The same patient 6 years later with a normal chest film and no physical complaint.*

cases. Pleural punch biopsy is a useful diagnostic procedure because both the finding of typical tubercles on histologic study and the culture of the tiny "plug" from the trocar are much more likely to establish the diagnosis than is culture of the pleural fluid.[289, 304]

The prognosis for children with tuberculous effusion in contrast with adults[416] always has been relatively good compared with that for other overt forms of tuberculosis, even in the days before chemotherapy.[289, 304] Permanent impairment of pulmonary function is surprisingly uncommon after pleural effusion.[155] The development of scoliosis is a remote possibility and should be guarded against while the patient recovers.

Progressive Pulmonary Tuberculosis

This is a serious complication of the primary complex in which the primary pulmonary focus, instead of resolving or calcifying, enlarges steadily and develops a large caseous center. This center then liquefies and empties into an adjacent bronchus, thus creating a "primary cavity" (Fig. 101–12)[505]; the liquefaction is associated with particularly large numbers of tubercle bacilli.[109] The stage then is set for further dissemination of tubercle bacilli to other parts of the lobe and to the entire lung, where other foci of infection form. On rare occasions, an enlarging primary focus ruptures into the pleural cavity, creating a pneumothorax, bronchopleural fistula, or caseous pyopneumothorax, or into the pericardial sac or the mediastinum.

Whereas clinical symptoms often are minimal when the primary focus is uncomplicated, a progressive lesion often is accompanied by more severe fever, cough, malaise, and weight loss, as well as by classic signs of cavitation, such as egophony. As readily can be surmised, before chemotherapy the inability to contain the primary focus was associated with a grave outlook: 25 to 65 per cent of patients so affected died. Now, with appropriate treatment, the prognosis is good.

It may be difficult to distinguish between progressive pulmonary tuberculosis and a simple tuberculous focus with a superimposed acute bacterial pneumonia caused by *Staphylococcus, Klebsiella*, or possibly anaerobes. Antimicrobial agents effective against these pathogens may be indicated in addition to appropriate antituberculosis drugs. Sometimes, especially during convalescence from pulmonary parenchymal lesions, bullous lesions appear and persist for several months. They seem to be associated, in children as in adults, either with "tears" in damaged alveolar walls or with the emptying of caseum out of cavities.[322]

Chronic Pulmonary Tuberculosis

Chronic pulmonary tuberculosis, sometimes referred to as adult or reactivation tuberculosis, is the type of disease seen in pulmonary tissue sensitized and immunized by an earlier tuberculosis infection. For many years, there was ongoing argument about whether the lesions of chronic pulmonary tuberculosis, more localized than those of the initial tuberculous lesion and less likely to spread to lymph nodes and blood stream, were due to "endogenous reinfection." Evidence has accumulated during subsequent decades that endogenous reinfection is the usual event.[486, 525] However, reinfection with a different strain of *M. tuberculosis* has been documented and may be more common in areas where tuberculosis is quite prevalent.[456]

Careful long-term studies of children hospitalized at the High Wood Sanatorium in England revealed that there is a continuum in many cases: first the primary focus, followed within a few years in some patients by infraclavicular small round foci, in the lung apices often calcified (Assmann foci, Simon foci) and thought to result from hematogenous spread at the time of initial infection. Later, these foci disappear spontaneously or remain visible as tiny calcifications or as larger "round foci," which may, if untreated, progress to the typical lesions of chronic pulmonary tuberculosis.

Even before the discovery of antituberculosis drugs, chronic pulmonary tuberculosis was rare in children (6 to 7 per cent among Lincoln and colleagues'[295] series of closely followed patients at Bellevue Hospital). It appears more frequently among children in the lower socioeconomic strata of society and is more frequent in girls than in boys. It has been noted that children who survive with a healed, untreated tuberculosis infection acquired before 2 years of age rarely develop chronic pulmonary tuberculosis, but it is much more frequent among children who acquire their initial infection after 7 years of age and particularly if they become infected close to the onset of puberty. In the latter case, the "adult" type of lesion often develops in the very lobe where the primary lesion occurred. In this situation, progressive pulmonary tuberculosis cannot be differentiated from chronic pulmonary tuberculosis. Now, with effective treatment, the differentiation is unimportant.[189]

Cough, fever of unknown origin, chest pain, hemoptysis, and supraclavicular adenitis are the most common clinical manifestations. Essential diagnostic procedures are the tuberculin skin test and appropriate chest roentgenograms, often including such special procedures as tomograms or lordotic views. An intense search for tubercle bacilli must be made in sputum, gastric washings, and, if necessary, secretions obtained by bronchoscopy. In serious lesions of this nature, tubercle bacilli must be obtained for drug susceptibility testing before any chemotherapy is begun.

Myocardial and Pericardial Tuberculosis

Tubercles often are found in the heart in miliary tuberculosis, and although it is exceedingly rare, myocardial caseation has been described, usually secondary to direct spread from mediastinal glands and accompanied by paroxysmal tachycardia or arrhythmias.[541]

Tuberculous pericarditis, although more common than symptomatic tuberculous myocarditis, occurred in only 0.4 per cent of 2500 children followed by Lincoln and Sewell[298] at Bellevue and in 4 per cent of 200 children in Boyd's series.[51] It is more common in males than in females. In most cases, it probably arises by direct invasion or by lymphatic drainage from caseous lymph nodes in the subcarinal area or from nodes close to the ductus arteriosus, with resulting exudation of hemorrhagic fluids and development of granulation tissue on both parietal and visceral surfaces of the pericardium.[415] Pericardial fluid, if aspirated, may be serofibrinous or hemorrhagic; tubercle bacilli rarely are found on smear.[218] Sometimes extensive fibrosis leads to obliteration of the pericardial sac, with development, usually years later, of constrictive pericarditis.

The presenting symptoms usually are nonspecific: low-grade fever, poor appetite, failure to gain weight, and, rarely, chest pain. On examination, a pericardial friction rub may be

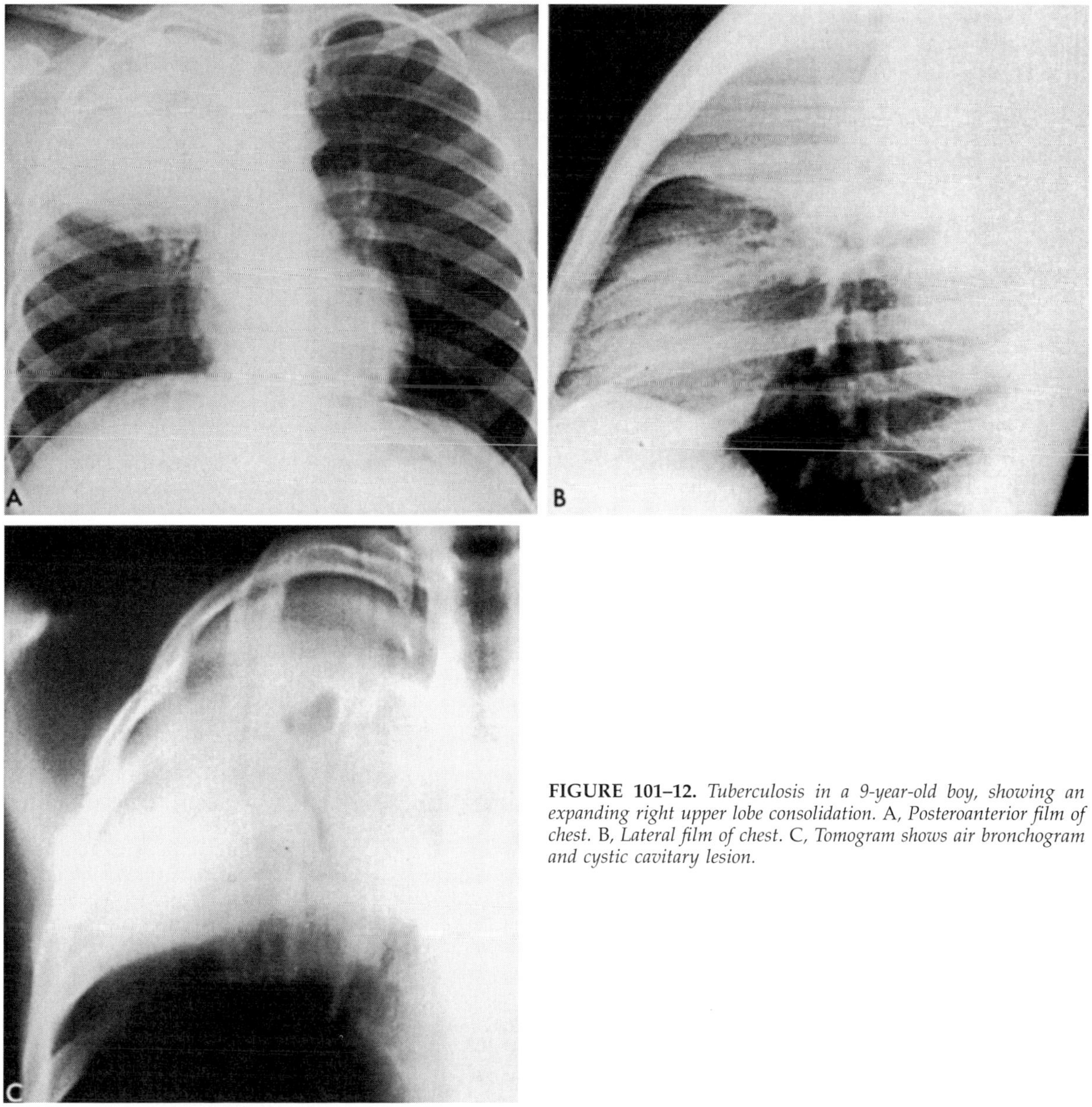

FIGURE 101–12. *Tuberculosis in a 9-year-old boy, showing an expanding right upper lobe consolidation.* A, *Posteroanterior film of chest.* B, *Lateral film of chest.* C, *Tomogram shows air bronchogram and cystic cavitary lesion.*

heard, or if a large effusion already is present, distant heart sounds, tachycardia, and narrow pulse pressure may suggest the diagnosis. The diagnosis then is confirmed by roentgenography, echocardiography, electrocardiography, tuberculin skin test, and aspiration of fluid for culture. In the past, approximately half of the patients succumbed before chemotherapy. Now, with appropriate drugs and possibly corticosteroids to diminish the size of the effusion[495] and also occasional partial pericardiectomy, the outlook is excellent.

Lymphohematogenous Spread

Tubercle bacilli from the lymphadenitis of the primary complex probably are disseminated during the incubation period in all cases of tuberculosis infection. In experiments with guinea pigs, Strom[497] found that local injection of radioactive-labeled BCG was followed by systemic dissemination within hours. The results of liver biopsies of young asymptomatic tuberculin converters (indicating recent infection) show that the liver always is involved.[88] It is clear that tubercle bacilli can reach deep, distant organs via the blood stream or lymphatic channels. Autopsies on individuals who have died soon after initial infection show that the bacilli often are deposited in the liver, spleen, skin, and apical pulmonary tissue.

The clinical picture produced by the lymphohematogenous spread probably is determined by host susceptibility at the time of spread and by the quantity of tubercle bacilli released.[530] Three clinical forms can be recognized:

1. The lymphohematogenous spread may be occult, in which case it usually remains so, or it may be occult initially with metastatic, extrapulmonary lesions appearing months or years later (for example, renal tuberculosis).[541]
2. So-called protracted hematogenous tuberculosis, rarely seen today, is characterized by high, spiking fever, marked leukocytosis, hepatomegaly and splenomegaly, and general glandular enlargement, sometimes with repeated evidence of metastatic seeding in the choroid, kidneys, and skin. Calcifications may appear subsequently, often in large numbers, in the pulmonary apices (Simon foci) and in the spleen, attesting to the earlier dissemination of tubercle bacilli via the blood. The tuberculin skin test usually is strongly positive. Bone marrow biopsy may confirm the clinical impression, but treatment often must be started on a presumptive diagnosis. Although this type of tuberculosis in past years often ended tragically in tuberculous meningitis, today it is completely treatable if diagnosed in time.
3. The third form of lymphohematogenous spread, analogous to sepsis with pyogenic bacteria, is miliary tuberculosis.[220] It usually arises from discharge of a caseous focus, often a lymph node, into a blood vessel such as a pulmonary vein; it may be self-propagating, with repeated discharge arising at various sites. Most common during the first 2 to 6 months after infection in infancy, it can arise even in adults who have apparently well-healed, calcified lesions or in those who have recovered, thanks to chemotherapy, from a recent attack of miliary tuberculosis or from an attack that occurred many years earlier.[264, 433, 551]

Miliary disease provides a striking illustration of the difference in susceptibility of tissue to tubercle bacilli; tubercles tend to be larger and more numerous in lung, spleen, liver, and bone marrow than in the heart, pancreas, and brain. The number of fixed intravascular phagocytes, as well as the relative tortuosity of the smaller blood vessels themselves, must play an important role in determining tissue susceptibility. In acute caseating miliary tuberculosis, the lesions are likely to be numerous and sometimes almost coalescent.

The clinical picture of miliary tuberculosis varies greatly, probably depending on the number of bacilli in the blood stream. Sometimes, the patient almost is afebrile, appears to be well, and is diagnosed by chance as a contact of another individual with infectious tuberculosis. The onset can be insidious, often occurring after the patient has had measles, pertussis, or other precipitating infection. In rare cases, the onset is abrupt. Drowsiness, loss of weight and appetite, persistent fever, weakness, rapid breathing with a rustling sound on auscultation of the lungs, occasionally cyanosis, and almost always a palpable spleen are the clinical manifestations that lead the clinician to obtain a chest roentgenogram.

Usually within no more than 3 weeks after the onset of symptoms, tubercles, sometimes tiny and sometimes large, can be seen evenly distributed throughout both lung fields[375]; in the early stages, they often are detected best on a lateral view of the retrocardiac space (Fig. 101–13). The reported incidence of choroidal tubercles varies greatly; it has been reported variously as 13 and 87 per cent. Recurrent pneumothorax, subcutaneous emphysema, pneumomediastinum, and pleural effusion are less serious but well-recognized complications of miliary tuberculosis. Second attacks have been reported.[551] Cutaneous lesions, including painful nodules, papulonecrotic tuberculids, and purpuric lesions, may appear in crops.[258]

Diagnosis usually is established by means of the clinical picture and a chest roentgenogram; sometimes it is confirmed by a liver or skin biopsy; by culturing *M. tuberculosis* from the gastric aspirate, urine, or bone marrow[88, 193]; or by fiberoptic bronchoscopy and transbronchial biopsy.[60] Treatment usually is very successful.

Extrathoracic Spread

Central Nervous System Tuberculosis

Tubercle bacilli are distributed by the blood stream into all parts of the central nervous system during lymphohematogenous spread.[297] Surprisingly, they do not multiply as well in nervous tissue as in other areas, such as the lung. Thus, central nervous system tuberculosis, although an early manifestation of infection, usually does not appear simultaneously with miliary spread, but days later. The tubercle bacilli can affect the central nervous system in various ways,[110, 522, 535] producing tuberculous meningitis,[225, 499] serous meningitis,[292, 522] tuberculoma,[367, 522] or tuberculous brain abscess, or it can affect mainly the spinal cord, causing spinal tuberculous leptomeningitis.[515]

Tuberculous meningitis arises from caseous foci, often very small ones, situated in the brain or meninges.[410] In time, the caseous foci discharge tubercle bacilli directly in the subarachnoid space. The thick, gelatinous exudate lies in the meshes of the pia-arachnoid, in the brain, where it infiltrates the walls of meningeal arteries and veins, producing inflammation, caseation, and obstruction, and extends along small vessels into the cortex, occluding them and producing infarcts. This same exudate interferes with the normal flow of the cerebrospinal fluid in and out of the ventricular system and with its absorption by the pacchionian bodies. The predilection of the exudate for the base of the brain accounts for frequent involvement of the third, sixth, and seventh nerves and the optic chiasm. The combination of vascular lesions producing infarcts,[288] interference with cerebrospinal fluid flow resulting in hydrocephalus, and direct cranial nerve involvement, especially of the eye, causes the devastating damage that all too often results from tuberculous meningitis.

Tuberculous meningitis has been estimated to occur in 1 of

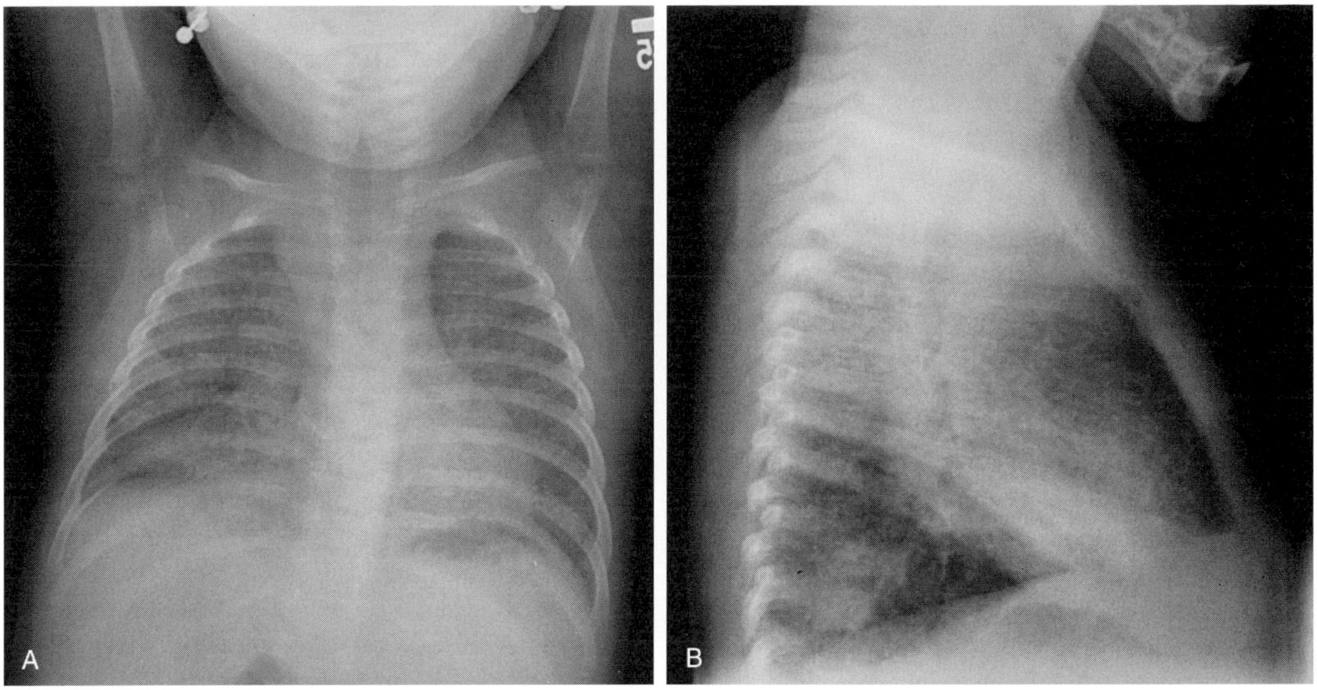

FIGURE 101–13. *Miliary tuberculosis in an infant. The numerous tubercles can be seen on both the posteroanterior* (A) *and lateral* (B) *views.*

every 300 untreated infections.[235] Practically never seen in infants younger than 4 months of age, it is most common in children younger than 6 years of age, appears usually within 2 to 6 months after initial infection, and accompanies miliary tuberculosis in about 50 per cent of cases. Currently, in many U.S. urban children's hospitals, tuberculous meningitis is more frequent than *Haemophilus influenzae* type b meningitis, containing both the best and worst of public health in one sentence! Tuberculosis should be suspected as the cause of meningitis that is accompanied by cranial nerve involvement, hydrocephalus, or evidence of inflammation at the base of the brain.

The onset of tuberculous meningitis usually is gradual, occurring over a period of about 3 weeks, and seems in some cases to be precipitated by a viral infection, a fall, or a blow on the head. Occasionally, the onset is abrupt and marked by a convulsion. It is convenient for the clinician to divide the course into three stages.[225] The first stage is characterized by personality change, irritability, anorexia, listlessness, and some fever. After 1 or 2 weeks, the disease passes into the second stage, when signs of increased intracranial pressure and cerebral damage appear: drowsiness, stiff neck, cranial nerve palsies (especially of the third, sixth, and seventh nerves), inequality of the pupils, vomiting, tache cérébrale, absence of the abdominal reflexes, and convulsions that may be tonic or clonic, focal, or generalized. The third stage is characterized by coma, irregular pulse and respirations, and rising fever. Occasionally, papilledema is noted.

Aids in diagnosis are a history of contact with an adult with tuberculosis (however, the family history for tuberculosis often is "negative" because the incubation period of meningitis is short and the contagious adult has not been discovered yet[122]); a tuberculin skin test (positive in only 50 per cent of cases); positive tuberculin skin tests in siblings; a chest roentgenogram, which often reveals changes (although Zarabi and his associates[552] found that chest roentgenograms were normal in 43 per cent of 180 children they treated); and the characteristic findings from spinal fluid. However, ventricular cerebrospinal fluid may be relatively normal because it is obtained proximal to the site of inflammation. The lumbar spinal fluid usually is clear and under substantially increased pressure. It will contain 50 to 500 white blood cells per mm^3, with polymorphonuclear leukocytes predominant early and lymphocytes predominant later. The spinal fluid glucose level may be at the lower limits of normal if the patient is examined early in the second stage, and it falls by 5 mg or so each day; by the third stage it usually is very low. The protein content may be normal at the time of the first spinal tap, but it rises steadily to very high concentrations, at which time the fluid will develop a pellicle on standing. Tubercle bacilli may be found in the pellicle but are scarce at best. Only about 50 per cent of cases of tuberculous meningitis in children can be confirmed by spinal fluid culture. Examination of the spinal fluid by means of an enzyme-linked immunosorbent assay (ELISA) for IgG antibody to purified protein derivative has been used in a few cases with good results.[249] Gastric washings should be cultured, not only to confirm the diagnosis in retrospect, but also to permit drug susceptibility testing of the organisms in case the patient's progress is not satisfactory.

Computed tomography or magnetic resonance imaging[182, 371] is recommended for evaluation of all patients with tuberculous meningitis. Both permit the recognition and follow-up of tuberculomas,[521, 550] infarct or vasculitis, and hydrocephalus that might require shunting.[101, 240, 494]

Profound abnormalities in the electrolyte pattern of intra- and extracellular fluids and the spinal fluid have been reported in patients with tuberculous meningitis.[399] These consist mainly of low sodium and chloride levels, with low or normal plasma potassium levels, accompanied by high sodium levels in red cells and skeletal muscle.[130, 190] High levels of antidiuretic hormone (syndrome of "inappropriate" antidiuretic hormone secretion) may cause hypotonic expansion of the extracellular fluid. Because intense vomiting and dehydration usually accompany tuberculous meningitis, the electrolyte disturbances usually include severe hypochloremia. Determination of the spinal fluid chloride concentration is useless because it merely reflects the plasma level.[432]

A good prognosis depends on immediate treatment without awaiting epidemiologic and bacteriologic confirmation of the diagnosis.[219] Before chemotherapy was used, every case of true tuberculous meningitis was fatal within 3 to 4 weeks, whereas today, appropriate treatment during the first stage allows survival in nearly every case, although the patient's intelligence may never return to its previous level. Initiated during the second stage, treatment results in survival in 75 per cent or more of patients. If patients are in coma when treatment is begun, they rarely recover unscathed. Very young age and the occurrence of convulsions generally are poor prognostic factors. Hydrocephalus, usually of the communicating type, occurs frequently (38 per cent in one series) and largely is responsible for poor outcome. Relieving the hydrocephalus surgically appears to improve the sensorium, vision, and neurologic deficit. One study advocates the early use of ventriculoperitoneal shunting in patients severely ill at the time of admission.[378] Infarcts caused by vasculitis also can leave catastrophic residua. The role of corticosteroids in the treatment of intracranial tuberculosis is discussed later in this chapter.

A realistic estimate of the effectiveness of current therapy is hard to establish because the incidence of tuberculous meningitis in the Western world is low.[124]

The long-term sequelae of tuberculous meningitis are numerous and include blindness, deafness, intracranial calcification, diabetes insipidus, obesity, paraplegia, and mental retardation.[305]

Serous tuberculous meningitis is uncommon (13 per cent of 500 cases in the experience of Udani and associates).[522] Apparently, it develops when a tuberculous focus close to the subarachnoid space causes a lymphocytic reaction in the subarachnoid space without the actual presence of tubercle bacilli.[555] In the days before chemotherapy, "serous" meningitis was differentiated readily from "true" tuberculous meningitis because the former was the only nonfatal form of tuberculous meningitis. Today, this differentiation no longer is possible because treatment is begun immediately, so that true tuberculous meningitis does not develop.

Tuberculoma is manifested clinically as a brain tumor.[18, 112, 448] As many as 30 per cent of brain tumors are tuberculomas, depending on the incidence of tuberculosis in the particular population under study (in India, for instance). Tuberculomas occur most often in children younger than 10 years of age and often are located at the base of the brain around the cerebellum.[538] In contrast, tuberculomas in adults more often are supratentorial. Headache, convulsions, fever, and other symptoms and signs usually associated with brain abscess or tumor also characterize tuberculoma. Only careful evaluation, including inquiry about exposure to tuberculosis, a tuberculin skin test, chest roentgenography, and computed tomography, will permit recognition of these cases in time to begin appropriate chemotherapy before neurosurgical intervention. A fairly recently recognized phenomenon is the symptomatic intracranial tuberculoma appearing and enlarging during treatment of meningeal, miliary, and even pulmonary tuberculosis.[5, 286, 445, 510] This phenomenon appears to be mediated immunologically; it usually responds to corticosteroids and does not necessitate a change in antituberculosis chemotherapy. Also, some small children with severe pulmonary or disseminated tuberculosis have one or several tuberculomas but a normal spinal fluid evaluation.[122] Computed tomography or magnetic resonance imaging of the head should be performed when neurologic signs or symptoms accompany tuberculosis.

Tuberculous brain abscess is a rarely reported form of central nervous system tuberculosis that tends to occur at an older age than tuberculoma.[547] Pathologically, the lesion lacks the giant cell and granulomatous reaction associated with tuberculoma. Focal neurologic signs occur commonly. Computed tomography and magnetic resonance imaging, if used routinely in cases of tuberculous meningitis, may permit more frequent recognition of this type of abscess, which requires surgical intervention as well as chemotherapy. Intramedullary tuberculoma of the spinal cord is exceedingly rare.[241, 312] It can be manifested by recurrent abdominal pain.[39, 367]

Spinal tuberculous leptomeningitis occurs more often in older children and adults than in infants[306]; in Udani and coworkers'[522] series of 500 cases, only 2 per cent fell into this last age group. There is a substantial elevation of protein in the spinal fluid and sometimes partial or total block on myelography. Exudate almost completely may surround the spinal cord.

Cutaneous Tuberculosis[48, 437]

The manifestations of cutaneous tuberculosis can be classified in children according to a modification of the classifications earlier designed for adults: (1) lesions by inoculation from an exogenous source[390] (a) in a previously uninfected child, (b) in a previously infected child, or (c) caused by inoculation with BCG vaccine; (2) lesions due to hematogenous dissemination[258]; (3) lesions arising from an endogenous source; and (4) erythema nodosum. A newer classification has been proposed and perhaps is more useful for adults than for children.[38, 48]

The skin lesions associated with the primary complex may be caused by direct inoculation of tubercle bacilli into a traumatized area such as a lesion on the sole of a child's bare foot, a mosquito bite on the face, an abraded elbow, or the foreskin at the time of ritual circumcision. The initial skin focus usually is a small, painless nodule, sometimes with tiny satellite lesions that soon turn into indolent ulcers without surrounding inflammation. The most striking feature is regional lymphadenitis, which often is what convinces the patient to see a physician. Fever and systemic reactions usually are minimal; low-grade pyogenic infection and cat-scratch fever (*Bartonella* infection) always must be considered in the differential diagnosis. A strongly positive tuberculin skin test usually is present. Needle aspiration and culture may differentiate disease due to *M. tuberculosis* from that due to environmental mycobacteria.

Scrofuloderma indicates tuberculosis of the skin overlying a caseous lymph node (most often in the cervical area) that has ruptured to the outside, leaving either a shallow ulcer or a deep sinus, sometimes surrounded by a cluster of nodules. In the past, scrofuloderma was a frequent manifestation of tuberculosis in children and usually left extensive scars. Today, it is rare because the diagnosis usually is made before node rupture. Chemotherapy often forestalls the need for surgical excision.

Manifestations that result from hematogenous dissemination are papulonecrotic tuberculids and tuberculosis verrucosa cutis. Papulonecrotic tuberculids[453] are miliary tubercles in the skin that usually appear as tiny papules with "apple-jelly" centers, most often on the trunk, thighs, and face. They often are similar to papular urticaria or early varicella lesions, or they may be confused with the skin lesions of Letterer-Siwe disease. Skin biopsy provides a reliable diagnosis. Lupus vulgaris is a rare form of chronic, indolent tuberculosis, usually on the face, which often seems to evolve from tuberculids, very rarely at the site of BCG inoculation.

Tuberculosis verrucosa cutis is a condition characterized by large (several centimeters in diameter) papulonecrotic tuberculids. The lesions usually appear on the arms, legs, or buttocks, suggesting that trauma may play some part in their causation. Fungal infection is the main consideration in differential diagnosis.

Erythema nodosum formerly was a common manifestation of hypersensitivity to tuberculin. It occurs mostly in young teenage girls. Usually beginning with fever and systemic toxicity soon after initial infection, it is characterized by large, deep, painful, indurated nodules on the shins and sometimes on the thighs, elbows, and forearms. The nodules gradually change from light pink to a bruise-like color. Erythema nodosum is not specific for tuberculosis but occurs in streptococcal and meningococcal infections, histoplasmosis, coccidioidomycosis, sarcoidosis, drug-sensitivity reactions, and perhaps cat-scratch disease. Tuberculin hypersensitivity is pronounced in children with tuberculosis underlying erythema nodosum, and tuberculin skin testing should be performed with caution. These patients may or may not have associated tuberculous lesions, but some clinicians believe that these patients have a greater chance of suffering complications. Skin biopsy reveals only nonspecific changes regardless of cause and is, therefore, useless in diagnosis. Both fever and nodules clear within 2 or 3 weeks.

Skeletal Tuberculosis

Bone and joint tuberculosis can be expected in 1 to 5 per cent of children whose initial infection with tubercle bacilli is untreated. Usually, the tubercle bacilli are disseminated to skeletal structures during the lymphohematogenous spread of initial infection.[27] The disease becomes symptomatic during the first 1 to 3 years after infection. Each of the most frequently involved bones and joints has a characteristic "incubation period": for example, 1 month for dactylitis but about 30 months for tuberculosis of the hip. In very young children, blood flow through growing bone is intense; consequently, they suffer from skeletal tuberculosis more often than do older children. The lesion usually starts as an area of endarteritis in the metaphysis of the long bone, where the blood supply particularly is abundant; lesions can be single or multiple.[444] There are two other mechanisms by which bone infection can be initiated, particularly in the vertebrae: (1) direct extension via the lymphatics from a caseous paravertebral lymph node[61] and (2) direct local hematogenous or lymphatic extension from a neighboring bone. As bone is destroyed progressively by pressure necrosis and cold abscess formation, a nearby joint may become involved.[401, 527, 537]

The bones most often affected are the vertebrae.[374] Tuli's[519] experience with skeletal tuberculosis is typical. Of 1074 patients with the disease, 440 had involvement of the vertebrae; 89, the knee; 81, the hip; and 51, the elbow. The upper extremities and non–weight-bearing bones, such as the skull, the clavicle, and the mandible, rarely are involved.[191, 195]

There often is a history of trauma, which may play some part in activating an underlying lesion or may serve simply to draw attention to the process.

Tuberculous spondylitis, or tuberculosis of the vertebrae, often affects the thoracic vertebrae, particularly the twelfth one.[199, 200] In one series of 64 cases of spinal tuberculosis in children, the lesions were in the thoracic area in 24 children, in the lumbar area in 19, and in both areas in 13. Cervical involvement is rare.[214] Most often, 2 vertebrae are involved; but sometimes 3, 4, or even as many as 11 (usually contiguous, but sometimes with "skips") are affected. The body of the vertebra is affected far more often than are the spinous processes or the arch.

The progression of tuberculous spondylitis, as seen on roentgenograms, is from slight narrowing of the disk space only to minimal disk involvement with slight collapse and "wedging" of the vertebral body; to marked narrowing of the disk space with collapse, wedging of the bodies, and resulting angulation of the spine (gibbus); to extensive destruction of the bodies with severe kyphosis (Pott disease).

Paravertebral abscess (Pott abscess), retropharyngeal abscess, psoas abscess, and neurologic lesions are serious complications to be expected in 10 to 30 per cent of cases of spondylitis. Neurologic complications most often arise from cervical and lumbar vertebral lesions and comprise various degrees of neuroplegia, paraplegia, or even quadriplegia. The complications are caused by inflammation of the spinal cord secondary to a neighboring cold abscess, by caseum or granuloma in the extradural space, or by spinal vessel thrombosis.

The signs and symptoms of spondylitis include "night cries" and restless sleep, a low-grade daily fever, and peculiar position (such as torticollis with cervical lesions) or gait. Findings on physical examination may include marked "guarding" because of dorsal muscle spasm, pain when the back is "pounded," a deformity (such as gibbus), or reflex changes (including clonus). Occasionally, the presence of referred chest pain leads to discovery of a paravertebral abscess on the chest roentgenogram. With chemotherapy and, when necessary, surgery, the outlook for both eventual clinical healing and neural recovery is in the range of 80 to 90 per cent, although the patient may not gain his or her full expected height.

Tuberculosis of the knee can be divided into several clinical types: (1) effusion into the joint without bone erosion and with little restriction of motion; (2) thickening and fibrosis of the synovial membrane without bone erosion but often with considerable restriction of motion; (3) synovial disease and a bone focus but an intact joint space; and (4) synovial disease with diminished range of motion.[34, 537] Some degree of pain, stiffness, and limping, usually intermittent in the milder cases, first calls attention to the problem.

Tuberculosis of the hip, in some series of patients more common than tuberculosis of the knee, should be considered in the differential diagnosis when a child refuses to walk or develops a limp. Nowadays, when the disease still is limited at the time of discovery to the acetabulum or to the head of the femur and there is no intra-articular disease, good mobility of the joint usually can be preserved.

Tuberculous dactylitis (spina ventosa)[187] is the most common form of skeletal tuberculosis in infants. Endarteritis is followed by swelling (often painless), and cystic bone lesions are seen on roentgenograms. A cold abscess may form and drain spontaneously. Prognosis for recovery without deformity is surprisingly good and was so even before chemotherapy was available.

Tuberculous arthritis is rare in children.[103] Usually monarticular, it involves primarily the weight-bearing joints and only exceptionally the joints of the upper extremities.[34] Bacterial cultures and histologic examinations of the synovium establish the diagnosis.[537]

The diagnosis of skeletal tuberculosis should be considered immediately in any child who is known to have been infected with tubercle bacilli and in whom a bone or joint lesion develops and in any child with a persistent, not otherwise explained bone or joint lesion.[533] Differential diagnosis must include low-grade infections caused by *Staphylococcus, H. influenzae, Salmonella,* and *Brucella*; fungal infections; rheumatoid arthritis; malignant disease of bone; eosinophilic granuloma (particularly with skull or pelvic lesions); and osteochondrosis resulting from aseptic necrosis of bone (particularly Legg-Calvé-Perthes disease and tuberculosis of the hip).

Children with bone and joint tuberculosis usually react strongly to tuberculin. Although the number of tubercle bacilli in an active bone lesion is much lower than in a lung lesion, the organisms almost invariably can be recovered on culture, and a great effort to do so should be made by means of aspiration or open biopsy.[181]

Treatment of skeletal tuberculosis includes both chemotherapeutic and orthopedic interventions, the former by far the more important. Orthopedic procedures can be used for several purposes: (1) diagnosis, (2) evacuation of caseum and necrotic bone, (3) immobilization of a joint, and (4) reconstruction or strengthening of damaged bone. Since the advent of chemotherapy, any indicated surgical procedure can be done without fear of consequent sinus formation. However, the trend has been toward reliance on drug therapy with increasingly conservative surgical management. Controlled trials of treatment undertaken in different parts of the world by the Medical Research Council Working Party on Tuberculosis of the Spine and others have demonstrated the remarkable effectiveness of ambulatory treatment in children and adults on different regimens of chemotherapy,[227, 329–331] including short-course chemotherapy.[185]

Tuberculosis of the Superficial Lymph Nodes (Scrofula)

Striking enlargement of the superficial regional lymph nodes is an integral part of the primary tuberculous complex. The tonsillar and submandibular nodes are involved most often and probably represent extension from the paratracheal lymph nodes (and not from a primary lesion in the tonsil, as once was thought); occasionally, these nodes are involved when the primary lesion occurs in the mucous membranes of the mouth, a rare event. Enlarged supraclavicular nodes may accompany a primary pulmonary lesion in the upper lung fields. Enlarged axillary and epitrochlear nodes can result from a primary skin lesion of the elbow or hand, often a small, rather insignificant-looking area that has, however, been present for some time. Preauricular adenitis suggests a focus on the scalp or forehead or in the lacrimal sac, sometimes attributed to an insect bite. With inguinal adenitis, careful examination of the sole of the foot may reveal a small ulcer, often at the base of the toes.

When the superficial lymph nodes are involved early in the course of infection—the normal event—the enlargement usually is painless and the node or nodes rubbery and discrete. Low-grade fever usually is present, sometimes unnoticed by the parents. Occasionally, acute respiratory infections seem to precipitate or aggravate superficial tuberculous lymphadenitis, and the patient has high fever, some local pain, and perilymphadenitis. Rarely, the patient is seen first with a fluctuant mass, and the overlying skin is shiny and erythematous.[106]

The diagnosis usually is not obvious, so it is wise in all cases of superficial cervical and supraclavicular lymphadenitis to perform a throat culture, roentgenography of the chest, and a Mantoux tuberculin test. If the node is fluctuant, it should be aspirated and cultured for mycobacteria as well as for pyogenic bacteria.[283] In preauricular, axillary, and inguinal adenitis, a possible primary skin lesion should be sought diligently. If a lesion is found, a biopsy should be performed, in addition to a tuberculin skin test, chest roentgenography, and a careful history.

Currently, in addition to pyogenic infection, cat-scratch disease, tularemia, malignant tumors, sarcoid, and mycobacteria other than *M. tuberculosis* also must be considered as the possible cause.[25, 277] If the adenitis is due to infection with *M. tuberculosis*, the induration from a Mantoux tuberculin skin test usually is greater than 15 mm, whereas the mycobacteria other than *M. tuberculosis* produce a less intense reaction. The key to distinguishing tuberculosis from infection by another mycobacterium usually is epidemiologic—has the child been exposed to tuberculosis?

Because infection with pyogenic bacteria often enhances mycobacterial adenitis, it frequently is wise, while awaiting the results of skin test, chest roentgenography, and cultures, to institute therapy with a conventional antibacterial agent. If the adenitis persists and evidence of mycobacterial infection is elicited, antituberculosis drug therapy should be initiated and surgical excision seriously considered.[277, 434] Surgical excision currently is the treatment of choice for adenitis due to mycobacteria other than *M. tuberculosis*. In the case of lymphadenitis due to *M. tuberculosis*, the response to antituberculosis drugs is likely to be good. On the other hand, the adenitis is more likely to extend down into the mediastinum and be difficult to remove. Under these circumstances, surgical excision probably is unwise, whereas a few weeks of corticosteroid and antituberculosis therapy may be very effective.[65, 237, 277]

Superficial tuberculous lymphadenitis sometimes occurs early in the course of lymphohematogenous spread, in which case it often presents as "general glandular enlargement," accompanied by swinging fever, malaise, and weight loss. The tuberculin test almost always is positive in immunocompetent patients and should be included in the investigation of every patient with general glandular enlargement.

Finally, tuberculous adenitis, either localized or generalized, can occur in adolescents or young adults who were infected months or even years earlier and whose infection has been quiescent and in whom the appearance of lymphadenitis heralds reactivation of the tuberculosis infection.[276]

Ocular Tuberculosis

Ocular tuberculosis is uncommon in children.[121] When it does occur, the conjunctiva and the cornea are the areas most often involved.

The conjunctiva can serve as the initial portal of entry for tubercle bacilli, especially after trauma. Unilateral lacrimation and reddening may lead to the discovery of yellowish-gray nodules, usually on the palpebral conjunctiva. Preauricular adenitis appears early; submandibular and cervical nodes also may enlarge. A tuberculin skin test and biopsy with culture can be performed to confirm the diagnosis.

Phlyctenular conjunctivitis probably is one of the hypersensitivity phenomena of childhood tuberculosis. Tubercle bacilli have, on rare occasions, been isolated from the small, grayish, jelly-like nodules usually clustered on the limbus and surrounded by dilated conjunctival vessels. Pain and photophobia are intense, and the lesions may recur in crops for weeks, affecting one or both eyes. In the differential diagnosis, foreign body, herpes simplex virus conjunctivitis, vernal conjunctivitis, and trachoma should be considered. Tuberculin sensitivity is apt to be pronounced, and it is best to use 1 tuberculin unit of purified protein derivative in the initial tuberculin skin test. Fortunately, hydrocortisone drops are effective in controlling both a strong local reaction to the diagnostic tuberculin test and the discomfort from the underlying disease. The prognosis for complete recovery is excellent, provided the phlyctenules do not ulcerate and leave corneal scars. Systemic chemotherapy should be started immediately after the diagnostic procedures.

Although tuberculosis of the ciliary body and iris has been reported rarely in children, tubercles of the choroid often have been found in patients with miliary tuberculosis (up to 70 per cent of patients in some series) and occasionally in children with a seemingly uncomplicated infection.[350, 372] Often multiple, the tubercles heal slowly with deposition of retinal pigment; residual scarring apparently can be prevented with steroid therapy. Tuberculous uveitis and tuberculosis presenting as an orbital mass are rare clinical entities.[446]

Tuberculosis of the Middle Ear

Tuberculosis of the middle ear is a relatively rare manifestation of the disease.[150, 308, 311, 352, 422] It occurs as a primary focus in the area of the eustachian tube (due to reflux up the tube) in neonates who have aspirated infected amniotic fluid or in older infants who have ingested tuberculous material. It can occur as a metastatic lesion in older children who have a primary focus elsewhere. If it is a primary focus, regional lymphadenitis involves the preauricular lymph node or the anterior cervical chain, and facial paralysis is frequent. The primary focus always is unilateral. Otorrhea is common and painless but may become foul-smelling because of bacterial contamination with enteric organisms. Older patients may complain of tinnitus and "funny noises." The eardrum often is damaged extensively. A large central perforation or several perforations are characteristic. A tuberculin skin test, biopsy, and careful cultures for tubercle bacilli are essential. Once greatly feared for the almost inevitable loss of hearing and the frequent occurrence of tuberculous meningitis, tuberculous otitis media now heals well with appropriate chemotherapy.[352]

Gastrointestinal and Abdominal Tuberculosis

Tuberculosis of the mouth seems to have been more common in the days of bovine tuberculosis than it is today; at that time, scrofula often represented a primary complex in the mouth or tonsil, with associated submandibular or cervical lymphadenitis.[339] A primary focus in the mouth generally consists of a painless ulcer or mass of granulation tissue around a tooth socket or in the gingivolabial sulcus, with enlarged submental or submandibular nodes. Primary tuberculosis of the tonsil begins as a painless swelling of one tonsil, sometimes with an ulcer or yellowish node and, of course, with enlargement of the regional lymph nodes. If tubercles found on histologic examination of a tonsil removed at tonsillectomy are unaccompanied by lymphadenitis, the lesion is considered a metastatic rather than a primary lesion. Tuberculosis of the esophagus occurs rarely, if ever, in children; sometimes dysphagia is produced by a mass of mediastinal nodes, which may rupture into the lumen and later heal, possibly leaving an esophageal diverticulum.

Abdominal tuberculosis may occur after ingestion of tubercle bacilli or as a part of generalized lymphohematogenous spread, but tuberculous enteritis always has been uncommon.[40, 503] When tubercle bacilli penetrate the gut wall, it usually is via the Peyer patches or the appendix, giving rise to local ulcers followed by mesenteric lymphadenitis and sometimes peritonitis. Occasionally, especially in older children, tuberculous enteritis accompanies extensive pulmonary cavitation. Symptoms and signs include vague abdominal pain, intussusception, blood in the stools, and sinus formation after a seemingly routine appendectomy.

The spleen probably always is seeded during the initial lymphohematogenous spread. Only rarely are the tubercles numerous enough and large enough to undergo caseation and calcify.[197, 269] The reticuloendothelial system of the liver probably always is involved also. Symptoms are rare except in miliary tuberculosis, in which the liver may be enlarged markedly, or in congenital tuberculosis, in which both liver and spleen usually are enlarged.[315]

Mesenteric lymphadenitis can arise as part of an intra-abdominal primary complex or by extension from tuberculous thoracic or pelvic lymph nodes; often asymptomatic, it may be discovered later when calcified. It can cause ascites and dilatation of the superficial abdominal veins, but the symptom most frequently attributed to mesenteric lymphadenitis is colicky abdominal pain after exercise, probably because adhesions are stretched.

Tuberculous peritonitis can result from direct extension from a primary intestinal focus, adjacent mesenteric lymph nodes, or tuberculous salpingitis.[85, 120, 163] It may be "plastic" or accompanied by a serous effusion. On palpation, a mass of lymph nodes often can be felt and the abdomen may have a characteristic "doughy" feeling. Paracentesis should be done with care because the intestine may be immobilized by adhesions. Even with a large effusion, absorption usually occurs within a month. Malignancy must, of course, be strongly considered in the differential diagnosis, and biopsy may be necessary even if the tuberculin skin test is positive. Laparoscopy frequently is useful, as is fine-needle aspiration[302] and ultrasonography.[252] The ascitic/blood glucose ratio of the aspirated peritoneal fluid can be helpful in the differentiation of tuberculous peritonitis from ascites due to other causes.[549]

Renal Tuberculosis

Renal tuberculosis is a late and uncommon complication of pulmonary disease, rarely occurring less than 4 or 5 years after primary infection and likely, therefore, to be diagnosed during adolescence.[144, 457, 525] However, tubercle bacilli can be recovered from the urine in many cases of miliary tuberculosis and some cases of pulmonary tuberculosis in young children. Hematogenous dissemination can give rise to tubercles in the glomeruli, with resultant caseating, sloughing lesions, however tiny, which then discharge tubercle bacilli into the tubules. Occasionally, in the zone between the renal pyramid and cortex, an encapsulated caseous mass develops that may calcify in situ or discharge into the pelvis of the kidney, forming a cavity quite analogous to a pulmonary cavity. Infection can be unilateral or bilateral and can spread downward to involve the bladder. Frequently, dysuria, hematuria, and "sterile" pyuria are the presenting findings in the urine; they may occur grossly but often not until late in the course of a disease that causes strikingly few symptoms. Appropriate examination and culture of single early-morning urine specimens rarely fail to reveal tubercle bacilli. Intensive chemotherapy makes surgical intervention rare.[457] It should be remembered that urine from patients with renal tuberculosis is highly infectious and that such children should be isolated until their urine is sterile.

Dialysis and Renal Transplant–Associated Tuberculosis

Infections are a common cause of morbidity and mortality in patients with end-stage renal disease. Depressed cellular immunity, as manifested by cutaneous anergy, delayed homograft rejection, and depressed lymphocyte count, has been demonstrated in uremic patients, whereas cell-mediated immunity appears to recover in stable patients on long-term hemodialysis. Thus, it is not surprising that tuberculosis is more frequent in patients on dialysis than in the general population and that, when it does become active, it does so prior to or early in the course of dialysis. Extrapulmonary involvement (mediastinal, meningeal, pleural, osseous, and renal) and miliary tuberculosis appear relatively frequently in this group. In these patients, fever of unknown origin should lead to the suspicion of active tuberculosis.[14, 261] Tuberculosis also can originate in the transplanted organ.

Any individual with chronic renal disease and a positive

or doubtful tuberculin skin test should be placed on chemotherapy, usually with INH. Limited experience shows that adults tolerate 300 mg/day satisfactorily, so that children probably tolerate 10 mg/kg/day. Should treatment of tuberculosis disease become necessary, rifampin (RIF) can be used in the usual dosage because its metabolism is not dependent on renal function. Ethambutol (EMB), which depends on renal excretion, should be avoided if possible. There is very limited information about pyrazinamide (PZA), but it appears to be safe. It probably should be given at the rate of 15 to 20 mg/kg/day. The appropriate duration of therapy is a matter of speculation, and it is not clear whether it should be prescribed for 9 or 12 months.

Genital Tuberculosis

Tuberculosis of the genital tract is uncommon in both sexes before puberty.[457] It usually arises as a metastatic lesion during lymphohematogenous spread and occasionally by direct extension from an adjacent lesion of bone, gut, or the urinary tract. Genital tuberculosis is a particular hazard for adolescent girls with tuberculosis infection. Frequently, other forms of tuberculosis associated with initial infection, such as a pleural effusion, also are present. The fallopian tubes are involved in 90 to 100 per cent of cases, the endometrium in 50 per cent, the ovaries in 20 to 30 per cent, and the cervix in 2 to 4 per cent.[429] With tubal involvement, peritoneal tuberculosis is frequent.

Lower abdominal pain and amenorrhea usually prompt the patient to seek medical care. A lower abdominal mass, free peritoneal fluid, and constitutional symptoms may or may not be present. Chemotherapy is effective, but infertility remains a potential sequela of the disease.

Tuberculosis of the external genitalia has been seen as a manifestation of child abuse.

Genital tuberculosis can occur in males as primary tuberculosis of the penis after ritual circumcision; many such instances were reported in the past.[203] Massive inguinal lymphadenopathy in a circumcised infant should arouse suspicion of a possible tuberculous etiology. Epididymitis or epididymo-orchitis can occur in early childhood.[174] These disorders are characterized by nodular, painless swelling of the scrotum and a dragging pain in the groin and have a gradual onset rather than the acute onset that results after trauma, torsion of the testis, mumps orchitis, or epididymitis associated with bacterial infection.

Inoculation Tuberculosis

More than 200 cases of syringe-transmitted tuberculosis have been described in the world literature, many by Debré and his associates.[114, 196] These have become more common since the widespread use of injectable penicillin and routine childhood immunization and have occurred usually as a result of contamination of the syringe or the solution by an individual with infectious sputum. If the recipient has not been infected previously, the lesion in the muscle or subcutaneous tissue will be the primary focus and the regional lymph nodes will enlarge, caseate, and, under favorable circumstances, calcify. However, at least 10 infants so infected have died as a result of generalized tuberculosis, and in others bone tuberculosis has developed. If the recipient already is tuberculin-positive, a tuberculous abscess will form without regional lymphadenitis. In this case, an injection abscess must be differentiated from a deep tuberculous abscess arising in the stage of hematogenous dissemination.

Perinatal Tuberculosis (Congenital and Postnatal)

Transmission of tuberculous infection from mother to infant via the placenta or amniotic fluid has been reported in about 300 patients.[66] Infection of the placenta has been demonstrated, and tubercle bacilli have been grown from the tissues of stillborn infants and from living infants within a few days of birth. The occurrence of true congenital tuberculous infection in humans strongly is attested to by its fairly common occurrence in calves when bovine tuberculosis was prevalent, probably because cows are quite susceptible to tuberculous endometritis.[267]

Perinatal tuberculosis can be acquired by the infant via one of several routes:[464]

1. By transplacental spread via the umbilical vein from a mother with primary hematogenous tuberculosis occurring during pregnancy (i.e., true congenital tuberculosis). The liver is enlarged, enlarged lymph nodes may be present at the porta hepatis, and there may be evidence of widespread miliary disease in the infant (i.e., there may be a primary liver complex or primary lung complexes).
2. By aspiration in utero of amniotic fluid infected from endometritis in the mother or from the placenta. This also constitutes true congenital tuberculosis. In both of these situations, clinical onset of signs and symptoms is apt to be rapid (by 2 to 3 weeks of age) and include failure to thrive, fever, respiratory distress, and hepatosplenomegaly.
3. By ingestion of infected amniotic fluid or secretions during delivery. This would seem to be less well documented than numbers 1 and 2, but it certainly is a possibility.
4. By inhalation of tubercle bacilli at or soon after birth, from the mother, other relatives, or attendants with infectious pulmonary tuberculosis. This is the most common mode of transmission to newborns.
5. By ingestion of infected breast milk or cow's milk.
6. By contamination of traumatized skin or mucous membranes, as for example, in ritual circumcision.

It is not always possible to be sure of the type of infection in a particular neonate: only clear-cut evidence of a primary complex in the liver establishes a definite diagnosis of congenital tuberculosis. However, the presence of early forms of tuberculosis (such as pleural, miliary, or meningeal) in the mother during pregnancy or the puerperium also is strong evidence of true congenital tuberculosis in the infant.

Numbers 4, 5, and 6 really are "postnatally" acquired tuberculosis and need, for epidemiologic purposes, to be distinguished from numbers 1 and 2. Neonates with these types of tuberculosis usually lack striking clinical features until 1 or 2 months of age.

Diagnosis of perinatal tuberculosis is apt to be difficult and often delayed. In the first place, disease in the mother often is overlooked; the mother may have pleural effusion, fever of unknown origin, cough, endometritis, and other symptoms without the tuberculous etiology being recognized. The early symptoms and signs in the neonate likewise often are overlooked and may be similar to those caused by other congenital infections. Once the diagnosis is suspected, treatment should be started immediately, and diagnostic procedures should be carried out rapidly and aggressively.

The clinical manifestations vary, probably depending on the size of the infecting dose of bacilli, the site and size of the caseous lesions, and so on.[323, 359] In many of the reported cases, tuberculosis disease was discovered only at autopsy.[217] Symptoms usually appeared during the second week of life and included loss of appetite and failure to gain weight, fever, nasal or ear discharge, cough, bronchopneumonia, jaundice, hepatomegaly, and splenomegaly occurring later.[66] Wasting has been noted frequently and, in one case, clearly was shown to be caused by hypoadrenocorticism.[348]

Because the tuberculin skin test is very rarely positive in infants, demonstration of tubercle bacilli in gastric washings, middle ear fluid, lymph node biopsy, lung biopsy, skin biopsy, bone marrow aspirate, endotracheal aspirate, or lung biopsy is essential.[184] Examination of the placenta for organisms or characteristic histopathologic changes can be extremely helpful and should be done when a mother is diagnosed with tuberculosis around the time of delivery. Successful treatment of congenital tuberculosis has been reported by several investigators, although clinical response may be very slow and extensive calcification of lungs, liver, spleen, and muscles may result.[253, 257, 359, 465, 477]

TUBERCULOSIS IN ADOLESCENTS

Tuberculosis in adolescents has become relatively more important as the incidence of infection in childhood has lessened.[24, 358, 462] Logically, it should be considered in two ways: first, tuberculosis acquired as an initial infection during the adolescent years, and second, tuberculosis infection acquired in early life and reactivated during adolescence.[361] In actual practice, it often is difficult or impossible to separate the two, and most clinical reports and studies do not.

Tuberculosis in adolescents may occur exactly as it does in young children, or a classic primary complex may progress rapidly to chronic pulmonary tuberculosis while the hilar lymph node involvement characteristic of childhood tuberculosis still is present. The Medical Research Council published in 1963 a report on 504 cases of tuberculosis in adolescents, including 316 cases of pulmonary tuberculosis, 44 cases of pleural effusion, 44 with hilar lymph node enlargement, 6 cases of miliary and 5 of meningeal tuberculosis, 13 with bone and joint disease, and 8 with genitourinary tuberculosis. In their series of cases of primary tuberculosis in adults, Stead and his associates[486, 487] included 11 adolescents, 2 with simple primary tuberculosis, 5 with pleurisy with effusion, and 1 with progressive pulmonary tuberculosis.

From the extensive clinical experience of Lincoln and Sewell[298] and others, several observations emerge. Tuberculosis infection in early infancy rarely leads to pulmonary tuberculosis in adolescence, perhaps because it has several years in which to heal, whereas a tuberculosis infection acquired after 7 years of age and particularly acquired after 10 years of age is prone to progress. When *M. tuberculosis* is acquired during adolescence, chronic pulmonary tuberculosis may develop within 1 to 3 years. Moreover, the risk of pulmonary tuberculosis is two to six times greater for adolescent girls than for adolescent boys. In both sexes, the adolescent growth spurt is the time of greatest risk. The work of Johnston[243] suggests that, at least in girls, the depressant effect of puberty on calcium and nitrogen retention may be correlated with the failure of tuberculosis infection to heal. A group of Danish epidemiologists clearly showed that the larger the tuberculin skin reaction, the greater the risk of developing chronic pulmonary tuberculosis.

These considerations lead clearly to the thought that screening high-risk adolescents for tuberculosis infection and disease is important. This particularly is so because adolescents often are unaware of having had contact with tuberculous individuals and because adolescents respond particularly well to appropriate chemotherapy.

TUBERCULOSIS AND PREGNANCY

In the era before chemotherapy, there was an ongoing controversy as to whether pregnancy and tuberculosis affected each other adversely. Since the advent of chemotherapy, however, the prognosis has improved greatly. The main problems now are serious unrecognized tuberculosis in the pregnant woman, sometimes with fatal outcome, or serious unrecognized disease in her infant. Another problem is whether pregnancy influences the risk of progression of tuberculosis infection to disease; the data are conflicting in this regard. Tuberculin skin testing probably is valid during pregnancy; chest roentgenograms (with shielding) should be obtained for all tuberculin-positive pregnant patients. Therapy, when indicated, can safely include INH, which crosses the placenta, but apparently without ill effects, RIF, and EMB. The safety of PZA in pregnancy has not been established, but a growing number of experts recommend it because anecdotal data have not shown it to be harmful to the mother or fetus. Streptomycin (STM), because of fetal ototoxicity, is not recommended.[473]

Should a mother on antituberculosis therapy breastfeed?[474] It probably is safe for her to do so because the drugs, although present in milk, are present only in small amounts.

TUBERCULOSIS AND HIV INFECTION

In adults infected with both HIV and *M. tuberculosis*, the rate of progression from asymptomatic infection to disease is increased greatly.[424] The clinical manifestations of tuberculosis in HIV-infected adults are typical when the CD4+ cell count is more than 500 per mm^3.[23] As the CD4+ cell count falls, manifestations become "atypical." Extrapulmonary foci occur in up to 60 per cent of profoundly immunocompromised patients.[19] Pulmonary cavities are rare; lower lobe infiltrates or nodules often accompanied by thoracic adenopathy are common, especially if the patient's tuberculosis infection is recent. Of course, many patients have a nonreactive tuberculin skin test. Sputum is less likely to be produced or to contain visible acid-fast organisms on stained smear; more invasive procedures, such as bronchoscopy, often are required to isolate *M. tuberculosis* and to rule out other causes of opportunistic lung disease. Malabsorption of antituberculosis drugs in HIV-infected patients can lead to prolonged symptoms and disease.[387]

When HIV-infected children develop tuberculosis, the clinical features tend to be fairly typical of childhood tuberculosis in immunocompetent children, although the disease often progresses more rapidly and clinical manifestations are more severe.[83, 262, 351] There may be an increased tendency for extrapulmonary disease. Diagnosis can be very difficult; a diligent search for an infectious adult in the child's environment may yield the best clues to the correct diagnosis.

DIAGNOSIS

How Children with Tuberculosis Are Discovered

In the developing world, the only way children with tuberculosis disease are discovered is when they present with a profound illness that is consistent with one presentation of tuberculosis. Having an ill adult contact is an obvious clue to the correct diagnosis. The only available laboratory test usually is an acid-fast smear of sputum, which the child rarely produces. In many regions, chest roentgenography is not available. To aid in diagnosis, a variety of scoring systems have been devised based on available tests, clinical signs and symptoms, and known exposures.[338] However, the sensitivity and specificity of these systems can be very low, leading to both over- and underdiagnosis of tuberculosis.[260, 338]

In industrial countries, children with tuberculosis usually are discovered in one of two ways.[131, 265, 427] Obviously, one way is consideration of tuberculosis as the cause of a symptomatic illness. Discovering an adult contact with infectious tuberculosis is an invaluable aid to diagnosis; the "yield" from a contact investigation usually is higher than that from cultures from the child. The culture from the infectious adult case may yield the only drug susceptibility results for the child because cultures from children with tuberculosis frequently are negative. The second way is discovery of a child with pulmonary tuberculosis during the contact investigation of an adult with tuberculosis. Typically, the affected child has few or no symptoms, but investigation reveals a positive tuberculin skin test and an abnormal chest roentgenogram. In some areas of the United States, up to 50 per cent of children with pulmonary tuberculosis are discovered in this manner, before significant symptoms have begun. It is rare to find tuberculosis disease in a child as the result of a community- or school-based tuberculin skin testing program.[132]

Tuberculin Sensitivity and the Skin Test

Sensitization to tuberculin is induced by infection with living tubercle bacilli or, to a lesser degree, by inoculation with dead tubercle bacilli, particularly if the latter are incorporated into a complex adjuvant mixture as described by Freund. Specific tuberculin sensitivity to either *M. tuberculosis* or to other mycobacteria can be transferred in humans by injection of lymphocytes from sensitized donors and also by injection of certain purified mycobacterial protein antigens.

The time of appearance of sensitivity in animals after infection with tubercle bacilli depends on the number of tubercle bacilli in the infective dose and on the virulence—that is, the rate of multiplication of the organisms—and there is no reason to doubt that this is so in humans.[20] For all practical purposes in humans, tuberculin reactivity seems to appear in 3 to 6 weeks, rarely a few days earlier, and occasionally as long as 3 months after initial infection.

The tuberculin sensitivity reaction has been studied best in the skin, although it can be elicited in any tissue of a sensitive subject (conjunctiva, lung, meninges, kidney, and so on) on injection of tuberculoprotein. At first, an inflammatory reaction appears at the site of injection, with predominance of segmented neutrophils, followed by immigration of macrophages and T lymphocytes, until the entire area of induration consists of mononuclear cells.

The size of the induration depends on the amount of tuberculoprotein injected and the availability of sensitized T lymphocytes in sufficient numbers. Multiple tuberculin skin tests given simultaneously result in smaller individual reactions, probably because of a finite number of sensitized cells in the body. Corticosteroids,[50, 313, 430] adrenocorticotropic hormone, nitrogen mustard, irradiation, and viral infections, such as measles, influenza, and mumps, diminish tuberculin reactivity, perhaps simply by inducing lymphopenia.[485] The size of the induration seems to depend on at least two further factors: the local behavior of the skin (the disappearance time for wheals of normal saline solution, the so-called Aldrich-McClure test, is accelerated during fever, pregnancy, cachexia, and extreme malnutrition) and the number of actively multiplying tubercle bacilli in the body, which can be demonstrated in animals and probably so in humans as well.[355] That there must be yet other factors involved is clear because 10 to 20 per cent of immunocompetent patients with proven tuberculosis are tuberculin-negative during initial disease, often regaining tuberculin sensitivity during treatment.[246, 392] Decreased T-lymphocyte blastogenesis has been demonstrated in some cases, and inhibition by B lymphocytes may play a role.

Temporary desensitization to tuberculin occurs most strikingly during measles and has been studied carefully. Full reactivity diminished during the incubation period and returned within approximately 1 month after appearance of the exanthem.[194] Influenza and administration of influenza and measles vaccines tend to depress sensitivity but rarely suppress it entirely.[58, 557] Whether other viral diseases and vaccines regularly are less active in this regard and what the important factors may be is not known in detail.[33] If a temporary desensitizing effect occurs in bacterial infections such as scarlet fever, it probably depends on factors such as hyperthermia and dehydration.

Sensitization to tuberculin due to infection by *M. tuberculosis* tends to persist undiminished for life.[143, 186, 211] The likelihood of tuberculin sensitivity disappearing seems to be greater when the lesion is negligible. It also is clear that low degrees of sensitivity to *M. tuberculosis* are induced by mycobacteria other than *M. tuberculosis* and that sensitivity of this kind diminishes within months. Previous receipt of a BCG vaccine can cause increased reactivity to tuberculin, but the association is weaker than many clinicians suspect.[156, 251, 440] Less than 50 per cent of infants given BCG vaccination have a reactive tuberculin skin test at 9 to 12 months of age, and the great majority will have a nonreactive skin test by 5 years of age.[290] Older children and adults who receive BCG vaccination develop a reactive skin test and keep it longer, but by 10 to 15 years post vaccination, most individuals have lost tuberculin skin test reactivity.[95, 337] Repeated administration of BCG vaccines can maintain tuberculin reactivity.[226] Repeated tuberculin skin tests in a person sensitized previously by a BCG vaccine, infection with *M. tuberculosis,* or probably infection by an environmental mycobacterium may increase the reaction to subsequent tuberculin skin tests (called the booster phenomenon).[439, 512]

In the first tuberculin test developed by von Pirquet in 1907, the skin was scarified with a scalpel between two drops of old tuberculin. This test no longer is used, nor are the Calmette and Wolff-Eisner conjunctival tests, the Moro percutaneous test, and the Vollmer patch test. The reference test used at present is the Mantoux intracutaneous test, which originally made use of old tuberculin but now employs 5 tuberculin units of purified protein derivative.

The antigens currently used in tuberculin testing are crude extracts indeed, consisting actually of a mixture of many antigens, some species-specific, some shared among many species. Standardized, isolated, purified mycobacterial antigens are badly needed in clinical practice.[377, 425] The antigens employed in tuberculin testing are as follows:

1. Old tuberculin, a filtrate prepared from sterilized concentrated broth cultures of tubercle bacilli, preserved with phenol, available as a stable liquid filtrate, to be diluted in a special isotonic fluid.
2. Purified protein derivative, obtained from filtrates of heat-killed tubercle bacilli. Batch 49608, prepared by Dr. Florence Seibert in 1939, has been designated by the WHO as the international standard tuberculin, the only one to be called PPD-S. All other purified protein derivative preparations are referred to simply as PPD or as PPD-T. However, each batch now must be stabilized with Tween 80 at 5 ppm to minimize adherence to glass and plastic and must be identified by manufacturer and lot number.[279]

In the past, antigens derived from other mycobacteria were available and of considerable help in diagnosis. However, no standardization was possible until species-specific antigens could be isolated, and so they were withdrawn.

A tuberculin unit is the activity contained in a specified weight of PPD-S. The standard test dose, 5 tuberculin units, refers to the equivalence of biologic activity, determined in the guinea pig, of a commercial purified protein derivative preparation with that contained in 5 tuberculin units of PPD-S. Products labeled 1 tuberculin unit and 250 tuberculin units are calculated dilutions based on 5 tuberculin units. However, it long has been recognized that the potency of purified protein derivative doses varies from batch to batch.[548]

The tuberculin skin tests in use at present are the following:

1. The Mantoux test is the reference test. A graduated syringe and a 26- or 27-gauge needle are used for injection of 0.1 mL of purified protein derivative into the most superficial layer of the epidermis of the forearm, which raises an immediate wheal (Fig. 101–14). Under optimal circumstances, the needle should not be withdrawn for a few seconds to minimize leakage. The reference test employs a dose of 5 tuberculin units. One tuberculin unit very rarely should be used, for example, if extreme hypersensitivity is suspected as when a tuberculous eye lesion or erythema nodosum is present. The reading should be made at 48 to 72 hours, with the forearm slightly flexed. Any induration (not erythema) should be measured, preferably with calipers, and the diameter at right angles to the axis of administration recorded in millimeters.[246] Use of the words "negative" and "positive" should be avoided because interpretation can change as more epidemiologic information becomes known.

2. Several multiple-puncture tests are used widely because of the speed and ease with which they can be administered, even by unskilled personnel.[128] However, several problems with multiple-puncture tests severely limit their usefulness. The exact dose of tuberculin introduced into the skin cannot be controlled precisely, so interpretation of the reaction size can not be standardized. As a result, any "positive" multiple-puncture test result (except blistering) must be verified by a Mantoux test. However, this second test can lead to boosting, which can create a false-positive Mantoux result by increasing the reaction size over that which would have occurred with only the Mantoux test. Unfortunately, multiple-puncture tests have variable and, in some cases, poor sensitivity and specificity compared with the Mantoux test.[71] Finally, the previous widespread use of multiple-puncture tests led to the practice of allowing parents to interpret the results and report them to the clinician. This practice assumes parental knowledge of and adherence to a broad range of motivational behaviors and skills. No study has demonstrated that parents can read positive skin tests accurately, but it has been well documented that they may not report positive results.[86, 178, 209] Virtually all experts, the CDC, and the American Academy of Pediatrics (AAP) agree that multiple-puncture tests no longer should be used in any clinical situation.

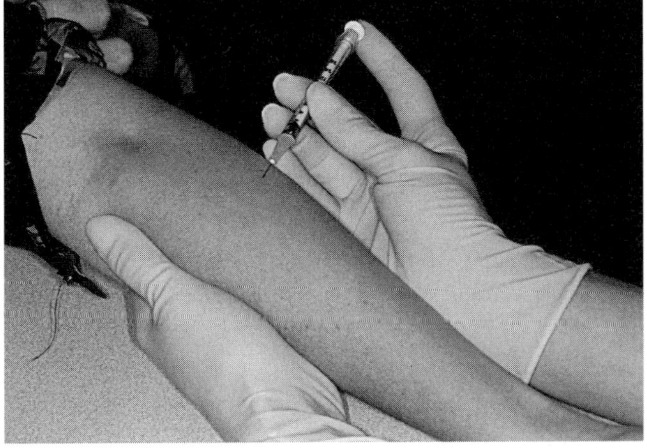

FIGURE 101–14. *A useful technique for placing a Mantoux tuberculin skin test on a child. The needle is applied perpendicular to the long axis of the arm to attain better control.*

Variability in Mantoux test reading has been shown by several studies to be great.[29, 128] It can be minimized only by ongoing training of both testers and readers and by concentrating the responsibility of testing and reading to a small number of trained individuals.

The importance of the tuberculin test cannot be overemphasized as the main criterion for diagnosing tuberculosis infection in the individual child.[256] Only rarely is the tuberculin test negative in an infected child, as a result of anergy from overwhelming infection, from viral infection, from HIV infection, from the use of immunosuppressive drugs, or because of factors not yet understood.[493] A simultaneous skin test, using a common antigen such as *Candida* to which almost all children are sensitive, is useful in determining the presence of anergy. However, anergy in tuberculosis can be selective for tuberculin; "control" skin tests may be positive but the Mantoux test negative in a child with tuberculosis disease.[484]

There have been several changes in recommendations for interpretation of the Mantoux test, which has a sensitivity and specificity of only around 90 per cent.[215] When a test with these characteristics is applied to a population with a 90 per cent prevalence of tuberculosis infection, the positive predictive value of the skin test is 99 per cent, an excellent result. However, if the same test is applied to a population with only a 1 per cent prevalence of infection, the positive predictive value drops to 8 per cent; 92 per cent of the "positive" results are false-positives, created by biologic variability, nonspecific reactions, and infection by environmental mycobacteria. Because the skin test is the only test to detect tuberculosis infection, true positives can not be distinguished from false-positive results by further testing. These false-positive results lead to unnecessary treatment, costs, and anxiety for the patient, family, and clinician. In short, the low sensitivity and specificity of the tuberculin skin test make the test undesirable for use in persons from low-prevalence groups. The trend in the United States is to reduce or eliminate the routine testing of low-risk children but target children with specific risk factors for one-time or periodic tuberculosis skin testing.[10–12, 79, 347]

The CDC and AAP have recommended varying the size of induration considered positive in various groups, according to risk factors (Table 101–8). This is an attempt to minimize false-negative results among children most likely to have rapid progression of asymptomatic tuberculosis infection to disease and minimize the false-positive results in persons with no known risk factors for tuberculosis. In general in the United States, prior receipt of a BCG vaccine should not influence the interpretation of the initial tuberculin skin test of a child.[242]

Diagnostic Mycobacteriology in Children[421]

The demonstration of acid-fast bacilli in stained smears of sputum is presumptive evidence of pulmonary tuberculosis in most patients. However, in children, tubercle bacilli usually are relatively few in number, and sputum cannot be obtained from children younger than about 10 years of age.

TABLE 101–8. Amount of Induration in Reaction to a Mantoux Tuberculin Skin Test Considered Positive (Indicating Likely Infection with *Mycobacterium tuberculosis*)

Reaction Size	Risk Factors
≥5 mm	Contacts to infectious cases Abnormal chest radiograph HIV infection or other immunocompromise
≥10 mm	Birth or previous residence in a high-prevalence country Residence in long-term care or corrections facility Certain medical risk factors: diabetes mellitus, silicosis, renal disease Occupation in health care field, exposure to tuberculosis patients Member of a local high-risk group Close contact to a high-risk adult (except health care workers) Age < 4 years
≥15 mm	No risk factors

Gastric washings, which often are used in lieu of sputum, can be contaminated with acid-fast organisms from the mouth. However, fluorescence microscopy of gastric washings has been found useful, particularly in a setting where malnutrition and tuberculin-negative tuberculosis are rampant.[284] Tubercle bacilli in cerebrospinal fluid, pleural fluid, lymph node aspirate, and urine are sparse; thus, only rarely are direct-stained smears for tubercle bacilli of any use in pediatric practice. When they are, it usually is for examination of a large amount of spinal fluid in a laboratory skilled in the fluorochrome staining method of Truant. Cultures for tubercle bacilli are of great importance, not only to confirm the diagnosis, but increasingly to permit testing for drug susceptibility. If culture and drug susceptibility data are available from the associated adult case and the child has a classic presentation of tuberculosis (positive skin test, consistent abnormal chest roentgenogram), obtaining cultures from the child adds little to the management.

Painstaking collection of specimens is essential for diagnosis in children because fewer organisms usually are present than in adults. Gastric lavage should be performed in the very early morning, when the patient has had nothing to eat or drink for 8 hours and before the patient has a chance to wake up and start swallowing saliva, tears, and so on; these presumably would dilute the bronchial secretions that were brought up during the night and that made their way into the stomach. Inhalation of superheated nebulized saline prior to gastric lavage has been reported to increase the bacteriologic yield.[167] The stomach contents should be aspirated first. Then, no more than 50 to 75 mL of sterile distilled water (not saline) should be injected through the stomach tube and the aspirate added to the first collection. The gastric acidity (poorly tolerated by tubercle bacilli) should be neutralized immediately, either with 10 per cent sodium carbonate added by dropper to a pH of 7 as indicated by phenol red or with 40 per cent anhydrous sodium phosphate to green with bromothymol blue as indicated. Concentration and culture should be performed as soon as possible after collection. However, even with optimal, in-hospital collection of three early-morning gastric aspirate samples, *M. tuberculosis* can be isolated from only 30 to 40 per cent of children and 70 per cent of infants with pulmonary tuberculosis.[484, 526] The yield from random outpatient gastric aspirate samples is exceedingly low.

Bronchial secretions obtained by stimulating cough with an aerosol solution of propylene glycol in 10 per cent sodium chloride can be used in older children.[69] The aerosol is heated in a nebulizer at 46° to 52° C (114.8° to 125.6° F) and administered to the patient for 15 to 30 minutes. This method gives good results and may be superior to gastric lavage both in yield of positive cultures and in patient acceptance.[69] Bronchial aspirate obtained at bronchoscopy often is thick, and the laboratory will process it using a mucolytic agent, such as *N*-acetyl-L-cysteine. In most studies, the yield of *M. tuberculosis* from bronchoscopy specimens has been lower than from properly obtained gastric aspirates.[1, 82]

Cerebrospinal fluid, pleural fluid, and synovial fluid (as much fluid as possible should be collected) usually are centrifuged, and the sediment is used for stained smear and culture. An overnight urine specimen should be obtained in the early morning and taken immediately to the laboratory for processing because the organisms tolerate the low pH of urine poorly. Lymph node aspirates and bits of biopsy tissue can be inoculated directly into a fluid medium, such as Middlebrook 7H9.

The staining and examination of smears, as well as the inoculation of special media, incubation in a carbon dioxide environment, strain differentiation based on many cultural characteristics, and drug susceptibility testing, all require equipment, skills, and experience beyond those available in the usual clinic or hospital laboratory. Thus, most laboratories will depend on regional or reference laboratories for procedures beyond their scope.

Despite an enormous amount of research and thousands of publications on the subject, the only definite way to diagnose active tuberculosis is by demonstration of the tubercle bacilli in tissues or secretions. No single species-specific antigen of *M. tuberculosis* ever has been identified. The search for quick, simple, inexpensive, specific, sensitive immunologic and chemical detection techniques is ongoing.

Nucleic Acid Amplification

The main form of nucleic acid amplification studied in children with tuberculosis is the polymerase chain reaction (PCR), which uses specific DNA sequences as markers for microorganisms.[146, 175, 319] Various PCR techniques, most using the mycobacterial insertion element IS6110 as the DNA marker for *M. tuberculosis* complex organisms,[72] have a sensitivity and specificity of more than 90 per cent compared with sputum culture for detecting pulmonary tuberculosis in adults. However, test performance varies even among reference laboratories.[365, 431] The test is relatively expensive, requires fairly sophisticated equipment, and requires scrupulous technique to avoid cross-contamination of specimens.

Use of PCR in childhood tuberculosis has been limited. Compared with a clinical diagnosis of pulmonary tuberculosis in children, sensitivity of PCR has varied from 25 to 83 per cent and specificity has varied from 80 to 100 per cent.[118, 393, 459] The PCR of gastric aspirates may be positive in a recently infected child even when the chest roentgenogram is normal, demonstrating the occasional arbitrariness of the distinction between tuberculosis infection and disease in children. The PCR may have a useful but limited role in evaluating children for tuberculosis. A negative PCR never eliminates tuberculosis as a diagnostic possibility, and a positive result does not confirm it. The major use of PCR will be in evaluating children with significant pulmonary disease when the diagnosis is not established readily by clinical or epidemiologic grounds. PCR particularly may be helpful in evaluating immunocompromised children with pulmonary disease, especially in children with HIV infection, although published reports of its performance in such children are lacking. PCR also may aid in confirming the diagnosis of extrapulmonary tuberculosis, although only a few case reports have been published.[318, 342]

Serology and Antigen Detection

Despite hundreds of studies published over the past century, serology has found little place in the routine diagnosis of tuberculosis in adults or children.[496] Some studies have used ELISA to detect antibodies to whole bacterial cells or to various purified or complex antigens of *M. tuberculosis* in children.[107, 248] In general, both the sensitivity and specificity of the various tests have been unacceptably low.[36, 221] Tests using the mycobacterial antigen A60 have shown both good[116] and bad[520] results in children. No available serodiagnostic test for tuberculosis is adequate under various clinical conditions to be useful for children.

Mycobacterial antigen detection has been evaluated in clinical samples from adults but rarely from children.[272, 419] Most of these techniques require technically advanced equipment (such as high-pressure liquid chromatography apparatus) and expertise that are not available where tuberculosis in children is common.

TREATMENT

Management of Tuberculous Children

The treatment of cavitary tuberculosis in the adult is one of the most scientifically accurate areas in all of medicine and one of the finest examples of international professional cooperation in all of history. Because tubercle bacilli in adult patients with active tuberculosis can be seen and cultured, their numbers quantified, and size of the cavities they produce measured and because there are so many cases of tuberculosis in the world, it has been possible to ask precise questions about treatment and to design prospective cooperative studies that yield accurate answers about the effect of individual drugs, multiple drug regimens, drug dosage, duration of chemotherapy, rest, and surgical procedures on the course of the disease. Although chemotherapy without doubt has been extremely effective in childhood tuberculosis, the recommendations for treatment historically have been based to a great extent on analogy with adults, on "custom," and on "experience" because in children the tubercle bacilli are fewer in number and not readily accessible and the lesions are not so easy to evaluate as are cavities. However, during the past decade, a large number of treatment trials for children have been reported, leading to dramatic changes in the therapeutic approach to childhood tuberculosis.

As recently as the early 1980s, the recommended treatment duration for children with tuberculosis disease was 12 to 18 months.[324] Although those regimens are effective when used properly, the actual failure rates are high because of poor adherence over the long period of treatment. Newer regimens often are called "short-course" chemotherapy because treatment durations as short as 6 months routinely are successful. However, the key to the new approach is not the short duration but the intensive initial therapy with three or more antituberculosis drugs.

Antituberculosis Drugs (Tables 101–9 and 101–10)

INH is the mainstay of treatment for tuberculosis in children. Cheap, highly effective in preventing the multiplication of tubercle bacilli, of low molecular weight and therefore readily diffusible to all tissues in the body,[125] and relatively nontoxic to children, it is one of the most nearly perfect drugs in the pediatrician's armamentarium. It can be administered orally or intramuscularly. When it is taken orally, high plasma, sputum, and spinal fluid levels are reached within a few hours and persist at least 6 to 8 hours.[281, 373] Because of the slow multiplication of *M. tuberculosis*, the total daily dose

TABLE 101–9. Commonly Used Drugs for the Treatment of Tuberculosis in Children

Drug	Dosage Forms	Daily Dose (mg/kg/day)	Twice Weekly Dose (mg/kg/dose)	Maximum Daily Dose
Ethambutol	Tablets: 100 mg 400 mg	15–25	50	2.5 g
Isoniazid*‡	Scored tablets: 100 mg 300 mg Syrup:† 10 mg/mL	10–15‡	20–30	Daily 300 mg Twice weekly: 900 mg 2 g
Pyrazinamide	Scored tablets: 500 mg	20–40	50	
Rifampin*	Capsules: 150 mg 300 mg Syrup: formulated in syrup from capsules	10–20	10–20	Daily 600 mg Twice weekly: 900 mg
Streptomycin (IM administration)	Vials: 1 g 4 g	20–40	20–40	

*Rifamate is a capsule containing 150 mg of isoniazid and 300 mg of rifampin. Two capsules provide the usual adult (>50 kg body weight) daily doses of each drug.
†Most experts advise against the use of isoniazid syrup due to instability and a high rate of gastrointestinal adverse reaction (diarrhea, cramps).
‡When isoniazid is used in combination with rifampin, the incidence of hepatotoxicity increases if the isoniazid dose exceeds 10 mg/kg/day.

TABLE 101–10. Drugs for Treatment of Drug-Resistant Tuberculosis in Children

Drugs	Dosage Forms	Daily Dosage (mg/kg/day)	Maximum Daily Dose
Capreomycin	Vials: 1 g	15–30 (IM)	1 g
Ciprofloxacin	Tablets: 250 mg 500 mg 750 mg	Adults: 500–1500 mg in 2 divided doses	1.5 g
Clofazamine	Capsules: 50 mg 100 mg	50–100 mg/day	200 mg
Cycloserine	Capsules: 250 mg	10–20	1 g
Ethionamide	Tablets: 250 mg	15–20, given in 2 or 3 divided doses	1 g
Kanamycin	Vials: 75 mg/2 mL 500 mg/2 mL 1 g/3 mL	15–30 (IM)	1 g
Ofloxacin	Tablets: 200 mg 300 mg 400 mg	Adults: 400–800 mg total/day	800 mg
Paraaminosalicylic acid	Packets: 4 g	200–300 given in 2 to 4 divided doses	12 g

can be given at one time. The usual level necessary to inhibit multiplication of tubercle bacilli is 0.02 to 0.05 μg/mL.

Human variation in the acetylation rate of INH to an inactive compound is known to be determined genetically.[321] Rapid acetylation occurs more frequently among black people and Asians than among whites. Although there now is a simple method, using a urine sample, of classifying patients as slow or rapid inactivators of INH, the normal way of coping with the problem in children has been to give a sufficiently large dose of INH to ensure an adequate level even in rapid inactivators.[398, 532]

The principal toxic effects of INH are peripheral neuritis and hepatitis. Peripheral neuritis, resulting from competitive inhibition of pyridoxine utilization, essentially is unknown in North American children because both milk and meat are the main dietary sources of pyridoxine.[42] In some well-nourished children, serum pyridoxine concentrations mildly are depressed by INH, but clinical signs are not apparent.[386] In the case of most children, therefore, it is not necessary to use supplementary pyridoxine. However, in teenagers whose diets may be inadequate, in children from ethnic groups with a low milk and meat intake, and in breast-fed babies, pyridoxine supplementation (25 to 50 mg/day) is important. Peripheral neuritis, when it does occur, usually is manifested by "pins and needles" sensations in the hands and feet.

Hepatotoxicity from INH, rare in children, increases in frequency with age.[30, 70, 271, 300, 354, 369, 400, 476, 488] Its cause is unclear.[273] Rapid acetylators are no more susceptible than slow acetylators.[147, 320] Simultaneous use of alcohol, phenytoin, piperazine, and especially RIF seems to increase the likelihood of hepatotoxicity.[70, 275] Monitoring of serum glutamic-oxaloacetic transaminase and serum glutamic-pyruvic transaminase sometimes reveals transient increases during treatment with INH, but the levels usually return spontaneously to normal without interruption of treatment. Liver enzyme abnormalities in adolescents receiving INH likewise are rather common and usually disappear spontaneously, but severe hepatitis can occur.[160, 301, 379, 466, 529]

The possible occurrence of hepatitis raises the question of routine monitoring of liver enzyme levels once a month in all children receiving INH. The advantage of doing so has to be weighed not only against the expense, but particularly against the difficulty of assuring regular monthly visits if patient and parents know that every clinic visit entails a venipuncture. Most experts prefer to substitute routine questions about appetite and well-being, determination of weight, and a check of the appearance of the sclera and the size of the liver.[63] Patients should be counseled to stop the INH and contact the clinician immediately if significant nausea, vomiting, abdominal pain, or jaundice occurs during the use of INH.

Allergic manifestations of INH hypersensitivity are extraordinarily rare. Convulsions have been reported after doses of 100 mg/kg or more.[326, 363, 380, 443] Adverse reactions to INH also have been reported rarely after ingestion of fish with a high histamine content, apparently because of the fact that INH is a potent inhibitor of histamine.[523]

The usual dosage in children is 10 to 20 mg/kg/day, to a maximum of 300 mg/day. INH is available in tablets of 100 and 300 mg. The original liquid preparation of INH in syrup was abandoned when it was found that the drug was unstable in sucrose.[45] A syrup of INH in sorbitol (10 mg/mL) now is on the market and appears to be satisfactory; however, it is unstable at 37° C (98.6° F) and should be kept cool. Many children develop significant gastrointestinal intolerance (nausea, vomiting) while taking the INH suspension. If tablets are used, they easily are crushed in a dessert spoon, to which then is added in the same spoon a vehicle such as applesauce, mashed banana, thawed undiluted frozen orange juice, or another palatable medium. The child then is encouraged to lick the spoon well! The crushed tablets must never be added to the nursing bottle or offered in milk or water because they will be ingested only partially. If INH is given concurrently with RIF, the dose should not exceed 10 mg/kg/day.[369] If the intramuscular form is used, for example, in a child with meningitis who is vomiting, the daily dose is the same as the daily oral dose but usually is divided and given every 8 to 12 hours. INH can interact with several other drugs, particularly theophylline, and the dosage of each may need modification in a patient taking several drugs.[17] INH also can increase serum phenytoin levels, leading to toxicity by blocking its metabolism in the liver.[341]

RIF is a semisynthetic drug derived from *Streptomyces mediterranei.* Active against a wide variety of both intracellular and extracellular organisms, it is more effective against mycobacteria than any other drug except INH. Most clinical isolates are susceptible to 5 μg/mL or less. The drug is absorbed readily from the gastrointestinal tract in the fasting state; peak serum levels of 6 to 10 μg/mL are achieved within 2 hours, and the drug is distributed widely in body fluids and tissues, including spinal fluid.[123] Excretion mainly is via the biliary tract; however, effective levels are achieved in the kidneys and urine. In many patients receiving RIF treatment, the tears, saliva, urine, and stool turn orange as a result of a harmless metabolite, but patients always must be warned in advance. Drawbacks include (1) the relatively high cost of treatment; (2) the rare occurrence of explosive hypersensitivity reactions with hemolytic anemia, which, however, usually accompany intermittent (separated by weeks or months) rather than daily RIF therapy; (3) the occasional occurrence of leukopenia or thrombocytopenia while the patient is taking daily RIF[169]; (4) the fact that RIF can render birth control pills inactive when both are used (an alternative method of birth control must be employed); and finally—most serious of all for children—(5) a "therapeutic orphan" clause in the United States for children younger than 5 years of age, which also means that there is no commercially available formulation for young children. However, RIF can be made into a suspension easily for use in children. Because of the effectiveness of the drug and because it has been used widely and satisfactorily throughout Europe since it first was isolated in the late 1950s, virtually all experts, including the AAP,[9] recommend its routine use in children, despite the warning on the package insert.

RIF should be used alone only when treating tuberculosis infection due to an INH-resistant organism. If one uses INH, 20 mg/kg, and RIF, 15 to 20 mg/kg, there is an appreciable incidence of hepatotoxicity. Therefore, when using the two together, one would be wise to approximate INH, 10 mg/kg, and RIF, 15 to 20 mg/kg. Rifamate is a capsule containing both INH (150 mg) and RIF (300 mg). Two capsules supply the usual adult (more than 50 kg) daily dose of each drug. Rifamate may be appropriate for older children and adolescents.[3] Rifater contains INH, RIF, and PZA together in one pill in varying concentrations.

PZA contributes to the killing of *M. tuberculosis,* particularly at a low pH such as that within macrophages.[420] The exact mechanism of action of PZA is a subject of controversy. PZA has no effect on extracellular tubercle bacilli in vitro but clearly contributes to the killing of intracellular bacilli. Primary resistance is very rare, except that *M. bovis* is resistant. The drug diffuses readily into all areas, including the spinal fluid.[148] The usual adult daily dose is 30 to 40 mg/kg. The optimal dose for children has not been established firmly because no formal pharmacokinetic studies have been reported. The adult dose is tolerated well by children, results in high cerebrospinal fluid concentrations, and clearly is effective in therapy trials for active tuberculosis in children.[126, 479] PZA appears to exert its maximum effect during the first 2 months of therapy. Hepatotoxicity can occur at high doses but is rare at the usual adult dose. PZA routinely causes an increase in the serum uric acid concentration by inhibiting its excretion through the kidneys. Toxic reactions in adults include flushing, cutaneous hypersensitivity, arthralgia, and overt gout; however, the considerable experience with this drug in children in Latin American countries, Hong Kong, and the United States has revealed few problems. It plays a major role in intensive, short-course treatment regimens.[170, 479]

EMB has been used for many years as a companion drug for INH in adults. The usual oral dose is 15 mg/kg/day. At this dose, the drug primarily is bacteriostatic, its major role being to prevent emergence of resistance to other drugs. However, at doses of 25 mg/kg/day or 50 mg/kg given twice a week, EMB has some bactericidal action.[99, 162] Unfortunately, at these higher doses, optic neuritis or red-green color blindness has occurred in some adults. Regular visual field and color chart testing should discover these reversible effects early. Although the incidence of ophthalmologic toxicity in children is extremely low, if it occurs at all, EMB is not recommended for routine use in young children in whom visual field and color discrimination tests are difficult and inaccurate. However, it is used frequently and safely in children with life-threatening forms of tuberculosis or with drug-resistant tuberculosis.

Ethionamide is a very effective and well-tolerated drug in children at a dose of 15 to 20 mg/kg/day divided into two or three doses given after meals. Children rarely complain about its sulfurous taste, which is repulsive to adults. Related to INH, it likewise diffuses readily into the spinal fluid.[127, 216] It is used in cases of drug-resistant tuberculosis. Unfortunately, no convenient pediatric dosage form is available.

STM is a valuable drug to be used in conjunction with INH and RIF in life-threatening forms of tuberculosis. It is bactericidal and tolerated well in children in the usual dose of 20 to 40 mg/kg/day intramuscularly up to 1 g. Usually, STM can be discontinued within 1 to 3 months if clinical improvement is definite, whereas the other two or three drugs are continued by mouth.

Para-aminosalicylic acid, either the sodium or the potassium salt, formerly was part of the standard treatment of tuberculosis. However, it is a purely bacteriostatic drug that has been superseded completely by more powerful drugs (RIF, PZA). It is used only for treatment of drug-resistant tuberculosis.

Other antituberculosis drugs that may be needed for patients whose mycobacteria are resistant to INH or RIF are the aminoglycosides kanamycin, amikacin, and capreomycin, each of which has a spectrum of activity that differs from that of STM with respect to individual mycobacterial strains.[370] Cycloserine and viomycin are other drugs sometimes used in patients with multidrug resistance. Clofazimine[236] and rifabutin (related to RIF) are newer drugs that have antimycobacterial activity but have been used mainly in children who have AIDS and are suffering from *M. avium-intracellulare* infections.[97, 104] Clofazimine also is used for infections due to *M. leprae.*[219]

Several of the fluoroquinolones, especially ofloxacin and ciprofloxacin, have significant antituberculosis activity,[259, 346] but they cannot be used routinely in children because of the possible destruction of growing cartilage seen in a puppy model.[517] However, the dire consequences of drug-resistant tuberculosis lead many experts to use them in children with multidrug-resistant tuberculosis disease.[222]

Microbiologic Basis for Treatment[480]

Laboratory observations of *M. tuberculosis* and results of clinical therapy trials have led to a hypothesis concerning the actions of various drugs and drug combinations.[141, 161, 179, 343, 344] The tubercle bacillus can be killed only during replication, which occurs among organisms that are active metabolically. In one model, bacilli in a host exist in different populations (Table 101–11). They are active metabolically and replicate freely where oxygen tension is high and the pH is neutral or alkaline. Environmental conditions for growth are best within cavities, leading to a large bacterial population.

TABLE 101–11. In Vivo Location of *Mycobacterium tuberculosis*: A Model

	Population Size	Metabolism and Replication	pH	Most Effective Drugs
Cavity	10^7–10^9	Active and rapid	Neutral or alkaline	INH, RIF, STM
Closed caseous lesions	10^5–10^7	Slow and intermittent	Neutral	RIF, INH
Within macrophages	10^4–10^6	Very slow	Acid	PZA, RIF, INH

INH, isoniazid; PZA, pyrazinamide; RIF, rifampin; STM, streptomycin.

Adults with reactivation-type pulmonary tuberculosis usually have all three populations of tubercle bacilli. Children with pulmonary tuberculosis and patients of all ages with only extrapulmonary tuberculosis are infected with a much smaller number of tubercle bacilli because the cavitary population is not present.

Naturally occurring drug-resistant mutant organisms occur within large populations of tubercle bacilli even before chemotherapy is started.[180] All known genetic loci for drug resistance in *M. tuberculosis* are located on the chromosome; no plasmid-mediated resistance is known. The rate of resistance within populations of organisms is related to the rate of mutations at these loci.[8, 334, 501, 504, 506, 553, 554] Although a large population of bacilli as a whole may be considered drug-susceptible, a subpopulation of drug-resistant organisms occurs at a fairly predictable rate. The mean frequency of these drug-resistant mutants is about 10^{-6} but varies among drugs: STM, 10^{-5}; INH, 10^{-6}; and RIF, 10^{-7}.[111] A cavity containing 10^9 tubercle bacilli has thousands of single drug–resistant mutant organisms, whereas a closed caseous lesion contains few, if any, resistant mutants.

The two microbiologic properties of population size and drug resistance mutation explain why single antituberculosis drugs can not cure cavitary tuberculosis. In the mid 1940s, STM alone was given to adults with cavitary pulmonary tuberculosis.[327] Within 3 months, 80 per cent of patients had significant numbers of STM-resistant organisms. This phenomenon has been observed for every antituberculosis drug developed subsequently. However, the natural occurrence of resistance to one drug is independent of resistance to any other drug because the resistance loci are not linked. The chance of having even one organism "naturally" resistant to two drugs is on the order of 10^{-11} to 10^{-13}. Populations of this size in patients are extremely rare, and mutants naturally resistant to two drugs essentially are nonexistent.

The population size of tubercle bacilli within a patient determines the appropriate therapy. For patients with large bacterial populations (adults with cavities or extensive infiltrates), many single drug–resistant mutants are present, and at least two antituberculosis drugs must be used. Conversely, for patients with tuberculosis infection but no disease, the bacterial population is very small (about 10^3 to 10^4 organisms), drug-resistant mutants are rare, and a single drug can be used. Children with pulmonary tuberculosis and patients of all ages with extrapulmonary tuberculosis have medium-sized populations where drug-resistant mutants may or may not be present. In general, these patients should be treated with at least two drugs.

Some antituberculosis drugs, such as INH, RIF, and STM, are bactericidal against *M. tuberculosis*. Other drugs, including ethionamide, para-aminosalicylic acid, and low-dose EMB, are bacteriostatic. The earliest treatment regimens for tuberculosis combined the killing action of a bactericidal drug with a bacteriostatic drug that would suppress replication of drug-resistant mutant organisms.[328] A small number of organisms survived despite chemotherapy, and 18 to 24 months of treatment were necessary to permit host defenses to eliminate persisting organisms. Despite the prolonged treatment period, relapse rates were 5 to 15 per cent, mostly due to poor adherence with treatment.

The availability of RIF and the rediscovery of PZA in the early 1970s effected radical change in antituberculosis chemotherapy. These two drugs have the most potent sterilizing action, the ability to kill tubercle bacilli within lesions as quickly as possible.[239] The addition of RIF to INH for the treatment of pulmonary tuberculosis leads to cure rates approaching 100 per cent with only 9 months of treatment.[137, 239] The further addition of PZA shortens the necessary treatment duration to only 6 months.

TREATMENT OF THE STAGES OF TUBERCULOSIS

Exposure

In the United States, children exposed to potentially infectious adults with pulmonary tuberculosis should be started on treatment, usually INH only, if the child is younger than 5 years of age or has other risk factors for the rapid development of tuberculosis disease, such as immunocompromise of some kind. Failure to do so may result in development of severe tuberculosis disease even before the tuberculin skin test becomes reactive; the "incubation period" of disease may be shorter than that for the skin test. The child is treated for a minimum of 3 months after contact with the infectious case is broken (by physical separation or by effective treatment of the case). After 3 months, the tuberculin skin test is repeated. If the second test is positive, infection is documented and INH should be continued for a total duration of 9 months; if the second skin test is negative, the treatment can be stopped. If the exposure was to a case with an INH-resistant but RIF-susceptible isolate, RIF is the recommended treatment.

Two special circumstances of exposure deserve special attention. A difficult situation arises when exposed children are anergic because of HIV infection. These children particularly are vulnerable to rapid progression of tuberculosis, and it will not be possible to tell if infection has occurred. In general, these children should be treated as if they have tuberculosis infection (for 12 months in this group).[10]

The second situation is potential exposure of a newborn to a mother (or other adult) with a positive tuberculin skin test or, rarely, a nursery worker with contagious tuberculosis.[291, 492] The management is based on further evaluation of the mother:

1. *Mother has a normal chest roentgenogram*. No separation of the infant and mother is required. Although the mother should receive treatment of tuberculosis infection and other household members should be evaluated for tuberculosis infection or disease, the infant needs no further work-up or treatment unless a case of disease is found.
2. *Mother has an abnormal chest roentgenogram*. The mother

and child should be separated until the mother has been evaluated thoroughly. If the roentgenograph, history, physical examination, and analysis of sputum reveal no evidence of active pulmonary tuberculosis in the mother, it is reasonable to assume the infant is at low risk of infection. The roentgenographic abnormality is due to another cause or a quiescent focus of previous tuberculosis infection. However, if the mother remains untreated, she later may develop contagious tuberculosis and expose her infant. Both mother and infant should receive appropriate follow-up care, but the infant does not need treatment. If the roentgenogram and clinical history are suggestive of pulmonary tuberculosis, the child and mother should remain separated until both have begun appropriate chemotherapy. The infant should be evaluated for congenital tuberculosis. The placenta should be examined. If the mother has no risk factors for drug-resistant tuberculosis, the infant should receive INH and close follow-up care. The infant should have a tuberculin skin test at 3 or 4 months after the mother is judged no longer to be contagious; evaluation of the infant at this time follows the guidelines for other exposures of children. If no infection is documented at this time, it would be prudent to repeat the tuberculin skin test in 6 to 12 months. If the mother has tuberculosis caused by a multidrug-resistant isolate of *M. tuberculosis* or she has poor adherence to therapy, the child should remain separated from her until she no longer is contagious or the infant can be given a BCG vaccine and be kept separated until the vaccine "takes" (marked by a reactive tuberculin skin test).

Infection

The recommendation for so-called preventive therapy of tuberculosis,[468] that is, the treatment of asymptomatic tuberculin-positive individuals (previously untreated), is based on data from several well-controlled studies; it applies particularly to children and adolescents who are at high risk for the development of overt disease but at very low risk for the development of the main toxic manifestation of INH therapy, which is hepatitis.[54, 129, 154, 360, 369] The large, carefully controlled U.S. Public Health Study of 1955, followed by others both in this country and abroad, demonstrated beyond a shadow of a doubt the favorable effect of 12 months of INH on the incidence of complications due to both lymphohematogenous and pulmonary spread.[213] The younger the tuberculin reactor, the greater the benefit.[97]

The American Thoracic Society and the CDC[13] recommend that INH treatment of tuberculosis infection be given to the following groups, listed in order of priority determined by the likelihood of developing tuberculosis disease:

1. Household members and other close associates of potentially infectious tuberculosis cases. All contacts of any age with a Mantoux tuberculin skin test reading of 5 mm or greater and without a documented history of reaction in the past should be considered recently infected and receive therapy.
2. Newly infected people regardless of age who have had a tuberculin skin test conversion within the past 2 years.
3. People with HIV infection or at risk for HIV infection who have a reaction of 5 mm or greater to a Mantoux test.
4. People of any age with past tuberculosis who received inadequate treatment.
5. People of any age with a significant tuberculin reaction and an abnormal but stable chest roentgenogram.
6. People with significant tuberculin reactions who have special clinical situations, including silicosis, diabetes mellitus, prolonged corticosteroid therapy, immunosuppressive therapy, hematologic malignancy, and end-stage renal disease.
7. Tuberculin skin test reactors younger than 35 years of age with none of the aforementioned risk factors.

The question arises as to how long the protective effect can be expected to last. Comstock and associates,[94] in their final report on INH prophylaxis in Alaska, demonstrated the protective effect of 1 year of chemoprophylaxis to be 19 years at least. Hsu[212] reported on 2494 patients followed for up to 30 years and showed that adequate drug prophylaxis prevented reactivation of tuberculosis infection during adolescence and into young adulthood. There seems reason to hope that the decreased risk of active tuberculosis after INH in fact may be lifelong in individuals infected with INH-susceptible tubercle bacilli. Failure of INH after exposure to INH-resistant *M. tuberculosis* has been documented. No controlled study of an alternative regimen has been reported. RIF alone is recommended and widely used, although one failure has been reported.[303]

The dosage of INH to be used has had little study. Most investigators have used a regimen based on 4 to 8 mg/kg of body weight/day, usually taken all at once, for a period of 6 to 12 months. A dose of 5 mg/kg/day was found satisfactory in one study.[96] Some clinicians prescribe a dose of 10 to 15 mg/kg/day to a total of 300 mg/day for treatment of infection to be sure of achieving therapeutic levels even among patients who inactivate the drug rapidly by acetylation.

The duration of INH treatment initially was set arbitrarily at 12 months.[229] A large trial was conducted on adults in Eastern Europe with old fibrotic lesions caused by tuberculosis, comparing regimens of daily INH taken for 12, 24, and 52 weeks with a placebo for their ability to prevent tuberculosis disease. Therapy for 1 year was most effective, especially if patients were adherent. However, therapy for 24 weeks afforded a fairly high level of protection. A subsequent analysis concluded that the 24-week duration of preventive therapy was more cost-effective for adults than the 52-week duration.[467] Subsequently, many health departments have accepted 6 months of INH preventive therapy as their standard regimen for adults. However, the cost-effectiveness analysis does not apply to children. There are no similar data for INH therapy in children. A duration of 9 months is recommended for children by the AAP and CDC.[10] INH is taken daily under self-supervision or can be taken twice weekly under directly observed therapy. When the child is infected with an INH-resistant but RIF-susceptible strain of *M. tuberculosis*, RIF should be substituted for INH. If the infecting strain is resistant to both INH and RIF, usually two other drugs are used; an expert in tuberculosis should be consulted in this situation.

Disease in Adults

There are several reasons why shorter durations of antituberculosis chemotherapy are desirable: (1) it may be significantly less expensive than traditional therapy[157, 316]; (2) the patient is exposed to potentially toxic drugs for shorter periods; (3) more time and resources can be allotted to ensuring adherence with treatment; and (4) if a patient absconds from treatment, there will be a greater likelihood that bacteriologic cure already has been achieved as a result of the early and rapid sterilizing activity of the newer regimens.

It is well established that a 9-month regimen of INH and RIF cures more than 98 per cent of cases of drug-susceptible pulmonary tuberculosis in adults.[137, 454] Both drugs are given daily for the first 2 weeks to 2 months and then can be given daily or twice weekly under directly observed therapy (see later) for the remaining 7 to 8 months with equivalent results and rates of adverse reactions.[139] When given twice weekly, the RIF dose is the same as the daily dose, but the INH dose is increased to 900 mg in adults. Twice-weekly administration is supported by pharmacologic and animal model data determining the area-under-the-curve characteristics for these antituberculosis drugs.[4] Unfortunately, durations of therapy of less than 9 months using INH and RIF are unacceptable because the failure and relapse rates exceed 10 per cent.

When three or more antituberculosis drugs are used initially, treatment durations of 6 months routinely are successful.[89] Regimens using INH, RIF, PZA, and STM during the initial phase (2 months) followed by INH and RIF in the continuation phase (4 months) routinely yield cure rates greater than 98 per cent and relapse rates below 4 per cent.[15, 56, 451] If PZA is excluded from the initial phase, the rate of bacteriologic failure rises to 7 to 10 per cent.[205] However, the exclusion of STM does not affect the cure or relapse rates appreciably.[92, 205, 469] Use of PZA beyond the first 2 months of therapy does not add any benefit.[206] Regimens of 4 months' total duration have unacceptably high relapse rates of 10 per cent or greater. On the basis of all reported studies, the American Thoracic Society and CDC currently recommend for the treatment of pulmonary tuberculosis in adults a 6-month regimen using INH, RIF, and PZA for 2 months, followed by 4 months of daily or twice-weekly doses of INH and RIF.[13] EMB is added to the initial regimen if the risk of INH resistance is high (greater than 4 per cent incidence in the community or the patient already has been treated for tuberculosis).

Chemotherapy for Children

Clinical trials of antituberculosis drugs in children are difficult to perform, mostly because of the difficulty in obtaining positive cultures at diagnosis or relapse and the need for very long-term follow-up.[479] Historically, recommendations for treating children with tuberculosis have been extrapolated from clinical trials of adults with pulmonary tuberculosis.[461] However, during the past decade, a large number of clinical trials involving only children have been reported. In 1983, Abernathy and colleagues[2] reported successful treatment of 50 children with tuberculosis in Arkansas using INH and RIF daily for 1 month, then twice weekly for 8 months. The success rate virtually was 100 per cent. Most pulmonary infiltrates cleared by the end of therapy, but hilar adenopathy usually still was present radiographically, then gradually cleared over 2 to 3 years. Patients with only hilar adenopathy can be treated successfully with INH and RIF for 6 months.[233, 405]

Several major studies of 6-month therapy in children using at least three drugs in the initial phase have been reported.[15, 41, 224, 263, 274, 388, 483, 516, 531] The most commonly used regimen was 6 months of INH and RIF supplemented during the first 2 months with PZA. The overall success rate has been greater than 98 per cent and the incidence of clinically significant adverse reactions less than 2 per cent. Regimens not using STM were as successful as those that included it. Using twice-weekly medications (under directly observed therapy) during the continuation phase was as effective and safe as daily administration. Two studies used twice-weekly therapy throughout the treatment regimen with excellent success.[274, 531] The 6-month, three-drug regimen is successful, tolerated well, and less expensive.[518] It also effects a cure faster, so that there is a greater likelihood of successful treatment if the child becomes nonadherent later in therapy.

Extrapulmonary Tuberculosis

Controlled treatment trials for various forms of extrapulmonary tuberculosis are rare. In most reports, extrapulmonary cases have been combined with pulmonary cases and often are not analyzed separately. Several of the 6-month, three-drug trials in children included extrapulmonary cases.[41, 274] Most non–life-threatening forms of extrapulmonary tuberculosis respond well to a 9-month course of INH and RIF[140, 142] or to a 6-month regimen including INH, RIF, and PZA.[237] One exception may be bone and joint tuberculosis, which may have a high failure rate when 6-month chemotherapy is used, especially when surgical intervention has not occurred.[140]

Tuberculous meningitis usually is not included in trials of extrapulmonary tuberculosis therapy because of its serious nature and low incidence. Treatment with INH and RIF for 12 months generally is effective.[534] In the 1950s, Lorber[306] treated children with tuberculous meningitis for only 6 months with good results. Kendig[256] reported 15 children who absconded from therapy for tuberculous meningitis between 4 and 9 months of therapy; only 2 children died, and the majority of survivors had a good outcome. A more recent study from Thailand showed that a 6-month regimen including PZA for serious tuberculous meningitis led to fewer deaths and better outcomes than did longer regimens that did not contain PZA.[234] Most children are treated initially with four drugs (INH, RIF, PZA, and EMB or STM). The PZA and fourth drug are stopped after 2 months, and INH and RIF are continued for a total of 9 to 12 months.

Drug-Resistant Tuberculosis in Children

The incidence of drug-resistant tuberculosis is increasing in the United States and the world due to poor adherence by the patient, the availability of some antituberculosis drugs in noncontrolled over-the-counter formulations, and poor management by physicians.[43, 159, 316, 366] In the United States, about 10 per cent of *M. tuberculosis* isolates are resistant to at least one drug.[46, 74, 75] Initial drug resistance rates up to 80 per cent have been noted in adults with pulmonary tuberculosis in some countries,[317] and rates of 20 to 30 per cent are common. Resistance is most common to STM and INH and still is relatively rare for RIF.[115, 207, 345, 556] Certain epidemiologic factors—disease in an Asian or Hispanic immigrant to the United States, homelessness in some communities, and history of prior antituberculosis therapy—correlate with drug resistance in adult patients.[6, 22, 382] Patterns of drug resistance in children tend to mirror those found in adult patients in the population.[73, 413, 442, 471, 489, 491] Outbreaks of drug-resistant tuberculosis in children occurring at schools have been reported.[73, 407] Individual cases also have been recognized.[228] The key to determining drug resistance in childhood tuberculosis usually comes from the drug susceptibility results of the infectious adult contact case's isolate.

Therapy for drug-resistant tuberculosis is successful only when at least two bactericidal drugs to which the infecting strain of *M. tuberculosis* is susceptible are given.[172, 381, 490, 507] If only one effective drug is given, secondary resistance will develop. When INH resistance is considered a possibility, on the basis of epidemiologic risk factors or the identification of an INH-resistant source case isolate, an additional drug—usually EMB or STM—should be given initially to the child until the exact susceptibility pattern is determined and a more specific regimen can be designed. Exact treatment regimens must be tailored to the specific pattern of drug resistance. Duration of therapy usually is extended to at least 9 to 12 months if either INH or RIF can be used and to at least 18 to 24 months if resistance to both drugs is present.[230] Occasionally, surgical resection of a diseased lung or lobe is required.[232, 395] An expert in tuberculosis always should be involved in the management of children with drug-resistant tuberculosis infection or disease.

Adherence and Directly Observed Therapy

Nonadherence with drug treatment by patients is a major problem in tuberculosis control because of the long-term nature of treatment.[336, 498] As treatment regimens become shorter in duration, adherence assumes an even greater importance.[37, 426] *Suspected* cases of tuberculosis must be reported to the local health department so that it can perform necessary contact investigations and assist both patients and health care providers to overcome barriers to adherence.[100] In order to comply, the patient and family must know the expectations of them through verbal and written instructions in the patient's first language. An assessment of potential nonadherence should be made at the beginning of therapy.[28] Missed appointments quickly should be brought to the attention of the responsible public health officials, who may be able to use incentives/enablers, behavior modification, or rarely confinement to ensure adherence. The success of twice-weekly therapy, especially after a period of daily administration of medications, allows directly observed therapy to be given by a health care professional in cases of proven or suspected nonadherence.[84, 231] Most experts feel that twice-weekly medication should be used only under the direct observation of a health care worker present as the medication is taken.[270, 544] Direct observation means that a health care worker or other nonrelated third party (e.g., teacher, school nurse, social worker) physically is present while the patient ingests the medication. Up to 50 per cent of patients taking long-term antituberculosis medications will have significant nonadherence, and its occurrence is not predictable by the physician. In many communities in the United States, directly observed therapy is the standard of care for all patients with tuberculosis disease.

Summary of Treatment Recommendations

1. A regimen of INH and RIF for 6 months, supplemented with PZA during the first 2 months, is standard therapy for children with drug-susceptible intrathoracic tuberculosis in the United States and Canada.
2. An alternative regimen is INH and RIF for 9 months. The disadvantages of this regimen include a longer duration, the potential for increased drug resistance occurring during therapy, and less effectiveness if the patient absconds from treatment. This regimen should be used only if PZA cannot be tolerated.
3. After an initial 2 weeks to 2 months of daily drug administration, drugs can be given twice weekly under directly observed therapy with excellent effectiveness.[391] For patients for whom social or other restraints prevent reliable daily self-administration even during the initial phase of therapy, drugs can be given two or three times per week from the beginning under directly observed therapy.
4. In most cases, extrapulmonary tuberculosis can be treated with the same regimens as are used for pulmonary tuberculosis, although data for tuberculous meningitis and bone or joint disease are relatively lacking.
5. In cases of possible initial INH resistance, EMB or STM should be added to the initial phase of all regimens until drug susceptibilities are known.[77]
6. Optimal therapy of tuberculosis in children with HIV infection has not been established. Most HIV-infected adults with tuberculosis respond well to antituberculosis drugs but may require longer durations of treatment.[244, 307, 500] Immunosuppressed patients with tuberculosis, including those with HIV infection, should be treated with at least three drugs initially, and treatment should be continued for at least 9 to 12 months. HIV testing is recommended for all infants and children with tuberculosis disease.
7. Tuberculosis disease occurring during pregnancy should be treated with a 9-month regimen of INH and RIF supplemented during the initial phase by EMB (STM should not be used). The use of PZA in pregnant patients is controversial, although probably safe.

Corticosteroids

Corticosteroids have a place in the treatment of patients with tuberculosis. They should never be used except under cover of effective antituberculosis drugs. Because the probable drug susceptibility of the tubercle bacilli infecting a particular child can only be guessed at early in the illness, when corticosteroids are likely to be most needed, their use often is restricted. The most useful information is gleaned from the history of the probable infector. Were his or her tubercle bacilli found by culture or by treatment response to be susceptible to a particular drug regimen? This information can be obtained from the infector's physician or from the Health Department.

Corticosteroids would be expected to be beneficial in situations when the host inflammatory reaction is contributing to tissue damage or is impairing function.

Corticosteroids often are a useful addition to antituberculosis drugs if suppression of inflammatory reaction is desired, such as in the following situations:[460]

1. In patients with tuberculous meningitis in whom increased intracranial pressure is present. The major actions are to reduce vasculitis, inflammation, and, ultimately, intracranial pressure. Not only is reduction of pressure per se desirable, but also lowering the pressure probably favors the circulation of chemotherapeutic drugs through the brain and meninges.[153, 168] One study demonstrated lower rates of mortality and long-term neurologic sequelae among patients with tuberculous meningitis treated with corticosteroids, compared with non–steroid-treated control patients.[168]
2. In patients with acute pericardial effusion in whom tamponade is occurring. Relief of symptoms takes place within hours.[415, 495]
3. In patients with pleural effusion in whom there is shift of the mediastinum with acute respiratory embarrassment.[285, 463] The long-term course probably is the same with or without steroids, but symptomatic improvement usually is dramatic.
4. In patients with miliary tuberculosis if the inflammatory reaction is so severe as to produce alveolocapillary block with cyanosis.
5. In patients with enlarged mediastinal lymph nodes that are causing (1) respiratory difficulty or (2) a severe collapse-consolidation lesion, particularly in the middle or lower lobes, where bronchiectasis is likely to be a troublesome sequela.[356, 357] Under either of these circumstances, a course of corticosteroids is warranted, with the realization that it will be more successful in the younger infection because

inflammation characterizes the early stages of tuberculosis. If caseation already is advanced, steroids will be of little benefit.

The dosage of corticosteroids should be in the anti-inflammatory range, that is, prednisone 1 to 2 mg/kg/day for 4 to 6 weeks with gradual withdrawal. Some experts prefer dexamethasone, but no comparative trials have been published.

Activity

Activity need not be restricted in children with tuberculosis, except as it is inevitable for a particular complication (shortness of breath in pleural effusion, immobilization for a vertebral lesion). During the early months of treatment, patients probably should avoid competitive sports, excessive study, fatigue, and sunburn.

Isolation

Isolation should be maintained for children with cavitary lesions, draining sinuses, or renal tuberculosis until their secretions are negative on smear and preferably on culture. Other children may continue or return to their usual activities as soon as their symptoms have disappeared. It long has been known that children practically are noninfectious because they rarely cough and because their bronchial secretions contain few bacilli compared with those of adults with tuberculosis. Guidelines issued by the CDC state that most children with typical tuberculosis do not require isolation in the hospital.[78] Children with possible pulmonary tuberculosis should be treated as potentially infectious if they have a cavity or extensive upper lobe infiltrate, if they have a productive cough (especially if the sputum is acid-fast smear-positive), or during high-risk procedures, such as bronchoscopy.

Follow-up

Follow-up of children treated with antituberculosis drugs has become somewhat more streamlined in recent years. While receiving chemotherapy, the patient should be seen monthly, both to encourage regular taking of the prescribed drugs and to check, by a few simple questions (concerning appetite, well-being) and a few observations (weight gain; appearance of skin and sclerae; palpation of liver, spleen, and lymph nodes), that the disease is not spreading and that toxic effects of the drugs are not appearing. Repeat chest roentgenograms probably should be obtained 1 to 2 months after the onset of chemotherapy to ascertain the maximal extent of disease before chemotherapy takes effect; thereafter, roentgenograms rarely are necessary. Chemotherapy has been so successful that follow-up beyond its termination is not necessary, except for children with serious disease, such as tuberculous meningitis, or those with extensive residual chest roentgenogram findings at the end of chemotherapy.

Case Reporting

Every case of definite or suspected tuberculosis must, by law,[76] be reported immediately by telephone to the Health Department[171] to ensure (1) prompt contact investigation[210] and (2) free antituberculosis drugs, which are available for diagnosed cases and for intimate contacts in almost every state of the United States.

PREVENTION

Prevention of tuberculosis can be subdivided logically to consider the following circumstances:

1. Protection against exposure to the disease.
2. Use of antituberculosis drugs in tuberculin-negative individuals at high risk of infection.
3. Immunization of tuberculin-negative individuals.

Protection against exposure to disease is the ideal form of prevention. It presupposes thorough pre-employment and ongoing case-finding programs among all who come in contact with children, including day care center and school personnel, Sunday school personnel, music and art teachers, hospital nurses, babysitters, household servants, food handlers, beauticians, and barbers. Numerous epidemics, mini-epidemics, and mass exposures in newborn nurseries have been traced to such infected individuals. Removal of neonates at birth from a tuberculous mother or from a tuberculous home is a measure extensively and successfully used in France in the early part of this century but, fortunately, rarely indicated today.

Immunization

Immunization against tuberculosis theoretically would be a tremendous boon to humanity, but in practice it has been fraught with very great difficulties. Various strains of mycobacteria and diverse nonliving immunogenic fractions have been studied.[509] The impossibility of standardizing vaccines in the early days, the lack of any clinically useful test reflecting the immune status of the individual, and the relatively slow course of the disease greatly have handicapped epidemiologic studies. Furthermore, the very lack of adequate scientific data has intensified national and individual emotional responses to the point where rational approaches to data gathering and interpretation often are impossible. Although the use of tuberculosis vaccines for control of tuberculosis has waned in recent years in industrialized countries because of the falling incidence of the disease, new interest in them has cropped up because of their beneficial effect in certain types of malignancy. The new insights obtained into their mode of action may prove fruitful in the long run in understanding immunity to tuberculosis, as well as to neoplasia, and might lead to a greatly improved and clinically useful vaccine.

BCG was developed at the Institut Pasteur in Paris by Calmette and Guérin, who, starting in 1908, made 231 passages of a strain of *M. bovis* on a beef bile medium, thereby producing marked attenuation.[145] Injected into laboratory animals, this strain was shown to increase resistance to challenge with virulent *M. tuberculosis*. In 1921, it first was administered orally to newborn infants and since then has been given to more than 3 billion people.

BCG vaccine attempts to replace the potentially dangerous primary infection due to *M. tuberculosis* with an innocuous primary infection due to the bacillus of Calmette and Guérin, thus activating host cell-mediated immunity with minimal chance of progressive disease, so that an infection with *M. tuberculosis* will be of the "reinfection" type.[299]

Strain variation and lack of standardization are basic problems in evaluating the results of immunization.[176, 508] BCG was maintained for many years by serial passage at the Institut Pasteur and distributed to hundreds of laboratories all over the world. Not until 1966 did the WHO Expert Committee on Biological Standardization adopt formal requirements for the maintenance of frozen "seed lots" to minimize the inevitable mutations that have produced BCGs with widely varying characteristics. The routine quality-control measures carried out by the production laboratory include identity test, test for contamination, safety test in guinea pigs, estimate of total bacillary mass, viability, and test of heat stability. Periodic assessment of the allergenic capacity in humans is part of quality-control testing. The WHO, through its International Reference Preparation for BCG Vaccine and through quality-control testing on request carried out in its several cooperating laboratories, has helped to decrease the gross variations in BCG vaccine found until quite recent years.

Pre-BCG vaccination tuberculin testing is widely recommended. Theoretically desirable in order to avoid severe reactions from BCG administration, it has been found very impractical in mass immunization programs. Many potential vaccinees do not return for reading of the test and for the actual vaccination. For this reason, so-called direct BCG vaccination (i.e., without prior tuberculin testing) was looked into carefully in WHO-assisted projects and was recommended finally by the WHO Committee on Tuberculosis in 1964. Although the local BCG vaccination reactions are, on the average, larger in reactors than in nonreactors, they very rarely are severe. In the United States, where BCG is given to only one or a few individuals at one time, pre-BCG tuberculin testing seems advisable.

Vaccination techniques and dosages are quite variable. Intradermal injection is the most precise technique. Multiple puncture techniques are popular because they are easy, but reported results consistently are inferior to those obtained with intradermal injection. Oral vaccination, the original method of administration, largely has been abandoned because of poor results. The actual dose of BCG at present usually is about 10^6 culturable particles. Because, in animals, large doses produce better resistance to challenge than small ones, the largest convenient dose is used. However, in neonates, who have a higher incidence of untoward reactions, it is customary to halve the dose usually employed in older infants and children, to prevent local complications.

The usual local reaction to intradermal BCG vaccine is the development of a papule at the site of vaccination, and this papule reaches its maximum diameter (10 to 20 mm) in the sixth week. A small crust that may form on the papule detaches at about this time, leaving a small ulcer that may discharge a surprising amount of pus. Most ulcers are healed by the tenth week. A small scar is visible in almost all BCG-vaccinated individuals. Enlargement of the regional lymph nodes occurs regularly and is painless, sometimes ending in calcification. Abscess formation with breakdown is rare, occurring more often in infants.

Untoward reactions to BCG rarely have been a problem. Fatalities due to progressive disease have been reported in no more than 30 vaccine recipients (out of an estimated 3+ million), usually (but not always) children with well-documented immunodeficiency.[68, 152, 173, 385, 389] No return of the attenuated strain to virulence has ever been noted. In countries where BCG routinely is used for immunization of neonates, osteomyelitis has been diagnosed in some 5 per 100,000 neonates. It usually becomes manifest between 5 and 33 months of age, when a tender swelling is noted near a joint; bone destruction is localized well and responds to conservative treatment. On the whole, BCG is one of the safest vaccines in use.

In many countries where BCG is given routinely, the incidence of HIV infection in adults and children is high.[55, 418] Reports of local and systemic complications due to BCG in HIV-infected people are increasing, but the true magnitude of the interaction is not known yet.[35, 208, 368, 404] In most cases, BCG complications occur shortly after vaccination, but in one man with AIDS, adenitis due to BCG occurred 30 years after inoculation.[408] It is not recommended to treat patients routinely with prior BCG vaccination who subsequently become immunocompromised, but the clinician should be aware of prior BCG vaccination if signs or symptoms of mycobacterial infection occur.

The sensitivity of BCG to INH occasionally comes into question (1) if a BCG vaccinee develops a rather severe reaction with an indolent draining ulcer, a draining lymph node, or osteomyelitis or (2) when it appears desirable to use simultaneously INH prophylaxis and BCG (e.g., in the neonate of a mother with active tuberculosis). *M. bovis* and the various strains known as BCG *are* susceptible to approximately the same concentration of INH as *M. tuberculosis*. As a matter of fact, the therapeutic dose of INH in bovines is 10 mg/kg, as in humans.[267] Despite the effectiveness of INH, BCG organisms apparently do multiply sufficiently, when a large immunizing dose is given, to induce tuberculin sensitivity and, presumably, cell-mediated immunity. Canetti and his group in the 1950s developed an INH-resistant strain of BCG for immunization, but it turned out to be excessively attenuated and its use was abandoned.

Post-BCG sensitivity to tuberculin develops in a high percentage of vaccinated subjects—the exact percentage depends on the many factors previously listed. In mass BCG campaigns, it often is not possible to retest; however, when one or several individuals are vaccinated, it is desirable to retest 10 to 12 weeks later. It usually is assumed that increased resistance to disease accompanies hypersensitivity. If the follow-up tuberculin test is nonreactive, another dose of BCG may be given.

The need for revaccination has never been evaluated clearly.

The efficacy of BCG vaccines in humans has been evaluated in several large, well-controlled studies (Table 101–12).[145] Three of these trials showed excellent protection, two showed mediocre protection, and two showed little or no effect of BCG. Another study, not tabulated because its numbers are relatively small, is the "experiment of nature" reported by Hyge in 1957.[223] Hyge observed an epidemic of tuberculosis in a school for girls, where 105 girls initially were tuberculin-negative, 130 tuberculin-positive, and 133 BCG-immunized. In this group, the total incidence of tuberculosis was 23 times as high among the tuberculin-negative as among the BCG-immunized girls. Explanations for these differences in outcome between trials must be sought in (1) the quality and characteristics of the BCG vaccine used in the particular trial, (2) the possible immunizing effect (in Georgia and Alabama) of infections due to other mycobacteria,[458] (3) the possible greater effectiveness of BCG vaccine in areas of high tuberculosis prevalence, and (4) methodologic variations among the trials.

The most recent large study of BCG effectiveness is the Chingleput Study, started in 1968 in Chingleput District near Madras, South India, an area where sensitization with environmental mycobacteria is prevalent. People of all ages were vaccinated with one of two BCG vaccines or a placebo; only the incidence of adult-type pulmonary tuberculosis in the three groups was compared (i.e., not the forms usually found in children). Over the ensuing years, there was no difference in incidence between the three groups. This disturbing result has been the subject of several WHO investigations because BCG is one of the vaccines recommended for all children in the Expanded Program of Immunization sponsored by the WHO itself.[406] Another study of neonatal vaccination with BCG in England reports very favorable results with BCG.[102]

A group at the Harvard School of Public Health reviewed

TABLE 101–12. Summary of Seven Large Controlled Trials of Bacillus Calmette-Guérin (BCG) Immunization Against Tuberculosis

Trial	Investigators	Intake Period	Vaccine Laboratory	Duration of Observation (Years)	% Protection from BCG
North America: Native Americans	Stein and Aronson, 1953	1935–1938	Phipps	9–11	80
Chicago: Infants	Rosenthal et al., 1961	1937–1948	Tice	12–23	75
Britain: School children	Medical Research Council, 1971	1950–1952	Copenhagen	15	78
South India: Rural population	Frimodt-Moller et al., 1964	1950–1955	Madras	2.5–7	60/31*
Puerto Rico: Children	Palmer et al., 1958	1949–1951	New York State	5.5–7.5	31
Georgia, Alabama: Population	Comstock and Palmer, 1966	1950	Tice	14	14
Georgia: School children	Comstock and Webster, 1969	1947	Tice	20	0

*The initial estimate of efficacy was 60 per cent. Subsequently, when follow-up was extended to 9 to 14 years, the efficacy figure declined to 31 per cent.

Adapted from Sutherland. Quoted by Eickhoff, T. C.: The current status of BCG immunization against tuberculosis. Annu. Rev. Med. *28*:411–423, 1977.

all published studies of BCG efficacy in a meta-analysis.[91] Most published trials were not analyzed due to serious flaws in their experimental design or reporting. Among all included trials and case-control studies, the average protection against tuberculosis disease by various BCG preparations was 50 per cent. The protective levels were higher for disease in children, particularly for meningitis and tuberculosis-associated death.[90] However, ascertainment bias and lack of standardized case definitions make the results of these analyses very difficult to interpret. The BCG vaccines prevent many cases of tuberculosis in children, but the effect is quite variable. It also has become apparent that BCG vaccines are not an instrument of tuberculosis control because they do not prevent infection with *M. tuberculosis*, their protective effect is short-lived, and vaccinating infants does little to prevent future cases of contagious tuberculosis among adults in a community.

The role of BCG vaccine in the United States today is very limited. Rouillon and Waaler[417] have suggested that BCG immunization is justified only where the annual tuberculin conversion rates are 0.5 to 1 per cent or more. The Advisory Committee on Immunization Practices of the U.S. Public Health Service and Advisory Council for the Elimination of Tuberculosis recommend BCG only for tuberculin-negative infants and children in the United States who (1) are at high risk for intimate and prolonged exposure to persistently untreated or ineffectively treated adults with infectious pulmonary tuberculosis, cannot be removed from the source of infection, and cannot be placed on long-term preventive therapy or (2) continuously are exposed to people with tuberculosis resistant to INH and RIF.[81] A few observers, however, are more inclined toward the use of BCG in neonates who are at any risk of exposure to tuberculosis whatsoever.[254, 255, 452, 513]

Contraindications to the use of BCG for prevention of tuberculosis include congenital immunodeficiency, known HIV infection (in the United States; WHO recommends giving BCG to asymptomatic HIV-infected infants who reside in areas with high tuberculosis rates), leukemia, lymphoma, and generalized malignancy, as well as, treatment with corticosteroids, alkylating agents, antimetabolites, and radiation.

Selected Readings

1. Brailey, M. E.: Tuberculosis in White and Negro Children. II. The Epidemiologic Aspects of the Harriet Lane Study. Cambridge, MA, Harvard University Press, 1958.
2. Clinics in Chest Medicine. Vol. 10, No. 3, 1989 (entire volume devoted to mycobacterial diseases).
3. Dubos, R., and Dubos, J.: The White Plague: Tuberculosis, Man and Society. Boston, Little, Brown, 1952. Reissued by Rutgers University Press, 1987.
4. Friedman, L. N. (ed.): Tuberculosis: Current Concepts and Treatment. Boca Raton, CRC Press, 1994.
5. Gerbeaux, J.: Primary Tuberculosis in Childhood. Springfield, IL, Charles C Thomas, 1970.
6. Grange, J. M.: Mycobacteria and Human Disease. London, Edward Arnold, 1988.
7. Hardy, J. B.: Tuberculosis in White and Negro Children. I. The Roentgenologic Aspects of the Harriet Lane Study, Cambridge, MA, Harvard University Press, 1958.
8. Kubica, G. P., and Wayne, L. G.: The Mycobacteria. Parts A and B. New York, Marcel Dekker, 1984.
9. Lincoln, E. M., and Sewell, E. M.: Tuberculosis in Children. New York, McGraw-Hill, 1963.
10. Miller, F. J. W., Seal, R. M. E., and Taylor, M. D.: Tuberculosis in Children. Boston, Little, Brown, 1963.
11. Miller, F. J. W.: Tuberculosis in Children. New York, Churchill Livingstone, 1981.
12. Reichman, L. B., and Hershfield, E. S. (eds.): Tuberculosis: A Comprehensive International Approach. New York, Marcel Dekker, 1993.
13. Seminars in Pediatric Infectious Disease. Vol. 10, No. 4, 1993 (entire volume devoted to tuberculosis in children).

References

1. Abadco, D., and Steiner, P.: Gastric lavage is better than bronchoalveolar lavage for isolation of *Mycobacterium tuberculosis* in childhood pulmonary tuberculosis. Pediatr. Infect. Dis. J. *11*:735–738, 1992.
2. Abernathy, R. S., Dutt, A. K., Stead, W. W., et al.: Short-course chemotherapy for tuberculosis in children. Pediatrics *72*:801–806, 1983.
3. Acocella, G.: The use of fixed dose combinations in antituberculous chemotherapy: Rationale for their application in daily, intermittent and pediatric regimes. Bull. Int. Union Tuberc. Lung Dis. *65*:77–83, 1990.
4. Acocella, G., and Angel, S. H.: Short-course chemotherapy of pulmonary tuberculosis: A new approach to drug dosages in the initial intensive phase. Am. Rev. Respir. Dis. *134*:1283–1286, 1986.
5. Afghani, B., and Lieberman, J. M.: Paradoxical enlargement or development of intracranial tuberculomas during therapy: Case report and review. Clin. Infect. Dis. *19*:1092–1099, 1994.
6. Aitken, M. L., Sparks, R., Anderson, K., et al.: Predictors of drug resistant diseases: *Mycobacterium tuberculosis*. Am. Rev. Respir. Dis. *130*:831–833, 1984.
7. Alland, D., Kolkut, G. E., Moss, A., et al.: Transmission of tuberculosis in New York City: An analysis by DNA fingerprinting and conventional epidemiologic methods. N. Engl. J. Med. *330*:1710–1716, 1994.
8. Altamirano, M., Marostenmaki, J., Wong, A., et al.: Mutations in the catalase-peroxidase gene from isoniazid-resistant *Mycobacterium tuberculosis* isolates. J. Infect. Dis. *169*:1162–1165, 1994.
9. American Academy of Pediatrics, Committee on Infectious Diseases: Chemotherapy for tuberculosis in infants and children. Pediatrics *89*:161–165, 1992.
10. American Academy of Pediatrics, Committee on Infectious Diseases: Screening for tuberculosis in infants and children. Pediatrics *93*:131–134, 1994.
11. American Academy of Pediatrics, Committee on Infectious Diseases: Update on tuberculosis skin testing of children. Pediatrics *97*:282–284, 1996.

12. American Thoracic Society: Control of tuberculosis in the United States. Am. Rev. Respir. Dis. *146*:1623– 1633, 1993.
13. American Thoracic Society: Treatment of tuberculosis and tuberculosis infection in adults and children. Am. J. Respir. Crit. Care. Med. *144*:1359–1374, 1994.
14. Andrew, O. T., Schoenfeld, R. Y., Hopewell, P. C., et al.: Tuberculosis in patients with end-stage renal disease. Am. J. Med. *68*:59–65, 1980.
15. Aquinas, S. M.: Short-course therapy for tuberculosis. Drugs *24*:118–132, 1982.
16. Aznar, J., Safi, H., Romero, J., et al.: Nosocomial transmission of tuberculosis infection in pediatrics wards. Pediatr. Infect. Dis. J. *14*:44–48, 1995.
17. Baciewicz, A. M., and Self, T. H.: Isoniazid interactions. South. Med. J. *78*:714–718, 1985.
18. Bagga, A., Kalra, V., and Ghai, O. P.: Intracranial tuberculoma evaluation and treatment. Clin. Pediatr. *27*:487–490, 1988.
19. Barber, T. W., Craven, D. E., and McCabe, W. R.: Bacteremia due to *Mycobacterium tuberculosis* in patients with human immunodeficiency virus infection: A report of 9 cases and a review of the literature. Medicine *69*:375–383, 1990.
20. Barclay, W. R.: Does a positive tuberculin test indicate the presence of live tubercle bacilli? J. A. M. A. *232*:755, 1975.
21. Barksdale, L., and Kim, K. S.: *Mycobacterium*. Bacteriol. Rev. *41*:217–372, 1977.
22. Barnes, P. F.: The influence of epidemiologic factors on drug resistance rates in tuberculosis. Am. Rev. Respir. Dis. *136*:325–328, 1987.
23. Barnes, P. F., Bloch, A. B., Davidson, P. T., et al.: Tuberculosis in patients with human immunodeficiency virus infection. N. Engl. J. Med. *324*:1644–1650, 1991.
24. Barry, M. A., Shirley, L., Grady, M. T., et al.: Tuberculosis infection in urban adolescents: Results of a school-based testing program. Am. J. Public Health *80*:439–441, 1990.
25. Barton, L. L., and Feigin, R. D.: Childhood cervical lymphadenitis: A reappraisal. J. Pediatr. *84*:846–852, 1974.
26. Bates, J. E., Stead, W. W., and Rado, T. A.: Phage type of tubercle bacilli isolated from patients with two or more sites of organ involvement. Am. Rev. Respir. Dis. *114*:353–358, 1976.
27. Bavadekan A. V.: Osteoarticular tuberculosis in children. Prog. Pediatr. Surg. *15*:131–151, 1982.
28. Bayer, R., and Wilkinson, D.: Directly observed therapy for tuberculosis: History of an idea. Lancet *345*:1545– 1548, 1995.
29. Bearman, J. E., Kleinman, H., Glyer, V. V., et al.: Study of variability in tuberculin skin reading. Am. Rev. Respir. Dis. *90*:913–919, 1964.
30. Beaudry, P. H., Brickman, H. F., and Wise, M. B.: Liver enzyme disturbances during isoniazid chemoprophylaxis in children. Am. Rev. Respir. Dis. *110*:581–584, 1974.
31. Beck-Sague, C., Dooley, S. W., Hutton, M. D., et al.: Hospital outbreak of multidrug-resistant *Mycobacterium tuberculosis* infections: Factors in transmission to staff and HIV infected patients. J. A. M. A. *268*:1280–1286, 1992.
32. Bellin, E. Y., Fletcher, D. D., and Safyer, S. M.: Association of tuberculosis infection with increased time in or admission to the New York City jail system. J. A. M. A. *269*:2228–2231, 1993.
33. Belsey, M. A.: Tuberculosis and varicella infections in children. Am. J. Dis. Child. *113*:444–448, 1967.
34. Berney, S., Goldstein, M., and Bishko, F.: Clinical and diagnostic features of tuberculous arthritis. Am. J. Med. *53*:36–42, 1972.
35. Besnard, M., Sauvion, S., Offredo, C., et al.: Bacillus Calmette-Guerin infection after vaccination of human immunodeficiency virus-infected children. Pediatr. Infect. Dis. J. *12*:993–997, 1993.
36. Beyazova, U., Rota, S., Ceuheroglu, C., et al.: Humoral immune response in infants after BCG vaccination. Tubercle Lung Dis. *76*:248–253, 1995.
37. Beyers, N., Gie, R., Schaaf, H., et al.: Delay in the diagnosis, notification and initiation of treatment and compliance in children with tuberculosis. Tubercle Lung Dis. *75*:260–265, 1994.
38. Beyt, B. E., Jr., Ortbals, D. W., Santa Cruz, D. J., et al.: Cutaneous mycobacteriosis: Analysis of 34 cases with a new classification of the disease. Medicine *60*:96–109, 1980.
39. Bhagwati, S. N.: Spinal intramedullary tuberculoma in children. Childs Brain *5*:568, 1979.
40. Bhansali, S. K.: Abdominal tuberculosis: Experience with 300 cases. Am. J. Gastroenterol. *67*:324–337, 1977.
41. Biddulph, J.: Short-course chemotherapy for childhood tuberculosis. Pediatr. Infect. Dis. J. *9*:794–801, 1990.
42. Biehl, J. P., and Vilter, R. W.: Effects of isoniazid on pyridoxine metabolism. J. A. M. A. *156*:1549–1552, 1954.
43. Bifani, P. J., Plikaytis, B. B., Kapur V., et al.: Origin and interstate spread of a New York City multidrug-resistant *Mycobacterium tuberculosis* clone family. J. A. M. A. *275*:452–457, 1996.
44. Blacklock, J. W. S.: Tuberculous Disease in Children. Medical Research Council Special Report. Series No. *172*. London, HMSO, 1932.
45. Blake, M. J., Bode, D., and Rhodes, H. J.: Comparison of analysis of isoniazid and its dosage forms by several methods. J. Pharm. Sci. *63*:60–63, 1974.
46. Bloch, A., Cauthen, G., Onorato, I., et al.: Nationwide survey of drug-resistant tuberculosis in the United States. J. A. M. A. *271*:665–671, 1994.
47. Bloch, A. B., and Snider, D. E., Jr.: How much tuberculosis in children must we accept? Am. J. Public Health *76*:14–15, 1986.
48. Bluefarb, S. M., and Caro, W. A.: Cutaneous manifestations of tuberculosis. Modern Medicine, March *23*, 1970, pp. 80–85.
49. Blumberg, H. M., Watkins, D. L., Berschling, J. D., et al.: Preventing the nosocomial transmission of tuberculosis. Ann. Intern. Med. *122*:658–663, 1995.
50. Bovornkitti, S., Kangsdal, P., Sathirapat, P., et al.: Reversion and reconversion rate of tuberculin skin test reactions in correlation with the use of prednisone. Dis. Chest *38*:51–55, 1960.
51. Boyd, G. L.: Tuberculosis pericarditis in children. Am. J. Dis. Child. *86*:293–300, 1953.
52. Braden, C. R., and an Investigative Team: Infectiousness of a university student with laryngeal and cavitary tuberculosis. Clin. Infect. Dis. *21*:565–570, 1995.
53. Brailey, M. E.: Observations on the development of intrathoracic calcification in tuberculin-positive infants. Bull. Johns Hopkins Hosp. *61*:258–271, 1937.
54. Brailey, M. E.: Tuberculosis in White and Negro Children. II. The Epidemiologic Aspects of the Harriet Lane Study. Cambridge, MA, Harvard University Press, 1958.
55. Braun, M. M., Byers, R. H., Heyward, W. L., et al.: Acquired immunodeficiency syndrome and extrapulmonary tuberculosis in the United States. Arch. Intern. Med. *150*:1913–1916, 1990.
56. British Thoracic Society: A controlled trial of 6 months' therapy in pulmonary tuberculosis. Final report: Results during the 36 months after the end of chemotherapy and beyond. Br. J. Dis. Chest *78*:330–336, 1984.
57. Brock, R. C.: Post-tuberculous bronchostenosis and bronchiectasis of the middle lobe. Thorax *5*:5–39, 1950.
58. Brody, J. A., and McAlister, R.: Depression of tuberculin sensitivity following measles vaccination. Am. Rev. Respir. Dis. *90*:607–611, 1964.
59. Brudney, K., and Dobkin, J.: Resurgent tuberculosis in New York City: Human immunodeficiency virus, homelessness and the decline of tuberculosis control programs. Am. Rev. Respir. Dis. *144*:745–749, 1991.
60. Burk, J. R., Viroslav, J., and Bynum, L. J.: Miliary tuberculosis diagnosed by fiberoptic bronchoscopy and transbronchial biopsy. Tubercle *59*:107–109, 1978.
61. Burke, H. E.: Pathogenesis of Pott's disease. Trans. Am. Clin. Climatol. Assoc. *59*:122–137, 1948.
62. Burke, R. M.: An Historical Chronology of Tuberculosis. 2nd ed. Springfield, IL, Charles C Thomas, 1955.
63. Byrd, R. B., Horn, B. R., Solomon, D. A., et al.: Toxic effects of isoniazid in tuberculous chemoprophylaxis: Role of biochemical monitoring in 1,000 patients. J. A. M. A. *241*:1239–1241, 1979.
64. Caffey, J.: Pediatric X-Ray Diagnosis. 7th ed. Chicago, Year Book Medical Publishers, 1978.
65. Campbell, I. A., and Dyson, A. J.: Lymph node tuberculosis: A comparison of various methods of treatment. Tubercle *58*:171–179, 1977.
66. Cantwell, M., Shehab, Z., Costello. A., et al.: Brief report: Congenital tuberculosis. N. Engl. J. Med. *330*:1051–1054, 1994.
67. Cantwell, M., Snider, D.E., Jr., Cauthen, G., et al.: Epidemiology of tuberculosis in the United States, 1985 through 1992. J. A. M. A. *272*:535–539, 1994.
68. Carlgren, L. E., Hansson, C. G., Henricsson, L., et al.: Fatal BCG infection in an infant with congenital lymphocytopenic agammaglobulinemia. Acta Paediatr. Scand. *55*:636–644, 1966.
69. Carr, D. T., Karlson, A. G., and Stilwell, G. G.: A comparison of cultures of induced sputum and gastric washings in the diagnosis of tuberculosis. Mayo Clin. Proc. *42*:23–25, 1967.
70. Casteels-Van Daele, M., Igodt-Ameye, L., Corbeel, L., et al.: Hepatotoxicity of rifampin and isoniazid in children. J. Pediatr. *86*:739–741, 1975.
71. Catanzaro, A.: Multiple-puncture skin test and Mantoux test in Southeast Asian refugees. Chest *87*:346–350, 1985.
72. Cave, M., Eisenach, K., McDermott, P., et al.: IS6110: Conservation of sequence in the *Mycobacterium tuberculosis* complex and its utilization in DNA fingerprinting. Mol. Cell. Probes *5*:73–80, 1991.
73. Centers for Disease Control: Interstate outbreak of drug-resistant tuberculosis involving children: California, Montana, Nevada, Utah. M. M. W. R. *32*:516–518, 1983.
74. Centers for Disease Control: Primary resistance to antituberculosis drugs. M. M. W. R. *32*:521–523, 1983.
75. Centers for Disease Control and Prevention: National action plan to combat multidrug-resistant tuberculosis. M. M. W. R. *41*:5–50, 1992.
76. Centers for Disease Control and Prevention: Tuberculosis control laws: United States, 1993. M. M. W. R. *42*(RR 15):1–28, 1993.
77. Centers for Disease Control and Prevention: Initial therapy for tuberculosis in the era of multidrug resistance. M. M. W. R. *42*(RR-7):1–8, 1993.
78. Centers for Disease Control and Prevention: Guidelines for preventing the transmission of *Mycobacterium tuberculosis* in health-care facilities, 1994. M. M. W. R. *43*(RR-13):1–133, 1994.
79. Centers for Disease Control and Prevention: Screening for tuberculosis and tuberculosis infection in high-risk populations. M. M. W. R. *44*(RR-11):19–34, 1995.
80. Centers for Disease Control and Prevention: Tuberculosis morbidity: United States, 1995. M. M. W. R. *45*:365–370, 1996.

81. Centers for Disease Control and Prevention: The role of BCG vaccine in the prevention and control of tuberculosis in the United States: A joint statement by the Advisory Council for the Elimination of Tuberculosis and the Advisory Committee on Immunization Practices. M. M. W. R. *45*(RR-4):1–18, 1996.
82. Chan, S., Abadco, D., and Steiner, P.: Role of flexible fiberoptic bronchoscopy in the diagnosis of childhood endobronchial tuberculosis. Pediatr. Infect. Dis. J. *13*:506–509, 1994.
83. Chan, S. P., Birnbaum, J., and Rao, M.: Clinical manifestation and outcome of tuberculosis in children with acquired immunodeficiency syndrome. Pediatr. Infect. Dis. J. *15*:443–447, 1996.
84. Chaulk, C. P., Moore-Rice, K., Rizzo, R., et al.: Eleven years of community-based directly observed therapy for tuberculosis. J. A. M. A. *274*:945–951, 1995.
85. Chavalittamvong, B., and Talalak, P.: Tuberculous peritonitis in children. Prog. Pediatr. Surg. *15*:161–167, 1982.
86. Cheng, T. L., Ottolin, M., Getson, P., et al.: Poor validity of parent reading of skin test induration in a high risk population. Pediatr. Infect. Dis. J. *15*:90–91, 1996.
87. Chintu, C., Bhat, G., Luo, C., et al.: Seroprevalence of human immunodeficiency virus type 1 infection in Zambian children with tuberculosis. Pediatr. Infect. Dis. J. *12*:499–504, 1993.
88. Choremis, C., Vlachos, J., Vlachou, C. A., et al.: Needle biopsy of the liver in various forms of childhood tuberculosis. J. Pediatr. *62*:203–207, 1963.
89. Cohn, D. L., Catlin, B. J., Peterson, K. C., et al.: A 62-dose, 6-month therapy for pulmonary and extrapulmonary tuberculosis. Ann. Intern. Med. *112*:407–415, 1990.
90. Colditz, G., Berkey, C. S., Mosteller, F., et al.: The efficacy of bacillus Calmette-Guérin vaccination of newborns and infants in the prevention of tuberculosis: Meta-analysis of the published literature. Pediatrics *96*:29–35, 1995.
91. Colditz, G., Brewer, T., Berkey, C., et al.: Efficacy of BCG vaccine in the prevention of tuberculosis: Meta-analysis of the published literature. J. A. M. A. *271*:698–702, 1994.
92. Combs, D. L., O'Brien, R. J., and Geiter, L. J.: USPHS tuberculosis short-course chemotherapy trial 21: Effectiveness, toxicity and acceptability. Ann. Intern. Med. *112*:397–406, 1990.
93. Comstock, G. W.: Variability of tuberculosis trends in a time of resurgence. Clin. Infect. Dis. *19*:1015–1022, 1994.
94. Comstock, G. W., Baum, C., and Snider, D. E., Jr.: Isoniazid prophylaxis among Alaskan Eskimos: Final report of the Bethel isoniazid studies. Am. Rev. Respir. Dis. *119*:827–830, 1979.
95. Comstock, G. W., Edwards, L. B., and Nabangxang, H.: Tuberculin sensitivity eight to fifteen years after BCG vaccination. Am. Rev. Respir. Dis. *103*:572–575, 1971.
96. Comstock, G. W., Hammes, L. M., and Pio, A.: Isoniazid prophylaxis in Alaskan boarding schools: Comparison of two doses. Am. Rev. Respir. Dis. *100*:773–779, 1969.
97. Comstock, G. W., Livesay, V. T., and Woolpert, S. F.: Prognosis of a positive tuberculin reaction in childhood and adolescence. Am. J. Epidemiol. *99*:131–138, 1974.
98. Courtice, F. C., and Simmonds, W. J.: Physiological significance of lymph drainage of the serous cavities and lungs. Physiol. Rev. *34*:419–442, 1954.
99. Crowle, A. J., Sbarbaro, J. A., Judson, F. N., et al.: The effect of ethambutol on tubercle bacilli within cultured human macrophages. Am. Rev. Respir. Dis. *132*:742–745, 1985.
100. Cuneo, W. D., and Snider, D. E., Jr.: Enhancing patient compliance with tuberculosis therapy. Clin. Chest Med. *10*:375–380, 1989.
101. Curless, R. G., and Mitchell, C. D.: Central nervous system tuberculosis in children. Pediatr. Neurol. *7*:270–274, 1991.
102. Curtis, H. M., Bamford, F. N., and Leck, I.: Incidence of childhood tuberculosis after neonatal BCG vaccination. Lancet *1*:145–148, 1984.
103. Dall, L., Long, L., and Stanford, J.: Poncet's disease: Tuberculosis rheumatism. Rev. Infect. Dis. *11*:105–107, 1989.
104. Dalme, P., McClatchy, J. K., Gangadharam, P. R. J., et al.: Antimycobacterial activity of some potential chemotherapeutic compounds. Tubercle *59*:135–138, 1978.
105. Daly, J. F., Brown, D. S., Lincoln, E. M., et al.: Endobronchial tuberculosis in children. Dis. Chest. *22*:380–398, 1952.
106. Dandapat, M. C., Mishra, B. M., Dash, S. P., et al.: Peripheral lymph node tuberculosis: Review of 80 cases. Br. J. Surg. *77*:911–912, 1990.
107. Daniel, T., and Debanne, S.: The serodiagnosis of tuberculosis and other mycobacterial diseases by enzyme-linked immunosorbent assay. Am. Rev. Respir. Dis. *135*:1137–1151, 1987.
108. Dannenberg, A. M., Jr.: Delayed-type hypersensitivity and cell-mediated immunity in the pathogenesis of tuberculosis. Immunol. Today *12*:228–234, 1991.
109. Dannenberg, A. M., Jr., and Sugimoto, M.: Liquefaction of caseous foci in tuberculosis. Am. Rev. Respir. Dis. *113*:257–259, 1976.
110. Dastur, H. M., and Desai, A. D.: Comparative study of brain tuberculosis and gliomas based upon 107 case records of each. Brain *88*:375–396, 1965.
111. David, H. L.: Probability distribution of the drug-resistant mutants in unselected populations of *Mycobacterium tuberculosis*. Appl. Microbiol. *20*:810– 814, 1970.
112. De Angelis, L. M.: Intracranial tuberculoma: Case report and review of the literature. Neurology *31*:1133–1136, 1981.
113. de Blic, J., Azevedo, I., Burren, C., et al.: The value of flexible bronchoscopy in childhood pulmonary tuberculosis. Chest *100*:188–192, 1991.
114. Debré, R., Brissaud, H. E., and Canloube, P.: Les tuberculoses primaires par injection chez les jeunes enfants. Arch. Fr. Pediatr. *8*:49, 1951.
115. Debré, R., Noufflard, H., Brissaud, H. E., et al.: Infection of children by strains of tubercle bacilli initially resistant to streptomycin or to isoniazid. Am. Rev. Respir. Dis. *80*:326–331, 1959.
116. Delacourt, C., Gobin, J., Gaillard, J., et al.: Value of ELISA using antigen 60 for the diagnosis of tuberculosis in children. Chest *104*:393–398, 1993.
117. Delacourt, C., Mani, T. M., Bonnerot, V., et al.: Computed tomography with normal chest radiograph in tuberculous infection. Arch. Dis. Child. *69*:430–432, 1993.
118. Delacourt, C., Poveda, J. D., Churean, C., et al.: Use of polymerase chain reaction for improved diagnosis of tuberculosis in children. J. Pediatr. *126*:703–709, 1995.
119. Diagnostic Standards and Classification of Tuberculosis: Joint Statement of the American Thoracic Society and the Centers for Disease Control. Am. Rev. Respir. Dis. *142*:725–735, 1990.
120. Dineen, P., Homan, W. P., and Grafe, W. R.: Tuberculous peritonitis: 43 years' experience in diagnosis and treatment. Ann. Surg. *184*:717–722, 1976.
121. Dinning, W. J., and Mauston, S.: Cutaneous and occular tuberculosis: A review. J. R. Soc. Med. *78*:576–581, 1985.
122. Doerr, C. A., Starke, J. R., and Ong, L. T.: Clinical and public health aspects of tuberculous meningitis in children. J. Pediatr. 127:27–33, 1995.
123. D'Oliveira, J. J. G.: Cerebrospinal fluid concentrations of rifampin in meningeal tuberculosis. Am. Rev. Respir. Dis. *106*:432–437, 1972.
124. Domingo, Z., and Peter, J. C.: Intracranial tuberculomas: An assessment of a therapeutic 4-drug trial in 35 children. Pediatr. Neurosci. *15*:161–167, 1989.
125. Donald, P. R., Gent, W. L., Seifart, H., et al.: Cerebrospinal fluid isoniazid concentrations in children with tuberculous meningitis: The influence of dosage and acetylation status. Pediatrics *89*:247–250, 1992.
126. Donald, P. R., and Seifart, H.: Cerebrospinal fluid pyrazinamide concentrations in children with tuberculous meningitis. Pediatr. Infect. Dis. J. *7*:469–471, 1988.
127. Donald, P. R., and Seifart, H. I.: Cerebrospinal fluid concentrations of ethionamide in children with tuberculous meningitis. J. Pediatr. *115*:483–486, 1989.
128. Donaldson, J. C., and Elliott, R. C.: Study of co-positivity of three multipuncture techniques with intradermal PPD tuberculin. Am. Rev. Respir. Dis. *118*:843–846, 1978.
129. Dormer, B. A., Harrison, I., Swart, J. A., et al.: Prophylactic isoniazid protection of infants in a tuberculosis hospital. Lancet *2*:902–903, 1959.
130. Doxiadis, S. A., Goldfinch, M. K., and Philipott, M. G.: Electrolyte imbalance in tuberculous meningitis. Br. Med. J. *1*:1406–1410, 1954.
131. Driver, C., Luallen, J., Good, W., et al.: Tuberculosis in children younger than five years old: New York City. Pediatr. Infect. Dis. J. *14*:117–121, 1995.
132. Driver, C. R., Valway, S. E., Cantwell, M. E., et al.: Tuberculin skin test screening of school children in the United States. Pediatrics *98*:97–102, 1996.
133. Drolet, G. J.: Tuberculosis among different nationalities in New York. N. Y. Tuberc. Assoc. Bull. *4*:3, 1923.
134. Drucker, E., Alcabes, P., Bosworth, W., et al.: Childhood tuberculosis in the Bronx, New York. Lancet *343*:1482–1485, 1994.
135. Dubos, R., and Dubos, J.: The White Plague: Tuberculosis, Man and Society. New Brunswick, NJ, Rutgers University Press, 1987.
136. Dunlap, N. E., Harris, R. H., Benjamin, W. H., Jr., et al.: Laboratory contamination of *Mycobacterium tuberculosis* cultures. Am. J. Respir. Crit. Care Med. *152*:1702–1704, 1995.
137. Dutt, A. K., Jones, L., and Stead, W. W.: Short-course chemotherapy for tuberculosis with largely twice-weekly isoniazid-rifampin. Chest *75*:441–447, 1979.
138. Dutt, A. K., Mehta, J. B., Whitaker, B. J., et al.: Outbreak of tuberculosis in a church. Chest *107*:447–452, 1995.
139. Dutt, A. K., Moers, D., and Stead, W. W.: Undesirable side effects of isoniazid and rifampin in largely twice-weekly short-course chemotherapy for tuberculosis. Am. Rev. Respir. Dis. *128*:419–424, 1983.
140. Dutt, A. K., Moers, D., and Stead, W. W.: Short-course chemotherapy for extrapulmonary tuberculosis. Ann. Intern. Med. *107*:7–12, 1986.
141. Dutt, A. K., and Stead, W. W.: Present chemotherapy for tuberculosis. J. Infect. Dis. *146*:698–704, 1982.
142. Dutt, A. K., and Stead, W. W.: Tuberculous pleural effusion: 6-month therapy with isoniazid and rifampin. Am. Rev. Respir. Dis. *145*:1429–1432, 1992.
143. Edwards, L. B., and Hardy, J. B.: Relation of the degree of sensitivity to tuberculin to the persistence of sensitivity and to prognosis in young children. Bull. Johns Hopkins Hosp. *78*:13–20, 1946.
144. Ehrlich, R. M., and Lattimer, J.: Urogenital tuberculosis in children. J. Urol. *105*:461–465, 1971.
145. Eickhoff, T. C.: The current status of BCG immunization against tuberculosis. Annu. Rev. Med. *28*:411–423, 1977.
146. Eisenach, K. D., Sifford, M. D., Cave, M. D., et al.: Detection of *Mycobacte-*

rium tuberculosis in sputum samples using a polymerase chain reaction. Am. Rev. Respir. Dis. *144*:1160–1163, 1991.

147. Ellard, G. A.: Hepatic toxicity of isoniazid among rapid and slow acetylators of the drug. Am. Rev. Respir. Dis. *118*:628–629, 1978.
148. Ellard, G. A., Humphries, M. J., Gabriel, M., et al.: Penetration of pyrazinamide into the cerebrospinal fluid in tuberculous meningitis. Br. Med. J. *294*:284–285, 1987.
149. Ellner, J. J.: Pleural fluid and peripheral blood lymphocyte function in tuberculosis. Ann. Intern. Med. *89*:932–933, 1978.
150. Emmett, J. R., Fischer, N. D., and Biggers, W. P.: Tuberculous mastoiditis. Laryngoscope *87*:1157–1163, 1977.
151. Enarson, D. A.: The International Union Against Tuberculosis and Lung Disease model national tuberculosis programs. Tubercle Lung Dis. *76*:95–99, 1995.
152. Esterly, J. R., Sturner, W. Q., Esterly, N. B., et al.: Disseminated BCG in twin boys with presumed chronic granulomatous disease of childhood. Pediatrics *48*:141–144, 1977.
153. Excobar, J. A., Belsey, M. A., Dueñas, A., et al.: Mortality from tuberculous meningitis reduced by steroid therapy. Pediatrics *56*:1050–1055, 1975.
154. Ferrebee, S. H.: Controlled chemoprophylaxis trials in tuberculosis: A general review. Adv. Tuberc. Res. *17*:28–106, 1969.
155. Filler, J., and Porter, M.: Physiologic studies of the sequelae of tuberculous pleural effusion in children treated with antimicrobial drugs and prednisone. Am. Rev. Respir. Dis. *88*:181–188, 1963.
156. Fox, A. S., and Lepow, M. L.: Tuberculin skin testing in Vietnamese refugees with a history of BCG vaccination. Am. J. Dis. Child. *137*:1093–1094, 1983.
157. Fox, W., and Nunn, A. J.: The cost of anti-tuberculous drug regimens. Am. Rev. Respir. Dis. *120*:503–509, 1979.
158. Frieden, T. R., Fujiwara, P. I., Washko, R. M., et al.: Tuberculosis in New York City: Turning the tide. N. Engl. J. Med. *333*:229–233, 1995.
159. Frieden, T. R., Sterling, T., Pablos-Mendez, A., et al.: The emergence of drug-resistant tuberculosis in New York City. N. Engl. J. Med. *328*:521–526, 1993.
160. Gal, A. A., and Klatt, E. C.: Fatal isoniazid hepatitis in a child. Pediatr. Infect. Dis. J. *5*:490–491, 1986.
161. Gangadharam, P. R. J.: Drug Resistance in Mycobacteria. Boca Raton, CRC Press, 1984.
162. Gangadharam, P. R. J., Pratt, P. F., Perumal, U. K., et al.: The effects of exposure time, drug concentration, and temperature on the activity of ethambutol versus *Mycobacterium tuberculosis*. Am. Rev. Respir. Dis. *141*:1478–1482, 1990.
163. Gaur, S., Kesarwala, H., and Frenkel, L. D.: Tuberculous peritonitis in an adolescent female. Pediatr. Infect. Dis. J. *18*:859–862, 1987.
164. George, R. H., Gully, P. R., Gill, O. N., et al.: An outbreak of tuberculosis in a children's hospital. J. Hosp. Infect. *8*:129–142, 1986.
165. Ghon, A.: The Primary Lung Focus of Tuberculosis in Children. London, J. A. Churchill, 1916.
166. Ghon, A., and Kuedlich, H.: Die eintrittspforten der infektion. *In* Engel, S., and Pirquet, C. (eds.): Handbuch der Kindertuberkulose. Stuttgart, Georg Thieme Verlag, 1930.
167. Giammona, S. T., and Zelkowitz, P. S.: The use of superheated nebulized saline and gastric lavage to obtain bacterial cultures in primary pulmonary tuberculosis in children. Am. J. Dis. Child. *117*:198–200, 1969.
168. Girgis, N. I., Fariz, Z., Kilpatrick, M. E., et al.: Dexamethasone adjunctive treatment for tuberculous meningitis. Pediatr. Infect. Dis. J. *10*:179–182, 1991.
169. Girling, D. J: Adverse reactions to rifampicin in antituberculosis regimens. J. Antimicrob. Chemother. *3*:115, 1977.
170. Girling, D. J.: Role of pyrazinamide in primary chemotherapy for pulmonary tuberculosis. Tubercle *65*:1–4, 1984.
171. Glassroth, J., Bailey, W. C., Hopewell, P. C., et al.: Why tuberculosis is not prevented. Am. Rev. Respir. Dis. *141*:1236–1240, 1990.
172. Goble, M., Iseman, M. D., Madsen, L. A., et al.: Treatment of 171 patients with pulmonary tuberculosis resistant to isoniazid and rifampin. N. Engl. J. Med. *328*:527–532, 1993.
173. Gonzalez, B., Moreno, S., Burdach, R., et al.: Clinical presentation of bacillus Calmette-Guérin infections in patients with immunodeficiency syndromes. Pediatr. Infect. Dis. J. *8*:201–206, 1989.
174. Gorse, G. J., and Belshe, R. B.: Male genital tuberculosis: A review of the literature with instructive case reports. Rev. Infect. Dis. *7*:511–524, 1985.
175. Grange, J. M.: Rapid diagnosis of paucibacillary tuberculosis. Tubercle *70*:1–4, 1989.
176. Grange, J. M., Gibson, J., Osborn, T. W., et al.: What is BCG? Tubercle *64*:129–139, 1983.
177. Grange, J. M., and Redmond, W. B.: Host-phage relationships in the genus *Mycobacterium* and their clinical significance. Tubercle *59*:203–225, 1978.
178. Graziani, A. L., and MacGregor, R. R.: Self-reading of tuberculin testing vs. physician reading. Infect. Dis. Clin. Pract. *4*:72–74, 1995.
179. Grosset, J.: Bacteriologic basis for short-course chemotherapy for tuberculosis. Clin. Chest Med. *1*:231–241, 1980.
180. Grosset, J. H.: Present status of chemotherapy for tuberculosis. Rev. Infect. Dis. *11*(Suppl. 2):S342– S347, 1989.
181. Grosskopf, I., David, A., Charach, G., et al.: Bone and joint tuberculosis: A 10-year review. Isr. J. Med. Sci. *30*:278–283, 1994.
182. Gupta, R., Gupta, S., Dingh, D., et al.: MR imaging and angiography in tuberculous meningitis. Neuroradiology *36*:87–92, 1994.
183. Gutman, L., Moye, J., Zimmer, B., et al.: Tuberculosis in human immunodeficiency virus-exposed or -infected United States children. Pediatr. Infect. Dis. J. *13*:963–968, 1994.
184. Hageman, J., Shulman, S., Schreiber, M., et al.: Congenital tuberculosis: Critical reappraisal of clinical findings and diagnostic procedures. Pediatrics *66*:980–984, 1980.
185. Hannachi, J., Martin, M., Boulabal, F., et al.: Comparison of three daily short-course regimens in osteoarticular tuberculosis in Algiers. Bull. Int. Union Tuberc. *57*:46–47, 1982.
186. Hardy, J. B.: Persistence of hypersensitivity to old tuberculin following primary tuberculosis in childhood: A long-term study. Am. J. Public Health *36*:1417–1426, 1946.
187. Hardy, J. B., and Hartmann, J. R.: Tuberculous dactylitis in childhood. J. Pediatr. *30*:146–156, 1947.
188. Harries, A. D.: Tuberculosis and human immunodeficiency virus infection in developing countries. Lancet *335*:387–390, 1990.
189. Harris, V. J., Dida, F., Lander, S. S., et al.: Cavitary tuberculosis in children. J. Pediatr. *90*:660–661, 1977.
190. Harrison, H. E., Finberg, L., and Fleischman, E.: Disturbances of ionic equilibrium of intracellular and extracellular electrolytes in patients with tuberculous meningitis. J. Clin. Invest. *31*:300–308, 1952.
191. Haygood, T., and Williamson, S.: Radiographic findings of extremity tuberculosis in childhood: Back to the future? Radiographics *14*:561–570, 1994.
192. Heifetz, L.: Drug Susceptibility in the Chemotherapy of Bacterial Infections. Boca Raton, CRC Press, 1991, pp. 124–127.
193. Heinle, E. W., Jr., Jensen, N. N., and Westerman, M. P.: Diagnostic usefulness of marrow biopsy in disseminated tuberculosis. Am. Rev. Respir. Dis. *91*:701–705, 1965.
194. Helms, S., and Helms, P.: Tuberculin sensitivity during measles. Acta Tuberc. Scand. *35*:166–171, 1956.
195. Heney, C., Baise, T., and Cohen, M. A.: Tuberculosis of the mandible: A case report. Pediatr. Infect. Dis. J. *7*:74–76, 1988.
196. Heycock, J. B., and Noble, T. C.: Four cases of syringe-transmitted tuberculosis. Tubercle *42*:25–27, 1961.
197. High, R. H.: Calcifications in the spleen: Occurrence in histoplasmin and tuberculin reactors. Public Health Rep. *61*:1782–1786, 1946.
198. Hinman, A. R., Judd, J. M., Kolnik, J. P., et al.: Changing risks in tuberculosis. Am. J. Epidemiol. *103*:486–497, 1976.
199. Hodgson, A. R., Wong, W., and Yau, A. C. M. A.: X-ray Appearances of Tuberculosis of the Spine. Springfield, IL, Charles C Thomas, 1969.
200. Hoffman, E. B., Crosier, J. H., and Cremin, B. J.: Imaging in children with spinal tuberculosis. J. Bone Joint Surg. *75*(B):233–239, 1993.
201. Hoffman, N. D., Kelly, C., and Futterman, D.: Tuberculosis infection in human immunodeficiency virus-positive adolescents and young adults: A New York City cohort. Pediatrics *97*:198–203, 1996.
202. Hoge, C., Fisher, L., Donnell, D., et al.: Risk factors for transmission of *Mycobacterium tuberculosis* in a primary school outbreak: Lack of racial difference in susceptibility to infection. Am. J. Epidemiol. *139*:520–530, 1994.
203. Holt, L. E.: Tuberculosis acquired through ritual circumcision. J. A. M. A. *61*:99–102, 1913.
204. Holt, L. E., Jr., and McIntosh, R.: Diseases of Infancy and Childhood. New York, Appleton-Century-Crofts, 1940.
205. Hong Kong Chest Service/British Medical Research Council Fifth Collaborative Study: Controlled clinical trial of five 6-month regimens of chemotherapy for pulmonary tuberculosis. Am. Rev. Respir. Dis. *136*:1339–1342, 1987.
206. Hong Kong Chest Service/British Medical Research Council: Controlled trial of 2, 4 and 6 months of pyrazinamide in 6-month, three times weekly regimens for smear positive pulmonary tuberculosis, including an assessment of a combined preparation of isoniazid, rifampin and pyrazinamide: Results at 30 months. Am. Rev. Respir. Dis. *143*:700–706, 1991.
207. Honore, N., and Cole, S.: Streptomycin resistance in mycobacteria. Antimicrob. Agents Chemother. *38*:238– 241, 1994.
208. Houde, C., and Dery, P.: *Mycobacterium bovis* sepsis in an infant with human immunodeficiency virus infection. Pediatr. Infect. Dis. J. *7*:810, 1988.
209. Howard, T. P., and Soloman, D. A.: Reading the tuberculin skin test: Who, when and how? Arch. Intern. Med. *148*:2457–2459, 1988.
210. Hsu, K. H. K.: Contact investigation: A practical approach to tuberculosis eradication. Am. J. Public Health *53*:1761–1769, 1963.
211. Hsu, K. H. K.: Tuberculin reaction in children treated with isoniazid. Am. J. Dis. Child. *137*:1090–1092, 1983.
212. Hsu, K. H. K.: Thirty years after isoniazid: Its impact on tuberculosis in children and adolescents. J. A. M. A. *251*:1283–1285, 1984.
213. Hsu, K. H. K., and Starke, J. R.: Diagnosis and treatment of tuberculous infection. Semin. Pediatr. Infect. Dis. *4*:283–290, 1993.
214. Hsu, L. C. S., and Leong, J. C. Y.: Tuberculosis of the lower cervical spine (C2 to C7). J. Bone Joint Surg. *66*:1–5, 1984.
215. Huebner, R. E., Schein, M. F., and Bass, J. B.: The tuberculin skin test. Clin. Infect. Dis. *17*:968–975, 1993.

216. Hughes, I. E., Smith, H., and Kane, P. O.: Ethionamide: Its passage into the cerebrospinal fluid in man. Lancet *1*:616–617, 1962.
217. Hughesdon, M. R.: Congenital tuberculosis. Arch. Dis. Child. *21*:121–138, 1946.
218. Hugo-Hamman, C. T., Scher, H., and DeMoor, M. M. A.: Tuberculous pericarditis in children: A review of 44 cases. Pediatr. Infect. Dis. J. *13*:13–18, 1994.
219. Humphries, M. J., Teoh, R., Lau, J., et al.: Factors of prognostic significance in Chinese children with tuberculous meningitis. Tubercle *71*:161–168, 1990.
220. Hussey, G., Chisholm, T., and Kibel, M.: Miliary tuberculosis in children: A review of 94 cases. Pediatr. Infect. Dis. J. *10*:832–836, 1991.
221. Hussey, G., Kibel, M., and Dempster, W.: The serodiagnosis of tuberculosis in children: An evaluation of an ELISA test using IgG antibodies to *M. tuberculosis*, strain H37RV. Ann. Trop. Paediatr. *11*:113–118, 1991.
222. Hussey, G., Kibel, M., and Parker, N.: Ciprofloxacin treatment of multiply drug-resistant extrapulmonary tuberculosis in a child. Pediatr. Infect. Dis. J. *11*:408–409, 1992.
223. Hyge, T. V.: Efficacy of BCG vaccination: Epidemic of tuberculosis in a state school with an observation period of 12 years. Acta Tuberc. Scand. *32*:89–107, 1956.
224. Ibanez, S., and Ross, G.: Quimioterapia abreviada de 6 meses en tuberculosis pulmonar infantil. Rev. Chil. Pediatr. *51*:249–252, 1980.
225. Idriss, Z. H., Sinno, A., and Kronfol, N. M.: Tuberculous meningitis in childhood: Forty-three cases. Am. J. Dis. Child. *130*:364–367, 1976.
226. Ildirim, I., Hacimustafaoglu, M., and Ediz, B.: Correlation of tuberculin induration with the number of bacillus Calmette-Guérin vaccines. Pediatr. Infect. Dis. J. *14*:1060–1063, 1995.
227. Ingalhalikar, V. T., Deostale, D. A., and Abhyankar, V. K.: Nonimmobilization of surgically treated tuberculosis of spine in children. Prog. Pediatr. Surg. *15*:153–157, 1982.
228. Inselman, L. S., Delavega, C. E., and Evans, H. E.: Drug-resistant tuberculosis of the hip in a child. N.Y. State J. Med. *84*:84–85, 1984.
229. International Union Against Tuberculosis Committee on Prophylaxis: Efficacy of various durations of isoniazid preventive therapy for tuberculosis: Five years of follow-up in the IUAT trial. Bull. W. H. O. *60*:555–564, 1982.
230. Iseman, M. D.: Treatment of multidrug-resistant tuberculosis. N. Engl. J. Med. *329*:784–791, 1993.
231. Iseman, M. D., Cohn, D. L., and Sbarbaro, J. A.: Directly observed treatment of tuberculosis: We can't afford not to try it. N. Engl. J. Med. *328*:576–578, 1993.
232. Iseman, M. D., Madsen, L., Goble, M., et al.: Surgical intervention in the treatment of pulmonary disease caused by drug-resistant *Mycobacterium tuberculosis*. Am. Rev. Respir. Dis. *141*:623–625, 1990.
233. Jacobs, R. F., and Abernathy, R. S.: The treatment of tuberculosis in children. Pediatr. Infect. Dis. *4*:513–517, 1985.
234. Jacobs, R. F., Sunakorn, P., Chotpitayasunonah, T., et al.: Intensive short course chemotherapy for tuberculous meningitis. Pediatr. Infect. Dis. J. *11*:194–198, 1992.
235. Jaffe, I. P.: Tuberculous meningitis in childhood. Lancet *1*:738, 1982.
236. Jagannath, C., Reddy, M. V., Kailasam, S., et al.: Chemotherapeutic activity of clofazamine and its analogues against *Mycobacterium tuberculosis*. Am. J. Respir. Crit. Care Med. *151*:1083–1086, 1995.
237. Jawahar, M. S., Sivasubramanian, S., Vijayan, V. K., et al.: Short course chemotherapy for tuberculous lymphadenitis in children. Br. Med. J. *301*:359–362, 1990.
238. Jereb, J., Kelly, G., and Porterfield, D.: The epidemiology of tuberculosis in children. Semin. Pediatr. Infect. Dis. *4*:220–231, 1993.
239. Jindani, A., Aber, V. R., Edwards, E. A., et al.: The early bactericidal activity of drugs in patients with pulmonary tuberculosis. Am. Rev. Respir. Dis. *121*:939–949, 1980.
240. Jinkins, J. R.: Computed tomography of intracranial tuberculosis. Neuroradiology *33*:126–135, 1991.
241. John, J. F., and Douglas, R. G.: Tuberculous arachnoiditis. J. Pediatr. *86*:235–237, 1975.
242. Johnson, H., Lee, B., Doherty, E., et al.: Tuberculin sensitivity and the BCG scar in tuberculosis contacts. Tubercle Lung Dis. *76*:122–125, 1995.
243. Johnston, J. A.: Nutritional Studies in Adolescent Girls and Their Relation to Tuberculosis. Springfield, IL, Charles C Thomas, 1953.
244. Jones, B. E., Otaya, M., Antoniskis, D., et al.: A prospective evaluation of antituberculosis therapy in patients with human immunodeficiency virus infection. Am. J. Respir. Crit. Care Med. *150*:1499–1502, 1994.
245. Jones, D., Malecki, J., Bigler, W., et al.: Pediatric tuberculosis and human immunodeficiency virus infection in Palm Beach County, Florida. Am. J. Dis. Child. *146*:1166–1170, 1992.
246. Jones, H. E., Miller, S. D., and Greenberg, J. H.: Measurement of tuberculin reactions. Corres. N. Engl. J. Med. *287*:721, 1972.
247. Jones, W. D., Jr., Good, R. L., Thompson, N. J., et al.: Bacteriophage types of *Mycobacterium tuberculosis* in the United States. Am. Rev. Respir. Dis. *125*:640–643, 1982.
248. Kalish, S. B., Radiu, R. C., Phair, J. P., et al.: Use of an enzyme-linked immunosorbent assay technique in the differential diagnosis of active pulmonary tuberculosis in humans. J. Infect. Dis. *147*:523–530, 1983.
249. Kalish, S. B., Rodin, R. C., Levitz, D., et al.: Enzyme-linked immunosorbent assay method for IgG antibody to purified protein derivative in cerebrospinal fluid of patients with tuberculous meningitis. Ann. Intern. Med. *99*:630–633, 1983.
250. Kallmann, I. J., and Reisner, D.: Twin studies on the genetic factors in tuberculosis. Am. Rev. Tuberc. *47*:549, 1943.
251. Karalliede, S., Katugha, L. P., and Uragoda, C. G.: The tuberculin response of Sri Lankan children after BCG vaccination at birth. Tubercle *68*:33–38, 1987.
252. Kedar, R. P., Shah, P. P., Shivde, R. S., et al.: Sonographic findings in gastrointestinal and peritoneal tuberculosis. Clin. Radiol. *49*:24–29, 1994.
253. Kendig, E. L., Jr.: Tuberculosis in the very young: Report of three cases of infants less than one month of age. Am. Rev. Tuberc. *70*:161–165, 1954.
254. Kendig, E. L., Jr.: Prognosis of infants born of tuberculous mothers. Pediatrics *26*:97–100, 1960.
255. Kendig, E. L., Jr.: The place of BCG vaccine in the management of infants born of tuberculous mothers. N. Engl. J. Med. *281*:520–523, 1969.
256. Kendig, E. L., Jr.: Tuberculosis among children in the United States. Pediatrics *62*:269–271, 1978.
257. Kendig, E. L., Jr., and Rodgers, W. L.: Tuberculosis in the neonatal period. Am. Rev. Tuberc. Pulm. Dis. *77*:418–422, 1958.
258. Kennedy, C., and Knowles, G. K.: Miliary tuberculosis presenting with skin lesions. Br. Med. J. *3*:356, 1975.
259. Kennedy, N., Fox, R., Kisyombe, G. M., et al.: Early bactericidal and sterilizing activities of ciprofloxacin in pulmonary tuberculosis. Am. Rev. Respir. Dis. *148*:1547–1551, 1993.
260. Khan, E. A., and Starke, J. R.: Diagnosis of tuberculosis in children: Increased need for better methods. Emerg. Infect. Dis. *1*:115–123, 1995.
261. Khan, M. A., Chandrasekaran, B., and Needle, M.: Tuberculosis in chronic renal failure. Corres. Arch. Intern. Med. *141*:1554, 1981.
262. Khouri, Y., Mastrucci, M., Hutto, C., et al.: *Mycobacterium tuberculosis* in children with human immunodeficiency virus type 1 infection. Pediatr. Infect. Dis. J. *11*:950–955, 1992.
263. Khubchandani, R. P., Kumta, N. B., Bharucha, N. B., et al.: Short-course chemotherapy in childhood pulmonary tuberculosis. Am. Rev. Respir. Dis. *141*(Suppl.):A338, 1990.
264. Kim, J. H., Langston, A. A., and Gallis, H. A.: Miliary tuberculosis: Epidemiology, clinical manifestations, diagnosis and outcome. Rev. Infect. Dis. *12*:583–590, 1990.
265. Kimerling, M. E., Vaughn, E. S., and Dunlap, N. E.: Childhood tuberculosis in Alabama: Epidemiology of disease and indicators of program effectiveness, 1983 to 1993. Pediatr. Infect. Dis. J. *14*:678–684, 1995.
266. Klausner, J. D., Ryder, R. W., Baende, E., et al.: *Mycobacterium tuberculosis* in household contacts of human immunodeficiency virus type-1-seropositive patients with active pulmonary tuberculosis in Kinshasa, Zaire. J. Infect. Dis. *168*:106–111, 1993.
267. Kleeberg, H. H.: Chemotherapy and chemoprophylaxis of tuberculosis in cattle. Adv. Tuberc. Res. *15*:189–258, 1966.
268. Kochi, A.: The global tuberculosis situation and the new control strategy of the World Health Organization. (Leading article.) Tubercle *72*:1–6, 1991.
269. Kohli, V., Kumar, L., and Kataria, S.: Multiple hepatosplenic tuberculous abscesses in an eight-year-old boy. Pediatr. Infect. Dis. J. *15*:178–179, 1996.
270. Kohn, M. R., Arden, M. R., Vasilakis, J., et al.: Directly observed preventive therapy: Turning the tide against tuberculosis. Arch. Pediatr. Adolesc. Med. *150*:727–729, 1996.
271. Kopanoff, D. E., Snider, D. E., and Caras, G. J.: Isoniazid-related hepatitis: A United States Public Health Service Cooperative Surveillance Study. Am. Rev. Respir. Dis. *117*:991–1001, 1978.
272. Krambovitis, E., McIllmurray, M. B., Lock, P. E., et al.: Rapid diagnosis of tuberculous meningitis by latex particle agglutination. Lancet *2*:1229–1231, 1984.
273. Kumar, A., Misra, P. K., Mehotra, R., et al.: Hepatotoxicity of rifampin and isoniazid: Is it all drug-induced hepatitis? Am. Rev. Respir. Dis. *143*:1350–1352, 1991.
274. Kumar, L., Dhand, R., Singhi, P. D., et al.: A randomized trial of fully intermittent vs. daily followed by intermittent short-course chemotherapy for childhood tuberculosis. Pediatr. Infect. Dis. J. *9*:802–806, 1990.
275. Kutt, H., Brennan, R., Dehejia, H., et al.: Diphenylhydantoin intoxication: A complication of isoniazid therapy. Am. Rev. Respir. Dis. *101*:377–384, 1970.
276. Lai, K. K., Stottmeier, K. D., Sherman, I. H., et al.: Mycobacterial cervical lymphadenopathy: Relation of etiologic agents to age. J. A. M. A. *251*:1286–1288, 1984.
277. Lake, A. M., and Oski, F. A.: Peripheral lymphadenopathy in childhood: Ten-year experience with excisional biopsy. Am. J. Dis. Child. *132*:357–359, 1978.
278. Lamont, A., Cremin, B., and Pettenet, B.: Radiologic patterns of pulmonary tuberculosis in the pediatric age group. Pediatr. Radiol. *16*:2–7, 1986.
279. Landi, S., and Held, H. R.: Stability of dilute solutions of tuberculin purified protein derivative. Tubercle *59*:121–133, 1978.
280. Lange, W. R., Warnock-Eckhart, E., and Bean, M. E.: *Mycobacterium tuberculosis* infection in foreign born adoptees. Pediatr. Infect. Dis. J. *8*:625–629, 1989.
281. Lanier, V. S., Russell, W. F., Jr., Heaton, A., et al.: Concentrations of active isoniazid in serum and cerebrospinal fluid of patients with tuberculosis treated with isoniazid. Pediatrics *21*:910–915, 1958.

282. Larmola, E.: Two cases of sudden death in infants recovering from primary tuberculosis. Acta Tuberc. Scand. *21*(Suppl.):67, 1949.
283. Lau, S. K., Kwan, S., Lee, J., et al.: Source of tubercle bacilli in cervical lymph nodes: A prospective study. J. Laryngol. Otol. *105*:558–561, 1991.
284. Laven, G. T.: Diagnosis of tuberculosis in children using fluorescence microscopic examination of gastric washings. Am. Rev. Respir. Dis. *115*:743–749, 1977.
285. Lee, C., Wang, W., Lan, R., et al.: Corticosteroids in the treatment of tuberculous pleurisy: A double-blind, placebo-controlled randomized study. Chest *94*:1256–1259, 1988.
286. Lees, A., Macleod, A., and Marshall, J.: Cerebral tuberculoma developing during treatment of tuberculous meningitis. Lancet *1*:1208–1211, 1980.
287. Leggiadro, R. J., Collery, B., and Dowdy, S.: Outbreak of tuberculosis in a family day care home. Pediatr. Infect. Dis. J. *8*:52–54, 1989.
288. Leiguarda, R., Berthier, M., Starkstein, S., et al.: Ischemic infarction in 25 children with tuberculous meningitis. Stroke *19*:200–204, 1988.
289. Levine, H., Metzger, W., Lacera, S., et al.: Diagnosis of tuberculous pleurisy by culture of pleural biopsy specimen. Arch. Intern. Med. *126*:269–271, 1970.
290. Lifschitz, M.: The value of the tuberculin skin test as a screening test for tuberculosis among BCG-vaccinated children. Pediatrics *36*:624–627, 1965.
291. Light, I. J., Saidleman, M., and Sutherland, J. M.: Management of newborns after nursery exposure to tuberculosis. Am. Rev. Respir. Dis. *109*:415–419, 1974.
292. Lincoln, E. M.: Tuberculous meningitis in children: With special reference to serous meningitis. Am. Rev. Tuberc. *56*:75–94, 95–109, 1947.
293. Lincoln, E. M.: Epidemics of tuberculosis. Adv. Tuberc. Res. *14*:159–197, 1965.
294. Lincoln, E. M., Davies, P. A., and Bovornkitti, S.: Tuberculous pleurisy with effusion in children. Am. Rev. Tuberc. *77*:271–289, 1958.
295. Lincoln, E. M., Gilbert, L., and Morales, S. M.: Chronic pulmonary tuberculosis in individuals with known previous primary tuberculosis. Dis. Chest *38*:473–482, 1960.
296. Lincoln, E. M., Harris, L. C., Bovornkitti, S., et al.: Endobronchial tuberculosis in children. Am. Rev. Tuberc. Pulm. Dis. *77*:39–61, 1958.
297. Lincoln, E. M., Sabato, V. R., and Davies, P. A.: Tuberculous meningitis in children. J. Pediatr. *57*:807–823, 1960.
298. Lincoln, E. M., and Sewell, E. M.: Tuberculosis in Children. New York, McGraw-Hill, 1963.
299. Lindgren, I.: Pathology of tuberculous infection in BCG-vaccinated humans. Adv. Tuberc. Res. *14*:203–231, 1965.
300. Linna, O., and Uhari, M.: Hepatotoxicity of rifampicin and isoniazid in children treated for tuberculosis. Eur. J. Pediatr. *134*:227–229, 1980.
301. Litt, I. F., Cohen, M. I., and McNamara, H.: Isoniazid hepatitis in adolescents. J. Pediatr. *89*:133–135, 1976.
302. Liu, K. W., Chan, Y. L., Tseng, R., et al.: Childhood abdominal tuberculosis: The role of echo-guided fine-needle aspiration in its management. Surg. Endosc. *8*:326–328, 1994.
303. Livengood, J. R., Sigler, T. G., Foster, L. R., et al.: Isoniazid-resistant tuberculosis: A community outbreak and report of a rifampin prophylaxis failure. J. A. M. A. *253*:2847–2849, 1985.
304. Loddenkemper, R.: Prospective individual comparison of blind needle biopsy and of thoroscopy in the diagnosis and differential diagnosis of tuberculous pleurisy. Scand. J. Respir. Dis. *102*(Suppl.):196–198, 1978.
305. Lorber, J.: Intracranial calcification following tuberculous meningitis in children. Am. Rev. Tuberc. Pulm. Dis. *78*:38–61, 1958.
306. Lorber, J.: Isoniazid and streptomycin in tuberculous meningitis. Lancet *1*:1140–1142, 1964.
307. Louie, E., Rice, L. B., and Holzman, R. S.: Tuberculosis in non-Haitian patients with acquired immunodeficiency syndrome. Chest *90*:542–545, 1986.
308. Lucente, F. E., Tobias, G. W., Parisier, S. C., et al.: Tuberculous otitis media. Laryngoscope *88*:1107–1116, 1978.
309. Luo, C., Chintu, C., Bhat, G., et al.: Human immunodeficiency virus type-1 infection in Zambian children with tuberculosis: Changing seroprevalence and evaluation of a thiacetazone-free regimen. Tubercle Lung Dis. *75*:110–115, 1994.
310. Lurie, M. B.: Resistance to Tuberculosis: Experimental Studies in Native and Acquired Defense Mechanisms. Cambridge, MA, Harvard University Press, 1964.
311. MacAdam, A. M., and Rubio, T.: Tuberculous otomastoiditis in children. Am. J. Dis. Child. *131*:152–156, 1977.
312. MacDonnell, A. H., Baird, R. W., and Bronze, M. S.: Intramedullary tuberculomas of the spinal cord: Case report and review. Rev. Infect. Dis. *12*:432–439, 1990.
313. MacGregor, R. R., Sheagren, J. N., Lipsett, M. B., et al.: Alternate-day prednisone therapy: Evaluation of delayed hypersensitivity response, control of disease and steroid side effects. N. Engl. J. Med. *280*:1427–1431, 1969.
314. Mackaness, G. B.: Cellular immunity in tuberculosis. *In* Johnson, J. E. (ed.): Rational Therapy and Control of Tuberculosis. Gainesville, University of Florida Press, 1970.
315. Maharaj, B., Leary, W. P., and Pudifin, D. J.: A prospective study of hepatic tuberculosis in 41 black patients. Q. J. Med. *242*:517–522, 1987.
316. Mahmoudi, A., and Iseman, M.: Pitfalls in the care of patients with tuberculosis: Common errors and their association with the acquisition of drug resistance. J. A. M. A. *270*:65–68, 1993.
317. Manalo, F., Tan, F., Sbarbaro, J. A., et al.: Community-based short-course treatment of pulmonary tuberculosis in a developing nation: Initial report of an eight-month, largely intermittent, regimen in a population with a high prevalence of drug resistance. Am. Rev. Respir. Dis. *142*:1301–1305, 1990.
318. Mancao, M. Y., Nolte, F. S., Nahmias, A. J., et al.: Use of polymerase chain reaction for diagnosis of tuberculous meningitis. Pediatr. Infect. Dis. J. *13*:154–155, 1994.
319. Manjunath, N., Shankar, P., Rajan, L., et al.: Evaluation of a polymerase chain reaction for the diagnosis of tuberculosis. Tubercle *72*:21–27, 1991.
320. Martinez-Roig, A., Cami, J., Llorens-Terol, J., et al.: Acetylation phenotype and hepatotoxicity in the treatment of tuberculosis in children. Pediatrics *77*:912–915, 1986.
321. Mason, E., and Russell, D. W.: Isoniazid acetylation rates (phenotypes) of patients being treated for tuberculosis. Bull. W. H. O. *45*:617–624, 1971.
322. Matsaniotis, N., Kattanis, C., Economou-Mavrou, C., et al.: Bullous emphysema in childhood tuberculosis. J. Pediatr. *71*:703–708, 1967.
323. McCray, M. K., and Esterly, M. B.: Cutaneous eruptions in congenital tuberculosis. Arch. Dermatol. *117*:460– 464, 1981.
324. McDermott, W.: The chemotherapy of tuberculosis. Am. Rev. Respir. Dis. *86*:323–335, 1962.
325. McKenna, M. T., McCray, E., and Onorato, I. M.: The epidemiology of tuberculosis among foreign-born persons in the United States, 1986 to 1993. N. Engl. J. Med. *332*:1071–1076, 1995.
326. McKenzie, S. A., McNab, A. J., and Katz, G.: Neonatal pyridoxine responsive convulsions due to isoniazid therapy. Arch. Dis. Child. *51*:567–568, 1976.
327. Medical Research Council Investigation: Streptomycin treatment of pulmonary tuberculosis. Br. Med. J. *2*:769–782, 1948.
328. Medical Research Council-Tuberculosis Chemotherapy Trials Committee: Long-term chemotherapy in the treatment of chronic pulmonary tuberculosis with cavitation. Tubercle *43*:201–267, 1962.
329. Medical Research Council Working Party on Tuberculosis of the Spine: Five-year assessment of controlled trials of inpatient and outpatient treatment and of plaster-of-paris jackets for tuberculosis of the spine in children on standard chemotherapy: Studies in Masan and Pusan, Korea. J. Bone Joint Surg. (Br.) *58*:399–411, 1976.
330. Medical Research Council Working Party on Tuberculosis of the Spine: Five-year assessment of controlled trials of ambulatory treatment, debridement and anterior spinal fusion in the management of tuberculosis of the spine; Studies in Bulawayo (Rhodesia) and in Hong Kong. J. Bone Joint Surg. (Br.) *60*:163–177, 1978.
331. Medical Research Council Working Party on Tuberculosis of the Spine: Twelfth report: Controlled trial of short-course regimens of chemotherapy in the ambulatory treatment of spinal tuberculosis. J. Bone Joint Surg. *75*(B):240–248, 1993.
332. Medlar, E. M.: Behavior of pulmonary tuberculous lesions: A pathological study. Am. Rev. Tuberc. *71*:31, 1955.
333. Mehta, J. B., and Bentley, S.: Prevention of tuberculosis in children: Missed opportunities. Am. J. Prev. Med. *8*.283–286, 1992.
334. Meier, A., Kirschner, P., Bange, F., et al.: Genetic alterations in streptomycin-resistant *Mycobacterium tuberculosis*: Mapping of mutations conferring resistance. Antimicrob. Agents Chemother. *38*:228–233, 1994.
335. Menzies, R., Fanning, A., Yuan, L., et al.: Tuberculosis among healthcare workers. N. Engl. J. Med. *332*:92–98, 1995.
336. Menzies, R., Rocher, I., and Vissandjee, B.: Factors associated with compliance in treatment of tuberculosis. Tubercle Lung Dis. *74*:32–37, 1993.
337. Menzies, R., and Vissandjee, B.: Effect of bacille Calmette-Guérin vaccination on tuberculin reactivity. Am. Rev. Respir. Dis. *141*:621–625, 1992.
338. Migliori, G. B., Borghesi, A., Rossanigo, P., et al.: Proposal of an improved score method for the diagnosis of pulmonary tuberculosis in childhood in developing countries. Tubercle Lung Dis. *73*:145–149, 1992.
339. Miller, F. J. W., Seale, R. M. E., and Taylor, M. D.: Tuberculosis in Children. Boston, MA, Little, Brown, 1963, p. 214.
340. Miller, R. A., Lanza, L. A., Kline, J. N., et al.: *Mycobacterium tuberculosis* in lung transplant recipients. Am. J. Respir. Crit. Care Med. *152*:374–376, 1995.
341. Miller, R. R., Porter, J., and Greenblatt, D. J.: Clinical importance of the interaction of phenytoin and isoniazid: A report from the Boston Collaborative Drug Surveillance Program. Chest *75*:356–358, 1979.
342. Miorner, H., Sjobring, U., Nayak, P., et al.: Diagnosis of tuberculous meningitis: A comparative analysis of 3 immunoassays, an immune complex assay and the polymerase chain reaction. Tubercle Lung Dis. *76*:381–386, 1995.
343. Mitchison, D. A.: Basic mechanisms of chemotherapy. Chest *76*(Suppl.):771–781, 1979.
344. Mitchison, D. A.: The action of anti-tuberculous drugs in short-course chemotherapy. Tubercle *66*:219–225, 1985.
345. Mitchison, D. A., and Nunn, A. J.: Influence of initial drug resistance on the response to short-course chemotherapy of pulmonary tuberculosis. Am. Rev. Respir. Dis. *133*:423–428, 1986.
346. Mohanty, K. C., and Dhamgaye, T. M.: Controlled trial of ciprofloxacin in

short-term chemotherapy for pulmonary tuberculosis. Chest *104*:1194–1198, 1993.
347. Mohle-Boetani, J. C., Miller, B., Halpern, M., et al.: School-based screening for tuberculous infection: A cost benefit analysis. J. A. M. A. *274*:613–619, 1995.
348. Morens, D. M., Baublis, J. V., and Heidelberger, K. P.: Congenital tuberculosis and associated hypoadrenocorticism. South. Med. J. *72*:160–161, 165, 1979.
349. Morrison, J. B.: Natural history of segmental lesions in primary pulmonary tuberculosis. Arch. Dis. Child. *48*:90–98, 1973.
350. Morse, M. L., Karr, D. J., and Menddman, P. M.: Ocular tuberculosis in a five-month-old. Pediatr. Infect. Dis. J. *7*:514–516, 1988.
351. Moss, W. J., Dedyo, T., Suarez, M., et al.: Tuberculosis in children infected with human immunodeficiency virus: A report of five cases. Pediatr. Infect. Dis. J. *11*:114–120, 1992.
352. Mumtaz, M. A., Schwartz, R. H., Grundfast, K. M., et al.: Tuberculosis of the middle ear and mastoid. Pediatr. Infect. Dis. *2*:234–236, 1983.
353. Murray, J. F.: Cursed duet: HIV infection and tuberculosis. Respiration *57*:210–220, 1990.
354. Nakajo, M. M., Rao, M., and Steiner, P.: Incidence of hepatotoxicity in children receiving isoniazid chemoprophylaxis. Pediatr. Infect. Dis. J. *8*:649–650, 1989.
355. Narain, R., Naganna, K., Chandrasekhar, R., et al.: Crude mortality by size of tuberculin reaction. Am. Rev. Respir. Dis. *101*:897–906, 1970.
356. Nemir, R. L., Cardona, J., Lacoius, A., et al.: Prednisone therapy as an adjunct in the treatment of lymph node–bronchial tuberculosis in childhood: A double-blind study. Am. Rev. Respir. Dis. *88*:189–198, 1963.
357. Nemir, R. L., Cardona, J., Vaziri, F., et al.: Prednisone as an adjunct in the chemotherapy of lymph node–bronchial tuberculosis in childhood: A double-blind study. II. Further term observation. Am. Rev. Respir. Dis. *95*:402–410, 1967.
358. Nemir, R. L., and Krasinski, K.: Tuberculosis in children and adolescents in the 1980's. Pediatr. Infect. Dis. J. *7*:375–379, 1988.
359. Nemir, R. L., and O'Hare, D.: Congenital tuberculosis. Am. J. Dis. Child. *139*:284–287, 1985.
360. Nemir, R. L., and O'Hare, D.: Tuberculosis in children 10 years of age and younger: Three decades of experience during the chemotherapeutic era. Pediatrics *88*:236–241, 1991.
361. Nemir, R. L., and Teichner, A.: Management of tuberculin reactors in children and adolescents previously vaccinated with BCG. Pediatr. Infect. Dis. 2:446–451, 1983.
362. Nolan, C. M., and Elarth, A. M.: Tuberculosis in a cohort of Southeast Asian refugees. Am. Rev. Respir. Dis. *137*:805–809, 1988.
363. Nolan, C. M., Elarth, A. M., and Barr, H. W.: Intentional isoniazid overdose in young Southeast Asian refugee women. Chest *93*:803–806, 1988.
364. Nolan, R., Jr.: Childhood tuberculosis in North Carolina: A study of the opportunities for intervention in the transmission of tuberculosis in children. Am. J. Public Health *76*:26–30, 1986.
365. Noordhoek, G., Kolk, A., Bjune, G., et al.: Sensitivity and specificity of PCR for detection of *Mycobacterium tuberculosis*: A blind comparison study among seven laboratories. J. Clin. Microbiol. *32*:277–284, 1994.
366. Nunn, P., and Felten, M.: Surveillance of resistance to antituberculosis drugs in developing countries. Tubercle Lung Dis. *75*:163–167, 1994.
367. Obaegbulam, S. C.: Spinal extraosseous extradural tuberculoma. Tubercle *58*:97, 1977.
368. O'Brien, K., Ruff, A., Louis, M., et al.: Bacillus Calmette-Guérin complications in children born to HIV-1-infected women with a review of the literature. Pediatrics *95*:414–418, 1995.
369. O'Brien, R. J., Long, M. W., Cross, F. S., et al.: Hepatotoxicity from isoniazid and rifampin among children treated for tuberculosis. Pediatrics *72*:491– 499, 1983.
370. O'Brien, R. J., and Snider, D. E., Jr.: Tuberculosis drugs: Old and new. Am. Rev. Respir. Dis. *131*:309–311, 1985.
371. Offenbacher, H., Fazekas, F., Schmidt. R., et al.: MRI in tuberculous meningoencephalitis: Report of four cases and review of the neuroimaging literature. J. Neurol. *238*:340–344, 1991.
372. Olazabal, F.: Choroidal tubercles: A neglected sign. J. A. M. A. *200*:104–107, 1967.
373. Olson, W. A., Pruitt, A. W., and Dayton, P. G.: Plasma concentration of isoniazid in children with tuberculous infections. Pediatrics *67*:876–878, 1981.
374. Omari, B., Robertson, J. M., Nelson, R. J., et al.: Pott's disease: A resurgent challenge to the thoracic surgeon. Chest *95*:145–150, 1989. (See also follow-up letters, Chest *96*:955–956, 1989.)
375. Optican, R. J., Ost, A., and Ravin, C. E.: High-resolution computed tomography in the diagnosis of miliary tuberculosis. Chest *102*:941–943, 1992.
376. Orme, I. M., Andersen, P., Boom, W. H.: T cell response to *Mycobacterium tuberculosis*. J. Infect. Dis. *167*:1481–1497, 1993.
377. Palmer, C. E., and Edwards, L. B.: Identifying the tuberculous infected: The dual test technique. J. A. M. A. *205*:167–169, 1968.
378. Palur, R., Rajohekhar, V., Chandy, M. J., et al.: Shunt surgery for hydrocephalus in tuberculous meningitis: A long-term follow-up study. J. Neurosurg. *74*:64–69, 1991.
379. Paluschi, V. J., O'Hare, D., and Lawrence, R. M.: Hepatotoxicity and transaminase measurement during isoniazid chemoprophylaxis in children. Pediatr. Infect. Dis. J. *14*:144–148, 1995.
380. Parish, R. E., and Brownstein, D.: Emergency department management of children with acute isoniazid poisoning. Pediatr. Emerg. Care *2*:88–90, 1986.
381. Park, M. M., Davis, A. L., Schluger, N. W., et al.: Outcome of MDR-TB patients, 1983-1993: Prolonged survival with appropriate therapy. Am. J. Respir. Crit. Care Med. *153*:317–324, 1996.
382. Passannante, M., Gallagher, C., and Reichman, L.: Preventive therapy for contacts of multidrug-resistant tuberculosis: A Delphi study. Chest *106*:431–434, 1994.
383. Payne, M., quoted by Miller, F. J. W., Seale, R. M. E., and Taylor, M. D.: Tuberculosis in Children. Boston, MA, Little, Brown, 1963.
384. Pearson, M. L., Jereb, J. A., Frieden, T. R., et al.: Nosocomial transmission of multidrug-resistant *Mycobacterium tuberculosis:* A risk to patients and healthcare workers. Ann. Intern. Med. *117*:191–196, 1992.
385. Pederson, F. K., Schiotz, P. O., Valerius, N. H., et al.: Fatal BCG infection in an immunocompetent girl. Acta Paediatr. Scand. *67*:19–23, 1978.
386. Pellock, J. M., Howell, J., Kendig, E. L., Jr., et al.: Pyridoxine deficiency in children treated with isoniazid. Chest *87*:658–661, 1985.
387. Peloquin, C. A., MacPhee, A. A., and Berning, S. E.: Malabsorption of antimycobacterial medications. N. Engl. J. Med. *329*:1122–1123, 1993.
388. Pelosi, F., Budani, H., Rubenstein, C., et al.: Isoniazid, rifampin and pyrazinamide in the treatment of childhood tuberculosis with duration adjusted to clinical status. Abstract. Am. Rev. Respir. Dis. *131*(Suppl.):A229, 1985.
389. Peltola, H., Salmi, I., Vahvanen, V., et al.: BCG vaccination as a cause of osteomyelitis and subcutaneous abscess. Arch. Dis. Child. *59*:157–161, 1984.
390. Pereira, C. A., Webber, B., and Orson, J. M.: Primary tuberculous complex of the skin. J. A. M. A. *235*:942, 1976.
391. Perry, S., and Starke, J. R.: Adherence to prescribed treatment and public health aspects of tuberculosis in children. Semin. Pediatr. Infect. Dis. *4*:291–298, 1993.
392. Pesanti, E.: The negative tuberculin skin test: Tuberculin, HIV and anergy panels. Am. J. Respir. Crit. Care Med. *149*:1699–1709, 1994.
393. Pierre, C., Olivier, C., Lecossier, D., et al.: Diagnosis of primary tuberculosis in children by amplification and detection of mycobacterial DNA. Am. Rev. Respir. Dis. *147*:420–424, 1993.
394. Pineda, P., Leung, A., Muller, N., et al.: Intrathoracic pediatric tuberculosis: A report of 202 cases. Tubercle Lung Dis. *74*:261–266, 1993.
395. Pomerantz, M., Madsen, L., Goble, M., et al.: Surgical management of resistant mycobacterial tuberculosis and other mycobacterial pulmonary infections. Ann. Thorac. Surg. *52*:1108–1112, 1991.
396. Pray, L. G.: Obstructive emphysema in infancy due to tuberculous mediastinal glands. J. Pediatr. *25*:253–256, 1944.
397. Pospelov, L. E., Matrakshin, A. G., Chernousova, L. N., et al.: Association of various genetic markers with tuberculosis and other lung disease in Tuvinian children. Tubercle Lung Dis. *77*:77–80, 1996.
398. Rao, K. V. N., Mitchison, D. A., Nair, N. G. K., et al.: Sulphadimidine acetylation test for classification of patients as slow or rapid inactivators of isoniazid. Br. Med. J. *3*:495–497, 1970.
399. Rao, P. T., Chitra, D. R., and Krishniah, H. G.: A study of the early clinical signs and biochemical values of cerebro-spinal fluid in the course of tuberculous meningitis during treatment and other factors influencing the prognosis. Indian J. Pediatr. *26*:178–186, 1959.
400. Rapp, R. S., Campbell, R. W., Howell, J. C., et al.: Isoniazid hepatotoxicity in children. Am. Rev. Respir. Dis. *118*:794–796, 1978.
401. Rasool, M., Govender, S., and Naidoo, K.: Cystic tuberculosis of bone in children. J. Bone Joint Surg. *76*:113–117, 1994.
402. Raviglione, M. C., Rieder, H. L., Styblo, K., et al.: Tuberculosis trends in Eastern Europe and the former USSR. Tubercle Lung Dis. *75*:400–416, 1994.
403. Raviglione, M. C., Snider, D., Jr., and Kochi, A.: Global epidemiology of tuberculosis: Morbidity and mortality of a worldwide epidemic. J. A. M. A. *273*:220–226, 1995.
404. Reichman, L. B.: Why hasn't BCG proved dangerous in HIV-infected patients? J. A. M. A. *261*:3246, 1989.
405. Reis, F. J., Bedran, M. B., Mowra, J. A., et al.: Six-month isoniazid-rifampin treatment for pulmonary tuberculosis in children. Am. Rev. Respir. Dis. *142*:996–999, 1990.
406. Report of a WHO Study Group: BCG vaccination policies. WHO Technical Report Series No. 652, 1980–1981.
407. Reves, R., Blakey, D., Snider, D. E., Jr., et al.: Transmission of multiple drug-resistant tuberculosis: Report of a school and community outbreak. Am. J. Epidemiol. *113*:423–435, 1981.
408. Reynes, J., Perez, C., Lamaury, I., et al.: Bacille Calmette-Guérin adenitis 30 years after immunization in a patient with AIDS. J. Infect. Dis. *160*:727, 1989.
409. Rich, A. R.: The Pathogenesis of Tuberculosis. 2nd ed. Springfield, IL, Charles C Thomas, 1951.
410. Rich, A. R., and McCordock, H. A.: The pathogenesis of tuberculous meningitis. Bull. Johns Hopkins Hosp. *52*:5–35, 1933.
411. Ridgeway, A. L., Warner, G. S., Phillips. P., et al.: Transmission of *Mycobac-*

terium tuberculosis to recipients of single lung transplants from the same donor. Am. J. Respir. Crit. Care Med. *153*:1166–1168, 1996.

412. Rieder, H. L., Cauthen, G. M., Comstock, G. W., et al.: Epidemiology of tuberculosis in the United States. Epidemiol. Rev. *11*:79–98, 1989.
413. Riley, L. W., Arathoon, E., and Loverde, V. D.: The epidemiologic patterns of drug-resistant *Mycobacterium tuberculosis* infections: A community-based study. Am. Rev. Respir. Dis. *139*:1282–1285, 1989.
414. Riley, R. L.: Airborne transmission. *In* Johnson, J. E. (ed.): Rational Therapy and Control of Tuberculosis. Gainesville, University of Florida Press, 1970.
415. Rooney, J. J., Crocco, J. A., and Lyons, H. A.: Tuberculous pericarditis. Ann. Intern. Med. *72*:73–78, 1970.
416. Roper, W. H., and Waring, J. J.: Primary serofibrinous pleural effusion in military personnel. Am. Rev. Tuberc. *71*:616–634, 1955.
417. Rouillon, A., and Waaler, H.: Vaccination and epidemiological situation: A decision-making approach to the use of BCG. Adv. Tuberc. Res. *19*:64–126, 1976.
418. Ryder, R. W., Oxtoby, M. J., Mvula, M., et al.: Safety and immunogenicity of bacille Calmette-Guérin, diphtheria-tetanus-pertussis, and oral polio vaccines in newborn children in Zaire infected with human immunodeficiency virus type 1. J. Pediatr. *122*:697–702, 1993.
419. Sada, E., Aguilar, D., Torres, M., et al.: Detection of lipoarabinomannan as a diagnostic test for tuberculosis. J. Clin. Microbiol. *30*:2415–2418, 1992.
420. Salfinger, M., Crowle, A. J., and Reller, L. B.: Pyrazinamide and pyrazinoic acid activity against tubercle bacilli in cultured human macrophages and in the BACTEC system. J. Infect. Dis. *162*:201–207, 1990.
421. Salfinger, M., and Pfyfler, G. E.: The new diagnostic mycobacteriology laboratory. Eur. J. Clin. Microbiol. *13*:961–979, 1994.
422. Saltzman, S. J., and Feigin, R. D.: Tuberculous otitis media and mastoiditis. J. Pediatr. *79*:1004–1006, 1971.
423. Sassan-Morokro, M., DeCock, K. M., Ackah, A., et al.: Tuberculosis and HIV infection in children in Abidjon, Cote d'Ivoire. Trans. R. Soc. Trop. Med. Hyg. *88*:178–181, 1994.
424. Sathe, S. S., and Reichman, L. B.: Mycobacterial disease in patients infected with human immunodeficiency virus. Clin. Chest Med. *10*:445–463, 1989.
425. Sbarbaro, J. A.: Skin test antigens: An evaluation whose time has come. Am. Rev. Respir. Dis. *118*:1–5, 1978.
426. Sbarbaro, J. A.: Compliance: Inducements and enforcements. Chest *76*(Suppl.):750–756, 1979.
427. Schaaf, H. S., Beyers, N., Gie, R. P., et al.: Respiratory tuberculosis in childhood: The diagnostic value of clinical features and special investigations. Pediatr. Infect. Dis. J. *14*:189–194, 1995.
428. Schaaf, H. S., Gie, R. P., Beyers, N., et al. Tuberculosis in infants less than 3 months of age. Arch. Dis. Child. *69*:371–374, 1993.
429. Schaefer, G.: Tuberculosis in Obstetrics and Gynecology. Boston, MA, Little, Brown, 1956.
430. Schick, B., and Dolgin, J.: The influence of prednisone on the Mantoux reaction in children. Pediatrics *31*:856–859, 1963.
431. Schluger, N., Kinney, D., Harkin, T., et al.: Clinical utility of the polymerase chain reaction in the diagnosis of infections due to *Mycobacterium tuberculosis*. Chest *105*:1116–1121, 1994.
432. Schoen, E. J.: Spinal fluid chloride: A test 40 years past its time. J. A. M. A. *251*:37–38, 1984.
433. Schuit, K. E.: Miliary tuberculosis in children. Am. J. Dis. Child. *133*:583–585, 1979.
434. Schuit, K. E., and Powell, D. A.: Mycobacterial lymphadenitis in childhood. Am. J. Dis. Child. *132*:675–677, 1978.
435. Schwartz, P.: Lymph node tuberculosis: A decisive factor in pulmonary pathology. Arch. Pediatr. *74*:159–177, 201–218, 1957.
436. Seal, R. M. E., and Thomas, S. M. E.: Endobronchial tuberculosis in children. Lancet *2*:995–996, 1956.
437. Sehgal, V. N., and Wagh, S. A.: Cutaneous tuberculosis. Int. J. Dermatol. *29*:237–252, 1990.
438. Selwyn, P., Hartel, D., Lewis, V., et al.: A prospective study of the risk of tuberculosis among intravenous drug users with human immunodeficiency virus infection. N. Engl. J. Med. *320*:545–550, 1989.
439. Sepulveda, R. L., Burr, C., Ferrer, X., et al.: Booster effect of tuberculosis testing in healthy 6-year-old school children vaccinated with bacille Calmette-Guérin at birth in Santiago, Chile. Pediatr. Infect. Dis. J. *7*:578–582, 1988.
440. Sepulveda, R. L., Heiba, I. M., King, A., et al.: Evaluation of tuberculin reactivity in BCG-immunized siblings. Am. J. Respir. Crit. Care Med. *149*:620–624, 1994.
441. Sepulveda, R. L., Heiba, I. M., Navarrete, C., et al.: Tuberculin reactivity after newborn BCG immunization in mono- and dizygotic twins. Tubercle Lung Dis. *75*:138–143, 1994
442. Shafer, R., Small, P., Larkin, C., et al. Temporal trends and transmission patterns during the emergence of multidrug-resistant tuberculosis in New York City: A molecular epidemiologic assessment. J. Infect. Dis. *171*:170–176, 1995.
443. Shah, B. R., Santucci, K., Sinert, R., et al.: Acute isoniazid neurotoxicity in an urban hospital. Pediatrics *95*:700–704, 1995.
444. Shannon, F. B., Moore, M., Houkom, J. A., et al.: Multifocal cystic tuberculosis of bone. J. Bone Joint Surg. (Am.) *72*:1089–1092, 1990.
445. Shepard, W. E., Field, M. L., James, D. H., et al.: Transient appearance of intracranial tuberculomas during treatment of tuberculous meningitis. Pediatr. Infect. Dis. J. *5*:599–601, 1986.
446. Sheridan, P. H., Edman, J. B., and Starr, S. E.: Tuberculosis presenting as an orbital mass. Pediatrics *67*:874–875, 1981.
447. Shimokata, K., Kawachi, H., Kishumoto, H., et al.: Local cellular immunity in tuberculous pleurisy. Am. Rev. Respir. Dis. *126*:822–824, 1982.
448. Sibley, W. A., and O'Brien, J. L.: Intracranial tuberculomas: Review of clinical features and treatment. Neurology *6*:157–165, 1956.
449. Siddiqi, S. H., Hwangbo, C. C., Silcox, V., et al.: Rapid radiometric methods to detect and differentiate *Mycobacterium tuberculosis/M. bovis* from other mycobacterial species. Am. Rev. Respir. Dis. *130*:634–640, 1984.
450. Silverman, F. N.: Pulmonary calcification: Tuberculosis? Histoplasmosis? Am. J. Roentgenol. Radium Ther. *64*:747–764, 1950.
451. Singapore Tuberculosis Service/British Medical Research Council: Five-year follow-up of a clinical trial of three 6-month regimens of chemotherapy given intermittently in the continuation phase in the treatment of pulmonary tuberculosis. Am. Rev. Respir. Dis. *137*:1147–1150, 1988.
452. Sirinavin, S., Chotpitayasunondh, T., Suwanjutha, S., et al.: Efficacy of neonatal bacillus Calmette-Guérin vaccination against tuberculosis. Pediatr. Infect. Dis. J. *10*:359–365, 1991.
453. Sloan, J. B.: Papulonecrotic tuberculid in a 9-year-old American girl: Case report and review of the literature. Pediatr. Dermatol. *7*:191–195, 1990.
454. Slutkin, G., Schecter, G. F., and Hopewell, P. C.: The results of 9-month isoniazid-rifampin therapy for pulmonary tuberculosis under program conditions in San Francisco. Am. Rev. Respir. Dis. *138*:1622–1624, 1988.
455. Small, P., Hopewell, P., Singh, S., et al.: The epidemiology of tuberculosis in San Francisco: A population-based study using conventional and molecular methods. N. Engl. J. Med. *330*:1703–1709, 1994.
456. Small, P. M., Shafer, R. W., Hopewell, P. C., et al.: Exogenous reinfection with multidrug-resistant *Mycobacterium tuberculosis* in patients with advanced HIV infection. N. Engl. J. Med. *328*:1137–1144, 1993.
457. Smith, A. M., and Lattimer, J. K.: Genitourinary tract involvement in children with tuberculosis. N. Y. State J. Med. *73*:2325–2328, 1973.
458. Smith, D., Reeser, P., and Musa, S.: Does infection with environmental mycobacteria suppress the protective response to subsequent vaccination with BCG? Tubercle *66*:17–23, 1985.
459. Smith, K. C., Starke, J. R., Eisenach, K., et al.: Detection of *Mycobacterium tuberculosis* in clinical specimens from children using a polymerase chain reaction. Pediatrics *97*:155–160, 1996.
460. Smith, M. H. D.: The role of adrenal steroids in the treatment of tuberculosis. Pediatrics *22*:774–776, 1958.
461. Smith, M. H. D.: What about short course and intermittent chemotherapy for tuberculosis in children? Pediatr. Infect. Dis. *1*:298–303, 1982.
462. Smith, M. H. D.: Tuberculosis in children and adolescents. Clin. Chest Med. *10*:381–395, 1989.
463. Smith, M. H. D., and Matsaniotis, N.: Treatment of tuberculous pleural effusions with particular reference to adrenal corticosteroids. Pediatrics *22*:1074–1087, 1959.
464. Smith, M. H. D., and Teele, D. W.: Tuberculosis. *In* Remington, J. S., and Klein, J. O. (eds.): Infectious Diseases of the Fetus and Newborn. 3rd ed. Philadelphia, W. B. Saunders, 1990.
465. Snider, D. E., Jr., and Block, A. B.: Congenital tuberculosis. Tubercle *65*:81–82, 1984.
466. Snider, D. E., Jr., and Caras, G. J.: Isoniazid-associated hepatitis deaths: A review of available information. Am. Rev. Respir. Dis. *145*:494– 497, 1992.
467. Snider, D. E., Jr., Caras, G. J., and Kaplan, J. P.: Preventive therapy with isoniazid: Cost-effectiveness of different durations of therapy. J. A. M. A. *255*:1579–1583, 1986.
468. Snider, D. E., Jr., and Farer, L. S.: Preventive therapy for tuberculous infection: An intervention in need of improvement. Am. Rev. Respir. Dis. *130*:35–356, 1984.
469. Snider, D. E., Graczyk, J., Bek, E., et al.: Supervised six-months treatment of newly diagnosed pulmonary tuberculosis using isoniazid, rifampin, and pyrazinamide with and without streptomycin. Am. Rev. Respir. Dis. *130*:1091–1094, 1984.
470. Snider, D. E., Jr., Jones, W. D., and Good, R. C.: The usefulness of phage typing *Mycobacterium tuberculosis* isolates. Am. Rev. Respir. Dis. *130*:1095–1099, 1984.
471. Snider, D. E., Jr., Kelly, G. D., Cauthen, G. M. et al.: Infection and disease among contacts of tuberculosis cases with drug-resistant and drug-susceptible bacilli. Am. Rev. Respir. Dis. *132*:125–128, 1985.
472. Snider, D. E., Jr., and LaMontagne, J.: The neglected global tuberculosis problem: A report of the 1992 World Congress on Tuberculosis. J. Infect. Dis. *169*:1189–1196, 1994.
473. Snider, D. E., Jr., Layde, P. M., Johnson, M. W., et al.: Treatment of tuberculosis during pregnancy. Am. Rev. Respir. Dis. *122*:65–79, 1980.
474. Snider, D. E., Jr., and Powell, K. E.: Should women taking antituberculosis drugs breastfeed? Arch. Intern. Med. *144*:589–590, 1984.
475. Snider, W. R., Cohen, D., Reif, J. S., et al.: Tuberculin sensitivity in a high risk canine population. J. Epidemiol. *102*:185–190, 1975.
476. Spyridis, P., Sinaniotis, C., Papadea, I., et al.: Isoniazid liver injury during chemoprophylaxis in children. Arch. Dis. Child. *54*:65–67, 1979.
477. Stallworth, J. R., Brasfield, D. M., and Tiller, R. E.: Congenital miliary

tuberculosis proved by open lung biopsy specimen and successfully treated. Am. J. Dis. Child. *134*:320–321, 1980.
478. Stansberry, S. D.: Tuberculosis in infants and children. J. Thorac. Imag. *5*:17–27, 1990.
479. Starke, J. R.: Multidrug therapy for tuberculosis in children. Pediatr. Infect. Dis. J. *9*:785–793, 1990.
480. Starke, J. R.: Current chemotherapy for tuberculosis in children. Infect. Dis. Clin. North Am. *6*:215–238, 1992.
481. Starke, J. R., and Correa, A. G.: Management of mycobacterial infection and disease in children. Pediatr. Infect. Dis. J. *14*:455–470, 1995.
482. Starke, J. R., Jacobs, R., and Jereb, J.: Resurgence of tuberculosis in children. J. Pediatr. *120*:839–855, 1992.
483. Starke, J. R., and Taylor-Watts, K. T.: Six-month chemotherapy of intrathoracic tuberculosis in children. Am. Rev. Respir. Dis. *139*(Suppl.):A314, 1989.
484. Starke, J. R., and Taylor-Watts, K. T.: Tuberculosis in the pediatric population of Houston, Texas. Pediatrics *84*:28–35, 1989.
485. Starr, S., and Berkovich, S.: Effects of measles, gammaglobulin-modified measles and vaccine measles on the tuberculin test. N. Engl. J. Med. *270*:386–391, 1964.
486. Stead, W. W.: Pathogenesis of a first episode of chronic pulmonary tuberculosis in man: Recrudescence of residuals of the primary infection or exogenous reinfection? Am. Rev. Respir. Dis. *95*:729–745, 1967.
487. Stead, W. W., Kerby, G. R., Schlueter, D. P., et al.: Clinical spectrum of primary tuberculosis in adults. Ann. Intern. Med. *68*:731–744, 1968.
488. Stein, M. T., and Liang, D.: Clinical hepatotoxicity of isoniazid in children. Pediatrics *64*:499–505, 1979.
489. Steiner, M., Steiner, P., and Schmidt, H.: Primary drug-resistant tuberculosis in children: A continuing study of the incidence of disease caused by primarily drug-resistant organisms in children observed between the years 1965 and 1968 at the Kings County Medical Center of Brooklyn. Am. Rev. Respir. Dis. *102*:75–82, 1970.
490. Steiner, P., and Rao, M.: Drug-resistant tuberculosis in children. Semin. Pediatr. Infect. Dis. *4*:275–282, 1993.
491. Steiner, P., Rao, M., and Mitchell, M.: Primary drug-resistant tuberculosis in children: Correlation of drug-susceptibility patterns of matched patient and source-case strains of *Mycobacterium tuberculosis.* Am. J. Dis. Child. *139*:780–782, 1985.
492. Steiner, P., Rao, M., Victoria, M. S., et al.: Miliary tuberculosis in two infants after nursery exposure: Epidemiologic, clinical, and laboratory findings. Am. Rev. Respir. Dis. *113*:267–271, 1976.
493. Steiner, P., Rao, M., Victoria, M. S., et al.: Persistently negative tuberculin reactions: Their presence among children culture positive for *Mycobacterium tuberculosis*. Am. J. Dis. Child. *134*:747–750, 1980.
494. Stevens, D. L., and Everett, E. D.: Sequential computerized axial tomography in tuberculous meningitis. J. A. M. A. *239*:642, 1978.
495. Strang, J. I. G., Kakaza, H. H. S., Gibson, D. G., et al.: Controlled trial of prednisolone as adjunct in treatment of tuberculous constrictive pericarditis in Transkei. Lancet 2:1418–1422, 1987.
496. Stroebel, A. B., Daniel, T. M., Lau, J. H., et al.: Serologic diagnosis of bone and joint tuberculosis by an enzyme-linked immunosorbent assay. J. Infect. Dis. *146*:280–283, 1982.
497. Strom, L.: Experiments with radioactive Calmette BCG vaccine. Acta Tuberc. Scand. Suppl. 21, 1950.
498. Sumartojo, E.: When tuberculosis treatment fails: A social behavior account of patient adherence. Am. Rev. Respir. Dis. *147*:1311–1320, 1993.
499. Sumaya, C. V., Simek, M., and Smith, M. H. D.: Tuberculous meningitis in children during the isoniazid era. J. Pediatr. *87*:43–49, 1975.
500. Sunderam, G., McDonald, R. J., Maniatis, T., et al.: Tuberculosis as a manifestation of the acquired immunodeficiency syndrome (AIDS). J. A. M. A. *256*:362–366, 1986.
501. Swanson, D. S., and Starke, J. R.: Drug-resistant tuberculosis in pediatrics. Pediatr. Clin. North Am. *42*:553–581, 1995.
502. Sweany, H. C.: Studies on the pathogenesis of primary tuberculous infection. Am. Rev. Tuberc. *27*:559–588, 1933.
503. Tabrisky, J., Lindstrom, R. R., Peters, R., et al.: Tuberculous enteritis. Am. J. Gastroenterol. *63*:49–57, 1975.
504. Takiff, H., Salazar, L., Guerrero, C., et al.: Cloning and nucleotide sequence of *Mycobacterium tuberculosis gyrA* and *gryB* genes and detection of quinoline resistance mutations. Antimicrob. Agents Chemother. *38*:773–780, 1994.
505. Teeratkulpisarn, J., Lumbigagnon, P., Pairojkul, S., et al.: Cavitary tuberculosis in a young infant. Pediatr. Infect. Dis. J. *13*:545–546, 1994.
506. Telenti, A., Imboden, P., Marchesi, F., et al. Detection of rifampin-resistance mutations in *Mycobacterium tuberculosis*. Lancet *341*:647–650, 1993.
507. Telzak, E. E., Sepkowitz, K., Alpert, P., et al.: Multidrug-resistant tuberculosis in patients without HIV infection. N. Engl. J. Med. *333*:907–911, 1995.
508. tenDam, H. G.: Research on BCG vaccination. Adv. Tuberc. Res. *21*:79–106, 1984.
509. tenDam, H. G., Toman, K., Hitze, K. L., et al.: Present knowledge of immunization against tuberculosis. Bull. WHO *54*:255–269, 1976.
510. Teoh, R., Humphries, M. J., and Sister Gabriel O'Mahony: Symptomatic intracranial tuberculoma developing during treatment of tuberculosis: Report of 10 patients and review of the literature. Q. J. Med. *63*:449–460, 1987.
511. Terplan, K.: Anatomical studies on human tuberculosis. Am. Rev. Tuberc. *42*(Suppl.):3–176, 1940.
512. Thompson, W. J., Glassroth, J. L., Snider, D. E., Jr., et al.: The booster phenomenon in serial tuberculin testing. Am. Rev. Respir. Dis. *119*:587–597, 1979.
513. Tidjani, O., Amedome, A., and tenDam, H. G.: Protective effect of BCG vaccination of the newborn against childhood tuberculosis in an African community. Tubercle *67*:269–281, 1986.
514. Toppet, M., Malfroot, A., Derde, M. P., et al.: Corticosteroids in primary tuberculosis with bronchial obstruction. Arch. Dis. Child. *65*:1222–1226, 1990.
515. Traub, M., Colchester, A. C., Kingsley, D. P., et al.: Tuberculosis of the central nervous system. Q. J. Med. *53*:81–100, 1984.
516. Tsakalidis, D., Pratsidou, P., Hitoglou-Makedou, A., et al.: Intensive short course chemotherapy for treatment of Greek children with tuberculosis. Pediatr. Infect. Dis. J. *11*:1036–1042, 1992.
517. Tsukamura, M.: In vitro antituberculosis activity of a new antibacterial substance ofloxacin (DL8280). Am. Rev. Respir. Dis. *131*:348–351, 1985.
518. Tuberculosis in Children: Guidelines for diagnosis, prevention and treatment (Statement of the Scientific Committee of the International Union Against Tuberculosis and Lung Diseases). Bull. Int. Union Tuberc. Lung Dis. *66*:61–67, 1991.
519. Tuli, S. M.: Tuberculosis of the Spine. New Delhi, Amerind Publishing Co., 1975.
520. Turneer, M., VanNerom, E., Nyabenda, J., et al.: Determination of humoral immunoglobulins M and G directed against mycobacterial antigen 60 failed to diagnose primary tuberculosis and mycobacterial adenitis in children. Am. J. Respir. Crit. Care Med. *150*:1508–1512, 1994.
521. Tyler, B., Bennett, H., and Kim, J.: Intracranial tuberculomas in a child: Computed tomographic scan diagnosis and nonsurgical management. Pediatrics *71*:952–954, 1983.
522. Udani, P. M., Parekh, U. C., and Dastur, D. K.: Neurological and related syndromes in CNS tuberculosis: Clinical features and pathogenesis. J. Neurol. Sci. *14*:341–357, 1971.
523. Uragoda, C. G.: Histamine poisoning in tuberculous patients after ingestion of tuna fish. Am. Rev. Respir. Dis. *121*:157–159, 1980.
524. Ussery, X. T., Valway, S. E., McKenna, M., et al.: Epidemiology of tuberculosis among children in the United States. Pediatr. Infect. Dis. J. *15*:697–704, 1996.
525. Ustvedt, H. J.: The relationship between primary and adult tuberculosis. Br. J. Tuberc. *40*:85–92, 1946.
526. Vallejo, J., Ong, L., and Starke, J.: Clinical features, diagnosis and treatment of tuberculosis in infants. Pediatrics *94*:1–7, 1994.
527. Vallejo, J., Ong, L. T., and Starke, J. R.: Tuberculous osteomyelitis of the long bones in children. Pediatr. Infect. Dis. J. *14*:542–546, 1995.
528. Vallejo, J. G., and Starke, J. R.: Tuberculosis and pregnancy. Clin. Chest Med. *13*:693–707, 1992.
529. Vanderhoof, J. A., and Ament, M. E.: Fatal hepatic necrosis due to isoniazid chemoprophylaxis in a 15-year old girl. J. Pediatr. *88*:867–868, 1976.
530. Van Zwanenberg, D.: Influence of the number of bacilli on the development of tuberculous disease in children. Am. Rev. Respir. Dis. *82*:31–44, 1960.
531. Varudkar, B. L.: Short-course chemotherapy for tuberculosis in children. Indian J. Pediatr. *52*:593– 597, 1985.
532. Venkataraman, P., Menon, N. K., Nair, N. G. B., et al.: Classification of subjects as slow or rapid inactivators or isoniazid based on the ratio of urinary excretion of acetylisoniazid to isoniazid. Tubercle *53*:84–91, 1972.
533. Versfeld, G. A., Soloman, A.: A diagnostic approach to tuberculosis of bones and joints. J. Bone Joint Surg. *64*:446–449, 1982.
534. Visudhiphan, P., and Chiemchanya, S.: Tuberculous meningitis in children: Treatment with isoniazid and rifampin for twelve months. J. Pediatr. *114*:875–879, 1989.
535. Waeker, N. J., Jr., and Connor, J. D.: Central nervous system tuberculosis in children: A review of 30 cases. Pediatr. Infect. Dis. J. *9*:539–543, 1990.
536. Walker, C. H. M.: Pulmonary primary tuberculosis in childhood. Lancet *1*:218–224, 1955.
537. Wallace, K., and Cohen, A. S.: Tuberculous arthritis: Report of two cases with review of biopsy and synovial fluid findings. Am. J. Med. *61*:277–282, 1976.
538. Wallace, R. C., Burton, E. M., Barrett, F. F., et al.: Intracranial tuberculosis in children: CT appearance and clinical outcome. Pediatr. Radiol. *21*:241–246, 1991.
539. Wallgren, A.: On contagiousness of childhood tuberculosis. Acta Paediatr. *22*:229–234, 1937.
540. Wallgren, A.: Pulmonary Tuberculosis in Adults and Children. New York, Thomas Nelson and Sons, 1939.
541. Wallgren, A.: Tuberculous heart disease. Acta Med. Scand. *196*(Suppl.): 132–144, 1947.
542. Wallgren, A.: The time-table of tuberculosis. Tubercle *29*:245–251, 1948.
543. Weinstein, J., Barrett, C., Baltimore, R., et al.: Nosocomial transmission of tuberculosis from a hospital visitor on a pediatrics ward. Pediatr. Infect. Dis. J. *14*:232–234, 1995.
544. Weis, S., Slocum, P., Blais, F., et al.: The effects of directly observed therapy on the rates of drug resistance and relapse in tuberculosis. N. Engl. J. Med. *330*:1179–1184, 1994.

545. Werhane, M. J., Snukst-Torbeck, G., and Schraufnagel, D. E.: The tuberculosis clinic. Chest *96*:815–818, 1989.
546. Whalen, C., Horsburgh, C., Hom, D., et al.: Accelerated course of human immunodeficiency virus infection after tuberculosis. Am. J. Respir. Crit. Care Med. *151*:129–135, 1995.
547. Whitener, D. R.: Tuberculous brain abscess. Arch. Neurol. *35*:148–155, 1978.
548. Wijsmuller, G.: The problem of comparing tuberculins for potency. Bull. W. H. O. *45*:633–648, 1971.
549. Wilkins, E. G. L.: Tuberculous peritonitis: Diagnostic value of the ascitic/blood glucose value. Tubercle *65*:47–52, 1984.
550. Witrak, B. J., and Ellis, G. T.: Intracranial tuberculosis: Manifestations on computerized tomography. South. Med. J. *78*:386–392, 1985.
551. Wright, F. W., and Hamilton, W. S.: Miliary tuberculosis twice. Br. J. Dis. Chest *68*:210–212, 1974.
552. Zarabi, M., Sane, S., and Girdany, B. R.: Chest roentgenogram in the early diagnosis of tuberculous meningitis in children. Am. J. Dis. Child. *121*:389–392, 1971.
553. Zhang, Y.: Genetic basis of isoniazid resistance of *Mycobacterium tuberculosis*. Rev. Microbiol. *144*:143–150, 1993.
554. Zhang, Y., Heym, B., Allen, B., et al.: Catalase-peroxidase gene and isoniazid resistance of *Mycobacterium tuberculosis*. Nature *358*:591–593, 1992.
555. Zinneman, H. H., and Hall, W. H.: Transient tuberculous meningitis. Am. Rev. Respir. Dis. *114*:1185–1188, 1976.
556. Zitrin, C. M., and Lincoln, E. M.: Initial tuberculous infection due to drug-resistant organisms: With a review of the world literature on initial infection due to isoniazid-resistant tubercle bacilli. J. Pediatr. *58*:219–223, 1961.
557. Zweiman, B., Pappano, J. E., Jr., and Hildrath, E. A.: Effect of influenza vaccine administration on tuberculin skin sensitivity. Dis. Chest. *52*:46–49, 1967.

102

OTHER MYCOBACTERIA

J. Thomas Cross, Jr., and Richard F. Jacobs

The definition of mycobacteria other than tubercle bacilli is quite confusing. Ernest Runyon, in his address to the International Conference on Atypical Mycobacteria, probably defined them best: "Tubercle bacilli include *Mycobacterium tuberculosis, Mycobacterium bovis,* and *Mycobacterium africanum.* Together with *Mycobacterium microti* (not pathogenic for humans), these organisms constitute the tubercle bacillus complex."[107] Any mycobacterium not listed in this group is considered to be in the "other" grouping. Mycobacteria other than tuberculosis and leprosy were not recognized as causes of diseases in humans until the 1950s.[132] The incidence of disease due to these organisms remained fairly stable until the AIDS epidemic began in the 1980s. The most common forms of the disease are chronic pulmonary disease resembling tuberculosis (occurring mainly in adults), cervical adenopathy in children, skin and soft tissue infection, and disseminated disease in immunocompromised persons.[96] In the mid-1980s, the incidence of infections due to atypical mycobacteria increased markedly. The incidence likely has increased because of the increased prevalence of immunocompromised patients (AIDS, transplant, etc.), and the microbiologic methods for cultivating these organisms have improved significantly in the last 30 years.[154, 156]

EPIDEMIOLOGY

The atypical mycobacteria are ubiquitous in nature. They are found in soil, animals, milk,[37] and food. Of importance in some hospital-acquired infections or infections in immunocompromised hosts is the presence of the organisms in common tap water.[14, 48, 86, 125] Exposure to environments (especially soil) that colonize these organisms seems important for acquisition of disease in children. Organisms commonly found in the soil include *M. scrofulaceum, M. flavescens, M. avium-intracellulare, M. gastri, M. terrae, M. fortuitum,* and *M. chelonae.* Water is an important source for all of the previously named organisms and also for *M. kansasii, M. marinum, M. gordonae,* and *M. xenopi.* In contrast, humans are the only known reservoirs for *M. tuberculosis.* In a survey from the Centers for Disease Control and Prevention, 35 per cent of mycobacteria isolated in laboratories were nontuberculous.[43] *M. avium-intracellulare* accounted for 66 per cent of the nontuberculous isolates, followed by *M. fortuitum* (19 per cent), *M. kansasii* (9 per cent), and *M. scrofulaceum* (6 per cent). These data were collected in 1980 before the present AIDS epidemic and before the rapid increase in the number and types of immunocompromised patients; therefore, the current rates are likely much higher.

Geography also appears to have some bearing on the prevalence of these infections. The southeastern United States has much higher rates in children than are seen in the Northeast or Northwest. *M. avium* complex (MAC) was seen most commonly along coastal borders of the United States and states bordering Canada. Highest rates were seen in Hawaii (10.9 cases per 100,000 population), Connecticut (8.9 cases per 100,000 population), and Florida (8.4 cases per 100,000 population). High rates, however, also were seen in Kansas and the desert Southwest, demonstrating the widespread nature of this organism in causing disease. In contrast, *M. kansasii* was seen most commonly in the midwestern United States and almost never was seen in parts of the southeastern United States.[43] States with rates of *M. kansasii* higher than 0.75 cases per 100,000 included Missouri, Illinois, Kentucky, Indiana, Kansas, Nebraska, Louisiana, Texas, Arizona, and Florida. North Carolina, a state with one of the highest rates of *M. avium* complex (>4.8 cases per 100,000 population), had very few cases of *M. kansasii* (0.00 to 0.25 cases per 100,000 population). *M. marinum* was isolated frequently from coastal areas, whereas *M. xenopi* was scattered across the United States, with 50 per cent of cases being found in just three states (Connecticut, Wisconsin, and California). For all the nontuberculous species, males and rural residents also had a much higher incidence of infection.[113] The use of these rates for determining disease patterns cannot be extrapolated easily, however. The number of mycobacterial isolates easily could be skewed by the presence of multiple isolates from a single patient or may just represent colonization. These rates, however, can help predict which species of nontuberculous mycobacterium is most likely to be encountered in a particular geographic region while the physician awaits final identification and sensitivity testing on an isolated nontuberculous organism.

TABLE 102–1. Characteristics of Slow-Growing Pathogenic Mycobacteria

Organism	Growth Present °C 25	37	45	Growth Rate (Days)	Niacin	Nitrate Reduction	Pigment Dark	Pigment Light	Growth 5% NaCl
M. tuberculosis	–	+	–	12–28	+	+	–	–	–
M. bovis	–	+	–	21–40	–	–	–	–	–
Photochromogens									
Runyon group I									
M. kansasii	+	+	–	10–21	–	+	–	+	–
M. marinum	+	±	–	7–14	–	–	–	+	–
Scotochromogens									
Runyon group II									
M. scrofulaceum	+	+	–	10–28	–	–	+	+	–
M. szulgai	+	+	–	12–28	–	+	+	+	–
M. gordonae	+	+	–	10–28	–	–	+	+	–
Nonchromogens									
Runyon group III									
M. avium	+	+	+	10–21	–	–	–	–	–
M. intracellulare	+	+	–	10–21	–	–	–	–	–
M. ulcerans	–	–	–	28–60	–	–	–	–	?
M. xenopi	–	+	–	14–28	–	–	–	–	–

The site of isolation from the human source can be helpful in determining the type of mycobacteria that may be involved in the disease process. *M. avium* and *M. intracellulare* are responsible for lymphadenitis, particularly in children. These two organisms also are responsible for pulmonary disease and disseminated disease to bones and occasionally to the meninges. *M. kansasii* is associated most commonly with infections of pulmonary origin and disseminated lesions in adults; rarely, it is associated with adenitis and skin granuloma in children. *M. scrofulaceum* is responsible also for lymphadenitis in children, and *M. marinum* is responsible for skin granuloma and ulcers after exposure to certain saltwater beaches, swimming pools, and tropical fish tanks. The rapid growers (*M. fortuitum* and *M. chelonae*) are responsible rarely for pulmonary and disseminated disease in adults and children.

A familial immune defect predisposing to disseminated atypical mycobacterial infection in childhood has been reported.[76] The six children studied had disseminated infection with atypical mycobacterium without obvious evidence of immunodeficiency. Clinical and immunologic features seem to indicate that these children acquire infections similarly to Lsh/Ity/Bcg–susceptible mice. Studies that are ongoing to determine the defect may provide insights into the mechanisms by which certain children are susceptible to mycobacterial infections while others exposed to the same environmental factors do not develop disseminated disease.

MICROBIOLOGY

Runyon and Timpe in their monumental work on atypical mycobacteria suggested a useful classification system based upon three characteristics of the organisms: pigment production, rate of growth, and colonial characteristics.[106, 108, 132] The four groups are group I—photochromogens, which produce bright yellow to red pigment in the presence of light; group II—scotochromogens, which produce yellow to orange pigment in the dark; group III—nonphotochromogens, which are nonpigment producers; and group IV—rapid growers, which grow generally in less than a week. Kubica, in 1978, published an updated version of Runyon's classification, and it became useful for many years.[70] After this, a more "simplified" classification was proposed based on the growth rates of the organisms alone.[154]

The atypical mycobacteria today still are differentiated by most clinical laboratories on the basis of a variety of morphologic, physiologic, and biochemical characteristics (Tables 102–1 and 102–2). The difficulty with identifying many of these organisms is their slow growth rates with standard techniques. It is useful to begin sensitivity testing as soon as an organism is cultivated and felt to be the pathogen responsible, because it can take several months for proper identification and susceptibility testing to be determined. Serologic tests can be useful for identifying some of the organisms.[31, 71, 106, 133, 138, 151, 154, 156] However, in clinical medicine, they are rarely of value in diagnosing individual patients. A study using humoral immunoglobulins against mycobacterial antigens failed to diagnose tuberculosis or nontuberculous adenitis in children.[134]

Blood cultures for mycobacteria are performed best using the Isolator lysis-centrifugation system (Wampole Laboratories, Cranbury, NJ) or the radiometric BACTEC 13A blood culture bottle (Becton-Dickenson Diagnostic Instrument Systems, Cockeysville, MD).[1, 63, 64] Blood collected in ethylenediaminetetraacetic acid or coagulated blood is not acceptable. Body fluids, such as cerebrospinal fluid, pleural fluids, and peritoneal fluids, can be inoculated directly into BACTEC or

TABLE 102–2. Characteristics of the Rapid Growers

Runyon Group IV	Optimum Temperature	Growth Rate	Niacin	Nitrate Reduction	Growth 5% NaCl
M. fortuitum	37° C	3–7 days	–	+	+
M. abscessus	37° C	3–7 days	–	–	+
M. chelonae	37° C	3–7 days	–	–	–

Septi-Chek (Becton-Dickinson) broth, particularly if only small volumes are available. Gene probes became commercially available in the late 1980s. These involve DNA probes complementary to species-specific sequences of rRNA for the identification of *M. tuberculosis*, MAC, *M. gordonae*, and *M. kansasii* (AccuProbe; Gen-Probe, San Diego, CA).[45] Polymerase chain reaction (PCR) has been evaluated for the routine detection of *M. tuberculosis* in the clinical laboratory and compared with fluorochrome smear and culture. Two large studies were published that compared PCR with the standard technique and found that the sensitivity of PCR was 84 per cent in both studies.[24, 41] PCR testing offered by commercial laboratories at the present is not approved by the Food and Drug Administration for use as an in vitro diagnostic test. The sensitivity and specificity for this test vary widely between laboratories.[94]

MANIFESTATIONS OF NONTUBERCULOUS MYCOBACTERIA IN CHILDREN

Lymphadenitis

Lymphadenitis is the most common manifestation of atypical mycobacterial infection in children. It also rarely can occur in adults.[33, 75, 81] All nodes in the cervical chain can be affected, but the nodes of the submandibular region appear to be most commonly involved.[35] The parotid gland also can be affected.[78] The differential diagnosis frequently centers on deciding if a malignant process versus a nonmalignant process is present. Nonmalignant processes to consider include mononucleosis, bacterial adenitis, cat-scratch disease, toxoplasmosis, and *M. tuberculosis* infection. Most mycobacterial cases of lymphadenitis are due to the nontuberculous organisms. However, the clinician also must consider the possibility of *M. tuberculosis*.[26] There are no clinical features to help the clinician discern between the nontuberculous mycobacteria and tuberculosis. Reports postulate the use of histopathology to help differentiate between atypical and tuberculous infections.[98] In this retrospective study, the findings of ill-defined (nonpalisading) granulomas, irregular or serpiginous granulomas, a predominantly nonspecific granulomatous response, predominantly sarcoid-like granulomas, or lack of significant caseation were seen more commonly with nontuberculous lymphadenitis. Additionally, the nontuberculous infections had neutrophils predominantly in the center of the necrosis compared with the tuberculous infections, in which neutrophils were scattered throughout the specimen. A prospective study looking at these findings has not been published to date. Other authors have not noted similar patterns.[9]

In a Canadian study, the rate of atypical mycobacterium as a cause of lymphadenitis was 1.21 cases per 100,000 children compared with 0.3 cases per 100,000 children due to tuberculosis.[117] Authors from San Diego report a marked increase in the number of infections in children.[99] Other authors around the world have reported a markedly increased incidence in infection with these organisms in immunocompetent children.[42] In one study, the incidence increased from 1 case in 1987 to 1990 to 85 cases in 1991 to 1993.[74] In the large study compiled by Lincoln and Gilbert involving 243 children, more than 50 per cent were younger than 3 years of age and 80 per cent were younger than 5 years of age.[80] In contrast, one study showed that the mean age had increased to 5.2 years.[148] Most patients have no systemic symptoms and normal chest roentgenograms; other laboratory studies generally are unhelpful. Mean duration of swelling is about 6 weeks. Cervical nodes are the nodes most commonly affected in children. Infections mainly are due to *M. avium-intracellulare* and *M. scrofulaceum*. A large prospective study spanning 32 years from 1958 to 1990 showed that MAC has become the predominant etiologic agent compared with *M. scrofulaceum* from earlier in the study.[153] Case reports involving *M. fortuitum* also have been published.[104] Five immunocompetent children were diagnosed with lymphadenitis due to *M. haemophilum* in Australia.[5]

Usefulness of mycobacterial antigens in skin testing for the diagnosis of atypical mycobacteria versus tuberculous lymphadenitis is controversial. The use of purified protein derivative (PPD)-B (*M. intracellulare*), PPD-Y (*M. kansasii*), PPD-G (*M. scrofulaceum*), and PPD-T (*M. tuberculosis*) was compared to discern if children with active lymphadenitis due to the atypical mycobacteria could be distinguished from those with tuberculosis.[59] Patients with confirmed nontuberculous adenitis were six times more likely to have greater than 10 mm induration to PPD-B than were children with negative culture/biopsy results. In all groups, except those with confirmed *M. tuberculosis*, the responses to PPD-T were significantly smaller compared with those to the nontuberculous mycobacterial antigens. The results of the study seem to indicate that the use of the nontuberculous mycobacterial antigens could be useful in diagnosing mycobacterial cervical adenopathy. However, the specificity for nontuberculous organisms is unknown.

Needle aspiration of an affected node can be a valuable diagnostic tool. Cultures for bacterial and mycobacterial etiologies should be sought. Recovery rates for cervical lymphadenitis range from 60 to 88 per cent.[7, 12, 62, 158] The aspirate should be inoculated onto aerobic and anaerobic media as well as Sabouraud agar and mycobacterial media (Löwenstein-Jensen slants or Middlebrook media). The use of the BACTEC system can be very helpful. Mycobacteria can be isolated as early as 12 to 17 days after inoculation.[121]

The best treatment for atypical mycobacterium causing lymphadenitis is complete excision of the involved lymph node.[137] Incision and drainage without excision result in a high rate of secondary drainage, requiring subsequent excision of the remaining tissue for cure.[4, 110, 115]

AIDS and Atypical Mycobacteria

Surveys have noted an increasing rate of nontuberculous infection in children with AIDS.[58] About 6 per cent of adults and 4 per cent of children with AIDS reported to the Centers for Disease Control and Prevention had disseminated MAC infection as their AIDS-defining disease.[17] Autopsy studies show that MAC infection is present in 20 to 50 per cent of HIV-infected patients.[102, 147, 150] MAC was the most commonly isolated nontuberculous mycobacteria. *M. kansasii* and *M. scrofulaceum* were found in one case each. In adult studies, the incidence of infection due to *M. kansasii* and *M. scrofulaceum* also is quite low.[34, 57] More than 70 per cent of the children with MAC and AIDS had evidence of disseminated disease. Almost all had CD4 counts less than 100 cells/mm^3. Clinical findings included failure to maintain growth curves, anorexia, fever, abdominal pain, and anemia. Median age at diagnosis was 46 months with a median time between symptom onset and positive culture of 9 months. Once these patients were diagnosed with nontuberculous mycobacteria infection, they survived less than 10 months. Blood cultures have a 90 to 95 per cent sensitivity in detecting disseminated MAC in adult patients with AIDS.[51]

M. genavense has been shown to cause infection in children with HIV.[93] The children presented with fever, abdominal cramps, and diarrhea. CD4 lymphocytes were less than 400/mm³. The organism was found in numerous stool samples and lymph node biopsies. Multiple-drug regimens including amikacin, ethambutol, rifampin, and clarithromycin may be useful in treating this infection.

Clarithromycin and azithromycin have been utilized extensively in the adult population for the treatment of atypical mycobacteria. Clarithromycin, due to its liquid form, has become available therapy for many infections in pediatric patients, including otitis media, pharyngitis, and skin infections.[67] Many pediatric specialists also recommend these agents for the treatment of susceptible atypical mycobacterial infections in children with AIDS. The dose of clarithromycin recommended for disseminated MAC is 30 mg/kg divided every 12 hours, to a maximum daily dose of 2 g. The macrolide usually is combined with another agent (ethambutol 15/mg/kg/day, with a maximum dose of 2.5 g/day, or rifabutin, 300 mg total daily dose for adults).[78] The use of rifabutin for prophylaxis has been recommended based on adult studies in an attempt to delay and prevent MAC bacteremia in adults with CD4 cell counts less than 100 cells/mm³.[135] Use of agents for mycobacterial prophylaxis in children is not recommended routinely at this time.

Pulmonary Infections

Reviews from the late 1970s showed that pulmonary disease due to atypical mycobacteria most commonly was due to *M. kansasii* and MAC.[22, 44, 105] Infection due to MAC most commonly occurred during the sixth decade compared with infection due to *M. kansasii,* which occurred in individuals a decade younger. Men most commonly were affected in ratios as high as 4 to 1. Chronic obstructive pulmonary disease as noted by roentgenographic findings was found in 50 to 60 per cent of patients with atypical mycobacterial pulmonary infections. Bullous lung disease was seen in 24 to 39 per cent. The lobar distribution and severity of disease were similar between the atypical mycobacterial agents and *M. tuberculosis* with one exception: *M. kansasii* was much more prone to produce unilateral disease. This occurred in *M. kansasii* nearly 60 per cent of the time compared with 35 per cent of infections due to MAC or *M. tuberculosis*. Typically, disease begins in the posterior portions of the upper lobes. Progression to cavitary disease occurred in 87 per cent of patients with *M. tuberculosis* and MAC infections and 96 per cent of patients with *M. kansasii* infection.

Hilar and mediastinal adenopathy were uncommon, particularly with MAC (4 per cent) and *M. kansasii* (0.5 per cent). Pleural effusions were rare, occurring in 6 per cent of patients with MAC and 4 per cent with *M. kansasii*. Treatment at that time generally involved three to four courses of drug therapy including regimens of isonicotinic acid hydrazide, *p*-aminosalicylic acid, streptomycin, and rifampin. The American Thoracic Society recommends a four-drug regimen for MAC pulmonary infection in adults: isoniazid (300 mg), rifampin (600 mg), ethambutol (25 mg/kg for 2 months, then 15 mg/kg), and streptomycin (0.5 to 1.0 g five times each week for 8 to 12 weeks, then 0.5 to 1.0 g two or three times each week for 3 months, as tolerated).[142] Drugs are administered for 18 to 24 months, with a minimum of 12 months of culture negativity required on therapy. A previous clinical investigation revealed success rates between 25 and 80 per cent, with the best response rate using a three-drug regimen of ethambutol, ethionamide, and cycloserine.[39] Resectional surgery appeared to have poor outcomes. For *M. kansasii* pulmonary infection, the American Thoracic Society recommendations include isoniazid (300 mg/day), ethambutol (15 mg/kg/day), and rifampin (600 mg/day) for 18 months for adults.

Patients with cystic fibrosis have been noted to have an increased incidence of infection with nontuberculous mycobacteria. Prevalence rates from 2 to 20 per cent have been reported in the early 1990s.[3, 52, 53, 66] Organisms most commonly found are MAC, *M. kansasii, M. fortuitum,* and *M. chelonae*. Bacterial contamination, particularly with *Pseudomonas aeruginosa,* of the acid-fast bacilli cultures from cystic fibrosis patients has been a major problem, making it more difficult to isolate mycobacterium.[119] Another confounding problem is the difficulty in discerning infection from colonization in cystic fibrosis patients.[66] The American Thoracic Society recommends roentgenographic changes, isolation of multiple colonies of the same species, and the absence of other potential pathogens as criteria for the diagnosis of pathogenic infection with nontuberculous mycobacteria.[2] This is even more difficult in the setting of chronic lung disease seen in cystic fibrosis patients. Kilby and associates[66] suggest that repeated isolation of nontuberculous mycobacterium associated with pulmonary cavities or infiltrates that do not improve with aggressive standard antibacterial treatment could indicate active mycobacterial disease in patients with cystic fibrosis.

M. xenopi has been described in adults as a cause of infection of the pulmonary tract.[118] Mean age of infection was 62 years and occurred in a mainly Canadian population. Eighty-six per cent of the patients had underlying pulmonary pathology, including chronic obstructive pulmonary disease, previous pulmonary tuberculosis, carcinoma of the lung, sarcoidosis, and cystic fibrosis.

M. simiae has been isolated in adults with underlying pulmonary abnormalities.[8, 69] *M. simiae* is the most drug-resistant of all the nontuberculous mycobacteria. Some isolates are resistant to all drugs tested.

M. szulgai has been described in several case series as a cause of lung disease.[85, 145] Disease occurred in elderly white men and resembled chronic tuberculosis. Therapeutic regimens effective against *M. avium* appeared to provide good clinical outcomes.

Skin Infections

Mycobacterium marinum

M. marinum is photochromogenic and was identified as a pathogen in fish in 1926 by Aronson.[80] The skin lesions usually occur secondarily to light trauma (abrasions) in swimming pools or other bodies of water when the surfaces of the pools are colonized with *M. marinum*.[30, 90] Fish tanks also have been implicated and usually involve a finger.[130] Most cases occur in children between the ages of 10 and 16 years. The most common sites are the elbows, knees, and ankles. Cooler superficial portions of the body most commonly are affected. Other exposed body areas can be involved, depending upon what part of the body has made contact with the surface containing the mycobacterium (e.g., the nose in divers).[91]

The incubation period from exposure to formation of a small indurated area that ulcerates generally is 3 weeks. The lesion then crusts and forms a granuloma with a small crater. The lesions are painless usually and resolve in several months; occasionally, they can last longer. Unlike other mycobacterial diseases, regional nodes are not involved.

Infection with this organism usually is benign. A main consequence, however, is that patients with infection due to *M. marinum* frequently will have conversion of their PPD-T to positive.[80] The natural reservoir for *M. marinum*, which requires a cool incubator (32° C), is in fish and other cold-blooded animals. Generally, only small numbers of organisms may be isolated in some granulomas.

M. marinum treatment modalities have been successful with rifampin and ethambutol.[136, 155] One report showed good results with rifampin alone.[36] An accompanying editorial, however, cautioned against the use of rifampin alone and recommended using rifampin with ethambutol.[15] Duration of therapy in the literature varies from several weeks to 18 months. In general, response to therapy is rapid, and treatment should be continued for 4 to 6 weeks after clinical resolution.[36]

Mycobacterium ulcerans

MacCallum[84] reported the first cases of disease due to *M. ulcerans* in 1948. Most cases since have occurred in remote, tropical, or subtropical areas of the world, including parts of Africa and Australia.[83, 103] In a 1-year period, 23 cases of Buruli ulcers due to *M. ulcerans* occurred in Lambarene (Gabon).[16] Reports also have been made in Mexico.[80] The natural reservoir for *M. ulcerans* is unknown, although one report suggests the spines of a tall prickly grass known as *Echinocloa pyrimidalis*.[123] The lesions due to *M. ulcerans* occur mainly on the cooler superficial portions of the body. Patients harboring this organism are in otherwise good health without underlying immunodeficiency.[23] Scraping of the skin by thorns or pieces of wood has been implicated as the route of inoculation in many of the cases. The organism is very fastidious, with growth seen only between 30° C and 35° C.

The incubation period for this painless infection also is about 3 weeks. Regional lymphadenitis is rare with this organism. The infection has three distinct stages, and knowing them can be helpful in diagnosis and treatment. The disease begins as a hard, mobile nodule. It frequently is associated with pruritus and in Zaire is termed *mputa matadi* (the itching stone). This is known as the preulcerative stage.

In some patients, the infection resolves on its own, but in others, it progresses to the ulcerative stage. In contrast to *M. marinum*, in which the lesions are relatively short-lived and do not progress past the ulcerative stage, the lesions of *M. ulcerans* usually last 6 to 9 months and frequently can progress, leading to deformities of limbs that may require amputation.[80] The organisms can be isolated in large numbers from the periphery of the ulcers adjacent to normal tissues. This again contrasts with infection seen with *M. marinum*, in which very few organisms are found in the lesions.

The infection generally involves the subcutaneous adipose tissue and leads to areas of fat necrosis. This then proceeds to overlying necrosis of the adjacent skin. The lesions can grow enormous, sometimes involving a complete limb. Even though numerous organisms are seen in the progressing edge of the infection, little evidence is seen of cellular immune response. Additionally, anergy to skin reagents prepared from *M. ulcerans* (Burulin) frequently is seen at this stage.[124] Finally, the next stage, called the reactive phase, is reached. Cellular infiltrates with granuloma formation occur in the lesion. The number of organisms in the lesion decreases dramatically, and the patient develops a positive skin test reaction to the Burulin. Infection with *M. ulcerans* also can cause conversion of a patient's PPD response to positive but only in about 50 per cent of cases.[23] Finally, healing may take place but with fibrosis in its wake.

Treatment of infections due to *M. ulcerans* is anecdotal at best. Treatment choices are based on the stage of infection. Lesions in the preulcerative stage are treated best with excision and primary closure.[46] Successful therapy in the anergic progressive stage is felt to be the most difficult and involves appropriate antimycobacterial therapy for the infection. Success has been reported using both isonicotinic acid hydrazide and streptomycin or diaminodiphenylsulfone and oxytetracycline combinations,[23] as well as sulfamethoxazole, rifampin, minocycline,[122] and clofazimine.[83] In the final stage, healing should be promoted with as little deformity or loss of function as possible with the use of skin grafting and splinting and the excision of fibrous tissue.[46, 103] Disseminated infection in an immunocompetent child has been described with the development of multifocal osteomyelitis.[54]

Other Mycobacteria in Skin Disease

M. haemophilum has produced painful subcutaneous nodules in immunocompromised patients, particularly those with renal transplants.[32, 152] Additionally, *M. haemophilum* has produced disseminated disease, including bacteremia, osteomyelitis, and pulmonary disease in immunocompromised patients.[128] *M. chelonae* has been found to be a cause of disseminated cutaneous infection.[140] Steroid use is the predisposing factor for infection due to this organism. *M. fortuitum* has been implicated in cutaneous lesions in a child involved in a motor scooter accident, with the subsequent development of lesions at the site of knee lacerations; he also developed regional adenopathy of the inguinal nodes.[116] *M. fortuitum-chelonae* complex has been responsible for superficial skin abscesses in children.[11] *M. fortuitum* in adult studies also has been implicated in severe infections in immunocompromised hosts; these infections usually are rapidly disseminating, with high mortality.[152] *M. avium* has been isolated from an eyelid abscess with drainage.[114] Treatment of cutaneous disease due to these organisms is difficult at best. Four- or five-drug therapy has been tried but with poor results.

ORGANISMS SEEN IN CHILDREN

Specific organisms and treatment guidelines are discussed in the following sections. Table 102–3 provides a quick guide to some of the more commonly used antimycobacterial agents.

Mycobacterium avium-intracellulare Complex

MAC consists of *M. avium* and *M. intracellulare.* These organisms are slow-growing, obligate aerobes that require 2 to 6 weeks for colony formation on solid media. Colonies usually are smooth but may be rough and can be transparent or opaque. These organisms will grow on routine bacterial media, but growth is achieved best using selective mycobacterial media, such as Löwenstein-Jensen medium or Middlebrook 7K10 and 7K11 agar. Nucleic acid hybridization probes using target sequences of ribosomal RNA are commercially available for rapid identification of clinical isolates.[79, 92] MAC infection is diagnosed most commonly by culture of blood or bone marrow.

M. avium was recognized in 1890 as the causative agent of disease in chickens.[152] *M. intracellulare* became designated in 1967 and at the time was difficult to distinguish routinely from *M. avium*, thus the designation of *M. avium-intracellulare.* Today, with the use of DNA probes, most seroagglutination types have been discerned between the two groups. *M. avium* is the most common nontuberculous mycobacterium causing disease in humans. Isolates found from environmental sources are more likely to be *M. intracellulare.* Both of these

TABLE 102–3. Antimycobacterial Agents*

Drug	Dosage	Form
Amikacin (A)	15–20 mg/kg/day divided q 8 hours	IV or IM
Azithromycin (Z)	500 mg bid (adults/adolescents); 10–12 mg/kg/day (children)	PO
Cefoxitin (X)	80–160 mg/kg/day divided q 4–6 hours	IV or IM
Ciprofloxacin (C)	20–30 mg/kg/day divided q 12 hours (adults only in U.S.)	PO or IV
Clarithromycin (CL)	15–30 mg/kg/day divided q 12 hours	PO
Clofazimine (CLO)	1–2 mg/kg/day	PO
Doxycycline (D)	2–4 mg/kg/day divided q 12 hours (older than 8 years of age)	PO, IV
Ethambutol (ETB)	15–25 mg/kg/day	PO
Ethionamide (ETH)	10–20 mg/kg/day divided q 12 hours	PO
Isoniazid (I)	10–14 mg/kg/day	PO
Pyrazinamide (PZA)	15–30 mg/kg/day	PO
Rifabutin (RIB)	5–10 mg/kg/day; maximum 300 mg/day (adults)†	PO
Rifampin (RIF)	10–20 mg/kg/day divided q 12–24 hours	PO or IV
Streptomycin (S)	20–30 mg/kg/day	IM

Infections

Disseminated MAC: HIV-infected: CL (or Z) + ETB (± RIB)
Disseminated MAC: HIV-negative, immunocompromised: RIF + ETB + INH + S or A
M. kansasii: RIF + ETB + INH
M. marinum: ETB + RIF, or D or TMP-SMZ
M. chelonae: A ± CLO, or CL alone
M. fortuitum: A + X + Probenicid or A + C + sulfonamide
M. abscessus: CL alone or A alone

*Data based on references 49, 58, 72, 77, 78, 109, 136, 142, 144, 152, 155.
†Not approved for use in children.
MAC, *M. avium* complex.

organisms are likely to be found in birds, soil, dust, and fresh or salt water. Infections due to MAC strains isolated from adult AIDS patients could be identified as either serotype 4 or 8, in contrast to non-AIDS patients, in whom no predominant serotype has been identified.[65, 157] Nearly all isolates of MAC from AIDS patients have been identified as *M. avium*, compared with those from non-AIDS patients, in whom the rate of *M. avium* falls to about 55 per cent and that of *M. intracellulare* to 32 to 40 per cent.[49, 157]

Lung disease has been the major manifestation of MAC infection in the nonimmunocompromised adult. Most investigators felt that MAC infection occurred mainly in patients with deficient immunity or underlying lung disease. Later reports, however, seemed to indicate that normal adult hosts are at risk for infection with MAC and that the rates are increasing.[61, 100] Case reports involving children are lacking in details because they usually appear within discussions of adult patients.[101]

Pediatric case reports of disseminated disease due to *M. avium-intracellulare*/MAC have appeared in the literature. Children have presented with ulcerative lesions of their colon[29]; mesenteric disease with abscess formation[114]; hematogenous spread to liver, spleen, kidneys, and adrenal cortex; epididymis[120]; bone lesions[139]; and skin lesions. Disseminated osteomyelitis rarely is due to nontuberculous mycobacteria, but if it occurs, *M. intracellulare* most commonly is isolated.[21, 68] Immunocompromised patients with disseminated infection with *M. avium-intracellulare* historically require multiple-drug therapy including isoniazid, ethambutol, clofazimine, and rifabutin in four-drug combination therapy.[77] However, some reports indicate that disseminated disease in HIV-infected patients may respond to only two agents, as mentioned earlier in the AIDS section. The addition of other agents may be necessary because of the high incidence of resistant organisms. A preliminary report showed that interferon gamma may be effective when combined with conventional therapy in some patients who are refractory to standard chemotherapy alone.[56]

Bacterial peritonitis is common in patients undergoing chronic ambulatory peritoneal dialysis for chronic renal failure. Reports of nontuberculous mycobacteria causing peritonitis have been noted.[50, 97, 149] Cases involving nontuberculous mycobacteria with foreign bodies, such as Tenckhoff catheters, frequently result in the development of sinus tracts. Additionally, antituberculous drug regimens in these cases generally are unsuccessful. Even though the mycobacteria were sensitive to the agents used, the patients continued to have sinus tract drainage without improvement, even with removal of the foreign body.

Mycobacterium scrofulaceum

M. scrofulaceum has many characteristics similar to *M. avium* and *M. intracellulare*. This organism most commonly is associated with lymphadenitis in children 1 to 5 years of age. It also can be found in soil, water, and dairy products. It rarely causes other manifestations in humans. Skin and bony lesions have been reported in two cases of children chronically infected with *M. scrofulaceum* for up to 10 years.[38, 146] Few data are available on chemotherapeutic agents for treatment of infections due to this organism. Based on susceptibility patterns, three or more drugs may be necessary for serious disease. Lymphadenitis can be cured with complete excision of the lymph node.

Mycobacterium kansasii

Of the photochromogens, *M. kansasii* is the most commonly isolated in humans. In contrast to *M. avium-intracellulare* and *M. scrofulaceum*, *M. kansasii* rarely is isolated in soil but has been cultured from water[6] and milk.[19, 20] Chronic pulmonary infection is the most common manifestation of this disease and is seen mainly in adults, particularly those with AIDS. Pulmonary disease in children is infrequent. Some of the children present as adults do, with underlying pulmonary disease due to previous tuberculosis or chronic pulmonary disease.[10, 89] In contrast, some children present with acute symptoms of classic bacterial pneumonia with abrupt onset of fever and sputum production, as well as the finding of consolidation on physical examination and roentgenograms.[10, 18] Pleural effusions also can occur. In contrast to some of the other nontuberculous organisms, *M. kansasii* is sensitive to most of the antituberculous drugs, particularly rifampin. Thus, treatment of infections due to this organism is accomplished easily. Most authorities recommend the use of three drugs including rifampin, isoniazid, and ethambutol. The treatment course usually requires a minimum of 12 months, with some requiring therapy as long as 24 months. Patients with AIDS and infection with *M. kansasii* have responded to this three-drug regimen, but total duration of therapy is unknown at this time. In children with AIDS, the diagnosis of infection due to *M. kansasii* is rare and clinical response to therapy has been poor.[58] Other immunocompromised children have been reported in the literature, including a 7-month-old boy from Texas with disseminated *M. kansasii* infection with numerous organisms found in the spleen at autopsy.[88] Meningitis due to this organism also has been described; the patients died despite the use of antimycobacterial therapy.[60, 112]

Mycobacterium malmoense

This organism, which frequently is overlooked on standard Löwenstein-Jensen egg medium, particularly in children with lymphadenitis, grows at between 25° C and 37° C. The organism is slow growing and may require 8 to 12 weeks for colonies to become visible on solid media. The BACTEC system (Becton Dickinson, Sparks, MD) was shown to be superior in one study of children with lymphadenitis in isolating *M. malmoense*.[55] A case with bone marrow involvement also was described in a patient with chronic granulocytic leukemia.[40] Most strains of *M. malmoense* are sensitive to ethambutol and cycloserine.

Mycobacterium chelonae *and* Mycobacterium fortuitum

M. chelonae is the most important rapidly growing pathogenic mycobacteria, but its taxonomy is quite confusing.[47] Since Grange's presentation in 1981, the organism's taxonomy has continued to be in flux. The *M. chelonae* group consists of *M. chelonae* (formerly *M. chelonae* subsp. *chelonae*), *M. abscessus* (formerly *M. chelonae* subsp. *chelonae*), and a third biovariant known as *M. chelonae*-like organisms.[73] The *M. fortuitum* group consists of *M. fortuitum*, *M. peregrinum*, and a third unnamed biovariant.[73] *M. fortuitum* is associated closely with *M. chelonae*. The two groups can be separated on the biochemical basis of nitrate reduction and iron uptake. Wallace and associates[140] provided the largest series of patients with skin, soft tissue, and bone involvement due to *M. chelonae*. Steroid use seemed to be the factor associated most commonly with development of disease.

M. fortuitum and *M. chelonae* have been implicated in sternal wound infections and endocarditis and have occurred in outbreak-type settings.[72, 109] Patients responded to surgical débridement and amikacin with cefoxitin. A case series from Hong Kong reported on successful treatment of *M. fortuitum* sternotomy infections with the use of single daily dose ofloxacin as monotherapy in three patients.[159] Adult renal transplant patients also have been described with skin and subcutaneous tissue involvement due to *M. chelonae*.[27] *M. chelonae* also has been described as an etiology for otitis media, likely due to contamination of ear, nose, and throat instruments with colonized water sources.[82]

M. abscessus, as stated earlier, is related closely to *M. chelonae* and should be designated as a separate species.[73] Manifestations of infection due to this organism usually are related to pulmonary, cutaneous, or disseminated infections.[143] Clarithromycin may be effective for infection due to *M. chelonae*.[144] Maxson and associates[87] reported on a case of osteomyelitis due to *M. abscessus* that was controlled successfully with long-term monotherapy with clarithromycin.

M. smegmatis, which resembles *M. fortuitum* except for the absence of a positive 3-day arylsulfatase test, is a rapid grower that is responsible for skin and soft tissue infections.[141]

OTHER SITES OF INFECTION

Carpal tunnel syndrome in adults has been reported as being caused by *M. szulgai*, an uncommon scotochromogenic mycobacterium.[127] Effective treatment included débridement, ethambutol, and rifampin. Other infections in humans include choroiditis,[25] panniculitis,[111] genitourinary tract infection,[13, 131] and synovitis.[129] Ear infections due to nontuberculous mycobacteria also have been reported, as well as mastoiditis.[95, 126]

With the continued proliferation of immunocompromised patients due to AIDS as well as new treatment modalities that induce the patient to be immunocompromised (organ transplant, new immunosuppressive drugs, etc.), the atypical mycobacteria likely will continue to remain important pathogens. With newer isolation techniques and new technology, such as DNA probes, our ability to diagnose these infections and our understanding of the pathogenesis of the infections that these organisms produce should improve. It is hoped that our ability to treat these infections also will continue to improve.

References

1. Agy, M. B., Wassis, C. K., Plorde, J. J., et al.: Evaluation of four mycobacterial blood culture media: BACTEC 13A, Isolator/BACTEC 12B, Isolator/Middlebrook Agar and a biphasic medium. Diagn. Microbiol. Infect. Dis. *12*:303–308, 1989.
2. Ahn, C. H., McLarty, J. W., Ahn, S. S., et al.: Diagnostic criteria for pulmonary disease caused by *Mycobacterium kansasii* and *Mycobacterium intracellulare*. Am. Rev. Respir. Dis. *125*:388–391, 1982.
3. Aitken, M. L., Burke, W., McDonald, G., et al.: Nontuberculous mycobacterial disease in adult cystic fibrosis patients. Chest *103*:1096–1099, 1993.
4. Altman, R. P., and Margileth, A. M.: Cervical lymphadenopathy from atypical mycobacteria: Diagnosis and surgical treatment. J. Pediatr. Surg. *10*:419–422, 1975.
5. Armstrong, K. L., James, R. W., Dawson, D. J., et al.: *Mycobacterium haemophilum* causing perihilar or cervical lymphadenitis in healthy children. J. Pediatr. *121*:202–205, 1992.
6. Bailey, R. K., Wyles, S., Dingley, M., et al.: The isolation of high catalase *Mycobacterium kansasii* from tap water. Am. Rev. Resp. Dis. *101*:430, 1970.
7. Barton, L. L., and Feigin, R. D.: Childhood cervical lymphadenitis: A reappraisal. J. Pediatr. *84*:846–852, 1974.
8. Bell, R. C., Higuchi, J. H., Donovan, W. N., et al.: *Mycobacterium simiae:* Clinical features and follow-up of twenty-four patients. Am. Rev. Resp. Dis. *127*:35–38, 1983.
9. Benjamin, D. R.: Granulomatous lymphadenitis in children. Arch. Pathol. Lab. Med. *111*:750–753, 1987.
10. Bialkin, G., Pollak, A., and Weil, A. J.: Pulmonary infection with *Mycobacterium kansasii*. Am. J. Dis. Child. *101*:739, 1961.
11. Blacklock, Z. M., and Dawson, D. J.: Atypical mycobacteria causing non-pulmonary disease in Queensland. Pathology *11*:283–287, 1979.
12. Brook, I.: Aerobic and anaerobic bacteriology of cervical adenitis in children. Clin. Pediatr. *19*:693–696, 1980.
13. Brooker, W. J., and Aufderheide, A. C.: Genitourinary tract infections due to atypical mycobacteria. J. Urol. *124*:242–244, 1980.
14. Brooks, R. W., Parker, B. C., Gruft, H., et al.: Epidemiology of infection by nontuberculous mycobacteria. Am. Rev. Resp. Dis. *130*:630–633, 1984.
15. Brown J. W., III, and Sanders, C. V.: *Mycobacterium marinum* infections: A problem of recognition, not therapy? Arch. Intern. Med. *147*:817–818, 1987.
16. Burchard, G. D., and Bierther, M.: Buruli ulcer: Clinical pathological study of 23 patients in Lambarene, Gabon. Trop. Med. Parasitol. *37*:1–8, 1986.
17. Centers for Disease Control and Prevention: HIV/AIDS Surveillance Rep. *Feb*:1–23, 1993.
18. Chapman, J. S.: Varieties of tuberculosis in children. Minn. Med. *42*:1773, 1959.
19. Chapman, J. S., Bernard, J. S., and Speight, M.: Isolation of mycobacteria from raw milk. Am. Rev. Resp. Dis. *91*:351, 1965.
20. Chapman, J. S., and Speight, M.: Isolation of atypical mycobacteria from pasteurized milk. Am. Rev. Resp. Dis. *98*:1052, 1968.
21. Chicoine, L., La Pointe, N., Simoneau, R., et al.: "Anonymous" mycobacterial infection causing disseminated osteomyelitis and skin lesions. Can. Med. Assoc. J. *98*:1059, 1968.
22. Christensen, E. E., Dietz, G. W., Ahn, C. H., et al.: Initial roentgenographic manifestations of pulmonary *Mycobacterium tuberculosis, M. kansasii, and M. intracellularis* infections. Chest *80*:132–136, 1981.

23. Clancy, J. K., Dodge, O. G., Lunn, H. F., et al.: Mycobacterial skin ulcers in Uganda. Lancet 2:951–954, 1961.
24. Clarridge, J., Shawar, R., Shinnick, T., et al.: Large-scale use of polymerase chain reaction for detection of *Mycobacterium tuberculosis* in a routine mycobacteriology laboratory. J. Clin. Microbiol. *31*:2049–2056, 1993.
25. Clever, V. G.: Choroidal involvement with *Mycobacterium intracellulare*. Ann. Ophthalmol. *12*:1409–1411, 1980.
26. Colville, A.: Retrospective review of culture-positive mycobacterial lymphadenitis cases in children in Nottingham, 1979–1990. Eur. J. Clin. Microbiol. Infect. Dis. *12*:192–195, 1993.
27. Cooper, J. F., Lichtenstein, M. J., Graham, B. S., et al.: *Mycobacterium chelonae:* A cause of nodular skin lesions with a proclivity for renal transplant recipients. Am. J. Med. *86*:173–177, 1989.
28. Currarino, G., Votteler, T. H., and Weinberg, A.: Atypical mycobacterial infection of intraparotid lymph nodes: Clinical and sialographic observations. Pediatr. Radiol. *6*:10–12, 1977.
29. Cuttino, J. T., and McCabe, A. M.: Pure granulomatous nocardiosis: A new fungus disease distinguished by intracellular parasitism. Am. J. Pathol. *25*:1, 1949.
30. Dailloux, M., Morlot, M., and Sirbat, C.: Etude des facteurs intervenant sur la presence des Mycobacteries atypiques dans l'eau d'une piscine. Rev. Epidemiol. Sante Publique *28*:299–306, 1980.
31. Davidson, P. T.: Introduction (international conference on atypical mycobacteria). Rev. Infect. Dis. *3*:816–818, 1981.
32. Davis, B. R., Brumbach, M. T., Sanders, W. J., et al.: Skin lesions caused by *Mycobacterium haemophilum*. Ann. Intern. Med. *97*:723–724, 1982.
33. Deepe, G. S., Jr., Capparell, R., and Coonrod, J. D.: Atypical mycobacterial lymphadenitis in an adult. Chest *78*:882–883, 1980.
34. Delabie, J., DeWolfe-Peeters, C., Bobbaers, H., et al.: Immunophenotypic analysis of histocytes involved in AIDS-associated *Mycobacterium scrofulaceum* infection: Similarities with lepromatous lepra. Clin. Exp. Immunol. *85*:214–218, 1991.
35. Dhooge, I., Dhooge, C., De-Baets, F, et al.: Diagnostic and therapeutic management of atypical mycobacterial infections in children. Eur. Arch. Otorhinolaryngol. *250*:387–391, 1993.
36. Donta, S. T., Smith, P. W., Levitz, R. E., et al.: Therapy of *Mycobacterium marinum* infections. Arch. Intern. Med. *146*:902–904, 1986.
37. Dunn, B. L., and Hodgson, D. J.: Atypical mycobacteria in milk. J. Appl. Bacteriol. *52*:373–376, 1982.
38. Dustin, P., Demol, P., Derks-Jacobovitz, D., et al.: Generalized fatal chronic infection by *Mycobacterium scrofulaceum* with severe amyloidosis in a child. Pathol. Res. Pract. *168*:237–248, 1980.
39. Dutt, A. K., and Stead, W. W.: Long-term results of medical treatment in *Mycobacterium intracellulare* infection. Am. J. Med. *67*:449–453, 1979.
40. Engervall, P., Bjorkholm, M., Petrini, B., et al.: Disseminated *Mycobacterium malmoense* infection in a patient with chronic granulocytic leukaemia. J. Intern. Med. *234*:231–233, 1993.
41. Forbes, B., and Hicks, K.: Direct detection of *Mycobacterium tuberculosis* in respiratory specimens in a clinical laboratory by polymerase chain reaction. J. Clin. Microbiol. *31*:1688–1694, 1993.
42. Gill, M. J., Fanning, E. A., and Chomyc, S.: Childhood lymphadenitis in a harsh northern climate due to atypical mycobacteria. Scand. J. Infect. Dis. *19*:77–83, 1987.
43. Good, R. C., and Snider, D. E., Jr.: Isolation of nontuberculous mycobacteria in the United States, 1980. J. Infect. Dis. *146*:829–833, 1982.
44. Gorse, G. J., Fairshter, R. D., Friedly, G., et al.: Nontuberculous mycobacterial disease: Experience in a southern California hospital. Arch. Intern. Med. *143*:225–228, 1983.
45. Goto, M., Oka, S., Okuzumi, K., et al.: Evaluation of acridinium ester-labeled DNA probes for identification of *Mycobacterium tuberculosis* and *Mycobacterium avium-Mycobacterium intracellulare* complex in culture. J. Clin. Microbiol. *29*:2473–2476, 1991.
46. Grange, J. M.: Mycobacteria and the skin. Int. J. Dermatol. *21*:497–503, 1982.
47. Grange, J. M.: *Mycobacterium chelonae*. Tubercle *62*:273–276, 1981.
48. Gruft, H., Falkinham, J. O., III, and Parker, B. C.: Recent experience in the epidemiology of disease caused by atypical mycobacteria. Rev. Infect. Dis. *3*:990–996, 1981.
49. Guthertz, L. S., Damsker, B., Bottone, E. J., et al.: *Mycobacterium avium* and *Mycobacterium intracellulare* infections in patients with and without AIDS. J. Infect. Dis. *160*:1037–1041, 1989.
50. Hakim, A., Hisam, N., and Reuman, P. D.: Environmental mycobacterial peritonitis complicating peritoneal dialysis: Three cases and review. Clin. Infect. Dis. *16*:426–431, 1993.
51. Havlir, D., Kemper, C. A., and Deresinski, S. C.: Reproducibility of lysis-centrifugation cultures for quantification of *Mycobacterium avium* complex bacteremia. J. Clin. Microbiol. *31*:1794–1798, 1993.
52. Hjelt, K., Hojlyng, N., Howitz, P., et al.: The role of mycobacteria other than tuberculosis (MOTT) in patients with cystic fibrosis. Scand. J. Infect. Dis. *26*:569–576, 1994.
53. Hjelte, L., Petrini, B., Kallenius, G., et al.: Prospective study of mycobacterial infections in patients with cystic fibrosis. Thorax *45*:397–400, 1990.
54. Hofer, M., Hirschel, B., Kirschner, P., et al.: Brief report: Disseminated osteomyelitis from *Mycobacterium ulcerans* after a snakebite. N. Engl. J. Med. *328*:1007–1009, 1993.
55. Hoffner, S. E., Henriques, B., Petrini, B., et al.: *Mycobacterium malmoense*: An easily missed pathogen. J. Clin. Microbiol. *29*:2673–2674, 1991.
56. Holland, S. M., Eisenstein, E. M., Kuhns, D. B., et al.: Treatment of refractory disseminated nontuberculous mycobacterial infection with interferon gamma. N. Engl. J. Med. *330*:1348–1355, 1994.
57. Horsburgh, C. R., and Selik, R. M.: The epidemiology of disseminated nontuberculous mycobacterial infection in the acquired immunodeficiency syndrome (AIDS). Am. Rev. Resp. Dis. *139*:4–7, 1989.
58. Hoyt, L., Oleske, J., Holland, B., et al.: Nontuberculous mycobacteria in children with acquired immunodeficiency syndrome. Pediatr. Infect. Dis. J. *11*:354–360, 1992.
59. Huebner, R. E., Schein, M. F., Cauthen, G. M., et al.: Usefulness of skin testing with mycobacterial antigens in children with cervical lymphadenopathy. Pediatr. Infect. Dis. J. *11*:450–456, 1992.
60. Huempfner, H. R., Kingsolver, W. R., and Deuschle, K. W.: Tuberculous meningitis caused by both *Mycobacterium tuberculosis* and atypical mycobacteria. Am. Rev. Resp. Dis. *94*:612, 1966.
61. Iseman, M. D.: *Mycobacterium avium* complex and the normal host: The other side of the coin. N. Engl. J. Med. *321*:896–897, 1989.
62. Kent, D. C.: Tuberculous lymphadenitis: Not a localized disease process. Am. J. Med. Sci. *254*:866–873, 1967.
63. Kiehn, T. E., and Cammarata, R.: Comparative recoveries of *Mycobacterium avium-M. intracellulare* from isolator lysis-centrifugation and BACTEC 13A blood culture systems. J. Clin. Microbiol. *26*:760–761, 1988.
64. Kiehn, T. E., and Cammarata, R.: Laboratory diagnosis of mycobacterial infections in patients with acquired immunodeficiency syndrome. J. Clin. Microbiol. *24*:708–711, 1986.
65. Kiehn, T. E., Edwards, F. F., Brannon, P., et al.: Infections caused by *Mycobacterium avium* complex in immunocompromised patients: Diagnosis by blood culture and fecal examination, antimicrobial susceptibility tests, and morphological and seroagglutination characteristics. J. Clin. Microbiol. *21*:168–173, 1985.
66. Kilby, J., Gilligan, P., Yankaskas J., et al.: Nontuberculous mycobacteria in adult patients with cystic fibrosis. Chest *102*:70–75, 1992.
67. Klein, J. O.: Clarithromycin: Where do we go from here? Pediatr. Infect. Dis. J. *12*:S148–S151, 1993.
68. Koenig, M. G., Collins, R. D., and Heyssel, R. M.: Disseminated mycobacteriosis caused by Battey-type mycobacteria. Ann. Intern. Med. *64*:145, 1966.
69. Krasnow, I., and Gross, W.: *Mycobacterium simiae* infection in the United States. Am. Rev. Resp. Dis. *111*:357–360, 1975.
70. Kubica, G. P.: Current nomenclature of the mycobacteria. Bull. Int. Union Tuberc. *53*:192, 1978.
71. Kubica, G. P., and Wayne, L. G.: The Mycobacteria: A Sourcebook, Part A. New York, Marcel Dekker, 1984, pp. 38–41.
72. Kuritsky, J. N., Bullen, M. G., Broome, C. V., et al.: Sternal wound infections and endocarditis due to organisms of the *Mycobacterium fortuitum* complex. Ann. Intern. Med. *98*:938–939, 1983.
73. Kusunoki, S., and Ezaki, T.: Proposal of *Mycobacterium peregrinum* sp. nov., nom. rev., and elevation of *Mycobacterium chelonae* subsp. *abscessus* (Kubica et al.) to species status: *Mycobacterium abscessus* comb. nov. Int. J. Syst. Bacteriol. *42*:240–245, 1992.
74. Kuth, G., Lamprecht, J., and Haase, G.: Cervical lymphadenitis due to mycobacteria other than tuberculosis: An emerging problem in children? J. Otorhinolaryngol. Relat. Spec. *57*:36–38, 1995.
75. Lai, K. K., Stottmeier, K. D., Sherman, I. H., et al.: Mycobacterial cervical lymphadenopathy: Relation of etiologic agents to age. J. A. M. A. *251*:1286–1288, 1984.
76. Levin, M., Newport, M. J., D'Souza, S., et al.: Familial disseminated atypical mycobacterial infection in childhood: A human mycobacterial susceptibility gene? Lancet *345*:79–83, 1995.
77. Levin, R. H., and Bolinger, A. M.: Treatment of nontuberculous mycobacterial infections in pediatric patients. Clin. Pharm. *7*:545–551, 1988.
78. Lewis, L. L.: Nontuberculous mycobacterial infections. *In* Pizzo, P. A., and Wilfert, C. M. (eds.): Pediatric AIDS: The Challenge of HIV Infection in Infants, Children, and Adolescents. 2nd ed. Baltimore, Willliams & Wilkins, 1994, pp. 308–320.
79. Lim, S. D., Lopez, J., Ford, E., et al.: Genotypic identification of pathogenic *Mycobacteria* species by using a nonradioactive oligonucleotide probe. J. Clin. Microbiol. *29*:1276–1278, 1991.
80. Lincoln, E. M., and Gilbert, L. A.: Disease in children due to mycobacteria other than *Mycobacterium tuberculosis*. Am. Rev. Resp. Dis. *105*:683–714, 1972.
81. Lindberg, M. C., and Thomas, G. G.: Lymphadenitis due to atypical mycobacteria. Ala. Med. *59*:19–21, 1989.
82. Lowry, P. W., Jarvis, W. R., Oberle, A. D., et al.: *Mycobacterium chelonae* causing otitis media in an ear-nose-and-throat practice. N. Engl. J. Med. *319*:978–982, 1988.
83. Lunn, H. F., and Rees, R. J. W.: Treatment of mycobacterial skin ulcers in Uganda with a riminophenazine derivative (B663). Lancet *i*:246, 1964.
84. MacCallum, P.: A new mycobacterial infection in man. I. Clinical aspects. J. Pathol. Bact. *60*:93, 1948.
85. Maloney, J. M., Gregg, C. R., Stephens, D. S., et al.: Infections caused by *Mycobacterium szulgai* in humans. Rev. Infect. Dis. *9*:1120–1126, 1987.

86. Mankiewicz, E., and Majdaniw, O.: Atypical mycobacteria in tapwater. Can. J. Public Health *73*:358–360, 1982.
87. Maxson, S., Schutze, G. E., and Jacobs, R. F.: *Mycobacterium abscessus* osteomyelitis: Treatment with clarithromycin. Infect. Dis. Clin. Pract. *3*:203–206, 1994.
88. McCracken, G. H., Jr., and Reynolds, R. C.: Primary lymphopenic immunologic deficiency: Disseminated *Mycobacterium kansasii* infection. Am. J. Dis. Child. *120*:143, 1970.
89. Merckx, J. J., Soule, E. H., and Karlson, A. G.: The histopathology of lesions caused by infection with unclassified acid-fast bacteria in man. Am. J. Clin. Pathol. *41*:244, 1964.
90. Mollohan, C. S., and Romer, M. S.: Public health significance of swimming pool granuloma. Am. J. Public Health *51*:883, 1961.
91. Morgan, J. K., and Blowers, R.: Swimming pool granuloma in Britain. Lancet *1*:1034, 1964.
92. Musial, C. E., Tice, L. S., Stockman, L., et al.: Identification of mycobacteria from culture by using the Gen-Probe rapid diagnostic system for *Mycobacterium avium* complex and *Mycobacterium tuberculosis* complex. J. Clin. Microbiol. *26*:2120–2123, 1988.
93. Nadal, D., Caduff, R., Kraft, R., et al.: Invasive infection with *Mycobacterium genavense* in three children with the acquired immunodeficiency syndrome. Eur. J. Clin. Microbiol. Infect. Dis. *12*:37–43, 1993.
94. Noordhoek, G. T., Kolk, A. H. J., Bjune, G., et al.: Sensitivity and specificity of PCR for detection of *Mycobacterium tuberculosis*: A blind comparison study among seven laboratories. J. Clin. Microbiol. *32*:277–284, 1994.
95. Nylen, O., Alestig, K., Fasth, A., et al.: Infections of the ear with nontuberculous mycobacteria in three children. Pediatr. Infect. Dis. J. *13*:653–656, 1994.
96. O'Brien, R. J.: The epidemiology of nontuberculous mycobacterial disease. Clin. Chest Med. *10*:407–418, 1989.
97. Perlino, C. A.: *Mycobacterium avium* complex: An unusual cause of peritonitis in patients undergoing continuous ambulatory peritoneal dialysis. Clin. Infect. Dis. *17*:1083–1084, 1993.
98. Pinder, S. E., and Colville, A.: Mycobacterial cervical lymphadenitis in children: Can histological assessment help differentiate infections caused by non-tuberculous mycobacteria from *Mycobacteria tuberculosis*? Histopathology *22*:59–64, 1993.
99. Pransky, S. M., Reismann, B. K., Kearns, D. B., et al.: Cervicofacial mycobacterial adenitis in children: Endemic to San Diego? Laryngoscope *100*:920–925, 1990.
100. Prince, D. S., Peterson, D. D., Steiner, R. M., et al.: Infection with *Mycobacterium avium* complex in patients without predisposing conditions. N. Engl. J. Med. *321*:863–868, 1989.
101. Reich, J. M., and Johnson, R. E.: *Mycobacterium avium* complex pulmonary disease: Incidence, presentation, and response to therapy in a community setting. Am. Rev. Resp. Dis. *143*:1381–1385, 1991.
102. Reichert, C. M., O'Leary, T. J., Levens, D. L., et al.: Autopsy pathology in the acquired immune deficiency syndrome. Am. J. Pathol. *112*:357–382, 1983.
103. Reid, I. S.: *Mycobacterium ulcerans* infection: A report of 13 cases at the Port Moresby General Hospital, Papua. Med. J. Aust. *1*:427, 1967.
104. Rivron, M. J., Hughes, E. A., Sibert, J. R., et al.: Cervical lymphadenitis in childhood due to mycobacteria of the Fortuitum group. Arch. Dis. Child. *54*:312–313, 1979.
105. Rosenzweig, D. Y.: Pulmonary mycobacterial infections due to *Mycobacterium intracellulare-avium* complex: Clinical features and course in 100 consecutive cases. Chest *75*:115–119, 1979.
106. Runyon, E. H.: Anonymous mycobacteria in pulmonary disease. Med. Clin. North Am. *43*:273–290, 1959.
107. Runyon, E. H.: Mycobacteria: An overview. Rev. Infect. Dis. *3*:819–821, 1981.
108. Runyon, E. H.: Pathogenic mycobacteria. Adv. Tuberc. Res. *14*:235–287, 1965.
109. Safranek, T. J., Jarvis, W. R., Carson, L. A., et al.: *Mycobacterium chelonae* wound infections after plastic surgery employing contaminated gentian violet skin-marking solution. N. Engl. J. Med. *317*:197–201, 1987.
110. Salyer, K. E., Votteler, T. P., Dorman, G. W.: Surgical management of cervical adenitis due to atypical mycobacteria in children. J. A. M. A. *204*:1037–1040, 1968.
111. Sanderson, T. L., Moskowitz, L., Hensley, G. T., et al.: Disseminated *Mycobacterium avium-intracellulare* infection appearing as a panniculitis. Arch. Pathol. Lab. Med. *106*:112–114, 1982.
112. Sanford, J. P., and Barnett, J. A.: Atypical mycobacterial organisms as encountered in a general hospital and its clinics. *In* Chapman, J. S. (ed.): The Anonymous Mycobacteria in Human Disease. Springfield, IL, Charles C Thomas, 1960, p. 98.
113. Schaefer, W. B.: Incidence of the serotypes of *Mycobacterium avium* and atypical mycobacteria in human and animal diseases. Am. Rev. Resp. Dis. *97*:18–23, 1968.
114. Schonell, M. E., Crofton, J. W., Stuart, A. E., et al.: Disseminated infection with *Mycobacterium avium*. I. Clinical features, treatment and pathology. Tubercle *49*:12, 1968.
115. Schuit, K. E., and Powell, D. A.: Mycobacterial lymphadenitis in childhood. Am. J. Dis. Child. *132*:675–677, 1978.
116. Shocket, E., Drosd, R. E., Tate, C. F., Jr.: Granuloma of the skin due to *Mycobacterium fortuitum*. South. Med. J. *57*:1352, 1964.
117. Sigalet, D., Lees, G., and Fanning, A.: Atypical tuberculosis in the pediatric patient: Implications for the pediatric surgeon. J. Pediatr. Surg. *27*:1381–1384, 1992.
118. Simor, A. E., Salit, I. E., and Vellend, H.: The role of *Mycobacterium xenopi* in human disease. Am. Rev. Resp. Dis. *129*:435–438, 1984.
119. Smith, M. J., Efthimiou, J., Hodson, M. E., et al.: Mycobacterial isolations in young adults with cystic fibrosis. Thorax *39*:369–375, 1984.
120. Snijder, J.: Morphological aspect of atypical mycobacterioses. *In* Selected Papers. Royal Netherlands Tuberculosis Association, The Hague, *10*:99, 1967.
121. Sommers, H. M., and Good, R. C.: Mycobacterium. *In* Lennette, E. H., Balows, A., Hausler, W. J., Jr., et al. (eds.): Manual of Clinical Microbiology. 4th ed. American Society for Microbiology, 1985, pp. 216–240.
122. Song, M., Vincke, G., Vanachter, H., et al.: Treatment of cutaneous infection due to *Mycobacterium ulcerans*. Dermatologica *171*:197–199, 1985.
123. Stanford, J. L., and Paul, R. C.: A preliminary report on some studies of environmental mycobacteria. Ann. Soc. Belg. Med. Trop. *53*:321, 1973.
124. Stanford, J. L., Revill, W. D. L., Gunthorpe, W. J., et al.: The production and preliminary investigation of Burulin, a new skin test reagent for *Mycobacterium ulcerans* infection. J. Hyg (Camb.) *74*:7, 1975.
125. Steadham, J. E.: High catalase strains of *Mycobacterium kansasii* isolated from water in Texas. J. Clin. Microbiol. *11*:496–498, 1980.
126. Stewart, M. G., Troendle-Atkins, J., Starke, J. R., et al.: Nontuberculous mycobacterial mastoiditis. Arch. Otolaryngol. Head Neck Surg. *121*:225–228, 1995.
127. Stratton, C. W., Phelps, D. B., and Reller, L. B.: Tuberculoid tenosynovitis and carpal tunnel syndrome caused by *Mycobacterium szulgai*. Am. J. Med. *65*:349–351, 1978.
128. Straus, W. L., Ostroff, S. M., Jernigan, D. B., et al.: Clinical and epidemiologic characteristics of *Mycobacterium haemophilum*, an emerging pathogen in immunocompromised patients. Ann. Intern. Med. *120*:118–125, 1994.
129. Sutker, W. L., Lankford, L. L., and Tompsett, R.: Granulomatous synovitis: The role of atypical mycobacteria. Rev. Infect. Dis. *1*:729–735, 1979.
130. Swift, S., and Cohen, H.: Granulomas of the skin due to *Mycobacterium balnei* after abrasions from a fish tank. N. Engl. J. Med. *267*:1244, 1962.
131. Thomas, E., Hillman, B. J., and Stanisic, T.: Urinary tract infection with atypical mycobacteria. J. Urol. *124*:748–750, 1980.
132. Timpe, A., and Runyon, E. H.: Relationship of "atypical" acid-fast bacilli to human disease: Preliminary report. J. Lab. Clin. Med. *44*:202–209, 1954.
133. Tsukamura M.: A review of the methods of identification and differentiation of mycobacteria. Rev. Infect. Dis. *3*:841–861, 1981.
134. Turneer, M., Van-Nerom, E., Nyabenda, J., et al.: Determination of humoral immunoglobulins M and G directed against mycobacterial antigen 60 failed to diagnose primary tuberculosis and mycobacterial adenitis in children. Am. J. Resp. Crit. Care Med. *150*:1508–1512, 1994.
135. U. S. Public Health Service Task Force on Prophylaxis and Therapy for *Mycobacterium avium* Complex: Recommendations for prophylaxis and therapy for *Mycobacterium avium* complex for adults and adolescents infected with human immunodeficiency virus. M. M. W. R. *42*:14–20, 1993.
136. Van Dyke, J. J., and Lake, K. B.: Chemotherapy for aquarium granuloma. J. A. M. A. *233*:1380–1381, 1975.
137. Venkatesh, V., Everson, N. W., and Johnstone, J. M.: Atypical mycobacterial lymphadenopathy in children: Is it underdiagnosed? J. R. Coll. Surg. Edinburgh *39*:301–303, 1994.
138. Vestal, A. L.: Procedures for the isolation and identification of mycobacteria. CDC Publication No. 76-8230. Washington, D.C., Department of Health, Education and Welfare, 1975.
139. Vollini, F., Cotton, R., and Lester, W.: Disseminated infection caused by Battey type mycobacteria. Am. J. Clin. Pathol. *43*:39, 1965.
140. Wallace, R. J., Brown B. A., and Onyi, G. O.: Skin, soft tissue, and bone infections due to *Mycobacterium chelonae*: Importance of prior corticosteroid therapy, frequency of disseminated infections, and resistance to oral antimicrobials other than clarithromycin. J. Infect. Dis. *166*:405–412, 1992.
141. Wallace, R. J., Nash, D. R., Tsukamura, M., et al.: Human disease due to *Mycobacterium smegmatis*. J. Infect. Dis. *158*:52, 1988.
142. Wallace, R. J., Jr., O'Brien, R., Glassroth, J., et al.: Diagnosis and treatment of disease caused by nontuberculous mycobacteria. Am. Rev. Resp. Dis. *142*:940–953, 1990.
143. Wallace, R. J., Swenson, J. M., Silcox, V. A., et al.: Spectrum of disease due to rapidly growing mycobacteria. Rev. Infect. Dis. *5*:657–679, 1983.
144. Wallace, R. J., Tanner, D., Brennan, P. J., et al.: Clinical trial of clarithromycin for cutaneous (disseminated) infection due to *Mycobacterium chelonae*. Ann. Intern. Med. *119*:482–486, 1993.
145. Wayne, L. G., and Sramek, H. A.: Agents of newly recognized or infrequently encountered mycobacterial diseases. Clin. Microbiol. Rev. *5*:1–25, 1992.
146. Weed, L. A., Karlson, A. G., Ivins, J. C., et al.: Recurring migratory chronic osteomyelitis associated with saprophytic acid-fast bacilli: Report of a case of 10 years' duration apparently cured by surgery. Proc. Staff Meeting, Mayo Clin. *31*:238, 1956.
147. Welch, K., Finkbeiner, W., Apers, C. E., et al.: Autopsy findings in the acquired immune deficiency syndrome. J. A. M. A. *252*:1152–1159, 1984.

148. White, M. P., Bangash, H., Goel, K. M., et al.: Non-tuberculous mycobacterial lymphadenitis. Arch. Dis. Child. *61*:368–371, 1986.
149. White, R., Abreo, K., Flanagan, R., et al.: Nontuberculous mycobacterial infections in continuous ambulatory peritoneal dialysis patients. Am. J. Kidney Dis. *22*:581–587, 1993.
150. Wilkes, M. S., Fortin, A. H., Felix, J. C., et al.: Value of necropsy in acquired immunodeficiency syndrome. Lancet *2*:85–88, 1988.
151. Wolinsky, E.: Mycobacteria: Significance of speciation and sensitivity tests. *In*: Lorian, V. (ed.): Significance of Medical Microbiology in the Care of Patients. Baltimore, Williams & Wilkins, 1982, pp. 103–110.
152. Wolinsky, E.: Mycobacterial diseases other than tuberculosis. Clin. Infect. Dis. *15*:1–10, 1992.
153. Wolinsky, E.: Mycobacterial lymphadenitis in children: A prospective study of 105 nontuberculous cases with long-term follow-up. Clin. Infect. Dis. *20*:954–963, 1995.
154. Wolinsky, E.: Nontuberculous mycobacteria and associated diseases. Am. Rev. Resp. Dis. *119*:107–159, 1979.
155. Wolinsky, E., Gomez, F., and Zimpfer, F.: Sporotrichoid *Mycobacterium marinum* infection treated with rifampin-ethambutol. Am. Rev. Resp. Dis. *105*:964–967, 1972.
156. Woods, G. L., and Washington, J. A., II: Mycobacteria other than *Mycobacterium tuberculosis*: Review of microbiologic and clinical aspects. Rev. Infect. Dis. *9*:275–294, 1987.
157. Yakrus, M. A., and Good, R. C.: Geographic distribution frequency and specimen source of *Mycobacterium avium* complex serotypes isolated from patients with acquired immunodeficiency syndrome. J. Clin. Microbiol. *28*:926–929, 1990.
158. Yamauchi, T., Ferrieri, P., and Anthony, B. F.: The aetiology of acute cervical adenitis in children: Serological and bacteriological studies. J. Med. Microbiol. *13*:37–43, 1980.
159. Yew, W. W., Kwan, S. Y. L., Ma, W. K., et al.: Single daily-dose ofloxacin monotherapy for *Mycobacterium fortuitum* sternotomy infection. Chest *96*:1150–1152, 1989.

103

LEPROSY

Wayne M. Meyers

Leprosy is a chronic infectious disease, caused by *Mycobacterium leprae*, affecting principally the cooler parts of the body, especially the skin, upper respiratory tract, testes, eyes, and superficial segments of peripheral nerves. The geographic origin of this infection is unknown, but nearly every part of the world has been affected at some time. The World Health Organization reports that in 1995 there were 2.4 million patients with active leprosy and that there are 600 to 800 thousand new patients annually. In the Middle Ages, leprosy was common in Europe and may have been transported to the Western Hemisphere by Portuguese and Spanish explorations beginning in the fifteenth century and later by slaves from Africa. At least two foci, however, were established in the United States in the nineteenth century by specific immigrations: Oriental peoples brought leprosy to the Hawaiian Islands and started an epidemic among the highly susceptible Hawaiians,[126] and Scandinavians introduced leprosy into the northern Midwest United States.[101]

The stigmata suffered by patients with leprosy frequently are severe and, in Western cultures, at least partially are attributable to a misunderstanding of what is called leprosy in the Old Testament.[10] Other cultures not influenced by Judaic laws and traditions, however, have similar or more severe attitudes toward leprosy patients. For example, Chinese literature illustrates that as early as the eighth century B.C., patients with symptoms now recognized as leprosy were stigmatized.[158] Because of enduring irrational attitudes based on the premise that the Old Testament references are to the same single disease now called leprosy, a brief explanation of "Old Testament leprosy" is offered.

The Hebrew word *tsara'ath* was rendered *lepra* when the Old Testament was translated into Greek about 100 B.C. In preparing the Latin Vulgate version in A.D. 405, Jerome used the word *lepra* directly from the Greek. In the first English translation from the Vulgate in 1384, Wycliffe translated *lepra* as *leprosy*, perhaps because leprosy, then common in Europe and Great Britain, seemed to portray an image of an unholy and loathsome human condition. In the original text, *tsara'ath* was not a specific disease but probably a group of diseases, the identities of which are obscure, and the word referred more generally to ceremonial uncleanness. Old Testament *tsara'ath*, as described, for example, in Leviticus 13 and 14, had none of the distinctive clinical features of leprosy. There is thus no rationale for attitudes toward leprosy that are based on Old Testament *tsara'ath*. A continuing effort must be made to minimize the stigmata peculiarly associated with leprosy. To help achieve this goal, the Fifth International Leprosy Congress in 1948 adopted a resolution to abandon the word leper for leprosy patient.[96] Hansen's disease is preferred by some as a synonym for leprosy. Because of the stigmata of leprosy, the physician must consider carefully the social implications of a diagnosis of leprosy, especially in children.

THE ORGANISM

M. leprae is a species in the order Actinomycetales and the family Mycobacteriaceae. This bacillus was seen first by Hansen in 1873 in Bergen, Norway, in lepromas from Norwegian patients, and this organism was the first reported bacterium causing chronic disease in humans.

M. leprae is an acid-fast bacillus, 0.3 to 0.5 μm wide by 4 to 7 μm long. The acid-fastness of *M. leprae* is weaker than that of other mycobacteria; but as in other mycobacteria, the acid-fastness is related to mycolic acid in the cell wall.[1] Viable undamaged *M. leprae* stain solidly, but degenerating organisms first stain irregularly, then become granular, and eventually lose acid-fastness completely. The persistence of bacillary carcasses can be verified by silver staining techniques.[172] Staining quality, therefore, provides a rapid method for determining the effectiveness of therapy. The in vitro cultivation of *M. leprae* frequently is claimed, but all claims have been refuted or are as yet unsubstantiated.[86] Because *M. leprae* still is noncultivable, identification depends on criteria other than those used routinely for cultivable mycobacteria. The current criteria for *M. leprae* are the following: (1) does not grow on routine laboratory media; (2) infects the footpads of mice in a characteristic manner[155]; (3) acid-fastness is extractable with pyridine[22]; (4) invades nerves of the host; (5) suspensions of dead bacilli produce a characteristic pattern of reactions when injected into the skin of patients (lepromin reaction) with the various clinical forms of leprosy; (6) produces the species-specific antigen, phenolic glycolipid-1 (PGL-1)[44]; and (7) demonstrates species-specific DNA sequences.[184]

Electron micrographs of *M. leprae* reveal a cell wall 15 to 20 nm thick around a cytoplasmic membrane that gives rise to mesosomes extending into the cytoplasm. *M. leprae* divides by transverse fission. Cell walls contain arabinogalactan, mycolates, peptidoglycan, and protein.[106]

In experimental animals, *M. leprae* multiplies slowly; for example, in footpads of immunologically intact mice, the generation time during the logarithmic phase is approximately 13 days. In humans, this characteristic may account, at least in part, for the long incubation periods often encountered. Generation time of *M. leprae* in nude mice may, however, be as short as 26 hours,[61] which suggests that in environments more optimal than the normal mouse footpads, the generation time of *M. leprae* may be near that of other mycobacteria (e.g., the generation time of *M. tuberculosis* is 18 hours). This could explain the obviously short incubation periods observed in a few infants younger than 1 year of age.[12, 50] Localization of infections to the cooler parts of the body,[8] the selective growth in footpads of immunologically intact mice and in ears of hamsters, and the high susceptibility of the armadillo (central body temperature of 32° to 35° C [89.6° to 95° F]) to disseminated infections all suggest that the optimal temperature for growth of *M. leprae* is below 37° C (98.6° F).[109]

Transmission

The modes of transmission of *M. leprae* in nature have not been established. The frequency in children of a single early lesion in skin that usually is covered by clothing argues against the development of such lesions at the site of contact with *M. leprae*.[2] For many years, skin-to-skin contact between patient and healthy subjects was considered the most important means of transmission, and this concept cannot be abandoned readily[95]; however, it has been challenged in recent years. Intact skin of heavily infected patients discharges small numbers of *M. leprae*, but ulcers in the skin may be a source of large numbers of bacilli. Thus, skin-to-skin contact and fomites containing *M. leprae* could be sources of infection. That the nasal mucosa of lepromatous patients harbors massive numbers of *M. leprae* has been known since Hansen's original discovery, and studies suggest that the respiratory passages could be a source of infecting bacilli.[28] *M. leprae* may bind to nasal mucosal cells by first binding fibronectin and attaching to fibronectin receptors on mucosal cells.[17] *M. leprae* organisms ejected in nose-blows remain viable for up to 1 week,[25] and immunosuppressed mice develop disseminated leprosy after the inhalation of aerosols that contain *M. leprae*.[142] Breast tissue and milk from lepromatous patients contain *M. leprae*, and infants may acquire infections from this source.[138]

Placental transmission of leprosy long has been a subject of conjecture, but there is growing evidence for a significant influence of leprosy on fetal development and for intrauterine infection of the fetus. In a study of 116 pregnant leprosy patients in Ethiopia, the placentas were small, birth weights were low, and growth rates of the infants were retarded.[32] Mean birth weights of infants of lepromatous and healthy control mothers were 2558 g and 3280 g, respectively. Estrogen excretion levels at 32 to 40 weeks' gestation are reduced in leprosy patients, which suggests fetoplacental dysfunction.[34] There are IgA and IgM antibodies for *M. leprae* in the cord blood of 30 to 50 per cent of babies from mothers with lepromatous leprosy.[107] This is strong evidence for fetal antibody synthesis to *M. leprae* or antigens thereof. *M. leprae* has been demonstrated in placentas and cord blood on occasion.[66, 167] *M. leprae*–specific IgA and IgM levels rose in infants of lepromatous mothers during the 3- to 24-month period after birth,[108] and two of such infants had clinical leprosy at 9 and 17 months.[33] Leprosy in young infants may be common in areas of high endemicity. In a report combining cases on file in the Leprosy Registry at the Armed Forces Institute of Pathology, cases cited in the literature, and personal observations by experienced leprologists, a total of at least 49 leprosy patients younger than 1 year of age were identified.[12] In only half of these infants did the mother have leprosy or a history of leprosy. The youngest infant was 2½ months old at diagnosis. The fact that many of the mothers never had clinical leprosy suggests that they had an evanescent *M. leprae* bacteremia during gestation. A substantial bacteremia is common in multibacillary disease[31] and is detectable in as many as 15 per cent of paucibacillary patients.[87]

With the discovery of a naturally acquired leprosy-like disease in recently captured wild armadillos in Louisiana,[175] in chimpanzees,[30, 53] and a mangabey monkey from West Africa,[117] there is reason to believe that leprosy is a zoonosis.[111, 174] In all three species, the histopathologic changes resemble those in leprosy in humans, and the bacilli that cause the infection cannot be distinguished from *M. leprae*.[8, 112, 116] Leprosy has been transmitted successfully from the mangabey monkey to other mangabey, rhesus, and African green monkeys.[77, 186]

Some authorities suggest that insects may ingest *M. leprae* during a blood meal from lepromatous patients and harbor viable bacteria, but the natural transmission of leprosy by insects remains unproven and widely is disregarded.

EPIDEMIOLOGY

Highest prevalences are in tropical Africa, South America, India, Southeast Asia, the Philippines, and some South Pacific islands.[132] Approximately 73 per cent of all patients live in Southeast Asia (65 per cent in India), 12 per cent in Africa, and 8 per cent in the Americas. Based on limited whole population surveys in endemic areas, the total number of active patients may exceed by a significant margin the 2.4 million reported by the World Health Organization. The stigma of the disease and inefficiencies in health care delivery systems contribute to this disparity of statistics.[94] In 1995, there were approximately 6000 patients in the United States,[69] with 136 new patients reported in 1994, down from an annual high in recent times of 361 in 1985.[120] Most are immigrants, but a few indigenous patients regularly come from Hawaii, Louisiana, and Texas. There has been no documentation of secondary transmission from imported cases within the United States; thus, immigrants with leprosy present no known public health risk to the population of the United States. The same probably is true for other nonendemic countries.

Hansen's discovery of the leprosy bacillus developed from his conviction that leprosy was a specific contagious disease. This conviction was based on clinical and anatomic findings and, more importantly, on epidemiologic observations. In 1871 and 1872, Hansen studied 69 families with several members with leprosy in western Norway. The prevailing concept of that era was that leprosy was hereditary, but from data gathered on these families, Hansen showed that patients had always had contact with another leprosy patient. Members of the same families with no such contacts were free of leprosy.[58] Hansen thus reasoned, after his pioneering observation of the leprosy bacillus in 1873, that the spread of leprosy depended on the dissemination of this etiologic agent in a susceptible population.

The leprosy epidemic in Nauru in the central Pacific demonstrates how rapidly leprosy can spread in a leprosy-naive population.[54] Leprosy was introduced into this small island in 1912, and by 1924, one-third of the 2500 inhabitants had leprosy.

The prevailing concept has been that an individual becomes infected only after repeated exposure. This concept now is doubted, and a single exposure under optimal conditions may be sufficient. It may be true, however, that in any patient-contact situation, the number of viable *M. leprae* being shed by the patient and the degree of susceptibility of the contact both vary. Thus, long periods of association may be necessary before there are optimal conditions for infection.

Lymphocyte transformation studies show that occupational contacts of leprosy patients in Ethiopia have the highest rate of sensitization (58 per cent) to *M. leprae*, followed closely by household contacts (47 per cent). Noncontacts living in endemic areas have a lower rate of sensitization, but still approximately 29 per cent of the population is sensitized.[51]

Geographic, ethnic, and socioeconomic factors may contribute to the spread of leprosy by affecting the number of untreated or ineffectively treated bacillary-positive patients and the opportunities for exposure. The percentage of patients who harbor large numbers of bacilli—generally, those with lepromatous leprosy—is related to ethnic background. In some Asian populations, for example, 50 per cent or more of those with leprosy have lepromatous leprosy; in Africans, this figure is 5 to 10 per cent. Socioeconomic factors are difficult to assess, and their relationship to prevalence or clinical severity of leprosy is unknown. Nutritional status may or may not be important. The Nauru leprosy epidemic, indolent from 1912 through 1920, became rampant after a devastating epidemic of influenza (30 per cent mortality) left a debilitated population with marked dietary deficiencies. During the next 4 years, the annual incidence of leprosy rose from 4 to 346, but the role played by malnutrition is obscure.[54] Ryrie[147] in Malaya noted that during the Japanese occupation, the severity of leprosy worsened, and he attributed this to a combination of malnutrition and psychic trauma. Skinsnes and Higa[159] drew similar conclusions from a study of mortality in leprosaria in China during World War II. Nevertheless, convincing evidence that the prevalence of leprosy is unusually high in chronically malnourished populations is lacking.

Improvements in housing and other living conditions may play a role in the prevalence of leprosy. There is, for instance, no other satisfactory explanation for the virtual disappearance of leprosy from northern Europe after the Middle Ages and from Scandinavia in the twentieth century, long before there was any effective chemotherapy. If the disease is airborne, then the construction of dwellings that provided less-confined sleeping quarters could have contributed in a major way to the disappearance of leprosy there. Consistent with this concept is the inadequate housing that prevails in all geographic areas where leprosy is common today.

The presumed increased susceptibility of children is difficult to establish and may depend more on exposure to contagious patients than on other factors. The proportion of children among all detected patients is 20 to 30 per cent.[45, 133] Of the 615 known patients who became infected in Louisiana between 1855 and 1970, 5 per cent had onset at 0 to 9 years of age and 19 per cent were in the 10- to 19-year age group.[38] Lara,[92] in a study of 2000 children who lived in a leprosarium in the Philippines in an era when effective chemotherapy was not available, noted that 470 (23 per cent) developed leprosy. Of these 470 patients, 254 were followed closely, and in about 75 per cent, the lesions healed spontaneously. Thus, approximately 6 per cent of the children who were heavily exposed to leprosy developed active, persistent disease.

In adults, leprosy is more common in men than in women (2:1 to 3:1); in children, the sex ratio is approximately 1:1.

Genetic factors may influence the susceptibility of an individual to leprosy.[157] If one twin has leprosy, the chance that a monozygotic twin will develop leprosy is 60 to 85 per cent, compared with a 15 to 25 per cent risk for dizygotic twins.[59] Certain human leukocyte antigen (HLA)-DR antigens appear to be associated with specific forms of leprosy. In Surinam, HLA-DR3 is frequent in mixed African-Caucasians with tuberculoid leprosy and rare in lepromatous patients; however, in Indians with tuberculoid leprosy, HLA-DR2 predominates.[170] DR antigens may influence the presentation of antigens of *M. leprae* to T cells and thus affect the immune response to leprosy.[135]

In Texas and Louisiana, the ratios of autochthonous to imported leprosy patients are the highest in the continental United States. Indigenous leprosy is highly prevalent in armadillos only in those two states,[7, 160, 165, 174, 175] and contact with such wild-infected armadillos probably transmits leprosy to humans.[98, 180] There are no reports of transmission of leprosy to humans from naturally infected mangabey monkeys or chimpanzees, but there is this potential.[53, 113]

PATHOGENESIS AND PATHOLOGY

M. leprae causes disease by its ability to survive and multiply in macrophages (Fig. 103–1). If macrophages of the host digest the bacilli early, disease is not detectable or there are only minimal lesions. If the macrophages totally are incapable of destroying the organisms, a widely disseminated lepromatous leprosy will follow. Survival of *M. leprae* in macrophages depends on the immune response of the patient, which makes a knowledge of immunity to *M. leprae* necessary background for understanding the mechanism of pathologic changes in leprosy.

Immunity

The ability of an individual to resist *M. leprae* is assessed readily by the induration provoked by the intradermal injection of a suspension of killed *M. leprae* prepared from lepromatous tissue. Lepromatous nodules of patients were

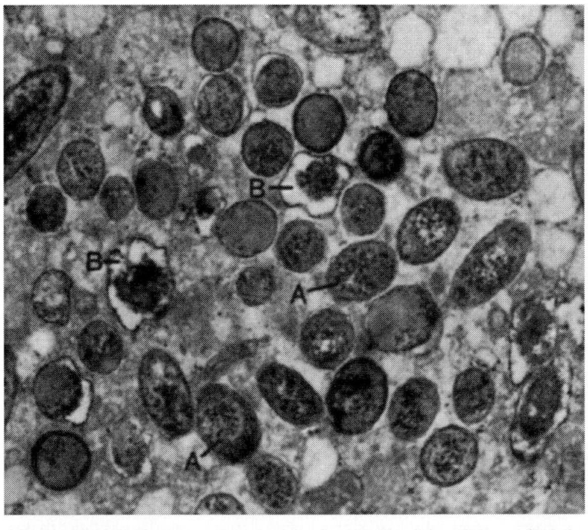

FIGURE 103–1. *Electron micrograph of a portion of a globus of* M. leprae *within a histiocyte in a leproma in the skin. There are cross sections of both well-preserved (A) and degenerated (B) bacilli. (× 45,000.) (Courtesy of Dr. S. C. Chang.)*

the traditional source, but infected tissue from armadillos now is used commonly.[114] The reagent is known as *lepromin* and the response as the lepromin reaction. This reaction, first studied by Hayashi and later evaluated by Mitsuda,[118] has two components: an early response at 48 hours (Fernandez reaction) and a late response at 3 to 4 weeks (Mitsuda reaction). The Mitsuda reaction is the most consistent and is used by clinicians as an aid in the classification of the clinical forms of leprosy. Mitsuda reactions are strongly positive (more than 5 mm in diameter) in tuberculoid patients, weak or negative (0 to 2 mm) in lepromatous patients, and intermediate (3 to 5 mm) in borderline patients. The reactions are a direct measure of delayed hypersensitivity or cell-mediated immunity (CMI) to *M. leprae* antigens; hence, lepromatous patients are anergic to *M. leprae*. The lepromin reaction has no value in diagnosis because a high percentage of any population is Mitsuda-positive. Even in children without leprosy, the Mitsuda reaction is positive in 20 per cent of those younger than 5 years of age and two-thirds of those 7 to 9 years of age.[56] Modifications of the lepromin reaction, with use of concentrated lepromin, show that macrophages at the test site in lepromatous patients cannot clear *M. leprae* from the skin, whereas in tuberculoid patients the bacilli are destroyed efficiently.[21]

Nonspecific factors participate in host defense against *M. leprae*. Complement, for example, promotes phagocytosis of leprosy bacilli.[152] After phagocytosis, there is phagolysosomal fusion and intracellular killing, perhaps by oxygen-independent mechanisms.

Although precise mechanisms of specific immunity remain elusive, abundant experimental evidence indicates that in the lepromatous patient, CMI to *M. leprae* markedly is suppressed. Skin test reactions to many antigens often are depressed, but they are depressed most consistently and most severely to *M. leprae*.[13] The degree of suppression gradually is less pronounced in clinical forms of disease that are progressively nearer tuberculoid leprosy.

There is a continuous decrease in the sensitivity of peripheral blood lymphocytes to *M. leprae* that proceeds from tuberculoid to lepromatous patients.[129] Many investigators believe that the defect in CMI to *M. leprae* is in T-lymphocyte function or in the interaction of T lymphocytes with macrophages. Total numbers of circulating T lymphocytes are decreased in lepromatous patients,[35] but there is no consistent alteration in the percentage distribution of circulating T-cell subsets, particularly in the suppressor-helper ratio.[141] T-lymphocyte subsets in lesions of leprosy in the skin, however, show marked differences in suppressor-helper distributions in the different forms of leprosy.[123, 124, 140] In tuberculoid lesions, helper cells are plentiful and distributed within the granulomas, whereas suppressor cells are in the mantle of the granuloma. In lepromatous lesions, the helper and suppressor cells are admixed among the macrophages. Suppressor activity is generated by lepromin in vitro in peripheral leukocytes from lepromatous patients but not in cells from tuberculoid patients.[105] This suppressor activity also may be induced by the unique species-specific antigen, phenolic glycolipid (PGL-1) of *M. leprae*[63, 104] but is unrelated to the type of leprosy.[139] This PGL abounds in the tissues of lepromatous patients. Secondary immunosuppression in advanced lepromatous leprosy may result from a blockade of thymus-dependent areas of lymph nodes by *M. leprae*-laden macrophages.[166] Specific suppressor T-cell activity in immunosuppression in leprosy remains controversial.[82]

Macrophages of lepromatous patients are believed to have the capacity to kill, digest, and clear *M. leprae* if they are activated.[62] Lepromatous leprosy patients, however, fail to produce interleukin-2 (IL-2), but IL-2 restores proliferation of lymphocytes in response to specific antigens.[60] There also is defective interferon (IFN-γ) production by lymphocytes from lepromatous patients on stimulation by *M. leprae* antigens.[131] IL-2–bearing lymphocytes are reduced markedly in lepromatous infiltrations in tissues.[122] Thus, suppressor T cells may influence IL-2 production in situ and reduce proliferation of specifically sensitized T cells to release IFN-γ, with the result that macrophages are not activated. The injection of IFN-γ into the skin of lepromatous patients causes a local influx of $CD4^+$ T cells with the formation of epithelioid and giant cells and the reduction of bacillary load.[81] IL-2 and IFN-γ, when available in quantity, thus may prove to be important immunotherapeutic agents for lepromatous leprosy. Therapy with these cytokines, however, provokes tumor necrosis factor–α (TNF-α). Activity of this toxic molecule may be inhibited by thalidomide or pentoxifylline.[80, 163]

Immunoglobulin production (IgG, IgA, and IgM) usually is elevated only slightly in tuberculoid patients but is elevated markedly in lepromatous patients.[15] There are corresponding rises in circulating antibody to mycobacterial antigens.[130] The total number of B lymphocytes is increased in the blood of lepromatous patients.[42]

The role of immunologic processes in damage to nerves in leprosy is unknown. Some observations suggest that antineural antibodies in the sera of many patients, especially those with lepromatous disease, are related to such damage.[136] TNF-α is associated with macrophage infiltration of peripheral nerves in reversal reactions.[89]

Histopathology

Biopsy specimens from well-defined lesions of leprosy should be taken from the active border and fixed in buffered 10 per cent formalin or other suitable fixative. The Fite-Faraco staining method is employed because the Ziehl-Neelsen stain does not demonstrate *M. leprae* optimally in tissue sections. DNA probes specific for *M. leprae* are available and are useful in the identification of leprosy bacilli in tissue or nasal secretions.[28, 184] Specimens for DNA studies should be preserved in ethyl alcohol.[39] A histopathologic diagnosis of leprosy must not be made unless the evidence is convincing. The pathologist must avoid ambiguous evaluations, such as "consistent with leprosy."

Indeterminate Leprosy

In indeterminate leprosy (Fig. 103–2), the immune potential of the patient is not portrayed clearly in the cellular reaction. There is only a mild chronic inflammation with small infiltrations of lymphocytes or histiocytes along neurovascular channels and sometimes around appendages (Fig. 103–3). If leprosy is suspected, all nerves in the dermis and subcutaneous tissue in numerous sections of the biopsy specimen must be searched for acid-fast bacilli, even though there are no inflammatory changes within them (Fig. 103–3). Sometimes acid-fast bacilli appear only in the arrectores pilorum muscles or subepidermal zone.[143] A histopathologic diagnosis of leprosy cannot be made unreservedly in indeterminate leprosy without demonstrating acid-fast bacilli.

Tuberculoid Leprosy

Tuberculoid patients (Fig. 103–4) possess a high level of CMI to *M. leprae*, and this is reflected in the cellular reaction. There are granulomas composed of epithelioid cells, Langhans giant cells, and lymphocytes in the dermis or subcutaneous tissue (Fig. 103–5*A*). Frequently, the upper dermal granu-

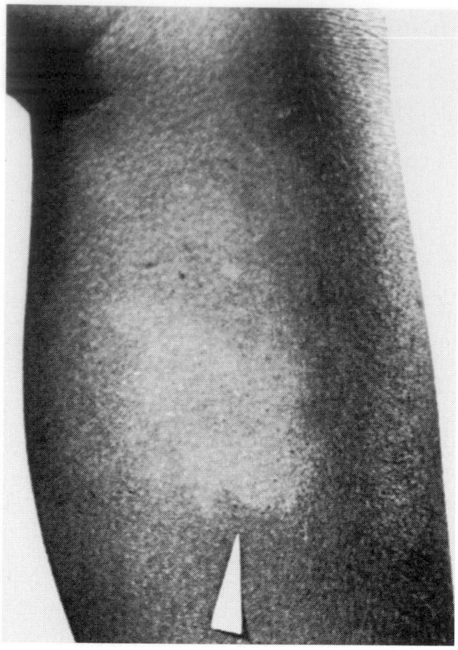

FIGURE 103–2. *Hypopigmented macule of indeterminate leprosy on the calf of a Filipino. (AFIP 74-9029-1.)*

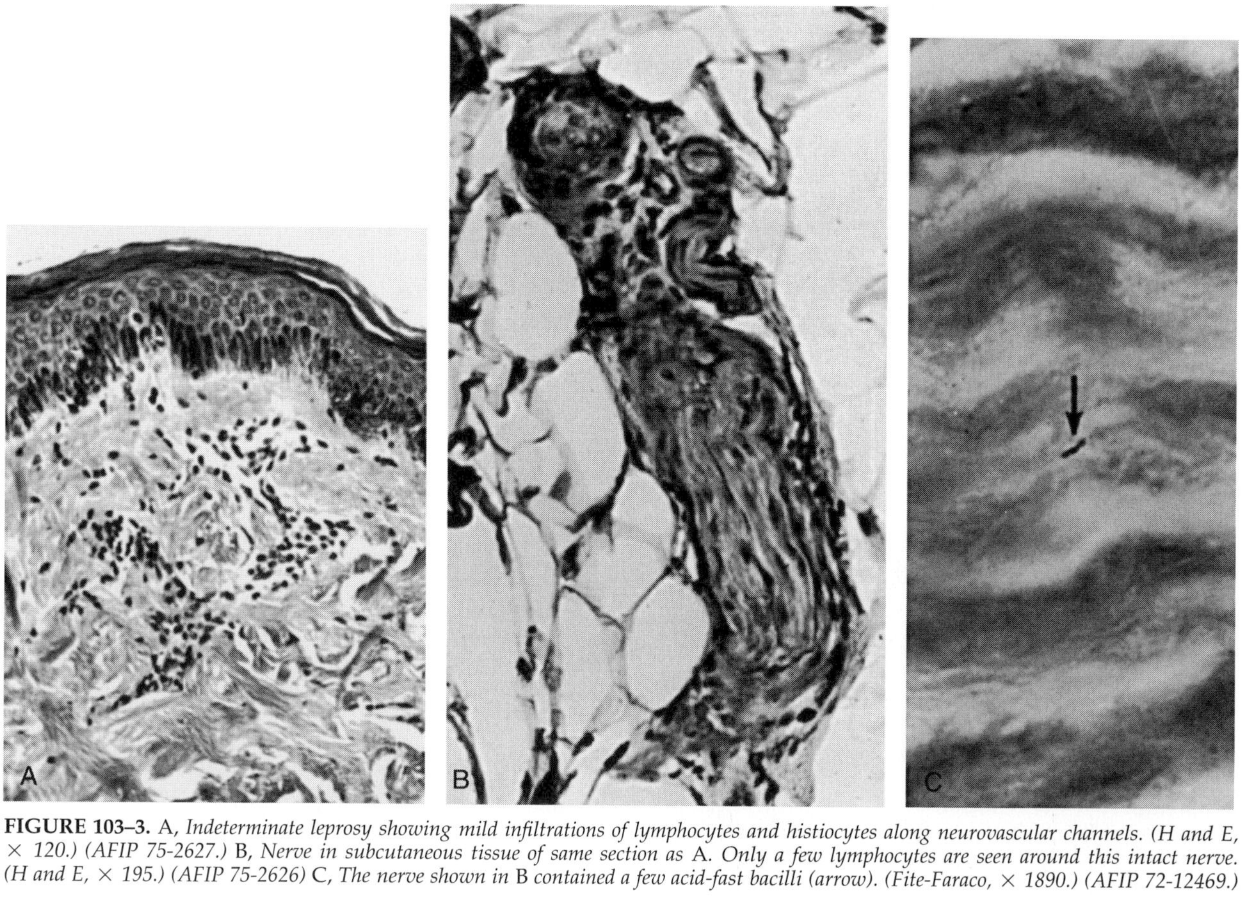

FIGURE 103–3. A, *Indeterminate leprosy showing mild infiltrations of lymphocytes and histiocytes along neurovascular channels. (H and E, × 120.) (AFIP 75-2627.)* B, *Nerve in subcutaneous tissue of same section as* A. *Only a few lymphocytes are seen around this intact nerve. (H and E, × 195.) (AFIP 75-2626)* C, *The nerve shown in* B *contained a few acid-fast bacilli (arrow). (Fite-Faraco, × 1890.) (AFIP 72-12469.)*

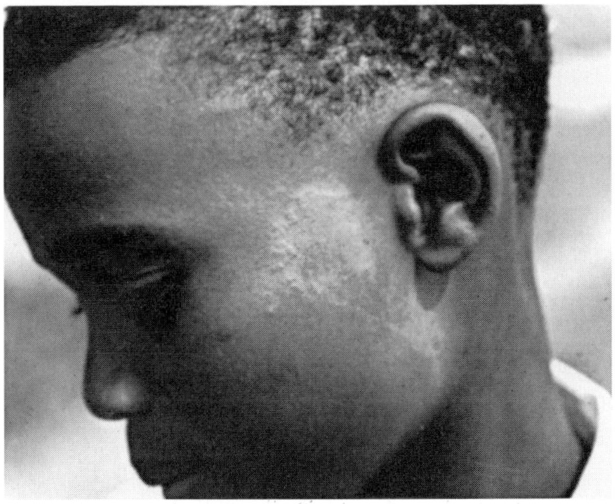

FIGURE 103–4. *Tuberculoid leprosy in a 12-year-old Zairian boy. This was the only lesion, and it has a well-defined papulated border with central healing. (AFIP 75-15598.)*

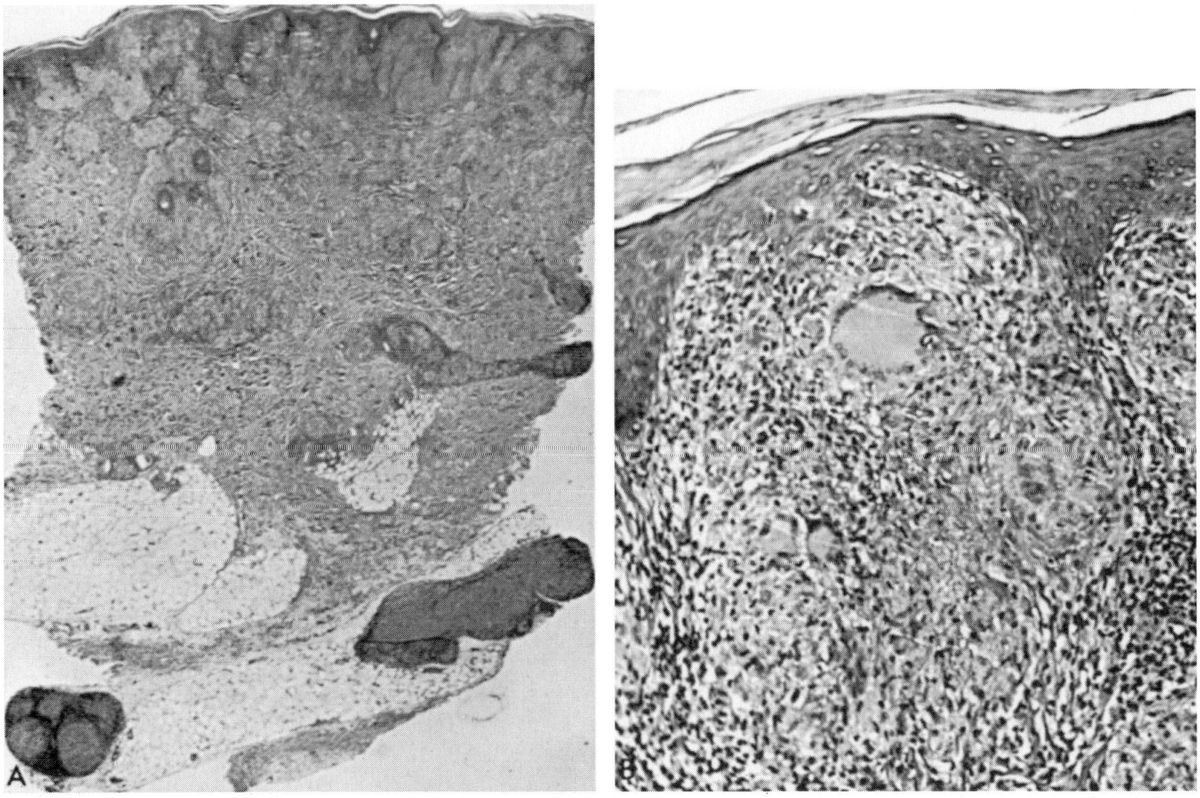

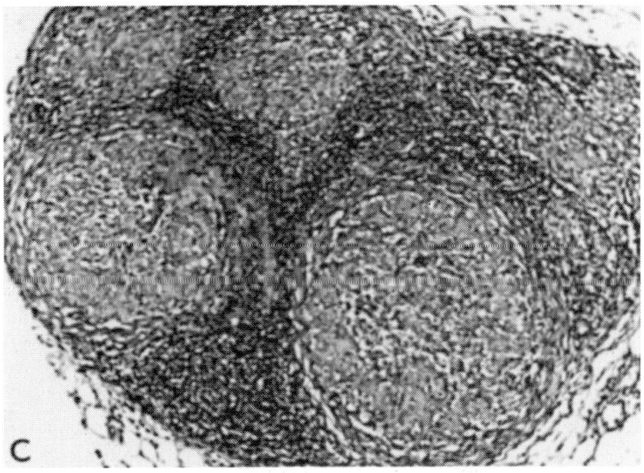

FIGURE 103–5. A, *Tuberculoid leprosy, demonstrating a dense granulomatous infiltration in the middle and upper dermis and in and around nerves in the subcutaneous tissue. (H and E, × 19.) (AFIP 72-12492.)* B, *Same section as A; the granulomas are composed of epithelioid cells, Langhans giant cells, and lymphocytes and invade the epidermis. (H and E, × 115.) (AFIP 72-12465.)* C, *High magnification of nerve in subcutaneous tissue seen in A. Nerves are replaced nearly completely by granulomas. Rare bacilli were in remaining remnants of nerves. (H and E, × 130.) (AFIP 72-12463.)*

lomas invade the lower layers of the epidermis (Fig. 103–5*B*). Damage to nerves is a distinctive feature; in old advanced lesions, all cutaneous nerves may be damaged beyond recognition (Fig. 103–5*C*). Schwann cells are increased in number in early lesions, and the nerves are invaded by mononuclear cells. Bacilli are rare, and often many sections must be searched for a single bacillus to be found. The bacilli usually are within remnants of dermal nerves but sometimes are just beneath the epidermis.

When major nerve trunks are involved, they contain typical tuberculoid infiltrates that eventually may replace the entire nerve. Occasionally, in large nerves, there are caseous "abscesses," but this is rare in children.

Borderline Leprosy

Borderline leprosy represents a broad spectrum of clinical (Fig. 103–6) and histopathologic (Table 103–1) variations. In

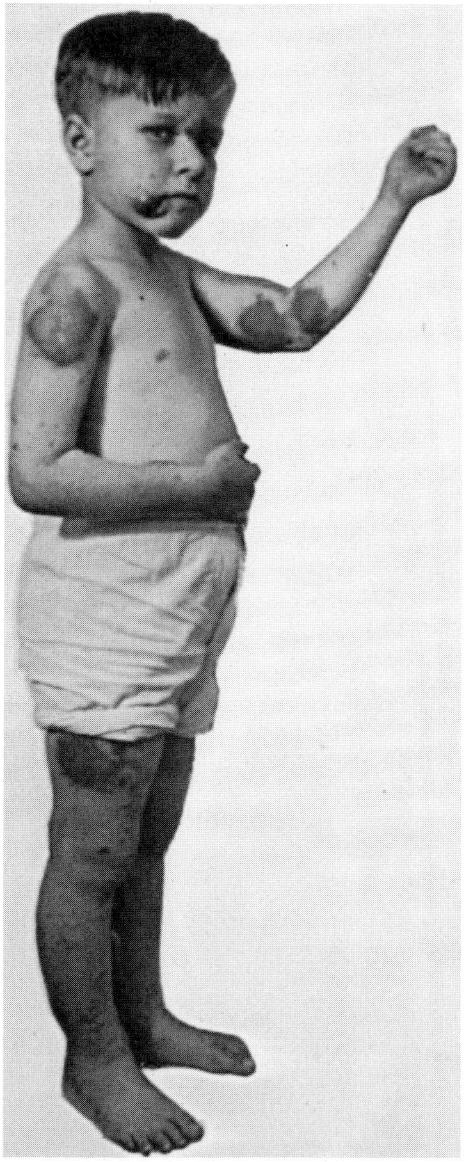

FIGURE 103–6. *Borderline lepromatous leprosy in a 6-year-old boy. There are many small papular lesions and a few larger erythematous plaques undergoing reversal reaction. (AFIP 77-9195[A]-1.)*

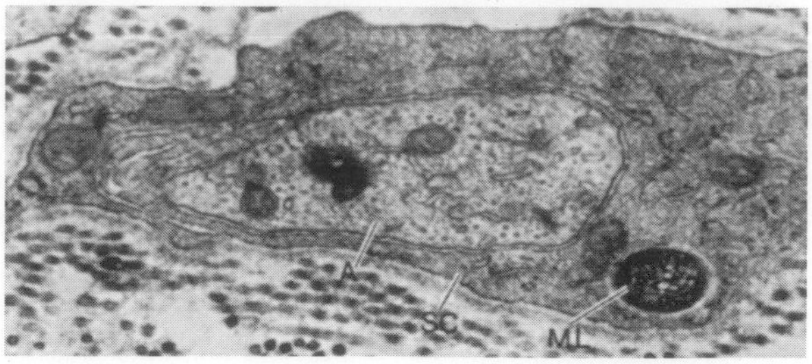

FIGURE 103–7. *Electron micrograph of a portion of a damaged dermal nerve in borderline leprosy. A nonmyelinated axon (A) is surrounded by a Schwann cell (SC) that contains a single* M. leprae *bacillus (ML). (× 60,000.) (Courtesy of Dr. S. C. Chang.)*

the borderline-tuberculoid area, strong CMI still is evident by the large numbers of epithelioid cells and lymphocytes. The nerves usually are damaged less and more readily are identifiable than in tuberculoid leprosy. Usually, *M. leprae* are found easily in the Schwann cells of nerves (Fig. 103–7) or in the subepidermal zone. In borderline leprosy, the epithelioid cells are not surrounded by large numbers of lymphocytes, and Langhans giant cells are not common. The subepidermal area is free of infiltrating cells, and nerves are not severely damaged, but the perineurium often is laminated by invading epithelioid cells. Some histopathologists do not recognize mid-borderline leprosy as an entity because usually there are features that suggest that the lesion is either on the borderline-tuberculoid or on the borderline-lepromatous side of the spectrum of the disease.[76] Borderline-lepromatous lesions reveal a low level of CMI. The granulomas are composed mostly of macrophages but contain irregularly distributed lymphocytes. A few nests of epithelioid cells are in the granu-

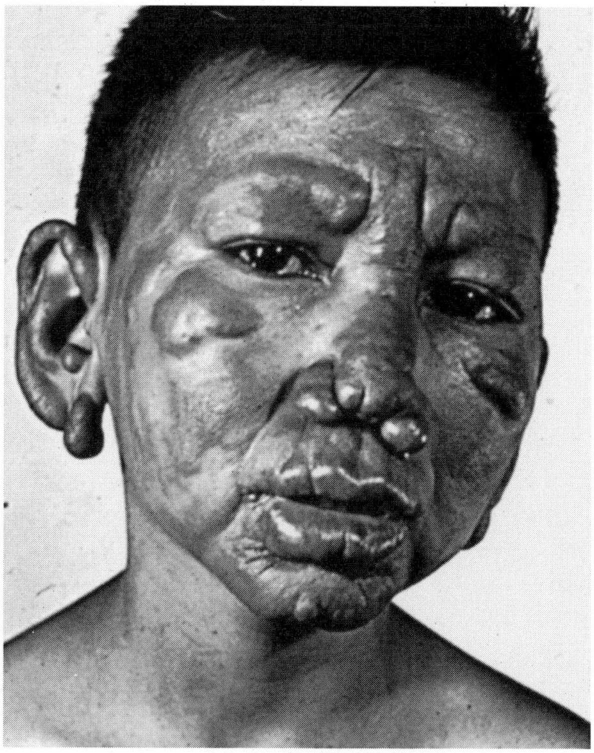

FIGURE 103–8. *Advanced lepromatous leprosy in an adolescent Filipino boy. Note the loss of eyebrows and the thickening of the ears. (AFIP 77-9359-2.)*

TABLE 103–1. Criteria for Classification of Leprosy

Group	Clinical Features	Histologic Features	Lepromin Reaction (Mitsuda)	Bacillary Density
Tuberculoid (TT)	A single or few anesthetic macules or plaques Borders well defined Peripheral nerve involvement common	Epithelioid–lymphocyte granulomas, with or without giant cells, in skin and nerves No subepidermal clear zone Bacilli in nerves, but rare	Strongly positive	Rare
Borderline–tuberculoid (BT)	Lesions similar to TT but more numerous Borders of lesions less distinct Satellite lesions sometimes present around larger lesions Peripheral nerve involvement common	Granulomas similar to TT Nerves are infiltrated Bacilli frequently found in nerves	Positive	Scanty
Borderline (BB)	More lesions than BT Borders more vague Satellite lesions often seen Peripheral nerve involvement common	Epithelioid cells and histiocytic infiltrations focalized by lymphocytes Nerves show increased cellularity Bacilli readily found in nerves	Negative or weakly positive	Moderate
Borderline–lepromatous (BL)	Lesions are numerous and similar to BB Some nerve damage	Histiocytic infiltrations show a tendency to evolve toward both epithelioid cells and foamy cells Lymphocytes present Nerves have less cellular infiltration Bacilli plentiful in nerves	Negative	Heavy
Lepromatous (LL)	Multiple, nonanesthetic, macular or papular, symmetrically distributed lesions No neural lesions until late Late complications of madarosis, leonine facies, testicular damage, etc.	Foamy histiocytes containing large numbers of bacilli Few or no lymphocytes Subepidermal clear zone Numerous bacilli in nerves and perineurium without significant intraneural cellular infiltration	Negative	Very heavy
Indeterminate (I)	Vaguely defined hypopigmented or erythematous macule	Often indistinguishable from "mild nonspecific dermatitis" Lymphocytes and histiocytes around skin appendages and nerves	Weakly positive or negative	Negative or scanty

lomas. The perineurium of the nerves is infiltrated with cellular exudates. Nerves are identified easily and contain many bacilli.

Lepromatous Leprosy

The prelepromatous lesion shows only a mild proliferation of macrophages around vessels, nerves, and appendages. Acid-fast bacilli are few and often difficult to demonstrate.

Anergy to *M. leprae* becomes apparent early in the lepromatous lesion (Fig. 103–8), with the bacilli-laden macrophage (Virchow cell or lepra cell) as the predominant inflammatory cell. In early lesions, they tend to accumulate around vessels, nerves, and appendages, but they eventually replace the entire dermis in a fully developed leproma (Fig. 103–9*A*). The infected macrophages are supported by a delicate stroma and supplied by a rich network of capillaries. As the macrophages age, they become vacuolated (foamy), largely because of their lipid content. In developing lesions, the intracellular bacilli are arranged in small bundles (Fig. 103–9*B*); in advanced lesions, dense masses of bacilli, called globi, may replace nearly the entire cytoplasm of the macrophage. Infiltrating cells do not invade the epidermis but leave a narrow subepidermal clear zone. There are many bacilli in the dermal nerves and frequently in endothelial cells and walls of blood vessels,[128] arrectores pilorum muscles, and epithelial cells of hair follicles. Plasma cells vary in numbers and proba-

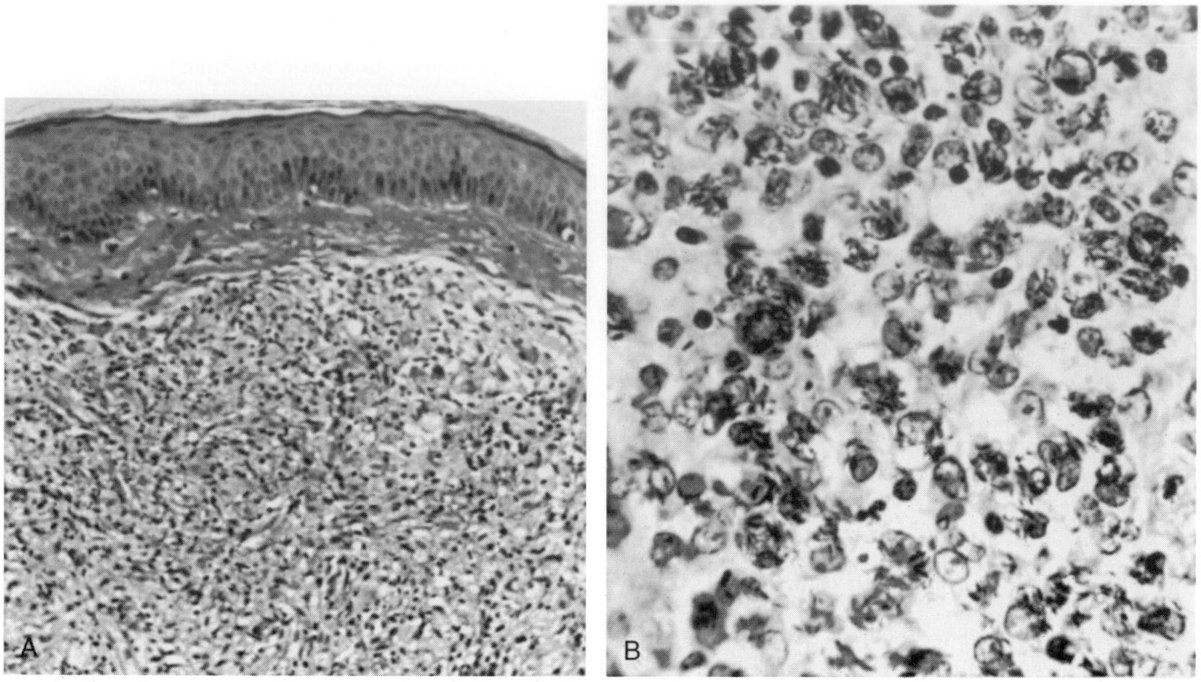

FIGURE 103–9. A, *Advanced lepromatous leprosy showing replacement of dermis by foamy histiocytes (lepra cells) and a thin subepidermal clear zone. (H and E, × 208.) (AFIP 65-1653.)* B, *Higher magnification showing clumps of* M. leprae *in histiocytes in a leproma in the skin. (Fite-Faraco, × 657.) (AFIP 56-19549.)*

bly reflect B-lymphocyte hyperactivity.[42] There are few lymphocytes in a lepromatous lesion. Large nerve trunks may show typical lepromatous infiltrations.

Occasionally in lepromatous leprosy patients, elevated firm nodules form in the skin, especially in relapsing disease. Because of the characteristic histologic pattern of these lesions in which the histiocytes resemble fibrocytes, this form is called histoid leprosy.[173]

Lepromatous leprosy is disseminated widely, and frequently there are lepromatous infiltrations in the upper respiratory tract as far down as the larynx and in the sclera, liver, and testes. In adults, the testes frequently are infiltrated, which results in sterility and gynecomastia, but these complications are rare in children.

Lymph nodes often are infiltrated by bacilli-laden macrophages, especially in the medulla and paracortical areas (Figs. 103–10 and 103–11).

CLINICAL MANIFESTATIONS

The incubation period varies (usually 2 to 5 years), and there are no well-established prodromal manifestations. Some experienced clinicians working in areas of high prevalence recognize early signs of nerve involvement (localized paresthesia, itching, or numbness) before there are any visible lesions.

After the incubation period, lesions of varying description

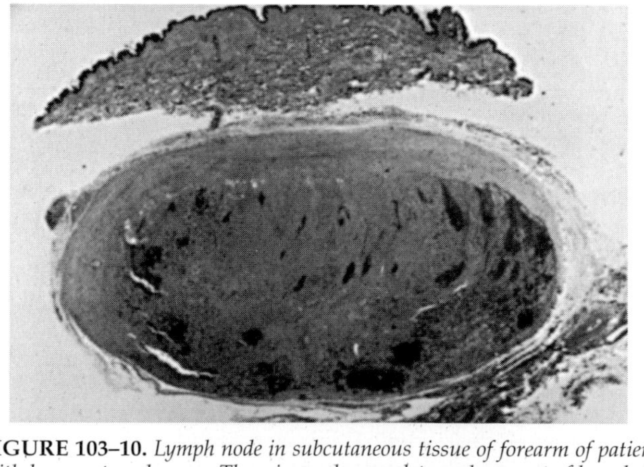

FIGURE 103–10. *Lymph node in subcutaneous tissue of forearm of patient with lepromatous leprosy. There is nearly complete replacement of lymphoid tissue (dark-staining areas) by lepra cells. (H and E, × 11.) (AFIP 72-12502.)*

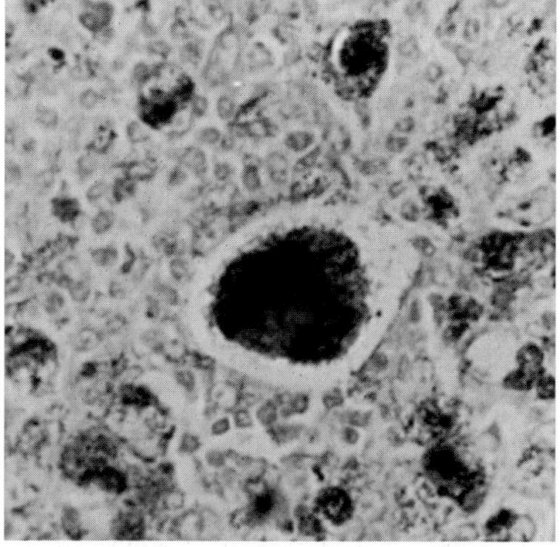

FIGURE 103–11. *High magnification of lymph node in Figure 103–10, demonstrating globi of* M. leprae *in histiocytes. (Fite-Faraco, × 645.) (AFIP 72-12509.)*

appear. The nature of the lesions depends on the immune response of the patient to *M. leprae*. Thus far, no strain variations of the bacillus, except in drug sensitivity, have been detected.[183] Most clinicians today follow the classification scheme outlined by Ridley and Jopling,[144] and Table 103–1 summarizes their criteria. Classification is important because it aids in establishing prognosis and treatment programs for the patient.

Virtually all leprosy patients have peripheral neuropathy, if cutaneous sensory changes are included, and approximately 25 per cent have significant deformity. Detailed discussions of peripheral neuropathy in leprosy may be consulted for further coverage of this important topic.[148]

Ocular complications in leprosy are well known. Therefore, all leprosy patients should be evaluated by an ophthalmologist at diagnosis and periodically reevaluated, especially during any reactional episodes.

Indeterminate Leprosy

The indeterminate lesion is the first manifestation in most patients and may heal spontaneously, remain unchanged for months or years, or gradually progress toward tuberculoid or lepromatous leprosy. Patients with indeterminate leprosy have a single or a few macules in the skin (see Fig. 103–2). The macule is defined poorly and mildly hypopigmented in deeper pigmented skins and slightly erythematous in lighter skins. Skin texture, sensation, and sweating within early macules are normal or only slightly altered. There is no damage to peripheral nerves, and skin smears from the lesions rarely contain bacilli. Diagnosis can be made only by finding acid-fast bacilli in histopathologic sections.

Tuberculoid Leprosy

Patients with tuberculoid leprosy have a single or several asymmetrically distributed hypopigmented skin lesions (Fig. 103–4). Tuberculoid lesions arise de novo or evolve from indeterminate macules. The lesion may be macular or infiltrated, but the borders always are demarcated sharply from the surrounding normal skin and frequently are papulated finely. Lesions range in size from less than 1 cm to those that cover entire regions, such as the thigh or buttock. Many tuberculoid lesions heal spontaneously. In large, active lesions, the centers often are healed and repigmented, although somewhat atrophic.

In tuberculoid lesions, there is sensory loss with impaired sweating and eventual loss of hair. On the face, because of a rich innervation, the detection of hypesthesia in early lesions requires discriminating tests. Conversely, clinicians mistakenly may diagnose leprosy in areas of the body that normally are hypesthetic (e.g., over the elbows or knees).

Involvement of peripheral nerves is common in tuberculoid leprosy (Fig. 103–12), and cutaneous nerves often can be palpated adjacent to or within lesions. The regional nerve trunks most commonly enlarged are the ulnar from the olecranon groove to midarm, the lateral popliteal just distal to the head of the fibula, and the posterior tibial in the medial aspect of the ankle. Enlarged or tender nerves anywhere should alert the clinician to the possibility of leprosy. Any readily palpable cutaneous nerve probably is enlarged, but the evaluation of nerve trunk size requires experience because of the wide range of normal sizes.

Borderline Leprosy

Borderline leprosy, sometimes called dimorphous or intermediate leprosy, has features of both the lepromatous and the tuberculoid forms and represents a continuous spectrum of disease ranging from near-tuberculoid to near-lepromatous. This is an unstable form of leprosy and gradually may evolve toward tuberculoid leprosy by undergoing reversal reactions or be downgraded toward lepromatous leprosy. Table 103–1 describes the three major subgroups of borderline leprosy: borderline-tuberculoid, borderline, and borderline-lepromatous.

In borderline-tuberculoid leprosy, the number of lesions usually is greater than in tuberculoid leprosy, and the borders of each lesion, macule, or plaque are defined less sharply

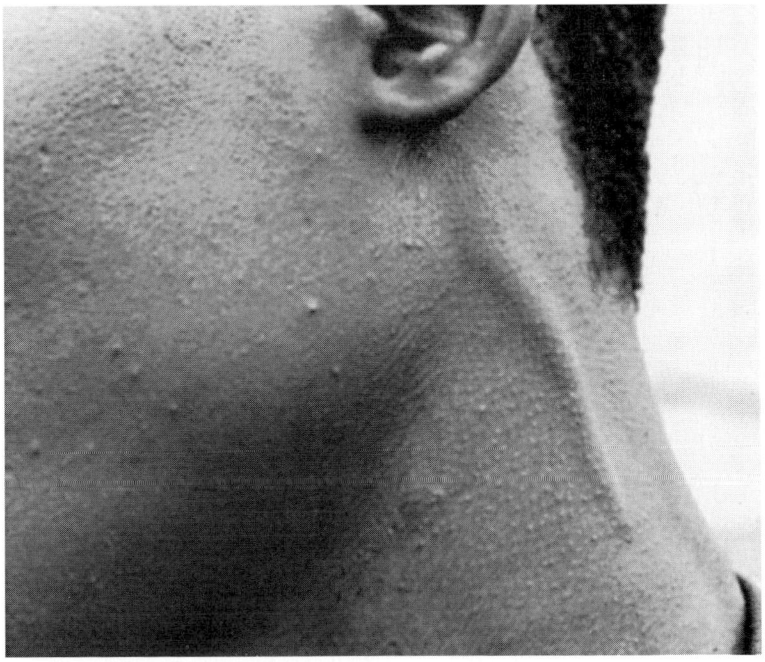

FIGURE 103–12. *Enlargement of the great auricular nerve in an adolescent Zairian boy. A large macule of tuberculoid leprosy in the area of the angle of the mandible is now nearly inactive and barely visible. (AFIP 77-9359-5.)*

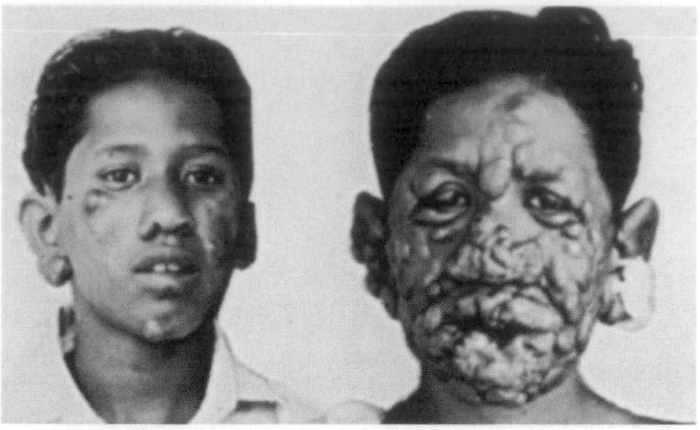

FIGURE 103–13. *Advance of lepromatous leprosy in a Hawaiian boy. The photograph on the left was taken in 1931, when the patient was 13 years old, and the photograph on the right was taken 2 years later. In that era, there was no effective chemotherapy. (AFIP 75-2479[A]-2.)*

than in tuberculoid leprosy. Often there are small satellite lesions around larger macules or plaques. In borderline-lepromatous leprosy, there are widespread nodular infiltrations or plaques of varying sizes (Fig. 103–6).

Damage to nerves and resulting deformity occur early and often are widespread. Pain in nerves or neurotropic changes (e.g., sensory changes that lead to damaged hands or feet or a muscular weakness such as footdrop) frequently bring the patient to the physician. Severe damage to nerves is infrequent in early childhood but can be disastrous. Prevention of this complication is an important goal of leprosy detection programs and of every clinician treating a leprosy patient.

Lepromatous Leprosy

In lepromatous leprosy, the bacilli multiply freely and the disease disseminates widely, often before there are striking cutaneous manifestations, in contrast to the strict localization of lesions in tuberculoid leprosy. Lepromatous leprosy may evolve from indeterminate or borderline leprosy or may be the first recognizable form. In its earliest form, lepromatous leprosy presents as "juvenile leprosy," a clinical entity delineated from observations of large numbers of children in homes for children of leprosy patients in India.[127] This form, also called prelepromatous leprosy, is difficult to detect and frequently goes unrecognized until a more advanced stage develops. Skin texture may be altered slightly, but the vague macules with indistinct borders are detected only under appropriate lighting, preferably daylight. There are no changes in sensation or sweating in the macules, and acid-fast bacilli frequently are not detectable in smears from skin. Histopathologic sections may reveal a few bacilli to confirm the diagnosis; however, if there is a suspicion of leprosy, the patient should be followed until an explanation for the mild skin changes is found. If leprosy is present and not detected and treated, many of these patients will develop advanced forms of lepromatous leprosy (Fig. 103–13).

The hypopigmented or slightly erythematous macules of early lepromatous leprosy, like those of juvenile leprosy, easily are missed because they also are vague and have slight if any sensory changes. These macules usually are small but gradually may coalesce and cover large areas of skin, even nearly the entire body. Clinical diagnosis then is difficult, and over a few years, the patient will develop advanced lepromatous leprosy. If skin smears or biopsy specimens are taken in the macular stage, diagnosis almost always is assured. If the disease is not diagnosed and treated in the macular stage, the infiltration of the skin will increase gradually, and nodules may develop. The skin is infiltrated most heavily in the cooler portions of the body, notably the ears (pinnae) and face. By this time, nerves usually are enlarged and there are early signs of sensory loss in the hands and feet. The eyebrows are thinned and eventually lost, beginning at the lateral edges. These advanced changes of lepromatous leprosy are not common in young children but are well-known (Fig. 103–14).

In patients of Latin American ancestry, especially those from Mexico and Costa Rica, there is the highly anergic diffuse form of lepromatous leprosy called Lucio leprosy, so diffuse that the disease often is not recognized until the patient begins to have sensory changes of the hands and feet and the eyebrows and other body hair begin to disappear. In advanced forms of Lucio leprosy, there is a marked obstruc-

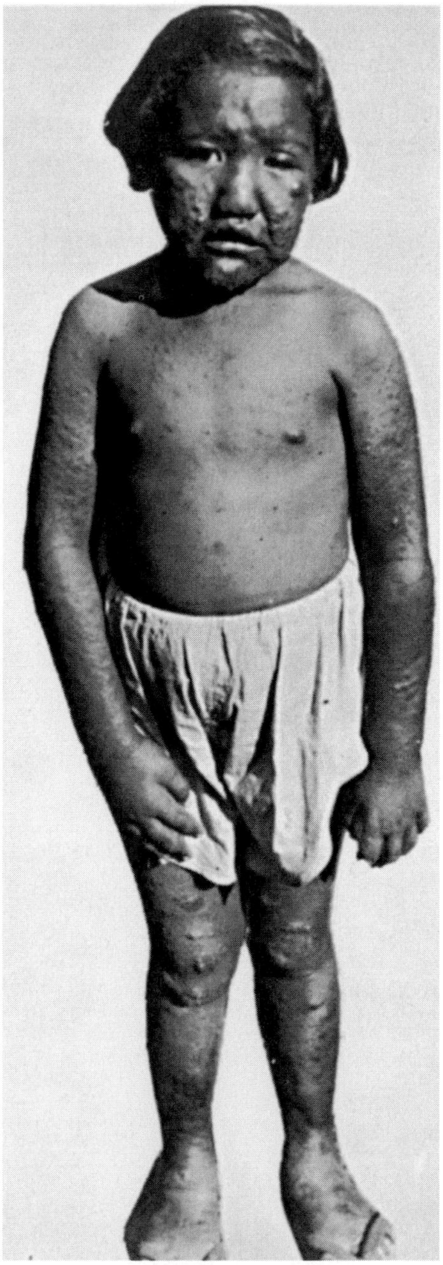

FIGURE 103–14. *Advanced lepromatous leprosy in a 6-year-old Hawaiian girl. There is diffuse infiltration of the skin and many nodules. (AFIP 75-15806-A.)*

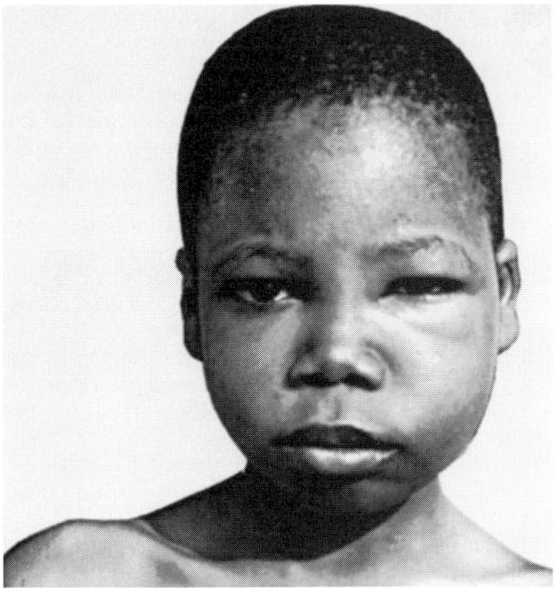

FIGURE 103–15. *Reversal reaction in an 8-year-old Zairian boy with borderline-tuberculoid leprosy. The left side of the face is swollen, and there is mild palsy due to facial nerve damage. The patient responded rapidly to steroid therapy. (AFIP 77-9359[A]-1.)*

tive vasculitis in the skin with production of dermal infarcts and irregular ulcers (Lucio phenomenon).[93] Lucio leprosy has been reported in children as young as 7 years of age.[151]

Neuritic Leprosy

Rarely, leprosy involves one or more major nerve trunks unaccompanied by cutaneous lesions. These patients have anesthesia, paresis, or wasting of muscles in the affected area. Nerve trunks frequently are painful, enlarged, and tender. Leprosy thus must be suspected in any peripheral neuritis with these features.

Reactions

The course of leprosy, treated or nontreated, often is interrupted by acute episodes. These are called reactions and fall into two general categories: reversal reactions (or type 1) and erythema nodosum leprosum (ENL) (or type 2).

Reversal Reactions

Reversal reactions complicate borderline leprosy and represent delayed hypersensitivity reactions with an upgrading of the CMI toward tuberculoid leprosy. Lesions become erythematous and edematous, and neuritis is common (Fig. 103–15). Patients who are lepromin-positive and have IgM antibodies to PGL-1 are most at risk for reversal reactions.[145] Proliferation of sensitized T lymphocytes initiates reversal reactions, releasing lymphokines that amplify the inflammatory response, calling in and activating macrophages.[146] There is immunohistopathologic evidence that effective chemotherapy of both paucibacillary and multibacillary patients activates CMI and provokes clinical or subclinical reversal reactions. There is, for example, increased expression of HLA-DR that may enhance IFN-γ production by lymphocytes in granulomas.[24] This is expressed histopathologically by edema accompanied by an increase in numbers of lymphocytes, often with epithelioid cells and giant cells. In severe reactions, there may be necrosis within the granulomas. An increase in levels of TNF-α during reactions partially may explain this necrosis.[153] Patients undergoing such reactions must be observed closely so that sensory loss and deformities are minimized. By repeated reversal reactions, borderline leprosy, even those forms near lepromatous disease, gradually may upgrade to tuberculoid leprosy.

Differentiation of reversal reactions from relapsing lesions often is difficult and requires careful correlation of clinical and histopathologic findings. This is becoming increasingly important in endemic areas where shorter-term chemotherapeutic regimens of fixed duration are employed.[40]

Erythema Nodosum Leprosum

Approximately 50 per cent of lepromatous patients have ENL after a few months of chemotherapy. There is a rapid onset of tender subcutaneous nodules that become erythematous (Fig. 103–16); often they are accompanied by fever and occasionally by synovitis and iridocyclitis. ENL resembles the Arthus reaction and is thought to result from immune complex formation. This concept is suggested by the detection of immune complexes in the sera of patients with ENL.[46] Immune complexes may form within lesions by the local release of antigens of *M. leprae* and could modulate the development of T-cell populations in situ. For example, there are increased numbers of OKT4 (helper) lymphocytes within lesions of ENL.[121] Serum TNF-α is elevated in ENL.[150, 153] In the nodule, there is an infiltration of neutrophils and sometimes an intense vasculitis. Ulceration of the skin frequently accom-

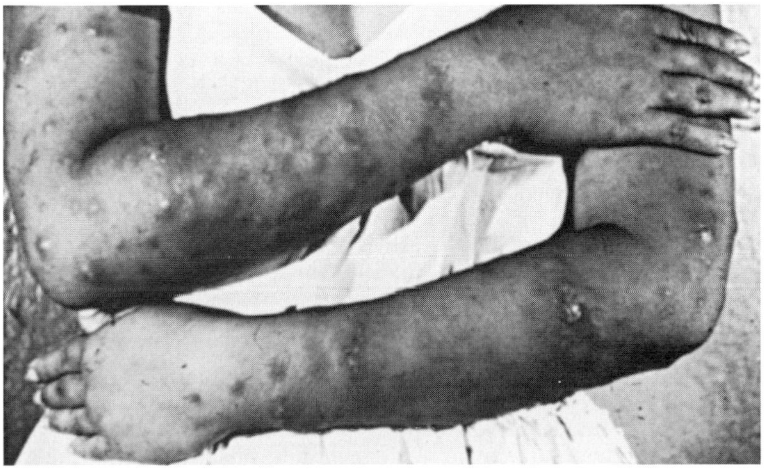

FIGURE 103–16. *Erythema nodosum leprosum in a Filipino adolescent girl with lepromatous leprosy. (AFIP 74-9029-7.)*

panies severe ENL. Glomerulonephritis sometimes complicates ENL; secondary amyloidosis is a late sequela of repeated reactions and may be a consequence of the neutrophilic leukocytosis.[100] Although neutrophilic infiltration is considered by many as the hallmark of the tissue reaction, tissues of some patients with typical ENL clinically do not show neutrophils. In such patients, demonstration of serum amyloid A and C-reactive protein may aid in establishing ENL.[64]

DIAGNOSIS AND DIFFERENTIAL DIAGNOSIS

The cardinal signs of leprosy are hypesthetic lesions of the skin, enlarged peripheral nerve(s), and acid-fast bacilli in skin smears. In the absence of another clear explanation, any one of these signs strongly suggests leprosy.

The experienced observer can diagnose most patients clinically, except those with early leprosy, with a high degree of accuracy. Histopathologic evaluation, however, strongly is recommended for accurate classification and for documentation.

Leprosy patients may be found in almost any geographic area. An awareness of this will minimize missed and delayed diagnoses, especially in areas of low prevalence. In the United States, the usual delay in diagnosis after the first visit to a physician for symptoms related to leprosy is approximately 1.5 to 2 years. This delay often significantly worsens prognosis.

History is important. Contact with leprosy patients or residence in an endemic area raises suspicion of leprosy in a patient with a chronic lesion of the skin. Sensory loss in or unexplained damage to hands or feet suggests damage to nerve trunks. Sometimes a footdrop will bring the patient to a physician. Occasionally, lepromatous patients first will consult an otolaryngologist because of a chronic stuffy nose.

The clinician must evaluate sensory changes in a lesion by using the precautions already mentioned. Sensory changes are detected readily in cooperative older children. The modalities usually tested are light touch with the use of a few fibers of cotton or calibrated nylon threads and heat-cold discrimination with the use of warm and cold water in test tubes. Much patience and repeated testing often are necessary in young children. Spontaneous sweating can be observed directly, or induced sweating can be evaluated.[99] Hair may be preserved completely in early lesions but lost in advanced lesions.

Main nerve trunks must be palpated for tenderness and enlargement. Skin in the area of discrete lesions also must be palpated gently to detect enlargement of cutaneous nerves. In the world population, leprosy is the most common cause of peripheral neuropathy and thus must be considered in any patient with peripheral neuropathy.[148]

Obtaining and examining smears for acid-fast bacilli is an important diagnostic procedure and should be controlled carefully by experienced laboratories. Briefly, smears are made from the edge of discrete macules or plaques, nodules, earlobes, and nasal mucosa. Skin smears are made by squeezing and holding a fold of skin between the thumb and forefinger to avoid blood in the smear and making a short, shallow slit in the skin with a razor blade or scalpel. The instrument then is turned at a right angle to the slit, and the edges of the incision are scraped. The cells and fluid thus obtained are spread on a slide, heat-fixed, and stained by the Ziehl-Neelsen method.[171] Evaluation of smears should not be done by those unfamiliar with their interpretation. An occasional acid-fast bacillus may, for example, be a harmless contaminant on the patient or in the reagents.

The lepromin reaction is useless for the diagnosis of leprosy. Currently available skin tests with soluble *M. leprae* antigens are unreliable.[57] There are enzyme-linked immunosorbent and gelatin particle agglutination tests for antibodies to the PGL-1 of *M. leprae*.[18, 52, 67] Although specificity for *M. leprae* is high, these tests detect antibodies to PGL-1 in only about 50 per cent of paucibacillary patients. Other serologic tests for antibodies to *M. leprae*–specific epitopes on protein moities of the bacillus are under evaluation.[137] PGL-1 antigen is detectable in the serum and urine of most multibacillary patients.[134, 187]

Reliance on DNA probes and polymerase chain reaction technology may prove useful in the diagnosis of leprosy in tissue sections, skin smears, and nasal smears.[28, 162, 184] Because these methods can detect a single leprosy bacillus, interpretation of results, particularly in highly endemic areas, is difficult. Careful clinicopathologic correlation is essential in basing diagnosis on DNA findings.[168]

The differential diagnosis of leprosy in children is an extensive subject and can be discussed only briefly here. Superficial mycoses and postinflammatory changes commonly are confused with early leprosy. Changes in pigmentation may be caused, for instance, by scars, birthmarks, and actinic dermatitis. In areas where dermal filariasis is endemic, vague macules in the black-skinned patient may appear identical to early macules of leprosy.[11, 102, 110] Among the many infiltrated lesions of the skin that can resemble leprosy are leishmaniasis, lymphoma, granuloma annulare, granuloma multiforme (Mkar disease), lupus erythematosus, psoriasis, pityriasis rosea, sarcoidosis, and neurofibromatosis. Peripheral neuropathies that may simulate leprosy are those seen in Morvan disease, syringomyelia, lead intoxication, diabetes mellitus, primary amyloidosis of nerves, and familial hypertrophic neuropathy.

Sera from patients with advanced lepromatous leprosy frequently give false-positive reactions for syphilis with the use of cardiolipin antibody assays.

PROGNOSIS

Without chemotherapy, prognosis in all patients except those with limited and self-healing disease potentially is poor. Those with borderline or advanced tuberculoid leprosy frequently become mutilated because of damage to nerves. Borderline leprosy can downgrade toward lepromatous leprosy. In lepromatous patients, the disease is progressive and can cause death from laryngeal obstruction. Secondary amyloidosis is a frequent late sequela. Blindness may result from lagophthalmic keratitis or repeated episodes of iridocyclitis. General debility and deformity eventually prevent gainful employment in many patients.

With adequate specific chemotherapy and control of reactions, prognosis is good in nearly all patients. If therapy is started early, prognosis usually is excellent and deformity and mutilation are prevented. Even after successful chemotherapy, however, some patients continue to suffer significant neuritis and loss of peripheral nerve function. Sometimes this "silent neuropathy" goes unnoticed by both the patient and physician.[27, 169] Appropriate early attention to anesthetic hands and feet and restoration of function by reconstructive surgery can prevent most mutilation.

The lepromin test is a valuable prognostic tool[75] because it measures the CMI potential of the host to infection by *M. leprae*. Patients with early macular lesions who are lepromin-negative have a poorer prognosis than do those who are lepromin-positive if treatment cannot be administered. Histopathologic evaluation before chemotherapy is important for prognosis and, if available, should not be neglected.

TREATMENT

Once a diagnosis of leprosy is established, chemotherapy must be initiated and appropriate measures instituted for preventing or correcting deformity in patients with neurotrophic changes.[19, 41, 91] The three most commonly used chemotherapeutic agents are dapsone, clofazimine, and rifampin. The effectiveness of chemotherapy is assessed readily in lepromatous or near-lepromatous patients by the staining quality of *M. leprae* in skin smears. Skin smears are recommended after the first 3 months of therapy and thereafter every 6 months to 1 year until the smears are negative. Response to chemotherapy in tuberculoid patients and most borderline patients is assessed by clinical response and by histopathologic evaluation. Viability of *M. leprae* in tissues is assessed in the mouse footpad.

There is increasing acceptance of combined chemotherapy for all forms of active leprosy. Although there are few experimental data,[156] the growing body of clinical data indicates that multidrug therapy rapidly is replacing monotherapy.[29, 68, 94] In fact, monotherapy with any chemotherapeutic agent no longer is advised. The currently recommended regimens for multidrug therapy are given later, after a brief discussion of the most used individual drugs.

Dapsone

In 1941, Faget and associates at Carville, Louisiana, introduced the sulfones as the first regularly effective chemotherapy for leprosy and thus revolutionized the care of the leprosy patient. The sulfone in common use is dapsone (4,4′-diaminodiphenylsulfone). Dapsone is an antimetabolite for *M. leprae* and is a bacteriostatic agent. The drug usually is given orally at 6 to 10 mg/kg body weight per week, divided into equal daily doses. The effect of dapsone on the bacilli is slow; 3 to 6 months of treatment is necessary to render bacilli from lepromatous patients noninfectious for the mouse footpad. Sulfone-resistant strains of *M. leprae* are being detected with increasing frequency,[177, 178] and monotherapy with dapsone is not recommended.

Dapsone usually is well tolerated but may provoke one or more of the following side reactions: dermatitis, anemia, hepatitis, or psychosis.

Clofazimine

Clofazimine (Lamprene) is a bacteriostatic riminophenazine dye that has both anti–*M. leprae* and anti-inflammatory activities, which make it a useful drug for the treatment of patients who are prone to ENL reactions. The mechanism of bacteriostasis may involve enhancement of oxygen-dependent killing of *M. leprae* and binding to bacterial DNA. Optimal dosage of clofazimine for children has not been determined, but the adult dose ranges from 50 to 300 mg daily. The lower dosages are used for maintenance therapy once a good clinical response has been achieved, and the higher dosages may be needed to control ENL. The major side reactions to clofazimine are hyperpigmentation of skin and enteritis. Enteritis is experienced only at the higher dosages usually employed for ENL. The hyperpigmentation subsides with the clinical improvement of leprosy, and both hyperpigmentation and enteritis resolve after drug withdrawal. Only two instances of clofazimine-resistant *M. leprae* have been reported.[83, 176] Clofazimine long has been considered safe in pregnancy, but there is a report of three neonatal deaths in 15 observed pregnancies.[37] Association between the drug and the deaths was not established. Monotherapy with clofazimine is not recommended.

Rifampin

Rifampin is an antibiotic that inhibits bacterial DNA-dependent RNA polymerase and is rapidly bactericidal for *M. leprae*. A single large dose can render a highly positive lepromatous patient noninfectious within 1 week. Dosages of 15 to 20 mg/kg/day have been given to children (maximum dose, 600 mg/day). Optimal doses for children with leprosy have not been reported. Adult doses range from 300 to 600 mg daily.[181] Many side reactions to rifampin have been described, and the relevant literature must be consulted.[14] Rifampin-resistant leprosy has been reported.[70, 185] Monotherapy with rifampin is not recommended.

Multidrug Treatment

Because of drug-resistant *M. leprae*, combined drug regimens are mandatory for the treatment of all forms of leprosy.[36, 156, 177, 178] The first large-scale multidrug therapy of leprosy was carried out in Malta, beginning in 1972. Rifampin, dapsone, prothionamide, and isoniazid were employed. Evaluation of the patients approximately 20 years later revealed a single relapse; however, presumed "persisting" *M. leprae* were detected.[43, 79]

Combined drug therapy minimizes drug-resistant strains of *M. leprae* and may eliminate some "persisting" organisms. Persisting *M. leprae* are viable bacilli that can be isolated in small numbers from patients who are responding well clinically to therapy. These persisting *M. leprae* bacilli are sensitive to the drug in question when tested in the mouse footpad and may account for relapses when treatment is discontinued. Persisting *M. leprae* have been detected after up to 5 years of rifampin, 6 years of clofazimine, and 22 years of dapsone therapy.

In 1982, a World Health Organization Study Group recommended the multidrug therapy regimens described as follows.[182] Patients were divided into paucibacillary and multibacillary groups. Paucibacillary patients (usually indeterminate, tuberculoid, and borderline-tuberculoid) now are defined as those with negative skin smears at all sites or who have fewer than four lesions and no clinical peripheral neuritis. All other patients are multibacillary.

The multidrug therapy regimens were designed primarily for field programs, employing, for example, pulsed supervised monthly rather than daily rifampin.[4] Multidrug therapy is well tolerated, and compliance in large-scale control programs has been satisfactory. Efficacy of multidrug therapy has been promising[68, 179]: In two surveys involving approximately 112,000 multibacillary patients followed up to 9 years post-therapy, the cumulative risk of relapse was 0.77 per cent. There are, however, anecdotal reports of certain groups of highly bacilliferous patients with relapse rates up to 20 per cent, with recurrences developing 5 years or more post-therapy.[72] These and other results suggest that therapeutic regimens for multibacillary patients should be given for longer than 2 years. In most reports, relapse rates in paucibacillary patients exceed those in multibacillary patients. In the author's experience in evaluating histopathologic specimens, many patients classified clinically as paucibacillary were, in fact, multibacillary. Potential for relapse after multidrug therapy regimens must await long-term, large-scale follow-up results.[71]

Regimen for Paucibacillary Patients (Indeterminate, Tuberculoid, and Borderline-Tuberculoid)

In adults, rifampin, 600 mg once a month, plus dapsone, 100 mg daily, is given for 6 months, and treatment is stopped. After the conclusion of multidrug therapy, the patient must be seen every 3 to 6 months. All apparent relapses require histopathologic examination for establishing whether the lesions represent relapses or reversal reactions. Relapsing patients must be treated again. Multidrug therapy is not used alone in patients with concurrent tuberculosis.

Regimen for Multibacillary Patients (Lepromatous, Borderline-Lepromatous, and Borderline)

In adults, rifampin, 600 mg monthly, dapsone, 100 mg daily, and clofazimine, 50 mg daily, are given. If patient compliance is questionable, the rifampin and 300 mg of clofazimine should be given monthly under supervision in addition to the 50 mg daily. These drugs must be given for at least 2 years and continued until skin smears are negative. For patients in whom the hyperpigmentation is unacceptable, daily doses of 250 to 375 mg of prothionamide or ethionamide may be substituted for clofazimine.

Recommendations for the United States

The Gillis W. Long Hansen's Disease Center, Carville, Louisiana, recommends the following variations of the World Health Organization–recommended multidrug regimens for adult patients in the United States[68]:

- Paucibacillary disease: dapsone, 100 mg daily, plus rifampin, 600 mg daily (or monthly) for 6 months, followed by dapsone monotherapy for a total of 3 years (indeterminate and tuberculoid) or 5 years (borderline-tuberculoid).
- Multibacillary disease: dapsone, 100 mg daily, plus rifampin, 600 mg daily (or monthly), for a total of 3 years, followed by dapsone monotherapy for 10 years (borderline) or life (borderline-lepromatous and lepromatous).
- Clofazimine (50 mg daily) may be added to the multibacillary regimen and should be used if any uncertainty exists as to whether the patient's bacilli are fully sulfone-sensitive.
- Multibacillary patients infected with dapsone-resistant bacilli are treated with clofazimine plus rifampin for 3 years, followed by clofazimine monotherapy indefinitely or rifampin plus ethionamide (250 mg daily) indefinitely if the patient will not take clofazimine.
- Other drugs: potent antileprosy drugs that now are undergoing advanced clinical evaluation and may soon gain general usage include fluoroquinolones (pefloxacin and ofloxacin), the macrolide clarithromycin, and the tetracycline minocycline.[47, 49, 55, 74]

Dosages of Multidrug Treatment for Children

Table 103–2 indicates appropriate adjustment of adult drug doses for children.[78]

Treatment of Reactions

Patients in reaction should be observed daily in the early stages and hospitalized if symptoms are severe. Formerly, specific therapy was stopped or the dosage reduced during reactions, but these measures no longer are recommended.[181] Damage to eyes and neurotrophic changes may ensue rapidly without immediate attention. Nerve tenderness and function must be assessed frequently during reactions. Acute inflammation of isolated lesions without damage to nerves is likely to be of little consequence except for cosmetic considerations, but the patient should be followed closely.

Reversal (Type 1) Reaction

Patients with painful, tender nerves must receive immediate care, usually in the hospital. Analgesics are given, and the affected area is put at rest. Large daily doses of corticosteroids are started and tapered to a minimum effective dose until the reaction subsides. Conversion to alternate-day steroid regimens may be attempted when long-term treatment is necessary. Some clinicians use clofazimine for chronic reversal reactions, but this is not recommended for the initial treatment of reactions with acute neuritis. Clofazimine is probably consistently efficacious only for ENL.[65]

Erythema Nodosum Leprosum (Type 2) Reaction

Mild ENL is treated with analgesics; more severe ENL is treated with thalidomide or corticosteroids. Pediatric doses of thalidomide in ENL have not been established; the initial adult dose is 100 mg four times daily followed by a minimal effective dose, usually 100 mg daily. The teratogenic action of thalidomide demands that appropriate measures be taken in the treatment of fertile females. For the rare patient who does not respond to thalidomide or in fertile females, corticosteroids or clofazimine is used. Corticosteroids, if employed, are given in the usual dosage schedules, beginning with large doses and tapering to a minimum effective level. Some clinicians use an alternate-day regimen when long-term steroid therapy is necessary, thus minimizing the well-known side effects.

Clofazimine is effective in most patients with ENL and does not have the disadvantages of thalidomide or corticosteroids. The anti-inflammatory action of clofazimine is not manifest until after 4 to 6 weeks of continuous use. Dosage must be adjusted to the minimum effective level.

Iridocyclitis requires emergency measures. Local corticoste-

TABLE 103–2. Multidrug Treatment for Children

Weight (kg)	Percentage of Adult Dose
Less than 15	25
15–30	50
30–45	75
More than 45	100

Adapted from Jopling, W. H.: Handbook of Leprosy. London, William Heinemann Medical Books LTD, 1984.

roids must be added to systemic anti-inflammatory regimens and ophthalmologic consultation obtained.

PREVENTION

Precise recommendations for the prevention of leprosy in individuals have never been formulated. Control programs today are based on the general principles that (1) the number of contagious patients is reduced by chemotherapy and (2) the surveillance of contacts will detect early leprosy. To accomplish these goals, there must be appropriate education of the public and medical personnel and population surveys in areas of higher prevalence. In endemic areas, improved housing is probably a highly important preventive measure by its reducing close contact of patients with healthy individuals.

The most important obstacles to improving control of leprosy include persistence of *M. leprae* in treated patients, cost and toxicity of antileprotics, long terms of therapeutic regimens, patient compliance, and social stigma of leprosy.[119]

For the eradication of leprosy, zoonotic sources of *M. leprae* must be taken into account.[113]

Chemoprophylaxis

Chemoprophylaxis of close contacts with dapsone has limited usefulness[26] and is not recommended for large populations. This recommendation is based on the probability that long-term usage would be irregular and that dapsone-resistant *M. leprae* may develop.[181]

Vaccination, Immunoprophylaxis, and Immunotherapy

The World Health Organization initiated an Immunology of Leprosy Program (IMMLEP) in 1974 with two primary goals: (1) the development of a vaccine against leprosy and (2) the development of reagents for detecting subclinical leprosy. Achievement of both goals could diminish profoundly the incidence of leprosy. *M. leprae*, or specific antigens thereof, for the IMMLEP studies are obtained from experimentally infected armadillos. Vaccines composed of heat-killed whole *M. leprae* alone, or in combination with live bacille Calmette-Guérin (BCG), have been found safe and induce delayed-type hypersensitivity to *M. leprae* in a high percentage of lepromin-negative individuals. Several other vaccines based on cultivable mycobacteria (*M. vaccae, Mycobacterium "w,"* and the ICRC bacillus) induce similar responses.[5, 84, 161] Field trials of these vaccines for immunoprophylaxis of leprosy are in progress; however, because of the chronicity and low prevalence of the disease, meaningful evaluations of their efficacy will require extended follow-up observations.[6] Because an infection-induced immunity is not observed regularly in leprosy, there is reasonable doubt that vaccines containing only *M. leprae* will be protective. In view of this, combined vaccines of killed *M. leprae* and live BCG have been studied. Such vaccines convert lepromin-negative contacts of leprosy patients to positive reactors,[20] and upgrade lepromatous patients toward the tuberculoid area of the spectrum of the disease.[115] Vaccines based on cell-wall fractions of *M. leprae* are under study.[48] The World Health Organization does not recommend BCG vaccination for the prevention of leprosy.[3] This decision was based on the highly variable results of extensive studies in Burma, New Guinea, and Uganda.[181] Another trial in India involving 270,000 individuals confirmed that over a 12½-year follow-up, BCG vaccination was only about 25 per cent effective against leprosy.[164]

Initial evaluations of a large-scale immunoprophylaxis trial of heat-killed *M. leprae* plus BCG vaccine in humans in Venezuela showed no better protection than BCG at 5 years' postvaccination.[23]

LEPROSY AND AIDS

Because *M. tuberculosis, M. avium-intracellulare*, and *M. kansasii* are frequent opportunistic pathogens in patients with AIDS, there is interest in observing this syndrome in leprosy patients. In one study in Zambia, antibodies to HIV were found in 33 per cent of new leprosy patients, compared with 7 per cent in controls.[103] Perhaps positivity of some of these leprosy patients can be explained by the cross-reactivity between antibodies to HIV-1 and to the lipoarabinomannan of *M. leprae*.[85] More recent prospective studies show that HIV infection may not be a risk factor for leprosy in some populations.[88, 154] In other populations in Africa, HIV infection constituted an overall risk factor of 2.2 for leprosy, with 4 to 23 per cent of multibacillary leprosy attributable to HIV coinfection.[9] There are only a few detailed clinicopathologic reports on individuals coinfected with *M. leprae* and with HIV.[73, 90, 125] In these patients, there was no consistent deleterious effect of HIV infection on the clinical or pathologic findings of leprosy. These observations are supported by a study of parameters of CMI in coinfected patients in Brazil.[149] In these patients with borderline leprosy, despite low CD4+ T-cell counts, the quality of the granulomas in the infiltrations of leprosy was not altered significantly. The incidence of reversal (type 1) reactions and neuritis is increased in multibacillary patients coinfected with HIV.[16] Perhaps, as previously suggested,[97] the observations of patients coinfected with HIV and *M. leprae* will lead to some revisions of the immunopathogenesis of leprosy.

References

1. Barksdale, L., and Kim, K. S.: *Mycobacterium*. Bacteriol. Rev. *41*:217–372, 1977.
2. Bechelli, L. M., Gallego Garbajosa, P. G., Gyi, M. M., et al.: Site of early skin lesions in children with leprosy. Bull. W. H. O. *48*:107–111, 1973.
3. Bechelli, L. M., Gallego Garbajosa, P. G., Gyi, M. M., et al.: BCG vaccination of children against leprosy: Seven-year findings of the controlled WHO trial in Burma. Bull. W. H. O. *48*:323–334, 1973.
4. Becx-Bleuminck, M.: Operational aspects of multidrug therapy. Int. J. Lepr. *57*:540–551, 1989.
5. Bhatki, W. S., Chulawala, R. G., Bapat, C. V., et al.: Reversal reaction in lepromatous patients induced by a vaccine containing killed ICRC bacilli: A report of five cases. Int. J. Lepr. *51*:466–472, 1983.
6. Bhutani, L. K., Nath, I., Mehra, N. K., et al.: Grand round: Leprosy. Lancet *345*:697–703, 1995.
7. Binford, C. H., Meyers, W. M., Walsh, G. P., et al.: Naturally acquired leprosy-like disease in the nine-banded armadillo *(Dasypus novemcinctus)*: Histopathologic and microbiologic studies of tissues. J. Reticuloendothel. Soc. *22*:377–388, 1977.
8. Binford, C. H., Meyers, W. M., and Walsh, G. P.: Leprosy: State of the art. J. A. M. A. *247*:2283–2292, 1982.
9. Borgdorff, M. W., van den Broek, J., Chum, H. J., et al.: HIV-1 infection as a risk factor for leprosy: A case-control study in Tanzania. Int. J. Lepr. *61*:556–562, 1993.
10. Brody, S. N.: The Disease of the Soul: Leprosy in Medieval Literature. Ithaca, NY, Cornell University Press, 1974.
11. Browne, S. G.: Onchocercal depigmentation. Trans. R. Soc. Trop. Med. Hyg. *54*:325–334, 1960.
12. Brubaker, M. L., Meyers, W. M., and Bourland, J.: Leprosy in children one year of age and under. Int. J. Lepr. *53*:517–523, 1985.
13. Bullock, W. E.: Studies of the immune mechanism in leprosy. N. Engl. J. Med. *278*:298–304, 1968.

14. Bullock, W. E.: Rifampin in the treatment of leprosy. Rev. Infect. Dis. *5*(Suppl. 3):S606–S613, 1983.
15. Bullock, W. E., Ho, M. F., and Chen, M. J.: Studies of immune mechanisms in leprosy. II. Quantitative relationships of IgG, IgA, and IgM immunoglobulins. J. Lab. Clin. Med. *75*:863–870, 1970.
16. Bwire, R., and Kawuma, H. J. S.: Type 1 reactions in leprosy, neuritis and steroid therapy: The impact of the human immunodeficiency virus. Trans. R. Soc. Trop. Med. Hyg. *88*:315–316, 1994.
17. Byrd, S. R., Gelber, R., and Bermudez, L. E.: Roles of soluble fibronectin and β_1 integrin receptors in the binding of *Mycobacterium leprae* to nasal epithelial cells. Clin. Immunol. Immunopathol. *69*:266–271, 1993.
18. Cho, S.-N., Chatterjee, D., and Brennan, P. J.: A simplified serological test for leprosy based on a 3,6-di-*O*-methylglucose-containing synthetic antigen. Am. J. Trop. Med. Hyg. *35*:167–172, 1986.
19. Cochrane, R. G., and Davey, T. F. (eds.): Leprosy in Theory and Practice. 2nd ed. Bristol, England, John Wright & Sons, 1964.
20. Convit, J., Aranzazu, N., Ulrich, M., et al.: Immunotherapy with a mixture of *Mycobacterium leprae* and BCG in different forms of leprosy and in Mitsuda-negative contacts. Int. J. Lepr. *50*:415–424, 1982.
21. Convit, J., Avila, J. L., Goihman, M., et al.: A test for the determination of competency in clearing bacilli in leprosy patients. Bull. W. H. O. *46*:821–826, 1972.
22. Convit, J., and Pinardi, M. E.: A simple method for the differentiation of *Mycobacterium leprae* from other mycobacteria through routine staining technics. Int. J. Lepr. *40*:130–132, 1972.
23. Convit, J., Sampson, C., Zuniga, M., et al.: Immunoprophylactic trial with combined *Mycobacterium leprae*/BCG vaccine against leprosy: Preliminary results. Lancet *339*:446–450, 1992.
24. Cree, I. A., Coghill, G., Subedi, A. M. C., et al.: Effects of treatment on the histopathology of leprosy. J. Clin. Pathol. *48*:304–307, 1995.
25. Davey, T. F., and Rees, R. J. W.: The nasal discharge in leprosy: Clinical and bacteriological aspects. Lepr. Rev. *45*:121–134, 1974.
26. Dayal, R., and Bharadwaj, V. P.: Prevention and early detection of leprosy in children. J. Trop. Ped. *41*:132–138, 1995.
27. de Rijk, A. J., Gabre, S., Byass, P., et al.: Field evaluation of WHO-MDT of fixed duration, at ALERT, Ethiopia: The AMFES project—II. Reaction and neuritis during and after MDT in PB and MB leprosy patients. Lepr. Rev. *65*:320–332, 1994.
28. de Wit, M. Y. L., Douglas, J. T., McFadden, J., et al.: Polymerase chain reaction for detection of *Mycobacterium leprae* in nasal swab specimens. J. Clin. Microbiol. *31*:502–506, 1993.
29. Dietrich, M., Gaus, W., Kern, P., et al.: An international randomized study with long-term follow-up of single versus combination chemotherapy of multibacillary leprosy. Antimicrob. Agents Chemother. *38*:2249–2257, 1994.
30. Donham, K. J., and Leininger, J. R.: Spontaneous leprosy-like disease in a chimpanzee. J. Infect. Dis. *136*:132–136, 1977.
31. Drutz, D. J., Chen, T. S. N., and Lu, W. H.: The continuous bacteremia of lepromatous leprosy. N. Engl. J. Med. *287*:159–164, 1972.
32. Duncan, M. E.: Babies of mothers with leprosy have small placentae, low birth weights and grow slowly. Br. J. Obstet. Gynecol. *87*:471–479, 1980.
33. Duncan, M. E., Melsom, R., Pearson, J. M. H., et al.: A clinical and immunological study of four babies of mothers with lepromatous leprosy, two of whom developed leprosy in infancy. Int. J. Lepr. *51*:7–17, 1983.
34. Duncan, M. E., and Oakey, R. E.: Estrogen excretion in pregnant women with leprosy: Evidence of diminished fetoplacental function. Obstet. Gynecol. *60*:82–86, 1982.
35. Dwyer, J. M., Bullock, W. E., and Fields, J. P.: Disturbances of the blood: T:B lymphocyte ratio in lepromatous leprosy. N. Engl. J. Med. *288*:1036–1039, 1973.
36. Ellard, G. A.: Rationale of the multidrug regimens recommended by a World Health Organization Study Group on Chemotherapy of Leprosy for Control Programs. Int. J. Lepr. *52*:395–401, 1984.
37. Farb, H., West, D. P., and Pedvis-Leftick, A.: Clofazimine in pregnancy complicated by leprosy. Obstet. Gynecol. *59*:122–123, 1982.
38. Feldman, R. A., and Sturdivant, M.: Leprosy in Louisiana 1855–1970: An epidemiologic study of long-term trends. Am. J. Epidemiol. *102*:303–310, 1975.
39. Fiallo, P., Williams, D. L., Chan, G. P., et al.: Effects of fixation on polymerase chain reaction detection of *Mycobacterium leprae*. J. Clin. Microbiol. *30*:3095–3098, 1992.
40. Flaguel, B., Wallach, D., Vignon-Pennamen, M., et al.: Late onset of reversal reaction in borderline leprosy. J. Am. Acad. Dermatol. *20*:857–860, 1989.
41. Fritschi, E. P.: Reconstructive Surgery in Leprosy. Bristol, England, John Wright & Sons, 1971.
42. Gajl-Peczalska, K. J., Lim, S. D., Jacobson, R. R., et al.: B lymphocytes in lepromatous leprosy. N. Engl. J. Med. *288*:1033–1035, 1973.
43. Gatt, P. The Malta experience, 1972–1992: 20 years after starting the eradication project in Malta. Int. J. Lepr. *61*:304, 1993.
44. Gaylord, H., and Brennan, P. J.: Leprosy and the leprosy bacillus: Recent developments in characterization of antigens and immunology of the disease. Annu. Rev. Microbiol. *41*:645–675, 1987.
45. Gehr, E.: Leprosy in childhood. Doc. Med. Geog. Trop. *9*:101–124, 1957.
46. Gelber, R. H., Drutz, D. J., Epstein, W. V., et al.: Clinical correlates of C1q-precipitating substances in the sera of patients with leprosy. Am. J. Trop. Med. Hyg. *23*:471–475, 1974.
47. Gelber, R. H., Fukuda, K., Byrd, S., et al.: A clinical trial of minocycline in lepromatous leprosy. Br. Med. J. *304*:91–92, 1992.
48. Gelber, R. H., Mehra, V., Bloom, B., et al.: Vaccination with pure *Mycobacterium leprae* proteins inhibits *M. leprae* multiplication in mouse footpads. Infection Immunity *62*:4250–4255, 1994.
49. Gelber, R. H., Murray, L. P., Siu, P., et al.: Efficacy of minocycline in single dose and at 100 mg twice daily for lepromatous leprosy. Int. J. Lepr. *62*:568–573, 1994.
50. Girdhar, B. K., Girdhar, A., Ramu, G., et al.: Borderline leprosy (BL) in an infant: Report of a case and a brief review. Lepr. India *55*:333–337, 1983.
51. Godal, R.: Growing points in leprosy research. (3) Immunological detection of sub-clinical infection in leprosy. Lepr. Rev. *45*:22–30, 1974.
52. Gonzalez-Abreu, E., Mora, N., Perez, M., et al.: Serodiagnosis of leprosy in patients' contacts by enzyme-linked immunosorbent assay. Lepr. Rev. *61*:145–150, 1990.
53. Gormus, B. J., Xu, K., Alford, P. L., et al.: A serologic study of naturally-acquired leprosy in chimpanzees. Int. J. Lepr. *59*:450–457, 1991.
54. Grant, A. M. B.: Leprosy at Nauru since 1928. Int. J. Lepr. *2*:305–310, 1934.
55. Grosset, J. H.: Progress in the chemotherapy of leprosy. Int. J. Lepr. *62*:268–277, 1994.
56. Guinto, R. S., Doull, J. A., and Mabalay, E. B.: The Mitsuda reaction in persons with and without household exposure to leprosy. Int. J. Lepr. *23*:135–138, 1955.
57. Gupte, M. D., Anantharaman, D. S., Nagaraju, B., et al.: Experiences with *Mycobacterium leprae* soluble antigens in a leprosy endemic population. Lepr. Rev. *61*:132–144, 1990.
58. Harboe, M.: The work and concepts of Armauer Hansen: How do they stand today? Ethiop. Med. J. *21*:123–126, 1983.
59. Harboe, M.: The immunology of leprosy. *In* Hastings, R. C. (ed.): Leprosy (Medicine in the Tropics Series). Edinburgh, Churchill Livingstone, 1985, pp. 53–87.
60. Haregewoin, A. T., Godal, T., Mustafa, A. S., et al.: T-cell conditioned media reverse T-cell unresponsiveness in lepromatous leprosy. Nature *303*:342–344, 1983.
61. Hastings, R. C., and Morales, M. J.: Observations, calculations, and speculations on the growth and death of *M. leprae* in vivo. Int. J. Lepr. *50*:579–582, 1982.
62. Horwitz, M. A., Levis, W. R., and Cohn, Z. A.: Defective production of monocyte-activating cytokines in lepromatous leprosy. J. Exp. Med. *159*:666–678, 1984.
63. Hunter, S. W., Fujiwara, T., and Brennan, P. J.: Structure and antigenicity of the major specific glycolipid antigen of *Mycobacterium leprae*. J. Biol. Chem. *257*:15072–15078, 1982.
64. Hussain, R., Lucas, S. B., Kifayet, A., et al.: Clinical and histological discrepancies in diagnosis of ENL reactions classified by assessment of acute phase proteins SAA and CRP. Int. J. Lepr. *63*:222–230, 1995.
65. Imkamp, F. M. J. H.: Clofazimine (Lamprene or B663) in lepra reactions. Lepr. Rev. *52*:135–140, 1981.
66. Inaba, T.: Ueber die Histopathologischen und Bakteriologischen Untersuchungen der Plazenta bei Leprosen. La Lepro. *9*(Suppl. III), 1938.
67. Izumi, S., Fujiwara, T., Ikeda, M., et al.: Novel gelatin particle agglutination test for serodiagnosis of leprosy in the field. J. Clin. Microbiol. *28*:525–529, 1990.
68. Jacobson, R. R.: Treatment of leprosy. *In* Hastings, R. C. (ed.): Leprosy. 2nd ed. (Medicine in the Tropics Series). Edinburgh, Churchill Livingstone, 1994, pp. 317–349.
69. Jacobson, R. R.: Carville and Hansen's disease control: Past, present and future. Int. J. Lepr. *63*:272–273, 1995.
70. Jacobson, R. R., and Hastings, R. C.: Rifampin-resistant leprosy. Lancet *2*:1304–1305, 1976.
71. Jakeman, P.: Risk of relapse in multibacillary leprosy. Lancet *345*:4–5, 1995.
72. Jamet, P., Ji, B., and the Marchoux Chemotherapy Study Group: Relapse after long-term follow up of multibacillary patients treated by WHO multidrug regimen. Int. J. Lepr. *63*:195–201, 1995.
73. Janssen, F., Wallach, D., Khuong, M. A., et al.: Association de maladie de Hansen et d'infection par le virus de l'immunodéficience humaine: Deux observations. Presse Med. *17*:1652–1653, 1988.
74. Ji, B., Jamet, P., Perani, E. G., et al.: Powerful bactericidal activities of clarithromycin and minocycline against *Mycobacterium leprae* in lepromatous leprosy. J. Infect. Dis. *168*:188–190, 1993.
75. Job, C. K.: The Kellersberger Memorial Lecture, 1983: The lepromin test and its role in the management of leprosy. Ethiop. Med. J. *21*:233–242, 1983.
76. Job, C. K., and Chacko, C. J. G.: A simplified 6 group classification of leprosy. Lepr. India *54*:26–32, 1982.
77. Johnstone, P. A. S., Meyers, W. M., Binford, C. H., et al.: Recent advances in the development of nonhuman primates as animal models for leprosy. Scand. J. Lab. Anim. Sci. *16*(Suppl. 1):102–105, 1989.
78. Jopling, W. H.: Handbook of Leprosy. London, William Heinemann Medical Books LTD, 1984.
79. Jopling, W. H., Ridley, M. J., Bonnici, E., et al.: A followup investigation of the Malta project. Lepr. Rev. *55*:247–253, 1984.

80. Kaplan, G.: Recent advances in cytokine therapy of leprosy. J. Infect. Dis. *167(Suppl)*:S18–S22, 1993.
81. Kaplan, G., Mathur, N. K., Job, C. K., et al.: Effect of multiple interferon-γ injections on the disposal of *Mycobacterium leprae*. Proc. Natl. Acad. Sci. U. S. A. *86*:8073–8077, 1989.
82. Kaplan, G., Sampaio, E. P., Walsh, G. P., et al.: Influence of *Mycobacterium leprae* and its soluble products on the cutaneous responsiveness of leprosy patients to antigen and recombinant interleukin 2. Proc. Natl. Acad. Sci. U. S. A. *86*:6269–6273, 1989.
83. Kar, H. K., Bhatia, V. N., and Harikrishnan, S.: Combined clofazimine- and dapsone-resistant leprosy: A case report. Int. J. Lepr. *54*:389–391, 1986.
84. Kar, H. K., Sharma, A. K., Misra, R. S., et al.: Reversal reaction in multibacillary leprosy patients following MDT with and without immunotherapy with a candidate for an antileprosy vaccine, *Mycobacterium w*. Lepr. Rev. *64*:219–226, 1993.
85. Kashala, O., Marlink, R., Ilunga, M., et al.: Infection with human immunodeficiency virus type 1 (HIV-1) and human T cell lymphotropic viruses among leprosy patients and contacts: Correlation between HIV-1 cross-reactivity and antibodies to lipoarabinomannan. J. Infect. Dis. *169*:296–304, 1994.
86. Kato, L.: Leprosy associated mycobacteria: Implications. Acta Leprol. *7*:1–6, 1989.
87. Kaur, I., Kaur, S., Sharma, V. K., et al.: Bacillaemia and *Mycobacterium leprae* cell wall antigen in paucibacillary leprosy. Indian J. Lepr. *65*:283–288, 1993.
88. Kawuma, H. J. S., Bwire, R., and Adatu-Engwau, F.: Leprosy and infection with the human immunodeficiency virus in Uganda: A case-control study. Int. J. Lepr. *62*:521–526, 1994.
89. Khanolkar Young, S., Rayment, N., Brickell, P. M., et al.: Tumour necrosis factor-alpha (TNF-α) synthesis is associated with the skin and peripheral nerve pathology of leprosy reversal reactions. Clin. Exp. Immunol. *99*:196–202, 1995.
90. Lamfers, E. J., Bastiaans, A. H., Mravunac, M., et al.: Leprosy in the acquired immunodeficiency syndrome. Ann. Intern. Med. *107*:111–112, 1987.
91. Languillon, J., and Carayon, A.: Précis de Léprologie. Paris, Masson et Cie, 1969.
92. Lara, C. B.: Leprosy in children: General considerations: Initial and early changes. Philipp. J. Lepr. *1*:22–57, 1966.
93. Latapi, F., and Zamora, A. C.: The "spotted" leprosy of Lucio: An introduction to its clinical and histological study. Int. J. Lepr. *16*:421–429, 1948.
94. Lechat, M. F.: Global evaluation of the introduction of multidrug therapy. Leprosy Epidemiology Bulletin. WHO Collaborating Center for the Epidemiology of Leprosy, Brussels, Belgium. Bulletin Number 4, January 1990.
95. Leiker, D. L.: On the mode of transmission of *Mycobacterium leprae*. Lepr. Rev. *48*:9–16, 1977.
96. Leprosy News and Notes: Fifth International Leprosy Congress—1948: The words "leper" and "leprosy." Int. J. Lepr. *16*:243, 1948.
97. Lucas, S. B.: Human immunodeficiency virus and leprosy. Lepr. Rev. *64*:97–103, 1993.
98. Lumpkin, L. R., III, Cox, G. F., and Wolf, J. E., Jr.: Leprosy in five armadillo handlers. J. Am. Acad. Dermatol. *9*:899–903, 1983.
99. Mathur, N. K., Pasricha, J. S., Pal, D., et al.: Comparison of cutaneous autonomic and somatic nervous functions in the lesions of leprosy. Int. J. Lepr. *39*:146–150, 1971.
100. McAdam, K. P. W. J., Anders, R. F., Smith, S. R., et al.: Association of amyloidosis with erythema nodosum leprosum reactions and recurrent neutrophil leucocytosis in leprosy. Lancet 2:572–576, 1975.
101. McCoy, W.: History of leprosy in the United States. Am. J. Trop. Med. *18*:19–34, 1938.
102. McDougall, A. C., and Waudby, H.: Dermal microfilariasis and leprosy. Lepr. Rev. *48*:161–168, 1977.
103. Meeran, K.: Prevalence of HIV infection among patients with leprosy and tuberculosis in rural Zambia. Br. Med. J. *298*:364–365, 1989.
104. Mehra, V., Brennan, P. J., Rada, E., et al.: Lymphocyte suppression in leprosy induced by unique *M. leprae* glycolipid. Nature *308*:194–196, 1984.
105. Mehra, V., Mason, L. H., Rothman, W., et al.: Delineation of a human T-cell subset responsible for lepromin-induced suppression in leprosy patients. J. Immunol. *125*:1183–1188, 1980.
106. Melancon-Kaplan, J., Hunter, S. W., McNeil, M., et al.: Immunologic significance of *Mycobacterium leprae* cell walls. Proc. Natl. Acad. Sci. U. S. A. *85*:1917–1921, 1988.
107. Melsom, R., Harboe, M., Duncan, M. E., et al.: IgA and IgM antibodies against *Mycobacterium leprae* in cord sera and in patients with leprosy: An indication of intrauterine infection in leprosy. Scand. J. Immunol. *14*:343–352, 1981.
108. Melsom, R., Harboe, M., and Duncan, M. E.: IgA, IgM and IgG anti-*M. leprae* antibodies in babies of leprosy mothers during the first two years of life. Clin. Exp. Immunol. *49*:532–542, 1982.
109. Meyers, W. M., Binford, C. H., Walsh, G. P., et al.: Animal models of leprosy. *In* Microbiology—1984. Washington, D.C., American Society for Microbiology, 1984, pp. 307–311.
110. Meyers, W. M., Connor, D. H., Harman, L. E., et al.: Human streptocerciasis: A clinico-pathologic study of 40 Africans (Zairians), including identification of the adult filaria. Am. J. Trop. Med. Hyg. *21*:528–545, 1972.
111. Meyers, W. M., Gormus, B. J., and Walsh, G. P.: Nonhuman sources of leprosy. Int. J. Lepr. *60*:477–481, 1992.
112. Meyers, W. M., Gormus, B. J., and Walsh, G. P.: Experimental leprosy. *In* Hastings, R. C. (ed.): Leprosy. 2nd ed. (Medicine in the Tropics Series). Edinburgh, Churchill Livingstone, 1994, pp. 385–408.
113. Meyers, W. M., Gormus, B. J., Walsh, G. P., et al.: Naturally acquired and experimental leprosy in nonhuman primates. Am. J. Trop. Med. Hyg. *44*(Suppl.):24–27, 1991.
114. Meyers, W. M., Kvernes, S., and Binford, C. H.: Comparison of reactions to human and armadillo lepromins in leprosy. Int. J. Lepr. *43*:218–225, 1975.
115. Meyers, W. M., McDougall, A. C., Fleury, R. H., et al.: Histologic responses in sixty multibacillary leprosy patients inoculated with *Mycobacterium leprae* and live BCG. Int. J. Lepr. *56*:302–309, 1988.
116. Meyers, W. M., Walsh, G. P., Brown, H. L., et al.: Naturally acquired leprosy-like disease in the nine-banded armadillo *(Dasypus novemcinctus)*: Reactions in leprosy patients to lepromins prepared from naturally infected armadillos. J. Reticuloendothel. Soc. *22*:369–375, 1977.
117. Meyers, W. M., Walsh, G. P., Brown, H. L., et al.: Leprosy in a mangabey monkey: Naturally acquired infection. Int. J. Lepr. *53*:1–14, 1985.
118. Mitsuda, K.: On the value of a skin reaction to a suspension of leprous nodules. Hifuka Hinyoka Zasshi (Jpn. J. Dermatol. Urol.) *19*:697–708, 1919. In Japanese. English translation in Int. J. Lepr. *21*:347–358, 1953.
119. MMWR: Recommendations of the International Task Force for Disease Eradication. U. S. Department of Health and Human Services, Centers for Disease Control *42*:1–38, 1993.
120. MMWR: U. S. Department of Health and Human Services, Centers for Disease Control *44*:539, 1995.
121. Modlin, R. L., Gebhard, J. F., Taylor, C. R., et al.: *In situ* characterization of T-lymphocyte subsets in the reactional states of leprosy. Clin. Exp. Immunol. *53*:17–24, 1983.
122. Modlin, R. L., Hoffman, F. M., Horowitz, D. A., et al.: *In situ* identification of cells in human leprosy granulomas with monoclonal antibodies to interleukin-2 and its receptor. J. Immunol. *132*:3085 3090, 1984.
123. Modlin, R. L., Hoffman, F. M., Taylor, C. R., et al.: T lymphocyte subsets in the skin lesions of patients with leprosy. J. Am. Acad. Dermatol. *8*:182–189, 1983.
124. Modlin, R. L., Melancon-Kaplan, J., Young, S. M. M., et al.: Learning from lesions: Patterns of tissue inflammation in leprosy. Proc. Natl. Acad. Sci. U. S. A. *85*:1213–1217, 1988.
125. Moran, C. A., Nelson, A. M., Tuur, S. M., et al.: Leprosy in five human immunodeficiency virus-infected patients. Modern Pathol. *8*:662 664, 1995.
126. Mouritz, A. A. M.: The Path of the Destroyer: A History of Leprosy in the Hawaiian Islands. Honolulu, Honolulu Star-Bulletin, Ltd., 1916.
127. Muir, E.: Juvenile leprosy. Int. J. Lepr. *4*:45–48, 1936.
128. Mukherjee, A., and Meyers, W. M.: Endothelial cell bacillation in lepromatous leprosy: A case report. Lepr. Rev. *58*:419–424, 1987.
129. Myrvang, B., Godal, T., Ridley, D. S., et al.: Immune responsiveness to *Mycobacterium leprae* and other mycobacterial antigens throughout the clinical and histopathological spectrum of leprosy. Clin. Exp. Immunol. *14*:541–553, 1973.
130. Navalkar, R. G., Norlin, M., and Ouchterlony, O.: Characterization of leprosy sera with various mycobacterial antigens using double diffusion-in-gel analysis. Int. Arch. Allergy *28*:250–260, 1965.
131. Nogueira, N., Kaplan, G., Levy, E., et al.: Defective γ-interferon production in leprosy: Reversal with antigen and interleukin-2. J. Exp. Med. *158*:2165–2170, 1983.
132. Noordeen, S. K., Lopez Bravo, L., and Sundaresan, T. K.: Estimated number of leprosy cases in the world. Bull. W. H. O. *70*:7–10, 1992.
133. Noussitou, F. M.: Leprosy in Children. Geneva, World Health Organization, 1976.
134. Olcen, P., Harboe, M., Warndorff, T., et al.: Antigens of *M. leprae* and anti-*M. leprae* antibodies in the urine of leprosy patients. Lepr. Rev. *54*:203–216, 1983.
135. Ottenhoff, T. H. M.: State of the art lectures: Immunology of leprosy: Lessons from and for leprosy. Int. J. Lepr. *62*:108–121, 1994.
136. Park, J. Y., Cho, S. N., Youn, J. K., et al.: Detection of antibodies to human nerve antigens in sera from leprosy patients by ELISA. Clin. Exp. Immunol. *87*:368–372, 1992.
137. Parkash, O. M., Chaturvedi, V., Girdhar, B. K., et al.: A study on performance of two serological assays for diagnosis of leprosy patients. Lepr. Rev. *66*:26–30, 1995.
138. Pedley, J. C.: The presence of *M. leprae* in human milk. Lepr. Rev. *38*:239–242, 1967.
139. Prasad, H. K., Mishra, R. S., and Nath, I.: Phenolic glycolipid-I of *Mycobacterium leprae* induces general suppression of in vitro concanavalin A responses unrelated to leprosy type. J. Exp. Med. *165*:239–244, 1987.
140. Rangdaeng, S., Scollard, D. M., Suriyanon V., et al.: Studies of human leprosy lesions in situ using suction-induced blisters. 1. Cellular components of new, uncomplicated lesions. Int. J. Lepr. *57*:492–498, 1989.
141. Rea, T. H., Bakke, A. C., Parker, J. W., et al.: Peripheral blood T lymphocyte subsets in leprosy. Int. J. Lepr. *52*:311–317, 1984.

142. Rees, R. J. W., and McDougall, A. C.: Airborne infection with *Mycobacterium leprae* in mice. J. Med. Microbiol. *10*:63–68, 1977.
143. Ridley, D. S.: Skin Biopsy in Leprosy. 2nd ed. Basel, Doc. Geigy, 1985.
144. Ridley D. S., and Jopling, W. H.: Classification of leprosy according to immunity: A five-group system. Int. J. Lepr. *34*:255–273, 1966.
145. Roche, P. W., Theuvenet, W. L., and Britton, W. J.: Risk factors for type-1 reactions in borderline leprosy patients. Lancet *338*:654–657, 1991.
146. Rook, G. A. W.: The immunology of leprosy. Tubercle *64*:297–312, 1983.
147. Ryrie, G. A.: Some impressions of Sungei Buloh Leper Hospital under Japanese occupation. Lepr. Rev. *18*:10–17, 1947.
148. Sabin, T. D., and Swift, T. R.: Leprosy. *In* Dyck, P. J., Thomas, P. K., Lambert, E. H., et al. (eds.): Peripheral Neuropathy. Philadelphia, W. B. Saunders, 1984, pp. 1955–1987.
149. Sampaio, E. P., Caneshi, J. R. T., Nery, J. A. C., et al.: Cellular immune response to *Mycobacterium leprae* infection in human immunodeficiency virus-infected individuals. Infect. Immun. *63*:1848–1854, 1995.
150. Sarno, E. N., Grau, G. E., Vieira, L. M. M., et al.: Serum levels of tumor necrosis factor-alpha and interleukin-1B during leprosy reactional states. Clin. Exp. Immunol. *84*:103–108, 1991.
151. Saul, A., and Novales, J.: La lèpre de Lucio-Latapi et le phénomène de Lucio. Acta Leprol. *92*:115–132, 1983.
152. Schlesinger, L. S., and Horwitz, M. A.: Complement receptors and complement component C3 mediate phagocytosis of *Mycobacterium tuberculosis* and *Mycobacterium leprae*. Int. J. Lepr. *58*:200–201, 1990.
153. Sehgal, V. N., Bhattacharya, S. N., Chattopadhya, D., et al.: Tumor necrosis factor: Status in reactions in leprosy before and after treatment. Int. J. Dermatol. *32*:436–439, 1993.
154. Sekar, B., Jayasheela, M., Chattopadhya, D., et al.: Prevalence of HIV infection and high-risk characteristics among leprosy patients of South India: A case-control study. Int. J. Lepr. *62*:527–531, 1994.
155. Shepard, C. C.: The experimental disease that follows the injection of human leprosy bacilli into foot pads of mice. J. Exp. Med. *112*:445–454, 1960.
156. Shepard, C. C.: Combinations involving dapsone, rifampin, clofazimine, and ethionamide in the treatment of *M. leprae* infections in mice. Int. J. Lepr. *44*:135–139, 1976.
157. Shields, E. D., Russell, D. A., and Pericak-Vance, M. A.: Genetic epidemiology of the susceptibility to leprosy. J. Clin. Invest. *79*:1139–1143, 1987.
158. Skinsnes, O. K.: Leprosy in society. II. The pattern of concept and reaction to leprosy in Oriental antiquity. Lepr. Rev. *35*:106–122, 1964.
159. Skinsnes, O. K., and Higa, L. H.: The role of protein malnutrition in the pathogenesis of ulcerative "lazarine" leprosy. Int. J. Lepr. *44*:346–358, 1976.
160. Smith, J. H., Folse, D. S., Long, E. G., et al.: Leprosy in wild armadillos *(Dasypus novemcinctus)* of the Texas Gulf Coast: Epidemiology and mycobacteriology. J. Reticuloendothel. Soc. *34*:75–88, 1983.
161. Stanford, J. L., Rook, G. A. W., Bahr, G. M., et al.: *Mycobacterium vaccae* in immunoprophylaxis and immunotherapy of leprosy and tuberculosis. Vaccine *8*:525–530, 1990.
162. Sung, K. J., Kim, S. B., Choi, J. H., et al.: Detection of *Mycobacterium leprae* DNA in formalin-fixed, paraffin-embedded samples from multibacillary and paucibacillary leprosy patients by polymerase chain reaction. Int. J. Dermatol. *32*:710–713, 1993.
163. Talhari, S., Orsi, A. N., Talhari, A. C., et al.: Pentoxifylline may be useful in the treatment of type 2 leprosy reactions. Lepr. Rev. *66*:261–263, 1995.
164. Tripathy, S. R.: BCG trial in leprosy. Indian J. Lepr. *56*:686–687, 1984.
165. Truman, R. W., Kumaresan, J. A., McDonough, C. M., et al.: Seasonal and spatial trends in the detectability of leprosy in wild armadillos. Epidemiol. Infect. *106*:549–560, 1991.
166. Turk, J. L.: Cell-mediated immunological processes in leprosy. Lepr. Rev. *41*:207–222, 1970.
167. Valla, M. C.: Lèpre et grossesse: Thèse de Médecine. Lyon, France, 1976.
168. van Beers, S. M., Izumi, S., Madjid, B., et al.: An epidemiological study of leprosy infection by serology and polymerase chain reaction. Int. J. Lepr. *62*:1–9, 1994.
169. Van Brakel, W. H., and Khawas, I. B.: Silent neuropathy in leprosy: An epidemiological description. Lepr. Rev. *65*:350–360, 1994.
170. VanEden, W., DeVries, R. R. P., Deamaro, J., et al.: HLA-DR associated genetic control of the type of leprosy in a population from Surinam. Hum. Immunol. *4*:343–350, 1982.
171. Vettom, L., and Pritze, S.: Reliability of skin smear results: Experiences with quality control of skin smears in different routine services in leprosy control programmes. Lepr. Rev. *60*:187–196, 1989.
172. Wabitsch, K. R., and Meyers, W. M.: Histopathologic observations on the persistence of *Mycobacterium leprae* in the skin of multibacillary leprosy patients under chemotherapy. Lepr. Rev. *59*:341–346, 1988.
173. Wade, H. W.: The histoid variety of lepromatous leprosy. Int. J. Lepr. *31*:129–142, 1963.
174. Walsh, G. P., Meyers, W. M., Binford, C. H., et al.: Leprosy as a zoonosis: An update. Acta Leprol. *6*:51–60, 1988.
175. Walsh, G. P., Storrs, E. E., Meyers, W. M., et al.: Naturally acquired leprosy-like disease in the nine-banded armadillo *(Dasypus novemcinctus)*: Recent epizootiologic findings. J. Reticuloendothel. Soc. *22*:363–367, 1977.
176. Warndorff-van Diepen, T.: Clofazimine-resistant leprosy: A case report. Int. J. Lepr. *50*:139–142, 1982.
177. Waters, M. F. R.: The diagnosis and management of dapsone-resistant leprosy. Lepr. Rev. *48*:95–105, 1977.
178. Waters, M. F. R.: The treatment of leprosy. Tubercle *64*:221–232, 1983.
179. Waters, M. F. R.: Relapse following various types of multidrug therapy in multibacillary leprosy. Lepr. Rev. *66*:1–9, 1995.
180. West, B. C., Todd, J. R., Lary, C. H., et al.: Leprosy in six isolated residents of northern Louisiana: Time-clustered cases in an essentially non-endemic area. Arch. Intern. Med. *148*:1987–1992, 1988.
181. WHO Expert Committee on Leprosy: W. H. O. Tech. Rep. Ser. No. 607, 1977.
182. WHO: Chemotherapy of leprosy for control programmes. W. H. O. Tech. Rep. Ser. No. 675, 1982.
183. Williams, D. L., and Gillis, T. P.: A study of relatedness of *Mycobacterium leprae* isolates using restriction fragment length polymorphism analysis. Acta Leprol. 7(Suppl. 1):226–230, 1989.
184. Williams, D. L., Gillis, T. P., Booth, R. J., et al.: The use of a specific DNA probe and polymerase chain reaction for the detection of *Mycobacterium leprae*. J. Infect. Dis. *162*:193–200, 1990.
185. Williams, D. L., Waguespack, C., Eisenach, K., et al.: Characterization of rifampin resistance in pathogenic mycobacteria. Antimicrob. Agents Chemother. *38*:2380–2386, 1994.
186. Wolf, R. H., Gormus, B. J., Martin, L. N., et al.: Experimental leprosy in three species of monkeys. Science *227*:529–531, 1985.
187. Young, D. B., Harnisch, J. P., Knight, J., et al.: Detection of phenolic glycolipid-1 in sera from patients with lepromatous leprosy. J. Infect. Dis. *152*:1078–1080, 1985.

104

NOCARDIA

Toni Darville and Richard F. Jacobs

Nocardia species are obligate aerobic bacilli that exist throughout the world as soil and dust saprophytes. These organisms are non–spore-forming, thin, branching, gram-positive, partially acid-fast, filamentous bacteria. Humans become infected with *Nocardia* by two primary routes: inhalation of contaminated airborne dust particles or traumatic implantation of the bacterium into the subcutaneous tissues. Pulmonary disease caused by *N. asteroides* is the form of nocardiosis recognized most commonly in the United States. The pulmonary event may be subclinical or transient, or it may provoke an acute or chronic process mimicking staphylococcal or fungal pneumonia, tuberculosis, or carcinoma. Hematogenous dissemination may occur, especially in immunocompromised hosts. The central nervous system is the most common site of dissemination, manifesting most often as a brain abscess. Cutaneous nocardiosis may be acute, subacute, or chronic. This form of disease is seen predominantly in immunocompetent hosts, with *N. brasiliensis* being the agent identified most frequently.

In 1888, Nocard noted an aerobic actinomycete in bovine

farcy, a chronic wasting disease in cattle characterized by pulmonary abscesses and draining cutaneous sinus tracts. Eppinger first described human disease in 1890. The first pediatric case was documented in 1895 in a boy with pulmonary and subcutaneous infection.[4] Lesions of nocardiosis, whether in the lung or in subcutaneous tissues, notably are suppurative, involving primarily a proliferation of polymorphonuclear neutrophils rather than the formation of granulomas.

THE ORGANISM

Nocardia species are included among the aerobic actinomycetes. They are gram-positive bacteria that are more filamentous and branched and grow more slowly than other aerobic and facultatively anaerobic bacteria. They commonly produce a fungus-like mycelium that fragments or breaks up into rod-shaped and short coccoid forms. *Nocardia* species grow well aerobically on a variety of simple media (e.g., blood agar, brain-heart infusion agar); added carbon dioxide (10 per cent) promotes more rapid growth. They are inhibited by antibiotics and antifungal agents, so media containing such agents do not support the growth of *Nocardia*. Because of their growth on commonly used fungus media (e.g., Sabouraud dextrose agar) as well as on some mycobacterial media (e.g., Löwenstein-Jensen medium), many *Nocardia* samples may be misdirected to the mycology or mycobacteriology sections of clinical laboratories for identification. *N. asteroides* is the predominant pathogenic species, accounting for more than 90 per cent of cases of nocardiosis. Other pathogenic species include *N. brasiliensis, N. otitidiscavarium (caviae),* and *N. farcinica*. Microscopic and colonial morphology, various biochemical tests, and thin-layer chromatography are among the current laboratory methods used for speciation.

Nocardia species grow in temperatures from 25° to 45° C; growth at higher temperatures may be used in differentiation. In pure culture, small, chalky white, heaped, wrinkled, or verrucose colonies appear in 3 to 5 days. Mature colonies are most commonly light orange and have a velvety appearance due to production of rudimentary aerial mycelia. They have the odor of a musty basement or freshly turned soil. It is important to note that it may take 2 to 4 weeks to detect colonies from clinical specimens such as respiratory secretions. In mixed cultures, rapidly growing bacteria may obscure small *Nocardia* colonies. Modified Thayer-Martin medium may enhance recovery.[25]

Gram stain of a portion of a colony shows delicate, branching filaments no more than 1 μm in diameter. The delicate filaments may fragment, producing bacillary or coccoid forms. Many *Nocardia* species partially are acid-fast (i.e., compared with *Mycobacterium* species they retain fuchsin less tenaciously). A modified Ziehl-Neelson or Kinyoun stain that decolorizes with 1 per cent sulfuric acid instead of the more active acid alcohol is best for demonstrating acid-fast *Nocardia* in clinical specimens. Acid-fastness is characteristic of nocardiae in tissue or primary colonial isolates but is lost quickly on subculture; not all pathogenic strains of *Nocardia* are acid-fast.[7] *N. asteroides* often survives the *N*-acetylcysteine digestion procedure (without sodium hydroxide) that is performed on sputum or bronchial washings, and yet some positive sputum specimens may be rendered falsely negative.[24] Thus, cultures of sputum and bronchial washings for isolation of *Nocardia* species should be performed both before and after the digestion procedure.

EPIDEMIOLOGY, TRANSMISSION, AND PATHOGENESIS

Nocardia species occasionally can be skin contaminants or respiratory tract saprophytes.[14, 29, 34] Bronchial obstruction or decreased bronchociliary clearance predisposes to colonization.[29] Most infections occur in the lungs, presumably via inhalation, with dissemination to the central nervous system occurring in up to a third of patients. Although nocardiosis occurs in immunocompetent persons, up to 70 per cent of patients are immunosuppressed by medication or underlying disease.[15] The typical patient has compromised cellular immunity (steroids, organ transplantation, cytotoxic chemotherapy, AIDS). Communicability from human to human has not been a problem. The incidence of nocardiosis in the United States has been estimated to be around 1000 new cases per year.[11]

Systemic nocardiosis is caused most commonly by the bacterium *N. asteroides*. Pulmonary and systemic infection with *N. otitidiscavarium (caviae)* has been documented in both normal and immunocompromised hosts.[9, 11] *N. farcinica* has been reported as a human pathogen in the United States.[31, 39] In the series of 200 cases of *Nocardia* species infections presented by Wallace and associates,[39] the isolates designated *N. farcinica* were from patients with severe illness, 56 per cent of whom had disseminated infections. *N. farcinica* isolates were characterized by their resistance to third-generation cephalosporins.

Traumatic implantation of aerobic actinomycetes into the deep subcutaneous tissues may result in an indolent condition called actinomycotic mycetoma, to distinguish it from the eumycotic mycetomas caused by true fungi. Actinomycotic mycetomas usually involve the lower extremities and are caused most commonly by *Actinomadura madurae*, a non–acid-fast aerobic actinomycete. "Madura foot" is a chronic infection of the deep subcutaneous tissues and bone. Mycetomas, the cause of which may be *N. brasiliensis*, have been described in Mexican and South American field workers. This *Nocardia* species also has been documented as an opportunistic pathogen prevalent in Florida, with a predilection for diabetics.[32]

In addition to the classic mycetoma, traumatic introduction of *Nocardia* species from soil may result in wound infections that follow more of an acute or subacute course. Posttraumatic endophthalmitis[13] and poststernotomy mediastinitis[35, 40] have been described. The organism can be introduced into the skin by tick[22] and other insect bites[26] or by a cat scratch,[30] resulting in cellulitis, pustules, or pyoderma; these conditions occasionally disseminate in immunocompromised persons.[18, 19]

Nocardiosis once was considered a rare disease in humans; however, it is being recognized more and more frequently.[23] It has been diagnosed in persons ranging from 4 weeks to 82 years of age, and, except in cases of localized cellulitis, almost all patients have one or more severe underlying diseases (e.g., lupus erythematosus, asthma, glomerulonephritis, ulcerative colitis, bronchiectasis, tuberculosis, rheumatoid arthritis, sarcoidosis). Patients with lymphoreticular neoplasm and transplant recipients seem to be particularly at risk. In addition, the risk of infection is increased in those with chronic pulmonary disease and in any patient who is receiving long-term corticosteroid treatment. Children with chronic granulomatous disease may develop severe infection with this catalase-positive organism.[16] Although not a surveillance organism for AIDS, patients with AIDS may present with nocardiosis.[17]

The immune response to *Nocardia* species is multifaceted.[2] Neutrophils are mobilized to the site of infection and are the predominant cell type found in lesions. However, neutrophils only inhibit the organisms limiting the spread of infection until an adequate cell-mediated immune response develops or until effective antimicrobial agents are given. Immune T cells are vital in clearing *Nocardia* species from the lung and preventing dissemination; thus, it is not surprising that many predisposing conditions for nocardiosis involve inadequate cell-mediated immunity. Activated macrophages induce cytotoxic T cells effective against *N. asteroides. Nocardia* species may survive inside neutrophils and macrophages by inhibiting phagosome-lysosome fusion and by the production of catalase and superoxide dismutase, which inactivate the myeloperoxidase system. *Nocardia* organisms exhibit differential abilities to evade phagosome-lysosome fusion based on their state of growth, possibly related to specific cell-wall mycolic acids detected only in log-phase cells.[3] Differential cell-wall characteristics also may influence the ability of nocardiae to exhibit specific organ tropism (e.g., the brain).[6] Antibody may play a role in host defense through enhancement of macrophage activities. Thus, although antecedent conditions of nocardiosis frequently involve dysfunctional cellular immunity, other preconditions include neutrophil and immunoglobulin disorders.

PATHOLOGY

The lesions of nocardiosis are suppurative, involving primarily a proliferation of neutrophils rather than the formation of granulomas. Pulmonary nocardiosis in immunocompetent patients often resembles pulmonary actinomycosis, in that it forms a chronic localized pneumonia that often abuts the pleura.[14] Indolent progressive fibrosis resembling fibronodular tuberculosis may occur. Nocardiosis is more aggressive in immunocompromised patients, occurring as multifocal necrotizing pneumonia with confluent abscess formation. *Nocardia* species tend to invade the pleura and chest wall, disregarding tissue planes in the process. Little evidence of encapsulation is characteristic of all organs invaded and probably accounts for the ready dissemination of organisms from the initial pulmonary focus.

N. asteroides appear as delicate, beaded, branching filaments in tissue stained with Gram stain or modified acid-fast stain (Fig. 104–1). *Nocardia* species are not visible in hematoxylin and eosin preparations or in sections stained with periodic acid–Schiff for fungi. Methenamine-silver preparations sometimes detect tissue organisms; overstaining with silver enhances visualization.

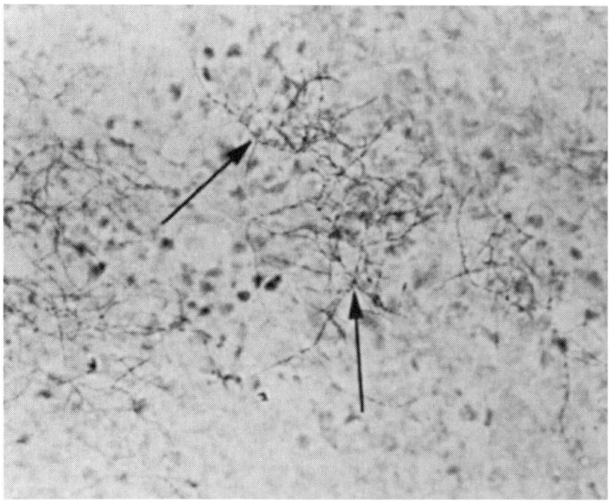

FIGURE 104–1. *Appearance of* N. asteroides *and* N. brasiliensis *(arrows) in a properly decolorized acid-fast smear. Organisms appear as fragmented bacilli with stain concentrated in a beaded fashion along portions of the filaments (× 160).*

CLINICAL MANIFESTATIONS AND DIAGNOSIS

The most common presentation of nocardiosis in the United States is that of pulmonary disease in a patient with underlying immunosuppression.[10] Infection may remain localized to the lung or may disseminate hematogenously to the central nervous system and skin and, more rarely, to almost any organ of the body. In high-risk patients, the diagnosis should be suspected when central nervous system manifestations, particularly signs of a brain tumor or abscess or soft tissue swellings or abscesses, develop in conjunction with a current or recent subacute or chronic pulmonary infection.

Clinical manifestations are not specific and include anorexia, weight loss, productive cough, pleural pain, dyspnea, and occasionally hemoptysis.[11] Untreated pulmonary nocardiosis usually runs a chronic course, much like tuberculosis, but it also may clear spontaneously, obscuring the source of subsequent metastatic infection. The diverse clinical and radiographic manifestations, including acute bronchopneumonia, lobar pneumonia or necrotizing pneumonia with single or multiple abscesses, and pleural empyema, may mimic more common pulmonary infections, such as mycobacterial, staphylococcal, and fungal pneumonia. Normal hosts or patients with only slightly impaired host defenses may present with only mild respiratory tract symptoms of several months' duration.[12]

The central nervous system is the most common secondary site of infection, occurring in up to a third of patients. Most experts recommend routine cranial computed tomography in patients with pulmonary nocardiosis, even when asymptomatic, because of the frequency of central nervous system involvement. Brain abscesses are the most common presentation; meningitis is reported less frequently, often (in 43 per cent of cases) associated with an abscess.[8]

Other clinical manifestations reported include tracheitis, peritonitis, iliopsoas abscess, hematogenous endophthalmitis, endocarditis, mediastinitis, septic arthritis, and osteomyelitis.[11] Traumatic inoculation may result in localized disease presenting as cellulitis, subcutaneous abscess, or a lymphocutaneous syndrome in which one or more cutaneous nodules are associated with regional adenopathy or suppurative lymphadenitis.[21] *Nocardia* species may cause cervicofacial disease and cervical adenitis in children.[20]

The diagnosis of nocardiosis is established in one-third of cases by sputum analysis and culture. Although *Nocardia* species at times can be respiratory saprophytes, it is difficult to withhold therapy in immunocompromised persons when cultures are repeatedly positive. Bronchoalveolar lavage or lung biopsy may be required to establish the diagnosis. The demonstration of tissue invasion confirms active infection. Humoral methods to diagnose nocardiosis generally lack specificity because of the high degree of serologic cross-reactivity among the *Nocardia* species and between *Mycobacterium* and *Streptomyces* species.[7] However, an enzyme immunoassay using a 55-kDa protein that has apparent specificity for *N. asteroides* is encouraging.[1, 7] Further work is required before a serologic test for nocardiosis is commercially available.

TREATMENT AND PROGNOSIS

Sulfonamides are the most effective and best-studied drugs for the treatment of nocardiosis.[33, 37] Sulfisoxazole

(150 mg/kg/day every 4 to 6 hours) therapy for 3 to 6 months is standard. More recently, trimethoprim-sulfamethoxazole (TMP-SMX), the only available intravenous sulfonamide formulation in the United States, has been used successfully in doses of 15 mg/kg/day of TMP, 75 mg/kg/day of SMX, either parenterally or orally.[35, 36] Toxicity of the combination exceeds that of sulfonamides alone, especially in patients receiving myelosuppressive therapy. Sulfonamides used alone remain the treatment of choice for nocardiosis.

The use of drugs other than sulfonamides always must be supported by susceptibility testing. Disk diffusion testing is practical for most antibiotics,[38] so alternative therapies can be selected when sulfonamides fail or cannot be given because of patient intolerance or allergy. Clinical experiences with minocycline and amikacin are encouraging. Amoxicillin–clavulanic acid holds promise as an alternative oral β-lactam antibiotic for treating infections due to *N. brasiliensis*, commonly a β-lactamase producer.[36] Combinations of amikacin and imipenem with cefotaxime and TMP-SMX display synergy for most *Nocardia* strains, although the value of and need for combined therapy remain an unsettled issue. The variable and chronic course of nocardiosis precludes sharp therapeutic end-points. Metastatic lesions can appear during or after an otherwise effective course of sulfonamide therapy with maintenance of the recommended 100 to 150 μg/mL level in serum or plasma. Because of the tendency for relapse or the late appearance of metastatic disease, therapy often is continued for many months. AIDS patients probably should be treated indefinitely. Surgical drainage of abscesses is important; metastatic abscesses can appear in the face of adequate therapy until surgical drainage is achieved.[14] Brain abscesses may respond to antimicrobial treatment without surgery.

Despite specific therapy, the mortality rate is 25 to 40 per cent.[27, 28] Most reported cases involving dissemination to the central nervous system have been fatal. Factors associated with increased mortality in one reported patient series were treatment with corticosteroids or antineoplastic agents, underlying Cushing disease, disseminated disease involving two or more noncontiguous organs or the central nervous system, and the presence of symptoms for less than 3 weeks prior to presentation.[28]

References

1. Angeles, A. M., and Sugar, A. M.: Rapid diagnosis of nocardiosis with an enzyme immunoassay. J. Infect. Dis. *155*:292–296, 1987.
2. Beaman, B. L., and Beaman, L.: *Nocardia* species: Host-paarasite relationships. Clin. Microbiol. Rev. *7*:213–264, 1994.
3. Beaman, B. L., and Moring, S. E.: Relationship among cell wall composition, state of growth, and virulence of *Nocardia asteroides* GUH-2. Infect. Immun. *56*:557–563, 1988.
4. Beckmeyer, W. J.: Nocardiosis: Report of a successfully treated case of cutaneous granuloma. Pediatrics *23*:33–39, 1959.
5. Berd, D.: Laboratory identification of clinically important aerobic actinomycetes. Appl. Microbiol. *25*:665–681, 1973.
6. Black, C. M., Paliescheskey, M., Beaman, B. L., et al.: Acidification of phagosome in murine macrophages: Blockage by *Nocardia asteroides*. J. Infect. Dis. *154*:952–958, 1986.
7. Boiron, P., and Stynen, D.: Immunodiagnosis of nocardiosis. Gene *115*:219–222, 1992.
8. Bross, J. E., and Gordon, G.: Nocardial meningitis case reports and review. Rev. Infect. Dis. *3*:160–165, 1991.
9. Brown, R. A., Janda, W. M., and Hellermen, D. V.: Pulmonary *Nocardia caviae* infection. Clin. Microbiol. Newsletter *4*:65–66, 1982.
10. Causey, W. A.: *Nocardia caviae*: A report of 13 new isolations with clinical correlation. Appl. Microbiol. *28*:193–198, 1974.
11. Curry, W. A.: Human nocardiosis: A clinical review with selected case reports. Arch. Intern. Med. *140*:818–826, 1980.
12. Feigin, D. S.: Nocardiosis of the lung: Chest radiographic findings in 21 cases. Radiology *159*:9–14, 1986.
13. Ferry, A. P., Font, R. L., Weinberg, R. S., et al.: Nocardial endophthalmitis: Report of two cases studied histopathologically. Br. J. Ophthalmol. *72*:55–61, 1988.
14. Frazier, A. R., Rosenow, E. C., III, and Roberts, G. D.: Nocardiosis: A review of 25 cases occurring during 24 months. Mayo Clin. Proc. *50*:657–663, 1975.
15. Heffner, J. E.: Pleuropulmonary manifestations of actinomycosis and nocardiosis. Semin. Respir. Infect. *3*:352–361, 1988.
16. Idriss, Z. H., Cunningham, R. J., and Wilfert, C. M.: Nocardiosis in children. Pediatrics *55*:479–484, 1975.
17. Javalry, K., Horowitz, H. W., and Wormser, G. P.: Nocardiosis in patients with human immunodeficiency virus infection: Report of 2 cases and review of the literature. Medicine *71*:128–138, 1980.
18. Kahn, F. W., Gornick, C. C., and Tofte, R. W.: Primary cutaneous *Nocardia asteroides* infection with dssemination. Am. J. Med. *70*:859–863, 1981.
19. Kalb, R. E., Kaplan, M. H., and Grosman, M. E.: Cutaneous nocardiosis. J. Am. Acad. Dermatol. *13*:125–133, 1985.
20. Lampe, R. M., Baker, C. J., Septimus, E. J., et al.: Cervicofacial nocardiosis in children. J. Pediatr. *99*:593–595, 1981.
21. Law, B. L., and Marks, M. I.: Pediatric nocardiosis. Pediatrics *70*:560–564, 1982.
22. Leggiadro, R. J., and Miller, R. B.: Cutaneous nocardiosis presenting as a tick-borne infection. Pediatr. Infect. Dis. J. *6*:421–422, 1987.
23. Murray, J. F., Finegold, S. M., Froman, S., et al.: The changing spectrum of nocardiosis. Am. Rev. Respir. Dis. *83*:315–330, 1961.
24. Murray, P. R., Neeren, R. L., and Niles, A. C.: Effect of decontamination procedures on recovery of *Nocardia* spp. J. Clin. Microbiol. *25*:2010–2011, 1987.
25. Murray, P. R., Niles, A. C., and Heeren, R. L.: Modified Thayer Martin medium for recovery of *Nocardia* species from contaminated specimens. J. Clin. Microbiol. *26*:1219–1220, 1988.
26. O'Conner, P. T., and Dire, D. J.: Cutaneous nocardiosis associated with insect bites. CUTIS *50*:301–302, 1992.
27. Palmer, D. L., Harvey, R. L., and Wheeler, J. K.: Diagnostic and therapeutic considerations in *Nocardia asteroides* infection. Medicine *53*:391–401, 1974.
28. Present, C. A., Wiernik, P. H., and Serpick, A. A.: Factors affecting survival in nocardiosis. Am. Rev. Respir. Dis. *108*:1444–1451, 1973.
29. Rosett, W., and Hodges, G. R.: Recent experiences with nocardial infections. Am. J. Med. Sci. *276*:279–285, 1978.
30. Sachs, M. K.: Lymphocutaneous *Nocardia brasiliensis* infection acquired from a cat scratch: Case report and review. Clin. Infect. Dis. *15*:710–711, 1992.
31. Schiff, T. A., McNeil, M. M., and Brown, J. M.: Cutaneous *Nocardia farcinica* infection in a nonimmunocompromised patient: Case report and review. Clin. Infect. Dis. *16*:756–760, 1993.
32. Smego, R. A., Jr., and Gallis, H. A.: The clinical spectrum of *Nocardia brasiliensis* infection in the United States. Rev. Infect. Dis. *6*:164–180, 1984.
33. Smego, R. A., Jr., Moeller, M. G., and Gallis, H. A.: Trimethoprim-sulfamethoxazole therapy for *Nocardia* infections. Arch. Intern. Med. *143*:711–718, 1983.
34. Stropnik, Z.: Isolation of *Nocardia asteroides* from human skin. Sabouradia *4*:41–44, 1965.
35. Thaler, F., Gotainer, B., Teodori, G., et al.: Mediastinitis due to *Nocardia asteroides* after cardiac transplantation. Intensive Care Med. *18*:127–128, 1992.
36. Wallace, R. J., Nash, D. R., Johnson, W. K., et al.: β-Lactam resistance in *Nocardia barasiliensis* is mediated by β-lactamase and reversed in the presence of clavulanic acid. J. Infect. Dis. *156*:959–966, 1987.
37. Wallace, R. J., Septimus, E. J., Williams, T. W., et al.: Use of trimethoprim-sulfamethoxazole for treatment of infections due to *Nocardia*. Rev. Infect. Dis. *4*:315–325, 1982.
38. Wallace, R. J., and Steele, L. C.: Susceptibility testing on *Nocardia asteroides* for the clinical laboratory. Diagn. Microbiol. Infect. Dis. *9*:155–166, 1988.
39. Wallace, R. J., Jr., Tsukamura, M., Brown, B. A., et al.: Cefotaxime-resistant *Nocardia asteroides* strains are isolates of the controversial species *Nocardia farcinica*. J. Clin. Microbiol. *28*:2726–2732, 1990.
40. Yew, W. W., Wong, P. C., Kwan, S. Y. L., et al.: Two cases of *Nocardia asteroides* sternotomy infection treated with ofloxacin and a review of other active antimicrobial agents. J. Infect. Dis. *23*:297–302, 1991.

105

MISCELLANEOUS GRAM-POSITIVE BACILLI

William C. Gruber and Randall G. Fisher

The gram-positive rods encompass a vast number of species. They are widespread in the environment and are part of the normal flora of animals and humans. This chapter focuses on gram-positive bacilli encountered uncommonly as pathogens in healthy persons. Many of these organisms show increasing prominence as causes of disease in the immunocompromised patient.[16] Bacteria from the following genera are discussed: *Corynebacterium* (other than *C. diphtheriae*), *Arcanobacterium*, *Rhodococcus*, and *Bacillus*.

CORYNEBACTERIUM

This genus comprises a wide number of organisms possessing little pathogenic potential, with some notable exceptions. The most infamous member of this genus, *C. diphtheriae* (see Chapter 95), is a cause of a potentially lethal pharyngeal infection with systemic manifestations. *C. jeikeium* (formerly *Corynebacterium* group JK) can be a major nosocomial agent of bacteremia and endocarditis; other species commonly are associated with infections in animals and rarely cause invasive infection in humans.[79, 105]

Bacteriology

Corynebacterium species derive their name from their club-like shape. Because of their resemblance to *C. diphtheriae*, they are included in the heterogeneous group of diphtheroids. Snapping division produces the angular and palisade arrangement of cells responsible for their characteristic gram-positive, "Chinese letters" microscopic appearance.[30] Organisms are facultatively anaerobic or aerobic and do not produce spores. They are nonmotile and catalase-positive and contain mycolic acid in their cell walls. Clinically relevant species include *C. diphtheriae*, *C. jeikeium*, *C. pseudotuberculosis*, *C. xerosis*, *C. pseudodiphtheriticum*, *C. minutissimum*, *C. striatum*, *C. ulcerans*, and *C. urealyticum*. Species can be differentiated according to biochemical tests and fermentation of sugars.[30, 103]

Epidemiology

Corynebacterium species commonly are recovered as normal flora in hospitalized patients. Nosocomial acquisition of *C. jeikeium* has been characterized most completely. Up to 35 per cent of hospitalized patients may be colonized with *C. jeikeium*, and the organism may be isolated at the time of admission.[56] The skin, groin, and rectum are common sites of recovery. Wounds and suppurative sites quickly become colonized.[56] Hospital personnel caring for oncology patients have higher rates of hand colonization with pathogenic *Corynebacterium* species than do nurses caring for dermatology patients.[71] Not surprisingly, transmission from patient to patient in the hospital environment can occur, and selective antibiotic pressure has been shown to augment colonization with *Corynebacterium* species.[78, 85, 134] Outbreaks of bacteremic infection have been reported in hematology wards,[100, 116] and DNA restriction fragment analysis and hybridization techniques have been used to document spread.[78, 97]

Pathophysiology

Corynebacterium species, particularly *C. jeikeium*, possess lipophilic properties that may account for their ability to proliferate on skin that has a higher lipid content; organisms have been isolated from sebum-filled eccrine gland biopsies in an adolescent with malignancy.[72] Breach of skin integrity is clearly an important risk factor for local infection and bacteremia with *Corynebacterium*. Plastic intravascular catheters increase the risk of infection.[101] Certain isolates of *C. pseudotuberculosis* and *C. ulcerans* can express diphtheria-like toxins,[133] which may confer virulence.

Some *Corynebacterium* species, notably *C. jeikeium* and *C. urealyticum*, commonly show resistance to penicillins, cephalosporins, aminoglycosides, erythromycin, and tetracycline.[42, 56, 79, 85, 90, 103, 112] Strains with a significant DNA relationship to the *C. jeikeium* type strain demonstrate penicillin resistance.[102] Resistant organisms have been noted to have significantly thickened cell walls compared with susceptible strains, but the functional importance of this feature is unknown.[17]

Clinical Manifestations

Systemic infections with *Corynebacterium* species generally are not clinically distinguishable from serious infections due to other pathogens. Immunocompromised patients are at the highest risk of disease due to *Corynebacterium*,[64, 104] but infections also have been described in neonates and immunocompromised older children.[42, 74] Risk factors include male gender, neutropenia, broad-spectrum antibiotic exposure, and prolonged hospital stay.[100, 116] Catalase production may be responsible for the rare infection with non-JK *Corynebacterium* species in children with chronic granulomatous disease.[74]

C. jeikeium is a pathogen of particular concern. In 1976, this agent first was described as a cause of serious infection in four patients, including an 11-year-old boy with a ventriculoatrial shunt.[64] Immunocompromised patients, particularly those with leukemia, are vulnerable to bacteremia. These high-risk subjects may demonstrate a local inflammatory lesion at the site of infection or a disseminated, hemorrhagic, or necrotic papular exanthem. Up to 25 per cent of neutropenic patients with septicemia have associated skin manifestations[36]; *C. jeikeium* has been recovered from disseminated lesions in a 14-year-old boy with leukemia.[72]

Infections with *C. jeikeium* also have been reported after trauma, ventriculoperitoneal shunting procedures,[5, 76] orthopedic procedures,[27] bone marrow aspiration,[42] and central venous catheter placement.[42] *C. jeikeium* now is recognized to be one of the most common causes of prosthetic valve endocarditis in adults.[90] Curiously, cutaneous findings of bacteremia so commonly observed in cancer patients generally are absent in patients with endocarditis.[36]

Although primarily a pathogen in sheep and goats, *C. pseudotuberculosis* can cause localized granulomatous lymphadenitis in humans[79]; almost all cases are associated with animal contact.[58]

C. xerosis is a rare cause of endocarditis, arthritis, and ventriculoperitoneal shunt infection.[8, 18] Most persons with endocarditis have a prosthetic heart valve.[47, 80]

C. pseudodiphtheriticum, a commensal of the oropharynx, can cause pneumonia, bronchitis, or tracheitis.[3, 31, 34] Lung disease usually occurs in the circumstance of underlying cardiopulmonary pathology. Onset typically is acute, but fever may be noticeably absent.[82] At least 18 cases of *C. pseudodiphtheriticum* endocarditis have been reported, including three infections in children with congenital heart disease.[89] Infection of allograft material is common; native heart valves may be involved, but usually in the context of preexisting lesions or intravenous drug abuse.

C. minutissimum is the cause of the mild cutaneous disease erythrasma. It now is recognized as a rare nosocomial infectious complication of malignancy and dialysis and has been implicated in a case of pyelonephritis in an 8-month-old child with posterior urethral valves.[33]

C. striatum has been recovered from purulent sputum of hospitalized patients and from infected central venous catheter sites.[129] It has been reported as a cause of fatal pulmonary infection and endocarditis.[78, 84, 105]

C. ulcerans derives its name from its association with ulcerative pharyngitis. Although more commonly a pathogen of nonhuman primates,[96] infection can occur in humans after animal contact or consumption of contaminated raw milk.[12, 39]

C. urealyticum (formerly *Corynebacterium* group D2) is a cause of alkaline-encrusted cystitis, primarily in the elderly.[50, 112] It is associated less commonly with infection at other sites and with bacteremia.[113]

Diagnosis

Diagnosis of *Corynebacterium* infection is based on isolation of the organism from clinical material. This organism commonly is accompanied by other pathogens. Like *Mycobacterium* and *Nocardia* species, *Corynebacterium* organisms have mycolic acids in their cell wall. However, the chains are shorter, and the organisms are not acid-fast. *Corynebacterium* species may be difficult to distinguish from some *Rhodococcus* species.[30] Colonies of *C. jeikeium* may demonstrate a metallic sheen when grown on agar.[64] Most *Corynebacterium* species can be differentiated quickly from each other by sugar fermentation, hydrolysis of urea, and reduction of nitrate.[122] Selective media containing kanamycin or trimethoprim-sulfamethoxazole have been useful in the recovery of multidrug-resistant strains of *Corynebacterium*.[63]

Treatment

Empiric therapy of infection must account for the frequency of *C. jeikeium* infection. In some series of immunocompromised patients, this organism is the most common *Corynebacterium* species encountered.[114, 132] Hence, vancomycin is recommended for empiric therapy of suspected *Corynebacterium* infection until susceptibilities are known. Treatment can be changed to a penicillin or cephalosporin, if appropriate. Two-drug therapy generally is recommended for treatment of *Corynebacterium* endocarditis; for gentamicin-susceptible strains, penicillin-gentamicin combinations have been shown to be synergistic, regardless of whether the strains are susceptible to penicillin.[90] Rarely, resistance to vancomycin is encountered. A woman with prosthetic valve endocarditis due to a vancomycin-resistant *Corynebacterium* species was treated successfully with imipenem and ciprofloxacin.[10] Removal of infectious sources, such as central nervous system shunts and central venous catheters, may be required for cure. Scrupulous attention to skin hygiene may reduce colonization of hospital personnel and the incidence of patient-to-patient transmission of pathogenic strains.[45, 100]

ARCANOBACTERIUM (see also Chapter 98, *Arcanobacterium haemolyticum*)

The genus *Arcanobacterium* has one clinically relevant species, *A. haemolyticum* (formerly *Corynebacterium haemolyticum*). Although first identified in 1946, the organism was recognized only a few years ago as a cause of exudative pharyngitis and maculopapular rash in adolescents and young adults.[127] Wound infections and visceral disease are less common.

Bacteriology

A. haemolyticum is an asporogenous, facultatively anaerobic, catalase-negative, gram-positive rod. It resembles *C. diphtheriae* but lacks metachromatic granules and grows poorly on tellurite-containing media. In contrast with the cell wall of *Corynebacterium* species, that of *A. haemolyticum* lacks mycolic acids.[29, 127]

Epidemiology

A. haemolyticum is recovered from 0.5 to 10 per cent of children and adolescents presenting with pharyngitis[25, 75, 88]; in one series, group A streptococci were recovered from nearly half of such subjects.[25] More than 90 per cent of cases occur in patients older than 11 years of age.[88]

Pathophysiology

The propensity for *A. haemolyticum* to colonize the pharynx and cause disease almost selectively in adolescents is unexplained. The capacity for organisms to survive intracellularly may explain in part the difficulty encountered in eradicating penicillin-susceptible organisms from the oropharynx.[95]

Clinical Manifestations

A. haemolyticum pharyngitis generally is indistinguishable from pharyngitis due to other causes, but palatal petechiae and strawberry tongue usually are absent. Approximately half of subjects infected with *A. haemolyticum* have a maculopapular rash.[51] The rash may mimic that of scarlet fever but typically is confined to extensor surfaces and spares the trunk, palms, and soles.[75] Pharyngeal infection is the primary manifestation of *A. haemolyticum* infection and may be complicated by the development of a tonsillar abscess.[11] Associations with brain abscess,[26] paravertebral abscess,[41] wound infection,[49] orbital cellulitis,[54] sepsis,[57] septic arthritis,[70] and cavitary pneumonia[128] have been described.

Diagnosis

Coccoid forms may predominate in clinical material.[29] Beta-hemolysis is less striking on blood agar than that due to group A streptococci and may be overlooked in cultures with heavy growth of commensal flora. Incubation on trypticase soy agar for 48 to 72 hours may be required prior to the appearance of characteristic beta-hemolysis and agar pitting.[35] The organism grows poorly on tellurite medium, which helps to distinguish it from *C. diphtheriae*. Colonies may show a "smooth" (predominant in wound infections) or "rough" (predominant in respiratory specimens) phenotype.[24] *Actinomyces pyogenes* (*Corynebacterium pyogenes*) is a common animal pathogen and a rare cause of pharyngitis in humans, mimicking that caused by *A. haemolyticum*. The ability to hydrolyze gelatin, produce beta-glucuronidase, react with antisera against group G streptococci, and produce acid from xylose differentiates *A. pyogenes* from *Arcanobacterium*.[55] A 4-hour alpha-mannosidase test, a catalase test, and a reverse cAMP test are useful in further differentiating *A. haemolyticum* strains from *Corynebacterium* species, *Rhodococcus equi*, *Erysipelothrix rhusiopathiae*, *A. pyogenes*, and *Listeria*.[22]

Treatment

Therapy with erythromycin is the treatment of choice.[95, 127] *A. haemolyticum* is variably susceptible to penicillins but is insensitive to trimethoprim-sulfamethoxazole.[23] Despite minimal inhibitory concentrations of 0.0015 to 1.0 μg/mL for penicillin, penicillin tolerance may limit the ability of this agent to clear *A. haemolyticum* from the oropharynx.[93]

RHODOCOCCUS

The genus *Rhodococcus* contains at least 15 species, of which *R. equi* is the most clinically relevant to humans. This organism derives its name from its role as a cause of pyogranulomatous pneumonia in young horses.[99] It has assumed a prominent role as a cause of human pulmonary disease in immunocompromised patients, particularly in those with HIV infection.[48, 65, 108]

Bacteriology

R. equi is a catalase-positive, urease-positive, oxidase-negative, gram-positive rod. The organism assumes a more coccoid morphology in solid media and a more bacillary form in liquid media. Its cell wall contains mycolic acid, making it acid-fast when grown on Löwenstein-Jensen media and stained with Kinyoun stain.[59]

Epidemiology

R. equi is a soil organism, and its growth is enriched by the manure of herbivores. Despite the common occurrence of this pathogen as a cause of veterinary infections, exposure to animals does not appear necessary for human infection[99]; most reported human patients have not had farm or animal exposure.[65] Hospital outbreaks of infection associated with patient-to-patient transmission have not been reported.

Pathophysiology

The prominence of pulmonary infection suggests that the respiratory tract is a common portal of entry. After gaining access to the lower respiratory tract, organisms are taken up by alveolar macrophages; Mac-1 macrophage receptors and complement are required for binding.[68] The appearance of pyogranulomatous lesions is consistent with the role of *R. equi* as an intracellular parasite containing mycolic acid, a possible virulence factor in the cell wall.[61, 98] Surface 15-kd and 17-kd antigens expressed by an 85-kb plasmid appear to confer virulence in mice and foals,[118] and virulent strains seem to have an increased capacity for intracellular survival in macrophages.[69] However, most isolates obtained from human infections in one series did not contain the 85-kb virulence plasmid.[119] Hence, other factors may play a role in promoting *Rhodococcus* disease in humans.[120] Death of parasitized macrophages may release enzymes, which further contribute to tissue damage. CD4+ lymphocytes are essential for pulmonary clearance of *R. equi* in a mouse model,[73] which may help to explain the high risk of infection associated with cellular immunodeficiency.

Clinical Manifestations

Infection typically presents as a subacute pneumonia developing over several weeks. Symptoms such as cough and fever are common, but disease progression may be relatively silent. Although most infections currently occur in patients with AIDS, malignancy and transplantation also pose risks. Pulmonary infection in children with leukemia has been described.[6, 86] Infection may be accompanied by other pathogens, particularly in AIDS patients.

Pulmonary infection often is pleural-based and associated with cavitation.[65] Empyema may occur as a complication. An unusual-appearing granulomatous inflammation, called *malakoplakia*, in lung tissue from a child or adult should raise suspicion of *R. equi* infection.[21, 106]

Extrapulmonary disease is seen at diagnosis in 7 per cent of patients with pneumonia.[126] Manifestations of infection include abscesses,[52] osteomyelitis,[92] peritonitis,[19] meningitis,[40] and endophthalmitis.[46] The organism has been grown from a biopsy of a granulomatous skin lesion in an immunocompetent 7-year-old girl.[83]

Diagnosis

Diagnosis relies on isolation of *Rhodococcus* from clinical material. Although sputum specimens may be positive, bronchoalveolar lavage or lung biopsy may be required. The physician should be alert to the possible coexistence of *R. equi* with other pathogens. In the laboratory, confusing this organism with *Corynebacterium*, acid-fast organisms, and other gram-positive cocco-bacilli has been shown to delay diagnosis.[43] Positive findings on Gram stain and Kinyoun stain should be interpreted in the context of clinical information.[108] Organisms appear salmon-pink when grown on blood agar and orange on Löwenstein-Jensen medium.[16] Differentiation from acid-fast bacteria on smear sometimes can be difficult. Combined use of a siderophore detection medium, ethylene glycol degradation, and beta-galactosidase activity may help differentiate *Rhodococcus* from *Nocardia* and rapid-growing mycobacteria.[53] DNA restriction fragment analysis and ribotyping show promise in aiding the identification and tracking of *Rhodococcus* species.[77]

Treatment

Clinical isolates commonly are resistant to penicillins and cephalosporins. Erythromycin, clindamycin, rifampin, aminoglycosides, vancomycin, fluoroquinolones, and imipenem are active against *R. equi*.[91] Synergy has been demonstrated with various combinations of these agents. Including rifampin or erythromycin in a two-drug combination has been recommended because of penetrance of macrophages.[16, 110] Combinations of antibiotics that included vancomycin were found to be most effective in clearing infection in a mouse model.[91] Cure rates in adults with lung infection are approximately 60 per cent when antibiotic therapy alone is employed but may reach 75 per cent when combined with surgical resection of infected pulmonary tissue.[65] Pediatric patients generally have fared better than adults, but most reported cases in children have been in non-AIDS patients.[16] Relapse has been reported to occur at extrapulmonary sites in 13 per cent of immunocompromised patients,[126] often without reappearance of pulmonary disease.

BACILLUS

Most *Bacillus* species other than *B. anthracis*, the cause of anthrax (see Chapter 96), are uncommon causes of infection in the immunocompetent host. *B. cereus* is a noteworthy exception because it may cause wound infections, bacteremia, endophthalmitis, and gastroenteritis.

Bacteriology

Members of the genus *Bacillus* are large, straight, endospore-forming, gram-positive rods.[28] Organisms are catalase positive and aerobic or facultatively anaerobic. Endospores are resistant to adverse conditions. Clinically relevant species include *B. anthracis* and the closely related *B. cereus*. Properties of *B. cereus* not possessed by *B. anthracis* include motility, beta-hemolysis of blood agar, penicillin resistance, and resistance to bacteriophage gamma.[28, 44] Less frequent pathogens are *B. brevis, B. licheniformis, B. subtilis, B. sphaericus,* and *B. thuringiensis*.[44]

Epidemiology

Organisms are found widely in nature, partly because of the ability of spores to spread far away from their natural soil habitat.[28] Hospital outbreaks of local and systemic infection have been associated with contamination of scrub suits or bed linens,[13] ventilators,[20] and gauze impregnated with plaster of paris.[4] Foodborne outbreaks of gastrointestinal illness are the most common manifestation of significant *B. cereus* infections. Diarrhea due to enterotoxin is a common complication of infection from contaminated meat.[38, 44] Rice contaminated with *B. cereus* is associated more commonly with vomiting illness due to elaboration of emetic toxin.[7, 62, 87] Fried rice has been implicated most commonly in epidemics.[7, 44] Fried rice that has been allowed to cool slowly and then kept at room temperature to avoid clumping may pose the greatest risk of *B. cereus* spore germination and toxin elaboration.[44]

Pathogenesis

B. cereus colonization of intravenous catheters may be favored by localization in adherent biofilms.[9] Elaboration of toxins and other extracellular products is important to the virulence of *Bacillus* species. *B. cereus* produces several extracellular products, including a necrotizing enterotoxin, an emetic toxin, phospholipases, proteases, and hemolysins.

Thermolabile enterotoxin is composed of three 38- to 57-kd protein components, which act to produce the clinical syndrome of diarrhea.[60, 62, 115, 123, 125] The toxin can produce an increased vascular permeability reaction in the skin of rabbits, necrosis and toxicity in tissue culture, and fluid accumulation in rabbit and mouse intestinal loops.[62, 115] Progress has been made in identifying genes associated with this biologic activity.[1]

The emetic toxin is a clearly distinguishable, stable peptide of less than 10 kd.[125] A novel dodacadepsipeptide, ceruilide, has emerged as the leading candidate for this emetic toxin. This peptide, purified from an emetic strain, displays the same properties as culture supernatants expressing the toxin (i.e., it produces cytotoxicity in HEp2 cells and causes a vomiting illness in a mouse model).[2]

At least four hemolysins and several phospholipases are elaborated and believed to be virulence factors for local infection.[62] For example, a hemolysin that binds and lyses cells (hemolysin BL) contributes to virulence in an endophthalmitis model,[14] and neutrophils exposed to phospholipase C of *B. cereus* degranulate, which may increase tissue damage.[130]

Clinical Manifestations

Bacillus species can cause local and disseminated infection after traumatic injury, burns, or surgery. Patients undergoing orthopedic procedures seem to be particularly susceptible to disease. In one series, organisms were isolated from a quarter of patients with wound infection after hip arthroplasty.[4] Local infection may be indolent, marked only by increased drainage at wound sites. Osteomyelitis, necrotizing fasciitis, shunt infections, and endocarditis have been reported.[44, 107, 117, 124] In most cases, bacteremia is unassociated with disease and is cleared spontaneously. However, tissue necrosis and profound morbidity are common to localized infection, such as pneumonia, visceral abscess, and musculoskeletal infections.[111]

Eye infection with *B. cereus* deserves special mention because it is common and devastating. Keratitis, endophthalmitis, and panophthalmitis can be caused by this organism; *B. cereus* now is believed to be second only to *Staphylococcus epidermidis* as a cause of serious ophthalmic infection after traumatic injury.[37] Endophthalmitis also has been reported as a complication of bacteremic illness in patients infected with HIV and in intravenous drug abusers.[32] Contamination of injection equipment is the likely source in the latter circumstance.[109]

A corneal ring abscess is the classic manifestation of eye infection. Findings include pain, chemosis, proptosis, and retinal hemorrhage.[32] Eye infections are aggressive, partly because of the elaboration of extracellular toxins and enzymes in the closed space of the globe.

In the 1950s, Hauge[66] experienced diarrhea after consuming vanilla sauce purposely contaminated with more than 10^6 organisms/mL. This experiment established *B. cereus* as a cause of food poisoning, and two syndromes, characterized by either diarrhea or vomiting, now are recognized. The diarrheal syndrome is due to effects of enterotoxin and usually occurs in the absence of vomiting. Classically, infected persons experience an afebrile illness marked by profuse diarrhea, abdominal pain, and cramps, which begins approximately 8 to 16 hours after consumption of contaminated food (usually meat). However, in one outbreak related to contaminated pork at a university gathering, one-third of suspect cases occurred more than 24 hours after exposure and nearly one-quarter of subjects experienced fever.[81] Diarrhea usually is self-limited and resolves within 12 hours. The emetic toxin elaborated by growth of *B. cereus* in rice or pasta produces an illness similar to that of *Staphylococcus aureus* food poisoning (see Chapter 52). After toxin ingestion and a short incubation period of 1 to 5 hours, nausea, vomiting, and occasionally diarrhea occur. Patients typically recover within 24 hours with minimal or supportive care.

Diagnosis

Diagnosis relies on identification of the organism in clinical material. Confirmation of bacteremia is made difficult because *Bacillus* species are common contaminants of blood cultures. Therefore, appreciation of the clinical significance of a blood isolate may occur only after clinical deterioration forces a reappraisal of the patient. Differentiation of individual species can be difficult. *B. cereus* usually can be distinguished from *B. anthracis* by phenotypic features of motility, beta-hemolysis, and penicillin resistance. However, some *B. cereus* variants are nonmotile; conversely, some *B. anthracis* organisms may be weakly hemolytic.[44] Organisms grown in sheep blood at 37° C for 8 hours may be examined for a *B. anthracis*–specific capsule with India ink or methylene blue. Anthrax toxin can be identified immunologically. *B. cereus* strains responsible for epidemics can be characterized further by spore, somatic, and flagellar antigens.[121] Other speciation requires use of additional biochemical or serologic tests.

Treatment

Vancomycin and clindamycin are of value in the treatment of serious *Bacillus* species infection; organisms commonly are resistant to penicillins and cephalosporins.[111, 131] Removal of an intravenous catheter may be sufficient to cure bacteremia. However, in immunocompromised patients, antibiotic therapy is recommended.[9] In the circumstance of tissue necrosis, effective débridement may be required for cure. Although endophthalmitis almost always is associated with blindness, successful therapy and visual recovery have been reported in a child.[15] Combination therapy with clindamycin and gentamicin or vancomycin has been the most promising regimen for eye infection.[37, 67, 94] Systemic and topical administration of these agents may ensure good antibiotic levels in the anterior eye compartment, but therapeutic levels of effective agents are difficult to achieve in the vitreous by these methods.[37] An ophthalmologist should be consulted early for application of topical and intravitreal antibiotics.

References

1. Agata, N., Ohta, M., Arakawa, Y., et al.: The *bceT* gene of *Bacillus cereus* encodes an enterotoxic protein. Microbiology *141*:983–988, 1995.
2. Agata, N., Ohta, M., Mori, M., et al.: A novel dodecadepsipeptide, cereulide, is an emetic toxin of *Bacillus cereus*. FEMS Microbiol. Lett. *129*:17–20, 1995.
3. Ahmed, K., Kawakami, K., Watanabe, K., et al.: *Corynebacterium pseudodiphtheriticum*: A respiratory tract pathogen. Clin. Infect. Dis. *20*:41–46, 1995.
4. Akesson, A., Hedstrom, S. A., and Ripa, T.: *Bacillus cereus*: A significant pathogen in postoperative and post-traumatic wounds on orthopaedic wards. Scand. J. Infect. Dis. *23*:71–77, 1991.
5. Allen, K. D., and Green, H. T.: Infections due to a "group JK" *Corynebacterium*. J. Infect. *13*:41–44, 1986.
6. Allen, V. D., Niec, A., Kerem, E., et al.: *Rhodococcus equi* pneumonia in a child with leukemia. Pediatr. Infect. Dis. J. *8*:656–658, 1989.
7. Anonymous: *Bacillus cereus* food poisoning associated with fried rice at two child day care centers: Virginia, 1993. M. M. W. R. *43*:177–178, 1994.
8. Arisoy, E. S., Demmler, G. J., and Dunne, W. M. J.: *Corynebacterium xerosis* ventriculoperitoneal shunt infection in an infant: Report of a case and review of the literature. Pediatr. Infect. Dis. J. *12*:536–538, 1993.
9. Banerjee, C., Bustamante, C. I., Wharton, R., et al.: *Bacillus* infections in patients with cancer. Arch. Intern. Med. *148*:1769–1774, 1988.
10. Barnass, S., Holland, K., and Tabaqchali, S.: Vancomycin-resistant *Corynebacterium* species causing prosthetic valve endocarditis successfully treated with imipenem and ciprofloxacin. J. Infect. *22*:161–169, 1991.
11. Barnham, M., and Bradwell, R. A.: Acute peritonsillar abscess caused by *Arcanobacterium haemolyticum*. J. Laryngol. Otol. *106*:1000–1001, 1992.
12. Barrett, N. J.: Communicable disease associated with milk and dairy products in England and Wales: 1983–1984. J. Infect. *12*:265–272, 1986.
13. Barrie, D., Hoffman, P. N., Wilson, J. A., et al.: Contamination of hospital linen by *Bacillus cereus*. Epidemiol. Infect. *113*:297–306, 1994.
14. Beecher, D. J., Pulido, J. S., Barney, N. P., et al.: Extracellular virulence factors in *Bacillus cereus* endophthalmitis: Methods and implication of involvement of hemolysin BL. Infect. Immun. *63*:632–639, 1995.
15. Beer, P. M., Ludwig, I. H., and Packer, A. J.: Complete visual recovery after *Bacillus cereus* endophthalmitis in a child. Am. J. Ophthalmol. *110*:212–213, 1990.
16. Berkowitz, F. E.: The gram-positive bacilli: A review of the microbiology, clinical aspects, and antimicrobial susceptibilities of a heterogeneous group of bacteria. Pediatr. Infect. Dis. J. *13*:1126–1138, 1994.
17. Blom, J., and Heltberg, O.: The ultrastructure of antibiotic-susceptible and multi-resistant strains of group JK diphtheroid rods isolated from clinical specimens. Acta Pathol. Microbiol. Immunol. Scand. *94*:301–308, 1986.
18. Booth, L. V., Richards, R. H., and Chandran, D. R.: Septic arthritis caused by *Corynebacterium xerosis* following vascular surgery. Rev. Infect. Dis. *13*:548–549, 1991.
19. Brown, E., and Hendler, E.: *Rhodococcus* peritonitis in a patient treated with peritoneal dialysis. Am. J. Kidney Dis. *14*:417–418, 1989.
20. Bryce, E. A., Smith, J. A., Tweeddale, M., et al.: Dissemination *of Bacillus cereus* in an intensive care unit [see comments]. Infect. Control Hosp. Epidemiol. *14*:459–462, 1993.
21. Byard, R. W., Thorner, P. S., Edwards, V., et al.: Pulmonary malacoplakia in a child. Pediatr. Pathol. *10*:417–424, 1990.
22. Carlson, P., and Kontiainen, S.: Alpha-mannosidase: A rapid test for identification of *Arcanobacterium haemolyticum* [see comments]. J. Clin. Microbiol. *32*:854–855, 1994.
23. Carlson, P., Kontiainen, S., and Renkonen, O. V.: Antimicrobial susceptibility of *Arcanobacterium haemolyticum*. Antimicrob. Agents Chemother. *38*:142–143, 1994.
24. Carlson, P., Lounatmaa, K., and Kontiainen, S.: Biotypes of *Arcanobacterium haemolyticum*. J. Clin. Microbiol. *32*:1654–1657, 1994.
25. Carlson, P., Renkonen, O. V., and Kontiainen, S.: *Arcanobacterium haemolyticum* and streptococcal pharyngitis. Scand. J. Infect. Dis. *26*:283–287, 1994.
26. Chhang, W. H., Ayyagari, A., Sharma, B. S., et al.: *Arcanobacterium haemolyticum* brain abscess in a child (a case report). Indian J. Pathol. Microbiol. *34*:145–148, 1991.
27. Claeys, G., Vershchraegen, G., DeSmet, L., et al.: *Corynebacterium* JK (Johnson-Kay strain) infection of a Kuntscher-nailed tibial fracture. Clin. Orthop. Related Res. *202*:227–229, 1986.
28. Claus, D., and Berkeley, R. C. W.: *Bacillus*. *In* Sneath, P. H. A., Mair, N. S., Sharpe, M. E., et al. (eds.): Bergey's Manual of Systematic Bacteriology. Vol. 2. Baltimore, Williams & Wilkins, 1986, pp. 1105–1134.
29. Collins, M. D., and Cummins, C. S.: *Arcanobacterium*. *In* Sneath, P. H. A., Mair, N. S., Sharpe, M. E., et al. (eds.): Bergey's Manual of Systematic Bacteriology. Vol. 2. Baltimore, Williams & Wilkins, 1986, pp. 1261–1287.
30. Collins, M. D., and Cummins, C. S.: *Corynebacterium*. *In* Sneath, P. H., Mair, N. S., Sharpe, M. E., et al. (eds.): Bergey's Manual of Systematic Bacteriology. Vol. 2. Baltimore, Williams & Wilkins, 1986, pp. 1266–1276.
31. Colt, H. G., Morris, J. F., Marston, B. J., et al.: Necrotizing tracheitis caused by *Corynebacterium pseudodiphtheriticum*: Unique case and review. Rev. Infect. Dis. *13*:73–76, 1991.
32. Cowan, C. L. J., Madden, W. M., Hatem, G. F., et al.: Endogenous *Bacillus cereus* panophthalmitis. Ann. Ophthal. *19*:65–68, 1987.
33. Craig, J., Grigor, W., Doyle, B., et al.: Pyelonephritis caused by *Corynebacterium minutissimum*. Pediatr. Infect. Dis. J. *13*:1151–1152, 1994.
34. Craig, T. J., Maguire, F. E, and Wallace, M. R.: Tracheobronchitis due to *Corynebacterium pseudodiphtheriticum*. South. Med. J. *84*:504–506, 1991.
35. Cummings, L. A., Wu, W. K., Larson, A. M., et al.: Effects of media, atmosphere, and incubation time on colonial morphology of *Arcanobacterium haemolyticum*. J. Clin. Microbiol. *31*:3223–3226, 1993.
36. Dan, M., Somer, I., Knobel, B., et al.: Cutaneous manifestations of infection with *Corynebacterium* group JK. Rev. Infect. Dis. *10*:1204–1207, 1988.
37. Davey, R. T. J., and Tauber, W. B.: Posttraumatic endophthalmitis: The emerging role of *Bacillus cereus* infection. Rev. Infect. Dis. *9*:110–123, 1987.
38. DeBuono, B. A., Brondum, J., Kramer, J. M., et al.: Plasmid, serotypic, and enterotoxin analysis of *Bacillus cereus* in an outbreak setting. J. Clin. Microbiol. *26*:1571–1574, 1988.
39. de Carpentier, J. P., Flanagan, P. M., Singh, I. P., et al.: Nasopharyngeal *Corynebacterium ulcerans*: A different diphtheria. J. Laryngol. Otol. *106*:824–826, 1992.
40. DeMarais, P. L., and Kocka, F. E.: *Rhodococcus* meningitis in an immunocompetent host. Clin. Infect. Dis. *20*:167–169, 1995.
41. Dieleman, L. A., de Marie, S., Mouton, R. P., et al.: Paravertebral abscess due to nondiphtheria coryneform bacteria as a complication of ingrown toenails. Infection *17*:26–27, 1989.
42. Dietrich, M. C., Watson, D. C., and Kumar, M. L.: *Corynebacterium* group JK infections in children. Pediatr. Infect. Dis. J. *8*:233–236, 1989.

43. Doig, C., Gill, M. J., and Church, D. L.: *Rhodococcus equi*: An easily missed opportunistic pathogen. Scand. J. Infect. Dis. *23*:1–6, 1991.
44. Drobniewski, F. A.: *Bacillus cereus* and related species. Clin. Microbiol. Rev. *6*:324–338, 1993.
45. Eagan, J. A., Blevins, A., and Armstrong, D.: Prevention of skin colonization and subsequent bacteremia with CDC-JK organisms in patients with cancer [published erratum appears in Cancer Pract. 2:15, 1994]. Cancer Pract. *1*:325–328, 1993.
46. Ebersole, L. L., and Paturzo, J. L.: Endophthalmitis caused by *Rhodococcus equi* Prescott serotype 4. J. Clin. Microbiol. *26*:1221–1222, 1988.
47. Eliakim, R., Silkoff, P., Lugassy, G., et al.: *Corynebacterium xerosis* endocarditis. Arch. Intern. Med. *143*:1995, 1983.
48. Emmons, W., Reichwein, B., and Winslow, D. L.: *Rhodococcus equi* infection in the patient with AIDS: Literature review and report of an unusual case. Rev. Infect. Dis. *13*:91–96, 1991.
49. Esteban, J., Zapardiel, J., and Soriano, F.: Two cases of soft-tissue infection caused by *Arcanobacterium haemolyticum*. Clin. Infect. Dis. *18*:835–836, 1994.
50. Estorc, J. J., de La Coussaye, J. E., Viel, E. J., et al.: Teicoplanin treatment of alkaline encrusted cystitis due to *Corynebacterium* group D2. Eur. J. Med. *1*:183–184, 1992.
51. Fell, H. W., Nagington, J., Naylor, G. R., et al.: *Corynebacterium haemolyticum* infections in Cambridgeshire. J. Hyg. *79*:269–274, 1977.
52. Fierer, J., Wolf, P., Seed, L., et al.: Non-pulmonary *Rhodococcus equi* infections in patients with acquired immune deficiency syndrome (AIDS). J. Clin. Pathol. *40*:556–558, 1987.
53. Fiss, E., and Brooks, G. F.: Use of a siderophore detection medium, ethylene glycol degradation, and beta-galactosidase activity in the early presumptive differentiation of *Nocardia, Rhodococcus, Streptomyces*, and rapidly growing *Mycobacterium* species. J. Clin. Microbiol. *29*:1533–1535, 1991.
54. Ford, J. G., Yeatts, R. P., and Givner, L. B.: Orbital cellulitis, subperiosteal abscess, sinusitis, and septicemia caused by *Arcanobacterium haemolyticum*. Am. J. Ophthalmol. *120*:261–262, 1995.
55. Gahrn-Hansen, B., and Frederiksen, W.: Human infections with *Actinomyces pyogenes* (*Corynebacterium pyogenes*). Diagn. Microbiol. Infect. Dis. *15*:349–354, 1992.
56. Gill, V. J., Manning, C., Lamson, M., et al.: Antibiotic-resistant group JK bacteria in hospitals. J. Clin. Microbiol. *13*:472–477, 1981.
57. Givner, L. B.: *Arcanobacterium haemolyticum* sepsis and Epstein-Barr virus infection. Pediatr. Infect. Dis. J. *11*:417–418, 1992.
58. Goldberger, A. C., Lipsky, B. A., and Plorde, J. J.: Suppurative granulomatous lymphadenitis caused by *Corynebacterium ovis* (*pseudotuberculosis*). Am. J. Clin. Pathol. *76*:486–490, 1981.
59. Goodfellow, M.: *Rhodococcus*. *In* Williams, S. T., Sharpe, M. E., and Holt, J. G. (eds.): Bergey's Manual of Systematic Bacteriology. Vol. 4. Baltimore, Williams & Wilkins, 1989, pp. 2362–2371.
60. Corina, L. G., Fluer, F. S., Olovnikov, A. M., et al.: Highly sensitive determination of *Bacillus cereus* exo-enterotoxin using the method of aggregate haemagglutination. J. Hyg. Epidemiol. Microbiol. Immunol. *21*:361–367, 1976.
61. Gotoh, K., Mitsuyama, M., Imaizumi, S., et al.: Mycolic acid-containing glycolipid as a possible virulence factor of *Rhodococcus equi* for mice. Microbiol. Immunol. *35*:175–185, 1991.
62. Granum, P. E.: *Bacillus cereus* and its toxins. Soc. Appl. Bacteriol. Symp. Ser. *23*:61S–66S, 1994.
63. Hamilton, D. J., Ulness, B. K., Baugher, L. K., et al.: Comparison of a novel trimethoprim-sulfamethoxazole-containing medium (XT80) with kanamycin agar for isolation of antibiotic-resistant organisms from stool and rectal cultures of marrow transplant patients. J. Clin. Microbiol. *25*:1886–1890, 1987.
64. Hande, K. R., Witebsky, F. G., Brown, M. S., et al.: Sepsis with a new species of *Corynebacterium*. Ann. Intern. Med. *85*:423–426, 1976.
65. Harvey, R. L., and Sunstrum, J. C.: *Rhodococcus equi* infection in patients with and without human immunodeficiency virus infection. Rev. Infect. Dis. *13*:139–145, 1991.
66. Hauge, S.: Food poisoning caused by aerobic spore-forming bacilli. J. Appl. Bacteriol. *18*:591–595, 1955.
67. Hemady, R., Zaltas, M., Paton, B., et al.: *Bacillus*-induced endophthalmitis: New series of 10 cases and review of the literature [published erratum appears in Br. J. Ophthalmol. *75*:255, 1991]. Br. J. Ophthalmol. *74*:26–29, 1990.
68. Hondalus, M. K., Diamond, M. S., Rosenthal, L. A., et al.: The intracellular bacterium *Rhodococcus equi* requires Mac-1 to bind to mammalian cells. Infect. Immun. *61*:2919–2929, 1993.
69. Hondalus, M. K., and Mosser, D. M.: Survival and replication of *Rhodococcus equi* in macrophages. Infect. Immun. *62*:4167–4175, 1994.
70. Hoosen, A. A., Rasool, M. N., and Roux, L.: Posttraumatic ankle joint infection with *Arcanobacterium haemolyticum*: A case report. J. Infect. Dis. *162*:780–781, 1990.
71. Horn, W. A., Larson, E. L., McGinley, K. J., et al.: Microbial flora on the hands of health care personnel: Differences in composition and antibacterial resistance. Infect. Control Hosp. Epidemiol. *9*:189–193, 1988.
72. Jerdan, M. S., Shapiro, R. S., Smith, N. B., et al.: Cutaneous manifestations of *Corynebacterium* group JK sepsis. J. Am. Acad. Dermatol. *16*:444–447, 1987.
73. Kanaly, S. T., Hines, S. A., and Palmer, G. H.: Failure of pulmonary clearance of *Rhodococcus equi* infection in CD4+ T-lymphocyte-deficient transgenic mice. Infect. Immun. *61*:4929–4932, 1993.
74. Kaplan, A., and Israel, F.: *Corynebacterium aquaticum* infection in a patient with chronic granulomatous disease. Am. J. Med. Sci. *296*:57–58, 1988.
75. Karpathios, T., Drakonaki, S., Zervoudaki, A., et al.: *Arcanobacterium haemolyticum* in children with presumed streptococcal pharyngotonsillitis or scarlet fever. J. Pediatr. *121*:735–737, 1992.
76. Keren, G., Geva, T., Bogokovsky, B., et al.: *Corynebacterium* group JK pathogen in cerebrospinal fluid shunt infection: Report of two cases. J. Neurosurg. *68*:648–650, 1988.
77. Lasker, B. A., Brown, J. M., and McNeil, M. M.: Identification and epidemiological typing of clinical and environmental isolates of the genus *Rhodococcus* with use of a digoxigenin-labeled rDNA gene probe. Clin. Infect. Dis. *15*:223–233, 1992.
78. Leonard, R. B., Nowowiejski, D. J., Warren, J. J., et al.: Molecular evidence of person-to-person transmission of a pigmented strain of *Corynebacterium striatum* in intensive care units. J. Clin. Microbiol. *32*:164–169, 1994.
79. Lipsky, B. A., Goldberger, A. C., Tompkins, L. S., et al.: Infections caused by nondiphtheria corynebacteria. Rev. Infect. Dis. *4*:1220–1235, 1982.
80. Lortholary, O., Buu-Hoi, A., Fagon, J. Y., et al.: Mediastinitis due to multiple resistant *Corynebacterium xerosis*. Clin. Infect. Dis. *16*:172, 1993.
81. Luby, S., Jones, J., Dowda, H., et al.: A large outbreak of gastroenteritis caused by diarrheal toxin-producing *Bacillus cereus*. J. Infect. Dis. *167*:1452–1455, 1993.
82. Manzella, J. P., Kellogg, J. A., and Parsey, K. S.: *Corynebacterium pseudodiphtheriticum*: A respiratory tract pathogen in adults. Clin. Infect. Dis. *20*:37–40, 1995.
83. Martin, T., Hogan, D. J., Murphy, F., et al.: *Rhodococcus* infection of the skin with lymphadenitis in a nonimmunocompromised girl. J. Am. Acad. Dermatol. *24*:328–332, 1991.
84. Martinez-Martinez, L., Suarez, A. I., Ortega, M. C., et al.: Fatal pulmonary infection caused by *Corynebacterium striatum*. Clin. Infect. Dis. *19*:806–807, 1994.
85. McGowan, J. E. J.: JK coryneforms: A continuing problem for hospital infection control. J. Hosp. Infect. *11*:(Suppl. A):358–366, 1988.
86. McGowan, K. L., and Mangano, M. F.: Infections with *Rhodococcus equi* in children. Diagn. Microbiol. Infect. Dis. *14*:347–352, 1991.
87. Melling, J., Capel, B. J., Turnbull, P. C., et al.: Identification of a novel enterotoxigenic activity associated with *Bacillus cereus*. J. Clin. Pathol. *29*:938–940, 1976.
88. Miller, R. A., Brancato, F., and Holmes, K. K.: *Corynebacterium hemolyticum* as a cause of pharyngitis and scarlatiniform rash in young adults. Ann. Intern. Med. *105*:867–872, 1986.
89. Morris, A., and Guild, I.: Endocarditis due to *Corynebacterium pseudodiphtheriticum*: Five case reports, review, and antibiotic susceptibilities of nine strains. Rev. Infect. Dis. *13*:887–892, 1991.
90. Murray, B. E., Karchmer, A. W., and Moellering, R. C. J.: Diphtheroid prosthetic valve endocarditis: A study of clinical features and infecting organisms. Am. J. Med. *69*:838–848, 1980.
91. Nordmann, P., Kerestedjian, J. J., and Ronco, E.: Therapy of *Rhodococcus equi* disseminated infections in nude mice. Antimicrob. Agents Chemother. *36*:1244–1248, 1992.
92. Novak, R. M., Polisky, E. L., Janda, W. M., et al.: Osteomyelitis caused by *Rhodococcus equi* in a renal transplant recipient. Infection *16*:186–188, 1988.
93. Nyman, M., Banck, G., and Thore, M.: Penicillin tolerance in *Arcanobacterium haemolyticum*. J. Infect. Dis. *161*:261–265, 1990.
94. O'Day, D. M., Smith, R. S., Gregg, C. R., et al.: The problem of *Bacillus* species infection with special emphasis on the virulence of *Bacillus cereus*. Ophthalmology *88*:833–838, 1981.
95. Osterlund, A.: Are penicillin treatment failures in *Arcanobacterium haemolyticum* pharyngotonsillitis caused by intracellularly residing bacteria? Scand. J. Infect. Dis. *27*:131–134, 1995.
96. Panaitescu, M., Maximescu, P., Michel, J., et al.: Respiratory pathogens in non-human primates with special reference to *Corynebacterium ulcerans*. Lab. Anim. *11*:155–157, 1977.
97. Pitcher, D., Johnson, A., Allerberger, F., et al.: An investigation of nosocomial infection with *Corynebacterium jeikeium* in surgical patients using a ribosomal RNA gene probe. Eur. J. Clin. Microbiol. Infect. Dis. *9*:643–648, 1990.
98. Prescott, J. F., Johnson, J. A., and Markham, R. J.: Experimental studies on the pathogenesis of *Corynebacterium equi* infection in foals. Can. J. Comp. Med. *44*:280–288, 1980.
99. Prescott, J. F.: *Rhodococcus equi*: An animal and human pathogen. Clin. Microbiol. Rev. *4*:20–34, 1991.
100. Quinn, J. P., Arnow, P. M., Weil, D., et al.: Outbreak of JK diphtheroid infections associated with environmental contamination. J. Clin. Microbiol. *19*:668–671, 1984.
101. Riebel, W., Frantz, N., Adelstein, D., et al.: *Corynebacterium* JK: A cause of nosocomial device-related infection. Rev. Infect. Dis. *8*:42–49, 1986.
102. Riegel, P., de Briel, D., Prevost, G., et al.: Genomic diversity among *Corynebacterium jeikeium* strains and comparison with biochemical charac-

teristics and antimicrobial susceptibilities. J. Clin. Microbiol. *32*:1860–1865, 1994.
103. Riley, P. S., Hollis, D. G., Utter, G. B., et al.: Characterization and identification of 95 diphtheroid (group JK) cultures isolated from clinical specimens. J. Clin. Microbiol. *9*:418–424, 1979.
104. Rozdzinski, E., Kern, W., Schmeiser, T., et al.: *Corynebacterium jeikeium* bacteremia at a tertiary care center. Infection *19*:201–204, 1991.
105. Rufael, D. W., and Cohn, S. E.: Native valve endocarditis due to *Corynebacterium striatum*: Case report and review. Clin. Infect. Dis. *19*:1054–1061, 1994.
106. Scannell, K. A., Portoni, E. J., Finkle, H. I., et al.: Pulmonary malacoplakia and *Rhodococcus equi* infection in a patient with AIDS. Chest *97*:1000–1001, 1990.
107. Schricker, M. E., Thompson, G. H., and Schreiber, J. R.: Osteomyelitis due to *Bacillus cereus* in an adolescent: Case report and review. Clin. Infect. Dis. *18*:863–867, 1994.
108. Scott, M. A., Graham, B. S., Verrall, R., et al.: *Rhodococcus equi*: An increasingly recognized opportunistic pathogen: Report of 12 cases and review of 65 cases in the literature. Am. J. Clin. Pathol. *103*:649–655, 1995.
109. Shamsuddin, D., Tuazon, C., Levy, C., et al.: *Bacillus cereus* panophthalmitis: Source of the organism. Rev. Infect. Dis. *4*:97–103, 1982.
110. Sirera, G., Romeu, J., Clotet, B., et al.: Relapsing systemic infection due to *Rhodococcus equi* in a drug abuser seropositive for human immunodeficiency virus. Rev. Infect. Dis. *13*:509–510, 1991.
111. Sliman, R., Rehm, S., and Shlaes, D. M.: Serious infections caused by *Bacillus* species. Medicine *66*:218–223, 1987.
112. Soriano, F., Ponte, C., Santamaria, M., et al.: *Corynebacterium* group D2 as a cause of alkaline-encrusted cystitis: Report of four cases and characterization of the organisms. J. Clin. Microbiol. *21*:788–792, 1985.
113. Soriano, F., Ponte, C., Ruiz, P., et al.: Non-urinary tract infections caused by multiply antibiotic-resistant *Corynebacterium urealyticum*. Clin. Infect. Dis. *17*:890–891, 1993.
114. Soriano, F., Zapardiel, J., and Nieto, E.: Antimicrobial susceptibilities of *Corynebacterium* species and other non-spore-forming gram-positive bacilli to 18 antimicrobial agents. Antimicrob. Agents Chemother. *39*:208–214, 1995.
115. Spira, W. M., and Goepfert, J. M.: Biological characteristics of an enterotoxin produced by *Bacillus cereus*. Can. J. Microbiol. *21*:1236–1246, 1975.
116. Stamm, W. E., Tompkins, L. S., Wagner, K. F., et al.: Infection due to *Corynebacterium* species in marrow transplant patients. Ann. Intern. Med. *91*:167–173, 1979.
117. Steen, M. K., Bruno-Murtha, L. A., Chaux, G., et al.: *Bacillus cereus* endocarditis: Report of a case and review. Clin. Infect. Dis. *14*:945–946, 1992.
118. Takai, S., Iie, M., Watanabe, Y., et al.: Virulence-associated 15- to 17-kilodalton antigens in *Rhodococcus equi*: Temperature-dependent expression and location of the antigens. Infect. Immun. *60*:2995–2997, 1992.
119. Takai, S., Sasaki, Y., Ikeda, T., et al.: Virulence of *Rhodococcus equi* isolates from patients with and without AIDS. J. Clin. Microbiol. *32*:457–460, 1994.
120. Tan, C., Prescott, J. F., Patterson, M. C., et al.: Molecular characterization of a lipid-modified virulence-associated protein of *Rhodococcus equi* and its potential in protective immunity. Can. J. Vet. Res. *59*:51–59, 1995.
121. Taylor, A. J., and Gilbert, R. J.: *Bacillus cereus* food poisoning: A provisional serotyping scheme. J. Med. Microbiol. *8*:543–550, 1975.
122. Thompson, J. S., Gates-Davis, D. R., and Yong, D. C.: Rapid microbiochemical identification of *Corynebacterium diphtheriae* and other medically important corynebacteria. J. Clin. Microbiol. *18*:926–929, 1983.
123. Thompson, N. E., Ketterhagen, M. J., Bergdoll, M. S., et al.: Isolation and some properties of an enterotoxin produced by *Bacillus cereus*. Infect. Immun. *43*:887–894, 1984.
124. Tuazon, C. U., Murray, H. W., Levy, C., et al.: Serious infections from *Bacillus* sp. J. A. M. A. *241*:1137–1140, 1979.
125. Turnbull, P. C., Kramer, J. M., Jorgensen, K., et al.: Properties and production characteristics of vomiting, diarrheal, and necrotizing toxins of *Bacillus cereus*. Am. J. Clin. Nutr. *32*:219–228, 1979.
126. Verville, T. D., Huycke, M. M., Greenfield, R. A., et al.: *Rhodococcus equi* infections of humans: 12 cases and a review of the literature. Medicine *73*:119–132, 1994.
127. Waagner, D. C.: *Arcanobacterium haemolyticum*: Biology of the organism and diseases in man. Pediatr. Infect. Dis. J. *10*:933–939, 1991.
128. Waller, K. S., Johnson, J., Wood, B. P.: Radiological case of the month: Cavitary pneumonia due to *Arcanobacterium hemolyticum*. Am. J. Dis. Child. *145*:209–210, 1991.
129. Watkins, D. A., Chahine, A., Creger, R. J., et al.: *Corynebacterium striatum*: A diphtheroid with pathogenic potential. Clin. Infect. Dis. *17*:21–25, 1993.
130. Wazny, T. K., Mummaw, N., and Styrt, B.: Degranulation of human neutrophils after exposure to bacterial phospholipase C. Eur. J. Clin. Microbiol. Infect. Dis. *9*:830–832, 1990.
131. Weber, D. J., Saviteer, S. M., Rutala, W. A., et al.: *In vitro* susceptibility of *Bacillus* spp. to selected antimicrobial agents. Antimicrob. Agents Chemother. *32*:642–645, 1988.
132. Williams, D. Y., Selepak, S. T., and Gill, V. J.: Identification of clinical isolates of nondiphtherial *Corynebacterium* species and their antibiotic susceptibility patterns. Diagn. Microbiol. Infect. Dis. *17*:23–28, 1993.
133. Wong, T. P., and Groman, N.: Production of diphtheria toxin by selected isolates of *Corynebacterium ulcerans* and *Corynebacterium pseudotuberculosis*. Infect. Immun. *43*:1114–1116, 1984.
134. Young, V. M., Meyers, W. F., Moody, M. R., et al.: The emergence of coryneform bacteria as a cause of nosocomial infections in compromised hosts. Am. J. Med. *70*:646–650, 1981.

❑ ❑ ❑

SUBSECTION FOUR

ENTEROBACTERIA

106

CITROBACTER

William C. Gruber and Randall G. Fisher

Citrobacter, a genus of enteric gram-negative rods closely related to *Salmonella*, has been associated increasingly with human disease. *Citrobacter* strains are found infrequently as normal inhabitants of the intestinal tract of humans and animals[22, 31, 44]; they have been associated with urinary tract infections,[4, 12, 22, 27, 29, 30] osteomyelitis,[24, 29] diarrhea,[7, 17, 48] and invasive disease in the immunocompromised host.[21, 22, 29, 30] *Citrobacter* has been associated commonly with sepsis and meningitis of the newborn.[13]

BACTERIOLOGY

In 1931, Werkman and Gillen[44] proposed the generic term *Citrobacter* for citrate-positive coliaerogenes intermediates isolated from stool. This genus includes *Citrobacter freundii (Escherichia freundii)*, *C. amalonaticus*, and *C. diversus (C. koseri, Levinea malonatica)*. In addition to utilization of citrate, these motile organisms hydrolyze urea and ferment glucose, with production of gas.[36] They grow on ordinary media as gray, opaque, round colonies producing a strong, fetid odor. Unlike *Salmonella*, *Citrobacter* grows in the presence of potassium cyanide. Indole-negative strains that produce hydrogen sulfide are classified as *C. freundii*. Indole-positive, hydrogen sulfide–negative strains are differentiated by their ability to ferment malonate; *C. diversus* ferments malonate, whereas *C. amalonaticus* does not.[1] Antigenic schemata have been developed to classify the O somatic antigens of *Citrobacter*[13, 16, 48]; these antigens show cross-reactivity with O antigens of other Enterobacteriaceae.

EPIDEMIOLOGY

Meningitis due to *Citrobacter* first was reported in 1960, with two cases of *C. freundii*.[20] In the decade of 1970 to 1979, 69 cases of *Citrobacter* meningitis were reported,[14] and 4 per cent of neonatal meningitis cases reported in the First Neonatal Meningitis Cooperative Study Group were due to *Citrobacter*.[34] *C. diversus* is the species usually isolated with meningitis; central nervous system infection caused by *C. freundii* is less common.[14] Most of the cases in the United States are reported from southern states; biotype d or serotypes O2 and O1[14] are the most common isolates of *C. diversus* encountered.

Most cases of neonatal meningitis due to this organism have been sporadic, but occasional clusters of meningeal infection have been reported.[8] Numerous attempts have been made to define the mode of introduction and spread of this organism in nursery outbreaks.[9, 13, 35, 41, 48] Maternal transmission to the infant and contaminated infant formula have been implicated as a source of *Citrobacter* introduction into the nursery.[2, 9, 41] Once *Citrobacter* is introduced into the neonatal nursery, colonization may exceed 79 per cent.[13] Parry and associates[35] described a nursery outbreak in which 11 of 128 infants were colonized with *C. diversus* over an observation period of 3 months; two of the colonized infants developed meningitis. Additional colonization of neonates appeared to be eliminated by removal of a nurse with persistent hand carriage of the organism. Curiously, the bacteria were isolated more frequently from the umbilicus than from the stool of colonized infants, which implicated umbilicus to nurses' hands to umbilicus as the possible mode of spread.

In another outbreak,[48] introduction of *C. diversus* into the nursery was linked to an infant admitted with meningitis. Thirty-one per cent of infants in the nursery subsequent to the index case were found to be colonized with *C. diversus* of the same serotype and biotype. A second infant from this study developed meningitis with the organism during the observation period. Umbilical colonization of infants in this cluster was more common than rectal colonization, but rectal colonization was more persistent, lasting as long as 4 months. Two nurses were found to have hand colonization with the organism, and the reintroduction of these bacteria into the nursery was linked to a pregnant nurse who had perineal cultures at delivery yielding the epidemic strain. She was implicated in the colonization of her own infant as well as three other neonates. Corresponding culture data from a reference hospital revealed an overall neonatal colonization rate with *Citrobacter* of 1 to 10 per cent over a 5-year period, with no invasive disease.

Although *Citrobacter* has been isolated increasingly from debilitated adult patients,[45] particularly as a urinary tract,[22, 29, 30] soft-tissue,[15, 29, 30] and bone[30] pathogen, *Citrobacter* infection in children is unusual after the first several months of life. In the older infant and child, *Citrobacter* is almost exclusively an opportunistic pathogen.

PATHOPHYSIOLOGY

Citrobacter infrequently colonizes the intestinal tract and perineum of humans.[22] Epidemiologic data and onset of some *Citrobacter* infections within 24 hours of birth suggest that the newborn can acquire colonization at the time of passage through the birth canal of a colonized mother. Onset of disease beyond the first week of life is related commonly to colonization of the infant in the nursery. As with other types of gram-negative neonatal meningitis, central nervous system infection results from bacteremia in a colonized infant, leading to seeding of the meninges. The basis for the particular invasiveness of *Citrobacter* in the neonate and its propensity to cause multiple brain abscesses are unexplained. Many strains of *C. diversus* appear to be able to produce brain pathology in the mouse, but the degree of damage appears related to strain virulence and mouse age.[26, 37] Strain differences, related to the presence of an outer-membrane protein with a molecular weight of 32,000, have been associated with differences in brain histopathology in one infant rat model of *C. diversus* meningitis.[25] Strains isolated from cerebrospinal fluid of infants with meningitis more commonly possess this outer-membrane protein than do strains isolated from other body sites.[26]

In the immunocompromised patient, broad use of antimicrobial agents may produce selective pressure, leading to increased colonization with *Citrobacter*. Increased bacterial density combined with a blunted immune response may result in invasive disease.

CLINICAL MANIFESTATIONS

Citrobacter, like other neonatal pathogens, can cause early- as well as late-onset infection. In a review of 74 cases of neonatal meningitis due to these bacteria,[14] the mean age of onset reported for early disease was 7 days; 85 per cent of patients were included in this group. Fifteen per cent of cases occurred after 3 weeks of age. Twenty-three of 74 patients were younger than 36 weeks gestational age at birth, which suggests that the preterm infant is at increased risk for *Citrobacter* infection.

Clinical signs and symptoms are those typical of neonatal sepsis. Fever, lethargy, poor feeding, vomiting, irritability, bulging fontanelle, seizures, and jaundice are common presenting features. Umbilical infection and surgical manipulation of colonized umbilical stumps occasionally have preceded bacteremia and meningitis.[35] White blood cell count may show leukocytosis or leukopenia. Cerebrospinal fluid findings are consistent with most types of neonatal bacterial meningitis and usually show polymorphonuclear cell elevation, elevated protein, and depressed glucose; gram-negative rods may be seen on smear. In 35 per cent of *Citrobacter* meningitis cases, these bacteria are isolated concurrently from the blood.[14]

Citrobacter is a particularly devastating cause of neonatal meningitis. Central nervous system infection with this organism produces multiple brain abscesses with unusually high frequency.[14, 18, 23, 26, 28] In the extensive review by Graham and Band,[14] three quarters of *Citrobacter* meningitis cases resulted in intracerebral abscesses. The incidence of abscess formation in non-*Citrobacter* gram-negative meningitis is reported to be as low as 10 per cent.[14] The case-fatality rate for *Citrobacter* meningitis varies from 30 to 50 per cent, and at least three-quarters of surviving infants are delayed in development. The presence of brain abscess appears to contribute significantly to morbidity and mortality.[6, 13, 14]

In adults, *Citrobacter* is isolated most commonly from the urinary tract.[22, 29, 30] Five to 12 per cent of bacterial isolates from urinary tract infections in adult patients are due to *Citrobacter*,[27, 46] and *C. diversus* has been isolated from a perinephric abscess in a diabetic kidney transplant recipient.[47] *Citrobacter* urinary tract infection in children is extremely rare but has been documented in a 6-week-old male with bilateral hydronephrosis and a 7-year-old catheterized female who was impaired neurologically.[12] Sputum is the second most common clinical specimen to yield *Citrobacter* in adults[22]; lung abscess,[11] pneumonia,[29, 30] bronchitis,[21] and septic arthritis[29] have been reported.

Gastrointestinal disease occasionally has been attributed to *Citrobacter*, but frequent isolation of this agent from normal stools often makes this diagnosis equivocal. This genus first was implicated in an outbreak of mild gastroenteritis by Barnes and Cherry[3] in 1946, and an outbreak of watery diar-

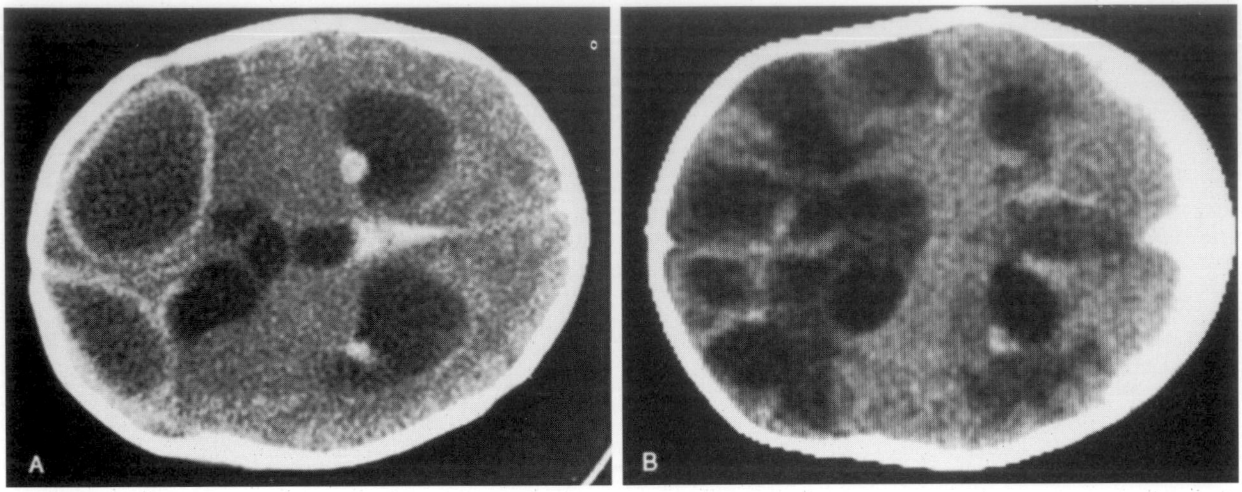

FIGURE 106–1. *Computed tomogram demonstrating progressive abscess formation and encephalomalacia in an infant at 3 weeks of age* (A) *and 6 weeks of age* (B), *despite bacteriologic "cure" of* Citrobacter *meningitis.*

rhea in a Virginia infant care unit included two infants in whom isolates of enterotoxin-liberating *Citrobacter* were obtained from the stool.[17] Some studies have found higher incidences of *Citrobacter* isolation from the stool of enterocolitis syndrome patients than from stools of control patients.[48] Verotoxigenic *C. freundii* isolated from butter was associated with an outbreak of diarrhea and hemolytic-uremic syndrome in a day care setting.[42] *C. freundii* has been found as a cause of appendicitis in a healthy adult, peritonitis in adults with liver disease or pancreatitis,[29] and meningitis in adults[40] as a complication of neurosurgery. Bone and soft-tissue infections occur[5]; 3 per cent of *Citrobacter* pathogens were isolated from joint or bone in one adult series.[29] A 3-year-old child treated with multiple antibiotics and corticosteroids for a variety of medical problems developed *Citrobacter* osteomyelitis of multiple bones of the lower extremities.[31]

DIAGNOSIS

Biochemical characteristics of *C. diversus* include lack of hydrogen sulfide production on triple sugar iron agar, negative Voges-Proskauer reaction, utilization of citrate, motility, production of indole, decarboxylation of ornithine but not lysine, and production of acid from adonitol.[1, 38] Identification of this organism as a pathogen in a nursery setting should heighten suspicion of its possible role in subsequent neonatal infections.

C. freundii is indole-negative and hydrogen sulfide–positive, which differentiates it from *C. diversus. C. amalonaticus* differs from *C. diversus* because of the former's inability to ferment malonate. *C. freundii* and *C. amalonaticus* account for a significant portion of disease due to *Citrobacter* in immunocompromised persons and should be suspected particularly in this group of patients.[21]

TREATMENT

Most *C. diversus* organisms are resistant to ampicillin (97 per cent in one series),[29] but approximately 40 per cent of *C. freundii* organisms are ampicillin-sensitive.[43] Most species are sensitive to aminoglycosides and third-generation cephalosporins. However, a 4-year experience with neonatal septicemia due to *C. diversus* has been described in which all of 13 isolates were resistant to gentamicin but susceptible to third-generation cephalosporins.[10]

Treatment of meningitis often requires a multidisciplinary effort involving the neurosurgeon as well as the pediatrician. Antibiotic therapy for gram-negative neonatal meningitis generally has proved disappointing (see Chapter 77).[32, 33] Once the identity of the infecting gram-negative organism is known, the standard of therapy is an intravenously administered aminoglycoside, a third-generation cephalosporin, or both.[33] Poor meningeal penetration of aminoglycoside in addition to the presence of intracranial abscesses makes antibiotic therapy for *Citrobacter* meningitis especially difficult. The ability of this organism to persist in the brain is demonstrated by its recovery 4 years after neonatal infection.[7] Addition of systemic chloramphenicol,[6, 13, 19] imipenem,[19] or intraventricular gentamicin[23, 32, 35, 39] has been tried in individual cases, but improved outcome has not been documented consistently. Cranial computed tomography often is essential for evaluation of complications such as hydrocephalus and multicystic encephalomalacia (Fig. 106–1). Real-time cranial ultrasonography has shown good correlation with computed tomography.[28] Ventriculostomy and craniectomy with open drainage of abscesses have been required in some children to effect bacteriologic "cure," and shunt placement for hydrocephalus often is required. Scrupulous attention to preventive infection-control practices has been recommended to stem nursery outbreaks.[13, 35, 48] These prophylactic measures include skin and umbilical cord care, elimination of crowding with isolation of infected infants and carriers, and good hand washing practices. Exclusion of colonized personnel and temporary closing of the nursery have been followed by a reduction in neonatal *C. diversus* colonization. Although cohorting of colonized infants is a reasonable practice, multiple sources of *Citrobacter* introduction may limit the efficacy of this approach in some outbreaks.[12]

Treatment of *Citrobacter* infection beyond the neonatal period requires choice of an appropriate antibiotic, with drainage of abscesses and appropriate débridement of wounds. Therapy should be guided by antimicrobial susceptibility testing. Outcome largely depends on the preceding debility of the host and location of the infection. Significant mortality is associated with immunocompromised persons with septicemia or pulmonary disease.[21, 22, 29, 30]

References

1. Altmann, G., Sechter, I., Cahan, D., et al.: *Citrobacter diversus* isolated from clinical material. J. Clin. Microbiol. 3:390–392, 1976.

2. Ashbaugh, J. A., and Barlow, J. F.: Neonate with jaundice and leukopenia. South. Med. J. 35:17–21, 1982.
3. Barnes, L. A., and Cherry, C. B.: A group of paracolon organisms having apparent pathogenicity. Am. J. Public Health 36:481–483, 1946.
4. Barton, L. L., and Walentik, C.: *Citrobacter diversus* urinary tract infection. Am. J. Dis. Child. 136:467–468, 1982.
5. Bruehl, C. L., and Listernick, R: *Citrobacter freundii* septic arthritis. J. Paediatr. Child Health 28:402–403, 1992.
6. Curless, R. G.: Neonatal intracranial abscess: Two cases caused by *Citrobacter* and a literature review. Ann. Neurol. 8:269–272, 1980.
7. Eppes, S. C., Woods, C. R., Mayer, A. S., et al.: Recurring ventriculitis due to *Citrobacter diversus*: Clinical and bacteriologic analysis. Clin. Infect. Dis. 17:437–440, 1993.
8. Feng-Ying, C., Devoe, W. F., Morrison, C., et al.: Outbreak of neonatal *Citrobacter diversus* meningitis in a suburban hospital. Pediatr. Infect. Dis. J. 6:50–55, 1987.
9. Finn, A., Talbot, G. H., Anday, E., et al.: Vertical transmission of *Citrobacter diversus* from mother to infant. Pediatr. Infect. Dis. J. 7:293–294, 1988.
10. Giacoia, G. P., and West, K.: Sepsis with *Citrobacter diversus* in sick newborns. Am. J. Perinatol. 6:49–54, 1989.
11. Gilman, R. M., Irwin, R. S., Garrity, F. L., et al.: Community-acquired *Citrobacter diversus* infections. Respir. Care 25:66–71, 1980.
12. Goering, R. V., Ehrenkranz, N. J., Sanders, C. C., et al.: Long-term epidemiological analysis of *Citrobacter diversus* in a neonatal intensive care unit. Pediatr. Infect. Dis. 11:99–104, 1992.
13. Graham, D. R., Anderson, R. L., Arier, F. E., et al.: Epidemic nosocomial meningitis due to *Citrobacter diversus* in neonates. J. Infect. Dis. 144:203–209, 1981.
14. Graham, D. R., and Band, J. D.: *Citrobacter diversus* brain abscess and meningitis in neonates. J. A. M. A. 245:1923–1925, 1981.
15. Grant, M. D., Horowitz, H. I., and Lorian, V.: Gangrenous ulcer and septicemia due to *Citrobacter*. N. Engl. J. Med. 280:1286–1287, 1969.
16. Gross, R. J., Rowe, B., and Easton, J. A.: Neonatal meningitis caused by *Citrobacter koseri*. J. Clin. Pathol. 26:138–139, 1973.
17. Guerrant, R. L., Dickens, M. D., Wenzel, R. P., et al.: Toxigenic bacterial diarrhea: Nursery outbreak involving multiple bacterial strains. J. Pediatr. 89:885–891, 1976.
18. Gwynn, C. M., and George, R. H.: Neonatal citrobacter meningitis. Arch. Dis. Child. 48:455–458, 1973.
19. Haimi-Cohen, Y., Amir, J., Weinstock, A., et al.: The use of imipenem-cilastatin in neonatal meningitis caused by *Citrobacter diversus*. Acta Paediatr. 82:530–532, 1993.
20. Harris, D., and Cone, T. E., Jr.: *Escherichia freundii* meningitis: Report of two cases. J. Pediatr. 56:774–777, 1960.
21. Hodges, G. R., Degener, C. E., and Barnes, W. G.: Clinical significance of *Citrobacter* isolates. Am. J. Clin. Pathol. 70:37–40, 1978.
22. Jones, S. R., Ragsdale, A. R., Kutscher, E., et al.: Clinical and bacteriologic observations on a recently recognized species of Enterobacteriaceae, *Citrobacter diversus*. J. Infect. Dis. 128:563–565, 1973.
23. Kaplan, A. M., Itabashi, H. H., Yoshimori, R., et al.: Cerebral abscesses complicating neonatal *Citrobacter freundii* meningitis. West. J. Med. 127:418–422, 1977.
24. Kleint, W., and Herwig, H.: Septische osteomyelitis durch *Citrobacter*, zugleich ein beitrag zum problem der cortison-wendung bei bacteirellen infectionen. Arzneimittel Wochenschr. 13:965–969, 1958.
25. Kline, M. W., Kaplan, S. L., Hawkins, E. P., et al.: Pathogenesis of brain abscess formation in an infant rat model of *Citrobacter diversus* bacteremia and meningitis. J. Infect. Dis. 157:106–112, 1988.
26. Kline, M. W., Mason, E. O., and Kaplan, S. L.: Characterization of *Citrobacter diversus* strains causing neonatal meningitis. J. Infect. Dis. 157:101–105, 1988.
27. Lesseva, M. I., and Hadjiski, O. G.: Analysis of bacteriuria in patients with burns. Burns 21:3–6, 1995.
28. Levine, R. S., Rosenberg, H. K., Zimmerman, R. A., et al.: Complications of *Citrobacter* neonatal meningitis: Assessment by real-time cranial sonography correlated with CT. Am. J. Neuroradiol. 4:668–671, 1983.
29. Lipsky, B. A., Hook, E. W., III, Smith, A. A., et al.: *Citrobacter* infections in humans: Experience at the Seattle Veterans Administration Medical Center and a review of the literature. Rev. Infect. Dis. 2:746–760, 1980.
30. Madrazo, A., Geiger, J., and Lauter, C. B.: *Citrobacter diversus* at Grace Hospital, Detroit, Michigan. Am. J. Med. Sci. 270:497–501, 1975.
31. Marklein, G., Waschkowski, G., and Reichertz, C.: *Erwinia herbicola* bei sepsis im kindesalter. Klin. Pediatr. 193:394–397, 1981.
32. McCracken, G. H., Jr.: New developments in the management of children with bacterial meningitis. Pediatr. Infect. Dis. 3:S32–S34, 1984.
33. McCracken, G. H., Jr., and Mize, S. G.: A controlled study of intrathecal antibiotic therapy in gram-negative enteric meningitis of infancy: Report of the Neonatal Meningitis Cooperative Study Group. J. Pediatr. 89:66–72, 1976.
34. McCracken, G. H., Jr., Mize, S. G., and Threlkeld, N.: Intraventricular gentamicin therapy in gram-negative bacillary meningitis of infancy: Report of the Second National Meningitis Cooperative Study Group. Lancet 1:787–791, 1980.
35. Parry, M. F., Hutchinson, J. H., Brown, N. A., et al.: Gram-negative sepsis in neonates: A nursery outbreak due to hand carriage of *Citrobacter diversus*. Pediatrics 65:1105–1109, 1980.
36. Smith, R. F., Dayton, S. L., and Chipps, D. D.: Recognition of *Citrobacter diversus* in the clinical laboratory. Appl. Microbiol. 25:157–158, 1973.
37. Soriano, A. L., Russell, R. G., Johnson, D., et al.: Pathophysiology of *Citrobacter diversus* neonatal meningitis: Comparative studies in an infant mouse model. Infect. Immun. 59:1352–1358, 1991.
38. Spirer, Z., Jurgenson, U., Lazewnick, R., et al.: Complete recovery from an apparent brain abscess treated without neurosurgery: The importance of early CT scanning. Clin. Pediatr. 21:106–109, 1982.
39. Tamborlane, W. V., Jr., and Soto, E. V.: *Citrobacter diversus* meningitis. A case report. Pediatrics 55:739–741, 1975.
40. Tang, L. M., Chen, S. T., and Lui, T. N.: *Citrobacter* meningitis in adults. Clin. Neurol. Neurosurg. 96:52–57, 1994.
41. Thurm, V., and Gericke, B.: Identification of infant food as a vehicle in a nosocomial outbreak of *Citrobacter freundii*: Epidemiological subtyping by allozyme, whole-cell protein and antibiotic resistance. J. Appl. Bacteriol. 76:553–558, 1994.
42. Tschape, H., Prager, R., Streckel, W., et al.: Verotoxinogenic *Citrobacter freundii* associated with severe gastroenteritis and cases of haemolytic uraemic syndrome in a nursery school: Green butter as the infection source. Epidemiol. Infect. 114:441–450, 1995.
43. Tullus, K., Olsson Liljequist, B., Lundstrom, G., et al.: Antibiotic susceptibility of 629 bacterial blood and CSF isolates from Swedish infants and the therapeutic implications. Acta Paediatr. Scand. 80:205–212, 1991.
44. Werkman, C. H., and Gillen, G. F.: Bacteria producing trimethylene glycol. J. Bacteriol. 23:167–182, 1932.
45. Werthamer, S., and Weiner, M.: Subacute bacterial endocarditis due to *Flavobacterium meningosepticum*. Am. J. Clin. Pathol. 57:410–412, 1972.
46. Wientzen, R. L., McCracken, G. H., Jr., Petruska, M. L., et al.: Localization and therapy of urinary tract infections of childhood. Pediatrics 63:467–473, 1979.
47. Williams, R. D., and Simmons, R. L.: *Citrobacter* perinephric abscess presenting as pneumoscrotum in transplant recipient. Urology 3:478–480, 1974.
48. Williams, W. W., Mariano, J., Spurrier, M., et al.: Nosocomial meningitis due to *Citrobacter diversus* in neonates: New aspects of the epidemiology. J. Infect. Dis. 150:229–235, 1984.

107

ENTEROBACTER

William C. Gruber and Randall G. Fisher

Enterobacter is a genus of Enterobacteriaceae that is an increasingly frequent cause of nosocomial pediatric infection. *Enterobacter* can cause infection of postsurgical wounds, meningitis, and infection of the gastrointestinal, urinary, and respiratory tracts. Development of resistance to antibiotics commonly used for treatment of infection is an increasingly common challenge.

BACTERIOLOGY

Enterobacter species are named for their enteric recovery as gram-negative bacteria.[57] They commonly are found in soil, water, and sewage. These organisms are anaerobic facultatively and motile by peritrichous flagella. They yield positive results on malonate, citrate, and Voges-Proskauer tests. Taxonomic studies have led to several classifications of species contained in this genus. With the reclassification of *E. agglomerans* as *Pantoea agglomerans* (see Chapter 118), *E. cloacae, E. aerogenes,* and *E. sakazakii* are the most common species recovered from clinical material.[2, 11, 15, 20, 26, 36, 65, 66] Additional species in the *Enterobacter* genus rarely recovered from human infections include *E. amnigenus, E. asburiae, E. gergoviae, E. intermedium, E. taylorae, E. dissolvens,* and *E. nimipressuralis.*[29] *E. hormaechei* has been proposed as a new species.[52]

EPIDEMIOLOGY

Enterobacter is encountered most commonly as a hospital-acquired pathogen in patients with chronic illness.[2, 11, 15, 20, 36, 65, 66] In some series, less than one-third of infections are community-acquired.[12] In a Centers for Disease Control and Prevention survey, *Enterobacter* was one of the five most commonly encountered pathogens in intensive care units and accounted for 8.6 per cent of reported infections.[36] In one pediatric hospital, *Enterobacter* species (primarily *E. cloacae*) were the most common cause of enteric bacteremia and accounted for 14 per cent of all bacteremic episodes over a 3-year period.[2] Up to one-third of *Enterobacter* bacteremias are polymicrobial.[12, 26] At least one burn unit has noted an increased incidence of *Enterobacter* infection in recent years.[18]

Vertical spread of *Enterobacter* from mother to infant may occur at the time of birth.[25] Environmental sources implicated in outbreaks of infection have included intravenous fluids,[44] nonsterile blood collection tubes,[4] chronic hand dermatitis of a care provider,[6] contaminated infant formula,[8, 16, 50] and blood-gas machines.[1, 39]

Plasmid typing, pulsed-field electrophoresis, and restriction-fragment polymorphism analysis of DNA from clinical isolates have been useful in discriminating possible sources of contamination and patient-to-patient transfer of individual strains.[9, 15, 16, 32, 34, 40] Endogenous origin of infection also has been documented by sequential isolation of the same organism in stool, blood, and cerebrospinal fluid from an infected neonate.[40]

PATHOPHYSIOLOGY

Newborn infants often are colonized by *Enterobacter* species in the gastrointestinal tract soon after birth,[7] and acquisition of hospital strains in immunocompromised newborn infants is common.[7, 24] *Enterobacter* then may contaminate the compromised respiratory tract. The oropharynx commonly is colonized by *Enterobacter* by 1 month of age; colonization rates generally are lower in breast-fed infants.[5] Enteric organisms are recovered less commonly from the oropharynx of healthy older children and adults, but increased colonization is noted during illness (see also *Klebsiella*, Chapter 109).

The ability of *Enterobacter* species to develop resistance to cephalosporins increases their pathogenic potential. Most enteric and related organisms contain an *ampC* gene coding for a class C β-lactamase.[17, 51] In *E. cloacae,* this β-lactamase is inducible by β-lactam antibiotics because of the presence of an additional regulatory gene, *ampR,* which is lacking in noninducible species.[42] β-Lactam antibiotics may bind to penicillin-binding proteins and produce a peptidoglycan fragment that acts directly or indirectly on *ampR.*[51] The *ampR* regulator functions as a transcriptional activator in the presence of β-lactam inducer; induction is down-regulated by *ampD.*[38, 51] Hence, depending on the genetic makeup, the induction of chromosomal β-lactamase expression can vary in *Enterobacter* species.[61] In general, antibiotic therapy quickly increases the risk of acquiring resistant organisms in infants, children, and adults.[1, 2, 15, 21, 35, 42, 49, 53, 58, 69]

In one study, gram-negative fecal aerobic flora was eradicated completely after 24 hours of ceftriaxone therapy, only to be replaced within 10 days (mean, 6.7 days) of therapy by *Pseudomonas aeruginosa, Enterobacter,* and *Citrobacter* resistant to all β-lactam antibiotics.[33] The combination of reduced outer-membrane permeability and high-level β-lactamase production renders some clinical isolates of *Enterobacter* resistant to imipenem.[41, 64]

Other factors responsible for the virulence of *Enterobacter* species are less well defined. In vitro, it is possible to transfer and express an *Escherichia coli* enterotoxigenic plasmid in *Enterobacter,* implicating the potential for transfer of virulence factors to *Enterobacter* from other species.[70] Like other organisms associated with central venous catheter infections, *Enterobacter* species may adhere irreversibly to catheter material, promoting colonization and infection.[54] Certain ribotypes have been encountered more commonly as community or blood stream isolates, indicating the presence of as yet undefined factors affecting virulence.[67] The propensity of *Enterobacter sakazakii* to produce neonatal meningitis complicated by abscesses and cerebral infarction is unexplained.[8, 16, 68]

CLINICAL MANIFESTATIONS

Infection due to *Enterobacter* commonly is indistinguishable from illness due to other enteric pathogens. Sources of infection include central venous catheters and the respiratory, urinary, and biliary tracts.[2, 3, 26, 36, 43] Neonatal infection deserves special mention because of the prominence of *E. sakazakii* as a cause of devastating meningitis.

Like *Citrobacter diversus* (see Chapter 106), *E. sakazakii* causes neonatal meningitis complicated by cerebral abscesses or infarctions.[8, 16, 37, 68, 69] Poor feeding, irritability, jaundice, a full anterior fontanelle, and fever or hypothermia are presenting features that are shared with other gram-negative causes of bacterial meningitis. However, the mortality rate reaches 50 per cent, and almost all survivors suffer severe neurologic complications.[68] This severe morbidity is consistent with the development of multiple cystic lesions of the brain in 50 per cent of surviving neonates. Serial computed tomography commonly reveals evolution of lesions most consistent with cerebral infarction, rather than primary abscess formation.[27, 68] *Enterobacter* also may be associated with necrotizing enterocolitis in the newborn; *Enterobacter* species were the third most common isolate recovered in peritonitis in a series of patients with necrotizing enterocolitis.[48]

In older immunocompromised children, bacteremia complicated by sepsis is a significant risk. Central venous catheterization and gastrointestinal tract pathology appear to pose greater risks for bacteremia than does infection of the urinary tract.[2, 15, 26, 43] Bacteremia is accompanied by shock in close to one-third of patients, but disseminated intravascular coagulation occurs in less than 5 per cent.[10, 12, 26] In some series, overall mortality rates with bacteremia approach 50 per cent[10]; factors associated with a poor prognosis include age younger than 18 months, inadequacy of antimicrobial chemotherapy, septic shock, type of underlying disease, presence of pulmonary infection, thrombocytopenia, and requirement for intensive care.[10, 12, 26] Absence of fever during the course of infection may be a particularly ominous sign; indeed, four of five afebrile subjects died in one series.[10]

Some *Enterobacter* species recovered from children with diarrhea have been reported to produce enterotoxin.[13] Other recent presentations of *Enterobacter* infection include endophthalmitis,[46, 47] endometritis,[30] wound infections,[26] discitis,[60] and osteomyelitis.[19, 62]

DIAGNOSIS

Diagnosis of infection due to *Enterobacter* relies primarily on isolation of the organism in culture from clinical material. The ability to detect pathogens directly in tissue using biotinylated probes offers promise for rapid diagnosis.[45] Motility, ornithine decarboxylase production, and the absence of deoxyribonuclease help to distinguish the genus from *Klebsiella* and *Serratia*. Patterns of sugar fermentation and decarboxylase production also distinguish the species. Ribotyping is a highly discriminatory and reproducible method for the typing of *E. cloacae*, the most common cause of infection, but may offer little increase in discrimination over biotyping, serotyping, and phage susceptibility for characterization of outbreaks.[28]

TREATMENT

Treatment of *Enterobacter* infection is made problematic by resistance to cephalosporins. Antibiotic resistance may be present at the time of initial isolation or may develop during therapy.[15, 35] This problem is compounded by the common observation of resistance to extended-spectrum penicillins and aminoglycosides. The risks for development of resistance to cephalosporins, piperacillin, and aminoglycosides have been reported to be higher at a tertiary care center than at a primary care hospital.[23] Previous administration of third-generation cephalosporins increases the risk of multiresistant *Enterobacter* isolates in an initial, positive blood culture.[7, 14] However, hospitalized newborns quickly may acquire multiresistant strains, even though they themselves have not been treated with cephalosporins.[7] In turn, isolation of multiresistant *Enterobacter* in blood culture is associated with a higher death rate, compared with mortality after isolation of a more sensitive *Enterobacter*.[14, 58] Although less common, possible resistance to imipenem should be anticipated.[22, 41, 63]

Some investigators recommend combination therapy that includes an aminoglycoside wherever cephalosporin resistance is common. When strains are resistant to gentamicin and tobramycin, amikacin may be a suitable alternative. Good responses to therapy and return of the gentamicin susceptibility of hospital *Enterobacter* strains have followed routine substitution of amikacin for gentamicin.[56, 59] Trimethoprim-sulfamethoxazole alone (or combined with an aminoglycoside) and quinolones appear to be good alternatives for the treatment of *Enterobacter* infections, including meningitis.[2, 31, 69]

Meningitis creates special concerns. As is common with other forms of neonatal enteric meningitis, even susceptible organisms often persist in cerebrospinal fluid for 5 days or longer.[37] The physician should anticipate the potential development of abscesses, infarctions, and cysts in newborn infants with *E. sakazakii* infection. Serial computed tomography should be considered, and a neurosurgeon should be sought for drainage of abscesses or management of fluid accumulation.

References

1. Acolet, D., Ahmet, Z., Houang, E., et al.: *Enterobacter cloacae* in a neonatal intensive care unit: Account of an outbreak and its relationship to use of third generation cephalosporins. J. Hosp. Infect. *28*:273–286, 1994.
2. Andresen, J., Asmar, B. I., and Dajani, A. S.: Increasing *Enterobacter* bacteremia in pediatric patients. Pediatr. Infect. Dis. *13*:787–792, 1994.
3. Ashkenazi, S., Even-Tov, S., Samra, Z., et al.: Uropathogens of various childhood populations and their antibiotic susceptibility. Pediatr. Infect. Dis. *10*:742–746, 1991.
4. Astagneau, P., Gottot, S., Gobin, Y., et al.: Nosocomial outbreak of *Enterobacter agglomerans* pseudobacteraemia associated with non-sterile blood collection tubes. J. Hosp. Infect. *27*:73–75, 1994.
5. Baltimore, R. S., Duncan, R. L., Shapiro, E. D., et al.: Epidemiology of pharyngeal colonization of infants with aerobic gram-negative rod bacteria. J. Clin. Microbiol. *27*:91–95, 1989.
6. Beck-Sague, C. M., Chong, W. H., Roy, C., et al.: Outbreak of surgical wound infections associated with total hip arthroplasty. Infect. Control Hosp. Epidemiol. *13*:526–534, 1992.
7. Berkowitz, F. E., and Metchock, B.: Third-generation cephalosporin-resistant gram-negative bacilli in the feces of hospitalized children. Pediatr. Infect. Dis. *14*:97–100, 1995.
8. Biering, G., Karlsson, S., Clark, N. C., et al.: Three cases of neonatal meningitis caused by *Enterobacter sakazakii* in powdered milk. J. Clin. Microbiol. *27*:2054–2056, 1989.
9. Bingen, E., Denamur, E., Lambert-Zechovsky, N., et al.: Rapid genotyping shows the absence of cross-contamination in *Enterobacter cloacae* nosocomial infections. J. Hosp. Infect. *21*:95–101, 1992.
10. Bodey, G. P., Elting, L. S., and Rodriguez, S.: Bacteremia caused by *Enterobacter*: 15 years of experience in a cancer hospital. Rev. Infect. Dis. *13*:550–558, 1991.
11. Bonadio, W. A., Margolis, D., and Tovar, M.: *Enterobacter cloacae* bacteremia in children: A review of 30 cases in 12 years. Clin. Pediatr. *30*:310–313, 1991.
12. Bouza, E., Garcia de la Torre, M., Erice, A., et al.: *Enterobacter* bacteremia: An analysis of 50 episodes. Arch. Intern. Med. *145*:1024–1027, 1985.
13. Chatterjee, B. D., Thawani, G., and Sanyal, S. N.: Etiology of acute childhood diarrhoea in Calcutta. Trop. Gastroenterol. *10*:158–166, 1989.
14. Chow, J. W., Fine, M. J., Shlaes, D. M., et al.: *Enterobacter* bacteremia: Clinical features and emergence of antibiotic resistance during therapy [see comments]. Ann. Intern. Med. *115*:585–590, 1991.
15. Chow, J. W., Yu, V. L., and Shlaes, D. M.: Epidemiologic perspectives on *Enterobacter* for the infection control professional [see comments]. Am. J. Infect. Control *22*:195–201, 1994.
16. Clark, N. C., Hill, B. C., O'Hara, C. M., et al.: Epidemiologic typing of *Enterobacter sakazakii* in two neonatal nosocomial outbreaks. Diagn. Microbiol. Infect. Dis. *13*:467–472, 1990.
17. Dever, L. A., and Dermody, T. S.: Mechanisms of bacterial resistance to antibiotics. Arch. Intern. Med. *151*:886–895, 1991.
18. Donati, L., Scamazzo, F., Gervasoni, M., et al.: Infection and antibiotic therapy in 4000 burned patients treated in Milan, Italy, between 1976 and 1988. Burns *19*.345-348, 1993.
19. Dubey, L., Krasinski, K., and Hernanz-Schulman, M.: Osteomyelitis secondary to trauma or infected contiguous soft tissue. Pediatr. Infect. Dis. *7*:26–34, 1988.
20. Ehni, W. F., Reller, L. B., and Ellison, R. T.: Bacteremia in granulocytopenic patients in a tertiary-care general hospital. Rev. Infect. Dis. *13*:613–619, 1991.
21. Ehrhardt, A. F., and Sanders, C. C.: Beta-lactam resistance amongst *Enterobacter* species. J. Antimicrob. Chemother. *32*(Suppl. B):1–11, 1993.
22. Ehrhardt, A. F., Sanders, C. C., Thomson, K. S., et al.: Emergence of resistance to imipenem in enterobacter isolates masquerading as *Klebsiella pneumoniae* during therapy with imipenem/cilastatin. Clin. Infect. Dis. *17*:120–122, 1993.
23. Ellner, P. D., Fink, D. J., Neu, H. C., et al.: Epidemiologic factors affecting antimicrobial resistance of common bacterial isolates. J. Clin. Microbiol. *25*:1668–1674, 1987.
24. Fryklund, B., Tullus, K., and Burman, L. G.: Epidemiology of enteric bacteria in neonatal units: Influence of procedures and patient variables. J. Hosp. Infect. *18*:15–21, 1991.
25. Fryklund, B., Tullus, K., Berglund, B., et al.: Importance of the environment and the faecal flora of infants, nursing staff and parents as sources of gram-negative bacteria colonizing newborns in three neonatal wards. Infection *20*:253–257, 1992.
26. Gallagher, P. G.: *Enterobacter* bacteremia in pediatric patients. Rev. Infect. Dis. *12*:808–812, 1990.
27. Gallagher, P. G., and Ball, W. S.: Cerebral infarctions due to CNS infection with *Enterobacter sakazakii*. Pediatr. Radiol. *21*:135–136, 1991.
28. Garaizar, J., Kaufmann, M. E., and Pitt, T. L.: Comparison of ribotyping with conventional methods for the type identification of *Enterobacter cloacae*. J. Clin. Microbiol. *29*:1303–1307, 1991.
29. Gaston, M. A.: *Enterobacter*: An emerging nosocomial pathogen. J. Hosp. Infect. *11*:197–208, 1988.
30. Gibbs, R. S., Blanco, J. D., and Bernstein, S.: Role of aerobic gram-negative bacilli in endometritis after cesarean section. Rev. Infect. Dis. *7*(Suppl.):S690–S695, 1985.
31. Goepp, J. G., Lee, C. K., Anderson, T., et al.: Use of ciprofloxacin in an infant with ventriculitis. J. Pediatr. *121*:303–305, 1992.
32. Grattard, F., Pozzetto, B., Berthelot, P., et al.: Arbitrarily primed PCR, ribotyping, and plasmid pattern analysis applied to investigation of a

nosocomial outbreak due to *Enterobacter cloacae* in a neonatal intensive care unit. J. Clin. Microbiol. *32*:596–602, 1994.
33. Guggenbichler, J. P., Kofler, J., and Allerberger, F.: The influence of third-generation cephalosporins on the aerobic intestinal flora. Infection *13*(Suppl. 1):S137–S139, 1985.
34. Haertl, R., and Bandlow, G.: Epidemiological fingerprinting of *Enterobacter cloacae* by small-fragment restriction endonuclease analysis and pulsed-field gel electrophoresis of genomic restriction fragments. J. Clin. Microbiol. *31*:128–133, 1993.
35. Heusser, M. F., Patterson, J. E., Kuritza, A. P., et al.: Emergence of resistance to multiple beta-lactams in *Enterobacter cloacae* during treatment for neonatal meningitis with cefotaxime. Pediatr. Infect. Dis. *9*:509–512, 1990.
36. Jarvis, W. R., and Martone, W. J.: Predominant pathogens in hospital infections. J. Antimicrob. Chemother. *29*(Suppl. A):19–24, 1992.
37. Kaplan, S. L., and Patrick, C. C.: Cefotaxime and aminoglycoside treatment of meningitis caused by gram-negative enteric organisms. Pediatr. Infect. Dis. *9*:810–814, 1990.
38. Korfmann, G., Sanders, C. C., and Moland, E. S.: Altered phenotypes associated with ampD mutations in *Enterobacter cloacae*. Antimicrob. Agents Chemother. *35*:358–364, 1991.
39. Lacey, S. L., and Want, S. V.: An outbreak of *Enterobacter cloacae* associated with contamination of a blood gas machine. J. Infect. *30*:223–226, 1995.
40. Lambert-Zechovsky, N., Bingen, E., Denamur, E., et al.: Molecular analysis provides evidence for the endogenous origin of bacteremia and meningitis due to *Enterobacter cloacae* in an infant. Clin. Infect. Dis. *15*:30–32, 1992.
41. Lee, E. H., Nicolas, M. H., Kitzis, M. D., et al.: Association of two resistance mechanisms in a clinical isolate of *Enterobacter cloacae* with high-level resistance to imipenem. Antimicrob. Agents Chemother. *35*:1093–1098, 1991.
42. Lindberg, F., and Normark, S.: Contribution of chromosomal beta-lactamases to beta-lactam resistance in enterobacteria. Rev. Infect. Dis. *8*(Suppl. 3):S292–S304, 1986.
43. Lohr, J. A., Donowitz, L. G., and Sadler, J. E.: Hospital-acquired urinary tract infection. Pediatrics *83*:193–199, 1989.
44. Matsaniotis, N. S., Syriopoulou, V. P., Theodoridou, M. C., et al.: *Enterobacter* sepsis in infants and children due to contaminated intravenous fluids. Infect. Control *5*:471–477, 1984.
45. Matsuhisa, A., Saito, Y., Sakamoto, Y., et al.: Detection of bacteria in phagocyte-smears from septicemia-suspected blood by in situ hybridization using biotinylated probes. Microbiol. Immunol. *38*:511–517, 1994.
46. Milewski, S. A., and Klevjer-Anderson, P.: Endophthalmitis caused by *Enterobacter cloacae*. Ann. Ophthalmol. *25*:309–311, 1993.
47. Mirza, G. E., Karakucuk, S., Doganay, M., et al.: Postoperative endophthalmitis caused by an *Enterobacter* species. J. Hosp. Infect. *26*:167–172, 1994.
48. Mollitt, D. L., Tepas, J. J., and Talbert, J. L.: The microbiology of neonatal peritonitis. Arch. Surg. *123*:176–179, 1988.
49. Neu, H. C., and Winshell, E. B.: Relation of β-lactamase activity and cellular location to resistance of *Enterobacter* to penicillins and cephalosporins. J. Antimicrob. Chemother. *1*:107–111, 1972.
50. Noriega, F. R., Kotloff, K. L., Martin, M. A., et al.: Nosocomial bacteremia caused by *Enterobacter sakazakii* and *Leuconostoc mesenteroides* resulting from extrinsic contamination of infant formula. Pediatr. Infect. Dis. *9*:447–449, 1990.
51. Normark, S., Bartowsky, E., Lindquist, S., et al.: The molecular basis of β-lactamase induction in enterobacteria. *In* Neu, H. C. (ed.): Frontiers of Infectious Diseases: New Antibacterial Strategies. New York, Churchill Livingstone, 1990, pp. 161–173.
52. O'Hara, C. M., Steigerwalt, A. G., Hill, B. C., et al.: *Enterobacter hormaechei*, a new species of the family Enterobacteriaceae formerly known as enteric group 75. J. Clin. Microbiol. *27*:2046–2049, 1989.
53. Olson, B., Weinstein, R. A., Nathan, C., et al.: Broad-spectrum β-lactam resistance in *Enterobacter*: Emergence during treatment and mechanisms of resistance. J. Antimicrob. Chemother. *11*:299–310, 1983.
54. Penner, J., Allerberger, F., Dierich, M. P., et al.: In vitro experiments on catheter-related infections due to gram-negative rods. Chemotherapy *39*:336–354, 1993.
55. Raimondi, A., Traverso, A., and Nikaido, H.: Imipenem- and meropenem-resistant mutants of *Enterobacter cloacae* and *Proteus rettgeri* lack porins. Antimicrob. Agents Chemother. *35*:1174–1180, 1991.
56. Raz, R., Sharir, R., Shmilowitz, L., et al.: The elimination of gentamicin-resistant gram-negative bacteria in a newborn intensive care unit. Infection *15*:32–34, 1987.
57. Richard, C.: *Enterobacter*. *In* Krieg, N. R., and Holt, J. G. (eds.): Bergey's Manual of Systematic Bacteriology. Vol. 1. Baltimore, Williams & Wilkins, 1984, pp. 465–467.
58. Shlaes, D. M.: The clinical relevance of *Enterobacter* infections. Clin. Ther. *15*:(Suppl. A):21–28, 1993.
59. Shulman, S. T., and Yogev, R.: Treatment of pediatric infections with amikacin as first-line aminoglycoside. Am. J. Med. *79*:43–50, 1985.
60. Solans, R., Simeon, P., Cuenca, R., et al.: Infectious discitis caused by *Enterobacter cloacae*. Ann. Rheum. Dis. *51*:906–907, 1992.
61. Stoorvogel, J., van Gestel, M. H., Ketelaar-van Gaalen, P. A., et al.: Variation in induction of chromosomal beta-lactamase expression in strains of *Enterobacter cloacae*. Chemotherapy *37*:175–185, 1991.
62. Syrogiannopoulos, G. A., McCracken, G. H. J., and Nelson, J. D.: Osteoarticular infections in children with sickle cell disease. Pediatrics *78*:1090–1096, 1986.
63. Thomson, K. S., Sanders, C. C., and Chmel, H.: Imipenem resistance in *Enterobacter*. Eur. J. Clin. Microbiol. Infect. Dis. *12*:610–613, 1993.
64. Tzouvelekis, L. S., Tzelepi, E., Kaufmann, M. E., et al.: Consecutive mutations leading to the emergence in vivo of imipenem resistance in a clinical strain of *Enterobacter aerogenes*. J. Med. Microbiol. *40*:403–407, 1994.
65. Watanakunakorn, C., and Weber, J.: *Enterobacter* bacteremia: A review of 58 episodes. Scand. J. Infect. Dis. *21*:1–8, 1989.
66. Weischer, M., and Kolmos, H. J.: Retrospective 6-year study of *Enterobacter* bacteraemia in a Danish university hospital. J. Hosp. Infect. *20*:15–24, 1992.
67. Weischer, M., and Kolmos, H. J.: Ribotyping of selected isolates of *Enterobacter cloacae* and clinical data related to biotype, phage type, O-serotype, and ribotype. APMIS *101*:879–886, 1993.
68. Willis, J., and Robinson, J. E.: *Enterobacter sakazakii* meningitis in neonates. Pediatr. Infect. Dis. *7*:196–199, 1988.
69. Wolff, M. A., Young, C. L., and Ramphal, R.: Antibiotic therapy for *Enterobacter* meningitis: A retrospective review of 13 episodes and review of the literature. Clin. Infect. Dis. *16*:772–777, 1993.
70. Yamamoto, T., Honda, T., Miwatani, T., et al.: A virulence plasmid in *Escherichia coli* enterotoxigenic for humans: Intergenetic transfer and expression. J. Infect. Dis. *150*:688–698, 1984.

108

DIARRHEA- AND DYSENTERY-CAUSING *ESCHERICHIA COLI*

David W. K. Acheson and Gerald T. Keusch

The concept that certain *Escherichia coli* are enteric pathogens is not new. With information derived from the limited techniques available 75 years ago, Adam[3] postulated the existence of a group of *E. coli* "dyspepsia" bacteria responsible for neonatal and infantile diarrheas. However, the technical limitations proved too severe for proof, and because all *E. coli* appeared alike under the microscope and upon routine culture, it was impossible to make distinctions between them and to separate the "bad" from the "good."

Proof of Adam's concept required the development of serologic typing techniques for bacterial surface antigens by Kauffman and the adroit use of the human nose by Bearan and Bray in London. In the 1940s, Bearan and Bray were interested in acute infantile gastroenteritis, a disease with high mortality affecting otherwise healthy bottle-fed babies, from whom recognizable enteric pathogens were not recovered. After culture of the fecal specimens, all that Bray[15] found was "the normal *Bacterium coli* that appear on every culture plate of a faecal specimen." Bearan and Bray settled upon the term *cholera infantum* for this disease because, as in

TABLE 108–1. Serologic Specificities of Diarrheagenic *Escherichia coli*

Classic Enteropathogenic	Enterotoxigenic	Enteroinvasive	Enterohemorrhagic	Enteroaggregative
O44:H34	O6:H−,12, 16, 40	O28:H−	O26:H11	Nontypable
O55:H6, 7, 32	O8:H−, 9	O29:H−	O103:H2	Rough
O86:H2, 34	O25:H−, 42	O32:H−	O104:H21	O3:H2
O111:H2, 7, 12	O27:H7	O42:H−	O128:H2	O6:H1
O114:H2	O29:H21	O112:H−	O145:H−	O11:H16
O119:H6	O63:H−, 12	O121:H−	O157:H−, 7	O15:H21
O124:H?	O78:H11, 12	O124:H−	Many others	O44:H18
O125:H21	O117:H4	O136:H−		O77:H18
O126:H2, 5	O128:H21	O143:H−		O89:H−
O127:H4, 6, 21	O153:H45	O144:H−		O92:H23
O128:H2	O159:H4, 21	O152:H−		O111:H21
O142:H6, 34	Others	Others		O125:H30
O158:H23				O126:H10, 27
				O127:H2
				O128:H8, 35
				O146:H39
				O148:H28

true Asiatic cholera, "children apparently not in danger one minute were, in an hour or two more, in extremis." This analogy to cholera, at least for some forms of *E. coli* diarrhea, has proved to be more correct than ever anticipated, as is documented later in this discussion.

Bearan, a clinician, noted that patients with cholera infantum often had a distinctive and discernible "seminal smell." When this was brought to the attention of Bray, a microbiologist, he began to smell the cultures obtained from these patients and found that he could identify an odor in the *E. coli* from cholera infantum patients but not in other *E. coli* organisms cultured on the same medium. Bray classified these organisms initially as *Bact. coli* smellers.

In what now must be appreciated as an historic moment in medical history, Bray took a culture plate of an odoriferous *Proteus* and one of the *E. coli* "smellers" up to the ward and asked the nurse in charge to sniff the two. To her unbiased nose, the *Proteus* had a nasty smell, much like glue; but when the "smeller" was exposed, she immediately cried out in recognition, "Why, that smells just like Baby Wickens!" To this, Dr. Bray replied, "Sister, that is Wickens," for it was indeed Wickens' organism.

Bray carried his investigation an important step further by preparing rabbit antiserum to the Wickens bacterium and determining that many, but not all, isolates from cholera infantum were agglutinated, whereas *E. coli* organisms from other sources were not. Somewhat later, the Wickens "smeller" organism was serotyped by the Kauffman scheme as O111:B4, one of the now classic groups of enteropathogenic *E. coli* (EPEC) (Table 108–1). Anticipating the problems later associated with EPEC serotyping, Bray noted that "agglutination tests sometimes failed to show the hoped-for results, or else the supposed malefactors were found in apparently healthy children or again were not isolated from cases thought to have the disease."[15] The first outbreak of infantile gastroenteritis associated with a specific *E. coli* in the United States occurred in 1947, and it was caused by a O111:B4 strain.[56]

THE CAUSATIVE ORGANISMS

Over the past 45 years, a restricted number of *E. coli* bearing certain of the approximately 180 known somatic O antigens of the genus have been shown to be associated with intestinal infections (see Table 108–1). The association of serotype and virulence is even more striking when the combination of O and the 60 or so H (flagellar) antigens is employed.[35] Only a small percentage of the approximately 10,000 O:H serotypes possible are known to be enteric pathogens. Five well-defined groups of *E. coli* have been characterized on the basis of clinical, biochemical, and molecular/genetic criteria and accepted by most workers in the field: (1) enterotoxigenic *E. coli* (ETEC), which produce one or both types of secretory enterotoxins known as LT (heat-labile toxin) and ST (heat-stable toxin); (2) EPEC, defined by their pattern of adherence to tissue culture cells, ability to polymerize cellular actin, and ability to produce a characteristic alteration in the microvillus membrane, termed the *attaching and effacing* (A/E) lesion; (3) the enterohemorrhagic *E. coli* (EHEC), which produce cytotoxins (Stx) related to Shiga toxin (also termed *Shiga-like toxins* [SLTs], or *verotoxins* [VTs]) and may cause bloody diarrhea, hemorrhagic colitis (HC), and hemolytic uremic syndrome (HUS) or thrombotic thrombocytopenic purpura (TTP); (4) enteroinvasive *E. coli* (EIEC), which are capable of invading intestinal epithelial cells and causing a dysenteric illness; and (5) enteroaggregative *E. coli* (EAggEC), which adhere in vitro to HEp-2 cells in a characteristic autoaggregative manner and are associated with persistent diarrhea in infants.[62]

As described later, virulence of diarrheagenic *E. coli* is polygenic and determined by genes encoding colonization factors or adhesins, invasins, toxins, and factors that alter the cellular cytoskeleton.

TRANSMISSION AND EPIDEMIOLOGY

Diarrhea-causing *E. coli* are worldwide in distribution. The route of infection is, in the last analysis, fecal-oral; however, several additional factors may be interposed between the two orifices, including person-to-person contact transmission; transmission via water, milk, or food; and even the intercession of flies or other insects as intermediate vectors. Unfortunately, few epidemiologic investigations are germane to the question of transmission.

Enterotoxigenic *Escherichia coli*

Spurred by the remarkable progress in understanding the role of a protein enterotoxin in the pathogenesis of cholera and careful thorough studies of ETEC diarrhea in animals, Sack and colleagues[104] provided the first evidence for ETEC diarrhea in humans. Numerous studies since then involving both pediatric and adult populations have established the importance of ETEC as a cause of diarrheal disease. They account for approximately 20 to 30 per cent of diarrhea episodes in the developing world and are the most common bacterial pathogen in visitors to these countries (traveler's diarrhea). They are encountered less frequently in technically advanced nations, such as the United States, except in certain populations living in more primitive conditions, for example, Native Americans on reservations.[105]

Among children in developing countries, ETEC often cause two to three episodes of diarrhea per year and may represent more than 25 per cent of diarrheal episodes in such children.[12] Forty per cent of food fed to children in Bangladesh has been shown to be contaminated with ETEC.[13] ETEC are acquired by ingesting contaminated water or food, and as many as 10^8 bacteria may be required for clinical illness.[29] The incubation period is from 14 to 50 hours.[77] In one prospective study involving a group of U.S. physicians and their families traveling to Mexico, food—raw salad in particular—was implicated by classic epidemiologic methods correlating eating history and disease incidence.[72] A domestic U.S. outbreak of diarrhea at Crater Lake National Park in Oregon was traced to ETEC organisms in the water supply.[102] The few environmental surveillance studies that have been done indicate that ETEC can be found in both water[104] and food. Mehlman and colleagues[71] and Sack and associates[106] have found ETEC in a number of food samples in the United States, including cheese, hamburger, sausage, and seafood. This suggests that a variety of foodstuffs may be capable of supporting growth and facilitating transmission of ETEC. Because large numbers of organisms are required for experimental infections, transmission probably would require multiplication of the inoculum, and food is a good vehicle for this to occur.

Enteropathogenic *Escherichia coli*

Neter and associates[86] initially used the term *EPEC* to denote a limited group of *E. coli* serotypes associated with nursery outbreaks of diarrheal disease, separable from other *E. coli* serogroups causing urinary tract infection, septicemia, peritonitis, or meningitis. However, in recent years, specific virulence markers of EPEC have been discovered that are independent of serotype. More specifically, serotype is associated with but does not define the virulence of an isolate. In addition, the epidemiology of EPEC has changed, and the original classic serotypes no longer are found primarily in neonatal nursery outbreaks, providing an epidemiologic clue for the diagnosis of EPEC infection; rather, they are associated more commonly with sporadic or endemic diarrhea during the first year of life,[121] although they may cause nonspecific watery diarrhea in adults as well.[110]

The impossibility of diagnosing EPEC infections by serotyping methods alone has made it difficult to carry out good studies of EPEC epidemiology in the United States. EPEC are important enteric pathogens in children in developing countries. However, establishing the prevalence of these infections is difficult without the use of sophisticated methods of investigation. In developing countries, the association between EPEC and diarrhea in children is strongest in infants younger than 6 months of age.[23, 41] Levels of EPEC infection in young children may be even higher than those of rotavirus infection.[23, 41, 100] Breast feeding offers some level of protection against EPEC, attributable to the presence in breast milk of both immune factors and oligosaccharides that inhibit EPEC adherence to epithelial cells.[24] In the industrialized countries, such as the United States, EPEC generally are not considered to be as frequent a cause of childhood diarrhea as in the past, although EPEC still are identified in this setting.[28]

Enterohemorrhagic *Escherichia coli*

Since their discovery in 1977, EHEC have been identified as important and increasingly common human pathogens. These organisms are commensals in cattle, and it is not surprising that large outbreaks of human infection have been associated with ingestion of undercooked hamburger, especially associated with fast-food restaurants. In meat processing plants where bulk ground beef is prepared for the fast-food industry, meat from one contaminated carcass can contaminate and distribute the organisms in a huge number of beef patties. Careful prospective epidemiologic surveillance in Minnesota has revealed an increase in incidence of EHEC from 0.5 to 2.0 per 100,000 children younger than 18 years of age during the period 1979 to 1988,[67] similar to the incidence of EHEC determined in the state of Washington in the late 1980s, 2.1 per 100,000. Very young children are not a target group of EHEC. Rather, severe and complicated illness occurs most often among children from 2 to 10 years of age or in the elderly. Ground beef is the most common identified source of EHEC infection. However, several other food sources of transmission have been documented, including apple cider, mayonnaise, milk, dry fermented sausage, lettuce, and water, and both person-to-person and cattle-to-person routes have been implicated. Many of these unusual modes of transmission also are linked with cattle, poorly washed apples dropped in cow pastures and used to make cider, or surface water supplies in proximity to cattle grazing.

The epidemiology of EHEC-associated HUS is of current interest because these episodes account for the majority of acute renal failure cases in children in the United States and approximately 250 deaths per year. Although Shiga toxin–producing *Shigella dysenteriae* type 1 were associated with HUS in the mid 1970s in Bangladesh, this organism rarely is encountered in the United States. The etiology of the majority of cases of HUS in the United States was unexplained until the Stx-producing EHEC was identified. Strong epidemiologic evidence associates EHEC with HUS. In one series of patients from Canada, 60 per cent of HUS patients had either neutralizable free Stx or Stx-producing *E. coli* in their stool, and 75 per cent had serum antibody against Stx.[95] Cases in the United States have been associated almost exclusively with EHEC serotype O157:H7. However, this may be due primarily to the fact that it is the only Stx-producing *E. coli* for which clinical microbiology laboratories test. During a large outbreak of *E. coli* O157:H7 infection on the West Coast of the United States in 1993 associated with fast-food restaurant hamburgers, 732 affected individuals were identified, of whom 195 were admitted to the hospital, 55 (7.5 per cent) developed HUS, and 4 died.[42] Investigation of this outbreak demonstrated that small numbers of bacteria (in the range of a few hundred) constituted an infectious dose. Among 93 cases reported in Washington State in 1987, HUS or TTP developed in 11 (12 per cent), for an approximate incidence of 0.23 per 100,000.[93] The highest incidence of HUS is in children younger than 5 years of age, among whom the age-specific incidence ranges from 2.6 to 5.8 per 100,000 in Minnesota,[67] Washington,[93] and Oregon.[101] The incidence of HUS in Argentina, 21.7 per 100,000, is four to eight times greater and primarily is due to non-O157:H7 Stx-producing EHEC serotypes.[63] In fact, more than 100 non-O157:H7 serotypes have been associated with HC or HUS in Canada. Many of these serotypes have been implicated in both sporadic and outbreak disease in the United States (e.g., an outbreak due to O104:H21 acquired from contaminated milk[76]).[14]

HUS is seasonal in the United States and Canada (most common during the summer months), although no specific seasonal risk factor(s) for infection with Stx-producing *E. coli* are known. Other epidemiologic data suggest that poor children are at lower risk for the development of HUS, perhaps because they already have immunity to EHEC or Stx toxins through early contact with the organisms in their environment.[20] It also has been suggested that the risk of HUS is increased in patients treated with the antimicrobial agent trimethoprim-sulfamethoxazole (TMP-SMX) (relative risk, 3.1; confidence limits, 0.6 to 9.8).[59] A similar association between antibiotic use and HUS due to *S. dysenteriae* type 1 also has been suggested.[16] However, neither study used a randomized placebo-controlled design, and the association may reflect selection bias because both antibiotic use and systemic complications are associated with more severe disease. Other studies have found no association.[93] In vitro data suggest that subinhibitory concentrations of TMP-SMX may increase Stx expression,[53] perhaps related to increased release of toxin from damaged organisms.[5] The relevance of these observations is, however, uncertain. The prolonged use of antimotility agents is reported to be associated with more serious systemic complications of EHEC infection.[18, 19]

In the United Kingdom and the United States, HUS and TTP particularly are associated with Stx2-producing *E. coli* O157:H7.[67, 94] In Buenos Aires, Argentina, which has the highest reported incidence of HUS in the world, non-O157:H7 Stx2-producing strains are isolated most commonly.[63] Similarly, in Australia, other serotypes, especially O111, have been associated with major outbreaks and significant levels of HUS.[17]

Enteroinvasive *Escherichia coli*

As with EPEC, there are few studies on the epidemiology of EIEC. In retrospect, one of the earliest outbreaks occurred during World War II when an *E. coli* O124 strain was found to be the cause of bloody diarrhea.[36] A food-borne outbreak of EIEC in an English school also was reported in 1947.[44] The outbreak that led to the definition of EIEC occurred in 1971, in which bloody diarrhea was traced to consumption of French Camembert cheese contaminated with *E. coli* O124.[66] Small outbreaks or sporadic cases involving a limited number of serotypes have been reported from a number of countries, including the United States, France, Japan, and Brazil.[66, 90, 115, 123, 124] Prospective studies in Thailand using cDNA probes for EIEC invasion genes indicate that as many as 5 per cent of sporadic diarrheal episodes and 10 per cent of bloody diarrhea cases may be caused by EIEC strains. The epidemiology of the cases is complicated by the fact that, in contrast to the initial descriptions of EIEC-associated disease, most EIEC infections probably are neither dysenteric nor characterized by bloody diarrhea but, rather, remain a mildly febrile watery diarrhea. In this sense, EIEC infection resembles *Shigella sonnei* infection more than it does the more virulent *S. dysenteriae* or *Shigella flexneri* clinical presentations. Because these manifestations also are similar to ETEC diarrhea, the role of EIEC would be overlooked without the use of routine screening for EIEC virulence traits, which is not practical at present.

Multiplication to high numbers of EIEC organisms may be important for the transmission of these organisms, for it has been demonstrated that infection with 10^8 bacteria is required to cause experimental dysentery in human volunteers.[29] In this regard, EIEC infection appears to differ epidemiologically from *Shigella* species, for which 10^4 or fewer organisms are sufficient to cause disease, and suggests that EIEC are likely to be food-borne. In food, they can multiply to a sufficient inoculum and are unlikely to be transmitted by direct contact. This is consistent with the finding in a food-borne outbreak due to a nontypable EIEC that secondary person-to-person transmission, so commonly observed in *Shigella* infection, did not occur in EIEC infection.[115]

Enteroaggregative *Escherichia coli*

EAggEC first were recognized by their ability to aggregate in a "stacked-brick" appearance on epithelial cells in tissue culture. Epidemiologic evidence, human volunteer studies, and animal models all associate organisms that demonstrate this property with diarrheal disease.[9, 69] The full epidemiology of these strains is not known yet because it remains difficult to establish EAggEC as the cause of disease. This is in large part because the major means of detection has been to observe the pattern of adherence of isolates to HEp-2 cells.[68] DNA-based methods are available, using a gene probe to a segment of DNA associated with the EAggEC phenotype but probably distinct from the gene mediating this property itself. Moreover, at least one-third of *E. coli* showing aggregative phenotypes in tissue culture do not hybridize with this probe and are polymerase chain reaction–negative using primers currently available. Even so, a particular clinical association of EAggEC with persistent diarrhea in infants younger than 1 year of age has been suggested. In prospective cohort studies in India, EPEC strains were isolated more frequently in patients with acute diarrhea, whereas EAggEC strains were isolated more frequently in patients with diarrhea persisting for more than 14 days.[50] Patients with EAggEC had a mean duration of diarrhea of 17.0 ± 14.4 days, significantly longer than that of other pathogens isolated in this setting. EAggEC, however, frequently are found in any appropriately studied population, and asymptomatic excretion rates can be as high as 28 per cent.[78] This makes epidemiologic studies of EAggEC even more difficult to interpret.[119]

CLINICAL MANIFESTATIONS

Diarrhea-causing *E. coli* may result in a variety of clinical syndromes because virtually all known mechanisms of diarrhea are present in *E. coli,* including secretory toxins, cytotoxic toxins, invasion, and pathogenic adherence. The clinical manifestations are determined largely by the pathogenic mechanisms employed by the different classes of *E. coli,* as determined by their complement of virulence genes (Table 108–2). Thus, invasive strains (EIEC) produce inflammatory diarrhea with fever, abdominal pain, nausea, vomiting, and leukocytes and blood in the stool. The noninvasive cytotoxin-producing EHEC strains cause a frankly bloody diarrhea, associated with leukocytosis but without pus cells in stool or fever. Secretory LT- or ST-producing organisms cause less fever but result in brisk, watery diarrhea with the potential to cause significant dehydration. The adherent EPEC and EAggEC strains also cause noninflammatory and otherwise nonspecific watery diarrhea.

There are age-specific predilections of the various *E. coli* pathogens (Table 108–3). *E. coli* diarrhea in the first year of life generally is due to EPEC or EAggEC, although ETEC also can be responsible. The clinical presentations of each

TABLE 108–2. Relationship of *Escherichia coli* Virulence Genes to Clinical Patterns of Diarrhea

Pathogen Group	Virulence Genes									Clinical Disease
	EAF	*A/E*	*LA*	*AA*	*LT/ST*	*CFA*	*Invasion Plasmid*	*Stx*	*ShET-2*	
ETEC	–	–	–	–	+	+	–	–	–	Watery
EPEC	+	+	+	–	–	–	–	–	–	Watery
EHEC	–	+	–	–	–	–	–	+	–	Bloody (hemorrhagic colitis)
EIEC	–	–	–	–	–	–	+	–	+	Bloody (dysentery)
EAggEC	–	–	–	+	+*	–	–	–	–	Watery (persistent)

*Enteroaggregative stable toxin (EAST) is a member of the ST family. EAF, EPEC adherence factor; A/E, attaching and effacing changes; LA, localized adherence pattern; AA, autoaggregative attaching pattern; LT/ST, heat-labile and heat-stable toxins; CFA, colonization factor antigens; invasion, chromosomal and plasmid factors mediating cell invasion; Stx, Shiga family cytotoxins; ShET-2, plasmid-encoded *Shigella* enterotoxin-2, highly homologous to the plasmid-encoded EIEC toxin; ETEC, enterotoxigenic *E. coli*; EPEC, enteropathogenic *E. coli*; EHEC, enterohemorrhagic *E. coli*; EIEC, enteroinvasive *E. coli*; EAggEC, enteroaggregative *E. coli*.

often are similar, and their most characteristic feature is the lack of characteristic features, unless a dysentery-like illness or HC is noted.

Enterotoxigenic *Escherichia coli*

ETEC cause watery, nonmucoid, nonbloody diarrhea in infants, older children, and adults and are a common cause of traveler's diarrhea. Stool frequency varies from a few to more than 10 per day, and there is a striking absence of leukocytes when the diarrheal stool is examined by light microscopy. These patients may or may not be vomiting, but they commonly are febrile (38° to 40° C), except in the case of adults with traveler's diarrhea. In older children, ETEC disease can not be distinguished clinically from the multiple other causes of acute nonspecific watery diarrhea. The illness usually is self-limiting in 3 to 5 days but occasionally lasts beyond a week. Severely dehydrating illness that resembles clinical cholera can occur but is not common. Variability in the clinical picture may be due to age differences and preexisting immunity but also can be attributed to differences in the infecting inoculum. DuPont and colleagues[29] produced mild diarrhea (three watery stools per day for 2 to 3 days) when 10^8 bacteria were fed to adult volunteers, whereas 10^{10} organisms caused more pronounced diarrhea (more than five stools per day for 4 to 5 days), with mucus but no blood observed in some subjects. Some also had abdominal cramping, but there was no tenesmus, and all remained afebrile. This is the typical clinical picture of traveler's diarrhea in adults.[72] Although the illness usually is self-limiting, the diarrhea can result in severe dehydration, requiring aggressive fluid therapy.

Enteropathogenic *Escherichia coli*

Much of the published data on the clinical aspects of infection with EPEC are historical and are based solely on serotype diagnosis. There is a paucity of documented EPEC infection using contemporary criteria, especially in developed countries, in recent years. Although nursery outbreaks no longer are common, infants infected with EPEC still can develop severe illness,[50] with high mortality rates ranging from 25 to 70 per cent, depending on the study.[28] In contrast, limited investigations using an experimental EPEC infection model in adult volunteers show that mild watery diarrhea occurs 3 to 16 hours after inoculation and generally lasts less than 2 days. Diarrhea occasionally was copious and in some was associated with abdominal cramps, nausea, vomiting, malaise, and fever.[27] This clinical picture is consistent with the disease caused by outbreaks of EPEC in adults or traveler's diarrhea due to EPEC. EPEC also has been implicated in chronic diarrhea in the United States and elsewhere, with serious nutritional consequences that may require total parenteral nutrition with hospital stays up to 120 days.[103] In prospective studies of EPEC diarrhea among young infants in Brazil[41] and Ethiopia,[120] fever, vomiting, and dehydration all commonly were observed. The clinical significance of chronic diarrhea may be increased by the underlying malnutrition in infants in developing countries. In many settings, especially where effective oral rehydration programs are in place, chronic diarrhea and associated malnutrition now are more important causes of diarrheal deaths than are acute diarrhea and dehydration.[11]

These manifestations of EPEC infection are distinct from the classic epidemic nursery outbreaks of cholera infantum of the past. In this setting, the first signs and symptoms may be mild and nonspecific but commonly are followed by

TABLE 108–3. Age-Related Patterns of *Escherichia coli* Diarrhea

Pathogen Classification	Age at Highest Risk	Characteristics of Diarrhea		
		Bloody	*Watery*	*Inflammatory*
EAggEC	<6 months	–	+ + +	–
EPEC	<1 year	–	+ + +	–
ETEC	>1 year	–	+ + +	–
EIEC	>2 years	+ +	+	+ + +
EHEC	2–10 years	+ + +	+	–

EAggEC, enteroaggregative *E. coli*; EHEC, enterohemorrhagic *E. coli*; EIEC, enteroinvasive *E. coli*; EPEC, enteropathogenic *E. coli*; ETEC, enterotoxigenic *E. coli*.

vomiting and diarrhea of increasing severity. The stools contain neither mucus nor blood, and the volume tends to fluctuate over a period of weeks. Plain abdominal radiographs show only nonspecific dilation of small bowel loops, although severe ileus not attributable to hypokalemia develops in many patients. During periods of profuse watery diarrhea, infants may lose as much as 15 per cent of their body weight, leading to profound electrolyte disturbances and severe dehydration, with central nervous system manifestations, such as irritability, hypertonicity, convulsions, and coma. Fluid requirements seldom drop below 300 mL/kg/day, increasing to 500 mL/kg/day during relapses. Circulatory collapse can occur and recur despite adequate fluid replacement and achievement of electrolyte balance. In an earlier epidemic in Virginia, Belnap and O'Donnell[7] described fatal infections due to *E. coli* O111:B4 occurring after 3 weeks of illness and associated with renal failure, coma, and signs of disseminated intravascular coagulation, although blood cultures typically remained negative. The fatality rate was age-dependent; although the overall mortality was 16 per cent, it was 40 per cent for neonates. This study and others have noted that breast-fed infants are relatively protected against infection by these organisms.

Enterohemorrhagic *Escherichia coli*

As early as 1971, a distinctive clinical diarrheal syndrome characterized by bloody diarrhea, associated with cramping and colonic inflammatory changes, usually right-sided, was recognized.[98] In 1983, this illness was associated with an otherwise rare *E. coli* serotype, O157:H7, and a characteristic syndrome, HC, was defined.[99] The organisms causing this syndrome, grouped together as EHEC, initially were identified in 1977 because of their ability to produce cytotoxins. EHEC now have been shown to cause a wide spectrum of diseases that may be confined to the gastrointestinal tract or, in a sizable proportion (typically between 5 and 10 per cent), can become systemic. The local gastrointestinal illness usually begins with nonbloody diarrhea that can progress to a bloody diarrhea after 1 or 2 days. There may be further progression over the next day or two, resulting in the passage of frank blood, the pathognomonic clinical feature of HC. Associated manifestations include vomiting in about 50 per cent of patients and abdominal pain. Fever may occur but typically is low-grade. This clinical picture may be confused with other conditions, such as appendicitis, intussusception, inflammatory bowel disease, ischemic colitis, and diverticulitis. The difficulty in making the diagnosis can lead to inappropriate drug therapy or even surgery.[43, 48] A serious complication is the development of HUS or TTP.[43] HUS is characterized by the triad of acute renal failure, thrombocytopenia, and hemolytic anemia. The acute mortality rate is approximately 5 per cent, and many more will go on to develop chronic renal failure over the next several decades. TTP shares the same clinical features as HUS but generally occurs in older adults and is associated with prominent neurologic findings, including behavioral changes, altered consciousness or coma, and seizures, as well as fever.[45]

A prospective study in Canada identified *E. coli* O157:H7 in 15 per cent of 125 patients presenting with grossly bloody diarrhea over a 6-month period.[95] The age range was 15 months to 73 years; however, almost half were younger than 10 years of age. The illness was similar to that described earlier, with a mean duration of 7.8 days, but was significantly longer in children (9.1 ± 2 days), compared with adults (6.6 ± 1.1 days). Sigmoidoscopy was abnormal in seven of eight adults examined, with hyperemic mucosa in six and superficial ulcerations in one. Biopsies showed mild mucosal inflammation in four of five patients. Because both local and systemic manifestations in EHEC infection are, at least partially, due to Stx, the presence of these same toxins in the intestinal lumen in patients with non-O157:H7 infection puts them at risk of developing HC and HUS. No comparative data are available to assess the relative risk in O157:H7 and non-O157:H7 EHEC infection.

Enteroinvasive *Escherichia coli*

Naturally acquired EIEC infection causes a mild to moderately severe dysentery syndrome, with fever, malaise, diarrhea, tenesmus, and abdominal cramping.[29, 124] Watery diarrhea usually occurs at the onset of the illness and progresses to mucoid diarrhea with streaks of blood or microscopic hematochezia but rarely to the classic small-volume, grossly bloody, dysenteric stool seen with *Shigella* infection. Of 204 cases reported in one study, grossly bloody stool occurred in only 4.[41] In two of these cases, sigmoidoscopy revealed superficial ulcerations in one and hyperemia alone in the second. As in *Shigella* infection, however, the stool is loaded with inflammatory cells, indicative of the invasive nature of the organism. Vomiting and dehydration can occur, the latter generally being mild. Fever of 38° to 39.5° C is typical, occurring early in association with malaise, myalgia, and headache and lasting for 2 to 3 days. In most instances, diarrhea ceases in a week or less but in a few patients may continue for 2 weeks or more. In adult volunteers with experimentally induced EIEC disease, febrile illness developed approximately 11 hours (range, 8 to 24 hours) after ingestion of the inoculum.[29] Chills, myalgia, headache, and profuse diarrhea or abdominal cramps and tenesmus rapidly followed. In 2 of 13 subjects, this was associated with systemic toxicity and transient hypotension consistent with bacteremia, even though blood cultures were negative in all. Clinical dysentery, with bloody stools, occurred in several subjects, and reddened, friable mucosa with multiple bleeding points was seen by sigmoidoscopy. Clinical illness was controlled quickly with parenteral ampicillin therapy.

Enteroaggregative *Escherichia coli*

Few studies describe the clinical features of EAggEC infection. However, EAggEC are associated with watery diarrhea, which may continue to persistent diarrhea and last 14 days or longer,[9, 78] and have been associated with some cases of persistent diarrhea in HIV–positive patients.[70] Clinical manifestations in these patients may be aggravated by secondary lactase deficiency and progressive nutritional deterioration. In at least two studies, EAggEC isolates from clinical isolates have been inoculated experimentally in adult volunteers and have resulted in clinical manifestations including diarrhea, abdominal cramps, and borborygmi in some but not all volunteers, even in doses as large as 10^{10} bacteria. EAggEC have been associated with bloody diarrhea in some studies,[30] although this does not appear to be the typical presentation.

PATHOGENESIS

Enterotoxigenic *Escherichia coli*

Spurred by the remarkable progress in understanding the pathogenesis of human cholera after the discovery of cholera enterotoxin and based on precedents from veterinary medicine for similar toxins in watery *E. coli* diarrhea in animals, Sack and colleagues[104] provided the first evidence that *E. coli* diarrhea in humans also could be related to secretory enterotoxins. ETEC make ST and/or LT. Studies of ST have revealed these to be of two major types: STa (sometimes called ST-I or STh, for human ST), of importance in human infections, and STb (sometimes called ST-II or STp, for porcine ST), of importance in veterinary infections. STa is a small peptide (approximately 2 kDa) without subunit structure, contains three disulfide bonds, which accounts for its heat stability, is methanol-soluble, and causes gut fluid secretion in suckling mice. ST is made as a larger precursor molecule, which is modified posttranslationally and by extracellular processing.[97, 116] STa, which causes intestinal fluid and electrolyte secretion, has an immediate and reversible onset of action and activates guanylate cyclase,[39, 73, 111] although other pathways, including protein kinase C, may participate in the guanylate cyclase response.[22, 125] A putative STa receptor molecule now has been identified,[21] but its precise nature and distribution remain to be clarified. The in vivo suckling mouse model for fluid secretion has been the standard assay for STa. However, other quantitative methods now are available, including quantitating the activation of particulate guanylate cyclase in tissue culture of intestinal cell lines, radioimmunoassays, and enzyme-linked immunosorbent assays (ELISAs). STa also is 50 per cent homologous with an endogenous mammalian ligand, guanylin, that binds to and activates guanylate cyclase C.[25] Guanylin is present in intestinal epithelial cells and is thought to play a role in regulating fluid and electrolyte secretion in the intestine. As described in greater detail later, EAggEC also make an enterotoxin (known as EAST-1) that has significant homology with STa.

The second ST, STb, described in 1970,[75] is methanol-insoluble and inactive in the suckling mouse model but does cause intestinal fluid secretion in weaned pigs. The host susceptibility to STb may be related to the sensitivity of STb to protease because the administration of trypsin inhibitors can make mice susceptible to the effects of STb.[126] Like STa, STb is made as a large precursor molecule that is processed and secreted from the bacterium as a 5.2-kDa mature 48–amino acid protein containing two disulfide bonds.[60] There is no homology between STa and STb, and the two toxins are not cross-neutralizable. STb does not lead to alterations in sodium or chloride flux but instead probably affects bicarbonate excretion. STb also may open a receptor-operated calcium channel in the plasma membrane. Although STb-producing strains have been isolated from humans with diarrhea,[64, 91] it is not clear yet whether or not they may be responsible for human disease.

The LT family of toxins includes LTI, which is similar structurally and functionally to cholera toxin, with about 80 per cent homology at the amino acid level. LTI can be subdivided into LThI and LTpI, which are antigenic variants of human and porcine origin.[46] These toxins are composed of one A subunit enzyme that activates adenylate cyclase and five B subunit monomers that form a multivalent pentameric structure responsible for receptor recognition and binding to susceptible cells. LTI binds to GM1 ganglioside, like cholera toxin, as well as a glycoprotein receptor present on the intestinal brush border membrane.[21] LT and cholera toxin share the identical adenosine diphosphate–ribosyl transferase enzymatic activity for the same target. Both covalently transfer the adenosine diphosphate–ribosyl moiety from nicotine adenine dinucleotide to the guanosine 5′-triphosphate–binding regulatory component of the adenylate cyclase enzyme complex. This leads to permanent activation of the cyclase enzyme and continuous production of cyclic adenosine monophosphate (cAMP). In turn, high levels of cAMP activate chloride secretory mechanisms in crypt cells and inhibit sodium absorptive mechanisms in villus cells. For these reasons, diarrhea due to LT^+ *E. coli* is similar pathophysiologically to cholera. The combination of increased chloride secretion and diminished sodium absorption leads to the accumulation of large amounts of isotonic fluid in the gut lumen, exceeding the intestinal absorptive capacity and resulting in watery diarrhea. Otherwise similar LTs but not neutralized with antisera raised to cholera toxins are designated LTII, including LTIIa and LTIIb. The A subunit of LTIIa is approximately 50 per cent homologous with LThI, although the B subunits are quite different. In contrast, LTIIb is distinct both antigenically and chemically from LTIIa.

After the discovery of *E. coli* enterotoxins in animal strains, it was realized quickly that enterotoxin production by ETEC, although necessary, was not sufficient to explain their virulence. The pioneering studies were carried out by veterinarians who were studying *E. coli* infections (colibacillosis) in newborn piglets. As early as 1963, Smith and Halls[113] observed the marked proliferation of *E. coli* in the proximal small bowel of animals with spontaneous colibacillosis. Strains isolated from infected animals when fed to newborn piglets also heavily colonized the proximal gut and caused diarrhea, whereas isolates from healthy animals failed to do either. Smith and Halls suggested that virulent colibacillosis strains of *E. coli* adhered to the intestinal mucosa and evaded clearance mechanisms of the gut, allowing multiplication to very high numbers. Additional studies soon confirmed this for the porcine pathogens and further suggested that a surface antigen, K-88, was responsible for adhesion.[61, 112] This was consistent with the already known properties of K-88, a fimbrial protein mediating hemagglutination in the presence of mannose (termed mannose-resistant *hemagglutination*), which distinguished it from type 1 pili that result in mannose-sensitive hemagglutination.[112]

Because the two properties, toxin and adhesin, were controlled by plasmid genes, Smith and Linggood[114] could create mutants expressing none, one, or both proteins by inserting or removing the two plasmids independently. They showed convincingly that K-88 was the adherence (colonization) factor and that a noncolonizing toxigenic organism virtually was avirulent when fed to intact animals (Table 108–4). Both factors were, in fact, required for full virulence, unless the intestine first was ligated to prevent clearance of nonadhering toxigenic strains.

Adherence of human ETEC to intestinal epithelial cells also is due to the presence of microbial surface antigens that intimately interact with as yet unknown constituents on the gut cell surface (Fig. 108–1). The adherence antigens of these strains, known as CFAs (colonization factor antigens), are different from those present on animal strains (K-88, K-99, and others), establishing the basis for host range specificity. The best characterized and most frequently encountered adhesins from human strains are CFA I and CFA II.[33, 34] The latter actually is composed of three distinct antigens designated coli-surface–associated antigens 1 to 3 (cs 1, 2, 3). CFA I and CFA II, except for cs3, are synthesized as long, slender fimbriae on the bacterial surface (Fig. 108–2). In contrast, cs 3 (and a few other adhesins) are nonfimbriate in nature. Whereas fimbriate CFAs mediate mannose-resistant hemagglutination of human and/or bovine erythrocytes, which aids in their detection, nonfimbriate antigens may not be detectable as hemagglutinins. However, these proteins all impart a high surface hydrophobicity to the organisms, allowing hydrophobic interactions to overcome the repulsive electrostatic charges of the epithelial cell.[37] Other CFAs include CFA III and IV, the latter composed of a family of antigens: cs4, cs5, and cs6.[57]

TABLE 108–4. Conversion of an Avirulent *Escherichia coli* O9:H19 into an Enterovirulent Strain by Insertion of Plasmids Mediating K-88 Adhesin and Enterotoxin Production

Plasmid Present		Colonization (Log_{10}/g)		Clinical Response
K-88	*Enterotoxin*	*Jejunum*	*Colon*	*No. with Diarrhea/Total*
No	No	5.3	8.4	0/8
Yes	No	8.3	9.7	3/11 (mild)
No	Yes	4.4	6.9	0/6
Yes	Yes	9.5	9.5	12/16

Data from reference 114.

CFA genes are present on plasmids. Of particular interest and possible epidemiologic importance is the observation that the genes for CFA I and II usually are on plasmids containing ST genes or sometimes ST and LT genes. This association of colonization and ST genes may explain why ST appears to be the more frequently encountered of the two *E. coli* enterotoxins. These plasmids also are found primarily in a limited number of serotypes of ETEC from patients (Table 108–5), presumably because they are stable in the genetic environment of these strains. Such organisms have been called reservoir serotypes because they are responsible for most endemic ETEC disease.[35] LT-only ETEC generally do not produce CFA I or II, may be of diverse serotype, and readily lose the *ent* (enterotoxin) gene in vitro.

Further work has extended these observations to many other strains virulent for humans[3, 16] and has established a consistent principle: noninvasive diarrhea-causing ETEC strains require at least two virulence attributes, including (1) adhesins to allow colonization of the intestine to occur, presumably leading to (2) enterotoxin production, which actually causes secretion of water and electrolytes and leads to diarrhea.

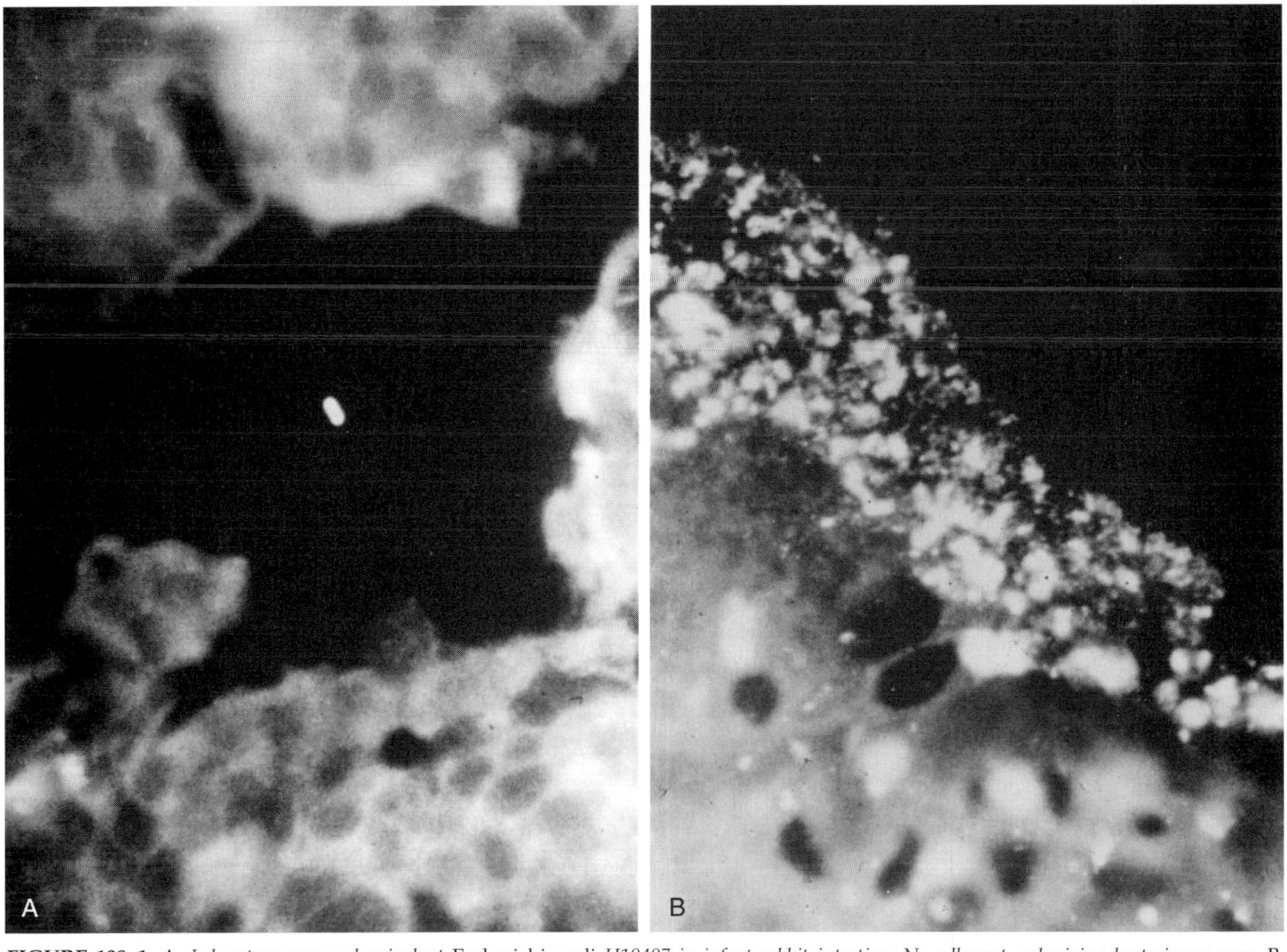

FIGURE 108–1. A, *Laboratory-passaged avirulent* Escherichia coli *H10407 in infant rabbit intestine. No adherent, colonizing bacteria are seen.* B, *Fresh, virulent H10407 at the same time interval in infant rabbit intestine closely are adherent to the brush border. (Indirect immunofluorescent stained section, × 1000.) (Courtesy of Drs. Dolores and Doyle Evans, Department of Microbiology, Baylor College of Medicine.)*

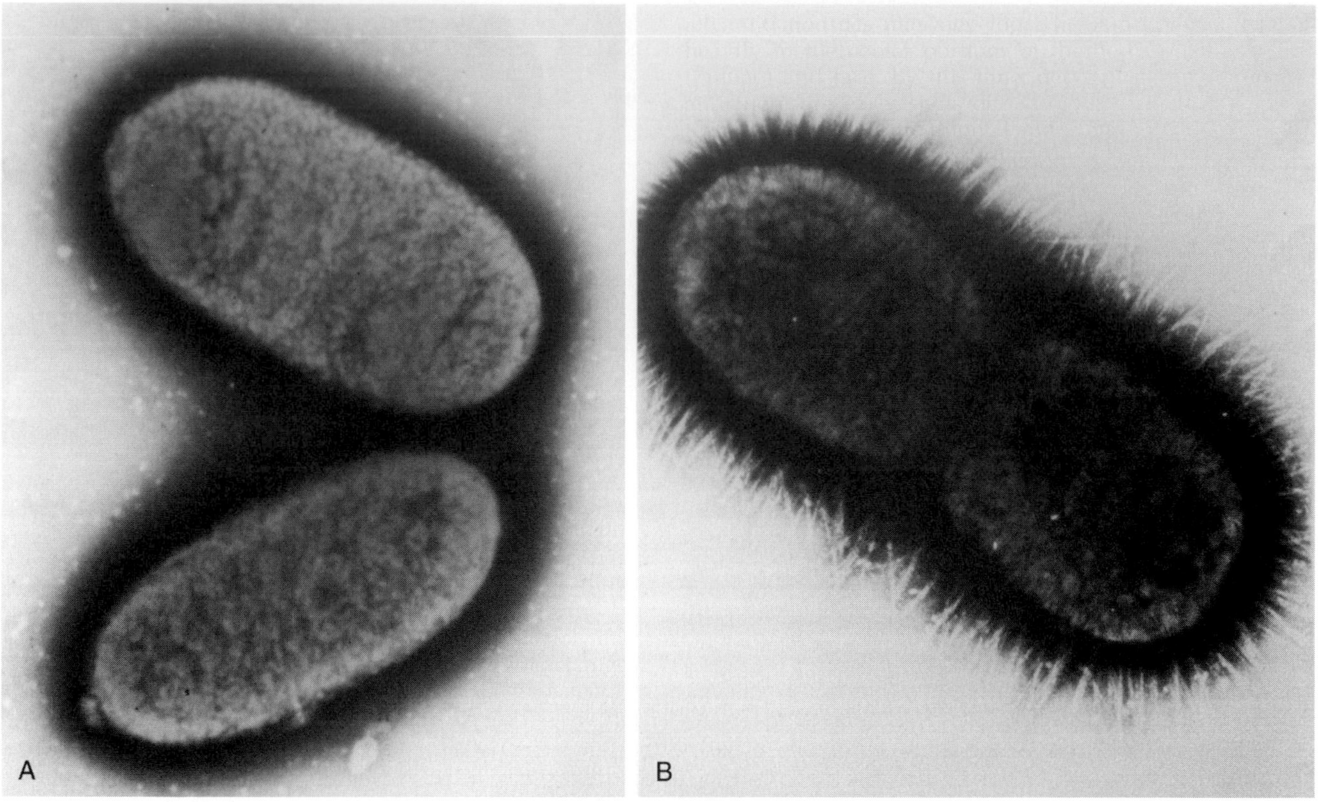

FIGURE 108–2. A, *Electron micrograph of negatively stained cells of avirulent* Escherichia coli *H10407. Note the bald appearance of the outer surface of the organism.* B, *Similar view of virulent, fresh* E. coli *H10407. Note the hairy surface of the organism due to colonization factor. (× 20,000.) (Courtesy of Drs. Dolores and Doyle Evans, Department of Microbiology, Baylor College of Medicine.)*

Enteropathogenic *Escherichia coli*

Although serotype remains the most commonly used criterion for identification of EPEC, true virulence attributes have been discovered that define the pathogenic potential of these organisms. Among these are the ability to adhere to HEp-2 cells in a characteristic localized adherence (LA) pattern, in which the bacteria grow as a microcolony on one region of the HEp-2 cell membrane (Fig. 108–3).[28] Demonstration of the LA phenotype in tissue culture cells or hybridization with an EPEC adherence factor (EAF) DNA probe is sufficient for the putative identification of EPEC.[51] EPEC cause actin polymerization of target cells at sites of attachment, a virulence property readily detected in tissue culture (e.g., HEp-2 cells) by a fluorescent actin staining test (FAST).[56] In this procedure, HEp-2 cells are infected with the organism and subsequently exposed to a fluorescein-labeled mushroom toxin specific for filamentous polymerized actin. Under the microscope, the brightly fluorescing actin beneath the organism easily is seen outlining the microbe (Fig. 108–4).

EPEC infection results in villus atrophy that frequently is accompanied by crypt hypertrophy. Bacteria can be found attached intimately to epithelial cells, and the microvilli disappear (or become effaced), the so-called A/E lesion. Pathogenesis is considered to involve three distinct stages.[28] Localized adherence of the EPEC to epithelial cells appears to be the first event, and this is mediated initially by the plasmid-encoded EAF.[28] Other plasmid-associated fimbriae subsequently were identified and termed *bundle-forming pili* for their characteristic bundled appearance by electron microscopy.[40] Although bundle-forming pili are essential for localized adherence, they are not sufficient, and other gene products clearly are involved.[28] The second step is the intimate attachment of EPEC to intestinal epithelial cells. During this process, epithelial cell microvilli disappear directly below the attached bacteria and appear to elongate adjacent to the

TABLE 108–5. Correlation of Production of Toxin and Colonization Factor with Virulence in Human *Escherichia coli*

Strain Studied	Virulence*	Toxin†	Colonization	Colonization Factor Antigen Production‡
H10407 passaged	No	Yes	No	No
H10407 fresh	Yes	Yes	Yes	Yes
H10407 revertant	No	Yes	No	No

*Experimental diarrhea in animal models.
†Small bowel fluid secretion response to cell-free toxins.
‡Electron microscopic visualization of colonization factor.
Data from reference 34.

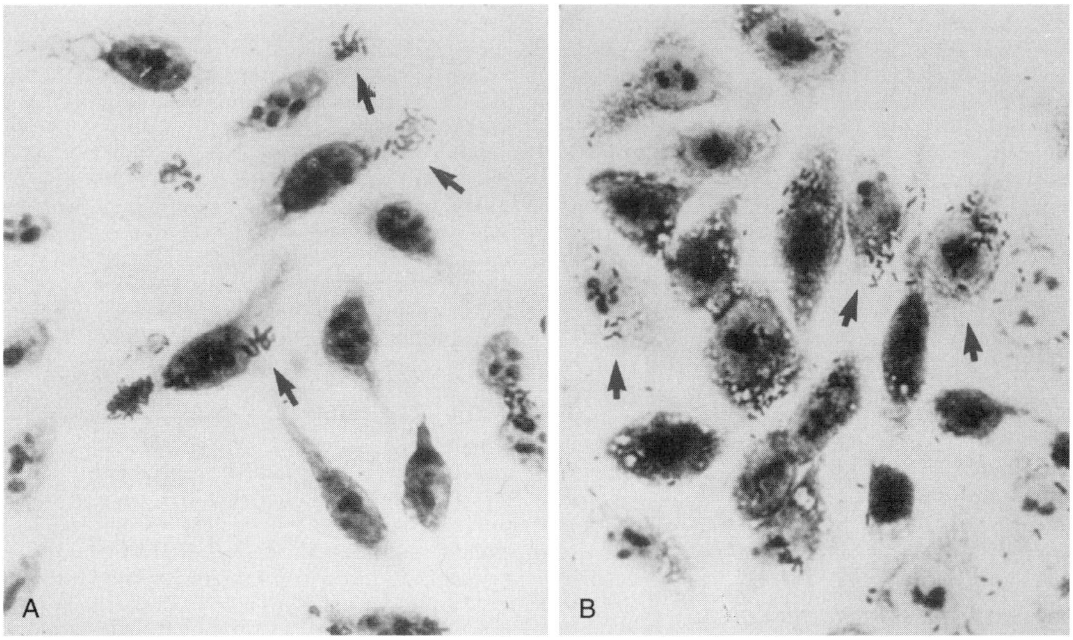

FIGURE 108–3. *Patterns of adherence of* Escherichia coli *to HEp-2 cells in tissue culture. Typical enteropathogenic* E. coli *associate with HEp-2 cells in the pattern shown in* A, *termed* localized adherence *(LA). The arrows point to cells where microcolonies of bacteria are growing attached to focal areas of the cell membrane. Other* E. coli *organisms isolated from patients with diarrhea adhere over the entire HEp-2 cell membrane, shown in the cells identified with arrows in* B. *This pattern of interaction is termed* diffuse adherence *(DA). Whereas the LA phenotype has been associated definitively with the capacity to induce diarrhea in experimental models, no convincing evidence of virulence in DA strains has been obtained to date.*

organisms. To make the resulting cup-like pedestal, which defines the A/E lesion (Fig. 108–5), epithelial cells must reorganize the various cytoskeletal elements, including actin, the light chain of myosin, a-actinin, talin, and ezrin.[78] One gene required for these physiologic events to proceed, *eaeA*, is situated in a 35-kb region of the chromosome termed the *locus of enterocyte effacement*.[52] The *eaeA* gene product is a 94-kDa outer-membrane protein named *intimin*, although its precise function is unknown. A highly homologous *eaeA* gene has been identified in EHEC strains as well, which also are associated with A/E lesions. Homology between *eaeA* and the *inv* (invasin) gene product of *Yersinia* strains, which recognizes membrane proteins of the integrin family and results in cell invasion, suggests that *eaeA* also may bind to cell integrins. Although there are a few reports that EPEC are invasive in vitro, they are not invasive to the same degree as

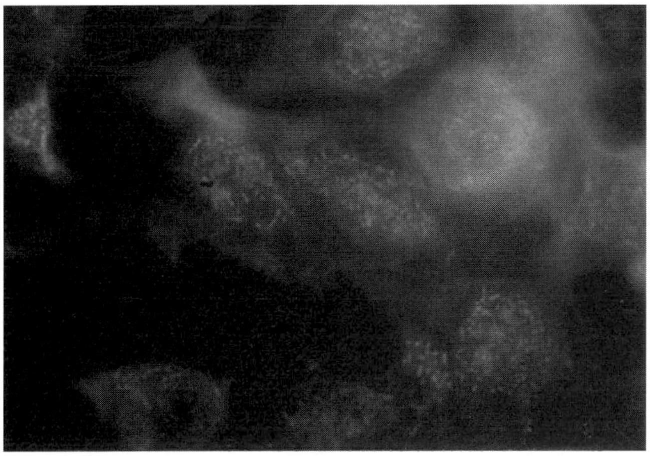

FIGURE 108–4. *Some* Escherichia coli *strains have the capacity to attach to the eukaryotic cell membrane and induce the polymerization of actin beneath the membrane. This may be demonstrated by the fluorescent actin staining test (FAST), in which polymerized F-actin is detected by a fluorescein-tagged mushroom toxin specific for this form of actin. In this figure, the bacteria are attached to HEp-2 cells, and the induced actin polymerization revealed by the fluorescent reagent highlights the organisms seen as bright rods on the infected cells.*

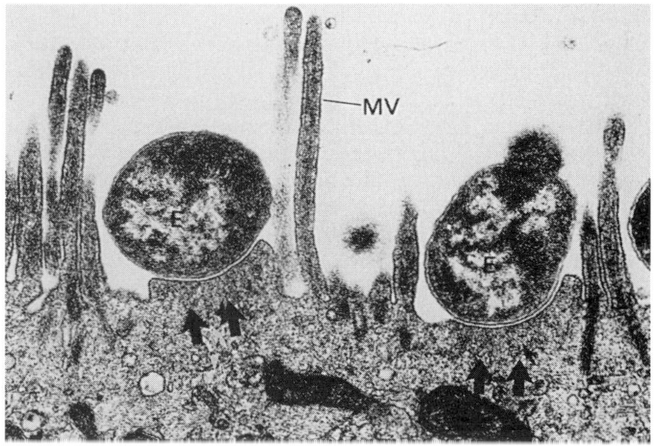

FIGURE 108–5. *High-power electron micrograph of intestinal epithelium infected by classic enteropathogenic* Escherichia coli *strains (E), with occasional intact microvilli (MV) and the pedestal formation shown by the double arrows. This figure shows not only the structural alterations and loss of the brush border but also the close apposition of the organisms to the epithelial cells. (Courtesy of Ralph A. Gianella, Department of Medicine, University of Cincinnati School of Medicine.)*

EIEC or *Shigella*, and the relevance of this to pathogenesis is not known. A second gene in the locus of enterocyte effacement region, *eaeB*, encodes a 33-kDa secreted protein essential for developing A/E lesions. EPEC alter the epithelial cell signal transduction pathways, particularly the protein kinase/phosphatase pathways, and cause an elevation of intracellular calcium levels.[28]

Despite the detailed knowledge of the interaction of EPEC with epithelial cells in vitro, it is not clear how EPEC cause diarrhea in vivo. It has been suggested that loss of microvilli results in malabsorption. However, sometimes the diarrhea begins 3 hours after oral delivery of EPEC in volunteers, thus suggesting the initiation of a secretory process.[28]

Other *E. coli* adhere to HEp-2 cells with a second pattern of interaction called diffuse adherence (DA), in which the organisms attach over the entire cell surface, rather than at just a localized region (see Fig. 108–3). The pathogenic significance of these DA strains still is unclear,[117] and because DA strains usually are not classic EPEC serotypes, they are not considered further in this chapter.

Enterohemorrhagic *Escherichia coli*

Although O157:H7 is the prototypic EHEC isolated from patients with typical hemorrhagic colitis,[98] approximately 100 other serotypes also cause this clinical syndrome.[42] Some of these may, in some settings, be more prevalent, for example, O26:H11, formerly included in the classic EPEC serotypes but now reclassified as EHEC because of its ability to produce high levels of Stx toxins.[61] EHEC typically are LT/ST- and EAF-negative and therefore distinct from ETEC and EPEC, but, like the latter, many but not all polymerize actin, are FAST-positive, possess a 60-mDa plasmid encoding a fimbrial adhesin involved in attachment to epithelial cell lines, contain a homologue of the *eae* gene, and cause the A/E lesion.[122] EHEC also produce large amounts of bacteriophage-encoded Stx,[8] which may account for many of the clinical manifestations of HC.

Stx were discovered approximately 20 years ago by Konowalchuk and associates,[58] who reported finding cytotoxic activity in culture filtrates of certain strains of *E. coli* isolated from patients with diarrhea. The activity was heat-labile, could not be neutralized by antisera to LT, and was toxic to Vero cells. It therefore was designated Verotoxin and the strains producing it were called verotoxigenic *E. coli*. A few years later, O'Brien and Holmes[87] observed that Verotoxins were neutralized by antisera to Stx from *Shigella*, and they were renamed *SLTs*. These toxins now more correctly are designated Stx. They constitute a family of proteins that share the identical enzymatic action and target cell–binding specificity. In addition to the originally described *E. coli* Stx1 (originally named *SLT-1*), it soon became apparent that there was a second related toxin not neutralized by Shiga antibody and now known as Stx2.[87] Subsequently, at least two other members of the Stx2 family have been described, Stx2c and Stx2e, the first from human diarrhea patients and the second from swine with a characteristic toxin-mediated illness: edema disease.[65]

In contrast to Stx of *S. dysenteriae* type 1, encoded by chromosomal genes, and LT and ST, carried by plasmids, Stx in *E. coli* are encoded by genes present on temperate bacteriophages. The *stx1* gene differs from the *Shigella stx* gene encoding Stx by three nucleotide changes, resulting in a single conservative amino acid substitution in the A subunit: threonine[45] to serine[45]. The *stx2* genes are organized in an operon like the *stx* and *stx1* genes but share approximately 56 to 58 per cent nucleotide and amino acid homology with the *stx* and *stx1 A* and *B* subunit genes.[49] All three toxins are composed of a single A subunit and five noncovalently linked B subunits responsible for toxin binding to neutral glycolipid receptors on susceptible cells. All Stx have an identical mechanism of action, cleavage of the N-glycosidic bond in a specific adenosine of the 28S rRNA in the 60S ribosomal subunit.[31] This single cleavage event results in irreversible cessation of protein synthesis and ultimately leads to cell death. Intestinal villus cells are susceptible to the action of toxin and may be defective in the absorption of sodium as a result, possibly contributing to the diarrhea. Evidence suggests that Stx induces local inflammatory cytokine production, with potential effects on epithelial cell and mucosal integrity.

Epidemiologic evidence strongly links Stx-producing strains to HC and, in addition, to the associated systemic complications HUS and TTP.[42, 54, 99] The mechanisms underlying HUS and TTP are not certain but appear to be due to toxin effects on vascular endothelial cells, possibly in concert with lipopolysaccharide and a variety of cytokines. This initiates events resulting in endothelial cell injury and platelet thrombi, resulting in the characteristic thrombotic microangiopathy.[20, 55, 89] Other possible initiation factors include abnormal von Willebrand factor, but it is not known whether this is a cause or consequence of disease.[74] Stx1 has been shown to decrease production of prostacyclins; however, the role of this in the pathogenesis of HUS remains uncertain.[55]

Enteroinvasive *Escherichia coli*

In 1967, Trabulsi and coworkers[123] in Brazil and Sakazaki and associates[107] in Japan described the isolation of certain *E. coli* serotypes from patients with a disease resembling bacillary dysentery but with negative cultures for *Shigella*. These isolates possessed a critical virulence hallmark associated with *Shigella*, namely, the ability to invade intestinal and other epithelial cells (Fig. 108–6).[90] Hence, they have been called EIEC, and a limited number of serotypes, distinct from the EPEC O groups but often cross-reactive with *Shigella* O antigens, have been found to possess this property (see Table 108–1). The genetic and molecular basis of invasion by *Shigella* has been well defined over the past decade, and the same plasmid and chromosomal genes encoding invasion properties and mechanisms appear to be present in EIEC as well.[47, 61, 96, 108] The invasive process for EIEC is considered to be the same as that for *Shigella* species. This has been well characterized and involves four main steps: (1) initial entry into cells, (2) intracellular multiplication, (3) intra- and intercellular spread; and (4) host-cell killing. The process is complex and involves multiple genes on both the invasion plasmid and the chromosome.[2] EIEC produces toxins reported to be structurally distinct from Stx of *S. dysenteriae* type 1 and Stx1 and Stx2 made by EHEC.[38] Nonetheless, studies suggest that EIEC toxins possess many properties in common with the Shiga family of toxins, including the ability to cause fluid secretion in animal models.[38] A 63-kDa protein that is thought to be the EIEC enterotoxin has been purified.[81]

Enteroaggregative *Escherichia coli*

When the HEp-2 cell adherence assay was applied to the study of *E. coli* isolated from infants with diarrhea and carried out in a specified manner, a third pattern of adherence, called aggregative (or autoaggregative), was observed.[79] In contrast to LA or DA, in which organisms are found almost exclusively in association with cells, the aggregative strains

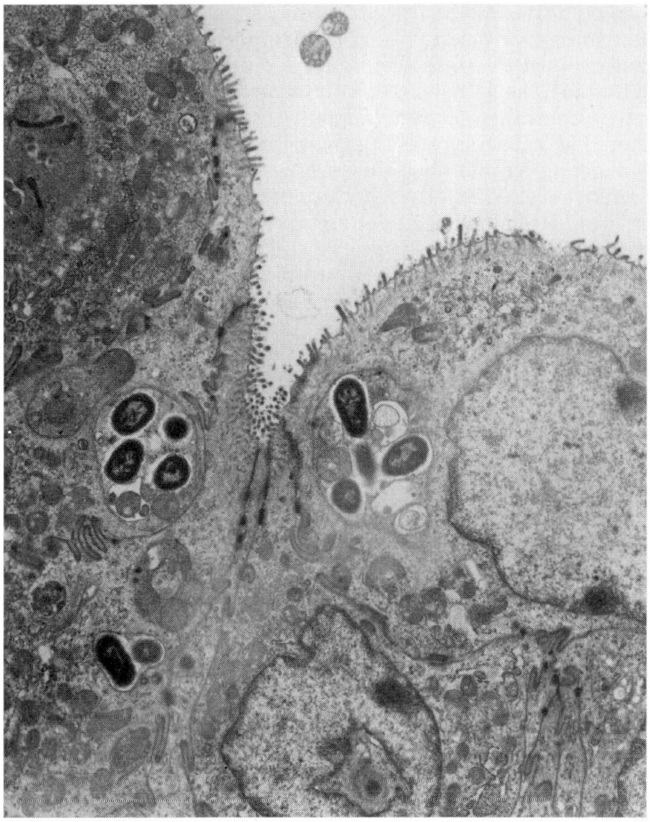

FIGURE 108–6. *Electron micrograph of enteroinvasive* Escherichia coli *infection of intestinal mucosa. The intracellular location of the bacteria clearly is seen within membrane-bound vesicles in two adjacent infected cells. The pathogenesis of enteroinvasive* Escherichia coli *infection involves the invasion of intestinal cells and local cell-to-cell spread, as shown here, by a mechanism identical to that of* Shigella *species. (Courtesy of Saul Tzipori, D.V.M., Department of Comparative Medicine, Tufts University School of Veterinary Medicine.)*

autoagglutinate in a typical "stacked-brick" pattern on the edges of the HEp-2 cells as well as in between them. Because LA and DA strains sometimes have been called enteroadherent *E. coli* (EAEC), the term *EAggEC* has been suggested to refer specifically to the autoaggregative isolates. Perhaps in the future this term will be simplified to *EAEC* because the other clinically important adherent but nontoxigenic *E. coli* group, the LA strains, now are grouped together as EPEC.

The serotypes of EAggEC isolates often are nontypable or rough and when typable are distinct from those of other diarrhea-causing *E. coli* (see Table 108–1). They are negative with probes for other *E. coli* virulence factors; however, they possess a 60- to 65-mDa plasmid that can transfer the aggregative phenotype to rough *E. coli* K-12. Initial data indicate that EAggEC may produce a novel low-molecular-weight ST (EAST, for enteroaggregative stable toxin), which, like classic ST, increases cyclic guanosine monophosphate within target cells.[109] However, in contrast to ST, EAST appears to be inactive in the well-known infant mouse test, and $EAST^+$ strains fail to hybridize with ST probes. EAST 1 is a 38-amino-acid protein with four cysteine residues. The role of EAST in EAggEC pathogenesis is unknown and has been found in several different types of enteric *E. coli* that do not have an aggregative phenotype.

The in vivo significance of the EAggEC phenotype is indicated by the ability of the organisms to cause diarrhea in the gnotobiotic pig model, in which they are found associating with the villus tip in the characteristic aggregative fashion (S. Tzipori, personal communication) (Fig. 108–7). Experimental infections in human adult volunteers using four different EAggEC strains resulted in symptomatic disease in three of five individuals infected with one of these strains, whereas the other three failed to elicit diarrhea.[80] No single putative virulence factor predicted clinical response to these isolates. EAggEC have been isolated frequently from infants with persistent diarrhea, and a specific association is suggested. EAggEC strains have been shown to cause a destructive lesion with shortening of the villi, hemorrhagic necrosis of the villus tips, a mild inflammatory response with edema, and mononuclear infiltration when injected into rabbit loops.[78] The adherence of EAggEC to HEp-2 cells has been associated with fimbriae designated adherence fimbriae I.[80, 83] The genes for these fimbriae are organized as two separate clusters on the plasmid. Widespread use of a DNA probe for the aggregative phenotype[6] has demonstrated that not all phenotypically aggregative strains are probe-positive. A specific probe that will hybridize with all EAggEC has yet to be defined but will facilitate the study of these organisms in the future.

DIAGNOSIS AND DIFFERENTIAL DIAGNOSIS

Specialized laboratory tests are required to identify enterovirulent *E. coli*. Most diagnostic microbiology laboratories do not perform these studies routinely; hence, pathogenic *E. coli* will be called either normal flora or an EPEC strain, depending upon whether or not they agglutinate with commercially available EPEC typing sera. There still is some value in serotyping *E. coli* isolates from diarrhea patients because clinical isolates of ETEC, EPEC, EHEC, and EIEC usually are restricted to a limited number of serogroups distinctive for each. Unfortunately, except for EPEC and a few EHEC serotypes, the antisera needed are not commercially available. Many virulence factors have been identified that, as discussed earlier, define different groups of *E. coli* enteric pathogens. Although it is feasible to detect these factors in the

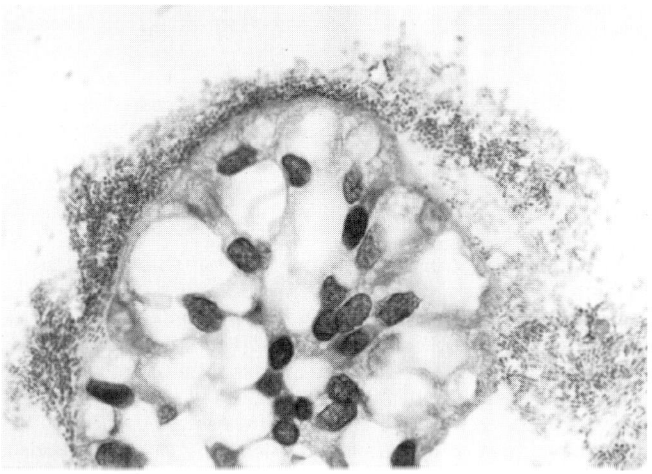

FIGURE 108–7. *Enteroaggregative* Escherichia coli *infection of the gnotobiotic pig intestine. This photomicrograph shows the characteristic "stacked-brick" appearance of the aggregative organisms over the surface of the intestinal epithelium in vivo in the same manner described for EAggEC adherence to HE-2 cells in tissue culture. (Courtesy of Saul Tzipori, D.V.M., Department of Comparative Medicine, Tufts University School of Veterinary Medicine.)*

laboratory by gene probes or polymerase chain reaction, by ELISA, or in some instances by phenotyping a physiologic assay (e.g., cell culture), for the next several years at least, specific identification will not be available to clinicians except in unusual circumstances.

Because of the potential of EHEC infection to cause systemic microangiopathic complications, specific diagnosis is of clinical importance. Currently, the laboratory can use sorbitol-MacConkey agar to screen colonies for sorbitol fermentation and/or the methylumbelliferylglucuronide test for β-glucuronidase production because *E. coli* O157:H7 is almost uniquely sorbitol- and glucuronidase-negative. However, there are sorbitol-fermenting O157:H7 isolates, as well as a large number of other sorbitol-fermenting EHEC, capable of causing severe illness and HUS that are missed by sorbitol-MacConkey agar. New ELISAs for O157 lipopolysaccharide and other outer-membrane proteins have been developed, but the former is specific for just one serotype and the value of outer-membrane protein markers for non-O157:H7 EHEC is not established. A commercial enzyme immunoassay for Stx was approved by the Food and Drug Administration for either confirmation of isolates as toxin producers or rapid direct diagnosis based on detecting the presence of Stx1 or Stx2 in the stool. This approach may be exceedingly useful because it is a rapid test that can recognize any EHEC and not just O157:H7 EHEC infections. At present, early diagnosis of EHEC may be of major epidemiologic importance. It also can serve to alert clinicians to the potential of systemic microangiopathy and, when improved therapeutic measures now being developed become available, to signal early initiation of therapy, which should improve the outcome measurably.

Diagnosis of ETEC would require identifying the LT or ST genes in an isolate or, after isolation and growth in vitro, detecting their products by ELISA. A retrospective diagnosis can be made by detecting a rise in antitoxin antibody, especially for LT. ELISA for CFA antigens of ETEC also could be useful. EPEC can be detected reliably by DNA probes for the 60-mDa EAF adherence plasmid or by tissue culture assay for the LA pattern or the FAST$^{\pm}$ phenotype. The only way to confirm EAggEC at present is by tissue culture assay for the aggregative adherence phenotype. DNA probes are available for an aggregative adherence–associated DNA sequence, but a significant proportion of clinical isolates from all regions of the world are probe-negative. EIEC are, in general, responsible for only a fraction of diarrheal illnesses. Detection relies primarily on detection of invasion genes or gene products, as in *Shigella* species, which share these virulence factors. Tissue culture also can be used to demonstrate the invasive capacity of these strains. Although some other enterovirulent *E. coli* can invade mammalian cells to a limited extent, there is no overlap with the invasive capacity of an EIEC.

In sum, this is a sorry state that is amenable to change as more sophisticated methods become available, but only if sufficient priority is given to rapid diagnosis to incur the cost involved. Diagnosis is important to avoid the danger of inappropriate therapy and to increase the likelihood that necessary therapy will be started early in the course of the illness. Other identifiable agents that should be treated differently may cause similar illnesses, including human rotavirus strains in children younger than 2 years of age; *Vibrio cholerae, Vibrio parahaemolyticus,* or related marine vibrios; *Salmonella* and *Shigella* species; *Campylobacter* species, especially in adolescents in the United States; and *Yersinia enterocolitica.* Rotavirus can be diagnosed readily by commercially available ELISA, but this is not in routine use, primarily because of cost. Although there is an endemic focus of cholera in the United States along the Louisiana/Texas Gulf Coast, only a few indigenous cases occur, probably because the risk factor, ingestion of raw shellfish, is limited and a high inoculum is required. The same is true of infection with *V. parahaemolyticus. Salmonella* and *Shigella* both cause an exudative stool like that caused by EIEC, with many polymorphonuclear leukocytes visible, and this simple test can be of diagnostic significance, especially when routine stool culture for *Salmonella* and *Shigella* is negative. *Campylobacter* usually is not isolated from infants or young children in the United States but may cause watery or blood-tinged diarrhea in older children and young adults. The laboratory must use special selective media cultured at 42° C under 10 per cent carbon dioxide in order to isolate these organisms. *Y. enterocolitica* infection is rare in the United States but can masquerade as ETEC because both are likely initially to be considered a normal stool coliform to be discarded by the laboratory. Unlike ETEC, however, special tests to demonstrate its virulence attributes are not necessary for *Y. enterocolitica;* rather, a high index of suspicion and additional classic diagnostic microbiologic testing will suffice.

PROGNOSIS

EPEC, EAggEC, and ETEC do not cause systemic infections or complications except those due to dehydration or the consequences of nutritional depletion. Thus, prognosis is related directly to availability and adequacy of fluid therapy. When this is dealt with correctly in the otherwise healthy and well-nourished patient, the principal complication is the rare instance of monosaccharide intolerance. In infants or young children in developing countries with protein-energy malnutrition, however, chronic diarrhea and progressive worsening of nutritional status commonly are observed, sometimes terminating fatally. When food is withheld from either well- or poorly nourished youngsters, hypoglycemia may occur, producing seizures, coma, or even death. Rarely, loss of water in excess of salt causes hypertonic dehydration with serum sodium concentrations above 160 mEq/L, a situation that may cause seizures, coma, and death as well.

EAggEC has been associated with persistent diarrhea greater than 14 days in young infants and children, which may result in part from feeding lactose-containing diets in the presence of secondary lactase deficiency. Persistent diarrhea, however, leads to nutritional deterioration, may be difficult to control, and may lead to death due to sepsis or other infections. Inflammatory diarrhea due to EIEC also results in nutritional deterioration, with significant protein losses occurring via the gut.

EHEC is associated significantly with HUS and, especially in adults, TTP. As many as 10 per cent of the patients may die early in the course of the systemic phase of either HUS or TTP. Although the renal failure of HUS generally is reversible with good management of fluid and electrolytes and use of dialysis as needed, permanent damage to the kidneys is, contrary to earlier more optimistic assessments, likely to occur in 50 per cent or more over one or two decades, and many will require permanent dialysis or transplantation in the future. Prognosis in TTP is related directly to initiation of plasmapheresis, which has been documented to reduce mortality significantly. No such benefit has been noted in HUS.

TREATMENT

In all age groups, the principal treatment for the intestinal manifestations of *E. coli* enteric infection is replacement of fluid and electrolytes; with maintenance of fluid balance, the disease is self-limited to a week or less in most patients and lasts no more than 2 weeks in nearly all. The earlier fluid replacement therapy is begun, the better is the prognosis, particularly when one considers that clinical signs of dehydration do not develop until there is a 5 per cent loss of body weight, whereas sustained loss of more than 10 per cent of body weight is incompatible with survival. This does not allow much of a margin of safety and mandates close attention to fluid balance.

When shock is present (usually with altered consciousness and absent or thready pulse) or oral rehydration is not successful because of persistent vomiting, patients must be rehydrated by intravenous infusion of an electrolyte solution, such as Ringer lactate solution. For the patient in shock, a volume of 30 mL/kg body weight should be given over 1 hour, followed by an additional 40 mL/kg body weight in the next 2 hours. When dehydration is less severe, initial replacement of losses usually can be accomplished by oral rehydration. Patients not in shock, who may have a normal physical examination or may manifest poor skin turgor, tachycardia, postural hypotension, and oliguria (along with irritability and a sunken fontanelle in the very young), should receive 50 to 120 mL/kg in fluid, depending on the severity of dehydration, as rapidly as they can be encouraged to drink over a period of 4 hours. Pulse, blood pressure, urine volume, skin turgor, general appearance, and thirst are followed as indicators of response. Adults may need up to a liter an hour to establish rehydration, and they, as well as youngsters, may tire of drinking and fail to keep up with requirements. Thus, several prerequisites must be defined for oral therapy: (1) the patient is not in shock; (2) the patient is fully conscious; (3) the patient is able to drink (vomiting, particularly common in youngsters, is not an absolute contraindication, for frequent small oral feedings usually largely are retained; once the metabolic abnormality begins to reverse toward normal, vomiting ceases); (4) bowel sounds are present; and (5) renal function is normal. Current recommendations in the United States and Europe suggest use of a hypotonic fluid containing 30 to 60 mEq of sodium per liter. In the developing world, where cholera is common, the World Health Organization recommends that a solution containing 90 mEq of sodium be used for all diarrhea because of the large sodium losses in cholera and the desire to avoid the need to choose among formulations because of the difficulty of making etiological diagnoses. Current studies to evaluate a new solution with reduced sodium and glucose content are under way, and the results are likely to influence future recommendations.

Although rehydration therapy is the cornerstone of management, antibiotic therapy should be considered in some cases. In most *E. coli*–associated diarrheal illnesses, the disease is mild and of relatively short duration, and therefore no specific antimicrobial therapy is required. Studies to address this issue have found the effects of antibiotics beneficial in some circumstances. For example, in traveler's diarrhea secondary to ETEC, antibiotic therapy can shorten the duration of the illness and decrease its severity.[32, 84] Prophylactic antibiotic therapy, however, probably carries more risk than benefit and generally is not recommended. When antibiotics are used, TMP-SMX therapy presently is recommended for adults and children with traveler's diarrhea, the new 4-fluoroquinolones being an alternative for adults. Antimotility agents, such as loperamide, generally are not needed but should be used cautiously if prescribed, with great attention to dosage, especially in the very young.[118] Dysentery is a contraindication to the use of antimotility agents, which may be a risk factor for the development of ileus and abdominal distention. Current Food and Drug Administration recommendations preclude giving 4-fluoroquinolones to infants and children younger than 17 years of age because the possibility of causing cartilage damage has been raised by animal toxicology studies, although no convincing evidence exists that this is a real risk in humans.

Children in developing countries with ETEC diarrhea also may benefit from antibiotic therapy.[88] Resistance of ETEC to TMP-SMX was noted among United States troops in Saudi Arabia, where 44 per cent of isolates were resistant.[92] EIEC infection theoretically would benefit even more from antibiotic therapy, given its pathogenic similarity to shigellosis and the known benefits of early use of antibiotics. However, there are no controlled studies to validate this for EIEC. In experimentally induced disease, DuPont and colleagues[29] reported that parenteral ampicillin, 2 g/24 hours for 3 days, produced bacteriologic cure and rapid clinical response with defervescence and improvement of diarrhea in adults. TMP-SMX and ampicillin are the current drugs of choice, unless resistance is a problem.

Epidemic EPEC infection, especially in the newborn, appears to be affected favorably by antibiotic therapy.[85] The potential for this pathogen to cause prolonged disease and a history of high rates of mortality in neonates suggest the need for antibiotic trials in this age group. Based on limited data, either TMP-SMX or oral nonabsorbable antibiotics, such as gentamicin or colistin, usually are recommended.[5]

Antibiotic treatment of EHEC still is controversial because of the lack of controlled studies in etiologically confirmed cases and conflicting reports on efficacy. The important question of whether or not antibiotics increase the likelihood of HUS or TTP remains controversial and unanswered.[4, 10, 18] Large, probably multicenter, double-blind, placebo-controlled studies will be needed to address this problem.

Persistent diarrhea due to EAggEC appears to be as much a nutritional problem as it is a specific infection treatable with antibiotics. By the time the prolonged symptoms are noted, however, antibiotics may have been tried already, with little impact on the diarrhea, and the problem now is secondary to damage to the brush border of the gut cell. Nutritional management, focused first on reduction and possibly removal of lactose and then on elemental diets per os or parenterally if necessary in the event of continuing illness, remains the therapeutic strategy of choice.

Immunocompromised hosts, especially children with acquired immunodeficiency syndrome, may require prolonged antibiotic therapy for prolonged or recrudescent diarrhea, even when caused by bacteria that normally cause only self-limited disease. Malnourished children and children with other serious underlying illness also fit this category. In these patients, systemic invasion may develop, with associated complications, including shock and renal failure. In addition, prolonged carrier states are common, with frequent relapses requiring chronic antibiotic therapy for suppression of relapse.

Practically speaking, in most instances of *E. coli* diarrhea, the clinician is left to make therapeutic decisions without knowing the etiologic agent responsible. For the reasons already outlined, routine diagnostic microbiology laboratories cannot distinguish pathogenic from nonpathogenic *E. coli*, with the exception of classic EPEC serotypes and O157:H7 EHEC. There is no system of national referral laboratories available for sporadic isolates, and even when there is an outbreak investigated by local or national public health laboratories, several days or more likely weeks are required. Clinical decisions regarding antibiotic therapy therefore are made on purely clinical grounds with criteria such as the history, duration, and severity of the illness; the age and immunologic competence of the patient; and the nature of the diarrheal stool (for example, watery, inflammatory, bloody, or dysenteric). Empiric antimicrobial therapy is more justifiable in immunocompromised hosts; in patients with prolonged or severe illness and those with a history of relevant risk factors (specific food ingestion, travel, exposure to known contacts, etc.); and in cases of inflammatory or dysenteric illness.

PREVENTION

The nature of protective immunity still is not well understood, and no vaccines are available for clinical use. Of interest, however, is the modest protective effect against ETEC diarrhea observed in the first few months after an immunization trial in Bangladesh using a killed whole-cell cholera vaccine plus cholera toxin B subunit, which has homology with the *E. coli* LT B subunit. This is encouraging because, experimentally, antitoxin can prevent symptoms of disease due to ETEC. Although ST by itself does not stimulate an immune response, coupling to a protein carrier induces a protective response to challenge with ST or ST-producing ETEC in experimental animals. Synthetic ST, modified so as to be biologically inactive, also has been coupled to LT B subunit epitopes by genetic fusion or chemical coupling of the two peptides and used as an experimental vaccine to stimulate antibody to both toxins.

Other approaches to ETEC vaccines follow the approach being used for cholera as well. For example, the use of CFAs as vaccine antigens is analogous to the exploitation of the TcpA adherence pilus antigen in *V. cholerae*. Unfortunately, protection afforded by ETEC CFAs in experimental models is specific, and multiple CFAs are known now, suggesting the need for a multicomponent vaccine. The observation that some of these antigens (CFA I, II, and IV) appear to predominate in nature may limit the number of CFA antigens needed for an effective vaccine. Unfortunately, most ST-only isolates of ETEC do not express fimbriate colonization factors and would be unaffected by a CFA-based vaccine.

Vaccine development for other enterovirulent *E. coli* strains lags behind that for ETEC. The identification of virulence molecules, such as EAF, the *eae* genes that encode the ability to cause the A/E lesions in the brush border, the invasive genes of EIEC, and the Stx of EHEC, suggests that future vaccine development for these other classes of diarrhea-causing *E. coli* now can proceed with clearly defined target antigens available. Experimental data in rabbits suggest that either parenteral immunization with recombinant Stx1 B subunit or oral administration of a live cholera vaccine expressing recombinant Stx1 B subunit can induce protective immune responses.[1] Antibody raised to a flagellin-like 30-kDa outer-membrane protein of EAggEC encoded by the 60-mDa plasmid blocks enteroaggregative adherence to HEp-2 cells in vitro, suggesting a potential in vivo immunization strategy.[26]

Epidemic nursery outbreaks of diarrhea of the newborn can be controlled by the application of antique but still perfectly valid principles of preventive medicine. Prompt diagnosis and treatment and scrupulous attention to details of hand washing and environmental sanitation to eliminate person-to-person transmission still are effective, whereas prophylactic antimicrobials have no role to play. Outbreaks in neonatal nurseries can be contained by epidemiologic control measures, such as cohorting, by screening staff for carriage and if necessary by closing the unit until it is decontaminated. In contrast, prevention of sporadic *E. coli* diarrhea is difficult. In communities with obvious deficits in water supply and feces disposal, correction of these problems will lead to a diminished incidence of diarrheal diseases in general. For the diarrhea of travelers, several studies indicate that prophylactic use of doxycycline (100 mg/day) or TMP-SMX (160 and 800 mg, respectively, twice daily) can protect adult travelers, at least for a limited time. However, this is no magic bullet to eliminate the problem, and the risk of selection of resistant organisms and drug side effects limits the use of antibiotic prophylaxis to short-term travelers with business or diplomatic missions that would be limited significantly by an episode of diarrhea. Use of tetracyclines is not recommended for children younger than 8 years of age because of deposition in teeth and bones, and no studies of TMP-SMX have been done in children. Some evidence has been presented for the efficacy of bismuth compounds, such as bismuth subsalicylate, for prevention of ETEC diarrhea in adults. However, the concern for bismuth toxicity with prolonged use in young children would make this a problematic solution for pediatric *E. coli* diarrhea and its prevention.

References

1. Acheson, D. W. K., Levine, M. M., Kaper, J. B., et al.: Protective immunity to Shiga-like toxin I following oral immunization with Shiga-like toxin I B-subunit–producing *Vibrio cholerae* CVD 103-HgR. Infect. Immun. *64*:355–357, 1996.
2. Acheson, D. W. K., and Keusch, G. T.: *Shigella* and enteroinvasive *Escherichia coli*. *In* Blaser, M. J., Smith, P. D., Ravdin J. I., et al.: Infections of the Gastrointestinal Tract. New York, Raven Press, 1995, pp. 763–784.
3. Adam, A.: Biology of colon bacillus in dyspepsia, and its relation to pathogenesis and to intoxication. J. Kinderheilk. *101*:295–314, 1923.
4. Al-Qarawi, S., Fontaine, R. E., and Al-Qahtani, M-S.: An outbreak of hemolytic uremic syndrome associated with antibiotic treatment of hospital inpatients for dysentery. Emerg. Infect. Dis. *1*:138–140, 1995.
5. Ashkenazi, S., and Cleary, T. G.: Antibiotic treatment of bacterial gastroenteritis. Pediatr. Infect. Dis. J. *10*:140–148, 1991.
6. Baudry, B., Savarino, S. J., Vial, P., et al.: A sensitive and specific DNA probe to identify enteroaggregative *Escherichia coli*, a recently discovered diarrheal pathogen. J. Infect. Dis. *161*:1249–1251, 1990.
7. Belnap, W. D., and O'Donnell, J. J.: Epidemic gastroenteritis due to *Escherichia coli* O-111: A review of the literature with the epidemiology, bacteriology, and clinical findings of a large outbreak. J. Pediatr. *47*:178–193, 1955.
8. Bettelheim, K. A., Brown, J. E., Lolekha, S., et al.: Serotypes of *Escherichia coli* that hybridized with DNA probes for genes encoding Shiga-like toxin I, Shiga-like toxin II, and serogroup O157 enterohemorrhagic *E. coli* fimbriae isolated from adults with diarrhea in Thailand. J. Clin. Microbiol. *28*:293–295, 1990.
9. Bhan, M. K., Raj, P., Levine, M. M., et al.: Enteroaggregative *Escherichia coli* associated with persistent diarrhea in a cohort of rural children in India. J. Infect. Dis. *159*:1061–1064, 1989.
10. Bin Saeed, A. A. A., El Bushra, E., and al-Hamdan, N. A.: Does treatment of bloody diarrhea due to *Shigella dysenteriae* type 1 with ampicillin precipitate hemolytic uremic syndrome? Emerg. Infect. Dis. *1*:134–137, 1995.
11. Black, R. E.: Persistent diarrhea in children of developing countries. Pediatr. Infect. Dis. *12*:751–761, 1993.
12. Black, R. E., Brown, K. H., Becker, S., et al.: Longitudinal studies of infectious diseases and physical growth of children in rural Bangladesh. II. Incidence of diarrhea and association with known pathogens. Am. J. Epidemiol. *115*:315–324, 1982.
13. Black, R. E., Merson, M. H., Rahman, A. S. M. M., et al.: A two-year study of bacterial viral and parasitic agents associated with diarrhea in rural Bangladesh. J. Infect. Dis. *142*:660–665, 1980.
14. Bokete, T. N., O'Callahan, C. M., Clausen, C. R., et al.: Shiga-like toxin–producing *Escherichia coli* in Seattle children: A prospective study. Gastroenterology *105*:1724–1731, 1993.
15. Bray, J. S. B.: Bray's discovery of pathogenic *Esch. coli* as a cause of infantile gastroenteritis. Arch. Dis. Child. *48*:923–926, 1973.
16. Butler, T., Islam, M. R., Azad, M. A. K., et al.: Risk factors for development of hemolytic uremic syndrome during shigellosis. J. Pediatr. *110*:894–897, 1987.
17. Cameron, A. S., Beers, M. Y., Walker, C. C. et al.: Community outbreak of hemolytic uremic syndrome attributable to *Escherichia coli* O111:NM—South Australia, 1995. M. M. W. R. *44*:550–558, 1995.
18. Cimolai, N., Carter, J. E., Morrison, B. J., et al.: Risk factors for the progression of *Escherichia coli* O157:H7 enteritis to hemolytic-uremic syndrome. J. Pediatr. *116*:589–592, 1990.
19. Cimolai, N., Morrison, B. J., and Carter, J. E.: Risk factors for the central nervous system manifestations of gastroenteritis-associated hemolytic-uremic syndrome. Pediatrics *90*:616–621, 1992.

20. Cleary, T. G., and Lopez, E. L.: The Shiga-like toxin producing *Escherichia coli* and hemolytic uremic syndrome. Pediatr. Infect. Dis. J. *8*:720–724, 1989.
21. Cohen, M. B., and Giannella, R. A.: Enterotoxigenic *Escherichia coli*. *In* Blaser, M. J., Smith, P. D., Ravdin J. I., et al. (eds.): Infections of the Gastrointestinal Tract. New York, Raven Press, 1995, pp. 691–707.
22. Crane, J. K. Weehner, M. S., Bolen E. J., et al.: Regulation of intestinal guanylate cyclase by the heat stable enterotoxin of *Escherichia coli* (STa) and protein kinase C. Infect. Immun. *60*:5004–5012, 1992.
23. Cravioto, A., Reyes, R., Ortega, R., et al.: Prospective study of diarrhoeal disease in a cohort of rural Mexican children: Incidence and isolated pathogens during the first two years of life. Epidemiol. Infect. *101*:123–134, 1988.
24. Cravioto, A., Tello, A., Villagan, H., et al.: Inhibition of localized adhesion of enteropathogenic *Escherichia coli* to Hep-2 cells by immunoglobulin and oligosaccharide fractions of human colostrum and breast milk. J. Infect. Dis. *163*:1247–1255, 1991.
25. Currie, M. G., Fok, K. F., Kato, J. et al.: Guanylin: An endogenous activator of intestinal guanylate cyclase. Proc. Natl. Acad. Sci. U. S. A. *89*:947–951, 1992.
26. Debroy, C., Yearly, J., Wilson, R. C. A., et al.: Antibodies raised against the outer membrane protein interrupt adherence of enteroaggregative *Escherichia coli*. Infect. Immun. *63*:2873–2879, 1995.
27. Donnenberg, M. S., Tacket, C. O., James, S. P., et al.: The role of the *eaeA* gene in experimental enteropathogenic *Escherichia coli* infection. J. Clin. Invest. *92*:1412–1417, 1993.
28. Donnenberg, M. S.: Enteropathogenic *Escherichia coli*. *In* Blaser, M. J., Smith, P. D., Ravdin J. I., et al. (eds.): Infections of the Gastrointestinal Tract. New York, Raven Press, 1995, pp. 709–726.
29. DuPont, H. L., Formal, S. B., Hornick, R. B., et al.: Pathogenesis of *Escherichia coli* diarrhea. N. Engl. J. Med. *285*:1–9, 1971.
30. Embaye, H., Hart, C. A., Getty, B., et al.: Effects of enteropathogenic *Escherichia coli* on microvillar membrane proteins during organ culture of rabbit intestinal mucosa. Gut *33*:1184–1189, 1992.
31. Endo, Y., Tsurugi, K., Yutsudo, T., et al.: Site of action of a Verotoxin (VT2) from *Escherichia coli* O157:H7 and of Shiga toxin on eukaryotic ribosomes: RNA N-glycosidase activity of the toxin. Eur. J. Biochem. *171*:45–50, 1988.
32. Ericsson, C. P., DuPont, H. L., Mathewson, J., et al.: Treatment of traveler's diarrhea with sulfamethoxazole and trimethoprim and loperamide. J. A. M. A. *263*:257–261, 1990.
33. Evans, D. G., Evans, D. J., Jr., and DuPont, H. L.: Virulence factors of enterotoxigenic *Escherichia coli*. J. Infect. Dis. *136*:S118–S123, 1977.
34. Evans, D. G., Silver, R. P., Evans, D. J., Jr., et al.: Plasmid-controlled colonization factor associated with virulence in *Escherichia coli* enterotoxigenic for humans. Infect. Immun. *12*:656–667, 1975.
35. Evans, D. J., Jr., and Evans, D. G.: Classification of pathogenic *Escherichia coli* according to serotype and the production of virulence factors, with special reference to colonization-factor antigens. Rev. Infect. Dis. *5*:S692–S701, 1983.
36. Ewing, W. H., and Gravatti, J. L.: *Shigella* types encountered in the Mediterranean area. J. Bacteriol. *53*:191–195, 1947.
37. Faris, A., Wadstrom, T., and Freer, J. H.: Hydrophobic adsorptive and hemagglutinating properties of *Escherichia coli* possessing colonization factor antigens (CFA/I or C FA/II), type 1 pili, or other pili. Curr. Microbiol. *5*:67–72, 1981.
38. Fasano, A., Kay, B., Russell, R. G., et al.: Enterotoxin and cytotoxin production by enteroinvasive *Escherichia coli*. Infect. Immun. *58*:3717–3723, 1990.
39. Giannella, R. A., Luttrell, M., and Thompson, M.: Binding of *Escherichia coli* heat-stable enterotoxin to receptors on rat intestinal cells. Am. J. Physiol. *243*:G36–G41, 1983.
40. Giron, J. A., Ho, A. S. Y., and Schoolnik, G. K.: An indelible bundle-forming pilus of enteropathogenic *Escherichia coli*. Science *254*:710–713, 1991.
41. Gomes, T. A. T., Rassi, V., Macdonald, K. L., et al.: Enteropathogens associated with acute diarrheal disease in urban infants in São Paulo, Brazil. J. Infect. Dis. *164*:331–337, 1991.
42. Griffin, P. M.: *Escherichia coli* O157:H7 and other enterohemorrhagic *Escherichia coli*. *In* Blaser, M. J., Smith, P. D., Ravdin J. I., et al. (eds.): Infections of the Gastrointestinal Tract. New York, Raven Press, 1995, pp. 739–761.
43. Griffin, P. M., and Tauxe, R. V.: The epidemiology of infections caused by *Escherichia coli* O157:H7, other enterohemorrhagic *E. coli* and the associated hemolytic uremic syndrome. Epidemiol. Rev. *13*:60–98, 1991.
44. Hobbs, B. C., and Thomas, M. E. M.: School outbreak of gastroenteritis associated with a pathogenic paracolon bacillus. Lancet 2:530–532, 1949.
45. Hofmann, S. L.: Southwestern internal medicine conference: Shiga-like toxin in hemolytic-uremic syndrome and thrombotic thrombocytopenic purpura. Am. J. Med. Sci. *306*:398–406, 1993.
46. Honda, T., Tsuji, T., Takeda, Y., et al.: Immunological non-identity of heat-labile enterotoxins from human and porcine enterotoxigenic *Escherichia coli*. Infect. Immun. *33*:677–682, 1981.
47. Hromockyj, A. E., and Maurelli, A. T.: Identification of an *Escherichia coli* gene homologous to virR, a regulator of *Shigella* virulence. J. Bacteriol. *171*:2879–2881, 1989.
48. Hunt, C. M., Harvey, J. A., Youngs E. R., et al.: Clinical and pathological variability of infection by enterohaemorrhagic (Verocytotoxin producing) *Escherichia coli*. J. Clin. Pathol. *43*:847–852, 1989.
49. Jackson, M. P., Newland, J. W., Holmes, R. K., et al.: Nucleotide sequence analysis of the structural gene for Shiga-like toxin I by bacteriophage 933J from *Escherichia coli*. Microbiol. Pathogenesis *2*:147–153, 1987.
50. Jacobs, S. I., Holzel, A., Wolman, B., et al.: Outbreak of infantile gastroenteritis caused by *Escherichia coli* O114. Arch. Dis. Child. *45*:656–663, 1970.
51. Jerse, A. E., Martin, W. C., Galen, J. E., et al.: Oligonucleotide probe for detection of the enteropathogenic *Escherichia coli* (EPEC) adherence factor of localized adherent EPEC. J. Clin. Microbiol. *28*:2842–2844, 1990.
52. Kaper, J. B.: Molecular genetics of attaching and effacing *E. coli*. *In* Karmali, M. A., and Goglio, A. G. (eds.): Recent advances in Verocytotoxin-producing *Escherichia coli* infections. Amsterdam, Elsevier, 1994, pp. 223–231.
53. Karch, H.: Growth of *Escherichia coli* in the presence of trimethoprim/sulfamethoxazole facilitates detection of Shiga like toxin producing strains by colony blot assay. FEMS Microbiol. Lett. *35*:141–145, 1986.
54. Karmali, M. A., Petric, M., Lim, C., et al.: The association between idiopathic hemolytic uremic syndrome and infection by Verotoxin-producing *Escherichia coli*. J. Infect. Dis. *151*:775–782, 1985.
55. Kavi, J., and Wise, R.: Causes of the haemolytic uraemic syndrome. Br. Med. J. *298*:65–66, 1989.
56. Knutton, S., Baldwin, T., Williams, P. H., et al.: Actin accumulation at sites of bacterial adhesion to tissue culture cells: Basis of a new diagnostic test for enteropathogenic and enterohemorrhagic *Escherichia coli*. Infect. Immun. *57*:1290–1298, 1989.
57. Knutton, S., McConnell, M. M., Rowe, B., et al.: Adhesion and ultrastructural properties of human enterotoxigenic *Escherichia coli* producing colonization factor antigens III and IV. Infect. Immun. *57*:3364–3371, 1989.
58. Konowalchuk, J., Speirs, J. I., and Stavric, S.: Vero response to a cytotoxin of *Escherichia coli*. Infect. Immun. *18*:775–779, 1977.
59. Kovacs, M. J., Roddy, J., Gregoire, S., et al.: Thrombotic thrombocytopenic purpura following hemorrhagic colitis due to *Escherichia coli* O157:H7. Am. J. Med. *88*:177–179, 1990.
60. Kupersztoch, Y. M., Tachias, K., Moonman, C. R., et al.: Secretion of methanol-insoluble heat-stable enterotoxin (STb): Energy and secA dependent conversion of pre-STb to an intermediate indistinguishable from the extracellular toxin. J. Bacteriol. *172*:2427–2432, 1990.
61. Levine, M. M., Xu, J. G., Kaper, J. B., et al.: A DNA probe to identify enterohemorrhagic *Escherichia coli* of O157:H7 and other serotypes that cause hemorrhagic colitis and hemolytic uremic syndrome. J. Infect. Dis. *156*:175–182, 1987.
62. Levine, M. M.: *Escherichia coli* infections. N. Engl. J. Med. *313*:445–447, 1985.
63. Lopez, E. L., Diaz, M., Grinstein, S., et al.: Hemolytic uremic syndrome and diarrhea in Argentine children: The role of Shiga-like toxins. J. Infect. Dis. *160*:469–475, 1989.
64. Lortie, L. A. Dubreuil, J. D., and Harel, J.: Characterization of *Escherichia coli* strains producing heat-stable enterotoxin b (STb) isolated from humans with diarrhea. J. Clin. Microbiol. *29*:656–659, 1991.
65. MacLeod, D. L., and Gyles, C. L.: Purification and characterization of an *Escherichia coli* Shiga like toxin II variant. Infect. Immun. *58*:1232–1239, 1990.
66. Marier, R., Wells, J. G., Swanson, R. C., et al.: An outbreak of enteropathogenic *Escherichia coli* foodborne disease traced to imported French cheese. Lancet *2*:1376–1378, 1973.
67. Martin, D. L., MacDonald, K. L., White, K. E., et al.: The epidemiology and clinical aspects of the hemolytic uremic syndrome in Minnesota. N. Engl. J. Med. *323*:1161–1167, 1990.
68. Mathewson, J. J., and Cravioto, A.: HEp-2 cell adherence as an assay for virulence among diarrheagenic *Escherichia coli*. J. Infect. Dis. *159*:1057–1060, 1989.
69. Mathewson, J. J., Johnson, P. C., DuPont, H. L., et al.: Pathogenicity of enteroadherent *Escherichia coli* in adult volunteers. J. Infect. Dis. *154*:524–527, 1986.
70. Mayer, H. B., Acheson, D. W. K., and Wanke, C. A.: Enteroaggregative *Escherichia coli* are a potential cause of persistent diarrhea in adult HIV patients in the United States. Abstracts of the Thirty-first US-Japan cholera and related diarrheal disease conference. 1995.
71. Mehlman, I. J., Fishbein, M., Gorbach, S. L., et al.: Pathogenicity of *Escherichia coli* recovered from food. J. Assoc. Anal. Chem. *59*:67–80, 1976.
72. Merson, M. H., Morris, G. K., Sack, D. A., et al.: Travelers' diarrhea in Mexico: A prospective study of physicians and family members attending a congress. N. Engl. J. Med. *294*:1299–1305, 1976.
73. Mezoff, A. G., Giannella, R. A., Eade, M. N., et al.: *Escherichia coli* entero toxin (STa) binds to receptors, stimulates guanyl cyclase and impairs absorption in rat colon. Gastroenterology *102*:816–822, 1992.
74. Moake, J. L.: Haemolytic-uraemic syndrome: Basic science. Lancet *343*:393–397, 1994.
75. Moon, H. W., and Whipp, S. C.: Development of resistance with age by swine intestine to effects of enteropathogenic *Escherichia coli*. J. Infect. Dis. *122*:220–223, 1970.
76. Moore, K., Damrow, T., and Jankowski, S.: Outbreak of acute gastroenteri-

tis attributable to *Escherichia coli* serotype O104:H21—Helena, Montana, 1994. M. M. W. R. *44*:501–503, 1995.

77. Nalin, D. R., McLaughlin, J. C., Rahaman, M., et al.: Enteropathogenic *Escherichia coli* and idiopathic diarrhoea in Bangladesh. Lancet *2*:1116–1119, 1975.
78. Nataro, J. P., Kaper, J. B., Robins-Browne, R., et al.: Patterns of adherence of diarrheagenic *Escherichia coli* to HEp-2 cells. J. Pediatr. Infect. Dis. *6*:829–831, 1987.
79. Nataro, J. P. Deng, Y., Maneval D. R., et al.: Aggregative adherence fimbriae I of enteroaggregative *Escherichia coli* mediate adherence to HEp-2 cells and hemagglutination of human erythrocytes. Infect. Immun. *60*:2297–2304, 1992.
80. Nataro, J. P., Deng, Y., Cookson, S., et al.: Heterogeneity of enteroaggregative *Escherichia coli* virulence demonstrated in volunteers. J. Infect. Dis. *171*:465–468, 1995.
81. Nataro, J. P., Seriwatana, J., Fasano, A., et al.: Identification and cloning of a novel plasmid-encoded enterotoxin of enteroinvasive *Escherichia coli* and *Shigella* strains. Infect. Immun. *63*:4721–4728, 1995.
82. Nataro, J. P., Yikang, D. Giron, J. A., et al.: Aggregative adherence fimbria I expression in enteroaggregative *Escherichia coli* requires two unlinked plasmid regions. Infect. Immun. *61*:1126–1131, 1993.
83. Nataro, J. P.: Enteroaggregative and diffusely adherent *Escherichia coli*. *In* Blaser, M. J., Smith, P. D., Ravdin J. I., et al. (eds.): Infections of the Gastrointestinal Tract. New York, Raven Press, 1995, pp. 727–737.
84. National Institutes of Health Consensus Development Conference: Travelers' diarrhea. Rev. Infect. Dis. *8*(Suppl. 2):S109–S233, 1986.
85. Nelson, J. D.: Duration of neomycin therapy for enteropathogenic *Escherichia coli* diarrheal disease: A comparative study of 113 cases. Pediatrics *48*:248–258, 1971.
86. Neter, E., Krons, R. F., and Trussel, R. E.: Association of *Escherichia coli* serotype O111 with two hospital outbreaks of epidemic diarrhea of the newborn infant in New York State during 1947. Pediatrics *12*:377–383, 1953.
87. O'Brien, A. D., and Holmes, R. K.: Shiga and Shiga-like toxins. Microbiol. Rev. *51*:206–220, 1987.
88. Oberhelman, R. A., de la Cabada, F. J., Garibay, E. V., et al.: Efficacy of trimethoprim-sulfamethoxazole in treatment of acute diarrhea in a Mexican pediatric population. J. Pediatr. *110*:960–965, 1987.
89. Obrig, T. G., Vecchio, P. H. D., Brown, E. J., et al.: Direct cytotoxic action of Shiga toxin on human vascular endothelial cells. Infect. Immun. *56*:2373–2378, 1988.
90. Ogawa, H., Nakamura, A., and Sakazaki, R.: Pathogenic properties of "enteropathogenic" *Escherichia coli* from diarrheal children and adults. Jpn. J. Med. Sci. Biol. *21*:333–349, 1968.
91. Okamoto, K., Fujii, Y., Akashi, N., et al.: Identification and characterization of heat-stable enterotoxin-II producing *Escherichia coli* from patients with diarrhea. Microbiol. Immunol. *37*:411–414, 1993.
92. Oldfield, III, E. C., Wallace, M. R., Hyams, K. C., et al.: Endemic infectious diseases of the Middle East. Rev. Infect. Dis. *13*:S199–S217, 1991.
93. Ostroff, S. M., Kobayashi, J. M., and Lewis, J. H.: Infections with *Escherichia coli* O157:H7 in Washington State: The first year of statewide disease surveillance. J. A. M. A. *262*:355–359, 1989.
94. Ostroff, S. M., Tarr, P. I., Neill, M. A., et al.: Toxin genotypes and plasmid profiles as determinants of systemic sequelae in *Escherichia coli* O157:H7 infections. J. Infect. Dis. *160*:994–998, 1989.
95. Pai, C. H., Gordon, R., Sims, H. V., et al.: Sporadic cases of hemorrhagic colitis associated with *Escherichia coli* O157:H7: Clinical, epidemiologic and bacteriologic features. Ann. Intern. Med. *101*:738–742, 1984.
96. Pal, T., Formal, S. B., and Hale, T. L.: Characterization of virulence marker antigen of *Shigella* spp. and enteroinvasive *Escherichia coli*. J. Clin. Microbiol. *27*:561–563, 1989.
97. Rasheed, J. K., Buzman-Verduzco, L. M., and Kupersztoch, Y. M.: Two precursors of the heat-stable enterotoxin of *Escherichia coli*: Evidence of extracellular processing. Mol. Microbiol. *4*:265–273, 1990.
98. Riley, L. W.: The epidemiologic, clinical, and microbiological features of hemorrhagic colitis. Ann. Rev. Microbiol. *41*:383–407, 1987.
99. Riley, L. W., Remis, R. S., Helgerson, S. D., et al.: Hemorrhagic colitis associated with a rare *E. coli* serotype. N. Engl. J. Med. *308*:681–685, 1983.
100. Robins-Browne, R., Still, C. S., Miliotis, M. D., et al.: Summer diarrhoea in African infants and children. Arch. Dis. Child. *55*:923–928, 1980.
101. Rogers, M. F., Rutherford, G. W., Alexander, S. R., et al.: A population-based study of hemolytic uremic syndrome in Oregon, 1979–1982. Am. J. Epidemiol. *123*:137–142, 1986.
102. Rosenberg, M. L., Koplan, J. P., Wachsmuth, I. K., et al.: Epidemic diarrhea at Crater Lake from enterotoxigenic *Escherichia coli:* A large waterborne outbreak. Ann. Intern. Med. *86*:714–718, 1977.
103. Rothbaum, R., McAdams, A. J., Ginnella, R., et al.: A clinicopathological study of enterocyte-adherent *Escherichia coli*: A cause of protracted diarrhea in infants. Gastroenterology *83*:441–454, 1982.
104. Sack, R. B., Gorbach, S. L., Banwell, J. G., et al.: Enterotoxigenic *Escherichia coli* isolated from patients with severe cholera-like disease. J. Infect. Dis. *123*:378–385, 1971.
105. Sack, R. B., Hirschhorn, N., Brownlee, I., et al.: Enterotoxigenic *Escherichia coli*–associated diarrheal disease in Apache children. N. Engl. J. Med. *292*:1041–1045, 1975.
106. Sack, R. B., Sack, D. A., Mehlman, I. J., et al.: Enterotoxigenic *Escherichia coli* isolated from food. J. Infect. Dis. *135*:313–317, 1977.
107. Sakazaki, R., Tamura, L., and Saito, M.: Enteropathogenic *Escherichia coli* associated with diarrhea in children and adults. Jpn. J. Med. Sci. Biol. *20*:387–399, 1967.
108. Sansonetti, P. J.: Genetic and molecular basis of epithelial cell invasion by *Shigella* species. Rev. Infect. Dis. *13*:S285–S292, 1991.
109. Savarino, S., Fasano, A., Watson, J., et al.: Enteroaggregative *Escherichia coli* heat stable enterotoxin 1 represents another subfamily of *E. coli* heat-stable toxin. Proc. Natl. Acad. Sci. U. S. A. *90*:3093–3097, 1993.
110. Schroeder, S. A., Caldwell, J. R., Vernon, T. M., et al.: A water borne outbreak of gastroenteritis in adults associated with *Escherichia coli*. Lancet *i*:737–740, 1968.
111. Schulz, S., Green, C. K., Yuen, P. S. T., et al.: Guanyl cyclase is a heat-stable enterotoxin receptor. Cell *63*:941–948, 1990.
112. Smith, H. W.: Neonatal *Escherichia coli* infections in domestic mammals: Transmissibility of pathogenic characteristics. *In* Knight, K., and Elliot, J. (eds.): Acute Diarrhea in Childhood. New York, Elsevier, 1976, pp. 45–64.
113. Smith, H. W., and Halls, S.: Observations by the ligated intestinal segment and oral inoculation methods on *Escherichia coli* infections in pigs, calves, lambs, and rabbits. J. Pathol. Bacteriol. *93*:499–529, 1967.
114. Smith, H. W., and Linggood, M. A.: Observations on the pathogenic properties of the K 88, Hly and Ent plasmids of *Escherichia coli* with particular reference to porcine diarrhea. J. Med. Microbiol. *4*:467–485, 1971.
115. Snyder, J. D., Wells, J. G., Yashuk, J., et al.: Outbreak of invasive *Escherichia coli* gastroenteritis on a cruise ship. Am. J. Trop. Med. Hyg. *33*:281–284, 1984.
116. So, M., and McCarthy, B. J.: Nucleotide sequence of the bacterial transposon TN1981 encoding a heat-stable enterotoxin (ST) and its identification in enterotoxigenic *Escherichia coli* strains. Proc. Natl. Acad. Sci. U. S. A. *77*:4011–4015, 1980.
117. Tacket, C. O., Moseley, S. L., Kay, B., et al.: Challenge studies in volunteers using *Escherichia coli* strains with diffuse adherence to HEp-2 cells. J. Infect. Dis. *162*:550–552, 1990.
118. Taylor, D. N., Sanchez, J. L., Candler, W., et al.: Treatment of travelers' diarrhea: Ciprofloxacin plus loperamide compared with ciprofloxacin alone: A placebo-controlled, randomized trial. Ann. Intern. Med. *114*:731–734, 1991.
119. Thea, D. T., St. Louis, M. E., Atido, U., et al.: A prospective study of diarrhea and HIV-1 infection among 429 Zairian infants. N. Engl. J. Med. *329*:1696–1702, 1993.
120. Thorén, A., Stintzing, G., Tufvesson, B., et al.: Aetiology and clinical features of severe infantile diarrhoea in Addis Ababa, Ethiopia. J. Trop. Pediatr. *28*:127–131, 1982.
121. Toledo, M. R. F., Alvariza, M. C. B., Murahovschi, J., et al.: Enteropathogenic *Escherichia coli* serotypes and endemic diarrhea in infants. Infect. Immun. *39*:586–589, 1983.
122. Toth I., Cohen, M. L., Rumschlag, H. S., et al.: Influence of the 60 megadalton plasmid on adherence of *Escherichia coli* O157:H7 and genetic derivatives. Infect. Immun. *58*:1223–1231, 1990.
123. Trabulsi, L. R., Fernandes, M. R., and Zuliani, M. E.: Novas bacterias patogenicas para o intestino do homen. Rev. Inst. Med. Trop. São Paulo *9*:31–39, 1967.
124. Tulloch, E. F., Ryan, K. J., Formal, S. B., et al.: Invasive enteropathic *Escherichia coli* dysentery: An outbreak in 28 adults. Ann. Intern. Med. *79*:13–17, 1973.
125. Weikel, C. S., Spann, C. L., Chambers, C. P., et al.: Phorbol esters enhance the cyclic GMP response of T84 cells to the heat-stable enterotoxin of *Escherichia coli* (STa). Infect. Immun. *58*:1402–1407, 1990.
126. Whip, S. C.: Protease degradation of *Escherichia coli* heat-stable, mouse-negative, pig-positive enterotoxin. Infect. Immun. *55*:2057–2060, 1987.

109

KLEBSIELLA

William C. Gruber and Randall G. Fisher

Klebsiella is a genus of Enterobacteriaceae that is a frequent cause of nosocomial pediatric infection. Classically described by Friedländer[24] as a cause of pneumonia, *Klebsiella* can cause infections of the urinary tract, lung, and central venous catheters in the high-risk newborn and immunocompromised older child.[12]

BACTERIOLOGY

Klebsiella organisms were named for Edwin Klebs, the noted German bacteriologist.[59] Distinguishing features of *Klebsiella* species include the absence of motility and the presence of a polysaccharide capsule that gives rise to large mucoid colonies on solid media. The organisms are oxidase-negative and citrate-positive; they ferment inositol and hydrolyze urea but do not produce ornithine decarboxylase or hydrogen sulfide. Acetoin and 2,3-butanediol predominate over acidic end-products during sugar fermentation (positive result on the Voges-Proskauer test). Four species of *Klebsiella* commonly are agreed on by microbiologists: *K. pneumoniae* (the most common human pathogen), *K. oxytoca* (a less common human pathogen), and *K. terrigena* and *K. planticola* (almost exclusively recovered from soil and aquatic environments). Organisms are defined serologically by their capsular polysaccharide (K antigens) and lipopolysaccharide (O antigens). There is significant cross-reactivity between the capsule of some pneumococci (e.g., 19F) and *Klebsiella*.[46]

EPIDEMIOLOGY

Friedländer[24] proposed that *K. pneumoniae* was the most common cause of community pneumonia, an observation that was refuted by Fraenkel's[23] observations on pneumococcal pneumonia. *K. pneumoniae* accounts for less than 10 per cent of hospitalized cases of pneumonia in adults.[14] *Klebsiella* species now are in greatest evidence as opportunistic nosocomial pathogens of the urinary tract, respiratory tract, biliary tract, and blood stream. In one Centers for Disease Control and Prevention survey, the nosocomial *K. pneumoniae* infection rate was 16.7 infections per 10,000 patients discharged.[36] Hand carriage generally is regarded as the common mode of transmission.[26] Recent environmental sources have included contaminated blood pressure monitoring equipment,[65] ventilator traps,[26] and dialysate.[43] The emergence of plasmid-mediated β-lactamase resistance can be responsible for the rapid spread of resistant organisms to susceptibles in intensive care settings.[6, 8] Outbreaks may be complex; patient-to-patient transmission of epidemic strains containing different plasmids may be interspersed with sporadic, nonepidemic *Klebsiella* infections.[8] *Klebsiella* species are second only to *Escherichia coli* as causes of sepsis,[25] with the highest rates of infection reported from larger hospitals affiliated with medical schools.

Klebsiella species commonly are highlighted as pathogens of debilitated adults and alcoholics,[41] but by 1985, nearly 50 per cent of reported *Klebsiella* outbreaks were in neonatal intensive care units.[36] Newborn outbreaks continue to be frequent worldwide.[1, 3, 17, 22, 32, 61, 66] Most such outbreaks have been associated with *K. pneumoniae* infection, but scattered nursery outbreaks of *K. oxytoca* infection also have been reported.[2, 69] A high percentage of infants in intensive care settings may become colonized with hospital strains of *Klebsiella*.[29] Infecting organisms have been isolated from care providers and from mothers of colonized infants.[17] *Klebsiella* may spread from newborn units to adult units; interhospital and international spread of resistant strains has been described.[16, 22] Different ribotypes that share plasmids conferring antibiotic resistance can be responsible for pediatric infections in a particular institution.[8]

PATHOPHYSIOLOGY

Pneumonias due to *Klebsiella* most commonly arise from colonization of the upper respiratory tract, followed by aspiration of organisms to the lower respiratory tract. Some degree of gram-negative oropharyngeal colonization is a normal finding in newborns. The oropharynx of nearly one-third of healthy newborns is colonized by gram-negative rods, including *Klebsiella*, by 1 month of age; colonization rates generally are lower in breast-fed infants.[5] Antibiotic pressure in high-risk newborns and older children has been observed to promote overgrowth of *Klebsiella*.[7, 67] Enteric organisms are recovered less commonly from the oropharynx of healthy older children and adults; oral colonization with gram-negative rods is increased during illness,[38] after postoperative viral infections,[39, 64] and in debilitated adults.[48] Increased adherence of gram-negative rods to oropharyngeal cells contributes to increased colonization.[39] Elastase made by polymorphonuclear cells contributes to such colonization by reducing the fibronectin coating of sugar receptors.[19] Adherence properties may be affected by plasmid content[21] and may be transferred between *E. coli* and *K. pneumoniae*.[35]

In animal models of sepsis, capsular polysaccharide (K antigens) is a virulence factor; monoclonal antibodies to the K antigens reduce illness severity in mice.[45] In a mouse model of urinary tract infection, the K antigens appear to be more important in infection than the lipopolysaccharide (O antigens).[13] In one series of adult human subjects, capsular type K2 was associated commonly with asymptomatic bacteruria and cystitis but not pyelonephritis; the presence of type 1 fimbriae bore a closer relationship to upper urinary tract infection.[62]

CLINICAL MANIFESTATIONS

Klebsiella infection shows little clinical distinction from diseases produced by other enteric pathogens. The organism generally is less common than group B *Streptococcus* or *E. coli* as a cause of "early-onset" or "late-onset" newborn infection.[27, 51] However, investigators from Spain[32] reported one 7-year interval in which *K. pneumoniae* was the most common cause of newborn bacteremia. Risk factors for neonatal *Klebsiella* infection include prematurity, presence of indwelling catheters, previous antibiotic treatment, and parenteral nutrition.[66] Newborn infection is characterized by typical features of pneumonia, sepsis, and meningitis.[51] In one surgical series of 86 infants with necrotizing enterocolitis complicated by peritonitis, *Klebsiella* species were recovered more commonly from the peritoneum than were *E. coli* organisms.[54] Less common manifestations in infants include toxic epidermal necrolysis,[30, 60] conjunctivitis,[44] parotitis,[15] retropharyngeal abscess,[18] and renal abscess.[68]

Klebsiella is an unusual cause of infection in the otherwise healthy older child. The classic Friedländer pneumonia of the debilitated adult[24] is rare in children. The identification of pulmonary infection should suggest the possibility of underlying immunodeficiency or significant malnutrition, if not suspected previously.[34, 40] If pneumonia due to *Klebsiella* does occur, progression to lung abscesses should be anticipated.

Lung abscesses may develop within days to weeks after *Klebsiella* infection. Abscess formation is more common during *Klebsiella* pulmonary infection than during any other community-acquired infection.[14] A rare but devastating outcome is massive pulmonary gangrene—the rapid total destruction of part of the lung presumed to be due to vascular compromise. This complication is heralded by radiographs that show small cavities that later coalesce into a large cavity with an intracavitary mass of necrotic lung.[56, 58] There is speculation that *Klebsiella* lung infection is accompanied by coincident anaerobic infection that contributes to or primarily is responsible for the pathology.[14]

Catheterization of the urinary tract can be associated with urinary tract *Klebsiella* infection, but bacteremia is an uncommon complication in the immunocompetent child.[20, 47] Approximately 10 per cent of nosocomial urinary tract infections observed in infants after surgery are due to *Klebsiella*.[20] *K. pneumonia* bacteremia has been associated with lesions of the gastrointestinal tract, presence of an indwelling central venous catheter, and neutropenia. Curiously, patients with short-bowel syndrome seem to be at greater risk than patients with inflammatory bowel disease or malignancy for catheter-associated *Klebsiella* or *Enterobacter* bacteremia. *K. pneumoniae* was a constituent of polymicrobial bacteremia in 15 such patients (26 per cent).[10] Mortality rates have ranged from 5 to 20 per cent, with higher death rates occurring in children infected with an aminoglycoside-resistant strain.[9, 36] Pneumonia, shock, and disseminated intravascular coagulation are poor prognostic factors in children with underlying malignancy. Rare clinical presentations include multifocal osteomyelitis[42] and endopthalmitis.[49]

DIAGNOSIS

Klebsiella species characteristically grow as large mucoid colonies on MacConkey agar. Citrate-containing media can be used to facilitate isolation of *Klebsiella* strains because these organisms can use citrate as a sole carbon source.[59] Serotyping with specific antisera usually is determined by countercurrent immunoelectrophoresis or a Quellung test.[4] In situ hybridization techniques have been used to identify *Klebsiella* in phagocytes from blood specimens,[50] and restriction-enzyme analysis and ribotyping of clinical isolates have been used to characterize nosocomial spread of antibiotic-resistant strains.[8, 28] However, conventional, commonly used microbiologic methods may misidentify some *Klebsiella* species, particularly *K. planticola* and *K. terrigena*.[55] Rarely, blood cultures have required longer than 72 hours of incubation for radiometric detection of *Klebsiella*.[52]

TREATMENT

Empiric antimicrobial therapy should be guided by an understanding of antimicrobial susceptibilities of *Klebsiella* in the hospital. Therapy with a cephalosporin plus an aminoglycoside (rather than a cephalosporin alone) has been associated with a more favorable outcome in patients with cancer who are infected with susceptible strains.[9] However, antimicrobial therapy of *Klebsiella* species is made problematic by the common emergence of plasmid-mediated resistance to penicillins and cephalosporins conferred by extended-spectrum β-lactamases.[6, 8, 11, 31] Plasmid-mediated resistance to aminoglycosides also is common.[2, 17, 25, 57] Antibiotic pressure is important in increasing the risk for resistant isolates.[63] In some nursery outbreaks, switching from gentamicin to amikacin has been associated with return of the gentamicin susceptibility of *Klebsiella* isolates.[2, 33] Imipenem or the combination of piperacillin and tazobactam may demonstrate good antimicrobial activity against multiply resistant organisms.[37, 63] Strict adherence to infection control policies that promote restricted antibiotic use, cohorting, and hand washing may help to prevent the spread of resistant *Klebsiella* strains.[2, 17, 29, 53]

References

1. Akindele, J. A, and Gbadegesin, R. A.: Outbreak of neonatal *Klebsiella* septicaemia at the University College Hospital, Ibadan, Nigeria: Appraisal of predisposing factors and preventive measures. Trop. Geogr. Med. *46*:151–153, 1994.
2. Aronsson, B., Eriksson, M., Herin, P., et al.: Gentamicin-resistant *Klebsiella* spp. and *Escherichia coli* in a neonatal intensive care unit. Scand. J. Infect. Dis. *23*:195–199, 1991.
3. Arredondo-Garcia, J. L., Diaz-Ramos, R., Solorzano-Santos, F., et al.: Neonatal septicaemia due to *K. pneumoniae*: Septicaemia due to *Klebsiella pneumoniae* in newborn infants: Nosocomial outbreak in an intensive care unit. Revista Latinoamericana de Microbiologia *34*:11–16, 1992.
4. Ayling-Smith, B., and Pitt, T. L.: State of the art in typing: *Klebsiella* spp. J. Hosp. Infect. *16*:287–295, 1990.
5. Baltimore, R. S., Duncan, R. L., Shapiro, E. D., et al.: Epidemiology of pharyngeal colonization of infants with aerobic gram-negative rod bacteria. J. Clin. Microbiol. *27*:91–95, 1989.
6. Bauernfeind, A., Rosenthal, E., Eberlein, E., et al.: Spread of *Klebsiella pneumoniae* producing SHV-5 beta-lactamase among hospitalized patients. Infection *21*:18–22, 1993.
7. Bennet, R., Eriksson, M., Nord, C. E., et al.: Fecal bacterial microflora of newborn infants during intensive care management and treatment with five antibiotic regimens. Pediatr. Infect. Dis. *5*:533–539, 1986.
8. Bingen, E. H., Desjardins, P., Arlet, G., et al.: Molecular epidemiology of plasmid spread among extended broad-spectrum beta-lactamase-producing *Klebsiella pneumoniae* isolates in a pediatric hospital. J. Clin. Microbiol. *31*:179–184, 1993.
9. Bodey, G. P., Elting, L. S., Rodriquez, S., et al.: *Klebsiella* bacteremia: A 10-year review in a cancer institution. Cancer *64*:2368–2376, 1989.
10. Bonadio, W. A.: *Klebsiella pneumoniae* bacteremia in children: Fifty-seven cases in 10 years. Am. J. Dis. Child. *143*:1061–1063, 1989.
11. Bradford, P. A., Cherubin, C. E., Idemyor, V., et al.: Multiply resistant *Klebsiella pneumoniae* strains from two Chicago hospitals: Identification of the extended-spectrum TEM-12 and TEM-10 ceftazidime-hydrolyzing beta-lactamases in a single isolate. Antimicrob. Agents Chemother. *38*:761–766, 1994.
12. Brown, R. B., Cipriani, D., Schulte, M., et al.: Community-acquired bacteremias from tunneled central intravenous lines: Results from studies of a single vendor. Am. J. Infect. Control *22*:149–151, 1994.
13. Camprubi, S., Merino, S., Benedi, V. J., et al.: The role of the O-antigen lipopolysaccharide and capsule on an experimental *Klebsiella pneumoniae* infection of the rat urinary tract. FEMS Microbiol. Lett. *111*:9–13, 1993.
14. Carpenter, J. L.: *Klebsiella* pulmonary infections: Occurrence at one medical center and review. Rev. Infect. Dis. *12*:672–682, 1990.
15. Coban, A., Ince, Z., Ucsel, R., et al.: Neonatal suppurative parotitis: A vanishing disease? Eur. J. Pediatr. *152*:1004–1005, 1993.
16. Cookson, B., Johnson, A. P., Azadian, B., et al.: International inter- and intrahospital patient spread of a multiple antibiotic-resistant strain of *Klebsiella pneumoniae*. J. Infect. Dis. *171*:511–513, 1995.
17. Coovadia, Y. M., Johnson, A. P., Bhana, R. H., et al.: Multiresistant *Klebsiella pneumoniae* in a neonatal nursery: The importance of maintenance of infection control policies and procedures in the prevention of outbreaks. J. Hosp. Infect. *22*:197–205, 1992.
18. Coulthard, M., and Isaacs, D.: Retropharyngeal abscess. Arch. Dis. Child. *66*:1227–1230, 1991.
19. Dal Nogare, A. R., Toews, G. B., and Pierce, A. K.: Increased salivary elastase precedes gram-negative bacillary colonization in postoperative patients. Am. Rev. Respir. Dis. *135*:671–675, 1987.

20. Davies, H. D., Jones, E. L., Sheng, R. Y., et al.: Nosocomial urinary tract infections at a pediatric hospital. Pediatr. Infect. Dis. *11*:349–354, 1992.
21. Denoya, C. D., Trevisan, A. R., and Zorzopulos, J.: Adherence of multiresistant strains of *Klebsiella pneumoniae* to cerebrospinal fluid shunts: Correlation with plasmid content. J. Med. Microbiol. *21*:225–231, 1986.
22. Eisen, D., Russell, E. G., Tymms, M., et al.: Random amplified polymorphic DNA and plasmid analyses used in investigation of an outbreak of multiresistant *Klebsiella pneumoniae*. J. Clin. Microbiol. *33*:713–717, 1995.
23. Fraenkel, A.: Bakteriologische mitteilungen. Leitsch. F. Klin. Med. *10*:401–411, 1886.
24. Friedländer, C.: Über die schizomyceten bei der acuten fibrosen pneumonie. Arch. Pathol. Anat. Physiol. Klin. Med. *87*:319–324, 1882.
25. Garcia de la Torre, M., Romero-Vivas, J., Martinez-Beltran, J., et al.: *Klebsiella* bacteremia: An analysis of 100 episodes. Rev. Infect. Dis. *7*:143–150, 1985.
26. Gorman, L. J., Sanai, L., Notman, A. W., et al.: Cross infection in an intensive care unit by *Klebsiella pneumoniae* from ventilator condensate. J. Hosp. Infect. *23*:27–34, 1993.
27. Grauel, E. L., Halle, E., Bollmann, R., et al.: Neonatal septicaemia: Incidence, etiology and outcome: A 6-year analysis. Acta Paediatr. Scand. *360*(Suppl.):113–119, 1989.
28. Haertl, R., and Bandlow, G.: Use of small fragment restriction endonuclease analysis (SF-REA) for epidemiological fingerprinting of *Klebsiella oxytoca*. Int. J. Med. Microbiol. Virol. Parasitol. Infect. Dis. *280*:312–318, 1994.
29. Hambraeus, A., Lagerqvist-Widh, A., Zettersten, U., et al.: Spread of *Klebsiella* in a neonatal ward. Scand. J. Infect. Dis. *23*:189–194, 1991.
30. Hawk, R. J., Storer, J. S., and Daum, R. S.: Toxic epidermal necrolysis in a 6-week-old infant. Pediatr. Dermatol. *2*:197–200, 1985.
31. Heritage, J., Hawkey, P. M., Todd, N., et al.: Transposition of the gene encoding a TEM-12 extended-spectrum beta-lactamase. Antimicrob. Agents Chemother. *36*:1981–1986, 1992.
32. Hervas, J. A., Alomar, A., Salva, F., et al.: Neonatal sepsis and meningitis in Mallorca, Spain, 1977–1991. Clin. Infect. Dis. *16*:719–724, 1993.
33. Hesseling, P. B., Mouton, W. L., Henning, P. A., et al.: A prospective study of long-term use of amikacin in a paediatrics department: Indications, administration, side-effects, bacterial isolates and resistance. S. Afr. Med. J. *78*:192–195, 1990.
34. Hughes, W. T.: Pneumonia in the immunocompromised child. Semin. Resp. Infect. 2:177–183, 1987.
35. Jallat, C., Darfeuille-Michaud, A., Girardeau, J. P., et al.: Self-transmissible R plasmids encoding CS31A among human *Escherichia coli* strains isolated from diarrheal stools. Infect. Immun. *62*:2865–2873, 1994.
36. Jarvis, W. R., Munn, V. P., Highsmith, A. K., et al.: The epidemiology of nosocomial infections caused by *Klebsiella pneumoniae*. Infect. Control *6*:68–74, 1985.
37. Jett, B. D., Ritchie, D. J., Reichley, R., et al.: In vitro activities of various beta-lactam antimicrobial agents against clinical isolates of *Escherichia coli* and *Klebsiella* spp. resistant to oxyimino cephalosporins. Antimicrob. Agents Chemother. *39*:1187–1190, 1995.
38. Johanson, W. G., Pierce, A. K., and Sanford, J. P.: Changing bacterial flora of hospitalized patients. N. Engl. J. Med. *281*:1137–1140, 1969.
39. Johanson, W. G., Higuchi, J. H., Chaudhuri, T. R., et al.: Bacterial adherence to epithelial cells in bacillary colonization of the respiratory tract. Am. Rev. Respir. Dis. *121*:55–63, 1980.
40. Johnson, A. W., Osinusi, K., Aderele, W. I., et al.: Bacterial aetiology of acute lower respiratory infections in pre-school Nigerian children and comparative predictive features of bacteraemic and non-bacteraemic illnesses. J. Trop. Pediatr. *39*:97–106, 1993.
41. Jong, G. M., Hsiue, T. R., Chen, C. R., et al.: Rapidly fatal outcome of bacteremic *Klebsiella pneumoniae* pneumonia in alcoholics. Chest *107*:214–217, 1995.
42. Kishan, J., Mir, N. A., Elzouki, A. Y., et al.: Radiological case of the month: *Klebsiella* multifocal osteomyelitis. Am. J. Dis. Child. *142*:687–688, 1988.
43. Kolmos, H. J.: *Klebsiella pneumoniae* in a nephrological department. J. Hosp. Infect. *5*:253–259, 1984.
44. Krohn, M. A., Hillier, S. L., Bell, T. A., et al.: The bacterial etiology of conjunctivitis in early infancy: Eye Prophylaxis Study Group. Am. J. Epidemiol. *138*:326–332, 1993.
45. Lang, A. B., Bruderer, U., Senyk, G., et al.: Human monoclonal antibodies specific for capsular polysaccharides of *Klebsiella* recognize clusters of multiple serotypes. J. Immunol. *146*:3160–3164, 1991.
46. Lee, C. J.: Bacterial capsular polysaccharides: Biochemistry, immunity and vaccine. Mol. Immunol. 24:1005–1019, 1987.
47. Lohr, J. A., Donowitz, L. G., and Sadler, J. E.: Hospital-acquired urinary tract infection. Pediatrics *83*:193–199, 1989.
48. Mackowiak, P. A., Martin, R. M., Jones, S. R., et al.: Pharyngeal colonization by gram-negative bacilli in aspiration-prone persons. Arch. Intern. Med. *138*:1224–1227, 1978.
49. Margo, C. E., Mames, R. N., and Guy, J. R.: Endogenous *Klebsiella* endophthalmitis: Report of two cases and review of the literature. Ophthalmology *101*:1298–1301, 1994.
50. Matsuhisa, A., Saito, Y., Sakamoto, Y., et al.: Detection of bacteria in phagocyte-smears from septicemia-suspected blood by in situ hybridization using biotinylated probes. Microbiol. Immunol. *38*:511–517, 1994.
51. McCracken, G. H. J., Mize, S. G., and Threlkeld, N.: Intraventricular gentamicin therapy in gram-negative bacillary meningitis of infancy: Report of the Second National Meningitis Cooperative Study Group. Lancet *1*:787–791, 1980.
52. Meadow, W. L., and Schwartz, I. K.: Time course of radiometric detection of positive blood cultures in childhood. Pediatr. Infect. Dis. *5*:333–336, 1986.
53. Meyer, K. S., Urban, C., Eagan, J. A., et al.: Nosocomial outbreak of *Klebsiella* infection resistant to late-generation cephalosporins [see comments]. Ann. Intern. Med. *119*:353–358, 1993.
54. Mollitt, D. L., Tepas, J. J., and Talbert, J. L.: The microbiology of neonatal peritonitis. Arch. Surg. 123:176–179, 1988.
55. Monnet, D., Freney, J., Brun, Y., et al.: Difficulties in identifying *Klebsiella* strains of clinical origin. Int. J. Med. Microbiol. 274:456–464, 1991.
56. Moon, W. K., Im, J. G., Yeon, K. M., et al.: Complications of *Klebsiella* pneumonia: CT evaluation. J. Comput. Assist. Tomogr. 19:176–181, 1995.
57. Nathoo, K. J., Mason, P. R., Gwanzura, L., et al.: Severe *Klebsiella* infection as a cause of mortality in neonates in Harare, Zimbabwe: Evidence from postmortem blood cultures. Pediatr. Infect. Dis. *12*:840–844, 1993.
58. O'Reilly, G. V., Dee, P. M., and Otteni, G. V.: Gangrene of the lung: Successful medical management of three patients. Diagn. Radiol. *126*:575–579, 1978.
59. Orskov, I.: *Klebsiella*. *In* Krieg, N. R., and Holt, J. G. (eds.): Bergey's Manual of Systematic Bacteriology. Vol. 1. Baltimore, Williams & Wilkins, 1984, pp. 461–465.
60. Picard, E., Gillis, D., Klapholz, L., et al.: Toxic epidermal necrolysis associated with *Klebsiella pneumoniae* sepsis. Pediatr. Dermatol. *11*:331–334, 1994.
61. Pierce, J. R., Merenstein, G. B., and Stocker, J. T.: Immediate postmortem cultures in an intensive care nursery. Pediatr. Infect. Dis. *3*:510–513, 1984.
62. Podschun, R., Sievers, D., Fischer, A., et al.: Serotypes, hemagglutinins, siderophore synthesis, and serum resistance of *Klebsiella* isolates causing human urinary tract infections. J. Infect. Dis. *168*:1415 1421, 1993.
63. Quinn, J. P.: Clinical significance of extended-spectrum beta-lactamases. Eur. J. Clin. Microbiol. Infect. Dis. *13*(Suppl. 1):S39 S42, 1994.
64. Ramirez-Ronda, C. H., Fuxench-Lopez, Z., and Nevarez, M.: Increased pharyngeal bacterial colonization during viral illness. Arch. Intern. Med. *141*:1599–1603, 1981.
65. Ransjo, U., Good, Z., Jalakas, K., et al.: An outbreak of *Klebsiella oxytoca* septicemias associated with the use of invasive blood pressure monitoring equipment. Acta Anaesthesiol. Scand. 36:289–291, 1992.
66. Reish, O., Ashkenazi, S., Naor, N., et al.: An outbreak of multiresistant *Klebsiella* in a neonatal intensive care unit. J. Hosp. Infect. *25*:287–291, 1993.
67. Sakata, H., Fujita, K., and Yoshioka, H.: The effect of antimicrobial agents on fecal flora of children. Antimicrob. Agents Chemother. *29*:225–229, 1986.
68. Sood, S. K., Mulvihill, D., and Daum, R. S.: Intrarenal abscess caused by *Klebsiella pneumoniae* in a neonate: Modern management and diagnosis. Am. J. Perinatol. *6*:367–370, 1989.
69. Tullus, K., Ayling-Smith, B., Kuhn, I., et al.: Nationwide spread of *Klebsiella oxytoca* K55 in Swedish neonatal special care wards. APMIS *100*:1008–1014, 1992.

110

MORGANELLA MORGANII

William C. Gruber and Randall G. Fisher

Like *Proteus* and *Providencia* species, *Morganella morganii* has emerged as an important nosocomial pathogen, most often associated with urinary tract or wound infection. Although most descriptions of infection are in adult populations, infections in children do occur.

BACTERIOLOGY

M. morganii (formerly *Proteus morganii*) is a motile gram-negative bacillus commonly found in the feces of humans, other mammals, and reptiles.[21] The organism was elevated to genus rank because of genetic differences from *Proteus,* with which it is otherwise biologically similar.[6] Most strains do not ferment lactose. *M. morganii, Proteus,* and *Providencia* are distinguished from other Enterobacteriaceae by their ability to deaminate phenylalanine and lysine. Organisms are indole-positive and ornithine decarboxylase–positive. Like *Proteus* and *Providencia, M. morganii* produces urease, but this enzyme is unrelated genetically and serologically to those of the other two genera.[16, 21] Unlike *Proteus, M. morganii* does not demonstrate swarming activity on 1.5 per cent agar.[21] (This organism liquefies gelatin and does not produce hydrogen sulfide.)

EPIDEMIOLOGY

Like *Proteus* and *Providencia* species, *Morganella* organisms commonly are found in soil, sewage, and manure. Like *Proteus mirabilis, M. morganii* commonly invades the instrument-fitted urinary tract and surgical wounds; adults in inpatient surgical units have the greatest risk for colonization and infection.[1] The institutionalized elderly also have frequent infection with these organisms. Urinary tract colonization with *Morganella* accompanying groin-skin colonization in elderly persons may account for the greater frequency of urinary tract infections in this population.[12] *M. morganii* accounted for nearly 10 per cent of 145 consecutive complicated, multidrug-resistant urinary tract infections.[9] *Escherichia coli* and *P. mirabilis* account for the vast majority of urinary tract infections in childhood, but *M. morganii* has been implicated in some cases of cystitis and pyelonephritis. In contrast with well-described nursery epidemics of *P. mirabilis* infection,[3, 8] no *M. morganii* neonatal outbreaks have been described, and central nervous system infections are rare in newborns.[11, 25]

PATHOPHYSIOLOGY

Factors that predispose the urinary tract to invasion by *P. mirabilis* and *Providencia* species also may favor *M. morganii* colonization and infection. These organisms all split urea, forming ammonium hydroxide and increasing local pH, which results in toxicity to renal cells and potentiation of urolithiasis.[5, 20] The ability of *P. mirabilis* to regenerate more rapidly in urine with faster generation of alkaline pH, when compared with *M. morganii,* may provide a selective advantage for the former organism in establishing itself as a urinary tract pathogen.[24]

CLINICAL MANIFESTATIONS

Urinary tract infection with *M. morganii* often is associated with an elevated urinary pH. Urolithiasis can occur, although perhaps less frequently than during *P. mirabilis* infection.[4] *M. morganii* has been recovered from less than 10 per cent of adult bacteremic episodes, but mortality rates have exceeded 20 per cent.[1] Other reported complications identified in immunocompromised or instrument-fitted patients include meningitis,[14, 19] arthritis,[13] empyema,[23] peritonitis,[15] and skin infection.[2] *M. morganii* has been recovered alone or in combination with other organisms from surgical wounds[9] and soft-tissue abscesses in children.[7]

DIAGNOSIS

M. morganii produces a reddish-brown pigment when cultured on nutrient media supplemented with 5 per cent tryptophan.[21] Urease production and deamination of tryptophan help to distinguish this bacteria from other organisms. Unlike the closely related *Proteus* and *Providencia* species, *M. morganii* generally ferments only glucose and mannose and does not produce a red color on lysine iron agar.[21] *M. morganii* may be missed or mistaken for other organisms in the common circumstance of polymicrobial infection in the catheterized patient. In one series, *M. morganii* actually was among the most common bacteriuric species in patients on long-term catheterization but commonly was missed by reference laboratories.[10] The clinical laboratory should be directed to look for this organism, particularly in circumstances of nosocomial urinary tract infection and sepsis.

TREATMENT

Effective treatment of local infections or septicemia relies on appropriate antibiotic choice, often including an aminoglycoside, combined with surgical débridement and drainage of abscesses as necessary. Variability in antimicrobial susceptibility can be wide among *M. morganii* and the related *Proteus* and *Providencia* strains, emphasizing the importance of species identification and susceptibility testing.[22] Fortunately, most urinary tract infections respond to ampicillin or third-generation cephalosporins, but failure to clear bacteria should alert the physician to the possibility of urolithiasis or structural abnormality[4]; stone removal or surgical correction of anatomic defects often is required for cure. Aztreonam has shown effectiveness in therapy for up to 98 per cent of multidrug-resistant strains.[9]

References

1. Adler, J. L., Burke, J. P., Martin, D. F., et al.: *Proteus* infection in a general hospital. II. Some clinical and epidemiological characteristics. Ann. Intern. Med. *75*:531–536, 1971.

2. Bagel, J., and Grossman, M. E.: Hemorrhagic bullae associated with *Morganella morganii* septicemia. J. Am. Acad. Dermatol. *12*:575–576, 1985.
3. Becker, A. H.: Infection due to *Proteus mirabilis* in a newborn nursery. Am. J. Dis. Child. *104*:355–359, 1962.
4. Bensman, A., Roubach, L., Allouch, G., et al.: Urolithiasis in children: Presenting signs, etiology, bacteriology and localisation. Acta Paediatr. Scand. *72*:879–883, 1983.
5. Braude, A. I., and Siemienski, J.: Role of bacterial urease in experimental pyelonephritis. J. Bacteriol. *80*:171–179, 1960.
6. Brenner, D. J., Farmer, J. J., III, Fanning, G. R., et al.: Deoxyribonucleic acid relatedness of *Proteus* and *Providencia* species. Int. J. Syst. Bacteriol. *28*:269–282, 1978.
7. Brook, I., and Martin, W. J.: Aerobic and anaerobic bacteriology of perirectal abscess in children. Pediatrics *66*:282–284, 1980.
8. Burke, J. P., Ingall, D., Klein, J. O., et al.: *Proteus mirabilis* infections in a hospital nursery traced to a human carrier. N. Engl. J. Med. *284*:115–121, 1971.
9. Cox, C. E.: Aztreonam therapy for complicated urinary tract infections caused by multidrug-resistant bacteria. Rev. Infect. Dis. *7*(Suppl. 4):S767–S771, 1985.
10. Damron, D. J., Warren, J. W., Chippendale, G. R., et al.: Do clinical microbiology laboratories report complete bacteriology in urine from patients with long-term urinary catheters? J. Clin. Microbiol. *24*:400–404, 1986.
11. Darby, C. P., and Hill, O.: *Proteus morganii* meningitis treated with trimethoprim-sulfamethoxazole (co-trimoxazole). Clin. Pediatr. *14*:669–672, 1975.
12. Ehrenkranz, N. J., Alfonso, B. C., Eckert, D. G., et al.: *Proteeae* species bacteriuria accompanying *Proteeae* species groin skin carriage in geriatric outpatients. J. Clin. Microbiol. *27*:1988–1991, 1989.
13. Haddad, J. J., Inglesby, T. V. J., and Addonizio, L.: Head and neck infections in pediatric cardiac transplant patients. Ear Nose Throat J. *74*:422–425, 1995.
14. Isaacs, R. D., and Ellis-Pegler, R. B.: Successful treatment of *Morganella morganii* meningitis with pefloxacin mesylate. J. Antimicrob. Chemother. *20*:769–770, 1987.
15. Isobe, H., Motomura, K., Kotou, K., et al.: Spontaneous bacterial empyema and peritonitis caused by *Morganella morganii*. J. Clin. Gastroenterol. *18*:87–88, 1994.
16. Jones, B. D., and Mobley, H. L.: Genetic and biochemical diversity of ureases of *Proteus*, *Providencia*, and *Morganella* species isolated from urinary tract infection. Infect. Immun. *55*:2198–2203, 1987.
17. Kaslow, R. A., Lindsey, J. O., Bison, A. L., et al.: Nosocomial infection with highly resistant *Proteus rettgeri*: Report of an epidemic. Am. J. Epidemiol. *104*:278–286, 1976.
18. Katz, L. M., Lewis, R. J., and Borenstein, D. G.: Successful joint arthroplasty following *Proteus morganii* (*Morganella morganii*) septic arthritis: A four-year study. Arthritis Rheum. *30*:583–585, 1987.
19. Mastroianni, A., Coronado, O., and Chiodo, F.: *Morganella morganii* meningitis in a patient with AIDS. J. Infect. *29*:356–357, 1994.
20. Musher, D. M., Griffith, D. P., Yawn, D., et al.: Role of urease in pyelonephritis resulting from urinary tract infection with *Proteus*. J. Infect. Dis. *131*:177–181, 1975.
21. Penner, J. L.: *Morganella*. *In* Krieg, N. R., and Holt, J. G. (eds.): Bergey's Manual of Systematic Bacteriology. Vol. 1. Baltimore, Williams & Wilkins, 1984, pp. 497–498.
22. Piccolomini, R., Cellini, L., Allocati, N., et al.: Comparative in vitro activities of 13 antimicrobial agents against *Morganella-Proteus-Providencia* group bacteria from urinary tract infections. Antimicrob. Agents Chemother. *31*:1644–1647, 1987.
23. Schonwetter, R. S., and Orson, F. M.: Chronic *Morganella morganii* arthritis in an elderly patient. J. Clin. Microbiol. *26*:1414–1415, 1988.
24. Senior, B. W.: *Proteus morganii* is less frequently associated with urinary tract infections than *Proteus mirabilis*: An explanation. J. Med. Microbiol. *16*:317–322, 1983.
25. Verboon-Maciolek, M., Vandertop, W. P., Peters, A. C., et al.: Neonatal brain abscess caused by *Morganella morganii*. Clin. Infect. Dis. *20*:471, 1995.

111

PROTEUS

William C. Gruber and Randall G. Fisher

Proteus species are pathogens that are associated increasingly with pediatric illness. Neonatal meningitis and pediatric urinary tract infections are the most common childhood settings in which these organisms are isolated, but infections of other organ systems have been described.

BACTERIOLOGY

Proteus species are motile, gram-negative bacilli that do not ferment lactose and are distinguished from other Enterobacteriaceae by their ability to deaminate phenylalanine and lysine. Rapid and abundant urease production further differentiates *Proteus* from *Providencia*.[20] *Proteus vulgaris* and *Proteus mirabilis* tend to form a thin, spreading growth (swarm) on the surface of moist agar media, often overgrowing other bacterial isolates. They also produce hydrogen sulfide and liquefy gelatin. *P. mirabilis* is distinguished from other *Proteus* species (e.g., *P. vulgaris*) by its inability to produce indole from tryptophan. Disparate DNA content and anomalous biochemical and serologic reactions have caused *Proteus morganii* to be renamed *Morganella morganii* (see Chapter 110),[20] and both terms for this organism appear in the clinical literature.

EPIDEMIOLOGY

Proteus species commonly are found in soil, sewage, and manure. Although they are normal inhabitants of the colon and perineum, their numbers can be increased in persons receiving antibiotic therapy.[17]

First reported by Buisine and Henninot in 1949,[8] neonatal meningitis due to *P. mirabilis* accounts for approximately 4 per cent of all neonatal meningitis cases.[26] Nursery outbreaks have been attributed to contaminated equipment as well as human carriers. Vertical transmission from mother to infant has been confirmed by DNA fingerprinting and ribotyping methods.[6] In Becker's series[4] of *P. mirabilis* neonatal meningitis, all affected infants came from the same nursery and all were exposed to mist from an apparatus that yielded *P. mirabilis*. The importance of hand carriage was well documented by Burke and associates[9]; newborn umbilical colonization and invasive disease were linked to a single nurse from whom *P. mirabilis* was cultured from hands, rectum, and vagina.

Proteus infection after the first few months of life most commonly involves the urinary tract. Although *Escherichia coli* accounts for the vast majority of urinary tract infections in childhood, *Proteus* species commonly are implicated in reported series of cystitis and pyelonephritis[5, 13, 18, 38]; *P. mirabilis* is the most common species of *Proteus* isolated. *P. mirabilis* has been cultured more frequently from the urethra of uncircumcised than of circumcised male infants and has replaced *E. coli* as the most prevalent pathogen in one consecutive series of male patients presenting with initial urinary tract infection.[18, 39]

Proteus urinary tract infection is one of the most common presenting signs of urolithiasis in childhood,[11] and *P. mirabilis* supplants *E. coli* as the major urinary tract pathogen in children prone to renal stone formation.[5] Diagnosis of greater than 50 per cent of pediatric urolithiasis cases is based on preceding urinary tract infection, and *Proteus* is responsible for up to 65 per cent of these infections.[5] Isolation of this organism as a pathogen on urine culture should alert the physician to the possible presence of a urinary tract stone.

PATHOPHYSIOLOGY

Most cases of central nervous system infection due to *Proteus* occur in neonates and are thought to arise by bacteremic spread of the organism to the brain or meninges. Contiguous spread to the brain from localized infections is reported occasionally.[25] As is the case with *Citrobacter* meningitis, a propensity for central nervous system abscess formation remains unexplained. Rabbit models of *P. mirabilis* meningitis have shown that in vivo concentrations of gentamicin necessary to produce bacterial killing are 10 to 30 times higher than those predicted from in vitro susceptibility testing.[37] Reduced aminoglycoside effect may be secondary to depressed cerebrospinal fluid pH associated with *P. mirabilis* infection.[37] Whatever the mechanism, lack of effective antimicrobial activity in the ventricles accounts in part for the persistence of organisms at these sites.

A number of factors may predispose the urinary tract to invasion by *Proteus. Proteus* splits urea, forming ammonium hydroxide and increasing local pH, which results in toxicity to renal cells and potentiation of urolithiasis.[7, 27] The ability of *P. mirabilis* to regenerate more rapidly in urine with faster generation of alkaline pH, when compared with *M. morganii (P. morganii),* may provide a selective advantage for the former organism in establishing itself as a urinary tract pathogen.[32] Biochemically complex struvite ($MgNH_4PO_4$) stones provide a refuge for *Proteus* organisms and form a barrier to effective antimicrobial therapy.[5] Struvite stone formation is a major cause of urinary bacterial persistence in adult women without azotemia,[36] and a similar case probably can be made for the pediatric patient with urolithiasis. *P. mirabilis* ureases demonstrated lower affinities for substrate but hydrolyzed urea 6 to 25 times faster than did enzymes from other species, which may explain the frequent association of this species with stone formation.[15] Pili may enhance the virulence of *Proteus* in pyelonephritis by increasing adherence of organisms to the renal pelvis.[33] Flagella have been implicated in the spread of this organism in the urinary tract[28]; the ability to invade host urothelial cells is coupled closely with the ability of *P. mirabilis* to differentiate into hyperflagellated, filamentous swarm cells capable of rapid spread on the surface of moist agar media.[1] Swarming behavior might inherently assist ascending colonization of the urinary tract, as demonstrated in a mouse model of infection.[2] The role of fimbriae as a factor predisposing to ascending infection is less clear.[3, 24]

CLINICAL MANIFESTATIONS

P. mirabilis can produce a broad spectrum of symptoms associated with neonatal infection. Most patients present with typical symptoms of early-onset neonatal sepsis, including nonspecific lethargy, fever, and poor feeding; manifestations of sepsis may include septic arthritis and osteomyelitis. A minority of patients present after the first week of life. Meningitis may occur with either early- or late-onset disease. Brain abscesses associated with subtle clinical abnormalities rarely develop for weeks to months prior to presentation.[10] *Proteus* brain abscesses are associated with a high degree of mortality, frequent complications, and increased risks of neurologic deficits in survivors.[16, 22, 34] Hydrocephalus is a particularly frequent complication and should be anticipated. Brain destruction may progress to porencephaly or compartmentalization of ventricles and often requires surgical intervention.[16] Computed tomography is useful, especially in diagnosing and following progression of cerebral complications.[34]

Urinary tract infection with these bacteria predominantly involves younger patients and often is associated with an elevated urinary pH; clinical findings and urine abnormalities often are less striking than in patients with *E. coli* urinary tract infections.[18] Up to 30 per cent of patients demonstrate recurrent infection during the 12 months after initial treatment.[18] Indwelling urinary catheters increase the risk of *Proteus* colonization and infection. Long-term indwelling urinary catheters may become blocked by encrustations of aggregated struvite crystals; prolonged colonization with urease-producing *P. mirabilis* is associated with this complication.[21]

Proteus species often are implicated as agents of septicemia in adult patients and account for approximately 8 per cent of gram-negative bacteremias in this group.[12, 19] In 60 per cent of *Proteus* bacteremic episodes in adults, the urinary tract has been determined to be the source[12]; no anatomic source is identified in 20 per cent of cases of *Proteus* bacteremia. *P. mirabilis* followed by *P. vulgaris* are the species responsible for the vast majority of cases of *Proteus* bacteremia. The overall incidence of gram-negative enteric bacteremia in the pediatric age group is lower than that of adults; 5 per cent of such cases are due to *Proteus.*[12] As in adults, the genitourinary tract is the most common identified source.[12] Mortality averages less than 40 per cent and strongly depends on the severity of underlying disease in the host.[12, 19]

Osteomyelitis,[29, 37] pneumonia,[12, 19, 30] mastoiditis,[25] and wound infections[19] also occur. In particular, pediatric osteomyelitis secondary to contiguous infection of traumatized soft tissue often is polymicrobial, and *Proteus* has been implicated as a copathogen in at least 10 per cent of such cases.[29]

DIAGNOSIS

Proteus is suspected readily because of its ability to swarm on the surface of moist agar. A selective medium developed for the isolation of proteae relies on the ability of all members to produce a dark brown pigment in medium containing DL-tryptophan.[14] Urease production, lack of indole production from tryptophan, and a positive result with ornithine decarboxylase testing distinguish *P. mirabilis* from *Providencia* and other *Proteus* species.[20]

TREATMENT

Treatment of meningitis due to *Proteus* should conform itself to standard regimens recommended for gram-negative meningitis. However, *P. mirabilis* usually is sensitive to ampicillin, and this drug alone or combined with an aminoglycoside often is suitable therapy once the identity and susceptibilities of the infecting organism are known.[31] A third-generation cephalosporin often is an alternative. Consecutive lumbar punctures should be performed for *Proteus* meningitis until cerebrospinal cultures are sterile. A minimum of 2 weeks of antibiotic therapy is recommended after bacteriologic cure. Ventricular aspiration or drainage of abscesses may be required to direct therapy, based on persistence of organisms at these sites. Open drainage of abscesses often is necessary, but resolution of abscess formation on antibiotic therapy alone has been reported.[35] Intraventricular antibiotics are not of proven benefit in terms of mortality or morbidity but have been used to clear ventricular colonization. A 15-year-old boy with *Proteus* mastoiditis and meningitis has been treated successfully with intravenous trimethoprim-sulfamethoxazole.[25]

Effective treatment of local infections or septicemia relies on appropriate antibiotic choice, often including an aminoglycoside, combined with surgical débridement and drainage of abscesses as necessary. Most *P. mirabilis* urinary tract infections respond to ampicillin, but some organisms have been shown to acquire a plasmid-mediated β-lactamase.[23] Failure to clear bacteria should alert the physician to the possibility of urolithiasis or structural abnormality; stone removal or surgical correction of anatomic defects often is required for cure.

References

1. Allison, C., Coleman, N., Jones P. L., et al.: Ability of *Proteus mirabilis* to invade human urothelial cells is coupled to motility and swarming differentiation. Infect. Immun. *60*:4740–4746, 1992.
2. Allison, C., Emody, L., Coleman, N., et al.: The role of swarm cell differentiation and multicellular migration in the uropathogenicity of *Proteus mirabilis*. J. Infect. Dis. *169*:1155–1158, 1994.
3. Bahrani, F. K., Massad, G., Lockatell, C. V., et al.: Construction of an MR/P fimbrial mutant of *Proteus mirabilis*: Role in virulence in a mouse model of ascending urinary tract infection. Infect. Immun. *62*:3363–3371, 1994.
4. Becker, A. H.: Infection due to *Proteus mirabilis* in a newborn nursery. Am. J. Dis. Child. *104*:355–359, 1962.
5. Bensman, A., Roubach, L., Allouch, G., et al.: Urolithiasis in children: Presenting signs, etiology, bacteriology and localisation. Acta Paediatr. Scand. *72*:879–883, 1983.
6. Bingen, E., Boissinot, C., Desjardins, P., et al.: Arbitrarily primed polymerase chain reaction provides rapid differentiation of *Proteus mirabilis* isolates from a pediatric hospital. J. Clin. Microbiol. *31*:1055–1059, 1993.
7. Braude, A. I., and Siemienski, J.: Role of bacterial urease in experimental pyelonephritis. J. Bacteriol. *80*:171–179, 1960.
8. Buisine, A., and Henninot, E.: Les meningites a *Proteus* chez l'enfant. Ann. Biol. Clin. *7*:448, 1949.
9. Burke, J. P., Ingall, D., Klein, J. O., et al.: *Proteus mirabilis* infections in a hospital nursery traced to a human carrier. N. Engl. J. Med. *284*:115–121, 1971.
10. Darby, C. P., Conner, E., and Kyong, C. U.: *Proteus mirabilis* brain abscess in a neonate. Dev. Med. Child Neurol. *20*:366–375, 1978.
11. Diamond, D. A.: Clinical patterns of paediatric urolithiasis. Br. J. Urol. *68*:195–198, 1991.
12. duPont, H. L., and Spink, W. H.: Infections due to gram-negative organisms: An analysis of 860 patients with bacteremia at the University of Minnesota Medical Center, 1958–1966. Medicine *48*:307–329, 1969.
13. Ginsburg, C. M., and McCracken, G. H., Jr.: Urinary tract infections in young infants. Pediatrics *69*:409–412, 1982.
14. Hawkey, P. M., McCormick, A., and Simpson, R. A.: Selective and differential medium for the primary isolation of members of the Proteeae. J. Clin. Microbiol. *23*:600–603, 1986.
15. Jones, B. D., and Mobley, H. L.: Genetic and biochemical diversity of ureases of *Proteus, Providencia,* and *Morganella* species isolated from urinary tract infection. Infect. Immun. *55*:2198–2203, 1987.
16. Kalsbeck, J. E., DeSousa, A. L., Kleiman, M. B., et al.: Compartmentalization of the cerebral ventricles as a sequela of neonatal meningitis. J. Neurosurg. *52*:547–552, 1980.
17. Kaslow, R. A., Lindsey, J. O., Bison, A. L., et al.: Nosocomial infection with highly resistant *Proteus rettgeri*: Report of an epidemic. Am. J. Epidemiol. *104*:278–286, 1976.
18. Khan, A. J., Ubriani, R. S., Bombach, E., et al.: Initial urinary tract infection caused by *Proteus mirabilis* in infancy and childhood. J. Pediatr. *93*:791–793, 1978.
19. Kreger, B. E., Craven, D. E., Carling, P. C., et al.: Gram-negative bacteremia. III. Reassessment of etiology, epidemiology and ecology in 612 patients. Am. J. Med. *68*:332–343, 1980.
20. Krieg, N. R., and Holt, J. G. (eds.): Bergey's Manual of Systematic Bacteriology. Baltimore, Williams & Wilkins, 1984, pp. 491–494.
21. Kunin, C. M.: Blockage of urinary catheters: Role of microorganisms and constituents of the urine on formation of encrustations. J. Clin. Epidemiol. *42*:835–842, 1989.
22. Levy, H. L., and Ingall, D.: Meningitis in neonates due to *Proteus mirabilis*. Am. J. Dis. Child. *114*:320–324, 1967.
23. Mariotte, S., Nordmann, P., and Nicolas, M. H.: Extended-spectrum beta-lactamase in *Proteus mirabilis*. J. Antimicrob. Chemother. *33*:925–935, 1994.
24. Massad, G., Lockatell, C. V., Johnson, D. E., et al.: *Proteus mirabilis* fimbriae: Construction of an isogenic pmfA mutant and analysis of virulence in a CBA mouse model of ascending urinary tract infection. Infect. Immun. *62*:536–542, 1994.
25. McConville, J. H., and Manzella, J. P.: Parenteral trimethoprim/sulfamethoxazole for gram-negative bacillary meningitis. Am. J. Med. Sci. *287*:43–45, 1984.
26. McCracken, G. H., Jr.: New developments in the management of children with bacterial meningitis. Pediatr. Infect. Dis. *3*:S32–S34, 1984.
27. Musher, D. M., Griffith, D. P., Yawn, D., et al.: Role of urease in pyelonephritis resulting from urinary tract infection with *Proteus*. J. Infect. Dis. *131*:177–181, 1975.
28. Pazin, G. J., and Braude, A. I.: Immobilizing antibodies in urine. 2. Prevention of ascending spread of *Proteus mirabilis*. Invest. Virol. *122*:129–133, 1974.
29. Pichichero, M. E., and Friesen, H. A.: Polymicrobial osteomyelitis: Report of three cases and review of the literature. Rev. Infect. Dis. *4*:86–96, 1982.
30. Pine, J. R., and Hollman, J. L.: Elevated pleural fluid pH in *Proteus mirabilis* empyema. Chest *84*:109–111, 1983.
31. Scherzer, A. L., Kaye, D., and Shinefield, H. R.: *Proteus mirabilis* meningitis: Report of two cases treated with ampicillin. J. Pediatr. *68*:731–740, 1966.
32. Senior, B. W.: *Proteus morganii* is less frequently associated with urinary tract infections than *Proteus mirabilis*: An explanation. J. Med. Microbiol. *16*:317–322, 1983.
33. Silverblatt, F. J.: Host-parasite interaction in the rat renal pelvis: A possible role for pili in the pathogenesis of pyelonephritis. J. Exp. Med. *140*:1696–1711, 1974.
34. Smith, M. L., and Mellor, D.: *Proteus mirabilis* meningitis and cerebral abscess in the newborn period. Arch. Dis. Child. *55*:308–310, 1980.
35. Spirer, Z., Jurgenson, U., Lazewnick, R., et al.: Complete recovery from an apparent brain abscess treated without neurosurgery: The importance of early CT scanning. Clin. Pediatr. *21*:106–109, 1982.
36. Stamey, T. A.: Pathogenesis and Treatment of Urinary Tract Infections. Baltimore, Williams & Wilkins, 1980.
37. Strausbaugh, L. J., and Sande, M. A.: Factors influencing the therapy of experimental *Proteus mirabilis* meningitis in rabbits. J. Infect. Dis. *137*:251–260, 1978.
38. Wientzen, R. L., McCracken, G. H., Jr., Petruska, M. L., et al.: Localization and therapy of urinary tract infections of childhood. Pediatrics *63*:467–473, 1979.
39. Wiswell, T. E., Miller, G. M., Gelston, H. M., et al.: Effect of circumcision status on periurethral bacterial flora during the first year of life. J. Pediatr. *113*:442–446, 1988.

112

PROVIDENCIA

William C. Gruber and Randall G. Fisher

The genus *Providencia* comprises pathogens most commonly associated with urinary tract infection. *Providencia* species are encountered most often as pathogens in hospitals or chronic care facilities and can be responsible for outbreaks of multidrug-resistant infection.[22]

BACTERIOLOGY

Providencia species, named after the city of Providence, Rhode Island, are motile gram-negative bacilli that do not ferment lactose and are distinguished from other Enterobacteriaceae by their ability to deaminate phenylalanine and lysine.[7, 20] The genus distinguishes "urease-negative" organisms *P. rettgeri*, *P. stuartii*, *P. alcalifaciens*, *P. rustigianii*, and *P. heimbachae* from the otherwise biochemically similar "urease-positive" *Proteus* species.[14, 20] Urease is produced by most strains of *P. rettgeri* and by 15 per cent or less of *P. stuartii* strains.[20] *Providencia* also differs from other Proteae in its ability to produce acid from inositol. Strains are differentiated further by reactivity with straight-chain hydroxy alcohols.[20]

EPIDEMIOLOGY

Providencia organisms are recovered uncommonly from stool in healthy human subjects but frequently colonize indwelling or condom urinary catheters, particularly in persons receiving antibiotic therapy.[4, 9, 15, 22, 23] *Providencia* species have been recognized as pathogens for more than 50 years[7]; *P. rettgeri* and *P. stuartii* are the most common species implicated in urinary tract infection.[9, 11, 12, 17, 23] Multiple biotypes of *P. stuartii* have been identified in hospital outbreaks, indicating the probability of multiple sources of colonization.[2]

PATHOPHYSIOLOGY

P. stuartii does not appear to have greater access to the urinary tract compared with other bacteria; in chronically catheterized patients, the incidence of bacteruria caused by this organism is equivalent to that caused by other uropathogens.[22] Rather, *P. stuartii* manifests an extraordinary ability to persist within the catheterized urinary tract.[23] Bacteruria may take weeks to months to clear. A mannose-resistant, *Klebsiella*-like hemagglutinin may play an important role in the persistence and adherence of *P. stuartii* to urinary tract catheters.[18]

Despite the similarities between *Proteus mirabilis* (the major pathogen responsible for urolithiasis in children)[3] and urease-producing *Providencia* species, the latter organisms rarely are associated with stone formation. *P. stuartii* occasionally produces urease with a higher affinity for substrate, but *P. mirabilis* ureases hydrolyze urea 6 to 25 times faster.[13] Restriction-enzyme analysis of genes coding for the respective enzymes shows significant divergence.[13] These differences may explain the more frequent association of *P. mirabilis* with stone formation.

Some strains of *Providencia alcalifaciens* have been reported to cause diarrhea, and enteropathogenicity has been demonstrated in a rabbit model.[1]

CLINICAL MANIFESTATIONS

Although *Escherichia coli* and *Proteus* species account for the vast majority of urinary tract infections in childhood, *Providencia* species have been reported as a cause of infection in children with spinal injury and long-term urinary tract catheterization.[16, 17] Most infections, however, have been described in the elderly or adult spinal injury patient who requires chronic urinary tract catheterization.[22] Clinical findings are typical of those associated with urinary tract infection. In the rare setting of bacteremia, vascular collapse may occur.[16]

DIAGNOSIS

Providencia should be suspected when indole-positive, urease-negative, gram-negative rods, which oxidatively deaminate tryptophan, are isolated in culture. Because chronically catheterized patients may be colonized with multiple organisms, it is common for *Providencia* species to be overlooked or misidentified.[6] Therefore, clinical laboratories should be encouraged to identify all bacterial colonies in chronically catheterized individuals in whom infection is suspected. Identification particularly is important because of the marked differences in susceptibility of uropathogens.[21]

TREATMENT

Empiric therapy should be guided by antimicrobial susceptibility testing of the patient's isolate and a knowledge of susceptibilities of previously identified *Providencia* within the care facility. Removal of urinary tract catheters speeds eradication of these pathogens. Strains of *P. stuartii* and *P. rettgeri* commonly are resistant to many antibiotics. Since the 1970s, multidrug resistance has emerged[19]; many strains are resistant to sulfonamides, trimethoprim, nitrofurantoin, nalidixic acid, penicillins, cephalosporins, and aminoglycosides; some singular strains are resistant to most antibiotics in common use.[21] Much of the observed resistance appears to be plasmid-based[10]; quinolones and aztreonam have shown some promise in the treatment of such cases.[5, 8] Organisms that are resistant to gentamicin and tobramycin may remain susceptible to amikacin.

References

1. Albert, M. J., Ansaruzzaman, M., Bhuiyan, N. A., et al.: Characteristics of invasion of HEp-2 cells by *Providencia alcalifaciens*. J. Med. Microbiol. *42*:186–190, 1995.
2. Albert, M. J., Alam, K., Ansaruzzaman, M., et al.: Pathogenesis of *Providencia alcalifaciens*–induced diarrhea. Infect. Immun. *60*:5017–5024, 1992.
3. Bensman, A., Roubach, L., Allouch, G., et al.: Urolithiasis in children: Presenting signs, etiology, bacteriology and localisation. Acta Paediatr. Scand. *72*:879–883, 1983.

4. Breitenbucher, R. B.: Bacterial changes in the urine samples of patients with long-term indwelling catheters. Arch. Intern. Med. *144*:1585–1588, 1984.
5. Cox, C. E.: Aztreonam therapy for complicated urinary tract infections caused by multidrug-resistant bacteria. Rev. Infect. Dis. *7*(Suppl. 4):S767–S771, 1985.
6. Damron, D. J., Warren, J. W., Chippendale, G. R., et al.: Do clinical microbiology laboratories report complete bacteriology in urine from patients with long-term urinary catheters? J. Clin. Microbiol. *24*:400–404, 1986.
7. Ewing, W. H., Tanner, K. E., and Dennard, D. A.: The providence group: An intermediate group of enteric bacteria. J. Infect. Dis. *94*:134–140, 1954.
8. Fang, G. D., Brennen, C., Wagener, M., et al.: Use of ciprofloxacin versus use of aminoglycosides for therapy of complicated urinary tract infection: Prospective, randomized clinical and pharmacokinetic study. Antimicrob. Agents Chemother. *35*:1849–1855, 1991.
9. Fierer, J., and Ekstrom, M.: An outbreak of *Providencia stuartii* urinary tract infections: Patients with condom catheters are a reservoir of the bacteria. J. A. M. A. *245*:1553–1555, 1981.
10. Hawkey, P. M.: *Providencia stuartii*: A review of a multiply antibiotic-resistanct bacterium. J. Antimicrob. Chemother. *13*:209–226, 1984.
11. Hawkey, P. M., Penner, J. L., Potten, M. R., et al.: Prospective survey of fecal, urinary tract, and environmental colonization by *Providencia stuartii* in two geriatric wards. J. Clin. Microbiol. *16*:422–426, 1982.
12. Hollick, G. E., Nolte, F. S., Calnan, B. J., et al.: Characterization of endemic *Providencia stuartii* isolates from patients with urinary devices. Eur. J. Clin. Microbiol. *3*:521–525, 1984.
13. Jones, B. D., and Mobley, H. L.: Genetic and biochemical diversity of ureases of *Proteus, Providencia,* and *Morganella* species isolated from urinary tract infection. Infect. Immun. *55*:2198–2203, 1987.
14. Jones, B. D., and Mobley, H. L.: *Proteus mirabilis* urease: Genetic organization, regulation, and expression of structural genes. J. Bacteriol. *170*:3342–3349, 1988.
15. Kaslow, R. A., Lindsey, J. O., Bison, A. L., et al.: Nosocomial infection with highly resistant *Proteus rettgeri*: Report of an epidemic. Am. J. Epidemiol. *104*:278–286, 1976.
16. Keren, G., and Tyrrel, D. L.: Gram-negative septicemia caused by *Providencia stuartii*. Int. J. Pediatr. Nephrol. *8*:91–94, 1987.
17. McHale, P. J., Walker, F., Scully, B., et al.: *Providencia stuartii* infections: A review of 117 cases over an eight-year period. J. Hosp. Infect. *2*:155–165, 1981.
18. Mobley, H. L., Chippendale, G. R., Tenney, J. H., et al.: MR/K hemagglutination of *Providencia stuartii* correlates with adherence to catheters and with persistence in catheter-associated bacteriuria. J. Infect. Dis. *157*:264–271, 1988.
19. Overturf, G. D., Wilkins, J., and Ressler, R.: Emergence of resistant *P. stuartii* to multiple antibiotics: Specification and biochemical characterization of *Providencia*. J. Infect. Dis. *129*:353–357, 1974.
20. Penner, J. L.: *Providencia*. *In* Krieg, N. R., and Holt, J. G. (eds.): Bergey's Manual of Systematic Bacteriology. Vol. 1. Baltimore, Williams & Wilkins, 1984, pp. 494–496.
21. Piccolomini, R., Cellini, L., Allocati, N., et al.: Comparative in vitro activities of 13 antimicrobial agents against *Morganella-Proteus-Providencia* group bacteria from urinary tract infections. Antimicrob. Agents Chemother. *31*:1644–1647, 1987.
22. Warren, J. W.: *Providencia stuartii*: A common cause of antibiotic-resistant bacteriuria in patients with long-term indwelling catheters. Rev. Infect. Dis. *8*:61–67, 1986.
23. Warren, J. W., Tenney, J. H., Hoopes, J. M., et al.: A prospective microbiologic study of bacteriuria in patients with chronic indwelling urethral catheters. J. Infect. Dis. *146*:719–723, 1982.

113

SHIGELLA

Henry F. Gomez and Thomas G. Cleary

Shigellosis, or bacillary dysentery, is characterized by acute febrile diarrhea with abdominal pain, often with mucus or blood in the feces. The patient typically is toxic and not infrequently develops extraintestinal manifestations of infection.

HISTORICAL BACKGROUND

The term dysentery classically has been used to describe the frequent painful passage of stools containing blood and mucus. The syndrome has been recognized since the time of Hippocrates. The differentiation of dysentery into bacillary and amebic forms followed the recognition by Shiga in 1898 that one form of dysentery was associated with a bacterium in the stools of affected individuals; their sera also was found to agglutinate the bacillus. In recognition of his achievement, the genus was named after Shiga.

The most important subsequent advance has been the recognition of the molecular basis of *Shigella* virulence. Forty years ago, it was demonstrated that shigellae invade the corneal epithelium of guinea pigs and cause keratoconjunctivitis (Sereny test). Subsequently, Formal and colleagues[63] showed that *S. flexneri* invades the intestinal epithelium. Since 1980, Sansonetti, Maurelli, and other investigators[169, 170, 172] have identified multiple plasmid and chromosomal virulence genes and their associated protein products. The 120- to 140-megadalton virulence plasmid absolutely is necessary (but not sufficient) for a strain to cause disease; chromosomal genes also are necessary for full virulence. *Shigella*-like enteroinvasive *Escherichia coli* have the same genes and produce a similar clinical syndrome.

THE ORGANISM

Shigellae are small, nonencapsulated gram-negative rods that are members of the family Enterobacteriaceae. Technically, they are *E. coli*, but for reasons of tradition and clinical usefulness, the designation has been preserved. The shigellae do not ferment lactose or do so slowly and are nonmotile (lack the H [flagellar] antigen). They lack urease and do not produce hydrogen sulfide on triple sugar iron media or gas during carbohydrate metabolism.[55] Their core lipopolysaccharide antigens are shared with other members of Enterobacteriaceae. The somatic antigen (or O antigen) side chains that determine serotype/serogroup are attached as multiple repeating units to the lipid A core and core oligosaccharides. Envelope or K antigens that are heat-labile also have been described, although their clinical relevance is uncertain.

Serogroup Classification

Four serogroups, or species, of *Shigella* are defined based on serologic similarities and biochemical reactions. Group A (*S. dysenteriae*), the mannitol nonfermenters, includes 13 serotypes that do not cross-react immunologically. There are two additional provisional serovars, types 14 and 15, that also are pathogenic.[9] Serogroup D (*S. sonnei*), the ornithine decarboxylase-positive, slow lactose fermenters, all share the same lipopolysaccharide. *Shigella* strains that ferment mannitol (unlike *S. dysenteriae*) but do not decarboxylate ornithine or ferment lactose (unlike *S. sonnei*) are classified as serogroups B and C; of these, the strains that express lipopolysaccharides that are related to each other immunologically are group B (*S. flexneri*), whereas those whose O antigens are unrelated to each other or to other shigellae are group C (*S. boydii*). There are multiple serotypes of *S. flexneri* (1a, 1b, 2a, 2b, 3a, 3b, 4a, 4b, 5a, 5b, 6, X variant, and Y variant) and of *S. boydii* (18 serotypes).

EPIDEMIOLOGY

Because shigellae are spread through a fecal-oral route, they especially are prevalent where hygiene is poor. The organisms can be cultured from around toilets in homes where shigellae have caused disease. Toilet paper does not prevent contamination of fingers. Thus, handwashing and wearing gloves are mandatory procedures for those caring for patients with bacillary dysentery. Shigellae are transmitted easily from person to person because the inoculum size required to cause disease is as few as 10 organisms in the case of *S. dysenteriae* serotype 1[52] and a few hundred organisms in the case of *S. sonnei* and *S. flexneri*.[49] Patients who lack the acid barrier provided by a normally functioning stomach because of prior gastrectomy or antacid use are at increased risk of infection. Shigellae survive for up to 30 days in such foods as milk, whole eggs, oysters, shrimp, and flour.[118] Epidemics usually are associated with contaminated water or food exposures,[193] although, as might be predicted from the inoculum size, outbreaks related to swimming also occur.[112] Houseflies can be colonized with shigellae in their guts without illness and pass shigellae in their feces. Feces adherent to their legs can lead to contamination of food. Flies have been implicated in epidemics of shigellosis, particularly where the fly population is large. *Shigella* infection shows seasonal variation. In North America, there are relatively few cases in the winter, whereas in tropical regions, the peak is during the rainy season. Thus, shigellae are worldwide and thrive where susceptible individuals are grouped together (including institutions for the retarded or mentally ill, prisoner-of-war camps, Indian reservations, the military, day care centers, and the developing world).[93, 151, 183] Spread within family groups is typical.

There are regional variations in the species of *Shigella* causing most infections. In the developed countries, *S. sonnei* is the most common species, followed by *S. flexneri* (about 70 per cent *S. sonnei* and 25 per cent *S. flexneri*); however, in the developing world, this pattern is reversed, and in addition there are occasional outbreaks of *S. dysenteriae* serotype 1. The developing world pattern of infection was seen in the United States early in the twentieth century.

Humans and other primates can be infected with shigellae. There is an age-related risk of acquiring symptomatic shigellosis. Unlike *Salmonella* species, which are most frequent in the first few months of life, shigellae infrequently cause illness in the first 6 months of life. The peak incidence occurs between 1 and 4 years of age, with fewer cases between 5 and 9 years of age. Adults account for a minority of cases, although young mothers are at risk, presumably because they care for susceptible infants and because they traditionally handle fecal material more regularly than do men. Women thus may be exposed to larger inocula that overcome partial immunity.

PATHOGENESIS

Invasiveness

The ability to invade mammalian cells is the most important virulence trait of *Shigella* species.[65, 101, 104, 130, 144] Invasion of M cells overlying Peyer's patches may be the earliest event. Uptake of organisms by macrophages under the M cells induces cytokine production and recruitment of polymorphonuclear leukocytes. Apoptosis is induced in macrophages after ingestion of *Shigella*; these events are accompanied by release of interleukin 1 (IL-1), which in turn triggers other inflammatory events.[196, 197] Polymorphonuclear leukocytes enter the gut lumen by moving between epithelial cells. The gaps between epithelial cells may be the portal of entry of bacteria into the epithelium. After penetration of intestinal epithelial cells, shigellae are located in vacuoles derived from the cytoplasmic membrane of the mucosal cells. The bacteria lyse these vacuoles, move intracellularly, multiply, kill the epithelial cells, and infect adjacent cells. Cell death is followed by formation of ulcerations and microabscesses in the colon. Unlike *Salmonella* infection, *Shigella* infection rarely spreads beyond the lamina propria, so that bacteremia and metastatic infections are very uncommon.

The genetic basis of virulence has been studied extensively in the last 15 years. Invasiveness is the result primarily of genes on a large 120- to 140-megadalton (200- to 220-kb) virulence plasmid (Fig. 113–1).[72, 73, 81, 169–172] The invasive plasmid antigen (ipa) region includes genes for four polypeptides needed for invasion; these genes are *ipaA, ipaB, ipaC*, and *ipaD*. The proteins produced by these loci are recognized by the humoral immune system. The product of the *ipaB* locus is essential for induction of apoptosis in macrophages.[198] The inv region of the virulence plasmid is necessary for orientation of the ipa-encoded proteins into the outer membrane of the bacteria. The *virG* gene encodes a protein that causes intracellular and intercellular spread of shigellae after invasion of epithelial cells. The *virF* gene regulates a locus (*virB*) that is responsible for positive regulation of the *ipa* genes.[165] Although less important, chromosomal loci also regulate virulence.[148] Lipopolysaccharides are encoded by chromosomal genes; the lipopolysaccharides probably play a role in resistance to nonspecific host defense mechanisms that are encountered during tissue invasion. Smooth colonies express the complete complex of lipopolysaccharide O side chains required for full virulence, that is, ability to invade epithelial cells, multiply within them, and also resist phagocytosis.[68, 145] Rough colonial variants that lack complete lipopolysaccharides do not penetrate epithelial cells efficiently and are avirulent. Chromosomal loci also regulate expression of the virulence plasmid. The keratoconjunctivitis provocation (*kcpA*) gene is a positive regulator of the *virG* virulence plasmid gene that determines ability to spread within and between cells. The chromosomal *virR* gene is a temperature regulator that represses expression of *ipa* genes at 30° C but not at 37° C. Other chromosomal (i.e., mannitol-arginine–related) loci and plasmid/chromosomal (i.e., *ipaH*) genes also are related to virulence, although their role is not understood.

Some strains of *Shigella* produce toxins that injure mammalian cells. There is a chromosomal locus in *S. dysenteriae* serotype 1 that encodes for a protein synthesis–inhibiting exotoxin (Shiga toxin) that clearly is a major virulence factor in this serotype (and in the enterohemorrhagic *E. coli* serotypes that have the same or closely related genes).[21, 178] This toxin is composed of a single copy of an A subunit (32,000 daltons) that is linked to five copies of B subunits (7790 daltons).[142] The B subunits bind to a glycolipid cell receptor, globotriaosylceramide, followed by internalization of the enzymatically active A subunit. The A subunit cleaves an adenine residue from the eukaryotic 28S ribosomal subunit. The resulting block in elongation factor 1–dependent binding of aminoacyl tRNA to the ribosome causes cell death through inhibition of protein synthesis.[142] Shiga toxin once was considered to be a neurotoxin because its administration to mice

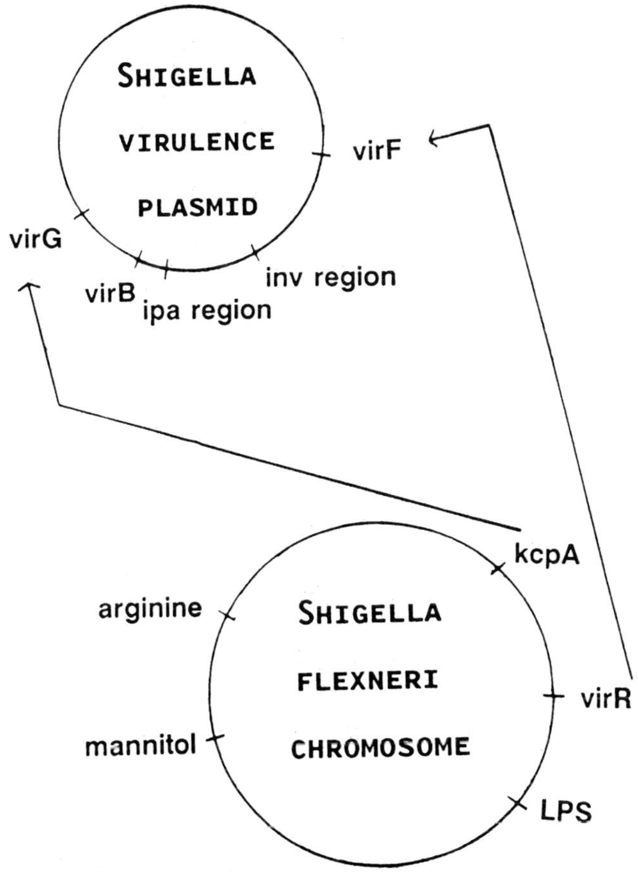

FIGURE 113–1. *Major plasmid and chromosomal genes of* Shigella *that are related to virulence. Plasmid loci include the invasive plasmid antigens (ipa), which encode surface proteins that are necessary for invasion;* virG *gene, which is necessary for intracellular and intercellular spread; inv region, which is necessary for orientation of the ipa proteins in the outer membrane; and* virB, *which is a positive regulator of the* ipa *genes. Important chromosomal loci include genes encoding for the lipopolysaccharide (LPS); the keratoconjunctivitis provocation* (kcpA) *gene, which is a positive regulator of the plasmid* virG *gene; and the* virR *gene, which suppresses the expression of* ipa *genes at 30° C. Also shown is the location of the genes for biosynthesis of arginine and degradation of mannitol. Arginine- and mannitol-linked genes also are necessary for full virulence.*

or rabbits caused paralysis and death[33, 41, 84]; it now is thought to target primarily the vascular endothelium. It causes fluid accumulation in rabbit ileal loops,[57, 94] probably related to reduced fluid uptake by damaged villus cells.

The severity of *S. dysenteriae* serotype 1 infection relative to other *Shigella* serotypes is thought to be due to production of Shiga toxin. Enterohemorrhagic *E. coli,* such as *E. coli* O157:H7, produce an identical (Shiga-like toxin I) or similar (Shiga-like toxin II) toxin and, like *S. dysenteriae* serotype 1, cause bloody diarrhea and hemolytic uremic syndrome. Enteroinvasive *E. coli* do not produce these toxins.[43] *Shigella* serotypes other than *S. dysenteriae* serotype 1 produce little or no Shiga toxin, although other exotoxins are made.[21]

S. flexneri 2a strains make an enterotoxin referred to as ShET1. All *S. flexneri* 2a produce this enterotoxin, whereas only 3.3 per cent of other *Shigella* serotypes and no enteroinvasive *E. coli* serotypes possess the gene for this toxin.[139] Genes of an additional toxin, designated *Shigella* enterotoxin, or Sen, have been found in 75 per cent of enteroinvasive *E. coli* and 83 per cent of *Shigella* strains.[128] These new enterotoxins may be the cause of the watery diarrhea often seen early in the course of shigellosis.

Immune Response

Serum IgG, IgM, and IgA responses occur both to the lipopolysaccharide and invasion plasmid antigens of shigellae.[141] Secretory IgA to both of these sets of antigens occurs in both human milk and feces.[42] Many investigators believe that protection primarily is serotype-specific. The level of IgG antibodies to lipopolysaccharide present in an individual prior to infection appears to determine whether or not symptomatic shigellosis develops.[46] No clear proof currently exists regarding the role of antibodies to the invasion plasmid virulence proteins or to the toxins. Cell-mediated immunity against shigellae also may play a role in resolution of infection. Antibody-dependent cellular cytotoxicity against shigellae has been demonstrated.

The levels of cytokines (tumor necrosis factor–α [TNF-α], IL-1β, IL-1ra, IL-6, IL-8, and granulocyte macrophage colony-stimulating factor [GM-CSF]) in stool correlate with the severity of shigellosis. Interferon-γ levels are depressed early and rise during recovery. Fecal concentrations of TNF-α, IL-1β, IL-1ra, IL-6, IL-8, and GM-CSF are significantly higher in patients with *S. dysenteriae* serotype 1 than in those with *S. flexneri*.[160] Elevated TNF-α and IL-6 levels in stool and serum have been associated with complications during *S. dysenteriae* serotype 1 infection.[78] Infiltration of polymorphonuclear leukocytes and lymphocytes into the intestine is controlled by these cytokines. T lymphocytes with both suppressor/cytotoxic and helper/inducer phenotypes are recruited into the epithelium and lamina propria during *Shigella* infection related in part to the induction of HLA-DR expression in the rectal mucosa.[159]

PATHOLOGY

The main morphologic changes of shigellosis (superficial ulcerations, focal hemorrhages, mucosal edema, erythema, and friability) occur in the colon where the organisms invade.[87, 179] The rectosigmoid and distal colons typically are involved more severely than the proximal colon. The epithelial cell damage may cause development of a pseudomembrane composed of thick, fibropurulent exudate tightly adherent to the necrotic ulcerated colonic mucosa. Pseudopolyposis also has been reported.[38] Microscopically, there is damage to epithelial cells, ulcerations, goblet cell depletion, and intense polymorphonuclear and mononuclear infiltration with crypt abscesses. Vessels in the lamina propria are congested or thrombosed. Perforation of the colon usually does not occur as part of the colitis.[19] Histologic changes in general are more severe with *S. dysenteriae* than with *S. flexneri*.[8] Evidence of inflammation and proinflammatory cytokines persists for at least a month after clinical resolution.[158]

CLINICAL MANIFESTATIONS

The incubation period may be as short as 12 hours up to a few days (if a low number of organisms are ingested). Onset of high fever, toxicity, and crampy abdominal pain is sudden. During the first 48 hours, high-volume watery diarrhea (small bowel phase of disease) may occur; subsequently, small volume, bloody, and mucousy diarrhea develops, associated with urgency and tenesmus (large bowel disease). In some, the watery diarrhea persists for several days, without subsequent development of dysentery. Other children present with bloody or mucousy diarrhea.

Physical examination shows fever, signs of toxicity, tenderness over the lower abdominal quadrants, and hyperactive bowel sounds. Signs of dehydration may be present. Rectal examination reveals severe tenderness. Rectal prolapse may be present, particularly when diarrhea is associated with malnutrition.

The course without therapy typically lasts 7 to 10 days. Protein-losing enteropathy occurs during shigellosis; this enteropathy is severe with *S. dysenteriae* serotype 1.[28] In addition, anorexia related in part to fever and abdominal pain further contributes to malnutrition; anorexia particularly is problematic in *S. dysenteriae* type 1 infection.[157] These facts partly may explain the hypoproteinemia and adverse effect on growth of severe shigellosis. Malnutrition is associated with a more severe course of shigellosis. Fever may not develop, even when severe dysentery is present. Chronic infection may last for months, despite appropriate antibiotic therapy. This may cause further deterioration of the nutritional status, which, together with other complications (such as ileus, bacteremia, and pneumonia), is associated with overall increased mortality from shigellosis.

Although the organism usually is excreted for only a few days or weeks (range, 1–30 days), carriage for many months is well documented.[44, 105] Although the illness usually is acute, a chronic carrier state can occur in the malnourished individual. Surprisingly, asymptomatic infection of toddlers living in an endemic area is very common; for example, the majority of *Shigella* infections in Mexican children cultured each week from birth are not associated with illness.[70]

Extraintestinal Manifestations and Complications

Seizures have been reported in 10 to 45 per cent of hospitalized children with culture-proven shigellosis.[15, 18, 20, 48, 61] In outpatient settings, the frequency of seizures is very low. Those children who develop neurologic complaints may have lethargy, severe headache, disorientation, hallucinations, or self-limited convulsions lasting less than 15 minutes.[13, 16, 18, 124] Seizures are most likely in the very young, those with a high peak body temperature, and those with a family history of convulsive disorders.[15, 97] Seizures can be focal, although usually they are generalized. When symptoms related to the nervous system occur, they are likely to be very early in the illness, often even preceding development of diarrhea. Death rarely has been described[83]; most children recover completely with no residual neurologic deficits.[16] The pathogenesis of neurologic signs and symptoms during shigellosis is unclear. Hypoglycemia and electrolyte abnormalities are found in a few patients.[16] Direct invasion of the central nervous system during *Shigella* bacteremia is very rare.[194] Simple febrile seizures might explain convulsions in a few children with dysentery, but some children with seizures during shigellosis do not experience seizures during other febrile infections and are outside the age range usually associated with febrile seizures.[16] Shigatoxin formerly was thought to cause the neurologic symptoms because it was considered to be a neurotoxin. However, data now clearly demonstrate that Shiga toxin is not responsible.[14]

Severe toxic encephalopathy has been described. This syndrome (Ekiri), as originally described in Japan, was characterized by dysentery with hyperpyrexia, convulsions, sensory disturbances, and rapid progression to death.[166] The children died with cerebral edema early in the course of disease (6 to 48 hours after onset). Mild hyponatremia has been very common.[67] The children with Ekiri did not have sepsis, disseminated intravascular coagulation, hemolytic uremic syndrome, or severe dehydration. This toxic encephalopathy is rare. It is not clear whether this syndrome is part of a continuum of central nervous system dysfunctions with seizures and other encephalopathic symptoms or whether it has a completely different pathogenesis.

Hemolytic uremic syndrome (microangiopathic hemolytic anemia, thrombocytopenia, and acute renal failure) or isolated hemolysis has been reported, mainly after infections with *S. dysenteriae* 1 and rarely after *S. flexneri* infection.[155] Vascular endothelial cell damage by Shiga toxin is considered to be the initial event, although endotoxin absorbed from the gut also may play a role.[96]

Ileus that progresses to toxic megacolon with distended loops and eventual intestinal perforation[19] is seen mainly with *S. dysenteriae* serotype 1.

Septicemia in shigellosis is rare, except in malnourished children, young infants, and those with *S. dysenteriae* serotype 1 infections.[75, 115, 174] The mortality rate is at least twice as high in dysentery-associated sepsis as in shigellosis uncomplicated by bacteremia. The serogroup-related mortality risk in shigellemia has been reported to be 85 per cent for *S. dysenteriae*, 43 per cent for *S. flexneri*, and 25 per cent for *S. sonnei*; bacteremia rarely is reported for *S. boydii*.[113] In Bangladesh, *Shigella* bacteremia was found in 4 per cent of patients.[184] When bacteremia occurs with dysentery, it is as likely to be due to other enteric bacteria as to the *Shigella* itself. The occurrence of *Klebsiella, E. coli,* and other enteric pathogens in blood cultures of children with shigellosis presumably reflects the loss of the barrier function of the intestinal mucosa that occurs during severe colitis.[129] *Shigella* bacteremia may be complicated by disseminated intravascular coagulation and multiorgan failure. Bronchopneumonia may develop in septicemic children,[4] but its pathogenesis is unclear. Children who die with shigellosis often have pneumonia at autopsy.[38]

Other extraintestinal infections rarely are caused by *Shigella*. Vaginitis with a bloody discharge (sometimes lasting for months in the absence of specific therapy) may occur, usually without concurrent or recent diarrhea.[47, 126] *Shigella* cystitis, not always associated with diarrhea, has been described, usually in girls.[20] Conjunctivitis, keratitis, corneal ulcers, and iritis are other very uncommon manifestations of shigellosis that usually are assumed to follow autoinoculation.[20, 187] Reactive arthritis or Reiter syndrome (arthritis, urethritis, conjunctivitis) may develop after shigellosis,[39] especially in adults who are HLA-B27–positive; reactive arthritis is very uncommon in children. Hepatitis with mildly abnormal liver function tests has been described.[182] Myocarditis manifest clinically by hypotension, despite fluid replacement, arrhythmia, heart block, or decreased voltage on electocardiogram, and pathologically by interstitial lymphocytic infiltrates and focal necrosis has been described.[163]

Shigellosis in the Neonatal Period

Bacillary dysentery is rare in newborns.[22, 54, 59, 74, 102] More than half of the reported neonatal cases occurred during the first 3 days of life, consistent with fecal-oral transmission during delivery,[69, 136] usually from a symptomatic mother. Although the neonate with shigellosis usually has only low-grade fever with diarrhea of variable severity,[5, 99, 121] both septicemia[103, 156] and chronic diarrhea are more common than in older children. Intestinal perforation has been reported in neonatal shigellosis.[181] Diarrhea more often is nonbloody in infants; fever also is less common than in older children.[85] Data on age-related mortality due to shigellosis in developing countries suggest that the mortality rate in the neonate is more than twice as high as that in older children.

Shigellosis in AIDS

Unlike the usual short self-limited course of shigellosis, *Shigella* infection in patients also infected with HIV may be chronic and relapsing, despite appropriate antibiotic treatment,[177] or it may be complicated by bacteremia.[23]

LABORATORY FINDINGS

The fecal leukocyte examination is helpful in evaluation of the patient with febrile diarrhea. Direct microscopic examination of fecal mucus stained with methylene blue shows many polymorphonuclear leukocytes in patients with colitis, including most patients with shigellosis.[80] The blood leukocyte count in patients with shigellosis often is within normal limits, although leukopenia or leukocytosis may occur.[11] The differential of the blood leukocyte count typically shows an increased percentage of band forms (a shift to the left). About a third of children with shigellosis have more bands than segmented neutrophils in their peripheral blood smear. A leukemoid reaction, with a peripheral leukocyte count greater than 50,000/mm^3, has been reported, mainly with *S. dysenteriae* serotype 1 infections[37]; a leukemoid reaction has been reported in as many as 10 per cent of the patients infected with the Shiga bacillus. When cerebrospinal fluid examination is performed in children with neurologic symptoms, normal results usually are obtained, although some have a mild lymphocytic pleocytosis. Likewise, when electroencephalography is performed, the results usually are within normal limits.[16]

DIAGNOSIS

Bacillary dysentery usually is suspected in children who present with bloody diarrhea, high fever, and generalized toxicity. However, about half of the children do not develop bloody diarrhea during the course of their disease. This especially is relevant in developed countries, where most of the infections are caused by *S. sonnei*. Thus, the presence of only watery diarrhea does not exclude the possibility of shigellosis in an ill patient with high fever.

Isolation Techniques

Proof of the diagnosis of suspected bacillary dysentery often is problematic. Definite diagnosis of *Shigella* infection depends on isolation of the organism from stool specimens or rectal swabs. However, the bacteria may not survive in fecal specimens during transit; furthermore, special selective media are necessary for isolation. Recovery of shigellae is easier early in the course of the disease than later because the number of viable organisms in stools decreases significantly during late stages of the disease. Even in adult volunteer studies, when appropriate stool cultures were obtained daily, cultures still failed to isolate shigellae in about 20 per cent of those who had ingested the organism and developed diarrhea. Several measures increase the likelihood of isolating the *Shigella*. Specimens should be processed without delay. If a specimen can not be processed immediately, a transport medium, such as buffered glycerol saline, should be used. It is recommended that more than one stool culture or rectal swab be obtained and inoculated promptly onto at least two different culture media. Specimens should be plated lightly onto MacConkey, xylose-lysine-deoxycholate, or eosin-methylene blue agars, whereas a heavier plating is necessary for the more inhibitory *Shigella-Salmonella* medium.[123, 186] After overnight incubation at 37° C, lactose-negative colonies are transferred to triple sugar iron and lysine iron agar slants and incubated again overnight. Slants showing characteristic reactions of alkaline red slants, acid butt, and no gas production are tested biochemically for presumptive identification and then serologically for definitive identification. Because many of the O antigens of *Shigella* and those of *E. coli* have antigenic similarities, serologic techniques cannot be utilized as the sole determinant in identifying *Shigella* strains.

Other Diagnostic Methods

Because presumptive identification of *Shigella* takes at least 48 hours and definite identification about 72 hours, attempts to develop rapid diagnostic methods are being made, especially because institution of early treatment is important in shigellosis. Latex agglutination assays that detect *Shigella* antigens now are commercially available. They usually are used for identification of colonies suspected of being shigellae or for testing enrichment broth cultures.[119] The assays detect the four *Shigella* serogroups and are based on color reactions. These assays are not used for direct identification of shigellae in stool specimens.

Identification of shigellae by specific DNA probes using either restriction fragments or synthetic oligonucleotides[137] based on detecting virulence genes located on the 120- to 140 megadalton plasmid has been described. Because the invasion plasmids of shigellae, like other plasmids, may be lost spontaneously, a DNA probe derived from *S. flexneri ipaH* gene, a multicopy element that is found both on the chromosome and on the invasion plasmid of shigellae, has been developed and found to be more sensitive than previous probes.[190] The use of these probes is not practical for clinical settings. Use of the polymerase chain reaction, in vitro amplification of nucleic acids, to detect shigellae directly from stool specimens has been reported.[64] Polymerase chain reaction can detect as few as 10 colony-forming units of *S. flexneri* in stool specimens, whereas the sensitivities of DNA probe hybridization (with no amplification) and standard biochemical methods are 10^3 and 10^6 colony-forming units, respectively.

Serologic studies are not helpful in establishing the diagnosis of shigellosis in the individual patient; humoral antibodies develop after clinical recovery. Serologic studies, however, may be helpful in epidemiologic studies to define spread of the disease in a population.[20]

Sigmoidoscopy and barium enema are not necessary unless they are indicated to rule out other conditions. When these procedures are performed in patients with a possibility of shigellosis, caution is necessary because of the diffuse acute colitis.

DIFFERENTIAL DIAGNOSIS

Colitis of any etiology presenting with acute onset of bloody diarrhea with fever and abdominal cramps can be confused with shigellosis. Etiologic agents to be considered include *Campylobacter* species, *Salmonella* species, *Clostridium difficile*, *Yersinia enterocolitica*, *Shigella* species, *Vibrio parahaemolyticus*, enteroinvasive *E. coli*, enterohemorrhagic *E. coli* (such as serotype O157:H7), and *Entamoeba histolytica*. The initial presentation of inflammatory bowel disease can mimic shigellosis. Etiologic diagnosis of the acute colitis syndrome on the basis of clinical presentation is difficult, although some data suggest a specific causative agent. In developed countries, *Campylobacter* is the most common cause of acute infectious colitis. Shigellosis should be suspected when there is evidence of person-to-person spread and when convulsions or other neurologic symptoms develop. In the first few months of life, *Salmonella* is the most common cause of bloody diarrhea and *Shigella* is very rare. A history of previous antibiotic treatment is suggestive of *C. difficile*–related diarrhea, and previous seafood consumption suggests *V. parahaemolyticus* disease. *Yersinia* infections are found mainly in the cooler regions of Europe and North America; the disease may mimic acute appendicitis because of the right lower quadrant pain associated with mesenteric lymphadenitis. The enterohemorrhagic *E. coli* often cause bloody diarrhea with little or no fever, in contrast to shigellosis, in which high fever is typical. Negative stool cultures for the mentioned bacterial pathogens may suggest infection by enteroinvasive *E. coli.* Amebiasis causes a colitis similar to that caused by *Shigella,*[180] although it is of slower onset, with a lower degree of fever; the fecal leukocyte examination is negative. The involvement of the colon with amebiasis is less diffuse than in shigellosis; there are areas of normal mucosa between ulcerations. A prolonged course with negative cultures should raise the possibility of either ulcerative colitis or Crohn disease. When watery diarrhea is present, the list of possible etiologic agents is even longer, although many of the agents causing watery diarrhea are associated with little or no fever and thus are not confused with those causing shigellosis. Diagnosis usually cannot be made by clinical presentation alone and depends on culture results or other specific laboratory assays.

TREATMENT

Fluid Administration

Dehydration is less of a problem with shigellosis than with rotavirus or toxigenic *E. coli.* However, some children with shigellosis, particularly young infants, develop dehydration during the course of the disease. The high-volume watery diarrhea seen early in the course of the disease may cause excess fluid and electrolyte losses; likewise, in those with severe colitis, the systemic toxicity and vomiting may cause enough anorexia to interfere with fluid intake. Assessment of the hydration status of the patients on admission is mandatory, with early institution of appropriate fluid and electrolyte therapy. The World Health Organization's oral rehydration therapy with glucose-electrolyte solutions usually is effective.[127] This solution contains 90 mEq/L of Na^+, 20 mEq/L of K^+, 80 mEq/L of Cl^-, 30 mEq/L of bicarbonate or citrate, and 20 g/L of glucose. Oral rehydration therapy should be given with additional water containing no electrolytes to prevent hypernatremia; this particularly is important in children too young to express their need for additional free water. In infants, two parts of oral rehydration therapy should be followed by one part of water without electrolytes. Intravenous fluid therapy is necessary in children who are comatose, have an ileus, or are in shock when first seen. Early (12 to 24 hours after beginning oral fluids) reinstitution of breast milk or other food is mandatory.

Antibiotic Therapy

Therapy of shigellosis is controversial because of concern that treatment selects for emergence of resistant organisms. However, it is unclear whether the increasing resistance is due to treatment of symptomatic shigellosis or to irrational use of antibiotics for colds, ill-defined fevers, and other inadequately evaluated illnesses. Treatment with an agent to which the *Shigella* is susceptible results in rapid improvement. Shedding of the organisms in stools stops within 1 to 2 days, so that intrafamilial spread may be decreased. It is unclear whether antibiotic treatment prevents complications, such as hemolysis, seizures, and hemolytic uremic syndrome. Although use of antibiotics may favor emergence of resistant organisms, most authorities recommend that early empiric antibiotic treatment be given to all patients with a diagnosis of presumptive shigellosis, even if the illness is relatively mild. Antibiotics should be started when shigellosis first is suspected clinically, before culture confirmation of the infection is obtained. Therapy should be stopped or changed based on culture results (e.g., another pathogen or a resistant *Shigella* is isolated) and clinical response.

The choice of antimicrobial agent is complicated by the increasing frequency of antibiotic-resistant shigellae.[56, 60, 168] Multiresistant *Shigella* species particularly are likely in those who are exposed to multiple antibiotics (e.g., patients with AIDS)[91] and those who recently have traveled to areas with known high resistance (e.g., the Middle East,[1, 6, 10, 17, 57, 79, 90, 195] Africa,[1, 40, 114] South America,[128, 107, 138] Spain,[191] Eastern Europe and Russia,[31, 92, 98] Asia,[7, 29, 106, 108, 110]). Likewise, children in day care centers are at risk of having resistant organisms because the frequent use of antibiotics for otitis media may favor selection and emergence of resistant enteric organisms and because crowding and poor hygiene facilitate transmission.[32]

For many years, ampicillin was the drug of choice for shigellosis.[76, 77, 131, 147] Since the mid 1970s, increased rates of resistance of shigellae to ampicillin have been reported throughout the world.[162] In the United States, about half of *S. sonnei* are resistant to ampicillin; *S. flexneri* remains relatively susceptible. In developed countries, trimethoprim-sulfamethoxazole (TMP-SMX) has been the recommended empiric treatment for suspected shigellosis.[133–135, 146] However, in certain areas of Southeast Asia, North and South America, and Africa, *Shigella* strains that are resistant to TMP-SMX are common.[82] Thus, local resistance patterns, history of travel to an area of frequent resistance,[185] and severity of illness should determine whether TMP-SMX or an alternate agent should be administered. For those settings in which TMP-SMX still is appropriate, the usual dose is 10 mg TMP plus 50 mg SMX per kilogram per day in two divided doses; the maximal dose is 160 mg per dose of TMP and 800 mg per dose of SMX given twice daily. This treatment can be given orally or intravenously. Cefixime (8 mg/kg/day given orally in two divided doses for 5 days[12]) or ceftriaxone (50 mg/kg/day [maximum, 1.5 g] as a single intramuscular dose daily for 5 days[189]) represents effective treatment in many settings and should be the first-line approach in most of the world at present. However, one study suggests that cefixime may not be adequate therapy for adults with shigellosis.[167] Other oral third-generation cephalosporins also may be effective, although most have not been studied. Ceftibuten is effective therapy[164] but has not been approved for this indication. Some data suggesting that even a 2-day course of ceftriaxone may be adequate therapy.[53] Pivmecillinam also is effective therapy for susceptible organisms.[154]

Use of the quinolones has been problematic in children. Nalidixic acid (55 mg/kg/day in four divided doses) is effective treatment,[164] although plasmid-mediated resistance to nalidixic acid of *S. dysenteriae* serotype 1 strains in Bangladesh[24, 26, 125] has emerged and spread rapidly. However, nalidixic acid is not approved by the Food and Drug Administration for the treatment of shigellosis. Various other quinolones have been effective in adult patients with shigellosis, but they are not approved for use in children younger than 17 years of age because of potential damage to the cartilage of epiphyseal plates.[161] However, recent data suggest that nalidixic acid does not cause arthropathy or limit growth when used for a short time.[140] It is likely that as resistance continues to increase there will be situations in which a quinolone is the only option for treatment of a child with severe shigellosis. A recent consensus panel suggested that shigellosis is one of the illnesses for which use of a fluoroquinolone can be justified in some patients.[173] Limited data in children suggest that norfloxacin at a dose of 10 to 15 mg/kg/day for 5 days is effective therapy.[111] In adults, short-course therapy (1 or 2 days) with ciprofloxacin has been effective for *Shigella* species other than *S. dysenteriae,* for which a 10-dose, 5-day regimen is superior.[27]

Because the patterns of antibiotic resistance of shigellae change, susceptibility testing should be performed on all clinical isolates, and the treatment should be changed accordingly. The recommended duration of antibiotic therapy for shigellosis usually is 5 days. However, studies in adults and children older than 2 years of age have shown that a single-dose treatment is nearly as effective as multiple doses in terms of symptomatic improvement,[66] although eradication of the organism from stools is less likely with a single-dose regimen.[88] Because a major goal of antibiotic therapy is to reduce person-to-person transmission, multiple doses are preferred.

After initiation of therapy, a resistant organism can be suspected if there is persistence of fever, grossly bloody stools, or unchanged stool frequency by day 3 of therapy.[86] Persistence of large numbers of fecal leukocytes (>50/hpf) and erythrocytes (>5/hpf) at day 5 also suggests resistance. These findings are important because both morbidity and mortality are higher when the organism is not susceptible to the initial drug of choice.[90] Protein-losing enteropathy is more likely with resistant *Shigella* if an inadequate agent has been used.[28]

Adjunctive Therapy

As with other forms of infectious colitis, antimotility agents should be avoided. Antimotility drugs, such as diphenoxylate (Lomotil), prolong the duration of fever, diarrhea, and excretion of the organism.[51] It has been speculated that intestinal motility and the constant fluid flow actually may be important host defense factors for rapid clearing of the organism and recovery from the infection.

A high-protein diet given during convalescence may be important, particularly in settings in which malnutrition, growth retardation, and hypoproteinemia are major complications of shigellosis.[89]

PROGNOSIS

Most patients recover eventually with or without specific antimicrobial therapy, although illness may be prolonged and severe if not treated.[36] The mortality rate in developed countries is less than 1 per cent, and life-threatening complications are rare. With appropriate antibiotic therapy, defervescence usually occurs within 24 hours, and the diarrhea decreases dramatically in 2 to 3 days. If left untreated, the disease usually lasts a week or more. In developing countries, childhood shigellosis is associated with significant morbidity and mortality (10 to 30 per cent),[25] particularly if caused by *S. dysenteriae* serotype 1. Children with malnutrition particularly are likely to have a complicated course. Shigellosis in malnourished children often causes a vicious cycle of further impaired nutrition and repeated infections that may be associated with impaired growth. Young infants and children whose course is complicated by bacteremia also are at increased risk of death.[143]

PREVENTION

In developed countries where person-to-person transmission of shigellae is the major mode of infection, personal hygiene measures are most important.[95] Special attention should be given in day care centers, which sometimes play a central role in community-wide outbreaks of shigellosis.[120] The close contact among children too young to control their excretions makes this setting ideal for fecal-oral spread of the organism. Moreover, children attending day care centers frequently transmit infection to their families. Handwashing after defecation and before meals is important and helpful in preventing spread.[95] Day care personnel who prepare food should avoid diaper-changing duties. Sick children should be excluded from the day care center or cohorted, and mothers should be educated as to the possibility of being infected by their children and use of the necessary precautions. Proper cooking of potentially infected food, appropriate refrigeration, and exclusion of persons with diarrhea from food handling are important. Education of staff members in proper hygiene is essential to infection control.[150]

Patients with diarrhea in institutional and hospital settings should be isolated for prevention of outbreaks. Aggressive investigation and early initiation of appropriate antibiotic therapy in cases of bacillary dysentery are important in reducing excretion of virulent shigellae and stopping spread of the disease. Use of antibiotics for prophylaxis is, however, not recommended.

In developing countries, a safe water supply and appropriate sanitation systems are important measures for reducing the risk of shigellosis. Chlorination of drinking water is important. Water stored in vessels that permit hand dipping has been defined as a risk factor.[188] Food prepared by street vendors also has been recognized as a risk factor. Prolonged breast feeding is the best practical strategy for prevention of shigellosis (and most other enteric infections) in infants in most of the developing world.[3, 45, 116] Educational efforts to promote breast feeding in these areas are key to child survival. Human milk contains specific secretory IgA antibodies against both *Shigella* lipopolysaccharides and virulence plasmid-coded antigens.[42] Nonspecific (nonantibody) factors in human milk, the effect of human milk on the type of intestinal flora, and the supply of an uncontaminated food source all may contribute to the protective effect of breast feeding against diarrheal disease.

Epidemiologic data suggest that prior infection with shigellae confers resistance to subsequent illness caused by organisms of the same serotype. Serotype-specific (lipopolysaccharide based) vaccines have been made.[62, 63] Although early studies showed that immunization by the parenteral route with killed vaccines was not effective, there continues to be interest in this approach. Several oral, live organism–based *Shigella* vaccines have been studied. Avirulent mutants of *S. flexneri* that lack the ability to invade the intestinal mucosa are safe and effective in monkeys. However, multiple doses of large numbers of organisms were required to protect humans. Attenuated vaccines prepared from streptomycin-dependent mutant strains were effective but somewhat unstable.[117] Genetically attenuated *S. flexneri* strains conferred protection but caused diarrhea when fed to some volunteers. Vaccines based on understanding the molecular basis of *Shigella* virulence have been developed. Initially, the genes encoding the *Shigella* somatic antigen were transferred to an avirulent strain of *S. typhi.* Although effective, lot-to-lot variation in the efficacy of this product has precluded its use so far. No effective, licensed vaccine against shigellosis is available.[109]

References

1. Adeleye, I. A.: Conjugal transferability of multiple antibiotic resistance in three genera of Enterobacteriaceae in Nigeria. J. Diarrhoeal Dis. Res. *10*:93–96, 1992.
2. Admoni, O., Yagupsky, P., Golan, A., et al.: Epidemiological, clinical and microbiological features of shigellosis among hospitalized children in northern Israel. Scand. J. Infect. Dis. *27*:139–144, 1995.
3. Ahmed, F., Clemens, J. D., Rao, M. R., et al.: Community-based evaluation of the effect of breast feeding on the risk of microbiologically confirmed or clinically presumptive shigellosis in Bangladeshi children. Pediatrics *90*:406–411, 1992.
4. Alam, A. N., Chowdhurg, A. A. K. M., Kabir, I. A. K. M., et al.: Association of pneumonia with under-nutrition and shigellosis. Indian Pediatr. *21*:609–613, 1984.
5. Aldrich, J. A., Flowers, R. P., and Hall, F. K.: *S. sonnei* septicemia in a neonate: A case report. J. Am. Osteopath. Assoc. *79*:93–98, 1979.
6. al-Eissa, Y., al-Zamil, F., al-Kharashi, M., et al.: The relative importance of *Shigella* in the aetiology of childhood gastroenteritis in Saudi Arabia. Scand. J. Infect. Dis. *24*:347–351, 1992.
7. Aleksic, S., Katz, A., Aleksic, V., et al.: Antibiotic resistance of *Shigella* strains isolated in the Federal Republic of Germany 1989–1990. Int. J. Med. Microbiol. Virol. Parasitol. Infect. Dis. *279*:484–493, 1993.
8. Anand, B. S., Malhotra, V., Bhattacharya, S. K., et al.: Rectal histology in acute bacillary dysentery. Gastroenterology *90*:654–660, 1986.
9. Ansaruzzaman, M., Kibriya, A. K. M. G., Rahman, A., et al.: Detection of provisional serovars of *S. dysenteriae* and designation as *S. dysenteriae* serotypes 14 and 15. J. Clin. Microbiol. *33*:1423–1425, 1995.
10. Araj, G. F., Uwaydah, M. M., and Alami, S. Y.: Antimicrobial susceptibility patterns of bacterial isolates at the American University Medical Center in Lebanon. Diagn. Microbiol. Infect. Dis. *20*:151–158, 1994.
11. Ashkenazi, S., Amir, J., Dinari, T., et al.: The differential leukocyte count in acute gastroenteritis: An aid to early diagnosis. Clin. Pediatr. *22*:356–358, 1983.
12. Ashkenazi, S., Amir, J., Waisman, Y., et al.: A randomized double-blind study comparing cefixime and TMP/SMX in the treatment of childhood shigellosis. J. Pediatr. *123*:817–821, 1993.
13. Ashkenazi, S., Bellah, G., and Cleary, T. G.: Hallucinations as an initial manifestation of childhood shigellosis. J. Pediatr. *114*:95–97, 1989.
14. Ashkenazi, S., Cleary, K. R., and Pickering, L. K., et al.: The association of Shiga toxin and other cytotoxins with the neurologic manifestations of shigellosis. J. Infect. Dis. *161*:961–965, 1990.
15. Ashkenazi, S., Dinari, G., Weitz, R., et al.: Convulsions in shigellosis: Evaluation of possible risk factors. Am. J. Dis. Child. *137*:985–987, 1983.
16. Ashkenazi, S., Dinari, G., Zevulunov, A., et al.: Convulsions in childhood shigellosis: Clinical and laboratory features in 153 children. Am. J. Dis. Child. *141*:208–210, 1987.
17. Ashkenazi, S., May-Zahav, M., Sulkes, J., et al.: Increasing antimicrobial resistance of *Shigella* isolates in Israel during the period 1984 to 1992. Antimicrob. Agents Chemother. *39*:819–823, 1995.
18. Avital, A., Maayan, C., and Goitein, K. J.: Incidence of convulsions and encephalopathy in childhood *Shigella* infections. Clin. Pediatr. *21*:645–648, 1982.
19. Azad, M. A., Islam, M., and Butler, T.: Colonic perforation of *S. dysenteriae* 1 infection. Pediatr. Infect. Dis. *5*:103–104, 1986.
20. Barrett-Connor, E., and Connor, J. D.: Extraintestinal manifestations of shigellosis. Am. J. Gastroenterol. *53*:234–245, 1970.
21. Bartlett, A. V., III, Prado, D., Cleary, T. G., et al.: Production of Shiga toxin and other cytotoxins by serogroups of *Shigella*. J. Infect. Dis. *154*:996-1002, 1986.
22. Barton, L. L., and Pickering, L. K.: Shigellosis in the first week of life. Pediatrics *52*:437–438, 1973.
23. Baskin, D. H., Lax, J. D., and Barenberg, D.: *Shigella* bacteremia in patients with the acquired immunodeficiency syndrome. Am. J. Gastroenterol. *82*:338–341, 1986.
24. Bennish, M., Eusof, A., and Kay, B.: Multiresistant *Shigella* infections in Bangladesh. Lancet *2*:441, 1985.
25. Bennish, M. L., Harris, J. R., Wojtyniak, B. J., et al.: Death in shigellosis: Incidence and risk factors in hospitalized patients. J. Infect. Dis. *161*:500–506, 1990.
26. Bennish, M. L., Salam, M. A., Hossain, M. A., et al.: Antimicrobial resistance of *Shigella* isolates in Bangladesh, 1983–1990: Increasing frequency of strains multiply resistant to ampicillin, trimethoprim-sulfamethoxazole, and nalidixic acid. Clin. Infect. Dis. *14*:1055–1060, 1992.
27. Bennish, M. L., Salam, M. A., Khan, W. A., et al.: Treatment of shigellosis. III. Comparison of one- or two-dose ciprofloxacin with standard 5-day therapy. Ann. Intern. Med. *117*:727–734, 1992.
28. Bennish, M. L., Salam, M. A., and Wahed, M. A.: Enteric protein loss during shigellosis. Am. J. Gastroenterol. *88*:53–57, 1993.
29. Bhattacharya, M. K., Bhattacharya, S. K., Paul, M., et al.: Shigellosis in Calcutta during 1990–1992: Antibiotic susceptibility pattern and clinical features. J. Diarrhoeal Dis. Res. *12*:121–124, 1994.
30. Boehme, C., Rodriguez, G., Illesca, V., et al.: Shigellosis in children of the IX region of Chile: Clinical and epidemiologic aspects and antibiotic sensitivity. Revista Medica Chile *120*:1261–1266, 1992.
31. Bratoeva, M. P., John, J. F., and Barg, N. L. Molecular epidemiology of trimethoprim–resistant *Shigella boydii* serotype 2 strains from Bulgaria. J. Clin. Microbiol. *30*:1428–1431, 1992.
32. Brian, M. J., Van, R., Townsend, I., et al.: Evaluation of the molecular epidemiology of an outbreak of multiply resistant *Shigella sonnei* in a day-care center by using pulsed-field gel electrophoresis and plasmid DNA analysis. J. Clin. Microbiol. *31*:2152–1256, 1993.
33. Bridgwater, F. A. J., Morgan, R. S., Rowson, K. E. K., et al.: The neurotoxin of *Shigella shigae:* Morphological and functional lesions produced in the central nervous system of rabbits. Br. J. Exp. Pathol. *36*:447, 1955.
34. Brown, J. E., Griffin, D. E., Rothman, S. W., et al.: Purification and biological characterization of Shiga toxin from *Shigella dysenteriae* 1. Infect. Immun. *36*:996–1005, 1982.
35. Brown, J. E., Rothman, S. W., and Doctor, B. P.: Inhibition of protein synthesis in intact HeLa cells by *Shigella dysenteriae* 1 toxin. Infect. Immun. *29*:98–107, 1980.
36. Burry, V. F., Thurn, A. N., and Co, T. G.: Shigellosis: An analysis of 239 cases in a pediatric population. Mo. Med. *65*:671–674, 1968.
37. Butler, T. C., Islam, M. R., and Bardhan, P. K.: The leukemoid reaction in shigellosis. *In* Rahaman, M. M., Greenough, W. B., Novak, N. R., et al. (eds.): Shigellosis: A Continuing Global Problem. Bangladesh, International Centre for Diarrhoeal Disease Research, 1983, p. 154.
38. Butler, T., Dunn, D., Dahms, B., et al.: Causes of death and the histopathologic findings in fatal shigellosis. Pediatr. Infect. Dis. J. *8*:767–772, 1989.
39. Calin, A., and Fries, J. F.: An "experimental" epidemic of Reiter's syndrome revisited: Follow-up evidence on genetic and environmental factors. Ann. Intern. Med. *84*:564–566, 1976.
40. Casalino, M., Nicoletti, M., Salvia, A., et al.: Characterization of endemic *Shigella flexneri* strains in Somalia: Antimicrobial resistance, plasmid profiles, and serotype correlation. J. Clin. Microbiol. *32*:1179–1183, 1994.
41. Cavanagh, J. B., Howard, J. G., and Whitby, J. L.: The neurotoxin of *Shigella shigae:* A comparative study of the effects produced in various laboratory animals. Br. J. Exp. Pathol. *37*:272–276, 1956.
42. Cleary, T. G., Winsor, D. K., Reich, D., et al.: Human milk immunoglobulin A antibodies to *Shigella* virulence determinants. Infect. Immun. *57*:1675–1679, 1989.
43. Cleary, T. G., and Murray, B. E.: Lack of shiga-like cytotoxin production by enteroinvasive *E. coli*. J. Clin. Microbiol. *26*:2177–2179, 1988.
44. Clemens, D., Ellis, C. J., and Allan, R. N.: Persistent shigellosis. Gut *29*:1277–1278, 1988.
45. Clemens, J. S., Stanton, B., Stohl, B., et al.: Breast-feeding as a determinant of severity of shigellosis. Am. J. Epidemiol. *123*:710–720, 1986.
46. Cohen, D., Green, M. S., Block, C., et al.: Serum antibodies to lipopolysaccharide and natural immunity to shigellosis in an Israeli military population. J. Infect. Dis. *157*:1068–1071, 1988.
47. Davis, T. C.: Chronic vulvovaginitis in children due to *S. flexneri.* Pediatrics *56*:41–44, 1975.
48. Donald, W. D., Winkler, C. H., Jr., and Bargeron, L. M., Jr.: The occurrence of convulsions in children with *Shigella* gastroenteritis. J. Pediatr. *48*:323–327, 1956.
49. DuPont, H. L., Hornick, R. B., Dawkins, A. T., et al.: The response of man to virulent *Shigella flexneri* 2a. J. Infect. Dis. *119*:296–299, 1969.
50. DuPont, H. L., Hornick, R. B., Snyder, M. J., et al.: Immunity in shigellosis. II. Protection induced by oral live vaccine or primary infection. J. Infect. Dis. *125*:12–16, 1972.
51. DuPont, H. L., and Hornick, R. B.: Adverse effect of Lomotil therapy in shigellosis. J. A. M. A. *226*:1525–1528, 1973.
52. DuPont, H. L., Levine, M. M., Hornick, R. B., et al.: Inoculum size in shigellosis and implications for expected mode of transmission. J. Infect. Dis. *159*:1126–1128, 1989.
53. Eidlitz-Marcus, T., Cohen, Y. H., Nussinovitch, M., et al.: Comparative efficacy of two- and five- day courses of ceftriaxone for treatment of severe shigellosis in children. J. Pediatr. *123*:822–824, 1993.
54. Emanuel, B., and Sherman, J. O.: Shigellosis in a neonate. Clin. Pediatr. *14*:725–726, 1975.
55. Ewing, W. H.: Edwards and Ewing's Identification of Enterobacteriaceae. 4th ed. New York, Elsevier Science Publishing, 1986.
56. Farrar, W. E., Eidson, M., Guerry, P., et al.: Interbacterial transfer of R-factor in the human intestine: In vitro acquisition of R-factor mediated kanamycin resistance by a multi-resistant strain of *S. sonnei.* J. Infect. Dis. *126*:27–33, 1972.
57. Fernandez, A., Sninsky, C. A., O'Brien, A. D., et al.: Purified *Shigella* enterotoxin does not alter intestinal motility. Infect. Immun. *43*:477–481, 1984.
58. Finkelman, Y., Yagupsky, P., Fraser, D., et al.: Epidemiology of *Shigella* infections in two ethnic groups in a geographic region in southern Israel. Eur. J. Clin. Microbiol. Infect. Dis. *13*:367–73, 1994.

59. Floyd, T., Higgins, A. R., and Kader, M. A.: Studies in shigellosis. V. The relationship of age to the incidence of *Shigella* infections in Egyptian children, with special reference to shigellosis in the newborn and infant in the first six months of life. Am. J. Trop. Med. Hyg. *5*:119–130, 1956.
60. Fontaine, O.: Antibiotics in the management of shigellosis in children: What role for the quinolones? Rev. Infect. Dis. *11*:S1145-S1150, 1989.
61. Forbes, G.: Neurologic complications of systemic disease. Postgrad. Med. *15*:157, 1954.
62. Formal, S. B., Hale, T. L., and Kapfer, C.: *Shigella* vaccines. Rev. Infect. Dis. *11*:S547–S551, 1989.
63. Formal, S. B., Kent, T. H., Austin, S., et al.: Fluorescent-antibody and histological studies of vaccinated control monkeys challenged with *Shigella flexneri.* J. Bacteriol. *91*:2368–2376, 1966.
64. Frankel, G., Riley, L., Giron, J. A., et al.: Detection of *Shigella* in feces using DNA amplification. J. Infect. Dis. *161*:1252–1256, 1990.
65. Gemski, P., Jr., Takeuchi, A., Washington, O., et al.: Shigellosis due to *S. dysenteriae.* 1. Relative importance of mucosal invasion versus toxin production in pathogenesis. J. Infect. Dis. *126*:523–530, 1972.
66. Gilman, R. H., Spira, W., Rabbani, H., et al.: Single dose ampicillin therapy for severe shigellosis in Bangladesh. J. Infect. Dis. *143*:164–169, 1981.
67. Goren, A., Freier, S., and Passwell, J. H.: Lethal toxic encephalopathy due to childhood shigellosis in a developed country. Pediatrics *89*:1189–1193, 1992.
68. Gots, R. E., Formal, S. B., and Gianella, R. A.: Indomethacin inhibition of *Salmonella typhimurium, Shigella flexneri,* and cholera-mediated rabbit ileal secretion. J. Infect. Dis. *130*:280–284, 1974.
69. Greenberg, M., Frant, S., and Shapiro, R.: Bacillary dysentery acquired at birth. J. Pediatr. *17*:363–366, 1940.
70. Guerrero, L., Calva, J. J., Morrow, A. L., et al.: Asymptomatic *Shigella* infections in a cohort of Mexican children younger than two years of age. Pediatr. Infect. Dis. J. *13*:597–602, 1994.
71. Haider, K., Huq, M. I., Samadi, A. R., et al.: Plasmid characterization of *Shigella* spp. isolated from children with shigellosis and asymptomatic excretors. J. Antimicrob. Chemother. *16*:691–698, 1985.
72. Hale, T. L., Oaks, E. V., and Formal, S. B.: Identification and characterization of virulence-associated, plasmid-coded proteins of *Shigella* spp. and enteroinvasive *E. coli.* Infect. Immun. *50*:620–623, 1985.
73. Hale, T. L., Sansonetti, P., Schad, P. A., et al.: Characterization of virulence plasmids and plasmid-mediated outer membrane proteins in *Shigella flexneri, Shigella sonnei* and *Escherichia coli.* Infect. Immun. *40*:340–350, 1983.
74. Haltalin, K. C.: Neonatal shigellosis. Am. J. Dis. Child. *114*:603–611, 1967.
75. Haltalin, K. C., and Nelson, J. D.: Coliform septicemia complicating shigellosis in children. J. A. M. A. *192*:441–443, 1965.
76. Haltalin, K. C., Nelson, J. D., Kusmiesz, H. T., et al.: Optimal dosage of ampicillin in shigellosis. J. Pediatr. *74*:626–631, 1969.
77. Haltalin, K. C., Nelson, J. D., and Kusmiesz, H. T.: Comparative efficacy of nalidixic acid and ampicillin for severe shigellosis. Arch. Dis. Child *48*:305–312, 1973.
78. Harenda de Silva, D. G., Mendis, L. N., Sheron, N., et al.: Concentrations of IL-6 and TNF in serum and stools of children with *S. dysenteriae* 1 infection. Gut *34*:194–198, 1993.
79. Harnett, N.: High-level resistance to trimethoprim, cotrimoxazole and other antimicrobial agents among clinical isolates of *Shigella* species in Ontario, Canada: An update. Epidemiol. Infect. *109*:463–472, 1992.
80. Harris, J. C., DuPont, H. L., and Hornick, R. B.: Fecal leukocytes in diarrheal illness. Ann. Intern. Med. *76*:697–703, 1972.
81. Harris, J. R., Wachsmuth, I. K., Davis, B. R., et al.: High molecular weight plasmid correlates with *Escherichia coli* enteroinvasiveness. Infect. Immun. *37*:1295–1298, 1982.
82. Heikkila, E., Siitonen, A., Jahkola, M., et al.: Increase of trimethoprim resistance among *Shigella* species 1975–1988: Analysis of resistance mechanisms. J. Infect. Dis. *161*:1242–1248, 1990.
83. Hoefnagel, D.: Fulminating, rapidly fatal shigellosis in children. N. Engl. J. Med. *258*:1256–1257, 1958.
84. Howard, J. G.: Observations on the intoxication produced in mice and rabbits by the neurotoxin of *Shigella shigae.* Br. J. Exp. Pathol. *36*:439–443, 1955.
85. Huskins, W. C., Griffiths, J. K., Faruque, A. S. G., et al.: Shigellosis in neonates and young infants. J. Pediatr. *125*:14–22, 1994.
86. Islam, M. R., Alam, A. N., Hussain, M. S., et al.: Effect of antimicrobial (nalidixic acid) therapy in shigellosis and predictive values of outcome variables in patients susceptible or resistant to it. J. Trop. Med. Hyg. *98*:121–125, 1995.
87. Islam, M. M., Azad, A. K., Bardhan, P. K., et al.: Pathology of shigellosis and its complications. Histopathology *24*:65–71, 1994.
88. Kabir, I., Butler, T., and Khanam, A.: Comparative efficacies of single intravenous doses of ceftriaxone and ampicillin for shigellosis in a placebo-controlled trial. Antimicrob. Agents Chemother. *29*:645–648, 1986.
89. Kabir, I., Butler, T., and Underwood, L. E., et al.: Effects of a protein rich diet during convalescence from shigellosis on catch up growth, serum proteins, and insulin like growth factor I. Pediatr. Res. *32*:689–692, 1992.
90. Kagalwalla, A. F., Khan, S. N., Kagalwalla, Y. A., et al.: Childhood shigellosis in Saudi Arabia. Pediatr. Infect. Dis. J. *11*:215–219, 1992.
91. Kariuki, S., Gilks, C., Brindle, R., et al.: Antimicrobial susceptibility and presence of extrachromosomal deoxyribonucleic acid in *Salmonella* and *Shigella* isolates from patients with AIDS. East Afr. Med. J. *71*:292–296, 1994.
92. Kaminski, N., Bogomolski, V., and Stalnikowicz, R.: Acute bacterial diarrhoea in the emergency room: Therapeutic implications of stool culture results. J. Accident Emerg. Med. *11*:168–171, 1994.
93. Keusch, G. T., and Bennish, M. L.: Shigellosis: Recent progress, persisting problems and research issues. Pediatr. Infect. Dis. J. *8*:713–719, 1989.
94. Keusch, G. T., and Jacewicz, M.: The pathogenesis of *Shigella* diarrhea. V. Relationship of Shiga enterotoxin, neurotoxin, and cytotoxin. J. Infect. Dis. *131*:S33, 1975.
95. Khan, M. U.: Interruption of shigellosis by handwashing. Trans. R. Soc. Trop. Med. Hyg. *76*:164–165, 1982.
96. Koster, F., Levin, J., Walker, L., et al.: Hemolytic-uremic syndrome after shigellosis: Relation to endotoxemia and circulating immune complexes. N. Engl. J. Med. *298*:927–933, 1978.
97. Kowlessar, M., and Forbes, G. B.: The febrile convulsion in shigellosis. N. Engl. J. Med. *258*:520–523, 1958.
98. Kozlova, N. S.: Plasmids of antibiotic-resistant strains of *Shigella* isolated in Leningrad and Leningrad region. Antibiot. Khimioter. 38:9–14, 1993.
99. Kraybill, E. N., and Controni, G.: Septicemia and enterocolitis due to *S. sonnei* in a newborn infant. Pediatrics *42*:529–531, 1968.
100. LaBrec, E. H., and Formal, S. B.: Experimental *Shigella* infections. IV. Fluorescent antibody studies of an infection in guinea pigs. J. Immunol. *87*:562–572, 1961.
101. LaBrec, E. H., Schneider, H., Magnani, T. J., et al.: Epithelial cell penetration as an essential step in the pathogenesis of bacillary dysentery. J. Bacteriol. *88*:1503–1518, 1964.
102. Landsberger, M.: Bacillary dysentery in a newborn infant. Arch. Pediatr. *59*:330–332, 1942.
103. Levin, S. E.: *Shigella* septicemia in the newborn infant. J. Pediatr. *71*:917–918, 1967.
104. Levine, M. M., DuPont, H. L., Formal, S. B., et al.: Pathogenesis of *Shigella dysenteriae* 1 (Shiga) dysentery. J. Infect. Dis. *127*:261–270, 1973.
105. Levine, M. M., DuPont, H. L., Khodabandebou, M., et al.: Long-term *Shigella*-carrier state. N. Engl. J. Med. *288*:1169–1171, 1973.
106. Lim, Y. S., and Tay, L.: Serotype distribution and antimicrobial resistance of *Shigella* isolates in Singapore. J. Diarrhoeal Dis. Res. *9*:328–331, 1991.
107. Lima, A. A., Lima, N. L., Pinho, M. C., et al.: High frequency of strains multiply resistant to ampicillin, trimethoprim-sulfamethoxazole, streptomycin, chloramphenicol, and tetracycline isolated from patients with shigellosis in northeastern Brazil during the period 1988 to 1993. Antimicrob. Agents Chemother. *39*:256–259, 1995.
108. Lin, S. R., and Chang, S. F.: Drug resistance and plasmid profile of shigellae in Taiwan. Epidemiol. Infect. 108:87–97, 1992.
109. Lindberg, A. A., and Pal, T.: Strategies for development of potential candidate *Shigella* vaccines. Vaccine *11*:168–179, 1993.
110. Ling, J. M., Shaw, P. C., Kam, K. M., et al.: Molecular studies of plasmids of multiply-resistant *Shigella* spp. in Hong Kong. Epidemiol. Infect. *110*:437–446, 1993.
111. Lolekha, S., Vibulbandhitkit, S., and Poonyarit, P.: Response to antimicrobial therapy for shigellosis in Thailand. Rev. Infect. Dis. *13*:S342–S346, 1991.
112. Makintubee, S., Mallonee, J., and Istre, G. R.: Shigellosis outbreak associated with swimming. Am. J. Public Health *77*:166–168, 1987.
113. Martin, T., Habbick, B. F., and Nyssen, J.: Shigellosis with bacteremia: A report of two cases and a review of the literature. Pediatr. Infect. Dis. 2:21–26, 1983.
114. Mason, P. R., Nathoo, K. J., Wellington, M., et al.: Antimicrobial susceptibilities of *Shigella dysenteriae* type 1 isolated in Zimbabwe: Implications for the management of dysentery. Cent. Afr. J. Med. *41*:132–137, 1995.
115. Mata, L. G.: The Children of Santa Maria Cauque: A Prospective Field Study of Health and Growth. Cambridge, MIT Press, 1978.
116. Mata, L. J., Urrutia, J. J., Garcia, B., et al.: *Shigella* infections in breast fed Guatemalan Indian neonates. Am. J. Dis. Child. *117*:142–146, 1969.
117. Mel, D. M., Terzin, A. L., and Vuksic, L.: Studies on vaccination against bacillary dysentery. 3. Effective oral immunization against *Shigella flexneri* 2a in a field trial. Bull. W. H. O. *32*:647–655, 1965.
118. Merson, M. H., Goldmann, D. A., Boyer, K. M., et al.: An outbreak of *Shigella sonnei* gastroenteritis on Colorado River raft trips. Am. J. Epidemiol. *100*:186–196, 1974.
119. Metzler, J., and Nachamkin, I.: Evaluation of latex agglutination test for the detection of *Salmonella* and *Shigella* spp. by using broth enrichment. J. Clin. Microbiol. *26*:2501–2504, 1988.
120. Mohle-Boetani, J. C., Stapleton, M., Finger, R., et al.: Community-wide shigellosis: Control of an outbreak and risk factors in child day care centers. Am. J. Public Health *85*:812–816, 1995.
121. Moore, E. E.: *Shigella sonnei* septicemia in a neonate. Br. Med. J. *1*:22–23, 1974.
122. Morgan, D. R., DuPont, H. L., Wood, L. V., et al.: Cytotoxicity of leukocytes from normal and *Shigella*-susceptible (opium-treated) guinea pigs against virulent *Shigella sonnei.* Infect. Immun. *46*:22–24, 1984.
123. Morris, G. K., Koehler, J. A., Gangarosa, E. J., et al.: Comparison of media for direct isolation and transport of shigellae from fecal specimens. Appl. Microbiol. *19*:434–437, 1970.

124. Mulligan, K., Nelson, S., Friedman, H. S., et al.: Shigellosis-associated encephalopathy. Pediatr. Infect. Dis. J. 11:889–890, 1992.
125. Munshi, M. H., Sack, D. A., Haider, K., et al.: Plasmid-mediated resistance to nalidixic acid in *Shigella dysenteriae* type 1. Lancet 2:419–421, 1987.
126. Murphy, T. V., and Nelson, J. D.: *Shigella* vaginitis: Report on 38 patients and review of the literature. Pediatrics *63*:511–516, 1979.
127. Nalin, D. R., and Cash, R. A.: Oral or nasogastric maintenance of cholera and other severe diarrhea in children. J. Pediatr. *78*:355–358, 1971.
128. Nataro, J. P., Seriwatana, J., Fasano, A., et al.: Identification and cloning of a novel plasmid encoded enterotoxin of enteroinvasive *E. coli* and *Shigella* strains. Infect. Immun. *63*:4721–4728, 1995.
129. Neglia, T. G., Marr, T. J., and Davis, A. T.: *Shigella* dysentery with secondary *Klebsiella* sepsis. J. Pediatr. *63*:253–254, 1976.
130. Neill, R. J., Gemski, P., Formal, S. B., et al.: Deletion of Shiga toxin gene in a chlorate-resistant derivative of *Shigella dysenteriae* type 1 that retains virulence. J. Infect. Dis. *158*:737–741, 1988.
131. Nelson, J. D., and Haltalin, K. C.: Amoxicillin less effective than ampicillin against *Shigella* in vitro and in vivo: Relationship of efficacy to activity in serum. J. Infect. Dis. *129*:S222–S227, 1974.
132. Nelson, J. D., and Haltalin, K. C.: Comparative efficacy of cephalexin and ampicillin for shigellosis and other types of acute diarrhea in infants and children. Antimicrob. Agents Chemother. *7*:415–420, 1975.
133. Nelson, J., Kusmiesz, H., Jackson, L., et al.: Trimethoprim-sulfamethoxazole therapy for shigellosis. J. A. M. A. *235*:1239–1243, 1976.
134. Nelson, J. D., Kusmiesz, H., and Jackson, L. H.: Comparison of trimethoprim/sulfamethoxazole and ampicillin for shigellosis in ambulatory patients. J. Pediatr. *89*:491–493, 1976.
135. Nelson, J. D., Kusmiesz, H., and Shelton, S.: Oral or intravenous trimethoprim/sulfamethoxazole therapy for shigellosis. Rev. Infect. Dis. *4*:546–550, 1982.
136. Neter, E.: *S. sonnei* infection at term and its transfer to the newborn. Obstet. Gynecol. *17*:517–519, 1961.
137. Newland, J. W., and Neill, R. J.: DNA probes for Shiga-like toxins I and II and for toxin-converting bacteriophages. J. Clin. Microbiol. *26*:1292–1297, 1988.
138. Notario, R., Morales, E., Carmelengo, E., et al.: Enteropathogenic microorganisms in children with acute diarrhea in 2 hospitals of Rosario, Argentina. Medicina *53*:289–299, 1993.
139. Noriega, F. R., Liao, F.M., Formal, S.B., et al.: Prevalence of *Shigella* enterotoxin 1 among *Shigella* clinical isolates of diverse serotypes. J. Infect. Dis. *172*:1408–1410, 1995.
140. Nuutinen, M., Turtinen, J., and Uhari, M. Growth and joint symptoms in children treated with nalidixic acid. Pediatr. Infect. Dis. J. *13*:798–800, 1994.
141. Oaks, E. V., Hale, T. L., and Formal, S. B.: Serum immune response to *Shigella* protein antigens in rhesus monkeys and humans infected with *Shigella* spp. Infect. Immun. *53*:57–63, 1986.
142. O'Brien, A. D., and Holmes, R. K.: Shiga and Shiga-like toxins. Microbiol. Rev. *51*:206–220, 1987.
143. O'Connor, H. J., and O'Callaghan, U.: Fatal *S. sonnei* septicemia in an adult complemented by marrow aplasia and intestinal perforation. J. Infect. *3*:277–279, 1981.
144. Ogawa, H.: Experimental approach in studies on pathogenesis of bacillary dysentery: With special reference to the invasion of bacilli into intestinal mucosa. Acta. Pathol. Jpn. *20*:261-77, 1970.
145. Okamura, N., Nagai, T., and Nakaya, R., et al.: HeLa cell invasiveness and O antigen of *Shigella flexneri* as separate and prerequisite attributes of virulence to evoke keratoconjunctivitis in guinea pigs. Infect. Immun. *39*:505–513, 1983.
146. Orenstein, W. A., Ross, L., and Overturf, G. D., et al.: Antibiotic treatment of acute shigellosis: Failure of cefamandole compared to trimethoprim/sulfamethoxazole and ampicillin. Am. J. Med. Sci. *282*:27–33, 1981.
147. Ostrower, V. G.: Comparison of cefaclor and ampicillin in the treatment of shigellosis. Postgrad. Med. J. *55*:82–84, 1979.
148. Pal, T., Newland, J. W., Tall, B. D., et al.: Intracellular spread of *Shigella flexneri* associated with the *kcpA* locus and a 140-kilodalton protein. Infect. Immun. *57*:477–486, 1989.
149. Patton, C., Gangarosa, E. J., Weissman, J., et al.: Diagnostic value of indirect hemagglutination in the seroepidemiology of *Shigella* infections. J. Clin. Microbiol. *3*:143–148, 1976.
150. Pickering, L. K., Bartlett, A. V., and Woodward, W. E.: Acute infectious diarrhea among children in day care: Epidemiology and control. Rev. Infect. Dis. *8*:539–547, 1986.
151. Pickering, L. K., and Woodward, W. E.: Diarrhea in day care centers. Pediatr. Infect. Dis. *1*:47–52, 1982.
152. Prado, D., Cleary, T. G., Pickering, L. K., et al.: The relation between production of cytotoxin and clinical features in shigellosis. J. Infect. Dis. *154*:149–155, 1986.
153. Prado, D., Lopez, E., Liu, H., et al.: Ceftibuten and TMP/SMX for treatment of *Shigella* and enteroinvasive *E. coli* disease. Pediatr. Infect. Dis. J. *11*:644–647, 1992.
154. Prado, D., Liu, H., Valasquez, T., et al.: Comparative efficacy of pivmecillinam and cotrimoxazole in acute shigellosis in children. Scand. J. Infect. Dis. *25*:713–719, 1993.
155. Rahaman, M. M., JamiulAlam, A. K. M., Islam, M. R., et al.: Shiga bacillus dysentery associated with marked leukocytosis and erythrocyte fragmentation. Johns Hopkins Med. J. *136*:65–70, 1975.
156. Raderman, J. W., Stoller, K. P., and Pomerance, J. J.: Bloodstream invasion with *S. sonnei* in an asymptomatic newborn infant. Pediatr. Infect. Dis. *5*:379–380, 1986.
157. Rahman, M. M., Kabir, I., Mahalanabis, D., et al.: Decreased food intake in children with severe dysentery due to *S. dysenteriae* 1 infection. Eur. J. Clin. Nutr. *46*:833–838, 1992.
158. Raqib, R., Lindberg, A. A., Wretlind, B., et al.: Persistence of local cytokine production in shigellosis in acute and convalescent stages. Infect. Immun. *63*:289–296, 1995.
159. Raqib, R., Reinholt, F. P., Bardhan, P. K., et al.: Immunopathological patterns in the rectal mucosa of patients with shigellosis: Expression of HLA-DR antigens and T lymphocyte subsets. A. P. M. I. S. *102*:371–380, 1994.
160. Raqib, R., Wretlind, B., Andersson, J., et al.: Cytokine secretion in acute shigellosis is correlated to disease activity and directed more to stool than to plasma. J. Infect. Dis. *171*:376–384, 1995.
161. Rogerie, F., Ott, D., Vandepitte, J., et al.: Comparisons of norfloxacin and nalidixic acid for treatment of dysentery caused by *S. dysenteriae* type 1 in adults. Antimicrob. Agents Chemother. *29*:883–886, 1986.
162. Ross, S., Controni, G., and Khan, W.: Resistance of shigellae to ampicillin and other antibiotics: Its clinical and epidemiological implications. J. A. M. A. *221*:45–47, 1972.
163. Rubenstein, J. S., Noah, Z. L., Zales, V. R., et al.: Acute myocarditis associated with *S. sonnei* gastroenteritis. J. Pediatr. *122*:82–84, 1993.
164. Salam, M. A., and Bennish, M. L.: Therapy of shigellosis. 1. Randomized, double-blind trial of nalidixic acid in childhood shigellosis. Pediatrics *113*:901–907, 1988.
165. Sakai, T., Sasakawa, C., Makino, S., et al.: DNA sequence and product analysis of the *virF* locus responsible for Congo red binding and cell invasion in *Shigella flexneri* 2a. Infect. Immun. *54*:395–402, 1986.
166. Sakamoto, A., and Kamo, S.: Clinical, statistical observations on Ekiri and bacillary dysentery: A study of 785 cases. Ann. Paediatr. *186*:1–18, 1956.
167. Salam, M. A., Seas, C., Khan, W. A., et al.: Treatment of shigellosis. IV. Cefixime is ineffective in shigellosis in adults. Ann. Intern. Med. *123*:505–508, 1995.
168. Salzman, T. C., Scher, C. D., and Moss, R.: Shigellae with transferable drug resistance: Outbreak in a nursery for premature infants. J. Pediatr. *71*:21–26, 1967.
169. Sansonetti, P. J., Hale, T. L., Dammin, G. I., et al.: Alterations in the pathogenicity of *Escherichia coli* K-12 after transfer of plasmids and chromosomal genes from *Shigella flexneri*. Infect. Immun. *39*:1392–1402, 1983.
170. Sansonetti, P. J., Kopecko, D. J., and Formal, S. B.: *Shigella sonnei* plasmids: Evidence that a large plasmid is necessary for virulence. Infect. Immun. *34*:75–83, 1981.
171. Sansonetti, P. J., Kopecko, D. J., and Formal, S. B.: Involvement of a plasmid in the invasive ability of *Shigella flexneri*. Infect. Immun. *35*:852–860, 1982.
172. Sasakawa, C., Kamata, K., Sakai, T., et al.: Molecular alteration of the 140-megadalton plasmid-associated with the loss of virulence and Congo red binding activity in *Shigella flexneri*. Infect. Immun. *51*:470–475, 1986.
173. Schaad, U. B., Salam, M. A., Aujard, Y., et al.: Use of fluoroquinolones in pediatrics: Consensus report of an International Society of Chemotherapy commission. Pediatr. Infect. Dis. J. *14*:1–9, 1995.
174. Scragg, J. N., Rubidge, C. J., and Appelbaum, P. C.: *Shigella* infection in African and Indian children with special reference to *Shigella* septicemia. J. Pediatr. *93*:796–797, 1978.
175. Sereny, B.: Experimental *Shigella* keratoconjunctivitis. Acta. Microbiol. Acad. Sci. Hung. *2*:293–296, 1955.
176. Sharp, T. W., Thornton, S. A., Wallace, M. R., et al.: Diarrheal disease among military personnel during Operation Restore Hope, Somalia, 1992–1993. Am. J. Trop. Med. Hyg. *52*:188–193, 1995.
177. Simor, A. E., Poon, R., and Borczyk, A.: Chronic *Shigella flexneri* infection preceding development of acquired immunodeficiency syndrome. J. Clin. Microbiol. *27*:353–355, 1989.
178. Smith, H. R., Scotland, S. M., Chart, H., et al.: Vero cytotoxin production and presence of VT genes in strains of *Escherichia coli* and *Shigella*. FEMS Microbiol. Lett. *42*:173, 1987.
179. Speelman, P., Kabir, I., and Islam, M.: Distribution and spread of colonic lesions in shigellosis: A colonoscopic study. J. Infect. Dis. *150*:899–903, 1984.
180. Speelman, P., McGlaughlin, R., Kabir, I., et al.: Differential clinical features and stool findings in shigellosis and amoebic dysentery. Trans. R. Soc. Trop. Med. Hyg. *81*:549–551, 1987.
181. Starke, J. R., and Baker, C. J.: Neonatal shigellosis with bowel perforation. Pediatr. Infect. Dis. *4*:405-407, 1985.
182. Stern, M. S., and Gitnick, G. L.: *Shigella* hepatitis. J. A. M. A. *235*:2628, 1976.
183. Stoll, B. J., Glass, R. I., Huq, M. I., et al.: Surveillance of patients attending a diarrhoeal disease hospital in Bangladesh. Br. Med. J. *285*:1185–1188, 1982.
184. Struelens, M. J., Patte, D., Kabir, I., et al.: *Shigella* septicemia: Prevalence, presentation, risk factors, and outcome. J. Infect. Dis. *152*:784–790, 1985.
185. Tauxe, R. V., Puhr, N. D., Wells, J. G., et al.: Antimicrobial resistance of

Shigella isolates in the USA: The importance of international travelers. J. Infect. Dis. *162*:1107–1111, 1990.
186. Taylor, W. I., and Harris, B.: Isolation of shigellae. II. Comparison of plating media and enrichment broths. Am. J. Clin. Pathol. *44*:471–475, 1965.
187. Tobias, J. D., Starke, J. R., and Tosi, M. F.: *Shigella* keratitis: A report of two cases and a review of the literature. Pediatr. Infect. Dis. *6*:79–81, 1987.
188. Tuttle, J., Ries, A. A., Chimba, R. M., et al.: Antimicrobial resistant epidemic *S. dysenteriae* type 1 in Zambia: Modes of transmission. J. Infect. Dis. *171*:371–375, 1995.
189. Varsano, I., Eidlitz-Marcus, T., Nussinovitch, M., et al.: Comparative efficacy of ceftriaxone and ampicillin for treatment of severe shigellosis in children. J. Pediatr. *118*:627–632, 1991.
190. Venkatesan, M. M., Buyssee, J. M., and Kopecko, D. J.: Use of *Shigella flexneri ipaC* and *ipaH* gene sequences for the general identification of *Shigella* spp. and enteroinvasive *Escherichia coli*. J. Clin. Microbiol. *27*:2687–2691, 1989.
191. Vila, J., Gascon, J., Abdalla, S., et al.: Antimicrobial resistance of *Shigella* isolates causing traveler's diarrhea. Antimicrob. Agents Chemother. *38*:2668–2670, 1994.
192. Watanabe, H., Nakamura, A., and Timmis, K.: Small virulence plasmid of *Shigella dysenteriae* 1 strain W30864 encodes a 41,000-dalton protein involved in formation of specific lipopolysaccharide side chains of serotype 1 isolates. Infect. Immun. *46*:55–63, 1984.
193. Weissman, J. B., Williams, S. V., Hinman, A. R., et al.: Foodborne shigellosis at a country fair. Am. J. Epidemiol. *100*:178–185, 1974.
194. Whitfield, C., and Humphries, J. M.: Meningitis and septicemia due to shigellae in a newborn infant. J. Pediatr. *70*:805–806, 1967.
195. Yolken, R. H., Ojeh, C., Khatri, I. A., et al.: Intestinal mucins inhibit rotavirus replication in an oligosaccharide-dependent manner. J. Infect. Dis. *169*:1002–1006, 1994.
196. Zychlinsky, A., Fitting, C., Cavaillon, J. M., et al.: IL-1 is released by murine macrophages during apoptosis induced by *S. flexneri*. J. Clin. Invest. *94*:1328–1332, 1994.
197. Zychlinsky, A., Perdomo, J. J., and Sansonetti, P. J. Molecular and cellular mechanisms of tissue invasion by *S. flexneri*. Ann. N. Y. Acad. Sci. *730*:197–208, 1994.
198. Zychlinsky, A., Kenny, B., Menard, R., et al.: *IpaB* mediates macrophage apoptosis induced by *S. flexneri*. Mol. Microbiol. *11*:619–627, 1994.

114

SERRATIA

William C. Gruber and Randall G. Fisher

Like other members of Enterobacteriaceae, the genus *Serratia* contains species increasingly associated with opportunistic infection in the compromised host. One of the oldest bacterial organisms to be named,[87] *Serratia marcescens* is the chief species associated with disease in humans and has been associated with infection of the urinary tract, the respiratory tract, local wounds, and central venous catheters. Illness may be complicated by bacteremia and meningitis. Treatment of infection may be made exceptionally difficult due to frequent resistance of these organisms to penicillins, cephalosporins, and aminoglycosides.

BACTERIOLOGY

S. marcescens can produce a red pigment resembling blood on contaminated foodstuffs. As early as the sixth century the "miraculous" appearance of blood on food provoked both superstition and scientific investigation. Troops were goaded into battle, and religious beliefs gained support due to the fortuitous growth of the saprophyte in bread.[87] In 1819, *S. marcescens* was named by Bizio, who correctly interpreted the discoloration of cornmeal to be due to a living organism.[57] The genus name honors the Italian physicist Serrafino Serrati, who Bizio thought had been slighted in favor of Robert Fulton as inventor of the steamboat; *marcescens* was drawn from the Latin word meaning "to decay."

We now recognize the genus *Serratia* as straight, motile, catalase-positive, gram-negative rods. Colonies are opaque, iridescent, and white, pink, or red on solid agar. Organisms are Voges-Proskauer test–positive.[43] The genus may be distinguished from other enterobacteria (genera) by its utilization of caprylate or L-fucose as a sole carbon source and its hydrolysis of gelatin.[43, 82] Clinically relevant strains include *S. marcescens*, *S. liquefaciens*, *S. odorifera*, *S. ficara*, and *S. plymuthica*.[15, 32]

EPIDEMIOLOGY

S. marcescens was felt to be nonpathogenic in earlier times and was used as a biologic marker of transmission as early as 1906. In that year, M. H. Gordon, commissioned to study the atmospheric hygiene of the British House of Commons, gargled a liquid culture of *S. marcescens* and then quoted Shakespeare to an audience of agar plates in the otherwise empty House.[38, 87] The organism subsequently was recovered from the plates, documenting the possibility of aerosol transmission of bacteria. (Gordon reported no ill effects.) The importance of *S. marcescens* as a biologic marker for hand-to-hand bacterial transmission, ascension of bacteria in the urinary tract in catheterized patients, and bacteremia after dental extraction is reviewed in detail by Yu.[87] Most remarkably, in investigations in 1950 and 1952 to judge the threat of biological warfare to the United States, the Navy released *S. marcescens* into the Pacific, where it became aerosolized and drifted as far as 80 meters inland.[6] Although an epidemic of *S. marcescens* infection in a San Francisco hospital coincided with this event, subsequent serotype and biotype analyses cast doubt on any relationship to the Navy experiments.[31] Rather, the early San Francisco hospital experience heralded the increased frequency of nosocomial infections that would be observed in subsequent years.[87]

Sporadic nosocomial outbreaks of infection first were reported in the 1950s and 1960s.[54, 68, 85] Early outbreaks in a pediatric ward and neonatal nursery were attributed to contaminated intravenous solution and caps of bottles containing saline used to moisten umbilical cords.[54] As reviewed by Yu,[87] environmental sources before 1979 included disinfectants, water from ultrasonic nebulizers, respirators, arterial pressure monitors, and fiberoptic bronchoscopes. Environmental sources since have included suction traps,[61] intra-aortic pressure transducers,[9, 83] contaminated handwashing brushes,[5] illicit intravenous drug paraphernalia,[24] contaminated urologic instruments,[29] colonized disinfectants or soaps,[30, 52, 55] contaminated infant parenteral nutrition fluid,[33] contaminated whole blood,[37] and inadequately sterilized breast-milk pumps.[40] However, hand-to-hand transmission appears to be the primary mechanism of nosocomial spread. In one dramatic outbreak, spread of an organism with the same serotype, phage type, and antimicrobial sensitivity pattern was documented between four geographically separated teaching hospitals in the same region[73]; spread was likely due to passive carriage of *S. marcescens* on the hands of rotating personnel. By 1979, it was apparent that nosocomial increase in *S. marcescens* infection was becoming a worldwide concern.[15] Outbreaks in neonatology units and pediatric wards have been widespread, persistent, and associated with high morbidity and mortality.[5, 12, 61, 62, 79] At the peak of one epidemic of invasive *S. marcescens* disease in a neonatal nursery, more than 90 per cent of infants were colonized with the epidemic strain.[28] Increased rates of colonization have been associated with nearly 10-fold increases in rates of *S. marcescens* bacteremia and meningitis.[89] Outbreaks of multidrug-resistant strains have been especially troublesome in surgical subspecialty wards.[16]

Biotyping may be successful in characterizing isolates, which then can be traced in the hospital environment.[42, 78] Ribotyping or identification of a unique biochemical characteristic has proved useful for demonstrating cross-contamination across hematology, gastroenterology, and neonatology units in a pediatric hospital.[10, 34] Use of typing methods may be particularly important because drug-resistant and drug-susceptible isolates of *Serratia* may cocirculate.[22] DNA amplification techniques offer promise for characterizing isolates in future outbreaks.[52]

PATHOPHYSIOLOGY

Pathologic findings of sepsis are similar to those of other gram-negative enteric bacilli. Postmortem examination of the lungs of patients with radiologic findings of *S. marcescens* pneumonia reveals a focal necrotizing pneumonia in most and hemorrhagic manifestations in some.[8]

Several properties may enhance virulence of *Serratia* in human infection. The 56-kd protease of *S. marcescens* appears to possess properties of a virulence factor. It enhances vascular permeability through activation of the Hageman factor–kallikrein-kinin pathway in vivo.[53] The protease also has the capacity to degrade host proteins important in humoral immune response, such as immunoglobulins and fibronectin,[60] and inactivates the chemotactic effect of C5a.[64] *Serratia* hemolysin indirectly may increase vascular permeability, local edema, and granulocyte accumulation. Compared with some enteric organisms, *Serratia* adheres better to bladder epithelial cells, which may facilitate urinary tract infection.[26]

Both cell-mediated immunity and humoral immunity may be important in protection from *Serratia* infection and illness. In a murine model of immunization against *S. marcescens,* only the transfer of both antiserum and spleen cells from vaccinated mice increased bacterial clearance from the liver and survival after infection.[49]

Resistance of *S. marcescens* to aminoglycosides generally is plasmid-mediated. Resistance to aminoglycosides may be conferred by one of several genes producing acetylating, phosphorylating, or adenylating enzymes.[1, 2, 16, 44, 58] Risk of infection with aminoglycoside resistance increases with exposure to these agents.[39, 88] However, in some patients, repeated hospitalizations have shown greater importance than aminoglycoside use as a risk factor for infection with resistant strains.[7] High levels of resistance to penicillins and cephalosporins are mediated by one or more plasmids. Cephalosporin resistance also may be derived chromosomally (see also Chapter 107, *Enterobacter*).[22, 35, 56, 67] Chromosomally mediated β-lactam resistance may be inducible in the presence of high levels of penicillin, particularly when plasmid-derived β-lactamase is blocked by clavulanic acid.[17] Transposable plasmid elements may seem in part responsible for the rapid spread of multiple drug resistance.[69, 70, 75] Plasmids conferring multiple drug resistance are transferable from *S. marcescens* to *Klebsiella* and may be responsible for sequential nosocomial outbreaks of different genera sharing common drug resistance patterns.[81]

CLINICAL MANIFESTATIONS

First described in a patient with bronchiectasis as a cause of "blood-tinged" sputum colored by the organism,[86] *S. marcescens* commonly is associated with urinary tract, respiratory tract, central venous catheter, and bacteremic infections.[2] Other species, including *S. liquefaciens, S. ficara, S. odorifera,* and *S. plymuthica,* are less common causes of disease.[11, 20, 27, 32, 76]

Chromogenic *S. marcescens* was responsible for the historically interesting and reportedly benign "red diaper syndrome," which persisted for 7 months in the infant of a genetics professor.[84] However, in at least one series, the organism has been identified as one of the top five causes of neonatal sepsis[41] and now is recognized as a major pathogen of the compromised newborn. Disease in newborn intensive care units is associated commonly with high rates of underlying respiratory illness.[62] Other preexisting risk factors include necrotizing enterocolitis, intravenous catheters, and cardiac disease. Clinical illness shares features in common with other neonatal enteric pathogens; apnea, hypotension, and respiratory distress are frequent. Meningitis may occur as a complication, and antibiotic resistance may emerge during therapy for bacteremia or localized infection.[18] Significant brain injury caused by ventriculitis, brain abscesses, or porencephalic cysts is observed in the majority of infants with meningitis.[18, 50]

In older children and adults, *Serratia* species are isolated most frequently from the urinary tract.[2, 73] Instrumentation, catheterization, and clustering of susceptibles are important risk factors.[7, 19, 44, 71, 74] By the 1970s, increased frequencies of serious infection, such as endocarditis, were noted in intravenous drug abusers.[24] In some series of respiratory and urinary tract infections, *S. marcescens* was observed to be associated more commonly with the complication of bacteremia than was any other enteric pathogen.[45, 48] As is true of other causes of gram-negative sepsis, *Serratia* sepsis characterized by shock, pneumonia, or hemorrhage confers a substantially poorer prognosis.[13, 72] However, the risk of these complications in cancer patients was observed by Saito and associates[72] to be somewhat lower than their previous experience with other pathogens, such as *Escherichia coli* and *Pseudomonas aeruginosa*. When predictive factors of mortality were sought in 385 subjects with nosocomial bacteremia, *S. marcescens* was not an independent predictor of death.[59] Other infections caused by *Serratia* include soft tissue infections, abscesses, endophthalmitis (including a case occurring after septicemia in an infant),[3, 4] osteomyelitis and arthritis,[80] and peritonitis in dialysis patients.[23]

DIAGNOSIS

The diagnosis of *Serratia* infection primarily relies on isolation of organisms from clinical material. Nonspecific laboratory tests occasionally may be misleading. For example, *Serratia* meningitis in the neonate may be accompanied by a normal cerebrospinal fluid white blood cell count or only a modest cerebrospinal fluid pleocytosis.[18] Although *S. marcescens* is famous historically because of its chromogenic potential, most strains are nonpigmented. Hydrolysis of gelatin distinguishes *S. marcescens* from *Klebsiella* and *Enterobacter* in the clinical microbiology laboratory. The presence of ornithine decarboxylase and fermentation of sorbitol but not arabinose helps to differentiate further *S. marcescens* from other *Serratia* species.[43] Biotyping,[42] DNA and RNA detection techniques,[52] and antimicrobial susceptibilities[78] can be used to characterize strains.

TREATMENT

Empiric decisions about antibiotic treatment of *Serratia* infection should rely on knowledge of hospital flora. Therapy should be tailored once susceptibilities are known. In the newborn, meningitis and its complications should be suspected, and interventions should be guided by imaging of the central nervous system. Imaging techniques may be useful in guiding needle aspiration of abscesses.[63] Recommended antibiotic therapy for neonatal meningitis is a cephalosporin and an aminoglycoside for susceptible strains. Still, mortality remains high (>45 per cent), even with appropriate antibiotic management.[18]

In older children and adults, reported response rates for bacteremic infection have been 75 per cent for patients who received appropriate antibiotics, 22 per cent for those who received inappropriate antibiotics, and 29 per cent for those who received no antibiotics.[72] Patients who continue to have positive blood culture results while receiving appropriate antibiotic therapy have a poor prognosis. Inclusion of a penicillin or cephalosporin for susceptible strains should be considered. In Saito's review[72] of 118 patients with *Serratia* bacteremia, patients who received only an aminoglycoside had the poorest response rate among those who received appropriate therapy; those who received a cephalosporin, alone or in combination, fared better. However, the physician needs to be wary of potential resistance to cephalosporins and penicillins due to the production of extended-spectrum β-lactamases. An extended-spectrum metallo–β-lactamase mediating resistance to imipenem has been described.[66]

Amikacin historically has been effective in the treatment of gentamicin-resistant strains.[25, 51] As recently as 1985, amikacin was recommended as a first-line antibiotic for treatment of pediatric nosocomial infection when *Serratia* or other enterics with resistance potential were suspected.[77] However, since the 1980s, outbreaks of *S. marcescens* infections due to amikacin-resistant strains have been reported.[65] Quinolones have been used with some success for treatment of organisms resistant to other agents,[36] but resistance to these drugs also has been identified.[47]

Cohorting and attempts to remove environmental sources of infection have been successful in ending epidemics but typically require several months.[21] Rarely, neonatal intensive care units have been closed to admissions to halt epidemics.[14, 61]

References

1. Acar, J. F., Witchitz, J. L., Goldstein, F., et al.: Susceptibility of aminoglycoside-resistant gram-negative bacilli to amikacin: Delineation of individual resistance patterns. J. Infect. Dis. *134*(Suppl.):S280–S285, 1976.
2. Acar, J. F.: *Serratia marcescens* infections. Infect. Control. *7*:273–278, 1986.
3. al Hazzaa, S. A., Tabbara, K. F., and Gammon, J. A.: Pink hypopyon: A sign of *Serratia marcescens* endophthalmitis. Br. J. Ophthalmol. *76*:764–765, 1992.
4. Alvarez, R., Adan, A., Martinez, J. A., et al.: Haematogenous *Serratia marcescens* endophthalmitis in an HIV-infected intravenous drug addict. Infection *18*:29–30, 1990.
5. Anagnostakis, D., Fitsialos, J., Koutsia, C., et al.: A nursery outbreak of *Serratia marcescens* infection: Evidence of a single source of contamination. Am. J. Dis. Child. *135*:413–414, 1981.
6. Anonymous: Biologic testing involving human subjects by the Department of Defense, 1977: Hearings before the Subcommittee on Health and Science Research of the United States Senate. Washington, D.C., Government Printing Office, 1977.
7. Arroyo, J. C., Milligan, W. L., Postic, B., et al.: Clinical, epidemiologic and microbiologic features of a persistent outbreak of amikacin-resistant *Serratia marcescens*. Infect. Control *2*:367–372, 1981.
8. Balikian, J. P., Herman, P. G., and Godleski, J. J.: *Serratia* pneumonia. Radiology *137*:309–311, 1980.
9. Beck-Sague, C. M., and Jarvis, W. R.: Epidemic bloodstream infections associated with pressure transducers: A persistent problem. Infect. Control Hosp. Epidemiol. *10*:54–59, 1989.
10. Bingen, E. H., Mariani-Kurkdjian, P., Lambert-Zechovsky, N. Y., et al.: Ribotyping provides efficient differentiation of nosocomial *Serratia marcescens* isolates in a pediatric hospital. J. Clin. Microbiol. *30*:2088–2091, 1992.
11. Bollet, C., Grimont, P., Gainnier, M., et al.: Fatal pneumonia due to *Serratia proteamaculans* subsp. *quinovora*. J. Clin. Microbiol. *31*:444–445, 1993.
12. Bollmann, R., Halle, E., Sokolowska-Kohler, W., et al.: Nosocomial infections due to *Serratia marcescens*: Clinical findings, antibiotic susceptibility patterns and fine typing. Infection *17*:294–300, 1989.
13. Bouza, E., Garcia de la Torre, M., Erice, A., et al.: *Serratia* bacteremia. Diagn. Microbiol. Infect. Dis. *7*:237–247, 1987.
14. Braver, D. J., Hauser, G. J., Berns, L., et al.: Control of a *Serratia marcescens* outbreak in a maternity hospital. J. Hosp. Infection *10*:129–137, 1987.
15. Brooks, H. J., Chambers, T. J., and Tabaqchali, S.: The increasing isolation of *Serratia* species from clinical specimens. J. Hyg. *82*:31–40, 1979.
16. Bullock, D. W., Bidwell, J. L., Reeves, D. S., et al.: Outbreaks of hospital infection in southwest England caused by gentamicin-resistant *Serratia marcescens*. J. Hosp. Infect. *3*:263–273, 1982.
17. Bush, K., Flamm, R. K., Ohringer, S., et al.: Effect of clavulanic acid on activity of beta-lactam antibiotics in *Serratia marcescens* isolates producing both a TEM beta-lactamase and a chromosomal cephalosporinase. Antimicrob. Agents Chemother. *35*:2203–2208, 1991.
18. Campbell, J. R., Diacovo, T., and Baker, C. J.: *Serratia marcescens* meningitis in neonates. Pediatr. Infect. Dis. J. *11*:881–886, 1992.
19. Cann, K. J., Johnstone, D., and Skene, A. I.: An outbreak of *Serratia marcescens* infection following urodynamic studies. J. Hosp. Infect. *9*:291–293, 1987.
20. Chmel, H.: *Serratia odorifera* biogroup 1 causing an invasive human infection. J. Clin. Microbiol. *26*:1244–1245, 1988.
21. Christensen, G. D., Korones, S. B., Reed, L., et al.: Epidemic *Serratia marcescens* in a neonatal intensive care unit: Importance of the gastrointestinal tract as a reservoir. Infect. Control *3*:127–133, 1982.
22. Coleman, D., Falkiner, F. R., Carr, M. E., et al.: Simultaneous outbreaks of infection due to *Serratia marcescens* in a general hospital. J. Hosp. Infect. *5*:270–282, 1984.
23. Connacher, A. A., Old, D. C., Phillips, G., et al.: Recurrent peritonitis caused by *Serratia marcescens* in a diabetic patient receiving continuous ambulatory peritoneal dialysis. J. Hosp. Infect. *11*:155–160, 1988.
24. Cooper, R., and Mills, J.: *Serratia* endocarditis. A follow-up report. Arch. Intern. Med. *140*:199–202, 1980.
25. Craven, P. C., Jorgensen, J. H., Kaspar, R. L., et al.: Amikacin therapy of patients with multiply antibiotic-resistant *Serratia marcescens* infections: Development of increasing resistance during therapy. Am. J. Med. *62*:902–910, 1977.
26. Daifuku, R., and Stamm, W. E.: Bacterial adherence to bladder uroepithelial cells in catheter-associated urinary tract infection. N. Engl. J. Med. *314*:1208–1213, 1986.
27. Darbas, H., Jean-Pierre, H., and Paillisson, J.: Case report and review of septicemia due to *Serratia ficaria*. J. Clin. Microbiol. *32*:2285–2288, 1994.
28. Duggan, T. G., Leng, R. A., Hancock, B. M., et al.: *Serratia marcescens* in a newborn unit: Microbiological features. Pathology *16*:189–191, 1984.
29. Echols, R. M., Palmer, D. L., King, R. M., et al.: Multidrug-resistant *Serratia marcescens* bacteriuria related to urologic instrumentation. South. Med. J. *77*:173–177, 1984.
30. Ehrenkranz, N. J., Bolyard, E. A., Wiener, M., et al.: Antibiotic-sensitive *Serratia marcescens* infections complicating cardiopulmonary operations: Contaminated disinfectant as a reservoir. Lancet 2:1289–1292, 1980.
31. Farmer, J. I., Davis, B. R., and Grimont, P. A. D.: Source of American *Serratia*. Lancet 2:459–460, 1977.
32. Fitzgerald, P., Drew, J. H., and Kruszelnicki, I.: *Serratia*: A problem in a neonatal nursery. Aust. Paediatr. J. *20*:205–207, 1984.
33. Frean, J. A., Arntzen, L., Rosekilly, I., et al.: Investigation of contaminated parenteral nutrition fluids associated with an outbreak of *Serratia odorifera* septicaemia. J. Hosp. Infect. *27*:263–273, 1994.
34. Geiseler, P. J., Harris, B., and Andersen, B. R.: Nosocomial outbreak of nitrate-negative *Serratia marcescens* infections. J. Clin. Microbiol. *15*:728–730, 1982.
35. Gianneli, D., Tzelepi, E., Tzouvelekis, L. S., et al.: Dissemination of cephalosporin-resistant *Serratia marcescens* strains producing a plasmidic SHV type beta-lactamase in Greek hospitals. Eur. J. Clin. Microbiol. Infect. Dis. *13*:764–767, 1994.
36. Goldstein, E. J., Alpert, M. L., Najem, A., et al.: Norfloxacin in the treatment of complicated and uncomplicated urinary tract infections: A comparative multicenter trial. Am. J. Med. *82*:65–69, 1987.
37. Gong, J., Hogman, C. F., Hambraeus, A., et al.: Transfusion-associated

Serratia marcescens infection: Studies of the mechanism of action. Transfusion 33:802–808, 1993.
38. Gordon, W. H.: Report on an investigation of the ventilation of the debating chamber of the House of Commons. Parliamentary Command Paper, p. 3035, 1906.
39. Graham, D. R., Clegg, H. W. D., Anderson, R. L., et al.: Gentamicin treatment associated with later nosocomial gentamicin-resistant *Serratia marcescens* infections. Infect. Control 2:31–37, 1981.
40. Gransden, W. R., Webster, M., French, G. L., et al.: An outbreak of *Serratia marcescens* transmitted by contaminated breast pumps in a special care baby unit. J. Hosp. Infect. *7*:149–154, 1986.
41. Grauel, E. L., Halle, E., Bollmann, R., et al.: Neonatal septicaemia: Incidence, etiology and outcome: A 6-year analysis. Acta Paediatr. Scand. *360*(Suppl.):113–119, 1989.
42. Grimont, P. A., and Grimont, F.: Biotyping of *Serratia marcescens* and its use in epidemiological studies. J. Clin. Microbiol. *8*:73–83, 1978.
43. Grimont, P. A. D., and Grimont, F.: *Serratia*. *In* Krieg, N. R., and Holt, J. G. (eds.): Bergey's Manual of Systematic Bacteriology. Vol. 1. Baltimore, Williams and Wilkins, 1984, pp. 476–484.
44. John, J. F. J., and McNeill, W. F.: Characteristics of *Serratia marcescens* containing a plasmid coding for gentamicin resistance in nosocomial infections. J. Infect. Dis. *143*:810–817, 1981.
45. Karnad, A., Alvarez, S., and Berk, S. L.: Pneumonia caused by gram-negative bacilli. Am. J. Med. *79*:61–67, 1985.
46. Konig, W., Faltin, Y., Scheffer, J., et al.: Role of cell-bound hemolysin as a pathogenicity factor for *Serratia* infections. Infect. Immun. *55*:2554–2561, 1987.
47. Korner, R. J., Nicol, A., Reeves, D. S., et al.: Ciprofloxacin-resistant *Serratia marcescens* endocarditis as a complication of non-Hodgkin's lymphoma. J. Infect. *29*:73–76, 1994.
48. Krieger, J. N., Kaiser, D. L., and Wenzel, R. P.: Urinary tract etiology of bloodstream infections in hospitalized patients. J. Infect. Dis. *148*:57–62, 1983.
49. Kumagai, Y., Okada, K., and Sawae, Y.: The effect of humoral and cell-mediated immunity in resistance to systemic *Serratia* infection. J. Med. Microbiol. *36*:245–249, 1992.
50. Lam, A. H., Berry, A., deSilva, M., et al.: Intracranial *Serratia* infection in preterm newborn infants. Am. J. Neuroradiol. *5*:447–451, 1984.
51. Leonard, J. M., McGee, Z. A., and Alford, R. H.: Gentamicin-resistant bacillary infection: Clinical features and amikacin therapy. Arch. Intern. Med. *138*:201–205, 1978.
52. Liu, P. Y., Lau, Y. J., Hu, B. S., et al.: Use of PCR to study epidemiology of *Serratia marcescens* isolates in nosocomial infection. J. Clin. Microbiol. *32*:1935–1938, 1994.
53. Matsumoto, K., Yamamoto, T., Kamata, R., et al.: Pathogenesis of serratial infection: Activation of the Hageman factor-prekallikrein cascade by serratial protease. J. Biochem. *96*:739–749, 1984.
54. McCormack, R. C., and Kunin, C. M.: Control of a single source nursery epidemic due to *Serratia marcescens*. Pediatrics *37*:750–755, 1966.
55. McNaughton, M., Mazinke, N., and Thomas, E.: Newborn conjunctivitis associated with triclosan 0.5 per cent antiseptic intrinsically contaminated with *Serratia marcescens*. Can. J. Infect. Control *10*:7–8, 1995.
56. Medeiros, A. A., and O'Brien, T. F.: Contributions of R factors to the antibiotic resistance of hospital isolates of *Serratia*. Antimicrob. Agents Chemother. *8*:30–35, 1968.
57. Merlino, C. P.: Bartolomeo Bizio's letter to the most eminent priest, Angelo Bellani, concerning the phenomenon of the red-colored polenta. J. Bacteriol. *9*:527–543, 1924.
58. Meyer, R. D.: Patterns and mechanisms of emergence of resistance to amikacin. J. Infect. Dis. *136*:449–452, 1977.
59. Miller, P. J., and Wenzel, R. P.: Etiologic organisms as independent predictors of death and morbidity associated with bloodstream infections. J. Infect. Dis. *156*:471–477, 1987.
60. Molla, A., Matsumoto, K., Oyamada, I., et al.: Degradation of protease inhibitors, immunoglobulins, and other serum proteins by *Serratia* protease and its toxicity to fibroblast in culture. Infect. Immun. *53*:522–529, 1986.
61. Montanaro, D., Grasso, G. M., Annino, I., et al.: Epidemiological and bacteriological investigation of *Serratia marcescens* epidemic in a nursery and in a neonatal intensive care unit. J. Hyg. *93*:67–78, 1984.
62. Newport, M. T., John, J. F., Michel, Y. M., et al.: Endemic *Serratia marcescens* infection in a neonatal intensive care nursery associated with gastrointestinal colonization. Pediatr. Infect. Dis. *4*:160–167, 1985.
63. Obana, W. G., Cogen, P. H., Callen, P. W., et al.: Ultrasound-guided aspiration of a neonatal brain abscess. Child. Nerv. Sys. *7*:272–273; discussion 274, 1991.
64. Oda, T., Kojima, Y., Akaike, T., et al.: Inactivation of chemotactic activity of C5a by the serratial 56-kilodalton protease. Infect. Immun. *58*:1269–1272, 1990.
65. Okuda, T., Endo, N., Osada, Y., et al.: Outbreak of nosocomial urinary tract infections caused by *Serratia marcescens*. J. Clin. Microbiol. *20*:691–695, 1984.
66. Osano, E., Arakawa, Y., Wacharotayankun, R., et al.: Molecular characterization of an enterobacterial metallo beta-lactamase found in a clinical isolate of *Serratia marcescens* that shows imipenem resistance. Antimicrob. Agents Chemother. *38*:71–78, 1994.
67. Pagani, L., Luzzaro, F., Ronza, P., et al.: Outbreak of extended-spectrum beta-lactamase–producing *Serratia marcescens* in an intensive care unit. FEMS Immunol. Med. Microbiol. *10*:39–46, 1994.
68. Rabinowitz, K., and Schiffrin, R.: A ward contamination by *Serratia marcescens*. Acta Med. Orient. *11*:181–184, 1952.
69. Rubens, C. E., McNeill, W. F., and Farrar, W. E. J.: Evolution of multiple-antibiotic-resistance plasmids mediated by transposable plasmid deoxyribonucleic acid sequences. J. Bacteriol. *140*:713–719, 1979.
70. Rubens, C. E., Farrar, W. E. J., McGee, Z. A., et al.: Evolution of a plasmid mediating resistance to multiple antimicrobial agents during a prolonged epidemic of nosocomial infections. J. Infect. Dis. *143*:170–181, 1981.
71. Rutala, W. A., Kennedy, V. A., Loflin, H. B., et al.: *Serratia marcescens* nosocomial infections of the urinary tract associated with urine measuring containers and urinometers. Am. J. Med. *70*:659–663, 1981.
72. Saito, H., Elting, L., Bodey, G. P., et al.: *Serratia* bacteremia: Review of 118 cases. Rev. Infect. Dis. *11*:912–920, 1989.
73. Schaberg, D. R., Alford, R. H., Anderson, R., et al.: An outbreak of nosocomial infection due to multiply resistant *Serratia marcescens*: Evidence of interhospital spread. J. Infect. Dis. *134*:181–188, 1976.
74. Schaberg, D. R., Haley, R. W., Highsmith, A. K., et al.: Nosocomial bacteriuria: A prospective study of case clustering and antimicrobial resistance. Ann. Intern. Med. *93*:420–424, 1980.
75. Schaberg, D. R., Rubens, C. E., Alford, R. H., et al.: Evolution of antimicrobial resistance and nosocomial infection: Lessons from the Vanderbilt experience. Am. J. Med. *70*:445–448, 1981.
76. Serruys-Schoutens, E., Rost, F., and Depre, G.: A nosocomial epidemic of *Serratia liquefaciens* urinary tract infection after cystometry. Eur. J. Clin. Microbiol. *3*:316–317, 1984.
77. Shulman, S. T., and Yogev, R.: Treatment of pediatric infections with amikacin as first-line aminoglycoside. Am. J. Med. *79*:43–50, 1985.
78. Sifuentes-Osornio, J., Ruiz-Palacios, G. M., and Groschel, D. H.: Analysis of epidemiologic markers of nosocomial *Serratia marcescens* isolates with special reference to the Grimont biotyping system. J. Clin. Microbiol. *23*:230–234, 1986.
79. Stamm, W. E., Kolff, C. A., Dones, E. M., et al.: A nursery outbreak caused by *Serratia* marcescens: Scalp-vein needles as a portal of entry. J. Pediatr. *89*:96–99, 1976.
80. Svensson, O., Parment, P. A., and Blomgren, G.: Orthopaedic infections by *Serratia marcescens*: A report of seven cases. Scand. J. Infect. Dis. *19*:69–75, 1987.
81. Thomas, F. E., Jackson, R. T., Melly, A., et al.: Sequential hospitalwide outbreaks of resistant *Serratia* and *Klebsiella* infections. Arch. Intern. Med. *137*:581–584, 1977.
82. Verrall, R.: *Serratia marcescens*. Infect. Control *4*:469–471, 1983.
83. Villarino, M. E., Jarvis, W. R., O'Hara, C., et al.: Epidemic of *Serratia marcescens* bacteremia in a cardiac intensive care unit. J. Clin. Microbiol. *27*:2433–2436, 1989.
84. Waisman, H. A., and Stone, W. H.: The presence of *Serratia marcescens* as the predominating organism in the intestinal tract of the newborn: The occurrence of the "red diaper syndrome." Pediatrics *21*:8–12, 1958.
85. Wheat, R. P., Zuckerman, A., and Rantz, L. A.: Infection due to chromobacteria: Report of eleven cases. Arch. Intern. Med. *88*:461–466, 1951.
86. Woodward, H. M. M., and Clarke, K. B.: A case of infection in man by the *Bacterium prodigiosum*. Lancet *1*:314–315, 1913.
87. Yu, V. L.: *Serratia marcescens*: Historical perspective and clinical review. N. Engl. J. Med. *300*:887–893, 1979.
88. Yu, V. L., Oakes, C. A., Axnick, K. J., et al.: Patient factors contributing to the emergence of gentamicin-resistant *Serratia marcescens*. Am. J. Med. *66*:468–472, 1979.
89. Zaidi, M., Sifuentes, J., Bobadilla, M., et al.: Epidemic of *Serratia marcescens* bacteremia and meningitis in a neonatal unit in Mexico City. Infect. Control Hosp. Epidemiol. *10*:14–20, 1989.

115

SALMONELLA

Henry F. Gomez and Thomas G. Cleary

Salmonella species are ubiquitous human and animal pathogens. In humans, they are responsible for a variety of clinical syndromes, including asymptomatic carriage, self-limited gastroenteritis, bacteremia, enteric fever, and metastatic focal infections.

MICROBIOLOGY

Salmonella are motile (due to peritrichous flagellae), nonencapsulated, gram-negative bacilli of the Enterobacteriaceae family. Most ferment glucose, maltose, and mannitol but do not utilize lactose or sucrose. All pathogenic *Salmonella* other than *S. typhi* produce gas. *Salmonella* species are facultative anaerobes. Blood agar or chocolate agar support their growth when they are present as the sole organisms in blood, cerebrospinal fluid, or joint fluid. For specimens containing mixed flora (e.g., stool), selective media such as *Salmonella-Shigella* (SS agar) or bismuth sulfate agar must be used.

The classification of *Salmonella* is confusing because multiple nomenclature systems are used. In hospital laboratories, three "species" of *Salmonella* (*S. choleraesuis*, *S. typhi*, and *S. enteritidis*) are distinguished biochemically. Serogroup, based on O (somatic) antigen, also usually is determined on initial isolation, and organisms that are not *S. typhi* or *S. choleraesuis* are reported as *Salmonella* serogroup A, B, C1, D1, etc. Common *Salmonella* and their serogroups are shown in Table 115–1. *Salmonella* serotype is defined by the somatic or lipopolysaccharide (O) antigens, the flagellar (H) antigens, and the virulence (Vi) antigen. H antigens can be either phase 1 (nonspecific) or phase 2 (specific). The Vi antigen is a heat-labile polysaccharide found on *S. typhi*, *S. dublin*, and *S. paratyphi* C, which may block O antigen-antibody agglutination. Serotyping generally is done in state or county public health department laboratories. Although serotyping is an important epidemiologic tool that is useful in defining outbreaks, it is much more useful when an unusual type is disease associated. When a common serotype is associated with an outbreak (e.g., *S. typhimurium*), plasmid characterization,[321] bacteriophage typing,[73] outer-membrane polypeptide analysis, biochemical phenotype, and antibiogram[2] may help determine whether a single-strain, common-source outbreak is in progress.

TABLE 115–1. *Salmonella* Species Included in Major Serogroups

Serogroup	Representative Serotypes
A	*S. paratyphi* A
B	*S. paratyphi* B
	S. saintpaul
	S. agona
	S. derby
	S. typhimurium
	S. heidelberg
C1	*S. paratyphi* C
	S. choleraesuis
	S. montevideo
	S. infantis
C2	*S. newport*
C3	*S. santiago*
D1	*S. typhi*
	S. enteritidis
	S. dublin
D2	*S. strasbourg*
E1	*S. anatum*
E2	*S. newington*
E3	*S. illinois*

*Human infections with organisms in serogroups E4, F, G1, G2, H, and I and the O antigens not given serogroup designation (O17 through O67) are relatively uncommon.

Six subgroups of *Salmonella* have been proposed based on DNA relatedness. Most serotypes, including almost all of the serotypes important in human and animal disease, belong to subgroup 1. *Salmonella* in subgroups 2 to 5 usually are found in cold-blooded animals and the environment. *Arizona* now is considered part of the genus *Salmonella*.

The multiple systems for naming *Salmonella* can confuse the clinician because, for example, an organism initially may be identified as *Salmonella* not *typhi*, not *choleraesuis* by a hospital laboratory. The hospital laboratory then may identify it as *Salmonella* serogroup B. A state health department then may determine it to be serotype *heidelberg*. This same organism may be referred to by taxonomists as *Salmonella* serotype *heidelberg* or *Salmonella* subgroup 1 (*choleraesuis*) serotype 1, 4, 5, 12:r:1, 2.

EPIDEMIOLOGY

Nontyphoidal *Salmonella*

PUBLIC HEALTH ISSUES. In most of the world, the prevalence of *Salmonella* varies depending on the water supply, waste disposal, food preparation practices, and climate. However, the incidence of nontyphoidal salmonellosis in the United States has been increasing steadily over the last four decades, despite good public health measures. Over the last 40 years, there has been a more than sixfold increase in reported nontyphoidal *Salmonella* infection in the United States; more than 50,000 cases are reported each year.[29] This reflects industrial-scale food production, misuse of antimicrobial agents (in both humans and animals) that alter the gastrointestinal flora, thereby increasing host susceptibility to *Salmonella*, and probably an increasing number of immunocompromised persons in the population.

THE SIGNIFICANCE OF ANIMAL RESERVOIRS. Unlike *Shigella* species, which infect only primates, nontyphoidal *Salmonella* species infect a variety of animals (including poultry, livestock, and pets). Thus, animals and animal products (including meat and dairy products), water, and infected humans can be the source of infection. *Salmonella* species have been isolated from up to 50 per cent of poultry,[23] 16 per cent of pork, 5 per cent of beef, and 40 per cent of frozen egg products in retail stores. Undercooked eggs (e.g., in Caesar salad, egg-dipped bread, homemade eggnog) may be contaminated by organisms on the shell surface or be contaminated transovarially directly via the egg yolk. Grade A shell eggs have been implicated in more than 80 per cent of recent outbreaks.[147] Even in the absence of recognized outbreaks, eggs probably are important vehicles of infection; sporadic cases are more likely to have consumed undercooked egg-containing foods during the 3 days prior to illness than are controls.[98]

The risk of outbreaks was demonstrated when *S. typhimurium*–contaminated milk was distributed in Chicago, Illinois. It was estimated that more than 150,000 became ill, with more than 16,000 culture-confirmed cases, 2777 persons hospitalized, and 14 fatalities.[19] Ice cream, cream cakes, and mayonnaise commonly have been incriminated as the source of infections. Fruits and vegetables rarely are vehicles.[31]

Some serotypes are associated with particular reservoirs. For example, *S. dublin* is associated with dairy cattle and thus frequently is found in those who drink raw milk.[211] *S. choleraesuis* is associated with pigs. Infection with *S. marina* is associated with contact with pet iguanas. *Salmonella* group F, *S. typhimurium, S. muenchen,* and *S. java* infections have been traced to pet turtles. Reptiles, including rattlesnakes, are important *S. arizona* reservoirs.

HUMANS AS A RESERVOIR. After infection, nontyphoidal *Salmonella* species are excreted in feces for a median of 5 weeks. Children younger than 5 years of age may excrete the organisms for 20 weeks after illness, but older children and adults usually excrete *Salmonella* less than 8 weeks. *S. typhi* may be excreted chronically, particularly in the presence of gall bladder disease. Food handlers who are excreting *Salmonella* species represent an important risk group.

BACTERIAL CHARACTERISTICS FAVORING SURVIVAL. *Salmonella* species are hardy. They survive refrigeration and sometimes heating; they may remain viable at ambient or reduced temperatures for weeks. When contaminated foods are cooked for less than 12 minutes at temperatures less than 150° F (65.5° C), *Salmonella* may remain viable. *Salmonella* species are killed by heating to 130° F (54.4° C) for 1 hour or 140° F (60° C) for 15 minutes. *Salmonella* survive for hours on the hands of slaughterhouse workers.[164] They have been found to survive in flour for nearly a year.[141] *S. tennessee* has been reported to remain viable for 2 to 8 days on glass, stainless steel, enameled surfaces, rubber mattress, linen, and a rubber tabletop.[226] Nosocomial infections have been related to contaminated medical equipment (e.g., endoscopes) and diagnostic or pharmacologic preparations, particularly those of animal origin (e.g., pituitary extracts, bile salts, pancreatic extracts, pepsin, vitamins).

THE RELATIONSHIP OF AGE TO RISK OF DISEASE. The highest incidence rates occur in children younger than 5 years of age, especially those younger than 1 year of age, and in individuals older than 70 years of age. There is little gender difference in children.

Nursery outbreaks often can be traced to an infected mother,[1, 2, 14, 119] with subsequent spread via health care personnel.[226, 194] The mother of the index case can be symptomatic[68, 136, 185, 258] or asymptomatic,[22] recovering from recent infection,[2, 156, 196] or a chronic carrier.[191] Low birth weight infants appear to be at higher risk of acquiring *Salmonella* than do full-term infants.[17, 194] The source of infection occasionally is contaminated food but more often fomites (delivery room resuscitators,[186] rectal thermometers,[107, 139] suction devices,[115] waterbaths for heating formula,[178] soap dispensers,[146] scales,[5, 18, 226] tables,[226] air conditioning filters,[226] and plumbing[143]). Nursery outbreaks often are extraordinarily difficult to stop. They have been reported to last several months[139, 160, 226] to several years.[68, 143, 205] Contamination sometimes can become so widespread that other areas of the hospital also experience cases.[137, 195] Nursery outbreaks are far more common with *Salmonella* than with other bacterial enteropathogens. Such outbreaks sometimes are due to multiresistant *Salmonella*.[119]

SEASONALITY. *Salmonella* infection occurs in warm months, when there are more food-borne outbreaks related to contaminated food, contaminated hands of food handlers, or contaminated fomites. Between 1985 and 1991, there were 380 outbreaks of *S. enteritidis* infection in the United States reported to the Centers for Disease Control and Prevention; these outbreaks involved 13,056 ill persons and resulted in 50 deaths.[147]

INOCULUM SIZE REQUIRED TO CAUSE DISEASE. The estimated inoculum size required to cause symptomatic disease in healthy adult volunteers is 10^5 to 10^{10} organisms,[21] but the number of organisms required to cause symptoms in infants and children probably is much lower. In contrast, large inocula are not required for *Shigella* infection, which occurs in human volunteers exposed to as few as 10 organisms. In some outbreaks, it appears that very low inocula of *Salmonella* have caused disease. Within a given serotype, there are strain-related differences in dose needed to cause illness. Large inocula (e.g., 10^9) may cause severe symptoms, even in healthy children.[210] The incubation period usually is less than 24 hours but, depending on inoculum size,[105] bacterial virulence, and host immunocompetence, ranges from 6 to 72 hours. Communicability parallels the duration of fecal excretion; nontyphoidal *Salmonella* may be carried for several months. The probability of salmonellosis is increased when a member of the household is infected. Infants especially may be prone to acquiring *Salmonella* infection directly or indirectly from ill family members. In a retrospective review of 187 infants younger than 1 year of age with *Salmonella* gastroenteritis, 39 per cent had at least one family contact with diarrhea, and 71 per cent of the contacts had stool cultures positive for *Salmonella*.[227] *Salmonella* species rarely have been isolated during studies of gastroenteritis in day care centers, perhaps suggesting that larger inocula are required to cause illness in toddlers and older children.[34, 126, 166]

ANTIBIOTIC SELECTION PRESSURE. Since the mid 1960s, *Salmonella* species increasingly have become resistant to ampicillin, chloramphenicol, and trimethoprim-sulfamethoxazole (TMP-SMX). Multiresistant strains have included *S. typhimurium*, which is the most common serotype in Europe and the United States, as well as *S. heidelberg, S. agona, S. muenchen, S. enteritidis,* and *S. hadar.* Antibiotic resistance usually is transferable between organisms via plasmids that carry genes encoding resistance factors.[83] Exposure to prior antibiotics is significantly more common in those who develop both antibiotic-resistant and antibiotic-susceptible salmonellosis. Patients who are infected with antibiotic-resistant strains are more likely to be hospitalized, to be very young, to be black, and to have been exposed recently to antibiotic agents.[120] Previous use of antimicrobial agents for treatment of other illnesses is a significant risk factor for acquiring multiresistant *Salmonella* infection.[131, 179] Perhaps the most important factor is the overuse and misuse of antibiotics in animals raised for food.[37, 102, 103, 125, 202] Subtherapeutic concentrations of antibiotics used to enhance growth and prevent infection promote intestinal colonization by antibiotic-resistant bacteria, including *Salmonella;* these organisms may be found in feces and may contaminate meat at the time of slaughter. Plasmid analysis and antibiotic susceptibility patterns have linked *Salmonella* outbreaks to specific farms and slaughterhouses.[102, 103, 159]

Salmonella typhi

It is estimated that there are approximately 12.5 million cases annually in the world, with an incidence of 365 cases per 100,000 persons. *S. typhi* is the most common *Salmonella* isolate in many developing countries; the incidence in these countries is estimated at 10 to 540 cases per 100,000 persons. In developed countries, the annual incidence is 0.2 to 3.7 cases per 100,000 persons in Western Europe, the United States, and Japan and 4.3 to 14.5 cases per 100,000 persons in Southern Europe.[56] In the United States, there were approximately 1700 total cases reported (1.0 case per 100,000 persons) in 1955. In 1988, there were approximately 400 total cases reported (.018 cases per 100,000 persons). Only about 28 per cent of infections occurred in individuals 19 years of age or younger.[29] In developing countries, the incidence is highest in 5- to 25-year-olds. In the United States, persons traveling to developing countries are a high-risk group; 62 to 70 per cent of infections are related to foreign travel, especially to Mexico or India.[30, 56, 189]

THE RESERVOIR. Humans are the reservoir for *S. typhi*; infection implies direct or indirect contact with an infected person. Animal products transmit *S. typhi* if contaminated by infected humans during processing. The most common mode of transmission is food or water contaminated by human feces. Water-borne typhoid fever epidemics especially are important. Congenital transmission can occur from a bacteremic mother to her fetus transplacentally or at the time of delivery via the fecal-oral route.

THE RELEVANCE OF INOCULUM SIZE TO DISEASE. As with nontyphoidal *Salmonella*, more than 10^5 organisms are required to cause clinical illness in adults.[105] The incubation period is 7 to 14 days but may be from 3 to 60 days.

ANTIBIOTIC RESISTANCE. The worldwide frequency of antibiotic-resistant *S. typhi* has been increasing since the 1960s[199] but remains much lower than that for nontyphoidal *Salmonella*. Extensive protracted outbreaks have been reported throughout Asia, the Middle East, and Central and South America. Epidemic enteric fever in Mexico caused by chloramphenicol-resistant strains lasted for 2 years in the early 1970s.[221] These outbreaks may have been related to widespread availability and inappropriate use of antimicrobial agents (especially chloramphenicol) as over-the-counter drugs in these areas.

PATHOPHYSIOLOGY

Host susceptibility is understood most easily in terms of specific events in pathogenesis. Tables 115–2 and 115–3 show the relevance of specific host and bacterial virulence factors in salmonellosis. The outcome of *Salmonella* ingestion depends on both the bacteria and the host.

Various *Salmonella* strains can (1) adhere to, invade, and multiply in intestinal epithelium; (2) produce cholera toxin–like enterotoxin that increases cyclic adenosine monophosphate levels within intestinal crypt cells, causing a net efflux of electrolytes and water into the intestinal lumen; (3) uptake by M cells overlying Peyer's patches of the distal ileum and proximal colon; (4) survive in macrophages of Peyer's patches, mesenteric lymph nodes, and the extraintestinal reticuloendothelial system; and (5) survive in the blood stream. Specific genes (often on virulence plasmids) encode for virulence factors necessary for each step in these processes. Table 115–4 shows an overview of *Salmonella* pathogenesis and the genetic elements related to each process. Pathologic findings include hypertrophy and hyperplasia of the intestinal and mesenteric lymphoid tissues, liver, and spleen in *S. typhi*. In contrast, *S. typhimurium* and other nontyphoidal serotypes cause diffuse colitis, mucosal edema, and crypt abscesses as the major pathologic abnormalities.[23, 45] Some of these virulence genes are shared by all *Salmonella*, whereas others are serotype-specific. There are differences in invasiveness of various serotypes. For example, *S. typhi, S. choleraesuis, S. heidelberg*,[106, 141] and *S. dublin*[211] are more likely to enter the blood and seed distant sites. Virulence plasmids have been identified in *S. typhi, S. typhimurium*, and *S. dublin*.[15]

Although it commonly is said that any *Salmonella* occasionally can cause severe disease such as enteric fever, this may not be true. Nursery *Salmonella* outbreaks dramatically have demonstrated the variability in severity of illness related to strain or serotype. For example, in nursery outbreaks of *S. oranienburg*[205] and *S. newport*,[119] grossly bloody stools were found in 76 to 90 per cent of infected infants, with 10 to 11 per cent febrile and only 9 to 11 per cent asymptomatic. Watery, green, nonbloody diarrhea has been common with

TABLE 115–2. Susceptibility to *Salmonella* Species Infection

Patient Group at Risk	Mechanism
Newborn	Achlorhydria/rapid gastric emptying Poorly developed cell-mediated immunity Complement deficiency Immunoglobulin deficiency in premature infants
Sickle-cell anemia	Reticuloendothelial system overload Functional asplenia Tissue infarcts Defective opsonization
Neutropenia (congenital or acquired)	Polymorphonuclear neutrophils needed for killing
Chronic granulomatous disease	Defective killing by polymorphonuclear neutrophils
AIDS	Low CD4 ? effects of malnutrition on cell-mediated immunity Survival of organisms in macrophages (PhoP/PhoQ, spvA–D, R)
Organ transplantation immunosuppression	Defective cell-mediated immunity
Gastrectomy	Loss of stomach acid barrier
Malaria	Reticuloendothelial overload during hemolysis Abnormal complement levels Abnormal macrophage function
Bartonellosis	Reticuloendothelial overload during hemolysis
Schistosomiasis	*Salmonella* sequestered in schistosomes so that neither host defenses nor antibiotics are effective

TABLE 115–3. Physiologic Basis of Clinical Features of *Salmonella* Species Infection

Clinical Feature	Mechanism
Watery diarrhea	Enterotoxin (cholera toxin–like) ? role of neutrophils
Bacteremia	Vi capsular antigen (*S. typhi, S. dublin,* and *S. paratyphi* C) interferes with C3 binding Lipopolysaccharides (*S. typhi, S. choleraesuis*) Prevent formation of C5b-9 membrane attack complex (*S. dublin, S. typhimurium, S. enteritidis*) Virulence plasmids (*S. typhimurium*) Leukopenia increases bacteremic relapses in nontyphoidal *Salmonella*
Typhoid fever (relapses, prolonged fever, failure of certain antibiotics) Relapse of meningitis in nontyphoidal *Salmonella* species infection	Survival of organisms in macrophages (PHoP/PHoQ, spvA–D, R)
Chronic fecal excretion	Biliary tract disease (*S. typhi*)

S. typhimurium,[2] *S. virchow,*[183] and *S. nienstedten.*[195] A high frequency of asymptomatic infections has been seen during nursery outbreaks with *S. heidelberg* (38 per cent asymptomatic),[17] *S. virchow* (42 per cent asymptomatic),[183] and *S. tennessee* (100 per cent asymptomatic).[226]

Specific bacterial virulence genes are relevant to the intestinal phase of illness. The *invA–H* chromosomal genes are necessary for adherence to and invasion of intestinal mucosal cells[66]; most of the genes described so far appear to be involved in secretion or transport of virulence proteins.[87, 220] Recently, genes closely related to the *Shigella* invasion plasmid antigens (ipaA–D) have been described in *Salmonella* species[111, 112]; these *Salmonella* genes (*sipA–D*) probably play a role similar to their role in *Shigella*.

For most nontyphoidal *Salmonella*, infection does not extend beyond the lamina propria and the local lymphatics. In contrast, *S. typhi, S. dublin,* and *S. choleraesuis* rapidly invade the blood stream with relatively little intestinal involvement. Some virulence genes confer a survival advantage to the organisms if they get into the extraintestinal milieu. Vi capsular antigen present in *S. typhi, S. dublin,* and *S. paratyphi* C interferes with C3 binding. Mutations in lipopolysaccharide genes decrease invasiveness of *S. typhi* and *S. choleraesuis* but not *S. typhimurium.*[67, 149] *S. dublin, S. typhimurium,* and *S. enteritidis* have virulence genes that confer resistance to complement by preventing the formation and insertion of the C5b-9 membrane attack complex. Sickle-cell anemia patients have complement defects and defects in opsonization of *S. typhimurium.*[95] Newborns also have complement deficiencies that may explain their high frequency of *Salmonella* infection and their susceptibility to bacteremic complications seldom seen in normal hosts.

The role of host cells in the invasion process is complex. After *S. typhimurium* comes in contact with epithelial cells, there is activation of epidermal growth factor receptor, which then activates a kinase that turns on phospholipase A2 so that arachidonic acid is generated. Arachidonic acid is converted to leukotriene LTD_4, which opens Ca^{2+} channels and causes membrane ruffling, cytoskeletal changes, and uptake of bacteria.[66] Nonphagocytic cells, including epithelial cells, are adapted poorly for killing of internalized bacteria. *Salmonella* species not only survive in vacuoles within epithelial cells, but they also can replicate actively.[67] In contrast, *S. typhimurium* does not appear to be able to replicate after being ingested by macrophages.[26] There are several sets of genes that appear to allow *Salmonella* to survive within the hostile environment of macrophages. The PhoP/PhoQ system and the *spvA–D* and *spvR* plasmid loci seem to be key to this process.[89, 90] The presence of virulence plasmids appears to be more common in blood isolates of *S. typhimurium*

TABLE 115–4. Relationship Between Specific Virulence Genes and Pathophysiology

	Salmonella Genes Involved	Effect on Animal Host
Intestinal Epithelial Phase		
Adherence	*invA–H*	Endocytosis of organisms
Invasion	*invE, sipA–D*	
Replication		
Enterotoxin	*stx*	Fluid secretion
Intestinal Macrophage Phase		
Uptake by M cells	*prgH*	Bacteria persist in gut lymphoid tissue
Survival in macrophages	*PhoP/PhoQ*	
Extraintestinal Phase		
Spread beyond Peyer's patches to mesenteric nodes, liver, spleen	*spvA–D, spvR*	Reticuloendothelial system Hyperplasia Bacteremia
Resistance to complement	*rfb* (lipopolysaccharide synthesis)	Persistent bacteremia
	viaB (Vi synthesis)	Metastatic foci of infection
	rck	

than in fecal isolates (76 per cent vs. 42 per cent).[65] However, *S. typhi* and *S. paratyphi* A do not contain virulence plasmids and yet are invasive.

The development of diarrhea depends on host and pathogen factors. There must be an influx of polymorphonuclear leukocytes into the mucosa to develop diarrhea.[223] Neutropenic animals fail to develop fluid secretion when infected with *Salmonella*[224]; it is thought that infiltration of leukocytes triggers prostaglandin production because fluid secretion can be blocked by indomethacin.[77] A cholera toxin–like enterotoxin is made by about two-thirds of *Salmonella* strains, including *S. typhimurium* and *S. typhi*.[109]

Multiple host defense strategies have evolved to deal with these virulence factors; host susceptibility often can be related directly to defects in these defense mechanisms. The host tries to kill ingested organisms in the stomach, to inhibit their growth in the gut, to limit their spread beyond the intestine, and to clear them by immune mechanisms.

At a pH of 2.0, most *Salmonella* species are killed rapidly.[74] When gastric pH is raised by oral administration of antacid, susceptibility increases.[75, 105, 179] Slow gastric emptying also is protective. *Salmonella* ingested in water passes through the stomach more rapidly than when the same inoculum is ingested in food. Rapid transit through the small bowel decreases the contact time of organisms with the mucosa. Patients with decreased intestinal motility due to medication or anatomic factors have increased severity and complications and may have a prolonged carrier state. In experimental animals, bacterial interference is a major host defense. The normal flora may compete for substrates, lower the local pH by production of short-chain fatty acids, and produce antibacterial substances such as colicins. Some patients with gastroenteritis have progression or exacerbation of symptoms when antibiotics are given.[182] Prior antimicrobial exposure increases the risk of infection with both antimicrobial-susceptible and -resistant strains of *Salmonella*.[163]

Salmonella are able to survive in macrophages but not in polymorphonuclear leukocytes. Thus, patients with neutropenia (e.g., congenital, related to chemotherapy) or neutrophil dysfunction (e.g., chronic granulomatous disease) are at high risk of disseminated infection. Patients who have been bacteremic with a nontyphoidal *Salmonella* are at increased risk of relapse if leukopenia is present.[70]

Although the bulk of the evidence suggests that humoral immunity is less important, there are data demonstrating that preterm neonates who are infected with *S. typhimurium* have a lower risk of complications (e.g., intestinal perforation, meningitis, endophthalmitis, sepsis, pyelitis) if given intravenous immunoglobulin plus cefoperazone than do controls given cefoperazone alone (16 per cent vs. 82 per cent); mortality also is decreased (12 per cent vs. 41 per cent).[82]

Cell-mediated immunity generally is thought to be more important than is humoral immunity in clearance of *Salmonella*. T-cell activation of macrophages is necessary for killing of intracellular *Salmonella*.[133] Oral immunization with an attenuated typhoid vaccine primes lymphocytes to produce cytokines typical of a TH1 response (high interferon-gamma/low interleukin-4) to the flagellar antigen.[206] Healthy individuals vaccinated with either oral or parenteral typhoid vaccines develop antibody-dependent cellular cytotoxicity mediated by IgA and/or IgG.[43] However, studies of serum and secretory antibodies to O, H, and Vi antigens have not demonstrated protection; relapses of typhoid fever have occurred despite high antibody titers. Immunity may be short lived. In a study of 14 individuals (17 to 28 years of age) with acute typhoid fever, cell-mediated immunity persisted for 16 weeks; intestinal secretory IgA persisted for 48 weeks; and IgG, IgM, and anti-O and anti-H agglutinins persisted for 2 years, 16 weeks, 16 weeks, and 36 weeks, respectively.[193]

There is an increased risk of disease in settings in which there is impaired[152, 201] or immature[155] reticuloendothelial function or cell-mediated immunity. For example, hemolytic anemias are thought to cause reticuloendothelial overload. Children with sickle-cell anemia commonly become bacteremic and develop osteomyelitis.[135, 231] Sickle-C and S-Thal also sometimes develop osteomyelitis.[36]

Impaired cell-mediated immunity probably explains the high frequency of bacteremia with nontyphoidal *Salmonella* in children with HIV infection.[187] Cell-mediated immunity also is defective in malnutrition, and this fact further contributes to the susceptibility of persons with malnutrition,[198] including HIV-infected patients.[92] Defective cell-mediated immunity can be congenital or acquired (tumors,[94] collagen vascular disease, organ transplantation,[58] chemotherapy, glucocorticosteroids).[175] Patients with complicated typhoid fever do not develop a cell-mediated immune response as well as do those with uncomplicated infections. Patients with inflammatory bowel disease are at risk of developing toxic megacolon.

Malaria predisposes to salmonellosis by multiple mechanisms.[130] During the rainy season, when malaria is most common, 50 per cent of blood cultures taken from West African children younger than 5 years of age with pneumonia are positive for *Salmonella* or coliform species.[158]

Schistosomiasis predisposes to *Salmonella* infections and prolonged bacteremia[180]; reticuloendothelial cell killing of *Salmonella* is impaired, and *Salmonella* colonizes the schistosomes. Pili on *Salmonella* adhere to the surface of *Schistosoma mansoni* and *Schistosoma haematobium*.[128] In Gabonese children with bacteremic nontyphoidal *Salmonella*, rectal biopsies show the eggs of *Schistosoma intercalatum* in 90 per cent of cases.[72]

CLINICAL MANIFESTATIONS

Salmonella may cause acute or chronic asymptomatic infection. Symptomatic infections include acute gastroenteritis, bacteremia with or without local suppuration, and enteric fever. Specific serotypes are associated more commonly with certain clinical syndromes. *S. typhimurium*, the most common isolate in the United States, causes acute intestinal infection, sometimes without symptoms. *S. choleraesuis* almost always is isolated only from the blood. *S. typhi* and *S. paratyphi* A, B, and C cause enteric fever.

Acute Asymptomatic Infection

The inoculum required to infect infants and children probably is smaller than that required to infect adults. Asymptomatic infections usually are identified by stool cultures obtained during epidemiologic investigations. A study of Mexican infants showed that 74 per cent of nontyphoidal *Salmonella* infections were asymptomatic.[42]

Acute Gastroenteritis

The most common clinical illness caused by *Salmonella* is gastroenteritis. Nausea, vomiting, and crampy abdominal pain begin 6 to 72 hours (median, 24 hours) after ingestion of contaminated food or water. The abdominal pain may be severe enough to suggest appendicitis. Diarrhea usually is moderate in volume and, depending on the serotype, may contain blood. Headaches, malaise, myalgias, and fevers are common. These symptoms usually resolve in about a week without antibiotic therapy; symptoms may persist in the very young and those with underlying diseases. In neonates, loose, green, mucous stools or less often bloody diarrhea is seen; fever is common in *Salmonella* gastroenteritis during the first months of life.[106] Reactive arthritis develops in some adults after otherwise uncomplicated *Salmonella* gastroenteritis; this complication is rare in children.

Bacteremia With or Without Metastatic Focal Infection

Some *Salmonella* serotypes (e.g., *S. typhi; S. choleraesuis; S. paratyphi* A, B, and C; *S. heidelberg; S. typhimurium; S. enteritidis; S. saint-paul; S. newport; S. panama; S. dublin*) have a propensity to invade the blood stream; others (e.g., *S. tennessee, S. weltevreden*[229]) seem to cause bacteremia rarely. Fever, chills, diaphoresis, myalgias, anorexia, and weight loss may last for days or weeks. Stool cultures may be negative; diarrhea may not precede the fever. A child sometimes can have afebrile diarrhea and yet be bacteremic for several days.[113] The true frequency of bacteremia is uncertain. Depending on the patient's age, geographic location, and nature of the study (prospective vs. retrospective), 2 to 45 per cent of infections are bacteremic.[44, 106, 141, 155, 198, 214, 229, 230] Bacteremia probably is more common in the newborn (in some studies as high as 30 to 50 per cent) than in the older child,[76, 106] although not all studies have reached this conclusion.[141] It is likely that the true risk of bacteremia in the first year of life is in the 2 to 6 per cent range.[44, 214] Hemolytic anemia, especially sickle-cell anemia, is associated with a high risk of *Salmonella* bacteremia. Persistent or recurrent bacteremia occurs in patients with AIDS, schistosomiasis, and intravascular focal infection. Adults who become bacteremic with *Salmonella* are more likely to do so without a preceding gastroenteritis and to have a high mortality rate, presumably because they so often are immunocompromised. Children more typically are relatively immunocompetent, most often develop bacteremia associated with diarrhea, and have a much better prognosis.[121, 141] Even children with neoplastic disease seem to have a relatively benign course when bacteremic with *Salmonella* species.[157]

Focal suppurative infections may occur almost anywhere; the most common sites are bones (particularly in sickle-cell anemia)[22, 204] and meninges.[24, 52, 116, 129, 181] Meningitis has a high morbidity, with acute hydrocephalus, seizures, ventriculitis, abscesses, subdural empyema, and long-term neurologic sequelae (e.g., mental retardation, hemiparesis, chronic hydrocephalus, epilepsy, visual impairment, athetosis).[36] Mortality from meningitis has been as high as 40 to 60 per cent in the past, even with appropriate treatment; recent data suggest that mortality now is much lower. Relapses even after prolonged therapy are common (presumably reflecting the intracellular localization of *Salmonella* and the difficulty of achieving adequate levels of antibiotics within central nervous system macrophages). Fifty to 75 per cent of nontyphoidal *Salmonella* meningitis occurs in the first 4 months of life.[36] The serotypes causing meningitis, including *S. typhimurium, S. heidelberg, S. enteritidis, S. saint-paul, S. havana, S. oranienburg, S. newport*, and *S. panama*,[36, 227] are serotypes commonly associated with bacteremia. In infants, complications include pneumonia,[17] osteomyelitis,[49, 118] septic arthritis,[17, 194] pericarditis,[93, 140] pyelitis,[207] peritonitis,[2] otitis media,[2] mastitis,[154] cholecystitis,[91] endophthalmitis,[41] cutaneous abscesses,[172] and infected cephalhematoma.[49] In adults and occasionally in older children, femoral and distal aorta (mycotic aneurysms),[36] heart valves,[36] scrotum,[217] testicles,[36] prostate,[192] ovaries,[36] and fallopian tubes[192] also may be infected.

Hemolytic uremic syndrome associated with *S. typhimurium*[53, 138] and *S. typhi*[16] has been reported. Because the cytotoxins produced by various *Salmonella* strains are distinct immunologically from Shiga toxin produced by *Shigella dysenteriae* 1 and the Shiga-like toxins produced by enterohemorrhagic *Escherichia coli*,[11] the association of hemolytic uremic syndrome and salmonellosis in the some patients may be a coincidence.

Enteric Fever

Enteric fever usually is caused by *S. typhi* and, less often, other invasive *Salmonella*, including *S. paratyphi* and *S. choleraesuis*. In contrast to sepsis caused by other gram-negative bacilli, the onset of symptoms in enteric fever is insidious.[105] After an incubation period of 10 to 14 days (range, 6 to 21 days), which generally is related to the inoculum size, fever, malaise, anorexia, and abdominal pain develop over a 2- to 3-day period. The incubation period tends to be somewhat shorter in paratyphoid fever. The fever rises in small increments, usually reaching 40° to 40.5° C (104° to 105° F) by the end of the first week of illness. The temperature does not return to normal but rather rises to higher peaks each afternoon, with higher nadirs each subsequent morning during the first week. Eventually, the fever is unremittent; there are spikes in temperature without any return to normal.

Constipation is more common than is diarrhea; it occurs in approximately 50 per cent, whereas diarrhea occurs in about 30 per cent of patients. When diarrhea develops, it usually is after the patient has been febrile for several days; it is small-volume, resembles pea soup, and contains erythrocytes but usually is not grossly bloody. Fecal leukocytes are present in nearly all patients with diarrhea.[184] Diarrhea is more common with paratyphoid than with typhoid fever.[216] Vomiting is mild and not sustained.

A dull, continuous frontal headache begins during the first 2 days of fever; headache is present in about 75 per cent of patients. Confusion or delirium is more common than is a normal mental status in adults. Children commonly complain of headache; they often are drowsy, irritable, or delirious.[48] Mild arthralgia involving multiple joints and vague, poorly localized back pain occurs in nearly 60 per cent of patients.

Physical examination during the first week may show a relative bradycardia for the degree of fever. The patient has a dull, expressionless, toxic facies; there is a coated tongue, a musty "damp hay–like" odor, and a tender, doughy abdomen with slight guarding. Occasionally, a child may have a cough; it tends to be minimal and unimpressive. The skin is dry with little sweating. Meningismus may occur early in the illness.

During the second week, rose spots may appear on the abdomen or chest and less often on the back, upper arms, and thighs. They typically begin between days 7 and 10 as crops of 10 to 15 lesions measuring 2 to 4 mm. There may be more lesions in paratyphoid. They are blanching, erythematous, very slightly raised lesions that last about 3 days. Rose spots occur in a minority of patients and are difficult to recognize in dark-skinned individuals. New crops of rose spots may continue for 1 to 2 weeks.

The spleen becomes palpable, soft, and tender by early in the second week of illness. Respiratory symptoms may progress, and epistaxis occasionally may occur. If left untreated, enteric fever has a prolonged course, with continuous high fever of 39.5° to 40.5° C (103° to 105° F) for up to 4 weeks, followed by a gradual return to normal beginning during the third or fourth week. A rapid drop in temperature late in illness suggests intestinal hemorrhage or perforation[20]; such a drop in temperature typically is followed by a rise a few hours later as peritonitis develops. Intestinal hemorrhage and intestinal perforation[20, 28, 78] may occur in the second to fourth week in up to 3 per cent of patients with typhoid fever.[28] Late in the course of untreated typhoid, the mental status changes to a "coma vigil," in which the patient lies with open eyes, mutters, and is oblivious to the surroundings.

Most complications develop during the second or third week of illness. Complications include cholecystitis,[228] hepatitis,[174] osteomyelitis,[161] arthritis, parotitis, myocarditis, pneumonia, meningitis, pyelonephritis, and orchitis.[124] Suppurative lymphadenitis,[151] tonsillitis,[110, 192] infected prosthetic heart valves,[8] and pancreatitis[138, 269] are rare. Patients who have thalassemia or G6PD deficiency may have hemolysis during typhoid fever.[216] The relapse rate is 5 to 20 per cent, even when appropriate therapy has been given. Relapses typically are milder than is the initial illness.

In some geographic areas, such as Indonesia, where an exceptionally virulent *S. typhi* is endemic, toxemia, delirium, obtundation, coma, and shock sometimes occur.[105, 124] Some serotypes in Indonesia (e.g., H1-j) appear to be less virulent than do others, suggesting that properties of the flagellar antigen may be important to virulence.[88]

Typhoid fever is quite variable in its clinical course; patients commonly lack some of the features. Variations on the classic theme include a completely afebrile course occurring in debilitated patients, high spiking fever from the first day (particularly in children), a focal presentation (e.g., pneumonia, nephritis), and a severe course during relapses. Infants are said to be at higher risk of developing massive hepatomegaly, thrombocytopenia, and other complications.[173] The mortality is high in the neonatal period.[176] Infants and toddlers often have a nondescript febrile illness misinterpreted as a "viral syndrome." In children younger than 2 years of age, the fever may last for as little as 1 to 5 days, despite the presence of *S. typhi* or *S. paratyphi* in the blood; low-grade fever (38.3° to 38.8° C; 101° to 102° F) and cough may be the only findings in such children.[63] Prolonged hypothermia during convalescence occurs in some children.

Both typhoid and nontyphoidal *Salmonella* infections during pregnancy increase the risk of aborting the fetus.[146, 203] Spontaneous abortion and/or premature labor usually can be prevented by early treatment.[197] Transmission of *S. typhi* rarely occurs in utero.[33] Typically, premature delivery occurs during the second to fourth week of untreated maternal typhoid fever.[86] In the preantibiotic era, 40 per cent of women with typhoid delivered prematurely; the rest carried to term, although only 17 per cent of infants survived.[47] If infection occurs late in gestation and is treated appropriately, the infant may survive intact.

Asymptomatic Chronic Carrier State

Chronic carriers excrete *Salmonella* in stools for more than 1 year after gastroenteritis/enterocolitis or enteric fever. Approximately 1 to 4 per cent of patients who recover from enteric fever due to *S. typhi* chronically excrete the organism[32, 144]; less than 1 per cent of patients with nontyphoidal *Salmonella* excrete for such a prolonged period.[25, 32] Nontyphoidal infection is associated with excretion for a mean of 5 weeks, although children younger than 5 years of age,[25] females, the elderly, and patients with biliary tract disease are more likely to become carriers. The biliary tract is infected in almost all chronic carriers of *S. typhi*. Up to 10^6 organisms per gram of feces may be excreted.[144] The significance of chronic excretion is that such patients serve as a source of infection to their contacts. Chronic carriers represent an epidemiologically important reservoir of *S. typhi*; they often are the source of typhoid fever outbreaks. In the United States, although typhoid fever generally is imported, up to 30 per cent of infections result from exposure to previously diagnosed or newly diagnosed chronic carriers.[189]

Patients who have a history of *S. haematobium* or tuberculosis infections of the urinary tract may develop chronic urinary carriage[59, 180] after a bout of typhoid fever. Other predisposing conditions include hydronephrosis, strictures, and kidney stones.

DIAGNOSIS

The symptoms in *Salmonella* gastroenteritis overlap sufficiently with those seen in other diarrheal illnesses that laboratory studies generally are required to prove the diagnosis. Young children with diarrhea may develop dehydration and electrolyte abnormalities. The fecal leukocyte examination is positive for polymorphonuclear leukocytes in 36 to 82 per cent[96, 167] of nontyphoidal cases, but this finding is nonspecific. On the rare occasions when proctoscopy has been done, typical findings have included mucosal edema, hyperemia, friability, and hemorrhages.[45] Definitive diagnosis only can be made by isolation of the organism. In patients with gastroenteritis, cultures of stool or rectal swabs are positive in the majority of infected individuals. Stool culture is preferable to swab culture, particularly for evaluation of long-term carriers.[117]

Salmonella usually can be isolated readily from blood using conventional media if the patient is bacteremic. In patients with extraintestinal focal nontyphoidal infection, specimens from the affected areas may have positive Gram stains and grow the organism.

Enteric fever should be suspected based on the setting and clinical course. Laboratory abnormalities are common but nonspecific. There often is a normocytic, normochromic anemia and leukopenia and/or neutropenia, perhaps due to hemophagocytosis in the bone marrow.[134] Clotting abnormalities consistent with disseminated intravascular coagulation (e.g., thrombocytopenia, hypofibrinogenemia) may occur[27] but usually are transient and not associated with clinically significant bleeding. In enteric fever, electrolyte values usually are normal, but increases in alkaline phosphatase, serum lactic acid dehydrogenase, serum aspartate aminotransferase, and serum cholesterol are frequent. A transient proteinuria sometimes occurs during the first week of enteric fever. Cultures from multiple sites should be submitted for suspected enteric fever; culture of bone marrow has the highest yield,[99, 101, 218] particularly if there has been antibiotic pretreatment. During the first week of typhoid fever, approximately 90 per cent of patients have positive blood and bone marrow cultures but negative stool and urine cultures. During subsequent weeks, the yield of blood and bone marrow cultures decreases as the yield of stool and urine cultures increases. Culture of duodenal fluid obtained by string capsules can be as sensitive as culture of bone marrow aspirates can.[13, 101, 218] One study found that in those children able to tolerate the string test, it was positive in 85 per cent, compared with blood test (positive in 62 per cent).[9] The overall frequency of positive cultures during the course of typhoid is blood (40 to 54 per cent), urine (7 to 10 per cent), stool (approximately 35 per cent), bone marrow (80 to 90 per cent), rose spots (approximately 65 per cent), and duodenal string test culture (58 to 85 per cent).[79, 101]

The Widal test measures antibodies against the O and H

antigens of *S. typhi*. Although many patients with enteric fever may develop a fourfold rise in the titer of paired sera during the second week of illness, both false-negative and false-positive tests occur. Those with acute or chronic liver disease as well as patients infected with other gram-negative enteric bacilli may develop cross-reacting antibodies. Recipients of the typhoid vaccine show positive Widal test results, which can be misleading. These titers may be more useful in children with typhoid who are living in a nonendemic area, such as the United States. Although those who have a negative titer early in infection tend to keep a negative titer, the vast majority develop titers of 1:80 or more.[38] Interpretation of Widal tests is aided by information about seropositivity in the population to which the patient belongs.[435]

A variety of new diagnostic kits have been developed including serologic tests such as passive hemagglutination, passive bacterial agglutination, latex particle agglutination slide tests, counter immunoelectrophoresis, radioimmunoassay, and enzyme-linked immunosorbent assay using monoclonal antibodies. Molecular techniques used primarily in epidemiologic studies include DNA hybridization studies, phage typing, chromosome analysis, and plasmid analysis. Other methods based on early detection of *Salmonella* in feces have been described and shown to have good sensitivity and specificity[6, 71, 145] but have not been used widely.

DIFFERENTIAL DIAGNOSIS

Salmonella gastroenteritis cannot be distinguished reliably clinically from other infectious causes of acute diarrhea, although history and epidemiology sometimes may suggest an etiologic agent. Bloody diarrhea with mucus can be due to *Salmonella, Shigella*, enteroinvasive *E. coli*, enterohemorrhagic *E. coli, Campylobacter* species, *Yersinia enterocolitica, Clostridium difficile, Trichura trichuris,* and *Entamoeba histolytica*. Watery diarrhea may be due to rotavirus or other viral enteropathogens or, less commonly, enterotoxin-producing bacterial pathogens. When abdominal pain and tenderness are severe, appendicitis, perforated viscus, and mesenteric adenitis are in the differential diagnosis.

Enteric fever can mimic other infections of the reticuloendothelial system, including Epstein-Barr virus infection, disseminated histoplasmosis, tuberculosis, ehrlichiosis, brucellosis, leptospirosis, tularemia, plague, malaria, systemic *Bartonella henselae* infection, and typhus. Noninfectious illnesses with prolonged fever that sometimes can be confused with typhoid include juvenile rheumatoid arthritis and other collagen vascular diseases, Kawasaki syndrome, and lymphomas. An early diagnosis often is very difficult because the findings are nonspecific. Findings that particularly are helpful in discriminating typhoid fever from other prolonged febrile illnesses include severe cough and chest pain (more typical of lobar pneumonia), diarrhea with grossly obvious blood (more typical of dysentery), acute onset of chills (more typical of malaria), and marked lower abdominal pain early in the febrile illness (more typical of bacillary dysentery, *Y. enterocolitica* infection, and salpingitis).

TREATMENT

For those children with salmonellosis for whom antibiotic treatment is appropriate, the interpretation of antimicrobial susceptibility studies is important. Drugs such as aminoglycosides, polymyxins, tetracyclines, and first- and second-generation cephalosporins (e.g., cephalothin, cefazolin, cefuroxime, cefamandole) have a very poor clinical track record, despite apparent in vitro susceptibility. The drugs that typically are useful in treating children with *Salmonella* infections are shown in Table 115–5; the usual range of minimum inhibitory concentration values is shown in Table 115–6.

TABLE 115–5. Antibiotics Commonly Useful in the Treatment of *Salmonella* Infections

Drug	Dose
Ampicillin	200 mg/kg/day in 4 doses PO, IM, or IV
TMP-SMX	10 mg/kg/day TMP, 50 mg/kg/day SMX in 2 doses PO or IV
Cefotaxime	150–200 mg/kg/day in 3 doses IM or IV
Ceftriaxone	100 mg/kg/day in 1 to 2 doses IM or IV
Chloramphenicol	75 mg/kg/day in 4 doses PO

TMP-SMX, trimethoprim-sulfamethoxazole.

Gastroenteritis

As with all forms of gastroenteritis, fluid and electrolyte replacement and maintenance are the first order of business. For most patients, oral rehydration is all that is necessary to treat *Salmonella* gastroenteritis. The role of antibiotics is secondary. It generally is agreed that *Salmonella* gastroenteritis should not be treated with antibiotics because these agents do not shorten the course of illness but, rather, lengthen the period of excretion. Multiple agents have been shown to be ineffective, including ampicillin-amoxicillin,[114, 165, 153] neomycin,[12] chloramphenicol,[132] TMP-SMX,[114] and ciprofloxacin.[10, 190] Antibiotics prolong excretion of *Salmonella*.[10, 12, 50, 114, 153, 165] However, it should be noted that *Salmonella* species typically have been grouped together for these treatment studies as though they were all the same organism. Given the variability in expression of virulence genes, it remains an open question whether treatment may be useful for some serotypes that possess particular virulence traits.

Exceptions to the generalization that *Salmonella* gastroenteritis should not be treated include children at high risk of complications, including those with underlying diseases or therapies that impair host defenses. Examples of children who probably ought to be given antibiotics include infants in the first 3 months of life; those ill with AIDS or malignancies; and children with hemolytic anemias, particularly sickle-cell anemia. Treatment of these patients is debatable; the data from neonates suggest that antibiotics make little difference to the course.[2, 57, 114, 177, 205] However, because the risk of bacteremia is high, it is likely that antibiotics will continue to be used in such settings. Because bacteremia occurs in a relatively small fraction of infections, it is impossi-

TABLE 115–6. Susceptibility (MIC_{90}) of *Salmonella* Species

Drug	MIC_{90}
Ampicillin	4–8 μg/mL
TMP-SMX	<0.5 and 9.5 μg/mL
Cefotaxime	<0.003–0.25 μg/mL
Ceftriaxone	0.07–0.19 μg/mL
Chloramphenicol	8 μg/mL

MIC, minimum inhibitory concentration; TMP-SMX, trimethoprim-sulfamethoxazole.

ble to determine whether treatment of gastroenteritis prevents bacteremia without a massive study. Because it is debatable whether treatment is indicated, it also is debatable how long it should be done when elected. Probably no more than 5 days of antibiotics is indicated, barring complications. Although antibiotic resistance is an increasingly important problem, those who require antibiotic therapy for *Salmonella* gastroenteritis not thought to be life-threatening usually should be given ampicillin or amoxicillin, pending susceptibility testing.

Extraintestinal Infections

Any child who appears to be toxic enough that bacteremia is suspected also should be started on antibiotic treatment until blood cultures exclude the diagnosis. For children with bacteremic *Salmonella* and focal extraintestinal complications, a third-generation cephalosporin (e.g., ceftriaxone, cefotaxime) or chloramphenicol is an appropriate choice. If the patient appears to have a life-threatening infection, ampicillin should be used only if there is evidence that the pathogen is not ampicillin-resistant. Children at high risk of bacteremia recurrence (those with congenital or acquired immunodeficiencies, such as AIDS) may require a third-generation cephalosporin or a fluoroquinolone to achieve cure; frequent recurrences of life-threatening infection sometimes necessitate use of lifelong maintenance therapy.[39, 104]

Meningitis should be treated with a third-generation cephalosporin because these agents have good penetration into cerebrospinal fluid; ampicillin and chloramphenicol use has been associated with higher relapse rates and lower cure rates than have third-generation cephalosporins.[116] Meningitis must be treated for at least 4 weeks; approximately three-fourths of those who have relapses have been treated for 3 weeks or less.[36]

A bactericidal agent, such as ampicillin or a third-generation cephalosporin, is preferred for treatment of endovascular infections (e.g., endocarditis, mycotic aneurysm).

For extraintestinal infections, the duration of antibiotic treatment usually is 10 to 14 days in children with bacteremia, 4 to 6 weeks in those with acute osteomyelitis, and 4 weeks in those with meningitis. Collections of pus should be drained. Schistosomiasis, when present, must be treated to achieve resolution of the coincident *Salmonella* infection.

Typhoid Fever

For the child with enteric fever, chloramphenicol, ampicillin, TMP-SMX, a third-generation cephalosporin, or, in selected cases, a fluoroquinolone (e.g., ciprofloxacin, ofloxacin, norfloxacin) are the choices. The response to treatment with antibiotics is relatively slow. Fever may persist for many days, even after bacteremia has resolved. Although diarrhea due to nontyphoidal *Salmonella* is not responsive to antibiotics, when *S. typhi* causes diarrhea, treatment with chloramphenicol is effective.[184] *S. typhi* usually is treated for at least 2 weeks with chloramphenicol, ceftriaxone, cefotaxime, or TMP-SMX. Data suggest that TMP-SMX may not be as effective as is ampicillin or chloramphenicol in typhoid fever.[80]

In the United States, multiresistant *S. typhi* is less of a problem than it is elsewhere; most strains are sensitive to ampicillin and chloramphenicol.[189] However, when there is a history of recent travel to an area with antibiotic-resistant *S. typhi* or when there is contact with a person returning from such an area, the choice of empiric treatment should take this information into account. Third-generation cephalosporins are effective against both *S. typhi* and nontyphoidal *Salmonella* strains resistant to ampicillin, chloramphenicol, and TMP-SMX[61, 108, 116, 142, 148, 162, 200, 213] and are appropriate for children with suspected or proven multiresistant *Salmonella*. Some studies suggest that cefoperazone may have advantages in typhoid fever over chloramphenicol treatment (more rapid sterilization and defervescence),[162] perhaps related to its biliary excretion.[46] A short course of ceftriaxone (once daily for 3 to 5 days) is as effective and safe as is a 2- to 3-week course of chloramphenicol in adults, and based on relatively small numbers, this probably also is true in children.[3, 148] There are reports of successfully using aztreonam in typhoid fever, although defervescence is slow compared with reports of chloramphenicol use.[60, 84, 209] However, a 5-day course of ceftriaxone (50 to 70 mg/kg/day as a single dose) was associated with a significantly more rapid defervescence (average, 3.9 days until afebrile) than was oral cefixime (7.5 mg/kg/dose twice daily for 14 days) or intramuscular aztreonam (50 to 70 mg/kg/dose every 8 hours for 7 days); relapses rates were similar (about 5 per cent).[81]

Concerns about toxicity of fluoroquinolones in children have limited their use to exceptional situations in which infection is caused by an organism proved to be resistant to all of the usual antibiotics but sensitive to a fluoroquinolone. Unfortunately, such isolates are becoming all too common. Ciprofloxacin (500 mg twice daily for 10 days in adults) causes defervescence in an average of 4.2 days with infrequent relapses, even with multiresistant organisms.[7] Children with resistant organisms who have been treated with ciprofloxacin (10 mg/kg/day) became afebrile in 3.3 days, and 94 per cent achieved clinical cure, with no relapses or carriers detected on follow-up.[54] Very short courses (3 to 5 days) of ofloxacin have been effective in treating both adults and children with multiresistant *S. typhi*; a 3-day course (15 mg/kg per day) is safe and effective.[215]

Other agents have been described that occasionally may be useful. Furazolidone (7.5 mg/kg/day) is nearly as effective as is chloramphenicol in strains susceptible to both drugs (86 per cent vs. 90 per cent cure).[55]

A variety of nonantimicrobial measures should be considered as part of the management of *S. typhi* infections. Antipyretics are said to be potentially deleterious in enteric fever, although this recommendation is based on observations of five patients who received aspirin and developed dramatic drops in temperature with bradycardia, sweating, profound weakness, and prostration.[51] The mechanism responsible for these observations and their relevance to other antipyretics remain open questions. No reports in the last 30 years have reexamined this issue.

Dexamethasone, although potentially increasing the relapse rate,[40] is indicated for those with severe typhoid fever presenting with delirium, stupor, shock, or coma; the dose is 3 mg/kg initially and then eight doses of 1 mg/kg every 6 hours for 48 hours. This therapy lowers mortality from 35 to 55 per cent to 10 per cent.[100, 171]

Intestinal hemorrhage or perforation during enteric fever generally is considered to be an indication for surgical intervention.[20, 28, 78, 127] Antibiotic coverage should be broadened to include anaerobes and gram-negative enterics when perforation occurs.[20]

Chronic Carriers

In general, those who are not food handlers probably should not be cultured or given special treatment after a bout of gastroenteritis due to a nontyphoidal *Salmonella*. On the other hand, carriers of *S. typhi* should be decolonized to decrease the risk to close contacts. Those who have a normal gallbladder can be treated with high-dose intravenous ampicillin, oral ampicillin, or amoxicillin combined with probenecid for 6 weeks or, when a multiresistant organism is present, with a fluoroquinolone, such as norfloxacin[85] or ciprofloxacin.[64] Chronic carriers who cannot be decolonized are treated with cholecystectomy if cholelithiasis or cholecystitis is present; such patients should receive ampicillin intravenously for 7 to 10 days before and 30 days after cholecystectomy.

PREVENTION

Public Health Measures

Recognition of an increased frequency of human infections with an unusual serotype should be followed by an epidemiologic investigation aimed at detecting the source and vehicle. Intervention to stop such outbreaks then can be attempted. Judicious use of antibiotics in dairy and livestock animals,[102] careful food processing and storage, and proper preparation of foods all are helpful in decreasing transmission of infection. Appropriate sewage disposal, assurance of a safe water supply, prevention of sale of pet turtles, inspection of cosmetics for contamination, and adequate cleaning of medical equipment are important public health strategies.

Personal Hygienic Measures

Person-to-person spread can be decreased by attention to hand washing after defecation or diaper changing, frequent hand washing during preparation of foods that might be contaminated (e.g., meat), and exclusion of infected individuals from food-handling tasks.

Infection Control

Hospitalized children with *Salmonella* gastroenteritis should be isolated (enteric precautions) until stool cultures are negative. Children with extraintestinal infections should be isolated until stool studies exclude intestinal infection/colonization.

Nursery Outbreaks

Neonatal *Salmonella* infection outbreaks should be investigated to determine the source. Cultures of fomites sometimes reveal a removable focus. Neonates and the staff caring for them should be cohorted during outbreaks, using enteric precautions when dealing with those infants who are excreting the organism. Surveillance cultures should be done on feces not only of sick infants but also of well babies in order to cohort more appropriately. With current early postpartum discharge policies, reporting of *Salmonella* infections in infants is important in detecting outbreaks. Isolation and cohorting can be effective in controlling such outbreaks.[177]

Breast Feeding

In the developing world, breast feeding is key because human milk contains secretory IgA and other factors that protect infants from *Salmonella* species.[62, 69, 168, 169]

Vaccination

Several vaccines have been developed for typhoid fever. Vaccination of children is indicated when the risk of typhoid fever is high (e.g. living with a chronic carrier or in an endemic area [e.g., Latin America, Asia, Africa]). There are three vaccines currently available: (1) heat-phenol–inactivated whole-cell vaccine (Typhoid vaccine, Wyeth-Ayerst) and an acetone-inactivated vaccine, which has greater efficacy but is only available for use by the military, (2) oral live attenuated Ty21a vaccine[30] (Vivotif Berna™, Swiss Serum and Vaccine Institute), and (3) a parenteral purified Vi capsular polysaccharide vaccine (Typhim Vi, Pasteur Merieux).[122–124] None of these vaccines has been compared with the others in a controlled trial.

The heat-phenol–inactivated vaccine has an efficacy of 51 to 67 per cent protection for 4 to 7 years. Adverse side effects (e.g., fever [14 to 29 per cent], headaches [9 to 30 per cent], local pain and swelling [6 to 50 per cent]) are too frequent to warrant routine use. If there have been severe local or systemic reactions, no further doses should be administered. The only current use for this vaccine in children is in the very young child in whom the other vaccines (which are safer and equally effective) have not been tested adequately. Two doses (0.5 mL if 10 years of age or older, 0.25 mL if 6 months to 9 years of age) are given subcutaneously at least 4 weeks apart. When there is not enough time to give two doses 4 weeks apart, a regimen of three doses separated by 1 week each has been used commonly. A booster, given intradermally rather than subcutaneously, should be administered every 3 years if the risk of disease continues. This vaccine can be used in children 6 months of age or older, unlike the other two vaccines, which cannot be used until the child is 2 years of age (Vi capsular vaccine) or 6 years of age (oral live attenuated Ty21a vaccine).

The Ty21a vaccine has been evaluated in both liquid and capsule forms. Ty21a oral vaccine is well tolerated; abdominal pain, nausea, vomiting, and rashes occur rarely. A randomized, placebo-controlled trial of more than 32,000 school children 6 to 7 years of age demonstrated that three doses of a liquid vaccine preparation given over a 1-week period, preceded by a 1-g tablet of $NaHCO_3$ to neutralize gastric acid, had a 3-year protective efficacy of 96 per cent.[222] However, children younger than 2 years of age fail to develop either humoral or cellular immunity.[123, 150] Randomized, placebo-controlled studies of a gelatin capsule formulation containing $NaHCO_3$ and an enteric-coated capsule without bicarbonate given at three doses in 1 week or three doses over a 21-day interval were performed in children older than 6 years of age.[123] The enteric-coated capsule formulation given at three doses in 1 week had an efficacy of 65 per cent over a 5-year period; this was not improved by giving the doses every 21 days; $NaHCO_3$ lowers efficacy. The liquid formulation appears to be more protective than does the enteric-coated capsule.[122] The form licensed in the United States is an enteric-coated capsule preparation meant to be given in four separate doses on alternate days taken 1 hour before meals. Revaccination using the entire four-dose series is recommended every 5 years in high-risk settings. Because the Ty21a oral vaccine is a live attenuated *Salmonella*, it should not be used in immunocompromised hosts or in those taking antibiotics at the time of vaccination.[30] The antimalarial mefloquine inhibits growth of the attenuated organism, and thus vaccine should be delayed for 24 hours after its use.

Several large field trials suggest that the Vi capsular vaccine as a single 25-μg dose has an efficacy of 55 and 75 per cent in adults and children older than 5 years of age, respectively.[4, 170] Although fever, malaise, local pain, and tenderness occur with this vaccine, it has two major advantages over the Ty21a oral vaccines: It does not require refrigeration, and only a single dose is required for protection. It has the advantage of being safer than the whole cell vaccine and may be used in children as young as 2 years of age.

Other vaccines under development include virulence polysaccharide conjugated to tetanus toxoid,[122] an oral, bivalent *S. typhi–Shigella sonnei* vaccine,[219] and an *S. typhi* strain Ty21a used as a carrier in a typhoid-cholera hybrid vaccine.[208]

PROGNOSIS

Salmonella gastroenteritis usually is a self-limited disease in the normal host, although chronic diarrhea sometimes develops after an acute episode. Extraintestinal focal infections with nontyphoidal *Salmonella* are difficult to cure, particularly if they involve the meninges or occur in compromised hosts. *Salmonella* species meningitis routinely relapses if too short a course of treatment is given. Likewise, bacteremia as well as focal infection recurs after treatment in severely compromised hosts, particularly those with AIDS. Relapse after typhoid fever long has been recognized as a risk.

References

1. Abramson, H.: Infections with *S. typhimurium* in the newborn. Am. J. Dis. Child. *74*:576–586, 1947.
2. Abroms, I. F., Cochran, W. D., Holmes, L. B., et al.: A *Salmonella newport* outbreak in a premature nursery with a one-year follow-up. Pediatrics *37*:616–623, 1966.
3. Acharya, G., Butler, T., Ho, M., et al.: Treatment of typhoid fever: Randomized trial of a three-day course of ceftriaxone versus a fourteen-day course of chloramphenicol. Am. J. Trop. Med. Hyg. *52*:162 165, 1995.
4. Acharya, I. L., Lowe, C. U., Thapa, R., et al.: Prevention of typhoid fever in Nepal with the Vi capsular polysaccharide of *Salmonella typhi*. N. Engl. J. Med. *317*:1101–1104, 1987.
5. Adler, J. L., Anderson, R. L., Boring, J. R., et al.: A protracted hospital-associated outbreak of salmonellosis due to a multiple antibiotic-resistant strain of *S. Indiana*. J. Pediatr. *77*:970–975, 1970.
6. Aguirre, P. M., Cacho, J. B., Folgueira, L., et al.: Rapid fluorescence method for screening *Salmonella* spp. from enteric differential agars. J. Clin. Microbiol. *28*:148–149, 1990.
7. Alam, M. N., Haq, S. A., Das, K. K., et al: Efficacy of ciprofloxacin in enteric fever. Comparison of treatment duration in sensitive and multi-drug resistant *Salmonella*. Am. J. Trop. Med. Hyg. *53*:306–311, 1995.
8. Alvarez-Elcoro, S., Soto-Ramirez, L., and Mateos Mora, M.: *Salmonella* bacteremia in patients with prosthetic heart valves. Am. J. Med. *77*:61–66, 1984.
9. Antony, T. J., Patwari, A. K., Anand, V. K., et al.: Duodenal string test in typhoid fever. Indian Pediatr. *30*:643–647, 1993.
10. Aserkoff, B., and Bennett, J. V.: Effect of antibiotic therapy in acute salmonellosis on the fecal excretion of salmonellae. N. Engl. J. Med. *281*:636–40, 1969.
11. Ashkenazi, S., Cleary, T. G., Murray, B. E., et al.: Quantitative analysis and partial characterization of cytotoxin production by *Salmonella* strains. Infect. Immun. *56*:3089–3094, 1988.
12. Association for Study of Infectious Diseases: Effect of neomycin in noninvasive salmonella infections of the gastrointestinal tract. Lancet *2*:1159–1161, 1970.
13. Avendano, A., Herrera, P., Horwitz, I., et al.: Duodenal string cultures: Practicality and sensitivity for diagnosing enteric fever in children. J. Infect. Dis. *153*:359–362, 1986.
14. Baine, W. B., Gangarosa, E. J., Bennett, J. V., et al.: Institutional salmonellosis. J. Infect. Dis. *128*:357–360, 1973.
15. Baird, G. D., Manning, E. J., and Jones, P. W.: Evidence for related virulence sequences in plasmids of *Salmonella dublin* and *Salmonella typhimurium*. J. Gen. Microbiol. *131*:1815–1823, 1985.
16. Baker, N. M., Mills, A. E., Rachman, I., et al.: Hemolytic uraemic syndrome in typhoid fever. Br. Med. J. *2*:84–87, 1974.
17. Bannerman, C.H.: *S. heidelberg* enteritis: An outbreak in the neonatal unit of Harare Central Hospital. Cent. Afr. J. Med. *31*:1–4, 1985.
18. Bate, J. G., and James, U.: *Salmonella typhimurium* infection dust-borne in a children's ward. Lancet *2*:713, 1958.
19. Bean, N. H., Griffin, P. M., Goulding, J. S., et al.: Foodborne disease outbreaks, 5-year summary, 1983–1987. M. M. W. R. *39*(SS-1):15–57, 1990.
20. Bitar, R., and Tarpley, J.: Intestinal perforation in typhoid fever: A historical and state-of-the-art review. Rev. Infect. Dis. *7*:257–270, 1985.
21. Blaser, M. J., and Newman, L. S.: A review of human salmonellosis. I. Infective dose. Rev. Infect. Dis. *4*:1096–1106, 1982.
22. Borecka, J., Hocmannova, M., and van Leeuwen, W. J.: Nosocomial infection of nurslings caused by multiple drug-resistant strain of *S. typhimurium* utilization of a new typing method based on lysogeny of strains. Zentralbl. Bakteriol. 1. Abt. Orig. A *2336*:262, 1976.
23. Boyd, J. F.: Pathology of the alimentary tract of *S. typhimurium* food poisoning. Gut *26*:935–944, 1985.
24. Bryan, J. P., Rocha, H., and Scheld, W. M.: Problems in salmonellosis: Rationale for clinical trials with newer β-lactam agents and quinolones. Rev. Infect. Dis. *8*:189–207, 1986.
25. Buchawald, D. S., and Blaser, M. J.: A review of human salmonellosis. II. Duration of excretion following infection with non-typhi *Salmonella*. Rev. Infect. Dis. *6*:345–356, 1984.
26. Buckmeier, N. A., and Heffron, F.: Intracellular survival of wild type *Salmonella typhimurium* and macrophage sensitive mutants in diverse populations of macrophages. Infect. Immun. *57*:1–7, 1989.
27. Butler, T., Bell, W. R., Levin, J., et al.: Typhoid fever: Studies of blood coagulation, bacteremia, and endotoxemia. Arch. Intern. Med. *138*:407–410 1978.
28. Butler, T., Knight, J., Nath, S. K., et al.: Typhoid fever complicated by intestinal perforation: A persisting fatal disease requiring surgical management. Rev. Infect. Dis. *7*:244–256, 1985.
29. Centers for Disease Control: Multistate outbreak of *Salmonella poona* infections: United States and Canada. M. M. W. R. *40*:549, 1991.
30. Centers for Disease Control: Typhoid immunization: Recommendations of the Immunization Practices Advisory Committee (ACIP). M. M. W. R. *39*:1–5, 1990.
31. Centers for Disease Control: Update: *Salmonella enteritidis* infections and grade A shell eggs: United States 1989. M. M. W. R. *37*:490, 1989.
32. Challapalli, M., Cherubin, C., and Cunningham, D. G.: Lack of chronic carriage of *Salmonella typhimurium*. Pediatr. Infect. Dis. J. *8*:539–540, 1989.
33. Chin, K. C., Simmons, E. J., and Tarlow, M. J.: Neonatal typhoid fever. Arch. Dis. Child. *61*:1228–1230, 1986.
34. Chorba, T. L., Meriwether, R. A., Jenkins, B. R., et al.: Control of a non-foodborne outbreak of salmonellosis: Day care in isolation. Am. J. Public Health *77*:979–981, 1987.
35. Chow, C. B., Wang, P. S., Cheung, M. W., et al.: Diagnostic value of the Widal test in childhood typhoid fever. Pediatr. Infect. Dis. J. *6*:914–917, 1987.
36. Cohen, J. I., Bartlett, J. A., and Corey, G. R.: Extra-intestinal manifestations of *Salmonella* infections. Medicine *66*:349–388, 1987.
37. Cohen, M. L., and Tauxe, R. V.: Drug-resistant *Salmonella* in the United States: An epidemiologic perspective. Science *234*:964–969, 1986.
38. Colon, A. R., Gross, D. R., and Tamer, M. A.: Typhoid fever in children. Pediatrics *56*:606–609, 1975.
39. Connolly, M. J., Snow, M. N., and Ingham, H. R.: Ciprofloxacin treatment of recurrent *Salmonella* septicemia in a patient with acquired immune deficiency syndrome. J. Antimicrob. Chemother. *18*:647–648, 1986.
40. Cooles, P.: Adjuvant steroids and relapse of typhoid fever. J. Trop. Med. Hyg. *89*:229–231, 1986.
41. Corman, L. I., Poirier, R. H., Littlefield, C. A., et al.: Endophthalmitis due to *S. enteritidis*. J. Pediatr. *95*:1001–1002, 1979.
42. Cravioto, A., Reyes, R. E., Trujillo, F., et al.: Risk of diarrhea during the first year of life associated with initial and subsequent colonization by specific enteropathogens. Am. J. Epidemiol. *131*:886–904, 1990.
43. D'Amelio, R., Tagliabue, A., Nencioni, L., et al.: Comparative analysis of immunological responses to oral (Ty21a) and parenteral (TAB) typhoid vaccines. Infect. Immun. *56*:2731–2735, 1988.
44. Davis, R. C.: *Salmonella* sepsis in infancy. Am. J. Dis. Child. *135*:1096–1099, 1981.
45. Day, D. W., Mandal, B. K., and Morson, B. C.: The rectal biopsy appearances in *Salmonella* colitis. Histopathology *2*:117–131, 1978.
46. Demmerich, B., Lode, H., Borner, K., et al.: Biliary excretion and pharmacokinetics of cefoperazone in humans. J. Antimicrob. Chemother. *12*:27–37, 1983.
47. Diddle, A. W., and Stephens, R. L.: Typhoid fever in pregnancy. Am. J. Obstet. Gynecol. *38*:300–305, 1939.
48. Dietrich, H. F.: Typhoid fever in children. J. Pediatr. *10*:191–201, 1937.
49. Diwan, N., and Sharma, K.B.: Isolation of *S. typhimurium* from cephalohematoma and osteomyelitis. Indian J. Med. Res. *67*:27–29, 1978.
50. Dixon, J. M. S.: Effect of antibiotic treatment on duration of excretion of *S. typhimurium* by children. Br. Med. J. *2*:1343–1345, 1965.
51. Dowdle, E.: The reaction of patients with typhoid fever to the administration of aspirin. S. Afr. Med. J., May 19, 1956, pp. 474–477.
52. Dunn, D. W., McAllister, J., and Craft, J. C.: Brain abscess and empyema caused by *Salmonella*. Pediatr. Infect. Dis. *3*:54–57, 1984.
53. Dutta, P., Bhattacharya, S. K., Dutta, D., et al.: Hemolytic uremic syndrome following *Salmonella typhimurium* enteritis. Indian J. Pediatr. *56*:409–410, 1989.
54. Dutta, P., Rasaily, R., Saha, M. R., et al.: Ciprofloxacin for treatment of severe typhoid fever in children. Antimicrob. Agents Chemother. *37*:1197–1199, 1993.
55. Dutta, P., Rasaily, R., Saha, M. R., et al.: Randomized clinical trial of furazolidone for typhoid fever in children. Scand. J. Gastroenterol. *28*:168–172, 1993.
56. Edelman, R., and Levine, M. M.: Summary of an international workshop on typhoid fever. Rev. Infect. Dis. *8*:329–349, 1986.

57. Edgar, W. M., and Lacey, B. W.: Infection with *S. heidelberg*: An outbreak presumably not foodborne. Lancet *1*:161, 1963.
58. Ejlertsen, T., and Aunsholt, N. A.: *Salmonella* bacteremia in renal transplant recipients. Scand. J. Infect. Dis. *21*:241–244, 1989.
59. Farid, Z., Bassily, S., Kent, D. C., et al.: Chronic urinary *Salmonella* carriers with intermittent bacteremia. J. Trop. Med. Hyg. *73*:153–157, 1970.
60. Farid, Z., Girgis, N., and Abu El Ella, A., et al.: Aztreonam in the treatment of enteric fevers. Ann. Trop. Med. Parasitol. *81*:725–756, 1987.
61. Farid, Z., Girgis, N., and Abu El Ella, A.: Successful treatment of typhoid fever in children with parenteral ceftriaxone. Scand. J. Infect. Dis. *19*:467–468, 1987.
62. Feachem, R. G., and Koblinsky, M. A.: Interventions for the control of diarrhoeal diseases among young children: Promotion of breastfeeding. Bull W. H. O. *62*:271, 1984.
63. Ferreccio, C., Levine, M. M., Manterola, A., et al.: Benign bacteremia caused by *S. typhi* and *paratyphi* in children younger than 2 years. J. Pediatr. *104*:899–901, 1984.
64. Ferreccio, C., Morris, J. G., and Valdivieso, C., et al.: Efficacy of ciprofloxacin in the treatment of chronic typhoid carriers. J. Infect. Dis. *157*:1235–1239, 1988.
65. Fierer, J., Krause, M., Tauxe, R., et al.: *Salmonella typhimurium* bacteremia: Association with the virulence plasmid. J. Infect. Dis. *166*:639–642, 1992.
66. Finlay, B. B.: Molecular and cellular mechanisms of *Salmonella* pathogenesis. Curr. Top. Microbiol. Immunol. *192*:163–185, 1994.
67. Finlay, B. B., and Falkow, S.: Comparison of the invasion strategies used by *S. choleraesuis*, *S. flexneri*, and *Y. enterocolitica* to enter cultured animal cells. Biochimie *70*:1089–1099, 1988.
68. Foley, A. R.: An outbreak of paratyphoid B fever in a nursery of a small hospital. Can. J. Public Health *38*:73, 1947.
69. France, G. L., Marmer, D. J. and Steele, R. W.: Breast-feeding and *Salmonella* infection. Am. J. Dis. Child. *134*:147–152, 1980.
70. Galofre, J., Moreno, A., Mensa, J., et al.: Analysis of factors influencing the outcome and development of septic metastasis or relapse in *Salmonella* bacteremia. Clin. Infect. Dis. *18*:873–878, 1994.
71. Geers, T. A., and Backes, B. A.: Evaluation of two rapid methods to screen pathogens from stool specimens. Am. J. Clin. Pathol. *91*:327–330, 1989.
72. Gendrel, D., Kombila, M., Beaudoin-Leblevec, G., et al.: Nontyphoidal salmonellal septicemia in Gabonese children infected with *Schistosoma intercalatum*. Clin. Infect. Dis. *18*:103–105, 1994.
73. Gershman, M.: Single phage typing set for differentiating *salmonella*. J. Clin. Microbiol. *5*:302–314, 1977.
74. Giannella, R. A., Broitman, S. A., and Zamcheck, N.: Influence of gastric acidity on bacterial and parasitic enteric infections: A perspective. Ann. Intern. Med. *78*:271–276, 1973.
75. Giannella, R. A., Broitman, S. A., and Zamcheck, N.: *Salmonella* enteritis. I. Role of reduced gastric secretion in pathogenesis. Dig. Dis. *16*:1000–1006, 1971.
76. Giannella, R. A., Formal, S. B., Dammin, G. J., et al.: Pathogenesis of salmonellosis: Studies of fluid secretion, mucosal invasion, and morphologic reaction in the rabbit ileum. J. Clin. Invest. *52*:441–453, 1973.
77. Giannella, R. A., Gots, R. E., Charney, A. N., et al.: Pathogenesis of *Salmonella*-mediated intestinal fluid secretion: Activation of adenylate cyclase and inhibition by indomethacin. Gastroenterology *69*:1238–1245, 1975.
78. Gibney, E. J.: Typhoid perforation. Br. J. Surg. *76*:887–889, 1989.
79. Gilman, R. H., Terminel, M., and Levine, M. M.: Relative efficacy of blood, urine, rectal swab, bone marrow, and rose spot cultures for recovery of *S. typhi* in typhoid fever. Lancet *i*:1211–1213, 1975.
80. Gilman, R. H., Terminel, M., Levine, M. M., et al.: Comparison of trimethoprim/sulfamethoxazole and amoxicillin in therapy of chloramphenicol-resistant and chloramphenicol-sensitive typhoid fever. J. Infect. Dis. *132*:630–636, 1975.
81. Girgis, N. I., Sultan, Y., Hammad, O., et al.: Comparison of the efficacy, safety and cost of cefixime, ceftriaxone and aztreonam in the treatment of multidrug resistant *S. typhi* septicemia in children. Pediatr. Infect. Dis. J. *14*:603–605, 1995.
82. Gokalp, A. S., Toksoy, H. B., Turkay, S., et al.: Intravenous immunoglobulin in the treatment of *Salmonella typhimurium* infections in preterm neonates. Clin. Pediatr. *33*:349–352, 1994.
83. Goldstein, F. W., Chumpitaz, J. C., Guevara, J. M., et al.: Plasmid-mediated resistance to multiple antibiotics in *Salmonella typhi*. J. Infect. Dis. *153*:261–266, 1986.
84. Gotuzzo, E., Echevarria, J., Carrillo, C., et al.: Randomized comparison of aztreonam and chloramphenicol in treatment of typhoid fever. Antimicrob. Agents Chemother. *38*:558–562, 1994.
85. Gotuzzo, E., Guerra, J. G., Benavente, L., et al.: Use of norfloxacin to treat chronic typhoid carriers. J. Infect. Dis. *157*:1221–1225, 1988.
86. Griffith, J. P. C., and Ostheimer, M.: Typhoid fever in children. Am. J. Med. Sci. *124*:868–888, 1902.
87. Groisman, E. A., and Ochman, G.: Cognate gene clusters govern invasion of host epithelial cells by *S. typhimurium* and *Shigella flexneri*. EMBO J. *12*:3779–3787, 1993.
88. Grossman, D. A., Witham, N., Burr, D. H., et al.: Flagellar serotypes of *S. typhi* in Indonesia: Relationships among motility, invasiveness, and clinical illness. J. Infect. Dis. *171*:212–216, 1995.
89. Gulig, P. A., and Curtiss, R.: Plasmid-associated virulence of *Salmonella typhimurium*. Infect. Immun. *55*:2891–2900, 1987.
90. Gulig, P. A., Danbara, H., Guiney, D. G., et al.: Molecular analysis of *spv* virulence genes of the *Salmonella* virulence plasmids. Mol. Microbiol. *7*:825–830, 1993.
91. Guthrie, K. J., and Montgomery, G. I.: Infections with *Bacterium enteritidis* in infancy with the triad of enteritis, cholecystitis and meningitis. J. Pathol. Bacteriol. *49*:393, 1939.
92. Hadfield, T. L., Monson, M. H., and Wachsmoth, I. K.: An outbreak of antibiotic-resistant *Salmonella enteritidis* in Liberia, West Africa. J. Infect. Dis. *151*:790–795, 1985.
93. Haggman, D. L., Rehm, S. J., Moodie, D. S., et al.: Non-typhoidal *Salmonella* pericarditis: A case report and review of the literature. Pediatr. Infect. Dis. J. *5*:259–264, 1986.
94. Han, T., Sokal, J. E., and Neter, E.: Salmonellosis in disseminated malignant diseases: A seven-year review (1959–1963). N. Engl. J. Med. *276*:1045, 1967.
95. Hand, W. L., and King, N. L.: Serum opsonization of *Salmonella* in sickle cell anemia. Am. J. Med. *64*:388–395, 1978.
96. Harris, J. C., DuPont, H. L. and Hornick, R. B.: Fecal leukocytes in diarrheal illness. Ann. Intern. Med. *76*:697–700, 1972.
97. Hearne, S. E., Whigham, T. E., and Brady, C. E.: Pancreatitis and typhoid fever. Am. J. Med. *86*:471–473, 1989.
98. Hedberg, C. W., David, M. J., White, K. E., et al.: Role of egg consumption in sporadic *Salmonella enteritidis* and *Salmonella typhimurium* infections in Minnesota. J. Infect. Dis. *167*:107–111, 1993.
99. Hoffman, S. L., Edman, D. C., Punjabi, N. H., et al.: Bone marrow aspirate culture superior to streptokinase clot culture and 8 ml 1:10 blood-to-broth ratio blood culture for diagnosis of typhoid fever. Am. J. Trop. Med. Hyg. *35*:836–839, 1986.
100. Hoffman, S. L., Punjabi, N. H., Kumala, S., et al.: Reduction of mortality in chloramphenicol-treated severe typhoid fever by high dose dexamethasone. N. Engl. J. Med. *310*:82–88, 1984.
101. Hoffman, S. L., Punjabi, N. H., Rockhill, R. C., et al.: Duodenal string-capsule culture compared with bone marrow, blood, and rectal swab cultures for diagnosing typhoid and paratyphoid fever. J. Infect. Dis. *149*:157–161, 1984.
102. Holmberg, S. D.: Drug-resistant *Salmonella* species from animals fed antimicrobics. Infect. Dis. Newsletter *5*:25, 1986.
103. Holmberg, S. D., Osterholm, M. T., Senger, K. A., et al.: Drug-resistant *Salmonella* from animals fed antimicrobials. N. Engl. J. Med. *311*:617–622, 1984.
104. Hoppe, J. E., Dopfer, R., Huber, S., et al.: Eradication of *Salmonella dublin* in an immunodeficient child by combined use of ceftriaxone and ciprofloxacin after failure of either agent alone. Infection *17*:399–400, 1989.
105. Hornick, R. B., Griesman, S. E., Woodward, T. E., et al.: Typhoid fever. Pathogenesis and immunologic control. Parts I and II. N. Engl. J. Med. *283*:686–691 and 739–746, 1970.
106. Hyams, J. S., Durbin, W. A., Grand, R. J., et al.: *Salmonella* bacteremia in the first year of life. J. Pediatr. *96*:57–59, 1980.
107. Im, S. W. K., Chow, K., and Chau, P. Y.: Rectal thermometer-mediated cross-infection with *S. wadsworth* in a pediatric ward. J. Hosp. Infect. *2*:171–174, 1981.
108. Isomaki, O., Vuento, R., and Granfors, K.: Serological diagnosis of *Salmonella* infections by enzyme immunoassay. Lancet *1*:1411–1414, 1989.
109. Jiwa, S. F.: Probing for enterotoxigenicity among the salmonellae: An evaluation of biological assays. J. Clin. Microbiol. *14*:463–472, 1981.
110. Johnson, P. C., and Sabbaj, J.: Typhoid tonsillitis. J. A. M. A. *244*:362, 1980.
111. Kaniga, K., Trollinger, D., Galan, J. E.: Identification of two targets of the type III protein secretion system encoded by the *inv* and *spa* loci of *Salmonella typhimurium* that have homology to the *Shigella* IpaD and IpaA proteins. J. Bacteriol. *177*:7078–7085, 1995.
112. Kaniga, K., Tucker, S., Trollinger, D., Galan, et al.: Homologs of the *Shigella* IpaB and IpaC invasins are required for *Salmonella typhimurium* entry into cultured epithelial cells. J. Bacteriol. *177*:3965–3971, 1995.
113. Katz, B. Z., and Shapiro, E. D.: Predictors of persistently positive blood cultures in children with "occult" *Salmonella* bacteremia. Pediatr. Infect. Dis. *5*:713–714, 1986.
114. Kazemi, M., Bumpert, T. G., and Marks, M. I.: A controlled trial comparing trimethoprim/sulfamethoxazole, ampicillin, and no therapy in the treatment of *Salmonella* gastroenteritis in children. J. Pediatr. *83*:646–650, 1973.
115. Khan, M. A., Abdur-Rab, M., Israr, N., et al.: Transmission of *S. worthington* by oropharyngeal suction in hospital neonatal unit. Pediatr. Infect. Dis. J. *10*:668–672, 1991.
116. Kinsella, T. R., Yoger, R., Shulman, S. T., et al.: Treatment of *Salmonella* meningitis and brain abscess with the new cephalosporins: Two case reports and a review of the literature. Pediatr. Infect. Dis. J. *6*:476–480, 1987.
117. Klugman, K. P., Gilbertson, I. T., Koornhof, H. J., et al.: Protective activity of Vi capsular polysaccharide vaccine against typhoid fever. Lancet *2*:1165–1169, 1987.
118. Konzert, W.: *Salmonella* osteomyelitis in reference to *S. typhimurium* epidemics in a newborn infant ward. Wien. Klin. Wochenschr. *81*:713–716, 1969.

119. Lamb, V. A., Mayhall, C. G., Spadora, A. C., et al.: Outbreak of *Salmonella typhimurium* gastroenteritis due to an imported strain resistant to ampicillin, chloramphenicol and trimethoprim/sulfamethoxazole in a nursery. J. Clin. Microbiol. *20*:1076–1079, 1984.
120. Lee, L. A., Puhr, N. D., Maloney, E. K., et al.: Increase in antimicrobial-resistant *Salmonella* infections in the US, 1989–1990. J. Infect. Dis. *170*:128–134, 1994.
121. Lee, S. C., Yang, P. H., Shieh, W. B., et al.: Bacteremia due to non-typhi *Salmonella*: Analysis of 64 cases and review. Clin. Infect. Dis. *19*:693–696, 1994.
122. Levine, M. M.: Modern vaccines: Enteric infections. Lancet *335*:958–961, 1990.
123. Levine, M. M., Taylor, D. N., and Ferereccio, C.: Typhoid vaccines come of age. Pediatr. Infect. Dis. J. *8*:374–381, 1989.
124. Levine, M. M.: Typhoid fever and enteric fever. *In* Kass, E., and Platt, R. (eds.): Current Therapy in Infectious Diseases. Toronto, B. C. Decker, 1986.
125. Levy, S. B.: Man, animals, and antibiotic resistance. Pediatr. Infect. Dis. *4*:3–5, 1985.
126. Lieb, S., Gunn, R. A., and Taylor, D. N.: Salmonellosis in a day care center. J. Pediatr. *100*:1004, 1982.
127. Lizarralde, E.: Typhoid perforation of the ileum in children. J. Pediatr. Surg. *16*:1012–1016, 1981.
128. LoVerde, P. T., Amento, C., and Higashi, G. I.: Parasite-parasite interaction of *Salmonella typhimurium* and *Schistosoma*. J. Infect. Dis. *141*:177–185, 1980.
129. Low, L. C., Lam, B. C., Wong, W. T., et al.: *Salmonella meningitis* in infancy. Aust. Paediatr. J. *20*:225–228, 1984.
130. Mabey, D. C., Brown, A., and Greenwood, B. M.: *Plasmodium falciparum* malaria and *Salmonella* infections in Gambian children. J. Infect. Dis. *155*:1319, 1987.
131. MacDonald, K. L., Cohen, M. L., Hargrett-Bean, N. T., et al.: Changes in antimicrobial resistance of *Salmonella* isolated from humans in the United States. J. A. M. A. *258*:1496–1499, 1987.
132. MacDonald, W. B., Friday, F., and McEacharn, M.: The effect of chloramphenicol in *Salmonella enteritis* in infancy. Arch. Dis. Child. *29*:238, 1954.
133. Mackaness, G. B., Blander, R. V., and Collins, F. M.: Host-parasite relations in mouse typhoid. J. Exp. Med. *124*:573–583, 1966.
134. Mallouh, A. A., and Sadi, A. R.: White blood cells and bone marrow in typhoid fever. Pediatr. Infect. Dis. J. *6*:527–529, 1987.
135. Mallouh, A. A., and Salamah, M. M.: Pattern of bacterial infections in homozygous sickle cell disease. Am. J. Dis. Child. *139*:820–826, 1985.
136. Martyn-Jones, D. M., and Pantin, G. C.: Neonatal diarrhea due to *S. paratyphi*. B. J. Clin. Pathol. *9*:128, 1956.
137. Marzetti, G., Laurenti, F., deCaro, M., et al.: *Salmonella münchen* infections in newborns and small infants. Clin. Pediatr. (Phila.) *12*:93–97, 1973.
138. Maudgil, A., Bhan, M. K., and Khoshoo, V.: Hemolytic uremic syndrome associated with *Salmonella typhimurium*. Indian Pediatr. *24*:608–609, 1987.
139. McAllister, T. A., Roud, J. A., and Marshall, A., et al.: Outbreak of *Salmonella eimsbuettel* in newborn infants spread by rectal thermometers. Lancet *1*:1262–1264, 1986.
140. McKinlay, B.: Infectious diarrhea of the newborn caused by an unclassified species of *Salmonella*. Am. J. Dis. Child. *54*:1252, 1937.
141. Meadow, W. L., Schneider, H., and Beem, M.: *Salmonella enteritidis* bacteremia in childhood. J. Infect. Dis. *152*:185–189, 1985.
142. Meloni, T., Marinaro, A. M., Desole, M. G., et al.: Ceftriaxone treatment of *Salmonella* enteric fever. Pediatr. Infect. Dis. J. *7*:734–735, 1986.
143. Mendis, N. M. P., de la Motte, P. U., Gunatillaka, P. D. P., et al.: Protracted infection with *S. bareilly* in a maternity hospital. J. Trop. Med. Hyg. *79*:142–150, 1976.
144. Merselis, J. G., Kaye, D., Connolly, C. S., et al.: Quantitative bacteriology of the typhoid carrier state. Am. J. Trop. Med. Hyg. *13*:425, 1964.
145. Metzler, J., and Nachamkin, I.: Evaluation of a latex agglutination test for the detection of *Salmonella* and *Shigella* spp. by using broth enrichment. J. Clin. Microbiol. *26*:2501–2504, 1988.
146. Michel, J., Malpuach, G., Godeneche, P., et al.: Clinical and bacterological study of a salmonellosis epidemic in a hospital (*Salmonella oranienburg*). Pediatrie *25*:13–19, 1970.
147. Mishu, B., Koehler, J., Lee, L. A., et al.: Outbreaks of *Salmonella enteritidis* infections in the US, 1985–1991. J. Infect. Dis. *169*:547–552, 1994.
148. Moosa, A., and Rubidge, C. J.: Once daily ceftriaxone vs. chloramphenicol for treatment of typhoid fever in children. Pediatr. Infect. Dis. J. *8*:696–699, 1989.
149. Mroczenski-Wildey, M. J., Di, F. J. L., and Cabello, F. C.: Invasion and lyssi of HeLa cell monolayers by *S. typhi*: The role of lipopolysaccharide. Microb. Pathogen. *6*:143–152, 1989.
150. Murphy, J. R., Grez, L., Schlesinger, L., et al.: Immunogenicity of *S. typhi* Ty21a vaccine for young children. Infect. Immun. *59*:1291–1293, 1991
151. Naqvi, S. H., Thobani, S., Moazam, F., et al.: Generalized suppurative lymphadenitis with typhoidal salmonellosis. Pediatr. Infect. Dis. J. *7*:882–883, 1988.
152. Nelson, J. D., and McCracken, G. H.: What next? J. Pediatr. Infect. Dis. *16*:10–16, 1990.
153. Nelson, J. D., Kusmiesz, H., Jackson, L. H., et al.: Treatment of *Salmonella* gastroenteritis with ampicillin, amoxicillin, or placebo. Pediatrics *65*:1125–1130, 1980.
154. Nelson, J. D.: Suppurative mastitis in infants. Am. J. Dis. Child. *125*:458–459, 1973.
155. Nelson, S. J., and Granoff, D.: *Salmonella* gastroenteritis in the first three months of life. Clin. Pediatr. *21*:709–712, 1982.
156. Neter, E.: Observation on the transmission of salmonellosis in man. Am. J. Public Health *40*:929, 1950.
157. Novak, R., and Feldman, S.: Salmonellosis in children with cancer. Am. J. Dis. Child. *133*:298–300, 1979.
158. O'Dempsey, T. J., McArdle, T. F., Lloyd-Evans, N., et al.: Importance of enteric bacteria as a cause of pneumonia, meningitis and septicemia among children in a rural community in The Gambia, West Africa. Pediatr. Infect. Dis. J. *13*:122–128, 1994.
159. Olsvik, O., Sorum, H., Birkness, K., et al.: Plasmid characterization of *Salmonella typhimurium* transmitted from animals to humans. J. Clin. Microbiol. *22*:336–338, 1985.
160. Omland, T., and Gardborg, O.: *Salmonella enteritidis* infections in infancy with special reference to a small nosocomial epidemic. Acta Paediatr. Belg. *49*:583–590, 1960.
161. Ortiz-Neu, C., Marr, J. S., Cherubin, C. E., et al.: Bone and joint infections due to *Salmonella*. J. Infect. Dis. *138*:820–828, 1978.
162. Pape, J. W., Gerdes, H., Oriol, L., et al.: Typhoid fever: Successful therapy with cefoperazone. J. Infect. Dis. *153*:272–276, 1986.
163. Pavia, A. T., Shipman, L. D., Wells, J. G., et al.: Epidemiologic evidence that prior antimicrobial exposure decreases resistance to infection by antimicrobial-sensitive *Salmonella*. J. Infect. Dis. *161*:255–260, 1990.
164. Pether, J. V., and Gilbert, R. J.: The survival of salmonellas on finger-tips and transfer of the organisms to foods. J. Hyg. (Camb.) *69*:673–681, 1971.
165. Pettersson, T., Klemola, E., and Wager, O.: Treatment of acute cases of *Salmonella* infection and *Salmonella* carriers with ampicillin and neomycin. Acta Med. Scand. *175*:185, 1964.
166. Pickering, L. K.: Bacterial and parasitic enteropathogens in day care. Semin. Pediatr. Infect. Dis. *1*:263, 1990.
167. Pickering, L. K., DuPont, H. L., Olarte, J., et al.: Fecal leukocytes in enteric infections. Am. J. Clin. Pathol. *68*:562–565, 1977.
168. Pickering, L. K., Kohl, S., and Cleary, T. G.: Humoral factors in breast milk that protect against diarrhea. *In* Jensen, R. G. and Neville, M. C. (eds.): Human Lactation. New York, Plenum Publishing Corp., 1985, p. 63.
169. Pickering, L. K., and Ruiz-Palacios, G.: Antibodies in milk directed against specific enteropathogens. *In* Hamosh, A., and Goldman, A. S. (eds.): Human Lactation 2. New York, Plenum Publishing Corp., 1986, p. 499.
170. Plotkin, S. A., and Bouveret-Le, Cam. N.: A new typhoid vaccine composed of the Vi capsular polysaccharide. Arch. Intern. Med. *155*:2293–2299, 1995.
171. Punjabi, N. H., Hoffman, S. L., Edman, D. C., et al.: Treatment of severe typhoid fever in children with high dose dexamethasone. Pediatr. Infect. Dis. J. *7*:598–600, 1988.
172. Puri, V., Thirupuram, S., Khalil, A., et al.: Nosocomial *S. typhimurium* epidemic in a neonatal special care unit. Indian Pediatr. *17*:233–239, 1980.
173. Rajajee, S., Anandi, T. B., Subha, S., et al.: Patterns of resistant *S. typhi* infection in infants. J. Trop. Pediatr. *41*:52–54, 1995.
174. Ramachandran, S., Godfrey, J. J., and Perera, M. V.: Typhoid hepatitis. J. A. M. A. *230*:236–240, 1974.
175. Ramos, J. M., Garcia-Corbeira, P., Aguado, J. M., et al.: Clinical significance of primary vs. secondary bacteremia due to nontyphoid *Salmonella* in patients without AIDS. Clin. Infect. Dis. *19*:777–780, 1994.
176. Reed, R. P., and Klugman, K. P.: Neonatal typhoid fever. Pediatr. Infect. Dis. J. *13*:774–777, 1994.
177. Rice, P. A., Craven, P. C., and Wells, J. G.: *Salmonella heidelberg* enteritis and bacteremia: An epidemic on two pediatric wards. Am. J. Med. *60*:509–516, 1976.
178. Riley, L. W., and Cohen, M. L.: Plasmid profiles and *Salmonella* epidemiology. Lancet *1*:573, 1982.
179. Riley, L. W., Cohen, M. L., Seals, J. E., et al.: Importance of host factors in human salmonellosis caused by multi-resistant strains of *Salmonella*. J. Infect. Dis. *149*:878–883, 1984.
180. Rocha, H., Kirk, J. W., and Hearey, C. D.: Prolonged *Salmonella* bacteremia in patients with *Schistosoma mansoni* infection. Arch. Intern. Med. *128*:254–257, 1971.
181. Rodriguez, R. E., Valero, V., and Watanakunakorn, C.: *Salmonella* focal intracranial infections: Review of the world literature (1884–1984) and report of an unusual case. Rev. Infect. Dis. *8*:31–41, 1986.
182. Rosenthal, S. L.: Exacerbation of *Salmonella* enteritis due to ampicillin. N. Engl. J. Med. *280*:147–148, 1969.
183. Rowe, B., Giles, C., and Brown, G. L.: Outbreak of gastroenteritis due to *S. virchow* in a maternity hospital. Br. Med. J. *3*:561–564, 1969.
184. Roy, S. K., Speelman, P., Butler, T., et al.: Diarrhea associated with typhoid fever. J. Infect. Dis. *151*:1138–1143, 1985.
185. Rubinstein, A. D., Feemster, R. F., and Smith, H. M.: Salmonellosis as a public health problem in wartime. Am. J. Public Health *34*:841, 1944.
186. Rubinstein, A. D., and Fowler, R. N.: Salmonellosis of the newborn with transmission by delivery room resuscitators. Am. J. Public Health *45*:1109, 1955.
187. Ruiz-Contreras, J., Ramos, J. T., Hernandez-Sampelayo, T., et al.: Sepsis in children with HIV infection: The Madrid HIV Pediatric Infection Collaborative Study Group. Pediatr. Infect Dis. J. *14*:522–526, 1995.

188. Russell, I. J., Forgacs, P., and Geraci, J. E.: Pancreatitis complicating typhoid fever. J. A. M. A. *235*:753–754, 1976.
189. Ryan, C. A., Hargrett-Bean, N. T., and Blake, P. A.: *Salmonella typhi* infections in the United States, 1975–1984: Increasing role of foreign travel. Rev. Infect. Dis. *11*:1-8, 1989.
190. Sanchez, C., Garcia Restoy, E., Garau, J., et al.: Ciprofloxacin and TMP/SMX versus placebo in acute uncomplicated *Salmonella* enteritis: A double-blind trial. J. Infect. Dis. *168*:1304–1307, 1993.
191. Sanders, D. Y., Sinal, S. H., and Morrison, L.: Chronic salmonellosis in infancy. Clin. Pediatr. (Phila.) *13*:640–643, 1974.
192. Saphra, I., and Winter, J. W.: Clinical manifestations of salmonellosis in man: An evaluation of 7779 human infections identified at the New York *Salmonella* Center. N. Engl. J. Med. *256*:1128, 1957.
193. Sarasombath, S., Banchuin, N., Sukosol, T., et al.: Systemic and intestinal immunities after natural typhoid infection. J. Clin. Microbiol. *25*:1088–1093, 1987.
194. Sasidharan, C. K., Rajagopal, K. C., Jayaram, C. K., et al.: *S. typhimurium* epidemic in newborn nursery. Indian J. Pediatr. *50*:599–605, 1983.
195. Seals, J. E., Parrott, P. L., McGowan, J. E., et al.: Nursery salmonellosis: Delayed recognition due to unusually long incubation period. Infect. Control *4*:205–208, 1983.
196. Seligman, E.: Mass invasion of salmonellae in a babies ward. Ann. Paediatr. *172*:406, 1949.
197. Seoud, M., Saade, G., Uwaydah, M., et al.: Typhoid fever in pregnancy. Obstet. Gynecol. *71*:711–714, 1988.
198. Sirinavin, S., Jayanetra, P., Lolekha, S., et al.: Predictors for extraintestinal infection in *Salmonella* enteritis in Thailand. Pediatr. Infect. Dis. J. *7*:44–48, 1988.
199. Smith, S. M., Palumbo, P. E., and Edelson, P. J.: *Salmonella* strains resistant to multiple antibiotics: Therapeutic implications. Pediatr. Infect. Dis. *3*:455–460, 1984.
200. Soe, G. B., and Overturf, G. D.: Treatment of typhoid fever and other systemic salmonellosis with cefotaxime, ceftriaxone, cefoperazone, and other newer cephalosporins. Rev. Infect. Dis. *9*:719–736, 1987.
201. Sperber, S. J., and Schleupner, C. J.: Salmonellosis during infection with human immunodeficiency virus. Rev. Infect. Dis. *9*:925–934, 1987.
202. Spika, J. S., Waterman, S. H., Soo Hoo, G. W., et al.: Chloramphenicol-resistant *Salmonella newport* traced through hamburger to dairy farms. N. Engl. J. Med. *316*:565–570, 1987.
203. Stuart, B. M., and Pullen, R. L.: Typhoid: Clinical analysis of 360 cases. Arch. Intern. Med. *78*:629, 1946.
204. Syrogiannopoulos, G. A., McCracken, G. H., and Nelson, J. D.: Osteoarticular infections in children with sickle cell disease. Pediatrics *78*:1090–1096, 1986.
205. Szanton, V. L.: Epidemic salmonellosis: A 30-month study of 80 cases of *S. oranienburg* infection. Pediatrics *20*:794–808, 1957.
206. Sztein, M. B., Wasserman, S. S., Tacket, C. O., et al.: Cytokine production patterns and lymphoproliferative responses in volunteers orally immunized with attenuated vaccine strains of *S. typhi*. J. Infect. Dis. *170*:1508–1517, 1994.
207. Szmuness, W., Sikorska, J., Szymanek, E., et al.: The microbiological and epidemiological properties of infections caused by *S. enteritidis*. J. Hyg. (London) *64*:9–21, 1966.
208. Tacket, C. O., Forrest, B., Morona, R., et al.: Safety, immunogenicity, and efficacy against cholera challenge in humans of a typhoid-cholera hybrid vaccine derived from *Salmonella typhi* Ty21a. Infect. Immun. *58*:1620–1627, 1990.
209. Tanaka-Kido, J., Ortega, L., and Santos, J. I.: Comparative efficacies of aztreonam and chloramphenicol in children with typhoid fever. Pediatr. Infect. Dis. J. *9*:44–48, 1990.
210. Taylor, D. N., Bopp, C., Birkness, K., et al.: An outbreak of salmonellosis associated with a fatality in a healthy child: A large dose and severe illness. Am. J. Epidemiol. *119*:907–912, 1984.
211. Taylor, D. N., Beid, J. M., Munro, J. S., et al.: *Salmonella dublin* infections in the United States, 1979–1980. J. Infect. Dis. *146*:322–327, 1982.
212. Taylor, D. N., Bopp, C., Birkness, K., et al. An outbreak of salmonellosis associated with a fatality in a healthy child: A large dose and severe illness. Am. J. Epidemiol. *119*:907–912, 1984.
213. Ti, T. Y., Monteiro, E. H., Lam, S., et al.: Ceftriaxone therapy in bacteremic typhoid fever. Antimicrob. Agents Chemother. *28*:540–543, 1985.
214. Torrey, S., Fleisher, G., and Jaffe, D.: Incidence of *Salmonella* bacteremia in infants with *Salmonella* gastroenteritis. J. Pediatr. *108*:718–721, 1986.
215. Tsang, R. S., Chau, P. Y., Lam, S. K., et al.: Antibody response to the lipopolysaccharide and protein antigens of *Salmonella typhi* during typhoid infection. Clin. Exp. Immunol. *46*:508–514, 1981.
216. Thisyakorn, U., Mansuwan, P., and Taylor, D. N.: Typhoid and paratyphoid fever in 192 hospitalized children in Thailand. Am. J. Dis. Child. *141*:862–865, 1987.
217. Uwyyed, K., and Uromen, A.: Scrotal abscess with bacteremia caused by *Salmonella* group D after ritual circumcision. Pediatr. Infect. Dis. J. *9*:65–66, 1990.
218. Vallenas, C., Hernandez, H., Kay, B., et al.: Efficacy of bone marrow, blood, stool, and duodenal contents cultures for bacteriologic confirmation of typhoid fever in children. Pediatr. Infect. Dis. *4*:496–498, 1985.
219. Van de Verg, L., Herrington, D. A., Murphy, J. R., et al.: Specific immunoglobulin A–secreting cells in peripheral blood of humans following oral immunization with a bivalent *Salmonella typhi–Shigella sonnei* vaccine or infection by pathogenic *S. sonnei*. Infect. Immun. *58*:2002–2004, 1990.
220. Van Gijsegem, F., Genin, S., and Boucher, C.: Conservation of secretion pathways for pathogenecity determinants of plant and animal bacteria: Trends Microbiol. *1*:175–180, 1993.
221. Vazquez, V., Calderon, E., and Rodriguez, R. S.: Chloramphenicol-resistant strains of *Salmonella typhi*. N. Engl. J. Med. *286*:1220, 1972.
222. Wahdan, M. H., Serie, C., and Cerisier, Y.: A controlled field trial of live *Salmonella typhi* strain Ty21a oral vaccine against typhoid: Three-year results. J. Infect. Dis. *145*:292–295, 1982.
223. Wallis, T. S., Starkey, W. G., Stephen, J., et al.: The nature and role of mucosal damage in relation to *Salmonella typhimurium* induced fluid secretion in the rabbit ileum. J. Med. Microbiol. *22*:39–49, 1986.
224. Wallis, T. S., Hawker, R. J., Candy, D. C., et al.: Quantification of the leucocyte influx into rabbit ileal loops induced by strains of *S. typhimurium* of different virulence. J. Med. Microbiol. *30*:149–156, 1989.
225. Watt, J., and Carlton, E.: Studies of the acute diarrheal diseases. XVI. An outbreak of *S. typhimurium* infection among newborn premature infants. Public Health Rep. *60*(Part I):734–810, 1945.
226. Watt, J., Wegman, M. E., Brown, O. W., et al.: Salmonellosis in a premature nursery unaccompanied by diarrheal diseases. Pediatrics *22*:689–705, 1958.
227. Wilson, R., Feldman, R. A., Davis, J., et al.: Salmonellosis in infants: the importance of intrafamilial transmission. Pediatrics *69*:436–438, 1982.
228. Winkler, A. P., and Gleich, S.: Acute acalculous cholecystitis caused by *Salmonella typhi* in an 11-year-old. Pediatr. Infect. Dis. *7*:125–128, 1988.
229. Wittler, R. R., and Bass, J. W.: Non-typhoidal *Salmonella* enteric infections and bacteremia. Pediatr. Infect. Dis. J. *8*:364–367, 1989.
230. Yamamoto, L. G., and Ashton, M. J.: *Salmonella* infections in infants in Hawaii. Pediatr. Infect. Dis. J. *7*:48–52, 1988.
231. Zarkovsky, H. S., Gallagher, D., and Gill, F. M.: Bacteremia in sickle hemoglobinopathies. J. Pediatr. *109*:579–585, 1986.

116

PLAGUE (*YERSINIA PESTIS*)

Maria D. Goldstein

HISTORY

Yersinia pestis has been responsible for the most devastating epidemics in human history. Possibly the first mention of plague dates to 1320 B.C., in 1 Samuel, Chapters 5 and 6. The next recorded outbreak was in A.D. 542 during Justinian's reign, when an estimated 100 million people died.[39] This epidemic was followed by a quiescent period lasting until 1346, when plague appeared during the siege of the city of Kaffa in the Crimea. The epidemic quickly spread through most of Europe, becoming known as the black death. One-third of the population of Europe died in its aftermath. Between the 14th and 20th centuries, plague remained endemic in most of Europe and Russia, with resultant frequent outbreaks.[35]

In 1894, Yersin and Kitasato,[38] working independently, first described the bacillus responsible for plague. At about that time, the role played by rats and fleas in the spread of the disease became known. In 1900, plague was introduced to San Francisco by rats aboard ships docking there. The disease spread to ground squirrels and then to other wild animals of the American Southwest.[37] In 1943, effective antibiotics against *Y. pestis* became available.[35] Thanks to these advances, plague is rare today, and when it occurs, its prognosis is not as grave as it used to be. Early diagnosis and treatment are essential.

BACTERIOLOGY

Y. pestis belongs in the family Enterobacteriaceae. It is a small, pleomorphic, nonmotile, gram-negative bacillus. With Wayson, Giemsa, and Gram stains, the bacillus takes on bipolar or safety-pin morphologic features.[13]

Y. pestis grows at temperatures ranging from 0° to 40° C (32° to 104° F); the optimal temperature is 28° C (82.4° F). On first isolation at 35° C (95° F) on 5 per cent blood agar, the colonies are pinpoint in size, growing to 1 to 2 mm after 2 days. They are nonhemolytic on 5 per cent sheep blood agar.

Depending on the clinical nature of the disease, blood cultures, sputum samples, or aspirates of enlarged nodes should be examined for typical bacilli. The isolated bacilli can be identified by the following criteria: *Y. pestis* is nonmotile at 37° and 22° C (98.6° and 71.6° F). The organism usually is negative for urea hydrolysis but may be positive in freshly isolated strains. The organism is positive for esculin, β-galactosidase, catalase, and methyl red. The oxidase, indole, and Voges-Proskauer reactions are negative. It ferments glucose, maltose, salicin, xylose, arabinose, dextrin, trehalose, and mannitol. It does not produce acid from lactose, sucrose, rhamnose, melibiose, adonitol, cellobiose, sorbose, or dulcitol. It does not utilize citrate, and it does not grow in potassium cyanide. *Y. pestis* is negative for lysine, ornithine decarboxylase, and arginine dihydrolase.[36, 43]

Definitive identification may be based on the following tests: (1) lysis of the isolate by known strains of bacteriophage, (2) fluorescent antibody staining, (3) agglutination test with specific *Y. pestis* antiserum, and (4) animal inoculation.[43]

Y. pestis strains vary in their degree of virulence. The following determinants of virulence are chromosomally mediated: (1) an antiphagocytic capsular material known as fraction 1, (2) the endogenous purine synthesis that allows the organism to grow within macrophages, and (3) the ability to absorb iron from the medium. Several plasmids have been implicated in the development of other virulence factors. A plasmid of 9-kb pairs contains the determinant of secretory protein that kills other bacterial strains. A plasmid of 72-kb pairs that all pathogenic *Y. pestis* strains contain confers the requirement for environmental Ca^{2+} to be present in order for the organism to grow at 37° C (98.6° F). When grown under this condition, *Y. pestis* produces V and W antigens that are necessary for virulence.[17] Toxins have been produced by all fully virulent strains. Both an exotoxin and an endotoxin have been found to contribute to the lethal effects of plague.[43]

TRANSMISSION

Host

Historically, epidemics of plague usually were transmitted by the fleas of infected rats. This form of spread is more likely in urban, rat-infested, and crowded dwellings and may result in epidemics. In the United States, plague is transmitted sporadically to humans after contact with an enzootic sylvatic focus.[23] Infected wild rodents perpetuate the plague bacillus in a given ecosystem by virtue of their ability to withstand an inoculum of *Y. pestis* many times larger than that necessary to cause disease in humans or domestic animals. After becoming inoculated, the wild rodent may become bacteremic and infect the fleas that feed on it; these in turn transmit the plague bacillus to another rodent. Hibernating animals especially are resistant to clinical infection. Animals inoculated before going into hibernation may survive through the winter and not succumb until after coming out of their burrows, thus reintroducing the bacillus in the new season.[23] Carnivores are relatively resistant to infection but contribute to the spread of the organism by transporting infected fleas from one area to another.[23]

The role of domestic animals in bridging the gap between sylvatic plague and human infection has been studied extensively.[33, 38, 42] Cats and dogs are susceptible to both natural and experimental plague. Epizootics in cats have been observed in conjunction with plague epidemics in humans.[38] Experimentally infected cats develop severe systemic illness, with bacteremia and abscess formation at the site of the inoculum. Between 1977 and 1985, there were 60 confirmed cases of feline plague in New Mexico. Five of the 60 cases resulted in human infection. In four of these five cases, *Y. pestis* probably was transmitted by direct inoculation via draining abscesses, bites, or pneumonic discharges of the infected cats. A total of 10 other cases reported in the literature of feline plague transmission to humans involved four veterinarians.[15] Dogs also are susceptible, but their disease is milder.[42] Swine are resistant to plague, the only evidence of subclinical infection being the presence of antibodies to the fraction 1 antigen of *Y. pestis*. It appears, then, that domestic animals, by virtue of their intimate contact with both wildlife and humans, may be responsible for some cases of human plague. This danger is accentuated by a dearth of symptoms in some animals.[33]

Vector

Plague is transmitted to humans by the bite of an infected flea, the skinning and evisceration of infected animals,[29] or the inhalation of infected droplets from a case of pneumonic plague.[27] Infrequent portals of entry include the conjunctiva[38] and the pharynx.[40, 32]

The efficiency of the flea as a vector for human disease depends on the likelihood that the infected flea will feed on a person and that, in the process of feeding, the flea will regurgitate the bacillus into the victim's blood stream.[23] Flea species vary in both of these attributes. Wild rodent fleas, for example, are reluctant to feed on humans and do it only under duress (e.g., when the natural host dies). Fleas of domestic animals are more likely to bite humans. The Oriental rat flea, *Xenopsylla cheopsis*, is the most efficient plague transmitter because of its willingness to bite people and its propensity for regurgitating large numbers of bacilli in the process.[23] When the Oriental rat flea ingests infected blood, the actions of a coagulase produced by *Y. pestis* and a trypsin-like enzyme present in the flea's stomach result in the formation of an infected clot that blocks the flea's proventriculus. In obstructing the flea's intestinal tract, the clot allows further replication of bacteria. When the flea tries to feed again, it regurgitates large numbers of plague bacilli. The formation and dissolution of the fibrin clot are temperature-dependent. At temperatures above 27° C (80.6° F), a fibrinolytic enzyme is activated that dissolves the clot and allows the flea to dispose of the bacillus. It has been postulated that this temperature-dependent phenomenon is responsible for the observed cyclic nature of urban plague epidemics, which tend to subside with the advent of hot weather.[5]

In contrast, fleas in which the intestinal tracts do not become blocked contribute to the endemicity of plague by harboring the organism and transmitting it in sublethal dosages.[10] Sylvatic plague depends on the rodent flea as the vector. This flea, although not as efficient as the rat flea in transmitting the bacillus, may itself become a reservoir of *Y. pestis* by surviving for 12 to 15 months after the original host dies. In the new season, it reintroduces the plague bacillus into the new rodent population.[39] The observation that *Y. pestis* can survive in the soil during interepizootics suggests another mechanism of plague transmission.[18]

EPIDEMIOLOGY

The plague bacillus exists in enzootic cycles involving wild animals or domestic rats. In urban plague, the course of events usually is initiated by the introduction of the plague bacillus from an enzootic focus into a susceptible rat population. With humans and rats living in close proximity, an epizootic in rats then may be followed by an epidemic in people.[39] The epidemic may subside with the advent of hot, humid weather[5] or the obliteration of the rat population.[39] Such epidemics are rare today but have been described in South Vietnam[3, 25] and most recently in India.[11] In 1992, 1582 cases of human plague were reported to the World Health Organization from nine countries, including Brazil, Madagascar, Myanmar (formerly Burma), Tanzania, Vietnam, and the United States.[46]

In the United States today, people become infected most frequently by direct contact with a sylvatic reservoir of infection. Sporadic human cases usually result from working or hunting in a plague-infested area[23] and increasingly from living near foci of infection as suburban spread encroaches on the natural habitats of rodents.[12] In recent years, domestic animals, especially cats, have been responsible for a significant proportion of human cases. Since 1977, 15 human cases have resulted from contact with infected cats.[12]

Sylvatic plague epizootics occur in the summer seasons. Most cases of rural plague occur between April and September. The rare occurrence of human plague in the winter months usually is associated with hunting and direct exposure to infected tissues.[9, 24]

The continental United States has a large enzootic focus that includes 130 counties in 15 western states. Surveillance for plague in rodents during the 1990s has identified infected animals farther east than ever before. The plague bacillus now has been isolated in wild rodents in eastern Montana, western Nebraska, western North Dakota, and eastern Texas.[12] Between 1925 and 1965, the number of reported cases in the United States averaged between two and three per year.[6, 7] During the 1970s, 105 cases were reported.[24] The number of cases reported in 1980 through 1982 showed a similar increasing trend.[7] Between 1970 and 1979, 53 per cent of cases were in females, in contrast with the period 1926 to 1969, when only 27 per cent were in females. About 60 per cent of cases occur in persons younger than 20 years of age.[24] However, of 10 confirmed cases reported in the United States in 1993, the age distribution was 22 to 96 years. Five of the patients were older than 65 years of age.[12] Native Americans living on reservations in the states of Arizona, New Mexico, and Utah are at increased risk. In the period 1970 to 1979, 35 per cent of cases in these three states occurred in Native Americans.[7, 24] Many of the patients were infected within 1 mile of their residence and almost all within their state of residence.[24] Seven of the 10 patients reported in 1993 were exposed in their homesites, and one, a veterinarian, was exposed at work.[12] Occasionally, plague has been acquired by a traveler in an endemic area who then traveled during the incubation period to a plague-free region of the country. This set of circumstances shows why all physicians need to be aware of the presenting symptoms and signs of plague as well as the need to obtain an accurate travel history.[26]

PATHOGENESIS AND PATHOLOGY

The portal of entry of the plague bacillus determines, to some extent, the form the disease will take. By far the most common portal of entry is the skin when it is bitten by an infected flea. Broken skin may provide access for direct inoculation while infected animals are being handled. After overcoming the skin barrier, the organisms move via the lymphatics to the regional lymph nodes, where they elicit an inflammatory response. The infection may be localized at this site, with subsequent antibody formation and recovery. This clinical form is known as pestis minor. Commonly, the bacillus is disseminated via the blood stream. Distant organ involvement may include the liver, spleen, kidneys, lungs, and meninges. Disseminated intravascular coagulation is common in fatal cases. Coagulation defects, including thrombocytopenia and elevated fibrin split products,[3] as well as fibrin deposits in the glomeruli,[16, 38] may be present. Bacteremia is not synonymous with severe disease and is common in relatively mild cases.[38]

The major determinant of severity seems to be the presence of high levels of endotoxin. The toxin of *Y. pestis* has the biologic properties of typical endotoxin. When injected in experimental animals, it can cause the clinical symptoms and signs and pathologic changes characteristic of endotoxic shock and death. The quantity of endotoxin necessary to kill is estimated to be comparable with that present in a lethal dose of live bacteria.[1, 45] The murine toxin of *Y. pestis* has a direct inhibitory effect in vitro on the respiration of heart mitochondria of rats and mice, whereas it has little or no effect on the mitochondria of rabbits, chimpanzees, dogs, and monkeys. The differing sensitivities in vitro correlate with the susceptibilities in vivo of these species to *Y. pestis* infection.[41]

Achieving high levels of toxin depends on the ability of the bacillus to replicate in the infected host. Resistance to phagocytosis had been assumed to be related to virulence. More recent experimental evidence has shown that virulent *Y. pestis* organisms are phagocytized but, in contrast with avirulent ones, are not killed. They continue to replicate freely in macrophages, allowing the accumulation of endotoxin.[22, 41]

When the lung is the portal of entry, the disease usually is more fulminant. After being inhaled, bacilli replicate freely in the alveolar spaces. Severe pneumonia, endotoxemia, and septicemia ensue and, if untreated, cause death. In fatal cases, the thoracic lymph nodes show infarction, necrosis, and liquefaction, with pus formation. Edema and inflammation of the surrounding tissue are common.[38] The mucosa of trachea and bronchi is covered by bloody, frothy exudate. Submucosal hemorrhages and areas of necrosis may surround the trachea. The pleural surfaces contain hemorrhagic lesions and fibrinous adhesions. The lung parenchyma may be consolidated or show signs of acute edema.[38] The predominant histologic feature is an alveolar exudate consisting of histiocytes and polymorphonuclear leukocytes.[16]

Other organs are involved as well. The kidneys may appear grossly hemorrhagic and contain areas of necrosis. Microscopic examination reveals leukocytic infiltrates of congested veins and capillaries. Glomeruli with fibrin thrombi frequently are found in patients with disseminated intravascular coagulation.[16] Biopsy of purpuric skin lesions reveals subepithelial hemorrhages and fibrin deposit in the capillaries. These changes are indistinguishable from those seen in a generalized Shwartzman reaction.[3]

CLINICAL MANIFESTATIONS

The incubation period of *Y. pestis* generally is 3 to 4 days but may be as short as a few hours or as long as 10 days. The onset of illness usually is abrupt, beginning with fever, malaise, weakness, and headache.[38, 39] Fever is high, frequently accompanied by shaking chills.[38] The appearance of a visible and palpable bubo may be preceded by pain and tenderness at that site.[39]

On physical examination, the patient is "toxic," apprehensive, and tachycardic. The inoculation site in the skin may not be evident or may be marked by a carbuncle. In bubonic plague, typical large, fixed, edematous, and exquisitely tender nodes are present at one anatomic site.[25] In decreasing order of frequency, the areas of nodal involvement are the groin (including femoral and inguinal nodes), axilla, and neck.[38] Any lymph node may suppurate, sometimes presenting an atypical picture (e.g., if intra-abdominal nodes are involved, an acute abdominal emergency may be suspected).[39] Septicemia as an initial presentation of *Y. pestis* infection is not rare.[20] Twenty-five per cent of the 71 confirmed cases of plague in New Mexico from 1980 to 1984 presented without adenopathy. All patients with septicemic presentation had fever and chills, and most had tachycardia, tachypnea, and relative hypotension. Seventy-two per cent had gastrointestinal symptoms. Plague pneumonia was twice as likely among septicemic than among bubonic plague patients. Septicemic patients were significantly older and more likely to die than were patients with a bubonic presentation. Although septicemic plague occurred more often in older patients, those younger than 30 years of age with septicemic presentation were more likely to die.[20]

As a result of its nonspecific presentation, septicemic plague is difficult to diagnose early. Of 27 patients with plague admitted to Indian Medical Center in Gallup, New Mexico, between 1965 and 1989, 5 presented with a nonspecific febrile syndrome with upper respiratory symptoms. They were prescribed penicillin. Three of the five patients died. Another five patients presented with a nonspecific febrile syndrome associated with chills, myalgias, and anorexia. These patients were not treated initially with antibiotics, and three of the five died.[14] The index of suspicion, therefore, must be high because early diagnosis is imperative for avoiding a high mortality rate. Persons presenting with what appears to be community-acquired, gram-negative sepsis and who reside in or have a history of recent travel to endemic areas of plague must be evaluated for and treated with antibiotics effective against *Y. pestis*.[31]

Gastrointestinal symptoms occur in patients with plague, especially those with septicemic plague.[19] Between 1980 and 1984, more than half of the 71 patients with plague reported in New Mexico presented with gastrointestinal symptoms that sometimes preceded the appearance of the buboes in the bubonic cases. Common symptoms are abdominal pain, nausea, vomiting, and diarrhea. These symptoms are thought to be a general response of the body to gram-negative septicemia. On occasion, hepatosplenomegaly and mesenteric or retroperitoneal lymphadenopathy have masqueraded as an acute abdomen.[21, 26]

Neurologic manifestations due to the effects of toxin on the brain are common. The patient with plague may suffer from insomnia, delirium, stupor, weakness, staggering gait, vertigo, disorders of speech, and loss of memory.[38] *Y. pestis* meningitis is relatively rare, but it does occur. Children younger than 15 years of age seem to be more susceptible, and septicemic patients are four times more likely to develop it than are patients with bubonic plague. It often manifests itself while the patient is well into a course of antibiotic therapy for bubonic or septicemic plague.[2] When intravascular coagulation supervenes, renal involvement may manifest itself by acute cortical or tubular necrosis. Hepatic involvement may be evidenced by mildly elevated liver enzymes.[38]

Primary pneumonic plague has identical constitutional symptoms but follows a fulminant course with a more pronounced pulmonary component. Within 20 to 24 hours after the onset of the illness, tachypnea, dyspnea, and cough productive of bloody mucopurulent sputum supervene. If early and effective treatment is not instituted, the patient usually dies.[38]

DIFFERENTIAL DIAGNOSIS

Because of the rarity of plague today, the diagnosis often is delayed or missed. Bubonic plague may be confused with other diseases affecting the skin and lymph nodes. The diagnosis of staphylococcal or streptococcal adenitis can be established easily by culture. Lymphogranuloma venereum is more indolent, has milder systemic symptoms, and is associated with anogenital ulcer. Syphilitic adenitis usually is nontender. With cat-scratch disease and *Pasteurella multocida* infections, the constitutional symptoms are few and there is a typical history of animal exposure. Tularemia has a more gradual onset.[39] In their later stages, the ulcerated skin lesions of plague may resemble anthrax.[25]

The buboes of plague are exquisitely tender. Bacterial staining of lymph node material by Gram, Wayson, or Wright stain often shows the typical bipolar plague organisms. In the septicemic form of the disease, similar bacterial staining of venous blood frequently permits visualization of the plague bacillus.[28] Fluorescent antibody staining of direct smears and tissues may provide a rapid, presumptive diagnosis of plague.[44]

TREATMENT

In all cases of plague, the definitive diagnosis can be made only by culture of *Y. pestis* from an infected tissue or body fluid. Therapeutic decisions, however, cannot await culture results, and all patients suspected of having plague should receive prompt antimicrobial therapy after appropriate blood and tissue have been obtained for cultures, fluorescent antibody staining, and serologic testing.

The sulfonamides and streptomycin proved effective when first introduced in the 1940s. Resistant strains to one or the other of these antibiotics soon appeared.[4, 40] In areas in which streptomycin-resistant *Y. pestis* is found, chloramphenicol is given concurrently to critically ill patients.[25]

The Centers for Disease Control and Prevention[7] recommends treatment of suspected cases of plague. Patients who do not require hospitalization should receive tetracycline or chloramphenicol after appropriate cultures are obtained. Tetracycline should be given to patients older than 8 years of age at a dose of 25 to 50 mg/kg/day every 4 to 6 hours up to a total daily dose of 1 g in children and 2 g in adults. When outpatient treatment is given, the patient should be followed closely for the first 3 days so that resolution of the disease is ensured.[11]

For acutely ill patients suspected of plague infection, streptomycin is the drug of choice. (At the time of this writing, it is available in the United States only through Pfizer Laboratories Compassionate Use Program. It may be obtained by calling 1-800-254-4445 or faxing 1-800-251-4445.) Streptomycin should be given intramuscularly in the dosage of 20 to 30 mg/kg/day in two divided doses.[30] Other intravenous antibiotics that may be useful in the presence of hypotension are kanamycin 15 mg/kg/day in three divided doses up to a maximum adult dose of 1.5 g/day and gentamicin 7.5 mg/kg/day in children and 3 to 5 mg/kg/day in adults in three divided doses. When plague meningitis develops, chloramphenicol 50 to 100 mg/kg/day intravenously in four divided doses is the treatment of choice. The duration of therapy should be determined by the length and severity of the illness. Treatment should be continued for at least 7 days in patients with uncomplicated disease.[11]

PROGNOSIS

In outbreaks of untreated plague, the mortality rate has ranged between 40 and 70 per cent. Pneumonic plague almost invariably is fatal without treatment. With prompt specific antimicrobial therapy, the overall mortality rate for plague has dropped to 5 per cent.[27] Complications during convalescence include polyarthritis, small lung abscesses, delayed suppuration of buboes,[25] and meningitis. *Staphylococcus aureus* and *Pseudomonas* species may superinfect involved lymph nodes.[39] Immunity usually ensues after clinical or asymptomatic infection, but natural reinfection rarely has been observed.[39]

PREVENTION AND CONTROL

Hygienic measures and eradication of rats from areas of human habitations have all but eliminated epidemics of urban plague. When epizootics occur in wild rodents, control measures must be directed against rodents and fleas. Vector control can be achieved by the use of insecticides in fields and housing areas. Rodent control must be carried out by poisoning, trapping, and fumigation of burrows.[44] In plague-endemic areas, the public must be instructed to avoid burrows, not to handle sick or dead rodents, to deflea household pets, and to eliminate trash near living areas.[8] The immune status of domestic animals can be used as a surveillance tool to ascertain the presence of *Y. pestis* in the community. Dogs, cats, and swine develop antibodies to the fraction 1 antigen of *Y. pestis*.[33, 42]

Plague victims should be isolated with respiratory precautions until they are bacteriologically sterile. Contacts of pneumonic plague victims should receive chemoprophylaxis with tetracycline at 25 to 50 mg/kg/day up to 2 g in adults and up to 1 g in children and streptomycin 20 mg/kg/day in two divided doses if younger than 8 years of age. Trimethoprim-sulfamethoxazole at 40 mg/kg/day (sulfamethoxazole) in two equal doses orally also has been used. The 6-day quarantine period for international travel for contacts of patients with plague does not guarantee the clearance of the bacillus from asymptomatic pharyngeal carriers.[4] Public and professional education in endemic zones is of paramount importance for ensuring prompt reporting of human and animal cases.

Plague vaccines have been used since the late 19th century. Although not fully effective, they decrease the prevalence and severity of the disease. The plague vaccine licensed in the United States consists of formaldehyde-inactivated *Y. pestis* preserved in 0.5 per cent phenol. The Centers for Disease Control and Prevention[10] recommends plague vaccine for (1) laboratory and field personnel regularly working with *Y. pestis* or plague-infected rodents and (2) workers who reside in or visit areas of enzootic or epidemic plague where avoidance of rodents or fleas is impossible.

Primary vaccination of adults and children 11 years of age or older consists of three doses of vaccine. A first dose of 1.0 mL is followed by a second dose of 0.2 mL 4 weeks later and a third dose of 0.2 mL 6 months after the first dose. Three booster doses follow at 6-month intervals. Additional doses are given at 1- to 2-year intervals. No vaccine trials have tested the safety and efficacy of the vaccine in children younger than 11 years of age. Present recommendations are as follows: children younger than 1 year of age receive one-fifth the adult dose; 1 to 4 years of age, two-fifths the adult dose; and 5 to 10 years of age, three-fifths the adult dose, following the same time schedule.

Vaccinated persons who definitely are exposed to plague should receive chemoprophylaxis because the vaccine may not be completely protective, even in the presence of high antibody levels.[10]

References

1. Albizo, J. M., and Surgalla, M. J.: Isolation and characterization of *Pasteurella pestis* endotoxin. Infect. Immun. *2*:229–236, 1970.
2. Becker, T. M., Poland, J. D., Quan, T. J., et al.: Plague meningitis: A retrospective analysis of cases reported in the United States, 1970–1979. West. J. Med. *147*:554–557, 1987.
3. Butler, T.: A clinical study of bubonic plague. Am. J. Med. *53*:268–276, 1972.
4. Cantey, J. R.: Plague in Vietnam. Arch. Intern. Med. *133*:280–283, 1974.
5. Cavanaugh, D. C.: Specific effect of temperature upon transmission of the plague bacillus by the Oriental rat flea, *Xenopsylla cheopsis*. Am. J. Trop. Med. Hyg. 20:264–273, 1971.
6. Centers for Disease Control: Plague: United States, 1976. M. M. W. R. *28*:159, 1977.
7. Centers for Disease Control: Plague in the United States, 1982. M. M. W. R. *32*:19SS–24SS, 1983.
8. Centers for Disease Control: Plague: Human plague in the United States, 1983. M. M. W. R. *32*:329–330, 1983.
9. Centers for Disease Control: Plague: Winter plague—Colorado, Washington, Texas, 1983–1984. M. M. W. R. *33*:145–148, 1984.
10. Centers for Disease Control: Plague vaccine. M. M. W. R. *31*:301–303, 1982.
11. Centers for Disease Control and Prevention: Plague Treatment Guidelines. Bacteriologic Zoonoses Branch, Division of Vector-Borne Infectious Diseases, Fort Collins, CO, 80522.
12. Centers for Disease Control and Prevention: Human plague: United States, 1993–1994. M. M. W. R. *43*:242–246, 1994.
13. Chen, T. H., and Elberg, S. S.: *Yersinia, Pasteurella*, and *Francisella*. *In* Braude, A. I., Davis, C. E., and Fierer, J. (eds.): Medical Microbiology and Infectious Diseases. Philadelphia, W. B. Saunders, 1981, pp. 393–399.
14. Crook, D., and Tempest, B.: Plague: A review of 27 cases. Arch. Intern. Med. *152*:1253–1256, 1992.
15. Eidson, M., Tierney, L., Rollag, O. J., et al.: Feline plague in New Mexico: Risk factors and transmission to humans. Am. J. Public Health *78*:1333–1335, 1988.
16. Finegold, M. J.: Pathogenesis of plague. Am. J. Med. *45*:549–555, 1968.
17. Ganem, D. E.: Plasmids and pestilence: Biological and clinical aspects of bubonic plague. West. J. Med. *144*:447–451, 1986.
18. Goldenberg, M. I., and Kartman, L.: Role of soil in the ecology of *Pasteurella pestis*. Bacteriol. Proc. *66*:54–57, 1966.
19. Hull, H. F., Montes, J. M., and Mann, J. M.: Plague masquerading as gastrointestinal illness. West. J. Med. *145*:485–487, 1986.
20. Hull, H. F., Montes, J. M., and Mann, J. M.: Septicemic plague in New Mexico. J. Infect. Dis. *155*:113–118, 1987.
21. Humphrey, M., McGiuney, R., Perkins, C., et al.: *Yersinia pestis:* A case of mistaken identity. Pediatr. Infect. Dis. J. *7*:365–366, 1988.
22. Janssen, W. A., and Surgalla, M. J.: Plague bacillus: Survival within host phagocytes. Science *163*:950–952, 1969.
23. Kartman, L., Goldenberg, M. I., and Hubbert, W. T.: Recent observations on the epidemiology of plague in the United States. Am. J. Public Health *56*:1554–1569, 1966.
24. Kaufmann, A. F., Boyce, J. M., and Martone, W. J.: Trends in human plague in the United States. J. Infect. Dis. *141*:522–524, 1980.
25. Legters, L. J., Cottingham, A. J., and Hunter, D. H.: Clinical and epidemiologic notes on a defined outbreak of plague in Vietnam. Am. J. Trop. Med. Hyg. *19*:639–652, 1970.

26. Leopold, J. C.: Septicemic plague in a 14-month old. Pediatr. Infect. Dis. J. *5*:108–110, 1986.
27. Maegraith, B. G.: Plague. *In* Adams, A. R., and Maegraith, B. G. (eds.): Clinical Tropical Diseases. Oxford, Blackwell Scientific, 1970, pp. 325–336.
28. Mann, J. M., Hull, H. F., Schmid, G. P., et al.: Plague and the peripheral smear. J. A. M. A. *251*:953, 1984.
29. Mann, J. M., Martone, W. J., Boyce, J. M., et al.: Endemic human plague in New Mexico: Risk factors associated with infection. J. Infect. Dis. *140*:397–401, 1979.
30. Mann, J. M., Schaudler, L., and Cushing, A.: Pediatric plague. Pediatrics *69*:762–767, 1982.
31. Mann, J. M., Schmid, G. P., Stoesz, P. A., et al.: Peripatetic plague. J. A. M. A. *247*:47–48, 1982.
32. Marshall, J. D., Guy, D. V., and Gibson, F. L.: Asymptomatic pharyngeal plague infection in Vietnam. Am. J. Trop. Med. Hyg. *16*:175–177, 1967.
33. Marshall, J. D., Harrison, D. N., Murr, J. A., et al.: The role of domestic animals in the epidemiology of plague. III. Experimental infection in swine. J. Infect. Dis. *125*:556–559, 1972.
34. Martin, A. R., Hurtado, F. P., Plessak, R. A., et al.: Plague meningitis. Pediatrics *40*:610–616, 1967.
35. McNeill, W. H. (ed.): Plagues and People. Garden City, NY, Anchor Press of Doubleday, 1976.
36. Mollaret, H. H., and Thal, E.: *Yersinia*. *In* Buchanan, R. E., and Gibbons, N. E. (eds.): Bergey's Manual of Determinative Bacteriology. 8th ed. Baltimore, Williams & Wilkins, 1974, pp. 330–332.
37. Plague, Historical Notes. Can. Med. Assoc. J. *119*:10, 1978.
38. Pollitzer, R.: Plague. W. H. O. Monogr. No. 22. Geneva, 1954.
39. Reed, W. P., Palmer, D. L., Williams, R. C., et al.: Bubonic plague in the southwestern United States. Medicine (Baltimore) *49*:465–486, 1970.
40. Reiley, C. G., and Kates, E. D.: The clinical spectrum of plague in Vietnam. Arch. Intern. Med. *126*:990–994, 1970.
41. Rust, J. H., Jr., Cavanaugh, D. C., Kadis, S., et al.: Plague toxin: Its effect in vitro and in vivo. Science *142*:408–409, 1963.
42. Rust, J. H., Cavanaugh, D. C., O'Shita, R., et al.: The role of domestic animals in the epidemiology of plague. I. Experimental infection of dogs and cats. J. Infect. Dis. *124*:522–526, 1971.
43. Sonnenwirth, A. C.: *Yersinia*. *In* Lennette, E. H., Spaulding, E. H., and Trauant, J. P. (eds.): Manual of Clinical Microbiology. 2nd ed. Washington, D. C., American Society for Microbiology, 1974, pp. 222–229.
44. Tirador, D. F., Miller, B. E., Stacy, J. W., et al.: An emergency program to control plague. Public Health Rep. *82*:1094–1099, 1967.
45. Walker, R. V., Bomes, M. G., and Thiggins, E. D.: Composition of and physiopathology produced by plague endotoxins. Nature *209*:1246, 1966.
46. World Health Organization: Weekly Epidemiological Record, *69*:5–12, 1994.

117

OTHER *YERSINIA* SPECIES

Charles R. Woods

Yersinia are gram-negative, coccobacillary organisms that primarily are zoonotic. The genus is a member of the family Enterobacteriaceae and consists of 11 species, 3 of which clearly are human pathogens[49]: *Y. pestis*, *Y. pseudotuberculosis* (both formerly included in the genus *Pasteurella*), and *Y. enterocolitica*. *Y. pestis*, the causative agent of plague, is found in rodents and insect vectors and is discussed in Chapter 116. *Y. enterocolitica* and *Y. pseudotuberculosis* are responsible for a variety of syndromes, some of which originally were called pseudotuberculosis. Infections caused by the nonpestis *Yersinia* now collectively are called yersiniosis, which is the focus of this chapter.

During the past three decades, *Y. enterocolitica* has become recognized as an important human pathogen worldwide and has emerged as the second or third most common cause of gastroenteritis in some pediatric populations of the industrialized world.[33, 39, 87] It also has drawn attention because of its immunologic or postinfectious manifestations, which include reactive arthritis and erythema nodosum.[33] *Y. pseudotuberculosis*, although widespread in nature, is a much less common cause of human disease.[49]

HISTORICAL ASPECTS

In 1883, Mallasez and Vignal[96] described a bacterium that produced a disease that they named pseudotuberculosis. When injected into guinea pigs, the organism produced tuberculosis-like lesions. It grew at 4° C and multiplied better at 22° C than at 37° C. This observation was confirmed in 1910 by Albrecht,[5] who labeled the disease enteritis follicularis suppurativa. The first case of mesenteric adenitis, the most common syndrome produced by *Y. pseudotuberculosis*, was reported in 1913 by Saisawa.[128] A second instance of disease that indicated its capacity to produce death (bacteremia and multiple hepatic abscesses) was recorded in 1949 by Hassig and colleagues.[55] Masshoff[98] was the first to recover the organism from a culture of mesenteric lymph nodes of a patient with the clinical picture of acute appendicitis. Masshoff and Dolle[99] subsequently described the histologic picture produced by *Y. pseudotuberculosis*. In 1954, Knapp and Masshoff[80] first reported the clinical features of infection produced by this organism. Only 14 cases of this infection had been described up to that time.[38]

The existence of a species of *Yersinia* other than that causing pseudotuberculosis was suggested in 1933 by Gilbert,[44] who reported an unusual infection in animals. Schleitstein and Coleman[129, 130] examined a number of organisms isolated between 1933 and 1957 from stool cultures of human cases of diarrhea from which *Salmonella* and *Shigella* could not be recovered and that resembled the infections in animals reported by Gilbert. They identified an organism that had not been described previously and named it *Bacterium enterocoliticum*. It later was named *Y. enterocolitica* by Frederiksen.[42]

The genus is named for A. J. Yersin, the French bacteriologist who first isolated the plague bacillus.[139] Over the past 40 years, an extensive literature detailing the microbiology, pathology, epidemiology, molecular pathogenesis, and clinical features of disease caused by *Y. pseudotuberculosis* and *Y. enterocolitica* has been developed.[7, 15, 16, 33, 38, 57, 58, 63, 68, 77–80, 87, 92, 109, 124, 136, 138, 139, 150]

MICROBIOLOGY

Yersinia organisms are relatively large (0.5 to 1.0 by 1 to 2 μm or larger), gram-negative, ovoid or rod-shaped organisms. Both *Y. enterocolitica* and *Y. pseudotuberculosis* are motile at 22° to 25° C but not at 37° C. Like other members of Enterobacteriaceae, *Yersinia* organisms are facultative anaerobes and grow well on ordinary media. On Gram staining, *Y. pseudotuberculosis* appears as a large coccobacillus. Staining with methylene blue and carbol fuchsin discloses a bipolar ("safety pin") morphology of most but not all strains.

Y. enterocolitica is somewhat smaller and shows little, if any, bipolarity.[136, 139]

Yersinia organisms may be confused with coliforms such as *Escherichia coli*, *Morganella*, *Proteus*, *Shigella*, *Salmonella*, or *Providencia* or with *Y. pestis*, *Brucella*, and *Achromobacter*, unless careful biochemical and physiologic studies are conducted. *Yersinia* reduce nitrates and are oxidase-negative, catalase-positive, urease-positive, and citrate-negative. They ferment glucose, maltose, mannitol, glycerol, xylose, and fructose, producing acid but no gas with each sugar. *Yersinia* organisms usually do not ferment lactose but produce alpha-D-galactosidase. They do not ferment dulcitol, inositol, raffinose, and rhamnose. On lysine iron agar slants, *Yersinia* organisms produce an alkaline slant with an acid butt. They do not produce hydrogen sulfide. The Voges-Proskauer reaction is negative at 37° C but may be positive at 25° C for some strains of *Y. enterocolitica*. All strains of *Y. pseudotuberculosis* and most strains of *Y. enterocolitica* isolated in Europe are indole-negative. Most strains of *Y. enterocolitica* found in the United States have been indole-positive.[35, 48, 65, 107, 109, 136, 139]

Although these two species of *Yersinia* share many properties, they are distinguishable on the basis of several biochemical activities, antigenic structure, and sensitivity to various *Yersinia* phages.[125] *Y. enterocolitica* produces an acid slant and acid butt on triple-sugar iron agar due to fermentation of sucrose, whereas *Y. pseudotuberculosis* produces an alkaline slant and an acid butt.[139] *Y. enterocolitica* elaborates ornithine decarboxylase and ferments sucrose and amygdalin. *Y. pseudotuberculosis* does none of these, but ferments adonitol, which *Y. enterocolitica* does not.[65, 139]

Typing of *Yersinia* Strains

Biotyping and serotyping have been the predominant methods used to characterize strains of *Y. enterocolitica*. At least 54 serotypes of *Y. enterocolitica* exist on the basis of variability of somatic O antigens.[16, 39, 49, 148] Five biotypes of *Y. enterocolitica* have been defined based on biochemical properties.[24, 146] Four can be distinguished by the presence or absence of lecithinase activity, indole production, lactose oxidation, and xylose fermentation. Strains of the fifth biotype produce negative reactions for these tests and do not reduce nitrates, ferment trehalose, or exhibit ornithine decarboxylase or beta-galactosidase activities, as do the majority of *Y. enterocolitica* strains.

Tests for pyrazinamidase activity, esculin hydrolysis, and salicin fermentation have been used as means to distinguish pathogenic from nonpathogenic strains. Pathogenic strains, which carry virulence plasmids, generally do not express these activities, whereas nonpathogenic strains do.[30, 37, 73]

Strains of *Y. enterocolitica* can be typed genetically by repetitive element-based (interrepeat) polymerase chain reaction (PCR) and arbitrarily primed PCR techniques[108] and by pulsed-field gel electrophoresis.[105] These methods allow distinction between strains within biotypes and serotypes and may be useful for outbreak and other epidemiologic investigations.

At least 11 antigenic groups of *Y. pseudotuberculosis* exist on the basis of variation of somatic O antigens. These have been labeled 1a, 1b, 2a, 2b, 2c, 3, 4a, 4b, 5a, 5b, and 6.[60, 67, 95] Type 2 is related antigenically to *Salmonella* group B and type 4 to *Salmonella* groups D and H.[48] *Y. pseudotuberculosis* strains also can be typed by arbitrarily primed PCR.[95]

EPIDEMIOLOGY

Although most of the early reports of yersiniosis caused by *Y. pseudotuberculosis* and *Y. enterocolitica* emanated from northern Europe, the presence of these microbes has been identified with increasing frequency in all parts of the world,[6] with the possible exception of South America.

Yersinia enterocolitica

Y. enterocolitica is distributed worldwide but is isolated most frequently in cooler climates.[103] It is unclear whether such geographic differences reflect differences in reservoirs or culinary practices that may enhance the risk of acquisition of this organism or rather represent differences in surveillance for the disease and use of more sensitive culturing techniques in these areas.[33] Increased frequency of infections during fall and winter months has been reported from Europe,[143] but no seasonality is evident among outbreaks of disease where more than three cases of *Y. enterocolitica* disease have been identified.[33]

Geographic differences in serotype distribution and frequency also exist. Sporadic infections due to serotypes O:3 and O:9 are common in Europe,[3, 61] but outbreaks have been rare.[33] In North America, multiple serotypes have been responsible for sporadic disease,[11, 14, 24, 75, 132, 134] but serotype O:3 more recently has become predominant.[24, 36, 87] Five outbreaks in the United States have been caused by serotype O:8 and two in Canada by serotypes O:5 and O:5,27.[33] Disease caused by serotype O:8 has been reported in Europe.[61]

The true incidence and prevalence of *Y. enterocolitica* infection are not known.[33] The reported proportional frequency of isolation of *Y. enterocolitica* from stool cultures from patients with diarrhea has ranged from 0 to 3.2 per cent in series from Europe, the United States, and New Zealand (Table 117–1).[34, 39, 61, 87, 97, 101, 132] Symptomatic infection is more common in children. Most series demonstrate a slight male predominance of about 1.3:1.[36, 39, 97, 146]

Animals and water sources are the primary environmental reservoirs for *Y. enterocolitica*, but the biotypes and serotypes of the strains found in them usually differ from those causing human disease.[24, 33, 132] Blood transfusions also may be a source of *Y. enterocolitica* infection.[25]

Animal Reservoirs

Y. enterocolitica strains have been isolated from a wide variety of mammals (dogs, pigs, sheep, rabbits, guinea pigs, cows, horses, chinchillas, monkeys),[65, 92] frogs, fish, flies, fleas, snails, crabs, and oysters.[33] Birds do not appear to be a major reservoir for *Y. enterocolitica*,[65] although avian isolates have been reported.[33]

Pigs appear to be an important reservoir for the human pathogenic serotypes O:3 and O:9 in Europe and Japan and serotype O:3 in North America and South Africa.[33, 87, 117] The biochemical and phage typing profiles of isolates from pigs are similar to those of strains commonly responsible for human infections.[150] *Y. enterocolitica* has been isolated from the tongue, tonsils, and cecal contents of swine and from pork, ham, and butchershop cutting boards.[33, 48] In Belgium, the country with the highest numbers of cases of yersiniosis in the world, ingestion of raw pork is common: a case-control study demonstrated that infection caused by serotypes O:3 and O:9 was associated highly with ingestion of raw pork during the 2 weeks preceding the illness.[143] Pig farmers in Finland have relative risks of 3.0 and 2.4 for seropositivity to serotypes O:3 and O:9, respectively, compared with berry farmers.[131]

Wild rodents captured in areas of Japan where human infections caused by *Y. enterocolitica* serotype O:8 had occurred were shown to harbor isolates of the same serotype.[32]

TABLE 117–1. Percentage of Stool Cultures Yielding *Yersinia enterocolitica*

Country	Year(s)	Population	Total Cultures	Per Cent *Y. enterocolitica*
Canada[97]	1977–1978	Symptomatic children	6364	2.8
The Netherlands[61]	1982–1984	Enteritis patients <40 years of age	827	2.9
Italy[101]	1981–1985	Children with diarrhea	2500	1.4[a]
New Zealand[39]	1988–1993	Patients with gastroenteritis	231,128	0.6
United States (Detroit, MI)[34]	May–November 1977	Children with diarrhea	1262	0
United States (New York State)[132]	1976–1980	Survey of cultures from a state laboratory, six hospitals, and several day care centers	2487	0.9[b]
United States[c] (7 cities)[87]	November 1989–January 1990	All stool cultures submitted to seven hospitals	4841	0.8

[a]Yearly percentages over the 5 years ranged from 0 to 4.4 per cent.
[b]This increased to 4.0 per cent of 3035 isolates when cultures from an outbreak and other screenings were included.
[c]Includes Detroit, MI.

Two distinct serotype O:8 strains, defined by restriction enzyme analysis of the virulence plasmids, were isolated from both humans and rodents. This suggests that rodents are a potential source of sporadic human infection in Japan.

Apparent transmission to humans from dogs and cats also has been reported. A fecal-oral or oral-oral route has been postulated but not confirmed. There is little evidence to support airborne or insect vector-borne transmission.[33]

Water and Foods

Ingestion of water contaminated with serotype O:8 has led to sporadic cases and outbreaks.[33] Bean sprouts that had been immersed in contaminated water were the source of an outbreak among members of a Brownie troop in Pennsylvania in 1982. Ingestion of tofu (bean curd) packed in untreated spring water that subsequently was found to be contaminated with *Y. enterocolitica* caused 44 cases of symptomatic infection in Washington state in 1981 and 1982.[142] Serotypes commonly found in water samples, however, rarely are isolated from humans with symptomatic disease.[24]

Contaminated milk has been implicated as the source of several large outbreaks of *Y. enterocolitica* infection.[12, 33, 148] Whipped cream and ice cream may harbor the organism. Contamination of milk products after pasteurization has been documented.[33] *Y. enterocolitica* has been found in raw milk samples from cows and goats.[48] Samples of beef, lamb, poultry, oysters, and a variety of vegetables also have been found to be contaminated with *Y. enterocolitica*.[22, 33]

Serotypes O:3; O:4,33; O:5,27; O:7,8; O:8; O:10; O:13; and O:16 cause the majority of human disease in North America but rarely are isolated in surveillance of water or food samples.[24, 132, 148] Serotype O:8 strains have been cultured from cattle, milk, and water samples[132]; serotype O:4,33 strains have been isolated from pigs and cattle[132]; and serotype O:4,32 strains have been found in cheese, ham, sausage, raw beef, and one pancake specimen.[24]

Incubation, Carriage, and Transmission in Humans

The incubation period of *Y. enterocolitica* enterocolitis ranges from 1 to 14 days.[33, 87] The minimal infective dose of *Y. enterocolitica* is not known. Ingestion of 3.5×10^9 organisms by a volunteer resulted in diarrhea in less than a day, but such large inocula are unlikely to be encountered clinically. The duration of excretion of the organism after infection in children ranges from 14 to 97 days (mean, 42 days).[97] The impact, if any, of antibiotic treatment on the duration of carriage is not known.

Transmission to household members is uncommon, even among young children, who appear to be at higher risk for development of symptomatic disease.[12, 97, 142] Six per cent of household contacts developed disease in one outbreak,[142] but several large outbreaks with no secondary household cases have been reported.[33]

Yersinia enterocolitica *and Blood Transfusion–Related Sepsis*

Sporadic cases of *Y. enterocolitica* sepsis related to contamination of red blood cell transfusions have been recognized since 1987 and have occurred in the United States, Europe, and Australia.[25] *Y. enterocolitica* is the most common cause of transfusion-related sepsis.[72] Among 20 cases from the United States, chills occurred in 16, fever in 14, hypotension in 13, and disseminated intravascular coagulation in 7.[31] Death attributable to *Y. enterocolitica* infection occurred in 12, and half of these occurred within 25 hours of receipt of the contaminated transfusion. Among the 20 donors, 13 had had gastrointestinal symptoms within the month before blood donation and 16 had titers ≥1:128 (considered positive).

In many cases of transfusion-related sepsis, the contaminated red blood cell units had been stored for 25 days or more.[56] After experimental inoculation of small numbers of *Y. enterocolitica* into packed cells kept at 4° C, the organisms continue to replicate, reaching concentrations of 100 colony-forming units (cfu)/mL in 7 days and 10^6 cfu/mL in 21 days. High levels of endotoxin can result from such replication and have been documented in samples from red blood cell units that led to transfusion-related sepsis.[31]

Human Outbreaks

Outbreaks of *Y. enterocolitica* disease have involved communities, families (with interfamily spread), hospitals, and schools. The sources of the organism have been various foods and animals, especially dogs. A review of these outbreaks demonstrates that *Y. enterocolitica* readily is communicable and that infection may be more common than has been recognized. Yersiniosis also resembles disease caused by *Salmonella* and *Shigella* in many respects, including environmental sources of the organisms, the clinical syndromes, and the occurrence of asymptomatic infection.

OUTBREAKS IN SCHOOLS AND COMMUNITIES. A community outbreak due to a serotype O:8 strain occurred in New York State in 1976.[12] At least 222 children and employees had a yersiniosis-like illness during a 10-week period. An epidemiologic investigation showed that illness was associated with drinking chocolate milk purchased in school cafeterias. Thirty-six children were hospitalized, 16 of whom had appendectomies. The milk apparently was contaminated after pasteurization during hand mixing of the milk with chocolate syrup. Transmission of infection from ill children to household contacts was not observed.

School-related outbreaks also have occurred in Japan.[8, 159] In one school, 182 children were affected, and most had abdominal pain and fever.[8] *Y. enterocolitica* was cultured from 48 of 113 stool specimens (42 per cent). Of 993 children and 49 adults at risk at another school, 542 (52.6 per cent) developed enteritis. *Y. enterocolitica* was recovered from the stools of 75 per cent of the cases. The duration of the disease was as short as 12 to 18 hours in some cases. In a third school outbreak of diarrhea, fever, and abdominal pain, *Y. enterocolitica* serotype O:3 was recovered from the stools of 122 patients and 17 asymptomatic individuals.[159]

In the summer of 1982, it was estimated that several thousand persons in several southern states who consumed milk from a single dairy developed yersiniosis. A total of 172 culture-positive infections were confirmed, many as a result of hospitalization for illness. Seventeen patients underwent appendectomy; 24 others suffered extraintestinal spread of infection. The strain involved was designated serotype O:13a,13b.[148]

FAMILY EPIDEMICS. Twenty-one persons were involved in an outbreak of yersiniosis involving four families in North Carolina in which there was an unusually high attack rate and a poor response to antimicrobial therapy.[50] Eighteen were children who ranged in age from 3 to 13 years; 16 of the 21 had diarrhea and fever, and 5 were asymptomatic. *Y. enterocolitica* was recovered from the spleen of the youngest child at autopsy. The diagnosis was established serologically in the other patients. A dog that had given birth to nine puppies, five of which had died of a diarrheal illness a week before the families became ill, appeared to be the source of the infection.

NOSOCOMIAL OUTBREAKS. A young child who was hospitalized in Finland with acute gastroenteritis was the source case of infection in a housekeeping worker and four nurses who cared for her.[145] The infecting strain was serotype O:9. Another hospital outbreak involved nine patients in Canada.[119] This was caused by a serotype O:5 strain. Person-to-person contact was considered the likely mode of transmission.

Prevention of Disease

During outbreaks, efforts should be made to identify both environmental sources and vehicles of transmission.[33] A single environmental source can harbor multiple serotypes of *Y. enterocolitica*, such that resulting outbreaks may be polyclonal in nature.[142] Enteric precautions should be used for hospitalized patients with diarrhea caused by *Y. enterocolitica* (as with other causes of gastroenteritis).[33] At the population level, decreased consumption of raw or undercooked pork products potentially could reduce the incidence of infection.[143]

Yersinia pseudotuberculosis

Y. pseudotuberculosis may infect individuals of all ages, but at least 75 per cent of patients with clinically apparent disease are children younger than 15 years of age.[67, 125] Infection in young infants has been reported.[67, 154] Of 130 cases diagnosed in Great Britain from 1959 to 1970, boys were involved three times more frequently than girls.[92] Infections occur more commonly during the cold months of the year.[67, 125] The seasonal winter peak of human infection produced by *Y. pseudotuberculosis* is similar to that seen in wild and domesticated animals.[77, 78, 125]

The attack rates for children living in rural and urban areas appear to be the same.[125] *Y. pseudotuberculosis* occasionally has been recovered from healthy persons. Exposure to the organism appears to be uncommon; antibody to *Y. pseudotuberculosis* was detected in only 1 of 2000 sera from individuals with no history of yersiniosis.[42]

Y. pseudotuberculosis is distributed worldwide in a large variety of animals and birds, but infection is uncommon.[45] Guinea pigs, rodents, and rabbits most often are infected[92] and may suffer a plague-like illness.[45, 65] Lesions in guinea pigs easily may be confused with those caused by *Y. pestis*. Rats and other rodents also may have plague-like disease caused by *Y. pseudotuberculosis*. Infection has been reported in a variety of domestic animals (cattle, sheep, goats, cats, dogs, hamsters), commercially raised fur bearers (chinchillas, mink, coypu), and other wild or captive animals (rabbits, raccoons, foxes, deer, beavers, monkeys, puma, kangaroos). *Y. pseudotuberculosis* has been found in more than 50 species of birds,[54, 74, 92] and epizootics have occurred among turkeys, ducks, pigeons, and doves and in aviaries of canaries and finches.[92, 125] Strains obtained from animals and birds in the United States predominantly are of serotypes 1a, 1b, and 3.[65]

The incubation period for human disease may be as short as 41 hours or as long as 20 days.[67] The organism can survive in fresh tap water for 46 days at room temperature and for 8 months at 4° C. It can survive at 4° C in meat for up to 145 days and in milk and bread for 2 to 3 weeks.[92]

A family outbreak of mesenteric adenitis caused by *Y. pseudotuberculosis* that involved four siblings ages 7, 9, 12, and 14 years has been reported.[118] A pet dog was shown to have rising antibody titers at the time the children were ill.

Three outbreaks in Japan have been described.[67] Eating sandwiches prepared by a single bakery at an athletic event was the primary risk factor for 67 cases that occurred in a 3-week period. Two additional outbreaks occurred in small villages where the only risk factor appeared to be drinking unchlorinated well water or mountain stream water. Samples of the water sources yielded isolates of the same serotypes causing disease. Two or more serotypes were present in each village outbreak. Children were much more likely to have clinical disease than adults.

PATHOLOGY

The diseases produced by *Y. enterocolitica* and *Y. pseudotuberculosis* are similar and share the histopathologic theme of involvement of the lymphoid tissues of the intestinal mucosa and mesentery.

Yersinia enterocolitica

Y. enterocolitica infection predominantly affects the gastrointestinal tract. The most severe clinical symptoms correlate with an acute terminal ileitis. The mucosal surface of the ileum and other involved sites may be inflamed diffusely.

Ulcerations may occur throughout the gastrointestinal tract and may be small and superficial or extend to the muscularis propria. Mucosal and submucosal hyperplasia of the Peyer patches occurs with scattered micbroabscess formation.

Ulcers occur primarily over the sites of lymphoid tissue within the mucosa. This accounts for their more longitudinal appearance in the small intestine and an oval or punctate appearance in the stomach and colon. Ulcerations are characterized by necrosis of the epithelial layer. In the colon, the necrosis also may extend through the superficial third of the crypts. Large colonic ulcerations covered by pseudomembranes or mucoid debris are seen occasionally. Ulcerations may progress to perforation with subsequent peritonitis or gastrointestinal hemorrhage in severe cases.[19, 46, 149, 150]

The inflammatory response in the mucosa consists mainly of neutrophils and mononuclear cells. Lymphocytes and plasma cells also may be seen. Giant cells are not seen, although a granulomatous appearance can be imparted by the presence of plump epithelioid histiocytes.[46, 149, 150]

The appendix usually appears normal on gross inspection, but small focal ulcerations frequently are present.[1] Large areas of necrosis are found occasionally, and acute, suppurative appendicitis has been reported.[19, 71, 97] Periappendicular inflammation may result from a true appendicitis or an adjacent terminal ileitis.[150]

Mesenteric adenitis, the hallmark of infection by *Y. pseudotuberculosis*, also is a common feature of enterocolitis caused by *Y. enterocolitica*. The lymph nodes usually show numerous large pyroninophilic cells and mitotic figures in the cortical area and marginal sinuses. Small collections of leukocytes in the germinal centers are seen in some cases and suggest microabscess formation. In severe cases, extensive areas of necrosis circumscribed by a neutrophilic infiltrate may be seen. The sinusoids can become filled with neutrophils and mononuclear cells. The germinal centers often appear reactive.

The necrotizing epitheloid granulomas that may be present in the mesenteric adenitis caused by *Y. pseudotuberculosis* have not been described in *Y. enterocolitica* infection. The histopathologic appearance of the mesenteric adenitis of *Y. enterocolitica* infection can resemble the adenitides caused by cat-scratch disease *(Bartonella henselae)*, toxoplasmosis, infectious mononucleosis, and *Y. pseudotuberculosis*.[1, 150, 155]

Numerous colonies of gram-negative bacteria often can be seen beneath the mucosal ulcerations and within the microabscesses that occur in the lymphoid tissues.[46]

Yersinia pseudotuberculosis

A number of reports collectively have described the pathology of infection caused by *Y. pseudotuberculosis*.[35, 38, 40, 63, 78, 91, 98, 99, 104, 118, 153] Grossly enlarged, soft, and inflamed mesenteric lymph nodes are the predominant finding on laparotomy. These frequently are located at the ileocecal angle. Punctate hemorrhages and small, yellow microabscesses may be present on the surfaces of the nodes at the height of infection. The appendix usually appears normal, but the terminal ileum and cecum occasionally appear inflamed. A necrotic purulent mass sometimes is seen in the mesentery.

Histopathologic findings in the mesenteric lymph nodes include enlarged follicles and small abscesses; hyperplasia of reticulum cells; necrosis of the nodes with infiltrates of neutrophilic leukocytes and plasma cells; and, in some instances, punctate hemorrhages. Scattered clusters of neutrophils may be seen within the sinusoids and germinal centers without abscess formation or necrosis. Atypical mononuclear cells, some of which may be mitotic, may be present in the sinusoids. When necrosis is absent, large numbers of eosinophilic leukocytes sometimes are seen surrounding reticulogranulocytic infiltrates in the nodes. Giant cells can occur and may cause the histologic picture to be confused with tuberculosis.

The mesenteric adenitis produced by *Y. pseudotuberculosis* appears to progress through four histopathologic stages[35, 51]: stage 1—infiltration of reticulocytes alone; stage 2—reticulogranulocytic infiltration with formation of abscesses, stage 3—retinogranulocytic infiltration with the development of abscesses, and stage 4—organization of the infiltrates with clearing of the abscesses. The inflammatory process of *Y. pseudotuberculosis* appears to remain confined to the lymph nodes without rupture through the nodal capsule.

Focal mucosal ulcerations may be seen in the ileum and are more likely to be found at the site of Peyer patches. Aggregates of neutrophilic leukocytes similar to those in mesenteric nodes may be seen in germinal centers within mucosal lymphoid tissue. Fibrinoid material may be a prominent feature at these sites. Small areas of necrosis surrounded by reticulum cells and leukocytes also may be present in the submucosal follicles.[40, 78, 98, 153] Ulcerated lymphoid follicles in the intestinal wall are connected to the regional lymph nodes by a lymphangitis. This anatomic situation is analagous to the primary complex of tuberculosis.

Despite a clinical picture of acute appendicitis as the presenting feature of infection by *Y. pseudotuberculosis*, the appendix typically is grossly and microscopically normal. Inflammatory changes, when present, usually are in the form of a periappendicitis. Phlegmonous appendicitis can result from *Y. pseudotuberculosis* infection but is rare.[35, 60]

PATHOGENESIS

The pathogenesis of infection by *Y. enterocolitica* has been well studied. After reaching the intestinal tract, *Y. enterocolitica* penetrate into the lamina propria by passing through the cytoplasm of mucosal epithelial cells. While within the epithelial cells, the bacteria are enclosed in membrane-limited vesicles. After reaching the lamina propria, the microbes multiply in lymph follicles and Peyer patches. Neutrophils and macrophages infiltrate these sites in response to the infection, but *Y. enterocolitica* is able to resist intracellular killing by macrophages and phagocytosis by neutrophils. The microbes then drain to the mesenteric lymph nodes. Infection usually is contained at this point, but systemic spread occurs occasionally and is more common with infection by serotype O:8 strains.[32] Infection by *Y. enterocolitica* induces a T-cell response that appears to play a protective role in restriction of bacterial growth in infected organs through cytokine-mediated activation of macrophages and stimulation of production of *Yersinia*-specific antibody.

Only a few of the many serotypes of *Yersinia* are capable of infecting humans. A number of virulence factors have been identified among these "pathogenic" strains. Much of this knowledge has been gained through mouse and rabbit models of human infection and observations of interactions of *Yersinia* with in vitro cell culture models.[18, 32, 58, 93, 115]

Virulence Plasmid

Pathogenic strains of *Y. enterocolitica* harbor a plasmid that consists of ~70 kb (denoted pYV) and encodes for outer-membrane proteins (designated Yops), secreted proteins, regulatory proteins, and proteins that function as a secretion machinery. Transcription of plasmid proteins is governed by environmental signals such as temperature and calcium concentration. A related plasmid is harbored in *Y. pseudotuberculosis* and *Y. pestis*. At least 16 proteins are encoded by pYV, among which at least 5 are located on the outer membrane.[32]

The Yop designated *Yersinia* adhesin A (YadA) is a putative multifunctional virulence factor of *Y. enterocolitica*. YadA is about 50 kDa and likely forms tetrameric fibrillae on the microbial surface. It can bind to extracellular matrix proteins, such as collagen, and mediate adhesion to cells. YadA also inhibits the terminal complement attack complex (this inhibition accounts for resistance to killing by serum), enables the microbe to resist phagocytosis by neutrophils, and contributes to the ability of *Y. enterocolitica* to resist killing by antimicrobial polypeptides of human granulocytes. YadA knock-out mutants are far less virulent in mice than the parent wild-type strain.[58, 152]

Functions of other Yops also have been characterized partially. YopM is able to bind to thrombin and von Willebrand factor and may be able to inhibit thrombin-induced platelet aggregation. YopH is a tyrosine phosphatase that may play a role in cytotoxicity and phagocytosis resistance. Other Yops function as calcium sensors, cytotoxins, and protein kinases.[58]

Pathogenic strains of *Y. enterocolitica* require calcium concentrations equivalent to those of serum and extracellular fluids in humans for growth at body temperature. Plasmid proteins, however, are synthesized maximally at 37° C under conditions of low calcium concentrations, such as those found intracellularly. These regulatory effects of environmental calcium concentration may permit free growth of *Yersinia* during extracellular life and production of factors protective against the host immune system after ingestion by granulocytes.[32, 58]

Plasmid-encoded factors are required for survival and extracellular multiplication after reaching the Peyer patches. Plasmid-cured derivatives are ingested rapidly and killed by neutrophils in the Peyer patches, whereas the virulent parent strain is able to proliferate and spread through the lamina propria to adjacent villi. Plasmid-encoded factors are not required for *Y. enterocolitica* to penetrate the intestinal mucosa.[58]

Mucosal Invasion

Two outer-membrane proteins encoded by chromosomal genes permit entry into a variety of mammalian cell types in vitro and likely are responsible for the ability of *Yersinia* to invade into and through the intestinal mucosal epithelium. These have have been named invasin and the attachment invasin locus protein (Ail). All isolates of *Y. enterocolitica* that are virulent in humans contain DNA sequences that encode for invasin and Ail. Nonpathogenic strains do not contain the genetic code for Ail, but most contain invasin genes that can not be expressed due to chromosomal rearrangements. These proteins appear unique to the genus *Yersinia*.[68, 100, 112]

Invasin attaches to receptors in the beta-1 integrin family and induces an actin-mediated endocytosis of the microbe. Invasin is expressed maximally at ambient temperatures when the organism is in stationary phase. *Y. enterocolitica* microbes living in the environment likely exist in a stationary phase-like state and thus may be primed maximally for host invasion after ingestion. Invasin expression also can remain elevated at 37° C when the pH is 5.5, and such conditions are encountered during passage through the intestinal tract. Ail is expressed maximally at 37° C, functions both as an adhesin and an invasion factor, and plays a role in the resistance of *Y. enterocolitica* to the bactericidal activity of human serum.[68, 69, 112]

American versus European Strains

There also are differences in virulence properties among the human pathogenic serotypes. Serotypes O:8; O:4,32; O:13; O:18; O:20; and O:21 (historically considered the "American" strains) are mouse-virulent after intraperitoneal injection and are able to evoke a keratoconjunctivitis after inoculation into the conjunctival sac of guinea pigs (the positive Sereny test). Oral infection in mice produces predominantly the features of mesenteric adenitis and systemic infection rather than simple gastroenteritis. This picture is characteristic of human infection by American strains.

The "European" serotypes, O:3; O:9; and O:5,27, yield a negative Sereny test and cause mild diarrhea but not death in mice. These virulence differences are chromosomally rather than plasmid-mediated and may be the result of differences in iron metabolism among serotypes (vide infra).[32, 58, 100]

Enterotoxin Production

All enteropathogenic strains of *Y. enterocolitica* produce a heat-stable enterotoxin that closely resembles the heat-stable toxin of *E. coli*. Both enterotoxins induce increases in cyclic guanylic acid levels in intestinal epithelial cells. The *Y. enterocolitica* enterotoxin is not plasmid-encoded, and its presence does not correlate with the expression of other virulence phenotypes.[58] Because the enterotoxin is not produced in vitro at temperatures exceeding 30° C, it was believed that production in the gastrointestinal tract, and thus a causative role in diarrhea, was unlikely.[33] However, observations in the young rabbit oral infection model have shown that enterotoxin-negative mutants did not induce diarrhea and the wild-type strain did. This suggests that the enterotoxin indeed may cause the diarrhea frequently associated with *Y. enterocolitica* infection in children.[58, 111]

Iron Metabolism

Iron is an essential growth factor for most bacteria, many of which release siderophores (high-affinity chelators) that bind ferric iron and then are reuptaken via receptors by the microbe. The European serotypes of *Y. enterocolitica* do not produce siderophores but are able to use those synthesized by other organisms. The American serotype O:8 strains synthesize a chromosomally encoded siderophore that sits on the outer membrane of the bacterium. The presence of this siderophore decreases the environmental iron concentration required for optimal growth and likely accounts for the increased virulence observed for serotype O:8 strains.[33, 58]

The increased availability of ferric iron that exists in iron-overload states such as hemachromatosis and diseases such as thalassemia that require frequent red blood cell transfusions facilitates survival and growth of *Y. enterocolitica*. Deferoxamine, a *Streptomyces*-derived siderophore used clinically to treat iron-overload states, also can be used by *Y. enterocolitica* as an iron source. Thus, iron overloading and deferoxamine are independent risk factors for systemic disease after intestinal infection with *Y. enterocolitica*.[33]

Gastric Acidity

Although *Y. enterocolitica* is able to grow under conditions at pH 5.0 to 9.0, optimal growth occurs at pH 7.0 to 8.0.

Gastric acidity thus may play a protective role against some *Yersinia* inocula. Therapeutic agents or clinical conditions that result in reduced reduced gastric acidity therefore may predispose patients to infection. *Y. enterocolitica* bacteremia has been reported after gastrectomy.[33]

CLINICAL MANIFESTATIONS

Clinical disease caused by *Y. enterocolitica* occurs far more frequently than that caused by *Y. pseudotuberculosis*.[39, 88, 89] Historically, diarrheal illness has been considered the hallmark of *Y. enterocolitica* and the pseudoappendicular syndrome of mesenteric adenitis indicative of *Y. pseudotuberculosis*. However, each species can cause enterocolitis and/or mesenteric adenitis. A variety of other clinical infections and postinfection syndromes also are caused by these microbes. In series of patients presenting with acute abdominal pain suggestive of appendicitis, the incidence of serologic evidence of *Yersinia* infection has ranged from 7 to 31 per cent.[9]

Yersinia enterocolitica

The clinical features of the disease caused by *Y. enterocolitica*, primarily an acute enteritis, have been described by a number of investigators.[10, 27, 33, 36, 53, 83, 86, 87, 93, 94, 97, 119, 122, 146] The clinical manifestations depend to a degree on the age and physiologic condition of the host.[33, 97, 118] Enterocolitis is the most common presentation and occurs most often in young children. The pseudoappendicular syndrome, which results primarily from mesenteric adenitis and mimics acute appendicitis, is more common in older children and young adults.[12, 33, 62, 71, 106, 122] Asymptomatic infection can occur, but the relative frequency compared with symptomatic disease is unknown. The predominant clinical features of *Y. enterocolitica* infection in children are summarized in Table 117–2.

Enterocolitis

Y. enterocolitica enterocolitis is characterized by diarrhea and abdominal pain. The diarrhea usually usually persists for 7 to 14 days.[87, 97, 150] A range of 1 to 46 days of diarrhea has been reported.[97] Up to 10 per cent of cases may persist for 30 days or more,[12] and chronic diarrhea persisting for several months has been described.[36]

During the first week of symptoms, 3 to 10 stools per day are common, with a gradual decrease in frequency thereafter. Stools typically are greenish, exhibit variable consistency (usually watery or mucoid), and are not remarkably malodorous. Gross blood is noted in about one quarter of patients. Vomiting occurs in 38 per cent of cases. Nausea is common. The abdominal pain can be colicky, diffuse, or localized to the right lower quadrant or epigastrium. Fever is common and usually of low grade but may exceed 40° C; it usually resolves within a week.[94]

Most cases are self-limited, but some children require hospitalization. Among 14 children hospitalized in the United States in a case series from 1989 and 1990, the median number of hospital days required was 3.5 (range, 2 to 12 days).[87]

Fecal leukocytes are present commonly but not universally. The peripheral white blood cell count may range from 5600 to more than 30,000. Mean values of 12,400 and 18,800 have been reported. Infants frequently exhibit an immature:total neutrophil ratio greater than 0.5.[87, 94]

Radiologic examination using upper gastrointestinal barium studies in 24 adult patients with severe diarrhea caused by *Y. enterocolitica* showed abnormalities of the terminal ilium in 21 cases.[149] Diffuse thickening of the mucosal folds was seen in 16 and nodular filling defects in 11. The radiographic appearance suggested the presence of one or more ulcerations of the terminal ileum in 11 patients. Dilation of the terminal ileum was noted in 12 patients, and extrinsic compression, presumably from enlarged lymph nodes, was present in 4. In some instances, the findings were suggestive of the terminal ileitis of Crohn disease. Follow-up studies 2 months after acute illness showed decreased but persistent thickening of mucosal folds in eight patients. Barium enemas were performed in 15 patients and showed no striking abnormalities other than mucosal ulcerations, which were seen best on air-contrast studies.[150]

Colonoscopy and/or sigmoidoscopy was performed in 13 adults with severe diarrhea caused by *Y. enterocolitica*.[149] Abnormalities were seen in eight: the mucosa appeared diffusely swollen, erythematous, and friable in six; two had only small, 1- to 2-mm aphthoid ulcerations. Serial procedures showed both macroscopic and microscopic healing of ulcers within 4 to 5 weeks.

Pseudoappendicitis–Mesenteric Adenitis

The syndrome of pseudoappendicitis, characterized in most cases by a normal appendix and an intense suppurative mesenteric adenitis, has attracted considerable attention since it first was reported in 1953.[98, 99] The first recognized cases were caused by *Y. pseudotuberculosis*, but the majority of cases

TABLE 117–2. Clinical Features of *Yersinia enterocolitica* Infection in Children

	Sweden[10] 1967–1973	Canada[36] 1972	Finland[94] 1974–1978	Canada[97] 1977–1978	United States[87] 1989–1990	Combined Totals
N	31	35	40	57	37[a]	200
Age ≤ 5 years	28	26	19	NS[b, c]	28+	101+/143 (≥71%)
Fever (>38° C)	15	6	36	39	35	92/200 (66%)
Diarrhea	31	26	32	56	37	126/200 (91%)
Grossly bloody	2	NS	7	NS	14	23/108 (21%)
Abdominal pain	4	6	20	31/48	NS	61/154 (40%)
Vomiting	NS	12	12	22	18	64/169 (38%)
Rash[d]	NS	2	2	NS	NS	4/75 (5.3%)
Appendectomy	0	0	4	1	0	5/200 (2.5%)
Serotype O:3	31	NS	34	57	34	156/165 (94%)

[a]All were black children; seven different cities, 3-month period.
[b]NS = not specified.
[c]More than half of these children were younger than 2 years of age.
[d]Maculopapular rash or urticaria.

reported in recent years have been caused by *Y. enterocolitica*.[20, 70, 86]

Fever, abdominal pain, right lower quadrant tenderness, and leukocytosis are the primary features of *Y. entercolitica*–induced pseudoappendicular syndrome.[33, 71] Some patients also will have features of enterocolitis: nausea, vomiting, and diarrhea. The clinical presentation often is highly suggestive of acute appendicitis, such that laparotomy is required. Among a series of 581 patients in Scandinavia who underwent laparotomy for suspected appendicitis, 3.8 per cent of cultures of stool or operative specimens yielded *Y. enterocolitica*.[106] Another 284 patients with similar symptoms were observed, and 5.6 per cent of stool cultures from these cases yielded *Y. enterocolitica*. In a similar Scandinavian series of 205 patients who underwent appendectomy, 22 subsequently were diagnosed as having *Y. enterocolitica* infection by serology.[71] The findings on laparotomy usually are mesenteric lymphadenitis, terminal ileitis, and a normal or slightly inflamed appendix.[12, 33, 71, 106]

Asymptomatic Infection

In an unknown number of cases, infection by *Y. enterocolitica* entirely is asymptomatic. In a study of the distribution of antibodies to *Y. enterocolitica* in sera collected for various purposes from 4209 persons who had no evidence of infection by this organism, specific antibody was present in 199 (serotype O:3 in 158 and serotype O:9 in 41).[146]

Other Presentations of Acute Infection

Y. enterocolitica may cause focal infections in many extraintestinal sites, even in the absence of detectable bacteremia. Bacteremia can occur[23, 28, 33, 102] and may result in spread of infection to virtually any body site. Such events are uncommon and are seen more often in adults than in children. Bacteremias may be transient and asymptomatic or lead to septic shock and death. Septic cases tend to occur in patients with underlying illnesses and are associated with mortality rates of 34 to 50 per cent.[33]

Pharyngitis has been reported and occurs primarily in adults. Cervical adenopathy may be associated with *Y. enterocolitica* pharyngitis, and gastrointestinal symptoms may be absent.[33] One adult with pharyngitis died of associated septic shock.[123] Conjunctivitis and panophthalmitis due to *Y. enterocolitica* have been described. Parinaud oculoglandular syndome,[29] inguinal adenopathy,[154] and suppurative lymphadenitis[147] have been reported.

Cellulitis, soft tissue abscesses, and wound infections have been reported. Cellulitis may have associated vesiculobullous lesions. An erysipelas-like rash, maculopapular rash, and urticaria also have been described in association with *Y. enterocolitica* infection.[10, 20, 33, 52, 84, 142, 157]

Pancreatitis, cholecystitis, diverticulitis, and intestinal perforation have been described.[89, 116] Peritonitis also has occurred but is extremely rare, especially considering the frequency of mesenteric adenitis. Pneumonia, pleural empyema, lung abscess, hepatic and splenic abscesses, urinary tract infection, and renal abscess have been reported.[33] Cases of meningitis, osteomyelitis, septic arthritis, pyomyositis (including psoas muscle abscess), endocarditis, mycotic aneurysm, and intravenous catheter–related infection due to *Y. enterocolitica* have been described.[21, 33, 59, 137, 139] Thrombocytopenia[47] and hemolytic anemia[81] have occurred in association with *Y. enterocolitica* infection.

Underlying Conditions That Predispose to Bacteremia

Y. enterocolitica bacteremias occur most often in patients with chronic illnesses or iron-overload states. Thalassemias are the most common such conditions in children.[27, 41, 76] Among 144 Italian children with thalassemia who were receiving deferoxamine therapy and frequent blood transfusions, 14 developed *Y. enterocolitica* infection during a 12-month period.[27] Septicemia occurred in 5 of the 14 and was preceded by enterocolitis or mesenteric adenitis in each case. All 14 recovered after 2 weeks of therapy with intravenous trimethoprim-sulfamethoxazole.

Hemachromatosis, cirrhosis, and other liver diseases may facilitate *Y. enterocolitica* bacteremia, also on the basis of excess availability of serum iron. Deferoxamine therapy itself is a risk factor for *Y. enterocolitica* sepsis because of the ability of the microbe to extract iron from this compound. Immunosuppressive therapies, diabetes mellitus, and malnutrition also may predispose to *Y. enterocolitica* bacteremia.[33]

Postinfectious Syndromes

A reactive arthritis may occur 1 to 14 (usually 4 to 10) days after the cessation of acute illness.[1, 2, 4, 6, 59, 62, 122, 144, 149, 158] Most such events occur in adults with a slight female predominance, but 8 of 74 cases in one series from Sweden were in children 11 to 20 years of age (5 males, 3 females).[158] In a series from the Netherlands, 10 per cent of children with yersiniosis developed arthritis.[62] Most were 7 years of age or older. The knees, ankles, and wrists most commonly are affected, and in about half of cases, only one or two joints are involved. Hands, fingers, toes, shoulders, hips, and elbows also may be involved. Pain usually is severe, and the arthritis is additive and usually not migratory. The inflammatory process is self-limited and may persist for 2 months or more in two-thirds of cases, with one-third persisting for 4 months or longer.

Erythema nodosum also occurs as a postinfectious manifestation and is more common in adults than children. It can occur alone or in association with arthritis.[62] Tendinitis, myositis, myocarditis, urethritis, uveitis, and conjunctivitis also can occur in association with arthritis. Many but not all patients who develop these postinfectious reactions are HLA-B27–positive.[1] Some patients manifest the full Reiter syndrome.[62, 82, 126, 135]

The erythrocyte sedimentation rate exceeds 60 mm/hour in about half of cases. Joint effusions usually are inflammatory, but cell counts and differentials are variable and occasionally mimic septic arthritis. Immune complexes have been found in joint fluid. Nonsteroidal anti-inflammatory agents and corticosteroids, both intra-articular and systemically administered, have been used for symptomatic relief for this process.[121]

Yersinia antigens but not intact bacteria have been found in synovial tissue obtained several weeks to months after onset of reactive arthritis. *Y. enterocolitica* is able to survive within in vitro cultures of human synovial cells for up to 6 weeks with resultant deposition of residual antigen aggregates within the cells.[66] T-cell clones from HLA-B27–positive patients who developed *Y. enterocolitica*–induced reactive arthritis are able to recognize a region of the plasmid-encoded tyrosine phoshatase YopH that is highly homologous to the catalytic domain of eukaryotic protein tyrosine phosphatases.[85] The urease beta subunit of *Y. enterocolitica* also has been identified as a potential target antigen in the induction of a reactive arthritis.[114] Epitopes on *Yersinia*-produced proteins thus may be able to trigger cross-reactive immunologic recognition of host proteins that leads to chronic inflammation in susceptible persons.[85]

Antibodies against *Y. enterocolitica* have been detected in patients with disorders of the thyroid, including Graves disease, thyroid adenoma, and Hashimoto thyroiditis.[133] Antibodies induced in mice by two low-molecular-weight outer-membrane proteins cross-react with the thyrotropin receptor.[90] These observations may reflect autoantibodies that cross-react with *Yersinia* epitopes rather than a causal link between yersiniosis and thyroid disease.[33, 120]

Brachial plexus neuropathy and transverse myelitis have been described in one patient each after the resolution of gastrointestinal symptoms caused by *Y. enterocolitica*.[140]

A variety of chronic ailments have been described among a group of 160 Scandinavian patients followed for 4 to 14 years after acute yersiniosis.[127] These included persistent joint complaints, ankylosing spondylitis (in HLA-B27–positive patients), iridocyclitis, chronic hepatitis, chronic abdominal pain, rheumatoid arthritis, chronic nephritis, thyroid disease, and neurologic ailments. Observed deaths among these patients exceeded the expected number. These findings require confirmation before causal links can be considered, however.

Yersinia pseudotuberculosis

The pseudoappendicular syndrome that results from mesenteric adenitis is the primary disease produced by *Y. pseudotuberculosis*.[13, 35, 38, 40, 48, 60, 64, 77, 78, 91, 109, 124, 125, 151, 153] The chief complaint is abdominal pain, either diffuse or localized to the right lower quadrant. Fever of varying degree (38° to 40° C) almost always is present. There usually is tenderness over the McBurney point. All of these are highly suggestive of acute appendicitis. Diarrhea may occur but often is absent. Mild leukocytosis occurs, but white blood cell counts usually are less than 20,000/mm^3. The clinical course almost always is benign, with recovery usually beginning about the fifth day of illness. On laparotomy, the appendix is normal in most cases but occasionally appears inflamed or suppurative. The mesenteric lymph nodes are enlarged and may appear necrotic.

Efforts have been made to distinguish the pseudoappendicular syndrome caused by *Y. pseudotuberculosis* from that due to *Y. enterocolitica*.[15, 48] *Y. pseudotuberculosis* adenitis is less likely to have associated enterocolitis and may have a shorter febrile course, but no clear distinction can be made on clinical grounds alone.

A fulminant typhoidal or septicemic form of *Y. pseudotuberculosis* infection can occur but appears to affect primarily older adults with debilitating conditions, such as diabetes or liver disease. This syndrome often is fatal.[78, 125] Isolated cervical adenitis and terminal ileitis have been described.[153] Subacute and recurrent disease can occur.[91] Hepatic abscess,[55] erythema nodosum,[125] and nonsuppurative arthritis[26] also have been reported in association with *Y. pseudotuberculosis* infection.

In Korea and Japan, *Y. pseudotuberculosis* strains have been responsible for a clinical syndrome mimicking Kawasaki disease.[26] This manifestation of disease occurs primarily in outbreaks and may be accompanied by acute interstitial nephritis. It also has been described as scarlet fever–like.[109]

DIFFERENTIAL DIAGNOSIS

The differential diagnosis of yersinial enterocolitis includes both viral and other bacterial causes of acute gastroenteritis. When the symptoms of mesenteric adenitis are predominant and severe, appendicitis and other causes of an acute abdomen must be considered. The acute terminal ileitis caused by *Yersinia* infections also can be similar to the gastrointestinal manifestations of Crohn disease, ulcerative colitis, cat-scratch disease, anisakiasis, amebiasis, actinomycosis, typhoid fever, and lymphoma.[46, 62, 109, 150, 153]

DIAGNOSIS

The most effective approach to the diagnosis of yersiniosis is isolation of the organism from the stool of patients with enteritis caused by *Y. enterocolitica* or from the infected mesenteric lymph nodes of those infected by *Y. pseudotuberculosis*. *Y. enterocolitica* occasionally can be recovered from involved mesenteric lymph nodes or the distal ileum.[33] Cultures of feces from individuals with acute suppurative mesenteric adenitis usually fail to grow either organism.

Isolation of *Yersinia* from extraintestinal specimens such as lymph nodes and blood is not difficult, because these grow on ordinary media (e.g., blood agar) and several selective and differential media employed for enteric bacteria. Isolation from fecal specimens, however, is more difficult because *Yersinia* multiply more slowly than other enteric bacteria at 37° C and have no characteristic colonial morphology. Selective media have been developed, but many clinical laboratories culture stool specimens for *Yersinia* species only on request due to the costs of these media and the relatively low frequencies of these pathogens in the community.

Strains of *Y. enterocolitica* grow well on MacConkey agar but are much smaller than those of other enteric bacteria after standard incubation at 37° C. Cefsulodin-irgasan-novobiocin agar plates have been designed specifically for the isolation of *Yersinia* species from stool specimens. After incubation for 48 hours, *Yersinia* colonies appear dark pink with translucent borders and occasionally are surrounded by a zone of precipitated bile. Cefsulodin-irgasan-novobiocin agar inhibits the growth of most other bacteria, except for *Citrobacter* species (whose positive citrate reactions allow their distinction). If a dedicated medium for *Yersinia* isolation is not used, MacConkey agar can be examined after 24 hours at 35° to 37° C for small colorless colonies that become much larger after an additional 24 hours of incubation at room temperature. The majority of *Y. enterocolitica* strains are lactose-negative.[49]

Y. enterocolitica strains grow faster at 37° C than at room temperature. However, growth occurs readily at 22° to 28° C, and these lower temperatures are recommended for primary isolation.[49] Because of the abilitiy of *Yersinia* to grow at even colder temperatures, specimens can be inoculated into phosphate-buffered saline, refrigerated at 4° to 6° C, and subcultured periodically (up to 4 weeks) if the routine plates that were inoculated with the specimen remain negative. Such "cold enrichment" greatly enhances the isolation rate of *Yersinia* species and may be the most reliable method for isolating these organisms from fecal specimens. However, many of the *Yersinia* isolates recovered by cold enrichment represent either *Y. enterocolitica* serotypes that usually are not associated with human disease or other *Yersinia* species whose role as pathogens is unclear.

In the laboratory, the presence of a non–lactose-fermenting gram-negative rod that is oxidase-negative, hydrogen sulfide–negative on triple-sugar iron agar, urease-positive but phenylalanine-negative, and motile only at room temperature should raise suspicion for a *Yersinia*. *Yersinia* can be differentiated readily from *Salmonella* because the latter are motile at 37° C, urease-negative, citrate-positive, and lysine-positive. Most *Salmonella* strains also produce gas during fermentation and produce hydrogen sulfide. *Shigella* are urease-negative and lack motility at room temperature.[139]

Pathologic or virulent strains of *Y. enterocolitica* can be distinguished in most instances from nonpathogenic strains by three biochemical tests that are associated with absence of the virulence plasmid. The virulent strains lack pyrazinamidase activity, do no ferment salicin, and do not hydrolyze esculin. On Congo red-magnesium oxalate agar during incubation at 36° C, fresh pathologic isolates (but not those that have been subcultured serially) grow as small red colonies, demonstrating the virulence plasmid–determined properties of Congo red dye uptake and calcium-dependent growth.[37]

Serology

Serology can be performed using microtiter techniques and is most reliable for serotypes O:3 and O:9 of *Y. enterocolitica*.[17, 150] Antibody to the infecting serotype usually is absent at the onset of disease. Peak titers usually are reached 3 to 4 weeks after onset of clinical illness and fall over the next 3 to 5 months. Low postconvalescent titers may persist for months.[150] Microhemagglutination, complement fixation, and enzyme immunoassays are available in a few commercial laboratories.[49]

Agglutinin titers 1:128 or higher for *Y. entercolitica* in previously normal healthy individuals are suggestive of infection.[17] Titers of 1:200 or higher were present within 3 weeks of onset of illness in 62 of 65 Canadian children who suffered infection with serotype O:3.[97] Fourfold rises in titer rarely were seen. Negative or minimal titers (1:32 or lower) do not rule out yersiniosis in infants or immunosuppressed patients. Serologic responses are more common and of higher titer in patients with extraintestinal systemic infection. Prozone reactions may occur at dilutions of 1:32 or lower. There is marked cross-agglutination between *Y. enterocolitica* serotype O:9 and *Brucella abortus*, *Morganella morganii*, and *Salmonella*.[17]

Antibodies to *Y. pseudotuberculosis* often are detectable at the onset of clinical signs of infection and may be highest during the acute phase of illness.[60]

Molecular Techniques

A nested PCR assay has been developed for *Y. pseudotuberculosis* and was able to identify the organism in blood and water samples.[26]

TREATMENT

Most patients with yersiniosis do not require treatment, because the disease usually is self-limited. Seriously ill patients generally have responded to treatment with chloramphenicol, gentamicin, or tetracyclines, but clinical success has not been uniform. Of these agents, tetracyclines have been the traditional agent of choice.[48, 150] However, *Y. enterocolitica* isolates resistant to the tetracyclines have been reported in recent years. Two per cent of a sample of *Y. enterocolitica* isolates from Canada in 1992 were resistant to tetracycline,[113] and 10 per cent of a sample of *Y. enterocolitica* isolates from the Netherlands from 1982 to 1991 were resistant to doxycycline.[141]

More than 99 per cent of 1060 isolates of *Y. enterocolitica* collected in Canada in the years 1972 to 1976, 1980, 1985, and 1990 were susceptible in vitro to piperacillin, cefotaxime, aztreonam, gentamicin, tobramycin, amikacin, trimethoprim-sulfamethoxazole, chloramphenicol, and ciprofloxacin.[113] There was no evidence of decreasing susceptibility to any of these agents across the periods that were sampled. These results were mirrored by a study of 335 isolates obtained in The Netherlands from 1982 to 1991.[141] All of these were susceptible to ceftazidime, cefepime, imipenem, trimethoprim-sulfamethoxazole, ciprofloxacin, and ofloxacin. Aminoglycosides were effective against more than 99 per cent, chloramphenicol against 94 per cent, and cefuroxime against 90 per cent. Seven multidrug-resistant isolates were present among the isolates from Canada,[113] but none were found among those from the Netherlands.[141]

The vast majority of *Y. enterocolitica* isolates, regardless of serotype, are resistant to ampicillin, ticarcillin, and first-generation cephalosporins.[113, 141] Most also are resistant to amoxicillin-clavulanic acid. Azithromycin was active in vitro against half of the 335 isolates in the Netherlands, but almost all isolates were resistant to erythromycin and clarithromycin.[141]

The decreasing in vitro effectiveness of tetracyclines raises the question of whether these agents should be the first choice for treatment of *Y. enterocolitica*. A retrospective review of 43 cases (with patient ages ranging from 3 to 89 years) treated for *Y. enterocolitica* septicemia in France between 1985 and 1991 showed that third-generation cephalosporins were effective in 85 per cent of cases in which these were used, although aminoglycosides or fluoroquinolones usually were administered concurrently.[43] Fluoroquinolones alone or in combination with other agents cured 15 of 15 patients.

In a double-blind, placebo-controlled trial of trimethoprim-sulfamethoxazole as treatment for children with gastroenteritis caused by *Y. enterocolitica*, the clinical course of illness was not shortened.[110] The children had been ill for a mean of 12 days before treatment was begun, however.

Systemic infections, extraintestinal focal infections, and enterocolitis in compromised hosts should be treated with antibiotics.[33] The in vitro susceptibilities and limited clinical data suggest that children with such infections should be treated with a third-generation cephalosporin and/or an aminoglycoside. Trimethoprim-sulfamethoxazole also may be used.[27, 62] Fluoroquinolones are not approved for use in children, but agents in this class may become available and appropriate for use against *Yersinia* infections in children in the future.

Even less clinical and in vitro susceptibility data are available for *Y. pseudotuberculosis*. These infections likely can be managed identically to *Y. enterocolitica*. All isolates of *Y. enterocolitica* and *Y. pseudotuberculosis* should be examined for susceptibiltiy to a variety of antibacterial drugs.

OTHER *YERSINIA* SPECIES

The other eight "nonpestis" *Yersinia* species (*Y. frederiksenii, Y. intermedia, Y. kristensenii, Y. aldovae, Y. bercovieri, Y. mollaretti, Y. rohdei*, and *Y. ruckeri*) occasionally have been isolated from clinical specimens, but their roles as human pathogens remain unclear.[49, 132] These organisms are similar biochemically to one another and have been termed atypical *Y. enterocolitica*.[33] None contain the *Yersinia* virulence plasmid.[100] These *Yersinia* species can grow at 4° C and on cefsulodin-irgasan-novobiocin agar and can multiply in refrigerated foods. Use of cold enrichment techniques may enhance recovery of these organisms. Their isolation from clinical specimens should not be disregarded or deemed causative of clinical disease without careful epidemiologic considerations.[49]

References

1. Ahlqvist, J., Ahvonen, P., Räsänen, J. A., et al.: Enteric infection with *Yersinia enterocolitica*: Large pyroninophilic cell reaction in mesenteric lymph nodes associated with early production of specific antibodies. Acta Pathol. Microbiol. Scand. *79A*:109–122, 1971.
2. Aho, K., Ahvonen, P., Lassus, A., et al.: HL-A 27 in reactive arthritis: A study of *Yersinia* arthritis and Reiter's disease. Arthritis Rheum. *17*:521–526, 1974.
3. Ahvonen P.: Human yersiniosis in Finland. 1. Bacteriology and serology. Ann. Clin. Res. *4*:30–38; 1972.
4. Ahvonen, P., Sievers, K., and Aho, K.: Arthritis associated with *Yersinia enterocolitica* infection. Acta Rheum. Scand. *15*:232–253, 1969.
5. Albrecht, H.: Zur aetiologie der enteritis follicularis suppurativa. Wien. Klin. Wochenschr. *23*:991, 1910.
6. Anonymous: Worldwide spread of infection with *Yersinia enterocolitica*. WHO Chron. *30*:494–496, 1976.
7. Arvastson, B., Damgaard, K., and Winblad, S.: Clinical symptoms of infection with *Yersinia enterocolitica*. Scand. J. Infect. Dis. *3*:37–40, 1971.
8. Asakawa, Y., Akahane, S., Kheata, N., et al.: Two community outbreaks of human infection with *Yersinia enterocolitica*. J. Hyg. (Camb.) *71*:715–723, 1973.
9. Attwood, S. E., Healy, K., Caffarkey, M. T., et al.: *Yersinia* infection and abdominal pain. Lancet *1*:529–533, 1987.
10. Bergstrand, C. G., and Winblad, S.: Clinical manifestations of infection with *Yersinia enterocolitica* in children. Acta Paediatr. Scand. *63*:875–877, 1974.
11. Bissett, M. L.: *Yersinia enterocolitica* isolates from humans in California, 1968–1975. J. Clin. Microbiol. *4*:137–144, 1976.
12. Black, R. E., Jackson, R. J., Tsai, T., et al.: Epidemic *Yersinia enterocolitica* infection due to contaminated chocolate milk. N. Engl. J. Med. *298*:76–79, 1978.
13. Blattner, R. J.: Acute mesenteric lymphadenitis. J. Pediatr. *74*:479–481, 1969.
14. Bottone, E. J.: Current trends of *Yersinia enterocolitica* isolates in the New York City area. J. Clin. Microbiol. 17:63–67, 1983.
15. Bottone, E. J., Chester, B., Malowany, M. S., et al.: Unusual *Yersinia enterocolitica* isolates not associated with mesenteric lymphadenitis. Appl. Microbiol. *27*:858–861, 1974.
16. Bottone, E. J.: *Yersinia enterocolitica*: A panoramic view of a charismatic microorganism. CRC Crit. Rev. Microbiol. *5*:211–241, 1977.
17. Bottone, E. J., and Sheehan, D. J.: *Yersinia enterocolitica*: Guidelines for serologic diagnosis of human infections. Rev. Infect. Dis. *5*:898–906, 1983.
18. Bovallius, A., and Nilsson, G.: Ingestion and survival of *Y. pseudotuberculosis* in HeLa cells. Can. J. Microbiol. *21*:1997–2007, 1975.
19. Bradford, W., Noce, P., and Gutman, L.: Pathologic features of enteric infection with *Yersinia enterocolitica*. Arch. Pathol. *98*:17–22, 1974.
20. Braunstein, H., Tucker, E. B., and Gibson, B. C.: Mesenteric lymphadenitis due to *Yersinia enterocolitica*: Report of a case. Am. J. Clin. Pathol. *55*:506–510, 1971.
21. Brennessel, D. J., Robbins, H., and Hindman, S.: Pyomyositis caused by *Yersinia enterocolitica*. J. Clin. Microbiol. *20*:293–294, 1984.
22. Brocklehurst, T. E., Zaman-Wong, C. H., and Lund, B. M.: A note on the microbiology of retail packs of prepared salad vegetables. J. Appl. Bacteriol. *63*:409–415, 1987.
23. Caplan, L. M.: *Yersinia enterocolitica* septicemia. Am. J. Clin. Pathol. *69*:189, 1978.
24. Caprioli, T., Drapeau, A. J., and Kasatiya, S.: *Yersinia enterocolitica*: Serotypes and biotypes isolated from humans and the environment in Quebec, Canada. J. Clin. Microbiol. *8*:7–11, 1978.
25. Centers for Disease Control: *Yersinia enterocolitica* bacteremia and endotoxin shock associated with red blood cell transfusions—United States, 1991. M. M. W. R. *40*:176–178, 1991.
26. Cheong, H. I., Park, H. W., Koo, J. W., et al.: Diagnosis of *Yersinia pseudotuberculosis* infection by polymerase chain reaction. Pediatr. Infect. Dis. J. 15:596–599, 1996.
27. Cherchi, G. B., Pacifico, L., Cossellu, S., et al.: Prospective study of *Yersinia enterocolitica* infection in thalassemic patients. Pediatr. Infect. Dis. J. *14*:579–584, 1995.
28. Chessum, B., Frengley, J. D., Fleck, D. G., et al.: Case of septicemia due to *Yersinia enterocolitica*. Br. Med. J. *3*:466, 1971.
29. Chin, G. N., and Noble, R. C.: Ocular involvement in *Yersinia enterocolitica* infections presenting as Parinaud's oculoglandular syndrome. Am. J. Ophthalmol. *83*:19–23, 1977.
30. Cimolai, N., Trombley, C., and Blair, G.: Implications of *Yersinia enterocolitica* biotyping. Arch. Dis. Child. *70*:19–21, 1994.
31. Cookson, S. T., Arduino, M. J., Aguero, S. M., et al.: *Yersinia enterocolitica*–contaminated red blood cells (RBCs): An emerging threat to blood safety. Abstracts of the 36th Interscience Conference on Antimicrobial Agents and Chemotherapy, New Orleans, LA, American Society for Microbiology, p. 237 (Abstract J99), 1996.
32. Cornelis, G., Laroche, Y., Balligand, et al.: *Yersinia enterocolitica*, a primary model for bacterial invasiveness. Rev. Infect. Dis. *9*:64–86, 1987.
33. Cover, T. L., and Aber, R. C.: *Yersinia enterocolitica*. N. Engl. J. Med. *321*:16–24, 1989.
34. Dajani, A., and Maurer, M.: Is *Yersinia enterocolitica* gastroenteritis a Canadian disease? J. Pediatr. *97*:165–166, 1980.
35. Daniels, J. J. H.: Enteric infections with *Pasteurella pseudotuberculosis*: An acute abdominal syndrome. J. Int. Coll. Surg. *38*:397–411, 1962.
36. Delorme, J., Laverdiere, M., Martineau, B., et al.: Yersiniosis in children. Can. Med. Assoc. J. *110*:281–284, 1974.
37. Farmer, J. J., III, Carter, G. P., Miller, V. L., et al.: Pyrazinamidase, CR-MOX agar, salicin fermentation-esculin hydrolysis, and D-xylose fermentation for identifying pathogenic serotypes of *Yersinia enterocolitica*. J. Clin. Microbiol. *30*:2589–2594, 1992.
38. Feldman, W. H., and Karlson, A. G.: Pseudotuberculosis. *In* Hull, T. (ed.): Diseases Transmitted from Animals to Man. 5th ed. Springfield, Charles C Thomas, 1963.
39. Fenwick, S. G., and McCarthy, M. D.: *Yersinia enterocolitica* is a common cause of gastroenteritis in Auckland. N.Z. Med. J. *108*:269–271, 1995.
40. Finlayson, N. B., and Fagundes, B.: *Pasteurella pseudotuberculosis* infection: Three cases in the United States. Am. J. Clin. Pathol. 55:24–29, 1971.
41. Fontani, C., Valeri M., and Pifferesi, M.: *Yersinia enterocolitica* septicemia in a girl with thalassemia major. Pediatr. Med. Clin. *10*:657–658, 1988.
42. Frederiksen, W.: Human pseudotuberculosis in Denmark. Symp. Series Immunobiol. Stand. *9*:137, 1968.
43. Gayraud, M., Scavizzi, M. R., Mollaret, H. H., et al.: Antibiotic treatment of *Yersinia enterocolitica* septicemia: A retrospective review of 43 cases. Clin. Infect. Dis. *17*:405–410, 1993.
44. Gilbert, R.: Interesting cases and unusual specimens. Annual Report of the Division of Laboratory Research. Albany, New York, New York State Department of Health, 1933, p. 57.
45. Gillespie, J. H., and Timoney, J. F.: Hagan and Bruner's Infectious Diseases of Domestic Animals. 7th ed. Ithaca, Comstock, 1981, pp. 96–97.
46. Gleason, T. H., and Patterson, S. D.: The pathology of *Yersinia enterocolitica* ileocolitis. Am. J. Surg. Pathol. *6*:347–355, 1982.
47. Glud, T. K., and Laursen, B.: *Yersinia enterocolitica* infection complicated by severe thrombocytopenia resistant to high-dose intravenous immunoglobulin. Acta Med. Scand. *217*:233–234, 1985.
48. Goodwin, C. S.: *Yersinia* infections including mesenteric adenitis, and gastrointestinal tuberculosis. *In* Goodwin, C. S. (ed.): Microbes and Infection of the Gut. Melbourne, Blackwell Scientific Publications, 1984, pp. 241–251.
49. Gray, L. D.: *Escherichia, Salmonella, Shigella*, and *Yersinia*. *In* Murray, P. R. (ed.): Manual of Clinical Microbiology. 6th ed. Washington, D.C., ASM Press, 1995, pp. 450–456.
50. Gutman, L. T., Ottesen, E. A., Quan, T. J., et al.: An inter-familial outbreak of *Yersinia enterocolitica* enteritis. N. Engl. J. Med. *288*:1372–1377, 1973.
51. Haenselt, V.: Zur kenntnis der abscedierenden reticulocytaren lymphadenitis (Masshoff). Arzt. Wochenschr. *12*:509, 1957.
52. Hagan, A. G., Lassen, J., and Berge, L. N.: Erysipelas-like disease caused by *Yersinia enterocolitica*. Scand. J. Infect. Dis. *6*:101–102, 1974.
53. Hallstrom, K., Sairanen, E., and Ohela, K.: A pilot clinical study of yersinioses in South-Eastern Finland. Acta Med. Scand. *191*:485–491, 1972.
54. Hamasaki, S., Hayashidani, H., Keneko, K., et al.: A survey for *Yersinia pseudotuberculosis* in migratory birds in coastal Japan. J. Wildl. Dis. *25*:401–403, 1989.
55. Hassig, A., Karrer, J., and Pusterla, F.: Über pseutuberculoses beim menschen. Schweiz. Med. Wochenschr. *79*:791, 1949.
56. Hastings, J. G. M., Batta, K., Gourevitch, D., et al.: Fatal transfusion reaction due to *Yersinia enterocolitica*. J. Hosp. Infect. *27*:75–79, 1993.
57. Hayashidani, H., Ohtomo, Y., Toyokawa, Y., et al.: Potential sources of sporadic human infection with *Yersinia enterocolitica* serovar O:8 in Aomori Prefecture, Japan. J. Clin. Microbiol. *33*:1253–1257, 1995.
58. Heesemann, J., Gaede, K., and Autenrieth, I. B.: Experimental *Yersinia enterocolitica* infection in rodents: A model for human yersiniosis. APMIS *101*:417–429, 1993.
59. Hewstone, A. S., and Davidson, G. P.: *Yersinia enterocolitica* septicaemia with arthritis in a thalassaemic child. Med. J. Aust. *1*:1035–1038, 1972.
60. Hnatko, S. I., and Rodin, A. E.: *Pasteurella pseudotuberculosis* infection in man. Can. Med. Assoc. J. *88*:1108–1112, 1963.
61. Hoogkamp-Korstanje, J. A. A., De Koning, J., and Samsom, J. P.: Incidence of human infection with *Yersinia enterocolitica* serotypes O3, O8, and O9 and the use of indirect immunofluorescence in diagnosis. J. Infect. Dis. 153:138-141, 1986.
62. Hoogkamp-Korstanje, J. A. A., and Stolk-Engelaar, V. M. M.: *Yersinia enterocolitica* infection in children. Pediatr. Infect. Dis. J. *14*:771–775, 1995.
63. Horstebrock, R.: Zur frage der "abscedierenden, retikulocytaren lymphadenitis (Masshoff)." Zentralbl. Allg. Pathol. *91*:221, 1954.
64. Hubbert, W. T., Petenyi, C. W., Glasgow, L. A., et al.: *Yersinia tuberculosis* infection in the United States: Septicemia, appendicitis, and mesenteric lymphadenitis. Am. J. Trop. Med. Hyg. *20*:679–684, 1971.
65. Hubbert, W. T.: Yersiniosis in mammals and birds in the United States: Case reports and review. Am. J. Trop. Med. Hyg. *21*:458–463, 1972.
66. Huppertz, H., and Heesemann, J.: Experimental *Yersinia* infection of hu-

man synovial cells: Persistence of live bacteria and generation of bacterial antigen deposits including "ghosts," nucleic acid-free bacterial rods. Infect. Immun. *64*:1484–1487, 1996.
67. Inoue, H., Nakashima, H., Ishida, T., et al.: Three outbreaks of *Yersinia pseudotuberculosis* infections. Zentralbl. Bakteriol. Mikrobiol. Hyg. *186*:504–511, 1988.
68. Isberg, R. R.: Mammalian cell adhesion functions and cellular penetration of enteropathogenic *Yersinia* species. Mol. Microbiol. *3*:1449–1453, 1989.
69. Isberg, R. R., Voorhis, D. L., and Falkow, S.: Identification of invasin: A protein that allows enteric bacteria to penetrate cultured mammalian cells. Cell *50*:769–778, 1987.
70. Jansson, E., Wallgren, G. R., and Ahvonen, P.: *Yersinia enterocolitica* as a cause of acute mesenteric lymphadenitis. Acta Paediatr. Scand. *57*:448–450, 1968.
71. Jepsen, O. B., Korner, B., Lauritsen, K. B., et al.: *Yersinia enterocolitica* infection in patients with acute surgical abdominal disease: A prospective study. Scand. J. Infect. Dis. 8:189–194, 1976.
72. Jones, B. L., and Hanson, M. F.: Prevention of transfusion of *Yersinia enterocolitica*. J. Hosp. Infect. *28*:236–238, 1994.
73. Kandolo, K., and Wauters, G.: Pyrazinamidase activity in *Yersinia enterocolitica* and related organisms. J. Clin. Microbiol. *21*:980–982, 1985.
74. Kato, Y., Ito, K., Kubo, Y., et al.: Occurrence of *Yersinia enterocolitica* in wild-living birds. App. Environ. Microbiol. *49*:198–200, 1985.
75. Kay, B. A., Wachsmuth, K., Gemski, P., et al.: Virulence and phenotypic characterization of *Yersinia enterocolitica* isolated from humans in the United States. J. Clin. Microbiol. *17*:128–138, 1983.
76. Kelly, D. A., Price, E., Jani, B., et al.: *Yersinia enterocolitis* vs. iron overload. J. Pediatr. Gastroenterol. Nutr. *6*:643–645, 1987.
77. Knapp, W.: *Pasteurella pseudotuberculosis* als erreger einer mesenterialen lymphadenitis beim menschen. Zentralbl. Bakteriol. *161*:422–424, 1954.
78. Knapp, W.: Mesenteric adenitis due to *Pasteurella pseudotuberculosis* in young people. N. Engl. J. Med. *259*:776–778, 1958.
79. Knapp, W., and Steuter, W.: Untersuchungen über den nachweis komplementbindender und agglutinierender antikorper gegen *Pasteurella* pseudotuberculosis in sera infizierter und immunisierter menschen and tiere. Z. Immunitatsforsch. Exp. Ther. *113*:370–374, 1956.
80. Knapp, W., and Masshoff, W.: Zur ätiologie der abszedierenden retikulozytaren lymphadenitis: Einer praktisch wichtigen, vielfach unter dem bilde einer akuten appendizitis verlaufenden erkrankung. Dtsch. Med. Wochenschr. *79*:1266–1271, 1954.
81. von Knorring, J., and Petterson, T.: Haemolytic anaemia complicating *Yersinia enterocolitica* infection: Report of a case. Scand. J. Haematol. *9*:149, 1972.
82. Kobayashi, S., Ogasawara, M., Maeda, K., et al.: Antibodies against *Yersinia enterocolitica* in patients with Reiter's syndrome. J. Lab. Clin. Med. *105*:380–389, 1985.
83. Kohl, S., Jacobson, J. A., and Nahmias, A.: *Yersinia enterocolitica* infections in children. J. Pediatr. *89*:77–79, 1976.
84. Krogstad, P., Mendelman, P. M., Miller, et al.: Clinical and microbiologic characteristics of cutaneous infection with *Yersinia enterocolitica*. J. Infect. Dis. *165*:740–743, 1992.
85. Lahesmaa, R., Soderberg, C., Bliska, J., et al.: Pathogen antigen- and superantigen-reactive synovial fluid T cells in reactive arthritis. J. Infect. Dis. *172*:1290–1297, 1995.
86. Larsen, J. H.: Human yersiniose. Ugeskr. Laeger. *134*:431, 1972.
87. Lee, L. A., Taylor, J., Carter, G. P., et al.: *Yersinia enterocolitica* O:3: An emerging cause of pediatric gastroenteritis in the United States. J. Infect. Dis. *163*:660–663, 1991.
88. Leino, R., and Kalliomaki, J. L.: Yersiniosis as an internal disease. Ann. Intern. Med. *81*:458–461, 1974.
89. Leino, R., Granfars, K., Havia, T., et al.: Yersiniosis as a gastrointestinal disease. Scand. J. Infect. Dis. *19*:63–68, 1987.
90. Luo, G., Seetharamaiah, G. S., Niesel, D. W., et al.: Purification and characterization of *Yersinia enterocolitica* envelope proteins which induce antibodies that react with human thyrotropin receptor. J. Immunol. *152*:2555–2561, 1994.
91. Mair, N. S., Mair, H. J., Stirk, E. M., et al.: Three cases of acute mesenteric lymphadenitis due to *Pasteurella pseudotuberculosis*. J. Clin. Pathol. *13*:432–439, 1960.
92. Mair, N. S.: Yersinosis (infections due to *Yersinia pseudotuberculosis* and *Yersinia enterocolitica*). *In* Hubbert, W. T., McCollough, W. F., and Schnurrenberger, P. R. (eds.): Diseases Transmitted from Animals to Man. 6th ed. Springfield, Charles C Thomas, 1975, pp. 174–185.
93. Maki, M., Gronroos, P., and Vesikari, T.: In vitro invasiveness of *Yersinia enterocolitica* isolated from children with diarrhea. J. Infect. Dis. *138*:677–680, 1978.
94. Maki, M., Vesikari, T., Rantala, I., et al.: Yersiniosis in children. Arch. Dis. Child. *55*:861–865, 1980.
95. Makino, S., Okada, Y., Maruyama, T., et al.: PCR-based random amplified polymorphic DNA fingerprinting of *Yersinia pseudotuberculosis* and its practical applications. J. Clin. Microbiol. *32*:65–69, 1994.
96. Mallasez, L., and Vignal, W.: Tuberculos zoologique (forme ou aspect ou tuberculose sans bacillus). Arch. Physiol. Norm. Pathol. *53*:2, 1883.
97. Marks, M. I., Pai, C. H., Lafleur, L., et al.: *Yersinia enterocolitica* gastroenteritis: A prospective study of clinical, bacteriologic, and epidemiologic features. J. Pediatr. *96*:26–31, 1980.
98. Masshoff, W.: Eine neuartige form der mesenterialen lymphadenitis. Dtsch. Med. Wochenschr. *78*:532–535, 1953.
99. Masshoff, W., and Dolle, W.: Über eine besondere form der sog. mesenterialen lymphadenopathie: "Die abscedierende reticulocytare lymphadenitis." Virchows Arch. Pathol. Anat. *323*:664–684, 1953.
100. Miller, V. L., Farmer, J. J., III, Hill, W. E., et al.: The *ail* locus is found uniquely in *Yersinia enterocolitica* serotypes commonly associated with disease. Infect. Immun. *57*:121–131, 1989.
101. Mingrone M. G., Fantasia M., Figura N., et al.: Characteristics of *Yersinia enterocolitica* isolated from children with diarrhea in Italy. J. Clin. Microbiol. *25*:1301–1304, 1987.
102. Mollaret, H.-H., et al.: Les septicemies humaines à "*Yersinia enterocolitica*": Propos de dix-sept cas recents. Presse Med. *19*:345, 1971.
103. Mollaret, H. H., Bercovier, H., and Alonso, J. M.: Summary of the data received at the WHO Reference Center for Yersinia enterocolitica. Contrib. Microbiol. Immunol. *5*:174–184, 1979.
104. Mollaret, H.-H.: Un domaine pathologique nouveau. Ann. Biol. Clin. *30*:1–5, 1972.
105. Najdenski, H., Iteman, I., and Carniel, E.: Efficient subtyping of pathogenic *Yersinia enterocolitica* strains by pulsed-field gel electrophoresis. J. Clin. Microbiol. *32*:2913–2920, 1994.
106. Nilehn, B., and Sjostrom, B.: Studies on *Yersinia enterocolitica*: Occurrence in various groups of acute abdominal disease. Acta Pathol. Microbiol. Scand. *71*:612–628, 1967.
107. Nilehn, B.: Studies on *Yersinia enterocolitica*: With special reference to bacterial diagnosis and occurrence in human enteric disease. Acta Pathol. Microbiol. Scand. *206* (Suppl.):1–48, 1969.
108. Odinot, P. T., Meis, J. F. G. M., Van Den Hurk, P. J. J. C., et al.: PCR-based characterization of *Yersinia enterocolitica*: Comparison with biotyping and serotyping. Epidemiol. Infect. *115*:269–277, 1995.
109. Paff, J. R., Triplett, D. A., and Saari, T. N.: Clinical and laboratory aspects of *Yersinia pseudotuberculosis* infection with a report of two cases. Am. J. Clin. Pathol. *66*:101–110, 1976.
110. Pai, C. H., Gillis, F., Tuomanen, E., et al.: Placebo-controlled double-blind evaluation of trimethoprim-sulfamethoxazole treatment of *Yersinia enterocolitica* gastroenteritis. J. Pediatr. *104*:308–311, 1984.
111. Pai, C. H., and Mors, V.: Production of enterotoxin by *Yersinia enterocolitica*. Infect. Immun. *19*:908–911, 1978.
112. Pepe, J. C., Badger, J. L., and Miller, V. L.: Growth phase and low pH affect the thermal regulation of the *Yersinia enterocolitica inv* gene. Mol. Microbiol. *11*:123–125, 1994.
113. Preston, M. A., Brown, S., Borczyk, A. A., et al.: Antimicrobial suseptibility of pathogenic *Yersinia enterocolitica* isolated in Canada from 1972 to 1990. Antimicrob. Agents Chemother. *38*:2121–2124, 1994.
114. Probst, P., Hermann, E., Hermann-Meyer zum Buschenfelde, K., et al.: Identification of the *Yersinia enterocolitica* urease B subunit as a target antigen for human synovial T lymphocytes in reactive arthritis. Infect. Immun. *61*:4509–4509, 1993.
115. Quan, T. J., Meek, J. L., Tsuchiya, K. R., et al.: Experimental pathogenicity of recent North American isolates of *Yersinia enterocolitica*. J. Infect. Dis. *129*:341–344, 1974.
116. Rabinovitz, M., Stremple, T. H., Granforo, K., et al.: *Yersinia enterocolitica* infections complicated by intestinal perforation. Arch. Intern. Med. *147*:1062–1063, 1987.
117. Rabson, A. R., and Koornhof, H. J.: *Yersinia enterocolitica* infections in South Africa. S. Afr. Med. J. *46*:798–803, 1972.
118. Randall, K. J., and Mair, N. S.: Family outbreak of *Pasteurella pseudotuberculosis* infection. Lancet *1*:1042–1043, 1962.
119. Ratman, S., Mercer, E., Picco, B., et al.: A nosocomial outbreak due to Yersinia enterocolitica serotype O:5, biotype 1. J. Infect. Dis. *145*:242–247, 1982.
120. Resetkova, E., Notenboom, R., Arreaza, G., et al.: Seroreactivity to bacterial antigens is not a unique phenomenon in patients with autoimmune thyroid diseases in Canada. Thyroid *4*:269–274, 1994.
121. Rodnan, G. P., Schumacher, H. R., and Zvaifler, N. J.: Primer on the Rheumatic Diseases. 8th ed. Atlanta, Arthritis Foundation, 1983, pp. 93–94.
122. Rodriguez, W. J., Controni, G., Cohen, G. J., et al.: *Yersinia enterocolitica* in children. J. A. M. A. *242*:1978–1980, 1979.
123. Rose, E. B., Camp, C. J., and Antes, E. J.: Family outbreak of fatal *Yersinia enterocolitica* pharyngitis. Am. J. Med. *82*:636–637, 1987.
124. Ryser, R. J., and Hornick, R. B.: A review of "new" bacterial strains causing diarrhea. *In* Remington, J. S., and Swartz, M. N. (eds.): Clinical Topics in Infectious Diseases. New York, McGraw-Hill, 1981, pp. 184–210.
125. Saari, T. N., and Tripplet, D. A.: *Yersinia pseudotuberculosis* mesenteric adenitis. J. Pediatr. *85*:656–659, 1974.
126. Saari, M., Make, M., Paivonsal, T., et al.: Acute anterior uveitis and

conjunctivitis following *Yersinia* infection in children. Int. Ophthalmol. Med. 9:237–241, 1986.
127. Saebo, A., and Lassen, J.: *Yersinia enterocolitica*: An inducer of chronic inflammation. Int. J. Tiss. Reac. 16:51–57, 1994.
128. Saisawa, K.: Ueber die pseudotuberkulose beim menschen. Zeitschr. Hyg. 73:353, 1913.
129. Schleifstein, J., and Coleman, M. B.: An identified microorganism resembling *B. ligneri* and *Past. pseudotuberculosis* and pathogenic for man. N. Y. State J. Med. 39:1749, 1939.
130. Schleifstein, J., and Coleman, M. B.: *Bacterium enterocoliticum*. Annual Report, Revision of Laboratories and Research. Albany, State Department of Health, 1943, p. 56.
131. Seuri, M., and Granfors, K.: Antibodies against *Yersinia* among farmers and slaughterhouse workers. Scand. J. Work Environ. Health 18:128–132, 1992.
132. Shayegani, M., DeForge, L., McGlynn, D. M., et al.: Characteristics of Yersinia enterocolitica and related species isolated from human and environmental sources. J. Clin. Microbiol. 14:304–312, 1981.
133. Shenkman, L., and Bottone, E. J.: Antibodies to *Yersinia enterocolitica* in thyroid disease. Ann. Intern. Med. 85:735–739, 1976.
134. Snyder, J. D., Christenson, E., and Feldman, R. A.: Human *Yersinia enterocolitica* infections in Wisconsin: Clinical, laboratory and epidemiologic features. Am. J. Med. 72:768–774, 1982.
135. Solem, J., and Lassen, J.: Reiter's disease following *Yersinia enterocolitica* infection. Scand. J. Infect. Dis. 3:83, 1971.
136. Sonnenwirth, A. C.: *Yersinia*. *In* Lennett, E. H., Spaulding, E. H., and Truant, J. P. (eds.): Manual of Clinical Microbiology. 2nd ed. Washington, D.C., American Society of Microbiology, 1954, pp. 222–229.
137. Sonnenwirth, A. C.: *Yersinia enterocolitica* as an etiologic agent in meningitis. Bact. Proc. Abstr. M. 128:87, 1969.
138. Sonnenwirth, A. C.: *Yersinia enterocolitica*. N. Engl. J. Med. 283:1468, 1970.
139. Sonnenwirth, A. C.: Isolation and characterization of *Yersinia enterocolitica*. Mt. Sinai. J. Med. 43:736–745, 1976.
140. Sotaniemi, K. A.: Neurologic complications associated with yersiniosis. Neurology 33:95–97, 1983.
141. Stolk-Engelaar, V. M. M., Meis, J. F. G. M., Mulder, J. A., et al.: In-vitro antimicrobial susceptibility of Yersinia enterocolitica isolates from stools of patients in The Netherlands from 1982–1991. J. Antimicrob. Chemother. 36:839–843, 1995.
142. Tackett, C. O., Ballard, J., Harris, N., et al.: An outbreak of *Yersinia enterocolitica* infections caused by contaminated tofu (soybean curd). Am. J. Epidemiol. 121:705–711, 1985.
143. Tauxe, R. V., Vandepitta, J., Mautero, G., et al.: *Yersinia enterocolitica* infections and pork: The missing link. Lancet 1:1129–1133, 1987.
144. Thomas, A. F., Solomon, L., and Rabson, A.: Polyarthritis associated with *Yersinia enterocolitica* infection. S. Afr. Med. J. 49:18–20, 1975.
145. Toivanen, P., Toivanen, A., Olkkonen, L. et al.: Hospital outbreak of *Yersinia enterocolitica* infection. Lancet 1:801–803, 1973.
146. Toma, S.: Survey on the incidence of *Yersinia enterocolitica* in the province of Ontario. Can. J. Public Health 64:477–487, 1973.
147. Toshniwal, R., Kocka, F. E., and Kallick, C. A.: Suppurative lymphadenitis with *Yersinia enterocolitica*. Eur. J. Clin. Microbiol. 4:587–588, 1985.
148. Toma, S., Wauters, G., McClure, H. M., et al.: O:13a, 13b, a new pathogenic serotype of *Yersinia enterocolitica*. J. Clin. Microbiol. 20:843–845, 1984.
149. Vantrappen, G., Ponette, E., Geboes, K., et al.: *Yersinia* enteritis and enterocolitis: Gastroenterological aspects. Gastroenterology 72:220–227, 1977.
150. Vantrappen, G., Geboes, K., and Ponette, E.: *Yersinia* enteritis. Med. Clin. North Am. 66:639–653, 1982.
151. Vilinskas, J., Tilton, R. C., and Kriz, J. J.: A new clinical entity: Human infection with *Yersinia* presenting as an acute abdomen. Am. J. Surg. 7:568, 1971.
152. Visser, L. G., Hiemstra, P. S., Van Den Barselaar, M. T., et al.: Role of YadA in resistance to killing of *Yersinia enterocolitica* by antimicrobial polypeptides of human granulocytes. Infect. Immun. 64:1653–1658, 1996.
153. Weber, J., Finlayson, N. B., and Mark, J. B. D.: Mesenteric lymphadenitis and terminal ileitis due to *Yersinia pseudotuberculosis*. N. Engl. J. Med. 283:172–174, 1970.
154. Wilson, H. D., McCormick, J. S., and Feely, J. C.: *Yersinia enterocolitica* infection in a 4-month-old infant associated with infection in household dogs. J. Pediatr. 89:767–769, 1976.
155. Winblad, S., Nilehn, B., and Jonsson, M.: Two further cases, bacteriologically verified, of human infection with "*Pasteurella X*" (syn. *Yersinia enterocolitica*). Acta Pathol. Microbiol. Scand. 67:537–541, 1966.
156. Winblad, S., Nilehn, B., and Sternby, N. H.: *Yersinia enterocolitica* (*Pasteurella X*) in human enteric infections. Br. Med. J. 2:1363–1366, 1966.
157. Winblad, S.: Erythema nodosum associated with infection with *Yersinia enterocolitica*. Scand. J. Infect. Dis. 1:11–16, 1969.
158. Winblad, S.: Arthritis associated with *Yersinia enterocolitica* infections. Scand. J. Infect. Dis. 7:191–195, 1975.
159. Zen-Yoji, H., Maruyama, T., Sakai, S., et al.: An outbreak of enteritis due to *Yersinia enterocolitica* occurring at a junior high school. Jpn. J. Microbiol. 17:220–222, 1973.

118

MISCELLANEOUS ENTEROBACTERIA

Randall G. Fisher and William C. Gruber

This chapter focuses on three less commonly isolated organisms of the family Enterobacteriaceae—*Edwardsiella tarda*, *Hafnia alvei*, and *Pantoea agglomerans*. Each of these organisms, although uncommon, can cause significant disease in certain clinical circumstances.[31]

EDWARDSIELLA TARDA

Bacteriology

E. tarda is a non–lactose-fermenting, gram-negative bacillus that is indole-positive and produces hydrogen sulfide. It ferments only glucose and maltose. The species name *tarda* reflects its biochemical inactivity. It usually is lysine- and ornithine-decarboxylase–positive.[15] The organism resembles *Salmonella* both biochemically and clinically.[20] *Salmonella*, however, usually ferments mannitol, sorbitol, and rhamnose. *Edwardsiella's* innate resistance to colistin also distinguishes it from *Salmonella*.[33]

E. tarda grows well on usual differential media in the laboratory and produces smooth, glistening, semitranslucent colonies.

Epidemiology

E. tarda is an organism associated with fresh water and marine life and has been isolated from turtles, fish, pelicans, alligators, seals, and toads.[20] It also is found often in reptiles, including snakes and lizards. Case reports of human disease have implicated ornamental fish,[47] pet turtles,[34] snakes,[39] and catfish[9, 18] as sources of infection.

Patients with chronic liver disease, chronic ethanol abuse, steroid therapy, and hemoglobinopathy particularly are prone to infection with *E. tarda*.[20] Any condition associated with iron overload also is a potential risk factor.

Invasiveness of the organism in both HeLa and HEp-2 cells, siderophore production, the elaboration of a cell-associated hemolysin, and resistance to complement-mediated lysis may contribute to virulence, although no clear associations have been made.[19]

Infection with *E. tarda* is global but more common in tropical and subtropical climates. The elderly and the very young seem to be at increased risk for severe illness.[5]

Asymptomatic carrier states have been documented well,[38]

but no true epidemic has been reported, and person-to-person transmission has not been established directly.[11]

Clinical Manifestations

Infections with *E. tarda* can be divided broadly into two types: intestinal and extraintestinal. Gastrointestinal infection usually causes a secretory self-limited enteritis, with intermittent watery diarrhea and low-grade fever.[21] Nausea and vomiting usually are not seen. Occasionally, enterocolitis or a dysentery-like illness is noted.[28]

Wound infection is the most common extraintestinal infection. Most of the wounds were caused by fish fins or snakes; wounds sustained in automobile accidents also have been implicated.[20] Cellulitis or abscesses may be produced. Coinfection with other organisms, particularly *Aeromonas hydrophila*,[18] has been noted.

Septicemia with *E. tarda* is a rare but serious infection that carries a mortality rate of about 45 per cent. Most patients with septicemia have underlying conditions, such as liver disease, iron overload, and immune suppression. Septicemia occasionally follows a mild diarrheal illness.[9] Infants without other risk factors have been reported.[48] Septicemia presents with high fever, shock, and often disseminated intravascular coagulation. Meningitis also has been reported.[37, 42] Death sometimes occurs despite appropriate antimicrobial therapy.

Other syndromes associated with *E. tarda* infection include an enteric fever-like illness,[9] multiple liver abscesses,[55] osteomyelitis,[39] and peritonitis.[9] Patients with sickle-cell disorders may be predisposed to bony infection with *E. tarda*, as they are with *Salmonella*.[42, 53] Interestingly, reported cases are all in patients with SC hemoglobinopathy rather than homozygous sickle-cell disease.

Diagnosis and Treatment

Diagnosis rests on identification of *E. tarda* in culture. The major pitfall is mistaking it for *Salmonella*.

E. tarda is sensitive in vitro to most antibiotics used routinely in the treatment of gram-negative infections, including β-lactams, cephalosporins, aminoglycosides, and fluoroquinolones.[8] It also is sensitive to chloramphenicol. Resistance has been demonstrated to polymyxin B, colistin, and, occasionally, penicillin.[8, 9] The organism almost universally elaborates a β-lactamase, but no resistance to β-lactams other than penicillin has been reported.[8]

Gastrointestinal disease does not require treatment. Severe disease, such as septicemia or meningitis, probably should be treated with the combination of a β-lactam and an aminoglycoside,[20] even though synergy has not been demonstrated.

HAFNIA ALVEI

Bacteriology

H. alvei is a facultatively anaerobic, gram-negative bacillus, formerly referred to as *Enterobacter hafnia*.[43] This indole-negative, catalase-positive, and oxidase-negative organism is positive for both lysine and ornithine decarboxylases. It is motile at lower temperatures but may be immotile at 35° C and above. *H. alvei* ferments mannitol, maltose, and sucrose. It grows well on blood or MacConkey agar as a nonlactose fermenter, producing gray-white, slightly elevated, glistening colonies.[12]

Epidemiology

H. alvei has been found in soil, dairy products, sewage, and the feces of humans and animals. There is some question as to whether it is part of the endogenous microflora of the gut[40] or whether an asymptomatic "carrier" state exists. One study from Japan cultured *H. alvei* from as many as 13 per cent of healthy subjects[30]; other epidemiologic surveys, however, have shown the incidence to be less than 2 per cent.[41]

Long regarded as a nonpathogen, *H. alvei* now has been associated clearly with enteritis and rarely has been isolated in pure culture from other sites, including blood, cerebrospinal fluid, peritoneal fluid, and urine. Infection appears to be opportunistic.

Pathophysiology

The pathophysiology of *H. alvei* has been investigated most thoroughly with regard to its production of gastrointestinal symptoms.[22] Albert and associates[2] showed that, although *H. alvei* had neither enterotoxins nor a Shiga-like toxin and was not invasive in HeLa cell assays or by Sereny test, it did produce diarrhea in experimental animals whether given parenterally or by mouth. Sections of intestines from infected animals showed lesions indistinguishable from those caused by enteropathogenic *Escherichia coli*. Because attachment effacement was the known mechanism of pathology in enteropathogenic *E. coli* infection, clinical strains of *H. alvei* were tested for homology with *E. coli*. Genes encoding for attachment effacement were found in *H. alvei* by this method.[2] Some strains that do not produce attachment effacement lesions also have been reported.

Clinical Manifestations

Most patients with gastroenteritis secondary to *H. alvei* report 6 to 12 episodes of watery diarrhea per day, low-grade or no fever, and nausea with or without vomiting. Mucus sometimes is found in stools, but blood is not.[40, 52] In most patients, symptoms last for a few days, but in some patients, symptoms persist for more than a week.[40] One patient with a reactive arthritis from *H. alvei* enteritis has been reported.[35]

One 20-day-old premature baby with necrotizing enterocolitis grew *H. alvei* from blood and stool.[16] Yeager and associates[54] reported four cases of pneumatosis intestinalis in patients after bone marrow transplantation, and one of the four grew *H. alvei* in pure culture from blood.[54] Approximately nine cases of septicemia due to *H. alvei* occur each year in the United States. Signs and symptoms are indistinguishable from sepsis due to other causes. Septic arthritis has been documented.[23] One case of meningitis in a 1-year-old infant without known predisposing risk factors has been reported.[32] An interesting case of a woman with rheumatoid arthritis who contracted endophthalmitis with *H. alvei* in mixed culture has been described; the woman used snake powder as a food seasoning.[7] There are two case reports in the older literature of persistent bacteremia with this organism, alone and in mixed cultures. One of these patients was a previously well 13-year-old girl.[17]

Diagnosis and Treatment

Diagnosis is made by isolation of the organism from stools or from normally sterile body fluids.

No comprehensive antibiotic susceptibility studies are available for *H. alvei*. It is constitutively cephalothin-resistant.[52] Case reports show that most isolates are resistant to ampicillin.[16, 40] Most are sensitive to aminoglycosides, second- and third-generation cephalosporins, aztreonam, imipenem, chloramphenicol, and trimethoprim-sulfamethoxazole. One report describes an inducible β-lactamase that rendered one isolate ceftazidime-resistant.[45]

Treatment probably is not necessary for most cases of gastroenteritis. Treatment for invasive infection should be based on susceptibility testing; empiric therapy with a third-generation cephalosporin and an aminoglycoside is reasonable pending results.

PANTOEA AGGLOMERANS

First identified as a plant pathogen and named after Erwin Smith in 1917, the genus *Erwinia* has an extended domain as an infectious microbe, including production of disease in humans.[6, 44, 49] A member of this group of organisms, *P. agglomerans (Enterobacter agglomerans, Erwinia herbicola)* has been established as a cause of conjunctivitis,[6] central nervous system infections,[6, 50] urinary tract infections,[44, 49] pneumonia,[1] and nosocomial infections secondary to contaminated intravenous fluids.[25]

Bacteriology

Species definition within *Erwinia* has been controversial and confusing. It has been suggested that the anaerogenic clinically relevant *Erwinia* of the *herbicola-lathryi* group be renamed *E. agglomerans* or *P. agglomerans*.[13, 21, 51] In clinical microbiology, both of the latter terms tend to be used interchangeably. This species consists of facultatively anaerobic, fermentative, hydrogen sulfide–negative, gram-negative rods; they do not possess oxidase, phenylalanine deaminase, proteinase, or arginine dehydrolase.[13] None decarboxylate ornithine.[24] They are motile, have peritrichous flagella, and produce a yellow pigment. Strains grow well at 37° C (98.6° F) on standard agar. When colonies are viewed microscopically after growth for 18 to 20 hours, characteristic biconvex spindle-shaped bodies and bacterial aggregates often can be seen.[6, 49] Almost all strains isolated from clinical specimens and grown on agar slants show characteristic elongated, spheroidal aggregates,[49] called symplasmata, by Cruickshank,[10] who first described them.

Epidemiology

Microorganisms of the genus *Erwinia* long have been recognized as phytopathogens producing dry necrosis, wilts, and soft rots in plants, and they more recently have been associated with disease in trout and leafhoppers.[44, 49] *P. agglomerans (E. herbicola)* first was isolated in humans from stool specimens of typhoid fever patients in the 1920s and given the name *Bacterium typhi flavum* because of the organism's alleged capacity to be transformed into *Salmonella typhi* in subculture. Identification of saprophytic human strains followed, and the biochemical and cultural identity of *B. typhi flavum* with the *E. herbicola-lathryi* group finally was established.[13]

The first reports of *P. agglomerans* as a human pathogen appeared in the 1960s. Subsequently, a nationwide outbreak of infection due to this organism was traced to contaminated liners from caps of parenteral solution bottles.[25, 26] The importance of this organism as a nosocomial cause of bacteremia is emphasized by the 17 per cent mortality rate in patients receiving an infusion with the contaminated intravenous fluid.[26] There was a trend for increased mortality rate in infected individuals younger than 20 years of age. Lipid-based medications support rapid bacterial growth at room temperature and, in the absence of strict aseptic handling, have been implicated in recent nosocomial *P. agglomerans* blood stream infections.[4] *Pantoea* outbreaks also have been traced to contaminated blood products; prolonged storage of packed red blood cells at 4° C provides conditions that allow these *P. agglomerans* organisms to grow and subsequently produce high concentrations of endotoxin.[3] Cotton used to filter heroin has been implicated as a source of infection in intravenous drug users.[14]

Outbreaks in pediatric hospitals due to contaminated intravenous solutions also have been described.[29] At least one retrospective review of *Erwinia* organisms isolated from clinical specimens suggested a predisposition to infection in the pediatric age group[6]; however, other studies have noted no preference based on season, sex, age, or residence in hospitals.[49]

Pathophysiology

The true incidence of clinical infection due to *P. agglomerans* is difficult to ascertain because of the common association of this microbe with other organisms when obtained from clinical specimens. Nonetheless, accumulation of case reports in which this organism is isolated in pure culture from infected material leaves little doubt that *P. agglomerans* can be a human pathogen, apart from its role as a nosocomial contaminant. This organism has little inherent invasiveness. Evidence for animal pathogenicity of *Erwinia* strains isolated from plants and humans is limited; 10^{13} washed organisms injected intraperitoneally into mice or guinea pigs do not cause symptoms, whereas inoculation of 10^{25} organisms leads to death within 36 hours.[10]

Most strains appear to act as saprophytes in humans,[49] but the organism has been isolated from purulent wounds of the extremities acquired through lacerations or thorn pricks, which suggests agricultural injury as a possible mode of infection.[49] Most serious infection has occurred in individuals with a breakdown or breach of host defenses, e.g., immunocompromised individuals or patients who received contaminated intravenous fluid.

Clinical Manifestations

P. agglomerans bacteremia often is associated with fever, shaking chills, and systemic toxicity characteristic of gram-negative sepsis. However, these symptoms frequently have been misinterpreted in hospitalized patients who unknowingly were administered contaminated intravenous fluids.[25]

Eye and skin infections due to *P. agglomerans* particularly are prominent. Bottone and Schneierson[6] included six cases of conjunctivitis, five of which occurred in infants, from whom this organism was isolated. However, only two of the isolates were in pure culture, and a description of the clinical course of these children was not included in the report. *Erwinia* endophthalmitis has been associated with foreign body penetration of the eye in a 14-year-old boy.[36] Skin infection in association with a casted fracture has been described in an elderly patient,[49] and wound infections from which this organism was isolated have been described subsequently, most often in association with agricultural injury.[49] Four isolates were obtained in mixed cultures from skin lesions of children younger than 5 years of age, but their possible role in those infections was not confirmed.[6] *P. agglomerans* was the only organism isolated from six consecutive blood cultures in a 9-year-old boy with osteomyelitis.[27]

Primary lung disease due to these bacteria is extremely uncommon and has been reported in an adult with chronic bronchitis.[1] This organism is a very rare cause of meningitis. A contaminated incubator has been implicated in two cases of neonatal central nervous system infection,[46] and a cisternal tap revealed the presence of *P. agglomerans* in an unrelated newborn case whose clinical course was not described.[6] A 57-year-old man with tetralogy of Fallot and cyanosis had a brain abscess in which *P. agglomerans* organisms grew in pure culture.[50] Presenting manifestations included headaches, seizures, and left-sided weakness, which occurred over a 2-week period prior to admission. The patient recovered after drainage of the abscess and gentamicin therapy.

Diagnosis

Difficulty in identifying this organism is common; in March 1972, as part of a quality control program, *P. agglomerans* was sent as an unknown organism to 250 United States hospitals and was identified incorrectly 45 per cent of the time.[25] Even when fully identified in isolates from human sources, *P. agglomerans* often is considered a contaminant or saphrophyte. The organisms have been identified mistakenly as *Citrobacter, E. coli, Flavobacterium,* and *Klebsiella*. In addition to routine microbiologic studies, identification of yellow-pigmented colonies and observation of the characteristic spindle-shaped bodies and symplasmata can aid in this differentiation. Symplasmata (elongated, spheroid aggregates) are seen best in the condensation water of slant cultures.[49] Spindle-shaped bodies termed "Wetzsteinformen" by German authors are observed best on standard agar with a low-power microscope lens.[49]

Treatment

Most localized infections respond to treatment that includes an aminoglycoside. The presence of persistent localized infection with this organism should prompt a search for an organic foreign body, given the organism's tendency to live as a saprophyte or as a pathogen in vegetable material. In addition to appropriate antimicrobial therapy, treatment of bacteremia should include removal of any potentially contaminated intravenous access. The physician should be alert to the possibility of a common source of infection in nosocomial outbreaks.[25] In view of the rarity of bacteremia due to *P. agglomerans*, single sporadic cases should be investigated, and clusters of two or more cases should lead to immediate inquiry into possible sources of contamination. Formal surveillance programs have been the key to early recognition and abortion of epidemics.[25]

References

1. Al-Damluji, S., Dickinson, C. M., and Beck, A.: *Enterobacter agglomerans*: A new cause of primary pneumonia. Thorax *37*:865, 1982.
2. Albert, M. J., Faruque, S. M., Ansaruzzaman, M., et al.: Sharing of virulence-associated properties at the phenotypic and genetic levels between enteropathogenic *Escherichia coli* and *Hafnia alvei*. J. Med. Microbiol. *37*:310–314, 1992.
3. Arduino, M. J., Bland, L. A., Tipple, M. A., et al.: Growth and endotoxin production of *Yersinia enterocolitica* and *Enterobacter agglomerans* in packed erythrocytes. J. Clin. Microbiol. *27*:1483–1485, 1989.
4. Bennett, S. N., McNeil, M. M., Bland, L. A., et al.: Postoperative infections traced to contamination of an intravenous anesthetic, propofol. N. Engl. J. Med. *333*:147–154, 1995.
5. Bockemuhl, J., Pan-Urai, R., and Burkhardt, E.: *Edwardsiella tarda* associated with human disease. Pathol. Microbiol. *37*:393–401, 1971.
6. Bottone, E., and Schneierson, S. S.: *Erwinia* species: An emerging human pathogen. Am. J. Clin. Pathol. *57*:400–405, 1972.
7. Caravalho, J., Jr., McMillan, V. M., Ellis, R. B., et al.: Endogenous endophthalmitis due to *Salmonella arizonae* and *Hafnia alvei*. South. Med. J. *83*:325–327, 1990.
8. Clark, R. B., Lister, P. D., and Janda, J. M.: In vitro susceptibilities of *Edwardsiella tarda* to 22 antibiotics and antibiotic-beta-lactamase-inhibitor agents. Diagn. Microbiol. Infect. Dis. *14*:173–175, 1991.
9. Clarridge, J. E., Musher, D. M., Fainstein, V., et al.: Extraintestnal human infection caused by *Edwardsiella tarda*. J. Clin. Microbiol. *11*:511–514, 1980.
10. Cruickshank, J. C.: A study of the so-called bacterium *Typhii flavum*. J. Hyg. *35*:354–371, 1935.
11. Desenclos, J. C., Conti, L., Junejo, S., et al.: A cluster of *Edwardsiella tarda* infection in a day-care center in Florida. J. Infect. Dis. *162*:782, 1990.
12. Englund, G. W.: Persistent septicemia due to *Hafnia alvei*: Report of a case. Am. J. Clin. Pathol. *51*:717–719, 1969.
13. Ewing, W. H., and Fife, M. A.: *Enterobacter agglomerans* (Beijerinck) comb. nov. (the *herbicola-lathryi* bacteria). Int. J. Syst. Bacteriol. *22*:4–11, 1972.
14. Ferguson, R., Feeney, C., and Chirurgi, V. A.: *Enterobacter agglomerans*–associated cotton fever. Arch. Intern. Med. *153*:2381–2382, 1993.
15. Gilchrist, M. J. R.: Enterobacteriaceae: Opportunistic pathogens and other genera. *In* Murray, P. R., Baron, E. J., Pfaller, M. A., et al. (eds.): Manual of Clinical Microbiology. 6th ed. Washington, D.C., ASM Press, 1995, pp. 457–464.
16. Ginsberg, H. G., and Goldsmith, J. P.: *Hafnia alvei* septicemia in an infant with necrotizing enterocolitis. J. Perinatol. *8*:122–123, 1988.
17. Grajupa, L. A., Mukhopadhyay, D., and Grossman, B. J.: Chronic polymicrobial bacteremia. Clin. Pediatr. *14*:280–283, 1975.
18. Hargreaves, J. E., and Lucey, D. R.: Life-threatening *Edwardsiella tarda* soft-tissue infection associated with catfish puncture wound. J. Infect. Dis. *162*:1416–1417, 1990.
19. Janda, J. M., Abbott, S. L., Kroske-Bystrom, S., et al.: Pathogenic properties of *Edwardsiella* species. J. Clin. Microbiol. *29*:1997–2001, 1991.
20. Janda, J. M., and Abbott, S. L.: Infections associated with the genus *Edwardsiella*: The role of *Edwardsiella tarda* in human disease. Clin. Infect. Dis. *17*:742–748, 1993.
21. Kourany, M., Vasquez, M. A., and Saenz, R.: Edwardsiellosis in man and animals in Panama: Clinical and epidemiological characteristics. Am. J. Trop. Med. Hyg. *26*:1183–1190, 1977.
22. Albert, M. J., Alam, K., Islam, M., et al.: *Hafnia alvei*: A probable cause of diarrhea in humans. Infect. Immun. *59*:1507-1513, 1991.
23. LeFrock, J. L., Klainer, A. S., and Zuckerman, K.: *Edwardsiella tarda* bacteremia. South. Med. J. *69*:188–190, 1976.
24. Lindh, E., Kjaeldgaard, P., and Frederiksen, W., et al.: Phenotypical properties of *Enterobacter agglomerans* (*Pantoea agglomerans*) from human, animal and plant sources. APMIS *99*:347–352, 1991.
25. Maki, D. G., Rhame, F. S., Mackel, D. C., et al.: Nationwide epidemic of septicemia caused by contaminated intravenous products. I. Epidemiologic and clinical features. Am. J. Med. *60*:471–485, 1976.
26. Maki, D. G., and Martin, W. T.: Nationwide epidemic of septicemia caused by contaminated infusion products. IV. Growth of microbial pathogens in fluids for intravenous infusion. J. Infect. Dis. *131*:267–272, 1975.
27. Marklein, G., Waschkowski, G., and Reichertz, C.: *Erwinia herbicola* bei sepsis im kindesalter. Klin. Pädiatr. *193*:394–397, 1981.
28. Marsh, P. K., and Gorbach, S. L.: Invasive entercolitis caused by *Edwardsiella tarda*. Gastroenterology *82*:336–338, 1982.
29. Matsaniotis, N. S., Syriopoulou, V. P., Theodoridou, M. C., et al.: *Enterobacter* sepsis in infants and children due to contaminated intravenous fluids. Infect. Control *5*:471–477, 1984.
30. Matsumoto, H.: Studies on the *Hafnia* isolated from normal human. Jpn. J. Microbiol. *7*:105–114, 1963.
31. Mayer, K. H., and Zinner, S. H.: Bacterial pathogens of increasing significance in hospital-acquired infections. Rev. Infect. Dis. *7*:S371–S379, 1985.
32. Mojtabaee, A., and Siadati, A.: *Enterobacter hafnia* meningitis. J. Pediatr. *93*:1062–1063, 1978.
33. Muyembe, T., Vandepitte, J., and Dismuter, J.: Natural colistin resistance in *Edwardsiella tarda*. Antimicrob. Agents Chemother. *4*:521–524, 1973.
34. Nagel, P., Serritella, A., and Layden, T. J. *Edwardsiella tarda* gastroenteritis associated with a pet turtle. Gastroenterology *82*:1436–1437, 1982.
35. Newmark, J. J., Hobbs, W. N., and Wilson, B. E.: Reactive arthritis associated with *Hafnia alvei* enteritis. Arthr. Rheum. *37*:960, 1994.
36. Oesterle, C. S., Kronenberg, H. A., and Peyman, G. A.: Endophthalmitis caused by an *Erwinia* species. Arch. Ophthalmol. *95*:824–825, 1977.
37. Okubadejo, O. A., and Alausa, K. O.: Neonatal meningitis caused by *Edwardsiella tarda*. Br. Med. J. *3*:357–358, 1968.
38. Onogawa, T., Terayama, T., Zen-yogi, H., et al.: Distribution of *Edwardsiella tarda* and hydrogen-sulfide producing *Escherichia coli* in healthy persons. Jpn. Assoc. Infect. Dis. *50*:10–17, 1976.
39. Rao, K. R., Shah, J., Rajashekaraiah, K. R., et al.: *Edwardsiella tarda* osteomyelitis in a patient with SC hemoglobinopathy. South. Med. J. *74*:288–292, 1981.
40. Reina, J., Hervas, J., and Borrell, N.: Acute gastroenteritis caused by *Hafnia alvei* in children. Clin. Infect. Dis. *16*:443, 1993.

41. Ridell, J., Siitonen, A., Paulin, L., et al.: *Hafnia alvei* in stool specimens from patients with diarrhea and healthy controls. J. Clin. Microbiol. *32*:2335–2337, 1994.
42. Sachs, J. M., Pacin, M., and Counts, G. W.: Sickle hemoglobinopathy and *Edwardsiella meningitis*. Am. J. Dis. Child. 128:387–388, 1974.
43. Sakazaki, R.: Genus IX. *Hafnia*. *In* Krieg, N. R., and Holt, J. C. (eds.): Bergey's Manual of Systematic Bacteriology. Vol. 1. Baltimore, Williams & Wilkins, 1984, pp. 484–486.
44. Starr, M. P., and Chatterjee, A. K.: The genus *Erwinia*: Enterobacteria pathogenic to plants and animals. Ann. Rev. Microbiol. *26*:389–426, 1972.
45. Thomson, K. S., Sanders, C. C., and Washington, J. A., II.: Ceftazidime resistance in *Hafnia alvei*. Antimicrob. Agents Chemother. *37*:1375–1376, 1993.
46. Urmenyi, A. M. C., and Franklin, A. W.: Neonatal death from pigmented coliform infection. Lancet *1*:313–315, 1961.
47. Vandepitte, J., Lemmens, P., and DeSmert, L.: Human edwardsiellosis traced to ornamental fish. J. Clin. Microbiol. 17:165–167, 1983.
48. Vohra, K., Torrijos, E., Jhaveri, R., et al.: Neonatal sepsis and meningitis caused by *Edwardsiella tarda*. Pediatr. Infect. Dis. J. *7*:814–815, 1988.
49. von Graevenitz, A.: *Erwinia* species isolates. Ann. N. Y. Acad. Sci. *174*:436–443, 1970.
50. Wechsler, A., Bottone, E., and Lasser R, et al.: Brain abscess caused by an *Erwinia* species: Report of a case and review of the literature. Am. J. Med. *51*:680–684, 1971.
51. Werkman, C. H., and Gillen, G. F.: Bacteria producing trimethylene glycol. J. Bacteriol. *23*:167–182, 1932.
52. Westblom, T. U., and Milligan, T. W.: Acute bacterial gastroenteritis caused by *Hafnia alvei*. Clin. Infect. Dis. *14*:1271–1272, 1992.
53. Wilson, J. P., Waterer, R. R., Wofford, J. D., Jr., et al.: Serious infections with *Edwardsiella tarda*: A case report and review of the literature. Arch. Intern. Med. *149*:208–210, 1989.
54. Yeager, A. M., Kanof, M. E., Kramer, S. S., et al.: *Pneumatosis intestinalis* in children after allogeneic bone marrow transplantation. Pediatr. Radiol. *17*:18–22, 1987.
55. Zigelbohm, J., Williams, T. W., Jr., Bradshaw, M. W., et al.: Successful medical management of a patient with multiple hepatic abscesses due to *Edwardsiella tarda*. Clin. Infect. Dis. *14*:117–120, 1992.

119

AEROMONAS

Ralph D. Feigin

Originally, *Aeromonas* was recognized as a cause of human disease by Sanarelli in 1891.[88] In general, *Aeromonas* species have been considered opportunistic pathogens for humans; however, with increasing frequency these organisms have been identified as primary pathogens in the normal individual as well as in the compromised host.

Aeromonas organisms are found as normal flora in nonfecal sewage and are isolated from tap water, canals, streams, and rivers. Aeromonads are pathogens for cold-blooded animals (fish, amphibians, and reptiles).

EPIDEMIOLOGY

Ewing and associates[22] as well as other investigators have isolated *Aeromonas* from tap water and from the water or sediments of rivers, especially during periods when the water temperature was relatively warm.[40, 57, 94] Hazen and colleagues[34] recovered *A. hydrophila* from 135 of 147 natural water sources in 30 states of the United States and reported that its density was higher in flowing (lotic) than in calm (lentic) water systems and lower in fresh water systems than in saline; however, *Aeromonas* could not be recovered from waters where the saline content approached that of sea water or from extremely polluted waters. Leclerc and Buttiaux[46] found *Aeromonas* in 30 per cent of more than 9000 samples of drinking water in France. *Aeromonas* also has been recovered from hospital water supplies.[57, 73, 74] More recently, *A. hydrophila* has been isolated from bottled water, prompting the development of regulations in Canada to prevent contamination of bottled water by this organism.[107]

Aeromonas survives readily on surfaces such as bench tops and moistened paper towels. Slotnick[97] recovered *Aeromonas* from a moistened paper towel that had been allowed to dry 24 hours after its application. When the towel was placed in a humidified closed environment, the period was extended to 2 weeks.

A. hydrophila may be found in the mouths of fish, alligators, turtles, tadpoles, and frogs.[37] It also has been found in the feces of guinea pigs and laboratory mice.[19] Ticks are another source of *Aeromonas*. Unusual sources of *Aeromonas* infection include contamination of home or hospital hemodialysis equipment,[39, 78] tornado-associated wound contamination,[28] and contamination of blood or blood products.[76, 79]

San Joaquin and colleagues[86] noted that *Aeromonas* organisms also have been found in ornamental aquaria belonging to patients with *Aeromonas*-associated gastroenteritis; however, they found that isolates from the aquaria differed in susceptibility testing from the gastrointestinal isolates, and thus the aquaria probably were not the sources of infection.

In 1988, California made infection by *Aeromonas* a reportable condition, thereby permitting the first population-based study of the epidemiology of infection caused by this organism. The overall incidence rate for *Aeromonas* isolation was 10.6 cases per 1 million population. The gastrointestinal tract was the most common site of infection (81 per cent of cases), followed by wounds (9 per cent). Five (2 per cent) of 219 patients with *Aeromonas* infection died; all had serious underlying medical conditions.[43]

ETIOLOGIC AGENT

Aeromonas organisms are motile, asporogenous gram-negative rods that contain a single polar flagellum. The organisms are oxidase- and catalase-positive and produce acid and/or gas during carbohydrate fermentation. They can grow between 0° and 41° C. Growth may occur within a pH range of 5.5 to 9. Lipase, gelatinase, DNAase, and other exoenzymes are formed by these organisms.[21, 93, 103]

Aeromonads grow well on blood agar; most strains produce a large zone of beta-hemolysis on this medium, although nonhemolytic strains exist. *Aeromonas* colonies on blood agar have a ground-glass appearance and a fruity odor.[108] Aeromonads also grow on MacConkey, eosin–methylene blue, *Salmonella-Shigella*, and triple sugar iron media.

The sensitivity and specificity of various media for detection of *Aeromonas* species in fecal specimens have been evaluated.[65, 82, 104] Isolation is achieved readily on any of the following: pril-xylose-ampicillin agar, xylose-sodium, deoxycholate citrate agar, alkaline peptonic water, inositol–brilliant green bile salts agar, trypticase soy broth with ampicillin, and dextrin-fuchsin-sulfite agar.[104] The colonies appear almost colorless on these media with the exception of growth on dextrin-fuchsin-sulfite agar, on which they appear dark red.

Mishva and associates[60] evaluated five selective agars. Of these, sheep blood agar with 30 mg ampicillin/L (ASBA 30) permitted the greatest number of *Aeromonas* colonies to grow while also inhibiting the competing fecal flora. They recommend that ASBA 30 be used with DNAase–toluidine blue agar (DNTA) to detect the ampicillin-susceptible strains and the nonhemolytic strains. The combination of ASBA 30–DNTA allowed detection of 98 per cent of all isolates.

Strains of motile *Aeromonas* isolates can be identified to species level using the following tests: esculin production, formation of gas from glucose, production of acetoin, production of acid from mannitol and arabinase; decarboxylation of lysine and ornithine, dihydrolation of arginine; and pyrazinamide hydrolysis in a semisolid medium.[106] *A. caviae* and *A. hydrophila* hydrolyze pyrazinamide, whereas all strains of *A. sobria* show no pyrazinamide production. This absence of pyrazinamidase is a convenient phenotype marker for *A. sobria.*

Detection of *Aeromonas* by using strain-specific fluorescent antibody has been described.[103] The technique is not satisfactory; only a small percentage of isolates react with prepared antisera, which suggests the presence of a number of serogroups. For typing of *Aeromonas* strains, restriction endonuclease analysis of whole-cell DNA appears to be quite valuable.[45]

Aeromonas is a member of the Vibrionaceae family, which includes the genera *Vibrio* and *Plesiomonas.* Several classifications within the genus are in use. The genus has been classified as follows: *A. hydrophila* (including biovars, *hydrophila,* and *anaerogenes*), *A. sobria,* and *A. salmonicida.* Schubert[92] classified *Aeromonas* into *A. hydrophila* (subspecies *hydrophila, anaerogenes,* and *proteolytica*); *A. punctata* (subspecies *punctata* and *caviae*); and *A. salmonicida, achromogenes,* and *masoucida. A. hydrophila* is the proposed type species. *A. proteolytica* and *A. salmonicida* have not been isolated from humans. According to the latest edition of *Bergey's Manual of Systematic Bacteriology,*[77] the genus *Aeromonas* consists of four species: *A. hydrophila, A. sobria, A. caviae,* and *A. salmonicida* (subspecies *salmonicida, achromogenes,* and *masoucida*). In addition, four new species—*A. media* (similar to *A. salmonicida*),[2] *A. veronii,*[36] *A. schubertii,*[11, 35] and *A. eucrenophila*[93]—have been described.

Aeromonas is confused most frequently with Enterobacteriaceae. The oxidase test always should be performed to aid in differentiation; *Aeromonas* organisms generally are oxidase-positive, whereas Enterobacteriaceae organisms are oxidase-negative. McGrath and associates[55] described oxidase-variable strains of *A. hydrophila.* These strains are oxidase-positive when grown on nonselective media but are oxidase-negative when grown on differential or gram-negative media. Organic acid end-products of lactose fermentation can inhibit the oxidase reaction. Paik[70] also has shown that a platinum wire loop should be used for oxidase testing; use of an iron-containing loop can cause false-positive oxidase results.

Aeromonas is susceptible to cefamandole (8 μg/mL), chloramphenicol (2 to 4 μg/mL), gentamicin (0.5 to 2 μg/mL), streptomycin (16 μg/mL), and trimethoprim-sulfamethoxazole (<0.5/9.5 μg/mL).[22, 23, 69, 80, 104] *Aeromonas* appears to be particularly susceptible to moxalactam, with a 90 per cent minimal inhibitory concentration (MIC) of less than 0.006 to 0.39 μg/mL. Reinhardt and George[81] determined that the most active on a weight basis were ciprofloxacin, enoxacin, and norfloxacin; nalidixic acid and trimethoprim-sulfamethoxazole also possessed good activity. Neither sulfamethoxazole nor trimethoprim alone was active. In addition, they did not note appreciable differences in susceptibility between species or in susceptibility between fecal versus nonenteric isolates. In contrast, Motyl and colleagues[64] noted higher levels of resistance to various antibiotics among *A. hydrophila* strains when compared with *A. sobria* or *A. caviae* as judged by MIC. Susceptibility to cephalothin may serve as a useful criterion in the identification of *A. sobria.*[64, 87] *Aeromonas* organisms consistently are resistant to penicillin, ampicillin, carbenicillin, cephalothin, erythromycin, clindamycin, and vancomycin. Sawai and associates[91] demonstrated that resistance to β-lactam antibiotics is caused by the production of a species-specific chromosome-mediated β-lactamase. It is not R plasmid–mediated. In 1980, McNicol and coworkers[56] reported the recovery of *Aeromonas* from the Chesapeake Bay that was resistant to tetracycline and polymyxin B. They also noted that 57 per cent of isolates from Bangladesh had a multiple streptomycin-chloramphenicol-tetracycline resistance phenotype that correlated with the presence of a larger plasmid.

PATHOGENESIS

A. hydrophila produces a number of extracellular toxins and enzymes. Alpha- and beta-hemolysins may be significant virulence factors in the pathogenesis of *A. hydrophila* infection. The majority of clinical isolates are beta-hemolytic, and hemolysis is a common feature of infection caused by *Aeromonas.*

Alpha-hemolysin is released from cells during a stationary growth phase. Alpha-hemolysin has a molecular weight of 50,000[49, 51] to 65,000[51] and is stable at room temperature between pH 3.5 and pH 9.5. It is heat-labile. Alpha-hemolysin is cytotoxic to HeLa cells and human embryonic lung fibroblasts.[101] When injected into rabbit skin, it causes dermonecrosis. Intraperitoneal injection of alpha-hemolysin is lethal for rabbits and mice.

Beta-hemolysin has a molecular weight of 49,000 to 53,000 and is released near the end of the logarithmic phase of growth of the *Aeromonas* organism. It is heat-labile and resists destruction by trypsin and pronase.[51] It causes dermonecrosis of rabbit skin and is lethal for rabbits, rats, and mice. It is cytotoxic to HeLa cells and to human diploid lung fibroblasts.[101]

Both alpha- and beta-hemolysin in high concentration produce hemorrhagic enteritis in a rabbit ileal loop; however, neither hemolysin is established as a virulence factor in diarrheal disease.[50] Antibodies to either hemolysin neutralize both toxins.

In 1975, Sanyal and associates[89] demonstrated that the enterotoxins from *A. hydrophila* were enterotoxigenic. Subsequently, enterotoxigenic *A. hydrophila* has been isolated from humans,[10, 30–32, 40, 105] water sources, fish, and pigs.[7, 69] *Aeromonas* enterotoxin has a molecular weight of 15,000 to 20,000 and is heat-labile.

Enterotoxins can be divided into two types: cytotonic and cytotoxic.[41] Cytotonic enterotoxins are those that stimulate the cyclic AMP–mediated sequence of events in cells. Cytotoxic enterotoxins cause cell damage or death. *Aeromonas* enterotoxin induces fluid accumulation in mouse, rat, or rabbit ileal loops and does not injure mucosal cells.[48] It also increases the intracellular content of cyclic AMP in rabbit intestinal epithelial cells. Thus, *Aeromonas* enterotoxin is classified as a cytotonic enterotoxin.[47] Chlopromazine, an inhibitor of cyclic AMP, decreases fluid secretion into intestinal loops induced by *Aeromonas* enterotoxin by 60 per cent.[48]

Aeromonas also produces a heat-stable enterotoxin, proteinase A and B, endopeptidase, staphylolytic enzyme, fibrinolysin, and leukocidin.[49] The precise relationship of these toxins and enzymes to the pathogenesis of human infection is not clear.

Antihemolysin and agglutinating and precipitating antibodies to *A. hydrophila* have been detected in patients with systemic *Aeromonas* infections but not in those with superficial infections. Increases in the antihemolysin titer to as high as 1:1280 and in the agglutinin titer to 1:640 have been noted.[12]

Burke and colleagues[9] found that many strains associated with diarrhea were able to hemagglutinate cells from human, horse, rat, and guinea pig; 68 per cent of these strains displayed fucose-resistant hemagglutination. They suggested that these properties may contribute to virulence.

Ketover and associates[41] showed that normal serum promotes phagocytosis and intracellular killing of *Aeromonas* by normal white blood cells. In contrast, sera from two patients with fatal *Aeromonas* infections failed to do so. One patient had a rise in the serum opsonic antibody titer from less than 1:5 in the acute stage of disease to 1:5120 in the convalescent stage. These studies suggest that a specific opsonizing antibody that is present in normal serum and normal bactericidal activity of neutrophils are required to prevent invasive *A. hydrophila* infections.

Of interest is the lack of correlation between known virulence properties and enteropathogenicity in humans. Morgan and coworkers[61] challenged 57 volunteers with five strains of *A. hydrophila* known to produce cytotoxin, hemolysin, enterotoxin, lysine decarboxylase, acetyl methylcarbinol, and DNAase. All strains produced purulent hemorrhagic fluid accumulation in rabbit ileal loops, but they induced diarrhea in only 2 of 57 human volunteers. Similarly, Kindschuh and colleagues[42] found that the majority of *A. hydrophila* strains produce a cytotoxin and that there is no correlation between the production of cytotoxin and gastroenteritis. In addition, Mégraud[58] noted that only 11 of 44 strains isolated from the feces of children with diarrhea yielded virulence factors, such as cytotoxin, hemolysin, and hemagglutinin.

Kuijper and colleagues[44] also found that correlation between cytotoxigenic strains and the presence of diarrhea was not significant and that the development of diarrhea was associated strongly with host factors such as age.

CLINICAL MANIFESTATIONS

Aeromonas has been implicated as a cause of septicemia, gastroenteritis, peritonitis, skin and wound infections, osteomyelitis, septic arthritis, ocular infections, myositis, urinary tract infections, pneumonia, meningitis, and hemolytic uremic syndrome in children. Most of these manifestations of infection have been noted in both normal and compromised hosts.[6, 24]

Sepsis caused by *Aeromonas* has been reported in at least 38 children.[8, 15, 16, 38, 41, 67, 71, 83, 90, 96, 108–110] Because *Aeromonas* infection is not a reportable disease, the total number of afflicted children is not known. Although septicemia caused by *Aeromonas* has occurred in normal children, most of those affected have had a disorder known to impair the normal host response to infection. *Aeromonas* has been noted in children with leukemia (particularly those with neutropenia), aplastic anemia, cirrhosis, hemoglobinopathies, malnutrition, and renal failure. The clinical manifestations of septicemia are similar to those noted in other gram-negative enteric blood stream infections with high fever and shock. During the course of septicemia in some of these patients, ecthyma gangrenosum also has been noted. The reported case fatality rate of 50 per cent despite antibiotic therapy presumably is related to the severity of the underlying disorders and not to an unusual virulence of the organism. The propensity for infection in the compromised host suggests, in fact, that *Aeromonas* organisms are of low virulence for the human host. Bacteremia with *A. sobria* and *A. punctata* also has been described.[39, 79]

Meningitis due to *Aeromonas* also has been reported in children.[25, 26, 109] In one reported review of 20 years' experience with gram-negative bacillary meningitis, *Aeromonas* species accounted for 2 per cent of the cases.[102] The course was fulminant, and the patients died despite antibiotic therapy. All of these children could be considered immunocompromised as a result of sickle-cell anemia (a 23-month-old child) or age (neonates).

Gastrointestinal infections due to *Aeromonas* have been reported more commonly than septicemia. *A. hydrophila, A. sobria, A. caviae,* and *A. punctata* have been recovered from stool specimens of patients with gastroenteritis.[10, 14, 27, 39, 63] In 1961, Martinez-Silva and colleagues[53] described an epidemic of enteritis in a newborn nursery affecting nine infants (eight as newborns and one 7-day-old baby). *Aeromonas* was found in the stools of six of these infants. One newborn infant died, the only patient with a pure growth of *Aeromonas* in a stool specimen. In 1964, Rosner[84] reported severe gastroenteritis in a child with growth of *A. hydrophila* from four stool cultures.

In an attempt to assess the role of *Aeromonas* in diarrheal disease, a number of investigators have evaluated the fecal carriage rate of the organism.[33] Freij[26] described a study performed by other investigators who recovered *Aeromonas* from 0 of 300 adults and from 31 of 4426 (0.7 per cent) children younger than 2 years of age. Pitarangsi and coworkers[75] reported carrier rates of between 16 and 27 per cent in various districts in Thailand and noted the same frequency of *A. hydrophila* in stools of Thais with and without diarrhea. In contrast, *A. hydrophila* was recovered from the stools of American Peace Corps volunteers more frequently when they had diarrhea than when their stool frequency was normal. Only three *Aeromonas* isolates were reported from 1685 rectal swab cultures obtained from 1217 children hospitalized for gastroenteritis in Manitoba, Canada. Bhat and colleagues[4] recovered *Aeromonas* from 7 of 133 patients with acute diarrhea in a valley in India and found both *Aeromonas* and *Plesiomonas shigelloides* in the well water commonly used by these individuals.

Gracey and associates[31, 32] described a prospective study in Australia of 1156 children with diarrhea and an equal number of age- and sex-matched controls. Enterotoxigenic *Aeromonas* organisms were isolated from 10.2 per cent of children with diarrhea compared with 0.6 per cent of children who were well. *Aeromonas* was the only potential pathogen recovered in 6.5 per cent of children with diarrhea. Cases of *Aeromonas* infection peaked during the summer months. The mean duration of diarrhea was 15.3 days, and 33 per cent of the children required hospitalization. These investigators described three clinical syndromes of *Aeromonas* gastroenteritis: (1) watery diarrhea, vomiting, low-grade fever in 41 per cent; (2) diarrhea with blood and mucus in 22 per cent; and (3) prolonged diarrhea of more than 2 weeks' duration in 37 per cent.

Many investigators[1, 13, 66, 68, 85] have attempted to describe gastrointestinal infections due to *Aeromonas*. A 15-year study of the rate of *Aeromonas* species in gastroenteritis in hospitalized children was performed by Gluskin and associates.[29] One hundred forty-six strains of *Aeromonas* species were isolated from 32,810 fecal specimens from 13,820 hospitalized patients. These isolates constituted 4 per cent of all pathogenic bacterial strains cultured. Most of the cases of diarrhea (94 per cent) occurred in children younger than 3 years of age. The peak incidence was between 2 and 6 months of age. Bloody diarrhea occurred in 7 per cent of children. Several investigators[1, 85] have detected a larger number of cases of *Aeromonas*-associated diarrhea in the summer months than in other months, whereas Challapali and colleagues[13] found no seasonal patterns of *Aeromonas* isolation. The greatest number of cases occurred in children younger than 12 months to 3 years of age.

Symptoms included diarrhea, bloody stools, vomiting, abdominal cramps, mild dehydration, and fever. *Aeromonas*-associated diarrhea resembled other types of bacterial diarrhea, except that fecal leukocytes were absent in children with *Aeromonas*-associated diarrhea, whereas fecal leukocytes were found in 60 per cent of children with other types of bacterial enteritis.[13] A cholera-like illness caused by enterotoxigenic *A. sobria* has been described.[14] Gastroenteritis caused by *A. sobria* and *A. hydrophila* tended to be acute, whereas diarrhea associated with *A. caviae* frequently was chronic, lasting 4 to 6 weeks in untreated patients.

Interestingly, San Joaquin and colleagues[85] described three patients with *A. caviae* diarrhea that originally presented with failure to thrive presumed to be secondary to formula intolerance. These patients' diarrhea improved after administration of trimethoprim-sulfamethoxazole. Moyer[66] noted that although *A. caviae* is considered nonpathogenic, five pediatric patients with otitis media who were treated with penicillin or ampicillin subsequently developed diarrhea in which *A. caviae* was the only potential enteric pathogen. The prior therapy with antibiotics to which *Aeromonas* species are known to be resistant probably contributed to colonization of the gastrointestinal tract with *A. caviae* and subsequent development of diarrhea. These four patients also were treated successfully with trimethoprim-sulfamethoxazole.

Outbreaks of diarrhea associated with *Aeromonas* in day care centers have been described.[18] *A. caviae, A. hydrophila*, and *A. sobria* were the strains recovered most commonly.

Complications of *Aeromonas* intestinal infection included gram-negative bacteremia, intussusception, internal hernia strangulation, hemolytic-uremic syndrome, and failure to thrive.

Peritonitis has been reported in a 5-year-old patient with a ruptured appendix.[38] No additional clinical information about this patient was provided.

A. hydrophila has been recovered from the skin or from wound infections of children.[3, 5, 17, 24, 38, 41, 54, 67, 72, 83, 95, 100, 104] Most of these patients have been normal hosts; three had leukemia. In 40 per cent of these cases, *Aeromonas* was not recovered from the lesion in pure culture. The lower extremity was involved in 75 per cent of these cases. Exposure to water was noted in 40 per cent of these cases; alligator bite, snake bites, stepping on glass, and burns were other presumed predisposing factors. Clinical manifestations included cellulitis, hemorrhagic blebs, and purulent diarrhea with fever and leukocytosis. Secondary bacteremia and osteomyelitis have been reported.[5]

I have recovered *Aeromonas* from skin lesions that have been the result of tick bites. In each of these cases, a circumscribed area of purple discoloration has surrounded the bite, and nonpurulent drainage from the center of the lesion yielded the organism. These patients sought medical attention because the local lesion had persisted or had increased in size over a period of 1 to 2 weeks. *A. schubertii* also has been isolated from traumatic wound infections.[11]

Ecthyma gangrenosum due to *A. hydrophila* has been described in several children with leukemia.[41, 67, 95] I have seen ecthyma gangrenosum in several children with *Aeromonas* septicemia who have had malignancy or hepatobiliary disease.

Lopez and associates[52] described an 8-year-old child with acute myelogenous leukemia with bacteremia and osteomyelitis; *Aeromonas* grew from a bone aspirate of this patient. Blatz[5] reported osteomyelitis and *Aeromonas* bacteremia in a previously healthy 16-year-old patient; a bone aspirate was not attempted. Septic arthritis due to *A. hydrophila* also has been described in a child with leukemia; the organism was recovered from the second metacarpophalangeal joint at autopsy.[16]

Aeromonas has been recovered from the conjunctiva of a previously healthy 7-year-old boy whose eye had been penetrated by a safety pin and from the anterior chamber of an 8-year-old boy who developed endophthalmitis after a corneal laceration from a fish hook.[15, 98]

Although there are a number of reported *Aeromonas* urinary tract infections in adults, only two cases have been reported in children. McCracken and Barkley[54] reported the recovery of *A. hydrophila* in pure culture from the urine of a 5-month-old male with diarrhea. Bartolomé and colleagues[3] described a case of urinary tract infection associated with diarrhea in a male neonate with bilateral ureterohydronephrosis and bladder involvement from posterior urethral valves.

Myositis due to *Aeromonas* also has been described in children. A 9-year-old girl and a 16-year-old boy both required amputation of their legs as a result of *Aeromonas* myositis.[17, 99] Necrosis of muscle was noted in both cases, and gas was seen on the radiographs prior to amputation in the 9-year-old girl.

Aeromonas has been recovered from the throat and sputum of two children with pneumonia. In one of those patients, both *A. hydrophila* and *Streptococcus pneumoniae* were obtained from sputum of a patient who had been hospitalized after a near-drowning accident.

A. hydrophila has been isolated from lung abscess at autopsy of a 16-year-old girl with *A. hydrophila* septicemia and leukemia.[16]

DIAGNOSIS AND DIFFERENTIAL DIAGNOSIS

Aeromonas should be considered as a possible cause of infection in children with any of the disorders previously noted. It always should be included as a possible cause of gastroenteritis, bacteremia, and skin infection in the compromised host.

Generally, *Aeromonas* organisms are recognized only when they grow from body fluids or tissues that normally are sterile. The best methods for isolation of *Aeromonas* have been described (see Etiologic Agent).

A. hydrophila in food can be detected using an enzyme-linked immunosorbent assay.[59] These organisms also have been identified in environmental samples using 16S rDNA–targeted oligonucleotide primers.[20]

TREATMENT AND PROGNOSIS

Infection with *Aeromonas* occurs infrequently; controlled studies to permit recommending one antibiotic in preference to all others are not available. Penicillin-hydrolyzing β-lactamases have been detected in most strains of *Aeromonas*, rendering those strains resistant to ampicillin.[62] Piperacillin shows variable activity against *Aeromonas* species, whereas the ticarcillin-clavulanate combination generally is active. In vitro, *Aeromonas* generally is susceptible to chloramphenicol, aminoglycosides, trimethoprim-sulfamethoxazole, aztreonam, and the third-generation cephalosporins. In my experience, chloramphenicol or third-generation cephalosporins have proved efficacious. A drug to which the organism is sensitive should be provided (usually intravenously). The duration of administration depends upon the site of infection and the clinical response to therapy. The occurrence of *Aeromonas* infections predominantly in the compromised host accounts for the high case fatality rate despite therapy with an antibiotic agent to which the organism is susceptible.

References

1. Agger, W. A., McCormick, J. D., and Gurwith, M. J.: Clinical and microbial features of *Aeromonas hydrophila*–associated diarrhea. J. Clin. Microbiol. *21*:909–913, 1985.
2. Allen, D. A., Austin, B., and Colwell, R. R.: *Aeromonas media*, a new species isolated from river water. Int. J. Syst. Bacteriol. *33*:599, 1983.
3. Bartolomé, R. M., Andreu, A., Xercavins, M., et al.: Urinary tract infection by *Aeromonas hydrophila* in a neonate. Infection *17*:172–173, 1989.
4. Bhat, P., Shanthakumari, S., and Rajan, D.: The characterization and significance of *Plesiomonas shigelloides* and *Aeromonas hydrophila* isolated from an epidemic of diarrhoea. Indian J. Med. Res. *62*:1051–1060, 1974.
5. Blatz, D. J.: Open fracture of the tibia and fibula complicated by infection with *Aeromonas hydrophila*: A case report. J. Bone Joint Surg. (Am.) *61*:790–791, 1979.
6. Bogdanovic, R., Cobeljic, M., Markovic, M., et al.: Haemolytic-uraemic syndrome associated with *Aeromonas hydrophila* enterocolitis. Pediatr. Nephrol. *5*:293–295, 1991.
7. Boulanger, Y., Lallier, R., and Cousineau, G.: Isolation of enterotoxigenic *Aeromonas* from fish. Can. J. Microbiol. *23*:1161–1164, 1977.
8. Bulger, R. J., and Sherris, J. C.: The clinical significance of *Aeromonas hydrophila*: Report of two cases. Arch. Intern. Med. *118*:562–564, 1966.
9. Burke, V., Cooper, M., and Robinson, J.: Haemagglutination patterns of *Aeromonas* spp. related to species and source of strains. Aust. J. Exp. Biol. Med. Sci. *64*:563–570, 1986.
10. Burke, V., Gracey, M., Robinson, J., et al.: The microbiology of childhood gastroenteritis: *Aeromonas* species and other infective agents. J. Infect. Dis. *148*:68–74, 1983.
11. Carnahan, A. M., Marii, M. A., Fanning, G. R., et al.: Characterization of *Aeromonas schubertii* strains recently isolated from traumatic wound infections. J. Clin. Microbiol. *27*:1826–1830, 1989.
12. Caselitz, F. H., Freitag, V., and Jannasch, G.: Demonstration of specific antibodies in sera of patients with infections caused by *Aeromonas hydrophila*. Zentralbl. Bakteriol. Mikrobiol. Hyg. (A) *233*:347–354, 1975.
13. Challapalli, M., Tess, B. R., Cunningham, D. G., et al.: *Aeromonas*-associated diarrhea in children. Pediatr. Infect. Dis. *7*:693–698, 1988.
14. Champsaur, H., Andremont, A., Mathieu, D., et al.: Cholera-like illness due to *Aeromonas sobria*. J. Infect. Dis. *145*:248–254, 1982.
15. Cohen, K. L., Holyk, P. R., McCarthy, L. R., et al.: *Aeromonas hydrophila* and *Plesiomonas shigelloides* endophthalmitis. Am. J. Ophthalmol. *96*:403–404, 1983.
16. Dean, H. M., and Post, R. M.: Fatal infection with *Aeromonas hydrophila* in a patient with acute myelogenous leukemia. Ann. Intern. Med. *66*:1177–1179, 1967.
17. Deepe, G. S., and Coonrod, J. D.: Fulminant wound infection with *Aeromonas hydrophila*. South. Med. J. *73*:1546–1547, 1980.
18. de la Morena, M. L., Van, R., Singh, K., et al.: Diarrhea associated with *Aeromonas* species in children in day care centers. J. Infect. Dis. *168*: 215–218, 1993.
19. Dobrescu, L.: Enterotoxigenic *Aeromonas hydrophila* from a case of piglet diarrhea. Zentralbl. Veterinarmed. (B) *25*:713–718, 1978.
20. Dorsch, M., Ashbolt, N. J., Cox, P. T., et al.: Rapid identification of *Aeromonas* species using 16S rDNA targeted oligonucleotide primers: A molecular approach based on screening of environmental isolates. J. Appl. Bacteriol. *77*:722–726, 1994.
21. Ewing, W. H., and Hugh, R.: *Aeromonas*. *In* Lennette, E. H., Spaulding, E. H., and Truant, J. P. (eds.): Manual of Clinical Microbiology. 2nd ed. Washington, D.C., American Society for Microbiology, 1974, pp. 230–237.
22. Ewing, W. H., Hugh, R., and Johnson, J. G.: Studies on the *Aeromonas* group. Public Health Service, Communicable Disease Center, 1961, pp. 1–8.
23. Fainstein, V., Weaver, S., and Bodey, G. P.: In vitro susceptibilities of *Aeromonas hydrophila* against new antibiotics. Antimicrob. Agents Chemother. *22*:513–514, 1982.
24. Fraire, A. E.: *Aeromonas hydrophila* infection. J. A. M. A. *239*:192, 1978.
25. Freij, B. J.: *Aeromonas*: Biology of the organism and diseases in children. Pediatr. Infect. Dis. *3*:164–175, 1984.
26. Freij, B. J.: Human disease other than gastroenteritis caused by *Aeromonas* and *Plesiomonas*. *Aeromonas* Symposium, Manchester, England, September 5–6, 1986, pp. 19–20.
27. Fritsche, D., Dahn, R., and Hoffmann, G.: *Aeromonas punctata* subsp. *caviae* as the causative agent of acute gastroenteritis. Zentralbl. Bakteriol. Mikrobiol. Hyg. (A) *233*:232–235, 1975.
28. Gilbert, D. N., Sanford, J. P., Kutscher, E., et al.: Microbiologic study of wound infections in tornado casualties. Arch. Environ. Health *26*:125–130, 1973.
29. Gluskin, I., Batash, D. D., Shoseyov, et al.: A 15-year study of the role of *Aeromonas* spp. in gastroenteritis in hospitalised children. J. Med. Microbiol. *37*:315–318, 1992.
30. Goodwin, C. S., Harper, W. E. S., Steward, J. K., et al.: Enterotoxigenic *Aeromonas hydrophila* and diarrhoea in adults. Med. J. Aust. *1*:25–26, 1983.
31. Gracey, M., Burke, V., and Robinson, J.: *Aeromonas*-associated gastroenteritis. Lancet *2*:1304–1306, 1982.
32. Gracey, M., Burke, V., Rockhill, R. C., et al.: *Aeromonas* species as enteric pathogens. Lancet *1*:223–224, 1982.
33. Gurwith, M. J., and Williams, T. W.: Gastroenteritis in children: A two-year review in Manitoba. I. Etiology. J. Infect. Dis. *136*:239–247, 1977.
34. Hazen, T. E., Fliermans, C. B., and Hirsch, R. P.: Prevalence and distribution of *Aeromonas hydrophila* in the United States. Appl. Environ. Microbiol. *36*:731–738, 1978.
35. Hickman-Brenner, F. W., Fanning, G. R., Arduino, M. J., et al.: *Aeromonas schubertii*, a new mannitol-negative species found in human clinical specimens. J. Clin. Microbiol. *26*:1561–1564, 1988.
36. Hickman-Brenner, F. W., MacDonald, K. L., Steigerwalt, A. G., et al.: *Aeromonas veronii*, a new ornithine decarboxylase–positive species that may cause diarrhea. J. Clin. Microbiol. *25*:900–906, 1987.
37. Hird, D. W., Diesch, S. L., McKinnel, R. G., et al.: *Aeromonas hydrophila* in wild-caught frogs and tadpoles *(Rana pipiens)* in Minnesota. Lab. Anim. Sci. *31*:166–169, 1981.
38. Hunter, W. F., and Atkinson, H. M.: Infection due to *Aeromonas hydrophila*. Med. J. Aust. *1*:565, 1968.
39. Janda, J. M., Bottone, E. J., and Reitano, M.: *Aeromonas* species in clinical microbiology: Significance, epidemiology and speciation. Diagn. Microbiol. Infect. Dis. *1*:221–228, 1983
40. Kaper, J. B., Lockman, H., and Colwell, R. R.: *Aeromonas hydrophila*: Ecology and toxigenicity of isolates from an estuary. J. Appl. Bacteriol. *50*:359–377, 1981.
41. Ketover, B. P., Young, L. S., and Armstrong, D.: Septicemia due to *Aeromonas hydrophila*: Clinical and immunologic aspects. J. Infect. Dis. *127*:284–290, 1973.
42. Kindschuh, M., Pickering, L. K., Cleary, T. G., et al.: Clinical and biochemical significance of toxin production by *Aeromonas hydrophila*. J. Clin. Microbiol. *25*:916–921, 1987.
43. King, G. E., Werner, S. B., and Kizer, K. W.: Epidemiology of *Aeromonas* infections in California. Clin. Infect. Dis. *15*:449–452, 1992.
44. Kuijper, E. J., Peeters, M. F., Steigerwalt, A. G., et al.: Clinical and epidemiologic aspects of members of *Aeromonas* DNA hybridization groups isolated from human feces. J. Clin. Microbiol. *27*:1531–1537, 1989.
45. Kuijper, E. J., van Alphen, L., Leenders, E., et al.: Typing of *Aeromonas* strains by DNA restriction endonuclease analysis and polyacrylamide gel electrophoresis of cell envelopes. J. Clin. Microbiol. *27*:1280–1285, 1989.
46. Leclerc, H., and Buttiaux, R.: Fréquence des *Aeromonas* dans les eaux d'alimentation. Ann. Inst. Pasteur. *103*:97–100, 1962.
47. Ljungh, A., Eneroth, P., and Wadstrom, T.: Cytotonic enterotoxin from *Aeromonas hydrophila*. Toxicon *20*:787–794, 1982.
48. Ljungh, A., and Kronevi, T.: *Aeromonas hydrophila* toxins: Intestinal fluid accumulation and mucosal injury in animal models. Toxicon *20*:397–407, 1982.
49. Ljungh, A., and Wadstrom, T.: *Aeromonas* toxins. Pharmacol. Ther. *15*:339–354, 1982.
50. Ljungh, A., and Wadstrom, T.: *Aeromonas* and *Plesiomonas* as possible causes of diarrhea. Infection *13*:169–173, 1985.
51. Ljungh, A., and Wadstrom, T.: Toxins of *Vibrio para-haemolyticus* and *Aeromonas hydrophila*. J. Toxicol. Toxin Rev. *1*:257–307, 1982–1983.
52. Lopez, J. F., Quesada, J., and Saied, A.: Bacteremia and osteomyelitis due to *Aeromonas hydrophila*: A complication during treatment of acute leukemia. Am. J. Clin. Pathol. *50*:587–591, 1968.
53. Martinez-Silva, V. R., Guzmann-Urrego, M., and Caselitz, F. H.: Zur frage der bedeutung aeromonasstammen bei sauglingsenteritis. Z. Tropenmed. Parasitol. *12*:445–451, 1961.
54. McCracken, A. W., and Barkely, R.: Isolation of *Aeromonas* species from clinical sources. J. Clin. Pathol. *25*:970–975, 1972.
55. McGrath, V. A., Overman, S. B., and Overman, T. L.: Media-dependent oxidase reaction in a strain of *Aeromonas hydrophila*. J. Clin. Microbiol. *5*:112–113, 1977.
56. McNicol, L. A., Aziz, K. M. S., Huq, I., et al.: Isolation of drug-resistant *Aeromonas hydrophila* from aquatic environments. Antimicrob. Agents Chemother. *17*:477–483, 1980.
57. Meeks, M. V.: The genus *Aeromonas*: Methods for identification. Am. J. Med. Technol. *29*:361–378, 1963.
58. Mégraud, F.: Incidence and virulence of *Aeromonas* species in feces of children with diarrhea. Eur. J. Clin. Microbiol. *5*:311–316, 1986.
59. Merino, S., Camprubi, S., and Tomas, J. M.: Detection of *Aeromonas hy-*

drophila in food with an enzyme-linked immunosorbent assay. J. Appl. Bacteriol. *74*:149–154, 1993.

60. Mishva, S., Nair, G. B., and Bhadra, R. K.: Comparison of selective media for primary isolation of *Aeromonas* species from human and animal feces. J. Clin. Microbiol. *25*:2040–2043, 1987.
61. Morgan, D. R., Johnson, P. C., DuPont, H. L., et al.: Lack of correlation between known virulence properties of *Aeromonas hydrophila* and enteropathogenicities for humans. Infect. Immun. *50*:62–65, 1985.
62. Morita, K., Watanabe, N., Kurata, S., et al.: β-Lactam resistance of motile *Aeromonas* isolates from clinical and environmental sources. Antimicrob. Agents Chemother. *38*:353–355, 1994.
63. Motyl, M. R., and Janda, J. M.: *Aeromonas* gastroenteritis: A two-year survey. Presented at the 23rd Interscience Conference on Antimicrobial Agents and Chemotherapy, Las Vegas, October 24–26, 1983.
64. Motyl, M. R., McKinley, G., and Janda, J. M.: In vitro susceptibilities of *Aeromonas hydrophila, Aeromonas sobria,* and *Aeromonas caviae* to 22 antimicrobial agents. Antimicrob. Agents Chemother. *28*:151–153, 1985.
65. Moulsdale, M. T.: Isolation of *Aeromonas* from faeces. Lancet *1*:351, 1983.
66. Moyer, N. P.: Clinical significance of *Aeromonas* species isolated from patients with diarrhea. J. Clin. Microbiol. *25*:2044–2048, 1987.
67. Moyes, C. D., Sykes, P. A., and Rayner, J. M.: *Aeromonas hydrophila* septicaemia producing ecthyma gangrenosum in a child with leukaemia. Scand. J. Infect. Dis. *9*:151–153, 1977.
68. Nygaard, G. S., Biosett, M. L., and Wood, R. M.: Laboratory identification of aeromonads from man to other animals. Appl. Microbiol. *19*:618–620, 1970.
69. Olivier, G., Lallier, R., and Lariviere, S.: A toxigenic profile of *Aeromonas hydrophila* and *Aeromonas sobria* isolated from fish. Can. J. Microbiol. *27*:330–333, 1981.
70. Paik, G.: Reagents, stains, and miscellaneous test procedures. *In* Lennette, E. H., Balows, A., Hausler, W. J., Jr., et al. (eds.): Manual of Clinical Microbiology. 3rd ed. Washington, D.C., American Society for Microbiology, 1980, pp. 1006–1007.
71. Pearson, T. A., Mithchell, C. A., and Hughes, W. T.: *Aeromonas hydrophila* septicemia. Am. J. Dis. Child. *123*:579–582, 1972.
72. Phillips, J. A., Bernhardt, H. E., and Rosenthal, S. G.: *Aeromonas hydrophila* infections. Pediatrics *53*:110–112, 1974.
73. Picard, B., Arlet, G., and Goullet, P.: Origin hydrique d'infections hospitalieres a *Aeromonas hydrophila*. Presse Med. *12*:700, 1983.
74. Picard, B., and Goullet, P.: Seasonal prevalence of nosocomial *Aeromonas hydrophila* infection related to *Aeromonas* in hospital water. J. Hosp. Infect. *10*:152–155, 1987.
75. Pitarangsi, C., Escheverria, P., Whitmire, R., et al.: Enteropathogenicity of *Aeromonas hydrophila* and *Plesiomonas shigelloides*: Prevalence among individuals with and without diarrhea in Thailand. Infect. Immun. *35*:666–673, 1982.
76. Pittman, M.: A study of bacteria implicated in transfusion reactions and of bacteria isolated from blood products. J. Lab. Clin. Med. *42*:273–288, 1953.
77. Popoff, M.: Genus III: *Aeromonas* Kluyver and van Niel 1936. *In* Krieg, N. R., and Holt, J. G. (eds.): Bergey's Manual of Systematic Bacteriology. Baltimore, Williams & Wilkins, 1984, p. 545.
78. Ramsey, A. M., Rosenbaum, B. J., Yarbrough, C. L., et al.: *Aeromonas hydrophila* sepsis in patient undergoing hemodialysis therapy. J. A. M. A. *239*:128–129, 1978.
79. Raszeja, S., Krynski, S., Krueger, A., et al.: Blood contamination with *Aeromonas hydrophilus* as a cause of lethal post-transfusion complications. Pol. Tyg. Lek. *28*:1159–1162, 1973.
80. Reines, H. D., and Cook, F. V.: Pneumonia and bacteremia due to *Aeromonas hydrophila*. Chest *80*:264–267, 1981.
81. Reinhardt, J. F., and George, W. L.: Comparative in vitro activities of selected antimicrobial agents against *Aeromonas* species and *Plesiomonas shigelloides*. Antimicrob. Agents Chemother. *27*:643–645, 1985.
82. Rogol, M., Sechter, I., Grinberg, L., et al.: Prilxylose-ampicillin agar, a new selective medium for the isolation of *Aeromonas hydrophila*. J. Med. Microbiol. *12*:229–231, 1979.
83. Rosenthal, S. G., Bernhardt, H. E., and Phillips, J. A.: *Aeromonas hydrophila* wound infection. Plast. Reconstr. Surg. *53*:77–79, 1974.
84. Rosner, R.: *Aeromonas hydrophila* as the etiologic agent in a case of gastroenteritis. Am. J. Clin. Pathol. *42*:402–404, 1964.
85. San Joaquin, V. H., and Pickett, D. A.: *Aeromonas*-associated gastroenteritis in children. Pediatr. Infect. Dis. *7*:53–57, 1988.
86. San Joaquin, V. H., Pickett, D. A., Welch, D. F., et al.: *Aeromonas* species in aquaria: A reservoir of gastrointestinal infections? J. Hosp. Infect. *13*:173–177, 1989.
87. San Joaquin, V. H., Scribner, R. K., Pickett, D. A., et al.: Antimicrobial susceptibility of *Aeromonas* species isolated from patients with diarrhea. Antimicrob. Agents Chemother. *30*:794–795, 1986.
88. Sanarelli, G.: Ueber einem neuen mikroorganismus des wassers, welcher fuer tieren mit veranderlichen und konstanter temperatur pathogen ist. Zentralbl. Bakteriol. Parasitenk. *9*:193–199, 222–228, 1891.
89. Sanyal, S. C., Singh, S. J., and Sen, P. C.: Enteropathogenicity of *Aeromonas hydrophila* and *Plesiomonas shigelloides*. J. Med. Microbiol. *8*:195–198, 1975.
90. Sasu, D., and Apostica, E.: On a strain of *Aeromonas liquefaciens* isolated from blood. Microbiologia (Bucur) *12*:437–441, 1967.
91. Sawai, T., Takahashi, I., Nakagawa, H., et al.: Immunochemical comparison between an oxacillin-hydrolyzing penicillinase of *Aeromonas hydrophila* and those mediated by R plasmids. J. Bacteriol. *135*:281–282, 1978.
92. Schubert, R. H. W.: Genus II: *Aeromonas*. *In* Buchanan, R., and Gibbons, N. (eds.): Bergey's Manual of Determinative Bacteriology. 8th ed. Baltimore, Williams & Wilkins, 1974, pp. 345–348.
93. Schubert, R. H. W., and Hegazi, M.: *Aeromonas eucrenophila* species nova *Aeromonas caviae*: A later and illegitimate synonym of *Aeromonas punctata*. Zentralbl. Bakteriol. Mikrobiol. Hyg. (A) *268*:34–39, 1988.
94. Seidler, R. J., Allen, D. A., Bockman, H., et al.: Isolation, enumeration and characterization of *Aeromonas* from polluted waters encountered in diving operations. Appl. Environ. Microbiol. *39*:1010–1018, 1980.
95. Shackelford, P. G., Ratzan, S. A., and Shearer, W. T.: Ecthyma gangrenosum produced by *Aeromonas hydrophila*. J. Pediatr. *83*:100–101, 1973.
96. Sirinavin, S., Likitnukul, S., and Lolekha, S.: *Aeromonas* septicemia in infants and children. Pediatr. Infect. Dis. *3*:122–125, 1984.
97. Slotnick, I. J.: *Aeromonas* species isolates. Ann. N. Y. Acad. Sci. *174*:503–510, 1970.
98. Smith, J. A.: Ocular *Aeromonas hydrophila*. Am. J. Ophthalmol. *89*:449–451, 1980.
99. Smith, J. A.: *Aeromonas hydrophila*: Analysis of 11 cases. Can. Med. Assoc. J. *122*:1270–1272, 1980.
100. Stephens, S., Rao, K. N. A., Kumar, M. S., et al.: Human infection with *Aeromonas* species: Varied clinical manifestations. Ann. Intern. Med. *83*:368–369, 1975.
101. Thelestam, M., and Ljungh, A.: Membrane-damaging and cytotoxic effects on human fibroblasts of alpha- and beta-hemolysins from *Aeromonas hydrophila*. Infect. Immun. *34*:949–956, 1981.
102. Unhanand, M., Mustafa, M. M., McCracken, G. H., Jr., et al.: Gram-negative enteric bacillary meningitis: A twenty-one-year experience. J. Pediatr. *122*:15–21, 1993.
103. von Graevenitz, A.: *Aeromonas* and *Plesiomonas*. *In* Lennette, E. H., Balows, A., Hausler, W. H., et al. (eds.): Manual of Clinical Microbiology. 3rd ed. Washington, D.C., American Society for Microbiology, 1980, pp. 220–225.
104. von Graevenitz, A., and Bucher, C.: Evaluation of differential and selective media for isolation of *Aeromonas* and *Plesiomonas* spp. from human feces. J. Clin. Microbiol. *77*:16–21, 1983.
105. Wadstrom, T., Aust-Kettis, A., Habte, D., et al.: Enterotoxin-producing bacteria and parasites in stools of Ethiopian children with diarrhoeal disease. Arch. Dis. Child. *51*:865–870, 1976.
106. Wakabongo, M., Bortey, E., Meier, F. A., et al.: Rapid identification of motile *Aeromonas*. Diagn. Microbiol. Infect. Dis. *15*:511–515, 1992.
107. Warburton, D. W., McCormick, J. K., and Bowen, B.: Survival and recovery of *Aeromonas hydrophila* in water: Development of methodology for testing bottled water in Canada. Can. J. Microbiol. *40*:145–148, 1994.
108. Washington, J. A., II: The role of *Aeromonas hydrophila* in clinical infection. *In* Holloway, W. J. (ed.): Infectious Disease Reviews. Vol. 2. Mount Kisco, NY, Futura Publishing, 1973, pp. 75–86.
109. Yadava, R., Seeler, R. A., Kalelkar, M., et al.: Fatal *Aeromonas hydrophila* sepsis and meningitis in a child with sickle cell anemia. Am. J. Dis. Child. *133*:753–754, 1979.
110. Zajc-Satler, J.: Morphological and biochemical studies of 27 strains belonging to the genus *Aeromonas* isolated from clinical sources. J. Med. Microbiol. *5*:263–265, 1972.

120

PASTEURELLA MULTOCIDA

Barbara W. Stechenberg

In 1878, Kitt first isolated a bacterium of the *Pasteurella* group from wild hogs during an epidemic; 2 years later, Pasteur described the organism that causes fowl cholera. Since that time, the same organism has been implicated in rabbit septicemia, swine plague, hemorrhagic septicemia, and wildseuche (a fatal disease in deer). Hueppe applied the term *hemorrhagic septicemia* to this group of infectious diseases in lower animals because of the characteristic hemorrhagic areas scattered throughout most of the viscera. Original names for the causative organisms included *Pasteurella aviseptica, boviseptica, suiseptica*, and *lepiseptica*, but these now are classified under the name *Pasteurella multocida*, a small, nonmotile, gram-negative rod.[35]

Although *P. multocida* primarily is a pathogen in the animal world, there has been increasing recognition of its potential for infection in humans. Brugnatelli reported the first bacteriologically proven case in a human in 1913. Schipper[31] made an extensive review of the literature from 1930 through 1947 and reported only 40 cases of *P. multocida* infection. Subsequently, an increasing number of reports of human infection with *P. multocida* have been reported.

THE ORGANISM

P. multocida generally appears as a short, ovoid, gram-negative rod; however, the form may vary from this to coccobacilli with convex sides and rounded ends. The length ranges from 0.3 to 1.25 μm and the diameter from 0.15 to 0.25 μm. It may appear singly or in pairs, chains, or clusters. Healthy organisms stain easily with aniline dyes and are gram-negative. They may show bipolar staining, especially when smears are made directly from animal tissue or fluids. They become increasingly pleomorphic on subculture and may resemble enterics in broth. They do not grow on eosin–methylene blue agar, MacConkey, deoxycholate, or any other bile-containing agar. They do not require X or V factor for growth, an important differential point in distinguishing them from *Haemophilus influenzae*. Some strains require serum, and some may grow primarily on solid media because of a requirement for a low oxidation-reduction potential for primary isolation.

Colonies are nonhemolytic and translucent, usually 1 to 2 mm in diameter, and generally low, convex, and butyrous. Occasionally, they may be larger and mucoid. In a study of 30 strains isolated from humans, Heddleston and Wessman[12] reported that 9 of the cultures produced watery mucoid colonies, 4 produced iridescent colonies, 10 produced blue colonies, and 3 produced a mixture of iridescent and blue colonies. Colonies on blood agar are smaller, opaque, and grayish-white. In broth cultures, there is turbidity, often with a flocculent sediment.

Cultures tend to autoagglutinate in saline and have a peculiar odor described as musty, like semen or burning hair. They are catalase-positive, usually oxidase-positive, and indole-positive. They usually ferment galactose, glucose, fructose, mannitol, mannose, and sucrose without gas production. There is some variability in the fermentation of other sugars. They reduce nitrates but have negative results for urease, methyl red, and Voges-Proskauer reactions. Using fermentation reactions, Oberhofer[22] developed a biotyping system in which there was correlation of biotype, 61 per cent A and B, with cat-bite isolates but not with dog-bite isolates.

The pathogenicity of the organism is variable; most mucoid and smooth colony-forming strains produce a capsule and usually are highly pathogenic for mice and rabbits. Some smooth, nonencapsulated variants and rough variants have low pathogenicity for mice.

By use of the indirect hemagglutination test with capsular antigens absorbed onto human type O erythrocytes, five serotypes (A, B, C, D, and E) were selected. A and D are the most common in cultures of human origin. A newer capsule serogroup, serogroup F, has been isolated from turkeys.[28] Nielsen and Rosdahl[20] have developed a bacteriophage typing system for typing toxigenic and nontoxigenic strains. DNA hybridization studies have allowed a reclassification of the genus *Pasteurella*. *P. multocida* now includes three subspecies—*P. multocida* subspecies *multocida*, P. *multocida* subspecies *septica*, and *P. multocida* subspecies *gallicida*. Of 159 strains recovered from 46 infected humans, 95 were identified as *P. multocida* subspecies *multocida* and 21 as *P. multocida* subspecies *septica*, the rest being divided among multiple other species.[13] The use of serology in conjunction with DNA fingerprinting can classify isolates for epidemiologic studies.[42]

Immunity to *P. multocida* can be demonstrated in many animals, and vaccines have been developed with known efficacy, especially in birds and cattle. However, the precise mechanisms involved in this immunity and, more important, in natural immunity have not been elucidated. Woolcock and Collins[43] have developed models in pathogen-free mice that may help uncover these mechanisms. The efficacy of heat-killed vaccine has been shown to be considerable when multiple doses are used. However, with the use of an aerogenic mouse model for the stimulation of respiratory spread, the protection is reduced. Local instillation of the vaccine can be used with this model to develop local antibodies, but preliminary results show protection only with very modest challenge doses.[3] A footpad inoculation model may help elucidate the mechanisms in local human infections.

TRANSMISSION

The organism is found in the oral flora of many different animals. As many as 67 per cent of cats may harbor this organism in their mouths or throats. Smith[32] found that *P. multocida* could be recovered from the tonsils of 54 per cent and from the nose of 10 per cent of dogs. Schipper[31] grew it from 14 per cent of wild rats trapped in the Baltimore area. Hansmann and Tully[11] demonstrated that *P. multocida* may remain as a commensal for prolonged periods in the mouth of a cat. They described a patient who had been bitten on two occasions 3 years apart by the same healthy pet cat; each time, an abscess due to *P. multocida* developed. It has been isolated also from lion, panther, buffalo, mink, and opossum.[14]

Although it has been easiest to verify the mode of transmission when there has been an infection related specifically to a pet or farm animal, many cases of infection due to *P. multocida* have been documented despite a negative history of such exposure. Respiratory infection with this organism has been described in veterinarians, farmers, milkmen, and persons employed where animal tissues are processed. Meningitis due to *P. multocida* has been described in a patient after brain surgery in which rabbit muscle was used for hemostasis.

The possibility of a reservoir of infection in humans with resultant interhuman transmission rarely has been considered. In a study of veterinary students, Smith[32] reported 2 of 71 with positive throat isolations. The organisms were present in one for a few days and in the other for the full 4 months of the study; both were asymptomatic. There have been several other cases of isolation of the organism from the human respiratory tract, many without associated symptoms or known animal contact.

In addition, interhuman spread by nasopharyngeal excretions, feces, and urine also is a possibility, because the organism has been recovered from these sites. The female genital tract is another potential source, especially for cases of septicemia and meningitis during pregnancy and in the newborn period.

Investigators of an outbreak in a chronic disease hospital showed that *P. multocida* may be viable on a hand towel for up to 24 hours; although the source in this outbreak was not proved, this may have implications for spread in other situations, particularly for pet owners.[16]

EPIDEMIOLOGY

P. multocida has been isolated from humans in all areas of North America and Europe, with some reports from other areas. In the United States, it is not a reportable organism, so incidence and prevalence data are unavailable. Lee and Buhr[19] have cited a seasonal variation in the number of reported dog bite–related cases, with the highest incidence being in the fall and winter months, possibly related to increased nasal carriage in dogs during that period. Other investigators, however, have found no seasonal differences.[7, 15]

There appears to be no difference in attack rate between the sexes. The attack rate is higher in individuals of both sexes in the very young (0 to 4 years of age) and in older individuals (>55 years of age).

PATHOGENESIS AND PATHOLOGY

In animals that are stressed, a benignly parasitic strain may invade the mucous membrane on which it is carried. With highly virulent strains, a picture of hemorrhagic septicemia may develop. This may be characterized by high fever, cardiac weakness, toxemia, and early death. Organisms can be cultured from the blood; autopsy findings may be minimal or include petechial hemorrhages on mucosal and serosal surfaces and in various organs. Less acute forms, such as a pneumonia with serofibrinous exudate in the interlobular septa of the lungs, a hemorrhagic gastroenteritis, and subacute and chronic infections, such as otitis in the rabbit, may occur.

In humans, there are three major types of infection.[41] In the first and most common type, there is local infection after a cat bite or scratch, a dog bite, or, rarely, the bite of another animal. Usually, these are characterized by a rapidly progressive, acute cellulitis with lymphangitis, local lymphadenitis, or both. In the case of cat bites, these may progress to osteomyelitis of the underlying bone. This is not because of any known predilection of *P. multocida* for the bone but because the sharp fangs of the cat deposit the organism on or under the periosteum.

The secondary type includes cases of chronic pulmonary infection in which the organism may be the only isolate or one of several organisms. Cases of bronchiectasis and empyema have been reported, usually in patients with underlying pulmonary disease. In a series of 28 cases of bronchiectasis in which the organism was recovered, it usually appeared as a secondary invader. It appears to have low pathogenicity in the respiratory tract until some other infection or physiologic disturbance decreases the natural resistance of the host, which enables active infection to occur.

Pasteurella infection also may be septicemic or occur with meningitis. The pathology and pathogenesis are not unlike those of other organisms.

CLINICAL MANIFESTATIONS

In cases of local infection from a scratch or bite, the usual clinical pattern shows swelling, erythema, and tenderness within a few hours of the bite; the majority of symptoms are manifest within the first 24 hours. There may be a gray-colored serous or sanguinopurulent discharge from the puncture sites. Signs of systemic toxic effects, such as chills and fever, may or may not be present; regional lymphadenopathy often is evident. Less commonly, the infection may be more low-grade and smoldering.[26] As noted, osteomyelitis and tenosynovitis most often occur after cat bites because of the sharpness of their teeth.

Lee and Buhr[19] found *P. multocida* to be the most common infecting organism in a report of 69 dog bites that had been cultured; 20 of the bites became grossly infected, and *P. multocida* was isolated from 10. Of 30 wounds that were sutured, 14 (47 per cent) were infected with *P. multocida*.

Other unusual localized infections include chronic skin ulcers, secondary infection of a gouty joint, and infection of a compound fracture site and an amputation site.[38]

Clinical manifestations of those patients having respiratory complaints are not unusual. Most of the isolates have been associated with chronic bronchitis, bronchiectasis, chronic sinusitis and/or otitis media, and pneumonia. Several cases of massive pulmonary abscesses, pleural effusion, and empyema also have been reported. Larsen and Holden[18] described a 14-year-old girl with chronic otitis media for 2 years who developed a *P. multocida* cerebellar abscess. One case of epiglottitis due to this organism has been reported in an adult.[17]

In a report of 136 cases of *P. multocida* infection that were not related to animal bites, the most common site of infection after the respiratory tract was the abdomen; the organism was recovered from 10 patients with appendicitis. Eight isolates were from the female reproductive tract, four from the urine, and one from a chronic sacral abscess.[15] Whether these cases are secondary to ingestion of the organism or to hematogenous spread has not been determined. Raffi and colleagues[25] described three children with appendiceal peritonitis associated with *P. multocida*.

The disseminated infections are the other major clinical group of *Pasteurella* infections. Isolated bacteremia may be present[24]; however, the majority of these have been cases of meningitis, many of which were mistaken for cases of *H. influenzae* or *Neisseria meningitidis* infection because of the morphologic similarities among these organisms. In a review of the subject in 1967, Controni and Jones[5] noted 14 confirmed cases of *Pasteurella* meningitis; 11 occurred in adults,

3 in children. Eight of the 14 cases had a history of accidental or surgical trauma. The mortality rate was 50 per cent, but only five patients were treated with antibiotics. Evaluation of the cerebrospinal fluid showed white blood cell counts from 580 to 5200/mm^3, all with a predominance of polymorphonuclear leukocytes.

That review included one newborn infant who died of *Pasteurella* meningitis at 88 hours of age.[1] The mother had a fever in the postpartum period, but her pretreatment cultures were lost, so verification of the source was impossible.[7] Since then, there has been a report of *Pasteurella* chorioamnionitis associated with premature delivery and neonatal sepsis and death within 1.5 hours of delivery.[34] Gingival cultures of a pet cat that had scratched a mother numerous times during pregnancy also yielded *P. multocida*. Subsequently, several young infants with septicemia and meningitis due to this organism have survived without apparent sequelae after treatment with penicillin or ampicillin and gentamicin.[2, 8, 27, 37] Another report of neonatal infection was that by Pizey[23] of a 3-week-old infant with septic arthritis. *P. multocida* infection may take a rapidly fatal course even in an older infant.[36] Clapp and associates[4] described two infants whose disease was associated with nontraumatic facial licking by pets, an avoidable exposure. In another report, a case of in utero infection at 12 weeks' gestation was described.[40]

DIAGNOSIS AND TREATMENT

Although *P. multocida* is one of the more likely pathogens to cause infection of cat or dog bites, its clinical manifestations are not unusual. Diagnosis of *P. multocida* infection can be made definitively only by culture. It may resemble several other organisms morphologically, but its identification should not be difficult. The fact that it does not require X and V factors for growth should distinguish it from *H. influenzae*. Its production of indole should differentiate it from the *Neisseria* group, and its inability to grow on MacConkey or a bile salt medium should distinguish it from *Acinetobacter* species and the enteric organisms.

The drug of choice for *P. multocida* infection is penicillin, to which the organism is exquisitely sensitive. This feature may be used as a rapid means of distinguishing it from *H. influenzae* or the enterics. Rare strains producing β-lactamase and thus resistant to penicillins have been recovered.[29] Usually, the organism is sensitive to a wide variety of other antibiotics, including ampicillin, other broad-spectrum penicillins (e.g., ticarcillin, piperacillin, mezlocillin), ampicillin–clavulanic acid,[9] tetracyclines, parenteral cephalosporins (particularly second- and third-generation),[21] and chloramphenicol. Semisynthetic penicillins (e.g., nafcillin, methicillin, dicloxacillin), erythromycin, orally administered cephalosporins (cephalexin, cefaclor), clindamycin, and aminoglycosides have relatively low activity against *P. multocida*.[6, 10, 33] The newer macrolide azithromycin appears to have acceptable activity.[6] Trimethoprim-sulfamethoxazole may be an alternative, particularly for those unable to take a β-lactam antibiotic.[30] Surgical drainage or débridement also may be necessary. The duration of treatment depends on the primary disease process.

Proper cleansing and débridement of wounds caused by animal bites or scratches are important in prevention of this infection. Lee and Buhr[19] found that suturing of wounds due to dog bite was associated with a higher incidence of infection. No vaccine for human use is available.

Prognosis depends on the particular site of infection. With appropriate treatment, resolution usually occurs, but the healing process may be very slow, particularly in local infections with extension to the bone or tendons.[7, 39]

References

1. Bates, H. A., Controni, G., Elliott, N., et al.: Septicemia and meningitis in a newborn due to *Pasteurella multocida*. Clin. Pediatr. *4*:668–670, 1965.
2. Bhave, S. A., Guy, L. M., and Rycroft, J. A.: *Pasteurella multocida* meningitis in an infant with recovery. Br. Med. J. *2*:741–742, 1977.
3. Branson, D., and Bunkfeldt, F.: *Pasteurella multocida* in animal bites of humans. Am. J. Clin. Pathol. *48*:552–555, 1967.
4. Clapp, W. C., Kleiman, M. B., Reynolds, J. K., et al.: *Pasteurella multocida* meningitis in infancy. Am. J. Dis. Child. *140*:444–446, 1986.
5. Controni, G., and Jones, R. S.: Pasteurella meningitis: A review of the literature. Am. J. Med. Technol. *33*:379–386, 1967.
6. Fass, R. J.: Erythromycin, clarithromycin and azithromycin: Use of frequency, distribution, curves, scattergrams and regression analyses to compare in vitro activities and describe cross-resistance. Antimicrob. Agents Chemother. *37*:2080–2086, 1993.
7. Francis, D. P., Holmes, M. A., and Brandon, G.: *Pasteurella multocida*: Infection after domestic animal bites and scratches. J. A. M. A. *233*:42–45, 1975.
8. Frutos, A. A., Levitsky, D., Scott, E. G., et al.: A case of septicemia and meningitis in an infant due to *Pasteurella multocida*. J. Pediatr. *92*:853, 1978.
9. Goldstein, E. J. C., and Citron, D. M.: Comparative activities of cefuroxime, amoxicillin–clavulanic acid, ciprofloxacin, enoxacin, and ofloxacin against aerobic and anaerobic bacteria isolated from bite wounds. Antimicrob. Agents Chemother. *32*:1144–1148, 1988.
10. Goldstein, E. J. C., Citron, D. M., and Rechwald, G. A.: Lack of in vitro efficacy of oral forms of certain cephalosporins, erythromycin and oxacillin against *Pasteurella multocida*. Antimicrob. Agents Chemother. *32*:213–215, 1988.
11. Hansmann, G. H., and Tully, M.: Cat bite and scratch wounds with consequent *Pasteurella* infection of man. Am. J. Clin. Pathol. *15*:312–318, 1945.
12. Heddleston, K. L., and Wessman, G.: Characteristics of *Pasteurella multocida* of human origin. J. Clin. Microbiol. *1*:377–383, 1975.
13. Holst, E., Rollof, J., Larsson, L. et al.: Characterization and distribution of *Pasteurella* species recovered from humans. J. Clin. Microbiol. *30*:2984–2987, 1992.
14. Hubbert, W. T., and Rosen, M. N.: *Pasteurella multocida* infection due to animal bite. Am. J. Public Health *60*:1103–1108, 1970.
15. Hubbert, W. T., and Rosen, M. N.: *Pasteurella multocida* infection in man unrelated to animal bite. Am. J. Public Health *60*:1109–1117, 1970.
16. Itoh, M., Tierno, P. M., Milstoc, M., et al.: A unique outbreak of *Pasteurella multocida* in a chronic disease hospital. Am. J. Public Health *70*:1170–1173, 1980.
17. Johnson, R. H., and Rumans, L. W.: Unusual infections caused by *Pasteurella multocida*. J. A. M. A. *237*:146–147, 1977.
18. Larsen, T. E., and Holden, F. A.: Isolation of *Pasteurella multocida* from an otogenic cerebellar abscess. Can. Med. Assoc. J. *101*:629–630, 1969.
19. Lee, M. L. H., and Buhr, A. J.: Dog bites and local infection with *Pasteurella septica*. Br. Med. J. *1*:169–171, 1960.
20. Nielsen, J. P., and Rosdahl, V. T.: Development and epidemiological applications of a bacteriophage typing system for typing *Pasteurella multocida*. J. Clin. Microbiol. *28*:103–107, 1990.
21. Noel, G. T., and Teele, D. W.: In vitro activities of selected new and long-acting cephalosporins against *Pasteurella multocida*. Antimicrob. Agents Chemother. *29*:344–345, 1986.
22. Oberhofer, T. R.: Characteristics and biotypes of *Pasteurella multocida* isolated from humans. J. Clin. Microbiol. *13*:566–577, 1981.
23. Pizey, N. C. D.: Infection with *Pasteurella septica* in a child aged three weeks. Lancet *2*:324–326, 1953.
24. Raffi, F., Barrier, J., Baron, D., et al.: *Pasteurella multocida* bacteremia: Report of thirteen cases over twelve years and review of the literature. Scand. J. Infect. Dis. *19*:385–393, 1987.
25. Raffi, F., David, A., Mouzard, A., et al.: *Pasteurella multocida* appendiceal peritonitis: Report of three cases and review of the literature. Pediatr. Infect. Dis. *5*:695–698, 1986.
26. Reinert, P., Canet, J., Pesnel, G., et al.: Une cause souvent ignorée d'arthrite subaiguë chez l'enfant; la pasteurellose à *P. multocida*. Arch. Fr. Pediatr. *29*:99–104, 1972.
27. Repice, J. P., and Neter, E.: *Pasteurella multocida* meningitis in an infant with recovery. J. Pediatr. *86*:91–93, 1975.
28. Rimler, R. B., and Phoades, K. R.: Serogroup F, a new capsule serogroup of *Pasteurella multocida*. J. Clin. Microbiol. *25*:615–618, 1987.
29. Rosenau, A., Labigne, A., Escande, F. et al.: Plasmid-mediated ROB-1 β-lactamase in *Pasteurella multocida* from a human specimen. Antimicrob. Agents Chemother. *35*:2419–2422, 1991.
30. Sands, M., Ashley, R., and Brown, R.: Trimethoprim-sulfamethoxazole therapy of *Pasteurella multocida* infection. J. Infect. Dis. *160*:353–354, 1989.
31. Schipper, G. J.: Unusual pathogenicity of *Pasteurella multocida* isolated from the throats of common wild rats. Bull. Johns Hopkins Hosp. *81*:333–356, 1947.

32. Smith, J. E.: Studies on *Pasteurella septica*. I. Occurrence in nose and tonsils of dogs. J. Comp. Pathol. *65*:239–245, 1955.
33. Stevens, D. L., Higbee, J. W., Oberhofer, T. R., et al.: Antibiotic susceptibilities of human isolates of *Pasteurella multocida*. Antimicrob. Agents Chemother. *16*:322–324, 1979.
34. Strand, C. L., and Helfman, L.: *Pasteurella multocida* chorioamnionitis associated with premature delivery and neonatal sepsis and death. Am. J. Clin. Pathol. *55*:713–716, 1971.
35. Swartz, M. N., and Kunz, L. J.: *Pasteurella multocida* infection in man. N. Engl. J. Med. *261*:889–893, 1959.
36. Tessin, I., Brorson, J. E., and Trollfors, B.: Rapidly fatal *Pasteurella multocida* septicemia in infant following cat scratch. Pediatr. Infect. Dis. *6*:425–426, 1987.
37. Thompson, C. M., Pappu, L., Levkoff, et al.: Neonatal septicemia and meningitis due to *Pasteurella multocida*. Pediatr. Infect. Dis. *3*:559–561, 1984.
38. Tindall, J. P., and Harrison, C. M.: *Pasteurella multocida* infections following animal injuries, especially cat bites. Arch. Dermatol. *105*:412–416, 1972.
39. Torphy, D. E., and Ray, C. G.: *Pasteurella multocida* in dog and cat bite infections. Pediatrics *43*:295–297, 1969.
40. Waldor, M., Roberts, D., and Kazanjian, P.: In utero infections due to *Pasteurella multocida* in the first trimester of pregnancy: Case report and news. Clin. Infect. Dis. *14*:497–500, 1992.
41. Weber, D. J., Wolfson, J. S., Swartz, M. N., et al.: *Pasteurella multocida* infections: Report of 34 cases and review of the literature. Medicine *63*:133–154, 1984.
42. Wilson, M. A., Rimbler, R. B., and Hoffman, L. J.: Comparison of DNA fingerprints and somatic serotypes of serogroup B and E *Pasteurella multocida* isolates. J. Clin. Microbiol. *30*:1518–1524, 1992.
43. Woolcock, J. B., and Collins, F. M.: Immune mechanism in *Pasteurella multocida*–infected mice. Infect. Immun. *13*:949–958, 1976.

121

CHOLERA

Gerald T. Keusch and Michael L. Bennish

Cholera is a disease associated with prodigious acute diarrhea, and it is possible to lose a volume of fluid and fecal material equivalent to one's body weight during the course of the illness. Without replacement of water and electrolytes, this obviously is lethal. However, with proper fluid therapy alone, no individual should die of cholera. Yet, well into the twentieth century, cholera frequently was a lethal disease, despite the diversity of therapies that were tried.[18, 40] Indeed, it was not until approximately 40 years ago,[163] when the physiologic basis of treating cholera dehydration was defined by systematic clinical investigations, that mortality really dropped, and it is 30 years since a simple oral rehydration therapy was proved effective.[110]

The history of cholera is studded with medically notable events (Table 121–1). These include one of the more successful outbreak investigations when, during the 1850 pandemic in London, John Snow concluded that the "morbid material producing cholera must be introduced into the alimentary canal accidentally for persons would not take it intentionally . . . [and] material which passes from the sick to the healthy and which increases and multiplies in the systems of persons attacked . . . must necessarily have some sort of structure, most likely that of a cell."[139] This was before bacteria were known and 35 years before Robert Koch proved that a specific organism, *Vibrio cholerae*, was the etiologic agent of the disease. Surmising that water transmitted the illness, Snow acted to halt the use of the contaminated water, with a sharp drop in cases thereafter. Studies of cholera also resulted in the first use of intravenous fluids,[40] the first use of the science of diagnostic microbiology to contain the spread of an infection, fulfillment of Koch's third postulate by voluntary human experimentation, discovery of complement-mediated bacteriolysis and immune agglutination, the first systematic studies of acid-base balance and fluid therapy of dehydration, discovery of the first secretory enterotoxin[47] leading to the uncovering of normal small intestinal chloride secretion pathways,[46] and the development of oral rehydration therapy of diarrhea.[66, 129] Cholera has become the model par excellence for the study of toxigenic bacterial diarrheas and is the best understood of them all.[13]

Despite our abundant knowledge of cholera, it remains a major killer of children.[88] Even though rarely diagnosed in the United States and other developed countries, cholera continues to kill tens of thousands of children in poor countries. The ever-present threat posed by cholera was demonstrated dramatically by the deaths of more than 20,000 people from epidemic cholera in less than 4 weeks during the 1994 Rwandan refugee crisis.[58] Social breakdown can lead to a resurgence of cholera in nonrefugee settings as well, as evidenced by the cholera epidemics that have occurred since the dissolution of the Soviet Union.[72] The emergence of a new serogroup of *V. cholerae*, O139 Bengal, the first serogroup of *V. cholerae* other than O1 shown to cause epidemic severe cholera, has raised additional concerns about our ability to control this often deadly disease.[1, 31, 78, 146]

THE ORGANISM

Cholera is caused by a gram-negative, curved bacillus that is highly motile by means of a single flagellum. Originally called the *Kommabacillus* by Koch because of its shape, the genus name *Vibrio* relates to its active motility in unfixed wet preparations that creates the impression that the organism is vibrating. On Gram stain, motility cannot be observed, and the curved comma shape of the organism is not as readily apparent.

V. cholerae is not fastidious in nutritional requirements for growth. It does need an adequate buffering system if fermentable carbohydrate is present, however, because viability is severely compromised below pH 6.0, often resulting in autosterilization of the culture. Many of the selective media used to differentiate enteric pathogens do not support the growth of all *V. cholerae*. Colonies are lactose-negative, a common feature of intestinal pathogenic bacteria, but sucrose-positive, and when plated onto triple sugar iron agar to screen for *Salmonella* and *Shigella*, the organism gives the nonpathogen pattern of an acid (yellow) slant and acid butt due to fermentation of the sucrose contained in triple sugar iron agar. In contrast to most other Enterobacteriaceae, *V. cholerae* is oxidase-positive. Thus, any motile, oxidase-positive, gram-negative rod isolated on routine differential media from the stool of a patient with diarrhea that gives an acid-acid reaction on triple sugar iron agar should be suspected of being *V. cholerae*.

Intentional culturing for *V. cholerae* takes advantage of the

TABLE 121-1. Medical Milestones Associated with Cholera

Year	Event	Comment
1832	Use of intravenous fluids for rehydration by Latta	Patients initially improved but inevitably succumbed—a case of "too late."
1854	John Snow's monograph on the epidemiology of cholera during the Third World pandemic	Clear, logical thought can solve medical mysteries. Ironically, this epidemic of diarrhea was stopped by turning off the water rather than increasing the supply for hygienic purposes.
1883	Robert Koch isolates *Vibrio cholerae*	In the controversy that followed, Koch elaborated the famous set of postulates to document the etiologic association of a microorganism with a specific disease.
1888	Microbiologic identification and quarantine of cases among sailors on incoming vessel in New York harbor prevent epidemic spread to United States	This established the rational, scientific basis for practice of public health medicine.
1894	Fulfillment of Koch's third postulate	Continuing to doubt the significance of Koch's isolate, Pettenkofer and Emmerich publicly drank a culture of *V. cholerae.* One passed a few loose stools and the other nearly died of dehydrating cholera, and the doubt disappeared.
1894	Discovery of in vivo bacteriolysis by Pfeiffer, who injected live vibrios intraperitoneally into immunized guinea pigs	The first complement-mediated host defense mechanism was uncovered.
1896	Discovery of immune agglutination of bacteria by Gruber and Durham	This established the principle of serologic diagnosis of bacterial infections.
1910	Systematic studies of acid-base balance	This was important in developing an understanding of normal physiology and homeostasis.
1949	Systematic studies of fluid and electrolyte therapy of severe dehydration	It took more than a century to prove that cholera is basically a self-limited nonfatal illness.
1967	Documentation of 3′, 5′-cyclic adenosine monophosphate–mediated small bowel electrolyte secretion	A normal secretory process in the intestine was uncovered.

organism's ability to grow at a high pH or in bile salts, which are inhibitory to many Enterobacteriaceae. Thus, alkaline enrichment media, such as peptone water (pH, 8.5–9.0), or selective media containing bile salts, such as thiosulfate-citrate-bile-sucrose agar (pH, 8.6), are recommended to facilitate isolation and laboratory diagnosis. On thiosulfate-citrate-bile sucrose agar, the sucrose-fermenting *V. cholerae* grow as characteristic large, smooth, round yellow colonies that stand out against the blue-green agar. The rare sucrose-negative variant of the cholera vibrio would, however, be missed on this agar.[6] Almost instantaneous diagnosis can be made by direct darkfield examination of stool, which shows the characteristically motile vibrios.[11] The diagnosis of cholera can be confirmed immediately by adding *Vibrio* antisera, which results in cessation of motility of only the homologous organism. Darkfield examination is not likely to be attempted in countries where cholera is not endemic, however, and *V. cholerae* antisera for confirmation of the diagnosis generally are not available in clinical laboratories in nonendemic areas.

V. cholerae are grouped on the basis of their somatic O antigens.[105] Until recently, serogroup O1 was the only one of the 138 serogroups of *V. cholerae* known to cause epidemic cholera. Although infection with some non-O1 *V. cholerae* serogroup organisms caused diarrhea, none was known to produce cholera toxin, and none caused epidemic cholera. However, the appearance of a new non-O1 epidemic serogroup in 1992, O139 Bengal, has changed this belief irrevocably.[1, 31, 78]

There are two serotypes of *V. cholerae* O1, termed *Ogawa* and *Inaba*, distinguishable by agglutination in specific antisera. These serotypes of *V. cholerae* are equally virulent. However, serotype not only is a useful epidemiologic marker for investigations but also helps in the rapid darkfield diagnosis of infection. If antisera to both serotypes are used in the immobilization test, only the antiserum specific for the vibrio type present will give a positive immobilization test; the second serves as a negative control. In addition, there are two biotypes, known as classic and El Tor vibrios. Each biotype can express either Ogawa or Inaba antigens; hence, there are four distinct *V. cholerae* O1. Biotype also is a useful marker for epidemiologic study.

Regardless of serotype and biotype, *V. cholerae* O1 produce three important metabolites, each of which may relate to pathogenesis: (1) a protein enterotoxin called cholera toxin (CTX); (2) neuraminidase, otherwise known as receptor-destroying enzyme for its action on the influenza virus receptor of the erythrocyte; and (3) protease, an enzyme complex capable of hydrolyzing mucin and other substrates.[80] Virulent organisms produce a critical adhesin known as the toxin-coregulated pilus (Tcp) because its synthesis is regulated coordinately with CTX, and several other putative virulence attributes, including an accessory cholera enterotoxin (Ace), zona occludens toxin (Zot), which disrupts tight junctions between intestinal epithelial cells, and a second adhesin, core-encoded pilus (Cep). The genes for these factors are grouped together in a region of the chromosome termed the *cholera genetic element*, an integrated filamatous phage.[95, 160a]

TRANSMISSION AND EPIDEMIOLOGY

Cholera can be an endemic, an epidemic, or a pandemic disease. *V. cholerae* is a saltwater organism, with an established niche in the marine ecosystem, where it lives in intimate association with plankton.[39, 152] Humans are infected incidentally, but the chances of this happening can be facilitated by seasonal increases in the number of organisms, possibly associated with changes in water temperature and algal blooms.[45] Where sanitary water and sewage systems are lacking, secondary transmission through contaminated water and food can result in explosive epidemics. This occurred in 1991, when the first outbreak of cholera in the twentieth century in South America began along the coast of Peru.[17] Carried first by fishermen and then by travelers, the *V. cholerae* O1 organism rapidly spread through South and Central America and into Mexico (Fig. 121–1). Almost half a million cases occurred in 1991 alone.[145]

Periodic global, or pandemic, spread of cholera from its endemic reservoir in the Indian subcontinent was recognized as a characteristic of cholera when the second pandemic reached England in 1831.[158] Five of the six nineteenth-century pandemics affected Europe, and four reached the United States, causing more than 150,000 deaths in 1832 and 50,000 deaths in 1866. The seventh pandemic of cholera, and the first in the twentieth century, began in 1961 and by 1991 had affected five continents.[158] This was the first pandemic recognized to be caused by the El Tor biotype of *V. cholerae* O1. *V. cholerae* O1 El Tor was named for the El Tor quarantine station in the Sinai desert where it originally was isolated from pilgrims returning to Egypt from the annual Haj to Mecca. The organism was identified only sporadically during the next 50 years, usually in asymptomatic persons, and it was not considered to be a human pathogen until 1958, when an outbreak of severe El Tor disease occurred in Thailand. After its spread in Asia in the 1960s, *V. cholerae* O1 El Tor entered Africa in the early 1970s, causing epidemic cholera and establishing itself as a significant endemic infection.[55] Cholera epidemics in Africa now occur on a regular basis, sometimes facilitated by social disruption, as in the camps set up for refugees fleeing the Rwandan civil war in 1994[58] and among Mozambican refugees in Malawi.[104] It was this organism that in 1991 finally gained a foothold in South America.

The number of patients with cholera worldwide is uncertain because most cases go unreported. In 1990, fewer than 30,000 cases were reported to the World Health Organization.[25] Reported cases increased more than 10-fold with the beginning of the Latin American epidemic in 1991.[4, 28] In 1994, the number of cases (384,403) and countries (94) reporting cholera was the largest ever registered at the World

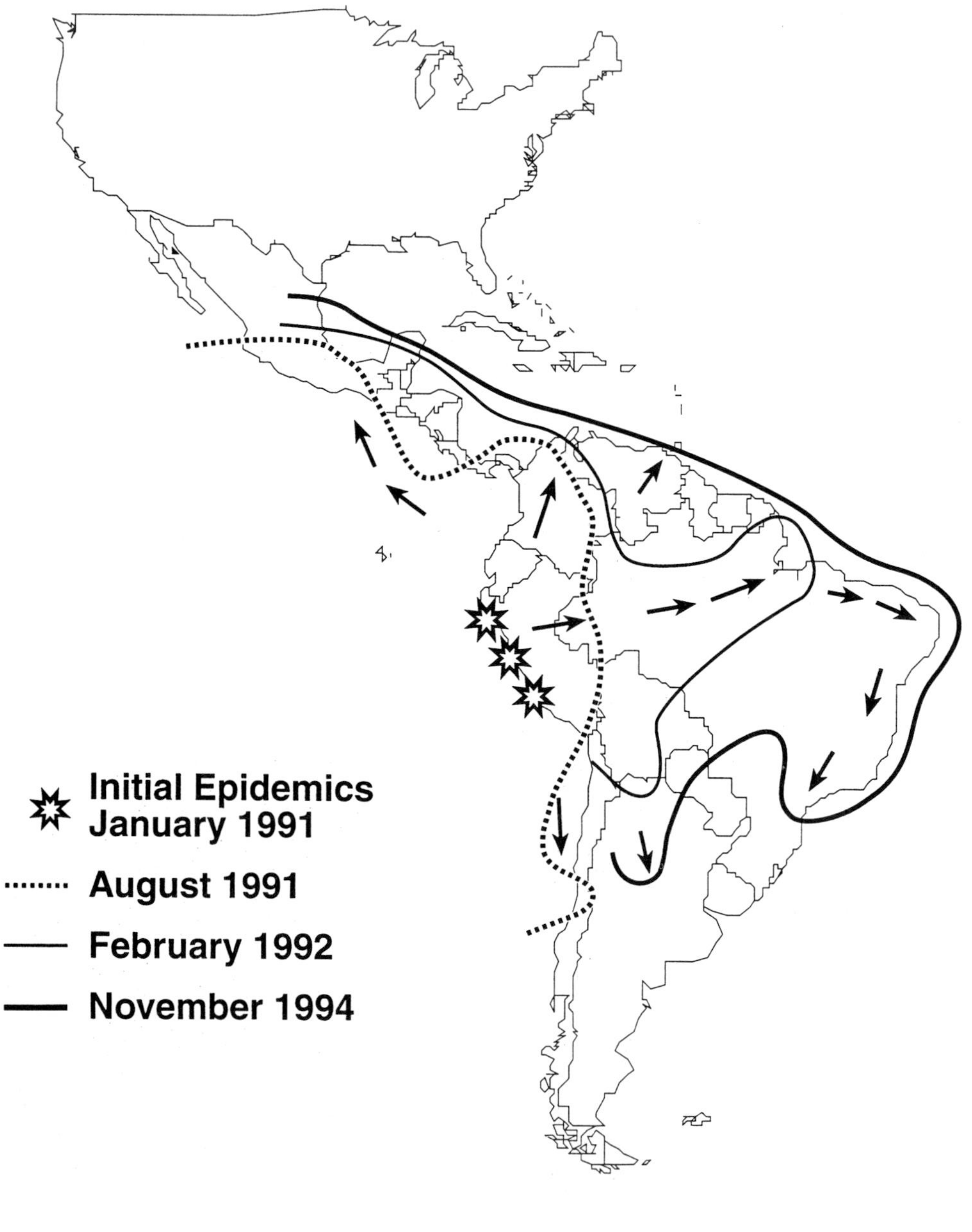

FIGURE 121–1. *The time course of the spread of* Vibrio cholerae *O1 in the Americas, 1991–1994, is shown in this map of the Western Hemisphere. (Courtesy of Dr. Robert V. Tauxe, Centers for Disease Control and Prevention, Atlanta, GA.)*

Health Organization.[4] Even Europe experienced a 30-fold increase in cholera from 1993 to 1994, with reported cases increasing from 73 to 2339 and deaths from 2 to 47.[3]

Without doubt, the global figures are a gross understatement of the actual number of cases and deaths. In Bangladesh alone, where the annual incidence of cholera is 3 to 5 per 1000 persons and the population is 120 million, approximately 360,000 to 600,000 infections occur annually, of which 90,000 to 150,000 are likely to be clinical cholera.[35] There are several reasons for the underreporting of cases to the World Health Organization: most cases occur in remote areas of developing countries where definitive diagnosis is not possible; in such regions, reporting systems often are nonexistent; the stigma of reporting cholera has important consequences for commercial trade and tourism, let alone national self-esteem; and many countries with known endemic cholera report no cases at all.

Cholera has two main reservoirs—man and water. *V. cholerae* rarely is isolated from domestic animals,[133] and they do not play a role in transmission of infection. In endemic areas, most primary infections result from ingestion of contaminated water. Secondary cases then occur by fecal-oral spread of the organism through person-to-person contact or through food or domestic water supplies.[74, 98, 108, 145] Such secondary spread commonly occurs in households,[93] but it also can occur in clinics or hospitals where cholera patients are treated.[97, 130] Infection rates predictably are highest in communities where water is not potable and where personal and community hygiene standards are low. Even in communities where cholera is endemic, infection rates can differ within groups, depending upon habits and practices. For instance, people with occupations that bring them into contact with water or other sources of infection, such as fishing, are at greater risk.[17, 92]

In the United States, an aquatic reservoir of *V. cholerae* O1 in the Gulf of Mexico has been known since 1973, and a handful of cases traceable to this reservoir occur annually, usually due to ingestion of uncooked shellfish.[17] Because seafood often is shipped to distant sites, cases of cholera may occur in any state. Serologic studies indicate that asymptomatic infection among residents of areas along the Gulf of Mexico, especially those in marine-related work, is considerably more common than is disease.[69] No large-scale outbreaks of cholera have occurred, presumably because of the general adequacy of environmental sanitation and chlorination of water supplies. The Gulf strain of *V. cholerae* O1, biotype El Tor, differs from the strain responsible for the seventh pandemic in several ways, such as its ribotype being based on restriction fragment length polymorphisms.[157] This makes it possible to trace domestic versus imported cases by molecular epidemiologic techniques.

Travelers or expatriate residents in cholera-endemic areas have been considered to be at minimal risk of acquiring infection, so long as they observe basic precautions regarding the food and water they ingest.[26, 140] Outbreaks of *V. cholerae* among American and British tourists on a passenger cruise during a stopover in Bangkok[19] and among passengers on an airline flight from South America to the United States[15] raise questions about the validity of this view. It also had been thought that international shipments of food were not a source of cholera transmission.[2] Cases of cholera in the United States caused by the legal importation of canned coconut milk from Thailand[153] and the illegal importation of seafood or other foodstuff from South America[29, 49] also have changed this concept. Indeed, the majority of the 192 cases of cholera reported in the United States from 1990 to 1994 were imported by travel or via food, rather than acquired domestically.[30, 163]

Compared with other enteric pathogens, such as *Shigella*, the infective dose of cholera is high—10^8 to 10^{10} organisms are required to establish infection in volunteers.[23] The infective dose may be reduced if, as usually is the case, food and organisms are ingested at the same time. Two factors are known to put persons at increased risk for infection—achlorhydria[51] and O blood group.[54] The mechanism whereby achlorhydric patients, regardless of the cause (including gastric surgery,[51] vagotomy, use of H2 blockers for ulcer disease, smoking of cannabis,[111] or *Helicobacter pylori* infection[35]), are at increased risk is easily discernible—gastric acid quickly can render an inoculum of *V. cholerae* O1 noninfectious before it reaches the site of colonization in the small bowel. The role of O blood group is less certain, but in cholera-endemic areas, people with the O blood group have twice the risk of having severe cholera than those of other blood groups.[54, 147] This predisposition to severe cholera may account for the relative paucity of people with the O blood group living in the Ganges delta, where cholera is endemic, and it may have played a role in the severity of the outbreak in Latin America, where the majority of the population is O blood group–positive.[147]

The role of asymptomatic carriers in sustaining the disease in endemic areas is uncertain. In areas where *V. cholerae* is endemic but seasonally epidemic, it is difficult to isolate the organism from water sources during intraepidemic periods. In some studies, it was assumed that asymptomatic carriers were responsible for maintaining the organism in the community.[7, 92, 98] Other evidence suggests that the organism persists in a noncultivatable state in association with plankton.[71, 152] When aquatic conditions are conducive to growth, *V. cholerae* proliferates.[39] Thus, it is the aquatic reservoir that is essential for maintaining endemicity and is the source of seasonal increases in disease incidence.

Asymptomatic carriers may play a more important role in introducing cholera into areas where cholera is not endemic, especially for El Tor vibrios, because serosurveys have found that asymptomatic infection with the El Tor biotype is more common than with the classic biotype.[8] The ratio of asymptomatic to symptomatic El Tor infections may be as high as 5 to 1 and is at least twice the ratio for the classic biotype. Although carriage usually is short-lived, a few individuals may excrete the organism for a prolonged period.[7] Thus, efforts to halt the spread of infection by quarantine of symptomatic patients are unlikely to be effective.

Infection rates of household contacts of cholera patients range from 20 to 50 per cent.[93] Rates are lower where infection is endemic and there are preexisting vibriocidal antibodies from previous encounters with the organism, especially in adults. For this reason, infected adults also less frequently are symptomatic than are children.[89] Second infections rarely occur,[166] and they are less likely to be symptomatic than are first infections.[24] In nonendemic areas, the incidence of infection is similar for all age groups,[36] although adults are less likely to become symptomatic than are children.[62] The exception to this is breast-fed children, who are protected against severe disease both because of a lesser exposure and because of the antibodies to cholera they obtain in breast milk.[33, 52]

In 1992, an epidemic of typical clinical cholera occurred in South India, in and around the port city of Madras.[78] What was unusual about this outbreak, however, was that although *V. cholerae* was isolated readily, the organisms did not agglutinate in antibody to the O1 serogroup antigen.[109] The causative vibrio turned out to be a new non-O1 serogroup, now designated O139 Bengal in recognition of its emergence and initial spread along the Bay of Bengal from South India to Bangladesh.[1] This organism behaved as if it had been introduced into a virgin population with respect to prior exposure to *V. cholerae*, and the majority of cases occurred in adults.[1, 31, 109] Aside from this difference in age-specific incidence, the transmission pattern and the clinical manifestations of the new organism were the same as for *V. cholerae* O1.[1]

This is the first example of epidemic cholera due to a non-O1 serogroup organism. The concern quickly was raised that the eighth pandemic might have begun,[146] and indeed in the year after the emergence of cholera due to serotype O139 Bengal, the organism spread to neighboring countries[1, 78] (Fig. 121–2), and imported cases were reported in a number of western countries, including the United States.[3, 27] For unknown reasons, however, after virtually replacing the O1 serogroup in Bangladesh in the first year after the recognition of serotype O139 Bengal, most cholera infections in Bangladesh once again are caused by *V. cholerae* O1 (Fig. 121–3), although in some parts of India the O139 serogroup still accounts for a substantial proportion of cholera cases.[77]

PATHOGENESIS

V. cholerae are ingested by mouth and must reach and colonize the small intestine in order to cause disease. Gastric acid rapidly kills ingested vibrios, and the infectious dose is reduced by 10,000-fold or more when an experimental inoculum is administered to adults with sodium bicarbonate or food to buffer gastric acid.[23, 24] The relationship of achlorhydria and cholera susceptibility is well-described.[51]

Once past the stomach, organisms must colonize the upper small bowel and multiply, or they will be cleared rapidly by specific and nonspecific host defenses, including secretory antibody and peristalsis. Experimental studies suggest that a vibrio must be capable of adhering to the brush border of the jejunal epithelial cell to be virulent. Several properties of the organism have been shown to enhance colonization, including motility, chemotaxis, and the production of a hemagglutinin/protease, which facilitates penetration of the mucus overlying the epithelium.[48, 128] In experimental models, protease-defective *V. cholerae* strains are less virulent.[48] Attachment to intestinal epithelial cells is mediated by the TcpA pilus,[143] which is synthesized in parallel with CTX because both genes are regulated at the transcriptional level by the same "master-switch" regulatory gene, *toxR*.[95] Antibodies to TcpA inhibit attachment of vibrios to in vitro–cultured epithelial cells and protect infant mice from in vivo challenge with virulent *V. cholerae* strains.[143] Expression of TcpA is essential for virulence in humans as well, and although a poor antigen itself, TcpA increases antibody responses to other vibrio antigens.[65]

In vivo–grown cholera vibrios also express surface antigens not produced in vitro, which suggests that they might

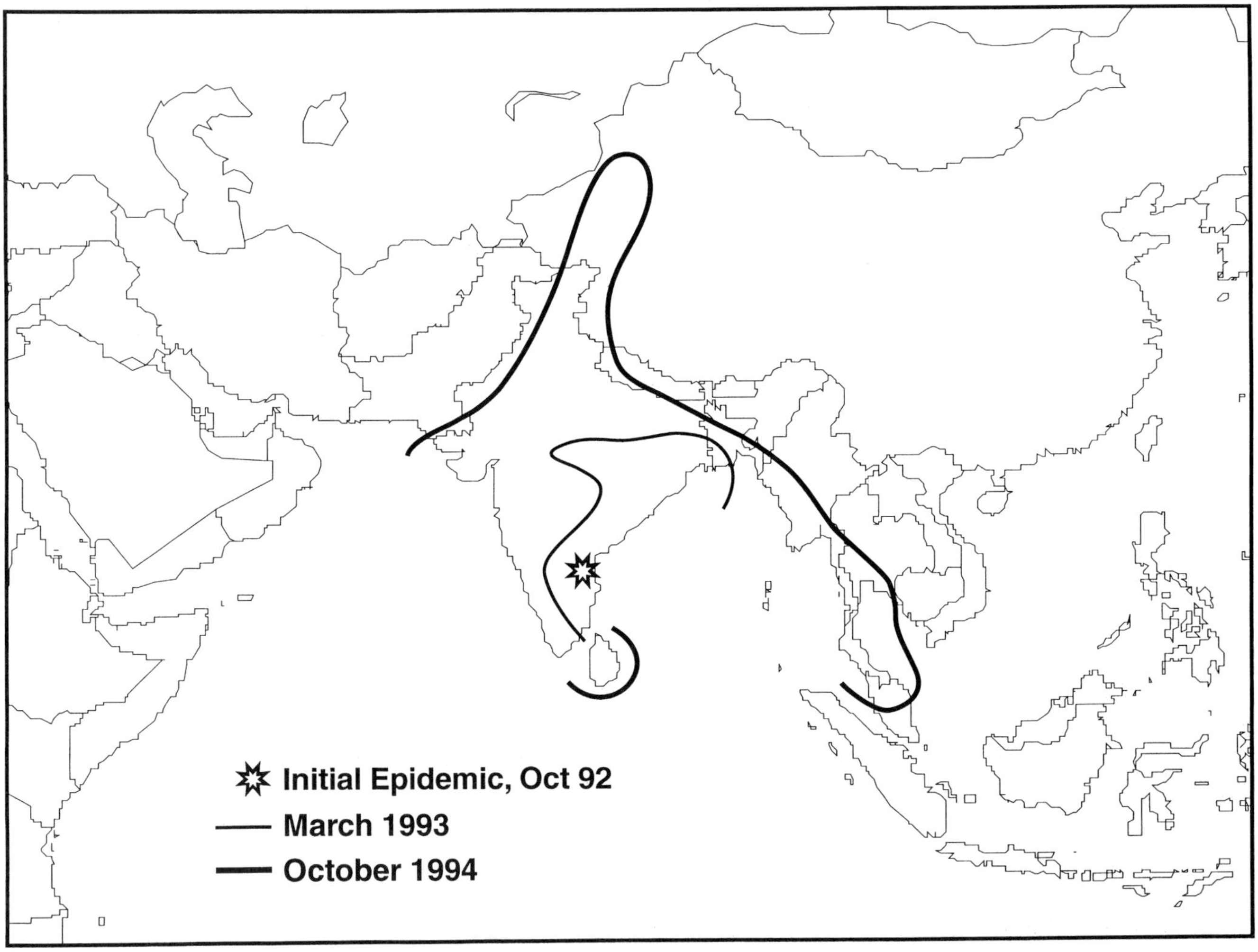

FIGURE 121–2. *The time course of the spread of* Vibrio cholerae *O139 in the Indian subcontinent and adjacent Asian countries, 1992–1994, is shown in this map of Asia. (Courtesy of Dr. Robert V. Tauxe, Centers for Disease Control and Prevention, Atlanta, GA.)*

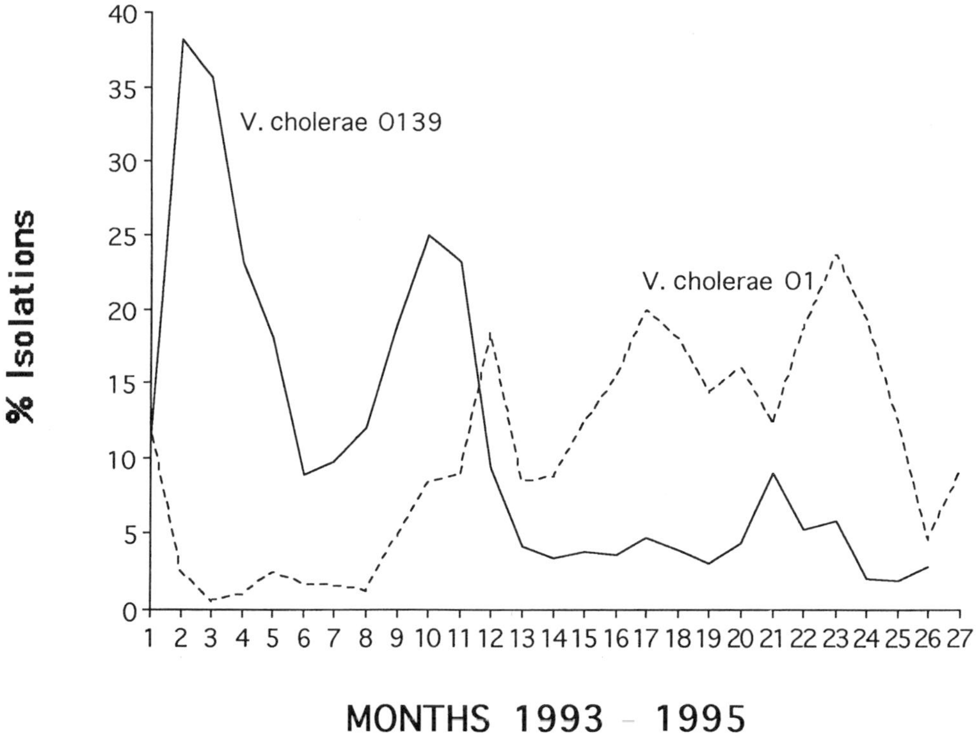

FIGURE 121–3. *The relative percentage of* Vibrio cholerae *O1 and O139 among identified diarrheal pathogens isolated in Dhaka, Bangladesh, 1993–1995. (Courtesy of Drs. John Albert and A. S. G. Faruque, International Centre for Diarrhoeal Disease Research, Bangladesh.)*

be virulence factors.[79] Some *V. cholerae* outer-membrane proteins also are synthesized when iron availability is restricted, as normally occurs in vivo.[56] Low iron therefore may serve as an environmental signal that indicates to the organism that it is in a suitable host and needs to produce its complement of virulence factors. Iron-regulated surface constituents are potential vaccine antigens.

Within the gut lumen, *V. cholerae* multiplies and produces the protein enterotoxin CTX. Proof of the role of CTX in the pathogenesis of human cholera comes from the experiments of Levine and colleagues[87] and more recently Hunt and coworkers,[70] who documented jejunal fluid secretion after perfusion of CTX in human volunteers. CTX binds to a membrane receptor on the intestinal epithelial cell, monosialosyl G_{M1} ganglioside.[47] *V. cholerae* neuraminidase can convert disialosyl gangliosides, which do not bind CTX into the neuraminidase-resistant G_{M1} toxin receptor and possibly augment virulence in this way.

CTX is an 84-kDa protein consisting of an enzymatically active 27-kDa A subunit and a cluster of five B subunit monomers, each with a molecular weight of 11,600.[47] The pentameric B subunit is arranged in a doughnut shape and mediates binding to the target cell surface. The A subunit consists of a 22-kd A1 subunit enzyme and a 5400-Da A2 component, which serves noncovalently to associate the A subunit with the B subunit pentamer and to shield a highly hydrophobic stretch of active site amino acids in the A1 portion of the molecule. This maintains the A1 component in an inactive form until it proteolytically is cleaved and activated. CTX is related closely to the heat-labile toxin (LT) produced by *Escherichia coli*. Indeed, these toxins form a large family of related toxins, including several allelic variants of CTX and LT.[95, 167]

The events leading to electrolyte and fluid secretion are turned on by brief (5–10 minutes) exposure of intestinal mucosa to toxin.[80] Binding of toxin to the intestinal cell surface G_{M1} ganglioside receptor results in the endocytosis of the toxin and delivery of the CTX A1 enzyme to the basolateral intestinal cell membrane,[85, 86] where it encounters its target, the 42-kDa guanosine 5′-triphosphate–binding protein of the regulatory portion of the adenylate cyclase enzyme complex.[46] The A1 enzyme is one of a class of bacterial adenosine diphosphate–ribosylating enzymes that hydrolyze nicotinamide adenine dinucleotide and covalently link its adenosine diphosphate–ribosyl moiety to the target substrate.[47] The function and regulation of adenylate cyclase are complex and involve a number of distinct regulatory elements. In essence, adenosine diphosphate ribosylation of the guanosine 5′-triphosphate–binding protein prevents the subsequent hydrolysis of bound guanosine 5′-triphosphate to guanosine 5′-diphosphate. This effectively locks the catalytic unit of the cyclase into the "on" position, and adenosine triphosphate thereafter for the life of the affected cell continuously is converted into 3′, 5′-cyclic adenosine monophosphate. The resultant increase in the intracellular level of this monophosphate in intestinal epithelial cells[83] turns on electrolyte secretory pathways through activation of protein kinases, which phosphorylate and activate target membrane proteins involved in ion transport.[46] CTX affects both villus and crypt cells, reducing sodium absorption and enhancing chloride secretion, respectively, and greatly increasing the content of sodium and chloride in the bowel lumen. Because water passively follows these electrolytes to maintain iso-osmolarity, the volume of fluid in the small intestine quickly overwhelms the absorptive capacity of the rest of the gastrointestinal tract, resulting in prodigious choleraic diarrhea.[46] Studies also suggest that CTX may activate prostaglandin synthetic pathways and/or neural mechanisms that increase electrolyte accumulation in the lumen.[155] The existence of such secretory pathways in human cholera and their relative importance remain to be determined but could lead to new antisecretory therapies.

Because the O139 Bengal strain of *V. cholerae* is related closely to the seventh pandemic O1 El Tor strain, it has the

TABLE 121–2. Classification of Dehydration and Fluid Deficit Based on Clinical Signs and Symptoms

	Degree of Dehydration		
Sign or Symptom	***Mild or None***	***Some or Moderate***	***Severe***
Mentation	Alert	Restless or lethargic Lethargic	Infants or young children may be comatose Children may be comatose; older children and adults are apprehensive
Thirst	Present	Present	Present
Radial pulse	Normal	Rapid	Rapid and feeble or impalpable
Respiratory pattern	Normal	Tachypneic	Tachypneic, labored
Blood pressure	Normal	Normal	Hypotensive
Mucous membranes	Moist	Dry	Dry
Elasticity of subcutaneous tissues	Pinch retracts immediately	Pinch retracts slowly	Pinch retracts very slowly
Eyes	Normal	Sunken	Sunken
Urine flow	Normal	Scant and dark	Scant or absent
Approximate fluid deficit	≤50 mL/kg	51–90 mL/kg	>90 mL/kg

identical virulence factors and pathogenic mechanisms of O1 El Tor vibrios, including the CTX genetic element, Tcp, and the *toxR* regulon.[159] It differs in two significant ways. First, it has a distinct O antigen, and second, like many non-O1 cholera vibrios, it produces a carbohydrate capsule that in O139 Bengal shares structural features with the O139 somatic antigen. The evidence suggests that O139 Bengal has arisen from O1 El Tor by a deletion of the central region of the O1 antigen biosynthetic complex and horizontal gene transfer of a large segment of new DNA encoding the O139 lipopolysaccharide.[160] At least one gene within this region is required for synthesis of both the O139 lipopolysaccharide and capsule. Based on colonization studies in a mouse model, both antigens may be virulence factors. In addition, the capsule confers serum resistance to the organism and may explain the anecdotal reports of bacteremia in patients with *V. cholerae* O139 Bengal infection.[76] O139 Bengal infection leads to a specific protective vibriocidal antibody response[106] that does not cross-react with vibriocidal antibodies to O1 cholera vibrios.[1] This largely may explain the apparent lack of immunity conferred by prior exposure to *V. cholerae* O1 El Tor.[31]

Cholera vibrios do not invade or structurally damage the intestinal mucosa, and CTX affects only the regulation of normal physiologic intestinal processes. Previous evidence of marked histologic changes in cholera was artifactual due to postmortem changes not present in vivo.[50] Ultrastructural studies revealed alterations of the zonula occludens and widening of the paracellular space, consistent with an action of the Zot toxin.[90]

CLINICAL MANIFESTATIONS

Diarrhea and Vomiting

Profuse watery diarrhea is the hallmark of cholera.[13] Stool volume during cholera is greater than that of any other infectious diarrhea.[101] Patients with severe disease may have a stool volume of more than 250 mL/kg body weight in a 24-hour period.[101, 122] Although early in the course of illness the stool may contain fecal material, the characteristic cholera stool is an opaque white liquid that is not malodorous. Cholera stool often is described as having a rice water appearance, that is, in color and consistency it resembles water that has been used to wash or cook rice. *V. cholerae* does not invade enterocytes and does not elicit an inflammatory response, and cholera stool contains few leukocytes and no erythrocytes.

Because of the large volume of diarrhea, patients with cholera have frequent, often uncontrolled bowel movements. Although the passage of stool is not painful, abdominal cramps are common, presumably due to distention of loops of small bowel as a result of the large volume of intestinal secretions. Vomiting is a prominent manifestation of illness, both early in the course of disease, when the vomiting presumably is due to decreased gastric and intestinal motility,[37] as well as later in the course of illness, when acidemia is the more likely cause.[63] If untreated, the diarrhea and vomiting lead to isotonic dehydration and, in patients with severe disease, vascular collapse, shock, and death.[13] Dehydration can develop with remarkable rapidity, within hours after the onset of symptoms. This contrasts with disease produced by infection with either rotavirus or enterotoxigenic *E. coli*, the other common infectious causes of profuse watery diarrhea, in which dehydration usually develops only 24 or more hours after the onset of symptoms. Because the dehydration is isotonic, the water loss is proportional between the three body compartments—intracellular, intravascular, and interstitial.

Dehydration and Its Categorization

To facilitate patient management, dehydration has been classified into three categories: severe, some (previously termed *moderate* in the World Health Organization criteria for the classification of dehydration), and none (previously termed *mild* by the World Health Organization).[165] Table 121–2 shows the clinical findings associated with these three categories of dehydration. Patients with severe dehydration have a characteristic clinical appearance that is attributable to the loss of ~p15 per cent of total body water (~p10 per cent of total body weight). Intracellular and intravascular dehydration is manifested in decreased skin turgor (Fig. 121–4), sunken eyes, and wrinkled ("washer woman") hands. Decreased intravascular volume is manifested by tachycardia, peripheral pulses that are absent or barely palpable, and hypotension. Tachypnea and hypercapnia also are part of the clinical picture and are attributable to the metabolic acidosis that invariably is present in cholera patients who are dehydrated.[13]

Patients with severe dehydration from cholera make an indelible impression on the observer (Fig. 121–4). Once seen, it is an image and a diagnosis that is never forgotten. No better description exists of the severely dehydrated cholera

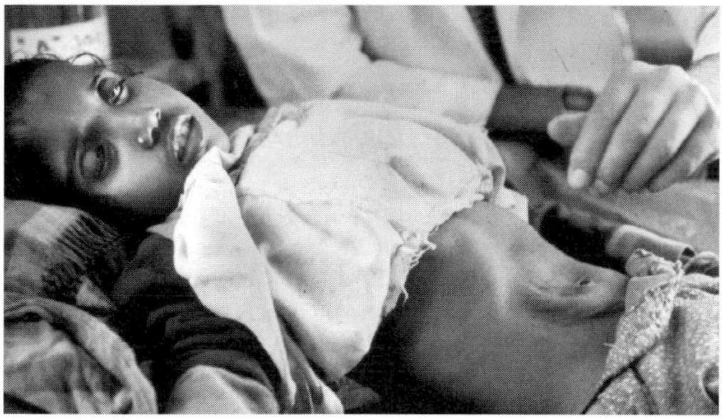

FIGURE 121–4. *An adolescent girl with severe dehydration due to cholera. Characteristic features include obtundation, sunken eyes, and "tenting" of the abdominal skin and subcutaneous tissues after firmly pinching the abdomen.*

patient than that written by Dr. William O'Shaughnessy in 1831, during the second cholera pandemic:

> On the floor . . . lay a girl of slender make and juvenile height . . . but with the face of a superannuated hag. She uttered no moan, gave no expression of pain, but she languidly flung herself from side to side . . . her eyes were sunk deep into her sockets, as though they had been driven an inch behind their natural position; her mouth was squared; her features flattened; her eyelids black; her fingers shrunk, bent and inky in their hue. All pulse was gone at the wrist, and a tenacious sweat moistened her bosom. In short, Sir, that face and form I can never forget, were I to live beyond the period of man's natural age.[40]

Children with some (or moderate) dehydration have lost approximately 7 to 10 per cent of body water (~p5 per cent of body weight).[165] In these patients, cardiac output and vascular resistance are normal, and changes in interstitial and intracellular volume are the primary manifestations of illness.[13] They have decreased skin turgor, as manifested by prolonged skin tenting in response to a skin pinch (the most reliable sign of isotonic dehydration), but normal pulses. Children without clinically significant dehydration (<5 per cent loss of body weight) may have increased thirst without other signs of dehydration.

Metabolic and Systemic Manifestations of Cholera

When first seen, children with cholera often are surprisingly alert, given the severity of their dehydration. Alterations in consciousness can occur because of diminished cerebral blood flow in patients with severe dehydration or because of metabolic abnormalities, of which hypoglycemia[12] and acidemia[63] are the most important.

After dehydration, hypoglycemia is the most common lethal complication occurring during cholera in children.[13] The mortality rate in children with cholera and hypoglycemia admitted to a diarrhea treatment center in Bangladesh was 15 per cent, compared with less than 1 per cent in cholera patients who did not have hypoglycemia.[13] Hypoglycemia in these children was a result of diminished food intake during the acute illness, exhaustion of glycogen stores, and defective gluconeogenesis secondary to insufficient stores of gluconeogenic substrates in fat and muscle. How specific this is for cholera is uncertain because hypoglycemia also has been found to occur with other acute infections in children in the tropics.[81] It also is not restricted to children who severely are malnourished. Acidosis in cholera is a result of bicarbonate loss in stools, accumulation of lactate because of diminished perfusion of peripheral tissues, and hyperphosphatemia.[161] Severely dehydrated children invariably will have serum bicarbonate concentrations of less than 15 mmol/L and often less than 5 mmol/L.[122] Acidemia occurs when respiratory compensation is unable to sustain a normal blood pH.

Hypokalemia also results from potassium loss in the stool, with a mean potassium concentration of ~30 mmol/L (Table 121–3). Because of the coexisting acidosis, however, children often have normal serum potassium concentrations when first seen, despite severe total body potassium depletion, and hypokalemia develops only after the acidosis is corrected and intracellular hydrogen ion is exchanged for extracellular potassium.[122, 127, 163] Hypokalemia is most severe in children with preexisting malnutrition who have diminished body stores of potassium and may be manifested as paralytic ileus. Although electrocardiographic changes of hypokalemia frequently are seen, severe cardiac arrhythmias rarely are observed.

Rehydration therapy with bicarbonate-containing fluids also can produce hypocalcemia by decreasing the proportion of serum calcium that is ionized. Chvostek's and Trousseau's

TABLE 121–3. Electrolyte Concentration in Cholera Stool and in Fluids Used for Rehydration and Replacement of Stool Losses

	Electrolyte Concentration (mmol/L)				
	Na^+	Cl^-	K^+	HCO_3	Osmolality
Cholera Stool					
Adults	130	100	20	44	300*
Infants and children	100	90	33	30	300*
Hydration Solutions					
WHO oral rehydration	90	80	20	30†	220‡
Intravenous					
Dhaka	133	98	13	48	273
Lactated Ringer	130	109	4	28§	251
5:4:1	129	97	11	44	281

*Osmolality includes unmeasured osmotically active molecules (primarily organic acids) in addition to electrolytes.
†As citrate.
‡From electrolytes only; also contains 111 mmol/L of glucose.
§As lactate.
WHO, World Health Organization.

signs often are present, and spontaneous tetanic contractions can occur.[13] Muscle cramping not related to calcium derangements, but presumably related to other metabolic derangements, also can occur.

Cholera patients with some or severe degrees of dehydration have a prerenal azotemia and may be anuric when first seen.[122] Urine flow will resume after restoration of intravascular volume. Even with rapid administration of rehydration fluids, 4 or more hours usually are required before urine is produced. Renal failure can occur as a result of prolonged hypotension but is extremely rare. Most often what is perceived to be renal failure, however, simply is continued volume depletion.[94]

Because *V. cholerae* O1 and O139 infections, unlike infection with non-O1 vibrios,[131] are contained within the intestinal lumen and do not cause systemic or soft tissue infection, symptoms other than those attributable to fluid and electrolyte derangements are uncommon. Dehydrated patients are more likely to be hypothermic than febrile, and leukocytosis, which occurs, is related more likely to the stress response elicited by hypovolemia and subsequent demargination of leukocytes, rather than to inflammation.[61] Occasional cases of *V. cholerae* O1 or O139 bacteremia have been reported anecdotally,[75, 76, 126] but specific therapy is not indicated unless the patient is immunocompromised. In treatment centers in cholera-endemic countries, nosocomial bacteremia from contaminated intravenous solutions or infusion apparatus is a more common problem[142] and should be suspected in any patient who develops an appreciable fever (>38.5° C) while receiving therapy.

Laboratory Findings

The major laboratory derangements in cholera patients derive from the alterations in intravascular volume and electrolyte concentrations.[13] Hematocrit, serum specific gravity, and serum protein are elevated in dehydrated patients due to the resulting hemoconcentration. Serum sodium usually is 130 to 135 mmol/L, reflecting the substantial loss of sodium in the stool that has accompanied the loss of water.[122] As noted earlier, serum potassium most often is normal in the acute phase of illness, reflecting the exchange of intracellular potassium for extracellular hydrogen ion in an effort to correct the acidosis. Bicarbonate concentration usually is less than 15 mmol/L in severely dehydrated patients and often is nondetectable.[161] Blood urea nitrogen and serum creatinine are elevated, reflecting the decrease in glomerular filtration. The extent of their elevation is dependent upon the degree and duration of dehydration but usually is more than 100 μmol/L in the severely dehydrated patient.[122] Patients generally have a leukocytosis without a "left shift" when first seen.

DIAGNOSIS AND DIFFERENTIAL DIAGNOSIS

Definitive diagnosis currently depends upon isolation of *V. cholerae* in stool. A sensitive immediate direct diagnostic method pioneered by the International Centre for Diarrhoeal Disease Research, Bangladesh, utilizes darkfield microscopy to demonstrate the characteristically motile organism in stool,[11] but virtually no laboratory outside of cholera-endemic regions will have experience with this method. Latex agglutination tests have been developed, but their sensitivity has not been satisfactory.[38, 135] New and simple enzyme immunoassay kits[21] for both O1 and O139 organisms, such as the SMART test, have been created and compare very favorably with culture methods, but these are unlikely to be available in United States clinical microbiology laboratories and they undoubtedly will be too expensive to use in poor countries, where cholera is endemic.[64, 116, 123] DNA-based methods also have been developed, including polymerase chain reaction and oligoprobes.[100, 156] Use of an oligoprobe at the Osaka Airport in Japan allowed more rapid diagnosis of travelers with *V. cholerae* infection either by direct stool examination or after alkaline peptone water enrichment culture.[100]

The clinical picture of severe cholera, however, is such that it is unlikely to be confused with any other disease.[13] Even in children, no other diarrheal infection dehydrates so rapidly, and few infections produce the degree of dehydration that is seen in severe cholera. This especially is true for adults, among whom other infections causing watery diarrhea, such as enterotoxigenic *E. coli* or rotavirus, rarely result in profound life-threatening dehydration. Thus, in any community where adults with dehydrating diarrhea are being seen in appreciable numbers, it must be suspected that cholera is present. Unfortunately, in the United States this may not trigger a diagnosis of cholera because medical personnel are not accustomed to thinking of this possibility. Thus, when an airliner from South America touched down in Los Angeles, California, with cholera-infected patients, the diagnosis generally was missed when those with severe diarrhea sought medical help,[15] even though the Latin American epidemic still was very much in the news. In addition, the intravenous fluid management was found to be inadequate upon subsequent assessment by the team from the Centers for Disease Control and Prevention, and most of the facilities did not have adequate oral rehydration solutions available.[15] Definitive diagnosis, however, is not a prerequisite for the management of patients with cholera. The treatment of any watery diarrhea is basically the same—replacing the lost fluids and electrolytes and providing an antimicrobial agent when indicated.

TREATMENT

Fluid Therapy

The primary objective of the treatment of cholera patients is to correct dehydration if present and then maintain hydration.[13] The principles of cholera therapy succinctly were stated by O'Shaughnessy when he wrote to *The Lancet* in 1831 ". . . the indications of cure . . . are two in number—viz. 1st to restore the blood to its natural specific gravity; 2nd to restore its deficient saline matters. The ingredients deficient in the blood were detected in the dejections, or in other words, the addition of the dejection to the blood, in due proportion, would have restored the latter to its normal constitution."[40] Despite this sound assessment of the physiologic derangements in cholera and the effective intravenous hydration of cholera patients by O'Shaughnessy and Latta using a goose trachea as intravenous tubing, it was only in the 1950s and 1960s, after studies by Phillips, Watten, Carpenter, and others,[22, 113, 162] that an intravenous fluid containing the proper concentration of electrolytes came into routine use for the treatment of cholera. Fluid therapy of cholera is relatively simple and can be done without laboratory studies and with the simplest of supplies.

Intravenous Fluids

If fluid replacement is initiated early in the course of illness, dehydration can be prevented. If it is started after dehydration has occurred, both preexisting and continuing fluid losses have to be treated. There are two possible routes of fluid administration: oral and parenteral. All patients with severe dehydration ideally should be rehydrated with intravenous fluids because these produce a more rapid and more predictable expansion of intracellular volume in hypovolemic patients than do oral solutions. Intravenous solutions also should be used to maintain hydration in patients who are purging heavily (i.e., ≥10 mL/kg body weight/hour) because oral fluids will fail to sustain hydration in a majority of such patients.[112]

Despite the marked vascular collapse that has occurred in patients with severe dehydration, it almost always is possible to infuse intravenous fluids through a peripheral vein. At the International Centre for Diarrhoeal Disease Research, Bangladesh, which treats thousands of patients with cholera yearly, venous cutdowns or central lines are never used. If an intravenous line cannot be established in a vein in an extremity, fluids can be infused through scalp veins. Because stool losses become relatively low once a child has become severely dehydrated, fluids infused through a scalp vein will be sufficient to prevent further vascular collapse. In time, as vascular volume is re-established, a larger needle or catheter can be introduced into a peripheral vein.

Many field facilities treating cholera patients, especially during epidemics, will not have the benefit of having staff experienced in treating severely dehydrated patients, and establishing intravenous lines in these situations on occasion will be problematic. Parenteral fluids also can be given effectively via intraosseous infusion, a method now gaining increasing acceptance in pediatric emergency units throughout the world.[57] Although the intraperitoneal route also has been used, it is not recommended.[125] If intravenous fluids cannot be provided immediately, oral fluids should be administered without delay. Oral fluids can be given via a nasogastric tube in severely dehydrated patients who are obtunded or unconscious.[119]

Rehydration of severely dehydrated patients with intravenous fluids can be accomplished within 2 to 4 hours.[66, 122] There is no advantage in using slower rehydration regimens, such as those still recommended by many standard pediatric textbooks. In epidemic situations, such slow regimens simply limit the number of persons to whom care can be provided. The volume of fluid to be administered is determined by the rate of stool losses and the degree of preexisting dehydration (Table 121–4). Patients with severe dehydration initially require 100 mL/kg body weight, and patients with some (or moderate) dehydration require 60 to 80 mL/kg body weight.

The volume of ongoing stool losses can be monitored by keeping patients on a cholera cot covered by a plastic sheet with a hole in the center to allow the stool to collect in a calibrated bucket underneath. Use of such a cot allows minimally trained health workers to calculate fluid losses and replacement needs (Fig. 121–5). The volume of stool is measured every 2 to 4 hours, and the volume of fluid administered is adjusted accordingly. In the initial phase of therapy, urine losses will account for only a small proportion of total fluid losses, and the amount of fluid in the bucket is an adequate reflection of stool losses.[13] With rehydration, an effort to collect urine separately is useful, or otherwise a vicious circle of supplying ever greater amounts of fluid to replace urine losses will ensue. There is a risk of overhydration with intravenous fluids, and this usually is first manifest as puffiness around the eyes. Continued excessive administration of intravenous fluids can lead to pulmonary edema, even in children with normal cardiovascular reserve. Thus, it is important to monitor patients who are receiving intravenous rehydration hourly. Serum specific gravity is an additional measure of the adequacy of rehydration. Severely dehydrated patients have a serum specific gravity of greater than 1.030, often greater than 1.035. With appropriate rehydration, this soon returns to the normal value of 1.025 or less.[113, 162]

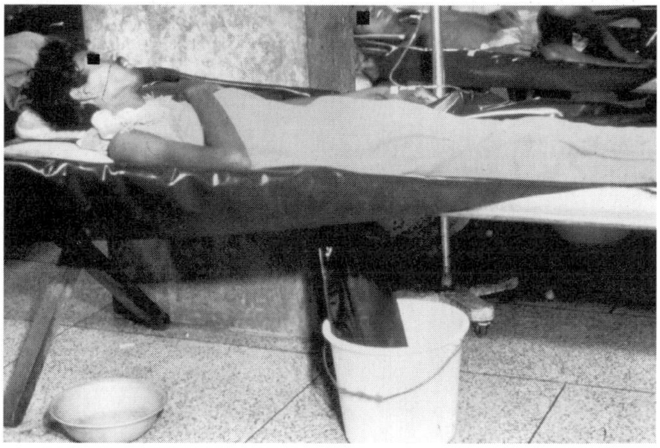

FIGURE 121–5. *A cholera cot—a simple folding cot, covered with plastic and with a hole and bucket for collecting the stool output, as used for the care of cholera patients at the International Centre for Diarrhoeal Disease Research in Bangladesh. The bucket is calibrated, and the volume of stool (and replacement fluids required) can be calculated easily. The plastic sheet is cleaned daily and between patients.*

The ideal intravenous solution for the treatment of children with cholera contains electrolytes in concentrations similar to those found in cholera stools.[66, 165] It also should contain dextrose to prevent hypoglycemia. A number of solutions that approximate these requirements are available (see Table 121–3). Although normal saline has been used to treat cholera patients, it does not correct the severe acidosis that accompanies cholera as quickly as bicarbonate-containing solutions and does not replace potassium.[16] Because of the inevitable fall in serum potassium that accompanies the administration of bicarbonate-rich fluids in cholera patients, potassium should be included in the initial fluid regimen, even though urination might not occur for 4 or more hours.[122, 163]

Oral Therapy

Oral rehydration therapy was made possible by the discovery that despite the reduction in sodium absorption across the small intestine due to the action of CTX, the glucose-coupled sodium chloride cotransport mechanism remains intact.[46, 66, 129] Thus, solutions that contain sodium chloride and glucose or glucose-yielding carbohydrates, such as sucrose[112] or oligosaccharides derived from cereal starches,[115] can be used to replace the fluid losses that occur during cholera. Oral rehydration therapy can be provided in a number of different forms: as prepackaged sachets containing glucose and electrolytes, which then are dissolved in water; as ready-to-use glucose-electrolyte solutions; or as a rice polymer-based electrolyte solution.[10] Oral rehydration solution also can be prepared from home ingredients—either as a solution of sucrose and salt or as a suspension of a powdered cereal (rice, wheat, maize, and sorghum all have been used successfully), water, and salt. The choice of which solution to use is entirely pragmatic because there is little difference in efficacy between preparations if they are used appropriately. Although some studies have suggested that cereal-based suspensions reduce diarrhea in children with cholera better than

TABLE 121–4. Treatment of Cholera

Fluid Therapy

	Replacement Fluids		*Maintenance Fluids*	
Degree of Dehydration	Type of Fluid to Use	Volume of Fluid to Administer	Type of Fluid to Use	Volume of Fluid to Administer
Severe	Intravenous	100–120 mL/kg over 2–4 hours	Intravenous if purging >10 mL/kg body weight/hr: oral if purging ≤10 mL/kg	To match stool output and insensible loss
Some or moderate	Intravenous or oral	60–80 mL/kg over 2–4 hours	Intravenous if purging >10 mL/kg body weight/hr: oral if purging ≤10 mL/kg	To match stool output and insensible loss
None or mild	—	—	Oral	Provide frequently, using thirst and stool frequency as a guide

Antimicrobial Therapy*

Agent	***Single Dose***	***Multiple Dose***
Doxycycline†	7 mg/kg; maximum dose, 300 mg‡	Two doses of 2 mg/kg on day 1; single dose of 2/mg/kg on days 2 and 3; maximum single dose, 100 mg
Tetracycline†	25 mg/kg; maximum dose, 1 g‡	40 mg/kg/day divided into 4 doses for 3 days; maximum dose, 2 g/day
Furazolidone	7 mg/kg; maximum dose, 300 mg	5 mg/kg/day divided into 4 doses for 3 days; maximum dose, 400 mg/day
Ciprofloxacin§	30 mg/kg; maximum dose, 1 g‡	30 mg/kg/day divided into 2 doses for 3 days; maximum dose, 1 g/day
Trimethoprim-sulfamethoxazole	Not evaluated	8 mg of trimethoprim, 40 mg of sulfamethoxazole/kg/day divided into 2 doses for 3 days; maximum doses, 320 mg trimethoprim and 1.6 g sulfamethoxazole daily
Ampicillin	Not evaluated	50 mg/kg day divided into 4 doses for 3 days; maximum dose, 2 g/day
Erythromycin	Not evaluated	40 mg/kg/day erythromycin base divided into 3 doses for 3 days; maximum dose, 1 g/day

*Antimicrobial therapy is an adjunct to fluid therapy of cholera and is not an essential component. It will, however, reduce diarrhea volume and duration by approximately 50 per cent. The choice of antimicrobial agent is determined by the susceptibility pattern of local strains of *Vibrio cholerae* O1 or O139. Resistance to all agents except fluroquinolones, such as ciprofloxacin, has been reported and is commonplace in some areas.

†Both tetracycline and doxycycline can discolor permanent teeth of children younger than 8 years of age. The risk of this is small when these drugs are used for short courses of therapy, especially if used in a single dose.

‡Single-dose therapy of these drugs has not been evaluated systematically in children, and recommendations are extrapolated from experience in adults.

§The fluoroquinolones, such as ciprofloxacin, are not approved for use in children younger than 18 years of age in the United States because when given in high doses to juvenile animals, they cause arthropathy. Clinical experience indicates that this risk is very small in children when used for short courses of therapy.

glucose-containing solutions do,[59] the latter remains more readily available in most cholera-endemic regions.

The electrolyte concentration of the oral solution currently recommended by the World Health Organization for use in the treatment of cholera is shown in Table 121–3.[165] The use of solutions with lower sodium concentrations, such as the solutions containing 60 mmol/L or less of sodium routinely used in the United States and in Europe and that now are being evaluated by the World Health Organization for wider use,[5] may not be appropriate for use in cholera patients because they cannot replace adequately the high sodium loss in cholera stools. Patients treated with such solutions are at risk of developing clinically important hyponatremia. Oral rehydration solutions can have an enormous impact on the logistics of treating cholera patients, especially under epidemic conditions. The routine use of oral, rather than intravenous, solutions to maintain hydration at cholera treatment facilities can reduce requirements for intravenous solutions by up to 80 per cent.[136] Sole reliance on oral solutions, however, will result in a higher mortality rate.[137]

For oral therapy to be used effectively, an adult (ideally the parents or another caretaker) must remain with the child to provide oral rehydration and encourage its intake.[10, 13] Parents need to be instructed in the appropriate use of oral rehydration solution, including the caveats that occasional vomiting is not a contraindication to beginning or continuing its use and that if necessary the oral rehydration solution should be offered in smaller amounts more frequently. It also is important that the staff believe in the efficacy of oral rehydration solution because in many settings intravenous fluids are perceived by both staff and parents as being more advanced therapy and thus more effective and a more desirable choice.

Antimicrobial Therapy

The administration of effective antimicrobial agents decreases the duration and volume of diarrhea by half and shortens the duration of excretion of *V. cholerae*.[14, 61] As such, antibiotic therapy is an important, but not essential, adjunct to fluid therapy of cholera, particularly during epidemics. Tetracycline and its long-acting congener, doxycycline, were the earliest agents used to treat adults with cholera.[61] Because tetracyclines can cause discoloration of both deciduous and permanent teeth, they have not been used routinely to treat children with cholera, even though this risk is small with the relatively short courses of therapy required. This especially is true for doxycycline, which causes less staining than tetracycline. However, on this basis, furazolidone has been the agent routinely used in the treatment of cholera in children.[121]

Increasing resistance has limited the utility of both tetracycline and furazolidone for the treatment of cholera.[14, 168] *V. cholerae* O1 strains resistant to these drugs have been reported from all regions in which cholera is endemic, and resistant strains now predominate in many areas.[20, 124, 168] Strains resistant to tetracycline also will be resistant to doxycycline in vivo, even if they test susceptible in vitro.[82a] Almost all *V. cholerae* O139 strains also are resistant to furazolidone and trimethoprim-sulfamethoxazole, although most strains have been susceptible to tetracycline.[1] Potentially effective alternative agents include ampicillin, erythromycin, and the fluoroquinolones.[14, 20, 60, 82]

Where tetracycline-resistant strains are uncommon, single-dose therapy with doxycycline or furazolidone, because of their low cost and efficacy, probably remains the treatment of choice; where tetracycline resistance is common, ampicillin, sulfamethoxazole-trimethoprim, erythromycin, and single-dose ciprofloxacin are possible options.[14, 20, 82, 82a] Although there are concerns about the use of fluroquinolones in children because of toxicity studies in juvenile animals that show damage to joint cartilage when these drugs are used in high doses, there is little evidence that short courses of therapy in children cause this problem.[134] Specific recommendations for antimicrobial therapy are shown in Table 121–4.

Antimicrobial agents typically have been given for 3 to 5 days.[14, 61] However, single-dose therapy with tetracycline, doxycycline, furazolidone, and ciprofloxacin has been shown since to be effective in reducing the duration and volume of diarrhea.[14, 82a] Single-dose ciprofloxacin appears to be the most effective of these agents in shortening the duration of excretion of *V. cholerae*.[82a] Antimicrobial therapy for cholera should be given when the patient first is seen and cholera is suspected. There is little reason to wait for culture and susceptibility results because by the time susceptibility results are available 48 to 72 hours later, the worst of the diarrhea will have abated. This means that the decision on which antimicrobial agent to use must be based upon knowledge of the resistance patterns of the *V. cholerae* strains circulating in the community.[14] These data, unfortunately, often are not available to practioners in cholera-endemic areas.

Nonantimicrobial Therapy for Diarrhea

A variety of nonantimicrobial therapies also have been evaluated for use in the treatment or prevention of cholera. These include agents that block CTX receptors (the nontoxic B subunit)[53] or bind to and inactivate CTX (G_{M1} ganglioside)[141]; agents that stimulate gut mucosal alpha-adrenergic receptors and enhance sodium and chloride absorption (clonidine)[120]; agents that inhibit adenylate cyclase (berberine, chlorpromazine, and nicotinic acid)[117–119]; agents that affect intestinal hormone release (somatostatin)[103]; aspirin to block the effect of prostaglandins[73]; bovine colostrum with high titers of anti-CTX antibodies[91]; and probiotics, that is, live organisms to restore a normal fecal flora and prevent further intestinal colonization by the pathogen.[99] None of these agents produces a decrease in diarrhea volume or duration of a sufficient magnitude to warrant their routine use.

Management of Hypoglycemia and Nutritional Support

After hypovolemia, hypoglycemia is the major cause of death of cholera patients. The best way to address this is to administer dextrose-containing solutions to all patients with cholera.[12] Providing dextrose selectively to those with documented hypoglycemia is not a realistic option in endemic regions because it is difficult clinically to identify which severely dehydrated cholera patients are obtunded from shock and which have serious hypoglycemia. In addition, adding dextrose to intravenous fluids at the bedside brings with it the risk of contamination because sterile technique is difficult to maintain in a developing country, especially during a cholera epidemic.[142] If nosocomial bacteremia is suspected, the entire intravenous apparatus should be replaced. There usually is no need for additional antimicrobial therapy beyond that used for *V. cholerae* treatment.

Because *V. cholerae* does not cause systemic infection and does not damage intestinal epithelium,[13, 50, 80] recovery is not complicated by late sequelae of disease. Once the diarrhea stops and fluids are replaced, the disease is over. Unlike dysentery due to *Shigella* or watery diarrhea due to rotavirus infection, malnutrition after infection is not a major problem.

The catabolic cost of infection is relatively low, anorexia is neither profound nor persistent, and intestinal enzyme activity remains intact after infection; hence, intestinal absorption of nutrients is near normal.[102] Thus, there is no reason to withhold food from cholera patients. For children not yet weaned, breast feeding should continue; those who have been weaned should be encouraged to eat as soon as they are capable of doing so after the dehydration has been corrected.

Site of Treatment

To reduce cholera mortality maximally, patients must have ready access to a treatment center skilled in the simple measures required to treat dehydration.[136] Severely ill cholera patients cannot be managed in the household with oral solutions alone, and the rapidity with which dehydration occurs precludes traveling long distances for care. During epidemics, makeshift treatment centers with a limited set of supplies, including cholera cots, oral and intravenous rehydration solutions, and an effective antimicrobial agent, are sufficient.[136] It is important that individuals treating cholera patients be instructed in the magnitude of fluid losses that can occur with cholera because medical care personnel inexperienced in the therapy of cholera often do not appreciate the large volumes of replacement fluids required; the consequences of inadequate therapy are, potentially, death of the patient.[137]

PROGNOSIS

Before the development of effective regimens for replacing fluid and electrolyte losses, the mortality in severe disease was more than 50 per cent.[22, 113] With the development of effective intravenous and oral rehydration solutions, no patient who reaches a cholera treatment center alive should die of the disease. Mortality will be lowest where intravenous therapy is available—less than 1 per cent of severely dehydrated patients at the Treatment Centre of the International Centre for Diarrhoeal Disease Research, Bangladesh, die.[13] Although mortality rates in Africa remain higher, low case-fatality rates also have been achieved in South America, presumably because of the availability of adequate treatment facilities and trained personnel.[4, 28]

PREVENTION

The precise immune response responsible for recovery from, as well as prevention of, cholera remains unclear. Vibriocidal and agglutinating IgM antibodies increase sharply, peaking 1 to 2 weeks after the onset of disease.[80, 144] These antibodies gradually wane over a period of months, most rapidly in young children. Vibriocidal antibody titers in populations in endemic regions are associated with resistance to cholera, and the height of the titer is related inversely to age. This may be why endemic cholera largely is a pediatric disease, with the peak age of illness between 5 and 10 years of age. The susceptibility of adults with vibriocidal antibody to O1 *V. cholerae* to the O139 Bengal serotype demonstrates the importance and specificity of the vibriocidal antibody response.[1]

Nonetheless, many individuals older than 15 years of age in cholera-endemic regions remain susceptible to infection and disease. Clinical infection provides substantial immunity to rechallenge.[24] Most patients convalescent from clinical cholera have circulating antitoxin antibodies, indicating a systemic immune response to cholera enterotoxin.[114, 144] There is no evidence, however, that this antibody protects against the clinical manifestations of cholera infection, and it is more likely that protective immunity is expressed at the intestinal mucosal surface itself.[67, 68, 144] A number of antigens, alone or in combination, may be responsible for protective immunity, including the O antigens, outer-membrane proteins, CTX, TcpA pilus, and soluble hemagglutinin/protease.[68]

Better understanding of virulence in *V. cholerae* and the methods of modern molecular genetics currently are being used to guide vaccine development.[80, 96] The previous parenteral killed cholera vaccines had little efficacy[68] and are not recommended for use in endemic areas, during outbreaks, or in people traveling to endemic areas.[107, 140] Contemporary efforts at vaccine development have focused on oral immunization, using three general approaches: (1) killed bacterial vaccines; (2) live, genetically engineered mutants deleted of CTX genes; and (3) avirulent vectors genetically engineered to express protective cholera antigens.[43]

It has been suggested that oral killed vaccines have some merit, at least to enhance immunity in individuals living in a cholera-endemic area.[34] The initial large-scale field trial in Bangladesh utilized an oral vaccine containing killed *V. cholerae* O1, with or without addition of the CTX B subunit,[32] which not only serves as a potential antigen for antitoxin immunity, but also seems to have adjuvant properties for other antigens simultaneously presented.[67] This trial showed protection against cholera, with the combined vaccine being significantly more effective for the first 6 months after immunization.[32] The importance of prior priming of the immune response in this cholera-exposed population is suggested by the reduced efficacy of the vaccine in those younger than 5 years of age. This finding, in addition to the requirement for multiple doses and the apparent waning of immunity after 6 months, especially in the very young most in need of protection, substantially limits the utility of this vaccine preparation. The strain used in the test vaccine did not, however, express the TcpA pilus antigens, and it is possible that inclusion of this antigen would improve substantially the results. A subsequent trial of the oral killed vaccine in Peru was much more immunogenic in young children[9] and was protective in adults.[132] Moreover, immunization of mothers with this "first-generation" oral killed vaccine was associated with significant protection of breast feeding infants. The mechanism of this protection is uncertain because increases in milk antibodies could not be demonstrated.[33] Use of strains hyperexpressing B subunit and TcpA pilus but deleted of the genes for the A subunit of CTX could be the basis for a simple, inexpensive, locally produced vaccine for cholera-endemic areas.[87]

Live vaccine strains have been the subject of intense investigation, and a number have been tested in humans.[80, 95, 96] The general approach has been to delete the genes for CTX, especially for the A subunit, without altering surface antigens of potential importance. Some of these candidate strains were effective immunogens but produced mild diarrhea in many recipients, possibly because they express accessory virulence factors.[87] The most advanced of the current candidates, CVD 103-HgR, licensed for sale in Switzerland, is a toxin A subunit deletion mutant containing a mercury resistance gene insert in the hemolysin gene, which allows its distinction from wild-type cholera vibrios.[80] CVD 103-HgR appears to be safe and to induce protective immunity as soon as 8 days after immunization,[149] even after a single oral dose in adults. It now has been shown to be similarly immunogenic in children as young as 2 years of age.[138] It remains to be seen whether or not this candidate strain will be safe and effective in both adults and children from nonendemic areas and in those previously exposed to the organism. Interestingly, although blood group O individuals have a predilection to develop severe cholera,[147] blood group O subjects also developed greater protective immune responses after immunization.[84] Because CVD 103-HgR is less effective in protecting vaccinees from an El Tor challenge compared with classic strain challenge, promising El Tor–based vaccines have been developed and tested.[150, 154] Based on the experience garnered in the development of *V. cholerae* O1 vaccines, prototypic vaccines for the O139 Bengal strain were produced rapidly after the initial outbreak.[151, 159]

The third approach, expression of protective antigens by insertion of the cloned genes into avirulent carrier organisms, also is eliciting great interest.[42] The genes controlling the expression of the Inaba O antigen have been cloned into a plasmid. This may be introduced stably into the live oral typhoid vaccine strain, Ty21a, which then expresses complete O1-Inaba lipopolysaccharide on its surface.[148] The hybrid vaccine strain, EX 645, appears to be well tolerated and is immunogenic in humans.

These approaches are likely to yield improved cholera vaccines in the next decade. If so, immunization in early childhood could be used to prevent clinical disease in endemic areas. For a vaccine to be useful in areas with endemic cholera, however, it must produce long-lasting immunity and be compatible with the schedule of the expanded program on immunization in use for children in most of the world. To be useful during epidemics, a cholera vaccine rapidly must induce a protective response, ideally after a single dose. It also is important that the vaccine protects against both O1 and O139 *V. cholerae*, if both organisms are present in the community.[41] To accomplish these goals probably will require production of a combined cholera vaccine composed of classic and El Tor O1 strains as well as O139 Bengal, regardless of whether the vaccine is a killed or live oral preparation.

Nonvaccine approaches to prevention of illness also have been considered. Because attack rates are higher in family members of a patient with cholera, selective antimicrobial prophylaxis of household contacts of patients with cholera has been attempted. Although this has had some success in at least one study,[44] it is not feasible as a routine public health measure.[60] Unfortunately, cholera vibrios are natural marine organisms, and eradication is not a possibility, as might be the case with other human-specific pathogens. Universal access to potable water would, in contrast, effectively end the threat of cholera as a major public health problem. This has been the case in the rich countries of North America, Europe, and eastern Asia, where cholera epidemics have not occurred since the beginning of the twentieth century. That the majority of the world's population will remain at risk of epidemic cholera at the beginning of the twenty-first century is an indictment of the increasing gap in wealth and social conditions between rich and poor nations and rich and poor children. Thus, as we approach the millennium, the major measure for control of mortality from cholera remains effective case management, with the continued hope that an effective vaccine and adequate water and sewage systems will become available to those at risk.

References

1. Albert, M. J. Minireview: *Vibrio cholerae* O139 Bengal. J. Clin. Microbiol. *32*:2345–2349, 1994.
2. Anonymous: Cholera: Small risk of cholera transmission by food imports. Wkly. Epidemiol. Rec. *66*:55–56, 1991.
3. Anonymous: Cholera in Europe. Wkly. Epidemiol. Rec. *69*:322–323, 1994.
4. Anonymous: Cholera in 1994: Part 1. Wkly. Epidemiol. Rec. *70*:201–208, 1995.
5. Anonymous: Multicentre evaluation of reduced-osmolarity oral rehydration salts solution: International Study Group on Reduced-Osmolarity ORS Solutions. Lancet *345*:282–285, 1995.
6. Ansaruzzaman, R. M., Rahman, M., Kibriya, A. K., et al.: Isolation of sucrose late-fermenting and nonfermenting variants of *Vibrio cholerae* O139 Bengal: Implications for diagnosis of cholera. J. Clin. Microbiol. *33*:1339–1340, 1995.
7. Azurin, J. C., Kobari, K., Barua, D., et al.: A long-term carrier of cholera: Cholera Delores. Bull. W. H. O. *37*:745–749, 1967.
8. Bart, K. J., Huq, Z., Khan, M., et al.: Seroepidemiologic studies during a simultaneous epidemic of infection with El Tor Ogawa and classical Inaba *Vibrio cholerae*. J. Infect. Dis. *121*:S17–S24, 1970.
9. Begue, R. E., Castellares, G., Ruiz, R., et al.: Community-based assessment of safety and immunogenicity of the whole cell plus recombinant B subunit (WC/rBS) oral cholera vaccine in Peru. Vaccine *13*:691–694, 1995.
10. Behrens, R. H.: Diarrhoeal disease: Current concepts and future challenges: The impact of oral rehydration and other therapies on the management of acute diarrhoea. Trans. R. Soc. Trop. Med. Hyg. *87*(Suppl. 3):35–38, 1993.
11. Benenson, A. S., Islam, M. R., and Greenough, W. B., III: Rapid identification of *Vibrio cholerae* by darkfield microscopy. Bull. W. H. O. *30*:827–831, 1964.
12. Bennish, M. L., Azad, A. K., Rahman, O., et al.: Hypoglycemia during diarrhea: Prevalence, pathophysiology, and outcome. N. Engl. J. Med. *322*:1357–1363, 1990.
13. Bennish, M. L.: Cholera: Pathophysiology, clinical features, and treatment. *In* Wachsmuth, I. K., Blake, P. A., and Olsvik, O. (eds.): *Vibrio cholerae* and Cholera: Molecular to Global Perspectives. Washington, D.C., American Society of Microbiology, 1994, pp. 229–255.
14. Bennish, M. L., and Levy, S. B.: Antimicrobial resistance of enteric pathogens. *In* Blaser, J. M., Smith, P. D., and Ravdin, J. I. (eds.): Infections of the Gastrointestinal Tract. New York, Raven Press, 1995, pp. 1499–1523.
15. Besser, R. E., Feikin, D. R., Eberhart-Phillips, J. E., et al.: Diagnosis and treatment of cholera in the United States: Are we prepared? J. A. M. A. *272*:1203–1205, 1994.
16. Biesel, W. R., Watten, R. H., Blackwell, R. Q., et al.: The role of bicarbonate pathophysiology and therapy in Asiatic Cholera. Am. J. Med. *35*:58–66, 1963.
17. Blake, P. A.: Epidemiology of cholera in the Americas. Gastroenterol. Clin. North Am. *22*:639–660, 1993.
18. Bonnici, W.: The blue epidemic cholera: Some aspects of treatment in the mid 19th century. J. R. Army Med. Corps *139*:76–78, 1993.
19. Boyce, T. G., Mintz, E. D., Greene, K. D., et al.: *Vibrio cholerae* O139 Bengal infections among tourists to southeast Asia: An intercontinental foodborne outbreak. J. Infect. Dis. *172*:1401–1404, 1995.
20. Burans, J. P., Podgore, J., Mansour, M. M., et al.: Comparative trial of erythromycin and sulpha-trimethoprim in the treatment of tetracycline-resistant *Vibrio cholerae* O1. Trans. R. Soc. Trop. Med. Hyg. *83*:836–838, 1989.
21. Carillo, L., Gilman, R. H., Mantle, R. E., et al.: Rapid detection of *Vibrio cholerae* O1 in stools of Peruvian cholera patients by using monoclonal immunodiagnostic kits: Loyaza Cholera Working Group in Peru. J. Clin. Microbiol. *32*:856–857, 1994.
22. Carpenter, C. C. J., Mondal, A., Sack, R. B., et al.: Clinical studies in Asiatic cholera. II. Development of 2:1 saline:lactate regimen: Comparison of this regimen with traditional modes of treatment, April and May, 1963. Bull. Johns Hopkins Hosp. *118*:174–196, 1966.
23. Cash, R. A., Music, S. I., Libonati, J. P., et al.: Response of man to infection with *Vibrio cholerae*. I. Clinical, serologic, and bacteriologic responses to a known inoculum. J. Infect. Dis. *129*:45–52, 1974.
24. Cash, R. A., Music, S. I., Libonati, J. P., et al.: Response of man to infection with *Vibrio cholerae*. II. Protection from illness afforded by previous diseases and vaccine. J. Infect. Dis. *130*:325–333, 1974.
25. Centers for Disease Control: Cholera: Worldwide. M. M. W. R. *39*:365–367, 1990.
26. Centers for Disease Control: Cholera associated with international travel, 1992. M. M. W. R. *41*:664–667, 1992.
27. Centers for Disease Control: Imported cholera associated with a newly described toxigenic *Vibrio cholerae* O139 strain: California, 1993. M. M. W. R. *42*:501–503, 1993.
28. Centers for Disease Control and Prevention: Update: *Vibrio cholerae* O1—Western Hemisphere, 1991–1994, and *V. cholerae* O139—Asia, 1994. M. M. W. R. *44*:215–219, 1995.
29. Centers for Disease Control and Prevention: Cholera associated with food transported from El Salvador: Indiana, 1994. M. M. W. R. *44*:385–386, 1995.
30. Centers for Disease Control and Prevention: Summary of notifiable diseases, United States, 1994. M. M. W. R. *43*:70, 1994.
31. Cholera Working Group, International Centre for Diarrhoeal Disease Research, Bangladesh: Large epidemic of cholera-like disease in Bangladesh caused by *Vibrio cholerae* 0139 synonym Bengal. Lancet *342*:387–390, 1993.
32. Clemens, J. D., Sack, D. A., Harris, J. R., et al.: Field trial of oral cholera vaccines in Bangladesh: Results from long-term follow-up. Lancet *1*:270–273, 1990.
33. Clemens, J. D., Sack, D. A., Harris, J. R., et al.: Breast feeding and the risk of severe cholera in rural Bangladeshi children. Am. J. Epidemiol. *131*:400–411, 1990.

34. Clemens, J. D., Sack, D. A., Rao, M. R., et al.: Evidence that inactivated oral cholera vaccines both prevent and mitigate *Vibrio cholerae* O1 infections in a cholera-endemic area. J. Infect. Dis. *166*:1029–1034, 1992.
35. Clemens, J., Albert, M. J., Rao, M., et al.: Impact of infection by *Helicobacter pylori* on the risk and severity of endemic cholera. J. Infect. Dis. *171*:1653–1656, 1995.
36. Cohen, J., Schwartz, T., Klasmer, R., et al.: Epidemiologic aspects of cholera El Tor outbreak in a nonendemic area. Lancet *2*:86–89, 1971.
37. Collins, B. J., Van Loon, F. P. L., Molla, A., et al.: Gastric emptying of oral rehydration solutions in acute cholera. J. Trop. Med. Hyg. *92*:290–294, 1989.
38. Colwell, R. R., Hasan, J. A., Huq, A., et al.: Development and evaluation of a rapid, simple, sensitive, monoclonal antibody-based co-agglutination test for direct detection of *Vibrio cholerae* O1. FEMS Microbiol. Lett. *76*:215–219, 1992.
39. Colwell, R. R., and Huq, A.,: Environmental reservoir of *Vibrio cholerae*: The causative agent of cholera. Ann. N.Y. Acad. Sci. *740*:44–54, 1994.
40. Cosnet, J. E.: The origins of intravenous fluid therapy. Lancet *1*:768–771, 1989.
41. Coster, T. S., Killeen, K. P., Waldor, M. K., et al.: Safety, immunogenicity, and efficacy of live attenuated *Vibrio cholerae* O139 vaccine prototype. Lancet *345*:949–952, 1995.
42. Cryz, S. J., Jr., Que, J. U., Levine, M. M., et al.: Safety and immunogenicity of a live oral bivalent typhoid fever (*Salmonella typhi* Ty21a) cholera (*Vibrio cholerae* CVD103-HgR) vaccine in healthy adults. Infect. Immun. *63*:1336–1339, 1995.
43. Anonymous: Development of vaccines against cholera and diarrhoea due to enterotoxigenic *Escherichia coli*: Memorandum from a WHO meeting. Bull. W. H. O. *68*:303–312, 1990.
44. Echevarría, J., Seas, C., Carrillo, C., et al.: Efficacy and tolerability of ciprofloxacin prophylaxis in adult household contacts of patients with cholera. Clin. Infect. Dis. *20*:1480–1484, 1995.
45. Epstein, P. R.: Algal blooms in the spread and persistence of cholera. Biosystems *31*:209–221, 1993.
46. Field, M., Rao, M. C., and Chang, E. B.: Intestinal electrolyte transport and diarrheal diseases. N. Engl. J. Med. *321*:800–806, 879–883, 1989.
47. Finkelstein, R. A.: Cholera, the cholera enterotoxins, and the cholera enterotoxin-related enterotoxin family. *In* Owen, P., and Foster, T. J. (eds.): Immunochemical and Molecular Genetic Analysis of Bacterial Pathogens. New York, Elsevier, 1988, pp. 85–102.
48. Finkelstein, R. A., Boesman-Finkelstein, M., Chang, Y., et al.: *Vibrio cholerae* hemagglutinin-protease, colonial variation, virulence, and detachment. Infect. Immun. *60*:472–478, 1992.
49. Finelli, L., Swerdlow, D., Mertz, K., et al.: Outbreak of cholera associated with crab brought from an area with epidemic disease. J. Infect. Dis. *166*:1433–1435, 1992.
50. Gangarosa, E. J., Beisal, W. R., Benyajati, C., et al.: The nature of the gastrointestinal lesion in Asiatic cholera and its relation to pathogenesis: A biopsy study. Am. J. Trop. Med. *9*:125–135, 1960.
51. Gitelson, S.: Gastrectomy, achlorhydria and cholera. Isr. J. Med. Sci. *7*:663–667, 1971.
52. Glass, R. I., Svennerholm, A.-M., Stoll, B. J., et al.: Protection against cholera in breast-fed children by antibodies in breast milk. N. Engl. J. Med. *308*:1389–1392, 1983.
53. Glass, R. I., Holmgren, J., Khan, M. R., et al.: A randomized, controlled clinical trial of the toxin-blocking effects of B subunit in family members of patients with cholera. J. Infect. Dis. *149*:495–500, 1984.
54. Glass, R. I., Holmgren, J., Haley, C. E., et al.: Predisposition for cholera of individuals with O blood group: Possible evolutionary significance. Am. J. Epidemiol. *121*:791–796, 1985.
55. Glass, R. I., Claeson, M., Blake, P. A., et al.: Cholera in Africa: Lessons on transmission and control for Latin America. Lancet *338*:791–795, 1991.
56. Goldberg, M. B., diRita, V. J., and Calderwood, S. B.: Identification of an iron-regulated virulence determinant in *Vibrio cholerae*, using Tn*pho*A mutagenesis. Infect. Immun. *58*:55–60, 1990.
57. Goldstein, B., Doody, D., and Briggs, S.: Emergency intraosseous infusion in severely burned children. Pediatr. Emerg. Care *6*:195–197, 1990.
58. Goma Epidemiology Group: Public health impact of Rwandan refugee crisis: What happened in Goma, Zaire, in July, 1994? Lancet *345*:339–344, 1995.
59. Gore, S. M., Fontaine, O., and Pierce, N. F.: Impact of rice-based oral rehydration solution on stool output and duration of diarrhoea: Meta-analysis of 13 clinical trials. Br. Med. J. *304*:287–291, 1992.
60. Gottuzo, E., Seas, C., Echevarría, J., et al.: Ciprofloxacin for the treatment of cholera: A randomized, double-blind, controlled clinical trial of a single daily dose in Peruvian adults. Clin. Infect. Dis. *20*:1485–1490, 1995.
61. Greenough, W. B., III., Gordon, R. S., Rosenberg, I. S., et al.: Tetracycline in the treatment of cholera. Lancet *1*:355–357, 1964.
62. Harris, J. R., Holmberg, S. D., Parker, R. D. R., et al.: Impact of epidemic cholera in a previously uninfected island population: Evaluation of a new seroepidemiologic method. Am. J. Epidemiol. *123*:424–430, 1986.
63. Harvey, R. M., Enson, Y., Lewis, M. L., et al.: Hemodynamic studies on cholera: Effects of hypovolemia and acidosis. Circulation *37*:709–728, 1968.
64. Hasan, J. A., Huq, A., Tamplin, M. L., et al.: A novel kit for rapid detection of *Vibrio cholerae* O1. J. Clin. Microbiol. *32*:249–252, 1994.
65. Herrington, D. A., Hall, R. H., Losonsky, G. A., et al.: Toxin, toxin-coregulated pili and the *tox*R regulon are essential for *Vibrio cholerae* pathogenesis in humans. J. Exp. Med. *168*:1487–1492, 1988.
66. Hirschhorn, N.: The treatment of acute diarrhea in children: An historical and physiological perspective. Am. J. Clin. Nutr. *33*:637–663, 1980.
67. Holmgren, J., Czerkinsky, C., Lycke, N., et al.: Strategies for the induction of immune responses at mucosal surfaces making use of cholera toxin B subunit as immunogen, carrier, and adjuvant. Am. J. Trop. Med. Hyg. *50*(Suppl. 5):52–54, 1994.
68. Hone, D., and Hackett, J.: Vaccination against enteric bacterial diseases. Rev. Infect. Dis. *6*:853–877, 1989.
69. Hunt, M. D., Woodward, W. E., Keswick, B. H., et al.: Seroepidemiology of cholera in Gulf Coastal Texas. Appl. Environ. Microbiol. *54*:1673–1677, 1988.
70. Hunt, J. B., Thillainayagam, A. V., Carnaby, S., et al.: Absorption of a hypotonic oral rehydration solution in a human model of cholera. Gut *35*:211–214, 1994.
71. Huq, A., Colwell, R. R., Rahman, R., et al.: Detection of *Vibrio cholerae* O1 in the aquatic environment by fluorescent-monoclonal antibody and culture methods. Appl. Environ. Microbiol. *56*:2370–2373, 1990.
72. Ingram, M.: Cholera epidemic hits former Soviet states. B.M.J. *311*:528–529, 1995.
73. Islam, A., Bardhan, P. K., Islam, M. R., et al.: A randomized double blind trial of aspirin versus placebo in cholera and non-cholera diarrhoea. Trop. Geogr. Med. *38*:221–225, 1986.
74. Islam, M. S., Hasan, M. K., Miah, M. A., et al.: Isolation of *Vibrio cholerae* O139 synonym Bengal from the aquatic environment in Bangladesh: Implications for disease transmission. Appl. Environ. Microbiol. *60*:1684–1686, 1994
75. Jamil, B. A., Ahmed A., and Sturm, A. W.: *Vibrio cholerae* O1 septicemia. Lancet *340*:910–911, 1992.
76. Jesudason, M. V., Cherian, A. M., and John, T. J.: Blood stream invasion by *Vibrio cholerae* O139. Lancet *342*:431, 1993.
77. Jesudason, M. V., Samuel, R., and John, T. J.: Reappearence of *Vibrio cholerae* O1 and concurrent prevalence of O1 and O139 in Vellore, South India. Lancet *344*:335–336, 1994.
78. Jesudason, M. V., and John, T. J.: The appearance and spread of *Vibrio cholerae* O139 in India. Ind. J. Med. Res. *99*:97–100, 1994.
79. Jonson, G., Svennerholm, A.-M., and Holmgren, J.: *Vibrio cholerae* expresses cell surface antigens during intestinal infection which are not expressed during in vitro cell culture. Infect. Immun. *57*:1809–1815, 1989.
80. Kaper, J. B, Morris, J. G., Jr., and Levine, M. M.: Cholera. Clin. Microbiol. Rev. *8*:48–86, 1995.
81. Kawo, N. G., Msengi, A. E., Swai, A. B. M., et al.: Specificity of hypoglycaemia for cerebral malaria in children. Lancet *336*:454–457, 1990.
82. Khan, W. A., Begum, M., Salam, M. A., et al.: Comparative trial of five antimicrobial compounds in the treatment of cholera in adults. Trans. R. Soc. Trop. Med. Hyg. *89*:103–106, 1995.
82a. Khan, W. A., Bennish, M. L., Seas, C., et al.: Randomised, controlled comparison of single-dose ciprofloxacin and doxycycline for cholera caused by *Vibrio cholerae* O1 or O139. Lancet *348*:296–300, 1996.
83. Kimberg, D. V., Field, M., Johnson, J., et al.: Stimulation of intestinal mucosal adenyl cyclase by cholera enterotoxin and prostaglandins. J. Clin. Invest. *50*:1218–1230, 1971.
84. Lagos, R., Avendano, A., Prado, et al.: Attenuated live cholera vaccine strain CVD 103-HgR elicits significantly higher serum vibriocidal antibody titers in persons of blood group O. Infect. Immun. *63*:707–709, 1995.
85. Lencer, W. I., Delp, C., Neutra, M. R., et al.: Mechanism of cholera toxin action on a polarized human intestinal epithelial cell line: Role of vesicular traffic. J. Cell. Biol. *117*:1197–1209, 1992.
86. Lencer, W. I., de Almeida, J. B., Moe, S., et al.: Entry of cholera toxin into polarized human intestinal epithelial cells: Identification of an early brefeldin A sensitive event required for A1-peptide generation. J. Clin. Invest. *92*:2941–2951, 1993.
87. Levine, M. M., Kaper, J. B., Herrington, D., et al.: Volunteer studies of deletion mutants of *Vibrio cholerae* O1 prepared by recombinant techniques. Infect. Immun. *56*:161–167, 1988.
88. Lindenbaum, J. L, Gordon, R. S., Jr., Hirschhorn, N., et al.: Cholera in children. Lancet *i*:1066–1068, 1966.
89. Martin, A. R., Mosley, W. H., Sau, B. B., et al.: Epidemiologic analysis of endemic cholera in urban East Pakistan, 1964–1966. Am. J. Epidemiol. *89*:572–582, 1969.
90. Mathan, M. M., Chandy G., and Mathan, V. I.: Ultrastructural changes in the upper small intestinal mucosa in patients with cholera. Gastroenterology *109*:422–430, 1995.
91. McClead, R. E., Butler, T., and Rabbani, G. H.: Orally administered bovine colostral anti-cholera toxin antibodies: Results of two clinical trials. Am. J. Med. *85*:811–816, 1988.
92. McCormack, W. M., Chowdhury, A. M., Jahangir, N., et al.: Tetracycline prophylaxis in families of cholera patients. Bull. W. H. O. *38*:787–792, 1968.
93. McCormack, W. M., Islam, M. S., Fahimuddin, M., et al.: A community study of inapparent cholera infections. Am. J. Epidemiol. *89*:658–664, 1969.

94. McDonald, J. J., Chanduvi, B., Velarde, G., et al.: Bioimpedance monitoring of rehydration in cholera. Lancet *341*:1049–1051, 1993.
95. Mekalanos, J. J., Swartz, D. J., Pearson, G. D. N., et al.: Cholera toxin genes: Nucleotide sequence, deletion analysis, and vaccine development. Nature *306*:551–557, 1983.
96. Mekalanos, J. J., and Sadoff, J. C.: Cholera vaccines: Fighting an ancient scourge. Science *265*:1387–1389, 1994.
97. Mhalu, F. S., Mtango, F. D. E., and Msengi, A. E.: Hospital outbreaks of cholera transmitted through close person to person contact. Lancet *2*:82–84, 1984.
98. Miller, C. J., Feachem, R. G., and Drasar, B. S.: Cholera epidemiology in developed and developing countries: New thoughts on transmission, seasonality, and control. Lancet *1*:261–263, 1985.
99. Mitra, A. K., and Rabbani, G. H.: A double-blind, controlled trial of bioflorin (*Streptococcus faecium* SF68) in adults with acute diarrhea due to *Vibrio cholerae* and enterotoxigenic *Escherichia coli*. Gastroenterology *99*:1149–1152, 1990.
100. Miyagi, K., Matsumoto, Y., Hayashi, K., et al.: Successful application of enzyme-labeled oligonucleotide probe for rapid and accurate cholera diagnosis in a clinical laboratory. Microbiol. Immunol. *38*:301–304, 1994.
101. Molla, A. M., Rahman, M., Sarker, S. A., et al.: Stool electrolyte content and purging rates in diarrhea caused by rotavirus, enterotoxigenic *E. coli*, and *V. cholerae* in children. J. Pediatr. *98*:825–838, 1981.
102. Molla, A., Molla, A. M., Rahim, A., et al.: Intake and absorption of nutrients in children with cholera and rotavirus infection during acute diarrhea and after recovery. Nutr. Res. *2*:233–242, 1982.
103. Molla, A. M., Gyr, K., Bardhan, P. K., et al.: Effect of intravenous somatostatin on stool output in diarrhea due to *Vibrio cholerae*. Gastroenterology *87*:845–847, 1984.
104. Moren, A., Stefanaggi, S., Antona, D., et al.: Practical field epidemiology to investigate a cholera outbreak in a Mozambican refugee camp in Malawi, 1988. J. Trop. Med. Hyg. *94*:1–7, 1991.
105. Morris, J. G., Jr.: Non-O group 1 *Vibrio cholerae* strains not associated with epidemic disease. *In* Wachsmuth, I. K., Blake, P. A., and Olsvik, O. (eds.): *Vibrio cholerae* and Cholera: Molecular to Global Perspectives. Washington, D.C., American Society of Microbiology, 1994, pp. 103–115.
106. Morris, J. G., Jr., Losonsky, G. E., Johnson, J. A., et al.: Clinical and immunological characteristics of *Vibrio cholerae* O139 Bengal infection in North American volunteers. J. Infect. Dis. *171*:903–908, 1995.
107. Morger, H., Steffen, R., and Schar, M.: Epidemiology of cholera in travellers, and conclusions for vaccination recommendations. Br. Med. J. *286*:184–186, 1983.
108. Mujica, O. J., Quick, R. E., Palacios, A. M., et al.: Epidemic cholera in the Amazon: The role of produce in disease risk and prevention. J. Infect. Dis. *169*:1381–1384, 1994.
109. Nair, G. B., Ramamurthy, T., Bhattacharya, S. K., et al.: Spread of *Vibrio cholerae* O139 in India. J. Infect. Dis. *169*:1029–1034, 1994.
110. Nalin, D. R., Cash, R. A., and Rahaman, M.: Oral (or nasogastric) maintenance therapy for cholera patients in all age groups. Bull. W. H. O. *43*:361–363, 1970.
111. Nalin, D. R., Levine, M. M., Rhead, J., et al.: Cannabis, hypochlorhydria, and cholera. Lancet *ii*:859–862, 1978.
112. Palmer, D. L., Koster, F. T., Islam, A. F. M. R., et al.: Comparison of sucrose and glucose in the oral electrolyte therapy of cholera and other severe diarrheas. N. Engl. J. Med. *297*:1107–1110, 1977.
113. Phillips, R. A.: Twenty years of cholera research. J. A. M. A. *202*:610–613, 1967.
114. Pierce, N. F., Banwell, J. G., Sack, R. B., et al.: Magnitude and duration of antitoxin response to human infection with *Vibrio cholerae*. J. Infect. Dis. *121*:S31–S35, 1970.
115. Pizzaro, D., Posada, G., Sandi, L., et al.: Rice-based oral electrolyte solutions for the management of infantile diarrhea. N. Engl. J. Med. *324*:517–521, 1991.
116. Qadri, F., Hasan, J. A., Hossain, J., et al.: Evaluation of the monoclonal antibody-based kit Bengal SMART for rapid detection of *Vibrio cholerae* O139 synonym Bengal in stool samples. J. Clin. Microbiol. *33*:732–734, 1995.
117. Rabbani, G. H., Greenough, W. B., III, Holmgren, J., et al.: Controlled trial of chlorpromazine as an antisecretory agent in patients with cholera hydrated intravenously. Br. Med. J. *284*:1361–1364, 1982.
118. Rabbani, G. H., Butler, T., Bardhan, P. K., et al.: Reduction of fluid-loss in cholera by nicotinic acid: A randomized controlled clinical trial. Lancet *2*:1439–1442, 1983.
119. Rabbani, G. H., Butler, T., Knight, J., et al.: Randomized, controlled trial of berberine sulfate therapy for diarrhea due to enterotoxigenic *Escherichia coli* and *Vibrio cholerae*. J. Infect. Dis. *155*:979–984, 1987.
120. Rabbani, G. H., Butler, T., Patte, D., et al.: Clinical trial of clonidine hydrochloride as an antisecretory agent in cholera. Gastroenterology *97*:321–325, 1989.
121. Rabbani, G. H., Butler, T., Shahrier, M., et al.: Efficacy of single dose of furazolidone for treatment of cholera in children. Antimicrob. Agents Chemother. *35*:1864–1867, 1991.
122. Rahman, O., Bennish, M. L., Alam, A. N., et al.: Rapid intravenous rehydration by means of a single polyelectrolyte solution with or without dextrose. J. Pediatr. *113*:654–660, 1988.
123. Ramamurthy, T. S., Bhattacharya, S. K., Uesaka, Y., et al.: Evaluation of the bead enzyme-lined immunosorbent assay for detection of cholera toxin directly from stool specimens. J. Clin. Microbiol. *30*:1783–1786, 1992.
124. Ramamurthy, T. S., Pal, A., Bhattacharya, M. K., et al.: Serovar, biotype, phagetype, toxigenicity and antibiotic susceptibility patterns of *Vibrio cholerae* isolated during two consecutive cholera seasons (1989–90) in Calcutta. Ind. J. Med. Res. [A] *95*:125–129, 1995.
125. Ransome-Kuti, O., Elebute, O., Agusto-Odutola, T., et al.: Intraperitoneal fluid infusion in children with gastroenteritis. Br. Med. J. *3*:500–503, 1969.
126. Rao, A., and Stockwell, B. A.: The Queensland cholera incident of 1977. Bull. W. H. O. *58*:661–664, 1980.
127. Rapoport, S. M., Dodd, M., Clark, M., et al.: Postacidotic state of infantile diarrhea: Symptoms and chemical data: Postacidotic hypocalcemia and associated decreases in levels of potassium, phosphorus, and phosphatase in the plasma. Am. J. Dis. Child. *73*:391–441, 1947.
128. Richardson, K., Nixon, L., Mostow, P., et al.: Transposon-induced nonmotile mutants of *Vibrio cholerae*. J. Gen. Microbiol. *136*:717–725, 1990.
129. Ruxin, J. N.: Magic bullet: The history of oral rehydration therapy. Med. Hist. *38*:363–397, 1994.
130. Ryder, R. W., Rahman, M. A. S. M., Alim, A. R. M., et al.: An outbreak of nosocomial cholera in a rural Bangladesh hospital. J. Hosp. Infect. *8*:275–282, 1986.
131. Safrin, S., Morris, J. G., Adams, M., et al.: Non-O:1 *Vibrio cholerae* bacteremia: Case report and review. Rev. Infect. Dis. *10*:1012–1017, 1988.
132. Sanchez, J. L., Vasquez, B., Begue, R. E., et al.: Protective efficacy of oral whole-cell/recombinant-B-subunit cholera vaccine in Peruvian military recruits. Lancet *344*:1273–1276, 1994.
133. Sanyal, S. C., Singh, S. J., Tiwari, I. C., et al.: Role of household animals in maintenance of cholera infection in a community. J. Infect. Dis. *130*:575–579, 1974.
134. Schaad, U. B., Salam, M. A., Aujard, Y., et al.: Use of fluroquinolones in pediatrics: Consensus report of an International Society of Chemotherapy commission. Pediatr. Infect. Dis. J. *14*:1–9, 1995.
135. Shaffer, N., Silva do Santos, E., Andreason, P. A., et al.: Rapid laboratory diagnosis of cholera in the field. Trans. R. Soc. Trop. Med. Hyg. *83*:119–120, 1989.
136. Siddique, A. K., Mutsuddy, P., Islam, Q., et al.: Makeshift treatment centre during a cholera epidemic in Bangladesh. Trop. Doct. *20*:83–85, 1990.
137. Siddique, A. K., Salam, A., Islam, M. S., et al.: Why treatment centres failed to prevent cholera deaths among Rwandan refugees in Goma, Zaire. Lancet *345*:359–361, 1995.
138. Simanjuntak, C. H., O'Hanley, P., Punjabi, N. H., et al.: Safety, immunogenicity, and transmissibility of single-dose live oral cholera vaccine strain CVD 103-HgR in 24- to 59-month-old Indonesian children. J. Infect. Dis. *168*:1169–1176, 1993.
139. Snow, J.: On the Mode of Communication of Cholera. 2nd ed. London, Churchill, 1855.
140. Snyder, J. D., and Blake, P. A.: Is cholera a problem for US travelers? J. A. M. A. *247*:2268–2269, 1982.
141. Stoll, B. J., Holmgren, J., Bardhan, P. K., et al.: Binding of intraluminal toxin in cholera: Trial of GM1 ganglioside charcoal. Lancet *2*:888–891, 1980.
142. Struelens, M. J., Bennish, M. L., Mondal, G., et al.: Bacteremia during diarrhea: Incidence, etiology, risk factors, and outcome. Am. J. Epidemiol. *133*:451–459, 1991.
143. Sun, D., Mekalanos, J. J., and Taylor, R. K.: Antibodies directed against the toxin-coregulated pilus isolated from *Vibrio cholerae* provide protection in the infant mouse experimental cholera model. J. Infect. Dis. *161*:1231–1236, 1990.
144. Svennerholm, A. M., Jertborn, M., Gothefors, L., et al.: Mucosal antitoxic and antibacterial immunity after cholera disease and after immunization with a combined B subunit whole cell vaccine. J. Infect. Dis. *149*:884–893, 1983.
145. Swerdlow, D. L., Mintz, E. D., Rodriguez, M., et al.: Waterborne transmission of epidemic cholera in Trujillo, Peru: Lessons for a continent at risk. Lancet *340*:28–33, 1992.
146. Swerdlow, D. L., and Ries, A. A.: *Vibrio cholerae* non-01: The eighth pandemic? Lancet *342*:382–383, 1993.
147. Swerdlow, D. L., Mintz, E. D., Rodriguez, M., et al.: Severe life-threatening cholera associated with blood group O in Peru: Implications for the Latin American epidemic. J. Infect. Dis. *170*:468–472, 1994.
148. Tacket, C. O., Forrest, B., Morona, R., et al.: Safety, immunogenicity, and efficacy against cholera challenge in man of a bivalent typhoid-cholera hybrid vaccine derived from Ty21A. Infect. Immun. *58*:1620–1627, 1990.
149. Tacket, C. O., Losonsky, G., Nataro, J. P., et al.: Onset and duration of protective immunity in challenged volunteers after vaccination with live oral cholera vaccine CVD 103-HgR. J. Infect. Dis. *166*:837–841, 1992.
150. Tacket, C. O., Losonsky, G., Nataro, J. P., et al.: Safety and immunogenicity of live oral cholera vaccine candidate CVD 110, a delta *ctxA* delta *zot* delta *ace* derivative of El Tor Ogawa *Vibrio cholerae*. J. Infect. Dis. *168*:1536–1540, 1993.
151. Tacket, C. O., Losonsky, G., Nataro, J. P., et al.: Initial clinical studies of CVD 112 *Vibrio cholerae* O139 live oral vaccine: Safety and efficacy against experimental challenge. J. Infect. Dis. *172*:883–886, 1995.
152. Tamplin, M. L., Gauzens, A. L., Huq, A., et al.: Attachment of *Vibrio*

cholerae serogroup O1 to zooplankton and phytoplankton of Bangladesh waters. Appl. Environ. Microbiol. *56*:1977–1980, 1990.
153. Taylor, J. L., Tuttle, J., Pramukul, T., et al.: An outbreak of cholera in Maryland associated with imported commercial frozen fresh coconut milk. J. Infect. Dis., *167*:1330–1335, 1993.
154. Taylor, D. N., Killeen, K. P., Hack, D. C., et al.: Development of a live, oral, attenuated vaccine against El Tor cholera. J. Infect. Dis. *170*:1518, 1523, 1994.
155. van Loon, F. P., Rabbani, G. H., Bukhave, K., et al.: Indomethacin decreases jejunal fluid secretion in addition to luminal release of prostaglandin E_2 in patients with acute cholera. Gut *33*:643–645, 1992.
156. Varela, P., Pollevick, G. D., Rivas, M., et al.: Direct detection of *Vibrio cholerae* in stool samples. J. Clin. Microbiol. *32*:1246–1248, 1994.
157. Wachsmuth, I. K., Evins, G. M., Fields, P. I., et al.: The molecular epidemiology of cholera in Latin America. J. Infect. Dis. *167*:621–626, 1993.
158. Wachsmuth, I. K., Blake, P. A., and Olsvik, O. (eds.): *Vibrio cholerae* and Cholera: Molecular to Global Perspectives. Washington, D.C., American Society of Microbiology, 1994.
159. Waldor, M. K., and Mekalanos, J. J.: Emergence of a new cholera pandemic: Molecular analysis of virulence determinants in *Vibrio cholerae* O139 and development of a live vaccine prototype. J. Infect. Dis. *170*:278–283, 1994.
160. Waldor, M. K.. Colwell, R., and Mekalanos, J. J.: The *Vibrio cholerae* O139 serogroup antigen includes an O-antigen capsule and lipopolysaccharide virulence determinants. Proc. Natl. Acad. Sci. U. S. A. *91*:11388, 1994.
160a. Waldor, M. K., and Mekalanos, J. J.: Lysogenic conversion by a filamentous phage encoding cholera toxin. Science *272*:1910–1914, 1997.
161. Weber, J. T., Levine, W. C., Hopkins, D. P., et al.: Cholera in the United States, 1965–1991: Risks at home and abroad. Arch. Intern. Med. *154*:551–556, 1994.
162. Wang, F., Butler, T., Rabbani, G. H., et al.: The acidosis of cholera: Contributions of hyperproteinemia, lactic acidemia, and hyperphosphatemia to an increased anion gap. N. Engl. J. Med. *315*:1591–1595, 1986.
163. Watten, R. H., Morgan, F. M., Songkhla, Y. N., et al.: Water and electrolyte studies in cholera. J. Clin. Invest. *38*:1879–1889, 1959.
164. Watten, R. H., and Phillips, R. A.: Potassium in the treatment of cholera. Lancet *2*:999–1001, 1960.
165. World Health Organization Programme for Control of Diarrhoeal Disease: Guidelines for cholera control. Geneva, World Health Organization, 1991.
166. Woodward, W. E.: Cholera reinfection in man. J. Infect. Dis. *123*:61–66, 1971.
167. Yamamoto, T., Gojobori, T., and Yakota, T.: Evolutionary origin of pathogenic determinants in enterotoxigenic *Escherichia coli* and *Vibrio cholerae* O1. J. Bacteriol. *169*:1352–1357, 1987.
168. Yamamoto, T., Nair, G., Albert, M. J., et al.: Survey of in vitro susceptibilities of *Vibrio cholerae* O1 and O139 to antimicrobial agents. Antimicrob. Agents Chemother. *39*:241–244, 1995.

122

VIBRIO PARAHAEMOLYTICUS

Enrique Caceres and Thomas G. Cleary

Vibrio parahaemolyticus is recognized worldwide as a cause of food-borne disease associated with consumption of seafood, in particular crustaceans and mollusks, and occasionally as a cause of wound infections and sepsis in immunocompromised hosts.

Not surprisingly, the first association of *V. parahaemolyticus* seafood-related diarrhea was reported almost 45 years ago in Japan; 40 to 60 per cent of food-borne outbreaks in Japan are due to this pathogen.[29] Almost 10 years after the first description, the organism correctly was classified in the genus *Vibrio*,[6] and its distribution in coastal waters and estuaries of temperate climates around the world was recognized. The regional differences in the incidence of this disease clearly are related to patterns of consumption of marine products and the food preparation practices. In Japan, fish and shellfish are a major source of dietary protein and customarily are eaten raw; in the United States, where sporadic outbreaks have been reported,[3, 4, 14] seafood more typically is cooked.[11] Nevertheless, the potential risk for infectious and toxic syndromes with marine products exists in the United States.[20]

BACTERIOLOGY

V. parahaemolyticus belongs to the group of 12 species of the genus *Vibrio* that are human pathogens and have brackish water as their natural habitat. Vibrios are gram-negative, non–spore-forming, straight or curved rods with rounded ends that possess a polar flagellum.[36] When grown on solid media, *V. parahaemolyticus* has additional shorter lateral peritrichous flagella. It is a facultative anaerobe with both respiratory and fermentative metabolism. Like most vibrios, it is an oxidase-positive nonfermenter of lactose.[5] It is arginine-dihydrolase–negative and ornithine-decarboxylase–positive. The requirement of sodium and enhancement of growth in a specific range of concentration differentiate it from *V. cholerae* and *V. mimicus*. The optimal sodium concentration range is from 2 to 4 per cent; a concentration higher than 8 per cent inhibits its growth.[54]

V. parahaemolyticus produces round, blue-green colonies on the widely used *Vibrio*-selective thiosulfate citrate bile salts sucrose. This medium inhibits most fecal flora by the presence of bile salts and a highly alkaline pH. Direct plating on thiosulfate citrate bile salts sucrose may be used for feces and other clinical specimens, but food samples that are not contaminated heavily require enrichment either in alkaline peptone water supplemented with 3 per cent sodium chloride or in a strongly selective medium, such as glucose salt teepol broth.[54] The optimum pH for growth is in the neutral range, but *V. parahaemolyticus* can survive in alkaline media. It may survive storage at 5° C. Growth beyond 44° C is inhibited, and inactivation is greater with increased temperatures; for example, there is a millionfold decline in viable bacteria in shrimp homogenate kept at 100° C for only 1 minute.[52] Growth is remarkable in conventional media and foodstuff, with generation times as low as 8 minutes[29]; thus, a significant number of organisms can be found after a short period of inappropriate storage.

Serologically, *V. parahaemolyticus* can be grouped into 11 O and 71 K serotypes. K antigens associate with specific somatic antigens[11]; so, for example, serotypes K 3 and K 28 associate with the 2 O group. Environmental and clinical isolates do not differ in biochemical characteristics or in the presence of plasmids.[32] Plasmid carriage appears to be sporadic and not related to virulence but can be associated with resistance to multiple antibiotics.[28]

EPIDEMIOLOGY

In the United States, *V. parahaemolyticus* is found along the East, West, and Gulf Coasts.[15, 29] Water, sediments, suspended particulates, plankton, fish, and shellfish all have been shown to harbor the organism.[2, 38] The organisms are present in highest numbers in water between 17° C and 35° C containing 0.5 to 2.5 per cent salinity.[28] There is marked seasonal and geographic variation, with maximal mean concentrations during late summer and spring along the Gulf Coast.[15] The seasonal distribution correlates with the occurrence of outbreaks predominantly between June and October.[1]

Finfish and all types of shellfish products, including oysters, clams, crabs, and shrimp, may be involved in the transmission of the infection (Table 122–1).[28] The risk of infection is highest with seafood able to concentrate contaminants,[28] and, in general, shellfish are more contaminated than finfish.[2, 21] The density of *V. parahaemolyticus* may be 100 times greater in oysters than in water.[15] There is no association with water pollution, aerobic plate count, or fecal coliform density.[15] The levels of contamination of seafood generally are low in freshly collected oysters, with the highest mean density of only 160 bacteria/g found in the United States.[15] In market shellfish, higher counts (up to 10^3 to 10^4/g) have been reported in Japan.[11] The minimum infective dose is thought to be in the range of 10^5 to 10^7 organisms, based on volunteer feeding studies.[19]

During the period 1973 to 1987, only 23 of 1869 food-borne disease outbreaks with known bacterial etiology reported to the Centers for Disease Control and Prevention were caused by *V. parahaemolyticus*[3]; these accounted for 535 cases and represented less than 1 per cent of the total cases. In 18 of these outbreaks, a shellfish was recognized as the food vehicle; only 1 outbreak was related to finfish. There were no fatal cases reported. Contributing factors included inadequate cooking (92 per cent), improper holding temperature (75 per cent), and food acquired from an unsafe source (75 per cent).[3, 4] Attack rates ranged from 24 per cent to 86 per cent, with a medium of 51 per cent in 13 outbreaks in the United States.[1] Most of the affected people were adults, and no patterns of unusual susceptibility by age group or gender were noted. There was no evidence of secondary spread among family members. *Vibrio* surveillance in four Gulf Coast states (Alabama, Florida, Louisiana, and Texas) found that 67 per cent of patients with primary *Vibrio* septicemia and 74 per cent with gastroenteritis had eaten raw oysters in the week before illness began.[35]

PATHOGENESIS

The ability of certain strains to produce beta-hemolysis on Wagatsuma agar containing human red blood cells is related to the virulence of the bacteria; this so-called Kanagawa phenomenon is produced by a thermostable direct hemolysin (TDH).[37] This substance, unlike other hemolysins produced by *V. parahaemolyticus*, is not inactivated by heating at 100° C for 10 minutes. The hemolytic activity is not enhanced by the addition of lecithin, indicating a direct action on erythrocytes.[50] TDH has been characterized and purified, but the exact role and mechanism of action in the production of diarrhea still are under investigation.[18] The biologic activities include hemolysis of erythrocytes from various species, cytotoxicity, lethality to small experimental animals, and increased vascular permeability in rabbit skin.[50] The association of TDH and virulence first was based on epidemiologic grounds. Kanagawa phenomenon is observed in 88 to 96 per cent of strains from clinical specimens and in 1 to 2 per cent of strains from environmental sources.[19, 29, 51] After the epidemiologic association was made, Kanagawa phenomenon–positive strains were found to cause fluid accumulation in rabbit ileal loop assays, adherence to epithelial cells in tissue cultures, and invasion of intestinal mucosa.[13, 53] TDH has a molecular weight of 42,000 daltons, consisting of two subunits of 21,000 daltons.[38] It can be inactivated by trypsin or pepsin. The hemolytic activity is inhibited by neuraminidase-sensitive gangliosides, especially GT1. Cultured mouse heart cells show abnormal conduction, suggesting cardiotoxic activity in TDH and a possible explanation for changes in electrocardiograms of humans with intestinal infection.[29, 50] Reports of outbreaks produced by Kanagawa phenomenon–negative organisms[25] and contradictory studies of highly concentrated culture filtrates containing TDH[46] have caused doubts about the significance of Kanagawa phenomenon. The inability of antiserum to TDH to eliminate the fluid accumulation in the rabbit ileal loop assay and the requirement of unusually high doses of purified TDH to produce pathologic results have raised questions about the role of TDH.[11] A TDH-related hemolysin (TRH) immunologically and structurally similar to TDH is present in some Kanagawa phenomenon–negative strains.[26, 48] Likewise, some variants closely related to the original TDH by molecular analysis (Vp

TABLE 122–1. Selected Outbreaks of *Vibrio parahaemolyticus* Infection

Setting	Persons Ill/ Exposed	Symptoms	Incubation	Resolution	Medical Attention/ Hospitalization	Vehicle	Risk Factor
Picnic[14]	351/631 (56%)	D (95%), C (82%), N (68%), V (61%), HA (41%), F (27%)	16 hr (4–42 hr)	4 d (<1–10 d)	60%/2%	Steamed crab	Cross-contamination, unrefrigerated food
Chronic hospital[14]	24/100 (24%)	D (100%), C (89%), N (72%), V (44%), HA (56%), F (33%)	18 hr (4–60 hr)	3 d (<1–7 d)	No data available	Crab salad	No data available
Shrimp boil[49]	ca. 600/ 1200 (50%)	D, C, V, HA, F	23 hr (5–92 hr)	(few hr–1 wk)	1%/0%	Boiled shrimp	Storage temperature
International flight[43]	12/134 (9%)	D, C, V	(8–20 hr)	No data available	40%/25%	Cooked crab	Cross-contamination
Parish dinner[11]	ca. 1000/ 1700 (59%)	D (95%), C (92%), N (72%), HA (47%), P (47%), V (12%)	16 hr (3–76 hr)	4.6 d (<1–8 d)	26%/7.4%	Shrimp	Cross-contamination, storage temperature

D, diarrhea; C, cramps; N, nausea; V, vomiting; HA, headache; F, fever.

TDH/I and Vp TDH/II) have been isolated from Kanagawa phenomenon–negative strains.[39]

After the *tdh* gene had been cloned and sequenced, it became clear that certain strains possess the genetic material but are phenotypically incomplete. Eighty-six per cent of strains with weak hemolysis in Wagatsuma agar carry the *tdh* gene but in only one copy; a smaller proportion of Kanagawa phenomenon–negative strains contains both copies.[42] Low-level expression of the *tdh* genes may be the reason for the Kanagawa phenomenon–negative phenotype.[41] Less than half of *trh* gene–positive strains produce TRH when examined by enzyme-linked immunosorbent assay.[48] Gene probe hybridization analysis indicates that most of the environmental Kanagawa phenomenon–negative strains do not carry DNA encoding TDH.[31] The expression of the *tdh* genes is controlled by the Vp-*tox RS* operon. The basal production of mRNA and the degree of transcriptional activation seem related to differences in the nucleotide sequences and strength of the promoter region.[41] The *tdh* genes are chromosomal, but some variants are found on plasmids.[39] Isogeneic *tdh* gene–negative mutants lose the ability to produce fluid accumulation in the rabbit ileal loop assay.[40] Thermostable direct hemolysin may induce intestinal chloride secretion using GT1b as a receptor and calcium as a second messenger.[45]

Some studies suggest virulence mechanisms in addition to TDH.[53] *V. parahaemolyticus* requires intestinal colonization factors to cause disease. A variety of pili and other potential colonization factors are present, but there is poor evidence to implicate any of the candidate adhesins in virulence.[11] Adherence of *V. parahaemolyticus* to intestinal epithelial cells of rabbits[12] and human small intestine[23, 55] appears to require binding to complex carbohydrates or hemagglutinins of the host.

The occurrence of cases with grossly bloody stools[27] is indirect evidence of either invasiveness or cytotoxin production. Both Kanagawa phenomenon–positive and Kanagawa phenomenon–negative strains from clinical specimens can invade and colonize the mucosal cells of the rabbit ileum, producing acute inflammation, degeneration, and erosion of the villi.[5] Vibrios can be cultured from tissue specimens of spleen, liver, and heart in experimental animals, indicating spread via the lymphatic or circulatory systems.[8]

CLINICAL MANIFESTATIONS

The spectrum of disease varies from a mild gastroenteritis to a full-blown dysenteric syndrome. The incubation period typically is 15 hours to 24 hours, with extremes of 4 hours to 96 hours[1, 49]; the variability presumably is related to the number of organisms ingested. Resolution is expected in about 3 days,[38] but it varies from several hours to more than 10 days.[1, 9] Fatigue may persist for a few days. Diarrhea (96 per cent) and crampy abdominal pain (95 per cent) are the most frequent and earliest symptoms, accompanied by nausea, vomiting, and headache in 40 to 70 per cent of cases. Chills and moderate fever are less frequent (20 per cent).[1, 14] The diarrhea is watery and explosive,[10] with up to 15 stools during the first day. Shock due to fluid loss is an exceptional event.[15] Mucus is not observed infrequently, but grossly bloody stool is uncommon.[6, 27, 35] Small superficial ulcerations on sigmoidoscopy may be present.[6] There is no difference in symptoms in cases associated with Kanagawa phenomenon–negative strains.[25]

Extraintestinal infections occur. During the *Vibrio* Surveillance Program that started in 1989 in four Gulf Coast states, 18 per cent of *V. parahaemolyticus* isolates were found to come from wound infections and 3 per cent were found to be associated with septicemia.[35] Wound infection occurs after contamination of skin lacerations with seawater or after direct trauma with pieces of shellfish, fish hooks, or utensils contaminated with seawater.[7] Superficial infection can extend to deeper soft tissue and may require radical surgical débridement. Septicemia is a concern in immunocompromised patients, particularly leukemia patients[17] and those with liver disease.[16, 24] Bacteremia may occur after either wound infections[7, 17] or ingestion of seafood.[24, 44] Skin bullae,[24] intravascular hemolysis,[17] and disseminated intravascular coagulation[24] may complicate both wound and bacteremic infections.

COMPLICATIONS

The acute diarrheal episode requires medical attention in as many as 25 to 50 per cent of cases during an outbreak but infrequently requires hospitalization.[9, 14, 35, 49] There usually are no long-term sequelae. Severe dehydration, shock,[27, 43] and even death (0.04 per cent of cases in Japan) can occur.[5, 54] On the other hand, primary septicemia,[33, 35, 44] septicemia secondary to wound infection,[7, 17, 33] or septicemia secondary to gastroenteritis[24, 33] in immunosupressed patients or in those with liver diseases may cause death.[7]

DIAGNOSIS

Epidemiologic data are the basis for the presumptive diagnosis. In a patient with compatible symptoms, a history of recent consumption of seafood should raise suspicion of this diagnosis. Leukocytosis and fecal leukocytes may be found.[6, 27] A positive stool culture on selective media, such as thiosulfate citrate bile salts sucrose, can confirm the clinical impression. Routine use of thiosulfate citrate bile salts sucrose is not cost-effective, even in coastal areas, unless there is an appropriate clinical setting.[7, 35, 36] The use of a transport medium, such as Cary-Blair, is necessary if a delay in processing the sample is expected. Isolation of more than 10^5 *V. parahaemolyticus* from epidemiologically implicated food supports the diagnosis and identifies the vehicle.[36] A correlation between the serotype of the food and patient isolates is not present always, because multiple strains can contaminate a single food.[1] Adding an enrichment broth to the processing increases the yield of isolation.

For testing of blood specimens, use of routine culture media followed by selective media is appropriate.[24, 44] Immunoassays (enzyme-linked immunosorbent assay, immunoprecipitation in agar medium, reversed passive latex agglutination) are available in research laboratories and commercially in Japan (KAP-RPLA: Denka Seiken, Tokyo; and BT test: Nissui Pharm, Tokyo) to detect the TDH. Strains producing TRH may be detected by cross-reactions.[56] Serologic methods (slide agglutination) can detect H antigens in lateral flagellae.[47] Gene probe hybridization[42] and polymerase chain reaction using a sequence of a highly conserved DNA fragment[34] or targeting the *tdh* gene can be used to detect low numbers of the organism in environmental and clinical specimens.

TREATMENT

Only supportive therapy and careful control of the fluid and electrolyte balance are required for the management of gastroenteritis. Oral rehydration usually is appropriate, although intravenous fluids may be required if massive fluid losses occur.[6, 27, 43] Antibiotic therapy is unnecessary for this short-lived disease. In the unusual protracted episode, tetracycline may be of benefit for adults and older children.[5, 6, 29]

For wound infections and septicemia, antibiotics always

are indicated. *V. parahaemolyticus* usually is susceptible to tetracycline. In addition, there are only a few strains resistant to chloramphenicol, trimethoprim-sulfamethoxazole, third-generation cephalosporins, aztreonam, imipenem, quinolones, and aminoglycosides.[7, 17, 22, 24] Penicillins are ineffective because of the presence of β-lactamases in up to 50 per cent of isolates.[22, 30] The older cephalosporins also have poor activity.[30]

PREVENTION AND CONTROL

Although it is impossible to ensure the lack of contamination of seafood, avoiding food-handling errors should diminish the risk of infection. A recommendation for an acceptable upper limit of 100 colony-forming units per gram of *V. parahaemolyticus* in raw shrimp has been made by the International Commission on Microbiological Specification for Foods.[28] Thorough cooking eliminates the organism.[52] Heating seafood to 60° C for 15 minutes[19] or boiling for 7 minutes[9] appears to be adequate to reduce the risk of infection. When undercooked or raw seafood is consumed, adequate prior refrigeration to avoid multiplication of organisms is important. During the preparation of seafood, special attention should be paid to possible cross-contamination. Using the same utensils, board surfaces, or containers for fresh and recently cooked seafood should be avoided.[43, 52] Raw seafood consumption should be discouraged, particularly in those at high risk for developing septicemia.[16, 33, 35]

References

1. Barker, W. H., Jr.: *Vibrio parahaemolyticus* outbreaks in the United States. Lancet *i*:551–554, 1974.
2. Baross, J., and Liston, J.: Occurrence of *Vibrio parahaemolyticus* and related hemolytic vibrios in marine environments of Washington State. Appl. Microbiol. *20*:179–186, 1970.
3. Bean, N. H., and Griffin, P. M.: Foodborne disease outbreaks in the United States, 1973 1987: Pathogens, vehicles and trends. J. Food Protect. *53*:804–817, 1990.
4. Bean, N. H., Griffin, P. M., Goulding, J. S., et al.: Foodborne disease outbreaks, 5-year summary, 1983–1987. M. M. W. R. CDC Surveillance Summaries *39*:15–57, 1990.
5. Blake, P. A.: Disease of humans (other than cholera) caused by vibrios. Ann. Rev. Microbiol. *34*:341–367, 1980.
6. Bolen, J. L., Zamiska, S. A., and Greenough, W. B.: Clinical features in enteritis due to *Vibrio parahaemolyticus*. Am. J. Med. *57*:638–641, 1974.
7. Bonner, J. R., Coker, A. S., Berryman, C. R., et al.: Spectrum of *Vibrio* infections in a gulf coast community. Ann. Intern. Med. *99*:464–469, 1983.
8. Boutin, B. K., Townsend, S. F., Scarpino, P. V. et al.: Demonstration of invasiveness of *Vibrio parahaemolyticus* in adult rabbits by immunofluorescence. Appl. Environ. Microbiol. *37*:647–653, 1979.
9. Caraway, C. T., Gregg, J., and McFarland, L.: *Vibrio parahaemolyticus* foodborne outbreak, Louisiana. M. M. W. R. *27*:345–346, 1978.
10. Carpenter, C. J.: More pathogenic vibrios. N. Engl. J. Med. *300*:39–41, 1979.
11. Chai, T. J., and Pace, J.: *Vibrio parahaemolyticus*. *In* Hui, Y., Gorham, J. R., and Murrel, K. D. (eds.): Foodborne Disease Handbook. New York, Marcel Dekker, 1994, pp. 395–425.
12. Chakrabarti, M. K., Sinha, A. K., and Biswas, T.: Adherence of *Vibrio parahaemolyticus* to rabbit intestinal epithelial cells *in vitro*. FEMS Microbiol. Lett. *84*:113–118, 1991.
13. Chatterjee, B. D., Mukherjee, A., and Sanyal, S. N.: Enteroinvasive model of *Vibrio parahaemolyticus*. Indian J. Med. Res. *79*:151–158, 1984.
14. Dadisman, T. A., Nelson, R., Molenda, J. R. et al.: *Vibrio parahaemolyticus* gastroenteritis in Maryland. I. Clinical and epidemiological aspects. Am. J. Epidemiol. *96*:414–426, 1973.
15. DePaola, A., Hopkins, L. H., Peeler, J. T. et al.: Incidence of *Vibrio parahaemolyticus* in U. S. coastal waters and oysters. Appl. Environ. Microbiol. *56*:2299–2302, 1990.
16. Desenclos, J. A., Klontz, K. C., Wolfe, L. E., et al.: The risk of *Vibrio* illness in the Florida raw oyster eating population, 1981–1988. Am. J. Epidemiol. *134*:290–297, 1991.
17. Dobroszycki, J., Sklarin, N. T., Szilagy, G., et al.: *Vibrio parahaemolyticus* septicemia in a patient with neutropenic leukemia. Clin. Infect. Dis. *15*:738–739, 1992.
18. Douet, J. P., Castroviejo, M., Dodin, A. et al.: Purification and characterization of Kanagawa hemolysin from *Vibrio parahaemolyticus*. Res. Microbiol. *143*:569–577, 1992.
19. Doyle, M. P.: Pathogenic *Escherichia coli, Yersinia enterocolitica*, and *Vibrio parahaemolyticus*. Lancet *336*:1111–1115, 1990.
20. Eastaugh, J., and Shepherd, S.: Infectious and toxic syndromes from fish and shellfish consumption. Arch. Intern. Med. *149*:1735–1740, 1989.
21. Franca, S. M., Gibbs, D. L., Samuels, P., et al.: *Vibrio parahaemolyticus* in Brazilian coastal waters. J. A. M. A. *244*:587–588, 1980.
22. French, G. L., Woo, M. L., Hui, Y. W., et al.: Antimicrobial susceptibilities of halophilic vibrios. J. Antimicrob. Chemother. *24*:183–194, 1989.
23. Gingras, S. P., and Howard, L. V.: Adherence of *Vibrio parahaemolyticus* to human epithelial cell lines. Appl. Environ. Microbiol. *39*:369–371, 1980.
24. Hally, R. J., Rubin, R. A., Fraimow, H. S., et al.: Fatal *Vibrio parahaemolyticus* septicemia in a patient with cirrhosis. Dig. Dis. Sci. *40*:1257–1260, 1995.
25. Honda, S. I., Goto, I., Minematsu, I., et al.: Gastroenteritis due to Kanagawa negative *Vibrio parahaemolyticus*. Lancet *i*:331–332, 1987.
26. Honda, T., Ni, Y., and Miwatani, T.: Purification and characterization of a hemolysin produced by a clinical isolate of Kanagawa phenomenon–negative *Vibrio parahaemolyticus* and related to the thermostable direct hemolysin. Infect. Immun. *56*:961–965, 1988.
27. Hughes, J. M., Boyce, J. M., Aleem, A. R., et al.: *Vibrio parahaemolyticus* enterocolitis in Bangladesh: Report of an outbreak. Am. J. Trop. Med. Hyg. *27*:106–112, 1978.
28. Janda, J. M., Powers, C., Bryant, R. G., et al.: Current perspective on the epidemiology and pathogenesis of clinically significant *Vibrio* spp. Clin. Microbiol. Rev. *1*:245–267, 1988.
29. Joseph, S. W., Colwell, R. R., and Kaper, J. B.: *Vibrio parahaemolyticus* and related halophilic vibrios. CRC Crit. Rev. Microbiol. *10*:77–124, 1983.
30. Joseph, S. W., DeBell, R. M., and Brown, W. P.: *In vitro* response to chloramphenicol, tetracycline, ampicillin, gentamicin and beta-lactamase production by halophilic vibrios from human and environmental sources. Antimicrob. Agents Chemother. *13*:244–248, 1978.
31. Kaper, J. B., Campen, R. K., Seidler, R. J., et al.: Cloning of the thermostable direct or Kanagawa phenomenon–associated hemolysin of *Vibrio parahaemolyticus*. Infect. Immun. *45*:290–292, 1984.
32. Kelly, M. T., and Dan Stroh, E. M.: Urease-positive, Kanagawa-negative *Vibrio parahaemolyticus* from patients and the environment in the Pacific Northwest. J. Clin. Microbiol. *27*:2820–2822, 1989.
33. Klontz, K. C.: Fatalities associated with *Vibrio parahaemolyticus* and *Vibrio cholerae* non-O1 infections in Florida (1981 to 1988). South. Med. J. *83*:500–502, 1990.
34. Lee, C. Y., Pan, S. F., and Chen, C. H.: Sequence of a cloned pR72H fragment and its use for detection of *Vibrio parahaemolyticus* in shellfish with the PCR. Appl. Environ. Microbiol. *61*:1311–1317, 1995.
35. Levine, W. C., and Griffin, P. M.: *Vibrio* infections on the Gulf Coast. Results of first year of regional surveillance. J. Infect. Dis. *167*:479–483, 1993.
36. McLaughlin, J. C.: *Vibrio*. *In* Murray, P. R., Baron, E. J., and Pfaller, M. A. (eds.): Manual of Clinical Microbiology. 6th ed. Washington, D.C., American Society for Microbiology, 1995, pp. 465–476.
37. Miyamoto, Y., Kato, T., Obara, Y., et al.: *In vitro* hemolytic characteristic of *Vibrio parahaemolyticus*: Its close correlation with human pathogenicity. J. Bacteriol. *100*:1147–1149, 1969.
38. Morris, Jr., J. G., and Black, R. E.: Cholera and other vibrioses in the United States. N. Engl. J. Med. *312*:343–350, 1985.
39. Nagayama, K., Yamamoto, K., Mitawani, T., et al.: Characterization of a haemolysin related to Vp-TDH produced by a Kanagawa phenomenon–negative clinical isolate of *Vibrio parahaemolyticus*. J. Med. Microbiol. *42*:83–90, 1995.
40. Nishibuchi, M., Fasano, A., Russell, R. G., et al.: Enterotoxigenicity of *Vibrio parahaemolyticus* with and without genes encoding thermostable direct hemolysin. Infect. Immun. *60*:3539–3545, 1992.
41. Nishibuchi, M., and Kaper, J. B.: Thermostable direct hemolysin gene of *Vibrio parahaemolyticus*: A virulence gene acquired by a marine bacterium. Infect. Immun. *63*:2093–2099, 1995.
42. Nishibuchi, M., Ishibashi, M., Takeda, Y., et al.: Detection of the thermostable direct hemolysin gene and related DNA sequences in *Vibrio parahaemolyticus* and other *Vibrio* species by the DNA colony hybridization test. Infect. Immun. *49*:481–486, 1985.
43. Peffers, A. S., Bailey, J., Barrow, G. I., et al.: *Vibrio parahaemolyticus* gastroenteritis and international air travel. Lancet *i*:143–145, 1973.
44. Rabinowitch, B. L., Nam, M. H., Levy, C. S., et al.: *Vibrio parahaemolyticus* septicemia associated with water skiing. Clin. Infect. Dis. *16*:339–340, 1993.
45. Raimondi, F., Kao, J. P., Kaper, J. B., et al.: Calcium-dependent intestinal chloride secretion by *Vibrio parahaemolyticus* thermostable direct hemolysin in a rabbit model. Gastroenterology *109*:381–386, 1995.
46. Sakasaki, R., Tamura, K., Nakamura, A., et al.: Studies on enteropathogenic activity of *Vibrio parahaemolyticus* using ligated gut loop model in rabbits. Jpn. J. Med. Sci. Biol. *27*:35–43, 1974.
47. Shinoda, S., Nakahara, N., Ninomiya, Y., et al.: Serological method for identification of *Vibrio parahaemolyticus* from marine samples. Appl. Environ. Microbiol. *45*:148–152, 1983.
48. Shirai, H., Ito, H., Hirayama, T., et al.: Molecular epidemiologic evidence for association of thermostable direct hemolysin (TDH) and TDH-related hemolysin of *Vibrio parahaemolyticus* with gastroenteritis. Infect. Immun. *58*:3568–3573, 1990.

49. Spearman, J. G., Tronca, E. L., Nichlos, E. M., et al.: Epidemiologic notes and reports, *Vibrio parahaemolyticus*, Louisiana. M. M. W. R. *21*:341–343, 1972.
50. Takea, Y.: Thermostable direct hemolysin of *Vibrio parahaemolyticus*. Pharmacol. Ther. *19*:123–146, 1983.
51. Thompson, C. A., and Vanderzant, C.: Serological and hemolytic characteristics of *Vibrio parahaemolyticus* from marine sources. J. Food Sci. *41*:204–205, 1976.
52. Twedt, R. M.: *Vibrio parahaemolyticus*. *In* Doyle, M. P. (ed.): Foodborne Bacterial Pathogens. New York, Marcel Dekker, 1989, pp. 543–568.
53. Twedt, R. M., Peerler, J. T., and Spaulding, P. L.: Effective ileal loop dose of Kanagawa-positive *Vibrio parahaemolyticus*. Appl. Environ. Microbiol. *40*:1012–1016, 1980.
54. Varmam, A. H.: *Vibrio*. *In* Varmam, A. H., and Evans, M. G. (eds.): Foodborne Pathogens. London, Wolfe Publishing Ltd., 1991, pp. 157–183.
55. Yamamoto, T., and Yokota, T.: Adherence targets of *Vibrio parahaemolyticus* in human small intestines. Infect. Immun. *57*:2410–2419, 1989.
56. Yoh, M., Kawakami, N., Funakoshi, Y., et al.: Evaluation of two assay kits for thermostable direct hemolysin (TDH) as an indicator of TDH-related hemolysin (TRH) produced by *Vibrio parahaemolyticus*. Microbiol. Immunol. *39*:157–159, 1995.

123

VIBRIO VULNIFICUS

Randall G. Fisher and William C. Gruber

BACTERIOLOGY

Vibrio vulnificus is a small, curvilinear, gram-negative rod of the family Vibrionaceae.[6] This facultative anaerobe is oxidase- and lysine-positive like other species of the genus *Vibrio*. Its major difference is that it ferments lactose, a feature that accounts for its original name, Lac + *Vibrio*. *V. vulnificus* is arginine-negative and ornithine-variable. This halophilic (salt-loving) organism grows in concentrations of sodium chloride of from 1 to 8 per cent and seems to grow best at about 3 per cent.[24]

EPIDEMIOLOGY

V. vulnificus, like *V. parahemolyticus*, is a marine organism that is a common inhabitant of off-shore waters, especially estuarial waters.[33] It has been isolated from sediment, plankton, water, finfish, crabs, and oysters, with peak recovery in the summer and early fall.[11] This may be because at higher water temperatures *V. vulnificus* is released and rises to surface waters. There it attaches to plankton and shorefish and then is taken up and concentrated by filter-feeding mollusks and crustaceans.

V. vulnificus has been isolated from both wild and commercial oysters all over the world. It especially is prevalent in warm coastal waters. Reports about the survival of the organism in oysters stored at low temperatures are conflicting. However, Nilsson and associates[32] revealed that even if *V. vulnificus* is rendered nonculturable by storage at low temperatures, it can be "resuscitated" by allowing the oysters to come up to room temperature; this cycle could be carried out twice without any reduction in bacterial count. Hence, there probably is no way of ensuring that commercial shellfish do not contain viable *V. vulnificus* because of the ubiquity of the organism in the marine environment and its ability to thrive under even the most careful conditions of sanitation, storage, and transport.[10, 22]

Disease in humans is initiated by contact with the organism either through marine contamination of a wound or through the gastrointestinal tract after ingestion of the organism in raw shellfish, most commonly oysters.[6]

PATHOPHYSIOLOGY

V. vulnificus causes three distinct diseases in humans: wound infection and gastrointestinal infection, which may be self-limited or progress to septicemia. Local infection occurs after wound exposure to contaminated seawater. Wound infections with *V. vulnificus* are marked by rapid spread, the formation of bullae, and necrosis of involved tissues.[6] Marked edema and vascular thromboses occur in both experimental[15] and natural infection. *V. vulnificus* elaborates a cytolysin,[14, 15, 24] a collagenase,[39] and a protease,[30] which enhance its rapid spread in tissues. The protease activates the plasma kallikrein-kinin system to produce bradykinin,[29] and histamine also is released locally. These factors account for the intense inflammatory reaction seen in these lesions. In otherwise healthy individuals, a mild, self-limited gastrointestinal illness similar to that caused by *V. parahemolyticus* has been described.[23] However, the most serious infection produced by *V. vulnificus* is primary septicemia, which occurs most commonly in patients with liver disease, after ingestion of the organism in raw shellfish.[5, 35, 36]

For patients with hepatic disease, the risk of acquiring septicemia is 40 to 80 times greater and the case fatality rate 2.5 times higher then for otherwise healthy individuals.[17] *V. vulnificus*, like many other gram-negative organisms, requires iron for growth and grows better in an excess of iron.[46] It is able to extract iron from hemoglobin, even if it is complexed completely to haptoglobin.[46, 49] Liver damage, excess iron, and deferoxamine therapy all have been shown to decrease the median lethal dose (LD_{50}) of *V. vulnificus* in experimental animals. Deferoxamine alone decreased the LD_{50} by four orders of magnitude.[8] Iron overload almost certainly underlies *V. vulnificus* septicemia in patients who require repeated transfusions and deferoxamine therapy for anemia.[19, 48] There is some evidence that alcoholism, even in the absence of demonstrable liver disease, is a risk factor for sepsis.[35] Fatal septicemia also has been reported in patients with other chronic diseases, such as diabetes mellitus and lymphomas.[35]

Virulence factors of the organism also have been described.[47] Virulent strains are resistant to the bactericidal activity of human serum,[25] probably because of the presence of a polysaccharide capsule.[1] Poor uptake of virulent strains into phagocytes[42] and opaqueness of the colony on agar have been correlated with the presence of the capsule.[38, 47] There is no difference in the lipopolysaccharide of virulent versus avirulent strains.[4]

The production of recalcitrant shock in patients with septicemia is secondary to toxins, loss of vascular tone, capillary leak, and possibly negative inotropy, as in other forms of gram-negative sepsis.

CLINICAL MANIFESTATIONS

Patients commmonly present with wound infection or primary septicemia. Wound infection occurs after injury in seawater or after the contamination of a recently acquired wound with seawater. Often, the wound is caused by the shell of a crustacean or mollusk. Many patients with wound infections work in shellfish-related industries. Cellulitis may develop and spread rapidly. Overlying skin often is covered with tense bullae. At débridement, the extent of necrosis may exceed presurgical expectations.[45] Primary wound infection may progress to systemic infection; for this reason, wound infection with *V. vulnificus* carries a mortality rate of from 7[6] to 24 per cent.[23]

Patients with primary septicemia generally will give a history of recent (6 to 72 hours) consumption of raw seafood. Illness is marked by the rapid onset of fever, hypotension, and septic shock. Prodromal symptoms, such as malaise, chills, and fever, are common. Vomiting and diarrhea are seen in about 20 per cent of patients.[5] Shock progresses quickly and is difficult to reverse. Secondary skin lesions develop in about half the patients[6] and may be bullous, petechial, or maculopapular. It frequently is possible to isolate *V. vulnificus* from cultures of secondary lesions, providing evidence of septicemic spread to those sites.[6] Mortality from primary septicemia has been reported to be from 46 per cent[6] to 79 per cent.[35]

In addition to the above two syndromes, *V. vulnificus* has been reported as a cause of corneal ulcer,[12] myositis,[21] adult epiglottitis,[28] osteomyelitis,[44] endocarditis,[43] peritonitis,[18] and meningitis.[19, 35]

Ninety per cent of reported patients are 40 years of age or older.[6, 35] Childhood cases of septicemia have been associated with thalassemia major,[19] for which frequent transfusions and deferoxamine therapy are required. Wound infections in previously healthy children and adolescents have been reported. *V. vulnificus* also has been isolated from a premature baby's stool sample obtained on the infant's first day of life; the baby's mother worked as an oyster shucker.[3]

DIAGNOSIS

The diagnosis of *V. vulnificus* infection is made by isolating the organism from blood or tissue culture. It also may be recovered from stool specimens.[3, 36] *V. vulnificus* tends to grow best in thiocitrate bile salts agar[6] but also may be recovered from ordinary blood agar plates[2, 37] or MacConkey plates.[6]

Hill and colleagues[16] have described a polymerase chain reaction method, and Tamplin and associates[41] have developed an enzyme immunoassay. Both of these methods are experimental and not yet routinely available for clinical use.

The diagnosis of *V. vulnificus* wound infection or septicemia can be suspected on clinical grounds and appropriate therapy initiated while awaiting culture results. A history of raw shellfish ingestion or wound contamination with either seawater or brackish inland waters[40] should be sought. *V. vulnificus* infection should be given high consideration in patients with hemosiderosis, anemia with transfusion therapy, liver disease, or other chronic diseases.

TREATMENT

In severe wound infections, rapid surgical therapy is of paramount importance. In primary septicemia, support of the patient's airway, along with aggressive pressor support and other adjunctive therapies for severe septic shock, is of primary concern. Secondarily, appropriate antibiotic treatment for *V. vulnificus* should be started as early as possible. In vitro, the organism is susceptible to many antibiotics, including ampicillin, third-generation cephalosporins, tetracycline, chloramphenicol, and gentamicin.[6] Bowdre and associates[7] reported that, in mice, the minimum inhibitory concentrations (MIC) obtained in the laboratory did not seem to correspond with response to therapy. In particular, the organism appeared to be exquisitely sensitive to cefotaxime in vitro (MIC $\leq$ 0.06 μg/mL); however, 9 of 10 mice treated with cefotaxime succumbed to overwhelming infection. There is anecdotal evidence that this puzzling phenomenon may occur in humans as well: four of five patients reported by Chuang and associates[9] died, despite therapy with third-generation cephalosporins at appropriate dosages. Similarly, although the organism is almost universally sensitive to gentamicin in the laboratory, case reports show a lack of response to this antibiotic. Of all the antibiotics to which the organism was sensitive in vitro, only tetracycline led to mouse survival in Bowdre's study; all 12 of the mice treated with tetracycline survived the infection.[7] Case reports also show favorable outcomes with tetracycline or doxycyline,[9] as well as chloramphenicol[9] and ciprofloxacin.[27] The available evidence suggests that tetracycline should be the drug of choice for known or suspected *V. vulnificus* infection.[13, 31]

PREVENTION

Patients with severe anemia, liver disease, hemosiderosis, or other debilitating chronic diseases or those on deferoxamine therapy should be advised against eating raw seafood of any kind. Patients with open wounds probably should avoid contact with seawater or brackish inland waters.

References

1. Amako, K., Okada, K., and Miake, S.: Evidence for the presence of a capsule in *Vibrio vulnificus*. J. Gen. Microbiol. *130*:2741–2743, 1984.
2. Armstrong, C. W., Lake, J. L., and Miller, G. B., Jr.: Extraintestinal infections due to halophilic *Vibrios*. South. Med. J. *76*:571–574, 1983.
3. Bachman, B., Boyd, W. P., Jr., Lieb, S., et al.: Marine noncholera *Vibrio* infections in Florida. South. Med. J. *76*:296–299, 1983.
4. Bahrani, K., and Oliver, J. D.: Studies on the lipopolysaccharide of a virulent and an avirulent strain of *Vibrio vulnificus*. Biochem. Cell. Biol. *68*:547–551, 1990.
5. Blake, P. A., Weaver, R. E., and Hollis, D. G.: Disease of humans (other than cholera) caused by *Vibrios*. Ann. Rev. Microbiol. *34*:341–367, 1980.
6. Blake, P. A., Merson, M. H., Weaver, R. E., et al.: Disease caused by a marine *Vibrio*: Clinical characteristics and epidemiology. N. Engl. J. Med. *300*:1–5, 1979.
7. Bowdre, J. H., Hull, J. H., and Cocchetto, D. M.: Antibiotic efficacy against *Vibrio vulnificus* in the mouse: Superiority of tetracycline. J. Pharmacol. Exp. Ther. *225*:595–598, 1983.
8. Brennaman, B., Soucy, D., and Howard, R. J.: Effect of iron and liver injury on the pathogenesis of *Vibrio vulnificus*. J. Surg. Res. *43*:527–531, 1987.
9. Chuang, Y. C., Yuan, C. Y., Lin, C. Y., et al.: *Vibrio vulnificus* infection in Taiwan: Report of 28 cases and review of clinical manifestations and treatment. Clin. Infect. Dis. *115*:271–276, 1992.
10. Cook, D. W.: Effect of time and temperature on multiplication of *Vibrio vulnificus* in postharvest Gulf Coast shellstock oysters. Appl. Environ. Microbiol. *60*:3483–3484, 1994.
11. DePaola, A., Capers, G. M., and Alexander, D.: Densities of *Vibrio vulnificus* in the intestines of fish from the U. S. Gulf Coast. Appl. Environ. Microbiol. *60*:984–988, 1994.
12. DiGaetano, M., Ball, S. F., and Straus, J. G.: *Vibrio vulnificus* corneal ulcer: Case reports. Arch. Ophthalmol. *107*:323–324, 1989.
13. Fang, F. C.: Use of tetracycline for treatment of *Vibrio vulnificus* infections. Clin. Infect. Dis. *15*:1071–1072, 1992.
14. Gray, L. D., and Kreger, A. S.: Purification and characterization of an extracellular cytolysin produced by *Vibrio vulnificus*. Infect. Immun. *48*:62–72, 1985.
15. Gray, L. D., and Kreger, A. S.: Mouse skin damage caused by cytolysin from *Vibrio vulnificus* and by *Vibrio vulnificus* infection. J. Infect. Dis. *155*:236–241, 1987.
16. Hill, W. E., Keasler, S. P., Trucksess, M. W., et al.: Polymerase chain reaction

identification of *Vibrio vulnificus* in artificially contaminated oysters. Appl. Environ. Microbiol. *57*:707–711, 1991.
17. Hlady, W. G., Mullen, R. C., and Hopkin, R. S.: *Vibrio vulnificus* from raw oysters: Leading cause of reported deaths from foodborne illness in Florida. J. Florida Med. Assoc. *80*:536–538, 1993.
18. Holcombe, D. J.: *Vibrio vulnificus* peritonitis: A unique case. J. Louisiana State Med. Soc. *143*:27–28, 1991.
19. Katz, B. Z.: *Vibrio vulnificus* meningitis in a boy with thalassemia after eating raw oysters. Pediatrics *82*:784–786, 1988.
20. Kaysner, C. A., Tamplin, M. L., Wekell, M. M., et al.: Survival of *Vibrio vulnificus* in shellstock and shucked oysters (*Crassostrea gigas* and *Crassostrea virginica*) and effects of isolation medium on recovery. Appl. Environ. Microbiol. *55*:3072–3079, 1989.
21. Kelly, M. T., and McCormick, W. F.: Acute bacterial myositis caused by *Vibrio vulnificus*. J. A. M. A. *246*:72–73, 1981.
22. Kizer, K. W.: *Vibrio vulnificus* hazard in patients with liver disease. West. J. Med. *161*:64–65, 1994.
23. Klontz, K. C., Lieb, S., Schreiber, M., et al.: Syndromes of *Vibrio vulnificus* infections: Clinical and epidemiologic features in Florida cases, 1981–1987. Ann. Intern. Med. *109*:318–323, 1988.
24. Koga, T., and Kawata, T.: Composition of the major outer membrane proteins of *Vibrio vulnificus* isolates: Effect of different growth media and iron deficiency. Microbiol. Immunol. *30*:193–201, 1986.
25. Kreger, A., DeChatelet, L., and Shirley, P.: Interaction of *Vibrio vulnificus* with human polymorphonuclear leukocytes: Association of virulence with resistance to phagocytosis. J. Infect. Dis. *144*:244–248, 1981.
26. Kreger, A. S., Kothary, M. H., and Gray, L. D.: Cytolytic toxins of *Vibrio vulnificus* and *Vibrio damsela*. Methods Enzymol. *165*:176–189, 1988.
27. Meadors, M. C., and Pankey, G. A.: *Vibrio vulnificus* wound infection treated successfully with oral ciprofloxacin. J. Infect. *20*:88–89, 1990.
28. Mehtar, S., Bangham, L., Kalmanovitch, D., et al.: Adult epiglottitis due to *Vibrio vulnificus*. Br. Med. J. Clin. Res. *296*:827–828, 1988.
29. Miyoshi, N., Miyoshi, S., Sugiyama, K., et al.: Activation of the plasma kallikrein-kinin symstem by *Vibrio vulnificus* protease. Infect. Immun. *55*:1936–1939, 1987.
30. Miyoshi, S., and Shinoda, S.: Role of the protease in the permeability enhancement by *Vibrio vulnificus*. Microbiol. Immunol. *32*:1025–1032, 1988.
31. Morris, J. G., Jr., and Tenney, J.: Antibiotic therapy for *Vibrio vulnificus* infection. J. A. M. A. *253*:1121–1122, 1985.
32. Nilsson, L., Oliver, J. D., and Kjelleberg, S.: Resuscitation of *Vibrio vulnificus* from the viable but nonculturable state. J. Bacteriol. *173*:5054–5059, 1991.
33. Oliver, J. D., Warner, R. A., and Cleland, D. R.: Distribution of *Vibrio vulnificus* and other lactose-fermenting *Vibrios* in the marine environment. Appl. Environ. Microbiol. *45*:985–998, 1983.
34. Oliver, J. D.: Lethal cold stress of *Vibrio vulnificus* in oysters. Appl. Environ. Microbiol. *41*:710–717, 1981.
35. Park, S. D., Shon, H. S., and Joh N. J.: *Vibrio vulnificus* septicemia in Korea: Clinical and epidemiologic findings in seventy patients. J. Am. Acad. Dermatol. *24*:397–403, 1991.
36. Pollak, S. J., Parrish, E. F., III, Barrett, T. J., et al.: *Vibrio vulnificus* septicemia: Isolation of organism from stool and demonstration of antibodies by indirect immunofluorescence. Arch. Intern. Med. *143*:837–838, 1983.
37. Saraswathi, K., Barve, S. M., and Deodhar, L. P.: Septicaemia due to *Vibrio vulnificus*. Trans. R. Soc. Trop. Med. Hyg. *83*:714, 1989.
38. Simpson, L. M., White, V. K., Zane, S. F., et al.: Correlation between virulence and colony morphology in *Vibrio vulnificus*. Infect. Immun. *55*:269–272, 1987.
39. Smith, G. C., and Merkel, J. R.: Collagenolytic activity of *Vibrio vulnificus*: Potential contribution to its invasiveness. Infect. Immun. *35*:1155–1156, 1982.
40. Tacket, C. O., Barrett, T. J., Mann, J. M., et al.: Wound infections caused by *Vibrio vulnificus*, a marine *Vibrio*, in inland areas of the United States. J. Clin. Microbiol. *19*:197–199, 1984.
41. Tamplin, M. L., Martin, A. L., Ruple, A. D., et al.: Enzyme immunoassay for identification of *Vibrio vulnificus* in seawater, sediment, and oysters. Appl. Environ. Microbiol. *57*:1235–1240, 1991.
42. Tamplin, M. L., Specter, S., Rodrick, G. E., et al.: *Vibrio vulnificus* resists phagocytosis in the absence of serum opsonins. Infect. Immun. *49*:715–718, 1985.
43. Truwit, J. D., Badesch, D. B., Savage, A. M., et al.: *Vibrio vulnificus* bacteremia with endocarditis. South. Med. J. *80*:1457–1459, 1987.
44. Vartian, C. V., and Septimus, E. J.: Osteomyelitis caused by *Vibrio vulnificus*. J. Infect. Dis. *161*:363, 1990.
45. Woo, M. L., Patrick, W. G., Simon, M. T., et al.: Necrotising fasciitis caused by *Vibrio vulnificus*. J. Clin. Pathol. *37*:1301–1304, 1984.
46. Wright, A. C., Simpson, L. M., and Oliver, J. D.: Role of iron in the pathogenesis of *Vibrio vulnificus* infections. Infect. Immun. *34*:503–507, 1981.
47. Yoshida, S., Ogawa, M., and Mizuguchi, Y.: Relation of capsular materials and colony opacity to virulence of *Vibrio vulnificus*. Infect. Immun. *47*:446–451, 1985.
48. Yoshida, S., Tanabe, T., Chiba, S., et al.: Fatal *Vibrio vulnificus* infection in a patient with aplastic anemia. Sangyo Ika Daigaku Zasshi *5*:95–100, 1983.
49. Zakaria-Meehan, Z., Massad, G., Simpson, L. M., et al.: Ability of *Vibrio vulnificus* to obtain iron from hemoglobin-haptoglobin complexes. Infect. Immun. *56*:275–277, 1988.

124

MISCELLANEOUS NON-ENTEROBACTERIACEAE FERMENTATIVE BACILLI

Randall G. Fisher and William C. Gruber

This chapter discusses fermentative bacilli that are not of the family Enterobacteriaceae. Specifically, it will examine *Chromobacterium violaceum*, *Plesiomonas shigelloides*, and other *Pasteurella* organisms.

CHROMOBACTERIUM VIOLACEUM

C. violaceum is a facultatively anaerobic, gram-negative rod that is a saprophyte of soil and water, especially in tropical and subtropical climates. It causes occasional illness in animals and, rarely, in humans. Infection with *C. violaceum*, when it does occur, is a serious disease with a high mortality rate.

Bacteriology

C. violaceum is a long, motile, gram-negative bacillus that appears singly or in pairs on Gram stain. It has a polar flagellum and one to four subpolar or lateral flagella, which antigenically are distinct from the polar flagellum.[40] Most isolates produce an insoluble pigment, violacein. This pigment is intense and makes colonies appear from dark purple to black, especially on blood agar. *C. violaceum* grows readily on standard agar (any medium that contains tryptophan supports growth). The colonies are low convex, violet, smooth, and not gelatinous. Colonies produce hydrogen cyanide, so a faint almond odor may be present.[40]

C. violaceum is catalase-positive and oxidase-positive, although the latter may be difficult to interpret due to the production of pigment. Growing the organism anaerobically inhibits pigment formation.[22] Pigment also may be lost on subculture[35] or as effective treatment is initiated. *C. violaceum* has a fermentative, not oxidative, attack on carbohydrates.

C. violaceum produces antimicrobial agents that have been shown to have activity against bacteria and trypanosomes.

Epidemiology

C. violaceum commonly is found in soil and water of areas with tropical or subtropical weather patterns. It also has been recovered from soil as far north as New Jersey.[6]

Ten of the first 12 cases reported in the United States occurred in Florida; the other 2 were in Louisiana. Subsequently, one case from New Jersey[32] and one from Ohio[42] have been reported, along with more from southeastern states. All but one case occurred during the summer months.[35] Patients tend to be young, with a median age of 14 years.[35]

Pathophysiology

Although *C. violaceum* is a common inhabitant of soil and water, human infection is relatively rare. Disorders of neutrophil function are important risk factors. A disproportionately high number of *C. violaceum* infections have been in patients with chronic granulomatous disease.[26] There also is a report of a child with another disorder of neutrophil function, polymorphonuclear leukocyte glucose-6-phosphate dehydrogenase deficiency.[27] Organisms may demonstrate variable virulence, and there are observed differences in endotoxin activity, resistance to phagocytosis, and production of catalase and hydrogen peroxide between clinical and soil isolates.[30]

The organism usually gains entrance to the body through cuts or abrasions that come in contact with contaminated soil or water. After entrance, there usually is a localized infection at or around the site of entry, followed by dissemination of infection via the blood stream to distant sites. Two cases occurred in near-drowning victims. One case report describes fulminant infection and death in an immunocompetent host from *C. violaceum* sepsis that began as conjunctivitis after a fall that splattered mud into the patient's eye.[9]

Numerous microabscesses are found in multiple organs, especially liver, lung, and kidneys. Spread to bone, joints, and the central nervous system also has been described.

Clinical Manifestations

The pattern of illness in all reported patients is fairly similar, with a contaminated inoculation site, localized disease, regional lymphadenopathy, and then hematogenous spread to visceral organs. Progression of symptoms tends to be rapid after a varying incubation period.

Most patients have cutaneous lesions,[26] which are described as being nodular or pustular and sometimes with surrounding cellulitis.[45] They may progress to suppuration and drainage, or ulceration. Regional lymphadenopathy is common; some of the nodes suppurate and require surgical drainage or removal.

Severe disease is heralded by high fever (39° C to 41° C), confusion or lethargy, abdominal pain, headaches, nausea and vomiting, and sometimes myalgias. Patients with systemic illness are toxic in appearance. Hepatosplenomegaly is frequent, and jaundice may be present. Progression from high fever and moderate toxicity to septic shock with disseminated intravascular coagulation and multisystem organ failure is precipitous. After the liver, the lung is the most common site of dissemination of infection, and evidence of pneumonia often is found. Adult respiratory distress syndrome is a rare complication.[23] The overall mortality rate is 65 per cent.[26] Rarely, recurrence may occur and prove fatal.[22, 35]

Diagnosis

Diagnosis is made by recovery of the organism from blood, lymph nodes, skin lesions, or abscesses. Gram-negative bacilli sometimes can be seen in smears of material from skin lesions. Laboratory values reveal either very low or very high white blood cell counts with marked left shifts. Mild to moderate anemia is common. There may be elevated liver enzymes; evidence of early renal failure sometimes is present. The organism grows readily and is easy to identify if it produces the characteristic violet pigment. Nonpigmented forms exist in soil and have similar virulence in mice[39] but only have been recovered from clinical specimens on one occasion.[42] Other cases may have been missed, however, because the nonpigmented forms often are misidentified as *Aeromonas hydrophila* or as pseudomonads.[39] A clinical history of contamination of a wound with water or soil, especially in the southeastern United States or in Southeast Asia, with subsequent local infection, lymph node suppuration, and lack of response to conventional antibiotic therapy, should arouse suspicion of *C. violaceum* infection. The clinician particularly should be aware of the possibility of *C. violaceum* infection in patients with chronic granulomatous disease.

Treatment

C. violaceum is sensitive in vitro to chloramphenicol, gentamicin, fluorinated quinolones, tetracyclines, imipenem, trimethoprim-sulfamethoxazole, and semisynthetic penicillins. It often is resistant to cephalosporins, penicillin, ampicillin, and the antistaphylococcal penicillins. All isolates are resistant to vancomycin and rifampin.[3] Some strains have been shown to elaborate a β-lactamase, which is chromosomal, and are inducible in vitro.[8] At least one case report gives in vivo evidence of inducible resistance to ceftazidime.[45] Laboratory evidence of susceptibility to erythromycin cannot be relied upon. In vitro, the fluorinated quinolones have the highest activity,[3] but these drugs have not been employed clinically.

Because infection with *C. violaceum* is rare and often rapidly fatal, optimal antimicrobial therapy is not known. Most survivors have been treated with chloramphenicol, gentamicin, or both. Duration of therapy also is not known, but because of late recurrences, some authors recommend 3 to 4 weeks of intravenous therapy followed by a month or more of oral trimethoprim-sulfamethoxazole.[35]

PLESIOMONAS SHIGELLOIDES

The genus *Plesiomonas* has only one species: *P. shigelloides*. These organisms are facultatively anaerobic, motile, gram-negative rods that are common inhabitants of surface water and fish. They have been implicated in gastrointestinal infections and, rarely, have been recovered from extraintestinal sites.

Bacteriology

These facultatively anaerobic, gram-negative rods are members of the family Vibrionaceae, although some authorities believe they are related more closely to Enterobacteriaceae.[25] They are motile by means of a polar flagellum. They are lysine-, ornithine-, and arginine decarboxylase–positive. They can be distinguished from Enterobacteriaceae by oxidase positivity. They also are catalase- and indole-positive. They grow well on MacConkey agar but not on thiosulfate citrate–bile salts sucrose. Growth may be enhanced by the use of selective media, such as trypticase soy broth with ampicillin[36] and inositol brilliant green–bile salts agar. Growth is maximal at 40° C to 44° C and completely inhibited at 8° C. One- to 1.5-mm grayish, shiny, opaque colonies with a slightly raised center and a smooth surface usually are visible within 24 hours. A few isolates of *P. shigelloides* share a common O antigen with *Shigella sonnei*.

Epidemiology

The organism is a ubiquitous fresh-water inhabitant at temperatures higher than 8° C. It sometimes also is found in estuarial waters in temperate or tropical climates and can exist in seawater during the summer months. It has been cultured from finfish, shellfish, pigs, birds, and dogs.[46] Although infection with *P. shigelloides* has been associated with ingestion of raw or improperly cooked fish (especially oysters), it is not known what role, if any, other animals play in the ecology of the organism.

Asymptomatic carriage of *P. shigelloides* is rare in developed countries[38] but may be as high as 15 per cent in some parts of China.[46]

Pathophysiology

Despite the ubiquity of the organism in nature, human infection is relatively uncommon and has been recognized only recently. Most often, infection is associated with gastroenteritis. Evidence for the role of *P. shigelloides* in the production of gastrointestinal symptoms is that (1) it has been isolated much more frequently from patients with diarrhea than from healthy controls[15]; (2) there have been some outbreaks, especially in Japan; (3) it often is the only organism detected in the stools of patients with gastroenteritis[29]; and (4) patients who have *P. shigelloides* growing from a stool culture recover more quickly with antibiotic therapy than without.[20] Acquisition of disease specifically has been linked to consumption of raw seafood or untreated water and to foreign travel, especially to Mexico.[20, 28] The mechanism by which the organism produces disease, however, is somewhat elusive. It is not enteroinvasive by laboratory tests; most investigators fail to find either a shiga toxin or an enterotoxin[1, 14]; there is no animal model of gastrointestinal disease[4]; patients in the recovery phase do not show serologic evidence of infection; and inoculation of volunteers fails to produce illness.[14] Even in a suckling gnotobiotic piglet model in which the animals became septic, histology of the gastrointestinal tract showed neither destruction of cells nor invasion of tissues.[14] Some potential virulence factors, i.e., a cholera-like toxin, a weak cytolysin, serum resistance, and a large (>150-kDa) plasmid, have been described, but their exact roles in pathogenesis are uncertain; attempts to correlate these features with virulence have been fruitless.[1]

P. shigelloides rarely, but more clearly, is a pathogen in extraintestinal sites. Osteomyelitis, endophthalmitis, cholecystitis, pseudoappendicitis, meningitis,[43] and septicemia have been reported sporadically.[4] Most patients with septicemia have been immunocompromised hosts, but the organism has been isolated from blood cultures in otherwise healthy persons.[17, 34] The mode of infection in extraintestinal sites is not clear.

Clinical Manifestations

Patients with *P. shigelloides* gastroenteritis complain of diarrhea, crampy abdominal pain, nausea and vomiting, headache, and fever. Symptoms usually begin 24 hours to 4 days after contact with the organism.[15] Diarrhea tends to be secretory, although some patients have symptoms more consistent with colitis.[20] Passage of blood, mucus, or both in the stools is not uncommon, nor is the presence of white blood cells by Wright stain.[15] Patients with *P. shigelloides* gastroenteritis tend to have disease that is more acute, associated with more severe abdominal pain, and of longer duration than do patients with diseases caused by other enteropathogens.[20] In one case-control study, 76 per cent of patients were sick for more than 2 weeks and 32 per cent for more than a month.[20]

Septicemia, meningitis, or both usually occur in immunecompromised hosts. Newborns make up most of the reported cases of *P. shigelloides* meningitis, in whom the mortality rate is 80 per cent.[1] Septicemia also has a high mortality rate in adults, although otherwise well patients may recover with appropriate antimicrobial therapy.

Diagnosis

A clinical history of foreign travel or of ingestion of raw seafood or untreated water should raise suspicion of possible *P. shigelloides* infection, especially when the clinical illness matches the description just mentioned. Oxidase tests should be performed on any predominant or solitary organisms to distinguish them from Enterobacteriaceae organisms.[15] They can be shown not to be aeromonads or pseudomonads by production of ornithine decarboxylase and fermentation of inositol. Selective medium can be used if the index of suspicion is high.

Treatment

Most strains of *P. shigelloides* produce a β-lactamase,[37] which seems to be specific for the penicillins. In one study, all isolates were resistant to ampicillin, ticarcillin, carbenicillin, and piperacillin.[19] *P. shigelloides* is universally susceptible to trimethoprim-sulfamethoxazole, the fluoroquinolones, most cephalosporins, and chloramphenicol. It is variably susceptible to the aminoglycosides and mostly resistant to erythromycin.

P. shigelloides gastroenteritis resolves with therapy but typically after prolonged illness. Treatment seems to shorten the course.[20]

Extraintestinal infections carry a poor prognosis and should be treated aggressively. For meningitis, the cephalosporins have good cerebrospinal fluid penetration and are effective therapy against most isolates.

OTHER *PASTEURELLA* ORGANISMS

The genus *Pasteurella* consists of a group of pleomorphic, gram-negative coccobacilli that are part of the normal flora of many animals. These organisms are frequent animal pathogens. *P. multocida* is not an uncommon human pathogen; it is discussed elsewhere (see Chapter 120). The other species of the genus *Pasteurella* are rare but occasionally serious causes of infection in humans.

Bacteriology

These organisms, like *P. multocida*, grow readily on most common laboratory media, including blood agar. Most of the species do not grow on MacConkey. They are non–spore-forming, nonmotile, aerobic, and facultatively anaerobic. These glucose-fermenting organisms are all oxidase-positive. Most are nitrate- and catalase-positive, and all except *P. gallinarum* produce indole. They are small, coccoid or rod-shaped bacilli that may show prominent bipolar staining on Gram stain. Colonies are small, translucent, and gray. They may be smooth or rough. A browning discoloration may develop around them. Colonies are nonhemolytic. They have a distinctive musty or "mushroom" odor.[5]

The taxonomy of these organisms is confusing and has been revised as recently as 1985. It has been suggested that *P. ureae*, *P. haemolytica*, and *P. pneumotropica* be moved into the genus *Actinobacillus*. *P. dagmatis* is the name now given to what formerly was called *P.* new species, or *P.* gas.[31] Clinically recovered species other than *P. multocida* include *A. ureae*, *A. haemolytica*, *A. pneumotropica*, *P. dagmatis*, *P. canis*, *P. aerogenes*, and *P. stomatis*. *P. gallinarum* has been recovered from only one patient.[2]

Pathophysiology

Infection with *Pasteurella* species has been divided clinically into three types: infection (1) from animal bites, (2) from animal contact, and (3) without known animal contact.[10] Infections from animal bites include cellulitis, abscesses, tenosynovitis, or bone and joint infection but can become generalized, especially in patients with immune compromise. Infection due to animal contact can be similar to those described earlier and is caused by animals licking broken skin or wounds. Sometimes pulmonary infections occur, possibly related to aerosolization of organisms. Cases without known animal contact history make up from 3[16] to 30 per cent[18] of all cases.

Infection usually occurs when the organisms are inoculated into deeper tissues either on animal teeth that break the skin or in animal saliva that comes in contact with nonintact skin. Infection in cases without known animal contact is harder to explain, but some species, such as *A. ureae*, may be an occasional commensal of the human respiratory tract.[21] Most cases of serious infection occur in patients with underlying diseases, such as diabetes mellitus, chronic alcoholism, and other types of liver disease.[33] Central nervous system infection with these organisms has occurred after head trauma or neurosurgery in 10 of 11 reported cases.[21] One intrauterine death of the fetus of a 20-year-old who worked at a pig farm has been attributed to *P. aerogenes*.[44]

Clinical Manifestations

Pasteurella infections produce pain, swelling, pus, and sometimes abscess formation at the site of inoculation beginning within 24 to 36 hours. Clinically, these infections are not distinguishable from wound infections with *Staphylococcus aureus* or other gram-positive organisms. Gram stain may show the characteristic pleomorphic bacilli with bipolar staining. Growth on standard agar is rapid.

Patients with peritonitis,[33] meningitis,[21] osteomyelitis,[11] or infectious endocarditis[2] have symptoms typical of these diagnoses. Risk factors, such as household pet exposure, animal contact, and animal bites, should heighten suspicion of possible *Pasteurella* infection.

Diagnosis

Diagnosis of *Pasteurella* infection can be difficult, not because the organism is fastidious or slow growing, but because it often is misidentified. Other organisms of the same family, i.e., *Actinobacillus* species and *Haemophilus* species, have similar biochemical profiles and can be misidentified by commonly used systems, such as API. Lester and associates[24] reported that of 30 species firmly identified as *Pasteurella* by biochemical means, only 3 were identified correctly by the API 20E system. Additionally, Hamilton-Miller[13] reported that four strains of *Haemophilus influenzae* and three strains of *Haemophilus parainfluenzae* were identified falsely as *Pasteurella* species by API and suggested that if the clinical history makes *Pasteurella* infection unlikely, tests for X and V factor requirements should be performed (see Chapter 139). Clinical case reports corroborate these laboratory observations.[7, 33, 41] Notifying the bacteriology laboratory of suspicion of *Pasteurella* infection is helpful.

Treatment

Penicillin has been considered the drug of choice for *Pasteurella* infection in the past and, despite some reports of penicillin resistance, still is effective against most strains. *Pasteurella* species also are susceptible to ampicillin, β-lactamase inhibitor combination drugs, tetracycline, and chloramphenicol. The aminoglycosides, erythromycin, clindamycin, cefadroxil, and cefaclor are not recommended. Dicloxacillin and cephalexin, two drugs prescribed very commonly for wound infections, have poor activity against *Pasteurella* species and should not be used as monotherapy for animal bite wounds.[12]

References

1. Abbott, S. L., Kokka, R. P., and Janda, J. M.: Laboratory investigations on the low pathogenic potential of *Plesiomonas shigelloides*. J. Clin. Microbiol. *29*:148 153, 1991.
2. al-Fadel Saleh, M., al-Madan, M. S., Erwa, H. H., et al.: First case of human infection caused by *Pasteurella gallinarum* causing infective endocarditis in an adolescent ten years after surgical correction for truncus arteriosus. Pediatrics *95*:944–948, 1995.
3. Aldridge, K. E., Valainis, G. T., and Sanders, C. V.: Comparison of the in vitro activity of ciprofloxacin and twenty-four other antimicrobial agents against clinical strains of *Chromobacterium violaceum*. Diagn. Microbiol. Infect. Dis. *10*:31–38, 1988.
4. Brendan, R. A., Miller, M. A., and Janda, J. M.: Clinical disease spectrum and pathogenic factors asssociated with *Plesiomonas shigelloides* infections in humans. Rev. Infect. Dis. *10*:303–316, 1988.
5. Citron, D. M., Edelstein, M. A., Garcia, L. S., et al.: *In* Baron E. J., Peterson L. R., and Finegold, S. M. (eds.): Bailey and Scott's Diagnostic Microbiology. 9th ed. St. Louis, C. V. Mosby, 1994, pp. 420–423.
6. Duma, R. J.: Aztreonam, the first monobactam. Ann. Intern. Med. *106*:766, 1987.
7. Fajfar-Whetsone, C. J. T., Coleman, L., Biggs, D. R., et al.: *Pasteurella mutocida* septicemia and subsequent *Pasteurella dagmatis* septicemia in a diabetic patient. J. Clin. Microbiol. *33*:202–204, 1995.
8. Farrar, W. E., Jr., and O'Dell, N. M.: Beta-lactamase activity in *Chromobacterium violaceum*. J. Infect. Dis. *134*:290–293, 1976.
9. Feldman, R. B., Stern, G. A., and Hood, I.: *Chromobacterium violaceum* infection of the eye. Arch. Ophthalmol. *102*:711–713, 1984.
10. Furie, R. A., Cohen, R. P., Hartman, B. J., et al.: *Pasteurella multocida* infection: Report in urban setting and review of spectrum of human disease. N. Y. State Med. J. *80*:1597–1602, 1980.
11. Gadberry, J. L., Zipper, R., Taylor, J. A., et al.: *Pasteurella pneumotropica* isolated from bone and joint infections. J. Clin. Microbiol. *19*:926–927, 1984.
12. Goldstein, E. J. C., and Citron, D. M.: Comparative activities of cefuroxime, amoxicillin–clavulanic acid, ciprofloxacin, enoxacin, and ofloxacin against aerobic and anaerobic bacteria isolated from bite wounds. Antimicrob. Agents Chemother. *32*:1143–1148, 1988.
13. Hamilton-Miller, J. M.: A possible pitfall in the identification of *Pasteurella* spp. with the API system. J. Med. Microbiol. *39*:78–79, 1993.
14. Herrington, D. A., Tzipori, S., Robins-Browne, R. M., et al.: *In vitro* and *in vivo* pathogenicity of *Plesiomonas shigelloides*. Infect. Immun. *55*:979–985, 1987.
15. Holmberg, S. D., Wachsmuth, K., Hickman-Brenner, F. W., et al.: *Plesiomonas* enteric infections in the United States. Ann. Intern. Med. *105*:690–694, 1986.

16. Holst, E., Rollof, J., Larsson, L., et al.: Characterization and distribution of *Pasteurella* species recovered from infected humans. J. Clin. Microbiol. *30*:2984–2987, 1992.
17. Ingram, C. W., Morrison, A. J., Jr., and Levitz, R. E.: Gastroenteritis, sepsis, and osteomyelitis caused by *Plesiomonas shigelloides* in an immunocompetent host: Case report and review of the literature. J. Clin. Microbiol. *25*:1791–1793, 1987.
18. Jones, Jr., F. L., and Smull, C. E.: Infections in man due to *Pasteurella multocida*: Importance of human carrier. PA Med. J. *76*:41–44, 1985.
19. Kain, K. C., and Kelly, M. T.: Antimicrobial susceptibilities of *Plesiomonas shigelloides* from patients with diarrhea. Antimicrob. Agents Chemother. *33*:1609–1610, 1989.
20. Kain, K. C., and Kelly, M. T.: Clinical features, epidemiology, and treatment of *Plesiomonas shigelloides* diarrhea. J. Clin. Microbiol. *27*:998–1001, 1989.
21. Kaka, S., Lunz, R., and Klugman, K. P.: *Actinobacillus (Pasteurella) ureae* meningitis in an HIV-positive patient. Diagn. Microbiol. Infect. Dis. *20*:105–107, 1994.
22. Kaufman, S. C., Ceraso, D., and Schugurensky, A.: First case report from Argentina of fatal septicemia caused by *Chromobacterium violaceum*. J. Clin. Microbiol. *23*:956–958, 1986.
23. Leet, S., and Wright, B. D.: Fulminating chromobacterial septicemia presenting as respiratory distress syndrome. Thorax *36*:557–559 1981.
24. Lester, A., Jarlov, J. O., Westh H., et al.: *Pasteurella haemolytica* diagnosis questioned. J. Infect. *25*:334–335, 1992.
25. MacDonell, M. T., and Colwell, R. R.: Phylogeny of the Vibrionaceae, and recommendation for two new genera, *Listonella* and *Shewanella*. System. Appl. Microbiol. *6*:171–182, 1985.
26. Macher, A. M., Casale, T. B., and Fauci, A. S.: Chronic granulomatous disease of childhood and *Chromobacterium violaceum* infections in the southeastern United States. Ann. Intern. Med. *97*:51–55, 1982.
27. Mamlok, R. J., Mamlok, V., Mills, G. C., et al.: Glucose-6-phosphate dehydrogenase deficiency, neutrophil dysfunction, and *Chromobacterium violaceum* sepsis. J. Pediatr. *111*:852–854, 1987.
28. Martin, D. L., and Gustafson, T. L.: *Plesiomonas* gastroenteritis in Texas. J. A. M. A. *15*:2063, 1985.
29. McNeely, D., Ivy, P., Craft, J. C., et al.: *Plesiomonas*: Biology of the organism and disease in children. Pediatr. Infect. Dis. *3*:176–181, 1984.
30. Miller, D. P., Blevins, W. T., Steele, D. B., et al.: A comparative study of virulent and avirulent strains of *Chromobacterium violaceum*. Can. J. Microbiol. *32*:249–255, 1988.
31. Mutters, R., Ihm, P., Pohl, S., et al.: Reclassification of the genus *Pasteurella* Trivisan 1887 on the basis of deoxyribonucleic acid homology, with proposals for the new species *Pasteurella dagmatis, Pasteurella canis, Pasteurella stomatis, Pasteurella anatis*, and *Pasteurella langaa*. Int. J. Syst. Bacteriol. *35*:309, 1985.
32. Myers, J., Ragasa, D. A., and Eisole, C.: *Chromobacterium violaceum* septicemia in New Jersey. J. Med. Soc. N. J. *79*:213–214, 1982.
33. Noble, R. C., Marek, B. J., and Overman, S. B.: Spontaneous bacterial peritonitis caused by *Pasteurella ureae*. J. Clin. Microbiol. *25*:442–444, 1987.
34. Paul, R., Siitonen, A., Karkkainen, P.: *Plesiomonas shigelloides* bacteremia in a healthy girl with mild gastroenteritis. J. Clin. Microbiol. *28*:1445–1446, 1990.
35. Ponte, R., and Jenkins, S. G.: Fatal *Chromobacterium violaceum* infections associated with exposure to stagnant waters. Pediatr. Infect. Dis. J. *11*:583–586, 1992.
36. Rahim, Z., and Kay, B. A.: Enrichment for *Plesiomonas shigelloides* from stools. J. Clin. Microbiol. *26*:789–790, 1988.
37. Reinhardt, J. F., and George, W. L.: Comparative *in vitro* activities of selected antimicrobial agents against *Aeromonas* species and *Plesiomonas shigelloides*. Antimicrob. Agents Chemother. *27*:643–645, 1985.
38. Rolston, K. V. I., and Hopfer, R. L.: Diarrhea due to *Plesiomonas shigelloides* in cancer patients. J. Clin. Microbiol. *20*:597–598, 1984.
39. Sivendra, R., and Tan, S. H.: Pathogenicity of unpigmented cultures of *Chromobacterium violaceum*. J. Clin. Microbiol. *5*:514–516, 1977.
40. Sneath, P. H. A. Genus *Chromobacterium*. *In* Krieg N. R., and Holt, J. G. (eds.): Bergey's Manual of Systematic Bacteriology. Baltimore, Williams & Wilkins, 1984, pp. 580–582.
41. Sorbello, A. F., O'Donnell, J., Kaiser-Smith, J., et al.: Infective endocarditis due to *Pasteurella dagmatis*: Case report and review. Clin. Infect. Dis. *18*:336–338, 1994.
42. Sorenson, R. U., Jacobs, M. R., and Shurin, S. B.: *Chromobacterium violaceum* adenitis acquired in the northern United States as a complication of chronic granulomatous disease. Pediatr. Infect. Dis. J. *4*:701–702, 1985.
43. Terpeluk, C., Goldman, A., Bartmann, P., et al.: *Plesiomonas shigelloides* sepsis and meningoencephalitis in a neonate. Eur. J. Pediatr. *151*:499–501, 1992.
44. Thorsen, P., Moller, B. R., Arpi, M., et al.: *Pasteurella aerogenes* isolated from stillbirth and mother. Lancet *343*:485–486, 1994.
45. Ti T. Y., Tan, W. C., Chong, A. P. Y., et al.: Nonfatal and fatal infections caused by *Chromobacterium violaceum*. Clin. Infect. Dis. *17*:505–507, 1993.
46. Wang, S.: A study of the ecology of *Plesiomonas shigelloides*. (Chinese.) Chung-Hua Liu Hsing Ping Hsueh Tsa Chih Chinese J. Epidemiol. *12*:295–298, 1991.

125

ACINETOBACTER

Armando G. Correa

First recognized as a human pathogen in 1908,[52] the ubiquitous organism *Acinetobacter* has emerged as a rather common cause of nosocomial infections among immunocompromised hosts.[6] Some of the confusion regarding this organism may be attributed to the many changes in nomenclature that the members of this genus have undergone over the years. Names that have been used in the past to identify this genus include *Herrella, Bacterium, Mima, Achromobacter, Alcaligenes, Neisseria, Micrococcus, Diplococcus, Moraxella,* and *Cytophaga*. Treatment of infection due to *Acinetobacter* is complicated by its widespread, multidrug resistance and the difficulty in eradicating the organism.

THE ORGANISM

The genus *Acinetobacter* belongs to the Neisseriaceae family, which also includes the *Neisseria, Moraxella,* and *Kingella* genera. *Acinetobacter* is a gram-negative bacterium that typically appears as a rod 0.9 to 1.6 μm in diameter and 1.5 to 2.5 μm in length but may become spherical in the stationary phase of growth. It frequently occurs in pairs or short chains. Many strains are encapsulated. The organism has a strictly aerobic respiratory metabolism and does not grow under anaerobic conditions. It does not form spores or exhibit swimming mobility. It grows well between 20° C and 30° C, with optimal growth between 33° C and 35° C, in all common complex media and displays no growth factor requirements.

Convex, grayish-white colonies 1 to 2.5 mm in diameter are typical. The colonies may appear mucoid if the strain is encapsulated. *Acinetobacter* is catalase-positive and may be differentiated readily from other closely related genera by virtue of its negative reaction to oxidase.

Until recently, the genus *Acinetobacter* contained the single species *A. calcoaceticus* subdivided into two subspecies or biovars: *anitratus* and *lwoffii*.[25] However, in 1986 the taxonomy of the genus *Acinetobacter* was changed extensively on the basis of DNA hybridization studies,[9] and there now are seven recognized species: *A. baumannii, A. calcoaceticus, A. haemolyticus, A. johnsonii, A. junii, A. lwoffii*, and the recently described *A. radioresistens*.[14] There also are several unnamed genospecies.[14] These species may be differentiated in the clinical laboratory on the basis of their growth characteristics and biochemical activity. Under the new classification, most

A. baumannii strains represent organisms that were classified formerly as biovar *anitratus*, whereas *A. junii* and *A. lwoffii* previously were under biovar *lwoffii*.

EPIDEMIOLOGY

Acinetobacter strains are distributed widely in nature and can be found in soil, fresh water, and sewage.[8, 23] *Acinetobacter* also can be isolated from many animals, fresh meats, poultry, contaminated milk, and frozen foods.[8, 23] *Acinetobacter* can be part of the bacterial flora of the skin in healthy individuals,[8, 11] and the skin frequently becomes a reservoir for *Acinetobacter* among hospitalized patients and the health care staff.[6, 8] It occasionally forms part of the normal flora of the oral cavity and the upper respiratory, genital, and lower gastrointestinal tracts.[8, 11] Colonization by *Acinetobacter* particularly is common among patients who have undergone a tracheostomy.[39] The organism frequently can be found in the hospital environment, particularly in moist areas, such as in humidifiers, water sinks, and ventilators.[8] Nosocomial outbreaks have been linked to colonized medical equipment, such as ventilator tubing and other respiratory equipment,[1, 22] intravenous catheters,[8] gloves,[34] and mattresses.[45]

The frequency of nosocomial infections caused by *Acinetobacter* is not easy to assess, because the pathogenic role of this organism often has been underestimated. However, a national surveillance study conducted from 1974 to 1977 identified *Acinetobacter* as a pathogen in 0.76 per cent of nosocomial infections.[37] The estimated rate of nosocomial infections caused by this organism was 3.11 per 10,000 patients discharged, and approximately 15 per cent of 1372 reported episodes occurred in the pediatric age group.[37] By 1978, this rate increased by 14 per cent, accounting for 1 per cent of the bacterial isolates associated with nosocomial infections.[11] Of interest, an unusual seasonal pattern was observed, with most infections occurring in late summer.[11, 37] The cause for this increase is unknown. Pneumonia, tracheobronchitis, and infections of the urinary tract and surgical wounds were the entities observed most frequently.[37] Among the pediatric age group, neonates appear to be particularly susceptible to nosocomial infection due to this organism (Table 125–1).

PATHOGENESIS

There is limited information regarding the pathogenesis of *Acinetobacter* infections, and specific virulence factors have not been identified. Except for the presence of lipopolysaccharide, a normal constituent of the outer membrane of gram-negative bacteria capable of eliciting multiple pathogenic host responses, no cytotoxic products have been identified. In animal models, *Acinetobacter* can enhance the virulence of other bacteria in mixed infections, perhaps by slime-induced inhibition of neutrophils.[32] It has been speculated that the ability to grow in an acidic pH at lower temperatures may enhance its ability to invade devitalized tissue.[2] The organism also may survive in a dry environment for up to a week.[12]

CLINICAL MANIFESTATIONS

Acinetobacter can cause suppurative infection of virtually any organ, and the clinical manifestations typically are similar to those seen with other bacterial infections because there are no unique features suggesting *Acinetobacter* infection. The clinical manifestations also may depend on the underlying immune status of the compromised host. Infections due to *Acinetobacter* are rare in normal children.[16]

Intracranial Infection

Most cases of *Acinetobacter* meningitis are the result of a penetrating injury or occur after a neurosurgical procedure, although sporadic cases of meningitis have been reported in the absence of these factors. A cluster of eight children who developed *Acinetobacter* meningitis after the administration of intrathecal methotrexate has been reported.[26] All patients presented with fever, headache, nausea, and vomiting, and the lumbar puncture revealed cerebrospinal fluid pleocytosis.

Earlier literature contains several reports of *Acinetobacter* meningitis occurring in apparently normal children.[13, 15, 21, 49, 53] Cerebrospinal fluid pleocytosis with a predominance of segmented forms was common.[15] Because up to 30 per cent of those patients had a petechial rash and the finding of gram-negative diplococci on the smear of the cerebrospinal fluid, the diagnosis of meningococcal meningitis was made erroneously in the majority of these cases, leading to a delay in the institution of appropriate therapy and possibly contributing to a mortality rate as high as 27 per cent.[15]

Siegman-Igra and associates,[46] in a review of 25 cases of *Acinetobacter* meningitis secondary to invasive procedures that included some children, found that fever, leukocytosis, and neck stiffness along with other clinical signs of central nervous system infection were common features. The cerebrospinal fluid in these patients showed pleocytosis with a predominance of polymorphonuclear leukocytes, elevated protein concentration, and a low glucose concentration. The majority of infections were associated with indwelling ventriculostomy tubes or a fistula into the cerebrospinal fluid space.

TABLE 125–1. Nosocomial Clusters of *Acinetobacter* Infection Among Pediatric Patients

Country	Year	Type of Unit	Infected Children	Colonized Children	Presentation	Mortality (%)	Suspected Source
United Kingdom[30]	1981	NICU	4	0	Meningitis	0	None identified
United Kingdom[47]	1983	NICU	9	1	Pulmonary infection	22	Ambu bag
Japan[40]	1983–1986	NICU	19	52	Sepsis	11	Multiple sources
India[26]	1988	Oncology	8	N/A	Meningitis	38	Intrathecal needle
Germany[42]	1988	NICU	3	41	Sepsis	100	Humidifier
Israel[36]	1988–1990	NICU	9	N/A	Sepsis	44	None identified
United Kingdom[31]	1989	NICU	7	N/A	Sepsis	0	Intravenous fluids

NICU, neonatal intensive care unit; N/A, data not available.

It has been suggested that an inherited or acquired complement deficiency may be associated with meningitis due to *Acinetobacter*[17] because it is seen with *Neisseria meningitidis* and other related species. Treatment of central nervous system infections due to *Acinetobacter* requires a minimum of 3 weeks of parenteral antibiotics.

Bacteremia

Acinetobacter bacteremia may occur as an isolated event or be secondary to a primary infected site, such as the respiratory or urinary tract or a wound. Primary bacteremia appears to be more common among immunocompromised neonates, and its clinical manifestations can vary from the absence of clinical signs of infection to fulminant septic shock and disseminated intravascular coagulation.[31, 42] Thrombocytopenia has been reported to be a prominent feature among these neonates.[31, 36] Predisposing factors include low birth weight,[40, 42] prior antibiotic therapy,[36, 40, 42] and the presence of indwelling catheters.[40]

Acinetobacter bacteremia among children with malignancies also has been noted to occur rarely. Fuchs and colleagues[18] reported 29 episodes of sepsis due to this organism over a 12-year period in an oncology center. All of these children were febrile and appeared ill at the time of diagnosis, and there was a high association of *Acinetobacter* sepsis with the presence of intravascular catheters. Surprisingly, there was no association with the level of neutropenia.[18]

Respiratory Tract

Because *Acinetobacter* may be a transient colonizer of the pharynx in 7 per cent of healthy children[5] and adults[19] and this rate is increased among hospitalized patients, the relative importance of *Acinetobacter* compared with other potential pathogens isolated from sputum is difficult to ascertain. Tracheobronchitis and pneumonia attributed to *Acinetobacter* mostly are nosocomial infections associated with the presence of an endotracheal tube or tracheostomy.[19] Pneumonias frequently are multilobar and occasionally may lead to cavitary destruction or pleural empyema.[19]

Community-acquired pneumonia due to *A. baumannii* has been reported to occur among adults in the Northern Territory of Australia and other tropical regions.[4] This entity generally occurs in patients with diminished host defenses due to alcoholism, cigarette smoking, or underlying pulmonary disease and is characterized by the rapid onset of fever, dyspnea, pleuritic chest pain, and purulent sputum. The mortality rate has been as high as 53 to 64 per cent.[4]

Miscellaneous

Urinary tract infections occur almost exclusively in patients with indwelling bladder catheters, usually are limited to the bladder, and generally are mild in nature.[19] Burns, as well as traumatic and surgical wounds, frequently become colonized by *Acinetobacter* as a result of its ability to thrive on compromised tissue and foreign material.[19] Bacteremia may occur as a consequence of this colonization, which often is polymicrobial. *Acinetobacter* is a prominent cause of peritonitis among children receiving peritoneal dialysis when due to gram-negative organisms.[54]

Other rare infections due to *Acinetobacter* that have been reported include suppurative otitis media,[38, 49] cellulitis (frequently in association with trauma, foreign body, or animal bite),[19, 38] synergistic necrotizing fasciitis,[3] native and prosthetic value endocarditis,[21] septic arthritis,[38] osteomyelitis,[49] and liver abscesses.[19] Ocular infections also have been documented.[28, 35] A case of osteomyelitis occurring after a hamster bite in a child has been described.[29]

DIAGNOSIS

The diagnosis of *Acinetobacter* infection is made by culture of appropriate body fluids or tissue specimen. There are no serologic or antigen detection tests available. A selective media containing MacConkey agar with cephaloridine has been used to sample skin during investigation of outbreaks[47] because of its ability to inhibit most of the skin flora but not *Acinetobacter*.

Biotyping, phage typing, electrophoretic analysis of isoenzyme and cell wall proteins, plasmid analysis, and restriction-endonuclease digestion of DNA have been used for investigation of nosocomial outbreaks.[7] Antibiogram typing no longer is considered an effective method in the investigation of *Acinetobacter* epidemics, because the susceptibility pattern may change rapidly within the same outbreak.[7, 10]

TREATMENT

As with many other opportunistic gram-negative organisms, treatment of infections due to *Acinetobacter*, particularly among *A. baumannii*,[43, 51] has become more complicated by the rapid increase of resistance to antibiotics used commonly in hospitals. Selection of an antibiotic regimen should be based on in vitro susceptibility testing and ideally should include both a β-lactam and an aminoglycoside, which may have synergistic activity[19] and prevent the emergence of resistance.[6]

In recent years, *A. baumannii* has shown decreased susceptibility to ampicillin, broad-spectrum penicillins, cephalosporins, aminoglycosides, and ciprofloxacin.[43] Resistance to extended-spectrum cephalosporins may be the result of the presence of cephalosporinases, broad-spectrum β-lactamases, or changes in the outer membrane porins and penicillin-binding proteins.[33] Resistance to aminoglycosides is mediated by aminoglycoside-modifying enzymes.[51] Imipenem appears to be the most active agent against *A. baumannii*,[43, 51] but some reports have found up to 5 per cent of these strains to be resistant to this antibiotic,[43] and nosocomial outbreaks of imipenem-resistant *Acinetobacter* have been reported.[20, 50, 57] Caution should be exercised when using imipenem at high dosage in children for treatment of meningitis (i.e., 100 mg/kg/day) because of an unusually high rate of seizures.[56] The role of meropenem, a new carbapenem antibiotic with good in vitro activity against *Acinetobacter*, in the treatment of these infections has not been established. Combinations of a β-lactam antibiotic with a β-lactamase inhibitor, such as ampicillin/sulbactam or ticarcillin/clavulanate, or the polymyxins have been used for infections due to imipenem-resistant strains.[20, 50, 57]

Imipenem, amikacin, ciprofloxacin, ceftazidime, and ceftriaxone have exhibited good in vitro activity against isolates identified as species other than *A. baumannii*.[43] In addition to antimicrobial therapy, prompt drainage of focal suppurative sites and removal of infected indwelling catheters are essential. Intraventricular administration of amikacin has been used in the treatment of central nervous system infections due to this organism.[55]

PROGNOSIS

Because *Acinetobacter* strains often are resistant to antibiotics used commonly, prompt recognition of the specific etiology and institution of effective antibiotic therapy are critical to a successful outcome. The reported mortality rate among series of pediatric patients has ranged from 0 per cent to more than 50 per cent (see Table 125–1), and the outcome appears to correlate more closely with the underlying condition than with other factors, such as polymicrobial bacteremia.[48] In a series of 58 infections due to this organism that occurred over a 2-year period from 1973 through 1974 at the Massachusetts General Hospital, the mortality rate was 23 per cent.[19]

The nosocomial acquisition of multiresistant *A. baumannii* has been associated with high mortality rates and prolonged hospitalization among adult patients in intensive care units,[27, 41] compared with the more benign clinical outcome that usually is seen with other species of *Acinetobacter*.[44]

PREVENTION

Nosocomial acquisition of *Acinetobacter* by high-risk, compromised hosts can be prevented by placing emphasis on control measures routinely used for endemic infections, such as careful hand washing by personnel, limitations of the frequency and duration of use of devices, proper isolation of colonized and infected patients, application of strict techniques for invasive procedures, and restricted use of antibiotics.[12, 27, 46]

References

1. Ahmed, J., Brutus, A., D'Amato, R. F., et al.: *Acinetobacter calcoaceticus anitratus* outbreak in the intensive care unit traced to a peak flow meter. Am. J. Infect. Control 22:319–321, 1994.
2. Allen, D. M., and Hartman, B. J.: *Acinetobacter* species. *In* Mandell, G. L., Bennett, J. E., and Dolin, R. (eds.): Mandell, Douglas and Bennett's Principles and Practice of Infectious Diseases. 4th ed. New York, Churchill Livingstone, 1995, pp. 2009–2013.
3. Amsel, M. B., and Horrilleno, E.: Synergistic necrotizing fasciitis: A case of polymicrobial infection with *Acinetobacter calcoaceticus*. Curr. Surg. 42:370–372, 1985.
4. Anstey, N. M., Currie, B. J., and Withnall, K. M.: Community-acquired *Acinetobacter* pneumonia in the Northern Territory of Australia. Clin. Infect. Dis. *14*:83–91, 1992.
5. Baltimore, R. S., Duncan, R. L., Shapiro, E. D., et al.: Epidemiology of pharyngeal colonization of infants with aerobic gram-negative rod bacteria. J. Clin. Microbiol. *27*:91–95, 1989.
6. Bergogne-Berezin, E.: *Acinetobacter* spp., saprophytic organisms of increasing pathogenic importance. Int. J. Med. Microbiol. Virol. Parasitol. Infect. Dis. *281*:389–405, 1994.
7. Bergogne-Berezin, E., and Joly-Guillou, M. L.: Hospital infection with *Acinetobacter* spp.: An increasing problem. J. Hosp. Infect. *18*(Suppl. A):250–255, 1991.
8. Bergogne-Berezin, E., Joly-Guillou, M. L., and Vieu, J. F.: Epidemiology of nosocomial infections due to *Acinetobacter calcoaceticus*. J. Hosp. Infect. *10*:105–113, 1987.
9. Bouvet, P. J. M., and Grimont, P. A. D.: Taxonomy of the genus *Acinetobacter* with the recognition of *Acinetobacter baumannii* sp. nov., *Acinetobacter haemolyticus* sp. nov., *Acinetobacter johnsonii* sp. nov., and *Acinetobacter junii* sp. nov. and the emended descriptions of *Acinetobacter calcoaceticus* and *Acinetobacter lwoffii*. Int. J. Syst. Bacteriol. *36*:228–240, 1986.
10. Carlquist, J. F., Conti, M., and Burke, J. P.: Progressive resistance in a single strain of *Acinetobacter calcoaceticus* recovered during a nosocomial outbreak. Am. J. Infect. Control *10*:43–48, 1982.
11. Centers for Disease Control. Nosocomial infections caused by *Acinetobacter calcoaceticus*—United States, 1978. M. M. W. R., *28*:177–179, 1979.
12. Crombach, W. H. J., Dijkshoorn, L., van Noort-Klaassen, M., et al.: Control of an epidemic spread of a multi-resistant strain of *Acinetobacter calcoaceticus* in a hospital. Intensive Care Med. *15*:166–170, 1989.
13. DeBord, G. G.: *Mima polymorpha* in meningitis. J. Bacteriol. *55*:764–765, 1948.
14. Dijkshoorn, L., and van der Toorn, J.: *Acinetobacter* species: Which do we mean? Clin. Infect. Dis. *15*:748–749, 1992.
15. Donald, W. D., and Doak, W. M.: Mimeae meningitis and sepsis. J. A. M. A. *200*:111–113, 1967.
16. Feigin, R. D., and Shearer, W. T.: Opportunistic infection in children: III. In the normal host. J. Pediatr. *87*:852–866, 1975.
17. Fijen, C. A. P., Kuijper, E. J., Tjia, H. G., et al.: Complement deficiency predisposes for meningitis due to nongroupable meningococci and *Neisseria*-related bacteria. Clin. Infect. Dis. *18*:780–784, 1994.
18. Fuchs, G. J., Jaffe, N., and Pickering, L. K.: *Acinetobacter calcoaceticus* sepsis in children with malignancies. Pediatr. Infect. Dis. *5*:545–549, 1986.
19. Glew, R. H., Moellering R. C., and Kunz L. J.: Infections with *Acinetobacter calcoaceticus* (*Herrella vaginicola*): Clinical and laboratory studies. Medicine *56*:79–97, 1977.
20. Go, E. S., Urban, C., Burns, J., et al.: Clinical and molecular epidemiology of *Acinetobacter* infections sensitive only to polymyxin B and sulbactam. Lancet *344*:1329–1332, 1994.
21. Gradon, J. D., Chapnick, E. K., and Lutwick, L. I.: Infective endocarditis of a native valve due to *Acinetobacter*: Case report and review. Clin. Infect. Dis. *14*:1145–1148, 1992.
22. Hartstein, A. I., Rashad, A. L., Liebler, J. M., et al.: Multiple intensive care unit outbreak of *Acinetobacter calcoaceticus* subspecies *anitratus* respiratory infection and colonization associated with contaminated, reusable ventilator circuits and resuscitation bags. Am. J. Med. *85*:624–631, 1988.
23. Henriksen, S. D.: *Moraxella*, *Acinetobacter*, and the Mimeae. Bacteriol. Rev. *37*:522–561, 1973.
24. Hermann, G., and Melnick, T.: *Mima polymorpha* meningitis in the young. Am. J. Dis. Child. *110*:315–318, 1965.
25. Juni, E.: *Acinetobacter*. *In* Krieg, N. R. (ed.): Bergey's Manual of Systematic Bacteriology. Baltimore, Williams & Wilkins, 1984, pp. 303–306.
26. Kelkar, R., Gordon, S. M., Giri, N., et al.: Epidemic iatrogenic *Acinetobacter* spp. meningitis following administration of intrathecal methotrexate. J. Hosp. Infect. *14*:233–243, 1989.
27. Lortholary, O., Fagon, J. Y., Hoi, A. B., et al.: Nosocomial acquisition of multiresistant *Acinetobacter baumannii*: Risk factors and prognosis. Clin. Infect. Dis. *20*:790–796, 1995.
28. Marcovich, A., and Levartovsky, S.: *Acinetobacter* exposure keratitis. Br. J. Ophthalmol. *78*:489–490, 1994.
29. Martin, R. W., Martin, D. L., and Levy, C. S.: *Acinetobacter* osteomyelitis from a hamster bite. Pediatr. Infect. Dis. J. *5*:364–365, 1988.
30. Morgan, M. E. I., and Hart, C. A.: *Acinetobacter* meningitis: Acquired infection in a neonatal intensive care unit. Arch. Dis. Child. *657*:557–559, 1982.
31. Ng, P. C., Herrington, R. A., Beane, C. A., et al.: An outbreak of *Acinetobacter* septicaemia in a neonatal intensive care unit. J. Hosp. Infect. *14*:363–368, 1989.
32. Obana, Y.: Pathogenic significance of *Acinetobacter calcoaceticus*: Analysis of experimental infection in mice. Microbiol. Immunol. *30*:645–657, 1986.
33. Obara, M., and Nakae, T.: Mechanisms of resistance to β-lactam antibiotics in *Acinetobacter calcoaceticus*. J. Antimicrob. Chemother. *28*:791–800, 1991.
34. Patterson, J. E., Vecchio, J., Pantelick, E. L., et al.: Association of contaminated gloves with transmission of *Acinetobacter calcoaceticus* var. *anitratus* in an intensive care unit. Am. J. Med. *91*:479–483, 1991.
35. Peyman, G. A., Vastine, D. W., and Diamond, J. G.: Vitrectomy and intraocular gentamicin management of *Herrella* endophthalmitis after incomplete phacoemulsification. Am. J. Ophthalmol. *56*:764–765, 1975.
36. Regev, R., Dolfin, T., Zelig, I., et al.: *Acinetobacter* septicemia: A threat to neonates? Special aspects in a neonatal intensive care unit. Infection *21*:394–396, 1993.
37. Retailliau, H. F., Hightower, A. W., Dixon, R. E., et al.: *Acinetobacter calcoaceticus*: A nosocomial pathogen with an unusual seasonal pattern. J. Infect. Dis. *139*:371–375, 1979.
38. Reynolds, R. C., and Cluff, L. E.: Infection of men with Mimeae. Ann. Intern. Med. *58*:759–767, 1963.
39. Rosenthal, S. L.: Sources of *Pseudomonas* and *Acinetobacter* species found in human culture materials. Am. J. Clin. Pathol. *62*:807–811, 1974.
40. Sakata, H., Fujita, K., Maruyama, S., et al.: *Acinetobacter calcoaceticus* biovar *anitratus* septicaemia in a neonatal intensive care unit: Epidemiology and control. J. Hosp. Infect. *14*:15–22, 1989.
41. Scerpella, E. G., Wanger, A. R., Armitige, L., et al.: Nosocomial outbreak caused by a multiresistant clone of *Acinetobacter baumannii*: Results of the case-control and molecular epidemiologic investigations. Infect. Control Hosp. Epidemiol. *16*:92–97, 1995.
42. Schloesser, R. L., Laufkoetter, E. A., Lehners, T., et al.: An outbreak of *Acinetobacter calcoaceticus* infection in a neonatal care unit. Infection *18*:230–233, 1990.
43. Seifert, H., Baginski, R., Schulze, A., et al.: Antimicrobial susceptibility of *Acinetobacter* species. Antimicrob. Agents Chemother. *37*:750–753, 1993.
44. Seifert, H., Strate, A., Schulze, A., et al.: Bacteremia due to *Acinetobacter* species other than *Acinetobacter baumannii*. Infection 22:379–385, 1994.
45. Sherertz, R. J., and Sullivan, M. L.: An outbreak of infections with *Acinetobacter calcoaceticus* in burn patients: Contamination of patients' mattresses. J. Infect. Dis. *151*:252–258, 1985.
46. Siegman-Igra, Y., Bar-Yosef, S., Gorea, A., et al.: Nosocomial *Acinetobacter* meningitis secondary to invasive procedures: Report of 25 cases and review. Clin. Infect. Dis. *17*:843–849, 1993.
47. Stone, J. W., and Das, B. C.: Investigation of an outbreak of infection

with *Acinetobacter calcoaceticus* in a special care baby unit. J. Hosp. Infect. *6*:42–48, 1985.

48. Tilley, P. A. G., and Roberts, F. J.: Bacteremia with *Acinetobacter* species: Risk factors and prognosis in different clinical settings. Clin. Infect. Dis. *18*:896–900, 1994.
49. Torregrosa, M. V., and Ortiz, A.: Severe infections in children due to rare gram-negative bacilli (*Mima polymorpha* and *Bacillus anitratum*). J. Pediatr. *59*:35–41, 1961.
50. Urban, C., Go, E., Mariano, N., et al.: Effect of sulbactam on infections caused by imipenem-resistant *Acinetobacter calcoaceticus* biotype *anitratus*. *167*:448–451, 1993.
51. Vila, J., Marcos, A., Marco, F., et al.: *In vitro* antimicrobial production of β-lactamases, aminoglycoside-modifying enzymes, and chloramphenicol acetyltransferase by and susceptibility of clinical isolates of *Acinetobacter baumannii*. Antimicrob. Agents Chemother. *37*:138–141, 1993.
52. Von Lingelsheim, W.: Beitrage zur ätiologie der epidemischen genickstarre nach den ergebnissen der letzten jahre. Z. Hyg. Infektionskrankheiten *59*:457–460, 1908.
53. Waite, C. L., and Kline, A. H.: *Mima polymorpha* meningitis. Am. J. Dis. Child. *98*:121–126, 1959.
54. Warady, B. A., Campoy, S. F., Gross, S. P., et al.: Peritonitis with continuous ambulatory peritoneal dialysis and continuous cycling peritoneal dialysis. J. Pediatr. *105*:726–729, 1984.
55. Wirt, T. C., McGee, Z. A., Oldfield, E. H., et al.: Intraventricular administration of amikacin for complicated gram-negative meningitis and ventriculitis. J. Neurosurg. *50*:95–99, 1979.
56. Wong, V. K., Wright, H. T., Ross, L. A., et al.: Imipenem/cilastatin treatment of bacterial meningitis in children. Pediatr. Infect. Dis. J. *10*:122–125, 1991.
57. Wood, C. A., and Reboli, A. C.: Infections caused by imipenem-resistant *Acinetobacter calcoaceticus* biotype *anitratus*. J. Infect. Dis. *168*:1602–1603, 1993.

126

ALCALIGENES

Randall G. Fisher and William C. Gruber

Organisms of the genus *Alcaligenes* are gram-negative bacilli that live in aqueous environments. Originally considered commensals, they increasingly are recognized as important, although rare, hospital pathogens. *Alcaligenes* can be especially problematic in immunocompromised patients and in neonates, in whom infection can be life-threatening. They have been isolated from such diverse clinical specimens as sputum, urine, feces, blood, cerebrospinal fluid, and peritoneal and pleural fluids.

BACTERIOLOGY

Alcaligenes species are gram-negative, motile, indole-negative, obligate aerobes that are oxidase- and catalase-positive. They are considered to be nonfermenters because of their extremely limited action on carbohydrates. Most ferment xylose, and some ferment glucose. All reduce nitrate to nitrite. They are urease-, lysine-, and ornithine-negative. They grow well on both blood and MacConkey agar and produce colonies that are smooth and glistening and have a distinct edge. They alkalinize organic salts and amides; hence the name *Alcaligenes*, which means alkali producing. *A. faecalis* has a distinct, sweet odor that has been described as resembling that of green apples.[15]

Bacteriologically, they may be confused with other nonfermenting gram-negative organisms, especially *Pseudomonas* species. Morphologically, however, they can be distinguished easily from pseudomonads by the presence of peritrichous flagella. *Pseudomonas* species have polar flagella.[11]

The taxonomy of these organisms is confusing and undergoes frequent changes. They were classified formerly as *Achromobacter* species. The genus *Alcaligenes* consists of many species but clinically important ones are as follows: (1) *A. xylosoxidans*, which has two subspecies—*xylosoxidans* and *dentrificans*. The former is the most common cause of clinically recognizable infection. (2) *A. faecalis*, which is a less common pathogen but has a distinct antimicrobial susceptibility pattern.[1] (3) *A. piechaudii*, which has been isolated from clinical specimens[22] but is of doubtful significance.

EPIDEMIOLOGY

Like *Pseudomonas* species, *Alcaligenes* are water organisms and prefer aqueous environments and moist soil. They do not survive long on porous surfaces or fomites or if they become desiccated.[25] They also may be part of the normal flora of the gastrointestinal and respiratory tracts of some people. These organisms establish a niche within the hospital environment and have been recovered from ventilators, humidifiers, "sterile" saline, intravenous fluids, and irrigation and dialysis solutions. *Alcaligenes* species also have been recovered from infant formula,[8] children's soap bubbles,[20] well water,[28] and swimming pools.[13] Organisms also survive many disinfectants and have been cultured from chlorhexidine,[27] 1 per cent eosin,[2] and alcohol- or quarternary amine–containing compounds.[25, 27] Shigeta and associates[27] reported an outbreak of *A. xylosoxidans* ventriculitis secondary to contaminated chlorhexidine used on a surgical ward. Foley and colleagues[9] reported an outbreak accompanied by deaths in a neonatal intensive care unit secondary to contamination of saline used as an eyewash. Boukadida and coworkers[2] reported a neonatal death due to meningitis contracted by dissemination after treatment of a diaper rash with 1 per cent eosin. An outbreak of 37 cases (with two fatalities) was described by Reverdy and associates[23] that was caused by bacterial contamination of deionized water in a hemodialysis system. Surgical wound infection also has occurred, wherein infection was suspected to be secondary to contaminated irrigation fluids used in surgery.[30]

PATHOPHYSIOLOGY

Alcaligenes species are weakly virulent bacteria. Medical care commonly provides the conduit through which organisms are introduced into their host, by way of indwelling catheters, endotracheal tubes, etc. The bacteria may take advantage of a weakened immune system and disseminate, causing sepsis, meningitis, and death. Preterm or small-for-gestational-age term infants are at particular risk for such severe *Alcaligenes* infections.[9] Although most neonatal infections are considered to be nosocomial, vertical transmission from mother to baby may occur.[11] An increased incidence of infection has been reported for patients with neoplasms[16] and those receiving chronic steroid therapy.[14] There also are sporadic case reports of *Alcaligenes* infection in patients with idiopathic immunoglobulin M deficiency,[7] Waldenström macroglobulinemia,[29] and systemic lupus erythematosus.[24] We have seen *Alcaligenes* recurrently recovered from a boy with hyper-IgM syndrome. *Alcaligenes* infections occur in patients with AIDS,[3, 10] but it is unclear whether this syndrome is an independent risk factor for *Alcaligenes* infection.

In unusual circumstances, patients with neither overt underlying disease nor obvious immune deficiency will develop infection with *Alcaligenes* species. Most of these cases involve penetrating trauma.

CLINICAL MANIFESTATIONS

Signs of sepsis or meningitis caused by *A. xylosoxidans* in the newborn are difficult to differentiate from other causes of bacterial sepsis. However, some babies may develop a distinctive rash in association with this infection, in which 1- to 2-cm, sharply demarcated red patches appear, especially in the head and neck region. This rash was noted in 29 of 33 newborns with *A. xylosoxidans* infection reported by Doxiadis and associates in 1960[6] and was seen again in a case reported in 1993.[2] *A. xylosoxidans* sepsis/meningitis tends to present later in life than do infections with the usual vertically acquired pathogens and may have a more insidious onset.[18] In some cases, cerebrospinal fluid profiles may resemble those usually associated with viral meningitis, with white blood cell counts in the hundreds and with monocytic predominance.[26] Neonatal *Alcaligenes* sepsis or meningitis has an extremely poor prognosis; one series noted a mortality rate that approached 75 per cent, and 36 per cent of survivors had severe neurologic deficits.[9] The incidence of intracranial hemorrhage also was high.

One child developed osteomyelitis due to *A. xylosoxidans* after stepping on a nail through old sneakers (a clinical situation classically associated with *Pseudomonas* infection)[12, 13]; another got *Alcaligenes* infection as a consequence of a gunshot wound.[4, 5] In the setting of a patient with an artificial heart valve, *A. xylosoxidans* endocarditis has been described.[21] *A. xylosoxidans* infection in older patients usually is not suspected on clinical grounds, but either in the context of a common source outbreak or because of microbiologic clues. *A. faecalis* infection is less common and usually is part of a polymicrobial process.

DIAGNOSIS AND TREATMENT

The diagnosis of *Alcaligenes* infections rests on recovery of the organism from clinical samples. These organisms often are mistaken for pseudomonads, and the clinician should suspect *A. xylosoxidans* when the laboratory reports an organism as a *Pseudomonas* species that is resistant to all aminoglycosides.[25] Key differentiation features include the antibiogram and the morphology of the organism, with its distinctive peritrichous flagella.

Alcaligenes species typically are resistant to a large number of antibiotics, including ampicillin, aztreonam, aminoglycosides, first- and second-generation cephalosporins, tetracyclines, and rifampin. They variably are resistant to chloramphenicol, fluoroquinolones, macrolides, ureidopenicillins, and β-lactamase combination drugs.[1] *Alcaligenes* species have been shown to produce β-lactamases, some of which are chromosomal, constitutive, and inducible[5] and some of which are on plasmids.[17] Some isolates overproduce β-lactamase,[5] which stoichiometrically can render β-lactamase inhibitors useless. In addition, their porins are small, making antibiotic entry difficult. Although there is no antibiotic to which all isolates have been shown to be sensitive,[21] most are sensitive in vitro to trimethoprim-sulfamethoxazole, imipenem, ceftazidime, and cefoperazone. Two case reports describe treatment failures of ceftazidime[19] and piperacillin[5] in clinical isolates that were sensitive at the time of isolation but developed resistance during the course of therapy.

Because resistance patterns vary from isolate to isolate, the combination of a third-generation cephalosporin, piperacillin, or imipenem with trimethoprim-sulfamethoxazole is reasonable empiric therapy for suspected *Alcaligenes* infection, pending susceptibilty results. In general, in vitro susceptibilities seem to correlate well with in vivo results,[16] but the risk of inducible resistance to β-lactam antibiotics should be acknowledged. One report describes synergy in microbial killing with an aminoglycoside, despite the fact that the isolate was resistant to the same aminoglycoside when it was tested alone.[3]

Removal of infected catheters may speed recovery, although some patients have been treated successfully through indwelling lines.[3]

References

1. Bizet, C., Tekaia, F., and Phillipon, A.: In vitro susceptibility of *Alcaligenes faecalis* compared with those of other *Alcaligenes* species to antimicrobial agents including seven beta-lactams. J. Antimicrob. Chemother. *32*:907–910, 1993.
2. Boukadida, J., Monastiri, K., Snoussi, N., et al.: Nosocomial neonatal meningitis by *Alcaligenes xylosoxicans* transmitted by aqueous eosin. Pediatr. Infect. Dis. J. *12*:696–697, 1993.
3. Cieslak, T. J., and Raszka, W. V.: Catheter-associated sepsis due to *Alcaligenes xylosoxidans* in a child with AIDS. Clin. Infect. Dis. *16*:592–593, 1993.
4. D'Amato, R. F., Salemi, M., Mathews, A., et al.: *Achromobacter xylosoxidans* (*Alcaligenes xylosoxidans* subsp. *xylosoxidans*) meningitis associated with a gunshot wound. J. Clin. Microbiol. *26*:2425–2426, 1988.
5. Decre, D., Arlet, G., Danglot, C., et al.: A beta-lactamase overproducing strain of *Alcaligenes dentrificans* subsp. *xylosoxidans* isolated from a case of meningitis. J. Antimicrob. Chemother. *30*:769–779, 1992.
6. Doxiadis, S. A., Pavlatou, M., and Chryssostomidou, O.: *Bacillus foecalis alcaligenes* septicemia in the newborn. J. Pediatr. *56*:648–654, 1960.
7. Dworzack, D. L., Murray, C. M., Hodges, G. R., et al.: Community acquired bacteremic *Achromobacter xylosoxidans* type IIIa: Pneumonia in a patient with idiopathic IgM deficiency. Am. J. Clin. Pathol. *70*:712–717, 1978.
8. Edwards, L. D., Tan-Gatue, L. G., Levin, S., et al.: The problem of bacteriologically contaminated infant formulas in a newborn nursery. Clin. Pediatr. *13*:63–65, 1974.
9. Foley, J. F., Gravelle, C. R., Englehard, W. E., et al.: *Achromobacter* septicemia fatalities in prematures. Am. J. Dis. Child. *101*:279–288, 1961.
10. Gradon, J. D., Mayrev, A. R., and Hayes, J.: Pulmonary abscess associated with *Alcaligenes xylosoxidans* in a patient with AIDS. Clin. Infect. Dis. *17*:1071–1072, 1993.
11. Hearn, Y. R., and Gander, R. M.: *Achromobacter xylosoxidans*: An unusual neonatal pathogen. Am. J. Clin. Pathol. *96*:211–214, 1991.
12. Hoddy, D. M., and Barton, L. L.: Puncture wound–induced *Achromobacter xylosoxidans* osteomyelitis of the foot. Am. J. Dis. Child. *145*:599–600, 1991.
13. Holmes, B., Snell, J. J. S., and Lapage, S. P.: Strains of *Achromobacter xylosoxidans* from clinical material. J. Clin. Pathol. *30*:595–601, 1977.
14. Igra-Siegman, Y., Chmel, H., and Cobbs, C.: Clinical and laboratory characteristics of *Achromobacter xylosoxidans* infection. J. Clin. Microbiol. *11*:141–145, 1980.
15. Kersters, K., and DeLey, J.: Genus *Alcaligenes*. *In* Krieg, N. R., and Holt, J. C. (eds.): Bergey's Manual of Systematic Bacteriology. Baltimore, Williams & Wilkins, 1984, pp. 361–373.
16. Legrand, C., and Anqissie, E.: Bacteremia due to *Achromobacter xylosoxidans* in patients with cancer. Clin. Infect. Dis. *14*:479–484, 1992.
17. Levesque, R., Royu, P. H., Letarte, R., et al.: A plasmid-mediated cephalosporinase from *Achromobacter* species. J. Infect. Dis. *145*:753–761, 1982.
18. Mandell, W. F., Garvey, G. J., and Neu, H. C.: *Achromobacter xylosoxidans* bacteremia. Rev. Infect. Dis. *9*:1001–1005, 1987.

19. Manjra, A. I., Moosa, A., and Bhamjee, A.: Fatal neonatal meningitis and ventriculitis caused by multi-resistant *Achromobacter xylosoxidans*: A case report. S. Afr. Med. J. *76*:571–573, 1989.
20. McGarrity, G. J., and Coriell, L. L.: Bacterial contamination of children's soap bubbles. Am. J. Dis. Child. *125*:224–226, 1973.
21. Olson, D. A., and Hoeprich, P. D.: Postoperative infection of an aortic prosthesis with *Achromobacter xylosoxidans*. West. J. Med. *136*:153–157, 1982.
22. Peel, M. M., Hibberd, A. J., King, B. M., et al.: *Alcaligenes piechaudii* from chronic ear discharge. J. Clin. Microbiol. *26*:1580–1581, 1988.
23. Reverdy, M. E., Freney, J., Fleurette, J., et al.: Nosocomial colonization and infection by *Achromobacter xylosoxidans*. J. Clin. Microbiol. *19*:140–143, 1984.
24. San-Miguel, V. V., Lavery, J. P., York, J. C., et al.: *Achromobacter xylosoxidans* septic arthritis in a patient with systemic lupus erythematosus. Arthritis Rheum. *34*:1484–1485, 1991.
25. Schoch, P. E., and Cunha, B. A.: Nosocomial *Achromobacter xylosoxidans* infections. Infect. Control Hosp. Epidemiol. *9*:84–87, 1988.
26. Sepkowitz, D. V., Bostic, D. E., and Maslow, M. J.: *Achromobacter xylosoxidans* meningitis: Case report and review of the literature. Clin. Pediatr. *26*:483–485, 1987.
27. Shigeta, S., Yasunaga, Y., Honsumi, K., et al.: Cerebral ventriculitis associated with *Achromobacter xylosoxidans*. J. Clin. Pathol. *70*:712–717, 1978.
28. Spear, J. B., Fuhrer, J., and Kirby, B. D.: *Achromobacter xylosoxidans* (*Alcaligenes xylosoxidans* subsp. *xylosoxidans*) bacteremia associated with well-water source: Case report and review of the literature. J. Clin. Microbiol. *26*:598–599, 1988.
29. Taylor, P., and Fischbein, L.: Prosthetic knee infection due to *Achromobacter xylosoxidans*. J. Rheumatol. *19*:992–993, 1992.
30. Walsh, R. D., Klein, N. C., and Cunha, B. A.: *Achromobacter xylosoxidans* osteomyelitis. Clin. Infect. Dis. *16*:176–178, 1993.

127

EIKENELLA CORRODENS

Randall G. Fisher and William C. Gruber

Eikenella corrodens is a facultatively anaerobic, fastidious gram-negative rod that is part of the normal flora of the mouth and gastrointestinal and genitourinary tracts. Long regarded as a commensal, its pathogenicity no longer is in doubt. It frequently is a pathogen of periodontitis in both adults and children and is a common isolate from wounds that have been contaminated by oral secretions. It also has been recovered from pleuropulmonary infections, central nervous system infections, orbital cellulitis, peritonsillar abscesses, abdominal infections, osteomyelitis, and blood stream infections, including endocarditis.

BACTERIOLOGY

In 1948, Hendriksen[16] described the organism and called it the corroding bacillus because it pitted the agar. It was characterized more fully in 1958 by Eiken,[10] who named it *Bacteroides corrodens*. In 1972, Jackson and Goodman[18] separated two species of corroding bacteria; the strict anaerobe kept the name *B. corrodens* (now called *B. urealyticus*), and the facultative anaerobe was classified as *Eikenella*. It is a small, straight, nonmotile gram-negative rod that occasionally is coccobacillary. It is oxidase-positive and catalase-negative. Most strains are lysine- and ornithine decarboxylase–positive. The organism is nonfermentative, reduces nitrate to nitrite, and is urease- and indole-negative. *E. corrodens* cell surface components vary from isolate to isolate; these differences probably relate to virulence.[6]

E. corrodens will grow either aerobically or anaerobically, but its growth is not rapid. Growth can be enhanced by 3 to 10 per cent carbon dioxide. It grows on blood or chocolate agar but poorly or not at all on MacConkey agar. Selective medium, which contains clindamycin, may increase yield. Colonies are small and grayish. They look slightly yellow when they are old. Although *E. corrodens* is nonhemolytic, there may be a faint green appearance on blood agar. About 50 per cent produce the characteristic pitting. They elaborate an odor that resembles that of bleach or hypochlorite.[17]

E. corrodens is a member of the so-called HACEK family of organisms, which have the following in common: (1) slow growth, (2) a requirement for carbon dioxide, and (3) a predilection for infecting heart valves. The other members of the family are *Haemophilus aphrophilus*, *Actinobacillus actinomycetemcomitans*, *Cardiobacterium hominis*, and *Kingella kingae*.

EPIDEMIOLOGY

Infection with *E. corrodens* occurs when mucosal or skin barriers are disrupted and the organism gains access to deeper tissues. Infection commonly occurs after clenched-fist injury as a result of fistfighting.[13] Intravenous drug abusers are at risk for injection site and soft tissue abscesses,[14] bacteremia, and endocarditis.[9, 26] The elderly and people with advanced carcinomas are the other high-risk groups. However, it now is recognized that children are at particularly high risk for serious *E. corrodens* infections.[31] Reports of thyroid abscesses[7, 39] and purulent thyroiditis[30] all have been in children. In one review,[21] more than 20 per cent of *E. corrodens* pleuropulmonary infections occurred in children younger than 14 years of age, and more than 50 per cent of abdominal infections were reported in patients younger than 25 years of age.[8] *E. corrodens* orbital cellulitis,[15] empyema,[36] peritonsillar abscess,[22] paronychia,[1] and osteomyelitis[28, 33] have been observed in children.

PATHOPHYSIOLOGY

E. corrodens infections often are polymicrobial[37] and may include other anaerobes or gram-negative rods. However, *E. corrodens* is accompanied most frequently by recovery of alpha-hemolytic streptococci. In most reports, the streptococci are not speciated further, but Jacobs and associates[19] made a case for the *Streptococcus anginosus* group because of similarities between the two organisms, i.e., both are found in the mouth and gastrointestinal tract, both produce local suppurative infection, and both thrive in carbon dioxide–rich, oxygen-poor environments. Brooks and colleagues[4] also reported synergy of the two organisms in a rabbit model of skin infection.

E. corrodens has a propensity toward abscess formation in any location, whether alone or in concert with other organisms. Abscess formation is a hallmark of central nervous system infection.[3] Of intra-abdominal infections reported by

Danziger and associates,[8] 15 of 19 had abscesses. In two cases of orbital cellulitis reported by Hemady and coworkers,[15] both had subperiosteal abscesses. Deep or superficial skin abscesses reported in drug addicts[14] or in clenched-fist injury from fistfighting[13] often recur, even after presumed adequate drainage.[29]

CLINICAL MANIFESTATIONS

Infections with *E. corrodens* are indolent. The time from inoculation to onset of symptoms generally is 1 week or longer.[4] Many cases show initial improvement with therapy but relapse days later, even with appropriate therapy.[15, 22, 27, 31]

Infection of periodontal sites may be associated with rapid progression and bone resorption thought to be secondary to surface-associated materials of *E. corrodens* and other organisms of periodontitis.[25] Craniofacial and neck infections tend to have prolonged morbidity; many require repeated drainage procedures and long courses of antimicrobial agents.[31] Central nervous system infections often are preceded by sinus infections but also have been seen in children with congenital heart disease.[2, 38]

Pleuropulmonary infections are marked by fever, cough, and chest pain. Necrotizing pneumonia with multiple abscesses sometimes is seen. Effusions or empyema are noted in 30 per cent, and cavitation is seen in 8 per cent. Children with a predisposition toward aspiration may be at higher risk.[21]

Endocarditis is associated with large, friable vegetations and frequent emboli and often requires valve replacement.[11] Intravenous drug use has been implicated in about half of reported cases.

Abdominal *E. corrodens* infections are seen most commonly as complications of ruptured appendicitis but also have been associated with abdominal trauma and surgery. The clinical course is protracted.[8]

Chorioamnionitis leading to premature delivery has been documented infrequently.[20, 35]

Soft tissue infections tend to be severe. Many require wide débridement and skin grafting. Infection of underlying joints, tendons, or bones is not infrequent and can be necrotizing and even lead to amputation.[29]

DIAGNOSIS

Definitive diagnosis rests upon recovery of *E. corrodens* in culture. This can be a difficult task, however, because of the organism's slow growth. *Eikenella* tends to be overgrown by heartier species when it is part of a polymicrobial process and may be missed, especially if it does not pit the agar. All of the HACEK organisms can pit agar,[5] although not with the regularity of *E. corrodens*.

Many bacteriology laboratories have difficulty identifying and separating catalase-negative, oxidase-positive, gram-negative rods. Not surprisingly, one report noted that of 100 isolates of *E. corrodens* identified by the National Collection of Type Cultures, only 21 were sent in as probable *E. corrodens*.[5] Organisms that *E. corrodens* may be mistaken for include the other HACEK organisms, *H. paraphrophilus*, *Moraxella atlantae*, and *Pasturella ureae*.

TREATMENT

E. corrodens has a very unusual antimicrobial susceptibility pattern, in that although most isolates are sensitive to penicillin and ampicillin, they are resistant to semisynthetic penicillins, such as methicillin and nafcillin.[34] Additionally, they uniformly are resistant to clindamycin and metronidazole,[17] drugs commonly used to treat anaerobic infections. They also variably are resistant to aminoglycosides.

Most isolates are sensitive to carbenicillin, second- and third-generation cephalosporins, and tetracycline. Although penicillin often is cited as the drug of choice, some strains produce β-lactamases. One report associates the β-lactamase with a transposon[23] and another with a plasmid[32]; one finds a chromosomal enzyme that is not inducible.[24] In addition, there are reports of intermediate resistance to penicillin, even in isolates that do not produce a β-lactamase.[12]

Incision and drainage of abscesses and débridement of necrotic tissue are essential to recovery from these infections. Therapy should be prolonged after patients apparently have recovered because early cessation of antibiotic therapy tends to be associated with relapse. If patients continue to have fever or other signs of infection days after appropriate therapy has been started, reimaging of the infected area may be prudent to detect early reaccumulation of purulence.

References

1. Barton, L. L., and Anderson, L. E.: Paronychia caused by HB-1 organisms. Pediatrics *54*:372–373, 1974.
2. Brill, C. B., Pearlstein, L. S., Kaplan, M., et al.: Central nervous system infections caused by *Eikenella corrodens*. Arch. Neurol. *39*:431–432, 1982.
3. Bronitsky, R., Heim, C. R., and McGee, Z. A.: Multifocal brain abscesses: Combined medical and neurosurgical therapy. South. Med. J. *75*:1261–1263, 1982.
4. Brooks, G. F., O'Donoghue, J. M., and Rissing, J. P.: *Eikenella corrodens*: A recently recognized pathogen: Infections in medical-surgical patients and in association with methyphenidate abuse. Medicine *53*:325 342, 1974.
5. Chadwick, P. R., Malnick, H., and Ebizie, A. O.: *Haemophilus paraphrophilus* infection: A pitfall in laboratory diagnosis. J. Infect. *30*:67–69, 1995.
6. Chen, C-K. C., and Wilson, M. E.: Outer membrane protein and lipopolysaccharide heterogeneity among *Eikenella corrodens* isolates. J. Infect. Dis. *162*:664–671, 1990.
7. Cheng, A. F., Man, D. W. K., and French, G. L.: Thyroid abscess caused by *Eikenella corrodens*. J. Infect. *16*:181–185, 1988.
8. Danziger, L. H., Schoonover, L. L., Kale, P., et al.: *Eikenella corrodens* as an intra-abdominal pathogen. Am. Surg. *60*:296–299, 1994.
9. Decker, M. D., Graham, B. S., Hunter, E. B., et al.: Endocarditis and infections of intravascular devices due to *Eikenella corrodens*. Am. J. Med. Sci. *292*:209–212, 1986.
10. Eiken, M.: Studies on an anaerobic, rod-shaped, gram-negative microorganism: *Bacteroides corrodens*. Acta Pathol. Microbiol. Scand. *43*:391–406, 1958.
11. Ellner, J. J., Rosenthal, M. S., Lerner, P. I., et al.: Infectious endocarditis caused by slow-growing, fastidious, gram negative bacteria. Medicine *58*:145–158, 1979.
12. Goldstein, E. J. C., and Citron, D. M.: Sensitivity of *Eikenella corrodens* to penicillin, apalcillin, and twelve new cephalosporins. Antimicrob. Agents Chemother. *26*:947–948, 1984.
13. Goldstein, E. J. C., Miller, T. A., Citron, D. M., et al.: Infections following clenched-fist injury: A new perspective. J. Hand Surg. *3*:455–457, 1978.
14. Gonzalez, M. H., Garst, J., Nourbush, P., et al.: Abscesses of the upper extremities from drug abuse by injection. J. Hand Surg. *18*:868–870, 1993.
15. Hemady, R., Zimmerman, A., Katzen, B. W., et al.: Orbital cellulitis caused by *Eikenella corrodens*. Am. J. Ophthalmol. *114*:584–588, 1992.
16. Hendriksen, S. D.: Studies in gram-negative anaerobes. II. Gram-negative anaerobic rods with spreading colonies. Acta Pathol. Microbiol. Scand. *25*:368–375, 1948.
17. Jackson, F. L., and Goodman, Y.: Genus *Eikenella*. *In* Krieg, N. R., and Holt, J. G. (eds.): Bergey's Manual of Systematic Bacteriology. Baltimore, Williams & Wilkins, 1984, pp. 591–597.
18. Jackson, F. L., and Goodman, Y. E.: Transfer of the facultatively anaerobic organism *Bacteroides corrodens Eiken* to a new genus, *Eikenella*. Int. J. Syst. Bacteriol. *22*:73–77, 1972.
19. Jacobs, J. A., Algie, G. D., Cie, G. H., et al.: Association between *Eikenella corrodens* and streptococci. Clin. Infect. Dis. *16*:173, 1993.
20. Jeppson, K. G., and Reimer, L. G.: *Eikenella corrodens* amnionitis. Obstet. Gynecol. *78*:503–505, 1991.
21. Joshi, N., O'Bryan, T., and Appelbaum, P. C.: Pleuropulmonary infections caused by *Eikenella corrodens*. Rev. Infect. Dis. *13*:1207–1212, 1991.
22. Knudsen, T. D., and Simke, E. J.: *Eikenella corrodens*: An unexpected pathogen causing a persistent peritonsillar abscess. Ear Nose Throat J. *74*:114–117, 1995.

23. Lacroix, J.-M., and Walker, C. B.: Identification of a streptomycin resistance gene and a partial Tn3 transposon coding for a beta-lactamase in a periodontal strain of *Eikenella corrodens*. Antimicrob. Agents Chemother. *36*:740–743, 1992.
24. Lacroix, J.-M., and Wallar, C.: Characteristics of a beta-lactamase found in *Eikenella corrodens*. Antimicrob. Agents Chemother. *35*:886–891, 1991.
25. Meghji, S., Wilson, M., Barber, P., et al.: Bone resorbing activity of surface-associated material from *Actinobacillus actinomycetemcomitans* and *Eikenella corrodens*. J. Med. Microbiol. *41*:197–203, 1994.
26. Patrick, W. D., Brown, W. D., Bowmer, M. I., et al.: Infectious endocarditis due to *Eikenella corrodens*: Case report and review of the literature. Can. J. Infect. Dis. *1*:139–142, 1990.
27. Perez-Pomata, M. T., Dominguez, J., Hercajo, P., et al.: Spleen abscess caused by *Eikenella corrodens*. Eur. J. Clin. Microbiol. Infect. Dis. *11*:162–163, 1992.
28. Polin, K., and Shulman, S. T.: *Eikenella corrodens* osteomyelitis. Pediatrics *70*:462–463, 1982.
29. Pollner, J. H., Khan, A., and Tuazon, C. U.: Severe soft tissue infection caused by *Eikenella corrodens*. Clin. Infect. Dis. *15*:740–741, 1992.
30. Queen, J. S., Clegg, H. W., Council, J. C., et al.: Acute suppurative thyroiditis caused by *Eikenella corrodens*. J. Pediatr. Surg. *23*:359–361, 1988.
31. Raffensperger, J. G.: *Eikenella corrodens* infections in children. J. Pediatr. Surg. *21*:644–646, 1986.
32. Rotger, R. E., Garcia-Valdes, E., and Trallero, E. P.: Characterization of a beta-lactamase–specifying plasmid isolated from *Eikenella corrodens* and its relationship to a commensal *Neisseria* plasmid. Antimicrob. Agents Chemother. *30*:508–509, 1986.
33. Sagerman, S. D., and Lourie, G. M.: *Eikenella* osteomyelitis in a chronic nail biter: A case report. J. Hand Surg. *20*:71–72, 1995.
34. Sofianou, D., and Kolokotronis, A.: Susceptibility of *Eikenella corrodens* to antimicrobial agents. J. Chemother. 2:156–158, 1990.
35. Sporken, J. M. J., Muyfjens, H. L., and Vemer, H. M.: Intrauterine infection due to *Eikenella corrodens*. Acta Obstet. Gynecol. Scand. *64*:683–684, 1985.
36. St. John, A., Belda, A. A., Matlow, A., et al.: *Eikenella corrodens* empyema in children. Am. J. Dis. Child. *135*:415–417, 1981.
37. Suwanagool, S., Rothkopf, M. M., Smith, S. M., et al.: Pathogenicity of *Eikenella corrodens* in humans. Arch. Intern. Med. *143*:2265–2268, 1983.
38. Swanston, W. H., Cameron, E. S., and Ramchaunder, V.: *Eikenella corrodens* brain abscess in a child with congenital heart disease. W. Indian Med. J. *37*:243–245, 1988.
39. Vichyanond, P., Howard, C. P., and Olson, L. C. *Eikenella corrodens* as a cause of thyroid abscess. Am. J. Dis. Child. *137*:971–973, 1983.

128

FLAVOBACTERIUM

William C. Gruber and Randall G. Fisher

Members of the genus *Flavobacterium* uncommonly are associated with human infection, with most disease occurring after exposure to a contaminated environmental source. In 1944, Shulmann and Johnson[36] reported a case of meningitis due to a previously unidentified, gram-negative bacillus isolated from a 9-day-old premature infant. The term "*Flavobacterium meningosepticum*" was proposed for this organism by King[23] in 1959, based on her studies of bacterial isolates primarily associated with neonatal meningitis and septicemia. Although neonatal meningitis is the most common manifestation of human disease due to this genus,[12, 41] flavobacteria-associated sepsis,[11, 18, 31, 38] endocarditis,[43] pneumonia,[40] and skin infection[16] occur in individuals beyond the newborn period.[3]

BACTERIOLOGY

Taxonomic classification of *Flavobacterium* is considered to be uncertain, with seven species assigned to the genus, according to *Bergey's Manual of Systematic Bacteriology*.[22] These organisms are long, thin, catalase-positive, gram-negative rods with slightly swollen ends; they are nonmotile, oxidase-positive, weakly fermentative, proteolytic, and grow on solid agar as 1-mm, yellow-pigmented, convex, glistening colonies of buttery consistency.[23] Colonies do not demonstrate hemolysis on blood agar but may produce a lavender-green color in the surrounding media as a result of extensive proteolytic enzyme activity. *Flavobacterium* is unable to grow on *Salmonella-Shigella* agar or Simmons citrate and lacks motility. These characteristics distinguish *Flavobacterium* from *Pseudomonas*, with which it often is confused.[12] Similarly, utilization of glucose in an open tube of oxidation-fermentation media distinguishes *Flavobacterium* from *Alcaligenes faecalis*.[12] The clinically relevant species *F. meningosepticum* and *Flavobacterium IIB* (renamed *F. balustinum*) are differentiated by the former's consistent liquefaction of gelatin and early utilization of mannitol and maltose and the latter's lack of these abilities.[23] *F. odoratum*, which has been identified most commonly as a saphrophyte in skin wounds,[21] characteristically is nonsaccharolytic and produces a fruity odor when grown on standard media.

EPIDEMIOLOGY

Flavobacteria are distributed widely as saprophytes in fresh and salt water. *F. meningosepticum* has been identified as a pathogen in birds.[42] In hospitals, flavobacteria have been found to be ubiquitous colonizers of the patient's environment and have been isolated from flower vases,[40] ice machines,[38] vials of intravenous drugs,[31] and nebulizers.[13] In addition, tap water,[13] eyewashes,[32] tube feedings,[13] sink traps,[7] and hand cultures of hospital personnel[13] have yielded this organism. In some instances, these reservoirs of flavobacteria have been implicated in nosocomial outbreaks of patient colonization and invasive disease.

Neonatal infection due to *F. meningosepticum* has been reported frequently in the literature, often in association with nursery epidemics.[2, 6, 34] As with other neonatal pathogens, infants who are premature and small for gestational age seem to be at particular risk. Greater than 50 per cent of infected infants weigh less than 2500 g. Almost all cases occur within 3 weeks of birth, with greater than 50 per cent manifesting illness prior to 7 days of age.[12]

Nosocomial epidemics have occurred sporadically since the nursery outbreak reported by Brody and colleagues in 1958.[2, 4, 6, 7] Cabrera and Davis[7] reported such an outbreak in detail in 1960. Over a 3-month period, the bacteria were isolated from a total of 44 infants, of whom 14 had overt infection. Most colonized infants had organisms isolated from the nasopharynx. The only reservoir of infectious bacteria discovered was a faulty sink trap, beneath which cleaning materials for the nursery were stored. Repair of the defective trap and thorough cleansing and repainting of the nursery coincided with termination of the epidemic.

F. meningosepticum nursery outbreaks have been traced to saline used to flush infants' eyes after silver nitrate administration,[32] and organisms have been recovered from washbasins, sinks, disinfectants, and suction devices in other epidemics.[7] Colonization of patients in a surgical intensive care unit has been associated with tap water, sinks, ice machines, and washbasins yielding the bacteria.[13] Ribotyping offers promise for more precise characterization of epidemics.[10]

PATHOPHYSIOLOGY

Flavobacteria generally are of low virulence. Rabbits administered 1-mL intravenous injections of 24-hour-old broth cultures demonstrated no mortality or morbidity; death rates were less than 30 per cent in mice inoculated intracerebrally with "barely turbid" preparations.[23]

Most cases of invasive human disease are believed to be due to environmental contamination with high numbers of *F. meningosepticum*, with spread to the compromised newborn or debilitated older patient. Some neonatal infections may be due to colonization of the infant during passage through the birth canal of a colonized mother.[10] Intrapartum infection is supported by occurrence of symptoms as early as 10 hours after birth.[12] However, only 0.3 per cent of genital swabs submitted from patients with suspected venereal disease yielded the organism.[30] It has been speculated that continuing reports of flavobacteria as a cause of neonatal infection in underdeveloped countries may be related to use of contaminated groundwater for bathing of newborn infants and feminine genital hygiene.[17] The propensity for this organism to produce meningitis in the newborn is not understood, but infection may occur in association with heavy nasopharyngeal colonization, leading to subsequent bacteremia and seeding of the meninges.

In older individuals, flavobacteria primarily play the role of opportunists.[28] Heavy nosocomial colonization combined with a blunted immune response probably accounts for the immunocompromised patient's poor capacity to handle this otherwise noninvasive bacteria.

CLINICAL MANIFESTATIONS

Neonatal sepsis and meningitis due to *F. meningosepticum* share signs and symptoms in common with other forms of neonatal bacterial infection. However, development of meningitis may be insidious, and several days of illness often pass prior to its presentation[12, 34]; this is consistent with the low virulence of *F. meningosepticum* in comparison with other agents of neonatal sepsis. Prognosis is extremely poor, and mortality rates may exceed 60 per cent.[26] Fifty per cent of survivors develop significant neurologic complications, often in association with hydrocephalus.[24]

Flavobacteria are uncommon pathogens in adults, and childhood disease beyond the newborn period is extremely rare. Among the 24 initial isolates of *F. meningosepticum* identified by King,[23] organisms were identified in a throat culture from an adult patient and in cerebrospinal fluid from an 8-month-old infant. Bacteria classified as *Flavobacterium IIB (F. balustinum)* were isolated from the blood and cerebrospinal fluid of several adult patients without clinical information.[22] Since their initial identification in 1959, flavobacteria have been implicated as agents of meningitis,[28, 34] postoperative bacteremia,[3, 30] bacterial endocarditis,[43] pneumonia,[39, 40] and skin infection.[16] *F. meningosepticum* is the species most commonly isolated, but *F. odoratum, Flavobacterium IIB (F. balustinum)*, and other *Flavobacterium* species have been implicated in human disease.

F. meningosepticum meningitis beyond the neonatal period typically occurs in immunocompromised patients. Adults with preexisting leukemia,[34] glomerulonephritis,[28] and squamous cell carcinoma[18] have been described as having meningitis due to this organism. In a 56-year-old woman, meningitis with *F. meningosepticum* developed after transsphenoidal hypophysectomy[8]; in an 8-month-old male with preceding severe neurologic damage, meningitis developed with bacteria designated by the Centers for Disease Control and Prevention as *Flavobacterium*-like organisms (IIE). In a 6-week-old infant, *F. meningosepticum* bacteremia and meningitis developed in association with a strangulated hernia.[11]

Flavobacterium species were isolated commonly from tracheal aspirates of intensive care patients during a 70-month observation period; yet during that time, none of more than 2000 critically ill individuals developed pneumonia attributable to these microbes.[12] However, *Flavobacterium* respiratory tract infection has been identified in an intubated pediatric patient and in adults receiving aerosolized medications.[5, 40]

Sporadic cases of bacteremia have been reported in adult patients.[18, 25] Infection in immunocompromised patients can occur as a complication of relatively benign invasive procedures or as a localized infection.[25, 37] Endocarditis has been documented in intravenous drug abusers and dialysis patients.[15, 43] Postoperative bacteremia in eight adult patients has been linked to flavobacteria-contaminated intravenous medications infused during anesthesia.[31] Contaminated arterial catheters were implicated in an epidemic of *Flavobacterium* bacteremia.[38] Four patients, including a 7-year-old boy, became bacteremic in an outbreak associated with *Flavobacterium* contamination at the time of intracardiac surgery.[3] This organism also has been associated with bacteremia in pediatric burn patients.[35]

Flavobacterium species have been isolated from infected skin lesions presenting as papules, sheet-like lesions, plaques, and deep panniculitis.[16] Infection may have been related to wound contamination during repair of an orthopedic injury. Flavobacteria have been isolated from amputation stumps but may have been playing a largely saprophytic role at these sites.[21]

DIAGNOSIS

Rapid identification of *Flavobacterium* infection is urgent, not only to ensure proper therapy for the patient, but also to hasten appropriate infection control to forestall epidemic outbreaks. Identification of *F. meningosepticum* is hindered by characteristically long periods required for oxidation of carbohydrates and weak or delayed indole production. Cultures may be misidentified as species of *Alcaligenes* or *Pseudomonas*.[12] Clinical isolation of an unidentified gram-negative rod that is catalase- and oxidase-positive and that shows multiple antibiotic resistance should raise suspicion of *F. meningosepticum* infection. Cultures should be kept for several days for observation for typical carbohydrate reactions, which confirm the diagnosis.[12, 33]

TREATMENT

Unfortunately, treatment of *F. meningosepticum* meningitis represents an especially difficult challenge for the physician. Delay in specific identification of the organism is common. This often leads to prolonged periods of suboptimal therapy because recommended empiric antimicrobial treatment of gram-negative neonatal meningitis usually consists of ampicillin and an aminoglycoside, two drugs to which *F. meningo-*

septicum almost uniformly is resistant. Moreover, antimicrobial susceptibilities determined by disk diffusion must be interpreted with caution. Aber and associates[1] found clinical isolates in which specific strains were sensitive to gentamicin and rifampin by disk diffusion but were resistant by agar gel dilution susceptibility testing. Therefore, more direct methods of measuring the minimal inhibitory concentration than disk diffusion sensitivity should be used to determine the optimal microbial agents for therapy.

No doubt as a consequence of difficulties encountered in providing rapid and effective antibacterial therapy, persistence of organisms for prolonged periods in cerebrospinal fluid is common. Average persistence of *Flavobacterium* in cerebrospinal fluid is 19 days,[12] which can be compared with the 3.9 days described by McCracken[29] for most cases of gram-negative neonatal bacterial meningitis.

Drugs that have been used alone or in combination with some success have included erythromycin, vancomycin, trimethoprim-sulfamethoxazole, and rifampin. Some of these agents have the potential disadvantage of poor cerebrospinal fluid penetration. Combined use of many of these drugs makes interpretation of therapeutic response difficult. The 3 survivors in the 12 patients reported by George and associates[17] all received vancomycin intravenously, intrathecally, or both as a part of their regimen. Hawley and Gump[19] reported a case of *F. meningosepticum* meningitis in a neonate who responded to systemic vancomycin after unsuccessful treatment with multiple antibiotics, including erythromycin.

Intraventricular erythromycin[14, 34] or rifampin[9, 24, 26, 34] has been used in conjunction with systemic administration of these drugs. In particular, Lee and associates[24] reported no deaths in seven infants with *F. meningosepticum* meningitis treated with intraventricular rifampin through an Ommaya reservoir at a dose of 2 to 5 mg every 24 hours combined with 40 mg/kg/day administered intravenously. Intraventricular administration continued until the cerebrospinal fluid was sterile. However, colonization of the Ommaya reservoir was common, and formation of a porencephalic cyst occurred in one patient. Chandrika and Adler[9] reported sterilization of ventricles in one afflicted neonate within 48 hours after institution of therapy with intraventricular and intravenous rifampin. Erythromycin has been used intraventricularly with limited success at 5 to 10 mg/day.[14, 34] Rios and associates[34] reported the successful addition of intraventricular rifampin to a failing regimen of intravenous and intraventricular erythromycin. Development of resistance while undergoing therapy has been demonstrated with erythromycin and rifampin[14, 34]; persistence of cerebrospinal fluid organisms despite presumably adequate therapy should alert the physician to test for this possibility. Addition of trimethoprim-sulfamethoxozole may be of benefit with such an occurrence; this agent effected a bacteriologic cure in eight of nine infants with meningitis.[27] This agent usually is not recommended in the neonatal period because of possible displacement of bilirubin from albumin-binding sites. Bacterial eradication was achieved in 48 hours in two meningitis patients treated with clindamycin, rifampin, and cefotaxime systemically and rifampin intraventricularly.[6]

As with other types of gram-negative meningitis, antimicrobial therapy should be continued for at least 2 weeks after sterilization of ventricular fluid. Complications of hydrocephalus and the potential use of intraventricular therapy make the neurosurgeon an essential part of the management team. Historically, mortality has been in excess of 70 per cent, no doubt in part because of delays in identifying the organism and the limited antibiotic spectrum available for effective therapy. More recent series of patients, although small, suggest some improvement in this statistic, but the morbidity of hydrocephalus and neurologic deficits remains high.

Recovery has been the rule in immunocompetent older individuals infected with contaminated materials, often despite treatment with antibiotics to which *Flavobacterium* is insensitive.[31] However, significant mortality and morbidity often occur in immunocompromised individuals with bacteremia or meningitis. Use of chloramphenicol, vancomycin, ciprofloxacin, erythromycin, or rifampin has shown some success in these individuals, but the antibiotic choice should be based on a detailed examination of the organism's susceptibility.[20, 35]

References

1. Aber, R. C., Wennersten, C., and Moellering, R. C., Jr.: Antimicrobial susceptibility of flavobacteria. Antimicrob. Agents Chemother. *14*:483–487, 1978.
2. Abrahamsen, T. G., Finne, P. H., and Lingaas, E.: *Flavobacterium meningosepticum* infections in a neonatal intensive care unit. Acta Paediatr. Scand. *78*:51–55, 1989.
3. Berry, W. B., Morrow, A. G., Harrison, D. C., et al.: *Flavobacterium* septicemia following intracardiac operations. J. Thorac. Cardiovasc. Surg. *45*:476–481, 1963.
4. Brody, J. A., Moore, H., and King, E. O.: Meningitis caused by an unclassified gram-negative bacterium in newborn infants. Am. J. Dis. Child. *96*:1–5, 1958.
5. Brown, R. B., Phillips, D., Barker, M. J., et al.: Outbreak of nosocomial *Flavobacterium meningosepticum* respiratory infections associated with use of aerosolized polymyxin B. Am. J. Infect. Control *17*:121–125, 1989.
6. Bruun, B., Jensen, E. T., Lundstrom, K., et al.: *Flavobacterium meningosepticum* infection in a neonatal ward. Eur. J. Clin. Microbiol. Infect. Dis. *8*:509–514, 1989.
7. Cabrera, H. A., and Davis, G. H.: Epidemic meningitis of the newborn caused by flavobacteria. I. Epidemiology and bacteriology. Am. J. Dis. Child. *101*:289–295, 1961.
8. Chan, K. H., Chau, P. Y., Wang, R. Y. C., et al.: Meningitis caused by *Flavobacterium meningosepticum* after transsphenoidal hypophysectomy with recovery. Surg. Neurol. *20*:294–296, 1983.
9. Chandrika, T., and Adler, S. P.: A case of neonatal meningitis due to *Flavobacterium meningosepticum* successfully treated with rifampin. Pediatr. Infect. Dis. *1*:40–41, 1982.
10. Colding, H., Bangsborg, J., Fiehn, N. E., et al.: Ribotyping for differentiating *Flavobacterium meningosepticum* isolates from clinical and environmental sources. J. Clin. Microbiol. *32*:501–505, 1994.
11. Coyle-Gilchrist, M. M., Crew, P., and Roberts, G.: *Flavobacterium meningosepticum* in the hospital environment. J. Clin. Pathol. *29*:824–826, 1976.
12. Dooley, J. R., Nims, L. J., Lipp, V. H., et al.: Meningitis of infants caused by *Flavobacterium meningosepticum*. J. Trop. Pediatr. *26*:24–30, 1980.
13. du Moulin, G. C.: Airway colonization by *Flavobacterium* in an intensive care unit. J. Clin. Microbiol. *10*:155–160, 1979.
14. Ferlauto, J. J., and Wells, D. H.: *Flavobacterium meningosepticum* in the neonatal period. South. Med. J. *74*:757–759, 1981.
15. Ferrer, C., Jakob, E., Pastorino, G., et al.: Right-sided bacterial endocarditis due to *Flavobacterium odoratum* in a patient on chronic hemodialysis. Am. J. Nephrol. *15*:82–84, 1995.
16. Findlay, G. H., Hull, P. R., Smith, H. E., et al.: Cutaneous flavobacteriosis: Polymorphous skin granulomas from *Flavobacterium capsulatam*. S. Afr. Med. J. *64*:247–250, 1983.
17. George, R. M., Cochran, C. P., and Wheeler, W. E.: Epidemic meningitis of the newborn caused by flavobacteria. II. Clinical manifestations and treatment. Am. J. Dis. Child. *101*:296–304, 1961.
18. Harrington, S. P., and Perlino, C. A.: *Flavobacterium meningosepticum* sepsis: Disease due to bacteria with unusual antibiotic susceptibility. South. Med. J. *74*:764–766, 1981.
19. Hawley, H. B., and Gump, D. W.: Vancomycin therapy of bacterial meningitis. Am. J. Dis. Child. *126*:261–264, 1973.
20. Hirsh, B. E., Wong, B., Kiehn, T. E., et al.: *Flavobacterium meningosepticum* bacteremia in an adult with acute leukemia: Use of rifampin to clear persistent infection. Diagn. Microbiol. Infect. Dis. *4*:65–69, 1986.
21. Holmes, B., Snell, J. J. S., and Lapage, S. P.: *Flavobacterium odoratum*: A species resistant to a wide range of antimicrobial agents. J. Clin. Pathol. *32*:73–77, 1979.
22. Holmes, B., Owen, R. J., and McMeekin, T. A.: Genus *Flavobacterium*. *In* Krieg, N. R., and Holt, J. G. (eds.): Bergey's Manual of Systematic Bacteriology. Vol. 1. Baltimore, Williams & Wilkins, 1984, pp. 353–360.
23. King, E. O.: Studies on a group of previously unclassified bacteria associated with meningitis in infants. Am. J. Clin. Pathol. *31*:241–247, 1959.
24. Lee, E. L., Robinson, M. J., Thong, M. L., et al.: Intraventricular chemotherapy in neonatal meningitis. J. Pediatr. *91*:991–995, 1977.

25. Lee, M., and Munoz, J.: Septicemia occurring after colonoscopic polypectomy in a splenectomized patient taking corticosteroids. Am. J. Gastroenterol. *89*:2245–2246, 1994.
26. Lee, E. L., Robinson, M. J., Thong, M. L., et al.: Rifamycin in neonatal flavobacteria meningitis. Arch. Dis. Child. *51*:209–213, 1976.
27. Linder, N., Korman, S. H., Eyal, F., et al.: Trimethoprim-sulphamethoxazole in neonatal *Flavobacterium meningosepticum* infection. Arch. Dis. Child. *59*:582–584, 1984.
28. Mani, R. M., Kuruvila, K. C., Batliwala, P. M., et al.: *Flavobacterium meningosepticum* as an opportunist. J. Clin. Pathol. *31*:220–222, 1978.
29. McCracken, G. H., Jr.: New developments in the management of children with bacterial meningitis. Pediatr. Infect. Dis. *3*:S32–S34, 1984.
30. Olsen, H., and Raun, T.: *Flavobacterium meningosepticum* isolated from the genitals. Acta Pathol. Microbiol. Immunol. Scand. *79*:102–106, 1971.
31. Olsen, H., Frederiksen, W. C., and Siboni, K. E.: *Flavobacterium meningosepticum* in 8 non-fatal cases of postoperative bacteraemia. Lancet *1*:1294–1296, 1965.
32. Plotkin, S. A., and McKitrick, J. C.: Nosocomial meningitis of the newborn caused by *Flavobacterium*. J. A. M. A. *198*:662–664, 1966.
33. Ratner, H.: *Flavobacterium meningosepticum*. Infect. Control *5*:237–239, 1984.
34. Rios, I., Klimek, J. J., Maderazo, E., et al.: *Flavobacterium meningosepticum* meningitis: Report of selected aspects. Antimicrob. Agents Chemother. *14*:444–447, 1978.
35. Sheridan, R. L., Ryan, C. M., Pasternack, M. S., et al.: Flavobacterial sepsis in massively burned pediatric patients. Clin. Infect. Dis. *17*:185–187, 1993.
36. Shulmann, B. H., and Johnson, M. S.: A case of meningitis in a premature infant due to a proteolytic gram-negative bacillus. J. Lab. Clin. Med. *29*:500–507, 1944.
37. Skapek, S. X., Jones, W. S., Hoffman, K. M., et al.: Sinusitis and bacteremia caused by *Flavobacterium meningosepticum* in a sixteen-year-old with Shwachman Diamond syndrome. Pediatr. Infect. Dis. *11*:411–413, 1992.
38. Stamm, W. F., Colella, J. J., Anderson, R. L., et al.: Indwelling arterial catheters as a source of nosocomial bacteremia. N. Engl. J. Med. *292*:1099–1102, 1975.
39. Sundin, D., Gold, B. D., Berkowitz, F. E., et al.: Community-acquired *Flavobacterium meningosepticum* meningitis, pneumonia and septicemia in a normal infant. Pediatr. Infect. Dis. *10*:73–76, 1991.
40. Teres, D.: ICU-acquired pneumonia due to *Flavobacterium meningosepticum*. J. A. M. A. *228*:732, 1974.
41. Thong, W. L., Puthucheary, S. D., and Lee, E. L.: *Flavobacterium meningosepticum* infection: An epidemiological study in a newborn nursery. J. Clin. Pathol. *34*:429–433, 1981.
42. Vancanneyt, M., Segers, P., Hauben, L., et al.: *Flavobacterium meningosepticum*, a pathogen in birds. J. Clin. Microbiol. *32*:2398–2403, 1994.
43. Werthamer, S., and Weiner, M.: Subacute bacterial endocarditis due to *Flavobacterium meningosepticum*. Am. J. Clin. Pathol. *57*:410–412, 1972.
44. Wientzen, R. L., McCracken, G. H., Jr., Petruska, M. L., et al.: Localization and therapy of urinary tract infections of childhood. Pediatrics *63*:467–473, 1979.

129

PSEUDOMONAS AND RELATED SPECIES

Michael T. Brady and Ralph D. Feigin

Pseudomonas and related species are aerobic, motile, non-spore-forming, nonfermentative, gram-negative bacilli that live in soil, in water, and on plants and animals. Most organisms of these genera are ubiquitous and rarely pathogenic in humans. Although the pseudomonads may produce disease in any individual, they usually are opportunists that more commonly cause disease in patients with burns, cystic fibrosis, malignancies, and immunodeficiency conditions; in recipients of immunosuppressive therapy; or in malnourished persons. The most important of the opportunistic pseudomonads is *Pseudomonas aeruginosa*. However, a number of the other pseudomonads cause specific clinical syndromes in children. Some species formerly classified in the genus *Pseudomonas* were reclassified taxonomically. Table 129–1 provides changes in taxonomy for some of the more clinically important pseudomonads.[48]

ETIOLOGY

Pseudomonas species usually are obligate aerobes, but they can grow anaerobically in the presence of nitrates. They lack the phosphoenolpyruvate-hexose-phosphotransferase system and catabolize carbohydrates by the Entner-Doudoroff pathway. Because pseudomonads can utilize a wide variety of carbon sources, they can survive and multiply in almost any moist environment containing minimal amounts of organic compounds.

P. aeruginosa is the most clinically important species of the genus *Pseudomonas*. It is an oxidase-positive, gram-negative rod varying in size from 0.5 to 0.8 μm × 1.5 to 3.0 μm. Most strains are motile by polar, monotrichous flagella and display fine projections (pili or fimbriae). *P. aeruginosa* grows readily on standard laboratory media. It grows optimally at 37° C but not at 4° C. It does not ferment carbohydrates but does oxidize sugars, such as glucose and xylose, but not maltose. Strains from clinical specimens may produce beta-hemolysis on blood agar. More than 90 per cent of *P. aeruginosa* organisms produce a bluish-green phenazine pigment (pyocyanin-blue pus) as well as fluorescein, a yellow-green fluorescent pigment. These pigments diffuse into and color the medium surrounding the colonies. Strains of *P. aeruginosa* can be differentiated from one another for epidemiologic purposes by serologic typing, phage typing, ribotyping, and pyocin (bacteriocin) typing.

EPIDEMIOLOGY

P. aeruginosa is a ubiquitous environmental organism found in soil, in water, and on vegetation, including the surface

TABLE 129–1. Recent Taxonomic Changes in the Genus *Pseudomonas*

Previous Designation	Current Designation
Pseudomonas cepacia	*Burkholdeia cepacia*
Pseudomonas gladioli	*Burkholderia gladioli*
Pseudomonas mallei	*Burkholderia mallei*
Pseudomonas picketti	*Burkholderia picketti*
Pseudomonas pseudomallei	*Burkholderia pseudomallei*
Pseudomonas oryzihabitans	*Flavimonas oryzihabitans*
Pseudomonas acidovorans	*Commomonas acidovorans*
Pseudomonas testosteroni	*Commomonas testosteroni*
Pseudomonas putrefaciens	*Shewanella putrefaciens*
Pseudomonas paucimobilis	*Sphingomonas paucimobilis*
Pseudomonas maltophila (*Xanthomonas maltophilia*)	*Stenotrophomonas maltophilia*

Data from Gilligan, P. H.: *Pseudomonas* and *Burkholderia*. *In* Murray, P. R., Baron, E. J., Pfaller, M. A., et al. (eds.): Manual of Clinical Microbiology. 6th ed. Washington, D.C., ASM Press, 1995, pp. 509–519.

of many raw fruits and vegetables. Its minimal nutritional requirements and ability to grow in a wide variety of physical environments enhance the organism's ability to survive in a number of ecologic niches. *P. aeruginosa* usually is not found as normal microflora of healthy humans. As many as 5 to 30 per cent of normal persons have *P. aeruginosa* in their gastrointestinal tract, although rarely as the predominant organism. The large intestine is the most frequent site of transient colonization after ingestion. *P. aeruginosa* frequently enters the hospital environment on the clothes, skin, respiratory tract, or shoes of patients or hospital personnel; colonization of any moist environment ensues. Thus, these organisms may be found growing in distilled water, hospital kitchens and laundries, mops, showerheads, whirlpools, antiseptic solutions, eye drops, irrigation fluids, dialysis fluids, and equipment used for dialysis and respiratory care or inhalation therapy. Transmission of *P. aeruginosa* from patient to patient or from hospital personnel to patient often is assumed but rarely documented.[33, 141] In hospitalized patients, the likelihood of *Pseudomonas* colonization increases with the duration of the hospitalization. Sources of *Pseudomonas* outside of the hospital that may result in colonization with subsequent infection include swimming pools, waterslides, hot tubs, contact lens solutions, cosmetics, illicit injectable drugs, and the inner soles of sneakers.

The environmental distribution of many of the other pseudomonads is similar to that of *P. aeruginosa*. *Burkholderia cepacia* is a multiresistant, gram-negative bacterium that has been identified as a cause of sporadic nosocomial outbreaks of infection in medical intensive care units. Outbreaks have been traced to contamination of automated peritoneal dialysis machines, contaminated blood gas analyzers, contaminated povidone-iodine, and contaminated chlorhexidine.[13, 14, 52, 127] Colonization of the respiratory tract, sometimes associated with endobronchial infection in patients with cystic fibrosis, is becoming more common and is associated with increased morbidity and mortality. This organism also has become a more important agent for infections in patients with chronic granulomatous disease.

Stenotrophomonas maltophilia (formerly *Xanthomas maltophilia*) is being isolated with increasing frequency in hospitalized patients. Colonization of nonsterile sites, such as the respiratory tract and wounds in the absence of clinical disease, is common in hospitalized patients receiving long-term or broad-spectrum antibiotics. However, clinical illnesses such as pneumonia, urinary tract infections, endocarditis, bacteremia, meningitis, and peritonitis have been reported.[9, 36, 42, 84, 136] Isolation of *S. maltophilia* from the respiratory tract of patients with cystic fibrosis is increasing; in some centers, it is the second most frequent gram-negative bacterium isolated from sputum.[7, 67]

Burkholderia pseudomallei is most prevalent in tropical and subtropical areas of Southeast Asia and northern Australia. *B. pseudomallei* has been recovered frequently from rice paddy surface water in rice-growing areas of northern Thailand.[30, 128]

PATHOGENESIS[10, 76]

The requirement of oxygen for growth may account for the lack of invasiveness of these organisms after they have colonized and even infected the skin. *P. aeruginosa* possesses a variety of virulence factors, including an endotoxin, an enterotoxin, and a number of extracellular enzymes. *P. aeruginosa* endotoxin is not as potent as endotoxins produced by other gram-negative organisms (2 to 3 mg is needed to kill a 20-g mouse). This endotoxin may produce a diarrheal syndrome. A *Pseudomonas* enterotoxin also has been described, but its role in causing diarrhea in humans remains unclear.

The extracellular enzymes of *P. aeruginosa* include lecithinase, collagenase, lipase, elastase, caseinase, gelatinase, fibrinolysin, hemolysin, phospholipase C, and exotoxin A. The proteolytic enzymes may be responsible for localized necrosis of skin or lung and for corneal ulceration. Exotoxin A is an adenosine 5′-diphosphate-ribosyltransferase enzyme that inhibits eukaryotic cell protein synthesis. Specific exotoxin A–deficient mutants of *P. aeruginosa* have a reduced virulence for producing infection of the cornea or lung in mice or rats.[90, 143] Passive or active immunization against exotoxin A significantly protects against experimental infection with exotoxin-producing strains of *P. aeruginosa*. Phospholipase C degrades phospholipids, which are plentiful in eukaryotic but not prokaryotic cell membranes. Hemolysis due to *P. aeruginosa* may be caused by heat-labile phospholipase C and by a heat-stable moiety.

The various proteases also can degrade numerous plasma proteins, such as complement and coagulation factors.[144] Solubilization and destruction of lecithin (surfactant) may play a role in the atelectasis seen in pulmonary infections caused by *P. aeruginosa*. A leukocidin also has been described that may, in part, be capsular material. Exotoxin S has been identified and is suggested as still another virulence factor. The purified slime from *Pseudomonas* is nontoxic. Pigments produced by *P. aeruginosa* also are nontoxic.

Surface structures, such as the pili or fimbriae, are involved in attachment of *P. aeruginosa* to mucosal surfaces. *P. aeruginosa* binds preferentially to normal respiratory mucin, in contrast with some members of the family Enterobacteriaceae.[137] The glycocalyx (extracellular slime layer) is important in allowing *P. aeruginosa* organisms to adhere to each other and form microcolonies. The microcolonies impair phagocytosis and antibody and antibiotic activity.

The pathogenicity of *P. aeruginosa* also depends on its ability to resist phagocytosis. Fick and Reynolds[41] noted that, in patients with cystic fibrosis, the opsonic function of IgG was reduced as a result of a molecular change in the Fc portion of the IgG molecule. This deficit was magnified in the lung of the patient with cystic fibrosis infected with *P. aeruginosa* because bacterial proteases can fragment IgG and further impair its opsonic activity, which already may be marginal. Persistence of *P. aeruginosa* in the lungs of patients with cystic fibrosis also may be related to the presence of one or more factors in their sputum that interfere with the bactericidal activity of fresh normal human serum against *P. aeruginosa*. These blocking factors have been shown to be IgG antibody that blocks the normal bactericidal IgM activity of human sera.[96, 118]

The concentrations of IgG subclass immunoglobulins have been studied in patients with cystic fibrosis and compared with values obtained in age-matched healthy children and adults. Pressler and associates[100] noted that, in 52 per cent of patients with cystic fibrosis, at least one of the four IgG subclasses had an elevated serum concentration compared with controls. There was a significant correlation of elevated serum concentrations of IgG2 (and to a lesser extent of IgG3) with decreased forced expiratory volume at 1 second. Moss[83] noted that patients with cystic fibrosis who are infected with *P. aeruginosa* have markedly elevated serum concentrations of IgG antibodies to the opsonic immunodeterminant, type-specific lipopolysaccharide. This elevation was distributed among all four IgG subclasses, with a significant shift toward IgG3. Sera from cystic fibrosis patients who were colonized with *P. aeruginosa* had diminished opsonic capacity, but complement-dependent human neutrophil phagocytosis was not impaired. Serum concentrations of IgG4 but not of IgG1,

IgG2, or IgG3 correlated inversely with opsonic capacity. On the basis of these data, Moss[83] suggested that high levels of IgG4 antibodies to opsonic immunodeterminants may inhibit normal pulmonary clearance of *P. aeruginosa* by pulmonary macrophages in vivo.

Berger and associates[11] noted that elastase treatment of isolated polymorphonuclear leukocytes severely impaired their ability to kill opsonized *P. aeruginosa*. They demonstrated proteolytic degradation of C3b receptors and suggested that this may contribute to the inability of patients with cystic fibrosis to eradicate *P. aeruginosa* from their lungs. Because several cell types, including macrophages, monocytes, B lymphocytes, and some T lymphocytes, all carry the same C3b receptor, the proteolytic activity may cleave this molecule from all of these cells, thereby decreasing the phagocytic activity of monocytes and macrophages in these patients. Berger and associates[11] demonstrated that optimal intervention between complement-derived opsonic ligands, C3b and iC3b, and their respective receptors does not occur in the milieu of the lung of patients with cystic fibrosis who are infected with *Pseudomonas*. They suggested that both *Pseudomonas* and host proteases may contribute to the initiation of a cycle of events in which neutrophils entering the infected lung actually impair phagocytosis rather than eradicate the source of these infections.

The mucoid strains of *P. aeruginosa* isolated from respiratory secretions of patients with cystic fibrosis produce large quantities of alginate (composed of acetylated D-mannuronic acid and L-guluronic acid).[23, 129] This polysaccharide polymer not only gives *P. aeruginosa* a mucoid appearance on agar but also has antiphagocytic activity. Alginate also can elicit a significant inflammatory immune response in the lungs of patients with cystic fibrosis, which may contribute to the lung damage that follows chronic *P. aeruginosa* lung infection.[80] Because of its viscous nature, alginate contributes to the thick bronchial secretions in the lungs of children with cystic fibrosis, obstructing small airways and impairing mucociliary clearance and movement of phagocytic cells.

The role of lipopolysaccharide in the virulence of *P. aeruginosa* also has been studied. The virulence of several strains of *P. aeruginosa* for burned mice was found to be related directly to lipopolysaccharide integrity.[26] Deficiency of the O-side chain of lipopolysaccharide reduced virulence markedly.

CLINICAL MANIFESTATIONS

P. aeruginosa can produce disease in healthy, normal children.[39] Generally when this occurs, the organism has been introduced into a minor wound contaminated with water or soil; this is followed by the development of cellulitis as a localized abscess that exudes green or blue pus. The skin lesions (whether due to direct inoculation or secondary to septicemia) may begin as pink macules that progress to small cutaneous hemorrhagic nodules and eventually to areas of necrosis with eschar formation, surrounded by an intense red areola (ecthyma gangrenosum, Fig. 129–1). Bacteria multiply locally, and rarely (in normal children), *P. aeruginosa* causes septicemia, endocarditis, corneal infection, otitis externa, mastitis, mastoiditis, meningitis, pneumonia, peritonitis, and urinary tract infections. *Pseudomonas* osteomyelitis may develop after puncture wounds, particularly of the foot.[59]

Outbreaks of dermatitis (folliculitis), otitis externa, mastitis, and urinary tract infections caused by *P. aeruginosa* have been reported in normal, healthy children after the use of community swimming pools, water slides, recreational whirlpools, or family-owned hot tubs.[38, 39, 50, 113, 126, 138] Pruritic or painful skin lesions (5 to 30 mm) develop several hours to 5 days or longer (mean, 48 hours) after contact with these water sources. Skin lesions may be erythematous, macular, or pustular. In some cases, nodules have been observed. Illness may vary from a few scattered lesions in one patient to extensive truncal involvement in others. The rash is most severe in areas occluded by snug-fitting bathing suits. In some children, malaise, fever, otitis externa, vomiting, sore throat, conjunctivitis, rhinitis, pyuria, abdominal cramps, and swollen breasts may be associated with the dermal lesions.

Multiple serotypes of *P. aeruginosa* have been associated with these outbreaks. Use of whirlpool baths usually involves soaking in water for variable periods. Superhydration of skin and exposure to *P. aeruginosa* results in primary cutaneous infection.[54] Whirlpool water is heated to temperatures above 37.8° C (100° F) and frequently is not filtered, allowing for the persistence of desquamated skin. Both of these factors are conducive to growth of *P. aeruginosa*.

Otitis externa caused by *P. aeruginosa* also has been reported in healthy competitive swimmers who swim repetitively in a pool contaminated with *P. aeruginosa*.[103] The organism also has been associated with a more malignant form of otitis externa presenting with high fever, necrosis of portions of the external ear, facial nerve paralysis, mastoiditis, and temporal bone and basilar skull osteomyelitis.[57, 86] Rarely, *P. aeruginosa* meningitis results from progression of this infection.[99] This condition usually is associated with some predisposing factors, such as malnutrition; leukopenia, a disorder of leukocyte function; malignancy; or diabetes mellitus. Successful management of this condition requires aggressive surgical débridement in addition to appropriate systemic antibiotic therapy.

P. aeruginosa is a common agent for chronic suppurative otitis media (with or without cholesteatoma) and chronic mastoiditis.[63] Chronic suppurative otitis media is a complication of inadequately treated acute otitis media and manifests as a perforated tympanic membrane with persistent otorrhea. Chronic suppurative otitis media also occurs in children with surgically induced perforations of the tympanic membrane with tympanostomy tubes, complicated by incompletely or inadequately treated otitis media. Outpatient therapy with oral antibiotics frequently is unsuccessful because of a lack of oral antimicrobial agents with antipseudomonal activity. Intravenous antibiotics targeting the bacterial agents isolated from middle ear aspirates usually cure the chronic suppurative otitis media. This may avoid tympanomastoid surgery, which becomes essential when there is extensive granulation tissue and osteitis in the mastoid.

P. aeruginosa infection of the eye usually occurs after trauma or deposition of a large inoculum. Using contaminated contact lens solution, using tap water during contact lens care, and endotracheal suctioning without covering the eyes of sedated or comatose patients have been implicated.[53, 56] Infection of the cornea can result in ulceration, which may progress to more invasive disease, including endophthalmitis. Loss of vision may result, even if appropriate antimicrobial therapy is administered promptly.

P. aeruginosa may produce serious infections during the neonatal period. Septicemia may be noted in the earliest hours of life and is associated with high morbidity and mortality. In utero acquisition of the organism has been described.[111] The clinical course is similar to that of any other form of gram-negative septicemia, with hypotension, respiratory distress, and skin lesions as the predominant presentations. Late-onset neonatal *P. aeruginosa* infection usually occurs as nosocomial infection (bacteremia, urinary tract infection, and pneumonia) associated with a foreign-body (e.g., indwelling urinary or vascular catheter or endotracheal tube) in hospitalized infants.

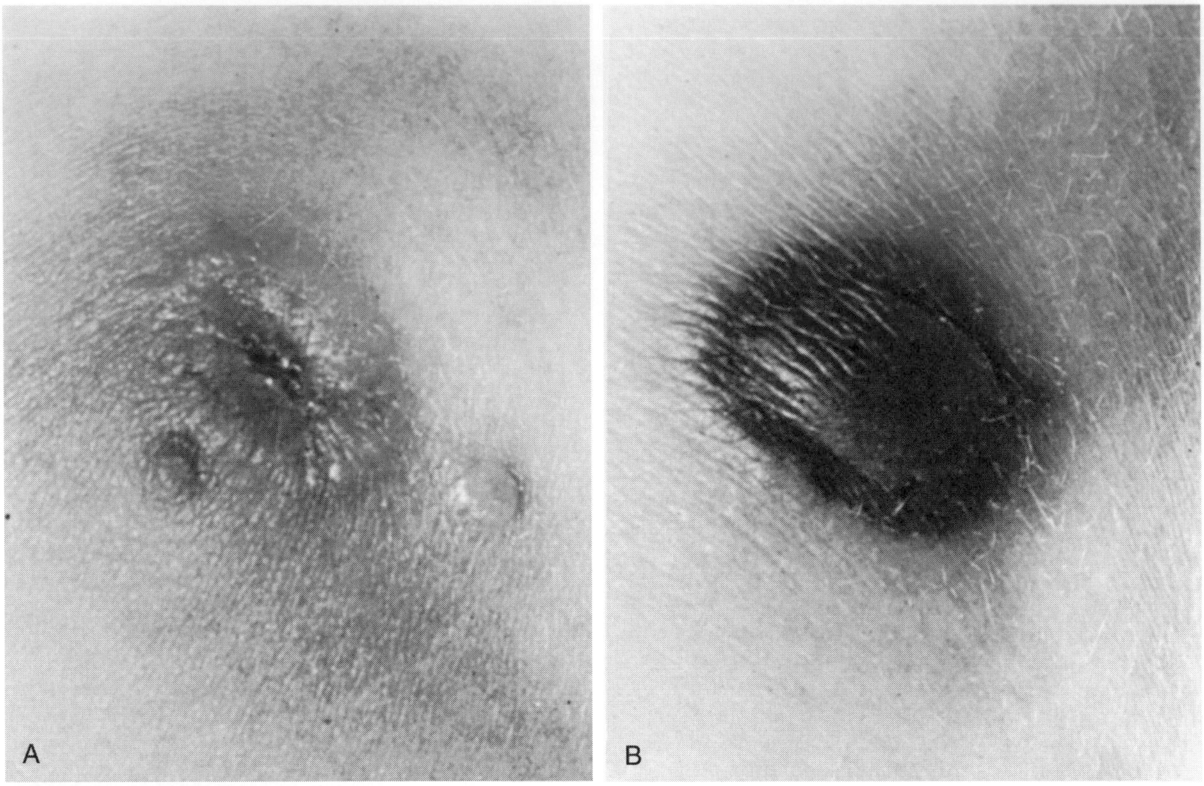

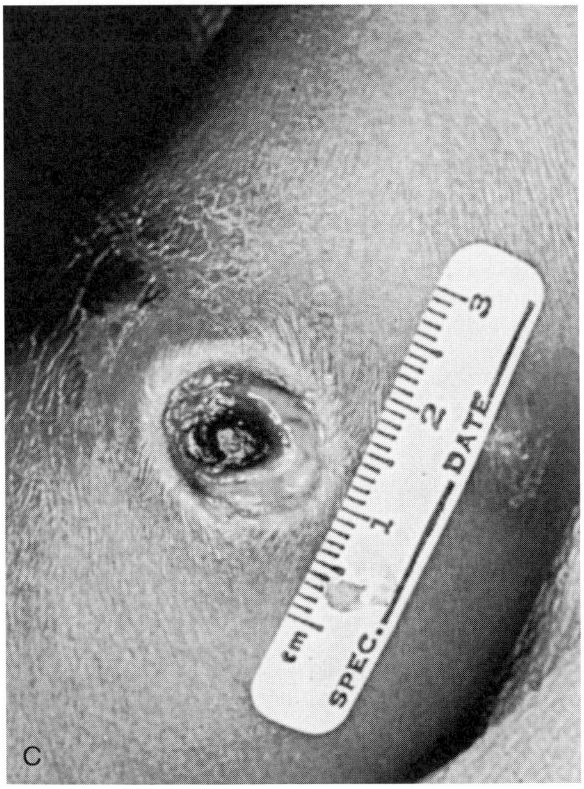

FIGURE 129–1. A, *Skin lesion due to septicemic* Pseudomonas aeruginosa *infection. A large macule has begun to undergo central necrosis and is surrounded by two smaller macules.* B, *A small cutaneous nodule representing the skin lesion of septicemic* P. aeruginosa. C, *A final stage of ecthyma gangrenosum in which a cutaneous hemorrhagic nodule has undergone central necrosis and eschar formation.*

Other pseudomonads (except *B. pseudomallei*) rarely cause disease in healthy persons. Reports in normal, healthy children, particularly when these children have been hospitalized in an intensive care unit,[16, 119] include pneumonia, keratitis,[74] and abscesses due to *B. cepacia*; otitis media due to *Shewanella putrefaciens*; abscesses due to *P. fluorescens*; otitis media, pneumonia, and osteomyelitis[21, 109] due to *P. stutzeri*; posttraumatic leg ulcers[95] and brain abscess[135] due to *Sphingomonas paucimobilis*; and cellulitis, pneumonia, septicemia, endocarditis, peritonitis, and meningitis due to *S. maltophilia*.

Septicemia and endocarditis due to *S. maltophilia* have been associated with intravenous abuse of illicit drugs.[147]

Peritonitis and septicemia caused by *B. cepacia*, *S. putrefaciens*, and *S. paucimobilis* have been associated with contamination of equipment used for peritoneal dialysis.[6, 14, 28, 49]

Burns and Wound Infection[39]

The surfaces of wounds or burns frequently are populated by pseudomonads and other gram-negative organisms. Colonization does not imply infection necessarily but is a necessary prerequisite to invasive disease. Septicemia with *P. aeruginosa* is a major problem in the burn patient. This may be related to multiplication of organisms in devitalized surface areas, followed by invasion, or it can be associated with prolonged intravenous or urinary catheterization required for the care of these persons. Antibiotics may diminish the susceptible microbiologic flora but permit more resistant selected strains of *P. aeruginosa* to flourish.

In burn patients, abnormalities of neutrophil function have been described that precede the onset of septicemia.[2] Killing of *Pseudomonas* by neutrophils is impaired. Burn injury also is associated with abnormal responses to antigens, delayed rejection of homografts, abnormal vascular responses, impaired delayed hypersensitivity responses, diminished uptake of particles by the reticuloendothelial system, and altered antimicrobial pharmacokinetics. Wound contamination with high concentrations of bacteria ($>10^5$ colony-forming units/g of tissue) impedes wound contraction and healing.[93] In addition, *P. aeruginosa* produces a number of substances that can further inhibit the natural healing process of burns and wounds. Secretion of exogenous plasminogen activators and proteases breaks down proteins such as fibrin and halts the contraction process.[98] *P. aeruginosa* exotoxin A, a protein synthesis inhibitor, also is a potent cause for retardation of wound healing.[51]

P. aeruginosa is the most common cause of osteomyelitis after puncture wounds of the foot, accounting for more than 90 per cent of cases.[18, 37, 81] The calcaneus or metatarsal bones commonly are affected.[25] Symptoms may be present for 2 to 40 days (mean, 9 days) prior to diagnosis and hospitalization.[25] Pain and swelling are the most common. Fever and wound drainage rarely are noted. Leukocytosis (white blood cell count $>10{,}000/mm^3$) and an elevated erythrocyte sedimentation rate are present in most patients. Radiographs of the affected foot usually show evidence of osteomyelitis at some time during the period of evaluation and treatment. Bone scan results are abnormal almost universally and frequently yield evidence of osteomyelitis prior to positive findings on radiographs. The inner pad of the sneaker has been implicated as a possible source of *P. aeruginosa* in these patients.[43] However, *P. aeruginosa* osteomyelitis of the foot bones has occurred when the puncture occurred through other types of footwear or while the child was barefoot.

Cystic Fibrosis[39]

Cystic fibrosis is one of the most common lethal inherited diseases of children. It is a generalized disorder of salt and water transport affecting exocrine glands and is caused by mutations in the cystic fibrosis transmembrane conductance regulator gene.[68, 108] The course and prognosis largely are determined by chronic infections of the airways with opportunistic bacteria. Death usually results from chronic obstructive pulmonary disease. *P. aeruginosa* can be recovered from cultures of most children with cystic fibrosis. Recovery of *P. aeruginosa* from the sputum of the child with cystic fibrosis does not necessarily imply infection and destructive pneumonitis related to this organism. In patients with cystic fibrosis, mucociliary clearance is impeded and results in a failure to cleanse the bronchopulmonary epithelium of inhaled particles, including bacteria.[68, 82] Colonization of the sputum of patients with cystic fibrosis may reflect the use of mist tents, inhalation therapy, and continuous broad-spectrum antibiotic therapy.[146] Once *P. aeruginosa* is in the respiratory tract, eradication by antibiotic therapy is rare.

Some observations, however, suggest that the relationship between *Pseudomonas* and the patient with cystic fibrosis is more specific. Patients with cystic fibrosis almost always harbor an unusual mucoid *P. aeruginosa* phenotype, which produces an excessive amount of capsular slime.[104] The tracheobronchial tree of 70 to 80 per cent of these patients is colonized chronically, and the organism is eradicated infrequently either spontaneously or by antibiotic therapy.[47, 124] The peculiar lung environment of the patient with cystic fibrosis is believed to trigger a switch to a cluster of genes that encode for the abundant production of the mucoid polysaccharide (alginate), giving rise to the mucoid phenotype.[23, 129] In contrast, mucoid strains of *P. aeruginosa* are recovered from only 0.5 to 1.7 per cent of patients without cystic fibrosis.

Persistence of *P. aeruginosa* within the respiratory tract is aided by growth of the organism in microcolonies embedded in a biofilm of alginate.[55, 94] This biofilm allows nutrients to pass through while protecting the organism from host defense mechanisms, antibodies, and probably antibiotics.[68] It also has been noted that rabbit alveolar macrophages fail to phagocytize and kill the organism in the presence of serum of patients with cystic fibrosis. This suggests the presence of a specific, local defect in pulmonary resistance to *P. aeruginosa* in these patients.

There also is a clustering of *P. aeruginosa* serotypes among isolates obtained from patients with cystic fibrosis. Homma type 8 strains may be recovered from 50 to 93 per cent of patients with cystic fibrosis.

Bacterial infection in cystic fibrosis is limited almost entirely to the respiratory tract. Pulmonary exacerbations with endobronchial disease are common in patients with cystic fibrosis. Infection of the pulmonary parenchyma is rare. Rather, the epithelium of the airways and submucosa are edematous and contain infiltrates of chronic inflammatory cells. Documentation of a pulmonary exacerbation in cystic fibrosis relies heavily on clinical impression (e.g., increase in frequency of productive cough; increase in volume or change in characteristic of sputum; increase in respiratory rate or dyspnea; and decreased appetite, activity, or exercise tolerance). Fever and leukocytosis are present in a minority of patients, and they are associated with poorer pulmonary function test results and a worse prognostic score.[125] Concentrations of *P. aeruginosa*, DNA (derived from polymorphonuclear leukocytes and to a lesser extent from respiratory epithelial cells), and total protein in sputum are increased during pulmonary exacerbations and decrease significantly after antimicrobial therapy.[125] Pulmonary infection in patients with cystic fibrosis generally is chronic. Bronchitis, bronchiolitis, and bronchiectasis can occur. Eventually, local necrotizing pneumonitis may be noted that contrasts with the overwhelming generalized necrotizing pneumonitis seen in immunosuppressed patients. Septicemia is rare. However, bacteremia may occur in patients with indwelling venous catheters.

B. cepacia also has emerged as an increasingly frequent agent of asymptomatic colonization, pneumonia, and septicemia in patients with cystic fibrosis. Rates of colonization have been as high as 40 per cent in some centers.[112] The frequency of colonization of the respiratory tract with *B. cepacia* in patients with cystic fibrosis has been associated with increased morbidity and mortality rates in some cystic fibrosis centers since the 1980s. The risk of colonization with *B. cepacia* increases with the severity of underlying disease and increasing age.[133] The source or mode of transmission of the organism has not been defined adequately.[75, 134] However, more recent information supports person-to-person transmission.[61] Nosocomial transmission (patient-to-patient and contaminated inhalation therapy equipment) within cystic fibrosis centers and social contact, particularly at summer camps, appear to be important in new infection with *B. cepacia*. Once colonization with *B. cepacia* has been identified in patients with cystic fibrosis, three distinct clinical patterns have been noted: (1) chronic asymptomatic carriage (usually in association with *P. aeruginosa*), (2) progressive deterioration over many months, with recurrent acute pulmonary exacerbations, accompanied by fever, progressive weight loss, leukocytosis, and elevated erythrocyte sedimentation rate, and (3) rapid, usually fatal, deterioration in pulmonary function.[58] The last presentation even can occur in patients who were affected only mildly prior to *B. cepacia* infection.

Malignancy[39]

Children with leukemia, particularly those receiving immunosuppressive therapy and who are neutropenic, are extremely susceptible to septicemia due to *P. aeruginosa* and other pseudomonads. Most pseudomonads have been reported as causes of septicemia in children with malignancy, including *P. putida*.[3] Generally, infection results from invasion of the blood stream by a colonizing *Pseudomonas* organism (e.g., from the gastrointestinal tract). Anorexia, malaise, nausea, vomiting, diarrhea, and fever may be noted. Generalized vasculitis develops, and hemorrhagic necrotic lesions can be found in all organs, including the skin, where they appear as purple nodules or ecchymotic areas that become gangrenous.[102] Hemorrhagic or gangrenous perirectal cellulitis or abscess may be noted, as well as ileus and profound hypotension.

Children undergoing treatment for malignancies particularly are vulnerable to bacterial infection. Chemotherapy and radiation therapy can disrupt mucocutaneous barriers and result in moderate to severe immunosuppression. Fergie and associates[40] described 98 children and adolescents with cancer who developed *P. aeruginosa* bacteremia; the rate of bacteremia was highest for patients with leukemia. Most cases occurred when patients had absolute neutrophil counts of less than $100/mm^3$. Mortality associated with *P. aeruginosa* bacteremia was higher for patients with solid tumors, an absolute neutrophil count of less than $100/mm^3$, perineal skin lesions, and bacteremia during remission or induction therapy rather than during a relapse.

The single most important factor that predisposes children with cancer to infection is granulocytopenia. The bactericidal capacity of children with leukemia and other neoplasms also may be impaired. Heat-stable opsonins specific for *P. aeruginosa* also may fall precipitously in children with acute leukemia who are receiving intensive combination chemotherapy. Fatal infections with *P. aeruginosa* may be related, in part, to deficiency of this specific opsonin.

Immunosuppression

Immunosuppressive agents may be employed in the management of malignancies, transplantation, or collagen-vascular disease. The location of the infectious process and the causative organisms depend somewhat on the underlying disease. Infection by *P. aeruginosa*, particularly pneumonia and septicemia, is more common in children receiving immunosuppressive therapy than in the normal, healthy population.

Other Conditions that Predispose to *Pseudomonas* Infection

P. aeruginosa is a major cause of hospital-acquired infections in children. It is the leading cause of nosocomial respiratory tract infection in children on mechanical ventilation or receiving inhalation therapy. Asymptomatic colonization of the upper and lower airways is common and should be distinguished from respiratory tract disease, tracheitis, or pneumonia. A predominance of gram-negative bacilli with an abundance of polymorphonuclear leukocytes on Gram stain of lower respiratory tract secretions, in conjunction with a positive culture for *P. aeruginosa*, strongly supports the role of *P. aeruginosa* as the causative agent for the lower respiratory tract infection. Absence of *P. aeruginosa* from lower respiratory tract secretions markedly reduces the likelihood that *P. aeruginosa* is in the lower respiratory tract.

Septicemia due to *P. aeruginosa* also occurs with increased frequency in children with indwelling vascular or urinary catheters.[131] Septicemia also may occur in children with congenital or acquired neutropenia or in persons with a functional deficit in polymorphonuclear leukocyte function. Urinary tract infections also have been associated with cystoscopic examination. *Pseudomonas* is a common cause of abscesses and meningitis in children with dermoid sinus tracts or dermoids extending down to or communicating with the meninges or neural tissue and in children with meningomyeloceles. *P. aeruginosa* may produce acute or subacute endocarditis in children with congenital cardiac lesions before or after cardiac surgery and in adolescents who inject illicit drugs intravenously. *P. aeruginosa* supraglottitis has been reported in a 6-month-old child with severe combined immunodeficiency syndrome.[70]

Severe *P. aeruginosa* infections have been reported in children infected with HIV, primarily after severe immunodeficiency has occurred.[44, 107] Bacteremia may occur with or without the presence of an indwelling vascular catheter. Fever, hypotension, skin lesions (papules or ecthyma gangrenosum), and pneumonia are common.[44] Mortality can be high, particularly when empiric antimicrobial therapy is inadequate for treatment of severe, invasive *Pseudomonas* infection.

Disease Due to Other Pseudomonads

Melioidosis is a rare disease of Southeast Asia that has increased in frequency in the United States in Americans who returned from Vietnam or, rarely, in Southeast Asian immigrants.[91] The causative agent is *B. pseudomallei*, an inhabitant of soil and water in the tropics. *B. pseudomallei* is a small, pleomorphic, gram-negative rod without a capsule that exhibits bipolar staining. It is an obligate aerobe that grows best at pH 7 and at 37° C (98.6° F). Infection occurs after contact of abrasions or wounds with contaminated soil or water or inhalation of contaminated dust.

Transmission from animal to human has not been reported. The rat flea and the *Aedes aegypti* mosquito have been reported to infect animals with *B. pseudomallei*, but this route of infection has not been documented in human cases.[92]

Melioidosis can present with a broad spectrum of clinical signs, and symptoms may be latent for months or years before the disease becomes manifest clinically. The initial clinical finding may be a single primary skin lesion (vesicle, pustule, bulla, urticaria) in a patient with no underlying disease. Septicemia occasionally occurs, and multiple abscesses may be noted in every organ of the body. The mortality rate associated with fulminant sepsis approaches 90 per cent. Meningitis, encephalitis, and endophthalmitis have been observed in both the normal and the compromised host after or concomitant with an episode of septicemia. The acute septicemic illness is indistinguishable from other types of septicemia caused by gram-negative organisms.

B. pseudomallei can cause myocarditis, pericarditis, endocarditis, intestinal abscess, cholecystitis, acute gastroenteritis, urinary tract infections, septic arthritis, paraspinal abscess, osteomyelitis, hilar lymphadenopathy, and cervical lymphadenopathy. Parotitis was documented in 38 per cent of 126 children with melioidosis in Thailand.[29] None of the 126 children with melioidosis had any apparent predisposition to infection.

Subacute melioidosis generally is characterized by an illness lasting weeks to months. Pulmonary infection in this form of disease is common and may mimic tuberculosis.

Neonatal melioidosis has been reported in Thailand.[77] Five infants with neonatal septicemia, meningitis, or both due to *B. pseudomallei* were described. The mode of transmission of this organism to these newborn infants was not elucidated.

Chronic melioidosis is more common in whites than in Asians.[79] Chronic melioidosis may involve every organ in the body except for the brain. Melioidosis may become dormant, with exacerbations occurring years after primary infection when host defenses are impaired as a result of steroids, burns, diabetes mellitus, or other processes. The longest latent period (24 years) was reported by Kingston.[66]

Melioidosis should be considered in any person with fever of unknown origin, overwhelming sepsis, single or multiple abscesses, or any tuberculosis-like illness who has been to Southeast Asia or northern Australia at any time. Diagnosis is established by culture of blood, skin lesions, or purulent material from an abscess cavity or from other sites of infection.[71] The organism grows in media commonly employed for isolation of gram-negative bacteria. On solid media, the colonies develop slowly (over a week) and have a characteristic daisy-head appearance. Alpha-hemolysis is noted on sheep blood agar. A selective medium ("Ashdown medium") can increase the recovery rate of *B. pseudomallei* from clinical specimens containing mixed bacterial flora, such as throat, rectal, and sputum specimens.[4] *B. pseudomallei* produces a dry, wrinkled, and violet-purple colony on Ashdown medium, with a pungent, earthy odor.[48]

Serologic tests are more useful in establishing the diagnosis of melioidosis in latent or asymptomatic forms of this disease.[1, 78, 88] Hemagglutination (HA), indirect HA, and complement-fixation (CF) tests and an enzyme-linked immunosorbent assay (ELISA) are available. Diagnostic titers are 1:40 or greater for the HA test and 1:10 or greater for the CF test. Because the sensitivity of these serologic tests varies, both should be performed. The HA antibodies generally are present within 7 to 14 days after the onset of the illness; the CF test yields positive results in 4 to 6 weeks. Maximal titers for both tests are reached in 4 to 6 months. Both HA and CF antibodies persist for 9 months to 2 years after the onset of disease. The indirect HA test is used by the Centers for Disease Control and Prevention for the diagnosis of melioidosis. An ELISA that detects specific IgG and IgM antibody to *B. pseudomallei* has been developed.[5] This test proved more suitable than an IgG–indirect fluorescent antibody test as a screening test for melioidosis and also was more sensitive than the indirect HA test for melioidosis. Gold-blot detection of IgM- and IgG-specific antibodies has been developed.[69] This allows a more rapid serodiagnosis of melioidosis. *B. pseudomallei* can be detected in serum by an ELISA method.[142]

DIAGNOSIS AND DIFFERENTIAL DIAGNOSIS

Diagnosis of *Pseudomonas* infection depends on recovery of the organism from the blood, cerebrospinal fluid, and urine obtained in a manner that avoids contamination by cutaneous flora (suprapubic aspiration or urethral catheterization usually is required for young children), joint fluid, peritoneal dialysis fluid, or purulent material obtained by aspiration of subcutaneous abscesses or areas of cellulitis. A diagnosis of *Pseudomonas* pneumonia can be made by needle aspirate of the lung and, less convincingly, by recovery of the organism from sputum obtained by postural drainage of a child with cystic fibrosis. Recovery of the organism from the surface of the skin or the throat, tracheal aspirate, or bronchial secretions may reflect colonization and is not necessarily diagnostic of infection.

Pseudomonas and *Burkholderia* grow well on most standard laboratory media. All members of both genera grow in broth blood culture systems.[48] Isolation of *Pseudomonas* and *Burkholderia* from specimens with mixed bacterial flora is enhanced by using selective media, such as MacConkey agar. Cetrimide or eosin-methylene blue agars can be used for isolation of *P. aeruginosa* from clinical as well as environmental specimens. Two media, PC (for *P. cepacia*)[48] and OFPBL (for oxidative-fermentative base-polymyxin B-bacitracin-lactose)[139] agar, inhibit *P. aeruginosa* and are useful for recovery of *B. cepacia* from sputum of patients with cystic fibrosis.

The bluish, nodular skin lesions and the ulcers with ecchymotic and gangrenous centers and bright areolae (ecthyma gangrenosum) have been considered to be virtually pathognomonic of *P. aeruginosa* infection. Rarely, skin lesions that clinically are indistinguishable from those caused by *P. aeruginosa* develop after septicemia due to *Aeromonas hydrophila*.[122] Cutaneous or disseminated infections with *Aspergillus* and *Fusarium* in immunocompromised patients also can cause the necrotic skin lesions of ecthyma gangrenosum.

Immunoglobulin antibodies to *P. aeruginosa* surface antigens in serum have been detected reliably by ELISA.[19] Detection of specific IgG and IgA antibodies is not clinically useful for diagnosis of acute *P. aeruginosa* infection. However, antibody titer increases were associated with active disease due to *P. aeruginosa* in patients with cystic fibrosis. Antibody titers returned to baseline when *Pseudomonas* infection was controlled by effective antimicrobial therapy. Thus, this assay appears to help in differentiating between early infection and colonization. Antibodies to *P. aeruginosa* also may be detected by immunoblotting (Western blotting).[123] These methods may be sensitive and useful for determining the onset of *P. aeruginosa* infection in patients with cystic fibrosis.

PREVENTION

Prevention of infection with pseudomonads depends, in part, on a continuous surveillance program of the hospital environment that is designed to identify and subsequently eradicate sources of pseudomonads as quickly as possible. Pseudomonads can grow to a concentration of 10^6 organisms/mL in distilled water that appears to be perfectly clear. Growth of pseudomonads in distilled water, disinfectants, and medications is the factor incriminated most commonly in single-source outbreaks of *Pseudomonas* infection in hospitals. Prevention of follicular dermatitis caused by *P. aeruginosa* contamination of whirlpools or hot tubs should be possible by maintenance of pool water at a pH of 7.2 to 7.8 and the free allowable chlorine concentrations at 0.4 to 1.5 ppm.[22]

Outbreaks of *Pseudomonas* infection in newborn nurseries have been reported.[16] Generally, infection has been transmitted by the hands of personnel from washbasin surfaces and suction catheter rinse solution to the newborn infants. Strict attention to hand washing before and between contacts with the newborn infant, particularly with a liquid iodophor hand washing agent, may prevent or interdict epidemic disease. Growth of *Pseudomonas* on suction catheters can be prevented by rinsing the catheter in an acetic acid solution.

Daily replacement of all apparatus used for intravenous administration greatly reduces the hazard of extrinsic contamination by *Pseudomonas* and other gram-negative organisms. When intravenous administration is indicated, a small metal needle is preferable to a plastic catheter because these needles have been associated with a lower rate of septicemia and phlebitis.

Meticulous care is required in the preparation of solutions for total parenteral alimentation and in the insertion and care of catheters.

Some studies have demonstrated the efficacy of active immunization of the burned patient with specific strains of *Pseudomonas* or the administration of hyperimmunoglobulin in the prevention of *Pseudomonas* septicemia.[2, 62] *Pseudomonas* infection in the burn patient also can be minimized by careful protective isolation and by the topical application of silver nitrate (0.5 per cent) solution or 10 per cent mafenide acetate cream. Débridement for removal of devitalized tissue also is imperative. *P. aeruginosa* vaccine also has been suggested as a possible method for preventing this disease in patients with acute leukemia or cystic fibrosis.[97]

Pseudomonas infection of dermal abnormalities that communicate with the cerebrospinal axis can be prevented by careful evaluation and early surgical repair. Antibiotic prophylaxis of *Pseudomonas* urinary tract infection is difficult without a suitable oral antipseudomonal antibiotic for children. Identification and corrective surgery of obstructive lesions of the urinary tract minimize or prevent *Pseudomonas* infection of the urinary tract.

Cohorting and isolating patients with cystic fibrosis who are colonized with multiresistant strains of *P. aeruginosa* or *B. cepacia* have been suggested as means of reducing nosocomial transmission of these organisms. However, the proper manner of handling patients with these organisms has not been established. Any attempt to reduce transmission should be based on measures with proven efficacy and also must consider the potential consequences of strict isolation or segregation on this population, which spends so much time at health care facilities.

TREATMENT[105]

Systemic infections with *Pseudomonas* should be treated promptly with antibiotics, to which the organism is susceptible in vitro. Nosocomially acquired *P. aeruginosa* is more likely to be antibiotic-resistant than community-acquired strains. Response to treatment may be impaired, and prolonged treatment may be required when systemic infection occurs in the compromised host.

Table 129–2 provides dosages of some of the more commonly prescribed antipseudomonal antibiotics.[85] These dosages provide only guidelines because doses of some of these antibiotics may vary with different clinical situations and patient populations. Once-daily aminoglycoside dosing is being evaluated as a way to decrease nephrotoxicity and improve clinical efficacy. Aminoglycoside doses must be decreased, preferably by increasing the dosing interval, in patients with diminished creatinine clearance (e.g., renal impairment, neonates). Significantly higher doses (e.g., 7 to 12 mg/kg/day for gentamicin or tobramycin) may be required for patients with increased total plasma clearance, such as patients with cystic fibrosis and burns. Therefore, aminogly-

TABLE 129–2. Dosages of Commonly Prescribed Antipseudomonal Antibiotics

Generic Name	Dosage	Route	Interval	Pediatric Precautions
Antipseudomonal penicillins				
Carbenicillin indanyl sodium	30–50 mg/kg/day	PO	q 6 h	SNE
Ticarcillin disodium	200–300 mg/kg/day	IV	q 4–6 h	
Mezlocillin sodium	200–300 mg/kg/day	IV	q 4–6 h	
Piperacillin	200–300 mg/kg/day	IV	q 4–6 h	PDNE
Cephalosporins				
Ceftazidime	75–200 mg/kg/day	IV	q 8 h	
Aminoglycosides				
Gentamicin sulfate	3–7.5 mg/kg/day	IV, IM	q 8 h	
Tobramycin sulfate	3–7.5 mg/kg/day	IV, IM	q 8 h	
Netilmicin sulfate	3–7.5 mg/kg/day	IV, IM	q 8 h	
Amikacin sulfate	15–22.5 mg/kg/day	IV, IM	q 8 h	
Quinolones				
Ciprofloxacin	20–30 mg/kg/day	PO	q 12 h	> 18y
	10–15 mg/kg/day	IV	q 12 h	> 18y
Monobactams				
Aztreonam	90–120 mg/kg/day	IV, IM	q 6–8 h	SNE
Carbapenems				
Imipenem	40–60 mg/kg/day	IV	q 6 h	SNE

>18 y = safety in children younger than 18 years of age is not established, and use is not recommended. SNE = safety in children not yet established.

PDNE = pediatric dose not yet established.

Data from Nelson, J. D.: Pocketbook of Pediatric Antimicrobial Therapy. 12th ed. Baltimore, Williams & Wilkins, 1996–1997, pp. 68–83.

coside therapy must be individualized and doses guided by pharmacokinetic information.

Invasive infections, including septicemia due to proven or suspected *P. aeruginosa* infection, should be treated with an aminoglycoside (gentamicin, tobramycin, netilmicin, or amikacin) combined with a β-lactam antibiotic (antipseudomonal penicillin, third- or fourth-generation cephalosporin or carbapenem).[64] The combination of an aminoglycoside and a β-lactam antibiotic may be synergistic against the organism. Rifampin may be added to the combination therapy if the clinical response is not adequate. Monotherapy with the cell-wall–active β-lactam antibiotics as well as the fluoroquinolones frequently results in the development of antibiotic resistance during therapy as a result of a mutation.[8, 120]

Aztreonam, a monobactam antibiotic, and the fluoroquinolones are antibiotics with excellent antipseudomonal activity but currently are not approved for use in pediatric patients. Polymyxin B and colistin (polymyxin E), used previously, largely have been superseded by less toxic agents but may be useful in selected patients who are infected with strains resistant to the other agents. However, all *Burkholderia* species are resistant to polymyxin B.

Ciprofloxacin and the other quinolones have been evaluated for the treatment of acute and chronic *P. aeruginosa* infection in teenage children and adults with cystic fibrosis.[60, 110, 130, 132] These antibiotics, which may be given orally or intravenously, proved to be effective, as judged by clinical scores and results of pulmonary function tests. In the United States, quinolone use is restricted until after puberty because these antibiotics may bind cartilage and produce growth arrest. Information available from clinical trials in Europe suggests that ciprofloxacin and the other quinolones may not be as harmful for children as they are for other immature animal species.[24, 115, 116] Ciprofloxacin may be considered in selected children when the risks associated with use of this antibiotic are outweighed by the potential benefits associated with its clinical efficacy (e.g., multiresistant strains of *Pseudomonas*, substitution of an oral quinolone for long-term intravenous therapy requiring an indwelling catheter). If ciprofloxacin is used, it may be administered in a dosage of 10 to 15 mg/kg every 12 hours orally or 5 to 7.5 mg/kg twice a day intravenously. Oral dosage should not exceed 1000 mg/day in patients who weigh less than 40 kg or 1500 mg/day in patients who weigh more than 40 kg.

P. aeruginosa meningitis or brain abscess should be treated with ceftazidime (200 mg/kg/day in four divided doses every 6 hours) and an aminoglycoside given intravenously. The initial empiric choice of the aminoglycoside should be guided by local susceptibility patterns. Concomitant intraventricular or intrathecal treatment with gentamicin may be required if initial intravenous therapy fails to sterilize the cerebrospinal fluid. Gentamicin can be placed into the ventricular or lumbar cerebrospinal fluid in a total dose of 1 or 2 mg once each day (dose is independent of body weight). Fluoroquinolones, such as parenteral ciprofloxacin or pefloxacin, and aztreonam are possible alternatives in the treatment of *P. aeruginosa* central nervous system infections if more conventional therapy has failed. However, the experience with these agents in central nervous system infections is limited.[65, 73, 89, 121]

Skin abscesses or abscesses due to *P. aeruginosa* in other locations should be incised and drained.[102] Failure to do so may cause a poor response, despite prolonged systemic antibiotic treatment. Osteomyelitis of foot bones requires surgical débridement in every case. Ten to 14 days of appropriate antibiotics appears to be adequate if surgery effectively has removed infected tissue.[59] Adequacy of surgical débridement and clinical improvement can be monitored with serial sedimentation rates.[25] *P. aeruginosa* infections of foreign bodies (vascular, peritoneal, and central nervous system catheters) may need to be removed to cure the infection. This particularly is true if a tunnel or exit-site infection exists.

Pseudomonas folliculitis usually is self-limited and usually does not require specific antimicrobial therapy. More severe cases can be treated with topical application of any of the following: 2.5 per cent acetic acid (vinegar is 5 per cent acetic acid) compresses, gentamicin ointment, or silver sulfadiazine (Silvadene).

The β-lactam antibiotics (antipseudomonal penicillins, cephalosporins, carbapenems), monobactams, and ciprofloxacin are rapidly bactericidal to *P. aeruginosa*.[45] The combination of an aminoglycoside with any of these antibiotics is unlikely to affect significantly the initial clinical response rate. However, a reduction in the emergence of drug-resistant *P. aeruginosa* clones is the major benefit of combination therapy including an aminoglycoside. Combination therapy with two β-lactam antibiotics is inappropriate for serious *Pseudomonas* infections because the induction of β-lactamase may result in resistance to both antibiotics.

Antibiotic resistance is an important factor in patients with serious *Pseudomonas* infections that do not respond to antibiotic therapy. As the quintessential opportunist, *Pseudomonas* has developed various means to resist the activity of antibiotics. *P. aeruginosa* produces a number of different β-lactamase enzymes. The most clinically relevant β-lactamases produced by *P. aeruginosa* are encoded primarily chromosomally rather than located on plasmids. Cephalosporinases, classified as class I β-lactamases,[106] produced by *P. aeruginosa* increase on exposure to any of the β-lactam antibiotics (derepression of the β-lactamase gene).[114] However, the propensity to induce β-lactamase varies among the β-lactam antibiotics.[27] Imipenem and cefoxitin are strong inducers of β-lactamase.[34] All antipseudomonal penicillins, cephalosporins, and aztreonam are susceptible to the class I β-lactamase produced by *P. aeruginosa*.[87]

Clavulanate and tazobactam are β-lactamase inhibitors effective against plasmid-encoded class III and V β-lactamases and chromosomally encoded class II β-lactamases found in *P. aeruginosa* and some other gram-negative bacteria. However, these β-lactamase inhibitors not only are ineffective against the common class I β-lactamase of *Pseudomonas* but also are potent inducers of the β-lactamase gene. Use of these β-lactamase inhibitors will not enhance activity of ticarcillin (Timentin) or piperacillin (Zosyn) against *Pseudomonas* and actually might increase the likelihood of emergence of resistant strains.

Pseudomonas strains with chromosomally encoded class I β-lactamase may not produce detectable β-lactamase until they are exposed to β-lactam antibiotics. These β-lactamase–encoded strains may appear sensitive to β-lactam antibiotics with in vitro sensitivity testing prior to antibiotic use. However, administration of β-lactam antibiotics to patients colonized or infected with these strains results in induction of β-lactamase production and emergence of resistance. For this reason, repeat in vitro sensitivity testing of clinical isolates of *Pseudomonas* a few days after administration of β-lactam antibiotics might reveal reduced sensitivity to β-lactams.

Whereas imipenem resists β-lactamases produced by *Pseudomonas*, resistance to imipenem can result through the loss of an outer-membrane porin that allows imipenem to enter *Pseudomonas*.[20] The permeability of other β-lactam antibiotics also may be reduced when this outer-membrane porin is lost. Although chemically distinct from imipenem, fluoroquinolones such as ciprofloxacin may induce decreased permeability to both antibiotics.[101] *S. maltophilia* innately is resistant to imipenem.

Resistance to aminoglycosides usually results from enzyme-mediated antibiotic modification.[32] The various aminoglycoside-modifying enzymes have different substrate affinities. Therefore, resistance to one aminoglycoside does not predict resistance to others necessarily. Resistance to amikacin is less common than to other aminoglycosides.[46, 145] Aminoglycoside-modifying enzymes usually are plasmid-mediated.[32] This allows transference of plasmid-encoded resistance rapidly among strains within an institution. *P. aeruginosa* also can develop resistance to aminoglycosides by decreasing the intracellular uptake of aminoglycosides or by modification of intracellular ribosomal attachment.[31, 34]

In addition to antibiotic resistance, other clinical factors can affect aminoglycoside activity against *Pseudomonas* adversely. The acidic environment in tissue infected with *P. aeruginosa* can inactivate aminoglycosides.[17] Aminoglycosides may fail to reach therapeutic tissue levels because of poor penetration into bronchial secretions and lung tissue.[12] For patients with tracheitis (e.g., intubated patients) or endobronchial disease (e.g., cystic fibrosis), aminoglycosides and less frequently colistin have been administered by aerosol.[117] This route of delivery allows for greater availability of the antibiotic at the site of the infection, with enhanced safety due to negligible absorption into the systemic circulation. Doses of gentamicin and tobramycin of 2.5 to 8 mg/kg can be given safely by aerosol three times a day. Resistance may emerge after prolonged courses.

Ciprofloxacin, a bacterial DNA gyrase inhibitor, is the most effective of the quinolones against *P. aeruginosa*. Alteration of the binding site of DNA gyrase and decreased penetration of ciprofloxacin through the *Pseudomonas* cell membrane can result in resistant strains.[34, 72] Decreased membrane permeability is the more important mechanism for *Pseudomonas* resistance to ciprofloxacin.

Antibiotic therapy for *B. cepacia* infections also should be guided by results of in vitro susceptibility testing. Unfortunately, *B. cepacia* frequently is resistant to many commonly used antipseudomonal antibiotic agents, particularly the aminoglycosides. Antibiotics that may have activity against *B. cepacia* include ceftazidime, cefoperazone, azlocillin, piperacillin, trimethoprim-sulfamethoxazole, and chloramphenicol. Susceptibility to imipenem and minocycline varies. Combination therapy with two or three antibiotics may be required to achieve a clinical response. Combinations of β-lactam agents with aminoglycosides might provide synergy clinically, even when the *B. cepacia* isolated is aminoglycoside-resistant.

S. maltophilia also exhibits significant antibiotic resistance to the common antipseudomonal agents. Trimethoprim-sulfamethoxazole, chloramphenicol, moxalactam, ceftazidine, cefoperazone, ticarcillin plus clavulanic acid, and ciprofloxacin may be active against this organism alone or in combinations. *S. maltophilia* is resistant to antipseudomonal penicillins, imipenem, and aminoglycosides. For patients with catheter-related infections, catheter removal offers the greatest opportunity for cure.[36]

The most active antibiotics against *B. pseudomallei* are imipenem, piperacillin-tazobactam, piperacillin, ceftazidime, ticarcillin-clavulanate, ampicillin-sulbactam, tetracycline, and chloramphenicol.[128] Piperacillin, ceftazidime, and imipenem are not bactericidal in vitro.[128] Ciprofloxacin seems to be of limited value because of a high rate of resistance.

Chronic melioidosis can be treated with chloramphenicol over a period of many months or with tetracycline. Trimethoprim-sulfamethoxazole was recommended previously, but most strains currently are resistant.

For acute systemic melioidosis, ceftazidime 120 mg/kg/day or chloramphenicol 50 to 75 mg/kg/day plus an aminoglycoside (kanamycin 20 to 30 mg/kg/day or amikacin 15 to 20 mg/kg/day) and sulfisoxazole 120 to 150 mg/kg/day should be administered for a period of 4 weeks. When third-generation cephalosporins have been utilized, cefoperazone and ceftazidime have shown greater activity against *B. pseudomallei* than have other third-generation cephalosporin agents. Ceftazidime was compared with chloramphenicol, doxycycline, and trimethoprim plus sulfamethoxazole for the treatment of severe melioidosis.[140] Ceftazidime treatment in a dosage of 120 mg/kg/day intravenously in three divided doses every 8 hours was associated with a 50 per cent lower overall mortality rate, compared with other forms of therapy. These results suggest that ceftazidime combined with an aminoglycoside and sulfisoxazole now should be considered the treatment of choice for severe melioidosis. Soft-tissue infections should be treated for 4 to 6 months with tetracycline (in children older than 8 years of age) provided in a dosage of 50 mg/kg/day in four divided doses. In younger children, trimethoprim-sulfamethoxazole (8 mg/kg/day of trimethoprim and 40 mg/kg/day of sulfamethoxazole) in two divided doses may be utilized. Therapy may be supplemented with sulfonamides. Duration of therapy must be guided by clinical and laboratory findings; therapy for 4 weeks to many months may be required in patients with osteomyelitis. Most penicillins are ineffective.[35, 128]

PROGNOSIS

Prognosis depends largely on the nature of the underlying disease process. Septicemia is the leading cause of death in children with leukemia; *Pseudomonas* is responsible for one-half of these deaths. Four variables independently influence the outcome of *Pseudomonas* septicemia: (1) development of septic shock, (2) inappropriate antibiotic therapy, (3) granulocyte counts less than 500/mm^3, and (4) development of septic metastases.[10] Most deaths in children with cystic fibrosis are due to pulmonary insufficiency. *Pseudomonas* can be recovered from the lungs in almost every one of these patients and in many has been responsible for their death.

References

1. Alexander, A. D., Huxsoll, D. L., Warner, A. R., et al.: Serological diagnosis of human melioidosis with indirect hemagglutination and complement fixation titers. Appl. Microbiol. *20*:825–833, 1970.
2. Alexander, J. W., and Fisher, M. W.: Immunization against *Pseudomonas* in infection after thermal injury. J. Infect. Dis. *130*:S152–S158, 1974.
3. Anaissie, E., Fainstein, V., Miller, P., et al.: *Pseudomonas putida*: Newly recognized pathogen in patients with cancer. Am. J. Med. *82*:1191–1194, 1987.
4. Ashdown, L. R.: An improved screening technique for isolation of *Pseudomonas pseudomallei* from clinical specimens. Pathology *1*:293–297, 1979.
5. Ashdown, L. R., Johnson, R. W., Koehler, J. M., et al.: Enzyme-linked immunosorbent assay for the diagnosis of clinical and subclinical melioidosis. J. Infect. Dis. *160*:253–260, 1989.
6. Baddour, L. M., Kraus, A. P., Jr., and Smalley, D. L.: Peritonitis due to *Pseudomonas paucimobilis* during ambulatory peritoneal dialysis. South. Med. J. *78*:336, 1985.
7. Bauernfeind, A., Bertele, R. M., Harms, K., et al.: Qualitative and quantitative microbiological analysis of sputa of 102 patients with cystic fibrosis. Infection *15*:270–277, 1987.
8. Bell, S. M., Pham, J. M., and Lanzarone, J. Y. M.: Mutation of *Pseudomonas aeruginosa* to piperacillin resistance mediated by β-lactamase production. J. Antimicrob. Chemother. *15*:665–670, 1985.
9. Berbari, N., Johnson, D. H., and Cunha, B. A.: *Xanthomonas maltophilia* peritonitis in a patient undergoing peritoneal dialysis. Heart Lung *22*:282–283, 1993.
10. Bergan, T.: Pathogenetic factors of *Pseudomonas aeruginosa*. Scand. J. Infect. Dis. *29*(Suppl.):7–12, 1981.
11. Berger, M., Sorensen, R. U., Tosi, M. F., et al.: Complement receptor expression on neutrophils at an inflammatory site, the *Pseudomonas*-infected lung in cystic fibrosis. J. Clin. Invest. *84*:1302–1313, 1989.

12. Bergogne-Berezin, E.: Pharmacokinetics of antibiotics in respiratory secretions. *In* Pennington, J. E. (ed.): Respiratory Infection: Diagnosis and Management. 2nd ed. New York, Raven Press, 1988, p. 608.
13. Berkelman, R. L., Lewis, S., Allen, J. R., et al.: Pseudobacteremia attributed to contamination of povidone-iodine with *Pseudomonas cepacia*. Ann. Intern. Med. *95*:32–36, 1981.
14. Berkelman, R. L., Godley, J., Weber, J. A., et al.: *Pseudomonas cepacia* peritonitis associated with contamination of automatic peritoneal dialysis machines. Ann. Intern. Med. *96*:456–458, 1982.
15. Bisbe, J., Gatell, J. M., Puig, J., et al.: *Pseudomonas aeruginosa* bacteremia: Univariate and multivariate analyses in 133 episodes. Rev. Infect. Dis. *10*:629–635, 1988.
16. Bobo, R. A., Newton, E. J., Jones, L. F., et al.: Nursery outbreak of *Pseudomonas aeruginosa*: Epidemiologic conclusions from five different typing methods. Appl. Microbiol. *25*:414–420, 1973.
17. Bodem, C. R., Lampton, L. M., Miller, D. P., et al.: Relevance to aminoglycoside activity in gram-negative bacillary pneumonia. Am. Rev. Respir. Dis. *127*:39–41, 1983.
18. Brand, R. A., and Black, H: *Pseudomonas* osteomyelitis following puncture wounds in children. J. Bone Joint Surg. [Am.] 56:1637–1642, 1974.
19. Brett, M. M., Ghoneim, A. T. M., and Littlewood, J. M.: Prediction and diagnosis of early *Pseudomonas aeruginosa* infection in cystic fibrosis: A follow-up study. J. Clin. Microbiol. *26*:1565–1570, 1988.
20. Buscher, K. H., Cullman, W., Dick, W., et al.: Imipenem resistance in *Pseudomonas aeruginosa* resulting from diminished expression of an outer membrane protein. Antimicrob. Agents Chemother. *31*:703–708, 1987.
21. Carratala, J., Salazar, A., Mascaro, J., et al.: Community-acquired pneumonia due to *Pseudomonas stutzeri*. Clin. Infect. Dis. *14*:792, 1992.
22. Centers for Disease Control: Swimming pools: Safety and disease control through proper design and operation [DHHS publication number (CDC) 98–411]. Washington, D.C., U.S. Government Printing Office, 1979.
23. Chitnis, C. E. and Ohman, D. E.: Genetic analysis of the alginate biosynthetic gene cluster of *Pseudomonas aeruginosia* shows evidence of an operonic structure. Mol. Microbiol. *8*:583–590, 1993.
24. Chysky, V., Kapila, K., Hullmann, R., et al.: Safety of ciprofloxacin in children: Worldwide clinical experiences based on compassionate use: Emphasis on joint evaluation. Infection *19*:289–296, 1991.
25. Crosby, L. A., and Powell, D. A.: The potential value of the sedimentation rate in monitoring treatment outcome in puncture-wound–related *Pseudomonas* osteomyelitis. Clin. Orthop. Related Res. *188*:172–176, 1984.
26. Cryz, S. J., Jr., Pitt, T. L., Furer, E., et al.: Role of lipopolysaccharides in virulence of *Pseudomonas aeruginosa*. Infect. Immun. *44*:508–513 1984.
27. Cullman, W., Buscher, K. H., and Dick, W.: Selection and properties of *Pseudomonas aeruginosa* variants resistant to beta-lactam antibiotics. Eur. J. Clin. Microbiol. 6:467–473, 1987.
28. Dan, M., Gutman, R., and Biro, A.: Peritonitis caused by *Pseudomonas putrefaciens* in patients undergoing continuous ambulatory peritoneal dialysis. Clin. Infect. Dis. *14*:359–360, 1992.
29. Dance, D. A., Davis, T. M. E., Wattanagoon, Y., et al.: Acute suppurative parotitis caused by *Pseudomonas pseudomallei* in children. J. Infect. Dis. *159*:651–660, 1989.
30. Dance, D. A.: Melioidosis: The tip of the iceberg? Clin. Microbiol. Rev. 4:52–60, 1991.
31. Davis, B. D.: Mechanism of bactericidal action of aminoglycosides. Microbiol. Rev. *51*:341–350, 1987.
32. Dever, L. A., and Dermody, T. S.: Mechanisms of bacterial resistance to antibiotics. Arch. Intern. Med. *151*:886–895, 1991.
33. Döring, G., Hörz, M., Ortelt, J., et al.: Molecular epidemiology of *Pseudomonas aeruginosa* in an intensive care unit. Epidemiol. Infect. *110*:427–436, 1993.
34. Dunn, M., and Wunderink, R. G.: Ventilator-associated pneumonia caused by *Pseudomonas* infection. Clin. Chest Med. *16*:95–109, 1995.
35. Eickhoff, T. C., Bennett, J. V., and Hayes, P. J.: *Pseudomonas pseudomallei*: Susceptibility to chemotherapeutic agents. J. Infect. Dis. *121*:95–102, 1970.
36. Elting, L. S., and Bodey, G. P.: Septicemia due to *Xanthomonas* species and non-aeruginosa *Pseudomonas* species: Incidence of catheter-related infections. Medicine *69*:296–306, 1990.
37. Faden, H., and Grossi, M.: Acute osteomyelitis in children: Reassessment of etiologic agents and their clinical characteristics. Am. J. Dis. Child. *145*:65–69, 1991.
38. Feder, H. M., Jr., Grant-Kels, J. M., and Tilton, R. C.: *Pseudomonas* whirlpool dermatitis. Clin. Pediatr. *22*:638–642, 1983.
39. Feigin, R. D., and Shearer, W. T.: Opportunistic infection in children: Parts I, II, and III. J. Pediatr. *87*:507–514, 677–694, 852–866, 1975.
40. Fergie, J. E., Sherma, S. J., Lott, L., et al.: *Pseudomonas aeruginosa* bacteremia in immunocompromised children: Analysis of factors associated with a poor outcome. Clin. Infect. Dis. *18*:390–394, 1994.
41. Fick, R. B., and Reynolds, H. Y.: *Pseudomonas* respiratory infection in cystic fibrosis: A possible defect in opsonic IgG antibody? Bull. Eur. Physiopathol. Respir. *19*:151–161, 1983.
42. Fisher, M. C., Long, S. S., Roberts, E. M., et al.: *Pseudomonas maltophilia* bacteremia in children undergoing open heart surgery. J. Am. Med. Assoc. *246*:1571–1574, 1981.
43. Fisher, M. C., Goldsmith, J. F., and Gilligan, P. H.: Sneakers as a source of *Pseudomonas aeruginosa* in children with osteomyelitis following puncture wounds. J. Pediatr. *106*:607–609, 1985.
44. Flores, G., Stavola, J. J., and Noel, G. J.: Bacteremia due to *Pseudomonas* aeruginosa in children with AIDS. Clin. Infect. Dis. *16*:706–708, 1993.
45. Fox, R. C., Williams, G. J., Wunderink, R. G., et al.: Followup bronchoscopy predicts therapeutic outcome in ventilated patients with nosocomial pneumonia. Am. Rev. Respir. Dis. *143*:A109, 1991.
46. Gerding, D. N., and Larson, T. A.: Aminoglycoside resistance in gram-negative bacilli during increased amikacin use. Am. J. Med. *79*(1A):1–7, 1985.
47. Gilligan, P. H.: Microbiology of airway disease in patients with cystic fibrosis. Clin. Microbiol. Rev. *4*:35–51, 1991.
48. Gilligan, P. H.: *Pseudomonas* and *Burkholderia*. *In* Murray, P. R., Baron, E. J., Pfaller, M. A., et al. (eds.): Manual of Clinical Microbiology. 6th ed. Washington D.C., ASM Press, 1995, pp. 509–519.
49. Glupczynski, Y., Hansen, W., Dratwa, M., et al.: *Pseudomonas paucimobilis* peritonitis in patients treated by peritoneal dialysis. J. Clin. Microbiol. *20*:1225–1226, 1984.
50. Gustafson, T. L., Band, J. D., Hutcheson, R. H., Jr., et al.: *Pseudomonas* folliculitis: An outbreak and review. Rev. Infect. Dis. *5*:1–8, 1983.
51. Heggers, J. P., Haydon, S., Ko, F., et al.: *Pseudomonas aeruginosa* exotoxin A: Its role in retardation of wound healing: The 1992 Lindberg Award. J. Burn Care Rehab. *13*:512–518, 1992.
52. Henderson, D. K., Baptiste, R., Parillo, J., et al.: Indolent epidemic of *Pseudomonas cepacia* bacteremia and pseudobacteremia in an intensive care unit traced to a contaminated blood gas analyzer. Am. J. Med. *84*:75–81, 1988.
53. Hilton, E., Adams, A. A., Uliss, A., et al.: Nosocomial bacterial eye infections in intensive-care units. Lancet *1*:1318–1320, 1983.
54. Hioyo-Tomoka, M. T., Marples, R. R., and Klingman, A. M.: *Pseudomonas* infection in superhydrated skin. Arch. Dermatol. *107*:723–727, 1973.
55. Hoiby, N., and Koch, C.: *Pseudomonas aeruginosa* infection in cystic fibrosis and its management. Thorax *45*:881–884, 1990.
56. Holland, S. P., Pulido, J. S., Shires, T. K., et al.: *Pseudomonas aeruginosa* ocular infections. *In* Fick, R. B., Jr. (ed.): *Pseudomonas aeruginosa*: The Opportunist. Boca Raton, CRC Press, 1993, pp. 159–176.
57. Horn, K. L., and Gherini, S.: Malignant external otitis of childhood. Ann. J. Otol. *2*:402–404, 1981.
58. Isles, A., Maclusky, I., Corey, M., et al.: *Pseudomonas cepacia* infection in cystic fibrosis: An emerging problem. J. Pediatr. *104*:206–210, 1984.
59. Jacobs, R. F., McCarthy, R. E., and Elser, J. M.: *Pseudomonas* osteochondritis complicating puncture wounds of the foot in children: A 10-year evaluation. J. Infect. Dis. *160*:657–661, 1989.
60. Jensen, T., Pedersen, S. S., Nielsen, C. H., et al.: The efficacy and safety of ciprofloxacin and ofloxacin in chronic *Pseudomonas aeruginosa* infection in cystic fibrosis. J. Antimicrob. Chemother. *20*:585–594, 1987.
61. John, M., Ecclestone, E., Hunter, E., et al.: Epidemiology of *Pseudomonas cepacia* colonization among patients with cystic fibrosis. Pediatr. Pulmonol. *18*.108–113, 1994.
62. Jones, C. E., Alexander, J. W., and Fisher, M. W.: Clinical evaluation of *Pseudomonas* hyperimmune globulin. J. Surg. Res. *14*:87–96, 1973.
63. Kenna, M. A., Bluestone, C. D., Reilly, J. S., et al.: Medical management of chronic suppurative otitis media without cholesteatoma in children. Laryngoscope *96*:146–151, 1986.
64. Kercsmar, C. M., Stern, R. C., Reed, M. D., et al.: Ceftazidime in cystic fibrosis: Pharmacokinetics and therapeutic response. J. Antimicrob. Chemother. *12*(Suppl. A):289–295, 1983.
65. Kilpatrick, M., Girgis, N., Farid, Z., et al.: Aztreonam for treating meningitis caused by gram-negative rods. Scand. J. Infect. Dis. 23:125–126, 1991.
66. Kingston, C. W.: Chronic or latent melioidosis. Med. J. Aust. 2:618–621, 1971.
67. Klinger, J. D., and Thomassen, M. J.: Occurrence and antimicrobial susceptibility of gram-negative nonfermentative bacilli in cystic fibrosis patients. Diagn. Microbiol. Infect. Dis. *3*:149–158, 1985.
68. Kock, C., and Koiby, N.: Pathogenesis of cystic fibrosis. Lancet *341*:1065–1069, 1993.
69. Kynakorn, M., Petchlai, B., Khupulsup, K., et al.: Gold blot for detection of immunoglobulin M (IgM)-specific antibodies for rapid serodiagnosis of melioidosis. J Clin. Microbiol. *29*:2065–2067, 1991.
70. Lacroix, J., Gauthier, M., Lapointe, N., et al.: *Pseudomonas aeruginosa* supraglottitis in a six-month-old child with severe combined immunodeficiency syndrome. Pediatr. Infect. Dis. J. *7*:739–741, 1988.
71. Leelarasamee, A., and Bovornkitti, S.: Melioidosis: Review and update. Rev. Infect. Dis. *11*:413–425, 1989.
72. Legakis, N. J., Tzouvelekis, L. S., Makris, A., et al.: Outer membrane alterations in multiresistant mutants of *Pseudomonas aeruginosa*. Antimicrob. Agents Chemother. *33*:124–127, 1989.
73. Lentnek, A. L. and Williams, R. R.: Aztreonam in the treatment of gram-negative bacterial meningitis. Rev. Infect. Dis. *13*(Suppl. 7):S586–S590, 1991.
74. Levy, J. H., and Katz, H. R.: *Pseudomonas cepacia* keratitis. Cornea *8*:67–71, 1989.
75. LiPuma, J. J., Mortensen, J. E., Dasen, S. E., et al.: Ribotype analysis of *Pseudomonas cepacia* from cystic fibrosis treatment centers. J. Pediatr. *113*:859–862, 1988.

76. Liu, P. V.: Biology of *Pseudomonas aeruginosa*. Hosp. Pract. *82*:139–147, 1976.
77. Lumbiganon, P., Pengsaa, K., Puapermpoonsiri, S., et al.: Neonatal melioidosis: A report of 5 cases. Pediatr. Infect. Dis. J. *7*:634–636, 1988.
78. Malizia, W. F., West, G. A., Brundage, W. G., et al.: Melioidosis: Laboratory studies. Health Lab. Sci. *6*:27–39, 1969.
79. Mayer, J. H., and Finnlayson, M. H.: Chronic melioidosis: A case with bone and pulmonary lesions. S. Afr. Med. J. *18*:109, 1944.
80. McCubbin, M., and Fick, R. B., Jr.: Pathogenesis of *Pseudomonas* lung disease in cystic fibrosis. *In* Fick, R. B., Jr. (ed.): *Pseudomonas aeruginosa*: The Opportunist. Boca Raton, CRC Press, 1993, pp. 189–211.
81. Minnefor, A. B., Olson, M. I., and Cawer, D. H.: *Pseudomonas* osteomyelitis following puncture wounds of the foot. Pediatrics *47*:598–601, 1971.
82. Mortensen, J., Hansen, A., Falk, M., et al.: Reduced effect of inhaled beta-2-adrenergic agonists on lung mucociliary clearance in patients with cystic fibrosis. Chest *103*:805–811, 1993.
83. Moss, R. B.: The role of IgG subclass antibodies in chronic infection: The case of cystic fibrosis. N. Engl. Regional Allergy Proc. *9*:57–61, 1988.
84. Muder, R. R., Yu, V. L., Dummer, J. S., et al.: Infections caused by *Pseudomonas maltophilia*: Expanding clinical spectrum. Arch. Intern. Med. *147*:1672–1674, 1987.
85. Nelson, J. D.: Pocketbook of Pediatric Antimicrobial Therapy. 12th ed. Baltimore, Williams & Wilkins, 1996–1997, pp. 68–83.
86. Neu, H. C.: The role of *Pseudomonas aeruginosa* in infections. J. Antimicrob. Chemother. *11*(Suppl. B):1–13, 1983.
87. Neu, H. C.: Carbapenems: Special properties contributing to their activity. Am. J. Med. *78*(6A):33–40, 1985.
88. Niggs, C., and Johnston, M. M.: Complement fixation test in experimental clinical and subclinical melioidosis. J. Bacteriol. *82*:159–168, 1961.
89. Norby, S. R.: 4-quinolones in the treatment of infections of the central nervous system. Rev. Infect. Dis. *10*(Suppl. 1):S253–S255, 1988.
90. Ohman, D. E., Burns, R. P., and Iglewski, B. H.: Corneal infections in mice with toxin A and elastase mutants of *Pseudomonas aeruginosa*. J. Infect. Dis. *142*:547–555, 1980.
91. Patamasucon, P., Pitchyangkura, C., and Fischer, G. W.: Melioidosis in childhood. J. Pediatr. *87*:133–136, 1975.
92. Patamasucon, P., Schaad, U. B., and Nelson, J. D.: Melioidosis. J. Pediatr. *100*:175–182, 1982.
93. Peacock, E. E.: Wound Repair. 3rd ed. Philadelphia, W. B. Saunders, 1984, pp. 38–55.
94. Pedersen, S. S.: Lung infection with alginate-producing, mucoid *Pseudomonas aeruginosa* in cystic fibrosis. Apmis. Suppl. *28*:1–79, 1992.
95. Peel, M. M., Davis, J. M., Armstrong, W. L. H., et al.: *Pseudomonas paucimobilis* from a leg ulcer on a Japanese seaman. J. Clin. Microbiol. *9*:561–564, 1979.
96. Penketh, A. R., Pitt, T. L., Hodson, M. E., et al.: Bactericidal activity of serum from cystic fibrosis patients for *Pseudomonas aeruginosa*. J. Med. Microbiol. *16*:401–408, 1983.
97. Pennington, J. E., Reynolds, H. Y., Wood, R. E., et al.: Use of *Pseudomonas aeruginosa* vaccine in patients with acute leukemia and cystic fibrosis. Am. J. Med. *58*:629–636, 1975.
98. Perry, A. W., Sutkin, H. S., Gottlieb, L. D., et al.: Skin graft survival: The bacterial answer. Ann. Plast. Surg. 22:479–483, 1989.
99. Pollack, M.: *Pseudomonas aeruginosa*. *In* Mandell, G. L., Douglas, R. G., Jr., and Bennett, J. E. (eds.): Principles and Practice of Infectious Diseases. 3rd ed. New York, Churchill Livingstone, 1990, pp. 1673–1691.
100. Pressler, T., Mansa, B., Jensen, T., et al.: Increased IgG2 and IgG3 concentration is associated with advanced *Pseudomonas aeruginosa* infection and poor pulmonary function in cystic fibrosis. Acta Pediatr. Scand. *77*:576–582, 1988.
101. Radberg, G., Nilsson, L. E., and Svensson, S.: Development of quinolone-imipenem cross resistance in *Pseudomonas aeruginosa* during exposure to ciprofloxacin. Antimicrob. Agents Chemother. *34*:2142–2147, 1990.
102. Reed, R. K., Larter, W. E., Sieber, O. F., Jr., et al.: Peripheral nodular lesions in *Pseudomonas* sepsis: The importance of incision and drainage. J. Pediatr. *88*:977–979, 1976.
103. Reid, T. M. S., and Porter, I. A.: An outbreak of otitis externa in competitive swimmers due to *Pseudomonas aeruginosa*. J. Hyg. (Camb.) *86*:357–362, 1981.
104. Reynolds, H. Y., DiSant'Agnese, P. A., and Zierdt, C. H.: Mucoid *Pseudomonas aeruginosa*. J. A. M. A. *236*:2190–2192, 1976.
105. Reynolds, H. Y., Levine, A. S., Wood, R. E., et al.: *Pseudomonas aeruginosa* infections: Persisting problems and current research to find new therapies. Ann. Intern. Med. *82*:819–831, 1975.
106. Richmond, H. M., and Sykes, R. B.: The β-lactamases of gram-negative bacilli and their possible physiologic role. Adv. Microb. Physiol. *9*:31–88, 1973.
107. Roiliders, E., Butler, K. M., Husson, R. N., et al.: *Pseudomonas* infections in children with human immunodeficiency virus infection. Pediatr. Infect. Dis. J. *11*:547–553, 1992.
108. Römling, V., Fiedler, B., Bosshammer, J., et al.: Epidemiology of chronic *Pseudomonas aeruginosa* in cystic fibrosis. J. Infect. Dis. *170*:616–621, 1994.
109. Rowley, A. H., Dias, L. D., Chadwick, E. G., et al.: *Pseudomonas stutzeri*: An unusual cause of calcaneal *Pseudomonas* osteomyelitis. Pediatr. Infect. Dis. J. *6*:296–297, 1987.
110. Rubio, T. T.: Ciprofloxacin: Comparative data in cystic fibrosis. Am. J. Med. *82*(Suppl. 4A):185–188, 1987.
111. Ruvalo, C., and Bauer, C. R.: Intrauterinely acquired *Pseudomonas* infection in the neonate. Clin. Pediatr. *21*:664–667, 1982.
112. Sajjan, U. S., Karmali, M. A., and Forstner, J. F.: Binding of *Pseudomonas cepacia* to normal human intestinal mucin and respiratory mucin for patients with cystic fibrosis. J. Clin. Invest. *89*:648–656, 1992.
113. Salmen, P., Dwyer, D. M., Vorse, H., et al.: Whirlpool-associated *Pseudomonas aeruginosa* urinary tract infections. J. A. M. A. *15*:2025–2026, 1983.
114. Sanders, C. C., and Sanders, W. E.: Type I β-lactamases of gram-negative bacteria: Interactions with β-lactam antibiotics. J. Infect. Dis. *154*:792–800, 1986.
115. Schaad, U. B., Sander, E., Wedgwood, J., et al.: Morphologic studies for skeletal toxicity after prolonged ciprofloxacin therapy in two juvenile cystic fibrosis patients. Pediatr. Infect. Dis. J. *11*:1047–1049, 1992.
116. Schaad, U. B., Stoupis, C., Wedgwood, J., et al.: Clinical, radiologic and magnetic resonance monitoring for skeletal toxicity in pediatric patients with cystic fibrosis receiving a three-month course of ciprofloxacin. Pediatr. Infect. Dis. J. *10*:723–729, 1991.
117. Schaad, U. B., Wedgwood-Krucko, J., Suter, S., et al.: Efficacy of inhaled amikacin as adjunct to intravenous combination therapy (ceftazidime and amikacin) in cystic fibrosis. J. Pediatr. *111*:599–605, 1987.
118. Schiller, N. L., and Millard, R. L.: *Pseudomonas*-infected cystic fibrosis patient sputum inhibits the bactericidal activity of normal human sputum. Pediatr. Res. *17*:747–752, 1983.
119. Schoch, P. E., and Cunha, B. A.: *Pseudomonas maltophilia*. Infect. Control *8*:169–172, 1987.
120. Scully, B. E., Parry, M. F., Nev, H. C., et al.: Oral ciprofloxacin therapy of infections due to *Pseudomonas aeruginosa*. Lancet *1*:819–822, 1986.
121. Sesev, S., Rosen, N., Joseph, G., et al.: Pefloxacin efficacy in gram-negative bacillary meningitis. J. Antimicrob. Chemother. *26*(Suppl. B):187–192, 1990.
122. Shackelford, P. G., Ratzan, S. A., and Shearer, W. T.: Ecthyma gangrenosum produced by *Aeromonas hydrophila*. J. Pediatr. *83*:100–101, 1973.
123. Shand, G. H., Pedersen, S. S., Tilling, R., et al.: Use of immunoblot detection of serum antibodies in the diagnosis of chronic *Pseudomonas aeruginosa* lung infection in cystic fibrosis. J. Med. Microbiol. *27*:169–177, 1988.
124. Sharma, G. D., Tosi, M. F., Stern, R. C., et al.: Progression of pulmonary disease after disappearance of *Pseudomonas* in cystic fibrosis. Am. J. Respir. Crit. Care Med. *152*:169–173, 1995.
125. Smith, A. L., Redding, G., Doershuk, C., et al.: Sputum changes associated with therapy for endobronchial exacerbation in cystic fibrosis. J. Pediatr. *112*:547–554, 1988.
126. Smith, G. L.: Methods for preventing *Pseudomonas* folliculitis. Cutis *29*:378–381, 1982.
127. Sobel, J. D., Hashman, N., Reinherz, G., et al.: Nosocomial *Pseudomonas cepacia* infection associated with chlorhexidine contamination. Am. J. Med. *73*:183–186, 1982.
128. Sookpranee, T., Sookpranee, M., Mellencamp, M. A., et al.: *Pseudomonas pseudomallei*, a common pathogen in Thailand that is resistant to bactericidal effects of many antibiotics. Antimicrob. Agents Chemother. *35*:484–489, 1991.
129. Speert, D. P., Farmer, S. W., Campbell, M. E., et al.: Conversion of *Pseudomonas aeruginosa* to the phenotype characteristic of strains from patients with cystic fibrosis. J. Clin. Microbiol. *28*:188–194, 1990.
130. Steen, H. J., Scott, E. M., Stevenson, M. I., et al.: Clinical and pharmacokinetic aspects of ciprofloxacin in the treatment of acute exacerbations of *Pseudomonas* infection in cystic fibrosis patients. J. Antimicrob. Chemother. *24*:787–795, 1989.
131. Strand, C. L., Bryant, J. K., Morgan, J. W., et al.: Nosocomial *Pseudomonas aeruginosa* urinary tract infections. J. A. M. A. *248*:1615–1618, 1982.
132. Strandvik, B., Hjelte, L., Lindblad, A., et al.: Comparison of efficacy and tolerance of intravenously and orally administered ciprofloxacin in cystic fibrosis patients with acute exacerbations of lung infection. Scand. J. Infect. Dis. *60*(Suppl.):84–88, 1989.
133. Tablan, O. C., Martone, W. J., Doershuk, C. F., et al.: Colonization of the respiratory tract with *Pseudomonas cepacia* in cystic fibrosis: Risk factors and outcomes. Chest *9*:527–532, 1987.
134. Tablan, O. C., Martone, W. J., and Jarvis, W. R.: The epidemiology of *Pseudomonas cepacia* in patients with cystic fibrosis. Eur. J. Epidemiol. *3*:336–342, 1987.
135. Tiffany, K. K., and Kline, M. W.: Mixed flora brain abscess with *Pseudomonas paucimobilis* after a penetrating lawn dart injury. Pediatr. Infect. Dis. J. *7*:667–669, 1988.
136. Victo, M. A., Arpi, M., Bruun, B., et al.: *Xanthomonas maltophilia* bacteremia in immunocompromised hematologic patients. Scand. J. Infect. Dis. *26*:163–170, 1994.
137. Vishwanath, S., and Ramphal, R.: Adherence of *Pseudomonas aeruginosa* to human tracheobronchial mucin. Infect. Immun. *45*:197–202, 1984.
138. Vogt, R., LaRue, D., Parry, M. F., et al.: *Pseudomonas aeruginosa* skin infections in persons using a whirlpool in Vermont. J. Clin. Microbiol. *15*:571–574, 1982.

139. Welch, D. F., Muszynski, M. J., Pai, C. H., et al.: Selective and differential medium for recovery of *Pseudomonas cepacia* from the respiratory tracts of patients with cystic fibrosis. J. Clin. Microbiol. *25*:1730–1734, 1987.
140. White, N. J., Dance, D. A., Chaowagul, W., et al.: Halving of mortality of severe melioidosis by ceftazidime. Lancet *2*:697–701, 1989.
141. Widmer, A. F., Wenzel, R. P., Trilla, A., et al.: Outbreak of *Pseudomonas aeruginosa* infections in a surgical intensive care unit: Probable transmission via hands of a health care worker. Clin. Infect. Dis. *16*:372–376, 1993.
142. Wongratanacheewin, S., Tattawasart, U., and Lulitanond, V.: An avidin-biotin enzyme-linked immunosorbent assay for the detection *Pseudomonas pseudomallei* antigens. Trans. Royal Trop. Med. Hyg. *84*:429–430, 1990.
143. Woods, D. E., Cryz, S. J., Friedman, R. L., et al.: Contribution of toxin A and elastase to virulence of *Pseudomonas aeruginosa* in chronic lung infections of rats. Infect. Immun. *36*:1223–1228, 1982.
144. Wretlind, B., and Pavlovskis, O. R.: The role of proteases and exotoxin A in the pathogenicity of *Pseudomonas aeruginosa* infections. Scand. J. Infect. Dis. *29*(Suppl.):13–19, 1981.
145. Young, E. J., Sewell, M. C., Koza, M. A., et al.: Antibiotic resistance patterns during aminoglycoside restriction. Am. J. Med. *290*:223–227, 1985.
146. Zimakoff, J., Hoiby, N., Rosendal, K., et al.: Epidemiology of *Pseudomonas aeruginosa* infection and the role of contamination of the environment in a cystic fibrosis clinic. J. Hosp. Infect. *4*:31–40, 1983.
147. Zuravleff, J. J., and Yu, V. L.: Infections caused by *Pseudomonas maltophilia* with emphasis on bacteremia: Case reports and review of the literature. Rev. Infect. Dis. *4*:1236–1246, 1982.

130

STENOTROPHOMONAS (XANTHOMONAS) MALTOPHILIA

Randall G. Fisher and William C. Gruber

Stenotrophomonas is a new genus with only one species: *maltophilia.*[13] This organism until recently was known as *Xanthomonas maltophilia* and prior to that, as *Pseudomonas maltophilia*. It is recognized increasingly as a nosocomial pathogen, mostly in debilitated patients and those with long-term indwelling central venous catheters.

BACTERIOLOGY

S. maltophilia is an aerobic, straight to slightly curved, gram-negative bacillus that usually occurs singly or in pairs. It is oxidase-negative and lysine decarboxylase–positive. Methionine and cysteine are required for growth. *S. maltophilia* is motile by means of polar multitrichous flagella. Optimum growth occurs at 35° C on standard laboratory media as large, smooth, glistening colonies that are lavender-green to gunmetal gray. Colonies may be slightly alpha-hemolytic and have a distinct ammonia-like odor.[18]

EPIDEMIOLOGY

S. maltophilia is a ubiquitous organism whose natural habitat is water and soil. It also has been cultured from milk, sewage, frozen fish, and hospital disinfectants.[9] These organisms have developed an ecologic niche in the hospital environment and have been found in dialysis fluids,[1] ventilators and other respiratory equipment,[8] preoperative surgical brushes,[12] and taps and sinks in intensive care units.[8] Ninety-seven per cent of *S. maltophilia* infection is hospital acquired.[5]

Infections with *S. maltophilia,* an opportunistic pathogen, are most common in patients with cancer, leukemia, debilitating disease, neutropenia, central venous catheters, or a combination of these risk factors.[8] Prior treatment with broad-spectrum antibiotics also is a significant predisposing feature.[4] The incidence of *S. maltophilia* infection has been increasing steadily, probably secondary to more frequent use of indwelling catheters and broad-spectrum antimicrobials to which the organism is not sensitive. In some hospitals, isolation of *S. maltophilia* has doubled or even tripled in the past 10 years.[9]

PATHOPHYSIOLOGY

Like many pseudomonads, *S. maltophilia* is an organism of low virulence and limited invasiveness. An intact host immune system is an important deterrent to severe and even life-threatening infection; most cases of septicemia and death occur in patients with underlying debilitating illnesses. Colonization with *S. maltophilia* is not uncommon, especially in the respiratory tract. Infection occurs when a change in the environment causes overgrowth of colonizing organisms or when the organisms gain access to sterile body sites. *S. maltophilia* infections are seen most commonly in patients with central venous catheters, which are presumed to be the portals of infection. In other cases, intravenous drug use has introduced the organism.[20] Infection with *S. maltophilia* also has followed surgical procedures,[6] clean intermittent catheterization,[10] etc. A few cases of community-acquired infection, including meningitis in newborns, have been described.[11] Risk factors for these infections are poorly understood.

CLINICAL MANIFESTATIONS

Infections with *S. maltophilia* separate broadly into two categories. First, and most common, is bacteremia or septicemia related to indwelling catheters, especially in patients with neutropenia. Patients have nonspecific signs, such as hectic or intermittent fevers, for a mean of 2 days before blood cultures become positive. Exit site infection is rare. Catheter-related infection, in general, has a good prognosis. The second form of infection is septicemia complicated by pneumonia, shock, or both. Pneumonia is an ominous clinical sign. In one series,[4] only 36 per cent of patients with pneumonia survived their *S. maltophilia* infection, compared with 99 per cent of those without. Not surprisingly, the presence of clinical signs of shock at the onset of fever also is a poor prognostic sign; only 38 per cent of these patients survived. Precipitous decline in clinical status and death sometimes are seen in this group of patients before the organism has been identified by the laboratory.

Endocarditis has occurred, almost exclusively in intravenous drug abusers, and carries a mortality rate that approaches 40 per cent.[20]

Meningitis is a rare occurrence. Signs and symptoms do not differ from those seen in meningitis due to more common bacterial pathogens. Central nervous system white blood cell counts, however, are disproportionately low. In a review of all reported cases,[6] the highest cerebrospinal fluid white blood cell count noted was 650/mm^3. Most were from 100/mm^3 to 300/mm^3.

Skin and soft tissue infections, including ecthyma gangrenosum, have been described and made up 15 per cent of *S. maltophilia* infections in one series.[17] A syndrome of metastatic nodular skin lesions that mimicked those seen in disseminated fungal infections also may occur.[17]

Pyelonephritis, peritonitis, mastoiditis, epididymitis, conjunctivitis, liver abscess,[3] and epidural abscess[19] also have been reported.

DIAGNOSIS

Diagnosis is made by isolating the organism from blood, pus, or other body fluids. Because nosocomial outbreaks have been reported, isolation of *S. maltophilia* from other patients in a hospital setting should alert the physician to the possibility of *Stenotrophomonas* infection. Infection control should be notified upon isolation of the organism.

Occasionally, *Pseudomonas cepacia* is misidentified as *S. maltophilia*, especially in patients with cystic fibrosis.[2] *S. maltophilia* is oxidase-negative and DNase-positive. These tests should be repeated in cases in which the identification of the organism is in doubt.

TREATMENT

S. maltophilia is a multidrug-resistant organism. It particularly is resistant to β-lactam antibiotic agents. It elaborates two inducible chromosomal β-lactamases. The first is a cephalosporinase, and the second is a metallo–β-lactamase capable of hydrolyzing both penicillins and carbapenems.[15] Production of these enzymes is derepressed rapidly in the presence of β-lactams.[9] Thus, virtually all isolates of *S. maltophilia* are resistant to penicillins and cephalosporins, and all are highly resistant to imipenem. Therapy with broad-spectrum cephalosporins and penicillins, especially empiric therapy in neutropenic patients, is a risk factor for infection.[8] Imipenem therapy has been shown to be a predisposing factor for both de novo infection[8, 15] and the conversion to infection in patients colonized with *S. maltophilia*.[4]

S. maltophilia also is resistant to aminoglycosides. The mechanism of this resistance is less well understood but in some cases appears to be plasmid mediated.[9] Resistance also has been transferred to other gram-negative organisms in vitro.[20]

In the laboratory, many isolates appear to be sensitive to fluoroquinolones by disk diffusion. Unfortunately, correlation between this method and agar dilution is poor,[7] and clinical experience with these agents, particularly in children, is limited.

Ninety-eight to 100 per cent of isolates of *S. maltophilia* are sensitive to trimethoprim-sulfamethoxazole. Doxycycline and minocycline are effective in about 60 per cent. Ticarcillin-clavulanate has some in vitro activity. Most authorities agree that trimethoprim-sulfamethoxazole is the drug of choice for *S. maltophilia* infection. Some advocate the addition of ticarcillin-clavulanate because trimethoprim-sulfamethoxazole is not bactericidal.[16]

In cases of catheter-related infection, removal of the catheter was noted to be curative, even without appropriate antimicrobial therapy, whereas treatment through the catheter, even with proper agents, was less successful.[4] Additionally, recurrence of infection, at a mean of 3 weeks later, was common in patients whose lines were not removed. In contrast, Roilides and associates[14] reported that they achieved a 65 per cent success rate in human immunodeficiency virus–infected children without catheter removal.

References

1. Berbari, N., Johnson, D. H., and Cunha, B. A.: *Xanthomonas maltophilia* peritonitis in a patient undergoing peritoneal dialysis. Heart Lung *22*:282–283, 1993.
2. Burdge, D. R., Noble, M. A., Campbell, M. E., et al.: *Xanthomonas maltophilia* misidentified as *Pseudomonas cepacia* in cultures of sputum from patients with cystic fibrosis: A diagnostic pitfall with major clinical implications. Clin. Infect. Dis. *20*:445–448, 1995.
3. Doerr, C. A., Demmler, G. J., Garcia-Prats, J. A., et al.: Solitary pyogenic liver abscess in neonates: Report of three cases and review of the literature. Pediatr. Infect. Dis. *13*:64–69, 1994.
4. Elting, L. S., and Bodey, G. P.: Septicemia due to *Xanthomonas* species and non-aeruginosa *Pseudomonas* species: Increasing incidence of catheter-related infections. Medicine *69*:296–306, 1990.
5. Gardner, P., Griffin, W. B., Swartz, M. N., et al.: Nonfermentative gram negative bacilli of nosocomial interest. Am. J. Med. *48*:735–749, 1970.
6. Girijaratnakumari, T., Raja, A., Ramani, R., et al.: Meningitis due to *Xanthomonas maltophilia*. J. Postgrad. Med. *39*:153–155, 1993.
7. Hohl, P., Frei, R., and Aubry, P.: In vitro sensitivity of 33 clinical case isolates of *Xanthomonas maltophilia*: Inconsistent correlation of agar dilution and of disk diffusion test results. Diagn. Microbiol. Infect. Dis. *14*:447–450, 1991.
8. Khardori, N., Elting, L., Wong, E., et al.: Nosocomial infections due to *Xanthomonas maltophilia* (*Pseudomonas maltophilia*) in patients with cancer. Rev. Infect. Dis. *12*:997–1003, 1990.
9. Marshall, W. F., Keating, M. R., Anhalt, J. P., et al.: *Xanthomonas maltophilia*: An emerging nosocomial pathogen. Mayo Clin. Proc. *64*:1097–1104, 1989.
10. McDonald, G. R., and Pernenkil, R.: Community-acquired *Xanthomonas maltophilia* pyelonephritis. South. Med. J. *86*:967–968, 1993.
11. Nguyen, M. H., and Muder, R. R.: Meningitis due to *Xanthomonas maltophilia*: Case report and review. Clin. Infect. Dis. *19*:325–326, 1994.
12. Oie, S., and Kamiya, A.: Microbial contamination of brushes used for preoperative shaving. J. Hosp. Infect. *21*:103–110, 1992.
13. Palleroni, N. J., and Bradbury, J. F.: *Stenotrophomonas*, a new bacterial genus for *Xanthomonas maltophilia*. Int. J. Syst. Bacteriol. *43*:606–609, 1993.
14. Roilides, E., Butler, K. M., Husson, R. N., et al.: *Pseudomonas* infections in children with human immunodeficiency virus infection. Pediatr. Infect. Dis. *11*:547–553, 1992.
15. Sanders, C. C., and Sanders, Jr., W. E.: Beta-lactam resistance in gram negative bacteria: Global trends and clinical impact. Clin. Infect. Dis. *15*:824–839, 1992.
16. Vartivarian, S., Anaissie, E., Bodey, G., et al.: A changing pattern of sensitivity of *Xanthomonas maltophilia* to antimicrobial agents: Implications for therapy. Antimicrob. Agents Chemother. *38*:624–627, 1994.
17. Vartivarian, S. E., Papadakis, K. A., Palacios, J. A., et al.: Mucocutaneous and soft tissue infections caused by *Xanthomonas maltophilia*. A new spectrum. Ann. Intern. Med. *121*:969–973, 1994.
18. von Graevenitz, A.: *Acinetobacter, Alcaligenes, Moraxella*, and other nonfermentative gram negative bacteria. *In* Murray, P. R., Baron, E. J., Pfaller, M. A., et al. (eds.): Manual of Clinical Microbiology. 6th ed. Washington, ASM Press, 1995, pp. 520–532.
19. Wagn, P., Hansen, H. M., Duun, P. S., et al.: *Xanthomonas maltophilia*: A cause of epidural abscess in a patient with epidural catheterization. (Danish.) Ugeskrift Laeger *156*:7229–7230, 1994.
20. Yu, V. L., Rumans, L. W., Wing, E. J., et al.: *Pseudomonas maltophilia* causing heroin-associated infective endocarditis. Arch. Intern. Med. *138*:1667–1671, 1978.

INDEX

❑ ❑ ❑

Note: Page numbers in *italics* refer to illustrations; page numbers followed by t refer to tables.